Oxford Textbook of
Medicine

VOLUME 2

Oxford Textbook of
Medicine

FIFTH EDITION
Volume 2: Sections 13–19

Edited by

David A. Warrell

Emeritus Professor of Tropical Medicine, Nuffield Department of Clinical Medicine; Honorary Fellow, St Cross College, University of Oxford, Oxford, UK

Timothy M. Cox

Professor of Medicine, University of Cambridge; Honorary Consultant Physician, Addenbrooke's Hospital, Cambridge, UK

John D. Firth

Consultant Physician and Nephrologist, Addenbrooke's Hospital, Cambridge, UK

Sub-editor Immunological Mechanisms and Disorders of the Skin
Graham S. Ogg
Reader in Cutaneous Immunology, MRC Senior Clinical Fellow; Consultant in Dermatology, Churchill Hospital, Oxford, UK

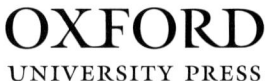

OXFORD

UNIVERSITY PRESS

Great Clarendon Street, Oxford OX2 6DP

Oxford University Press is a department of the University of Oxford.
It furthers the University's objective of excellence in research, scholarship,
and education by publishing worldwide in

Oxford New York

Auckland   Cape Town   Dar es Salaam   Hong Kong   Karachi
Kuala Lumpur   Madrid   Melbourne   Mexico City   Nairobi
New Delhi   Shanghai   Taipei   Toronto
With offices in
Argentina   Austria   Brazil   Chile   Czech Republic   France   Greece
Guatemala   Hungary   Italy   Japan   Poland   Portugal   Singapore
South Korea   Switzerland   Thailand   Turkey   Ukraine   Vietnam

Oxford is a registered trade mark of Oxford University Press
in the UK and in certain other countries

Published in the United States
by Oxford University Press Inc., New York

© Oxford University Press, 2010

British Library Cataloguing in Publication Data
Data available
Library of Congress Cataloging in Publication Data
Data available
Typeset by Cepha Imaging Pvt. Ltd., Bangalore
Printed in Italy by LegoPrint s.p.A.
9780199204854 (three volume set)
volume 1: 9780199592852
volume 2: 9780199592869
volume 3: 9780199592876
Available as a three volume set only
1 3 5 7 9 10 8 6 4 2

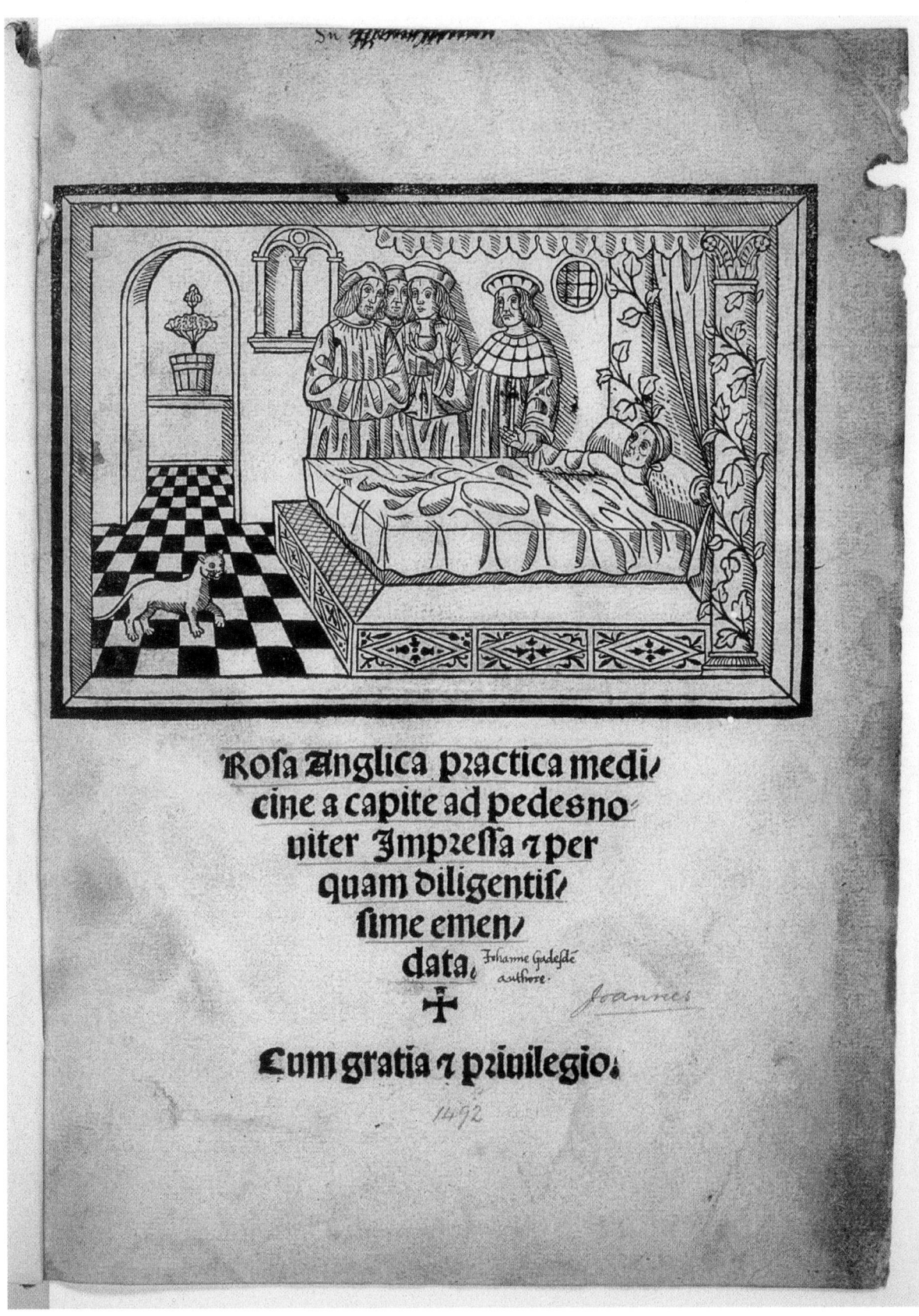

The title page of the 1492 edition of *Rosa Anglica* by John of Gaddesden (1280–1361), which was probably written in 1314. The author was a well known physician attached to Merton College, Oxford in the early part of the 14th century. His famous book was probably the first 'Oxford Textbook of Medicine'. The author was the model for the unsavoury Doctor of Physick in Chaucer's *Canterbury Tales*.

Foreword

by Professor Sir Aaron Klug OM FRS

Since it first appeared 25 years ago, the *Oxford Textbook of Medicine* has established itself as an authoritative source for doctors to consult in everyday practice, particularly when questions arise outside their experience. The coverage is comprehensive and covers diseases and problems that occur anywhere in the world. It is very respected and has become a standard reference in the United Kingdom for journalists and for legal disputes in the courts.

In a book with such wide coverage, it is important for the practising physician to be able to find the topic of current interest speedily. The book seems to me to be less discursive than, say, *Harrison's Principles of Internal Medicine*. Indeed, the layout of the book is such that one can efficiently look up something specific. This is facilitated by a good index, with the right degree of cross-referencing.

The book begins with the basic biological science underlying medicine, cell and molecular biology, and the genomic basis of medicine. Despite these big issues, the text does not lose sight of the clinical implications of the science being presented, in keeping with the underlying philosophy of the book that the material must be of practical value to the physician. Thus the advances in understanding the modification of proteins by kinases, which add phosphate groups to selected amino acids, has led to the development of chemical inhibitors of the kinases. An example of such a successful designer drug is imatinib for chronic myologenous leukaemia.

A totally new modality for the treatment has appeared in recent years, namely monoclonal antibodies with high selectivity against protein targets. Originally developed in mice, they could not be used in patients because of the anaphylactic response to a foreign protein, but over the years they have been 'humanized', i.e. their relatively small, specific antigen- or immunogen-recognition regions have been fused to a human framework, which make up most of the antibody. Examples include palivizumab, against respiratory syncytial virus, and bevacizumab, against colorectal cancer, now in widespread use. Even more striking is the development of fully human antibodies, synthesized out of the cloned repertoire of the human genes making up the constituent antibody domains. The antibody adalimumab, released a few years ago, not only relieves the pain of rheumatoid arthritis, but also stops the progress of the disease.

These new modalities are of course costly, as are many of the new anticancer drugs such as Herceptin: their introduction is changing the setting in which medicine is practised, particularly in the United Kingdom where the National Health Service (NHS) is free at the point of delivery, and in the United States of America where the Health Maintenance Organizations (HMOs) are insurance based. As recognized by David Weatherall in his foreword to the fourth edition of this textbook, none of the richer countries has got to grips with the problem of financing the increasing number and costs of new treatments. In the United Kingdom where the decision to allow the use of a licensed drug is made by the local Health Authority, there is no uniformity of practice, so leading to the term 'postcode availability' of a drug. There is also the question of individuals receiving treatment under the NHS but wishing to top up privately with other or new drugs not available under the NHS. Despite much controversy, this practice has recently been allowed by the NHS.

Another issue likely to arise out of the sequencing of the human genome is the prospect of personalized and preventive medicine. This is fast becoming a potential reality with the decreasing cost of rapid DNA sequencing to determine an individual genome. The supporting clinical data to interpret individual susceptibility to disease is likely to come from 'genome-wide association' studies. These represent a powerful approach to the identification of genetic variations involved in common human diseases. In 2007, there appeared in the journal *Nature* a genomic study of seven common diseases, including coronary artery disease, type 1 and type 2 diabetes, hypertension, and bipolar disorders. This large study involved 14 000 cases and 3000 shared controls. Similar studies have been carried out in several forms of cancer. The association of a particular locus in the genome with a disease is still very modest. The overall increase in risk conferred by the genetic factors identified is of the order of 1.2- to 1.5-fold, and so thus far does not provide a clinically useful prediction of disease. But the work must be recognized as an important first step towards dissecting the genomic basis of common diseases. By the time of the next edition of the *Oxford Textbook of Medicine*, we may well see the results of these powerful genomic tools becoming available or already in use.

Preface

The fruits of medical research

Publication of this new edition of the *Oxford Textbook of Medicine* prompts consideration of the precepts and practices of medicine in a world that faces unprecedented challenges. There is much to celebrate, and—with many new contributors—we have sought throughout the book to reflect the revolutionary effects of discovery in the medical sciences on clinical practice. Spectacular advances have been made at the most fundamental level and these continue to inspire our belief that improved prevention, diagnosis and treatment of disease will eventually relieve suffering. The popular term, 'translational medicine', reflects the shared optimism of many research agencies.

The Fifth edition has been rigorously revised and updated. It differs most blatantly from previous editions in having the gift of colour throughout and the inclusion of 'Essentials' (mostly written and all edited by John Firth) that summarize the main points of each chapter. The introductory Sections 2 and 3 include eight new chapters on topics ranging from the future of clinical trials, the evaluation and provision of effective medicines, to health promotion. This expansion reflects the ever burgeoning successes, constraints and frustrations of modern medicine. New sciences like stem cell biology, and emerging pathogens such as SARS, H1N1 and drug-resistant bacteria and malaria parasites, are well represented in our pages, and we have introduced some highly topical themes, notably Darwinian Medicine and the context of Human Disasters

Darwinian Medicine

Evolutionary medicine has a firm place in this book (Randolph Nesse and Richard Dawkins—Evolution: medicine's most basic science—Chapter 2.1.2), consistent with the 200th anniversary of Charles Darwin's birth and the 150th anniversary of the publication of *On the Origin of Species* in 2009. Darwin's remarkable synthesis (subtended in part by Gregor Mendel's later discoveries in heredity) has salient implications for understanding disease, rendering outmoded the crude analogy of the diseased body as a 'broken machine'. Much illness results from conflict between a person and the external influences to which he or she is uniquely maladapted at a particular time. Given that genetic and environmental variations are biological characteristics, the evolutionary concept has profound implications for any full description and understanding of disease.

But while we have prodigious methods for determining genetic variation, our ability to measure environmental changes and interactions—or predict environmental disasters—is rudimentary.

Human disasters: political, sociological, and historical context

Human populations are dependent on the natural environment for food and water but exquisitely vulnerable to its storms, earthquakes and tsunamis. As demonstrated by one of our Nobel Laureate authors, Amartya Sen (Human disasters—Chapter 3.5), the effects of natural disasters are, irrespective of their origin, invariably magnified by dire socioeconomic circumstances resulting from human conquest. An agonising recent example was the seismic horror in Haiti, affecting a society dysfunctional and impoverished as an historical consequence of the European slave trade and more recent political interferences. Such disasters, including those attributable to wars, are also the province of medicine: in such catastrophes, doctors are needed to provide emergency treatment but, through proper involvement with governments, they are also critical for public health planning and the restoration of appropriate infrastructure and clinical services. In response to another human tragedy, the AIDS pandemic, and to mounting pressure on the industry, one of the world's largest pharmaceutical companies has recently agreed to cut the prices of its medicines in the poorest countries and to donate some of its profits to local hospitals and clinics. This initiative might be a bit late but is a significant first step taking other 'Big Pharmas' in a direction that improves access to treatments for stricken patients in poor countries.

The teaching and practice of medicine: a fine tradition betrayed

Irrespective of the political dimension of medicine, the care of patients and the prevention of disease depend on practising clinicians; the medicine of the future relies not only on scientific advances but on the education of doctors. Since the last edition, leaders of our profession in Britain have presided over, and in some cases acquiesced to the partial dismantling of arguably one of the finest systems of medical education. The implementation of a national process for the appointment of junior doctors has disaffected many trainees and their clinical mentors, who feel that they have become pawns in a bureaucratic political game. More important, if they understood the full implications, we believe that the British public and patients would be horrified. Within Europe, matters have been compounded by implementation of the European Working Time Directive, which threatens the professional apprenticeship and mentoring relationships between junior and senior doctors that best nurture young colleagues. The frequently heard mantra of the 'consultant-led service' is all very well, but the ideal will be short-lived if training is put in jeopardy.

We, the editors of this textbook, learnt how to practise as clinicians from such 'hands-on' apprenticeships and ask: how can young doctors accumulate adequate working knowledge and acquire essential skills if their clinical work is restricted to 48 hours each week? One might pose the question: would a patient prefer to be treated by a fully rested but inexperienced doctor whom they had never seen before, or a tired doctor with immense medical experience who knew them and their illness? We know whom we would prefer, as does Christopher Booth (On being a patient—Chapter 1.1). Short hours and other radical changes in the organization of clinical teams impair the continuity of medical care, an element of key importance for the patient but also critical for clinical education through time-honoured individual experience. Many countries are seeking to improve their systems of medical education, but for those who might consider adopting the current UK training timetables, we humbly offer advice—don't. It would be better to provide their medical students and young doctors with sufficient time and resources to acquaint themselves with the principles and practice of modern scientific medicine that are emphasized in this book.

Decline and fall of clinical trials evidence

How the profession responds to these old and new threats to the practice of medicine will influence the translation of new knowledge and scientific understanding into clinical benefit. Our contemporary environment is contaminated by countless man-made chemicals, including drugs and other medicinal products: many of the latter have untested effects on human health. One foundation of good practice is the evidence provided by clinical trials, but this is under threat from powerful self-interest groups. On one hand are those promoting alternative and so-called traditional treatments, which are ineffective and supported at best by what Robert Park has termed 'Voodoo Science', and who mount sustained attacks on anyone who might be brave enough to say so, including one of our authors, Edzard Ernst (Complementary and alternative medicine—Chapter 2.5). On the other hand are those who promote expensive health care, of which they take a financial cut: scaremongering occurs at every opportunity, and with the intensity that only billions of dollars can bring. Already most clinical trials are sponsored by pharmaceutical companies and instances where prompt release of all the results has been suppressed for commercial reasons continue to scandalize the profession.

Clinical trials require proper regulation, but burgeoning bureaucracy has become disproportionate; it is stifling the discipline and greatly discourages investigator-led clinical trials. Yet another vacuous meta-analysis, performed in the absence of sufficient data and therefore allowing of no conclusions, will be no substitute. We plead also for simplification of the legal and regulatory framework in which therapeutic trials and medical research can be conducted by individual doctors; for without the freedom ethically to test hypotheses prompted by the immediacy of clinical necessity, many imaginative advances will be thwarted.

Inalienable personal liberty versus the public good

The tension between the right to personal liberty and the desire for public good is ever more acute and is manifest in many ways. For the world as whole, population control (or lack thereof), is the most pressing issue. Even when we thought medicine might have solved a problem, the activities of the anti-vaccination lobby that resulted in the anti-MMR scandal reminded us that old battles sometimes need to be fought again. Many people in diverse populations are suffering because of this phenomenon and from the misguided public assessment of risk and disregard for specialist advice.

Bureaucratic targets

Well chosen targets are a good way of managing complex systems, but there is grave danger when those who set targets for clinical practice are intrinsically suspicious of doctors, take very selective advice, choose inappropriate limits, and compound the error by specifying crude and inappropriate mechanisms by which they should be achieved. What is being measured becomes of overwhelming importance, and the patient with the most pressing clinical need may not get the priority that he or she deserves. Many will suffer unless this state of affairs is remedied.

The future

Against a background of such uncertainty, we believe that sound clinical experience, combined with knowledge of the subject, based on authoritative books and peer-reviewed publications, remain the rocks upon which clinical management is based. The doctor whom doctors want to see, when they or their family are ill, is the one they recognize as having great knowledge, great experience, and good judgement, of patients and their disease. We have asked such doctors to write for this book, so that it will be of most value to those seeking a 'higher medicine'. Despite the many adverse factors detailed above, we are reassured that many bright young men and women training in medicine are motivated, hungry for knowledge, and prepared to challenge dogma in the struggle to provide the best care for their patients. We trust that this edition of the book hits the mark and will help those who use it to achieve this aim.

Our debts

This edition is a tribute to our long-suffering but ever-patient contributors who, faced by delays in publication, had to update their work or risk instant obsolescence.

We remember with gratitude seven authors who have died since publication of the 4th edition, but who contributed to the present edition, Richard S. Doll (Chapter 6.1), Ernest Beutler (Chapter 22.5.11), Philip A. Poole-Wilson (Chapter 16.1.2), Pauline de la Motte Hall (Chapter 15.22.7), Peter ('PK') Thomas (Chapter 24.16),

M. Monir Madkour (Chapter 7.6.21), and Richard Edwards (Chapter 24.24.4). Sir Richard S. Doll, who died in 2005, a giant of Oxford and World Medicine and a marvellous friend and inspiration to many, was a great supporter of this book. As a guest of the popular radio programme 'Desert Island Discs', he delighted us by choosing the *Oxford Textbook of Medicine* for his reading material.

Graham S. Ogg contributed his special skills and experience to the planning and editing of the sections on Immunological mechanisms and Disorders of the skin for which we are most grateful. We thank our wives, Mary, Sue, and Helen, and dedicated secretaries, Eunice Berry and Joan Grantham. In the publication team, we are particularly grateful to Helen Liepman, Anna Winstanley, Kate Wilson, Kathleen Lyle, and Aparna Shankar.

David A. Warrell
Timothy M. Cox
John D. Firth

Oxford and Cambridge
February 2010

Contents

SECTION 19
Rheumatological disorders

Contributors

P. Aaby Bandim Health Project, National Institute of Health, Guinea-Bissau
7.5.6: Measles

Steven G. Achinger Attending Nephrologist, Watson Clinic, Lakeland, Florida, USA
21.2.1: Disorders of water and sodium homeostasis

Dwomoa Adu Consultant Nephrologist, Department of Medicine, Korle Bu Hospital, Accra, Ghana
21.8.3: Minimal-change nephropathy and focal segmental glomerulosclerosis; 21.8.4: Membranous nephropathy; 21.10.3: The kidney in rheumatological disorders

Raymond M. Agius Professor of Occupational and Environmental Medicine and Honorary Consultant in Occupational Medicine, University of Manchester, Manchester, UK
9.4.1: Occupational and environmental health

Syed M. Ahmed Health Manager UK, Mediterranean & Shipping, Shell International, London, UK
9.5.10: Noise

Michael J. Aldape Assistant Research Scientist, Infectious Diseases Section, Veterans Affairs Medical Center, Boise, Idaho, USA
7.6.24: Botulism, gas gangrene, and clostridial gastrointestinal infections

Graeme J.M. Alexander Consultant Hepatologist, Cambridge University Hospitals, Cambridge, UK
15.22.5: Liver transplantation

Michael E.D. Allison Consultant Hepatologist, Cambridge University Hospitals, Cambridge, UK
15.22.5: Liver transplantation

Chris Andrews Mt Ommaney Family Clinic, Brisbane, Australia
9.5.7: Lightning and electrical injuries

Emmanouil Angelakis Faculté de Médecine et de Pharmacie, Université de la Méditerranée, Marseille Cedex, France
7.6.42: Bartonellas excluding B. bacilliformis

Gregory M. Anstead Associate Professor, Division of Infectious Diseases, Department of Medicine, University of Texas Health Science Center at San Antonio, and Medical Director, Immunosuppression and Infectious Diseases Clinics, South Texas Veterans Healthcare System, San Antonio, Texas, USA
7.7.3: Coccidioidomycosis

Clive B. Archer Consultant Dermatologist and Honorary Clinical Senior Lecturer, University Hospitals Bristol NHS Foundation Trust; The University of Bristol, UK
23.15: Skin and systemic diseases

Mark J. Arends University Reader and Honorary Consultant in Histopathology, Division of Histopathology, Department of Pathology, University of Cambridge, Addenbrooke's Hospital, Cambridge, UK
4.6: Apoptosis in health and disease

J. Arendt Professor Emeritus of Endocrinology, School of Biological Sciences, University of Surrey, Guildford, UK
13.13: The pineal gland and melatonin

Alison Armitage Consultant in Nephrology, The Richard Bright Renal Unit, Southmead Hospital, Bristol, UK
21.13: Urinary tract infection

James O. Armitage The Joe Shapiro Professor of Medicine, Section of Oncology/Hematology, University of Nebraska Medical Center, Nebraska Medical Center, Omaha, Nebraska, USA
22.4.3: Lymphoma

Frances M. Ashcroft Royal Society Research Professor, Department of Physiology, Anatomy and Genetics, University of Oxford, Oxford, UK
4.4: Ion channels and disease

Caroline Ashley Lead Specialist Pharmacist, Centre for Nephrology, Royal Free Hospital, London, UK
21.19: Drugs and the kidney

S.Q. Ashraf Academic Clinical Lecturer and Specialty Registrar, John Radcliffe Hospitals, Oxford UK
15.14: Colonic diverticular disease

Tar-Ching Aw Head of Department of Community Medicine, Faculty of Medicine & Health Sciences, United Arab Emirates University, Al-Ain, United Arab Emirates
9.5.10: Noise; 9.5.11: Vibration

Juan Carlos Ayus Director of Clinical Research, Renal Consultants of Houston, Texas, USA
21.2.1: Disorders of water and sodium homeostasis

Trevor Baglin Consultant in Haematology, Department of Haematology & Eastern Region Haemophilia Comprehensive Care Centre, Cambridge University Hospitals NHS Trust, Addenbrooke's Hospital, Cambridge, UK
22.6.2: Evaluation of the patient with a bleeding tendency

M. Bagshaw Director of Aviation Medicine, King's College, London, UK
9.5.5: Aerospace medicine

C. Baigent Clinical Trial Service Unit & Epidemiological Studies Unit (CTSU), University of Oxford, UK
2.3.3: Large-scale randomized evidence: trials and meta-analyses of trials

I. Banerjee Department of Paediatric Endocrinology, Royal Manchester Children's Hospital, UK
13.9.2: Puberty

Adrian P. Banning Consultant Cardiologist, John Radcliffe Hospital, Oxford, UK
16.3.2: Echocardiography; 16.14.1: Thoracic aortic dissection

George Banting Department of Biochemistry, University of Bristol, Bristol, UK
4.1: The cell

T.M. Barber Oxford Centre for Diabetes, Endocrinology and Metabolism, Churchill Hospital, Oxford, UK
13.12: Hormonal manifestations of nonendocrine disease

D.J.P. Barker Professor of Clinical Epidemiology, University of Southampton; Professor in Cardiovascular Medicine, Oregon Health & Science University
16.13.3: Influences acting in utero *and in early childhood*

Roger A. Barker University Reader in Clinical Neuroscience & Honorary Consultant, Cambridge Centre for Brain Repair and Department of Neurology, University Department of Clinical Neuroscience, Addenbrooke's Hospital, Cambridge, UK
24.3.1: Lumbar puncture; 24.7.3: Movement disorders other than Parkinson's disease

D. Barlow Consultant Physician, Department of Genitourinary Medicine, Guy's and St Thomas' Hospitals, London, UK
7.6.6: Neisseria gonorrhoeae

M.P. Barnes Professor of Neurological Rehabilitation, Hunters Moor Neurorehabilitation Ltd
24.13.2: Spinal cord injury and its management

Jonathan Barratt Senior Lecturer, University of Leicester; Honorary Consultant Nephrologist, University Hospitals of Leicester, UK
21.8.1: Immunoglobulin A nephropathy and Henoch–Schönlein purpura

John G. Bartlett Professor of Medicine, Johns Hopkins University School of Medicine, Baltimore, Maryland, USA
7.6.23: Clostridium difficile; 18.4.2: Pneumonia in the normal host; 18.4.3: Nosocomial pneumonia

Buddha Basnyat Oxford University Clinical Research Unit, Patan Hospital, Nepal
7.6.8: Typhoid and paratyphoid fevers; 9.5.4: Diseases of high terrestrial altitudes

M.F. Bassendine Professor of Hepatology, Institute of Cellular Medicine, Newcastle University, Newcastle upon Tyne, UK
15.21.3: Primary biliary cirrhosis

D.N. Bateman Professor in Clinical Toxicology, National Poisons Information, Edinburgh, UK
9.1: Poisoning by drugs and chemicals

David Bates Professor of Clinical Neurology, Newcastle University, UK
24.5.5: The unconscious patient; 24.9: Brainstem syndromes

Robert P. Baughman University of Cincinatti Medical Center, Cincinatti, Ohio, USA
18.12: Sarcoidosis

Peter J. Baxter Institute of Public Health, University of Cambridge, Cambridge, UK
9.5.12: Disasters: earthquakes, volcanic eruptions, hurricanes, and floods

Harald Becher Consultant Cardiologist and Honorary Senior Lecturer, Department of Cardiology, John Radcliffe Hospital, Oxford, UK
16.3.3: Cardiac investigation—nuclear and other imaging techniques

Diederik van de Beek Department of Neurology, Center of Infection and Immunity Amsterdam (CINIMA), University of Amsterdam, Amsterdam, The Netherlands
24.11.1: Bacterial infections

D. Gareth Beevers Professor of Medicine, University Department of Medicine, City Hospital, Birmingham, UK
16.17.5: Hypertensive urgencies and emergencies

John R. Benson Consultant Surgeon, Cambridge Breast Unit, Addenbrooke's Hospital, Cambridge, UK; Fellow and Director of Clinical Studies, Selwyn College, Cambridge, UK
6.2: The nature and development of cancer

Malcolm K. Benson Oxford Pleural Unit, Oxford Centre for Respiratory Medicine, John Radcliffe Hospital, Oxford, UK
18.19.4: Mediastinal cysts and tumours

Anthony R. Berendt Consultant Physician, Bone Infection Unit, Nuffield Orthopaedic Centre NHS Trust, Oxford, UK
19.7: Pyogenic arthritis; 20.3: Osteomyelitis

David de Berker Department of Dermatology, Bristol Royal Infirmary, Bristol, UK
23.13: Hair and nail disorders

Nancy Berliner Chief, Division of Hematology, Brigham and Women's Hospital, Professor of Medicine, Harvard Medical School, Baltimore, Maryland, USA
22.4.1: Leucocytes in health and disease; 22.4.2: Introduction to the lymphoproliferative disorders

Gordon R. Bernard Melinda Owen Bass Professor of Medicine, Division of Allergy, Pulmonary, and Critical Care Medicine; Associate Vice Chancellor for Research, Senior Associate Dean for Clinical Sciences, Vanderbilt University School of Medicine, Nashville, Tennessee, USA
7.1.2: Physiological changes, clinical features, and general management of infected patients

J.M. Best Emeritus Reader in Virology, King's College London, UK
7.5.13: Rubella

Delia B. Bethell Armed Forces Research Unit of Medical Sciences, Bangkok, Thailand (Clinical Trials Investigator); Oxford Radcliffe Hospital NHS Trust, Oxford, UK (Honorary Consultant Paediatrician)
7.6.1: Diphtheria

Ernest Beutler[†] Molecular and Experimental Medicine, The Scripps Research Institute, La Jolla, California, USA
22.5.11: Erythrocyte enzymopathies

Kaustuv Bhattacharya Staff Specialist, Metabolic Genetics Department, Western Sydney Genetics Program, The Children's Hospital at Westmead, Australia, NSW
12.3.1: Glycogen storage diseases

Rudolf Bilous Professor of Clinical Medicine, Newcastle University, Academic Centre, James Cook University Hospital, Middlesbrough, UK
21.10.1: Diabetes mellitus and the kidney

D. Bilton Consultant Physician, Royal Brompton Hospital and Honorary Senior Lecturer, Imperial College, London, UK
18.9: Bronchiectasis

A.E. Bishop Reader, Stem Cells & Regenerative Medicine, Department of Experimental Medicine & Toxicology, Imperial College Faculty of Medicine, Hammersmith Hospital, London, UK
15.9: Hormones and the gastrointestinal tract

Carol M. Black Professor of Rheumatology, Royal Free and University College Medical School, London, UK
19.11.3: Systemic sclerosis

S.R. Bloom Professor of Medicine, Imperial College, London, UK
13.10: Pancreatic endocrine disorders and multiple endocrine neoplasia; 15.9: Hormones and the gastrointestinal tract

Lotta von Boehmer Department of Oncology, University Hospital Zurich, Zurich, Switzerland
6.4: Cancer immunity and clinical oncology

Roland M. du Bois National Jewish Health, Denver, Colorado, USA
18.11.5: The lung in vasculitis

Christopher Booth Wellcome Centre for the History of Medicine, University College, London, UK
1.1: On being a patient

T.C. Boswell Consultant Medical Microbiologist, Nottingham University Hospitals, Nottingham, UK
7.6.38: Legionellosis and legionnaires' disease

Marina Botto Professor of Rheumatology, Rheumatology Section, Imperial College London, London, UK
5.1.2: The complement system

[†] It is with regret that we report the death of Professor Ernest Beutler during the preparation of this edition of the textbook.

S.J. Bourke Consultant Physician, Royal Victoria Infirmary, Newcastle upon Tyne, UK
18.14.5: Pulmonary Langerhans' cell histiocytosis;
18.14.6: Lymphangioleiomyomatosis; 18.14.12: Radiation pneumonitis;
18.14.13: Drug-induced lung disease

I.C.J.W. Bowler Consultant Microbiologist and Clinical Lead, Department of Medical Microbiology, Oxford Radcliffe Hospitals NHS Trust, Oxford, UK
7.2.3: Nosocomial infections

Paul Bowness Consultant Rheumatologist, Nuffield Orthopaedic Centre NHS Trust and Reader in Immunology, Nuffield Department of Medicine, Oxford University, UK
5.1.1: The innate immune system

S.M. Bradberry National Poisons Information Service and West Midlands Poisons Unit, City Hospital, Birmingham, UK
9.1: Poisoning by drugs and chemicals

Marcus Bradley Consultant in Radiology, Frenchay Hospital, Bristol, UK
24.3.3: Imaging in neurological diseases

Thomas Brandt Klinikum Groshadem, Neurologische Klinik, Munchen, Germany
24.6.2: Eye movements and balance

P. Brandtzaeg Department of Paediatrics, Oslo University Hospital, Oslo, Norway
7.6.5: Meningococcal infections

H.R. Branley Consultant in Respiratory Medicine, Whittington Hospital, London, UK
18.11.4: The lung in autoimmune rheumatic disorders

Philippe Brasseur Emeritus Professor of Parasitology, Faculty of Medicine of Rouen (France) and Research Unit (UMR 198), Institute of Research for Development, Dakar, Senegal
7.8.3: Babesiosis

J. Braun Rheumazentrum Ruhrgebiet, Herne, Germany; Ruhr University, Bochum, Germany
19.6: Ankylosing spondylitis, other spondyloarthritides, and related conditions

Sydney Brenner The Salk Institute, University of California, San Diego, California, USA
4.2.1: The human genome sequence

J.A. Bridgewater University College London Cancer Institute and UCLH/UCL Comprehensive Biomedical Centre, London, UK
15.16: Cancers of the gastrointestinal tract

F. Bridoux Department of Nephrology, Hopital Jean Bernard, Poitiers, France
21.10.4: Renal involvement in plasma cell dyscrasias, immunoglobulin-based amyloidoses, and fibrillary glomerulopathies, lymphomas, and leukaemias

Paul H. Brion Rheumatologist in Private Practice, Vista, California, USA
19.9: Osteoarthritis

Maries van den Broek Department of Oncology, University Hospital Zurich, Zurich, Switzerland
6.4: Cancer immunity and clinical oncology

Anthony F.T. Brown Professor of Emergency Medicine, Discipline of Anaesthesiology and Critical Care, School of Medicine, University of Queensland, Brisbane, Australia; Senior Staff Specialist, Department of Emergency Medicine, Royal Brisbane and Women's Hospital, Brisbane, Australia
17.2: Anaphylaxis

Arthur E. Brown Colonel, U.S. Army, Armed Forces Research Institute of Medical Sciences, Bangkok, Thailand
7.6.20: Anthrax

Kevin E. Brown Consultant Medical Virologist, Virus Reference Department, Centres for Infection, Health Protection Agency, London, UK
7.5.20: Parvovirus B19

Michael Brown Senior Lecturer, Department of Infectious & Tropical Diseases, London School of Hygiene & Tropical Medicine, London, UK
7.9.4: Strongyloidiasis, hookworm, and other gut strongyloid nematodes

Morris J. Brown Professor of Clinical Pharmacology, University of Cambridge, Addenbrookes Centre for Clinical Investigation (ACCI), Addenbrookes Hospital, Cambridge, UK
16.17.3: Secondary hypertension

Amy E. Bryant Research Scientist, Infectious Diseases Section, Veterans Affairs Medical Center, Boise, Idaho; Affiliate Assistant Professor, University of Washington School of Medicine, Seattle, Washington, USA
7.6.24: Botulism, gas gangrene, and clostridial gastrointestinal infections

A.D.M. Bryceson London School of Hygiene and Tropical Medicine, London, UK
7.8.12: Leishmaniasis

Camilla Buckley MRC Clinician Scientist and Honorary Consultant, Department of Clinical Neurology, University of Oxford, Oxford, UK
24.22: Autoimmune limbic encephalitis and Morvan's syndrome

Susan Burge Consultant Dermatologist, Oxford Radcliffe Hospitals NHS Trust, UK
23.7: Cutaneous vasculitis, connective tissue diseases, and urticaria

David J. Burn Professor in Movement Disorder & Neurology & Honorary Consultant, Institute for Ageing and Health, Newcastle University; Director, Clinical Ageing Research Unit, Campus for Ageing and Vitality, Newcastle upon Tyne, UK
24.7.3: Movement disorders other than Parkinson's disease

Alan Burnett Co-Director of the Center for Refugee and Disaster Response, Johns Hopkins, Department of Haematology, University of Wales College of Medicine, Cardiff, UK
22.3.4: Acute myeloid leukaemia

Gilbert Burnham Co-Director of the Center for Refugee and Disaster Response, Johns Hopkins, Department of International Health, Baltimore, Maryland, USA
7.9.1: Cutaneous filariasis

Aine Burns Consultant Nephrologist and Director of Postgraduate Medical Education, Centre for Nephrology, Royal Free NHS Trust and University College Medical School, London, UK
21.19: Drugs and the kidney

Jacky Burrin Department of Endocrinology, St Bartholomew's and the Royal London School of Medicine and Dentistry, London, UK
13.1: Principles of hormone action

N.P. Burrows Consultant Dermatologist and Associate Lecturer, Department of Dermatology, Addenbrooke's NHS Trust, Cambridge, UK
20.2: Inherited defects of connective tissue: Ehlers–Danlos syndrome, Marfan's syndrome, and pseudoxanthoma elasticum

Andrew Bush Consultant Physician, Royal Brompton and Harefield NHS Trust, London, UK
18.10: Cystic fibrosis

K. Bushby Professor of Neuromuscular Genetics, Institute of Human Genetics, International Centre for Life, Newcastle upon Tyne, UK
24.24.2: Muscular dystrophy

Valai Bussaratid Assistant Professor of Tropical Medicine, Department of Clinical Tropical Medicine, Mahidol University, Bangkok, Thailand
7.9.7: Gnathostomiasis

Anthony Busuttil Regius Professor of Forensic Medicine Emeritus, Forensic Medicine Section, University of Edinburgh, Edinburgh, UK
27.1: Forensic medicine and the practising doctor

Geoffrey A. Butcher The Malaria Centre, Department of Life Sciences, Imperial College London, London, UK
7.8.2: Malaria

Gary Butler Consultant in Paediatric and Adolescent Medicine and Endocrinology, University College London Hospital; Honorary Professor in Paediatric Endocrinology, UCL Institute of Child Health, Hospital for Children, London, UK
13.9.1: Normal growth and its disorders

W.F. Bynum Professor Emeritus of History of Medicine, Wellcome Trust Centre for the History of Medicine at University College London, UK
2.1.1: Science in medicine: when, how, and what

S.M. Cacciò Department of Infectious, Parasitic and Immunomediated Diseases, Istituto Superiore di Sanità, Viale Regina Elena, Rome, Italy

7.8.5: Cryptosporidium and cryptosporidiosis

P.M.A. Calverley Professor of Respiratory Medicine, School of Clinical Sciences, University of Liverpool, UK

18.15: Chronic respiratory failure

Louis R. Caplan Professor of Neurology, Harvard Medical School; Senior Neurologist, Beth Israel Deaconess Medical Center, Boston, Massachusetts, USA

2.3.2: Evidence-based medicine—does it apply to my particular patient?

Jonathan R. Carapetis Director, Menzies School of Health Research, Charles Darwin University, Darwin, Australia

16.9.1: Acute rheumatic fever

Simon Carette Professor of Medicine, University of Toronto; Deputy Physician-in-Chief, Education UHN/MSH; Head, Division of Rheumatology UHN/MSH, Toronto, Ontario, Canada

19.4: Back pain and regional disorders

M. Cariati Lecturer in Surgery, King's College London, UK

13.8.3: Breast cancer

R. Carter Consultant Surgeon, Lister Department of Surgery, Royal Infirmary, Glasgow, UK

15.24.1: Acute pancreatitis

Tim E. Cawston Professor of Rheumatology, Musculoskeletal Research Group, Institute of Cellular Medicine, The Medical School, Newcastle University, Newcastle upon Tyne, UK

19.1: Structure and function: joints and connective tissue

Bruce A. Chabner Clinical Director, Massachusetts General Hospital Cancer Center and Professor of Medicine, Harvard Medical School, Boston, Massachusetts, USA

6.6: Cancer chemotherapy and radiation therapy

Richard E. Chaisson Professor of Medicine, Epidemiology and International Health, Johns Hopkins University School of Medicine and Bloomberg School of Public Health, Baltimore, Maryland, USA

7.6.25: Tuberculosis

S.J. Challacombe Consultant in Oral Medicine, Guy's Hospital, London, UK

15.6: The mouth and salivary glands

Siddharthan Chandran MRC Centre for Regenerative Medicine, University of Edinburgh, UK

4.8: Stem cells and regenerative medicine; 24.10.2: Demyelinating disorders of the central nervous system

Badrinath Chandrasekaran Specialty Registrar in Cardiology, Wessex Cardiothoracic Unit, Southampton General Hospital, Southampton, UK

16.5.1: Clinical features and medical treatments

R.W. Chapman Consultant in Gastroenterology, Department of Gastroenterology, John Radcliffe Hospital, Oxford, UK

15.21.4: Primary sclerosing cholangitis

V. Krishna Chatterjee Professor of Endocrinology, Institute of Metabolic Science and Department of Medicine, University of Cambridge, Addenbrooke's Hospital, Cambridge, UK

13.1: Principles of hormone action

K. Ray Chaudhuri Co-director National Parkinson Foundation Centre of Excellence, Lead Neuroscience Research and Development Strategy, London South Representative, NIHR Nervous Systems Committee, Kings College/University Hospital Lewisham, Kings College and Institute of Psychiatry, London, UK

24.7.2: Parkinsonism and other extrapyramidal diseases

P.F. Chinnery Professor of Neurogenetics and Director of Newcastle, NIHR Biomedical Research Centre for Ageing and Age-related Disease, Institute for Ageing and Health, Newcastle University, Newcastle upon Tyne, UK

24.24.5: Mitochondrial encephalomyopathies

Lydia Chwastiak Assistant Professor, Department of Psychiatry, Yale University, Connecticut, USA

26.5.5: Anxiety and depression

Stefan O. Ciurea Assistant Professor, Department of Stem Cell Transplantation, Division of Cancer Medicine, The University of Texas MD Anderson Cancer Center, Houston, Texas, USA

22.3.8: The polycythaemias; 22.3.10: Thrombocytosis

P. Jane Clarke Consultant Breast Surgeon, Oxford Radcliffe Trust, Oxford, UK

13.8.4: Benign breast disease

P.E. Clayton Consultant in Paediatrics, Royal Manchester Children's Hospital, Manchester, UK

13.9.2: Puberty

S.M. Cobbe Consultant Cardiologist, Glasgow Royal Infirmary; former BHF Walton Professor of Medical Cardiology, University of Glasgow, Scotland

16.2.2: Syncope and palpitations; 16.4: Cardiac arrhythmias

Fredric L. Coe Professor of Medicine, Nephrology Section MC5100, University of Chicago, Chicago Illinois, USA

21.14: Disorders of renal calcium handling, urinary stones, and nephrocalcinosis

J. Cohen Dean of Medicine and Professor of Infectious Diseases, Brighton & Sussex Medical School, Brighton, UK

7.2.4: Infection in the immunocompromised host

R.D. Cohen Emeritus Professor of Medicine, University of London; Queen Mary University of London, Centre for Diabetes, Blizard Institute of Cell & Molecular Science, Bart's & The London School of Medicine & Dentistry, London, UK

12.11: Disturbances of acid–base homeostasis

J. Collier Consultant in General Medicine, John Radcliffe Hospital, Oxford, UK

7.5.22: Hepatitis C

R. Collins Clinical Trial Service Unit & Epidemiological Studies Unit (CTSU), University of Oxford, UK

2.3.3: Large-scale randomized evidence: trials and meta-analyses of trials

Alastair Compston Professor of Neurology, University of Cambridge, Cambridge, UK

24.1: Introduction and approach to the patient with neurological disease; 24.10.2: Demyelinating disorders of the central nervous system

Juliet Compston Professor of Bone Medicine, University of Cambridge School of Clinical Medicine, Cambridge, UK

20.4: Osteoporosis

C.P. Conlon Reader in Infectious Diseases and Tropical Medicine, University of Oxford; Consultant Physician, John Radcliffe Hospitals, Nuffield Department of Medicine, John Radcliffe Hospital, Oxford, UK

7.4: Travel and expedition medicine; 7.5.23: HIV/AIDS

Graham Cooper Consultant Cardiac Surgeon, Sheffield Teaching Hospitals NHS Foundation Trust, UK

16.13.7: Coronary artery bypass surgery

John E. Cooper The University of the West Indies, St Augustine, Trinidad & Tobago, West Indies; Department of Veterinary Medicine, University of Cambridge, Cambridge, UK

7.8.7: Sarcocystosis (sarcosporidiosis)

Susan J. Copley Consultant Radiologist and Reader in Thoracic Imaging, Imperial NHS Trust, London, UK

18.3.2: Thoracic imaging

Minerva Covarrubias Division of Allergy, Pulmonary and Critical Care Medicine, Vanderbilt University School of Medicine, Nashville, Tennessee, USA

14.8: Chest diseases in pregnancy

Philip J. Cowen Professor of Psychopharmacology, Warneford Hospital, Oxford, UK

26.6.1: Psychopharmacology in medical practice

Martin R. Cowie Professor of Cardiology, Imperial College London; Honorary Consultant Cardiologist, Royal Brompton Hospital, London, UK

16.5.1: Clinical features and medical treatments

Timothy M. Cox Professor of Medicine, University of Cambridge, Honorary Consultant Physician, Acting Head of Department, Addenbrooke's Hospital, Cambridge, UK

12.1: The inborn errors of metabolism: general aspects; 12.3.2: Inborn errors of fructose metabolism; 12.3.3: Disorders of galactose, pentose, and pyruvate metabolism; 12.5: The porphyrias; 12.7.1: Hereditary haemochromatosis; 12.8: Lysosomal diseases; 13.13: The pineal gland and melatonin; 15.10.5: Disaccharidase deficiency; 22.5.4: Iron metabolism and its disorders; 33.1: Acute medical presentations; 33.2: Practical procedures

S.E. Craig Research Fellow and Respiratory Medicine Specialty Registrar, Oxford Sleep Unit, Churchill Hospital, Oxford, UK

18.1.1: The upper respiratory tract; 18.5.1: Upper airways obstruction; 18.5.2: Sleep-related disorders of breathing

Robin A.F. Crawford Consultant Gynaecological Oncologist, Addenbrooke's Hospital, Cambridge, UK

14.17: Malignant disease in pregnancy

Adrian Crisp Consultant in Rheumatology and Metabolic Bone Diseases, Addenbrooke's Hospital, Cambridge, UK

20.5: Osteonecrosis, osteochondrosis, and osteochondritis dissecans

Nigel Crisp Independent Member of the House of Lords and London School of Hygiene and Tropical Medicine (formerly NHS Chief Executive and Permanent Secretary of Department of Health)

2.4.3: Priority setting in developed and developing countries

Derrick W. Crook Infectious Disease and Clinical Microbiology, Nuffield Department of Medicine, John Radcliffe Hospital, Oxford, UK

7.6.12: Haemophilus influenzae

Paul Cullinan Faculty of Medicine, Imperial College, London, UK

18.7: Asthma

Peter F. Currie Consultant Cardiologist & Clinical Lead for Cardiology, Perth Royal Infirmary & Ninewells Hospital, Perth, UK

16.9.3: Cardiac disease in HIV infection

Tim Dalgleish Senior Scientist, Medical Research Council, Cognition and Brain Sciences Unit, Cambridge, UK

26.5.1: Grief, stress, and post-traumatic stress disorder

Chi V. Dang Professor of Medicine, Cell Biology, Oncology & Pathology;Professor Vice Dean for Research, Johns Hopkins University School of Medicine, Baltimore, Maryland, USA

22.3.7: Myelodysplasia

Norman Daniels Mary B Saltonstall Professor and Professor of Ethics and Population Health in the Department of Global Health and Population at Harvard School of Public Health, Massachusetts, USA

2.4.2: Reasonableness and its definition in the provision of health care

Christopher J. Danpure Professor of Molecular Cell Biology, University College London, London, UK

12.10: Hereditary disorders of oxalate metabolism—the primary hyperoxalurias

A. Davenport Centre for Nephrology, University College London Medical School, London, UK

21.4: Clinical investigation of renal disease

Gail Davey Associate Professor, School of Public Health, Addis Ababa University, Ethiopia

9.5.8: Podoconiosis (nonfilarial elephantiasis)

Alun Davies Professor of Vascular Surgery, Imperial College School of Medicine, London, UK

16.14.2: Peripheral arterial disease

P.D.O. Davies Consultant Physician, Liverpool Heart and Chest Hospital and Aintree University Hospital, Liverpool, UK

7.6.26: Disease caused by environmental mycobacteria

R. Rhys Davies Consultant in Anaesthesia, Frenchay Hospital, Bristol, UK

24.3.1: Lumbar puncture

Robert J.O. Davies Professor of Respiratory Medicine, Oxford Centre for Respiratory Medicine, NIHR Oxford Biomedical Research Centre, University of Oxford and John Radcliffe Hospital, Oxford, UK

18.17: Pleural diseases; 18.19.3: Pleural tumours; 18.19.4: Mediastinal cysts and tumours

Simon Davies Professor of Nephrology and Dialysis Medicine, Institute of Science and Technology in Medicine, Keele University; Consultant Nephrologist, University Hospital of North Staffordshire, Stoke-on-Trent, UK

21.7.2: Peritoneal dialysis

Richard Dawkins Charles Simonyi Professor for the Understanding of Science, University of Oxford, Oxford, UK

2.1.2: Evolution: medicine's most basic science

Chris P. Day Institute of Cellular Medicine, Newcastle University, Newcastle upon Tyne, UK

15.22.1: Alcoholic liver disease; 15.22.2: Nonalcoholic steatohepatitis

Colin Dayan Head of Clinical Research and Reader in Medicine, Henry Wellcome Laboratories for Integrative Neuroscience and Endocrinology, University of Bristol, UK

13.11.1: Diabetes

Linda Dayan Senior Staff Specialist and Director of Sexual Health Services, Royal North Shore Hospital, Sydney; Clinical Lecturer, School of Public Health, University of Sydney, Sydney, Australia

7.6.36: Syphilis

Marc E. De Broe Professor of Medicine, Laboratory of Pathophysiology, University of Antwerp, Belgium

21.9.2: Chronic tubulointerstitial nephritis

Kevin M. De Cock Centers for Disease Control and Prevention, Nairobi, Kenya

7.5.24: HIV in the developing world

Menno D. De Jong Department of Medical Microbiology, Academic Medical Center, University of Amsterdam, Amsterdam, The Netherlands

24.11.2: Viral infections

Pauline de la Motte Hall† Late Professor, Division of Science, Murdoch University, Murdoch, Australia

15.22.7: Hepatic granulomas

P.B. Deegan Consultant in Metabolic Medicine, Department of Medicine, Addenbrooke's Hospital, Cambridge, UK

12.8: Lysosomal diseases

Barbara A. Degar Assistant Professor of Pediatrics, Dana-Farber Cancer Institute, Children's Hospital Boston, Harvard Medical School, Boston, Massachusetts, USA

22.4.2: Introduction to the lymphoproliferative disorders

D.M. Denison Emeritus Professor of Clinical Physiology, Royal Brompton Hospital and Imperial College London, London, UK

9.5.5: Aerospace medicine; 9.5.6: Diving medicine

Christopher P. Denton Professor of Experimental Rheumatology, Centre for Rheumatology, Division of Medicine, UCL Medical School, Royal Free Hospital, London, UK

19.11.3: Systemic sclerosis

Ulrich Desselberger Director of Research, Department of Medicine, Addenbrooke's Hospital, Cambridge, UK

7.5.8: Enterovirus infections; 7.5.9: Virus infections causing diarrhoea and vomiting

Michael Doherty Professor of Rheumatology, University of Nottingham, UK

19.3: Clinical investigation; 19.10: Crystal-related arthropathies

Richard S. Doll†† Emeritus Professor of Medicine and Honorary Member, Cancer Studies Unit, Nuffield Department of Medicine, Radcliffe Infirmary, Oxford, UK

6.1: Epidemiology of cancer

† It is with regret that we report the death of Professor Pauline de la Motte Hall during the preparation of this edition of the textbook; †† it is with regret that we report the death of Professor Richard S. Doll during the preparation of this edition of the textbook.

Clare Dollery Divisional Clinical Director, Consultant Cardiologist, The Heart Hospital, UCLH NHS Foundation Trust, London, UK
16.13.1: Biology and pathology of atherosclerosis

Michael Donaghy Department of Clinical Neurology, John Radcliffe Hospital, Oxford, UK
24.15: The motor neuron diseases

Basil Donovan Professor of Sexual Health, National Centre in HIV Epidemiology and Clinical Research, University of New South Wales; Senior Staff Specialist, Sydney Sexual Health Centre, Sydney Hospital, Sydney, Australia
7.6.36: Syphilis

Philip Dormitzer Senior Director, Senior Project Leader, Viral Vaccine Research, Novartis Vaccines and Diagnostics, Cambridge, Massachusetts, USA
7.5.9: Virus infections causing diarrhoea and vomiting

H.M.P. Dowson Consultant General and Laparoscopic Surgeon, Frimley Park Hospital, Surrey, UK
15.4.2: Gastrointestinal bleeding

Tilman B. Drüeke Division of Nephrology and Inserm U845, Necker Hospital, Paris, France
21.6: Chronic kidney disease

Patrick C.A. Dubois MRC Clinical Research Training Fellow, Specialty Registrar in Gastroenterology, Barts and The London School of Medicine and Dentistry, Queen Mary University of London, London, UK
15.10.3: Coeliac disease

Christopher Dudley Consultant Renal Physician. The Richard Bright Renal Unit, Southmead Hospital, North Bristol NHS Trust, Bristol, UK
16.14.3: Cholesterol embolism

D.W. Dunne Department of Pathology, University of Cambridge, Cambridge, UK
7.11.1: Schistosomiasis

Stephen R. Durham Professor of Allergy and Respiratory Medicine; Head, Section of Allergy and Clinical Immunology, National Heart and Lung Institute, Imperial College and Royal Brompton Hospital, London
18.6: Allergic rhinitis

P.N. Durrington Professor of Medicine, Cardiovascular Research Group Division of Clinical and Laboratory Sciences, University of Manchester Core Technology Facility, Manchester, UK
12.6: Lipid and lipoprotein disorders

J. Dwight Consultant Cardiologist, John Radcliffe Hospital, Oxford, UK
16.2.1: Chest pain, breathlessness, and fatigue

Patrick C. D'Haese Associate Professor, Laboratory of Pathophysiology, University of Antwerp, Belgium
21.9.2: Chronic tubulointerstitial nephritis

Ian Eardley Consultant Urologist, Leeds Teaching Hospital Trust, Leeds, UK
13.8.5: Sexual dysfunction

M. Eastwood Post-Retirement Honorary Fellow, Department of Medical Sciences, Western General Hospital, Edinburgh, UK
11.2: Vitamins and trace elements

Tim Eden Honorary Professor of Paediatric and Adolescent Oncology, University of Manchester, UK
22.3.3: Acute lymphoblastic leukaemia

Mark J. Edwards Sobell Department of Motor Neuroscience and Movement Disorders, Institute of Neurology, University College London; National Hospital for Neurology and Neurosurgery, London, UK
24.7.1: Subcortical structures: the cerebellum, basal ganglia, and thalamus

Richard Edwards‡ Late Emeritus Professor of Medicine, Liverpool University, UK
24.24.4: Metabolic and endocrine disorders

Rosalind A. Eeles Professor of Oncogenetics, The Institute of Cancer Research; Honorary Consultant in Cancer Genetics & Clinical Oncology, Royal Marsden NHS Foundation Trust, Sutton, UK
6.3: The genetics of inherited cancers

Perry Elliott The Heart Hospital, University College London, UK
16.7.2: The cardiomyopathies: hypertrophic, dilated, restrictive, and right ventricular; 16.7.3: Specific heart muscle disorders

Christopher J. Ellis Consultant Physician, Department of Infection and Tropical Medicine, Heartlands Hospital, Birmingham, UK
7.2.1: Clinical approach

Monique M. Elseviers Associate Professor, Department of Nursing Sciences, University of Antwerp, Belgium
21.9.2: Chronic tubulointerstitial nephritis

Caroline Elston Consultant Physician, Respiratory Medicine and Adult Cystic Fibrosis, King's College Hospital, London, UK
18.10: Cystic fibrosis

M.A. Epstein Nuffield Department of Clinical Medicine, John Radcliffe Hospital, Oxford, UK
7.5.3: Epstein–Barr virus

Wendy N. Erber Consultant Haematologist and Clinical Director of Haematology, Addenbrooke's Hospital, Cambridge, UK
22.3.2: The classification of leukaemia

E. Ernst Professor of Complementary Medicine, Peninsula Medical School, Universities of Exeter and Plymouth, Exeter, UK
2.5: Complementary and alternative medicine

David Eschenbach Professor and Chair, Department of Obstetrics and Gynecology, University of Washington, Seattle, Washington, USA
8.5: Pelvic inflammatory disease

Andrew P. Evan Chancellor's Professor, Department of Anatomy and Cell Biology, Indiana University School of Medicine, Indianapolis, Indiana, USA
21.14: Disorders of renal calcium handling, urinary stones, and nephrocalcinosis

Martin J. Evans School of Biosciences, Cardiff University, Cardiff, UK
4.7: Discovery of embryonic stem cells and the concept of regenerative medicine

Timothy Evans Professor of Intensive Care Medicine, Imperial College; Department of Anaesthesia and Intensive Care Medicine, Royal Brompton Hospital, UK
17.5: Acute respiratory failure

Pamela Ewan Consultant Allergist, Department of Medicine, Addenbrooke's Hospital, Cambridge, UK
5.3: Allergy

Christopher G. Fairburn Wellcome Principal Research Fellow and Professor of Psychiatry, Department of Psychiatry, University of Oxford, Oxford, UK
26.5.6: Eating disorders

Jeremy Farrar Oxford University Clinical Research Unit, Wellcome Trust Major Overseas Programme Vietnam; South East Asia Infectious Disease Clinical Research Network, Ho Chi Minh City, Vietnam
7.5.15: Dengue; 24.11.1: Bacterial infections; 24.11.2: Viral infections

Ken Farrington Consultant Nephrologist, Lister Hospital, Stevenage, UK
21.3: Clinical presentation of renal disease; 21.7.1: Haemodialysis

John Feehally Consultant Nephrologist, University Hospitals of Leicester; Honorary Professor of Renal Medicine, University of Leicester, UK
21.8.1: Immunoglobulin A nephropathy and Henoch–Schönlein purpura; 21.8.2: Thin membrane nephropathy

Eleanor Feldman Consultant Liaison Psychiatrist, John Radcliffe Hospital Oxford; Consultant in Eating Disorders, Warneford Hospital Oxford; Honorary Senior Clinical Lecturer in Psychiatry, University of Oxford, UK
26.2: Taking a psychiatric history from a medical patient; 26.3: Acute behavioural emergencies

Peter J. Fenner Associate Professor, School of Public Health, Tropical Medicine and Rehabilitation Sciences, James Cook University, Townsville, Australia
9.5.3: Drowning

---

‡ It is with regret that we report the death of Professor Richard Edwards during the preparation of this edition of the textbook.

Robert Ferrari Department of Medicine, University of Alberta, Edmonton, Alberta, Canada

19.2: Clinical presentation and diagnosis of rheumatic disease

C. ffrench-Constant Professor of Medical Neurology, MRC Centre for Regenerative Medicine, Centre for Multiple Sclerosis Research, The University of Edinburgh, Queen's Medical Research Institute, Edinburgh, UK

24.18: Developmental abnormalities of the central nervous system

Richard E. Fielding Locum Consultant Nephrologist, Brighton and Sussex University Hospital Trust, Brighton, UK

21.3: Clinical presentation of renal disease

R.G. Finch Professor of Infectious Diseases, Nottingham University Hospitals NHS Trust, Nottingham, UK

7.2.5: Antimicrobial chemotherapy

H.V. Firth Consultant Clinical Geneticist, Addenbrooke's Hospital, Cambridge, UK

24.18: Developmental abnormalities of the central nervous system

John D. Firth Consultant Physician and Nephrologist, Cambridge University Hospitals NHS Foundation Trust, Cambridge, UK

14.5: Renal disease in pregnancy; 14.12: Neurological disease in pregnancy; 16.15.3: Pulmonary oedema; 16.16.1: Deep venous thrombosis and pulmonary embolism; 16.19: Idiopathic oedema of women; 17.3: The clinical approach to the patient who is very ill; 21.2.2: Disorders of potassium homeostasis; 21.5: Acute kidney injury; 21.6: Chronic kidney disease; 21.10.9: Atherosclerotic renovascular disease; 33.1: Acute medical presentations; 33.2: Practical procedures

Rebecca Fitzgerald Honorary Consultant Gastroenterologist, Cambridge University Hospitals NHS Foundation Trust, Cambridge, UK

15.7: Diseases of the oesophagus

R. Andres Floto Wellcome Trust Senior Clinical Fellow, Cambridge Institute for Medical Research, University of Cambridge; Honorary Respiratory Consultant, Papworth & Addenbrooke's Hospitals, Cambridge, UK

4.5: Intracellular signalling

Edward D. Folland Chief of Clinical Cardiology, UMassMemorial Medical Center, Worcester, Massachusetts; Professor of Medicine, University of Massachusetts Medical School, Worcester, Massachusetts, USA

16.3.4: Cardiac catheterization and angiography; 16.13.6: Percutaneous interventional cardiac procedures

Keith A.A. Fox British Heart Foundation Professor of Cardiology, Centre for Cardiovascular Sciences, University of Edinburgh, Edinburgh, UK

16.13.5: Management of acute coronary syndrome

Ross S. Francis Transplantation Research Immunology Group, Nuffield Department of Surgery, University of Oxford, John Radcliffe Hospital, Oxford, UK

5.5: Principles of transplantation immunology

Stephen Franks Professor of Reproductive Endocrinology, Imperial College London, Hammersmith Hospital, London, UK

13.8.1: Ovarian disorders

Keith N. Frayn Professor of Human Metabolism, Oxford Centre for Diabetes, Endocrinology and Metabolism, University of Oxford, Oxford, UK

11.1: Nutrition: macronutrient metabolism

A.H. Freeman Consultant Radiologist, Addenbrooke's Hospital, Cambridge, UK.

15.3.3: Radiology of the gastrointestinal tract

Izzet Fresko Professor, Division of Rheumatology, Department of Medicine, Cerrahpasa Medical Faculty, University of Istanbul, Istanbul, Turkey

19.11.5: Behçet's syndrome

Peter S. Friedmann Emeritus Professor of Dermatology, University of Southampton, Southampton, UK

23.6: Dermatitis/eczema; 23.16: Cutaneous reactions to drugs

Peggy Frith Consultant Ophthalmic Physician, John Radcliffe Hospital, Oxford and University College Hospital London, UK

25.1: The eye in general medicine

David A. Gabbott Consultant Anaesthetist, Gloucestershire Hospitals NHS Foundation Trust UK; Chairman, Research subcommittee, Resuscitation Council (UK) Executive Committee Resuscitation Council (UK)

17.1: Cardiac arrest

Patrick G. Gallagher Professor of Pediatrics and Genetics, Yale University School of Medicine, New Haven, Connecticut, USA

22.5.10: Disorders of the red cell membrane

Hector H. Garcia Professor, Department of Microbiology, Universidad Peruana Cayetano Heredia, Lima, Peru; Head, Cysticercosis Unit, Instituto de Ciencias Neurológicas, Lima, Peru

7.10.1: Cystic hydatid disease (Echinococcus granulosus); 7.10.3: Cysticercosis

Lawrence B. Gardner Assistant Professor of Medicine and Pharmacology, Division of Hematology and the NYU Cancer Institute, New York University School of Medicine, New York, USA

22.3.7: Myelodysplasia

J.S. Hill Gaston Consultant in Rheumatology, Department of Rheumatology, University of Cambridge, Cambridge, UK

19.8: Reactive arthritis

Sarah Germain Senior Registrar in Obstetric Medicine, Guy's & St Thomas' Foundation Trust, London, UK

14.14: Autoimmune rheumatic disorders and vasculitis in pregnancy

G.J. Gibson Emeritus Professor of Respiratory Medicine, Newcastle University Newcastle upon Tyne, UK

18.3.1: Respiratory function tests

J. van Gijn Emeritus Professor of Neurology, University Medical Centre, Utrecht, The Netherlands

24.10.1: Stroke: cerebrovascular disease

I.P. Giles Centre for Rheumatology, Department of Medicine, University College London, London, UK

19.11.1: Introduction

Robert H. Gilman Professor, Department of International Health, Johns Hopkins Bloomberg School of Hygiene and Public Health, Baltimore, Maryland, USA

7.10.3: Cysticercosis

Ian Gilmore President, Royal College of Physicians, London, UK

15.24.3: Tumours of the pancreas

Alexander Gimson Consultant Physician and Hepatologist, Liver Transplantation Unit, Cambridge University Hospitals Foundation NHS Trust, Cambridge, UK

14.9: Liver and gastrointestinal diseases in pregnancy; 15.19: Structure and function of the liver, biliary tract, and pancreas; 15.26: Miscellaneous disorders of the bowel and liver

Paul P. Glasziou Department of Primary Health Care, University of Oxford, Oxford, UK

2.3.1: Bringing the best evidence to the point of care

Fergus V. Gleeson Oxford Pleural Unit, Oxford Centre for Respiratory Medicine, John Radcliffe Hospital, Oxford, UK

18.17: Pleural diseases

M.A. Glover Medical Director, Hyperbaric Medicine Unit, St Richard's Hospital, Chichester, UK

9.5.6: Diving medicine

Peter J. Goadsby Headache Group, Department of Neurology, University of California, San Francisco, California, USA

24.8: Headache

D. Goldblatt Professor of Vaccinology and Immunology, Consultant in Paediatric Immunology, Head, Immunobiology Unit, Director, Clinical Research and Development and, Director, NIHR Biomedical Research Centre, Great Ormond Street Hospital for Children NHS Trust and Institute of Child Health, University College London, UK

7.3: Immunization

Ann-Marie J. Golden Research Worker, Medical Research Council, Cognition and Brain Sciences Unit, Cambridge, UK

26.5.1: Grief, stress, and post-traumatic stress disorder

John M. Goldman Professor of Haematology (Emeritus), Imperial College, London, UK
22.3.6: Chronic myeloid leukaemia

Armando E. Gonzalez Dean, School of Veterinary Medicine, Universidad Nacional Mayor de San Marcos, Lima, Peru
7.10.1: Cystic hydatid disease (Echinococcus granulosus)

Timothy H.J. Goodship Professor of Renal Medicine, Newcastle University, UK
21.10.5: Haemolytic uraemic syndrome

Sherwood L. Gorbach Tufts University, Nutrition/infection Unit, Boston, Massachusetts, USA
15.18: Gastrointestinal infections

E.C. Gordon-Smith Emeritus Professor of Haematology, St George's, University of London, London, UK
22.3.11: Aplastic anaemia and other causes of bone marrow failure; 22.8.2: Haemopoietic stem cell transplantation

Eduardo Gotuzzo Instituto de Medicina Tropical Alexander von Humboldt Universidad Peruana Cayetano Heredia Av. Honorio Delgado, San Martín de Porres, Lima, Peru
7.5.25: HTLV-1, HTLV-2, and associated diseases

P. Goulder Wellcome Senior Clinical Fellow & Honorary Consultant Paediatrician, University of Oxford, Oxford, UK
7.5.23: HIV/AIDS

Jan Tore Gran Professor and Head, Department of Rheumatology, Oslo University Hospital, Rikshospitalet, Oslo, Norway
19.11.4; Polymyalgia rheumatica and temporal arteritis

J.M. Grange Visiting Professor, University College London, Centre for Infectious Diseases and International Health, London, UK
7.6.26: Disease caused by environmental mycobacteria

Alison D. Grant Department of Paediatrics, University of Auckland, Auckland, New Zealand
7.5.24: HIV in the developing world

Cameron Grant Department of Paediatrics, University of Auckland, Auckland, New Zealand
7.6.14: Bordetella infection

David Gray Reader in Medicine & Honorary Consultant Physician, Department of Cardiovascular Medicine, Nottingham University Hospitals NHS Trust, Nottingham, UK
16.3.1: Electrocardiography

R. Gray Clinical Trial Service Unit & Epidemiological Studies Unit (CTSU), University of Oxford, UK
2.3.3: Large-scale randomized evidence: trials and meta-analyses of trials

John R. Graybill Professor Emeritus, Division of Infectious Diseases, Department of Medicine, University of Texas Health Science Center at San Antonio, San Antonio, Texas, USA
7.7.3: Coccidioidomycosis

Manfred S. Green Professor and Head, School of Public Health, University of Haifa, Haifa, Israel
9.5.13: Bioterrorism

Roger Greenwood Consultant Nephrologist, Lister Hospital, Stevenage, UK
21.7.1: Haemodialysis

I.A. Greer Professor of Obstetric Medicine & Dean, Hull York Medical School, UK
14.7: Thrombosis in pregnancy

Christopher Griffiths Professor of Dermatology, Salford Royal NHS Foundation Trust, The University of Manchester, Manchester, UK
23.5: Papulosquamous disease

William J.H. Griffiths Consultant Hepatologist, Department of Hepatology, Addenbrooke's Hospital, Cambridge, UK
12.7.1: Hereditary haemochromatosis; 15.22.6: Liver tumours—primary and secondary

David I. Grove Formerly Director of Clinical Microbiology and Infectious Diseases, The Queen Elizabeth Hospital, Woodville and Clinical Professor, University of Adelaide, South Australia, Australia
7.9.5: Gut and tissue nematode infections acquired by ingestion; 7.10.4: Diphyllobothriasis and sparganosis; 7.11.2: Liver fluke infections; 7.11.4: Intestinal trematode infections

J.P. Grünfeld Université Paris Descartes, Department of Nephrology, Necker Hospital, Paris, France
21.12: Renal involvement in genetic disease

D.J. Gubler Director, Program on Emerging Infectious Disease, Duke-NUS Graduate Medical School, Singapore; Asian Pacific Institute of Tropical Medicine and Infectious Diseases, University of Hawaii, Honolulu
7.5.12: Alphaviruses; 7.5.14: Flaviviruses excluding dengue

Richard L. Guerrant Hunter Professor of International Medicine, Division of Infectious Diseases and International Health; Director, Center for Global Health, University of Virginia, Charlottesville, Virginia, USA
7.6.11: Cholera

John Guillebaud Emeritus Professor of Family Planning and Reproductive Health, University College, London, UK
8.6: Principles of contraception; 14.19: Benefits and risks of oral contraception

Mark Gurnell University Lecturer in Endocrinology, Institute of Metabolic Science and Department of Medicine, University of Cambridge, Addenbrooke's Hospital, Cambridge, UK
13.1: Principles of hormone action

Alejandro Gutierrez Instructor of Pediatrics, Harvard Medical School, Dana-Farber Cancer Institute and Children's Hospital Boston, Massachusetts, USA
22.3.1: Cell and molecular biology of human leukaemias

M.R. Haeney Consultant Immunologist, Salford Royal NHS Foundation Trust, Salford, UK
15.5: Immune disorders of the gastrointestinal tract

Davidson H. Hamer Associate Professor of International Health and Medicine, Boston University Schools of Public Health and Medicine; Director, Travel Clinic, Boston Medical Center, Adjunct Associate Professor of Nutrition, Tufts University Friedman School of Nutrition Science and Policy, Center for International Health and Development, Boston, Massachusetts, USA
15.18: Gastrointestinal infections

P.J. Hammond Consultant in Endocrinology, Harrogate District Hospital, Harrogate, UK
15.9: Hormones and the gastrointestinal tract

Y. Han Staff Physician, Transfusion Medicine, City of Hope Medical Center, Duarte, California, USA
22.8.1: Blood transfusion

M.G. Hanna Consultant Neurologist, National Hospital for Neurology and Institute of Neurology, London, UK
24.24.1: Structure and function of muscle

David M. Hansell Consultant Radiologist and Professor of Thoracic Imaging, Royal Brompton and Harefield NHS Trust, London, UK
18.3.2: Thoracic imaging

J.M. Harrington Emeritus Professor of Occupational Medicine, The University of Birmingham, Birmingham, UK
9.4.1: Occupational and environmental health

Nicholas K. Harrison Respiratory Unit, Morriston Hospital, Swansea, Wales, UK
18.11.3: Bronchiolitis obliterans and cryptogenic organizing pneumonia

Tina Hartert Associate Professor of Medicine, Vanderbilt University School of Medicine, Institute for Medicine and Public Health, Center for Health Services Research, Nashville, Tennessee, USA
14.8: Chest diseases in pregnancy

Adrian R.W. Hatfield Hepatobiliary Unit, The Middlesex Hospital, London, UK
15.3.2: Upper gastrointestinal endoscopy

Philip N. Hawkins Professor of Medicine, National Amyloidosis Centre and Centre for Acute Phase Proteins, UCL Medical School, London, UK

12.12.2: Hereditary periodic fever syndromes; 12.12.3: Amyloidosis

Keith Hawton Professor of Psychiatry, Centre for Suicide Research, Department of Psychiatry, University of Oxford, Oxford, UK

26.5.2: The patient who has attempted suicide

Roderick J. Hay Professor of Cutaneous Infection, Dermatology Department, King's College Hospital, London, UK

7.6.30: Nocardiosis; 7.7.1: Fungal infections; 23.10: Infections and the skin

Catherine E.G. Head Consultant Cardiologist, Guy's and St Thomas' NHS Foundation Trust, London, UK

14.6: Heart disease in pregnancy

Eugene Healy Professor of Dermatology, Dermatopharmacology, University of Southampton, Southampton General Hospital, UK

23.8: Disorders of pigmentation; 23.16: Cutaneous reactions to drugs

Nick Heather Emeritus Professor of Alcohol & Other Drug Studies, School of Psychology & Sport Sciences, Northumbria University, UK

26.7.2: Brief interventions against excessive alcohol consumption

David W. Hecht The John W. Clarke Professor and Chairman, Department of Medicine, Loyola University Medical Center, Maywood, Illinois, USA

7.6.10: Anaerobic bacteria

David A. van Heel Professor of Gastrointestinal Genetics, Honorary Consultant Gastroenterologist, Barts and The London School of Medicine and Dentistry, Queen Mary University of London, London, UK

15.10.3: Coeliac disease

Harry Hemingway Professor of Clinical Epidemiology, Department of Epidemiology and Public Health, University College London Medical School, London, UK

16.13.2: Coronary heart disease: epidemiology and prevention

Janet Hemingway Director, Liverpool School of Tropical Medicine, Liverpool, UK

7.8.2: Malaria

D.J. Hendrick Emeritus Professor, University of Newcastle upon Tyne, Consultant Physician Royal Victoria Infirmary, Newcastle upon Tyne, UK

18.14.1: Pulmonary haemorrhagic disorders; 18.14.2: Eosinophilic pneumonia; 18.14.3: Lymphocytic infiltrations of the lung; 18.14.4: Extrinsic allergic alveolitis; 18.14.5: Pulmonary Langerhans' cell histiocytosis; 18.14.6: Lymphangioleiomyomatosis; 18.14.7: Pulmonary alveolar proteinosis; 18.14.8: Pulmonary amyloidosis; 18.14.9: Lipoid (lipid) pneumonia; 18.14.10: Pulmonary alveolar microlithiasis; 18.14.11: Toxic gases and aerosols; 18.14.12: Radiation pneumonitis; 18.14.13: Drug-induced lung disease

Michael Henein Professor of Cardiology, Umea University, Sweden; Canterbury Christ Church University, UK

16.6: Heart valve disease; 16.8: Pericardial disease

Martin F. Heyworth Staff Physician and Adjunct Professor of Medicine, VA Medical Center and University of Pennsylvania, Philadelphia, Pennsylvania, USA

7.8.8: Giardiasis, balantidiasis, isosporiasis, and microsporidiosis

Tran Tinh Hien Vice Director, Centre for Tropical Diseases (Cho Quan Hospital), Ho Chi Minh City, Vietnam

7.6.1: Diphtheria

Katherine A. High Professor of Pediatrics, University of Pennsylvania School of Medicine, Children's Hospital of Philadelphia, Abramson Research Center, Philadelphia, Pennsylvania, USA

22.6.4: Genetic disorders of coagulation

Sharon Hillier Professor, Department of Obstetrics, Gynecology and Reproductive Sciences, University of Pittsburgh School of Medicine, Pittsburgh, Pennsylvania, USA

7.8.13: Trichomoniasis

David Hilton-Jones Clinical Director, Muscular Dystrophy Campaign, Muscle & Nerve Centre, Department of Clinical Neurology, John Radcliffe Hospital, Oxford, UK

24.23: Disorders of the neuromuscular junction; 24.24.3: Myotonia; 24.24.4: Metabolic and endocrine disorders

N. Hirani Consultant in Respiratory Medicine, Royal Infirmary, Edinburgh, UK

18.11.2: Idiopathic pulmonary fibrosis

Gideon M. Hirschfield Assistant Professor of Medicine, University of Toronto Liver Centre, Toronto Western Hospital, Toronto, Ontario, Canada

15.22.5: Liver transplantation

Moshe Hod Director, Division of Maternal Fetal Medicine, Helen Schneider Hospital for Women, Rabin Medical Center, Sackler Faculty of Medicine, Tel Aviv University, Petah-Tiqva, Israel

14.10: Diabetes in pregnancy

John R. Hodges Federation Fellow and Professor of Cognitive Neurology, Prince of Wales Medical Research Institute, Sydney, Australia

24.4.1: Disturbances of higher cerebral function; 24.4.2: Alzheimer's disease and other dementias

H.J.F. Hodgson Sheila Sherlock Chair of Medicine, University College London, London, UK

15.10.6: Whipple's disease; 15.21.1: Viral hepatitis—clinical aspects; 15.21.2: Autoimmune hepatitis

H. Hof Labor Limbach, Heidelberg, Germany

7.6.37: Listeriosis

A.V. Hoffbrand Consultant in Haematology. Department of Haematology, Royal Free Hospital, London, UK

22.5.6: Megaloblastic anaemia and miscellaneous deficiency anaemias

Ronald Hoffman Albert A. and Vera G. List, Professor of Medicine, Division of Hematology/Oncology, Director, Myeloproliferative Disorders Program, Tisch Cancer Institute, Departments of Medicine, Mount Sinai School of Medicine, New York, USA

22.3.8: The polycythaemias; 22.3.10: Thrombocytosis

Georg F. Hoffmann Chairman, University Children's Hospital, Department of General Pediatrics, Heidelberg, Germany

12.2: Protein-dependent inborn errors of metabolism

P. Holloway Consultant Chemical Pathologist and Honorary Senior Lecturer in Metabolic Medicine, Site Lead Clinician in Chemical Pathology and Immunology, St Mary's Hospital, Imperial College Healthcare NHS Trust, Medical School, London, UK

32.1: Biochemistry in medicine—reference intervals: the use of biochemical analysis for diagnosis and management

L. Holmberg Professor of Cancer Epidemiology, King's College London, UK

13.8.3: Breast cancer

Tony Hope Professor of Medical Ethics, University of Oxford; Fellow of St Cross College; and Honorary Consultant Psychiatrist

2.2: Medical ethics

Julian Hopkin Rector, Medicine & Health, School of Medicine, Swansea University, UK

18.2: The clinical presentation of respiratory disease

Bala Hota Division of Infectious Diseases, Department of Medicine, John H. Stroger Jr. Hospital of Cook County; Assistant Professor, Rush University Medical Center, Chicago, Illinois, USA

7.6.4: Staphylococci

Andrew R. Houghton Consultant Physician & Cardiologist, Grantham & District Hospital, Grantham, UK, and Visiting Fellow, University of Lincoln, Lincoln, UK

16.3.1: Electrocardiography

Laurence Huang Professor of Medicine, University of California San Francisco; Chief, AIDS Chest Clinic, HIV/AIDS Division, San Francisco General Hospital, San Francisco, California, USA

7.7.5: Pneumocystis jirovecii

H.C. Hughes Specialty Registrar (Infectious diseases/Microbiology), University Hospital of Wales, UK
7.5.29: Newly discovered viruses

I.A. Hughes Head of Department, Department of Paediatrics, Addenbrooke's Hospital, Cambridge, UK
13.7.2: Congenital adrenal hyperplasia; 13.9.3: Normal and abnormal sexual differentiation

R.A.C. Hughes Emeritus Professor of Neurology, King's College, London; Visiting Professor of Neurology, University College London; Cochrane Neuromuscular Disease Group, MRC Centre for Neuromuscular Disease
24.12: Disorders of cranial nerves; 24.16: Diseases of the peripheral nerves

P.J. Hutchinson Honorary Consultant Neurosurgeon and Senior Academy Fellow, Addenbrooke's Hospital, Cambridge, UK
24.5.6: Brain death and the vegetative state

Lawrence Impey Consultant in Obstetrics and Fetal Medicine, The John Radcliffe Hospital, Oxford, UK
14.15: Infections in pregnancy

C.W. Imrie Consultant Surgeon, Lister Department of Surgery, Royal Infirmary, Glasgow, UK
15.24.1: Acute pancreatitis

P.G. Isaacson Consultant in Histopathology, Department of Histopathology, Royal Free and University College Medical School, London, UK
15.10.4: Gastrointestinal lymphoma

David A. Isenberg Professor of Rheumatology, Centre for Rheumatology, Department of Medicine, University College London, London, UK
19.11.1: Introduction; 19.11.2: Systemic lupus erythematosus and related disorders

C. Ison Director, Sexually Transmitted Bacteria Reference Laboratory, Health Protection Agency Centre for Infections, London, UK
7.6.6: Neisseria gonorrhoeae

Alan A. Jackson Consultant in General Medicine, Southampton General Hospital, Southampton, UK
11.3: Severe malnutrition

Robin Jacoby Professor Emeritus of Old Age Psychiatry, University of Oxford; Department of Psychiatry, The Warneford Hospital, Oxford, UK
29.2: Mental disorders of old age

Dean Jamison Professor of Global Health, Department of Global Health, University of Washington, Seattle, Washington, USA
3.1: Global burden of disease: causes, levels, and intervention strategies

David Jayne Consultant in Nephrology and Vasculitis, Renal Unit, Department of Medicine, Addenbrooke's Hospital, Cambridge, UK
21.10.2: The kidney in systemic vasculitis

K.J.M. Jeffery Consultant Virologist, Oxford Radcliffe NHS Trust, John Radcliffe Hospital, Oxford, UK
7.5.22: Hepatitis C

Jørgen Skov Jensen Mycoplasma Laboratory, Copenhagen, Denmark
7.6.45: Mycoplasmas

D.P. Jewell Emeritus Professor of Gastroenterology, University of Oxford; Honorary Consultant Physician, John Radcliffe Hospital, Oxford, UK
15.12: Ulcerative colitis

Vivekanand Jha Additional Professor of Nephrology; Co-ordinator, Stem Cell Research Facility, Postgraduate Medical Institute, Chandigarh, India
21.11: Renal diseases in the tropics

Alexis J. Joannides Department of Clinical Neurosciences, University of Cambridge, UK
4.8: Stem cells and regenerative medicine

Anne M. Johnson Professor of Infectious Disease Epidemiology, Centre for Sexual Health and HIV Research, Research Department of Infection and Public Health, University College London, London, UK
8.2: Sexual behaviour

D. Joly Université Paris Descartes, Department of Nephrology, Necker Hospital, Paris, France
21.12: Renal involvement in genetic disease

E. Anthony Jones Former Chief of Hepatology, Academic Medical Center, Amsterdam, The Netherlands
15.22.4: Hepatocellular failure

Islam Junaid Consultant Urologist Barts and London NHS Trust Hospitals
21.17: Urinary tract obstruction

Summerpal S. Kahlon Melbourne Internal Medicine Associates, Melbourne, Florida, USA
7.5.16: Bunyaviridae

P.A. Kalra Consultant in Nephrology, Salford Royal NHS Foundation Trust, Salford, UK
21.10.9: Atherosclerotic renovascular disease

Kenneth C. Kalunian Professor of Medicine, Division of Rheumatology, Allergy and Immunology, University of California, San Diego School of Medicine, La Jolla, California, USA
19.9: Osteoarthritis

Eileen Kaner Institute of Health and Society, Newcastle University, UK
26.7.2: Brief interventions against excessive alcohol consumption

Niki Karavitaki Locum Consultant in Endocrinology, Department of Endocrinology, Oxford Centre for Diabetes, Endocrinology and Metabolism, Churchill Hospital, Oxford, UK
13.2: Disorders of the anterior pituitary gland; 13.3: Disorders of the posterior pituitary gland

Fiona E. Karet Professor of Nephrology, Honorary Consultant in Renal Medicine, University of Cambridge, UK
21.15: The renal tubular acidoses

Wayne J. Katon Professor and Vice-Chair, Department of Psychiatry & Behavioral Sciences, University of Washington, Washington, USA
26.5.5: Anxiety and depression

David Keeling Oxford Haemophilia & Thrombosis Centre, Churchill Hospital, Oxford, UK
16.16.2: Therapeutic anticoagulation

Jonathan Kell Department of Haematology, University Hospital of Wales and Cardiff University, Cardiff, UK
22.3.4: Acute myeloid leukaemia

David P. Kelsell Centre for Cutaneous Research, Blizard Institute of Cell and Molecular Science, Barts and the London School of Medicine and Dentistry, Queen Mary University of London, London, UK
23.3: Inherited skin disease

John G. Kelton McMaster University Medical Center, Hamilton, Ontario, Canada
22.6.3: Disorders of platelet number and function

Christopher Kennard Professor of Clinical Neurology, Head of Department, Department of Clinical Neurology, John Radcliffe Hospital, Oxford, UK
24.6.1: Visual pathways

R.S.C. Kerr Neurosurgery Consultant, John Radcliffe Hospital, Oxford, UK
24.11.3: Intracranial abscesses

M.G.W. Kettlewell Emeritus Consultant Colorectal Surgeon, John Radcliffe Hospital, Oxford, UK
15.14: Colonic diverticular disease

Maurice King Honorary Research Fellow, University of Leeds, Leeds, UK
3.4.2: A sinister pathogen corrupts two disciplines: the demographic entrapment of Middle Africa

Paul Klenerman Nuffield Department of Medicine, University of Oxford, Oxford, UK
5.1.3: Adaptive immunity; 7.5.22: Hepatitis C

Steve Knapper Department of Haematology, University Hospital of Wales and Cardiff University, Cardiff, UK
22.3.4: Acute myeloid leukaemia

Richard Knight Associate Professor of Parasitology (retired), Department of Microbiology, University of Nairobi, Kenya
7.8.1: Amoebic infections; 7.8.9: Blastocystis hominis infection; 7.9.2: Lymphatic filariasis; 7.9.3: Guinea worm disease (dracunculiasis); 7.9.6: Parastrongyliasis (angiostrongyliasis); 7.10.2: Cyclophyllidian gut tapeworms

Daniël Knockaert General Internal Medicine, University Hospital Gasthuisberg, Leuven, Belgium
7.2.2: Fever of unknown origin

Nine V.A.M. Knoers Professor in Clinical Genetics, Department of Human Genetics, Radboud University, Nijmegen Medical Centre, Nijmegen, The Netherlands
21.16: Disorders of tubular electrolyte handling

Alexander Knuth Department of Oncology, University Hospital Zurich, Zurich, Switzerland
6.4: Cancer immunity and clinical oncology

Yasushi Kobayashi Department of Immunobiology, Yale University School of Medicine, New Haven, Connecticut, USA
16.14.4: Takayasu's arteritis

G.C.K.W. Koh Honorary Specialist Registrar, Department of Medicine, University of Cambridge, Cambridge, UK
7.6.7.2: Pseudomonas aeruginosa

Stefan Kölker Consultant, Pediatric Metabolic Medicine, University Children's Hospital, Heidelberg, Department of General Pediatrics, Division of Inborn Metabolic Diseases, Heidelberg, Germany
12.2: Protein-dependent inborn errors of metabolism

Edwin H. Kolodny Bernard A. and Charlotte Marden Professor and Chairman, Department of Neurology, New York University School of Medicine, New York, USA
24.17: Inherited neurodegenerative diseases

Michael D. Kopelman Professor of Neuropsychiatry, Consultant Neuropsychiatrist, King's College London, St Thomas' Hospital, London, UK
26.4: Neuropsychiatric disorders

Christian Krarup Professor of Clinical Neurophysiology, Department of Clinical Neurophysiology, Rigshospitalet; Faculty of Health Science, University of Copenhagen, Copenhagen, Denmark
24.3.2: Electrophysiology of the central and peripheral nervous systems

D. Kumararatne Addenbrooke's Hospital, Cambridge, UK
5.2: Immunodeficiency

Robert A. Kyle Mayo Clinic, Rochester, Minnesota, USA
22.4.5: Myeloma and paraproteinaemias

Helen J. Lachmann Senior Lecturer, National Amyloidosis Centre and Centre for Acute Phase Proteins, University College London Medical School, London, UK
12.12.2: Hereditary periodic fever syndromes

R. Lainson Ex Director, The Wellcome Parasitology Unit, and research-worker, Department of Parasitology, Instituto Evandro Chagas, Rodovia, Bairro Levilândia, Ananindeua, Pará, Brazil
7.8.6: Cyclospora and cyclosporiasis

Peter C. Lanyon Consultant Rheumatologist, Nottingham University Hospitals Trust, UK
19.3: Clinical investigation

A.J. Larner Consultant Neurologist, Cognitive Function Clinic, Walton Centre for Neurology and Neurosurgery, Liverpool, UK
24.5.4: Syncope; 24.13.1: Diseases of the spinal cord

Malcolm Law Professor of Epidemiology and Preventive Medicine, Wolfson Institute of Preventive Medicine, St Bartholomews' and the Royal London School of Medicine and Dentistry, Queen Mary University of London, UK
3.3.2: Medical screening

T.P. Lawrence Neurosurgery Registrar, John Radcliffe Hospital, Oxford, UK
24.11.3: Intracranial abscesses

Stephen Lawrie Consultant in Psychiatry, Royal Edinburgh Hospital, Edinburgh, UK
26.5.7: Schizophrenia, bipolar disorder, obsessive–compulsive disorder, and personality disorder

N.F. Lawton Consultant Neurologist, Wessex Neurological Centre, Southampton General Hospital; Honorary Senior Lecturer, University of Southampton, UK
24.10.5: Idiopathic intracranial hypertension

Ramanan Laxminarayan Senior Fellow and Director, Center for Disease Dynamics, Economics, and Policy, Resources for the Future, Washington, DC, USA
3.1: Global burden of disease: causes, levels, and intervention strategies

Alison Layton Harrogate District Hospital, Harrogate, UK
23.11: Sebaceous and sweat gland disorders

John H. Lazarus Emeritus Professor of Clinical Endocrinology, Centre for Endocrine and Diabetes Sciences, School of Medicine, Cardiff University, Cardiff, UK
14.11: Endocrine disease in pregnancy

J.W. LeDuc Professor, Microbiology and Immunology, Robert E. Shope M.D. and John S. Dunn Distinguished Chair in Global Health, Deputy Director, Galveston National Laboratory, University of Texas Medical Branch, Galveston, USA
7.5.16: Bunyaviridae

Susannah Leaver Clinical Research Fellow/Specialty Registrar Respiratory and Intensive Care Medicine, Imperial College and Royal Brompton Hospital, London, UK
17.5: Acute respiratory failure

Philip Lee Lately Reader, Charles Dent Metabolic Unit, The National Hospital for Neurology and Neurosurgery, London, UK
12.3.1: Glycogen storage diseases

Y.C. Gary Lee Oxford Pleural Unit, Oxford Centre for Respiratory Medicine, John Radcliffe Hospital, Oxford, UK
18.17: Pleural diseases; 18.19.3: Pleural tumours

T. Lehner Professor of Basic & Applied Immunology, Kings College London at Guy's Hospital, London, UK
15.6: The mouth and salivary glands

Irene M. Leigh Vice Principal and Head of College, College of Medicine, Dentistry and Nursing, Ninewells Hospital and Medical School, Dundee, UK
23.3: Inherited skin disease

G.G. Lennox Consultant in Neurology, Addenbrooke's Hospital, Cambridge, UK
14.12: Neurological disease in pregnancy

Elena N. Levtchenko Pediatric Nephrologist, Radbound University Nijmegen Medical Centre, Nijmegen, The Netherlands
21.16: Disorders of tubular electrolyte handling

Jeremy Levy Imperial College Kidney and Transplant Institute, Imperial College Healthcare NHS Trust, London, UK
21.8.7: Antiglomerular basement membrane disease

Siong-Seng Liau Specialty Registrar in Hepatopancreatobiliary (HPB), Surgery, HPB Unit, Department of Surgery, Addenbrooke's Hospital Cambridge, UK
6.2: The nature and development of cancer

Peter Libby Chief, Cardiovascular Medicine, Brigham and Women's Hospital, Mallinckrodt Professor of Medicine, Harvard Medical School, Massachusetts, USA
16.13.1: Biology and pathology of atherosclerosis

Oliver Liesenfeld Professor of Medical Microbiology and Infection Institute for Microbiology and Hygiene, Charité Medical School Berlin, Berlin, Germany
7.8.4: Toxoplasmosis

Aldo A.M. Lima Professor of Medicine and Pharmacology, Faculty of Medicine, Federal University of Ceará, Fortaleza, CE, Brazil
7.6.11; Cholera

D.C. Linch Head of Department of Haematology, University College London, London, UK; Director of CRUK Cancer Centre at University College London, UK
22.2.2: Haemopoietic stem cell disorders

M.J. Lindop Consultant, John Farman Intensive Care Unit, Addenbrooke's Hospital, Cambridge, UK
17.8: Discontinuing treatment of the critically ill patient; 17.9: Brainstem death and organ donation

Gregory Y.H. Lip Consultant Cardiologist and Professor of Cardiovascular Medicine, Director, Haemostasis Thrombosis & Vascular Biology Unit, University of Birmingham Centre for Cardiovascular Sciences, City Hospital, Birmingham, UK
16.17.5: Hypertensive urgencies and emergencies

P. Little Professor of Primary Care Research, School of Medicine, University of Southampton, UK
18.4.1: Upper respiratory tract infections

William A. Littler Consultant Cardiologist, The Priory Hospital, Birmingham, UK
16.9.2: Infective endocarditis

A. Llanos-Cuentas School of Public Health & Administration and School of Medicine, Universidad Peruana Cayetano Heredia, Lima, Peru
7.6.43: Bartonella bacilliformis infection

Diana N.J. Lockwood Professor of Tropical Medicine, London School of Hygiene and Tropical Medicine, and Consultant Leprologist, Hospital for Tropical Diseases, London, UK
7.6.27: Leprosy (Hansen's disease); 7.8.12: Leishmaniasis

Jay Loeffler Herman and Joan Suit Professor, Harvard Medical School; Chair, Department of Radiation Oncology, Massachusetts General Hospital, Boston, Massachusetts, USA
6.6: Cancer chemotherapy and radiation therapy

Thomas Lom Senior Director, BBDO NY, New York, USA
3.3.3: The importance of mass communication in promoting positive health

David A. Lomas Department of Medicine, University of Cambridge; Cambridge Institute for Medical Research, Wellcome Trust, Cambridge, UK
12.13: α_1-Antitrypsin deficiency and the serpinopathies

Martin Lombard Liver and Pancreato-Biliary Unit, Royal Liverpool University Hospital, Liverpool, UK
15.24.3: Tumours of the pancreas

A. Thomas Look Professor of Pediatrics, Harvard Medical School; Vice Chair for Research, Department of Pediatric Oncology, Dana-Farber Cancer Institute, Boston, Massachusetts, USA
22.3.1: Cell and molecular biology of human leukaemias

Elyse E. Lower University of Cincinnati Medical Center, Ohio, USA
18.12: Sarcoidosis

Katharine Lowndes Specialty Registrar, Department of Haematology, Salisbury District Hospital, Wiltshire, UK
14.16: Blood disorders specific to pregnancy

James R. Lupski Baylor College of Medicine, Houston, Texas, USA
4.2.2: The genomic basis of medicine

Linda M. Luxon Professor of Audiovestibular Medicine, UCL Ear Institute and Consultant Neuro-otologist, National Hospital for Neurology and Neurosurgery, London, UK
24.6.3: Hearing

Lucio Luzzatto Chairman, Department of Human Genetics, Memorial Sloan-Kettering Cancer Center, New York, USA
22.3.12: Paroxysmal nocturnal haemoglobinuria;
22.5.12: Glucose-6-phosphate dehydrogenase (G6PD) deficiency

Graz A. Luzzi Consultant in Genitourinary Medicine and Honorary Senior Clinical Lecturer, University of Oxford, Wycombe Hospital, High Wycombe, UK
7.5.23: HIV/AIDS; 8.3: Sexual history and examination

David Mabey Professor of Communicable Diseases, Department of Infectious and Tropical Diseases, London School of Hygiene and Tropical Medicine, London, UK
7.6.44: Chlamydial infections; 8.1: Epidemiology of sexually transmitted infections

J.T. Macfarlane Lately Professor of Respiratory Medicine, University of Nottingham, and Consultant Respiratory Physician, Nottingham University Hospitals, Nottingham, UK
7.6.38: Legionellosis and legionnaires' disease

Kenneth T. MacLeod Reader in Cardiac Physiology, National Heart and Lung Institute (NHLI) Division, Faculty of Medicine, Imperial College London, London, UK
16.1.2: Cardiac myocytes and the cardiac action potential

William MacNee Professor of Respiratory and Environmental Medicine/Honorary Consultant ELEGI Colt Laboratories, MRC Centre for Inflammation Research, The Queen's Medical Research Institute, Edinburgh, UK
18.8: Chronic obstructive pulmonary disease

M. Monir Madkour‡ Consultant Physician, Military Hospital, Riyadh, Saudi Arabia
7.6.21: Brucellosis

C. Maguiña-Vargas Instituto de Medicina Tropical Alexander von Humboldt, Universidad Peruana Cayetano Heredia, Lima, Peru
7.6.43: Bartonella bacilliformis infection

Hadi Manji Consultant Neurologist and Honorary Senior Lecturer, National Hospital for Neurology and Neurosurgery, London, UK
24.11.4: Neurosyphilis and neuro-AIDS

J.I. Mann Professor of Human Nutrition and Medicine, University of Otago, Dunedin, New Zealand
11.4: Diseases of overnourished societies and the need for dietary change

J. Mansi Consultant Medical Oncologist, Guy's & St Thomas NHS Foundation Trust, London, UK
13.8.3: Breast cancer

David Mant Professor of General Practice, Department of Primary Health Care, University of Oxford, Oxford, UK
3.3.1: Preventive medicine

Vincent Marks Professor of Clinical Biochemistry Emeritus, Postgraduate Medical School, University of Surrey, Guildford, UK
13.11.2: Hypoglycaemia

Michael Marmot Professor of Epidemiology, Director of International Institute for Society and Health at University College London, Research Department of Epidemiology and Public Health, London, UK
16.13.2: Coronary heart disease: epidemiology and prevention

T.J. Marrie Dean, Faculty of Medicine, Dalhousie University, Clinical Research Centre, Halifax, Nova Scotia, Canada
7.6.41: Coxiella burnetii infections (Q fever)

C.D. Marsden* Late Professor of Neurology, National Hospital for Neurology and Neurosurgery, London, UK
24.19: Acquired metabolic disorders and the nervous system

Judith C.W. Marsh Professor of Clinical Haematology/Honorary Consultant Haematologist, Department of Haematology, St George's Hospital, St George's University of London, London, UK
22.3.11: Aplastic anaemia and other causes of bone marrow failure

Kevin Marsh Director, KEMRI Wellcome Research Programme, Kilifi, Kenya
7.8.2: Malaria

Steven B. Marston Professor of Cardiac Biochemistry, National Heart and Lung Institute (NHLI) Division, Faculty of Medicine, Imperial College London, London, UK
16.1.2: Cardiac myocytes and the cardiac action potential

N.M. Martin Consultant in Endocrinology, Hammersmith Hospital, London, UK
13.10: Pancreatic endocrine disorders and multiple endocrine neoplasia

Duncan J. Maskell Head of Department and Marks & Spencer Professor of Farm Animal Health, Food Science & Food Safety, Department of Veterinary Medicine, University of Cambridge, Cambridge, UK
7.1.1: Biology of pathogenic microorganisms

Jay W. Mason Professor of Medicine, Cardiology Division, University of Utah College of Medicine, Salt Lake City, Utah, USA
16.7.1: Myocarditis

‡ It is with regret that we report the death of Dr M. Monir Madkour during the preparation of this edition of the textbook.
*Deceased.

V.I. Mathan Vice-Dean and Campus Director, ICDDR.B, Dhaka, Bangladesh
15.10.8: Malabsorption syndromes in the tropics

Christopher J. Mathias Professor of Neurovascular Medicine and Consultant Physician, Imperial College at St Mary's and the National Hospital for Neurology and Neurosurgery, Institute of Neurology, University College London, UK
24.14: Diseases of the autonomic nervous system

Peter W. Mathieson Dean of the Faculty of Medicine & Dentistry, University of Bristol, Professor of Medicine and Honorary Consultant Nephrologist at North Bristol NHS Trust, UK
21.8.5: Proliferative glomerulonephritis; 21.8.6: Mesangiocapillary glomerulonephritis

Mary E. McCaul Professor, Department of Psychiatry & Behavioral Sciences, Johns Hopkins University School of Medicine, Baltimore, Maryland, USA
26.7.1: Alcohol and drug dependence

Brian W. McCrindle Professor of Pediatrics, University of Toronto, Staff Cardiologist, The Hospital for Sick Children, Toronto, Canada
19.11.8: Kawasaki's disease

A.D. McGavigan Associate Professor of Cardiovascular Medicine, Flinders University, South Australia, Australia
16.2.2: Syncope and palpitations; 16.4: Cardiac arrhythmias

John A. McGrath Professor of Molecular Dermatology, St John's Institute of Dermatology, King's College London (Guy's Campus), London, UK
23.1: Structure and function of skin

Jane McGregor Senior Lecturer and Honorary Consultant Dermatologist, Barts and the London NHS Trust, UK
23.9: Photosensitivity

Iain B. McInnes Professor of Experimental Medicine and Honorary Consultant Rheumatologist, Glasgow Biomedical Research Centre, University of Glasgow, Glasgow, UK
4.3: Cytokines

William J. McKenna The Heart Hospital, University College London, UK
16.7.2: The cardiomyopathies: hypertrophic, dilated, restrictive, and right ventricular; 16.7.3: Specific heart muscle disorders

A.J. McMichael Professor and NHMRC Australia Fellow, National Centre for Epidemiology and Population Health, ANU College of Medicine, Biology and Environment, Australian National University, Canberra, Australia
3.2: Human population size, environment, and health

Martin McNally Consultant Orthopaedic Surgeon, Nuffield Orthopaedic Centre NHS Trust, Oxford, UK
20.3: Osteomyelitis

K. McNeil Professor of Medicine, University of Queensland, CEO Metro North Health Service, Brisbane, Australia
18.16: Lung transplantation

Henry McQuay Nuffield Department of Anaesthetics, University of Oxford, Oxford, UK
30.1: Dealing with pain

Jill Meara Deputy Director/Public Health Consultant, Health Protection Agency Centre for Radiation, Chemical and Environmental Hazards, Chilton, UK
9.5.9: Radiation

David K. Menon Head, Division of Anaesthesia, University of Cambridge; Consultant, Neurosciences Critical Care Unit, BOC Professor, Royal College of Anaesthetists, Professorial Fellow, Queens' College, Cambridge, Senior Investigator, National Institute for Health Research
17.6: Management of raised intracranial pressure

Catherine H. Mercer Senior Lecturer in Sexual Health Research, Centre for Sexual Health and HIV Research, Research Department of Infection and Public Health, University College London, London, UK
8.2: Sexual behaviour

Vinod K. Metta Research and Clinical Registrar for Neurology and Movement Disorders, Kings College Hospital NHS Trust and University Hospital, London, UK
24.7.2: Parkinsonism and other extrapyramidal diseases

J. ter Meulen Executive Director Vaccine Basic Research, Merck Research Laboratories, West Point, Pennsylvania, USA
7.5.17: Arenaviruses; 7.5.18: Filoviruses

Wayne M. Meyers Visiting Scientist, Department of Environmental and Infectious Disease Sciences, Armed Forces Institute of Pathology, Washington DC, USA
7.6.28: Buruli ulcer: Mycobacterium ulcerans infection

Anna Rita Migliaccio Dirigente de Ricerca in Transfusion Medicine, Laboratory of Clinical Biochemistry, Istituto Superiore doi Sanità, Rome, Italy
22.5.1: Erythropoiesis and the normal red cell

M.A. Miles Professor of Medical Protozoology, Pathogen Molecular Biology Unit, Department of Infectious and Tropical Diseases, London School of Hygiene and Tropical Medicine, London, UK
7.8.11: Chagas disease

Robert F. Miller Professor, Reader in Clinical Infection, Centre for Sexual Health and HIV Research, University College London, London, UK
7.7.5: Pneumocystis jirovecii

Dawn S. Milliner Division of Nephrology, Departments of Pediatrics and Internal Medicine, Mayo Clinic, Rochester, Minnesota, USA
12.10: Hereditary disorders of oxalate metabolism—the primary hyperoxalurias

K.R. Mills Department of Clinical Neurophysiology, King's College Hospital, London, UK
24.3.4: Investigation of central motor pathways: magnetic brain stimulation

Philip Minor Division of Virology, National Institute for Biological Standards and Control, South Mimms, UK
7.5.8: Enterovirus infections

Pramod K. Mistry Department of Pediatrics, Yale School of Medicine, New Haven, Connecticut, USA
12.7.2: Inherited diseases of copper metabolism: Wilson's disease and Menkes' disease

Andrew R.J. Mitchell Consultant Cardiologist, Jersey General Hospital, Jersey, UK
16.3.2: Echocardiography; 16.14.1: Thoracic aortic dissection

Andrew J. Molyneux Consultant in Neuroradiology, The Manor Hospital, Oxford, UK
24.3.3: Imaging in neurological diseases

D.H. Molyneux Centre for Neglected Tropical Diseases, Liverpool School of Tropical Medicine, Pembroke Place, Liverpool, UK
7.9.2: Lymphatic filariasis

Kevin Moore Professor of Hepatology, Department of Medicine, University College London, London, UK
15.22.3: Cirrhosis and ascites

Marina S. Morgan Consultant Medical Microbiologist, Royal Devon & Exeter Foundation NHS Trust, UK
7.6.18: Pasteurella

Pedro L. Moro Immunization Safety Office, Centre for Disease Control and Prevention, Atlanta, Georgia, USA
7.10.1: Cystic hydatid disease (Echinococcus granulosus)

Nicholas W. Morrell British Heart Foundation Professor of Cardiopulmonary Medicine, University of Cambridge School of Clinical Medicine, Addenbrooke's and Papworth Hospitals, Cambridge, UK
16.15.1: Structure and function; 16.15.2: Pulmonary hypertension; 16.15.3: Pulmonary oedema

Emma Morris Senior Lecturer and Honorary Consultant, UCL Medical School, University College London, London, UK
22.8.2: Haemopoietic stem cell transplantation

N.J. McC. Mortensen Professor of Colorectal Surgery, University of Oxford and Consultant Colorectal Surgeon, John Radcliffe Hospitals, Oxford, UK
15.14: Colonic diverticular disease

Peter S. Mortimer Professor of Dermatological Medicine to the University of London, Consultant Skin Physician to St George's Hospital, London and the Royal Marsden Hospital, London, UK
16.18: Chronic peripheral oedema and lymphoedema; 23.12: Blood and lymphatic vessel disorders

Tariq I. Mughal Professor of Medicine and Hematology/Oncology, University of Texas Southwestern School of Medicine, Dallas, Texas, USA
22.3.6: Chronic myeloid leukaemia

David R. Murdoch Professor and Head of Pathology, University of Otago, Christchurch, New Zealand
9.5.4: Diseases of high terrestrial altitudes

Jean B. Nachega Associate Scientist, Department of International Health, Johns Hopkins University, Bloomberg School of Public Health, Baltimore, Maryland, USA; Extraordinary Professor, Department of Medicine, and Director, Centre for Infectious Diseases, Stellenbosch University, Tygerberg, Cape Town, South Africa
7.6.25: Tuberculosis

Robert B. Nadelman Division of Infectious Diseases, Department of Medicine, New York Medical College, Valhalla, New York, USA
7.6.32: Lyme borreliosis

N.V. Naoumov Immunology and Infectious Diseases, Novartis Pharma AG, Basel, Switzerland, and Honorary Professor of Hepatology, University College London, UK
7.5.21: Hepatitis viruses (excluding hepatitis C virus)

Ravinder Nath Maini Emeritus Professor of Rheumatology, The Kennedy Institute of Rheumatology Division, Imperial College London, UK
19.5: Rheumatoid arthritis

David Neal Professor of Surgical Oncology, Honorary Consultant Urological Surgeon, University of Cambridge; Department of Oncology, Addenbrooke's Hospital, Cambridge, UK
21.18: Malignant diseases of the urinary tract

Graham Neale Department of Surgery, Imperial College, London, UK
15.2: Symptomatology of gastrointestinal disease; 15.17: Vascular and collagen disorders

Catherine Nelson-Piercy Consultant Obstetric Physician, Guy's & St Thomas' Foundation Trust and Imperial College Healthcare Trust, UK
14.14: Autoimmune rheumatic disorders and vasculitis in pregnancy

Randolph M. Nesse Professor of Psychiatry and Psychology, Research Professor, Research Center for Group Dynamics, ISR, Director, Evolution and Human Adaptation Program, The University of Michigan, Ann Arbor, Michigan, USA
2.1.2: Evolution: medicine's most basic science

Peter J. Nestor University Lecturer in Cognitive Neurology, University of Cambridge, Department of Clinical Neurosciences, Cambridge, UK; Honorary Consultant Neurologist, Addenbrooke's Hospital, Cambridge, UK
24.4.1: Disturbances of higher cerebral function

J. Neuberger Honorary Consultant Physician, Liver Unit, Queen Elizabeth Hospital, Birmingham, UK; Honorary Professor of Medicine, University of Birmingham, UK; Associate Medical Director, Organ Donation and Transplantation, NHS Blood and Transplant, Bristol, UK
15.22.8: Drugs and liver damage; 15.22.9: The liver in systemic disease

A.J. Newman Taylor Consultant in Respiratory Medicine, Faculty of Medicine, Imperial College, London, UK
18.7: Asthma

A.G. Nicholson Consultant Histopathologist, Royal Brompton and Harefield NHS Trust; Professor of Respiratory Pathology, National Heart and Lung Institute, Imperial College School of Medicine, London, UK
18.11.2: Idiopathic pulmonary fibrosis

Perry Nisen Senior Vice President, Cancer Research, GlaxoSmithKline, Philadelphia, Pennsylvania, USA
2.3.4: The future of clinical trials

Jerry P. Nolan Consultant in Anaesthesia and Intensive Care Medicine, Royal United Hospital Bath, UK; Co-Chair International Liaison Committee on Resuscitation
17.1: Cardiac arrest

John Nowakowski Division of Infectious Diseases, Department of Medicine, New York Medical College, Valhalla, New York, USA
7.6.32: Lyme borreliosis

Paul Nyirjesy Professor of Obstetrics and Gynecology and of Medicine, Drexel University College of Medicine, Philadelphia, Pennsylvania, USA
8.4: Vaginal discharge

Kunle Odunsi Professor and Research Program Director, Roswell Park Cancer Institute, Buffalo, New York, USA
6.4: Cancer immunity and clinical oncology

Graham S. Ogg Reader in Cutaneous Immunology, MRC Senior Clinical Fellow; Consultant in Dermatology, Churchill Hospital, Oxford, UK
23.7: Cutaneous vasculitis, connective tissue diseases, and urticaria

Yngvild K. Olsen Assistant Professor, Department of Medicine, Johns Hopkins University School of Medicine, Baltimore, Maryland, USA
26.7.1: Alcohol and drug dependence

Petra C.F. Oyston Defence Science and Technology Laboratories in the Biomedical Sciences Department, Dstl Porton Down, Salisbury, UK; Chair at the University of Leicester in the Department of Infection, Immunity and Inflammation
7.6.19: Francisella tularensis infection

Nigel O'Farrell Consultant Physician, Ealing Hospital, London, UK
7.6.13: Haemophilus ducreyi and chancroid

Donncha O'Gradaigh Consultant Rheumatologist, Waterford Regional Hospital, Ireland
19.12: Miscellaneous conditions presenting to the rheumatologist; 20.5: Osteonecrosis, osteochondrosis, and osteochondritis dissecans

Kevin O'Shaughnessy Senior Lecturer/Consultant, Clinical Pharmacology Unit, Department of Medicine, Addenbrooke's Hospital, Cambridge, UK
10.1: Principles of clinical pharmacology and drug therapy

Edel O'Toole Centre for Cutaneous Research, Blizard Institute of Cell and Molecular Science, Barts and the London School of Medicine and Dentistry and Department of Dermatology, Barts and the London NHS Trust, London, UK
23.14: Tumours of the skin

Aparna Pal Centre for Diabetes, Oxford Endocrinology and Metabolism, Churchill Hospital, Oxford, UK
13.3: Disorders of the posterior pituitary gland

Jacqueline Palace Consultant in Neurology, The Horton Hospital, Banbury, UK
24.23: Disorders of the neuromuscular junction

Thalia Papayannopoulou Professor of Medicine (Hematology), University of Washington, Division of Hematology, Seattle, USA
22.5.1: Erythropoiesis and the normal red cell

Jayan Parameshwar Consultant Cardiologist, Transplant Unit, Papworth Hospital, Cambridge. UK
16.5.2: Cardiac transplantation and mechanical circulatory support

S. Parish Clinical Trial Service Unit, University of Oxford, Oxford, UK
2.3.3: Large-scale randomized evidence: trials and meta-analyses of trials

Gilbert Park Consultant in Anaesthesia and Intensive Care, Addenbrooke's Hospital, Cambridge, UK
17.7: Sedation and analgesia in the critically ill

P. Parker Head of Division of Cancer Studies, King's College London, UK
13.8.3: Breast cancer

David Parkes SGDP Research Centre, Institute of Psychiatry and Neurosciences Department, King's Healthcare, Denmark Hill, London, UK
24.5.2: Narcolepsy

Miles Parkes Consultant Gastroenterologist, Inflammatory Bowel Disease Genetics Research Unit, Addenbrooke's Hospital, Cambridge, UK
15.11: Crohn's disease

Philippe Parola Unité de Recherche en Maladies Infectieuses et Tropicales Emergentes, WHO Collaborative Centre for Rickettsioses and other Arthropod borne Bacteria, Faculté de Médecine, Université de la Mediterraníe, Marseilles, France

7.6.39: Rickettsioses

C.M. Parry Oxford University Clinical Research Unit, Hospital for Tropical Diseases, Ho Chi Minh City, Vietnam

7.6.8: Typhoid and paratyphoid fevers

J. Paul Regional Microbiologist, Health Protection Agency, South East Region, Regional Microbiologist's Office, Royal Sussex County Hospital, Brighton, UK

7.6.46: A check list of bacteria associated with infection in humans; 7.12: Nonvenomous arthropods

S.J. Peacock Professor of Clinical Microbiology, Department of Medicine, University of Cambridge Cambridge, UK

7.6.7.2: Pseudomonas aeruginosa; 7.6.15: Melioidosis and glanders

Roger Pedersen MRC Centre for Stem Cell Biology and Regenerative Medicine, University of Cambridge, UK

4.8: Stem cells and regenerative medicine

Malik Peiris Department of Microbiology, The University of Hong Kong, Queen Mary Hospital Pokfualm, Hong Kong SAR

7.5.1: Respiratory tract viruses

Hugh Pennington Emeritus Professor of Bacteriology, University of Aberdeen, UK

7.6.7.1: Enterobacteria and bacterial food poisoning

M.B. Pepys Head, Division of Medicine, Royal Free Campus, University College London; Director, UCL Centre for Amyloidosis & Acute Phase Proteins; UK NHS National Amyloidosis Centre, UK

12.12.1: The acute phase response and C-reactive protein; 12.12.3: Amyloidosis

S.P. Pereira Senior Lecturer in Gastroenterology, University College, London Medical School, London, UK

15.16: Cancers of the gastrointestinal tract

G.D. Perkin Emeritus Consultant Neurologist, Charing Cross Hospital, London, UK

24.5.1: Epilepsy in later childhood and adulthood

P.L. Perrotta Associate Professor of Pathology, Director of Clinical Laboratories, West Virginia School of Medicine, West Virginia, USA

22.8.1: Blood transfusion

David J. Perry Consultant Haematologist, Department of Haematology, Addenbrooke's Hospital, Cambridge, UK

14.16: Blood disorders specific to pregnancy

Hans Persson Senior Consultant Physician, Swedish Poisons Centre, Stockholm, Sweden

9.3.1: Poisonous plants and fungi

Michael C. Petch Consultant Cardiologist, Queen Elizabeth Hospital, Kings Lynn, UK

16.13.8: The impact of coronary heart disease on life and work

Eskild Petersen Department of Infectious Diseases, Aarhus University Hospital, Skejby, Aarhus, Denmark

7.8.4: Toxoplasmosis

L.R. Petersen Director, Division of Vector-borne Infectious Diseases, Centers for Disease Control and Prevention, Fort Collins, Colorado, USA

7.5.12: Alphaviruses; 7.5.14: Flaviviruses excluding dengue

R. Peto Clinical Trial Service Unit & Epidemiological Studies Unit (CTSU), University of Oxford, UK

2.3.3: Large-scale randomized evidence: trials and meta-analyses of trials; 6.1: Epidemiology of cancer

T.E.A. Peto Professor of Infectious Diseases, University of Oxford; Consultant Physician, Oxford Radcliffe Hospitals, Nuffield Department of Medicine, John Radcliffe Hospital, Oxford, UK

7.5.23: HIV/AIDS

A.O. Phillips Consultant in Nephrology, University Hospital of Wales, Cardiff, UK

21.1: Structure and functions of the kidney

Wendy Phillips Specialty Registrar in Neurology, Cambridge University Hospitals Foundation Trust, Cambridge, UK

24.3.1: Lumbar puncture

G. Pichert Consultant Clinical Geneticist, Guy's & St Thomas' NHS Foundation Trust, London, UK

13.8.3: Breast cancer

J.D. Pickard Professor of Neurosurgery, Academic Neurosurgery Unit, Department of Clinical Neurosciences, University of Cambridge, Addenbrooke's Hospital, Cambridge, UK

24.5.6: Brain death and the vegetative state

V.V. Pillay Chief, Poison Control Centre, Head, Analytical Toxicology, Amrita Institute of Medical Sciences, Cochin, Kerala, India

9.3.2: Common Indian poisonous plants

S. Pinder Professor of Breast Histopathology, King's College London, Consultant Histopathologist, Guy's & St Thomas NHS Foundation Trust, London, UK

13.8.3: Breast cancer

Michael R. Pinsky Professor of Critical Care Medicine, Pittsburgh, Pennsylvania, USA

17.4: Circulation and circulatory support in the critically ill

Mervi L.S. Pitkanen Consultant Neuropsychiatrist, Neuropsychiatry and Memory Disorders Clinic, Adamson Centre, London, UK

26.4: Neuropsychiatric disorders

R.J. Playford Professor of Medicine, Clinical Gastroenterologist, Vice Principal NHS Liaison and Deputy Warden, Barts and The London School of Medicine and Dentistry, UK

15.10.7: Effects of massive small bowel resection

J.M. Polak Emeritus Professor, Division of Investigative Science, Imperial Colllege London, London, UK

15.9: Hormones and the gastrointestinal tract

Eleanor S. Pollak Associate Professor, Hospital of the University of Pennsylvania, Children's Hospital of Philadelphia and the Philadelphia VA Medical Center, Abramson Research Center, Philadelphia, Pennsylvania, USA

22.6.4: Genetic disorders of coagulation

Andrew J. Pollard Professor of Paediatric Infection and Immunity, Department of Paediatrics, University of Oxford, Oxford, UK

9.5.4: Diseases of high terrestrial altitudes

Aaron Polliack Emeritus Professor of Hematology, and Head of Lymphoma, Leukemia Unit, Department of Hematology, Hadassah University Hospital and, Hebrew University Medical School Jerusalem, Israel; Senior Consultant, Emeritus Professor of Hematology, Department of Hematology and Bone Marrow Transplantation, Tel Aviv Sourasky Medical Center, Tel Aviv, Israel

22.3.5: Chronic lymphocytic leukaemia and other leukaemias of mature B and T cells

Philip A. Poole-Wilson† British Heart Foundation Simon Marks Professor of Cardiology, National Heart and Lung Institute (NHLI) Division, Faculty of Medicine, Imperial College London, London, UK

16.1.2: Cardiac myocytes and the cardiac action potential

Françoise Portaels Mycobacteriology Unit, Department of Microbiology, Institute of Tropical Medicine Nationalestraat, Antwerpen, Belgium

7.6.28: Buruli ulcer: Mycobacterium ulcerans infection

Jerry Posner Evelyn Frew American Cancer Society Clinical Research Professor—George C. Cotzias Chair of Neuro-oncology—Professor of Neurology and Neuroscience, Weil Medical School of Cornell University Department of Neuro-oncology, Memorial Sloan-Kettering Cancer Center, New York City, New York, USA

24.21: Paraneoplastic neurological syndromes

---

† It is with regret that we report the death of Professor Philip A. Poole-Wilson during the preparation of this edition of the textbook.

William G. Powderly Professor of Medicine and Therapeutics, Dean of Medicine, UCD School of Medicine and Medical Sciences, University College Dublin, Dublin, Ireland

7.7.2: Cryptococcosis

J. Powell-Tuck Emeritus Professor of Clinical Nutrition, Barts and the London School of Medicine and Dentistry, UK

11.2: Vitamins and trace elements

Janet Powell Department of Surgery & Cancer, Imperial College, London, UK

16.14.2: Peripheral arterial disease

Amy Powers Instructor, Harvard Medical School and Beth Israel Deaconess Medical Center, Boston, Massachusetts, USA

22.5.9: Haemolytic anaemia—congenital and acquired

J.W. Powles Department of Public Health and Primary Care, University of Cambridge, Cambridge, UK

3.2: Human population size, environment, and health

Michael B. Prentice Professor of Medical Microbiology, Department of Microbiology, University College Cork, Cork, Ireland

7.6.16: Plague: Yersinia pestis; 7.6.17: Other yersinia infections: yersiniosis

A. Purushotham Professor of Breast Cancer, King's College London, Consultant Breast Surgeon, Guy's & St Thomas NHS Foundation Trust, London, UK

13.8.3: Breast cancer

Charles Pusey Imperial College Kidney and Transplant Institute, Imperial College London, UK

21.8.7: Antiglomerular basement membrane disease

Anisur Rahman Professor of Rheumatology, University College London, UK

19.11.2: Systemic lupus erythematosus and related disorders

S. Vincent Rajkumar Professor of Medicine, Division of Hematology, Mayo Clinic, Rochester, Minnesota, USA

22.4.5: Myeloma and paraproteinaemias

M. Ramsay Consultant Epidemiologist, Immunisation, Hepatitis and Blood Safety Department, HPA Centre for Infections, London, UK

7.3: Immunization

A.C. Rankin Professor of Medical Cardiology, BHF Glasgow Cardiovascular Research Centre, University of Glasgow, UK

16.2.2: Syncope and palpitations; 16.4: Cardiac arrhythmias

Didier Raoult Faculté de Médecine et de Pharmacie, Université de la Méditerranée, Marseille Cedex, France

7.6.39: Rickettsioses; 7.6.42: Bartonellas excluding B. bacilliformis

Michael D. Rawlins National Institute for Health and Clinical Excellence, London, UK

2.4.1: The evaluation and provision of effective medicines

Paul J. Reading Consultant in Neurology, Department of Neurology, The James Cook University Hospital, Middlesbrough, UK

24.5.3: Sleep disorders

C.W.G. Redman Emeritus Professor of Obstetric Medicine, University of Oxford; Honorary Research Fellow, Lady Margaret Hall, Oxford Nuffield Department of Obstetrics and Gynaecology, John Radcliffe Hospital Oxford, UK

14.4: Hypertension in pregnancy

Jeremy Rees Consultant Neurologist, National Hospital for Neurology and Neurosurgery, London, UK

24.10.4: Intracranial tumours; 24.21: Paraneoplastic neurological syndromes

Shelley Renowden Consultant in Neuroradiology, Frenchay Hospital, Bristol, UK

24.3.3: Imaging in neurological diseases

Todd W. Rice Assistant Professor of Medicine, Division of Allergy, Pulmonary, and Critical Care Medicine, Vanderbilt University School of Medicine, Nashville, Tennessee, USA

7.1.2: Physiological changes, clinical features, and general management of infected patients

J. Richens Centre for Sexual Health and HIV Research, Research Department of Infection & Population Health, University College London, London, UK

7.6.9: Intracellular klebsiella infections (donovanosis and rhinoscleroma)

A.B. Rickinson Institute for Cancer Studies, University of Birmingham, Birmingham, UK

7.5.3: Epstein–Barr virus

B.K. Rima Deputy Head of the School of Medicine, Dentistry and Biomedical Sciences, Belfast, Ireland

7.5.5: Mumps: epidemic parotitis

Eberhard Ritz Department of Internal Medicine, Division of Nephrology, Heidelberg, Germany

21.6: Chronic kidney disease

Harold R. Roberts Sarah Graham Kenan Distinguished Professor of Medicine, Department of Medicine; Division of Hematology/Oncology, University of North Carolina, Chapel Hill NC and Attending Physician, University of North Carolina Hospitals, North Carolina, USA

22.6.1: The biology of haemostasis and thrombosis

T.A. Rockall Director MATTU, University of Surrey, Guildford, UK

15.4.2: Gastrointestinal bleeding

Kenneth Rockwood Professor of Geriatric Medicine, Dalhousie University, Halifax, Nova Scotia, Canada

29.1: Medicine in old age

Edward Roddy Specialty Registrar in Rheumatology, Nottingham City Hospital, Nottingham, UK

19.10: Crystal-related arthropathies

Simon D. Roger Director of Renal Medicine, Gosford Hospital, Gosford, NSW, Australia; Clinical Associate Professor, Department of Medicine & Health Sciences, Newcastle University, Newcastle, NSW, Australia

21.9.1: Acute interstitial nephritis

Jean-Marc Rolain Faculté de Médecine et de Pharmacie, Université de la Méditerranée, Marseille Cedex, France

7.6.42: Bartonellas excluding B. bacilliformis

P. Ronco Professor of Renal Medicine, University Pierre et Marie Curie, Tenon Hospital, and Inserm Unit UMR_S702

21.10.4: Renal involvement in plasma cell dyscrasias, immunoglobulin-based amyloidoses, and fibrillary glomerulopathies, lymphomas, and leukaemias

Antony Rosen Mary Betty Stevens Professor of Medicine, Professor of Pathology, Director, Division of Rheumatology, Johns Hopkins University School of Medicine, Baltimore, Maryland, USA

5.4: Autoimmunity

Mark J. Rosen Chief, Division of Pulmonary, Critical Care and Sleep Medicine, North Shore University Hospital and Long Island Jewish Medical Center, Professor of Medicine, Hofstra University School of Medicine, New York, USA

18.4.4: Pulmonary complications of HIV infection

Peter Rubin Professor of Therapeutics, Division of Therapeutics & Molecular Medicine, University of Nottingham, Nottingham, UK

14.18: Prescribing in pregnancy

Simon M. Rushbrook Consultant Hepatologist, Department of Hepatology Norfolk and Norwich University Hospitals NHS Foundation Trust, Norfolk, UK

15.19: Structure and function of the liver, biliary tract, and pancreas; 15.22.6: Liver tumours—primary and secondary

Anthony S. Russell Professor Emeritus, Rheumatic Disease Unit, University of Alberta, Edmonton, Alberta, Canada

19.2: Clinical presentation and diagnosis of rheumatic disease

Nikant Sabharwal Consultant Cardiologist, Department of Cardiology, John Radcliffe Hospital, Oxford, UK

16.3.3: Cardiac investigation—nuclear and other imaging techniques

I. Sadaf Farooqi Metabolic Research Laboratories, Institute of Metabolic Science, Addenbrooke's Hospital, University of Cambridge, Cambridge, UK

11.5: Obesity

Hesham Saleh Consultant Rhinologist/Facial Plastic Surgeon, Charing Cross Hospital and Royal Brompton Hospital, Honorary Senior Lecturer, Imperial College, London, UK

18.6: Allergic rhinitis

Nilesh J. Samani British Heart Foundation Professor of Cardiology, Department of Cardiovascular Sciences, University of Leicester, Leicester, UK

16.17.4: Mendelian disorders causing hypertension

Swati Sathe Assistant Professor of Neurology, New York University School of Medicine, New York, USA

24.17: Inherited neurodegenerative diseases

Brian P. Saunders Wolfson Unit for Endoscopy, St Mark's Hospital for Colorectal Disorders, Harrow, London, UK

15.3.1: Colonoscopy and flexible sigmoidoscopy

S.J. Saunders Division of Hepatology, University of Cape Town Medical School, University of Cape Town, South Africa

15.22.7: Hepatic granulomas

E. Sawyer Consultant Clinical Oncologist, Guy's & St Thomas NHS Foundation Trust, London, UK

13.8.3: Breast cancer

K.P. Schaal Emeritus Professor of Medical Microbiology; Member of the Expert Committee of the Federal Ministry of Labour and Social Affairs Institute for Medical Microbiology, Immunology and Parasitology, University Hospital, Bonn, Germany

7.6.29: Actinomycoses

Michael L. Schilsky Associate Professor of Medicine, Medical Director, Adult Liver Transplant, Yale-New Haven Transplantation Center, Department of Internal Medicine, Yale School of Medicine, New Haven, Connecticut, USA

12.7.2: Inherited diseases of copper metabolism: Wilson's disease and Menkes' disease

Neil Scolding University of Bristol Institute of Clinical Neurosciences, Department of Neurology, Frenchay Hospital, Bristol, UK

24.19: Acquired metabolic disorders and the nervous system; 24.20: Neurological complications of systemic disease

Anthony Scott Wellcome Trust Senior Research Fellow in Clinical Science, KEMRI Wellcome Trust Research Programme, Kilifi, Kenya; Nuffield Department of Clinical Medicine, University of Oxford, Oxford, UK

7.6.3: Pneumococcal infections

A. Seaton Honorary Senior Consultant, Institute of Occupational Medicine, Edinburgh, UK and Emeritus Professor of Environmental and Occupational Medicine, University of Aberdeen, Aberdeen, UK

18.13: Pneumoconioses

Amartya Sen Lamont University Professor and Professor of Economics and Philosophy, Harvard University, Cambridge, Massachusetts, USA

3.5: Human disasters

G.R. Serjeant University of West Indies, Kingston, Jamaica

21.10.6: Sickle-cell disease and the kidney

Nicholas J. Severs Professor of Cell Biology, National Heart and Lung Institute (NHLI) Division, Faculty of Medicine, Imperial College London, London, UK

16.1.2: Cardiac myocytes and the cardiac action potential

Keerti V. Shah Department of Molecular Microbiology and Immunology, Johns Hopkins Bloomberg School of Public Health, Baltimore, Maryland, USA

7.5.19: Papillomaviruses and polyomaviruses

Pallav L. Shah Consultant Physician, Royal Brompton Hospital, London, UK, Chelsea & Westminster Hospital, London, UK

18.3.3: Bronchoscopy, thoracoscopy, and tissue biopsy

Michael Sharpe Professor of Psychological Medicine, Psychological Medicine Research, School of Molecular and Clinical Medicine, University of Edinburgh, UK

26.1: General introduction; 26.5.3: Medically unexplained symptoms in patients attending medical clinics; 26.5.4: Chronic fatigue syndrome (postviral fatigue syndrome, neurasthenia, and myalgic encephalomyelitis); 26.6.2: Psychological treatment in medical practice

Maire P. Shelly Consultant in Intensive Care, Wythenshawe Hospital, Manchester, UK

17.7: Sedation and analgesia in the critically ill

Jackie Sherrard Consultant in Genitourinary Medicine, Churchill Hospital, Oxford, UK

7.6.6: Neisseria gonorrhoeae; 8.3: Sexual history and examination

M.A. Shikanai-Yasuda Professor of Department of Infectious and Parasitic Diseases, Endemic Diseases Group/Infections in Immunosupressed Host Programme, Faculdade de Medicina, University of São Paulo, Brazil

7.7.4: Paracoccidioidomycosis

John M. Shneerson Director, Respiratory Support & Sleep Centre, Papworth Hospital, Cambridge, UK

18.18: Disorders of the thoracic cage and diaphragm

C.A. Sieff Division of Hematology, Karp 080006C, Children's Hospital Boston, Boston, Massachusetts, USA

22.2.1: Stem cells and haemopoiesis

J. Sieper Free University, Berlin, Germany

19.6: Ankylosing spondylitis, other spondyloarthritides, and related conditions

Udomsak Silachamroon Assistant Professor of Tropical Medicine, Department of Clinical Tropical Medicine, Faculty of Tropical Medicine, Mahidol University, Bangkok, Thailand

7.11.3: Lung flukes (paragonimiasis)

Leslie Silberstein Professor, Harvard Medical School, Children's Hospital Boston, Dana-Farber Cancer Institute, Brigham and Women's Hospital, and Harvard Stem Cell Institute, Boston, Massachusetts, USA

22.5.9: Haemolytic anaemia—congenital and acquired

Rod Sinclair Professor of Dermatology, University of Melbourne, Director of Dermatology, St. Vincent's Hospital, Director of Research and Training, Skin and Cancer Foundation, Fitzroy, Australia

23.17: Management of skin disease

Robert E. Sinden The Malaria Centre, Department of Life Sciences, Imperial College London, London, UK

7.8.2: Malaria

Joseph Sinning Harold Leever Regional Cancer Center, Waterbury, Connecticut, USA

22.4.1: Leucocytes in health and disease

Thira Sirisanthana Professor of Medicine, Chiang Mai University, Thailand

7.6.20: Anthrax; 7.7.6: Penicillium marneffei infection

J.G.P. Sissons Regius Professor of Physic, Director, Cambridge University Health Partners, School of Clinical Medicine, University of Cambridge, Cambridge, UK

7.5.2: Herpesviruses (excluding Epstein–Barr virus)

Geoffrey L. Smith Wellcome Principal Research Fellow, Section of Virology, Faculty of Medicine, Imperial College London, London, UK

7.5.4: Poxviruses

R. Smith Emeritus Professor of Rheumatology, Nuffield Orthopaedic Centre NHS Trust, Oxford, UK

20.1: Skeletal disorders—general approach and clinical conditions

Robert W. Snow Head, Malaria Public Health Group, KEMRI/Wellcome Trust Programme and Advisor, National Malaria Control Programme, Ministry of Health, Nairobi, Kenya

7.8.2: Malaria

E.L. Snyder Professor, Laboratory Medicine, Yale University School of Medicine, New Haven, Connecticut, USA

22.8.1: Blood transfusion

Jasmeet Soar Consultant in Anaesthesia and Intensive Care Medicine, Southmead Hospital Bristol, UK; Chair, Resuscitation Council (UK)

17.1: Cardiac arrest

Krishna Somers Consultant Physician in Cardiovascular Medicine, Royal Perth Hospital, Perth, Australia

16.9.4: Cardiovascular syphilis

M.W. Sonderup Division of Hepatology, University of Cape Town Medical School, University of Cape Town, South Africa

15.22.7: Hepatic granulomas

R.L. Souhami Emeritus Professor of Medicine, University College London, London, UK

6.5: Cancer: clinical features and management

C.W.N. Spearman Division of Hepatology, University of Cape Town Medical School, University of Cape Town, South Africa.
15.22.7: Hepatic granulomas

G.P. Spickett Consultant Clinical Immunologist, Regional Department of Immunology, Royal Victoria Hospital, Newcastle upon Tyne, UK
18.14.1: Pulmonary haemorrhagic disorders; 18.14.2: Eosinophilic pneumonia; 18.14.4: Lymphocytic infiltrations of the lung

S.G. Spiro Professor of Respiratory Medicine and Honorary Consultant Physician Royal Brompton Hospital, London, UK
18.19.1: Lung cancer; 18.19.2: Pulmonary metastases

Jerry L. Spivak Division of Hematology. The Johns Hopkins University School of Medicine, Baltimore, Maryland, USA
22.3.9: Idiopathic myelofibrosis

U. Srinivas-Shankar Consultant Physician, Department of Diabetes & Endocrinology, St Helens & Knowsley Teaching Hospitals NHS Trust, St Helens, UK
13.8.2: Disorders of male reproduction

Paweł Stankiewicz Assistant Professor, Department of Molecular and Human Genetics, Baylor College of Medicine
4.2.2: The genomic basis of medicine

Paul D. Stein Visiting Professor, Department of Internal Medicine, Michigan State University, College of Osteopathic Medicine, East Lansing, Missouri, USA
16.16.1: Deep venous thrombosis and pulmonary embolism

Dennis L. Stevens Chief, Infectious Diseases Section, Veterans Affairs Medical Center, Boise, Professor of Medicine, University of Washington School of Medicine, Seattle, Washington, USA
7.6.2: Streptococci and enterococci; 7.6.24: Botulism, gas gangrene, and clostridial gastrointestinal infections

Tom Stevens Consultant Psychiatrist, Lambeth Hospital, South London and Maudsley NHS Foundation Trust, London, UK
26.4: Neuropsychiatric disorders

J.C. Stevenson Department of Metabolic Medicine, Imperial College London, Royal Brompton Hospital, London, UK
14.20: Benefits and risks of hormone replacement therapy

P.M. Stewart Professor of Medicine and Director of Research and Knowledge Transfer, University of Birmingham, Birmingham, UK
13.7.1: Disorders of the adrenal cortex

Stephen F. Stewart Institute of Cellular Medicine, Newcastle University, Newcastle upon Tyne, UK
15.22.1: Alcoholic liver disease; 15.22.2: Nonalcoholic steatohepatitis

August Stich Department of Tropical Medicine, Medical Mission Institute, Würzburg, Germany
7.8.10: Human African trypanosomiasis

Heather Stoddart Principal Clinical Scientist, Department of Chemical Pathology and Immunology, St Mary's Hospital, Imperial College Healthcare NHS Trust, London, UK
32.1: Biochemistry in medicine—reference intervals: the use of biochemical analysis for diagnosis and management

John H. Stone Associate Professor of Medicine, Harvard Medical School, Director, Clinical Rheumatology, Massachusetts General Hospital, Massachusetts, USA
19.11.7: Polymyositis and dermatomyositis

J.R. Stradling Professor of Respiratory Medicine & Consultant Respiratory Physician, Oxford Centre for Respiratory Medicine, John Radcliffe Hospitals, Oxford, UK
18.1.1: The upper respiratory tract; 18.5.1: Upper airways obstruction; 18.5.2: Sleep-related disorders of breathing

Frank J. Strobl Director of Scientific Affairs, Therakos, Inc. RandCD, Exton, Pennsylvania, USA
22.5.9: Haemolytic anaemia—congenital and acquired

M.A. Stroud Senior Lecturer in Medicine, University of Southampton, UK
9.5.1: Heat; 9.5.2: Cold

Michael Strupp Department of Neurology, Ludwig-Maximilians University, Munich, Germany
24.6.2: Eye movements and balance

Peter H. Sugden Professor of Cellular Biochemistry, National Heart and Lung Institute (NHLI) Division, Faculty of Medicine, Imperial College London, London, UK
16.1.2: Cardiac myocytes and the cardiac action potential

J.A. Summerfield St Mary's Hospital, London, UK
15.23: Diseases of the gallbladder and biliary tree; 15.25: Congenital disorders of the liver, biliary tract, and pancreas

Joseph Sung Professor of Medicine, Head, Shaw College, Associate Dean (General Affairs), Chairman, Department of Medicine & Therapeutics, Director, Institute of Digestive Disease, Faculty of Medicine, The Chinese University of Hong Kong
15.8: Peptic ulcer disease

Pravan Suntharasamai Mahidol University, Bangkok, Thailand
7.9.7: Gnathostomiasis

P. Sweny Emeritus Consultant Nephrologist, Royal Free NHS Trust, London, UK
21.7.3: Renal transplantation

A.J. Swerdlow Professor of Epidemiology, Institute of Cancer Research, University of London, UK
6.1: Epidemiology of cancer

D. Swirsky Consultant Haematologist, St James's University Hospital, Leeds, UK
22.4.4: The spleen and its disorders

Penelope Talelli Sobell Department of Motor Neuroscience and Movement Disorders, Institute of Neurology, University College London; National Hospital for Neurology and Neurosurgery, London, UK
24.7.1: Subcortical structures: the cerebellum, basal ganglia, and thalamus

C.T. Tan Professor, Department of Medicine, University of Malaya, Kuala Lumpur, Malaysia
7.5.7: Nipah and Hendra virus encephalitides

David Taylor-Robinson Emeritus Professor of Genito-Microbiology and Medicine, Imperial College London, Division of Medicine, London, UK
7.6.44: Chlamydial infections; 7.6.45: Mycoplasmas

Henri A. Termeer Chairman and Chief Executive Officer, Genzyme Corporation, Cambridge, Massachusetts, USA
2.4.4: Sustaining innovation in an era of specialized medicine

R.V. Thakker May Professor of Medicine, Academic Endocrine Unit, Nuffield Department of Clinical Medicine, University of Oxford; Oxford Centre for Diabetes, Endocrinology and Metabolism, Churchill Hospital, Oxford, UK
13.6: Parathyroid disorders and diseases altering calcium metabolism

David G.T. Thomas Department of Neurological Surgery, Institute of Neurology, London, UK
24.10.3: Traumatic injuries to the head

P.K. Thomas[‡] Emeritus Professor of Neurology, Royal Free Hospital School of Medicine and Institute of Neurology, London, UK
24.12: Disorders of cranial nerves; 24.16: Diseases of the peripheral nerves

D.G. Thompson Professor of Gastroenterology, Epithelial Sciences Research Group, School of Translational Medicine, University of Manchester, Clinical Sciences Building, Salford Royal Hospitals Salford, UK
15.1: Structure and function of the gut; 15.13: Irritable bowel syndrome and functional bowel disorders

R.P.H. Thompson Gastrointestinal Laboratory, The Rayne Institute, St Thomas's Hospital, London, UK
15.20: Jaundice

S.A. Thorne Consultant Cardiologist, University Hospital, Birmingham, UK
16.12: Congenital heart disease in the adult

---

† It is with regret that we report the death of Professor P.K. Thomas during the preparation of this edition of the textbook.

C.L. Thwaites Oxford University Clinical Research Unit, Ho Chi Minh City, Vietnam
7.6.22: Tetanus

Guy E. Thwaites Department of Microbiology, Imperial College, London, UK
24.11.1: Bacterial infections

Adam D. Timmis Professor of Clinical Cardiology, London Chest Hospital, London, UK
16.13.4: Management of stable angina

Charles Tomson Consultant Nephrologist, Richard Bright Renal Unit, Southmead Hospital, Bristol, UK
21.13: Urinary tract infection

P.A. Tookey Senior Lecturer, MRC Centre of Epidemiology for Child Health, UCL Institute of Child Health, London, UK
7.5.13: Rubella

Peter Topham Consultant Nephrologist, John Walls Renal Unit, University Hospitals of Leicester NHS Trust Leicester, UK
21.8.2: Thin membrane nephropathy

P.P. Toskes Professor of Medicine, University of Florida College of Medicine, Gainesville, Florida, USA
15.10.2: Small-bowel bacterial overgrowth; 15.24.2: Chronic pancreatitis

G. Touchard Professor, Department of Nephrology, Poitiers University Hospital, Poitiers, France
21.10.4: Renal involvement in plasma cell dyscrasias, immunoglobulin-based amyloidoses, and fibrillary glomerulopathies, lymphomas, and leukaemias

Thomas A. Traill Adult Cardiology Faculty, Johns Hopkins, Hospital, Baltimore, Maryland, USA
16.10: Tumours of the heart; 16.11: Cardiac involvement in genetic disease

A.S. Truswell Emeritus Professor of Human Nutrition,University of Sydney, Australia
11.4: Diseases of overnourished societies and the need for dietary change

Wai Y. Tse Consultant Nephrologist and Senior Lecturer, Renal Unit, Derriford Hospital, Plymouth, UK
21.10.3: The kidney in rheumatological disorders

D.M. Turnbull Professor of Neurology and Director Newcastle Centre for Brain Ageing and Vitality, Institute for Ageing and Health, Newcastle University, Newcastle upon Tyne, UK.
24.24.5: Mitochondrial encephalomyopathies

A. Neil Turner Consultant in Nephrology, Royal Infirmary, Edinburgh, UK
21.10.7: Infection-associated nephropathies; 21.10.8: Malignancy-associated renal disease

J.A. Vale Director, National Poisons Information Service (Birmingham Unit) and West Midlands Poisons Unit; City Hospital, Birmingham, UK
9.1: Poisoning by drugs and chemicals

Patrick Vallance Senior Vice President Drug Discovery, GlaxoSmithKline, London, UK
2.3.4: The future of clinical trials; 16.1.1: Blood vessels and the endothelium

Steven Vanderschueren General Internal Medicine, University Hospital Gasthuisberg, Leuven, Belgium
7.2.2: Fever of unknown origin

Sirivan Vanijanonta Emeritus Professor of Tropical Medicine, Department of Clinical Tropical Medicine, Faculty of Tropical Medicine, Mahidol University, Bangkok, Thailand
7.11.3: Lung flukes (paragonimiasis)

Patrick J.W. Venables Professor of Viral Immunorheumatology, Kennedy Institute of Rheumatology. Imperial College, London, UK
19.11.6: Sjögren's syndrome

B.J. Vennervald DBL-Centre for Health Research and Development, Faculty of Life Sciences University of Copenhagen, Thorvaldsensvej, Denmark
7.11.1: Schistosomiasis

Vanessa Venning Consultant Dermatologist, Department of Dermatology, Churchill Hospital, Oxford, UK
23.2: Clinical approach to the diagnosis of skin disease

Anilrudh A. Venugopal Clinical Instructor, Division of Infectious Diseases, St. John Hospital and Medical Center, Detroit, Missouri, USA
7.6.10: Anaerobic bacteria

Kristien Verdonck Institute of Tropical Medicine Antwerp Nationalestraat, Antwerp, Belgium; Instituto de Medicina Tropical Alexander von Humboldt Universidad Peruana Cayetano Heredia Av. Honorio Delgado, San Martín de Porres Lima, Peru
7.5.25: HTLV-1, HTLV-2, and associated diseases

C.M. Verity Consultant Paediatric Neurologist, Child Development Centre, Addenbrooke's Hospital, Cambridge, UK
24.18: Developmental abnormalities of the central nervous system

Angela Vincent Consultant in Immunology, John Radcliffe Hospital, Oxford, UK
24.21: Paraneoplastic neurological syndromes; 24.22: Autoimmune limbic encephalitis and Morvan's syndrome

Raphael P. Viscidi Department of Pediatrics, Johns Hopkins University School of Medicine, Baltimore, Maryland, USA
7.5.19: Papillomaviruses and polyomaviruses

Peter D. Wagner Professor of Medicine & Bioengineering, Department of Medicine, University of California, San Diego, La Jolla, California, USA
18.1.2: Airways and alveoli

Nicholas Wald Professor of Environmental and Preventive Medicine, Wolfson Institute of Preventive Medicine, St Bartholomews' and the Royal London School of Medicine and Dentistry, Queen Mary University of London, UK
3.3.2: Medical screening

J.A. Walker-Smith Professor of Paediatric Gastroenterology, University Department of Paediatric Gastroenterology, Royal Free and University College Medical School, London, UK
15.15: Congenital abnormalities of the gastrointestinal tract

Mark J. Walport Director, The Wellcome Trust, London, UK
5.1.2: The complement system

Julian R.F. Walters Consultant Gastroenterologist and Reader, Imperial College, London UK
15.3.4: Investigation of gastrointestinal function; 15.10.1: Differential diagnosis and investigation of malabsorption

Gary S. Wand Professor, Department of Medicine Johns Hopkins University School of Medicine, Baltimore, Maryland, USA
26.7.1: Alcohol and drug dependence

T.E. Warkentin Professor, Department of Pathology and Molecular Medicine and Department of Medicine, Michael G. DeGroote School of Medicine, McMaster University, Hamilton, Ontario, Canada
22.6.5: Acquired coagulation disorders

David A. Warrell Emeritus Professor of Tropical Medicine, Nuffield Department of Clinical Medicine; Honorary Fellow, St Cross College, University of Oxford, Oxford, UK
7.4: Travel and expedition medicine; 7.5.10: Rhabdoviruses: rabies and rabies-related lyssaviruses; 7.5.11: Colorado tick fever and other arthropod-borne reoviruses; 7.5.27: Orf; 7.5.28: Molluscum contagiosum; 7.6.31: Rat-bite fevers; 7.6.33: Relapsing fevers; 7.6.35: Nonvenereal endemic treponematoses: yaws, endemic syphilis (bejel), and pinta; 7.8.2: Malaria; 7.13: Pentastomiasis (porocephalosis, linguatulosis/linguatuliasis); 9.2: Injuries, envenoming, poisoning, and allergic reactions caused by animals; 24.11.2: Viral infections; 24.24.6: Primary (tropical) pyomyositis; 33.1: Acute medical presentations; 33.2: Practical procedures

M. J. Warrell Oxford Vaccine Group, University of Oxford, Centre for Clinical Vaccinology & Tropical Medicine, Churchill Hospital, Oxford, UK
7.5.10: Rhabdoviruses: rabies and rabies-related lyssaviruses; 7.5.11: Colorado tick fever and other arthropod-borne reoviruses

Paul Warwicker Consultant in Nephrology, Lister Hospital, Stevenage, UK
21.10.5: Haemolytic uraemic syndrome

John A.H. Wass Professor of Endocrinology, University of Oxford Department of Endocrinology Oxford Centre for Diabetes, Endocrinology and Metabolism, Churchill Hospital, Oxford, UK
13.2: Disorders of the anterior pituitary gland; 13.3: Disorders of the posterior pituitary gland; 13.12: Hormonal manifestations of nonendocrine disease

Lawrence Waterman Director, Sypol Limited, Aylesbury; Head of Health and Safety, Olympic Delivery Authority, London
9.4.2: Occupational safety

Laurence Watkins Consultant in Neurosurgery, The National Hospital for Neurology and Neurosurgery, London, UK
24.10.3: Traumatic injuries to the head

Chris Watson Reader in Surgery and Honorary Consultant Surgeon, University of Cambridge Department of Surgery, Addenbrooke's Hospital, Cambridge, UK
15.4.1: The acute abdomen

George Watt Associate Professor of Medicine, University of Hawaii at Manoa, John A. Burns School of Medicine, Hawaii, USA
7.6.34: Leptospirosis; 7.6.40: Scrub typhus

Richard W.E. Watts Retired Professor & Honorary Consultant Physician, Imperial College School of Medicine, Hammersmith Hospital, London, UK
12.1: The inborn errors of metabolism: general aspects; 12.4: Disorders of purine and pyrimidine metabolism

D.J. Weatherall Regius Professor of Medicine Emeritus, University of Oxford; Weatherall Institute of Molecular Medicine, Oxford, UK
22.1: Introduction; 22.5.2: Anaemia: pathophysiology, classification, and clinical features; 22.5.3: Anaemia as a challenge to world health; 22.5.5: Normochromic, normocytic anaemia; 22.5.7: Disorders of the synthesis or function of haemoglobin; 22.7: The blood in systemic disease

D.K.H. Webb Consultant Paediatric Haematologist, Great Ormond Street Hospital for Children, London, UK
22.4.7: Histiocytoses

Lisa J. Webber Consultant in Reproductive Medicine, St Mary's Hospital, London, UK
13.8.1: Ovarian disorders

Kathryn E. Webert Assistant Professor, Haematology and Thromboembolism, McMaster University, Hamilton, Ontario, Canada
22.6.3: Disorders of platelet number and function

Bee Wee Consultant and Senior Clinical Lecturer in Palliative Medicine, Oxford Radcliffe Hospitals NHS Trust, and Fellow of Harris Manchester College, University of Oxford, UK
31.1: Palliative care

Anthony P. Weetman Professor of Medicine, Department of Human Metabolism, University of Sheffield, Sheffield, UK
13.4: The thyroid gland and disorders of thyroid function; 13.5: Thyroid cancer

Robert A. Weinstein The C. Anderson Hedberg Professor of Internal Medicine, Rush Medical College, Interim Chair, Department of Medicine, John H. Stroger Jr. Hospital of Cook County, Professor, Rush University Medical Center, Chicago, Illinois, USA
7.6.4: Staphylococci

R.A. Weiss Professor of Viral Oncology, Division of Infection and Immunity, University College London, London, UK
7.5.26: Viruses and cancer

Peter F. Weller Professor of Medicine, Harvard Medical School, Professor of Immunology and Infectious Diseases, Harvard School of Public Health, Chief, Infectious Disease and Allergy and Inflammation Divisions Beth Israel Deaconess Medical Center, Boston, Massachusetts, USA
22.4.6: Eosinophilia

A.U. Wells Interstitial Lung Disease Unit, Royal Brompton Hospital, London, UK
18.11.1: Diffuse parenchymal lung disease: an introduction; 18.11.2: Idiopathic pulmonary fibrosis; 18.11.3: Bronchiolitis obliterans and cryptogenic organizing pneumonia; 18.11.4: The lung in autoimmune rheumatic disorders; 18.11.5: The lung in vasculitis

Simon Wessely Professor, King's College, London, UK
26.6.2: Psychological treatment in medical practice

Gilbert C. White Executive Vice President for Research, Director, Blood Research Institute, Richard H. and Sara E. Aster Chair for Medical Research BloodCenter of Wisconsin; Associate Dean for Research, Professor of Medicine, Pharmacology, and Biochemistry Medical College of Wisconsin, USA
22.6.1: The biology of haemostasis and thrombosis

Joseph White Luxenberg Family Professor of Public Policy, Department of Political Science, Case Western Reserve University, Cleveland, Ohio, USA
3.4.1: The cost of health care in Western countries

H.C. Whittle Visiting Professor, London School of Hygiene and Tropical Medicine, MRC Laboratories, The Gambia, West Africa
7.5.6: Measles

Anthony S. Wierzbicki Department of Metabolic Medicine/Chemical Pathology Guy's & St Thomas Hospitals London, UK
12.9: Disorders of peroxisomal metabolism in adults

David E.L. Wilcken Emeritus Professor of Medicine, University of New South Wales, Prince of Wales Hospital, Sydney, Australia
16.1.3: Clinical physiology of the normal heart

Gordon Wilcock Professor of Clinical Geratology, University of Oxford, UK
29.1: Medicine in old age

James S. Wiley Professor of Haematology, Nepean Clinical School, University of Sydney, Penrith, Australia
22.5.8: Anaemias resulting from defective maturation of red cells

R.G. Will Professor of Clinical Neurology, Department of Clinical Neurosciences, University of Edinburgh, Edinburgh, UK
24.11.5: Human prion diseases

Bryan Williams Professor of Medicine, Department of Cardiovascular Sciences, University of Leicester School of Medicine, UK
16.17.1: Essential hypertension—definition, epidemiology, and pathophysiology; 16.17.2: Diagnosis, assessment, and treatment of essential hypertension

Christopher B. Williams Honorary Physician, Wolfson Unit for Endoscopy, St Mark's Hospital for Colorectal Disorders, London, UK
15.3.1: Colonoscopy and flexible sigmoidoscopy

David J. Williams Consultant Obstetric Physician, Institute for Women's Health, University College London Hospitals, London, UK
14.1: Physiological changes of normal pregnancy; 14.2: Nutrition in pregnancy; 14.3: Medical management of normal pregnancy

Gareth Williams Professor of Medicine, School of Clinical Science, University of Bristol, UK
13.11.1: Diabetes

J. David Williams Institute of Nephrology, University of Wales College of Medicine, Cardiff, UK
21.1: Structure and functions of the kidney

Bridget Wills Hospital for Tropical Diseases, Oxford University Clinical Research Unit, Wellcome Trust Major Overseas Programme, Vietnam, Ho Chi Minh City, Vietnam
7.5.15: Dengue; 24.11.2: Viral infections

R. Wilson Consultant Radiologist, Royal Marsden Hospital, London, UK
13.8.3: Breast cancer

Fenella Wojnarowska Professor Emeritus, University of Oxford, UK
14.13: The skin in pregnancy; 23.4: Vesiculobullous disease

Roger L. Wolman Consultant in Rheumatology and Sport and Exercise Medicine, Royal National Orthopaedic Hospital, Stanmore, UK
28.1: Sports and exercise medicine

Kathryn J. Wood Transplantation Research Immunology Group, Nuffield Department of Surgery, University of Oxford, John Radcliffe Hospital, Oxford, UK
5.5: Principles of transplantation immunology

Nicholas Wood Galton Professor of Genetics, Head of Department of Molecular Neuroscience, UCL Institute of Neurology, UK
24.7.4: Ataxic disorders

H.F. Woods Division of Molecular and Genetic Medicine, University of Sheffield School of Medicine, Sheffield, UK

12.11: Disturbances of acid–base homeostasis

Jeremy Woodward Consultant Gastroenterologist, Addenbrooke's Hospital, Cambridge, UK

11.6: Artificial nutrition support

Elaine M. Worcester Professor of Medicine, University of Chicago, Section of Nephrology, Chicago, Illinois, USA

21.14: Disorders of renal calcium handling, urinary stones, and nephrocalcinosis

B.P. Wordsworth Professor of Rheumatology, Nuffield Department of Orthopaedics, Rheumatology and Musculoskeletal Sciences, Nuffield Orthopaedic Centre, Oxford, UK

20.1: Skeletal disorders—general approach and clinical conditions

Gary P. Wormser Division of Infectious Diseases, Department of Medicine, New York Medical College, Valhalla, New York, USA

7.6.32: Lyme borreliosis

V.M. Wright Professor of Paediatric Gastroenterology, University Department of Paediatric Gastroenterology, Royal Free and University College Medical School, London, UK

15.15: Congenital abnormalities of the gastrointestinal tract

F.C.W. Wu Department of Endocrinology, Manchester Royal Infirmary, Manchester, UK

13.8.2: Disorders of male reproduction

Andrew H. Wyllie Head of Department, Department of Pathology, Cambridge, UK

4.6: Apoptosis in health and disease

Muhammad M. Yaqoob Professor of Nephrology, Barts and London NHS Trust Hospitals and School of Medicine and Dentistry, UK

21.17: Urinary tract obstruction

Hasan Yazici Professor and Chief, Department of Medicine and Division of Rheumatology, Cerrahpasa Medical Faculty, University of Istanbul, Istanbul, Turkey

19.11.5: Behçet's syndrome

Lam Minh Yen Hospital of Tropical Disease, Ho Chi Minh City, Vietnam

7.6.22: Tetanus

Jenny Yiend Research Scientist, Department of Psychiatry, University of Oxford, Oxford, UK

26.5.1: Grief, stress, and post-traumatic stress disorder

Yariv Yogev Director, Division of Maternal Fetal Medicine, Helen Schneider Hospital for Women, Rabin Medical Center, Sackler Faculty of Medicine, Tel - Aviv University, Petah-Tiqva, Israel

14.10: Diabetes in pregnancy

Sebahattin Yurdakul Professor, Division of Rheumatology, Department of Medicine, Cerrahpasa Medical Faculty, University of Istanbul, Istanbul, Turkey

19.11.5: Behçet's syndrome

A. Zeman Professor of Cognitive and Behavioural Neurology, Peninsula Medical School, Exeter, UK

24.2: Mind and brain: building bridges linking neurology, psychiatry, and psychology

Clive S. Zent Consultant Hematologist, Associate Professor of Medicine, Mayo Clinic, Rochester, Minnesota, USA

22.3.5: Chronic lymphocytic leukaemia and other leukaemias of mature B and T cells

SECTION 13

Endocrine disorders

13.1

Principles of hormone action

Mark Gurnell, Jacky Burrin, and
V. Krishna Chatterjee

Essentials

Hormones, produced by glands or cells, are messengers which act locally or at a distance to coordinate the function of cells and organs. Types of hormone include (1) peptides (e.g hypothalamic releasing factors) and proteins (e.g. insulin, growth hormone)—these generally interact with membrane receptors located on the cell surface, causing activation of downstream signalling pathways leading to alteration in gene transcription or modulation of biochemical pathways to effect a physiological response; (2) steroids (e.g. cortisol, progesterone, testosterone, oestradiol) and other lipophilic substances (e.g. vitamin D, retinoic acid, thyroid hormone)—these act by crossing the plasma membrane to interact with intracellular receptors, with hormone action via nuclear receptors altering cellular gene expression directly.

Hormone synthesis, processing and secretion—production of hormones can be regulated at many levels, including (1) gene transcription; (2) mRNA processing; (3) post-translational modification. Some hormones are not significantly concentrated within cells and are released via Golgi-derived transport vesicles that fuse with the plasma membrane (a 'constitutive' pathway of secretion).

By contrast, many endocrine cells contain an additional 'regulated' secretory pathway, which allows the export of high concentrations of hormone stored in cytoplasmic vesicles. Many hormones are released in a rhythmic or pulsatile manner.

Control of hormone production—the classical mechanism by which hormone-producing glands are controlled is by negative feedback, e.g. tri-iodothyronine (T_3) inhibits production of thyrotropin releasing hormone and thyroid stimulating hormone.

Physiological roles of hormones—these are enormously varied and include (1) control of growth and differentiation; (2) maintenance of homeostasis—energy balance, metabolic pathways; fluid, electrolyte and calcium balance; control of blood pressure; and (3) regulation of reproduction.

Clinical features of endocrine disorders—these comprise conditions of either hormone excess or hormone deficiency or hormone resistance, with germ-line or somatic defects in genes mediating hormone synthesis or action causing inherited syndromes or acquired endocrine cellular dysfunction.

Definition

Endocrinology is the study of hormones secreted by glands or cells which, acting locally or at a distance, facilitate communication between cells and different organs thus coordinating their activities.

Classically, the production of hormones has been associated with specialized glands or tissues including the hypothalamus, pituitary, thyroid, parathyroids, gonads, pancreatic islet cells, adrenal glands, and placenta. It is now recognized that hormones are also produced by a range of other organs and tissues which are not considered to be classical endocrine glands. The heart is the primary source of atrial natriuretic peptide factor which controls blood pressure and intravascular volume; endothelin and nitric oxide are derived from vascular endothelium and regulate vascular tone. Endocrine cells are distributed throughout the gastrointestinal tract and are a rich source of hormones such as cholecystokinin, gastrin, secretin, and vasoactive intestinal peptide; many of these gastrointestinal hormones are also produced in the brain and central nervous

system, where their role is less well understood. Erythropoietin, a circulating factor that stimulates erythropoiesis, is derived from the kidney. Adipose tissue produces leptin, a circulating hormone which acts centrally to control appetite.

However, as understanding of intercellular communication has advanced, the lines of division that separate different physiological systems have become blurred. For example, neuroendocrinology represents intimate connections between the nervous and endocrine systems: peptide hormones produced in the brain exert effects via the hypothalamus to control hormone secretion from the pituitary gland; in the periphery, the sympathetic nervous system modulates hormone production by the adrenal medulla and pancreatic islets. Similarly, there are complex inter-relationships between the immune and endocrine systems: e.g. glucocorticoid hormones exert powerful immunosuppressive effects; conversely, cytokines, e.g. tumour necrosis factor α and interleukin (IL)-6, produced by cells of the immune system markedly influence hormone secretion by glands such as the pituitary and adrenal.

Nature of hormones

In general, hormones can be classified into those that are based on proteins or peptides and those that are chemically derived. Small peptides include hypothalamic releasing factors produced by neuroendocrine cells, which act locally on the pituitary; larger polypeptides such as insulin or growth hormone (GH) are characteristically circulating hormones which act on more distant targets. Biogenic amines including catecholamines, dopamine, and serotonin are derived from amino acids. The majority of protein and peptide hormones interact with membrane receptors located on the cell surface. Binding to membrane receptors activates downstream signalling pathways leading to changes in cellular function which mediate responses to hormones.

A second class of hormones includes steroids and other lipophilic substances which act by crossing the plasma membrane to interact with intracellular receptors. Steroid hormones are derived from cholesterol and include cortisol, progesterone, testosterone, oestradiol. Vitamin D and retinoic acid, which are synthesized from dietary sources, and thyroid hormone produced by modification of tyrosines in thyroglobulin, are structurally dissimilar to steroids but also act via nuclear receptors.

Development of endocrine glands

The hypothalamus develops from forebrain tissue adjacent to the third ventricle. Neurons secreting releasing factors send cellular processes which terminate in portal capillaries that perfuse the pituitary gland. The latter develops from ectoderm to form the adenohypophysis or anterior pituitary; the posterior pituitary or neurohypophysis is formed directly from axonal terminals of hypothalamic neurons which grow downward. The thyroid gland develops from endoderm in the floor of the oropharynx with migration of cells caudally to its final position in the neck. During its descent, parafollicular C cells derived from neural crest tissue within the ultimobranchial body and parathyroid glands from the third and fourth pharyngeal pouches, become incorporated into the thyroid gland. The adrenal glands comprise a steroid-secreting cortex developing from mesoderm, together with a catecholamine-producing medulla composed of chromaffin cells derived from neural crest. Germ cells within indifferent gonadal primordia differentiate to form the ovary or, in the presence of the Y chromosome-encoded sex determining gene (*SRY*), develop into testes. Endocrine cells of the pancreas are derived from endoderm and differentiate to form the islets of Langerhans. Various transcription factors which control the development of cells within endocrine glands and their differentiation to hormone biosynthesis are listed in Table 13.1.1.

Hormone synthesis, processing, and secretion

The organization of endocrine genes is homologous to those encoding many other proteins, although there are some characteristic features. Gene transcription is usually regulated by the promoter, which is located in the upstream 5′ flanking region of the gene (Fig. 13.1.1). Typically, the promoter may contain three types of regulatory DNA sequence which are recognized by specific transcription factors; a hormone response element (HRE) is recognized by nuclear receptors; a tissue-specific element (TSE) binds cell-specific transcription factors (see Table 13.1.1), which enhance the transcription of the hormone gene in a tissue-specific manner; a third

Table 13.1.1 Some transcription factors involved in endocrine gland development

Gland	Transcription factor(s)
Pituitary	HESX-1, POU1F1, PROP-1, TBX19
Thyroid	TTF-1, TTF-2, PAX-8
Adrenal cortex	SF-1, DAX-1
Pancreatic islet cells	IPF-1
Testis	SRY, SF-1
Ovary	SF-1, DAX-1

DAX-1, *d*osage-sensitive sex reversal *a*drenal hypoplasia critical region on the X-chromosome 1; HESX-1, homeobox gene expressed in embryonic stem cells 1; IPF-1, insulin promoter factor 1; PAX-8, paired box gene 8; POU1F1, POU homeodomain containing pituitary transcription factor 1 (previously known as Pit-1); PROP-1, prophet of Pit-1; SF-1, steroidogenic factor 1; SRY, sex-determining region of the Y chromosome; TBX-19 (also known as TPIT), a T-box containing transcription factor; TTF-1, thyroid transcription factor 1; TTF-2, thyroid transcription factor 2.

class of response element mediates transcriptional activation in response to second-messenger signalling pathways. A rise in intracellular cAMP leads to phosphorylation of cAMP response element binding proteins (CREBs) which interact with CREs; cell signalling pathways which activate protein kinase C induce phosphorylation of the Fos-Jun (AP-1) transcription factor complex which binds its cognate DNA regulatory sequence. Binding of transcription factors

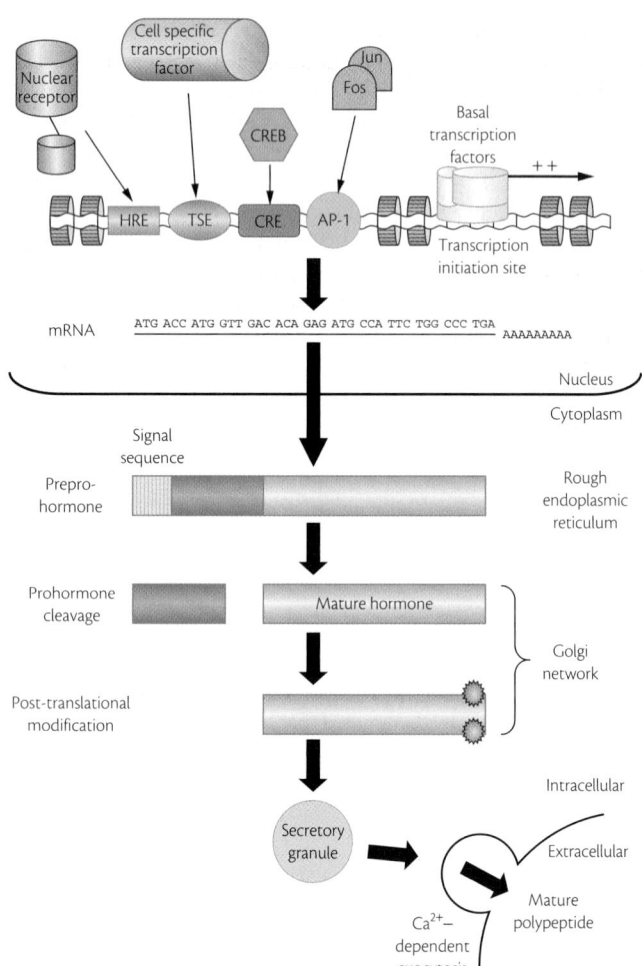

Fig. 13.1.1 Pathway of hormone synthesis, processing, and secretion.

to regulatory DNA response elements, activates and stabilizes basal transcription factors (BTFs), promoting gene transcription and mRNA synthesis (Fig. 13.3.1).

Transcription of the gene generates mRNA which undergoes translation in ribosomes leading to polypeptide synthesis. In some endocrine genes, alternative exon splicing allows substitution or removal of particular exons, such that peptides of differing sequence can be produced. For example, alternative splicing of the calcitonin gene in a tissue-specific manner directs the production of calcitonin in the C cells of the thyroid, whereas calcitonin gene-related peptide (CGRP) is produced preferentially in the brain.

Secreted polypeptide hormones incorporate a signal sequence at the amino terminus of the protein which directs its translocation across the endoplasmic reticulum where this sequence is cleaved (Fig. 13.1.1). Many hormones are synthesized as larger polypeptides (prohormones) which undergo proteolytic cleavage to generate smaller functional peptides. Such proteolytic processing is mediated by specific proteases, prohormone convertase 1 and 2 (PC1, PC2), which are highly expressed in cells of neuroendocrine lineage. Examples of hormone processing include the cleavage of proinsulin with removal of an internal C peptide to yield insulin, the active hormone. However, processing of the polypeptide precursor can also yield multiple functioning products. For example, pro-opiomelanocortin (POMC) is cleaved by endopeptidases to yield adrenocorticotropic hormone (ACTH), melanocyte-stimulating hormone (MSHα, β, γ), β-endorphin, and lipocortin.

Hormones may also undergo post-translational modification such as amidation of neuropeptides or glycosylation. Modification of amino acids by addition of carbohydrate side chains is a particular characteristic of the glycoprotein hormones—luteinizing hormone (LH), follicle-stimulating hormone (FSH), thyroid-stimulating hormone (TSH), and human chorionic gonadotropin (hCG)—and such glycosylation affects both their biological activity as well as their half-life in the circulation (see Fig. 13.1.1).

Hormones such as growth factors and cytokines are not concentrated within cells significantly but released via small, clear, Golgi-derived transport vesicles which fuse with the plasma membrane, representing a 'constitutive' pathway of secretion. In contrast, many endocrine cells contain an additional 'regulated' secretory pathway, which allows the export of high concentrations of hormone stored in cytoplasmic dense-core vesicles. Chromogranin B, an acidic

protein, and polypeptide proteases are additional constituents of secretory vesicles. Adrenal cells secreting catecholamine hormones contain chromaffin granules which include enzymes (e.g. dopamine β hydroxylase) that catalyse catecholamine biosynthesis. Dense-core vesicle exocytosis is mediated by a rise in intracellular calcium which activates cytoskeletal machinery, promoting vesicle translocation and docking with the plasma membrane (see Fig. 13.1.1). Cells secreting steroid hormones contain abundant mitochondrial and smooth endoplasmic reticulum which contain enzymes that mediate steroid biosynthesis. Mitochondrial side-chain cleavage enzyme converts cholesterol to pregnenolone and the latter is converted to glucocorticoid, mineralocorticoid, or sex steroids dependent on the cell specific expression of steroidogenic enzymes. Steroid hormones are not stored to any extent and are secreted constitutively.

Control of hormone production

The classic mechanism by which hormone-producing glands communicate is by endocrine pathways, whereby the products from one gland are secreted into the circulation (and exert effects on a different, distant target gland). Such endocrine pathways integrate the hypothalamus, pituitary and various end-organs to control the production of major hormones (Fig. 13.1.2). Thus, peptide-releasing factors (e.g. GnRH, TRH, GHRH, CRH) from the hypothalamus, stimulate production of tropic hormones from specific pituitary cell types; exceptions to this are somatostatin, which inhibits pituitary GH release, and dopamine, which is secreted continuously to inhibit prolactin secretion. The pituitary hormones act on end-organs to generate products which, in turn, exert a negative feedback effect at both hypothalamic and pituitary levels to regulate their own synthesis. Tri-iodothyronine (T_3) inhibits TRH and TSH production; gonadal steroids and inhibin negatively regulate hypothalamic GnRH and pituitary gonadotropins; cortisol suppresses CRH and ACTH generation; circulating insulin-like growth factor 1 (IGF-1) inhibits GHRH and GH secretion (Fig. 13.1.2). Osmoreceptors in the hypothalamus sense changes in serum osmolality to control the release of vasopressin from the posterior pituitary.

In addition to these endocrine control mechanisms, other types of local regulatory pathways are recognized. Paracrine regulation refers to factors that are released by one cell and act upon a nearby cell

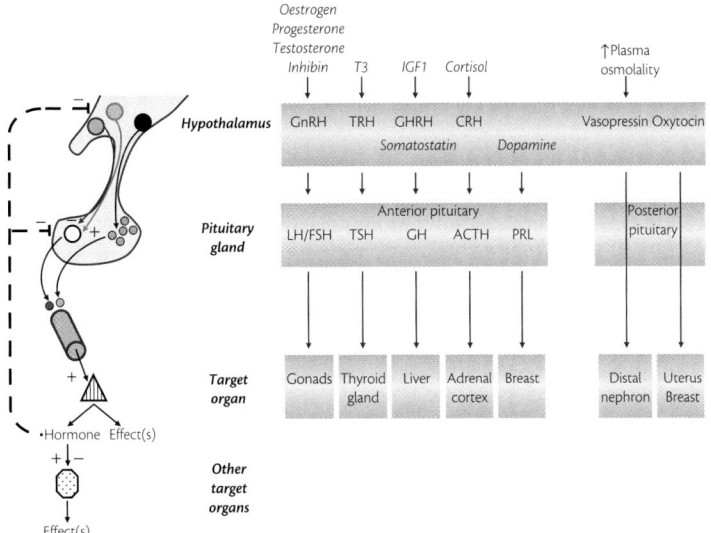

Fig. 13.1.2 Control of hormone production. Regulatory pathways integrating the hypothalamus, pituitary and various end organs. Hormones shown in italics exert inhibitory effects. Negative feedback regulation occurs at both hypothalamic and pituitary levels.

in the same tissue. For example, somatostatin produced by δ cells in pancreatic islets inhibits the local production of insulin from β cells; in the testis, testosterone produced from Leydig cells exerts an effect on nearby Sertoli cells to enhance spermatogenesis. Autocrine control refers to a factor which acts upon the same cell in which it is produced. Examples include gonadotroph secretion of activin which stimulates production of FSH from the same cell; similarly, T cells produce IL-2 which acts to promote their own proliferation.

In addition to discrete hormonal responses, endocrine systems can respond to environmental stimuli by the integrated production of multiple hormones. For example, stress activates an array of pathways, with sympathetic activation mediating catecholamine release from the adrenals, and stimulation of the hypothalamus inducing multiple axes, resulting in the production of cortisol, GH, prolactin, and vasopressin. The hormonal responses to starvation are also integrated by the hypothalamus. Here, diminished production of leptin from adipose tissue inhibits hypothalamic GnRH and TRH secretion with a consequent reduction in the production of both gonadal steroids and thyroid hormone to limit reproduction and energy expenditure.

In addition to the feedback regulatory mechanisms outlined above, many hormones are released in a rhythmic or pulsatile manner. Insulin is secreted in rapid (c. every 10 min) pulses in response to changes in glucose concentration in the pancreatic β cell. GnRH is secreted from the hypothalamus at a lower pulse frequency of every 1.5 to 3 h, stimulating similar pulses of pituitary LH and FSH release; another hypothalamic peptide (kisspeptin) can augment GnRH secretion in a paracrine manner. This hormonal rhythm controls ovarian folliculogenesis and steroid production to establish the female reproductive and menstrual cycle. Pituitary GH secretion is regulated by pulses of stimulatory GHRH and inhibitory somatostatin from the hypothalamus, which are out of phase with each other, corresponding to peaks and troughs of circulating GH.

Many hormonal pathways are influenced by the light–dark cycle, with circadian variation in their circulating levels. For example, the hypothalamic–pituitary–adrenal axis exhibits most activity in the early morning with peak cortisol production, followed by a nadir in glucocorticoid levels in the evening. Sleep is another environmental regulator: puberty is associated with nocturnal surges of LH; GH secretion is also enhanced nocturnally and the release of vasopressin during sleep inhibits renal diuresis.

Hormone binding proteins

Thyroid hormones and many steroids are transported in the circulation with serum binding proteins. Thus, thyroxine (T_4) and tri-iodothyronine (T_3) are bound to thyroxine binding globulin (TBG), albumin, and thyroxine binding prealbumin. Cortisol and progesterone are bound to cortisol binding globulin (CBG), while oestrogens and androgens are bound to sex hormone binding globulin (SHBG). The role of serum binding proteins is to provide a reservoir of circulating hormone. The interaction of hormones with binding proteins is relatively weak compared to their affinity for receptors, enabling them to dissociate easily. Only free hormone interacts with receptor to elicit a biological response. Hormone binding proteins are produced by the liver and their synthesis can be increased (e.g. by oestrogens or in pregnancy) or decreased (e.g. in liver disease), affecting the circulating concentration of total hormones. Accordingly, wherever possible, the concentration of free hormones in the circulation (e.g. T_4, T_3) or

urine (cortisol) is measured. Some protein hormones also circulate associated with binding proteins, which may modulate their action. A range of insulin-like growth factor binding proteins (IGFBPs) bind to IGF-1, with some inhibiting and others facilitating the action of this peptide on target tissue receptors. GH circulates bound to the extracellular domain of its receptor derived by cleavage from the membrane, with the complex prolonging the circulating half-life of the hormone.

Functions of hormones

The physiological roles of the major hormones can be broadly classified into three areas: control of growth and differentiation; maintenance of homeostasis; and regulation of reproduction. Some hormones have multiple functions and play a role in more than one area. In addition, some biological effects are mediated by the combined action of several different hormonal pathways. The principal actions of major hormones are outlined in Table 13.1.2.

Linear growth is dependent on a complex interplay of many hormones and growth factors. GH plays a key role and exerts many of its effects by stimulating the hepatic production of IGF-1. Thyroid hormone also stimulates the epiphyseal growth plate in childhood whereas, at puberty, production of sex steroids leads to epiphyseal closure. Other important actions of thyroid hormone include enhancement of myocardial contractility and differentiation of the central nervous system.

The maintenance of homeostasis includes the control of energy balance, metabolic pathways, fluid, electrolyte and calcium balance and regulation of blood pressure. Energy homeostasis involves regulation of food intake and energy expenditure. Leptin, an adipose tissue-derived hormone, acts via hypothalamic pathways (e.g. melanocortin 4) to reduce food intake; conversely, rising gastrointestinal production of ghrelin preprandially stimulates food intake. Thyroid hormone is an important determinant of resting energy expenditure or basal metabolic rate. Metabolic effects are mediated by several hormones: insulin lowers blood glucose by enhancing its cellular uptake and promotes glycogen synthesis; conversely, GH, cortisol, glucagon, and adrenaline act as counter-regulatory hormones to raise blood glucose. Glucagon and adrenaline stimulate glycogenolysis and, together with cortisol, promote gluconeogenesis. Other metabolic pathways are also influenced by these hormones: GH and cortisol are lipolytic whereas insulin mediates lipogenesis; insulin and GH are also anabolic by promoting protein biosynthesis, whereas cortisol increases protein breakdown. Adiponectin, another adipose tissue-derived hormone, enhances tissue insulin sensitivity.

Circulating concentrations of ions and water balance are also under hormonal control. Vasopressin promotes water reabsorption via membrane channels (aquaporins) in the distal collecting ducts of the kidney; aldosterone acts at the renal distal convoluted tubule to stimulate sodium reabsorption and potassium excretion. Both parathyroid hormone and vitamin D increase serum calcium levels; PTH mediates Ca^{2+} resorption from bone and kidney, whereas vitamin D acts on the gastrointestinal tract as well as these sites. Catecholamines and angiotensin II are potent vasoconstrictors and, together with cortisol, control blood pressure.

Hormones involved in reproduction exert effects from early in development. During embryogenesis, mullerian inhibiting substance (MIS) from the testis causes regression of female structures

Table 13.1.2 Major actions of hormones

Hormone	Action
Homeostasis	
Energy balance	
Leptin	Reduces food intake
Ghrelin	Increases hunger
Fluid and electrolyte balance	
Aldosterone	Renal Na^+/K^+ exchange
Vasopressin	↓Renal free water clearance
Metabolism	
Insulin	↑Cell glucose uptake; ↑glycogen synthesis; lipogenic; ↑protein synthesis
Glucagon	Glycogenolysis; gluconeogenic
Cortisol	Gluconeogenic; lipolysis; ↑protein breakdown
Growth hormone	Lipolysis; ↑protein synthesis
Testosterone	↑Protein synthesis
Calcium	
Parathyroid hormone	↑Ca^{2+} resorption from bone and kidney; ↑renal 1α hydroxylation of vitamin D
Vitamin D	↑Ca^{2+} absorption from gastrointestinal tract; ↑Ca^{2+} resorption from bone and kidney
Growth and development	
Growth hormone	Growth
Thyroid hormone	Growth, regulation of basal metabolic rate, central nervous system development
Retinoic acid	Embryonic development; morphogenesis
Reproduction	
Testosterone	Sexual differentiation, virilization, spermatogenesis
Dihydrotestosterone	Male external genitalia
Oestradiol	Female external genitalia; mammary gland development
Progesterone	Uterotrophic
Prolactin	Lactation
Oxytocin	Uterine contraction; milk reflex

(uterus, fallopian tube) and testosterone promotes the development of male structures (vas deferens, epididymis, seminal vesicles) which are derived from the wolffian duct. Dihydrotestosterone promotes development of the male external genitalia. In both sexes, the gonadal axes are quiescent in childhood and become reactivated at puberty. Testosterone mediates virilization, secondary sexual characteristics, and spermatogenesis in the male; in females, ovarian production of oestrogen and progesterone induces secondary sexual features and controls the menstrual cycle. In both sexes, gonadal steroids are required for the attainment of peak bone density at the end of puberty and its subsequent maintenance. During pregnancy, prolactin acts in concert with oestrogen to promote lactation; oxytocin stimulates uterine contraction at parturition and smooth muscle contraction in the mammary gland during suckling.

Hormone action

Hormones induce biological responses by interacting with receptors located either on the membrane or intracellularly in the cytoplasm or nucleus. Hormones bind to receptors with high affinity, such that low concentrations of free hormone associate and dissociate from receptors rapidly in a dynamic equilibrium. The interaction of hormones with receptors is usually highly specific, with individual receptors being highly selective for a single hormone even within a class of structurally related molecules (e.g. steroid hormones). However, there are exceptions to this: parathyroid hormone (PTH) and parathyroid hormone-related peptide (PTHrP) or LH and hCG share a common receptor, generating similar biological responses; insulin and IGF-1 exhibit some degree of cross-reactivity with their respective receptors; the mineralocorticoid receptor binds cortisol with equal or higher affinity than aldosterone.

Hormones that bind to membrane receptors act via effector proteins to activate second-messenger signalling pathways. In turn, the second messengers stimulate a cascade of kinases, which then act upon target substrates in the cell membrane, the cytoplasm or nucleus, to alter gene transcription or modulate a biochemical pathway, leading to a physiological response. Hormones that act through nuclear receptors are transported passively, or pumped actively, across the plasma membrane to interact with their targets. The hormone–receptor complex interacts with DNA sequences in target genes to either stimulate or repress their expression. The cellular actions of nuclear receptors are mediated by changes in target gene transcription, altering mRNA synthesis and, in turn, the levels of protein product.

Signalling by membrane receptors

Membrane receptors can be divided into several groups (Table 13.1.3) depending on the signalling pathways that they utilize.

Table 13.1.3 Membrane receptor families

G protein-coupled	
Glycoprotein hormones	FSH, TSH, LH/CG
Biogenic amines	Adrenaline, noradrenaline, serotonin, histamine, dopamine
Peptides	Calcitonin, PTH/PTHrP
	Ghrelin, GHRH, CRH, GnRH, kisspeptin, SRIF, TRH
	Vasopressin, oxytocin
	Angiotensin
	Glucagon, secretin, VIP, gastrin
Small molecules	Calcium, GABA
Tyrosine kinase	Insulin, IGF-1
Cytokine	GH, PRL, EPO, leptin
Serine/threonine kinase	Activin, inhibin, MIS

CG, chorionic gonadotrophin; CRH, corticotropin releasing hormone; EPO, erythropoietin; FSH, follicle stimulating hormone; GABA, γ-aminobutyric acid; GH, growth hormone; GHRH, growth hormone releasing hormone; GnRH, gonadotropin releasing hormone; IGF-1, insulin-like growth factor 1; LH, luteinizing hormone; MIS, mullerian inhibiting substance; PRL, prolactin; PTH, parathyroid hormone; PTHrP, parathyroid hormone-related peptide; SRIF, somatostatin; TRH, thyrotropin-releasing hormone; TSH, thyroid-stimulating hormone; VIP, vasoactive intestinal polypeptide.

The largest group consists of receptors with multiple transmembrane domains which are coupled to G proteins; a second class of receptor contains an intracellular domain with tyrosine kinase activity; a number of hormones signal via membrane proteins that are homologous to cytokine receptors; a fourth class of hormone receptor contains an intracellular domain with serine or threonine kinase activity.

G protein-coupled receptors (GPCRs) are characterized by seven separate hydrophobic domains that traverse the membrane phospholipid bilayer (Fig. 13.1.3a). They possess an extracellular domain of variable size, enabling further subclassification of these receptors: glycoprotein hormones or small molecule ligands (e.g. calcium, GABA) interact with large N-terminal extracellular domains; biogenic amines (e.g. catecholamines, serotonin) bind to residues that lie within the transmembrane domain; other polypeptide hormones interact with residues in both the extracellular and transmembrane domains. The intracellular domains of the receptor enable interaction with G proteins.

G proteins typically form a heterotrimeric complex of α, β, and γ subunits which bind the guanine nucleotides GTP and GDP. The complex transduces signals from the receptor to downstream effectors such as adenylate cyclase, phospholipase C or membrane voltage dependent calcium channels. A family of different G proteins (G_s, G_i, G_q and others) exists with the ability to couple to different receptors and effectors, allowing a large array of potential receptor–G protein–effector complexes, leading to diversity of cellular signalling.

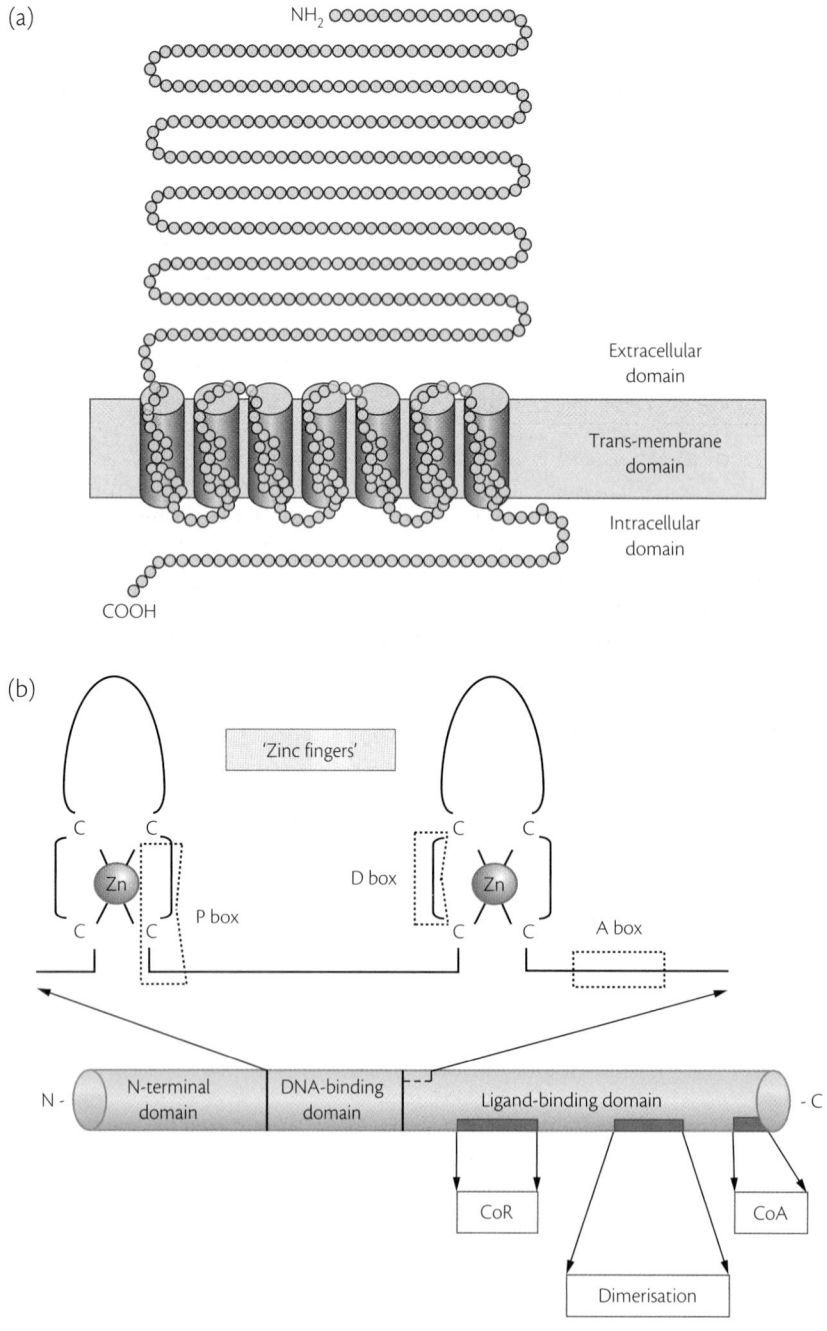

Fig. 13.1.3 Schematic representations of (a) G protein-coupled receptor and (b) nuclear receptor, illustrating their functional domains.

Table 13.1.4 Signalling pathways of membrane receptors

Signalling pathway	Hormone/receptor
$G_s\alpha$/cAMP↑	β-Adrenergic receptor
	CRH
	GHRH
	ACTH
$G_i\alpha$/cAMP↓	Somatostatin
	Dopamine
	α-Adrenergic receptor
$G_q\alpha$/IP$_3$ and DAG	TRH
	GnRH
$G_s\alpha$/cAMP↑ and $G_q\alpha$/IP$_3$ and DAG	LH
	FSH
	TSH
	PTH
	Calcitonin
JAK–STAT	GH
	PRL
	EPO
	Leptin
Tyrosine kinase/MAP kinase	Insulin
	IGF-1
Ser/Thr kinase/SMAD	Activin, inhibin, MIS

Abbreviations as for Table 13.1.3.

A number of hormones signal via the cAMP pathway (Table 13.1.4) and this mechanism is considered in further detail (Fig. 13.1.4). In the resting state, the G protein complex is inactive and bound to GDP (Fig. 13.1.4a). Following hormone binding to the receptor (Fig. 13.1.4b), the Gα subunit binds GTP, becomes activated and dissociates from the βγ complex, to interact with adenylate cyclase (Fig. 13.1.4c). The latter converts ATP to the second messenger, cAMP. This rise in intracellular cAMP activates protein kinase A (PKA), which can phosphorylate a number of cellular targets: phosphorylation of a transcription factor, CREB, stimulates transcription of genes containing CREs; other targets for PKA include enzymes in biochemical pathways or membrane ion channels.

Several mechanisms serve to terminate signalling via a hormone–receptor complex: first, hydrolysis of GTP to GDP by the Gα subunit promotes its reassociation with βγ subunits to reform an inactive complex; second, the hormone–receptor complex is internalized via cell surface vesicles and targeted for lysosomal degradation; third, following hormone binding, the GPCRs undergo phosphorylation of their intracellular domains by either PKA or other specific kinases (GRKs). Such phosphorylation prevents further coupling to G proteins and promotes receptor internalization desensitizing the cell to hormone action, until further surface receptor is expressed.

Activation of their receptors by hormones such as somatostatin or dopamine, is known to decrease intracellular cAMP. Here, the hormone–receptor complex associates with a G protein (G$_i$), whose α subunit inhibits adenylate cyclase. Although many GPCRs signal via cAMP, some receptors (e.g. TRH, GnRH, Table 13.1.4) are linked to different pathways. These receptors are coupled to G$_q$, whose α subunit activates membrane phospholipase C (PLC) (Fig. 13.1.5). This enzyme catalyses the hydrolysis of phosphatidylinositol 4,5-bisphosphate (PIP$_2$) to generate the second messengers inositol 1,4,5-triphosphate (IP$_3$) and 1,2-diacylglycerol (DAG). IP$_3$ interacts with a specific receptor located on smooth endoplasmic reticulum, inducing opening of intracellular channels leading to a rise in cytoplasmic calcium (Fig. 13.1.5). Interaction of calcium with calmodulin, a cytoplasmic calcium-binding protein, activates a specific kinase (CAM kinase), which regulates a number of processes including hormone secretion, gene transcription and metabolic enzymes. The rise in cellular calcium also facilitates DAG activation of protein kinase C (PKC), leading to phosphorylation of the Fos-Jun transcription factor complex, inducing target gene expression (Fig. 13.1.5). Hormones do not signal exclusively via a single pathway, with glycoprotein hormones and some peptides for example (Table 13.1.4) activating both cAMP and phosphoinositide signalling.

The tyrosine kinase class of receptors is a diverse family that transduces signalling by insulin and IGF-1 but also epidermal, nerve, fibroblast, and platelet-derived growth factors. Growth factor signalling differs from insulin and the latter pathway will be considered (Fig. 13.1.6). Hormone interaction with receptor promotes autophosphorylation of tyrosine residues in their cytoplasmic domains. In turn, this promotes phosphorylation of substrates, e.g. Shc and insulin receptor substrate 1 (IRS-1), followed by recruitment of adaptor proteins (Grb2/SOS). The Grb2/SOS complex recruits Ras, a GTP-binding protein. Ras activation induces signalling via a series of kinases (Raf, Mek, MAP kinase), culminating in the phosphorylation and activation of transcription factors which regulate target genes involved in mitogenesis or cellular differentiation. On the other hand, IRS-1 recruits phosphatidylinositol-3′-OH-kinase (PI3-kinase), which in turn activates the AKT cascade. The latter mediates a number of the metabolic effects of insulin, enhancing translocation of a glucose transporter to the membrane to promote cellular glucose uptake, and activating pathways involved in glycogen, lipid, or protein synthesis.

Hormones such as prolactin and GH interact uniquely with their receptors; a single polypeptide interacts simultaneously with two receptors promoting their dimerization (Fig. 13.1.7). The hormone–receptor complex recruits Janus kinases (JAKs) which phosphorylate STATs (signal transducers and activators of transcription). STATs translocate to the nucleus, interact with regulatory DNA elements and promote target gene transcription.

Activin and inhibin belong to the transforming growth factor (TGF) class of peptides which signal via a heterodimeric transmembrane receptor complex with intrinsic protein serine/threonine kinase activity (Fig. 13.1.8). Here, hormone binding promotes the association of two surface receptors (type I and type II) with differing properties. Subsequent transphosphorylation of the type I receptor by the intracellular kinase domain of the type II receptor leads to phosphorylation and dimerization of cytoplasmic Smad proteins. The Smad complex translocates to the nucleus to activate target gene expression (Fig. 13.1.8).

As described above, GPCR signalling is usually coupled to responses (e.g. hormone secretion) by Gα subunit activation of

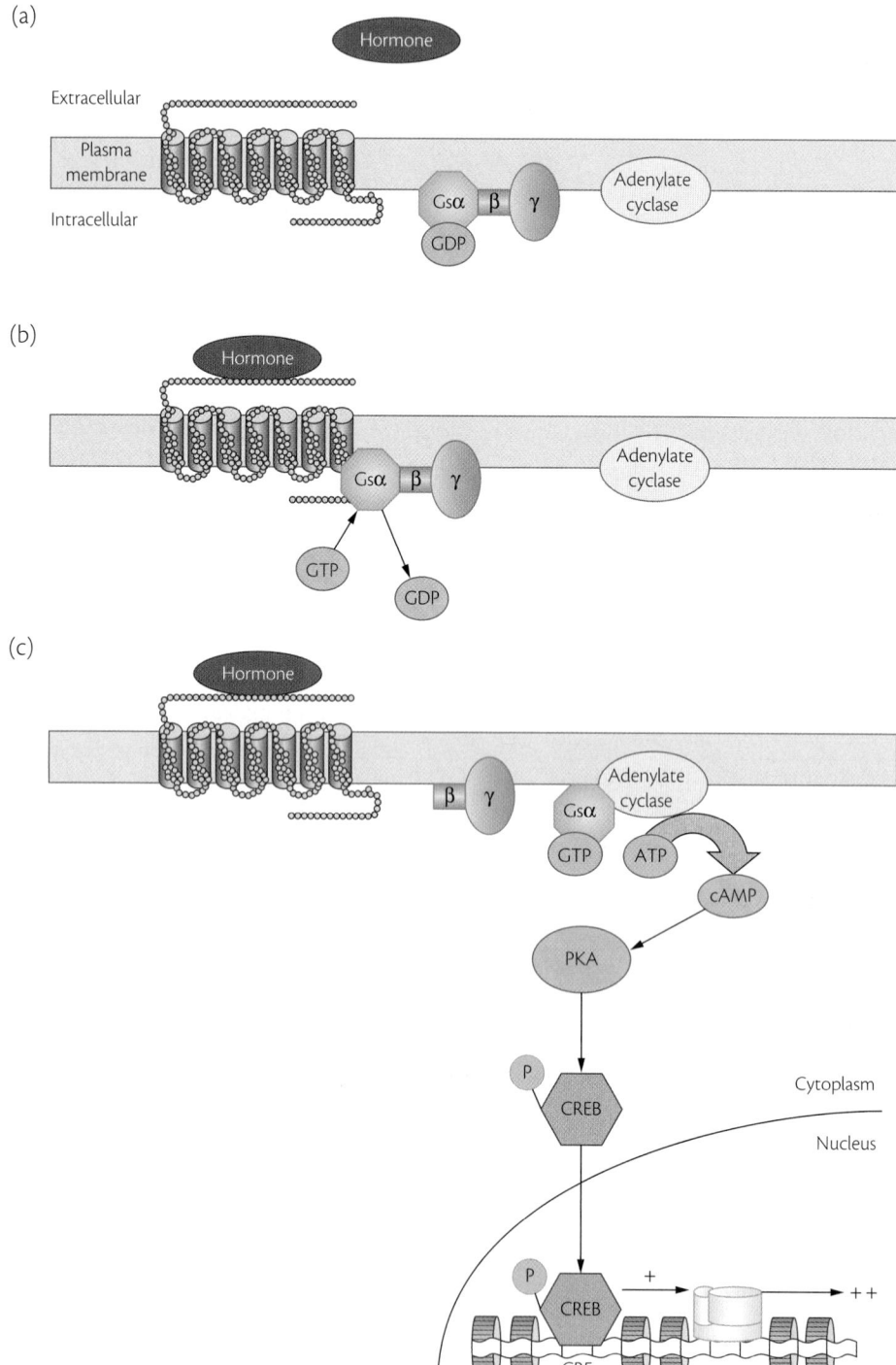

Fig. 13.1.4 G protein-coupled receptor signalling via the cAMP pathway.

cAMP or phosphoinositide pathways. However, following receptor activation in some cellular contexts, the dissociated Gβ/γ dimer subunit complex is also capable of stimulating effectors (e.g. Ras, PI3-kinase), to enhance MAPkinase activity and elicit a mitogenic response.

Nuclear receptor signalling

The nuclear receptors are a family of transcription factors which mediate the action of steroid and other lipophilic hormones.

The human genome encodes approximately 60 to 70 different receptors and it is clear that only a minority of these are targets for the action of major hormones (Table 13.1.5). The remainder comprise a large group classified as 'orphan receptors', reflecting the fact that either their ligands and/or physiological roles remain to be elucidated.

Based on homologies in their primary amino acid sequence, nuclear receptors can be divided into distinct domains which mediate specific functions (Fig. 13.1.3b). A central DNA binding domain contains cysteine-rich peptide motifs which chelate zinc

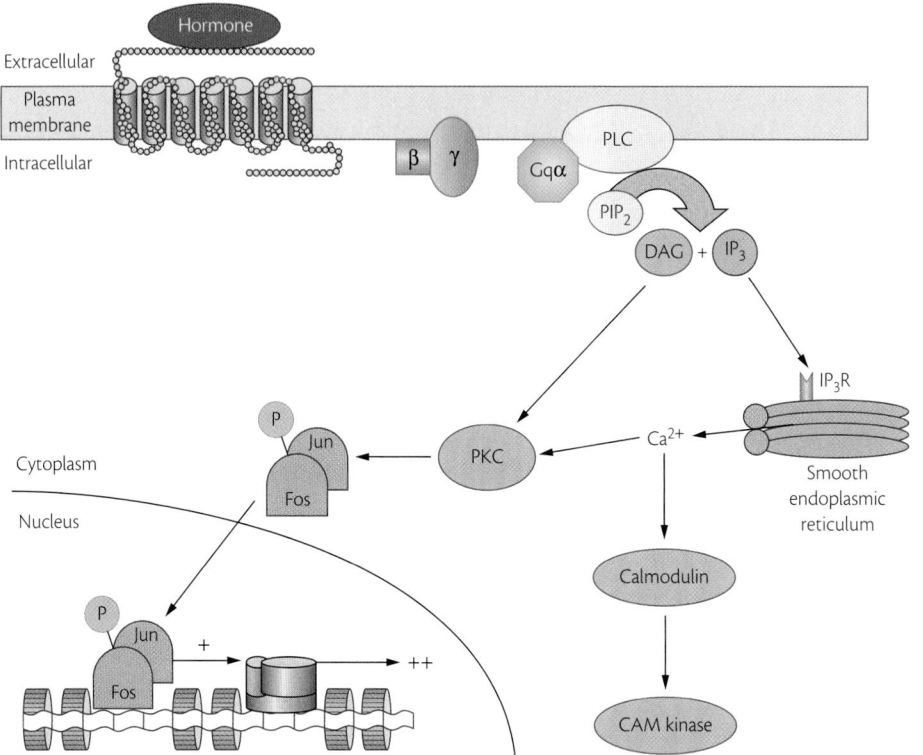

Fig. 13.1.5 G protein-coupled receptor signalling via the phosphoinositide pathway.

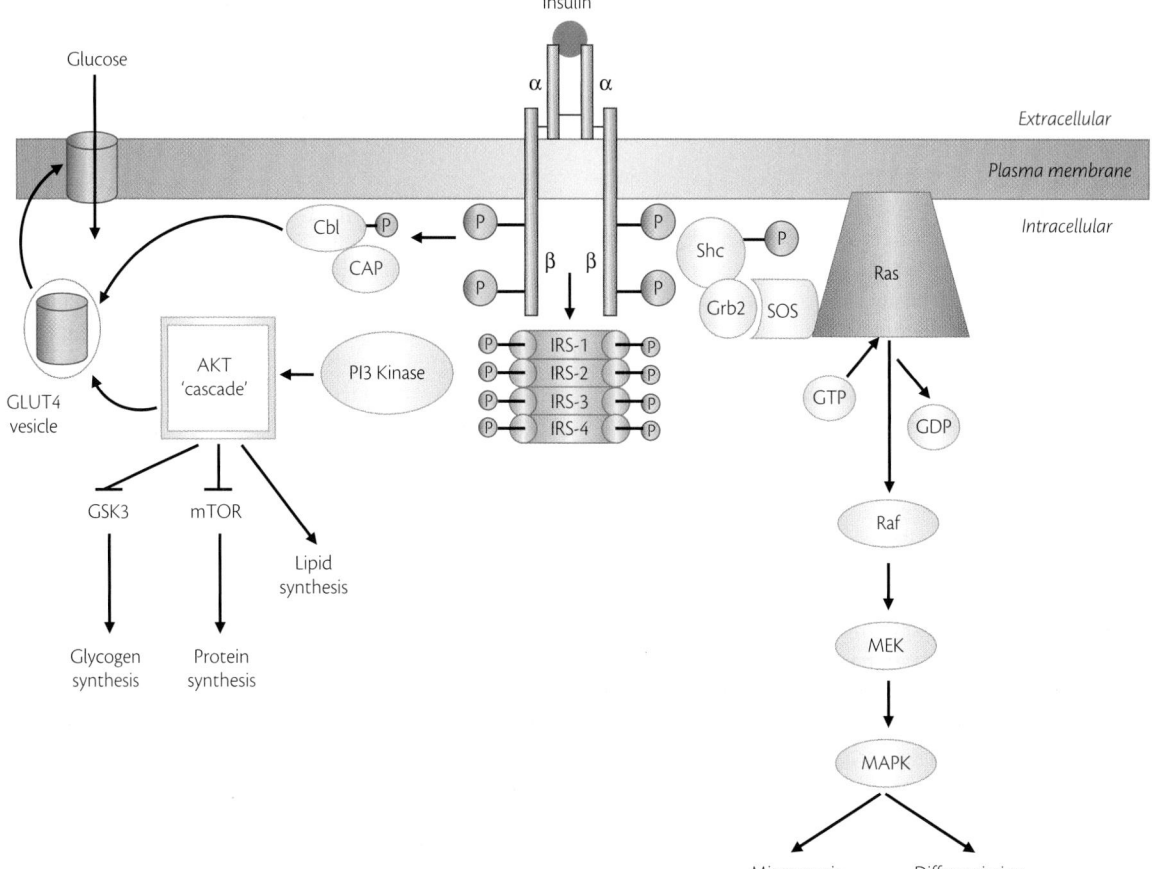

Fig. 13.1.6 Insulin action via its tyrosine kinase receptor and signalling cascade.

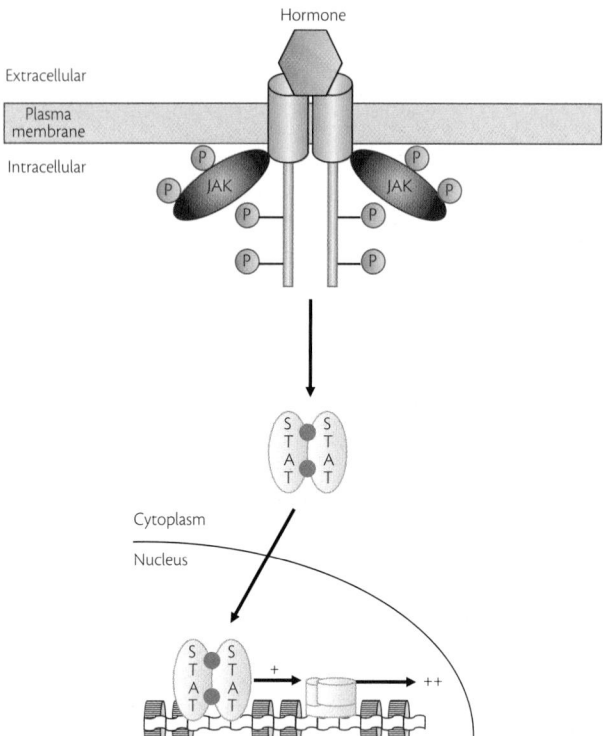

Fig. 13.1.7 Hormone signalling via the JAK-STAT pathway.

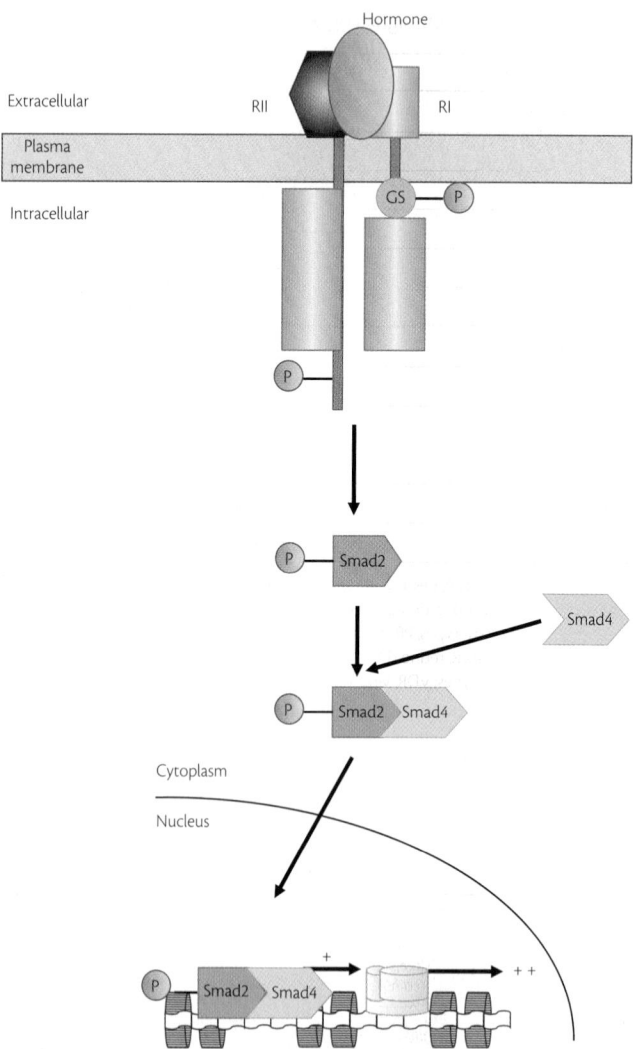

Fig. 13.1.8 Hormone signalling by the transforming growth factor peptide family.

to form two 'zinc fingers'. The latter mediate receptor binding to specific DNA sequences or hormone response elements, usually located in target gene promoters. The C-terminal region of receptors encompasses their hormone binding function as well as their ability to dimerize. Nuclear receptors can be divided into two major subclasses, the steroid receptors and heterodimeric receptors, which differ in their mode of action.

Steroid receptors (e.g. GR, MR, ER, PR, AR) bind to hormone response elements as homodimers (Fig. 13.1.9b). Some receptors (e.g. GR, PR, AR) are bound to cytosolic heat shock proteins. Hormone binding to receptors promotes their dissociation from these, enabling translocation to the nucleus, dimerization and interaction with DNA. In contrast, the thyroid, retinoid, and vitamin D receptors are constitutively nuclear and form heterodimers with a common partner (retinoid X receptor, RXR), to interact with DNA even in the absence of hormone or ligand (Fig. 13.1.9a). In some target gene contexts, RXR can also form homodimers to mediate retinoid signalling.

In contrast to other transcription factors whose activity is controlled by post-translational modification (e.g. phosphorylation), the hallmark of nuclear receptors is their ability to modulate gene expression in a hormone-dependent manner. Thus, in the absence of ligand, the thyroid and retinoic acid receptors actively silence target gene transcription by recruiting a corepressor complex of cofactors (Fig. 13.1.9a). For all nuclear receptors, hormone binding induces a conformational change with dissociation of corepressors and recruitment of coactivator proteins (Fig. 13.1.9b). This latter complex acts to relax the interaction between histone proteins and DNA in chromatin, thereby facilitating the access of basal transcription factors and RNA polymerase which induce gene transcription.

A further mechanism which controls signalling via nuclear receptors is regulation of the supply of their ligands to cells and tissues. A specific membrane transporter (MCT8) mediates cellular entry of thyroid hormone in the central nervous system. T_3, the ligand for TR, is generated from circulating thyroxine by the action of type 1 or type 2 deiodinase enzymes expressed in the liver and central nervous system respectively; the enzyme 5α reductase converts testosterone to dihydrotestosterone in tissues of the male external genitalia. In contrast, the enzyme 11β-hydroxysteroid dehydrogenase type 2 catabolizes cortisol in the renal cells, thereby enabling the mineralocorticoid receptor to respond selectively to aldosterone rather than to glucocorticoid, which it is also capable of binding with high affinity.

Finally, in contrast to classical effects of steroid hormones to modulate gene expression, recent evidence indicates that they can also modulate cellular functions such as hormone secretion or neuronal excitability within seconds or minutes. These rapid effects of steroid hormones occur independent of the genome and can occur either by hormone interaction with a cell surface receptor or by direct interaction of the nuclear receptor with cytoplasmic signalling molecules.

Table 13.1.5 Hormone signalling via nuclear receptors

Nuclear receptor	Hormone
Homodimeric	
GR	Cortisol
MR	Aldosterone
ERα/β	Oestradiol
PR	Progesterone
AR	Testosterone, dihydrotestosterone
Heterodimeric	
TRα/β	Triiodothyronine
RARα/β/γ	all-*trans*-Retinoic acid
RXRα/β/γ	9-*cis*-Retinoic acid
VDR	1,25-Dihydroxyvitamin D$_3$
PPARα/β/γ	Unsaturated fatty acids, eicosanoids

AR, androgen receptor; ER, oestrogen receptor α or β subtypes; GR, glucocorticoid receptor; MR, mineralocorticoid receptor; PPAR, peroxisome proliferator-activated receptor α, β, or γ subtypes; PR, progesterone receptor; RAR, retinoic acid receptor α, β or γ subtypes; RXR, retinoid X receptor α, β, or γ subtypes; TR, thyroid hormone receptor α or β subtypes; VDR, vitamin D receptor.

Genetic defects and endocrine disease

The majority of endocrine diseases can be divided into conditions of hormone excess, hormone deficiency and hormone resistance. Defects in genes involved in hormone synthesis and action give rise to a spectrum of disorders (Tables 13.1.6 and 13.1.7). Both germ-line gene defects causing inherited syndromes and somatic mutations leading to acquired endocrine cellular dysfunction have been described.

Defects in developmental transcription factors are usually associated with endocrine gland hypoplasia: mutations in HESX-1 cause optic and pituitary hypoplasia with agenesis of the corpus callosum; both Pit-1 (POU1F1) and PROP-1 mutations disrupt development of multiple pituitary cell types resulting in a combination of hormone deficiencies; defects in TTF-1, TTF-2, and PAX-8 result in thyroid dysgenesis manifesting as neonatal hypothyroidism; mutations in the *SRY* gene lead to failure of testis development and sex reversal in XY males.

Mutations in DAX-1 or SF-1, orphan members of the nuclear receptor family, disrupt both adrenal and gonadal development. Defects in other nuclear receptors (e.g. VDR, TR, GR) are characterized by tissue resistance to their respective hormone ligands. Vitamin D resistance leads to rickets together with abnormalities of skin differentiation, hair growth, and lymphocyte function, emphasizing its important extraskeletal actions. Point mutations in the androgen receptor are associated with a spectrum of phenotypes ranging from complete feminization of XY individuals to mildly impaired virilization in men. In addition, expansion of a polyglutamine repeat sequence in the N-terminal domain of AR is associated with adult-onset neuronal degeneration leading to spinal and bulbar muscular atrophy. A homozygous defect in the oestrogen receptor in a male led to failure of epiphyseal closure resulting in tall stature together with severe osteoporosis.

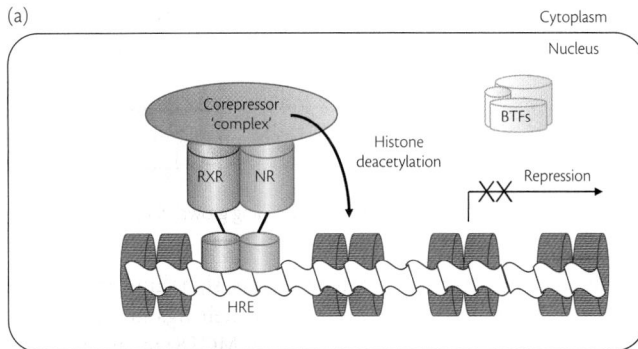

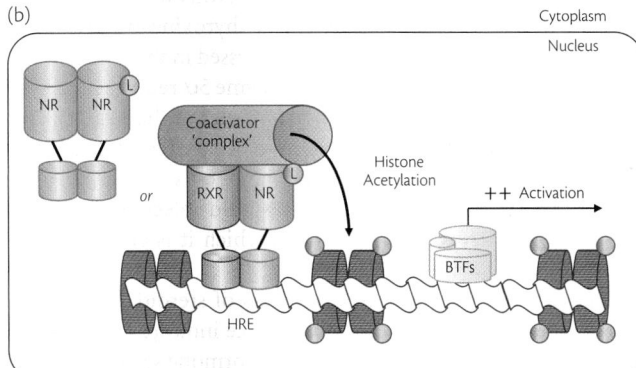

Fig. 13.1.9 Transcriptional regulation by nuclear receptors. (a) In the absence of hormone, a subset of heterodimeric nuclear receptors (thyroid, retinoic acid) recruit corepressors to inhibit gene transcription. (b) Hormone occupancy of homodimeric or heterodimeric receptors promotes their association with coactivators, leading to transcriptional activation.

Table 13.1.6 Genetic defects in transcription factors or nuclear receptors and endocrine disorders

Gene	Disorder or phenotype
Transcription factors	
HESX-1	Septo-optic dysplasia
POU1F1/PROP-1	GH, PRL, TSH deficiencies
TBX19	ACTH deficiency
TTF-1/TTF-2/PAX-8	Thyroid dysgenesis
SRY	XY female
Nuclear receptors	
DAX-1/SF-1	Adrenal insufficiency and hypogonadism
VDR	Hereditary vitamin D-resistant rickets
AR	Androgen insensitivity syndrome or spinal and bulbar muscular atrophy
ERα	Tall stature and osteoporosis
GR	Glucocorticoid resistance
TRβ	Resistance to thyroid hormone
PPARγ	Lipodystrophic insulin resistance

Table 13.1.7 Genetic defects in membrane receptors or signalling and endocrine disorders

Gene	Loss-of-function mutation	Gain-of-function mutation
G protein-coupled receptor		
GHRH	GH deficiency	
GnRH	Central hypogonadism	
Vasopressin V2	Nephrogenic diabetes insipidus	
ACTH	Isolated cortisol deficiency	
Ca^{2+}	Hypocalciuric hypercalcaemia	Hypercalciuric hypocalcaemia
TSH	TSH resistance	Thyroid adenomas or nonautoimmune hyperthyroidism
LH	Leydig cell hypoplasia	Male-limited precocious puberty
FSH	Ovarian dysgenesis	FSH-independent spermatogenesis
PTH/PTHrP	Blomstrand chondrodysplasia	Jansen's metaphyseal chondrodysplasia
Melanocortin 4	Obesity	
Tyrosine kinase receptor		
RET	Hirschprung's disease	MEN2: medullary thyroid carcinoma, phaeochromocytoma parathyroid neoplasia
Insulin	Insulin resistance	
Cytokine receptors		
GH	Laron dwarfism	
Leptin	Obesity	
Signalling pathway		
$G_s\alpha$	PTH, TSH, LH resistance Albright's hereditary osteodystrophy	Somatotroph adenomas, thyroid adenomas, McCune–Albright syndrome
$G_i\alpha$	Ovary, adrenal, thyroid tumours	
AKT2	Insulin resistance	

These manifestations suggest that testosterone effects on the male skeleton are, in part, mediated by its enzymatic conversion to oestrogens.

A growing number of disorders associated with defects in transmembrane receptors or their signalling intermediates have been described (Table 13.1.7). However, in addition to mutations which disrupt protein function, gain-of-function mutations causing constitutive activation of the receptor or signalling protein also occur. With GPCRs, diverse loss-of-function mutations, occurring most frequently in the extracellular domain, block hormone binding or signalling, leading to insensitivity to hormone action. Such hormone resistance can lead to both hypofunction (e.g. ACTH, TSH receptors) or hypoplasia (e.g. LH, FSH receptors) of target glands expressing the receptor. Conversely, gain-of-function mutations in GPCRs typically occur in the third intracellular loop, causing constitutive activation of the receptor in the absence of hormonal ligand. Again, the functional consequence is either autonomous hyperfunction (e.g. calcium, LH, FSH receptors) or excessive neoplastic proliferation (e.g. TSH receptor, RET tyrosine kinase receptor) of the target tissues in which the receptor is expressed (Table 13.1.7). Constitutive activation of signal transduction may also result from G protein mutations. Here, specific amino acid substitutions in $G_s\alpha$ inhibit its intrinsic GTPase activity, and the GTP-bound protein constitutively activates adenylate cylase leading to cAMP accumulation. Somatic $G_s\alpha$ mutations occur in a proportion of pituitary GH secreting and thyroid adenomas; more widespread expression of a somatic $G_s\alpha$ mutation occurring early in development, leads to polyostotic fibrous dysplasia, café au lait skin pigmentation, and hyperfunction of multiple endocrine glands, constituting the McCune–Albright syndrome. Similarly, germ-line loss-of-function mutations which reduce cellular $G_s\alpha$ activity, are associated with resistance to multiple hormones together with characteristic bone anomalies (Albright's hereditary osteodystrophy).

Further reading

Braverman LE, Utiger RD (eds) (2005). *Werner & Ingbar's the thyroid; a fundamental and clinical text*, 9th edition. Lippincott Williams & Wilkins, Phildelphia.

DeGroot LJ, Jameson JL (eds) (2010). *Endocrinology*, 6th edition. Elsevier Saunders, Philadelphia (in press).

Kronenberg HM, *et al.* (eds) (2008). *Williams' textbook of endocrinology*, 11th edition. Elsevier Saunders, Philadelphia.

Lodish H, *et al.* (2007). *Molecular cell biology*, 6th edition. W H Freeman, San Francisco.

Strauss JF, Barbieri RL (eds) (2004). *Yen & Jaffe's reproductive endocrinology*, 5th edition. Elsevier Saunders, Philadephia.

Disorders of the anterior pituitary gland

Niki Karavitaki and John A.H. Wass

Essentials

The anterior pituitary gland produces growth hormone (GH), luteinizing hormone (LH), follicle-stimulating hormone (FSH), adrenocorticotropic hormone (ACTH), thyroid-stimulating hormone (TSH), and prolactin. Their secretion is regulated by hypothalamic releasing and inhibitory factors delivered via portal capillaries, and by negative feedback inhibition of the cognate hormones produced by target endocrine glands such as the thyroid and adrenal cortex.

Clinical features—presentation of pituitary disease, mostly associated with a space-occupying lesion, may result from (1) local mass effects—often causing headache, visual field defects (most typically bitemporal hemianopia or upper temporal quadrantanopia) and ocular nerve palsies; (2) pituitary hormone deficits—producing wide-ranging effects as a result of single or multiple deficiencies, with GH and gonadotropins (LH and FSH) usually affected first, followed much later by ACTH and TSH; and/or (3) pituitary hormone hypersecretion, usually arising as a consequence of neoplastic proliferation of particular cell types within the gland, producing complex and disabling syndromes such as Cushing's disease or acromegaly.

Investigation—this includes testing for (1) hormonal hyper- or hyposecretion—measurements of basal levels of pituitary hormones with target gland hormone secretion are usually sufficient for assessment of TSH (thyroxine), FSH/LH (testosterone or oestradiol) and prolactin; dynamic testing is required for the ACTH/cortisol axis and determination of GH deficiency or excess; (2) radiological assessment—MRI is the modality of choice; and (3) neuro-ophthalmological evaluation, including assessment of visual acuity, visual fields and fundoscopy.

Management—the availability of sensitive hormonal assays, replacement hormones and hypothalamic peptides, together with refined neuroimaging methods and neurosurgical techniques, has increased our ability to identify precisely and treat successfully most patients with diseases of the anterior pituitary gland.

Growth hormone

GH deficiency—in children this causes growth failure, and in adults features including decreased energy and quality of life, and increase in fat mass/decrease in muscle mass. The insulin tolerance test is considered the 'gold standard' for diagnosis. Goals of GH treatment in adults are to achieve an appropriate clinical response whilst avoiding side effects, and an IGF-1 level in the middle of the reference range.

GH excess—this causes acromegaly, which develops insidiously with multiple clinical features, most notably including local tumour effects, and increase in size of hands, feet, jaw, and skull. Biochemical diagnosis is made by confirming absence of suppression of GH in the oral glucose tolerance test, and by increased serum IGF-1 levels. Management options include (1) surgery—with transsphenoidal surgery the treatment of choice for most patients; (2) drugs—including dopamine receptor agonists, somatostatin receptor ligands (e.g. octreotide, lanreotide) and GH receptor antagonists (e.g. pegvisomant); and (3) radiotherapy—generally offered for tumours that have recurred or persisted after surgery in patients with resistance to or intolerance of medical treatment.

FSH and LH

Gonadotropin deficiency—this presents in women with oligo/amenorrhoea, loss of libido, dyspareunia, hot flushes, and infertility; and in men with loss of libido; impaired sexual function; mood impairment; loss of facial, scrotal and trunk hair; decreased muscle bulk and energy. Diagnosis in women is based on clinical features in association with FSH and LH levels that are 'inappropriately normal' or low in premenopausal women and low in postmenopausal women; in men there is low morning serum testosterone with low or 'inappropriately normal' gonadotropins. Treatment comprises appropriate replacement therapy.

Prolactin

Prolactinomas are the most common pituitary adenomas and typically present with galactorrhoea and hypogonadism, manifesting in men as impotence, infertility, and decreased libido, and in women as oligo/amenorrhoea and infertility. Secondary causes of hyperprolactinaemia must be excluded in any patient with an elevated serum prolactin and serum prolactin levels usually parallel tumour size in those with prolactinomas. Dopaminergic agonists (e.g. cabergoline, bromocriptine, pergolide, quinagolide) are the primary therapy.

ACTH

Chronic ACTH deficiency is associated with fatigue, pallor, anorexia, weight loss, hypotension, hyponatraemia, hypoglycaemia, and eosinophilia. The insulin tolerance test is considered the 'gold standard' for diagnosis. Glucocorticoid deficiency can be life threatening and hence replacement with hydrocortisone (or other steroid) in a dose and timing to mimic the normal pattern of cortisol secretion should begin as soon as the diagnosis is confirmed.

Cushing's disease is caused by chronic exposure to endogenous glucocorticoids (Cushing's syndrome) produced by the adrenal cortex in response to excess ACTH production by a pituitary corticotroph adenoma. See Chapter 13.7.1 for further discussion.

TSH

Central hypothyroidism is diagnosed when the concentration of thyroxine is decreased and the level of TSH levels is usually normal or low. Clinical presentation is as for primary hypothyroidism (see Chapter 13.4). Treatment is with thyroxine.

Other conditions

Hypopituitarism—can be caused by a range of conditions including pituitary and nonpituitary tumours, hypophysitis, pituitary apoplexy, Sheehan's syndrome (postpartum), brain injury (traumatic, surgical, irradiation, postinfective), and granulomatous diseases.

Clinical manifestations depend mainly on the underlying disease, as well as the type and the degree of the hormonal deficits. Diagnosis and treatment of each pituitary hormone deficit is as described above.

Pituitary adenomas—the most common cause of pituitary disease; may be functioning (resulting in syndromes of hormonal excess) or nonfunctioning (presenting with mass effects). Treatment involves surgery, radiotherapy or medical therapy as described above. Pituitary carcinomas are very rare.

Pituitary apoplexy—occurs primarily in patients with pre-existing pituitary adenomas; results from acute haemorrhage or infarction of the pituitary gland and is characterized by sudden onset of headache, vomiting, visual disturbance, ophthalmoplegia, and altered consciousness. Initial management requires close monitoring of fluid and electrolyte balance and immediate replacement of deficient hormones, especially corticosteroids. Some authorities recommend urgent surgical decompression in some cases.

Craniopharyngiomas—these epithelial tumours can present with pressure effects and/or compomised hypothalamo-pituitary function. First-line treatment usually comprises surgery with or without adjuvant external beam irradiation.

Hypophysitis—may be primary (granulomatous, xanthomatous or lymphocytic) or secondary to a known agent/systemic disease. Differential diagnosis is from pituitary adenoma. Treatment is controversial and includes replacement of defective endocrine function and/or reducing the size of the pituitary mass.

Introduction

The pituitary gland or hypophysis cerebri was first described by Galen of Pergamon in the 2nd century AD, and is considered to be the 'master gland' integrating hormonal signals that control numerous endocrine and metabolic functions. Since the demonstration of the hypothalamic control of pituitary function by Harris in Oxford in the 1950s, our understanding of the physiology and pathophysiology of the pituitary gland has broadened. The development of radioimmunoassays in the 1960s, the extraction of hypothalamic factors principally by Schally and Guillemin in the 1970s, the advances in immunocytochemistry, electron microscopy, and *in situ* hybridization methods, as well as the expansion of molecular biology have increased this understanding. Finally, the advances in modern imaging techniques and in pituitary surgery combined with the development of medical treatments for pituitary tumours have greatly expanded the therapeutic possibilities, providing successful and safe outcomes in most patients.

Anatomy and embryology

The pituitary gland consists of the anterior lobe (adenohypophysis), the posterior lobe (neurohypophysis), and an intermediate zone. The adenohypophysis derives from the stomodeal ectoderm which invaginates by the 3rd week of gestation forming Rathke's pouch. In the 6th week of gestation it comes in contact with the infundibulum. A remnant of the pharyngohypophysis may be found in adults, forming the pharyngeal pituitary located in the midline of the nasopharynx. The posterior lobe originates from the neural primordium as an outpouching from the floor of the third ventricle at the 4th week of gestation. The intermediate lobe arises from the posterior portion of Rathke's pouch. This area normally contains microcytic remnants of Rathke's pouch, which rarely become clinically significant. The portal system starts developing at the 7th week and is completed at around the 20th week of gestation. The body of the sphenoid bone and the sella turcica arise from the fusion of hypophyseal cartilage plates on either side of the developing pituitary. The sella is well formed by the 7th week and matures by enchondral ossification.

The pituitary measures around 13 mm transversely, 9 mm anteroposteriorly, and 6 mm vertically. It weighs approximately 100 mg. It increases during pregnancy to almost twice its normal size, and decreases in older people. The gland is centrally located at the base of the brain in the sella turcica within the sphenoid bone. It is attached to the hypothalamus by the pituitary stalk and a fine vascular network. The gland lacks leptomeninges. The sella turcica is lined by periosteal dura mater; the dura properly covers the lateral aspects of the cavernous sinuses and constitutes the sellar diaphragm. The cavernous sinuses are on either side of the sella, lateral and superior to the sphenoid sinuses, and contain important neurovascular structures including the cavernous segments of the internal carotid arteries and the cranial nerves III, IV, V, and VI. The optic chiasm is located superiorly and is separated from the pituitary by the suprasellar cistern and the sellar diaphragm (Figs. 13.2.1, 13.2.2).

The anterior lobe comprises nearly 80% of the gland and includes the pars distalis, pars intermedia, and pars tuberalis. Staining characteristics divide the pars distalis into a central 'mucoid wedge' and two 'lateral wings'. On light microscopy the cells of the anterior lobe show variation in size, shape, and histochemical staining features. They are organized in nests and cords, and are separated by a complex capillary network. The pars intermedia is poorly developed in humans and lies between the pars distalis and the posterior pituitary. Large numbers of cells in the central zone are basophilic and produce adrenocorticotropic hormone (ACTH), luteinizing hormone (LH), follicle-stimulating hormone (FSH), and thyrotropic hormone (TSH). Most of the cells in the lateral wings are acidophilic and produce growth hormone (GH) and, less frequently, prolactin (PRL) (Table 13.2.1).

The pars tuberalis is an extension of the anterior lobe along the pituitary stalk. It is formed by normal acini of pituitary cells distributed around surface portal vessels. The anterior lobe also includes follicular cells, derived from secretory cells and constituting follicles within the gland, and folliculostellate cells (less than 5% of the adenohypophyseal cells), which have a physiological role that is not clear.

The anterior pituitary receives most of its blood supply from the hypothalamo-hypophyseal portal system (primary plexus, long portal venous system, and secondary plexus), which originates from the capillary plexus of the median eminence and superior stalk derived from the terminal ramifications of the superior and inferior hypophyseal arteries. This system carries blood and hypophysiotropic hormones down to the stalk. The remainder of the blood supply is through the pituitary capsular vessels originating from the superior hypophyseal arteries. The venous drainage from the anterior pituitary is through the cavernous sinuses into the petrosal sinuses and the internal jugular veins.

The anterior lobe has no direct innervation, apart from a few sympathetic nerve fibres spreading to the anterior lobe along blood vessels. The hypothalamic regulation is exerted via the neurohormonal link with the hypothalamic regulatory peptides reaching the pituitary via the portal vessels.

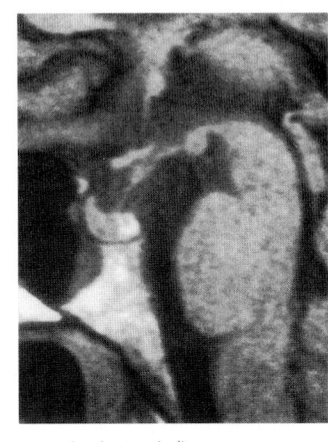

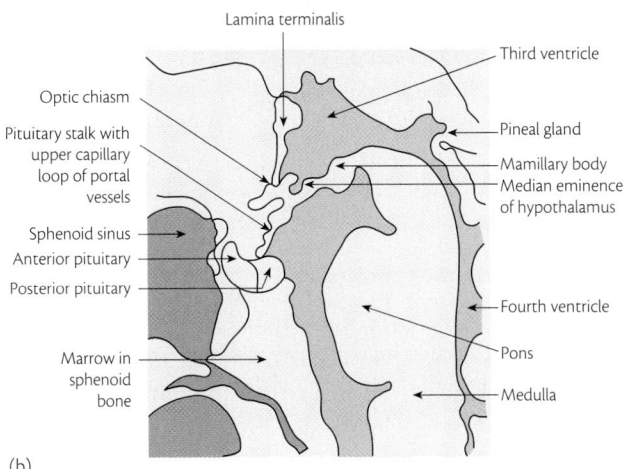

Fig. 13.2.1 Sagittal MRI scan of normal pituitary gland and an anatomical line drawing.

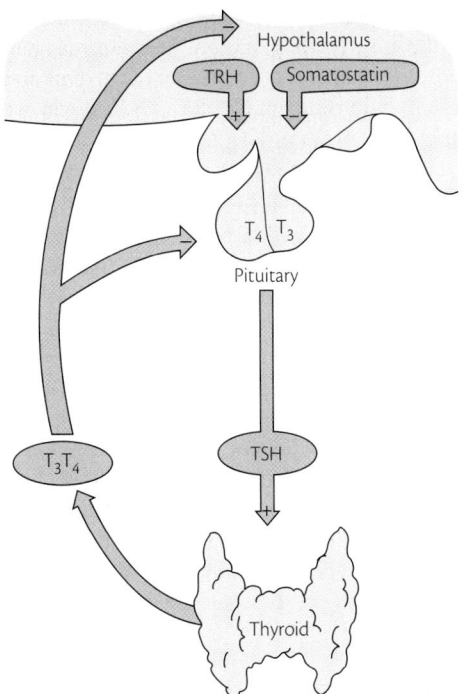

Fig. 13.2.2 Diagram of the hypothalamo-pituitary–thyroid axis showing negative feedback loops. TRH, thyrotrophin-releasing hormone; TSH, thyroid-stimulating hormone.

Table 13.2.1 Hormone-producing cells in anterior pituitary gland

Type of cell	Percentage of adenohypophyseal cells	Distribution
Somatotrophs or GH cells	c.50	Greatest density in lateral wings
Lactotrophs or PRL cells	c.20	Mainly in posterior portions of lateral wings
Corticotrophs or ACTH cells	c.15–20	Mainly middle and posterior portions of mucoid edge
Gonadotrophs or FSH and LH cells (produce FSH and LH in isolation or by the same cell)	c.10	Evenly distributed throughout anterior lobe
Thyrotrophs or TSH cells	c.5	Mainly in anterior part of mucoid edge

ACTH, adrenocorticotropic hormone; GH, growth hormone; FSH, follicle-stimulating hormone; LH, luteinizing hormone; PRL, prolactin; TSH, thyrotropic hormone.

General physiology

The secretion of the anterior pituitary hormones is under elegant regulation exerted by hypothalamic peptides and, with the exception of prolactin, by the negative feedback (at both the hypothalamic and pituitary level) of hormones from the target glands (Fig. 13.2.3). The hypothalamic peptides are secreted in the median eminence and are transferred to the anterior pituitary gland via the hypothalamic–pituitary portal system. They integrate environmental and neural information and bind to specific high affinity cell membrane receptors of the particular pituitary cell type. Failure of the target gland results in decreased negative feedback and increased hypothalamic and pituitary secretion. Primary overactivity of the target gland results in increased negative feedback and decreased hypothalamic and pituitary secretion. Additional 'short-loop' feedback, in which pituitary hormones affect the secretory activity of the hypothalamus, is also implicated in the network contributing to the meaningful function of the pituitary gland. Finally, the anterior pituitary synthesizes several peptides, growth factors, and cytokines that play an important part in autocrine and/or paracrine control of pituitary secretion and/or cell proliferation.

Clinical features of pituitary disease

The clinical features of pituitary disease, mostly associated with a space-occupying lesion, may result from local mass effects and/or pituitary hormone deficits or hypersecretion.

The local mass effects depend on the size of the tumour and its anatomical position. Headache is usually the consequence

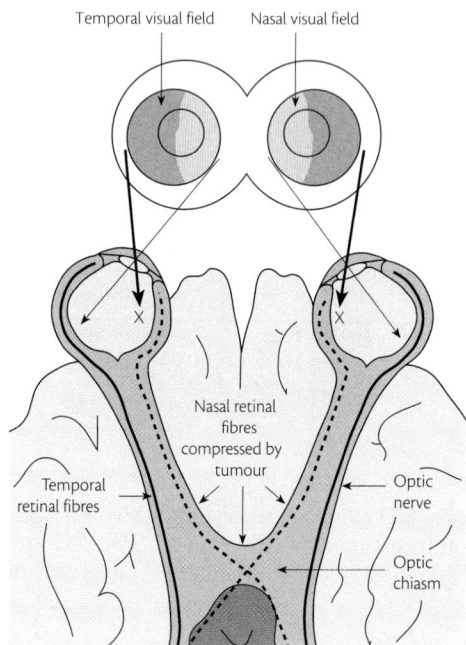

Fig. 13.2.4 Neuro-ophthalmological pathways and the classical bitemporal hemianopia that results from compression of the central optic chiasm by a pituitary tumour. However, any degree of unilateral or bilateral visual deficit can occur depending on the anatomical site of the lesion.

of dural stretching. It can be variable (occipital, retro-orbital, bitemporal) and is often nonspecific. The neuro-ophthalmological effects include visual field defects (usually bitemporal hemianopia or upper temporal quadrantanopia or any unilateral or bilateral visual field defect) from compression of the optic chiasm (Fig. 13.2.4) and squint from ocular nerve palsies caused by lateral tumour extension. Compression of the first or second branch of the trigeminal nerve may rarely result in facial pain. Very large pituitary tumours obstructing the fourth ventricle or the foramen of Monro cause hydrocephalus and expansion of the lateral ventricles. Inferior invasion and erosion of the sellar floor may result in recurrent sinusitis, cerebrovascular fluid rhinorrhoea, and recurrent meningitis. Extension into the temporal lobe may rarely be associated with temporal lobe epilepsy and to the cerebral peduncles with motor and/or sensory disturbances. Superior expansion to the hypothalamus may be associated with hypothalamic dysfunction including disorders of appetite, thirst, temperature regulation, and consciousness.

The pituitary hormone deficits attributed to a pituitary tumour tend to occur in a specific order, with GH and gonadotropins affected first, followed much later by ACTH and TSH. Diabetes insipidus is almost never a presenting feature of pituitary adenomas. The clinical manifestations of hypopituitarism are presented separately for each anterior pituitary hormone.

In case of a functioning pituitary adenoma, the clinical manifestations depend on the type or types of anterior pituitary hormone(s) hypersecreted and are also presented separately for each anterior pituitary hormone.

Pituitary assessment strategy

The investigation of suspected anterior pituitary disease includes testing for hormonal hyperfunction or hypofunction, radiological assessment, and neuro-ophthalmological evaluation.

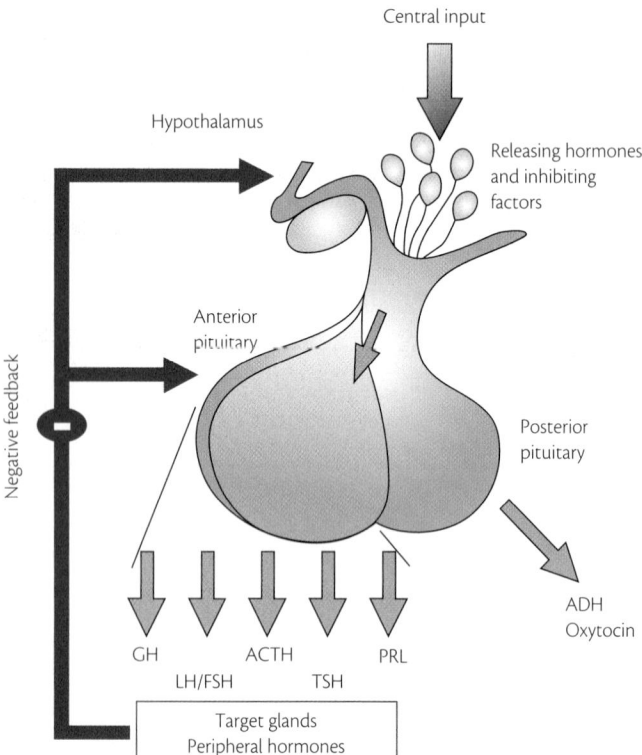

Fig. 13.2.3 Regulation of the hypothalamic–pituitary–peripheral function. The anterior pituitary produces GH, LH/FSH, ACTH, TSH, and PRL. The secretion of these hormones is regulated by hypothalamic-releasing and hypothalamic-inhibiting factors and by negative feedback inhibition of their peripheral hormones. (From Schneider HJ, et al. (2007). Hypopituitarism. *Lancet*, **369**, 1461–70, with permission. © (2007), with permission from Elsevier.)

Testing of pituitary function

The optimum methods for testing anterior pituitary function and the interpretation of the results are the subject of continuing debate. The diagnostic evaluation of pituitary hypofunction has many complementary limbs. First, it is necessary to demonstrate target organ hormonal insufficiency. Paired testing of both hormones in the pituitary–target organ feedback loop (e.g. serum testosterone and gonadotropins), sometimes in combination with provocative testing, will prove that target organ failure is consequent upon lack of stimulation by the relevant pituitary tropic hormone. Additional tests may be necessary to clarify whether the pituitary itself is at fault or whether the pituitary failure is secondary to understimulation by the hypothalamus.

Basal pituitary function tests

Measurements of basal levels of pituitary hormones with target gland hormone secretion are usually sufficient for cases of pituitary dysfunction involving TSH (thyroxine), FSH/LH (testosterone or oestradiol), and PRL. When interpreting basal measurements of pituitary hormones, several factors need to be taken into account:

♦ With the exception of PRL, the interpretation of the anterior pituitary hormonal levels should be done in relation to the level of the target hormone.

♦ The pulsatile secretion of the anterior pituitary hormones may make a single, random blood sample not representative of the total secretion (e.g. GH).

♦ Specific factors including time of day, stress, fed or fasting, asleep or awake, and stage of pubertal development may influence the results.

Currently, the modern chemiluminescent assays are used for measurement of hormone concentrations; these methods have the advantages of increased automation and sensitivity. They do not require radioisotopes and have a shorter assay time.

GH

The marked pulsatile secretion of GH results in values in a normal subject ranging from undetectable to more than 80 mU/litre. Furthermore, the GH secretion is influenced by several factors including nutritional status and stress. As a result of these variables, random levels are of limited value in clinical practice and dynamic endocrine tests are usually needed.

FSH/LH

Serum FSH and LH are secreted in a pulsatile manner. However, it is rare for tests other than basal measurements of gonadotropin hormones and sex steroid levels to be required for the evaluation of the pituitary–gonadal axis. The gonadotropins need to be interpreted taking into account the simultaneous levels of the target gland hormone, as well as the clinical picture of the patient. Thus, in men, a low serum testosterone in conjunction with low or 'inappropriately normal' gonadotropins suggests hypogonadotropic hypogonadism. In women, the interpretation is more complex because of the significant changes in the levels of the gonadotropins during the various phases of the menstrual cycle. A normal menstrual cycle with normal luteal phase serum progesterone (days 18–25 of the cycle) makes gonadotropin deficiency very unlikely. In cases of amenorrhoea, the measurements of gonadotropins, PRL, oestradiol, and human chorionic gonadotropin (possible pregnancy) are needed.

ACTH

The ACTH molecule undergoes rapid proteolytic degradation and, therefore, blood samples must be collected in a cold syringe, placed in an ethylenediaminetetraacetic acid (EDTA) tube at 4 °C, and immediately frozen. ACTH secretion is pulsatile with a circadian rhythm and it increases during stress. As a result, the interpretation of the measurements should take into account the time of sample collection, whether the sample was taken from an indwelling cannula in place for at least 30 min, and whether the patient was stressed. Simultaneous measurement of plasma cortisol is important to check the appropriateness of the ACTH levels. A 9.00 a.m. serum cortisol above 580 nmol/litre excludes adrenal insufficiency.

PRL

PRL is secreted in a pulsatile fashion and also shows an increase in the early morning hours. Stress may cause mild elevations of the hormone and, therefore, the stress of venepuncture should be taken into account when assessing the results.

TSH

The new ultrasensitive assays for TSH have made dynamic testing unnecessary and random sampling therefore provides meaningful information.

Dynamic endocrine tests

In general, the more dynamic the physiological system in health, the more likely will be the need for a dynamic test to investigate its possible malfunction in disease. The provocative tests include those that stimulate hormone release indirectly (e.g. insulin tolerance test) and those that stimulate hormone release directly by injecting pharmacological doses of synthetically manufactured peptides (e.g. short Synacthen test). Currently, the combined anterior pituitary function test with the administration of LH-releasing hormone (LHRH) and thyrotropin-releasing hormone (TRH) is not used in clinical practice, as basal hormone measurements provide the necessary diagnostic information. Thus, only disorders of ACTH and GH secretion need dynamic endocrine testing with stimulation or suppression tests, according the presenting picture.

The most commonly used tests in clinical practice are described below.

Insulin tolerance test

This test is considered the gold standard for assessing the integrity of the ACTH–cortisol axis, as well as the GH reserve. The hypoglycaemia induced by the intravenous injection of insulin is a powerful stimulus, which in the intact pituitary and hypothalamus induces ACTH and GH release, as well as a rise, therefore, in the serum cortisol levels. It has been proposed that the peak cortisol levels of patients undergoing major surgery are comparable to those achieved during the insulin-induced hypoglycaemia. The test should be undertaken only under close supervision at skilled centres. The patient should be fasted from midnight and the test started at 9.00 a.m. At 0 min, 0.1 to 0.15 IU/kg (or 0.3 IU/kg for those with acromegaly, Cushing's syndrome, or other conditions with insulin resistance) of soluble human insulin is injected intravenously and blood is drawn at times 0, 30, 45, 60, 90, and 120 min. During the procedure, pulse rate, blood pressure, and manifestations of hypoglycaemia should be recorded. Blood glucose must fall to less than 2.2 mmol/litre (to provide an adequate stimulus) in order to interpret the cortisol and GH levels. A normal cortisol response is a rise to 580 nmol/litre or above. Severe GH deficiency in adults is diagnosed if the peak GH is less than 3 µg/litre.

Contraindications include ischaemic heart disease, epilepsy or unexplained blackouts, severe long-standing hypoadrenalism, untreated hypothyroidism, and glycogen storage disease. Many physicians are uncomfortable with the use of this test in older people.

Short Synacthen test

This test has been advocated as an alternative to the insulin tolerance test for assessing the ACTH reserve. The rationale for its use is that chronic underexposure of the adrenal glands to ACTH (following prolonged corticosteroid therapy or due to hypothalamic–pituitary disease) will result in a blunted cortisol response to exogenously administered ACTH. It involves the injection of a pharmacological dose (250 μg) of ACTH with measurement of the cortisol response 30 min later. The correlation between cortisol levels 30 min after the injection of Synacthen and the peak cortisol achieved during the insulin tolerance test is excellent; stimulated cortisol concentrations of 580 nmol/litre or less suggest ACTH deficiency. This test does not differentiate primary from secondary adrenal insufficiency. It requires no specialist staff and the only reported side effect is allergy in patients with atopy. It cannot be used in cases of acute hypopituitarism as it takes at least 2 weeks for the adrenal zona fasciculata to involute following withdrawal of ACTH stimulation. In recent years, much interest has arisen in the use of a lower dose of ACTH (1 μg), as the injected bolus of 250 μg is considered supraphysiological; this has not gained widespread acceptance.

Glucagon stimulation test

The glucagon stimulation test is used as an alternative to the insulin tolerance test for assessment of the ACTH/cortisol and GH reserve. The subcutaneous injection of glucagon causes a transient rise in plasma glucose and, during the subsequent fall in glucose, ACTH and GH are released. The test involves the administration of 1 mg (or 1.5 mg if body weight >90 kg) glucagon subcutaneously with blood sampling for cortisol, GH, and glucose at times 0, 90, 120, 150, 180, and 210 min. The contraindications for this test include phaeochromocytoma or insulinoma, glycogen storage disease, and severe hypocortisolaemia. The interpretation of results relies on criteria established for the insulin tolerance test. The injection may cause nausea, abdominal pain, and vomiting. Glucagon is a less powerful stimulus to ACTH release and false-negative results may be seen in up to 20% of patients. In some false-negative results, no rise in the blood glucose is achieved after the glucagon injection.

Oral glucose tolerance test

The evaluation of GH hypersecretion requires a suppression test. Increased blood glucose levels inhibit GH secretion and the administration of oral glucose is used in suspected acromegaly. The test is performed at 9.00 a.m. with the patient fasted from midnight. Blood samples are drawn for measurement of glucose and GH at times 0, 30, 60, 90, and 120 min. Immediately after the first blood sample, 75 g of glucose are dissolved in water and given to the patient. In normal individuals serum GH should reach undetectable levels. Failure of suppression or a paradoxical rise in GH suggest acromegaly. False-positive results may be seen in uncontrolled diabetes mellitus, obesity, liver disease, renal insufficiency, malnutrition, or anorexia. During late adolescence, when GH secretion is maximal, GH may also fail to be suppressed.

Radiological assessment

Currently, the imaging modality of choice for patients with suspected pituitary pathology is MRI. CT is an acceptable alternative if MRI is contraindicated. The advantages of MRI are direct multiplanar scanning, lack of ionizing radiation, and good anatomical tissue discrimination without the need for pharmaceutical contrast agents. The evaluation of the pituitary and the hypothalamus is optimal in sagittal and coronal planes. The only disadvantage of MRI (apart from the cost) is its relative insensitivity to pathological calcification and lack of signal from corticated bone. CT or even plain film radiography may be required to demonstrate pathological calcification. The structures of the sellar region are best visualized using T_1-weighted sequences, which produce images with dark cerebrospinal fluid, grey brain and pituitary, and white fat. Corticated bone returns low signal and appears dark, but bone marrow fat returns high signal and appears white. The nuclei of the hypothalamus cannot be distinguished, but if phospholipid vesicles are present in the neurohypophysis they are apparent as high signal areas. The need for routine intravenous administration of paramagnetic agents is controversial (however, it increases the pick-up rate of pituitary microadenomas). These agents do not cross the blood–brain barrier and, therefore, the pituitary gland and stalk enhance and appear whiter on T_1-weighted images. The hypothalamus and the optic chiasm do not enhance if the blood–brain barrier is intact. Blood vessels, meninges, and mucosa of the paranasal sinuses will enhance. Dynamic MRI has been used to study the timing of intravenously administered gadolinium uptake by the hypophysis (see Figs. 13.2.1, 13.2.2).

Apart from its complementary role to MRI in detecting pathological calcification, CT scanning is the imaging modality of choice for patients who are unable to undergo MRI (extreme claustrophobia, presence of cardiac pacemakers or other implants such as intracranial aneurysm clips or traumatic metallic fragments). Multislice spiral CT scanners produce images of sufficient quality to demonstrate sellar anatomy on unenhanced images. Intravenous injection of iodinated contrast media is used to improve tissue contrast and it is taken up by the hypophysis in the same way as gadolinium. Thus, macroadenomas or craniopharyngiomas enhance and are better delineated, but demonstration of microadenomas within a morphologically normal pituitary depends on differential uptake rates.

Neuro-ophthalmological evaluation

The neuro-ophthalmological evaluation in suspected pituitary pathology includes assessment of the visual acuity (with the use of Snellen charts), assessment of the visual fields (by confrontation using a red pin and formally by the Goldmann perimetry test or by visual evoked responses), and fundoscopy (to check for optic atrophy, retinal vein engorgement, or papilloedema). Vision is usually lost gradually, except in cases of pituitary apoplexy when it may be sudden. Successful decompression of the optic nerves and chiasm achieved surgically or by medical therapy results in marked improvement of visual function; this becomes apparent within hours or days of surgery continuing thereafter for 6 months or more. The chance of complete reversal of any visual field defects is higher if the duration of compression of the optic chiasm is short (<1 year).

Pituitary surgery

Currently, the main aims of pituitary surgery are to cure any endocrine excess and to reverse the pressure effects (particularly the visual compromise and the pituitary dysfunction) without causing morbidity or mortality. For all pituitary tumours, except prolactinomas, surgery is the treatment of choice. It is also indicated when other therapies have not been successful or in case of tumour recurrence. The trans-sphenoidal approach (via the translabial or transethmoidal route) is most commonly used and, compared with the transfrontal route, it is less time consuming, less traumatic, and associated with less morbidity. The trans-sphenoidal approach is less successful for large tumours with significant invasion to neighbouring structures. In pituitary adenomas the tumour is usually soft and white and can be easily removed by curettes and suction. Other tumours may also be recognized during surgery, including meningiomas or craniopharyngiomas. Complications include cerebrospinal fluid leakage, impaired anterior pituitary function, diabetes insipidus (most commonly temporary), the syndrome of inappropriate secretion of antidiuretic hormone (usually transient), visual deterioration, meningitis, headache (attributed to haematoma in the air sinuses, meningitis, hyponatraemia, or abscess), vascular damage, epilepsy, frontal lobe damage, hypothalamic damage, and intracranial oedema/haemorrhage. The success and complication rates are mainly associated with the size and extensions of the tumour and any previous therapy, as well as the experience and expertise of the neurosurgeon.

Pituitary radiotherapy

After the improvement of trans-sphenoidal and microsurgery techniques and the availability of medical therapy for prolactinomas, pituitary irradiation is no longer prescribed routinely for the management of pituitary tumours. It is mainly reserved for patients who are not fit to undergo surgery, for those who have had an unsuccessful operation (nontotal tumour removal), or for those showing tumour recurrence.

Conventional irradiation uses a linear accelerator and is administered in a fractionated manner to a total dose of 4500 cGy in daily doses not exceeding 180 cGy over a 5- to 6-week period. Hormonal hypersecretion shows a rapid fall within the first 2 years with the decline continuing for up to 20 years. Radiotherapy is also considered an effective modality for decreasing the recurrence rates of pituitary tumours.

With modern technology and careful planning, the use of multiple fixed fields from linear accelerators, and careful fractionation, the risk of radiation-induced late complications is small. These include hypopituitarism and visual impairment; oncogenesis and cognitive impairment occur infrequently. With increasing time after irradiation, anterior pituitary function assessment will show compromised reserve in gonadotropins and GH, followed later by ACTH and TSH. It has been reported that by 10 years after radiotherapy, 47% of patients were hypogonadal, 30% were hypoadrenal, and 16% were hypothyroid. Therefore, any patient who has received pituitary irradiation needs lifelong follow-up aiming for the early diagnosis of hormonal deficits. Notably, the total dose and the dose per daily fraction influence the risk of hypopituitarism. Optic nerve/chiasmal damage can be avoided by keeping the daily fractionated dose to less than 200 cGy. From the available data, the incidence of late carcinogenesis cannot be estimated with certainty, but it is unlikely to be more than 1 to 2%.

Recently introduced techniques include stereotactic radiotherapy and stereotactic radiosurgery (producing a highly localized deposition of radiation on the target, at the perimeter of which there is a fast 'fall off' of the isodoses, thereby sparing the surrounding normal tissue from high doses of irradiation). Following stereotactic radiosurgery, there is a faster early reduction of the excessive secretory hormone product; hypopituitarism can also occur.

The selection of the optimal radiation treatment modality should be based on the size and extent of the adenoma, the postoperative endocrine situation for secretory tumours, and the immunohistochemical markers of aggression. For small, discrete tumours located in the fossa, radiosurgery seems to be a good option. This technique is also useful for patients with recurrence who have already received conventional radiotherapy.

Anterior pituitary hormones

GH

Human GH is a single chain protein of 191 amino acids containing two disulphide bonds. It is produced by the somatotroph cells and it has several similarities to prolactin and the placental lactogen molecule. Nearly 75% of the hormone circulates as a 22-kDa protein, 5 to 10% as a smaller 20-kDa isoform, and the remainder consists of glycosylated and sulphated isoforms. GH is secreted in an episodic manner (pulses occurring every 3–4 h) that is modified by age and sex. The most profound discharge occurs during deep sleep (phases III and IV). Its secretion is under complex neuroregulatory control. The hypothalamic participation is exerted through GH-releasing hormone (GHRH) and somatostatin, which reach the pituitary gland via the hypothalamo-pituitary portal vessels. GHRH stimulates both synthesis and secretion of GH, whereas somatostatin inhibits the release but not the synthesis of the hormone. Ghrelin, the endogenous ligand of the GH secretagogue receptor localized mainly in the stomach, may also be implicated in the control of GH secretion. The somatotroph cell is also regulated by negative feedback at the pituitary level by the circulating insulin-like growth factor 1 (IGF-1) and by 'short loop' feedback on the hypothalamus by GH. The secretion of GH is greater in women and it shows a decrease with age in both sexes. Amino acids (e.g. arginine, leucine), sleep, exercise, stress, a fall in blood glucose, poorly controlled diabetes mellitus type 1, hepatic cirrhosis, anorexia nervosa, central α-adrenergic agonists, and acetylcholine agonists enhance GH secretion. Oestrogens increase the pulse amplitude of GH. β-Antagonists augment the stimulatory effect of other stimuli. Agents lowering acetylcholine tone suppress GH release. Hyperglycaemia in normal subjects acutely suppresses GH secretion. Obesity is associated with decreased GH release and emotional deprivation may inhibit GH secretion in children. GH levels are decreased in pregnancy due to the negative feedback by the GH variant secreted by the placenta.

GH exerts its actions through a specific 638-amino acid receptor belonging to the class I haematopoietin or cytokine/GH/PRL receptor superfamily. It shows a wide distribution including muscle, adipose tissues, liver, mammary gland, bones, kidneys, brain, and embryonic stem cells. It is a single membrane-spanning type I glycoprotein with an extracellular ligand-binding domain, a single 24-amino acid hydrophobic transmembrane region, and an intracellular domain. The signal transduction requires dimerization of the receptor, which is facilitated by the GH binding. The downstream signalling pathways resulting in GH actions include, but are probably not limited to, the signal transducer and activator of transcription (STAT), mitogen-activated-kinase (MAP) and phosphoinositide 3-kinase (PI3) pathways. Abnormalities in the GH receptor occur in Laron's dwarfism, which is characterized by failure of growth, high levels of GH, and low IGF-1.

Up to 60% of the circulating serum GH is bound to the GH-binding protein, which corresponds to part of the extracellular domain of the GH receptor. The binding reduces the clearance rate of the hormone and thus prolongs its half-life.

The effects of GH are mediated either directly or mainly indirectly via the production of IGF-1 by the liver, bones, and other types of tissues. IGF-1 is a polypeptide of 70 amino acids and acts in an endocrine, paracrine, or autocrine fashion. It circulates bound to a group of binding proteins; IGF binding protein-3 is the main carrier of IGF-1 and plays an important role in regulating its bioactivity. IGF-1 induces cell proliferation and inhibits apoptosis. Its levels are determined by sex and genetic factors, are highest during late adolescence, and decline throughout adulthood. The production of IGF-1 is suppressed in malnourished patients, as well as in those with liver disease, hypothyroidism, or poorly controlled diabetes. Although IGF-1 levels usually reflect the integrated secretory activity of GH, subtly elevated GH levels may not uniformly induce high IGF-1.

The main actions of GH are the promotion of skeletal growth, mainly of long bones, and the regulation of several metabolic actions. In the muscles GH promotes the incorporation of amino acids and protein synthesis, and in the adipose tissue it promotes free fatty acid release.

Disorders of GH secretion

GH deficiency

The manifestations of GH deficiency are shown in Table 13.2.2. Given its pulsatile secretion, the measurements of random GH levels do not distinguish between normal and compromised GH secretion; multiple sampling for GH would be ideal but in clinical practice this is not a practical procedure. Therefore, the diagnosis of GH deficiency requires stimulation testing, unless all other pituitary hormones are deficient and the IGF-1 is low (in these patients the likelihood of GH deficiency is 99%). The biochemical criteria for the diagnosis of adult GH deficiency are complicated by the lack of normative data that are age-adjusted and sex-adjusted, by the assay variability, and by the stimulus used. Among the available

Table 13.2.2 Manifestations of GH deficiency

Children	Adults
Growth failure	Relative increase in fat mass
	Relative decrease in muscle mass
	Increased serum low-density lipoprotein cholesterol
	Decreased bone mineral density
	Increased risk of cardiovascular disease
	Increased inflammatory cardiovascular risk markers
	Decreased energy and quality of life

tests the insulin tolerance test is considered the gold standard. Severe GH deficiency in adults is diagnosed if the peak GH is less than 3 µg/litre. In children the secretory capacity of GH is higher and a cut-off of 10 µg/litre (20 mU/litre) is used. The GHRH plus arginine test (1 µg/kg GHRH intravenously as a bolus followed immediately by 30 g arginine as an infusion over 30 min) has been shown to reliably detect severe GH deficiency in a lean adult population when a cut-off of 9 µg/litre (18 mU/litre) is used. The response to this test declines greatly with increasing body mass index and the above cut-off in obese patients is associated with a high proportion of false-positive results. Furthermore, as GHRH directly stimulates the pituitary, it can give a falsely normal GH response in patients with GH deficiency of hypothalamic origin. Other alternative tests, but less commonly used in clinical practice, include the GHRH plus GH-releasing peptide-6 test, the glucagon test, the arginine test, the L-dopa test, and the clonidine test. Normal serum levels of IGF-1 do not exclude a diagnosis of GH deficiency.

The main targets of GH therapy in children with GH deficiency are to normalize height during childhood and to reach normal adult height. The benefits of treatment with GH among adult patients have been reported in several domains: body composition (decrease in total body fat content, increase in muscle mass), exercise capacity, bone health (increase in bone mineral density with greater effects at vertebral sites), cardiovascular risk factors (decrease in blood pressure, reduction of C-reactive protein, increase in high-density lipoprotein, and decrease in low-density lipoprotein and total cholesterol), and quality of life. In adults, the dosing plans have evolved from weight-based dosing to individualized dose-titration strategies with the goals being an appropriate clinical response, an avoidance of side effects, and an IGF-1 level in the middle of the age-adjusted reference range. In general, women require higher doses of GH to achieve the same IGF-1 response (much higher GH doses were also needed to achieve the same IGF-1 levels in women receiving oral oestrogen replacement, but this does not apply when oestrogens are offered as patches). Furthermore, as GH secretion normally decreases with age, older patients require lower doses of GH. The duration of GH replacement therapy in adults is unclear; if benefits are apparent, there is no particular reason to stop treatment. On the other hand, if there are no benefits following at least 1 year of treatment, discontinuing GH therapy may be appropriate. Most adverse effects are dose related and are attributed to fluid retention (paraesthesias, joint stiffness, peripheral oedema, arthralgia, and myalgia). In children, there is a risk of slipped capital femoral epiphysis. With the current dosing regimens, there may be a slight excess risk of diabetes mellitus. Other complications of GH therapy include retinopathy, benign intracranial hypertension, and gynaecomastia. GH replacement may cause a decrease of serum free thyroxine levels (perhaps due to increased deiodination of thyroxine) and of serum cortisol levels (revealing central hypoadrenalism that had been masked, probably due to enhanced conversion of cortisone to cortisol during the GH-deficient state). GH treatment is contraindicated in the presence of an active malignancy.

Acromegaly

Acromegaly is the syndrome resulting from GH hypersecretion. Its incidence is estimated to be approximately 3 cases per 1 million persons per year, and its prevalence is about 60 per million. More than 90% of patients with acromegaly have a benign monoclonal

GH-secreting pituitary adenoma surrounded by nonhyperplastic pituitary tissue. Co-secretion of PRL has been described in about 25% of GH-secreting adenomas. More than 70% of somatotroph tumours are macroadenomas at diagnosis. Younger patients usually present with more rapidly growing tumours. Rarely, acromegaly is associated with familial syndromes, including multiple endocrine neoplasia type I, the McCune–Albright syndrome, familial acromegaly, and Carney's syndrome. Excess production of GH-releasing hormone (as in central hypothalamic tumours, usually gangliocytomas, and peripheral neuroendocrine tumours, e.g. of the lung) can result in somatotroph hyperplasia and acromegaly.

Clinical features The clinical features of acromegaly are shown in Box 13.2.1. Disease features develop insidiously, and the diagnosis may often take 10 years from presentation. GH-secreting adenomas arising before the closure of epiphyseal bone are associated with accelerated growth and gigantism.

Whether acromegaly is associated with an increased relative risk of cancer is controversial and has been extensively reviewed. Prospective, controlled studies of colonoscopic screening suggest that the risk of colon cancer is nearly twice that in the general population; this probably reflects a tropic IGF-1 effect on the proliferation of epithelial cells. Screening colonoscopy should be performed when the diagnosis of acromegaly is made, with follow-up according to standard guidelines.

The overall standardized mortality ratio of patients with acromegaly is 1.48. Factors contributing to an increased mortality include the higher prevalence of hypertension, hyperglycaemia, or overt diabetes, cardiomyopathy, and sleep apnoea in this population. GH levels of less than 2.5 µg/litre (5 mU/litre) predict longer survival. In some studies, increased IGF-1 levels are associated with higher mortality. However, GH levels seem to be more consistently independent predictors of mortality than are IGF-1 levels.

Diagnosis The biochemical diagnosis is made by confirming absence of suppression of GH in the oral glucose tolerance test and by increased serum IGF-1 levels. With the use of most commercial assays, nadir GH levels of less than 1 µg/litre (2 mU/litre) during the oral glucose tolerance test rule out the diagnosis.

Treatment The goals of treatment in patients with acromegaly include the elimination of morbidities associated with the disease and normalization of the increased mortality. These aims are achieved by using safe approaches that decrease the mass effects and restore GH and IGF-1 secretion to normal. It should be noted that, with the currently available therapeutic options, normal GH secretion dynamics are only rarely achieved and it is, therefore, more appropriate to define disease control. Disease control implies nadir GH levels of less than 1 µg/litre (2 mU/litre) after the glucose tolerance test and a normal IGF-1 level (for sex and age). It has been recently proposed that for complete control of GH dynamics to be achieved, nadir GH values should be less than 0.4 µg/litre.

Management options include surgery, drugs, and radiotherapy. Trans-sphenoidal surgery remains the treatment of choice for most patients. The success rate depends on the size and extensions of the tumour, the presurgical GH levels, as well as the experience and expertise of the neurosurgeon. Biochemical control has been reported for up to 80% of microadenomas and for up to 40% of macroadenomas. Tumours that have invaded the cavernous sinus cannot be completely removed surgically and the hypersecretion

---

Box 13.2.1 Clinical features of acromegaly

Local tumour effects

- Pituitary enlargement
- Visual-field defects
- Cranial nerve palsy
- Headache

Somatic systems

- Acral enlargement including thickness of soft tissue of hands and feet

Musculoskeletal system

- Gigantism
- Prognathism
- Jaw malocclusion
- Arthralgias and arthritis
- Carpal tunnel syndrome
- Acroparesthesia
- Proximal myopathy
- Hypertrophy of frontal bones

Skin and gastrointestinal system

- Hyperhidrosis
- Oily texture
- Skin tags
- Colon polyps

Cardiovascular system

- Left ventricular hypertrophry
- Asymmetric septal hyptroptry
- Cardiomyopathy
- Hypertension
- Congestive heart failure

Pulmonary system

- Sleep disturbances
- Sleep apnoea (central and obstructive)
- Narcolepsy

Visceromegaly

- Tongue
- Thyroid gland
- Salivary glands
- Liver
- Spleen
- Kidney
- Prostate

Box 13.2.1 (*Cont'd*) Clinical features of acromegaly

Endocrine and metabolic systems

Reproduction
- Menstrual abnormalities
- Galactorrhea
- Decreased libido, impotence, low levels of sex hormone-binding globulin

Multiple endocrine neoplasia type 1
- Hyperparathyroidism
- Pancreatic islet cell tumors

Carbohydrate
- Impaired glucose tolerance
- Insulin resistance and hyperinsulinemia
- Diabetes mellitus

Lipid
- Hypertriglyceridemia

Mineral
- Hypercalciuria, increased levels of 25-hydroxyvitamin D_3
- Urinary hydroxyproline

Electrolyte
- Low renin levels
- Increased aldosterone levels

Thyroid
- Low thyroxine binding globulin levels
- Goitre

(From Melmed S (2006). Acromegaly. *N Engl J Med*, **355**, 2558–73, with permission. © 2006 Massachusetts Medical Society. All rights reserved.)

of GH almost invariably persists postoperatively in such patients. Although up to 10% of tumours recur, many recurrences probably represent persistent growth of residual nonresectable tumour tissue.

Medical treatment includes dopamine receptor agonists, somatostatin receptor ligands, and GH receptor antagonists. Dopamine receptor agonists are less costly than other agents, but are only occasionally effective in selected patients. The doses required are usually much higher than in prolactinomas and biochemical control has been reported in less than 15% of the patients. Somatostatin receptor ligands, such as octreotide and lanreotide, bind to somatostatin receptors resulting in suppression of GH secretion. They also act on the liver to block the synthesis of IGF-1. Octreotide and lanreotide are selective for somatostatin receptors type 2 and 5, which are expressed in more than 90% of the GH-secreting adenomas. Depot preparations—long-acting-release octreotide and a long-acting aqueous-gel preparation of lanreotide—allow for injections every 14 to 28 days maintaining highly effective drug levels. Biochemical control has been reported

in approximately 70% of the patients with the pretreatment GH levels affecting the efficacy of these agents (less effective when the GH level is higher). Shrinkage of tumour mass has been reported in about 50% of patients, and generally reverses when treatment is stopped. Surgical debulking of macroadenomas not amenable to total resection enhances the efficacy of subsequent somatostatin analogue treatment. Somatostatin analogues are indicated following unsuccessful surgery and after radiation therapy, during the period when GH levels remain elevated. They can also be offered as primary treatment to patients with large extrasellar tumours who have no evidence of central compressive effects, those who are too frail to undergo surgery, and those who decline an operation. Transient diarrhoea, nausea, and abdominal discomfort may occur, but typically resolve within 8 to 10 weeks. Blood glucose levels may rise in some patients. Gallbladder sludge or asymptomatic gallstones develop within 18 months in up to 20% of patients and these conditions should be managed according to standard guidelines. Selective activation of other somatostatin receptors by specific somatostatin receptor ligands results in additive suppression of GH; thus, the ligand pasireotide (SOM230), currently in clinical trials, suppresses levels of GH in patients with resistance to octreotide. Chimeric molecules that recognize both the dopamine D2 receptor and somatostatin receptors may also enhance receptor signalling and provide therapeutic synergy. Lastly, pegvisomant, a pegylated GH receptor analogue showing enhanced activity for the GH receptor, also prevents the functional GH-receptor signalling. As a result of this, it blocks the GH-mediated IGF-1 generation in nearly 90% of patients. It is indicated for patients whose GH levels are inadequately controlled with other modalities or in those experiencing significant drug side effects. During treatment with pegvisomant, GH levels increase and IGF-1 is the biomarker for monitoring the efficacy of treatment. Elevated hepatic aminotransferase levels have been reported requiring monitoring of the liver function tests monthly for the first 6 months of treatment and 6 monthly thereafter. Probable tumour size should be monitored at 6-month intervals to detect possible continued enlargement.

Radiotherapy (conventional or radiosurgery) is generally offered for tumours that have recurred or persisted after surgery in patients with resistance to or intolerance of medical treatment. Twenty-two per cent of patients achieved a level less than 2.5 ng/ml (5 mU/litre) by 2 years, 60% by 10 years, and 77% by 20 years. The interval to achieve this depends on the pre-irradiation GH level. Insulin-like growth factor-I levels normalize in 63% of patients by 10 years.

FSH/LH

The gonadotropins, TSH, and human chorionic gonadotropin β belong to the family of glycoprotein anterior pituitary hormones. They share a common α subunit and each has a unique β subunit conferring biological and immunological specificity. Both LH β subunit and FSH β subunit have 115 amino acids and two carbohydrate side chains. A terminal sialic acid may be present on the carbohydrate side chain of the FSH β subunit decreasing its metabolic clearance.

The regulation of FSH and LH secretion is exerted by the integration of the gonadotropin-releasing hormone (a hypothalamic decapeptide) signal and the (stimulatory and inhibitory) feedback effects of gonadal steroids and peptides. Gonadotropin-releasing hormone interacts with the membrane receptor and regulates the synthesis and release of gonadotropins. The major feature of the pituitary–gonadal axis is that its constituents exhibit a pulsatile pattern of hormonal release. The frequency and the amplitude of gonadotropin-releasing hormone pulses are important in differentially regulating LH and FSH secretion. The levels of gonadotropins are very low in children and the nocturnal augmentation of gonadotropin release marks the onset of sexual development.

In women, LH levels rise slightly during the follicular phase, peaking at the time of the midcycle surge and then decline during the luteal phase. The FSH levels start rising during the late luteal phase, increase during the early follicular phase of the next cycle, and decline just before the midcycle FSH surge. During the luteal phase, the FSH levels show a decline and increase again prior the next menses. In the follicular phase, most of the LH pulses are followed by a release of oestrogens from the ovary, whereas in the mid and late luteal phase the LH pulses induce progesterone secretion. Both oestradiol and progesterone inhibit the release of LH acting at the hypothalamic and pituitary level. However, in the follicular phase there is enhanced release of oestradiol, which acts in a stimulatory way and induces the large discharge of LH responsible for ovulation. During this surge, LH levels remain increased for 36 to 48 h, during which time ovulation occurs, oestradiol levels decline, and luteinization of the follicle results in increasing production of progesterone. The ovary exerts a negative feedback on FSH secretion mainly through the secretion of inhibin, a glycoprotein hormone synthesized in the granulosa cells of the ovarian follicle and counterbalanced by activin. In the late follicular phase, inhibin levels increase and, in combination with oestradiol, inhibit the synthesis and release of FSH, an inhibition that it is overcome at the preovulatory gonadotropin discharge. The hypothalamic control of FSH and LH secretion is very sensitive to environmental conditions, such as stress or changes to nutrition or energy homeostasis. Stress activates the corticotropin-releasing hormone pathways, which may inhibit the gonadotropin-releasing hormone neurons through opiate pathways. Reduction in the daily food intake leads to a reduction in the gonadotropin-releasing hormone secretion translated into a reduced and nonpulsatile secretion of FSH and LH into the circulation. The regulation of the gonadal axis is equally complex but more static in men. It is assumed that gonadotropin pulses in men follow the scarce pulses of gonadotropin-releasing hormone and, in fact, are highly variable and of small amplitude. Testosterone exerts a negative feedback on LH secretion, and Sertoli cells secrete activin and inhibin in order to regulate FSH secretion.

The gonadotropins are responsible for the gonadal sex-steroid production by the Leydig cells of the testis and the ovarian follicles, secondary sexual development, maintenance of secondary sexual characteristics, and fertility.

Disorders of FSH/LH secretion
FSH/LH deficiency
Gonadotropin deficiency presents with oligomenorrhoea/amenorrhoea, loss of libido, dyspareunia, hot flushes, and infertility in women, and with loss of libido, impaired sexual function, mood impairment, loss of facial, scrotal, and trunk hair, and decreased muscle bulk and energy in men. Hypogonadism in both sexes is associated with decreased bone mineral density. In children, gonadotropin deficiency causes delayed or arrested puberty.

The diagnosis in women is based on oligomenorrhoea/amenorrhoea combined with low or 'inappropriately normal' FSH

and LH levels. In postmenopausal women, the FSH and LH levels are inappropriately low. In men, there is low serum testosterone (9.00 a.m. sample, as levels show considerable diurnal variation) with low or 'inappropriately normal' gonadotropins.

The treatment consists of appropriate replacement therapy. In women, oestrogens are give orally or by transdermal patch or gel; when an intact uterus is present, additional progesterone is necessary. Given the findings of large studies of hormone replacement therapy in postmenopausal women without hypopituitarism showing increased risk of cardiovascular and neoplastic diseases, stopping treatment in hypogonadal women after the age of menopause is recommended. For induction of fertility, gonadotropins or pulsatile gonadotropin-releasing hormone (the latter only in hypothalamic dysfunction) are used. Serum androgen levels in women with hypopituitarism are low; the pros and cons of replacing androgens in such cases are under investigation. In men, testosterone replacement using one of the available preparations (gel, intramuscular injections, patch, buccal) is suggested. The dose is adjusted to normal testosterone concentrations. Serum LH cannot be used to monitor the adequacy of therapy. Monitoring for prostate-specific antigen, prostate size, and haematocrit (erythropoietin is stimulated by testosterone) are recommended annually. For the induction of fertility, human chorionic gonadotropin, human menopausal gonadotropin, FSH, or pulsatile gonadotropin-releasing hormone (the latter only in hypothalamic dysfunction) are available options.

Gonadotroph adenomas
Gonadotropinomas are pituitary adenomas secreting intact LH and/or FSH. They are rare, as most tumours expressing gonadotropins secrete a subunit without causing biological effects (nonfunctioning pituitary adenomas). Both types of tumours are most commonly diagnosed in middle-aged men and present with symptoms related to a pituitary mass. FSH-secreting tumours cause testicular enlargement in men and ovarian hyperstimulation syndrome in premenopausal women. Treatment includes surgical excision combined or not with radiotherapy.

PRL
PRL is released by the lactotroph cells of the adenohypophysis. It is composed of 199 amino acids and has three disulphide intramolecular bonds. Its molecular structure is similar to GH and to placental lactogen with which it shares a common phylogenetic origin. PRL physiology differs from that of other anterior pituitary hormones in that its secretion is mainly under tonic inhibition (affecting both synthesis and release) by dopamine released from the hypothalamus. Hypothalamic stressors, such as the insulin tolerance test, are able to release PRL and exogenous administration of TRH releases PRL in addition to TSH, operating through specific lactotroph receptors. Oestrogens induce hyperplasia of the lactotroph cells and enhance PRL secretion. The increase in pituitary volume in pregnant women may be in part due to the large oestrogenic production by the fetoplacental unit. In the third trimester, PRL concentrations may rise as high as 8000 mU/litre. During pregnancy, the development of the synthetic and secretory potential of the breast apparatus is under the influence of several hormones (oestrogen, insulin, cortisol, placental mammotropic hormones). Before delivery, lactation is inhibited by high levels of oestrogen and progesterone. The rapid fall of these hormones after

delivery allows PRL to initiate lactation. After delivery, maternal levels of PRL fall if there is no breast feeding, but remain increased in response to suckling. Conditions associated with hyperprolactinaemia are shown in Box 13.2.2.

PRL receptors have a wide distribution in the body. They are mostly found in the mammary gland and their activation is

---

Box 13.2.2 Causes of hyperprolactinaemia

Physiological
- Stress
- Pregnancy
- Lactation
- Nipple stimulation/suckling
- Sexual intercourse
- Sleep

Drugs (commonly used in clinical practice)
- Antipsychotics–neuroleptics (e.g. phenothiazines, butyrophenones)
- Antidepressants (e.g. tricyclic and tetracyclic antidepressants, monoamine oxidase inhibitors, selective serotonin reuptake inhibitors)
- Opiates
- Cocaine
- Antihypertensive medications (e.g. verapamil, methyldopa, reserpine)
- Gastrointestinal medications (e.g. metoclopramide, domperidone)
- Protease inhibitors?
- Oestrogens

Pathological
- Primary hypothyroidism
- Hypothalamic–pituitary disease
  - Hypothalamic tumours
  - Granulomatous disease (sarcoidosis, tuberculosis, Langerhans cell histiocytosis)
  - Cranial irradiation
  - Pituitary stalk section (e.g. following surgery)
  - Prolactinoma
  - Mixed GH/PRL-secreting adenoma
  - Tumours causing stalk compression
- Renal or hepatic failure
- Polycystic ovarian syndrome
- Chest wall stimulation (e.g. repeated breast self-examination, following herpes zoster infection)
- Ectopic secretion (e.g. bronchogenic carcinoma, hypernephroma)

---

responsible for the initiation and maintenance of physiological lactation. In mammary tissue primed with oestrogens and progesterone, PRL induces the synthesis of milk proteins. The actions of PRL at other sites have not been clarified; it has been suggested that PRL is involved in the immune functions and has probably antiapoptotic actions in several tissues.

Disorders of PRL secretion
PRL deficiency
A clinical syndrome associated with PRL deficiency is not recognized and the only known manifestation of PRL deficiency is the inability to lactate following delivery.

Prolactinomas
Prolactinomas are pituitary adenomas expressing and secreting PRL. They are the most common pituitary adenomas with an estimated prevalence in the adult population of 100 per million. Their frequency varies with age and sex; between the ages of 20 and 50 years they are most commonly diagnosed in women, whereas after the fifth decade of life their frequency is similar in both sexes. In the paediatric/adolescent age group, prolactinomas are rare but represent about half of all pituitary adenomas. Over 90% of prolactinomas are small, intrasellar tumours that rarely increase in size. Occasionally they can be aggressive or locally invasive and cause compression of vital structures. Malignant prolactinomas that are resistant to treatment and disseminate inside and outside the central nervous system are very rare. Mixed GH-secreting and PRL-secreting tumours are well recognized and are usually associated with acromegaly and hyperprolactinaemia. Rarely, PRL-secreting adenomas may also produce TSH or ACTH. Occasionally, prolactinomas may be a component of multiple endocrine neoplasia 1 (MEN1); they are the most common pituitary adenomas in this syndrome).

Presentation The clinical features of a prolactinoma predominantly result from hyperprolactinaemia. These include galactorrhoea and primary (in children) or secondary hypogonadism (in men, impotence, infertility, and decreased libido; in women, oligomenorrhoea/amenorrhoea and infertility). Hyperprolactinaemia interrupts the pulsatile secretion of gonadotropin-releasing hormone, inhibits the release of LH and FSH, and directly impairs gonadal steroidogenesis. In the case of large tumours, symptoms related to pressure effects may also be present. Most prolactinomas in women are microadenomas. Men usually present with larger tumours and neurological manifestations probably due to the delayed recognition of symptoms associated with the high PRL levels. Postmenopausal women with hyperprolactinaemia are often recognized only when a large adenoma produces mass effects.

Investigations When evaluating a patient with persistently elevated serum PRL, secondary causes of hyperprolactinaemia should first be ruled out by a careful clinical history, physical examination, pregnancy test, routine biochemical analysis (to assess kidney and liver function), and TSH measurement. If the patient is on a medication known to increase serum PRL, it is important to determine if the drug is indeed the cause by withdrawing it (if this can be done safely). When the drug cannot be stopped, the evaluation should include MRI of the sella to exclude a mass lesion. In the case of prolactinomas, serum prolactin levels usually parallel tumour size. PRL values between the upper limits of normal and 100 mg/litre (<2000 mU/L litre) may be due to psychoactive drugs, oestrogen, functional (idiopathic) causes, or microprolactinoma. Macroadenomas are typically associated with levels of more than 250 mg/litre (5000 mU/litre). It should be stressed, though, that such values are not absolute; prolactinomas may present with variable elevations in PRL and there may be dissociation between tumour mass and hormonal secretion. Furthermore, the interpretation of a moderate elevation of PRL in a patient with a pituitary macroadenoma needs to be done cautiously, as the hyperprolactinaemia may be attributed to compression of the pituitary stalk by a tumour other than a prolactinoma. Recent data suggest that serum PRL of more than 2000 mU/litre is almost never encountered in nonfunctioning pituitary macroadenomas. Values above this limit in the presence of a macroadenoma are probably associated with a prolactinoma (after acromegaly or Cushing's disease have been excluded). Alternatively, the empirical confirmation of the diagnosis can be obtained by treatment for several months with dopamine agonists with serial assessment of serum PRL levels and adenoma size. Normalization of PRL combined with a substantial reduction of the initial adenoma size confirms the diagnosis of a prolactinoma. Normalization of PRL with no change or only a small reduction in tumour volume may suggest a pituitary adenoma other than a prolactinoma. No change in serum PRL and no reduction in tumour volume indicate a drug-resistant prolactinoma (5% to 10% of cases).

Two potential pitfalls in the diagnosis of a prolactinoma should always be taken into account: (1) the presence of macroprolactin and (2) the 'hook effect'. Macroprolactin is a complex of PRL and, generally, an immunoglobulin G antibody. Serum PRL concentrations are increased due to the reduced rate of clearance of this complex. Macroprolactin has reduced bioactivity and is present in significant amounts in up to 20% of hyperprolactinaemic sera, resulting in pseudohyperprolactinaemia and the potential for misdiagnosis (thus, macroprolactinaemia is suggested in the presence of high PRL levels with no menstrual irregularities). For confirmation of macroprolactinaemia, polyethylene glycol precipitation is the most practical method. The 'hook effect' may be observed in cases of very high serum PRL concentrations, such as those observed in giant prolactinomas. The high levels of circulating PRL causes antibody saturation in the immunoradiometric assay, leading to artefactually low results. To overcome this effect, an immunoradiometric PRL assay should be performed at a serum dilution of 1:100 or, alternatively, should include a washout between the binding to the first antigen and the second step in order to eliminate excess unbound PRL. Currently, dynamic tests of PRL secretion are not used in clinical practice.

Treatment The primary goal of therapy in patients with microprolactinomas is to restore gonadal and sexual function by normalizing PRL levels. In patients with macroadenomas, reduction of tumour size is also important. Dopaminergic agonists such as cabergoline, bromocriptine, pergolide, and quinagolide are the primary therapy. Bromocriptine, pergolide, and cabergoline are all ergot derivatives. The only nonergot derivative that is used in clinical practice is quinagolide. These drugs normalize PRL levels and significantly reduce the volume of the tumour in most patients. Dopamine inhibition of PRL secretion is mediated by the D_2-dopamine receptors expressed by normal and tumorous lactotrophs. For microprolactinomas, bromocriptine is successful in 80% to 90% of patients in normalizing serum PRL levels, restoring gonadal function, and shrinking tumour mass. For macroprolactinomas, normalization of

serum PRL levels and tumour shrinkage occur in about 70% of patients. Tumour shrinkage can often be observed within a week or two after commencing treatment, but in some cases may not be observed for several months. Continued tumour shrinkage may occur for many months or even years. Visual field defects improve in the majority of patients. The therapeutic doses are in the range of 2.5 to 15 mg/day and most patients respond while on 7.5 mg/day or less. Cabergoline is effective in most patients, including those who did not previously respond to bromocriptine. Normalization of serum PRL has been reported in 86% of cases (92% with idiopathic hyperprolactinaemia or microprolactinoma, and 77% with macroprolactinoma). Following 12 to 24 months of treatment with cabergoline, a greater than 20% decrease of baseline tumour size has been reported in more than 80% of cases, with complete disappearance of tumour mass in 26% to 36% of them. The initial dose of cabergoline is 0.5 mg once weekly and doses up to 1 mg twice weekly are usually effective. Large comparative studies of cabergoline and bromocriptine have suggested the superiority of cabergoline in terms of patient tolerability and convenience, reduction in serum PRL, restoration of gonadal function, and decrease in tumour size. Although there is less experience with pergolide and quinagolide in the primary treatment of patients with prolactinomas, these drugs appear to have similar efficacy and adverse event profiles when compared with bromocriptine. The adverse effects of dopamine agonists may be grouped into gastrointestinal (most commonly nausea, vomiting, constipation, dry mouth, dyspepsia), cardiovascular (most commonly postural hypotension, digital vasospasm causing blanching of the extremities in response to cold), and neurological (headache and drowsiness). Other less common adverse effects are psychiatric manifestations (including psychosis and hypomania), cerebrospinal fluid rhinorrhoea (due to tumour shrinkage and an eroded pituitary sellar floor), leg cramps, flushing, and nasal congestion. Symptoms tend to occur after the initial dose and with dosage increases, but can be minimized by introducing the drug at a low dosage at bedtime, by taking it with food, and by very gradual dose escalation. Rarely, in patients with Parkinson's disease treated with very high doses of bromocriptine, pulmonary infiltrates, fibrosis, pleural effusions, pleural thickening, and retroperitoneal fibrosis have been reported; however, these effects are dose-dependent and are unlikely to occur at the low doses used for the treatment of prolactinomas. Recently, the occurrence of valvular insufficiency in patients who have been treated with high doses of cabergoline or pergolide for Parkinson's disease has been described. The significance of these findings for patients treated for prolactinomas needs to be investigated.

When a patient does not respond adequately to a dopamine agonist, the prolactinoma is considered resistant. For these patients possible treatment approaches include a trial of an alternative dopamine agonist, escalation of the dopamine agonist beyond conventional doses, surgical tumour resection, or radiotherapy. Trans-sphenoidal surgery does not reliably lead to a long-term cure, and recurrence of hyperprolactinaemia is frequent. The surgical outcomes are highly dependent on the experience of the neurosurgeon, the size of the tumour, and the serum PRL levels. The success rate of surgery in microadenomas is about 75% and for macroprolactinomas approximately 34%. The indications for surgery include unstable pituitary apoplexy, failure of medical therapy, inadequate reduction of PRL to restore gonadal function, tumour enlargement, tumour enlargement despite sufficient

PRL reduction, desire for pregnancy, previous pregnancy complicated by symptomatic tumour expansion, personal choice to avoid dopamine agonist therapy during gestation (in macroadenomas), and symptomatic tumour enlargement during pregnancy that does not respond to reinstitution of dopamine agonist treatment. The very high rate of efficacy of dopamine agonists combined with the high complication rates of radiotherapy render treatment with this modality rarely necessary; it is reserved for patients who do not respond to dopamine agonists, those who are not cured by surgery, or for malignant prolactinomas.

When beginning dopaminergic treatment, women must be warned that restoration of fertility may be immediate (even before their first normal menstruation). In women with a macroprolactinoma wishing to become pregnant, it is necessary to plan conception to occur after the normalization of the serum PRL and the significant reduction of the adenoma size. The considerable experience with patients taking bromocriptine during pregnancy suggests that the incidence of abortions, ectopic pregnancies, or congenital malformations is no higher than that in the general population. The experience with cabergoline is less, but there is no evidence to suggest that such treatment may be unsafe. The relevant information on pergolide and quinagolide is much more limited and, therefore, they should not be used in pregnancy or when pregnancy is desired. Given that for women with microprolactinomas the risk of clinically relevant tumour expansion is less than 2% during pregnancy, dopamine agonists can be safely stopped as soon as pregnancy has been confirmed. The patients need to be advised to report severe headaches or visual deterioration. In women with macroadenomas, symptomatic tumour expansion occurs in 20 to 30% of them; management options include stopping the dopamine agonist when pregnancy is confirmed with close surveillance thereafter, or continuing the dopamine agonist throughout the pregnancy. If visual field defects or progressive headaches develop, an MRI without gadolinium (not a CT) should be performed, and if the tumour has significantly increased in size, a dopamine agonist should be restarted. If the enlarged tumour does not respond to medical treatment, alternatives include delivery if the pregnancy is far enough advanced or trans-sphenoidal surgery. There are no data to suggest that breastfeeding leads to prolactinoma enlargement.

Treatment withdrawal When the serum PRL has been normal for at least 2 years and the size of the tumour decreased by more than 50%, the dose of the dopamine agonist can be gradually decreased, as at this stage low doses are likely to maintain stable PRL levels and tumour size. After pregnancy, normoprolactinaemia may occur. Women with hyperprolactinaemia who pass through the menopause may normalize their PRL requiring reassessment of the need for continuing treatment. If a patient has normal PRL levels after treatment with dopamine agonists for at least 5 years and the tumour volume is markedly decreased, a trial of tapering and discontinuation of these drugs may be initiated. In such cases, careful monitoring for detection of recurrence of hyperprolactinaemia and tumour enlargement in advised.

ACTH

ACTH is a single chain 39-amino acid peptide released by the corticotroph cells. The initial synthesis is of a larger 231-amino acid peptide (pro-opiomelanocortin, POMC) that following proteolytic cleavage produces several peptides and hormones, including ACTH, melanocyte-stimulating hormone (MSH), and β-endorphin. ACTH is secreted in a pulsatile manner. The secretion is under positive hypothalamic control by the corticotropin-releasing hormone, which exerts tropic and releasing actions on the corticotroph cells. Arginine vasopressin also stimulates ACTH release acting synergistically with corticotropin-releasing hormone. ACTH exerts a negative feedback effect at the hypothalamic level. ACTH and cortisol secretion follow a diurnal rhythm, with highest amounts in the early morning and lowest concentrations around midnight. The secretory bursts start at around 3.00 a.m. and are maximal in the last few hours before waking up. This pattern is mainly regulated by the light–dark and the sleep–wake cycles and may be altered by a major time shift. Any stressful event may induce a large discharge of ACTH into the circulation followed by a similar increase in the release of cortisol. Serum cortisol exerts feedback regulatory action on the pituitary but also at the hypothalamic level reducing ACTH release. This negative feedback may be imitated by synthetic glucocorticoids such as dexamethasone.

The first 24 amino acids of the ACTH are identical across species and are associated with its biological activity. ACTH acts through G protein-coupled receptors predominantly found in the fascicular and reticular zones in the adrenal cortex where it stimulates the secretion of glucocorticoids and androgens. It also contributes to the release of mineralocorticoids. ACTH is also responsible for the maintenance of the adrenal growth and size.

Disorders of ACTH secretion
ACTH deficiency
Chronic ACTH deficiency is associated with fatigue, pallor, anorexia, weight loss, hypotension, hyponatraemia, hypoglycaemia, and eosinophilia. Children may present with delayed puberty and failure to thrive. In its most severe form, when left untreated, it may be fatal due to vascular collapse especially during superimposed illness. In contrast to primary adrenal insufficiency, in which the ACTH levels are increased, there is no hyperpigmentation or hyperkalaemia.

Given the diurnal rhythm of ACTH and cortisol secretion, random serum cortisol measurements are not always helpful in the diagnosis of ACTH deficiency. It has been proposed that secondary adrenal insufficiency is present when morning cortisol concentrations are less than 100 nmol/litre; values greater than 580 nmol/litre exclude this diagnosis. Levels between these values need a stimulation test. Hypoglycaemia (blood glucose <2.2 mmol/litre) induced by the insulin tolerance test is considered the gold standard for the assessment of the entire hypothalamic–pituitary–adrenal axis. A maximum cortisol response to a peak concentration greater than 580 nmol/litre generally excludes adrenal insufficiency. ACTH deficiency causes adrenal atrophy and ACTH-receptor downregulation. Based on these, the standard 250 µg (1–24)ACTH (Synacthen) test may be useful for the diagnosis of secondary adrenal insufficiency, if done at least 4 weeks after the onset of ACTH deficiency. Stimulated cortisol concentrations at 30 min of 580 nmol/litre or less suggest ACTH deficiency. Other tests checking the ACTH reserve, which are less commonly used, include the glucagon and the metyrapone test.

Glucocorticoid deficiency can be life-threatening and, therefore, substitution should begin as soon as the diagnosis is confirmed.

The replacement involves the administration of hydrocortisone or other steroids (prednisolone or dexamethasone) in a dose and timing to mimic the normal pattern of cortisol secretion. The most commonly used regime involves 10 to 25 mg hydrocortisone/day; it is divided into two or three doses/day, e.g. 10 mg, 5 mg, and 5 mg. There is no reliable biochemical test to assess the adequacy of replacement and the least dose necessary to relieve clinical symptoms is recommended. All patients should be supplied with an emergency card or bracelet giving information about their diagnosis, and instructions on stress-related dose adjustments should be clearly offered. In case of vomiting or during the perioperative period, parenteral steroid administration is needed. GH replacement may unmask ACTH deficiency and glucocorticoid replacement may unmask underlying diabetes insipidus.

Cushing's disease
Cushing's disease refers to the chronic exposure to endogenous glucocorticoids (Cushing's syndrome) produced by the adrenal cortex caused by excess ACTH production by a pituitary corticotroph adenoma (see 'Pituitary adenomas' and 'Pituitary carcinomas', below).

Nelson's syndrome Nelson's syndrome is defined by the association of an expanding pituitary tumour and high levels of ACTH secretion after bilateral adrenalectomy for Cushing's disease. Its prevalence ranges from 8% to 29% with a time interval between adrenalectomy and the diagnosis of the syndrome of 0.5 to 24 years (most commonly thought to be within 2 years). Apart from high basal ACTH levels after adrenalectomy and the presence of a pituitary adenoma remnant after adrenalectomy, there is no general agreement on the predictive factors for the development of Nelson's syndrome. Notably, pituitary irradiation prior to adrenalectomy has been found to be protective in some studies, but not all. The clinical manifestations include those from the mass effect (headaches, deterioration of vision, ophthalmoplegia) and hyperpigmentation as a result of the increased ACTH levels. Early diagnosis is important and monitoring with measurement of ACTH levels and pituitary imaging at 6 months and yearly after the adrenalectomy are recommended. Cases of pituitary tumour with distant metastases have also been described. Treatment should be aggressive and includes surgical excision and pituitary irradiation.

TSH

TSH is a glycoprotein hormone consisting of two non-covalently bound subunits: the α subunit, which is common to all anterior pituitary glycoprotein hormones and the β subunit, which is unique for TSH and confers its biological specificity. The α subunit has a molecular weight of 20 to 22 kDa, is composed of 92 amino acid residues, and contains two N-linked carbohydrate groups. The β subunit has a molecular weight of 18 kDa, is composed of 110 amino acid residues, and contains one N-linked complex carbohydrate. The glycosylation is important for the normal bioactivity of TSH. TSH is secreted in a pulsatile manner (with low amplitude peaks), as well as in a circadian fashion (with elevation in the late hours of the evening). The hypothalamic tripeptide TRH stimulates TSH release, whereas thyroid hormones exert a negative feedback at the hypothalamic and pituitary levels. Somatostatin and dopamine inhibit TSH secretion. TSH binds to specific thyroid cell plasma membrane receptors and regulates both synthesis and secretion of thyroid hormones.

Disorders of TSH secretion
TSH deficiency
Central hypothyroidism is diagnosed when the concentrations of thyroxine are decreased and the TSH levels are usually normal or low. The clinical manifestations include tiredness, cold intolerance, constipation, hair loss, dry skin, hoarseness, cognitive slowing, lethargy, weight gain, bradycardia, facial puffiness, delayed relaxation phase of the deep tendon reflexes, and hypotension. In children, developmental delay and growth retardation are also present. TSH deficiency is treated with L-thyroxine with the aim of achieving normal serum free thyroxine levels (serum TSH cannot be used as a guide of adequate replacement). An increase in the dose of L-thyroxine may be necessary during pregnancy or new oestrogen or GH replacement. As thyroid hormone replacement increases the rate of metabolism of glucocorticoids and may therefore lead to an adrenal crisis in cases of coexisting hypoadrenalism, thyroxine should be administered after hydrocortisone substitution has been initiated.

Thyrotropinomas
TSH-secreting pituitary adenomas account for less than 1% of all pituitary adenomas with an overall prevalence of about 1 in 1 million of the population. They show no gender difference and the majority are diagnosed between the third and sixth decade of life. The signs of thyrotoxicosis may vary from severe to absent. More than 90% of the patients present with goitre. Compression features including headaches and visual field defects due to tumour invasion or suprasellar extension may be also present. In about 30% of TSH-secreting pituitary adenomas, coexistent oversecretion of other pituitary hormones may also occur resulting in additional symptoms. The biochemical profile of TSH-secreting pituitary adenomas includes elevated circulating thyroxine with normal or increased TSH levels (as opposed to undetectable levels of TSH in Graves' disease, which causes primary hyperthyroidism). Other markers of thyroid hormone action may be increased as well, such as sex hormone-binding globulin, cholesterol, angiotensin-converting enzyme, or C-terminal cross-linked telopeptide of type 1 collagen. Most tumours are macroadenomas.

Diagnosis It is essential to differentiate a TSH-secreting pituitary adenoma from the syndrome of pituitary resistance to thyroid hormone, in which mutations in the gene coding for the thyroid hormone receptor β prevent the detection of peripheral thyroid hormones by the pituitary resulting in increased levels of TSH and hyperthyroidism. While it is mainly the pituitary gland being insensitive to thyroid hormones, other tissues do not show resistance to thyroid hormones in this form of the syndrome. Detection of a mutation in the gene coding for thyroid hormone receptor β confirms the diagnosis. Nevertheless, in about 10% of patients, no mutations can be found. The combination of the TRH stimulation test, α subunit levels, and the α subunit/TSH ratio are helpful in the differential diagnosis. Thus, in cases of TSH-secreting pituitary adenoma, the α subunit level is increased, the molar ratio of α subunit to TSH is more than 1.0, and TRH administration is associated with a less than twofold increase of TSH.

Treatment The first-line therapy for patients with TSH-secreting pituitary adenoma is trans-sphenoidal resection of the tumour, after which about one-third of all patients will be cured. If surgery is contraindicated or declined, the administration of somatostatin analogues should be considered. About 85% of the patients respond to somatostatin analogues with decrease of thyroxine levels. Occasionally, external pituitary irradiation is indicated. Criteria of cure go beyond the establishment of euthyroidism and include the normalization of α subunit levels, α subunit/TSH ratio, peripheral markers of thyroid hormone action, and dynamic tests, as well as pituitary imaging. Long-term follow-up including clinical, biochemical, and radiological monitoring is mandatory.

Hypopituitarism

Hypopituitarism, first described by Simmonds in 1914, results from the decreased secretion of pituitary hormones. It is caused by an inability of the gland to produce hormones and/or an insufficient supply of hypothalamic-releasing hormones. It is associated with an increased mortality (with causes of premature mortality being cardiovascular and cerebrovascular disease) and its main causes are shown in Box 13.2.3.

The clinical manifestations of hypopituitarism depend mainly on the underlying disease, as well as the type and degree of the hormonal deficits. Tumoral masses in the sellar region with suprasellar extension may be associated with visual impairment, headaches, oculomotor nerve palsy, or damage to other cranial nerves within the cavernous sinus. Hypopituitarism may be sub-clinical, diagnosed only following hormonal investigations, or of acute and severe clinical onset requiring hospital admission. ACTH, TSH, and antidiuretic hormone deficiency are potentially life-threatening, whereas FSH/LH and GH deficiencies are associated with chronic morbidity. The clinical manifestations and the diagnosis and treatment of each pituitary hormone deficit are described in previous paragraphs. It should be noted that as thyroid hormone replacement increases the rate of metabolism of the glucocorticoids and may lead to an adrenal crisis, glucocorticoid substitution should begin before thyroid hormone treatment is offered.

Pituitary adenomas

Pituitary adenomas are the most common cause of pituitary disease. They are benign lesions arising from adenohypophyseal cells and account for up to 25% of intracranial tumours. Based on their secretory activity, they are classified as functioning (resulting in the syndromes of hormonal excess previously described) and nonfunctioning (presenting with mass effects). Tumours measuring less than 10 mm in diameter are considered microadenomas and those larger than 10 mm macroadenomas. Immunohistochemically they are grouped according to their hormone content; generally the clinical classification overlaps the histopathological one. On CT, macroadenomas are isodense or hypodense relative to brain tissue with variable patterns of enhancement after contrast administration. Calcification may be seen occasionally. On MRI, they have homogeneous low intensity on T_1-weighted images and, after contrast administration, homogeneous enhancement that is less intense than the enhancement in the adjacent pituitary. Cysts or areas of necrosis cause foci of moderate hypointensity on T_1-weighted sequences, foci of hyperintensity on T_2-weighted sequences, and heterogeneous enhancement with gadolinium. Haemorrhage in the subacute or chronic phase shows high signal on T_1-weighted images. On CT, microadenomas show little inherent contrast to the normal

---

Box 13.2.3 Causes of hypopituitarism

- ◆ Pituitary and nonpituitary tumours
  Pituitary adenomas
  Craniopharyngiomas
  Meningiomas
  Gliomas
  Chordomas
  Ependymomas
  Primary or metastatic (especially lung and breast) cancer
  Hamartomas
  Germinomas
  Optic gliomas
- ◆ Lymphocytic hypophysitis
- ◆ Pituitary apoplexy
- ◆ Sheehan's syndrome (postpartum hypopituitarism)
- ◆ Cranial irradiation
- ◆ Pituitary surgery
- ◆ Traumatic brain injury
- ◆ Subarachnoid haemorrhage
- ◆ Haemochromatosis
- ◆ Granulomatous diseases
  Sarcoidosis
  Tuberculosis
  Langerhans' histiocytosis
- ◆ Empty sella syndrome
- ◆ Genetic causes
  Mutations of genes encoding transcription factors including *HESX1* (homeobox gene expressed in embryonic stem cells 1), *LHX3* (LIM-domain homeobox gene 3), *LHX4* (LIM-domain homeobox gene 4), *PROP1* (prophet of Pit1), *POU1F1* (POU domain, class 1, transcription factor 1)
- ◆ Infections
  Abscess
  Meningitis
  Encephalitis

---

pituitary tissue and intravenous contrast demonstrates nonenhancement against a background of normal gland enhancement. On MRI, they are hypointense on T_1-weighted sequences and this contrast may or may not be amplified after gadolinium.

The treatment of pituitary adenomas involves surgery, radiotherapy, or medical therapy and has been described in previous sections.

Pituitary carcinomas

Pituitary carcinomas are defined as pituitary tumours with subarachnoid, brain, or systemic metastasis. They account for less than 0.5% of symptomatic pituitary tumours. They mainly arise from the transformation of initially large, but benign, adenomas. Their pathogenetic mechanism remains unclear; it has been proposed that under the influence of unknown growth-enhancing stimuli, an early proliferative stage of polyclonality is followed by monoclonal or multiclonal mutations, leading to selective growth advantage and a state of invasiveness. Alterations in the function of oncogenes and/or tumour suppressor genes may also be implicated. Their malignant nature is not usually obvious in their microscopic appearance and the reliable distinction between carcinoma and adenoma is impossible on the basis of standard histological criteria. Their clinical manifestations are similar to invasive and noninvasive pituitary adenomas (pressure effects to the surrounding tissues and/or consequences of hormonal hypersecretion). The great majority of pituitary carcinomas are hormonally active, most commonly ACTH-secreting or PRL-secreting. No differences in the hormone levels differentiating pituitary carcinomas from other invasive and/or noninvasive macroadenomas have been identified. Although on imaging pituitary carcinomas appear as invasive macroadenomas, there are no reliable features distinguishing tumours that could behave in a malignant manner from other types of invasive adenomas. Metastases can occur in every part of the central nervous system (usually cortex, cerebellum, and cerebellopontine angle) or in distant sites (usually liver, lymph nodes, bone, and lung).

The treatment of pituitary carcinomas is similar to that of large and aggressive pituitary tumours and includes surgery, external beam radiotherapy, and adjuvant medical treatment (chemotherapy). The therapy is mainly palliative and may not prolong survival to any major extent (mean survival after the development of metastatic disease is reported to be less than 4 years).

Pituitary apoplexy

Pituitary apoplexy is a clinical syndrome resulting from acute haemorrhage or infarction of the pituitary gland. It is potentially life-threatening and is characterized by the sudden onset of headache, vomiting, visual disturbance, ophthalmoplegia, and altered consciousness. This constellation of findings occurs primarily in patients with pre-existing pituitary adenomas and can be due to extensive tumour infarction or haemorrhage. The term has also been used to describe spontaneous infarction and haemorrhage within a nontumorous pituitary gland with similar clinical effects. The age range of occurrence is broad, from the first to the ninth decade. The incidence of pituitary apoplexy presenting with classic symptoms is reported to be in the order of 0.6 to 9.1% of surgically treated pituitary adenomas. However, clinically silent pathological evidence of pituitary haemorrhage ('subclinical pituitary apoplexy') has been reported in up to 25% of surgically removed pituitary adenomas. The clinical syndrome of pituitary apoplexy usually evolves fully within hours to 2 days and its pathophysiology remains uncertain. Predisposing factors for pituitary apoplexy include major surgery, warfarin, aspirin, arterial hypertension, oral contraceptive pill, gonadotropin-releasing hormone analogue, dynamic pituitary function tests, and head trauma. A variety of pituitary tumours, both endocrinologically active and inactive, have been documented in association with pituitary apoplexy, but opinions differ as to whether there is a predominance of a particular type of pituitary tumour. Following apoplexy, hypofunctioning (partial or complete) of normal pituitary tissue appears to be the rule. Hyponatraemia, noted in

44% of patients, may be caused either by inappropriate antidiuretic hormone secretion, hypocortisolism, or hypothyroidism or by a combination of these. MRI is the radiological investigation of choice; in the first 3 to 5 days, haemorrhage within the sella is isointense or hypointense on T_1-weighted images and hypointense on T_2-weighted sequences. When pituitary apoplexy is suspected, the initial management consists of close monitoring of fluid and electrolyte balance coupled with immediate replacement of deficient hormones, in particular corticosteroids. Although not widely accepted, it has been suggested that in patients with visual field or visual acuity defects, surgical decompression should be performed as soon as possible, preferably within the first week, as this appears to optimize visual outcome and to improve pituitary function. Following apoplexy, the risk of tumour recurrence is small, but careful follow-up initially with annual imaging is indicated.

Craniopharyngiomas

Craniopharyngiomas are epithelial tumours (grade I, World Health Organization classification) arising along the path of the craniopharyngeal duct (the canal connecting the stomodeal ectoderm with the evaginated Rathke's pouch). Their overall incidence is 0.13 per 100 000 person-years and they account for 2 to 5% of all the primary intracranial neoplasms (5.6–15% of the intracranial tumours in children). They may be diagnosed at any age (peak incidence rates between 5 and 14 years and 50 and 74 years). Histologically, two primary subtypes have been recognized, the adamantinomatous and the papillary, but transitional or mixed forms have also been described. The adamantinomatous craniopharyngioma is the most frequently reported and may be diagnosed at all ages. Macroscopically, it shows cystic and/or solid components, necrotic debris, fibrous tissue, and calcification. The liquid within the cysts ranges from 'machinery oil' to shimmering cholesterol-laden fluid and it is mostly composed of desquamated squamous epithelial cells, rich in membrane lipids and cytoskeleton keratin. In this subtype, the flat squamous epithelial cells may be desquamated in distinctive stacked clusters forming the pathognomonic nodules of 'wet' keratin. The papillary subtype has been almost exclusively found in adult patients. Macroscopically it is usually solid or mixed, calcification is rarely seen, and the cyst content is mostly viscous and yellow.

Presentation

Most of the craniopharyngiomas are detected in the sellar/parasellar region (a suprasellar component is present in 94–95% of cases). They may exert pressure effects to various brain structures resulting in multiple clinical features (neurological, visual, hypothalamo-pituitary); headaches, nausea/vomiting, visual disturbances, growth failure (in children), and hypogonadism (in adults) are the most frequently described symptoms. A substantial number of patients present with compromised hypothalamo-pituitary function; reported rates for pituitary hormone deficits include 35 to 95% for GH, 38 to 82% for FSH/LH, 21 to 62% for ACTH, 21 to 42% for TSH, and 6 to 38% for antidiuretic hormone. Useful imaging tools for the diagnosis of craniopharyngiomas include plain skull radiographs, CT, MRI, and, occasionally, cerebral angiography. The consistency of the tumours is purely or predominantly cystic in 46% to 64%, purely or predominantly solid in 18% to 39%, and mixed in 8% to 36%. Calcification is present in 45% to 57% and is probably more common in children (78–100%). Hydrocephalus has been reported in 20% to 38% and is probably more often seen in childhood populations (41–54%). Plain skull radiographs may show calcification and an abnormal sella. CT is helpful for the evaluation of the bony anatomy, the identification of calcifications, and the discrimination of the solid and the cystic components (the cystic fluid is hypodense and the solid portions, as well as the cyst capsule show enhancement following contrast administration). The MRI is useful for the topographic and structural analysis of the tumour. A solid lesion appears isointense or hypointense relative to the brain on precontrast T_1-weighted images, shows enhancement following gadolinium administration, and is usually of mixed hypointensity or hyperintensity on T_2-weighted sequences. Large amounts of calcification present as areas of low signal on both T_1-weighted and T_2-weighted images. A cystic element is usually hypointense on T_1-weighted sequences and hyperintense on T_2-weighted sequences. On T_1-weighted images a thin peripheral contrast-enhancing rim of the cyst is demonstrated. Protein, cholesterol, and methaemoglobin may cause high signal on T_1-weighted images. The differential diagnosis includes a number of sellar or parasellar lesions, including Rathke's cleft cyst, dermoid cyst, epidermoid cyst, pituitary adenoma, germinoma, hamartoma, suprasellar aneurysm, arachnoid cyst, suprasellar abscess, glioma, meningioma, sarcoidosis, tuberculosis, and Langerhans cell histiocytosis.

Treatment

Surgery combined or not with adjuvant external beam irradiation is currently the most widely used first therapeutic approach for these tumours. Craniopharyngiomas remain challenging tumours, even in the era of modern neurosurgery. This is mainly attributed to their sharp, irregular borders and to their tendency to adhere to vital neurovascular structures making surgical manipulations potentially hazardous to vital brain areas. Consequently, the attempted degree of excision has been a subject of long-standing debate. The advances in neuroimaging, microsurgical techniques, perioperative care, and hormone replacement therapy have significantly improved the perioperative mortality, which according to recent reports is between 1.7 and 5.4% for the primary operations. The mean interval for the diagnosis of recurrence following various primary treatment modalities ranges between 1 and 4.3 years. The recurrence rates following gross total removal range between 0 and 62% at 10 years follow-up and are significantly lower than those after partial or subtotal resection (25–100% at 10 years follow-up). In cases of limited surgery, adjuvant radiotherapy significantly improves the local control rates (recurrence rates 10–63% at 10 years follow-up). Finally, radiotherapy alone provides 10-year recurrence rates ranging between 0 and 23%. For predominantly cystic tumours, fluid aspiration provides relief of the obstructive manifestations and facilitates the consecutive removal of the solid tumour portion; the latter should not be delayed for more than a few weeks due to the significant risk of the cyst refilling. The management of recurrent tumours remains difficult, as scarring and/or adhesions from previous operations or irradiation decrease the chances of successful excision. In such cases, total removal is achieved at a substantially lower rate when compared with primary surgery (0–25%) and is associated with increased perioperative morbidity and mortality (10.5–24%). The beneficial effect of radiotherapy (preceded or not by second surgery) in recurrent lesions is well established. Other treatment modalities include brachytherapy (stereotactically guided instillation of β-emitting isotopes into cystic craniopharyngiomas), intracystic installation of the antineoplastic agent bleomycin, stereotactic radiosurgery or radiotherapy, and systemic chemotherapy.

Morbidity and mortality

Craniopharyngiomas are associated with significant long-term morbidity (mainly endocrine, visual, hypothalamic, neurobehavioural, and cognitive sequelae), which compromise normal psychosocial integration and quality of life. These complications are attributed to the damage to critical structures by the primary or recurrent tumour and/or to the adverse effects of the therapeutic interventions. In studies with variable follow-up periods and after different treatment modalities, the rates of individual hormone deficits range from 88 to 100% for GH, 80 to 95% for FSH/LH, 55 to 88% for ACTH, 39 to 95% for TSH, and 25 to 86% for ADH. Compromised vision has been reported in up to 62.5% of the patients treated by surgery combined or not with radiotherapy during observation periods of 10 years. Hypothalamic damage may result in hyperphagia and uncontrollable obesity, disorders of thirst and water/electrolyte balance, behavioural and cognitive impairment, loss of temperature control, and disorders in the sleep pattern. Among these, obesity is the most frequent (affecting 26–61% of the patients treated by surgery combined or not with radiotherapy) and is a consequence of the disruption of the mechanisms controlling satiety, hunger, and energy balance. Other rare long-term irradiation-attributed morbidities include vasculopathy and second brain tumours. The overall mortality rates of patients with craniopharyngioma have been reported to be 3 to 6 times higher than that of the general population. The 10-year survival rates range between 83 and 92.7% and are significantly lower in cases of recurrent disease. Apart from the deaths directly attributed to the tumour (pressure effects to critical structures) and to the surgical interventions, the risk of cardiovascular/cerebrovascular and respiratory mortality is increased.

Hypophysitis

Inflammatory processes of the hypophysis are classified as primary, when the inflammation is confined to the pituitary gland with no identifiable aetiological association, and secondary, when the inflammatory pituitary reaction is triggered by a definite aetiological agent or a known systemic disease (local lesions such as germinomas, Rathke's cleft cysts, craniopharyngiomas, or pituitary adenomas, or systemic diseases such as sarcoidosis, Langerhans cell histiocytosis, or tuberculosis). In the latter cases, the infiltrate is mainly lymphocytic or xanthogranulomatous and focuses around the lesion rather than diffusing to the entire gland.

Primary hypophysitis is histologically classified into three types: granulomatous, xanthomatous, and lymphocytic. Granulomatous hypophysitis has an unclear pathogenesis, affects men and women in equal proportions, and presents with nausea, vomiting, diabetes insipidus, and hyperprolactinaemia. It is characterized by diffuse collections of multinucleated giant cells and histiocytes with surrounding lymphocytes and plasma cells. Xanthomatous hypophysitis is an infiltrating process of the pituitary of unclear cause; it consists of cystic-like areas of liquefaction infiltrated by lipid-rich foamy histiocytes and lymphocytes. Lymphocytic hypophysitis is a rare condition, but insufficient population-based data exist to estimate its real incidence. Based on the published cases, women are affected more frequently than men in a ratio of about 5 to 1 or 8 to 1. It shows a striking temporal association with pregnancy, with most of these patients presenting in the last month of pregnancy (without causing complications to the fetus or the outcome of pregnancy) or in the first 2 months after delivery. Its clinical presentation is variable and comprises four categories of symptoms: sellar compression (headaches, visual disturbances, diplopia), hypopituitarism (mainly ACTH followed by TSH, gonadotropins, and PRL—it should be noted that the usual order of loss of anterior pituitary hormones does not occur in patients with hypophysitis), diabetes insipidus, and hyperprolactinaemia. The defining pathological feature is the infiltration of the pituitary gland with lymphocytes. The immune infiltrate also contains other cells including plasma cells, eosinophils, macrophages, histiocytes, and neutrophils. The role of antipituitary antibodies remains to be established but their detection has amplified the diagnostic criteria, also suggesting a possible pathogenetic role. The mechanisms by which the infiltrate causes loss of function/destruction of the endocrine cells or impairment of vasopressin release are not clear. It has been suggested that the disease progresses through various stages. Initially, the pituitary gland is inflamed, infiltrated by lymphocytes, and oedematous, causing mass effect symptoms; subclinical hypopituitarism may be present. If the inflammation resolves and the pituitary parenchyma is not destroyed, remission occurs. If the inflammation progresses, the pituitary is replaced by fibrotic tissue, becomes atrophic, and loses its function.

Even when using modern MRI studies, nearly 40% of the cases are misdiagnosed as pituitary adenomas. The typical precontrast MRI findings include a symmetrical enlargement of the pituitary gland, a thickened but rarely displaced stalk, and a usually intact sellar floor. The pattern of signal enhancement after gadolinium may be helpful in differentiating hypophysitis from macroadenoma. A strong and homogenous enhancement of the anterior pituitary gland is more suggestive of an inflammatory infiltrative process. A strip of enhanced tissue along the dura mater ('dural tail') has also been described. Macroadenomas enhance less or more slowly than the normal pituitary on dynamic MRI. If the infundibulo-neurohypophysis is involved, there is the loss of T_1 hyperintensity in the neurohypophysis, swelling of the posterior pituitary, and thickening of the pituitary stalk of more than 3 mm at the level of the median eminence of the hypothalamus.

The treatment of this condition is controversial and includes replacing the defective endocrine function and/or reducing the size of the pituitary mass. The role of surgery remains controversial; it should be performed only in the presence of serious and progressive deficits of visual fields, visual acuity, or ocular movements. It is also performed when a pituitary adenoma is suspected and the diagnosis is subsequently made by histology. Cases of spontaneous resolution without any treatment have been reported.

Rathke's cleft cysts

Rathke's cleft cysts are common benign sellar and/or suprasellar lesions, found in 13 to 33% of routine autopsies. Symptomatic cases are rare and they probably arise from remnants of Rathke's pouch, a structure apparent during the 3rd week of gestation and formed by the infolding of the simple ciliated columnar epithelium lining the roof of the stomodeum. Rathke's cleft cysts are smoothly marginated cysts with size usually ranging from a few millimetres to 1 to 2 cm. Their contents vary from a clear cerebrospinal fluid-like liquid to a thick mucoid material made up of cholesterol and protein. They are lined by single or pseudostratified cuboidal or columnar epithelium with or without cilia and with goblet cells. The presenting manifestations are the result of compression to adjacent structures. The most frequent ones include headaches, hypopituitarism of varying degrees, hyperprolactinaemia, visual disturbance, and diabetes insipidus. Their imaging features are highly variable. Forty per cent are completely intrasellar, whereas 60% have some suprasellar extension. On CT, the cyst density ranges from hypodense to isodense or is mixed. On MRI, they have a variable T_1 signal (hyperintense, hypointense, or isointense) depending on their biochemical content. Cysts with high protein concentration show high T_1 signal intensity and usually have a low intracystic water content leading to T_2 signal decrease. Small intracystic nodules corresponding to proteinaceous concentrations may be demonstrated presenting with lower T_2 and higher T_1 signal intensity than the rest of the cyst. The nodules do not enhance and are virtually pathognomonic for Rathke's cleft cysts.

Symptomatic cases are managed by surgery. The risk of recurrence following evacuation and biopsy ranges between 8 and 33%. Although not widely accepted, the extent of removal (gross total vs partial) may predict relapse.

Further reading

Assie G, et al. (2007). Corticotroph tumor progression after adrenalectomy in Cushing's disease: a reappraisal of Nelson's syndrome. *J Clin Endocrinol Metab*, **92**, 172–9.

Bellastella A, et al. (2003). Lymphocytic hypophysitis: a rare or underestimated disease?. *Eur J Endocrinol*, **149**, 363–76.

Byrne JV (2002). Imaging of the pituitary. In: Wass JAH, Shalet SM (eds) *Oxford textbook of endocrinology and diabetes*, pp. 136–45. Oxford University Press, Oxford.

Casanueva FF, et al. (2006). Guidelines of the Pituitary Society for the diagnosis and management of prolactinomas. *Clin Endocrinol*, **65**, 265–73.

Caturegli P, et al. (2005). Autoimmune hypophysitis. *Endocr Rev*, **26**, 599–614.

Couse M, et al. (2002). Pituitary anatomy and physiology. In: Wass JAH, Shalet SM (eds) *Oxford textbook of endocrinology and diabetes*, pp. 75–85. Oxford University Press, Oxford.

Drake WM, et al. (2002). Pituitary assessment strategy. In: Wass JAH, Shalet SM (eds) *Oxford textbook of endocrinology and diabetes*, pp. 127–36. Oxford University Press, Oxford.

Gillam MP, et al. (2006). Advances in the treatment of prolactinomas. *Endocr Rev*, **27**, 485–534.

Jenkins PJ, et al. (2006). Conventional pituitary irradiation is effective in lowering serum growth hormone and IGF-1 in patients with acromegaly. *J Clin Endocrinol Metab*, **91**, 1239–45.

Kaltsas GA, et al. (2005). Diagnosis and management of pituitary carcinomas. *J Clin Endocrinol Metab*, **90**, 3089–99.

Karavitaki N (2007). Benign cysts: Rathke's cysts, mucoceles, arachnoid cysts, and dermoid and epidermoid cysts. In: Wass JAH, Hay I (eds) *Clinical endocrine oncology*. Blackwell Publishing, Oxford.

Karavitaki N, et al. (2006). Craniopharyngiomas. *Endocr Rev*, **27**, 371–97.

Karavitaki N, et al. (2006). Do the limits of serum prolactin in disconnection hyperprolactinaemia need re-definition? A study of 226 patients with histologically verified non-functioning pituitary macroadenoma. *Clin Endocrinol*, **65**, 524–9.

Kienitz T, *et al*. (2007). Long-term management in five cases of TSH-secreting pituitary adenomas: a single center study and review of the literature. *Eur J Endocrinol*, **157**, 39–46.

Melmed S (2006). Acromegaly. *N Engl J Med*, **355**, 2558–73.

Melmed S, *et al*. (2005). Consensus statement: medical management of acromegaly. *Eur J Endocrinol*, **153**, 737–40.

Molitch ME, *et al*. (2006). Evaluation and treatment of adult growth hormone deficiency: an Endocrine Society Clinical Practice Guideline. *J Clin Endocrinol Metab*, **91**, 1621–34.

Plowman PN (2002). Pituitary radiotherapy. In: Wass JAH, Shalet SM (eds) *Oxford textbook of endocrinology and diabetes*, pp. 168–71. Oxford University Press, Oxford.

Randeva HS, *et al*. (1999). Classical pituitary apoplexy: clinical features, management and outcome. *Clin Endocrinol*, **51**, 181–8.

Schneider HJ, *et al*. (2007). Hypopituitarism. *Lancet*, **369**, 1461–70.

Wass JA, Karavitaki N (2009). Nonfunctioning pituitary adenomas: the Oxford experience. *Nat Rev Endocrinol*, **5**, 519–22.

Disorders of the posterior pituitary gland

Aparna Pal, Niki Karavitaki, and John A.H. Wass

Essentials

The posterior pituitary produces arginine vasopressin, which has a key role in fluid homeostasis, and oxytocin, which stimulates uterine contraction during birth and ejection of milk during lactation.

Cranial diabetes insipidus is the passage of large volumes (>3 litres/24 h) of dilute urine (osmolality <300 mOsm/kg) due to vasopressin deficiency, and most commonly occurs as a consequence of trauma or tumour affecting the posterior pituitary. Diagnosed by a water deprivation test revealing urine osmolality less than 300 mOsml/kg with concurrent plasma osmolality more than 290 mOsml/kg after dehydration, with urine osmolality rising to more than 750 mOsml/kg after desmopressin. MRI of the neurohypophysis is required to delineate the cause. Mild polyuria can be managed simply by ensuring adequate fluid intake; treatment with the long-acting vasopressin analogue, desmopressin (desamino, D-8 arginine vasopressin; DDAVP), is used for more severe cases.

Syndrome of inappropriate antidiuresis (SIADH)—diagnosed when there is hyponatraemia with hypotonic plasma (osmolality <270 mOsm/kg), inappropriate urine osmolality (>100 mOsm/kg) and urinary sodium >20 mmol/litre, together with (1) no evidence of volume overload or hypovolaemia, and (2) normal renal, adrenal, and thyroid function. Few patients satisfy these strict criteria, but many conditions, e.g. malignant diseases, chest diseases, central nervous system disorders and drugs, have been implicated. Aside from treatment (when possible) of the underlying cause, management requires fluid restriction and (rarely) infusion of hypertonic saline (see Chapter 21.2.1 for further discussion). Blockade of renal vasopressin receptors (V_2) would be a logical treatment, and several V_2 receptor antagonists are in clinical trials.

Anatomy

The posterior pituitary gland, lying dorsally and caudally to the anterior pituitary, is connected by the hollow pituitary stalk to the hypothalamus in the floor of the third ventricle and is sometimes referred to as the neurohypophysis as it acts as an extension of the nervous system.

In contrast to the anterior pituitary which develops from ectoderm, is highly cellular, and is connected to the hypothalamus via the circulatory system, the posterior pituitary is derived from forebrain and consists of nerve fibres which extend directly from the axonal terminals of hypothalamic neurons.

The posterior pituitary hormones are synthesized in the hypothalamic supraoptic nucleus (located just lateral to and above the optic chiasm) and the paraventricular nuclei (located on each side of the third ventricle). They then migrate along the axons of these neurons as neurosecretory granules in the supraoptic–hypophyseal tract to the posterior pituitary before release into the circulation via branches of the inferior hypophyseal artery. The sensory signals that affect release of vasopressin and oxytocin are accumulated from the afferent fibres of osmoreceptors close to the hypothalamic nuclei, the brainstem, and also from the vagus and glossopharyngeal nerves receiving input from the pharynx and baroreceptors of the heart and great vessels (Fig. 13.3.1).

The hypothalamic nuclei receive their blood supply from derivatives of the circle of Willis: the suprahypophyseal, anterior communicating, anterior cerebral, posterior communicating, and posterior cerebral arteries. The inferior and superior hypophyseal arteries, formed from branches of the internal carotid artery, supply the posterior pituitary. The venous supply of the system drains to the dural, cavernous, and inferior petrosal sinuses.

Structure and synthesis of vasopressin and oxytocin

Vasopressin and oxytocin have molecular weights of 1087 Da and 1007 Da, respectively, and are both nonapeptides with a disulphide bridge between the cysteine residues at positions 1 and 6 (Fig. 13.3.2). Oxytocin differs from vasopressin by only two amino acids with isoleucine for phenylalanine at position 3 and leucine for arginine at position 8. The genes for both these hormones

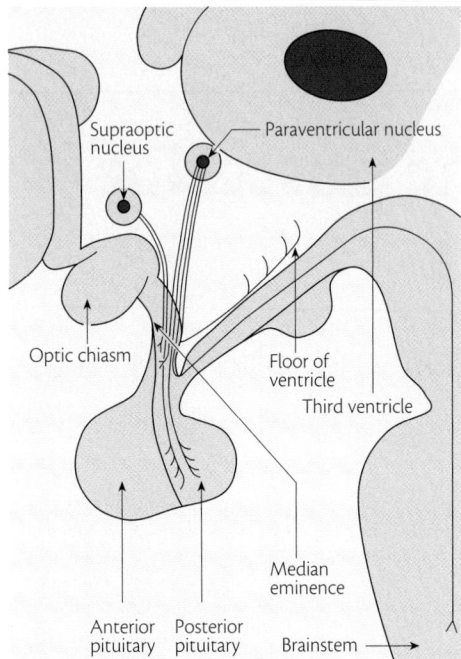

Fig. 13.3.1 Schematic representation of the neuronal pathways from the paraventricular and supraoptic nuclei. The nerves project to the posterior pituitary, the median eminence, the floor of the third ventricle, and the brainstem. Afferent fibres from the osmoreceptors and thirst centre are shown.
This article was published in *Clinical Endocrinology*, Besser GM, Thorner MO (eds) pp. 5.1–5.14, Mosby-Wolfe (2002).

lie 8 kb apart on chromosome 20q13. They encode 145-amino acid precursors comprising a signal peptide, the specific vasopressin or oxytocin sequence, a hormone-specific peptide called a neurophysin, and a C-terminal peptide. The vasopressin precursor also has a glycoprotein at the C-terminus. The hormones are initially packaged in granules as a precursor complex of neurophysin and oxytocin or vasopressin. During transport of these neurosecretory granules to the posterior pituitary, endopeptidases cleave off the active hormone from the neurophysin and the final products are stored in the nerve termini in the gland.

The synthesis of vasopressin and oxytocin occurs in separate neurons within the paraventricular and supraoptic nucleus which allows the individual release of hormones. On stimulus of the

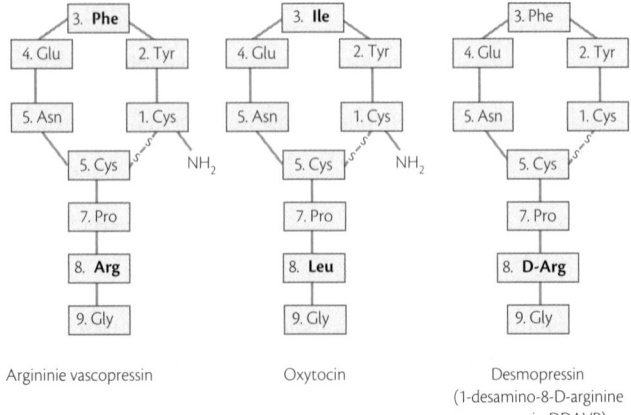

Argininie vasopressin   Oxytocin   Desmopressin (1-desamino-8-D-arginine casopressin DDAVP)

Fig. 13.3.2 The structure of vasopressin, oxytocin, and desmopressin. Amino acid differences are highlighted in bold.

appropriate magnocellular cell body, an action potential propagates along the axon, causing an influx of calcium at the axon terminal and releasing the hormone's neurosecretory granules into the perivascular space. Neurophysin is also released but has no further role after acting as a carrier protein in the neurons. The hormones are unbound in the circulation and their half-life is short, that of vasopressin being about 10 min. They are degraded by endothelial and circulating endopeptidases and aminopeptidases; vasopressin is mainly cleared in the liver and kidneys, while oxytocin is also cleared in the uterus.

Vasopressin

Physiology

Vasopressin is also known as antidiuretic hormone (ADH) and these two names relate to the two physiological entities regulated by this hormone: pressure/volume and osmosis. However, there are separate sensory inputs to these two systems and distinct receptors at the end-organs of response.

There are three known vasopressin receptors: V_1 receptors occur in vascular smooth muscle, V_2 receptors are expressed in the collecting tubules of the kidney, and V_3 receptors on anterior pituitary corticotrophs. The receptors are all seven-transmembrane-domain, G protein-coupled receptors; V_1 and V_3 signal by inositol phosphate pathways, while the V_2 receptor activates adenylate cyclase with an increase in intracellular cAMP.

The V_2 receptor mediates the principal physiological effect of vasopressin, that of regulation of water reabsorption in the distal nephron. The presence of selective water channel proteins (aquaporins) in the wall of the distal nephron allows reabsorption of water from the lumen along an osmotic gradient with excretion of concentrated urine. Eight aquaporins have been cloned so far. The V_2 receptor activation and subsequent release of intracellular cAMP results in the insertion of aquaporin-2 into the apical membrane of the collecting duct. The subsequent movement of water into the cell and renal interstitium accounts for the antidiuretic action of vasopressin.

The function of the remaining vasopressin receptors is summarized in Table 13.3.1. Activation of the V_1 receptor in vascular smooth muscle results in vasoconstriction and a rise in blood pressure with higher concentrations of vasopressin. The V_3 receptor acts as one of the central regulators of secretion of ACTH in synergy with corticotropin-releasing hormone. In addition, V_2 receptors stimulate the production of clotting factor VIII.

Regulation of vasopressin secretion

Vasopressin release occurs in response to three key stimuli: (1) a rise in plasma osmolality, (2) a drop in blood pressure, and (3) a stressful event. These changes are sensed by osmoreceptors in the hypothalamus and baroreceptors in the heart, aorta, and the great vessels.

The principal physiological stimulus is a rise in plasma osmolality detected in the osmoreceptor cells. Figure 13.3.3 illustrates the tight linear positive correlation between the plasma osmolality and release of vasopressin and thus the exquisite sensitivity of this system which maintains plasma osmolality within the narrow range of 285 to 295 mosmol/kg. This correlation also exists between osmolality and thirst, which is recognized in the

Table 13.3.1 Vasopressin receptor functions

	V₁	V₂	V₃
Location	Vascular smooth muscle	Basolateral membrane of distal nephron	Pituitary corticotroph
	Liver		
	Platelets		
	Central nervous system		
Function	Smooth muscle contraction	Increased production of aquaporin-2 and antidiuresis	Enhanced ACTH release
	Stimulation of glycogenolysis		
	Platelet adhesion		
	Neurotransmitter		

Adapted from Ball SG, Baylis PH (2002). The neurohypophysis. In: Wass JAH, Shalet SM (eds) *Oxford textbook of endocrinology and diabetes*. Oxford University Press, Oxford.

hypothalamus close to the osmoreceptor cells. A loss of extracellular water will stimulate vasopressin secretion to conserve water, accompanied by thirst and a drive to drink.

Like vasopressin, the regulation of thirst by osmolality is more important physiologically than that induced by hypovolaemia. Most humans consume the bulk of their ingested water as a result of relatively unregulated fluid intake such as consumption of drinks with food or in tea, coffee, and soft drinks. This explains why in the syndrome of inappropriate antidiuretic hormone described below, water intake must be consciously restricted to avoid overconsumption.

Hypotension stimulates vasopressin release through the activation of baroreceptors in the carotid sinus and aortic arch and low-pressure receptors in the atria and pulmonary venous system. A significant drop in circulating volume, i.e. falls of 5 to 10% of arterial blood pressure, are required to increase vasopressin concentrations. However, in contrast to osmoregulated vasopressin secretion, a progressive decrease in blood pressure produces an exponential increase in plasma vasopressin. The subsequent water retention helps to restore blood volume.

Vasopressin is also released under nonspecific stress. Although the precise role of vasopressin in the stress response is unknown, it is classified as a stress hormone as it is released, in response to e.g. neuroglycopenia, nausea, and emesis among other stimuli.

Modified normal physiological states

There are several normal physiological states where the system is modified. In pregnancy there is a resetting of the osmostat such that both increases and decreases in plasma vasopressin occur at an osmolality approximately 10 mosmol/kg less than the normal vasopressin concentration/plasma osmolality relationship. A similar but smaller change occurs in the luteal phase of the menstrual cycle.

Vasopressin concentrations increase with age, as does the response of vasopressin to osmotic stimulation. However, thirst recognition and thus fluid intake is reduced. These changes, along with a lessened ability to excrete a water load, predispose older people to both hypernatraemia and hyponatraemia.

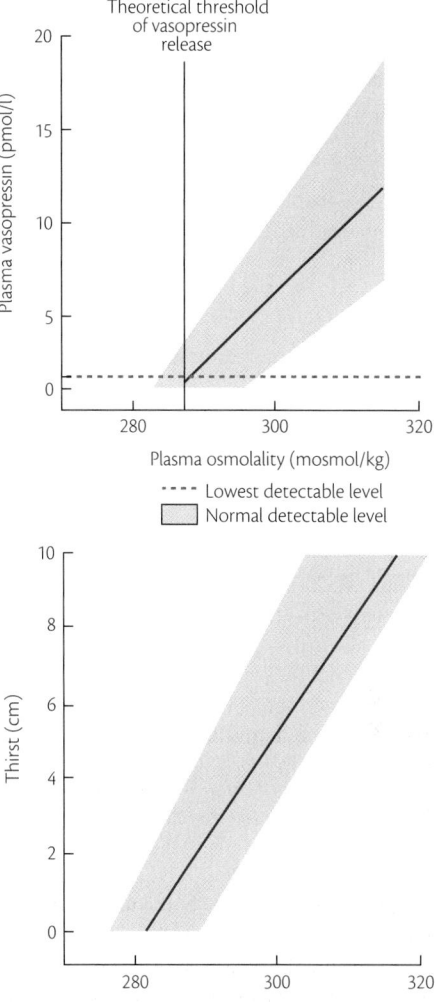

Fig. 13.3.3 The relationship between plasma osmolality and plasma arginine vasopressin concentration, and between plasma osmolality and thirst. AVP concentrations and thirst sensation rise in a linear fashion in relation to plasma osmolality.

This article was published in *Clinical Endocrinology*, Besser GM, Thorner MO (eds) pp. 5.1–5.14, Mosby-Wolfe (2002).

Disorders of vasopressin secretion

Diabetes insipidus

This is the passage of large volumes (>3 litres/24 h) of dilute urine (osmolality <300 mosmol/kg) and may be caused by: (1) vasopressin deficiency (cranial diabetes insipidus), (2) renal resistance to the actions of vasopressin (nephrogenic diabetes insipidus), and (3) excessive fluid intake (primary polydipsia) when the hypotonic polyuria is an appropriate physiological response. The causes of diabetes insipidus are listed in Box 13.3.1, and the clinical features of diabetes insipidus are polyuria, polydipsia, nocturia, and, in children, nocturnal enuresis and failure to thrive.

Differential diagnosis

Before the vasopressin axis is investigated, polyuria (>3 litres/24 h) should be confirmed and other aetiologies such as diabetes mellitus, renal failure, hypokalaemia, and hypercalcaemia should be excluded. Following this the most common investigation to discriminate normality from the various causes of diabetes insipidus is the water deprivation test (Box 13.3.2). This dynamic test assesses

---

Box 13.3.1 Causes of diabetes insipidus

Cranial diabetes insipidus

Familial

◆ Autosomal dominant (vasopressin gene)

◆ DIDMOAD syndrome (diabetes insipidus, diabetes mellitus, optic atrophy, deafness)

Acquired

◆ Trauma (head injury, neurosurgery, cerebral hypoxia)

◆ Tumours (craniopharyngioma, germinoma, pinealoma, metastases)

◆ Inflammatory conditions (sarcoidosis, Langerhans cell histiocytosis, tuberculosis, lymphocytic hypophysitis, Guillain–Barré syndrome)

◆ Infections (meningitis, encephalitis)

◆ Autoimmune (antivasopressin neuron antibodies)

◆ Vascular (aneurysm, arteriovenous malformations, infarction, Sheehan's syndrome, sickle cell disease)

◆ Idiopathic

Nephrogenic diabetes insipidus

Familial

◆ X-linked recessive (V2-receptor defect)

◆ Autosomal recessive (aquaporin-2 defect)

◆ Autosomal dominant (aquaporin-2 defect)

Acquired

◆ Drugs (lithium, demeclocycline)

◆ Metabolic (hypercalcaemia, hypokalaemia)

◆ Chronic renal disease (polycystic kidneys, obstructive uropathy)

◆ Osmotic diuresis (diabetes mellitus)

◆ Infiltrative (amyloid)

Primary polydipsia

Box 13.3.2 Water deprivation test

Preparation

◆ The patient is allowed fluids overnight (if primary polydipsia is suspected, consider fluid deprivation overnight to avoid morning overhydration).

◆ A light breakfast is taken at 6.30 a.m.; no tea, coffee, or smoking.

Fluid deprivation

◆ From 7.30 a.m. the patient is deprived of fluid for 8 h or until 5% of body weight is lost.

◆ The patient is weighed hourly.

◆ Plasma osmolality is measured at 4-h intervals, and urine volume and osmolality is measured every 2 h.

Desmopressin

◆ The patient is given 2 µg desmopressin intramuscularly.

◆ The patient is now allowed to drink freely.

◆ Plasma and urine osmolality are measured over the next 4 h.

In reality further investigation is sometimes required, particularly when patients have partial forms of the condition. Plasma vasopressin is measured directly in response to an infusion of 0.05 ml/kg per min of 5% hypertonic saline for 2 h. In cranial diabetes insipidus there is no increased vasopressin, whereas in nephrogenic diabetes insipidus the vasopressin level is high with no increased urine osmolality. Alternatively, the diagnosis of diabetes insipidus can be made with a therapeutic trial of desmopressin with monitoring of plasma and urine osmolality and plasma sodium. Patients with primary polydipsia develop progressive dilutional hyponatraemia, whereas those with nephrogenic diabetes insipidus remain unaffected. In cranial diabetes insipidus there is an improvement in polyuria and polydipsia. Imaging of the neurohypophysis with MRI should also be undertaken to identify any possible cause of cranial diabetes insipidus.

Cranial diabetes insipidus

In complete absence of vasopressin urine can reach a maximum dilution of 50 mosmol/kg and the deficiency will lead to passage of anywhere between 3 and 20 litres of urine in 24 h. With unrestricted access to water, normal circulating volume and sodium concentration are maintained by an intact thirst centre. Presentation with cranial diabetes insipidus implies destruction of more than 80% of the vasopressin cells. Cranial diabetes insipidus can be masked by cortisol deficiency as glucocorticoids are necessary for renal excretion of a water load. Therefore, diabetes insipidus may only become manifest with the introduction of corticosteroids.

The most common causes of cranial diabetes insipidus are trauma (head injury, neurosurgery) and tumours. Removal of or damage to the posterior pituitary usually results in temporary diabetes insipidus lasting 6 weeks to 6 months as the proximal nerve endings grow out to capillaries in scar tissue formed and resume secretion. As hormone synthesis actually occurs higher up in the hypothalamus, destruction here or at the level of the upper pituitary stalk or median eminence results in permanent diabetes insipidus.

the ability to concentrate urine during controlled water deprivation and is then followed by an assessment of response to exogenous vasopressin to confirm renal sensitivity. There is no contraindication to the test providing the patient is fully hydrated. Interpretation also relies on normal thyroid and adrenal function; if function is impaired, the patient must be adequately treated before undergoing the test.

Cranial diabetes insipidus can be diagnosed with paired urine osmolality less than 300 mosmol/kg and plasma osmolality more than 290 mosmol/kg after dehydration. Urine osmolality should rise above 750 mosmol/kg after desmopressin. However, if the urine osmolality does not rise above 300 mosmol/kg after dehydration and desmopressin, nephrogenic diabetes insipidus is confirmed. Patients with primary polydipsia should concentrate urine appropriately after dehydration, without a significant rise in plasma osmolality.

The most common solid tumour to produce diabetes insipidus is a craniopharyngioma. Suprasellar germinomas or pinealomas also commonly cause diabetes insipidus. Metastases to the pituitary hypothalamic area are more likely to cause diabetes insipidus than a deficiency of anterior pituitary hormones because they lodge in the portal system of the hypothalamus. Lymphoma and infiltration with leukaemia are rare causes of diabetes insipidus. If the thirst centre is destroyed as part of the hypothalamic lesion (whether a tumour or any other cause), dangerous dehydration may ensue.

Familial diabetes insipidus is rare, accounting for approximately 5% of cranial diabetes insipidus, and may be caused by an autosomal dominant mutation in the vasopressin gene in the sequence encoding the precursor molecule or the signal peptide but not the peptide hormone itself. It is postulated that this causes abnormal folding of the precursor protein which then accumulates within the neurons and leads to cell death. As the pathology develops over time diabetes insipidus becomes manifest when approximately 80% of the neurons have been destroyed. This is probably why symptoms are not present at birth but gradually develop between 1 and 6 years of age.

Treatment of cranial diabetes insipidus

Where polyuria is mild (<4 litres/24 h), patients with an intact thirst mechanism can be managed by advising an adequate fluid intake. With more severe symptoms the treatment is the long-acting vasopressin analogue desmopressin (1-desamino-8-D arginine vasopressin), which acts predominantly on the V_2 receptors in the kidney with almost no action at the V_1 receptors in vascular smooth muscle. Desmopressin is given orally (100–1000 µg daily), intranasally (10–40 µg daily), or parenterally (0.1–2 µg daily). There is wide individual variation in bioavailability and, therefore, dose required for symptom control. The main adverse effect is dilutional hyponatraemia, making monitoring of serum sodium and osmolality essential.

Nephrogenic diabetes insipidus

Until recently there were two known causes of congenital nephrogenic diabetes insipidus, an X-linked recessive mutation of the V_2 receptor, which accounts for 90% of cases, and an autosomal recessive mutation of the aquaporin-2 water channels. The two types can be discriminated by an infusion of desmopressin which leads to an increase in blood pressure, and in circulating von Willebrand factor and factor 8 in the autosomal recessive condition. These effects are expressed via V_2 receptor signalling and, therefore, will not be seen in the X-linked form. More recently an autosomal dominant mutation of the C-terminal intracellular tail of aquaporin-2 has been described. In all cases, in contrast to familial cranial diabetes insipidus, nephrogenic diabetes insipidus usually presents from birth with polyuria and hypernatraemia. Without recognition the hypernatraemia, polyuria, vomiting, constipation, fever, irritability, and a failure to thrive may result in long-term cognitive impairment. More commonly nephrogenic diabetes insipidus is due to acquired metabolic or pharmacological cauess (Box 13.3.1). The most common drugs causing nephrotoxicity leading to diabetes insipidus are lithium and demeclocycline.

Treatment of nephrogenic diabetes insipidus

Causative drugs should be withdrawn although the effects are not always reversible. High-dose desmopressin (up to 5 µg intramuscularly) can be effective in partial nephrogenic diabetes insipidus.

Thiazide diuretics which reduce urine output by increasing sodium excretion can be helpful. In addition, prostaglandin synthase inhibitors such as indomethacin may be effective as prostaglandins locally inhibit the renal actions of vasopressin.

Primary polydipsia

This is the inappropriate ingestion of excess fluid. It leads to a slight decrease in plasma osmolality and suppressed vasopressin secretion which results in polyuria. As the kidney can excrete up to 18 litres of dilute urine per day, serum osmolality is usually maintained in the normal range. The volumes of urine passing through the collecting duct reduce inner medulla osmolality and the sustained reduction in vasopressin release leads to less aquaporins in the collecting duct cells. These abnormalities lead to an inability to concentrate urine maximally. This dysfunction returns to normal within days to weeks of decreased fluid ingestion. The syndrome may occur as a behavioural abnormality in patients with psychiatric disease. Management is difficult, with reduced fluid intake being the only effective treatment; treatment of any underlying psychiatric condition is crucial.

Syndrome of inappropriate antidiuretic hormone (SIADH)

SIADH is a common cause of hyponatraemia and constitutes normovolaemic hyponatraemia as the increased water is dispersed though all compartments. The increased inappropriate vasopressin secretion leads to inappropriately concentrated urine, dilute plasma, and hyponatraemia with ongoing renal sodium excretion. The diagnosis is considered when renal, adrenal, and thyroid function are normal; there is no evidence of volume overload or hypovolaemia and the biochemistry is consistent, i.e. hyponatraemia and hypotonic plasma (osmolality <270 mosmol/kg), inappropriate urine osmolality (>100 mosmol/kg), and high urinary sodium (>20 mmol/litre). There are many causes (Box 13.3.3) and thus the diagnosis itself should prompt a hunt for underlying pathology.

Initially the condition is most often asymptomatic, as development of hyponatraemia is gradual. However, as sodium falls to 120 mmol/litre or less it is associated with confusion, drowsiness, and seizures; rapid reduction in sodium or severe hyponatraemia can cause coma and death.

The SIADH itself can be classified according to the pattern of abnormal vasopressin secretion (Table 13.3.2).

Treatment of SIADH

Management of the condition is the same whatever the cause or type of SIADH. The underlying cause should be treated appropriately and fluid restriction instituted to between 500 and 750 ml/24 h. This generally restores sodium levels and osmolality within a few days. Very rarely saline infusion may be required if the hyponatraemia is severe (c.100 mol/litre) or if drowsiness and seizures do not respond to fluid restriction. Rapid correction of hyponatraemia should be avoided because of the risk of central pontine myelinolysis; one should aim to increase plasma sodium by no more than 0.5 mmol/litre per hour. If the symptoms are not temporary and long-term fluid restriction is difficult for the patient, drugs such as demeclocycline that induce nephrogenic diabetes insipidus can be effective. The most specific treatment for SIADH is to block the V_2 receptor in the kidney. Several V_2 receptor antagonists are in phase 3 clinical trials. Tolvaptan, a V_2-receptor antagonist, and conivaptan, a combined V_1/V_2-receptor antagonist, are, respectively, in phase 3 clinical trials and approved for parenteral use in

Box 13.3.3 Causes of SIADH

Malignant disease

- Carcinoma (lung, duodenum, stomach, pancreas, bladder, ureter, prostate)
- Thymoma
- Lymphoma, leukaemia
- Mesothelioma
- Sarcoma
- Carcinoid

Chest disease

- Infection (pneumonia, tuberculosis, empyema)
- Pneumothorax
- Asthma
- Positive pressure ventilation
- Cystic fibrosis

Central nervous system disorders

- Head injury
- Infections (meningitis, encephalitis, abscess)
- Tumour
- Vascular disorders (haemorrhage, thrombosis)
- Guillain–Barré syndrome
- Acute intermittent porphyria
- Psychosis
- Hydrocephalus

Drugs

- Psychiatric drugs (phenothiazines, monoamine oxidase inhibitors, selective serotonin reuptake inhibitors)
- Chemotherapy (vincristine, vinblastine, cisplatin)
- Thiazides
- Anticonvulsants (carbamazepine)
- Clofibrate
- Chlorpropamide
- 3,4-Methylenedioxymethamphetamine (MDMA, 'ecstasy')
- Lansoprazole

Other

- Hypothyroidism
- Glucocorticoid deficiency
- Idiopathic
- Abdominal surgery

Table 13.3.2 Types of SIADH

Type	Characteristics
A	Erratic ADH secretion, unrelated to plasma osmolality, commonly associated with tumours; accounts for 40% of SIADH
B	Osmotic threshold for vasopressin release is reset to a lower plasma osmolality; accounts for 30% of SIADH
C	Inability to suppress vasopressin release at low plasma osmolality
D	Normal osmoregulated vasopressin release but inability to excrete a water load

ADH, antidiuretic hormone; SIADH, syndrome of inappropriate antidiuretic hormone.

the United States of America. Both tolvaptan and conivaptan are benzazepine derivatives (Fig. 13.3.4).

In a recent large multicentre randomized controlled trial, oral tolvaptan was shown to be effective in increasing serum sodium concentration at day 4 and day 30. Thus it showed not only a rapid increase in sodium but also that this increase was sustained weeks later. It shows promise for use in the outpatient setting provided there is adequate monitoring of plasma sodium.

A rare but important differential diagnosis of SIADH is cerebral salt wasting. This is a rare complication of pituitary surgery or more commonly occurs after subarachnoid haemorrhage. It tends to occur 5 to 10 days following a neurological event and is associated with hypovolaemia and hyponatraemia. It must be differentiated from SIADH as the treatments are quite different; fluid replacement in cerebral salt wasting and fluid restriction in SIADH. The diagnosis of cerebral salt wasting usually needs central venous pressure measurement as this demonstrates hypovolaemia compared with normovolaemia in SIADH. In cerebral salt wasting the urinary sodium is often extremely high and the plasma urate and haematocrit may be raised.

Oxytocin

The structure and synthesis of oxytocin is described above. The hormone binds to a G protein-coupled cell surface receptor on target cells to mediate a variety of physiological effects, but principally regulation of lactation, parturition, and reproductive behaviour.

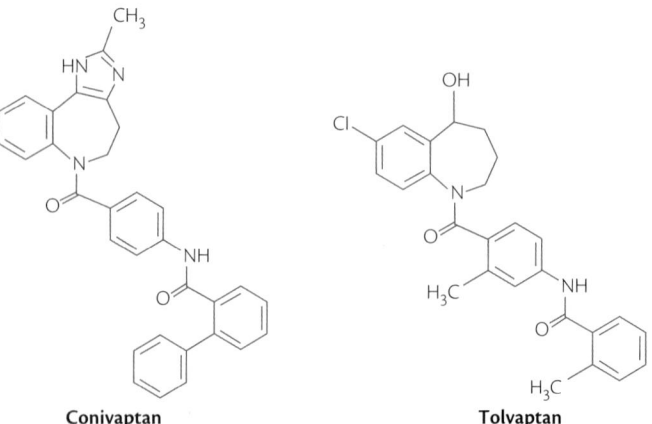

Conivaptan **Tolvaptan**

Fig. 13.3.4 Structures of tolvaptan and conivaptan.
(From Hays RM (2006). Vasopressin antagonists: progress and promise. *N Engl J Med*, **355**, 2146–8. © 2006 Massachusetts Medical Society. All rights reserved.)

It has no known role in men but has been postulated to aid contraction of the seminal vesicles. In women oxytocin receptors are expressed predominantly in uterine and breast myometrial cells. Their numbers are increased by oestrogen and during pregnancy. The hormone causes uterine contraction when cervical dilatation triggers oxytocin release during parturition. It is also released in response to suckling when breast duct smooth muscle contraction leads to ejection of breast milk during breastfeeding. The importance of oxytocin in maintaining milk secretion is demonstrated in transgenic mice with a knockout of oxytocin synthesis. These animals deliver their young normally, showing the involvement of several other hormones (prostaglandins, endothelins, adrenergic agonists, corticotropin-releasing hormone, glucocorticoids, and cytokines) in the initiation and completion of labour. They also produce their milk normally, demonstrating the role of prolactin. However, the mice are unable to release milk during suckling and the young die of dehydration. Administration of oxytocin to the knockout mothers restores milk secretion and the young survive.

Hypothalamic syndrome

This uncommon condition is usually caused by tumours of which the most common is craniopharyngioma. In older adults it is also caused by epidermoid and dermoid tumours as well as pinealomas. It is also a rare consequence of neurosurgery or can be due to infiltrative disease such as Langerhans cell histiocytosis. Typical symptoms are hyperphagia and weight gain, loss of thirst sensation, diabetes insipidus, somnolence, behaviour change, and disordered temperature regulation. Management is aimed at the causative lesion but other wise a pragmatic approach is taken to each individual symptom. For example, as mentioned above, diabetes insipidus with loss of thirst sensation may be managed by desmopressin and a prescribed regular fluid intake. These patients need to be monitored with daily weighing and fluid balance.

Further reading

Baylis PH (1994). The posterior pituitary. In: Besser GM, Thorner MO (eds) *Clinical endocrinology*, pp. 5.1–5.14. Mosby-Wolfe, London.

Buhimschi CS (2004). Endocrinology of lactation. *Obstet Gynecol Clin North Am*, **31**, 963–79.

Ellison DH, Berl T (2007). The syndrome of inappropriate antidiuresis. *N Engl J Med*, **356**, 2064–72.

Hays RM (2006). Vasopressin antagonists: progress and promise. *N Engl J Med*, **355**, 2146–8.

Knoers NVAM (2005). Hyperactive vasopressin receptors and disturbed water homeostasis. *N Engl J Med*, **352**, 1847–50.

Oksche A, Rosenthal W (1998). The molecular basis of nephrogenic diabetes insipidus. *J Mol Med*, **76**, 326–37.

Robinson AG, Verbalis JG (2003). The posterior pituitary gland. In: Larson PR, *et al.* (eds) *Williams' textbook of endocrinology*, 10th edition. Saunders, Philadelphia, PA.

Schrier RW, *et al.* (2006). Tolvaptan, a selective oral vasopressin V2-receptor antagonist, for hyponatraemia. *N Engl J Med*, **355**, 2099–112.

The thyroid gland and disorders of thyroid function

Anthony P. Weetman

Essentials

The iodine-containing thyroid hormones triodothyronine (T_3) and thyroxine (T_4) have diverse effects on metabolism and are essential for normal development, particularly of the fetal brain. The active principle, T_3, binds to nuclear receptor isoforms and serves as a transcriptional regulatory factor, thus explaining the protean actions.

Thyroid hormone release is regulated by thyrotropin (TSH) from the anterior pituitary, which is itself modulated by the hypothalamic tripeptide, thyrotropin-releasing hormone (TRH). Thyroid hormones exert negative feedback control on the pituitary gland and on the synthesis of TRH.

A normal TSH level rules out primary thyroid dysfunction, but when TSH levels are abnormal, or when pituitary or hypothalamic abnormalities are possible, it is essential to confirm thyroid status by measuring circulating thyroid hormone levels, which is best achieved by immunoassay of free T_3 and free T_4. Thyroid-antibody measurement and imaging by scintiscanning are useful in determining the aetiology of thyroid disease when this are not obvious clinically.

Goitre

Endemic goitre—which is particularly common in the Himalayas, the Andes, and parts of Africa—is mainly due to iodine deficiency, can cause massive thyroid enlargement, but rarely leads to compressive symptoms. Its main impact on health is the association with endemic cretinism, which can be prevented by iodine supplementation, achievable by iodization of salt or bread, intramuscular or oral iodized oil as a single annual dose, or iodination of drinking water.

Sporadic goitre—cause unknown; presentation is with neck swelling or sensation of pressure or discomfort; most patients are euthyroid and do not require treatment.

Hypothyroidism

Aetiology—iodine deficiency and neonatal hypothyroidism remain major challenges for public health in many countries, but the most frequent cause of thyroid dysfunction in iodine-sufficient areas is autoimmunity, where the follicular gland structure is destroyed by autoreactive T cells.

Clinical features—manifests in the adult with the gradual onset of a constellation of symptoms and signs including tiredness, feeling cold, weight gain, hoarseness of the voice, and slow-relaxing tendon reflexes. A goitre may (Hashimoto's thyroiditis) or may not (atrophic thyroiditis/primary myxoedema) be present. Biochemical diagnosis of primary hypothyroidism is confirmed by a high serum TSH and a low free T_4, with autoimmune hypothyroidism associated with the presence of thyroid peroxidase autoantibodies (against the 'microsomal' antigen). Treatment is with thyroxine (100–150 µg/day, but beginning with a low dose in older people or those with heart disease).

Myxoedema coma—this is the most dramatic presentation of hypothyroidism and a medical emergency with high mortality: management requires (1) supportive treatment; (2) identification and treatment of any precipitating condition, often infective; (3) parenteral thyroid hormone replacement.

Thyrotoxicosis

Aetiology—Graves' disease, which is caused by TSH receptor stimulating autoantibodies, is responsible for 60 to 80% of cases, and nodular thyroid disease (toxic multinodular goitre and toxic adenoma) accounts for most of the rest.

Clinical features—presents with a wide range of symptoms and signs including hyperactivity, palpitations, fatigue, weight loss (despite increased appetite), sinus tachycardia (or atrial fibrillation), tremor, and eye signs (including lid retraction and lid lag). Biochemical diagnosis of primary hyperthyroidism is confirmed by a low serum TSH and a high free T_4 and/or T_3, with autoimmune hyperthyroidism associated with the presence of thyroid peroxidase autoantibodies in most patients with Graves' disease. β-blockers can rapidly relieve symptoms, but definitive treatment requires antithyroid drugs (usually carbimazole or propythiouracil), radio-iodine (^{131}I), or surgery.

Thyroid-associated ophthalmopathy—this often causes anxiety and social embarrassment, but severe cases are a threat to vision and may require treatment with corticosteroids, radiotherapy, other immunosuppressive agents, or orbital decompression.

Thyrotoxic crisis or storm—this is the most dramatic presentation of hyperthyroidism and a medical emergency with high mortality. Manifestations include fever (>38.5 °C), delirium or coma, seizures, vomiting, diarrhoea and jaundice. Management requires (1) supportive treatment; (2) identification and treatment of any precipitating condition, including infection; (3) antithyroid treatment, e.g. loading dose of propylthiouracil, followed 1 h later by stable iodine (e.g. Lugol's iodine or ipodate).

Other conditions

Acute thyroiditis—usually caused by bacterial infection; presents with severe thyroid pain, fever and malaise; thyroid function is rarely disturbed.

Subacute (or de Quervain's) thyroiditis—due to viral infection and commonly presents with thyroid pain; there may be transient thyrotoxicosis, followed by hypothyroidism, before restoration of normal thyroid function; diagnosis depends on demonstration of raised inflammatory markers and low/absent radio-iodine uptake by the thyroid.

Amiodarone—inhibits T_4 deiodination and hence leads to free T_4 levels that are in the upper half of the reference range or mildly elevated; may cause hypothyroidism or hyperthyroidism, the latter being difficult to treat.

Structure of the thyroid gland
Development

The human thyroid develops as a diverticulum in the pharyngeal floor at around 3 weeks of gestation. This median anlage moves caudally and remains connected to the pharynx via the thyroglossal duct, which is subsequently obliterated when the thyroid begins to expand as two distinct lobes at around 2 months of gestation. The foramen caecum marks the point in the tongue where the thyroid develops and there is sometimes an upward extension of thyroid tissue from the isthmus, the pyramidal lobe, arising from the lower part of the thyroglossal duct. At the same time, the lateral anlage ultimobranchial bodies, derived from the fifth branchial pouches, fuse with the developing thyroid to which they contribute the parafollicular calcitonin-secreting clear cells. Synthesis of thyroid hormone begins at week 12, at the same time as TSH production by the pituitary. There is significant maternal-to-fetal T_4 transfer so that babies with no endogenous thyroid hormone production are nonetheless protected from the adverse effects of fetal hypothyroidism on development of the brain, lung, and skeleton. Preterm infants of less than 27 weeks gestation have immature thyroid function and their neurological development may be improved by temporary T_4 supplementation.

Anatomy and histology

The adult thyroid weighs 15 to 20 g; each lobe is around 4 cm long and 2 cm wide, although the right lobe is often larger than the left. The isthmus connecting the two lobes lies just below the cricoid cartilage. The blood supply on each side is derived from the external carotid artery via the superior thyroid artery and from the subclavian artery via the inferior thyroid artery. There is adrenergic and cholinergic innervation which regulates blood flow. The thyroid is attached to the trachea by connective tissue, and the recurrent laryngeal nerves lie between the trachea and the posterior aspect of the lobes.

The gland is made up of lobules each comprising 20 to 40 spherical follicles. The follicles vary considerably in size, but average 200 μm in diameter, and are made up of a single layer of thyroid follicular epithelial cells (Fig. 13.4.1). The cells are cuboidal when quiescent and columnar when active, and have a microvillous apical membrane. The follicular lumen contains colloid, the principal constituent of which is the glycoprotein thyroglobulin secreted by the thyroid cells. Each follicle is surrounded by a rich capillary network. Clear cells lie scattered between follicular epithelial cells or in the interstitium, and account for around 1% of the epithelial mass.

Thyroid hormone synthesis and metabolism
Synthesis and secretion

Thyroid hormone synthesis requires iodide uptake and oxidation, iodination of certain tyrosine molecules on thyroglobulin, and coupling of the iodotyrosines to form the thyroid hormones T_3 and T_4 (Fig. 13.4.2). Iodide is actively transported into the thyroid cell by the Na^+/I^- symporter, which is also expressed in breast tissue and the salivary glands. Perchlorate, thiocyanate, and pertechnetate are also transported by the same symporter and these anions can competitively inhibit iodide uptake. The recommended daily intake of iodine is 150 μg for adults (200 μg during pregnancy) but there is wide variation in actual intake with many countries having borderline or frankly deficient intakes of less than 50 to 100 μg, while in western Europe and North America intake may be excessive (up to 750 μg/day).

Iodide is oxidized by thyroid peroxidase, a haem-containing enzyme located at the apical border of the thyroid cell, and is rapidly incorporated into tyrosine residues to form monoiodotyrosine and di-iodotyrosine. Thyroid peroxidase is also responsible for the coupling of these iodotyrosines, with different sites in the thyroglobulin molecule being responsible for the formation of T_3 or T_4. Normally, each thyroglobulin molecule contains three or four T_4

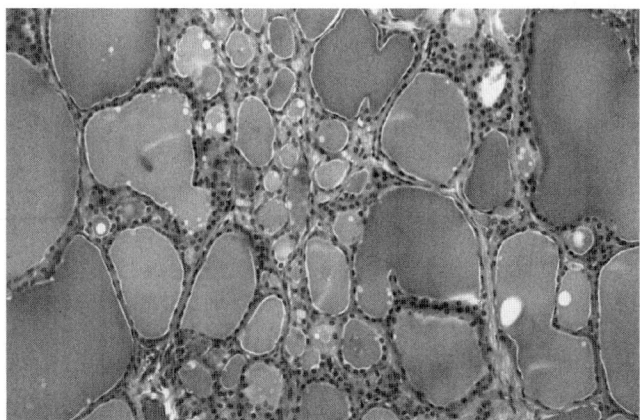

Fig. 13.4.1 Histology of a normal thyroid. Thyroid epithelial cells are arranged in follicles containing colloid. Original magnification ×200.
(Photomicrograph by courtesy of Dr K. Suvarna.)

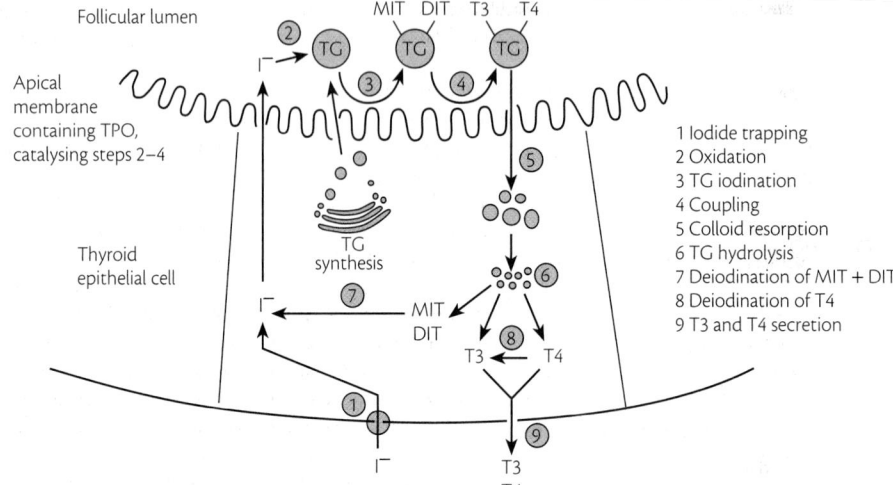

Fig. 13.4.2 Steps in the synthesis of thyroid hormones. DIT, di-iodotyrosine; MIT, monoiodotyrosine; TG, thyroglobulin; TPO, thyroid peroxidase.

molecules, but only 20% of thyroglobulin molecules contain a T_3 molecule. Thyroglobulin acts as slow turnover reservoir for thyroid hormone, thus ensuring maximum use is made of often scarce dietary iodine. Around a 7-week supply of T_4 is contained in the normal thyroid. Thyroid hormone is released from the gland after endocytosis of colloid and lysosomal hydrolysis of the thyroglobulin to yield T_4 and T_3, which are secreted from the basal membrane into the capillaries in a molar ratio of 14:1. Released iodotyrosines are deiodinated for iodide recycling.

Thyroid hormone transport

Up to 90% of the total T_3 in the circulation is derived from peripheral conversion of T_4 to T_3 by deiodinase enzymes (see below) rather than thyroid secretion. Only 0.03% of T_4 and 0.3% of T_3 in the circulation exist as free hormone that is able to diffuse into tissues; the remainder is protein bound. T_4 binds predominantly to T_4-binding globulin, and to a lesser extent to transthyretin (or prealbumin); a little is bound to albumin. T_3 binds to T_4-binding globulin and albumin, with little bound to transthyretin. Alteration in the concentration or binding capacity of thyroid hormone binding proteins can produce major changes in total but not free thyroid hormone levels (Table 13.4.1). Several transporters mediate thyroid hormone uptake by cells; monocarboxylate transporter 8 is particularly important in the uptake of T_3 by brain, and mutations in this gene cause severe psychomotor retardation due to brain-specific hypothyroidism during development.

Metabolism of thyroid hormone

The half-life of T_4 in the circulation is 7 days, contrasting with the much shorter half-life of T_3 of 24h. The most important metabolic pathway for T_4 is outer ring (5′) deiodination to T_3 (Fig. 13.4.3). This is catalysed by type I and type II deiodinase (EC 1.97.1.10), while type III deiodinase (EC 1.97.1.11) catalyses inner ring (5) deiodination leading to hormone inactivation. Type I deiodinase can also catalyse inner ring deiodination of T_3 and T_4. All three enzymes have a selenocysteine moiety as the active catalytic site. Type I deiodinase is expressed predominantly in the liver, kidney, thyroid, and brain, type II in the pituitary, brain, placenta, skeletal

Table 13.4.1 Conditions in which there is altered binding of thyroid hormones to binding proteins

TBG	
Increased binding	Genetic variation in TBG
	Oestrogens (pregnancy, oral contraception, hormone replacement therapy, tamoxifen)
	Other drugs (perphenazine, opiates, 5-fluorouracil, clofibrate, mitotane)
	Hepatitis, cirrhosis
	Acute intermittent porphyria
Decreased binding	Genetic variation in TBG
	Steroids (testosterone, anabolic steroids, glucocorticoids)
	Acromegaly
	Nephrotic syndrome
	Protein malnutrition
	Acute severe illness
	L-Asparaginase
Albumin	
Decreased binding	Any cause of hypoalbuminaemia
Increased binding	Genetic variation
Tranthyretin	
Increased binding	Genetic variation
Competition for binding sites	
Drugs	Phenytoin
	Carbamazepine
	Salicylates and nonsteroidal anti-inflammatory drugs
Nonesterified fatty acids	

TBG, thyroid-binding globulin.

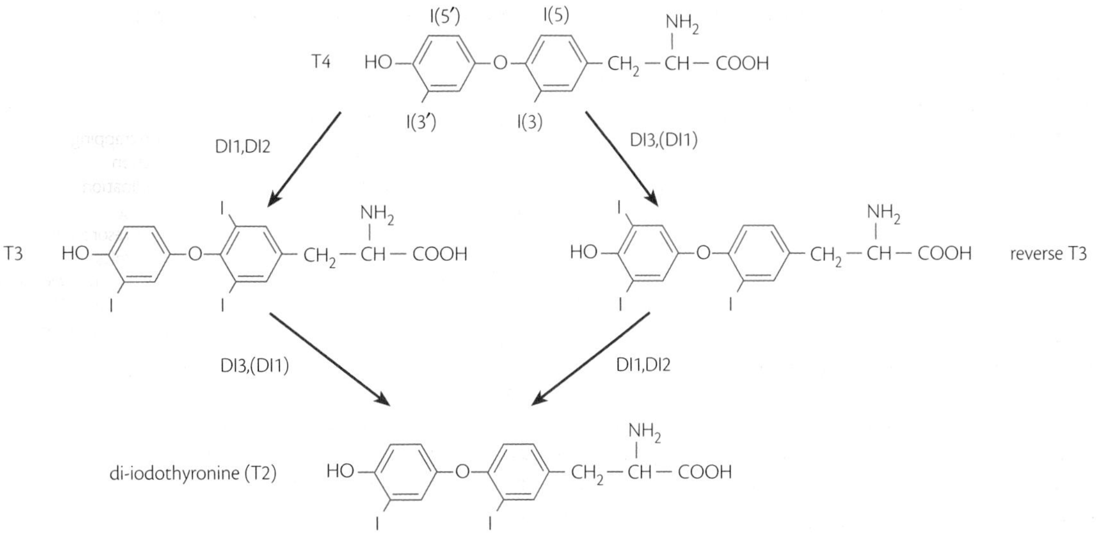

Fig. 13.4.3 Main deiodination pathway for thyroid hormones. DI, deiodinase enzyme; parentheses denote a minor contribution. Deiodination of T_3 also yields 3,5-T_2 and deiodination of reverse T_3 also yields 3′,5′-T_2. T_2 is further deiodinated to monoiodothyronine and thyronine.

muscle, and heart (tissues critically dependent on thyroid hormone for development or function), and type III in the brain, placenta, and skin. The type I deiodinase is largely responsible for the generation of circulating T_3 from T_4, whereas T_3 generated by the type II enzyme mainly provides intracellular T_3 at specific sites.

Around 40% of T_4 is metabolized to T_3 and 40% is converted to reverse T_3 by the type III deiodinase. This same enzyme is responsible for the main metabolic pathway for T_3 which is converted to 3,3′-di-iodothyronine. Starvation, trauma, and drugs (propylthiouracil, amiodarone, glucocorticoids, propranolol) impair T_4 to T_3 conversion and must be borne in mind when interpreting tests of thyroid function (see below). In addition to deiodination, a small proportion of thyroid hormone is metabolized by conjugation of the phenolic hydroxyl group with sulphate or glucuronic acid, which increases water solubility and allows urinary and biliary excretion. Biliary iodothyronine glucuronides can be reabsorbed, constituting an enterohepatic cycle.

Thyroid hormone action

Thyroid hormone acts primarily as a transcription regulatory factor, mediated by T_3 binding to nuclear receptor isoforms that belong to the same superfamily as steroid and retinoic acid receptors. All such receptors possess a conserved DNA-binding domain containing two zinc fingers, which interact with specific DNA response elements, and a hormone-binding domain. Alternative splicing results in two pairs of thyroid hormone receptors (Fig. 13.4.4) whose tissue expression varies during development. Thyroid hormone receptors bind to DNA as homodimers or heterodimers (with the retinoid X receptor). Without ligand, basal gene transcription is inhibited by a corepressor. When T_3 binds, homodimers dissociate releasing corepressor and allowing gene transcription; the stable heterodimer binds coactivators in the presence of T_3 with the same outcome. The α2 thyroid hormone receptor does not bind T_3 and may act as a natural inhibitor of receptor activity. A cell surface receptor for T_3, involving integrin αVβ3 and leading to protein kinase signal transduction, has recently been delineated and there may be further additional pathways for thyroid hormone action.

Regulation of thyroid function

The main regulator of thyroid function is TSH (thyrotropin), secreted by thyrotrophs in the anterior pituitary gland in response to the tripeptide thyrotropin-releasing hormone derived from the hypothalamic supraoptic and paraventricular nuclei. Thyroid hormones exert a classic negative feedback effect on thyrotrophs; the acute effect is mediated by T_3 in the pituitary which is derived from T_4 by type II deiodination. Thyroid hormones also inhibit hypothalamic thyrotropin-releasing hormone synthesis. TSH secretion stimulated by thyrotropin-releasing hormone is inhibited by dopamine and somatostatin, while α-adrenergic activation stimulates TSH release. Cytokines, particularly interleukin-1, interleukin-6, and tumour necrosis factor, inhibit TSH synthesis and may be responsible for the suppression of TSH seen in severe illness.

Within the thyroid, TSH binds to the G protein-coupled TSH receptor, leading to intracellular signalling predominantly via cAMP. TSH increases iodide transport and organification, endocytosis of colloid, and thyroid hormone secretion, as well as thyroid follicular epithelial cell division. Autoregulatory mechanisms can modulate thyroid function when TSH levels are constant. The most

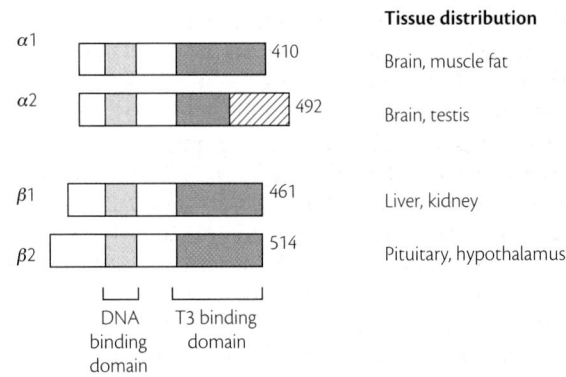

Fig. 13.4.4 Structure of the thyroid hormone receptors. The numbers indicate the amino acid content. Homologous areas are shaded; the lack of homology in the T_3-binding domain of the α2 receptor (hatched area) prevents T_3 binding and the function of this receptor is unknown.

important is iodine intake. Increased iodide transport transiently decreases organification and reduces thyroid hormone synthesis (the Wolff–Chaikoff effect); after several weeks under normal conditions, the thyroid escapes and resumes hormone production. Sudden increases in iodine intake can also acutely block thyroid hormone release. In iodine deficiency, thyroid hormone production is switched to preferential T_3 synthesis, but this effect is largely TSH-mediated rather than autoregulatory.

Laboratory investigation of thyroid function

Determining thyroid status

The introduction of sensitive immunoradiometric assays for circulating TSH, with a detection level of 0.1 mU/litre or less, has transformed the evaluation of thyroid status. A normal TSH level rules out primary thyroid dysfunction. Low levels of thyroid hormones elevate TSH as a result of negative feedback, while excessive thyroid hormone suppresses TSH. The thyrotropin-releasing hormone test for detecting low TSH levels is now redundant. As well as primary thyroid disorders, other conditions may alter TSH levels and must be borne in mind when using TSH as a screening test for thyroid dysfunction (Table 13.4.2), as must the possibility of secondary (pituitary or hypothalamic) disturbances of thyroid function.

It is, therefore, essential to confirm thyroid status when TSH levels are abnormal, or when pituitary or hypothalamic abnormalities are possible, by measuring circulating thyroid hormone levels. Methods which measure total T_3 or T_4 are prone to artefacts caused

Table 13.4.2 Causes of abnormal serum TSH concentrations

TSH level	Cause	Free thyroid hormone levels
Raised	Overt hypothyroidism	↓
	Subclinical hypothyroidism	N
	Sick euthyroid syndrome	↓ or N
	Dopamine antagonists (acute effect)	N
	TSH-secreting pituitary adenoma	↑
	Thyroid hormone resistance syndrome	↑
	Adrenal insufficiency	↓ or N
Lowered	Overt thyrotoxicosis	↑
	Subclinical thyrotoxicosis	N
	Recently treated hyperthyroidism	N
	Thyroid-associated ophthalmopathy without Graves' disease	N
	Excessive thyroxine treatment	N or ↑
	Sick euthyroid syndrome	↓ or N
	First trimester of pregnancy	N or ↑
	Pituitary or hypothalamic disease	N or ↓
	Anorexia nervosa	N or ↓
	Dopamine, somatostatin (acute effect)	N
	Glucocorticoids	N

N, normal; TSH, thyroid-stimulating hormone; ↑, increased; ↓, decreased.

by abnormal thyroid hormone binding (Table 13.4.1), although in the absence of such abnormalities these tests are reliable. When altered binding is suspected or found, compensation can be made by calculation of the free T_3 or free T_4 index. These indices are derived from the total hormone levels and measurement of the differential distribution of radiolabelled T_3 between unoccupied protein binding sites in the sample and an absorbent resin (hence the term 'resin uptake test'). T_4-binding globulin levels can also be measured directly.

However, the ready availability of immunoassays for free T_3 and free T_4 has generally supplanted these methods. The immunoassays rely on the ability of a radiolabelled thyroid hormone analogue to bind to thyroid hormone antibody but not to plasma binding proteins. The analogue then competes for antibody binding with the free thyroid hormone in the sample. Despite initial concerns about the theoretical basis and performance of such assays, recent improvements allow generally reliable estimation of free thyroid hormones. In cases of doubt, free hormone levels can be measured by physical separation from bound hormone using ultracentrifugation or equilibrium dialysis.

Several indirect methods can be used to determine thyroid status. The thyroidal uptake of radio-iodine (^{123}I, ^{131}I) or ^{99}Tcm pertechnetate is increased in hyperthyroidism and decreased in hypothyroidism, but can be affected by excessive dietary iodine and destructive processes in the thyroid so that uptake is low when the patient is thyrotoxic (see 'Destructive thyroiditis'). Serum thyroglobulin is raised in hyperthyroidism of all types but is also raised in destructive thyroiditis and thyroid cancer. Its main role in investigation is follow-up of treated thyroid cancer (see Chapter 13.5). Several nonspecific tests have also been used to determine end-organ responses to thyroid hormones, including basal metabolic rate, tendon relaxation time, and serum levels of cholesterol, ferritin, sex hormone-binding globulin, and liver enzymes.

Thyroid function in nonthyroidal illness and pregnancy

Assessing thyroid function in severely ill patients often reveals abnormalities termed the 'sick euthyroid syndrome'. Many of the changes are due to cytokine release, but therapeutic agents such as dopamine and glucocorticoids also contribute, as do unknown factors. Any major, acute illness or starvation can result in a decrease in circulating T_3 (total and free) with normal levels of T_4 and TSH. Reverse T_3 levels rise. The severity of the illness correlates with the magnitude of the fall in T_3, and in very sick patients total T_4 levels also fall. Analogue-based free T_4 assays generally produce normal results but sometimes high or low values occur. In 10 to 15% of sick individuals, TSH levels are abnormal (raised or lowered). Psychiatric illness can be associated with raised total and free T_4 levels with normal T_3.

There is no proven benefit from thyroid hormone administration in the sick euthyroid syndrome and the hormone changes may be protective by limiting catabolism (although this view is regularly challenged). The importance of these alterations lies in their potential to cause diagnostic confusion. Thyroid function tests should only be requested in ill patients when thyroid disease is genuinely suspected. Abnormal thyroid function tests due to the sick euthyroid syndrome return to normal after recovery and, therefore, repetition of testing is the simplest way to confirm the reason for unusual results.

Pregnancy also affects thyroid function testing. The most obvious change is the rise in T_4-binding globulin, which elevates total but not free T_3 and T_4 levels. In addition, the reference ranges for free T_3 and T_4 are higher than normal in the first half of pregnancy because placental human chorionic gonadotropin, at high levels, acts as a weak stimulator of the TSH receptor. There is a reciprocal fall in TSH levels during the first trimester, but TSH returns to normal in the second trimester as human chorionic gonadotropin levels decline. Occasionally, these changes are sufficient to cause transient 'gestational'hyperthyroidism, associated with hyperemesis during pregnancy. Antithyroid drugs are usually unnecessary in this condition, and attention should be directed to controlling the vomiting and giving parenteral fluids. Renal clearance of iodine is increased in pregnancy, leading to maternal and neonatal goitre and mild hypothyroidism in areas where iodine intake is marginal ($50\,\mu g$/day). These complications can be prevented by supplementing with iodine, 150 to $200\,\mu g$/day.

Determining the cause of thyroid dysfunction

The most frequent cause of thyroid dysfunction in iodine-sufficient areas is autoimmunity, and the simplest test for this is measurement of thyroid autoantibodies, particularly those directed against thyroid peroxidase (the 'microsomal'antigen). Antibodies against thyroglobulin are also easily measured but are almost always accompanied by thyroid peroxidase antibodies, so testing for the latter alone is usually adequate. Different methods, including haemagglutination, immunofluorescence, radioimmunoassay, and enzyme-linked immunosorbent assay, give different prevalence rates for thyroid autoantibodies. Almost all patients with autoimmune hypothyroidism and around 75% with Graves' disease have thyroid peroxidase antibodies. Generally lower levels are found in 5 to 15% of healthy women and 2% of men, and in slightly higher proportions of patients with nodular goitre and thyroid cancer, and results therefore need to be interpreted carefully. Individuals with positive thyroid autoantibodies but normal thyroid function are at increased risk of developing autoimmune hypothyroidism (c.2% per year).

Thyroid imaging by scintiscanning is useful in determining the aetiology of thyroid disease when this is not obvious clinically, particularly in hyperthyroidism and ectopic thyroid tissue. Its role in the evaluation of a solitary thyroid nodule is considered in Chapter 13.5. ^{99}Tcm pertechnetate is usually used as it has a short half-life (6 h) which allows safe administration of high activity and rapid scanning. ^{123}I is not as readily available but is preferable to ^{131}I, especially in children, as it too has a short half-life and does not emit β-radiation. Thyroid ultrasound is being increasingly used as an alternative to scintiscanning. The technique allows accurate determination of thyroid size, which may be useful in follow-up of goitre, and can help to determine the nature of an atypical neck mass. Its role in evaluating nodular thyroid disease is considered in Chapter 13.5. CT scanning is particularly valuable in determining the extent of a retrosternal goitre and assessing tracheal compression (Fig. 13.4.5). In contrast, a standard chest radiograph can be misleading in evaluating tracheal compression, particularly in the anterior–posterior plane.

Goitre

The distribution of thyroid size in any population forms a continuous, positively skewed curve, whose shape depends on the age, sex,

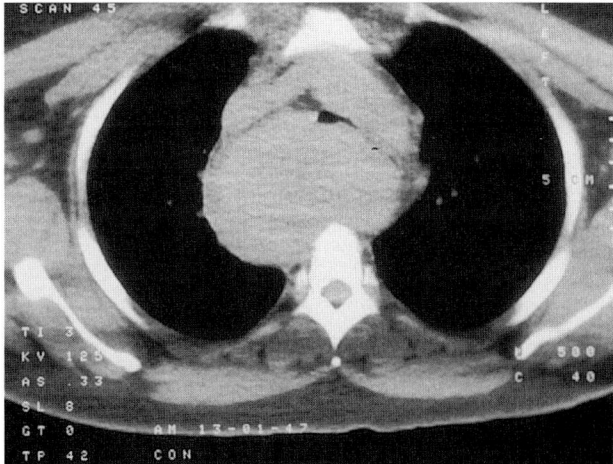

Fig. 13.4.5 CT scan of the chest of a patient with a large retrosternal goitre causing tracheal compression.

and country of residence of the individuals assessed. Hence a precise definition of goitre is impossible. Ultrasound is the most accurate method to assess thyroid size, and estimates of goitre prevalence based on inspection and palpation underestimate the true frequency. However, simple schemes, such as that shown in Box 13.4.1, are useful in field studies of goitre prevalence.

Of the many causes of goitre (Box 13.4.2), those associated with disturbances of thyroid function are considered later. The remainder can be classified broadly as endemic and sporadic nontoxic goitres.

Endemic goitre

Prevalence

Goitre is said to be endemic when the prevalence exceeds 10% in children aged 6 to 12 years, although this figure is arbitrary and it has recently been suggested that a prevalence of more than 5% should be used. Over 200 million people are affected worldwide, especially in the Himalayas, Andes, and parts of Africa, although Eastern and Southern Europe are also involved.

Aetiology

The main cause is iodine deficiency, with goitre prevalence exceeding 30% in areas with very low iodine intakes ($<30\,\mu g$/day). However, endemic goitre is not exclusively related to iodine deficiency. Naturally occurring goitrogens, such as those in vegetables of the cabbage family and in cassava, exaggerate the effects of iodine deficiency by the action of thiocyanates and cyanoglucosides, respectively, on iodine transport. Where selenium and iodine deficiency coincide, thyroid cell destruction and gland fibrosis minimize

Box 13.4.1 WHO/UNICEF grading of goitre
Grade 0 = no visible or palpable thyroid
Grade 1 = thyroid enlargement that is palpable but not visible when the neck is in the neutral position
Grade 2 = thyroid enlargement that is both visible and palpable when the neck is in the neutral position
Grade 3 = goitre visible at a considerable distance

Box 13.4.2 Causes of goitre

Endemic goitre

Iodine deficiency

Goitrogens, including drugs with an antithyroid action

Sporadic goitre

Simple, nontoxic goitre: diffuse or multinodular (colloid goitre)

Toxic multinodular goitre

Hashimoto's thyroiditis

Graves' disease

Destructive thyroiditis

    Postpartum thyroiditis

    Silent thyroiditis

    Subacute thyroiditis

    Amiodarone

Genetic disorders

    Dyshormonogenesis

    Thyroid hormone resistance syndrome

    McCune–Albright syndrome

    TSH receptor mutation

Infiltration

    Riedel's thyroiditis

    Amyloidosis

    Sarcoidosis

Secondary

    TSH-secreting pituitary tumour

    Excessive stimulation from human chorionic gonadotropin in pregnancy or choriocarcinoma

goitre formation. In Japan, endemic goitre actually results from iodine excess, as well as goitrogens in seaweed, and in Kentucky, chemically polluted water is goitrogenic.

Clinical presentation

Diffuse goitre is more frequent in girls, and gradually becomes nodular with age and increasing iodine deficiency. Endemic goitres can be massive but give few compressive symptoms. In areas of marginal iodine deficiency, such as Belgium, a modest goitre only appears when demands on thyroidal iodide metabolism are increased during puberty or in pregnancy.

The major impact of endemic goitre and iodine deficiency on health is the association with endemic cretinism. Two forms of cretinism can be delineated in separate geographical areas, but there is considerable overlap. First, when maternal iodine intake is severely reduced causing hypothyroidism there is reduced placental transfer of T_4 to the fetus, resulting in a profound neurological deficit in the infant, with mental deficiency, deafness, speech defects, and spastic gait. Second, hypothyroidism in the infant after birth produces the typical features of cretinism, in particular stunted growth.

The thyroid in such patients may be enlarged or atrophic and it is clear from field studies that iodine deficiency alone cannot account for the multiple forms of endemic cretinism.

Management

Iodine supplementation is perhaps the simplest and cheapest of all remedies and it prevents a condition that has devastating consequences; it is sobering that iodine deficiency still persists. There are few complications from iodine supplementation, although thyrotoxicosis may result in a variable proportion of individuals (the Jod–Basedow phenomenon) some of whom have avoided this previously through lack of sufficient iodine. Political, social, and economic inertia are at the heart of continuing iodine deficiency. Effective programmes are best targeted at children and women intending pregnancy. Iodization of salt or bread is widely used in developed countries, but intramuscular or oral iodized oil, as a single annual dose, or iodination of drinking water is preferable in areas where distribution of iodized foodstuffs is a problem.

Sporadic goitre

Prevalence

Goitre occurs in around 5% of the iodine-sufficient population and is 4 times more common in women. However, the prevalence varies with area and generally declines with age; over 60% of goitres found in adolescents regress over the next 20 years. The character also changes over time, from a diffuse (sometimes called simple) goitre to a multinodular goitre. The presentation of single thyroid nodules is dealt with in Chapter 13.5, but it is worth mentioning here that solitary thyroid nodules increase in frequency with age.

Aetiology

The aetiology of sporadic goitre is largely unknown. Unidentified goitrogens may be responsible in a few patients, and in others mild iodine deficiency in infancy may initiate goitrogenesis which persists despite a subsequently normal iodine intake. A large proportion are probably the result of mild defects in hormone synthesis; compensatory growth ensures normal thyroid function and current tests cannot identify the nature of the defect. Familial clustering of sporadic goitre supports this idea. Although TSH is the most obvious thyroid growth factor, TSH levels by definition are normal in sporadic goitre, which may therefore be the result of other autocrine and paracrine growth factors (e.g. insulin-like growth factor-1, epidermal growth factor, fibroblast growth factor).

Progression to a multinodular goitre occurs when unencapsulated nodules form in a long-standing diffuse goitre. These nodules contain colloid-rich polyclonal follicles and are usually distinct from adenomas, which are encapsulated and derived from a single thyroid follicular cell with a somatic mutation conferring growth advantage. However, some goitres contain both nodules and adenomas, suggesting a spectrum of pathological changes. Because thyroid follicular cells are heterogeneous, nodules generally develop with varying degrees of function, giving rise to 'hot' and 'cold' areas on scintiscanning with radio-iodine. Some nodules develop autonomy and may eventually cause hyperthyroidism, completing the evolution from nontoxic to toxic multinodular goitre (see below). Other nodules undergo degeneration with haemorrhage, fibrosis, and cyst formation.

Clinical presentation

Patients usually seek attention because of the appearance of the neck or a sensation of pressure or discomfort. Equally, they may be unaware of a long-standing small goitre which is noticed on examination. Careful palpation is sufficient to distinguish true goitre, which moves on swallowing, from a prominent pad of fat over the front of the neck. Very large goitres can cause dysphagia or even stridor when the trachea is compressed, but these symptoms are uncommon. Venous compression at the thoracic inlet is even rarer; this sign is exacerbated by asking the patient to raise his/her arms (Pemberton's sign). Pain in the thyroid, which radiates to the jaw, is uncommon and suggests either destructive thyroiditis (see below) or haemorrhage into a cyst in a multinodular goitre. In the latter, the pain is usually unilateral, acute, and associated with a rapid change in thyroid size; symptoms resolve spontaneously in a few days.

Investigations

Thyroid function should be assessed by checking TSH levels, and then free T_3 and T_4 levels if the TSH is abnormal to rule out goitre associated with thyroid dysfunction. The presence of thyroid peroxidase antibodies is also useful as a marker of an underlying autoimmune thyroiditis, which occurs in 10 to 20% of multinodular goitres. The use of imaging varies between centres. Ultrasound is useful in determining thyroid size and nodularity accurately and may reassure an anxious patient that the thyroid is not enlarging. Thyroidal uptake of radioisotopes (especially ^{99}Tcm pertechnetate) is indicated if destructive thyroiditis is suspected as a cause of goitre. Otherwise, the major role for imaging is to ensure there is no tracheal compression or intrathoracic/retrosternal component in a patient with suggestive symptoms, and a CT scan is then the preferred investigation (Fig. 13.4.5).

Treatment

Most patients with euthyroid sporadic goitre do not require treatment. Neck discomfort or cosmetic concerns may prompt intervention but it is necessary to take a careful history to ensure that discomfort or difficulty swallowing is indeed caused by the goitre. T_4, given at doses to maintain slightly suppressed TSH levels (0.1–0.3 mU/litre), leads to a reduction in goitre size in up to 60% of patients but is unlikely to have any effect on a very nodular goitre or when the TSH level is already low (so-called subclinical hyperthyroidism, discussed below). This treatment is now less used than previously as there are concerns about the long-term effects of suppressive doses of T_4 on the heart and skeleton, and treatment must be continued long-term to maintain any improvement.

Radio-iodine, by contrast, is increasingly being given to reduce goitre size. Doses of ^{131}I range from 600 to 3400 MBq (hospitalization is required for doses >800 MBq). Recent trials suggest that recombinant TSH administration may allow lower ^{131}I doses to be given, increasing the potential for outpatient treatment. Goitre size is usually reduced by more than 50% at 2 years, and most of the improvement occurs within 2 to 3 months. Long-term follow-up data are not yet available, although hypothyroidism certainly occurs in 20 to 40% by 5 years. Tracheal compression by a goitre can be treated with ^{131}I despite theoretical concerns over acute worsening due to a radiation thyroiditis.

Surgery is used in other centres and is particularly indicated for severe tracheal compression or retrosternal goitres and if there is any suspicion of malignancy. Thyroidectomy is the most effective treatment available for goitre, but there may be a recurrence in around 20% of patients within 10 years and is not avoidable by giving T_4 replacement. Complications, including recurrent laryngeal nerve damage, hypoparathyroidism, and hypothyroidism, are more likely with the biggest goitres, near total thyroidectomy, and reoperation.

Hypothyroidism

Impaired production of thyroid hormones is usually due to a primary abnormality of thyroid gland or iodine deficiency; occasionally it is secondary to pituitary or hypothalamic disorders, dealt with in Chapters 13.2 and 13.3. The onset of primary hypothyroidism is gradual and may be detected when the TSH is elevated (to compensate for impaired thyroid output) but the free thyroid hormone levels are normal. This state is subclinical hypothyroidism. As thyroid damage continues, TSH levels rise further but free T_4 levels fall. The TSH level at this stage is usually above 10 mU/litre, symptoms become apparent, and the patient is said to have overt or clinical hypothyroidism.

Aetiology

The causes of hypothyroidism are listed in Box 13.4.3. The commonest cause worldwide is iodine deficiency, discussed above. In iodine-sufficient areas, autoimmune hypothyroidism and thyroid damage after radio-iodine or surgical treatment for hyperthyroidism are the major causes.

Epidemiology

The prevalence of overt hypothyroidism in white populations is around 2% in women and 0.2% in men, with a mean age of 60 at diagnosis. Subclinical hypothyroidism is even more common (6–8% of women and 3% of men). Around 4% of these individuals progress to overt hypothyroidism annually if thyroid peroxidase antibodies accompany the elevated TSH. Half this number progress in the absence of thyroid peroxidase antibodies. Focal lymphocytic infiltration of thyroid associated with thyroid autoantibody positivity occurs in up to 15% of healthy women and 2% of men without an elevated TSH level, representing the earliest manifestation of thyroid autoimmunity; 2% of these people progress to overt hypothyroidism annually. Congenital hypothyroidism occurs in about 1 in 4000 births and this high frequency has led to the widespread introduction of neonatal screening.

Pathogenesis

Autoimmune hypothyroidism is primarily the result of autoreactive T-cell-mediated cytotoxicity directed against thyroid follicular cells. Cytokines derived from the locally infiltrating T cells, macrophages, and dendritic cells impair thyroid cell function and enhance T-cell-mediated cytotoxicity. The role of thyroid autoantibodies in thyroid cell destruction is unclear, but thyroid peroxidase antibodies fix complement and may cause secondary damage. In 10 to 20% of patients, antibodies which block the TSH receptor are partially or wholly responsible for hypothyroidism, and transplacental passage of these antibodies (but not thyroid peroxidase antibodies) occasionally causes transient neonatal hypothyroidism. Genetic and environmental factors are involved in the aetiology but, as with most autoimmune disorders, the complex interaction of these factors has so far prevented a full understanding.

Box 13.4.3 *Causes of hypothyroidism*

Primary

Iodine deficiency

Autoimmune hypothyroidism

  Hashimoto's thyroiditis

  Primary myxoedema

Iatrogenic

  ^{131}I treatment

  Subtotal or total thyroidectomy

  External irradiation for lymphoma or cancer involving the neck

Drugs

  Iodine-containing contrast media

  Amiodarone

  Lithium

  Antithyroid drugs

  p-Aminosalicylic acid

  Interferon-α and other cytokines

  Aminoglutethimide

Congenital hypothyroidism

  Absent or ectopic thyroid gland

  Dyshormonogenesis[a]

  TSH receptor mutation

Destructive thyroiditis

  Postpartum thyroiditis

  Silent thyroiditis

  Subacute thyroiditis

Infiltrative disorders

  Amyloidosis

  Sarcoidosis

  Haemochromatosis

  Scleroderma

  Cystinosis

  Riedel's thyroiditis

Secondary

Hypopituitarism

  Tumours

  Trauma

  Pituitary surgery or irradiation

  Infiltrative disorders

  Infarction

Isolated TSH deficiency or inactivity

Box 13.4.3 *(Cont'd) Causes of hypothyroidism*

Hypothalamic disease

  Tumours

  Trauma

  Infiltrative disorders

  Idiopathic

Drugs

  Bexarotene

[a] The following types of dyshormonogenesis are due to mutations in the genes given in parentheses: iodide transport defect (Na$^+$/I$^-$ symporter), defective iodide organification (thyroid peroxidase, pendrin), loss of iodide reutilization (dehalogenase), deficient thyroid hormone synthesis (thyroglobulin). Defects in monoiodotyrosine coupling also occur but are, so far, poorly characterized.

Polymorphisms in the *HLA-DR* and *CTLA4* genes are associated with autoimmune hypothyroidism, and a high iodine intake may be an important environmental factor in some cases.

Congenital hypothyroidism is caused by thyroid aplasia or hypoplasia in 60% of cases and in 30% there is an ectopic gland. Mutations in thyroid-specific transcription factors have been found in some of these cases. In the remaining 10%, hypothyroidism is due to dyshormonogenesis (see Box 13.4.3).

Clinical features

The cardinal features in adults with hypothyroidism are shown in Box 13.4.4. However, the ready availability of reliable screening tests for hypothyroidism, especially TSH assays, has led to the recognition of many patients in whom there are only vague or non-specific symptoms, such as tiredness, weight gain, and poor concentration. The differential diagnosis is accordingly vast but the high frequency of hypothyroidism should prompt its exclusion when any suggestive features are present, particular in middle-aged women with chronic fatigue or depression.

Autoimmune hypothyroidism may present with a goitre (Hashimoto's thyroiditis) or without (atrophic thyroiditis or primary myxoedema). When present, the goitre is of variable size but is often hard and irregular, sometimes giving rise to suspicion of a malignancy, which then requires exclusion by fine needle aspiration biopsy. Primary lymphoma of the thyroid is a rare but important association (Chapter 13.5). Thyroid pain due to autoimmune thyroiditis is also a rare complication. Patients may notice a Hashimoto goitre before any thyroid dysfunction has developed and annual follow-up is then needed.

The most dramatic presentation of hypothyroidism is myxoedema coma, which is fortunately rare. In addition to the usual features, there is hypothermia (as low as 23 °C) and coma, sometimes with seizures. Mortality is 50% even with intensive treatment. Patients are typically older and either previously undiagnosed or poorly compliant with medication. There is generally an additional precipitant, such as respiratory depression due to drugs, chest infection, heart failure, stroke, blood loss, or exposure to cold.

Autoimmune hypothyroidism is frequently associated with other autoimmune conditions. In the type 2 autoimmune polyglandular syndrome, autoimmune thyroid disease (hypothyroidism or Graves' disease) is associated with type 1 diabetes and/or Addison's disease.

Box 13.4.4 Clinical features of hypothyroidism

Symptoms

Tiredness, weakness

Dry skin

Altered facial appearance

Feeling cold

Hair dry, unmanageable, and thinning

Poor memory and concentration

Constipation

Weight gain with poor appetite

Dyspnoea

Hoarse voice

Menorrhagia (later, oligomenorrhoea or amenorrhoea), decreased libido

Paraesthesias

Deafness

Signs

Dry coarse skin

Cool peripheries

Puffy face, hands, and feet

Yellow skin due to carotene accumulation

Diffuse alopecia

Bradycardia

Peripheral oedema

Slow relaxing tendon reflexes

Carpal tunnel syndrome

Serous cavity effusions

Galactorrhoea (raised prolactin)

Enlarged salivary glands

Rarely: ataxia, dementia, psychosis, coma

This syndrome is autosomal dominant with variable penetrance. In the rare, autosomal recessive type 1 autoimmune polyglandular syndrome (chronic mucocutaneous candidiasis, Addison's disease, and hypoparathyroidism), autoimmune hypothyroidism is found in 5 to 10% of patients. Other common associations include pernicious anaemia, vitiligo, and alopecia areata and there is a significant excess of autoimmune hypothyroidism in coeliac disease, dermatitis herpetiformis, chronic active hepatitis, premature ovarian failure, rheumatoid arthritis, systemic lupus erythematosus, and Sjögren's syndrome. Breast cancer patients and individuals with Down's and Turner's syndromes have a higher than expected frequency of thyroid autoimmunity. Around 5% of patients with thyroid-associated ophthalmopathy, discussed later in this chapter, have autoimmune hypothyroidism and 15% of patients with Graves' disease successfully treated with antithyroid drugs develop hypothyroidism 10 to 20 years later. This relationship with Graves'

disease is further emphasized by rare patients who oscillate between hyperthyroidism and hypothyroidism over a period of months. The likely explanation is fluctuation in the relative levels of TSH receptor stimulating and blocking antibodies, but the cause of these changes is unknown.

Juvenile hypothyroidism is uncommon. The features of adult hypothyroidism (Box 13.4.4) may be present, but the diagnosis is usually suggested by retarded growth and dentition, and an infantile face. Myopathy with muscle enlargement is common. Puberty is usually delayed, although sometimes it is precocious. Congenital hypothyroidism is typically unrecognizable at birth but, if not identified by screening, gives rise to prolonged jaundice, failure to thrive, impaired growth, feeding difficulties, constipation, and hypotonia. Left untreated, even for a few weeks after birth, there is permanent neurological damage resulting in intellectual impairment.

Pathology

In Hashimoto's thyroiditis there is a prominent diffuse and focal lymphocytic infiltrate with germinal centre formation. The thyroid follicles show varying degrees of destruction and little or no colloid. The remaining thyroid follicular cells have an increased number of mitochondria, giving rise to oxyphil metaplasia (Askanazy or Hürthle cells). There is a variable degree of fibrosis. In atrophic thyroiditis, fibrosis is the most prominent feature, with a less obvious lymphocytic infiltrate than in Hashimoto's thyroiditis. Thyroid follicles are usually sparse, reflecting the later stage at which this form of autoimmune hypothyroidism is diagnosed. Whether there is a natural progression from Hashimoto's to atrophic thyroiditis is unclear, although the goitre usually decreases with T_4 replacement.

Laboratory diagnosis

Measuring serum TSH is the first step in diagnosing hypothyroidism, with the important caveat that this approach will miss most cases of secondary hypothyroidism in which the serum TSH measured by immunoassays may be low, normal, or even slightly raised, due to the secretion of bioactive forms of the hormone. If secondary hypothyroidism is suspected, for instance in the follow-up of a patient with treated pituitary disease, it is essential to check the free T_4 level. The TSH is elevated in other settings besides primary overt hypothyroidism (Table 13.4.2). It is therefore important to confirm the diagnosis by measuring the free T_4 in all samples in which the TSH is elevated. Measurement of free T_3 adds nothing to the diagnosis, especially as values may be within the reference range in a quarter of hypothyroid patients due to extrathyroidal conversion of T_4.

If myxoedema coma is expected, it is essential that treatment is initiated immediately without awaiting confirmation of the diagnosis. These patients often have dilutional hyponatraemia, hypoglycaemia, and electrocardiography changes (low voltage, prolonged QT interval, flat or inverted T waves, and heart block). Other nonspecific features which may be found in any patient with hypothyroidism are elevation in serum liver and muscle enzymes (the raised creatine phosphokinase particularly may cause unnecessary concern), raised cholesterol, and anaemia. The anaemia is usually normocytic or macrocytic, but microcytosis occurs when hypothyroidism is accompanied by menorrhagia.

The aetiology is usually easily established. In the absence of a history of treated hyperthyroidism or iodine exposure, the majority of juvenile or adult onset primary hypothyroidism in iodine-sufficient countries is due to autoimmune hypothyroidism. Transient hypothyroidism due to destructive thyroiditis is considered later. The diagnosis of autoimmune hypothyroidism is confirmed by the presence of thyroid peroxidase antibodies, usually at high levels, although occasionally these antibodies are absent. Cytological diagnosis of Hashimoto's thyroiditis is possible using fine needle aspiration biopsy, but is only necessary if there is uncertainty over the cause of a nodular goitre.

Once congenital hypothyroidism is diagnosed by routine testing after birth, it is usual to initiate T_4 immediately. Treatment can then be stopped without neurological consequences at age 3 to 4 years to establish whether life-long T_4 replacement is necessary. At this time, the aetiology can be established by scintiscanning and/or ultrasound. Dyshormonogenesis, suspected when there is detectable thyroid tissue and a family history, requires specialized investigation to establish the diagnosis and increasingly this is possible by direct analysis of gene mutations. The commonest of these defects is Pendred's syndrome in which there are mutations in the pendrin gene (*SLC26A4*) encoding a chloride/iodide transporter present in the thyroid and cochlea, leading to goitre, mild hypothyroidism, and deafness. The thyroid abnormalities usually appear in the second or third decade, rather than at birth. The diagnosis can be made easily by the perchlorate discharge test, which shows an excessive decline of radioactivity in the thyroid when potassium perchlorate is given 2 to 3 h after allowing the thyroid to take up a tracer dose of radio-iodine.

Treatment

In adult patients without heart disease and below the age of 60, treatment can begin with the estimated replacement dose of T_4. If there is no remaining thyroid tissue (indicated by a very high TSH level and very low or undetectable free T_4), the daily replacement dose is 1.6 µg T_4/kg body weight, which is around 100 to 150 µg/day. In practice, the typical starting dose is 50 to 100 µg T_4 daily, the lower dose being reserved for patients with mild to moderate biochemical abnormalities. Dosage changes should be based on TSH levels measured 2 to 3 months after starting treatment, the main goal of treatment being to normalize the TSH. A similar period is required to assess the effect of any change to the dosage, made as 25 or 50 µg increments or decrements depending on the degree of abnormality of the TSH. Treatment is usually straightforward, although if there is only partial thyroid failure when treatment is begun, the dose of T_4 may require adjustment over many months.

Once on a full replacement dose, TSH levels should be checked annually. Fluctuating or elevated TSH levels in a previously stable patient, or T_4 requirements in excess of 200 µg/day, usually indicate adherence problems. It is important to rule out malabsorption, including *Helicobacter pylori* infection, excessive soya intake, or drugs: cholestyramine, ferrous sulphate, lovastatin, aluminium hydroxide, rifampicin, amiodarone, carbamazepine, and phenytoin all alter the absorption or clearance of T_4. A common cause for poor adherence is worsening angina. Optimization of antianginal treatment is then required, although some patients may simply prove intolerant of full T_4 replacement if their coronary artery disease is extensive and irremediable. It is important to remind poorly adherent patients that, because of the long half-life of T_4, missed tablets should always be taken and that this is safe. It should be emphasized that, in the absence of coronary artery disease, T_4 has no adverse effects when given at doses that return TSH levels to normal.

In older patients or in individuals with heart disease, the usual starting dose is 25 µg T_4 daily (or on alternate days when there is severe angina). Dosage should be increased slowly with increments of 12.5 to 25 µg T_4. Proportionately higher doses of T_4 are needed during the first year of life than in adults, and the starting daily dose of T_4 for congenital hypothyroidism is 10 µg/kg body weight. There is a continuing debate on the benefit of T_4 in subclinical hypothyroidism. It is reasonable to commence T_4 when subclinical hypothyroidism is coupled with the presence of thyroid peroxidase antibodies, as there is a high risk of progression to overt hypothyroidism. Modest improvements in mental function and lipid levels occur when T_4 is given to some patients with subclinical hypothyroidism, but long-term studies on the benefits of treatment have not been conducted. At present, it seems reasonable to offer a 3-month trial of T_4 to thyroid peroxidase antibody-negative patients with subclinical hypothyroidism. If the patient notices an improvement in the symptoms which prompted thyroid function testing, T_4 is continued, but is stopped if there is no benefit. All patients with subclinical hypothyroidism or positive thyroid peroxidase antibodies should be offered annual testing for the development of overt hypothyroidism.

Another problem is posed by the occasional patient with overt hypothyroidism who continues to feel unwell or who fails to lose weight after the TSH is normalized with T_4 replacement. It can take around 3 months from achieving full replacement for all symptoms to disappear, and weight gained during hypothyroidism will generally only be lost by following an appropriate diet. It is sensible to ensure that the TSH level is in the lower half of the reference range and sometimes a small increment of T_4 can achieve this, improving symptoms but not suppressing the TSH. Higher doses of T_4 that suppress the TSH should be avoided, as there is an increased risk of atrial fibrillation due to subclinical thyrotoxicosis. The other recognized adverse effect of excessive T_4 is a decrease in bone mineral density, particularly in postmenopausal women who have previously had hyperthyroidism and therefore already have a low skeletal mass. However, the changes in bone mineral density are modest and no increase in fracture rate has been reported as a result of T_4 given at supraphysiological doses. There has been a revival of the concept that thyroid hormone replacement should consist of both T_4 and T_3, based on the observation that deiodinase activity varies between tissues, suggesting that in some organs the level of the active thyroid hormone, T_3, is insufficient when only T_4 is given. The short half-life of T_3 makes it alone unsuitable for replacement and a recent meta-analysis of all trials to date has shown no evidence of any benefit from combined T_4 and T_3 treatment.

Treatment of myxoedema coma is a medical emergency (see Box 13.4.5).

Prognosis

T_4 treatment is usually life-long and, properly taken, restores normal health and lifespan. Occasional patients may discontinue T_4 and remain euthyroid. Errors in initial diagnosis account for some of these; in others, a spontaneous decline in TSH receptor blocking antibody levels may be responsible. There is no easy means of ascertaining whether a patient continues to need T_4, short of stopping it and measuring the TSH 6 weeks later. Because remission is

---

Box 13.4.5 Treatment of myxoedema coma

- Thyroid hormone replacement
  - A single intravenous bolus of 500 µg T_4; thereafter 50 to 100 µg T_4 daily
  - An alternative strategy is 10 µg T_3 every 4 to 6 h, intravenously or by nasogastric tube
  - Some centres use 200 µg T_4 and 25 µg T_3 as a single bolus
- Supportive treatment
  - Ventilation usually required
  - Space blankets for hypothermia (avoid external warming)
  - Intravenous infusion of hypertonic saline or glucose as required
  - Parenteral hydrocortisone 50 mg every 6 h
- Identify and treat underlying precipitant (including chest or other site of infection, cardiac and renal failure, and myocardial infarction)
  - Broad-spectrum antibiotics if infection suspected

---

uncommon and of uncertain duration, few endocrinologists attempt T_4 withdrawal once started.

Special problems in pregnant women

Untreated hypothyroidism impairs fertility and increases the risk of miscarriage. Children born to such mothers have varying degrees of intellectual impairment. It is therefore essential that T_4 replacement is monitored closely in women with hypothyroidism who intend to become or who are pregnant. Ideally TSH and free T_4 should be checked prior to conception, once pregnancy is confirmed, and at the beginning of the second and third trimesters. The requirement for T_4 can increase by 50 to 100% during pregnancy but reverts to normal after delivery. There are no implications for breastfeeding.

Areas of uncertainty or needing further research

Although present preparations of T_3 and T_4 have shown no additional benefit compared to T_4 alone, development of a sustained release preparation of T_3 could be worth assessment. Because hypothyroidism is frequent, routine screening of certain groups or even the entire population has been advocated (Box 13.4.6), but the cost–benefit of setting up new screening programmes is unclear. If widely adopted, screening will turn up many individuals with subclinical hypothyroidism for whom the benefits of early treatment with T_4 have not yet been fully established. Recent data show that there is an increased risk of miscarriage in thyroid peroxidase antibody-positive women who are euthyroid and this may be reduced by T_4 treatment, but more work is needed to confirm this.

Thyrotoxicosis

Thyrotoxicosis is defined as the state produced by excessive thyroid hormone. Hyperthyroidism exists when thyrotoxicosis is caused by thyroid overactivity but there are several types of thyrotoxicosis that are not due to hyperthyroidism, the most obvious being administration of excessive T_4.

Box 13.4.6 Indications for screening for hypothyroidism

Established

Congenital hypothyroidism

Previous treatment for hyperthyroidism

Previous neck irradiation (e.g. for lymphoma)

Pituitary tumours, including follow-up after surgery or irradiation

Treatment with lithium or amiodarone

Subclinical hypothyroidism

Worthwhile

Antepartum[a] in type 1 diabetes

Three months postpartum after a prior episode of postpartum thyroiditis

Unexplained infertility

Nonspecific symptoms in women over 40 years of age

Refractory depression or bipolar affective disorder with rapid cycling

Turner's syndrome

Down's syndrome

Autoimmune Addison's disease

Uncertain

Patients with a family history of thyroid autoimmunity

Dementia or obesity without other evidence of thyroid disease

Antepartum to detect unsuspected hypothyroidism[b]

Breast cancer

[a] Also measure thyroid peroxidase antibodies; screen euthyroid antibody-positive women 3 months postpartum for postpartum thyroiditis.
[b] It is also uncertain whether all pregnant women should be checked for thyroid peroxidase antibodies as predictors of postpartum thyroiditis.

Aetiology

The causes of thyrotoxicosis are shown in Box 13.4.7. Graves' disease is responsible for 60 to 80% of cases and nodular thyroid disease (toxic multinodular goitre and toxic adenoma) accounts for most of the rest. Destructive thyrotoxicosis is dealt with in the next section.

Epidemiology

The prevalence of thyrotoxicosis in white people is 2 to 3% in women and 0.2 to 0.3% in men. The peak age of onset for Graves' disease is between 20 and 50 years of age, whereas toxic multinodular goitre occurs more often in later life.

Pathogenesis

Graves' disease is caused by TSH receptor stimulating antibodies, clearly demonstrated by the occurrence of transient, neonatal thyrotoxicosis in babies born to mothers with Graves' disease whose antibody levels are high enough for transplacental transfer to affect the fetus. As with autoimmune hypothyroidism, genetic

Box 13.4.7 Causes of thyrotoxicosis

Primary hyperthyroidism

Graves' disease

Toxic multinodular goitre

Toxic adenoma

Drugs: iodine excess (Jod–Basedow phenomenon), lithium, amiodarone

Thyroid carcinoma or functioning metastases

Activating mutation of the TSH receptor

Activating mutation of the Gsα protein (McCune–Albright syndrome)

Struma ovarii (ectopic thyroid tissue)

Thyrotoxicosis without hyperthyroidism

Ingestion of excess thyroid hormone (factitious thyrotoxicosis)

Subacute thyroiditis

Silent thyroiditis

Other causes of thyroid destruction: amiodarone, ^{131}I or external irradiation (acute effect), infarction of an adenoma

Secondary hyperthyroidism

TSH-secreting pituitary tumour

Chorionic gonadotropin-secreting tumours

Gestational thyrotoxicosis

Thyroid hormone resistance (usually euthyroid)

Box 13.4.8 Clinical features of thyrotoxicosis of any cause

Symptoms

Hyperactivity, irritability, altered mood

Heat intolerance, sweating

Palpitations

Fatigue, weakness

Weight loss with increased appetite

Diarrhoea, steatorrhoea

Polyuria

Oligomenorrhoea, amenorrhoea, loss of libido

Signs

Sinus tachycardia, atrial fibrillation in older patients

Fine tremor

Warm, moist skin

Goitre

Palmar erythema, onycholysis, pruritus, urticaria, diffuse pigmentation

Diffuse alopecia

Muscle weakness and wasting, proximal myopathy, hyper-reflexia

Eyelid retraction or lag

Gynaecomastia

Rarely: chorea, periodic paralysis (usually in Asian men), psychosis, impaired consciousness

---

factors, including *HLA-DR*, *CTLA4*, and *TSHR* gene polymorphisms, are associated with the disease; the concordance rate in monozygotic twins is about 20% and much less in dizygotic twins. A high iodine intake, smoking, and stress have all been identified as environmental factors, but in many patients the genetic and environmental triggers remain elusive. Smoking is a major risk factor for the development of thyroid-associated ophthalmopathy. These eye signs are due primarily to swelling of the extraocular muscles, the result of fibroblast activation by cytokines released by infiltrating T cells and macrophages, leading to glycosaminoglycan accumulation, oedema, and fibrosis. The close correlation between ophthalmopathy and thyroid disease is best explained by a shared orbital and thyroid autoantigen (possibly the TSH receptor).

Toxic multinodular goitre evolves from a nontoxic sporadic goitre (see above) and is particularly likely when iodine intake increases, either gradually as a result of changes in the diet, or acutely when iodine-containing agents (amiodarone, some contrast media) are given. More than 50% of toxic adenomas are due to a somatic activating mutation in the genes encoding the TSH receptor or the associated Gsα protein, and a similar but unknown mechanism leading to constitutive activation of a clone of thyroid cells must underlie the remainder.

Clinical features

The typical features of thyrotoxicosis from any cause are shown in Box 13.4.8, but their presence and severity depend on the duration of disease and the age of the patient. Occasionally there are paradoxical manifestations, such as the weight gain that can occur in up to 10% of patients when the increase in appetite exceeds the effects of increased metabolism, and apathetic or masked thyrotoxicosis in older patients which mimics depression. The most dramatic but rare presentation is thyrotoxic crisis or storm, with a mortality rate of 20 to 30% even with treatment. Patients typically are previously undiagnosed or partially treated and have an acute exacerbation of thyrotoxicosis precipitated by acute illness (infection, stroke, diabetic ketoacidosis) or trauma, especially directly to the thyroid (surgery or radio-iodine). Exact diagnostic criteria for thyrotoxic crisis are not agreed and its frequency is sometimes exaggerated. There is marked fever (>38.5°C), delirium or coma, seizures, vomiting, diarrhoea, and jaundice, with death being caused by arrhythmias, heart failure, or hyperthermia.

The differential diagnosis of thyrotoxicosis includes any cause of weight loss, anxiety, and phaeochromocytoma, but simple biochemical testing can readily distinguish thyrotoxicosis from these conditions. Once the diagnosis of thyrotoxicosis is made, it is essential to determine the cause (see Box 13.4.7), as this determines treatment. Graves' disease is usually clinically distinctive; there is a small to moderate, diffuse, firm goitre and around one-half of these patients have signs of thyroid-associated ophthalmopathy (Fig. 13.4.6 and Table 13.4.3). There may be evidence of another autoimmune disorder, in the patient or his/her family, with the

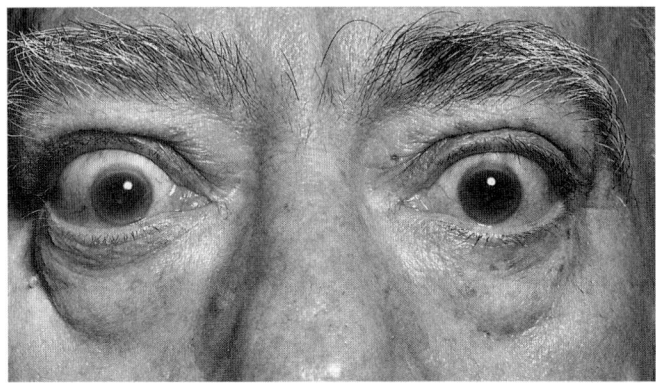

(a)

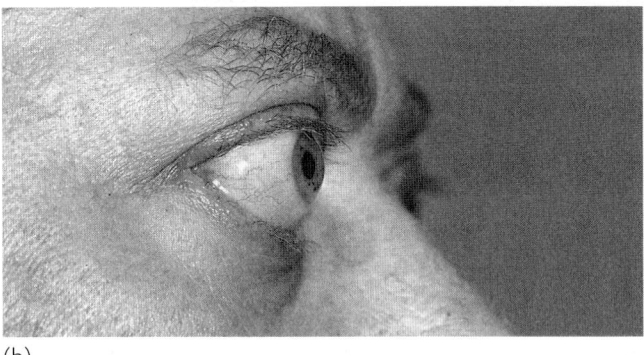

(b)

Fig. 13.4.6 Thyroid-associated ophthalmopathy. (a) Upper lid retraction, periorbital oedema, and scleral injection. (b) Chemosis (conjunctival oedema) and proptosis.

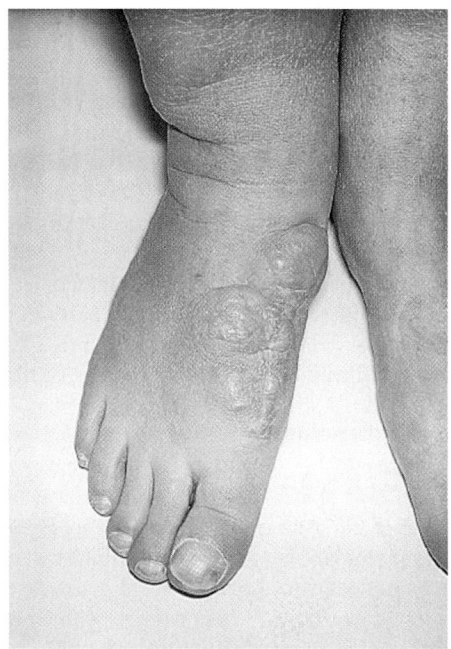

Fig. 13.4.7 Thyroid dermopathy (pretibial myxoedema) affecting the lateral aspect of the shin and the dorsum of the foot; the patient also had thyroid acropachy.

same associations as autoimmune hypothyroidism described above. Less than 5% of patients have pretibial myxoedema, which is better called thyroid dermopathy as it can occur anywhere, especially after trauma (Fig. 13.4.7). These patients almost always have moderate to severe ophthalmopathy and 10 to 20% have clubbing (thyroid acropachy). Thyroid dermopathy most commonly occurs as nonpitting plaques with a pink or purple colour but no inflammatory signs. Nodular and generalized forms, the latter mimicking

elephantiasis, also occur. Hyperplasia of lymphoid tissue, including splenomegaly and thymic enlargement, is sometimes found in Graves' disease.

The absence of these features of Graves' disease and the presence of a multinodular goitre strongly suggest toxic multinodular goitre, although nodular thyroid disease is so common that occasional patients with Graves' disease may cause confusion when their thyrotoxicosis arises in a pre-existing multinodular gland. In toxic adenoma, the solitary thyroid nodule is usually readily palpable. Other, rare causes of thyrotoxicosis can usually be easily identified from the history and biochemical investigations.

Pathology

In Graves' disease, there is thyroid hypertrophy and hyperplasia. The follicles show considerable folding, contain little colloid, and are composed of tall columnar cells. Gland vascularity increases. There is a focal and diffuse lymphocytic infiltrate and lymphoid hyperplasia may occur in the lymph nodes, spleen, and thymus. These changes are all reversed by antithyroid drugs. Toxic multinodular goitre comprises a mixture of areas of follicular hyperplasia and nodules filled with colloid. There is a variable degree of fibrosis, haemorrhage, and calcification. Toxic adenomas are encapsulated and cellular, sometimes with little evidence of follicle formation, and occasionally containing unusual cell forms suggesting malignant change. However, capsular invasion is absent and this is the cardinal feature which distinguishes a follicular adenoma from carcinoma.

Laboratory diagnosis

Measuring the serum TSH is the simplest way to exclude primary thyrotoxicosis. A normal or slightly raised TSH level can rarely be associated with secondary hyperthyroidism in the case of a

Table 13.4.3 Clinical features of thyroid-associated ophthalmopathy

Signs and symptoms	Assessment	Approximate frequency[a] (%)
Lid lag, lid retraction	Measure lid fissure width	50–60
Grittiness, discomfort, excessive tearing, retrobulbar pain, periorbital oedema	Self-assessment score by patient; activity score by clinician	40
Proptosis	Exophthalmometry or CT/MRI-based measurement	20
Extraocular muscle dysfunction (typically causing diplopia looking up and out)	Hess chart or similar; CT/MRI scan to detect muscle size	10
Corneal involvement, causing exposure keratitis	Rose bengal or fluorescein staining	<5
Loss of sight due to optic nerve compression	Visual acuity and fields, colour vision; CT/MRI scan	<1

[a] In patients with Graves' disease. Patients often have multiple signs and in 5–10% of them signs are unilateral.

TSH-secreting pituitary adenoma. A low TSH level is not always the result of thyrotoxicosis (see Table 13.4.2), therefore the diagnosis of thyrotoxicosis must be confirmed by measuring thyroid hormone levels. Free hormone assays are preferable to those for total hormone, to eliminate binding protein effects (see Table 13.4.1). Measuring free T_4 alone is adequate in most cases of thyrotoxicosis, which can be confirmed by the presence of a suppressed TSH and elevated free T_4 level. However, in up to 5% of patients, only free T_3 levels are elevated (T_3 toxicosis), especially during the earliest phase of the disorder. Therefore, if both free T_3 and T_4 are not measured routinely by a laboratory, it is essential to request free T_3 analysis in any sample showing a suppressed TSH but normal free T_4 level. Rarely, the free T_4 is elevated but the free T_3 is normal. This arises when Graves' disease or nodular thyroid disease is precipitated by the administration of excess iodine (the Jod–Basedow phenomenon).

Although it is possible to measure TSH receptor stimulating antibodies and thus prove the existence of Graves' disease in a thyrotoxic patient, these assays are cumbersome or expensive, and therefore, at present, are not widely used. Almost as much information can be gained by measuring thyroid peroxidase antibodies which are present in around 75% of patients with Graves' disease. In cases of diagnostic uncertainty, a thyroid scintiscan will demonstrate a diffuse goitre with high isotope intake in Graves' disease and reveal nodular thyroid disease, as well as ectopic thyroid tissue in the extremely rare struma ovarii. In destructive and factitious thyrotoxicosis, the thyroid scan shows virtually no isotope uptake and the diagnosis of factitious thyrotoxicosis can be confirmed by measuring serum thyroglobulin levels, which are suppressed in contrast to the raised levels in all other causes of thyrotoxicosis. When a TSH-secreting pituitary adenoma is suggested biochemically, the diagnosis is made by demonstrating both an elevated level of the α-subunit common to glycoprotein hormones including TSH and a pituitary tumour on CT, or preferably MRI. Prolonged thyrotoxicosis can cause several nonspecific biochemical abnormalities, especially abnormal liver function tests, hypercalciuria, and elevated serum levels of ferritin. Less commonly, serum calcium and phosphate may be raised, glucose intolerance or diabetes may occur, and rarely there may be a microcytic anaemia or thrombocytopenia.

Treatment

Definitive diagnosis is the most important determinant of treatment selection for thyrotoxicosis. In particular, antithyroid drugs only achieve a cure in Graves' disease. When due to a subacute or silent thyroiditis, discussed below, spontaneous resolution of thyrotoxicosis is expected and symptomatic treatment with β-blockers such as propranolol, 20 to 80 mg 3 times daily, is indicated. Although β-blockers will rapidly alleviate symptoms in all types of hyperthyroidism, definitive treatment is also necessary, and when euthyroidism is restored β-blockers can be gradually withdrawn.

There are three types of treatment for Graves' disease: antithyroid drugs, radio-iodine (^{131}I), and surgery. Local policy and patient age dictate the order of their use. For young or middle-aged adults, antithyroid drugs are generally used initially in Europe and Japan, whereas radio-iodine is preferred in North America. Surgery is particularly useful in patients with a large goitre, but is less frequently used in North America than elsewhere. The local

availability of an experienced surgeon is crucial. There is more international agreement over the preferential use of radio-iodine for a recurrence after antithyroid drugs and as first-line treatment in older people with Graves' disease.

The main antithyroid drugs used in Europe are carbimazole and its active metabolite methimazole, whereas propylthiouracil is preferred in North America. There is little to choose between them in normal practice, as all exert their principal action by inhibiting iodide oxidation and organification by thyroid peroxidase. Propylthiouracil additionally inhibits the activity of type I deiodinase, reducing T_3 formation in many tissues, but this activity is only of clinical importance in very severe hyperthyroidism, and more frequent dosing is necessary with this drug.

Two regimens are used to avoid antithyroid drug-induced hypothyroidism and achieve the best chance of remission, which occurs in 40 to 60% of patients and is inversely proportional to dietary iodine intake. The first method is to titrate the dose of antithyroid drug, giving carbimazole (or methimazole) 20 mg 2 or 3 times daily, and then lowering the dose every 3 to 4 weeks or so, based on free T_4 measurements, until a maintenance dose of 5 to 10 mg once daily is achieved. Equivalent starting and maintenance doses of propylthiouracil are 100 to 200 mg 3 times daily and 50 mg once or twice daily. Maximum remission rates occur after 18 to 24 months of treatment.

The second regimen is to start with the same dose of antithyroid drug but then to add 100 μg T_4 daily after 3 to 4 weeks when free T_4 levels are usually becoming normal, rather than lowering the dose of drug. Thereafter the patient is maintained on 40 mg carbimazole or methimazole once daily (alternatively, 100 to 150 mg propylthiouracil 3 times daily) and T_4, the latter being adjusted if necessary 4 weeks after starting to achieve normal free T_4 levels. The block–replace regimen achieves the same remission rate as the titration regimen within 6 months; continuation beyond this time is not necessary but can be used if a patient wishes to ensure euthyroidism for a particular period of time. Patients with the biggest goitres almost always relapse after antithyroid drug treatment, but unfortunately there are no reliable predictors of which other patients will relapse and therefore it is usual practice to follow patients closely (e.g. every 3 months) in the first year after stopping treatment. Thereafter, an annual check of thyroid function is warranted as recurrence occurs in 10 to 20% 1 to 5 years after treatment, and autoimmune hypothyroidism may supervene in around 15%.

The side effects of antithyroid drugs are shown in Box 13.4.9; most occur in the first 3 months of treatment and there is a moderate dose dependency. Substituting propylthiouracil for carbimazole or vice versa usually reverses the common side effects but further antithyroid drugs should be avoided if bone marrow disturbance develops. Lower doses of antithyroid drugs can be used in areas of low iodine intake. Lithium and potassium perchlorate have antithyroid actions and are alternatives when antithyroid drugs are not tolerated, but these drugs are difficult to use, their side effects are serious, and they are given as a last resort. Anticoagulation with warfarin should be considered in all patients with atrial fibrillation; only 50% of patients revert to sinus rhythm when euthyroidism is restored. In the remainder, attempts at cardioversion should be made, ideally when hyperthyroidism has been definitively treated with radio-iodine. Digoxin is useful to control atrial fibrillation acutely but higher doses than normal are needed in the thyrotoxic state.

<table>
<tr><td>

Box 13.4.9 Side effects of antithyroid drugs

Common

Rash (typically maculopapular)

Urticaria

Arthralgia

Fever, sometimes with malaise

Rare

Gastrointestinal symptoms

Abnormal taste and smell

Arthritis

Agranulocytosis[a]

Very rare

Thrombocytopenia

Aplastic anaemia

Hepatitis

Lupus-like syndrome, vasculitis

Hypoglycaemia due to the insulin autoimmune syndrome

[a] All patients must be warned in writing, before treatment commences, to seek medical advice and stop medication if features suggesting agranulocytosis (fever, mouth ulcers, sore throat) develop.

</td></tr>
</table>

Accurate dosimetry for radio-iodine administration, based on uptake tests, has now largely fallen out of favour as the results have been little or no better than more empirical methods of dose calculation. Typical ^{131}I doses are 400 to 600 MBq in uncomplicated Graves' disease, but local policies vary, not least because less ^{131}I is needed when iodine intake is low. Around 5 to 10% of patients treated this way require a second dose of ^{131}I, while hypothyroidism rates are 10 to 20% after 1 year and 5 to 10% annually thereafter. Close follow-up is needed in the first year after treatment, and an annual test of thyroid function thereafter is recommended. Transient cytoplasmic, rather than nuclear, damage may cause hypothyroidism in the first 2 to 3 months after ^{131}I treatment, which then resolves. It is usual to delay a second dose of ^{131}I for at least 4 to 6 months after the first, as hyperthyroidism is controlled only slowly by radiation-induced nuclear damage. Antithyroid drugs or β-blockers are useful in the interim.

Radio-iodine is contraindicated in pregnancy and breastfeeding. There are no teratogenic risks if men or women attempt conception 6 months or more after treatment. Overall mortality rates from cancer are not increased by radio-iodine, although there is a theoretical risk of an increase in the frequency and aggressiveness of thyroid cancer in children and adolescents, which makes many endocrinologists reluctant to use ^{131}I in this group, unless other treatments fail or are rejected. Another concern is the precipitation of thyrotoxic crisis by ^{131}I, but in practice this must be rare. To minimize the risk, antithyroid drugs can be given for up to 4 weeks or more prior to radio-iodine, particularly in older people who are at special risk. Thyroid-associated ophthalmopathy may appear or worsen after radio-iodine, especially if the patient smokes. A 3-month tapering course of prednisolone, starting with 40 mg

daily at the time of ^{131}I administration, will prevent such worsening but an extended course of antithyroid drugs, with scrupulous maintenance of euthyroidism, may well be preferable until the orbital disease becomes inactive.

Surgery for Graves' disease consists of subtotal or near total thyroidectomy, and in the best centres achieves cure in more than 98% of patients but with a hypothyroidism rate similar to radio-iodine. Lower rates of hypothyroidism are inevitably associated with a higher recurrence rate. Patient preference is the main determinant of when surgical treatment is used to treat relapses after antithyroid drugs. Euthyroidism must be achieved with a further course of these drugs prior to surgery to avoid thyrotoxic crisis. Stable iodine (e.g. Lugol's iodine three drops 3 times daily) is often also given for 7 to 10 days prior to surgery to block hormone synthesis acutely. Specific complications of surgery include haemorrhage leading to laryngeal oedema, damage to the recurrent laryngeal nerves, and hypoparathyroidism. These problems occur in less than 1% of patients in experienced hands and the last two problems are often transient.

The management of thyroid-associated ophthalmopathy is summarized in Box 13.4.10. Symptoms and signs are usually mild to moderate, although still capable of creating considerable anxiety and disturbance of social function. Severe ophthalmopathy is fortunately rare (1–5% of cases) and requires specialist ophthalmological management. Signs usually stabilize 12 to 18 months after onset, and may improve thereafter in 30 to 50% of patients, although improvement is less likely for marked proptosis

<table>
<tr><td>

Box 13.4.10 Treatment of thyroid-associated ophthalmopathy

Mild to moderate disease

Reassurance and explanation

Avoid hypothyroidism and hyperthyroidism

Stop smoking

Protect eyes from dust and bright light

Artificial tears; simple eye ointment at night

Sleep with more pillows or the head of the bed elevated

Diuretics

Stick-on prisms

Severe disease (worsening diplopia, exposure keratitis, sight loss)

Corticosteroids (e.g. prednisolone 40–80 mg daily, tapered over >3 months)

Radiotherapy (10 fractionated doses of 2 Gy)

Immunosuppressive agents (azathioprine, cyclosporin A)

Intravenous immunoglobulin

Orbital decompression (usually transantral)

Stable, burnt-out disease

Prisms

Surgery to extraocular muscle

Cosmetic eyelid surgery

</td></tr>
</table>

or diplopia. Corrective surgery for diplopia or cosmetic problems should only be considered in this stable phase. Thyroid dermopathy is left untreated and may resolve spontaneously. Surgical removal usually worsens the situation and, when troublesome, the best treatment is topical, high-potency corticosteroids.

Toxic multinodular goitre is usually managed by radio-iodine treatment. Antithyroid drugs will control the hyperthyroidism but relapse is inevitable when the drugs are stopped. Long-term use of antithyroid drugs may be indicated in the very old or frail, or when incontinence poses an insuperable problem for the safe disposal of excreta after ^{131}I. The therapeutic dose of ^{131}I used for toxic multinodular goitre is generally higher than for Graves' disease (500–800 MBq) because there is uneven uptake of the isotope and usually a large goitre. Surgery is sometimes used as an alternative in patients with a retrosternal goitre or if there is any suspicion of a malignancy. Toxic adenoma is also usually treated with ^{131}I and the rate of subsequent hypothyroidism is low because the function of the normal thyroid tissue is suppressed at the time the patient is hyperthyroid and therefore receives little irradiation. When there is a large (>5 cm) nodule or in young patients (<20 years) surgical excision is preferable and subsequent hypothyroidism is uncommon. Treatment of rare forms of primary hyperthyroidism is by surgical removal of the source of thyroid hormone or by radio-iodine. TSH-secreting pituitary adenomas causing secondary hyperthyroidism are usually treated by trans-sphenoidal surgery, with radiotherapy for any residual tumour. Octreotide can also be used to lower TSH secretion.

Thyrotoxic crisis is a medical emergency (Box 13.4.11).

Prognosis

Although spontaneous remission occurs in Graves' disease, its exact frequency is unknown and is unlikely to be more than 10%, with no guarantee of persistence. Remission does not occur in other types of hyperthyroidism. Mortality rates in untreated hyperthyroidism are also uncertain but are probably around 30%. Even after successful treatment, there is a threefold increased risk of death from osteoporotic fracture and a 1.3-fold increased risk of death from cardiovascular disease and stroke. It is important that the patient with Graves' disease understands that the course of ophthalmopathy is independent of the thyroid disorder; eye signs appear 1 or more years before or after the onset of hyperthyroidism in one-quarter of patients and progression of the orbital disease frequently occurs despite restoration of euthyroidism.

Special problems in pregnant women

Graves' disease during pregnancy is often treated with propylthiouracil, as carbimazole and methimazole have been associated with fetal aplasia cutis, but some dispute the significance of this association. The block–replace regimen is contraindicated in pregnancy, as preferential placental transfer of antithyroid drug will cause fetal hypothyroidism. Instead, the dose of antithyroid drug should be titrated to the lowest dose that results in maternal free T_4 levels in the upper part of the reference range. TSH receptor stimulating antibodies decline during pregnancy and it is usually possible to stop treatment at the beginning of the third trimester. Subtotal thyroidectomy can be performed in the second trimester for women intolerant of antithyroid drugs.

Transplacental passage of TSH receptor antibodies causes fetal and neonatal thyrotoxicosis in 1 to 5% of mothers with Graves'

Box 13.4.11 Treatment of thyrotoxic crisis ('thyroid storm')

♦ Antithyroid treatment

· Propylthiouracil 600 mg as a loading dose; then 250 mg every 6 h, given orally, by nasogastric tube, or per rectum

· Stable iodine given 1 h after starting propylthiouracil (e.g. Lugol's iodine five drops every 6 h; ipodate 500 mg every 12 h is an alternative with additional deiodinase blocking activity

· Propranolol 40 mg orally or 2 mg intravenously every 4 h to control heart rate; careful monitoring necessary in heart failure

· Severe cases may respond to plasmapheresis or dialysis

♦ Supportive treatment

· Oxygen

· External cooling

· Intravenous saline

· Dexamethasone 2 mg every 6 h

· Diuretics and digoxin for heart failure

♦ Identify and treat underlying precipitant (including trauma, infection, diabetic ketoacidosis, and myocardial infarction)

· Broad-spectrum antibiotics if infection suspected

---

disease and can be predicted by demonstrating a high level of these antibodies in the maternal circulation at the beginning of the third trimester. Poor intrauterine growth and a high fetal heart rate also suggest this diagnosis. Fetal thyrotoxicosis is treated by giving the mother antithyroid drugs and the neonate requires treatment for 1 to 3 months after delivery. Failure to treat intrauterine and neonatal thyrotoxicosis causes low birth weight, premature closure of the sutures, and intellectual impairment. Breastfeeding is safe with low doses of antithyroid drugs, but when high doses are needed (e.g. 20 mg or more carbimazole daily) thyroid function should be checked every 1 to 2 weeks in the baby. Patients with Graves' disease who have entered remission prior to or during pregnancy have an increased risk of relapse around 3 to 6 months after delivery and should be offered thyroid function testing at this time.

Areas of uncertainty or needing further research

The pathogenesis of thyroid-associated ophthalmopathy is poorly understood, and this remains an obstacle to developing better treatments. Outcome after antithyroid drug treatment in Graves' disease cannot yet be predicted, but improved assays for TSH receptor antibodies may permit better assessment in the near future. Antithyroid drugs modulate the autoimmune response favourably in those patients whose Graves' disease remits, indicating the potential for more specific immunotherapy aimed at the cause of the disease, which would be preferential to present treatments which merely block or destroy the thyroid.

The evolution of hyperthyroidism is gradual and patients with multinodular goitre in particular are now recognized at the stage of subclinical hyperthyroidism, i.e. with a low or suppressed TSH but normal free T_3 and T_4 levels. Their optimum management is uncertain. There is a twofold to threefold increased risk of atrial fibrillation over 10 years in subclinical thyrotoxicosis, as well as deleterious effects on bone mineral density, but no clinical trials have been performed to show a clear benefit from early intervention. Many endocrinologists simply follow such patients carefully, electing to treat when overt hyperthyroidism is shown by an abnormal free T_3 level (T_3 usually increases before T_4). However, in older patients with known cardiac disease there is an increasing tendency to use radio-iodine for sustained subclinical hyperthyroidism.

Destructive thyroiditis

Acute thyroiditis is rare and is usually caused by bacterial infection of the thyroid via a pyriform sinus connecting the gland with the oropharynx. There is severe thyroid pain with fever and malaise, but thyroid function is rarely disturbed. Diagnosis is made by fine needle aspiration biopsy with culture of the specimen, and treatment consists of antibiotics, surgical drainage of any abscess, and excision of the sinus which is identified by barium swallow.

Subacute (or de Quervain's) thyroiditis is due to thyroid infection by any of several viruses, especially mumps, Coxsackie, influenza, adenoviruses, and echoviruses. The most prominent symptom is pain in the thyroid, often radiating to the ears. A small, tender goitre can be palpated which is usually diffuse, but there can be asymmetrical involvement. Systemic upset with fever is variable but sometimes profound, and symptoms of a prodromal viral infection several weeks earlier may be recalled. There is a granulomatous thyroid inflammation with follicular destruction and the release of thyroid hormones often results in a transient thyrotoxicosis lasting 1 to 4 weeks. Continuing thyroid destruction then leads to a phase of hypothyroidism once stored hormone is depleted. This lasts 4 to 12 weeks before euthyroidism is restored, but relapses occur in 10 to 20% of patients. Sometimes only one phase of thyroid disturbance is seen. Confirmation of the clinical diagnosis is made by finding an elevated erythrocyte sedimentation rate and low or absent radio-iodine uptake by the thyroid. Thyroid function requires continuous monitoring as the disease evolves. Mild cases may resolve spontaneously with paracetamol or a nonsteroidal anti-inflammatory drug as symptomatic treatment, but most patients benefit from prednisolone 40 to 60 mg daily as this rapidly alleviates the pain. The dose is tapered over 6 to 8 weeks depending largely on symptoms. Propranolol may be useful for thyrotoxic symptoms, and temporary T_4 replacement is sometimes needed during the hypothyroid phase.

Silent thyroiditis is an autoimmune disorder in which there is a transient but painless thyroid destruction, giving rise to the same kind of thyroid function disturbances as subacute thyroiditis. As well as the absence of thyroid pain, there is no sign of a systemic inflammatory response (including a normal erythrocyte sedimentation rate) and the two conditions are therefore readily distinguished. The commonest setting for silent thyroiditis is in the postpartum period in women with positive thyroid peroxidase antibodies and a mild underlying autoimmune thyroiditis, exacerbated for unknown reasons at this time. Such postpartum thyroiditis is common, being detectable in up to 5% of women 3 to 6 months after delivery when repeated biochemical testing is done, although in many of these women the changes in thyroid function are mild and asymptomatic. Postpartum thyroiditis is 3 times more common in type 1 diabetes. Thyroid uptake tests are useful in the postpartum period to distinguish thyrotoxicosis due to postpartum thyroiditis from Graves' disease. ^{99}Tcm pertechnetate is used in preference to ^{131}I and only requires cessation of breastfeeding for a day. Treatment is with propranolol for thyrotoxic symptoms and T_4 for hypothyroidism. As 90% of women recover normal thyroid function, T_4 should be withdrawn 1 year after delivery and thyroid function tested 6 weeks later. However, annual follow-up is needed as around 20% of these women have permanent hypothyroidism 5 years later. The condition usually recurs in subsequent pregnancies.

Amiodarone inhibits T_4 deiodination, and in all amiodarone-treated patients free T_4 levels are in the upper half of the reference range or mildly elevated. Several months to years after starting amiodarone, however, effects on the thyroid may become manifest. In patients with mild thyroid dysfunction, especially autoimmune thyroiditis and positive thyroid peroxidase antibodies, the excessive iodine released from the drug causes hypothyroidism. This is treated as usual with T_4. Paradoxically, the high level of iodine causes hyperthyroidism in other subjects who are predisposed to this because of an underlying multinodular goitre or incipient Graves' disease (Jod–Basedow phenomenon). This is called type 1 amiodarone-induced thyrotoxicosis; type 2 amiodarone-induced thyrotoxicosis is due to thyroid destruction via drug-induced lysosomal activation. Colour-flow Doppler thyroid scanning shows an increase in vascularity in type 1 but not type 2 amiodarone-induced thyrotoxicosis, but mixed forms sometimes make an exact diagnosis impossible.

Treatment of amiodarone-induced thyrotoxicosis can be difficult and biochemical changes are often out of proportion to the symptoms. Amiodarone should be stopped if possible, but often this cannot be done and in any case the drug has a very long half-life. An antithyroid drug alone can be very slow to take effect in type 1 amiodarone-induced thyrotoxicosis and potassium perchlorate may need to be added, 200 mg 4 or 5 times daily. There is a high frequency of agranulocytosis (up to 1%) with this drug. Prednisolone can also be used at doses of 40 to 60 mg daily and is particularly helpful in type 2 amiodarone-induced thyrotoxicosis. Thyroidectomy is another alternative in severe cases.

Thyroid hormone resistance syndrome

Mutations in one allele of the β thyroid hormone receptor gene (Fig. 13.4.4) cause thyroid hormone resistance (the homozygous mutation is lethal). The mutations affect the hormone binding domain and the mutant receptor inhibits the activity of normally encoded receptors, so-called dominant negative inhibition, resulting in an autosomal dominant pattern of inheritance. The condition is usually discovered during screening for a goitre, but children may sometimes present with short stature, hyperactivity, or mild learning difficulties. Thyrotoxic features in some patients were originally ascribed to selective pituitary resistance to thyroid hormone, leading to increased thyroid hormone secretion and therefore thyrotoxicosis in the peripheral tissues. However, the same receptor mutations occur in generalized and pituitary resistance syndromes, and although differential tissue expression of receptor subtypes presumably underlies the occasional expression of thyrotoxic signs and symptoms, the exact molecular basis is unknown.

The diagnosis is suggested by the presence of a normal or elevated TSH level with elevated free T_3 and T_4 levels. Nonspecific biochemical changes of thyrotoxicosis such as elevated ferritin, sex hormone binding globulin, and liver enzymes are absent. The main differential diagnosis is a TSH-secreting adenoma. Thyroid hormone resistance can be confirmed by direct mutational analysis. Treatment is usually not required as reducing thyroid hormone levels to normal causes hypothyroidism. If thyrotoxic symptoms do occur, treatment is with β-blockers or thyroid hormone analogues (e.g. tri-iodothyroacetic acid) aimed at lowering TSH secretion.

Further reading

Amino N, *et al.* (1999). Screening for postpartum thyroiditis. *J Clin Endocrinol Metab*, **84**, 1813–21.

Anonymous (2006). Hypothyroidism in the pregnant woman. *Drug Ther Bull*, **44**, 53–6.

Association for Clinical Biochemistry, British Thyroid Foundation, British Thyroid Association (2006). *UK guidelines for thyroid function tests*. http://www.british-thyroid-association.org/TFT_guidelines_consultation_10_05.pdf.

Bartalena L, Pinchera A, Marcocci C (2000). Management of Graves' ophthalmopathy. *Endocr Rev*, **21**, 168–99.

Basaria S, Cooper DS (2005). Amiodarone and the thyroid. *Am J Med*, **118**, 706–14.

Beck-Peccoz P (1996). Thyrotropin-secreting pituitary tumors. *Endocr Rev*, **17**, 610–38.

Bianco AC, *et al.* (2002). Biochemistry, cellular and molecular biology, and physiological roles of the iodothyronine selenodeiodinases. *Endocr Rev*, **23**, 38–89.

Boelaert K, Franklyn JA (2005). Thyroid hormone in health and disease. *J Endocrinol*, **187**, 1–15.

Brabant G, *et al.* (2006). Is there a need to redefine the upper normal limit of TSH?. *Eur J Endocrinol*, **154**, 633–7.

Braverman LE, Utiger RD (eds) (2005). *Werner and Ingbar's the thyroid*, 9th edition. Lippincott-Raven, Philadelphia.

Brix TH, Kyvik KO, Hegedüs L (1998). What is the evidence of genetic factors in the etiology of Graves' disease? A brief review. *Thyroid*, **8**, 727–32.

Cheng SY (2005). Thyroid hormone receptor mutations and disease: beyond thyroid hormone resistance. *Trends Endocrinol Metab*, **16**, 176–82.

Cooper DS (2003). Hyperthyroidism. *Lancet*, **362**, 459–68.

Davis PJ, Davis FB, Cody V (2005). Membrane receptors mediating thyroid hormone action. *Trends Endocrinol Metab*, **16**, 429–35.

De Felice M, Di Lauro R (2004). Thyroid development and its disorders: genetics and molecular mechanisms. *Endocr Rev*, **25**, 722–46.

DeGroot LJ, *et al.* (2006). *Thyroid disease manager*. www.thyroidmanager.org.

Demers LM, Spencer CA (2002). *Laboratory support for the diagnosis and monitoring of thyroid disease. NACB guidelines*. http://www.nacb.org/lmpg/thyroid_lmpg_pub.stm.

Dohan O, *et al.* (2003). The sodium/iodide symporter (NIS): characterization, regulation, and medical significance. *Endocr Rev*, **24**, 48–77.

Escobar-Morreale HF, *et al.* (2005). Treatment of hypothyroidism with combinations of levothyroxine plus liothyronine. *J Clin Endocrinol Metab*, **90**, 4946–54.

European Group on Graves' Orbitopathy (EUGOGO) (2006). Clinical assessment of patients with Graves' orbitopathy: the European Group on Graves' Orbitopathy recommendations to generalists, specialists and clinical researchers. *Eur J Endocrinol*, **155**, 387–9.

Friesema EC, *et al.* (2006). Mechanisms of disease: psychomotor retardation and high T3 levels caused by mutations in monocarboxylate transporter 8. *Nat Clin Pract Endocrinol Metab*, **2**, 512–23.

Hegedüs L, *et al.* (2003). Management of simple nodular goiter: current status and future perspectives. *Endocr Rev*, **24**, 102–32.

Houghton DJ, Gray HW, MacKenzie K (1998). The tender neck: thyroiditis or thyroid abscess?. *Clin Endocrinol*, **48**, 521–4.

Kahaly GJ, Dillmann WH (2005). Thyroid hormone action in the heart. *Endocr Rev*, **26**, 704–28.

Krohn K, *et al.* (2005). Molecular pathogenesis of euthyroid and toxic multinodular goiter. *Endocr Rev*, **26**, 504–24.

Kung AW (2006). Clinical review: thyrotoxic periodic paralysis: a diagnostic challenge. *J Clin Endocrinol Metab*, **91**, 2490–5.

Laurberg P, *et al.* (1998). Guidelines for TSH receptor antibody measurements in pregnancy: results of an evidence-based symposium organized by the European Thyroid Association. *Eur J Endocrinol*, **139**, 584–6.

Milas M, *et al.* (2005). Ultrasonography for the endocrine surgeon: a valuable clinical tool that enhances diagnostic and therapeutic outcomes. *Surgery*, **138**, 1193–200.

Murphy E, Williams GR (2004). The thyroid and the skeleton. *Clin Endocrinol (Oxf)*, **61**, 285–98.

Newman CM, *et al.* (1998). Amiodarone and the thyroid: a practical guide to the management of thyroid dysfunction induced by amiodarone therapy. *Heart*, **79**, 121–7.

Peeters RP, *et al.* (2006). Changes within the thyroid axis during critical illness. *Crit Care Clin*, **22**, 41–55.

Roberts CGP, Ladenson PW (2004). Hypothyroidism. *Lancet*, **363**, 793–803.

Rose SR, *et al.* (2006). Update of newborn screening and therapy for congenital hypothyroidism. *Pediatrics*, **117**, 2290–303.

Surks MI, *et al.* (2004). Subclinical thyroid disease: scientific review and guidelines for diagnosis and management. *JAMA*, **291**, 228–38.

Surks MI, *et al.* (2005). The thyrotropin reference range should remain unchanged. *J Clin Endocrinol Metab*, **90**, 5489–96.

Weetman AP (2000). Medical progress: Graves' disease. *N Engl J Med*, **343**, 1236–48.

Wiersinga WM, Bartalena L (2002). Epidemiology and prevention of Graves' ophthalmopathy. *Thyroid*, **12**, 855–60.

Thyroid cancer

Anthony P. Weetman

Essentials

Thyroid cancers account for less than 1% of all malignancies but are much the most frequent cancers of endocrine organs.

Follicular epithelial cell cancer—the commonest type; may be induced by exposure to radiation; can be highly undifferentiated or differentiate into recognizable follicular cells, sometimes with retention of hormone biosynthesis; typically present with an asymptomatic thyroid nodule; usually diagnosed by fine needle aspiration biopsy; treatment is typically by total or near total thyroidectomy, with radio-iodine then administered to remove any remaining thyroid tissue (followed by long-term thyroid replacement therapy).

Medullary thyroid carcinoma—arises from parafollicular C cells; comprise 5 to 10% of all thyroid cancers; hereditary autosomal dominant forms associated with germ-line point mutations in the *RET* proto-oncogene occur as part of multiple endocrine neoplasia

(MEN) type 2A or 2B, or as isolated familial medullary carcinoma; typically present with a solitary thyroid nodule, accompanied in 50% of cases by cervical lymphadenopathy; can be associated with unusual hormonal effects, including secretory diarrhoea; diagnosis often made by fine needle aspiration biopsy, also by finding raised serum calcitonin; treatment is by total thyroidectomy, followed by monitoring of serum calcitonin levels (and long-term thyroid replacement therapy); testing for the presence of *RET* mutations (see Chapter 13.10) allows family testing, with prophylactic thyroidectomy recommended for affected individuals.

Rare thyroid tumours—include (1) anaplastic carcinomas—present as a rapidly enlarging and fixed thyroid mass, sometimes with local pain; rapidly fatal; (2) sarcomas; and (3) primary lymphomas—usually present as a rapidly enlarging thyroid mass in a patient with Hashimoto's thyroiditis.

Primary thyroid follicular epithelial tumours (Table 13.5.1)

Aetiology

Excessive stimulation of the thyroid by thyroid-stimulating hormone (TSH) accounts for the higher proportion of follicular carcinomas compared with papillary carcinomas in iodine-deficient areas. The thyroid-stimulating antibodies of Graves' disease do not increase the risk of developing thyroid cancer, but incidental thyroid tumours that arise in this disorder may behave more aggressively because of activation of TSH receptors. Low-dose external beam radiation (10–1500 cGy) to the head and neck increases the risk of papillary thyroid cancer over 10 to 30 years. Higher thyroid radiation doses, including those arising from radio-iodine given for treatment of hyperthyroidism, are not associated with an increased risk of malignancy because thyroid cells are destroyed rather than transformed. However, death from thyroid cancer, which is an unusual outcome, may be slightly increased by radio-iodine treatment, suggesting an effect of radiation on tumour dedifferentiation. In Belarus the incidence of papillary carcinomas in children and young adults has increased 60-fold after the disastrous release of radio-iodine and other radionuclides

from the Chernobyl nuclear reactor. The increase has been greatest in those aged less than 4 years at the time of exposure and is due to the potent mutagenic effects of radio-iodine on the growing thyroid gland.

Familial forms of papillary and follicular carcinomas exist but are unusual (less than 5% of cases). There are also associations with familial adenomatosis polyposis, including the Gardner syndrome variant (OMIM 175100), Cowden's disease (multiple hamartoma syndrome, OMIM 158350), Peutz–Jeghers syndrome (OMIM 175200), the Carney complex (OMIM 160980), and ataxia–telangiectasia (OMIM 208900).

Papillary carcinomas do not arise from hyperplastic nodules or adenomas. In about one-third of these tumours one of several distinct rearrangements of the *RET* proto-oncogene, a member of the receptor tyrosine kinase family, occurs. The resulting chimeric oncogenes are termed *RET/PTC* (for papillary thyroid carcinoma). *RET/PTC3* is particularly linked to radiation. Around 40% of papillary carcinomas have mutations in the *BRAF* gene which encodes a serine–threonine kinase, and these tumours tend to be more aggressive and present more often with extrathyroidal invasion. Less than 10% of papillary carcinomas have mutations in the *NTRK1* oncogene.

Table 13.5.1 Classification of thyroid malignancies

Primary thyroid follicular epithelial tumours	Differentiated (papillary, follicular)
	Poorly differentiated (insular, other)
	Undifferentiated (anaplastic)
C cell epithelial tumours (medullary carcinoma)	
Primary nonepithelial tumours	Lymphoid origin (lymphoma, plasmacytoma)
	Mesenchymal cell origin (sarcoma)
	Other (teratoma)
Secondary nonthyroidal tumours	Metastases
	Extension of tumour from adjacent structures

Follicular carcinomas probably arise, at least in some cases, from follicular adenomas. Activation of the *RAS* oncogene occurs in both these tumours (and in some papillary thyroid cancers) and they share cytogenetic abnormalities, especially on chromosome 3. Rarely follicular carcinomas are associated with activating mutations of the genes encoding the TSH receptor or $G_s\alpha$ protein, similar to those found in toxic adenoma. Anaplastic carcinoma may arise in a papillary or follicular carcinoma and is associated with inactivating mutations of the p53 tumour suppressor gene.

Epidemiology

Papillary microcarcinomas are tumours less than 1 cm in diameter that occur in up to 36% of autopsy specimens and up to 24% of surgical thyroidectomies. Clearly most of these do not become malignant. Excluding tumours that are found coincidentally, the annual incidence of thyroid follicular epithelial cancer is around 4 per 100 000. In iodine-sufficient countries, more than 80% of these are papillary carcinoma, about 10% are follicular carcinoma, and 5 to 10% are anaplastic carcinoma. Women are 2 to 4 times more likely to develop thyroid cancer than men, and the peak incidence is between 30 and 50 years of age.

Clinical features

Most patients present with an asymptomatic thyroid nodule; this may be noticed by themselves or their relatives, or sometimes the nodule is detected during physical examination for another complaint. The difficulty for diagnosis arises because thyroid nodules are frequent, and only about 5% of palpable thyroid nodules are malignant. Diffuse or multinodular thyroid enlargement occurs in around 10% of the population and is 4 times more common in women than in men. Solitary thyroid nodules occur in up to 5% of the population and are usually hyperplastic or colloid nodules; 5 to 20% of them are neoplastic, but this figure includes follicular adenomas as well as malignant tumours.

It can be seen that determining which thyroid nodules are malignant poses a dilemma that has been exacerbated by the widespread use of ultrasound examination of the neck. Up to 60% of adult thyroids have nodules detectable by high-resolution ultrasound scanning. Another problem is determining which nodules warrant investigation in a multinodular goitre. It seems reasonable to perform fine needle aspiration biopsy of so-called dominant nodules, as well as those nodules in which there are any suspicious ultrasonographic features (microcalcification, hypoechogenicity, and nodular hypervascularity) and any nodules that have demonstrated recent change in size.

There are usually no symptoms or signs to indicate that a solitary thyroid nodule is malignant because most tumours progress slowly and present before disease is advanced. Age and sex are important considerations, since a malignancy is more likely in a solitary nodule when the patient is a child or an adolescent, is over 60 years old, or is a man between the ages of 20 and 60 years. Previous exposure to radiation and a family history of thyroid cancer should also arouse suspicion. A carcinoma is more likely if the nodule has grown recently or is hard, irregular, or fixed on palpation. Clinical assessment should include careful examination of the cervical, submental, and supraclavicular lymph nodes. Late-presenting features include hoarseness, dysphagia, or dyspnoea which may indicate local invasion, but these symptoms can occasionally occur with an enlarging benign goitre. Rarely the diagnosis only becomes apparent when metastatic disease is detected in bone or lung.

The relatively indolent presentation of papillary and follicular thyroid carcinoma contrasts with that of anaplastic carcinoma in which a rapidly enlarging and fixed thyroid mass occurs, sometimes with local pain. Extension to the oesophagus, trachea, and/or recurrent laryngeal nerves is frequent, and the overlying skin may also be infiltrated.

Pathology

There are several variants of papillary thyroid carcinoma united by their characteristic cytological features. The nuclei are large, clear ('Orphan Annie', after the eyes of the cartoon character), and have longitudinal grooves and invaginations of cytoplasm (Fig. 13.5.1a). Two-thirds of tumours are unencapsulated and display papillary and follicular structures; the remainder are the encapsulated, follicular, tall cell, sclerosing, and clear cell variants.

The encapsulated variant has a better than average prognosis and the tall cell variant a worse prognosis. One-half of papillary carcinomas contain degenerate calcified papillae, termed psammoma bodies. The tumour is multicentric in up to 80% of cases if the resected thyroid is examined carefully. Metastasis is via the lymphatics, and local lymph nodes are infiltrated in 40 to 50% of cases (more in young patients). Distant metastases are found in less than 5% of patients at presentation, with the lung being the most common site.

Follicular carcinoma is characterized by follicular differentiation with a solid growth pattern and without the nuclear features of papillary carcinoma. The tumour is encapsulated, but there is invasion of the capsule and vessels (Fig. 13.5.1b). This invasion is the crucial feature which distinguishes follicular carcinoma from follicular adenoma, self-evidently a distinction only possible by histological examination. Minimally and widely invasive subtypes are recognized, the latter having a worse prognosis. When 75% or more of the tumour cells exhibit oxyphilic staining due to mitochondrial accumulation, it is called a Hürthle (or oncocytic) cell carcinoma, which probably also has a worse prognosis. Lymph node metastases are unusual, as is multicentricity in the thyroid. Metastasis occurs via the bloodstream, typically to bone and lungs.

When follicular differentiation is poor or absent, the tumour is classified as an insular carcinoma with a poor prognosis. In anaplastic

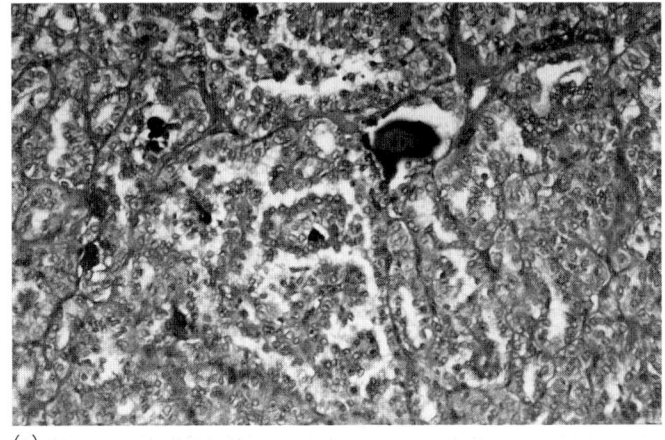

(a)

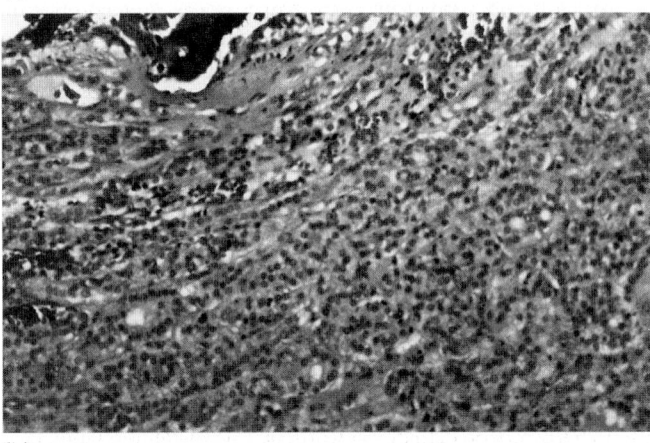

(b)

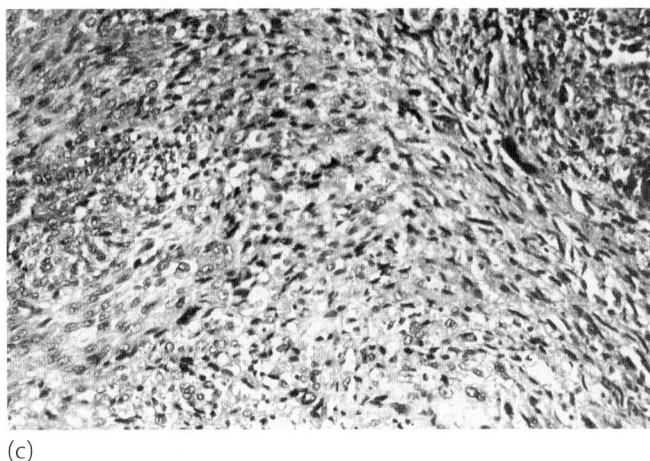

(c)

Fig. 13.5.1 Histopathological features of thyroid follicular epithelial carcinoma. (a) Papillary carcinoma, with psammoma bodies and typical nuclear appearance. (b) Metastatic follicular carcinoma, eroding vertebral bone. (c) Anaplastic carcinoma showing pleomorphic spindle cells. All sections, original magnification ×200. (Photomicrographs by courtesy of Dr K. Suvarna.)

carcinoma there is no capsule, the cells are atypical, including spindle, multinuclear, and squamoid forms, and mitoses are frequent (Fig. 13.5.1c).

Diagnosis

Thyroid epithelial cancers generally fail to affect thyroid function. However, this should be evaluated in all patients presenting with a thyroid nodule; a low circulating level of TSH strongly suggests an autonomous benign nodule. Anaplastic carcinoma may occasionally cause hypothyroidism, but the most frequent cause of an elevated level of TSH with a hard, nodular thyroid is Hashimoto's thyroiditis (OMIM 140300). Some of the glands in these cases are so irregular that a malignancy may be suspected. There is no increased or decreased risk of thyroid epithelial carcinoma in Hashimoto's thyroiditis, but thyroid lymphoma almost always occurs in association with autoimmune thyroiditis. Therefore, any dominant or atypical area in a Hashimoto's goitre requires careful evaluation. Thyroid peroxidase and/or thyroglobulin antibodies occur in about one-quarter of patients with thyroid follicular epithelial carcinoma, coincident with the presence of a lymphocytic infiltrate which, in turn, is associated with a slightly more favourable prognosis. Although the serum thyroglobulin concentration is extremely useful in follow-up, as discussed below, this investigation is useless in diagnosis; levels may not be elevated with some cancers and, even when elevated, cannot be causally distinguished from those that occur in benign adenoma, multinodular goitre, Graves' disease (OMIM 275000), or destructive thyroiditis.

Neither radionuclide nor ultrasound imaging is able to diagnose malignancy accurately. Radionuclide scanning can be performed with ^{99}Tcm pertechnetate or radio-iodine (^{123}I or ^{131}I), with similar information being obtained from either nuclide. Most thyroid cancers fail to take up radionuclide ('cold' nodules), but the more frequent benign lesions such as colloid nodules, cysts, adenomas, and thyroiditis behave similarly. About 20% of nodules have normal or increased radionuclide uptake. Malignancy cannot be excluded with these appearances, however. The only exception is when the nodule is 'hot' and the surrounding thyroid tissue fails to take up radionuclide, indicating the presence of a toxic adenoma which is almost invariably benign. This type of nodule will cause suppression of TSH and will be suspected from routine testing of thyroid function. In summary, radionuclide scanning usually adds little to the diagnosis.

The role of ultrasonography is more controversial but it is increasingly being used in the initial evaluation. Predicting the presence of malignancy based on the echo pattern of the tumour, and more recently using colour-flow Doppler imaging, may be successful in up to 80% of cases, but this depends on the operator having considerable experience. As well as the poor specificity of ultrasonography, the technique is so sensitive that many small unsuspected nodules will be uncovered, complicating the evaluation. Ultrasonography is useful for accurate measurement of thyroid and nodule size, which can be helpful in monitoring patients, for detecting lymphadenopathy, and for guiding biopsy, although this procedure is usually performed without imaging.

Fine needle aspiration biopsy is undoubtedly the current technique of choice for investigation of a thyroid nodule. Local anaesthetic is not needed because the procedure causes little discomfort. It is usual to take two to six biopsies to increase the sample yield. Essentially three diagnoses are possible: benign (65–75% of specimens), malignant (5%), and indeterminate (20–30%), but an experienced cytopathologist is needed to obtain reliable results. Papillary carcinoma is readily diagnosed by fine-needle aspiration biopsy, and medullary carcinoma and lymphoma can also be detected by the use of immunohistochemical staining, although lymphoma frequently requires core or open biopsy for confirmation.

Follicular carcinomas cannot be distinguished cytologically from follicular adenomas, and these tumours account for the bulk of needle aspiration specimens labelled indeterminate (or suspicious). Open biopsy is the only secure diagnostic method in this setting. About 15% of biopsies reported in experienced centres are considered unsuitable for diagnosis. It is relatively simple to repeat the biopsy, but a persistently equivocal biopsy should be grounds for considering surgery since malignant tumours will be found in about one-half of these cases. A cyst may be aspirated during biopsy. If this fails to reaccumulate and no lesion remains palpable, a malignancy is highly unlikely, but recurrence of a cyst may indicate malignant disease and require surgery for definitive diagnosis. Overall, the sensitivity and specificity of fine-needle aspiration biopsy is greater than 90%.

Treatment

Surgical excision

A total or near total thyroidectomy should usually be performed since thyroid carcinomas are often bilateral and removal of thyroid tissue facilitates subsequent ablation by radio-iodine. Unilateral total lobectomy is indicated for microcarcinoma. In papillary carcinoma, the central lymph nodes should be dissected, as should all palpable nodes. Central lymph node removal is also indicated in follicular carcinoma with histological evidence of extrathyroidal spread.

Radio-iodine therapy

After surgery, radio-iodine is usually administered to remove any remaining thyroid tissue, which then allows thyroglobulin or ^{131}I total body scanning to be used in follow-up to detect metastases. This treatment also destroys occult carcinoma and, by scanning after ablation, metastatic disease is revealed. Local policies vary, but in most centres an ^{131}I scan is performed 1 to 2 months after surgery and an ablation dose of 1100 to 3700 MBq ^{131}I is given, depending on the size of the remnant. In 15 to 30% of patients a second treatment dose of ^{131}I is necessary to achieve ablation. Iodine exposure, including iodine-containing contrast media, may prevent accumulation of ^{131}I during treatment. In patients whose tumour is less than 1.5 cm in diameter, excision alone without radio-iodine ablation is indicated. Whether all other patients require ablation is controversial, but there are persuasive arguments that low-risk patients with papillary carcinoma may not benefit from radio-iodine ablation and clinical staging scores (see below) may help to identify such patients.

High levels of stimulation by TSH are required to produce maximum uptake of ^{131}I; this is achieved by a period of 3 to 4 weeks without thyroxine replacement and can thus lead to the development of severe hypothyroid symptoms. The short action of tri-iodothyronine, 20 µg 3 times daily, as a replacement is therefore preferable in the weeks before scanning and ^{131}I treatment, because only 2 weeks are needed when this is stopped to increase endogenous TSH (which should be >30 mU/litre). Even this short period without thyroid hormone may be troublesome for the patient. Recombinant TSH suitable for intramuscular administration is now available and can be given without cessation of thyroid hormone replacement.

Long-term thyroid replacement therapy

The third aspect of treatment is to maintain the patient for life on thyroxine. This is given to high-risk patients at doses sufficient to suppress levels of TSH to below 0.1 mU/litre, because TSH is a growth factor for thyroid carcinoma. In almost all patients, satisfactory suppression of TSH can be achieved without inducing thyrotoxic symptoms. The effective thyroxine dosage is 2.2 to 2.8 µg/kg body weight. The optimum level of TSH is unknown, but higher levels of TSH (0.1–0.5 mU/litre) can be accepted in those low-risk patients known to be disease-free for several years.

Anaplastic carcinoma is rapidly fatal. The tumour does not take up radio-iodine. Surgery has a limited role in relieving obstructive symptoms, and external beam radiotherapy is useful in palliation. The place of chemotherapy (usually doxorubicin combined with other drugs) is unclear.

Follow-up

Lifelong follow-up is necessary for papillary and follicular cancer because they may recur many years after apparent cure. As well as monitoring the concentration of TSH and performing careful neck palpation, serum thyroglobulin should be measured. Detectable levels of thyroglobulin after thyroid ablation indicate persistent or recurrent disease. Measuring thyroglobulin levels is especially valuable when the patient is not taking thyroxine replacement or after recombinant TSH stimulation, as the rise in TSH will promote thyroglobulin production and exaggerate any increase. This is particularly useful in initial follow-up and in following high-risk patients; in those at low risk it is reasonable to measure thyroglobulin without withdrawing thyroxine.

If thyroglobulin is detectable, the patient should have a total body ^{131}I scan and any recurrent disease can then be treated with a therapeutic dose of 3700 to 5500 MBq ^{131}I. Many centres also perform a total body scan at 6 months after initial radio-iodine ablation, but repeated scans thereafter have now been superseded by measurement of thyroglobulin. The only exception is in the patient with thyroglobulin antibodies that interfere with many assays for thyroglobulin. If this is the case, repeated scans are the only way to ensure that the patient remains free of disease.

Ultrasonography is useful to confirm the presence of locoregional recurrence without distant metastases, and these tumour deposits are best dealt with surgically. For metastatic disease, usually in the lung, treatment with radio-iodine can be repeated every 4 to 6 months, but there is little benefit above a cumulative dose of 18 500 MBq. Bone metastases may respond to ^{131}I or external beam radiotherapy. The best survival in metastatic thyroid cancer occurs in young patients with small metastases, indicating the overall value of early treatment for this disease.

Prognosis

At least nine scoring systems have been advocated to assess prognosis in papillary and follicular carcinoma, of which the TNM classification system is now the most popular. These systems generally take into account the age and sex of the patient, tumour characteristics (especially size, extension, and metastases), and completeness of excision. An example of the predictive power of such scoring is shown in Box 13.5.1. The risk of death increases with age, especially after 60, while tumour recurrence is commonest in those aged under 20 and over 60. Men have a slightly worse prognosis than women.

With appropriate treatment the rate of recurrence of papillary carcinoma is about 15%, and the cause-specific death rate is approximately 5% at 20 years. In other words, 85% of these patients present with features of the group with the best prognosis, i.e. achieving a score of less than 6 in the system described in Table 13.5.2. In follicular carcinoma, the cause-specific survival rate is 80% at 20 years after treatment and 70% at 30 years. However, in the subgroup with metastases at presentation the

13.5 THYROID CANCER 1849

Box 13.5.1 The predictive value of a scoring system in determining outcome in papillary carcinoma

The scoring system is used to divide patients into four prognostic groups. The overall score is the sum of the following:

3.1 (if ≤39 years old) or 0.08 × patient age (if ≥40 years old)

0.3 × size of tumour in centimetres

1, if resection is incomplete

1, if there is extrathyroidal extension

3, if there are metastases

Score	20-year survival (%)
<6	99
6–6.99	89
7–7.99	56
≥8	24

Data from Hay ID, *et al.* (1993). Predicting outcome in papillary thyroid carcinoma: development of a reliable prognostic scoring system in a cohort of 1779 patients surgically treated at one institution during 1940 through 1989. *Surgery*, **114**, 1050–8.

10-year survival is only 20%. The median survival time for anaplastic carcinoma is 4 to 12 months and those with distant metastases at presentation have a median survival time of only 3 months.

Prevention

In the event of a nuclear accident, prompt administration of stable iodine prevents the uptake of inhaled and ingested radioactive iodine isotopes. Emergency arrangements should be in place close to nuclear installations to provide for distribution of potassium iodate tablets, and arrangements for the United Kingdom are detailed in the Department of Health document PL/CMO (1993) 1 (see 'Further reading').

Special problems in pregnancy

A solitary nodule in a pregnant woman should be evaluated by fine needle aspiration biopsy. If the biopsy suggests malignancy and the

nodule is growing significantly, surgery can be undertaken in the second trimester, but otherwise this is best deferred until after delivery. Women receiving radio-iodine ablation should avoid pregnancy and breast feeding for 6 to 12 months after treatment.

Medullary carcinoma of the thyroid (OMIM 155240)

This accounts for 5 to 10% of all thyroid cancers. About 80% are sporadic with a peak incidence at 40 to 50 years of age. Hereditary autosomal dominant forms occur as part of multiple endocrine neoplasia type 2A (MEN2A, OMIM 171400) or type 2B (MEN2B, OMIM 162300) or as isolated familial medullary carcinoma. These forms are associated with germ-line point mutations in the *RET* proto-oncogene (different from those in papillary carcinoma) and preneoplastic C-cell hyperplasia (Table 13.5.2).

The pathological findings are of an encapsulated tumour with round, spindle-shaped, or polyhedral cells arranged in a variety of patterns that have no prognostic significance. There is variable fibrosis and three-quarters of tumours show marked deposition of amyloid—a feature associated with a good prognosis. Heterogeneous staining for calcitonin, a hormone of C cells, is associated with a poorer outcome, reflecting dedifferentiation. Even the smallest medullary tumours may be associated with local lymph node metastases.

The presentation of sporadic medullary carcinoma is typically with a solitary thyroid nodule, accompanied by cervical lymphadenopathy in 50% of cases. Lung, liver, or bone metastases are present at diagnosis in 10% of cases. Symptoms due to local invasion or the paraneoplastic production of polypeptides and prostaglandins, such as flushing, diarrhoea, and Cushing's syndrome, are less common presenting features.

The diagnosis is often apparent from fine-needle aspiration biopsy. Basal serum calcitonin concentrations are almost invariably elevated and confirm the diagnosis. There is controversy over the utility of routine serum calcitonin measurement in the work-up of all thyroid nodules; most centres perform aspiration biopsy initially. Newly diagnosed patients should be screened for other evidence of MEN and a careful family history is also essential. In particular, phaeochromocytoma (OMIM 171300) occurring as part of an inherited cancer syndrome must be excluded before surgery.

Testing genomic DNA for *RET* mutations in the germ line is now widely available and should ideally be carried out on leucocyte DNA from all new patients. The absence of the most common mutations, coupled with a negative family history and the absence of C-cell hyperplasia or multicentric tumours in the resected thyroid, indicates that further family testing is not warranted. When a *RET* mutation is detected, there is a clear benefit from family testing, as prophylactic thyroidectomy in affected individuals improves outcome. However, there are some kindreds in whom familial medullary carcinoma occurs without a recognizable *RET* mutation and family screening must then be undertaken annually, up to the age of 35 to 40 years, using pentagastrin-stimulated serum calcitonin measurements as a guide to the presence of the inherited abnormality.

Medullary carcinoma should be treated by total thyroidectomy, with dissection of the central and other involved lymph nodes; this may require a second completion operation if the diagnosis is not

Table 13.5.2 Types of medullary carcinoma of the thyroid

Type	Frequency (%)	Associated lesions	RET gene mutation
Sporadic	80	None	Occasional somatic mutations in tumour tissue
MEN2A	10	Phaeochromocytoma, hyperparathyroidism	Germ line: codon 634, less commonly 609, 611, 618, 620
MEN2B	3	Phaeochromocytoma, mucosal neuromas, marfanoid habitus	Germ line: codon 918, less commonly 883
Familial medullary thyroid carcinoma	7	None	Usually germ-line mutation in codons 609, 611, 618, 620, or 634, or codons in exons 13, 14, and 15

MEN, multiple endocrine neoplasia.

made at the outset. Thyroxine replacement is needed at physiological doses rather than doses that suppress TSH. After surgery the patient should be monitored by measurement of serum calcitonin concentration. Cure, defined as a persistently normal calcitonin level, occurs in only about one-third of patients, but 80 to 90% of patients in whom there is an elevated calcitonin level and only nodal disease survive for 10 years. The best management of persistent disease is unclear, but local recurrence with identifiable lymph node involvement should be dealt with surgically. Radiotherapy and chemotherapy have a variable and at best partial effect. Profuse (secretory) watery diarrhoea is frequently a troublesome feature of extensive disease. This may respond to treatment with loperamide whereas somatostatin analogues have an inconsistent benefit.

Age, stage and size of tumour, and completeness of surgical removal are important prognostic features. Familial medullary carcinoma has the best outcome; in contrast, the tumour associated with MEN2B is very aggressive. The overall 10-year survival is around 70%, but is over 90% in those detected early by family screening.

Primary thyroid lymphoma

Less than 5% of thyroid malignancies are non-Hodgkin's B-cell lymphoma (OMIM 605027). The peak incidence is between 50 and 80 years of age, and women are affected 3 times more frequently than men. The typical presentation is a rapidly enlarging thyroid mass in a patient with Hashimoto's thyroiditis. The clinical features may suggest anaplastic carcinoma. The diagnosis can be made by fine-needle aspiration biopsy and confirmed by large-needle or open biopsy. Accurate staging is then necessary to plan treatment, which is with external beam radiotherapy and anthracycline-based chemotherapy. Intensive treatment has produced 8-year survival rates of over 90%.

Further reading

Al-Brahim N, Asa SL (2006). Papillary thyroid carcinoma: an overview. *Arch Pathol Lab Med*, **130**, 1057–62.

Braga-Basaria M, Ringel MD (2003). Beyond radioiodine: a review of potential new therapeutic approaches for thyroid cancer. *J Clin Endocrinol Metab*, **88**, 1947–60.

British Thyroid Association and the Royal College of Physicians of London (2002). *Guidelines for the management of thyroid cancer in adults*, pp. 1–70. Royal College of Physicians, London.

Cooper DS, *et al.* (2006). Management guidelines for patients with thyroid nodules and differentiated thyroid cancer. *Thyroid*, **16**, 1–33.

Department of Health (1993). *Potassium iodate (stable iodine) prophylaxis in the event of a nuclear accident*. PL/CMO(93) 1. Department of Health, London.

Diehl S, *et al.* (2005). Modern approaches to age-old questions about thyroid tumors. *Thyroid*, **15**, 575–82.

Hackshaw A, *et al.* (2007). [131]I activity for remnant ablation in patients with differentiated thyroid cancer: a systematic review. *J Clin Endocrinol Metab*, **92**, 28–38.

Hay ID (2006). Selective use of radioiodine in the postoperative management of patients with papillary and follicular thyroid carcinoma. *J Surg Oncol*, **94**, 692–700.

Kossev P, Livolsi V (1999). Lymphoid lesions of the thyroid: review in light of the revised European-American lymphoma classification and upcoming World Health Organization classification. *Thyroid*, **9**, 1273–80.

Leboulleux S, *et al.* (2004). Medullary thyroid carcinoma. *Clin Endocrinol (Oxf)*, **61**, 299–310.

Mazzaferri EL, *et al.* (2003). A consensus report of the role of serum thyroglobulin as a monitoring method for low-risk patients with papillary thyroid carcinoma. *J Clin Endocrinol Metab*, **88**, 1433–41.

Pacini F, *et al.* (2006). Radioiodine ablation of thyroid remnants after preparation with recombinant human thyrotropin in differentiated thyroid carcinoma: results of an international, randomized, controlled study. *J Clin Endocrinol Metab*, **91**, 26–32.

Pacini F, *et al.* (2006). European Thyroid Cancer Taskforce. European consensus for the management of patients with differentiated thyroid carcinoma of the follicular epithelium. *Eur J Endocrinol*, **154**, 787–803.

Sturgeon C, Clark O (2005). Familial nonmedullary thyroid cancer. *Thyroid*, **15**, 588–93.

Thieblemont C, *et al.* (2002). Primary thyroid lymphoma is a heterogeneous disease. *J Clin Endocrinol Metab*, **87**, 105–11.

13.6

Parathyroid disorders and diseases altering calcium metabolism

R.V. Thakker

Essentials

The control of body calcium involves a balance—chiefly under the control of parathyroid hormone (PTH)—between the amounts that are absorbed from the gut, deposited into bone and into cells, and excreted from the kidney. Under normal physiological circumstances PTH secretion from the parathyroid glands is increased by hypocalcaemia and diminished by hypercalcaemia.

Hypercalcaemia

Clinical presentation—this is very variable, ranging from a mild asymptomatic biochemical abnormality to (in extreme cases) a life-threatening medical emergency. Clinical manifestations can be renal (nephrocalcinosis, kidney stones), musculoskeletal (bone pain, muscular weakness), gastrointestinal (anorexia, nausea, vomiting, constipation, peptic ulceration, pancreatitis), neurological (depression, confusion, coma), and cardiac (arrhythmia).

Aetiology—primary hyperparathyroidism and malignancy account for >90% of patients with hypercalcaemia. Other causes include (1) excess vitamin D—exogenous or endogenous (e.g. granulomatous disorders); (2) drugs—e.g. thiazide diuretics, lithium, milk-alkali syndrome; (3) nonparathyroid endocrine disorders—e.g. thyrotoxicosis, immobilization; (4) inappropriate PTH levels due to altered set point—e.g. familial benign hypocalciuric hypercalcaemia.

Management—aside from appropriate treatment of the underlying condition, management of hypercalcaemia depends on its severity and the presence of symptoms. Asymptomatic patients with serum calcium less than 3.00 mmol/litre do not usually need urgent treatment. Patients with serum calcium below 3.50 mmol/litre, or above 3.00 mmol/litre with symptoms, require (1) vigorous hydration with 0.9% saline (assuming adequate renal function), with diuresis encouraged with a loop diuretic (e.g. furosemide) if necessary; (2) parenteral bisphosphonate (e.g. pamidronate, zoledronic acid); with (3) glucocorticoids—if the hypercalcaemia is mediated by the actions of 1,25-dihydroxy vitamin D, e.g. granulomatosis disease, lymphoma, myeloma; and in exceptional circumstances, (4) haemodialysis.

Specific diseases causing hypercalcaemia

Primary hyperparathyroidism—due to excessive secretion of PTH by parathyroid tumour(s); of unknown cause in most instances, but 10% of cases are associated with hereditary disorders, e.g. multiple endocrine neoplasia type 1 (MEN1, with combined occurrence of parathyroid, pancreatic islet cell and anterior pituitary tumours) and type 2 (MEN2, with association of medullary thyroid carcinoma, phaeochromocytoma and parathyroid tumours); biochemical diagnosis typically achieved by finding an elevated PTH concentration in the presence of hypercalcaemia; parathyroidectomy is the definitive cure, but cinacalcet—an allosteric activator of the calcium sensing receptor—can be effective.

Tertiary hyperparathyroidism—secondary hyperparathyroidism arises in the context of chronic kidney disease, but eventually the parathyroid cells become autonomous, secreting excessive PTH despite hypercalcaemia, which is known as tertiary hyperparathyroidism. See Chapter 21.6 for further discussion.

Malignancy—hypercalcaemia is usually due to increased bone resorption, which may either be directly due to skeletal metastases (most commonly from breast, lymphoma or multiple myeloma) or indirectly due to tumour-production of a humoral factor (usually parathyroid hormone related peptide, PTHrP, secreted from squamous carcinomas or other cancers) that stimulates osteoclastic bone resorption. Aside from measures described above, management involves reducing the tumour load by surgery, radiotherapy and/or chemotherapy.

Granulomatous disorders—hypercalcaemia is due to extrarenal synthesis of 1,25-dihydroxy vitamin D; most common diagnosis is sarcoidosis, when hypercalcaemia should respond within 10 days to treatment with glucocorticoids.

Familial benign hypocalciuric hypercalcaemia—autosomal dominant due to heterozygous inactivating mutation of the calcium sensing receptor; causes (usually) asymptomatic hypercalcaemia in association with an inappropriately low urinary calcium excretion and normal serum PTH.

Hypocalcaemia

Clinical presentation—this is variable, including (1) a mild, asymptomatic, biochemical abnormality; (2) in chronic cases with ectopic calcification, subcapsular cataract, papilloedema, and abnormal dentition; and (3) in severe cases with neuromuscular irritability.

Aetiology—may be associated with (1) low serum PTH—hypoparathyroidism, most often caused by autoimmune disease, surgical removal of the parathyroid glands, or hypomagnesaemia; or (2) high serum PTH—secondary hyperparathyroidism, most commonly due to vitamin D deficiency and/or renal failure.

Management—aside from appropriate treatment of the underlying condition, management of acute hypocalcaemia depends on its severity, rapidity of onset, and the degree of neuromuscular irritability. Patients with seizures or tetany may require intravenous calcium gluconate, as do asymptomatic patients with serum calcium below 1.90 mmol/litre as well as oral vitamin D.

Specific diseases causing hypocalcaemia

Pluriglandular autoimmune hypoparathyroidism—characterized by hypoparathyroidism, Addison's disease, and candidasis in the presence of other organ-specific autoimmune diseases; autosomal recessive inheritance due to mutation of an autoimmune regulator gene, with antibodies directed against the adrenal, thyroid, and parathyroid glands sometimes present.

Hypomagnesaemia—may be caused by malabsorption or renal tubular disorder; leads to functional hypoparathyroidism because magnesium is required for the release of PTH from the parathyroid gland and also for PTH action via adenyl cyclase.

A wide range of rare syndromes may cause hypoparathyroidism, and similar functional consequences can be caused by resistance to the effects of PTH, e.g. pseudohypoparathyroidism, of which there are five variants, some with somatic features such as shortening of one or more metacarpals.

Introduction

Calcium plays an important role in many physiological pathways that include muscle contraction, the secretion of neurotransmitters and hormones, and coagulation. The control of body calcium involves a balance between the amounts that are absorbed from the gut, deposited into bone and cells, and excreted from the kidney (Fig. 13.6.1). This fine balance, involving all these organs, is chiefly under the control of PTH, which is synthesized and secreted by the parathyroid glands. Thus, hypocalcaemia will lead to an increased secretion of PTH, whereas hypercalcaemia will result in diminished PTH secretion. Abnormalities of the parathyroid glands themselves will cause derangements of calcium homeostasis and several clinical disorders. PTH oversecretion due to parathyroid tumours, which affect 3 in 1000 of the population, is a major cause of hypercalcaemia which may be associated with kidney stones, osteoporosis, and peptic ulcers. PTH deficiency, which results in hypocalcaemia and occurs in 1 in 4000 live births, may be associated with epilepsy, tetany, cataracts, skeletal malformations, and abnormal dentition. This chapter will review the physiological and biochemical mechanisms underlying extracellular calcium homeostasis, the clinical features of hypercalcaemia and hypocalcaemia, the clinical disorders associated with abnormal calcium homeostasis and their management, and the genetic basis for disorders of calcium metabolism.

Historical perspective

The discovery of the parathyroids in the latter part of the 19th century and their function in regulating calcium homeostasis has evolved over 150 years and has involved studies in humans and other mammals (Table 13.6.1). In the past few decades with the advent of the advances in molecular biology, several cellular and molecular mechanisms involving G protein-coupled receptors, intracellular second messengers, and transcription factors have been shown to be involved in calcium homeostasis and in the aetiology of parathyroid disorders (Fig. 13.6.2). These advances have elucidated the roles of the parathyroids and PTH in regulating calcium. Moreover, these advances have helped in defining new

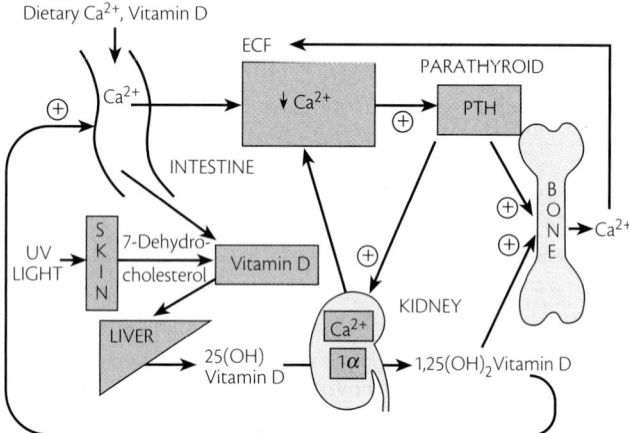

Fig. 13.6.1 Regulation of extracellular fluid (ECF) calcium (Ca^{2+}) by parathyroid hormone (PTH) action on kidney, bone, and intestine. A decrease in ECF Ca^{2+} is sensed by the calcium-sensing receptor (CaSR) (Fig. 13.6.2), and this leads to an increase in PTH secretion which predominantly acts directly on kidney and bone that possess the PTH receptor (PTHR, Fig. 13.6.2). The skeletal effects of PTH are to increase (+) osteoclastic bone reabsorption, but as osteoclasts do not have PTHRs, this action is mediated via the osteoblasts, which do have PTHRs and in response release cytokines and factors that activate osteoclasts. In the kidney, PTH stimulates (+) the 1α-hydroxylase (1α) to increase the conversion of 25-hydroxyvitamin D (25(OH)D) to the active metabolite 1,25-dihydroxyvitamin D (1,25(OH)$_2$D). In addition, PTH increases (+) the reabsorption of Ca^{2+} from the renal distal tubule and inhibits the reabsorption of phosphate from the proximal tubule, thereby leading to hypercalcaemia and hypophosphataemia. PTH also inhibits Na^+–H^+ antiporter activity and bicarbonate reabsorption, thereby causing a mild hyperchloraemic acidosis. The elevated 1,25(OH)$_2$D acts on the intestine to increase (+) absorption of dietary calcium and phosphate, and it is important to note that PTH does not appear to have a direct action on the gut. Thus, in response to hypocalcaemia and the increase in PTH secretion, all of these direct and indirect actions of PTH on the kidney, bone, and intestine will help to increase ECF Ca^{2+}, which in turn will act via the CaSR to decrease PTH secretion.

Table 13.6.1 Some historical landmarks elucidating the role of the parathyroids in calcium homeostasis

Date	Discovery
1852	Sir Richard Owen, curator of the Natural History Museum (London) discovers the parathyroids when dissecting a rhinoceros that had died in London Zoo
1880	Sandstrom, in Uppsala, describes parathyroids in man
1881	Weiss in Billroth's clinic (Vienna) reports tetany following thyroidectomy
1891	Gley shows that parathyroidectomy alone can cause tetany and death
1891	Von Recklinghausen reports first case of osteitis fibrosis cystica
1906	Erdheim describes parathyroid 'overgrowth' in calcium-deficient state of osteomalacia
1909	McCallum and Voegtlin demonstrate that postparathyroidectomy tetany and hypocalcaemia can be corrected by administration of parathyroid extract or calcium
1925	Collip establishes the role of parathyroids as endocrine glands that secrete PTH
1925	Mandl operates on a patient with severe bone demineralization and fractures and removes an enlarged parathyroid, resulting in a dramatic improvement of the patient's condition; this represents the first successful parathyroidectomy
1939	Drake et al. report six cases of idiopathic hypoparathyroidism
1942	Albright et al. report three cases of pseudohypoparathyroidism
1959	Aurbach, and Rasmussen and Craig independently isolate PTH
1978	Keutmann et al. report complete amino acid sequence of human PTH
1983	Vasicek et al. characterize nucleotide sequence of human PTH gene
1987	Mosely et al. Suva et al. and Strewler et al. independently identify PTHrP as the humoral factor causing the hypercalcaemia of malignancy
1991	Juppner et al. identify a G protein-coupled receptor that mediates actions of PTH and PTHrP
1993	Brown et al. identify the CaSR, a G protein-coupled receptor
2001	Neer et al. report that administration of PTH reduces the occurrence of osteoporotic vertebral and nonvertebral fractures in postmenopausal women
2004	Block et al. show that cinacalcet, a calcimimetic agent that acts on the CaSR, lowers PTH levels, and improves calcium and phosphate homeostasis in patients on dialysis and with uncontrolled secondary hyperparathyroidism
2005	Peacock et al. report that cinacalcet reduces serum calcium and PTH in patients with primary hyperparathyroidism, thereby providing a potential medical therapy for this condition

CaSR, calcium-sensing receptor; PTH, parathyroid hormone; PTHrP, parathyroid hormone-related peptide.

treatments for patients. For example, cinacalcet, which is an allosteric modulator of the calcium-sensing receptor (CaSR), is now used in the treatment of secondary hyperparathyroidism in dialysis patients with endstage renal disease and for the treatment of hypercalcaemia in parathyroid carcinoma, and PTH, which has been shown to reduce the incidence of vertebral and nonvertebral fractures, has now been approved as the first anabolic agent for the treatment of osteoporosis.

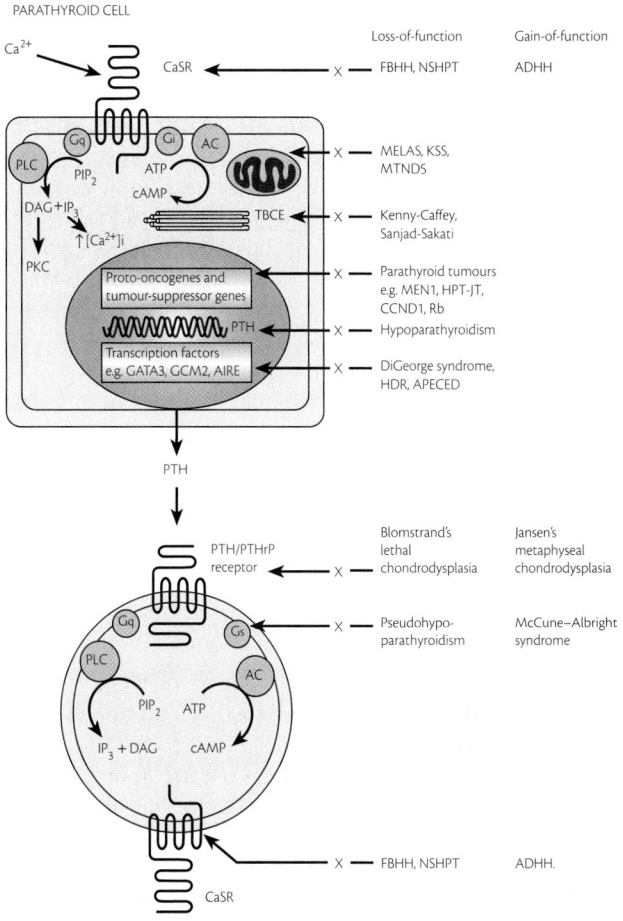

Fig. 13.6.2 Schematic representation of some of the components involved in calcium homeostasis. Alterations in extracellular calcium are detected by the calcium-sensing receptor (CaSR), which is a 1078 amino acid G protein-coupled receptor. The PTH/PTH-related peptide (PTHrP) receptor, which mediates the actions of PTH and PTHrP, is also a G protein-coupled receptor. Thus, Ca^{2+}, PTH, and PTHrP involve G protein-coupled signalling pathways, and interaction with their specific receptors can lead to activation of G_s, G_i, and G_q, respectively. G_s stimulates adenyl cyclase (AC) which catalyses the formation of cAMP from ATP. G_i inhibits AC activity. cAMP stimulates protein kinase A which phosphorylates cell-specific substrates. Activation of G_q stimulates phospholipase C (PLC), which catalyses the hydrolysis of the phosphoinositide (PIP_2) to inositol triphosphate (IP_3), which increases intracellular calcium, and diacylglycerol (DAG), which activates protein kinase C (PKC). These proximal signals modulate downstream pathways, which result in specific physiological effects. Abnormalities in several genes, which lead to mutations in proteins in these pathways, have been identified in specific disorders of calcium homeostasis (Table 13.6.1). ADHH, autosomal dominant hypocalcaemia with hypercalciuria syndrome; AIRE, autoimmune regulator protein; APECED, autoimmune polyendocrinopathy candidiasis ectodermal dystrophy syndrome; CCND1, cyclin D1; FBHH, familial benign hypocalciuric hypercalcaemia syndrome; GATA3, GATA binding protein 3; GCM2, glial cells missing homolog 2; HDR, hypoparathyroidism, deafness, and renal dysplasia syndrome; HPT-JT, hyperparathyroidism–jaw tumour syndrome; KSS, Kearns–Sayre syndrome; MELAS, mitochondrial encephalopathy, lactic acidosis, and stroke-like episodes; MEN1, multiple endocrine neoplasia type 1 syndrome; MT-ND5, mitochondrially encoded NADH dehydrogenase 5; NSHPT, neonatal severe primary hyperparathyroidism; Rb, retinoblastoma; TBCE, tubulin-specific chaperone.
(Adapted from Thakker RV (2000). Parathyroid disorders. Molecular genetics and physiology. In: Morris PJ, Wood WC (eds) *Oxford textbook of surgery*, 2nd edition, pp. 1121–9. Oxford University Press, Oxford.)

Calcium homeostasis

Most of the total of 1 kg of calcium in the healthy adult is present within the crystal structure of bone mineral and less than 1% is in soluble form in the extracellular and intracellular fluid compartments. In the extracellular fluid compartment about one-half of the total calcium is ionized and the rest is principally bound to albumin or complexed with counterions. Ionized calcium concentrations range from 1.17 to 1.33 mmol/litre, and the total serum calcium concentration ranges from 2.12 to 2.62 mmol/litre. Measurements of free ionized calcium are not often undertaken because they are difficult; most laboratories report total serum calcium concentration for routine clinical use. However, the usual 2:1 ratio of total to ionized calcium may be disturbed by disorders such as metabolic acidosis, which reduces calcium binding by proteins, or by changes in protein concentration caused by cirrhosis, dehydration, venous stasis, or multiple myeloma. In view of this, total serum concentrations are adjusted or 'corrected' to a reference albumin concentration; thus, the corrected serum calcium may be related to a reference albumin concentration of 41 g/litre and for every 1 g/litre of albumin above or below the reference value the calcium is adjusted by 0.016 mmol/litre up or down, respectively. For example, a total serum calcium of 2.70 mol/litre with an albumin concentration of 47 g/litre would be equivalent to a corrected serum calcium of 2.60 mmol/litre, thereby correcting the initial apparent hypercalcaemic value to a normal value.

The extracellular concentration of calcium is closely regulated within the narrow physiological range that is optimal for those cellular functions that are affected by calcium (Fig. 13.6.1). Indeed, both hypercalcaemia and hypocalcaemia impair the function of many different organ systems. Regulation of extracellular calcium takes place through complex interactions at the target organs of the major calcium-regulating hormone PTH (Fig. 13.6.2) and by vitamin D and its active metabolite 1,25-dihydroxyvitamin D. The parathyroid glands secrete PTH at a rate that is appropriate to and depending on the prevailing extracellular calcium ion concentration.

Aetiology and genetics

Parathyroid gland disorders cause either hypercalcaemia or hypocalcaemia, and these can be classified according to whether they arise from an excess of PTH, its deficiency, or an insensitivity to its effects (Table 13.6.2 and Fig. 13.6.2).

The PTH gene is located on chromosome 11p15 and consists of three exons (transcribed regions) which are separated by two introns. Exon 1 of the PTH gene is 85 bp in length and is untranslated whereas exons 2 and 3 code for the 115 amino acid pre-proPTH peptide. Exon 2 is 90 bp in length and encodes the initiation (ATG) codon, the prehormone sequence, and part of the prohormone sequence. Exon 3 is 612 bp in length and encodes the remainder of the prohormone sequence, the mature PTH peptide, and the 3' untranslated region. The 5' regulatory sequence of the human PTH gene contains a vitamin D response element 125 bp upstream of the transcription start site, which down-regulates PTH mRNA transcription in response to vitamin D receptor binding. PTH gene transcription (as well as PTH peptide secretion) is also dependent on the extracellular calcium concentration, although the presence of a specific upstream 'calcium response element' has not yet been demonstrated.

The mature PTH peptide is secreted from the parathyroid chief cell as an 84 amino acid peptide; however, when the PTH mRNA is first translated it is as pre-proPTH peptide. The 'pre' sequence consists of a 25 amino acid signal peptide (leader sequence) which is responsible for directing the nascent peptide into the endoplasmic reticulum to be packaged for secretion from the cell. The 'pro' sequence is 6 amino acids in length and, although its function is less well defined than that of the 'pre' sequence, it is also essential for correct PTH processing and secretion. After the 84 amino acid mature PTH peptide is secreted from the parathyroid cell, it is cleared from the circulation, with a short half-life of about 2 min, via nonsaturable hepatic uptake and renal excretion.

PTH shares a receptor with PTH-related peptide (PTHrP); this PTH/PTHrP receptor (Fig. 13.6.2) is a member of a subgroup of the G protein-coupled receptor family. The PTH/PTHrP receptor gene is located on chromosome 3p21–p24 and is expressed in kidney and bone, where PTH is its predominant agonist. Expression of the PTH/PTHrP receptor also occurs in the brain, heart, skin, lung, liver, and testis where it mediates the actions of PTHrP. Mutations involving the genes that encode these proteins and receptors in this calcium regulating pathway (Fig. 13.6.2) are associated with hypercalcaemic and hypocalcaemic disorders (Table 13.6.2).

Hypercalcaemia

Clinical features and investigations

The clinical presentation of hypercalcaemia varies from a mild, asymptomatic, biochemical abnormality detected during routine screening to a life-threatening medical emergency. In general, the presence or absence of symptoms correlates with the severity and rapidity of onset of the hypercalcaemia. Thus, symptoms do not usually develop when serum calcium is below 3.00 mmol/litre and are invariably present when the hypercalcaemia exceeds 3.50 mmol/litre. However, there is a considerable variability and some patients may be symptomatic with mild hypercalcaemia (2.65–2.90 mmol/litre). Although there are many causes of hypercalcaemia (Box 13.6.1), the signs and symptoms of hypercalcaemia are similar, regardless of aetiology. Indeed the clinical manifestations of hypercalcaemia involve several organ systems that include the renal, musculoskeletal, gastrointestinal, neurological, and cardiac systems (Box 13.6.2), and many of these have been referred to as 'moans, groans, pains, and stones'. Investigations should be directed at confirming the presence of hypercalcaemia and establishing the cause (Box 13.6.1).

The causes of hypercalcaemia can be classified according to whether serum PTH concentrations are elevated (i.e. primary hyperparathyroidism) or low (i.e. not due to a parathyroid tumour). Primary hyperparathyroidism and malignancy are the most common causes and account for more than 90% of patients with hypercalcaemia. Detailed clinical history and examination will usually help to differentiate between these two diagnoses. In primary hyperparathyroidism, the hypercalcaemia is often less than 3.00 mmol/litre, asymptomatic, and may have been present for months or years. If symptoms such as nephrolithiasis are present then they have usually been present for several months. However, in malignancy the patients are usually acutely ill, often with neurological symptoms, the hypercalcaemia is more than 3.00 mmol/litre, and the cancer (e.g. lung, breast, or myeloma) is often readily apparent. Hypercalcaemia from causes other than primary

Table 13.6.2 Parathyroid diseases and their chromosomal locations

Metabolic abnormality	Disease	Inheritance	Gene/gene product	Chromosomal location
Hypercalcaemia	MEN1 (OMIM 131100)	Autosomal dominant	Menin	11q13
	MEN2 (OMIM 171400)	Autosomal dominant	*RET*	10q11.2
	HPT-JT (OMIM 145001)	Autosomal dominant	Parafibromin	1q31.2
	Sporadic hyperparathyroidism (OMIM 145000)	Sporadic	*CCND1*	11q13
			Retinoblastoma	13q14
			Unknown	1p32-pter
	Parathyroid carcinoma (OMIM 608266)	Sporadic	Parafibromin	1q31.2
	FBH (OMIM 145980)		Retinoblastoma	13q14
	FBH1	Autosomal dominant	*CASR*	3q21.1
	FBH2	Autosomal dominant	Unknown	19p13
	FBH3	Autosomal dominant	Unknown	19q13
	NHPT (OMIM 239200)	Autosomal recessive	*CASR*	3q21.1
		Autosomal dominant		
	Jansen's disease (OMIM 156400)	Autosomal dominant	PTHR/PTHrPR	3p21.3
	William's syndrome (OMIM 194050)	Autosomal dominant	*ELN, LIMK1* (and other genes)	7q11.23
	McCune–Albright syndrome (OMIM 174800)	Mutations during early embryonic development?	$G_s\alpha$	20q13.3
Hypocalcaemia	Isolated hypoparathyroidism (OMIM 146200)	Autosomal dominant	*PTH*	11p15[a]
		Autosomal recessive	PTH, GCM2	11p15[a], 6p24.2
		X-linked recessive	SOX3	Xq26–27
	Hypocalcaemic hypercalciuria (OMIM 145980)	Autosomal dominant	CaSR	3q21.1
	Hypoparathyroidism associated with polyglandular autoimmune syndrome (APECED) (OMIM 240300)	Autosomal recessive	*AIRE1*	21q22.3
	Hypoparathyroidism associated with Kearns–Sayre (OMIM 530000) and MELAS (OMIM 540000) syndromes	Maternal	Mitochondrial genome	
	Hypoparathyroidism associated with complex congenital syndromes			
	DiGeorge syndrome (OMIM 188400)	Autosomal dominant	*TBX1*	22q11.2/10p
	HDR syndrome	Autosomal dominant	GATA3	10p15
	Blomstrand lethal chondrodysplasia (OMIM 215045)	Autosomal recessive	PTHR/PTHrPR	3p21.3
	Kenney–Caffey (OMIM 244460), and Sanjad–Sakati syndromes	Autosomal dominant	TBCE	1q42.3
	Barakat syndrome	Autosomal recessive[b]	Unknown	?
	Lymphoedema	Autosomal recessive	Unknown	?
	Nephropathy, nerve deafness	Autosomal dominant[b]	Unknown	?
	Nerve deafness without renal dysplasia	Autosomal dominant	Unknown?	?
	PHP (type Ia) (OMIM 103580)	Autosomal dominant parentally imprinted	GNAS exons 1–3	20q13.2
	PHP (type Ib) (OMIM 603233)	Autosomal dominant parentally imprinted	GNAS, upstream deletion	20q13.3

GATA3, GATA binding protein 3; GCM2, glial cells missing homolog 2; HDR, hypoparathyroidism, deafness, and renal dysplasia; MELAS, mitochondrial encephalopathy, lactic acidosis, and stroke-like episodes; PTHR, parathyroid hormone receptor; PTHrPR, parathyroid hormone-related peptide receptor; ? location not known.

[a] Mutations of PTH gene identified only in some families.

[b] Most likely inheritance.

Box 13.6.1 Causes of hypercalcaemia

High PTH levels

- Primary hyperparathyroidism[a] (adenoma, hyperplasia, or carcinoma): nonfamilial or familial, e.g. MEN1, MEN2, HPT-JT, FIHP
- Tertiary hyperparathyroidism (hyperplasia or adenoma in chronic renal failure)

Low PTH levels

Malignancy[a]

Primary

- PTH-related protein, PTHrP (carcinoma of lung, oesophagus, renal cell, ovary, and bladder)
- Excess production of 1,25-dihydroxyvitamin D (lymphoma)

Secondary

- Lytic bone metastases[a] (multiple myeloma[a] and breast carcinoma[a])
- Other location, ectopic factors (e.g. cytokines)
- Excess vitamin D
- Exogenous vitamin D toxicity by parent D compound, 25-hydroxyvitamin D_3, or 1,25-dihydroxyvitamin D_3 in vitamin preparations, cod liver oil, herbal medicines
- Endogenous production of 25-hydroxyvitamin D_3—William's syndrome
- Endogenous production of 1,25-dihydroxyvitamin D_3, e.g. granulomatous disorders (sarcoidosis, HIV, tuberculosis, histoplasmosis, coccidiomycosis, leprosy) and lymphoma

Drugs

- Thiazide diuretics
- Lithium
- Total parenteral nutrition
- Oestrogens/antioestrogens, testosterone
- Milk-alkali syndrome
- Vitamin A toxicity
- Foscarnet
- Aluminium intoxication (in chronic renal failure)
- Aminophylline

Nonparathyroid endocrine disorders

- Thyrotoxicosis
- Phaeochromocytoma
- Acute adrenal insufficiency
- Vasoactive intestinal polypeptide hormone producing tumour (VIPoma)
- Immobilization

Inappropriate PTH levels due to altered set point

- Familial benign hypocalciuric hypercalcaemia (FBH or FHH)

[a] Most common causes.

Box 13.6.2 Clinical features of hypercalcaemia

Renal

Stones (nephrolithiasis) and nephrocalcinosis

Polyuria

Polydipsia

Musculoskeletal

Bone pain

Osteopenia

Fractures

Muscular weakness, especially proximal myopathy

Gastrointestinal

Nausea

Vomiting

Lack of appetite

Constipation

Peptic ulcers

Pancreatitis

Neurological

Tiredness

Lethargy

Inability to concentrate

Increased sleepiness

Depression

Confusion

Coma

Cardiac

Bradycardia

First-degree AV block

Arrhythmias

Shortened QT interval

---

hyperparathyroidism or malignancy may also occur (Box 13.6.1) and a careful history (e.g. for vitamin D ingestion, drugs, renal disease) and examination (e.g. for thyrotoxicosis, adrenal disease, granulomatosis diseases), together with appropriate investigations (Box 13.6.3) are essential for establishing the diagnosis.

Management of hypercalcaemia

The management of hypercalcaemia depends on the severity of the hypercalcaemia and the presence of symptoms. Thus, asymptomatic patients with mild hypercalcaemia, i.e. serum calcium below 3.00 mmol/litre, do not usually need urgent treatment. However, a patient with severe hypercalcaemia, i.e. a serum calcium above 3.50 mmol/litre, would require treatment regardless of symptoms, while a patient with moderate hypercalcaemia, i.e. a serum calcium in the range 3.00 to 3.50 mmol/litre, would require urgent treatment

Box 13.6.3 Preliminary investigations for hypercalcaemia

Blood

Two or three estimations of serum calcium, phosphate, albumin, urea and electrolytes, creatinine, alkaline phosphatase, and liver function tests

PTH

Haemoglobin, full blood count, ESR

Electrophoretic protein strip

25-hydroxyvitamin D_3 (and, if indicated, 1,25-dihydroxy-vitamin D_3)

Thyroid function tests

Magnesium

Urine

Two or three estimations of 24-h urinary calcium and creatinine, and clearance ratios

Imaging

Chest radiograph

Radiograph of hands

Ultrasound of kidneys

---

if symptomatic. Before instituting treatment, it is always important to consider the underlying causes (Box 13.6.1) and to initiate investigations (Box 13.6.3). In addition, drugs such as thiazides and vitamin D compounds that cause hypercalcaemia should be discontinued and, if appropriate, dietary calcium restricted.

The acute management of hypercalcaemia involves general measures to enhance hydration and diuresis, and specific measures using drugs to lower serum calcium. Dehydration due to hypercalcaemic symptoms, e.g. anorexia, nausea, vomiting, and polyuria because of defective urinary concentration, is very common and patients may require 5 to 10 litres of 0.9% sodium chloride over a 24- to 48-h period. This vigorous hydration with normal saline may lower serum calcium by 0.25 to 0.75 mmol/litre; it enhances urinary calcium excretion by increasing glomerular filtration and reducing proximal and distal renal tubular reabsorption of calcium and sodium. The saline diuresis may need adjuvant therapy with a loop diuretic, e.g. furosemide 10 to 20 mg, as necessary, to control complications due to volume overload, especially in elderly people and those with impaired cardiovascular and renal function. It is important to note that excessive use of furosemide before intravascular volume has been restored may worsen the hypercalcaemia by exacerbating volume depletion. Saline diuresis may lead to hypokalaemia, hypomagnesaemia, and electrolyte imbalance, which will need correction.

If saline diuresis is not successful, and particularly if the hypercalcaemia is very severe, then more specific measures, e.g. dialysis and/or drugs, will be required. The drugs of choice are pamidronate or zoledronic acid, which are potent bisphosphonates that are administered parenterally. Recommended regimens are to administer pamidronate (60–90 mg) or zoledronic acid (4 mg) intravenously as a single infusion. Other bisphosphonates, e.g. etidronate

and clodronate, and other agents such as mithramycin, calcitonin, and gallium nitrate have also been used in the past. Glucocorticoid therapy (e.g. hydrocortisone 120 mg/day in three divided doses) is particularly effective when the hypercalcaemia is mediated by the actions of 1,25-dihydroxyvitamin D, e.g. in granulomatosis disease or lymphoma (Box 13.6.1), or myeloma. Dialysis using a low or zero calcium dialysate should be considered if these treatments are not effective or if the patient has renal failure. Once the acute management of hypercalcaemia has been completed, then appropriate treatment for the underlying cause, e.g. parathyroidectomy for primary hyperparathyroidism, needs to be undertaken.

Hypercalcaemic diseases

Hypercalcaemia may arise through one or more of three mechanisms: increased bone resorption, increased gastrointestinal absorption of calcium, and decreased renal calcium excretion (Fig. 13.6.1). For example, lytic bone metastases cause increased bone resorption, thiazide diuretics lead to a decrease in calcium excretion, and excessive PTH will either directly or indirectly, by increasing 1,25-dihydroxyvitamin D production, stimulate bone resorption and calcium absorption from the gut and renal tubules. The hypercalcaemic diseases may be classified according to whether serum PTH concentrations are elevated or reduced (Box 13.6.1). In addition, hypercalcaemia may be classified as being due to an excess of PTH (e.g. primary or tertiary hyperparathyroidism) from parathyroid tumours, an excessive production of PTHrP, a defect in the PTH receptor (i.e. the PTH/PTHrP receptor), an excess production of downstream mediators, e.g. 1,25-dihydroxyvitamin D, or an altered set point in the CaSR (Fig. 13.6.2).

Hyperparathyroidism

Hyperparathyroidism is characterized by high concentrations of serum immunoreactive PTH, and three types, referred to as primary, secondary, and tertiary, are recognized. Primary and tertiary hyperparathyroidism are associated with hypercalcaemia (Box 13.6.1), whereas secondary hyperparathyroidism is associated with hypocalcaemia (see below). Primary hyperparathyroidism may arise as an isolated endocrinopathy or as part of a multiple endocrine neoplasia (MEN) syndrome, and tertiary hyperparathyroidism usually arises in association with chronic renal failure.

Primary hyperparathyroidism

Primary hyperparathyroidism, which affects 3 in 1000 adults, is one of the two most common causes of hypercalcaemia and is due to an excessive secretion of PTH from one or more parathyroid tumours. Epidemiological studies have estimated that the global prevalence of parathyroid tumours is 4 million. In 80% of patients this tumour is a solitary parathyroid adenoma, and in 15 to 20% of patients hyperplasia involving all four parathyroids is present. Parathyroid carcinoma accounts for less than 0.5% of patients with primary hyperparathyroidism. Primary hyperparathyroidism usually occurs between the ages of 40 to 65 years, and is 3 times more common in women than men. The underlying causes of primary hyperparathyroidism are largely unknown, but abnormalities of several genes have been identified. Thus, abnormalities of the cyclin D1 (*CCND1*), retinoblastoma, CaSR (*CASR*), parafibromin, MEN type 1 (*MEN1*), and MEN type 2 (*MEN2*) genes, together with other genes yet to be identified, e.g. on chromosome 1p

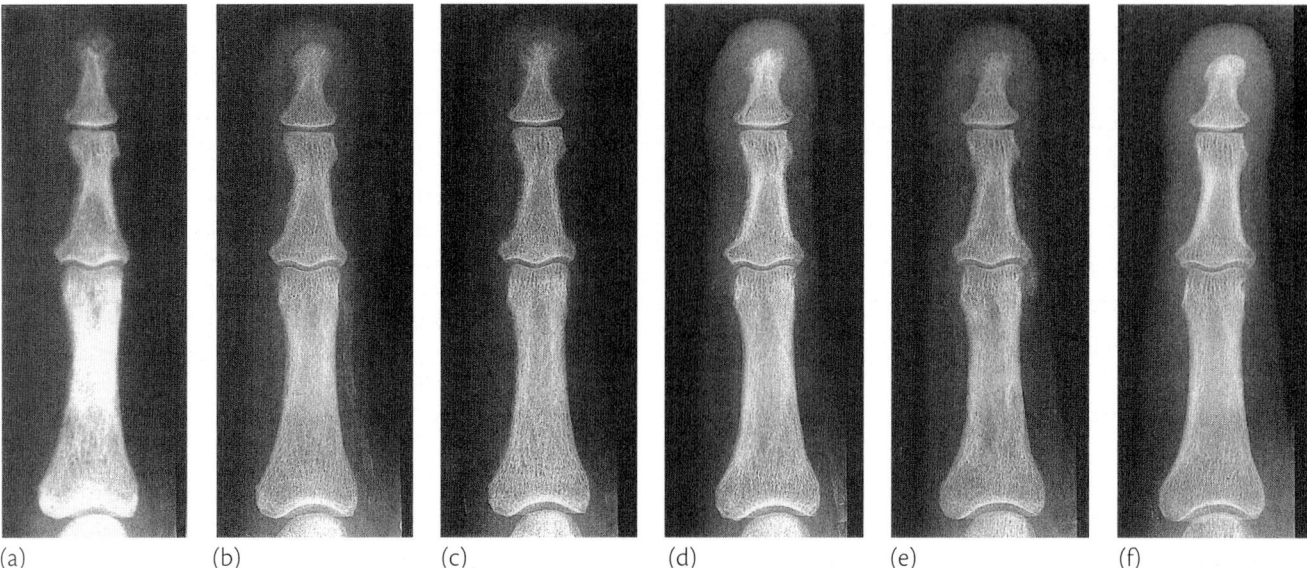

(a)   (b)   (c)   (d)   (e)   (f)

Fig. 13.6.3 Renal osteodystrophy over a 9-year period in a patient with chronic renal failure. Marked periosteal erosions were seen (a) despite treatment with 1α-hydroxycholecalciferol, and a resolution was observed following dialysis (b). Note the vascular calcification. One year later a relapse was noted with periosteal erosions (c) and the use of calcitriol resolved these (d). Unfortunately, a relapse occurred 2 years later (e), and following renal transplantation a marked resolution was observed (f).

(Table 13.6.2), are associated with the development of some parathyroid tumours.

Clinical features Many patients with primary hyperparathyroidism will be asymptomatic and the hypercalcaemia, which is usually mild, will have been detected by chance at the time of biochemical screening for other reasons. However, it is important to note that nearly one-half of the patients will have subtle neuromuscular symptoms such as fatigue and weakness and this becomes apparent only in retrospect after a successful parathyroidectomy.

Symptomatic hypercalcaemia (Box 13.6.2) predominantly affects the skeletal, renal, and gastrointestinal systems; peptic ulcers and pancreatitis may develop. The skeletal changes of osteitis fibrosa cystica due to subperiosteal resorption of the distal phalanges (Fig. 13.6.3), tapering of the distal clavicles, a 'salt and pepper' appearance of the skull, bone cysts, and brown tumours of the long bones are now identified in less than 5% of patients. However, osteopenia, as assessed by bone mineral density, occurs in 25% of patients. Renal stone disease (nephrolithiasis and nephrocalcinosis) occurs in 20% of patients and hypercalciuria occurs in 30% of patients; renal impairment may complicate this disease.

Investigations In the presence of hypercalcaemia, the finding of elevated circulating PTH concentrations establishes the diagnosis, as the PTH will be elevated in approximately 90% of patients with primary hyperparathyroidism who will invariably have hypercalcaemia. However, it is important to make sure that the immunoradiometric and immunochemiluminometric assays for PTH are used to measure the intact molecule, rather than the older radioimmunoassays which are not as reliable. The only other hypercalcaemic disorders in which PTH may occasionally be elevated are those related to FBH, immobilization, or lithium or thiazide use (Box 13.6.1), and a careful history and a cessation of drug use will help to exclude these possibilities. About one-third of patients with primary hyperparathyroidism will have a low serum phosphate and in the others it will be in the lower range of normal. In addition,

some patients will have a small increase in serum chloride concentration and a concomitant decrease in bicarbonate concentration. Serum alkaline phosphatase activity may be elevated in some patients, and urinary calcium excretion is increased in 30% of patients. The circulating 1,25-dihydroxyvitamin D concentration is elevated in some patients with primary hyperparathyroidism, although it is not of diagnostic value as it is also elevated in other hypercalcaemic disorders such as sarcoidosis and lymphomas. The serum 25-hydroxyvitamin D concentration is within the normal range. Densitometric scanning is of use in detecting early skeletal changes. Patients with primary hyperparathyroidism develop reduced bone mineral densities (osteopenia) primarily of the cortical bone (e.g. distal one-third of forearm) rather than the cancellous bone (e.g. lumbar spine). The hip bones, which are an equal mixture of cortical and cancellous bone, show intermediate reductions in bone mineral density. Overall, the risk of bone fractures in patients with mild primary hyperparathyroidism is similar to those in matched, normal controls. However, successful parathyroidectomy does lead to an increase in bone mineral density over a 6- to 12-month period and this continues for up to 10 years. Indeed, bone mineral density measurements are used in the evaluation of patients with primary hyperparathyroidism and in deciding on conservative as opposed to surgical management (Box 13.6.4).

Preoperative localization to define the site(s) of the parathyroid tumours may be undertaken. The noninvasive tests consist of ultrasonography, CT, MRI, and scintigraphy with technetium-99m sestamibi. Sestamibi scintigraphy has now become established as the best and most convenient localization test; this can be performed with CT techniques (single photon emission CT, SPECT) to give a three-dimensional image with greater anatomical resolution. It is important to note that there is an appreciable incidence of false-positive rates with all the noninvasive localization procedures and so a confirmation using two methods is preferable. Invasive localization tests consist of arteriography and selective venous sampling for PTH in the veins draining the thyroidal region. These tests are

---

Box 13.6.4 Guidelines for the management of primary hyperparathyroidism, recommended by the National Institutes of Health consensus conference (1990 and 2002)

Surgery is recommended if the patient meets any one of the following criteria:

- Serum calcium is >0.25 mmol/litre above upper limit of normal

- Any complication of primary hyperparathyroidism, e.g. nephrolithiasis, bone erosions of osteitis fibrosa cystica

- An episode of acute primary hyperparathyroidism with life-threatening hypercalcaemia

- Marked hypercalciuria (>9 mmol/litre per 24 h or >400 mg/24 h)[a]

- Significant reduction in creatinine clearance (>30% reduction when compared to age-matched and sex-matched controls)[a]

- Reduction in bone mass at any site as determined by bone densitometry; >2.5 standard deviations below age-matched and sex-matched controls

- Age <50 years

[a] These guidelines were revised in 2008, to state that urinary calcium excretion is no longer considered as a criteria, and that creatinine clearance < 60 ml/min is a criteria for surgery.

---

time-consuming, expensive, difficult, and dependent on the skill of the radiologist. It is generally accepted that these preoperative localization tests are indicated in those patients who have had previous neck surgery. However, their role in patients who have not had prior surgery remains to be established and at present the preferences and expertise of the local medical, radiology, and surgery teams usually determine the use of venous sampling procedures.

Management and treatment Parathyroidectomy, which is the definitive cure, is a generally successful and safe procedure if undertaken by an experienced surgeon. There have also been major advances in surgery that have facilitated a surgical approach to be undertaken under local, as opposed to general, anaesthesia. An example of this is the use of minimally invasive parathyroidectomy in the patient with single gland disease that has been successfully localized by the combined use of sestamibi scintigraphy and ultrasonography. Surgery is recommended for symptomatic patients and for those who have skeletal and renal complications. However, the decision to recommend surgery, which does have a small risk, may be difficult in asymptomatic patients, who may constitute over 50% of patients with primary hyperparathyroidism. The natural history of primary hyperparathyroidism in most patients is to progress slowly or not at all. For example, among asymptomatic patients only 25% will have progressive disease, which is usually manifested as a decrease in bone mineral density during a 10-year period. This has led to a controversy regarding the indications for surgery, and guidelines have been provided by the Consensus Development Conference on the Management of Asymptomatic Primary Hyperparathyroidism (Box 13.6.4). However, these guidelines may not exclusively influence the decision for or against surgery, and a careful evaluation and assessment of the risks and benefits is considered by most medical and surgical teams in

conjunction with the patient. Clearly, some patients will not wish to continue living with a curable disease and will prefer surgery despite the guidelines (Box 13.6.4), while other patients will decline surgery, despite having guideline indications for it, because they may have coexisting medical conditions that make them feel that the risks of surgery are too great.

Patients who do not undergo parathyroidectomy should be evaluated clinically, and also monitored for serum calcium, creatinine, and PTH at 6- to 12-month intervals, and for bone mineral density and nephrolithiasis at 12-month intervals. In addition, the following medical guidelines are recommended. First, they should avoid dehydration and remain ambulant. Second, the dietary intake of calcium should be moderate, i.e. at or below 1000 mg/day, and thiazide diuretics should be avoided. Finally, they should avoid herbal and tonic remedies that may contain vitamin D or vitamin A. These measures may help, and at present an effective and safe drug for the treatment of primary hyperparathyroidism is not available. Drugs that have been used include oral phosphate, oestrogens or selective oestrogen receptor modulators (SERMs) in postmenopausal women, and the bisphosphonates alendronate and clodronate. Phosphate is not used because of concerns related to soft tissue ectopic calcification. Oestrogens and SERMs such as raloxifene do increase bone density in postmenopausal women with primary hyperparathyroidism but they have only small effects on the serum calcium and PTH concentrations. The bisphosphonates inhibit bone resorption and do reduce serum calcium. However, these effects are not sustained. A more targeted approach using a calcimimetic drug such as cinacalcet, which increases the sensitivity of the parathyroid CaSR (see below) to extracellular calcium and thereby reduces PTH secretion, has been evaluated in a multicentre, randomized, double-blind, placebo-controlled clinical trial. Cinacalcet was effective in lowering serum calcium concentrations to normal values and reducing PTH levels in patients with primary hyperparathyroidism. These effects were maintained with long-term treatment without major adverse effects. Bone mineral density in the treated patients remained unchanged, but there was a reduction in biochemical markers for bone resorption and formation. Cinacalcet may therefore represent an effective nonsurgical treatment for the management of primary hyperparathyroidism. However, to date, the use of cinacalcet is approved only for patients on dialysis with uncontrolled secondary hyperparathyroidism or in patients with hypercalcaemia due to inoperable parathyroid carcinoma.

Uraemic hyperparathyroidism

Serum PTH levels rise in response to hypocalcaemia and this secondary hyperparathyroidism usually resolves with treatment of the underlying cause of hypocalcaemia (Box 13.6.5). However, in chronic renal failure the secondary hyperparathyroidism may persist for a longer time, and eventually the parathyroid cells gain an autonomous function, secreting excessive PTH despite hypercalcaemia; this state is referred to as tertiary hyperparathyroidism (Box 13.6.1). The cause of progression from the early, presumably polyclonal, secondary hyperplasia of the parathyroids to the later, presumably monoclonal, tumours is not understood and appears to involve genes other than those involved in the aetiologies of the sporadic and familial forms of primary hyperparathyroidism (Table 13.6.2).

Clinical features and treatment In chronic renal failure, the ensuing phosphate retention and decreased production of

Box 13.6.5 Causes of hypocalcaemia

Low PTH levels (hypoparathyroidism)

Parathyroid agenesis

Isolated or part of complex developmental anomaly (e.g. DiGeorge's syndrome)

Parathyroid destruction

Surgery[a]

Radiation

Infiltration by metastases or systemic disease (e.g. haemochromatosis, amyloidosis, sarcoidosis, Wilson's disease, thalassaemia)

Autoimmune

Isolated

Polyglandular (type 1)[a]

Reduced parathyroid function (i.e. PTH secretion)

PTH gene defects

Hypomagnesaemia[a]

Neonatal hypocalcaemia (may be associated with maternal hypercalcaemia)

Hungry bone disease (postparathyroidectomy)

CaSR mutations

High PTH levels (secondary hyperparathyroidism)

Vitamin D deficiency[a]

As a result of nutritional lack[a], malabsorption[a], liver disease, or vitamin D receptor defects

Vitamin D resistance (rickets)

As a result of renal tubular dysfunction (Fanconi's syndrome) or vitamin D receptor defects

PTH resistance

(e.g. pseudohypoparathyroidism, hypomagnesaemia)

Drugs

Calcium chelators (e.g. citrated blood transfusions, phosphate; cow's milk is rich in phosphate)

Inhibitors of bone resorption (e.g. bisphosphonates, calcitonin, plicamycin)

Altered vitamin D metabolism (e.g. phenytoin, ketoconazole)

Foscarnet

Miscellaneous

Acute pancreatitis

Acute rhabdomyolysis

Massive tumour lysis

Osteoblastic metastases (e.g. from prostate or breast carcinoma)

Toxic shock syndrome

Hyperventilation

[a] Most common causes.

1,25-dihydroxyvitamin D result in hypocalcaemia and secondary hyperparathyroidism. This combination of biochemical abnormalities results in a severe bone disease that shows combined features of hyperparathyroidism and vitamin D deficiency (i.e. osteomalacia). Thus in renal osteodystrophy, bone erosions (Fig. 13.6.3) and osteomalacia are simultaneously observed. Treatment is based on correcting the hypocalcaemia, e.g. with oral administration of calcium salts, which also ameliorates the hyperphosphataemia by chelating phosphate in the intestines, and with calcitriol (1,25-dihydroxyvitamin D). The use of the most appropriate phosphate binder is not well established but it is clear that aluminium-containing compounds are to be avoided. Aluminium in these preparations and as a contaminant of dialysis solutions contributed in the recent past to the osteomalacic osseous disease and other aspects of metal toxicity in patients with renal failure (e.g. hypochromic anaemia and encephalopathy). Early treatment of the metabolic disturbance will prevent or delay the onset of severe secondary hyperparathyroidism and tertiary hyperparathyroidism, which requires parathyroidectomy. For patients who have end-stage renal failure and are on dialysis, cinacalcet—the allosteric activator of the CaSR—can be used to treat the severe secondary hyperparathyroidism. Cinacalcet will reduce the PTH concentrations and may also have an antiproliferative effect.

Familial primary hyperparathyroidism

Primary hyperparathyroidism is most frequently encountered as a nonfamilial disorder. However, approximately 10% of patients with primary hyperparathyroidism will have a hereditary form which may either be part of the MEN type 1 (MEN1) and type 2 (MEN2) syndromes, or part of the hereditary hyperparathyroidism–jaw tumour (HPT-JT) syndrome. In addition, hereditary primary hyperparathyroidism may develop as a solitary endocrinopathy and this has also been referred to as familial isolated hyperparathyroidism (FIHP). Investigations of these hereditary and sporadic forms of primary hyperparathyroidism have helped to identify some of the genes and chromosomal regions that are involved in the aetiology of parathyroid tumours (Table 13.6.2). FIHP has been reported in several kindreds, and some have been shown to harbour mutations of the *MEN1* gene or the gene encoding parafibromin. These familial syndromes associated with parathyroid tumours will be briefly reviewed.

MEN1 MEN1 is characterized by the combined occurrence of tumours of the parathyroids, pancreatic islet cells, and anterior pituitary. Parathyroid tumours occur in 95% of MEN1 patients, and the resulting hypercalcaemia is the first manifestation of MEN1 in about 90% of patients. Pancreatic islet cell tumours occur in 40% of MEN1 patients, and gastrinomas, leading to the Zollinger–Ellison syndrome, are the most common type and also the important cause of morbidity and mortality in MEN1 patients. Anterior pituitary tumours occur in 30% of MEN1 patients, with prolactinomas representing the most common type. Associated tumours that may also occur in MEN1 include adrenal cortical tumours, carcinoid tumours, lipomas, angiofibromas, and collagenomas. The gene causing MEN1, which is located on chromosome 11q13 and represents a putative tumour suppressor gene, consists of 10 exons that encode a 610 amino acid protein, known as menin. Menin is predominantly a nuclear protein in nondividing cells, but in dividing cells it is found in the cytoplasm. Menin has been shown to interact with many proteins that are involved in transcriptional regulation, genome stability, and cell division. The majority (>80%) of the germ-line *MEN1* mutations in families are inactivating. Mutational analysis of the *MEN1* gene is helpful in the diagnosis and management of patients and their families.

MEN2 MEN2 describes the association of medullary thyroid carcinoma (MTC), phaeochromocytomas, and parathyroid tumours. Three clinical variants of MEN2 are recognized: MEN2a, MEN2b, and MTC-only. MEN2a is the most common variant, where the development of MTC is associated with phaeochromocytomas (50% of patients), which may be bilateral, and parathyroid tumours (20% of patients). MEN2b, which represents 5% of all MEN2 cases, is characterized by the occurrence of MTC and phaeochromocytoma in association with a marfanoid habitus, mucosal neuromas, medullated corneal fibres, and intestinal autonomic ganglion dysfunction leading to multiple diverticulae and megacolon. Parathyroid tumours do not usually occur in MEN2b. MTC-only is a variant in which MTC is the sole manifestation of the syndrome. The gene causing all three MEN2 variants was mapped to chromosome 10q11.2, a region containing the c-*RET* proto-oncogene which encodes a tyrosine kinase receptor with cadherin-like and cysteine-rich extracellular domains and a tyrosine kinase intracellular domain. Specific mutations of c-*RET* have been identified for each of the three MEN2 variants. Thus in 95% of patients, MEN2a is associated with mutations of the cysteine-rich extracellular domain and mutations in codon 634 (Cys→Arg) account for 85% of MEN2a mutations. MTC-only is also associated with missense mutations in the cysteine-rich extracellular domain and most mutations are at codon 618. MEN2b is associated with mutations in codon 918 (Met→Thr) of the intracellular tyrosine kinase domain in 95% of patients. Mutational analysis of c-*RET* to detect mutations in codons 609, 611, 618, 634, 768, and 804 in MEN2a and MTC-only, and codon 918 in MEN2b, has been used in the diagnosis and management of patients and families with these disorders.

HPT-JT The HPT-JT syndrome is an autosomal dominant disorder characterized by the occurrence of parathyroid tumours that may be carcinomas in approximately 15% of patients and ossifying fibromas that usually affect the maxilla and/or mandible. In addition, some patients may also develop Wilms' tumours, renal cysts, renal hamartomas, renal cortical adenomas, papillary renal cell carcinomas, uterine tumours that may be malignant, pancreatic adenocarcinomas, testicular mixed germ cell tumours with a major seminoma component, and Hürthle cell thyroid adenomas. It is important to note that the parathyroid tumours may occur in isolation and without any evidence of jaw tumours, and this may cause confusion with other hereditary hypercalcaemic disorders such as MEN1, FBH, and FIHP. HPT-JT can be distinguished from FBH, as in FBH serum calcium concentrations are elevated from the early neonatal or infantile period whereas in HPT-JT such elevations are uncommon in the first decade. In addition, HPT-JT patients, unlike those with FBH, will have associated hypercalciuria. The distinction between HPT-JT patients and MEN1 patients, who have only developed the usual first manifestation of hypercalcaemia (>90% of patients), is more difficult and is likely to be influenced by the operative and histological findings and the occurrence of other characteristic lesions in each disorder. It should be noted that HPT-JT patients will usually have single adenomas or a carcinoma, while MEN1 patients will often have multiglandular

parathyroid disease. The distinction between FIHP and HPT-JT in the absence of jaw tumours is difficult but important as HPT-JT patients may be at a higher risk of developing parathyroid carcinomas. These distinctions may be helped by the identification of additional features, and a search for jaw tumours and renal, pancreatic, thyroid, and testicular abnormalities may help to identify HPT-JT patients. The jaw tumours in HPT-JT are different from the brown tumours observed in some patients with primary hyperparathyroidism, and do not resolve after parathyroidectomy. Indeed ossifying fibromas of the jaw are an important distinguishing feature of HPT-JT from FIHP, and the occurrence of these may occasionally precede the development of hypercalcaemia in HPT-JT patients by several decades.

The gene causing HPT-JT is *CDC73*, located on chromosome 1q31.2 and consisting of 17 exons that encode a ubiquitously expressed 531 amino acid protein, parafibromin. This gene is also referred to as HRPT2 (i.e. hyperparathyroidism type 2). Parafibromin has been shown to be associated with the human homologue of the Paf1 protein complex which interacts with RNA polymerase II, and, as part of this protein complex, parafibromin may regulate post-transcriptional events and histone modification. The majority (>80%) of the germ-line mutations in HRPT-JT families are inactivating and are predicated to result in a functional loss of the parafibromin protein because of premature truncation. In addition, patients with nonfamilial parathyroid carcinomas may harbour germ-line mutations, and mutational analysis of the gene encoding parafibromin is now undertaken in patients who have nonfamilial parathyroid carcinoma, FIHP, and HPT-JT.

Malignancy

The hypercalcaemia of malignancy is usually due to increased bone resorption, which may be either directly due to skeletal metastases or indirectly due to tumour production of a humoral factor that stimulates osteoclastic bone resorption. The cancers that typically metastasize to produce lytic bone lesions are from the breast, lymphomas, or multiple myeloma (Box 13.6.1). The cancers that are typically associated with the humoral hypercalcaemia of malignancy (HHM) are squamous carcinomas of the lung, oesophagus, cervix, vulva, skin, head, or neck, but other types from the kidney, bladder, ovary, and breast may also occur. HHM accounts for up to 80% of patients with malignancy-associated hypercalcaemia. The most common factor causing HHM is PTHrP, which can be measured in the serum by immunoassay. However, these assays are relatively insensitive and the failure to detect serum PTHrP does not exclude the diagnosis of HHM. Patients with HHM generally have hypercalcaemia associated with lower or undetectable serum PTH levels, marked hypercalcaemia, and a reduced plasma 1,25-dihydroxyvitamin D level. Therapy of HHM is aimed at: (1) reducing the tumour load by surgery, radiotherapy, and/or chemotherapy; (2) reducing osteoclastic bone resorption by use of bisphosphonates or calcitonin; and (3) increasing renal calcium clearance by a saline diuresis.

Granulomatous disorders

Several granulomatous disorders are associated with hypercalcaemia (Box 13.6.1) and this is invariably associated with elevated circulating concentrations of 1,25-dihydroxyvitamin D, which is due to extrarenal synthesis. Sarcoidosis is the most frequently encountered granulomatous disorder associated with hypercalcaemia, and 10% of patients with sarcoidosis will have hypercalcaemia and about one-half will become hypercalciuric. The finding of raised serum angiotensin-converting enzyme activity may help in confirming the diagnosis. Glucocorticoids (e.g. 40–60 mg prednisolone) decrease 1,25-dihydroxyvitamin D production and restore the calcium concentration to normal. Failure to achieve normal serum calcium concentrations within 10 days of glucocorticoid therapy (e.g. hydrocortisone 40 mg, 3 times per day), which is referred to as the steroid suppression test, should suggest the coexistence of another cause for the hypercalcaemia, e.g. primary hyperparathyroidism or malignancy.

Endocrine causes of hypercalcaemia other than hyperparathyroidism

Several nonparathyroid disorders (Box 13.6.1) are associated with hypercalcaemia and these include thyrotoxicosis, phaeochromocytoma, Addison's disease, VIPomas, familial benign hypocalciuric hypercalcaemia, Jansen's disease, and William's syndrome.

Thyrotoxicosis

Mild hypercalcaemia (<3.00 mmol/litre) frequently accompanies thyrotoxicosis, which leads to increased bone turnover and resorption. The hypercalcaemia may respond to treatment with β-adrenergic blockers.

FBH and NHPT

FBH is an autosomal dominant disorder with a high degree of penetrance. It is characterized by lifelong asymptomatic hypercalcaemia in association with an inappropriately low urinary calcium excretion (i.e. ratio of calcium clearance to creatinine clearance <0.01). A normal circulating PTH concentration and mild hypermagnesaemia are also typically present. Although most patients with FBH are asymptomatic, chondrocalcinosis and acute pancreatitis have occasionally been observed. In addition, children of consanguineous marriages within FBH kindreds have been observed to have life-threatening hypercalcaemia due to neonatal primary hyperparathyroidism (NHPT). NHPT is defined as symptomatic hypercalcaemia with skeletal manifestations of hyperparathyroidism in the first 6 months of life. NHPT children often present in the first few days or weeks of life with failure to thrive, dehydration, hypotonia, constipation, rib cage deformities, and multiple fractures due to bony undermineralization. Children with NHPT often require urgent parathyroidectomy, which corrects the PTH-dependent hypercalcaemia and bone demineralization. FBH is due to heterozygous inactivating mutations of the CaSR and NHPT is often associated with inactivating homozygous CaSR mutations (Fig. 13.6.2). However, NHPT has also been observed in children where only one parent has clinically apparent FBH, and many other NHPT patients appear to be sporadic, i.e. both parents have normal serum calcium concentrations. In such NHPT patients with heterozygous CaSR mutations, the mutant CaSR may exert a dominant negative action on the normal CaSR. The human CaSR is a 1078 amino acid cell surface protein that is expressed in parathyroids, thyroid cells, and kidney, and is a member of the family of G protein-coupled receptors. The CASR gene is located on chromosome 3q21.1.

Jansen's disease

Jansen's disease is an autosomal dominant disease that is characterized by short-limbed dwarfism, due to metaphyseal chondrodysplasia, and severe hypercalcaemia and hypophosphataemia, despite normal or undetectable serum levels of PTH. These abnormalities are associated with activating mutations of the PTH receptor (Fig. 13.6.2)

and thus this represents a PTH-independent activation of the PTH receptor. Three different mutations of the PTH receptor have been identified, and these involve codon 223 (His→Arg), codon 410 (Thr→Pro), and codon 458 (Ile→Arg). Expression of the mutant receptors in COS-7 cells resulted in constitutive, ligand-independent accumulation of cAMP, while the basal accumulation of inositol phosphates was not increased. These findings provide a likely explanation for the abnormalities observed in mineral homeostasis and growth plate development in this disorder.

William's syndrome

William's syndrome is an autosomal dominant disorder characterized by supravalvular aortic stenosis, elfin-like facies, psychomotor retardation, and infantile hypercalcaemia. The underlying abnormality of calcium metabolism remains unknown but abnormal 1,25-dihydroxyvitamin D_3 metabolism or decreased calcitonin production have been implicated, although no abnormality has been consistently demonstrated. Hemizygosity due to a microdeletion at the ELN locus on chromosome 7q11.23 in over 90% of patients with the classic William's phenotype has been demonstrated. This microdeletion has been reported to involve another gene, designated LIMK1, that is expressed in the central nervous system. The calcitonin receptor gene has been localized to chromosome 7q21 and close to the region deleted in William's syndrome. However, the calcitonin receptor gene was not involved in the deletion found in four patients with William's syndrome, indicating that it is unlikely to be implicated in the hypercalcaemia of such children. While the involvement of the ELN and LIMK1 genes in the deletions of William's syndrome patients can explain the respective cardiovascular and neurological features of this disorder, it seems possible that another, as yet uncharacterized gene that is within this contiguously deleted region is likely to be involved to explain the abnormalities of calcium metabolism.

Drugs

Several drugs (Box 13.6.1) can cause hypercalcaemia by different mechanisms. Compounds containing vitamin D and vitamin A are common and frequently associated with hypercalcaemia. The use of thiazide diuretics is often associated with hypercalcaemia. The hypercalcaemia appears to be largely renal in origin, as thiazides enhance distal renal tubular calcium reabsorption. Hypercalcaemia reverses rapidly with discontinuation of the drug.

The milk-alkali syndrome was first described in the 1930s, generally in the context of ulcer treatment with large quantities of milk together with sodium bicarbonate. Today, the responsible agent is usually calcium carbonate, although consumption of large quantities of dairy products (milk, cheese, and yoghurt) may still contribute. Classic features include moderate to severe hypercalcaemia with alkalosis and renal impairment. The amount of calcium ingested by patients with this syndrome is usually 5 to 15 g/day. Treatment consists of: (1) discontinuing the ingestion of the calcium-containing compound(s) and antacids, (2) rehydration, and (3) saline diuresis.

Hypocalcaemia

Clinical features and investigations

The clinical presentation of hypocalcaemia (serum calcium <2.12 mmol/litre) ranges from an asymptomatic biochemical abnormality to a severe, life-threatening condition. In mild hypocalcaemia (serum calcium 2.00–2.12 mmol/litre), patients may be asymptomatic. Those with more severe (serum calcium <1.9 mmol/litre) and long-term hypocalcaemia may develop acute symptoms of neuromuscular irritability (Box 13.6.6), ectopic calcification (e.g. in the basal ganglia, which may be associated with extrapyramidal neurological symptoms), subcapsular cataract, papilloedema, and abnormal dentition.

Investigations should be directed at confirming the presence of hypocalcaemia and establishing the cause. Hypocalcaemia (Box 13.6.5) can be classified by cause, according to whether serum PTH concentrations are low (i.e. hypoparathyroid disorders) or high (i.e. disorders associated with secondary hyperparathyroidism). Hypocalcaemia is most commonly caused by hypoparathyroidism, a deficiency or abnormal metabolism of vitamin D, acute or chronic renal failure, or hypomagnesaemia. In hypoparathyroidism, serum calcium is low, phosphate is high, and PTH is undetectable; renal function and concentrations of the 25-hydroxy and 1,25-dihydroxy metabolites of vitamin D are usually normal. The features of pseudohypoparathyroidism are similar to those of hypoparathyroidism except for PTH, which is markedly increased. In chronic renal failure, which is the most common cause of hypocalcaemia, phosphate is high and alkaline phosphatase, creatinine, and PTH are elevated; 25-hydroxyvitamin D_3 is normal and 1,25-dihydroxyvitamin D_3 is low. In vitamin D deficiency osteomalacia, serum calcium, and phosphate are low, alkaline phosphatase and PTH are elevated, renal function is normal, and 25-hydroxyvitamin D_3 is low. The most frequent artefactual cause of hypocalcaemia is hypoalbuminaemia, such as occurs in liver disease or the nephrotic syndrome.

Management of acute hypocalcaemia

The management of acute hypocalcaemia depends on the severity of the hypocalcaemia, the rapidity with which it developed, and the degree of neuromuscular irritability (Box 13.6.6). Treatment should be given to symptomatic patients (e.g. with seizures or tetany) and asymptomatic patients with a serum calcium of less than 1.90 mmol/litre who are at high risk of developing complications. The preferred treatment for acute symptomatic

hypocalcaemia is calcium gluconate, 10 ml 10% weight per volume (w/v) (2.20 mmol calcium), diluted in 50 ml of 5% dextrose or 0.9% sodium chloride and given by slow intravenous injection (>5 min); this can be repeated as required to control symptoms. Serum calcium concentrations should be assessed regularly. Persistent hypocalcaemia may be managed acutely by administration of a calcium gluconate infusion as follows. Dilute 10 ampoules of calcium gluconate, 10 ml 10% w/v (22.0 mmol calcium), in 1 litre of 5% dextrose or 0.9% sodium chloride, start the infusion at 50 ml/h, and titrate to maintain serum calcium concentrations in the normal range. Generally, 0.3 to 0.4 mmol/kg elemental calcium infused over 4 to 6 h increases serum calcium by 0.5 to 0.75 mmol/litre. If hypocalcaemia is likely to persist, oral vitamin D therapy (see below) should also be administered. In hypocalcaemic patients who are also hypomagnesaemic, the hypomagnesaemia must be corrected before the hypocalcaemia will resolve. This may occur in the postparathyroidectomy period or in patients with severe malabsorption, e.g. those with established coeliac disease.

Management of persistent hypocalcaemia

The two main agents available for the treatment of hypocalcaemia are supplemental calcium (c.10–20 mmol calcium every 6–12 h), and vitamin D preparations. Patients with hypoparathyroidism seldom require calcium supplements after the early stages of stabilization with vitamin D. A variety of vitamin D preparations have been used. These include vitamin D_3 (cholecalciferol) or vitamin D_2 (ergocalciferol), 25 000 to 100 000 IU (1.25–5 mg/day); dihydrotachysterol (now seldom used), 0.25 to 1.25 mg/day; alfacalcidol (1α-hydroxycholecalciferol), 0.25 to 1.0 μg/day; and calcitriol (1,25-dihydroxycholecalciferol), 0.25 to 2.0 μg/day. In children, these preparations are prescribed in dosages based on body weight. Cholecalciferol and ergocalciferol are the least expensive preparations but have the longest durations of action and may result in prolonged toxicity. The other preparations, which do not require renal 1α-hydroxylation, have the advantage of shorter half-lives and thereby minimize the risk of prolonged toxicity. Calcitriol is probably the drug of choice because it is the active metabolite and, unlike alfacalcidol, does not require hepatic 25-hydroxylation. Close monitoring (at about 1- to 2-week intervals) of the patient's serum and urine calcium concentrations are required initially, and at 3- to 6-month intervals once stabilization is achieved. The aim is to avoid hypercalcaemia, hypercalciuria, nephrolithiasis, and renal failure. It should be noted that hypercalciuria may occur in the absence of hypercalcaemia.

Hypocalcaemic diseases

Hypocalcaemic diseases (Box 13.6.5) may arise because of destruction of the parathyroid glands, failure of parathyroid gland development, or reduced PTH secretion or PTH-mediated actions in target tissues. Thus, these diseases may be classified as being due to a deficiency of PTH, a defect in the PTH receptor (i.e. the PTH/PTHrP receptor), or an insensitivity to PTH caused by defects downstream of the PTH/PTHrP receptor (Fig. 13.6.2). The diseases may also be classified as being part of the hypoparathyroid disorders, of the CaSR abnormalities, or of the pseudohypoparathyroid disorders.

Hypoparathyroidism

Hypoparathyroidism is characterized by hypocalcaemia and hyperphosphataemia, which are the result of a deficiency in PTH secretion or action. Serum concentrations of immunoreactive PTH are low or undetectable and the concentrations of 1,25-dihydroxy-vitamin D$_3$ are usually in the low normal to low range, but alkaline phosphatase activity is unchanged. The daily urinary excretion of calcium is reduced, although the fractional excretion of calcium is increased. Nephrogenous cAMP excretion is low and renal tubular reabsorption of phosphate is elevated. Urinary cAMP, plasma cAMP, and urinary phosphate excretion increase markedly after administration of exogenous bioactive PTH (Chase–Aurbach and Ellsworth–Howard tests). Hypoparathyroidism may result from agenesis (e.g. DiGeorge's syndrome) or destruction of the parathyroid glands (e.g. following neck surgery, in autoimmune diseases), from reduced secretion of PTH (e.g. neonatal hypocalcaemia or hypomagnesaemia), or resistance to PTH (which may occur as a primary disorder (e.g. pseudohypoparathyroidism) or secondary to hypomagnesaemia). In addition, hypoparathyroidism may occur as an inherited disorder (Table 13.6.2) that may either be part of a complex congenital defect (e.g. DiGeorge's syndrome), or as part of a polyglandular autoimmune disorder, or as a solitary endocrinopathy, which has been referred to as isolated or idiopathic hypoparathyroidism. Hypoparathyroidism may also complicate iron storage disease, especially secondary haemochromatosis in children and adolescents. In thalassaemic children, destruction of the parathyroids is associated with ill health and frank tetany, which may elude diagnosis and effective treatment unless hypoparathyroidism is suspected.

Isolated hypoparathyroidism

Isolated hypoparathyroidism may either be inherited or it may be acquired by damage to the parathyroids at surgery, by infiltrating metastases, or following systemic disease (Box 13.6.5).

Inherited hypoparathyroidism Patients with inherited forms of hypoparathyroidism may develop hypocalcaemic seizures in the neonatal or infantile periods and require lifelong treatment with oral vitamin D preparations, e.g. calcitriol. Autosomal dominant, autosomal recessive, and X-linked recessive inheritances for hypoparathyroidism have been observed (Table 13.6.2). Some of the autosomal forms are due to mutations of the *PTH* gene, the CaSR (see below), and the transcription factor GCM2 (glial cells missing homologue 2).

Acquired forms of hypoparathyroidism Hypoparathyroidism may occur after neck surgery, irradiation, or because of infiltration by metastases or systemic disease, e.g. haemochromatosis, amyloidosis, sarcoidosis, Wilson's disease, or thalassaemia (Box 13.6.5). Surgical damage to the parathyroids occurs most commonly after a radical neck dissection, e.g. laryngeal or oesophageal carcinoma treatment, a total thyroid resection, or after repeated parathyroidectomies for multiglandular disease (e.g. in MEN1 or MEN2, see above). Hypocalcaemic symptoms begin 12 to 24 h postoperatively and may need treatment with oral or intravenous calcium. Parathyroid function often returns, but persistent hypocalcaemia requires treatment with vitamin D preparations.

Neonatal hypoparathyroidism resulting in hypocalcaemia may occur in the baby of a mother with hypercalcaemia caused by primary hyperparathyroidism. Maternal hypercalcaemia results in increased calcium delivery to the fetus, and this fetal hypercalcaemia suppresses fetal PTH secretion. Postpartum, the infant's suppressed parathyroids are unable to maintain normocalcaemia.

The disorder is usually self-limiting, but occasionally therapy may be required. In addition, the feeding to babies of cow's milk, which has a high phosphate content, may also result in hypocalcaemia in some infants.

Functional hypoparathyroidism may result from severe hypomagnesaemia (<0.40 mmol/litre), which may be due to a severe intestinal malabsorption disorder (e.g. Crohn's disease) or a renal tubular disorder. It is associated with hypoparathyroidism because magnesium is required for the release of PTH from the parathyroid gland and also for PTH action via adenyl cyclase. Magnesium chloride, 35 to 50 mmol intravenously in 1 litre of 5% glucose or other isotonic solution given over 12 to 24 h may be repeatedly required to restore normomagnesaemia.

Complex syndromes associated with hypoparathyroidism

Hypoparathyroidism may occur as part of a complex syndrome which may either be associated with a congenital developmental anomaly or with an autoimmune syndrome. The congenital developmental anomalies associated with hypoparathyroidism, which occurs in 1 in 4000 live births, include the DiGeorge, the HDR (hypoparathyroidism, deafness, and renal anomalies), the Kenney–Caffey, and the Barakat syndromes, and also syndromes associated with either lymphoedema or dysmorphic features and growth failure (Table 13.6.2).

DiGeorge's syndrome Patients with DiGeorge's syndrome (DGS) have neonatal hypoparathyroidism, T-cell immunodeficiency, congenital heart defects, and deformities of the ear, nose, and mouth (e.g. cleft lip and/or palate). Children with DGS often die from infections related to the immunodeficiency. The disorder arises from a congenital failure in the development of the derivatives of the third and fourth pharyngeal pouches with resulting absence or hypoplasia of the parathyroids and thymus. Most cases of DGS are sporadic but an autosomal dominant inheritance of DGS has been observed, and an association between the syndrome and an unbalanced translocation and deletions involving chromosome 22q11.2 have also been reported. In some patients, deletions of another locus on chromosome 10p13–p14 have been observed in association with DGS and this is referred to as DGS type 2 (DGS2), while patients with the 22q11.2 deletions are referred to as DGS type 1 (DGS1). Studies of the DGS1 deleted region on chromosome 22q11.2 have revealed four genes (*RNEX40*, *NEX2.2-NEX3*, *UDFIL*, and *TBX1*) to be involved. However, point mutations in DGS1 patients have been detected only in the *TBX1* gene, and *TBX1* is now considered to be the gene causing DGS1. *TBX1* encodes a DNA-binding transcriptional factor of the T-box family that is known to have an important role in vertebrate and invertebrate organogenesis and pattern formation. The *TBX1* gene is deleted in approximately 96% of all DGS1 patients, and some of those without deletions have been shown to harbour mutations of *TBX1*.

Hypoparathyroidism, deafness, and renal anomalies (HDR) syndrome HDR is an autosomal dominant disorder in which patients often have asymptomatic hypocalcaemia with undetectable or inappropriately normal serum concentrations of PTH, and normal brisk increases in plasma cAMP in response to the infusion of PTH. Bilateral, symmetrical, sensorineural deafness involving all frequencies occurs, and the renal abnormalities consist mainly of bilateral cysts that compress the glomeruli and tubules and lead to renal impairment. Cytogenetic abnormalities involving chromosome 10p14–10pter have been identified in HDR patients. HDR patients do not have immunodeficiency or heart defects, which are key features of DGS2, and indeed there are two nonoverlapping regions; thus, the DGS2 region is located on 10p13–14 and HDR on 10p14–10pter. HDR patients have deletions or mutations of the zinc finger transcription factor GATA3.

Mitochondrial disorders associated with hypoparathyroidism Hypoparathyroidism has been reported to occur in three disorders associated with mitochondrial dysfunction: the Kearns–Sayre syndrome (KSS), the mitochondrial encephalopathy, lactic acidosis, and stroke-like episodes syndrome (MELAS), and a mitochondrial trifunctional protein deficiency syndrome (MTPDS). Kearns–Sayre syndrome is characterized by progressive external ophthalmoplegia and pigmentary retinopathy before the age of 20 years, and is often associated with heart block or cardiomyopathy. The MELAS syndrome consists of a childhood onset of mitochondrial encephalopathy, lactic acidosis, and stroke-like episodes. In addition, varying degrees of proximal myopathy can be seen in both conditions. Both the Kearns–Sayre and MELAS syndromes have been reported to occur with insulin-dependent diabetes mellitus and hypoparathyroidism, and mitochondrial gene abnormalities have been identified in some patients. Mitochondrial trifunctional protein deficiency is a disorder of fatty acid oxidation that is associated with peripheral neuropathy, pigmentary retinopathy, and acute fatty liver degeneration in pregnant women who carry an affected fetus. Hypoparathyroidism has been observed in one patient with trifunctional protein deficiency.

Kenney–Caffey and Sanjad–Sakati syndromes Hypoparathyroidism has been reported to occur in over 50% of patients with the Kenney–Caffey syndrome, which is associated with short stature, osteosclerosis, and cortical thickening of the long bones, delayed closure of the anterior fontanel, basal ganglia calcification, nanophthalmos, and hyperopia. Parathyroid tissue could not be found in a detailed postmortem examination of one patient and this suggests that hypoparathyroidism may be due to an embryological defect of parathyroid development. In the Sanjad–Sakati syndrome, hypoparathyroidism is associated with severe growth failure and dysmorphic features. This has been reported in 12 patients, in whom consanguinity was noted in 11 of the 12 patients' families, the majority of which originated from the western province of Saudi Arabia. This syndrome, which is inherited as an autosomal recessive disorder, has also been identified in families of Bedouin origin, and homozygosity and linkage disequilibrium studies have located this gene to chromosome 1q42–q43. Molecular genetic investigations have identified mutations of the tubulin-specific chaperone (*TBCE*) to be associated with the Kenney–Caffey and Sanjad–Sakati syndromes. *TBCE* encodes one of several chaperone proteins required for the proper folding of α-tubulin subunits and the formation of α-β tubulin heterodimers.

Additional familial syndromes Single familial syndromes in which hypoparathyroidism is a component have been reported (Table 13.6.2). Thus, an association of hypoparathyroidism, renal insufficiency, and developmental delay has been reported in one Asian family in whom autosomal recessive inheritance of the disorder was established. The occurrence of hypoparathyroidism, nerve deafness, and a steroid-resistant nephrosis leading to renal failure, which has been referred to as the Barakat syndrome, has been reported in four brothers from one family, and an association of hypoparathyroidism with congenital lymphoedema, nephropathy, mitral valve prolapse, and brachytelephalangy has been observed in two brothers from another family. Molecular genetic studies have not been reported from these two families.

Blomstrand's disease Blomstrand's chondrodysplasia is an autosomal recessive disorder characterized by early lethality, dramatically advanced bone maturation, and accelerated chondrocyte differentiation. Affected infants, who usually have consanguineous unaffected parents, develop pronounced hyperdensity of the entire skeleton with markedly advanced ossification that results in extremely short and poorly modelled long bones. Mutations of the PTH/PTHrP receptor that impair its function are associated with Blomstrand's disease. Thus, it seems likely that affected infants will, in addition to the skeletal defects, have abnormalities in other organs, including secondary hyperplasia of the parathyroid glands, presumably due to hypocalcaemia.

Polyglandular autoimmune hypoparathyroidism This syndrome (Fig. 13.6.4) comprises hypoparathyroidism, Addison's disease, candidiasis, and two or three of the following: insulin-dependent diabetes mellitus, primary hypogonadism, autoimmune thyroid disease, pernicious anaemia, chronic active hepatitis, steatorrhoea (malabsorption), alopecia (totalis or areata), and vitiligo. The disorder has also been referred to as either the autoimmune polyendocrinopathy candidiasis ectodermal dystrophy (APECED) syndrome or the polyglandular autoimmune type 1 syndrome. Antibodies directed against the adrenal, thyroid, and parathyroid glands are detected in the sera of some patients. The polyglandular autoimmune type 2 syndrome is characterized by adrenal insufficiency, insulin-dependent diabetes mellitus, and thyroid disease, and does not involve hypoparathyroidism. APECED syndrome, which has an autosomal recessive inheritance, has a high incidence

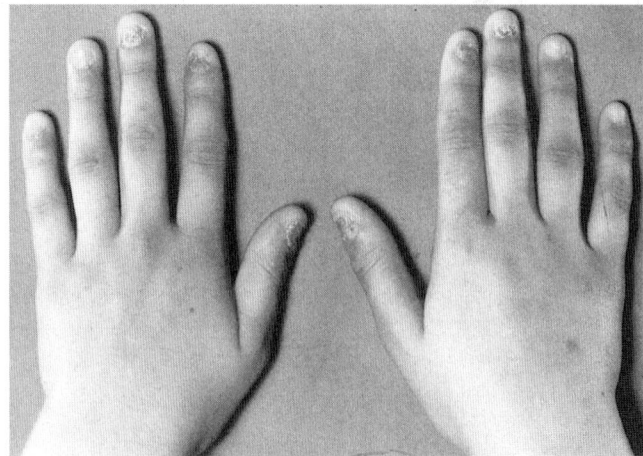

Fig. 13.6.4 Candidiasis and hyperpigmentation of the hands, particularly over the knuckles, are seen in this 8-year-old patient with hypoparathyroidism and Addison's disease. The patient also had vitiligo, and thus had some of the features of the polyglandular autoimmune syndrome type 1.
(Reproduced with permission from Thakker RV (1997). Hypocalcaemic disorders. In: Thakker RV, Wass JAH (eds) *Endocrine disorders, medicine*, vol. 25, pp. 68–70. The Medicine Group (Journals), Abingdon.)

in Finland and among Iranian Jews. The affected gene in APECED syndrome is the *AIRE* (autoimmune regulator) gene, which has been located to chromosome 21q22.3. It encodes a 545 amino acid protein that contains motifs suggestive of a transcriptional factor and includes a nuclear localization signal, two zinc-finger motifs, a proline-rich region, and three LXXLL motifs. Four *AIRE* mutations are commonly found in APECED families: Arg257Stop in Finnish, German, Swiss, British, and Northern Ireland families; Arg139Stop in Sardinian families; Tyr85Cys in Iranian Jewish families; and a 13-bp deletion in exon 8 in British, Dutch, German, and Finnish families. *AIRE1* has been shown to regulate the elimination of organ-specific T cells in the thymus, and APECED is likely to be caused by a failure of this specialized mechanism for deleting forbidden T cells and establishing immunological tolerance.

Calcium-sensing receptor abnormalities

The CaSR, which is located in the plasma membrane of the cell (Fig. 13.6.2), is at a critical site to enable the cell to recognize changes in extracellular calcium concentration. Thus, an increase in extracellular calcium leads to CaSR activation of the G protein signalling pathway, which in turn increases the free intracellular calcium concentration and leads to a reduction in transcription of the *PTH* gene. CaSR mutations that result in a loss of function are associated with familial hypocalciuric hypercalcaemia (see above). However, CaSR missense mutations that result in a gain of function (or added sensitivity to extracellular calcium) lead to hypocalcaemia with hypercalciuria. These hypocalcaemic individuals are generally asymptomatic and have serum PTH concentrations that are in the low to normal range, and because of the insensitivities of previous PTH assays in this range such patients have often been diagnosed to be hypoparathyroid. In addition, such patients may have hypomagnesaemia. Treatment with vitamin D or its active metabolites to correct the hypocalcaemia in these patients results in marked hypercalciuria, nephrocalcinosis, nephrolithiasis, and renal impairment. Thus, these patients need

to be distinguished from those with hypoparathyroidism and are referred to as having the condition of autosomal dominant hypocalcaemia with hypercalciuria.

Pseudohypoparathyroidism (PHP)

Patients with PHP, which may be inherited as an autosomal dominant disorder, are characterized by hypocalcaemia and hyperphosphataemia due to PTH resistance rather than PTH deficiency. Five variants are recognized on the basis of biochemical and somatic features (Table 13.6.3) and three of these—PHP type Ia (PHPIa), PHP type 1b (PHPIb), and pseudopseudohypoparathyroidism (PPHP)—will be reviewed in further detail.

Patients with PHPIa exhibit PTH resistance (hypocalcaemia, hyperphosphataemia, elevated serum PTH, and an absence of an increase in serum and urinary cAMP and urinary phosphate following intravenous human PTH infusion), together with the features of Albright's hereditary osteodystrophy (AHO), which includes short stature, obesity, subcutaneous calcification, mental retardation, round facies, dental hypoplasia, and brachydactyly (i.e. shortening of the metacarpals (Fig. 13.6.5), particularly the third, fourth, and fifth). In addition to brachydactyly, other skeletal abnormalities of the long bones and shortening of the metatarsals may also occur.

Patients with PHPIb exhibit PTH resistance only and do not have the somatic features of AHO, while patients with PPHP exhibit the somatic features of AHO in the absence of PTH resistance. The absence of a normal rise in urinary excretion of cAMP excretion after an infusion of PTH in PHPIa indicates a defect at some site of the PTH receptor–adenyl cyclase system (Fig. 13.6.2). This receptor system is regulated by at least two G proteins, one of which stimulates ($G_s\alpha$) and another which inhibits ($G_i\alpha$) the activity of the membrane-bound enzyme that catalyses the formation of the intracellular second messenger cAMP. Interestingly, patients with PHPIa may also show resistance to other hormones, e.g. thyroid-stimulating hormone, follicle-stimulating hormone, and luteinizing

Table 13.6.3 Clinical, biochemical, and genetic features of hypoparathyroid and pseudohypoparathyroid disorders

	Hypoparathyroidism	Pseudohypoparathyroidism				
		PHPIa	PPHP	PHPIb	PHPIc	PHPII
AHO manifestations	No	Yes	Yes	No	Yes	No
Serum calcium	↓	↓	N	↓	↓	↓
Serum PO$_4$	↑	↑	N	↑	↑	↑
Serum PTH	↓	↑	N	↑	↑	↑
Response to PTH:						
Urinary cAMP[a] (Chase–Aurbach test)	↑	↓	↑	↓	↓	↑
Urinary PO$_4$ (Ellsworth–Howard test)	↑	↓	↑	↓	↓	↓
G$_s\alpha$ activity	N	↓	↓	N	N	N
Inheritance	AD/AR/X	AD	AD	AD	AD	Sporadic
Molecular defect	PTH/CaSR/GATA3/GCM2/others	GNAS1	GNAS1	?GNAS1	?Adenyl cyclase	?cAMP targets
Other hormonal resistance	No	Yes	No	No	Yes	No

AD, autosomal dominant; AHO, Albright's hereditary osteodystrophy; AR, autosomal recessive; CaSR, calcium-sensing receptor; GATA3, GATA binding protein 3; GCM2, glial cells missing homolog 2; N, normal; PHP, pseudohypoparathyroidism; PPHP, pseudopseudohypoparathyroidism; X, X-linked; ↓, decreased; ↑, increased; ?, presumed, but not proven.

[a] Plasma cAMP responses are similar to those of urinary cAMP.

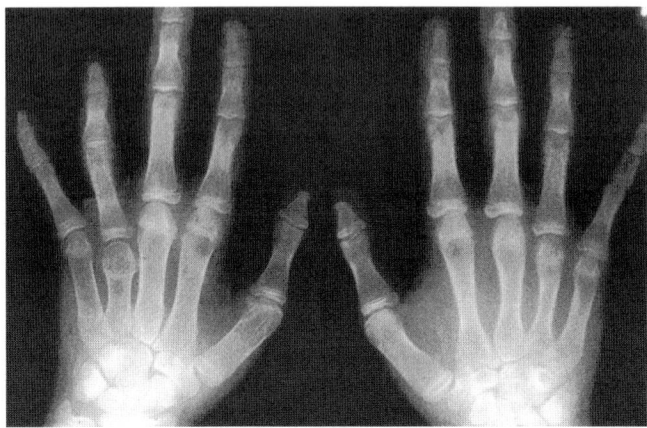

Fig. 13.6.5 Radiograph of both hands of a patient with pseudohypoparathyroidism type 1a. The patient has a normal right hand, but there is shortening of the left fourth metacarpal (brachydactyly). Metatarsals may be similarly shortened.
(Reproduced with permission from Thakker RV (1997). Hypocalcaemic disorders. In: Thakker RV, Wass JAH (eds) *Endocrine disorders, medicine*, vol. 25, pp. 68–70. The Medicine Group (Journals), Abingdon.)

hormone, that act via G protein-coupled receptors. Inactivating mutations of the $G_s\alpha$ gene (referred to as *GNAS1*), which is located on chromosome 20q13.2, have been identified in PHPIa and PPHP patients. However, *GNAS1* mutations do not fully explain the PHPIa or PPHP phenotypes, and studies of PHPIa and PPHP that occurred within the same kindred revealed that the hormonal resistance is parentally imprinted. Thus, PHPIa occurs in a child only when the mutation is inherited from a mother affected with either PHPIa or PPHP, and PPHP occurs in a child only when the mutation is inherited from a father affected with either PHPIa or PPHP. *GNAS1* mutations have not been detected in PHPIb, which has been considered to be due to a defect of the PTH/PTHrP receptor. However, studies of the PTH/PTHrP receptor gene and mRNA in PHPIb patients have not identified mutations, and linkage studies in four unrelated kindreds have mapped the PHPIb locus to chromosome 20q13.3, a location that also contains the *GNAS1* gene. In addition, parental imprinting of the genetic defect was observed and this is similar to the findings in kindreds with PHPIa and/or PPHP. Detailed analyses of the *GNAS1* gene in PHPIb families have revealed a large 3-kb deletion involving upstream exon(s) referred to as A/B. In affected individuals the deletion involved the maternal allele, whereas its occurrence on the paternal allele resulted in unaffected healthy carriers. This is consistent with parental imprinting of the *GNAS1* abnormality causing PHPIb.

Further reading

Arnold A (2006). Familial hyperparathyroid syndromes. In: Favus MJ (ed) *Primer on the metabolic diseases and disorders of mineral metabolism*, 6th edition, pp. 185–8. American Society for Bone and Mineral Research, Washington DC.

Bilezikian JP, Silversburg SJ (2006). Primary hyperparathyroidism. In: Favus MJ (ed) *Primer on the metabolic bone diseases and disorders of mineral metabolism*, 6th edition, pp. 181–5. American Society of Bone and Mineral Research, Washington, DC.

Block GA, *et al.* (2004). Cinacalcet for secondary hyperparathyroidism in patients receiving haemodialysis. *N Engl J Med*, **350**, 1516–25.

Bouillon R (2006). Vitamin D: from photosynthesis, metabolism, and action to clinical applications. In: DeGroot LJ, Jameson JL (eds) *Endocrinology*, 5th edition, pp. 1435–63. Elsevier Saunders, Philadelphia.

Bradley KJ, Thakker RV (2006). The hyperparathyroidism-jaw tumour (HPT-JT) syndrome. *Clin Cases Miner Bone Metab*, **3**, 167–74.

Bringhurst FR, Leder BZ (2006). Regulation of calcium and phosphate homeostasis. In: DeGroot LJ, Jameson JL (eds) *Endocrinology*, 5th edition, pp. 1465–98. Elsevier Saunders, Philadelphia.

Broadus AE, Nissenson RA (2006). Parathyroid hormone-related protein. In: Favus MJ (ed) *Primer on the metabolic diseases and disorders of mineral metabolism*, 6th edition, pp. 99–106. American Society for Bone and Mineral Research, Washington DC.

Diaz R, Brown EM (2006). Familial hypocalciuric hypercalcaemia and other disorders due to calcium-sensing receptor mutations. In: DeGroot LJ, Jameson JL (eds) *Endocrinology*, 5th edition, pp. 1595–609. Elsevier Saunders, Philadelphia.

Goltzman D, Cole EC (2006). Hypoparathyroidism. In: Favus MJ (ed) *Primer on the metabolic bone diseases and disorders of mineral metabolism*, 6th edition, pp. 216–19. American Society of Bone and Mineral Research, Washington DC.

Horwitz MJ, Stewart AF (2006). Hypercalcaemia associated with malignancy. In: Favus MJ (ed) *Primer on metabolic bone diseases and disorders of mineral metabolism*, 6th edition, pp. 195–9. American Society of Bone and Mineral Research, Washington DC.

Juppner H, *et al.* (2006). Parathyroid hormone and parathyroid hormone-related peptide in the regulation of calcium homeostasis and bone development. In: DeGroot LJ, Jameson JL (eds) *Endocrinology*, 5th edition, pp. 1377–417. Elsevier Saunders, Philadelphia.

Levine MA (2006). Parathyroid hormone resistance syndromes. In: Favus MJ (ed) *Primer on the metabolic bone diseases and disorders of mineral metabolism*, 6th edition, pp. 220–4. American Society of Bone and Mineral Research, Washington DC.

Marx SJ (2000). Hyperparathyroid and hypoparathyroid disorders. *N Engl J Med*, **343**, 1803–75.

Neer RM, *et al.* (2001). Effect of parathyroid hormone (1–34) on fractures and bone mineral density in postmenopausal women with osteoporosis. *N Engl J Med*, **344**, 1434–41.

Norton JA (2006). Surgical management of hyperparathyroidism. In: DeGroot LJ, Jameson JL (eds) *Endocrinology*, 5th edition, pp. 1583–94. Elsevier Saunders, Philadelphia.

Peacock M, *et al.* (2005). Cinacalcet hydrochloride maintains long-term normocalcemia in patients with primary hyperparathyroidism. *J Clin Endocrinol Metab*, **90**, 135–41.

Potts JT (2005). Parathyroid hormone: past and present. *J Endocrinol*, **187**, 311–25.

Prince RL (2006). Secondary and tertiary hyperparathyroidism. In: Favus MJ (ed) *Primer on the metabolic diseases and disorders of mineral metabolism*, 6th edition, pp. 190–5. American Society for Bone and Mineral Research, Washington DC.

Rubin MR, *et al.* (2003). Raloxifene lowers serum calcium and markers of bone turnover in postmenopausal women with primary hyperparathyroidism. *J Clin Endocrinol Metab*, **88**, 1174–8.

Shane E, Irani D (2006). Hypercalcaemia: pathogenesis, clinical manifestations, differential diagnosis and management. In: Favus MJ (ed) *Primer on the metabolic diseases and disorders of mineral metabolism*, 6th edition, pp. 176–80. American Society for Bone and Mineral Research, Washington DC.

Thakker RV (2000). Parathyroid disorders. Molecular genetics and physiology. In: Morris PJ, Wood WC (eds) *Oxford textbook of surgery*, pp. 1121–9. Oxford University Press, Oxford.

Thakker RV (2004). Diseases associated with the extracellular calcium-sensing receptor. *Cell Calcium*, **35**, 275–82.

Thakker RV (2006). Hypocalcaemia: pathogenesis, differential diagnosis and management. In: Favus MJ (ed) *Primer on the metabolic bone diseases and disorders of mineral metabolism*,

6th edition, pp. 213–15. American Society of Bone and Mineral Research, Washington DC.

Thakker RV (2006). Multiple endocrine neoplasia type 1. In: DeGroot LJ, Jameson JL (eds) *Endocrinology*, 5th edition, pp. 3509–31. Elsevier Saunders, Philadelphia.

Thakker RV, Juppner H (2006). Genetic disorders of calcium homeostasis caused by abnormal regulation of parathyroid hormone secretion or responsiveness. In: DeGroot LJ, Jameson JL (eds) *Endocrinology*, 5th edition, pp. 1511–31. Elsevier Saunders, Philadelphia.

Wysolmerski JJ (2006). Miscellaneous causes of hypercalcaemia. In: Favus MJ (ed) *Primer on the metabolic bone diseases and disorders of mineral metabolism*, 6th edition, pp. 203–8. American Society of Bone and Mineral Research, Washington DC.

13.7

Adrenal disorders

Contents

13.7.1 Disorders of the adrenal cortex

P.M. Stewart

Essentials

Three classes of steroid hormone are produced by the adrenal cortex after uptake of precursor cholesterol from the plasma: (1) mineralocorticoids—aldosterone, deoxycorticosterone; secreted in low amounts (100–150 µg aldosterone/day) from the zona glomerulosa, mainly under the control of angiotensin II; enhance uptake of sodium principally in the colon and kidney tubule by binding to receptors whose specificity for mineralocorticoids is established in these tissues by expression of 11 β-hydroxysteroid dehydrogenase 2, which converts cortisol to inactive cortisone; (2) glucocorticoids—cortisol, corticosterone; secreted in larger amounts (10–20 mg cortisol/day) from the zona fasciculata in response to stimulation by ACTH; have wide-ranging effects mediated by glucocorticoid receptors; and (3) sex steroids—principally dehydroepiandrosterone (DHEA) and its sulphated derivative (DHAS).

Classical endocrine feedback loops control secretion of these hormones: (1) aldosterone-induced retention of sodium inhibits secretion of renin; (2) cortisol inhibits secretion of both corticotropin-releasing factor (CRF) from the hypothalamus and ACTH from the pituitary.

Adrenocortical diseases are relatively uncommon, but their ease of diagnosis and the availability of effective treatment contribute to their importance in clinical practice. Hormonal deficiency or excess is usually the result of abnormal secretion, but similar functional defects may be caused by deranged metabolism of corticosteroids or by defective receptors. With increasing use of radiological investigations a frequent diagnosis is a patient with an underlying incidental tumour ('incidentaloma') of the adrenal: these are usually nonfunctional and benign.

Glucocorticoid excess

Cushing's syndrome may be (1) ACTH-dependent—usually due to a pituitary adenoma (Cushing's disease), but sometimes to nonpituitary tumours producing ACTH (most commonly small-cell carcinoma of the bronchus); (2) ACTH-independent—most often adrenal adenoma (rarely carcinoma).

Clinical features—typical presentation is with 'classical' manifestations of centripetal obesity, moon face, hirsutism, and plethora, with signs (when present) that best distinguish from simple obesity being bruising and muscle weakness (typically proximal).

Diagnosis of the presence of Cushing's syndrome—this can be confirmed by finding (1) elevated 24-h urinary free cortisol; and/or (2) raised midnight salivary/plasma cortisol; and/or (3) impaired plasma cortisol suppression (09.00 h sample) in response to a low-dose overnight dexamethasone suppression test.

Diagnosis of the cause of Cushing's syndrome—ACTH-dependent causes can be distinguished from ACTH-independent causes by measurement of plasma ACTH (09.00 h sample). Determining whether elevated ACTH is coming from the pituitary (Cushing's disease) or from an ectopic source can be difficult, but may be achieved by consideration of (1) plasma potassium—hypokalaemia is a typical feature of ectopic ACTH but not of Cushing's disease; (2) high-dose dexamethasone suppression test—which tends to suppress plasma cortisol in Cushing's disease but not ectopic ACTH; (3) CRF test—producing an exaggerated rise in ACTH and cortisol in Cushing's disease but not in ectopic ACTH; (4) inferior petrosal sinus sampling/selective venous catheterization—the most robust test to distinguish Cushing's disease from ectopic ACTH syndrome.

Imaging—pituitary MRI is the investigation of choice if biochemical testing suggests Cushing's disease, and abdominal CT scanning if biochemical testing suggests ACTH-independent Cushing's syndrome.

Management—drugs that interfere with cortisol synthesis (e.g. metyrapone, ketoconazole) can lower cortisol levels, but definitive treatment depends on the cause: (1) adrenal adenomas—unilateral adrenalectomy; (2) Cushing's disease—trans-sphenoidal removal of the pituitary tumour; (3) ectopic ACTH—surgical removal of the tumour is rarely possible but can lead to cure.

Glucocorticoid deficiency

Glucocorticoid deficiency can be due to adrenal disease (primary, in which case mineralocorticoids are also deficient) or because of deficiency of ACTH (secondary, in which case only glucocorticoids are deficient).

Aetiology—primary hypoadrenalism (Addison's disease) is most commonly caused by autoimmune disease (>70% cases in the Western world, associated with adrenal autoantibodies in many cases, and sometimes with other organ-specific autoimmune diseases) or infection, e.g. tuberculosis (the commonest cause worldwide). The commonest cause of secondary hypoadrenalism is stopping of exogenous glucocorticoid therapy or its inadequacy in stressful situations.

Clinical features—primary adrenal failure may present (1) acutely—with hypotension and acute circulatory failure (Addisonian crisis); or (2) chronically—with vague features of ill health, sometimes including gastrointestinal symptoms, features suggestive of postural hypotension, and salt craving. Skin pigmentation is nearly always present in primary adrenal insufficiency (but not in secondary).

Biochemical diagnosis—this depends on an ACTH stimulation test: plasma cortisol should rise to over 550 nmol/litre in response to injection of tetracosactrin (Synacthen, 250 μg) and failure to do so indicates adrenal insufficiency. In primary adrenal insufficiency the plasma ACTH level is disproportionately elevated in comparison with plasma cortisol.

Management—acute adrenal insufficiency is a medical emergency requiring volume resuscitation and parenteral steroid replacement, e.g. hydrocortisone 100 mg intravenously every 6 h, along with treatment of any precipitating condition, e.g. infection. Long-term treatment requires (1) glucocorticoid replacement—typically hydrocortisone, 20 mg on wakening and 10 mg at 18.00 h, to be doubled in the event of intercurrent stress or illness; (2) mineralocorticoid replacement—fludrocortisone, 0.05 to 0.1 mg/day, is usually required in primary adrenal failure. Every patient should be advised to wear a MedicAlert bracelet or necklace and to carry a 'steroid card'.

Mineralocorticoid excess

Primary aldosteronism (Conn's syndrome) is the commonest cause of mineralocorticoid hypertension and may be caused by an aldosterone-producing adenoma of the adrenal gland or by bilateral adrenal hyperplasia. The presence of primary aldosteronism is not easy to diagnose, but in the absence of confounding influences is suggested by a high random plasma aldosterone (PAC)/renin (PRA) ratio if PAC is over 400 pmol/litre (15 ng/dl). The cause of primary aldosteronism is also difficult to establish: adrenal MRI/CT scanning may demonstrate an adenoma; adrenal vein cannulation with sampling for estimation of aldosterone/cortisol ratio may be required in difficult cases. Treatment of adrenal adenoma is by surgical excision and of bilateral adrenal hyperplasia is medical, usually with spironolactone.

A number of single-gene defects can cause mineralocorticoid excess, including 17α-hydroxylase deficiency, 11β-hydroxylase deficiency, glucocorticoid-suppressible hyperaldosteronism (due to formation of a chimeric gene, 11β-hydroxylase/aldosterone synthase), and apparent mineralocorticoid excess (mutations in 11β-hydroxysteroid dehydrogenase type 2 gene).

Mineralocorticoid deficiency

This is most commonly seen in the context of primary hypoadrenalism (see above) but is also caused (rarely) by conditions including primary defects in aldosterone biosynthesis, defects in aldosterone action, and hyporeninaemic hypoaldosteronism (most commonly in the context of diabetic nephropathy).

Introduction

An initial rate-limiting step in adrenal steroidogenesis is the uptake of cholesterol from circulating cholesterol bound to low-density lipoprotein, by mitochondria in the adrenal cortex. This process is dependent upon steroidogenic acute regulatory protein. Thereafter, the functional zonation of the adrenal cortex is in part achieved through the discrete expression and regulation of the genes for the final steroidogenic enzymes: aldosterone synthase (EC 1.14.15.5) in the zona glomerulosa, and 11β-hydroxylase (EC 1.14.15.4) in the zona fasciculata (Fig. 13.7.1.1).

Aldosterone acts physiologically to stimulate sodium transport across epithelial cells in the distal nephron, colon, and salivary gland. This involves the interaction of aldosterone with the mineralocorticoid receptor, and the induction of the expression of the genes for the basolateral Na^+,K^+-ATPase pump and the apical sodium channel. This is mediated by the induction of $SGK1$, the gene for serum/glucocorticoid-regulated kinase 1. The mineralocorticoid receptor, however, is nonselective in vitro; paradoxically, cortisol and aldosterone have the same intrinsic affinity for this receptor, raising the question of why aldosterone is the preferred mineralocorticoid in vivo. This selectivity is achieved at a prereceptor level through the production of an enzyme, 11β-hydroxysteroid dehydrogenase type 2 (11β-HSD2; HSD11B2; EC 1.1.1.146), which efficiently inactivates cortisol to cortisone, allowing aldosterone to occupy the mineralocorticoid receptor. The inhibition of 11β-HSD2 results in cortisol, conventionally regarded as a glucocorticoid, acting as a potent mineralocorticoid.

Glucocorticoids have more diverse and extensive roles than mineralocorticoids, regulating sodium and water homeostasis, glucose and carbohydrate metabolism, inflammation, and stress. These effects are mediated by the interaction of cortisol with ubiquitous glucocorticoid receptors, and the induction or repression of target gene transcription.

Adrenocortical diseases are most readily classified by whether they are characterized by hormone excess or deficiency (Table 13.7.1.1).

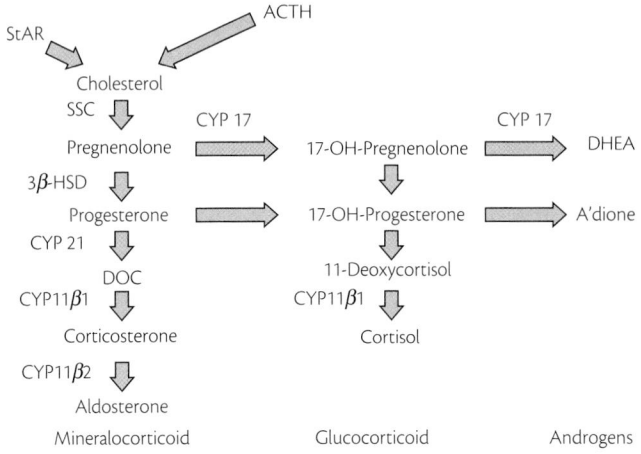

Fig. 13.7.1.1 Pathways of adrenocortical steroid biosynthesis.

Table 13.7.1.1 Adrenocortical diseases

Glucocorticoid excess
Cushing's syndrome
Glucocorticoid deficiency
Primary:
Congenital adrenal hyperplasia (21 hydroxylase, 3β-hydroxysteroid dehydrogenase, 17-hydroxylase, 11 β-hydroxylase, and StAR deficiencies)
Addison's disease
Hereditary adrenocortical unresponsiveness to ACTH
Secondary:
Post-corticosteroid therapy
Hypothalamic/pituitary disease
Mineralocorticoid excess
Aldosteronism
Other mineralocorticoids—monogenic forms of hypertension
Glucocorticoid resistance
Mineralocorticoid deficiency
Congenital adrenal hyperplasia
Congenital adrenal hypoplasia
Disorders of terminal part of aldosterone biosynthetic pathway
Pseudohypoaldosteronism
Hyporeninaemia
Addison's disease
Adrenal androgens
Excess:
Congenital adrenal hyperplasia (21-hydroxylase, 11 β-hydroxylase deficiency)
Polycystic ovary syndrome (PCOS), tumours
Deficiency:
Congenital adrenal hyperplasia (17-hydroxylase, 3β-hydroxysteroid dehydrogenase deficiency)
Adrenal incidentalomas and carcinomas

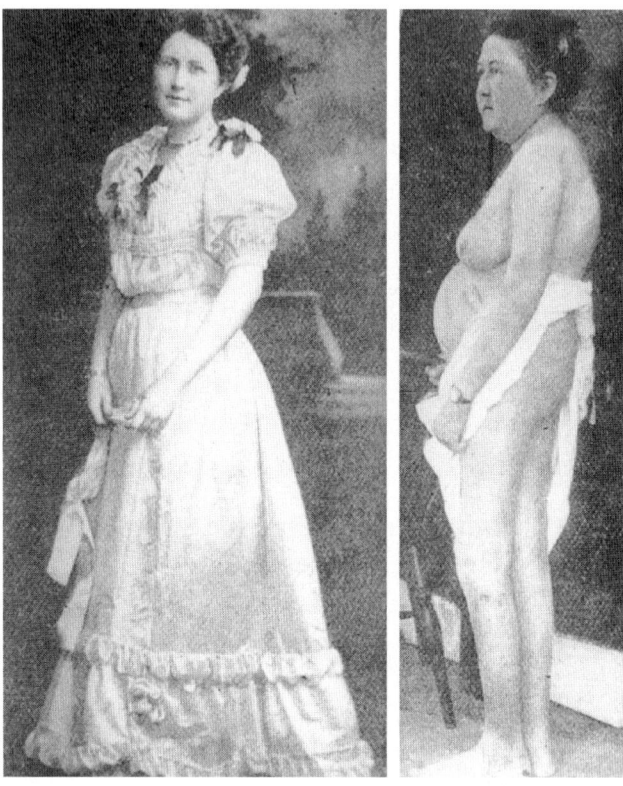

Fig. 13.7.1.2 H G Turney's case of Cushing's syndrome before and after developing the condition.

Glucocorticoid excess: Cushing's syndrome

Harvey Cushing first described a case of polyglandular syndrome secondary to pituitary basophilia in 1912, and several years later linked this to bilateral adrenal hyperplasia. The first case of an adrenal adenoma was probably reported by H G Turney in 1913 (Fig. 13.7.1.2).

Definition

Cushing's syndrome comprises the symptoms and signs associated with prolonged exposure to inappropriately elevated levels of free plasma glucocorticoids (Fig. 13.7.1.2). This definition thus takes into account the elevated corticosteroid levels that may be found in severely depressed patients, but which appear to be appropriate to the condition, and also the increased total (but normal free) glucocorticoid levels found when there is an increase in circulating cortisol-binding globulin (e.g. in patients on oestrogen therapy). The use of the term glucocorticoid in the definition covers both endogenous (cortisol) and exogenous steroid excess (e.g. prednisolone, dexamethasone).

The condition is most readily classified into ACTH-dependent and ACTH-independent causes (Table 13.7.1.2). The term 'Cushing's syndrome' is used to describe all causes, whereas 'Cushing's disease' is reserved for cases of pituitary-dependent Cushing's syndrome.

ACTH-dependent causes

Cushing's disease

When iatrogenic causes are excluded, the most frequent cause of Cushing's syndrome is Cushing's disease, which accounts for

Table 13.7.1.2 Classification of causes of Cushing's syndrome

ACTH-dependent
Iatrogenic (treatment with ACTH1–39 or Synacthen®, $ACTH_{1-24}$)
Cushing's disease (pituitary-dependent)
Ectopic ACTH syndrome
Ectopic corticotrophin-releasing factor syndrome
ACTH-independent
Iatrogenic (such as pharmacological doses of prednisolone or dexamethasone)
Adrenal adenoma
Adrenal carcinoma
Carney's syndrome
McCune–Albright syndrome
Aberrant receptor expression (gastric inhibitory polypeptide, interleukin 1β).
Alcohol

ACTH, adrenocorticotrophic hormone.

Table 13.7.1.3 Tumours associated with the ectopic ACTH syndrome

Tumour type	Approximate incidence (%)
Small-cell lung carcinoma	50
Non-small-cell lung carcinoma	5
Pancreatic tumours (including carcinoids)	10
Thymic tumours (including carcinoids)	5
Lung carcinoids	10
Other carcinoids	2
Medullary carcinoma of thyroid	5
Phaeochromocytoma and related tumours	3
Rare carcinomas of prostate, breast, ovary, gallbladder, colon	10

approximately 70% of cases. The adrenal glands show bilateral adrenocortical hyperplasia, with widening of the zona fasciculata and zona reticularis. Nodules may form within the hyperplastic glands.

Cushing himself raised the question of whether his disease was a primary pituitary condition or secondary to an abnormality of the hypothalamus. There is abundant evidence to indicate that the condition is related to the pituitary rather than the hypothalamus. In over 90% of cases the disease is caused by a pituitary adenoma of monoclonal origin; basophilic hyperplasia is very uncommon, and selective surgical removal of the microadenoma usually results in cure, with a low recurrence rate.

Ectopic production of corticotropin-releasing factor (CRF)

This is a very rare cause of pituitary-dependent Cushing's disease. However, cases have been described in which a tumour (e.g. medullary thyroid, prostate carcinoma) has been shown to produce CRF, but not ACTH.

Ectopic ACTH syndrome

Cushing's syndrome may be caused by nonpituitary tumours producing ACTH, most commonly a malignant small-cell carcinoma of the bronchus (Table 13.7.1.3). However, the most challenging diagnostic problems relate to ACTH secretion from more benign and indolent carcinoid tumours, which may present with Cushing's syndrome many years before the occult tumour manifests. These conditions are described further in Chapter 13.12.

ACTH-independent causes

Adrenal adenoma and carcinoma

With the exclusion of iatrogenic Cushing's syndrome, a solitary cortisol-secreting adrenal adenoma is the cause in about 10% of cases. Carcinomas are rarer, have a poor prognosis, and may be associated with the secretion of other hormones in addition to cortisol (usually adrenal androgens). The aetiology of these tumours is unknown.

Carney's syndrome (OMIM 160980)

This is an autosomal dominant condition involving mesenchymal tumours (especially atrial myxomas), spotty skin pigmentation, peripheral nerve tumours, and various endocrine tumours, one of which may lead to Cushing's syndrome. The adrenals then contain multiple small, pigmented nodules. The condition has been described as pigmented multinodular adrenocortical dysplasia, and results from mutations in the regulatory subunit R1A of protein kinase A, causing adrenal hyperfunction.

McCune–Albright syndrome (OMIM 174800)

In this condition, fibrous dysplasia and cutaneous pigmentation may be associated with pituitary, thyroid, adrenal, and gonadal hyperfunction. The adrenal hypersecretion may produce Cushing's syndrome. The underlying abnormality is a somatic mutation in the α subunit of the stimulatory guanine nucleotide-binding protein (G protein) that is linked to adenylate cyclase. The mutation results in the G protein being constitutively activated, which, in the adrenal gland, mimics constant ACTH stimulation. Adrenal nodular formation may occur.

Aberrant receptor expression (OMIM 219080)

Patients have been described with nodular hyperplasia, ACTH-independent Cushing's syndrome, and enhanced adrenal responsiveness to gastric inhibitory polypeptide (GIP). The biochemical clues are the presence of subnormal morning levels of plasma cortisol and a rise in cortisol after food. This food-dependent form of Cushing's syndrome results from the normal increase in GIP after eating. Not surprisingly, the clinical syndrome is related to food intake; fasting can produce adrenal insufficiency. It is now appreciated that a similar form of Cushing's syndrome can result from the aberrant expression of other receptors, including those for interleukin 1, luteinizing hormone, and serotonin.

Alcohol-associated pseudo-Cushing's syndrome

In the original description of this syndrome, urinary and plasma cortisol levels were elevated, but were not suppressed with dexamethasone. Plasma ACTH may be normal or suppressed. The frequency and pathogenesis of this condition remain unknown, but a two-hit hypothesis has been put forward to explain its aetiology. Chronic liver disease, irrespective of the cause, is associated with impaired cortisol metabolism, but in alcoholics this is associated with an increase in the cortisol secretion rate, rather than

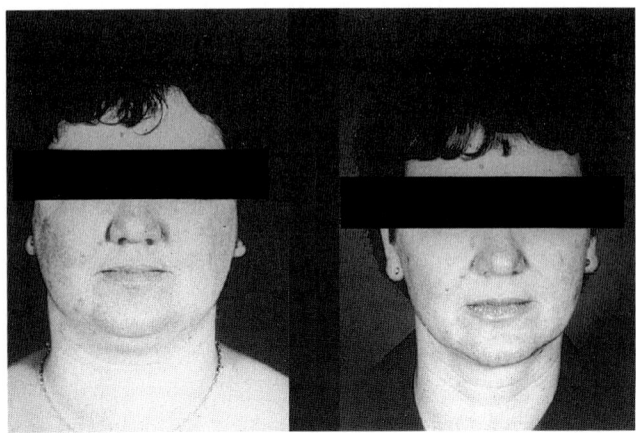

Fig. 13.7.1.3 Typical facies of a patient with Cushing's syndrome before and after treatment.

Table 13.7.1.4 Prevalence of symptoms and signs in Cushing's syndrome and discriminant index compared with prevalence of features in patients with simple obesity

	%	Discriminant index
Symptoms		
Weight gain	91	
Menstrual irregularity	84	1.6
Hirsutism	81	2.8
Psychiatric	62	
Backache	43	
Muscle weakness	29	8.0
Fractures	19	
Loss of scalp hair	13	
Signs		
Obesity	97	
Truncal	46	1.6
Generalized	55	0.8
Plethora	94	3.0
Moon face	88	
Hypertension	74	4.4
Bruising	62	10.3
Red/purple striae	56	2.5
Muscle weakness	56	
Ankle oedema	50	
Pigmentation	4	
Other findings		
Hypertension	74	
Diabetes	50	
Overt	13	
Impaired GTT	37	
Osteoporosis	50	
Renal calculi	15	

Data from Ross and Linch (1982).
GTT, glucose tolerance test.

concomitant suppression in the face of impaired metabolism. With abstinence from alcohol the biochemical abnormalities rapidly revert to normal.

Clinical features of Cushing's syndrome

The classical features of Cushing's syndrome—centripetal obesity, moon face, hirsutism, and plethora—are well known following Cushing's initial description in 1912 (Figs. 13.7.1.2 and 13.7.1.3). However, this gross clinical picture is not always present. The signs and symptoms in patients with Cushing's syndrome are listed in Table 13.7.1.4, together with the most discriminatory features distinguishing Cushing's syndrome from simple obesity. Weight gain and obesity are the most common symptom and sign, but the distribution of fat is not invariably centripetal—a 'buffalo hump' is present in about one-half of patients.

Gonadal dysfunction is very common, with menstrual irregularity in females and loss of libido in males, resulting from a suppressive effect of cortisol on gonadotropin secretion. Hirsutism is frequently found in female patients, as is acne, and reflects ACTH-stimulated hyperandrogenism.

Psychiatric abnormalities have been reported in all series of patients with Cushing's syndrome, regardless of cause. Depression and lethargy are among the most common problems, but poor concentration, paranoia, and overt psychosis are also well recognized. Lowering of plasma cortisol by medical or surgical therapy usually results in a rapid improvement in the psychiatric state.

Many patients with long-standing Cushing's syndrome have lost height because of osteoporotic vertebral collapse. Pathological fractures, either spontaneous or after minor trauma, are not uncommon. Rib fractures, by contrast with those of the vertebrae, are often painless. The radiographic appearance is typical, with exuberant callus formation at the site of the healing fracture.

The plethoric appearance of the patient with Cushing's syndrome results from thinning of the skin, not true polycythaemia. The typical red-purple livid striae of the syndrome are found most frequently on the abdomen, but may also be present on the upper thighs and arms. They are very common in younger patients, and less so in those over 50 years of age.

Myopathy and bruising are two of the most discriminatory features of the syndrome. The myopathy involves the proximal muscles of the lower limbs and the shoulder girdle. Complaints of weakness, such as an inability to climb stairs or get up from a deep chair, are relatively uncommon, but observation of whether the patient can rise from a crouching position often reveals the problem. Bruising of the skin is often extensive and occurs with unknown or trivial trauma.

Hypertension is another prominent feature. Even though epidemiological data show a strong association between blood pressure and obesity, hypertension is much more common in patients with Cushing's syndrome than in those with simple obesity.

Pigmentation is rare in Cushing's disease, but common in ectopic ACTH syndrome. However, in some pituitary tumours there is abnormal processing of the pro-opiomelanocortin (POMC) precursor molecule, with resulting pigmentation.

Infections are more common in patients with Cushing's syndrome than in unaffected individuals. In many instances these are asymptomatic, as the normal inflammatory response may be suppressed. Reactivation of tuberculosis has been reported. Fungal infection of the skin is frequently found. Glucose intolerance may be a predisposing factor, with overt diabetes being present in up to one-third of patients in some series.

Ocular effects may include raised intraocular pressure, chemosis, and exophthalmos (present in up to one-third of patients in Cushing's original series). Cataracts, a well recognized complication of exogenous corticosteroid therapy, seem to be uncommon, except as a complication of diabetes.

In patients with ectopic ACTH syndrome caused by small-cell lung carcinoma, the clinical presentation more commonly resembles Addison's disease than Cushing's syndrome. The patients are very commonly pigmented and have lost weight, but the association of these with hypokalaemic alkalosis and glucose intolerance should alert the clinician to the diagnosis. Patients with more indolent causes, such as bronchial carcinoids, present with the more typical features of Cushing's syndrome.

Special features of Cushing's syndrome

Cyclical Cushing's syndrome

Of particular clinical interest has been a group of patients with cyclical Cushing's syndrome, characterized by periods of excess cortisol production (e.g. 40 days), followed by intervals of normal cortisol production (e.g. 60–70 days). Some of these patients demonstrate a paradoxical rise in plasma ACTH and cortisol when treated with dexamethasone. Most patients have been thought to have pituitary-dependent disease, and in many of these patients basophil adenomas have been removed, some with long-term cure. However, cortisol secretion may show some evidence of cyclicity in other causes of Cushing's syndrome, notably ectopic ACTH syndrome.

Children

All the above features occur in children, but growth arrest is almost invariable. The dissociation between height and weight on the growth chart is obvious. If the child is growing along the same centile line then the diagnosis of Cushing's syndrome is highly unlikely. In addition to glucocorticoid-induced growth arrest, androgen excess may result in precocious puberty.

Pregnancy

Pregnancy is rare in women with Cushing's syndrome because of associated amenorrhoea resulting from androgen excess or hypercortisolism. However, approximately 100 such cases have been reported, 50% of which resulted from adrenal adenomas.

A few cases of true pregnancy-induced Cushing's syndrome have been reported, with postpartum regression. In these cases the aetiology is unknown. Establishing a diagnosis and cause can be difficult; normal pregnancy is associated with a threefold increase in plasma cortisol caused by increased production rates and increases in cortisol-binding globulin. Urinary free cortisol also rises, and dexamethasone does not suppress plasma cortisol to the same degree as in the nonpregnant state. Untreated, the condition has high maternal and fetal morbidity and mortality. Adrenal and/or pituitary adenomas should be excised. Metyrapone, which is not teratogenic, has been effective in controlling the hypercortisolism in many cases.

Adrenal carcinomas

In addition to the normal features of glucocorticoid excess the patient may present with other problems relating to: (1), the tumour, e.g. abdominal pain from the primary tumour or secondary deposits, or (2), the secretion of other steroids such as androgens or mineralocorticoids. Thus, in addition to hirsutism, there may be other features of virilization in females, including clitoromegaly, breast atrophy, deepening of the voice, temporal recession, and severe acne.

Investigation of patients with suspected Cushing's syndrome

There are two stages in the investigation of a patient with suspected Cushing's syndrome: (1), does the patient have Cushing's syndrome? (2), if the answer to (1) is yes, what is the cause? Unfortunately many investigators fail to make this distinction and ill-advisedly use tests that are relevant to question (2) to try to answer question (1). In particular, it is essential that appropriate radiological investigations are not undertaken until Cushing's syndrome has been confirmed biochemically. The principal diagnostic tests are listed in Table 13.7.1.5.

Diagnostic tests

Practically, three screening tests should be used to confirm Cushing's syndrome. Depending on the index of clinical suspicion these can be performed in isolation or combination.

Urinary free cortisol

For many years the diagnosis of Cushing's syndrome was based on the measurement of urinary metabolites of cortisol (24-h urinary 17-hydroxycorticosteroid or 17-oxogenic steroid excretion, depending on the method used). However, the sensitivity and

Table 13.7.1.5 Tests used in the diagnosis and differential diagnosis of Cushing's syndrome

Diagnosis
—does the patient have Cushing's syndrome?
Circadian rhythm of cortisol-late night plasma or salivary cortisol.
Urinary free cortisol excretion*
Low-dose dexamethasone suppression test*
Insulin tolerance test
Differential diagnosis
—what is the cause of the Cushing's syndrome?
Plasma ACTH
Plasma potassium
High-dose dexamethasone suppression test
Metyrapone test
Corticotrophin-releasing factor
Inferior petrosal sinus ± selective venous sampling for ACTH
MRI/CT scanning of pituitary/adrenals
Scintigraphy
Tumour markers

*Valuable outpatient screening tests (see text).

specificity of these methods is poor and these assays have now been replaced with the much more sensitive measurement of urinary free cortisol excretion. Urinary free cortisol is an integrated measure of plasma free cortisol. As cortisol secretion increases, the binding capacity of cortisol-binding globulin is exceeded, resulting in a disproportionate rise in urinary free cortisol. This is a useful screening test, but even so, it is accepted that urinary free cortisol may be normal in 7 to 10% of patients with Cushing's syndrome.

Measurement of the cortisol:creatinine ratio in the first urine specimen passed on waking obviates the need for a timed collection, and has been used by some as a sensitive screening test, particularly if cyclical Cushing's syndrome is suspected. Urine aliquots are stable at room temperature for up to 7 days, and can then be sent by post to the local endocrine laboratory.

Late night plasma/salivary cortisol

In normal subjects, plasma cortisol concentrations are at their highest first thing in the morning and reach a nadir at around midnight (up to 100 nmol/litre in the morning and <50 nmol/litre at midnight effectively excluding Cushing's syndrome). This circadian rhythm is lost in patients with Cushing's syndrome, such that in most patients the 09.00 level of plasma cortisol is normal, but nocturnal levels are raised. Random morning levels of plasma cortisol are therefore of little value in making the diagnosis. In addition, various factors, such as the stress of venepuncture, intercurrent illness, and admission to hospital, may result in normal subjects losing their circadian rhythm. It is therefore good practice not to measure plasma cortisol until the patient has been in hospital for 48 h. For this reason midnight plasma cortisol is not routinely used as a first-line screening test.

By contrast, midnight salivary cortisol can be collected at home and offers greater accuracy. A salivary cortisol value of more than 5.5 nmol/litre (2.0 ng/ml) has 100% sensitivity and 95% specificity in diagnosing Cushing's syndrome. Other screening and confirmatory tests may be required to evaluate false positive results.

Low-dose/overnight dexamethasone suppression tests

In normal subjects, administration of a supraphysiological dose of a glucocorticoid results in suppression of ACTH and hence cortisol secretion. In Cushing's syndrome of whatever cause there is failure of this suppression when low doses of the synthetic glucocorticoid dexamethasone are given. The overnight test is often used as an outpatient screening test. Various doses of dexamethasone have been used, usually given at midnight, but most experience is with a dose of 1 mg. A plasma cortisol of less than 50 nmol/litre between 08.00 and 09.00 the following morning has a sensitivity of 95% and specificity of 80% in excluding Cushing's syndrome. Thus the outpatient overnight test has high sensitivity but low specificity, and further investigation is often required.

The conventional low-dose 48-h test is more accurate, but usually requires inpatient admission. Here, plasma cortisol is measured at 09.00 on day 0 and 48 h later, following dexamethasone given at a dose of 0.5 mg every 6 h for 48 h. This test is reported as having a 97 to 100% true positive rate and a false positive rate of less than 1%. Certain drugs (phenytoin, rifampicin) may increase the metabolic clearance rate of dexamethasone, thereby giving false positive results. If pseudo-Cushing's syndrome is suspected, physicians in North America have modified this test slightly by administering CRF at the end of the dexamethasone suppression; ....

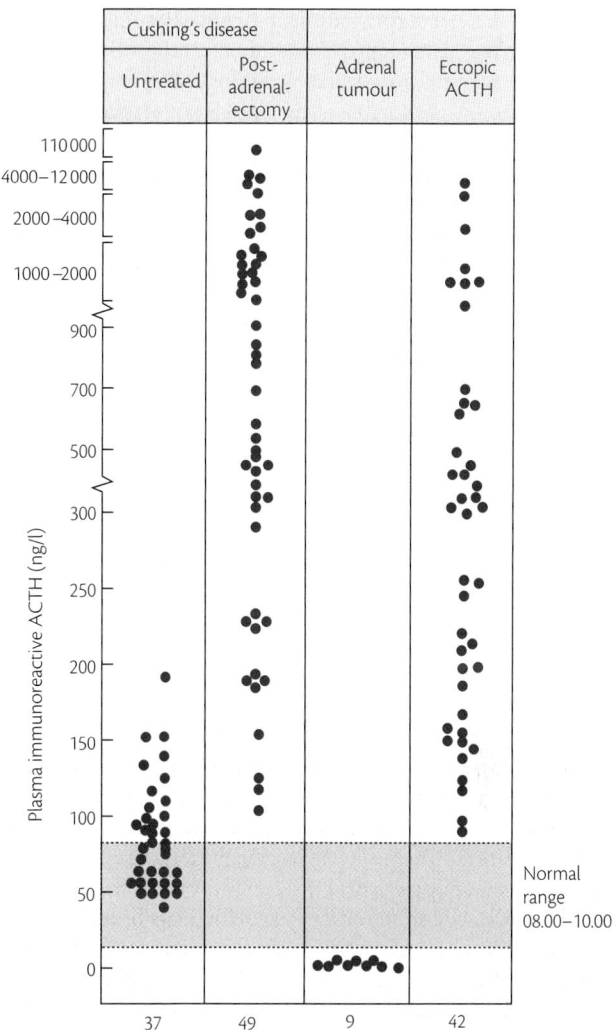

Fig. 13.7.1.4 Immunoreactive N-terminal ACTH levels in plasma samples taken between 08.00 and 10.00 in normal subjects (hatched area), and patients with Cushing's disease (either untreated or postadrenalectomy), adrenal tumours, or ectopic ACTH syndrome.
(Courtesy of Professor L H Rees.)

Differential diagnostic tests

Once the biochemical diagnosis has been made, other investigations are required to determine the cause of the Cushing's syndrome.

Plasma ACTH at 09.00

This will differentiate ACTH-dependent from ACTH-independent causes. ACTH is either within the normal reference range (50% of cases) or elevated in patients with Cushing's disease. ACTH levels in ectopic ACTH syndrome are high, but overlap the values seen in Cushing's disease in 30% of cases and cannot therefore be used to differentiate these two conditions (Fig. 13.7.1.4). The measurement of ACTH precursors (pro-ACTH, POMC) is not routinely available, but may be more useful in detecting an ectopic source of ACTH.

In patients with autonomous adrenal tumours, plasma ACTH is invariably undetectable. This can also occur with degradation of ACTH; consequently, nonhaemolysed blood samples should be taken on ice and immediately separated.

Diagnosis is a problem in those patients whose plasma ACTH levels are in the low normal range or intermittently detectable. This may occur in macronodular hyperplasia. The danger is that in some patients the asymmetry of the nodular hyperplasia may lead to a diagnosis of adrenal adenoma, the plasma ACTH is ignored, and an inappropriate adrenalectomy is performed. Conversely, in some patients with this syndrome an autonomous adrenal tumour develops and, despite detectable ACTH, unilateral adrenalectomy is required.

Plasma potassium

Hypokalaemic alkalosis is present in more than 95% of patients with ectopic ACTH syndrome, but in fewer than 10% of patients with Cushing's disease. Patients with the ectopic syndrome usually have higher cortisol secretion rates that saturate the renal protective 11β-HSD2 enzyme, resulting in cortisol-induced mineralocorticoid hypertension (see 'Apparent mineralocorticoid excess syndrome' below). In addition, these patients have higher levels of the ACTH-dependent mineralocorticoid deoxycorticosterone. See also Chapter 21.2.2.

High-dose dexamethasone suppression test

The rationale for this test is that in Cushing's disease there is negative feedback control of ACTH, but set at a higher level than normal. Thus, in this disease, cortisol levels are not suppressed with a low dose of dexamethasone, but are suppressed with a higher dose. The original test introduced by Liddle was based on giving dexamethasone at a dose of 2 mg every 6 h for 48 h and measuring urinary 17-oxogenic steroids. Suppression was defined as a greater than 50% fall in 24-h urinary 17-oxogenic steroids. In the modern test, plasma cortisol is measured at 0 and 48 h or, less commonly, plasma cortisol is measured at 08.00 (basal sample), 8 mg dexamethasone is given orally at 23.00 on the same day, and plasma cortisol is measured again at 08.00 on the following morning. In both these tests, greater than 50% suppression of plasma cortisol in comparison with the basal sample has been used to define a positive response. In Cushing's disease about 90% of patients have a positive 48-h test, compared with 10% with ectopic ACTH syndrome. With overnight high-dose testing, 89% sensitivity and 100% specificity has been reported for Cushing's disease.

Metyrapone test

Metyrapone is an 11β-hydroxylase inhibitor that blocks the conversion of 11-deoxycortisol to cortisol, and deoxycorticosterone to corticosterone (Fig. 13.7.1.1). This lowers plasma cortisol and, via negative feedback control, increases plasma ACTH. This in turn stimulates an increase in the secretion of adrenal steroids proximal to the block. When metyrapone is given in doses of 750 mg every 4 h for 24 h, patients with Cushing's disease exhibit an exaggerated rise in plasma ACTH, with 11-deoxycortisol levels at 24 h exceeding 1000 nmol/litre. In most patients with ectopic ACTH syndrome there is little or no response, but occasional patients (possibly those producing both ACTH and CRF) have an 11-deoxycortisol response that may be similar to that in Cushing's disease.

The metyrapone test was originally used to distinguish patients with Cushing's disease from those with a primary adrenal cause. However, these can be more reliably distinguished by measuring plasma ACTH and CT scanning of the adrenal glands. As indicated, the test does not reliably distinguish between Cushing's disease and ectopic ACTH syndrome, and the value of this test has been questioned. It should be reserved for patients in whom the results of other tests are equivocal.

CRF test

CRF is a peptide of 41 amino acids, identified by Vale in 1981 from ovine hypothalami. The ovine sequence differs by seven amino acid residues from that of the human peptide, but despite this stimulates the release of ACTH in humans. The test involves the intravenous injection of either ovine or human CRF at a dose of 1 μg/kg body weight or a single dose of 100 μg. The test can be performed in the morning or afternoon, and after basal sampling, blood samples for ACTH and cortisol are taken every 15 min for 1 to 2 h after administering CRF.

In normal subjects CRF elicits a rise in ACTH and cortisol, and this response is exaggerated in Cushing's disease. It is typically absent in ectopic ACTH syndrome and patients with adrenal tumours. In distinguishing pituitary-dependent Cushing's disease from ectopic ACTH syndrome, the response of ACTH to CRF has a specificity of 90%, and with cortisol as the endpoint, 95%. Using as an endpoint an ACTH increase of 100% over basal, or a cortisol rise of 50%, this positive response eliminates a possible diagnosis of ectopic ACTH syndrome.

Inferior petrosal sinus sampling/selective venous catheterization

This is the most robust test for distinguishing Cushing's disease from ectopic ACTH syndrome, but also the most costly and technically demanding. As blood from each half of the pituitary drains into the ipsilateral inferior petrosal sinus, catheterization of both sinuses with simultaneous sampling of venous blood can distinguish a pituitary from an ectopic source, and aid in the lateralization of a pituitary microadenoma (Fig. 13.7.1.5). In patients with ectopic ACTH syndrome there is no ACTH gradient between the inferior petrosal sinus samples and simultaneously drawn peripheral venous levels. In Cushing's disease the ipsilateral:contralateral ACTH ratio is usually greater than 1.4. However, because of the problem of intermittent ACTH secretion, it is useful to make measurements before and at intervals (e.g. 2, 5, and 15 min) after intravenous injection of 100 μg of synthetic ovine CRF. Using this approach, patients with Cushing's disease and bilateral inferior petrosal sinus ratios of less than 1.4 can readily be distinguished from those with the ectopic syndrome. The precise ratio that

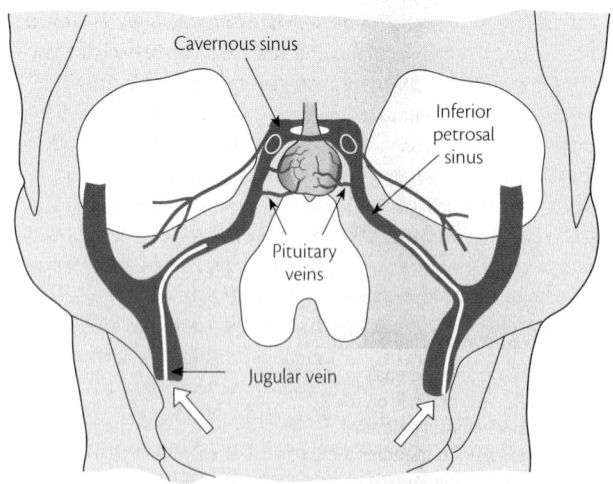

Fig. 13.7.1.5 Positions of bilateral catheters in inferior petrosal sinus sampling.

distinguishes Cushing's disease from the ectopic syndrome has been debated. Some authors use 2 rather than 1.4.

In our hands, petrosal sinus sampling is reserved for those cases where the differential diagnosis is still in doubt after high-dose dexamethasone, pituitary imaging, and peripheral CRF testing.

Rarely, selective catheterization of vascular beds may be required to identify the source of ectopic ACTH secretion, e.g. from a small pulmonary carcinoid or thymic tumour.

Tumour markers

Many tumours responsible for ectopic ACTH syndrome also produce peptide hormones other than ACTH or its precursors. Calcitonin, chromogranin A, and gut hormones such as gastrin and vasoactive intestinal polypeptide should be measured.

Imaging

There is no doubt that high-resolution contrast-enhanced imaging of thin sections of the pituitary and adrenals by either CT or MRI has revolutionized the investigation of Cushing's syndrome. However, if mistakes are to be avoided it is essential that the results of any imaging technique always be interpreted in the light of the biochemical results. In imaging the adrenals, asymmetrical nodular hyperplasia may lead to a false diagnosis of adrenal adenoma (Fig. 13.7.1.6). Owing to the presence of pituitary incidentalomas, pituitary MRI/CT scanning may produce false-positive results, particularly for lesions of less than 5 mm diameter (see 'Adrenal incidentalomas' below).

Pituitary MRI is the investigation of choice if the biochemical tests suggest Cushing's disease, and has a sensitivity of 70% and specificity of 87% (Figs. 13.7.1.7 and 13.7.1.8). About 90% of ACTH-secreting pituitary tumours are microadenomas, i.e. less than 10 mm in diameter. The classical features of a pituitary microadenoma are a hypodense lesion after contrast, associated with deviation of the pituitary stalk and a convex upper surface of the pituitary gland (Fig. 13.7.1.7). With such small tumours it is not surprising that the sensitivity of CT scanning is relatively low (20–60%), with a similar specificity.

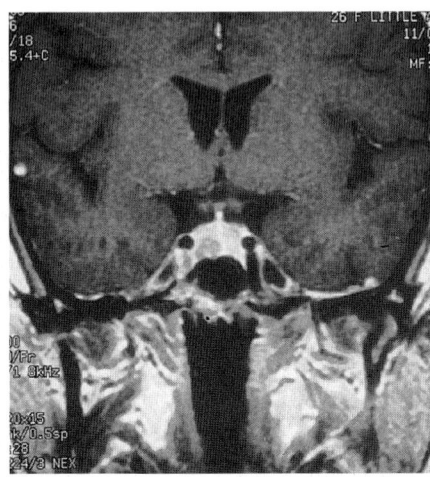

Fig. 13.7.1.7 MRI scan of pituitary demonstrating the typical appearance of a pituitary microadenoma. A hypodense lesion is seen in the left side of the gland, with deviation of the pituitary stalk away from the lesion. Following a biochemical diagnosis of Cushing's disease, this patient was cured following transsphenoidal hypophysectomy.

By contrast, CT scanning rather than MRI is the investigation of choice for adrenal imaging, offering better spatial resolution (Fig. 13.7.1.9). Once again it is stressed that adrenal incidentalomas are present in up to 5% of normal subjects, and thus adrenal imaging should not be performed unless biochemical investigation suggests a primary adrenal cause. Adrenal carcinomas are large and often associated with metastatic spread at presentation (Fig. 13.7.1.10).

In patients with occult ectopic ACTH syndrome, high-definition MRI/CT scanning of the neck, thorax, and abdomen/pelvis, with images every 0.5 cm, may be required to detect small ACTH-secreting carcinoid tumours.

Adrenal scintigraphy is of value in certain patients with primary adrenal pathology. The most commonly used agent is [131I]-6β-iodomethyl-19-norcholesterol, a marker of adrenocortical cholesterol uptake. In patients with adrenal adenomas the isotope is taken up by the adenoma, but not by the contralateral suppressed adrenal. Adrenal scintigraphy is useful in patients with suspected

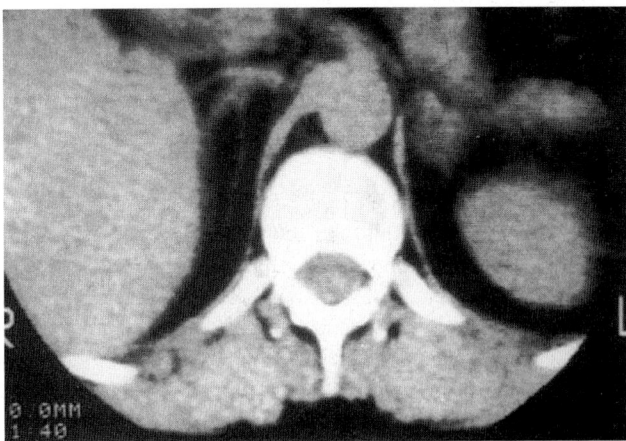

Fig. 13.7.1.6 CT scan of adrenals in patient with asymmetrical nodular hyperplasia. The macronodule on the left was initially thought to be an adrenal tumour. The biochemistry indicating ACTH-dependent Cushing's syndrome was ignored, and a unilateral adrenalectomy performed without cure of the hypercortisolism. Further investigation confirmed Cushing's disease, and a selective pituitary microadenomectomy resulted in cure.

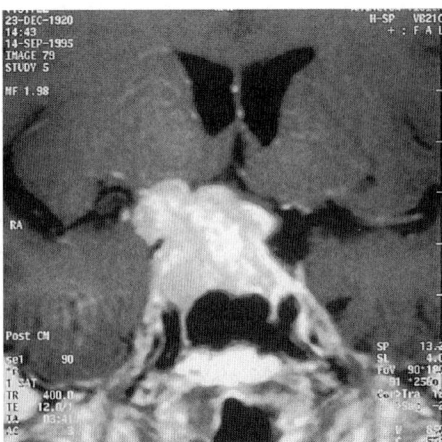

Fig. 13.7.1.8 MRI scan of the pituitary gland, demonstrating a large macroadenoma in a patient with Cushing's disease. By contrast with smaller tumours, these tumours are invariably invasive and recur following surgery.

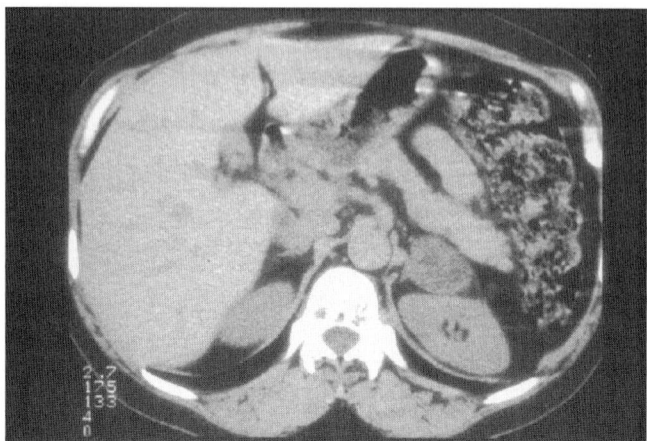

Fig. 13.7.1.9 Typical solitary left-sided adrenal adenoma on adrenal CT scanning.

adrenocortical macronodular hyperplasia, in which CT scanning may mislead by suggesting unilateral pathology, whereas with isotope scanning the bilateral adrenal involvement is identified (Fig. 13.7.1.11).

Treatment of Cushing's syndrome

Prognosis

Studies carried out before the introduction of effective therapy suggested that 50% of patients with untreated Cushing's syndrome

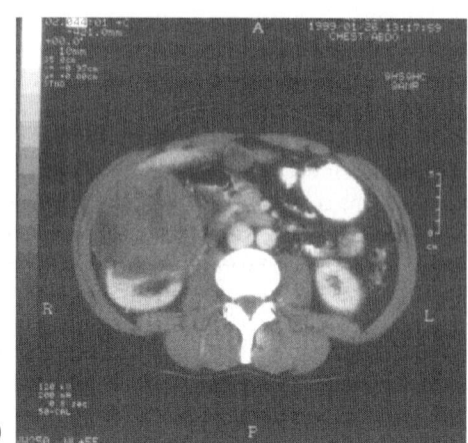

(a)

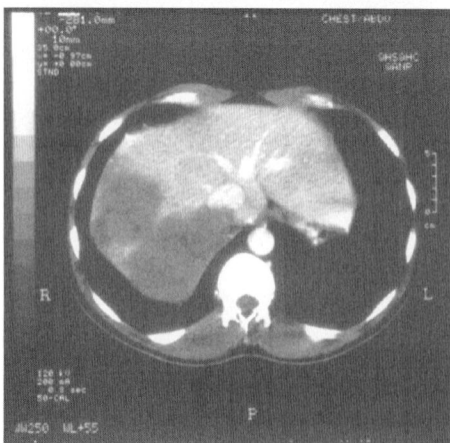

(b)

Fig. 13.7.1.10 CT scan of a patient with rapidly progressing Cushing's syndrome as a result of a right-sided adrenal carcinoma. An irregular right adrenal mass is shown (a) with a large liver metastasis (b).

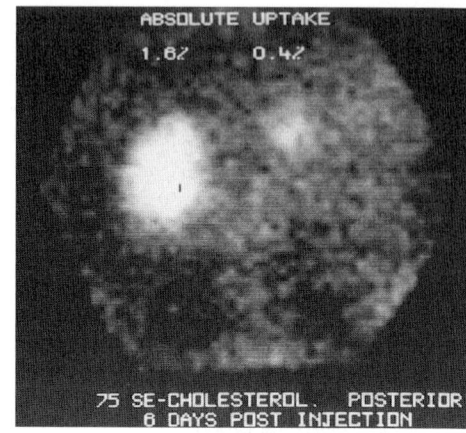

Fig. 13.7.1.11 Adrenal scintigraphy in a patient with Cushing's syndrome and macronodular hyperplasia. Note asymmetrical uptake in the adrenals, with 1.6% uptake on the left and 0.4% on the right.

died within 5 years, causing some physicians to label this the 'killing disease'. Even with modern management, an increased prevalence of cardiovascular risk factors persists for many years after an apparent cure. Close follow-up of all patients is recommended.

Adrenal causes

Adrenal adenomas should be removed by unilateral adrenalectomy, which has a 100% cure rate. With the increasing experience of laparoscopic adrenalectomy in most tertiary centres, this has now become the surgical treatment of choice for unilateral tumours, reducing surgical morbidity and postoperative hospital stay compared with traditional open approaches. After surgery it may take many months or even years for the suppressed adrenal to recover. It is wise therefore to give slightly suboptimal replacement therapy (<25–30 mg hydrocortisone/day or equivalent), with intermittent measurement of the 08.00 level of plasma cortisol after having omitted therapy for 24 h. When the morning plasma cortisol is above 180 nmol/litre a stimulation test such as an insulin tolerance test may then demonstrate whether or not the hypothalamic–pituitary–adrenal axis has recovered.

Adrenal carcinomas have a very poor prognosis and most patients are dead within 2 years. It is usual practice to try to remove the primary tumour, even though metastases may be present, so as to enhance the response to the adrenolytic agent mitotane (see 'Medical treatment of Cushing's syndrome' below). Radiotherapy to the tumour bed and to some metastases, such as those in the spine, may be of limited value.

Pituitary-dependent Cushing's disease

The treatment of Cushing's disease has been improved by transsphenoidal surgery conducted by an experienced surgeon. Before the selective removal of a pituitary microadenoma the treatment of choice was bilateral adrenalectomy. This had an appreciable mortality, even in the best centres (c.4%), as well as morbidity. The main risk was the subsequent development of Nelson's syndrome (postadrenalectomy hyperpigmentation with locally aggressive pituitary tumour) (Fig. 13.7.1.12). To avoid this, pituitary irradiation was often carried out following bilateral adrenalectomy. These patients required lifelong replacement therapy with hydrocortisone and fludrocortisone. Today, bilateral adrenalectomy is reserved for the occasional patient with Cushing's disease in whom

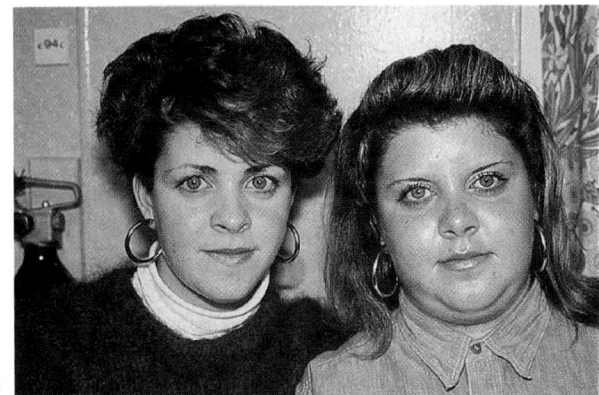

(a)

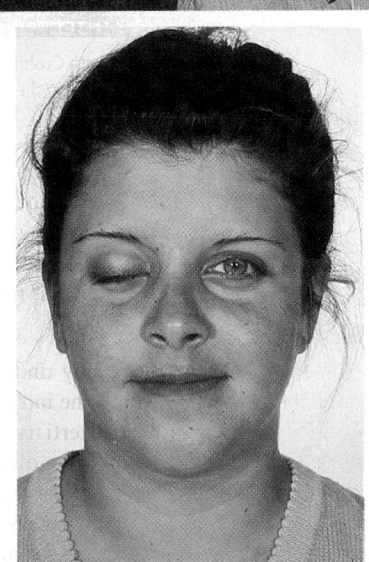

(b)

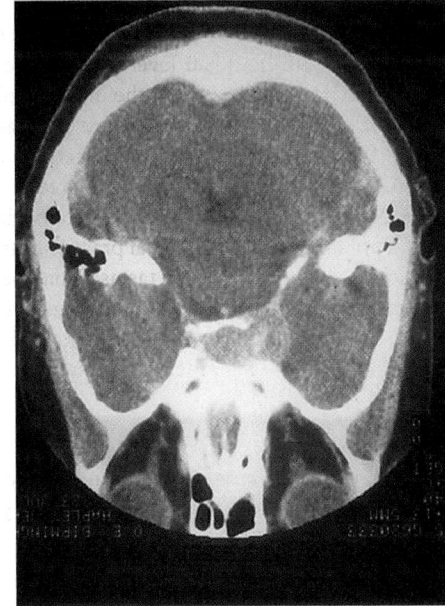

(c)

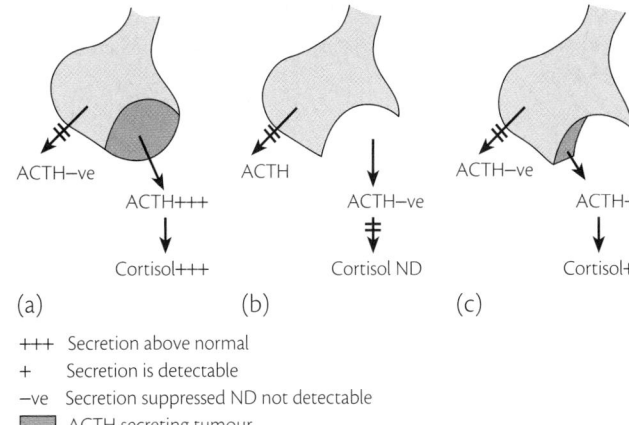

+++ Secretion above normal
+   Secretion is detectable
−ve Secretion suppressed ND not detectable
▧   ACTH secreting tumour

Fig. 13.7.1.13 Selective removal of a microadenoma and its effect on the hypothalamic–pituitary–adrenal axis. Because the surrounding normal pituitary corticotrophs are suppressed in a patient with an ACTH-secreting pituitary adenoma, successful removal of the tumour results in ACTH and hence adrenocortical deficiency with an undetectable (<50 nmol/litre) level of plasma cortisol. A plasma cortisol of more than 50 nmol/litre postoperatively implies that the patient is not cured.
(Courtesy of Professor P Trainer.)

no pituitary tumour can be found, or when pituitary surgery has failed or the condition has recurred.

After selective removal of a microadenoma, the surrounding corticotrophs are normally suppressed (Fig. 13.7.1.13). In these cases plasma cortisol concentrations are also suppressed postoperatively, and glucocorticoid replacement therapy is required, but gradual recovery of the hypothalamic–pituitary–adrenal axis can be anticipated (Fig. 13.7.1.14), particularly in patients with normal pituitary function as it relates to other endocrine axes. A nonsuppressed postoperative plasma cortisol suggests that the patient is not cured, even though cortisol secretion may have fallen to normal or subnormal values. Close follow-up of such individuals is required.

In the past, pituitary irradiation was often used in the treatment of Cushing's disease. However, improvements in pituitary surgery have resulted in far fewer patients being so treated. In children, pituitary irradiation appears to be effective. Radiotherapy is not recommended as a primary treatment, but is reserved for patients

Fig. 13.7.1.12 A young woman with Cushing's disease, photographed initially alongside her identical twin sister (a). In this case treatment with bilateral adrenalectomy was undertaken and several years later the patient re-presented with Nelson's syndrome and right third cranial nerve palsy following cavernous sinus infiltration from a locally invasive corticotropinoma.

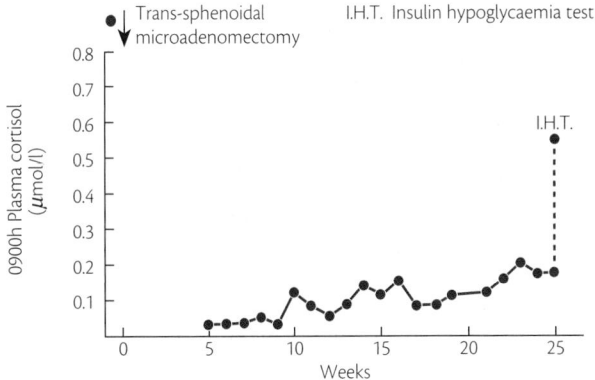

Fig. 13.7.1.14 Gradual recovery of function of the hypothalamic–pituitary–adrenal axis after removal of a pituitary ACTH-secreting microadenoma. The insulin hypoglycaemia test eventually demonstrated the return of a normal stress response.

not responding to pituitary microsurgery, when bilateral adrenalectomy has been performed, or in those with established Nelson's syndrome.

Ectopic ACTH syndrome

Treatment of ectopic ACTH syndrome depends on the cause. If the tumour can be found and has not spread, then its removal can lead to cure (e.g. bronchial carcinoid tumours, or thymomas). However, the prognosis for small-cell lung cancer associated with ectopic ACTH syndrome is poor. The cortisol excess and associated hypokalaemic alkalosis and diabetes mellitus can be ameliorated by medical therapy (see below). Treatment of the small-cell tumour itself will also, at least initially, produce improvement (see Chapter 18.19.3). Sometimes, if the ectopic source of ACTH cannot be found, it may be necessary to perform bilateral adrenalectomy and then follow the patient carefully (sometimes for several years) to find the primary tumour.

Medical treatment of Cushing's syndrome

Several drugs have been used in the treatment of Cushing's syndrome. Their site of action is shown in Fig. 13.7.1.15. Most commonly, metyrapone in Europe or ketoconazole in the United States of America has been given, often to lower cortisol concentrations before definitive therapy, or while awaiting benefit from pituitary irradiation. The daily dose has to be determined by measuring either plasma or urinary free cortisol. The aim should be to achieve a mean plasma cortisol of about 300 nmol/litre during the day, or a normal urinary free cortisol. Metyrapone is usually given in doses ranging from 250 mg twice daily to 1.5 g every 6 h. Nausea may be produced and can be alleviated (if not caused by adrenal insufficiency) by giving the drug with milk. Ketoconazole is an imidazole that has been widely used as an antifungal agent; it produces abnormal liver function tests signifying hepatitis in about 14% of patients. Ketoconazole blocks a variety of steroidogenic cytochrome P450-dependent enzymes and thus lowers plasma cortisol levels. For effective control of Cushing's syndrome, 400 to 800 mg ketoconazole daily is required.

Aminoglutethimide is a more toxic drug that in high doses blocks the initial steps in the biosynthetic pathway, and thus affects the secretion of steroids other than cortisol. In doses of 1.5 to 3 g daily (starting with 250 mg every 8 h) it commonly produces nausea, marked lethargy, and a skin rash. Trilostane, a 3β-hydroxysteroid dehydrogenase inhibitor, is ineffective in Cushing's disease since the block in steroidogenesis is overcome by the rise in ACTH. However, it can be effective in patients with adrenal adenomas.

Mitotane is an adrenolytic drug that is taken up by both normal and malignant adrenal tissue, causing adrenal atrophy and necrosis. Because of its toxicity, mitotane has been used mainly in the management of adrenal carcinoma. Doses of up to 8 g/day are required to control glucocorticoid excess, although evidence that it causes tumour shrinkage or improves long-term survival is scant. The drug will also produce mineralocorticoid deficiency, and both glucocorticoid and mineralocorticoid replacement therapy may be required. Side effects are common and include fatigue, skin rashes, and gastrointestinal disturbance.

Glucocorticoid deficiency: primary and secondary hypoadrenalism

Primary hypoadrenalism refers to glucocorticoid deficiency occurring in the setting of adrenal disease, whereas secondary hypoadrenalism arises from a deficiency of ACTH, the major trophic hormone controlling cortisol secretion. The principal distinction between these two conditions is that mineralocorticoid deficiency invariably accompanies primary hypoadrenalism, but this does not occur in secondary hypoadrenalism because only ACTH is deficient; the renin–angiotensin–aldosterone axis is intact.

Primary hypoadrenalism

Congenital adrenal hyperplasia

Various inherited enzyme defects have been identified in the synthetic pathway of adrenocortical hormones, which cause a spectrum of glucocorticoid and/or mineralocorticoid deficiency. Adrenal androgens may be increased or decreased, depending upon the underlying enzyme block. This group of conditions is addressed in Chapter 13.7.2.

Addison's disease

Thomas Addison described this condition in his classic monograph published in 1855. Addison worked with Bateman, a dermatologist who produced one of the first classifications of skin disease. It seems likely that this stimulated Addison's interest in the skin pigmentation that is so characteristic of this disease.

Aetiology

This is a rare condition, with an estimated incidence in the developed world of 0.8 cases per 100 000 population. The causes of Addison's disease are listed in Table 13.7.1.6.

Worldwide, infectious diseases are the most common cause of primary adrenal insufficiency. Leading causes include tuberculosis, fungal infections (histoplasmosis, cryptococcosis), and cytomegalovirus. Adrenal failure may occur in AIDS. In tuberculous Addison's disease the adrenals are initially enlarged, with extensive epithelioid granulomas and caseation. Calcification eventually ensues in most cases (Fig. 13.7.1.16). Both the cortex and the medulla are affected.

In the Western world, autoimmune adrenalitis accounts for over 70% of all cases of Addison's disease. Pathologically, the adrenal glands are atrophic, with loss of most of the cortical cells, but the medulla is usually intact. Adrenal autoantibodies can be detected

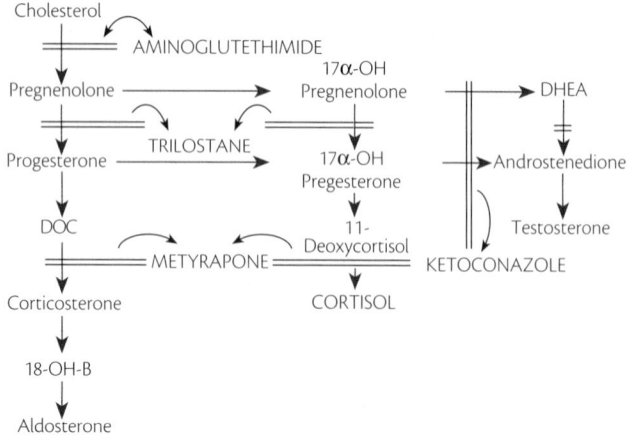

Fig. 13.7.1.15 Medical treatment of Cushing's syndrome: site of action of various drugs.

Table 13.7.1.6 Aetiology of adrenocortical insufficiency

Primary: Addison's disease

Tuberculosis

Autoimmune:

   Sporadic

   Polyglandular deficiency type I (Addison's disease, chronic mucocutaneous candidiasis hypoparathyroidism, dental enamel hypoplasia, alopecia, primary gonadal failure)

   Polyglandular deficiency type II (Schmidt's syndrome) (Addison's disease, primary hypothyroidism, primary hypogonadism, insulin-dependent diabetes, pernicious anaemia, vitiligo)

Metastatic tumour

Lymphoma

Amyloid

Intra-adrenal haemorrhage (Waterhouse–Friederichsen syndrome) following meningococcal septicaemia

Haemochromatosis

Adrenal infarction or infection other than tuberculosis (especially AIDS)

Adrenoleucodystrophies

Congenital adrenal hypoplasia (DAX-1 mutations)

Hereditary adrenocortical unresponsiveness to ACTH

Bilateral adrenalectomy

Secondary

Exogenous glucocorticoid therapy

Hypopituitarism:

   Selective removal of ACTH-secreting pituitary adenoma

   Pituitary tumours and pituitary surgery, craniopharyngiomas

   Pituitary apoplexy

   Granulomatous disease (tuberculosis, sarcoid, eosinophilic granuloma)

   Secondary tumour deposits (breast, bronchus)

   Postpartum pituitary infarction (Sheehan's syndrome)

   Pituitary irradiation (effect usually delayed for several years)

   Isolated ACTH deficiency

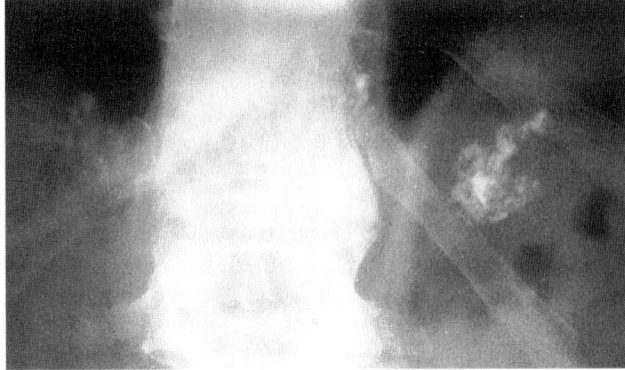

Fig. 13.7.1.16 Plain radiograph of the abdomen showing adrenal calcification in a patient with tuberculous Addison's disease.

in up to 75% of newly diagnosed cases, and have helped elucidate the cause of the disease. Fifty per cent of patients with Addison's disease have an associated autoimmune disease, and these polyglandular autoimmune syndromes have been classified into two distinct variants:

◆ Type I (OMIM 240300) is inherited as an autosomal recessive condition and comprises Addison's disease, chronic mucocutaneous candidiasis, and hypoparathyroidism. The condition is rare and usually presents in childhood with either candidiasis or hypoparathyroidism. Other autoimmune conditions, such as pernicious anaemia, thyroid disease, chronic active hepatitis, and gondal failure may occur, but are rare. Autoantibodies to the cholesterol side-chain cleavage enzyme and 17α-hydroxylase may be detected, but not to 21-hydroxylase. The condition occurs because of mutations in the autoimmune regulator gene, *AIRE*.

◆ Type II polyglandular autoimmune syndrome (OMIM 269200) is more common, comprising Addison's disease, autoimmune thyroid disease, diabetes mellitus, and hypogonadism. The condition has an inherited basis, with linkage to the HLA major histocompatibility complex, notably HLA DR3 and DR4. Autoantibodies to 21-hydroxylase are usually present, and are predictive for the development of adrenal destruction.

With the exception of tuberculosis and autoimmune adrenal failure, other causes of Addison's disease are rare (Table 13.7.1.6). Adrenal metastases (most commonly from primary lung and breast tumours) are often found at postmortem examinations, but adrenal insufficiency from these is uncommon. Necrosis of the adrenals following intra-adrenal haemorrhage should be considered in any severely ill patient, and may result from infection, trauma, or hypercoagulability. Intra-adrenal bleeding may be found in severe septicaemia of any cause, particularly in children. When this is caused by meningococci, the association with adrenal insufficiency is known as Waterhouse–Friederichsen syndrome. Adrenal replacement leading to glandular failure may also occur with amyloidosis and haemochromatosis. Congenital adrenal hypoplasia (OMIM 300200) is an X-linked disorder comprising congenital adrenal insufficiency and hypogonadotropic hypogonadism. The condition is caused by mutations in the *DAX1* (*NR0B1*) gene, a known member of the nuclear receptor family that is expressed in the adrenal cortex, gonads, and hypothalamus.

X-linked adrenoleukodystrophy causes adrenal insufficiency in association with demyelination within the nervous system, and results from a failure of β-oxidation of fatty acids within peroxisomes. Increased accumulation of very long-chain fatty acids (VLCFA) occurs in many tissues, and serum assays can be used diagnostically. Only male patients have the fully expressed condition, and female carriers are usually normal. Two forms are recognized, adrenoleukodystrophy and adrenomyeloneuropathy. Adrenoleukodystrophy (OMIM 300371) presents at 5 to 10 years of age, with progression eventually to a blind, mute, and severely spastic tetraplegic state. Adrenal insufficiency is usually present, but does not appear to correlate with the neurological deficit. X-linked adrenoleukodystrophy accounts for about 10% of cases of adrenocortical failure in boys and men. Adrenomyeloneuropathy by contrast presents later in life, with the gradual development of spastic paresis and peripheral neuropathy. Both the childhood and adult conditions result from mutations in the *ABCD1* gene on chromosome Xq28, which encodes an ATP-binding cassette peroxisomal membrane protein involved in the import of VLCFA into the peroxisome. Monounsaturated fatty acids that block the synthesis of saturated VLCFA have been used for treatment. A combination of erucic acid and oleic acid (Lorenzo's oil) has led to normal levels of VLCFA, but this has not altered the rate of neurological deterioration. Bone marrow transplantation appears to be more effective if undertaken in the early stages of the disease.

Familial glucocorticoid deficiency is a rare autosomal recessive cause of hypoadrenalism that usually presents in childhood. The renin–angiotensin–aldosterone axis is intact, and children usually present either with neonatal hypoglycaemia, or later with increasing pigmentation, often with enhanced growth velocity. Patients have glucocorticoid deficiency with very high plasma ACTH levels; this occurs because of mutations in the melanocortin 2 receptor (MC2R; ACTH receptor; OMIM 607397) or an accessory protein involved in the cellular trafficking of MC2R (OMIM 60916).

A variant syndrome is called the triple A or Allgrove's syndrome (OMIM 231550), and refers to a triad of adrenal insufficiency, namely ACTH resistance, achalasia, and alacrima. Mutations have not been found in the ACTH receptor and the molecular basis for this inherited syndrome is unknown.

Secondary hypoadrenalism (ACTH deficiency)

This is a common clinical problem and most often results from a sudden cessation of exogenous glucocorticoid therapy, or a failure to give glucocorticoid cover for intercurrent stress in a patient who has been on long-term glucocorticoid therapy. Such therapy suppresses the hypothalamic–pituitary–adrenal axis, with consequent adrenal atrophy that may last for months after stopping glucocorticoid treatment. Adrenal atrophy and subsequent deficiency should be anticipated in any subject who has taken more than the equivalent of 30 mg of oral hydrocortisone per day (approximately 7.5 mg/day prednisolone or 0.75 mg/day dexamethasone) for longer than 1 month. In addition to the magnitude of the dose of glucocorticoid, the timing of administration may affect the degree of adrenal suppression. Thus prednisolone in a dose of 5 mg at night and 2.5 mg in the morning will produce more marked suppression of the hypothalamic–pituitary–adrenal axis than 2.5 mg at night and 5 mg in the morning because the larger evening dose blocks the early morning surge of ACTH.

Other causes of secondary adrenal insufficiency are rare (Table 13.7.1.6), and reflect inadequate ACTH production from the anterior pituitary gland. In many of these, other pituitary hormones are deficient in addition to ACTH, so that the patient presents with partial or complete hypopituitarism. The clinical features of hypopituitarism make this a relatively easy diagnosis to make (see Chapter 13.4). However, if there is isolated ACTH deficiency this diagnosis may be readily missed. Lymphocytic hypophysitis and mutations in a transcription factor gene, Tpit (*TBX19*), involved in dictating the corticotroph lineage within the anterior pituitary, are rare diseases that may cause isolated ACTH deficiency (OMIM 604614).

Hypoadrenalism may also complicate critical illness, even in individuals with a previously intact hypothalamic–pituitary–adrenal axis. This functional adrenal insufficiency is usually transient and not caused by a structural lesion. Debate continues regarding its diagnosis and aetiology, but an inability to mount an adequate cortisol response to overwhelming stress and/or

sepsis encountered in intensive care units substantially increases the risk of death during acute illness. This can be reversed with supplementary corticosteroids.

Clinical features of adrenal insufficiency

The most obvious feature differentiating primary from secondary hypoadrenalism is skin pigmentation (Fig. 13.7.1.17), which is nearly always present in primary adrenal insufficiency (unless of short duration) and absent in secondary. The pigmentation is seen in sun-exposed areas, recent rather than old scars, axillae, nipples, palmar creases, pressure points, and in mucous membranes (buccal, vaginal, vulval, anal). The pigmentation reflects increased melanocyte activity induced by POMC-related peptides acting via the melanocortin 1 receptor (MC1R). In autoimmune Addison's disease there may be associated vitiligo (Fig. 13.7.1.17).

Patients with primary adrenal failure usually have both glucocorticoid and mineralocorticoid deficiency. By contrast, those with secondary adrenal insufficiency have an intact renin–angiotensin–aldosterone system. This accounts for differences in salt and water balance in the two groups of patients, which in turn result in different clinical presentations.

Primary adrenal failure may present with hypotension and acute circulatory failure (addisonian crisis). Anorexia may be an early feature that progresses to nausea, vomiting, diarrhoea, and sometimes, abdominal pain. These crises may be precipitated by intercurrent infection or by stress, such as surgery. Alternatively, the patient

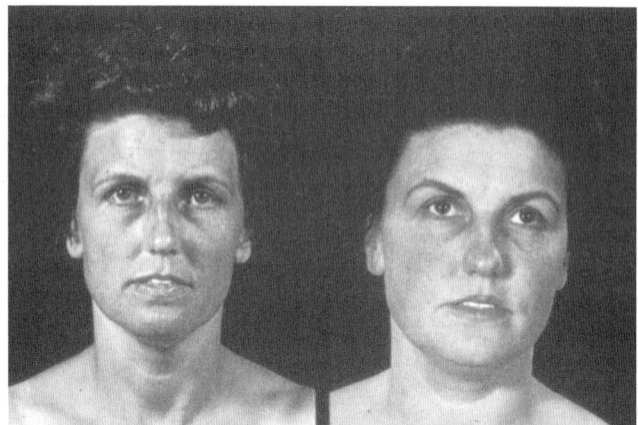
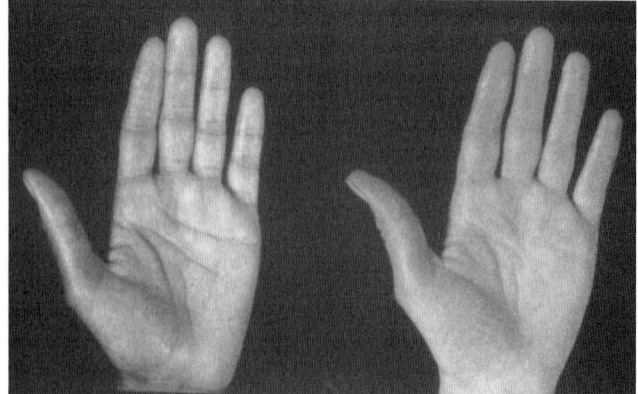

Fig. 13.7.1.17 Pigmentation in a patient with Addison's disease before and after treatment with hydrocortisone and fludrocortisone.
(Courtesy of Professor C R W Edwards.)

may present with vague features of chronic adrenal insufficiency—weakness, tiredness, weight loss, nausea, intermittent vomiting, abdominal pain, diarrhoea or constipation, general malaise, muscle cramps, and symptoms suggestive of postural hypotension. Salt craving may be a feature, and there may be a low-grade fever. The lying blood pressure is usually normal, but almost invariably there is a fall in blood pressure on standing.

In adrenal insufficiency secondary to hypopituitarism, the presentation may relate to deficiency of hormones other than ACTH, notably luteinizing hormone/follicle-stimulating hormone (infertility, oligo-/amenorrhoea, poor libido), thyroid-stimulating hormone (weight gain, cold intolerance), and growth hormone (hypoglycaemia). Patients with isolated ACTH deficiency present with malaise, weight loss, and other features of chronic adrenal insufficiency. By contrast with primary adrenal failure, patients are usually pale.

Laboratory investigation of hypoadrenalism

Routine biochemical profile

In established primary adrenal insufficiency, hyponatraemia is present in about 90% of cases and hyperkalaemia in 65%. The blood urea concentration is usually elevated. In secondary adrenal failure there may be dilutional hyponatraemia, with normal or low blood urea, because glucocorticoids are required to maintain the glomerular filtration rate and excrete a water load. Hypoglycaemia has been found in up to 50% of patients with chronic adrenal insufficiency.

Plasma cortisol/ACTH

Clinical suspicion of the diagnosis should be confirmed with definitive diagnostic tests. Basal plasma cortisol and urinary free cortisol levels are often in the low normal range and cannot be used to exclude the diagnosis. In primary adrenal insufficiency the simultaneous measurement of plasma cortisol and plasma ACTH reveals an ACTH level that is disproportionately elevated in comparison with plasma cortisol (Fig. 13.7.1.18).

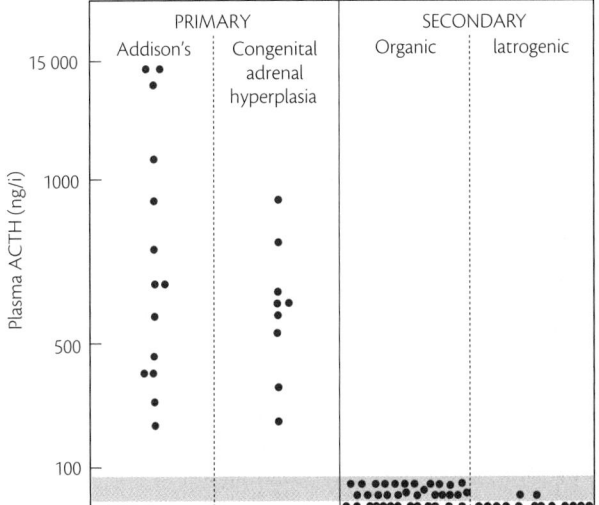

Fig. 13.7.1.18 Morning immunoreactive ACTH values in patients with hypoadrenalism. The reference range is indicated by the horizontal lines. (Courtesy of Professor L H Rees.)

Mineralocorticoid status

In primary hypoadrenalism there is usually mineralocorticoid deficiency, with elevated plasma renin activity and either low or low-normal plasma aldosterone. This aspect of investigation is all too frequently ignored in patients with Addison's disease. By contrast, in secondary adrenal failure, only ACTH drive to the adrenal cortex is lacking; the renin–angiotensin–aldosterone axis is intact.

Stimulation tests

In practice, all patients suspected of having adrenal insufficiency should have an ACTH stimulation test. This involves the intramuscular or intravenous administration of 250 μg of tetracosactrin (Synacthen), a peptide comprising the first 24 amino acids of normally secreted 1–39 ACTH. Plasma cortisol levels are measured at 0 and 30 min after tetracosactrin administration, and a normal response is defined by a peak plasma cortisol of more than 550 nmol/litre. Levels of less than 550 nmol/litre in response to tetracosactrin are found in both primary and secondary adrenal insufficiency, although false-positive results have occasionally been reported, particularly in cases of sudden-onset secondary hypoadrenalism. A low-dose ACTH stimulation test giving only 1 μg ACTH has been proposed to screen for adequate function of the hypothalamo–pituitary–adrenal axis, with the suggestion that it may be more sensitive than the conventional 250 μg test. At present there are insufficient data to support such a concept.

A prolonged ACTH stimulation test, involving the administration of depot tetracosactrin in a dose of 1 mg by intramuscular injection, with measurement of plasma cortisol at 0, 4, and 24 h will differentiate primary from secondary hypoadrenalism. However, the test is now rarely required if plasma ACTH has been appropriately measured at baseline.

The insulin-induced hypoglycaemia or insulin tolerance test remains one of the most useful in assessing ACTH and growth hormone reserves. It should not be performed in patients with ischaemic heart disease (check ECG before test), epilepsy, or severe hypopituitarism (i.e. plasma cortisol at 09.00 <180 nmol/litre). The test involves the intravenous administration of soluble insulin in a dose of 0.1 to 0.15 U/kg body weight, with measurement of plasma cortisol at 0, 30, 45, 60, 90, and 120 min. Adequate hypoglycaemia (blood glucose <2.2 mmol/litre, with signs of neuroglycopenia—sweating and tachycardia) is essential. In normal subjects the peak plasma cortisol exceeds 500 nmol/litre. However, the response to hypoglycaemia can be reliably predicted by the response to acute ACTH stimulation (see above); a safer, cheaper, and quicker test. If the ACTH test is normal, insulin-induced hypoglycaemia testing is not necessary in the vast majority of cases, unless there is a need to document endogenous growth hormone reserve in a patient with pituitary disease.

Other tests

Radioimmunoassays to detect autoantibodies, such as those against the 21-hydroxylase antigen, are available and should be undertaken in patients with primary adrenal failure. In autoimmune Addison's disease it is also important to look for evidence of other organ-specific autoimmune disease. In long-standing tuberculous adrenal disease there may be adrenal atrophy with calcification on plain radiographs or CT scanning. Early morning urine samples should be cultured for mycobacteria if tuberculosis is suspected.

Treatment of acute adrenal insufficiency

This is an emergency, and treatment should not be delayed while waiting for definitive proof of diagnosis. However, in addition to the measurement of plasma electrolytes and blood glucose, appropriate samples for ACTH and cortisol determination should be taken before giving corticosteroid therapy. If the patient is not critically ill, an acute ACTH stimulation test can be performed. However, if necessary, this can be delayed and carried out with the patient on corticosteroid therapy; provided the drug used does not interfere with the plasma cortisol assay (e.g. change from hydrocortisone to dexamethasone).

Intravenous hydrocortisone should be given at a dose of 100 mg every 6 h. If this is not possible then the intramuscular route should be used. In the patient with shock, 1 litre of normal saline should be given intravenously over the first hour. Because of possible hypoglycaemia, it is usual to give 5% dextrose saline. Subsequent intravenous fluid replacement will depend on biochemical monitoring and the patient's condition. Clinical improvement, especially in blood pressure, should be seen within 4 to 6 h if the diagnosis is correct. It is important to recognize and treat any associated condition, such as an infection, that may have precipitated the acute adrenal crisis.

After the first 24 h the dose of hydrocortisone can be reduced, usually to 50 mg intramuscularly every 6 h for the second 24 h and then, if the patient can take by mouth, to oral hydrocortisone, 40 mg in the morning and 20 mg at 18.00. This can then be rapidly reduced to the normal replacement dose of 20 mg on waking and 10 mg at 18.00. Some patients will require more than 30 mg/day, but most patients can cope with less than this (usually 15–25 mg/day in divided doses). In primary adrenal failure, cortisol day curves with simultaneous ACTH measurements may provide some insight into the adequacy of replacement therapy, but unfortunately there are no good objective tests in secondary adrenal failure. Nevertheless, crude objectives such as weight and body mass index, well-being, and blood pressure are important in this regard.

In primary adrenal failure, mineralocorticoid replacement is usually also required in the form of fludrocortisone at a dose of 0.05 to 0.1 mg/day. This has mineralocorticoid activity about 125 times that of hydrocortisone. After the acute phase has passed, the adequacy of mineralocorticoid replacement can be assessed by measuring electrolytes, supine and erect blood pressure, and plasma renin activity; too little fludrocortisone may cause postural hypotension with elevated plasma renin activity, and too much causes the converse.

Patients receiving glucocorticoid replacement therapy should be advised to double the dose in the event of an intercurrent febrile illness, accident, or mental stress such as an important examination. If the patient is vomiting and cannot take by mouth, parenteral hydrocortisone must be given urgently, as indicated above. For minor surgery, 50 to 100 mg of hydrocortisone hemisuccinate is given with the premedication. For major procedures this is then followed by the same regimen as for acute adrenal insufficiency.

Every patient on glucocorticoid therapy should be advised to register for a MedicAlert bracelet or necklace and must carry a steroid card giving information on the treatment being given.

For patients with both primary and secondary adrenal failure, beneficial effects have been reported for adrenal androgen replacement therapy with 25 to 50 mg/day DHEA. Benefit is principally confined to female patients and includes improvement in sexual function and well-being.

Mineralocorticoid excess

Blood pressure is a quantitative trait that significantly affects cardiovascular and cerebrovascular risk and mortality. Based on this, arbitrary cut-offs define a hypertensive population that, depending on age, constitutes 10 to 25% of the population. In most cases, no underlying cause for the patient's raised blood pressure can be found, and they are given a diagnosis of essential hypertension. Mineralocorticoid-based hypertension may account for secondary causes of hypertension, and classically refers to hypertension caused by increased sodium and water retention by the kidney, and expansion of the extracellular fluid compartment, resulting in suppression of endogenous plasma renin activity. The implicated mineralocorticoid is usually aldosterone.

Unlike most cases of secondary aldosteronism, which arise either in the setting of reduced oncotic pressure (nephrosis, cirrhosis) or in patients with cardiac failure, oedema is not a feature of primary aldosteronism, probably because of the aldosterone escape phenomenon. Nevertheless, in the short term, intravascular volume is reset to a higher level, and this leads to increased cardiac output and blood pressure. In the chronic state, hypervolaemia cannot be consistently demonstrated, and other mechanisms may be equally important in raising blood pressure. Mineralocorticoid receptors have been characterized in the vasculature and heart, and depending upon the activity of local 11β-HSD, either glucocorticoids or mineralocorticoids may increase vascular tone by potentiating catecholamine and angiotensin II-induced vasoconstriction, or by inhibiting endothelial relaxation. Mineralocorticoids can also modulate blood pressure centrally, independent of changes in renal electrolyte transport or vascular reactivity.

Mineralocorticoid hypertension: differential diagnosis

A comprehensive list of the causes of mineralocorticoid hypertension is given in Table 13.7.1.7.

Primary aldosteronism

First described by Conn in 1955, this is the most common cause of mineralocorticoid hypertension. Prevalence rates of 0.5 to 2% were widely reported in the literature, but an exciting development in recent years has been the realization that this might form a much more common cause of hypertension, with prevalence rates of 10%. This increased prevalence is due in part to the widespread implementation of the plasma aldosterone:renin ratio (ARR) as a screening tool.

Symptoms are often absent or nonspecific, but include tiredness, muscle weakness, thirst, polyuria, and nocturia resulting from hypokalaemia. Spontaneous hypokalaemia (<3.5 mmol/litre) is rare in untreated hypertension; when it is found in a patient on diuretics these should be withdrawn, and potassium stores replenished and remeasured 2 weeks later. Despite this, it is now accepted that most patients with confirmed primary aldosteronism will have normal serum potassium concentrations.

In approximately one-third of patients, primary aldosteronism results from a small (0.5–2 cm), solitary, aldosterone-producing adenoma of the adrenal, which is commoner in women than men (male:female ratio 1:3). Two-thirds of cases are caused by bilateral adrenal hyperplasia, and the remaining few (<2%) by glucocorticoid-suppressible hyperaldosteronism or adrenal carcinomas. The aetiology of aldosterone-producing adenomas is unknown, although rarely they may have a genetic basis and can occur as a component of multiple endocrine neoplasia type 1.

Table 13.7.1.7 Differential diagnosis of mineralocorticoid excess

Cause	Offending mineralocorticoid
Primary aldosteronism	Aldosterone
Congenital adrenal hyperplasia	Deoxycorticosterone
11β-Hydroxylase deficiency	
17α-Hydroxylase deficiency	
Glucocorticoid receptor resistance	Deoxycorticosterone
Glucocorticoid receptor mutations	
Metyrapone, RU486 ingestion	
Deoxycorticosterone-secreting adrenal tumour	Deoxycorticosterone
Liddle's syndrome	None
11β-Hydroxysteroid dehydrogenase deficiency	Cortisol
Apparent mineralocorticoid excess	
Liquorice and carbenoxolone ingestion	
Ectopic ACTH syndrome	

Diagnosis of primary aldosteronism

As with the diagnosis of Cushing's syndrome, this should be split into confirming the diagnosis, followed by establishing the differential diagnosis; again, inappropriate radiology before the diagnosis is biochemically confirmed can be misleading. The initial screening test should be the ARR (ratio of plasma aldosterone concentration (PAC) to plasma renin activity (PRA)). This can be performed in an outpatient setting with the patient in the sitting position. Primary aldosteronism is suspected by demonstrating a high ratio (see Table 13.7.1.8 for laboratory cut-off values). However, virtually all patients with suppressed plasma renin activity will have a high ratio; it is important to look also at the absolute aldosterone value, with an absolute aldosterone concentration of more than 400 pmol/litre (15 ng/dl) being highly suggestive in the face of a high ratio.

There are also important confounders: β-blockers, by suppressing PRA, increase the ARR, whereas ACE inhibitors and diuretics do the converse. α-Blockers, such as prazosin or doxazosin, interfere least with the renin–angiotensin–aldosterone axis and can be used as alternatives. Prevailing sodium intake and assay performance are vitally important issues that must be discussed with the local biochemist in establishing a normal reference range.

In each case a high ARR is insufficient to make the diagnosis. A confirmatory test must be performed to demonstrate autonomous aldosterone secretion, usually in the form of sodium loading; 30–50% of patients with a high ARR will suppress aldosterone secretion normally. Primary aldosteronism is confirmed if plasma aldosterone fails to be suppressed to below 140 pmol/litre (<5 ng/dl) following 2 litres of intravenous saline given over 4 h, or oral sodium supplementation (300 mmol/day) over 3 days. An alternative is to give fludrocortisone 0.1 mg four times daily for 4 days with a high salt diet.

Who should be screened? At present the recommendations are to screen any hypertensive with unexplained hypokalaemia, young patients with a family history of hypertension or stroke, patients with ongoing hypertension despite triple therapy, and patients referred with an adrenal incidentaloma (see 'Adrenal incidentalomas' below). However, it is now appreciated that elevated aldosterone is an important cardiovascular risk factor in its own right, independent of its effects upon blood pressure, mediating extrarenal effects including vascular inflammation and cardiac fibrosis. It seems likely therefore that the use of the ARR will increase.

Differential diagnosis of primary aldosteronism

The use of the ARR has seen a change in the breakdown of cases of primary aldosteronism, with an increased diagnosis of the ill-understood condition, bilateral adrenal hyperplasia. Unlike an autonomous adrenal adenoma, where aldosterone regulation by the normal secretagogue angiotensin II is lost, patients with hyperplasia show an exaggerated PAC response to any given level of angiotensin II.

Adrenal MRI/CT scanning should only be performed after a biochemical diagnosis has been made, because of the high incidence of nonfunctioning adrenal incidentalomas. CT has a better spatial resolution and may be more sensitive in detecting smaller aldosterone-producing adenomas (Fig. 13.7.1.19). Adopting the approach outlined in Fig. 13.7.1.20, few patients need selective adrenal vein sampling, although this may be required in an older patient if surgery is planned. Although technically difficult and not without risk, the demonstration of an aldosterone ratio of greater than 10:1 in one adrenal vein compared with the other remains the most sensitive diagnostic test. Simultaneous cortisol measurements ensure adrenal vein cannulation and, when expressed as an aldosterone:cortisol ratio, improve diagnostic accuracy.

In patients with a strong family history, glucocorticoid-suppressible hyperaldosteronism can be diagnosed by PCR sequencing of the cytochrome P450 11β-hydroxylase genes (see 'Glucocorticoid-suppressible hyperaldosteronism' below).

One reason for establishing a definitive diagnosis is that treatment is usually surgical excision in the case of an aldosterone-producing adenoma, but strictly medical for bilateral adrenal hyperplasia and glucocorticoid-suppressible hyperaldosteronism. The latter responds well to dexamethasone at 0.25 to 0.5 mg/day. Patients with an aldosterone-producing adenoma who are not suitable for surgery (or decline operation) and patients with bilateral adrenal hyperplasia should be treated with the mineralocorticoid receptor antagonist spironolactone at doses of 25 to 200 mg/day. Side effects are common and include painful gynaecomastia in men and menstrual irregularity in premenopausal women. Eplerenone is a more selective mineralocorticoid receptor antagonist and an effective alternative in such cases, but needs to be given twice daily.

To reduce surgical morbidity to a minimum, a laparascopic approach should be used for adrenalectomy wherever possible.

Table 13.7.1.8 Measurement of the plasma aldosterone:renin ratio (ARR), with suggested cut-off values indicative of primary aldosteronism, depending on whether renin is measured as plasma renin activity (PRA) or direct immunoreactivity (IrR), and the units used

Aldosterone	PRA		IrR	
	ng/ml per h	pmol/min	μU/ml	ng/litre
ng/dl	27	2.1	3.3	5.4
pmol/litre	750	59	90	150

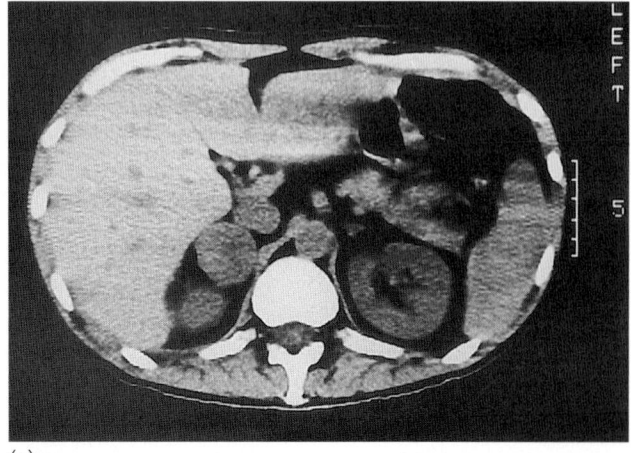

(a)

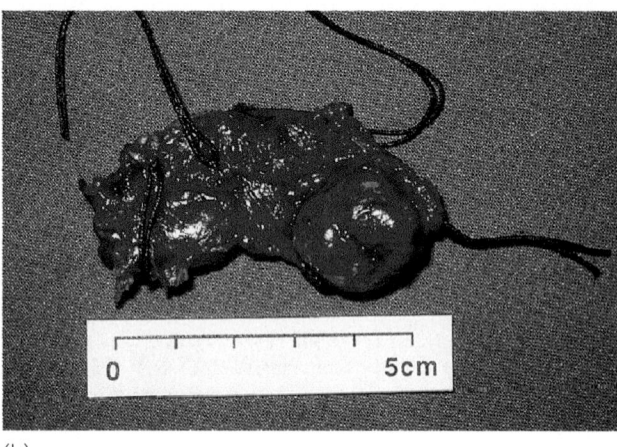

(b)

Fig. 13.7.1.19 (a) Adrenal CT scan demonstrating a solitary adrenal adenoma in a patients with Conn's syndrome and (b) the characteristic yellow appearance of the cut surface of the excised tumour reflecting the high cholesterol content of these tumours.

At risk group
Hypertension +/– low potassium
'resistant' hypertension
Family history
Stroke < 50 years of age
Adrenal incidentaloma and hypertension

PAC/PRA Ratio

>750 ng/ml/h / pmol/l ←——————————→ <750 ng/ml/h / pmol/l

Possible Primary Aldosteronism	Secondary Aldosteronism Essential Hypertension

Confirmatory Testing (Salt Loading)

High Resolution Adrenal CT

Unilateral Adenoma – Contralateral Gland Normal	Bilateral micro- or macronodular disease
Probable Aldosterone-producing Adenoma (APA)	AVS if Surgery considered as a therapeutic option >40 years of age (risk of co-existent incidentaloma)

Fig. 13.7.1.20 Suggested algorithm for a patient suspected of having primary aldosteronism. PAC, plasma aldosterone concentration; PRA, plasma renin activity.

Pre- and perioperative treatment should involve the coordinated management of surgeon and endocrinologist. Aldosterone secretion from the contralateral normal adrenal gland may be suppressed, and postoperative hypoaldosteronism should be anticipated and treated appropriately, by increasing sodium intake and/or giving transient fludrocortisone therapy. Overall, in patients treated surgically or effectively with specific medical therapy, normokalaemia is restored in 100% of patients postoperatively, and blood pressure falls to normal values in 70%.

Single gene defects resulting in mineralocorticoid excess

Hypertension is known to be a phenotype of some well-documented gene mutations; 17α-hydroxylase deficiency and 11β-hydroxylase deficiency cause forms of congenital adrenal hyperplasia in which mineralocorticoid excess occurs because of ACTH-driven deoxycorticosterone excess. A similar process is thought to explain the hypertension seen in patients with glucocorticoid resistance resulting from mutations in the glucocorticoid receptor gene (Table 13.7.1.1). More recently, a significant advance in our understanding of the molecular basis of cardiovascular disease has been the elucidation of other single gene defects causing mineralocorticoid hypertension (Fig. 13.7.1.21).

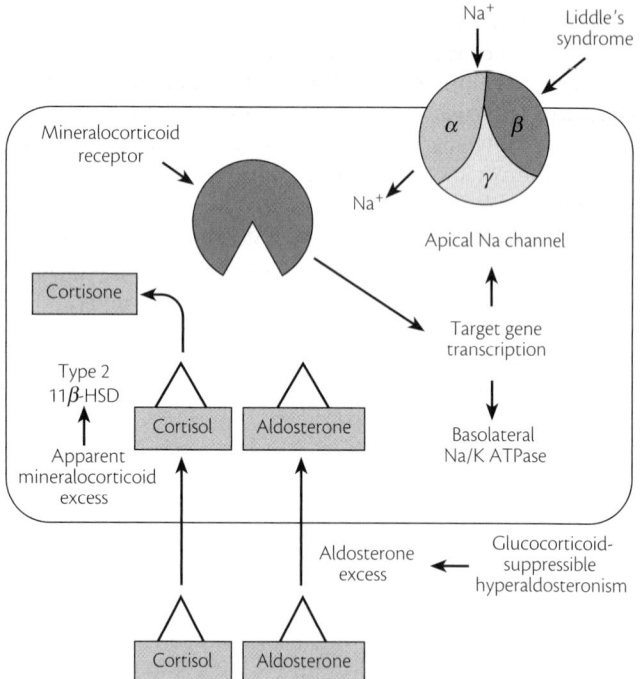

Fig. 13.7.1.21 A schematic diagram representing an epithelial cell in the distal colon or distal nephron. In normal physiology, aldosterone interacts with the mineralocorticoid receptor (MR) to stimulate sodium reabsorption via induction of the apical sodium channel and serosal Na^+,K^+-ATPase pump. GSH (glucocorticoid-suppressible hyperaldosteronism) is a cause of aldosterone excess that results from the production of a chimaeric gene, 11β-hydroxylase/ aldosterone synthase, within the adrenal cortex. Apparent mineralocorticoid excess results because cortisol cannot be inactivated to cortisone by the type 2 isoform of 11β-hydroxysteroid dehydrogenase (11β-HSD2); cortisol can then act as a potent mineralocorticoid. Liddle's syndrome occurs because of constitutively active mutations in the β- or γ-subunits of the apical sodium channel. Activating mutations in the MR can also lead to inappropriate sodium retention.

Glucocorticoid-suppressible hyperaldosteronism (OMIM 103900)

Glucocorticoid-suppressible hyperaldosteronism was first reported in 1966, and is an autosomal dominant form of low-renin hypertension characterized by aldosterone excess under the control of ACTH, rather than the normal principal secretogogue angiotensin II. There are two important consequences of this: first, there is dysregulation of aldosterone secretion because of the loss of the negative feedback loop (aldosterone does not suppress ACTH secretion), and second, the exogenous administration of a glucocorticoid such as dexamethasone, by decreasing ACTH secretion, results in the suppression of aldosterone secretion and can be used therapeutically. Long-term glucocorticoid therapy leads to reactivation and normal regulation of the renin–angiotensin–aldosterone axis. A further characteristic of glucocorticoid-suppressible hyperaldosteronism is the secretion of large quantities of 18-hydroxy- and 18-oxo-corticosterone/cortisol metabolites, again under the control of ACTH, and while there is some overlap with levels seen in aldosterone-producing adenoma, these provide a diagnostic marker for the condition.

The molecular basis for glucocorticoid-suppressible hyperaldosteronism was described by Lifton and colleagues following the cloning and characterization of the final two enzymes in the cortisol and aldosterone synthetic pathways, 11β-hydroxylase and aldosterone synthase, respectively. 11β-Hydroxylase converts 11-deoxycortisol to cortisol in the zona fasciculata, and aldosterone synthase converts corticosterone to aldosterone through an enzymatic step involving 11β-hydroxylation and 18-hydroxylation and oxidation. These enzymes are encoded by two genes, *CYP11B1* and *CYP11B2*, lying in tandem on chromosome 8. Despite the similarity in the coding sequences of 11β-hydroxylase and aldosterone synthase (>95%), their 5′ sequences differ, permitting the regulation of 11β-hydroxylase by ACTH through cAMP, and aldosterone synthase by angiotensin II through intracellular calcium ions, thereby establishing functional zonation of the adrenal cortex. In glucocorticoid-suppressible hyperaldosteronism a hybrid gene is formed at meiosis from unequal crossover of the *CYP11B1* and *CYP11B2* genes; this contains proximal components of *CYP11B1* and distal components of *CYP11B2*. As long as the breakpoint of the hybrid gene is in or 5′ to exon 4 of the *CYP11B1* gene, the product of this gene can synthesize aldosterone, but is now under the control of ACTH (Fig. 13.7.1.22). The chimaeric gene can be detected by Southern blotting or long polymerase chain reaction, providing a screening test for glucocorticoid-suppressible hyperaldosteronism and the facility for prenatal diagnosis.

Numerous kindreds with glucocorticoid-suppressible hyperaldosteronism have been reported, and an international register for such cases has been established (http://www.brighamandwomens.org/gra/). Interesting observations to come from these larger cohorts are that potassium may be normal in up to 50% of cases and there is poor correlation between genotype and phenotype (potassium, blood pressure), both between and within families. Severe mineralocorticoid excess has been reported in some individuals with this gene defect, but in other members of the same family the gene defect has not caused an abnormal phenotype. Patients with glucocorticoid-suppressible hyperaldosteronism are more susceptible to cerebrovascular haemorrhage.

Liddle's syndrome (OMIM 177200)

In 1963, Grant Liddle described a family with several siblings affected by early-onset hypertension and hypokalaemia associated

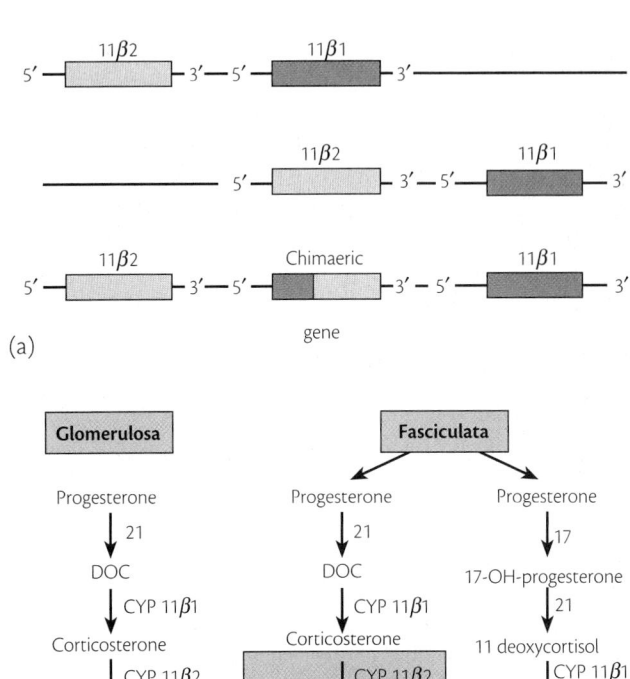

Fig. 13.7.1.22 (a) The chimaeric gene responsible for glucocorticoid-remediable hyperaldosteronism and its impact upon adrenal steroid secretion, and (b) the chimaeric gene is expressed in the zona fasciculata (boxed area) and can synthesize aldosterone, but is under the regulatory control of ACTH.

with low renin and low aldosterone levels. The condition responded well to inhibitors of epithelial sodium transport such as triamterene, but not to mineralocorticoid receptor antagonists such as spironolactone, and studies on erythrocytes suggested a generalized defect in sodium transport. Furthermore, in the proband of one of Liddle's original patients, renal transplantation resulted in blood pressure and potassium returning to normal levels, arguing against a circulating mineralocorticoid.

Mineralocorticoid-dependent epithelial sodium transport requires the activation of the apical sodium channel. Three subunits of this channel (α, β, and γ) have been cloned and characterized. Full sodium conductance requires the concerted action of α/β or α/γ subunits and cannot be sustained by any subunit in isolation. The β and γ subunits lie in close proximity on chromosome 16, and mutations in these subunits have been described in kindreds with Liddle's syndrome. In each case these cause deletions of the C-terminal part of the protein (45–75 amino acids), producing a sodium channel which is constitutively active. Liddle's syndrome is inherited as an autosomal dominant trait, and several other kindreds have been reported following the description of the genetic basis for the condition. As is the case with glucocorticoid-suppressible hyperaldosteronism, potassium has been reported to be normal in several patients.

Apparent mineralocorticoid excess and abnormalities of 11β-hydroxysteroid dehydrogenase type 2

Apparent mineralocorticoid excess (OMIM 218030) was first described in detail by Ulick and New in the late 1970s. This is an autosomal recessive form of low renin, low aldosterone hypertension, in which cortisol, conventionally regarded as a glucocorticoid, is able to act as a potent mineralocorticoid. The condition can be diagnosed by gas chromatography for cortisol metabolites in a 24-h urine collection. Affected individuals have a characteristic increase in urinary cortisol compared with cortisone metabolites (tetrahydrocortisol:tetrahydrocortisone ratio or urinary free cortisol:urinary free cortisone ratio). Serum cortisol levels are unhelpful because although patients with apparent mineralocorticoid excess have a prolonged plasma cortisol half-life, a reduction in the cortisol secretion rate mediated by the negative feedback mechanism ensures normal circulating concentrations. This defect in cortisol metabolism occurs because of the loss of 11β-HSD activity.

Two isozymes of 11β-HSD catalyse the interconversion of hormonally active cortisol (F) to inactive cortisone (E). 11β-HSD1 is predominantly found in the liver, adipose tissue, and gonads and acts principally as an oxoreductase generating F from E, but it is the 11β-HSD2 isoform, acting as an efficient dehydrogenase inactivating F to E, that is expressed in the mineralocorticoid target tissues kidney, colon, and salivary gland that is more important in modulating corticosteroid control of blood pressure. Aldosterone gains access to the mineralocorticoid receptor *in vivo* only when 11β-HSD2 activity is intact and F can be inactivated to E at a pre-receptor level (Fig. 13.7.1.23). Homozygous inactivating mutations and/or compound heterozygous mutations in the human *HSD11B2* gene have been identified in approximately 100 patients with apparent mineralocorticoid excess and result in cortisol-mediated mineralocorticoid hypertension. The condition is inherited as an autosomal recessive trait, and most heterozygotes, with a few notable exceptions, have a normal phenotype. Milder forms of apparent mineralocorticoid excess have been described, and there appears to be a close correlation between genotype and phenotype. Spironolactone or amiloride (often in higher doses than those used to treat primary aldosteronism) can be used therapeutically, as can dexamethasone, which suppresses endogenous cortisol secretion, but itself is not a good substrate for 11β-HSD2.

Liquorice has been associated with a mineralocorticoid excess state since the late 1940s, when Reevers, a Dutch physician, used a liquorice preparation, *succus liquoritiae*, to treat patients with dyspepsia. This was the origin of the antiulcer drug, carbenoxolone, which also results in mineralocorticoid side effects in up to 50% of patients. The active 'mineralocorticoids' in both cases are glycyrrhizic acid and its hydrolytic product, glycyrrhetinic acid, which themselves have little inherent mineralocorticoid activity, but cause hypertension and hypokalaemia by inhibiting 11β-HSD2. Such patients will also have an increase in the urinary ratio of cortisol to cortisone metabolites (THF+allo-THF/THE), although not to the same extent as patients with apparent mineralocorticoid excess.

Cortisol is also the offending mineralocorticoid in patients with some forms of Cushing's syndrome. In ectopic ACTH syndrome, for example, the high cortisol secretion rate overwhelms renal 11β-HSD2, resulting in spillover to the mineralocorticoid receptor. A high THF+allo-THF/THE ratio is also observed in some patients with pituitary-dependent Cushing's syndrome, and this may explain the hypertension in these cases.

Activating mutations in the mineralocorticoid receptor

One kindred has been reported with a homozygous point mutation in the mineralocorticoid receptor that results in a serine to leucine

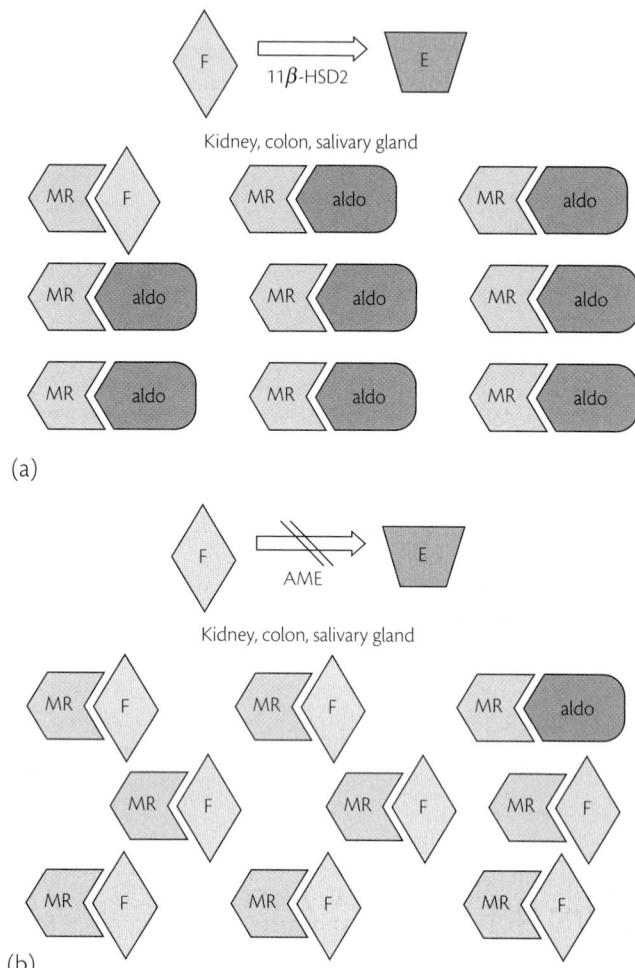

Fig. 13.7.1.23 (a) The role of 11β-hydroxysteroid dehydrogenase (11β-HSD2) in protecting the nonspecific mineralocorticoid receptor from cortisol, and (b) with congenital or acquired deficiency of the enzyme, F (cortisol) cannot be inactivated to E (cortisone) and acts as a potent mineralocorticoid.

change at amino acid 810. The phenotype is severe hypertension at a young age; an interesting facet of this mutation is that the mutated receptor is induced by progesterone and some of its hydroxylated derivatives, thereby explaining pregnancy-induced hypertension in affected female members of the kindred.

These unusual causes of mineralocorticoid hypertension have significantly enhanced our understanding of corticosteroid biosynthesis and hormone action. In addition they raise new questions as to the role of adrenal steroids in wider populations of patients with hypertension. Defects in the activity of 11β-HSD2, the epithelial sodium channel (ENaC), and CYP11β-hydroxylases have been reported in patients with essential hypertension, but have not consistently been associated with mineralocorticoid excess.

Glucocorticoid resistance

A small number of patients have been described who have increased cortisol secretion, but none of the stigmas of Cushing's syndrome. These patients are resistant to the suppression of cortisol with low-dose dexamethasone, but respond to high doses. ACTH levels are elevated and lead to increased adrenal production of androgens and deoxycorticosterone. Thus the patients may present with the features of androgen and/or mineralocorticoid excess.

Table 13.7.1.9 Causes of mineralocorticoid deficiency

Addison's disease
Adrenal hypoplasia
Congenital adrenal hyperplasia:
17-hydroxylase
3β-hydroxysteroid dehydrogenase deficiencies
Pseudohypoaldosteronism types I and II
Hyporeninaemic hypoaldosteronism
Aldosterone biosynthetic defects
Drug induced

Treatment with a dose of dexamethasone adequate to suppress ACTH (usually 3 mg/day) results in a fall in adrenal androgens and often the return of plasma potassium and blood pressure to normal levels. Many of these patients have been found to have point mutations in the steroid-binding domain of the glucocorticoid receptor, with consequent reduction of glucocorticoid-binding affinity.

Mineralocorticoid deficiency

These syndromes are listed in Table 13.7.1.9. They can be divided into those that are congenital and others that are acquired.

Adrenal insufficiency

Mineralocorticoid deficiency may occur in some forms of congenital adrenal hyperplasia and these are discussed elsewhere (see Chapter 13.7.2). Similarly, other causes of adrenal insufficiency (e.g. Addison's disease and congenital adrenal hypoplasia) are discussed above.

Primary defects in aldosterone biosynthesis

Before the characterization of the *CYP11B2* gene, the disease was termed corticosterone methyl oxidase type I (CMO I) deficiency (OMIM 203400) and corticosterone methyl oxidase type II (CMO II) deficiency (OMIM 124080). Subsequently, both variants were shown to be secondary to mutations in aldosterone synthase, and are now termed type I and type II aldosterone synthase deficiency. Both variants are rare and inherited as autosomal recessive traits. The type II deficiency is found most frequently among Jews of Iranian origin. Presentation is usually in neonatal life as a salt-wasting crisis with severe dehydration, vomiting, and failure to grow and thrive. Hyperkalaemia, metabolic acidosis, dehydration, and hyponatraemia are found. Plasma renin activity is elevated, and plasma aldosterone levels are low. Plasma 18-hydroxycorticosterone levels and the ratio of plasma 18-hydroxycorticosterone to aldosterone and their urinary metabolites are used to differentiate the type I and II variants. In most infants the disorders become less severe as the child ages; in older children, adolescents, and adults, the abnormal steroid pattern described may be present and may persist throughout life without clinical manifestations. Mineralocorticoids (fludrocortisone) are given during infancy and early childhood, but this therapy can be discontinued in most adults. Spontaneous normalization of growth can occur in untreated patients. Rarely, presentation can be in adulthood.

Defects in aldosterone action: pseudohypoaldosteronism

Pseudohypoaldosteronism (PHA) is a rare, inherited salt-wasting disorder characterized by a defective renal tubular response to mineralocorticoids. Patients present in the neonatal period with dehydration, hyponatraemia, hypokalaemia, metabolic acidosis, and failure to thrive, despite normal glomerular filtration and normal renal and adrenal function. Renin levels and plasma aldosterone are grossly elevated and patients fail to respond to mineralocorticoid therapy.

PHA type I can be divided into two distinct disorders. The first is an autosomal dominant form (OMIM 177735) that is usually less severe, with the patient's condition often improving spontaneously within the first several years of life, allowing discontinuation of treatment. This is explained on the basis of inactivating mutations in the mineralocorticoid receptor. By contrast, the second form (OMIM 264350) is a multiorgan disorder, with mineralocorticoid resistance seen in the kidney, sweat, and salivary glands, and the colonic mucosa. The condition does not spontaneously improve with age and is generally more severe. This arises because of inactivating mutations in the α, and to a lesser extent the β and γ subunits of ENaC (in effect this represents the opposite of Liddle's syndrome described above).

Two other variants of PHA have been described: types II and III. Type II PHA, or Gordon's syndrome (OMIM 145260), is in retrospect a misnomer. Patients with Gordon's syndrome share some of the features of patients with PHA type I, notably hyperkalaemia and metabolic acidosis, but exhibit salt retention (with mild hypertension and suppressed plasma renin activity) rather than salt wasting. The condition is explained by mutations in a serine threonine kinase family, *WNK1* and *WNK4*, resulting in increased expression of these proteins, with activation of the thiazide-sensitive Na^+,Cl^- cotransporter in the cortical and medullary collecting ducts. Type III PHA is an acquired and usually transient form of mineralocorticoid resistance seen in patients with underlying renal pathologies, including obstruction and infection, and in patients with excessive loss of salt through the gut or skin.

Hyporeninaemic hypoaldosteronism

Angiotensin II is a key stimulus for aldosterone secretion, and damage or blockade of the renin–angiotensin system may result in mineralocorticoid deficiency. Various renal diseases have been associated with damage to the juxtaglomerular apparatus and hence renin deficiency. These include systemic lupus erythematosus, myeloma, amyloidosis, AIDS, and the use of nonsteroidal anti-inflammatory drugs, but the most common (>75% of cases) is diabetic nephropathy.

The usual picture is of an older patient with hyperkalaemia, acidosis, and mild to moderate impairment of renal function. Plasma renin activity and aldosterone are low and fail to respond to sodium depletion, erect posture, or furosemide administration. By contrast with adrenal insufficiency, patients have normal or elevated blood pressure and no postural hypotension. Muscle weakness and cardiac arrhythmias may also occur. Other factors may contribute to the hyperkalaemia, including the use of potassium-sparing diuretics, potassium supplementation, insulin deficiency, and β-adrenoceptor blockers and prostaglandin synthase inhibitors that inhibit renin release.

The treatment of primary renin deficiency is with fludrocortisone in the first instance, together with dietary potassium restriction. However, these patients are not salt depleted and may become hypertensive with fludrocortisone. In such a scenario the addition of a loop-acting diuretic such as furosemide is appropriate. This will increase acid excretion and improve the metabolic acidosis.

Adrenal incidentalomas

With the more widespread use of high-resolution imaging procedures (CT, MRI), incidentally discovered adrenal masses have become a common problem. An adrenal mass will be uncovered in up to 4% of patients imaged for nonadrenal pathology. Over 80% of cases are nonfunctioning, with phaeochromocytomas and cortisol- or aldosterone-secreting adenomas making up the remainder. In addition, it is established that some incidentalomas may cause abnormal hormone secretion without obvious clinical manifestations of a hormone excess state; the best example of this relates to preclinical Cushing's syndrome, which may occur in up to 10% of all cases. This may explain why incidentalomas appear to be more common in patients with obesity and diabetes mellitus. As a result, all patients with incidentally discovered adrenal masses should undergo appropriate endocrine screening tests (24-h urinary catecholamines, urinary free cortisol, overnight dexamethasone suppression tests, plasma aldosterone:renin ratio, adrenal androgens) to exclude a functional lesion.

The possibility of malignancy should be considered in each case. In patients with a known extra-adrenal primary, the incidence of malignancy is obviously much higher (e.g. up to 20% of patients with lung cancer have adrenal metastases on CT scanning). Primary adrenal carcinoma is rare; in one study only 26 of 630 incidentalomas were found to be adrenal carcinomas. In true incidentalomas, size appears to be predictive of malignancy—a lesion of less than 5 cm diameter is most unlikely to be malignant. Nonfunctioning lesions of less than 5 cm can therefore be treated conservatively, and patients followed with annual imaging. Functional lesions, or tumours larger than 5 cm in diameter, should be removed by laparascopic adrenalectomy.

Further reading

Cushing's syndrome

Allolio B, *et al.* (2004). Management of adrenocortical carcinoma. *Clin Endocrinol (Oxf)*, **60**, 273–87.

Atkinson AB, *et al.* (1985). Five cases of cyclical Cushing's syndrome. *Br Med J*, **291**, 1453–7.

Findling JW, Raff H (2005). Screening and diagnosis of Cushing's syndrome. *Endocrinol Metab Clin North Am*, **34**, 385–402.

Kirschner LS, *et al.* (2000). Mutations of the gene encoding the protein kinase A type I-alpha regulatory subunit in patients with the Carney complex. *Nat Genet*, **26**, 89–92.

Lacroix A, *et al.* (1992). Gastric-inhibitory polypeptide-dependent cortisol hypersecretion—a new cause of Cushing's syndrome. *N Engl J Med*, **327**, 974–80.

Mampalam TJ, Tyrell B, Wilson CB (1988). Transsphenoidal microsurgery for Cushing's disease. A report of 216 cases. *Ann Intern Med*, **109**, 487–93.

Newell-Price J, *et al.* (1998). The diagnosis and differential diagnosis of Cushing's syndrome and pseudo-Cushing's states. *Endocr Rev*, **19**, 647–72.

Oldfield EH, *et al.* (1991). Petrosal sinus sampling with and without corticotropin releasing hormone for the differential diagnosis of Cushing's syndrome. *N Engl J Med*, **325**, 897–905.

Plotz CM, Knowlton AI, Ragan C (1952). The natural history of Cushing's syndrome. *Am J Med*, **13**, 597–614.

Ross EJ, Linch DC (1982). Cushing's syndrome—killing disease: discriminatory value of signs and symptoms aiding early diagnosis. *Lancet*, **2**, 646–9.

Wallace C, *et al.* (1996). Pregnancy-induced Cushing's syndrome in multiple pregnancies. *J Clin Endocrinol Metab*, **81**, 15–21.

Mineralocorticoids

Botero-Valez M, Curtis JJ, Warnock DG (1994). Brief report: Liddle's syndrome revisited—a disorder of sodium reabsorption in the distal tubule. *N Engl J Med*, **330**, 178–81.

Conn JW (1955). Primary aldosteronism: a new clinical syndrome. *J Lab Clin Med*, **45**, 6–17.

Edwards CRW, *et al.* (1988). Tissue localisation of 11β-hydroxysteroid dehydrogenase-tissue specific protector of the mineralocorticoid receptor. *Lancet*, **ii**, 986–9.

Fraser R, Davies DL, Connell JMC (1989). Hormones and hypertension. *Clin Endocrinol*, **31**, 701–46.

Gagner M, *et al.* (1997). Laparoscopic adrenalectomy: lessons learned from 100 consecutive procedures. *Ann Surg*, **226**, 238–46.

Gittler RD, Fajans SS (1995). Primary aldosteronism (Conn's syndrome). *J Clin Endocrinol Metab*, **80**, 3438–41.

Gordon RD, *et al.* (1992). Primary aldosteronism: hypertension with a genetic basis. *Lancet*, **340**, 159–61.

Hansson JH, *et al.* (1995). Hypertension caused by a truncated epithelial sodium channel γ subunit: genetic heterogeneity of Liddle syndrome. *Nat Genet*, **11**, 76–82.

Lamberts SWJ, *et al.* (1992). Cortisol receptor resistance. The variability of its clinical presentation and response to treatment. *J Clin Endocrinol Metab*, **74**, 313–21.

Lifton RP, *et al.* (1992). A chimaeric 11β-hydroxylase/aldosterone synthase gene causes glucocorticoid remediable aldosteronism and human hypertension. *Nature*, **355**, 262–5.

Mulatero P, *et al.* (2005). Diagnosis of primary aldosteronism: from screening to subtype differentiation. *Trends Endocrinol Metab*, **16**, 114–19.

Pascoe L, *et al.* (1992). Glucocorticoid-suppressible hyperaldosteronism results from hybrid genes created by unequal crossovers between CYP11B1 and CYP11B2. *Proc Natl Acad Sci USA*, **89**, 8327–31.

Rich GM, *et al.* (1992). Glucocorticoid-remediable aldosteronism in a large kindred: Clinical spectrum and diagnosis using a characteristic biochemical phenotype. *Ann Intern Med*, **116**, 813–20.

Shimkets RA, *et al.* (1994). Liddle's syndrome: heritable human hypertension caused by mutations in the α-subunit of the epithelial sodium channel. *Cell*, **79**, 407–14.

Stewart PM, *et al.* (1987). Mineralocorticoid activity of liquorice: 11β-hydroxysteroid dehydrogenase deficiency comes of age. *Lancet*, **2**, 821–4.

Stewart PM, *et al.* (1995). 11β-Hydroxysteroid dehydrogenase activity in Cushing's syndrome: Explaining the mineralocorticoid excess state of the ectopic ACTH syndrome. *J Clin Endocrinol Metab*, **80**, 3617–20.

White PC (2004). Aldosterone synthase deficiency and related disorders. *Mol Cell Endocrinol*, **217**, 81–7.

White PC, Mune T, Agarwal AK (1997). 11β-Hydroxysteroid dehydrogenase and the syndrome of apparent mineralocorticoid excess. *Endocr Rev*, **18**, 135–56.

Wilson FH, *et al.* (2001). Human hypertension caused by mutations in WNK kinases. *Science*, **293**, 1030.

Young WF (2007). Primary aldosteronism: renaissance of a syndrome. *Clin Endocrinol*, **66**, 607–18.

Zennaro MC, *et al.* (2004). Mineralcorticoid resistance. *Trends Endocrinol Metab*, **15**, 264–70.

Addison's disease

Arlt W, Allolio B (2003). Adrenal insufficiency. *Lancet*, **361**, 1881–93.

Arlt W, *et al.* (1999). Dehydroepiandrosterone replacement in women with adrenal insufficiency. *N Engl J Med*, **341**, 1013–20.

Betterle C, Greggio NA, Volpato M (1998). Clinical review 93: Autoimmune polyglandular syndrome type 1. *J Clin Endocrinol Metab*, **83**, 1049–55.

Cooper MS, Stewart PM (2003). Corticosteroid insufficiency in acutely ill patients. *N Engl J Med*, **348**, 727–34.

Erturk E, Jaffe CA, Barkan AL (1998). Evaluation of the integrity of the hypothalamo-pituitary adrenal axis by insulin hypoglycaemia test. *J Clin Endocrinol Metab*, **83**, 2350–4.

Oelkers W (1996). Adrenal insufficiency. *N Engl J Med*, **335**, 1206–12.

Stewart PM, *et al.* (1988). A rational approach for assessing the hypothalamo-pituitary adrenal axis. *Lancet*, **1**, 1208–10.

Miscellaneous

Kloos RT, *et al.* (1995). Incidentally discovered adrenal masses. *Endocr Rev*, **16**, 460–84.

Young WF (2007). Clinical practice: the incidentally discovered adrenal mass. *N Engl J Med*, **356**, 601–10.

13.7.2 Congenital adrenal hyperplasia

I.A. Hughes

Essentials

Congenital adrenal hyperplasia (CAH) results from enzymatic defects in the pathways of adrenal steroidogenesis, with over 90% of cases being due to 21-hydroxylase deficiency caused by autosomal recessive mutations in the *CYP21* gene.

Classical presentation—this is in the neonatal period with ambiguous genitalia/virilization of a female infant, with phenotype traditionally subdivided according to the presence (75%) or absence of salt wasting, which in affected males is the sole manifestation (and can, if unrecognized, be life-threatening). Delayed presentations can occur, manifest in women as hirsutism, oligomenorrhoea, and infertility and in men as infertility or testicular adrenal rest tumours.

Biochemical diagnosis—in the newborn this is made on the basis of an elevated plasma concentration of 17-OH progesterone; the diagnosis of late-onset CAH requires an ACTH stimulation test, with confirmation by sequencing of the *CYP21* gene for specific mutations.

Management—this requires glucocorticoid and mineralocorticoid replacement sufficient to replenish salt balance and suppress ACTH hyperstimulation without incurring steroid side effects. In the adolescent and young adult attention is focused on continuing optimal steroid replacement, with clinical endpoints being potential reproductive function rather than linear growth. Fertility in women is

compromised by scarring effects of surgery following genitoplasty in childhood, inadequate adrenal suppression that leads to anovulation, and an overall reduced maternal desire in women with CAH. Men with CAH should be screened for testicular adrenal rest tumours after puberty, and semen preservation should be considered in young adulthood. Genetic testing of the index case, their partner, and fetus allows prevention of major congenital malformation in an affected female infant by maternal treatment with dexamethasone during pregnancy.

Introduction

Congenital adrenal hyperplasia (CAH) comprises a family of inherited disorders of adrenal steroidogenesis, characterized by deficiency of cortisol and an accumulation of substrate precursors. A pathophysiological consequence of inadequate cortisol and aldosterone production is ACTH hypersecretion associated with hyperplastic adrenal glands. Genital abnormalities are not a universal feature of all forms of CAH, and the original adrenogenital syndrome nomenclature is now seldom used. Figure 13.7.2.1 shows the pathways of adrenal steroidogenesis. The rate-limiting step is the delivery of cholesterol from the outer to the inner mitochondrial membrane to act as substrate for P450scc, a mixed-function oxidase side-chain cleavage enzyme. The intracellular transport of cholesterol is controlled by a number of proteins, including steroidogenic acute regulatory protein (StAR). The synthesis of cortisol is predominantly controlled by ACTH, acting via a G-protein-coupled receptor activation of cAMP. Table 13.7.2.1 is a summary of the types of enzymes involved in adrenal steroidogenesis and the location of the genes that encode each enzyme. Deficiency of 21-hydroxylase activity is the cause of CAH in more than 90% of cases; it occupies the bulk of this chapter.

CAH resulting from 21-hydroxylase deficiency

Clinical presentation

CAH is a continuum of disorders that can manifest from birth to adult life (Table 13.7.2.2). The classical form presents in infancy, with ambiguous genitalia of the newborn. An affected female fetus becomes virilized *in utero* as a result of the effect of excess adrenal androgens, converted peripherally to testosterone, masculinizing the external genital anlagen. CAH is the commonest cause of ambiguous genitalia of the newborn, now classified as 46,XX DSD (disorder of sex development; see Chapter 13.9.3). Milder forms of virilization manifest either as isolated clitoromegaly or as isolated labial fusion. Aldosterone biosynthesis is deficient in at least 75% of cases; in affected males, salt loss is initially the sole manifestation, as the onset of virilization in males is delayed beyond infancy. Left unrecognized, this can lead to a life-threatening salt-losing crisis. The non-salt-losing male may not manifest until the second year of life or beyond, with signs of precocious sexual development, rapid growth, and tall stature. The testes remain prepubertal in size (<4 ml in volume), which is a useful distinguishing feature from precocious puberty associated with increased gonadotropin secretion.

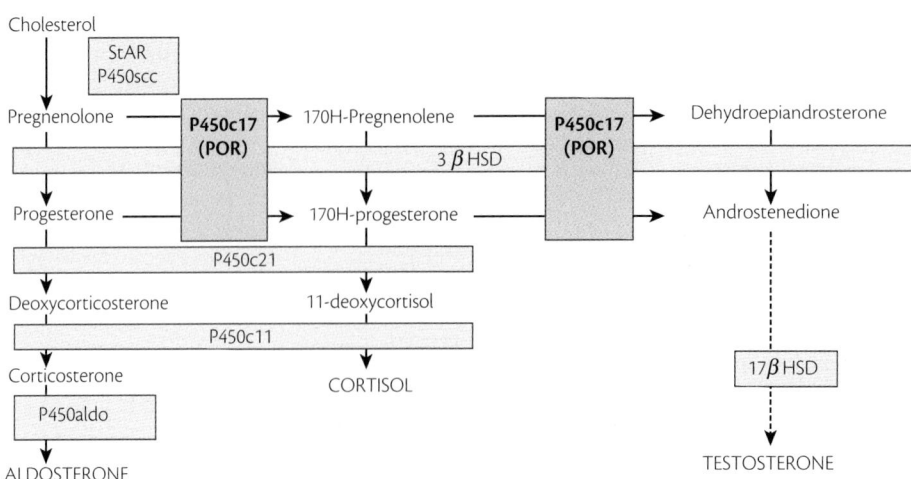

Fig. 13.7.2.1 Pathways of adrenal steroidogenesis. The enzymes involved are represented by the boxes; their cognate genes are listed in Table 13.7.2.1. The dashed line denotes extra-adrenal synthesis of testosterone, catalysed by 17β-hydroxysteroid dehydrogenase (17βHSD). 3βHSD, 3β-hydroxysteroid dehydrogenase; P450c11, 11β-hydroxylase; P450c21, 21-hydroxylase; P450scc, cytochrome P450 side-chain cleavage enzyme; POR, cytochrome P450 oxidoreductase; P450aldo, aldosterone synthase; StAR, steroidogenic acute regulatory protein.

Late-onset or nonclassical forms of CAH are also recognized, and have an incidence as high as 1 in 500 to 1 in 1000 among white populations. The nonclassical form in females may present with early onset of pubic hair growth, or after puberty with signs of hirsutism and symptoms of menstrual dysfunction. It is important to exclude an adrenal tumour as the cause of late-onset signs of virilization. In adult females the symptoms and signs are similar to those associated with polycystic ovary syndrome. Male infertility has also been ascribed to 21-hydroxylase deficiency. Tumours arising from the testicular adrenal rests may also be a presenting feature (see 'Reproductive function', below).

The characteristic biochemical hallmark is an elevated plasma concentration of 17-hydroxyprogesterone, generally greater than 300 nmol/litre (normal <10 nmol/litre). Plasma testosterone can reach adult male levels. The salt loser has hyponatraemia, hyperkalaemia, and elevated plasma renin levels. The newborn with salt-losing CAH may also have hypoglycaemia. The diagnosis of late-onset CAH requires an ACTH stimulation test. This is necessary to distinguish it from premature adrenarche, which is characteristically accompanied by elevated dehydroepiandrosterone sulphate (DHEAS) and androstenedione levels. Studies of women with signs of hyperandrogenism show only about 5% of hormone profiles consistent with late-onset CAH. Polycystic ovary syndrome

is a well recognized and more frequent cause of hirsutism and infertility, although ultrasonographic evidence of polycystic ovaries is common in CAH. The definitive diagnosis of idiopathic hirsutism as being the result of 21-hydroxylase deficiency can be confirmed by sequencing the *CYP21* gene for one of the mutations that specifically manifests as the late-onset form of CAH.

Management in infancy and childhood

Medical

For the infant in salt-losing crisis, treatment with intravenous saline and hydrocortisone is required. Blood glucose levels need monitoring for hypoglycaemia. Otherwise, the infant with CAH requires glucocorticoid replacement with oral hydrocortisone, and for the salt waster, mineralocorticoid replacement in the form of 9α-fludrocortisone. Since the majority of affected infants are salt wasters, it is reasonable to replace both steroid components from the outset, as confirming the presence of the more severe salt-wasting form of CAH can be undertaken at a later stage. The cortisol secretion rate is 6–8 mg/m² per day. Initially, a hydrocortisone dose of around 20 mg/m² per day may be used, which can subsequently be reduced to 15–20 mg/m² per day. The total dose is divided into three daily doses in view of the short half-life of hydrocortisone.

Table 13.7.2.1 Genes and proteins involved in adrenal steroidogenesis

Activity	Protein and synonyms	Site of protein	Gene/chromosome
Cholesterol transport	Steroidogenic acute regulatory protein StAR	Mitochondrial surface	STAR/8p11.2
Cholesterol side-chain cleavage	Cytochrome P450, subfamily XIA, polypeptide 1 P450scc	Mitochondrion	CYP11A/15q23-q24
3β-hydroxysteroid dehydrogenase/isomerase	3βHSD	Endoplasmic reticulum	HSD3B1, HSD3B2/1p11-p13
17α-hydroxylase and 17,20-lyase	Cytochrome P450, family 17, subfamily A, polypeptide 1 P450c17	Endoplasmic reticulum	CYP17/10q24-q25
Oxidoreductase	Cytochrome P450, oxidoreductase P450	Endoplasmic reticulum (membrane bound)	POR/7q11.2
21-hydroxylase	Cytochrome P450, subfamily XXIA, polypeptide 2 P450c21	Endoplasmic reticulum	CYP21A2, CYP21P/6p21.3
11β-hydroxylase	Cytochrome P450, subfamily XIB, polypeptide 1 P450c11	Mitochondrion	CYP11B1/8q21-q22
Aldosterone synthase	Cytochrome P450, subfamily XIB, polypeptide 2	Mitochondrion	CYP11B2/8q21-q22

Table 13.7.2.2 Clinical manifestations of 21-hydroxylase deficiency from birth to adulthood

Type	Female		Male	
	Age	Clinical signs	Age	Clinical signs
Classic	Neonatal	Ambiguous genitalia Occasional male phenotype Salt loss in 75%	Late neonatal	Occasional pigmented scrotum. Salt loss in 75% Unexpected death
			Early childhood	Penile growth. Pubic hair. Rapid linear growth Increased musculature
			Adult	Testicular adrenal rest tumour. Oligospermia
Nonclassic (late-onset)	Late infancy	Clitoromegaly	Late infancy	Occasional delayed salt loss
	Childhood	Pubic hair Rapid growth	Childhood	Pubic hair. Tall stature
	Adolescence	Abnormal menses Hirsutism Acne	Adolescence	Not known
	Adult	Hirsutism Oligomenorrhoea	Adult	Infertility

Fludrocortisone is given in doses ranging from 100 to 200 μg daily, a magnitude greater than conventional mineralocorticoid replacement in adulthood, in view of the reduced tubular sodium reabsorption capacity of normal infants. The addition of sodium chloride to the feeds is also usually required for the first few months.

The principle of longer-term medical treatment for CAH in childhood is to provide sufficient glucocorticoid (and, if necessary, mineralocorticoid) replacement for adequate homeostasis, but not at the expense of steroid side effects such as growth suppression. There is a tendency to overtreat during infancy, compounded by the need to increase the cortisol dose during episodes of intercurrent infection, which often occur at this time. This may result in later growth suppression and obesity, a problem more common in adolescent girls with CAH. Serial measurements of growth are thus the clinical mainstay of monitoring treatment for CAH in childhood. This is supplemented by calculating the bone age (undertaken by a scoring system based on 20 bones viewed on a radiograph of the left hand and wrist), at intervals of about 1 to 2 years. The assessment is particularly valuable as an index of undertreatment, where the resulting increase in adrenal androgens leads to an advanced bone age. If left unchecked, this will eventually lead to a significant reduction in adult height.

The child with late-onset CAH presenting in mid childhood usually already has a marked increase in bone age (often >3–4 years in advance of chronological age); final height will be considerably reduced. Furthermore, the advanced bone age is associated with an earlier puberty, thus further shortening the period for statural growth. Linear growth ceases when bony epiphyses fuse at the ends of the long bones. It had been assumed that this was mediated by androgens in males and oestrogens in females. However, it appears to be mediated by oestrogens in both sexes, based on studies of a rare male with a disrupted oestrogen receptor, and a number of reported males with aromatase deficiency. These individuals were excessively tall because of continued growth in young adulthood resulting from lack of closure of the growth plate. Oestrogen treatment was effective in fusing the epiphyses in aromatase-deficient patients, but not in the man with an oestrogen-receptor defect. These observations led to the use of aromatase inhibitors, such as letrozole and anastrozole, which inhibit the conversion of androgens to oestrogens in the growth plate, in order to enhance final height in children with advanced bone age and reduced predicted height.

There is a wide age range for the onset of puberty in normal children, but in girls with CAH the onset of menarche at a normal age (12–13 years) and subsequent regular menses is a reasonable index of adequate control. Hydrocortisone is the predominant glucocorticoid used in infancy and childhood. Later, when growth is mostly complete, a longer-acting glucocorticoid such as prednisolone is often substituted. Dexamethasone, which has a potency 80- to 100-fold greater than hydrocortisone in suppressing ACTH-induced steroidogenesis, can usefully restore regular menses in poorly controlled adolescent girls with CAH. However, the dose must be carefully titrated to avoid side effects such as weight gain, striae, and hypertension. Effective doses can be as small as 0.1 to 0.3 mg daily; its long half-life enables a single daily dose to be employed.

CAH requires biochemical monitoring to complement clinical indices of control, not dissimilar to the use of serial blood glucose and glycosylated haemoglobin measurements in diabetes. Figure 13.7.2.1 indicates that the equivalent analytes in CAH are 17-hydroxyprogesterone and testosterone. The former has a marked diurnal rhythm as well as responding to stress-induced increases in levels. Consequently, random single measurements can be misleading. A daily profile made up of samples collected in the early morning, at midday, in the late afternoon, and at bedtime is more appropriate and informative. Capillary blood spot and saliva assays of 17-hydroxyprogesterone enable families to undertake home sampling. Plasma testosterone is a longer-term marker of control, an age- and sex-related increase reflecting prolonged undertreatment, which in due course leads to excessive linear growth and an advancing bone age. Testosterone measurements are not reflective of CAH control in males from puberty onwards because of the predominance of testicular testosterone at this age. Androstenedione is also a useful marker of CAH control. Urinary steroid analysis by specific chromatographic techniques is primarily for diagnosis, but is also used in some centres to monitor treatment, as it avoids complete 24-h urine collections. The adequacy of mineralocorticoid replacement is best assessed by renin measurement. Renin values are normally higher in infants and young children than in adults.

Surgical

The degree of virilization of the external genitalia in female infants born with CAH can vary from mild clitoromegaly and some labial

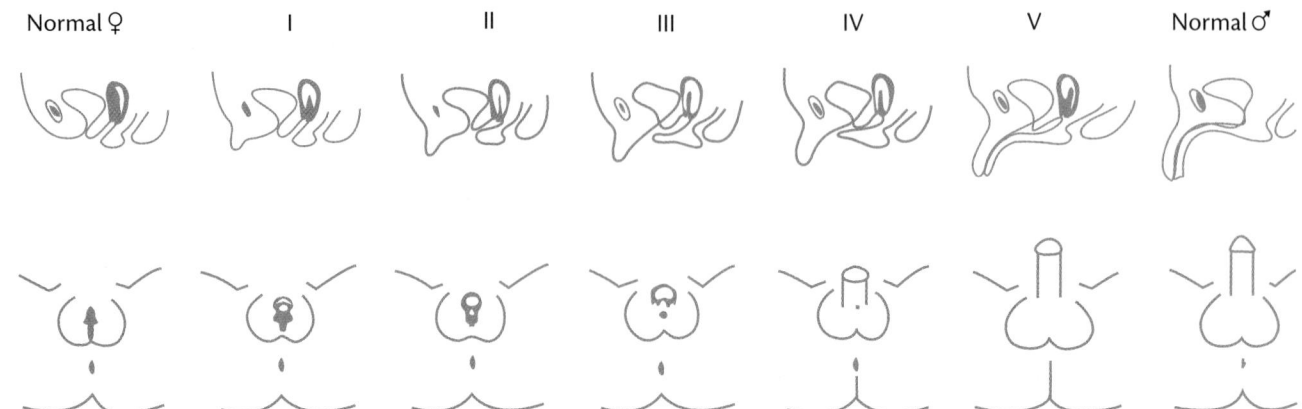

Fig. 13.7.2.2 Prader scoring system (reproduced from *Helv Paediatr Acta*). The upper panel denotes the stages of virilization, resulting in a penile urethra and high insertion of the vagina to a common urogenital sinus by Stage V. The lower panel depicts the degree of clitoral hypertrophy with Stage V resembling a penis.

fusion, to marked clitoromegaly, complete labial fusion resembling a scrotal sac, and a urethral opening on the tip of the phallus. In this circumstance the infant may initially be wrongly designated male. However, the absence of palpable gonads in the 'scrotal sac' on routine newborn examination should alert to the need for further investigation. A Prader scoring system, as shown in Fig. 13.7.2.2, is used to denote the degree of clitoromegaly and the site of insertion of the vagina into the common urogenital sinus. The surgery that is required is a reduction clitoroplasty and a vaginoplasty to enable separate urethral and vaginal openings to be exposed on the perineum.

There has been a change in policy regarding the threshold for deciding that the clitoris is too large and needs reducing in size. The current practice is not to operate on a clitoris of Prader stage less than III. Decisions about early surgery have been influenced by the results of studies in women with CAH who report dissatisfaction with sexual function, purported to be the result of clitoral surgery undertaken when they were infants. In the presence of marked clitoromegaly (Prader stages III–V), parents generally want surgery performed early to make the appearance consonant with the female sex of rearing, even though they understand this may have consequences for their daughter in adulthood. Technical details of clitoroplasty can be found in surgical texts, but it is vitally important to preserve as much of the highly innervated neurovascular bundle surrounding the clitoris. Any surgery in infancy is generally performed at 6 to 12 months. It is questionable whether vaginoplasty is needed before puberty, but many surgeons also undertake this procedure early to take advantage of favourable tissue healing at this age. A further examination under anaesthetic is usually required at puberty to assess the vaginal anatomy and the need for any revision surgery or the use of vaginal dilators. For those infants where a decision has been taken not to perform a clitoroplasty, medical treatment must be adequate to avoid further clitoral enlargement generated by elevated testosterone levels.

Genetics of 21-hydroxylase deficiency

CAH is an autosomal recessive condition. The *CYP21A2* gene (also known as *CYP21*) is closely linked to the highly polymorphic major HLA histocompatibility complex on chromosome 6p21.3.

It is 98% homologous with a pseudogene, *CYP21AP* (also known as *CYP21P*), which has accumulated several mutations that render it functionally inactive. The genes are in tandem repeat with neighbouring genes such as tenascin *TNXA/B*, complement *C4A/B*, and the serine/threonine nuclear protein kinase *RP*. The *CYP21A2* gene comprises 10 exons. Misalignment and unequal crossing over between sister chromatids during meiosis leads to a major gene deletion. This is always associated with the severe, salt-losing form of CAH. The frequency of gene deletions as a cause of 21-hydroxylase deficiency is about 25% and is highest in northern European populations. Another frequent genotype is associated with gene-conversion events, in which there is nonreciprocal transfer of multiple mutations from the pseudogene to the active gene. Such large-scale conversions may account for a further 10 to 15% of cases, all manifesting with the severe, salt-losing form. The majority of gene-conversion events are small-scale in nature. Several point mutations have now been identified, and linked microsatellites are useful for prenatal diagnosis when the family genotype has previously been ascertained.

There is close concordance between genotype and phenotype in CAH. The mutations that cause more than 90% of cases

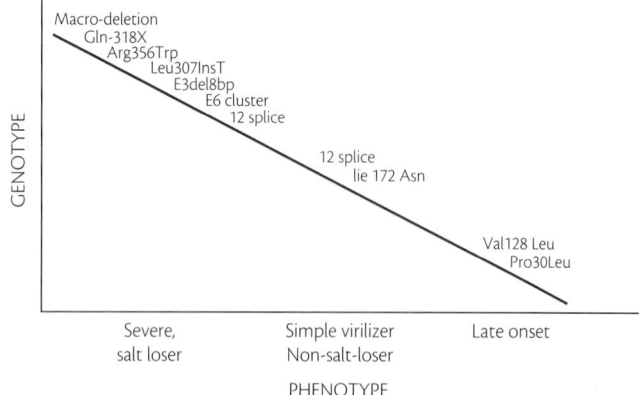

Fig. 13.7.2.3 Genotype–phenotype correlations for the 10 most frequent causes of 21-hydroxylase deficiency. E6 cluster refers to three mutations (Ile236Asp, Val237Glu, Met239Lys) in exon 6.

of 21-hydroxylase deficiency are shown in Fig. 13.7.2.3 in relation to the expected phenotype. A common mutation in classic 21-hydroxylase deficiency affects mRNA splicing and results from a nucleotide base change (A/C to G) in the second intron. A stretch of nucleotides that is normally spliced out is retained, so that the translational reading frame is altered and an inactive protein synthesized. Most patients with this mutation have the salt-losing form of CAH, but some patients who are homozygous for this mutation are salt replete. Presumably, enough normally spliced mRNA is generated to produce some enzyme activity (sometimes referred to as leaky transcription). Other examples leading to salt loss are shown in Fig. 13.7.2.3. *In vitro* functional assays of wild-type and mutant CYP21 enzymes using progesterone and 17-hydroxyprogesterone as substrates show total absence of enzyme activity for mutations leading to salt loss. A specific mutation not associated with salt wasting occurs in exon 4, changing isoleucine to asparagine (Ile172Asn). This mutation results in an enzyme with about 1 to 2% of normal activity, sufficient for adequate aldosterone production.

The nonclassical or late-onset form of 21-hydroxylase deficiency is associated with a mutant enzyme that displays 20 to 50% of normal activity in functional *in vitro* assays. An example is Val281Leu in exon 7; this single mutation accounts for the majority of nonclassical cases of CAH, and is most frequently found in Jews of eastern European origin. Other examples of nonclassical alleles include Pro30Leu, Arg339His, and Pro453Ser. The definitive diagnosis of late-onset CAH as a cause of premature adrenarche in a child or idiopathic hirsutism in a woman may not even be confirmed by a tetracosactide stimulation test, but only secured by *CYP21A2* analysis. Many patients with CAH are compound heterozygotes; in general, the phenotype reflects the less deleterious mutation.

Prenatal diagnosis and treatment

Chorionic villus sampling and molecular analysis of the *CYP21A2* gene has enabled an earlier and more reliable diagnosis to be made. Furthermore, there is the option of offering prenatal treatment to prevent virilization of an affected female fetus. Figure 13.7.2.4 outlines a protocol that may be used for the prenatal diagnosis and treatment of 21-hydroxylase deficiency. Dexamethasone is the chosen glucocorticoid as it crosses the placenta unmetabolized by the placental 11β-hydroxysteroid enzyme and is not protein-bound.

Maternal dexamethasone treatment needs to start once pregnancy is confirmed, as fetal adrenal steroidogenesis is established by 7 to 8 weeks of gestation. *CYP21A2* genotyping of the index case, parents, and unaffected siblings should have been performed previously. DNA analysis is then more reliable and can be coupled with using additional linked microsatellite markers. The conventional starting dose is 20 μg/kg per day based on prepregnancy body weight, administered in three divided doses. Once the diagnosis has been confirmed by molecular genetic analysis, treatment is only continued to term in the case of an affected female fetus. Thus, seven out of eight fetuses will be exposed unnecessarily to dexamethasone for about 6 weeks during early gestation. However, analysis of

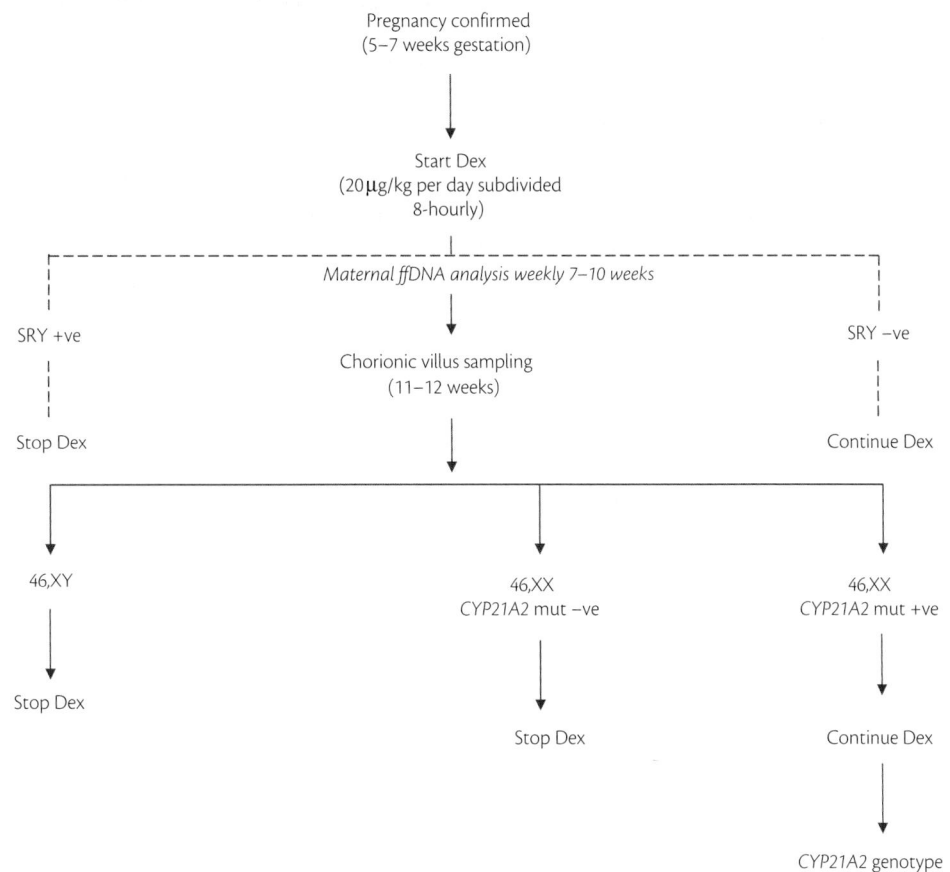

Fig. 13.7.2.4 Protocol for the prenatal treatment of 21-hydroxylase deficiency. The dashed lines indicate the management protocol that can be followed if free fetal DNA analysis is available. Dex, dexamethasone. ffDNA, free fetal DNA.

free fetal DNA in the maternal circulation enables Y chromosome material to be detected by specific probes (e.g. for *SRY*, the male sex-determining gene) as early as 7 weeks of gestation if the fetus is male. Thus, dexamethasone exposure would be avoided in male fetuses. Fetal adrenal suppression is monitored by serial measurement of maternal plasma or urinary oestriol concentrations. This steroid metabolite is formed as a result of placental aromatization of weak androgen substrates uniquely produced by the fetal adrenal gland. This monitoring also enables the dexamethasone dose to be lowered in later pregnancy. More direct evidence of adrenal suppression can be obtained by collecting amniotic fluid for measurement of 17-hydroxyprogesterone and testosterone.

The outcome of prenatal treatment is satisfactory in most cases when treatment is started early and continues uninterrupted to term. Thus the external genitalia in affected females are completely normal, or so mildly affected that surgery is not required. There have been isolated reports of other abnormalities in dexamethasone-exposed infants, but no cluster of anomalies that appear to be teratogenically specific to glucocorticoids. In animal studies, exposure to steroids has resulted in growth restriction, cleft palate, thymic hypoplasia, and features of metabolic syndrome, such as hypertension and impaired glucose tolerance. The hippocampus was also smaller in some species. Studies of cognitive function and verbal and visuospatial working memory, in a controlled study of children aged 7 to 17 years who had been prenatally exposed to dexamethasone, generally gave normal results, with perhaps poorer verbal working memory in the treated group. Maternal side effects occur in 10% of treated pregnancies, comprising excess weight gain, striae, and hypertension in some. Such treatment should only be conducted as part of clinical studies with longer-term follow-up procedures included.

Neonatal screening for CAH

It is possible to screen newborn infants for CAH by measurement of 17-hydroxyprogesterone in dried blood spots collected on the Guthrie card currently used for other conditions such as phenylketonuria and congenital hypothyroidism. Most centres use standard immunoassays, but improved positive predictive values can be achieved with the use of techniques such as tandem mass spectrometry. False-positive results may occur from sampling on the day of birth in low birth weight and sick preterm infants, and because of assay interference by cross-reacting steroids. It is essential that laboratories establish cut-off values of 17-hydroxyprogesterone that are specific for birth weight and gestational age. The classic form of CAH has an incidence of 1 in 10 000 to 1 in 15 000 live births, based on newborn screening. Nonclassical or late-onset CAH is much more common (at least 1 in 1000), but is not detected by newborn 17-hydroxyprogesterone measurement. A false-negative result can occasionally occur with the simple virilizing form of CAH, or if the mother has been treated with glucocorticoids during pregnancy.

The main benefit of newborn screening for CAH is the detection of affected males early enough to prevent a life-threatening salt-losing adrenal crisis. Retrospective case studies have shown a preponderance of females over males with CAH, suggesting an increased male mortality when screening is not employed. Other benefits include the avoidance of incorrect sex assignment (the Prader V virilized female thought to be a boy at birth) and earlier treatment, which may improve later growth and pubertal development. Not all countries, including the United Kingdom, have incorporated CAH in the panoply of conditions included in the newborn blood-spot screening programme.

Longer-term outcome in CAH

CAH is a disorder that extends across the lifespan, with management issues that vary according to development and maturation in adulthood (Fig. 13.7.2.5). It is during adolescence and young adulthood that the longer-term outcomes of treatment instigated during infancy, early childhood, and even before birth become manifest.

Adult stature and medical management

Management of CAH in childhood is primarily focused on growth. In turn, growth velocity is a dynamic biomarker of control, and is sensitive to any deviation in age-appropriate glucocorticoid replacement doses. Closure of the growth plate at around 16 to 17 years of age (or bone-age equivalent) signals the end of linear growth, and final height adjustment. Most adults with CAH are shorter than predicted from mean parental height, but are generally

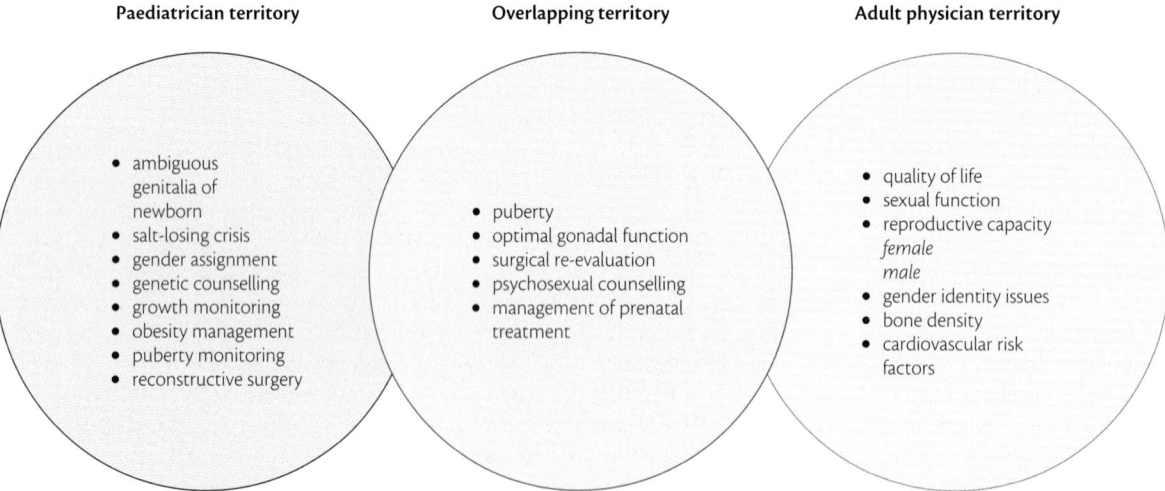

Fig. 13.7.2.5 A schema of the components of CAH as a lifelong disorder, and their management responsibilities.

within the normal population range for adult height. A meta-analysis that resulted in data on more than 500 patients with CAH gave a mean final height standard deviation score (SDS) of −1.37 which, when corrected for target height in a subgroup, gave a mean final height SDS of −1.21. Final height outcome was better in a single large clinic population based in Munich, Germany, where final height SDS corrected for target height was −0.6 for females and −0.9 for males with the salt-losing form of CAH. Much of the decrement in final height is attributed to a reduction in total pubertal growth and the use of longer-acting glucocorticoids such as prednisolone. There is also a relationship between total cumulative glucocorticoid dose and a reduction in bone mineral density, the impact being more pronounced during puberty. Paradoxically, the milder form of CAH that presents in later childhood has a worse outcome for final height because of the combination of advanced bone age and earlier onset of puberty. In such a situation, the addition of a long-acting gonadotropin-releasing hormone analogue to delay puberty, and supplementation with growth hormone, can have a beneficial effect on final height.

Glucocorticoid replacement is still provided as hydrocortisone in adulthood, but longer-acting glucocorticoid preparations, such as prednisolone and dexamethasone, are more often used. There is no fixed dose; the amount has to be calculated according to general well-being, the absence of steroid side effects, and biochemical monitoring using indices such as serum 17-hydroxyprogesterone, testosterone, and androstenedione. No current oral glucocorticoid preparation can replicate the normal diurnal cortisol rhythm, characterized by a rise in early morning levels. However, studies are underway to design delayed and sustained-release hydrocortisone preparations that can mimic the normal circadian rhythm of circulating cortisol. The requirement for mineralocorticoid replacement is lower in adulthood, so lower doses of fludrocortisone are used. Serial measurements of plasma renin are needed to adjust the dose to avoid hypertension.

There is a tendency for a higher body mass index in CAH, which is related to glucocorticoid dose. This can be associated with frank obesity, particularly occurring in the female during adolescence. At this time, control of CAH (as indicated by regularity of menses and measurements of 17-hydroxyprogesterone and testosterone) may be inadequate, yet increasing the glucocorticoid dose merely compounds the weight problem. This is also associated with insulin resistance, which perpetuates the irregular menses and anovulation. A problem of compliance may be the explanation, but medical manipulation with longer-acting steroids, the combined oral contraceptive pill, gonadotropin-releasing hormone analogues, or antiandrogens can all be to no avail in restoring control towards regular menses, ovulation, and reduced hyperandrogenism. Bilateral adrenalectomy is sometimes undertaken in these circumstances to good effect.

Reproductive function
Female
The overall fertility rate is reduced in women with CAH, an observation that is confined almost exclusively to the severe, salt-losing form of the condition. A number of factors appear to contribute to this outcome; these include vaginal stenosis and unsatisfactory sexual intercourse, ovulatory dysfunction from inadequate adrenal suppression, elevated progesterone levels acting like a contraceptive mini-pill, and a lower desire of women with CAH to become mothers.

Studies of clitoral sensation and measures of sexual function in adult women with CAH show impaired genital sensitivity and difficulties in sexual function (vaginal penetration and intercourse frequency) in those who had feminizing genitoplasty, compared with the minority of CAH women who did not have surgery and with non-CAH controls. Elevated progesterone levels during the follicular phase of the cycle are associated either with anovulatory cycles or a thin endometrium that is not receptive to blastocyst implantation. It is important to maintain androgen levels within the age-related range for females throughout childhood and adolescence, as permanent effects such as voice lowering can be a feature in adulthood.

Studies of psychosexual issues in women with CAH indicate overall satisfaction with their gender assignment, irrespective of the degree of prenatal masculinization. However, the rates of bisexual and homosexual orientation are increased, even in the milder forms of CAH. Women with CAH are less likely to have partners, are delayed in their sexual debut, and have decreased frequency of sexual intercourse. These features are more evident with higher Prader virilization scores. Even so, pregnancy rates in CAH have improved with better hormonal control, and rates in non-salt-losers are similar to those in women without CAH.

Glucocorticoid replacement for the mother should not be dexamethasone, as this steroid will readily cross the placenta unmetabolized. Prepregnancy doses of hydrocortisone or prednisolone can be used without the need to oversuppress slightly elevated levels of 17-hydroxyprogesterone and testosterone. The latter is efficiently converted to oestrogens by placental aromatase, thus protecting a female fetus from being virilized. Parenteral hydrocortisone is provided during labour, although most women are likely to need a caesarean section because of previous genital surgery. Women may have an increased risk of gestational diabetes, but the pregnancies are otherwise normal. The offspring have normal birthweight, no increased frequency of malformations, and normal development. Intriguingly, there is a 2:1 ratio of girls to boys born to mothers with CAH.

Male
The adult male with CAH is not devoid of problems of a reproductive nature. Noncompliance with treatment is prevalent, which can result in elevated adrenal androgen secretion and suppression of pituitary luteinizing hormone secretion following aromatization to oestrogens. Hypogonadotrophic hypogonadism with small testes may ensue, with consequent oligospermia. This can be rectified by reinstituting glucocorticoid replacement.

Adult males with CAH may develop testicular masses that are the result of hyperstimulation of adrenal rest cells by ACTH. The origin of such cells is the common site of adrenal and gonadal development at the urogenital ridge; it is not uncommon to observe a yellowish nodule of adrenal tissue adjacent to the testis when surgeons are performing an inguinal hernia repair or an orchidopexy. The prevalence of testicular adrenal rest tumours is reported to be more than 90% in males with CAH. They are evident on routine testicular ultrasound examination and, in severe cases, readily palpable. Histological examination shows sheets of polygonal cells separated by dense fibrous tissue with focal lymphocytic infiltrates. There is a decrease in diameter of the tubules and reduced spermatogenesis. Infertility is probably the result of long-standing obstruction of the seminiferous tubules. Testis-sparing surgery has not been successful in restoring normal pituitary–gonadal function. Ultrasound examination shows that nearly one-quarter of prepubertal boys with CAH have testicular adrenal rest tumours. It is now recommended that routine ultrasound screening should start at puberty. Semen preservation in young adulthood is an option to consider.

Other forms of CAH

Lipoid adrenal hyperplasia

Figure 13.7.2.1 indicates two key initial steps to enable cholesterol to be utilized as a substrate for steroidogenesis. Intracellular cholesterol needs to be transported from the outer to the inner mitochondrial membrane, mediated by the steroidogenic acute regulatory protein (StAR). Conversion of cholesterol to pregnenolone is then undertaken via three enzymatic reactions (20α-hydroxylation, 22-hydroxylation, and cleavage of the cholesterol side chain) via the mitochondrial enzyme, CYP11A1, also known as P450scc. These initial steps in steroidogenesis are rate limiting and ACTH dependent. StAR is not necessary for placental progesterone production, whereas P450scc is generally required to maintain sufficient progesterone synthesis in pregnancy.

Lipoid CAH is characterized by the accumulation of lipid within steroid-producing cells, resulting in large adrenals of yellow appearance. There is early onset of severe adrenal insufficiency, and none of the classes of steroid is detectable in plasma or urine after ACTH or human chorionic gonadotropin stimulation. Affected XY males have a female phenotype because of the lack of testosterone production by fetal Leydig cells. Affected XX females have normal genitalia and a uterus. Analysis of the *CYP11A1* gene initially showed no abnormality, but targeting the *STAR* gene revealed mutations that were particularly prevalent in Japanese and Korean populations. A common mutation is substitution of glutamine with a stop codon at amino acid 258, estimated to be carried by 1 in 300 of the Japanese population. The pathophysiology of StAR deficiency is explained by a 'two-hit' hypothesis, whereby there is reduced transport of cholesterol into the mitochondria which, under the continued stimulation of ACTH, leads to engorgement of steroid cells from cholesterol accumulation that ultimately severely disrupts cell function. Girls with StAR deficiency may start puberty spontaneously, but later develop hypergonadotrophic hypogonadism. It has been postulated that since fetal infant ovarian follicles are quiescent until puberty they are undamaged by the cholesterol accumulation effect. It is only after puberty, with elevated gonadotropins, that the ovarian cells become engorged and any cycles that occur will be anovulatory. Polycystic changes may also ensue.

As progesterone is essential to maintain pregnancy, this was considered to be the explanation for the *CYP11A1* gene being normal in lipoid adrenal hyperplasia. However, a few cases of P450scc deficiency as a result of mutations in *CYP11A1* have now been reported. The clinical presentation varies from prematurity and early onset of salt-losing adrenal failure, to adrenal failure presenting in later childhood. Affected XY male patients have female external genitalia, but sometimes with clitoromegaly. By contrast with StAR deficiency, the adrenals are not grossly enlarged.

3β-Hydroxysteroid dehydrogenase deficiency

3β-Hydroxysteroid dehydrogenase/isomerase (3βHSD) is a non-P450 membrane-bound enzyme which converts Δ^5 to Δ^4 steroids in the adrenals and gonads. Hence it is needed for the synthesis of glucocorticoids, mineralocorticoids, progesterone, androgens, and oestrogens. *HSD3B2* on chromosome Ip13.1 expresses the type II enzyme in the adrenals and gonads. The type I enzyme is expressed predominantly in the placenta and peripheral tissues, and is therefore essential for maintaining high levels of progesterone in pregnancy. Consequently, deficiency of 3βHSD activity is only associated with mutations in *HSD3B2*. Genital abnormalities occur, mainly in males, from inadequate masculinization resulting from the production of weak androgens by the testis. Affected females may be mildly virilized. Salt loss generally occurs. Diagnosis is confirmed by an elevated ratio of Δ^5 (17-hydroxypregnenolone) to Δ^4 (17-hydroxyprogesterone) steroids and analysis of urinary steroid metabolites.

Molecular studies show that the majority of patients have missense mutations in the *HSD3B2* gene, and many are compound heterozygotes. There is close concordance between genotype and phenotype with respect to salt-wasting forms. Significant conversion of Δ^5 to Δ^4 steroids occurs in peripheral tissues through the action of type I 3βHSD. Consequently, some patients have elevated levels of Δ^4 steroids (17-hydroxyprogesterone, androstenedione), which has led to a mistaken diagnosis of 21-hydroxylase deficiency. Spontaneous onset of puberty and menarche may occur in females, and gynaecomastia in males, presumably the result of conversion of Δ^5 to Δ^4 steroids by the type I enzyme.

17α-Hydroxylase deficiency

A single P450c17 (CYP17) microsomal enzyme catalyses 17α-hydroxylase and 17,20-lyase reactions. Both are required for the synthesis of sex hormones (C19 steroids), whereas only 17α-hydroxylase activity is required for the synthesis of cortisol (C21, 17-hydroxysteroids). The conversion of pregnenolone to 17-hydroxypregnenolone, and progesterone to 17-hydroxyprogesterone, is 17α-hydroxylase dependent, whereas the 17,20-lyase reaction converts 17-hydroxypregnenolone to DHEA and 17-hydroxyprogesterone to androstenedione. Mineralocorticoid biosynthesis is not dependent on the presence of the P450c17 enzyme, thus ACTH-stimulated, low-renin hypertension is a typical feature of the combined 17α-hydroxylase/17,20-lyase deficiency from excess production of C21,17-deoxysteroids such as deoxycorticosterone (DOC). There is an accompanying hypokalaemic metabolic alkalosis. Inadequate androgens in affected males cause a phenotype ranging from female genitalia to an ambiguous appearance or features of a hypospadic male. Female patients lack breast development and have primary amenorrhea; the prevalence is about 1 in 50 000. Male patients may only present at adolescence because of pubertal failure. The external genitalia are female in appearance, with a blind-ending vagina, testes that may be abdominal or inguinal in location, and absent pubic and axillary hair. The presentation is not unlike complete androgen insensitivity syndrome, apart from the lack of breast development.

Increased corticosterone, deoxycorticosterone, and progesterone and decreased levels of testosterone, oestradiol, and renin characterize this enzyme defect. Measurements of steroid metabolites delineate patterns indicative of 17α-hydroxylase or 17,20-lyase deficiency alone or combined. Isolated 17,20-lyase deficiency is rare; affected boys have genital anomalies, whereas in girls the presentation is one of delayed puberty.

The 6.5 kb human *CYP17* gene on chromosome 10q24.3 has eight exons. A frequent mutation is a 4 bp duplication in exon 8, which, as a result of altering the reading frame, leads to a shortened C-terminal sequence. Expression studies of the mutant protein show absence of both 17α-hydroxylase and 17,20-lyase activities. This mutation is shared by Mennonites and other individuals in the Friesland region of the Netherlands, suggesting a founder effect. There are other geographic clusters in South East Asia (in-frame deletion of residues 487–489) and Brazilians of Portuguese and Spanish ancestry (Arg362Cys and Trp406Arg, respectively). The differential catalytic activity of this enzyme is manifest at adrenarche, with the development of the zona reticularis and increased 17,20-lyase activity. This causes increased concentrations of DHEA and its sulphate, independent of any change in ACTH or cortisol levels. The increase in adrenal androgens may lead to premature adrenarche, characterized by early onset of pubic and axillary hair, body odour, and a moderate advance in skeletal maturation. Premature adrenarche must be differentiated from late-onset CAH or an adrenal tumour.

P450 oxidoreductase (POR) deficiency

Apparent combined deficiencies of the P450 17α-hydroxylase and 21-hydroxylase enzymes were reported in patients with ambiguous genitalia, but in whom analysis of the *CYP17* and *CYP21A2* genes revealed no mutations. The phenotypes comprised mild degrees of virilization of affected female infants (and their mothers during pregnancy), which was self-limiting after birth, and some undermasculinization in affected males. This diagnostic conundrum was resolved when mutations were found in P450 oxidoreductase (POR), which is a membrane-bound flavoprotein that functions to transfer electrons from NADPH to all P450 enzymes, including CYP17 and CYP21.

The dual deleterious effects of virilizing an affected girl and causing undermasculinization in an affected boy have two explanations. First, placental aromatase is also POR-dependent and thus requires this cofactor for adequate aromatization of fetal adrenal androgen. Mutations in *POR* would thus explain virilization of an affected female at birth, as well as the mother, and the self-limiting nature of the disorder. A second, more speculative, suggestion for the virilizing effect is the presence of a fetus-specific 'back door' pathway of dihydrotestosterone production from 17-hydroxyprogesterone, which does not utilize androstenedione and testosterone as intermediaries. Such a scheme has been documented in the tammar wallaby *Macropus eugenii*, and there is evidence that a similar pathway may be functional in the human fetus. The affected XY male is probably undermasculinized because of partial disturbance of 17,20-lyase activity.

Most patients with POR deficiency have associated skeletal abnormalities characteristic of Antley–Bixler syndrome (OMIM 207410). These include craniosynostosis, radiohumeral synostosis, choanal atresia, femoral bowing, and joint contractures, in addition to urogenital anomalies. The syndrome is distinct from the craniosynostosis syndromes associated with mutations in fibroblast growth factor receptors. Milder defects in POR can manifest as polycystic ovary syndrome in women or as gonadal dysfunction in men. More than 50 cases of POR deficiency have now been described since the human gene was first identified on chromosome 7q11.2. A range of different mutations has been described, which are distributed throughout all four functional domains of the POR protein. Most missense mutations are located within the central electron-transfer domain; Arg287Pro is prevalent in patients

of European ancestry, whereas Arg457His is common in Japan. Cortisol and mineralocorticoid deficiency is not common; responsiveness to ACTH is reduced, so steroid cover may be required as appropriate. The skeletal constituents of Antley–Bixler syndrome influence the morbidity and occasional mortality of this condition. A similar phenotype has been reported in association with prenatal exposure to the antifungal agent fluconazole. This is an inhibitor of lanosterol 14α-demethylase, which is also a P450 enzyme.

11β-Hydroxylase deficiency

Deficient 11β-hydroxylase activity accounts for 5 to 8% of cases of CAH, with an incidence of about 1 in 100 000. The enzyme is required for the terminal conversion of 11-deoxycortisol to cortisol, and DOC to corticosterone. The consequences of increased ACTH stimulation are salt and water retention, low-renin hypertension, and virilization, which appear to be more profound than in 21-hydroxylase deficiency. Prepubertal breast development may occur for no obvious reason. Hypertension is identified in late childhood or adolescence, the severity not necessarily correlating with plasma levels of DOC. Complications of longstanding hypertension include cardiomyopathy, retinal vein occlusion, and blindness.

There is typically hypernatraemia, hypokalaemia, and suppressed renin levels. The diagnosis is confirmed by elevated concentrations of 11-deoxycortisol and DOC in plasma, and their tetrahydro metabolites in urine. Plasma concentrations of androstenedione and testosterone are increased. Moderately elevated levels of 17-hydroxyprogesterone may lead to an erroneous diagnosis of 21-hydroxylase deficiency. Treatment requires only glucocorticoid replacement, although transient salt wasting may follow an initial fall in levels of the potent mineralocorticoid, DOC. Antihypertensive treatment may be necessary if hypertension has been long-standing. Milder or late-onset deficiency also occurs, and manifests similar features to the late-onset form of 21-hydroxylase deficiency.

11β-Hydoxylase activity is a function of the *CYP11B1* gene located on chromosome 8q21–22 in tandem with *CYP11B2*, which encodes aldosterone synthase, the enzyme involved in mineralocorticoid synthesis. *CYP11B1* is expressed in the zona fasciculata, whereas *CYP11B2* is exclusively expressed in the zona glomerulosa, where it not only catalyses the 11β-hydroxylation of DOC to corticosterone, but also catalyses the terminal steps of aldosterone synthesis.

More than 50 mutations causing 11β-hydroxylase deficiency are distributed throughout the *CYP11B1* gene. The majority are missense mutations, with some clustering occurring in exons 2, 6, 7, and 8. A higher incidence of this form of CAH occurs in Moroccan Jews, and is associated with an Arg448His mutation. This alters the haem-binding sequence that is a unique and conserved feature of all cytochrome P450 enzymes. Prenatal treatment with dexamethasone has been used successfully in this form of CAH to prevent virilization of an affected female fetus. A late-onset or nonclassic form of 11β-hydroxylase deficiency is described that can manifest as premature adrenarche, or hirsutism and infertility in adulthood.

Aldosterone synthase, encoded by *CYP11B2*, catalyses the terminal steps of aldosterone synthesis: the 11β-hydroxylation of DOC, 18-hydroxylation to 18-hydroxycorticosterone, and 18-oxidation to aldosterone. Aldosterone synthase deficiency is subdivided into two forms that can readily be distinguished by analysis of urinary steroid metabolites. Presentation is usually in infancy with severe salt wasting. Only 9α-fludrocortisone steroid replacement is required, the need for mineralocorticoid treatment lessening in later life.

A chimaeric form of the two *CYP11B* genes, under the control of the *CYP11B1* promoter, leads to an autosomal dominant form of hypertension that is suppressible with dexamethasone because of its ACTH dependence.

Further reading

Bidet M, *et al.* (2010). Fertility in women with nonclassical congenital adrenal hyperplasia due to 21-hydroxylase deficiency. *J Clin Endocrinol Metab*, **95**, [Epub ahead of print.]

Bonfig W, *et al.* (2007). Reduced final height outcome in congenital adrenal hyperplasia under prednisone treatment: deceleration of growth velocity during puberty. *J Clin Endocrinol Metab*, **92**, 1635–9.

Carroll AE, Downs SM (2006). Comprehensive cost-utility analysis of newborn screening strategies. *Pediatrics*, **117**, 5287–95.

Crouch NS, *et al.* (2008). Sexual function and genital sensitivity following feminizing genitoplasty for congenital adrenal hyperplasia. *J Urol*, **179**, 634–8.

Eugster EA, *et al.* (2001). Longitudinal analysis of growth and puberty in 21-hydroxylase deficiency patients. *J Pediatr*, **138**, 26–32.

Hagenfeldt K, *et al.* (2008). Fertility and pregnancy outcome in women with congenital adrenal hyperplasia due to 21-hydroxylase deficiency. *Hum Reprod*, **23**, 1607–13.

Hirvikoski T, *et al.* (2007). Cognitive functions in children at risk for congenital adrenal hyperplasia treated prenatally with dexamethasone. *J Clin Endocrinol Metab*, **92**, 542–8.

Hirvikoski T, *et al.* (2008). Long-term follow up of prenatally treated children at risk for congenital adrenal hyperplasia: does dexamethasone cause behaviour problems? *Eur J Endocrinol*, **159**, 309–16.

Hughes IA (2006). Prenatal treatment of congenital adrenal hyperplasia: do we have enough evidence? *Treat Endocrinol*, **5**, 1–6.

Hughes IA (2007). Congenital adrenal hyperplasia: a lifelong disorder. *Horm Res*, **68**, Suppl 5, 84–9.

Kim CJ, *et al.* (2008). Severe combined adrenal and gonadal deficiency caused by novel mutations in the cholesterol side chain cleavage enzyme, P450$_{ssc}$. *J Clin Endocrinol Metab*, **93**, 696–702.

Krone N, Arlt W (2009). Genetics of congenital adrenal hyperplasia. *Best Pract Res Clin Endocrinol Metab*, **23**, 181–92.

Meyer-Bahlburg HFL, *et al.* (2008). Sexual orientation in women with classical or non-classical congenital adrenal hyperplasia as a function of degree of prenatal androgen excess. *Arch Sex Behav*, **37**, 85–99.

Miller WL (2007). StAR search—what we know about the steroidogenic acute regulatory protein mediates mitochondrial cholesterol import. *Mol Endocrinol*, **21**, 589–601.

Nimkaru S, New MI (2008). Steroid 11β-hydroxylase deficiency congenital adrenal hyperplasia. *Trends Endocrinol Metab*, **19**, 96–9.

Nordenskjöld A, *et al.* (2007). Type of mutation and surgical procedure effect long-term quality of life for women with congenital adrenal hyperplasia. *J Clin Endocrinol Metab*, **93**, 380–6.

Nygren U, *et al.* (2009). Voice characteristics in women with congenital adrenal hyperplasia due to 21-hydroxylase deficiency. *Clin Endocrinol*, **70**, 18–25.

Prader A, Gurtner HP (1955). The syndrome of male pseudohermaphroditism in congenital adrenocortical hyperplasia without overproduction of androgens (adrenal male pseudohermaphrodism). *Helv Paediatr Acta*, **10**, 397–412.

Parajes S, *et al.* (2009). Functional consequences of seven novel mutations in the CYP11B1 gene: four mutations associated with nonclassic and three mutations causing classic II beta-hydroxylase deficiency. *J Clin Endocrinol Metab*, **95**, 779–88.

Ogilvie CM, *et al.* (2006). Congenital adrenal hyperplasia in adults: a review of medical, surgical and psychological issues. *Clin Endocrinol*, **64**, 2–11.

Rosa S, *et al.* (2007). P4SOC17 deficiency: Clinical and molecular characterization of sx patients. *J Clin Endocrinol Metab*, **92**, 1000–1007.

Scott RR, Willer WL (2008). Genetic and clinical features of P450 oxidoreductase deficiency. *Horm Res*, **69**, 266–75.

Speiser PW (2009). Nonclassic adrenal hyperplasia. *Rev Endocr Metab Disord*, **10**, 77–82.

Speiser PW, White PC (2003). Congenital adrenal hyperplasia. *N Engl J Med*, **349**, 776–88.

13.8

The reproductive system

Contents

13.8.1 Ovarian disorders

Stephen Franks and Lisa J. Webber

Essentials

The ovary produces (1) gametes—germ cells in the ovary have undergone the first meiotic division to become oocytes in primordial follicles by the time of birth, with about 400 of these ovulating during reproductive life; and (2) hormones—oestradiol, progesterone, androgens, and two nonsteroidal glycopeptides, inhibin A and B.

Ovulation and hormonal secretion is regulated by the pituitary gonadotropins, follicle-stimulating hormone (FSH) and lutenizing hormone (LH), production of which is controlled by pulsatile release of the decapeptide gonadotropin-releasing hormone (GnRH) from the hypothalamus. LH and FSH act on maturing ovarian follicles: LH inducing androgen secretion from the thecal layer, and FSH stimulating the inner granulosa cell layer to aromatize androgens to generate oestrogens. After ovulation, the corpus luteum produces oestradiol as well as progesterone: these two hormones, together with inhibins, exert feedback inhibition on gonadotropin release.

In the normal menstrual cycle, differential sensitivity to FSH leads to the further growth of a dominant follicle which becomes responsive to LH, with enhanced steroidogenesis and greatly increased oestradiol concentrations. These prevailing conditions trigger a surge in the production of LH, a unique positive feedback phenomenon that induces resumption of meiosis in the oocyte and ovulation by rupture of the follicle, which is then induced to secrete abundant progesterone. Progesterone suppresses gonadotrophin release and—if trophoblastic gonadotrophin secretion fails to occur (in the absence of fertilization and pregnancy)—the corpus luteum breaks down, inducing the onset of a new cycle.

Amenorrhoea

Involuntary infertility affects about one in six couples, with ovulatory disorders accounting for 25 to 30%.

Aetiology—the condition may be (1) primary—menarche delayed beyond 16 years, no previous periods; may be caused by developmental disorders (see Chapter 13.9.1); or (2) secondary—at least one previous spontaneous period; may be caused by primary ovarian failure, hypothalamic/pituitary dysfunction and polycystic ovary syndrome (PCOS). Oligomenorrhoea (more than 6 weeks between periods) is most commonly caused by polycystic ovary syndrome.

Premature (primary) ovarian failure—defined as ovarian failure at <40 years; cause unknown in most cases but may be associated with organ-specific autoimmune diseases and chromosomal abnormalities (e.g. Turner syndrome, 45X); high FSH, low oestrogen; often treated with hormone replacement therapy (HRT).

Hypothalamic/pituitary disorder—characterized by low FSH, low oestrogen; most commonly related to (a) weight loss—often associated with an underlying eating disorder that may benefit from specialist psychological/psychiatric treatment; GnRH or FSH is unwise until normal BMI has been achieved; or (b) hyperprolactinaemia—see Chapter 13.2.

PCOS—typically presents with amenorrhoea in association with clinical signs of hyperandrogenism (hirsutism, persistent acne, male pattern alopecia); wider definition requires two of (1) oligo- and/or anovulation, (2) clinical and/or biochemical signs (raised serum testosterone) of hyperandrogenism, and (3) polycystic ovaries.

PCOS is associated with a metabolic disorder including insulin resistance/hyperinsulinaemia/impaired glucose tolerance and dyslipidaemia. Management is mainly targeted at relief of symptoms with diet, antiandrogens (e.g. cyproterone acetate, spironolactone). Anovulatory women who wish to conceive usually respond to ovulation induction therapy (e.g. clomiphene).

Hirsutism

Mild to moderate long-standing hirsutism in women with regular menses is very likely to be associated with PCOS, which can be confirmed by finding normal/slightly elevated serum testosterone concentration and pelvic ultrasonography to determine ovarian morphology.

Patients with a short history of hirsutism (particularly if severe), symptoms suggesting other endocrine disorders (e.g. Cushing's syndrome), and/or serum testosterone above 5 nmol/litre (normal range 0.5–3.0) require further investigation including ovarian and/or adrenal imaging (for androgen-secreting tumour) and biochemical tests for Cushing's syndrome and congenital adrenal hyperplasia (see Chapter 13.7.2).

Introduction

Ovarian development and folliculogenesis

Ovarian development is essentially complete by about 6 months of fetal life, and at this time the ovaries contain some 6–7 million germ cells. By the time of birth, the number of germ cells has fallen to 1–2 million and the remaining germ cells have entered the first meiotic division to form oocytes. Each oocyte is surrounded by a single layer of flattened, somatic pregranulosa cells that forms the primordial follicle. It is the primordial follicles that constitute the resting pool, which must provide sufficient oocytes to last a normal reproductive lifespan.

Ovarian organogenesis and follicle formation

The fetal ovary is formed from three embryonic cell lineages: the coelomic epithelium, the mesenchyme of the mesonephros (primitive kidney), and primordial germ cells (which arise within the extraembryonic tissue of the yolk sac). Around embryonic day 35, the coelomic epithelium thickens over the mesial aspect of the mesonephros, forming the gonadal ridge. The underlying mesenchymal cells of the mesonephros also divide, and the gonadal ridge protrudes into the coelomic cavity as the gonadal anlagen or primordium. Concurrently, the primordial germ cells begin to migrate from the yolk sac using an amoeboid action. Before and during migration they divide by mitosis and an estimated maximum of 1700 enter the primordium. Once populated by primordial germ cells, the primordium becomes the indifferent gonad. This initial development of the ovary is identical to that of the testis until morphological changes occur at around day 39 of embryonic life that make the male and female gonads distinguishable. Evidence from the mouse indicates that once they have reached the gonad, primordial germ cells differentiate and lose their migratory ability; they are then known as oogonia.

Differentiation of the ovary occurs at embryonic day 40 to 42, a few days after that of the testis. Oogonia dramatically increase in number by mitosis, the number of germ cells reaching a maximum of about 7 million at mid gestation. Although mitosis can continue until birth, by the third trimester cell loss exceeds the rate of mitosis, and the number of germ cells falls. This loss occurs by apoptosis, or programmed cell death, and is mainly seen within the sex cords in oogonia and oocytes that have not formed follicles by association with somatic cells.

Proliferation of the coelomic epithelium forms protrusions into the mesenchyme, which gives rise to the primary sex cords, surrounding groups of primordial germ cells/oogonia. Shortly after, outgrowths of cells from the mesonephros form primordial sex cords containing the germ cells. At mid gestation, the sex cords intermingle and account for approximately 60% of the ovarian volume, falling to 14% by birth while the medulla of the ovary relatively enlarges. Meanwhile, oogonia begin to cease mitosis and enter meiosis at 10 to 12 weeks after conception, some weeks after sex-specific gonadal differentiation. This division is arrested 1 to 2 weeks later, at diplotene of the first meiotic division, resulting in the formation of oocytes. The oocyte remains arrested in the first meiotic division unless and until the follicle reaches the mature antral stage and is subjected to the gonadotropin surge preceding ovulation, which may be many decades later.

Newly formed oocytes become enclosed in a single flattened layer of somatic pregranulosa cells resting on a basement membrane, to form the primordial follicle (Fig. 13.8.1.1). Follicle formation begins close to the corticomedullary boundary, and primordial follicles appear to separate from the sex cords. The origin of granulosa cells is still not completely certain, and may vary from one species to another, but it is likely that they are derived from the ovarian surface epithelium.

Folliculogenesis in the normal ovary

Primordial follicles provide the stock of oocytes, which must last for up to 50 years. Initiation of follicle growth, i.e. progression of the follicle from the primordial to the early growth phase, must be tightly regulated to ensure a steady supply of oocytes for ovulation

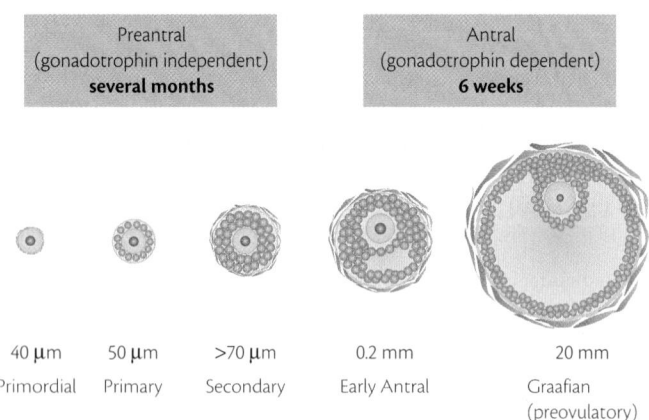

Fig. 13.8.1.1 Follicle development in the human ovary. The various stages of preantral and antral (gonadtropin-dependent) development of the follicle are depicted, ranging from the primordial (quiescent) stage, in which the oocyte is enclosed in a single layer of pregranulosa cells, to the preovulatory stage. This process takes several months.
(From Hardy K, et al. (2000). *In vitro* maturation of oocytes. *Br Med Bull*, **56**, 588–602. Copyright (2000), with permission from Oxford University Press.)

during a normal reproductive lifetime. However, the factors responsible for controlling the initiation of growth remain to be elucidated. The first indication of growth of the follicle is a change in shape of the granulosa cells, which become more cuboidal in appearance (Fig. 13.8.1.1). Follicles then pass through a transitional or intermediary stage, in which a proportion of the granulosa cells are cuboidal and the rest remain flattened. This is followed by the primary stage, in which the oocyte is enclosed in a single layer of completely cuboidal cells. By this stage the oocyte has increased significantly in volume. Follicle development progresses by formation of a second layer of granulosa cells, and at this stage the first theca cells, derived from surrounding stroma, begin to organize around the granulosa layer. This is followed by the formation of further layers of granulosa and theca cells (with enlargement of the oocyte) to form a multilayered preantral follicle. The outer layers of the theca comprise cells that are similar to those in surrounding stroma, and constitute the theca externa. The cells of the inner layers become polyhedral and form the theca interna, the site of androgen production in large preantral and antral follicles. Eventually, the theca interna of each follicle receives its own blood supply. Development of the follicle to the multilayered preantral stage can progress without the need for gonadotropins. It is unclear how long it takes for a follicle to progress from the primordial stage to a large preantral follicle, but estimates suggest that it may be at least 6 months.

Granulosa cells continue to proliferate, and a fluid-filled space (the antrum) eventually forms between them, and continues to enlarge. The follicle is now an antral follicle, the stage at which the endocrine system comes into play and gondaotropins take over control of folliculogenesis (Fig. 13.8.1.1). It is from this stage that the biggest expansion of the follicle occurs, in terms of granulosa and theca cell numbers, antrum size, oocyte growth, and overall follicle diameter. Follicles that reach this stage are considered to be part of a selectable pool of follicles from which the dominant follicle will arise (i.e. the one most likely to complete maturation and ovulate). This pool may number approximately 15 to 20 follicles between the 2 ovaries in young women, and declines with age, averaging 10 at 30 years and 5 at 40 years. It will be evident that only a small fraction of the total pool of follicles is destined to ovulate. The rest will undergo atresia (death by apoptosis). Although it is likely that follicle loss by atresia occurs at all stages of folliculogenesis, the highest proportion of atretic follicles is seen during the gonadotopin-dependent antral stages. As described below, selection of a single follicle for ovulation in the human menstrual cycle inevitably involves regression and demise of subsidiary follicles within the same cohort.

The hypothalamic–pituitary–ovarian axis

Like the testis, the ovary has two major functions: (1), the production of gametes and (2), the secretion of hormones (particularly sex steroids) that affect development and function of the reproductive tract, as well as having important peripheral affects on muscle, bone, and skin. Like all classic endocrine organs, the function of the ovary is dependent upon regulation by pituitary hormones, which in turn are regulated by hypothalamic signals (Fig. 13.8.1.2). Gonadotropin-releasing hormone (GnRH) is a decapeptide secreted by the hypothalamus in a pulsatile manner, the frequency

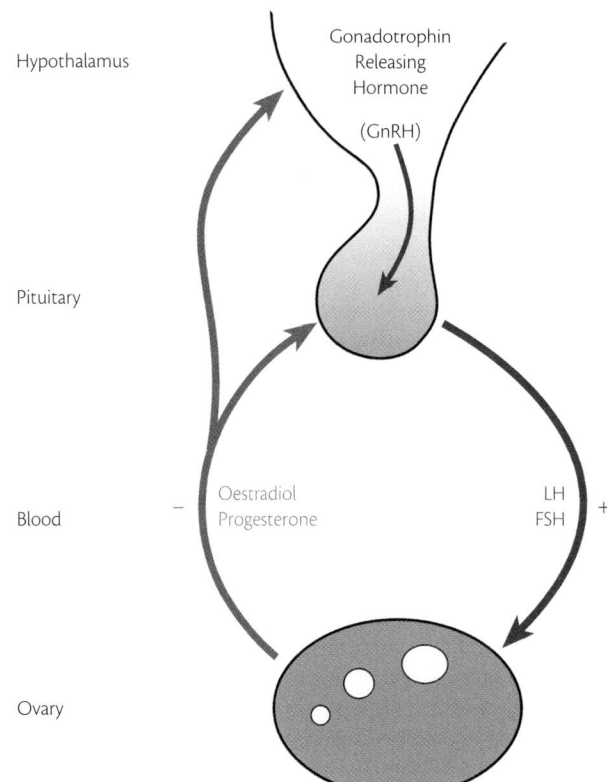

Fig. 13.8.1.2 The hypothalamic–pituitary–ovarian axis. (Courtesy of Prof K Hardy.)

of pulses (between 60 and 180 min, according to the stage of the menstrual cycle) having a profound influence on the response of the pituitary gonadotropins to GnRH. The episodic secretion of GnRH is reflected in the pattern of circulating gonadotropins, the pulses of luteinizing hormone (LH) being more discrete than those of follicle-stimulating hormone (FSH) because of the shorter half-life of LH in the circulation. LH and FSH, which are glycoproteins, act in concert on the maturing large ovarian follicles: LH stimulates the thecal layer of the follicle to produce androgens (androstenedione and testosterone), whereas FSH acts specifically on the inner, granulosa cell layer of the mature follicle, which lacks the capacity to synthesize androgens, to convert androgens to oestrogens—the so-called 'two cell, two gonadotropin' hypothesis. Following ovulation, oestradiol continues to be produced by the corpus luteum, but the principal circulating steroid at this stage of the cycle is progesterone. Oestradiol, during the mid follicular phase of the cycle (see 'The menstrual cycle', below), and progesterone (luteal phase) exert negative feedback on both the pituitary and the hypothalamus to inhibit the secretion of gonadotropins. The ovary also produces two closely related nonsteroidal glycopeptide hormones that selectively inhibit FSH and contribute to the negative feedback: inhibin B (produced by developing follicles in the follicular phase) and inhibin A (produced mainly by the corpus luteum). The extraordinary feature of the hypothalamic–pituitary–ovarian axis is the phenomenon of positive-feedback stimulation of gonadotropins by oestradiol in mid cycle, which results in the LH surge and ovulation, as described below.

The menstrual cycle

The endocrine events of the menstrual cycle are summarized in Fig. 13.8.1.3. At the beginning of each normal cycle (conventionally taken as the first day of menses), there is a cohort of follicles, ranging between 2 and 5 mm in diameter, that are dependent on and responsive to FSH. Between the late luteal phase of the previous cycle and the early follicular phase, the negative-feedback signal primarily provided by progesterone is removed, and the concentration of FSH rises. This intercycle increase in FSH exceeds a notional threshold level that encourages follicle maturation. Of the cohort of follicles that arrive at this FSH threshold, only one (or occasionally two) is destined to complete the journey to ovulation. This is the follicle that is most responsive to FSH. It is often the largest of the cohort, but not necessarily so. As the follicles grow in response to FSH, oestradiol (and inhibin B) levels rise in the circulation and exert a negative-feedback effect on FSH. As a result of the fall in FSH in the mid follicular phase, most of the follicles in the cohort will regress and die by atresia, leaving only the most FSH-sensitive, dominant follicle to continue to grow and to secrete oestradiol. By this time the granulosa cells of the dominant follicle have acquired LH receptors (the only time in the life of the follicle when this occurs) and are thus now responsive to LH. The dual effect of FSH and LH enhances granulosa cell differentiation and steroidogenesis, so that in the preovulatory phase of the cycle serum oestradiol levels in the circulation have increased more than 10-fold compared with the early follicular phase, 95% of circulating oestradiol being attributable to that single preovulatory follicle. The steeply rising levels of oestradiol (probably assisted by a small increase in circulating progesterone, signalling granulosa cell and perhaps oocyte maturation) then trigger the LH surge; the only

example of a positive-feedback effect of a target hormone on the hypothalamic–pituitary unit. The LH surge has three main functions: (1), it signals resumption of meiosis in the oocyte ready for fertilization, (2), it leads to follicle rupture and ovulation, and (3), it stimulates formation of the corpus luteum, converting the follicle from a mainly oestrogen-producing unit to a highly vascularized progesterone factory. Progesterone suppresses gonadotropins during the luteal phase and, if conception does not occur, luteolysis ensues after an apparently preprogrammed interval of 12 to 14 days, triggering the onset of a new cycle.

Disorders of ovulation

Clinical presentation and causes of anovulation

Disorders of ovulation usually result in perturbation of normal cyclical menses. It is uncommon to have regular but anovulatory cycles, the exception being during adolescence, when cyclical ovarian activity without ovulation (a feature of immaturity of the hypothalamic–pituitary–ovarian axis) is characteristic of the early months after menarche. Thus, anovulation is generally characterized by amenorrhoea, oligomenorrhoea (>6 weeks between periods), or very irregular menses. Amenorrhoea may be primary (i.e. no previous periods) or secondary (at least one previous spontaneous period). Primary amenorrhoea is less common, and although its causes overlap with those of secondary amenorrhoea, it is not surprising that disorders of development of the ovaries and/or reproductive tract are overrepresented in this category. In some cases, primary amenorrhoea (defined as menarche delayed beyond 16 years of age) is accompanied by delayed pubertal development (see Chapter 13.9.2). Menstrual disturbance may be accompanied

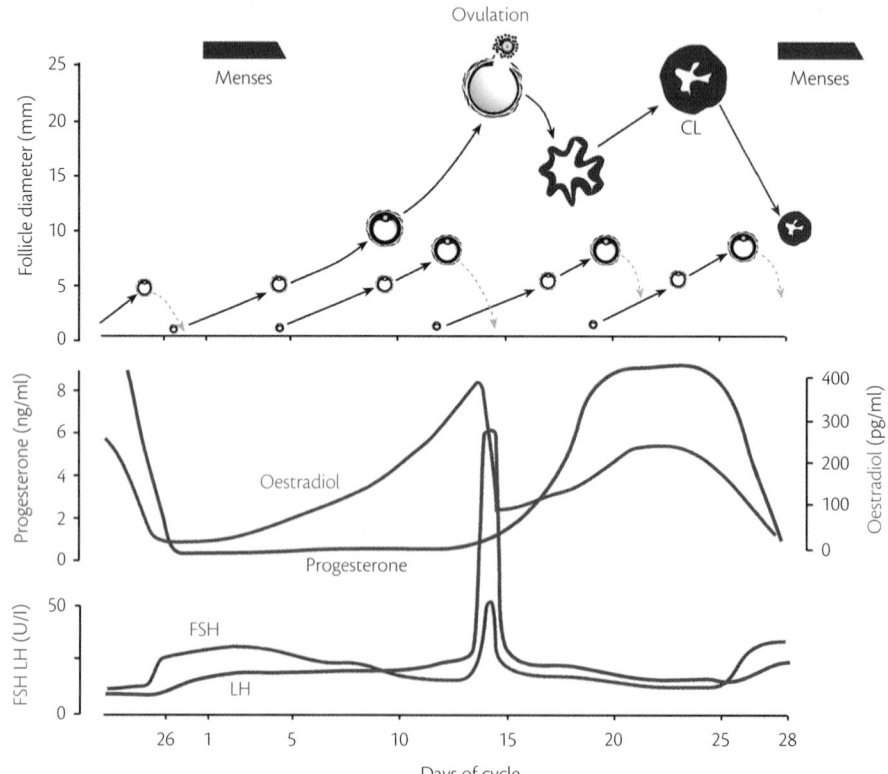

Fig. 13.8.1.3 The human menstrual cycle.
(Adapted by K. Hardy from Baird DT (1983). Prediction of ovulation: biophysical, physiological and biochemical coordinates. In: Jeffcoate SL (ed). *Ovulation: methods for its prediction and detection*, pp. 1–17, with permission from John Wiley and Sons Inc.)

Box 13.8.1.1 Causes of secondary amenorrhoea

♦ Primary ovarian failure (11%)

♦ Hypothalamic/pituitary dysfunction (55%)

  · Hyperproloactinaemia (11%)

  · Weight-loss related (35%)

  · Idiopathic (9%)

♦ PCOS (32%)

♦ Genital tract disorder (2%)

---

by symptoms of oestrogen deficiency, including vaginal dryness and hot flushes. Interestingly, vasomotor symptoms are common in women with primary ovarian failure, but not in those with oestrogen deficiency resulting from hypothalamic–pituitary dysfunction. Patients with hyperprolactinaemia may report inappropriate lactation (galactorrhoea), but it is important to recognize that this affects only 30 to 50% of women with hypersecretion of prolactin. Menstrual abnormalities accompanied by symptoms of androgen excess (hirsutism, acne, or alopecia) are typical of polycystic ovary syndrome (PCOS). Examination should include routine measurement of height and weight, and calculation of body mass index (BMI).

The causes of secondary amenorrhoea are summarized in Box 13.8.1.1.

The most prevalent cause of secondary amenorrhoea is hypothalamic and/or pituitary dysfunction. Hyperprolactinaemia, weight loss-related, and idiopathic amenorrhoea are all associated with a functional rather than structural hypothalamic disorder of gonadotropin regulation (see below). PCOS accounts for a further 32% of cases, and primary ovarian failure for 11%. Among women presenting with oligomenorrhoea (Box 13.8.1.2), the underlying cause is PCOS in the great majority of cases, making this the most common overall cause of anovulation, as discussed in more detail below.

Differential diagnosis of amenorrhoea and oligomenorrhoea

With the aid of a small number of endocrine investigations it is possible clearly to differentiate between the various causes of ovarian disorders, and to guide management (Table 13.8.1.1). Measurement of serum FSH will distinguish primary ovarian failure (wherein FSH is elevated) from other causes of amenorrhoea and oligomenorrhoea (in which FSH is normal or low). Assessment of oestrogen status is an important step in the investigation of women with amenorrhoea. This can be achieved by direct measurement of serum oestradiol, by ultrasonographic measurement of endometrial thickness, or by a progestagen challenge test. Serum oestradiol measurements are valuable if results are unequivocally low (i.e. lower than in the early follicular phase) or normal (equivalent to mid follicular phase levels), but concentrations in the early follicular phase range may not exclude chronic oestrogen deficiency. The advantage of ultrasonography or the progestagen challenge test is that these provide what amounts to an *in vivo* bioassay of endogenous oestrogen action (on the endometrium).

A combination of low oestrogen and low (or normal) FSH is indicative of hypothalamic/pituitary dysfunction. In such cases

---

Box 13.8.1.2 Causes of oligomenorrhoea

♦ PCOS (87%)

♦ Perimenopausal (3%)

♦ Recovered weight loss (9%)

♦ Uncertain cause (1%)

---

serum prolactin should be measured and, if it is elevated, pituitary imaging performed (see below and Chapter 13.2).

Overview of management of disorders of ovulation

A simple schema for the differential diagnosis of ovarian disorders provides a basis for the selection of appropriate treatment, as outlined in Table 13.8.1.1. Details of management of the individual disorders are given in the appropriate sections below. The first principle must always be to treat any underlying cause, if possible, e.g. helping women with weight loss-related amenorrhoea to gain weight. For primary ovarian failure (high FSH, low oestrogen), gamete donation is the only option for fertility treatment, but oestrogen/progestagen is required for the treatment of symptoms of oestrogen deficiency (see below). In women with a hypothalamic or pituitary cause of anovulation (low or normal FSH with low oestrogen), ovulation can be induced by gonadotropins or GnRH (or, in the case of hyperprolactinaemia, by dopamine agonists), but patients not requiring fertility treatment will, like those with primary ovarian failure, need sex-hormone replacement. Ovulation can be induced by antioestrogens in most women with PCOS (normal FSH, normal oestrogen), but some may require gonadotropin therapy. In those not wishing to conceive, management of erratic periods and treatment of attendant symptoms of androgen excess are important considerations.

Premature (primary) ovarian failure

Ovarian failure usually occurs after the end of the fifth decade and manifests as the menopause, defined as the last ever menstrual period (average age 51 years). It is described as being premature if it occurs under the age of 40 years, and this affects approximately 1% of women. Unfortunately, regardless of the cause, premature ovarian failure is irreversible, although it is not unusual to have episodes of spontaneous ovarian function after the menopause. In a very small proportion (1–2%) of women this may even result in pregnancy. The characteristic endocrine features are oestrogen

Table 13.8.1.1 Differential diagnosis and guide to management of women with amenorrhoea

Results of investigations	Diagnosis	Management
High FSH, low oestrogen	Primary ovarian failure	HRT
Normal/low FSH, low oestrogen (if prolactin high)	Hypothalamic/ pituitary disorder Hyperprolactinaemia	GnRH or FSH (or HRT) Dopamine agonists
Normal FSH, normal oestrogen (with or without high LH)	PCOS	Clomiphene, FSH Cyclical progestagen or oral contraceptive

FSH, follicle-stimulating hormone; GnRH, gonadotropin-releasing hormone; HRT, hormone replacement therapy; LH, luteinizing hormone; PCOS, polycystic ovary syndrome.

deficiency associated with elevated serum concentrations of FSH (and LH), sometimes referred to as hypergonadotrophic amenorrhoea.

Types

Idiopathic

Most cases of primary ovarian failure are idiopathic, and it is not clear if the underlying cause is related to an initially reduced population of primordial follicles within the fetal ovary, an increased rate of atresia throughout reproductive life, or a combination of both. It may be associated with autoimmune conditions and may be accompanied by ovarian, thyroid, adrenal, and antiendomysial autoantibodies. There is also an association with type 1 diabetes. The significance of ovarian autoantibodies in the aetiology of ovarian failure remains uncertain, however. 'Resistant ovary syndrome' refers to a state in which oestrogen-deficient amenorrhoea or oligomenorrhoea is associated with high serum FSH, but with the persistence of follicles in the ovary. This is now generally recognized as a stage of ovarian failure, inevitably culminating in further reduction and, finally, exhaustion of the follicle pool.

Chromosomal and genetic

It is important to investigate potential causes of premature ovarian failure, as these may be significant in counselling family members or any children of affected women. The commonest forms of gonadal dysgenesis are Turner's syndrome (45,X) and its mosaic forms. These women have a structurally normal vulva, vagina, uterus, fallopian tubes, and ovaries, although the latter may be small and will undergo premature failure. An oocyte requires an X chromosome to protect it from early atresia, and women with Turner's syndrome or mosaic Turner's syndrome are highly likely to experience premature ovarian failure. Indeed, many of these women will have primary amenorrhoea.

Other causes of gonadal dysgenesis include Swyer's syndrome (46, XY gonadal dysgenesis) which invariably results in delayed puberty and primary amenorrhoea. Approximately 30% of cases are caused by a deletion on the Y chromosome that results in non-functioning streak gonads, which are unable to secrete antimullerian hormone (normally a product of Sertoli cells in the fetal testis) and therefore the mullerian structures do not regress. The result is an anatomically normal vulva, vagina, uterus, and fallopian tubes. Mutations on autosomal chromosomes have also been described and although cases may be familial, the majority are caused by new mutations. The gonads are thought to be at increased risk of malignant change, and surgical removal is usually recommended. The gonads often lie high on the pelvic side-wall, or may even be found above the pelvis, and can be removed laparoscopically.

Autosomal dominant, autosomal recessive, and X-linked patterns of inheritance have also been described in primary ovarian failure. It is now recognized that the mutation responsible for fragile X syndrome, a cause of learning difficulties, can be associated with premature ovarian failure in carriers. The syndrome is caused by a full mutation in the *FMR1* gene and any of its unstable premutations can be associated with ovarian failure. These premutations are probably the commonest known genetic cause of ovarian failure.

Iatrogenic

Iatrogenic premature ovarian failure is increasingly seen in young adult survivors of childhood malignancies, especially haematological ones. The cause is loss of germ cells and follicles as a consequence of chemotherapy and/or irradiation. A second group seen with increasing frequency is young women who have had adjuvant chemotherapy for breast cancer. Not all chemotherapy regimens are equally toxic to the ovary and the effects are variable. Alkylating agents, especially cyclophosphamide and procarbazine, are particularly associated with reduced ovarian function and premature ovarian failure, although platinum-based agents are less so.

Treatment

Treatment of primary ovarian failure falls into four categories: (1), induction of puberty (using low-dose oestrogen) in girls with delayed puberty, (2), control of symptoms of oestrogen deficiency, (3), preservation (or improvement) of bone mineral density, and (4), improvement of fertility. Hypo-oestrogenic symptoms include hot flushes and night sweats, dyspareunia, urinary frequency, and loss of libido. There is also often a loss of a sense of general well-being, although that may be due in part to a reaction to the diagnosis. Bone mineral density is likely to be low in untreated ovarian failure, but can be preserved and increased with exogenous oestradiol. Oestrogen replacement is usually in the form of a sequential or continuous combined regimen, progesterone being required to protect the endometrium from the effects of unopposed oestrogen.

Some young women find the combined oral contraceptive pill a more acceptable form of oestrogen replacement. Compliance can be an issue, especially in those under 25 years, and the pill can be a useful alternative to conventional hormone replacement. Another advantage of relying on the pill for oestrogen replacement is that it is contraceptive, whereas conventional hormone replacement therapy is not. Although pregnancy after premature ovarian failure is uncommon, it can and does occur. Unplanned pregnancy for any woman can be traumatic, but when it occurs in one affected by premature ovarian failure the results can be particularly upsetting. An important part of the management is therefore contraceptive advice, if pregnancy is undesirable. By contrast, a woman who would welcome a pregnancy can be reassured that hormone replacement treatment will not decrease her chances of a pregnancy occurring.

Fertility

Once premature ovarian failure has occurred no fertility treatment will assist conception, and oocyte donation is the only option. It is an extremely successful treatment for many couples, but the main difficulty is finding an appropriate donor. Pelvic irradiation is associated with a poor outcome from oocyte donation because of attendant uterine abnormalities. The endometrium may be unable to support implantation, and even if pregnancy occurs the obstetric risks are increased, including miscarriage, premature delivery, and intrauterine growth restriction. The risks of pregnancy must also be seriously considered for women with Turner's syndrome, as maternal deaths from aortic arch dissection have occurred, and there appears to be an increased incidence of placental abruption.

Hypothalamic/pituitary dysfunction

Weight-loss related amenorrhoea

The majority of cases of amenorrhoea resulting from hypothalamic/pituitary dysfunction are of hypothalamic rather than pituitary origin, and most are a function of an underlying disorder. Weight loss-related amenorrhoea is very common. Nutritional status is an important determinant of reproductive function, and being

underweight (BMI <19 kg/m^2) is very likely to result in abnormalities in the pulsatile secretion of GnRH. This in turn leads to reduced frequency and amplitude of LH and FSH pulses, and oestrogen-deficient amenorrhoea. Cyclical ovarian function can be restored by weight gain, but this is not usually easy to effect. Most women with amenorrhoea related to weight loss have an underlying eating disorder and it is often necessary to seek the help of specialist psychological or psychiatric services. Fertility treatment is unwise in underweight women until they have reached a normal BMI. Although it is possible to induce ovulation with GnRH or gonadotropins, underweight women are at considerably increased risk of having a small baby. However, correction of oestrogen deficiency is appropriate while treatment to aid weight gain is under way.

Hyperprolactinaemia

Hyperprolactinaemia is another common cause of oestrogen-deficient amenorrhoea. It is discussed in greater detail in Chapter 13.2. Amenorrhoea is the typical presenting symptom of hyperprolactinaemia. It is important to exclude primary hypothyroidism or concurrent medication as possible causes before embarking upon pituitary radiology. In particular, dopamine antagonists (e.g. phenothiazines and metoclopramide) are well-recognized causes of elevated serum prolactin. MRI is the preferred method of detecting pituitary abnormalities. A microadenoma of the pituitary may be found in up to 50% of women with hyperprolactinaemic amenorrhoea. Larger tumours (≥ 10 mm) are much less common. Management of hyperprolactinaemic amenorrhoea, even in women with an obvious prolactinoma, is primarily by the use of long-acting dopamine agonists such as bromocriptine or cabergoline. These drugs lower prolactin, restore ovulatory function, and typically reduce the size of prolactin-secreting tumours. Pituitary surgery is rarely needed, even in women with large prolactinomas.

Idiopathic hypothalamic amenorrhoea

In about 10% of cases the underlying cause of hypothalamic amenorrhoea is uncertain. Recent studies of women with idiopathic (functional) hypothalamic amenorrhoea have suggested that this category of patients represent what is essentially a stress-related hypothalamic disorder. Such patients respond very well to cognitive behavioural therapy, which results in resumption of ovulatory cycles without the need for endocrine treatment. If cognitive behavioural therapy is unsuccessful, ovulation can be induced by GnRH or gonadotropins in women seeking fertility treatment (Fig. 13.8.1.4). Otherwise, oestrogen/progestagen replacement is desirable to treat symptoms of oestrogen deficiency and/or to maintain bone density. Finally, it is important to recognize that other hypothalamic–pituitary disorders, although themselves being rare causes of amenorrhoea, may first present with menstrual dysfunction. Congenital deficiency of GnRH, best illustrated by Kallmann's syndrome (in which gonadotropin deficiency is associated with anosmia), often presents as delayed puberty, but may manifest as primary amenorrhoea in girls who have completed pubertal development. Amenorrhoea is a common presenting symptom in women with acromegaly or Cushing's syndrome. Hypothalamic tumours or granulomas may cause deficiency of not only GnRH but also other hypothalamic hormones. It is not necessary routinely to screen for these rarer causes of amenorrhoea, but it is important to be alert to features in the history and examination that may suggest a more unusual diagnosis.

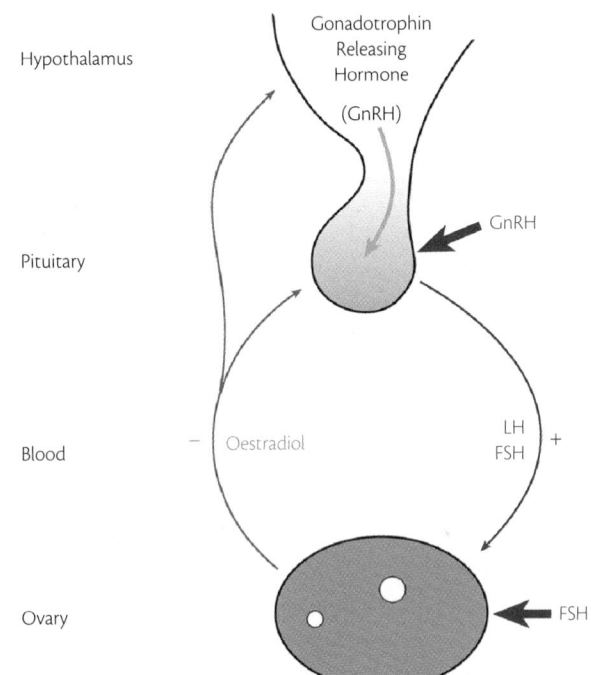

Fig. 13.8.1.4 Induction of ovulation in patients with hypothalamic amenorrhoea. Exogenous GnRH may be administered by pulsatile infusion pump, leading to restoration of gonadotropin secretion and normal negative feedback regulation of LH and FSH by ovarian steroids, thus limiting the risk of multiple follicle development. An alternative strategy is to give gondaotropins by daily injection, but the risk of hyperstimulation is greater than with GnRH.

PCOS

PCOS is the commonest of all the ovarian disorders and the commonest endocrine disorder in women of reproductive age, with a prevalence greater than 5% of the general population. The typical clinical presentation is the association of features of anovulation or oligo-ovulation (amenorrhoea or menstrual irregularity) with clinical and/or biochemical evidence of androgen excess (hirsutism, persistent acne, or male-pattern alopecia) in women with polycystic ovaries (Fig. 13.8.1.5). However, the recognition that there may be a broader spectrum of clinical and biochemical presentation has led to a recent revision of the diagnostic criteria for PCOS (see below). The aetiology of PCOS remains uncertain. There is strong evidence for an ovarian origin of androgen excess, although the hypersecretion of adrenal androgens can also be found, albeit in a minority of patients with PCOS. Genetic factors clearly play a part in the aetiology; there is clustering of cases of PCOS within families, and a recent twin study showed that the concordance of features of PCOS is significantly greater in identical than in nonidentical twins. The mode of inheritance is unclear, but it is unlikely to be a simple mendelian trait. Rather, like type 2 diabetes, it is a complex endocrine disorder in which several genes may play a part. In addition, as in type 2 diabetes, the phenotype is modified by environmental factors, and obesity clearly exacerbates endocrine and metabolic dysfunction, and is associated with more severe symptoms.

Definition and diagnostic criteria

The classic definition of PCOS, i.e. hyperandrogenism associated with chronic anovulation (in the absence of any confounding

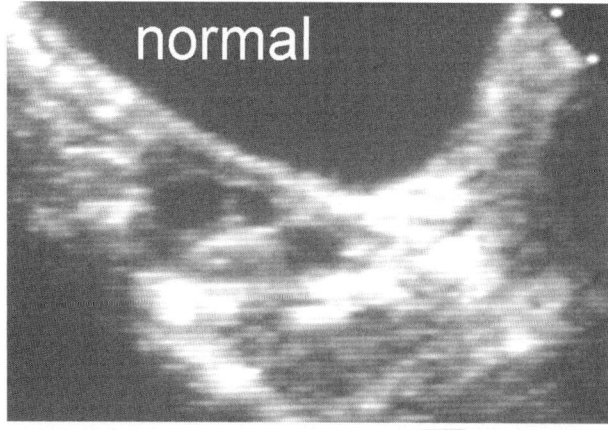

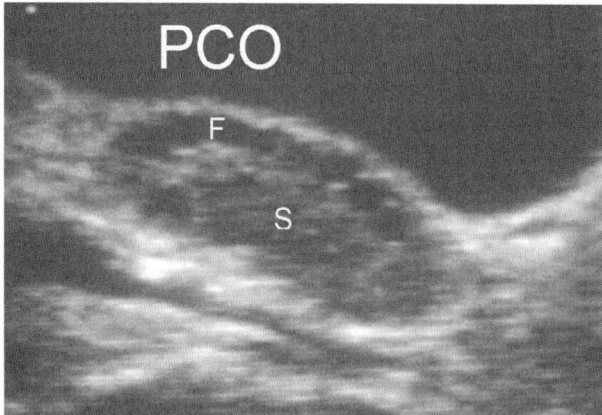

Fig. 13.8.1.5 Ultrasound images of a normal (A) and polycystic ovary (B). Note the numerous peripheral follicles (F) and extensive stromal area (S). (Courtesy of Ms J Adams.)

pituitary or adrenal disorders), is notable for its lack of reference to ovarian morphology, and yet almost all women who meet these criteria will have polycystic ovaries. In addition, polycystic ovaries can be found in women with symptoms of hyperandrogenism, but who have regular menstrual cycles, as well as in those with anovulation but no evidence of androgen excess. A consensus meeting held in 2003 revised the diagnostic criteria, allowing a more inclusive definition (Table 13.8.1.2). This revision has inevitably led to some controversy about the definition of PCOS, but there is ample evidence that women with polycystic ovaries who present with

Table 13.8.1.2 Diagnostic criteria for polycystic ovary syndrome

NIH 1990[a]	Rotterdam 2003[b]
Chronic anovulation	Oligo- and/or anovulation
Clinical and/or biochemical signs of hyperandrogenism	Clinical and/or biochemical signs of hyperandrogenism
	Polycystic ovaries

[a] Both criteria needed.

[b] Two of three criteria required.

Diagnosis using either set of criteria assumes that other aetiologies that may mimic PCOS (e.g. nonclassical 21-hydroxylase deficiency) have been excluded.

Source: NIH conference on PCOS 1990; Joint ESHRE/ASRM consensus conference, Rotterdam 2003.

hyperandrogenism, but have regular cycles, and those with oestrogen-replete amenorrhoea or oligomenorrhoea, but who have no features of androgen excess, simply have varying forms of the same underlying condition.

Endocrine features

The heterogeneity of the clinical features of PCOS extends to the endocrine abnormalities associated with it As a result, specific endocrine parameters are not a requirement for diagnosis, although measurement can be helpful to support it and, importantly, to exclude other conditions. Until the advent of widely available high-resolution ultrasonography, the diagnosis of PCOS was usually based on a combination of biochemical and clinical features.

Raised serum testosterone concentration is the most common biochemical abnormality in PCOS, occurring in about 70% of cases. The free androgen index, calculated from total testosterone and sex-hormone binding globulin (SHBG), has been found to be a useful marker by some clinicians. However, since SHBG is closely associated with BMI and, more particularly, abdominal circumference, the increased free androgen index found in PCOS is at least in part a reflection of increased abdominal adiposity. Serum concentrations of the weak androgen androstenedione are also elevated in PCOS. In practical terms, measuring serum testosterone is usually preferable to measuring androstenedione, as the process is automated in most clinical laboratories and therefore more cost-efficient. In 10 to 20% of patients with PCOS, serum levels of the weak adrenal androgen dehydroepiandrosterone sulphate (DHEAS) are also modestly elevated, suggesting that, at least in some patients with PCOS, there may be an adrenal contribution to increased circulating androgens.

Among women with PCOS, clinical signs of hyperandrogenaemia (e.g. hirsutism) are associated with higher testosterone levels than in those without. The presence or absence of features of hyperandrogenism, however, does not accurately predict serum androgen levels, as clinical expression depends on the peripheral conversion of testosterone to its active metabolite 5α-dihydrotestosterone by 5α-reductase, as well as on end-organ sensitivity (androgen receptor activity) (see 'Other causes of hyperandrogenism in women', below). Obesity in PCOS is associated with higher free testosterone levels than in lean counterparts, and in part reflects the lower SHBG levels found in the former group. In addition, obesity may have an independent effect on peripheral androgen metabolism since androsterone glucuronide levels, a marker for peripheral 5α-reductase activity, are raised in this group. Genetic factors may affect end-organ sensitivity, e.g. PCOS occurs in Chinese and Japanese women, but hirsutism is relatively uncommon in these populations. By contrast, hirsutism features commonly in women with PCOS from the Indian subcontinent.

Women with PCOS tend to have higher LH levels than those with normal ovaries. The highest prevalence of elevated LH levels is in those with anovulatory menses or amenorrhoea, but even in this group more than 40% will have normal LH. By contrast, FSH levels are normal but tend to be lower than in the normal early follicular phase. Many have cited a raised LH:FSH ratio (either 2.5:1 or 3:1) as a diagnostic feature of PCOS, but it is neither sensitive nor specific enough to be used as a reliable diagnostic criterion.

Oestrogen levels in women with all variants of PCOS are normal. As discussed previously, this can be used to distinguish between oligo/amenorrhoeic women with PCOS and those with other

causes of anovulation such as hypothalamic or pituitary disorders, or ovarian failure. Plasma oestradiol levels in PCOS lie within the range normally seen in the early to mid follicular phase of the menstrual cycle, but oestrone levels are significantly higher. This is probably because of the increased peripheral conversion of high levels of circulating androstenedione to oestrone in adipose tissue.

Hyperprolactinaemia has been described in association with PCOS, but this usually reflects spurious fluctuations in serum prolactin; it probably occurs no more commonly than in the normal population and is rarely a persistent problem.

Metabolic abnormalities

PCOS is not just a reproductive disorder, it is also associated with a characteristic metabolic abnormality, central to which are peripheral insulin resistance and compensatory hyperinsulinaemia. Insulin resistance is independent of body weight, but the difference between women with PCOS and controls is amplified with increasing body weight. Reduced insulin sensitivity is related to an abnormality in energy balance, specifically, reduced postprandial thermogenesis, which may contribute to the development of obesity. Interestingly, insulin resistance in PCOS appears to be confined to (or at least is most apparent in) the major subgroup of women who have both anovulation and hyperandrogenism (Box 13.8.1.3).

Typically, women with PCOS have increased abdominal adiposity and visceral fat accumulation, and this is correlated with insulin resistance. There is also an associated dyslipidaemia, characterized by lower than normal serum concentrations of high-density lipoprotein cholesterol and elevated levels of low-density lipoprotein cholesterol. Although glucose tolerance is often normal in these women, impaired glucose tolerance has been noted in 10 to 40% of young obese women with PCOS. The defect in insulin action associated with PCOS appears to be secondary to a defect in postreceptor signal transduction, and shows subtle differences from that found in other insulin-resistant states. The major defect associated with PCOS, independent of obesity, is in insulin signalling in classic insulin target tissues such as muscle. Suppression of hepatic gluconeogenesis is reduced, but only in obese PCOS women. By contrast, obesity alone has a smaller effect on the sensitivity of insulin-mediated glucose utilization, but a greater effect on the rate of glucose utilization.

There is some debate as to whether the insulin resistance in PCOS represents a primary defect in insulin action, or whether it is secondary to hyperandrogenism and/or the result of increased truncal–abdominal fat. The interaction of insulin and androgens is complex. Experimental data suggest that androgens affect the flux of free fatty acids from visceral fat deposits, which may in turn affect insulin sensitivity. However, therapeutic reduction of serum androgen levels does not appear to improve insulin sensitivity. On the other hand, hyperinsulinaemia clearly affects androgen production. Insulin has gonadotropic activity and can influence ovarian steroidogenesis by both theca and granulosa cells via an interaction with LH. In addition, hyperinsulinaemia reduces the hepatic production of SHBG and thereby raises levels of non-protein-bound (i.e. biologically available) testosterone.

Reproductive consequences

PCOS is by far the commonest cause of anovulatory infertility, accounting for more than 75% of cases. Anovulation is undoubtedly the principal reason for subfertility in women with polycystic ovaries, but there has been some speculation that polycystic ovaries, in the absence of the syndrome, may contribute to problems with fertility. Polycystic ovaries are found more commonly than in the general population in infertile ovulatory women with tubal disease (50%), in women whose partners have sperm dysfunction (53%), and in couples with unexplained infertility (44%). Women with polycystic ovaries are also over-represented among women with a history of recurrent miscarriage (three or more consecutive miscarriages). However, the live birth rate of ovulatory women with polycystic ovaries, after spontaneous conception, is the same as that in a well-matched population of women with normal ovaries.

Long-term consequences

The significance of PCOS for women's health at a population level is increasingly being recognized. Although management of symptoms such as infertility and hirsutism is important, consideration must also be given to management and, if possible, prevention of the long-term effects of the disorder. These include an increased risk of developing endometrial cancer and the consequences of metabolic abnormalities, namely diabetes and cardiovascular disease.

Endometrial carcinoma

PCOS has been recognized as a risk factor for endometrial carcinoma since the 1950s, and there are reports of the disease occurring in young (premenopausal) women with PCOS. In women with PCOS who have amenorrhoea or infrequent menses, the endometrium is exposed to prolonged stimulation with oestrogen in the absence of cyclical progesterone (unopposed oestrogen). This may lead to endometrial hyperplasia and, if untreated, to endometrial carcinoma. Obesity adds to the risk of developing endometrial cancer by a number of interrelated intermediary factors, including increased oestrogen production, hyperinsulinaemia, and reduced serum SHBG.

Gestational diabetes

The link between PCOS, insulin resistance, and impaired glucose tolerance suggests that women with PCOS are at increased risk of developing both type 2 diabetes and gestational diabetes. The physiological insulin resistance of pregnancy is added to that intrinsic to PCOS, and may unmask impaired pancreatic β-cell function. The evidence for an increased risk of gestational diabetes among women with PCOS is suggestive, but not yet compelling. Most of the studies to date have been small and retrospective, and involve ethnically mixed populations. However, a recent meta-analysis of the available data suggests a threefold increase in the risk of gestational diabetes in women with PCOS.

Box 13.8.1.3 Typical metabolic features of PCOS

- Insulin resistance and hyperinsulinaemia
- Abnormal energy expenditure (reduced postprandial thermogenesis)
- Dyslipidaemia
- Impaired glucose tolerance

Metabolic abnormalities are much more prevalent in women who have both anovulation and androgen excess, and are exacerbated by obesity.

Type 2 diabetes

As indicated above, impaired glucose tolerance and even frank diabetes are common in obese young women with PCOS. Longitudinal studies have been limited, both in number and in duration of follow-up, but those that are available indicate that the prevalence of both impaired glucose tolerance and diabetes increase, as might be predicted, with age and, inevitably, BMI. Likewise, population studies have been few, but the results support the view that PCOS is a significant risk factor for the development of type 2 diabetes. The relative risk is around twofold after adjustment for obesity, but rises to three- to sevenfold in obese women with PCOS.

Cardiovascular risk

PCOS is associated with well-recognized risk factors for cardiovascular disease, namely obesity, insulin resistance, dyslipidaemia, diabetes, and (in some but not all studies) hypertension. In addition, surrogate markers of cardiovascular disease have also been found to be abnormal. Endothelial function is impaired in young women with PCOS. Carotid artery intima–media wall thickness (associated with an adverse cardiovascular risk profile in middle-aged and older general populations) is increased in women with PCOS over the age of 45 years, and carotid plaques are more common. Coronary artery calcification is a marker for coronary atherosclerosis, and is also more common in women with PCOS than BMI-matched controls. Left ventricular mass index was found to be increased, and diastolic dysfunction present in obese and non-obese young women with PCOS, suggesting a detrimental effect on the cardiovascular system, although this is yet to be confirmed.

It might be expected from the presence of multiple risk factors for cardiovascular disease that women with PCOS, especially if obese, would have an increased morbidity and mortality from the condition. There are few epidemiological studies and no substantial longitudinal studies, but the data so far suggest that there are fewer cardiovascular events than would be predicted from the cluster of risk factors. The two largest studies give a similar odds ratio (1.5) for the risk of cardiovascular events. In both studies the populations were under 60 years of age, so it remains possible that the relative risk of heart attack (and stroke) will increase with age. An alternative explanation is that there are factors in women with PCOS that are protective against cardiovascular disease, e.g. as a result of unopposed oestrogen or even raised androgen levels. Perhaps most importantly of all, it must be appreciated that the presence of risk factors does not prove the presence of the disease, and that surrogate markers are not necessarily reliable predictors of outcome.

Management of PCOS

The management of PCOS is mainly targeted at the relief of symptoms. Symptoms of androgen excess, including hirsutism, acne, or alopecia, can be attenuated by the use of antiandrogens such as cyproterone acetate and spironolactone (which, in the absence of cyproterone acetate, is widely used in the United States of America). Flutamide is a pure antiandrogen (unlike cyproterone acetate it has no progestagenic activity), but its place is less secure in the management of symptoms of androgen excess because there are fewer studies to support its routine use and there have been reports of hepatic toxicity. Low-dose cyproterone acetate may be conveniently combined with ethinylestradiol (as co-cyprindiol) and this preparation is particularly useful in women with accompanying menstrual disturbance. It is also an effective contraceptive. For those in whom oestrogen is contraindicated cyproterone acetate can be given alone, but nonhormonal contraception should be advised in those at risk of pregnancy because of the theoretical risk of feminization of a male fetus. Women often seek medical help with hirsutism when beauty treatments such as waxing, plucking, electrolysis, and laser hair removal become inconvenient or too expensive. It is important to ensure a realistic expectation of treatment, which is that antiandrogens should be used as adjuncts, not replacements, to beauty treatments. In addition, hormone treatment may take 9 to 12 months to become fully effective; an improvement in hirsutism is often best judged by a reduced frequency of hair-removal treatment. Antiandrogen therapy is also effective for acne but, unfortunately, alopecia rarely improves with antiandrogen treatment, and the objective here is to limit further hair loss. It is therefore important to treat early signs of androgen-dependent hair loss.

Anovulatory women with PCOS who wish to conceive usually respond to ovulation induction therapy (Fig. 13.8.1.6). The principle is to raise serum FSH levels to encourage development of a single, healthy, dominant follicle (and therefore limit the risk of multiple pregnancy). The first-line treatment is the antioestrogen clomifene, to which 75 to 80% of women will ovulate in response. In those who do not respond or conceive after six or more ovulatory cycles, treatment with exogenous gonadotropin is appropriate. The modern approach is to start with a low dose of FSH and if necessary make small increments in dose to find the threshold for development of a single dominant follicle. Even low-dose FSH treatment requires close monitoring to reduce the risks of multiple pregnancy. An alternative to gonadotropin treatment is laparoscopic ovarian diathermy, a single, if invasive, procedure. However, surgery alone

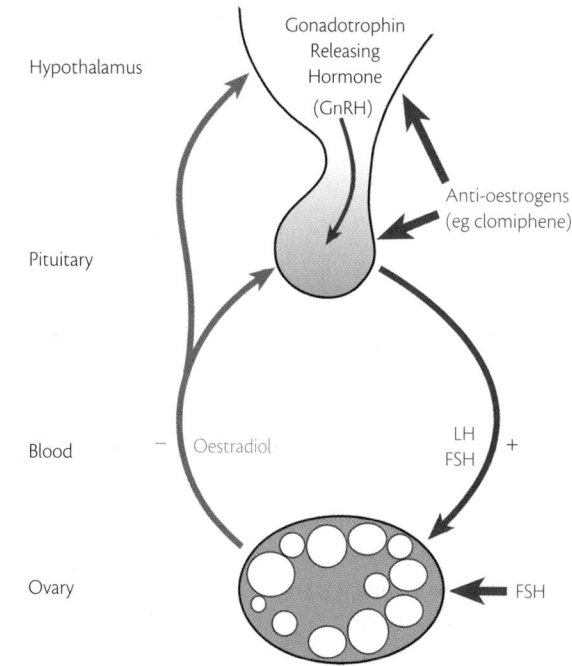

Fig. 13.8.1.6 Induction of ovulation in PCOS. The treatment of first choice is the antioestrogen clomifene, which leads to elevation of serum FSH. If this is ineffective, exogenous FSH can be given by daily low-dose injection.

will result in ovulatory cycles in less than 50% of subjects, and adjuvant clomifene or FSH treatment is often required.

In anovulatory women with PCOS who do not wish to conceive, regulation of menses can be ensured by treatment with a combined oral contraceptive or cyclical progestagen treatment. Because of the risk of endometrial hyperplasia or cancer it is important to offer such treatment, even in women with amenorrhoea or oligomenorrhoea who are not concerned about lack of periods.

In obese women with PCOS calorie restriction is not only desirable, but also surprisingly effective in improving the symptoms of PCOS, particularly menstrual pattern and fertility. Dietary restriction leading to merely a 5 to 10% reduction in weight is associated with much improved ovarian function. Overweight and obese women respond poorly to induction of ovulation, and from an obstetric viewpoint the risks of gestational diabetes and pregnancy-related hypertension are increased. Weight reduction before fertility treatment, though never easy to achieve, is therefore an important aspect of management. Evidence from the Diabetes Prevention Program, a prospective study of men and women with impaired glucose tolerance, suggests that calorie restriction coupled with lifestyle changes (including increased exercise) will reduce the risk of conversion to diabetes. Although there are, as yet, no such studies in women with PCOS, it is logical that such an approach will also reduce the chance of developing diabetes in this at risk group.

The Diabetes Prevention Program also showed that the biguanide metformin, which has long been used for the treatment of type 2 diabetes, was effective in reducing conversion from impaired glucose tolerance to diabetes (although significantly less so than diet and lifestyle changes). In recent years metformin has been enthusiastically advocated for the management of PCOS, even in the absence of impaired glucose tolerance. A large number of publications have supported its use in fertility treatment (particularly in combination with clomifene), menstrual regulation, and management of hirsutism. However, there have been few large randomized controlled trials of metformin in the management of PCOS, and those few adequately powered studies that have been performed to date have failed to support those claims. It remains to be seen whether metformin has a role in diabetes prevention in women with PCOS

Other causes of hyperandrogenism in women

Hyperandrogenism, in this context defined as clinical evidence of androgen excess in women, is a common and distressing problem. Hyperandrogenism manifests itself as hirsutism, persistent acne, or androgenic alopecia. Although PCOS is the commonest cause of androgen excess, it is important to consider other possible diagnoses.

Physiology of androgen-dependent hair growth and androgen production in women

During puberty circulating androgen concentrations rise, and the familiar pattern of androgen-dependent body (terminal) hair growth is seen. In normal premenopausal women the adrenal is the predominant source of androgens. Testosterone is the most important circulating androgen, and is secreted by both ovaries and adrenals. But about 50% of circulating testosterone is derived by conversion from androstenedione (a weak androgen) in peripheral tissues such as skin and adipose. More than 90% of circulating testosterone is bound either to SHBG or albumin. Only the unbound (and possibly albumin-bound) testosterone is available to target tissues. Testosterone is further metabolized within the hair follicle to the more potent androgen dihydrotestosterone by the enzyme 5α-reductase. Both testosterone and (with a higher affinity) dihydrotestosterone bind to specific androgen receptors within the hair follicle to affect the growth of terminal hair. The biological effect of androgens may also be regulated at the level of the androgen receptor itself. Recent evidence suggests that heterogeneity of the androgen receptor is conferred by epigenetic modification of the androgen-receptor gene, and that these modifications are related to clinical indices of androgenicity.

Causes of hirsutism

The causes of hirsutism are summarized in Box 13.8.1.4.

Hirsutism is most commonly caused by PCOS, which accounts for about 90% of cases, including those who might previously have been labelled as having idiopathic hirsutism. However, hirsutism may be a manifestation of other, much rarer but more serious endocrine disorders, such as Cushing's syndrome and adrenal or ovarian tumours. Careful clinical evaluation is the key to differential diagnosis. Long-standing mild to moderate hirsutism, with or without menstrual disturbance, is suggestive of PCOS or idiopathic hirsutism, whereas a short history of increasing hirsutism in a previously nonhirsute subject should alert the physician to the possibility of an alternative diagnosis. Hirsutism and menstrual disturbances are common presenting features in women with Cushing's syndrome or androgen-secreting tumours. In the case of Cushing's syndrome, the presence of additional features such as hypertension, easy bruising, and striae help to make the diagnosis more likely.

Hyperthecosis refers to the histological finding of islands of theca cells within dense ovarian stroma, and is almost certainly a variant of PCOS. Its clinical presentation is indistinguishable from that of PCOS, but it tends to be associated with severe hirsutism,

---

Box 13.8.1.4 Causes of hirsutism

Ovarian
- PCOS (>80%)
- Hyperthecosis (5–10%)
- Ovarian tumours (<1%)

Adrenal
- Congenital adrenal hyperplasia (classic 1%; nonclassic (late onset), 3%)
- Cushing's syndrome (<1%)
- Adrenal tumours (<1%)

Idiopathic
- With raised androgens (5%)
- Without raised androgens (7%)

and there is often also cutaneous evidence of significant insulin resistance (acanthosis nigricans).

Another well-recognized cause of hirsutism that may be difficult to distinguish clinically from PCOS is nonclassic (late-onset) congenital adrenal hyperplasia resulting from 21-hydroxylase deficiency (Chapter 13.7.2). Such cases tend to present during adolescence with symptoms of anovulation and androgen excess.

Androgen-secreting ovarian and adrenal tumours are rare. Causes, diagnosis, and management of adrenal tumours are described elsewhere (Chapter 13.7.1). Ovarian tumours may be benign or, less commonly, malignant and are classified as either sex cord-stromal tumours (Sertoli–Leydig cell tumours), or adrenal-like tumours (e.g. virilizing lipoid-cell tumours, adrenal rest tumours).

Investigation and diagnosis of hirsutism

A guide to the investigation of hirsutism is given in Table 13.8.1.3. Mild to moderate long-standing hirsutism in women with regular menses is very likely to be either idiopathic or, much more commonly, associated with polycystic ovaries. Serum testosterone concentrations are usually modestly elevated or within the normal range. It could be argued that no investigations are strictly necessary in this category of patient, but our practice is to measure serum testosterone and perform a pelvic ultrasound scan to determine ovarian morphology, so that a specific diagnosis can be offered to the patient. The principal reason for measuring testosterone in women with hirsutism is to screen for the more serious causes of androgen excess that will require further investigation. It is not measured to diagnose hyperandrogenism since this is already clinically manifested as hirsutism. In our clinic we have not found it necessary routinely to measure androstenedione, SHBG, or free testosterone. Some laboratories offer androstenedione as a reasonable alternative to testosterone assays.

In women with hirsutism and menstrual disturbance the most likely diagnosis is again PCOS. In such cases, however, it is legitimate to extend biochemical tests to include measurements of gonadotropins and, in amenorrhoeic women, prolactin and oestradiol. Further investigations are necessary in those patients with a short history of hirsutism (particularly if this is severe), those with symptoms suggesting other endocrine disorders (e.g. Cushing's syndrome), and

Table 13.8.1.3 Guide to the investigation of hirsutism

Presenting features	Investigations
Mild chronic hirsutism and regular cycles	Testosterone Ultrasonography of ovaries
Moderate hirsutism and/or cycle disturbance	Testosterone, LH, FSH Ultrasonography of ovaries
Severe hirsutism and/or short history and/or testosterone >5 nmol/litre	Dehydroepiandrosterone sulphate, 17-hydoxyprogesterone Dexamethasone suppression test 24-h urine free cortisol Ovarian and/or adrenal imaging Fasting glucose/insulin

those with a serum testosterone that exceeds 5 nmol/litre (normal range 0.5–3.0 nmol/litre). In patients with a serum testosterone concentration in the normal male range (>10 nmol/litre) the presence of an androgen-secreting tumour must be excluded. Imaging of the ovaries and adrenals by MRI is important. In experienced hands, ultrasonography of the adrenals and particularly the ovaries may also be helpful. Selective catheterization of adrenal or ovarian veins to localize a suspected tumour is difficult to execute and rarely informative. Measurement of DHEAS is a useful specific index of adrenal function in patients with a suspected androgen-secreting tumour, but it is less helpful as a routine test in hirsute patients.

The prevalence of nonclassic CAH in our clinic population is very low (<1% of cases of hirsutism), so we do not routinely measure basal and ACTH-stimulated concentrations of 17-hydroxyprogesterone to screen for this disorder. However, it is appropriate to do so in women with severe hirsutism and a serum testosterone greater than 5 nmol/litre.

Management of hirsutism

The management of women with hirsutism is described above in the section about PCOS. The principles of symptomatic management are similar in women with idiopathic hirsutism. In those with a specific underlying diagnosis, treatment is directed towards the primary disease or disorder. For example, removal of a pituitary corticotroph adenoma or an ovarian tumour is a very effective way of treating hirsutism.

Further reading

Baird DT (1983). Prediction of ovulation: biophysical, physiological and biochemical coordinates. In: Jeffcoate SL (ed). *Ovulation: methods for its prediction and detection*, pp. 1–17. John Wiley, Chichester.

Berga SL, Loucks TL (2005). The diagnosis and treatment of stress-induced anovulation. *Minerva Ginecol*, **57**, 45–54.

Chang RJ (2007). The reproductive phenotype in polycystic ovary syndrome. *Nat Clin Pract Endocrinol Metab*, **3**, 688–95.

Ehrmann DA (2005). Polycystic ovary syndrome. *N Engl J Med*, **352**, 1223–36.

Franks S (1995). Polycystic ovary syndrome. *N Engl J Med*, **333**, 853–61.

Gillam MP, *et al.* (2006). Advances in the treatment of prolactinomas. *Endocr Rev*, **27**, 485–534.

Goswami D, Conway GS (2005). Premature ovarian failure. *Hum Reprod Update*, **11**, 391–410.

Gougeon A (1996). Regulation of ovarian follicular development in primates: facts and hypotheses. *Endocr Rev*, **17**, 121–54.

Hardy K, *et al.* (2000). *In vitro* maturation of oocytes. *Br Med Bull*, **56**, 588–602.

Koulouri O, Conway GS (2008). A systematic review of commonly used medical treatments for hirsutism in women. *Clin Endocrinol (Oxf)*, **68**, 800–5.

Marshall JC, Eagleson CA, McCartney CR (2001). Hypothalamic dysfunction. *Mol Cell Endocrinol*, **183**, 29–32.

Norman RJ, *et al.* (2007). Polycystic ovary syndrome. *Lancet*, **370**, 685–97.

Venkatesan AM, Dunaif A, Corbould A (2001). Insulin resistance in polycystic ovary syndrome: progress and paradoxes. *Recent Prog Horm Res*, **56**, 295–308.

13.8.2 Disorders of male reproduction

U. Srinivas-Shankar and F.C.W. Wu

Essentials

Luteinizing hormone (LH) stimulates biosynthesis of androgenic steroids by binding to specific surface membrane receptors on the Leydig cells in the testis. Testosterone is essential for male sexual differentiation, growth and function of the male genital tract, secondary sexual characteristics, sexual potency, and production of spermatozoa.

Hypogonadism

Clinical features—male hypogonadism describes the clinical complex associated with testosterone deficiency due to pathological conditions affecting the hypothalamic–pituitary–testicular axis. Symptoms and signs depend on the age of onset of androgen deficiency. Prepubertal presentation is with sexual infantilism, delayed puberty, and eunuchoidal body proportions. Postpubertal presentation is with diminished sex drive and erection, loss of ejaculation, muscle atrophy, poor stamina, decreased secondary sexual hair, decreased shaving frequency, and regression of spermatogenesis (reduced testicular volume).

Diagnosis—hypogonadism is confirmed by low serum testosterone measured between 08.00 and 10.00 h. Measurement of LH, follicle-stimulating hormone (FSH), and prolactin is required to differentiate between primary (high gonadotrophins) and secondary (low gonadotrophins) hypogonadism. Patients with hypogonadotrophic hypogonadism without the stigmata of Kallmann's syndrome (anosmia, red–green colour blindness, synkinesis, nerve deafness, cleft lip or palate, and renal malformations) require full pituitary assessment to exclude an underlying pituitary tumour. Suspected Klinefelter's syndrome should be confirmed by chromosome karyotyping. Ultrasonography and MRI scan are useful in locating ectopic or intra-abdominal testes. DNA analysis can help confirm the diagnosis of androgen resistance syndromes and some other rare causes of hypogonadism.

Cryptorchidism—the absence of one or both testes from the scrotum and the commonest birth defect of the male genitals. It results from the failure of the testis to descend during fetal development from an abdominal position into the scrotum and is associated with increased risk of testicular cancer.

Klinefelter's syndrome (47,XXY)—the most common congenital cause of male hypogonadism and occurs due to the presence of an extra X chromosome derived from the meiotic nondisjunction of germ cells. Typically present with infertility in adulthood.

Management—the aims of treatment are to: (1) relieve the symptoms of androgen deficiency; (2) prevent the long-term consequences of androgen deficiency such as osteopenia; (3) reproduce physiological circulating and tissue levels of testosterone, dihydrotestoerone, and oestradiol; (4) induce fertility, if required, in hypogonadotrophic patients; (5) treat any specific underlying diseases. Before starting testosterone, patients over the age of 45 years should be checked for pre-existing occult prostatic cancer by digital rectal examination and measurement of prostate specific antigen. There are several testosterone formulations, each with specific advantages and disadvantages, with the choice depending on availability and the patient's age and preference.

Infertility

Male infertility is caused by a heterogeneous group of disorders and accounts for over one-third of a couple's infertility. The commonest cause is idiopathic azoo/oligozoospermia, which probably represents the end result of many conditions that disrupt normal seminiferous tubular functions, although discrete gene defects associated with impaired spermatogenesis are increasingly recognized, e.g. Klinefelter's syndrome, Y chromosome microdeletions, mutations in the ligand binding or DNA binding domains of the androgen receptor. Other causes include (1) male accessory gland infections, usually due to chlamydia, gonococcus, Gram-negative enterococci, and tubercle bacilli—a major cause of curable male infertility; (2) testicular tumours—the most common malignancy in young adult men; (3) obstructive azoospermia—usually due to vasectomy or previous genitourinary infections; may be amenable to surgical correction; (4) sperm autoimmunity.

Laboratory investigation—conventional parameters of the semen analysis such as sperm density, percentage of motile sperm, quality of sperm movements, and sperm morphology provide a semi-quantitative index of fertility potential. Testosterone and LH measurements are indicated only when there is clinical suspicion of androgen deficiency, Klinefelter's syndrome, or sex steroid abuse. Chromosome karyotyping and Y chromosome screening should be performed in all patients with nonobstructive azoospermia or severe oligozoospermia.

Management—(1) Intrauterine insemination (IUI) is first-line therapy for infertility due to the male factor, factors ascribed to the uterine cervix, minimal to mild endometriosis—and unexplained infertility. (2) *In vitro* fertilization (IVF) involves gonadotrophin stimulation of the female, suppression of spontaneous ovulation, and collection of multiple oocytes by laparoscopy or by ovarian puncture guided by transvaginal ultrasonography, with fertilization of eggs achieved by coincubation with prepared spermatozoa. (3) Microinjection of a single live spermatozoon directly into harvested oocytes (ICSI) is the treatment of choice for severe oligozoospermia in those who have failed IUI and IVF, but there is an increase in *de novo* chromosomal abnormalities, major congenital malformations, and imprinting disorders in children born as a result of such techniques, hence genetic counselling should be offered to all couples considering these treatments. (4) Cryopreservation of semen should be offered to all men of reproductive age before anticancer chemotherapy, orchidectomy, or testicular irradiation.

Introduction

The adult testis performs two functions—the secretion of androgens (principally testosterone) and the production of spermatozoa (Fig. 13.8.2.1). These functions are dependent on trophic hormones from the hypothalamus and anterior pituitary, which are

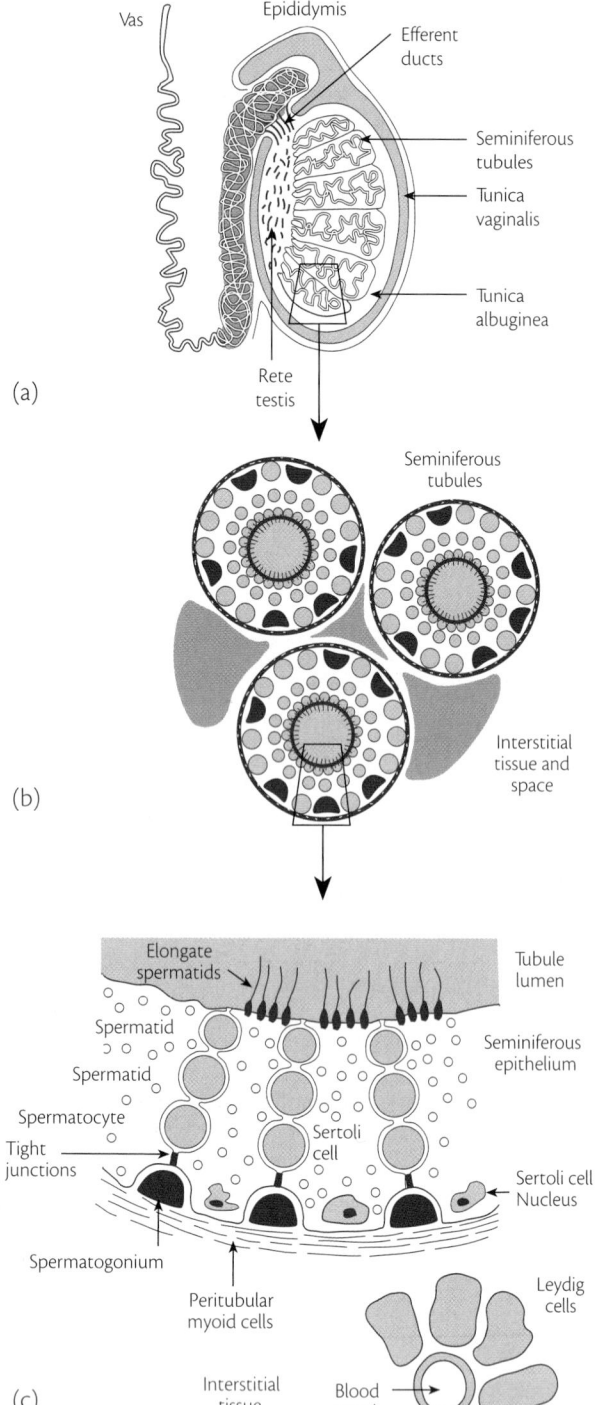

(a)

(b)

(c)

Fig. 13.8.2.1 (a) Human testis, epididymis, and vas deferens showing efferent ducts leading from the rete testis to the caput epididymis and the cauda epididymis, continuing to become the vas deferens; (b) cross-section through a seminiferous tubule showing central lumen, seminiferous epithelium, and interstitial space containing Leydig cells; (c) anatomical relationships in the seminiferous epithelium between germ cells (spermatogonia, spermatocytes, and spermatids), Sertoli cells, peritubular myoid cells, and Leydig cells.

responsive to the negative-feedback action of testicular hormones, thus forming a closed-loop functional axis (Fig. 13.8.2.2).

Gonadotropin-releasing hormone (GnRH) is synthesized in neurosecretory neurons in the hypothalamus and then released episodically into the pituitary portal circulation at a 1- to 2-hourly frequency. The neurophysiological control of GnRH secretion requires the integration of multiple internal and external cues acting upon a genetically determined process that remain unclear.

Luteinizing hormone (LH) stimulates the biosynthesis of androgenic steroids by binding to specific surface membrane receptors on the Leydig cells of the testis. This activates cAMP-dependent protein kinase and steroidogenic acute regulatory protein, which mobilize cholesterol substrate and transfer cholesterol from the outer to the inner mitochondrial membrane, where it is converted to pregnenolone by splitting the side chain at position C21. Figure 13.8.2.3 shows the principal steps in the steroidogenic pathway, in which the carbon skeleton of the parent compound, cholesterol, is progressively hydrolysed to form various androgenic steroids.

Testosterone is the main end product of the biosynthetic pathway in adult Leydig cells. The daily testicular production of testosterone is between 3 and 10 mg. As the principal circulating androgen secreted by the adult testes, testosterone exerts the major negative-feedback action on gonadotropin secretion, by restricting the frequency of GnRH release from the hypothalamus, and by reducing the amplitude of the LH response to GnRH.

Androgens are essential for the differentiation, growth, and function of the male genital ducts (epididymis) and accessory glands (seminal vesicles and prostate), for male secondary

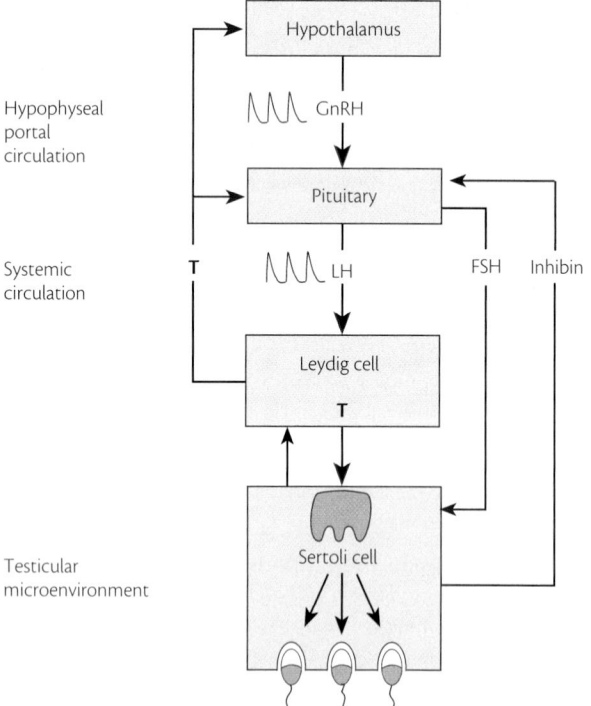

Fig. 13.8.2.2 Functional relationships in the hypothalamic–pituitary–testicular axis and testicular microenvironment. Gonadotropin-releasing hormone (GnRH) is secreted into the hypophysial circulation in an episodic manner, which is reflected by a luteinizing hormone (LH) pulse in the systemic circulation. Open arrows represent positive stimulation and closed arrows negative feedback.

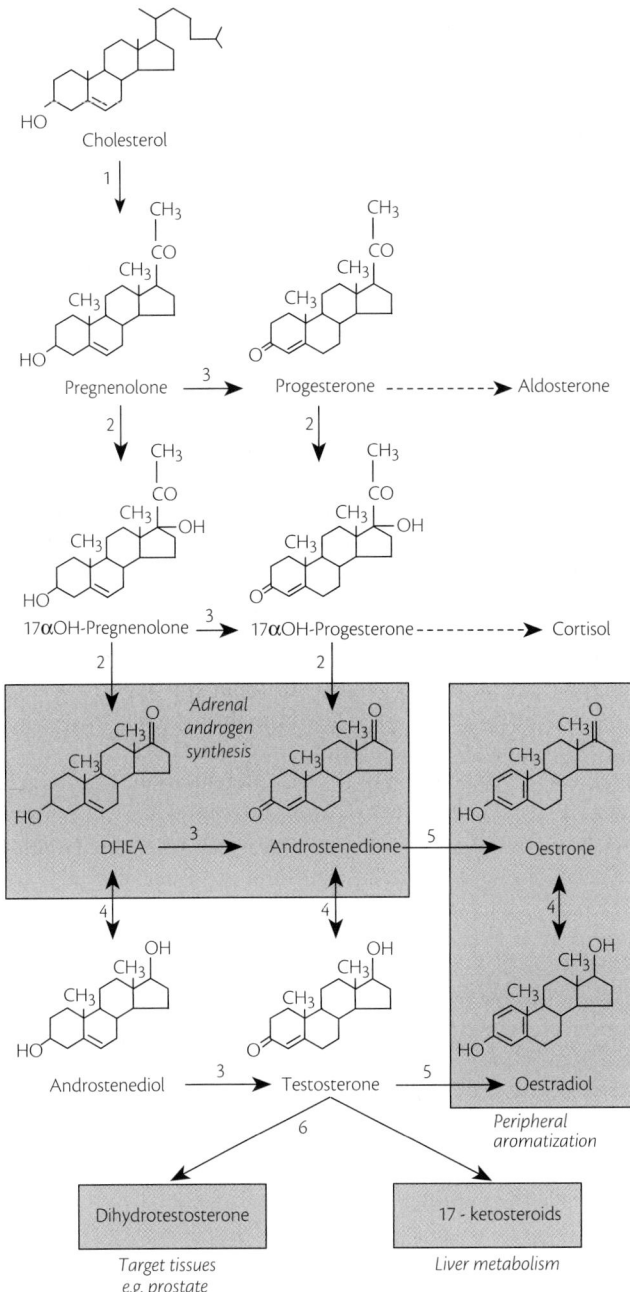

Fig. 13.8.2.3 Steroidogenic pathway from cholesterol to testosterone, and further conversion of testosterone: (1) cholesterol side-chain cleavage, (2) 17α-hydroxylase/17,20-lyase, (3) 3β-hydroxysteroid dehydrogenase, (4) 17β-hydroxysteroid dehydrogenase, (5) aromatase, and (6) 5α-reductase.

Table 13.8.2.1 Physiological action of androgens and clinical features of androgen deficiency

Physiological actions	Onset before puberty	Onset after puberty
Increase bone mass and density	Osteoporosis	Osteoporosis; female fat distribution
Fusion of long-bone epiphyses	Tall, eunuchoidal habitus	Decrease subcutaneous/ visceral fat
Female fat distribution	Female fat distribution	Laryngeal enlargement
Unbroken, high-pitched voice	Secondary sexual hair development	
Lack of pubic, axillary, and facial hair, no temporal recession	Decrease facial and pubic hair, no temporal recession	
Increase pilosebaceous activity	Lack of sebum, pale, smooth skin	Atrophy, fine wrinkles, pale
Stimulation of erythropoiesis	Moderate anaemia	Moderate anaemia
Increase muscle mass	Underdeveloped, poor physical stamina	Decrease strength and physical stamina
Penile growth	Infantile	
Prostate and seminal vesicle growth	Underdeveloped, no ejaculate	Atrophy, low volume or absence of ejaculate
Stimulation of spermatogenesis	Not initiated, very small testes	Regression of small testes
Stimulation of sexual interest	No development	Decreased
Stimulate erectile function	Low/ absent spontaneous erection	Decreased erection
Effects on mood and behaviour	Placid	Low moods, unassertive, tiredness

sexual characteristics, and for sexual potency (Table 13.8.2.1). Testosterone circulates in plasma bound to sex-hormone-binding globulin (SHBG) and albumin. In men, 60% of circulating testosterone is bound to SHBG, 38% to albumin, and 2% is unbound (free). Free testosterone represents the biologically active fraction of circulating testosterone.

Androgen action is primarily mediated through specific binding to intranuclear androgen receptors, which increase the transcription (genomic mechanism) of specific androgen-responsive genes in target cells. Transcription-independent signalling (nongenomic mechanism) through cell-surface membrane receptors is also recognized. Androgen action may also be influenced by genetic polymorphisms in the number of glutamine repeats (encoded by CAG trinucleotide repeats) in exon 1 of the androgen-receptor gene. Shorter CAG repeats are associated with higher androgenicity and vice versa.

In target organs such as the fetal external genitalia, prostate, and facial hair follicles, full activation requires the local metabolism of testosterone, by the enzyme 5α-reductase, to 5α-dihydrotestosterone, an androgen that is several-fold more potent than testosterone (Fig. 13.8.2.3).

Recently described males with a mutant oestrogen receptor gene (oestrogen resistance) or *CYP19* gene encoding P450 aromatase (oestrogen deficiency), and the corresponding knockout mouse models, have highlighted important roles for oestrogens in men. An increasing variety of androgen-dependent functions in males are now known to be mediated by the oestrogen receptors α and β, via conversion of testosterone to oestradiol by the widely distributed P450 aromatase in target tissues. These include the pubertal growth spurt, skeletal maturation, the fusion of epiphyses at the end of puberty, bone mass accrual and maintenance, some aspects of male-specific behaviour (in mouse models), fluid resorption from the testicular efferent ducts, and follicle-stimulating hormone (FSH) feedback regulation. Many of the actions of circulating testosterone are therefore diversified locally at different target tissues by the actions of 5α-reductase and aromatase. The relative contribution of circulating (endocrine action) compared with locally produced (paracrine or intracrine action) hormones, and the balance between androgen and oestrogen receptor activation, are crucial to the physiological effects of androgens in humans.

The endocrine (androgen synthesis) and gametogenic (spermatogenesis) functions of the testis are closely interlinked. Although testosterone is important as the principal circulating androgen, its local (paracrine) actions within the testis are crucial, together with FSH, for the initiation and maintenance of normal spermatogenesis and hence fertility (see Figs. 13.8.2.1 and 13.8.2.2). Since germ cells do not possess receptors for FSH or testosterone, these hormone signals are transduced through the Sertoli and peritubular cells. Sertoli cells create a microenvironment in the seminiferous tubules by providing a physical framework and elaborating ever-changing myriad chemical growth factors and cytokines for the developing germ cells enmeshed in their cytoplasm (Fig. 13.8.2.1). Sertoli cells also secrete inhibin B, a glycoprotein hormone that inhibits FSH secretion by the pituitary (Fig. 13.8.2.2).

Spermatogenesis is a complex, repetitive series of cytodifferentiation processes in the seminiferous epithelium, whereby cohorts of undifferentiated diploid germ cells (spermatogonia) proliferate and transform into greatly expanded populations of haploid spermatozoa (Fig. 13.8.2.1). The human testes produce around 200 million spermatozoa per day. Mitotic divisions of spermatogonial stem cells form subpopulations of spermatogonia, which at regular intervals of 16 days differentiate into primary preleptotene spermatocytes to initiate meiosis. Meiotic reduction divisions of spermatocytes generate round spermatids, which then transform (spermiogenesis) into compact, virtually cytoplasm-free, elongated spermatids. Condensed nuclear DNA forms the sperm head, with an overlying Golgi-derived acrosome cap, and a tail (containing nine pairs of microtubules arranged around a central pair) capable of propulsive flagellar movements. Mature spermatozoa are released from Sertoli cell cytoplasm into the tubular lumen some 74 days after their initial development from spermatogonia. The control systems regulating germ-cell division and development remain poorly understood.

Male hypogonadism

Male hypogonadism is a descriptive term for the clinical complex associated with androgen deficiency resulting from Leydig cell dysfunction. Concomitant impairment of spermatogenesis is likely, since the seminiferous tubules will also be androgen deficient or directly involved by the same pathological process. However, infertility is usually an isolated abnormality of spermatogenesis in which patients seldom show any clinical evidence of androgen deficiency. In the last 20 years an increasing number of specific genetic defects have been identified, by genomic DNA mapping, as being associated with abnormal gonadal function and development.

Aetiology

A large number of pathological conditions can lead to destruction or malfunction of the hypothalamic–pituitary–testicular axis (Table 13.8.2.2). It is important to identify the underlying cause of hypogonadism and distinguish between pituitary–hypothalamic (secondary or hypogonadotropic hypogonadism) and testicular (primary or hypergonadotropic hypogonadism) disorders. The causal conditions may require specific treatment of their own, e.g. pituitary tumour or haemochromatosis. Hypogonadotropic conditions are amenable to treatment aimed at inducing or restoring spermatogenesis, whereas primary testicular failure, which is usually irreversible, is not.

Diagnosis

Clinical features specific to hypogonadism

The age of onset of androgen deficiency critically influences the manifestation of hypogonadism (see Table 13.8.2.1). Prepubertal onset of testosterone deficiency gives rise to sexual infantilism, and patients present with delayed puberty. Eunuchoidal body proportions (arm span greater than height, and heel–pubis exceeding crown–pubis length by at least 5 cm; see Fig. 13.8.2.2) develop as a result of the continued growth of the long bones (mediated by growth hormone), allowed by the delayed closure of their epiphyses, and the lack of testosterone/oestradiol-induced spinal growth in late puberty.

Postpubertal onset of testosterone deficiency leads to diminished sex drive and erection, loss of ejaculation, muscle atrophy, poor stamina, decreased secondary sexual hair and shaving frequency, and regression of spermatogenesis (reduced testicular volume). However, no change is observed in body and penile proportions or voice (see Table 13.8.2.1). Symptoms and signs of hypogonadism usually develop and progress insidiously. It is therefore common for patients to present many years after the onset of hypogonadism. Furthermore, young patients who have never been adequately androgenized may not be aware, or may even deny, that secondary sexual function is subnormal. By contrast, after surgical or traumatic/inflammatory castration, adults may experience hot flushes from acute withdrawal of androgens. Fetal onset of defective androgen action because of androgen-receptor abnormalities or steroidogenic enzyme deficiency causes failure of masculinization of the genitalia resulting in intersexual states (see Table 13.8.2.2).

Additional clinical features associated with hypogonadism

Hypothalamic–pituitary tumours are suggested by headache, impairment of visual acuity or loss of visual field, polyuria and polydipsia, or evidence of pituitary hormone excess such as Cushing's disease, acromegaly, or hyperprolactinaemia. Hyperprolactinaemia causes loss of sex drive, even in the presence of normal testosterone. Primary testicular failure is suggested by a history of orchitis, testicular trauma, surgery, torsion, irradiation, or chemotherapy. An increasing number of chronic systemic diseases (see Table 13.8.2.2) are associated with compromised hypothalamic–pituitary–testicular function. With improved survival resulting from specific treatment, the role of gonadal dysfunction in the quality of life of these patients is increasingly important.

The use of recreational drugs and medications that interfere with pituitary–testicular function or androgen action should be sought (see Table 13.8.2.2). Evidence of alcohol abuse should be noted. Ethanol causes a lowering of plasma testosterone through a direct toxic effect on Leydig cell steroidogenesis. Testicular atrophy and gynaecomastia, found in 50% of men with hepatic cirrhosis, result from altered androgen metabolism, increased SHBG, and increased oestrogen production. These changes are usually irreversible.

Table 13.8.2.2 Classification and aetiology of male reproductive disorders

Condition	Cause/pathogenesis	Hypogonadism	Infertility
Hypothalamic/pituitary			
Isolated GnRH deficiency	Congenital GnRH deficiency	+	+
Kallmann syndrome (OMIM #147950)	Gene mutations in Xp22.3 (anosmin 1; KAL1), KISS-1 receptor (KISS1R; GPR54), fibroblast growth factor receptor1 (FGFR1), leptin receptor (LEPR), G-protein coupled receptor-54 (GPR-54), prohormone convertase 1 (PCSK1) and nuclear receptor DAX 1	+	+
GnRH insensitivity	4q13.1 GnRH receptor gene mutation	+	+
Fertile eunuch (Pasqualini's syndrome) (OMIM #228300)	Partial GnRH deficiency, low LH		
Hypogonadotrophic hypogonadism/ adrenal hypoplasia (OMIM #300200)	Xp21.2–3 DAX1 gene mutation	+	+
Constitutional delayed puberty	Functional GnRH deficiency—self limiting	+	+
Male anorexia nervosa	Weight-related, reversible, functional GnRH deficiency	+	+
Hyperprolactinaemia	Pituitary adenoma, drug-induced (see below)	+	+
Congenital hypopituitarism (OMIM 241540)	PROP1 gene mutation, combined deficiency of gonadotrophins, growth hormone, prolactin, TSH and ACTH	+	+
Acquired hypopituitarism	Pituitary adenoma, craniopharygioma, haemochromatosis, irradiation, transfusion siderosis, sarcoidosis, tuberculosis, histiocytosis X	+	+
Biologically inactive LH	19q13.32 LH β chain (LHB) gene mutation	+	+
Isolated FSH deficiency (OMIM #229070)	FSH β chain (FSHB) gene mutation	!	+
Testicular			
Klinefelter's syndrome	47XXY, 48XXXY, 47XXY/46XY, mosaic, etc.	+	+
46 XX male (OMIM #400045)	Translocation of SRY to X chromosome	+	+
Sex-chromosome or autosome abnormalities	Translocation, deletion	+	−
Mixed gonadal dysgenesis (OMIM #233420)	XY/XO mosaic, true hermaphroditism	+	+

Table 13.8.2.2 *(cont'd)* Classification and aetiology of male reproductive disorders

Condition	Cause/pathogenesis	Hypogonadism	Infertility
Testicular agenesis (congenital anorchia) (OMIM 273250)	Absence of testicular tissues postnatally	+	+
Testicular torsion	Destruction of testicular tissue	+	+
Surgical orchidectomy	Destruction of testicular tissue	+	+
Testicular trauma	Destruction of testicular tissue	+	+
Testicular tumour	Destruction of testicular tissue	+	+
Orchitis	Destruction of testicular tissue	!	+
Sickle-cell disease	Microinfarcts in testis from vascular occlusion	+	+
Noonan–Leopard syndrome	12q22 gene defect in autosomal dominant form, cryptorchidism, Turner's stigmata, e.g. short stature, webbed neck, pectus excavatum, hypertelorism, ptosis, right-sided congenital heart disease	+	+
Persistent mullerian duct syndrome (OMIM #261550)	Antimullerian hormone (AMH) or AMH type II receptor (AMHR2) gene mutation: fallopian tubes and uterus present with cryptorchidism		+
Congenital steroidogenic enzyme deficiencies	Mutation in 10q24.3 (17-hydroxylase/17,20 lyase; CYP17) or 9q22	+	+
	(17β-hydroxysteroid dehydrogenase; HSD17B3)	+	+
LH insensitivity	LH receptor gene mutation, pseudohermaphroditism	+	+
Idiopathic infertility	Defective spermatogenesis of uncertain aetiology	−	+
Varicocele	Reflux in spermatic vein	−	+
Microdeletions Yq chromosome (OMIM #415000)	Deletion of azoospermic factor (AZFs)	−	+
Cryptorchidism (OMIM #219050)	Congenital deficiency of testosterone or AMH action, dysgenetic gonads	±	+
Immotile cilia syndrome (Kartargener's syndrome) (OMIM #244400)	Absent dynein arms of sperm tail microtubules	−	+
Globozoospermia (OMIM #102530)	Absence of acrosome cap on sperm head	−	+
FSH insensitivity	2p21 FSH receptor (FSHR) gene mutation	?	+

(Continued)

Table 13.8.2.2 *(cont'd)* Classification and aetiology of male reproductive disorders

Condition	Cause/pathogenesis	Hypogonadism	Infertility
Post-testicular			
Immunological infertility	Sperm antibodies	–	+
Young's syndrome (OMIM 279000)	Obstruction of the epididymis by inspissated secretions	–	+
Congenital bilateral absence of vas deferens (OMIM #277180)	7q31.2 CBAVD/CFTR gene mutation and intronic variant	–	+
Genital tract obstruction	Postinfection, postvasectomy, herniorrhaphy	–	+
Accessory gland/prostate infection	Bacterial, chlamydial, abnormal seminal fluid	–	+
Retrograde ejaculation	Autonomic neuropathy, postprostatectomy	–	+
Coital insufficiency	Defective vaginal insemination	–	+
Target tissues			
Androgen insensitivity syndromes (OMIM #300068)	Xq11–12 androgen receptor (AR) gene mutation	+	+
Androgen receptor defects (OMIM *313700)	Xq11-12 androgen receptor (AR) gene CAG repeats expansion		
5α-reductase deficiency (OMIM *607306)	2p23 5α-reductase 2 (SRD5A2) gene mutation	+	+
Oestrogen insensitivity	ERα gene mutation	–	?
Aromatase deficiency (OMIM +107910)	CYP19 (15q21.1) gene mutation	–	?
Systemic diseases			
Acute critical illnesses	Cytokine or cortisol-induced multilevel dysfunction in HPT axis	+	–
Chronic debilitating illnesses including cardiac failure, neoplasia, uncontrolled diabetes	Cytokine or caloric deprivation-induced multilevel dysfunction in HPT axis	+	+
Liver cirrhosis	Primary testicular failure followed by gonadotropin deficiency	+	+
Chronic renal failure	Hypogonadotropic	+	+
Thyrotoxicosis	Increased SHBG, gonadotropins and oestradiol	+	+
Cushing's syndrome	Multilevel dysfunction in HPT axis	+	+
Haemochromatosis (OMIM +235200)	Hypogonadotropic	+	+

Table 13.8.2.2 *(cont'd)* Classification and aetiology of male reproductive disorders

Condition	Cause/pathogenesis	Hypogonadism	Infertility
HIV/AIDS	Hypogonadotropic	+	+
Obesity and metabolic syndrome	Hypogonadotropic, low SHBG, total, and free testosterone	+	+
Obstructive sleep apnoea	Hypogonadotropic	+	+
Rheumatoid arthritis	Suppression of testosterone during flare-up	+	?
Acute febrile illness	Temporary suppression of spermatogenesis	–	+
Cystic fibrosis (OMIM #219700)	Cystic fibrosis transmembrane conductance regulator (CFTR) gene mutation	–	+
Untreated congenital adrenal hyperplasia (OMIM +201910)	Suppression of gonadotropins	–	+
Neurological diseases			
Myotonic dystrophy	Myotonin protein kinase (DMPK) gene CTG repeats expansion	+	+
Prader–Willi syndrome (hypothalamic) (OMIM #176270)	Deletion/ mutation of imprinting centre in paternal 15q11–13, hypogonadotrophic, mental retardation, hypotonia, hyperphagia, obesity, short stature	+	+
Laurence–Moon syndrome (OMIM 245800)	Hypogonadotrophic, retinitis pigmentosa, mental retardation, obesity, paraplegia	+	+
Bardet–Biedl syndrome (OMIM #209900)	Defects in BBS loci 16q21, 15q22.3, or 3p12: hypogonadotrophic, retinitis pigmentosa, mental retardation, obesity, polydactyly	+	+
Familial cerebellar degeneration (Friedrich's) (OMIM # 229300)	9q13 frataxin (FXN) gene GAA repeats expansion: hypogonadotrophic, progressive ataxia	+	+
Kennedy's syndrome (OMIM #313200)	Xq11–12 androgen receptor (AR) gene CAG repeats expansion, late onset androgen resistance, progressive spinobulbar muscle atrophy	+	+
Temporal lobe epilepsy	Unknown	+	–
Spinal cord injury	Abnormal thermoregulation or neuroregulation of testis	–	+

Table 13.8.2.2 *(cont'd)* Classification and aetiology of male
reproductive disorders

Condition	Cause/pathogenesis	Hypogonadism	Infertility
Fragile X syndrome (OMIM # 300624)	Xq27.3 FMR1 gene CCG repeats expansion—mental retardation, macro-orchidism	–	–
Drugs/ chemical or physical agents			
Digitalis, spironolactone, cyproterone acetate flutamide, bicalutamide, cimetidine	Antiandrogenic	+	+
Corticosteroids	Multilevel dysfunction in HPT axis	+	+
Ketoconazole, aminoglutethimide	Inhibit steroidogenesis	+	+
Antipsychotics, sedatives	Hyperprolactinaemia, gonadotropin suppression	+	+
Anticonvulsants	Increase SHBG and decrease free testosterone	+	+
Ethanol	Direct suppression of testicular functions, hepatotoxic	+	+
Opiate, cocaine, cannabis abuse	Suppression of gonadotropins	+	+
Cytotoxic chemotherapy	Agent-specific, dose-related germ cell loss	–	+
Ionizing irradiation	Dose-dependent loss of spermatogonia, spermatocytes	–	+
Sulfasalazine	Abnormal sperm morphology and motility	–	+
Nitrofuratoin	Direct suppression of spermatogenesis	–	+
Anabolic steroids, oestrogens, progestins	Gonadotropin suppression or antiandrogenic	(+)	+
Lead, mercury, cadmium	Implicated adverse effects on spermatogenesis	–	+
Pesticides, fungicides, amoebicides	Direct toxic action on spermatogonia	–	+

HPT = hypothalamic–pituitary–testicular; FSH = follicle stimulating hormone; TSH = thyroid-stimulating hormone; ACTH = adenocorticotrophic hormone; SHBG = sex hormone binding globulin; AMH= antimullerian hormone.

Neurological diseases can be associated with hypogonadism. Postpubertal atrophy of the seminiferous tubules occurs in 80% of patients with myotonic dystrophy, an autosomal dominant disorder characterized by myotonia, distal muscle atrophy, lens opacity, and premature frontal balding. Varying degrees of androgen deficiency also exist. Hypogonadotropic hypogonadism is associated with familial cerebellar (Friedreich's) ataxia, Laurence–Moon, Bardet–Biedl, and Prader–Willi syndromes. Defective spermatogenesis is common in paraplegia or quadriplegia following spinal injury, resulting from the inability to maintain a low scrotal temperature.

Specific conditions
Klinefelter's syndrome
Klinefelter's syndrome is the most common cause of male hypogonadism, with an incidence of 2 in 1000 live births. It is a developmental disorder of the testis resulting from the presence of an extra X chromosome derived from the nondisjunction of parental (maternal origin in two-thirds of cases) germ cells during meiosis. The most common karyotype is 47,XXY (80–90%), but rarer variants include 46,XY/47,XXY mosaic, multiple X + Y, and the so-called XX male syndrome. Increased maternal age increases the risk of having a child with this syndrome. A high proportion (75%) of men with this condition remain undiagnosed. Most Klinefelter's patients are diagnosed in adulthood, presenting with infertility, whereas a few present prepubertally with educational or behavioural problems. Accelerated atrophy of germ cells before puberty, and hyalinization of the seminiferous tubules give rise to sterility and small, firm testes. Leydig cells appear relatively hyperplastic, but cell mass is in fact normal. The degree of Leydig cell steroidogenic defect (the mechanism of which remains uncertain) is very variable, ranging from the virilized adult male presenting with infertility (see below) to the eunuchoidal youth who fails to complete sexual maturation. In mid adulthood, 80% of patients have reduced testosterone, with elevated LH, FSH, and oestradiol. Other features include gynaecomastia, reduced body hair, long legs, tall stature, learning (verbal and cognitive) difficulties, poor school performance, behavioural disturbances, and autoimmune endocrinopathies including diabetes mellitus. There is also an increased incidence of osteopenia, breast and other cancers, testicular and extratesticular (especially mediastinal and retroperitoneal) germ-cell tumours, varicose veins, thromboembolism, and leg ulcers. Learning difficulties are associated with higher-order X-chromosome polysomy.

Kallmann's syndrome
Kallmann's syndrome, with an incidence of 1 in 7500 males, is a sporadic or familial (X-linked or autosomal dominant/recessive) form of congenital hypogonadotropic hypogonadism associated with a number of somatic congenital abnormalities, including anosmia or hyposmia (defective sense of smell), red–green colour blindness, synkinesis, nerve deafness, cleft lip or palate, and renal malformations. The X-linked variety is caused by deletion or mutation in the KAL1 gene in Xp22.3, which encodes anosmin 1, a secreted protein that has neural-cell adhesion molecule properties. Faulty embryonic migration of GnRH-secreting neurons from their site of origin in the nose to the hypothalamus prevents normal axonal secretion into the pituitary portal circulation in the median eminence. GnRH is thus unable to target the gonadotrophs in the anterior pituitary. The same migratory defect affects the olfactory neurons in the nose, resulting in aplasia of the olfactory bulb and anosmia.

Emerging evidence suggests that kisspeptin signalling plays a critical role in the control of GnRH secretion during the initiation of puberty. Kisspeptin, a 54 amino acid peptide encoded by the KISS1 gene, is the ligand for G-protein-coupled receptor 54 (GPR54), a member of rhodopsin family of G-protein-coupled receptors. Kisspeptin is expressed in several regions of the forebrain (arcuate nucleus, anteroventral periventricular nucleus, and infundibular nucleus) and its expression is increased during sexual maturation. Mutations in the *GPR54* gene and several others (see Table 13.8.2.2) are associated with phenotypes of hypogonadotropic hypogonadism.

Ageing

Total and free testosterone in men declines gradually but variably with age from the age of 40 years onwards. This is amplified by the age-related increase in SHBG, and exacerbated by concomitant nongonadal diseases and medications. In some older men testosterone may fall below the young adult physiological range. Differentiation of nonspecific symptoms of ageing such as frailty, decreased muscle strength, lack of stamina, and decline in libido from those of mild hypogonadism is difficult. Whether these functional changes, normally accepted as part of healthy ageing, are causally related to alterations in circulating testosterone is unclear. The existence and prevalence of a male climacteric remains controversial.

Clinical investigation

Confirmation of hypogonadism

A clinical suspicion or diagnosis of hypogonadism must be confirmed by demonstration of low circulating testosterone on two separate days (as significant intraindividual variation in levels can occur) before replacement therapy is commenced. Samples obtained between 08.00 and 10.00 h avoid the physiological diurnal trough levels of testosterone that occur later in the day.

Currently, the most popular method for testosterone measurement is by automated immunoassay platforms. Substantial interplatform variability in testosterone measurements emphasizes the need for determining reference ranges specific to each laboratory. Liquid chromatography–tandem mass spectrometry is the best method for testosterone measurement, and is increasingly being used.

Total testosterone levels are influenced by changes in SHBG concentration. Elevation in SHBG (resulting from ageing, obesity, diabetes, thyrotoxicosis, anticonvulsants, or liver disease) gives spuriously high levels of total testosterone, but reduces the fraction of free testosterone. Obesity and other insulin-resistant states are associated with low SHBG and apparently low total testosterone, but normal free testosterone. In such situations, free testosterone should be measured in addition to total testosterone. Free testosterone is most accurately measured by equilibrium dialysis, but this method is laborious and not widely available. Commercial direct (nonextraction) immunoassay kits for the measurement of free testosterone are unreliable and not recommended. Currently, calculations using total testosterone, SHBG, and albumin concentrations using a formula available at the International Society for the Study of the Aging Male website (http://www.issam.ch/freetesto.htm) is the most expedient way to derive free testosterone levels.

Assessment of the hypothalamic–pituitary–testicular axis and target-tissue resistance

Measurement of LH, FSH, and prolactin is required to differentiate between primary and secondary hypogonadism. The physiological basis for differentiating between hypogonadotropic and hypergonadotropic hypogonadism is illustrated in Fig. 13.8.2.1. Pathologies of the hypothalamus and pituitary will give rise to low or low to normal gonadotropins and low testosterone, i.e. a state of hypogonadotropic hypogonadism or secondary testicular failure, where the potential for stimulating testicular function by exogenous gonadotropin or GnRH replacement is maintained. Conditions affecting the testes will interrupt normal testicular negative feedback. This results in elevated gonadotropin levels with low testosterone, characteristic of hypergonadotropic hypogonadism or primary testicular failure. Failure of spermatogenesis with reduced testicular size is commonly associated with a rise in FSH alone. Patients with androgen insensitivity syndromes have elevated testosterone with high LH, but normal to low FSH. Increased LH or FSH is associated with the very rare LH and FSH resistance syndromes.

Human chorionic gonadotropin (hCG) stimulates Leydig cell steroidogenesis and plasma testosterone increases over 4 to 7 days. It is useful for detecting the presence of functional testicular tissue in infants with impalpable testes or ambiguous genital development, and in differentiating hypergonadotropic hypogonadism from rare cases who produce immunologically detectable, but biologically inactive, LH in excess. Stimulation tests of gonadotropin secretory reserve using clomifene and GnRH seldom give additional information, and have become largely obsolete since the availability of gonadotropin immunoassays with improved sensitivity.

Assessment of the pituitary

Patients with hypogonadotropic hypogonadism without the stigmata of Kallmann's syndrome should undergo full pituitary functional and anatomical assessment to exclude an underlying pituitary tumour. They require pharmacological tests of growth hormone and ACTH reserves, thyroid function tests, visual field charting, and MRI of the pituitary and hypothalamus.

Other investigations

Suspected Klinefelter's syndrome should be confirmed by chromosome karyotyping on peripheral blood lymphocytes. Ultrasonography and MRI are useful in locating ectopic or intra-abdominal testes. DNA analysis can help confirm the diagnosis of androgen resistance syndromes and an increasing number of rare causes of hypogonadism (see Table 13.8.2.2).

Treatment

The objectives of treatment are to:

+ relieve the symptoms of androgen deficiency
+ prevent the long-term consequences of androgen deficiency such as osteopenia
+ reproduce physiological circulating and tissue levels of testosterone, dihydrotestosterone, and oestradiol
+ induce fertility, if required, in hypogonadotropic patients
+ treat any specific underlying diseases

Since most of the specific underlying causes of hypogonadism are untreatable or irreversible, the mainstay of treatment of the hypogonadal male involves androgen replacement. Although hypogonadotropic patients have the potential for fertility, gonadotropin and pulsatile GnRH therapy should only be employed when there is a requirement for fertility, because of the expense and complexity of these regimens. Previous testosterone treatment does not jeopardize subsequent response to gonadotropin, so younger hypogonadotropic subjects should be treated by testosterone in the same manner as hypergonadotropic patients to initiate and maintain virilization and sexual function.

Androgen replacement
Testosterone preparations

The circulating half-life of free testosterone is short (10 min) because it is rapidly degraded by the liver. To achieve sustained physiological circulating concentrations, testosterone must be administered in a modified form or by a parenteral route, so that its rate of metabolism or absorption is retarded.

Injectable testosterone esters are the commonest first-line androgen preparations. A mixture of four different testosterone esters (propionate, phenylpropionate, isocaproate, and decanoate), 250 mg every 2 to 3 weeks, and testosterone enanthate, 200 mg every 2 weeks, are the most popular. Although undoubtedly effective, these preparations inevitably give rise to supraphysiological peak testosterone levels in the first week, which then fall sharply to the lower limits of normal before the next dose. Some patients are disturbed by fluctuations in libido, mood, and stamina associated with the repeated rise and fall of testosterone levels.

An intramuscular depot injection containing 1000 mg testosterone undecanoate in 4 ml of castor oil, with a terminal half-life of 33.9 days, has more recently become available. It is administered at 10 to 14 week intervals, and testosterone levels remain in the physiological range with fewer supra- and subphysiological peaks and troughs compared with shorter-acting preparations.

Crystalline testosterone compressed into cylindrical pellets, implanted subcutaneously under local anaesthesia, provide a depot source of testosterone. Peak testosterone levels are achieved after 2 to 4 weeks, followed by a gradual decline. The usual dose of 800 mg (4 × 200 mg implants) can maintain physiological concentrations of testosterone for 6 months. Side effects include extrusion, bleeding, and infection.

Oral testosterone undecanoate is absorbed from the gut through intestinal lymphatics, bypassing first-pass hepatic metabolism, but bioavailability is low (7%). This formulation is taken with or after meals, as food increases bioavailability by improving lipid-driven lymphatic absorption. To maintain testosterone consistently within the physiological range, two to three times daily administration of 80 mg (2 × 40 mg capsules) testosterone undecanoate is required. Intestinal 5α-reductase action gives rise to a disproportionate increase in dihydrotestosterone relative to testosterone. Oral testosterone undecanoate is useful in the induction of puberty in adolescents, where lower doses are preferable, and in adults who are intolerant to the other modes of administration of testosterone.

The 17α-alkylated androgens, e.g. oxandrolone, stanozolol, and oxymetholone, are relatively weak androgens, but some may have more potent anabolic effects. 17α-Alkylated compounds cause cholestatic jaundice in a reversible and dose-related manner, and long-term treatment is associated with peliosis hepatis (haemorrhagic cysts in the liver) and liver tumours. Consequently, 17α-methyltestosterone, oxymetholone, and fluoxymesterone have been withdrawn from the market in many countries. As a group, 17α-alkylated androgens are not recommended for clinical use, but they are the most commonly abused anabolic steroids. Mesterolone, which is not hepatotoxic, is a weak androgen with low clinical efficacy, but remains commercially available.

Transdermal testosterone preparations offer the advantages of stable physiological levels of testosterone without peaks and troughs, painless self-administration, minimal risk of overdosing, and low potential for abuse. A 60 cm² translucent membrane applied to the scrotum delivers testosterone at a rate of 4 or 6 mg/day. Daily renewal of the patch in the morning maintains plasma testosterone within the adult physiological range. Levels of 5α-dihydrotestosterone are elevated because of abundant 5α-reductase activity in genital skin. This does not seem to have any adverse consequences, even after several years of treatment. Local skin irritation is negligible (5–8%). Scrotal patches are not widely used because of the need to shave scrotal skin, difficulties with skin adherence, and the availability of newer, more acceptable transdermal systems.

A torso transdermal system delivers testosterone at 2.5 mg (6.5 cm diameter) or 5 mg (13 cm diameter) daily. These patches deliver testosterone via a permeation-enhancing vehicle and a gelling agent. They are applied to clean, dry skin on the back, abdomen, upper arm, or thigh and are changed after 24 h. These patches are effective in maintaining serum testosterone levels in the low to mid normal range. Although clinical efficacy is satisfactory, the major drawback of these patches is skin reaction at the application site, which occurs in 60 to 70% of cases. Pretreatment of the application site with triamcinolone acetonide cream (0.1%) decreases the incidence and severity of skin reactions, but acceptability is limited.

An open transdermal delivery system of testosterone dissolved in a hydroalcoholic gel can deliver physiological amounts of the hormone when applied thinly on the skin of the torso, shoulders, and upper arms. A dose of 50 mg of gel once daily delivers 5 mg of the hormone, maintaining stable testosterone levels in the middle of the normal range, with proven clinical efficacy. Skin irritation is less common than with testosterone patches (4–10%). Although there is a theoretical risk that the gel can be transferred to others through intensive skin contact, in practice significant interpersonal transfer is unlikely.

A sustained-release mucoadhesive buccal testosterone tablet, placed twice daily in the small depression above the upper incisor tooth, has more recently become available. First-pass hepatic metabolism is avoided, as testosterone enters the circulation directly via the superior vena cava. Stable physiological testosterone and dihydrotestosterone levels are achieved within 24 h of starting treatment. The commonest side effects are alterations in taste, and gum-related adverse events (reported in 16% of patients). This novel formulation is relatively expensive and acceptability is low.

Selective androgen-receptor modulators are novel, orally-active nonsteroidal synthetic compounds that reproduce the effects of testosterone with tissue selectivity, since they do not undergo 5α reduction or aromatization. The main advantage of these compounds is that they have anabolic effects on muscle without significant effects on the prostate. These compounds are currently in phase I and II clinical development.

Management of hypogonadal patients

The recent introduction of several newer testosterone formulations has increased the choice available to physicians and patients. While testosterone gel and long-acting testosterone undecanoate depot injections seem to have the best pharmacokinetic profiles, all formulations have specific advantages and disadvantages. The choice of testosterone preparation depends on the age of the patient, the patient's preference, the acceptability of injections, and the availability of expertise for surgical implants. For example, transdermal preparations may be preferred for the induction of secondary sexual development in testosterone-naive adolescent boys. Long-acting preparations are convenient for maintenance treatment in young adult men, and short-acting preparations are preferred in older men in whom the ability to withdraw treatment rapidly is advantageous, should prostate side effects develop.

Patients should be followed up for life and their treatment regime reviewed regularly, given that testosterone replacement is usually permanent. In the absence of a satisfactory biological marker for androgen action, monitoring of treatment is best gauged by the clinical response and verifying that plasma testosterone is within the lower normal range immediately before the next dose, so that appropriate adjustments to dosing intervals can be made.

Side effects from testosterone replacement are relatively rare and include acne, transient priapism, gynaecomastia, fluid retention, polycythaemia, obstructive sleep apnoea, and exacerbation of pre-existing behavioural disturbances. In older patients with benign prostatic hyperplasia, sleep apnoea, dyslipidaemia, cardiac failure, liver disease, and renal failure, a cautious approach with reduced doses of testosterone, careful dose titration, and close supervision or specific management of the coexisting problems usually allow patients to benefit from androgen replacement.

Safety considerations in hypogonadal patients over 45 years of age
Before starting testosterone, hypogonadal patients over the age of 45 years should be checked for pre-existing occult prostatic cancer by digital rectal examination and prostate specific antigen (PSA) measurement. There is no conclusive evidence that testosterone therapy increases the risk of prostate cancer, but raising testosterone levels can stimulate growth and aggravate symptoms in men with invasive and metastatic prostate cancer. Testosterone therapy should not be initiated in patients with palpable abnormalities of the prostate and PSA more than 4 ng/ml without further urological evaluation. Treatment is contraindicated in the presence of untreated carcinoma of the prostate or breast. Treatment with testosterone is also contraindicated in the presence of severe benign prostatic hyperplasia (International Prostate Symptom Score >21), haematocrit more than 52%, untreated obstructive sleep apnoea, or severe heart failure.

Prostate examination, and PSA and haematocrit measurement, should be repeated 3 to 6 months after initiating treatment and then annually. Erythrocytosis can develop, especially in older men treated with injectable testosterone preparations. If haematocrit is more than 55% treatment is stopped until it decreases to a safe level; therapy can be reinitiated at a reduced dose. Measurement of bone mineral density at the lumbar spine and/or femoral neck 1 to 2 years after the initiation of testosterone therapy in hypogonadal men with osteoporosis or low-trauma fracture can be informative.

Infertility

Infertility is defined as the inability of a couple to initiate a pregnancy after 12 months of unprotected intercourse. Some 8 to 15% of married couples experience involuntary infertility. Of these, male factors alone are estimated to be responsible in 30% and contributory in a further 20% of subfertile couples. Thus, male infertility may affect 5% of men of reproductive age. A secular trend of declining semen quality (sperm density) in men over the last 50 years has been reported in some but not all regions of Europe. This, together with a concurrent increase in the incidence of testicular cancer, hypospadias, and cryptorchidism, has raised the question of possible environmental endocrine disruptors with oestrogenic or antiandrogenic actions influencing prenatal or neonatal testicular and genital tract development. The concern has prompted the recent development of sensitive techniques for monitoring the potentially deleterious reproductive effects of environmental chemicals. However, there is currently no evidence that the incidence of male infertility is increasing.

Aetiologies

Male infertility, a term that includes a heterogeneous group of disorders (see Table 13.8.2.2), represents the male partner's contribution to a couple's failure to conceive. This implied failure to fertilize normal ova is usually associated with defective spermatogenesis, giving rise to absent (azoospermia) or low sperm output (oligozoospermia: <20 million/ml) and/or abnormal spermiogenesis, giving rise to spermatozoa with poor motility (asthenozoospermia: <50% of spermatozoa showing progressive motility) and abnormal morphology (teratozoospermia: <15% normal forms). The pathogenetic basis of defective spermatogenesis or spermiogenesis remains poorly understood. Testicular histology may show quantitative reduction in all germ-cell types (hypospermatogenesis), Sertoli cells only, or maturation arrest at the primary spermatocyte (premeiotic) or spermatid (postmeiotic) stage.

Idiopathic azoospermia/oligozoospermia

By far the most common form of male infertility (60%) is idiopathic azoospermia/oligozoospermia, usually associated with asthenozoopermia and teratozoospermia. This probably represents the end result of a multitude of ill-defined pathologies that disrupt normal seminiferous tubular functions. However, recent molecular analyses have revealed that a substantial proportion of the cases hitherto classified as idiopathic have discrete gene defects associated with impaired spermatogenesis (see 'Chromosome disorders' below).

Asthenozoospermia

Reduced velocity or vigour of sperm motility may result from metabolic/functional defects or ultrastructural malformations in the axonemal complex of the sperm tail, usually associated with oligozoospermia or a high percentage of dead and abnormally shaped sperm. The latter finding may indicate a rare condition, epididymal necro/asthenozoospermia; testicular spermatozoa are normal, the defects occurring during epididymal transit. Rarely, complete asthenozoospermia (with normal sperm density) may result from the absence of the dynein arms (site of Na^+,K^+-ATPase activity) linking individual microtubules. This is associated with similar defects in respiratory cilia, and a history of chronic respiratory infection, bronchiectasis, and sinusitis (immotile cilia syndrome). In addition, some of these patients have situs inversus (Kartagener's syndrome). Absence of the central pair of microtubules in the sperm tail is an even rarer cause of complete asthenozoospermia—the 9+0 syndrome.

Teratozoospermia

An extreme example of abnormal sperm morphology is the failure of acrosome cap development in the sperm head, leading to the formation of round-headed spermatozoa (globozoospermia), which are unable to bind to the zona pellucida of ova, a prerequisite for fertilization.

Chromosome disorders

Chromosome abnormalities identified by cytogenetic studies of peripheral blood lymphocytes are found in 15% of azoospermic patients; 90% of these have Klinefelter's syndrome. Other chromosomal abnormalities encountered include reciprocal X or Y autosomal translocations, XYY and XX males, reciprocal and robertsonian autosomal translocations, supernumerary autosomes, and inversion of autosomes.

Klinefelter's syndrome is the most common genetic abnormality and is diagnosed in approximately 14% of men with nonobstructive azoospermia. All patients with the classic form (47,XXY) are azoospermic. Spontaneous pregnancies have been reported in those with 46,XY/47,XXY mosaic forms, who may have limited sperm production. The mechanism by which an extra X chromosome gives rise to spermatogenic failure is not known. Inactivation of the X chromosome in primary spermatocytes is necessary for spermatogenesis to proceed normally through meiosis. Hyalinized seminiferous tubules devoid of germ cells are pervasive in the atrophic testes. Occasionally, isolated foci of tubules with preserved spermatogenesis can be identified in testicular biopsy of 47,XXY patients.

Y-chromosome microdeletions

A major breakthrough in the understanding of the molecular genetics of male infertility was the initial characterization of three nonoverlapping regions (designated azoospermic factors AZFa, AZFb, and AZFc) on the long arm of the Y chromosome (Yq11), which contain multiple genes involved in spermatogenesis. Three additional microdeletions have subsequently been recognized (gr/gr deletion, AZFbc, and AZFabc). AZFc is by far the most frequently (two-thirds) encountered deletion. Microdeletions in the AZF loci, identifiable by polymerase chain reaction (PCR) amplification of DNA (not by routine karyotyping), have been found in 3 to 37.5% of patients previously considered to have idiopathic azoospermia and severe oligozoospermia, but not in fertile control populations. Y-chromosome microdeletions are emerging as the second most common specific aetiology of male infertility (after varicoceles). Larger deletions (involving more than one AZF locus) are associated with more severe testicular phenotypes, and the incidence of microdeletions is highest among azoospermic patients with Sertoli cell-only histology.

Defects in target tissue

Mutations in the ligand-binding or DNA-binding domains of the androgen receptor cause defects in androgen action and varying degrees of failure of masculinization during primary sexual development (androgen insensitivity syndromes), despite raised levels of testosterone being produced by inguinal or intra-abdominal testes. These defects are, in descending order of severity:

- complete testicular feminization—female phenotype and female external genitalia, with absent uterus and fallopian tubes; presents with primary amenorrhoea
- incomplete testicular feminization—female phenotype and female external genitalia, with minimal virilization, such as clitoral hypertrophy and partial fusion
- Reifenstein's syndrome—ambiguous genitalia with perineoscrotal hypospadias, poor penile development, bifid scrotum, and gynaecomastia at puberty

By contrast with the above, expansion of the number of CAG polyglutamine repeats to more than 40 in the N-terminal domain of exon 1 of the androgen receptor gene causes X-linked spinal bulbar muscular atrophy (Kennedy's disease), associated with gynaecomastia, poor virilization, and azoospermia resulting from late-onset androgen resistance. Expansion of CAG glutamine repeats to between 25 and 40 is associated with a fourfold increased risk of oligozoospermia or azoospermia, without clinical evidence of neuromuscular degeneration. This may represent an exclusively testicular form of androgen insensitivity.

Deficiency in 5α-reductase 2 in genetic males (deficient 5α-dihydrotestosterone action in the genital tract) causes poor penile development (evident as clitoral hypertrophy) with perineoscrotal hypospadias and blind-ending pseudovagina, and inguinal testes with epididymis and vas deferens in a newborn with ambiguous external genitalia. Usually raised as girls, these patients virilize dramatically at puberty, without gynaecomastia.

Males with oestrogen resistance and aromatase deficiency are normally virilized at birth and have normal pubertal development, except for nonfusion of epiphyses resulting in extremely tall stature, and osteoporosis in adulthood. Effects on spermatogenesis and fertility are currently unclear.

Cryptorchidism

Cryptorchidism is the absence of one or both testes from the scrotum, and results from the failure of the testis to descend during fetal development from an abdominal position, through the inguinal canal, into the scrotum. Cryptorchidism has a prevalence of 2.5 to 5% at birth, declining to 1% by 1 year, and is one of the most common congenital abnormalities. Spontaneous descent rarely occurs after this age. Undescended testes can be a feature of many hypogonadotropic conditions and intersexual and dysgenetic states, such as androgen insensitivity syndromes and Noonan's syndrome. The lower temperature of the scrotum is a prerequisite for normal spermatogenesis. Undescended testes are therefore exposed to the harmful effects of the higher temperature of the abdomen and inguinal region. The testis that is not permanently in a low scrotal position by the age of 2 years will have sustained permanent damage to the seminiferous epithelium. Infertility is frequently observed in unilateral as well as bilateral forms of cryptorchidism. Orchidopexy after 2 years of age for undescended testes does not improve fertility. For these reasons, treatment should ideally be undertaken between 1 and 2 years of age. hCG or intranasal GnRH is used for the early initial treatment of cryptorchidism. If hormonal treatment is unsuccessful, orchidopexy can be carried out by the age of 2 years. The risk of testicular tumour in an adult patient with a history of undescended testis is four- to fivefold higher than the general population; however, there is evidence that treatment before puberty decreases this risk.

Testicular tumours

It is important to remember that infertility can be a presenting symptom of testicular tumours, the commonest malignancy in young adult men (15–34 years). With increasing use of testicular ultrasonography it has become clear that there is a significantly higher risk (up to 20 times) of testicular tumours in infertile men (in the absence of cryptorchidism) compared with the general population. There is good epidemiological evidence that the risk of testicular cancer among infertile men exceeds the frequency of cryptorchidism in the same population.

Varicocele

Varicocele is a dilatation of the scrotal portion of the pampiniform plexus resulting from reflux of blood in the internal spermatic veins, usually involving the left side from the renal vein. It usually gives rise to a reduction in ipsilateral testicular volume, but varying degrees of hypospermatogenesis are often seen in both testes. Although a varicocele is clinically detectable in up to 40% of male partners of infertile couples, its significance in male infertility remains controversial. Increased scrotal temperature, hypoxia, and exposure of the testes to adrenal metabolites have been postulated as possible mechanisms by which spermatic vein reflux can induce seminiferous tubular damage. Since varicoceles can be detected clinically in 15% of fertile young men, and their prevalence increases with age, it must not be assumed that this condition is invariably or solely responsible for infertility without actively excluding other possible aetiologies, including those in the female partner.

Sperm autoimmunity

Immunological infertility is a specific disorder caused by antisperm membrane-bound IgA antibodies found in around 5% of men presenting with infertility. Conditions predisposing to sperm autoimmunity include vasectomy, testicular injury/inflammation, genital tract infection/obstruction, and family history of autoimmune disease. The presence of sperm aggregates in the semen, oligospermia with normal hormone levels, and a history of predisposing conditions is an indication to look for antisperm antibodies. Male patients with significant antisperm antibody titres usually have severely suppressed fertility potential because of sperm agglutination, poor sperm transit through cervical mucus, and blocked sperm–oocyte fusion.

Genital tract infection

Infection in the lower genital tract is a major cause of curable male infertility in the global context. Urethritis, prostatitis, orchitis, and epididymitis are considered by the World Health Organization to be male accessory gland infections, and are usually caused by chlamydia, gonococci, Gram-negative enterococci, or tubercle bacilli. Although these pathogens are associated with increased prevalence of infertility, the evidence that these organisms have a direct negative influence on sperm quality is not strong. However, infection *per se*, its complications, and manipulations may contribute to obstruction, immune reactions, trauma, or ejaculatory disturbances, and contribute to infertility. Furthermore, chronic inflammatory changes in the seminiferous tubules may disrupt spermatogenesis. Leucocytes may have a detrimental effect on sperm function, and the presence of >1 million leucocytes/ml in the ejaculate indicates the possibility of genital tract infections.

Excurrent duct obstruction

Obstructive azoospermia occurs in 15 to 20% of men with azoospermia. Vasectomy and previous genitourinary infections, usually sexually transmitted or tuberculous, are common causes. Congenital bilateral agenesis of the wolffian duct-derived structures, corpus/cauda epididymis, vas deferens and seminal vesicles (characterized by impalpable scrotal vasa, distended caput epididymis, acidic noncoagulating semen of reduced volume (<2 ml) devoid of fructose and sperm) is present in 95% of males with cystic fibrosis. More commonly (6% of azoospermic men and 1–2% of infertile men), patients present with congenital bilateral absence of the vas deferens without frank respiratory tract disease or pancreatic insufficiency. They have milder heterozygous mutations and/or the *5T* variant in intron 8 of the *CFTR* gene, giving rise to a predominantly genital phenotype of cystic fibrosis. Renal and urinary tract abnormalities are common in these patients. In Young's syndrome, progressive epididymal obstruction results from progressive inspissation of amorphous secretion in the lumen. Ejaculatory duct obstruction may occur because of congenital cysts or inflammation following acute, nonacute, or chronic urethroprostatitis, and is found in 1 to 3% of cases of obstructive azoospermia.

Coital disorders

Erectile dysfunction, failure of ejaculation and retrograde ejaculation, inadequate coital frequency and technique (including the use of vaginal lubricants with spermicidal properties), and faulty timing of intercourse may contribute to continuing infertility.

Diagnosis

History

Particular attention should be paid to the following aspects. Previous surgery such as herniorrhaphy in childhood, trauma, or torsion suggests possible damage to the vas deferens or testis. A history of cryptorchidism or genitourinary infections is an important aetiological factor. Delayed onset of puberty may suggest the possibility of gonadotropin deficiency, and reduced libido, potency, and decreased frequency of shaving may suggest androgen deficiency. A history of recurrent chest infection, sinusitis, or bronchiectasis may be obtained in patients with epididymal obstruction (Young's syndrome), immotile cilia syndrome, and congenital bilateral absence of the vas deferens associated with cystic fibrosis. Chronic disorders such as renal failure, liver disease, malignancy, diabetes, and multiple sclerosis are associated with a variety of testicular and sexual dysfunctions. Each patient should be asked about episodes of pyrexia within the past 12 weeks because of transient suppression of spermatogenesis. Careful enquiry should also be made about occupational or environmental exposure to testicular toxins, radiation, current medications, previous treatment, or recreational drugs. Painful ejaculation, haemotospermia, and pain in the perineum are symptoms suggestive of chronic infection in the prostate and seminal vesicles. It is important to establish that vaginal intercourse takes place with appropriate frequency and timing, without the use of vaginal lubricants.

Clinical features

Assessment of height, weight, body habitus, and secondary sexual development should be carried out in all patients. Measurement of testicular volume by comparison with Prader's orchidometer provides a convenient clinical index of seminiferous tubular mass. Normal adult testicular volume is between 15 and 35 ml. Testicular volume is a key finding in differentiating between azoospermia resulting from seminiferous tubular failure (reduced volume) and that arising from excurrent duct obstruction (normal volume). Testicular size is also a useful indicator of the degree of testicular development in hypogonadotropic patients. If the testes are not in the scrotum, their lowest position should be defined with the patient upright. Irregular contour, induration, or abnormal consistency of the testis suggests previous orchitis, surgery, or malignancy. Special attention should also be paid to the palpation of the epididymis and scrotal vas. An enlarged and tense caput epididymis may be palpable in cases of obstructive azoospermia. Irregularity and induration of the epididymis and vas suggest previous infection. In congenital agenesis of wolffian duct-derived structures, the scrotal vasa are either impalpable or extremely thin. The patient should be examined standing, so that varicoceles can become visible (grade 3) or palpable (grade 2), or detected as a venous impulse in the spermatic cord during the Valsalva manoeuvre (grade 1). Rectal examination may reveal irregular contour, abnormal consistency, or tenderness in the prostate in the presence of chronic prostatitis and enlarged seminal vesicles following ejaculatory duct obstruction.

Laboratory investigation

Conventional parameters of semen analysis, such as sperm density, percentage of motile sperm, quality of sperm movements, and sperm morphology, provide a semiquantitative index of fertility potential. At least two semen analyses at 6- to 12-week intervals are recommended. Although a variety of tests of sperm function, such as computer-aided sperm movement analyses, cervical mucus penetration, acrosome reaction, sperm–zona binding, and hamster oocyte penetration have been devised, none are sufficiently reliable and accurate to be used routinely in clinical practice.

Infertile men with oligozoospermia produce spermatozoa harbouring abnormal DNA with strand breaks and redundant cytoplasm, which may produce excessive reactive oxygen species. Assays of chromatin structure, DNA strand breaks, and cytoplasmic enzymes (lactate dehydrogenase X and creatine kinase M) are being applied to assess the functional integrity of spermatozoa. They may provide more reliable quantitative biochemical measures of male fertility to guide management in the future.

Measurement of plasma FSH is useful in distinguishing primary from secondary testicular failure, and in identifying patients with obstructive azoospermia. In the presence of azoospermia or oligozoospermia an elevated FSH, particularly with reduced testicular volume, is presumptive evidence of severe and usually irreversible seminiferous tubular damage. Low or undetectable FSH (usually associated with low LH and testosterone, with clinical evidence of androgen deficiency) is suggestive of secondary hypogonadism, and full assessment of pituitary function, including an MRI scan of the pituitary and the hypothalamus, is indicated. Conversely, azoospermia with normal FSH and normal testicular volume usually indicates the presence of bilateral genital tract obstruction. The role of inhibin B measurement as a circulating marker of Sertoli cell function in routine diagnostic workup of male infertility remains unclear. Testosterone and LH measurements are only indicated in the assessment of the infertile male when there is clinical suspicion of androgen deficiency, Klinefelter's syndrome, or sex-steroid abuse. High LH and testosterone should raise the possibility of abnormalities in androgen receptors. Hyperprolactinaemia is not a recognized cause of male infertility, but prolactin measurement should be undertaken if there is clinical evidence of sexual dysfunction (particularly diminished libido) or pituitary disease leading to secondary testicular failure. Oestradiol measurement is rarely indicated, except in the presence of gynaecomastia.

Chromosome analysis by karyotyping or fluorescent in situ hybridization (FISH) should be carried out in patients with azoospermia, testicular atrophy, and elevated FSH, primarily to confirm the diagnosis of Klinefelter's syndrome. The FISH analysis of spermatozoa still, however, remains a research investigational tool. Screening for Y-chromosome microdeletions by PCR-based mapping of DNA markers should be considered in patients with nonobstructive azoospermia or severe oligozoospermia (sperm density <5 million/ml).

The need for diagnostic testicular biopsy to differentiate between primary testicular failure and obstructive lesions has largely been superseded by the measurement of plasma FSH. An undetectable or very low level of seminal fructose is used to confirm the clinical diagnosis of vasal and seminal vesicle agenesis, or blocked ejaculatory ducts in the presence of obstructive azoospermia. An increase in number (>1 million/ml) of peroxidase-positive or monoclonal antibody-detected leucocytes in the semen may indicate genital tract infection.

Semen culture for pathogens is difficult because of the bactericidal properties of seminal plasma and urethral and skin commensals. Antisperm antibodies can be detected in blood and semen by the mixed agglutination reaction, in which polyacrylamide beads are coated with rabbit antibodies to specific classes of human immunoglobulin. These will attach to motile spermatozoa carrying specific IgA on the surface of the sperm head or tail. Ultrasound examination of the testis has become a routine investigation for infertile males with nonobstructive azoospermia or severe oligospermia in order to detect occult testicular tumours. In patients with persistent or treated cryptorchidism, testicular ultrasonography should be carried out annually. Ultrasound examination of the urinary tract is indicated in patients with congenital bilateral absence of the vas deferens. Asymptomatic prostatitis arising from occult, usually focal infection is best diagnosed by transrectal ultrasound examination of the prostate.

Treatment

Pregnancies can occur in subfertile couples without treatment, albeit with a much reduced probability, depending on the duration of infertility, age, and coexisting subtle abnormalities in the female partner in addition to the defects in sperm quality. Since most patients with male infertility present no recognizable or reversible aetiologies, management remains largely empirical.

Subfertility resulting from idiopathic hypospermatogenesis

Although a wide variety of empirical medical treatments, including gonadotropins, androgens, and antioestrogens, have been tried in attempts to improve fertility in subfertile men, none have been shown to be effective when assessed in randomized controlled therapeutic trials, and are therefore not recommended. Instead, assisted conception techniques are now routinely employed to overcome idiopathic male infertility. This is based on the premise that placing a large number of prepared motile spermatozoa in close proximity to ovulated or retrieved oocytes in vivo or in vitro can enhance the probability of fertilization.

Intrauterine insemination of more than 1 million washed, motile spermatozoa (freed of seminal plasma, leucocytes, and abnormal/dead spermatozoa) is a relatively simple and inexpensive technique with few complications. It is the first-line therapy for male factor, cervical factor, minimal to mild endometriosis, and unexplained infertility, and can be performed with or without ovarian hyperstimulation. The addition of ovarian hyperstimulation improves live birth rates in couples with subfertility, but the risk of multiple pregnancies is increased. Pregnancy rates of 5 to 10% per cycle can be expected.

In vitro fertilization (IVF) involves more intensive gonadotropin stimulation of the woman, suppression of spontaneous ovulation, and collection of multiple oocytes by laparoscopy or transvaginal ultrasound-guided ovarian puncture. Fertilization of eggs is achieved by coincubation with prepared spermatozoa in culture medium, or by means of intracytoplasmic sperm injection (ICSI). In patients with moderate oligozoospermia, average fertilization rates of 30% and live birth rates of 5 to 12% per treatment cycle can be expected. In those with severe and multiple defects in semen parameters, standard IVF is less effective than ICSI.

Microinjection of a single live spermatozoon directly into a harvested oocyte (ICSI) has become the treatment of choice for severe oligozoospermia in those who have failed intrauterine insemination and IVF. This bypasses the sperm–oocyte interactions normally required for fertilization in natural conception or IVF, and can achieve remarkably high fertilization and live birth rates (55 and 26% per cycle, respectively) even with the most severely abnormal samples. Since only a few spermatozoa are required, ICSI has revolutionized the management of extreme oligozoospermia and azoospermia, irrespective of aetiology. Nonobstructive azoospermia is often intermittent, and careful examination of centrifuged deposits of semen to detect and harvest occasional ejaculated spermatozoa for ICSI should be attempted repeatedly before resorting to alternatives. One of these is direct testicular sperm extraction via multiple open biopsies (TESE) with microdissection of seminiferous tubules to harvest viable testicular spermatozoa for ICSI. This has proven to be successful, even in patients with persistent (nonobstructive) azoospermia where isolated foci of spermatogenesis may be preserved. For example, the sperm retrieval rate with TESE in men with Klinefelter's syndrome is between 50 and 70%. Although ICSI improves the fertilization rate compared with IVF alone, once fertilization is achieved the pregnancy rate is similar to that of IVF.

Specific treatable conditions

Removal or withdrawal of antispermatogenic agents or drug exposure may lead to an improvement in fertility. This is most commonly seen in patients with inflammatory bowel disease, on changing treatment from sulfasalazine to 5-aminosalicylic acid, which removes the offending moiety, sulfapyridine. Withdrawal from anabolic steroid abuse invariably leads to recovery of spermatogenesis, although this may take many months because of the long half-lives of some preparations. Cryopreservation of semen should be offered to all men of reproductive age before commencing anticancer chemotherapy, orchiectomy, or testicular irradiation.

When patients with hypogonadotropic hypogonadism desire fertility they can discontinue exogenous androgen replacement and start on hCG (1500–3000 IU subcutaneously twice weekly) for 6 to 12 months. This should maintain normal testosterone levels. Patients with postpubertally acquired gonadotropin deficiency (e.g. from a pituitary tumour) in whom spermatogenesis has previously been established usually respond to hCG treatment alone to reinitiate germ-cell development. If there are no spermatozoa in the ejaculate at the end of 6 months, human menopausal gonadotropin, which contains both FSH and LH, or recombinant or highly purified human FSH, should be added at 75 to 150 IU subcutaneously thrice weekly. Combined treatment may be required for a further 12 months. Most patients with congenital forms of hypogonadotropic hypogonadism will require FSH to stimulate Sertoli cell division and initiate spermatogenesis. In general, around 70% should show active spermatogenesis and 50% could be expected to achieve spontaneous pregnancies, even if sperm densities remain in the oligozoospermic range. Patients with hypothalamic GnRH deficiency can be treated by pulsatile GnRH delivered 2-hourly by a battery-driven portable infusion minipump, but many find this form of chronic therapy impractical and too demanding. The outcome of treatment is similar to that obtained with exogenous gonadotropin therapy.

The aim of treatment of male accessory gland infections is to cure infection, improve clinical symptoms, and prevent complications (infertility, testicular damage, and chronic pain). They should be treated early with appropriate antibiotics, anti-inflammatory agents, and surgical procedures (if necessary). Empirical therapy of acute urethritis with a single dose of a fluoroquinolone followed by a 2-week regimen of doxycycline is effective for gonococcal, chlamydial and ureaplasmal infections. Although treatment may improve sperm quality, there is no convincing evidence that treatment of these infections increases the probability of conception.

Obstructive azoospermia resulting from epididymal obstruction can be treated by end-to-end or end-to-side microsurgical epididymovasostomy, or vasovasostomy in the case of proximal vas deferens obstruction. High pregnancy rates can only be achieved by a few experienced microsurgeons. A more feasible and cheaper alternative is to obtain spermatozoa from the caput epididymis or efferent ducts proximal to the site of obstruction by microsurgical epididymal sperm aspiration or percutaneous epididymal sperm aspiration for use in assisted fertilization procedures (usually ICSI). Ejaculatory duct obstruction may be treated by transurethral resection of the ejaculatory ducts, and midline intraprostatic cysts causing ejaculatory duct obstruction are treated by incision or unroofing of the cyst.

Antisperm antibody production can be treated by immunosuppression with high-dose prednisolone 0.75 mg/kg per day or prednisolone 20 mg twice daily on days 1 to 10 and 5 mg on days 11 and 12 of the partner's cycle for three to six cycles. Side effects are common, including irritability, sleeplessness, arthralgia, muscle weakness, peptic ulceration, glucose intolerance, and bilateral aseptic necrosis of the femoral heads. The results of controlled trials of glucocorticoid treatment are conflicting. IVF and ICSI are increasingly being applied to manage immunological male infertility as they are safer and more effective.

Varicocele can be treated by open or laparoscopic surgical ligation, or transfemoral embolization of the internal spermatic veins. The results of treatment of varicocele from prospective controlled therapeutic trials are conflicting. Coexisting female factors contributing to infertility, insufficient sample size, high dropout rates, and lack of randomization/blinding or sham procedures are important confounding variables, which typify the difficulties of treatment trials in male infertility. Nevertheless, the Royal College of Obstetricians and Gynaecologists concluded that the treatment of varicocele in oligozoospermic, but not normospermic, subfertile men can significantly improve semen quality and pregnancy rate. The cost of varicocele treatment per live birth is less with surgical ligation (and embolization) than for assisted conception techniques.

Retrograde ejaculation can be treated medically with ephedrine, midodrine, α-adrenergic or anticholinergic agents, or imipramine.

If unsuccessful, spermatozoa can be recovered by bladder catheterization and irrigated with culture medium for artificial insemination, IVF or ICSI.

Untreatable sterility

Patients with persistent nonobstructive azoospermia without retrievable postmeiotic germ cells, unable to undergo ICSI or failing to be helped by it, should be counselled regarding the options of adoption and donor insemination.

Genetic screening and counselling

This has become important with the realization that genetic disorders could account for an increasing proportion of infertility previously believed to be idiopathic, and that there is a high probability of transmitting infertility to male offspring if assisted reproductive treatment is successful. Patients with obstructive azoospermia resulting from congenital bilateral absence of the vas deferens, and their partners, should undergo *CFTR* gene screening followed by genetic counselling if positive. Genetic counselling should also be carried out in all couples considering microassisted fertilization, including men with Klinefelter's syndrome. The risk of having a child with 47,XXY or 47,XXX may be higher after successful treatment, and preimplantation genetic diagnosis should be offered. It is also recommended that chromosome karyotyping and Y-chromosome screening be performed in patients with azoospermia and severe oligozoospermia (<5 million/ml) regardless of the coexistence of other clinical abnormalities such as varicocele or cryptorchidism. Increase in *de novo* chromosomal abnormalities, major congenital malformations, and imprinting disorders have been noted in children born with assisted reproductive technologies, necessitating long-term follow-up of these children.

Erectile dysfunction

Erectile failure may be caused by neurological disorders such as autonomic neuropathy (usually complicating diabetes), multiple sclerosis and spinal injuries, vascular disease, retroperitoneal and bladder-neck surgery, medications (commonly α- and β-adrenergic antagonists and psychotropic agents), alcohol abuse, severe systemic disease, psychological dysfunctions (including depression), relationship problems, androgen deficiency, and hyperprolactinaemia. Loss of libido characterizes androgen deficiency and hyperprolactinaemia, while preservation of spontaneous morning erection is suggestive of psychogenic impotence. Although the measurement of testosterone is recommended as part of the initial investigation of erectile dysfunction, testosterone deficiency is relatively uncommon (<5%) in these patients. Management should aim to correct any reversible underlying disease (e.g. prolactinoma) or substitute offending medications. Androgen replacement is only indicated in patients with testosterone in the hypogonadal range. Phosphodiesterase (PDE5) inhibitors such as sildenafil, tadalafil, and vardenafil improve erection by enhancing the neurovascular cGMP-mediated nitric oxide availability in the penile vasculature. These agents are now established as standard and very successful management of a wide variety of erectile disorders (a detailed description of the use of these medications is beyond the scope of this chapter). PDE5 inhibitors have largely superseded the use of vacuum devices and intracavernosal injection of vasodilators such as papaverine or prostaglandin E_1. These are reserved for cases with severe neurogenic impotence unresponsive to PDE5 inhibitors. In men presenting with erectile dysfunction and low testosterone, combination treatment with PDE5 inhibitors and testosterone can be effective when either treatment alone has failed.

Further reading

Hypogonadism

Bojesen A (2007). Klinefelter syndrome in clinical practice. *Nat Clin Pract Urol*, **4**, 192–204.

Bojesen A, Juul S, Gravholt CH (2003). Prenatal and postnatal prevalence of Klinefelter syndrome: a national registry study. *J Clin Endocrinol Metab*, **88**, 622–6.

Layman LC (2007). Hypogonadotropic hypogonadism. *Endocrinol Metab Clin North Am*, **36**, 283–96.

Seminara SB (2006). Mechanisms of disease: the first kiss—a crucial role for kisspeptin-1 and its receptor, G-protein-coupled receptor 54, in puberty and reproduction. *Nat Clin Pract Endocrinol Metab*, **2**, 328–34.

Testosterone replacement

Bhasin S, *et al.* (2006). Testosterone therapy in adult men with androgen deficiency syndromes: an endocrine society clinical practice guideline. *J Clin Endocrinol Metab*, **91**, 1995–2010.

Rosner W, *et al.* (2007). Position statement: Utility, limitations, and pitfalls in measuring testosterone: an Endocrine Society position statement. *J Clin Endocrinol Metab*, **92**, 405–13.

Srinivas-Shankar U, Wu FC (2006). Drug insight: testosterone preparations. *Nat Clin Pract Urol*, **3**, 653–65.

Infertility

Bhasin S (2007). Approach to the infertile man. *J Clin Endocrinol Metab*, **92**, 1995–2004.

Dohle GR, *et al.* (2005). EAU guidelines on male infertility. *Eur Urol*, **48**, 703–11.

Doria-Rose VP, Biggs ML, Weiss NS (2005). Subfertility and the risk of testicular germ cell tumors (United States). *Cancer Causes Control*, **16**, 651–6.

Jarow JP (2007). Diagnostic approach to the infertile male patient. *Endocrinol Metab Clin North Am*, **36**, 297–311.

Levinger U, *et al.* (2007). Is varicocele prevalence increasing with age? *Andrologia*, **39**, 77–80.

Mazumdar S, Levine AS (1998). Antisperm antibodies: etiology, pathogenesis, diagnosis, and treatment. *Fertil Steril*, **70**, 799–810.

Paduch DA (2006). Testicular cancer and male infertility. *Curr Opin Urol*, **16**, 419–27.

Pettersson A, *et al.* (2007). Age at surgery for undescended testis and risk of testicular cancer. *N Engl J Med*, **356**, 1835–41.

Schiff JD, Ramirez ML, Bar-Chama N (2007). Medical and surgical management male infertility. *Endocrinol Metab Clin North Am*, **36**, 313–31.

Van Voorhis BJ (2007). Clinical practice. In vitro fertilization. *N Engl J Med*, **356**, 379–86.

Verhulst SM, *et al.* (2006). Intra-uterine insemination for unexplained subfertility. *Cochrane Database Syst Rev*, 4, CD001838.

13.8.3 Breast cancer

M. Cariati, L. Holmberg, J. Mansi,
P. Parker, G. Pichert, S. Pinder, E. Sawyer,
R. Wilson, and A. Purushotham

Essentials

Epidemiology and aetiology—over 1 million women worldwide are diagnosed with breast cancer each year, with about 400 000 dying of the disease. Familial breast cancer, most commonly related to the *BRCA1* and *BRCA2* genes, accounts for only 5% of all cases. Many of the known risk factors are not modifiable because they are inherent or would require unrealistic lifestyle changes, but moderating alcohol consumption, avoiding obesity, and increasing physical activity are all possibly useful interventions.

Prevention—screening for breast cancer is an effective means of achieving earlier diagnosis and provides the opportunity for reducing mortality: X-ray mammography screening alone can be expected to reduce mortality by 30% in women aged 40 to 70 years who participate.

Clinical assessment

Diagnostic assessment of symptomatic breast problems and screen-detected abnormalities is best carried out by multidisciplinary teams following the principles of triple assessment, which involves (1) detailed history and clinical examination of both breasts, axillae and supraclavicular regions; (2) imaging; and (where indicated) (3) cytology/core biopsy. The primary imaging techniques are X-ray mammography and ultrasonography, with MRI when there is diagnostic uncertainty. Ultrasound-guided core needle biopsy is the preferred method for sampling abnormalities. Once the diagnosis has been made, further imaging is used to assess the extent of cancer in the breast and detect the spread of disease to the axilla.

The most significant histological predictors of prognosis are lymph node stage, histological grade, and histological assessment of tumour size, but evaluation of tumour type and the absence or presence of lymphovascular invasion provide additional information, and oestrogen receptor status and HER2 status are predictive markers for selection of therapy.

Management

Surgical treatment—(1) Breast: the main options are modified radical mastectomy, with or without immediate or delayed breast reconstruction, or breast-conserving surgery followed by adjuvant radiotherapy to the breast. (2) Axilla: metastatic involvement of these nodes is the best predictor of risk of recurrence and death, hence accurate assessment of axillary node status is important for staging, prognosis and guiding adjuvant treatment selection; many regard sentinel lymph node biopsy as the best technique.

Radiotherapy—this is an established means of reducing the risk of locoregional recurrence following surgery for invasive breast cancer and also improves survival. It can also be useful for palliation, particularly of bone and brain metastases.

Systemic therapy—(1) endocrine: hormone therapy is only of value in women in whom receptors have been identified histologically by immunohistochemistry; in premenopausal women reduction in oestrogen levels can be achieved by luteinizing hormone releasing hormone (LHRH) agonist or by oophorectomy, or by blocking oestrogen receptors with a SERM (selective oestrogen receptor modulator) such as tamoxifen; in postmenopausal women peripheral aromatization of androgens synthesized by the adrenal glands can be significantly reduced by aromatase inhibitors; (2) chemotherapy: many cytotoxic drugs with different mechanisms of action are available for the treatment of breast cancer (anthracyclines, alkylating agents, antimetabolites, tubulin-binding and platinum-based drugs); (3) biological therapy: Herceptin, a humanized monoclonal antibody against HER2, is active against breast cancers that express this receptor.

Early breast cancer—most women present with local disease confined to the breast, with or without axillary node involvement. Those with hormone-nonresponsive (oestrogen receptor/progesterone receptor, ER/PR –ve) disease should be offered chemotherapy. Those with hormone-responsive (ER/PR +ve) disease should be offered endocrine therapy, with the addition of chemotherapy to some intermediate-risk and all high-risk groups. Herceptin should be given to all women following chemotherapy if their tumours overexpress HER2.

Locally advanced (operable and inoperable), large or inflammatory breast cancers—chemotherapy is the initial treatment of choice, usually anthracycline based followed by a taxane, which can reduce the size of a tumour and render it operable.

Metastatic breast cancer—treatment is aimed at controlling symptoms, improving quality of life, and prolonging survival. Endocrine therapy is usually the treatment of first choice if the tumour is hormone-receptor positive. If the patient has exhausted all endocrine options, or has a hormone-receptor negative tumour, or has rapidly progressive disease, then chemotherapy is the treatment of choice.

Symptomatic treatment—patients with metastatic breast cancer may require pain control with appropriate analgesia; draining of ascites or pleural effusions; radiotherapy for bony pain, brain metastases, or spinal cord compression; and relief of obstructive jaundice by stenting. Symptoms due to bony involvement may be greatly helped by bisphosphonates.

Epidemiology
Disease burden

It is estimated that about 1.2 million women worldwide per year will be diagnosed with breast cancer in the decade 2000–2010, and about 400 000 women will die of the disease per year. About 4.5 million women are alive after a diagnosis of breast cancer. The incidence of the disease rises from a low level before 30 years of age to about 2 women per 1000 per year at the age of 50. After age 50 the risk in Western industrialized countries continues to rise, but less rapidly, and in developing countries the rise in risk after 50 years is substantially less than in the developed world. In countries currently adopting a Westernized lifestyle the risk after age 50 increasingly becomes similar to that in the industrialized world.

Since cancer monitoring with cancer registries started in the 1950s there has been a slow trend of increased breast cancer incidence (see 'Breast cancer screening' below). Thus breast cancer will become more common, both as the world's population ages and as the age-specific breast cancer incidence increases. Breast cancer therefore remains a large health problem, despite the fact that early diagnosis and more effective treatment has lowered the mortality rate in several countries.

Hereditary breast cancer

Women with a family history of breast cancer in first-degree relatives have an increased risk of breast cancer. Familial breast cancer accounts for ≤ 35% of all cases with about 5% due to a mutation in one of the high risk breast cancer genes and 20 to 30% due to a combination of genetic factors increasing the breast cancer risk slightly to moderately above the population risk.

Female reproductive hormones

Many breast cancer risk factors are associated with exposure to female reproductive hormones. Early menarche and late menopause increase the risk, whereas early first birth, high parity, and long duration of breast feeding are protective. Oral contraceptives increase the risk, but have a low population impact since they are taken at an age when underlying breast cancer risk is low. Hormone replacement therapy increases risk, especially if oestrogen is combined with progesterone. A high serum level of oestrogen is associated with a higher risk.

Anthropometric factors

Height is positively correlated with postmenopausal breast cancer risk. Body mass index is inversely correlated with breast cancer risk before the menopause, but high body mass index is a risk factor for postmenopausal breast cancer. Higher physical activity is protective, especially for postmenopausal breast cancer. These factors may partly act as modifiers of endogenous hormonal levels. Each of the hormonal factors and anthropometric factors has a modest impact on risk, but taken together they may account for a substantial part of the difference in incidence between countries.

Diet and other factors

Associations between diet and breast cancer risk have been extensively studied, but the only clear consistent finding has been that the consumption of each additional 10 g of alcohol per day increases the breast cancer risk by 9%, compared with no intake. Many other dietary components have attracted interest, but the findings are equivocal.

Ionizing radiation causes breast cancer, even at low doses, and especially if the exposure is around menarche. High breast density at mammography and previous benign breast disease (atypical hyperplasia) are markers of a higher risk of breast cancer, but it is not known why this is so.

Prevention

Modification of lifestyle

Many of the known risk factors for breast cancer are not modifiable because they are inherent (e.g. family history) or they would require unrealistic lifestyle changes (e.g. radically changing patterns of parity). However, moderating alcohol consumption, avoiding obesity, and increasing physical activity are all possible interventions. Even if there are many obstacles to modifying these factors, motivation for changes is enhanced by the fact that they would also help protect against other cancers, cardiovascular disease, and diabetes. Other modifiable factors include considering alternatives to oral contraceptives in older women, and restricting the use of hormonal replacement therapy for menopausal symptoms to those with severe symptoms, and to a few years of treatment.

Chemoprevention

Since the late 1990s it has been known that selective oestrogen receptor modifiers (SERMs) can reduce the risk of breast cancer by around 50%. However, the early SERM, tamoxifen, also has the side effects of increasing the risk of thromboembolic events, stroke, uterine cancer, and cataracts. The risk of side effects seems to be lower with newer generations of SERMs, but so far they have not been tested in prevention as extensively and for as long as tamoxifen. Chemoprevention is today only recommended for women at high risk, and there is ongoing research into how to best select these women (through epidemiological risk models and/or biomarkers) and which drugs to use.

Familial breast cancer

It is estimated that about 5% of all breast cancers result from a mutation in one of the high-risk breast cancer genes, and that a further 20 to 30% of all breast cancers arise from a combination of genetic factors that increase the breast cancer risk slightly to moderately above the population risk. Genes that confer a high risk for breast and other cancers, if mutated, are summarized in Table 13.8.3.1. The two genes most commonly involved in inherited breast and ovarian cancer are *BRCA1* and *BRCA2*. Other genes causing a high risk for breast cancer are *TP53*, *PTEN*, *STK11*, and the E-cadherin gene (*CDH1*).

Women with an average or slightly increased risk of breast cancer should be reassured in primary care and do not require enhanced breast surveillance. Women at moderately increased risk of breast cancer should be managed at secondary care level and referred for annual mammograms between the ages of 40 and 50 years. Women with a high risk of breast cancer because of their family history should be offered genetic counselling and testing, the key elements of which are as follows:

- Construction of a three-generation pedigree with verification of cancer diagnoses
- Clinical examination
- Cancer risk assessment based on family history of cancer
- Discussion of advantages and disadvantages of genetic testing
- Discussion of psychological issues and offer of psychological support
- Information about insurance implications
- Discussion of confidentiality
- Discussion of the genetic test result and its consequences for the affected individual and family members
- Discussion of options for surveillance and risk reduction, with and without a genetic test

Table 13.8.3.1 Inherited predisposition to breast and other cancers

Syndrome	Gene	Mode of inheritance	Significantly increased risk
Inherited breast/ ovarian cancer (OMIM #604370, #612555)	BRCA1 BRCA2	Autosomal dominant	Breast cancer Ovarian cancer Prostate cancer (BRCA2) Pancreatic cancer (BRCA2)
Li–Fraumeni syndrome	TP53	Autosomal dominant	Breast cancer Soft-tissue and bone sarcomas Adrenocortical cancer Brain tumours Leukaemias Other tumours
Cowden's syndrome (OMIM #158350)	PTEN	Autosomal dominant	Breast cancer Thyroid cancer Endometrial cancer Lhermitte–Duclos disease (dysplastic cerebellar gangliocytoma)
Peutz–Jeghers syndrome (OMIM #175200)	STK11	Autosomal dominant	Breast cancer Colon cancer Pancreatic cancer Stomach cancer Ovarian cancer Other tumours
Inherited stomach cancer (OMIM #192090)	CDH1	Autosomal dominant	Lobular breast carcinoma Diffuse stomach cancer

♦ Information on costs of genetic testing and surveillance, and risk-reducing measures

Testing of high-risk genes offers the opportunity to identify the cause of breast cancers in the family, to offer testing to family members to clarify their breast cancer risk, and to help individuals at risk to make appropriate decisions regarding surveillance and risk-reducing options. Women who carry a *BRCA1* or *BRCA2* mutation have a lifetime risk of breast cancer of up to 85%; their lifetime risk of ovarian cancer is also increased by up to 50% in *BRCA1* carriers and up to 30% in *BRCA2* carriers. Men with a *BRCA2* mutation have up to a 6% lifetime risk of breast cancer and an increased risk of prostate and other cancers.

Women at high risk of breast cancer because of their family history or a mutation in one of the breast cancer-associated genes should be offered digital mammograms and breast MRI. Prophylactic bilateral mastectomy has been shown to reduce the breast cancer risk by at least 90%, but reoperation rates of up to 30 to 49% have been reported.

At present there is no surveillance of proven benefit for women at high risk for ovarian cancer. There are ongoing trials designed to test the effectiveness of transvaginal ultrasonography and CA125 measurements for the early diagnosis of ovarian cancer. By contrast, prophylactic salpingo-oophorectomy has been proven to reduce the risk of ovarian cancer by up to 95%, and if performed premenopausally this also reduces the risk of breast cancer by up to 50%.

The future challenge is to a gain better understanding of the interaction of genetic and lifestyle/environmental factors in order to develop more effective surveillance and risk-reducing measures and treatments adapted to the biology of inherited cancers.

Clinical approach

Following a detailed history and clinical examination of both breasts, axillae, and supraclavicular regions, patients undergo imaging and cytology/core biopsy where indicated (triple assessment). Imaging is important in all aspects of the breast disease management pathway, with a key role in the early diagnosis of breast cancer through screening, the diagnostic assessment of breast symptoms and signs, the local and systemic staging of breast cancer, monitoring the response to treatment, and follow-up after treatment to detect recurrence.

Breast cancer screening

Population screening

Treatment of breast cancer at an early stage is more likely to prolong survival and may offer cure. Screening for breast cancer is an effective means of achieving early diagnosis, and provides the opportunity for reducing mortality. Randomized controlled trials indicate that X-ray mammography screening alone can be expected to reduce mortality by 30% in women aged 40 to 70 years who participate. The benefit is greatest in women aged 55 to 70 years (40%), with a lesser benefit in women aged 40 to 55 years (15%). Most developed countries offer mammographic breast screening to women aged 40 to 75 years every 1 to 3 years; this detects about 7 cancers per 1000 women screened, with 25% of these cancers being ductal carcinoma *in situ* (Fig. 13.8.3.1). To be effective, screening must be partnered with multidisciplinary assessment of screen-detected abnormalities and effective treatment of the cancers detected.

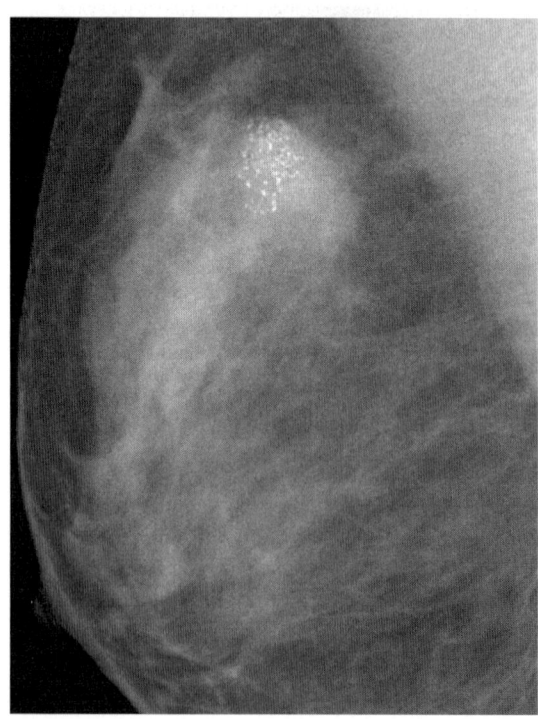

Fig. 13.8.3.1 Mediolateral view of mammogram showing malignant microcalcification characteristic of ductal carcinoma *in situ*.

High-risk group screening

In patients with a hereditary disposition, breast cancers usually develop at a much younger age and tend to be of a higher histological grade. The most effective management is prophylactic mastectomy, but early detection through screening is preferred by many women in this group. MRI must be combined with mammography for effective early detection in high-risk women.

Breast diagnosis

Diagnostic assessment of symptomatic breast problems and abnormalities detected at screening is best carried out by multidisciplinary teams following the principles of triple assessment. The primary imaging techniques used are X-ray mammography and ultrasonography (Figs. 13.8.3.2 and 13.8.3.3). MRI is used as a supplementary technique where there is diagnostic uncertainty. Ultrasound-guided core needle biopsy is the preferred method for sampling abnormalities. X-ray-guided core or vacuum-assisted mammotomy are used for impalpable abnormalities that are not visible on ultrasonography, these usually being microcalcifications detected at screening.

Results of the assessment process are discussed at prospective multidisciplinary meetings at which the clinical findings, imaging, and pathology are reviewed and clinical management decisions made before the treatment choices are discussed with the patient. This process ensures that patients with benign problems are provided with an accurate diagnosis and can be reassured rapidly, and those with breast cancer are provided with full information and advice on which to base their treatment choice.

Staging of breast cancer

Once the diagnosis has been made, further imaging is used to assess the extent of cancer in the breast and detect the spread of disease to

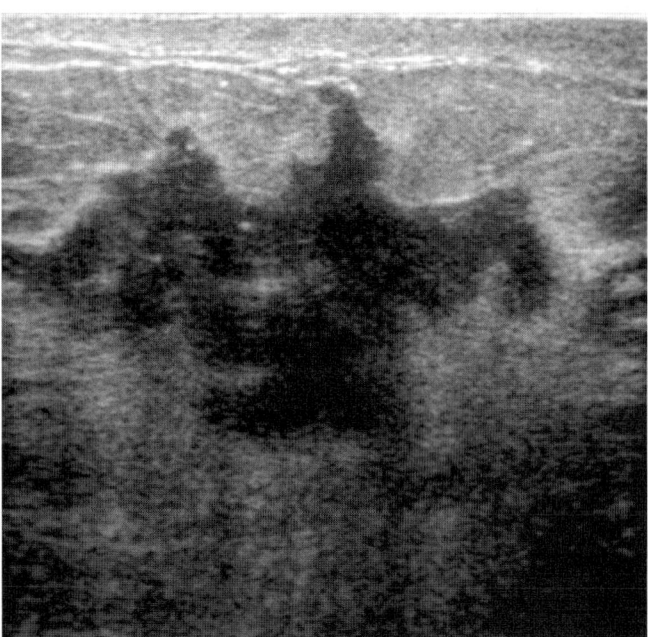

Fig. 13.8.3.3 Ultrasound scan showing characteristic appearance of invasive carcinoma with microcalcification.

the axilla. The extent of the disease is crucial for deciding if breast-conserving surgery is a viable option for treatment. Mammography provides an accurate assessment of disease extent in most cases, and axillary ultrasonography will detect around 40% of axillary node metastatic spread. For patients with dense breast tissue and those with invasive lobular carcinoma, MRI is the most reliable imaging technique for assessing the extent of disease and the presence of multifocality.

Axillary node involvement is a marker of possible spread of disease beyond the breast, and these patients may require additional staging. This involves skeletal scintigraphy to detect bone disease, and computed tomography of the chest and upper abdomen to detect lung, pleural, and visceral organ spread, prior to any further treatment.

Monitoring of treatment

Response to chemotherapy and hormone therapy, either primary or secondary, is best assessed with imaging. MRI provides the most accurate assessment of response in the breast, as it detects both anatomical and biological changes. To assess the response of systemic disease the imaging techniques used are the same as those used for staging.

Surveillance after treatment

Annual mammography is routine for the detection of ipsilateral breast recurrence and new primary malignancy in the opposite breast. Surveillance mammography is usually continued for 5 to 10 years after initial treatment, with the aim of reducing morbidity by earlier detection of recurrence of disease.

Histopathology of breast carcinoma

Ductal carcinoma *in situ*

Although it was previously believed that in some cases breast cancer arose in the ductules and in other cases in the lobules, it is now clear that this disease derives from the previously terminal duct lobular unit. However, two types of *in situ* carcinoma of the breast

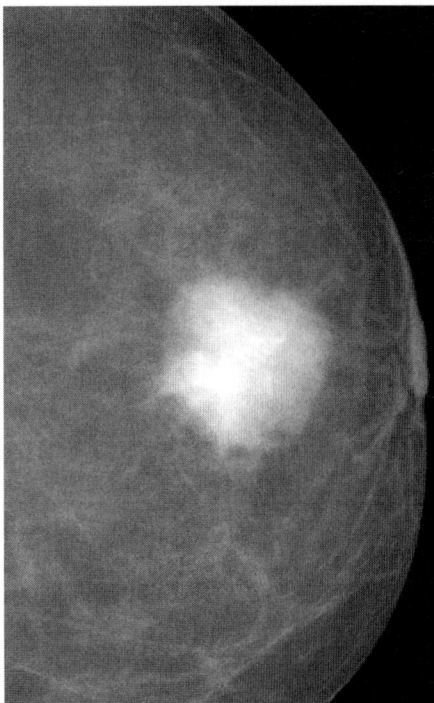

Fig. 13.8.3.2 Mediolateral view of mammogram showing a mass lesion characteristic of invasive carcinoma.

are conventionally described, ductal and lobular, and these have significant differences in morphology and clinical behaviour. Ductal carcinoma *in situ* (DCIS) is widely regarded as a true precursor of invasive breast cancer, but lobular carcinoma *in situ* is not generally accepted to be an invariable precursor of invasive disease. Histologically, DCIS can be recognized as a malignant proliferation of epithelial cells within the duct system, which has not breached the myoepithelial layer and basement membrane and therefore has not invaded into the breast stroma (Fig. 13.8.3.4). A variable number of ducts may be involved, but DCIS almost always involves a single duct system within the breast, although these vary significantly in size and distribution. As with invasive breast carcinoma, the microscopic appearance is highly variable, and DCIS is classified according to cytonuclear grade into high-, intermediate-, and low-grade forms, which are associated with differing risks of local recurrence and of harbouring an invasive tumour.

Invasive carcinoma

A large number of morphological variants of invasive breast carcinoma can be identified histologically, and it is clear that invasive breast carcinoma is a spectrum of disease with different appearances, protein profiles, and gene expression rather than a single entity. Despite recent interest in gene profiling of breast cancers, histological evaluation is clearly of importance as the inherent biological aggressiveness and likely clinical outcome can be predicted and influenced by selection of the most appropriate therapy based on these factors. According to national guidelines a minimum dataset of features provided in histological reports includes a number of factors. The most significant for prediction of prognosis remain histological examination of lymph node stage, histological grade, and histological assessment of tumour size, but evaluation of tumour type and the absence or presence of lymphovascular invasion provide additional information. Oestrogen receptor status and HER2 status are included as predictive markers for selection of therapy.

Lymph node stage must be determined by microscopic examination of the lymph nodes, as clinical and ultrasound assessment is not accurate. Histological grade is determined by assessing the amount of gland formation, the degree of nuclear pleomorphism, and the mitotic count of the tumour. Tumours are classified into three grades: grade 1 (equivalent to well differentiated) to grade 3 (poorly differentiated); 85% of patients with grade 1 tumours are alive 10 years after diagnosis, compared with 35% of patients with grade 3 tumours.

More than 50% of invasive breast carcinomas are classified as being of no special type (previously called ductal). These tumours are formed from cords and sheets of large malignant epithelial cells, which infiltrate in a disorganized fashion (Fig. 13.8.3.5). Infiltrating lobular carcinoma accounts for about 10 to 15% of invasive breast carcinomas, with linear cords of tumour cells classically infiltrating in a so-called targetoid or single-file pattern. Other forms of invasive carcinoma are less common, including medullary-like carcinoma, which is more commonly seen in women who have a *BRCA1* gene mutation. Other special types of invasive breast carcinoma include tubular and mucinous forms, which are of significance as they tend to have a more indolent course and a better prognosis. Mixed forms of invasive cancer, with more than one histological pattern, are also quite common. Other types of invasive breast carcinoma, such as metaplastic/spindle-cell or squamous-cell carcinoma, are rare.

There is increasing interest in subclassifying invasive carcinomas by the use of additional techniques such as immunohistochemistry panels and gene-array profiling. For example, the group of tumours categorized histologically as being of no special type can be further grouped with these techniques, and differing prognoses identified, e.g. some tumours express basal-type cytokeratins and appear, in general, to have a poorer outcome than those with luminal-type keratin expression. Recently, based on variations in gene expression, it has been shown that cancers can be classified into basal and luminal groups, a group overexpressing *ERBB2* (*HER2*), and a normal breast-like group. Furthermore, the luminal epithelial/oestrogen receptor-positive group could be divided into at least two subgroups, each with a distinctive expression profile. Survival analysis has shown significantly different outcomes for the patients belonging to the various groups, including a poor prognosis for the

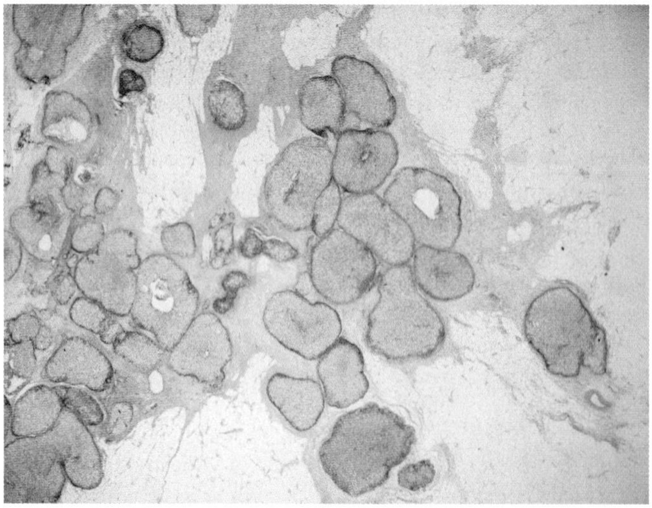

Fig. 13.8.3.4 Ductal carcinoma *in situ*. Low-power photomicrograph of sharply defined islands of malignant cells, with tumour retained within duct structures.

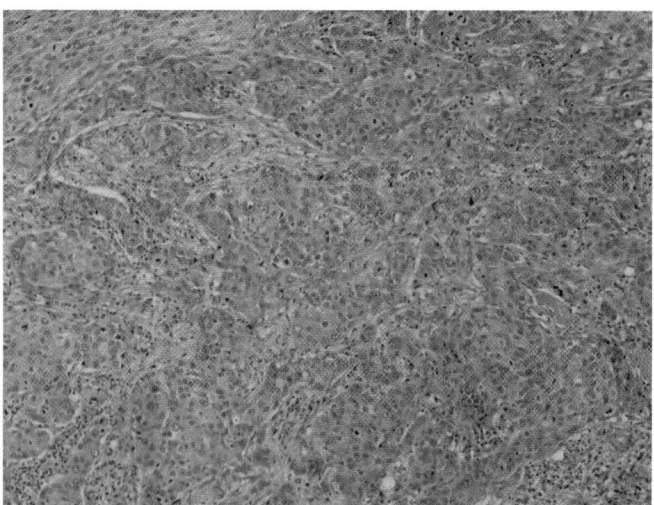

Fig. 13.8.3.5 Invasive breast cancer. Carcinoma of no special type (ductal), histological grade 3; the tumour is formed from sheets of large and pleomorphic malignant cells, with abundant mitoses present.

basal-like subtype and a significant difference in outcome for the two oestrogen receptor-positive groups.

Predictive markers

Alongside the increased use of targeted therapy there is a requirement for high-quality testing of markers that predict the value of a therapy for an individual patient. The oestrogen receptor competitor tamoxifen and aromatase inhibitors are frequently recommended for patients with tumours that express the oestrogen receptor. The degree of reactivity, in the form of the percentage and intensity of immunohistochemical staining (typically combined into a score from 0 to 8), approximates to the quantity of oestrogen receptor in the tumour-cell nucleus, and to the likelihood of a response to hormone therapy (Fig. 13.8.3.6).

HER2 (ERBB2) is a member of the human epidermal growth factor receptor family and is a transmembrane tyrosine kinase receptor. *HER2* is expressed in approximately 15 to 20% of early invasive breast cancers and is associated with poorer patient outcome. Humanized monoclonal antibodies against the HER2 protein have proven valuable in the treatment of the subgroup of patients who have cancers that overexpress *HER2* or have amplification of the gene. For this reason, all invasive breast cancers are now tested for the presence of excess protein on the cell surface by immunohistochemistry (scored 0 to 3) and/or for amplification of the gene by *in situ* hybridization (assessed as a ratio compared with chromosome 17 copy number) (Fig. 13.8.3.7).

Surgery

The surgical treatment of breast cancer has moved from radical to more conservative over the last century. Several randomized trials comparing different surgical procedures showed no difference in survival between radical mastectomy, modified radical mastectomy, and breast-conserving surgery with adjuvant radiotherapy.

Breast-screening programmes identify tumours at an earlier stage of disease, allowing locoregional treatment that, in some patients, results in complete cure. By contrast, patients

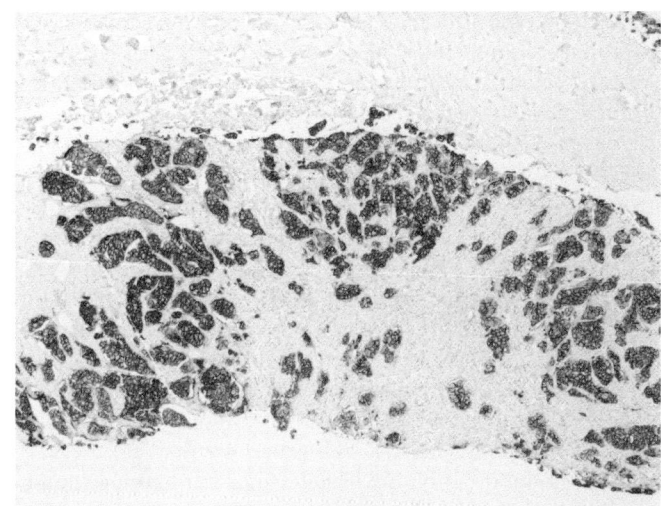

Fig. 13.8.3.7 HER2-positive invasive breast carcinoma. Core biopsy of invasive breast cancer showing strong complete membrane reactivity for HER2; score 3+ (range 0–3).

with aggressive tumours or those who present late often have locally advanced tumours with nodal involvement and sometimes systemic disease.

Surgical treatment for breast cancer is designed to achieve locoregional control and staging of disease in order to plan adjuvant therapy.

Surgery to the breast

Broadly speaking, two main surgical options are available to treat breast cancer. These are modified radical mastectomy with or without immediate or delayed breast reconstruction, or breast-conserving surgery followed by adjuvant radiotherapy to the breast. The purpose of adopting breast-conserving surgery is to minimize the psychological morbidity associated with mastectomy, hence in addition to removing the tumour with an adequate margin of normal tissue it is important to achieve a good cosmetic outcome. This has to be balanced against ensuring an adequate clearance (there is no absolute consensus on what constitutes an adequate margin of excision) in order to minimize the risk of local recurrence.

There is general agreement on the criteria used to select patients for breast-conserving surgery, some of these being size and extent of tumour (relative to size of breast), unifocal disease, and patient preference. With the advent of neoadjuvant chemotherapy and endocrine therapy, and the consequent downstaging of tumour size, more patients are now able to undergo breast-conserving surgery. Furthermore, with modern techniques larger volumes of tissue may be removed, with oncoplastic procedures adopted to remodel the breast, thereby providing excellent cosmesis.

Following breast-conserving surgery and adjuvant radiotherapy, an acceptable 5-year actuarial rate of local recurrence is in the order of 5 to 10%. Factors influencing risk of local recurrence include close/involved margins, young age, high grade, extensive DCIS, and the presence of vascular invasion.

Patients undergoing mastectomy should be offered breast reconstruction if clinically indicated, the options including immediate versus delayed, and prosthetic versus autologous. The choices will depend primarily on comorbidities, previous abdominal surgery, the likelihood of postoperative adjuvant radiotherapy to the chest

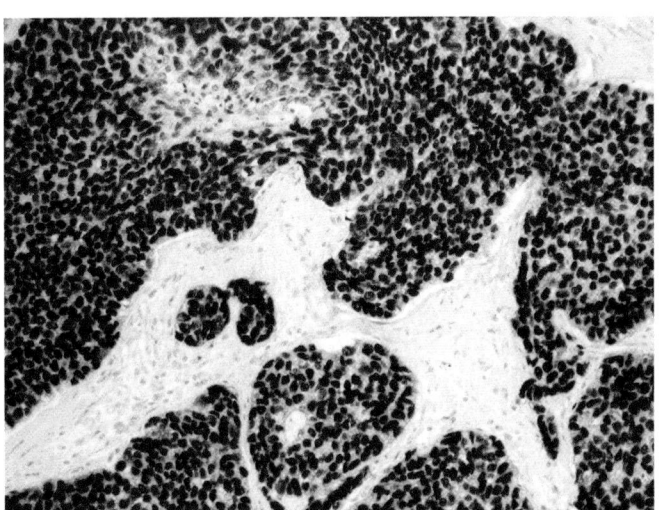

Fig. 13.8.3.6 Oestrogen receptor-positive invasive breast carcinoma. Sheets of invasive carcinoma cells all show strong nuclear immunoreactivity for oestrogen receptors (Allred score 8; range 0–8).

wall, and the patient's wishes. Broadly speaking, autologous immediate reconstruction offers the patient the best long-term cosmetic outcome. Breast reconstruction does not impact on the detection of subsequent locoregional tumour recurrence.

Surgery to the axilla

Approximately 30 to 40% of early breast cancers have axillary nodal involvement, the management of which has been a hot topic of debate. Metastatic involvement of these nodes has been shown to be the best predictor of risk of recurrence and death, hence accurate assessment of axillary node status is important for staging, prognosis, and guiding adjuvant treatment selection.

Axillary lymph node dissection may be performed to one of three levels based on the anatomical relationship of the nodes to the pectoralis minor muscle. This procedure may be associated with physical morbidity that includes shoulder stiffness, numbness/paraesthesia along the distribution of the intercostobrachial nerve, and breast cancer-related lymphoedema. The latter develops in approximately 25% of patients at some time, can be permanent and disfiguring, interferes with manual dexterity, and causes significant morbidity. Because of this, two alternative procedures have been explored, namely four-node axillary sampling and sentinel lymph node biopsy.

Four-node axillary sampling involves the removal of a number of nodes (usually four) that are identified by palpation of the axillary nodal tissue, and is associated with less physical morbidity than standard axillary lymph node dissection in node-negative patients. It has been shown by some that the incidence of positive nodes identified by axillary sampling does not differ from that identified by axillary lymph node dissection, but others have found that 24% of patients undergoing axillary sampling are erroneously staged.

Sentinel lymph node biopsy (Fig. 13.8.3.8) is a technique for identifying and then removing the first-draining lymph node (or nodes) of the breast. These so-called sentinel lymph node/s are then examined for the presence of tumour and, if metastases are present, the patient will require a completion axillary lymph node dissection. There are now three published prospective randomized controlled

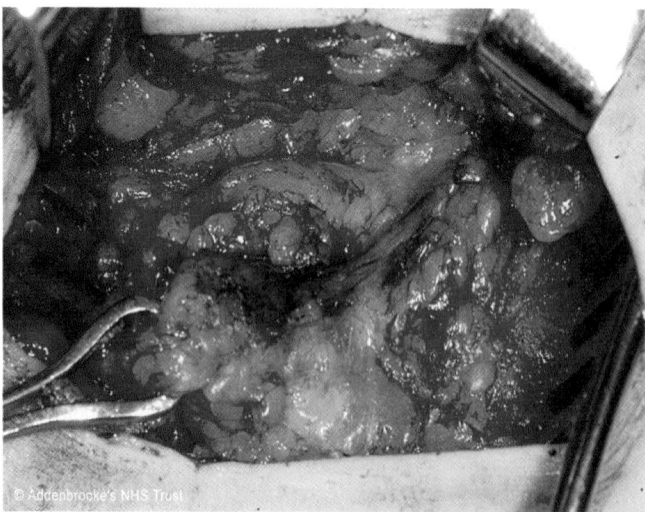

Fig. 13.8.3.8 Sentinel lymph node biopsy demonstrating lymphatics draining to the sentinel lymph node. A combined technique using isotope and patent blue dye is used.

trials in Europe comparing axillary lymph node dissection and sentinel lymph node biopsy for a variety of different parameters such as physical and psychological morbidity. All have shown significant decreases in measures of physical and psychological morbidity with sentinel lymph node biopsy. Of particular relevance for breast cancer-related lymphoedema, rates of arm swelling have been shown to be decreased compared with axillary lymph node dissection. The rate of axillary recurrence after negative sentinel lymph node biopsy is comparable with that following axillary lymph node dissection.

Radiotherapy

Radiotherapy is an established means of reducing the risk of locoregional recurrence following surgery for invasive breast cancer, and also improves survival. The prevention of four local tumour recurrences prevents one breast cancer death at 15 years.

Radiotherapy following breast-conserving surgery

Radiotherapy to the whole breast is recommended following breast-conserving surgery, in order to reduce the risk of local recurrence. Adjuvant radiotherapy reduces the risk of locoregional recurrence from 26% to 7% at 5 years, and decreases breast cancer and overall mortality at 15 years by 5.4% and 4.8%, respectively. Trials are assessing the use of partial breast irradiation in low-risk patients, but no group has as yet been identified in which breast-conserving surgery alone gives adequate local control. For patients at high risk of local recurrence (age <50 years, tumour grade 3, node-positive, large pT2 and T3 tumours, narrow excision margins, oestrogen receptor negative, presence of lymphovascular invasion) a boost to the tumour bed improves local control further. Three trials have shown that radiotherapy reduces the risk of recurrence following wide local excision of both high-grade and low-grade DCIS.

Postmastectomy radiotherapy

Postmastectomy radiotherapy to the chest wall, in combination with appropriate nodal irradiation (see below), has been demonstrated to improve locoregional control and survival in node-positive patients. Radiotherapy reduces the risk of locoregional recurrence from 23% to 6% at 5 years, and decreases breast cancer and overall mortality at 15 years by 6% and 3.5%, respectively. Patients with four or more involved lymph nodes get the most benefit from radiotherapy; the situation for those with one to three positive nodes is less clear, with current trials attempting to answer the question, particularly in the presence of more effective adjuvant systemic therapy. However, the 2005 Oxford overview of radiotherapy trials does show a decrease in local recurrence and breast cancer mortality in those with one to three positive nodes and those with four or more positive nodes.

Nodal irradiation following breast-conserving surgery or mastectomy

Axillary and supraclavicular fossa irradiation following a level 1 axillary node dissection or sentinel node biopsy

Following a negative sentinel node biopsy or level 1 axillary dissection, lymph node irradiation is unnecessary, as involvement of other nodes at higher levels is unlikely. If level 1 axillary nodes are involved and no further surgery is planned, irradiation may be given to the level 2 and 3 axillary and supraclavicular fossa nodes in order to reduce the risk of recurrence. The European Organisation for Research and Treatment of Cancer (EORTC) AMAROS trial is comparing complete axillary lymph node dissection with axillary radiotherapy in sentinel node-positive patients.

Axillary and supraclavicular fossa irradiation following level 3 axillary node dissection

Radiotherapy to the axilla is not recommended after a level 3 dissection as it is associated with a high incidence of lymphoedema. However, patients with four or more involved lymph nodes should be offered supraclavicular fossa irradiation because of the high risk of supraclavicular fossa nodal relapse (11% at 10 years).

Internal mammary nodes

Some of the radiotherapy trials that showed a survival advantage for postmastectomy irradiation (see above) irradiated both the supraclavicular fossa and internal mammary nodes. However, irradiating the internal mammary nodes increases the risk of cardiac toxicity, and trials (e.g. EORTC 22922) have evaluated the role of internal mammary irradiation. This is not currently recommended outside a clinical trial.

Practical issues

The most common fractionation schedule is 50 Gy in 25 fractions. A widely used fractionation regimen in the United Kingdom is 40 Gy in 15 fractions, and evidence from the START trial has shown its equivalence to 50 Gy in 25 fractions, both in terms of local control and cosmetic outcome.

Skin erythema and desquamation are common during radiotherapy and resolve within 4 weeks of completing treatment. Long term side effects are rare and include fibrosis, skin telangiectasia, lung fibrosis, rib fracture, ischaemic heart disease (left-sided tumours), and late malignancy (contralateral breast cancer, radiation-induced sarcoma, or lung cancer). They are uncommon in the first 5 years after treatment, but continue to occur 15 years or more after treatment. The excess mortality mainly results from heart disease and lung cancer.

Pregnancy, previous breast irradiation (including mantle irradiation for Hodgkin's disease), significant preexisting cardiac (for left-sided breast tumours) or lung disease, scleroderma, and limited shoulder mobility are contraindications for the use of radiotherapy.

Intensity-modulated radiotherapy (Fig. 13.8.3.9) can be used to optimize dose homogeneity and avoid unnecessary normal tissue irradiation. This will improve long-term cosmesis and reduce long-term side effects such as cardiac toxicity. Full-dose intraoperative radiotherapy with electrons during breast-conserving surgery is also under investigation.

Radiotherapy is useful for palliation, particularly of bone and brain metastases, both of which are common in breast cancer.

Systemic therapy

Considerable progress has been made in the management of breast cancer over the last two decades, with a marked decrease in recurrence and mortality. Endocrine therapy, chemotherapy, and, more recently, targeted therapy in both the early and advanced setting have all significantly contributed to this. Factors that profoundly affect decision-making in breast cancer include the hormone-receptor status (oestrogen receptor (ER) and progesterone receptor (PR)) and

overexpression of the HER2 receptor. The following section describes the rationale for treatment in these settings.

Endocrine therapy

The value of oestrogen deprivation in the treatment of breast cancer was first established in 1899 when Beatson removed the ovaries of premenopausal women with advanced breast cancer and noted regression of the tumour. Since then a large number of hormone therapies have been developed with different mechanisms of action (Table 13.8.3.2), but the aim of hormone therapy in breast cancer is to prevent the growth-stimulatory effects of oestrogen signalling in breast cancer cells. This can be achieved either by reducing the production of oestrogen or by blocking its receptors. It is clear that such therapy is only of value in women in whom receptors have been identified by immunohistochemistry, and the stronger the ER/PR expression the greater the benefit.

Premenopausal women

The main source of oestrogens in premenopausal women is the ovaries. A reduction in oestrogen levels can be achieved by preventing the ovaries from functioning, either medically with a luteinizing hormone-releasing hormone (LHRH) agonist or by oophorectomy (surgically or by radiotherapy). An alternative is to block the oestrogen receptors with a selective oestrogen-receptor modulator (SERM) such as tamoxifen, which is an antagonist with partial agonist activity, or one of the purer antioestrogens (Table 13.8.3.2).

Postmenopausal women

In postmenopausal women the major source of oestrogen is peripheral aromatization of androgens synthesized by the adrenal glands. This process can be significantly reduced by a group of drugs called the aromatase inhibitors (Table 13.8.3.2). Tamoxifen is also widely used.

Side effects

In general terms these agents are relatively well tolerated. The commonly recognized toxicities are shown in Table 13.8.3.2.

Chemotherapy

Breast cancer is a chemosensitive disease, and there are a large number of cytotoxic drugs with different mechanisms of action available for its treatment (Table 13.8.3.3). Because of the heterogeneous nature of breast cancer some of the regimens are given in combination, whereby drugs from different classes are administered together to achieve maximum cell kill and reduce the risk of drug resistance.

Side effects

Toxicities associated with chemotherapeutic drugs can cause significant short- and long-term morbidity and mortality. Short-term effects include nausea, vomiting, mucositis, alopecia, and myelosuppression with concomitant neutropenic sepsis. Long-term side effects include cardiotoxicity, infertility, and second malignancy. Every effort is made to reduce these side effects and all are explained to the patient before starting therapy.

Biological therapy

Overexpression of HER2 occurs in approximately 15 to 20% of women with breast cancer, and is associated with a more aggressive clinical course and poor outcome. Trastuzumab is a humanized

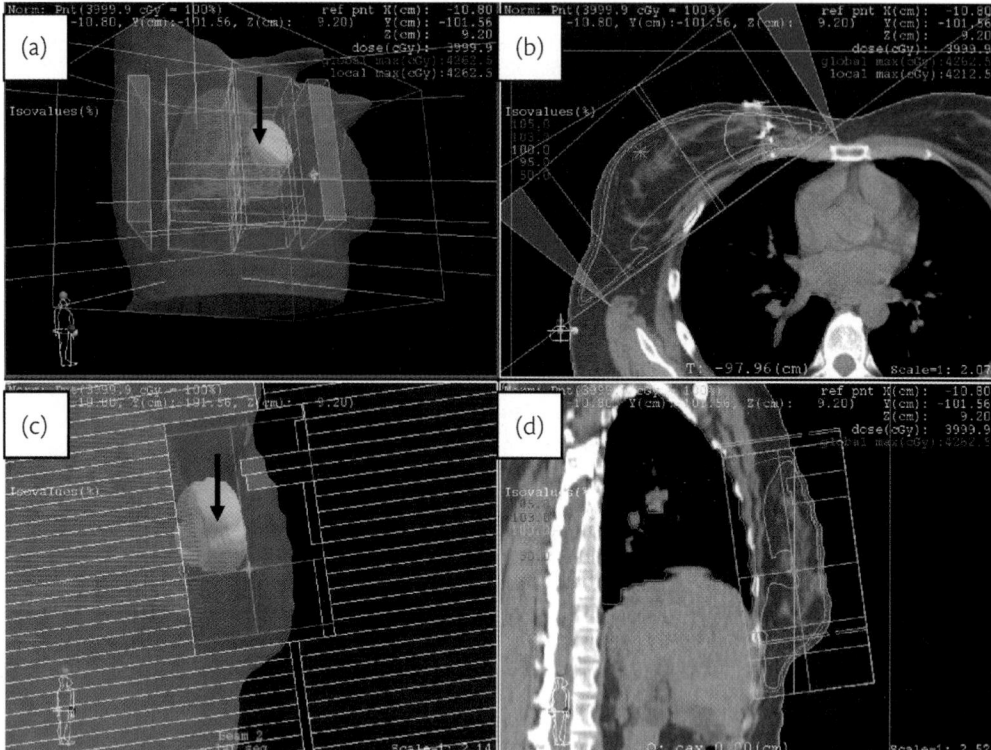

Fig. 13.8.3.9 Example of three-dimensional breast radiotherapy planning. A, multiplanar view; B, transverse and C, sagittal section showing homogenous dose distribution throughout the breast. Surgical clips can be seen on the transverse section delineating the tumour bed, and are used to define the boost volume (light brown volume in multiplanar and beam's-eye views [arrows]). D, beam's-eye view.

monoclonal antibody that has been created by inserting portions of the antigen-binding site of a mouse monoclonal antibody against HER2 into a human monoclonal antibody. This targeted agent is given intravenously on a 1- or 3-weekly basis, alone or in combination with chemotherapy, to patients whose tumours are strongly positive (3+ by immunocytochemistry or positive by fluorescence *in situ* hybridization). The major toxicity relates to cardiac dysfunction, hence close monitoring with regular assessment of ejection fraction is mandatory.

Lapatinib is an orally administered dual HER2 and EGFR (epidermal growth factor receptor; HER1) inhibitor that has shown significant activity in breast cancer, even in women who have progressed on trastuzumab. Bevacizumab is an intravenous vascular endothelial growth factor (VEGF) inhibitor that also has activity in breast cancer.

Systemic therapy in early breast cancer

Most women present with local disease confined to the breast, with or without axillary node involvement. The decision on the recommendation of adjuvant systemic therapy is based on the knowledge of various prognostic factors, which include the following: size and grade of the tumour, presence and number of axillary nodes, presence or absence of vascular invasion, hormone-receptor status, and HER2 overexpression. Other factors include menopausal status and comorbidities. Treatment guidelines are available to aid decision making. The National Institute of Health and Clinical Excellence has also produced guidelines to support recent developments in the use of many systemic therapies in the United Kingdom.

In general, women with hormone-nonresponsive (ER/PR-negative) disease should be offered chemotherapy. Those with hormone-responsive (ER/PR-positive) disease should be offered endocrine therapy, with the addition of chemotherapy to some intermediate-risk and all high-risk groups. Trastuzumab should be given to all women following chemotherapy if their tumours overexpress HER2.

Endocrine therapy

Tamoxifen has been the standard treatment of choice for many years for both pre- and postmenopausal women, with the recommendation that it is given for 5 years following surgery. In premenopausal women the uncertainty over whether ovarian function suppression provides additional benefit over and above endocrine therapy (with or without chemotherapy), is currently under investigation in large international randomized studies (SOFT, TEXT, PERCHE).

In postmenopausal women the third-generation aromatase inhibitors are playing an increasingly important role, and following the results of large randomized studies they are indicated either as initial therapy (ATAC, BIG 1–98) or after treatment with 2 to 3 years of tamoxifen (IES, BIG 1–98, ARNO) or following 5 years of tamoxifen (MA-17). The optimal timing and duration of aromatase inhibitor therapy has yet to be established. A disease-free survival advantage has been reported in all these trials, but an overall survival benefit only in the IES and MA-17 studies to date.

Chemotherapy

In general, all women with high-risk breast cancer will be offered chemotherapy, with the most benefit being gained in younger women and those with hormone-receptor negative tumours. Anthracycline-based chemotherapy is now standard of care. Treatment is given for six to eight courses in an outpatient setting, traditionally on a 3-weekly basis, but 2 weekly with growth-factor

Table 13.8.3.2 Hormone therapies in breast cancer

Hormone therapy	Route of administration	Indication	Main side effects
LHRH agonists			
Goserelin Leuprorelin	Subcutaneous, monthly/3 monthly	Premenopausal Adjuvant, metastatic	Menopausal symptoms[a]
Selective oestrogen-receptor modulators			
Tamoxifen	Oral, daily	Premenopausal	Endometrial cancer
		Postmenopausal	Thromboembolism
		Adjuvant, metastatic	Menopausal symptoms
Fulvestrant	Intramuscular, monthly	Postmenopausal	Menopausal symptoms
		Metastatic	Osteoporosis
Aromatase inhibitors			
Nonsteroidal			
Anastrozole Letrozole	Oral, daily	Postmenopausal Adjuvant[b]	Osteoporosis Joint aches, fractures
Steroidal			
Exemestane	Oral	Primary medical therapy, metastatic	Osteoporosis Joint aches, fractures
Progestogens			
Megestrol acetate	Oral, daily	Premenopausal	Weight gain
		Postmenopausal	Fluid retention
		Metastatic	Thromboembolism

LHRH, luteinizing hormonereleasing hormone.
[a] Hot flushes, sweats mood changes, vaginal dryness, osteoporosis.
[b] National Institute for Clinical Excellence approval: TA112, 2006.

Table 13.8.3.3 Chemotherapy in breast cancer

Chemotherapy	Indication	Class of cytotoxic	NICE approval
Doxorubicin	Adjuvant, PMT, metastatic	Anthracycline	Pre-NICE
Epirubicin	Adjuvant, PMT, metastatic	Anthracycline	Pre-NICE
Cyclophosphamide	Adjuvant, PMT, metastatic	Alkylating agent	Pre-NICE
5-Fluorouracil	Adjuvant, PMT, metastatic	Antimetabolite	Pre-NICE
Paclitaxel	Adjuvant, PMT, metastatic	Tubulin-binding	TA30, 2001 TA108, 2006
Docetaxel	Adjuvant, PMT, metastatic	Tublin-Binding	TA30, 2001 TA109, 2006
Capecitabine	Metastatic	Antimetabolite	TA62, 2003
Vinorelbine	Metastatic	Tubulin-binding	TA54, 2002
Gemcitabine	Metastatic	Antimetabolite	TA116, 2007
Carboplatin	Metastatic	Platinum	Pre-NICE

NICE, National Institute for Health and Clinical Excellence; PMT, primary medical therapy; TA, technology assessment and year of publication.

duration. Lapatinib and bevacizumab are also being investigated in the adjuvant setting.

Systemic therapy as primary medical therapy

For women with locally advanced (operable and inoperable) large or inflammatory breast cancers, treatment with systemic therapy, in particular chemotherapy, is given as the initial treatment of choice. This approach can reduce the size of the tumour and render it operable. For more than a decade this approach has been extended to women with earlier stage tumours so that they can choose primary chemotherapy as initial treatment to increase the potential for breast-conserving surgery and thus avoid a mastectomy. Randomized studies have shown that this approach, followed by definitive surgery, radiotherapy, and additional systemic therapy (e.g. endocrine or trastuzumab) has a similar outcome. Additional benefits include the opportunity to determine whether the patient has a chemosensitive tumour, with the option of changing to a different non-cross-resistant regimen or stopping early if there is no response or the disease progresses. This approach also offers the unique opportunity to study the biology of early breast cancer using the tumour as a model, which will ultimately lead to tailored therapy for particular molecular subsets.

Standard treatment is usually with initial anthracycline-based chemotherapy followed by a taxane. This sequential scheduling has been shown to increase the rate of pathological complete remission, which is strongly correlated with survival.

Metastatic breast cancer

Despite the major advances outlined above, many women develop distant metastases and die of their disease. The median survival is about 3 years, but some women may have a very protracted course over many years. The most common sites and clinical scenarios associated with metastatic disease are shown in Table 13.8.3.4.

support is also possible. For patients with hormone-receptor positive tumours endocrine therapy is traditionally given after the chemotherapy.

Taxanes are increasingly being used in the adjuvant setting, particularly for women with high-risk, node-positive disease. This is based on a number of large randomized studies, such as CALGB 9344, BCIRG 001, and PACS01, with small but significant differences for both disease-free survival and overall survival compared with the control group. Further information will be available with longer follow-up and with the reporting of recently completed or ongoing trials.

There are a number of agents which are still being evaluated in the adjuvant setting, including gemcitabine, capecitabine, and platinum compounds.

Biological therapy

Several trials have shown a significant benefit for the use of adjuvant trastuzumab in women whose tumours overexpress HER2. This is given for a period of a year following anthracycline-based chemotherapy, with several studies in progress to evaluate or report on a shorter (6 months, PERSEPHONE) or longer (2 years, HERA)

Table 13.8.3.4 Sites of metastatic disease and presentation

Site	Symptom/sign
Bone	Pain, fracture, hypercalcaemia, spinal cord compression
Soft tissue	Lymphadenopathy (with or without symptoms), skin nodules
Lung	Dyspnoea, cough, haemoptysis, pleural effusion(s), lung nodules, lymphangitis carcinomatosis
Liver	Anorexia, weight loss, abdominal pain, abdominal swelling, jaundice, ascites
Brain/CNS	Headaches, nausea, vomiting, visual disturbance, hemiparesis, carcinomatous meningitis
Heart	Dyspnoea, cardiac failure, pericardial effusion

Many of these can precipitate an acute medical emergency. If this is the first presentation of metastatic breast cancer the importance of taking a full medical history cannot be underestimated. Treatment is aimed at controlling symptoms, improving quality of life, and prolonging survival.

Endocrine therapy

In the absence of rapidly progressive or life-threatening metastatic disease, endocrine therapy is the treatment of first choice providing the tumour is hormone-receptor positive. The options available are shown in Table 13.8.3.2 and will depend on the type of endocrine therapy given in the adjuvant setting and the time interval between stopping therapy and the development of recurrence. Treatment is given on a continuous basis, providing the patient responds or shows evidence of disease stabilization. The median duration of response or stabilization is 18 months. Once the patient has become resistant to a particular endocrine therapy then a change to an alternative is appropriate, e.g. from a nonsteroidal aromatase inhibitor to a steroidal aromatase inhibitor in postmenopausal women. In premenopausal women the treatment of first choice is a combination of an LHRH agonist with tamoxifen, with a change to an aromatase inhibitor on progression while maintaining complete ovarian blockade.

Chemotherapy

If the patient has exhausted all endocrine options, or has a hormone receptor-negative tumour, or rapidly progressive disease, then chemotherapy is the treatment of choice. The regimen will depend on the type given in the adjuvant therapy (Table 13.8.3.3). For example, as most women will have received an anthracycline in the adjuvant setting, then a taxane (docetaxel 3 weekly or weekly paclitaxel) would be advised. Treatment is usually given for 4 to 6 months, with regular objective assessments by clinical evaluation and CT scan after 2 to 3 courses to ensure that the patient is responding. The median duration of response is about 8 months. Should the patient not respond, progress while on treatment, or relapse on follow-up, then additional second-line chemotherapy would be considered, e.g. capecitabine.

Biological therapy

Trastuzumab should be considered in combination with nonanthracycline chemotherapy for those women who are HER2-positive. A major advance in the management of metastatic disease has been the improvement in survival in HER2-positive women receiving trastuzumab with paclitaxel, compared with paclitaxel alone. Trastuzumab is advocated in combination with other types of chemotherapy such as capecitabine and vinorelbine. Lapatinib and bevacizumab are currently being evaluated in a number of metastatic settings. There are also a number of other small molecules that are being investigated either as single agents or in combination with endocrine therapy or chemotherapy.

Adjunctive therapies

The prompt treatment of symptoms related to metastatic breast cancer is essential as an adjunct to the systemic therapy outlined in the previous sections. These include pain control with appropriate analgesia; draining ascites or pleural effusions; radiotherapy for bone pain, brain metastases, or spinal cord compression; and relief of obstructive jaundice by stenting.

A major step forward in the management of symptoms related to bone involvement has been the use of bisphosphonates. Currently, these agents (e.g. zoledronic acid, ibandronic acid) are indicated in patients who have evidence of bone involvement (radiographs, CT scan, or MRI), whether they have developed symptoms or not. They are usually given intravenously 3 to 4 weekly, initially for 6 to 12 months, and then orally (with newer compounds that are relatively well absorbed such as ibandronic acid). This has resulted in a reduction in a number of the common morbidities associated with bone involvement (fractures, hypercalcaemia, and pain).

Future developments

Although significant improvements have been made there remain a number of unresolved issues. As many new genetic alterations involved in carcinogenesis are being unravelled and we gain greater understanding of previously identified molecular pathways, novel therapies are being introduced. Target-based therapies are widely considered to be the future of breast cancer treatment, and much attention has focused on developing agents directed against a number of pathways involving protein kinases, such as the EGFR–Ras–Raf–MEK–ERK–MAPK signalling pathway. A number of approaches have been employed in an attempt to target this and other pathways. These approaches include biological inhibitors (ribozymes, dominant-negative receptors, decoy receptors, peptides), antagonist antibodies, small-molecule inhibitors, and antisense inhibitors of expression.

Furthermore, as the cancer stem-cell hypothesis gains greater recognition, efforts have been made in an attempt to selectively target the cancer stem cell, believed to be resistant to conventional therapeutic approaches and to be responsible for local and systemic recurrence. A number of pathways involved in normal stem-cell regulation and believed to be disrupted in cancer have been the focus of attention, such as the Notch and Wnt signalling pathways. Table 13.8.3.5 summarizes and gives some examples of current and future attempts at target-based breast cancer treatment. These are all potentially useful, but trials in breast cancer are yet to be implemented for many.

Resistance to drug therapy is encountered regularly, hence further understanding of the mechanisms involved and the development of novel modulators to overcome resistance and target molecular subsets will contribute to increasing the survival in this disease and enable advances in tailor-made therapy.

Table 13.8.3.5 Current and future attempts at target-based breast cancer treatment

Pathway	Function	Disrupted/altered in	Current/potential future therapeutic agents
PI3K/Akt/mTOR	Proliferation Survival Growth Mobility	Renal cell carcinoma Breast cancer Prostate cancer Mantle cell lymphoma	Sirolimus Temsirolimus VQD-002 Perifosine Archexin
EGFR1–4	Growth Proliferation Survival Differentiation	Lung carcinoma Breast cancer Head–neck Gliomas	Lapatinib Gefitinib Erlotinib
HGF/cMet	Epithelial–mesenchymal transition Growth Angiogenesis Survival Morphogenesis Adhesion	Head–neck cancers Breast cancer Hepatocellular carcinoma Pancreatic cancer	NK4 PHA665752 U1 ribozyme Antibody antagonists (5D5)
Notch	Stem-cell maintenance Proliferation Differentiation Apoptosis Angiogenesis	T-cell acute lymphoblastic leukaemia Breast cancer Renal carcinoma Pancreatic cancer Colorectal cancer	LY450139
Wnt/apc/catenin	Cell proliferation Differentiation Cell motility Apoptosis	Colorectal cancer Medulloblastoma Breast cancer Wilm's tumour Prostate cancer Hepatocellular carcinoma	NSAIDs Imatinib mesilate Endostatin β-catenin antisense nucleotides Chimeric F-box protein TCF-restricted replicating viruses CGP049090
PLC/PKC	Cell proliferation Differentiation Apoptosis Angiogenesis	Breast cancer Pancreatic cancer Melanoma Haematological	Bryostatin 1 ISIS 3521 Enzastaurin
Ras/MEK	Cell proliferation Cell survival Differentiation	Colorectal cancer Pancreatic cancer Breast cancer Glioblastoma Papillary thyroid cancer	Antisense inhibitors of Raf expression LErafAON AZD6244 CI-1040
NFκB/IκBα	Transcription Apoptosis Cell cycle control Cell transformation Growth Differentiation	Breast cancer Colorectal cancer Hepatocellular carcinoma Myeloma	Parthenolide BAY 11–7082 Antioxidants Nucleotides (antisense)

Table 13.8.3.5 *(cont'd)* Current and future attempts at target-based breast cancer treatment

Pathway	Function	Disrupted/altered in	Current/potential future therapeutic agents
PDGFR	Embryonic development Cell proliferation Migration Angiogenesis	Gastrointestinal stromal tumours Renal cancer Small cell lung cancer Pancreatic cancer	Sunitinib Sorafenib Imatinib
CXCR/CCR7	Embryogenesis Angiogenesis Inflammation Cell migration	Breast cancer Ovarian cancer Prostate cancer Pancreatic cancer Melanoma	AMD3100 Bismacrocyclic analogues
VEGFR	Angiogenesis Increases vascular permeability	Colorectal cancer Renal cancer Prostate cancer Lung cancer Breast cancer	Bevacizumab Vatalanib Sunitinib AZD-2171

NSAIDs, nonsteroidal anti-inflammatory drugs.

Further reading

Aetiology

Collaborative Group on Hormonal Factors in Breast Cancer (1996). Breast cancer and hormonal contraceptives: collaborative reanalysis on individual data on 53 297 women with breast cancer and 100 239 women without breast cancer from 54 epidemiological studies. *Lancet*, **347**, 1713–27.

Collaborative Group on Hormonal Factors in Breast Cancer (1997). Breast cancer and hormone replacement therapy: collaborative reanalysis of data from 51 epidemiological studies of 52 705 women with breast cancer and 108 411 women without breast cancer. *Lancet*, **350**, 1047–59.

Cuzick J, et al. (2003). Overview of main outcomes in breast cancer prevention trials. *Lancet*, **361**, 296–300.

Easton DF, et al. (2007). Genome-wide association study identifies novel breast cancer susceptibility loci. *Nature*, **447**, 1087–93.

Ford D, Easton DF, Peto J (1995). Estimates of the gene frequency of *BRCA1* and its contribution to breast and ovarian cancer incidence. *Am J Hum Genet*, **57**, 1457–62.

Michels KB, et al. (2007). Diet and breast cancer: a review of the prospective observational studies. *Cancer*, **109** Suppl 12, 2712–49.

Rosman DS, Kaklamani V, Pasche B (2007). New insights into breast cancer genetics and impact on patient management. *Curr Treat Options Oncol*, **8**, 61–73.

Vainio H, Bianchini F (2002). *Breast cancer screening*. IARC handbooks of cancer prevention, vol 7. IARC Press, Lyon, France.

Walsh T, King MC (2007). Ten genes for inherited breast cancer. *Cancer Cell*, **11**, 103–5.

Wooster R, Stratton MR (1995). Breast cancer susceptibility: a complex disease unravels. *Trends Genet*, **11**, 3–5.

Yager JD, Davidson NE (2006). Mechanisms of disease. Estrogen carcinogenesis in breast cancer. *N Engl J Med*, **354**, 270–82.

Pathology

Harvey JM, et al. (1999). Estrogen receptor status by immunohistochemistry is superior to the ligand-binding assay for predicting response to adjuvant endocrine therapy in breast cancer. *J Clin Oncol*, **17**, 1474–81.

NHS Cancer Screening Programmes and The Royal College of Pathologists (2005). *Pathology reporting of breast disease*. http://www.cancerscreening.nhs.uk/breastscreen/publications/nhsbsp58.html.

Sørlie T, et al. (2001). Gene expression patterns of breast carcinomas distinguish tumor subclasses with clinical implications. *Proc Natl Acad Sci U S A.* **98**, 10869–74.

Treatment

Bartelink H, et al. (2007). Impact of a higher radiation dose on local control and survival in breast-conserving therapy of early breast cancer: 10-year results of the randomized boost versus no boost EORTC 228811–0882 trial. *J Clin Oncol*, **25**, 3259–65.

Bijker N, et al. (2006). Breast-conserving treatment with or without radiotherapy in ductal carcinoma-in-situ: ten-year results of European Organisation for Research and Treatment of Cancer randomized phase III trial 10853—a study by the EORTC Breast Cancer Cooperative Group and EORTC Radiotherapy Group. *J Clin Oncol*, **24**, 3381–87.

Clarke M, et al. (2005). Effects of radiotherapy and of differences in the extent of surgery for early breast cancer on local recurrence and 15-year survival: an overview of the randomised trials. *Lancet*, **366**, 2087–106.

Early Breast Cancer Trialists' Collaborative Group (EBCTCG) (2005). Effects of chemotherapy and hormonal therapy for early breast cancer on recurrence and 15-year survival: an overview of the randomised trials. *Lancet*, **365**, 1687–717.

Fernando SA, Edge SB (2007). Evidence and controversies in the use of post-mastectomy radiation. *J Natl Compr Canc Netw*, **5**, 331–8.

Fisher B, et al. (2002). Twenty-five-year follow-up of a randomized trial comparing radical mastectomy, total mastectomy, and total mastectomy followed by irradiation. *N Engl J Med*, **347**, 567–75.

Fisher B, et al. (2002). Twenty-year follow-up of a randomized trial comparing total mastectomy, lumpectomy, and lumpectomy plus irradiation for the treatment of invasive breast cancer. *N Engl J Med*, **347**, 1233–41.

Forrest AP, et al. (1995). The Edinburgh randomized trial of axillary sampling or clearance after mastectomy. *Br J Surg*, **82**, 1504–8.

Goldhirsch A, et al. (2007). Progress and promise: highlights of the international expert consensus on the primary therapy of early breast cancer 2007. *Ann Oncol*, **18**, 1133–44.

Kissin MW, et al. (1982). The inadequacy of axillary sampling in breast cancer. *Lancet*, **1**, 1210–2.

Lyman GH, et al. (2005). American Society of Clinical Oncology guideline recommendations for sentinel lymph node biopsy in early-stage breast cancer. *J Clin Oncol*, **23**, 7703–20.

Lynch MD, Cariati M, Purushotham AD. (2006). Breast cancer, stem cells and prospects for therapy. *Breast Cancer Res*, **8**, 211.

Veronesi U, et al. (2002). Twenty-year follow-up of a randomized study comparing breast-conserving surgery with radical mastectomy for early breast cancer. *N Engl J Med*, **347**, 1227–32.

Veronesi U, et al. (2005). Full-dose intraoperative radiotherapy with electrons during breast-conserving surgery: experience with 590 cases. *Ann Surg*, **242**, 101–6.

13.8.4 Benign breast disease

P. Jane Clarke

Essentials

Benign conditions of the breast are very common, but they cause great anxiety, often leading the patient to be concerned that she has breast cancer. Symptoms may include: (1) a mass in the breast, commonly due to fibroadenoma, benign cystic change, or macrocysts; (2) mastalgia; and (3) discharge from the nipple, which may be caused by hyperprolactinaemia, intraduct papilloma, or duct ectasia. Management involves exclusion of malignancy, often by triple assessment of any palpable abnormality (for clinical examination, radiological and pathological assessment, see Chapter 13.8.3), followed by reassurance, with appropriate specific treatment if required.

Introduction

Breast cancer is the most common malignancy in the United Kingdom and is a disease with a high media profile. As a result, breast symptoms often generate excessive patient anxiety, although most symptomatic patients have either benign conditions or have physical signs which are within normal limits.

Congenital abnormalities

Complete failure of breast development is rare (sometimes being associated with the absence of the pectoralis major muscle—Poland's syndrome), but varying degrees of hypoplasia are common, as are accessory nipples (most commonly seen at the inframammary crease) and accessory breast tissue (most commonly in the axilla).

Aberrations of normal breast development and involution

Fibroadenoma

This common aberration of normal lobular development occurs in adolescents and young women. Fibroadenomas are discreet lumps with a smooth or bosselated surface, are characteristically painless, without skin or deep fixation, and are extremely mobile within the breast tissue (they are sometimes referred to as 'breast mice') (see Fig. 13.8.4.1). They have a characteristic appearance on ultrasound scanning. The diagnosis can be confirmed by fine needle aspiration or core biopsy. The majority are asymptomatic and gradually involute with age. Rarely, they can achieve sufficient size to be called giant fibroadenomas. Surgical excision is indicated if there is diagnostic uncertainty or at the patient's request.

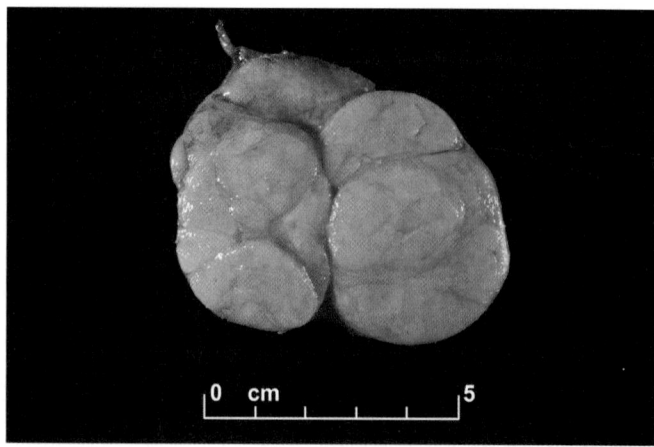

Fig. 13.8.4.1 Excised fibroadenoma, showing whorled surface.

Benign cystic change (benign breast change)

The monthly cycle of breast stimulation and involution frequently results in areas of nodularity which can be diffuse or discrete (benign breast change or benign cystic change). These areas can be tender, may become more prominent premenstrually, and resolve either completely or partially with menstruation. Areas of persistent asymmetrical nodularity, especially in women over the age of 35, should be assessed with imaging and biopsy to exclude malignancy.

Macrocysts

Palpable cysts are a common cause of a lump in the involuting, perimenopausal breast. They are well defined, with a smooth surface and are sometimes tender. The diagnosis is made by ultrasound or by aspiration of the fluid. The aspirate is classically serous, green, yellow, brown, or inky blue. Cysts which occur in the postmenopausal (involuted) breast are unusual, and an intracystic neoplasm should be excluded.

Other benign breast lumps

Fat necrosis

Because the breast has a predominantly fatty stroma, trauma to the breast can result in an entity known as fat necrosis. The resultant lump can be hard and irregular and needs to be differentiated from a cancer.

Phylloides tumours

Presenting as discrete solid masses, these tumours can be clinically and cytologically difficult to differentiate from fibroadenomas, but tend to occur in a slightly older age group. Histologically they have stromal and epithelial elements, and demonstrate a spectrum of behaviour from benign, through borderline, to frankly malignant. Treatment is by wide excision even for benign lesions as there is a high rate of local recurrence if they are simply enucleated. Mastectomy may be needed for the larger or malignant lesions.

Fibromatosis

The pathological features of this unusual condition are similar to those seen in desmoid tumours. Fibromatosis presents with a diffuse mass in the breast which can be locally invasive, infiltrating surrounding tissues. These features can mimic malignancy. Described treatments range from radical excision (including the chest wall), to more conservative approaches with nonsteroidal anti-inflammatory drugs.

Diabetic mastopathy

This condition (also known as lymphocytic lobulitis), characteristically occurs in insulin dependent diabetics. It presents with a diffuse rubbery thickening in the breast. There is no specific treatment other than to exclude malignancy.

Hamartoma

Hamartomas in the breast have physical findings similar to those of a fibroadenoma although they are frequently somewhat softer.

Benign problems of the nipple/areola complex

Nipple discharge (Fig. 13.8.4.2)

Nonphysiological lactation can be secondary to hyperprolactinaemia, rarely due to pituitary microprolactinomas. Once this is

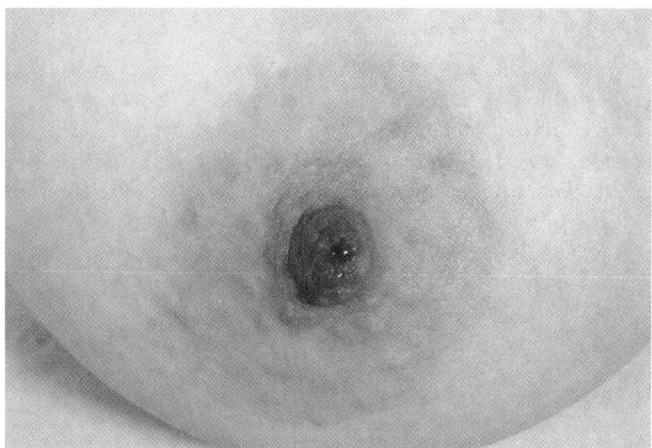

Fig. 13.8.4.2 Nipple showing discharge from two ducts.

excluded, aesthetically distressing discharge can be treated with bromocriptine.

Single duct serous or serosanguineous discharge is most commonly due to an intraduct papilloma, which is often excised to exclude papillary malignancy. In the peri- and postmenopausal age group investigations may include mammography and duct excision as preinvasive carcinoma may also present in this way.

Multicoloured discharge (green, yellow, brown, or inky blue) from multiple ducts is usually caused by duct ectasia. Duct excision is only necessary if the discharge is profuse and aesthetically unpleasant. Periductal fibrosis can result in nipple inversion (classically resulting in a linear, slit-like inversion).

Miscellaneous

Benign conditions of the nipple/areola complex include retention cysts of Montgomery's glands, benign pedunculated polyps, and nipple adenomas. The areola is a common site for eczema, which must be differentiated from Paget's disease as the latter is usually associated with underlying intraduct carcinoma.

Breast pain

Mastalgia can be classified as cyclical or noncyclical depending on its relationship to the menstrual cycle. Cyclical pain may need no treatment other than reassurance. If severe, danazol (a luteinizing hormone-releasing hormone analogue), bromocriptine, or tamoxifen may be used, but all have significant side effects. Noncyclical pain originating from the chest wall is treated with nonsteroidal anti-inflammatory drugs.

Breast inflammation

Obstruction to milk drainage can result in lactational mastitis or abscess. In young women who smoke, inflammation around ducts can present with a sterile inflammation (periductal or plasma cell mastitis), or with an abscess if secondary infection occurs. This can progress to form a mammillary fistula.

Granulomatous mastitis is uncommon, the diagnosis being made after excluding infection, especially tuberculosis, and other granulomatous conditions (e.g. sarcoidosis). Mondor's disease (superficial thrombophlebitis of a chest wall vein) results in a tender cord-like thickening running vertically in the subcutaneous tissues.

Benign conditions of the male breast

Hypertrophy of the ductal and stromal tissue (gynaecomastia) is a common finding at puberty and with failing testicular function, and is commonly unilateral. At other ages it may be idiopathic, but specific causes include drugs (e.g. digoxin, phenothiazines, spironolactone, and methyldopa), hormone secreting tumours (most commonly testicular or bronchial), and cirrhosis. Other benign conditions can occur in men, but are much less common than in women.

Further reading

Hughes LE, Mansel RE, Webster DJ (1987). Aberrations of normal development and involution (ANDI): a new perspective on pathogenesis and nomenclature of benign breast disorders. *Lancet*, **2**, 1316–19.

13.8.5 Sexual dysfunction

Ian Eardley

Essentials

Male sexual dysfunction

Erectile dysfunction—the inability to attain or maintain an erection satisfactory for sexual intercourse. It affects about 50% of men over the age of 40 years and can be caused by neurological, vascular, endocrine, and psychiatric diseases, and by drugs, with psychogenic and organic risk factors coexisting in most men. Specific remedies can cure erectile dysfunction in a few patients: the mainstay of treatment in most will be oral therapy using a phosphodiesterase type 5 inhibitor.

Penile deformity—usually due to Peyronie's disease: there is no licensed medical therapy and treatment is by surgical correction of any debilitating deformity.

Prolonged erection (priapism)—this is a medical emergency, requiring urgent therapy to prevent loss of erectile function. Most cases are caused by reduced venous drainage of the corpus cavernosum, most commonly due to intracavernosal injections, sickle cell disease, other hyperviscosity syndromes, or the use of some psychotropic drugs. Treatment initially involves aspiration via a wide bore cannula of enough blood to produce detumescence.

Premature ejaculation—a common but poorly understood condition that has no licensed medical therapies and is best treated with psychosexual therapy.

Female sexual dysfunction

Hypoactive sexual desire—may affect up to one-third of women under the age of 50 years: its aetiology is commonly multifactorial, including complex interaction with relationship issues, and the motivation for and success of treatment is low.

Sexual arousal disorders—affect up to one-quarter of women and may be caused by psychological or physical factors: treatment is directed towards the predominant aetiological issues.

Anorgasmia—reported by up to 37% of women in association with many psychological and cultural influences: therapy is primarily psychosexual, particularly when the problem is lifelong.

Dyspareunia—reported by up to 15% of sexually active women and can be caused by organic, psychological, or couple-related factors. Vaginismus affects less than 1%, with vulvar vestibulitis the most common cause: treatment is often unsatisfactory.

Male sexual dysfunction

Male sexual function is a complex neurovascular event that can be affected by a number of disease processes resulting in problems of penile erection, ejaculatory difficulties, and disorders of desire. Of these, the most common dysfunctions encountered in clinical practice are erectile dysfunction, penile deformity, prolonged erections, and rapid (or premature) ejaculation.

Erectile dysfunction

Erectile dysfunction is defined as the inability to attain or maintain an erection satisfactory for sexual intercourse. The first modern (and perhaps most important) epidemiological study was the Massachusetts Male Aging Study, which reported the age-related prevalence in North American men. It is a common symptom that affects around 50% of men over the age of 40 years. The prevalence increases with age, and there are associations with a range of conditions including diabetes, hypertension, dyslipidaemia, and depression.

The physiology of penile erection is complex and involves the coordinated interaction of the neurological, vascular, and endocrine systems. Hence, there are many diseases of these systems that can lead to the development of erectile dysfunction, some of which are listed in Table 13.8.5.1. It is now recognized that both

Table 13.8.5.1 Common causes of erectile dysfunction

System	Disease
Neurological disease	Multiple sclerosis
	Spinal cord injury
	Multiple system atrophy
	Lumbar disc prolapse
	Cauda equina syndrome
	Peripheral autonomic neuropathy (e.g. diabetes)
Vascular disease	Atherosclerosis
	Hypertension
	Hyperlipidaemia
	Diabetes
Endocrine disease	Diabetes mellitus
	Hypogonadism
	Hyperprolactinaemia
	Hyperthyroidism
Psychiatric disease	Depression
	Anxiety states
Iatrogenic	Pelvic surgery (with nerve damage)
	Pelvic radiotherapy
	Drugs (see Table 13.8.5.2)
Multifactorial aetiologies	Renal failure

psychogenic and organic risk factors coexist in most men with erectile dysfunction, albeit to varying degrees. Secondary performance related anxiety often complicates the pathophysiology of men who have a primary organic aetiology. The most common cause of erectile dysfunction is that which arises secondary to vascular disease, with erectile dysfunction being a common coexisting symptom in men with hypertension, diabetes, hyperlipidaemia, and cardiovascular disease. Indeed, there is emerging evidence that erectile dysfunction may be one of the very earliest features of systemic vascular disease.

Since erectile dysfunction is a self-declared symptom, the fundamental basis of diagnosis is the clinical history. Mild cases are characterized by a history of difficulty in maintaining an erection, while in more severe cases there may be difficulty in initiating an erection or even loss of erections altogether. Assessment should seek to identify treatable causes (see Tables 13.8.5.1 and 13.8.5.2) and remediable risk factors. A predominantly psychogenic aetiology is suggested by the continued presence of nocturnal or early morning erections. Current guidelines suggest a focused physical examination of the genitalia, assessment of secondary sexual characteristics, and assessment of blood pressure. More extensive genitourinary and vascular examination is only performed when clinically indicated. Baseline investigations should include a fasting blood sugar, a lipid screen, and measurement of serum testosterone. The role of routine measurement of serum prolactin is controversial. Further assessment is usually unnecessary, although in selected cases vascular investigations (including colour Doppler assessment of penile vasculature) and more complex endocrine investigations might be indicated.

Table 13.8.5.2 Drugs that can cause sexual dysfunction in men

Drug type	Drug or class of drug	Effect
Antihypertensive drugs	Diuretics	ED
	Beta-Blockers	ED
	Centrally acting anti-hypertensive agents e.g. clonidine, methyl DOPA	ED
Centrally acting agents	Phenothiazines	ED, Reduced libido, Ejaculatory dysfunction
	Butyrophenones	ED
	Serotonin reuptake inhibitors	ED, Ejaculatory dysfunction
	Tricyclic antidepressants	ED, Reduced libido
	Phenytoin	ED, Reduced libido
Endocrine drugs	LHRH analogues	ED, Reduced libido
	Antiandrogens	ED, Reduced libido
	Oestrogens	ED, Reduced libido
Recreational drugs	Alcohol	ED, Reduced libido, Ejaculatory dysfunction
	Marijuana	ED
	Cocaine	ED
	Opiates	ED, Reduced libido
	Amphetamines	Reduced libido, Ejaculatory dysfunction
	Anabolic steroids	ED, Reduced libido
Other drugs	Cimetidine	ED, Reduced libido
	Metoclopramide	ED, Reduced libido
	Digoxin	ED

Specific remedies can cure erectile dysfunction in a few patients. For instance, in men with a predominantly psychogenic aetiology, psychosexual counselling is often valuable. In men with an endocrine cause (such as hypogonadism or hyperprolactinaemia), appropriate therapy is also helpful. Finally, in men who have developed erectile dysfunction following pelvic or perineal trauma, reconstructive vascular surgery may be effective. In most men, however, treatment aims to treat the symptom, rather than curing the underlying problem. Given the prevalence of secondary psychogenic problems, patient education and counselling is always valuable, but in most men who present with erectile dysfunction the mainstay of therapy will be oral therapy using a phosphodiesterase-5 inhibitor (PDE5i). Sildenafil was the first such licensed preparation, and two other drugs—tadalafil and vardenafil—have been marketed in recent years. There appears to be little difference in efficacy and tolerability between these drugs, with the major differences relating to pharmacokinetics. The drugs are used on demand, with ingestion 1 to 2 h prior to sexual activity. They are ineffective in the absence of sexual stimulation and a heavy meal may delay absorption. Around 70 to 80% of men will respond to such therapy, although the response rate is lower in some patient groups, such as diabetics and men who have undergone radical pelvic surgery. Side effects include headache, flushing, indigestion, and nasal congestion, although these are usually mild and well tolerated. Prolonged erections are seen extremely rarely with these drugs. Extensive research has not identified any significant cardiac risk with this class of drugs, although they are contraindicated in men using nitrate medication, and sexual activity is inadvisable in men with unstable cardiac disease. A detailed summary of the management of erectile dysfunction in men with cardiac disease can be found in the Princeton Consensus Statements.

In men with identifiable risk factors for erectile dysfunction, or an identifiable aetiology, there is only limited evidence that treatment of the risk factors provides benefit. One randomized trial suggested that weight reduction in men who had a raised body mass index might be beneficial over a 2 year period, although the improvements seen were limited.

In men who fail to respond to oral PDE5i therapy, a number of approaches can be tried, although there is little evidence that use of a different PDE5i is beneficial. Regular (daily) dosing appears to help some patients, the rationale reflecting experimental evidence that a PDE5i might improve endothelial function when taken regularly. Alternatively, optimization of coexistent medical conditions is occasionally helpful in this respect. In men who fail to respond to these manoeuvres, alternative therapies such as vacuum erection devices or intracavernosal self-injection of alprostadil are often effective. In a few patients even these treatments are ineffective or poorly tolerated, and under these circumstances insertion of a penile prosthesis may be indicated.

Penile deformity and Peyronie's disease

Although young men or adolescents occasionally present with a lifelong penile deformity (congenital curvature of the penis), the most common cause of penile deformity is Peyronie's disease, which is a localized connective tissue disease of the penis leading to fibrotic plaque formation in the tunica albuginea of the corpus cavernosum. It was first described by Fallopius in 1561, although the condition is named after François Gigot de la Peyronie, surgeon to King Louis XV of France, who described it in 1743.

In pathological studies there is subclinical disease in over 20% of men, but the clinical prevalence is about 1%. In some cases the condition can be familial, and there are associations with Dupuytren's contracture, plantar fasciitis, and tympanosclerosis. The peak incidence occurs in the 6th decade, but cases have been reported throughout adult life. The pathophysiology is poorly understood, but the most commonly held view suggests that there is damage of the tunica albuginea associated with microvascular trauma. This leads to extravasation and perivascular inflammation with a round cell infiltrate, which in turn leads to fibrin deposition and subsequently fibrosis.

Patients present with a palpable plaque within the penis, most commonly felt on the dorsum, and there is a curvature of the penis, most commonly in the dorsal direction. The disease typically progresses over 9 to 18 months, during which time it is said to be active. During this time the erection may be painful, the size of the plaque typically increases, and the deformity worsens until the disease stabilizes. When this happens, up to 20% of patients will get significant resolution of their deformity, and in only 30% of cases is the deformity significant enough to justify surgery.

Numerous medical treatments have been tried in men with Peyronie's disease. The oral agents that are most commonly used in clinical practice are Vitamin E, tamoxifen, colchicine, and potassium aminobenzoate, but controlled studies have failed to demonstrate a consistent benefit for any of them. The most commonly used intralesional (injectable) agents are steroids, verapamil and collagenase, and although some recent data from controlled studies suggests that the latter may be beneficial, further controlled studies are awaited.

Surgical treatment is reserved for those patients whose penile deformity prevents sexual activity, or those in whom sexual activity is painful either for the patient or his partner. The disease must be stable prior to surgical intervention, since disease progression after corrective surgery should be avoided. The most common surgical approach is a Nesbit's procedure, which involves surgical excision of an ellipse of a tunica albuginea on the opposite side of the penis to the plaque. The edges of the ellipse are apposed. Occasionally, a grafting procedure can be performed whereby the plaque is incised and grafted, typically with a patch of saphenous vein. A penile prosthesis is indicated in severe cases associated with coexistent erectile dysfunction.

Priapism

A priapism is a penile erection which is unduly prolonged and which persists in the absence of a sexual stimulus. The classification of priapism divides cases into those where the aetiology is arterial (high flow priapism) and those cases where the aetiology reflects reduced venous drainage of the corpus cavernosum (low flow priapism).

Low flow priapism is by far the more common form and reflects stasis of blood within the penis, with sludging within the cavernosal sinusoids and subsequent thrombosis. Ischaemia, hypoxia, and acidosis develop as a consequence, and this in turn prevents contraction of the penile smooth muscle, which then exacerbates the condition. Low flow priapism is a medical emergency and requires urgent treatment to avoid irreversible damage to the vascular endothelium and smooth muscle of the penis and its erectile capacity. Although comprehensive evidence is lacking, there are data to suggest that if treatment is successful within 24 h, then 56% of men will recover erectile function, while if treatment is delayed beyond that only 11% will recover potency. Low flow priapism can arise under a number of circumstances (see Table 13.8.5.3), the most common causes including intracavernosal injections, sickle-cell disease, other hyperviscosity syndromes, and the use of some psychotropic drugs.

Men with low flow priapism typically present with a painful erection, in contrast to high flow priapism which is painless, but a careful assessment should seek to differentiate low flow from high flow disorders (Table 13.8.5.4) and to identify the underlying cause. Aspiration of penile blood in low flow priapism reveals thick dark venous blood, which on blood gas analysis shows hypoxia, hypercapnia, and acidosis. Doppler scanning confirms lack of blood flow within the penis.

Treatment for priapism initially involves aspiration via a wide bore cannula of enough blood to produce detumescence, followed if necessary by irrigation with warm heparinized normal saline (see Figs. 13.8.5.1 and 13.8.5.2). If the erection reappears, then intracavernosal injection of a smooth muscle α-agonist such as phenylephrine is appropriate, with concurrent monitoring of the systemic blood pressure. A surgical shunting procedure is appropriate if this fails. However, if treatment is delayed too long (see above), then even shunting procedures fail and the only hope for long-term potency is a penile prosthesis.

When there is a specific coexistent condition, such as sickle-cell disease, specific treatment may be appropriate alongside treatment of the priapism. However, the traditional regimen of oxygen, intravenous hydration, and analgesia is often unsuccessful, and only in selected cases is exchange transfusion indicated.

High flow or nonischaemic priapism develops following perineal trauma, when the penile artery is lacerated, resulting in a fistula between the artery and the sinusoidal spaces of the penis. The priapism may appear at the time of injury, but more commonly develops some time later following relief of spasm of the artery. Because the blood flowing through the penis is arterial (i.e. there is no ischaemia), there can be some circumspection in relation to treatment. The diagnosis is usually made by Doppler scanning and subsequent selective pudendal arteriography, which typically shows an arterial blush in the penile artery. The treatment of choice is embolization of the fistula with autologous blood clot.

Table 13.8.5.3 Causes of low flow priapism

Type	Example
Hypercoagulability disorders	Sickle-cell disease Myeloma Leukemia Thalassaemia Total parenteral nutrition
Drugs	Intracavernosal agents (e.g. alprostadil) Psychotropic agents (e.g. phenothiazines, butyrophenones, trazodone) Anticoagulants (e.g. warfarin, heparin) Antihypertensives (e.g. α-blockers, calcium channel blockers)
Miscellaneous	Lumbar disc disease Solid tumours affecting the base of the penis Genito-urinary sepsis Amyloidosis

Table 13.8.5.4 Features that help to differentiate low flow from high flow priapism

Findings	Low flow priapism	High flow priapism
History of perineal trauma	Rare	Common
History of coexistent blood disorder	Sometimes	Rare
History of recent intracavernosal injection	Sometimes	Rare
Corpora cavernosa rigid	Usually	Rare
Penile pain	Usually	Rare
Cavernosal blood gases	Hypoxia, hypercapnia, acidosis	Similar to arterial blood
Colour Doppler penis	Sluggish or absent flow	Normal flow with evidence of arterial turbulence

Rapid (premature) ejaculation

There is no universally accepted definition of premature ejaculation, which has plagued attempts to assess the prevalence of the condition, with some data suggesting that it is probably the most common of the male sexual dysfunctions, affecting between 21% and 32% of adult men. One approach to achieving an objective diagnosis has been to measure the intravaginal ejaculatory latency time, i.e. the time between vaginal penetration and ejaculation, but once again there is no clear consensus as to which time should be the cut-off between normal and abnormal, with 1 min and 2 min both being reported in the literature. Epidemiological data suggest that when the definition given to the condition by the American Psychiatric Association's *Diagnostic and Statistical Manual of Mental Disorders* (4th edition) is used, then men with a diagnosis of premature ejaculation have a much shorter intravaginal ejaculatory latency time than normal men (1.8 min vs 7.3 min).

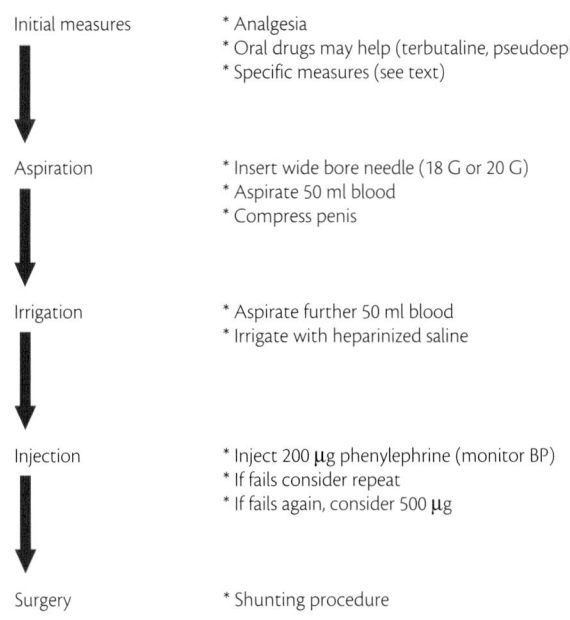

Fig. 13.8.5.1 Treatment of low flow priapism.

Initial measures
* Analgesia
* Oral drugs may help (terbutaline, pseudoephedrine)
* Specific measures (see text)

Aspiration
* Insert wide bore needle (18 G or 20 G)
* Aspirate 50 ml blood
* Compress penis

Irrigation
* Aspirate further 50 ml blood
* Irrigate with heparinized saline

Injection
* Inject 200 μg phenylephrine (monitor BP)
* If fails consider repeat
* If fails again, consider 500 μg

Surgery
* Shunting procedure

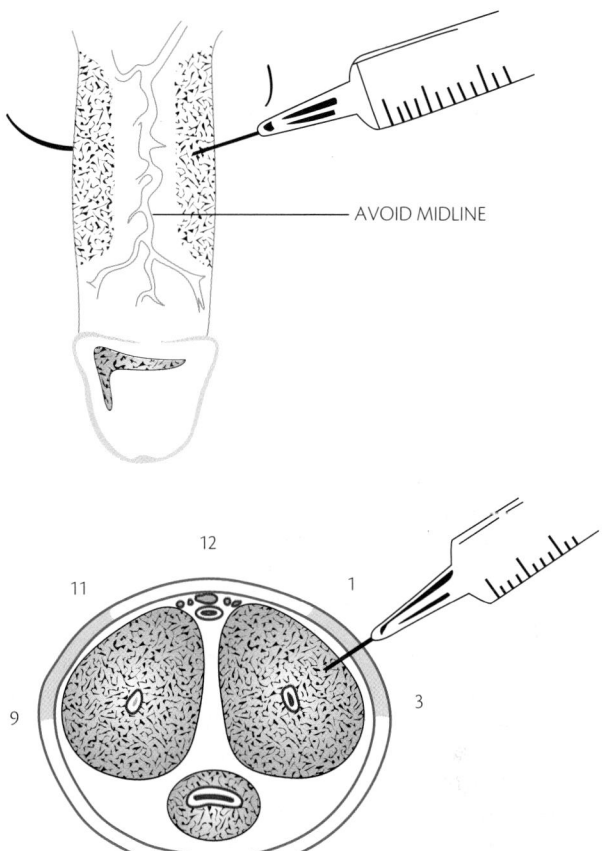

Fig. 13.8.5.2 Sites for safe aspiration of blood from the penis in low flow priapism are between 1 and 3 o'clock and between 9 and 11 o'clock.

Premature ejaculation is traditionally categorized into primary (lifelong) and secondary (acquired) types. The aetiology is poorly understood, with many potential pathophysiological mechanisms being proposed and none proven. Many men with premature ejaculation do not seek treatment, although there is evidence that there can be deleterious effects upon self-esteem, interpersonal relationships, and quality of life. When patients do seek medical attention, it is important to look for coexistent sexual dysfunctions (erectile dysfunction is commonly present) and to assess the degree to which relationship issues are important.

Therapy usually involves sex therapy and psychotherapy in the first instance. Although commonly successful in the short term, such approaches may not lead to a long-term cure. Currently there are no licensed pharmacological treatments for premature ejaculation, although there is some evidence that both selective serotonin re-uptake inhibitors and PDE5is may have a role. A number of pharmacological agents are currently undergoing development, including topical local anaesthetic sprays and short acting selective serotonin re-uptake inhibitors.

Female sexual dysfunction

The sexual problems of women have, until recently, received much less attention from the medical and scientific community than male sexual problems. This is reflected in a less well developed understanding of physiological and pathophysiological processes, in a less well defined classification of dysfunctions, and in a smaller

Table 13.8.5.5 A classification of female sexual dysfunction

Category	Subcategory
Disorders of desire	Interest desire disorders
	Sexual aversion disorders
Disorders of arousal	Subjective arousal disorders
	Genital arousal disorders
	Combined subjective and genital arousal disorders
	Persistent arousal disorder
Orgasmic disorders	
Pain disorders	Dyspareunia Vaginismus

range of therapeutic interventions. One classification of female sexual dysfunction is shown in Table 13.8.5.5. Epidemiological studies, although relatively immature, suggest that female sexual disorders are common and that they relate in part to age and to hormonal status. Comorbidities are common and should be identified, and the different sexual dysfunctions commonly coexist.

Sexual desire disorders

Hypoactive sexual desire disorder can be defined as absent or diminished feelings of sexual interest or desire, absent thoughts or fantasies, and a lack of responsive desire. This lack of interest will be greater than that which is normally seen with ageing and with the length of a relationship.

Epidemiological studies suggest that it affects up to 32% of women under the age of 50 years. It becomes more common with increasing age and with the onset of the menopause, whether natural or surgically induced. Around half of the women who have this condition are distressed by it, with the degree of distress diminishing with increasing age. Women with a surgically induced menopause are more likely to be distressed than those who have undergone a more natural menopause.

The physiology and pathophysiology of desire is poorly understood, but probably resides biologically in the limbic system of the brain, where hormonal influences, including oestrogens and androgens, are important. Other hormonal abnormalities including hyperprolactinaemia and thyroid dysfunction can also result in sexual desire disorders. The dominant neurotransmitters include dopamine, which is important in the seeking–appetite–lust system, and oxytocin, although as yet no pharmacological agents have any proven value. Other biological issues that are sometimes important include alcohol and recreational drug abuse. Psychological factors are also important in this condition, and their interaction with the biological issues makes this condition notoriously difficult to treat.

Clinical assessment includes a careful clinical history, which seeks to identify any psychological or physical issues. A full endocrine evaluation may be appropriate, which will include the measurement of serum testosterone, dehydroepiandrosterone sulphate, prolactin, 17β-oestradiol, and sex hormone-binding globulin.

Treatment is difficult and often unsuccessful, partly because the aetiology is commonly multifactorial, partly because of the complex interaction with relationship issues, but also because the motivation to be treated is often relatively low. Where physical causes can be identified, they should be treated, and indeed outcomes are best in the group of patients who have definite endocrine abnormalities and who are highly motivated. In other groups the results of therapy are often disappointing.

Sexual aversion disorders

Defined as severe anxiety or disgust at the thought of sexual activity, sexual aversion disorder may arise as a result of incest, rape, molestation, and psychological abuse. It may coexist with other anxiety disorders. Psychosexual therapy is the mainstay of treatment.

Sexual arousal disorders

Female sexual arousal includes the physiological responses of increased blood flow to the clitoris, the labia, and the vagina, leading to vasocongestion and engorgement. Vaginal lubrication appears to be a purely hydrostatic event, with transudation from the vaginal capillaries into the extracellular space. The physiology of these responses is poorly understood, but involves parasympathetic activation, with release of a number of neurotransmitters of which vasoactive intestinal peptide and nitric oxide are almost certainly the most important. There is concurrent relaxation of the vaginal smooth muscle with lengthening and dilation of the vagina. Systemically, there is an increase in the heart rate, flushing, and erection of the nipples.

There are three categories of arousal disorder. First, there is the so-called subjective arousal disorder, associated with a reduction in the feelings of sexual arousal (including sexual excitement and sexual pleasure), but with normal vaginal lubrication still occurring. Secondly, there may be genital sexual arousal disorder, when there is a definite and reduced degree of genital arousal in response to a sexual stimulus. Thirdly, the two may be found in combination.

Sexual arousal disorders are relatively common in the female population, affecting up to 24% of women. They are more common in older women, especially after the menopause, and the aetiology may be multifactorial. Psychological factors include reduced desire, sexual inhibition, anxiety, lack of intimacy, and male erection problems. Physical factors that may be important include endocrine abnormalities (e.g. reduced oestrogens, hyperprolactinaemia), vascular disease (e.g. diabetes), neuropathy (e.g. diabetes, multiple sclerosis), iatrogenic problems (e.g. post hysterectomy, post pelvic radiotherapy), and pain disorders (e.g. genital pain such as vaginismus, bladder pain due to recurrent urinary tract infection or interstitial cystitis).

Assessment should involve a careful history and examination, seeking to identify the range of risk factors that are present in an individual. Investigations might include an endocrine screen and, when indicated, Doppler assessment or plethysmography can evaluate vaginal and clitoral blood flow.

Treatment should be directed towards the predominant aetiological issues. Psychosexual methods are important for cases where subjective problems predominate. Physical treatments that may be of value include local lubricants, topical oestrogens (when vaginal atrophy and oestrogen deficiency are present), and local physical devices analogous to the vacuum erection devices used in male erection difficulties. Systemic hormone replacement therapy may be appropriate in some, but there are no licensed nonhormonal therapies for this condition. Given the physiological finding that nitric oxide is important in the control of vaginal blood flow, it was thought that the phosphodiesterase inhibitors such as sildenafil might have a role, but the results of clinical trials were relatively disappointing, and clinical development of these drugs for women has been halted.

Persistent sexual arousal disorder

This is a poorly documented but uncommon condition characterized by persistent genital arousal in the absence of a sexual stimulus.

The pathophysiology is unknown, and as such there is no recognized therapy.

Orgasmic disorders in women

Anorgasmia is reported in up to 37% of women, and in some women there may be marked delay or decrease in the intensity of the orgasm. The female orgasm is characterized by a transient sensation of intense pleasure, associated with rhythmic contractions of the pelvic floor musculature, often associated with uterine and anal muscular contractions. Although the nature of the orgasm changes with age (becoming shorter and less intense), there is no evidence that the prevalence of orgasmic disorders becomes more common with increasing age.

The physiology of the female orgasm is poorly understood, but in most cases involves clitoral stimulation, in association with an intact sacral reflex arc. Although it would seem logical that intact ascending neural pathways are necessary for a woman to experience an orgasm, patients with complete spinal cord transection can, on occasions, have the experience, hence it has been suggested that ascending fibres within the vagus nerve may be important.

There are multiple psychological and cultural influences on the ability of a woman to experience an orgasm. For instance, there is an inverse relationship between the degree to which a woman holds serious religious views and her ability to experience an orgasm. From a physical perspective, arousal disorders can result in delayed or absent orgasm. As such, therapy is primarily psychosexual, particularly when the problem is lifelong. When the problem is more recent in onset and associated with a physically induced sexual arousal disorder, then therapy should be directed at the arousal disorder. No pharmacological agents have shown any value in the treatment of this condition.

Sexual pain disorders in women

Dyspareunia is pain associated with attempted or complete vaginal entry; vaginismus indicates difficulties in the woman allowing entry of a penis (or any other object) into the vagina, despite her desire for this to happen. It is traditional to separate these two conditions, although in reality they may overlap, both in causality and in clinical presentation. Dyspareunia is reported by up to 15% of sexually active women, and it becomes much more common in the postmenopausal population. Vaginismus is far less common, affecting less than 1% of sexually active women.

Dyspareunia can be caused by a number of different conditions (see Table 13.8.5.6), and while these conditions can also cause vaginismus, there are cases where no clear organic aetiology appears to exist. Clinically, it is important to identify such causes when they do exist, and to identify and treat any sexual comorbidities.

Further reading

Male sexual dysfunction

Feldman HA, *et al*. (1994). Impotence and its medical and psychosocial correlates: results of the Massachusetts Male Aging Study. *J Urol*, **151**, 54–61.

Fonseca V, Jawa A (2005). Endothelial and erectile dysfunction, diabetes mellitus, and the metabolic syndrome: common pathways and treatments? *Am J Cardiol*, **96**(12B), 13M–18M.

Hatzimouratidis K, Hatzichristou DG (2005). A comparative review of the options for treatment of erectile dysfunction: which treatment for which patient? *Drugs*, **65**, 1621–50.

Hauck EW, *et al*. (2006). A critical analysis of nonsurgical treatment of Peyronie's disease. *Eur Urol*, **49**, 987–97.

Johannes CB, *et al*. (2000). Incidence of erectile dysfunction in men 40 to 69 years old: longitudinal results from the Massachusetts male aging study. *J Urol*, **163**, 460–3.

Kostis JB, *et al*. (2005). Sexual dysfunction and cardiac risk (the Second Princeton Consensus Conference). *Am J Cardiol*, **96**, 313–21.

McMahon CN, Smith CJ, Shabsigh R (2006). Treating erectile dysfunction when PDE5 inhibitors fail. *BMJ*, **332**, 589–92.

Montorsi F, Salonia A (2006). Medical therapy for premature ejaculation. *Lancet*, **368**, 894–896.

Padma-Nathan H, *et al*. (2004). Pharmacotherapy for erectile dysfunction. *J Sex Med*, **1**, 128–40.

Patrick DL, *et al*. (2005). Premature ejaculation: An observational study of men and their partners. *J Sex Med*, **2**, 358–67.

Pryor J, *et al*. (2004). Peyronie's disease. *J Sex Med*, **1**, 110–15.

Pryor J, *et al*. (2004). Priapism. *J Sex Med*, **1**, 116–20.

Rogers ZR (2005). Priapism in sickle cell disease. *Hematol Oncol Clin North Am*, **19**, 917–28.

Travison TG, *et al*. (2007). The natural progression and remission of erectile dysfunction: results from the Massachusetts Male Aging Study. *J Urol*, **177**, 241–6.

Wespes E, *et al*. (2006). EAU Guidelines on erectile dysfunction: an update. *Eur Urol*, **49**, 806–15.

Female sexual dysfunction

Basson R (2002). The complexities of female sexual arousal disorder: potential role of pharmacotherapy. World J Urol, 20(2), 119–26.

Basson R, *et al*. (2004). Women's sexual desire and arousal disorders and sexual pain. In: Lue TF, *et al*. (eds) *Sexual medicine: sexual dysfunctions in men and women: 2nd International Consultation on Sexual Dysfunctions*, pp. 851–974. Health Publications, Paris.

Basson R, *et al*. (2004). Revised definitions of women's sexual dysfunction. *J Sex Med*, **1**, 40–8.

Hatzichristou D, *et al*. (2004). Clinical evaluation and management strategy for sexual dysfunction in men and women. *J Sex Med*, **1**, 49–57.

Leiblum S, *et al*. (2005). Persistent sexual arousal syndrome: a descriptive study. *J Sex Med*, **2**(3), 331–7.

Meston CM, *et al*. (2004). Disorders of orgasm in women. *J Sex Med*, **1**, 66–8.

Segraves R, Woodard T (2006). Female hypoactive sexual desire disorder: History and current status. *J Sex Med*, **3**, 408–18.

Table 13.8.5.6 Causes of dyspareunia

Organic	Superficial and introital	Infections (vulvitis, vulvar vestibulitis, cystitis, vaginitis)
		Hormonal (vaginal atrophy)
		Anatomic (fibrous hymen, vaginal agenesis)
		Muscular (hyperactivity of levator ani)
		Iatrogenic (post surgical, post radiation)
		Neuropathic
	Deep	Endometriosis
		Pelvic inflammatory disease
		Chronic pelvic pain syndrome
		Iatrogenic (postsurgical, postradiation)
Psychological	Comorbidity with other disorders of female sexual function	
	Previous sexual abuse or rape	
	Depression and anxiety	
Couple related	Inadequate foreplay	
	Couple conflicts	
	Sexual dissatisfaction	
	Anatomical compatibility issues	

13.9

Disorders of growth and development

Contents

13.9.1 Normal growth and its disorders

Gary Butler

Essentials

Normal growth has three phases: rapid in infancy and adolescence, steady during mid childhood. Height should always be interpreted within the context of the family: short or tall stature is often familial; idiopathic short stature occurs when the height of a normal child is below their target range.

Failure of growth

Aetiology and investigation—constitutional growth delay is a common normal variant, but poor growth and/or weight gain may be associated with recognized and unrecognized chronic disease, and also with psychosocial deprivation. Investigation must exclude conditions including hypothyroidism, coeliac disease, inflammatory bowel disease and chronic kidney disease. Turner syndrome (karyotype 45,X) should be suspected in all girls presenting with growth failure, and skeletal dysplasia when a child is either short for their family or has one parent of significant short stature. Growth hormone (GH) deficiency—confirmed by a poor response to stimulation tests and low IGF-1 levels—may occur in isolation or in association with one or more additional pituitary hormone deficiencies, and may be genetic or acquired (usually from intracranial tumour).

Management—GH (given by daily subcutaneous injection) may restore growth potential completely in children with GH deficiency, and (usually in larger doses) can improve growth and may be appropriate for some children with conditions including, chronic kidney disease, Turner syndrome, Prader–Willi syndrome, *SHOX* deficiency, and those who were born small for gestational age.

Excessive growth

Aetiology and investigation—constitutional tall stature, often associated with obesity, is a common normal variant, but conditions that can present with tall stature include: (1) genetically identifiable syndromes – e.g. Marfan's syndrome, Klinefelter's syndrome (karyotype 47,XXY), 47, XYY boys; (2) any condition leading to precocious sexual maturation (see Chapter 13.9.2); (3) pituitary gigantism—a rare condition caused by a pituitary somatotroph macroadenoma secreting large quantities of GH.

Management—attempts at growth limitation with high dose sex steroids are not often effective and may have short- and long-term complications, but induction of early puberty with conventional hormone doses may offer some help. Absolute cessation of limb growth can only be obtained by epiphysiodesis.

Introduction: what is normal growth?

The growth of a person from a fertilized egg to a mature individual is a remarkable process involving many hundreds of thousands of synchronized steps, with size having increased a million-fold. Yet it is noteworthy that not only do the heights of adult men and women each fall within quite a narrow range, but so does the growth of children at each age. For growth, we usually mean height and weight. Therefore, it is relatively easy to define what is normal and this normal range for age is represented on standard growth charts (see Figs. 13.9.1.1 and 13.9.1.2). Even though some variability exists between people of different ethnic backgrounds, the pattern of growth is remarkably constant, which is why the World Health Organization has been able to produce for the first time truly

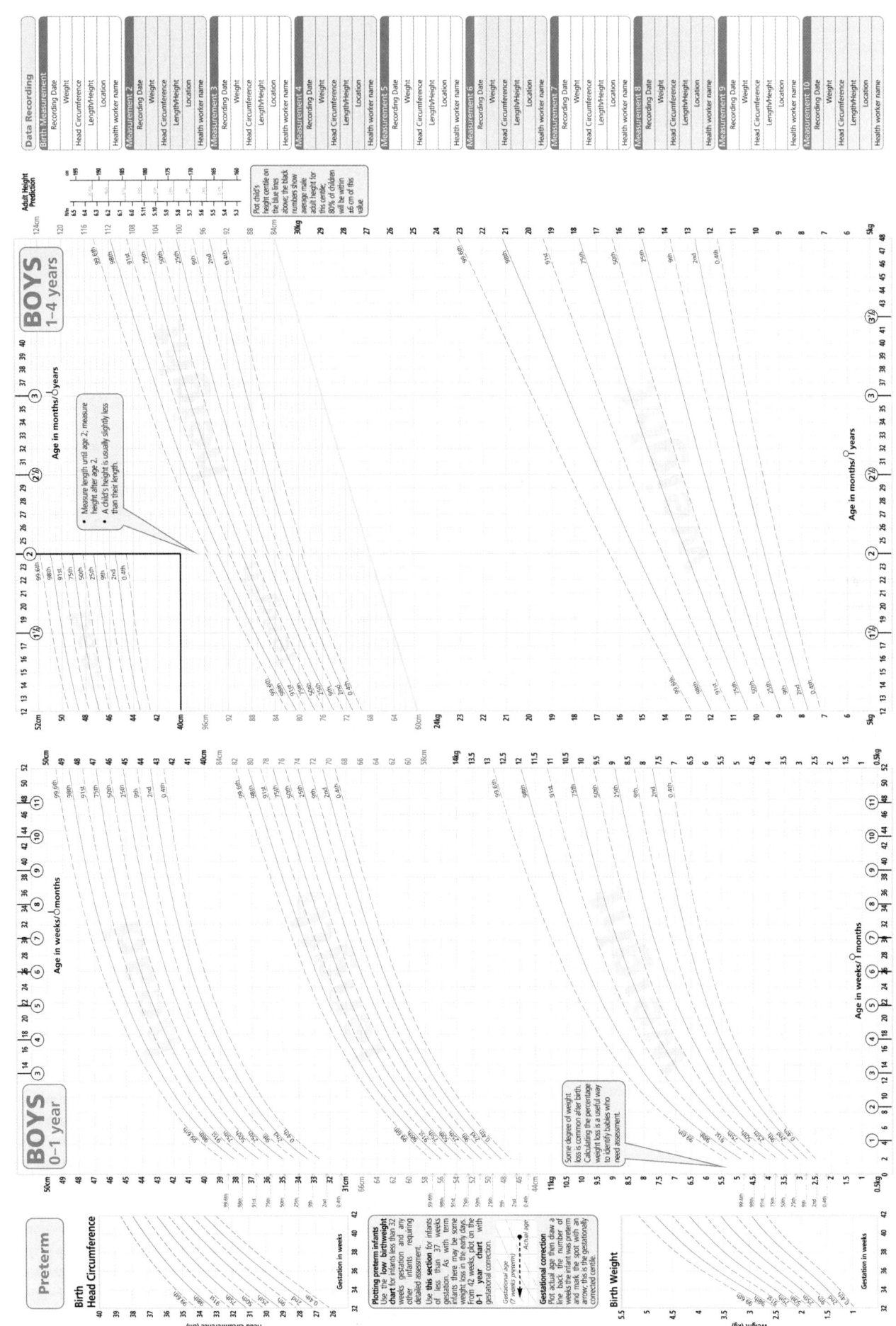

Fig. 13.9.1.1 UK-WHO growth standards 0–4 years in boys © 2009 Department of Health.

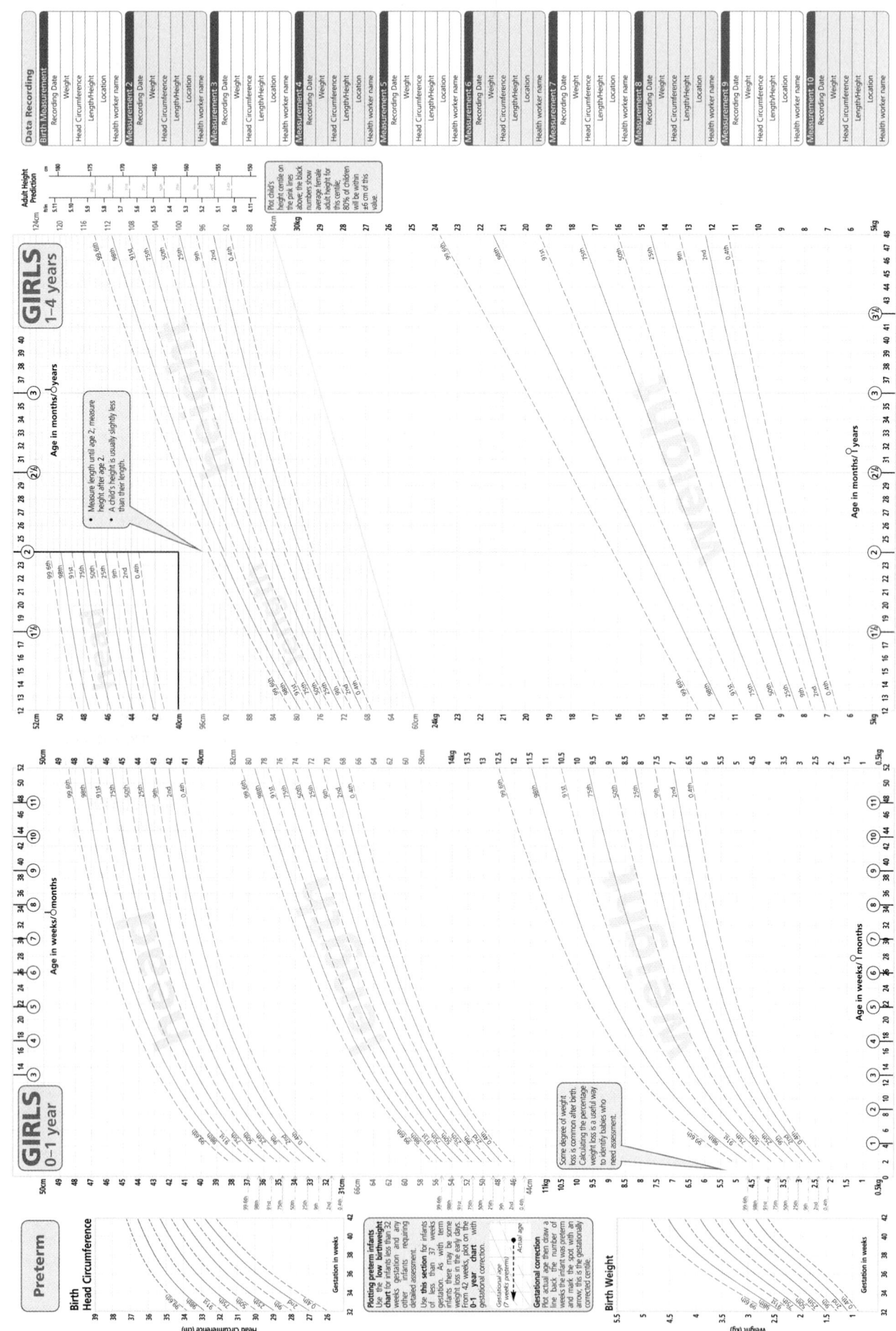

Fig. 13.9.1.2 UK-WHO growth standards 0–4 years in girls © 2009 Department of Health.

international growth reference standards. Of course, not all parts of the body grow at the same rate at the same time and spurts of growth can be seen at many different ages.

Before considering the problems of growth (summarized in Table 13.9.1.1), it is helpful to understand the three phases of postnatal growth separately: infancy, childhood, and adolescence.

Infancy

Growth is most rapid in the first year of life. Despite a normal weight loss of up to 10% in the first two weeks of life, weight will triple from a mean of 3.5 kg at birth to 10 kg and length increases by 50% from 50 cm to 75 cm, with a height velocity of 25 cm per year. Head circumference, which reflects brain growth, increases by one-third over the year, two-thirds of this occurring within the first 6 months.

Much tracking of growth measurements (movement upwards or downwards across centile bands) takes place over this first 6 months. Weight, length, and head circumference may each shift as much as two centile bands which, if a downwards move, may pose difficulties in the differential diagnosis of failure to thrive, but in normal growth variants this will cease once the genetic or preprogrammed centile has been attained. There are several reasons for this. First, size at birth principally tends to reflect maternal height and also placental function. Second, in the absence of disease, growth will follow a genetically determined trajectory. Adequate nutrition is a highly important factor in determining normal growth and has a fundamental influence during infancy.

A good example of shifts in growth centiles is catch-up growth exhibited by infants who have been subject to intrauterine growth retardation. Unless there are other constraints, more than 95% will show full catch-up of length and weight by the end of the first year and 98% by 2 years of age. This should not be confused with infants of preterm birth whose relative size may be attributed to their

Table 13.9.1.1 Principal causes of abnormalities in growth and stature

Short stature	Tall stature
Familial short stature	Familial tall stature
Constitutional delay of growth and/or puberty	Constitutionally advanced growth and/or puberty (constitutional tall stature)
Idiopathic short stature	Obesity
Small for gestational age/intrauterine growth retardation	Precocious sexual maturation
Psychosocial short stature	Supernumerary sex chromosomes, e.g. Klinefelter's, XYY, XXX
Chronic disease: recognized and unrecognized	Genetic/dysmorphic tall stature syndromes, e.g. Marfan's, Sotos, Beckwith–Wiedemann
Endocrine gland disorders including GH deficiency	
Genetic abnormalities of the GH axis	
Chromosomal variations including *SHOX* deletions	
Genetic/dysmorphic short stature syndromes, e.g. Turner's, Russell–Silver, Noonan's	
Skeletal dysplasias	

prematurity. Here, by convention, measurements are adjusted for gestational age up until their first birthday for those born after 32 weeks gestation and their second birthday for those below 32 weeks gestation.

Childhood

The childhood phase of growth lasts from the second year of life until the clinical onset of puberty. The rate of height and weight gain is less rapid than in infancy and is similar between boys and girls until the onset of puberty. This phase of growth is largely under the control of hormonal factors most notably growth hormone (GH) and insulin-like growth factor 1 (IGF-1). There are also environmental influences such as the seasons and health and endogenous rhythms which produce spurts of growth, the largest of which at around about 6 years of age is known as the mid-childhood growth spurt. This is one of a series of prepubertal growth spurts occurring approximately every 2 years. Although there is a temporal association with adrenarche which is the maturation of the adrenal cortex to produce adrenal androgens, there is no direct link between this new phase of adrenal physiology and growth as the prepubertal growth spurts are multiple and the mid-childhood spurt, although the most consistent, is not necessarily the largest prepubertal growth spurt.

Adolescence

The most marked difference in growth between the sexes starts during puberty. The total height gain in the male during this period is 25 to 30 cm, greater than in the female which is 20 to 25 cm. However, most of the 14 cm average difference between men and women occurs before the onset of the adolescent growth spurt. Approximately 11 to 12 cm is accounted for by boys continuing to grow at the prepubertal growth rate for a further 2 years until the onset of the faster pubertal growth spurt which contributes 2 to 3 cm more height than in girls.

Although the rapid acceleration in growth is coincident with the clinical and hormonal onset of puberty in both sexes, it is much more intense and hence more immediately noticeable in girls and they will attain the maximum growth rate (peak height velocity) 1 year after starting puberty, whereas in boys the acceleration is far more gradual and peak growth occurs 2 years after the onset of puberty.

Disorders of growth

Simple errors

Quite often children who are thought to have a growth disorder turn out not to; the apparent problem is due to an error in measurement or in plotting on a growth chart. Simply repeating these procedures if an odd pattern of growth is seen will usually reveal the problem. Genuine growth disorders demonstrate a continued trend, whether this is acceleration or deceleration of growth at inappropriate times or weight loss or gain when unexpected or at an unusual age.

Growth standards

Current UK-WHO charts aged 0-4 years are based on the WHO growth standards which are derived from prospectively collected data from over 8000 infants in 6 countries around the world until 5 years of age (see Figs. 13.9.1 and 13.9.2). These infants were breast fed and reared in optimal socioeconomic circumstances. They represent the ideal pattern of growth in health and are suitable for all ethnic groups. Charts are available in centile format (commonly used in the UK and US) and standard deviation format preferred in other European countries. Beyond age 4 years the UK 1990 growth charts (see Figs. 13.9.3 and 13.9.4) continue to be used until replaced by new data.

Familial short stature

From short parents generally come short children. The target centile range can generally be estimated from the information provided on national growth standards. In the United Kingdom a relatively simple formula is applied. The target or mid-parental height is a simple mean of the parents' height adjusted for the 14 cm mean male–female difference. Thus, target height for a boy is the parental mean plus 7 cm, and for a girl the target height is the parental mean minus 7 cm. The centile range within which most children of these biological parents will fall is 10 cm either side of the target height for boys and 8.5 cm for girls. Other formulae may include an adjustment for the secular trend towards increased intergenerational stature (c.1 cm per decade).

The term 'genetic short stature' should be avoided in this situation as it is imprecise and the meaning can be confused with small size from a chromosomal or single gene abnormality.

Children with short stature of familial origin grow normally with no deviation from their centile position. Assessment of height velocity over 1 year can confirm this. Clinical examination is unremarkable, children having normal body proportions, and pathological estimations are also normal. However, in real life situations, several causes of short stature may coexist or overlap, e.g. familial short stature and constitutional growth delay, causing a greater than expected slowing of growth. Experienced clinical judgment is often necessary in situations like this and investigations may need to be performed for reassurance purposes.

Once a familial cause of short stature is confirmed, the principal approach to management is reassurance of the child and their family. Some parents may wish to seek advantage for their child by requesting growth promoting treatments such as GH but evidence suggests that there is no significant height gain in either the short or the long term in these children.

Constitutional delay of growth and puberty

Although a delayed process of growth and maturation may present with short stature and delayed puberty, most often in boys, the process of slowing of growth starts much earlier and generally has a predictable pattern. Infants are of normal size at birth, but weight and length may begin decelerating in the first year, and can cause significant cause for concern as nonorganic failure to thrive may be considered. The rate of growth is low normal, rarely subnormal, but height and weight may show only barely acceptable gains, with the children remaining below the normal centile range until catch-up growth occurs during puberty. These children are phenotypically normal and in very good health, and the only usual finding on investigation is a moderately delayed bone age (1 to 3 years). When the height for bone age is plotted on the centile chart this often falls within the target centile range. Once identified, reassurance is all that is required, but a boost to growth and

sexual development may be given with low dose sex steroids if there is anxiety related to slow sexual development and growth in the mid-teenage years.

Idiopathic short stature

This term, more precisely defined as nonfamilial, non-GH deficient short stature, is inclusive of many pathologies. Children whose height lies 2.5 standard deviations below the mean and whose height falls below their target centile range are considered to have idiopathic short stature. Some children exhibit an appropriate height velocity and maintain their growth centile position, whereas others may grow slowly on the borderline of abnormal (c.4 cm/year). General investigations are unremarkable, and bone age may only be slightly delayed (<2 years). The GH response to stimulation tests is normal. The disparity between this normal response to GH provocation and an abnormal disorganized pattern of physiological secretion has been described as neurosecretory dysfunction, but in reality there may be many causes. One possibility is polymorphisms in the GH receptor with various alleles showing a different GH responsiveness.

If GH treatment is given to children whose abnormal growth pattern falls tightly within this definition, a good growth response to GH can be seen almost equivalent to that of true GH deficiency itself. Given diagnostic uncertainties in any case, there may be a case for GH treatment using the same dosage regimen, and this is an approved indication in the United States of America. However, there are inevitable accusations of advantage manipulation and social engineering which could be true if the precise definitions are not adhered to.

Small for gestational age

Infants born with weight and/or length 2 standard deviations below the mean (2nd centile) are stated to be small for gestational age. This usually arises by a process of intrauterine growth retardation, but the terms are not interchangeable and indeed definitions differ. Obstetric practice will usually refer to intrauterine growth retardation as fetal measurements falling below the 10th centile for gestational age and maternal size. The causes of intrauterine growth retardation may be extrinsic to the fetus such as placental dysfunction or twin–twin placental steal syndrome, or intrinsic such as insulin resistance or genetic reasons such as deletion of a paternally imprinted growth gene or the equivalent maternal uniparental disomy. This latter cause may account for approximately 10% of those children with clinical Russell–Silver syndrome (see below).

The diagnosis is reached from the obstetric history and subsequent postnatal growth pattern. In addition to intrauterine growth retardation there is often a sustained period of feeding difficulties and poor growth, often provoking much anxiety as general pathology investigations are normal and fears of child protection issues are often raised. The infants are usually thin with little adipose tissue and may have a disproportionately large head, head circumference being within the normal centile range, length and weight 2 standard deviations below the mean. In some cases, Russell–Silver syndrome may be defined clinically. These children show a typical triangular facies with frontal bossing, a pointed chin, clinodactyly of the fifth fingers and toes, and in about 50% there is some hemihypertrophy which may be quite subtle. In about 7 to 10%

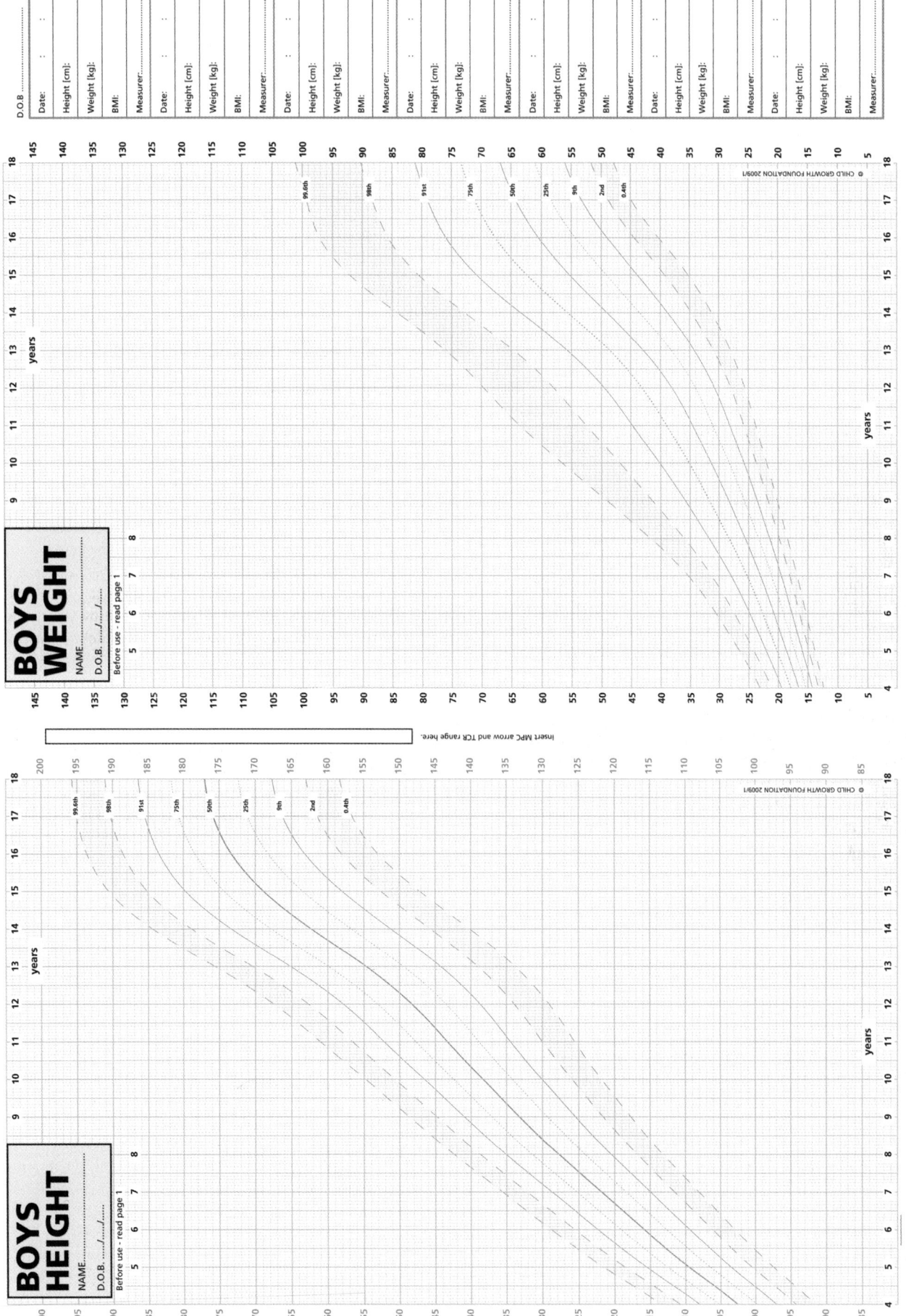

Fig. 13.9.1.3 United Kingdom 1990 standard centile chart for height, weight, years in boys 4–18. (© Child Growth Foundation).

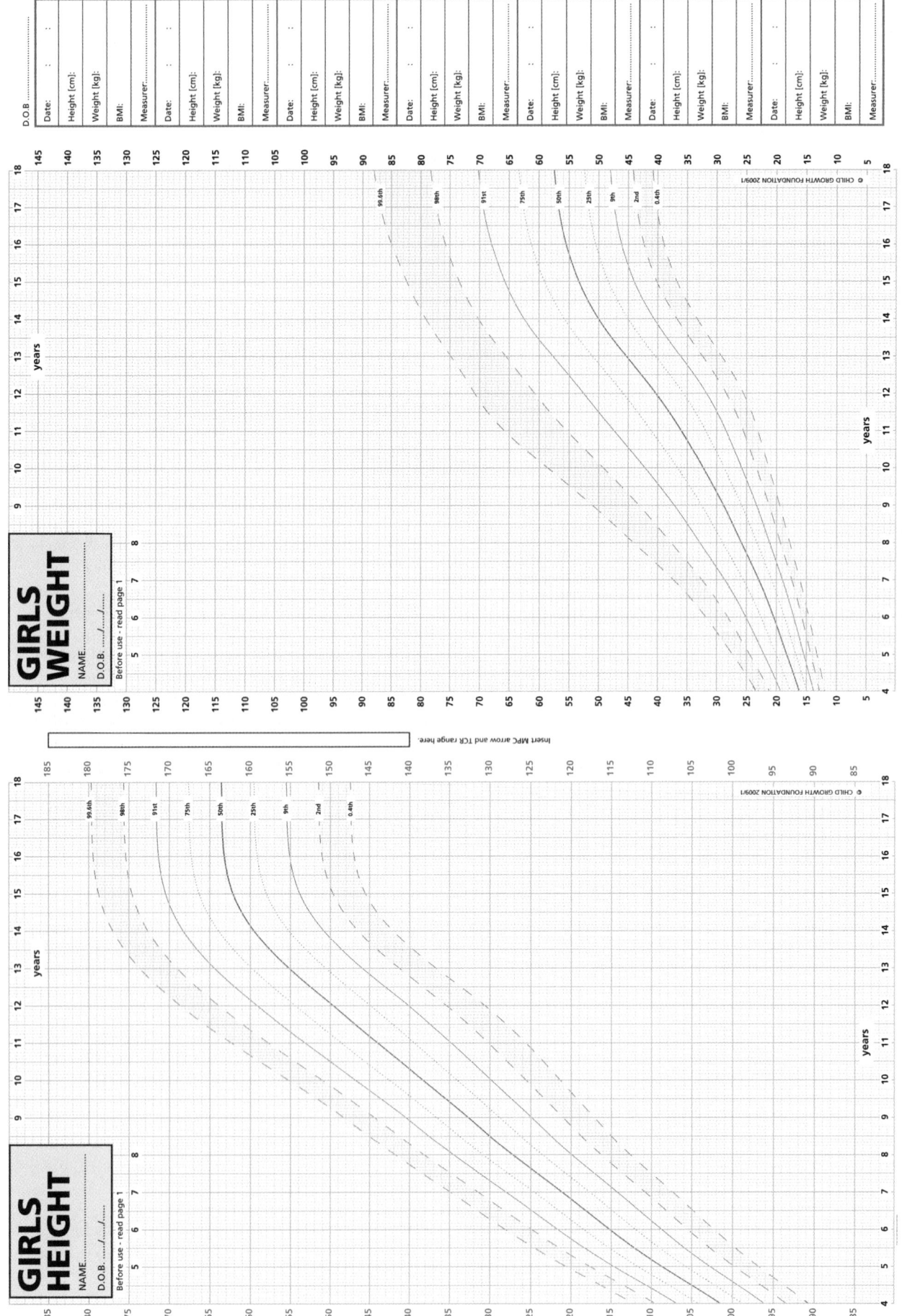

Fig. 13.9.1.4 United Kingdom 1990 standard centile chart for height, weight, years in girls 4–18. (© Child Growth Foundation).

of suspected cases, uniparental disomy of the maternal chromosome 7 can be identified, suggesting that it is an imprinted paternal gene which is required for normal growth. Recent studies have also suggested that imprinting defects within the 11p15 region play a role.

Bone age is often isochronological in children who do not show any catch-up growth, and consequently height prognosis is below the target centile range and often more than 2 standard deviations below the mean. For children over 4 years of age, GH treatment in doses between 35 and 67 µg/kg per day (1.0–1.7 mg/m^2 per day) have shown a dose dependent initial catch-up and gradual acceleration to adult heights within the normal range. Overall growth gain may be predicted from the first year response. Although some slight increase in insulin sensitivity and baseline glucose may be found, this is non progressive and reversible on stopping GH and long-term studies show continued benefits of having had GH treatment with lower blood pressure and an improved metabolic profile.

Pathological causes of growth failure

Recognized and unrecognized chronic disease

Part of the assessment process of any child presenting with an abnormality of growth is exclusion of other chronic conditions which may manifest initially as a variant of growth. Excess growth can result from overactivity of the thyroid gland as well as other nonendocrine causes of early puberty such as obesity. Slow growth is the more common, but usually less marked than it used to be in childhood diseases such as chronic renal insufficiency, cystic fibrosis, type 1 diabetes, and inflammatory bowel disease as a result of much improved nutrition and clinical management of these conditions.

Growth failure maybe the only presenting feature of conditions such as hypothyroidism, coeliac disease, inflammatory bowel disease, or chronic renal insufficiency, so an initial screen should always include a full biochemical profile including vitamin D levels, a full blood count, inflammatory markers, thyroid function, and coeliac antibodies.

Juvenile arthritis may, in its own right, and as a result of steroid treatment cause significant retardation of growth which may not be amenable to full catch-up if this is longstanding. However, GH treatment at standard doses may help restore growth in some children. Chronic eczema and other atopies may subtly slow the tempo of growth resulting in short stature and delayed puberty, but height usually catches up completely although this may not occur until the late teens or early twenties.

Excess endogenous glucocorticoid secretion in Cushing's syndrome (adrenal pathology) or Cushing's disease (ACTH secreting pituitary tumour) may present with slow or absent growth as well as other clinical signs such as central obesity, malar flushing, and striae. This can almost always be differentiated from children with exogenous obesity who usually grow faster than the norm and are taller than expected for their age.

GH treatment is indicated in children with chronic renal insufficiency in a high dose regimen of 50 µg/kg per day (1.4 mg/m^2 per day) as soon as growth failure occurs, as long as nutrition is optimized. The main benefit is abolishing or slowing the decline in height velocity resulting from the uraemia.

Juvenile hypothyroidism

Bone age is often markedly delayed in juvenile acquired hypothyroidism. This is usually due to autoimmune thyroiditis and may often present insidiously with growth failure alone. Early recognition and treatment with levothyroxine at an initial dose of 100 µg/m^2 per day, titrated consequently to normalize thyroid function, will usually result in complete catch-up of growth.

Psychosocial short stature

Psychosocial short stature occurs in children and adolescents in association with psychological harassment and/or emotional deprivation and may be associated with transient abnormalities of the GH–IGF-1 axis. The clinical features can be very similar to those of GH deficiency, but children suffering from this syndrome usually have a disturbed family environment with a history or current evidence of child abuse, most commonly occult sexual abuse. A child with psychosocial growth failure tends to be isolated and may not participate in family activities. Behavioural disturbance and bizarre eating habits are common, with a tendency to hyperphagia rather than undernourishment.

Two main subtypes of psychosocial short stature have been identified. Early-onset growth failure (type I or infantile psychosocial short stature) occurs during the first 2 years of life, is very common and the cause is thought to be undernutrition. This manifests clinically as failure to thrive. If sufficient nutrition is given, these children usually begin to grow normally again.

Type II or childhood psychosocial short stature occurs in children older than 3 years. There is often a greater psychological component compared with type I psychosocial short stature. Failure to thrive is not such a marked feature and there may be a component of this in some patients diagnosed with constitutional growth delay. Abnormalities of GH secretion can be demonstrated, and these often resolve when the child is removed from the home environment. The clinical presentation is often a short child with growth failure and a normal body mass index, but paradoxical hyperphagia. In some situations, growth may not recover. In such children, full investigation into the abnormality is needed and if inadequate GH secretion remains, replacement will be needed.

Turner's syndrome

Turner's syndrome should be suspected in all girls presenting with short stature and/or poor growth. The incidence of all karyotypes together with complete or partial absence of one X chromosome, or a structurally abnormal X is approximately 1 in 2500. Girls with karyotype 45, X are more likely to show more features of the syndrome, including peripheral oedema in infancy, webbed neck, low ears, low posterior hairline, cubitus valgus (increased carrying angle at the elbow), widely spaced nipples, a high arched palate, multiple small pigmented naevi, small convex nails, recurrent otitis media and deafness, delayed puberty, amenorrhea and infertility due to ovarian dysgenesis, a higher prevalence of autoimmune hypothyroidism, and congenital heart disease of which coarctation of the aorta is the most common form.

Growth is decreased *in utero* resulting in a slightly reduced size at birth, and remains slow during infancy. The height velocity is subnormal during childhood and there is no pubertal acceleration of growth due to the absence of spontaneous oestrogen secretion.

In untreated individuals with Turner's syndrome, mean final height is approximately 143 cm. The short stature may be partly associated with haploinsufficiency of a homeobox-containing gene *SHOX* located on the pseudoautosomal region of the X and Y chromosomes.

Treatment with GH is now the norm, starting as soon as possible after diagnosis, even in infancy. Most benefit is gained with an early initiation of treatment, and predicted when there is a good first year response. The target GH dose is 45 to 50 µg/kg per day (1.4 mg/m² per day). Significant height gain may thus occur, with some girls attaining adult heights within the predicted normal range. The link with family height is retained. Puberty may be induced with low dose oestrogen (ethinlylestradiol), starting at 1 to 2 µg daily, increasing over approximately 2 years to 20 µg daily, at which time a cyclical progestogen should be added often using the combined oral contraceptive pill for convenience, but the timing should be as close to normal as possible as delaying this does not bring additional height gains.

SHOX deficiency

Deletions or mutations of a homeobox-containing gene *SHOX* located on the pseudoautosomal region of the X and Y chromosomes are a rare cause of short stature which may respond to GH treatment. This gene also has a role in the aetiology of abnormal bone morphology (such as the radio-ulnar synostosis in Leri-Weill syndrome) and sensorineural hearing loss.

Prader–Willi syndrome

This condition is caused by either a deletion of the paternally imprinted genes on 15q or maternal uniparental disomy of chromosome 15. Although often presenting at birth with extreme hypotonia and feeding difficulties, it is more often known for its association with obesity and hyperphagia and other hypothalamic dysfunction such as delayed or absent puberty and slow growth due to a reduction in the numbers of gonadotropin releasing hormone and GH-releasing hormone secretory neurons. Although adult stature is only modestly reduced (155 cm in men, 147 cm in women), GH replacement at 35 µg/kg per day (1.0 mg/m² per day) may reverse the slowdown in growth, but additionally improves body composition with increased lean body mass and may enhance motor development. Caution should be exercised in treating children with extreme obesity as sudden death within the first 6 months of GH therapy due to obstructive sleep apnoea has been reported.

Skeletal dysplasia

Skeletal dysplasia may be suspected when a child is either short for their family or has one parent of significant short stature also. Body disproportion may exist, such as discrepancy between upper and lower segment measurements, short arms (span less than height) or a disproportionately large head circumference. Most of the skeletal dysplasias are monogenic. The most common of the nonlethal genetic defects is achondroplasia which is caused by mutations in the *FGFR3* gene in the region 4p16.3. Several skeletal dysplasias are caused by mutations in genes that encode the family of fibroblast growth factor receptors which are tyrosine kinases and mutations within these proteins are thought to slow the rate of endochondral bone growth. Approximately 90% of cases of this disorder arise from *de novo* mutations. GH treatment may slow deceleration in some conditions, and may produce height gains in milder phenotypes, but is less effective than surgical limb-lengthening procedures. Individual evaluation should be performed.

GH deficiency (secondary IGF-1 deficiency)

The prevalence of GH deficiency has been variously reported as from 1 in 4000 to 1 in 9000 live births. Childhood-onset GH deficiency may be congenital or acquired, and may occur in isolation (isolated GH deficiency) or in association with one or more additional pituitary hormone deficiencies (multiple pituitary hormone deficiency), male–female ratio 2.2:1. Congenital GH deficiency may be caused by an inherited mutation or by a developmental abnormality. Acquired GH deficiency most frequently results from an intracranial tumour (craniopharyngioma, pituitary adenomas, or destructive lesions arising close to the hypothalamo-pituitary axis such as optic glioma associated with neurofibromatosis or secondary to treatment with surgery or irradiation (doses >2400 cGy) which can damage the hypothalamus. Neurofibromatosis type 1 may directly affect pituitary function, leading to growth failure and/or precocious puberty.

Genetic causes of GH deficiency

Four distinct familial types of isolated GH deficiency are caused by mutations in the *GH1* gene: type IA is inherited in an autosomal recessive manner and results in a complete absence of endogenous GH; type IB is also inherited in an autosomal recessive manner; type II isinherited in an autosomal dominant manner; and type III is X-linked. Endogenous GH levels are diminished compared with normal in types IB, II and III.

The development of the pituitary gland is controlled by a large number of genes and transcription factors. Several mutations in the gene encoding POU1F1 (formerly known as PIT1), a pituitary-specific transcription factor responsible for pituitary development and hormone expression, have been shown to result in combined pituitary hormone deficiencies often of delayed onset. Other mutations in genes encoding pituitary transcription factors, such as *PROP1*, *HESX1*, *LHX3*, and *LHX4*, have also been described.

Clinical features

The severity and duration of GH deficiency is usually reflected by the height deficit and the clinical appearance. Although GH has effects on fetal growth, manifested by a slightly reduced birth length and size, children with congenital GH deficiency may not present with growth failure until after the second year of life.

Children with GH deficiency have skeletal proportions that are normal for their age and some are overweight for their height. Central adiposity if it occurs has a classical marbled appearance. Head circumference is within the normal range for age, but growth of the facial bones may be delayed, with a tendency for crowding of the facial features in the centre of the face, giving a doll-like facies. Dentition and skeletal maturity are also delayed. The voice may be high pitched due to the small size of the larynx.

Significant hypoglycaemia only occurs in children with severe isolated GH deficiency, and this tendency to hypoglycaemia usually wanes beyond the age of 5 years. However, if there is concurrent deficiency of ACTH (i.e. multiple pituitary hormone deficiency), hypoglycaemia will be exaggerated. In these cases, treatment with both GH and glucocorticoids is required.

The clinical features are less marked in children with milder or partial forms of GH deficiency. If a child's height velocity over 1 year is low and other causes of growth failure have been excluded, the GH status should be assessed, along with other aspects of hypothalamo-pituitary function.

Biochemical diagnosis

Measurements of random serum GH concentrations are not helpful in diagnosing GH deficiency, as GH is secreted in a pulsatile manner. Subnormal IGF-1 and IGFBP3 levels are only confirmatory of the diagnosis, as low levels are often found in short slowly growing children. The diagnosis is made on the basis of a provocation test, which assesses GH secretory reserve, in combination with an IGF-1 level which, if low, confirms an IGF-1 deficiency secondary to the GH deficiency.

Various stimuli may be used, including insulin, glucagon, arginine, clonidine, and levodopa. The tests should be done using a standardized protocol after a prescribed fast dependent on the child's age and only where there are experienced medical and nursing staff supervising the child constantly, and where full resuscitation facilities are immediately available.

A peak GH concentration of less than 10 μg/litre has traditionally been used to support the diagnosis of GH deficiency. This value depends on the assay used and the recombinant GH reference preparation, and when there are different conversion factors between international reference units and mass based units. Lower spontaneous levels are seen prior to puberty and in obesity, both of which can give false positive results if not correctly interpreted. Peripubertal patients should have sex steroid priming prior to testing.

It is clear, therefore, that diagnosing GH deficiency can be imprecise due to an overlap with the spectrum of normality. The growth response to a trial of GH therapy is ultimately the best diagnostic test.

Treatment with GH

GH treatment in the standard regimen of 25 to 35 μg/kg per day given by subcutaneous injection starting as soon as possible after diagnosis may allow complete catch-up of growth, with final heights in both idiopathic GH deficiency and multiple pituitary hormone deficiency falling between −1.0 and −1.6 standard deviations (−0.1 to −0.3 standard deviations below mid-parental height). Although physiological GH secretion increases during puberty, current recommendations for altering the GH dose during adolescence are unclear.

Primary IGF-1 deficiency (GH insensitivity, Laron's syndrome)

This is a very rare disorder which phenotypically may be similar to the much more common severe GH insufficiency, but the growth retardation is much more severe. In primary IGF-1 deficiency there is excessive secretion of GH by the pituitary gland; the fault lies in the GH receptor, which is either absent or nonfunctioning, leading to undetectable levels of IGF-1 and its acid-labile subunit before and after a brief course of GH (the IGF-1 generation test). The abnormality is due to one of several mutations in the receptor gene, which is inherited according to an autosomal recessive pattern. Recently recombinant IGF-1 has been licensed in Europe and in the United States of America, following successful clinical trials.

Tall stature

Given our 'heightist' society, which values tallness over shortness, and the tendency for a secular trend in increasing stature from one generation to the next (by c.1 cm per decade), referrals for concern about tall stature are far fewer than for short stature. By definition, the extremes of stature in men and women (i.e. the 99.6th centile) of 196 cm and 180 cm respectively, seem shorter than those actually tolerated and accommodated in society. As with short stature, diagnosis of a disorder depends on whether there is rapid growth for chronological age or not.

Causes of tall stature with rapid growth

Genetically identifiable syndromes will cause rapid growth from infancy, but the clue to diagnosis is in the phenotype, e.g. large head circumference, classic elongated facies, and mild developmental delay in Sotos syndrome; hemihypertrophy, hyperinsulinism, and Wilms' tumour (nephroblastoma) in Beckwith–Wiedemann syndrome.

Marfan's syndrome is an autosomal dominant condition affecting connective tissue where tall stature may be associated with scoliosis, chest deformities, high arched palate and arachnodactyly, dislocation of the lenses, and dissection of the aorta. Tall stature is noticed from infancy with general accelerated growth. Cardiac assessment and follow-up is essential in all suspected cases.

Klinefelter's syndrome (47,XXY) males are of normal size in infancy, but height acceleration throughout childhood is more rapid than usual. Extreme adult tall stature can be predicted early on as all the excess growth occurs in the prepubertal years, the adolescent growth spurt being of normal size and duration, which is in contrast with 47,XYY males who may exhibit tall stature during infancy and childhood, but in whom the adolescent growth spurt is exaggerated.

Precocious sexual maturation

Rapid growth may occur as a result of premature sexual maturation resulting from any cause, and it is essential that this is excluded in a child with tall stature and increased height velocity (see Chapter 13.9.2).

Familial tall stature

Children coming from tall parents are expected to be tall, and are often long at birth; the same approach to diagnosis and predicting adult height can be followed as for familial short stature (see above). Height velocities are not excessive for their age, but in general tall children grow more quickly than short children and secrete larger amounts of GH and IGF-1.

Constitutionally advanced growth and puberty

Just as growth delay is a variant of growth at one end of the normal range, so is constitutional tall stature. Assessments such as bone age and dental age are advanced toward the upper end of the predicted range and children usually enter puberty within the early normal range. Consequently, the adolescent growth spurt is accelerated and growth will cease according to the normal pattern of events. This can cause distress for someone who is used to being a tall child but who may end up at an average or below average height as an adult. As better nutrition is leading to obesity in contemporary children, this accelerated growth pattern is becoming more common.

Pituitary gigantism

Pituitary somatotroph macroadenomas secreting large quantities of GH are extremely rare, but may present insidiously at any age. The classic phenotype of the pituitary giant with acromegaloid features is a late finding, but this diagnosis should be suspected in children of any age who are taller than predicted for their family and who do not show the clinical and radiological features of constitutional advance. As random GH and IGF-1 levels have low specificity, a GH suppression test with glucose loading and a cranial MRI scan may be required. Treatment is with a combination of surgery and somatostatin analogues.

Treatment of tall stature

Attempts at growth limitation with high dose sex steroids have not in general been successful and may have short- and long-term complications. An early and rapid induction of puberty with conventional hormone doses may offer some help. Absolute cessation of limb growth can only be obtained by epiphysiodesis.

Further reading

Brook CGD, Clayton PE, Brown RS (eds) (2005). *Clinical pediatric endocrinology*, 5th edition. Blackwell, Oxford.

Kelnar CJH, *et al.* (eds) (2007). *Growth disorders*, 2nd edition. Hodder Arnold, London.

Kelnar CJH, Butler GE (2008).Endocrine Gland Disorders and Disorders of Growth and Development.In: N McIntosh,
P Helms, R Smyth, S Logan (eds) *Forfar and Arneil's Textbook of Pediatrics*, pp. 409–512. Elsevier, Edinburgh.

Ranke MB, Price DA, Reiter EO (eds) (2007). *Growth hormone therapy in pediatrics*. Karger, Basel.

Royal College of Paediatrics and Child Health, Department of Health, UK-WHO growth charts. http://www.growthcharts.rcpch.ac.uk

World Health Organization. *WHO Child Growth Standards*. http://www.who.int/childgrowth/en/index.html

13.9.2 **Puberty**

I. Banerjee and P.E. Clayton

Essentials

Puberty is characterized by well-defined physical changes as a child moves from the prepubertal state through the stages of puberty to full sexual development. The outward signs usually develop over 3 to 5 years, with significant variation both in the age that puberty starts and the pace at which development proceeds.

The events that lead to the triggering of puberty remain uncertain, but clinical presentations may arise because the process is abnor-

mally early (precocious puberty) or abnormally late (delayed or absent puberty). A number of variants of the normal processes may also present for clinical assessment, e.g. premature isolated thelarche (breast development) or adrenarche (pubic and axillary hair development), which do not require treatment.

Precocious puberty

Aetiology—this may be either (1) central gonadotropin dependent—due to congenital or acquired central nervous system abnormalities, prolonged exposure to sex steroids, ectopic human chorionic gonadotropin (hCG), prolonged hypothyroidism; or (2) peripheral gonadotropin independent—due to ovarian or testicular overactivity, exogenous sex steroids.

Investigation—this requires measurement of sex steroids, thyroid function, a gonadotropin-releasing hormone (GnRH) provocation test with additional pituitary function testing, usually combined with radiological imaging of the pituitary gland. A nondominant wrist radiograph for determination of bone age (advanced in precocious puberty) helps to define the extent of precocity and the possible impact on growth prognosis. In girls, a pelvic ultrasound scan is required to define ovarian and uterine dimensions.

Management—the goals are to stop pubertal progression, improve final height prognosis, reduce pubertal mood swings and behavioural changes, and diminish psychological distress. When possible any underlying cause should be treated. The treatment of choice for central precocious puberty is with a GnRH partial agonist.

Delayed or absent puberty

Aetiology—may be due to (1) hypogonadotrophic hypogonadism—with constitutional delay much the commonest cause of delayed/absent puberty; can be caused by a wide range of central nervous system syndromes or chronic medical conditions; or (2) hypergonadotrophic hypogonadism—due to gonadal failure, including chromosomal abnormalities (e.g. Turner's syndrome, Klinefelter's syndrome).

Investigation and management—investigation is largely as for precocious puberty. Treatment goals are to induce puberty, accelerate height gain, and improve self-confidence. When possible any underlying cause should be treated. Hormone replacement therapy is effective when used judiciously.

Introduction

Physiological mechanisms

The key point in the initiation of puberty is the reactivation of the gonadotropin-releasing hormone (GnRH) neurons in the hypothalamus. This leads to an increased frequency of high amplitude GnRH pulses being released into the vessels of the infundibulum to stimulate pituitary gonadotrophs to secrete follicle-stimulating hormone (FSH) and luteinizing hormone (LH). The GnRH neurons are active in fetal and very early postnatal life, but are then inhibited by poorly defined cortical pathways through childhood. It is the triggering of this reactivation of GnRH that is not fully understood. Recent evidence has implicated kisspeptin-1, secreted by hypothalamic kisspeptin neurons and acting through kisspeptin receptors (KISS1R), as a pivotal event in the reactivation and maintenance of GnRH secretion. There are, however, multiple neuronal pathways that impact directly or indirectly on GnRH neurons (including inhibitory factors such as γ-aminobutyric acid and excitatory factors such as glutamate and leptin) which are likely to modify the timing of the trigger event and the subsequent pace of puberty.

There are also many extrinsic and intrinsic factors that influence puberty. Body composition, in particular fat mass and its secreted adipokine leptin, can have a marked influence on pubertal development: anorexia nervosa with associated leptin deficiency is a potent stimulus both to the inhibition of pubertal initiation and to the arrest of an established puberty. Conversely, the recent rise in the incidence of childhood obesity may be leading to an earlier onset of puberty. In addition, specific growth patterns have been implicated in pubertal timing: children born small for their gestational age may have early adrenarche and/or puberty. A change in environment can also have a potent effect on pubertal timing. Thus, children from relatively impoverished countries who are adopted into families in affluent countries may have early pubertal onset.

Timing of puberty

The earliest sign of puberty in girls is breast development and in boys is an increase in testicular size to 4 ml associated with scrotal rugosity. However, these initial events in pubertal development may occur over a broad age range (Fig. 13.9.2.1). The age of onset of puberty follows a normal distribution: in the United Kingdom the average age at breast stage 2 in girls is 11 years and at genital stage 2 in boys is 12 years. In order to provide guidance for the identification of those children who may need evaluation for an abnormal puberty, it is necessary to define limits for normality. Two standard deviations either side of this average value ranges from 8.2 to 13.8 years in girls and 9.8 to 14.2 years in boys. In the United Kingdom, puberty commencing before 8 years of age in a girl and 9 years of age in a boy would be defined as precocious and commencing before 9 years in a girl and 10 years in a boy would be defined as early. Puberty commencing after 13.5 years in a girl and

after 14 years in a boy would be defined as delayed. However, these definitions may need to be revised to account for ethnic background: in particular, children of African origin are more likely to have an earlier age of onset of puberty. In addition, there is a strong familial component to the timing of the onset of puberty. Thus, evaluation in a clinical context must take account of these background variables.

Precocious puberty

Causes and evaluation (Table 13.9.2.1)

Precocious puberty is most commonly due to central activation of the hypothalamo–pituitary–gonadal axis, termed central precocious puberty or gonadotropin-dependent precocious puberty. Precocious puberty may also be induced by gonadotropin-independent mechanisms to give the much rarer clinical scenario of peripheral precocious puberty. This is due to autonomous sex steroid secretion from the gonads or adrenal glands, or due to the administration of exogenous sex steroids.

Central precocious puberty occurs in about 1 in 5000 children and is 10 times more common in girls than boys. In girls with central precocious puberty, the cause is often not determined and is presumed to be idiopathic. Conversely, in boys, the cause of central precocious puberty is more likely to be pathological. In both sexes, the appearance of pubertal signs before the age of 8 years in girls and 9 years in boys should prompt investigation to exclude an underlying pathology. It is important to define whether the puberty is of central or peripheral aetiology or whether the signs are consistent with a normal variant of puberty (isolated thelarche or adrenarche). Assessment over time will also reveal at what pace the clinical signs of puberty are progressing. Clinical evaluation should focus on risk factors, auxological assessment, pubertal staging, signs of an intracranial lesion, or signs of a syndrome (see Table 13.9.2.2).

Variants of normal pubertal development

Premature adrenarche is characterized by the development of pubic and/or armpit hair and/or acne and greasy skin in the absence

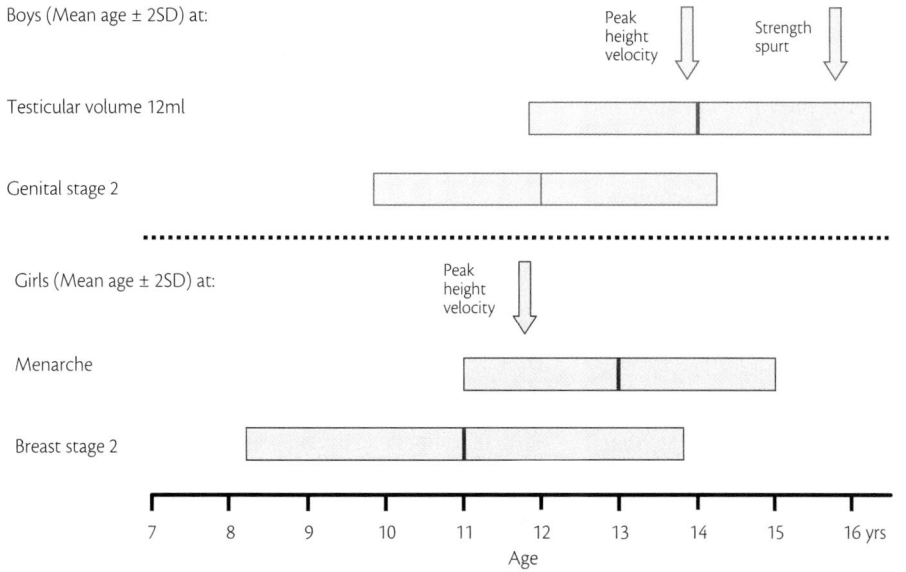

Fig. 13.9.2.1 Mean ages ± 2 standard deviations for the onset of puberty in both sexes, the attainment of 12 ml testicular volumes in boys and menarche in girls. The average age at which peak height velocity is achieved is also indicated.

Table 13.9.2.1 Causes of precocious puberty

Central gonadotropin-dependent

CNS abnormalities	Congenital/anatomical abnormalities
	Septo-optic dysplasia
	Arachnoid and pineal cysts
	Hamartoma
	Hydrocephalus
	Acquired abnormalities
	Hypothalamic–pituitary tumours
	Hamartoma
	Germinoma (can secrete hCG)
	Optic nerve glioma (± with
	neurofibromatosis type 1)
	CNS irradiation
	Hydrocephalus (associated with
	intraventricular haemorrhage or infection)
Cause not identified	Including familial (usually autosomal dominant) precocious puberty
Prolonged exposure to sex steroids	Late-onset congenital adrenal hyperplasia
Ectopic source of hCG	Hepatoblastoma
	Choriocarcinoma
Prolonged hypothyroidism	

Peripheral gonadotropin-independent

Ovarian overactivity	GSα activation in McCune–Albright syndrome
	Ovarian cysts and tumours
Testicular overactivity	Testotoxicosis (activating mutation of the LH receptor)
	$G_s\alpha$ activation in McCune–Albright syndrome
	Leydig cell or Sertoli cell tumours
Exogenous sex steroids	

CNS, central nervous system.

Table 13.9.2.2 Causes of delayed or absent puberty

Hypogonadotropic hypogonadism

Permanent	Kallmann's syndrome
	Isolated gonadotropin deficiency
	Congenital multiple pituitary hormone deficiency
	Unknown aetiology
	Transcription factor disorders, e.g. *PROP1, LHX3, HESX1*
	Midline abnormalities
	CNS tumours
	Craniopharyngioma
	Hypothalamic tumours
	Pituitary adenoma
	CNS irradiation (high dose)
	Infiltration
	Histiocytosis
	Traumatic brain injury
	Post CNS infection
	Syndromes
	Prader–Willi
	Bardet–Biedl
	CHARGE
Functional	Constitutional delay of growth and puberty
	Systemic disease
	Chronic renal failure
	Gastrointestinal disease
	Anorexia nervosa
	Chronic lung disease
	Blood disorders (e.g. thalassaemia)
	Arthritis, inflammatory disorders
	Hypothyroidism
	Hyperprolactinaemia
	Intensive exercise
	Syndromes
	Noonan's
	Down's

Hypergonadotropic hypogonadism (gonadal failure)

Chromosomal abnormalities	Turner's syndrome and variants
	Klinefelter's syndrome
	Disorders of sex development
	Gonadal dysgenesis
Ovarian failure	Idiopathic
	Autoimmune
	Metabolic (e.g. galactosaemia)
	Pelvic/spinal irradiation
	Chemotherapy
Testicular failure	Anorchia/vanishing testes
	Cryptorchidism
	Torsion
	Irradiation
	Chemotherapy
	Postinfection (e.g. mumps)
Disorders of steroid synthesis and action	Inactivating gonadotropin mutations
	Adrenal steroid enzyme defects

of gonadal activation before the age of 8 years in girls and 9 years in boys. Premature adrenarche is usually a benign process requiring no treatment. However, a very early onset of adrenarche (<5 years) or a very marked adrenarche could be consistent with late onset congenital adrenal hyperplasia or an androgen secreting tumour.

Premature thelarche is characterized by breast development in the absence of any other signs of puberty. It is classically seen in the first two years of life. Investigation is not required, but monitoring over time is reassuring to the parents. The thelarche variant is also recognized, in which breast development may be progressive with some other features of puberty (increased growth rate, some bone age advance, and/or some increase in uterine size). This condition merges into central precocious puberty and represents a spectrum of hypothalamic–pituitary–gonadal axis activation. Such patients will require evaluation and follow-up and may be treated if the full picture of central precocious puberty develops.

Investigation

Children with precocious puberty need biochemical and radiological investigations: a GnRH test (intravenous GnRH (100 μg bolus) with blood samples taken basally, 30 and 60 min after administration) should be performed with measurement of FSH and LH. This will aid in the differentiation between central precocious puberty and peripheral precocious puberty. Established central precocious puberty is associated with a significant rise in gonadotropins, in particular a peak LH greater than 10 IU/litre which is higher than the FSH peak. However, early breast development in girls can be associated with a much lower LH peak and higher FSH peak. Very low levels of gonadotropins throughout the test would be consistent with a gonadotropin-independent mechanism.

Serum testosterone or oestradiol should also be measured. Routine assays for oestradiol do not detect the low levels of oestrogen that are generated by the peripubertal ovary, and oestradiol can be undetectable even in the face of signs of breast development. An oestradiol level measurable in such an assay (usually >50 pmol/litre) would be consistent with pubertal development. High sex steroid levels with low gonadotropins would be consistent with peripheral precocious puberty. The tumour marker β-human chorionic gonadotropin (hCG) can be measured to aid in the detection of a hypothalamic germinoma.

In girls, a pelvic ultrasound examination is required to define ovarian and uterine dimensions and to identify ovarian follicles and cysts. Sizes should be compared to normative data. The scan may also detect the presence of an endometrial thickening indicative of exposure to oestrogen. In both sexes, a nondominant wrist radiograph for determination of bone age (advanced in precocious puberty) is a useful adjunct to define the extent of precocity and the possible impact on growth prognosis.

In those with confirmed central precocious puberty, an MRI scan of the brain with specific views of the hypothalamic–pituitary area should be undertaken. This may identify an aetiology; e.g. a hypothalamic hamartoma may be present or, rarely, a germinoma. Hydrocephalus may be present or there may be evidence of a general central nervous system pathology associated with central precocious puberty.

For those where the investigations for precocious puberty are not definitive, then clinical evaluation over time will reveal the speed at which puberty is advancing and aid in the decision about treatment.

Treatment

Precocious puberty often results in considerable anxiety for the child, the parents, and the family. In girls, parents are concerned at the occurrence or the prospect of menstrual bleeding at a relatively immature age. Children may exhibit sexualized behaviour causing embarrassment and distress. The goals of treatment are: (1) to stop pubertal progression, (2) to attenuate pubertal growth and bone maturation with the aim of improving final height prognosis (most effective in those <6 years of age), (3) to reduce mood swings and behavioural changes associated with puberty, and (4) overall to diminish the psychological distress caused by this condition.

Once puberty is established as precocious and progressive, the treatment of choice for central precocious puberty is a GnRH analogue (GnRHa). These agents are GnRH partial agonists, which cause a brief period of GnRH receptor activation followed by blockade and hence inhibition of gonadotropin secretion. Depot injections are available with durations of action up to 4 or 12 weeks. Close monitoring of clinical response to GnRHa treatment is required as central precocious puberty may progress and adjustments to the dose or frequency of administration may need to be made. Experience with GnRH analogues over the last decade has shown that they are effective and safe. Reports are now emerging that previous treatment with a GnRHa does not affect later fertility.

Children with precocious puberty are usually taller than expected with an advanced bone age. GnRHa treatment will slow epiphyseal fusion by inhibiting sex steroid secretion. However, their impact on preserving growth potential is greatest in those who develop central precocious puberty at the youngest ages.

Antagonists of sex steroid actions, e.g. cyproterone acetate at a dose of between 50 and 150 mg/m² for 4 to 6 weeks, can be used as an adjunct during the initial stimulatory phase of GnRHa treatment. This may be of particular use in the child who presents with a very rapid onset of central precocious puberty. In peripheral precocious puberty, such as McCune–Albright syndrome, cyproterone acetate and/or an aromatase inhibitor is required.

For all forms of precocious puberty, the underlying cause may need to be addressed. A hypothalamic germinoma will require treatment with chemotherapy and/or radiotherapy. An adrenal tumour or gonadal tumour needs removal. Congenital adrenal hyperplasia should be treated with glucocorticoids.

Delayed or absent puberty

Causes and evaluation (Table 13.9.2.2)

Delayed puberty is most often due to constitutional delay of growth and puberty, where the hypothalamic–pituitary–gonadal axis is slow to be reactivated. Boys are more commonly affected than girls (9:1). The presenting features are delayed puberty usually with short stature in the absence of any signs of system disease. This condition can cause significant anxiety, depression, and low self-esteem. These young people feel very different from their peer group and are excluded from age-appropriate activities due to their immature appearance. A positive family history of pubertal delay may be present in one or both parents, suggesting a familial predisposition. Although late, children with constitutional delay of growth and puberty will eventually go through puberty and reach an adult height that is usually within the normal range and within their parental target. Constitutional delay of growth and puberty is a state of temporary/functional hypogonadotropic hypogonadism. This is also seen in other conditions, e.g. some children with isolated growth hormone deficiency, autoimmune hypothyroidism, or those with poor weight gain in the peripubertal period due to anorexia nervosa or associated with systemic disease. Some syndromes are associated with inadequate pubertal development or functional hypogonadotropic hypogonadism, e.g. Prader–Willi, Bardet–Biedl, and Noonan's syndromes.

In contrast, delayed or absent puberty may be associated with permanent hypogonadotropic hypogonadism, due to a congenital or acquired defect in the hypothalamic–pituitary axis. Primary hypogonadotropic hypogonadism may be due to failure of GnRH neuronal migration in Kallmann's syndrome, often associated with anosmia and mutations in KAL1 or fibroblast growth factor receptor-1 (FGFR-1). Hypogonadotropic hypogonadism may also occur in those with a normal sense of smell, and in these cases mutations in the genes for FGFR-1 or the KISS1R receptor may be found. Hypogonadotropic hypogonadism occurs as part of congenital multiple pituitary hormone deficiency or it may be acquired in association with multiple pituitary hormone deficiencies caused by a suprasellar tumour, such as a craniopharyngioma.

Clinical evaluation should include auxological assessment, pubertal staging, the identification of signs of an intracranial lesion, or signs of a syndrome.

Investigation

The majority of cases presenting with delayed puberty will be boys who have constitutional delay of growth and puberty. To make this diagnosis, all other causes of permanent or functional hypogonadotropic hypogonadism need to be excluded. In most cases, a thorough history and clinical assessment with bone age estimation is adequate. However, in cases of severe pubertal delay (onset of puberty not occurred by age 15 years in boys or 14 years in girls) and/or the presence of signs of system or intracranial disease or signs of a syndrome, then investigations should be undertaken. These may include a gonadotropin-releasing hormone test, sex steroid levels, thyroid function, other pituitary function testing, and/or specific tests for system disease.

The distinction between constitutional delay of growth and puberty and permanent congenital hypogonadotropic hypogonadism based on stimulated gonadotropins during the gonadotropin-releasing hormone test may be difficult: although peak LH and FSH in hypogonadotropic hypogonadism are usually considerably lower than those in constitutional delay of growth and puberty, this is not always the case. In these cases, a trial of sex steroid treatment may need to be undertaken with a low dose of testosterone (intramuscular monthly injections of 50–100 mg testosterone esters or oral testosterone at a dose of 40–80 mg/day in males) or ethinyl oestradiol (2–4 μg/day orally in females) for a period of 4 to 6 months. In constitutional delay of growth and puberty this exposure to sex steroids is usually sufficient to induce spontaneous progression of pubertal development with increasing testicular volumes or ongoing breast development in the months after treatment. However in those with hypogonadotropic hypogonadism, pubertal signs do not progress.

An MRI scan of the pituitary may be considered in those with evidence of pituitary hormone deficiency to exclude the possibility of a space occupying lesion, e.g. a craniopharyngioma.

In children with gonadal failure who have reached the adolescent years, basal and GnRH-stimulated LH and FSH levels will usually be elevated (hypergonadotropic hypogonadism) and sex steroid levels low. The most common causes include direct damage to the gonad (e.g. testicular torsion, irradiation, or chemotherapy) or chromosomal disorders such as Turner's or Klinefelter's syndromes. Thus, a karyotype is an important test to consider.

In very rare cases, evaluation of the capacity of the testis to generate androgens may be needed. This can be done using a human chorionic gonadotropin (hCG) test (e.g. by administering 1500 IU of hCG by intramuscular injections on day 1) with measurement of androstenedione, testosterone, and dihydrotestosterone at baseline and on day 4. This may help to identify a disorder of sex development, such as a testosterone biosynthetic defect.

Treatment

Children, particularly boys, with constitutional delay of growth and puberty are often significantly distressed at the lack of pubertal features and short stature in relation to their peers. Many such children are keen to have treatment to improve growth and hasten puberty. The goals of treatment are: (1) to induce puberty and demonstrate spontaneous progression, (2) to accelerate height gain, and (3) to improve self-confidence.

Oxandrolone, a nonaromatizable anabolic derivative of testosterone (at a dose of 1.25–2.5 mg daily), may augment height gain but has no impact on puberty. Its use is confined to those children in the early peripubertal years (age 11–13 years) with constitutional delay in growth and a delayed bone age who are concerned about their short stature. Treatment can be given for 6 to 12 months. In children with constitutional delay of growth and puberty, treatment with low dose sex steroids for a short duration (as indicated above) may prime the pituitary to release gonadotropins, resulting in spontaneous progression of puberty. For those with hypogonadotropic hypogonadism, treatment with sex steroids needs to be sustained through puberty and maintained in adult life. In males, the dose of testosterone esters should start at 50 to 100 mg monthly increasing in increments dependent on clinical response and age at initiation of treatment over a 2 to 3 year period to an adult dose of 250 mg every 2–4 weeks. Induction of puberty can also be undertaken with a range of other preparations, including oral and transdermal testosterone. However, it is imperative that the initial dose is small and the increments in dose occur over a prolonged time frame. In females, a similar approach is recommended, starting at a low dose (e.g. 2–6 μg ethinyl oestradiol daily) and building the dose up over a 2 to 3 year period dependent on clinical response and age at initiation of treatment to a dose of 20 to 30 μg daily. Progesterone should be added to the regimen if there is breakthrough uterine bleeding or when the daily dose of ethinyl oestradiol is 10 μg. Adult regimens are most conveniently given in the form of an oral contraceptive pill. A number of alternative oestrogen preparations can be used, but in all cases a gradual increase in dose over a 2 to 3 year period is required.

In young males with hypogonadotropic hypogonadism, induction of testicular growth may be requested. This can be achieved to a limited extent with twice weekly hCG injections used in place of testosterone. The increase in testicular size is usually modest (up to 6–10 ml). If fertility is required, then treatment with hCG and FSH may be undertaken.

Further reading

Achermann JC, et al. (2002). Genetic causes of human reproductive disease. *J Clin Endocrinol Metab*, **87**, 2447–54.

Badaru A, et al. (2006). Sequential comparisons of one-month and three-month depot leuprolide regimens in central precocious puberty. *J Clin Endocrinol Metab*, **91**, 1862–7.

Gottsch ML, Clifton DK, Steiner RA (2006). Kisspepeptin-GPR54 signaling in the neuroendocrine reproductive axis. *Mol Cell Endocrinol*, **25**, 91–6.

Heger S, et al. (2006). Long-term GnRH agonist treatment for female central precocious puberty does not impair reproductive function. *Mol Cell Endocrinol*, **25**, 217–20.

Hughes IA, Kumanan M (2006). A wider perspective on puberty. *Mol Cell Endocrinol*, **25**, 1–7.

Leger J, Reynaud R, Czernichow P (2000). Do all girls with apparent idiopathic precocious puberty require gonadotropin-releasing hormone agonist treatment? *J Pediatr*, **137**, 819–25.

Nathan BM, Palmert MR (2005). Regulation and disorders of pubertal timing. *Endocrinol Metab Clin North Am*, **34**, 617–41.

Richmond EJ, Rogol AD (2007). Male pubertal development and the role of androgen therapy. *Nat Clin Pract Endocrinol Metab*, **3**, 338–44.

13.9.3 Normal and abnormal sexual differentiation

I.A. Hughes

Essentials

Human sex development follows an orderly sequence of embryological events coordinated by a cascade of gene expression and hormone production in a time- and concentration-dependent manner. Underpinning the entire process of fetal sex development is the simple mantra: sex chromosomes (XX or XY) dictate the gonadotype (ovary or testis), which then dictates the somatotype (female or male phenotype).

The constitutive sex in fetal development is female. Male development to form a testis from the indifferent gonad (sex determination) and the internal and external phenotype (sex differentiation) is due to (1) testis-determining genes, in particular *SRY* (sex chromosome related gene on the Y chromosome), which is first expressed in the XY gonad at 6 to 7 weeks of gestation; and (2) production by the testis of (a) antimullerian hormone—to repress mullerian ducts forming the uterus and fallopian tubes, (b) androgens (testosterone and dihydrotestosterone)—to stabilize the Wolffian ducts; and (c) insulin-like factor 3 (INSL3)—required for the migration of the testis from the urogenital ridge to its site at birth within the scrotum. An understanding of these basic principles is essential to formulate a logical approach to the diagnosis of disorders of sex development.

Disorders of sex development (DSD)—these can be classified into three broad categories based on the knowledge of the karyotype: (1) sex chromosome abnormality—e.g. XO/XY, mixed gonadal dysgenesis; (2) XX DSD—e.g. congenital adrenal hyperplasia (see Chapter 13.7.2); (3) XY DSD—e.g. partial androgen insensitivity syndrome.

Clinical features—the commonest presentations of DSD are (1) ambiguous genitalia of the newborn; and (2) development of secondary sexual characteristics at puberty discordant with the sex of rearing—generally signs of virilization occurring in a child hitherto assumed to be female.

Investigation and management—an extensive repertoire is available, but the choice of genetic, endocrine, and imaging tests should be based on the DSD classification (determined by sex chromosome analysis by fluorescent *in situ* hybridization (FISH) using X centromeric and SRY probes, followed by full karyotyping) and aimed at reaching a consensus about the choice of sex assignment. Any surgical procedure required to alter the external phenotype consonant with sex assignment need not be undertaken urgently. It is essential that families of children with DSD have the benefit of support and counselling by a multidisciplinary team that comprises at a minimum an endocrinologist, urologist/gynaecologist, geneticist, and psychologist.

Normal fetal sex development

The following key facts underpin the mechanism of dimorphic sex development:

* The constitutive sex is female.

* Male development requires the presence of a Y chromosome, a testis, and the production and action of testosterone during a critical time in early gestation.

* Fetal experiments in mammals indicate that early castration leads to a female phenotype, despite the presence of the Y chromosome (Jost's hypothesis).

* Absence of an ovary does not affect the female phenotype at birth (e.g. Turner syndrome).

* Oestrogen is not required for fetal female development, but androgen is essential for fetal male development.

The link between sex chromosomes, gonad determination and the expression of the phenotype (somatotype) is illustrated in simple configuration in Fig. 13.9.3.1. The events that occur during fetal male development are depicted in Fig. 13.9.3.2. The indifferent gonad develops in the urogenital ridge, where the kidney and adrenals also have their origins. This is germane to the frequent association of urinary tract anomalies with ambiguous genitalia and the occasional occurrence of nests of adrenal remnants found in the testis of males with congenital adrenal hyperplasia (see Chapter 13.7.2). Germ cells migrate from the yolk sac to take their position within the developing gonad. The testis is histologically defined initially by its seminiferous tubules and predates comparable maturation of the ovary by a few weeks. Three products of the somatic component of this testis are key to development of the male phenotype, i.e. sex differentiation. Anti-mullerian hormone (AMH), a product of Sertoli cells, acts on its type II receptor to repress mullerian ducts forming the uterus and fallopian tubes. This process is permitted to occur in the female because of the absence of AMH at this stage in gestation. Testosterone produced by Leydig cells under the control initially of placental human chorionic gonadotropin (hCG) acts locally in high concentration to

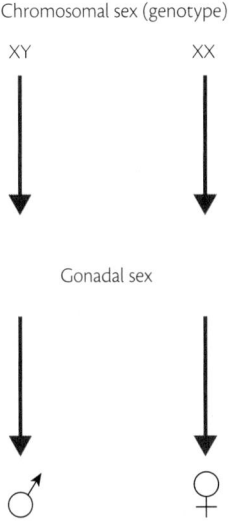

Fig. 13.9.3.1 The basic components of fetal sex development.

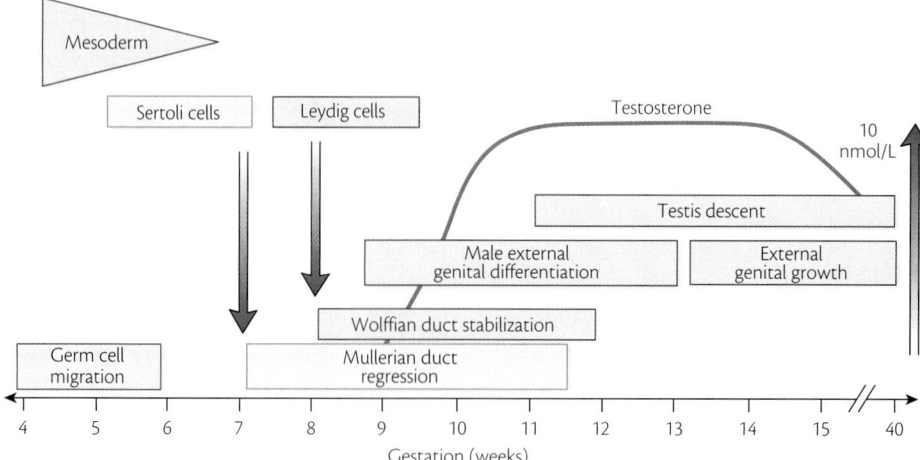

Fig. 13.9.3.2 The embryology of fetal sex development in the male. Mesoderm represents the tissue source for the somatic components of testis development. The solid line denotes the rise in fetal serum testosterone levels (nmol/litre).

stabilize the wolffian ducts. These form the vas deferens, epididymis, and seminal vesicles. A further product of the Leydig cells, insulin-like factor 3 (INSL3), is required for the transabdominal phase of migration of the testis from the urogenital ridge to its site at birth within the scrotum. The inguinoscrotal phase of testis descent in late gestation is under the control of androgens. All these events take place in a specific chronological order and are controlled by genes and hormones expressed at critical dosage thresholds and timing. The genetic and hormonal control of the events in male sex development is shown in Fig. 13.9.1.3. Not all the genes characterized for mammalian development are shown, but those identified in the human and relevant to disorders of sex development are emphasized. The formation of the urogenital ridge is dependent on factors such as WT1 and SF1, their role vividly illustrated by mouse gene knock-out studies (absence of gonads and kidneys or adrenals, respectively) and syndromes of urogenital anomalies (WAGR, Denys–Drash, Frasier syndromes) and combined gonadal dysgenesis/adrenal insufficiency in humans with inactivating mutations of *WT1* and *SF1* genes, respectively.

The master regulator of testis development (sex determination) is SRY (sex chromosome related gene on the Y chromosome) which is first expressed in the XY gonad at 6 to 7 weeks of gestation, just before the indifferent gonad differentiates as a testis. SRY is a 204 amino acid protein functioning as a high mobility group (HMG) box transcription factor. The HMG box of 79 amino acids is related to similar proteins such as SOX (SRY-like HMG box) which is also a key protein in the regulation of testis development. That SRY is essential for testis development is supported by the following observations: (1) translocation of *SRY* to the X chromosome during paternal meiosis is present in 90% of XX males (2) mutations in *SRY* in 15 to 20% of XY females with complete gonadal dysgenesis leads to complete sex reversal; (3) induction of a male phenotype occurs by transgenic insertion of *Sry* in XX mice. However, the observation that 10% of XX males lack *SRY* and the vast majority of XY gonadal dysgenic females have a normal *SRY* indicates that other genes must also be involved in testis determination. Candidates such as *SOX9* and *SF1* play some role, but their inactivation in humans leads to various syndromes of which gonadal dysgenesis is only one component. The role of clinicians recording detailed phenotypes in cases of disordered sex development is essential to continue the search for the multitude of genes that must be involved in testis determination. What is known in

the human is summarized in Fig. 13.9.3.3. The ovary is devoid of known factors, although genes such as *WNT4*, *RSPO1*, and *DAX1* may act in female development by suppressing testis-determining genes.

The differentiation of the internal genital ducts and external genitalia into male structures is entirely androgen dependent. For this to occur, an intact pathway of gonadotrophin-induced steroidogenesis is required to produce the potent androgens testosterone and dihydrotestosterone (DHT), which in turn promote androgen signalling by ligand activating the nuclear androgen receptor (AR) in target cells. The pathways of testicular steroidogenesis and the ligand-activated AR signalling are shown in Figs. 13.9.3.4 and 13.9.3.5, respectively.

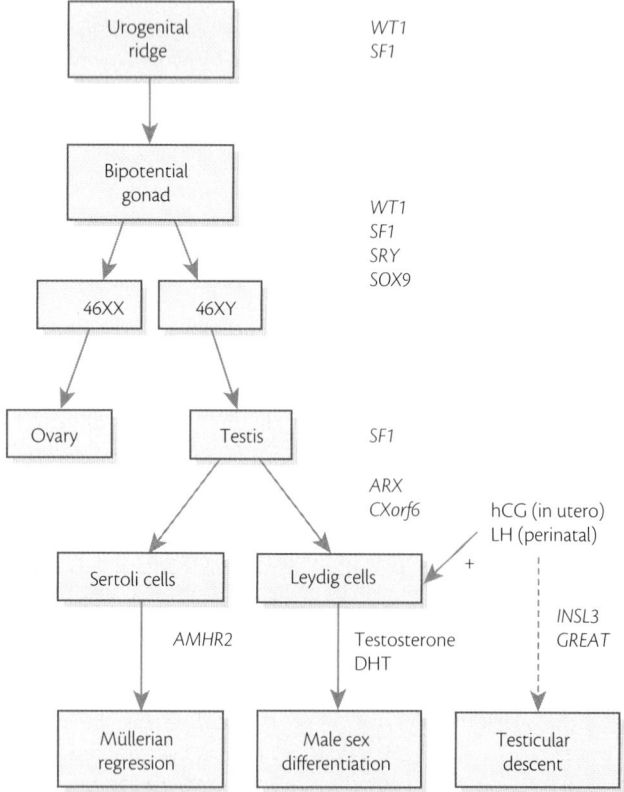

Fig. 13.9.3.3 Genetic and hormonal control of fetal sex development. Emphasis is placed on genes relevant to human development.

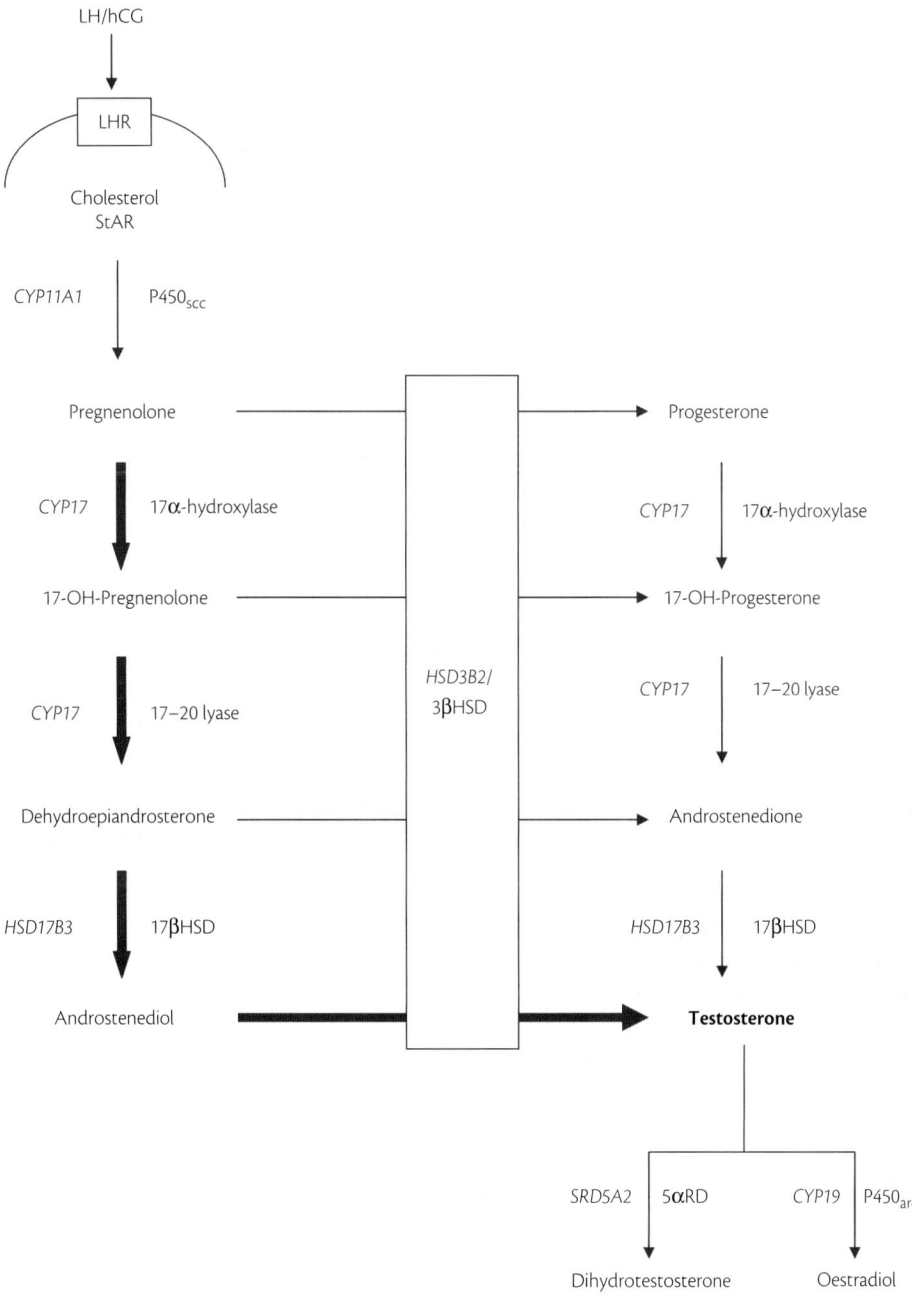

Fig. 13.9.3.4 Pathway of androgen biosynthesis, including aromatase conversion to estrogen. 3βHSD, 3β-hydroxysteroid dehydrogenase; 5αRD, 5α-reductase; 17βHSD, 17β-hydroxysteroid dehydrogenase; P450$_{arom}$, P450 aromatase. The cognate genes are depicted in italics.

The enzymatic steps in androgen production are encoded by genes, each of which, when mutated, results in syndromes of undermasculinization. Some of the more proximal enzyme defects also involve adrenal steroidogenesis and lead to syndromes that include adrenal insufficiency (see Chapter 13.7.1).

Androgen signalling is mediated by a single AR encoded by an X-linked gene at Xq11–12. The AR is a member of a large family of nuclear receptors that comprise four general functional domains: an N-terminal transactivation domain, a central DNA binding domain, a hinge region and a C-terminal domain to which the ligand binds (Fig. 13.9.3.6). Subdomains are involved in dimerization, nuclear localization and transcriptional regulation. Circulating androgens are bound to carrier proteins such as sex-hormone binding globulin (SHBG) and albumin but diffuse freely in to target cells where the ligand binds to cytoplasmic AR

complexed to heat shock proteins. The hormone–receptor complex translocates to the nucleus where it binds to DNA response elements as a homodimer. An added refinement in androgen signalling is provided by interaction with a number of coactivator proteins to enhance up-regulation of androgen-responsive genes via the general transcriptional machinery. Androgens have pleiotropic effects beyond fetal male development. These include the development of secondary sexual characteristics at puberty, muscle and skeletal growth, stimulation of sebaceous glands, and elongation and thickening of the vocal cords that give rise to the 'voice breaking' characteristic of the later stages of male puberty. Prostate development and growth is also androgen dependent, a feature that is countered by antiandrogenic forms of treatment for prostate cancer. It is also clear that androgens also have effects on brain development, with prenatal influences being especially

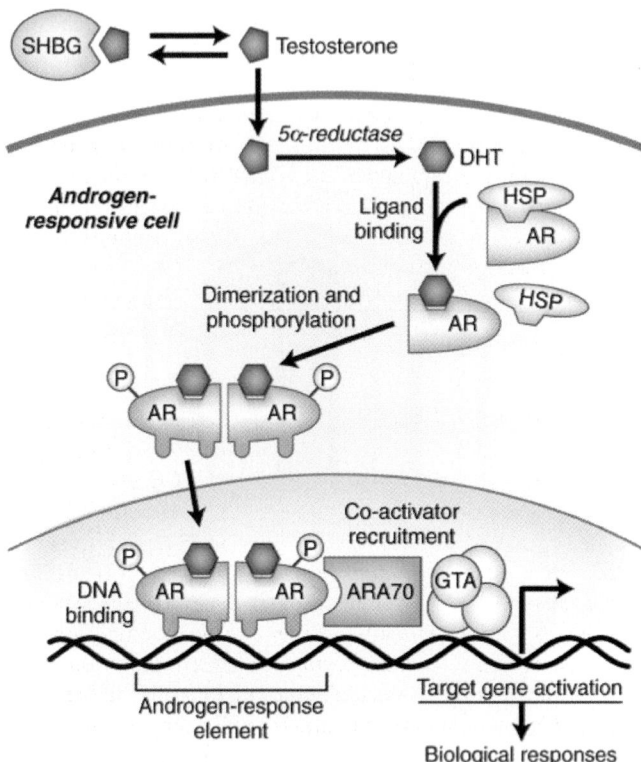

Fig. 13.9.3.5 Schematic of androgen action in a target cell. ARA70, an androgen receptor specific coactivator; GTA, general transcriptional apparatus; HSP, heat shock protein; P, phosphorylation; SHBG, sex hormone binding globulin.

relevant to the sex dimorphism in gender role behaviour. Much of the evidence for the role of androgens in psychosocial functioning has come from studies of females exposed to excess androgens (e.g. congenital adrenal hyperplasia) and syndromes associated with defects in androgen signalling (e.g. complete androgen insensitivity syndrome).

Definitions, terminology, and nomenclature

Clarity of thought is required when faced with a newborn infant whose external genitalia are so ambiguous in appearance that sex assignment is not instantaneously possible. The problem does not need compounding by the use of unclear, ambiguous terms such as 'true hermaphroditism' and 'pseudohermaphroditism'. The following definitions are relevant to the understanding of normal sex development, both somatic and psychosexual:

♦ sex determination—transformation of the indifferent gonad into a testis or an ovary

♦ sex differentiation—development of the phenotype (somatotype) as an expression of hormones produced by the gonad (in reality, testis only during fetal development)

♦ gender (sex) assignment—allocation of male or female at birth, usually instantaneous

♦ gender identity—the sense of self as being male or female

♦ gender role—sex-typical behaviours and preferences in which males and females differ (e.g. toy preferences, aggression)

♦ sexual orientation—refers to the target of sexual arousal

♦ gender attribution—assigning as male or female on first encounter with an individual

'Gender dysphoria' is a gender identity disorder characterized by a mismatch between the body habitus (phenotype as male or female) and gender identity as perceived by the affected individual ("I feel like a woman trapped in a man's body"). The desire to 'convert' from male to female, or vice versa, is a state of transsexualism. There is no direct evidence of a genetic or endocrine explanation for gender dysphoria. However, individuals with a disorder of sex development such as an androgen biosynthetic defect may express feelings of transsexualism in later life.

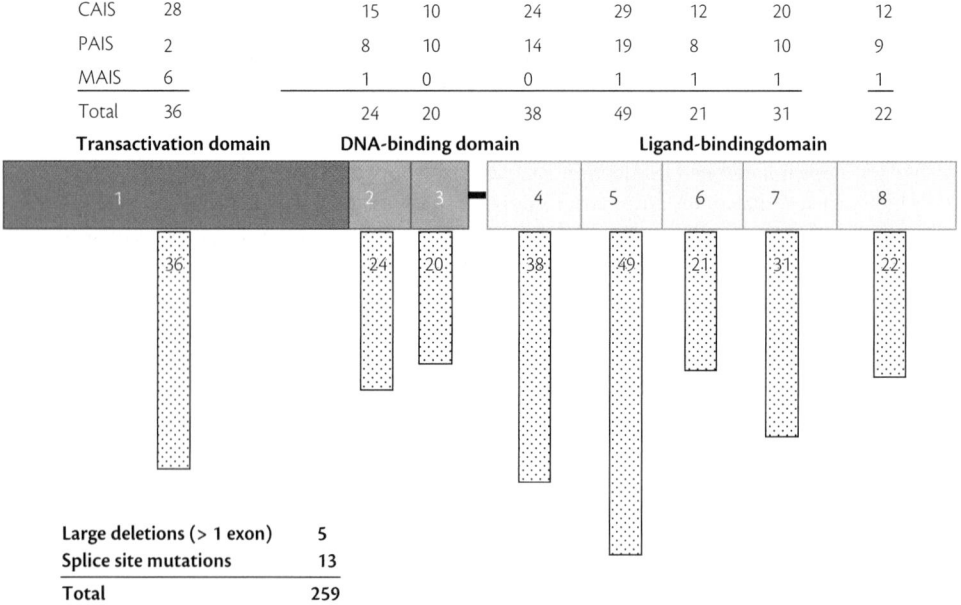

Fig. 13.9.3.6 Distribution of mutations in androgen insensitivity syndrome (AIS) as recorded on the Cambridge DSD Database. The three functional domains of the AR are indicated, encoded by their respective exons (1–8). The numbers within the vertical bars are a summation of nonsense and missense mutations and a breakdown according to type of AIS is denoted above the AR. MAIS, minimal/mild androgen insensitivity syndrome.

	Transactivation domain		DNA-binding domain		Ligand-binding domain				
CAIS	28		15	10	24	29	12	20	12
PAIS	2		8	10	14	19	8	10	9
MAIS	6		1	0	0	1	1	1	1
Total	36		24	20	38	49	21	31	22

Large deletions (> 1 exon)	5
Splice site mutations	13
Total	**259**

The term 'intersex' has traditionally been applied to the clinical scenario of an infant born with ambiguous genitalia and in whom the sex is indeterminate. That allocation has often strayed beyond this defined scenario to include conditions such as severe hypospadias, milder forms of congenital adrenal hyperplasia, and the complete androgen insensitivity syndrome, where intersex is an inappropriate term. Indeed, affected individuals representing a range of anomalies of the reproductive tract consider the term as pejorative and have clamoured for a change in terminology. In response, a consensus statement produced by a faculty of experts in genetics, endocrinology, surgery, and psychology has redefined the terminology that should now become the lexicon in this branch of medicine (Table 13.9.3.1).

A 'disorder of sex development' (DSD) is a wide-ranging term defined as a congenital condition in which development of chromosomal, gonadal, or anatomic sex is atypical. This broad definition enables a wide range of conditions to be considered as DSD. This would include the prototypic ambiguous genitalia of the newborn (e.g. due to congenital adrenal hyperplasia), simple hypospadias, cloacal exstrophy, the XX male, complete XY gonadal dysgenesis (Swyer's syndrome), undescended testes, and simple labial adhesions. Most of these examples could never be construed as intersex. Disorders of puberty are excluded by incorporating 'congenital' within the definition of DSD. Refining the terms to lead to specificity in definitions is achieved by subdividing according to knowledge of the sex chromosomes. Above all, the new consensus rids the medical literature of such confusing and ambiguous terminology as 'female pseudohermaphroditism' which purports to define a genetic female with virilized external genitalia at variance with the gonadal sex. Taking congenital adrenal hyperplasia as a common example, this becomes an example of XX DSD in which the sex chromosomes and gonads are congruent (female) but the virilized external genitalia are atypical. 'True hermaphroditism' had its adjectival preface to emphasize that the presence of both a testis and an ovary in the one individual was required to meet the definition of hermaphroditism. Why not precisely describe the morphology as being ovotesticular? The underlying karyotype may be 46,XX (the most frequent), 46,XY, or 46XX/XY.

DSD classification

Using the new nomenclature as a catalyst, it has been possible to derive a classification system which is simple, reflects procedures followed during initial investigation and is flexible enough to be adapted as new conditions are recognized and defined. Subtending the entire process is knowledge of the karyotype, a starting point which is now routine for the investigation of DSD. Since fertilization of the ovum with an X- or Y-bearing spermatozoon and sex chromosome aneuploidy or mosaicism are so fundamental to normal fetal sex development, it is logical to consider the causes of DSD in three broad categories. Table 13.9.3.2 contains a fairly comprehensive list of the causes of DSD; Table 13.9.3.3 focuses on the causes of ambiguous genitalia from a functional standpoint.

Sex chromosome DSD

It can be argued that Klinefelter's and Turner's syndromes are not examples of DSD in the context of abnormalities of the external genitalia. Klinefelter syndrome (47,XXY) has a genital component that typically comprises small, soft testes with oligo- or azoospermia and infertility. The syndrome affects 1 in 500 to 1 in 1000 live births. The problem of infertility is not absolute now that advances in artificial reproductive technologies have enabled some men with Klinefelter's syndrome to father children through testicular sperm extraction combined with intracytoplasmic sperm injection. Small testes are already evident in childhood and the penis may be small. Hypospadias may also occur and genitalia can be sufficiently undermasculinized to lead to ambiguity and even a sex-reversed phenotype. Klinefelter variants such as 48,XXXY and 49,XXXXY may have associated genital anomalies.

Turner's syndrome without evidence of Y chromosomal material is seldom associated with external genital abnormalities. The DSD classification has included this syndrome since it is a congenital disorder characterized by gonadal (ovarian) dysgenesis and a sex chromosome aneuploidy. Turner's syndrome has an incidence of 1 in 2500. The classic form is associated with a 45,XO karyotype, which accounts for more than 50% of cases. Genital anomalies are more evidenced in mosaic forms of Turner's syndrome characterized by a 45,X/46,XY karyotype. The external genitalia can range in appearance from normal female or mild clitoromegaly, through overt ambiguous genitalia to a male spectrum of simple hypospadias or normal male genitalia. Indeed, most individuals with this karyotype appear to be normal males based on amniocentesis analyses that have revealed fetuses with a 45,X/46,XY karyotype. The minority with ambiguous genitalia are detected at birth and can pose difficulties for assignment of gender. A multitude of factors need to be considered, including the genital appearance and urogenital anatomy, risk of gonadal tumour, fertility and reproductive options, gender identity, and psychosexual function. Those infants who are severely undermasculinized and have a uterine remnant are likely to be assigned female and any dysgenetic gonad should be removed. Infants assigned male will require a number of hypospadias procedures and removal of any dysgenetic gonads. Long-term outcome studies are not available. Furthermore, finding a 45,X/46,XY karyotype during investigations for male infertility or in men presenting with a tumour of the testis is rare.

Ovotesticular DSD (true hermaphroditism) is a rare cause of abnormal genital development and is characterized by the presence of testicular and follicle-containing ovarian tissue. The external genitalia can be variable, comprising ambiguous genitalia or just severe hypospadias. The gonadal distribution may be a testis on one side and an ovary on the other, bilateral ovotestes, or, most frequently,

Table 13.9.3.1 A revised nomenclature relating to disorders of sex development

Previous	Proposed
Intersex	Disorders of sex development (DSD)
Male pseudohermaphrodite Undervirilization of an XY male Undermasculinization of an XY male	46,XY DSD
Female pseudohermaphrodite Overvirilization of an XX female Masculinization of an XX female	46,XX DSD
True hermaphrodite	Ovotesticular DSD
XX male or XX sex reversal	46,XX testicular DSD
XY sex reversal	46,XY complete gonadal dysgenesis

Table 13.9.3.2 Classification of disorders of sex development (DSD)

Sex chromosome DSD	46,XY DSD	46,XX DSD
A: 47,XXY (Klinefelter's syndrome and variants) **B: 45,X** (Turner's syndrome and variants) **C: 45,X/46,XY** (mixed gonadal dysgenesis) **D: 46,XX/46,XY** (chimerism)	**A: Disorders of gonadal (testicular) development** 1. Complete or partial gonadal dysgenesis (e.g. *SRY, SOX9, SF1, WT1, DHH*, etc.) 2. Ovotesticular DSD 3. Testis regression	**A: Disorders of gonadal (ovary) development** 1. Gonadal dysgenesis 2. Ovotesticular DSD 3. Testicular DSD (eg *SRY+, dup SOX9, RSP01*)

	B: Disorders in androgen synthesis or action
	1. Disorders of androgen synthesis
	   LH receptor mutations
	   Smith–Lemli–Opitz syndrome
	   Steroidogenic acute regulatory protein mutations
	   Cholesterol side chain cleavage (*CYP11A1*)
	   3β-hydroxysteroid dehydrogenase 2 (*HSD3B2*)
	   17α-hydroxylase/17,20-lyase (*CYP17*)
	   P450 oxidoreductase (*POR*)
	   17β-OH steroid dehydrogenase (*HSD17B3*)
	   5α-reductase 2 (*SRD5A2*)
	2. Disorders of androgen action
	   Androgen insensitivity syndrome
	   Drugs and environmental modulators
		B: Androgen excess
		1. Fetal
		   3β-hydroxysteroid dehydrogenase 2 (*HSD3B2*)
		   21-hydroxylase (*CYP21A2*)
		   P450 oxidoreductase (*POR*)
		   11β-hydroxylase (*CYP11B1*)
		   Glucocorticoid receptor mutations
		2. Fetoplacental
		   Aromatase (*CYP19*) deficiency
		   Oxidoreductase (*POR*) deficiency
		3. Maternal
		   Maternal virilizing tumours (e.g. luteomas)
		   Androgenic drugs

	C: Other 1. Syndromic associations of male genital development (e.g. cloacal anomalies, Robinow, Aarskog, hand–foot–genital, popliteal pterygium) 2. Persistent mullerian duct syndrome 3. Vanishing testis syndrome 4. Isolated hypospadias (*CXorf6, MAMDL1*) 5. Congenital hypogonadotropic hypogonadism 6. Cryptorchidism (*INSL3, GREAT*) 7. Environmental influences	**C: Other** 1. Syndromic associations (e.g. cloacal anomalies) 2. Mullerian agenesis/hypoplasia (e.g. MURCS) 3. Uterine abnormalities (e.g. MODY5) 4. Vaginal atresias (e.g. McKusick–Kaufman) 5. Labial adhesions

an ovotestis on one side and a testis or ovary on the other. An ovary will be sited in its normal pelvic position whereas a testis or an ovotestis can be located anywhere along the migratory path to the scrotum, but usually in the inguinal region. The pattern of

Table 13.9.3.3 Causes of ambiguous genitalia: a functional classification

Type/cause	Illustrative examples
Masculinized female (46XX,DSD)	
Fetal androgens	CAH, placental aromatase deficiency
Maternal androgens	Ovarian and adrenal tumours
Undermasculinized male (46XY,DSD)	
Abnormal testis determination	Partial (XY) and mixed (XO/XY) gonadal dysgenesis
Androgen biosynthetic defects	LH receptor inactivating mutations 17β-OH-steroid dehydrogenase deficiency 5α-reductase deficiency
Resistance to androgens	Androgen insensitivity syndrome variants
Ovotesticular DSD	
Presence of testicular and ovarian tissue	Karyotypes XX, XY, XX/XY
Syndromal	Denys–Drash, Frasier's Smith–Lemli–Opitz

internal genital ducts can also be variable, but generally follows that of the ipsilateral gonad. A rudimentary uterus is often found adjacent to an ovary or ovotestis. The karyotype is 46,XX in most cases, but only in about 30% is the *SRY* gene X-translocated. Familial cases are reported, with evidence for both autosomal recessive and sex-limited autosomal dominant transmission.

The syndrome of XX male is similar to Klinefelter's syndrome where the external genitalia usually differentiate normally as male but the testes are small. Hypospadias may occur infrequently. The incidence is 1 in 20 000 male births and, unlike Klinefelter's syndrome, height is below average for normal males. Infertility is invariable; around 90% of XX males are *SRY* positive. However, the coexistence of ovotesticular DSD and XX male within families and the reported occurrence of 46,XX *SRY*-negative monozygotic twins with genital anomalies suggests that these two forms of DSD are manifestations of the same underlying disorder in gonad determination. Mutations in *RSPO1*, an ovarian-specific determining gene, results in female-to-male XX sex reversal and hence may explain the phenotype in some *SRY*-negative XX males. The phenotype is also replicated in a *Rspo1* (–/–) XX mouse model.

46,XX DSD (the masculinized female; female pseudohermaphroditism)

In most instances, this broad category of DSD is characterized by a list of conditions where the effect of an abnormal excess of endogenous or exogenous androgens is superimposed on the constitutive female sex development. Thus internal genital development is normal (ovaries, uterus, and fallopian tubes; absence of wolffian ducts) whereas the external genitalia are virilized to a variable degree. The prime example of XX, DSD is congenital adrenal hyperplasia.

Congenital adrenal hyperplasia (CAH)

This autosomal recessive disorder of adrenal steroidogenesis is covered in detail in Chapter 13.7.2. CAH is the commonest cause of ambiguous genitalia of the newborn, and mutations affecting the *CYP21A2* gene account for more than 90% of cases. The degree of external masculinization can be so extreme as to resemble a newborn male. However, routine newborn examination should reveal the absence of palpable testes, a sign that must prompt urgent investigation. The diagnosis is straightforward and must be undertaken promptly in view of the potential life-threatening consequences for the infant from glucocorticoid and mineralocorticoid deficiency. The much rarer enzyme deficiencies affecting early steps in adrenal steroidogenesis are also potentially life-threatening and are described in Chapter 13.7.2.

Other causes of endogenous fetal androgen excess

The fetal adrenals are unique in containing a large fetal zone which involutes after birth. Its peculiar role in producing large amounts of androgens does not become established again until late childhood when the zona reticularis differentiates functionally and is manifest as adrenarche. Large quantities of dehydroepiandrosterone (DHA) and its sulphated moiety (DHAS) are produced greatly in excess of the principle adrenal glucocorticoid, cortisol, yet the precise function of this steroid in both fetal and postnatal life remains a mystery.

DHEAS is 16-hydroxylated in the adrenals and liver before transfer to the placenta where the sulphate is cleaved by placental sulphatase. The substrates DHEA and 16-OH-DHEA are converted to more potent androgens such as androstenedione and testosterone and all three androgens are converted to oestrogens (oestrone, oestradiol, oestriol). This reaction is mediated by a single gene, *CYP19*, which encodes for placental aromatase enzyme via a tissue-specific promoter. Measurement of maternal serum or urinary oestriol was previously used as a rather nonspecific marker of placental dysfunction. However, the levels are specifically low in CAH, in placental sulphatase deficiency (as the sulphate moiety is uncleaved to allow substrate for aromatization), and as a marker of suppression of fetal adrenal steroidogenesis during prenatal treatment for CAH.

The effects of placental aromatase deficiency are profound on both the fetus and the mother. Exposing a female fetus to large amounts of adrenal-derived androgens leads to virilization of the external genitalia as severe as in CAH. Salt wasting is not an associated feature. The mother is also virilized during pregnancy, with evidence of hirsutism, acne, and sometimes clitoromegaly. These signs resolve postnatally but can recur in subsequent pregnancies. Affected girls in later life can present with delayed puberty due to primary gonadal failure where there are cystic ovarian changes and hypergonadotropism. A male fetus exposed to excess adrenal androgens, as with CAH, is not affected at birth. However, males with aromatase deficiency are very tall in young adulthood because of failure in oestrogen-induced closure of the growth plate. The aromatase enzyme has a massive capacity to convert androgens to oestrogens as the mother escapes virilization if only 1 to 2% activity

of mutant enzyme remains. The mechanism of virilization in a 46,XX infant with P450 oxidoreductase (POR) deficiency may also be partly related to a disturbance in aromatase deficiency as POR is also an electron donor for P450 aromatase. It has also been suggested that an alternative fetal pathway to DHT synthesis is adopted secondary to POR deficiency (see Chapter 13.7.2).

Maternal androgen excess

The fetus is protected against excess androgens because of a highly efficient placental aromatase enzyme that converts androgens to oestrogens. Women with CAH who become pregnant have relatively high serum androgen levels during pregnancy, yet virilization of a female fetus has not been observed. However, the enzyme can become overwhelmed by excess androgens originating from maternal adrenal or ovarian androgen-secreting tumours. Ovarian luteomas can be recurrent in pregnancies and are most common in multiparous women of Afro-Caribbean descent. Other virilizing ovarian tumours include hyperreactio luteinalis, arrhenoblastoma, hilar cell tumour, and a Krukenberg tumour. Occasionally, polycystic ovarian syndrome may result in fetal virilization. Danazol, a synthetic derivative of 17β-ethinyltestosterone with androgenic, antioestrogenic and antiprogestogenic properties, readily crosses the placenta. It is used for a number of conditions as diverse as endometriosis, benign fibrocystic breast disease, for unexplained female infertility, and in hereditary angioedema. A female fetus can become virilized and the use of danazol is contraindicated in pregnancy.

46,XY DSD (the undermasculinized male; male pseudohermaphroditism)

A lengthy list of causes is included in this category of DSD and the frequency is quite high if more common conditions such as hypospadias and cryptorchidism are included. Although the problem of XY DSD is more complex than XX DSD in terms of diagnosis and management, knowledge of the normal process of male fetal sex development allows the causes to be subdivided into (1) gonadal dysgenesis (defects in testis determination), (2) defects in androgen biosynthesis, and (3) resistance to androgens.

Defects in testis determination (gonadal dysgenesis)

The pivotal role of SRY in human testis development is vividly illustrated by the phenotype of complex XY sex reversal as a manifestation of an inactivating mutation of the *SRY* gene. There is complete gonadal dysgenesis with the histological appearance of streak gonads and no discernible testis development in the form of seminiferous tubules or Leydig cells. Lack of Sertoli cells and hence no AMH production leads to a uterine remnant and the external genitalia are female as a result of no androgen production. Presentation does not usually occur until adolescence on account of delayed puberty and primary amenorrhoea. The syndrome (Swyer's) may present in later adulthood because of a gonadal tumour, typically as a dysgerminoma. Other tumours include gonadoblastoma, teratoma, and embryonal carcinoma. The risk of gonadal tumours is in the range of 15 to 35%. Mullerian structures are preserved and the uterus increases in size when oestrogen replacement is started. Bone mineral density is reduced in the majority. Adult height in a United Kingdom series was 174 cm as compared with 164 cm in the normal female population. Successful pregnancies have been achieved following egg donation.

Mutations in the *SRY* gene are found in only 15 to 20% of cases of complete XY gonadal dysgenesis. The majority are located within the HMG box, a DNA binding domain which appears to function by modulating local chromatin structure in order to transcribe adjacent target genes. The majority of mutations are *de novo*, yet there is a curious subset of cases where the mutation is familial and found in the phenotypically normal and fertile father. Explanations for this paradox include expression of the gene to a sufficient threshold against a particular genetic background that is not present in the 46,XY daughter. Alternatively, paternal gonadal mosaicism may be an explanation for familial cases. Partial gonadal dysgenesis refers to evidence of some virilization in the form of clitoromegaly and partial labial fusion or a more male pattern of external genital development with severe hypospadias, bifid scrotum, and undescended gonads. This phenotype is common to many other causes of 46,XY DSD. Mutations in *SRY* are not identified in this form of gonadal dysgenesis but *SF1* mutations have been identified in some cases and without adrenal insufficiency.

A number of syndromes are described in association with XY gonadal dysgenesis where the genital anomalies can constitute complete sex reversal or varying degrees of external genital ambiguity. Denys–Drash syndrome (OMIM 194080) is characterized by gonadal dysgenesis, an early-onset nephropathy due to diffuse mesangial sclerosis and a high risk of Wilms' tumour. A related condition is Frasier's syndrome (OMIM 136680) which is also characterized by gonadal dysgenesis but of a greater severity (streak gonads), a later-onset nephropathy due to focal segmental glomerulosclerosis, and a high risk of gonadal tumours. The two syndromes may represent a continuum of phenotypes. Both have in common mutations in the Wilms' tumour-related gene, *WT1*, as the underlying cause. The gene encodes for a four-zinc-finger transcription factor expressed in the developing urogenital ridge, kidney, and gonads. A macro- deletion affecting the region on chromosome 11p13 where *WT1* resides causes the WAGR syndrome (Wilms' tumour, aniridia, genitourinary abnormalities and mental retardation; OMIM 194072). Denys–Drash and Frasier's syndromes are caused by heterozygous point mutations in *WT1* that have a dominant-negative effect on the wild-type protein. In the former syndrome, these affect the DNA-binding zinc-finger region of WT1. Most mutations causing Frasier's syndrome involve the donor splice site of exon 9. The use of an alternative splice donor site for exon 9 results in the addition of three amino acids—lysine (K), threonine (T), and serine (S)—between the third and fourth zinc fingers. The +KTS and –KTS isoforms are thought to have differential effects on gonad and renal development and an imbalance in the ratio of these isoforms may be the explanation for the phenotype of Frasier's syndrome. It has been proposed that all cases of XY DSD with external genital anomalies should have routine urinalysis for proteinuria and renal ultrasound to exclude a Wilms' tumour. Rarely, a *WT1* mutation has been identified in a case of isolated hypospadias but this does not justify routine *WT1* screening for this common genital anomaly.

Another syndrome associated with gonadal dysgenesis and genital anomalies is caused by mutations in *SOX9* which encodes for an SRY-related HMG box protein of 509 amino acids. The protein is expressed in the developing testis shortly after SRY expression. The protein is also expressed in cartilage; heterozygous mutations in *SOX9* (chromosome 17q24–25) cause campomelic dysplasia (long bone bowing, hypoplastic scapula and rib cage, deformed pelvis, cleft palate, macrocephaly, cardiac and renal defects) as well as the associated genital anomalies. *SOX9* mutations do not occur without the skeletal abnormalities. There are rare examples of gonadal dysgenesis occurring in association with mutations in desert hedgehog (*DHH*) and testis-specific protein-like-1 (*TSPYL1*) genes and with chromosomal deletions at 9p24-pter, 10q25-pter, and Xq13.3.

Defects in androgen biosynthesis

The steps in androgen production from LH-induced steroidogenesis via cholesterol through to testosterone and DHT are illustrated in Fig. 13.9.3.4. Many of the early steps in androgen biosynthesis are also essential for adrenal steroid biosynthesis and are described in Chapter 13.7. The same G-protein-coupled gonadotrophin receptor (LHR) on Leydig cells binds both placental hCG and later, fetal pituitary luteinizing hormone (LH) for the initiation of androgen biosynthesis. Inactivating mutations in the *LHR* gene in 46,XY DSD lead to a wide range of phenotypes that include complete sex reversal, ambiguous genitalia, severe hypospadias, or even just isolated micropenis. Why the phenotype should be so heterogeneous is not entirely clear, although partial loss-of-function mutations that result in a milder phenotype such as micropenis tend to localize within the seventh transmembrane domain of the receptor. The biochemical profile comprises elevated LHRH-stimulated LH and FSH levels and low androgen concentrations which do not respond to prolonged hCG stimulation. Leydig cells are absent or decreased in number on histological examination. Sertoli cells and seminiferous tubules are present but spermatogenic arrest attests to the importance of intracellular androgen concentrations in mediating the final stages of spermatogenesis. A range of homozygous or compound heterozygous mutations of the *LHR* gene are reported in this syndrome of Leydig cell hypoplasia. Their pathogenicity can be confirmed *in vitro* by demonstrating impaired hCG stimulation of intracellular cAMP due to disturbances in hCG binding, receptor stability or receptor trafficking. The extracellular N-terminal ligand binding domain of LHR consists of nine leucine-rich repeats flanked by cysteine-rich regions. The C-terminal cysteine-rich region is referred to as a hinge region of the receptor within which amino acid residues Asp330 and Tyr331 are key components of LH/hCG signalling. An XX female has been reported with an *LHR*-inactivating mutation. The phenotype comprised normal onset of puberty but associated primary amenorrhoea and elevated LH levels. Studies on a rare gene mutation in this context provides information to indicate that while the LHR is not required for oestrogen synthesis, it is necessary for the induction of ovulation and fertility, although some affected females may still have regular cycles.

Two penultimate steps in androgen biosynthesis essential for normal male sex differentiation are shown in Fig. 13.9.3.4. Both conversion steps are characterized by the respective substrates being the subject of catalysis by different isoenzymes and not involving steroid biosynthesis in the adrenals. The forms of XY DSD resulting from deficiencies in the two enzymatic steps have in common a severe degree of undermasculinization at birth but profound virilization at puberty. Thus, if unrecognized at birth and the affected infant is assigned female, the clinical presentation occurs at puberty with distressing signs of clitoromegaly, hirsutism, and deepening of the voice in a pubertal girl.

There are 14 known 17β-hydroxysteroid dehydrogenase (17HSD) isoenzymes, of which 12 are present in humans. They belong to a family of oxidoreductases involved in the metabolism of steroids, prostaglandins, and retinols. Of most relevance to XY DSD is 17HSD type 3, which is predominantly expressed in the testis and converts androstenedione to testosterone. The reaction is reversible and utilizes NADPH as a cofactor. The cognate gene, *HSD17B3*, is located on chromosome 9q22. A spectrum of mutations in this gene generally results in complete XY sex reversal at birth and can be mistaken for complete androgen insensitivity syndrome. Presentation in infancy may be in the form of an inguinal hernia or labial swelling where investigation reveals the presence of a testis. If sex assigned female, gonadectomy must be undertaken before puberty to avoid a pubertal girl becoming virilized. The mechanism of such profound androgenic effects is postulated to be the result of extraglandular conversion to androgens utilizing other isoenzymes such as types 1, 2, and 5. Some *17HSDB3* mutations are associated with retention of 15 to 20% of normal 17βHSD3 activity that leads to sufficient virilization of the external genitalia at puberty for sex reassignment. The biochemical profile shows elevated androstenedione and decreased testosterone levels so that the ratio of testosterone to androstenedione is typically 0.8 or less in this disorder. Wolffian ducts are stabilized to form the vas deferens, epididymis, and seminal vesicle which is presumably the result of high local concentrations of androstenedione. About 20 mutations in the *17HSDB3* gene are now reported, most being homozygous or compound heterozygous missense mutations. Females with 17βHSD type 3 deficiency are asymptomatic.

Testosterone is converted irreversibly to dihydrotestosterone (DHT) by the 5α-reductase type 2 enzyme which is expressed in the primordium of the prostate and external genitalia, but not in the wolffian ducts until after their differentiation to male internal genital ducts. As with 17βHSD deficiency, the male internal genital ducts develop normally in 5α-reductase deficiency. The phenotype is associated with some external virilization so that presentation is more frequent at birth because of ambiguous genitalia or severe hypospadias. This cause of XY DSD became well characterized through detailed descriptions of a genetic isolate in the Dominican Republic where males were born with severely undermasculinized external genitalia but then virilized to varying degrees at puberty. The testes enlarge appropriately at this stage, but the prostate gland remains hypoplastic, indicative of the DHT-dependent growth of this organ. Histology of the testes shows Leydig cell hyperplasia and decreased spermatogenesis due to maldescent of the testes. However, there are reports of male fertility occurring either following artificial reproductive techniques or even spontaneously after hypospadias repairs had been completed. Gender role changes occur frequently in this condition.

The biochemical profile is classically an elevated ratio of serum testosterone to DHT of more than 25:1 after puberty (or following hCG stimulation in a prepubertal child) and a reduced ratio of urinary 5α- to 5β-reduced C19 steroids. The 5α-reductase enzyme is also utilized in the metabolism of glucocorticoids, so C21 5α/5β steroids can usefully be analysed even when gonadectomy has already taken place. There are two isoenzymes of 5α-reductase, the type 2 enzyme being affected in this condition. *SRD5A2* is located on chromosome 2p23 and encodes for a 254 amino acid protein. The type 1 enzyme is expressed in skin and may contribute to the virilization which takes place at puberty. More than 40 mutations have been detected in the *SRD5A2* gene. The majority are missense mutations, including the Gly183Ser substitution observed in the Dominican Republic population. A complete gene deletion is found in an affected New Guinea population.

Defects in androgen action

Androgen resistance is defined as a failure in complete male sex differentiation despite the presence of a normal 46,XY karyotype in association with testes that produce age-appropriate circulating concentrations of androgens. The androgen insensitivity syndromes (AIS) are subdivided into complete (CAIS) and partial (PAIS) forms as defined by complete XY sex reversal (female phenotype) and partial virilization of the external genitalia. The degree of virilization in the latter category can vary from mild, isolated clitoromegaly to normal male development with oligospermia.

Total resistance to androgens leading to CAIS is the *sine qua non* of a hormone resistance syndrome and was previously labelled as the testicular feminization syndrome. Typical presentation is in adolescence with primary amenorrhoea. There is normal breast development as male-typical androgen levels are aromatized to oestrogens, but there is absent or scanty pubic and axillary hair growth. The external genitalia are female and a shortened vagina is blind-ending. The upper part of the vagina, together with the uterus and fallopian tubes, are structures derived from the mullerian duct, hence these are absent in CAIS as a result of normal AMH action by the testes. CAIS may also present in infancy because of the appearance of inguinal herniae which, at surgical repair, are found to contain testes. It is now recommended that the karyotype is checked in all female infants with an inguinal hernia. The increasing trend towards prenatal tests that reveal the karyotype is also a mode of presentation when the phenotype at birth is realized to be a mismatch with the prenatal genotype. Reference to Fig. 13.9.3.5 indicates that a defect in any one of the steps in androgen signalling may underlie the pathophysiology of CAIS. The problem is generally located with the AR where numerous mutations have been identified that cause CAIS or PAIS. These are recorded on an international database (http://androgendb.mcgill.ca/) and also by the author via the Cambridge DSD database (Fig. 13.9.3.5). Mutations are distributed throughout the coding region of the *AR* gene and includee deletions, insertions, premature stop codons, and splice-site as well as missense mutations. The majority are located within the ligand-binding domain and codons such as Arg840 and Arge855 appear to be relative 'hotspots' for mutagenesis. Mutations that are novel generally need re-creating by site-directed mutagenesis to determine their pathogenicity using reporter gene-based transactivation assays *in vitro*. Additional structural modelling studies can be used to predict the effect amino acid substitutions may have on the ligand-binding pocket. CAIS is an X-linked disorder and approximately 30% of *AR* gene mutations are spontaneous. The same mutation may manifest as different phenotypes, between and within affected families and to the extent of different sex assignments. The reasons for phenotypic variability are unclear but may include somatic mosaicism and differences in the lengths of the two AR trinucleotide repeats in the N-terminal domain, glutamine and glycine. The normal glutamine repeat range, (CAG) n, is approximately 10 to 31 and variations within this range are associated with several androgen-related disorders as shown in Table 13.9.3.4. Studies *in vitro* indicate a less transcriptionally active AR containing a longer CAG repeat. Hyperexpansion of the triplet repeat (>50) underlies the pathogenesis of spinal and bulbar muscular atrophy (Kennedy's disease). Males affected with this neurological disorder display signs of mild androgen insensitivity.

Gender assignment and sex of rearing in CAIS is female, as is later gender identity. Gonadectomy is recommended because of an

Table 13.9.3.4 Disease associations with variations in the AR glutamine repeat

Shortened (CAG)n	Increased (CAG)n
Prostate cancer	**Above normal range**
Ovarian hyperandrogenism	SBMA (Kennedy's disease)
Androgenetic alopecia	Hypospadias (one reported case)
Aspects of Klinefelter phenotype	**Within normal range**
Response to androgen treatment	Male infertility
Central obesity	Gynaecomastia
Mental retardation	Hypospadias
Endometrial cancer	Aspects of Klinefelter phenotype
Coronary artery disease severity	Bone density
	Breast cancer

approximately 5% risk of gonadal tumours. A precursor lesion to tumour development is intratubular germ cell neoplasia unclassified (ITGNU), also referred to as carcinoma *in situ* (CIS). This may subsequently lead to a gonadoblastoma, an occurrence which is rare before puberty. The timing of gonadectomy is variable but there is merit in delaying until young adulthood to enable spontaneous puberty to occur. There is no evidence that the slightly reduced bone mineral density in CAIS is ameliorated by this management approach, suggesting that androgens have a direct role in normal bone architecture. Oestrogen replacement needs to be started at about 11 years of age when gonadectomy is performed early. Ethinyl oestradiol starting at 2 μg/day is increased gradually, reaching 20 μg/day by 15 years of age. Final height rests between the average height of adult males and females.

Mutations are also distributed throughout the *AR* gene in PAIS, but are predominantly missense in nature. The partial androgenic effect can be verified by functional assays *in vitro* which demonstrate reporter gene responses close to the normal AR, but usually only after induction with very high concentrations of androgens. Such information can be valuable for predicting outcome at puberty in PAIS patients assigned male. Establishing a precise diagnosis in PAIS can be difficult as so many other disorders can be associated with the typical phenotype of severe hypospadias, micropenis, bifid scrotum, and undescended testes. These include androgen biosynthetic defects, partial gonadal dysgenesis, and mixed gonadal dysgenesis. In many instances, no single genetic cause can be found for a PAIS-like phenotype: external genitalia as described and normal androgen production. There is a strong association with low birth weight for gestational age in PAIS cases that have no *AR* gene mutation. This suggests placental dysfunction being a common link between early fetal growth restriction and inadequate placental hCG-induced early Leydig cell steroidogenesis. The infant with PAIS assigned male may require a number of surgical procedures to correct hypospadias, orchidopexy for undescended testes, and high supplemental androgen treatment to induce puberty. The risk of gonadal tumours is probably higher than in CAIS, but once in the scrotum, the testes can be monitored by self-examination and periodic testicular ultrasonography. Outcome data in adult males with PAIS are sparse but sexual function is reported to be impaired; fertility is rare. Those assigned female require genitoplasty procedures in infancy, gonadectomy before puberty, and oestrogen treatment to induce female secondary characteristics.

Other conditions within the XY DSD category

A number of disorders are associated with incomplete male development but do not raise any doubt that sex assignment at birth should be male. These include hypospadias, undescended testes, and the persistent mullerian duct syndrome (PMDS).

Isolated hypospadias has a birth prevalence of 3 to 4 per 1000 live births. The cause in the majority of cases is unknown, despite extensive analysis of the known genes involved in male reproductive tract development. Familial cases occur with a 7% incidence of one or more additional family members being affected with hypospadias. There is an association with increased maternal age, paternal subfertility, maternal vegetarian diet, maternal smoking, assisted reproductive techniques, exposure to pesticides, and twinning. The aforementioned low birth weight is also a further association, which is strong. Hypospadias is generally classified as mild to severe based on the site of the urethral meatus being subglanular, penile, or perineoscrotal (severe). There is often an associated chordee in the severe form. Numerous surgical techniques are described to resite the urethral opening on to the glans penis and may require several procedures. The initial procedure is usually undertaken in infancy. Complications include fistulas, meatal stenosis, and urethral strictures. Function is generally satisfactory in terms of urination and sexual intercourse, even though the cosmetic appearance may not be adequate.

Undescended testes or cryptorchidism is the commonest birth defect in boys, affecting 2 to 9% of male live births. Again, there is a strong association with low birth weight as well as disorders that affect pituitary–gonadal function and androgen action. These observations emphasize the importance of androgens in mediating complete descent of the testes into the scrotum by their action during the inguinoscrotal phase of descent. Other associations include maternal smoking or use of nicotine substitutes, alcohol use, and gestational diabetes. There is an association with intrauterine insemination, but not with other forms of artificial reproductive technology. Genetic factors also play a part, particularly for first-degree relatives among brothers and maternal half-brothers. Cryptorchidism can be unilateral or bilateral with the testis sited in the abdomen (nonpalpable), inguinal canal, suprascrotal, or high scrotal (where it is not possible to manipulate the testis to the bottom of the scrotum). Undescended testis must be distinguished from a retractile testis which ascends in response to a pronounced cremasteric reflex but can be manipulated completely into the scrotum. A testis may be descended at birth but found to be undescended at a later age. This has been termed the 'ascending' testis or an acquired form of cryptorchidism. Studies indicate that the phenomenon is more likely with a history of retractile testis, the processus vaginalis may be patent, and the testis is usually located in the inguinal region. Ascending testis accounts for nearly one-half of the cases of undescended testis and mostly explains why late orchidopexies occur around 7 years of age. It is recommended that orchidopexy for congenital cryptorchidism is undertaken between 6 to 12 months of age. Early surgery is associated with improved growth of the testis, less evidence of abnormal germ-cell development and a lower risk of developing a seminoma in adulthood. Hormonal treatment has low efficacy and stimulation with repeated injections of hCG may actually be harmful to future spermatogenesis by inducing apoptosis of germ cells. Despite evidence for the role of INSL3 and its receptor in testis descent, mutations in the genes that encode these proteins are found only in a minority of boys with cryptorchidism.

The components of a quartet of male reproductive tract disorders—hypospadias, cryptorchidism, abnormal spermatogenesis, testis cancer—are each interlinked, for which there is some epidemiological evidence to suggest an increase in frequency. Environmental factors have been proposed to explain the observation through the development of a testicular dysgenesis syndrome which has its origin in fetal life. Humans are exposed to more than 80 000 chemicals in the environment with any adverse effects assumed to be more profound on the developing fetus. Evidence that chemicals such as pesticides and phthalates can disrupt the androgen/oestrogen balance critical for normal fetal sex development is present in wildlife and in animal experiments. It is more difficult to prove similar effects in humans. However, such chemicals labelled as endocrine disruptors are reported to be present in higher concentrations in cord blood, placentas, and breast milk samples of mothers having male offspring with hypospadias or cryptorchidism, compared with normal control offspring. Furthermore, the anogenital distance, which is a sensitive index of androgen action used in rodent reproductive studies, is reduced in male infants of mothers who had higher prenatal exposure to phthalates.

Bilateral anorchia, also referred to as the vanishing testis syndrome, in an otherwise normal male infant indicates that testes were present and functioning normally in early gestation in order to programme normal male sex differentiation. It is hypothesized that interruption of the vascular supply to the testes must have occurred in later gestation (akin to bilateral torsion). This is supported by surgical findings which show a preserved vas deferens entering the internal inguinal ring at the end of which is only a nubbin of fibrous tissue containing haemosiderin-laden macrophages and dystrophic calcification. The diagnosis is confirmed by demonstrating elevated LH and FSH concentrations, no testosterone response to hCG stimulation, and an undetectable serum AMH. Even with this endocrine scenario, surgeons generally still perform a laparoscopy to ensure that any gonadal remnant is removed to avoid the risk of malignancy.

PMDS is also associated with testis maldescent but in this instance normal testes are prevented from descending to the scrotum because of being attached to a fallopian tube. The uterus and tubes in this syndrome are retained from early fetal development because of the lack of AMH action. This can either be the result of a mutation in the *AMH* gene with low or undetectable serum AMH, or serum AMH concentrations may be normal but the protein is unable to bind to its receptor because of a mutation in the gene coding for the AMH type II receptor. A mutation is found in the majority of cases with equal distribution between the two causative mutant genes. The phenotypes are identical. The external genitalia are otherwise normal; both testes may be descended to one hemiscrotum. Such transverse testicular ectopia is diagnostic of PMDS. The diagnosis is usually made at orchidopexy or for an inguinal hernia repair where the sac is found to contain a uterus or a fallopian tube. Care must be taken to re-site the testis to its normal position as such mobilization may damage the vas deferens. The uterus is often left in place.

Assessment of a DSD

Ambiguous genitalia of the newborn and development of secondary sexual characteristics at puberty discordant with the sex of rearing are the two key stages in life when a problem of DSD requires careful assessment based on clinical examination followed by a focused and logical investigation plan. It must also be recognized that while a definitive diagnosis may not be possible in some cases, this must not delay a decision on sex assignment unduly and lessen the importance for a management plan.

Examination

For the infant with ambiguous genitalia, the following details need to be recorded: the size of the phallus, presence of chordee, and whether the appearance is indicative of clitoromegaly or a micropenis; site of urethral opening; single or dual openings on the perineum; development of labioscrotal folds or a bifid scrotum; whether gonads are palpable and their site. Allied to the examination are salient points in the clinical history such as family history and exposure to potential reproductive tract teratogens. Problems arising only at the time of puberty are generally signs of virilization occurring in a child hitherto assumed to be female. These can include deepening of the voice, hirsutism, acne, and clitoromegaly. Delayed pubertal development and primary amenorrhoea are manifestations of gonadal dysgenesis, whereas primary amenorrhoea but normal breast development is more consistent with CAIS.

Investigations

Box 13.9.3.1 lists clinical problems presenting in infancy that merit further investigation. The tests to be performed and which protocols to use vary according to centres, but Box 13.9.3.2 lists the categories according to the relevant specialist areas. These investigations should enable a functional diagnosis to be achieved within days of birth for the infant with ambiguous genitalia. The leading causes are likely to be CAH, PAIS and XO/XY mixed gonadal dysgenesis. A provisional result on the sex chromosomes is now rapidly available using FISH analysis. The karyotype in turn will steer subsequent investigations in the appropriate direction.

Box 13.9.3.1 Newborn problems that merit DSD investigation

- Ambiguous genitalia
- Apparent female genitalia with:
  - Enlarged clitoris
  - Posterior labial fusion
  - Inguinal/labial mass
- Apparent male genitalia with:
  - Nonpalpable testes
  - Isolated perineoscrotal hypospadias
  - Severe hypospadias, undescended testes, micropenis
- Genital anomalies associated with syndromes
- Family history of DSD, such as CAIS
- Discordance between genital appearance and prenatal karyotype

---

Box 13.9.3.2 Investigating an infant with ambiguous genitalia

- Genetics
  - FISH (X centromeric and SRY probes)
  - Karyotype (high resolution; abundant mitoses)
  - Save DNA with consent
- Endocrine
  - 17-OH progesterone, 11-deoxycortisol (plus routine biochemistry; save serum) renin
  - ACTH, 24-h urinary steroids (also check proteinuria)
  - Testosterone, androstenedione, DHT
  - LH, FSH, AMH, inhibin B
  - hCG stimulation test (define dose, timing)
- Imaging
  - Pelvic, adrenal, renal US
  - MRI
  - Cystourethroscopy and sinogram
- Surgical
  - Laparoscopy
  - Gonadal biopsies
  - Genital skin biopsy (AR studies, extract DNA and RNA)

For example, a FISH analysis suggesting XX chromosomes and confirmed on full karyotype analysis, an ultrasound showing a uterus, and a markedly elevated serum 17-OH progesterone concentration clinches a diagnosis of CAH in an infant with ambiguous genitalia. For the XY or XO/XY infant with DSD, the hCG simulation test and AMH measurement will provide information about the presence of testes and whether they produce normal concentrations of testosterone. Imaging studies (ultrasonography and MRI) may locate the site of gonads but often laparoscopy is the only reliable method to identify gonads. This also provides the opportunity to obtain biopsies for histology, the only sure way to establish a diagnosis of ovotesticular DSD (true hermaphroditism).

Management

Only the principles of DSD management can be described since each cause of DSD has specific requirements, some of which have been covered for CAH in Chapter 13.7.2. The greatest challenges for the endocrinologist are to manage the newborn with ambiguous genitalia and the pubertal child who develops physical signs incongruent with the sex of rearing. It is axiomatic that management should only be undertaken by a multidisciplinary team that comprises, at a minimum, an endocrinologist, urologist, gynaecologist, a geneticist, and a clinical psychologist. There is consensus that all infants with DSD should have a gender assignment, but this may have to be delayed until the results of relevant investigations are available. Surgery required to make the genitalia concordant with gender assigned may be deferred, even to an age where the child is of sufficient cognitive development to be involved with the discussions. Psychological support is required for the family from the

outset, as misinformation given early can impact adversely in the longer term. As the child grows older preparations for disclosure must be carefully planned. In a female with XY DSD (CAIS, for example), this will entail explanation concerning the nature of the gonads, the presence of a Y chromosome, absence of a uterus, lack of menses, and future infertility. Such disclosure requires skilled counselling delivered as appropriate to the child's development. Transitional care from adolescence to young adulthood is a further level of complexity that requires the recruitment of adult specialists relevant to whether sex assignment has remained male or female. Longer-term studies in women with CAH are now being conducted and provide valuable information on surgical, endocrine, and psychosexual outcomes. In terms of XY DSD, outcome data are reasonably robust for miscellaneous conditions such as cryptorchidism, hypospadias, mixed gonadal dysgenesis (XO/XY), and CAIS. In contrast, data remain sparse in PAIS and some androgen biosynthetic defects, conditions where sex reassignment may arise in later childhood and adolescence.

Further reading

Audi L, et al. (2010). Novel (60%) and recurrent (40%) oncogene receptor gene mutations in a series of 59 patients with a 46,XY disorder of sex development. *J Clin Endocrinol Metab*, **95**, [Epub ahead of print.]

Baskin LS, Ebbers MB (2006). Hypospadias: anatomy, etiology, and technique. *J Pediatr Surg*, **41**, 463–72.

Blackless M, et al. (2000). How sexually dimorphic are we? Review and synthesis. *Am J Hum Biol*, **12**, 151–66.

Cohen-Kettenis PT (2005). Gender change in 46,XY persons with 5α-reductase-2 deficiency and 17β-hydroxysteroid dehydrogenase-3 deficiency. *Arch Sex Behav*, **34**, 399–410.

de Clemente N, Belville C (2006). Anti-Müllerian hormone receptor defect. *Best Pract Res Clin Endocrinol Metab*, **20**, 599–610.

Deeb A, et al. (2005). Correlation between genotype, phenotype and sex of rearing in 111 patients with partial androgen insensitivity syndrome. *Clin Endocrinol (Oxf)*, **63**, 56–62.

Greenland KJ, Zajac JD (2004). Kennedy's disease: pathogenesis and clinical approaches. *Int Med J*, **34**, 279–86.

Hagenfeldt K, et al. (2008). Fertility and pregnancy outcome in women with congenital adrenal hyperplasia due to 21-hydroxylase deficiency. *Hum Reprod*, **23**, 1607–13.

Han TS, et al. (2008). Comparison of bone mineral density and body proportions between women with complete androgen insensitivity syndrome and women with gonadal dysgenesis. *Eur J Endocrinol*, **159**, 179–85.

Hannema SE, Hughes IA (2008). Neoplasia and intersex states. In: Hay I, Wass J(eds) *Clinical Endocrine Oncology*, 2nd edition, pp. 86–96. Blackwell Publishing, Oxford.

Hirvikoski T, et al. (2008). Long-term follow-up of prenatally treated children at risk for congenital adrenal hyperplasia: does dexamethasone cause behavioural problems? *Eur J Endocrinol*, **159**, 309–16.

Hughes I, Acerini C (2008). Factors controlling testis descent. *Eur J Endocrinol*, **159** Suppl 1, S75–82.

Hughes IA, Achermann JC (2007). Disorders of sex differentiation. In: Kronenberg H, et al. (eds) *Williams' Textbook of Endocrinology*, 11th edition, pp. 783–48. Saunders Elsevier, Philadelphia.

Hughes IA, Deeb A (2006). Androgen resistance. *Best Pract Res Clin Endocrinol Metab*, **20**, 577–98.

Hughes IA, Houk C, Ahmed SF, Lee PA (2006). Consensus statement on management of intersex disorders. *Arch Dis Child*, **91**, 554–63.

Jones ME, et al. (2007). Recognising rare disorders: aromatase deficiency. *Nat Clin Pract Endocrinol Metab*, **3**, 414–421.

Lee YS, *et al.* (2007). Phenotypic variability in 17β-hydroxysteroid dehydrogenase-3 deficiency and diagnostic pitfalls. *Clin Endocrinol*, **67**, 20–8.

Lin L, *et al.* (2007). Heterozygous missense mutations in steroidogenic factor 1 (SF1/Ad4BP, NR5A1) are associated with 46,XY disorders of sex development with normal adrenal function. *J Clin Endocrinol Metab*, **92**, 991–9.

Looijenga LH, *et al.* (2007). Tumor risk in disorders of sex development (DSD). *Best Pract Res Clin Endocrinol Metab*, **21**, 480–95.

Looijenga, LHJ, *et al.* (2009). Disorders of sex development: update on the genetic background, terminology and risk for the development of germ cell tumors. *World J Pediatr*, **5**, 93–102.

Michala L, *et al.* (2009). 16 XY female. *Best Prac Res Clin Obstet Gynecol*, 1–10.

Ogilvy-Stuart AL, Brain CE (2004). Early assessment of ambiguous genitalia. *Arch Dis Child*, **89**, 401–7.

Paterski V, *et al.* (2009). Consequences of the Chicago consensus on disorders of sex development (DSD): Current practices in Europe. *Arch Dis Child* [Epub ahead of print.]

Pettersson A, *et al.* (2007). Age at surgery for undescended testis and risk of testicular cancer. *N Engl J Med*, **356**, 1835–41.

Royer-Pokara B, *et al.* (2004). Twenty-four new cases of WT1 germline mutations and review of the literature: genotype/phenotype correlations for Wilms tumour development. *Am J Med Genet*, **127A**, 249–57.

Scott RR, Miller WL (2008). Genetic and clinical features of p450 oxidoreductase deficiency. *Horm Res*, **69**, 266–75.

Sim H, Argentaro A, Harley VR (2008). Boys, girls and shuttling of SRY and SOX9. *Trends Endocrinol Metab*, **19**, 213–22.

Tomizuka K, Horikoshi K, Kitada R (2008). R-spondin1 plays an essential role in ovarian development through positively regulating Wnt-4 signaling. *Hum Mol Genet*, **17**, 1278–91.

Uhlenhaut NH, *et al.* (2009). Somatic sex reprogramming of adult ovaries to testes by FOXL2 ablation. *Cell*, **139**, 1130–42.

Verkauskas G, *et al.* (2007). The long-term follow up of 33 cases of true hermaphroditism: a 40 year experience with conservative gonadal surgery. *J Urol*, **177**, 726–31.

Vorona E, *et al.* (2007). Clinical, endocrinological, and epigenetic features of the 46,XX male syndrome, compared with 47,XXY Klinefelter patients. *J Clin Endocrinol Metab*, **92**, 3458–65.

Wang MH, Baskin LS (2008). Endocrine disruptors, genital development and hypospadias. *J Androl*, **29**, 499–505.

Wisniewski AB, Mazur T (2009). 46, XY DSD with female or ambiguous external genitalia at birth due to androgen insensitivity syndrome, 5α-reductase-2 deficiency, or 17β-hydroxysteroid dehydrogenase-3 deficiency: a review of quality of life outcomes. *Int J Ped Endocrinol* [Epub Sept 10].

Wünsch L, Schober JM (2007). Imaging and examination strategies of normal male and female sex development and anatomy. *Best Pract Res Clin Endocrinol Metab*, **21**, 367–79.

Pancreatic endocrine disorders and multiple endocrine neoplasia

N.M. Martin and S.R. Bloom

Essentials

Pancreatic neuroendocrine tumours (islet cell tumours) are rare and usually sporadic, but they may be associated with complex familial endocrine cancer syndromes. Recognized types of pancreatic neuroendocrine tumours are those that are nonfunctioning (often advanced at diagnosis due to the absence of symptoms attributable to hormone hypersecretion), insulinoma (the most frequent type, see Chapter 13.11.2), and others including:

Gastrinoma—90% located in the pancreatic region; present with severe, multiple peptic ulcers that are often associated with complications such as haemorrhage, perforation, and stricture formation (Zollinger–Ellison syndrome); diagnosis requires demonstration of a raised fasting plasma gastrin concentration associated with increased basal gastric acid secretion; symptomatic treatment is with high-dose proton pump inhibitors.

VIPoma—90% occur in the pancreas; present with large-volume diarrhoea without steatorrhoea (Verner–Morrison syndrome, pancreatic cholera); hypokalaemia may be profound; diagnosis can be confirmed by finding of an elevated plasma level of peptide histidine–methionine (PHM, produced from the prepro-VIP molecule); diarrhoea responds well to somatostatin analogues (octreotide, lanreotide).

Glucagonoma—rare α-cell tumours of the pancreas; presenting features include weight loss, diarrhoea, anorexia, abdominal discomfort (hepatomegaly from metastases), and diabetes, also necrolytic migratory erythema; diagnosis is made on the basis of an elevated fasting plasma glucagon in association with characteristic clinical features; skin rash and other symptoms may respond to somatostatin analogues; oral zinc sulphate supplementation may be of benefit and is usually given.

Management—the following should be considered in addition to the symptomatic treatments for pancreatic neuroendocrine tumours described above: (1) surgical resection—the only curative treatment, but not possible in many cases; (2) interferon-α and systemic chemotherapy (streptozotocin and either doxorubicin or 5-fluorouracil)—evidence of efficacy is limited, but some improvement in about 50% of cases; and—for patients with liver metastases—(3) surgical resection or other local ablative techniques; (4) radiopharmaceutical therapy—e.g. ^{90}Y-octreotide or ^{90}Y-lanreotide.

Multiple endocrine neoplasia (MEN)

There are two main MEN syndromes, which are rare hereditary conditions characterized by a predisposition to cancer development within two or more endocrine organs.

MEN 1—typical features are parathyroid adenomas, pancreatic neuroendocrine tumours (gastrinomas > insulinomas > others) and pituitary adenomas; caused by mutation of the *MEN1* gene, which encodes a nuclear protein (menin) that is presumed to be a tumour suppressor gene, with diagnosis confirmed by genetic analysis; following identification of an index case, genetic analysis in first-degree relatives allows identification of affected family members; minimal surveillance programme for individuals with MEN1 syndrome or a family-specific mutation of the *MEN1* gene should include annual measurement of serum prolactin (from age 5 years), fasting serum calcium and PTH (from age 8 years), and fasting serum gastrin concentration (from age 20 years).

MEN 2—there are three variants: (1) MEN 2A (Sipple's syndrome)—medullary thyroid carcinoma, phaeochromocytoma, and parathyroid hyperplasia/adenomas; (2) MEN 2B—medullary thyroid carcinoma and phaeochromocytoma, with other features including marfanoid habitus and mucosal neuromas; (3) familial medullary thyroid carcinoma. Caused by mutation in the *RET* oncogene, with diagnosis confirmed by genetic analysis and strong genotype–phenotype correlation informing management of index cases and affected family members, e.g. prophylactic thyroidectomy is recommended for those with mutations conferring the highest risk of aggressive medullary thyroid carcinoma; annual measurement of urinary catecholamines for those with high risk of phaeochromocytoma.

Other syndromes of MEN include (1) Carney complex, (2) McCune–Albright syndrome, (3) neurofibromatosis type 1, (4) von Hippel–Lindau syndrome.

Pancreatic neuroendocrine tumours

Pancreatic neuroendocrine tumours (islet cell tumours) are rare tumours representing 1 to 2% of all pancreatic neoplasms and have an incidence of approximately 1 per 100 000 per year. Although pancreatic neuroendocrine tumours may be associated with complex familial endocrine cancer syndromes such as multiple endocrine neoplasia (MEN), the majority are nonfamilial (sporadic) cases. Pancreatic neuroendocrine tumours have a wide range of clinical manifestations. Between 15 and 30% are clinically silent (nonfunctioning) and usually present with mass effect or metastatic disease. Those pancreatic neuroendocrine tumours associated with a specific endocrine hyperfunction syndrome are termed 'functional', with insulinomas and gastrinomas being the most common. The pancreas is an extremely rare site of carcinoid tumours, and the majority of carcinoids arise from extrapancreatic sites (carcinoid tumours are described in Chapter 15.9). This section will consider biochemical confirmation and localization of pancreatic neuroendocrine tumours, specific clinical presentations of functional tumour types, management options, and discussion of the clinical features of MEN types 1 and 2 (MEN1 and MEN2).

Introduction and definition

The gastrointestinal tract is the largest endocrine organ in the body, which includes endocrine cells of the gut and pancreas. The ability of these enteroendocrine cells to take up amine precursor substances and perform their decarboxylation to produce peptide hormones and biogenic amines led to their original description as APUD (amine precursor uptake and decarboxylation) cells. APUD cells were initially believed to arise from the embryological neural crest. However, this theory has been disproved, with current evidence suggesting that these cells are derived from endodermal, omnipotent stem cells. Since these enteroendocrine cells share many of the properties exhibited by neural cells, this has led to their description as neuroendocrine cells. Criteria for defining neuroendocrine cells include production of bioactive substances that provide transmitter functions, release of hormones via exocytosis from dense-core secretory vesicles following an external stimulus, and an absence of axons or synapses. These cells also share certain histological features with neural cells, including the presence of chromogranin-A, synaptophysin, and neuron-specific enolase.

Aetiology and genetics

Pancreatic neuroendocrine tumours are associated with complex familial endocrine neoplasia syndromes, including MEN1 and MEN2, von Hippel–Lindau (VHL) syndrome as well as the phacomatoses neurofibromatosis type 1 (NF-1) and tuberous sclerosis. Nevertheless, the majority of pancreatic neuroendocrine tumours are actually sporadic (i.e. non-inherited). Pancreatic neuroendocrine tumours are a principal feature of multiple endocrine neoplasia type 1. Over 95% of patients with MEN1 display germline-inactivating mutations in the *MEN1* gene, a presumed tumour suppressor gene located on chromosomes 11q13 which encodes for the menin protein. Of all these familial endocrine neoplasia syndromes, it is MEN1 that has the strongest association with pancreatic neuroendocrine tumours and these occur in up to 80% of MEN1 patients. Somatic mutations of the *MEN1* gene together with loss of heterozygosity on 11q13 have been associated

with nonfamilial malignant pancreatic neuroendocrine tumours. Approximately 14% of patients with VHL have pancreatic neuroendocrine tumours, which are usually nonfunctioning and often multiple. Products of the *VHL* gene inhibit transcription elongation, but the *VHL* gene does not appear to be involved in the pathogenesis of sporadic pancreatic neuroendocrine tumours.

Pancreatic neuroendocrine tumour markers

Serum markers

The chromogranins are acidic glycoproteins occurring in the dense-core secretory granules of neuroendocrine cells (see Chapter 15.9). Chromogranin A is released into the circulation and, to date, is considered to be the most useful nonspecific neuroendocrine tumour marker. Several commercial radioimmunoassays (RIAs) for the measurement of chromogranin A have been developed. Chromogranin A concentrations may correlate with tumour burden and can be also useful in monitoring response to treatment or recurrence of disease. Chromogranin A is elevated in patients with kidney, liver, or heart failure as well as with hypergastrinaemia, most notably due to the use of proton pump inhibitors. Chromogranin B coexists with chromogranin A, yet differs in its amino acid sequence and has been reported to be less influenced by renal failure and proton pump inhibitors. Chromogranin B may be more useful than chromogranin A in the diagnosis of insulinomas. The 74 amino acid C-terminal fragment of chronogranin B, known as GAWK, has been described as a particularly useful marker for pancreatic neuroendocrine tumours. Pancreatic polypeptide is produced by the F cells of the normal pancreas, although levels of pancreatic polypeptide may also be significantly increased in patients with pancreatic neuroendocrine tumours. Pancreatic polypeptide alone is a less sensitive neuroendocrine tumour marker than chromogranin A, yet its diagnostic sensitivity may be significantly increased when combined with chromogranin A. Pancreastatin, a cleavage product of chromogranin A, can also be measured by commercially available RIA, although it has been largely superseded by the measurement of chromogranin A. Although non- pancreatic neuroendocrine tumours are not associated with hypersecretion of a specific hormone, these tumours commonly secrete chromogranin A, pancreatic polypeptide, and α and β subunits of human chorionic gonadotrophin (hCG).

In addition to general pancreatic neuroendocrine tumour marker, specific gut hormones produced by these tumours can be measured by RIA using a single fasting plasma sample, and for certain syndromes a small number of confirmatory tests. As with chromogranins, several non-neoplastic conditions are associated with increased levels of specific circulating gut hormones (Table 13.10.1). Gut hormone RIAs are not well standardized, and there is considerable variation between laboratories. However, concentrations are usually of the same order of magnitude in all assays and show a similar percentage increase above normal.

Immunohistochemical markers

Assessment of pancreatic neuroendocrine tumours using immunohistochemistry involves general neuroendocrine tumour markers derived either from the cytosol such as neuron-specific enolase and the protein gene product 9.5 (PGP9.5), or granular markers such as chromogranin A and synaptophysin. The tumour should be stained for Ki-67 protein, to generate a proliferative index. Malignant neuroendocrine tumours are usually poorly differentiated,

Table 13.10.1 Causes of elevated gut hormones other than pancreatic endocrine tumours

All hormones	Nonfasting sample
	Renal failure
Gastrin	Hypercalcaemia
	Achlorhydria (most commonly proton pump inhibitor or other antacid therapy)
	Antral gastrin cell hyperfunction
VIP	Hepatic cirrhosis
	Bowel ischaemia
Glucagon	Hepatic failure
	Oral contraceptives and danazol
	Stress
	Prolonged fast
	Familial hyperglucagonaemia
PP	Elderly
	Pernicious anaemia
	Hypercalcaemia
	Neurotensin
	Fibrolamellar hepatoma

PP, pancreatic polypeptide; VIP, vasoactive intestinal polypeptide.

with cellular atypia, a high mitotic index, and a high proliferative status.

Imaging in pancreatic neuroendocrine tumours

Investigations used in the radiographic localization of pancreatic neuroendocrine tumours include ultrasonography, CT and MRI. Transabdominal ultrasonography may have limited use in the detection of small pancreatic neuroendocrine tumours, but can be used to take biopsies from metastases for histopathological analysis. In experienced hands, endoscopic ultrasonography may be more sensitive than conventional imaging, with a resolution of 2 mm and a detection rate of over 75% for tumours in the pancreatic head (Fig. 13.10.1). However, visualization using ultrasound is poorer for lesions in the pancreatic tail. Intraoperative ultrasonography

may be particularly effective in identifying pancreatic neuroendocrine tumours, especially when it is combined with palpation by the surgeon. Neuroendocrine tumour cells express somatostatin receptors, and hence somatostatin receptor scintigraphy with radiolabelled somatostatin analogues is the mainstay of imaging in most neuroendocrine tumours, particularly those arising from the pancreas. There are five somatostatin receptor subtypes (SSTRs 1–5) which all avidly bind endogenous somatostatin. The clinically used somatostatin analogues, octreotide and lanreotide, used for diagnosis and treatment, bind to SSTR-2 and SSTR-5. Only 50% of nonmetastatic insulinomas express SSTR-2, yet insulinomas with metastatic spread may be more likely to be positive for these receptors. Therefore, although somostatin receptor scintigraphy is recognized as the most sensitive imaging modality for pancreatic neuroendocrine tumours (80–90%), its role in nonmetastatic insulinomas is often limited. In cases of nonfunctioning pancreatic neuroendocrine tumours, somostatin receptor scintigraphy may be helpful in differentiating these from pancreatic adenocarcinomas. Somostatin receptor scintigraphy is also useful in detecting metastatic disease (Fig. 13.10.3), although the standard ^{99}Tc bone scan is the most sensitive imaging modality for bony metastases.

Somostatin receptor scintigraphy may be more limited in detecting small tumours, which is significant since 40% of gastrinomas and insulinomas are microadenomas (<1 cm). Such small pancreatic neuroendocrine tumours may be detected by selective angiography with secretagogue injection into the main pancreatic arteries (gastroduodenal, superior mesenteric, inferior pancreaticoduodenal, and splenic) (Fig. 13.10.2). In addition to anatomical localization, this enables biochemical localization. Previously, secretin was the secretagogue of choice, but this has now been replaced by calcium. Injection of calcium into the artery supplying the tumour causes a marked rise in hormone levels in the hepatic vein, and hence allows equivocal lesions to be verified. Visualization of a tumour blush on angiography prior to calcium stimulation further increases the sensitivity of this investigation. Furthermore, since the hepatic artery is cannulated at the end of the procedure, hepatic metastases may also be detected. Positron emission tomography (PET) utilizes uptake of certain radiolabelled tracers. The role of PET in pancreatic neuroendocrine tumours remains to be fully elucidated since most pancreatic neuroendocrine tumours do not

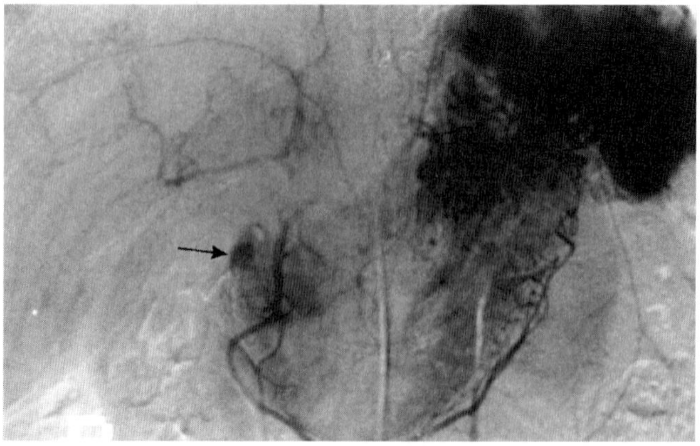

Fig. 13.10.1 Endoscopic ultrasound scan showing a 0.7 cm insulinoma in the head of the pancreas (arrowed).

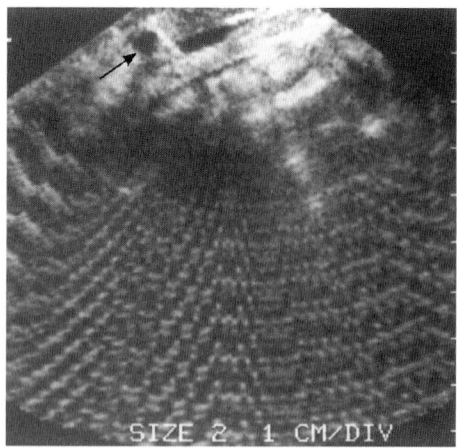

Fig. 13.10.2 Venous phase of coeliac axis angiogram demonstrating gastrinoma blush in duodenal wall (arrowed).

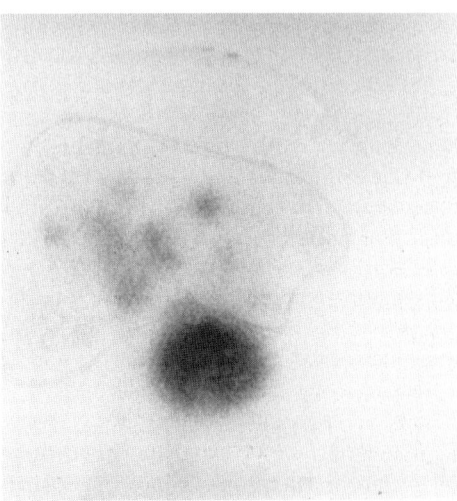

Fig. 13.10.3 ^{111}In-labelled SRS showing a large pancreatic glucagonoma and diffuse hepatic metastases.

show uptake with fluorodeoxyglucose PET owing to low metabolic activity.

Natural history

The spontaneous course of disease in pancreatic neuroendocrine tumours is difficult to ascertain because of their low incidence, heterogeneous behaviour, and an absence of controlled prospective clinical trials to assess the efficacy of different therapeutic strategies. Nonfunctioning pancreatic neuroendocrine tumours are often more advanced at diagnosis because of the absence of symptoms attributable to hormone hypersecretion. Poorly differentiated, large (>3 cm) tumours associated with metastases are indicators of a poor prognosis. Early in the disease, morbidity and mortality result from the effects of peptide hypersecretion rather than tumour bulk. Metastatic spread to liver and bone is a major cause of death in patients with pancreatic neuroendocrine tumours. The overall 5-year survival for pancreatic neuroendocrine tumours is 50 to 80%, with insulinomas and gastrinomas having up to 94% 5-year survival. Pancreatic neuroendocrine tumours associated with familial disease such as MEN1 may have a less favourable outcome than sporadic tumours, since these are frequently multiple and diffuse, which may limit surgical cure.

Specific tumour syndromes

Insulinomas

Insulinomas are the most frequent functional pancreatic neuroendocrine tumours and are discussed in Chapter 13.11.2.

Gastrinoma

Overall, gastrinomas are the second most frequent functionally active pancreatic neuroendocrine tumour. At the time of diagnosis, 50 to 60% are malignant. Over 90% of gastrinomas are in the pancreatic region of the 'gastrinoma triangle', an area bounded by the junction between the cystic duct and the common bile duct, the junction between the second and third parts of the duodenum, and the junction between the head and neck of pancreas. Those gastrinomas arising in the pancreas are most frequently situated in the pancreatic head. In MEN1 patients, gastrinomas are the most common functional pancreatic neuroendocrine tumour.

Approximately 25% of gastrinomas are associated with MEN1, although these tend to be situated in duodenum rather than the pancreas and are usually small and multifocal. The gastrinoma syndrome was first described in 1955 by Zollinger and Ellison, who reported the triad of fulminating ulcer diathesis, recurrent ulceration with a poor response to therapy, and pancreatic non-β-cell islet tumours. The syndrome, also known as Zollinger–Ellison syndrome, is the result of excess gastrin-stimulated gastric acid secretion. This causes severe, multiple peptic ulcers, which are usually duodenal, but may occur in the oesophagus and jejunum, and are often associated with complications such as haemorrhage, perforation, and stricture formation. The excess gastric acid secretion inactivates pancreatic enzymes and damages the intestinal mucosa, resulting in diarrhoea and steatorrhoea, which may be prominent features and may precede symptoms of peptic ulcer disease.

The diagnosis of the gastrinoma syndrome requires the demonstration of a raised fasting plasma gastrin concentration (>40 pmol/litre), associated with increased basal gastric acid secretion. Hypercalcaemia may increase plasma gastrin concentrations, which may be of consequence in patients with MEN1 and coexistent primary hyperparathyroidism. Since plasma gastrin levels in gastrinomas overlap with those seen with the use of antacids such as proton pump inhibitors, ideally patients should not take H_2-blockers for 3 days or proton pump inhibitors for 2 weeks before gastrin measurement. However, patients with true gastrinomas may be at risk of peptic ulcer perforation if anatacids are stopped for plasma gastrin measurements. Hypergastrinaemia and raised acid output may also arise from retained antrum following partial gastrectomy or the rare condition of antral gastrin cell hyperfunction. The intravenous secretin test distinguishes these conditions from gastrinoma and can aid diagnosis when other investigations are equivocal. Under normal physiological conditions, secretin inhibits serum gastrin. In contrast, secretin provokes a paradoxical rise in serum gastrin in patients with gastrinoma. Alternatively, an intravenous calcium infusion can be used diagnostically with a rise in plasma gastrin observed in gastrinoma patients. Since ingestion of food is a stimulus for gastrin secretion from the antral and duodenal mucosa, it has been proposed that a standard test meal may differentiate hypergastrinaemia of antral and tumoral origin. However, more recently the usefulness of this test has been questioned. If gastric acid output studies are not possible, a basal gastric pH above 2 virtually excludes the diagnosis of Zollinger–Ellison syndrome. Endoscopy may be valuable in demonstrating oesophageal and duodenal ulceration and hypertrophy of the gastric mucosa. Localization of microgastrinomas may be aided preoperatively by endoscopic ultrasound or selective visceral angiography and venous sampling. Survival depends on the presence of hepatic metastases at presentation, which is more commonly seen with pancreatic rather than duodenal gastrinomas. Overall, the 5-year survival rate is about 65%.

VIPoma

Tumours secreting vasoactive intestinal polypeptide (VIP) are termed VIPomas. Ninety per cent of VIPomas occur in the pancreas, most frequently arising from the pancreatic tail. Extrapancreatic VIPomas may be of neural origin, such as gangliomas or ganglioneuroblastomas which arise from the sympathetic chain or adrenal medulla, and these tumours are especially common in children. Most extrapancreatic tumours are benign, but more than 50% of pancreatic VIPomas have metastasized at the time of diagnosis, usually to local lymph nodes and the liver. Approximately 9% of VIPomas are associated with MEN1.

The features of the VIPoma (Verner–Morrison, pancreatic cholera) syndrome reflect the known biological actions of VIP. Large-volume diarrhoea without steatorrhoea is the cardinal symptom, with most patients excreting more than 3 litres per day. It is often intermittent at first, but in severe crises the volume loss coupled with the vasodilatory effects of VIP and the associated hypokalaemia may precipitate cardiovascular collapse. Hypokalaemia in the VIPoma syndrome may be profound, resulting from gastrointestinal losses and activation of the renin–angiotensin system. The loss of bicarbonate in the stool leads to a paradoxical acidosis, which may mask the true potassium deficit. Achlorhydria or hypochlorhydria occurs in more than 50% of patients and distinguishes this diarrhoeal syndrome from that associated with gastrinoma. Nevertheless, the absence of this feature in a significant proportion of VIPoma patients makes the acronym WDHA (watery diarrhoea, hypokalaemia, and achlorhydria) syndrome inappropriate. In up to 50% of cases there is glucose intolerance as a result of the glucagon-like actions of VIP. Other biochemical abnormalities include hypercalcaemia, probably due to secretion of parathyroid hormone-related peptide (PTHrP) and exacerbated by the dehydration and hypomagnesaemia, due to loss in stools. The vasodilatory action of VIP may cause flushing of the head and neck and, particularly on tumour palpation, may be associated with a marked fall in systemic blood pressure. In advanced cases, extreme weight loss may occur.

VIPomas are usually associated with markedly raised plasma VIP concentrations (>30 pmol/litre). Since the half-life of circulating VIP is only 2 min it may be difficult to always confirm an elevation in circulating VIP. Peptide histidine–methionine (PHM) produced from the prepro-VIP molecule, is more stable in plasma than VIP, and is cosecreted by VIPomas. Therefore, in patients with features consistent with VIPoma syndrome, the finding of an elevated PHM may confirm the diagnosis. Pancreatic polypeptide concentrations levels are elevated in 75% of cases and neurotensin in 10%. Primary pancreatic VIPomas are usually large (>2 cm) and so localization is rarely a problem. Occasionally, selective visceral angiography and venous sampling may be necessary to detect small pancreatic lesions. In those with nonmetastatic VIPomas, the 5-year survival rate is more than 90%; when metastases are present it is about 60%.

Glucagonoma

Glucagonomas are rare α-cell tumours of the pancreas which secrete various forms of glucagon and other peptides derived from the preproglucagon molecule. Primary glucagonomas most commonly arise in the pancreatic tail and extrapancreatic glucagonomas are rare. Glucagonomas are usually more than 2 cm in diameter at presentation. Smaller glucagonomas tend to be benign and increased tumour size correlates with risk of malignancy. In the majority of cases of sporadic glucagonomas, metastases have occurred at presentation. Up to 17% of glucagonomas are associated with MEN1 and these patients tend to present at a younger age.

Common presenting features of glucagonoma syndrome are weight loss, diarrhoea, anorexia, and abdominal discomfort, with the latter often reflecting tumour bulk from hepatomegaly.

Necrolytic migratory erythema is a frequent presenting feature of glucagonoma syndrome; it is cyclical in nature, consisting of macules, central bulla formation, and crusted plaques occurring mainly at friction sites such as perineum, buttocks, groin, lower abdomen, and lower extremities. The exact pathogenesis of this unusual skin eruption remains unclear and is likely to be multifactorial. Hypoaminoacidaemia, zinc deficiency, hypovitaminosis B, and hepatic dysfunction have all been implicated.

Diabetes mellitus is present in approximately two thirds of those with the glucagonoma syndrome and this may predate neurolytic migratory erythema. Other common presentations in glucagonoma syndrome include glossitis, angular cheilitis, and neurological and psychiatric symptoms. Thromboembolism has been described in up to 30% of all cases of glucagonoma syndrome, which is not a feature of other pancreatic neuroendocrine tumours and is a significant cause of death in glucagonoma syndrome.

The diagnosis of glucagonoma is made on the basis of an elevated fasting plasma glucagon (>50 pmol/litre), in association with characteristic clinical features and a demonstrable neuroendocrine tumour and/or metastatic deposits. Glucagonomas are usually of significant size at presentation to be identified by contrast-enhanced CT or MRI. Endoscopic ultrasonography may be of limited use in glucagonomas, as these are usually located in the pancreatic tail. Glucagonomas and their metastases are commonly hypervascular, making selective visceral angiography and venous sampling particularly useful in localizing the tumour and identifying small hepatic metastases. Although the majority of patients with glucagonoma syndrome present with evidence of metastases, the slow-growing nature of these tumours can result in a relatively good prognosis. The 5-year survival ranges from 66 to 85%.

Somatostatinoma

Somatostatinomas are extremely rare, with an estimated annual incidence of about 1 in 40 million per year. Fifty per cent of these tumours are pancreatic, the remainder arising in the duodenum. Unlike other functional pancreatic neuroendocrine tumours, somatostatinomas are rarely associated with MEN1. Pancreatic somatostatinomas are usually large, more than 2 cm at diagnosis, and thus present with local symptoms or features relating to excess somatostatin secretion. Somatostatin has been described as 'endocrine cyanide' because of its inhibitory effects on gut motility, transit and absorption, gallbladder contraction and secretion, and endocrine and exocrine pancreatic functions. The so-called somatostatin or 'inhibitory' syndrome resulting from somatostatin hypersecretion therefore consists of diarrhoea, steatorrhoea, cholelithiasis, hyperglycaemia, and hypochlorhydria. Hypoglycaemia has occasionally been described, possibly due to larger molecular forms of somatostatin having a greater inhibitory effect on counter-regulatory hormones than on insulin. In comparison to pancreatic somatostatinomas, duodenal somatostatinomas are smaller, frequently associated with neurofibromatosis type 1, seldom associated with a recognizable 'somatostatin syndrome' and often contain psammoma bodies. Duodenal somatostatinomas usually present with obstructive jaundice, pancreatitis, intestinal obstruction, or gastrointestinal haemorrhage. Diagnosis of a somatostatinoma is secured by demonstrating elevated plasma somatostatin levels (>150 pmol/litre) in the context of a relevant clinical history and the presence of a pancreatic mass. Multiple molecular weight forms of somatostatin may be demonstrated by column chromatography of plasma or tumour extracts, and these may explain unusual clinical features. Localization is rarely a problem due to the large size at presentation. Pancreatic and duodenal somatostatinomas appear to have similar rates of metastases and malignancy. The overall 5-year survival rate is 75%, or 60% if metastases are present.

Rare pancreatic neuroendocrine tumours

Ectopic ACTH production by pancreatic neuroendocrine tumours, resulting in Cushing's syndrome, is well documented in the literature and virtually all cases are highly malignant with a poor prognosis. Neurotensinomas are rare and truly difficult to separate from the symptom complex produced by VIP excess. There are reports of patients with acromegaly and gigantism as a result of ectopic GHRH secretion by pancreatic neuroendocrine tumours. Secretion of PTHrP by pancreatic neuroendocrine tumours resulting in hypercalcaemia has been rarely described. Other peptides produced by islet-cell tumours include neuropeptide Y, neuromedin B, calcitonin gene-related peptide, bombesin, and motilin, but these are not associated with recognized clinical syndromes.

Nonfunctioning pancreatic neuroendocrine tumours and pancreatic polypeptide-secreting tumours (PPomas)

Nonfunctional tumours represent 15 to 30% of pancreatic neuroendocrine tumours. These most frequently arise in the pancreatic head and are most often diagnosed in the fifth to sixth decades of life. Twenty to thirty per cent of these tumours are associated with MEN1. They usually present late with symptoms attributable to either tumour bulk, such as anorexia and weight loss, or to effects on local structures, such as obstructive jaundice or intestinal obstruction. Despite pancreatic polypeptide (PP) being secreted by up to 75% of pancreatic neuroendocrine tumours, PP itself has no recognized physiological role or associated tumour syndrome. Therefore, pure PPomas can also be regarded effectively as nonfunctioning tumours. Although diarrhoea may be a feature, PPomas are usually silent and present with pressure effects such as abdominal pain. Their malignant potential has not yet been defined. The clinical silence of these nonfunctioning pancreatic neuroendocrine tumours may also reflect secretion of neuropeptides at low circulating concentrations, biologically inactive molecular forms, down-regulation of peripheral receptors or simultaneous production of an inhibitor such as somatostatin. Nonfunctioning pancreatic neuroendocrine tumours are often mistakenly diagnosed as adenocarcinomas, but the presence of elevated circulating gut hormones, such as PP or neurotensin, negative uptake on somatostatin receptor scintigraphy and the use of immunocytochemical analysis can establish the correct diagnosis. The overall 5-year survival is about 50%.

Management of pancreatic neuroendocrine tumours

Surgical treatment

Surgery is the only curative treatment for pancreatic neuroendocrine tumours. In sporadic pancreatic neuroendocrine tumours, small isolated insulinomas or gastrinomas may be removed by enucleation. Larger functioning and nonfunctioning sporadic tumours may be removed by either a distal pancreatectomy or pancreato-duodenectomy depending on the location of the tumour. Surgical management of pancreatoduodenal neuroendocrine tumours in MEN1 remains controversial because of the multifocal nature of the associated pancreatic disease. In patients

with MEN1, surgical cure rates are high for insulinomas, but significantly lower for gastrinomas. Some centres advocate an aggressive surgical approach to MEN1-associated pancreatoduodenal neuroendocrine tumours, including distal subtotal pancreatectomy combined with preservation of the pancreatic head, enucleation of any neuroendocrine tumours remaining in the pancreatic head and in the duodenal wall. This approach may significantly reduce morbidity and mortality associated with pancreatic neuroendocrine tumours in MEN1 patients.

Symptomatic treatments
Somatostatin analogues

The inhibitory effects of somatostatin have therapeutic implications in pancreatic neuroendocrine tumours, although the clinical effectiveness of native somatostatin is limited by its short half-life of only minutes in the circulation. This necessitated the development of somatostatin analogues, which are the only proven treatment for control of symptoms in pancreatic neuroendocrine tumours and also control tumour growth, presumably because of their antiproliferative effects. The clinically available somatostatin analogues, octreotide and lanreotide, bind most avidly to SSTR-2 and -5 with a lower affinity for SSTR-3. SSTR-2 is believed to mediate the biochemical responses to somatostatin analogues, whereas both SSTR-2 and -5 subtypes are believed to mediate their antiproliferative effects.

Octreotide has a half-life of several hours in the circulation and is usually administered two to three times a day. Depot injections of somatostatin analogues have been developed more recently, allowing sustained release over a few weeks. Therefore, patients may be stabilized on short acting octreotide before converting to longer acting depot preparations. Tachyphylaxis often occurs with time which may necessitate dose escalation to control the clinical symptoms. Imaging using somatostatin scintigraphy can not only identify those who would benefit from somatostatin analogues, but also can be used to monitor the effects of treatment.

Specific tumour syndromes

Insulinomas Treatment of insulinomas is discussed in Chapter 13.11.2.

Gastrinomas Short- or long-term treatment with proton pump inhibitors, which inhibit gastric acid secretion, is highly effective for symptomatic relief and tachyphylaxis does not occur. Somatostatin analogues may be superfluous if symptomatic relief occurs with high-dose proton pump inhibitors, although these may be effective in metastatic disease.

VIPomas VIPomas are usually exquisitely sensitive to somatostatin analogues, with small doses often significantly reducing diarrhoeal symptoms. During acute crises, patients require aggressive intravenous rehydration combined with potassium and bicarbonate replacement if necessary.

Glucagonomas Octreotide is particularly useful as a prompt and effective treatment of necrolytic migratory erythema, providing improvement within 48 to 72 h of initiating treatment. Similarly, other symptoms such as diarrhoea and weight loss may also improve. Somatostatin analogues have a variable effect on glucose intolerance and adjuvant glucose-lowering therapy with oral hypoglycaemic agents or insulin may be required. Most patients with glucagonoma syndrome are treated empirically with oral zinc sulphate supplementation, regardless of plasma zinc levels. Patients should be anticoagulated because of the high incidence of thromboembolic disease.

Somatostatinomas There are a small number of cases reported demonstrating improvements of symptoms by administration of somatostatin analogues. Pancreatic enzyme supplementation and insulin for diabetes mellitus may also be necessary.

Nonfunctioning pancreatic neuroendocrine tumours These may also benefit from somatostatin analogues if somatostatin receptor imaging is positive and there is evidence of progressive disease.

Interferon-α and systemic chemotherapy Interferon-α has been used in the treatment of carcinoids and pancreatic neuroendocrine tumours with varying degrees of success and its efficacy may be improved by combining it with a somatostatin analogue. However, use of interferon-α may be limited by side effects including fatigue and flu-like symptoms. The efficacy of systemic chemotherapy in pancreatic neuroendocrine tumours is limited by the restricted number of prospective studies. The combination of streptozotocin and doxorubicin has been shown to be superior to a regimen of streptozotocin and 5-fluorouracil, although the use of doxorubicin may be limited by cardiotoxicity. These combinations produce symptomatic improvement in about 50% of cases and significant tumour regression is seen in up to a third of patients.

Management options for hepatic metastases Where hepatic metastases are confined to one lobe, surgical resection may be possible, aiming either at cure or at a significant reduction in tumour burden. Other local ablative techniques involve cryosurgery using liquid nitrogen and radiofrequency ablation using a slow-wave diathermy technique to destroy the tumour cells. In the presence of extensive hepatic metastases, debulking surgery may lead to palliation of symptoms. Although orthoptic liver transplantation has been performed for metastatic pancreatic neuroendocrine tumours, outcome is variable and hence it role has not been fully elucidated. Hepatic embolization exploits the fact that hepatic metastases are supplied by the hepatic artery, yet the liver parenchyma has a dual blood supply from the hepatic artery and portal vein. Embolization of these metastases can therefore occur via the hepatic arterial blood supply, resulting in devascularization and necrosis, while portal blood supply to the hepatic parenchyma is preserved. Hepatic artery embolization is achieved using polyvinyl alcohol or microspheres. Administration of somatostatin analogues is necessary before and after the procedure, since necrosis of hepatic metastases may be associated with massive release of neuropeptides. Hepatic chemoembolization combines this approach with the targeted local delivery of chemotherapy agents such as doxorubicin and cisplatin.

Radiopharmaceutical therapy Following the introduction of radiolabelled somatostatin analogues for diagnostic purposes, the next step was to develop radiopharmaceuticals as therapies. Such targeted radiotherapy acts systemically and is particularly useful palliative option for patients with inoperable or multisite disease. Prerequisites for treatment success include demonstration of high tumour uptake relative to nontarget tissues on quantitative diagnostic radionuclide imaging and stable haematological and biochemical function. Toxicity is generally low, being limited to reversible myelosuppression and nephrotoxicity. Radiopeptides emitting β-radiation rather than γ-radiation are superior in their therapeutic potential, since they emit particles with sufficient energy to cause cell damage without penetrating very far into surrounding tissue. Yttrium-90 (^{90}Y) is a pure β-emitter which is well suited to internal radiotherapy and may be coupled with octreotide or lanreotide. Administration of ^{90}Y-octreotide or ^{90}Y-lanreotide has been associated with regression of liver metastases and substantial symptomatic improvement.

External beam radiotherapy This may be effective in relieving pain from bone metastases and, in a small number of cases, has been curative in patients with locally unresectable pancreatic neuroendocrine tumours.

Multiple endocrine neoplasia

MEN refers to rare hereditary cancer syndromes characterized by a predisposition to tumour development within two or more endocrine organs. The two major forms of MEN, namely MEN1 and MEN2, are caused by germ-line mutations which display an autosomal dominant pattern of inheritance and a high degree of penetrance. MEN1 is associated with mutations in the *MEN1* gene, whereas MEN2 results from a *RET* (REarranged during Transfection) gene mutation. These MEN subtypes can either be sporadic, or more commonly, familial. Recent advances in our understanding of the molecular and clinical genetics of these syndromes have significantly altered the approach to diagnosis and management of these patients.

Multiple endocrine neoplasia type 1 (MEN1)
Clinical features and classification
The major components of MEN1 are parathyroid adenomas, pancreatic neuroendocrine tumours, and pituitary adenomas (see Table 13.10.2). Underdahl first described the association of these tumours in 1953, and Wermer subsequently proposed their autosomal dominant inheritance in 1954, with the latter providing the eponym for this syndrome. MEN1 occurs in approximately 1 in 30 000 individuals, with an equal sex distribution and may be defined as a case in which two of the three main MEN1-related endocrine tumours occur. Two different forms of MEN1, sporadic and familial, have been described. Familial MEN1 (OMIM 131100) is more prevalent, with an autosomal dominant pattern of inheritance, and is defined as an MEN1 case with at least one first-degree relative with one of these three characteristic endocrine tumours.

Table 13.10.2 Clinical features of MEN1 (Wermer's syndrome) with estimated prevalence in parentheses

Endocrine features	Associated nonendocrine features
Parathyroid hyperplasia/adenoma (>95%)	Facial angiofibromas (85%)
Pancreatic tumour (30–75%)	Collagenomas (70%)
(gastrinoma most common)	Lipomas (10–30%)
Anterior pituitary tumour (30%)	
(prolactinoma most common)	
Adrenal cortical tumour (nonfunctioning) (25%)	
Foregut carcinoid (3–4%)	

More than 95% of *MEN1* mutation carriers manifest clinical features of the syndrome by the age of 40 years.

Parathyroid hyperplasia/adenomas

Primary hyperparathyroidism is the most common presenting feature of MEN1, reaching almost 100% penetrance by age 50 years. The typical age of onset of primary hyperparathyroidism in MEN1 is 20 to 25 years, which is 30 years earlier than that of sporadic primary hyperparathyroidism. Patients present either with asymptomatic hypercalcaemia on biochemical screening or with features similar to those of sporadic primary hyperparathyroidism (see Chapter 13.6). In MEN1, hyperparathyroidism reflects hyperplasia of multiple parathyroid glands and supernumerary glands are common. There is a consensus that minimally invasive parathyroidectomy is not advisable, since it prevents the routine identification of all four glands. However, controversy exists regarding the most appropriate surgical approach. Subtotal parathyroidectomy with near total thymectomy (to remove ectopic parathyroid tissue in the thymus) is the most common approach. Some centres advocate total parathyroidectomy with autotransplantation of a fresh parathyroid gland into the forearm to avoid reoperative neck surgery if recurrent primary hyperparathyroidism in the transplanted hyperplastic gland occurs. An alternatively approach is a total parathyroidectomy followed by immediate replacement therapy with 1α-hydroxycholecalciferol.

Pancreatic neuroendocrine tumours

Pancreatic neuroendocrine tumours are the second most common clinical manifestation of MEN1, occurring in about 30 to 80% of MEN1 patients, with gastrinomas accounting for 60% of cases. Insulinomas represent about 30% of MEN1-associated pancreatic neuroendocrine tumours and coexist with gastrinomas in 10% of cases. Other functional tumour types such as VIPomas, glucagonomas, and somatostatinomas are rare. MEN1 patients with pancreatic neuroendocrine tumours usually manifest with symptoms of hormone hypersecretion by the age of 40 years, although these tumours may be detected earlier if asymptomatic carriers are having routine biochemical or imaging screening. The MEN1 pancreas characteristically contains numerous microadenomas which have the potential to grow to clinically relevant lesions. Tumours arise in any part of the pancreas, although MEN1 associated gastrinomas frequently arise within the duodenal submucosa. Surgical management of MEN1 associated pancreatic neuroendocrine tumours is described earlier in this chapter. Despite surgical options, MEN1-associated gastrinomas are associated with a high risk of recurrence and hence some centres advocate medical management with proton pump inhibitors. Pancreatic neuroendocrine tumours associated with MEN1 are less malignant than sporadic tumours and carry a better prognosis, with a median survival of 15 years compared to 5 years in patients with sporadic tumours. This may reflect more indolent disease or—since MEN1 patients usually participate in a surveillance programme—earlier diagnosis.

Pituitary adenomas

The incidence of pituitary adenomas in MEN1 patients varies from 10 to 60%. These adenomas are detected by screening in 30% of patients, but are found at autopsy in more than 50% of patients. The majority of these tumours are microadenomas (diameter <1 cm). Prolactinomas are the most common type of pituitary adenoma in MEN1 (60%), although tumours secreting growth hormone or ACTH are not uncommon. Double and even triple pituitary adenomas, which may secrete different pituitary hormones, have been described in MEN1. Imaging and treatment is the same as for sporadic pituitary tumours (see Chapter 13.2).

Other manifestations of MEN1

Carcinoid tumours occur in 3 to 4% of patients with MEN1. These originate in the foregut and are rarely associated with hypersecretion of hormones. MEN1 thymic carcinoid is seen mainly in men, whereas bronchial carcinoid is commoner in women. Gastric carcinoids in MEN1 are small and multiple, and their malignant potential remains uncertain. Adrenal cortical adenomas are present in up to 40% of patients with MEN1. These are often nonfunctioning and bilateral. Other forms of adrenal pathology associated with MEN1 are diffuse adrenal hyperplasia, adrenal nodular hyperplasia, and adrenal carcinoma. The presence of multiple facial angiofibromas, which consist of acneiform papules, is highly suggestive of MEN1. Collagenomas are another common feature and are multiple, skin-coloured, or occasionally hypopigmented cutaneous nodules, on the trunk, neck, and upper limbs. Subcutaneous or, rarely, visceral lipomas occur in 10 to 30% of MEN1 patients. Furthermore, MEN1 gene mutations have been demonstrated in individuals with atypical familial endocrine syndromes including phaeochromocytoma.

Genetics of MEN1

The *MEN1* gene was identified in 1997 by positional cloning and is a putative tumour suppressor gene, in keeping with the 'two-hit' model of hereditary cancer as originally postulated by Knudson for retinoblastoma. Knudson proposed that affected family members inherited a 'first hit' as an inactivating germ-line mutation in one allele of a tumour suppressor, resulting in a predisposition to tumour development. The 'second hit' is acquired as a stochastic somatic event in a susceptible cell type. The inactivation of the remaining functional allele results in progression to neoplasia. Therefore, to explain the apparent paradox of an autosomal dominant disease that is clearly recessive at the cellular level, there must be a relatively high frequency of such stochastic somatic events.

Sporadic cases of MEN1 involve distinct first and second 'hits' in somatic cells. There is an enormous diversity of mutations occurring in the *MEN1* gene, with over 400 different germ-line or somatic mutations currently reported in MEN1 families and sporadic cases. These mutations are dispersed throughout the entire coding region. Unlike the *RET* gene in MEN2, there is no significant correlation between the nature or position of the mutation in the *MEN1* gene and clinical status. Sequencing of the *MEN1* gene detects a germ-line mutation in about 70% of index cases for familial MEN1. The remaining 30% are mostly false negatives, reflecting mutations in the *MEN1* gene which are not detected by current gene sequencing techniques. More than 10% of *MEN1* mutations arise *de novo* and may be transmitted to subsequent generations. The *MEN1* gene encodes a 610 amino acid nuclear protein, menin, which has been shown to interact with several proteins, including the activator protein 1 transcription factor JunD. It has been proposed that menin may act in DNA repair or synthesis, although its exact function remains to be established.

Genetic screening and management

Mutational analysis of the *MEN1* gene is recommended for those in whom a diagnosis of MEN1 is suspected and requires a single blood sample. Following identification of an MEN1 mutation in an index case, genetic analysis in first-degree relatives allows identification of affected family members. Such early identification of MEN1 in asymptomatic carriers is particularly useful to allow subsequent periodic surveillance. This screening may detect the onset of the disease about 10 years before symptoms develop and thus provide an opportunity for earlier treatment. This early detection and treatment of the potential malignant neuroendocrine tumours should reduce the morbidity and mortality associated with MEN1 syndrome. Current guidelines suggest that the minimal surveillance programme for individuals known to have MEN1 syndrome or to have a family-specific mutation of the MEN1 gene should include annual measurement of: serum prolactin (from age 5 years), fasting serum calcium and PTH (from age 8 years), and fasting serum gastrin concentration (from age 20 years). Onset of MEN1 is rare before the age of 5 years, so screening does not need to occur before that age. Periodic radiological screening may include brain MRI, upper gastrointestinal endoscopy, abdominal CT, and somatostatin receptor scintigraphy imaging. In the 10 to 20% of cases of MEN1 where genetic analysis fails to detect a mutation, periodic biochemical testing is an alternative.

Multiple endocrine neoplasia type 2 (MEN2)

Clinical features and classification

MEN2 has at least three distinct variants: MEN2A, MEN2B and familial medullary thyroid carcinoma, and their clinical features are outlined in Table 13.10.3. Although MEN2 can arise sporadically, familial cases are more common. Familial MEN2 is defined as an MEN2 case with at least one of the characteristic endocrine tumours in a first degree relative. MEN2 has an estimated prevalence of 1:30 000. Each variant of MEN2 is caused by germline mutations in the *RET* proto-oncogene, which is located on chromosome 10.

MEN2A (OMIM 171400)

This may also be referred to as Sipple's syndrome and is characterized by medullary thyroid carcinoma, phaeochromocytoma and parathyroid hyperplasia/adenomas. MEN2A accounts for 80% of MEN2 cases. Medullary thyroid cancer is usually the first

neoplastic manifestation in MEN2, appearing between the ages of 5 and 25 years. Phenotypic variants of MEN2A include MEN2A plus megacolon and aganglionosis of the colon (Hirschprung's MEN2B disease) and MEN2A plus cutaneous lichen amyloidosis, a pruritic rash located on the upper back which usually arises before the onset of the thyroid cancer.

MEN2B (OMIM 162300)

Endocrine features of this subtype are medullary thyroid cancer and phaeochromocytoma, but not primary hyperparathyroidism. Medulary thyroid cancer associated with MEN2B occurs about 10 years earlier than MEN2B. Patients with this syndrome have a marfanoid habitus, skeletal abnormalities (kyphoscolisos or lordosis), mucosal neuromas, intestinal ganglioneuromas (which may cause chronic megacolon) and myelinated corneal nerves (Fig. 13.10.4). This variant represents about 5% of all cases of MEN2, and although MEN2B is often diagnosed earlier than MEN2A because of the characteristic associated physical features, it exhibits a higher morbidity and mortality than MEN2A.

Familial medullary thyroid carcinoma (OMIM 155240)

Medullary thyroid carcinoma (MTC) is the only clinical feature in this MEN2 subtype, although this may sometimes be associated with Hirschprung's disease. Since MTC is usually the first neoplasm to manifest in MEN2, because of its earlier and overall higher

Table 13.10.3 Clinical features of MEN2 with estimated prevalence in parentheses

MEN2A[a]	Medullary thyroid carcinoma (99%)
	Phaeochromocytoma (>50%)
	Parathyroid hyperplasia/adenoma (15–30%)
MEN2B	Medullary thyroid carcinoma (100%)
	Phaeochromocytoma (40–50%)
	Intestinal ganglioneuromatosis and mucosal neuromas (40%)
	Marfanoid habitus
	Megacolon
Familial medullary thyroid carcinoma	Thyroid tumour is sole manifestation

MEN, multiple endocrine neoplasia; MTC, medullary thyroid carcinoma.
[a] MEN2A accounts for >80% of all MEN2 cases.

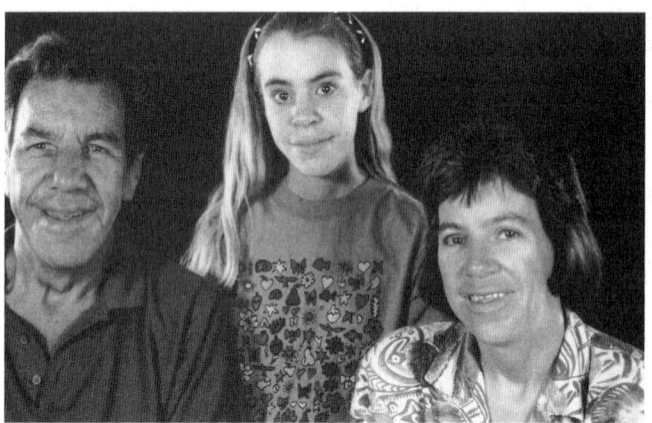

(a)

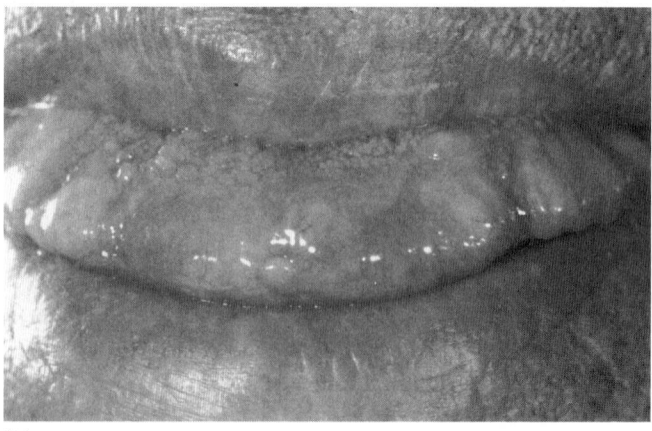

(b)

Fig. 13.10.4 (a) Characteristic phenotype of MEN2B showing facial appearance. (b) Characteristic phenotype of MEN2B showing mucosal neuromas on the tongue.

penetrance, it is essential to correctly classify familial medullary thyroid carcinoma. Misdiagnosis of familial medullary thyroid carcinoma in situations where the correct diagnosis is actually MEN2A may unintentionally exclude future screening for phaeochromocytoma, which may have catastrophic consequences. FMTC may be diagnosed where there are at least 10 carriers in the kindred, multiple carriers or affected members above the age of 50 years, and an family history adequate to exclude hyperparathyroidism and phaeochromocytoma.

Clinical features

Medullary thyroid carcinoma

Medullary thyroid carcinoma originates from the parafollicular cells (C cells) of the thyroid (see Chapters 13.4 and 13.5). These cells secrete calcitonin, which serves as a tumour marker. In MEN2, familial medullary thyroid carcinoma is the most benign, indolent form, whereas medullary thyroid carcinoma in association with MEN2B represents the most malignant form of the disease. C-cell hyperplasia is the precursor to hereditary MTC, with a variable progression to nodular hyperplasia and finally, through clonal progression, to malignancy. MTC occurs at a younger age in patients with MEN2 than does the sporadic form. Local invasion is common, with metastatic spread to lymph nodes in the neck and mediastinum occurring in up to 50% of cases. Distant metastases to liver, bone, and lung are seen in 15 to 25% of cases. Presentation in MTC may be with a neck mass, or symptoms from distant metastases (diarrhoea, flushing, weight loss, or bone pain). Rarely, ectopic ACTH secretion from MTC may cause Cushing's syndrome.

Calcitonin is elevated in all cases of clinically palpable MTC. In smaller tumours or cases of C-cell hyperplasia, basal calcitonin levels may be normal and stimulation with a secretagogue such as pentagastrin may be necessary to confirm the diagnosis. Genetic screening in MEN2-associated MTC has now largely replaced biochemical screening for MTC using the pentagastrin-stimulated calcitonin test. Cytological diagnosis using fine needle aspiration may be useful where MTC manifests in previously unidentified MEN2 carriers as a neck mass. Cross-sectional imaging of MTC using CT or MRI may be useful when planning surgery, and radioisotopes such as [131]I- metaiodobenzylguanidine (MIBG) and pentavalent ^{99m}Tc-dimercaptosuccininc acid are often valuable in detecting metastatic disease. As the tumour stage at presentation is the major prognostic factor, early diagnosis and surgical intervention before cervical lymph node metastases appear is necessary to improve survival. Current practice involves total thyroidectomy with central node dissection. Postoperatively, in addition to a diagnostic role, calcitonin is used to establish the presence of metastases or disease recurrence.

Phaeochromocytoma

Phaeochromocytomas are neuroendocrine neoplasias of neural crest origin. These occur in approximately 50% of patients with MEN2A or MEN2B, are usually benign, and are invariably confined to the adrenal glands. Phaeochromocytomas associated with MEN2A or MEN2B are bilateral in 50 to 80% of cases. Features and management of phaeochromocytomas are outlined in Chapter 16.17.3. Earlier detection and improved management has resulted in a significant reduction in the morbidity associated with phaeochromocytoma in MEN2. If MTC and phaeochromocytoma are diagnosed simultaneously in MEN2A or MEN2B individuals, adrenalectomy should be performed before thyroidectomy.

Parathyroid hyperplasia/adenomas

Primary hyperparathyroidism is a feature in 20 to 30% of MEN2A patients and is usually asymptomatic. Compared to MEN1, parathyroid disease in MEN2A is usually milder and has a later onset. Surgical management of primary hyperparathyroidism in MEN2A is similar to that in MEN1. During thyroidectomy in MEN2A, enlarged parathyroid glands in a normocalcaemic individual should be evaluated and removed if necessary.

Genetics of MEN2

In contrast to *MEN1*, which is a tumour suppressor gene, *RET* is an oncogene. *RET* has 21 exons and encodes a membrane tyrosine kinase receptor protein called RET. Normal RET is expressed mainly in developing and adult neural ectoderm and comprises extracellular, transmembrane, and intracellular regions. The extracellular region contains four cadherin-like domains and a juxtamembrane cysteine-rich region. Two tyrosine kinase domains located in the intracellular region are involved in the activation of numerous intracellular signal transduction pathways. Mutations involving exons 8, 10, 11, 13, 14, 15, and 16 have been identified in patients with MEN2A, MEN2B, and familial MTC. These exons should therefore be routinely screened for *RET* mutations. MEN2A and FMTC mutations usually affect the extracellular cysteine-rich domain, whereas those associated with MEN2B most frequently involve the intracellular tyrosine kinase domains of RET. In 85% of cases of MEN2A, codon 634 is affected and more than 95% of cases of MEN2B result from a mutation at codon 918. Generally, mutations associated with FMTC are distributed among the six cysteine codons. In contrast to MEN1, MEN2 displays a strong genotype–phenotype correlation and mutations are identified in more than 95% of patients.

Genetic screening and management

Early recognition of carriers of *RET* mutations can prevent and cure medullary thyroid cancer, by enabling prophylactic thyroidectomy before the clinical manifestation of the tumour. Genetic testing for germ-line *RET* mutations is performed in blood leucocytes. Since there is a strong correlation between the specific *RET* codon mutation and the aggressiveness of the tumour, decision regarding prophylactic thyroidectomy is based on the *RET* mutation identified. Genetic testing for germ-line *RET* mutations is recommended in all children with a parent known to have MEN2. Those children carrying MEN2B mutations (codon 883, 918, 922) have the highest risk of aggressive MTC and total thyroidectomy with central node dissection is recommended within the first 6 months of life. This surgery should be performed by age 5 years in carriers of *RET* codon mutations 611, 618, 620, and 634. Mutations affecting codons 609, 768,790, 791, 804, and 891 are associated with more indolent disease and may have prophylactic surgery by age 5 to 10 years or following first detection of abnormal stimulated calcitonin.

Genetic screening may also be useful in the management of MEN2-associated phaeochromocytoma. Individuals with *RET* mutations associated with a high risk of developing phaeochromocytoma should have annual measurement of urinary catecholamines.

Other MEN syndromes

In addition to MEN1 and MEN2, there are four other MEN syndromes. Carney complex (OMI 160980) is a rare syndrome characterized by myxomas (cutaneous, mucosal, and cardiac), spotty skin pigmentation (lentiginosis), primary pigmented adrenocortical disease, and pituitary adenomas. A diagnosis of McCune–Albright syndrome (OMIM 174800) requires at least two features of the triad of polyostotic fibrous dysplasia, café-au-lait skin pigmentation, and autonomous endocrine hyperfunction. Patients with Carney complex or McCune–Albright syndrome have mild hypersomatomammotropinemia (excess growth hormone secretion) starting in adolescence. In both disorders, pituitary hyperplasia appears to precede tumour development. Patients with neurofibromatosis type 1 (NF1; OMIM 162200) are predisposed to neuroendocrine tumours including phaeochromocytomas and duodenal somatostatinomas. Finally, as previously described, VHL syndrome (OMIM 193300) is associated with phaeochromoytomas and pancreatic neuroendocrine tumours.

Further reading

Akerstrom G, *et al.* (2005). Pancreatic tumours as part of the MEN-1 syndrome. *Best Pract Res Clin Gastroenterol*, **19**, 819–30.

Barakat MT, Meeran K, Bloom SR (2004). Neuroendocrine tumours. *Endocr Relat Cancer*, **11**, 1–18.

Brandi ML, *et al.* (2001). Guidelines for diagnosis and therapy of MEN type 1 and type 2. *J Clin Endocrinol Metab*, **86**, 5658–71.

Doherty GM (2005). Rare endocrine tumours of the GI tract. *Best Pract Res Clin Gastroenterol*, **19**, 807–17.

de Groot JW, *et al.* (2006). RET as a diagnostic and therapeutic target in sporadic and hereditary endocrine tumours. *Endocr Rev*, **27**, 535–60.

Dhillo WS, *et al.* (2006). Plasma gastrin measurement cannot be used to diagnose a gastrinoma in patients on either proton pump inhibitors or histamine type-2 receptor antagonists. *Ann Clin Biochem*, **43**(Pt 2), 153–5.

Kaltsas GA, Besser GM, Grossman AB (2004). The diagnosis and medical management of advanced neuroendocrine tumours. *Endocr Rev*, **25**, 458–511.

Lewington VJ (2003). Targeted radionuclide therapy for neuroendocrine tumours. *Endocr Relat Cancer*, **10**, 497–501.

Marini F, *et al.* (2006). Multiple endocrine neoplasia type 1. *Orphanet J Rare Dis*, **1**, 38.

Marini F, *et al.* (2006). Multiple endocrine neoplasia type 2. *Orphanet J Rare Dis*, **1**, 45.

Marx SJ (2005). Molecular genetics of multiple endocrine neoplasia types 1 and 2. *Nat Rev Cancer*, **5**, 367–74.

Oberg K, Eriksson B (2005). Endocrine tumours of the pancreas. *Best Pract Res Clin Gastroenterol*, **19**, 753–81.

Ramage JK, *et al.* (2005). Guidelines for the management of gastroenteropancreatic neuroendocrine (including carcinoid) tumours. *Gut*, **54** Suppl IV, iv1–16.

Taupenot L, Harper KL, O'Connor DT (2003). The chromogranin-secretogranin family. *N Engl J Med*, **348**, 1134–49.

Van Eeden S and Offerhaus GJ (2005). Historical, current and future perspectives on gastrointestinal and pancreatic endocrine tumours. *Virchows Arch*, **448**, 1–6.

13.11

Disorders of glucose homeostasis

Contents

13.11.1 Diabetes

Colin Dayan and Gareth Williams

Essentials

Diabetes mellitus can be defined as a state of chronic hypergly-caemia sufficient to cause long-term damage to specific tissues, notably the retina, kidney, nerves, and arteries. It is due to inadequate production of insulin and/or 'resistance' to the glucose-lowering and other actions of insulin, and is a significant and growing threat to global health, probably affecting 250 million people worldwide.

Definitions—normal fasting blood glucose concentration is in the range 3.5 to 5.5 mmol/litre, and even large carbohydrate loads do not raise the concentration above 8 mmol/litre. Widely accepted diagnostic criteria for diabetes and other hyperglycaemic states are (1) diabetes mellitus—fasting glucose more than 7.0 mmol/litre (126 mg/dl) and/or a value exceeding 11.1 mmol/litre (199 mg/dl), either at 2 h during a 75-g oral glucose tolerance test or in a random sample; (2) impaired glucose tolerance—2-h oral glucose tolerance test value between 7.8 and 11.1 mmol/litre (140–199 mg/dl); (3) impaired fasting glucose—fasting glucose 5.6 to 6.9 mmol/litre (100–125 mg/dl). The role of HbA1C as a diagnostic test is currently under review.

Impaired glucose tolerance is a not a stable state: within 5 years, about 25% of subjects deteriorate into type 2 diabetes, while a further 25% revert to normoglycaemia.

Type 1 diabetes

This condition, previously referred to as 'juvenile-onset' or 'insulin-dependent' diabetes, most commonly develops in childhood, with highest incidence in northern European countries, and accounts for 5 to 15% of all cases of diabetes.

Aetiology—Type 1 diabetes is caused by an autoimmune, predominantly T-cell-mediated process that selectively destroys the pancreatic β cells. Genetic factors explain 30 to 40% of total susceptibility: at least 10 loci are involved, with the HLA class II locus *IDDM2* having by far the greatest effect. Environmental factors that have been implicated include viral infection (particularly coxsackie B), bovine serum albumin from cow's milk (by immunological cross-reactivity) and other toxins. Notable β-cell selective autoantibodies that are commonly found are those that recognize GAD65 (a heat shock protein), IA-2 (a protein tyrosine phosphatase-like molecule), ZnT8 (a zinc transporter molecule) and insulin itself, but these are clearly not the immediate cause of the disease. Several years of progressive autoimmune damage usually precede the clinical onset of diabetes.

Pathogenesis—in untreated type 1 diabetes, insulin concentrations are generally 10 to 50% of nondiabetic levels in the face of hyperglycaemia which would normally greatly increase insulin secretion. Such severe deficiency cannot sustain the normal anabolic effects of insulin and leads to runaway catabolism in carbohydrate, fat, and protein metabolism. A similar clinical picture of insulin dependence can be caused by other forms of severe pancreatic damage.

Clinical features—classical presentation of untreated or poorly controlled type 1 diabetes is with onset over days or a few weeks of polyuria (caused by osmotic diuresis due to hyperglycaemia), thirst, weight loss, and general tiredness/malaise. Other features can include blurred vision (due to hyperglycaemia-related refractive changes in the lens), infection (particularly genital candidiasis), and diabetic ketoacidosis. Chronic diabetic complications are not seen at presentation.

Type 2 diabetes

Type 2 diabetes (previously referred to as 'non-insulin-dependent' or 'maturity-onset') is a heterogeneous condition, diagnosed empirically by the absence of features suggesting type 1 diabetes.

It is most commonly diagnosed in those >40 years of age, with peak incidence at 60 to 65 years, and it accounts for 85 to 90% of diabetes worldwide, but with striking geographical variation (prevalence <1% in rural China, 50% in Pima Indians of New Mexico).

Aetiology—type 2 diabetes is due to the combination of insulin resistance and β-cell failure. Genetic factors explain 60 to 90% of total susceptibility, with a polygenic pattern reflecting the inheritance of a critical mass of minor diabetogenic polymorphisms in genes that influence insulin secretion, insulin resistance, pancreatic development and obesity. An important specific risk factor for type 2 diabetes, which aggravates insulin resistance, is obesity—particularly if this develops after the early twenties, and especially around the waist. The mechanism of β-cell failure in human type 2 diabetes is not known.

Clinical features—in type 2 diabetes significant hyperglycaemia may have been present for several years at the time of diagnosis, hence cases are often discovered by screening or at routine health checks. Many cases present with classical symptoms of osmotic diuresis, blurred vision and genital candidiasis. The hyperosmolar nonketotic state can present with confusion or coma, but diabetic ketoacidosis is rare. Chronic diabetic complications may be a presenting feature.

Monogenic and other types of diabetes

Maturity-onset diabetes of the young (MODY)—most often caused by mutations in the genes for glucokinase (*MODY2*) and HNF-1α (*MODY3*). This diagnosis should be considered if there is a family history of young-onset diabetes in more than one generation, with at least one family member diagnosed under the age of 25; affected members are not markedly obese; there is no evidence of insulin resistance; fasting C-peptide is detectable and within the normal range; islet cell or anti-GAD autoantibodies are absent; other associated features are present.

Other types of diabetes include those related to pancreatic disease (chronic pancreatitis, cystic fibrosis, haemochromatosis) and gestational diabetes (see Chapter 14.10).

Management of diabetes

General aspects—management requires tackling cardiovascular risk factors and obesity in addition to hyperglycaemia. Important issues include (1) dietary modification—reducing total energy intake in patients who are overweight (body mas index >28 kg/m^2), improving dietary composition (fat <30% total energy intake, with saturated animal fat <10%; carbohydrates—preferably pulses, root/leaf vegetables and fruit—>55% total energy intake; sodium <6 g/day); (2) increasing physical activity; (3) smoking cessation; and in some patients (4) antiobesity drugs and/or bariatric surgery.

Glucose-lowering drugs—these include (1) insulin—soluble (regular, or short-acting) insulin injected subcutaneously begins to lower glucose within 30 min, has a peak effect between 1 and 2 h and lasts 3 to 5 h; long-acting preparations (e.g. isophane and lente insulins) are used to cover basal insulin requirements; (2) insulin analogues—have improved physicochemical characteristics for subcutaneous absorption and can be fast acting, e.g. insulin lispro and insulin aspart, or long acting, e.g. insulin glargine (Lantus) and insulin detemir (Levemir); (3) oral hypoglycaemic agents—(a) sulphonylureas and meglitinides—insulin secretagogues;

(b) metformin—a biguanide that acts primarily by inhibiting gluconeogenesis in the liver; (c) thiazolidinediones—act to improve insulin sensitivity; (d) α-glucosidase inhibitors—partly block digestion of complex carbohydrates and so damp post-prandial glycaemic rises, but are of low efficacy and poorly tolerated; (e) incretin mimetics—augment insulin secretion.

Type 1 diabetes—patients must be given insulin immediately and for life. Standard treatment involves giving a short-acting insulin 20 to 30 min before eating or a fast-acting insulin immediately before eating, and a twice (sometimes once) daily dose of a long-acting insulin. Common practice is to commence with low dosages of long-acting insulin, e.g. 8–12 U in the morning and 4–6 U at night, with short/fast-acting insulin then added to cover excessive prandial hyperglycaemia. Premixed insulins (e.g. 30% short-acting with 70% long-acting) can be given twice daily and are more convenient than giving short- and long-acting insulins separately, but they lack flexibility. Administration is usually by conventional syringes or pen injection devices, but pumps can be used to administer continuous subcutaneous infusions of insulin.

Type 2 diabetes—the first-line oral hypoglycaemic agent for socalled 'dietary failure' is metformin, with a (usually) sulphonylurea or (sometimes) thiazolidinedione added as second-line treatment. A once-daily dose of a long-acting insulin can be combined effectively with metformin. Insulin therapy can range from once- or twice-daily long-acting insulin in subjects with residual insulin, to the more intensified basal and prandial regimens used in type 1 diabetes (>200 U/day may be required in very obese, insulin-resistant patients).

Treatment targets for blood glucose—these have been selected to reduce the risk of chronic diabetic complications. Avoiding acute episodes of hyper- and hypoglycaemia is also important. Management should aim for fasting blood glucose below 5.5 mmol/litre, postprandial peak glucose below 7.5 mmol/litre, and HbA$_{1c}$ 6.5% or less ('good' control defined as below 7%, 'poor' control as over 8%).

Multidisciplinary care—diabetes is best managed by the combined efforts of a well-trained primary care team and a team of specialists with complementary and overlapping skills: physician, specialist diabetes nurse, dietitian, and chiropodist. Patients require education about diabetes, with key elements including (1) causes of hyperglycaemia and diabetic symptoms; (2) own treatment—diet and lifestyle; drawing up and injecting insulin; oral agents; recognizing and treating hypoglycaemia 'hypos'; (3) self-monitoring technique—targets and danger levels; how to respond to poor control; (4) 'sickday' rules—monitoring during intercurrent illness; how to adjust own treatment; when and how to call for help (never stop taking your insulin; check your blood glucose every 4 h; test your urine for ketones; call for help if you start vomiting, have glucose over 15 mmol/litre that does not come down after insulin, get hypos, get ketones in the urine, are worried, and don't know what to do).

Acute metabolic complications of diabetes

Diabetic ketoacidosis—uncontrolled hyperglycaemia with hyperketonaemia severe enough to cause metabolic acidosis. Precipitating factors include new presentation of type 1 diabetes, omission or underdosing of insulin by patients known to have type 1 diabetes, and intercurrent illness (compounded by failure to monitor blood glucose and take appropriate action). Usual presentation is with classical hyperglycaemic symptoms together with acidotic (Kussmaul) breathing and ketotic foetor, evidence of dehydration and hypovolaemia, and signs of any precipitating condition. Drowsiness and coma are late features. Diagnosis is confirmed with a finger-prick blood glucose measurement and urinalysis for ketones: other investigations should include a biochemical screen, full sepsis screen, arterial blood gas analysis and ECG. Management requires (1) fluid replacement—usually with 0.9% saline (typically 1–2 litres in 2 h, then 1 litre in 4 h, then 4 litres in next 24 h); (2) potassium replacement—typically 20 mmol of KCl to each litre of intravenous fluid if K$^+$ is normal (3.5–5.0 mmol/litre), but adjusted in response to frequent monitoring; (3) intravenous insulin—initially at a rate of 6 U/h, then titrated down according to a sliding scale; (4) treatment, when possible, of any precipitating condition. Intravenous fluids and insulin can be discontinued when the patient can eat and drink, and they can be restarted on their usual insulin regimen (or a typical maintenance regimen can be introduced).

Hyperosmolar non-ketotic state (HONK)—is distinguished from diabetic ketoacidosis by the absence (because circulating insulin levels are high enough to suppress lipolysis and ketogenesis) of marked hyperketonaemia and metabolic acidosis. Presentation is typically with classical hyperglycaemic symptoms; confusion, drowsiness and coma are commoner than in diabetic ketoacidosis. Typical biochemical features include severe hyperglycaemia (>30 mmol/litre) and hypernatraemia (sodium often >155 mmol/litre). Management is largely as for diabetic ketoacidosis, excepting that (1) 0.45% saline is often given if plasma sodium is over 150 mmol/litre or osmolality over 350 mosmol/kg; (2) intravenous insulin infusion at low doses rapidly controls hyperglycaemia in most cases; (3) the risk of thrombotic events is particularly high, hence prophylactic doses of low molecular weight heparin should be given.

Hypoglycaemia—an inevitable side-effect of antidiabetic drugs that raise circulating insulin levels. Typical features include (1) autonomic symptoms—pallor, sweating, tremor, and tachycardia, and (2) symptoms of neuroglycopenia—commonly drowsiness, confusion, incoordination, and dysarthria, but also automatic or disinhibited behaviour and focal neurological deficits. Diagnosis is confirmed with a finger-prick blood glucose measurement below 3.5 mmol/litre in an appropriate clinical context. Treatment is with (1) oral glucose or sucrose or other carbohydrate—if the patient can swallow safely; or (2) intravenous glucose (15–20 g as 10% or 50% solution) or intramuscular glucagon (1 mg)—if the patient is not able to swallow safely. For further discussion see Chapter 13.11.2.

Chronic complications of diabetes

Long-term tissue damage is the major burden of diabetes, the greatest source of fear for diabetic people, and the most expensive item in the diabetes health care budget. Microvascular complications—retinopathy, neuropathy, and nephropathy—are specific to diabetes and reflect damage inflicted on the microcirculation throughout the body. Macrovascular disease is atherosclerosis, which behaves more aggressively than in nondiabetic people, and causes typical coronary heart disease, stroke and peripheral arterial disease.

Pathogenesis—possible mechanisms for diabetic complications include glycation of proteins and macromolecules, overactivity of the polyol pathway, activation of protein kinase C and abnormal microvascular blood flow.

Diabetic eye disease—is the commonest cause of blindness in people of working age in most Westernized countries. Stages of diabetic retinopathy are (1) background—microaneurysms, hard exudates, haemorrhages (flame, dot, blot), cotton wool spots (<5); (2) preproliferative—rapid increase in microaneurysms, intraretinal microvascular abnormalities, multiple deep haemorrhages, cotton wool spots (>5), venous beading/loops/duplication; (3) proliferative—new vessels on the disc or elsewhere, fibrous proliferation on the disc or elsewhere, preretinal or vitreous haemorrhages; (4) advanced eye disease—retinal detachment, retinal tears, rubeosis iridis, neovascular glaucoma. Disease of the macula (maculopathy), serious enough to affect central vision, can accompany any stage of diabetic retinopathy including background, and may be present in newly diagnosed type 2 patients. Management requires (1) general preventive measures—tight glycaemic control, control of hypertension, stopping smoking, regular (annual) eye screening; and (2) specific treatments—laser photocoagulation can preserve useful vision in many cases of proliferative retinopathy and maculopathy.

Diabetic neuropathies—recognized clinically distinct syndromes include (1) diffuse symmetrical polyneuropathy—classically a distal 'glove and stocking' peripheral polyneuropathy that affects all sizes of sensory and motor fibres; (2) autonomic neuropathy—manifest as sexual difficulties (erectile failure, ejaculatory failure), postural hypotension, disturbed gastrointestinal motility, abnormal sweating, neuropathic bladder, abnormal blood flow, sudden unexplained death; (3) acute mononeuropathy; (4) diabetic amyotrophy; (5) cranial and other nerve palsies. Management is difficult: specific treatments have so far been disappointing. Numb feet are at greatly increased risk of ulceration and require sensible shoes and good foot care. Poor glycaemic control should be corrected. Pain may be difficult to treat: simple analgesics are generally ineffective; tricyclic drugs can suppress neurogenic pain; anticonvulsants may help. Autonomic neuropathic symptoms may be treated as follows: (1) erectile failure with oral phosphodiesterase type 5 inhibitors (e.g. sildenafil); (2) postural hypotension with compression stockings, fludrocortisone and/or midodrine; (3) gastroparesis with erythromycin, metoclopramide or domperidone; (4) excessive sweating with oral clonidine or topical glycopyrrolate cream; (5) neuropathic bladder with regular bladder training, but intermittent self-catheterization may be needed.

Diabetic nephropathy—see Chapter 21.10.1.

Macrovascular disease—(1) dyslipidaemia—first-line treatment is with statins, aiming for a 30 to 40% reduction in LDL and to achieve an LDL level below 2.6 mmol/litre in all patients and below 1.8 mmol/litre in those with overt cardiovascular disease; (2) hypertension—clinic blood pressure should be reduced to a target of 130/80 mmHg, with angiotension converting enzyme (ACE) inhibitors often recommended as first line; (3) coronary heart disease—there should be a low threshold for referring patients with diabetes presenting with typical or atypical chest pain suggestive of angina for further evaluation; (4) stroke—investigation and management are conventional; (5) peripheral vascular disease—investigation and management are conventional.

Diabetic foot disease—ulceration and severe ischaemia leading to gangrene of the toes or forefoot are the commonest problems. Many problems can be avoided by teaching the patients basic foot care, by regularly checking their feet and shoes, and by providing prophylactic podiatry and special footwear as appropriate. Typical manifestations include (1) neuropathic ulcers—occur at high-pressure sites (heel, metatarsal heads) and appear cleanly punched out of the surrounding callus; (2) ischaemic ulcers—tend to affect the edges of the foot and toes; (3) traumatic damage—e.g. symmetrical damage across the toes and margins of the feet from tight shoes; with (4) all lesions prone to be complicated by infection. Management requires the prevention of further trauma, treatment of infection, and optimization of the circulation. Charcot's arthropathy most commonly affects the ankle and joints in the mid- and forefoot, which in advanced cases degenerate (usually painlessly) into a 'bag of bones': treatment is often unsatisfactory—off-loading pressure with a plaster-cast boot may temporarily halt bone destruction; bisphosphonate infusions may slow the disease process by inhibiting osteoclast activity.

Introduction

Diabetes mellitus can be defined as a state of chronic hyperglycaemia sufficient to cause long-term damage to specific tissues, notably the retina, kidney, nerves, and arteries, but this functional label gives little insight into the long and colourful history of this disease, its clinical and scientific importance, or its immense personal and socioeconomic impact. Diabetes was recognized in antiquity, and its clinical features (with empirical treatment guidelines) were recorded over 3500 years ago in the Egyptian Ebers papyrus. Our understanding of the disease has advanced greatly, especially during the last two decades, but many aspects of its management remain imperfect. The American Diabetes Association has proposed a generally accepted classification of diabetes mellitus into three types: type 1 is associated with β-cell destruction leading to absolute deficiency of insulin, is immune-mediated and of unknown root cause; type 2 is associated with a relative insulin deficiency and insulin resistance—a range of abnormalities occur, and in some patients a secretory defect predominates; type 3 diabetes is used to encompass diabetes caused by specific defects, other endocrine abnormalities, and drug-induced diabetes, and accounts for about 5% of patients.

The incidence of all types of diabetes is rising, but in developed countries—once patients have been treated for ketoacidosis and with modern regimens for insulin treatment and systems in place for diabetic care—the prognosis is improved for those with type 1 disease and relates to glycaemic control. Extensive studies have shown a strong relationship between glycaemic control, the fraction of glycated haemoglobin (HbA$_{1c}$), and disease outcomes. Treatment of raised blood pressure and abnormal blood lipids has also contributed to the improved outcomes of nephropathy, retinopathy, myocardial infarction and stroke. In both type 1 and type 2 diabetes, there are compelling data to show that outcomes are improved by intensive therapy: better glycaemic control appears to have no overall effect on the macrovascular complications, but lowering blood pressure has significant benefits on both small vessel (microvascular) and macrovascular disease.

Diabetes is a significant and growing threat to global health. Worldwide, diabetes probably affects 250 million people. This number was eightfold less in 1985 (30 million) and the world prevalence is predicted to reach 380 million by 2025.

Diagnosis of diabetes

Blood glucose concentrations are normally tightly regulated: fasting values lie between 3.5 and 5.5 mmol/litre and even large carbohydrate loads do not raise the concentration more than 8 mmol/litre. It is logical to define diabetes by the blood glucose concentrations which cause the chronic complications of the disease but the choice of the diagnostic glucose levels has been contentious (and has stirred up much passion among epidemiologists). One difficulty is that some diabetic complications show a 'threshold' effect with the risk rising above a cut-off level (e.g. fasting plasma glucose of 6 to 7 mmol/litre for retinopathy), whereas macrovascular disease (atheroma) does not (see later). Another problem is that even the current criteria are not self-consistent: e.g. up to 30% of patients with a diagnostic raised fasting glucose will have a 2h value in the glucose tolerance test that is below the diagnostic cut-off.

The current diagnostic criteria for diabetes and other hyperglycaemic states (see Fig. 13.11.1.1) have been approved by the World Health Organization (WHO) and most national diabetes associations. All values refer to venous plasma glucose concentrations:

- Diabetes mellitus: fasting glucose greater than 7.0 mmol/litre (126 mg/dl) and/or a value exceeding 11.1 mmol/litre, either at 2h during a 75g oral glucose tolerance test or in a random sample. The corresponding levels in non-SI units are 126 and 200 mg/dl respectively. The diagnostic fasting glucose level was lowered from the previous value of 7.8 mmol/litre to reflect more accurately the risk of developing diabetic retinopathy

- Impaired glucose tolerance (WHO): 2h oral glucose tolerance test value between 7.8 and 11.1 mmol/litre (140–199 mg/dl)

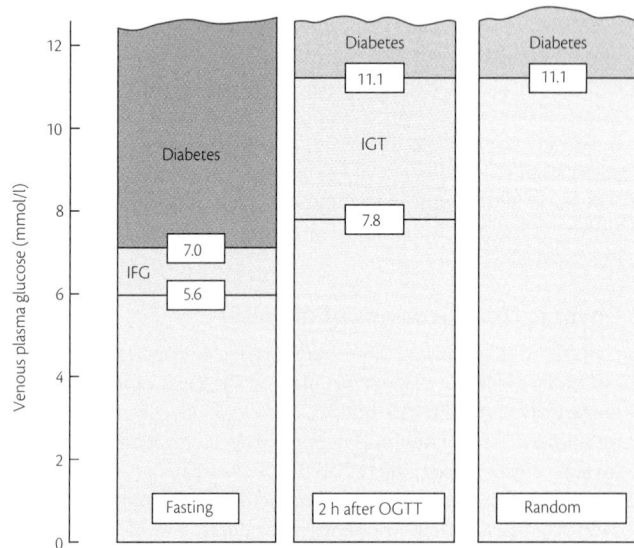

Fig. 13.11.1.1 Diagnostic thresholds for diabetes, impaired glucose tolerance (IGT), and impaired fasting glucose (IFG). For conversion to mg/dl, multiply values in mmol/litre by 18.
(From Genuth S, *et al.* (2003). Follow-up report on the diagnosis of diabetes mellitus. *Diabetes Care*, 26, 3160–67.)

♦ Impaired fasting glucose: fasting glucose 5.6 to 6.9 mmol/litre (100–125 mg/dl). The lower value for this range was reduced from 6.0 mmol/litre to 5.6 mmol/litre by the American Diabetes Association in 2003

Impaired glucose tolerance (IGT) and the recently distinguished impaired fasting glucose (IFG) are intermediate categories of hyperglycaemia that carry definite risks and so require follow-up and risk-factor management (see below). They are often transient stages and overlap to some extent: about one-third of subjects with impaired fasting glucose also have impaired glucose tolerance, while one-quarter of those with impaired glucose tolerance also show impaired fasting glucose.

The new criteria put much emphasis on the fasting plasma glucose concentration. However, the time-consuming oral glucose tolerance test is still required in some cases with borderline fasting hyperglycaemia, because the 2-h oral glucose tolerance test value in such patients may be high enough to put them at risk of microvascular complications. Moreover, the oral glucose tolerance test remains the only way to define impaired glucose tolerance.

Practical screening and diagnostic procedures

Figure 13.11.1.2 shows an algorithmic approach to screening for and diagnosis of diabetes and its associated hyperglycaemic states. Certain high-risk groups need to be actively screened for type 2 diabetes, which may be present (and causing complications) for several years before it is noticed. These include subjects predisposed to develop type 2 diabetes through genotype and/or phenotype, those affected by diabetogenic conditions such as pregnancy, endocrine disorders or certain drugs, and those with other cardiovascular risk factors in whom hyperglycaemia must not be missed.

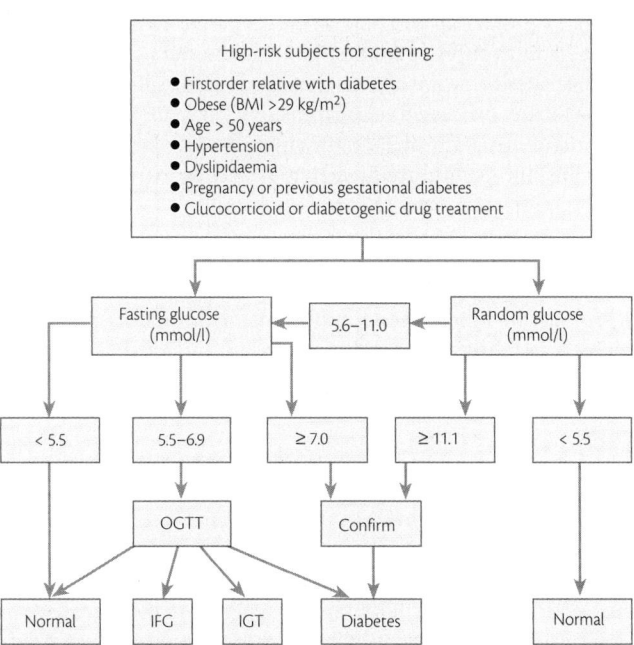

Fig. 13.11.1.2 Screening algorithm for diagnosing diabetes, impaired glucose tolerance, and impaired fasting glucose. All glucose values relate to venous plasma (mmol/litre).
(Adapted from data in Shaw JE, Zimmet P (2000). Do we know how to diagnose diabetes and do we need to screen for the disease? In: Gill GV, Pickup JC, Williams G, (eds) *Difficult diabetes*, pp. 3–21. Blackwell Science, Oxford.)

Diabetes is not a trivial diagnosis, and certain practical points must be carefully observed:

♦ Glucose should be measured in venous plasma using a quality-controlled laboratory method. Capillary (finger-prick) samples contain higher glucose levels than venous blood, from which glucose has been extracted by the tissue bed; whole-blood glucose levels are lower than in plasma, because red cells actively metabolize glucose and so contain only low concentrations. These differences may reach 0.5 to 1.0 mmol/litre. Portable glucose meters correlate well with laboratory glucose methods, but because of potential technical errors they should not be used to make or refute the diagnosis.

♦ An oral glucose tolerance test is indicated for borderline hyperglycaemia (Fig. 13.11.1.2). After an overnight fast, the subject drinks 75 g of anhydrous glucose dissolved in 250 ml water (or 419 ml of a glucose drink such as Lucozade Energy Original—73 kcal/100 ml); venous blood is sampled at baseline and 2h later. Food intake should be normal during the preceding few days: poor nutrition can cause delayed hyperglycaemia with a raised 2h value (the lag curve).

♦ Abnormal values need confirmation. Postchallenge glucose levels in particular can vary considerably. Because of this and possible laboratory error, the diagnosis of diabetes should be verified using a further sample on another day unless there is a clear history of symptoms of hyperglycaemia confirming that this value is not a one-off result.

♦ Diabetes is not currently diagnosed from indirect measures of hyperglycaemia such as raised HbA_{1c} or fructosamine levels in blood, or glycosuria. HbA_{1c} and fructosamine reflect average blood glucose concentrations, but the measurements are not sufficiently sensitive or standardized (several different methods are in use) to be used diagnostically although this recommendation is currently under review and is likely to change in the near future. Glycosuria depends on the renal threshold for glucose reabsorption and its presence does not necessarily indicate hyperglycaemia; conversely, glucose may be absent from the urine in diabetic subjects who also have a high renal threshold. However, abnormal results with any of these tests suggest diabetes and indicate the need for formal blood glucose screening.

Impaired glucose tolerance

Impaired glucose tolerance is a not a stable state: within 5 years, about 25% of subjects with impaired glucose tolerance deteriorate into type 2 diabetes, while a further 25% revert to normoglycaemia. The degree of hyperglycaemia in impaired glucose tolerance falls, by definition, below the threshold for microvascular complications but is enough to predispose to cardiovascular disease (see later).

Subjects found to have impaired glucose tolerance must be followed up because of the hazards of both diabetes and macrovascular disease. An oral glucose tolerance test should be repeated at least annually, and dietary and lifestyle advice given to decrease metabolic and cardiovascular risks; increased physical activity, a low-fat diet and weight loss convincingly reduce both the progression to type 2 diabetes (by 58%) and cardiovascular risk. Risk factors such as smoking, hypertension, dyslipidaemia, and obesity should be managed actively. Specific antihyperglycaemic treatments also reduce progression to type 2 diabetes—metformin (24%), rosiglitazone (60% risk reduction, but associated with weight gain)—in addition to pharmacological (orlistat) or physical (bariatric surgery) weight loss interventions (see Chapter 11.5). These measures should be used in combination with lifestyle intervention, which is recommended for all subjects with impaired glucose tolerance.

Impaired fasting glucose

As with impaired glucose tolerance, the 5-year risk of progressing to type 2 diabetes appears to be about 25%, and IFG predisposes to cardiovascular disease. Long-term monitoring and management should therefore be as for impaired glucose tolerance.

Metabolic basis of diabetes

Diabetes is due to inadequate production of insulin and/or 'resistance' to the glucose-lowering and other actions of insulin. To put this in context, key aspects of normal metabolism will be briefly reviewed.

The islets of Langerhans

There are about 1 million islets of Langerhans in the normal adult: insulin is produced by the β cells, which make up the bulky core of each islet; β cells also synthesize the peptide known as amylin or islet-associated polypeptide. The other islet cell types, mostly surrounding the β-cell core, are the α cells that produce glucagon, the δ cells that produce somatostatin, and the PP cells that synthesize pancreatic polypeptide. All islet cells are derived embryologically from the buds of gut endoderm which also give rise to the exocrine pancreatic tissue.

The various islet cell types communicate with each other through the hormones they secrete into the islet's rich capillary plexus and probably by paracrine effects on adjacent cells; these interactions presumably regulate hormone secretion. Insulin inhibits release of glucagon, while glucagon powerfully stimulates insulin secretion—an action exploited in the testing of β-cell reserve (see below). Somatostatin suppresses the secretion of insulin and glucagon. Amylin can inhibit insulin and glucagon secretion as well as reduce appetite and gastric emptying. Its physiological role is uncertain but amylin analogues when used as pharmacotherapy have been shown to reduce weight as well as blood glucose levels. Amylin also polymerizes outside the β cell to produce fibrils of amyloid material, which have been implicated in the progressive β-cell damage of type 2 diabetes.

Insulin

Insulin is a 5800 Da protein made up of an A chain (21 amino acid residues) and a B chain (30 residues), joined covalently by two disulphide bridges. The precursor molecule, proinsulin, consists of the A and B chains linked end-to-end through a connecting (C) peptide which is cleaved off during insulin processing. In the circulation, insulin is monomeric but in crystals and more concentrated solutions (e.g. in the insulin vial and the subcutaneous injection site), six insulin molecules self-associate around a central Zn^{2+} ion. Self-association influences the pharmacokinetic properties of subcutaneously injected insulin: the rate-limiting dissociation of hexamers into monomers slows the absorption of even fast-acting insulin.

Insulin regulates metabolism in birds, fish, and reptiles as well as mammals, and its structure is remarkably well conserved across the phyla. Three species of insulin are used therapeutically; the human sequence differs from porcine at a single residue (B30) and from bovine at two others. These differences affect the pharmacokinetic and immunogenic characteristics of the insulins (see below). The physicochemical behaviour of insulin has been successfully manipulated in synthetic 'designer' insulins that have improved absorption profiles: modification of the C terminus of the B chain, a region crucial for self-association, produces analogues that remain in the monomeric state and are therefore absorbed faster than the native soluble insulin (see below).

Insulin biosynthesis and processing

Insulin is a product of the *INS* gene, located on the short arm of chromosome 11, whose coding region contains three exons. Translation of *INS* mRNA in the rough endoplasmic reticulum produces preproinsulin, which is successively cleaved during its passage through the Golgi vesicles and secretory vesicles to yield first proinsulin and finally insulin and C-peptide. Proinsulin is converted into insulin by the proteolytic excision of the C-peptide chain; the two intermediate cleavage products (with either end of the C-peptide remaining attached to insulin) are called split products of proinsulin. Normally, almost all proinsulin is processed through this regulated pathway to yield equimolar amounts of insulin and C-peptide. However, a constitutive pathway may predominate in dysfunctional β cells (e.g. in type 2 diabetes and insulinoma), when processing is not complete and large quantities of proinsulin and split products may be released into the circulation.

C-peptide is generally regarded as an inert byproduct of insulin production. However, its structure is also conserved across species and it may have vasoactive and other properties.

Insulinopathies are point mutations in the *INS* gene which either produce a mutant insulin (e.g. insulin Chicago: a phenylalanine for leucine substitution at residue B25) or interfere with one of the cleavage sites of proinsulin so that the mutant split product cannot be further processed (e.g. proinsulin Tokyo). These conditions are inherited as autosomal dominant traits; circulating insulin-like or proinsulin-like immunoreactivities may be extremely high but glucose intolerance is often surprisingly mild.

Insulin secretion

Glucose is the main insulin secretagogue; this action of glucose is modulated by other ingested nutrients, by hormones released by the islets and the gut, and by the autonomic innervation of the islet. The process gives insight into the mode of action of the sulphonylureas and related drugs, and the cause of maturity-onset diabetes of the young (see below).

Glucose-stimulated insulin secretion

The amount of insulin released by the normal β cell is tightly coupled to blood glucose levels and begins to increase immediately when blood glucose rises. The ability of the β cell to sense ambient glucose levels accurately and rapidly depends on the glucose transporter isoform GLUT-2 and the glucose metabolizing enzyme glucokinase, while insulin release hinges on depolarization of the β-cell membrane which is controlled by a specific ion channel, the ATP-sensitive K^+ channel. The characteristics of GLUT-2 allow glucose at physiological concentrations to freely enter the β cell, where it is immediately converted by glucokinase into glucose 6-phosphate—the point of entry into the glycolytic pathway which ultimately yields ATP; ATP production within the β cell is therefore proportionate to extracellular glucose.

ATP binds to and closes the ATP-dependent K+ channel; when open, this channel allows K+ ions to leave the β cell along their concentration gradient and thus helps to maintain the negative charge inside the β-cell membrane. ATP-induced closure of the channel therefore causes K+ ions to accumulate within the cell and the membrane to depolarize, which triggers the opening of specific (voltage-gated) Ca²⁺ channels in the membrane. Ca²⁺ ions then flood into the β cell from the outside and activate the contractile proteins which drag the secretory vesicles containing insulin and C-peptide to the cell surface. Here, the vesicles fuse with the cell membrane and release their contents into the extracellular space (exocytosis), from where insulin and C-peptide enter the islet capillaries.

Other factors affecting insulin secretion

Sulphonylureas induce insulin secretion by closing the same ATP-sensitive K+ channel as glucose: they bind to a specific sulphonylurea receptor (SUR1) linked to the K+ channel protein (called Kir 6.2). Repaglinide also closes this K+ channel, but binds to a different site from the sulphonylureas. By contrast, diazoxide locks the channel open, hyperpolarizing the β-cell membrane and inhibiting insulin secretion—hence its use in treating insulinoma.

Glucagon and glucagon-like peptide 1 7–36 amide (GLP-1; a gut peptide with insulin secretagogue (incretin) actions) both stimulate insulin secretion by raising cytosolic Ca²⁺ concentrations; binding to their receptors increases generation of cAMP which blocks removal of Ca²⁺ into intracellular organelles. Conversely, somatostatin and possibly amylin act to decrease production of cAMP and inhibit insulin secretion. Arginine stimulates insulin secretion, possibly by depolarizing the β-cell membrane as it enters the cell (it is cationic).

The autonomic nervous system is an important modulator of insulin secretion; it is stimulated by the parasympathetic (vagal) outflow and inhibited by the sympathetic. Vagal stimulation is mediated by acetylcholine acting via muscarinic receptors, while the inhibitory sympathetic neurotransmitter is noradrenaline, interacting with α_2-adrenoceptors.

Defects in insulin secretion due to mutations affecting glucokinase are responsible for 20% of cases of maturity-onset diabetes of the young (MODY), i.e. glucokinase-dependent MODY (MODY 2). This impairs ATP production from glucose, blunting the insulin response of the β cell to rising glucose and resulting in variable hyperglycaemia (see below). By contrast, familial neonatal hyperinsulinism is caused by inactivating mutations in *ABCC8* (*SUR1*) or *KCNJ11* (*Kir6.2*) that result in closure of the ATP-sensitive K+ channel, leading to sustained insulin secretion and severe hypoglycaemia soon after birth. Activating mutations of *KCNJ11* (*Kir6.2*) cause impaired ATP-sensitive K+ channel closure and have recently been shown to be a cause of persistent neonatal diabetes that can be treated with high dose sulphonylureas.

Normal pattern of insulin secretion

Insulin concentrations in peripheral blood show basal levels of about 10 mU/litre (1 mU/litre is approximately equivalent to 6.5 pmol/litre) that tend to fall overnight, on which are superimposed prandial peaks reaching 80 to 100 mU/litre, roughly proportionate to the amount eaten. The prandial peaks are elicited by the insulin secretagogue effects of glucose and other nutrients, augmented by incretin gut peptides (such as GLP-1) and the vagal outflow (the early cephalic phase of insulin release).

Very frequent sampling (every minute) shows that 'basal' insulin secretion is in fact pulsatile, with clear but low-amplitude peaks every 9 to 13 min. This may help to keep the target tissues sensitive to insulin; loss of this pulsatility is an early sign of β-cell dysfunction in type 2 diabetes. An acute insulin secretagogue challenge (e.g. an intravenous glucose bolus) induces a sharp 'first-phase' insulin peak, loss of which is another early abnormality in type 2 diabetes.

The insulin response elicited by eating is larger than when an equivalent nutrient load is given intravenously. This is because glucose entering the gut stimulates neuroendocrine cells in the gut wall to release 'incretin' hormones which act on the β cell to enhance insulin secretion (the enteroinsular axis: see Chapter 15.9). An important incretin appears to be GLP-1, a product of alternative processing of the preproglucagon gene (glucagon itself is not produced, in contrast to the islet α cell). GLP-1 released from the small intestine augments insulin release in the presence of glucose, slows gastric emptying and acts on the central nervous system to generate a feeling of satiety, effects currently being exploited in the treatment of type 2 diabetes by use of long-acting GLP-1 analogues or inhibitors of GLP-1 breakdown (see below).

Peripheral insulin levels are lower than those in the portal vein, into which the islets drain, because up to 30 % of insulin is removed on its first pass through the liver—one of the main targets for insulin action. The kidney also actively clears and degrades insulin; the circulating half-life is only a few minutes.

C-peptide provides a robust measure of residual β-cell function, because it is cleared more slowly than insulin and its plasma concentrations are therefore more stable. C-peptide is generally measured after intense β-cell stimulation with the powerful insulin secretagogue glucagon; alternatives are a heavy oral load of carbohydrate, mixed meal stimulation including amino acids (such as Boost or Sustacal) or simply the measurement of 24-h secretion of C-peptide in urine (it is cleared largely intact through the kidneys). In normal subjects and most with type 2 diabetes, peak C-peptide concentrations at 6 min after 1 mg of intravenous glucagon are 1 to 4 nmol/litre, whereas type 1 diabetic individuals are typically C-peptide negative, with peak levels less than 0.2 nmol/litre after 5 years. However, at diagnosis of type 1 diabetes there may be overlap with levels in patients with type 2 diabetes and accordingly the test is not used diagnostically (see Fig. 13.11.1.6).

The insulin receptor and signal transduction

The insulin receptor belongs to the family that also includes the insulin-like growth factor 1 (IGF-1) receptor. Insulin receptors are found in the obvious insulin target tissues (fat, liver, and skeletal muscle) but also in unexpected sites, such as the brain and gonads, in which glucose uptake does not depend on insulin.

The insulin receptor is a 400-kDa heterotetramer composed of two α and two β glycoprotein subunits, interconnected by disulphide bridges (Fig. 13.11.1.3). Both α and β subunits are encoded within a complex gene (22 exons) on chromosome 19q. The α subunit (135 kDa) lies entirely extracellularly, while the β subunit (95 kDa) spans the cell membrane and extends into the cytoplasm. Part of the intracytoplasmic tail functions as a tyrosine kinase, attaching phosphate groups from ATP to tyrosine residues

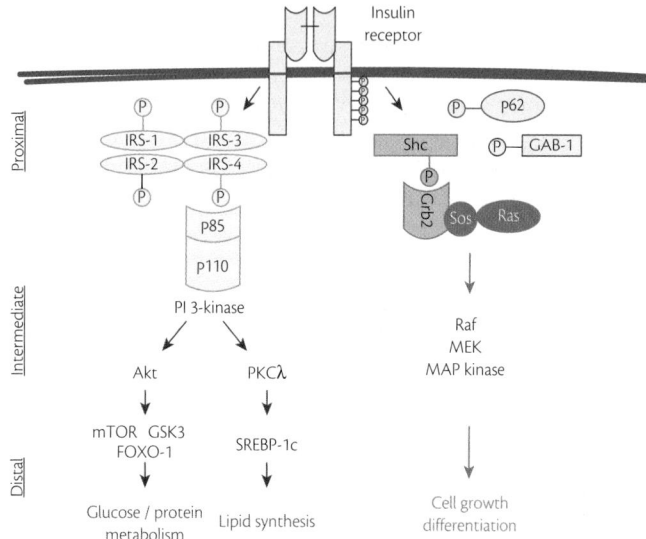

Fig. 13.11.1.3 The insulin receptor and signal transduction pathways within insulin's target cells. Binding of insulin to the extracellular α subunits of the receptor activates the tyrosine (Tyr) kinase domain of the intracellular β subunit. This results in phosphorylation of more than 10 substrate proteins including 4 structurally related proteins of the insulin receptor substrate (IRS) family which vary in their tissue distribution, as well as Shc, Cbl, p62dok and Gab-1. These activated proteins then trigger other reactions that result in the biological actions of insulin, including enhanced glucose uptake, anabolic effects, and cell growth. MAP kinase, mitogen-activated protein kinase; PI3 kinase, phosphatidylinositol-3-kinase. Akt is also known as protein kinase B (PKB). (Adapted from Biddinger SN, Kahn CR (2006). From mice to men: insights into the insulin resistance syndromes. *Annu Rev Physiol*, 68, 123–58.)

elsewhere on the receptor (autophosphorylation) and on other intracellular proteins. This tyrosine kinase activity is essential for insulin signalling and for insulin to exert its many effects on its target tissues. Insulin binds to a site on the extracellular α subunits, and binding triggers a conformational change in the receptor which activates the tyrosine kinase domain of the β subunits.

Postreceptor mechanisms

The activated receptor phosphorylates tyrosine residues on specific intracellular proteins which initiate the signal transduction pathway within the target cell. One group of proteins is the insulin receptor substrate family (IRS 1–4) that vary in their tissue distribution and subcellular localization. Additional substrates include Shc, Cbl, p62dok and Gab-1. All these substrates carry docking sites for proteins possessing specific src homology region SH2 domains. Docking of these proteins by the IRS molecules and other substrates begins a cascade of intracellular reactions that lead ultimately to the effects of insulin on glucose, lipid, and protein metabolism and its many other actions (see Fig. 13.11.1.3). A key element is the phosphatidylinositol 3-kinase pathway which appears to mediate almost all of insulin's effects on glucose transport, lipogenesis, and glycogenesis. The mitogen-activated protein kinase pathway, by contrast, is particularly relevant to insulin's actions on cell growth, with less relevance to its metabolic effects (see Fig. 13.11.1.3).

Receptor turnover

Receptors that bind insulin are internalized, i.e. taken up into the target cell by an invagination of the cell membrane that is coated with the protein clathrin. Bound insulin is degraded in the lysosomes, while most of the insulin receptors are carried back to the cell surface and reinserted into the membrane. The density of receptors on the cell surface is therefore a dynamic quantity, regulated partly by new receptor synthesis and partly by receptor recycling, which in turn is determined by insulin binding. Prolonged exposure to high insulin concentrations increases the proportion of internalized receptors and so decreases the density of receptors available on the cell surface. This down-regulation of receptors reduces the sensitivity of the target tissue to insulin.

Disorders due to insulin receptor defects

Many mutations have now been described in the insulin receptor, including point mutations that cause single-residue substitutions or truncation of the α or β subunits. The most severe mutations affect the insulin binding extracellular domain and result in so-called leprechaunism, while less severe mutations affect the tyrosine kinase domain and interfere with insulin signaling (Rabson–Mendenhall syndrome). Both syndromes are associated with severe insulin resistance (type A) as well as serious mental and physical abnormalities, confirming the importance of insulin in fetal development.

Antibodies may develop against the insulin receptor and usually cause insulin resistance with variable hyperglycaemia (the type B insulin resistance syndrome); rarely, hypoglycaemia results from antibodies that activate the receptor (analogous to thyrotoxicosis induced by antibodies to the thyroid-stimulating hormone receptor in Graves' disease).

Metabolic actions of insulin

Insulin functions as an anabolic hormone, favouring the uptake, utilization, and storage of glucose, the storage of lipids as triglyceride, and preventing the breakdown of protein.

Effects on carbohydrate metabolism

Insulin lowers blood glucose in two main ways (Fig. 13.11.1.4). At low basal concentrations (overnight and between meals) it shuts off the production of glucose by the liver, which is the main determinant of fasting glycaemia. Hepatic glucose output is fuelled by both glycogen breakdown (glycogenolysis) and gluconeogenesis (i.e. glucose synthesis from substrates including lactate, glycerol, and alanine and other amino acids); the rate-limiting enzymes for these processes are powerfully inhibited by insulin. Conversely, insulin stimulates glycogen synthesis.

At higher concentrations, such as after meals, insulin also stimulates glucose transport into skeletal muscle (where it is utilized to provide energy via glycolysis or stored as glycogen) and into fat (where it is used to synthesize triglycerides). In both these tissues, insulin enhances glucose uptake through a specific glucose transporter protein, GLUT-4 (Fig. 13.11.1.4). Insulin causes GLUT-4 units to be translocated rapidly to the cell surface and inserted into the membrane: there, GLUT-4 units act as hydrophilic pores through which glucose can cross the otherwise impermeable membrane into the cell, following its concentration gradient. Insulin also stimulates GLUT-4 synthesis. Overall, insulin acting via GLUT-4 can increase glucose uptake into muscle and fat by up to 40-fold over the basal, non-insulin-mediated, glucose uptake. Non-insulin-mediated glucose uptake occurs through other glucose transporter isoforms that operate in the absence of insulin, notably GLUT-1 in peripheral tissues and erythrocytes and GLUT-3 in brain.

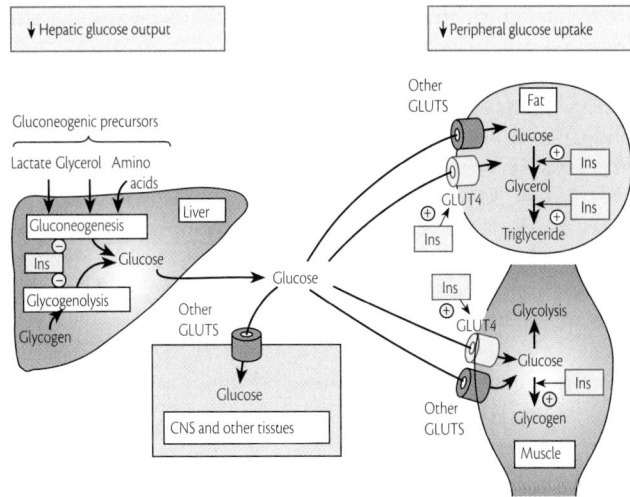

Fig. 13.11.1.4 Effects of insulin on glucose homeostasis. Insulin inhibits gluconeogenesis and glycogen breakdown in the liver, thus decreasing hepatic glucose output. Blood glucose is also lowered by increased glucose uptake into fat and skeletal muscle, mediated by the insulin-stimulated glucose transporter, GLUT-4. (Noninsulin mediated glucose uptake is effected by other GLUT proteins.)

Effects on lipid metabolism

Insulin inhibits triglyceride breakdown (lipolysis), while promoting its synthesis (lipogenesis). Lipolytic enzymes that split triglyceride into glycerol and free fatty acids are powerfully inhibited by insulin, even at low basal insulin concentrations. Profound insulin deficiency, such as in untreated type 1 diabetes, is therefore required before uncontrolled lipolysis occurs and generates enough free fatty acids to cause ketoacidosis (see below).

Effects on protein metabolism

Insulin inhibits protein catabolism and thus reduces the generation of amino acids which can act as gluconeogenic precursors to enhance glucose production by the liver and kidney. Insulin also promotes protein synthesis and cellular and tissue growth.

Other actions of insulin

These include vasodilatation, mediated by endothelial production of nitric oxide; growth and differentiation of the fetal nervous system; and enhanced tubular reabsorption of Na⁺ ions by the kidneys.

Measurements of insulin action

Glucose lowering is the most easily tested biological action of insulin, and forms the basis for most measurements of insulin resistance. Several methods are used in the research setting; theoretically, the simplest could be used in clinical diabetes care, to identify patients with marked insulin resistance who might benefit particularly from insulin-sensitizing drugs such as the thiazolidinediones:

♦ Homeostatic model assessment (HOMA) is an index derived by mathematical modelling of the relationship between the fasting glucose and insulin concentrations: with decreasing insulin sensitivity, insulin secretion increases in an attempt to maintain euglycaemia, resulting in compensatory hyperinsulinaemia. Homeostatic model assessment yields measures of both insulin resistance and β- cell function; the test can be performed on a single fasting blood sample and the results compare well with the insulin–glucose clamp.

♦ Insulin–glucose (hyperinsulinaemic–euglycaemic) clamp. Insulin is infused intravenously to achieve constant high concentrations and a separate infusion of glucose is adjusted to maintain blood glucose 'clamped' at a normal value. The more glucose required, the greater is the insulin sensitivity. The clamp is generally regarded as the gold standard method but demands blood glucose measurements every few minutes and takes some hours to perform.

♦ Intravenous glucose tolerance test. An intravenous glucose bolus stimulates insulin release, and mathematical modelling of the relationship between the insulin peak and the decay in blood glucose levels can yield indices of both insulin secretion and insulin sensitivity.

Insulin resistance

Insulin resistance (or insensitivity) is a poorly defined term signifying decreased biological activity of insulin, and which is usually equated with impaired glucose-lowering.

There is no universal normal range for insulin sensitivity, because the ability of insulin to lower glucose varies considerably between and within individuals—it is influenced e.g. by levels of physical activity and fitness. Subjects with 'insulin-resistant' conditions such as type 2 diabetes or essential hypertension commonly show reductions of 40 to 60% in glucose disposal (measured by the clamp technique), as compared with matched healthy controls, yet many apparently normal subjects also have comparable decreases in insulin sensitivity. There is no argument about extreme examples of insulin resistance: in some patients with leprechaunism, over 20 000 U/day of insulin have failed to control hyperglycaemia and ketosis. A working definition of clinically relevant insulin resistance in insulin-treated diabetic patients is a daily requirement of more than 1.5 U/kg.

Causes of insulin resistance

Inherited causes

Inherited causes include the very rare mutations affecting the insulin receptor or postreceptor signalling pathways which can lead to extreme insulin resistance (type A insulin resistance syndrome); milder polygenic defects contribute to the insulin resistance of type 2 diabetes (see below). Insulin receptor mutations cause clinically distinct syndromes, often with acanthosis nigricans and, in women, features of polycystic ovary disease and masculinization; hyperglycaemia is variable. Specific syndromes include the speculatively named leprechaunism and various inherited lipodystrophies in which fat is lost from subcutaneous and other depots in defined but unexplained anatomical patterns (see Chapter 11.5). Recently, mutations affecting the *PPARG* gene (the target for the thiazolidinedione drugs; see below) have been shown to modify insulin sensitivity. Several mutations in loci that predispose to obesity have recently been reported, but interestingly, only a subset of these also predispose to type 2 diabetes (e.g. *LEP*, *FTO*, and *TCF7L2*) suggesting that genetic influences in addition to obesity are required for the generation of diabetes.

Obesity

Obesity induces insulin resistance, especially in skeletal muscle, and weight loss can improve insulin sensitivity in the obese. Insulin resistance is particularly associated with truncal (central) obesity, where fat is deposited in and around the abdomen; both the subcutaneous and intra-abdominal (visceral) fat depots have been implicated to various degrees that may reflect ethnic and other differences.

It is still not clear how an increased fat mass can decrease whole-body insulin sensitivity, but circulating fat-derived products are presumed to be responsible. Intra-abdominal fat depots would secrete potentially diabetogenic mediators into the portal circulation—where they would be delivered directly to the liver—and this may explain the association of visceral adiposity with insulin resistance. Possible candidates include free fatty acids and the cytokine tumour necrosis factor-α (TNFα); both are secreted by adipocytes and, under experimental conditions at least, interfere with aspects of insulin action. Levels of free fatty acids are raised in obese subjects, apparently because lipolysis is enhanced, and free fatty acids may cause hyperglycaemia by competing with glucose metabolism in liver and muscle. In liver, free fatty acids enhance gluconeogenesis by stimulating the rate-limiting enzyme pyruvate carboxylase and so increase hepatic glucose production. In muscle, free fatty acids inhibit glycolysis at the level of phosphofructokinase and glucose oxidation via pyruvate dehydrogenase, causing a decrease in glucose utilization and a secondary reduction in glucose uptake (the glucose–fatty acid or Randle cycle). *In vitro*, TNFα inhibits the tyrosine kinase activity of the insulin receptor that is crucial for insulin signalling. Production of TNFα by adipose tissue is increased in obesity but its role as a mediator of insulin resistance in human obesity is uncertain. Recently, a novel adipocyte product, adiponectin, has been shown to enhance insulin sensitivity in rodents; intriguingly, circulating adiponectin concentrations are decreased in human obesity. Several other recently identified hormones released by adipose tissue (adipokines) also have effects on insulin action (e.g. resistin, visfatin, interleukin-6) but their role in type 2 diabetes is less well defined. Obesity is also accompanied by the ectopic deposition of triglyceride in liver and skeletal muscle, and the accumulation of triglyceride is correlated with impairment of insulin action in these tissues.

Physical inactivity strongly predisposes to obesity and also promotes insulin resistance which can be reversed by regular exercise. The mechanism is unknown but physical training is known to stimulate translocation of GLUT-4 glucose transporters to the surface of muscle cells independently of insulin. In addition, muscle contraction enhances expression of the enzyme AMP kinase which mediates improved glucose transport and fatty acid metabolism. AMP kinase has recently been shown to be a molecular target of two drugs known to reduce insulin resistance (metformin and rosiglitazone).

Other acquired causes

There are several other acquired causes of insulin resistance. Intrauterine growth retardation may contribute (see the Barker–Hales hypothesis below). Physiological states of insulin resistance, due to the appropriate oversecretion of the counter-regulatory hormones whose metabolic actions oppose those of insulin, are puberty and pregnancy (see gestational diabetes, Chapter 13.10). Endocrine diseases that induce insulin resistance and can cause glucose intolerance and overt diabetes through excessive production of anti-insulin hormones include acromegaly (prevalence of diabetes and impaired glucose tolerance each c.25%), Cushing's disease (diabetes c.30%), thyrotoxicosis, and the very rare glucagonoma (diabetes in >90% of cases). In these disorders, diabetes is

mostly nonketotic, although insulin may be needed to control hyperglycaemia.

Intercurrent illnesses, e.g. myocardial infarction, stroke, or severe infections, induce the secretion of counter-regulatory stress hormones that can cause marked insulin resistance—insulin-treated diabetic patients may need twice their usual insulin dosages during such episodes. Many drugs decrease insulin sensitivity, including glucocorticoids, β_2 adrenoceptor agonists (ritodrine, salbutamol), and certain oral contraceptive pills containing high-dose oestrogen or levonorgestrel; glucocorticoid-induced hyperglycaemia commonly requires insulin treatment. Acquired lipodystrophies, most notably that induced by drugs used to treat HIV, especially protease inhibitors (PIs) and nucleoside analogue inhibitors of viral reverse transcriptase (NRTIs), are also associated with insulin resistance and the development of diabetes.

The type B insulin resistance syndrome is due to the development of autoantibodies against the insulin receptor which interfere with insulin binding and/or signalling. Most patients are young women, usually with pre-existing autoimmune diseases such as lupus erythematosus, and masculinization often occurs. 'Immune insulin resistance' describes insulin-treated patients with very high insulin requirements (sometimes several thousand U/day) because of high titres of insulin-binding antibodies that bind and inactivate administered insulin. This has become very rare since the introduction of highly purified human-sequence insulin preparations with low immunogenicity (see below).

Metabolic and clinical features of insulin resistance

The metabolic disturbance due to insulin-resistant syndromes ranges from subclinical glucose intolerance to severely symptomatic hyperglycaemia, sometimes with ketosis. A crucial determinant is the capacity of the individual's β cells to secrete insulin in response to the rises in blood glucose that are due to impaired insulin action. The resulting hyperinsulinaemia is extremely variable, with plasma insulin levels ranging from twice normal in many obese subjects to 500 times normal in patients with defects of insulin receptors. Near normoglycaemia can be maintained as long as hyperinsulinaemia can compensate for the underlying defect in insulin signalling; diabetes occurs when β-cell failure supervenes and insulin secretion falls below a critical level. In the total absence of functional insulin receptors (e.g. in leprechaunism), massive endogenous hyperinsulinaemia or administration of industrial insulin dosages cannot prevent severe diabetes, although very high insulin concentrations may exert some metabolic actions through 'cross-talk' with the IGF-1 receptor.

Acanthosis nigricans, a characteristic skin manifestation of severe insulin resistance, may be due to high insulin concentrations activating growth factor receptors (perhaps the IGF1 receptor) that drive the proliferation of keratinocytes and melanocytes. Hyperplasia of these cells leads to a velvety thickening and variable darkening of the skin, especially in the axillae (often with proliferation of skin tags), groin, and nape of the neck (see Chapter 23.1). Widespread acanthosis nigricans can also accompany gut tumours, which may also secrete dermal growth factors.

Increased androgen concentrations may lead to hirsutism and occasionally virilization in women with severe insulin resistance; high insulin concentrations may stimulate androgen production by the ovaries, which often show a polycystic appearance. Insulin resistance is a feature of polycystic ovary syndrome, especially in obese patients (Chapter 13.8.1). Enhancing insulin sensitivity through weight loss or treatment with metformin or the thiazolidinediones can decrease androgen levels and improve hirsutism and menstrual dysfunction.

The metabolic syndrome

The metabolic syndrome (syndrome X) denotes the co-occurrence of insulin resistance and glucose intolerance (ranging from mild to overt type 2 diabetes), with truncal obesity, dyslipidaemia (raised triglycerides and a high low-density lipoprotein:high-density lipoprotein (HDL/LDL) ratio), and hypertension (see Fig. 13.11.1.5).

These abnormalities are all common in most Westernized populations, and it is still not clear whether or not this constellation of cardiovascular risk factors represents a genuine syndrome with a common underlying cause. Reaven and others have argued that insulin resistance is the central abnormality, and that the key features can be explained either by loss of specific actions of insulin or by the effects of the compensatory hyperinsulinaemia on organs that remain relatively insulin sensitive. For example, raised insulin levels could contribute to hypertension by enhancing retention of Na^+ by the kidney; conversely, blood pressure could also be raised through loss of the direct vasodilator action of insulin. The pattern of abnormalities would therefore require insulin resistance to affect certain tissues and specific actions of insulin but not others. Other proatherogenic defects identified in subjects with various features of syndrome X include increased coagulability of the blood (e.g. increased levels of plasminogen activator inhibitor-1) and impaired endothelial-mediated vasodilatation. The relationship of these abnormalities to insulin resistance is uncertain. Obesity, dyslipidaemia, hypertension, and glucose intolerance are all independent cardiovascular risk factors; any possible proatherogenic role of hyperinsulinaemia *per se* remains controversial.

The aetiology of syndrome X is unresolved; indeed it has been argued that it is not a distinct entity, but simply represents the variable association of several abnormalities that are relatively common in all populations, and especially those that generally overeat and are too sedentary. Adiposity, insulin sensitivity, and blood pressure show variable strengths of familial transmission that differ between populations and generally suggest polygenic inheritance of multiple minor genes. On the other hand, Barker and Hales have suggested that fetal malnutrition programmes insulin resistance, hypertension, and dyslipidaemia in middle to late adult life. The underlying mechanisms remain elusive. Because obesity leads to insulin resistance and glucose intolerance, dyslipidaemia, hypertension, and atheroma, weight gain in middle age may be particularly hazardous in subjects who were underweight at birth.

Clustering of these metabolic and cardiovascular risk factors is important clinically because it predisposes to atheroma formation and substantially increases the risk of dying prematurely from myocardial infarction or stroke. Treatment is currently based on correcting any factors (e.g. type 2 diabetes, hypertension, and dyslipidaemia) present in the individual patient. Lifestyle and dietary modification that achieves weight loss can improve most aspects of the syndrome. Several drugs have been shown to slow progression from impaired glucose tolerance to type 2 diabetes (e.g. metformin, rosiglitazone, and weight-loss drugs such as orlistat), although their role in treatment of the metabolic syndrome remains controversial and rosiglitazone, in particular, fails to decrease cardiovascular risk despite improving insulin sensitivity.

Types and classification of diabetes mellitus

The current WHO classification is based on aetiology (see Table 13.11.1.1). Type 1 and type 2 diabetes together account for 90 to 95% of cases and will be described in detail.

Type 1 diabetes

Type 1 diabetes—previously referred to as juvenile-onset or insulin-dependent diabetes—is due to autoimmune killing of the β cells (the type 1 process). A similar clinical picture of insulin dependence can be caused by other forms of severe pancreatic damage.

Epidemiology and demographic features

Type 1 diabetes is considerably rarer than type 2, accounting for between 5 and 15% of all diabetes and 30 to 50% of insulin-treated cases in various populations. It appears predominantly in childhood, with a peak age at presentation of about 11 years in girls and 14 years in boys—hence the old description of juvenile-onset. However, it can develop at any age; up to 50% of all cases are diagnosed over the age of 18 and about 5% of newly diagnosed white diabetic patients over 65 years are considered to have type 1 diabetes.

The prevalence of type 1 diabetes varies considerably throughout the world. Incidence is highest in northern European countries (about 30 to 35 cases per 100 000 children per year in Finland and Scotland) and declines progressively towards the equator; there are some isolated hot spots such as Sardinia, where the incidence is as high as in Finland. High susceptibility is found in European populations throughout the world, while African and East Asian populations are relatively spared (incidences of less than 1 per 100 000 per year). Superimposed on this geographical variation are time-related changes in incidence that hint at the importance of the environment in causing the disease. Type 1 diabetes presents more frequently during the winter months, particularly in children aged 10 to 14 years. In many countries (e.g. Norway, Poland, Sweden, and the United Kingdom), there have been sharp 30 to 50% increases in incidence over 10 to 20 year periods, although the explanation and significance of these secular trends are not clear. In particular, there seems to be a shift to diabetes at a younger age

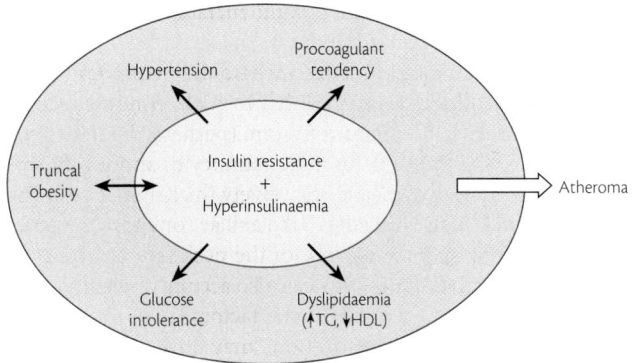

Fig. 13.11.1.5 Metabolic syndrome, a constellation of atherogenic risk factors which may each be related to insulin resistance and/or the hyperinsulinaemia that accompanies insulin-resistant states. ↓HDL, reduced high-density lipoprotein cholesterol; ↑TG, hypertriglyceridaemia;.

Table 13.11.1.1 Classification of diabetes mellitus according to aetiology

Type 1 diabetes	β-Cell destruction, usually leading to absolute insulin deficiency (10–15% of cases in Europe and USA):
	1A-Immune mediated
	1B-Idiopathic (e.g. fulminant Type 1 diabetes)
Type 2 diabetes	May range from predominantly insulin resistance with relative insulin deficiency to a predominantly secretory defect with insulin resistance (80–85% of cases in Europe and USA)
Other specific types (Type 3 diabetes)	Other types with specific causes (5% of cases in Europe and USA)
A *Genetic defects of β-cell function*	MODY: see Table 13.11.1.4
	Others, including mitochondrial DNA defects (MELAS syndrome)
	Neonatal diabetes: mutations in *KCNJ11*; imprinting abnormality in *ZAC* and *HYMAI*—may be transient
B *Genetic defects of insulin action*	Type A insulin resistance syndrome
	Leprechaunism
	Rabson–Mendenhall syndrome
	Congenital lipodystrophies
C *Diseases of the exocrine pancreas*	Pancreatitis, chronic and acute
	Carcinoma of the pancreas
	Haemochromatosis
	Cystic fibrosis
	Pancreatectomy, trauma
	Fibrocalculous pancreatopathy
D *Endocrinopathies*	Acromegaly
	Cushing's disease and syndrome
	Phaeochromocytoma
	Glucagonoma
	Hyperthyroidism
	Somatostatinoma
	Aldosteronoma
E *Drug- or chemically-induced*	Glucocorticoids
	β-Blockers
	Thiazides
	Diazoxide
	Others – phenytoin, pentamidine, nicotinic acid, interferon-α
F *Infections*	Congenital rubella
	Cytomegalovirus
G *Uncommon forms of immune-mediated diabetes*	Type B insulin resistance (insulin receptor antibodies)
	'Stiff man' syndrome

Table 13.11.1.1 *(cont'd)* Classification of diabetes mellitus according to aetiology

H *Other genetic syndromes*	Prader–Willi syndrome
	Wolfram's syndrome (DIDMOAD)
	Down's syndrome
	Turner's syndrome
	Klinefelter's syndrome
	Others, e.g. Laurence–Moon–Biedl syndrome
Type 4 diabetes	Gestational diabetes or glucose intolerance

DIDMOAD, diabetes insipidus, diabetes mellitus, optic atrophy, and deafness; MELAS, myopathy, encephalopathy, lactic acidosis, and stroke-like episodes (associated with type 1 or type 2 diabetes); MODY, maturity-onset diabetes of the young.

(Adapted from American Diabetes Association (2007). Diagnosis and classification of diabetes. *Diabetes Care*, **30**, S42–S47.)

with a particularly marked rise in cases being diagnosed under the age of 5.

Susceptibility to type 1 diabetes shows no gender bias in cases diagnosed before puberty, but in older individuals there is a male preponderance in new cases of 1.5:1 to 1.8:1

Aetiology

Type 1 diabetes is an autoimmune, predominantly T-cell-mediated process that selectively destroys the β cells. Susceptibility is multifactorial, resulting from the impact of environmental agents in a genetically disadvantaged subject. Of these two components, the environment appears more important; genetic factors explain only 30 to 40% of total susceptibility. Immunogenetic aspects are discussed in detail in Chapter 13.11.2.

Genetic factors (see also Chapter 13.11.2)

Over 20 genetic loci are associated with type 1 diabetes, at least 10 of which have been confirmed by repeated studies and genome-wide analyses with large cohorts. The best characterized are the HLA class II locus (*HLA-DQB1, IDDM1*) and the insulin gene promoter region (*IDDM2*), of which the HLA class II locus has by far the greatest effect (odds ratio for diabetes is 7–13:1 for susceptible alleles).

The HLA class II locus lies within the major histocompatibility complex region on chromosome 6, that encodes several proteins intimately involved in immune responses. Of particular importance is *HLA-DQB1*; this encodes the DQB1 peptide chain, which forms part of the cleft in the surface of the HLA class II molecule that is crucial in presenting peptide fragments of antigen to the T-helper lymphocyte. Changes in the structure of the DQB1 peptide could therefore influence the coupling between the class II molecule–peptide complex and the T-lymphocyte receptor, and thus modulate the immune response against the (auto)antigenic peptide. Specific DQB1 polymorphisms have been shown to predispose to type 1 diabetes (e.g. *DQB1*0302*), whereas others (e.g. *DQB1*0602*) are protective—at least in certain racial groups. The relationships of these polymorphisms to the long-recognized influences of the DR3 and DR4 class II antigens (which increase several-fold the risk of type 1 diabetes) and of the protective DR2 are discussed further in Chapter 13.12.2.

The HLA class II locus corresponds to the insulin gene (*INS*) whose uniqueness as a β-cell product makes it an obvious candidate gene. The insulin coding sequence is unchanged in type 1 diabetes. However, variation is observed in a region upstream of the insulin gene in which there is a variable number of repeats of the consensus sequence, 5′-ACAGGGGTGTGGGG-3′ one after another, known as the variable number of tandem repeats (VNTR) minisatellite. The short class I VNTR alleles (26–63 repeats) predispose to diabetes, while class III alleles (140–210 repeats) have a dominant protective effect (odds ratio for type 1 diabetes with class I vs class III alleles is 2.2:1). This protective effect appears to be mediated by a two- to threefold increased expression of insulin in the thymus. Insulin, like many other self proteins, is normally expressed at low level in the thymus as part of the process which promotes central tolerance to self antigens amongst T cells. The further increased levels associated with class III alleles thereby results in a relative reduction in the risk of autoimmunity.

Additional loci confirmed to predispose to type 1 diabetes show a strong predominance of genes affecting the immune system, including *PTPN22* and *CTLA4*, both negative regulatory molecules of the immune system, *IL2RA* (CD25), the high-affinity interleukin-2 receptor and *IFIH1*, a cytoplasmic helicase that mediates induction of interferon in response to viral RNA. Work is in progress to define more precisely how disease predisposition is increased by the high-risk alleles and should ultimately shed light on the pathogenesis of the disease.

Environmental factors

Viruses have long been popular candidates as an environmental trigger for diabetes. Some (e.g. mumps, Coxsackie, cytomegalovirus, and rubella) infect the pancreas but normally damage the entire gland, particularly the exocrine tissue, rather than causing selective β-cell injury. Certain viruses target the β cell in animals (e.g. the Kilham rat virus) and can cause insulin-dependent diabetes, either through their direct cytolytic effects or by provoking a type 1-like autoimmune process. Important contenders in humans are coxsackieviruses (especially B4), rubella, and rotaviruses.

Serological studies indicate that recent Coxsackie B infections are relatively common among newly diagnosed patients with type 1 diabetes; these could represent the final insult in the disease's long natural history, since the autoimmune process can be detected many years prior to this. Coxsackieviruses capable of damaging rodent β cells have also been isolated post-mortem from the islets of some type 1 diabetic subjects. About 20% of children who survive intrauterine rubella infection develop type 1 diabetes, with typical autoimmune markers. Endogenous retroviruses were previously implicated as aetiological agents but this has not been confirmed in further studies. For other viruses, the epidemiological data are conflicting: e.g. the eradication of rubella by vaccination has not reduced the incidence of type 1 diabetes in Finland while the prevalence of Coxsackie infections is lower in Finland than in the adjacent Russian Karelian population which is genetically related but has a substantially lower type 1 diabetes risk.

Viruses could trigger or maintain autoimmune β-cell damage in various ways. Acute or persistent viral infection of β cells could release β-cell antigens that are normally sequestered beyond the reach of the immune cells. Certain viral proteins may elicit an immune response which cross-reacts with specific β-cell antigens that happen to be similar (molecular mimicry): e.g. peptide sequences of the P2-C capsid protein of coxsackie B viruses may cross-react with glutamate decarboxylase-65 (GAD65) in the β-cell membrane.

Other environmental factors are suggested to include bovine serum albumin from cow's milk and various toxins. Bovine serum albumin contains a peptide sequence that may crossreact with a β-cell surface protein (see below); this was suggested as an explanation for an apparent excess risk of type 1 diabetes among children fed with cow's milk in the neonatal period, although a protective effect for breastfeeding remains controversial. Various toxins selectively damage β cells, including streptozotocin, a nitrosourea used to induce experimental diabetes in rodents. Related nitrosamine compounds have been blamed for the higher risk of type 1 diabetes in the children of women who eat fermented smoked mutton (a traditional delicacy in Iceland).

To try to resolve the controversies in this complex area, an international consortium—The Environmental Determinants of Diabetes in the Young (TEDDY; http://www.niddk.nih.gov/patient/TEDDY/TEDDY.htm)—has been established. This will follow several thousand children with high-risk HLA genotypes from birth until adolescence to identify infectious agents and dietary or other environmental factors that trigger β-cell autoimmunity in genetically susceptible people.

Autoimmune features

Type 1 diabetes has strong associations with endocrine and other autoimmune diseases, including Schmidt's syndrome (with hypothyroidism and adrenocortical failure) and the autoimmune polyendocrinopathy–candidiasis–ectodermal dystrophy (APECED) syndrome caused by mutations in the *AIRE* gene which controls self-tolerance by influencing thymic expression of autoantigens. Type 1 diabetes is also a feature of the IPEX syndrome (immunodysregulation, polyendocrinopathy, and enteropathy, X-linked syndrome) caused by mutations in the key T cell regulatory gene, *FOXP3*.

Most β-cell damage is probably inflicted by T lymphocytes. Insulitis—infiltration of the islets with immune cells, mostly cytotoxic/suppressor (CD8+) T lymphocytes—is a pathognomic feature of the disease, and circulating T-helper lymphocytes can be identified that react against β-cell antigens including proinsulin and GAD65.

Various circulating autoantibodies also occur. Some target antigens are unique to the β cell, while other autoantigens are shared by other islet cell types. Notable β-cell selective autoantibodies are those that recognize GAD65, a heat shock protein (hsp60), and insulin itself. GAD catalyses the conversion of glutamic acid to γ-aminobutyric acid, whose role in the β cell is uncertain. Studies in rodents with type 1 diabetes suggest that the level of GAD65 expression influences the intensity of the autoimmune attack on the β cells. The GAD67 isoform of the enzyme is also expressed in the central nervous system, and autoimmune damage of GABAergic neurons is presumed to explain the association of type 1 diabetes with the rare 'stiff man' syndrome (Chapter 24.19). High frequencies of autoantibodies to the protein tyrosine phosphatase-like molecule IA-2 are also seen. Most recently, autoantibodies against the cation efflux transporter, zinc transporter 8 (ZnT8) have been identified.

GAD65 antibodies are present in 70 to 90% of newly diagnosed type 1 patients, insulin antibodies in 40 to 70%, IA-2 autoantibodies in around 50 to 60% and ZnT8 antibodies in around 70%. Islet cell antibodies detected by immunofluorescence on tissue sections are present in 80 to 90% of newly diagnosed patients but are technically difficult to measure. Recent studies suggest that automated combined testing for GAD and IA-2 has equivalent sensitivity and specificity to islet cell antibodies (ICA) testing. This is increasingly replacing ICA assays, although undoubtedly ICA reactivity encompasses more (as yet undetermined) antigens than insulin, GAD 65, IA-2 and ZnT8 alone. These antibodies cannot explain the selective destruction of β cells: although some islet cell surface antibodies are complement-fixing the majority of the islet cell destruction is believe to be caused by T cells.

High titres of each of these classes of antibodies have some value in predicting diabetes in high-risk individuals—the combination of high titres of three autoantibodies (GAD, IA-2, and insulin or ICA) amongst family members of subjects with type 1 diabetes is 90% predictive of disease, although hyperglycaemia may not develop for 20 years or more. However, they are clearly not the immediate cause of the disease: single autoantibody-positive individuals rarely progress to disease, suggesting that these autoantibodies are general markers of autoimmunity against the β cell, rather than evidence of β-cell destruction, which is primarily cell mediated. Titres of all these antibodies tend to be high at presentation and (according to prospective studies of high-risk subjects) during the months leading up to this. Thereafter, antibody levels decline progressively and may even become undetectable, possibly through dwindling of the antigen load that perpetuates autoimmunity as any remaining β cells disappear.

Natural history of type 1 diabetes

The damage to β cells might be initiated by direct viral attack, environmental toxins, and/or a primary immune attack against specific β-cell antigens such as GAD65, perhaps via molecular mimicry. T-helper lymphocytes (CD4+) are activated by β-cell antigens presented together with diabetogenic class II antigens by antigen-presenting cells (dendritic cells). Activated T-helper cells produce cytokines that attract T and B lymphocytes and encourage them to proliferate in the islet, leading to insulitis. B lymphocytes might then damage β cells by producing antibodies against released β-cell antigens, while cytotoxic (CD8+) T lymphocytes directly attack β cells carrying the target autoantigens. Insulitis is a patchy and unpredictable process that might flare up after encounters with new environmental triggers such as viral infections, but which can also fade and abort for unknown reasons.

Several years of progressive autoimmune damage usually precede the clinical onset of diabetes. This long prediabetic phase is asymptomatic, although careful testing (e.g. with the intravenous glucose tolerance test) reveals loss of the first phase, then increasingly obvious disturbances of insulin and C-peptide secretion, and eventually glucose intolerance. Finally, when the β-cell mass has been eroded to a critical level (probably 5 to 10% of normal), falling insulin secretion can no longer restrain hyperglycaemia and clinical diabetes develops.

Residual β-cell mass is variable at presentation of type 1 diabetes: some newly diagnosed type 1 patients are C-peptide positive, and β-cell secretion may improve temporarily during the 'honeymoon period' that can follow the lowering of blood glucose when insulin treatment is started (see below). As a result, it is not possible to absolutely distinguish type 1 and type 2 diabetes by measurement of C-peptide at diagnosis although levels tend to be very much lower in type 1 diabetes (see Fig. 13.11.1.6, panel A). With continuing β-cell destruction, endogenous insulin production declines progressively, and more than 90% of type 1 patients become permanently C-peptide negative within 5 years of presentation. The loss of C-peptide is more rapid in individuals diagnosed in

childhood than in new onset disease in adults (see Fig. 13.11.1.6, panels B and C). Ultimately, insulitis burns itself out and the immune cells retreat, leaving islet remnants that are devoid of β cells but which still contain intact α, δ, and PP cells. Interestingly, there is a concomitant 50% reduction in the size of the exocrine pancreas in patients with long-standing type 1 diabetes: this appears not to result in clinically significant malabsorption and the mechanism by which it occurs is unknown.

The protracted prediabetic phase provides an opportunity to prevent subjects with active insulitis from developing clinical disease. A combination of autoantibody titres and genetic markers (HLA haplotypes) can be used to predict the chances of the disease developing in high-risk subjects, such as the siblings of children with type 1 diabetes; various immunosuppressive and immunomodulatory treatments are currently undergoing clinical trials as forms of early intervention or prevention.

Metabolic disturbances of type 1 diabetes

In untreated type 1 diabetes, insulin concentrations are generally 10 to 50% of nondiabetic levels in the face of hyperglycaemia which would normally greatly increase insulin secretion. Such severe deficiency cannot sustain the normal anabolic effects of insulin and leads to runaway catabolism in carbohydrate, fat, and protein metabolism. Each of these processes accelerates hyperglycaemia, while the oxidation of excess free fatty acids generated by triglyceride breakdown can result in diabetic ketoacidosis.

Carbohydrate metabolism

Basal hyperglycaemia is due mainly to unrestrained production of glucose by the liver and is accentuated after eating by the failure of glucose to be cleared peripherally (see Fig. 13.11.1.4). Hepatic glucose output is boosted, especially by increased gluconeogenesis: the normal inhibition of the process by insulin is lost, while the supply of gluconeogenic precursors (glycerol from lipolysis, amino acids such as alanine from protein breakdown) is increased. Enhanced gluconeogenesis in the kidney may also contribute. Postprandial glucose uptake into muscle and fat, mediated by insulin and GLUT-4, is greatly decreased; this is partly offset by increased non-insulin-dependent glucose uptake into peripheral tissues, via glucose transporters that do not require insulin. The overall result is hyperglycaemia, commonly in the range of 15 to 25 mmol/litre and higher after meals. Glucose concentrations of over 40 mmol/litre are not uncommon during intercurrent illness and especially when insulin treatment is omitted or not increased sufficiently.

Fat metabolism

Lipolysis is stimulated by severe insulin deficiency, generating glycerol (a gluconeogenic precursor) and free fatty acids, the substrate for ketone formation. Ketogenesis is particularly enhanced by concomitant glucagon excess (see below). Mobilization of body fat contributes to the marked weight loss in untreated type 1 diabetes.

Protein metabolism

Loss of the net anabolic effect of insulin encourages catabolism of proteins (primarily through the proteasome-mediated pathway), thus generating amino acids including gluconeogenic precursors such as alanine and glutamine. Muscle wasting may be prominent.

Role of counter-regulatory hormones

The effects of hypoinsulinaemia are compounded by the counter-regulatory hormones which are secreted in excess in response to

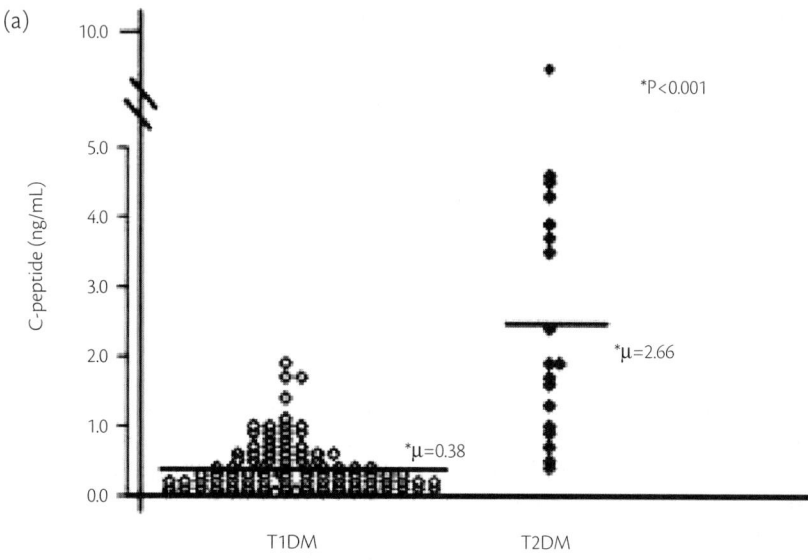

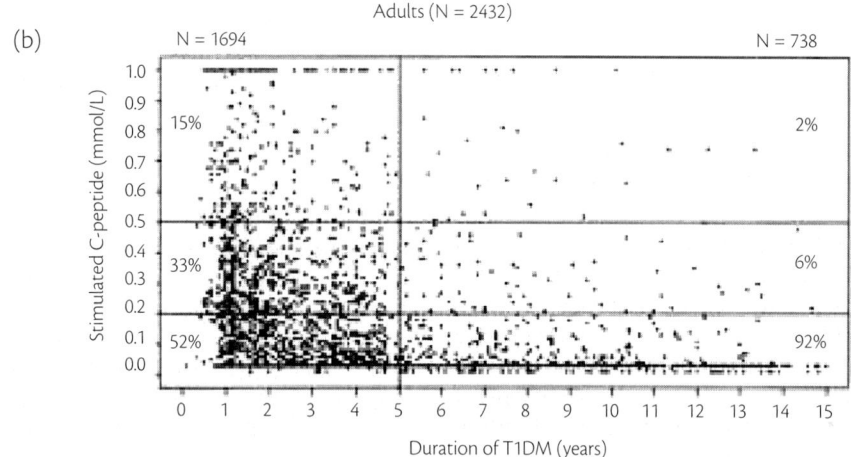

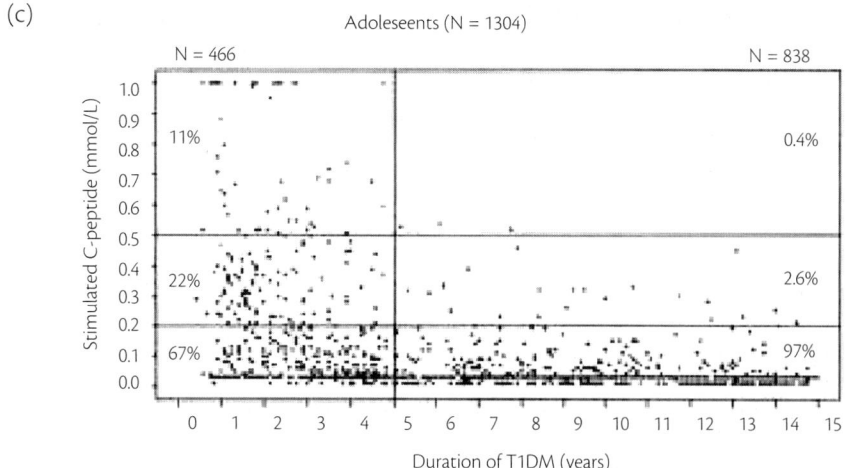

Fig. 13.11.1.6 Loss of insulin production in type 1 diabetes. Panel A compares fasting insulin C-peptide levels at diagnosis in children with type 1 vs type 2 diabetes showing that although the levels are very different, there is still some degree of overlap; the lower panels show the peak C-peptide during a mixed meal tolerance test in patients more than 18 years of age (panel B, adults) or less than 18 years of age (panel C) at onset of diabetes and when tested after 1 to 15 years duration of diabetes, as part of screening for entry into the DCCT study. Note that C-peptide levels fall faster in younger subjects so that after 5 years 8% of adults but only 3% of children have a peak C-peptide level > 200 nmol/litre.

(Panel A adapted from Katz LE, *et al.* (2007). Fasting C-peptide and insulin-like growth factor-binding protein-1 levels help to distinguish childhood type 1 and type 2 diabetes at diagnosis. *Pediatr Diabetes,* **8**, 53–9; panels B and C reproduced from Palmer JP, *et al.* (2004). C-peptide is the appropriate outcome measure for type 1 diabetes clinical trials to preserve beta-cell function: report of an ADA workshop, 21–22 October 2001. *Diabetes,* **53**, 250–64.)

stress (e.g. infections, myocardial infarction, trauma, surgery) and when circulating volume falls (e.g. in hyperglycaemic dehydrated patients). Insulin deficiency also leads to increased glucagon secretion, because insulin normally inhibits the α cells.

Glucagon increases hepatic glucose production, both by driving glycogen breakdown and by increasing uptake of glucogenic amino acids by the liver and enhancing gluconeogenesis. It also stimulates ketogenesis by increasing entry of free fatty acids (as their fatty acyl-CoA derivatives) into liver mitochondria (see Fig. 13.11.1.10 below). Glucagon excess is an important factor that promotes diabetic ketoacidosis, acting synergistically with insulin deficiency (see below).

Cortisol and catecholamines enhance gluconeogenesis. Cortisol, catecholamines, and growth hormone oppose the lipogenic action of insulin and favour lipolysis, in the presence of hypoinsulinaemia. Cortisol is a powerful inducer of proteolysis, whereas growth hormone cooperates with insulin to stimulate protein synthesis.

Clinical features of type 1 diabetes

The classical presentation of untreated or poorly controlled type 1 diabetes reflects the consequences of catabolism and hyperglycaemia (see Table 13.11.1.2). These features usually develop progressively and quite rapidly over a period of a few days to a few weeks.

Table 13.11.1.2 Typical features of type 1 and type 2 diabetes, with some distinguishing characteristics

	Type 1 diabetes	Type 2 diabetes
Osmotic and glycosuric symptoms: polyuria, nocturia, enuresis; thirst, polydipsia; blurred vision; genital candidiasis (pruritus vulvae, balanitis)	+ → ++	± → ++
Systemic symptoms: malaise, tiredness, lack of energy	+ → ++	0 → ++
Catabolic features: recent weight loss; muscle wasting and weakness	+ → ++	0 → +
Ketoacidosis	Spontaneous	Rare; mostly precipitated by intercurrent illness
Diabetic microvascular complications at presentation	–	±
Age at presentation	Young > old	Old > young
Obesity	Unusual	++ (almost invariable in white people)
Family history	±	+
Clinical insulin dependence (weight loss and hyperglycaemia without insulin replacement)	+	–
Special investigations:		
C peptide	low especially 5 years after diagnosis	normal or raised
HLA DR3 or DR4	++	–
Islet cell antibodies: ICA, GAD, IA-2	++	–

GAD, glutamic acid decarboxylase; HLA, human leukocyte antigen; ICA, islet cell antibodies; IA-2, insulinoma associated antigen-2.

Diuresis is due mainly to the osmotic effect of glucose remaining in the renal tubule, when its concentration exceeds the reabsorption threshold for glucose (corresponding generally to plasma glucose levels of about 10 mmol/litre). The osmotic loads of urinary ketones and of electrolytes that are obligatorily lost with glucose also contribute. Urine output may reach several litres per day, causing polyuria, nocturia, and in children, enuresis.

Thirst generally parallels urine output and can be very intense; it is characteristically made worse by sugar-rich drinks. Taking water to bed at night is a useful sign of pathological thirst. A high fluid intake is an important homeostatic response to diuresis, and patients unable to drink (e.g. through nausea in ketoacidosis) can rapidly become dehydrated and hypovolaemic.

Weight loss, due to loss of fat and muscle and later to dehydration, can be dramatic and reach several kilograms over a few weeks. The energy deficit caused by catabolism and urinary losses of glucose can amount to several hundred calories per day. Appetite is often increased; the mechanism in humans is not known; falls in circulating leptin and insulin, both of which act on the central nervous system to inhibit feeding, are probably responsible for hyperphagia in diabetic rodents.

Systemic symptoms include tiredness, malaise, lack of energy, and muscular weakness.

Blurred vision is commonly due to changes in the shape of the lens due to osmotic shifts, typically causing long-sightedness. Rarely, acute 'snowflake' cataracts develop because of reversible refractile changes, rather than the permanent denaturation of lens proteins in senile cataract.

Infections are often present because hyperglycaemia predisposes to infections and also because infections stimulate the secretion of stress hormones. Genital candida infections, causing recurrent pruritus vulvae in women and balanitis in men, are frequent and should always prompt testing for diabetes. Pyogenic skin infections and urinary tract infections, sometimes complicated by severe renal damage, are also common, and certain rare infections have a particular predilection for diabetic people (see below).

Diabetic ketoacidosis presents with hyperglycaemic symptoms, which are usually severe, together with nausea and vomiting, acidotic (Kussmaul) breathing, the smell of acetone on the breath, and, especially in children, altered mood and clouding of consciousness that may progress to coma. Diabetic ketoacidosis is described in detail later.

Unlike type 2 diabetes, which is often present for several years before diagnosis, hyperglycaemia in newly presenting type 1 patients develops too acutely for chronic diabetic complications to appear. Because obvious symptoms appear quickly, very few cases are picked up fortuitously, although doctors who have forgotten to think of diabetes in their differential diagnosis of weight loss or hyperventilation may be surprised when hyperglycaemia is detected by routine screening. With the rising incidence and awareness of diabetes in the general population (due to rising rates of type 2 diabetes), an increasing number of cases of type 1 diabetes are detected before ketosis develops—giving rise, especially in adults, to confusion over whether the diagnosis is type 1 or type 2 diabetes.

Prognosis of type 1 diabetes

Before the introduction of insulin during the early 1920s, type 1 diabetes was invariably fatal, usually within months. With various semistarvation diets, hyperglycaemic symptoms could be improved somewhat and life extended by a few miserable months.

With modern insulin treatment, type 1 diabetic patients can be rescued from diabetic ketoacidosis, although one-third of deaths in diabetic children and young adults are still due to metabolic emergencies, notably ketoacidosis. The main threat to survival with type 1 diabetes is now chronic tissue damage, particularly renal failure from nephropathy, and vascular disease, notably myocardial infarction and stroke. Throughout adult life, the overall risk of dying within 10 years is about fourfold higher for patients with type 1 diabetes than for their nondiabetic peers.

There is encouraging evidence from Europe and the United States of America that the outlook for type 1 diabetes has improved over the last 10 to 20 years, with definite declines in the incidence of microvascular complications and extended survival—at least in countries able to afford effective diabetes care. This is partly attributable to tighter control of hyperglycaemia, which can reduce by 30 to 40% the risks of nephropathy and retinopathy developing or progressing to a clinically significant degree (see below). Other measures have undoubtedly contributed, including better treatment of raised blood pressure and blood lipids.

Tragically, however, in many parts of the world patients with type 1 diabetes still die today as they did a century ago, simply because insulin is not available.

Type 2 diabetes

Type 2 diabetes is a heterogeneous condition, diagnosed empirically by the absence of features suggesting type 1 diabetes (see Table 13.11.1.2) and of the many other conditions that cause hyperglycaemia (see Table 13.11.1.1). Diagnostic accuracy may depend on the thoroughness of investigation: e.g. up to 10% of subjects with late-onset diabetes show evidence of autoimmune β-cell damage and thus probably have slowly evolving type 1 diabetes (so-called latent autoimmune diabetes in adults, LADA).

The term 'type 2' replaces 'non-insulin-dependent' and 'maturity-onset' which were both clumsy and misleading: many type 2 patients require insulin to control hyperglycaemia and increasingly type 2 diabetes is being diagnosed in (overweight) children.

Epidemiology and demographic features

Type 2 diabetes accounts for 85 to 90% of diabetes worldwide. It is very common, affecting at least 3 to 4% of the white populations in most countries, with rates rising to between 8 and 11% in eastern Europe and North America. The prevalence rises with age to well over 10% of those over 70 years. It is substantially more common in certain immigrant populations living in more affluent countries, e.g. 10 to 15% of adults in some Asian or Afro-Caribbean groups in the United Kingdom are affected, compared with a prevalence of 4% in the white population.

Type 2 diabetes is most commonly diagnosed in those over 40 years of age and the incidence rises to a peak at 60 to 65 years. However, much younger people are now presenting with type 2 diabetes, following the rapid rise in childhood obesity. Up to one-third of North Americans diagnosed as diabetic under 20 years of age have type 2 diabetes, with Afro-Caribbean and Hispanic populations being at particular risk. Maturity-onset diabetes of the young (MODY) due to single-gene defects, commonly presents before 25 years of age in more than one generation, and is now classified separately (see below for more details); clinically MODY is becoming increasingly difficult to distinguish from common (polygenic) type 2 diabetes.

The prevalence of type 2 diabetes shows striking geographical variation—entirely different from that of type 1—and ranges from less than 1% in rural China to 50% in the Pima Indians of New Mexico. Prevalence is also rising rapidly, especially in developing countries and, worldwide, will increase by at least 50% within 10 to 15 years. This pandemic can be largely explained by Westernization, and is following in the wake of the obesity that is spreading throughout the world. The Pima Indians illustrate this process especially vividly; most developed and developing countries are now showing the same phenomenon, albeit more slowly. Diabetes was rare while the Pima tribes led a frugal existence in desert conditions and were lean and physically active. Following urban resettlement and exposure to overnutrition and inactivity, there were rapid increases in the prevalence of obesity (currently 80% of adult Pima Indians have a body mass index (BMI) of over $30\,kg/m^2$) and later of type 2 diabetes. The Pima Indians' spectacular susceptibility to obesity and diabetes may be explained by the selection of thrifty genes, i.e. those encouraging the storage of excess energy as fat, which would favour survival in their original harsh environment. In a setting of readily available food, cars, and television, the same thrifty genes would lead to obesity and ultimately diabetes (see below).

There is a 3:2 male preponderance among subjects with type 2 diabetes in Western countries although worldwide there is a 10% excess of females.

Aetiology

Type 2 diabetes is due to the combination of insulin resistance and β-cell failure, the latter preventing sufficient insulin secretion to overcome insulin resistance. These two components vary in importance between different individuals, who may be clinically quite similar, and each has numerous possible causes. Susceptibility is determined by the interactions between genes and environment. The steeply rising prevalence of type 2 diabetes suggests that diabetogenic genes are common and are now enjoying an unparalleled opportunity to express themselves through the global spread of Westernized lifestyle and obesity.

Genetic factors

Overall genetic susceptibility to type 2 diabetes is probably 60 to 90%, rather less than was previously deduced from twin studies. Generally, transmission does not follow simple mendelian rules, and this polygenic pattern reflects the inheritance of a critical mass of minor diabetogenic polymorphisms which interfere with insulin action and/or insulin secretion. Having a first-order relative with the disease increases an individual's chances of developing it fivefold, representing a lifetime risk in white people of about 40%.

Much progress has been made recently in identifying the gene loci predisposing to type 2 diabetes by using genome-wide scanning in large population databases. Importantly, these findings have been verified by repeat analyses in other data sets to exclude spurious statistical findings arising from the very large number of statistical comparisons performed. At least 9 loci have been confirmed, with predicted effects on insulin resistance (*PPARG*) and obesity (*FTO*), but interestingly, a greater number of confirmed loci seem to relate to pancreas development and/or insulin secretion (*TCF7L2*, *KCNJ11*, *HHEX–IDE*, *CDKAL1*, *CDKN2*, *IGF2BP2*, and *SLC30A8*). Although confirmed, the influence of each locus is relatively weak: the strongest association is with *TCF7L2* (odds ratio for diabetes of high risk polymorphism is 1.5) with the remaining loci conferring odds ratios of 1.1 to 1.25. Taken together, the known loci still only explain a small proportion of the inheritance of type 2 diabetes, indicating that there are many more minor loci to be identified. Interestingly, none of the defined loci for common polygenic type 2 diabetes are the same as those identified to cause the much rarer monogenic diabetes syndromes of maturity-onset diabetes of the young (MODY, see below)

Environmental factors

These clearly play a critical part, because obesity and type 2 diabetes are spreading too rapidly to be explicable by changes in the genome; environmental factors are also important in practice because they may be modified to treat and prevent the disease. Known environmental diabetogenic factors mostly induce insulin resistance (e.g. obesity, pregnancy, intercurrent illness, certain drugs). Hyperglycaemia *per se* can both impair insulin sensitivity and inhibit insulin secretion (glucotoxicity).

Specific risk factors for type 2 diabetes

Obesity, itself determined by both genes and environment, is one of the most important risk factors, apparently due to aggravation of insulin resistance (see above). The diabetogenic properties of excess fat depend not only on its bulk but also on its anatomical distribution and the time of life at which it is laid down. The risks of developing type 2 diabetes begin to increase steeply once the BMI exceeds $28 \, \text{kg/m}^2$; some studies estimate the risk at a BMI over $35 \, \text{kg/m}^2$ to be 80-fold higher than for individuals with a BMI of less than $22 \, \text{kg/m}^2$—a lifetime risk of about 50%. Fat in the truncal (central) distribution is more diabetogenic than that deposited around the hips and thighs, and the visceral (intra-abdominal) depot is strongly associated with insulin resistance. Increasing adiposity after the early twenties, especially around the waist, aggravates the risk of a high BMI.

Physical inactivity, especially from the twenties onwards, is an independent predictor of diabetes in middle age, the risk increasing by about threefold for sedentary people as compared with regular athletes. This is due to worsening insulin resistance, which can be improved by physical training and may in part be due to changes in activity of the enzyme AMP kinase in skeletal muscle.

The Barker–Hales hypothesis suggests that poor fetal growth can programme enduring metabolic and vascular abnormalities that are manifested in adult life, especially in people who were underweight at birth but then become obese. These abnormalities include key features of the metabolic syndrome (hyperglycaemia, hypertension, dyslipidaemia), resulting in atheroma formation, myocardial infarction, and stroke (see above). Evidence, mainly from animals, suggests that maternal and therefore fetal malnutrition during a critical early phase of fetal development can reduce β-cell mass and permanently impair insulin secretory reserve; deficiencies of sulphur-containing amino acids may be responsible in experimental animals but the relevance to humans is unknown. Other studies suggest that insulin sensitivity may also be reduced into adult life.

β-Cell failure in type 2 diabetes

β-Cell failure is an obligatory defect in the pathogenesis of type 2 diabetes: near normoglycaemia can be maintained even in severe insulin resistance (e.g. due to mutations in the insulin receptor), as long as the β cell can respond to the challenge and secrete enough insulin to overcome the resistance.

Subtle abnormalities of insulin secretion, including loss of the physiological pulses and of the first-phase response to intravenous glucose injection, are seen in normoglycaemic subjects who later develop the disease. These defects presumably indicate that the β cell is already stressed in trying to produce enough insulin to overcome insulin resistance. Normoglycaemic first-order relatives of type 2 diabetic subjects also show loss of pulsatility of insulin secretion which might indicate an inherited tendency to β-cell failure. The key role of β-cell failure in predisposing to type 2 diabetes has recently been underlined by the finding that most of the confirmed genetic susceptibility loci for type 2 diabetes relate to islet cell function or development rather than insulin resistance (see above).

The mechanism of β-cell failure in human type 2 diabetes is not known. Histologically, the islets in type 2 diabetes show no features of type 1 autoimmune insulitis, and β-cell mass is not so dramatically reduced. Animal models of the disease suggest various causes, including synchronized β-cell apoptosis (possibly mediated by nitric oxide) in the Zucker diabetic fatty rat, and the deposition of amyloid fibrils (see above) in the rhesus monkey. Amyloid deposits are also prominent in the islets of some type 2 diabetic patients but may merely be due to dysfunctional β-cell hypersecretion rather than the cause of β-cell damage. Once hyperglycaemia is established, glucotoxicity *per se* may further worsen both insulin secretion and insulin resistance. Elevated free fatty acid levels resulting from insulin resistance have also been proposed to impair β-cell function—so-called lipotoxicity—but this remains controversial.

In established type 2 diabetes, insulin secretion is unequivocally subnormal and tends to decline progressively with time, as illustrated by the long-term follow-up data from the United Kingdom Prospective Diabetes Study. Initially, plasma insulin levels may be higher than in nondiabetic subjects but are still inappropriately low, as the normal pancreas would produce much higher insulin concentrations in response to diabetic levels of blood glucose. Conventional radioimmunoassays may overestimate insulin levels in type 2 diabetic patients because of cross-reaction with incompletely processed insulin precursors (proinsulin and its split products) released by the constitutive pathway which operates in the malfunctioning β cell (see above). Many type 2 patients ultimately need insulin replacement; this indicates relatively severe insulin deficiency, although still not as profound as in type 1 diabetes. Some type 2 patients who require insulin early have autoimmune markers characteristic of type 1 diabetes, suggesting that they in fact have an indolent variant of type 1 diabetes. Although patients with type 1 diabetes have significantly lower insulin C-peptide levels at diagnosis than in type 2 diabetes, there remains overlap in the ranges (see Fig. 13.11.1.6) such that C-peptide alone only has a sensitivity of 83% in diagnosing type 2 diabetes even in children.

Natural history

Longitudinal and cross-sectional studies indicate that insulin resistance develops first and that compensatory increases in insulin secretion can initially maintain near normoglycaemia. Worsening insulin resistance is thought to drive the β cells towards maximal insulin output, a metastable stage that probably corresponds to impaired glucose tolerance (see above). Rescue is still possible if insulin resistance is decreased, e.g. through weight loss or insulin-sensitizing drugs: about 25% of subjects with impaired glucose tolerance return to normoglycaemia within 5 years. However, if insulin resistance persists or worsens, the β cells fail and insulin production falls. At this point, the brake limiting hyperglycaemia is released and blood glucose rises into the diabetic range. The bell-shaped response of insulin secretion, initially increasing to compensate but ultimately failing, has been termed the 'Starling curve' of the β cells because it recalls the classical plot of cardiac output against preload in heart failure.

In common type 2 diabetes, these events usually take many years, and significant hyperglycaemia may have been present for several years at the time of diagnosis. The whole process can be greatly accelerated by acute increases in insulin resistance as those induced by steroid treatment or pregnancy, to give just two examples.

Metabolic disturbances in type 2 diabetes

Hyperglycaemia is the most obvious abnormality, the extreme case being the hyperosmolar nonketotic state. Lipid metabolism is also disturbed but true ketoacidosis occurs only exceptionally and is usually provoked by intercurrent events such as infections or myocardial infarction.

Blood glucose concentrations are raised both in the basal (fasting) state and after eating. This reflects the impairment of insulin action in both liver and skeletal muscle, where insulin respectively shuts off hepatic glucose production and stimulates glucose uptake after meals. Hepatic glucose output is increased, due mainly to unsuppressed gluconeogenesis, and this is largely responsible for hyperglycaemia overnight and before meals. In muscle, GLUT-4 activity and glycogen synthesis are especially decreased; this reduces insulin-stimulated glucose uptake into muscle after meals, although basal glucose uptake (noninsulin mediated glucose uptake; see above) is higher than in normal subjects because of the mass action effect of hyperglycaemia. The degree of hyperglycaemia varies widely: many patients have fasting plasma glucose levels of 8 to 13 mmol/litre with postprandial peaks of up to 20 mmol/litre, while values exceeding 60 mmol/litre are not uncommon in the hyperosmolar nonketotic state.

Insulin deficiency is less profound than in type 1 diabetes, so mobilization of triglyceride (loss of body fat, ketoacidosis) and catabolism of protein (muscle breakdown) are not usually pronounced. Diabetic ketoacidosis may develop in patients with apparently typical type 2 diabetes who can subsequently be controlled by oral hypoglycaemic agents rather than insulin (see 'Flatbush diabetes' below). Diabetic ketoacidosis is usually precipitated by severe intercurrent illness (e.g. myocardial infarction, stroke, or pneumonia) in which excessive secretion of counter-regulatory stress hormones exacerbates the metabolic disturbance caused by relative insulin deficiency.

Clinical features

Many cases present with classical symptoms of osmotic diuresis, blurred vision due to hyperglycaemia-related refractive changes in the lens, and genital candidiasis (see Table 13.11.1.2).

Weight loss may occur but is generally less dramatic than with newly presenting type 1 diabetes, and may not be obvious because many type 2 patients—over two-thirds in the United Kingdom—are obese. Rapid or severe weight loss in patients who otherwise appear to have type 2 diabetes should be regarded with suspicion as it may point to an early need for insulin replacement (and possibly type 1 diabetes itself) or to coexisting illness: a well-recognized

but unexplained association with recent onset type 2 diabetes is carcinoma of the pancreas.

The hyperosmolar nonketotic state can present with confusion or coma (see below); as mentioned above, diabetic ketoacidosis is rare.

Chronic diabetic complications may be a presenting feature, because hyperglycaemia severe enough to cause tissue damage may already have been present for several years. Extrapolating the numbers of microaneurysms (which only develop at diabetic glucose concentrations) in type 2 patients at various intervals after diagnosis suggests that significant hyperglycaemia is present for an average of 5 to 7 years before diagnosis. Common problems are arterial disease (myocardial infarction, stroke, and peripheral vascular disease), cataracts—which are especially common in the older population—and retinopathy, especially maculopathy, which can damage central vision, and foot ulceration.

Increasing numbers of people with diabetes are detected by screening, either in high-risk groups such as the obese and those with cardiovascular disease, or at routine health checks. Many of these are nominally asymptomatic but will admit to symptoms such as nocturia or perineal irritation if asked directly.

Prognosis of type 2 diabetes

A long-held and prevalent misconception is that type 2 diabetes is mild. Some patients do have relatively unexciting or asymptomatic hyperglycaemia but this can still be enough to cause complications which wreck the patient's life just as much as in type 1 diabetes. Moreover, hyperglycaemia can be as hard to control (even with insulin) as in type 1 patients.

Overall, life expectancy is shortened by up to a quarter in patients with type 2 diabetes presenting in their forties, with vascular disease (myocardial infarction and stroke) being the main cause of premature death. Renal failure from diabetic nephropathy is becoming more common in type 2 patients as their survival from vascular complications improves, and the disease is now the most frequent pathology among people waiting for renal replacement therapy in the United States of America and some European countries.

Type 2 diabetes is therefore an important threat to the patient's health and survival, and must be taken seriously by patients and their medical attendants, even if the blood glucose concentrations are not dramatically raised. Accordingly, treatment guidelines for the disease are rigorous (see Table 13.11.1.3).

Monogenic diabetes: maturity-onset diabetes of the young (MODY) and neonatal diabetes

Maturity-onset diabetes of the young (MODY)

While the vast majority of diabetes is polygenic in origin, there is now an expanding list of single-gene loci that are associated with diabetes either in the neonatal period, in childhood, or in early adulthood. In 1974, Tattersall described a rare familial form of non-insulin-dependent diabetes that he distinguished from the generality of cases by its early age of onset, autosomal dominant inheritance, and an apparently low risk of microvascular complications. The term 'maturity-onset diabetes of the young' (MODY) came to be applied to individuals in which (1) a diagnosis of type 2 diabetes had been made under the age of 25; (2) there is evidence of autosomal dominant inheritance (diagnosis under the age of 25 in more than one generation); and (3) subjects can be managed without insulin.

In 1992, the first conclusive evidence for the existence of monogenic diabetes was provided when a subset of MODY (now known as MODY 2) was linked to the glucokinase gene locus. There are now seven forms of MODY, accounting for around 1% of all cases of diabetes, in which the gene has been identified (see Table 13.11.1.4). Two forms predominate and have a distinctive clinical picture. MODY 2 (glucokinase mutations) is similar to the initial cases described by Tattersall with mild, nonprogressive fasting hyperglycaemia and a very low risk of long-term complications even without treatment. By contrast, MODY 3 (*HNF1A* mutations) is associated with progressive decline in glycaemic control. In addition, the renal threshold for glucose is low and there is a high risk of long-term complications. Of particular importance, MODY 3 is exquisitely sensitive to sulphonylureas and most patients wrongly diagnosed as having type 1 diabetes have been successfully transferred from insulin to sulphonylureas with improvement in glycaemic control. Doses required may be as low as one-quarter of the normal adult starting dose.

A diagnosis of MODY should be considered if:

◆ There is a family history of young-onset diabetes in more than one generation with at least one family member diagnosed under the age of 25.

◆ Affected members are not markedly obese or of normal weight.

◆ There is no evidence of insulin resistance—no acanthosis nigricans, low insulin doses if insulin treated, high-density lipoprotein greater than 1.2 mol/litre.

◆ Fasting C-peptide is detectable and within the normal range (not elevated).

◆ Islet cell or anti-GAD autoantibodies are absent.

◆ Other associated features are present (see Table 13.11.1.4).

None of these criteria are absolute and where doubt exists, advice from an expert centre should be sought before requesting genetic screening. Detection of MODY 3 is of particular importance because of the excellent response to treatment with sulphonylureas.

Neonatal diabetes

Diabetes diagnosed under the age of 6 months is very unlikely to be type 1 (autoimmune) diabetes and alternative causes should be sought. Neonatal diabetes is insulin-requiring diabetes, usually diagnosed with the first 3 months of life, and two subgroups have now been identified. Transient neonatal diabetes mellitus (TNDM) resolves around 3 months after birth although it can return in later life in up to 50% of cases. The most common cause is an imprinting abnormality in the *ZACN* (*ZAC*) and *HYMAI* genes on chromosome 6 at the 6q24 locus. Macroglossia occurs in 23% of cases and is the only nonpancreatic feature. Presenting blood glucose levels are high (from 12 to >50 mmol/litre) and insulin is required:

Table 13.11.1.3 Treatment targets for patients with diabetes

	Glycaemic control		
	Low risk	*Arterial risk*	*Microvascular risk*
Fasting blood glucose (mmol/litre)	< 5.5	> 6.5	> 6.0
Postprandial peak glucose (mmol/litre)	< 7.5	≥ 7.5	> 9.0
HbA$_{1c}$ (DCCT aligned)	≤ 6.5	> 6.5	> 7.5
	Serum lipids (mmol/litre)		
	Low risk	*Arterial risk*	*High arterial risk*
Total cholesterol	< 4.8	4.8–6.0	> 6.0
HDL cholesterol	> 1.2	1.0–1.2	< 1.0
LDL cholesterol	< 2.0	2.0–3.0	> 3.0
Fasting triglycerides	< 1.7	1.7–2.2	> 2.2
	Blood pressure (mmHg)		
	Low risk	*Unacceptable*	
General	< 130/80	> 140/90	
Patients with microalbuminuria	< 125/75		
	Body-mass index (kg/m^2)		
	Low risk	*Acceptable*	*Increased risk*
Men	< 25	25–27	> 27
Women	< 24	24–26	> 26

DCCT, Diabetes Control and Complications Trial; HDL, high-density lipoprotein; LDL, low-density lipoprotein.

'Ideal' treatment targets ('low-risk' values) may not be appropriate for some patients. Risks are stratified for arterial disease and/or microvascular complications.

Collated from various sources including: European Diabetes Policy Group (1999). A desktop guide to Type 2 diabetes mellitus. *Diabet Med*, **16**, 716–30; American Diabetes Association (2007). Standards of medical care in diabetes—2007. *Diabetes Care*, **30**, Suppl 1 S4–S41; Ramsay LE, *et al.* (1999). British Hypertension Society guidelines for hypertension management 1999: summary. *BMJ*, **319**, 630–5.

Table 13.11.1.4 Maturity-onset diabetes of the young (MODY)

Type	Genetic defect	OMIM	Frequency (% of MODY)	Clinical features	Sensitive to sulphonylureas
MODY 1	HNF-4α	125850	1%	Rare. Similar to MODY 3 but renal threshold normal. Consider if MODY 3 screen negative	May be sensitive
MODY 2	Glucokinase	125851	20%	Mild, nonprogressive fasting hyperglycaemia (5.5–8.5 mmol/litre, HbA_{1c} < 6%). Glucose increment < 3.5 mmol/litre on OGTT. Complications rarely develop. Frequently do not response well to drug treatment and do not require it	No
MODY 3	HNF-1α	600496	60%	Young-onset diabetes. Not particularly overweight and not insulin requiring (no ketosis) or surprisingly good control for several years on little insulin. Detectable C-peptide beyond 3 years post-diagnosis. Low renal threshold. Large glucose increment (> 5 mol/litre) on OGTT. Progressive deterioration in glycaemic control and high risk of complications	Extremely sensitive
MODY 4	IPF-1	606392	1%	Rare. Possibly later-onset disease. Some affected family members may not be diabetic	Not determined
MODY 5	HNF-1β(TCF2)	137920	1%	Renal cysts and diabetes. Renal, uterine and/or genital developmental abnormalities are typical initial presentation especially renal cysts. Gout, abnormal LFTs. Subclinical pancreatic exocrine insufficiency	No
MODY 6	NEUROD1	606394	<1%	Rare	Not determined
MODY 7	KLF11	610508	<1%	Rare	Not determined
MODY 8	CEL	609812	< 1	Associated pancreatic exocrine deficiency	Not determined
MODY 9	PAXA4	612225	< 1	Rare	Not determined
MODY X	Unknown		15%	Not defined	Not determined

HNF, hepatocyte nuclear factor; IPF-1, insulin promoter factor 1; LFT, liver function test; NEUROD1, neurogenic differentiation 1 transcription factor; OGTT, oral glucose tolerance test.

if relapse occurs, this is normally not insulin requiring, at least in the initial stages. MODY 5 and *KCNJ11* (*Kir6.2*) mutations (see below) occasionally also present as TNDM.

Permanent neonatal diabetes mellitus (PNDM) requires continual insulin treatment from diagnosis. The most common cause is a mutation in the *KCNJ11* gene, encoding the Kir6.2 subunit of the β-cell KATP channel. Ninety per cent of cases are due to spontaneous (new) mutations so there is no family history. Affected individuals may have a range of neurological abnormalities that in the most severe form are referred to as DEND syndrome (developmental delay, epilepsy, and neonatal diabetes). Patients with Kir6.2 mutations behave as insulin-deficient, with a 30% risk of ketoacidosis and low or undetectable C-peptide levels. However, the majority of patients respond well to high doses of sulphonylureas, given at up to 4 times the normal adult therapeutic dosage (e.g. glibenclamide 0.5–1 mg/kg per day), with the restoration of insulin secretion. Occasionally, MODY 2 and 4 may also present as PNDM as can other rare genetic syndromes (see below).

Other types of diabetes (see Table 13.11.1.1)

Diabetes in pancreatic disease

Chronic pancreatitis, most commonly due to alcohol abuse, causes diabetes that needs insulin in about one-third of cases. Widespread flecks of fine to medium calcification are often scattered through the pancreas, outlining it on a plain abdominal radiograph. Concomitant destruction of the islet α cells means that glucagon secretion is lost as well as insulin; diabetic ketoacidosis is therefore rare, while hypoglycaemia can be profound and prolonged—a particular hazard in those who continue to drink alcohol. Acute pancreatitis causes acute hyperglycaemia in 50% of cases but few develop permanent diabetes.

Carcinoma of the pancreas is associated with newly presenting type 2 diabetes, and should be suspected in older patients with weight loss (especially when accompanied by abdominal or back pain and jaundice). The mechanism is unknown but appears to be due to tumour products that cause insulin resistance rather than to β-cell loss.

Genetic diseases that cause diabetes through pancreatic damage include haemochromatosis and cystic fibrosis. In one-half of cases of haemochromatosis, heavy deposition of haemosiderin in the islets causes diabetes, usually requiring insulin; associated features are slate-grey skin pigmentation due to deposition of iron in the dermis ('bronze diabetes'), cirrhosis, secondary gonadal failure, and pyrophosphate arthropathy. MRI shows abnormal signals in the liver and pancreas, while serum ferritin concentrations are greatly elevated; diagnosis is usually possible by means of molecular analysis of the *HFE* gene but Perls' stain for iron deposition in a liver biopsy may be necessary (see Chapter 12.7.1). Diabetes due to excessive iron deposition in the pancreas is also seen in children surviving thalassaemia major. Cystic fibrosis causes pancreatic exocrine failure, with an increasing risk of diabetes (often requiring insulin) that approaches 25% in subjects who survive beyond 20 years of age.

Gestational diabetes

This includes all degrees of hyperglycaemia (impaired glucose tolerance as well as overt diabetes) diagnosed during pregnancy in previously normoglycaemic women. It is covered in Chapter 14.10.

Malnutrition-related diabetes

This controversial diagnostic category was omitted from the most recent WHO classification. It included 'fibrocalculous pancreatic diabetes' and 'protein-deficient diabetes mellitus'. Fibrocalculous pancreatic diabetes was identified by dense pancreatic fibrosis, the formation of discrete and often spectacularly large stones in the dilated pancreatic ducts, and recurrent abdominal pain; protein-deficient diabetes mellitus was a vaguer entity that lacked the pancreatic stones. Patients conforming to these 'syndromes' were rare even in the tropical zones where they were described (<5% of all diabetes), and the current consensus is that they represent type 2 diabetes or chronic pancreatitis superimposed on malnutrition.

Flatbush diabetes

This term has been used to refer to diabetes in young Afro-Caribbeans who present with profound diabetic ketoacidosis but later prove to be non-insulin-dependent. It appears that at diagnosis they have both marked insulin resistance and impaired insulin secretion but the latter later recovers, sometimes sufficiently for them to go into prolonged remission. In at least one report there was an excess of *HLA DR3* and *DR4* alleles, but anti-GAD autoantibodies are negative.

Fulminant type 1 diabetes

This form of diabetes was first described in 2000 in Japan and refers to presentation with severe diabetic ketoacidosis but low HbA_{1c} (<8.5%) relative to their initial marked hyperglycaemia, thus indicating an abrupt onset. Additional typical features include a short history of symptoms (2–10 days), raised pancreatic enzyme levels, and negative anti-GAD (and other) autoantibodies. Prevalence in Japanese and Korean populations may approach 20–30% of cases of rapid onset diabetes with ketosis, especially where the presentation is in adulthood and/or in pregnancy. It is rare in other races including white populations. Pancreatic biopsy reveals T-cell infiltrates in the exocrine pancreas, but without insulitis or features of acute pancreatitis.

Mitochondrial diabetes

Maternal transmission of mutations in mitochondrial DNA (mtDNA), especially the A3243G substitution in the leucine tRNA gene, can result in maternal inheritance of diabetes. Typical clinical presentation includes a presentation age of 20 to 50 with associated sensorineural deafness and short stature as in MIDD syndrome (maternally inherited diabetes and deafness). There is progressive nonautoimmune β-cell failure which may progress rapidly to insulin dependence (40% are insulin-dependent within 4 years) The same mutation occurs in MELAS syndrome (mitochondrial myopathy, encephalopathy, lactic acidosis, and stroke-like episodes) and both MIDD and MELAS can occur in the same family. The ratio of mutant to wild-type mtDNA in the blood (i.e. the degree of heteroplasmy) at diagnosis does not correlate with disease phenotype or severity, presumably because it does not reflect the degree of heteroplasmy in other tissues such as the pancreas.

Management of diabetes

The treatment of diabetes has traditionally concentrated on correcting hyperglycaemia, the most obvious and easily monitored biochemical abnormality and the cause of troublesome symptoms, as well as specific chronic diabetic complications. This approach has not been entirely successful, partly because it is difficult to normalize blood glucose but also because macrovascular disease—the principal cause of morbidity and premature death—is heavily dependent on other factors, notably hypertension and

dyslipidaemia. The current treatment targets for both type 1 and type 2 diabetes (see Table 13.11.1.3) are therefore more holistic, tackling cardiovascular risk factors and obesity in addition to hyperglycaemia.

This section describes the roles of lifestyle modification and antidiabetic drugs, followed by specific treatment strategies for type 1 and type 2 diabetes.

Diet and lifestyle modification and management of obesity

About 80% of patients with type 2 diabetes are obese, as are at least 30% of those with type 1 disease. Obesity is arguably one of the greatest obstacles to successful management of diabetes: it worsens insulin resistance, dyslipidaemia, and hypertension and is now recognized in its own right as a risk factor for coronary heart disease. Proven benefits of 10% weight loss in type 2 patients with a BMI of 30 to $40 kg/m^2$ include falls in fasting glucose of 2 to 4 mmol/litre and a 1% decrease in HbA_{1c}—comparable with sulphonylureas or metformin—and reduced dosages of antidiabetic drugs, including insulin. There may also be variable improvements in blood pressure and dyslipidaemia (decreased triglycerides and low-density lipoprotein cholesterol, increased high-density lipoprotein). The traditional focus on obesity has been on type 2 diabetes, but there is no reason to assume that the cardiovascular hazards of obesity do not also apply to type 1 diabetes.

Weight reduction is regarded as the cornerstone for treating obese type 2 diabetics but is often undermined by a lack of determination. Accordingly, doctors have little confidence in its efficacy and tend to assume that most obese patients will be 'dietary failures'. However, with clear advice, better understanding of the causes of obesity, and the use of realistic targets, the currently poor track record of diet and lifestyle therapy can be greatly improved. All members of the diabetes team must understand the principles (but not necessarily the detail) of lifestyle management so that a strong and unified message can be given to the patient.

The notion of the 'diabetic diet' must now finally be laid to rest. Traditionally, carbohydrate intake was restricted because of the simplistic assumptions that sugar alone raised blood glucose and might even be diabetogenic; this strategy favoured a high fat intake that undoubtedly helped to sustain obesity and probably predisposed to atheroma. Current advice is close to the healthy eating recommendations for the whole population and can therefore be suggested for the patient's entire family, which will greatly increase the chances of compliance.

The following diet and activity recommendations apply to both type 1 and type 2 diabetes. The aims are to:

- correct obesity, which worsens insulin resistance, reduces the efficacy of glucose-lowering, antihypertensive, and lipid-modifying drugs, and is an independent risk factor for macrovascular disease. (Management of obesity is discussed in detail in Chapter 11.5.)

- reduce cardiovascular risk, by limiting fat, cholesterol, sodium, and alcohol intakes

- avoid hypoglycaemia in patients receiving insulin or sulphonylureas by optimizing the timing and content of meals

The steps in designing dietary advice for the individual patient are shown in Fig. 13.11.1.7.

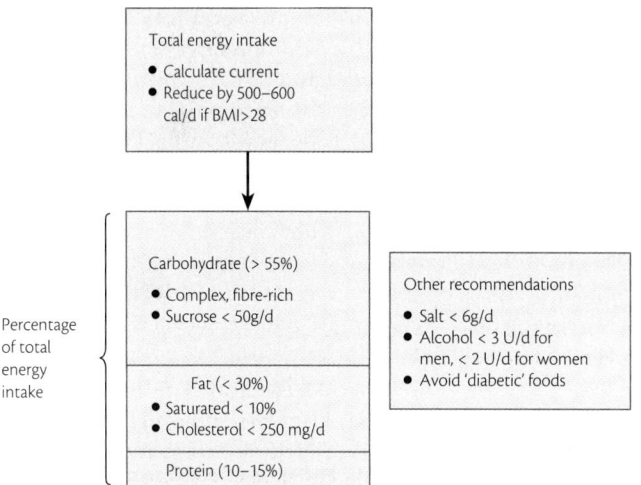

Fig. 13.11.1.7 Dietary recommendations for people with diabetes. These guidelines now reflect healthy eating for the general population, rather than a diabetic diet.

Reducing total energy intake

This should be reduced by 500 to 600 kcal/day (2100–2520 kJ/day) in patients who are overweight (BMI >28 kg/m²). This energy deficit mobilizes fat preferentially, whereas protein, glycogen, and water are also lost with more aggressive energy restriction; initially, the rate of weight loss will be 0.5 to 1.0 kg/week (adipose tissue contains *c*.7000 cal/kg or 29 400 J/kg).

The desired energy intake should be calculated from standard formulae that employ the subject's age, sex, weight, and level of physical activity to estimate energy expenditure, which must equal energy intake under steady state conditions. The standard dietary history is not useful for trying to assess energy intake, because overweight subjects consistently under-report how much they eat. Specific advice about how to cut energy intake is best left to the dietitian, but hinges on reducing fat intake—a simple message that can be reinforced by the entire diabetes care team. Fat-rich foods not only have the highest energy density (9 cal/g or 38 J/g, compared with 4 cal/g (17 J/g) for carbohydrate and protein), but also have poor satiating effects and so tend to encourage overeating.

The initial target should be a 10% loss of starting weight, not the 'ideal' body weight or BMI, which is only rarely attained by obese diabetic patients. When energy intake is cut acutely, type 2 patients often show an immediate fall in blood glucose, due to a drop in hepatic glucose output, even before weight loss begins.

Weight loss during an energy deficit of 500 to 600 cal/day (2100–2520 J/day) is a slow process: for a 100 kg patient, a 10% weight loss may take several months. Frequent contact and encouragement are the best predictors of success, and the patient should be reassured that weight loss by a small but tolerable change in lifestyle is much more likely to be maintained than weight lost by a crash diet. As weight falls, resting energy expenditure also declines: it is proportional to lean body mass, which also decreases, although at a slower rate than fat. This means that greater reductions in energy intake (>600 cal/day or 2520 J/day) will be needed to maintain the same rate of weight loss. If the 10% target is met, further loss towards an 'ideal' BMI of around 23 kg/m² may be feasible.

Weight loss is harder to achieve in diabetic patients than in their nondiabetic counterparts; possible reasons include fears about sugar rather than fat, and the adipogenic effects of insulin, sulphonylureas,

and thiazolidinediones. In practice, weight loss of even 10% is not commonly achieved by diet and lifestyle modification alone; only 15 to 30% of newly diagnosed type 2 diabetic patients can normalize glycaemia initially by this means, and fewer than 10% can sustain this for 5 years or more. The progressive β-cell dysfunction in type 2 diabetes (see above) makes it inevitable that the proportion of 'dietary failures' will increase steadily.

Improving dietary composition

Intakes of fat, salt, and refined sugar are generally too high in westernized populations. Current recommendations for healthy eating are based on evidence of beneficial effects on body weight, glycaemic control, lipids, and blood pressure (see Fig. 13.11.1.7). Fat should provide less than 30% of total energy intake (in most industrialized countries, it accounts for 40%). Polyunsaturated or monounsaturated fats (e.g. sunflower or olive oils respectively) are preferred to saturated animal fats, which should comprise less than 10% of total energy intake. Patients may need to be reminded that 'good' unsaturated fats still contain 9 cal/g (38 J/g) and therefore sustain obesity just as effectively as the others. Cholesterol should be limited to less than 250 mg/day (less if dyslipidaemia is present).

Carbohydrates should account for more than 55% of total energy intake, preferably in the form of foods rich in soluble fibre (e.g. pulses, root and leaf vegetables, and fruit); the current WHO recommendation for the general population is for the consumption of at least five portions of fruit or vegetables per day. Sugary drinks (especially fizzy glucose solutions that are supposed to give energy) should be avoided, except to treat hypoglycaemia. The present recommendation, which seems reasonable but is not based on evidence, is to limit added sucrose to less than 25 g/day and total sucrose intake to less than 50 g/day.

Protein should contribute 10 to 15% of total energy—close to current levels in the general population. (For patients with renal impairment, see Chapter 21.10.1) Sodium intake should be less than 6 g/day, and less in patients with hypertension.

Alcohol contains 7 cal/g (29 J/g), and beers and wines in particular can be fattening. Intake should not exceed three units (30 g) per day in men and two units (20 g) per day in women, and should be further limited or avoided in those with hypertension or obesity. Alcohol can delay recovery from hypoglycaemia (see below); 'diabetic' beers (low in sugar, but strong in alcohol) and spirits with sugar-free mixers are especially likely to provoke hypoglycaemia.

Moderate amounts of sucrose are acceptable (see above), and noncaloric sweeteners (such as aspartame) have no adverse metabolic effects. Diabetic sweets and foods contain sorbitol or fructose instead of glucose, and are an expensive way to get diarrhoea; they should be avoided by patients, and withdrawn by the manufacturers.

Optimizing meal patterns

Judging the size and content of meals so as to limit glycaemic excursions remains an art rather than a science, and a skill which some patients develop with experience. Dosages of glucose-lowering drugs that act acutely to cover meals (short-acting insulin and sulphonylureas) can be tailored reasonably accurately to meals of similar composition but may not be matched to other meals, even when the total weights of carbohydrate, fat, and protein are similar.

There has been much interest in the ability of various foods to raise blood glucose, usually measured as the 'glycaemic index', i.e. the area under the curve of the rise in plasma glucose after eating a standardized load (50 g) of the food, expressed as a percentage of the area under the glucose curve after ingesting 50 g of glucose. Foods with a low glycaemic index include pulses and cereals, probably because of their high fibre and complex carbohydrate contents, while bread has a surprisingly high index. The glycaemic index of many foods such as potatoes and pasta varies widely according to the method of cooking (and even the shape of the pasta), and mixing different foods in a real-life meal has unpredictable effects on the overall postprandial glucose rise. It may be sensible to base meals around components with a low glycaemic index but it is clearly not feasible to use the index to adjust dosages of antidiabetic medication.

Appropriate portion size in meals is also important in limiting overall calorie intake. Portion size has crept up inexorably in restaurants in many countries and probably contributes to the observed association between excessive weight gain and eating outside the family home.

Increasing physical activity

Short-term exercise and improved physical fitness both increase insulin sensitivity, partly through increased translocation of GLUT-4 units to the surface of skeletal muscle cells resulting in increased glucose uptake; this effect is independent of insulin, and can enhance glucose uptake (under clamp conditions) better than metformin or the thiazolidinediones. Physical training also improves muscle blood flow. Several studies, notably the Finnish and American Diabetes prevention trials, have demonstrated that regular physical exercise reduces by over 50% the risk of impaired glucose tolerance progressing to type 2 diabetes. There is also evidence that it significantly decreases cardiovascular events. Exercise must therefore be encouraged in all diabetic patients, but the advice must be realistic, achievable, and safe. Brisk walking for 30 to 40 min every day is better physiologically than a hectic workout in the gym once or twice a week, and is within almost everyone's reach.

Potential hazards of exercise include hypoglycaemia in patients on sulphonylureas or insulin, which may be delayed by several hours (see below), and cardiac disease. Patients at risk should have an ECG, with consideration for an exercise tolerance test and echocardiography, and appropriate treatment for ischaemic heart disease or heart failure. Exercise remains beneficial and important in these cases but should be built up gradually.

Antiobesity drugs and bariatric surgery in diabetes

Antiobesity drugs may be indicated in selected obese diabetic patients with a BMI over 28 kg/m² and who have demonstrated, by losing weight beforehand through diet and exercise alone, that they are prepared to make long-term changes in their lifestyle. Without this commitment, clinically useful weight loss is unlikely to be achieved or maintained beyond the period of drug prescription; the medical and pharmacoeconomic benefits of modest weight loss for a couple of years in the obese patient's middle age are not known but are probably not dramatic.

Drugs currently available in many countries are orlistat, a gastrointestinal lipase inhibitor, and sibutramine, a combined serotonin/noradrenaline reuptake inhibitor. With each of these, up to 30% of obese type 2 patients lose 10% or more of body weight within 6 to 12 months, HbA$_{1c}$ can fall by 1% or more, and dosages of glucose-lowering drugs, including insulin, may be decreased. More recently, the selective type 1 cannabinoid (CB1) receptor antagonist rimonabant was introduced; this reduces insulin resistance and

may have the additional benefit of promoting smoking cessation. However, the exacerbation of pre-existing depression or anxiety has resulted in the drug being withdrawn by the manufacturer.

Surgical treatment with gastric banding or gastric bypass operations is indicated in selected patients with a BMI over 40 kg/m² (Chapter 11.5). These operations are generally safe when performed by an experienced team and can achieve dramatic weight loss (up to 70% of excess fat, maintained for several years), often with an impressive reversal of glucose intolerance. Although randomized prospective studies have not been performed, reduction in medication and reversal of the diabetes state has been reported in 50 to 85% of subjects with type 2 diabetes undergoing bariatric surgery. Particularly dramatic results are seen with modern non-malabsorptive gastric by-pass procedures, perhaps because they increase GLP-1 secretion and reduced glucagon levels in addition to causing weight reduction. The cost-effectiveness and optimal indications for the use of weight-loss drugs or surgery in managing type 2 diabetes remain to be established.

Smoking

Smoking is at least as common among diabetic patients as in the general population. Smoking greatly amplifies macrovascular risk in diabetic subjects: 10-year mortality (mainly from myocardial infarction) is about 50% higher than in diabetic nonsmokers and twice as high as in nondiabetic nonsmokers. Smoking may also accelerate the progression of nephropathy and possibly retinopathy.

Many diabetic people, especially young women, continue to smoke as a means of keeping thin, and because they fear gaining weight if they stop. Nicotine reduces fondness for sweet, energy-dense, foods and may also be mildly thermogenic. Weight gain after stopping smoking averages 3 kg but about 20% of cases gain more than 6 kg; much of this weight is often lost within the following 1 to 2 years, and it can be limited or prevented by careful dietetic support beforehand and in the months after cessation. Moreover, the risks of continuing to smoke are much greater than this degree of weight gain, especially in diabetic people. Pharmacological support to overcome nicotine dependence including the use of nicotine replacement, antidepressants (e.g. bupropion, nortriptyline) and the nicotine receptor partial agonist varenicline each increases the chance of quitting by around two- to threefold.

Glucose-lowering drugs

Insulin

Insulin is the rational treatment for type 1 diabetes and the only drug that can normalize blood glucose in many type 2 diabetic patients. Unfortunately, subcutaneously injected insulin cannot match the physiological profile of normal insulin secretion (see Fig. 13.11.8) and is a poor substitute for the finely tuned β cell with its nearly instantaneous capacity for 'in-flight' adjustment. Moreover, insulin given subcutaneously is absorbed into the systemic circulation rather than secreted into the portal system where an immediate effect on the liver, and first pass clearance by that organ, are important in regulating the metabolic actions of insulin.

Insulin manufacture

Insulin was traditionally extracted from pork and beef pancreases in acid ethanol and purified by precipitation and recrystallization. Soluble (or 'crystalline') insulin prepared in this way was contaminated with other islet proteins, including glucagon and pancreatic polypeptide, which had an adjuvant-like effect and enhanced the

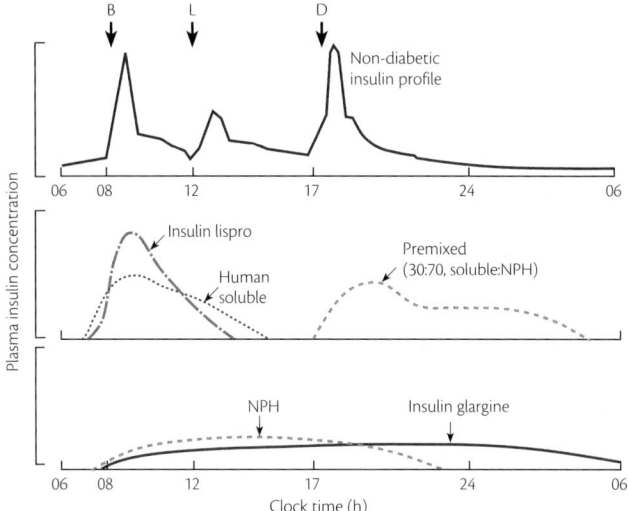

Fig. 13.11.1.8 Time course of insulin preparations, compared with the normal diurnal profile of plasma insulin concentrations in nondiabetic subjects (top). Breakfast (B), lunch (L), and dinner (D) were given as shown. Fast-acting analogues (such as lispro) act more rapidly than conventional soluble ones but are still sluggish compared with normal prandial insulin release. Premixed insulins injected in the early evening cover the evening meal adequately, but the long-acting component can cause hyperinsulinaemia and troublesome hypoglycaemia in the small hours. None of the conventional long-acting insulins reliably lasts 24 h; new long-acting analogues such as insulin glargine or insulin detemir may provide adequate background insulin levels with once-daily injections.

immunogenicity of the injected insulin; immune reactions were relatively common with the 'dirty' animal insulins in use until the 1970s (see below). More sophisticated purification techniques including gel filtration yield 'highly purified' or 'monocomponent' insulins which only rarely provoke immune reactions.

Biosynthetic human-sequence insulin, produced by recombinant DNA technology, entered clinical practice in the early 1980s and was the first genetically engineered protein to be used therapeutically. The current approach is to introduce a synthetic gene for recombinant proinsulin or a novel insulin precursor into yeast; the secreted product is then cleaved enzymatically to yield insulin and C-peptide.

There are some clinically relevant differences between the three species used therapeutically, although the shortcomings of insulin therapy relate mainly to the general pharmacokinetic misbehaviour of injected insulin. Human insulin is more lipophilic than porcine and bovine insulins and is slightly more rapidly absorbed: human soluble insulin especially may lower glucose faster and patients being transferred from other species should be warned of this and prandial doses reduced initially by one-third. Human ultralente has a shorter and steeper action profile than its animal counterparts, particularly the bovine preparation; in real life, human ultralente behaves similarly to lente or isophane insulins and does not provide adequate basal levels for a full 24 h. Human insulin has been suggested to interfere with awareness of hypoglycaemia but the balance of evidence does not support this view (see below). Early beef insulins were especially prone to cause immune reactions (see below), although highly purified preparations do not appear to be particularly immunogenic.

Most insulin manufacturers are now turning to biosynthetic production of human-sequence insulin. Some patients prefer to continue using animal insulins—for reasons that may or may not appear scientifically sound—and these wishes should be respected by both clinicians and the pharmaceutical industry.

Insulin absorption

Absorption of insulin injected subcutaneously is slow and unpredictable. Individual day-to-day variability in the amount absorbed within a few hours can exceed 50%. This means that small changes (<10%) in insulin dosage are unlikely to influence glycaemic control, and that insulin treatment should generally not be adjusted on a daily basis.

Insulin absorption is influenced by the physical state of the insulin (soluble or delayed action), its speed of dissociation into monomers, the lipophilicity of the insulin species, and by blood flow and other characteristics of the injection site. Absorption is accelerated, and may lead to noticeably faster falls in blood glucose, by stimulating general or local blood flow through exercise, hot climate, saunas, and/or massaging the injection site. Conversely, absorption is slowed when subcutaneous blood flow is reduced, e.g. in cold conditions or hypovolaemic states. Lipohypertrophy, which may develop at frequently used injection sites, can significantly delay absorption—another reason for avoiding such areas.

The anatomical site of injection also influences the rate of subcutaneous absorption. It is fastest in the abdomen (also a good site to limit any effects of exercise) and arm, and slower in the leg. These differences are often eclipsed by the overall variability in absorption. Absorption from muscle is faster, presumably because of its higher blood flow, and this route is preferred for the emergency treatment of hyperglycaemia or ketoacidos if the best option, controlled intravenous infusion, is not practicable.

Insulin preparations

Soluble (regular or short-acting) insulin injected subcutaneously begins to lower glucose within 30 min, has a peak effect between 1 and 2 h and lasts 3 to 5 h (see Fig. 13.11.1.7). This action profile is suitable for covering meals or hyperglycaemic emergencies and for use in insulin pumps or infusions. However, it would have to be injected several times per day to control hyperglycaemia around the clock, at the cost of frequent hypoglycaemia. Long-acting preparations are therefore used to cover basal insulin requirements.

Various approaches have been used to slow and prolong insulin absorption, especially the chemical combination of insulin into complexes that release it slowly. More recently, synthetic analogues have been designed whose structure promotes precipitation when injected subcutaneously (see Fig. 13.11.1.7).

Isophane insulins are also known as NPH (neutral protamine Hagedorn, from the director of the Danish laboratory where they were developed). They consist of a microcrystalline complex of insulin and the highly basic protein protamine (intriguingly isolated from fish sperm), together with trace amounts of Zn^{2+}. Isophanes were derived from protamine–zinc insulin which has a longer but highly unpredictable action profile. Isophanes produce peak plasma insulin levels at variable intervals between 4 and 8 h after injection, and their glucose-lowering action wears off rapidly after 10 to 12 h.

Insulin–zinc suspensions (lente insulins) employ higher Zn^{2+} concentrations which encourage insulin to form crystalline lattices. Varying the reaction pH can produce either larger crystals which are particularly slow to dissolve (ultralente) or the amorphous semilente which releases insulin faster; the familiar lente is a 70:30

mixture of ultralente and semilente. Ultralente made with bovine insulin has a long, relatively flat action profile that can last 24h or more, while human ultralente and the lente insulins of all three species have glucose-lowering profiles similar to that of isophane. These long-acting insulins have a cloudy appearance and need to be shaken before use to bring the insulin into suspension; visibly large particles or discoloration indicates that the insulin has become denatured and will have lost activity. Both lente and isophane insulins can be injected alone or mixed with soluble insulin.

Premixed insulins contain a short-acting soluble component together with a longer-acting lente or isophane. The aim is to provide prandial cover and then basal levels for several hours thereafter. Many preparations are available, with the proportion of short-acting insulin varying from 10 to 50%. Mixtures with a 30:70 ratio are popular.

All these insulin types have been produced with porcine-, bovine- and human-sequence insulins, and are available in catridges for pen injection devices.

Insulin analogues

The pharmacokinetic properties of native insulins of any species are poorly suited to subcutaneous injection: soluble insulins (despite their high-speed trade names) are too slow and prolonged in duration, while long-acting insulins do not provide reliable enough 24-h basal levels to be given once daily. Various synthetic insulin analogues, designed by molecular modelling, have improved physicochemical characteristics.

Fast-acting analogues are modified at the C-terminal end of the B chain, an area crucial in the self-association of insulin molecules, so as to resist dimerization and hexamerization. Insulin hexamers formed in the subcutaneous injection site, dissociate slowly into absorbable monomers, and this is a rate-limiting step in insulin absorption. Faster-acting analogues include insulin lispro (interchanging the B28 lysine and B29 proline residues of the normal human sequence) and insulin aspart, which carries aspartic acid at position B28 instead of the usual proline. They have an appreciably faster and shorter action profile (see Fig. 13.11.1.7), and day-to-day variability in absorption and glycaemic responses may also be decreased. They can therefore reduce both prandial hyperglycaemia and the risk of postprandial hypoglycaemia. Despite these theoretical advantages, meta-analyses show only very modest reductions in HbA_{1c} ($c.$ 0.1%) and reductions in hypoglycaemic episodes when a fast-acting analogue is substituted for soluble insulin, but there are significant improvements in quality of life generally attributable to the convenience of injecting immediately before or after meals rather than 30 min beforehand.

Long-acting insulin analogues have also been developed. These are designed to give a smoother 24-h profile than isophane ('peakless' insulin). At present two forms are available. Insulin glargine (A21 glycine, with two extra arginine residues extending the C-terminal of the B chain) has an altered isoelectric point such that it is soluble in the vial or cartridge at pH 4 but precipitates under the skin at pH 7. Insulin detemir has a delayed action due to the addition of a fatty acyl chain that binds to plasma proteins such as albumin. It has a slightly shorter half-life than glargine and can be given once or twice daily. Both analogues are clear in the vial or cartridge—potentially a source of confusion with rapidly acting insulin. Claims have been made for improved HbA_{1c} levels and less daytime hypoglycemia, as well as weight loss or neutrality for detemir in type 2 diabetes, but the most robust finding appears to be a reduction in nocturnal hypoglycaemia.

Side effects of insulin

Hypoglycaemia is the most common complication of insulin treatment and can be unpleasant, debilitating, and occasionally life-threatening.

Mild hypoglycaemia is common—many insulin-treated patients have at least one episode most weeks—but serious attacks causing unconsciousness or requiring the assistance of others are rare, about once every 3 patient years. Predictably, the frequency of both mild and severe attacks rises progressively when mean blood glucose levels are lowered by intensive insulin therapy; hypoglycaemia was three times more frequent in the tightly controlled group of the Diabetes Control and Complications Trial than in conventionally treated patients (see below).

The manifestations and treatment of hypoglycaemia are covered in detail later. As discussed there, there is no convincing evidence that the use of human as opposed to animal insulins specifically interferes with awareness of hypoglycaemic symptoms.

Weight gain is due to the anabolic effects of insulin, compounded by energy saved from glycosuria and sometimes by overeating after hypoglycaemia. Fear of weight gain discourages some patients, especially young women, from taking their full insulin dosages; surprisingly often, deliberate omission or underdosing of insulin may be used by patients wishing to stay thin.

Lipohypertrophy is the local thickening of subcutaneous tissue at frequently used injection sites, and is probably due to the lipogenic effects of high local insulin concentrations. Lipohypertrophy can be unsightly and can significantly delay insulin absorption. It can be prevented by rotating injections around several sites, and large lesions can be removed by liposuction.

Insulin allergy, now very rare with highly purified (especially human) insulins, can include local IgE-mediated erythematous reactions or even anaphylaxis. The commonest manifestation is repeated pain at the site of injection. Lipoatrophy (localized pitting of the skin due to loss of subcutaneous fat) is apparently related to a chronic immune response generated around insulin crystals. Immune insulin resistance was seen with impure animal and especially bovine insulins; high titres of insulin-binding antibodies mop up free insulin from the circulation, resulting in very high insulin requirements (occasionally more than 10 000 U/day), sometimes with unpredictable hypoglycaemia following the release of antibody-bound insulin.

Insulin oedema is rare, and is usually seen in patients recovering from ketoacidosis who have been deprived of insulin for long periods. Fluid retention is probably due to the sodium-conserving effects of insulin on the renal tubule, and may cause ankle or generalized oedema. It usually resolves within a few days, although treatment with diuretics or ephedrine may be required. Insulin neuritis refers to severe, persistent neuropathy following the use of insulin in individuals with very poor control glycaemic control; however, this is a consequence of the sudden improvement in metabolic state rather than a side effect of the insulin itself.

Insulin regimens

Different individuals may need quite different insulin regimens, depending on their residual insulin reserve and severity of insulin resistance, as well as the desired tightness of control and the inconvenience that the patient will accept. Specific insulin schedules used in type 1 and type 2 diabetes are described later.

Insulin dosage

The healthy pancreas secretes about 40 to 60 U of insulin daily. Therapeutic insulin requirements range from less than this in thin type 1 patients (notably during the 'honeymoon period') to more than 200 U/day in very obese, insulin-resistant type 2 patients. High insulin requirements are often due to insulin resistance (see above), whereas low or falling dosages may be caused by weight loss (including anorexia nervosa), coeliac disease, or loss of counter-regulatory hormones in Addison's disease or hypothyroidism—all these conditions being associated with type 1 diabetes. Changing dosages, especially in previously stable subjects, should prompt investigation of these possibilities. Some patients with 'brittle' diabetes or psychological maladaptation to life with diabetes may pretend to take very high or very low dosages (see later). Interestingly, insulin requirements via continuous subcutaneous infusion are typically 30% less than by intermittent injections.

Types of insulin

Formularies contain a bewildering assortment of insulins, many distinguished by imaginative claims about their action profile. Practically, prescribers should become familiar with regimens based on one or two preparations from the following broad classes:

♦ Fast-acting insulin: either a soluble (regular) insulin such as Humulin S or Actrapid, injected 20 to 30 min before eating, or a faster-acting analogue (e.g. lispro or aspart) which can be given immediately before or even shortly after eating

♦ Long-acting insulin: either a lente insulin (e.g.Humulin Zn or Insulatard) or an isophane (e.g.Humulin I or Monotard). With either, circulating insulin falls to below useful levels after 10 to 14 h; they therefore need to be given twice daily in C-peptide negative patients, although those with residual insulin secretion (or who are given three premeal injections of soluble insulin) may be able to maintain good glycaemic control with a single bedtime injection. Bovine (but not human) ultralente can last a full 24 h, but its absorption is erratic and it is rarely used. The long-acting analogues currently available (such as insulin glargine and detemir) have flat, steady action profiles that can provide basal insulin levels with a single daily injection. The timing of long-acting insulin injections does not have to be yoked to mealtimes as tightly as for soluble insulin. It is convenient to inject the dose at bedtime rather than together with the before-supper soluble dose. This is because the action profile of long-acting insulin clashes with the physiological changes in insulin sensitivity that occur overnight. Growth hormone is normally secreted in large spikes on entering deep sleep, typically between 24.00 and 02.00 h; this induces delayed insulin resistance which raises blood glucose during the hours leading up to breakfast. This 'dawn phenomenon' is accentuated if insulin levels are falling simultaneously—as happens if long-acting insulin is injected in the early evening. Another hazard with this timing is potentially dangerous nocturnal hypoglycaemia when insulin levels peak during the early morning (typically 02.00–04.00). Both problems can be reduced by delaying the long-acting injection until bedtime (22.00–23.00), when the risk of nocturnal hypoglycaemia is lower, and insulin levels generally persist long enough to counteract the insulin resistance of the dawn phenomenon. If a second injection is required, this can be given with the before-breakfast soluble insulin. Note that the long-acting analogue insulins (glargine and detemir) should not be mixed in the same syringe as short-acting insulin.

♦ Premixed insulins (e.g. 30% short-acting with 70% long-acting) are obviously more convenient than giving short- and long-acting insulins separately, but they lack flexibility. Premixed insulin injected 30 to 40 min before breakfast can achieve good glycaemic control through the morning and afternoon, but timing the evening dose is problematic: giving it before supper will tend to cause both early morning hypoglycaemia and fasting hyperglycaemia because of the time course of the long-acting component, and simply increasing the evening dosage often makes nocturnal hypoglycaemia worse while failing to lower the before-breakfast glucose. Premixed preparations including rapidly acting analogues such as insulin aspart or lispro and isophane are also available and may be of some advantage.

Insulin injections

Most insulin formulations are now available for both conventional syringes or pen injection devices. Pen injectors are compact, convenient, and easy to use: the required dose is 'dialled up' and injected by pressing the plunger; the ratchet mechanism of most pens gives an audible click that can help blind patients to count dosages.

Syringes and pens carry very fine (28–31 G) needles that allow insulin to be injected almost painlessly. The needle should be pushed in vertically and the insulin injected over a few seconds. Injecting into a pinched up fold of skin to avoid intramuscular injection is advisable in places where there is limited subcutaneous tissue. Backtracking of insulin to the skin surface, which can occasionally cause loss of several units of insulin, may be reduced by leaving the needle in place for a short while. A spot of bleeding may occur; very rarely, sudden hypoglycaemia may be due to direct injection of insulin into a subcutaneous vein.

Injections can be given into any site that is accessible and well padded with adipose tissue, especially the abdomen, thighs, buttocks, and upper arms. The abdomen has the advantage (theoretically at least) of relatively faster absorption that is less influenced by exercise, as compared with the limbs. Rotating injection sites, e.g. between the abdomen and leg, or around the quadrants of the abdomen, helps to avoid local reactions, especially lipohypertrophy which can make insulin absorption slow and erratic.

Jet injectors fire a metered dose of insulin as a high-pressure aerosol that penetrates the skin. These have obvious appeal to patients with needle phobia, although there may be bruising and delayed discomfort at the injection site. Jet injectors are bulky and expensive and do not offer any pharmacokinetic advantages over conventional injections.

Inhaled insulin

Several companies have developed an aerosol formulation of insulin that can be inhaled into the lower airways (insulin is not absorbed from the nasal passages). Inhaled insulin has almost identical pharmokinetic characteristics to subcutaneously injected soluble insulin and so its use might be considered to be predominantly a matter of convenience to avoid injections, especially in those with injection site problems or needle phobia. Sophisticated pharmaceutical preparation and delivery devices are required to ensure accurate dosing. It cannot be used by current smokers (as absorption is variably enhanced to an unpredictable degree) or subjects with chronic airways disease including asthma and chronic obstructive pulmonary disease. Transient cough may occur. Regular lung function testing is advised, as there is a progressive fall in lung function although in most people this is no more rapid than the reduction with age. An increase in insulin autoantibodies has been noted although the significance is uncertain. Inhaled insulin can be used in both type 1 and type 2 diabetes although in type 1 diabetes a subcutaneous injection of intermediate acting insulin is still required. The long-term risks of inhaling insulin over many years are not known and there is a theoretical concern of an increased risk of lung neoplasia. Currently no preparations of inhaled insulin are available. The marketed preparation was withdrawn due to poor sales as it was considerably more expensive than subcutaneous insulin.

Insulin pumps

Portable insulin pumps that administer continuous subcutaneous insulin infusion were developed by Pickup and colleagues in the late 1970s. Modern pumps are compact and light and worn in a belt or holster. Soluble insulin in a special cartridge is delivered through a fine-bore butterfly-type cannula, which is inserted subcutaneously in the anterior abdominal wall or other suitable site and generally left in place for 2 to 4 days; the pump can be safely removed for up to 60 min for bathing or other activities. Different basal rates can be preprogrammed, and mealtime boluses are selected and given by pressing a button. Typical basal rates are 0.5 to 1.5 U/h during the day and 0.5 to 1 U/h overnight, with mealtime boluses (given immediately before meals or snacks) amounting to about 50% of the total daily dose. Most centres use rapid acting analogues in pumps and there is trial evidence to support this.

Continuous subcutaneous insulin infusion (CSII)

CSII can achieve relatively steady insulin levels under laboratory conditions and can partly overcome the variability of subcutaneous insulin absorption seen with intermittent injections of larger doses. When used carefully by highly motivated patients who are supported by an experienced diabetes care team, continuous subcutaneous insulin infusion can achieve glycaemic control which is at least as good as that achieved with multiple injections; the two were used side by side in the Diabetes Control and Complications Trial. Insulin pumps are expensive (£2600–£3500 or US$5000–US$6000) as are consumables (another £1800 per year); medical backup can also be costly to provide. Continuous subcutaneous insulin infusion is indicated for well-informed patients with type 1 diabetes who are prepared to monitor their blood glucose frequently, learn carbohydrate counting, and take responsibility for adjusting the pump. It provides more flexibility for varied lifestyles than multiple daily doses. Randomized trials suggest modest reductions in HbA$_{1c}$ and reduced hypoglycaemia. Although not all randomized trials confirm this, with careful patient selection, these benefits are frequently seen in clinical practice and many patients refuse to return to conventionally delivered insulin. CSII appears to be most beneficial in patients striving hard to improve glycaemic control who are limited by recurrent hypoglycaemia. It is widely used in the United States of America and many European countries.

Infections at the infusion site with pyogenic skin commensals or unusual organisms (e.g. atypical mycobacteria) are uncommon but can be troublesome and cause rapid deterioration in glycaemic control. An increased rate of diabetic ketoacidosis was reported with earlier and less reliable pumps. With CSII, the subcutaneous insulin depot is only a few units, and any interruption of insulin delivery (e.g. with pump failure or cannula blockage) can lead to rapid rises in blood glucose and especially ketone levels. However, modern pumps carry no excess risk of diabetic ketoacidosis as compared with intensified injection therapy. Similarly, the risk of hypoglycaemia due to the pump overrunning is now very low.

With the advent of continuous glucose sensing technology, attempts have been made to develop a closed-loop system for CSII. However, to date, these have had limited success as the pump cannot respond rapidly enough to large meals or sudden exercise to avoid major swings of blood sugar. Wireless technology is now available to display glucose levels on the pump, thus allowing the operator to adjust the insulin delivery rate, but continuous sensing is currently twice as expensive as CSII itself because of the cost of the probes.

Continuous intraperitoneal infusion

The peritoneum is a good route for insulin administration: absorption is very rapid across its large surface area and insulin enters the portal circulation. Continuous intraperitoneal insulin infusion has been used in some cases, mostly employing a pump and reservoir implanted subcutaneously in the abdomen and delivering insulin through a flexible cannula sewn into the peritoneal cavity. The reservoir is filled with soluble insulin through an injection port lying just beneath the skin and is emptied by a liquid/gas compression system at a rate that can be varied by an external electromagnetic control. Continuous intraperitoneal insulin infusion can provide basal insulin; meals need to be covered by additional insulin, either injected subcutaneously or triggered by an external control device.

Intraperitoneal pumps are expensive, and convincing indications for their use are rare. They have been successful in some patients with apparently very high subcutaneous insulin dosages but surprisingly normal intravenous requirements. It is now clear that this situation is not due to a mysterious syndrome of 'subcutaneous insulin resistance', and that most of, if not all, these patients are interfering with their own treatment (see below). In this setting, continuous intraperitoneal insulin infusion is probably effective because these pumps are difficult to sabotage.

Oral hypoglycaemic agents
Sulphonylureas and meglitinides

The sulphonylureas were the first orally active glucose-lowering drugs to be used and were discovered in the 1930s when early sulphonamide antibiotics were found to cause hypoglycaemia. The first generation (chlorpropamide, tolbutamide) have since been superseded by the second generation (e.g. gliclazide and glibenclamide) and by newer agents such as glimepiride. Repaglinide acts in a similar way to the sulphonylureas.

Mode of action Sulphonylureas are insulin secretagogues but insulin synthesis is not stimulated. Insulin levels peak within 1 to 2 h and decline within 4 to 6 h for the short-acting drugs (such as gliclazide) but may remain elevated for much longer with chlorpropamide and glibenclamide, which therefore carry a greater risk of hypoglycaemia. An extrapancreatic action has also been attributed to sulphonylureas, i.e. improving insulin sensitivity. This effect is small and is probably explained by the nonspecific decrease in insulin resistance (glucotoxicity) when hyperglycaemia is corrected by any means.

Repaglinide acts in a similar way to the sulphonylureas but is structurally different. It is derived from the nonsulphonylurea part of the glibenclamide molecule (called meglitinide), which was found fortuitously to have glucose-lowering activity of its own. Nateglinide behaves in a similar fashion and both of these drugs are particularly effective at increasing insulin levels after meals, although the marketing title of postprandial glucose regulators is overstated.

Efficacy and potency The ability of these agents to lower glycaemia depends on how much insulin is available for release from the β cells (which are already stimulated by hyperglycaemia) and by the severity of insulin resistance. In practice, all sulphonylureas lower basal and postprandial glucose levels by no more than 2 to 4 mmol/litre and HbA_{1c} by 1 to 2%; mild hyperglycaemia may therefore be corrected but patients with fasting glucose in excess of 13 mmol/litre are very unlikely to achieve normoglycaemia (primary failure). Moreover, as β-cell function declines progressively in type 2 diabetes, many patients who initially respond well to sulphonylureas will subsequently need additional glucose-lowering drugs; this secondary failure overtakes 5 to 10% of patients per year, in a cumulative fashion. These limitations apply to all sulphonylureas and repaglinide: the more potent drugs have lower therapeutic dosages than the earlier agents but cannot lower glycaemia any further.

Pharmacokinetics Most are taken twice daily with meals; glimepiride is taken once daily and repaglinide with each meal. Chlorpropamide has a very long action profile, while glibenclamide shows variable and sometimes prolonged hypoglycaemic activity. Sulphonylureas and repaglinide bind to circulating proteins and may be displaced by other strongly protein-bound drugs, causing hypoglycaemia (see below). All these drugs are cleared through the kidneys and can accumulate in renal failure, causing frequent hypoglycaemia and other side effects. Gliquidone and tolbutamide are metabolized mainly in the liver and may be slightly less hazardous in patients with renal impairment, although insulin is usually indicated in these cases.

Side effects Weight gain is due to the anabolic effects of hyperinsulinaemia, compounded by reduced losses of energy through glycosuria. Weight gain is typically 2 to 3 kg greater than with diet alone or metformin.

Hypoglycaemia is rarer than with insulin, but the risk is greater with longer-acting sulphonylureas (glibenclamide, chlorpropamide), in renal failure, and especially in older people.

Sulphonylureas can cause allergic reactions including skin rashes (notably Stevens–Johnson syndrome) and marrow dyscrasias, and can precipitate acute intermittent porphyria. Side effects exclusive to chlorpropamide include the syndrome of inappropriate secretion of antidiuretic hormone (SIADH; see Chapter 21.2.1) and acetaldehyde-mediated facial flushing on drinking alcohol.

The cardiovascular safety of sulphonylureas has remained under a cloud since tolbutamide was associated with an excess of cardiovascular deaths during an essentially uninterpretable study (the University Group Diabetes Program or UGDP) conducted in the 1970s; the presence of the ABCC9 (SUR2) receptor on cardiomyocytes has recently reinforced suspicions that these drugs may trigger ischaemia and arrhythmias (by preventing preconditioning). However, the long-term United Kingdom Prospective Diabetes Study found no evidence that patients treated with sulphonylureas

suffered cardiovascular events more often than those treated with insulin. Glimepiride is highly selective for ABCC8 (SUR1).

Indications and contraindications These drugs can be used as first-line therapy for nonobese subjects with type 2 diabetes in whom lifestyle and dietetic measures have failed to control hyperglycaemia. However, because of their tendency to increase weight, in the overweight majority of type 2 diabetes patients, sulphonylureas are used as second-line agents, typically combined with metformin, which may partly offset the weight gain.

Insulin secretagogues are inappropriate for severely insulin-deficient patients or during intercurrent illness, when insulin is needed, and are unlikely to be effective if fasting glucose exceeds 13 mmol/litre. Sulphonylureas are contraindicated in renal failure: all should be stopped and insulin started if serum creatinine exceeds 250 µmol/litre. Pregnancy has been viewed as a contraindication, because sulphonylureas cross the placenta and could cause fetal hyperinsulinaemia and perhaps teratogenesis; however, a recent study with glibenclamide which has less transplacental passage, did not substantiate these concerns (see Chapter 14.10). Sulphonylureas are the therapy of first choice in patients with HNF1α MODY, since these subjects are exquisitely sensitive to these agents, and in patients with the Kir6.2 mutation, who may require very high doses (see above).

Many drugs interact with sulphonylureas, the most common outcome being hypoglycaemia due to displacement and/or decreased clearance of protein-bound sulphonylureas (e.g. by sulphonamides, fibrates, salicylates, and probenecid). Potential interactions must always be checked for any drug being contemplated in patients receiving sulphonylureas.

Choice of drug There is little to choose between the newer agents; chlorpropamide is now obsolete. Glibenclamide should be avoided in older people because of its unpredictable tendency to cause hypoglycaemia.

Metformin

Metformin and phenformin are biguanides, the class of compounds responsible for the mild hypoglycaemic action of goat's rue *Galega officinalis* (an otherwise undistinguished weed). Phenformin is no longer available in many countries because it carries a 10-fold greater risk of lactic acidosis, and metformin has only fairly recently entered clinical use in the United States of America.

Mode of action Metformin acts primarily by inhibiting gluconeogenesis in the liver, thus reducing the raised hepatic glucose output which underpins basal and overnight hyperglycaemia; this effectively enhances the action of insulin on the liver. AMP kinase, a key enzyme that balances anabolic and catabolic processes in the liver and other tissues, is an important target for metformin action. Peripheral glucose uptake may also be increased, while gastrointestinal side effects may help to reduce fondness for food. Metformin does not stimulate insulin secretion.

Overall, metformin lowers blood glucose (especially postprandial) by 2 to 4 mmol/litre and HbA_{1c} by 1 to 2%, which is comparable to the effect of sulphonylureas. On its own, metformin does not cause hypoglycaemia, although this can obviously occur when it is combined with either a sulphonylurea or insulin. Weight does not usually increase with metformin, and may fall.

Metformin may have beneficial cardiovascular effects, as the United Kingdom Prospective Diabetes Study found a reduction in vascular events in the metformin-treated group only (see below). It is not clear whether this is related to the specific metabolic effects of metformin (improved insulin sensitivity), to its mild antiobesity properties, or to other actions such as reported reductions in blood pressure and coagulability.

Pharmacokinetics Metformin is given twice or three times daily with meals. It is cleared mainly through the kidneys, and the increase in plasma levels in renal failure is a major risk factor for lactic acidosis. Recently, a slow-release preparation has been marketed which is taken once daily and appears to produce fewer gastrointestinal side effects.

Side effects Gastrointestinal symptoms (30% of cases) include altered taste, loss of appetite, heartburn, abdominal discomfort and bloating, and diarrhoea (metformin is the most common cause of this in the diabetic clinic). These problems are mostly mild, but may discourage the patient from taking the drug; they can be reduced by starting with a low dosage and increasing it slowly.

Lactic acidosis is very rare with metformin (about 3 cases per 100 000 patient-years) if it is carefully prescribed. This stems from the mode of action of metformin, namely the inhibition of hepatic gluconeogenesis—a process that constantly consumes the lactate produced by glycolysis. Blood lactate levels are modestly raised in patients receiving biguanides, and can escalate rapidly and cause life-threatening acidosis if lactate is overproduced (e.g. in respiratory or cardiac failure), or is not cleared by the liver (hepatic failure), or if metformin accumulates in renal failure. The risk is also increased in the presence of excessive amounts of alcohol. Lactic acidosis is described in detail later. Megaloblastic anaemia can occur due to impaired absorption of vitamin B_{12} and 5-yearly vitamin B_{12} estimations have been recommended.

Indications and contraindications Metformin is now considered the first-line treatment for type 2 diabetes in type 2 patients whose hyperglycaemia does not respond adequately to modification of diet and lifestyle; as it does not tend to cause weight gain, and may even reduce weight, it is especially valuable in obese patients. Recent American Diabetes Association guidelines propose starting metformin concurrently with lifestyle interventions, but this is not universally accepted. The addition of metformin can also be helpful in obese patients who are poorly controlled by sulphonylureas or insulin. Metformin has also proved beneficial in other insulin-resistant conditions such as polycystic ovary syndrome (resulting in improved fertility, reduced hirsutism and oligomenorrhoea) and impaired glucose tolerance where it reduces progression to diabetes by around 25%.

Contraindications include all the major organ failures—renal, hepatic, cardiac, and respiratory. It should not be used when serum creatinine concentration exceeds 150 μmol/litre or the estimated GFR is less than 30 ml/min. It must also be discontinued 2 days before giving radiographic contrast media, to reduce the risk of renal impairment.

Thiazolidinediones

Thiazolidinediones are a novel class of glucose-lowering drugs which improve insulin sensitivity. There are distinct differences between individual thiazolidinediones which influence their therapeutic spectrum and safety. Rosiglitazone and pioglitazone are currently available in many countries; troglitazone has been withdrawn because it caused rare but life-threatening hepatic damage.

Mode of action and pharmacokinetics Thiazolidinediones bind to specific receptors in the nucleus which have the cumbersome title of peroxisome proliferator activating receptor-γ (PPAR-γ). PPAR-γ and the related PPAR-α (the target for the fibrate class of lipid-lowering drugs) are ligand-activated transcription factors whose natural ligands appear to be fatty acid derivatives. PPAR-γ that has bound a thiazolidinedione forms a heterodimeric complex with another nuclear receptor, retinoid X receptor, bound to its own endogenous ligand, retinoic acid. The heterodimer then binds to specific recognition motifs found in the promoter sequences upstream of many genes, notably those involved in adipocyte and lipid metabolism.

The affinity of individual thiazolidinediones at PPAR-γ parallels their glucose-lowering ability in animal models of type 2 diabetes, but their precise mode of action remains uncertain. Thiazolidinediones exert concerted effects that encourage the storage of triglyceride in mature adipocytes, including the differentiation of preadipocytes into adipocytes and enhanced expression of lipogenic enzymes; overall, circulating levels of free fatty acids fall and this may reduce hepatic glucose production and increase glucose uptake into muscle as described earlier. The net effect is to enhance the action of insulin—hence their description as insulin sensitizers. Thiazolidinediones have negligible glucose-lowering action unless insulin resistance and hyperglycaemia are present. As with metformin, they do not cause hypoglycaemia when used alone, but can exaggerate the hypoglycaemic effects of insulin or sulphonylureas.

Efficacy and potency Alone, all thiazolidinediones lower glucose by 2 to 3 mmol/litre and HbA_{1c} by 1%, somewhat less than the sulphonylureas. However, in some individuals they can result in marked falls in HbA_{1c}, up to 4%. For unknown reasons, blood glucose declines slowly during thiazolidinedione treatment, and a maximal effect may not be reached for up to 6 months. In terms of dosage, rosiglitazone is the most potent thiazolidinedione but, as with the more potent sulphonylureas, cannot lower blood glucose further than the other thiazolidinediones.

Pharmacokinetics All are metabolized in the liver and cleared chiefly through the kidney. They are highly protein bound.

Side effects Weight gain, averaging 1 to 4 kg, is due mainly to subcutaneous fat deposition. This appears to spare the visceral depot associated with insulin resistance and does not negate the glucose-lowering action.

Fluid retention of unknown aetiology may cause a mild dilutional anaemia (haemoglobin typically falls by 1–2 g/dl) and ankle oedema (in 5–10% of cases); heart failure may also be precipitated in patients with pre-existing myocardial dysfunction, especially if they are also treated with insulin. Recent meta-analyses have suggested that rosiglitazone is associated with an increased risk of myocardial ischaemic events, but this has not been confirmed by prospective in a study.

Hepatic damage, ranging from subclinical elevations of hepatic enzymes to fulminant and fatal hepatic necrosis (about one case per 1000 patient-years), has been reported with troglitazone but does not appear to be a risk with rosiglitazone or pioglitazone. Indeed, early indications suggest that thiazolidinediones may be helpful in reducing and possibly reversing steatosis (fat deposition) in the liver that is associated with obesity and insulin resistance and can progress to cirrhosis.

An unexpected class side effect of the thiazolidinediones in clinical trials is an increase in fractures in the limbs rather than the axial skeleton. This is especially a concern in post-menopausal women. Mechanisms appear to include increased bone resorption and suppression of osteoblast formation from mesenchymal progenitors.

Indications and contraindications Thiazolidinediones are generally regarded as second- or third-line drugs for treating type 2 diabetes when sulphonylureas or metformin (or the combination of the two) are ineffective or unsuitable. They can be combined with either a sulphonylurea or metformin, when HbA_{1c} may fall by more than 1%; if HbA_{1c} has not fallen by more than 1% within 6 months of adding a thiazolidinedione, it should be discontinued especially in view of the recent concerns over heart failure and fractures. When used alone, they have a lower rate of failure than metformin or sulphonylureas alone, but cost and potential side-effect concerns argue against using them as monotherapy. When pioglitazone is used with insulin, insulin dosage can be reduced but weight gain may be problematic; rarely, heart failure may be precipitated (the combination of rosiglitazone with insulin is currently contraindicated). Subjects with impaired glucose tolerance treated with a thiazolidinedione have a lower risk of progressing to overt type 2 diabetes, and the drugs can improve hirsutism and menstrual dysfunction (sometimes inducing ovulation) in women with polycystic ovary syndrome.

Contraindications include congestive heart failure. Although there is no evidence of hepatotoxicity with thiazolidinediones other than troglitazone, it seems prudent to monitor liver enzymes periodically and to stop the drug if transaminases rise to more than 1.5 times the upper limit of normal, or if any other signs of hepatic dysfunction appear.

α-Glucosidase inhibitors

Acarbose (and the related miglitol and voglibose) are inhibitors of α-glucosidase, an enzyme of the brush border of the small intestine essential for the breakdown of dietary starch to disaccharides, which are then hydrolysed to the absorbable monosaccharides. They partly block digestion of complex carbohydrates and so damp postprandial glycaemic rises but the therapeutic effect is small: postprandial glucose may fall by 1 to 2 mmol/litre, with predictably little impact on overnight glucose, and HbA_{1c} by 0.5% or less. Side effects due to carbohydrate malabsorption (flatus, abdominal bloating, gassy diarrhoea) are common and probably damage compliance. Despite its poor efficacy and low tolerability, acarbose is still widely prescribed and in some countries is regarded as a first-line drug.

Incretin mimetics

These drugs mimic or enhance the action of the incretin hormones that augment insulin secretion. GLP-1 is an incretin that stimulates insulin secretion and may also induce satiety, particularly by delaying gastric emptying. Blood glucose can be lowered comparably to sulphonylureas with GLP-1 infused intravenously. Exenatide (exendin-4) is an analogue of GLP-1, first identified in the saliva and concentrated in the tail of the American venomous lizard, the Gila monster, which by an interesting coincidence lives alongside the diabetes-prone Pima Indians of Arizona. Exenatide shares 50% homology with GLP-1 but has a considerably longer half-life *in vivo* and is now available as a twice daily subcutaneous injection at a dose of 5 or 10 μg and can be used in combination with metformin or a sulphonylurea—only in the latter case is it associated with an increased risk of hypoglycaemia. Mean falls in HbA_{1c} of 0.8 to 1% are seen with the higher dose and direct comparison suggested that these were similar to the results of addition of insulin with less associated hypoglycaemia. In contrast to the weight gain seen with insulin, exenatide is associated with a modest weight loss of around 4 kg, due in part to direct inhibition of appetite. The main side effect is nausea, which occurs in more than 50% of patients, and precludes continuing therapy in around 10% of patients. Pancreatitis has been reported rarely and the use of these drugs is contraindicated in people who have had a previous of pancreatitis. Animal studies show that exenatide is trophic for β cells; confirmation of this very valuable effect in humans is awaited. An additional once daily GLP-1 analogue, liraglutide is currently available and appears to produce less nausea and equal if not greater glucose lowering. Additional analogues, including once weekly versions are in preparation.

The gliptin class of drugs (including sitagliptin, vildagliptin and saxagliptin) are oral selective inhibitors of dipeptidyl peptidase IV (DPP IV), the enzyme that causes the breakdown of circulating GLP-1. They therefore prolong the survival and enhance the action of endogenous GLP-1. These drugs are better tolerated than exenatide and lisaglutide but do not result in weight loss and have less impact on HbA1c levels. An unexpected side effect is an increase in infections, notably sinusitis which is linked to the expression of DPPIV on the surface of lymphocytes (CD26). The optimal place of the incretin mimetics in treatment of type 2 diabetes remains to be determined but currently they are attractive though expensive options to initiating insulin after failure of metformin and sulphonylureas.

Practical management of hyperglycaemia

Most newly diagnosed diabetic patients are easily allocated to either type 1 or type 2 on clinical criteria (see Table 13.11.1.2) and treatment is started accordingly. However, initial impressions may be misleading: a thin young patient may not need insulin because he has MODY, whereas a classical maturity-onset subject may lose weight rapidly and develop ketoacidosis because he has type 1 diabetes. Continuing monitoring and vigilance are therefore essential. The diagnostic pitfalls of Flatbush and fulminant type 1 diabetes have been mentioned above.

Type 1 diabetes

These patients must be given insulin immediately and for life. The insulin regimen will depend particularly on any remaining endogenous insulin, the patient's body weight, lifestyle, and motivation. Patients with residual insulin secretion, especially newly presenting and particularly during the 'honeymoon period' (see below), can often fill in gaps in insulin replacement and enjoy good glycaemic control with few injections and low insulin dosages. However, C-peptide negative patients will require exogenous insulin to cover both basal and prandial needs (see Fig. 13.11.1.7) to achieve good control. Regimens include:

◆ Twice daily long-acting insulin with preprandial short-acting insulin: lente or isophane is injected before breakfast (and can be mixed with prebreakfast short-acting insulin) and at bedtime (see above). Soluble insulin is injected 30 min before breakfast and the evening meal, or a fast-acting analogue (such as lispro or aspart) given with food. Midday meals, unless large, are usually covered satisfactorily by the morning's long-acting dose and do not need separate short-acting insulin.

♦ Once daily long-acting insulin with preprandial short-acting insulin (basal–bolus regimen) is currently unsatisfactory because both lente and isophane run out too quickly, but longer-lasting analogues such as glargine or detemir may be effective when injected once daily at bedtime or breakfast. Short-acting insulin is given separately to cover meals, as above.

♦ Premixed insulins injected before breakfast and before the evening meal suit some patients and many doctors, but often fail to control overnight and/or fasting glucose levels (see above).

Insulin dosages should be titrated according to blood glucose and HbA$_{1c}$ monitoring (see Table 13.11.1.3). Highly motivated patients may be suitable for continuous subcutaneous insulin infusion treatment as discussed above.

Starting insulin therapy

Patients at risk of ketoacidosis may need hospital admission, but most patients are clinically well and can start insulin as an outpatient, supervised by a specialist diabetes nurse. Good control can often be achieved with long-acting insulin injected at breakfast and bedtime, starting with low dosages (e.g. 8–12 U in the morning and 4–6 U at night) to avoid potentially demoralizing hypoglycaemia. Short-acting insulin can then be added to cover excessive prandial hyperglycaemia. Wherever practicable, patients should be encouraged to give their own injections as soon as possible.

Newly diagnosed patients starting insulin need to be warned about a possible 'honeymoon period' of good glycaemic control, when the fall in glucose levels allows partial though temporary recovery of the remaining β cells. Blood glucose can often be easily controlled with low insulin dosages (and exceptionally, without exogenous insulin) but the honeymoon ultimately ends usually within a few months: blood sugar levels and insulin requirements then escalate, because of the progressive loss of remaining β cells over the next 1–5 years.

Poor diabetic control and 'brittle' diabetes

In real life, relatively few type 1 patients approach the high-quality glycaemic control aspired to in Table 13.11.1.3. This largely reflects the pharmacokinetic shortcomings of current insulin preparations and the unpredictable nature of subcutaneous absorption. The patient's compliance is a crucial determinant of overall diabetic control; teenagers are notoriously resistant to advice about diabetes, as with other matters, and many have markedly elevated HbA$_{1c}$ concentrations. This clearly increases the risk of future diabetic complications.

A few patients have such poor metabolic control that they cannot live a normal life. Most have chronically high blood glucose and suffer recurrent hospital admissions with ketoacidosis; some suffer frequent hypoglycaemia, while others have an unstable or 'brittle' blood glucose profile that can swing rapidly between hyper- and hypoglycaemia. Occasionally, endocrine or intercurrent illnesses are found to be responsible (see Table 13.11.1.5), but most cases remain idiopathic after even intensive investigation. It is now clear that poor compliance, often aggravated by deliberate interference with treatment, is responsible in many of these patients. Most are young women who tend to be obese and are generally hyperglycaemic despite apparently high insulin dosages; when tested under

Table 13.11.1.5 Causes of poor glycaemic control in type 1 diabetic patients

Characteristics	Cause
High insulin requirements, chronic hyperglycaemia ± recurrent ketoacidosis	Obesity
	Puberty
	Endocrine diseases: Cushing's syndrome, thyrotoxicosis
	Drugs: especially glucocorticoids
	Immune insulin resistance
Low insulin requirements, recurrent hypoglycaemia	Weight loss
	Loss of hypoglycaemia awareness
	Endocrine diseases: adrenocortical failure, hypothyroidism, growth hormone deficiency, hypopituitarism
	Gastroparesis
	Coeliac disease
	Liver disease
Erratic glycaemic profile, frequent hyper- and hypoglycaemia ('brittle' diabetes)	Pancreatic damage
	Overtreating hypoglycaemia
	Gastroparesis
	Injection site problems (lipohypertrophy)
	Recurrent or chronic infections: tuberculosis, sinusitis

For all three characteristics, always consider: unsuitable insulin regime; poor diabetes education; deliberate noncompliance; appetite disorders (anorexia nervosa, food bingeing).

controlled conditions, however, their intravenous and subcutaneous insulin requirements are unremarkable. Many are probably omitting insulin or taking only small doses: common motives include escape from difficulties at school or home, or wanting to stay thin (disturbances of body image are common in this group). Coexistent eating disorders, such as anorexia and bulimia nervosa, are commonly seen in these individuals. Initially, such patients may appear to lead charmed lives despite frequent hospital admissions but many die prematurely (especially from ketoacidosis or hypoglycaemia); significant diabetic complications frequently develop during their twenties or thirties.

Management can be extremely difficult. Patients with sustained poor control should be admitted selectively for intensive education, observation, and exclusion of other possible causes (see Table 13.11.1.3). In some cases, it may be necessary to confirm that insulin is effective at conventional doses (for more information see the paper by Schade and Duckworth listed in 'Further reading'). Even close supervision in hospital does not exclude ingenious interference with insulin treatment or glucose monitoring. Intensified insulin schedules or continuous subcutaneous insulin infusion may help in some cases and increasingly whole pancreas transplantation is being considered as an option if patients are willing to take the associated risks (see below).

Experimental and future treatments for type 1 diabetes

Whole pancreatic transplantation, usually performed in conjunction with renal transplantation for patients with diabetic nephropathy, can achieve good results including long-term withdrawal of exogenous insulin (> 5 years) in up to 70% of cases. The whole gland or a segment is transplanted into the pelvis and anastomosed to the iliac vessels; to avoid damage from pancreatic exocrine secretions, the pancreatic duct is drained either into the gut or into the bladder (when urinary amylase excretion can indicate the health of the graft). Outcomes for both the pancreas and the kidney are better when simultaneous transplantation is performed as the early treatment of rejection, which is easier to identify in the kidney by serum creatinine and or biopsy, preserves both organs and the improved glycaemic control from the pancreas is beneficial to the kidney. Problems are the need for lifelong immunosuppression (required anyway for renal transplantation) and the global shortage of donor organs. An increasing number of pancreas transplants alone are being performed in type 1 diabetes but the balance of risks (especially of malignancy and infection from the immunosuppression) and benefits (from improved glycaemic control) is difficult to assess. The exact indication for this procedure, where available, remains but it is generally performed for persistent poor metabolic control with or without recurrent ketoacidosis. Although there are attendant risks from the surgery and immunosuppression, recurrent ketoacidosis and poor metabolic control itself carries a not insignificant risk of death.

Introduction of an improved immunosuppressive regimen (which omits glucocorticoids) by Shapiro and colleagues reported in 2000 has lead to a resurgence in pancreatic islet transplantation. The most widely used method is by transcutaneous injection into the portal vein of islets isolated from a donor pancreas; these colonize and function well in the liver, the first stop for insulin secreted physiologically. Even with less toxic immunosuppression, two or three donor pancreases are currently needed for each recipient, and only 10% of patients are insulin independent at 5 years. Nevertheless, up to 90% of patients report significant reductions in the rate of hypoglycaemia; hence recurrent severe hypoglycaemia unresponsive to changes in insulin therapy or the use of CSII remains the main indication for this procedure.

Prevention of type 1 diabetes by aborting insulitis during the long prediabetic phase by immunosuppression in high-risk subjects, or preserving islet cell function in newly diagnosed patients, is a major goal of current research. Trials in the 1980s demonstrated that ciclosporin can achieve this, but the cost in terms of side effects of continuous therapy is too high. Newer immunomodulatory agents, such as nondepleting anti-CD3, that regulate rather than suppress immune responses, may ultimately improve the risk–benefit ratio to the point of acceptability but are not currently available.

Much effort is also being invested in promoting the regeneration of β cells either from pancreatic tissue or more generic stem cells. These studies remain at a preliminary stage, but potentially offer a renewable therapy. Although they may not require immunosuppression for allograft rejection, it remains to be seen whether such new cells would be retargeted by the autoimmune process in subjects with type 1 diabetes.

Management of type 2 diabetes

Dietary and lifestyle measures form an essential foundation for the management of type 2 diabetes and must be maintained throughout, even though fewer than 10% of patients can be controlled satisfactorily for more than a year by these means alone.

Patients who fail to meet the glycaemic targets set out in Table 13.11.1.3 should generally follow the steps outlined below,

although compromises may be more appropriate in older people or those at risk of hypoglycaemia. Progress should be reviewed every 3 months or so if blood glucose is unacceptably high; the inexorable deterioration of β-cell function in type 2 diabetes means that there is no point in delaying decisions to increase drug doses or add insulin.

The first-line oral hypoglycaemic agent for dietary failure is metformin, particularly for obese patients (those with a BMI >30 kg/m^2). Full effect takes 3 or more months to be achieved, so doses should not be increased too rapidly.

The addition to metformin of a sulphonylurea or a thiazolidinedione represents second-line treatment. The place of triple therapy (typically with the addition a thiazolidinedione as the third drug) is uncertain but in some cases very marked and prolonged improvements are seen in glycaemic control. Some diabetologists would consider adding acarbose at this stage, although the chances of lowering glucose adequately are remote.

Long-acting insulin with a first-line oral agent: although seemingly illogical, a bedtime injection of isophane can control blood glucose overnight and before breakfast, and this apparently helps oral hypoglycaemic agents to act more effectively during the day. The combination of metformin (three times daily with meals) with bedtime isophane often achieves good glycaemic control, while limiting the weight gain that commonly follows the introduction of insulin in type 2 patients. Isophane with a sulphonylurea or pioglitazone may increase weight; the combination of rosiglitazone with insulin should be avoided because of the risk of heart failure from fluid retention.

Insulin therapy can range from once or twice daily long-acting insulin in subjects with residual insulin, to the more intensified basal and prandial regimens used in type 1 diabetes. Large dosages (150 to 300 U/day) may be needed to achieve good glycaemic control in obese, highly insulin-resistant subjects. Rapidly acting and very long-acting analogues have been promoted in type 2 diabetes but meta-analyses do not suggest a major advantage over conventional insulins. The recent 4T study (Treating to Target in Type 2 Diabetes) confirmed that intensified regimes with prandial insulin achieve lower HbA$_{1c}$ levels than once or twice daily therapy but, as expected, they are associated with an increased incidence of hypoglycaemia.

Obesity (and therefore insulin resistance) may worsen when insulin treatment is started. The average weight gain is around 6 kg; possible reasons include reduced loss of energy through glycosuria, a tendency to relax dietary restriction when a more effective means of lowering glycaemia is introduced, and sometimes overeating during hypoglycaemic episodes. Increasing insulin resistance may lead to escalating insulin dosages. The possible hazards of insulin-induced obesity are not clear but could theoretically include vascular disease, which may be hinted at by the lower frequency of cardiovascular events among patients treated with metformin in the United Kingdom Prospective Diabetes Study trial. At present, however, the consensus is probably to aim for the glycaemic targets set out in Table 13.11.1.3 (which will reduce the risks of microvascular complications) and to accept an increase in weight, while actively treating other cardiovascular risk factors. The increasing use of incretin mimetics in place of insulin conversion may challenge this practice, although the long-term safety and efficacy of these drugs is not known.

Antiobesity drugs (including orlistat, sibutramine) could have an important impact in many type 2 patients although their exact role remains to be determined. Rimonabant, a canabinoid receptor (CB1)antagonist which reduced appetite and increase insulin sensitivity, has been withdrawn because of exacerbation of depression and anxiety. Additional appetite modulating agents currently in preclinical testing include neuropeptide Y receptor (NPY5R) antagonists, melanocortin-4 receptor agonists, and low molecular weight leptin and peptide YY mimetics (see Chapter 11.5). Bariatric surgery is the most effective means of lowering weight and fat mass in obesity. Up to 80% of subjects with impaired glucose tolerance or established type 2 diabetes will revert to normoglycaemia following bariatric procedures. Those with long-standing type 2 diabetes requiring insulin treatment are the least likely to respond. The optimal place of this invasive approach in diabetes management remains to be defined.

Monitoring diabetic control

Treatment targets for blood glucose in type 1 and type 2 diabetes (see Table 13.11.1.3) have been selected to reduce the risk of chronic diabetic complications. Avoiding acute episodes of hyper- and hypoglycaemia is also important.

Blood glucose monitoring

Blood glucose concentration can be easily and quickly measured in small drops of blood (a few microlitres or less), using various test strips; the ability to perform such measurements is an essential skill for all professionals delivering diabetes care and for most diabetic patients. Test strips contain glucose oxidase (which catalyses the oxidation of glucose to gluconic acid) together with a detection system to measure specific reaction products, either electrochemically or colorimetrically (using dyes sensitive to hydrogen peroxide). The signal is read by a reflectance meter or electrically, and converted into the glucose concentration in the sample. Colour-based test strips can also be read by eye against a printed standard scale, although this may be difficult for partially sighted or colour-blind patients.

A drop of blood is obtained by pricking the sides of the fingertip, avoiding the sensitive pads; various lancets and automatic finger-pricking devices are available. Blood must cover the reaction area completely and be left in contact for exactly the period stipulated; modern meters read out automatically at this point, whereas older strips must be wiped dry and left for the colour to develop. Failure to follow the manufacturer's instructions is the main cause of inaccurate readings, which are disturbingly frequent. With attention to detail, readings correspond closely to laboratory measurements of glucose (which also employ the glucose oxidase reaction) but are not reliable enough to be used for diagnosing diabetes.

Monitoring schedules

Type 2 diabetes treated with diet and oral agents can be monitored using fasting glucose and values in the mid-afternoon or 2 h postprandially (both of which correlate with overall glucose level) measured once or twice per week. Recent trials indicate that glucose monitoring *per se* does not improve glycaemic control in type 2 diabetes and home monitoring is not essential in patients treated with diet alone or a single oral agent.

Insulin-treated patients need more frequent monitoring to adjust insulin dosages. Bed-time and pre-meal testing (4-point) as well as ideally 2 hour post-prandial (7-point) testing is recommended. Fasting glucose is determined by the previous evening's long-acting insulin, while values before the evening meal reflect mainly the morning's long-acting dose. Prandial short-acting insulin dosages can be titrated from the glucose rise 90 to 120 min after eating. Readings can be scattered across these time points on different days; most patients can be persuaded to check their glucose levels once or twice per day but to achieve tight glycaemic control targets without hypoglycaemia more frequent blood glucose testing is required.

Written records help to bring out general patterns in glucose control and many modern meters can be downloaded to display the pattern in different formats. Patients must also be encouraged to check their glucose if they feel unwell and, crucially, at frequent intervals during intercurrent illness. Occasional tests during the night (especially between 02.00 and 04.00) are useful in patients at risk of nocturnal hypoglycaemia, including those injecting long-acting or premixed insulins in the early evening.

Checking the self-monitoring technique and the patient's action plan when glucose levels fall outside the target range is a core part of the patient's diabetic education.

HbA$_{1c}$ and fructosamine

These tests measure the nonenzymatic reaction of glucose with circulating proteins (see below), and therefore reflect longer-term blood glucose levels. Glycated (glycosylated) haemoglobin (HbA$_1$) results from the combination of glucose with the N-terminal valine residue of the B chain of adult Hb (HbA), and can be separated from unaltered HbA by electrophoretic and other methods. HbA$_1$ includes the stable HbA$_{1c}$ fraction, which is most closely related to average blood glucose levels over the preceding 6 to 8 weeks.

The various assay methods for HbA$_{1c}$ are now standardized to match the methodology used in the Diabetes Control and Complications Trial (DCCT), which defined the long-term risks of diabetic microvascular complications (see below). For assays conforming to DCCT standards, nondiabetic HbA$_{1c}$ ranges from 3.5 to 5.5% of total HbA, with good control defined as values less than 7% and poor control as more than 8%; some poorly compliant patients have HbA$_{1c}$ concentrations of 14 to 16%. HbA$_{1c}$ measurements are a useful index of medium-term glycaemic control, but may be invalidated by abnormal red cell turnover (values are spuriously low in haemolysis, bleeding, and pregnancy), in renal failure (carbamylated HbA coelutes with HbA$_{1c}$, falsely raising levels), and with abnormal haemoglobins such as hetero- or homozygous sickle cell disease (HbF also comigrates with HbA$_1$). Modern analytical methods for HbA$_{1c}$ detect the presence of abnormal haemoglobins and hence spurious results are usually highlighted by the laboratory.

Serum albumin also undergoes glycation, which is measured by the fructosamine reaction. As albumin turns over faster than haemoglobin, the fructosamine concentration reflects mean blood glucose over the previous 1 to 2 weeks. Assays are cheap but not standardized between laboratories, and are generally less reliable and reproducible than measurements of HbA$_{1c}$.

Measurements of urinary glucose and ketones

Urinary glucose concentrations can be measured easily using glucose oxidase test strips, but are of limited use: urinary glucose concentration depends on the renal threshold (which can lie between 7 and 13 mmol/litre), urine output, and the time since the bladder was last emptied. Crucially, hypoglycaemia cannot be detected. Urinary glucose measurements are acceptable in type 2 diabetic patients with a normal renal threshold who are not receiving hypoglycaemic medication (insulin or sulphonylureas) and in patients who decline to prick their fingers.

Urinary ketone measurements can be useful for predicting impending ketoacidosis, particularly during intercurrent illness when blood glucose is high. Moderate ketonuria can be caused by fasting or undereating, including during infections. Some modern blood testing meters can also often also measure blood ketones with appropriate testing strips.

Structures for diabetes care

Diabetes is best managed by the combined efforts of a well-trained primary care team and a team of specialists with complementary and overlapping skills: physician, specialist diabetes nurse, dietitian, and chiropodist. The specialist diabetes nurse has a crucial role in educating patients about diabetes and its practical management, and in starting and adjusting therapy. Many patients are more receptive and responsive to information given by primary care teams and specialist nurses than by doctors. For complex cases, there must be frequent contact with and easy access to other specialists (ophthalmologist, vascular surgeon, renal physician, obstetrician, and clinical psychologist), ideally in the setting of combined clinics. Each member of the team has a particular niche but all must agree common strategies (such as dietary advice for obesity) to avoid giving the patients conflicting or inconsistent information.

Diabetes care can be delivered effectively by well-informed general practitioners or practice nurses, hospital-based clinics, community mini-clinics, or shared care schemes that bridge the primary and secondary sectors. Because of the unpredictable course and potential complications of diabetes, all patients must be thoroughly reviewed each year and be rapidly referred for specialist help if the need arises. A check list for the annual review is suggested in Table 13.11.1.6.

Diabetes education

Living and coping with diabetes is a considerable burden that is poorly appreciated by many doctors and nurses. Careful education about diabetes, its complications, and its practical management can provide great reassurance to patients and also reduce emergency hospital admissions and complications such as foot ulceration and amputation.

Diabetes education is most effectively provided by a trained practice nurse or specialist diabetes nurse, but all members of the diabetes care team should understand the key messages, and check and reinforce these whenever possible. Evidence suggests that education in a group setting is often more effective than on a one to one basis and may promote informal support networks. Key elements of the education programme include:

- causes of hyperglycaemia and diabetic symptoms

- own treatment: diet and lifestyle; drawing up and injecting insulin; oral agents; recognizing and treating hypoglycaemia

- self-monitoring technique; targets and danger levels; how to respond to poor control

- 'sick-day' rules: monitoring during intercurrent illness; how to adjust own treatment; when and how to call for help (Box 13.11.1.1)

Several very intensive training courses have been developed such as the Diabetes Adjustment For Normal Eating (DAFNE) course for type 1 diabetes; effectiveness when applied at a wide variety of training centres has been confirmed for some but not all courses and likely depends on the enthusiasm, skills and attention to detail of individual trainers.

Employment, driving, and insurance

Because of the risk of hypoglycaemia, patients treated with insulin (type 1 or 2) are generally barred from driving heavy goods and public service vehicles. Licensing for taxi drivers varies between local authorities. Until recently, insulin-treated individuals were also barred from active service in the police, fire service, or armed forces, and from work as airline pilots or cabin staff; but this policy is increasingly being revised in favour of individual case-based assessments, following new legislation regarding discrimination against people with disabilities. In the armed forces, although there remains reluctance to recruit subjects already on insulin, military personnel who develop diabetes can request to have their particular circumstances reviewed. Specific diabetic complications, notably sight-threatening retinopathy, may preclude particular jobs or pastimes.

Patients must inform the driving licence authorities and their driving insurer that they have diabetes, and those receiving insulin or with clinically significant retinopathy may require periodic medical confirmation of fitness to drive. Frequent hypoglycaemia, especially with decreased awareness of symptoms, is a bar to driving. Currently the use of GLP-1 agonists carries no specific restrictions in the UK except for heavy goods vehicle or public service vehicle drivers taking these agents in conjunction with sulphonylureas, in which case the driving authority will make an assessment on individual basis.

Special life insurance policies are available from companies endorsed by patient-centred organizations such as Diabetes UK and the American Diabetes Association. Many patients find it valuable to join these organizations.

Intercurrent events in diabetes and their management

Infections

People with diabetes probably have increased susceptibility to pyogenic bacterial infections, especially when diabetes is poorly controlled. Hyperglycaemia can impair the killing of microorganisms by neutrophils and macrophages and may also interfere with the function of T lymphocytes. Some infections particularly associated with poorly controlled diabetes include:

- recurrent and sometimes invasive candidiasis

- tuberculosis, often widespread and cavitating

- necrotizing fasciitis, rapidly spreading necrosis of subcutaneous tissues down to muscle, usually due to β-haemolytic streptococci with staphylococci and often anaerobes

- gas-forming infections with anaerobes and clostridia, including emphysematous pyelonephritis, cholecystitis, cystitis, and foot infections. plain radiography shows gas in the affected tissues

- diabetic foot ulcers (see below), which are often infected, with the risk of osteomyelitis and deep soft tissue spread

- recurrent oral and genital candida infections

Table 13.11.1.6 Routine annual review of a diabetic patient: key points include those specific to patients taking insulin

	History and discussion	Examination	Investigations
Diabetic treatment	Diet, physical activity	Weight, height, BMI	
	Weight and change	Waist–hip ratio	
	Glucose-lowering drugs	Insulin injection sites	
Diabetic control	Self-monitoring results (± check technique)		
	Hyperglycaemic symptoms		HbA$_{1c}$
	Hypoglycaemia frequency and awareness of symptoms		Liver function tests in type 2 diabetes if known fatty liver disease.
Diabetes education and skills (± family or associates)	General knowledge		
	Treatment targets		
	'Sick-day' rules, driving rules, pregnancy plans		
	Hypoglycaemia treatment		
	Insulin injection technique		
Diabetic complications:			
Macrovascular	Ischaemic heart disease (angina, MI, failure, arrhythmias)	Examine heart, including signs of failure. Blood pressure, lying and standing	Fasting lipid screen (total, HDL and LDL cholesterol; triglycerides). ECG (if other risk factors or age > 40)
	Peripheral vascular disease (claudication, stroke, TIA)	Peripheral pulses, strength and bruits	
	Smoking history		
	Other risk factors (hypertension, dyslipidaemia, family history)		
Eyes (retinopathy and cataract)	Altered acuity, loss of vision	Visual acuity (± corrected). Retinal examination (digitial imaging, fundoscopy through dilated pupils)	
Nephropathy			Blood electrolytes, urea, creatinine. Microalbumia screen (e.g. albumin:creatinine ratio) or timed urinary albumin excretion
Neuropathy	Altered or reduced sensation	Sensory testing screen as appropriate (feet: see below)	
	Pain	Postural blood pressure drop	
	Weakness in limbs		
	Autonomic symptoms (sweating, postural dizziness, gastrointestinal)		
Feet	Pain, numbness	General condition: posture, callus, footwear appropriate	
	Ulceration: current and previous	Pulses and perfusion	
	Footwear (sensible?)	Oedema	
	Foot care	Sensory deficits (vibration sense, pin prick, monofilament)	
Sexual function	Erectile and ejaculatory problems (men)		
Other illnesses	Other medication (possible effects on glycaemic control and interactions with antidiabetic drugs)		

BMI, body mass index; MI, myocardial infarction; HDL, high-density lipoprotein; LDL, low-density lipoprotein; TIA, transient ischaemic attack.

- urinary tract infections, which may be complicated by ascending infections with pyelonephritis and renal or perinephric abscess (sometimes with gas), and occasionally acute papillary necrosis; severe loin pain and systemic symptoms, with deteriorating renal function, should suggest these possibilities and the need for urgent imaging
- 'malignant' or necrotizing otitis externa, due to pseudomonas infection, which can invade the skull and facial nerve
- periodontal infections, sometimes causing tooth loss—these are common
- rhinocerebral mucormycosis, a highly invasive fungal infection that originates in the sinuses but often spreads into the orbit and cranial cavity; mortality is about 50%, even with debridement and high-dose intravenous amphotericin B

The bacterial infections often require aggressive intravenous antibiotic treatment with cover against anaerobes. Fastidious and rare organisms should be considered when standard antibiotic regimens are ineffective.

Diabetic control during infections

Minor viral infections rarely disturb diabetic control, but increased secretion of counter-regulatory stress hormones during severe infections, especially with fever, can rapidly worsen insulin resistance in both type 1 and 2 diabetes.

Type 1 patients may need twice as much insulin as usual, even if they are unable to eat. Failure to increase the insulin dosage will therefore allow glucose to rise, sometimes dramatically fast, and risk precipitating ketoacidosis. It is therefore essential to continue taking insulin, to monitor blood glucose frequently, and to increase insulin if sustained hyperglycaemia develops. An increase of 30 to 50% in long-acting insulin is often enough, but requirements will be determined by blood glucose levels and should be decided in consultation with the diabetes care team. Avoidable deaths still occur every year because poorly educated patients (sometimes advised by ignorant doctors) reduce or even stop taking insulin because they feel ill, are not eating, and are worried about becoming hypoglycaemic. Clear 'sick-day' rules (see Box 13.11.1.1) are a crucial part of diabetes education, which must be regularly checked and reinforced.

During severe infections, insulin requirements may fluctuate rapidly and the safest way to give insulin is by continuous intravenous infusion, backed up by frequent (hourly) blood glucose measurements (see below). Type 2 patients may similarly lose glycaemic control, and are best transferred temporarily to subcutaneous or intravenous insulin. It seems best to maintain blood glucose between 5 and 10 mmol/litre during intercurrent infections, although this is not firmly evidence-based.

Myocardial infarction

This is discussed in detail later (see pp. 2043–44).

Surgery

Surgery can be hazardous to diabetic patients: the counter-regulatory stress response to surgical trauma can rapidly lead to hyperglycaemia and ketoacidosis, especially in insulin-deficient patients, while poorly controlled diabetes accelerates catabolism and delays wound healing. Moreover, insulin and the sulphonylureas can cause severe hypoglycaemia in fasted or anorexic patients, which can be particularly dangerous during general anaesthesia.

Glycaemic control must therefore be meticulous throughout the perioperative period. A routine management policy should be agreed between the diabetes care team, surgeons, anaesthetists, and ward staff, and this will greatly reduce the risks of operating on diabetic people. Fitness for surgery should be carefully assessed, in view of cardiovascular or other complications. Patients may need to be admitted some days before operation to optimize their treatment.

For type 2 patients who are well controlled by diet or oral agents and undergoing minor surgery only, long-acting sulphonylureas (glibenclamide) should be changed to short-acting ones (e.g. gliclazide) some days before surgery to reduce the risk of hypoglycaemia. Oral agents and breakfast should be omitted on the morning of operation and blood glucose should be monitored closely. Persistent hyperglycaemia should be treated with the intravenous glucose–potassium–insulin regimen described below.

For all other diabetic patients, subcutaneous insulin should be stopped on the morning of surgery, and a continuous intravenous infusion of balanced amounts of glucose, potassium, and insulin should be given (Box 13.11.1.2). If the patient is in steady state, the

Box 13.11.1.1 'Sick-day' rules for patients with type 1 diabetes

If you feel unwell, and even if you think it is a minor infection:
- Never stop taking your insulin—you often need more when you are unwell
- Check your blood glucose every 4 h—glucose levels can rise very fast during infections
- Test your urine for ketones each time you pass some—ketones are an important warning sign
- Contact your doctor at once if you:
  - start vomiting
  - get high glucose levels (>15) that do not come down after insulin
  - get hypos (glucose <3)
  - get ketones in the urine
  - are worried and do not know what to do

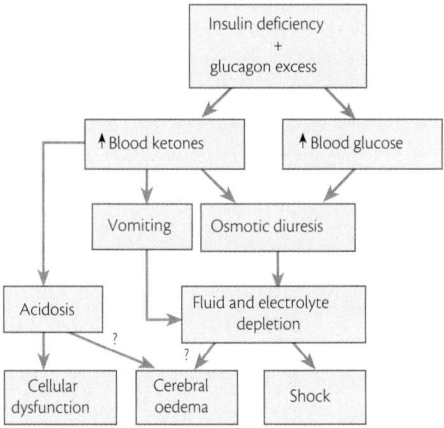

Fig. 13.11.1.9 Pathophysiological changes in diabetic ketoacidosis. Cellular dysfunction induced by intracellular acidosis, as well as cerebral oedema and shock are potentially life-threatening.

Box 13.11.1.2 Glucose–potassium–insulin infusion regime

Infusion (standard recipe)
- 500 ml of 10% dextrose plus
- 15 U soluble insulin plus
- 10 mmol KCl

Instructions
- Infuse at 100 ml/h
- Check blood glucose every hour
- If blood glucose deviates outside target range of 5–10 mmol/litre, then take down the bag and replace it as follows:
  - if blood glucose < 5 mmol/litre, put 10 U insulin in new bag with 10 mmol KCl
  - if blood glucose > 10 mmol/litre, put 20 U insulin in new bag with 10 mmol KCl
  - (lower or higher insulin dosages are occasionally needed)
- Check plasma K^+ every 6 h and adjust accordingly

Indications and contraindications
- Indications: temporary measure for diabetic patients in steady state, i.e. not eating and no other antidiabetic medication
- Contraindications: not for treatment of severe hyperglycaemia or ketoacidosis

---

glucose–potassium–insulin (GKI) infusion will both maintain satisfactory glycaemic control (5–10 mmol/litre) and prevent hypokalaemia (insulin enhances potassium entry into skeletal muscle). This regimen should be started on the morning of surgery and continued until the patient is able to eat and drink normally, when the usual treatment can be resumed. GKI bags must be changed if glucose levels are unsatisfactory. Alternatively, insulin may be given as a variable-rate intravenous infusion (sliding scale insulin) adjusted according to hourly blood glucose measurements, which provides greater flexibility.

Acute metabolic complications of diabetes and their treatment

Diabetic ketoacidosis

This is uncontrolled hyperglycaemia with hyperketonaemia severe enough to cause metabolic acidosis. It remains a major cause of death in patients with type 1 diabetes under 20 years of age, and episodes still carry an overall mortality of 5 to 10% (50% in older patients with diabetic ketoacidosis precipitated by infection or myocardial infarction). Prompt diagnosis and careful management can prevent many deaths.

Causes

Diabetic ketoacidosis only develops when severe insulin deficiency, compounded by an excess of glucagon, stimulates lipolysis and a massive increase in ketogenesis (see above). It therefore almost always occurs in untreated or poorly treated type 1 diabetes and is generally regarded as the hallmark of that disease. However, diabetic ketoacidosis can occur in subjects with type 2 diabetes who are relatively insulin deficient, especially when the secretion of counter-regulatory hormones (especially glucagon) is increased by severe intercurrent illness. Precipitating factors include:

- newly presenting type 1 diabetes
- omission or underdosing of insulin by established type 1 diabetic patients, which may be deliberate in patients with disturbances of body image
- intercurrent illness, such as infections, myocardial infarction, stroke, trauma, surgery, and burns; many patients (and their doctors) fail to increase insulin dosages or monitor blood glucose during such events

About 30 to 40% of episodes are unexplained; omitted or inadequate insulin treatment should always be suspected if no obvious infective or other cause is found.

Pathophysiology

Diabetic ketoacidosis is due to the accumulation of ketones, i.e. acetoacetate and its derivatives, 3-hydroxybutyrate (or β-hydroxybutyrate) and acetone (see Fig. 13.11.1.9). They are generated by β-oxidation of free fatty acids within the mitochondria of the liver. Free fatty acids enter the cytoplasm of hepatocytes and combine with coenzyme A (CoA) to form their fatty acyl-CoA derivatives. These are then transported into the mitochondria by the carnitine shuttle, a complex of two linked enzymes, carnitine palmitoyltransferase I (CPT I) on the outer mitochondrial membrane and carnitine palmitoyltransferase II (CPT-II) on the inner. CPT-I, and the overall activity of the shuttle, is powerfully inhibited by insulin and stimulated by glucagon. Once inside the mitochondria, free fatty acids undergo β-oxidation to yield ATP (the process of oxidative phosphorylation) and acetyl-CoA. The latter is converted to acetoacetate, which may be oxidized to 3-hydroxybutyrate or undergo condensation to produce acetone.

Ketones are transported out of the liver and are used as metabolic fuels by various tissues including the brain; they supply a few% of total energy needs after an overnight fast, but the proportion rises to over one-third during prolonged fasting. When produced in excess, they can accumulate rapidly, especially if plasma levels exceed 5 mmol/litre (about 10 times normal), when tissue uptake mechanisms become saturated. Ketogenesis is greatly enhanced in uncontrolled type 1 diabetes because of the combination of low insulin with increased glucagon concentrations: lipolysis is unrestrained, and the uptake into liver mitochondria of the increased amounts of fatty acyl-CoA is stimulated by the synergistic effects on CPT-I of high glucagon and low insulin. The main consequences of raised circulating ketone levels are shown in Fig. 13.11.1.9 and listed below:

- Acidosis: acetoacetate and 3-hydroxybutyrate are both moderately strong organic acids and lower the extracellular pH when the buffering capacity of plasma proteins is exceeded. Ion exchange across cell membranes leads to intracellular acidosis which compromises cellular metabolism because many crucial enzymes operate within a narrow pH range. Clinical measurements of acid–base status are confined to the extracellular fluid and may underestimate the severity of intracellular acidosis.
- Diuresis: ketones are filtered in the urine and are osmotically active. They therefore exacerbate the osmotic diuresis caused by glycosuria and the resulting polyuria, electrolyte losses, dehydration, and hypovolaemia.

◆ Nausea: through direct stimulation of the chemoreceptor trigger zone in the medulla.

Clinical features

Diabetic ketoacidosis usually presents with classical hyperglycaemic symptoms (see Table 13.11.1.2), together with features of acidosis and hyperketonaemia:

◆ Acidotic (Kussmaul) breathing is deep, sighing hyperventilation which has been mistaken for panic attacks, pulmonary embolism, and left ventricular failure.

◆ Nausea and vomiting are ominous signs, because dehydration develops quickly in polyuric patients unable to drink.

◆ Drowsiness and coma occur late and may indicate early cerebral oedema.

The patient generally looks ill and may show postural hypotension and other signs of dehydration and hypovolaemia. Acetone is volatile and may be smelled on the breath (ketotic foetor; 'nail varnish remover' odour). Some patients are hypothermic due to heat loss from peripheral vasodilation, and this may mask the pyrexia of infection. Children with diabetic ketoacidosis often complain of abdominal pain, sometimes mimicking acute appendicitis or other surgical emergencies. A full examination is essential to identify any intercurrent illness.

Investigations and diagnosis

Once suspected, the diagnosis can be confirmed on the spot with a finger-prick blood glucose measurement and urinalysis for ketones. Treatment with intravenous saline and insulin should begin immediately, and baseline investigations carried out. Venous blood is taken for biochemical screening and arterial blood for pH and acid–base status. Additional tests to identify the cause of the episode should include a full blood count, urine and blood culture, chest radiograph, and, especially in older patients, ECG and cardiac enzymes or troponin levels.

Typical values and some diagnostic pitfalls in diabetic ketoacidosis are shown in Fig. 13.11.1.10. Plasma ketone levels are measured by some laboratories or by test strips but are not usually needed for safe management. High ketone concentrations cause a large anion gap, i.e. plasma $[Na^+ + K^+]$ exceeds $[HCO_3^- + Cl^-]$ by more than 17 mmol/litre.

Management

Diabetic ketoacidosis is a potentially life-threatening medical emergency that requires urgent treatment with scrupulous clinical and biochemical monitoring: many avoidable and serious accidents still happen because the patient is abandoned once treatment has been started. Severe diabetic ketoacidosis is best managed initially on a high-dependency or intensive care unit.

The highest priority is to correct hypovolaemia and dehydration, which will often improve acidosis and hyperglycaemia. Insulin replacement must also be started urgently. However, it now appears likely that the high mortality of diabetic ketoacidosis has been partly due to overenergetic replacement of intravenous fluids (especially bicarbonate) and perhaps insulin, which may predispose to the development of cerebral oedema. The treatment guidelines below (see Fig. 13.11.1.10) are based on large studies that have reported very low mortality and morbidity.

Fluid replacement

Good intravenous access is crucial: a large peripheral vein may be used but a central venous cannula is safest for severely hypovolaemic patients and for older people or those at risk of heart failure, in whom monitoring of central venous pressure is essential.

Most patients recover rapidly with slower fluid replacement than was previously recommended. For those who are not shocked give:

◆ 1 to 2 litres in 2 h, then

◆ 1 litre over the next 4 h, then

◆ 4 litres over the next 24 h

Fluid losses in urine or vomit should be added to these volumes. Shocked or oliguric patients may require faster fluid repletion, possibly with plasma expanders rather than saline, while slower replacement is safer in those with signs of fluid overload, myocardial infarction, heart failure, or any suspicion of cerebral oedema. Urine output must be monitored closely, as must blood pressure, central venous filling, and signs of pulmonary or peripheral oedema.

Saline containing potassium is the logical fluid to replace the losses of Na^+, K^+, and Cl^- induced by the osmotic diuresis of diabetic ketoacidosis. The use of intravenous bicarbonate to try to correct acidosis is contentious, both in terms of biochemistry and clinical outcome (see below).

Isotonic (0.9%) saline is used initially. Half isotonic (0.45%) saline has been suggested to empirically replace 1 or 2 litres of isotonic saline, if severe hyperosmolarity (> 350 mosmol/kg) and/or hypernatraemia (> 150 mmol/litre) are present. However, the rationale may be flawed: 0.9% (normal) saline is already hypotonic with respect to the patient's hypertonic plasma, and the use of even more hypotonic solutions would seem likely to exacerbate the intracellular movement of water which may lead to cerebral oedema. Five% dextrose is generally substituted when plasma glucose has fallen to 10 to 14 mmol/litre to prevent hypoglycaemia (insulin is still required to prevent ketogenesis and promote glucose utilization in the tissues).

Intravenous sodium bicarbonate was previously recommended for severe acidosis. However, the hope that adding alkali will correct

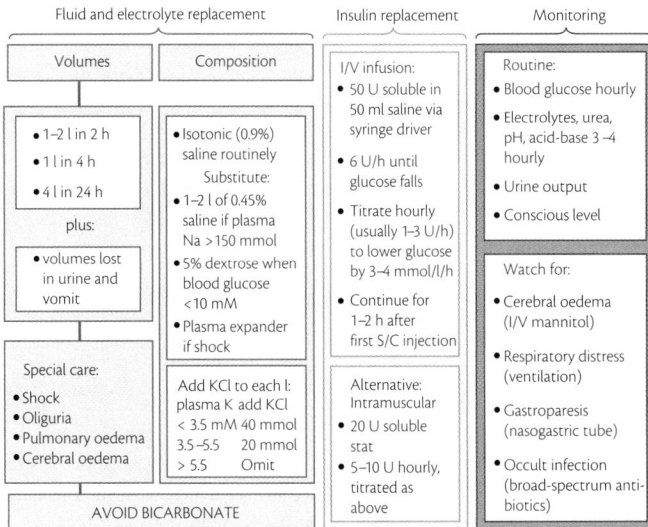

Fig. 13.11.1.10 Guidelines for the management of diabetic ketoacidosis.

acidosis may be oversimplistic. HCO_3^- and H^+ ions (from 3-hydroxybutyric and acetoacetic acids) combine extracellularly to produce H_2CO_3, which dissociates to produce water and CO_2; this may reduce extracellular acidosis, but as cell membranes are impermeable to HCO_3^- ions, the all-important intracellular acidosis is not improved. Indeed, CO_2 can enter cells where it can combine with water to produce H_2CO_3, itself a weak organic acid that can dissociate into H^+ and HCO_3^- ions. Paradoxically, therefore, intravenous bicarbonate administration could worsen intracellular acidosis and there is evidence from animal models of acidosis that this occurs. Worryingly, a recent study identified bicarbonate administration as the most important independent predictor of cerebral oedema in children with moderately severe diabetic ketoacidosis. Another problem with high strength (8.4%) sodium bicarbonate solution is the intense thrombophlebitis it causes when given intravenously, which can obliterate even large central veins. Extravasation can also cause severe tissue necrosis.

The current consensus is that bicarbonate is unlikely to do good but runs the risk of doing harm, and that it should not be used in the treatment of diabetic ketoacidosis

Potassium replacement

Diabetic ketoacidosis always depletes total body K^+ stores to a variable degree because of electrolyte losses through osmotic diuresis, but H^+/K^+ exchange across the plasma membrane encourages K^+ to leak out of cells in acidosis. Plasma K^+ levels can therefore be low, normal, or high, and dangerous hyperkalaemia can be present, especially if severe hypovolaemia causes prerenal failure. During insulin replacement, K^+ is carried intracellularly with glucose, and plasma K^+ levels can fall rapidly. Frequent monitoring of K^+ (every 3 to 4 h initially) is therefore essential in the safe management of diabetic ketoacidosis, and patients with marked K^+ disturbances should have continuous ECG monitoring.

Potassium replacement should be determined by current plasma K^+ levels:

* Add 20 mmol of KCl to each litre of intravenous fluid if K^+ is normal (3.5–5.0 mmol/litre).
* Add 40 mmol/litre of KCl to each litre if plasma K^+ is less than 3.5 mmol/litre.
* Omit KCl if plasma K^+ is more than 5.0 mmol/litre, because of the risk of precipitating arrhythmias.

Insulin replacement

Continuous intravenous infusion is the best way to give insulin in diabetic ketoacidosis; subcutaneous and intramuscular absorption are too erratic to be safe and the rate of fall of glucose (one of the factors implicated in cerebral oedema) cannot be easily controlled.

A dose of 50 U soluble insulin should be added to 50 ml isotonic saline (i.e. 1 U/ml) and delivered by a syringe driver pump, either into a separate vein or piggy-backed into the intravenous fluids line.

Because the half-life of insulin in the circulation is only a few minutes, blood glucose and ketone levels will rise rapidly if insulin delivery is interrupted; hourly monitoring of blood glucose is therefore mandatory during intravenous insulin. Failure of glucose to fall usually means that the pump has been turned off or that the infusion cannula is blocked. Initially, 6 U/h (i.e. 6 ml/h) should be given and once blood glucose has started to fall, the rate can then be titrated so that glucose falls by 3 to 4 mmol/litre every hour. Faster rates of fall are unnecessary, commonly cause hypoglycaemia, and are thought to predispose to cerebral oedema. Most patients need 1 to 3 U of insulin per hour, and the requirement will become clear after 3 to 4 h of blood glucose monitoring.

A typical intravenous sliding scale (based on hourly glucose measurements) is:

* blood glucose less than 4 mmol/litre: give 0.5 ml/h (along with dextrose)
* blood glucose 4.1 to 7 mmol/litre: give 1 ml/h
* blood glucose 7.1 to 11 mmol/litre: give 2 ml/h
* blood glucose 11.1 to 15 mmol/litre: give 4 ml/h
* blood glucose 15.1 to 20 mmol/litre: give 6 ml/h.
* blood glucose greater than 20 mmol/litre: revise sliding scale and review infusion regimen.

An alternative to the syringe driver is to dilute insulin into a larger volume (50 U soluble insulin into 500 ml of saline; 0.1 U/ml) and to regulate delivery (e.g. 20 ml/h (2 U/h)) using an electronic drip counter or a paediatric giving set with a burette.

The GKI infusion used for perioperative management of diabetic patients (see above) is not appropriate because it assumes that the patient is in steady state (which is not the case) and because K^+ disturbances may be exacerbated; moreover, making up and changing GKI infusion bags is time-consuming and in practice is very rarely done as often as is needed to control the fall in glucose.

If it is impossible to give a controlled intravenous infusion, then intramuscular soluble insulin can be injected every 4 h or so, starting with 20 U and attempting to titrate subsequent dosages (e.g. 5–10 U hourly).

Other complications

Intercurrent illness must be treated energetically. Broad-spectrum antibiotics are often given prospectively. Myocardial infarction (see below) has a poor prognosis if it causes diabetic ketoacidosis.

Shock may lead to prerenal failure and sometimes acute tubular necrosis. Plasma expanders and inotropes may occasionally be required for severe hypotension, although rehydration as above is usually adequate.

Cerebral oedema still accounts for 50% of fatalities in diabetic ketoacidosis, especially in children, although modern management protocols with slower fluid replacement and low-dose intravenous insulin infusion can markedly reduce its incidence. The cause is thought to be shifts of ions and water into the brain, particularly the movement of water into dehydrated, hypertonic cells when relatively hypotonic fluids reach the extracellular space. Such shifts would be predicted with the administration of isotonic and particularly with hypotonic fluids. Risk factors for cerebral oedema include over-rapid falls in blood glucose, excessive fluid replacement, and high insulin dosages. Insulin can affect various ion transport mechanisms in the brain, but its role remains mysterious and may simply reflect changes in extracellular osmolarity. Interestingly, CT scanning before fluid and insulin replacement has demonstrated subclinical cerebral oedema in children with diabetic ketoacidosis.

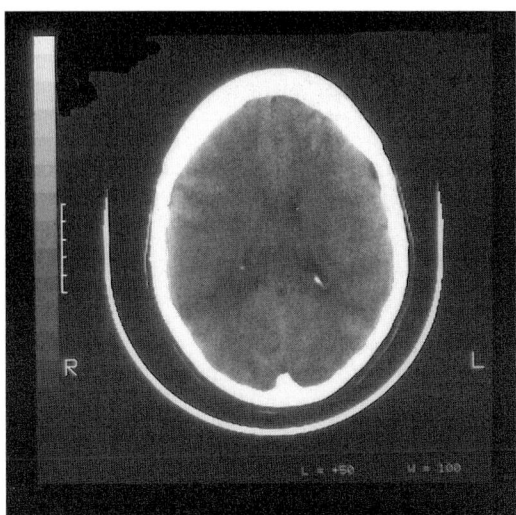

Fig. 13.11.1.11 Cerebral oedema in a patient recovering from diabetic ketoacidosis. The CT shows generalized swelling and loss of cortical detail with squashing of the cerebral ventricles.

Swelling of the brain within the cranium causes coning, leading to cardiorespiratory arrest. It presents as a decline in consciousness, usually rapid and often when the patient's metabolic state has been stabilized. Papilloedema may be present, and CT or MRI will show characteristic swelling, with loss of cortical features and squashing of the ventricular system (Fig. 13.11.1.11). It is usually fatal (in >90% of established cases), but intravenous mannitol (0.2 g/kg over 30 min, repeated hourly if there is no improvement) may help by raising the osmolality of extracellular fluid and drawing free water out of the brain; there is no firm evidence to support the use of dexamethasone.

Adult respiratory distress syndrome is due to accumulation of fluid in the alveoli, perhaps due to ionic and water shifts or to excessive leakiness of the pulmonary capillaries. Hypoxia is severe, and chest radiography shows an appearance like left ventricular failure but with a normal heart size. Risk factors include rapid fluid replacement. It carries a poor prognosis, but ventilation with high-concentration oxygen may be useful supportive treatment.

Acute gastric dilatation (gastroparesis) presents with vomiting and may produce a succussion splash and a ground-glass appearance on abdominal radiograph. Nasogastric drainage may be needed to prevent aspiration, especially in the unconscious patient.

Hypotension may persist or develop during treatment and generally reflects inadequate fluid replacement. Alternative causes of hypotension including septic shock and cardiogenic shock should also be considered. Polyuria secondary to continuing high glucose levels may occasionally give false reassurance that the patient's fluid replacement status is adequate.

Persisting acidosis despite correction of blood sugar levels and a fall in plasma (and later urine) ketones raises the possibility of lactic acidosis secondary to sepsis or metformin use (see below). Blood lactate levels should be measured. Plasma sodium levels may rise despite fluid replacement as the initial high glucose levels may have resulted in an erroneously low initial reading. Falling sodium levels may reflect the need for more saline and less dextrose-based fluid replacement.

Hypothermia indicates a poor outcome. It may respond to rewarming with a space blanket.

Subsequent management

When the patient can eat and drink, intravenous fluids and insulin can be discontinued. There is no need for a GKI regimen; instead, the patient can be restarted on their usual insulin regimen (or on twice-daily mixed insulin, if newly diagnosed). The intravenous insulin infusion should be maintained until the first injection has had time to act (3–4 h for long-acting insulin alone).

The causes of the episode must be determined if possible, and efforts made to prevent it from happening again. The patient's understanding of diabetes, including the 'sick-day' rules (Box 13.11.1.1), must be checked and reinforced if necessary. Recurrent diabetic ketoacidosis is a feature of brittle diabetes, and these patients need careful monitoring and counselling.

Hyperosmolar nonketotic state (HONK)

HONK is distinguished from diabetic ketoacidosis by the absence of marked hyperketonaemia and metabolic acidosis. Hyperglycaemia can be greater than in diabetic ketoacidosis and, together with a rise in urea due to dehydration and prerenal failure, may elevate the plasma osmolality to well over 350 mosmol/kg. HONK may be the first presentation of type 2 diabetes.

Ketosis does not develop because circulating insulin levels are high enough to suppress lipolysis and ketogenesis; these patients are therefore C-peptide positive, with type 2 diabetes which is often previously undiagnosed. It is more common in people of Afro-Caribbean origin. Precipitating factors include myocardial infarction, stroke, infection, and diabetogenic drugs such as glucocorticoids and thiazide diuretics; fizzy glucose drinks may also contribute.

Presentation is typically with classical hyperglycaemic symptoms (polyuria, intense thirst, weight loss, blurred vision), without the features of ketoacidosis. Confusion, drowsiness, and coma are more common than in diabetic ketoacidosis. At blood glucose levels over 30 mmol/litre, drowsiness can lead to a cycle of deterioration as fluid loss continues due to the osmotic diuresis but the patient is increasingly too lethargic to drink adequate replacement fluids. Progressive dehydration then leads to even higher glucose levels, more lethargy and a further decline in oral intake.

Complications include thrombotic events such as stroke and peripheral arterial occlusion, and deep venous thrombosis and pulmonary embolism, these being due apparently to increased blood viscosity. Mortality exceeds 30%, partly because these patients are old and often have a serious precipitating illness.

Biochemical features of HONK state are:

- hyperglycaemia: often over 50 mmol/litre, sometimes over 90 mmol/litre

- hypernatraemia: often over 155 mmol/litre (may be artefactually depressed by high glucose levels)

- uraemia due to dehydration, with or without renal failure

- hypersmolality: over 350 mosmol/kg

- blood and ketone levels are normal or only slightly raised (usually through anorexia)

- arterial pH, venous bicarbonate, and anion gap show no features of severe acidosis

Management is largely as for diabetic ketoacidosis:

- Saline replacement must be particularly cautious in older patients, in whom cardiac disease is common. Half isotonic (0.45%) solution is often given if plasma sodium exceeds 150 mmol/litre or osmolality exceeds 350 mosmol/kg; the rationale for preferring this to isotonic saline is not proven, but the risks of cerebral oedema appear to be lower than in diabetic ketoacidosis.

- Potassium levels must be carefully monitored and replaced as above.

- Intravenous insulin infusion at low doses rapidly controls hyperglycaemia in most cases.

- low-dose heparin (5000 U subcutaneously 8-hourly or low molecular weight heparin once daily) should be given prophylactically, but full anticoagulation should be reserved for proven thromboembolism as the risks of fatal gastrointestinal bleeding are high. Intercurrent illness must be sought and treated appropriately.

After recovery, many of these patients can be successfully weaned off insulin. Drugs and other precipitating factors must be identified and avoided if possible.

Lactic acidosis

Lactate is generated by glycolysis and its levels rise rapidly during tissue anoxia (e.g. during shock, cardiac failure, or pneumonia) or when the liver is prevented from utilizing it as a gluconeogenic substrate (e.g. in hepatic impairment). Lactic acidosis is best known in diabetic patients as a rare but often fatal complication of the biguanides, phenformin and metformin, which act mainly by inhibiting hepatic gluconeogenesis. The risk is about 10 times higher with phenformin than with metformin, and it is very rare during metformin treatment as long as other predisposing factors (the major organ failures) are avoided.

Lactic acidosis presents as coma with metabolic acidosis (reduced arterial pH and venous bicarbonate) and a wide anion gap due to hyperlactataemia. Blood glucose levels are usually raised.

Treatment is still unsatisfactory. Intravenous sodium bicarbonate may paradoxically aggravate intracellular acidosis, although forced ventilation to blow off carbon dioxide may help (see above). Haemodialysis may both clear lactate and hydrogen ions, and correct any sodium overload following bicarbonate administration. Sodium dichloroacetate, which stimulates pyruvate dehydrogenase to metabolize lactate, is undergoing evaluation.

Mortality remains high (>30%), partly because of the organ failures that commonly coexist.

Hypoglycaemia

Hypoglycaemia is an inevitable side effect of antidiabetic drugs that raise circulating insulin levels, namely insulin itself and sulphonylureas; it does not occur with metformin or thiazolidinediones alone, or with dietary restriction. Common contributory factors are:

- accelerated insulin absorption, e.g. due to exercise or hot surroundings

- unfavourable timing of insulin injection: injecting too soon before eating can cause late postprandial hypoglycaemia, while long-acting insulins injected in the early evening often cause nocturnal hypoglycaemia

- too much insulin injected: dosage errors are quite common, particularly in older people

- inadequate food intake: missed, delayed, or small meals; vomiting, including gastroparesis

- exercise: this hastens insulin absorption while enhancing insulin action; delayed hypoglycaemia may occur many hours later because muscle continues to take up glucose to replenish glycogen

- alcohol: this inhibits hepatic gluconeogenesis, preventing the increase in hepatic glucose output that is crucial for restoring euglycaemia

- impaired awareness of early warning symptoms (see below)

Progressively more frequent or severe attacks may be caused by various conditions, which should always be sought:

- weight loss, including anorexia nervosa and appetite disorders (relatively common in young women with type 1 diabetes)

- loss of counter-regulatory hormones: Addison's disease, hypothyroidism, hypopituitarism, blunted glucagon secretion in long-standing type 1 diabetes.

- intestinal malabsorption, notably coeliac disease (more common in type 1 diabetes)

- renal failure, which impairs the clearance of insulin

- deliberate inappropriate injection of insulin, often in the context of 'brittle' diabetes

Manifestations

Clinical features of hypoglycaemia are due to an autonomic discharge, predominantly sympathetic, together with the cerebral effects of neuroglycopenia. Falling glucose levels are sensed by glucose-sensitive neurons, which are found in the periphery (vagal sensory endings in the portal vein) and medulla as well as the hypothalamus. This triggers a powerful sympathetic discharge that releases adrenaline from the adrenal medulla and noradrenaline from sympathetic nerve endings, causing the familiar 'flight or fight' response. Features include pallor (cutaneous vasoconstriction), sweating (which can be very profuse), tremor (a β_2-adrenergic effect on skeletal muscle), and tachycardia; systolic blood pressure rises due to increased cardiac output while pulse pressure widens—giving the typical bounding pulse—because β_2-mediated vasodilatation in skeletal muscle causes peripheral resistance to fall.

Hypoglycaemia also triggers the secretion of counter-regulatory hormones, namely glucagon and adrenaline (both crucial to restoring euglycaemia), growth hormone, and cortisol. Collectively, these inhibit insulin secretion and raise blood glucose by enhancing hepatic glycogenolysis and gluconeogenesis, causing glucose to pour out of the liver. Defects in glucagon or adrenaline release (which occur in long-standing type 1 diabetes, for example), or in the ability of the liver to produce glucose (e.g. the presence of ethanol which inhibits gluconeogenesis, or a recent glucagon injection which depletes liver glycogen) will delay recovery of blood glucose.

The physiological and neurological features of hypoglycaemia usually develop in a fixed sequence when blood glucose is lowered in a controlled fashion in the laboratory. However, this hierarchy may not be apparent in real life, and some patients specifically lose their awareness of the early warning symptoms (see below). Key events as glucose falls are:

- at *c*.3.8 mmol/litre: increased glucagon and adrenaline secretion
- at *c*.3.0 mmol/litre: onset of hypoglycaemic symptoms
- at *c*.2.8 mmol/litre: neuroglycopenia and cognitive impairment
- <2 mmol/litre: coma.

Symptoms of hypoglycaemia

The symptom complex can be extremely variable, and hypoglycaemia should be suspected as the cause of any 'funny turn' in patients treated with insulin or sulphonylureas. Autonomic manifestations include sweating, tremor, tachycardia, and hunger, while neuroglycopenia can cause drowsiness, confusion, incoordination, dysarthria, and automatic or disinhibited behaviour; distinct neurological deficits include aphasia, diplopia, and hemiparesis. Nonspecific malaise and headache afterwards are also common. Nocturnal episodes may pass completely unnoticed by the patient, or may cause sweating and restlessness (often obvious to the patient's partner), vivid nightmares, nocturnal epilepsy, or a hung-over feeling the following morning.

Awareness of hypoglycaemic symptoms

Diabetic patients rely on the early autonomic symptoms (sweating, shaking, and hunger) to warn them of an impending hypoglycaemic attack, when corrective action can be taken. In some patients, the early warning symptoms are attenuated or not noticed at all; this clumsily named 'hypoglycaemia unawareness' is potentially dangerous because severe neuroglycopenia (confusion, fitting, irrational behaviour, coma) may suddenly incapacitate the patient. Reduced awareness of hypoglycaemia occurs particularly in two settings, which may coexist:

- Long-standing type 1 diabetes. Some 30 to 50% of patients with diabetes of more than 20 years' duration have decreased awareness of symptoms, and many also show a flat glucagon and adrenaline response to hypoglycaemia. Blunted recognition of hypoglycaemia by the central nervous system may be responsible.
- Excessively tight glycaemic control impairs awareness of hypoglycaemia; for unknown reasons, even a single episode can blunt perception of symptoms and counter-regulatory hormone responses for some days. Conversely, relaxing control and avoiding hypoglycaemia completely for several weeks can partially restore awareness of warning symptoms.

The use of human insulin has been suggested to impair awareness of hypoglycaemic symptoms. Human insulin is relatively lipophilic—hence its faster subcutaneous absorption—which could theoretically promote its entry into the brain. Insulin may act directly on the brain to affect various autonomic processes, but detailed comparisons of human and animal insulins, both in the laboratory and in real life, have not shown any species differences in counter-regulatory responses or the intensity of hypoglycaemic symptoms.

Sequelae of hypoglycaemia

Even the most dramatic neurological manifestations of acute hypoglycaemia—including aphasia, hemiparesis, fitting, and unconsciousness—usually resolve rapidly when blood glucose is normalized. Recovery from profound coma may take many hours or even days, and this is probably due to cerebral oedema. Patients who survive severe and prolonged hypoglycaemic coma may show permanent neurological damage, including memory loss, aphasia, and a vegetative state. There are concerns that repeated mild attacks, especially in children and perhaps particularly at night, can cause cumulative intellectual impairment, but this is not yet proven.

Severe hypoglycaemia has been implicated in precipitating myocardial infarction or stroke, particularly in older people; rises in blood pressure and increased coagulability of the blood following sympathetic stimulation may contribute. Like any convulsions, hypoglycaemic fits may cause injury, including limb and vertebral crush fractures.

Prolonged severe hypoglycaemia can be fatal and is one of the most common causes of death in young type 1 patients. Postmortem studies show neuronal damage and necrosis in the hippocampus and cerebral cortex. Hypoglycaemia has been suspected as a cause of death in patients found unexpectedly dead in bed; arrhythmias may be responsible.

Diagnosis and detection of hypoglycaemia

Hypoglycaemia is easy to diagnose but is also easily missed; differential diagnoses include transient ischaemic attacks, psychosis, drunkenness, epilepsy, and migraine. Symptoms may be instantly recognizable to some patients, but may present atypically. If suspected, the blood glucose levels should be checked, taking care to avoid under-reading artefacts with reagent test strips. Urinalysis is obviously of no use—hence all patients receiving insulin or sulphonylureas must be able to check their blood glucose. The patient's close associates should also know how to diagnose and treat hypoglycaemia.

Various experimental hypoglycaemia detectors are undergoing development including subcutaneous sensors and transcutaneous near-infrared spectroscopy. Subcutaneous sensors able to give a real-time display of blood glucose levels every few minutes are now available and may prove especially valuable in recurrent hypoglycaemia. Current limitations include cost (sensors require replacing every 3–6 days) and the fact that there is a delay of approximately 20 min before interstitial fluid and blood glucose levels equilibrate, which means that the sensor can underestimate the severity of hypoglycaemia when blood glucose levels are falling rapidly.

Prevention and treatment of hypoglycaemia

It has been shown that insulin-treated patients fear hypoglycaemia as much as blindness or renal failure; this may prevent them from tightening their diabetic control as much as their doctors would prefer. Many doctors underestimate the impact of hypoglycaemia; asking about it and trying actively to prevent it are an essential part of diabetes care. It should emphasized that a 'good' HbA_{1c} level can be misleading in this context, as it can be the result of a combination of high blood glucose levels and recurrent hypoglycaemia.

Attention to the factors listed above should help to reduce the frequency and severity of attacks. Advice about exercise, moderating alcohol intake, and timing of insulin injections and meals are particularly important. Nocturnal hypoglycaemia can be reduced by checking the blood glucose at bedtime, and by taking long-acting carbohydrate (e.g. bread or cereal) if the level is less than 6 mmol/litre. Long-acting analogue insulin and insulin pump therapy may also be of value in this situation (see above).

Blood glucose levels of less than 3 mmol/litre should be treated immediately (see Table 13.11.1.7). Oral glucose or sucrose or other carbohydrate should be given if the patient can swallow safely. Give 20 to 30 g (e.g. 3–6 Dextrosol tablets or 75–150 ml of a glucose drink such as Lucozade) initially; if possible, check the blood glucose 15 min later and repeat glucose administration if this has not risen. Taking too much carbohydrate—which is an understandable reaction, given the unpleasantness of hypoglycaemia—can cause marked rebound hyperglycaemia.

If the patient is unconscious, give either:

+ glucagon 1 mg (0.5 mg in children), subcutaneously or intramuscularly; with either route, glucose should rise within 10 to 15 min. Side effects of glucagon include malaise, nausea, and abdominal discomfort. Importantly, as glucagon acts primarily by breaking down hepatic glycogen (a limited resource), a second injection may be ineffective

+ intravenous glucose: 15 to 20 g intravenously, as a 50% or 10% solution (the former may cause painful thrombophlebitis, even if given into a large vein)

Glucose gels or jam can be smeared inside the mouth and cheeks in the unconscious patient, but these alone are unlikely to correct serious hypoglycaemia.

On recovery, blood glucose should be checked and oral glucose given as above. Slow recovery from coma may be due to cerebral oedema, which has a high mortality (*c.*10%) but may respond to intravenous mannitol and forced ventilation with high inspired oxygen concentration. Once the episode is treated, its cause must be identified if possible and corrective action taken to prevent it from happening again.

Options for intractable, recurrent hypoglycaemia

Recurrent, disabling hypoglycaemia often develops in patients who have maintained very tight glycaemic control over many years. The frequent hypoglycaemic episodes that often occur with tight control themselves result in loss of hypoglycaemia awareness and

Table 13.11.1.7 Management of hypoglycaemia

Immediate	
Patient conscious	Oral glucose (20–30 g) or sucrose
Patient unconscious	Intravenous glucose (30–50 ml of 50% solution. NB: risk of necrosis if extravasates) or Intramuscular or subcutaneous glucagon (1 mg; 0.5 mg in children)[a]
Then	Check blood glucose after 15–20 min
	Confirm recovery (glucose > 5 mmol/litre)
On recovery	Give long acting carbohydrate (e.g. sandwich, meal) Identify cause
	Re-educate patient to avoid future episodes
If recovery is delayed	
Patient unconscious	Set up infusion of 10% dextrose; transfer to hospital
Patient conscious	Take more oral glucose

[a] Caution with glucagon: it often causes nausea and malaise; depletes liver glycogen—a second injection may therefore be ineffective; contraindicated in hypoglycaemia caused by sulphonylureas (glucagon stimulates insulin secretion).

physiological defence mechanisms (e.g. glucagon and adrenaline). The result is more frequent hypoglycaemia—'hypoglycaemia begets hypoglycaemia'. Options for reversing this situation include careful inspection of injection sites and avoidance of areas of lipohypertrophy or potential for inadvertent intramuscular injection, attempting less tight glycaemic control, the use of analogue insulins and carbohydrate counting as part of intensive multiple-dose insulin therapy, and insulin pump therapy (with or without real-time glucose monitoring). If these measures fail and recurrent hypoglycaemia continues to impact very significantly on the patient's quality of life, islet transplantation remains an option as it generally achieves marked improvement in hypoglycaemia with a lower risk procedure than whole pancreas transplantation (see above). The patients are nonetheless exposed to immunosuppressive risks which need to be taken into account in weighing the risks and benefits.

Chronic complications of diabetes

Long-term tissue damage is now the major burden of the disease, the greatest source of fear for diabetic people, and the most expensive item in the diabetes health care budget. The list of possible complications is depressingly long but fortunately at least 40% of diabetic patients escape clinically significant complications, and improved diabetes care should reduce the risks even further.

Microvascular complications—retinopathy, nephropathy, and neuropathy—are specific to diabetes and reflect the damage inflicted on the microcirculation throughout the body. Retinopathy and nephropathy are obviously microvascular disorders; the microcirculation of nerves (vasa nervorum) is also damaged in diabetic neuropathy, although other functional and structural abnormalities in the nerves themselves probably contribute. Macrovascular disease is simply atherosclerosis. This causes typical coronary heart disease, stroke, and peripheral arterial disease, but often behaves more aggressively than in nondiabetic people.

Other complications are due to irreversible biochemical and structural changes in tissues chronically exposed to hyperglycaemia. These include cataract, whose formation during normal ageing is accelerated by diabetes, and specific soft tissue disorders such as limited joint mobility (diabetic cheiroarthropathy).

Causes of chronic diabetic complications

Role of hyperglycaemia

Tissue lesions are identical in all types of diabetes, indicating that hyperglycaemia (or a closely related metabolic abnormality) is likely to be responsible. Microvascular disease in the retina, kidneys, and nerves is generally determined by the severity and duration of hyperglycaemia, although individual susceptibility varies considerably. By contrast, macrovascular disease does not display a clear dose–response relationship with hyperglycaemia: instead, the risk is increased above glucose values that lie below the diabetic range (see above).

Recent intervention studies have confirmed that improving glycaemic control is rewarded by partial protection against microvascular complications but not atheroma. This principle is valid for both type 1 and type 2 diabetes, and is now embodied in their treatment targets (see Table 13.11.1.3). Two landmark studies are generally cited, although several smaller ones have also reached the same conclusion.

Type 1 diabetes

The Diabetes Control and Complications Trial (DCCT) was a 12 year North American study of over 1400 patients that compared intensive insulin treatment (aiming for an HbA_{1c} of 6%) with conventional (i.e. bad) regimens of once or twice daily injections (HbA_{1c} about 9%). Intensive treatment consisted of at least three daily injections or an insulin pump (CSII), and achieved a mean HbA_{1c} of 7%.

The trial concluded that improved glycaemic control reduced the risks of microvascular complications. In subjects who were initially free of complications, intensified treatment for 9 years decreased the prevalence of a defined degree of background retinopathy by 70% (i.e. from 55% with conventional treatment to 15% see Fig. 13.11.1.12), while the risks of developing microalbuminuria or clinical neuropathy fell by 33% and 70% respectively. In subjects who already had background retinopathy at baseline, intensified treatment reduced the overall progression of retinopathy by 50%; more importantly the risks of suffering sight-threatening retinopathy or requiring laser treatment were reduced by a similar degree. The development of clinical nephropathy (overt albuminuria) and neuropathy were each decreased by about 60%. By contrast, intensified insulin treatment did not reduce the prevalence of macrovascular disease. However, an 11 year follow-up of subjects after the end of the trial (the Epidemiology of Diabetes Interventions and Complications study, EDIC) showed a reduction in cardiovascular events in the subjects who had previously been in the intensive treatment arm, indicating that a prolonged period of good glycaemic control does confer a lasting cardiovascular protective effect. Persistent reductions in microvascular complications were also seen in those originally in the intensive therapy group, despite the fact that HbA1c levels were similar in the extended follow period, indicating that good glycaemic control in the early years can have very long-lasting benefits.

Type 2 diabetes

The United Kingdom Prospective Diabetes Study (UKPDS) was guided through its 20-year course by the late Robert Turner, who died shortly after it was completed. This very large trial followed the outcome of over 5000 patients treated with diet and lifestyle alone (termed 'conventional' treatment), or together with sulphonylureas, metformin, or insulin; confusingly, sulphonylureas and insulin treatments were both described as 'intensive' treatment. The trial confirmed the real-life difficulty of achieving good glycaemic control, especially against the progressive deterioration of type 2 diabetes: very few patients achieved and maintained the intensive target fasting plasma glucose of 6 mmol/litre. The trial has been criticized for its convoluted design (which diluted its statistical power) and both the lumping and splitting of data for outcome analysis. Nevertheless, it yielded useful messages about the importance of treating both hyperglycaemia and hypertension and about the natural history of the disease itself. Its conclusions were broadly similar to those of the DCCT study: improved glycaemic control decreased the risk of microvascular complications. Lowering HbA_{1c} from 7.9% (conventional) to 7.0% (intensive) decreased the lumped rate of microvascular events by 25% (see Fig. 13.11.1.13), including sight-threatening retinopathy (20%) and the development of microalbuminuria (33%). Across a reasonably wide range of HbA_{1c}, lowering HbA_{1c} by 1% reduced the risk of microvascular disease by about one-third. Improved glycaemic control had no overall effect on macrovascular disease, although metformin treatment significantly decreased cardiovascular events (see above). By contrast, blood pressure lowering had very significant benefits in terms of both micro- and macrovascular disease (see Fig. 13.11.1.12). Extended follow-up results of the UKPDS study have now been reported. These show that although the difference in HbA1c and blood pressure control between conventional and intensively treated groups was lost during period, intensively treated subjects still had lower myocardial infarction and death rate (for treatment with metformin, suphonylureas or insulin) and microvasular complications (for subjects treated with sulphonylureas or insulin) 10 years beyond the end of the study. This extended benefit from early tight control has been referred to as a "legacy effect" and similar benefits are seen in type 1 diabetes (see above). Note that by contrast no "legacy effect" was seen with blood pressure lowering - within 1–2 years of blood pressures equating between the conventional and intensively treated groups any benefit from earlier blood pressure lowering was lost.

Possible mechanisms of hyperglycaemic tissue damage

High glucose levels can damage the function and structure of many tissues. The mechanisms currently thought most relevant to human diabetic complications probably operate to different degrees in different tissues.

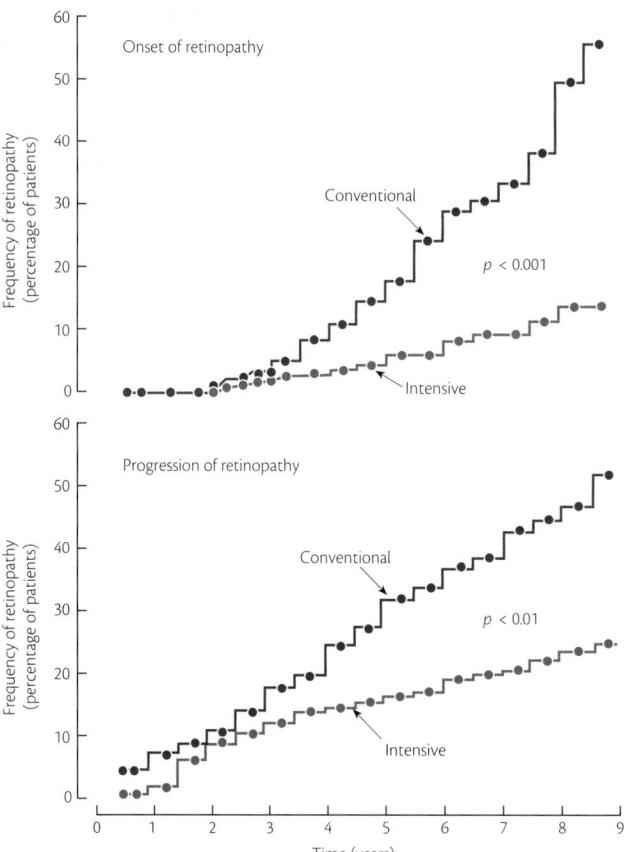

Fig. 13.11.1.12 Intensive insulin therapy and improved diabetic control in type 1 diabetes reduces the risks of developing retinopathy (upper panel) and of established retinopathy progressing (lower panel).
(Data from the Diabetic Control and Complications Trial (DCCT).)

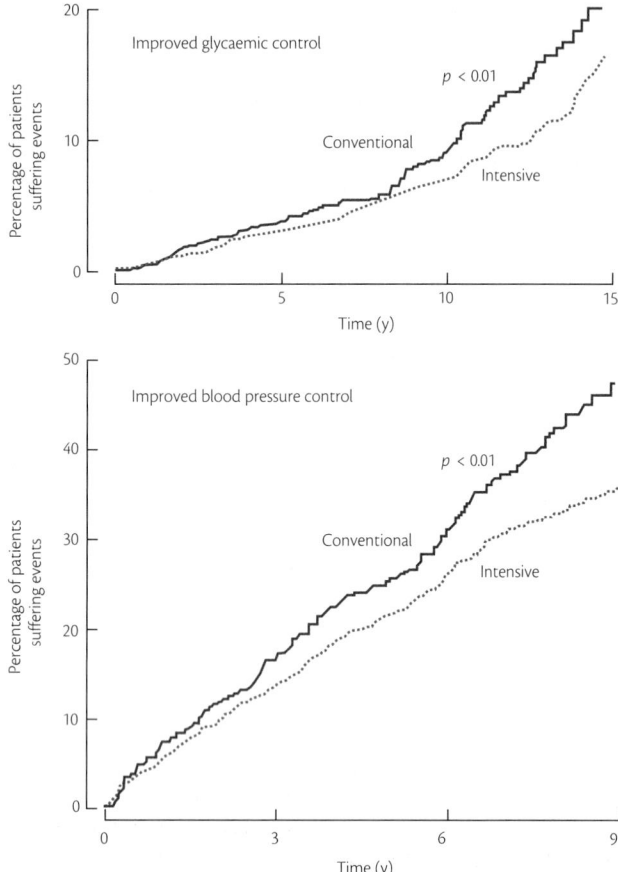

Fig. 13.11.1.13 Benefits of improving glycaemic and blood pressure control in type 2 diabetic patients. Upper panel: intensive treatment with glucose-lowering drugs reduces the risks of suffering any microvascular complication by about 25%. Lower panel: tighter control of blood pressure reduces the risks of suffering any diabetes-related complication (including micro- and macrovascular disease) by about 24%. Note the scale differences in both axes.
(Data from the United Kingdom Prospective Diabetes Study (UKPDS).)

Glycation of proteins and macromolecules

Glycation begins with the nonenzymatic combination of glucose and other reactive sugars with amino groups of proteins, and with acceptor groups of other long-lived macromolecules such as nucleic acids. Glycation is initially reversible, yielding a Schiff base which undergoes molecular rearrangement to form an Amadori product. Amadori products then undergo further reactions, including covalent cross-linking with the sugar groups in other glycated proteins. These irreversibly modified molecules, collectively termed advanced glycation endproducts, resist normal degradation mechanisms and thus accumulate.

Advanced glycation endproducts (AGE) can interfere with tissue structure and function in several ways. Stiffening of connective tissue in the limited joint mobility syndrome (see below) is related to cross-linking of collagen by AGE, while the same process in the proteins of the lens fibre (crystallins) causes cataract. AGE also damage blood vessels, and formation of AGE in the basement membrane increases vascular permeability. AGE in the arterial wall may bind low-density lipoprotein and promote atherogenesis. Curiously, endothelial cells carry specific receptors for AGE (RAGE); binding AGE to RAGE receptors generates oxygen free radicals that may induce oxidative damage and favour coagulation.

Overactivity of the polyol pathway

Polyols are sugar alcohols formed from their respective sugars (e.g. sorbitol from glucose) under the action of aldose reductase, the rate-limiting enzyme of the polyol pathway. This enzyme is expressed in various tissues susceptible to diabetic complications, notably the retina, glomerulus, lens epithelium, and Schwann cells of the nerves.

Glucose is preferentially shunted through the polyol pathway under hyperglycaemic conditions, generating sorbitol which is poorly diffusible and therefore accumulates intracellularly. This, together with reciprocal intracellular depletion of myoinositol (another polyol, involved in phosphatidylinositol metabolism) may lead to activation of protein kinase C (see below) and the production of highly reactive sugars that can glycate proteins. Increased glucose flux through the polyol pathway also generates oxygen free radicals and can deplete antioxidants which normally mop up free radicals.

At present, the importance of the polyol pathway in humans remains uncertain. Clinical trials of various aldose reductase inhibitors (e.g. sorbinil and ponalrestat) have failed to show any convincing benefits in human microvascular complications.

Protein kinase C activation

This enzyme is stimulated by diacylglycerol, which is generated intracellularly in hyperglycaemia. Protein kinase C may mediate adverse effects such as increased vascular permeability and enhanced basement membrane synthesis, although the mechanisms remain obscure.

Abnormal microvascular blood flow

Diabetes interferes with blood flow through the microcirculation, potentially impairing the supply of nutrients and oxygen to the tissues. Resting blood flow is increased in the retina, glomerulus, and other tissues, apparently in response to hyperglycaemia; this may damage the endothelium, favouring thrombogenesis (diabetes also enhances the coagulability of the blood) and perhaps the release of vasoconstrictors such as the endothelins, which may cause microvascular occlusion.

Other factors

Individual susceptibility to microvascular and macrovascular complications varies widely, to a degree that is not entirely explicable by differences in hyperglycaemia. Other risk factors include hypertension, which predisposes to atheroma and is also crucial in determining the rate of deterioration of diabetic nephropathy (see Chapter 21.10.1) and perhaps retinopathy. Smoking is implicated in retinopathy and nephropathy as well as macrovascular disease. Familial clustering of markers for nephropathy has been reported (Chapter 21.10.1), with preliminary evidence for polymorphisms in genes including the carnosinase 1 gene *CNDP1* on chromosome 18q, the adiponectin gene *ADIPOQ* on 3q, and the engulfment and cell motility gene *ELMO1* on 7p.

Diabetic eye disease

Eye complications are greatly feared by diabetic patients, with good reason: in the United Kingdom and most Westernized countries, diabetes (especially diabetic retinopathy) is the most common cause of blindness in people of working age. Annual screening is advisable, with prompt referral for laser treatment if appropriate.

Diabetic retinopathy

This is an easily demonstrated example of the microvascular damage that diabetes inflicts throughout the body. The retina is particularly vulnerable because of its high metabolic and oxygen demands and its dependence on an intact blood–retinal barrier; moreover, small lesions that would pass unnoticed in other vascular beds can have a devastating impact on patients and their quality of life.

Epidemiology

Minor background changes, especially the characteristic microaneurysms, are very common in type 1 patients. Microaneurysms begin to appear after 5 years, affecting about 50% of cases at 10 years and virtually all after 20 years. By contrast, the formation of new vessels that defines proliferative retinopathy emerges after 10 years, reaching a plateau at about 40% of all cases after 20 years. The incidence of maculopathy follows a similar curve, ultimately affecting 10 to 20% of cases (more in older subjects). These different patterns suggest that distinct processes are responsible, and that susceptibility to neovascularization and maculopathy may be determined by factors additional to hyperglycaemia.

In type 2 patients, background changes and sometimes maculopathy and proliferative retinopathy may be present at diagnosis, consistent with the generally long duration of subclinical hyperglycaemia.

All grades of retinopathy can complicate any type of diabetes of sufficiently long duration, with some provisos. Retinopathy may be slow to appear in the mildly hyperglycaemic variants of MODY, while some racial groups (e.g. Native Americans and Afro-Caribbeans) appear more susceptible. The sexes are equally affected.

Aetiology and pathogenesis

Progression of retinopathy is generally related to the severity and duration of hyperglycaemia, while lowering blood glucose can slow or even prevent the process (see above). Hyperglycaemia damages the retinal vessels in various ways; glycation of key proteins and overactivity of protein kinase C appear to be more important than abnormalities of the polyol pathway.

When differences in glycaemic control are allowed for, there remains considerable individual variability in susceptibility. Genetic factors appear less important than in nephropathy (see above), while hypertension and possibly cigarette smoking may accelerate progression.

Increased vascular permeability, which leads to macular oedema and hard exudates, is an early abnormality, demonstrable by fluorescein angiography. Likely causes include glycation and other changes in the basement membrane of the microvessels, abolishing the negative charge which normally repels plasma proteins such as albumin, and endothelial cell damage, which opens up the tight intercellular junctions that constitute the blood–retinal barrier. Local production of vascular endothelial growth factor, which enhances permeability, may also contribute. Fallout of pericytes, the specialized contractile cells that enclose the capillaries, may weaken the capillary wall, increasing retinal blood flow and leading to the formation of microaneurysms. Increased retinal blood flow, perhaps following pericyte loss and hyperglycaemia *per se*, may cause endothelial damage and thrombogenesis and also enhance protein extravasation. Capillary occlusion is probably due to the formation of microthrombi following endothelial damage and diabetes-related changes in coagulability. Closure produces areas of capillary nonperfusion, which can be surprisingly widespread when shown by fluorescein angiography, and ultimately foci of

ischaemia where the retina may infarct (causing cotton wool spots) and angiogenesis may be stimulated.

New vessel formation is thought to be stimulated by growth factors released by ischaemic tissues, which cause endothelial cells to proliferate. A currently favoured angiogenic factor is vascular endothelial growth factor, a 46-kDa dimeric protein which is expressed, together with its receptors, by retinal endothelial cells; its expression is enhanced by hypoxia and its effects include both increased vascular permeability and endothelial cell proliferation. New vessels sprout initially as solid buds of endothelial cells that later canalize. They can grow within the retina, forward into the vitreous, or across the iris, and are indirectly responsible for the main vision-threatening complications of diabetic retinopathy. They are fragile and rupture easily, causing retinal, preretinal (subhyaloid), vitreous, or anterior chamber haemorrhages, while the fibrous tissue that proliferates around them can cause retinal traction and detachment and lead to glaucoma.

Lesions, clinical stages, and natural history

The stages of diabetic retinopathy are summarized in Fig. 13.11.1.14.

Background retinopathy

Individual lesions may appear and regress but their total density tends to increase with lengthening duration of diabetes. Vision is not damaged unless maculopathy coexists; over 50% of patients do not progress beyond this stage.

Microaneurysms are outpouchings of capillaries, perhaps representing ballooning of the weakened capillary wall or endothelial buds attempting to revascularize the ischaemic retina. They appear as tiny red dots. Microaneurysms are not fixed features: about 50% disappear within 3 years. The sudden appearance of numerous microaneurysms often indicates worsening retinal ischaemia and can herald preproliferative and proliferative changes.

Hard exudates are due to the precipitation in the retina of lipoproteins and other circulating proteins that escape from abnormally leaky retinal vessels. They are yellow-white spots or streaks with a waxy or shiny appearance, and often form clusters or arcs (a circinate pattern) around the macula and foci of capillary leakage. Like microaneurysms, their distribution and extent can vary markedly with time.

Haemorrhages are due to the rupture of weakened capillaries, their size and shape depending on their situation. Small 'dot'

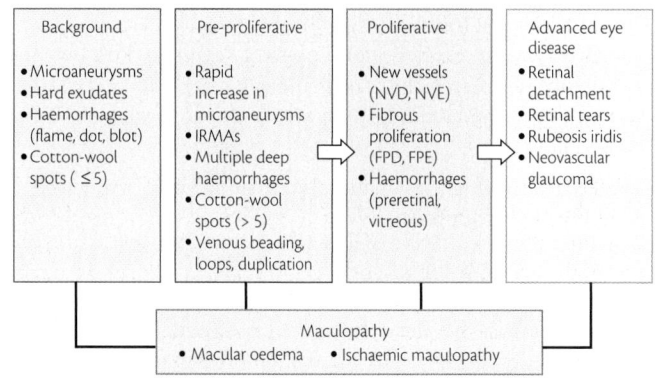

Fig. 13.11.1.14 Stages of diabetic retinopathy. Maculopathy may develop at any stage. FPD/FPE, fibrous proliferation on the disc/elsewhere; IRMAs, intraretinal microvascular abnormalities; NVD/NVE, new vessels on the disc/elsewhere.

and larger 'blot' haemorrhages are spheroidal because they are contained within the densely packed deeper layers of the retina, whereas 'flame' haemorrhages track along nerve fibre bundles in the more superficial layers. Haemorrhages outside the retina (preretinal or vitreous) generally originate from new vessels and therefore indicate proliferative change.

Maculopathy

Disease of the macula, serious enough to affect central vision, can accompany any stage of diabetic retinopathy including background, and may be present in newly diagnosed type 2 patients.

Macular oedema is due to extravasation of plasma proteins across abnormally leaky capillaries. It may cause only retinal thickening which may be undetectable by routine fundoscopy, even when advanced enough to reduce visual acuity. Exudates, often circinate, and spotty cystoid changes may occur.

Ischaemic maculopathy is the result of extensive capillary closure and can cause severe central visual loss. As with macular oedema, fundoscopy may appear deceptively normal; the macula may simply look featureless.

Maculopathy presents as progressive and painless loss of central vision. Testing of visual acuity is important in routine screening for maculopathy: poor acuity with no obvious explanation (e.g. cataract, vitreous haemorrhage) must always prompt specialist assessment for macular oedema or ischaemia. Retinal thickening can be identified easily by slit lamp examination, while fluorescein angiography will demonstrate both ischaemic areas (hypofluorescent) and sites of vascular leakage (hyperfluorescent).

Preproliferative retinopathy

This stage indicates worsening retinal ischaemia which, if left untreated, often leads to the formation of new vessels. It is defined by one or more of the following, of which intraretinal microvascular abnormalities and venous beading are the most ominous:

- multiple deep round haemorrhages, especially when appearing over a short period

- multiple (more than five) cotton wool spots, which are due to the accumulation of axoplasm at the edges of retinal infarcts. they appear as dead-white patches with vague borders

- intraretinal microvascular abnormalities (IRMA)—flat clusters of abnormal capillaries which, unlike new vessels, are confined to the retina and do not leak fluorescein

- venous abnormalities including dilatation (due to general retinal hyperaemia and the shunting of blood around infarcted or non-perfused areas), beading, looping, and reduplication; beading probably represents the terminations of occluded capillaries, while looping and reduplication may be due to local diversion of blood flow

Arterial abnormalities include occlusion, when the vessel is reduced to a thin white line.

Proliferative retinopathy

New vessels appear as fine fronds or arcades of abnormal structure, commonly arising on the optic nerve head (new vessels on disc) or elsewhere, especially at the bifurcation of veins. Greyish fibrous tissues and haemorrhages may be found in association.

Proliferative retinopathy threatens vision through the complications of the abnormal new vessels, namely haemorrhage, retinal detachment, and glaucoma. Overall, only 10% of untreated patients retain useful vision after 10 years. New vessels on the disc carry the worst prognosis: if left untreated, the chances of becoming blind within 5 years are over 50% (compared with 30% for new vessels elsewhere). Vitreous haemorrhages tend to recur, and 30% of eyes are blind within 1 year of the first bleed. Fortunately, laser photocoagulation has revolutionized the outlook for proliferative retinopathy.

Advanced diabetic eye disease

This represents endstage damage that commonly leads to blindness; vitreoretinal surgery has improved the prognosis somewhat.

- Vitreous and preretinal haemorrhages develop when new vessels grow forward from the retina, cross the potential preretinal (subhyaloid) space, and enter the vitreous. These vessels rupture easily: associated fibrous tissue contracts and tears them, as does the normal shrinkage of the vitreous with age. Vitreous haemorrhages appear as reddish or dark opacities that may completely fill the eye and block the view of the retina. Preretinal (subhyaloid) haemorrhages have a flat top (if the subject has been upright), because the red cells sediment within the haemorrhage cavity.

- Retinal detachment occurs: the retina is pulled off the underlying choroid by contracting strands of fibrous tissue associated with the formation of new vessels or previous vitreous haemorrhages. The retina may appear wrinkled (traction lines) or thrown into folds or bumps, sometimes with a visible tear.

- New vessels grow on to the iris (rubeosis iridis), usually in the context of widespread proliferative retinopathy. Fine vessels and diffuse reddening of the iris may be seen with the ophthalmoscope. The main complication is glaucoma, caused by proliferating fibrovascular tissue obstructing the filtration angle in the anterior chamber. Signs include circumcorneal injection, a fixed irregular pupil and corneal haze; the eye is often intensely painful.

Symptoms of diabetic retinopathy

There may be no visual symptoms, even with extensive proliferative changes, until sight-threatening complications occur.

- Vitreous haemorrhage and retinal detachment cause sudden loss of vision that is painless but often terrifying. Retinal detachment occurring behind a vitreous haemorrhage may be reported by the patient as a further deterioration in already poor vision.

- Maculopathy presents as a gradual painless decline in central vision, which may not be noticed by the patient but is picked up on routine eye screening.

- Rubeosis and particularly neovascular glaucoma cause worsening vision with pain and redness in the eye.

Other causes of visual loss need to be considered in diabetic patients, including cataract, stroke, retinal artery or vein occlusion, and hypoglycaemia and glaucoma.

Examination of the eyes in diabetic patients

This should be performed routinely on diagnosis, annually thereafter (or every 6 months if marked background or other changes are present), and immediately if the patient reports any change in vision. There should be close liaison with the ophthalmologist, and a low threshold for referral: indications for seeking expert advice are shown in Table 13.11.1.8.

Table 13.11.1.8 Indications and standards for ophthalmological referral in patients with diabetic retinopathy in the United Kingdom

Background retinopathy (R1)	Routine diabetes care
microaneurysm(s)	Arrange annual screening
retinal haemorrhage(s)	
Preproliferative retinopathy (R2)	Achievable standard:
venous beading, venous loop or	95% seen by ophthalmologist
reduplication	in <13 weeks
IRMA	Minimum standard:
multiple deep, round or blot	70% seen by ophthalmologist in
haemorrhages	<13 weeks
(CWS—careful search for above	100% seen by ophthalmologist
features)	in <18 weeks
Maculopathy (MI)	Achievable standard:
exudate within 1 DD of the centre	95% seen by ophthalmologist in
of the fovea	<13 weeks
circinate or group of exudates	Minimum standard:
within the macula	70% seen by ophthalmologist
retinal thickening within 1 DD of	in <13 weeks
the centre of the fovea	100% seen by ophthalmologist in
(if stereo available)	<18 weeks
any microaneurysm or	
haemorrhage within 1 DD of	
the centre of the fovea only if	
associated with a best VA of	
<6/12 (if no stereo)	
Proliferative retinopathy/rubeosis	Achievable standard:
iridis (R3)	95% seen by ophthalmologist <2 weeks
NVD	Minimum standard:
NVE	70% seen by ophthalmologist in
preretinal or vitreous	<2 weeks
haemorrhage	100% seen by ophthalmologist in
preretinal fibrosis ± tractional	<4 weeks
retinal detachment	
Very urgent	Emergency referral to ophthalmologist
sudden loss of vision	(same day)
retinal detachment	

DD, disc diameter; IRMA, intraretinal microvascular abnormality; NVD, new vessels on disc; NVE, new vessels elsewhere; VA, visual acuity.
Source: UK National Screening Committee for Diabetic Retinopathy (2006).

Visual acuity must be checked with a Snellen chart, with the pupils undilated, and both uncorrected and corrected for refraction errors (with the patient's spectacles or a pinhole). Poor visual acuity (worse than 6/12) that is not correctable and has no other obvious cause (cataract, vitreous haemorrhage) is usually due to maculopathy, and this must be actively excluded (see below).

The iris and pupil are examined for evidence of rubeosis or glaucoma. Pupillary reflexes should be checked: an afferent pupillary defect (see Section 25) indicates severe retinal or optic nerve disease, such as retinal detachment.

Fundoscopy, if used, must be performed through fully dilated pupils: peripheral new vessels may otherwise be invisible. Relative contraindications to mydriatics are intraocular lens implants; referral to the ophthalmologist is then advisable. The disc, entire retina, and macula must be carefully scanned. Current retinopathy screening programmes recommend two-field digital photography with standardized grading by trained staff, rather than fundoscopy by indirect ophthalmoscopy. Nonmydriatic cameras that allow photography of most of the retina, through partly dilated pupils (in a darkened room) are widely used in community screening for retinopathy. Binocular ophthalmoscopy provides good all-round and three-dimensional views, especially of vitreous haemorrhage, macular oedema, and retinal detachment. Slit lamp biomicroscopy is an alternative technique.

Additional specialist investigations include:

- slit lamp biomicroscopy,which is useful for examining the anterior chamber (for rubeosis and glaucoma) and assessing retinal thickness (for detecting macular oedema)
- fluorescein angiography: fluorescein injected intravenously binds to albumin and therefore only escapes outside abnormally permeable vessels; sites of leakage are highlighted by persistent fluorescence when the retina is photographed under ultraviolet light; this is useful for showing the foci of leakage (e.g. for targeting laser photocoagulation) and for the diagnosis of macular oedema
- B-scan ultrasound, which provides a cross-sectional image of the eye and can show retinal detachments that are invisible on fundoscopy because of a dense vitreous haemorrhage or cataract
- Optical coherence tomography (OCT), which uses optical reflectivity of near-infrared light to produce cross-sectional images of the retina, and is now the investigation of choice to assess macular oedema

In many areas, community retinal screening has been established using mobile camera units and the identification of patients through diabetes registers held by primary care physicians. There is little doubt that when performed well and graded by fully trained staff, this is the most robust form of retinopathy screening. In addition, the images can be used to plan laser therapy and diagnose nondiabetic lesions that are found incidentally.

Management of diabetic retinopathy

Specific treatments for sight-threatening retinopathy have improved greatly, but general preventative measures are still crucial. These include:

- tight glycaemic control, as highlighted by the DCCT and the UKPDS studies (Paradoxically, a rapid reduction in hyperglycaemia can provoke a transient deterioration in retinopathy, with worsening of the background condition or the development of preproliferative changes. This is probably due to an acute fall in retinal blood flow (which is elevated by hyperglycaemia), thus worsening ischaemia in already underperfused areas. Typically, the acute lesions resolve and the overall long-term outcome is improved if good glycaemic control can be maintained.)
- control of hypertension—likely to be important; the EUCLID study of enalapril showed beneficial effects which may reflect the inhibition of angiotensin-converting enzyme as well as lowering of blood pressure
- stopping smoking: smoking is thought to hasten the progression of retinopathy
- lipid lowering with fenofibrate (but not statins) appears to slow progression of diabetic retinopathy
- regular eye screening—essential, because even severe diabetic retinopathy may cause few or no symptoms

Specific treatments

Laser photocoagulation can preserve useful vision in many cases of proliferative retinopathy and maculopathy. The blue-green light of the argon laser is maximally absorbed by vascular structures. It has a spot size of 50 to 500 μm and can be used to target discrete lesions such as clusters of leaking vessels identified by fluorescein angiography, but is usually employed to destroy larger areas of generally diseased retina. Panretinal photocoagulation ablates the peripheral retina with 1500 to 2000 burns that spare only a horizontal keyhole-shaped central area that includes the disc, the macula, and the maculopapillary nerve bundle running between them. Panretinal photocoagulation effectively concentrates the remaining retinal blood flow on to this crucial region which serves central, high-resolution colour vision, at the expense of the periphery. It is indicated for the formation of new vessels (on the disc or elsewhere, and rubeosis), and can be very effective: the chance of blindness within 5 years is reduced from 50% to 25% in patients at risk. It is increasingly used in the preproliferative phase to prevent the formation of new vessels. Photocoagulation is also used to treat macular oedema, in a grid pattern around the central macula to destroy leaky capillaries; this reduces the 3-year risk of becoming blind from 30% to 15%.

Vitreoretinal surgery can now restore useful vision to some blind or severely impaired eyes. Techniques include vitrectomy (aspiration of vitreous haemorrhage and fibrovascular debris) and reattachment of detached or torn retina (using high-powered lasers to stitch down the retina). Easy and rapid access to ophthalmologists and surgeons is often critical: e.g. a detached retina must be repaired within a few weeks if it is to remain viable.

Practical aids for visual handicap range from pen injection devices and 'talking' blood glucose meters, to social support networks and national organizations for the visually impaired.

Clinical trials have shown that the protein kinase C β inhibitor ruboxistaurin appears unable to prevent progression from non-proliferative to proliferative diabetic retinopathy, but can reduce the development of macular oedema and the associated visual loss. Monoclonal anti-vascular endothelial growth factor (VEGF) treatment has also shown promise in improving vision in macular oedema in clinical trials. Neither treatment is currently licensed for use for this indication.

Cataract in diabetes

The normal lens transmits light because the fibre cells of the lens and the stacks of crystallin proteins which they contain are aligned in parallel. Normal ageing causes irreversible chemical modification (browning) of the crystallins, with cross-linking and distortion that interrupt transmission of light and thus cause clouding of the lens. Diabetes accelerates the formation of these senile cataracts, probably through nonenzymatic glycation and cross-linking of-modified crystallins.

Cataract is the most common cause of severe visual loss in diabetic patients over the age of 30, and is usually a typical 'senile' nuclear cataract with a characteristic radial spoke pattern. Much rarer is the 'snowflake' cataract with opacities scattered through the lens, which tends to occur in children presenting with severe hyperglycaemia. Here, the opacities are reversible and are presumably due to local pockets of osmotic imbalance which distort the alignment of the lens crystallins.

Treatment of cataracts is conventional, usually removal and replacement by an intracapsular plastic lens. The long-term outcome is often not as good as in nondiabetic patients, because of coexisting maculopathy or proliferative retinopathy.

Glaucoma is more common in diabetic subjects and is a complication of proliferative retinopathy.

Other ocular problems

Cranial nerve palsies, especially of the third and sixth nerves, cause typical limitations of eye movement, often with acute onset of pain and diplopia (see below and Chapter 24.12).

Eye infections include the rare but extremely destructive mucormycosis, which often spreads from the sinus to involve the orbit (see Chapter 25).

Diabetic neuropathies

Clinical syndromes

Diabetes damages nerves, both somatosensory and autonomic, in various ways that cause clinically distinct syndromes (see Fig. 13.11.1.15). Subclinical nerve damage is common among patients with diabetes, but significant neuropathic symptoms are fortunately unusual.

Diffuse symmetrical polyneuropathy

This is classically a distal 'glove and stocking' peripheral polyneuropathy that affects all sizes of sensory and motor fibres; a variant selectively picks off small C fibres (see below). Both forms may be accompanied by neuropathy involving the sympathetic and parasympathetic divisions of the autonomic nervous system.

Aetiology The diffuse nature of the nerve damage and its predilection for longer nerves is typical of toxic and metabolic neuropathies, and suggests cumulative damage that must reach a critical level before the function of a nerve is impaired. Both metabolic and vascular factors may contribute. The duration and severity of hyperglycaemia are generally related to the prevalence of neuropathy, while the DCCT study confirmed that good glycaemic control decreased by the risks of developing neuropathy by about 70%. Hyperglycaemia could damage nerves by glycation of key proteins. In the nerves of diabetic animals, polyol pathway

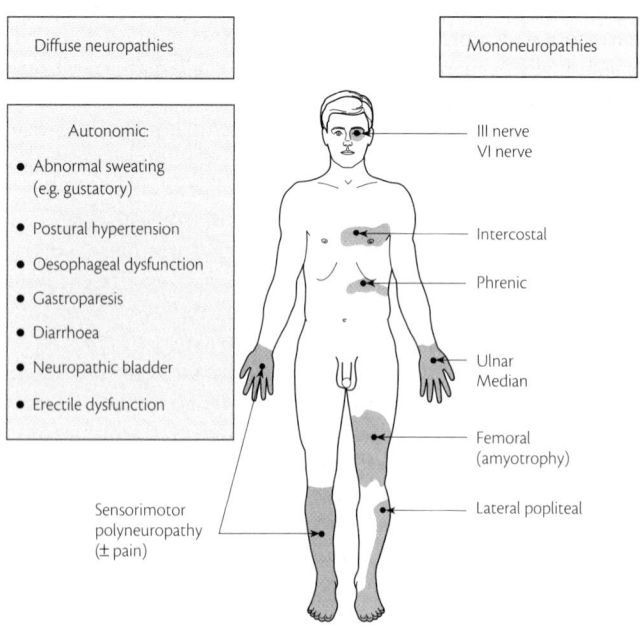

Fig. 13.11.1.15 Clinical manifestations of diabetic nerve damage.

overactivity has also been implicated (Schwann cells express aldose reductase), while myoinositol depletion may impair nerve conduction by inhibiting Na^+, K^+-ATPase activity; in human diabetic neuropathy, however, the roles of polyols are less convincing and aldose reductase inhibitors proved ineffective in clinical trials. There is some evidence of blockage of the vasa nervorum by microthrombi, which could follow the formation of AGE and the other mechanisms described earlier. Microvascular occlusion could contribute to intraneural hypoxia, demonstrated in the nerves of both animals and humans with diabetes.

Pathological changes affect both axons and Schwann cells. Axons fall out by dying back distally, sometimes accompanied by sprouting of regenerating nerve endings. Schwann cell damage leads to segmental demyelination. Nerve conduction velocity is slowed, in proportion to structural nerve damage.

Epidemiology and natural history About 30% of unselected patients with diabetes have evidence of neuropathy on formal testing, but only 10% suffer significant symptoms. Signs of neuropathy may be present in up to 10% of newly diagnosed type 2 diabetic patients.

Nerve function generally worsens progressively over months or years, and areas of numbness may advance up the legs and occasionally involve the hands. Symptoms, including pain, may be variable; pain in particular may develop acutely, especially after weight loss or periods of poor diabetic control. Acute flare-ups tend to resolve after weeks or months, especially if glycaemic control is improved.

Symptoms and signs Sensory symptoms are the most common manifestation; muscle weakness occasionally predominates. Sensory symptoms may include loss of sensation, which can be profound, as well as positive symptoms of pain (often described as 'walking on broken glass', worse at night-time), paraesthesiae, and allodynia (i.e. pain provoked by a normally innocuous stimulus, such as light touch or contact with bedclothes). Loss of the sense of touch and joint position may give the sensation of walking in thick socks, and Romberg's sign may be positive. Patients may report trips and falls due to reduced proprioception. Reduced pain sensation, which paradoxically may coexist with neurogenic pain, is potentially dangerous and an important cause of damage to neuropathic feet (see below). Horrifying examples include full-thickness burns to the soles after crossing a hot beach, pressure ulceration from a day's walking in tight new shoes, and transfixing the foot inside the shoe by stepping on a nail.

The mechanism of neuropathic pain is unknown; spontaneous firing of unstable regenerating nerves may be responsible. Pain is typically neurogenic, usually described as burning, shooting, or electric shock-like sensations, often with unpleasant pins and needles and allodynia. The feet and legs are usually affected, and the hands only rarely; neuropathic symptoms in the hands are usually due to damage to the ulnar and/or median nerves, which can be bilateral (see Fig. 13.11.1.16). Pain is characteristically worse at night, may be relieved by walking (in contrast to claudication), and can severely disturb sleep and cause depression (and suicide).

Examination may reveal symmetrical 'stocking' sensory loss affecting all modalities. Sensory deficits are frequently patchy and may be much less impressive than the symptoms suggest; clinical findings may even be normal in acute painful neuropathy. Tendon reflexes in the legs are often reduced or absent, and there may

occasionally be marked muscle wasting. Neuropathic foot problems due to somatosensory and autonomic nerve damage may also be obvious, including ulceration, increased skin blood flow, and Charcot's arthropathy. The hands are less commonly involved.

Diffuse small fibre neuropathy

This rare variant affects especially young women with type 1 diabetes, and may be autoimmune in origin. There is loss of temperature and pain sensation in a stocking distribution, other modalities remaining intact. Autonomic neuropathy is frequent, usually with postural hypertension, gustatory sweating, and diarrhoea. Ulceration and Charcot's arthropathy affecting the feet are common.

Autonomic neuropathy

Autonomic disturbances commonly accompany somatosensory neuropathy, because the autonomic nerves are damaged by the same mechanisms. Up to 40% of unselected people with diabetes have abnormal tests of autonomic neuropathy, but only a few of these suffer major symptoms; however, these can be very debilitating and these patients have a significantly reduced life expectancy. The sympathetic and parasympathetic divisions are both affected.

Clinically apparent features are most common in patients with long-standing diabetes and include the following.

◆ Sexual difficulties, which include failure of erection (a parasympathetic response mediated by the sacral nerves) and sometimes failure of ejaculation (a sympathetic reflex transmitted by the lumbosacral outflow). Erectile failure is relatively common in diabetic men, affecting about 50% of those over 55 years; as in the nondiabetic population, depression and anxiety (including fears about poor sexual performance) are common contributory factors. Arterial inflow to the corpora cavernosa may be compromised by atheromatous disease of the pudendal arteries or common iliac arteries, the latter causing the Leriche's syndrome of impotence with claudication pain affecting the buttocks. Interestingly erectile dysfunction has been associated with an increased incidence of cardiovascular disease.

◆ Postural hypotension, with a systolic fall exceeding 20 mmHg on standing, is due to failure of the normal sympathetically mediated increases in cardiac output and vasoconstrictor tone. This causes dizziness and blackouts, which may be mistaken for arrhythmias or myocardial ischaemia. Symptoms and the degree of postural drop may vary considerably with time. Postural hypotension may be exacerbated by the vasodilator effects of antihypertensives, nitrates, tricyclic antidepressants (used to treat neuropathic pain), and insulin.

◆ Disturbed gastrointestinal motility. Dysphagia may be due to oesophageal dysmotility. Gastric stasis, due to failure of the pylorus to relax when the antrum contracts, causes particular difficulties with emptying liquids and presents with recurrent vomiting. There may be obvious fullness in the epigastrium, sometimes with a succussion splash. Characteristically, bouts of vomiting, which can last for several days, are interspersed with long periods in apparent remission, thus resulting in a delay in making the correct diagnosis. Disturbances of motility in the colon most commonly lead to diarrhoea (characteristically but not always worse at night), which may be exacerbated by bacterial overgrowth in the relatively immotile small bowel. As with all these gastrointestinal symptoms, diarrhoea is often episodic and may alternate with constipation. Bacterial overgrowth can be

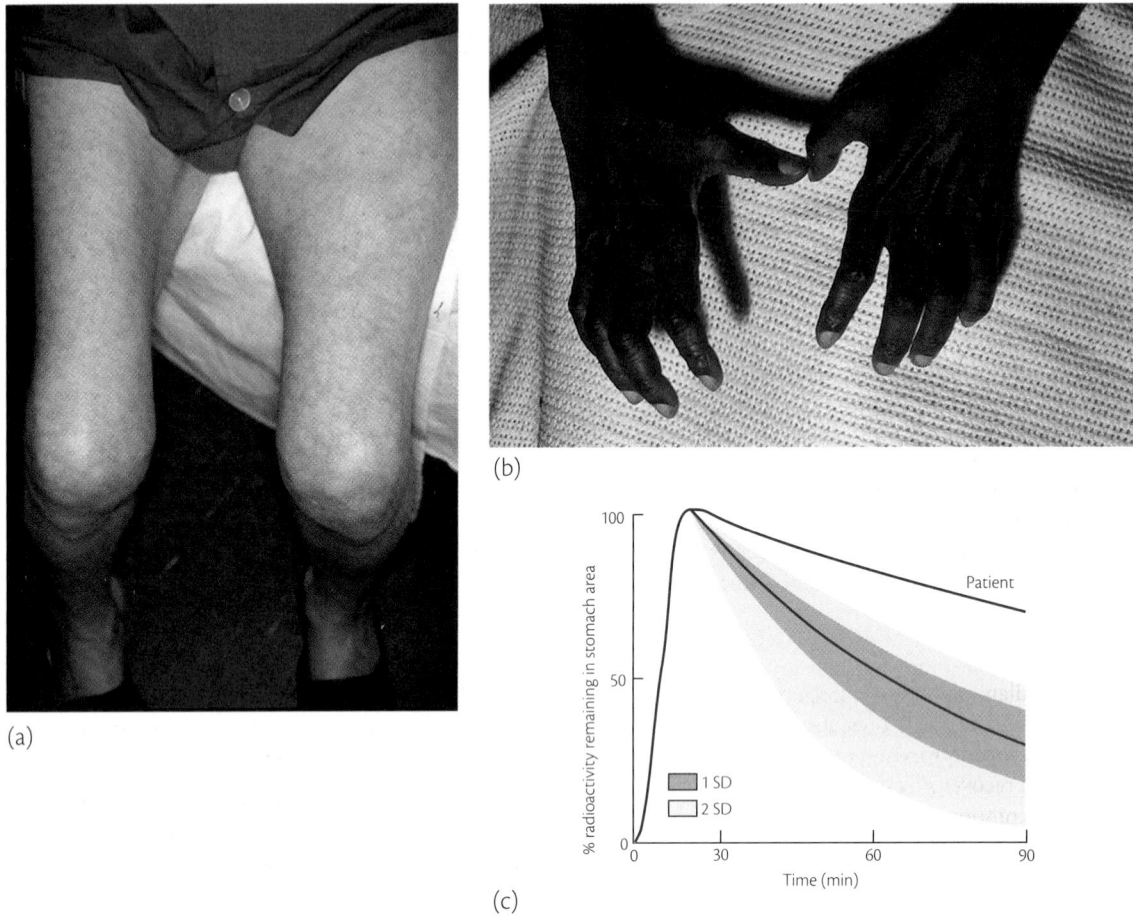

Fig. 13.11.1.16 (a) Diabetic amyotrophy: quadriceps (right) wasting due to femoral neuropathy. (b) Wasting of small muscles of the hands due to both ulnar and median nerve lesions. (c) Gastroparesis: grossly delayed gastric emptying. The normal range for clearance of the radiolabelled test meal from the stomach area is shown in the darker shade (50% confidence intervals) and lighter shade (95% confidence intervals).
((a) courtesy of Dr Geoff Gill, University Hospital Aintree, Liverpool.)

confirmed by a hydrogen breath test; it is an important diagnosis to make as it is easily treated with appropriate antibiotics (see below). Side-effects of metformin or statin therapy should also be considered in the differential diagnosis of diarrhoea in people with diabetes. Anorectal dysfunction from autonomic neuropathy is luckily rare, but can cause severe faecal incontinence.

◆ Abnormal sweating, mediated by cholinergic sympathetic nerves; this is one of the most common autonomic symptoms. Profuse gustatory sweating of the face and trunk (the area supplied by the superior cervical ganglion) may be provoked by eating, while sweating in the feet is often reduced.

◆ Neuropathic bladder, due to damage to the sacral nerves, prevents normal emptying and can lead to a permanently distended, sometimes palpable, bladder, with overflow incontinence. Hydroureter and hydronephrosis are other complications, and ascending urinary tract infections are common.

◆ Abnormal blood flow. Sympathetic denervation allows vasodilatation and relaxation of precapillary sphincters in the skin, hence the warm skin and distended veins characteristic of the neuropathic foot. Increased blood flow in bone may be an early abnormality in Charcot's arthropathy.

◆ Sudden unexplained death ("dead in bed") is more common in patients with severe autonomic symptoms. Possible causes

include cardiorespiratory arrest and arrhythmias triggered by hypoglycaemia, awareness of which is blunted in many patients with long-standing diabetes. Prolonged electrocardiographic QTc intervals are associated with an increased risk of cardiovascular mortality in both diabetic and nondiabetic populations, and QTc intervals are more commonly prolonged in patients with diabetes with autonomic neuropathy (31%) than in those without (24%).

Acute mononeuropathies

These syndromes are due to acute damage to isolated peripheral nerves, presumably due to a vascular event rather than metabolic damage. Limited histological studies show focal demyelination, probably consistent with this. Occasionally, two or more nerves can be affected more or less simultaneously (mononeuritis multiplex).

Diabetic amyotrophy

This is due to damage of one of the major nerve trunks or roots (radiculopathy) supplying the leg. The femoral nerve is most commonly involved, causing symptoms in the quadriceps muscle; other muscle groups are less often affected. Femoral neuropathy causes neurogenic pain of acute onset (burning or lancinating, and usually severe), with weakness and often surprisingly rapid wasting in the quadriceps, and loss of the knee tendon reflex (see

Fig. 13.11.1.16). For unknown reasons, some patients have extensor plantar reflexes, in which case a spinal or cauda equina lesion must be excluded. Associated acute weight loss (diabetic cachexia) may be seen prompting a suspicion of malignancy.

Amyotrophy most commonly presents in patients over 50 years of age, often following a period of poor diabetic control. Pain usually resolves spontaneously over several months, especially if diabetic control is improved, but muscle strength and tendon reflexes may take much longer to return.

Cranial and other nerve palsies

These are common, affecting the third and sixth nerves in particular. Third nerve palsy is often accompanied by pain behind the eye, and may need to be differentiated from an aneurysm of the posterior communicating artery; however, unlike in classical third nerve palsy, ptosis and pupillary dilatation are usually absent. Acute neuropathic damage may also affect the phrenic nerve (causing an elevated hemidiaphragm), and intercostal or truncal nerves, causing shingles-like pain and sometimes localized bulging of the abdominal wall. All these acute palsies tend to resolve spontaneously over a period of months.

Pressure palsies

These include the median, ulnar, and occasionally lateral popliteal nerves, and are thought to be due to pressure damage superimposed on hypoxic or otherwise compromised nerves. These present in the classical way, but often recover slowly and incompletely, and do not respond to surgical decompression as well as in nondiabetic subjects (see Fig. 13.11.1.16).

Insulin neuritis

This is a transient deterioration in nerve function, often with pain and dysaesthesiae which follows an acute improvement in glycaemic control, typically after starting insulin therapy. It may be due to an acute fall in nerve perfusion analogous to the decrease in retinal blood flow thought to explain a temporary deterioration in retinopathy under these circumstances (see above). The pain, which can be very severe, generally affects the legs symmetrically but can commence in any area of the body. Symptoms usually resolve within weeks or months.

Diagnosis of diabetic neuropathies
Peripheral sensorimotor neuropathies

A carefully taken history is usually diagnostic. The key qualities of neuropathic pain should distinguish it from claudication, night cramps and sciatica.

Sensory deficits should be mapped on the legs and hands, for both large-fibre (vibration with a 128 Hz tuning fork, joint position sense, light touch, temperature, e.g. with a cold tuning fork) and small-fibre modalities (pin prick, light touch); objective losses may not match the patient's symptoms. A useful test uses the Semmes–Weinstein nylon monofilament, which is pressed against the skin until it buckles; the patient's inability to feel the 10 g filament indicates neuropathy severe enough to predict foot ulceration. Various bedside instruments can be used to assess specific sensory modalities, such as the biothesiometer (for measuring vibration sense) and thermal threshold testers; age-related normal ranges are available for these methods but they are quite variable and add little to routine management. Muscle wasting and weakness should be sought, and the tendon reflexes checked.

Peripheral diabetic neuropathy must be differentiated from other metabolic neuropathies, including vitamin B_{12} deficiency (associated with metformin use), uraemia, and alcohol, all of which may affect diabetic patients.

Autonomic neuropathy

The most convenient tests are of cardiovascular autonomic function, which detect loss of the normal reflexes that modulate heart rate during respiration (mainly vagal) and that increase heart rate and blood pressure on standing (sympathetic). The simplest test is to measure heart rate (R-R interval) from an ECG tracing during controlled deep breathing (5 s inspiration, then 5 s expiration, repeated for 1 min); the physiological bradycardia on expiration is lost, with a difference of less than 10 beats/min between inspiration and expiration. Reflex bradycardia during the Valsalva manoeuvre is similarly abolished. More sophisticated measures employing spectral analysis of variability of heart rate during normal breathing are more sensitive.

Postural hypotension is defined as a drop of more than 20 mmHg in systolic blood pressure, measured 30 s after standing. Postural drops often vary considerably through the day and from week to week.

Abnormalities of cardiovascular autonomic tests are common in patients with long-standing diabetes, especially type 1, and do not necessarily indicate that symptoms such as vomiting, diarrhoea, or erectile dysfunction are due to autonomic neuropathy. Other specific tests include the following.

- Gastroparesis: a plain abdominal radiograph may show a 'ground glass' appearance in the epigastrium, while endoscopy (always indicated to exclude pyloric obstruction) shows a dilated, poorly contracting stomach with a closed pylorus. Gastric emptying studies using radiolabelled test meals show delayed disappearance of radioactivity, particularly of a liquid test meal; however, abnormalities may not be consistent with the severity of symptoms (see Fig. 13.11.1.16).

- Neuropathic bladder and associated hydroureter and hydronephrosis can be confirmed by ultrasound or intravenous urography.

- Erectile failure is often multifactorial (see above). If it is due to autonomic neuropathy, other signs of autonomic dysfunction, especially neuropathic bladder, may be present.

Treatment of diabetic neuropathies
General measures

Poor glycaemic control should be corrected. As well as helping to prevent the development of neuropathy, this may curtail pain in the acute syndromes; insulin neuritis is rare and usually self-limiting. Once established, chronic sensory motor neuropathy tends to progress, irrespective of glycaemic control. Specific treatments which aim to prevent or reverse diabetic nerve damage—aldose reductase inhibitors and aminoguanidine (which prevents the formation of AGE)—have so far been disappointing. Numb feet are at greatly increased risk of ulceration and require sensible shoes and good foot care (see below).

Pain may be difficult to treat; pain management programmes in specialized pain relief clinics may be helpful. Recently, there has been increased interest in the development of new drugs for neuropathic pain. The following should be tried in sequence.

- Simple analgesics (aspirin, paracetamol) are mostly unhelpful. Opiates were traditionally regarded as ineffective in diabetic neuropathy, but recent studies indicate that they can be of value, particularly as second- or third-line agents in combination with anticonvulsant derived drugs such as gabapentin.

- Tricyclic drugs suppress neurogenic pain, in addition to their antidepressant effects. Amitriptyline or imipramine can be started at 25 mg at bedtime (10 mg in older people), increasing weekly to a maximum of 75 to 150 mg. Duloxetine has been recently licensed as an alternative. Side effects, including postural hypotension, may limit the dosage. A phenothiazine such as fluphenazine (2.5–5 mg) is said to enhance the analgesic effect of tricyclics but its use is not evidence-based and it often exacerbates postural hypotension.

- Anticonvulsants, which stabilize the neuronal membrane and may prevent spontaneous firing of C fibres, may be substituted for tricyclics, or used in combination with them. Carbamazepine (initially 100 mg once or twice daily, up to 800 mg/day in divided doses) is often effective. Sodium valproate or phenytoin are time honoured alternatives. More recent additions, shown to be effective in clinical trials, of neuropathic pain include gabapentin and pregabalin. Gabapentin is given in divided doses totalling 900 to 3600 mg/day (rather more than the standard antiepileptic regimen but apparently well tolerated), and pregabalin at 75 mg twice daily increasing to a maximum total dose of 300 mg/day. Lacosamide has shown promise in clinical trials.

Pain in the feet may respond to topical application of capsaicin ointment; capsaicin causes the burning sensation of hot chillies, and depletes the pain-transmitting C fibres of the neurotransmitter substance P. Pain may be transiently worsened after application, but relief can last for many hours. Contact hypersensitivity (allodynia) can be helped simply with a bed cradle to prevent contact with bed clothes, or by applying adhesive plastic film such as Opsite to the skin.

Other drugs that have proved successful in some but not all trials include oral mexiletine (a class 1b antiarrhythmic agent that stabilizes nerve cell membranes; up to 450 mg/day in divided doses), intravenous lidocaine infusions (providing relief for several weeks); and oral clonazepam (0.5–3 mg) in patients whose sleep is disturbed by 'restless legs'. Some patients unresponsive to drug therapy may benefit from implantation of a dorsal column stimulator, designed to exploit the gate control of pain transmission.

Autonomic neuropathic symptoms may be treated as follows:

- Excessive sweating may be controlled by oral clonidine or topical 0.5 to 1% glycopyrrholate ointment; systemic anticholinergics such as poldine have also been effective but have many side effects, including urinary retention.

- Postural hypotension may be helped simply by raising the head of the bed at night. Additional simple measures include the use of compression stockings, taking time to rise in stages from lying down, and carrying a folding stool so that the subject can sit immediately on feeling faint, thereby avoiding a syncopal event. Fludrocortisone can be useful, but aggravates coexistent supine hypertension; very high doses (up to 1 mg/day) may be needed. The α_1-adrenergic agonist midodrine (2.5–10 mg daily) may also be helpful, but can also worsen hypertension.

- Vomiting due to gastroparesis often responds to metoclopramide or domperidone, and the prokinetic motilin agonist drug erythromycin (given intravenously or orally at 250 mg three times daily or less). Cisapride, an additional prokinetic drug has been withdrawn because of arrhythmias. Additional drugs that have been of benefit in uncontrolled trials include sulpiride, and the 5-HT4 antagonist tegaserod. Some patients unresponsive to drug therapy may require intrajejunal feeding, most conveniently by percutaneous endoscopic gastrostomy or jejunostomy; some patients benefit from surgical drainage procedures such as a Roux-en-Y gastrojejunostomy. Laparoscopically-placed gastric electrical pacing units have also been reported in controlled trials to be of benefit in refractory cases. Injections of botulinum toxin into the pylorus may also be beneficial, but the evidence is less robust.

- Diarrhoea is often improved or cured by erythromycin or tetracycline when bacterial overgrowth is a contributory factor.

- Neuropathic bladder may respond to regular bladder training, but intermittent self-catheterization may be needed.

- Erectile dysfunction can be treated with oral sildenafil 50 to 100 mg, which should be taken about 1 h before intercourse. It is effective in about 50% of diabetic patients but is absolutely contraindicated in those taking nitrates in any form, because of the risk of profound hypotension and circulatory collapse. Newer phosphodiesterase inhibitors include vardenafil, whose absorption is less affected by fatty food than sildenafil, and tadalafil, whose effects last for 24 h and thus allow more convenient dosing. Alternatives, if phosphodiesterase inhibitors are contraindicated or ineffective, include the injection of vasodilators such as papaverine or prostaglandin E_1 into the corpus cavernosum, intraurethral alprostadil, the use of vacuum tumescence devices, or inflatable penile implants. Coexistent contributory factors such as depression, alcohol, or drugs (including β-blockers and thiazides) should be sought and treated. Counselling of the couple is obviously important.

Diabetic nephropathy

This is covered in detail in Chapter 21.10.1.

Macrovascular disease

Diabetes of all types increases the background risk of atheroma, amplifying the hazards of additional cardiovascular risk factors such as hypercholesterolaemia, hypertension, and smoking. Atheroma appears earlier, spreads faster and more extensively, and carries greater morbidity and mortality than in people who do not have diabetes. Overall risks for myocardial infarction, stroke, and limb ischaemia are two to four times higher than in the general population, and women with diabetes lose the premenopausal protection which their euglycaemic counterparts normally enjoy. This increased level of risk is comparable with that in nondiabetic subjects who have already suffered a myocardial infarct. Accordingly, it has been argued that primary cardiovascular prevention for diabetic patients should be as active as secondary prevention in the nondiabetic population. Macrovascular disease, especially coronary heart disease, is the main cause of premature death in type 2 diabetes (two-thirds of all deaths).

As discussed earlier, cardiovascular risk is increased at glucose levels that lie below the diabetic range: impaired glucose tolerance also predisposes to coronary heart disease, but not to retinopathy. This relationship probably explains why tight glucose control has not yet been shown to fully prevent macrovascular disease, because none of the trials (e.g. the DCCT or the UKPDS) has managed to achieve even near normoglycaemia. Paradoxically, a recent trial of very aggressive glucose lowering in patients with type 2 diabetes (ACCORD) aiming for HbA1c < 6% should increased mortality, possibly due to hypoglycemia. There is a very strong relationship between microalbuminuria and premature death from cardiovascular disease (see Chapter 21.10.1). This presumably reflects widespread damage to the endothelium, which both predisposes to atheroma formation and enhances albumin leakage in the glomerulus.

Cardiovascular risk factors tend to cluster together with type 2 diabetes in metabolic syndrome X (see above). These risk factors are also common in the type 1 diabetic and the nondiabetic populations. Because their impact is worsened by diabetes, they require active management. Treatment of obesity and smoking is discussed in Chapters 11.5 and 3.3.1.

Dyslipidaemia in diabetes

Type 1 and type 2 diabetes are both commonly accompanied by lipid disorders that are strongly atherogenic but may appear deceptively trivial on routine screening (see Fig. 13.11.1.17).

In poorly controlled type 1 diabetes, the most obvious abnormality is hypertriglyceridaemia. This is due mainly to increased production of very low-density lipoprotein (LDL) by the liver, driven by high levels of free fatty acids resulting from enhanced lipolysis in fat; triglyceride levels can be lowered by improved insulin therapy. Total cholesterol concentrations are often 'normal', while high-density lipoprotein (HDL) may be increased, although this is predominantly the HDL3 subclass which does not confer protection against atheroma (see Chapter 12.6). As stressed below, a 'normal' cholesterol is not necessarily reassuring because modified LDL particles in diabetes are particularly atherogenic and because cardiovascular risk in diabetic people is increased at all levels of cholesterol.

Dyslipidaemia in type 2 diabetes is also subtle, and similar to that of obesity and the metabolic syndrome. High-density lipoprotein (HDL) cholesterol is reduced, increasing the ratio of LDL to HDL, while triglycerides are often modestly raised. The abnormalities are also due to excessive production of very low-density lipoprotein (VLDL) by the liver, due to insulin resistance rather than insulin deficiency: free fatty acid levels are raised by lipolysis (adipocytes are resistant to the normal antilipolytic action of insulin), while the inhibition by insulin of hepatic production of VLDL is lost. High levels of VLDL favour the production of two highly atherogenic cholesterol particles, namely intermediate-density lipoprotein (IDL) and small dense LDL, which is easily oxidized; both IDL and oxidized LDL are taken up, via specific receptors, by macrophages in the artery wall which are then transformed into foam cells (see Chapter 12.6). As mentioned above, high triglyceride levels also accelerate the removal of cholesterol ester (via cholesterol ester transfer protein) from HDL, ultimately reducing levels of HDL and producing the nonprotective HDL3 fraction.

Risks of dyslipidaemia

Cardiovascular events including fatal myocardial infarction are 3 to 4 times more common among diabetic patients than in the general population, across a wide range of cholesterol levels including normal values. The risks of the slightly raised triglyceride concentrations are less obvious. The FIELD study reported a relatively small (11%) relative reduction in coronary events (but with no reduction in total mortality) following a 28% reduction in triglyceride levels with fenofibrate.

Management

Recent trials indicate that people with diabetes benefit even more from cholesterol-lowering with statins than do people without diabetes, as their ischaemic heart disease event rates are higher. Clear-cut positive outcome data have been reported with simvastatin, atorvastatin and rosuvastatin. The high background risk of diabetes is reflected in the lower treatment thresholds for hypercholesterolaemia in the various risk factor tables (see Chapter 12.6), and lipid-lowering drugs are now used at ever lower cholesterol levels. Statin therapy arguably has more effect on survival than any other single treatment in diabetes and should be strongly promoted. The American Diabetes Association recommends treatment of all individuals with overt cardiovascular disease and individuals over 40 with one or more additional risk factor. A treatment goal of LDL levels of less than 2.6 mmol/litre is remmended in all patients and less than 1.8 mmol/litre in overt cardiovascular disease. First-line treatment is with statins, aiming for a 30 to 40% reduction in LDL. It seems reasonable at present to consider adding a fibrate if triglycerides then remain in excess of 2.3 mmol/litre, especially where there is a marked mixed hyperlipidaemia with very high triglyceride levels, although the lipid-lowering results are often disappointing. Ezetimibe, an inhibitor of cholesterol reabsorption, powerfully synergizes with statins in LDL lowering or can be used as an alternative if statins are not tolerated, but long-term outcome data with this drug to date have been disappointing.

Other factors that aggravate dyslipidaemia (and especially hypertriglyceridaemia)—obesity, alcohol excess, poor glycaemic control, and drugs such as thiazides and β-blockers—should be tackled if possible.

Hypertension

Hypertension commonly accompanies diabetes: about 40% of type 2 patients are hypertensive at diagnosis, and probably two-thirds of

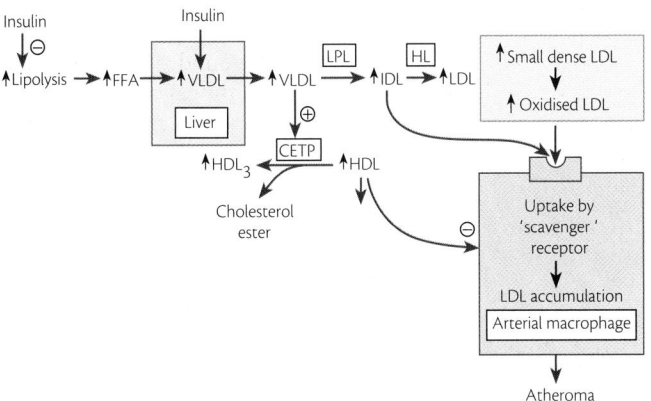

Fig. 13.11.1.17 Mechanisms of lipid abnormalities in diabetes. Insulin resistance or loss of insulin leads to increased lipolysis and hepatic secretion of very low-density lipoprotein (VLDL). High levels of VLDL stimulate cholesterol ester transfer protein which converts the antiatherogenic high-density lipoprotein (HDL) into HDL3, which lacks this protective effect. VLDLs are stripped of triglyceride by lipoprotein lipase to yield atherogenic intermediate-density lipoprotein (IDL), and then by hepatic lipase to produce low-density lipoprotein (LDL), including the highly atherogenic small dense oxidized fractions. These, with IDL, are taken up by arterial wall macrophages, forming the foam cells that initiate the atheromatous plaque.

the diabetic population are inadequately treated with respect to current management guidelines (see Table 13.11.1.3).

Causes

Essential hypertension is an integral feature of the metabolic syndrome, associated with obesity and insulin resistance. Possible mechanisms include enhanced central sympathetic tone (possibly mediated in part by raised insulin levels), and increased total body sodium and extracellular fluid volume, to which the Na^+-retaining effects of hyperinsulinaemia could contribute; loss of insulin-induced vasodilatation due to insulin resistance could also play a role. Secondary hypertension may also develop because of specific diabetic complications, notably nephropathy (loss of the normal nocturnal dip in blood pressure can be an early feature: see Chapter 21.10.1), stenosis of the renal artery due to atheroma, and stiffening of the larger conduit arteries causing isolated systolic hypertension. Supine hypertension can coexist with postural hypotension—a particularly difficult combination to treat effectively.

Treatment targets

The blood pressure thresholds for active management have fallen progressively, with wider appreciation of the damage inflicted by even modest hypertension in diabetic patients and of the benefits of control of blood pressure. The American Diabetes Association now recommends 130/80 mmHg (recorded in the clinic) as the treatment target for blood pressure, and that consistently higher values require active treatment; levels exceeding 140/90 mmHg are increasingly regarded as unacceptably poor. Ambulatory (or home) blood pressure readings are lower than those recorded in the clinic, and mean daytime levels of less than 130/75 mmHg are the current target. Target blood pressure (clinic readings) for patients with microalbuminuria is 125/75 mmHg.

Impact of hypertension in diabetes

Like all cardiovascular risk factors, the atherogenic hazards of hypertension are amplified in the diabetic population. Hypertension also plays a crucial role in accelerating the progression of diabetic nephropathy and also of retinopathy. Several studies have shown that treating hypertension reduces the risks of myocardial infarction and stroke by 30 to 70%; in the UKPDS, tight blood pressure control (averaging 144/82 mmHg compared with 154/87 mmHg in less tightly controlled subjects) reduced stroke by 40% and the need for photocoagulation by 30%, although strangely, no effect on myocardial infarction was observed (see Fig. 13.11.1.13).

Management

This should begin with lifestyle modifications, including restricting energy intake and increasing exercise in the obese, and reducing alcohol and sodium intakes. If actually carried out, these general measures can lower blood pressure at least as effectively as many antihypertensive drugs. Most patients, however, will require drugs and many need combination therapy. Antihypertensive drugs can be used in the conventional stepped approach (Chapter 16.17.2) to achieve the target blood pressure, ideally 130/80 mmHg; less stringent targets may be appropriate for older patients or those who cannot tolerate tight blood pressure control because of other problems.

The choice of hypotensive drugs is less important than the level of blood pressure achieved, although some agents have properties that are better suited to diabetes. All these drugs can worsen or precipitate postural hypotension in autonomic neuropathy. ACE inhibitors are often recommended as first-line in view of their additional benefits in reducing cardiovascular risk, improving myocardial function, and slowing the advance diabetic nephropathy.

ACE inhibitors

These can effectively control blood pressure when combined with low-dose diuretics and are useful in the many diabetic patients who also have heart failure or left ventricular dysfunction, especially following a myocardial infarct. They reduce proteinuria, by relaxing the efferent arterioles in the glomerulus, and slow the development of both nephropathy and retinopathy; some evidence points to specific beneficial effects in nephropathy, in addition to the lowering of blood pressure (see Chapter 21.10.1). ACE inhibitors do not worsen blood glucose or lipids, and may even improve insulin sensitivity. They are contraindicated in renal artery stenosis, which is relatively common in arteriopathic diabetic patients, and can cause dangerous hyperkalaemia in those with hyporeninaemic hypoaldosteronism (type 4 renal tubular acidosis) which can be associated with diabetic nephropathy. Renal function and electrolytes should be checked before and during therapy with these drugs.

Diuretics

High-dose thiazides (e.g. 5 mg bendrofluazide) can worsen hyperglycaemia in type 2 diabetes, apparently by impairing insulin secretion (a consequence of K^+ depletion) and possibly increasing insulin resistance. However, low dosages (e.g. 2.5 mg bendroflumethiazide) are effective at blood pressure lowering and do not appear to aggravate glucose intolerance. Diuretics can precipitate hyperosmolar nonketotic coma, while thiazides may also worsen dyslipidaemia. Loop diuretics (e.g. furosemide) can potentiate the effects of ACE inhibitors and are a valuable alternative in patients with cardiac failure.

Calcium channel antagonists

These have no adverse metabolic effects and are useful in patients with angina or tachyarrhythmia (diltiazem), but may cause dependent oedema.

β-Blockers

β-Blockers may also raise blood glucose in type 2 patients by increasing insulin resistance (possibly related to weight gain) and by interfering with insulin release (which is stimulated by β_2 adrenoceptors). β-Blockers can also aggravate dyslipidaemia and impotence, while noncardioselective agents can mask the sympathetically driven symptoms of hypoglycaemia. Low dosages of cardioselective β-blockers (e.g. atenolol or metoprolol) are safe, and are also indicated for treating angina and in the secondary prevention of myocardial infarction, as well as of being of benefit in cardiac failure (e.g. bisoprolol, carvedilol). Recent meta-analyses indicate that β-blockers may be less effective at preventing cardiovascular events (particularly stroke) than other agents and it has been suggested that they should be used as fourth line drugs after the above three categories. However, the differences are small and as many patients with diabetes will need multiple drugs to control their hypertension, β-blockers may be used in a combination which can be well tolerated by an individual patient.

Angiotensin-II receptor antagonists

These drugs (e.g. losartan, candesartan, irbesartan, valsartan, and telmisartan) are very well tolerated by patients, and an increasing body of evidence suggests they have comparable benefits to ACE inhibitors (including in diabetes nephropathy). They are indicated in patients intolerant of an ACE inhibitor due to cough. The benefits of combined ACE and angiotensin receptor treatment remain unproven.

Other drugs

Other drugs include α_1-adrenoreceptor antagonists (e.g. doxazosin), which may slightly improve insulin sensitivity; moxonidine, a centrally acting sympathetic drug acting on imidazoline I1 receptors; and the recently introduced direct renin inhibitors (e.g. aliskiren). Data on the last in diabetes are very limited.

Coronary heart disease

Compared with their nondiabetic counterparts, clinically significant coronary heart disease is over twice as common in diabetic men and postmenopausal women and 4 times more common in premenopausal women. It is the cause of death in two-thirds of patients.

Angina

Recent studies have confirmed that coronary artery stenting and, particularly, bypass grafting markedly reduce fatal myocardial infarction in diabetic patients. Clinicians should maintain a low threshold for referring patients with diabetes presenting with typical or atypical chest pain suggestive of angina, or unexplained shortness of breath on exertion for further evaluation, including exercise tolerance testing, stress echocardiography, CT angiography, cardiac MRI or coronary angiography. Relatively mild symptoms often belie very extensive triple-vessel disease with lesions that are too numerous or distal for angioplasty. Such patients are at high risk of major infarction even with blockage of only one branch vessel as there is little available flow for cross-perfusion from the other arteries. Although coronary artery disease is very common in diabetes, presentation with classical angina of effort seems relatively rare, presumably due to limited exertional activity or impairment of the sensation of myocardial ischaemia due to neuropathy. Once assessed, and if intervention is deemed unnecessary to improve prognosis, angina can be treated with conventional drugs, remembering the diabetogenic and other hazards of β-blockers and the potential of nitrates and calcium channel antagonists to aggravate postural hypertension. Worsening symptoms should prompt rapid re-evaluation, including angiography and angioplasty, which has a good outcome in diabetic subjects.

Myocardial infarction

The risk of fatal myocardial infarction is as high in people with diabetes as in people without diabetes who have already suffered an infarct. Mortality from myocardial infarction is over twice as high as in matched nondiabetic controls, whether or not thrombolytic agents are used. About 75% of diabetic patients are dead within 5 years of their first infarct, the main causes of death being heart failure and acute cardiogenic shock.

Primary and secondary prevention

Independent risk factors—hypertension, dyslipidaemia, smoking, and obesity—must be treated energetically in all diabetic patients, and poor glycaemic control should be tightened even though this alone is unlikely to protect against coronary heart disease. Specific prophylactic therapy, comparable to secondary prevention

measures (i.e. measures given after an initial infarct) in the nondiabetic population, is increasingly recommended for people with diabetes with any evidence of ischaemic heart disease, because their risk of infarction is so high. This includes a cardioselective β-blocker (e.g. atenolol or metoprolol) and/or an ACE inhibitor if echocardiography shows left ventricular dysfunction with an ejection fraction of less than 40%. β-Blockers are at least as effective as in the general population; the case for ACE inhibitors in patients with diabetes and increased cardiovascular risk is also proven. Some authorities recommend aspirin in all patients with diabetes over 40 years of age, although the dosage (75–300 mg/day) remains undecided and recent studies have suggested that the benefits in primary prevention may be limited.

Management of acute myocardial infarction

Acute myocardial infarction should be managed as follows (see Box 13.11.1.3).

* Thrombolytic drugs should be given if rapid access primary angioplasty is not available; survival is improved at least as much and probably more than in the nondiabetic population. Proliferative retinopathy is not a contraindication, and the risk of intraocular haemorrhage is very low.

* Glycaemic control should be optimized during the acute episode. Initial evidence suggested that long-term survival is improved if intensive insulin treatment is started on admission of a diabetic patient and continued for some months afterwards. The Diabetes Mellitus, Insulin Glucose Infusion in Acute

---

Box 13.11.1.3 Prevention and treatment of myocardial infarction in diabetic patients

Primary prevention
* Optimize glycaemic control
* Seek and treat hypertension
* Seek and treat dyslipidaemia
* Stop smoking
* Aspirin in patients >40 years

Acute myocardial infarction
* Primary angioplasty or Thrombolytic drugs (usual indications)
* Tight glycaemic control (glucose 5–10 mmol/litre) for at least 48 h: low-dose intravenous insulin infusion
* Aspirin
* β-Blocker or ACE inhibitor (if congestive heart failure or marked left ventricular dysfunction)

Secondary prevention
* Aspirin
* β-Blocker and ACE inhibitor (as above)
* Statin, to maintain total cholesterol < 4.0 (LDL<1.8 or 2.0) mmol/litre
* Optimize glycaemic control
* Tight blood pressure control
* Stop smoking
* If develop chest pain, low threshold for further evaluation (exercise testing, stress echo, angiography) and consider coronary revascularization (angioplasty plus stent, or bypass grafting)

Myocardial Infarction study (DIGAMI) showed that late (>1 year) cardiovascular deaths were significantly reduced by one-quarter (from 44% to 33% after 3 years) in hyperglycaemic patients who received an insulin–glucose infusion in the coronary care unit, followed by multiple daily subcutaneous insulin injections for 3 months. The follow-up study, DIGAMI 2, unfortunately did not recruit sufficient patients and the intensive insulin arm did not reduce glucose levels more than conventional therapy. In this setting, the benefits of glucose control with immediate insulin postacute coronary syndrome were not confirmed. Nonetheless, glucose levels are an independent predictor of mortality in this patient group and it is reasonable to control hyperglycaemia (aiming for 5–10 mmol/litre) during the first 48 h in all known diabetic patients, and in those diagnosed diabetic at admission (blood glucose >11 mmol/litre, with HbA$_{1c}$ in the diabetic range). This can be done most easily with a simple sliding scale continuous intravenous insulin infusion, as used to treat diabetic ketoacidosis (see above). Delivering insulin as a 1 U/ml solution with a syringe driver avoids unnecessary intravenous fluids—this is an important consideration, as heart failure is a common (and often fatal) complication of myocardial infarction in diabetic people. The optimal approach to glycaemic control after the acute episode (insulin vs oral hypoglycaemic medication or lifestyle alone) remains unresolved. Metformin may be stopped acutely if there is a risk of heart failure, but should be restarted where at all possible after the acute episode because of its longer term cardiovascular benefits.

♦ Secondary prevention must include aspirin with a β-blocker and/or ACE inhibitors, as discussed above, and these have proven to have a greater beneficial effect in the diabetic than in the nondiabetic population postinfarction. Total cholesterol should be reduced to less than 4.0 mmol/litre and LDL to less than 2.0 mmol/litre with a statin, with the option of adding a fibrate to control residual hypertriglyceridaemia. Early echocardiography and exercise testing or equivalent stress testing are needed, followed when appropriate by coronary angiography and ultimately referral for coronary angioplasty and stenting or bypass grafting.

Stress-induced hyperglycaemia and myocardial infarction
The intense sympathetic discharge triggered by an infarct can push blood glucose acutely into the diabetic range in previously normoglycaemic individuals. Stress-induced hyperglycaemia can be distinguished from previously undiagnosed diabetes because the HbA$_{1c}$ will be normal. The acute management of these individuals is uncertain; they were classified as diabetic in the DIGAMI Study and also enjoyed improved survival with intensive insulin therapy. Pending further information, a pragmatic strategy would be to control glycaemia tightly during the admission with intravenous insulin for 48 h as described above, and then to monitor blood glucose closely and treat any persistent hyperglycaemia with insulin. However, it should be noted that up to 30% of subjects with acute coronary syndrome have raised blood glucose levels and the majority of these will later be confirmed to have diabetes on retesting 6 weeks after the acute episode.

Heart failure
This is common in diabetic people with ischaemic heart disease and is a major cause of death in those who suffer an infarct. In addition to ischaemia from coronary artery disease, a specific diabetic cardiomyopathy may contribute to failure, as left ventricular function may be impaired in the absence of obvious atheroma on coronary angiography. Various defects in contractility and calcium flux within cardiomyocytes have been identified in diabetic animal models, but their relevance to humans is not clear. Echocardiography may show specific abnormalities early in diastole, as well as areas of dyskinesia and a reduced ejection fraction. Moderate or severe left ventricular dysfunction, with an ejection fraction of less than 40%, should be treated with an ACE inhibitor, cardioselective β-blockers, and spironolactone as for nondiabetic individuals.

Stroke
Cerebrovascular accidents, mostly embolic, are 2 to 5 times more common in people with diabetes than in the general population. They are managed conventionally. As with myocardial infarction, a stroke can acutely raise blood glucose in both diabetic and nondiabetic people. The recent UK Glucose Insulin in Stroke Trial (GIST) did not show any outcome benefits of acute glucose lowering in stroke patients with admission glucose levels of 6 to 17 mmol/litre (of whom only 17% had a previous diagnosis of diabetes), but the study recruited fewer than 50% of the number of participants required for adequate statistical power; for the moment it seems reasonable to keep blood glucose within the range 7 to 10 mmol/litre, with the early use of insulin (probably subcutaneously) if this proves difficult.

Peripheral vascular disease
This is very common in the legs, often with diffuse disease distally (infrapoliteal) as well as in the iliac and femoral arteries. Consequences include intermittent claudication, pain at rest, and gangrene which is usually dry and may lead to the loss of one or more toes. However, because of the coexistence of diabetic neuropathy and the high prevalence of infrapoliteal disease, very significant foot ischaemia is often present in asymptomatic patients. Severe atheroma in the iliac arteries can cause Leriche's syndrome, with buttock claudication and erectile failure; the latter may also be due to involvement of the pudendal arteries.

Investigation and management are conventional. Intermittent claudication may improve with the simple advice to stop smoking and keep walking, but a shortening claudication distance or pain at rest require urgent investigation. Angiography often shows widespread atheroma, and this may preclude reconstructive surgery. Otherwise, standard operations such as femoral–popliteal (or more commonly fem-distal by-pass to the tibial vessels is required) bypass and the use of the saphenous vein *in situ* for more distal disease can achieve good results and must not be withheld from people simply because they have diabetes. Nonetheless, diabetes still accounts for about one-half of all nontraumatic leg amputations.

Patients with diabetic renal failure or autonomic neuropathy may show calcification of the artery walls, often easily visible in the digital arteries on plain radiography of the feet (see Fig. 13.11.1.18). This medial sclerosis (Mönckeberg's) is not directly related to atheroma, although the two often coexist.

Other manifestations of peripheral vascular disease include angina-like abdominal pain after eating, which is due to narrowing of the mesenteric artery, and renal artery stenosis which can contribute to hypertension and precipitate acute renal impairment soon after starting an angiotensin converting enzyme inhibitor.

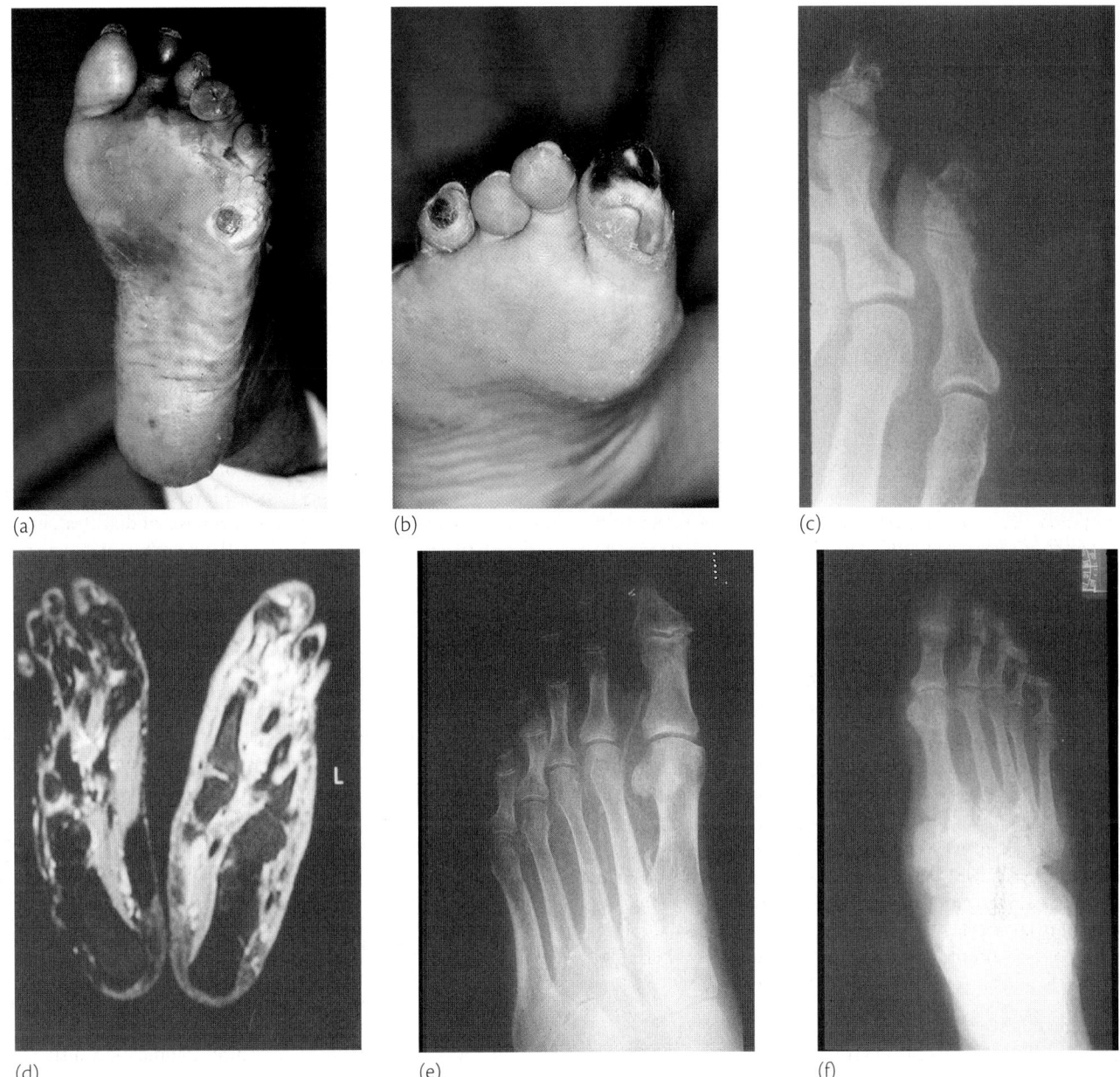

Fig. 13.11.1.18 The diabetic foot. (a) Typical punched-out neuropathic ulcer on the lateral aspect of the sole in an ischaemic foot with gangrene of the second, fourth, and fifth toes. (b) Ulceration and digital gangrene, caused by wearing tight shoes on a severely ischaemic foot. (c) Osteomyelitis in the diabetic foot. Early changes can be subtle: in this case, an erosion at the lateral edge of the distal end of the proximal phalanx of the fifth toe. ^{111}In-labelled white cell scanning showed an intense 'hot spot' at this site. (d) Osteomyelitis affecting the proximal phalanx of the left big toe and the adjacent metatarsophalangeal joint, visible as an abnormally high signal on MRI. Associated oedema shows as a high signal in the surrounding soft tissues. (e) Mönckeberg's medial sclerosis, outlining the digital arteries on this plain radiograph. (f) Charcot's arthropathy, showing massive destruction of the distal ankle joint.
(Part (c) courtesy of Dr Hans Laasch, Manchester Royal Infirmary; part (d) courtesy of Dr King Sun Leong, Whiston Hospital.)

Diabetic foot disease

The feet are at the mercy of various diabetic complications and problems such as ulceration, and resistant deep infections often cause long and expensive hospital admissions. Ulceration and severe ischaemia leading to gangrene of the toes or forefoot are the most common problems.

Diabetic foot disorders are best managed in a dedicated combined clinic. Prevention is extremely important. Many problems can be avoided by teaching the patients basic foot care, by regularly checking their feet and shoes, and by providing prophylactic podiatry and special footwear as appropriate. Charcot's arthropathy most commonly affects joints in the ankle or foot.

Neuropathy damages the foot through motor, sensory, and autonomic involvement. Distal motor neuropathy alters the posture of the foot by weakening its small intrinsic muscles and allowing the unopposed action of the long extensors to claw the foot, concentrating pressure on the heel and the metatarsal heads. Shear forces generated by walking and shoes cause the skin over pressure points to thicken into callus; eventually, pressure damage leads to foci of liquefactive necrosis deep within the callus, and these break through to the surface to form an ulcer (see Fig. 13.11.1.18).

Autonomic denervation opens up arteriovenous anastomoses, shunting blood to the skin—hence the warm skin and dilated veins of the neuropathic foot. Shunting may also deprive the tissue bed of oxygen and nutrients, thus worsening ischaemia from arterial disease. Increased blood flow may also be an initiating factor in Charcot's arthropathy (see below). Sensory denervation and loss of pain sensation can allow the foot to be damaged by agents such as overtight new shoes, a drawing pin, or sharp stones in the shoe.

Ischaemia, due to peripheral vascular disease and possibly microvascular damage, can lead to ischaemic ulceration and to gangrene of the toes or forefoot (see Fig. 13.11.1.18).

Foot ulceration

This is usually multifactorial, although one cause (e.g. neuropathy) may initiate or dominate the process.

Trauma includes the normal wear and tear of walking in shoes and damage from foreign bodies, often undetected because of neuropathy. Inexpert do-it-yourself chiropody is another cause.

Infection commonly complicates diabetic foot ulcers, and often penetrates deep into the soft tissues and bone. Mixed organisms are usually responsible, including staphylococci, streptococci, pseudomonas, and anaerobic organisms, sometimes gas-forming. Osteomyelitis is particularly ominous and requires urgent diagnosis and treatment (see Fig. 13.11.1.18).

Clinical features of diabetic foot ulcers

Primary neuropathy and ischaemic ulcers can generally be distinguished as below, but careful examination of the whole foot is essential so that all the possible contributory causes can be adequately treated.

- Primarily neuropathic ulcers occur at high pressure sites (heel, metatarsal heads) and appear cleanly punched out of the surrounding callus (see Fig. 13.11.1.18). The foot may be numb, with or without neuropathic pain, and the ulcer is often painless and may not have been noticed by the patient. Typical neuropathic features including clawed posture of the foot, warm skin, and sensory loss.

- Ischaemic ulcers tend to affect the edges of the foot and are often painful. There may be a history of intermittent claudication, absent foot pulses, and cold skin, sometimes with obviously ischaemic toes, the presence of areas of necrosis (gangrene), or previous amputation (see Fig. 13.11.1.18).

- There may be evidence indicating traumatic damage to the feet, e.g. symmetrical damage across the toes and margins of the feet from tight shoes (see Fig. 13.11.1.18).

- Infection may cause local signs of inflammation, although the skin may appear deceptively normal even over extensive and serious deep infection; characteristically, pain is absent. Anaerobes and pseudomonas characteristically produce a foul smell, while gas formation may occasionally cause crepitus in the subcutaneous tissues.

Investigation of diabetic foot ulcers

Effective treatment depends on identifying the cause(s) of ulceration. Neuropathy and ischaemia are assessed and managed as above. Swabs or curettings from deep in the ulcer should be cultured for both aerobic and anaerobic organisms. Plain radiography of the foot may show gas in the soft tissues or osteomyelitis, which can be difficult to distinguish from Charcot's arthropathy. ^{99}Tc bone scanning reveals changes several weeks before any alterations in plain radiographs, owing to osteomyelitis and Charcot's arthropathy. MRI is useful to delineate the extent of infected soft tissues but cannot always distinguish osteomyelitis from Charcot's arthropathy (see Fig. 13.11.1.18). Visible or palpable bone on probing ulcers that penetrate the deep tissues is almost invariably associated with the presence of osteomyelitis.

Management of diabetic foot ulcers

The principles of management of diabetic foot ulceration are the prevention of further trauma, treatment of infection, and optimization of the circulation. Predominantly neuropathic ulcers are treated by the chiropodist to remove callus, and ulcers underneath the foot may be protected from further trauma with a lightweight plaster cast to unload pressure from the affected area; this accelerates healing while keeping the patient mobile and may need to be worn for several weeks. Extra depth or custom-built shoes, or pressure-absorbing socks, will reduce pressure loading and help to prevent recurrence. Ischaemia is treated as above, aiming to avoid or limit amputation.

Infection must be treated with appropriate antibiotics and repeated cultures may be needed to ensure that mixed infections, especially including fastidious organisms and anaerobes, are completely covered. Soft tissue infections may respond to oral broad-spectrum antibiotics such as amoxicillin/flucloxacillin/metronidazole, co-amoxiclav, or ciprofloxacin/clindamycin. Treatment courses need to be considerably longer than in nondiabetic ulceration, as the absence of pain means the infection has often gone unnoticed for many days or weeks, resulting in more extensive infection. Minimum treatment is for 2 weeks and where osteomyelitis is suspected or confirmed, 3 months of antibiotic treatment is required. Severe, extensive, or unresponsive infections may require intravenous and surgical debridement. Amputation may be needed in refractory cases, but where ischaemia is absent remarkably extensive infections can heal after several weeks or months of conservative treatment. If ischaemia is present, revascularization should be attempted first to limit the extent of amputation required; if unsuccessful, primary amputation at the minimal viable level (which may be above or below the knee) is preferable, as an insufficiently extensive amputation is often followed by failure of wound healing. Successful healing of foot ulceration must be followed by very active preventive measures including regular podiatry, optimization of footwear, reduction of callous, and regular inspection as recurrence rates are very high; if peripheral vascular disease is present, aggressive cardiovascular risk factor management is required as up to 50% of patients die of cardiovascular disease over the 2 years following ischaemic ulceration.

Charcot's arthropathy

This is fortunately rare, affecting fewer than 0.5% of diabetic patients. It usually occurs in those with dense peripheral neuropathy and profound sensory loss, often with symptomatic autonomic damage. Reduced pain sensation is assumed to favour traumatic damage, and acute flare-ups are often preceded by injuries, which may be apparently trivial. Interestingly, blood flow to the affected area is increased early in the Charcot's process, possibly because sympathetic denervation allows dilation of arterioles supplying the bone; this may stimulate osteoclast activity and bone resorption.

The ankle and joints in the mid- and forefoot are most commonly affected; non-weight-bearing joints are very rarely involved. The natural history is variable but can lead to massive destruction of the articular surfaces and resorption of adjacent bone, often with a large effusion that can become acutely inflamed and mimic septic or inflammatory arthritis. In advanced cases, the joint degenerates into a 'bag of bones'. The process is generally painless, but acute flare-ups can cause discomfort. The most important differential diagnosis is from septic arthritis and osteomyelitis. Radiographic appearances are characteristic in advanced cases (see Fig. 13.11.1.18), but may be ambiguous early on; ⁹⁹Tc bone scans show increased uptake while the ¹¹¹In white blood cell scan is usu-

ally negative. An acutely inflamed joint may need to be aspirated to exclude infection, especially if systemic symptoms, neutrophilia, or raised erythrocyte sedimentation rate are present.

Treatment is often unsatisfactory. Nonsteroidal anti-inflammatory drugs can provide symptomatic relief, while offloading pressure with a plaster cast boot may temporarily halt bone destruction, but neither appears to improve the eventual outcome. Bisphosphonate infusions may slow the disease process by inhibiting osteoclast activity. Surgery should be avoided if possible, because the Charcot process may then spread to neighbouring joints. Occasionally, amputation is the only option for a dangerously unstable or painful foot.

Other tissue complications of diabetes

Limited joint mobility, also known as the diabetic hand syndrome or cheiroarthropathy, is probably due to glycation of collagen and other connective tissue proteins. It is particularly common in type 1 diabetes, and may develop during childhood. It causes worsening flexion deformities of the fingers so that their palmar surfaces cannot be opposed when the hands are pushed together (the 'prayer sign'), often with Dupuytren's contracture. Median and ulnar nerve lesions, presumably compressive, are often associated. Rarely, thickening of skin over the metacarpophalangeal and interphalangeal joints causes Garrod's knuckle pads (see Fig. 13.11.1.19).

Necrobiosis (lipoidica diabeticorum) is strongly associated with diabetes, although 25% of affected patients are normoglycaemic. Necrobiosis is the hyaline degeneration of collagen. The lesions present as trophic, nonscaling, yellowish areas, often with telangiectasias (see Fig. 13.11.1.20). They are most common on the shins but may appear elsewhere, slowly enlarge, and may perforate. Their progression is unrelated to glycaemic control. Topical or locally injected steroids may be helpful. The histologically

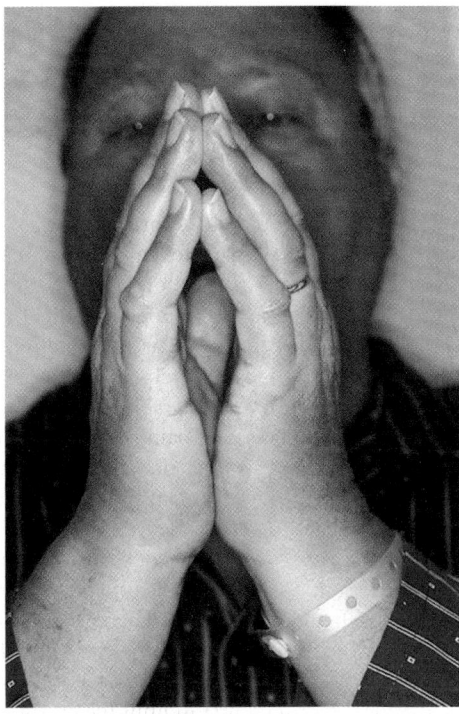

(a)

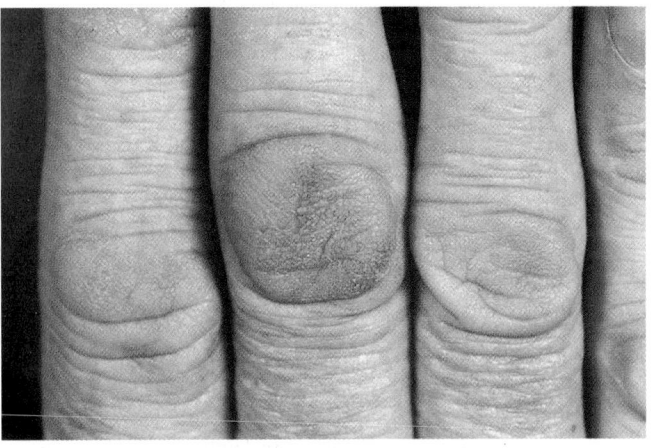

(b)

Fig. 13.11.1.19 The hands in long-standing diabetes. (a) Limited joint mobility (cheiroarthropathy), showing the 'prayer sign'. (b) Thickening of the skin over the knuckles and proximal interphalangeal joints (Garrod's pads).

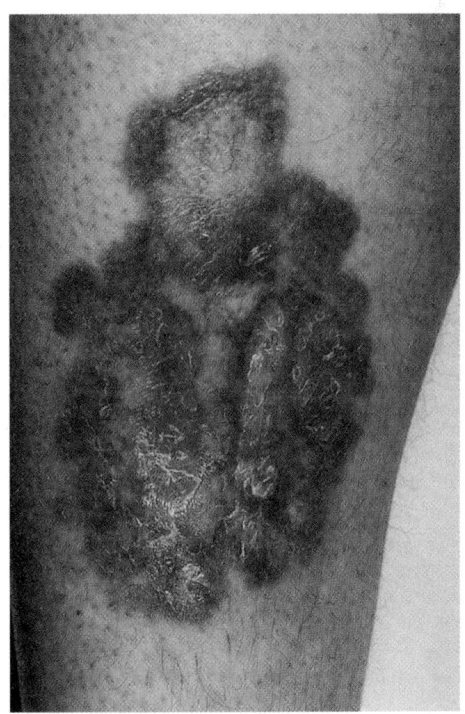

Fig. 13.11.1.20 Necrobiosis lipoidica diabeticorum. (Courtesy of Dr Geoff Gill, University Hospital, Aintree, Liverpool.)

similar granuloma annulare is not convincingly associated with diabetes.

Diabetic dermopathy ('shin spots') is the most common skin disorder in diabetic patients and is also seen in nondiabetic patients. These atrophic brownish or erythematous lesions, usually in the pretibial area, generally cause no problems and often resolve within a year or so.

Diabetic bullas (bullosis diabeticorum) are due to subepithelial splitting and present as tense and painful blisters which appear and heal within a few weeks. Differential diagnoses include bullous pemphigoid.

In diabetic osteopenia, poorly controlled type 1 diabetes causes general loss of bone mineral, although this does not appear to increase fracture rate significantly. Plain radiographs of the feet may show low-density phalanges that taper and may be smoothly eroded—an appearance imaginatively described as resembling partly sucked candy.

Further reading

Alberti K, Zimmet P, Shaw J (2005). The metabolic syndrome—a new worldwide definition. *Lancet*, **366**, 1059–62.

American Diabetes Association (2009). Diagnosis and classification of diabetes mellitus. *Diabetes Care*, **32**, **Supp l**, S151–S61.

American Diabetes Association (2009). Standards of Medical Care in Diabetes. *Diabetes Care*, **32 Suppl 1**, S13–61.

Biddinger SB, Kahn CR (2006). From mice to men: insights into the insulin resistance syndromes. *Annual Rev Physiol*, **68**, 123–58.

DECODE Study Group (2003). European Diabetes Epidemiology Group. Is the current definition for diabetes relevant to mortality risk from all causes and cardiovascular and noncardiovascular diseases? *Diabetes Care*, **26**, 688–96.

Diabetes Control and Complications Trial Research Group (1993). The effect of intensive treatment of diabetes on the development and progression of long-term complications in insulin-dependent diabetes mellitus. *N Engl J Med*, **329**, 977–86.

Diabetes Control and Complications Trial Research Group (1995). Adverse events and their associations with treatment regimens in the Diabetes Control and Complications Trial. *Diabetes Care*, **122**, 561–8.

Drucker DJ, Nauck MA (2006). The incretin system: glucagon-like peptide-1 receptor agonists and dipeptidyl peptidase-4 inhibitors in type 2 diabetes. *Lancet*, **368**, 1696–705.

Gale EAM (2002). The rise of childhood type 1 diabetes in the twentieth century. *Diabetes*, **51**, 3353–61.

Glaser N, *et al.* (2001). Risk factors for cerebral edema in children with diabetic ketoacidosis. *N Engl J Med*, **344**, 264–9.

Holman, R.R. *et al.* (2008). Long-term follow-up after tight control of blood pressure in type 2 diabetes. *N Engl J Med*, **359**, 1565–76.

Holman, R.R. *et al.* (2008). 10-year follow-up of intensive glucose control in type 2 diabetes. *N Engl J Med*, **359**, 1577–89.

International Expert Committee report on the role of the A1C assay in the diagnosis of diabetes. (2009). *Diabetes Care*, **32**, 1327–34.

JBS 2 (2005). Joint British Societies' guidelines on prevention of cardiovascular disease in clinical practice. *Heart*, **91** Suppl 5, v1–52.

Keech A, *et al.* (2005). Effects of long-term fenofibrate therapy on cardiovascular events in 9795 people with type 2 diabetes mellitus (the FIELD study): randomised controlled trial. *Lancet*, **366**, 1849–61.

Knowler WC, *et al.* (2002). Reduction in the incidence of type 2 diabetes with lifestyle intervention or metformin. *N Engl J Med*, **346**, 393–403.

Malmberg K for the DIGAMI (Diabetes Mellitus Insulin Glucose Infusion in Acute Myocardial Infarction) Study Group (1997), Prospective randomized study of intensive insulin treatment on long-term survival after acute myocardial infarction in patients with diabetes mellitus. *BMJ*, **314**, 1512–15.

Malmberg K, *et al.* (2005). Intense metabolic control by means of insulin in patients with diabetes mellitus and acute myocardial infarction (DIGAMI 2): effects on mortality and morbidity. *Eur Heart J*, **26**, 650–61.

Nathan DM, *et al.* (2005). Intensive diabetes treatment and cardiovascular disease in patients with type 1 diabetes. *N Engl J Med*, **353**, 2643–53.

Nathan DM, *et al.* (2006). Management of Hyperglycemia in Type 2 Diabetes: A Consensus Algorithm for the Initiation and Adjustment of Therapy: A consensus statement from the American Diabetes Association and the European Association for the Study of Diabetes. *Diabetes Care*, **29**, 1963–72.

Nathan, D.M. *et al.* (2009). Modern-day clinical course of type 1 diabetes mellitus after 30 years' duration: the diabetes control and complications trial/epidemiology of diabetes interventions and complications and Pittsburgh epidemiology of diabetes complications experience (1983–2005). *Arch Intern Med*, **169**, 1307–16.

Nathan, D.M. *et al.* (2009). Medical management of hyperglycemia in type 2 diabetes: a consensus algorithm for the initiation and adjustment of therapy: a consensus statement of the American Diabetes Association and the European Association for the Study of Diabetes. *Diabetes Care* **32**, 193–203.

Pickup JC, Williams G (eds) (2002). *Textbook of diabetes*, 3rd edition. Blackwell Science, Oxford.

Ryden L, *et al.* (2007). Guidelines on diabetes, pre-diabetes, and cardiovascular diseases: executive summary. The Task Force on Diabetes and Cardiovascular Diseases of the European Society of Cardiology (ESC) and of the European Association for the Study of Diabetes (EASD). *Eur Heart J*, **28**, 88–136.

Schade DS, Duckworth WC (1986). In search of the subcutaneous insulin resistance syndrome. *N Engl J Med*, **315**, 147–53.

Shapiro A, *et al.* (2000). Islet transplantation in seven patients with type 1 diabetes mellitus using a glucocorticoid-free immunosuppressive regimen. *N Engl J Med*, **343**, 230–8.

Tuomilehto J, *et al.* (2001). Prevention of type 2 diabetes mellitus by changes in lifestyle among subjects with impaired glucose tolerance. *N Engl J Med*, **344**, 1343–50.

Turnbull, F.M. *et al.* (2009). Intensive glucose control and macrovascular outcomes in type 2 diabetes. *Diabetologia*, **52**, 2288–98.

UK Prospective Diabetes Study Group (1998). Tight blood pressure control and risk of macrovascular and microvascular complications in type 2 diabetes. *BMJ*, **317**, 703–13.

UK Prospective Diabetes Study Group (1998). Intensive blood glucose control with sulphonylureas or insulin compared with conventional treatment and risk of complications in patients with type 2 diabetes (UKPDS 33). *Lancet*, **352**, 837–53.

Unwin N, *et al.* (2002). Impaired glucose tolerance and impaired fasting glycaemia: the current status on definition and intervention. *Diabet Med*, **19**, 708–23.

Useful websites

American Diabetes Association Home Page. http://www.diabetes.org

Diabetes UK Home Page. http://www.diabetes.org.uk

Hattersley A, *et al. The diagnosis and management of monogenic diabetes in children.* http://www.projects.ex.ac.uk/diabetesgenes/Monogenic%20diabetes%20ISPAD%20guidelines.doc

Diabetes Research Department and Centre for Molecular Genetics, Peninsula Medical School and Royal Devon and Exeter Hospital. *Genetic Types of Diabetes Including Maturity-Onset Diabetes of the Young (Mody).* http://www.diabetesgenes.org [Information for patients and professionals on research and clinical care in genetic types of diabetes]

English National Screening Committee for Diabetic Retinopathy. http://www.retinalscreening.nhs.uk/pages/

International Diabetes Federation Home Page. http://www.idf.org

Mendosa, D. *Online Diabetes Resources.* http://www.mendosa.com/faq.htm.
[Useful compendium of links covering clinical practice, research, and
patient-based organizations.]

United Kingdom Prospective Diabetes Study. http://www.dtu.ox.ac.uk/
index.php?maindoc=/ukpds/index.php

World Health Organization. *Diabetes Programme.* http://www.who.int/
diabetes/en/

13.11.2 Hypoglycaemia

Vincent Marks

Essentials

Hypoglycaemia is defined as a blood glucose concentration below
3.0 mmol/litre, which is clinically important because of its effect
on brain function. Much the commonest cause is excessive (in
relation to intake of food and drink) administration of insulin or
sulphonylurea drugs to patients known to have diabetes, but there
are many rarer causes including insulinoma, toxins (alcohol), organ
failure (hepatic), endocrine diseases (adrenal insufficiency, pituitary
insufficiency), non-islet cell tumour hypoglycaemia, autoimmune
insulin syndrome, factitious or felonious administration of insulin/
sulphonylureas, and infections (malaria).

Clinical features—patients classically present either to the
Emergency Department in a stuporose or comatose state with
concurrent hypoglycaemia, or to outpatient services with a normal blood glucose level but a history suggesting recurrent neuroglycopenic episodes or progressive neurological/psychological
dysfunction. Recognized clinical syndromes include: (1) acute
neuroglycopenia—profuse sweating, anxiety/nervousness, tremor,
tachycardia, hunger, and paraesthesiae, also speech and visual
disturbances, unsteady gait and confusion; (2) subacute neuroglycopenia—reduction in spontaneous movements and speech,
somnolence, inefficient cerebration, personality change, and amnesia of varying severity; (3) chronic neuroglycopenia—insidious
changes in personality, defective memory, psychosis, or mental
deterioration resembling dementia. The symptoms of acute and
subacute neuroglycopenia are ephemeral but—unless aborted
by restoration of normoglycaemia—can lead to stupor, coma or
(in exceptional cases) death.

Diagnosis and management—hypoglycaemia is usually detected by
point-of-care blood glucose determination and confirmed by formal laboratory blood glucose analysis. Treatment (in the patient
unable to drink or eat safely) is with intravenous glucose 25 g (50 ml
of 50% weight/volume) after (in cases where there is doubt as to the
cause) blood has been withdrawn for subsequent laboratory analysis, most importantly for total insulin immunoreactivity, C-peptide,
and proinsulin, and in some cases for alcohol, sulphonylureas and
other assays. Glucagon 1 mg may be given intramuscularly if venous
access is not available.

Particular causes of hypoglycaemia

Insulinoma—insulin-secreting β cell tumours are the most common endocrine neoplasm of the pancreas; most are benign and
solitary, but about 10% are multiple (often as part of the MEN1 syndrome) and about 10% are malignant. Diagnosis is made by demonstrating that symptoms are caused by hypoglycaemia (typically
provoked by fasting and/or rigorous exercise), relieved by intravenous glucose, and associated with inappropriately high plasma
concentrations of total immunoreactive insulin, C-peptide, proinsulin, and proinsulin-like fragments with regard to the prevailing
blood glucose concentration. No imaging technique is sufficiently
reliable to justify dismissing a diagnosis made on sound clinical and biochemical grounds. The treatment of choice is surgical
ablation. Localization by an experienced surgeon at laparotomy is
remarkably (96%) successful, but can be further improved by use of
intra-operative ultrasound.

Non-islet cell tumour hypoglycaemia—results from overproduction of an abnormally large form of IGF-2 or (rarely) IGF-1. Can
occur with almost every histological type of malignant tumour,
but least uncommonly with haemangiopericytomas, sarcomas, and
primary hepatomas.

Autoimmune insulin syndrome—due to polyclonal autoantibodies
to insulin that bind and sequester insulin secreted in response to a
meal, and then release it after absorption is complete, producing
an inappropriately high free plasma insulin level. Treatment is dietary and aimed at avoiding excessive insulin secretion in response
to meals until spontaneous remission occurs, usually within a few
years of onset.

Alcohol-induced hypoglycaemia—the most common cause of noniatrogenic hypoglycaemia, which typically develops within 6 to 36 h
of the ingestion of moderate to large amount of alcohol (>30 g) by a
fasting or malnourished subject.

Introduction

Hypoglycaemia means low blood glucose concentration
(<3.0 mmol/litre). It is a biochemical abnormality whose importance lies in its effects upon brain function. These are responsible,
directly or indirectly, for the signs and symptoms produced by
hypoglycaemia and often provide the first clue to the presence of
curable or preventable disease.

The brain obtains glucose from the blood by means of facilitated
transport and mainly utilizes the glucose-transporting protein
(GLUT1 or SLC2A1). The activity of this protein is increased by
hypoglycaemia and reduced by hyperglycaemia. It is not insulin-
dependent. Although blood glucose concentration is the single
most important factor determining glucose availability to the brain,
it is not the only one. Indeed there is a poor correlation between
blood glucose concentration and the severity and nature of cerebral
symptoms—especially in diabetic patients. It is therefore important
to distinguish hypoglycaemia, a description of blood glucose, from
neuroglycopenia, which is responsible for the signs and symptoms
to which hypoglycaemia gives rise. Several distinct, but not mutually exclusive, neuroglycopenic syndromes are recognized.

Acute neuroglycopenia, the most common, is normally associated with iatrogenic and experimental hypoglycaemia and is characterized by profuse sweating, anxiety/nervousness, tremor, tachycardia, hunger, and paraesthesia—all of which can be attenuated by adrenergic and cholinergic blockade—and by speech and visual disturbances, unsteady gait, confusion, and a sense of fatigue, which are independent of the autonomic nervous system.

Subacute neuroglycopenia occurs in most varieties of spontaneous hypoglycaemia and, when it occurs in insulin-treated diabetic subjects, is called hypoglycaemia unawareness. It is characterized by a reduction in spontaneous movements and speech, somnolence, inefficient cerebration and work performance, personality change, and amnesia of varying severity. Other signs and symptoms common to acute and subacute neuroglycopenia include transient hemiplegia, hypo- or hyperthermia, convulsions, diplopia, and strabismus. The symptoms of acute and subacute neuroglycopenia are ephemeral but, unless aborted by restoration of normoglycaemia, can lead to stupor, coma, or, in exceptional cases, death from cerebral oedema.

Chronic neuroglycopenia is rare and virtually confined to patients with hypoglycaemia due to insulinoma or diabetic patients overzealously treated with insulin. It is characterized by insidious changes in personality, defective memory, psychosis—often with paranoid features—or mental deterioration resembling dementia. Temporary elevation of the blood glucose level has no discernible effect on cerebral or neuronal function but removal of the causative agent often does over the course of a few years.

Hyperinsulin neuronopathy, the clinical features of which may be mistaken for motor neuron disease, is a form of chronic neuroglycopenia.

Normoglycaemic neuroglycopenia, postulated to occur as an acquired abnormality in adults with diabetes and as a possible explanation for symptomatic reactive hypoglycaemia was identified as a hereditary disorder in siblings with deficiency of the glucose transporter GLUT1. In infants it produces neurological deficits characterized by infantile seizures, spacisticy, ataxia, and hypoglycorrhachia. In adults it produces an acute neuroglycopenic reaction to lower than usual, but still normoglycaemic, blood glucose concentrations in susceptible subjects.

Physiological considerations

There is a hierarchy in the activation of brain centres as hypoglycaemia develops which is, however, not often observed in spontaneous hypoglycaemia. The tissue most sensitive to a falling blood glucose level is the normal pancreatic β cell which virtually ceases secreting insulin as blood glucose concentrations fall to about 4.0 to 4.2 mmol/litre. The sympathetic nervous system is activated and glucagon is secreted as the blood glucose concentration reaches about 3.7 mmol/litre. Stimulation of growth hormone secretion occurs at glucose levels of about 3.5 mmol/litre and that of ACTH and cortisol at about 3.3 mmol/litre. The threshold for vasopressin release has not been determined. Most subjects experience symptoms only after their blood glucose concentration has fallen to less than 3 mmol/litre, but objective evidence of minor cognitive impairment, of which the subject is usually completely unaware, occurs at concentrations nearer to 4 mmol/litre.

Patients, whether diabetic or not, with recent experience of hypoglycaemia often tolerate lower blood glucose levels before symptoms develop and counter-regulatory hormones are secreted. They remain, however, just as sensitive to the deleterious effect of hypoglycaemia on cognitive function.

Some of the cerebral symptoms of neuroglycopenia and effects upon neuronal viability are due to the liberation of the excitatory amino acids glutamate and aspartate, rather than solely to decreased intracellular energy production.

Definition

Hypoglycaemia is defined arbitrarily by the blood glucose concentration; it is not determined by whether symptoms are present or not. For most purposes, an arterial (or capillary) blood glucose concentration of less than 3.0 mmol/litre can be considered diagnostic of hypoglycaemia and one of 2.5 mmol/litre or less pathological and demanding of investigation as to cause. The possibility that a patient's symptoms are of neuroglycopenic origin should not be dismissed solely on the basis of blood glucose concentration. Normoglycaemic neuroglycopenia must be considered.

Classification

Iatrogenic hypoglycaemia as a consequence of insulin or sulphonylurea treatment for diabetes is common and accounts for most hypoglycaemia encountered in practice. It seldom presents diagnostic difficulties. There are, on the other hand some 100 or so causes of spontaneous hypoglycaemia, all of which are rare. Collectively, they are responsible for 0.1% of all patients arriving in emergency or medical investigation departments.

Table 13.11.2.1 lists the main causes of hypoglycaemia, which vary in frequency from country to country. Although all may occur in infants and children, the main causes of hypoglycaemia in this age group are not usually encountered in adults and not considered further in this chapter.

Table 13.11.2.1 Principal causes of hypoglycaemia

Induced	
Insulin: iatrogenic, accidental, factitious, felonious	
Sulphonylurea: iatrogenic, accidental, factitious, felonious	
Spontaneous	
Pancreatic causes	Insulinoma: benign, malignant, multiple, and microadenomatosis
	Insular hyperplasia: hyperinsulinaemic hypoglycaemia or functional hyperinsulinism
	Pluriglandular syndrome
	Pancreatitis
Extrapancreatic IGF-2 and IGF-1 secreting neoplasms	Mesenchymal tumours
	Haemangiopericytoma
	Primary hepatic carcinoma
	Adrenal tumour
	Various other carcinomas

Table 13.11.2.1 (cont'd) Principal causes of hypoglycaemia

Autoimmune hypoglycaemia	Autoimmune insulin syndrome (AIS) and insulin-binding paraprotein secreting myelomas
	Anti-insulin receptors
	Pancreatic Graves' disease
Toxic hypoglycaemia	Alcohol
	Drugs, e.g. pentamidine, quinine, paracetamol
	Poisons, e.g. mushrooms
Alimentary (reactive) hypoglycaemia	Postgastrectomy
	Alcohol-provoked reactive hypoglycaemia
	Noninsulinoma pancreatogenic hypoglycaemia
	Idiopathic postprandial syndrome
Organ failure	Septicaemia
	Acute and chronic hepatocellular disease
	Endstage kidney disease
	Congestive cardiac failure
	Acute respiratory failure
Endocrine disease	Pituitary insufficiency: generalized or specific, e.g. selective ACTH deficiency
	Adrenocortical insufficiency: congenital or acquired
	Hypothyroidism
	Selective hypothalamic insufficiency
	Phaeochromocytoma
Inborn errors of metabolism	Hepatic glycogen storage diseases
	Hereditary fructose intolerance (HFI) and galactosaemia
	Disorders leading to defective gluconeogenesis (e.g. fructose-1,6-bisphosphatase deficiency)
	Disorders of mitochondrial β-oxidation (e.g. medium-chain acyl-CoA dehydrogenase deficiency, MCAD).
Hypoglycaemia of the newborn	Transient hyperinsulinaemic hypoglycaemia
	Persistent hyperinsulinaemic hypoglycaemia
	Hypoinsulinaemic hypoglycaemia of the newborn
Miscellaneous causes	Bacterial, viral, and parasitic infections, especially malaria
	Diseases of the nervous system
	Prolonged carbohydrate deprivation: starvation, anorexia nervosa
	Excessive exercise (especially in combination with certain drugs)
	Chronic renal dialysis

Presentation

Patients classically present either to emergency departments in a stuporose or comatose state with concurrent hypoglycaemia, or to outpatient departments with a normal blood glucose level but a history suggestive of recurrent neuroglycopenic episodes or progressive neurological/psychological dysfunction.

Management of the stuporose/comatose hypoglycaemic patient

Hypoglycaemia should be suspected in any case of altered consciousness, coma, hemiplegia, apparent alcoholic intoxication, or epilepsy, and eliminated or supported (though not established) by a point-of-care blood glucose determination. The diagnosis is confirmed by formal laboratory blood glucose analysis. Hypoglycaemia may also be caused by, and contribute to the symptomatology of, congestive cardiac failure, liver or kidney disease, malaria, and other severe infections. Management falls quite clearly into two separate phases.

Emergency treatment

Glucose 25 g (50 ml of 50% w/vol) should be given intravenously to alleviate hypoglycaemia after sufficient venous blood (20–30 ml) has been withdrawn for subsequent laboratory analysis to determine its cause. Glucagon 1 mg may be given intramuscularly if venous access is not available, especially in cases of iatrogenic hypoglycaemia (in which it is usually effective).

Recovery of consciousness ordinarily occurs within 10 min. A further injection of 25 g glucose plus 100 mg hydrocortisone is indicated if recovery is delayed beyond 20 min. Overtreatment with intravenous glucose must be avoided. Specific measures to reduce brain swelling should be introduced if recovery does not occur within a further 20 min.

Prolonged, formerly called irreversible, hypoglycaemic coma is due to cerebral oedema and a consequence of profound hypoglycaemia generally lasting 5 h or more. Its treatment includes the use of intravenous mannitol and dexamethasone. Blood glucose must be monitored constantly and sufficient glucose infused to keep it within the range of 5 to 10 mmol/litre until consciousness is restored or permanent brain damage is established. In cases of suicidal insulin or sulphonylurea overdose, glucose in doses up to 80 g/h given as a 25 to 50% solution through a central line may be required.

Investigation

The second and third stages are similar to those employed in investigating patients suspected of suffering from a hypoglycaemic disorder but who are currently asymptomatic (Fig. 13.11.2.1).

Management of the asymptomatic patient suspected of having a hypoglycaemic disorder

Diagnosis takes place in three sequential stages:

1 Suspicion of hypoglycaemia and its confirmation by measurement of the blood glucose concentration during a spontaneous neuroglycopenic episode

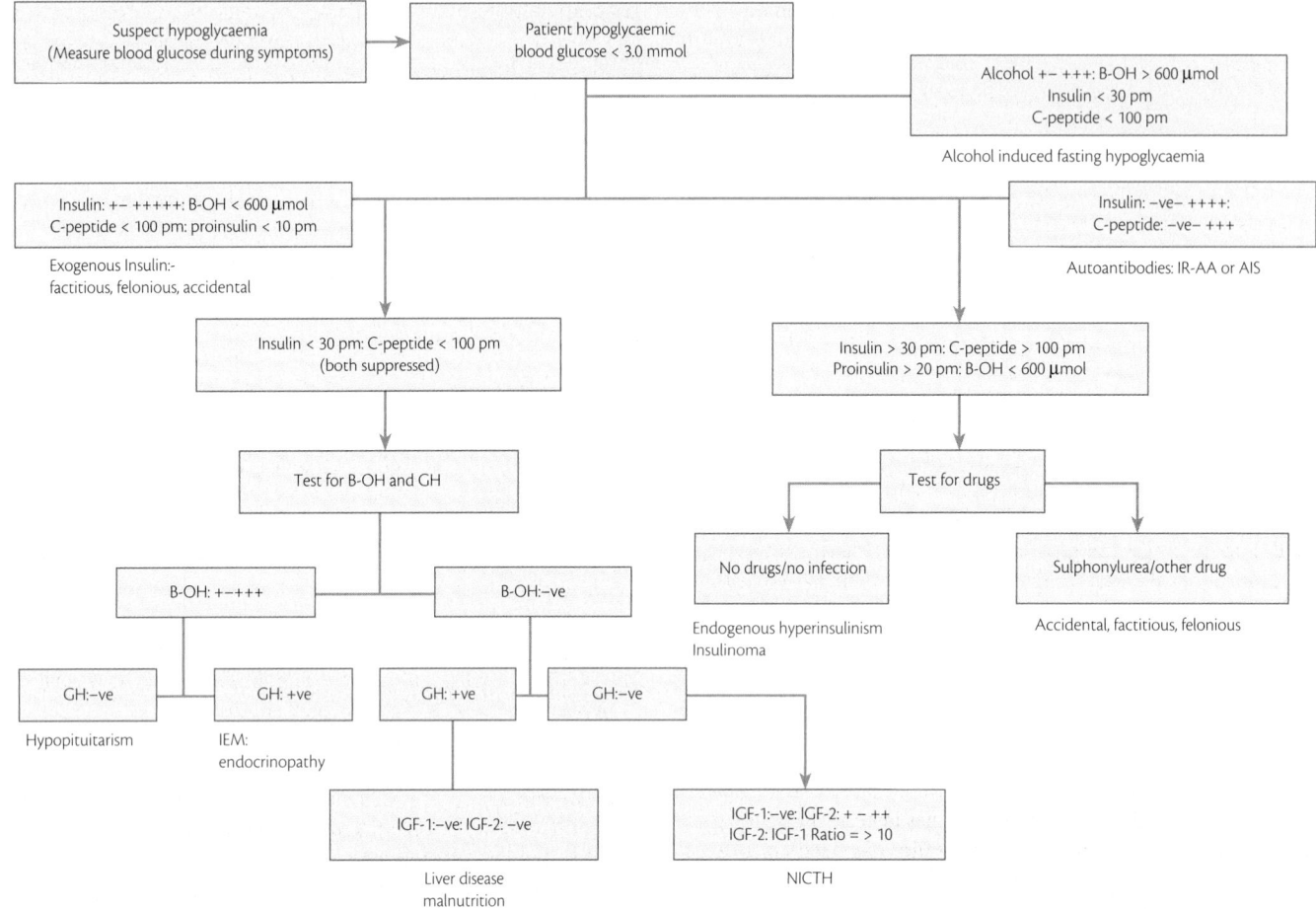

Fig. 13.11.2.1 Investigation of a patient suspected of suffering from hypoglycaemia who is hypoglycaemic but not unwell from some other cause, e.g. congestive cardiac failure, septicaemia, liver, or renal failure at the time of examination. It is customary to measure plasma total insulin immunoreactivity, C-peptide, proinsulin, β-hydroxybutyrate, growth hormone, IGF-1 and IGF-2, alcohol, and sulphonyureas simultaneously or sequentially on the initial hypoglycaemic blood sample. + to ++++: insulin >30 to 300000 pmol/litre; C-peptide >150 to 10000 pmol/litre; proinsulin >20 pmol/litre; GH ≥5 mU/litre; BHB >600 μmol/litre; alcohol ≥2 to 100 mmol/litre; −ve: insulin <25 pmol/litre; C-peptide <100 pmol/litre; GH <1 mU/litre; B-OH <600 μmol/litre; IGF-1 < 10 nmol/litre; IGF-2 <45 nmol/litre. AIS, autoimmune insulin syndrome; B-OH, β-hydroxybutyrate; GH, growth hormone; IEM, inborn errors of metabolism; IR-AA, insulin receptor autoantibodies; NICTH, non-islet-cell hypoglycaemia.

2 Determination of its aetiology on the basis of specific investigative procedures

3 Localization of the lesion responsible if the hypoglycaemia has an anatomico-pathological rather than a purely metabolic aetiology

Confirmation of hypoglycaemia

Most patients, except those presenting in a stupor or coma, are normoglycaemic and asymptomatic when first seen. Suspicion of hypoglycaemia is aroused by a history of subacute neuroglycopenia, e.g. episodes of altered behaviour or disturbed consciousness, or of symptoms suggestive of intermittent episodes of acute neuroglycopenia. Because amnesia is often a feature of their illness, patients may be unable to supply a reliable history.

Exclusion or confirmation that a patient's symptoms are hypoglycaemic in origin can often be achieved by teaching them, or their relatives, to collect capillary blood during spontaneous symptomatic episodes occurring in the course of everyday life. Blood collected into specially prepared tubes or filter paper should be sent to the laboratory for glucose analysis since point-of-care monitoring

systems are insufficiently reliable in the hypoglycaemic range to warrant initiation of detailed investigation and may cause confusion. A blood glucose concentration during a symptomatic episode greater than 3.5 mmol/litre effectively eliminates hypoglycaemia as its cause. Glucose concentrations lower than this are unusual and require further investigation.

Hyperinsulinism

This is a misnomer for the syndrome to which insulinoma and other β-cell abnormalities give rise. It would be better called dysinsulinism since its hallmark is inappropriate, rather than excessive, secretion of insulin or proinsulin.

Insulinoma

Insulin-secreting tumours (insulinomas) are the most common type of neoplasm affecting the endocrine tissues of the pancreas. They have an incidence of one case or more per million of the population. Eighty per cent of insulinomas are benign and solitary, 7 to 10% are multiple—often as part of multiple endocrine neoplasia type 1 (MEN1) syndrome—and 8 to 10% are malignant. They occur at any age but are rare before the age of 10 and infrequently diagnosed after the age of 70. The lack of cases after age 70 may be due to their mode of presentation, which is often that of progressive dementia, rather than to their rarity. There is a 6:4 ratio in favour of women for benign but not for malignant tumours.

Insulinomas are composed mainly, or exclusively, of β cells. Most are between 10 and 20 mm in diameter at diagnosis, though tumours as small as 5 mm in diameter have been associated with severe symptoms. Regardless of size, they occur at all sites in the pancreas with equal frequency.

Histological classifications, while valuable for the light they throw on insulin secretory mechanisms, contribute little to clinical management. Malignant insulin-secreting tumours are impossible to distinguish, clinically or histologically, from benign ones unless metastases are present. Some have the histological appearance of carcinoid tumours and both may contain and secrete other peptide hormones of which glucagon, somatostatin, ACTH, and GHRH are amongst the most common. Only rarely, however, do these biochemical endocrinopathies manifest themselves clinically. There is no evidence that malignant tumours ever begin as benign tumours or that benign tumours ever become malignant.

The average time between the onset of symptoms and diagnosis of insulinoma is currently about 1 year but symptoms persisting over 30 years or more without evidence of permanent brain damage are not unknown. Diagnostic delays are usually due to reluctance by patients to seek help or failure by clinicians to suspect hypoglycaemia, rather than any difficulties in confirming the presence of an insulinoma once the possibility has been considered. Only very rarely is an insulinoma found at autopsy as the cause of unexplained death.

In a minority, probably not exceeding 1 to 2%, functionally defective β cells are distributed throughout the pancreas rather than in discrete tumours. Clinically and biochemically, such patients are indistinguishable from patients with insulinomas. Biologically, such patients resemble infants with persistent hyperinsulinaemic hypoglycaemia of infants (formerly nesidioblastosis).

Chemical pathology

Endogenous hyperinsulinism is characterized by the failure of the abnormal β cells to stop secreting insulin in response to hypoglycaemia. This is ordinarily the most sensitive physiological response to a falling blood glucose concentration and becomes apparent at a level (4.2–4.0 mmol/litre) well above the threshold for neuroglycopenic symptoms. A consequence of insulin secretion persisting during fasting is inhibition of hepatic glucose release and a gradual fall in blood glucose to below the level capable of sustaining normal brain function.

Paradoxically, the functionally abnormal β cells are often insensitive to hyperglycaemia *per se* and so produce glucose intolerance as well as fasting hypoglycaemia. They do, however, respond, often excessively, to other insulin secretagogues including glucagon, sulphonylureas, L-leucine, and the intestinal incretins gastric inhibitory polypeptide and glucagon-like peptide-1, and may therefore present with reactive rather than fasting hypoglycaemia.

Typically, plasma cortisol and growth hormone levels in patients with insulinomas are normal even in the presence of hypoglycaemia. This would ordinarily be considered evidence of hypothalamic–pituitary insufficiency but responsiveness returns after restoration of permanent normoglycaemia. Plasma free fatty acid and β-hydroxybutyrate concentrations are typically suppressed (<600 μmol/litre) but rise, though not to expected levels, during prolonged fasting.

Diagnosis

Diagnosis is made by demonstrating that the symptoms are caused by hypoglycaemia, provoked by fasting and/or rigorous exercise, relieved by intravenous glucose, and are caused by inappropriate insulin and/or proinsulin secretion. Plasma concentrations of total immunoreactive insulin, C-peptide, proinsulin, and proinsulin-like fragments are all inappropriately high having regard to the prevailing blood glucose concentration but are not necessarily high in absolute (quantitative) terms.

Thus, in the presence of concurrent hypoglycaemia (blood glucose <3 mmol/litre), plasma total immunoreactive insulin concentrations of more than 30 pmol/litre and C-peptide concentrations of more than 100 pmol/litre are inappropriately high. When both peptide levels are inappropriately high, a diagnosis of endogenous hyperinsulinism is virtually certain, providing sulphonylurea ingestion and various rare autoimmune diseases and infections, such as malaria, can be excluded. If the patient was normo- or hyperglycaemic at the time of plasma sampling, the results of insulin, C-peptide, and proinsulin assays are uninterpretable.

Fasting combined with modest exercise under close observation for up to 48 h produces symptomatic hypoglycaemia with inappropriate hyperinsulinaemia (proinsulinaemia and C-peptidaemia) in over 95% of insulinoma patients but not in healthy men and women who, if they do become hypoglycaemic, do not experience symptoms or have inappropriately high plasma insulin levels. As an alternative to prolonged fasting, the overnight fasted patient can be exercised to exhaustion on a treadmill. In insulinoma patients, this fails to produce the normal suppression of plasma insulin and C-peptide secretion. It is, however, rarely necessary to subject a patients to these tests, especially if investigations are restricted to those who have blood glucose levels of less than 3 mmol/litre during spontaneous episodes occurring in everyday life. Dynamic function tests including oral glucose, tolbutamide, glucagon, L-leucine, and insulin–hypoglycaemia/C-peptide suppression tests are unnecessary for the diagnosis of hyperinsulinism.

Some 5 to 10% of insulinomas secrete only, or mainly, proinsulin and thus the diagnosis may be missed if an insulin-specific assay, rather than one capable of detecting total immunoreactive insulin, is used. Moreover, unusually efficient extraction of insulin by the liver can lead to low plasma total immunoreactive insulin concentrations in peripheral blood in the presence of genuinely inappropriate insulin secretion. This can occur in infants with hyperinsulinaemic hypoglycaemia as well as in adults with endogenous hyperinsulinism in whom inappropriately high plasma C-peptide levels will confirm the diagnosis. Hyperproinsulinaemia, e.g. a plasma proinsulin concentration greater than 20 pmol/litre, is found in some 95% of patients with endogenous hyperinsulinism; its absence should raise doubts about the accuracy of the diagnosis.

Pre- and intraoperative localization

A diagnosis of endogenous hyperinsulinism, established on the basis of inappropriate hyperinsulinaemia, is almost synonymous with one of insulinoma. The treatment of choice is surgical ablation. Localization by an experienced surgeon at laparotomy is remarkably successful (96%), but can be further improved by use of intraoperative ultrasound.

Though virtually every imaging technique has been advocated for preoperative localization of insulinoma, none is sufficiently reliable to justify dismissing a diagnosis made on sound clinical and biochemical grounds. Endoscopic ultrasonography, with a 90% prediction rate, and pancreatic intra-arterial calcium injection with hepatic venous sampling are currently the only imaging techniques that are useful for localization prior to operation. Hepatic venous sampling is especially indicated when surgery has failed to reveal a tumour and/or diffuse islet hyperplasia is suspected. It is the only way of establishing a diagnosis of noninsulinoma pancreatogenic hypoglycaemia preoperatively, which should never be made until sulphonylurea-induced hypoglycaemia has been demonstrably excluded.

Treatment

Surgical ablation ensures an excellent prognosis with no reduction in life expectancy except when the tumour is malignant. Even then, since these tumours grow slowly and rarely spread beyond the liver, removal of the primary tumour, and as many hepatic secondaries as possible, may add years of useful life. Operative mortality for adenomas is under 2%, except in older people. Benign tumours recur in up to 5% of patients.

In patients over 70 years of age, and others in whom surgery is impracticable, treatment with diazoxide (200–600 mg/day) combined with chlorothiazide (1 g/day) to increase its effectiveness, is well tolerated. It is the treatment of choice in hyperinsulinism due to diffuse islet hyperplasia, noninsulinoma pancreatogenic hypoglycaemia, and after surgical debulking in cases of metastatic insulinoma. Only when diazoxide/chlorothiazide treatment fails to relieve hypoglycaemia are other drugs, such as octreotide, β-blockers, or calcium channel blockers worth trying. In patients with malignant insulinomas, embolization or surgical debulking of hepatic metastases may produce remissions lasting several years—as may treatment with cytotoxic agents such as streptozotocin and 5-fluorouracil.

Non-islet-cell tumour hypoglycaemia (NICTH)

The symptoms of hypoglycaemia produced by non-islet cell tumours (NICTH) may be indistinguishable from that of insulinoma. The symptoms are almost invariably those of subacute neuroglycopenia and the features of autonomic nervous activation are absent. Biochemically, NICTH is characterized by fasting hypoglycaemia, hypoketonaemia, and low plasma total immunoreactive insulin, C-peptide, and proinsulin levels. Growth hormone, ACTH, and glucagon secretion are depressed during both hypo- and normoglycaemia and plasma levels of insulin-like growth factor 1 (IGF-1) are always low—unlike in insulinoma when they are normal or high.

NICTH can occur with almost every histological type of malignant tumour but is rare. Although sarcomas are disproportionately well represented, less than 1% of them develop hypoglycaemia. It is, however, common in patients with haemangiopericytomas, which are themselves rare. Amongst the carcinomas, no histological type is exempt from NICTH but only in primary hepatomas is it at all common.

Chemical pathology

Regardless of histological type, hypoglycaemia due to non-islet cell tumours (NICTH) results from overproduction of an abnormally large form of IGF-2 or, exceptionally, IGF-1.

'Big IGF-2' is generated by the removal of a 24 amino acid leader sequence from the N-terminal of prepro-IGF-2. Normally, it then undergoes cleavage at its C-terminal to produce regular IGF-2. Failure to do so leaves the E domain intact and leads to the appearance of big IGF-2 in the blood.

There is characteristically a marked reduction in the most plentiful of the plasma binding proteins, IGFBP3, and a partial compensatory increase in IGFBP2 the net effect of which is, however, to reduce IGF protein binding capacity. Consequently, plasma free (big) IGF-2 is increased without a corresponding increase in total immunoreactive IGF-2 which is often normal.

The exact mechanism by which big IGF-2 produces hypoglycaemia is unknown and may involve several steps, the most important of which is activation of insulin and IGF receptors on peripheral tissues and their increased uptake of glucose. The next most important step is the suppression of glucagon and growth hormone secretion resulting in reduced release of glucose by the liver.

Ectopic insulin secretion

Ectopic insulinomas are confined to the duodenum and are rare (<1%). Insulin production by non-islet cell tumours is even rarer, but does occur. The coincidence of an insulinoma and another type of tumour is more common.

Diagnosis

The diagnosis of NICTH is seldom in doubt once thorough investigations into the cause of hypoglycaemia have been initiated because:

◆ hypoglycaemia, once it has developed, seldom remits for more than very brief periods after meals

◆ the tumours are usually, though not invariably, sufficiently large to reveal themselves either on physical examination or as a result of comparatively straightforward imaging

In the laboratory, findings of low plasma insulin, C-peptide, and proinsulin concentrations (<30, <100, and <20 pmol/litre respectively) in the presence of hypoglycaemia and hypoketonaemia are highly suggestive of NICTH. Clinical laboratory assays that typically measure total IGF-2 are often reported as normal (50–100 nmol/litre) or high whereas IGF-1 levels are invariably low (<10 nmol/litre) except in IGF-1 secreting tumours. Consequently, plasma IGF-2:IGF-1 ratios, expressed on a molar basis, are abnor­mally high (>10) and not seen in any other condition except gross undernutrition and rare IGF-1 secreting tumours. Assays for the E domain of proIGF-2 have been developed. Although useful for establishing recurrence, they provide less accurate initial diagnostic information than the IGF-2:IGF-1 ratio.

Treatment

The treatment of choice is surgical. In rare cases of benign tumour NICTH, the cure is permanent. In malignant cases, ablation or debulking of secondaries may produce prolonged remissions. Prednisolone, in doses up to 60 mg/day, produces improvement in the biochemical profile and remissions from hypoglycaemia in many cases, but has no effect upon tumour growth itself.

Growth hormone and long-acting glucagon preparations also produce symptomatic relief given alone or with prednisolone. Benefit from diazoxide with chlorothiazide is less predictably than with insulinomas.

Postprandial syndrome

The appearance of symptoms suggestive of acute neuroglycopenia in relation to the ingestion of food has been called the postprandial syndrome. It has many causes, one of the less common being hypoglycaemia.

Reactive hypoglycaemia

Following an initial rise, venous blood glucose concentrations may decrease in normal healthy volunteers as far as 2 mmol/litre below fasting levels after ingestion of a liquid glucose load of 75 g or more on an empty stomach. A smaller fall in arterial blood glucose also occurs and may, in up to 50% of normal healthy subjects, be accompanied by mild symptoms. This phenomenon, referred to as reactive hypoglycaemia, rarely occurs in everyday life when normal mixed meals are eaten. When it does, diagnostic difficulties may arise since symptoms are usually vague, unspecific, and indistinguishable from those due to other illnesses, especially neurosis.

In the mid 20th century, the diagnosis of reactive hypoglycaemia, referred to by lay writers simply as hypoglycaemia, reached epidemic proportions in the United States of America. In most cases, the diagnosis was based on misattribution of a normal response to oral glucose to an illness. While some patients with postprandial syndrome may have a lower threshold to neuroglycopenia, experiencing symptoms at (arterial) blood glucose levels of 3.5 to 4.0 mmol/litre rather than the more customary level of 2.8 to 3.3 mmol/litre, most do not. Nor do they manifest any abnormalities of glucose homeostasis.

The criteria for the recognition and diagnosis of reactive hypoglycaemia were laid down at the Third International Symposium on Hypoglycaemia, adherence to which has greatly reduced the number of persons misdiagnosed. The criteria include a history of food-stimulated autonomic symptoms appropriate to acute neuroglycopenia—a capillary blood glucose concentration measured during a spontaneous symptomatic episode below 3 mmol/litre and rapid relief by oral glucose. Sometimes, when suspicion is high and blood collection during everyday life proves difficult, it may be necessary to give the patient a standard meal and observe the glycaemic, symptomatic, and electroencephalographic responses over the ensuing 5 h. The oral glucose load test is not appropriate.

The term 'reactive hypoglycaemia' is not a definitive diagnosis; it is only the first step towards determining causation. Almost every condition in which hypoglycaemia is induced by fasting may present as reactive hypoglycaemia. Therefore, organic causes, including acquired and inherited metabolic derangements, must be eliminated before making a diagnosis of idiopathic reactive hypoglycaemia—which is rare. Conditions in which patients experience only reactive, but not fasting, hypoglycaemia include partial gastrectomy and jejuno-oesophageal anastamosis (also referred to as alimentary hypoglycaemia) and, recently identified, noninsulinoma pancreatogenous hypoglycaemia. Reactive hypoglycaemia, unaccompanied by fasting hypoglycaemia, occurs in up to 2% of patients harbouring insulinomas. Autoimmune insulin syndrome usually produces only a reactive hypoglycaemia, but rarely develops

sufficiently long after eating to be mistaken for fasting hypoglycaemia. Prolonged fasting does not, however, reproduce it.

Clinical features

Typically, patients present with a history of transient episodes of dizziness, anxiety, palpitations, sweating, hot flushes, and even convulsions or brief periods of altered consciousness, and extending over a period of 1 to 30 years. Between episodes they are asymptomatic but rarely in robust health. They rarely notice any relationship of symptoms to food but may do so when prompted. Physical, including radiological, investigation is generally normal except in alimentary hypoglycaemia. In them, but few others, food-induced reactive hypoglycaemia may be of sufficient severity as to cause loss of consciousness.

Acute neuroglycopenia-like symptoms experienced by patients with the postprandial syndrome are rarely associated with any abnormality of glucose homeostasis or insulin secretion though exaggerated enteroglucagon, gastric inhibitory polypeptide, and glucagon-like peptide-1 amide response to food may occur. Some patients are unduly sensitive to modest reductions in blood glucose concentration to which most healthy subjects would be oblivious and in them the possibility of nonhypoglycaemic neuroglycopenia may be entertained.

Alcohol-induced reactive hypoglycaemia

Symptomatic reactive hypoglycaemia may occur in healthy young subjects after ingesting a mixture of alcohol, sucrose, and quinine given as gin and tonic and, less commonly, with other mixtures of alcohol and carbohydrate on an empty stomach. Simultaneous ingestion of carbohydrate-rich snacks increases the severity of the hypoglycaemia; snacks rich in fat reduce it.

Diagnosis

Diagnosis of reactive hypoglycaemia is suggested by the clinical history and confirmed or refuted by glucose measurements made on capillary blood collected during spontaneous symptomatic episodes. Other laboratory tests, including measurement of plasma insulin, C-peptide, proinsulin, and β-hydroxybutyrate are used to exclude conditions such as noninsulinoma pancreatogenous hypoglycaemia, autoimmune insulin syndrome, and other conditions that do not produce hypoglycaemia during fasting but do require specific treatment.

Capillary blood glucose concentrations of less than 3.5 mmol/litre, measured in an accredited laboratory on two or more occasions, establish hypoglycaemia as a factor in the symptomatology. The oral glucose load test, formerly the linchpin for diagnosis, may be misleading especially when conducted on individuals who have taken a self-prescribed low carbohydrate diet (<100 g/day) and should rarely be employed. A standard glucidic breakfast providing 100 g of readily assimilated starchy food has been advocated in its stead but is seldom indicated.

Treatment

Prevention of fluctuations in blood glucose is key to the management of reactive hypoglycaemia and is achieved by minimizing the intake of rapidly absorbed carbohydrates such as sucrose, bread, and potato starch. Frequent small meals, rich in dietary fibre—and taken without alcohol—offer the best chance of symptomatic relief. Incorporation of soluble dietary fibre supplements, such as guar and glucomannan, in meals and taking α-glucosidase inhibitors, such as acarbose and miglitol, with them reduce blood glucose excursions but their side effects are often worse than the discomfort from minimal hypoglycaemia.

Prognosis

Idiopathic postprandial syndrome is a self-limiting disorder but may be resistant to all physical treatments. Some patients respond well to psychotherapy and/or avoidance of alcohol.

Autoimmune hypoglycaemia

Autoimmune diseases are important causes of spontaneous hypoglycaemia. Three main types are recognized.

Autoimmune insulin syndrome

The autoimmune insulin syndrome occurs throughout the world, especially in East Asia, but is increasingly recognized in the West. It is due to polyclonal autoantibodies to insulin resembling those produced in response to exogenous insulin but more likely to bind proinsulin and its cleavage products including C-peptide.

Hypoglycaemia typically occurs as a late response to the ingestion of food. Insulin secreted early in response to a meal is sequestered by antibodies present in the plasma and rendered temporarily inactive. Dissociation of the insulin–antibody complex, after absorption is complete, produces an inappropriately high free plasma insulin level resulting in hypoglycaemia. This, though often profound, is of limited duration, rarely leading to coma and never to death.

There is often a history of autoimmune disease affecting other organs, especially the thyroid, and many patients have received treatment with methimazole, carbimazole, or other thiol-containing drugs.

Free plasma insulin concentrations are always inappropriately high and C-peptide is usually depressed during hypoglycaemia. C-peptide concentrations may, however, be normal or high depending on the binding characteristics of the autoantibody.

Treatment is dietary and aimed at avoiding excessive insulin secretion in response to meals until spontaneous remission occurs, usually within a few years of onset. Surgery, in the mistaken belief that the patient has islet hyperplasia or insulinoma, must be avoided. Myelomas associated with IgG or IgA insulin binding paraproteins may be confused with autoimmune insulin syndrome. Treatment is supportive and of the primary disorder.

Insulin receptor autoantibodies

Hypoglycaemia due to insulin receptor autoantibodies is rare but may be the first indication of the causative disease. More often it develops in a patient already known to be suffering from an autoimmune disease or a neoplasm—especially lymphoma. Typically, hypoglycaemia is intractable but occasionally occurs only in response to food. Its immediate cause is binding of stimulatory autoantibodies to insulin receptors on hepatic and peripheral cell membranes, simulating the effects of insulin itself.

Clinically, the symptoms are indistinguishable from that of insulinoma though usually of shorter duration and greater severity. Plasma C-peptide and proinsulin concentrations are low (<20 pmol/litre). Plasma insulin, though also often low, may be very high (>1000 pmol/litre) due to its delayed clearance from the blood. Diagnosis can usually be inferred from the clinical associations

and evidence suggestive of hyperinsulinism, e.g. coincident low blood glucose and β-hydroxybutyrate, but depressed plasma C-peptide, proinsulin (and usually insulin) concentrations rule it out. Definite diagnosis depends upon demonstrating antireceptor antibodies in the patient's plasma using *in vitro* bioassay techniques.

Treatment is that of the primary disease. Glucocorticoids and other immunosuppressants have been used with benefit in some cases but although remissions may occur, the prognosis is generally poor.

Islet-cell stimulating antibodies

Antibodies capable of stimulating insulin release from isolated pancreatic β cells *in vitro* have been held responsible for a form of hyperinsulinaemic hypoglycaemia analogous to Graves' disease of the thyroid. The evidence is, however, inconclusive and few documented cases have been published.

Drug and toxin-induced hypoglycaemia

Medicines and toxins, such as alcohol, paracetamol, quinine, amanita (fungi), and *Blighia sapida* (ackee) are collectively amongst the most frequent causes of noniatrogenic hypoglycaemia. They produce their effects in various ways, mostly by interfering with hepatic glucose production, counter-regulatory hormone action, or by stimulating insulin secretion.

Alcohol-induced hypoglycaemia

Alcohol-induced hypoglycaemia is the most common cause of noniatrogenic hypoglycaemia. The patient is usually stuporose or comatose. Sometimes they are aggressively uncooperative and their symptoms are attributed to alcoholic intoxication rather than to hypoglycaemia. Characteristically, hypoglycaemia develops within 6 to 36 h of the ingestion of moderate to large amounts of alcohol (>30 g) by fasting or malnourished subjects who may be, but often are not, habituated to alcohol. Hypothermia is more common than with other causes of hypoglycaemia and may provide the first clue to diagnosis. Children, in whom there is a 25% mortality rate, are particularly susceptible to this type of hypoglycaemia.

Blood glucose is less than 2.5 mmol/litre and alcohol is almost always present, generally at a concentration of less than 20 mmol/litre (100 mg/100 ml). Plasma and urinary ketones are high but often overlooked because traditional tests for ketones detect only acetone and acetoacetate rather than β-hydroxybutyrate—the redox pair member normally present in alcoholic ketoacidosis.

Once considered, the diagnosis is seldom in doubt and is due to the inhibition by alcohol of hepatic gluconeogenesis from lactate and glycerol. It can be confirmed by demonstrating hypoglycaemia, raised plasma β-hydroxybutyrate, and low plasma insulin, C-peptide, and proinsulin levels together with, in most cases, measurable amounts of alcohol.

Consciousness can be restored with intravenous glucose but not with glucagon, which is ineffective. Long-term treatment is avoidance of the predisposing factors.

Accidental, factitious, and felonious hypoglycaemia

In these states, although hypoglycaemia is due to exogenous hypoglycaemic agents, this fact is not revealed by the history. The correct diagnosis emerges only from critical examination of laboratory test results and other nonclinical or forensic evidence. Typically, the patient is hypoglycaemic and stuporose or comatose when first seen and—unless the possibility of drug-induced hypoglycaemia is suspected from the outset, and appropriate samples of blood and urine collected for insulin, C-peptide, proinsulin, and sulphonylurea assay—the correct diagnosis may never be made.

Sulphonylureas

Dispensing or prescription errors are an important cause of hypoglycaemia—a sulphonylurea being substituted for another drug with a similar name—e.g. Diabinese (chlorpropamide) for Diamox (acetazolamide). In hospital, victims of accidental hypoglycaemia often have received medication intended for someone else. Because patients are usually older people and slip slowly into hypoglycaemic coma without warning, the diagnosis may be delayed or missed completely.

Deliberate sulphonylurea overdose with suicidal or murderous intent is uncommon. It may be difficult to distinguish from accidental overdose in a diabetic patient unless the plasma sulphonylurea level is grossly abnormal or a suicide note is found. Treatment with diazoxide or octreotide and intravenous glucose may be required for many days to prevent recurrent hypoglycaemia.

Insulin

Factitious insulin-induced hypoglycaemia is as common in previously healthy subjects as in insulin-dependent diabetics and is due to deliberate, but concealed, injection of insulin. The history suggests insulinoma but is eliminated by the laboratory results which reveal high plasma insulin and low C-peptide (and proinsulin) concentrations during hypoglycaemia. In long-standing factitious hypoglycaemia, and in insulin-treated diabetics, insulin antibodies may be present in the plasma. Although once considered a strong pointer to factitious hypoglycaemia, the presence of insulin antibodies should nowadays suggest autoimmune insulin syndrome.

Suicidal overdosing with insulin is not confined to diabetic patients and is usually unsuccessful. Most patients are found within 12 h of injecting themselves and are restored to consciousness by appropriate treatment. Plasma C-peptide is unrecordably low and (free) insulin concentrations generally greater than 2000 pmol/litre. In factitious hypoglycaemia, plasma insulin concentrations are generally lower than this.

Murder or attempted murder with insulin is rare and virtually confined to infants, critically ill patients, and older people. The victims are often dead when first seen; if suspected, the diagnosis can be made retrospectively by demonstrating inordinately high concentrations of insulin in blood drawn from a peripheral blood vessel or in tissue removed from the putative injection site. Blood, cerebrospinal fluid, and vitreous glucose measurements are uninterpretable after death.

Organ failure

Hypoglycaemia can occur, sometimes as a dominant feature, in almost any serious and life threatening illness. Most notably are: congestive cardiac failure; acute liver failure; chronic renal failure; bacterial, viral, and parasitic infections (especially malarial); and terminal malnutrition. The cause of the hypoglycaemia is seldom in doubt but its recognition and the restoration of normoglycaemia sometimes dramatically alter the course of the illness.

Endocrine hypoglycaemia

Hypoglycaemia is a rare but important presenting sign of several endocrine disorders of which Addison's disease, panhypopituitarism, and isolated ACTH deficiency are the most common. The typical clinical features of endocrinopathy are inconspicuous and the diagnosis may be missed unless specifically sought through appropriate laboratory testing. Paradoxically, reactive hypoglycaemia is a rare manifestation of pheochromocytoma with which its symptomatology may be confused. Primary glucagon deficiency has only once been documented as a cause of hypoglycaemia.

Inborn errors of metabolism

Many inborn errors of carbohydrate metabolism—which usually present as hypoglycaemia in childhood—can first manifest themselves in adult life. Mild variants may be responsible for obscure cases of hypoglycaemia which occur only under very stressful conditions, such as prolonged fasting or exceptionally violent exercise, and for which no endocrine or organic cause can be found. Hereditary fructose intolerance causes hypoglycaemia as a dominant feature of the metabolic disturbance that characterizes the manifestations of this inborn error which are rapidly induced by consuming fruit, nuts, confectionery and meals containing fructose, sucrose and the related sugar alcohol, sorbitol. This condition is often undetected in infancy and many present for the first time with florid symptoms in adult life.

Further reading

Bolli GB, Fanelli CG (1999). Physiology of glucose counterregulation to hypoglycemia. *Endocrinol Metab Clin North Am*, **28**, 467–93.

Clark PM (1999). Assays for insulin, proinsulin(s) and C-peptide. *Ann Clin Biochem*, **36**, 541–64.

Cryer PE (1999). Symptoms of hypoglycemia, thresholds for their occurrence, and hypoglycemia unawareness. *Endocrinol Metab Clin North Am*, **28**, 495–500.

Cryer P E, *et al.* (2009). Evaluation and management of sdult hypoglycemic disorders: An Endocrine Society Clinical Practice Guideline. *J Clin Endocrinol Metab*, **94**, 709–28.

Cryer P (2007). Hypoglycemia, functional brain failure, and brain death. *J Clin Invest*, **117**, 868–70.

Grant CS (1999). Surgical aspects of hyperinsulinemic hypoglycemia. *Endocrinol Metab Clin North Am*, **28**, 533–54.

Halsall DJ, *et al.* (2007). Hypoglycemia due to an insulin binding antibody in a patient with an IgA-κ myeloma. *J Clin Endocrinol Metab*, **92**, 2013–16.

Kar P, *et al.* (2006). Insulinomas may present with normoglycaemia after prolonged fasting but glucose-stimulated hypoglycemia. *J Clin Endocrinol Metab*, **91**, 4733–36.

Koch CA, Rother KI, Roth J (1999). Tumor hypoglycemia linked to IGF-II. In: Rosenfeld R, Roberts C Jr (eds) *Contemporary endocrinology: the IGF system*, pp. 675–98. Humana Press, Totowa, New Jersey.

Kwong PYP, Teale JD (2002). Screening for sulphonylureas in the investigation of hypoglycaemia. *J R Soc Med*, **95**, 381–385.

Lteif AN, Schwenk WF (1999). Hypoglycemia in infants and children. *Endocrinol Metab Clin North Am*, **28**, 619–46.

Marks V, Richmond C (2007). *Insulin Murders; true-life cases*. RSM Press, London.

Marks V, Teale JD (1998). Tumours producing hypoglycaemia. *Endocr Relat Cancer*, **5**, 111–29.

Marks V, Teale JD (1999). Drug-induced hypoglycemia. *Endocrinol Metab Clin North Am*, **28**, 555–77.

Marks V, Teale JD (1999). Hypoglycemia: factitious and felonious. *Endocrinol Metab Clin North Am*, **28**, 579–601.

Nauck M, *et al.* (2007). Hypoglycemia due to paraneoplastic secretion of Insulin-Like Growth Factor-I in a patient with metastasizing large-cell carcinoma of the lung. *J Clin Endocrinol Metab*, **92**, 1600–1605.

Seckle MJ, *et al.* (1999). Hypoglycemia due to an insulin-secreting small-cell carcinoma of the cervix. *N Engl J Med*, **341**, 733–6.

Teale JD, Wark G (2004). The effectiveness of different treatment options for non-islet cell tumour hypoglycaemia. *Clin Endocrinol (Oxf)*, **60**, 457–60.

Vezzosi D, *et al.* (2007). Insulin, C-peptide and proinsulin for the biochemical diagnosis of hypoglycaemia related to endogenous hyperinsulinism *Europ J Endocrinol*, **157**, 75–83.

Wang D, *et al.* (2004). GLUT-1 deficiency syndrome: clinical, genetic, and therapeutic aspects. *Ann Neurol*, **57**, 111–118.

Won JGS, *et al.* (2006). Clinical features and morphological characterization of 10 patients with non-insulinoma pancreatogenous hypoglycemia syndrome (NNIPHS). *Clin Endocrinol (Oxf)*, **65**, 566–78.

Hormonal manifestations of nonendocrine disease

T.M. Barber and John A.H. Wass

Essentials

Tumours (usually but not invariably malignant), other 'nonendocrine conditions' and drugs can be associated with a wide variety of endocrine syndromes. 'Ectopic' hormone secretion, defined as the release of a hormone from a site different from the gland that normally produces it, has classically been recognized in the context of neoplasia, but it is now apparent that many hormones are synthesized by 'nonendocrine' tissue. Although a particular endocrinopathy may be associated with a specific type of tumour in a particular organ, the relationship is not invariable, and many neoplasms elaborate more than one hormonal substance at the same or at different times and thus produce a mixed endocrine picture.

Syndromes of ectopic hormone secretion

Most syndromes of ectopic hormone secretion are due to peptide hormones. Clinically evident syndromes are much less common than laboratory abnormalities, which are frequently found if extensive biochemical and hormonal assays are applied to patients with cancer. Well-described syndromes include the following:

Ectopic calciotropic hormones—hypercalcaemia in the absence of detectable bony metastases occurs in about 15% of patients with squamous cell carcinoma (usually bronchial), carcinoma of the kidney, ovary or breast. Parathyroid hormone related protein (PTHrP) is responsible for most cases, but sometimes increased production of 1,25-dihydroxyvitamin D_3 (lymphoproliferative tumours) or transforming growth factor α (TGFα) may be involved.

Syndrome of inappropriate antidiuresis (SIAD)—is reported in 40% of cases of small cell lung cancer; usually associated with high levels of circulating AVP, but other unidentified antidiuretic substances are sometimes involved. Presentation is with hyponatraemia, with diagnosis requiring exclusion of the very many other causes of this condition (see Chapter 21.2.1).

Ectopic ACTH secretion—pro-opiomelanocortin (POMC), the precursor for ACTH and other polypeptides, can be secreted by a variety of nonpituitary tumours (e.g. small cell lung cancer, carcinoids), which are responsible for about 20% of patients with Cushing's syndrome. Presentation is variable, but with rapid onset the physical manifestations of Cushing's syndrome may not have time to develop, and typical features include weight loss, proximal muscular weakness, oedema, diabetes and hypokalaemic alkalosis.

Ectopic secretion of insulin-like growth factors (IGFs)—IGF-2 is most typically (although rarely) secreted by large mesenchymal tumours; presentation is with symptoms of neuroglycopenia.

Endocrine manifestations of non-malignant nonendocrine diseases

Systemic disease of nonendocrine glands may influence endocrine function due to (1) a specific effect of the disease itself—e.g. hypercalcaemia in sarcoidosis driven by 1,25 dihydroxyvitamin D produced by alveolar macrophages; opportunistic infections, lymphoma, or Kaposi's sarcoma involving the adrenal glands in HIV/AIDS; and (2) as a general response to either acute or chronic illness—e.g. 'sick euthyroid syndrome', where reduced peripheral conversion of thyroxine (T_4) to tri-iodothyronine (T_3) is associated with a normal or reduced TSH in association with reduced T_3 and T_4.

Drug-induced endocrine manifestations

Drugs may (1) induce manifestations of endocrine disease—e.g. amiodarone may cause hyperthyroidism because of its high iodine content or due to a destructive thyroiditis—and (2) influence the results of hormonal assays and lead to mistaken diagnosis—e.g. oestrogen increases thyroid-binding globulin, hence women on the combined oral contraceptive pill have high total T_4 concentrations but are euthyroid.

Introduction

Several endocrine syndromes may develop in association with diseases that are not primarily disorders of an endocrine gland. In most the cause is a tumour, usually but not invariably malignant, that develops in tissue not normally looked upon as the site of the particular hormone synthesized. Other nonendocrine conditions may also be associated with either hormonal excess or deficiency, e.g. sarcoidosis and AIDS. Certain drugs may also modify hormonal biochemistry and cause hormonal imbalance syndromes. Albright suggested that the hypercalcaemia sometimes associated with malignant disease without osteolytic metastases might be due to the secretion by the tumour of a parathyroid hormone (PTH)-like peptide; we now know that this is true (parathyroid hormone related protein, PTHrP). Later it was shown that hypersecretion of ACTH, not from the pituitary but from an ectopic site, was the cause in about one-fifth of patients with Cushing's syndrome.

Syndromes of ectopic hormone secretion— general considerations

Although ectopic hormone secretion has classically been recognized in the context of neoplasia, and defined as the release of a hormone from a site different from the gland that normally produces the hormone, it is increasingly being recognized that many hormones are synthesized by nonendocrine tissue. Thus, the syndromes of neoplastic ectopic hormone secretion are actually due to the pathological oversecretion and/or inappropriate production of hormones. Increasing recognition of the importance of paracrine secretion of hormones such as insulin-like growth factors (IGF-1), their modulation by growth factors and binding proteins (e.g. IGFBP1, 2, and 3), and their role in progression of neoplasia adds greatly to these complexities.

Many different hormones are ectopically secreted by neoplasms arising in diverse organs, notably the bronchus, breast, pancreas, kidney, and ovary as well as in mesenchymal tissue. Although a particular endocrinopathy may be associated with a specific type of tumour in a particular organ, the relationship is not invariable. An example is the lung, where squamous cell carcinomas are often associated with hypercalcaemia due to PTHrP, while small cell lung cancer and bronchial carcinoid tumours are both associated with ectopic ACTH secretion, but with very different clinical manifestations. Many neoplasms elaborate more than one hormonal substance at the same or at different times and thus may produce a mixed endocrine picture (e.g. pancreatic endocrine tumours producing ACTH and insulin). The amount of ectopic hormone(s) produced may fluctuate from time to time (e.g. cyclical Cushing's syndrome in ectopic ACTH secretion). The changes induced by the ectopic hormone may mimic very closely, and be clinically indistinguishable, from those found in the true endocrinopathy. In others, the picture is less characteristic and dominated more by abnormalities of biochemistry or hormone levels. Thus, in many cases of ectopic ACTH production by small cell lung cancer, the downhill course of the illness may be too rapid for the classical features of florid Cushing's syndrome to develop, and hypokalaemic alkalosis with diabetes predominates.

Definition

The diagnosis of ectopic hormone production depends on a number of criteria, although it is seldom practicable or possible to confirm them all:

1 There is an association of the tumour with an endocrine syndrome.

2 Even though the endocrine syndrome may not be clinically florid, there is an elevated or inappropriately raised plasma level of the putative hormone.

3 Removal or suppression of the tumour induces a regression of the endocrinopathy and a fall in the hormone level.

4 The clinical picture and hormone levels are uninfluenced by removal of the gland that normally secretes the hormone.

5 The hormone level is higher in venous blood draining the tumour than in the arterial blood supplying it.

6 Extraction or immunohistochemical staining shows a higher concentration of the hormone in the tumour than in adjacent, noninvolved tissue.

7 Demonstration can be made of tumour cell synthesis of identifiable hormones *in vitro* or of mRNA coding for the hormone.

Chemical structure

Most syndromes of ectopic hormone secretion are due to peptide hormones. It is rare for tumours to secrete steroid hormones because of the complexity of the enzyme cascade required for steroid biosynthesis. Tumours may, however, be associated with altered steroid metabolism—e.g. increased aromatase activity in hepatocellular carcinoma leads to feminization and gynaecomastia due to androgen conversion to oestrogens.

The precise amino acid sequences of hormones of ectopic origin are being increasingly defined. In general, they appear to resemble closely those of their normally occurring counterparts (except PTH and PTHrP). There is a tendency for a greater proportion of higher molecular weight precursors, prohormones, subunits, and fragments to be associated with an ectopic origin than with true endocrinopathies, but it is not always clear whether this is due to differences in biosynthesis or in intracellular or extracellular processing. Minor differences in molecular structure are sometimes reflected in disparities between bioassay and immunoassay.

Prevalence

Clinically evident syndromes are less common than biochemical or hormonal abnormalities. The prevalence of ectopic production of ACTH, corticotrophin-releasing hormone (CRH), PTHrP, calcitonin, human chorionic gonadotrophin (hCG), prolactin, or growth hormone (GH), without clinical manifestations, is high when extensive biochemical and hormonal assays are applied to patients with cancer. These assays bring closer the prospect of finding a diagnostic marker for tumours in general and, in particular, as is already the case with the monitoring of hCG or its subunits, to determine the response of tumours to treatment.

Hypercalcaemia in the absence of detectable bony metastases is the most common abnormality. It occurs in about 15% of patients with squamous cell carcinoma (usually of the bronchus), carcinoma of the kidney, ovary, or breast. Next most common in neoplastic diseases is the syndrome of inappropriate antidiuresis, usually associated with a small cell lung cancer and reported in 40% of such cases. Cushing's syndrome due to ectopic ACTH or CRH secretion occurs in about 5% of patients with small cell lung cancer, and in association with other neoplasms. Biochemical accompaniments of Cushing's syndrome in the absence of the clinical features are much more common, occurring in 50% of patients with small cell lung cancer.

Pathogenesis

As techniques for molecular analyses have evolved, it has become clear that every somatic cell is capable of synthesizing every polypeptide hormone. However, only under pathological circumstances is that capability ever likely to be expressed. A variety of hypotheses for ectopic hormone synthesis and secretion have been made. None explains all of the observed facts. Fundamentally, all cells inherit an identical complement of DNA. They are therefore totipotential and have all the coded information required for the synthesis of all proteins and peptides, including protein hormones. The normal inability of nonendocrine tissue to synthesize hormones is ascribed to repressors that mask specific segments of the DNA molecule. It seems possible that when a cell becomes malignant this normal repression becomes ineffective, allowing the unmasked DNA to synthesize proteins or peptides foreign to the cell concerned. Such a de-repression hypothesis does not explain why certain tumours are more prone to secrete certain ectopic hormones. Neuroendocrine cells, characterized by the presence of peptide hormone granules, are likely to be the origin of some tumours associated with hormone secretion, such as small cell lung cancer and bronchial carcinoids. Another hypothesis suggests that there are a small number of special proliferative cells in normal mature tissues that have fetal characteristics with the ability to produce peptide hormones—a process of dysdifferentiation rather than de-repression. There is currently no unifying mechanism with supportive experimental evidence to explain ectopic hormone production. Further information on the control of gene expression and hormone production, the role of oncogenes, and paracrine growth factors may provide further insight.

Treatment

Treatment of the clinical or biochemical abnormalities associated with endocrinopathies of nonendocrine origin is best directed at the primary disorder. In neoplastic disease, this may involve surgical excision, radiotherapy, or chemotherapy. Sometimes, the tumour secreting the ectopic hormone is extremely difficult to locate even with the use of sophisticated imaging techniques such as MRI, radiolabelled isotope scanning (e.g. indium-111 penetreotide imaging), or using selective venous catheterization.

More specific therapy may be necessary to contain the metabolic abnormality until such time as the fundamental disorder can be controlled. For example, immediate measures may be required to reduce hypercalcaemia with fluids and bisphosphonates, or steps taken (administration of metyrapone) to diminish corticosteroid secretion from adrenal glands stimulated by ectopic ACTH secretion.

Particular syndromes of ectopic hormone secretion

Ectopic secretion of calciotropic hormones

Malignancy is the most common cause of hypercalcaemia in hospital inpatients and may be due to direct tumour spread to the bones or related to secreted calcium-releasing factors. Often several different mechanisms are involved in the same patient.

After its discovery in 1987, it was shown that PTHrP is responsible for hypercalcaemia in up to 70% of patients with this tumour-associated phenomenon. Most of these patients also have bone metastases. PTHrP shares amino acid homology with PTH between positions 2 and 13 of the 84 residues of PTH and acts via the PTH receptor, resulting in an elevation of extracellular calcium concentration. The *PTHRP* gene is located on the short arm of chromosome 12; that of PTH is on chromosome 11. The *PTHRP* gene may be activated by transactivation, hypomethylation (renal carcinomas), or the effect of growth factors and cytokines, including IGF-1 and epidermal growth factor, while glucocorticoids and vitamin D_3 suppress PTHrP levels. Unlike PTH-mediated hypercalcaemia, dihydroxycholecalciferol is suppressed in PTHrP-mediated hypercalcaemia. PTHrP is made by squamous carcinomas as well as renal, bladder, ovary, skin, pancreas, and breast carcinomas, and lymphomas.

Other factors can be involved in hypercalcaemia unassociated with osseous metastases. It is not uncommon for 1,25-dihydroxyvitamin D_3 to be made by lymphoproliferative tumours, which are either high grade or widely disseminated. Transforming growth factor-α (TGFα) which stimulates osteoclastic bone resorption, is also made by squamous carcinoma, and renal and breast carcinomas. Some tumours cosecrete both TGFα and PTHrP. Interleukin-1 (IL-1), which is a very powerful stimulator of osteoclastic bone resorption, is also made by squamous carcinomas as well as some haematological malignancies. Tumour necrosis factor (TNF) and lymphotoxin also stimulate osteoclastic bone resorption. These related cytokines cause hypercalcaemia *in vivo*; lymphotoxin is produced by cultured myeloma cells *in vitro* and accounts for the hypercalcaemia seen in this condition. Prostaglandins of the E series may also cause hypercalcaemia. Finally, vascular endothelial growth factor (VEGF) and IL-8 and IL-11 may be implicated in the development of hypercalcaemia of malignancy.

It is important to remember that primary hyperparathyroidism itself is common, particularly in older people; two diseases may coexist. For this reason, primary hyperparathyroidism should always be considered when hypercalcaemia occurs, even if it is in a patient within the setting of malignant disease. It is now possible to differentiate between these two conditions by using the PTH two-site radioimmunoassay.

Paraneoplastic hypercalcaemia may be either asymptomatic or dominate the clinical picture and be life-threatening as a consequence of dehydration and renal failure. The features of hypercalcaemia and its general management are discussed elsewhere (see Chapter 13.6).

Oncogenic osteomalacia, an acquired phenotype, is a rare syndrome characterized clinically by reduced mineralization of newly formed bone and the features of osteomalacia (including fractures, bone pain, and muscle weakness). It is usually associated with benign mesenchymal or mixed connective tissue tumours (particularly haemangiopericytomas) that have a propensity to arise in the head and neck. The use of imaging (including octreotide scintigraphy) is important in the localization of such tumours. Biochemical features of oncogenic osteomalacia include an excessive renal loss of phosphate that results in phosphaturia and hypophosphataemia. The serum calcium level is usually normal and serum alkaline phosphatase is usually elevated. Circulating levels of 1,25-dihydroxyvitamin D_3 are usually suppressed (despite ambient hypophosphataemia). Circulating levels of fibroblast growth factor 23 (FGF-23), a secretory product of tumours associated with oncogenic osteomalacia, are usually elevated. It is possible that FGF-23 plays an important role in renal phosphate wasting or impairs regulation of vitamin D metabolism, although there may be other unknown phosphaturic factors which also inhibit the 1α-hydroxylase enzyme. Removal of the causative tumour is the treatment of choice.

Syndrome of inappropriate antidiuresis (SIAD)

Syndrome of inappropriate antidiuresis is a disorder of sodium and water balance characterized by impaired water excretion, with resultant hyponatraemia, reduced plasma osmolality, and inappropriately high urine osmolality. A diagnosis of this syndrome requires the absence of hypovolaemia, hypotension, deficiency of cardiac, renal, thyroid or adrenal function, or any known stimulus for the secretion of AVP, an antidiuretic hormone. The syndrome is usually, but not invariably, associated with high levels of circulating AVP, although other, as yet unidentified antidiuretic substances are sometimes involved.

Inappropriate secretion of AVP can either be from an ectopic or eutopic (posterior pituitary) source. The most common ectopic source of AVP associated with a syndrome of inappropriate antidiuresis is bronchogenic carcinoma. Inappropriate eutopic secretion of AVP can be induced by a wide variety of diseases and drugs. Thus, although a syndrome of inappropriate antidiuresis in association with malignancy may be due to inappropriate ectopic secretion of AVP from the tumour itself, it may also result from inappropriate eutopic AVP secretion. The latter may be caused by treatment of the tumour (e.g. chemotherapy such as cyclophosphamide), an intercurrent illness such as pneumonia, a complication such as hydrocephalus or cerebrovascular accident, or even by the tumour itself (see Table 13.12.1). The treatment of this syndrome is restriction of fluid intake (e.g. 500 ml/24 h). Occasionally, it may also be necessary to administer hypertonic saline, or a V_2 receptor antagonist such as tolvaptan, that blocks AVP from binding to V_2 receptors within the distal nephron.

Ectopic ACTH secretion

Pro-opiomelanocortin (POMC) is a 31-kDa precursor for both ACTH and β-lipotrophin as well as for other polypeptides derived from it, including γ-lipotrophin and β-endorphin. A variety of non-pituitary tumours are capable of secreting POMC-derived peptides, accounting for about 20% of patients with Cushing's syndrome. Approximately 50% of ectopic ACTH-producing tumours are in the lung and the rest are present in a variety of other tissues (Table 13.12.2). Some tumours, particularly pancreatic islet cell tumours which are seldom (< 5%) associated with Cushing's syndrome, can, in addition to ACTH, also secrete a number of other hormones, including insulin, gastrin, and glucagon (see Chapter 13.10). This accounts for the usefulness, when screening for ectopic ACTH, of measuring other hormones (e.g. calcitonin, hCG) which may be cosecreted, the presence of which raises the suspicion of an ectopic hormone-secreting tumour. Very rarely, CRH is secreted ectopically in association with ACTH.

Neuroendocrine tumours are the most common source of ectopically-derived ACTH. These include bronchial carcinoid tumours most frequently, but also include carcinoids at other sites including the foregut, pancreas, and thymus. Other endocrine and non-endocrine tumours that can secrete ectopic ACTH include small cell lung carcinoma, phaeochromocytoma, medullary carcinoma

Table 13.12.1 Conditions associated with the syndrome of inappropriate antidiuresis (SIAD)

Malignancies
Carcinoma
Small cell lung
Pancreas—islet cell
Duodenum
Colon
Bladder
Prostate
Thymus
Cervix
Lymphoma

Lung diseases
Pneumonia
Viral
Bacterial
Fungal
Tuberculosis
Lung abscess
Asthma
Pneumothorax
Chest wall injury
Mechanical ventilation

Central nervous system diseases
Cerebral trauma
Cerebrovascular accident
Meningitis
Encephalitis
Brain tumours—primary or secondary (e.g. cerebellar haemangioblastoma)
Cerebral abscess
Hydrocephalus
Guillain-Barré syndrome
Delirium tremens
Acute intermittent porphyria

General surgery

Drugs
Vasopressin
Desmopressin (DDAVP)
Oxytocin
Thiazides
Vincristine, vinblastine
Cyclophosphamide
Phenothiazines
Tricyclic antidepressants
Carbamazepine
Chlorpropamide
Clofibrate
Serotonin-reuptake inhibitors

Metabolic causes
Porphyria

of the thyroid, mesothelioma, and small cell colorectal carcinoma (see Table 13.12.2).

The exact mechanism of synthesis of ectopic POMC-derived peptides is still debated. POMC mRNA can be found in the majority of tumours, but ACTH secretion is much less common, probably due to the lack of the signal sequence required for translocation. Changes in promoter usage and also in POMC processing may

Table 13.12.2 Types of neoplasm causing ectopic pro-opiomelanocortin (ACTH) secretion

Small cell carcinoma of the bronchus
Bronchial carcinoid
Thymic carcinoid
Islet cell pancreatic tumour
Phaeochromocytoma
Medullary carcinoma of the thyroid
Breast carcinoma
Tracheal carcinoma
Oesophageal carcinoma
Gastric carcinoma
Ileal carcinoma
Appendicular carcinoma
Colonic carcinoma
Ovarian carcinoma
Prostatic carcinoma
Squamous carcinoma of the cervix
Adrenal medullary paraganglioma
Melanoma
Mesothelioma

lead to ectopic secretion of ACTH. In addition, many tumours associated with ectopic ACTH secretion are of neuroendocrine morphology and may arise from progenitor cells associated with ACTH secretion.

Presentation
The clinical picture is variable and independent of the mass of the ectopically ACTH-secreting tumour. In patients with small cell lung cancer who have a rapidly progressive tumour, the physical features of Cushing's syndrome may not have time to develop. The major features are weight loss, proximal muscular weakness, polyuria, thirst, oedema, carbohydrate intolerance with glycosuria, and sometimes pigmentation due to ACTH. Hypokalaemic alkalosis is a characteristic finding; the plasma potassium is less than 3.2 mmol/litre and the bicarbonate greater than 30 mmol/litre, the urine potassium loss being the direct cause of most of the symptoms. This hypokalaemia is in part due to the very high cortisol levels, which have a mineralocorticoid action, and corticosterone and 11-deoxycorticosterone which may also be produced in excess. The 11β-hydroxysteroid dehydrogenase enzyme may also function abnormally, causing decreased inactivation of cortisol and corticosterone. The serum cortisol level is usually greatly elevated (>1000 nmol/litre) and the plasma ACTH level is also raised (>200 µg/litre). These high levels do not usually occur in pituitary-dependent Cushing's disease. However, there is some overlap between plasma ACTH levels between patients with ectopic ACTH secretion and patients with Cushing's disease, with very high ACTH levels having been reported in a cohort of patients with pituitary macroadenomas.

When the ectopic sources are other than a small cell lung cancer, the clinical manifestations may be quite indistinguishable from Cushing's disease, and cushingoid features (including proximal myopathy, thinning of the skin, bruising, and psychiatric disorders) may antedate by months or years any evidence of a tumour causing ectopic ACTH secretion. The degree of elevation of ACTH is less marked than with small cell lung cancer and is proportional to tumour size. Some carcinoid tumours may be small and difficult to locate. The real problem is to differentiate ectopic ACTH secretion from pituitary-dependent disease (Table 13.12.3). The presence of a hypokalaemic alkalosis (K<3.2 mmol/litre) is a very useful test in the differential diagnosis. Lack of suppression on high-dose dexamethasone testing is found in 90% of patients with ectopic disease, but also in up to 20% with pituitary disease. However, the CRH test is very useful in differentiation as patients with ectopic ACTH secretion show an absent rise in cortisol whereas pituitary dependent disease is associated with an exaggerated response in 95% of patients. Because most of the tumours secreting POMC are in either the chest or abdomen, MRI or CT scans will often reveal the source of ectopic hormone secretion. In patients in whom the lesion is not readily visible by imaging techniques, selective venous catheterization and sampling may help determine a source of ACTH by comparing levels at various sites within the venous system. Such sampling should include inferior petrosal sinuses in case of pituitary-dependent disease. Radionuclide imaging (including octreotide scintigraphy) may occasionally be helpful in localizing the source of ectopic ACTH secretion. In a significant minority of patients with presumed ectopic ACTH secretion, the source of ACTH cannot be identified.

Treatment
Rapid control of hypercortisolaemia is the initial aim of management following diagnosis. Removal or debulking of the primary tumour or its control with radiotherapy, chemotherapy or, in the case of neuroendocrine tumours, [131]I-*m*-iodobenzylguanidine therapy, will relieve the endocrine manifestations. A relapse may occur if metastases develop because these, too, usually secrete ACTH. When it proves impossible to control a primary tumour, or when the source of ectopic ACTH cannot be identified, adrenocortical hypersecretion may be reduced by medical adrenalectomy. This can usually be achieved through the administration of steroidogenesis inhibitors, including metyrapone (500–4000 mg/day), an 11β-hydroxylase inhibitor of the conversion of 11-deoxycortisol

Table 13.12.3 Response to tests used to differentiate ectopic ACTH secretion from Cushing's disease (from Howlett *et al.* 1986)

	Ectopic ACTH (% of cases)	Cushing's disease (% of cases)
Hypokalaemia <3.2 mmol/l	100	10
Diabetes mellitus	78	38
Dexamethasone 8 mg/day (no suppression)	89	22
CRH test excessive response	0	>90

CRH = corticotrophin-releasing hormone.

to cortisol. Aminoglutethimide (1000–1500 mg/day) may also be used but frequently causes a skin rash. Ketoconazole (400–800 mg/day), which can cause fatal liver damage, and the adrenolytic drug mitotane are also useful. Mifepristone (RU-486), a glucocorticoid antagonist at the receptor level, has been used as palliative therapy for some patients (10–30 mg/kg per day). Lastly, the long-acting somatostatin analogue, octreotide (0.3 mg/day, subcutaneously), has also been used in the treatment of ectopic ACTH syndrome.

Bilateral adrenalectomy is an alternative approach, but frequently it is not practical for patients with rapidly progressive metastatic disease. It may be possible to embolize the arterial supply of the adrenal gland if patients are not suitable surgical candidates for adrenalectomy. Medical treatment needs to be monitored carefully so that adrenal insufficiency is avoided.

The prognosis of patients with ectopic ACTH secretion is poor in patients with small cell lung carcinoma but can be excellent in patients with neuroendocrine tumours, depending on tumour histology and the presence of lymph node metastases.

Ectopic secretion of insulin-like growth factors

The insulin-like growth factors, IGF-1 and IGF-2, share some sequence homology and actions of insulin. IGF-2 is important in fetal growth, whereas IGF-1, synthesized in the liver, mediates most of the actions of GH. IGFs circulate bound to one of six binding proteins (IGFBPs). Of these, the most important is IGFBP3, which itself is GH-dependent and binds 75% of IGF-1 and IGF-2.

IGF-2 secretion from tumours may be associated with hypoglycaemia. Usually the tumour is large and of mesenchymal origin, arising in the abdomen or thorax. Symptoms are those of neuroglycopenia—sweating, tachycardia, disorientation, drowsiness, fits, and coma. Histology shows a mesothelioma, a fibrosarcoma, or other sarcoma such as a leiomyosarcoma. Other neoplasms associated with hypoglycaemia are haemangiopericytoma, hepatoma, adrenal carcinoma, lung carcinoma, Wilms' tumour, and colonic carcinoma.

IGF-2 secretion leads to suppression of GH and insulin, and reduced production of IGFBP3, IGF-1, and acid-labile subunit (ALS), leading to reduced formation of the IGF–IGFBP3–ALS complex which protects the IGFs from degradation. IGF-2 circulates as a smaller complex which has enhanced tissue and receptor bioavailability, allowing access to the insulin receptor. There is also an increase in the large molecular weight molecules and the increased amounts of big IGF-2 not detected on radioimmunoassay. GH deficiency, decreased gluconeogenesis, and increased glucose metabolism by the tumour, which is usually large, may also contribute to hypoglycaemia. Treatment of these tumours is difficult. The hypoglycaemia is often not responsive to diazoxide, glucagon, octreotide, or corticosteroids. However, administration of GH may be effective—increasing IGFBP3 and IGF-1 and antagonizing the effect of excess IGF-2. The underlying tumour may be resistant to radiotherapy; surgery, although effective if possible, is not always feasible.

IGF-1 and IGF-2 may also play an important role in tumour progression. Studies of breast cancer cells have suggested that IGF-1 may have local mitogenic effects, and a role for IGF-2 has recently been proposed in hepatocellular, colorectal, and adrenocortical tumours.

Ectopic hCG secretion

hCG is a glycoprotein consisting of an α and a β subunit. The α subunit is species specific and is the same for all glycoprotein hormones—luteinizing hormone (LH), follicle stimulating hormone (FSH), and thyroid stimulating hormone (TSH). The β-subunit determines receptor interaction and specific hormone activity. The β subunit of hCG is very similar to that of LH and this can cause problems with cross-reaction in assays: the LH value may be spuriously elevated in the presence of increased hCG levels. Clinically silent, ectopic secretion of hCG, with or without its free α and β subunits, occurs in many patients (Table 13.12.4).

Patients with ectopic secretion of gonadotrophins usually present with abnormalities in the reproductive system. In the first decade of life, ectopic hCG production may cause isosexual precocious puberty in boys with hepatoblastoma or a germ cell tumour. hCG, through its LH-like action, causes Leydig cell stimulation in the testes. In turn, testosterone levels reach those of a normal adult, and secondary sexual characteristics develop together with premature skeletal maturity. The testes remain small because there is no seminiferous tubule growth as this is dependent on FSH. Precocious puberty is rare in girls.

Intracranial teratoma, choriocarcinoma, and pinealoma are associated with ectopic hCG secretion. In some patients, cosecretion of ectopic hCG with oestrogen may be associated with gynaecomastia in men, and with dysfunctional uterine bleeding in women. Hirsutism and amenorrhoea are also presenting features of women with ectopic hCG secretion. Other tumours associated with ectopic hCG secretion include dysgerminomas, testicular tumours, ovarian adenocarcinoma, and stomach, pancreatic, bronchogenic, hepatic, and renal cell carcinomas. Rarely, ectopic LH secretion has been

Table 13.12.4 Human chorionic gonadotrophin (hCG) in sera of patients with malignant tumours (from Vaitukaitis 1991)

Tissue	Percentage of cases with ectopic secretion of hCG
Breast	21
Lung	10
Gastrointestinal tract	18
Pancreas (more commonly hCG -α)	33
Stomach	22
Liver	21
Small intestine	13
Large intestine	12
Biliary tract	11
Ovary (adenocarcinoma)	40
Testis	62
Seminoma	38
Embryonal cell carcinoma	58
Choriocarcinoma	100
Mixed	73

described in adrenal tumours and pancreatic neuroendocrine tumours.

hCG is a useful tumour marker in gestational trophoblastic disease (choriocarcinoma) and in some men with testicular tumours, and provides an early warning of recurrent disease. However, it is important to measure other tumour markers, e.g. α-fetoprotein, which may also be secreted by nonseminomatous germ cell tumours. Discordance of marker levels and tumour progress may be seen. In central nervous system disease, cerebrospinal fluid/plasma ratios may help in the correct localization of tumours, as hCG does not cross the blood–brain barrier and levels in cerebrospinal fluid remain undetectable in pregnancy. Thus, cerebrospinal fluid concentrations higher than plasma suggest primary central nervous system disease.

In some patients, most commonly with choriocarcinoma and massive elevation of hCG, the latter, through its weak TSH activity, due to its biochemical similarity to TSH, may cause goitre and hyperthyroidism. This most frequently occurs in women, is not associated with eye signs, and is usually associated with modest biochemical abnormalities. Treatment of the tumour results in a resumption of a euthyroid state but, if this is not possible, carbimazole or propylthiouracil may be required.

Ectopic human placental lactogen

Human placental lactogen (hPL), also called human chorionic somatomammotropin (hCS), is a trophoblastic hormone which may be secreted ectopically in association with lung tumours, testicular tumours, and trophoblastic disease. It is usually associated with gynaecomastia in men, and these tumours may also be associated with increased levels of oestradiol and hCG.

Ectopic GHRH and GH secretion

Most patients with acromegaly (98%) have benign GH-producing pituitary adenomas. Less than 2% of patients with acromegaly have ectopic growth hormone-releasing hormone (GHRH) production which causes hyperstimulation of the somatotroph cells within the anterior pituitary, and consequently increased GH secretion. Indeed, the presence of anterior pituitary somatotroph hyperplasia differentiates histologically the minority of acromegalic patients with ectopic GHRH syndrome from those with GH-producing pituitary adenomas. A patient with a carcinoid tumour of the pancreas producing GHRH enabled the final elucidation of the structure of this important hypothalamic peptide. Ectopic GHRH syndrome is caused most frequently by carcinoid tumours, especially of the lung and gastrointestinal tract. Although many carcinoid tumours express immunoreactive GHRH, the development of acromegaly is uncommon (although many of these patients may display abnormal GH secretory dynamics). Other tumours reported to secrete GHRH ectopically include small cell lung cancer, adrenal adenomas, endometrial tumours, and phaeochromocytoma. GHRH can also be secreted by hypothalamic hamartomas which also result in anterior pituitary somatotroph hyperplasia. Determination of the cause of acromegaly (pituitary GH excess versus ectopic GHRH syndrome) is extremely important in the management of acromegaly. Ectopically GHRH-secreting tumours are usually clinically apparent and GHRH levels in the circulation are elevated. Surgical resection of such tumours is the logical

approach to management. Long-acting somatostatin analogues can also be used in those patients with ectopic GHRH syndrome caused by disseminated or recurrent carcinoid tumours.

Ectopic GH secretion has been reported in patients with bronchial, pancreatic, and gastrointestinal carcinoma, and cells cultured from an undifferentiated lung cancer have been shown to synthesize GH *in vitro*. Breast carcinoma and ovarian tumours may also occasionally secrete GH but no clinical syndrome has been clearly identified as caused by ectopic GH.

Ectopic prolactin secretion

Prolactin may be secreted by bronchial carcinoma and renal cell carcinoma; the usual endocrine manifestation is galactorrhoea and there may be marked hyperprolactinaemia. These abnormalities are reversed if the tumour is controlled or removed. Difficulties in differential diagnosis may arise unless the underlying abnormality is clinically obvious or suspected, because in most instances the hyperprolactinaemia will be attributed to a prolactin-secreting adenoma. Suspicion of an ectopic source may only arise when the prolactin level is not lowered by treatment with dopamine agonists. An autocrine role for prolactin in breast and prostate cancer has recently been postulated.

Ectopic calcitonin secretion

Increased serum calcitonin levels are encountered in a variety of cancers apart from medullary carcinoma of the thyroid. The most common of these are small cell lung cancer, leukaemia, and neoplasms of the breast and pancreas. It is often produced as part of a multihormonal profile in conjunction with gastrin, ACTH, and somatostatin among others. Ectopic calcitonin may differ from the normal hormone in having more components of high molecular weight; it does not cause any apparent symptoms and does not produce hypocalcaemia.

Ectopic renin secretion

Although hypertension associated with hyper-reninism and increased aldosterone production is usually due to a renal lesion, ectopic secretion of renin has also been described in association with cancer of the lung, pancreas, ovary, and, rarely, testicle. The clinical picture is usually dominated by the underlying neoplasm but the patient has hypertension and the cause of this may be suspected from the associated hypokalaemia and its accompanying muscle weakness. Effective treatment of the primary lesion will reduce the increased renin and aldosterone levels and hence the raised blood pressure. When the underlying cause cannot be eradicated, the use of an angiotensin-converting enzyme (ACE) inhibitor will control the hypertension.

Ectopic aldosterone secretion

Hypertension and hypokalaemia related to ectopic secretion of aldosterone from a nonadrenal neoplasm have been described in patients with ovarian tumours. Its pathogenesis is different from the others described in this section. The aberrant production of a steroid, aldosterone, rather than a peptide, is presumably due to biochemical change in the ovarian steroidogenic cells. Attention is likely to be focused on a suspected lesion of the adrenal zona glomerulosa because the hyperaldosteronism is associated with low

2066 SECTION 13 ENDOCRINE DISORDERS

plasma renin activity. The ovarian lesion may initially be clinically silent and only revealed by pelvic imaging.

Endocrine manifestations of nonmalignant, nonendocrine diseases

Systemic disease of nonendocrine glands may influence endocrine function due to a specific effect of the disease itself, due to a general response to either acute or chronic illness, or due to drug therapy used to treat the illness itself (Table 13.12.5). Often, hormonal perturbations may be a complex mixture of all of these mechanisms, as may be seen in AIDS or critically ill patients on intensive therapy units. This section includes examples of systemic disease causing endocrine disorders.

A commonly observed hormonal disturbance encountered in many hospital inpatients is the sick euthyroid syndrome. Peripheral conversion of thyroxine (T_4) to tri-iodothyronine (T_3) is reduced, and typical thyroid function tests in this syndrome are a normal or reduced TSH in association with reduced T_3 and T_4 (and increased reverse T_3 if measured). Severe illness may also interfere with hypothalamopituitary function and lead to hypogonadotrophic hypogonadism. Possible mechanisms include increased cortisol levels, stress, cytokines, or opioids given as analgesia.

Disorders influencing hypothalamopituitary function

Anorexia nervosa is associated with complex changes in hypothalamopituitary function, with reduction in GnRH and gonadotrophin secretion leading to hypogonadotrophic hypogonadism, but increased GH secretion is associated with increased peripheral resistance to GH.

Iron overload due to haematological conditions such as β-thalassaemia major and to haemochromatosis may cause iron deposition in the anterior pituitary gland, and in particular in the gonadotrophs. This leads to hypogonadotrophic hypogonadism, which may be ameliorated to a degree by venesection and iron chelation therapy. Haemochromatosis may also lead to other hormonal changes due to pancreatic involvement causing diabetes mellitus, and cirrhosis associated with secondary hyperaldosteronism and hypogonadism.

Thyroid

Morning sickness in the first trimester of pregnancy may be associated with clinical and biochemical features of thyrotoxicosis, as the molecules hCG and TSH share very similar β subunits, allowing cross-reactivity when high levels of hCG occur.

Opportunistic infections of the thyroid gland may occur, in conditions associated with immunosuppression such as AIDS. Infections with cytomegalovirus, cryptococcus, and pneumocystis have been described. In addition, some patients with HIV infection have increased T_4 and T_3 due to increased thyroid binding globulin. As the disease progresses, T_4 and T_3 levels fall as patients develop biochemical features of sick euthyroidism.

Adrenal

Opportunistic infections (cytomegalovirus, atypical mycobacteria, cryptococci, toxoplasma, and pneumocystis), lymphoma, and Kaposi's sarcoma may involve the adrenal glands in HIV and AIDS.

Table 13.12.5 Hormonal abnormalities associated with non-endocrine disorders

Disease	Endocrine abnormality
Severe illness	Sick euthyroid syndrome ($\downarrow$TSH $\downarrow T_4$ $\downarrow$T3 $\uparrow$rT_3)
	Hypogonadism ($\downarrow$LH $\downarrow$testosterone/oestradiol)
Anorexia nervosa	Hypogonadotrophic hypogonadism ($\downarrow$GnRH $\downarrow$LH/FSH $\uparrow$GH)
Iron overload	Hypogonadotrophic hypogonadism ($\downarrow$LH/FSH $\downarrow$T or E_2)
Hyperemesis gravidarum	Thyrotoxicosis ($\downarrow$TSH $\uparrow t_4$, $\uparrow$hCG)
HIV infection and AIDS	$\uparrow T_4$ $\uparrow T_3$ $\uparrow$TBG(HIV)
	Opportunistic infections may cause goitre, hypo- or hyperthyroidism
	Adrenal infiltration (infection, lymphoma, and Kaposi's sarcoma), however Addison's rare
	Impaired aldosterone and adrenal androgen secretion, with preferential glucocorticoid production
Cytotoxic chemotherapy and radiotherapy	Hypogonadotrophic hypogonadism ($\downarrow$ LH/FSH $\downarrow$T/E_2)
	Premature ovarian and testicular failure due to direct cytotoxic effect
Coeliac disease	Reversible androgen resistance ($\uparrow$FSH/LH $\downarrow$testosterone)
Alcoholic liver disease	Androgen deficiency ($\downarrow$testosterone $\uparrow$SHBG $\uparrow E_2$)
Sarcoidosis and other granulomatous disorders	$\uparrow$1,25 DHCC $\uparrow$calcium
HTLV-1 infection	$\uparrow$PTHrP $\uparrow$calcium

The adrenal gland is the most commonly involved endocrine gland at autopsy. However, frank adrenal insufficiency is rare because this requires destruction of over 90% of the adrenal cortex.

Gonads

Chemotherapy and irradiation may be associated with gonadal failure due to hypothalamopituitary gonadotrophin deficiency, e.g. following cranial irradiation or due to testicular/ovarian damage following cytotoxic drug therapy such as cyclophosphamide, cisplatin, and busulfan.

Coeliac disease is associated with reversible male infertility due to androgen resistance, and improves on a gluten free diet. Alteration of gonadal steroid metabolism may occur in chronic liver disease, particularly if alcohol related. Elevated sex hormone binding globulin and oestradiol levels are associated with a reduction in bioavailable testosterone leading to testicular atrophy, gynaecomastia, and erectile impotence.

Gynaecomastia

Palpable breast glandular tissue is prevalent in population studies of men and boys. Subareolar glandular tissue of more than 2 cm in diameter is found in 35 to 60% of men. Gynaecomastia may occur as a result of different conditions (Table 13.12.6) as well as drug therapy, and results from an alteration in the ratio of oestrogen

Table 13.12.6 Non-endocrine conditions associated with gynaecomastia

Neoplasms
Ectopic production of human chorionic gonadotrophin or human placental lactogen
Liver disease (18%)
Starvation during recovery phase (refeeding)
Renal disease and dialysis (1%)
Drugs (10–20%)
Antiandrogens/inhibitors of androgen synthesis
Cyproterone
Flutamide
Spironolactone
Antibiotics
Ketoconazole
Antiulcer medication
Cimetidine
Omeprazole
Ranitidine
Cancer chemotherapeutic agents
Alkylating agents
Cardiovascular drugs
Captopril
Digoxin
Methyldopa
Nifedipine
Psychoactive drugs
Haloperidol
Phenothiazines
Drugs of abuse
Cannabis

to androgen. Gynaecomastia has been found in association with testicular and adrenal neoplasms, Klinefelter's syndrome, thyrotoxicosis, cirrhosis, primary hypogonadism, malnutrition, and ageing (see Table 13.12.6). An increase in free oestrogen, a decrease in free endogenous androgens, androgen receptor defects, and partially enhanced secretions of breast tissue may underlie these changes. Increased aromatization of oestrogen precursors occurs in patients with obesity, liver disease, and hyperthyroidism, and as a result of ageing.

Calcium

Hypercalcaemia in sarcoidosis is due to increased circulating 1,25-dihydroxyvitamin D_3. This is produced by alveolar macrophages in a dose-dependent fashion stimulated by γ-interferon, which is one factor responsible for the maintenance of the inflammatory process in sarcoidosis. Other granulomatous disorders (tuberculosis, histoplasmosis, coccidiomycosis, ruptured silicone breast implants) may rarely be associated with hypercalcaemia due to the same

mechanism. Treatment with glucocorticoids or hydroxychloroquine are effective in lowering 1,25-dihydroxycholecalciferol and calcium.

HTLV1 infection may be associated with hypercalcaemia, due to transactivation of the *PTHRP* gene on chromosome 12.

Drug-induced endocrine manifestations

Several pharmaceutical drugs may induce manifestations of endocrine disease. More commonly they may influence the results of hormonal assays and lead to mistaken diagnosis. It may not be a major problem when it is known that the patient is taking a particular compound and, from its molecular structure, it is appreciated that such a substance could influence the endocrine system or the results of hormonal assays. The problem is greater, however, when the drug in question has no clear relationship to a hormone and the mechanism by which it induces an endocrine manifestation, or interferes with an assay procedure, is not readily apparent.

Thyroid

Abnormalities of thyroid function test measurements

Drugs can interfere with thyroid function tests. Some act by inhibiting the conversion of T_4 to T_3, others by increasing thyroid-binding globulin. β-Blockers with membrane stabilizing properties, such as propranolol, inhibit peripheral conversion of T_4 to T_3. Oral cholecystographic agents and amiodarone, a heavily iodinated antiarrhythmic agent, are also potent inhibitors of T_4 to T_3 conversion and produce decreased serum T_3 concentrations and an increase in reverse T_3. Oestrogen increases thyroid-binding globulin, due to an increase in the sialic acid content of thyroxine-binding globulin, which prolongs its half-life in the circulation. Thus, women on oestrogens, e.g. the contraceptive pill, have high total T_4 concentrations but are euthyroid. Such results may also be seen on tamoxifen. Heroin and methadone addicts also have raised levels of thyroxine-binding globulin, as do patients on the lipid-lowering agent, clofibrate.

A decreased serum T_4 does not necessarily indicate the presence of hypothyroidism. Many pharmacological agents lower the total T_4 concentration by interfering with the binding of T_4 to one or more of the thyroid-binding proteins. Therapeutic levels of phenytoin lower the level of serum T_4 and high concentrations are capable of inhibiting the binding of T_4 and T_3 to thyroid-binding globulin. High doses of salicylates have the same effect. Diclofenac, a nonsteroidal anti-inflammatory drug structurally similar to thyroxine, also interferes with thyroid hormone binding. Phenylbutazone, anabolic steroids, and glucocorticoids may also be associated with a low total T_4 and normal thyroid function. Measurement of free thyroxine (FT_4) will obviate the problems of misleading results from the measurement of total T_4.

Drug-induced hyperthyroidism

Amiodarone may cause hyperthyroidism due to its high iodine content, or due to a destructive thyroiditis. Biochemically, there may be a marked elevation of total thyroxine, a relatively normal level of T_3, and a suppressed TSH. Often, thyrotoxicosis is masked by the β-blocking effect of the drug. Because of the large iodine load, it may be very difficult to treat with antithyroid drugs, and steroids may also be necessary to suppress thyroid hormone levels into the normal range. Even if amiodarone is stopped, its effects continue for many weeks because it is predominantly stored in adipose tissue. Contrast media and iodine-containing cough medicines may similarly induce hyperthyroidism (Jod–Basedow phenomenon).

Drug-induced hypothyroidism

Increased iodide intake may also lead to decreased iodide trapping and a decrease in synthesis of thyroid hormones, hypothyroidism, and goitre. Iodine is contained in a number of tonics and cough medicines. Amiodarone, besides producing thyrotoxicosis, may cause iodine-induced hypothyroidism in patients replete with iodine. Lithium blocks iodine uptake and the release of thyroid hormones. It also interferes with cAMP formation and thus inhibits the effects of TSH stimulation and may lead to goitre, although only 2% of patients on lithium actually develop clinical features of hypothyroidism.

Adrenal cortex

Abnormalities of adrenal hormone measurements

Drugs may interfere with tests of adrenal function. Thus, the drug phenytoin accelerates metabolism of dexamethasone, and patients on phenytoin may not suppress cortisol normally during dexamethasone suppression tests. Furthermore, during the assessment of adrenal reserve, chronic topical application of steroids, as well as inhalation of steroids for asthma, may suppress adrenal function. Oestrogens, by enhancing hepatic production of cortisol-binding globulin, which binds between 90 and 97% of circulating cortisol, increases cortisol-binding globulin two- to threefold. Thus, assessment of glucocorticoid replacement in patients on oestrogens is influenced by this effect and oestrogens should be stopped 6 weeks prior to the test.

Drug-induced Cushing's syndrome

Chronic, excessive intake of alcohol causes alcoholic pseudo-Cushing's syndrome. These patients behave biochemically as if they have Cushing's syndrome with absent dexamethasone suppression. This occurs through a centrally mediated mechanism with hypersecretion of pituitary ACTH and secondary secretion of cortisol by the adrenals.

Drug-induced primary aldosteronism

Primary aldosteronism can be mimicked by the mineralocorticoid effect of glycyrrhizic acid contained in both carbenoxolone and liquorice. Cortisol is normally inactivated by conversion to the inactive metabolite, cortisone, by the enzyme 11β-hydroxysteroid dehydrogenase but these compounds inhibit the enzyme, which is important in the kidney because it protects renal mineralocorticoid receptors from cortisol.

Drug-induced adrenal insufficiency

The antifungal agent, ketoconazole, and the short-acting anaesthetic, etomidate, are imidazole derivatives with significant inhibitory effects on 11β-hydroxylase. While they do not usually produce clinical insufficiency, they may do so in subjects with limited pituitary or adrenal reserve. Rifampicin and phenytoin, which both accelerate the metabolism of cortisol by inducing hepatic mixed-function oxygenase enzymes, can also provoke adrenal insufficiency in similar patients with limited pituitary or adrenal reserve. In such patients, increased doses of replacement therapy are necessary.

Gonads

Several drugs can affect testicular function, leading to hypogonadism and infertility. Mechanisms include the direct inhibition of testosterone synthesis or competitive inhibition of androgen action at receptor level. Spironolactone acts as a partial androgen receptor antagonist. Alcohol reduces testosterone levels acutely and chronically, by both a central and a gonadal effect on testosterone synthesis, secretion, and metabolism. Cimetidine has antiandrogen effects due to direct interaction with the androgen receptor and it may also exert antiandrogen effects at the pituitary and hypothalamus leading to gynaecomastia and impotence in males. Anticonvulsants, e.g. phenytoin, increase sex hormone-binding globulin and therefore decrease free testosterone levels. They also enhance testosterone to oestradiol conversion. Sulfasalazine causes reversible male infertility associated with oligospermia.

Infertility may occur as a result of cytotoxic therapy, caused in particular by alkylating agents such as cyclophosphamide. These produce depletion of the germinal epithelium and lead to a raised FSH level, and oligo- or azoospermia, but normal LH and testosterone levels in males, and may lead to premature ovarian failure in women.

In women, hirsutism can be caused by a number of drugs, including danazol, phenytoin, diazoxide, and minoxidil.

Pharmacological doses of glucocorticoids may lead to hypogonadism because of inhibited gonadotrophin release. Drugs such as tricyclics, benzodiazepines, antihypertensives, and antipsychotics may also lead to hypogonadotrophic hypogonadism in both sexes.

Prolactin

Prolactin is controlled predominantly by a hypothalamic inhibitory mechanism through dopamine secretion. A number of drugs can cause hyperprolactinaemia and galactorrhoea usually acting through a dopaminergic mechanism. They may elevate prolactin to a sufficient extent to cause a clinical suspicion of prolactinoma, and in such patients a careful drug history is particularly important. Metoclopramide, pimozide, and sulpiride all act as dopamine antagonists and may considerably elevate prolactin, with all the attendant effects thereof. Fluoxetine may also lead to elevated serum prolactin, although tricyclic antidepressants are not usually associated with hyperprolactinaemia.

Phenothiazines, chlorpromazine, perphenazine, and trifluoperazine also act as dopamine antagonists, as do haloperidol and butyrophenone. Reserpine and methyldopa both decrease catecholamine stores and may cause hyperprolactinaemia. Oestrogens, in high doses, may slightly elevate prolactin but normal contraceptive pills do not. Verapamil, by decreasing dopaminergic tone, may also increase prolactin levels.

Gynaecomastia

Gynaecomastia may occur due to treatment with various drugs (see Table 13.12.6). Drugs such as spironolactone and ketoconazole, which can displace steroids from sex-hormone binding globulin, displace oestrogens more easily than androgens. Activation of the oestrogen receptors in breast tissue may take place with drugs that have structural homology with oestrogen, such as digoxin; griseofulvin and cannabis may have the same effect. A decrease in androgen occurs in older men and with drugs such as spironolactone and ketoconazole that inhibit the biosynthesis of testosterone. The mechanism for the induction of gynaecomastia by captopril and calcium channel blockers (nifedipine) is unclear. With cimetidine and omeprazole, this effect may be due to a direct antiandrogen effect or the inhibition of liver cytochrome P450.

Posterior pituitary

The syndrome of inappropriate antidiuresis is characterized by normovolaemic hyponatraemia with persistent secretion of AVP, despite a reduced plasma osmolality. A number of drugs can cause this syndrome through the inappropriate stimulation of eutopic AVP secretion. These include thiazide diuretics, vincristine, vinblastine, cyclophosphamide, chlorpropamide, phenothiazines, carbamazepine, clofibrate, tricyclic antidepressants, and serotonin-reuptake inhibitors (see Table 13.12.1). The syndrome of inappropriate antidiuresis can also be caused by the administration of desmopressin (a V2 selective analogue of AVP) or oxytocin.

Nephrogenic diabetes insipidus can be induced by lithium in the therapeutic range, and up to 20% of patients receiving long-term therapy may develop this complication. Demethylchlortetracycline produces dose-dependent nephrogenic diabetes insipidus, and both the concentrating defect and the unresponsiveness to vasopressin are reversible on cessation of the drug.

Parathyroid

Lithium therapy can cause an increase in parathyroid gland size, either with hyperplasia or adenoma. This hyperparathyroidism leads to mild hypercalcaemia and sometimes osteoporosis. Thiazide diuretics, by causing haemoconcentration and hypocalciuria, may also result in mild hypercalcaemia but this is usually transient (4–6 weeks); after this time, other causes of hypercalcaemia should be sought. Vinblastine and colchicine inhibit parathyroid hormone secretion which may result in hypocalcaemia.

Further reading

Bell NH (1991). Endocrine complications of sarcoidosis. *Endocrinol Metab Clin North Am*, **20**, 645–654.

Braunstein GD (1993). Current concepts: gynecomastia. *N Engl J Med*, **328**, 490–5.

Carpenter TO (2003). Oncogenic osteomalacia–a complex dance of factors. *N Engl J Med*, **348**, 1705–8.

Chattopadhyay N (2006). Effects of calcium-sensing receptor on the secretion of parathyroid hormone-related peptide and its impact on humoral hypercalcemia of malignancy. *Am J Physiol Endocrinol Metab*, **290**, E761–E770.

Chopra IJ (1997). Clinical review 86: Euthyroid sick syndrome: is it a misnomer? *J Clin Endocrinol Metab*, **82**, 329–34.

Daughaday WH, Deuel TF (1991). Tumour secretion of growth factors. *Endocrinol Metab Clin North Am*, **20**, 539–63.

Docter R, et al. (1993). The sick euthyroid syndrome: changes in thyroid hormone serum parameters and hormone metabolism. *Clin Endocrinol (Oxf)*, **39**, 499–510.

Gola M, et al. (2006). Neuroendocrine tumors secreting growth hormone-releasing hormone: Pathophysiological and clinical aspects. *Pituitary*, **9**, 221–9.

Grinspoon SK, Bilezikian JP (1992). HIV disease and the endocrine system. *N Engl J Med*, **327**, 1360–5.

Guise TA, Mundy GR (1998). Cancer and bone. *Endocr Rev*, **19**, 18–54.

Hirshberg B, et al. (2003). Ectopic luteinizing hormone secretion and anovulation. *N Engl J Med*, **348**, 312–17.

Howlett TA, et al. (1986). Diagnosis and management of ACTH-dependent Cushing's syndrome: comparison of the features in ectopic and pituitary ACTH production. *Clin Endocrinol (Oxf)*, **24**, 699–713.

Hung W, et al. (1963). Precocious puberty in a boy with hepatoma and circulating gonadotropin. *J Pediatr*, **63**, 895–903.

Isidori AM, et al. (2006). The ectopic adrenocorticotropin syndrome: clinical features, diagnosis, management, and long-term follow-up. *J Clin Endocrinol Metab*, **91**, 371–7.

Kovacs L, Robertson GL (1992). Syndrome of inappropriate antidiuresis. *Endocrinol Metab Clin North Am*, **21**, 859–76.

Melmed S (1991). Extrapituitary acromegaly. *Endocrinol Metab Clin North Am*, **20**, 507–18.

Penny E, et al. (1984). Circulating growth hormone releasing factor concentrations in normal subjects and patients with acromegaly. *Br Med J*, **289**, 453–55.

Robertson GL (2006). Regulation of arginine vasopressin in the syndrome of inappropriate antidiuresis. *Am J Med*, **119**, Suppl 1, S36–S42.

Schrier RW, et al. (2006). Tolvaptan, a selective oral vasopressin V2-receptor antagonist, for hyponatremia. *N Engl J Med*, **355**, 2099–112.

Turner HE, Wass JAH (1997). Gonadal function in men with chronic illness. *Clin Endocrinol (Oxf)*, **47**, 379–403.

Vaitukaitis JL (1991). Ectopic hormonal secretion and reproductive dysfunction. In: Yen SSC, Jaffe RB (eds) *Reproductive endocrinology*, 3rd edition, pp. 795–806. WB Saunders, Philadelphia.

Vanderpump MPJ, Tunbridge WMG (1993). The effects of drugs on endocrine function. *Clin Endocrinol (Oxf)*, **39**, 389–97.

Wass JAH, et al. (1982). HCGB producing pineal choriocarcinoma. *Clin Endocrinol (Oxf)*, **17**, 423–31.

White A, Clark AJL (1993). The cellular and molecular basis of the ectopic ACTH syndrome. *Clin Endocrinol (Oxf)*, **39**, 131–41.

13.13

The pineal gland and melatonin

J. Arendt and Timothy M. Cox

Essentials

The pineal gland transduces light–dark cycles into body rhythms by secretion of melatonin, an endogenous indoleamine derived from tryptophan, the concentrations of which in plasma and cerebrospinal fluid are up to 100 times higher at night than in the daytime. This exerts its effects through transmembrane, G-protein coupled receptors (MT1 and MT2) and nuclear receptors in the pituitary gland and hypothalamus.

The natural period of the human circadian system is on average 24.2 to 24.3 h, and the principal resetting agent is light. Exogenous melatonin can shift the timing of the internal clock to earlier and later times, and synchronize a free-running clock that is not properly entrained to the 24-h day, hence it may have a therapeutic role for disorders of sleep rhythm including jet lag, in shift workers, and in blind people.

Introduction

The mammalian pineal gland is a secretory organ. Whereas in fish and amphibians it is directly photoreceptive, in reptiles and birds it has a mixed photoreceptor and secretory function. Although an endocrine function was considered for many years, this was only given credibility in 1958 by the pioneering work of Lerner, who isolated a small molecule from bovine pineal glands that he named melatonin because it caused blanching of melanophores in amphibian skin. The primary function of the pineal gland in all species studied to date is to transduce information concerning light–dark cycles to body physiology, particularly for the organization of body rhythms, via the secretion of its major hormone melatonin. In some birds and lower vertebrates it serves as a rhythm generating system, or biological clock. In mammals, it is concerned with the coordination of rhythm physiology without having the capacity to act as a rhythm generator. In humans, the gland has been known since antiquity. Many questions remain unanswered about the function of the human pineal gland, but its secretion of the chronobiotic molecule melatonin has prompted enormous interest in the fields of travel medicine, neurophysiology, and endocrine research.

The pineal gland

Structure

The pineal gland is less than 1 cm in its longest diameter and weighs less than 0.2 g; it lies above the posterior aspect of the third cerebral ventricle. The major cellular component of the normal mammalian pineal gland, the pinealocyte, is believed to have evolved from truly photoreceptive cells in lower vertebrates and structural remnants of the outer segments of photoreceptor cells are reported in higher vertebrates.

It also contains neuroglial components, principally of astrocytic type, which occasionally become malignant. Human pineal tissue calcifies with age but this does not necessarily diminish its secretory activity. The pineal gland is considered to reside outside the functional blood–brain barrier.

Pathology

Tumours of the pineal region in children are frequently associated with abnormal pubertal development. Much evidence suggests that precocious puberty in such cases is due to the production of human chorionic gonadotrophin (β-hCG) by germ cell tumours of the pineal gland. Delayed puberty has also been associated with pineal tumours. Pineal tumours are heterogeneous and may arise from germ cells (teratomas, germinomas, choriocarcinomas, endodermal sinus tumours, mixed germ cell tumours), pineal parenchymal cells (pineoblastoma and pineocytoma), and the supporting stroma (gliomas). Classification of pineal parenchymal tumours is complicated by the presence of mixed pineocytoma-pineoblastoma types, some with intermediate differentiation. A new classification has been proposed recently, based on histological features, which is closely related to patient survival.

Treatment of pineal tumours by surgical excision or radiation appears to suppress melatonin secretion leading to sleeping difficulties; melatonin replacement therapy has been reported to benefit such patients with defective melatonin release.

Melatonin

Melatonin, like serotonin, is an endogenous indoleamine derived from tryptophan. The first step in indoleamine synthesis is the 5-hydroxylation of tryptophan by tryptophan hydroxylase—an enzyme with requirements for dioxygen, iron, and tetrahydrobiopterin. The enzyme arylalkylamine N-acetyltransferase, regulated by the sympathetic transmitter noradrenaline, appears to be the rate-limiting step in melatonin synthesis. The enzyme is localized principally in the pineal gland but also in the retina, the skin, within specific cells in the upper gastrointestinal tract, and perhaps elsewhere. Melatonin binds to specific receptors including the seven transmembrane G-protein coupled MT1 and MT2 receptors, as well as nuclear receptors RZR/ROR orphan receptor family and downstream transcription factors that are associated with melatonin signalling. A third site named MT3 is in fact the enzyme quinone reductase, associated with detoxification mechanisms. Membrane G-protein receptors for melatonin are principally expressed in the nervous system but they have been found in numerous other locations. The nuclear transcription factor appears to be expressed in the periphery. There is emerging evidence that a nuclear signalling pathway with ligand-induced control of target gene transcription, mediates some functions of melatonin. Melatonin has been reported to control expression of the 5-lipoxygenase gene; the cognate enzyme is not implicated in circadian rhythms but is expressed principally in myeloid cells and participates in allergic and inflammatory reactions. Melatonin (formal chemical name, N-acetyl-5-methoxytryptamine) has been found within membrane-bound bodies in pinealocytes. In experimental animals these show light-dependent morphological changes associated with melatonin secretion under altered environmental light conditions. The pineal gland is the principal source of circulating melatonin in mammals, indeed pinealectomy leads to undetectable melatonin concentrations in blood. Synthesis elsewhere, e.g. in the retina, seems to change local concentrations only. Melatonin appears to exert its main effects through MT1 receptors in the infundibular part of the pituitary gland, through MT1 and MT2 receptors in the central biological rhythm generating system of the brain (the suprachiasmatic nuclei of the hypothalamus) and other regions of the hypothalamus that modulate the secretion of pituitary hormones, and that influence core body temperature and other functions.

The role of melatonin and the pineal gland in photoperiodism

In all species studied to date, melatonin is normally synthesized and secreted at night. This rhythm is circadian in nature, i.e. it is endogenously driven by the activity of the suprachiasmatic nuclei. Exposure to light influences the secretion of melatonin, and melatonin release is suppressed particularly under illuminance with short wavelength light. The length of the day (photoperiod) strongly influences melatonin secretion such that the longer the night the longer the duration of secretion. In humans, our manipulation of the light environment renders this relationship hard to show except under conditions of changing length of total darkness.

However, in animals that time their seasonal physiology according to the photoperiod this changing duration of melatonin secretion is the critical signal for induction of particular seasonal responses (e.g. reproduction, coat growth). Exogenous melatonin can be used as the photoperiodic signal and it has been commercialized for use in changing the timing of the breeding season in species such as sheep, mink, and goats. In animals and humans there is evidence that a new photoreceptive system, which does not depend on retinal rods or cones, mediates the nonvisual effects of light on physiology and is differentially responsive to short wavelength light.

Melatonin and circadian rhythms

Rhythmic melatonin secretion leads to concentrations in the plasma or cerebrospinal fluid that are up to 100 times higher at night than in the daytime, with very large interindividual variations but consistent intraindividual variations. It is extensively used to assess the timing of the human biological clock; its secretion profile provides, in the periphery, the most accurate and sensitive index of the activity of the suprachiasmatic nuclei. In the diagnosis of circadian rhythm disorders, blood and saliva measures are useful, in addition to measures of its principal metabolite 6-sulphatoxymelatonin (aMT6s) in urine. Maximum concentrations are observed in childhood and melatonin levels thereafter decline with age. The endogenous role of melatonin in humans is unclear. Peak night-time levels are closely associated with the nadirs of core temperature, alertness, performance, and metabolism. The profile of secretion is strongly associated with increasing sleep propensity and sleep is longer and of better quality when taken in phase with peak melatonin secretion (and with the nadir in core temperature). Melatonin is able to reinforce night-time physiology, e.g. in contributing to sleep propensity and the drop in core temperature at night. Melatonin appears to have a supporting role to that of the light–dark cycle in the synchronization of circadian rhythms to the 24-h day: the natural period of the human circadian system in the absence of time cues is on average 24.2 to 24.3 h and the principal resetting agent is light.

Exogenous melatonin is clearly able to shift the timing of the internal clock to earlier and later times and to synchronize a free-running clock that is not properly entrained to the 24-h day. Several syndromes associated with long-term insomnia in humans appear to result from slower, faster, or free-running sleep–wake cycles. These include the non-24-h sleep–wake cycle of blind people (with no light perception at all), delayed sleep-phase syndrome, advanced sleep-phase syndrome, and irregular sleep–wake cycles. In addition, abrupt shifts of time cues such as are found in shift work and jet lag lead to circadian asynchrony with resultant problems of sleep, fatigue, alertness, and with possible long-term health consequences. Melatonin has actual and potential therapeutic benefit in these circumstances due to its chronobiotic activity. Timed exposure to light at high luminance may improve disorders of the circadian rhythm that affect sleep. However, in many circumstances, the correct timing and intensity of light exposure (and avoidance) is hard to achieve. Notably, blind people cannot have access to light treatment and for the non 24-h sleep–wake disorder of the blind, melatonin, correctly timed, is the treatment of choice.

Pharmaceutical use of melatonin

In addition to its use in blind circadian rhythm disorder, melatonin has proved successful in normalizing delayed sleep timing in delayed sleep-phase syndrome, stabilizing irregular sleep–wake cycles in neurologically disabled children, and in treating the symptoms of jet lag. Melatonin treatment has also been suggested as a means to improve sleep in night shift workers, in older individuals with insomnia, and in patients with pineal tumours.

Many studies have been carried out to investigate the efficacy of melatonin as a chronobiotic agent for the alleviation of symptoms of jet lag. The results of one meta-analysis to assess the effectiveness of oral melatonin, taken in different dosing regimens for alleviating jet lag after travel across several time zones, showed that the agent is effective in preventing or reducing jet lag and that its short-term use appears to be safe on an occasional basis. Side-effect reporting has been low, except in patients with epilepsy or those who are taking warfarin in whom convulsant effects or increased bleeding, respectively, have been reported. Melatonin may theoretically influence reproductive development in children and reduce sexual activity, if overused, in adults. No evidence of these effects has yet been reported. Recent jet lag studies tend to recommend the use of preflight timed melatonin (0.5 mg) to initiate an advance or delay as required of the circadian system, and to use postflight higher doses (3–5 mg) again timed correctly, to reinforce the shift in timing and to acutely induce sleepiness.

Another meta-analysis was less positive. Melatonin is nevertheless recommended as a treatment for jet lag, delayed sleep-phase syndrome, and irregular sleep–wake cycles by the American Academy of Sleep Medicine. Its use in shift work has proved inconsistent, not all studies have been successful regarding its use in insomnia in older people, and there is insufficient data to evaluate properly its effect in pineal tumours. The timing of treatment with respect to internal circadian timing is very important and judging such timing is often not simple, especially in shift work and jet lag.

Melatonin is freely available in the United States of America, but only recently has a melatonin formulation been registered for use in insomnia in older people in Europe and a melatonin agonist (ramelteon) has been approved by the United States Food and Drug Administration, again for insomnia. Other formulations are under development and another agonist (agomelatine) is close to registration.

In summary, the evidence is that oral ingestion of melatonin may be indicated for occasional use after transmeridian flights that would induce daytime fatigue and sleep disturbance associated with gastrointestinal complaints, weakness, malaise, loss of mental efficiency, and other symptoms that typify with jet lag. Clearly, since the drug is not as yet licensed in all countries, routine pharmaceutical quality control must be established. Its use and safety in pregnancy has not yet been completely validated. At a time when prion-related diseases may result from the ingestion or injection of material derived from brain or other animal tissue, only pure biosynthetic melatonin should be considered for human use. Melatonin derived from bovine pineal or other biological sources should be avoided.

Melatonin is widely taken in certain communities, particularly in the United States of America, where it is claimed to provide indiscriminant protection against ageing, degenerative diseases, cancer, impaired immune function, and reproductive and psychiatric illnesses. Nonetheless, it should be acknowledged that melatonin does have diverse physiological actions in humans, as in other vertebrates, which are incompletely understood. At present, the principal indication for exogenous melatonin is for the control of sleep disorders and the treatment of symptoms associated with jet lag, rather than the many conditions for which our scientific understanding of its proposed benefits is as yet inchoate.

Further reading

Arendt J (1995). *Melatonin and the mammalian pineal gland*. Chapman & Hall, London.

Arendt J (2005). Melatonin: characteristics, concerns, and prospects. *J Biol Rhythms*, **4**, 291–303.

Arendt J (2005). *Chapter 15: The pineal gland and pineal tumours*. http://www.endotext.org/neuroendo/neuroendo15/ neuroendoframe15.htm.

Buscemi N, *et al.* (2006). Efficacy and safety of exogenous melatonin for secondary sleep disorders and sleep disorders accompanying sleep restriction: meta-analysis. *BMJ*, **332**, 385–93.

Carlberg, C, Wiesenberg, I (2007). The orphan receptor family RZR/ROR, melatonin and 5-lipoxygenase: An unexpected relationship. *Pineal Research*, **18**, 171–8.

Herxheimer A, Petrie KJ (2002). Melatonin for the prevention and treatment of jet lag. *Cochrane Database Syst Rev*, **2**, CD001520.

Morgenthaler TI, *et al.* (2007). Practice parameters for the clinical evaluation and treatment of circadian rhythm sleep disorders. An American Academy of Sleep Medicine report. *Sleep*, **30**, 1445–59.

SECTION 14

Medical disorders in pregnancy

Physiological changes of normal pregnancy

David J. Williams

Essentials

Almost every maternal organ system makes a physiological adaptation to pregnancy that is required for optimal pregnancy outcome. An understanding of these adaptations brings insight into the aetiology and management of gestational syndromes, and also helps the clinician to advise women with pre-existing chronic illness about the risks and consequences of a pregnancy.

Physiological adaptations in pregnancy—these include (1) cardiovascular—cardiac output increases 50%; (2) respiratory—oxygen consumption increases 20%; and (3) renal—glomerular filtration rate increases 55%.

Biochemical and endocrine changes in pregnancy—gestational changes alter the normal ranges for many important metabolic

and endocrine laboratory tests, including (1) serum creatinine, urea—both decreased; (2) cholesterol and triglycerides—both increased; (3) liver blood tests—alkaline phosphatase increased up to four fold; and (4) thyroid function tests—free thyroxine and tri-iodothyronine levels fall, thyroid-stimulating hormone (TSH) levels rise. Awareness of these changes is essential, both for recognition of disease in pregnancy and to prevent inappropriate pursuit of test results that are normal in pregnancy.

Long-term implications of pregnancy syndromes—conditions such as pre-eclampsia and gestational diabetes mellitus are abnormal responses to pregnancy that resolve after delivery, but herald similar complications, i.e. hypertension and diabetes mellitus, in later life.

Introduction

The physiological changes of pregnancy make extra demands on almost all maternal organs. Women unable to meet these demands put their own health at risk as well as compromise pregnancy outcome. Pregnancy syndromes such as pre-eclampsia and gestational diabetes mellitus are abnormal responses to pregnancy that resolve after delivery, but herald similar complications, i.e. hypertension and diabetes mellitus, in later life. In this respect pregnancy acts as a maternal 'stress test' that identifies a woman's vulnerability to future disease. An understanding of the normal physiological demands of pregnancy not only brings insight into the aetiology and management of gestational syndromes, but also helps the clinician advise women with pre-existing chronic illness about the risks and consequences of a pregnancy.

Preparing for pregnancy

The female body prepares for pregnancy during every menstrual cycle. It is not only the endometrium that anticipates implantation of a fertilized ovum, but the whole cardiovascular system. During the postovulatory or luteal phase of each menstrual cycle there is a decrease in systemic vascular resistance by approximately 20%, leading to a 10% fall in mean arterial pressure compared with the

follicular phase. Cardiac output increases by almost 20%, and renal vasodilatation increases both renal blood flow and glomerular filtration by approximately 10%. All of these changes resolve with involution of the corpus luteum and onset of menses.

Cardiovascular changes in pregnancy

If fertilization is successful the haemodynamic changes established in the menstrual cycle progress further, with systemic vascular resistance falling by almost 40% and creating a maximal decrease in mean arterial pressure by the end of the first trimester. Diastolic blood pressure falls between 5 and 15 mmHg, before rising to non-pregnancy levels at term, whilst systolic blood pressure remains unchanged throughout pregnancy. A gestational increase in heart rate from approximately 72 to 85 beats/min and of stroke volume by up to 30% combine with the reduction in systemic vascular resistance to increase cardiac output. By 24 weeks, cardiac output reaches a maximum of 50% above nonpregnant levels, which is sustained until term. During the third trimester, cardiac output falls in the supine position when the gravid uterus compresses the inferior vena cava. Left ventricular wall thickness and left ventricular mass increase progressively throughout pregnancy, by up to 30% and 50% respectively. Cardiac output returns almost completely to prepregnancy levels within 2 weeks of delivery.

Distribution of increased cardiac output

Although it is technically difficult to measure blood flow to particular maternal viscera during pregnancy, it is clear that the timing and extent of changes to blood flow varies between organs. This is summarized in Fig. 14.1.1. Mammary artery blood flow increases early in pregnancy, breast tenderness and swelling being amongst the first symptoms.

Mechanism of gestational cardiovascular change

The onset of physiological change during the menstrual cycle suggests that maternal rather than fetoplacental factors initiate gestational adaptation. Oestrogen, mainly in the form of 17β-oestradiol, is a potent vasodilator. It is produced by the corpus luteum during the luteal phase of each menstrual cycle and for the first 10 weeks of pregnancy. After 10 weeks, the placenta elaborates its own 17β-oestradiol, so that by term maternal oestradiol levels are approximately 250-fold higher than those found during the menstrual cycle. 17β-Oestradiol relaxes vascular smooth muscle through both endothelium-dependent and independent mechanisms, and all of the endothelium-derived vasodilators—nitric oxide, prostacyclin, and endothelial-derived hyperpolarizing factor—have been implicated in the gestational fall of systemic vascular resistance.

Much less is known about the vascular effects of progesterone, whose circulating levels increase by a similar amount to 17β-oestradiol and may play a role in reducing pressor responsiveness to angiotensin II.

Although the precise mechanism of maternal vasodilatation is likely to be different in different vascular beds, a healthy endothelium is essential for normal cardiovascular adaptation to pregnancy.

Fluid balance during pregnancy

Arterial dilatation creates a relatively 'underfilled' state, which stimulates the renin–angiotensin–aldosterone system. As a result, sodium and water retention throughout pregnancy leads to a 6 to 8 litre rise in total extracellular fluid volume. Plasma volume increases steadily until week 32, when it is 40% (or c.1.2 litres) above nonpregnant levels. This is partly mediated by a fall in the osmotic threshold for thirst, with a concomitant fall in the threshold for secretion of antidiuretic hormone (AVP) preventing a water diuresis and sustaining a low plasma osmolality (lower by 10 mosmol/kg) until term. During the second half of pregnancy, placental production of vasopressinase increases maternal AVP degradation, but plasma AVP levels remain stable as pituitary secretion of AVP normally increases fourfold. A failure of increased AVP secretion leads to transient diabetes insipidus of pregnancy. Plasma atrial

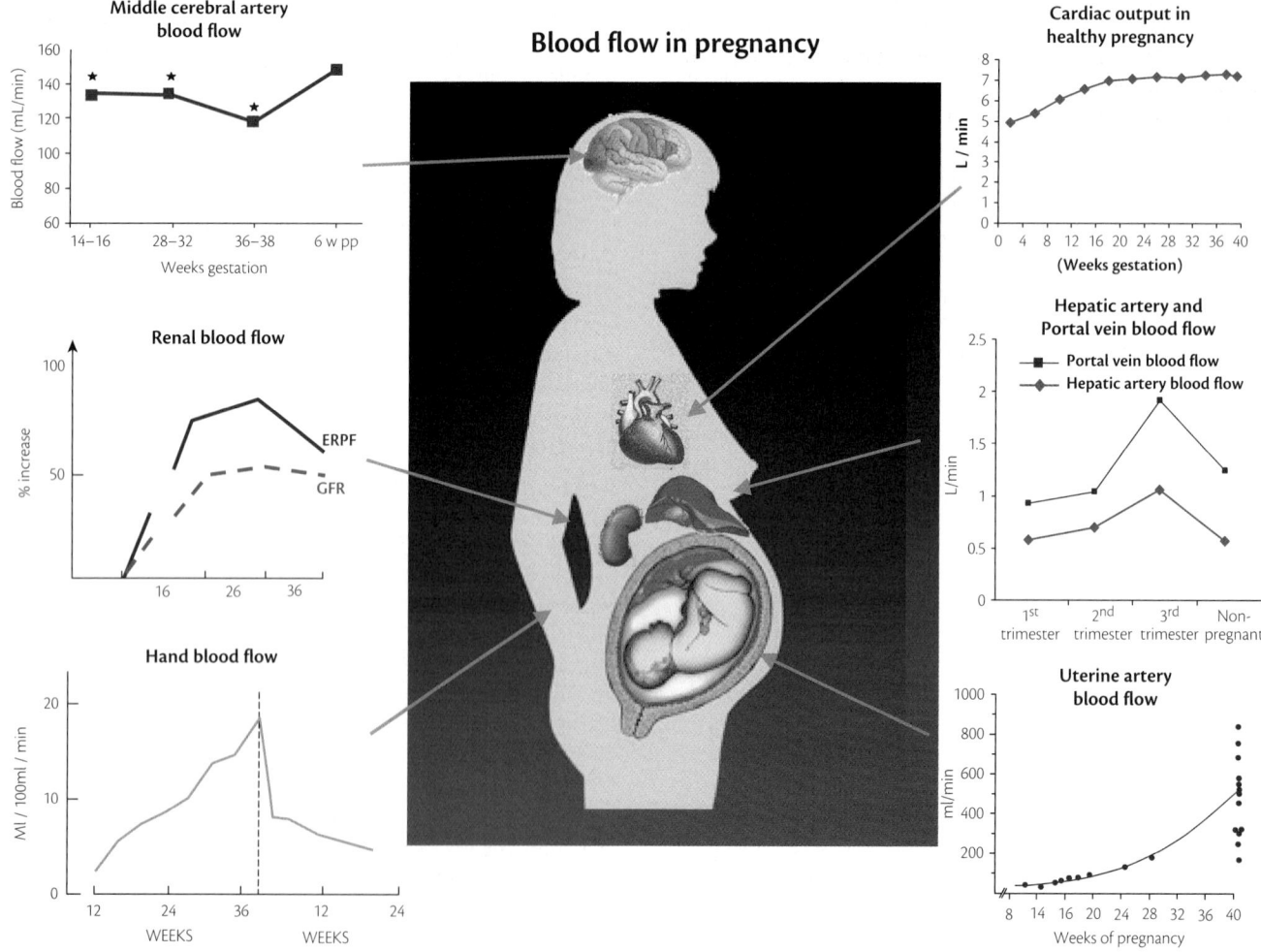

Fig. 14.1.1 Changes in maternal organ blood flow during healthy pregnancy (ERPF, estimated renal plasma flow; GFR, glomerular filtration rate).

natriuretic peptide levels are normal until the second trimester, when they rise by approximately 40%.

Immunological changes during pregnancy

It is often presumed that pregnant women are immunosuppressed in order that the fetal 'semiallograft' can survive. This is not true: certain aspects of maternal immunity are modulated, but it is the placenta that deserves most credit for eluding maternal immunity. Much harm is prevented by the physical separation of maternal and fetal blood, fetal haemolytic disease being an example of the harm that can follow a breach in this barrier, a rhesus-negative mother becoming isoimmunized against rhesus-positive fetal blood.

In normal pregnancy the placenta has to invade uterine tissue and become bathed in maternal blood. To avoid a hostile immune response the surface layers of placenta express a unique nonpolymorphic HLA G, rather than classical histocompatibility antigens. It is thought that HLA G confers resistance to lysis by maternal T cells and natural killer (NK) cells. The placenta also expresses a plethora of complement control systems to protect itself from the gestational rise in serum levels of maternal complement factors C3 and C4.

Innate immunity is modulated in pregnancy so that maternal NK cell activity at the uteroplacental interface promotes placental invasion, but intercurrent infection can activate latent NK cytolytic activity to harm fetal and maternal tissues. Fetal survival is also enhanced by a shift away from maternal T-helper 1 cytokine responses that promote cell-mediated immunity towards a stronger T-helper 2 cytokine response that promotes antibody production. In consequence, pregnant women are more prone to severe infections with intracellular pathogens such as malaria, tuberculosis, listeria, and *Salmonella typhimurium*, and they are also more likely to suffer reactivation of viruses such as Epstein–Barr.

Circulating levels of maternal immunoglobulin increase and, once transferred to the fetus, have a role in passive immunity. Neutrophils increase in number and develop a proinflammatory phenotype. Mean total white cell count increases to 9.0×10^9/litre and can rise as high as 40.0×10^9/litre during labour, returning to normal within 6 days. Erythrocyte sedimentation rate (ESR) rises as a consequence of increased fibrinogen and globulin: an ESR over 30 mm/h is usual, and up to 70 mm/h is within normal limits. Circulating levels of C-reactive protein do not change during healthy pregnancy. Anatomical changes to the maternal immune system include involution of the thymus and enlargement of the spleen.

Human chorionic gonadotropin (hCG) and progesterone play important roles in mediating some of these immune changes. Understanding gestational immune modulation and how it sometimes fails in pathological pregnancies will facilitate measures to improve pregnancy outcome.

Ventilatory changes during pregnancy

The increased metabolic demands of pregnancy lead to a progressive increase in oxygen consumption of up to almost 20% by term. Pregnant women breathe more deeply, but not more quickly, to achieve this. Tidal volume increases from approximately 500 to 700 ml, and effective alveolar ventilation actually surpasses the body's demand for oxygen, creating a respiratory alkalosis with P_{CO_2} falling from 5.0 to 4.0 kPa. Progesterone stimulates deeper breathing by a direct effect on the respiratory centre, particularly increasing sensitivity to CO_2.

Renal changes during pregnancy

By 16 weeks gestation renal blood flow has increased by 80% (Fig. 14.1.1) and glomerular filtration rate by 55%. The rise in renal blood flow causes the kidneys to swell so that they appear approximately 1 cm longer on ultrasonography. The renal pelvis and ureters dilate, sometimes appearing obstructed to those unaware of these changes.

Serum levels of creatinine and urea fall, so that levels considered normal outside pregnancy may reflect renal impairment during pregnancy. Proteinuria increases during pregnancy, but levels above 300 mg/24 h should be considered abnormal. Gestational glycosuria reflects reduced tubular glucose reabsorption and does not necessarily indicate abnormal carbohydrate metabolism. Furthermore, reduced tubular absorption of bicarbonate creates a metabolic acidosis that compensates for the respiratory alkalosis, keeping maternal pH at 7.4.

The production of erythropoietin, active vitamin D, and renin increases during healthy pregnancy, but their effects are masked by other physiological changes. In early pregnancy, peripheral vasodilatation exceeds the renin–aldosterone mediated plasma volume expansion, hence mean arterial pressure falls by 12 weeks. The 40% expansion of plasma volume exceeds the effect of a two- to fourfold increase in maternal serum erythropoietin levels, which stimulates only a 25% rise in red cell mass. This creates a 'physiological anaemia', which should not normally cause haemoglobin concentration to fall to less than 9.5 g/dl (see Chapter 14.16). Similarly, active vitamin D circulates at twice nongravid levels, but concomitant halving of parathyroid hormone levels, as well as hypercalciuria and increased fetal requirements, keeps plasma ionized calcium levels unchanged.

Liver metabolism during pregnancy

The size of the liver and its blood flow appear not to change during healthy pregnancy, but hepatic synthetic function and metabolism do alter such that there is an increase in serum concentrations of fibrinogen, ceruloplasmin, transferrin, and binding proteins such as thyroid-binding globulin, and a fall in serum albumin levels by approximately 25%. At term, serum cholesterol is raised by 50% and triglycerides by up to 300%. The normal ranges for aspartate transaminase, alanine transaminase, γ-glutamyl transferase, and bilirubin decrease by as much as 20% from the first trimester until term. After the fifth month, placental production of alkaline phosphatase increases maternal plasma levels by up to fourfold. Telangiectasia and palmar erythema are common signs of healthy pregnancy that resolve postpartum.

Gastrointestinal system in pregnancy

Nausea and vomiting affect about 60% of women during the first trimester. The rise and fall of hCG levels correlate chronologically with the onset and improvement of these symptoms, but the role of hCG in gestational nausea is unproven and the cause is likely to be multifactorial. Relaxation of intestinal smooth muscle by progesterone and relaxin creates many of the other pregnancy-induced gastrointestinal changes: gastric motility and small-bowel transit are slowed, especially during labour; the gallbladder enlarges and empties slowly in response to meals; a decrease in lower oesophageal pressure leads to gastro-oesophageal reflux in many women.

Endocrine changes in pregnancy

Thyroid function

The thyroid faces three challenges during pregnancy. First, increased renal clearance of iodide and losses to the fetus create a state of relative iodine deficiency, such that pregnancy stimulates growth of thyroid goitres in geographical areas where dietary iodine intake is low. Secondly, high oestrogen levels induce hepatic synthesis of thyroid binding globulin, but free thyroxine (T_4) and tri-iodothyronine (T_3) levels still fall during pregnancy, occasionally below the normal range for nonpregnant women. Thyroid-stimulating hormone (TSH) levels rise as pregnancy progresses, but generally remain within the normal range for nonpregnancy. Thirdly, placental hCG shares structural similarities with TSH and has weak TSH-like activity. Although hCG rarely stimulates free T_4 levels into the thyrotoxic range, trophoblastic disease and hyperemesis gravidarum are often associated with high hCG levels and can lead to hyperthyroxinaemia and suppression of TSH. In these circumstances, the mother remains clinically euthyroid.

Pituitary function

The maternal pituitary makes only a small contribution to a successful pregnancy once ovulation has occurred and the uterus is prepared for implantation. The only pituitary hormone to increase significantly during pregnancy (by c.10-fold) is prolactin, which is responsible for breast development and subsequent milk production.

Pituitary secretion of growth hormone (GH) is mildly suppressed during the second half of pregnancy by placental production of a GH variant, the role of which is unclear, but it may contribute to gestational insulin resistance.

Placental production of ACTH leads to an increase in maternal ACTH levels, but not beyond the normal range for nonpregnant subjects. Free cortisol levels double and in the second half of pregnancy may contribute to insulin resistance and striae gravidarum.

High oestrogen levels during pregnancy stimulate lactotroph hyperplasia and result in pituitary enlargement. These high levels, together with those of progesterone, suppress luteinizing hormone (LH) and follicular stimulating hormone (FSH). Plasma FSH levels recover within 2 weeks of delivery, but pulsatile luteinizing hormone release is only resumed in women who do not breastfeed. In suckling mothers, prolactin inhibits gonadotropin-releasing hormone (GnRH) and hence LH.

Carbohydrate metabolism

Women develop insulin sensitivity during the first half of pregnancy, but insulin resistance develops after 20 weeks gestation such that women in the second half of pregnancy respond to a glucose load by producing more insulin, but with less effect. Obese women who are already insulin resistant are more likely to develop gestational diabetes mellitus. Hormones that might mediate this insulin resistance include cortisol, progesterone, oestrogen, and human placental lactogen. Placental production of human placental lactogen, a GH-like protein, coincides temporally with insulin resistance.

Coagulation

In anticipation of haemorrhage at childbirth, normal pregnancy is characterized by low grade, chronic intravascular coagulation within both the maternal and uteroplacental circulation. There are increased levels of clotting factors (V, VIII, and X), decreased levels of the endogenous anticoagulant protein S, and decreased fibrinolytic activity. These changes lead to an acquired protein C resistance in nearly half of all pregnant women. However, postpartum contraction of the uterus by oxytocin is probably more effective at preventing haemorrhage than any changes to the coagulation system.

Skin and hair during pregnancy

Hyperpigmentation affects up to 90% of pregnant women. Areas that are normally hyperpigmented, such as the areolae and vulva, become darker. This may be mediated by oestrogen and progesterone, which are powerful melanogenic stimulants. Hair growth increases during pregnancy and hair loss is accelerated postpartum. The gestational rise in corticosteroids and ovarian androgens contributes to the number of hairs in the growing phase (anagen). The levels of these hormones fall postpartum and hairs move back into the resting phase (telogen).

Further reading

Casey BM, Leveno KJ (2006). Thyroid disease in pregnancy. *Obstet Gynecol*, **108**, 1283–92.

Chamberlain G, Broughton-Pipkin F (eds) (1998). *Clinical physiology in obstetrics*, 3rd edition. Blackwell Science, Oxford.

Chapman AB, *et al.* (1998). Temporal relationships between hormonal and hemodynamic changes in early human pregnancy. *Kidney Internat*, **54**, 2056–63.

James DK, *et al.* (eds) (2006). *High Risk pregnancy: management options*, 3rd edition. Elsevier Saunders, Philadelphia, PA.

Lindheimer MD, Davison JM (eds) (1994). Renal disease in pregnancy. *Baillière's Clin Obstet Gynaecol*, **8**, 209–527.

Poppas A, *et al.* (1997). Serial assessment of the cardiovascular system in normal pregnancy. *Circulation*, **95**, 2407–15.

Poston L, Williams DJ (2002). Vascular function in normal pregnancy and pre-eclampsia. In: Hunt BJ, *et al.* (eds) *An introduction to vascular biology*, pp. 398–427. Cambridge University Press, Cambridge.

Nutrition in pregnancy

David J. Williams

Essentials

Nutritional requirements for healthy pregnancy vary according to a woman's prepregnancy nutritional state and her access to food during pregnancy: there is no unifying nutritional advice that is appropriate for all pregnant women throughout the world, or even within nations.

The well-nourished mother—maternal adaptation to pregnancy requires few dietary changes during pregnancy. She should eat one or two portions of sea fish per week to -ensure intake of n-3 long-chain polyunsaturated fatty acids sufficient to provide at least 200 mg of docosahexaenoic acid per day, which is needed for the healthy development of the fetal central nervous system. Supplemental folic acid (400 μg/day) during the first trimester reduces the risk of neural tube defects, but with this exception extra vitamins and micronutrients are not necessary for well-nourished, healthy pregnant women who eat a balanced diet, and excessive amounts of some micronutrients can actually be harmful to the fetus. Thiamine replacement is essential for women with hyperemesis gravidarum.

The chronically undernourished pregnant woman—needs a balanced diet that is supplemented with (1) vitamins—including folic acid, vitamins A, B1 (thiamine) and others; and (2) micronutrients—iron, zinc, iodine. and others, to ensure that the fetus fulfils its growth potential. However, although protein and energy supplements given to such women of small stature and pelvis size improve fetal growth and perinatal outcome, they can lead to obstructed labour, a significant cause of maternal and perinatal death in the developing world.

Overeating and obesity—pregnancy complications due to poor nutrition in high-income countries tend to follow from these causes. Those who gain excessive weight in pregnancy double their risk of a poor outcome and increase their likelihood of postpartum weight retention, and women who retain weight after their first pregnancy have an increased risk of gestational diabetes, pre-eclampsia, caesarean delivery, stillbirth, and large for gestational age babies in subsequent pregnancies. Obesity during pregnancy fuels obesity in the next generation.

Introduction

There is no unifying nutritional advice that is appropriate for all pregnant women throughout the world, or even within nations. Nutritional advice must take account of maternal body size, lifestyle, and availability of food. In the developed world, where food is generally plentiful and obesity is more prevalent than undernourishment, dietary recommendations for a healthy pregnancy are often targeted to reduce excessive weight gain and pregnancy complications. By contrast, in nations where food is scarce, nutritional intake falls far below the average intake of women who eat to satisfy their appetite, and pregnancy adaptations—which are inevitably a compromise—attempt to maximize fetal growth. Micronutrients and vitamin supplements are given with good effect to chronically undernourished pregnant women in the developing world, but with few exceptions are unnecessary and can be harmful to well-nourished pregnant women in the developed world. Conversely, protein and energy supplements given to chronically malnourished pregnant women of small stature and

pelvis size improve fetal growth and perinatal outcome, but can lead to obstructed labour, a major cause of maternal and perinatal death in the developing world.

The ability of pregnant women to adapt to different environmental and nutritional conditions is a key requirement for reproductive success. Gestational metabolic adaptations minimize extra nutritional requirements and optimize fetal growth. However, millions of pregnant women are unable to provide enough nutrition for their fetus to thrive despite these adaptations. Poor prenatal nutrition not only affects perinatal outcome, but also dictates susceptibility to adult diseases and even the health of the next generation (see Chapter 16.13.3).

The liberal availability of food can also be harmful when it goes unchecked. In the United Kingdom between 1990 and 2002–2004 the prevalence of obesity doubled amongst pregnant women attending for their first antenatal appointment. In 2002, almost half of all women in the United State of America of child-bearing age (20–44 years) were either overweight or obese, with a body mass index (BMI) of more than 25kg/m^2. A similar rise in the prevalence of obesity has been seen worldwide, including in many developing countries, and is associated with an increased risk of pregnancy complications.

Weight gain in pregnancy

During pregnancy, well-nourished mothers with free access to food gain up to 30% of their prepregnancy weight, of which only 25% is fetal. By contrast, mothers with limited access to food gain as little as 10% of their prepregnancy weight, of which up to 60% is fetal. Excess weight gain increases birth weight, but also increases the rate of caesarean section, pre-eclampsia and gestational diabetes mellitus. Poor weight gain increases the incidence of low birth weight (defined as <2500 g at term). A World Health Organization study of maternal anthropometry on 110 000 births from 20 countries found that best pregnancy outcome was associated with a full-term baby weighing 3.1 to 3.6 kg (mean 3.3 kg) and maternal weight gain of 10 to 14 kg (mean 12 kg).

In 1990 the Institute of Medicine in the United States refined these observations with guidelines for weight gain in pregnancy, adjusted according to prepregnancy maternal weight (Table 14.2.1). These recommendations remain appropriate despite many subsequent analyses: they minimize the overall risk of adverse pregnancy outcome for both mother and neonate. Obese women are least able to keep within these guidelines. Those who gain excessive weight double their risk of a poor pregnancy outcome and increase their likelihood of postpartum weight retention. Women who retain weight after their first pregnancy have an increased risk of gestational diabetes, pre-eclampsia, caesarean delivery, stillbirth, and babies that are large for gestational age in subsequent pregnancies. Furthermore, obesity during pregnancy fuels obesity in the next generation: about one-third of infants of obese mothers are in the 90th centile for their age, and a child of an overweight mother is three times more likely to be overweight by age 7 years.

Maternal undernutrition in the developing world

Nutrition during pregnancy and until a child is 24 months of age is most critical to its future growth and development. Maternal and child undernutrition is the underlying cause of 3.5 million deaths around the world each year, mainly of children. Eighty per cent of the world's undernourished children live in just 20 countries, mainly in sub-Saharan Africa, and south-central and south-eastern Asia (Fig. 14.2.1). In these countries 20 to 40% of women aged 15 to 49 years are undernourished (BMI <18.5 kg/m^2). Chronically undernourished women are often of short stature, which increases their risk of an operative delivery due to cephalopelvic disproportion, and perioperative comorbidity is high even if caesarean section is available.

In these low-income countries, 16% of babies are of low birth weight (<2500 g), of which more than two-thirds are due to fetal growth restriction and less than one-third are due to prematurity. In comparison, in high-income nations only 5% of babies are of low birth weight, of which most (55%) are premature. Low birth weight increases an individual's risk of morbidity and mortality during all phases of life: neonatal, childhood, and adult.

Energy requirements during pregnancy

The rate of human fetal growth is slow and the daily incremental energy stress of human pregnancy is relatively low compared with that in other species (Fig. 14.2.2). This allows a mother time to adapt her metabolism and energy expenditure to diverse nutritional conditions and the fetus to develop a complex brain. The total energy cost of pregnancy for a woman with a mean weight gain of 12 kg is 325 MJ (77 000 kcal). Energy requirements increase gradually as pregnancy progresses. In the first trimester an estimated 375 kJ (90 kcal)/day is required, in the second trimester 1200 kJ (287 kcal)/day, and in the third 1950 KJ (466 kcal)/day. Energy requirements during lactation are similar to those of the third trimester.

The three major components of energy expenditure in an average well-nourished pregnant woman are growth of the fetus and reproductive tissues (c.18%), new maternal fat stores (c.38%), and increased maternal metabolism (c.44%). Poorly nourished women try to maintain fetal growth by depressing their basal metabolic rate until late pregnancy and by laying down less fat. Although such adaptations usually result in successful reproduction, they are inevitably a compromise with regards to perinatal health. However, attempts to quantify minimal energy requirements for good perinatal health will always be confounded by huge individual variability and the practical difficulties of attributing a single nutritional component to morbidity, which is a multifaceted problem.

Well-nourished women increase their basal metabolic rate most rapidly after 16 weeks gestation until term. During the middle trimester large amounts of maternal fat are laid down as energy stores, although women with the highest cumulative rise in basal metabolic rate lay down the least fat. If food intake becomes limited during late pregnancy, maternal fat can be mobilized to support the period of most rapid fetal growth. A similar strategy of fat storage before anticipated energy expenditure is used by birds before they migrate and by mammals before they hibernate. Well-nourished women with free access to food rarely need to utilize all their fat stores to support late fetal growth, and excess fat remains difficult to lose postpartum. Even poorly nourished women with low gestational weight gain lay down some extra fat, but they also suppress their basal metabolic rate until late in pregnancy in order to support fetal growth.

Studies of well-nourished women have found that maternal energy intake actually increases by little more than 25% of that required to fulfil energy needs. It is likely that much of this estimated shortfall is due to under-reporting of nutritional intake, while some is made up by an economy of energy expenditure, including reduced physical activity and diet-induced thermogenesis.

Table 14.2.1 Recommended weight gain in pregnancy (adapted from recommendations of the Institute of Medicine of the United States)

Maternal BMI (kg/m²)	Recommended weight gain (kg)
Low (<19.8 kg/m²)	12.5–18
Normal (19.8–26.0 kg/m²)	11.5–16
High (26.1–28.9 kg/m²)	7–11.5
Obesity (>29 kg/m²)	<7

BMI, body mass index.

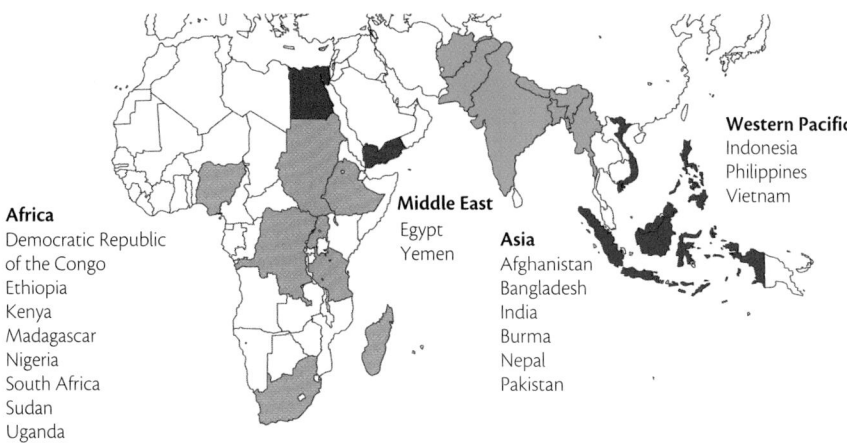

Fig. 14.2.1 The 20 countries with the highest burden of undernutrition. In these countries the prevalence of stunting is 20% or more in children under the age of 5 years, accounting for over 80% of the world's undernourished children.
(From Bryce J, et al. for the Maternal and Child Undernutrition Study Group (2008). Maternal and child undernutrition: effective action at national level. *Lancet*, **371**, 510–26.)

Metabolic changes in pregnancy

The mechanisms that control the diverse metabolic responses to pregnancy are not fully understood.

Fat metabolism

Leptin, a protein produced by adipose tissue and the placenta, circulates in increasing amounts during pregnancy and controls peripheral energy status and body fat. Ob/ob mice (deficient in leptin) become insensitive to exogenous leptin when pregnant, consistent with the build-up of maternal fat stores until the last trimester, but a precise role for leptin during pregnancy remains to be elucidated. Leptin is integrated with the hypothalamo–pituitary–gonadal axis and may explain why thin women with low leptin levels remain infertile until they have adequate fat stores.

There is no need for pregnant women to increase their total dietary fat as a percentage of energy intake during pregnancy or lactation. The only change that is recommended is an increase in consumption of n – 3 long-chain polyunsaturated fatty acid (LC-PUFA) sufficient to provide at least 200 mg of docosahexaenoic acid (DHA) per day, which can be achieved with the consumption of one or two portions of sea fish per week. DHA is needed for the healthy development of the fetal central nervous system and several small studies have shown that it appears to improve pregnancy outcomes for mother and neonate. Concerns that large predator fish contaminated by neurotoxic levels of methylmercury might be harmful to the fetus are easily outweighed by the benefits of DHA. Limiting fish intake to smaller oily fish such as herring, mackerel, and salmon will further diminish this concern.

Carbohydrate metabolism

During the first half of pregnancy women produce more insulin in response to a glucose load and are more sensitive to exogenous insulin than in the nonpregnant state. These changes affect carbohydrate and lipid metabolism to favour increased fat production and storage. During the second half of pregnancy a woman becomes resistant to insulin, so that at term the action of a particular circulating concentration of insulin is 50 to 70% lower than in the nongravid state. As a consequence, the fat stores laid down in the first half of pregnancy are mobilized and postprandial blood glucose levels remain higher for longer. Circulating levels of fatty acids and glycerol increase and are used by the mother as an energy source in

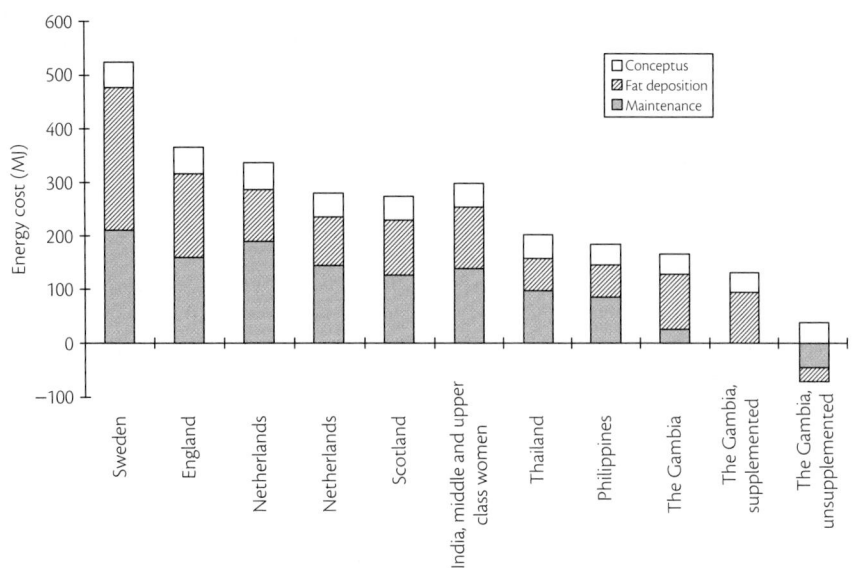

Fig. 14.2.2 Estimated total energy costs of pregnancy in different nutritional environments. The 'supplemented' women from the Gambia were given a balanced protein–energy diet.
(From Prentice AM, Goldberg GR (2000). Energy adaptations in human pregnancy: limits and long term consequences. *Am J Clin Nutr*, **71** Suppl, 1226–32S.)

preference to glucose and amino acids, which are left for the fetus. As a consequence, fasting pregnant women oxidize fat and produce ketones far sooner than they do when they are not pregnant, and women with an exaggerated peripheral resistance to insulin are at risk of gestational diabetes mellitus.

Protein metabolism

Pregnancy is an anabolic state. Protein and nitrogen metabolism adapt early and gradually throughout healthy pregnancy to provide for tissue growth. Well-nourished women are estimated to accumulate an extra 500 g to 1 kg of protein during pregnancy, almost half of which is maternal lean body mass, whilst the rest lies within the fetus and reproductive tissues.

In the United Kingdom the advised increment of dietary protein has been calculated to increase gradually throughout pregnancy to 8.5 g/day at term, but this does not take into account reduced hepatic metabolism of branched chain amino acids and hence reduced urea synthesis. The rate of urea synthesis declines by 30% during the first trimester and by 45% during the third trimester, hence serum urea concentration falls, providing more nitrogen for protein synthesis.

Vitamins and micronutrients

In many parts of the developing world micronutrient deficiencies are endemic and have serious consequences for fetal, neonatal, and maternal well-being, e.g. hypothyroidism due to iodine deficiency and night blindness due to vitamin A deficiency. Such deficiencies are rare in developed countries.

Calculated increments in the recommended daily allowance of specific nutrients are derived from estimates of the cost of fetal growth and increased maternal metabolism. However, these calculations do not usually take account of maternal metabolic adaptations aimed to minimize the need for extra nutrients. For example, intestinal absorption of calcium increases in well-nourished women and the need for an increase in dietary calcium diminishes. Conversely, increased folic acid excretion leads to an underestimate of folic acid requirements. Furthermore, individual micronutrients interact with each other and changes to one may have a detrimental effect on the activity of another.

It is now widely accepted that supplemental folic acid (400 µg/day) during the first trimester reduces the risk of neural tube defects. With this exception, extra vitamins and micronutrients are not necessary for well-nourished, healthy pregnant women who eat a balanced diet. Indeed, excessive amounts of certain micronutrients can be harmful to the fetus. The situation is quite different for undernourished women of countries in the developing world.

Vitamin A

Vitamin A is a lipid-soluble vitamin essential for healthy embryogenesis and fetal growth. Preformed vitamin A is found in dairy products and liver, the recommended daily allowance during pregnancy being 2000 to 2700 IU/day (670–899 retinol equivalents; RE). Vitamin A deficiency is endemic in some parts of the world and maternal vitamin A supplements of 6000 to 8000 IU/day (2000–2670 RE/day) result in a small increase in birth weight. However, excessive doses of vitamin A (>15 000 IU/day or 5000 RE/day) or supplements of more than 10 000 IU/day, are teratogenic, and drugs that are derived from vitamin A, such as the retinoids, are associated with an estimated 25-fold increased risk of

fetal malformation. It is therefore recommended that the daily dose of vitamin A should not exceed 5000 IU/day (1665 RE/day) during pregnancy.

The carotenoids (β-carotene), which are precursors to vitamin A, do not appear to be teratogenic and are now being substituted for preformed vitamin A in multivitamin preparations. In general, vitamin A supplements are unnecessary for well-nourished women and potentially harmful to the fetus. Breast milk is rich in vitamin A, and is important for neonatal immunity.

Thiamine (vitamin B₁)

Thiamine deficiency is endemic in some developing countries, but is also a global problem in women with hyperemesis gravidarum. Severe and persistent vomiting during pregnancy leads to thiamine deficiency and can cause Wernicke's encephalopathy, hence thiamine replacement is essential for women with this condition.

Vitamins C and E

Serum vitamin C levels fall by about 50% during pregnancy, hence it was previously recommended that this was supplemented. Furthermore, the antioxidant properties of vitamins C and E were thought to reduce the risk of pre-eclampsia, but this is not the case. Indeed, at high doses (vitamin C 1 g/day and vitamin E 400 IU/day) these vitamins increase the risk of babies being born with a low birth weight and their supplementation is not justified in pregnancy.

Iodine

More than 800 million people live in iodine-deficient areas. Inadequate dietary iodine leads to maternal hypothyroidism, which in turn is detrimental to *in utero* growth and development. Supplemental iodine, which is added to salt in most developed countries, can prevent these consequences.

Zinc

Zinc deficiency is associated with intrauterine growth restriction and teratogenesis. Maternal zinc levels remain stable during pregnancy through increased intestinal absorption. Excess iron supplements, smoking, alcohol abuse, or subsistence cereal diets high in phytate can all inhibit zinc absorption: under such conditions pregnant women may benefit from 25 mg zinc daily.

Iron

During pregnancy expansion in plasma volume exceeds the increase in red cell mass, causing a fall in haemoglobin concentration. Healthy pregnant women not taking iron supplements drop their haemoglobin from 13.3 g/dl to 11.0 g/dl by 36 weeks gestation. The minimum incidence of low birth weight (<2500 g at term) and preterm labour is associated with maternal haemoglobin in the range 9.5 to 10.5 g/dl, which in the nongravid state would indicate anaemia, but supplemental iron is probably unnecessary in pregnancy unless the mean corpuscular volume is less than 84 fl. A meta-analysis of randomized controlled trials examining the benefit of supplemental iron found a significant reduction in the proportion of women with haemoglobin levels less than 10 g/dl, but no effect—beneficial or harmful—on maternal or fetal outcome.

Anaemia of multiple causes is endemic in many developing nations, and the risk of maternal death is increased with severe anaemia (haemoglobin <7.0 g/dl), a condition where supplemental iron is unlikely to have much effect. However, in such countries mild to moderate anaemia can be prevented with iron and folate supplementation and has improved pregnancy outcome, and multiple micronutrient supplements may be even more beneficial. Many developing countries advocate a policy of iron and folic acid supplementation for all pregnant women. More studies are necessary to monitor the effects of this policy on maternal and perinatal outcome. Anaemia in pregnancy is discussed in more detail in Chapter 14.16.

Calcium

The growing fetus gains about 50 mg calcium per day by mid pregnancy and about 300 mg/day at term, and the breastfed infant receives about 250 mg of calcium in breast milk each day. The recommended daily allowance of calcium during pregnancy and lactation is 1.2 g/day, but women with much less dietary calcium undergo metabolic adaptations to meet the demands of pregnancy and lactation without any detriment to their health or that of the fetus.

During pregnancy, maternal calcium absorption increases twofold, stimulated by increased 1,25-dihydroxyvitamin D (calcitriol) activity due to placental synthesis of calcitriol and increased renal 1α-hydroxylase activity. Although urinary calcium excretion doubles during pregnancy, fasting urinary calcium excretion, corrected for increased creatinine clearance, is unchanged. The concentration of parathyroid hormone falls during pregnancy, suggesting that the pregnant woman receives enough calcium for her growing fetus. There are two caveats: one is the pregnant adolescent who needs to meet the demands of her own growth as well as that of the fetus; the other is the benefit of supplemental calcium for women on a low-calcium diet, but not those on a normal calcium diet, to prevent pre-eclampsia.

Following delivery, circulating calcitriol concentrations return to nonpregnant levels. During the first 3 to 6 months of breastfeeding mineralization of the maternal axial skeleton declines by about 3 to 5%, recovering after 6 months whether or not breastfeeding continues. Calcium supplements of 1 g/day given to lactating women do not prevent bone demineralization or improve the calcium concentration of breast milk, even if the woman is on a low-calcium diet. Furthermore, repeated long periods of breastfeeding in women with a low calcium intake do not contribute to osteoporosis in later life.

Fetal programming—the influence of fetal nutrition on adult disease

Epidemiological studies have found that low birth weight due to intrauterine growth restriction, rather than prematurity, is associated with an increased risk of cardiovascular disease in adulthood. It is hypothesized that a poorly growing fetus makes metabolic adaptations *in utero* to optimize growth and development. Despite these physiological adaptations, driven in part by insulin-like growth factors, birth weight remains low, and because of them the individual is indelibly programmed to insulin-resistance syndromes that are detrimental to long-term cardiovascular health. These issues are discussed further in Chapter 16.13.3.

Animal studies have shown that the composition of maternal diet can influence fetal growth and consequently blood pressure in her offspring. At present not enough is known about the mechanisms that control human fetal growth to give maternal nutritional advice that might eventually reduce the risk of cardiovascular disease in her children. Understanding these mechanisms may help to ameliorate the global epidemic of cardiovascular disease.

Foods to avoid during pregnancy

Food contaminated with *Listeria monocytogenes* can cause listeriosis. During pregnancy this organism has a predilection to replicate at the uteroplacental site, leading to septic abortion in early pregnancy, or neonatal listeriosis in later pregnancy. Pregnant women should avoid eating soft ripened cheeses, all types of pâté, and undercooked meats to reduce the risk of such infection, which is discussed in Chapters 7.6.37 and 14.15.

Acute maternal infection with *Toxoplasma gondii* can cross the placenta to the fetus. Congenital infection is least likely during early pregnancy, but more severe when it occurs. The risk of congenital infection can be kept to a minimum by not eating undercooked meat, taking care whilst handling raw meat, and avoiding contact with cat faeces. This infection is discussed in Chapters 7.8.4 and 14.15.

Food cravings during pregnancy

Common food cravings during pregnancy are for dairy products and occasionally for nonorganic material such as soil (pica). Common aversions are to alcohol, caffeine, and meats.

Further reading

American College of Obstetricians and Gynecologists (2005). ACOG Committee Opinion 315: Obesity in pregnancy. *Obstet Gynecol*, **106**, 671–5.

Black RE, *et al.* for the Maternal and Child Undernutrition Study Group (2008). Maternal and child undernutrition: global and regional exposures and health consequences. *Lancet*, **371**, 243–60.

Butte NF, King JC (2005). Energy requirements during pregnancy and lactation. *Public Health Nutr*, **8**, 1010–27.

Bryce J, *et al.* for the Maternal and Child Undernutrition Study Group (2008). Maternal and child undernutrition: effective action at national level. *Lancet*, **371**, 510–26.

DeVader SR, *et al.* (2007). Evaluation of gestational weight gain guidelines for women with normal pre-pregnancy body mass index. *Obstet Gynecol*, **110**, 743–4.

Gluckman PD, Hanson MA (2004). Living with the past: evolution, development, and patterns of disease. *Science*, **305**, 1733–6.

Hofmeyr GJ, Duley L, Atallah AN (2007). Dietary calcium supplementation for prevention of pre-eclampsia and related problems: a systematic review and commentary. *Br J Obstet Gynaecol*, **114**, 933–43.

Huxley R, *et al.* (2007). Is birth weight a risk factor for ischaemic heart disease in later life? *Am J Clin Nutr*, **85**, 1244–50.

Institute of Medicine (United States) Food and Nutrition Board (1990). *Nutrition during pregnancy. Report of the Committee on Nutritional Status during pregnancy and lactatio*. National Academies Press, Washington, DC.

Institute of Medicine of the National Academies (2006). *Dietary reference intakes: The essential guide to nutrient requirements*. National Academies Press, Washington, DC.

Kalhan SC (2000). Protein metabolism in pregnancy. *Am J Clin Nutr*, **71** Suppl, 1249S–1255S.

Kalkwarf HJ, Specker BL (2002). Bone mineral changes during pregnancy and lactation. *Endocrine*, **17**, 49–53.

Koletzko B, Cetin I, Thomas Brenna J for the Perinatal Lipid Intake Working Group (2007). Dietary fat intakes for pregnant and lactating women. Consensus statement. *Br J Nutr*, **98**, 873–7.

Pena-Rosas JP, Viteri FE (2006). Effects of routine oral iron supplementation with or without folic acid for women during pregnancy. *Cochrane Database Syst Rev*, **3**, CD004736.

Poston L, *et al.* for the vitamins in pre-eclampsia (VIP) Trial consortium (2006). Vitamin C and vitamin E in pregnant women at risk for pre-eclampsia (VIP trial): randomized placebo-controlled trial. *Lancet*, **367**, 1145–54.

Prentice A (2000). Calcium in pregnancy and lactation. *Annu Rev Nutr*, **20**, 249–72.

Prentice AM, Goldberg GR (2000). Energy adaptations in human pregnancy: limits and long term consequences. *Am J Clin Nutr*, **71** Suppl, 1226–32S.

Rothman KJ *et al.* (1995). Teratogenicity of high vitamin A intake. *N Engl J Med*, **333**, 1369–73.

Supplementation with multiple micronutrients intervention trial (SUMMIT) study group, Shankar AH, *et al.* (2008). Effect of maternal micronutrient supplementation on fetal loss and infant death in Indonesia: a double-blind cluster-randomised trial. *Lancet*, **371**, 215–27.

Vahratian A (2009). Prevalence of overweight and obesity among women of childbearing age: Results from the 2002 National Survey of Family Growth. *Matern Child Health J*, 13, 268–73.

Villamour E, Cnattingius S (2006). Inter-pregnancy weight change and risk of adverse pregnancy outcomes: a population-based study. *Lancet*, **368**, 1164–70.

World Health Organization (1995). Maternal anthropometry and pregnancy outcomes—a WHO collaborative study. *Bull WHO*, **73**, S1–69.

Medical management of normal pregnancy

David J. Williams

Essentials

Reducing the number of maternal deaths is one of the United Nation's eight Millennium Development Goals, yet despite this initiative maternal deaths are increasing in some parts of Africa, usually from readily preventable causes that would not occur in the presence of a skilled birth attendant.

Diagnosis of pregnancy—this can be achieved within a day of missing a menstrual bleed by identifying a rise in concentration of urinary human chorionic gonadotropin.

Antenatal checks—at the first antenatal visit a medical and obstetric history is combined with (1) cardiovascular examination; (2) urinalysis—proteinuria, bacteriuria; and (3) laboratory tests—HIV, hepatitis B, and syphilis; screening for sickle cell disease, thalassaemias, and rhesus antibodies. Further antenatal checks (obstetric, blood pressure, urinalysis) are usually performed around 16, 25, 28, 31, 34, 36, 38 and 40 weeks, then weekly until delivery.

Clinical features of pregnancy—aside from those obviously related to a growing fetus in the abdomen, symptoms of a healthy pregnancy include fatigue, palpitations, dizziness, syncope, dyspnoea, nausea, vomiting, headaches, and oedema, and signs include full and bounding arterial pulses and an ejection systolic flow murmur.

General management—pregnant women may require nutritional advice (see Chapter 14.2) and should be advised to take regular exercise, stop smoking, and avoid heavy alcohol consumption (but there is no evidence that 1 to 2 units of alcohol once or twice a week is harmful to the fetus).

Clinical priorities—when managing medical disorders in pregnancy, the clinician's priority is to treat the maternal condition, sometimes at the risk of fetal well-being.

Introduction

Until recently *Homo sapiens* thrived with nothing but the most primitive antenatal care, and the first introductions of hospital-based childbirth in the United Kingdom and elsewhere were disasters. In the mid 19th century it became clear to some that unhygienic medical practice was responsible for puerperal sepsis and a high maternal mortality rate, but not until the 1930s did the maternal mortality rate in the United Kingdom fall from more than 1 in 100 deliveries in the worst maternity hospitals to less than 1 in 7000 deliveries today. Lessons learnt over the last century in the developed world are still not being implemented around the world, and globally there are over 500 000 pregnancy-related maternal deaths each year, mostly in sub-Saharan Africa and Asia.

Reducing the number of maternal deaths is one of the United Nations Millennium Development Goals, yet despite this initiative maternal deaths are increasing in some parts of Africa. Women in Sierra Leone have a 1:6 chance of death during their reproductive lifetime. The tragedy is that these are usually deaths from readily preventable causes that would not occur in the presence of a skilled birth attendant. Added problems such as HIV/AIDS and health systems disrupted by war exacerbate the problem. Furthermore, for every maternal death there are at least 20 additional women who suffer serious pregnancy-related conditions that cause lifelong disabilities.

In the developed world, the dramatic reduction in the number of maternal deaths from obstetric complications has not been matched by a similar fall in deaths associated with pre-existing maternal disease. This is partly due to the success of modern medicine in helping more women with congenital or chronic disease to survive until reproductive age, and partly due to the inability of physicians to manage otherwise familiar medical conditions during pregnancy.

Misplaced concern about fetal welfare often denies the mother life-saving investigations and treatment, hence substandard care is responsible for many maternal deaths. By contrast, the general physician must be aware of the symptoms and signs of normal pregnancy and familiar with advice on how women should prepare for and maintain a healthy pregnancy, or else clinical anxiety may lead to meddlesome and sometimes harmful intervention when a doctor is presented with a healthy but symptomatic pregnant woman.

Maternal factors that influence pregnancy outcome

Maternal age

There is a trend among women in the developed world to delay childbearing. In Sweden, the mean maternal age at the birth of the first child increased between 1974 and 2001 from 24.4 years to 28.5 years. The number of women delaying pregnancy until after the age of 40 years has also increased, yet women over 35 years have an increased risk of pregnancy-induced hypertension, gestational diabetes, thrombosis, and adverse pregnancy outcome.

The risk of fetal aneuploidy, most notably trisomy 21 (Down's syndrome), also increases with maternal age: at 25 years of age it is 1:1250, at 35 years 1:385, and at 45 years 1:30. These risks can be refined between 11 weeks 0 days and 13 weeks 6 days of gestation by the 'combined test' (nuchal translucency, which is an ultrasound measurement of skin-fold thickness at the back of the fetal neck, combined with a maternal serum measure of β-human chorionic gonadotropin, and pregnancy-associated plasma protein A). For women who book for antenatal care the most clinically and cost-effective serum screening test is the triple or quadruple test that should be offered between 15 and 20 weeks gestation. Women found to be at high risk of a chromosomal abnormality can be offered diagnostic testing with amniocentesis, which carries a 0.5 to 1.0% risk of miscarriage.

Maternal weight

Maternal health is threatened by a high prepregnancy weight, as measured by the body mass index (BMI): pre-eclampsia, gestational diabetes mellitus, and late fetal death are all more common in overweight (BMI 25–30 kg/m^2) and obese women (BMI > 30 kg/m^2), and it is of concern that nearly half of all women of childbearing age in the developed world are now either overweight or obese. Conversely, underweight women (BMI <19 kg/m^2) are more prone to have babies with lower birth weights.

Weight gain during healthy pregnancy varies between 10 and 16 kg in Western societies, i.e. about 20% of prepregnancy weight. Lean, nulliparous, healthy, pregnant women who eat to appetite gain 0.65 kg to 1.1 kg during the first 10 weeks of pregnancy, about 0.45 kg/week during the second trimester, and about 0.36 kg/week during the last trimester. Maternal weight gain correlates poorly with fetal growth. Unless the mother is underweight before pregnancy (BMI <19) or has hyperemesis gravidarum, conditions that often coexist, regular antenatal measurements of maternal weight are not helpful and fetal growth is most accurately assessed by serial ultrasound measurements.

Past medical history

Pregnancy is a medical stress test for the woman, which is particularly evident in those with chronic medical disorders. A diseased maternal organ system may transiently lose residual function in attempting to accommodate the physiological demands of pregnancy. For example, women with classic risk factors for hypertension are more likely to develop pre-eclampsia, and women with subclinical insulin resistance are at increased risk of gestational diabetes. Similarly, women with inherited thrombophilias may develop thrombosis only in combination with the hypercoagulable environment of healthy pregnancy. These gestational syndromes are likely to be associated with an adverse fetal outcome, but the physiological changes of pregnancy are not always damaging: some conditions improve, while others deteriorate (Box 14.3.1).

Family history

Gestational conditions tend to run in families. Pre-eclampsia, gestational diabetes mellitus, obstetric cholestasis, and probably both hyperemesis gravidarum and postnatal depression have genetic components. Inherited thrombophilias also have a direct impact on pregnancy outcome.

Infertility and multiple pregnancies

In 1978 the first baby was born by *in vitro* fertilization (IVF), and she herself has now given birth to a healthy child following natural conception. Over the last 30 years well over 1 million babies have been born worldwide using IVF technology. One-quarter of these pregnancies have resulted in multiple births, compared with 11 per 1000 pregnancies following natural conception. In the United Kingdom this has led to a 66% increase in twin births, which itself has increased the frequency of maternal complications in often older mothers. The cause of infertility may also lead to problems in pregnancy, e.g. women with polycystic ovary syndrome are at increased risk of pregnancy-induced hypertension and gestational diabetes.

Box 14.3.1 Effect of pregnancy on pre-existing conditions

Conditions that tend to improve during pregnancy

- Mitral and aortic regurgitation
- Raynaud's phenomenon
- Mild hypertension (worsens towards term)
- Hyperthyroidism (may transiently worsen in first trimester)
- Sarcoid
- Rheumatoid arthritis
- Multiple sclerosis (may relapse postpartum)
- Peptic ulceration

Conditions that are unpredictable during pregnancy

- Asthma
- Systemic lupus erythematosus (may relapse postpartum)

Conditions that tend to deteriorate during pregnancy

Cardiovascular system

- Mitral and aortic stenosis
- Pulmonary hypertension (40% risk of maternal mortality)
- Congenital cyanotic heart disease
- Supraventricular arrhythmias (in third trimester)

Box 14.3.1 *(Cont'd)* Effect of pregnancy on pre-existing conditions

- Vascular aneurysms
- Haemolytic–uraemic syndrome/thrombotic thrombocytopenic purpura
- Epistaxis
- Varicose veins and haemorrhoids
- Venous thrombosis
- Antiphospholipid syndrome (deep vein thrombosis and recurrent miscarriage)

Respiratory system
- Viral pneumonia
- Pulmonary embolus

Gastrointestinal system
- Gastro-oesophageal reflux (especially in third trimester)
- Cholestatic liver disease (in third trimester)
- Inflammatory bowel disease, in some women
- Constipation

Genitourinary system
- Upper urinary tract infections (pyelonephritis)
- Reflux nephropathy
- Renal impairment (glomerular filtration rate <30 ml/min)

Musculoskeletal system
- Osteoporosis
- Osteoarthritis
- Back pain

Endocrine system
- Diabetes mellitus
- Diabetes insipidus
- Hypothyroidism
- Hyperlipidaemia
- Pituitary macroadenoma

Neurological system
- Epilepsy
- Cerebrovascular accidents, especially postpartum
- Depression (postnatal)
- Headache, in first and second trimester
- Carpal tunnel syndrome, third trimester

Haematological system
- Anaemia and thrombocytopenia
- Sickle cell disease
- Thrombophilias

Infections
- Intracellular pathogens (e.g. malaria, leprosy, listeria)

Ovarian hyperstimulation syndrome

To increase the yield of eggs, women receiving IVF undergo ovarian stimulation with gonadotropins, following which up to 10% develop an ovarian hyperstimulation syndrome that is severe in 1% of cases. This occurs when multiple follicles each develop into a corpus luteum, producing excessive amounts of progesterone and resulting in massive ovarian enlargement and increased vascular permeability. Protein-rich fluid shifts into serous cavities, causing ascites and (in more severe cases) pleural and pericardial effusions. Haemoconcentration and hypotension result, increasing the risk of thrombosis and reducing renal perfusion. Most cases are mild, but death has followed acute respiratory distress, hepatorenal failure, thromboembolism, and rupture of grossly enlarged ovaries. Management is mainly supportive, including careful fluid balance, thromboprophylaxis, analgesia, and adjustment of luteal stimulation under the guidance of a specialist in assisted conception. In some cases paracentesis can be used to transiently relieve abdominal pressure symptoms.

Diagnosis of pregnancy

Pregnancy can be diagnosed within a day of missing a menstrual bleed by identifying a rise in concentration of urinary human chorionic gonadotropin (hCG). At this time the embryo is 2 weeks old, but obstetric convention dictates that the gestation of pregnancy is calculated from the first day of the last menstrual period, i.e. 2 weeks earlier than embryonic age. Teratogenic drugs interfere with organ development in the 2 to 8 weeks postconception (embryonic period). After 9 weeks and until delivery, the conceptus is known as a fetus, but it is still vulnerable to the effects of drugs given to the mother.

Screening of maternal health during pregnancy

Pregnancy is an opportunity for women to be screened for occult disease. In the United Kingdom, healthy women are encouraged to register with an antenatal clinic by 10 weeks gestation. However, by this time they will have missed the opportunity to take folic acid prophylaxis against neural tube defects, and may not recognize the need to adjust social behaviour or stop regular medications.

At the first antenatal visit a medical and obstetric history is combined with cardiovascular examination, urinalysis, and laboratory tests. Identification of maternal infection with HIV, hepatitis B, or syphilis is crucial for the appropriate management of the mother and her partner, and to minimize the risk of vertical transmission to the infant. All women should be screened for sickle cell disease and thalassaemias as early as possible in pregnancy, and the father of the pregnancy should be strongly encouraged to undergo screening if a woman is found to be a carrier of a significant haemoglobinopathy. Rhesus antibody screening allows prophylactic measures to prevent haemolytic disease of the fetus.

Further antenatal checks are usually performed around 16 weeks to discuss the results of screening tests, and then at 25, 28 (in combination with a serum glucose check in those at high risk of gestational diabetes mellitus, and a full blood count), 31, 34, 36, 38, and 40 weeks, then weekly until delivery. At each visit, obstetric assessment is combined with a check of blood pressure and urinalysis.

Screening and treatment of asymptomatic bacteriuria during healthy pregnancy reduces the risk of maternal pyelonephritis and fetal morbidity. The cost-effectiveness of such screening depends on the prevalence of asymptomatic bacteriuria in the pregnant population. If this is less than 5%, as it is in many developed countries, then screening is not cost-effective, but in the developing world and in high-risk populations, e.g. women with renal disease and diabetes mellitus, asymptomatic bacteriuria is far more common and screening is worthwhile. As the recurrence rate of asymptomatic bacteriuria is about 30%, women identified with an occult infection should be screened every 4 to 6 weeks throughout the remainder of their pregnancy. See Chapter 14.5 for further discussion.

Symptoms and signs of healthy pregnancy

Fatigue

Fatigue is a common symptom that often begins early in healthy pregnancy, improves in the second trimester, and reappears towards term. Insomnia is caused in the third trimester by changes in maternal size and shape as well as nocturia. Anaemia or hypothyroidism should be excluded if daily living is significantly compromised.

Cardiovascular system

The hyperdynamic circulation of pregnancy causes cardiovascular symptoms that can mimic heart disease (see Chapter 14.6). Palpitations, dizziness, syncope, and dyspnoea are common symptoms of healthy pregnancy. Failure to distinguish between benign physiological change and significant pathology creates unnecessary anxiety and investigations. However, ischaemic heart disease is the most common cause of maternal death from cardiac disease in the United Kingdom, hence older and more obese women with symptoms suggestive of ischaemic heart disease should be investigated promptly and thoroughly, especially in the third trimester and immediately postpartum.

Palpitations

Transient sinus tachycardia, up to 130 beats/min, and premature atrial and ventricular ectopic beats are common features of healthy pregnancy, especially in women who complain of palpitations. As pregnancy may expose previously asymptomatic abnormalities of cardiac conducting tissue, investigations should include a 12-lead ECG. During healthy pregnancy, the QRS axis moves to the left as the diaphragm becomes elevated, and Q waves and inverted T waves are frequently seen in leads III and aVR. Pregnant women with syncope or presyncope coinciding with palpitations require further investigation. Thyrotoxicosis, anaemia, hypokalaemia, excess caffeine, or tobacco should be excluded.

Oedema

By the end of pregnancy 80% of healthy women will have some degree of oedema. This is associated with a fall in plasma albumin concentration of 5 to 10 g/litre and reduced venous return. Unless peripheral oedema is very severe, or is associated with pulmonary oedema, diuretics should be avoided as they attenuate the plasma volume expansion of healthy pregnancy and lead to fetal growth restriction. Severe and rapid onset of oedema, especially affecting hands and face, may herald pre-eclampsia and warrants further assessment.

Blood pressure

Peripheral vasodilatation leads to a slight fall in diastolic blood pressure by the end of the first trimester, which gradually returns to nonpregnant values during the third trimester. Systolic and diastolic readings are approximately 10 mmHg higher when measured sitting or standing as compared with the left lateral position, hence blood pressure should be measured with the mother in the same position at each antenatal visit. A blood pressure reading before 20 weeks gestation is important to discriminate between pre-existing hypertension and pregnancy-induced hypertension.

Clinical examination

During healthy pregnancy the peripheral pulses are full, bounding, and often collapsing, suggesting aortic regurgitation. From mid gestation onwards the jugular venous pressure becomes more obvious and may be raised, perhaps due to increased intra-abdominal pressure. The apex beat is more forceful and mildly displaced because of the increase in cardiac output, suggesting cardiomegaly in healthy pregnant women. An apex beat more than 2 cm outside the midclavicular line should be considered abnormal. On auscultation an ejection systolic flow murmur can be heard in up to 90% of healthy pregnant women, and increased mammary blood flow in the third trimester occasionally produces a bruit that varies with the pressure of the stethoscope.

In developed countries it is rare for new heart lesions to be identified during pregnancy, as most women with congenital heart disease are diagnosed early in life. By contrast, women in developing countries are more likely to present with previously unrecognized cardiac abnormalities.

Respiratory system

Dyspnoea

The physiological hyperventilation of pregnancy leads to a subjective feeling of breathlessness in about 70% of women. The maximum prevalence of breathlessness is between 28 and 31 weeks' gestation, but about 50% of women will feel breathless before 20 weeks. The early onset of dyspnoea and improvement towards term suggests that the gravid uterus has little influence on this physiological symptom. Women with gestational dyspnoea are more sensitive to CO_2 and hypoxia than asymptomatic women and respond with excessive ventilation. However, physiological dyspnoea does not usually interfere with daily activities: further investigations are only necessary if symptoms or signs suggest cardiorespiratory disease, e.g. chest infection, pulmonary embolus, or heart failure.

Radiological imaging in pregnancy

In general, the management of sick pregnant women should consider the health of the mother before that of the fetus. Nowhere is this consideration ignored more than with the use of X-rays. Although ionizing radiation is a known carcinogen, there is very little—if any—increased risk of childhood cancer following prenatal exposure to X-rays. Radiation from a chest radiograph is minimal (0.02 mSv), equivalent to 10 days of background radiation or a transatlantic air flight.

During healthy pregnancy the chest radiograph shows an increased cardiothoracic ratio and pulmonary vascular markings. If pulmonary embolus is suspected and the chest radiograph is normal, then a pregnant woman should not be denied a ventilation–perfusion scan (1.3 mSv), and a CT pulmonary angiogram should be performed if the chest radiograph is abnormal and pulmonary embolism is still suspected (see Chapter 14.7).

Gastrointestinal system

Nausea and vomiting

About 75% of all healthy women will feel nauseated and up to 50% will vomit during early pregnancy. Nausea usually begins around the fifth week; by 16 to 20 weeks it will have resolved in most women, but 10% of healthy pregnant women will still feel nauseated at 22 weeks. Contrary to popular belief, nausea is confined to the mornings in less than 2% of cases, and affects 80% of sufferers all day. Beneficial palliative measures include rest, eating carbohydrates, and drinking carbonated drinks.

Vomiting is severe and persistent in about 1.5% of pregnant women. Hyperemesis gravidarum is associated with dehydration, weight loss, and ketonuria (see Chapter 14.9). Ptyalism is a frequent accompaniment, due to an inability to swallow saliva. Biochemical changes often include elevated liver transaminases, elevated free thyroxine (T_4), and depressed thyroid-stimulating hormone (TSH). Hyperthyroxinaemia associated with hyperemesis gravidarum coincides with the rise and fall of serum hCG, which has thyroid-stimulating activity. Resolution of hyperemesis, not treatment of biochemical thyrotoxicosis, corrects the abnormal thyroid biochemistry.

Most antiemetics have not been fully evaluated in early pregnancy, and as with all prescribing in pregnancy the clinician must balance the potential risks to the fetus of maternal drug use against the risks of leaving the mother untreated. With regard to hyperemesis gravidarum, a woman is at risk of malnourishment, dehydration, and thrombosis, and most antiemetics have been used effectively during pregnancy for decades without apparent fetal harm. These include antihistamines, phenothiazines, metoclopramide, pyridoxine (vitamin B_6), and ginger. More severe cases have responded to steroid treatment (e.g. prednisolone 30 mg daily) or serotonin antagonists. Admission to hospital and intravenous rehydration is often beneficial. Parenteral nutrition is rarely necessary, but thiamine (vitamin B_1) supplementation is essential to prevent Wernicke's encephalopathy, as is thromboprophylaxis with low molecular weight heparin for women who are bed-bound.

New onset of nausea and vomiting during the second half of pregnancy suggests pathology unrelated to hyperemesis and may herald pre-eclampsia. Gastro-oesophageal reflux is a common problem of late pregnancy that usually improves with antacids or a change in diet. Persistent symptoms during pregnancy have been safely treated with H_2-receptor antagonists or proton pump inhibitors. Increased circulating progesterone levels relax intestinal smooth muscle and commonly provoke constipation, for which increased dietary fibre and avoidance of unnecessary iron supplements provide symptomatic relief.

Neurological system

Headaches are common in healthy pregnancy, and many pregnant women develop migrainous-type headaches for the first time in early pregnancy. If these are recurrent or do not respond to occasional paracetamol, then regular aspirin 75 mg daily or propranolol 10 to 20 mg three times daily are good prophylactic measures. Severe, persistent headache that presents for the first time in pregnancy, or is accompanied by focal neurological signs, requires investigation with MRI (see Chapter 14.12).

Introduction of an epidural catheter during labour can lead to accidental puncture of the dura and a cerebrospinal fluid leak which causes a postural headache that improves when lying flat. If there is no improvement within 24 h, then an injection of 2 to 3 ml of autologous blood at the site of dural puncture (blood patch) usually resolves the headache.

Carpal tunnel syndrome affects about 20% of women with healthy pregnancies. It begins during the second half of pregnancy and is associated with excessive weight gain and fluid retention. Pain and numbness in the distribution of the median nerve, affecting the first three fingers, can be severe. Wrist splints alleviate symptoms, usually making surgical intervention inappropriate as most cases recover within weeks of delivery.

Musculoskeletal system

Low back and pelvic pain affect about 50% of all pregnancies. A combination of mechanical stress on the lumbar spine and pelvis and the effects of relaxin, a hormone produced by the corpus luteum to relax ligaments in anticipation of childbirth, are believed to be responsible. Some women develop radicular symptoms affecting nerve roots and the lumbar sacral plexus, but only 1% develop true sciatica with a dermatomal distribution. Progressive neurological symptoms necessitate further investigations, often with MRI. Some relief can be gained from massage, exercises, or a maternity cushion. Others can obtain relief from transcutaneous electrical nerve stimulation (TENS) or a trochanteric support belt. Nonsteroidal anti-inflammatory drugs (NSAIDs) should be avoided in the third trimester and used sparingly in early pregnancy because of fetal effects.

Skin

Pruritus is a common symptom of late pregnancy, thought to relate to increased cutaneous blood flow and dryness. If there is an associated rash, then gestational skin conditions need to be considered (see Chapter 14.13). If there is no rash, then liver function should be checked to exclude obstetric cholestasis.

Dietary modification, vitamin/mineral supplementation, and treatments during pregnancy

Folic acid

In the United Kingdom and the United States of America spina bifida or anencephaly (neural tube defects) affect about 1 in 1000 pregnancies. The neural tube develops and then closes within 28 days of conception. Women who take 400 μg folic acid daily around the time of conception and for the first 2 months of pregnancy reduce their risk of a pregnancy complicated by neural tube defects by approximately 70%. In some countries the fortification of food with folic acid provides an extra 100 μg/day of folic acid, which appears to be effective in lowering rates of neural tube defects. Women who have had a baby affected by spina bifida are advised to take a higher dose of folic acid (5 mg/day).

Multivitamins and other supplements

Multivitamin preparations without folic acid do not reduce the risk of neural tube defects. Multivitamins taken periconceptually may reduce the risk of some congenital heart defects, but beyond the first trimester are of no proven benefit for healthy women on a balanced diet. Antioxidant vitamins (vitamin C 1000 mg and vitamin E 400 IU daily) taken from mid pregnancy do not reduce the incidence of pre-eclampsia and even increase the incidence of low birth weight babies.

Women should keep up adequate stores of vitamin D during pregnancy and when breast feeding. Women at high risk of vitamin D deficiency should be particularly encouraged to take supplemental vitamin D (10 µg/day).

Certain liver products and vitamin A supplementation above 700 µg daily increase the risk of embryonic teratogenesis and should be avoided. In the developing world where diet is poor, vitamin A supplements and zinc improve fetal outcome. See Chapter 14.2 for further discussion.

In the developed world, supplemental iron should be reserved for those who have a haemoglobin of less than 9.5 g/dl and a mean corpuscular volume of less than 84 fl in the third trimester. In the developing world, malnutrition and chronic infection diminish iron stores that are further exhausted during pregnancy. Under these conditions, routine supplemental iron and folate improves maternal and neonatal outcome. See Chapter 14.2 for further discussion.

Sea food, fish oils, and omega-3 fatty acids

There is conflicting information regarding the harm and benefit that may follow ingestion of seafood and its unsaturated fatty acids during pregnancy. Official guidance from United States federal agencies recommends that seafood intake should be limited to less than 340 g per week during pregnancy because of the fear of methylmercury ingestion. This consequence has not eventuated from the ingestion of fish outside Japan, indeed children born to mothers who eat less than 340 g seafood during pregnancy have a greater risk of being in the lowest quartile for verbal IQ and other scores for poor social development. As a consequence of this latter observation many women take omega-3 fatty acids to improve their child's intelligence, but whether this is an advisable strategy has yet to be proven. For example, cod liver oil, which contains high doses of long-chain polyunsaturated fatty acids, is associated with an increased odds ratio of pre-eclampsia and gestational hypertension.

Prophylaxis against pre-eclampsia

Pre-eclampsia is discussed in Chapter 14.4. At present, prophylactic measures to prevent the condition have proved only weakly beneficial or even harmful, e.g multivitamins. Low dose aspirin 60 to 150 mg daily, given to women at increased risk of pre-eclampsia, reduces the incidence by 17%. Calcium supplementation is beneficial to populations of women with a low dietary intake of calcium. However, our ability to prevent or treat this condition will remain inadequate until our understanding of its pathophysiology improves.

Iodine and thyroxine

Neurodevelopment of the fetus during the first trimester depends on thyroxine and maternal subclinical hypothyroidism has been associated with impaired neurodevelopment in the infant. It has therefore been suggested that all women should be screened for hypothyroidism before conception or in early pregnancy, but more easily applied public health measures to increase iodine intake are generally more practical, and the benefit of thyroxine replacement in women with 'low normal' thyroxine levels is not proven.

Behavioural habits during pregnancy

Exercise

Pregnancy outcome is improved by regular exercise throughout a healthy pregnancy. The gestational increases in both cardiac output and respiratory work are enhanced further by exercise, but the intensity of exercise should not exceed levels to which a woman is accustomed. In late pregnancy non-weight-bearing exercises such as swimming become easier. Exercise may be harmful to women with impaired cardiac or respiratory function who struggle to fulfil the physiological demands of pregnancy alone.

Alcohol

Heavy alcohol consumption during pregnancy leads to the 'fetal alcohol syndrome' in approximately one-third of offspring. The susceptibility of the fetus to alcohol depends on genetic vulnerability, the nutritional status of the woman, and her abuse of other drugs. The developmental and neurological abnormalities that make up the fetal alcohol syndrome affect approximately 1 to 2 per 1000 live births, but there is a spectrum of fetal alcohol disorder that includes infants with less marked neurological impairment, which is likely to be associated with lower levels of maternal alcohol consumption. It is not known whether there is a safe level of alcohol consumption in pregnancy, but evidence suggests that one or two units of alcohol once or twice a week is not harmful to the fetus.

Tobacco

Women should stop smoking during pregnancy as it impairs fetal growth and increases the risk of poor obstetric outcome. Nicotine gum contains less nicotine than cigarettes and none of the other toxins, making it preferable to continued smoking during pregnancy. Nicotine patches provide a constant release of nicotine throughout the day that exceeds that of periodic nicotine gum. Pregnant women are advised to remove nicotine patches before they go to bed. It is of interest that despite the negative effects on most pregnancy outcomes, women who smoke before and during pregnancy suffer less pre-eclampsia than nonsmokers.

Caffeine

Large quantities of caffeine, more than six cups of coffee a day, appear to increase the risk of miscarriage, but moderate caffeine consumption is unlikely to be harmful.

Travel

Aircraft are pressurized to an oxygen partial pressure equivalent to that found at 2440 m (8000 ft) above sea level. During a routine commercial flight healthy pregnant women (32–38 weeks gestation) increase their heart rate and blood pressure and drop their oxygen saturation, but fetal heart rate remains unchanged. Long-haul flights further increase a pregnant woman's risk of deep vein thrombosis. Simple thromboprophylaxis with antiembolic stockings, hydration and mobility—including calf muscle exercise—are sufficient for the overwhelming majority of pregnant women. Low dose aspirin is safe in pregnancy and may have an as yet unproven role in reducing the risk of thrombosis in pregnant women during travel. Airlines are reluctant to carry women after 36 weeks gestation for the obvious and sensible practical reason that they don't want to deliver a baby in flight.

Events after delivery

Lactation

Breastfeeding is beneficial to the infant. However, the mother who breastfeeds for 6 months or longer transiently loses 4 to 5% of bone density in her lumbar spine. Calcium supplementation does not prevent this transient loss of bone mineral density, which recovers spontaneously 6 months after delivery whether or not the mother continues to breastfeed. Calcium supplementation does not increase the concentration of calcium in breast milk or the bone mineral status of the infant in the first year of life.

Postnatal depression

Almost half of all women develop the 'maternity blues'. This is characterized by tearfulness, anxiety and irritability, starting around the third to fifth postpartum days and usually resolving with nothing more than reassurance by the tenth day. About 10% of women develop nonpsychotic postnatal depression 4 to 6 weeks postpartum, with a maximum incidence at 3 months postpartum. The depression is similar to that occurring at other times, but is often accompanied by thoughts of harming the baby. Although most women recover without treatment over 3 to 6 months, recovery can be hastened by counselling. Women who fail to respond to counselling or who have severe depression may benefit from antidepressant treatment. Small amounts of tricyclic antidepressants and selective serotonin reuptake inhibitors appear in breast milk, but not enough to recommend stopping breastfeeding. Nonetheless, the infant should be watched for possible unwanted effects. Women who have had postpartum depression are more likely to suffer depression in later life.

Future maternal health

'Gestational syndromes' must be monitored postpartum until they resolve or reveal occult disease. For example, proteinuria related to

pre-eclampsia can take up to 12 months to disappear, but may be the first sign of previously subclinical renal disease. Similarly, abnormal liver function that may have manifest as obstetric cholestasis in pregnancy needs to be followed up postpartum as it may be the first sign of nongestational liver disease.

Insulin resistance underlying gestational diabetes mellitus returns to prepregnancy levels immediately postpartum, but affected women have an almost sixfold relative risk of future type 2 diabetes in later life compared with women who had a normoglycaemic pregnancy. Similarly, both pregnancy-induced hypertension and pre-eclampsia are associated with a two-fold relative risk of maternal cardiovascular disease in later life (Fig. 14.3.1).

However, despite the demands of pregnancy, it must be remembered that most women complete an uncomplicated pregnancy and have a healthy baby. This bodes well for maternal health during subsequent pregnancies and for the mother and her offspring in future life.

Further reading

Annual vital statistics, part 4. (2002). Statistics Sweden, Orebro.

National Institute for Health and Clinical Excellence (2008) *Antenatal care. Routine care for the healthy pregnant woman. NICE clinical guideline 62*. National Institute for Health and Clinical Excellence, London.

Bhutta ZA, *et al.* (2008). Maternal and child undernutrition study group. What works? Interventions for maternal and child undernutrition and survival. *Lancet*, **371**, 417–40.

Busby A, *et al.* (2005). Preventing neural tube defects in Europe: A missed opportunity! *Reprod Toxicol*, **20**, 393–402.

Bellamy L, *et al.* (2007). Pre-eclampsia and risk of cardiovascular disease and cancer in later life: systematic review and meta-analysis. *BMJ*, **335**, 974–77.

Buchanan TA, *et al.* (2007). What is gestational diabetes? *Diabetes Care*, **30** Suppl 2, S105–11.

Castles A, *et al.* (1999). Effects of smoking during pregnancy. Five meta-analyses. *Am J Prev Med*, **16**, 208–15.

Confidential Enquiry into Maternal and Child Health (CEMACH) (2007). *Saving mother's lives—Reviewing maternal deaths to make motherhood safer 2003–05*. CEMACH, London.

Duley L, *et al.* (2007). Antiplatelet agents for preventing pre-eclampsia and its complications. *Cochrane Database Syst Rev*, **2**, CD004659.

Garcia-Rio F, *et al.* (1996). Regulation of breathing and perception of dyspnoea in healthy pregnant women. *Chest*, **110**, 446–53. [Thorough study of pattern and mechanism of dyspnoea during normal pregnancy.]

Henderson J, Gray R, Brocklehurst P (2007). Systematic review of effects of low-moderate prenatal alcohol exposure on pregnancy outcome. *Br J Obstet Gynaecol*, **114**, 243–52.

Hibbeln JR, *et al.* (2007). Maternal seafood consumption in pregnancy and neurodevelopmental outcomes in childhood (ALSPAC study): an observational cohort study. *Lancet*, **369**, 578–85.

Human Fertilisation and Embryology Authority (2007). *A long term analysis of the HFEA Register data 1991–2006*. HFEA, London.

Jacobsson B, Ladfors L, Milson I (2004). Advanced maternal age and adverse perinatal outcome. *Obstet Gynecol*, **104**, 727–33.

James DK, *et al.* (eds) (2005). *High risk pregnancy*, 3rd edn. WB Saunders, London. [Comprehensive review of management of normal and abnormal pregnancies.]

Jarjou LM, *et al.* (2006). Randomized placebo controlled, calcium supplementation study in pregnant Gambian women: effects on

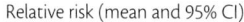

Relative risk (mean and 95% CI)

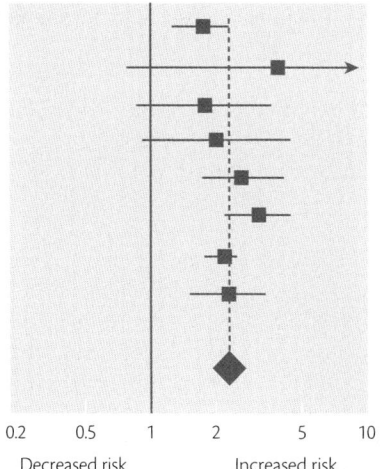

0.2 0.5 1 2 5 10

Decreased risk   Increased risk

Fig. 14.3.1 The relative risk of developing fatal or nonfatal ischaemic heart disease after a pregnancy affected by pre-eclampsia. Summary data are shown from eight studies comprising a total of 121 487 women with pre-eclampsia and 2 187 112 women without pre-eclampsia. Overall the relative risk of ischaemic heart disease in those who had pre-eclampsia was 2.16 (95% CI: 1.86–2.52). (From Bellamy L, *et al.* (2007). Pre-eclampsia and risk of cardiovascular disease and cancer in later life: systematic review and meta-analysis. *BMJ*, 335, 974–77.)

breast-milk calcium concentrations and infant birth weight, growth, and bone mineral accretion in the first year of life. *Am J Clin Nutr*, **83**, 657–66.

Lacroix R, Eason E, Melzack R (2000). Nausea and vomiting during pregnancy: a prospective study of its frequency, intensity and patterns of change. *Am J Obstet Gynecol*, **182**, 931–7.

Magnussen EB, *et al.* (2007). Pre-pregnancy cardiovascular risk factors as predictors of pre-eclampsia: population based cohort study. *BMJ*, **335**, 978–82.

Olafsdottir AS, *et al.* (2006). Relationship between high consumption of marine fatty acids in early pregnancy and hypertensive disorders in pregnancy. *Br J Obstet Gynaecol*, **113**, 301–9.

Pomp ER, *et al.* (2008). Pregnancy, the postpartum period and prothrombotic defects: risk of venous thrombosis in the MEGA study. *J Thromb Haemost*, **6**, 632–7.

Pop VJ, *et al.* (2003). Maternal hypothyroxinaemia during early pregnancy and subsequent child development: a 3 year follow-up study. *Clin Endocrinol*, **59**, 282–8.

Reece EA (2008). Perspectives on obesity, pregnancy and birth outcomes in the United States: the scope of the problem. *Am J Obstet Gynecol*, **198**, 23–7.

Steer PJ (2000). Maternal hemoglobin concentration and birth weight. *Am J Clin Nutr*, **71**, 1285S–1287S. [Review of relationship between maternal haemoglobin and clinical outcome.]

Vikse BE, *et al.* (2008). Preeclampsia and the risk of end-stage renal disease. *N Engl J Med*, **359**, 800–9.

Vlahos NF, Gregoriou O (2006). Prevention and management of ovarian hyperstimulation syndrome. *Ann N Y Acad Sci*, **1092**, 247–64.

Williams DJ (2003). Pregnancy: a stress test for life. *Curr Opin Obstet Gynecol*, **15**, 465–71.

Hypertension in pregnancy

C.W.G. Redman

Essentials

In normal pregnancy the arterial pressure falls in the second half of the first trimester: systolic pressure then remains unchanged throughout pregnancy, with diastolic pressure tending to rise gradually towards its prepregnancy level in the later weeks.

Definitions, epidemiology and clinical features—(1) Pregnancy-induced hypertension (PIH), transient hypertension of pregnancy, or gestational hypertension describe new hypertension, defined as blood pressure equal to or in excess of 140/90 mmHg, which without proteinuria affects up to 10% of women after mid term (20 weeks) and resolves after delivery. (2) Pre-eclampsia, which affects 3 to 5% of pregnancies, is defined by the presence of PIH and pregnancy-induced proteinuria arising after 20 weeks gestation that both improve after delivery. Other features include (a) renal insufficiency; (b) hepatocellular dysfunction and/or severe epigastric/right upper quadrant pain; (c) neurological problems—convulsions (eclampsia), severe headaches, persistent scotomata; (d) haematological disturbances—thrombocytopenia, disseminated intravascular coagulation, haemolysis; (e) fetal growth restriction.

Differential diagnosis—the main differential diagnosis of pre-eclampsia is from chronic hypertension, which in its pure form does not share the renal, coagulation, hepatic and placental abnormalities of pre-eclampsia. The perinatal risks of chronic hypertension in pregnancy result from superimposed pre-eclampsia.

Aetiology—the cause of pre-eclampsia is unknown, but it depends upon the placenta and is characterized by diffuse maternal endothelial dysfunction and a systemic inflammatory response.

Management before pregnancy and prevention—women with no more than moderate chronic hypertension should stop antihypertensive treatment before conception. There is no good method of preventing pre-eclampsia, but low-dose aspirin may be effective in some women.

Management during pregnancy—extreme hypertension (≥160/110 mmHg), whatever the underlying cause, is as dangerous as it is in any other medical situation and demands treatment, but there is no clear reason for treating more moderate hypertension on either maternal or fetal grounds, although most centres will initiate treatment at less extreme levels of blood pressure. As far as it is known the progression of moderate pre-eclampsia is not delayed, nor is the later superimposition of pre-eclampsia on moderate chronic hypertension prevented. Key aspects of management include (1) antihypertensive agents—methyldopa is the most thoroughly tested drug for use in pregnancy: no significant adverse reactions have been observed, but because of its side effect profile labetalol and nifedipine are popular alternatives. (2) Magnesium sulphate – this should be given to prevent eclampsia (grand-mal convulsions) in women with the HELLP syndrome (haemolysis, elevated liver enzymes and low platelet counts) and those who have had one eclamptic convulsion. (3) Delivery of the baby and placenta—this is the definitive treatment for pre-eclampsia.

Cardiovascular changes in pregnancy
(Box 14.4.1)

Cardiac output increases during the first trimester and remains steady in the second and early third trimesters but towards full term declines in the supine but not lateral recumbent position, owing to the pressure of the gravid uterus on the inferior vena cava, which reduces venous return to the heart. In the third trimester about two-thirds of the additional cardiac output is distributed to the placental circulation and to augment renal plasma flow. The increased output results from both a greater stroke volume and a higher pulse rate. Plasma volume increases progressively during the second and third trimesters and is significantly correlated with the birthweight of the conceptus. Arterial pressure falls in the second half of the first trimester while the cardiac output is increasing because peripheral resistance decreases relatively more than the cardiac output increases. The uteroplacental circulation is too small at this time to cause these changes, which must therefore result from generalized arteriolar dilatation.

In the later weeks of pregnancy diastolic pressure tends to rise slowly towards what it was before pregnancy, the systolic pressure remaining more or less unchanged. However, in the supine

> **Box 14.4.1** Cardiovascular changes in pregnancy
>
> ◆ Increased cardiac output
> ◆ Increased plasma volume
> ◆ Increase heart rate
> ◆ Increased stroke volume
> ◆ Reduced arterial pressure, (mainly in second trimester)
> ◆ Reduced peripheral resistance

position, with venocaval compression and reduced venous return, the arterial pressure may be atypically low with a narrowed pulse pressure and reflex vasoconstriction. This fall in systolic pressure may exceed 30% in 10% of cases and cause the 'supine hypotension syndrome'—evident as restlessness, faintness, breathlessness, and pallor.

Hypertension in pregnancy: definition, causes, and terminology

Causes and terminology

Hypertension in obstetric practice is conventionally recognized at or above an arbitrary threshold of 140/90. In the second half of pregnancy about one-quarter of all women will be, at least transiently, hypertensive by this criterion. About 2.5% have a maximum arterial pressure of 160/105 or more and about 1% of 170/110 or more.

Pregnancy-induced hypertension (PIH), transient hypertension of pregnancy, or gestational hypertension are terms used to describe new hypertension that appears after mid term (20 weeks) and resolves after delivery (Box 14.4.2). This is one of the components of pre-eclampsia, which is a syndrome comprising PIH and pregnancy-induced proteinuria. Pre-eclampsia (previously called pre-eclamptic toxaemia, PET) is so called because it may precede eclampsia, which is one of a number of possible crises of the condition. Eclampsia is characterized by grand-mal convulsions, but other crises (described below) may be as dangerous and occur more commonly. Not all cases of eclampsia are preceded by a prodromal illness of pre-eclampsia, so the terminology is simplistic. Toxaemia is an obsolete expression, previously used to describe

> **Box 14.4.2** Terminology
>
> ◆ Pregnancy-induced hypertension (PIH), also gestational hypertension: new hypertension after 20 weeks, regressing after delivery
> ◆ Pre-eclampsia (pre-eclamptic toxaemia or PET): a multisystem syndrome, defined by the presence of PIH combined with pregnancy-induced proteinuria, regressing after delivery
> ◆ Superimposed pre-eclampsia: pre-eclampsia occurring in association with chronic hypertension or renal disease or both.
> ◆ Eclampsia: Grand-mal convulsions associated with pre-eclampsia. The risk of convulsions quickly recedes after delivery

any hypertension or proteinuria in pregnancy, whether pregnancy-induced or not.

PIH on its own (a relatively common clinical presentation) is not pre-eclampsia; at least one more sign is required. The clusters of clinical features that comprise any syndrome are chosen for convenience; they describe outward appearances and embody no special truth about the underlying disease or diseases. When a syndrome such as pre-eclampsia is 'defined', rules are set that bring consistency to what is being discussed. The validity of the rules cannot be tested because there is no standard to which to refer. All the definitions of pre-eclampsia suffer from these limitations and none can be said to be the best. The conventional components of the cluster are PIH combined with new proteinuria that regress after delivery.

Almost all hypertension presenting before mid term (gestational age of 20 weeks) indicates pre-existing or chronic hypertension; the exceptions are women with rare very early-onset pre-eclampsia. However, normotension in the first half of pregnancy does not necessarily mean long-term normotension because the fall in blood pressure induced in early pregnancy may be exaggerated in some women. Many with relatively severe hypertension may have normal blood pressures by 12 weeks, without treatment; in one study as many as 60% of women with chronic hypertension defined before pregnancy were normotensive by the end of the first trimester. In other words, some women enjoy the benefits of pregnancy-induced normotension just as others suffer the disadvantages of PIH. Pregnancy-induced normotension tends to be lost in the third trimester. If the prepregnancy blood pressures are unknown then this may be misinterpreted as PIH rather than recognized for what it is, namely re-establishment of the normal, long-term blood pressure.

PIH thus represents at least two clinical situations: early pre-eclampsia or occult chronic hypertension. In many cases the signs of pre-eclampsia are not confirmed but nevertheless the blood pressure reverts to normal after delivery. It is possible that these are early unconfirmed stages of pre-eclampsia; an alternative is that an innate tendency to hypertension has been revealed in pregnancy but will become overt only many years later. The studies have not been done to confirm or refute this suggestion.

Pre-eclampsia

Pre-eclampsia becomes evident in the second half of pregnancy, during labour, or even—for the first time and without apparent preceding problems—in the immediate puerperium. It resolves after delivery. It is common, can be dangerous for both mother and baby, and of unknown cause. It has many signs that reflect widespread systemic disturbances, but few symptoms, which are suffered only late in its evolution. It is neither predictable nor preventable. The simple signs that are used for clinical screening are new hypertension and proteinuria, both regressing after delivery. The incidence of pre-eclampsia depends on how it is defined and how assiduously the signs are sought, but in the United Kingdom the incidence is of the order of 1 in 20 to 30 maternities.

Pre-eclampsia is primarily a placental problem. The presence of a placenta is necessary and sufficient to cause the disorder. A fetus is not required, as pre-eclampsia can occur with hydatidiform mole. A uterus is not required, as pre-eclampsia may develop with abdominal pregnancy (i.e. an ectopic pregnancy in the peritoneal cavity). Central to management is delivery, which removes the causative organ, namely the placenta.

Aetiology and pathogenesis of pre-eclampsia

The placental problem appears to be a relative insufficiency of the uteroplacental circulation. The clinical problem evolves in two stages: preclinical and clinical (Fig. 14.4.1). The first stage, in the first half of pregnancy, involves the development and expansion of the spiral end arteries supplying maternal blood to the placental intervillous space. With poor placentation, remodelling of the spiral arteries that normally occurs between weeks 6 and 18 (before there is clinical evidence of pre-eclampsia) is inadequate such that the arteries remain too small. This problem is later aggravated by obstructive lesions called 'acute atherosis', aggregates of fibrin, platelets, and lipid-loaded macrophages (foam cells) that partially or completely block the ends of the arteries. Neither change is specific to pre-eclampsia: they can also occur with intrauterine growth retardation without a maternal syndrome.

Once pre-eclampsia is established, uteroplacental blood flow is reduced. The ensuing damage from oxidative stress in the placenta, which may include tissue infarction, is thought to stimulate the vascular inflammatory response that characterizes women with pre-eclampsia. The second stage of pre-eclampsia includes all the features of the maternal syndrome, short of decompensation. The maternal syndrome is variable, in its time of onset, speed of progression, and the extent to which it involves different systems including arterial, coagulation, renal, central nervous, and hepatic.

The maternal endothelium is the primary target for pre-eclampsia. Diffuse endothelial dysfunction causes widespread circulatory disturbances in different organ systems as well as generalized arterial and coagulation abnormalities. In short, pre-eclampsia is more than a hypertensive problem. Endothelial dysfunction is associated with increased levels of anti-endothelial factors produced in excess by the oxidatively stressed placenta, namely the soluble vascular endothelial receptor 1 (sFlt-1) and soluble endoglin. Experimental rats, exposed to these factors separately, develop features of pre-eclampsia, and together the factors synergize in their effects in the best current experimental animal model of pre-eclampsia.

Recently it has been shown that the endothelial dysfunction is one facet of a broader dysfunction of a systemic maternal inflammatory response that affects circulating leukocytes and other components of the inflammatory system (e.g. the clotting system). Moreover, in comparison to nonpregnant women, women in the third trimester of normal pregnancy also display an increased inflammatory response, which is not different from that in pre-eclampsia except that it is milder. It seems that pre-eclampsia develops when a pregnancy-induced systemic inflammatory response causes one or other maternal system to decompensate. In other words, the disorder is not a separate condition but simply the extreme end of a continuum of maternal systemic inflammatory responses engendered by pregnancy itself. This concept has profound implications for clinical practice. If true, it is unlikely that there ever will be a single cause, single diagnostic test, or single preventive measure for pre-eclampsia.

Under certain circumstances the secondary disturbances of pre-eclampsia can become so severe that they cause decompensation or crises (Box 14.4.3), which is what makes the condition dangerous for the mother or baby.

Clinical characteristics of pre-eclampsia (Box 14.4.4)

The only consistent feature of pre-eclampsia is its inconsistency. Usually hypertension precedes proteinuria, although the converse can happen. It may fulminate suddenly or take weeks to evolve. Although pre-eclampsia is defined as presenting after 20 weeks, it may occur earlier or, at the other extreme, become evident only after delivery.

The hypertension of pre-eclampsia appears to be caused by an increased peripheral resistance secondary to generalized maternal endothelial dysfunction. There is not a single haemodynamic pattern. The blood pressure is typically unstable at rest, possibly owing to reduced baroceptor sensitivity. Circadian variation is altered with an initial loss of the normal fall in blood pressure at night then, in the worst cases, a reversed pattern with the highest readings during sleep. Since the disorder originates in the placenta, pre-eclampsia is a form of secondary hypertension, probably the most common in clinical practice.

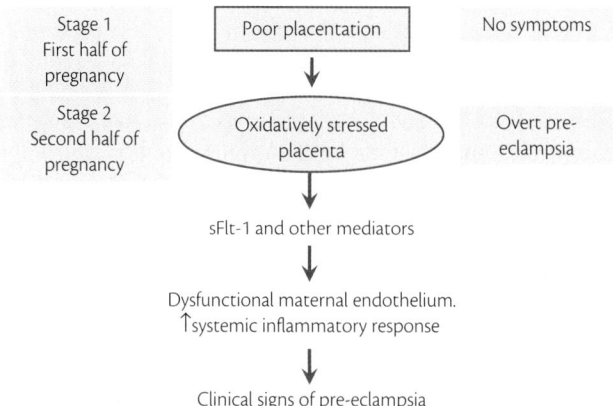

Fig. 14.4.1 The two stages of pre-eclampsia. The oxidatively stressed placenta is a source of of antiangiogenic factors such as sFlt-1 which is a soluble vascular endothelial growth factor receptor.

Box 14.4.3 Crises of pre-eclampsia

Maternal

+ Eclampsia
+ HELLP syndrome
+ Cerebral haemorrhage
+ Cortical blindness
+ Acute renal cortical necrosis
+ Acute renal tubular necrosis
+ Pulmonary oedema
+ Laryngeal oedema
+ Adult respiratory disress syndrome
+ Disseminated intravascular coagulation
+ Hepatic infarction
+ Hepatic rupture

Fetal (placental)

+ Intrauterine asphyxia
+ Intrauterine death
+ Placental abruption

Box 14.4.4 Possible features of pre-eclampsia

- PIH
- Generalized oedema and excessive weight gain (>1.0 kg/ week)
- Haemoconcentration and increased haematocrit
- Disturbances of renal function
  - Hyperuricaemia
  - Proteinuria
  - Raised plasma creatinine, reduced creatinine clearance
  - Hypocalciuria
- Increased circulating markers of endothelial dysfunction
  - Von Willebrand factor
  - Cellular fibronectin
- Excessive activation of the clotting system
  - Reduced plasma concentration of antithrombin III
  - Thrombocytopenia
  - Increased circulating D-dimer
- Increased plasma liver enzymes
  - Raised AST, ALT

Pre-eclampsia may cause arterial pressures that are well above the level (i.e. a mean pressure of *c.*140 mmHg) at which arterial and arteriolar damage would be expected. It is therefore not surprising that an important cause of maternal death from pre-eclampsia and eclampsia is cerebral haemorrhage, the pathology of which is similar to that seen in other hypertensive states. As far as it is known, cerebral haemorrhage is the only consequence of pre-eclampsia likely to be affected by antihypertensive treatment.

Renal involvement gives the defining feature of proteinuria. This usually develops after the onset of hypertension although in 10% of cases it is detected first. The proteinuria is moderately selective, increases until delivery and can exceed 10 g/24 h—pre-eclampsia being the commonest cause of nephrotic syndrome in pregnancy. It is associated with impaired glomerular perfusion and filtration, reflected in increased plasma creatinine and urea concentrations and reduced creatinine clearance. The typical and unique renal glomerular lesion of pre-eclampsia is glomerular endotheliosis: the endothelial cells of the glomeruli swell and block the capillary lumina so that the glomeruli appear enlarged and bloodless. Despite the specificity of the glomerular histology, renal biopsy is never indicated before delivery for clinical management (and after delivery the indications are the same as in general nephrological practice). Hyperuricaemia resulting from a reduced renal urate clearance is often an early feature of pre-eclampsia, preceding proteinuria and useful for diagnosis at that stage, but it is not consistently present so that its absence does not exclude the condition. It is associated with hypocalciuria, another early change in renal function. As the plasma urate rises, the plasma concentrations of urea and creatinine at first remain steady, tending to increase slowly after proteinuria has become established. The tertiary pathology of renal involvement in

pre-eclampsia is acute renal failure arising from either tubular or cortical necrosis.

Generalized oedema is an inconsistent feature. It may develop suddenly and be associated with accelerated weight gain. Ascites is not uncommon with severe disease. Laryngeal oedema can cause respiratory obstruction and difficulties with intubation when general anaesthesia is administered. Pulmonary oedema is a dangerous complication that in association with modern methods of ventilatory support may progress to the adult respiratory distress syndrome, which can cause maternal death.

The clotting system is often, but not invariably, disturbed in pre-eclampsia with accelerated intravascular generation of thrombin and parallel reductions in the platelet count ascribed to increased consumption. The time course is variable, but a fall in the platelet count may be a relatively early sign—antedating proteinuria, for example. However, even when eclampsia supervenes, most women have normal platelet counts at the time of presentation. The coagulation disturbances may decompensate to give overt disseminated intravascular coagulation (DIC), and a further complication is microangiopathic haemolysis that may cause a sudden drop in haemoglobin associated with haemoglobinuria, fragmented or distorted red cells (schistocytes) on the peripheral blood film, and reduced serum haptoglobin concentrations.

The severe clotting abnormalities of pre-eclampsia, particularly DIC, are usually associated with liver pathology. The acronym 'HELLP syndrome' has been used to label the concurrence of haemolysis, elevated liver enzymes, and low platelet counts, which is often not associated with marked hypertension or other conventional indices of severe pre-eclampsia (see Chapter 14.9).

Definition and diagnosis

The clusters of clinical features that comprise any syndrome are chosen for convenience. When a syndrome such as pre-eclampsia is 'defined', rules are set that bring consistency to what is being discussed. The validity of the rules cannot be tested, because there is no standard to which to refer. All definitions of pre-eclampsia suffer from these limitations and none can be said to be the best. A pragmatic approach has led to the suggestion of two definitions (Box 14.4.5): one for research and the other for clinical work. The former is stricter and enables researchers to ensure that they are dealing with comparable groups; the latter is wider and designed to guide clinicians in troublesome presentations that lead to morbidity but do not necessarily fit neat diagnostic categories. The advantage of the broad definition is that it includes the fetal syndrome of pre-eclampsia, which is secondary to placental disease, and other rarer variants are also encompassed. It is really an aid to alert the clinician to think about pre-eclampsia-like processes in appropriate contexts, but it may not be clear at the time how much of the problem is pregnancy induced, hence in the strict sense it is more a clinical alert signal than a definition. In terms of the broad definition hypertension is not required as a defining feature of pre-eclampsia, but considered to be one of several useful signs.

Pre-eclampsia is usually symptomless, hence its detection depends on signs or investigations. However, one symptom is crucially important because it is often misinterpreted. The epigastric pain, which reflects hepatic involvement and is typical of the HELLP syndrome, may be confused with heartburn, a very common problem of pregnancy. However, the abdominal pain of pre-eclampsia is not burning in quality, does not spread upwards towards the throat, is associated with hepatic tenderness, may radiate through to the back, and is not relieved by giving antacids. It is often very severe—described by sufferers as the worst pain that they have ever experienced. Affected women are not uncommonly referred to general surgeons as suffering from an acute abdomen with a working diagnosis of acute cholecystitis (or similar).

None of the signs of pre-eclampsia is specific; even convulsions in pregnancy are more likely to have causes other than eclampsia in modern practice. Diagnosis therefore depends on finding a coincidence of several pre-eclamptic features, the final proof being their regression after delivery. To make the diagnosis it is necessary to recognize the wide range of possible features, when they occur together, which are encompassed in the broad definition (Box 14.4.5). As with all syndromes, the more of the features that are clustered together the more certain is the diagnosis, but the absence of any one feature does not exclude the diagnosis. For example, eclampsia can occur without proteinuria, and even hypertension seems not to be an essential component.

In practical terms hypertension and proteinuria have to be the signs of interest for screening in routine antenatal clinics. Different definitions have been proposed as to what constitutes hypertension, the details being less important than the principle of an increment from an early baseline. Between weeks 20 and 30 the blood pressure is normally steady, so that even a small consistent rise is clinically important. Between week 30 and term the diastolic will normally rise by about 10 mmHg. In general the requirement

that the diastolic reaches at least 90 mmHg is more useful than using lower thresholds, but these are only guidelines; there is no clinical situation where rigid interpretation of the blood pressure is helpful.

The same applies to other measurements such as changes in the plasma urate. As a rough guide abnormal levels are in excess of 0.30, 0.35, 0.40, and 0.45 mmol/litre at 28, 32, 36, and 40 weeks respectively. Proteinuria and evidence of a reduced glomerular filtration rate are later signs. The changes in the measurements of renal function are usually within the normal range for nonpregnant women. In general concentrations of plasma creatinine and urea above 100 μmol/litre and 6.0 mmol/litre respectively are abnormal. The proteinuria of pre-eclampsia ranges from 0.5 to 15 g/24 h, depending on the individual case and the stage of evolution of the disorder. In terms of stick testing, 0.5 g/24 h corresponds to at least + in every specimen of urine tested: when this point is reached the disease, can be said to have entered its proteinuric phase.

Thrombocytopenia ($<100 \times 10^9$/litre) and increased plasma fibrin/fibrinogen degradation products (or specific fragments thereof such as the D-dimer) tend to develop late, if at all. The same is true for raised liver enzymes, and in regard to the latter it should be noted that measurement of plasma alkaline phosphatase is not a useful guide to hepatic disease because is always elevated in late pregnancy by the contribution from the placental isoenzyme. Serum bilirubin is rarely abnormal except in the context of haemolysis. γ-Glutamyl transferase is increased only late in the evolution of the HELLP syndrome. Therefore the best simple tests are plasma aspartate aminotransferase (AST) or alanine aminotransferase (ALT).

New hypertension and the de novo occurrence of one other sign allow the diagnosis to be made with reasonable certainty. PIH on its own is not pre-eclampsia although the term is commonly, but wrongly, used to mean mild or early pre-eclampsia. It is true that PIH maybe the first indication of the onset of pre-eclampsia, but this remains unconfirmed unless other signs appear. Often spontaneous or induced delivery prevents further developments so that a final certain diagnosis cannot be made.

Superimposed pre-eclampsia

Certain medical problems, including some (chronic hypertension, renal disease) that can mimic the disorder, also predispose to it. Superimposed pre-eclampsia refers to a mixed syndrome comprising pre-eclampsia in an individual with pre-existing hypertension or renal disease. In the absence of a specific diagnostic test for pre-eclampsia it can be difficult or impossible to disentangle what elements of proteinuric hypertension are caused by a chronic medical problem from those arising from superimposed pre-eclampsia. The conventional definitions of pre-eclampsia cease to apply. If a woman is permanently proteinuric there are, for example, no accepted criteria for diagnosing 'proteinuric pre-eclampsia'. There is no substitute for clinical experience in such situations.

Risk factors for pre-eclampsia

Risk factors include fetal-specific as well as maternal-specific components (Table 14.4.1). Primigravidae are several times more prone to the condition. In parous women, pre-eclampsia particularly affects those who have had the problem before. The predisposition to pre-eclampsia is, in part, familial or genetic, but the pattern of inheritance is not clear. Other factors must also be relevant, because pre-eclampsia does not affect identical twin sisters concordantly.

Table 14.4.1 Risk factors for pre-eclampsia

Maternal	Fetal
Primigravidity	Advancing gestational age
Primipaternity[a]	Multiple pregnancy
Increasing maternal age	Hydatidiform mole
Previous pre-eclampsia	Triploidy
Obesity (syndrome X, polycystic ovarian syndrome)	Trisomy 13
Medical disorders	Trisomy 16 mosaic
Diabetes	Placental hydrops
Chronic hypertension	
Chronic renal disease	
Thrombophilia and antiphosphopholipid antibody syndromes	
Migraines	
Asthma	
Family history of pre-eclampsia	
Stressful job	

[a] There is partner specificity also, hence it is not simply the first pregnancy that is important but the first by the current partner.

Chronically hypertensive women are three to seven times more likely to develop higher blood pressures and proteinuria ('superimposed pre-eclampsia') than normotensive women. Women with hypertension associated with chronic renal disease are particularly susceptible. Assessment of risk is an important part of antenatal care because pre-eclampsia is both symptomless and unpredictable. Hence 'high risk' women will be screened more often than low risk women after 20 weeks. It is important to recognize that primiparae are not the lowest risk: a first pregnancy itself bestows a substantial added risk.

Prevention of pre-eclampsia

Once pre-eclampsia becomes overt it cannot be reversed except by delivery. Reliable methods of primary prevention are therefore needed, although none that is completely effective is known. If the concepts of pathogenesis are correct it is unlikely that any single measure will be effective for all women, but specific measures of reducing the susceptibilities among subgroups of women may be identified (Table 14.4.2).

Table 14.4.2 Preventive measures for pre-eclampsia

Ineffective	May be effective for at least some women
Weight restriction	Low dose aspirin, other antiplatelet agents
Salt restriction	Calcium supplements
Diuretics	
Antihypertensive agents	
Fish oil	
Antioxidant vitamins (vitamins C and E)	

There is no evidence that blood pressure control attenuates the progression of early pre-eclampsia, or that it prevents superimposition of pre-eclampsia in chronically hypertensive women who are otherwise more susceptible to the disorder. The only clear advantage of antihypertensive treatment is where the hypertension is so severe that delivery is essential to preserve maternal safety. At early gestational ages antihypertensive treatment can allow prolongation of pregnancy in this context. The benefit is not from prevention but palliation, but the extent of the presumed benefit has not been measured because severe hypertension is a reason for exclusion from randomized trials of treatment. Hence in all contexts antihypertensive treatment helps to protect the mother from the consequences of her problem, not from the problem itself.

Trials of antiplatelet agents, in particular low doses of aspirin, have given mixed results. Meta-analyses confirm that they are safe and reduce the incidence of pre-eclampsia by about 10% and significantly reduce perinatal mortality. There is good evidence that the prophylactic use of antioxidant vitamins C and E does not help to prevent the condition when started in mid gestation in selected groups of women at risk.

Management of pre-eclampsia

The rationale for antihypertensive treatment

Since pre-eclamptic hypertension is secondary, control of the blood pressure is only part of patient management. The definitive treatment is always delivery, which removes the cause of the problem (the placenta). If delivery is expedited before there is irreversible maternal damage (such as cerebral haemorrhage) complete recovery is assured, hence the purpose of medical management is to protect the mother from the dangers of her illness during the relatively brief interval between onset of the disease and planned delivery. The criterion for antihypertensive treatment to prevent long-term degenerative arterial disease in middle aged and elderly people cannot be transposed to the specialized context of pregnancy, where the main objective is to prevent extreme hypertension. The threshold at which antihypertensive treatment should be started is a matter of opinion. A conservative criterion is to prevent maximum readings (systolic or diastolic) repeatedly reaching or exceeding 160 or 110 mmHg, respectively: lower thresholds are used in many centres, and some emphasize systolic more than diastolic readings.

Treatment with antihypertensive agents

The evidence on which drug selection is based is incomplete. Under these circumstances the skill and experience of the prescribing physician is more important than the precise medication that is selected. The choice of drugs is dictated by considerations of fetal safety (Table 14.4.3).

For many years methyldopa has been the preferred agent because its fetal effects have been defined more clearly than those of other agents. In adequate doses, typically a loading dose of 500–1000 mg followed by 250–500 mg two to four times a day, it can control the blood pressure within 6 to 12 h. However, its side effect profile is problematic. Sedation is the rule for the first 48 h and tiredness thereafter is common, and many patients simply say they feel awful on the drug, which has led to increased use of other agents, in particular labetolol and nifedipine. Postural hypotension is rarely a problem in antenatal patients.

Labetalol, a combined α- and β-adrenergic blocking agent, is given orally in doses rising from 100 mg twice daily to 400 mg

Table 14.4.3 Antihypertensive drugs in pregnancy

Trimester	Drugs to avoid		Possible agents
	Relatively contraindicated	Absolutely contraindicated	
First	–	ACE inhibitors	Methyldopa
		A-II receptor inhibitors	Labetalol
Second	β-Blockers	ACE inhibitors	Methyldopa
	Diuretics	A-II receptor inhibitors	Clonidine
			Prazosin
			Doxazosin
			Nifedipine
Third	Diuretics	ACE inhibitors	Methyldopa
		A-II receptor inhibitors	Clonidine
			Prazosin
			Doxazosin
			Nifedipine
			β-Blockers

three times a day. It also has the advantage that it can be given intravenously if the patient cannot take and absorb oral medication. In this circumstance it lowers the blood pressure smoothly but rapidly, without the tachycardia caused by hydralazine or other vasodilators. A typical intravenous regimen starts with 20 mg/h, which is doubled every 30 min until control has been gained, but there are no adequate trials of its parenteral use in pregnancy to show how it might affect perinatal outcome.

The calcium channel blocking agent nifedipine appears to be safe and is an effective vasodilator that acts rapidly when given by mouth. The modified-release tablets begin to act about 60 min after administration and may be repeated three or four times a day if necessary. Long acting, slow-release preparations, formulated for once a day administration, are inappropriate for acute blood pressure control. The commonest and most distressing side effect is headache. In theory, nifedipine could interact with parenteral magnesium sulphate given to prevent or treat eclampsia because the magnesium ion inhibits calcium channels, but in practice this is not a problem. Note that sublingual nifedipine should not be given: it can cause dangerously acute hypotension.

Common practice in many centres will be to initiate treatment with either labetolol or nifedipine if blood pressure exceeds threshold values, increasing the dose and then adding in the other agent if required, with methyldopa held in reserve, although many experienced obstetric physicians will prefer the more traditional approach that begins with methyldopa.

Antihypertensive agents to be avoided, or used only with great care

Diuretics are avoided because they exacerbate the hypovolaemia of pre-eclampsia, which may often be severe, but they are indicated if complications such as pulmonary or laryngeal oedema occur. Sodium nitroprusside and nitroglycerine are rapidly acting vasodilators that have been used to manage hypertensive emergencies in pregnancy: both should be reserved for use by specialists, usually in the context of intensive cardiovascular monitoring, their main danger being problems caused by extreme hypotension.

β-Blockers other than labetolol are safe for short-term use but have been associated with significant fetal growth retardation if administered throughout the second and third trimesters and should be avoided at this time. Angiotensin converting enzyme inhibitors (ACE inhibitors) and the related angiotensin II receptor inhibitors are contraindicated throughout pregnancy.

The effect of blood pressure control

Good blood pressure control in pre-eclampsia does not ameliorate its other features. The disease persists and progresses relentlessly until delivery, and escape from control is common. Adequate treatment does not prevent other complications such as eclampsia, the HELLP syndrome, abruption, or progressive fetal problems secondary to placental insufficiency. A persisting inability to control maternal arterial pressure is an indication for immediate delivery.

Recent evidence suggests that long-term lowering of the blood pressure has a modest but statistically significant effect in reducing the baby's birthweight. Whether this has any long-term implications is not known, but it is a good reason for using antihypertensive agents parsimoniously, only where there is clear evidence of a maternal risk.

Prevention of eclamptic convulsions.

Eclampsia is probably caused by focal cerebral vasoconstriction and ischaemia secondary to endothelial damage and therefore is neither the result of hypertension nor prevented by antihypertensive treatment. The best mode of prevention is well-timed delivery. It is debated whether anticonvulsant prophylaxis needs to be offered routinely in all cases of advanced pre-eclampsia and, if so, what it should be. To prevent convulsions either starting for the first time or recurring in a high risk situation, magnesium sulphate is superior to other anticonvulsants, but in developed countries with high-level antenatal care nearly 400 pre-eclamptic women need to be treated to prevent a first onset of eclampsia, and efficacy is not proved without doubt. Its use is appropriate only in the context of immediate delivery and its aftermath. However, two very high-risk groups for eclampsia comprise women who have had one eclamptic convulsion and those with the HELLP syndrome, of whom about 4% have eclamptic convulsions: these women certainly merit prophylaxis with magnesium sulphate (4–6 g, infused intravenously over 20 min, followed by maintainance 1 g/h, aiming for a therapeutic level of 4–7 mEq/l). Intravenous lorazepam (4 mg by slow intravenous injection) is available to stop eclamptic convulsions, although most are self-limiting.

Critical care

Obstetric patients comprise about 1% of all admissions for intensive care, and pre-eclampsia is the commonest problem. Pre-eclamptic women are admitted because of eclampsia, intracerebral haemorrhage, pulmonary oedema, renal insufficiency, liver failure or rupture, or placental abruption. The commonly used scoring systems (APACHE II, ASAPS II) for grading severity of admissions to intensive care units tend to overestimate mortality and do not account for variables reflecting liver damage or DIC, which are important for the outcome of pre-eclampsia.

Eclampsia

Eclampsia is the most dramatic evidence of involvement of the nervous system (Box 14.4.6). It presents before, during, or after delivery. Antepartum eclampsia is likely to occur earlier in gestation and is more dangerous than that presenting in labour or after delivery. Most postpartum crises develop in the first 12 h after delivery, but later occurrences (up to 22 days) are possible. Ten per cent of cases of eclampsia are totally unheralded, i.e. without a warning prodrome of hypertension and proteinuria.

Average blood pressures in eclampsia are high (170–195/110–120 mm Hg), but cases with much lower or normal blood pressures are not rare. Eclampsia is not associated with gross papilloedema or retinopathy. Although much clinical attention is naturally focused on the blood pressure, there is no good evidence that hypertension causes eclampsia and none that adequate medical control of the blood pressure prevents the condition. It is now generally agreed that eclampsia results from acute cerebral circulatory disturbances secondary to endothelial dysfunction. Cerebral vasospasm with focal ischaemia and oedema are major features that have been demonstrated by MRI and CT scanning. Eclampsia is one of the causes of 'reversible posterior leukoencephalopathy syndrome' or 'posterior leukoencephalopathy'. These terms refer to the appearance in imaging studies of areas of signal abnormality in the posterior regions of the cerebral hemispheres combined with headaches, vomiting, confusion, seizures, cortical blindness or other visual abnormalities, and motor signs. The terminology is misleading because the lesions are not necessarily confined to the posterior hemispheres; nor are they always reversible or restricted to the white matter.

Chronic hypertension complicating pregnancy

Pregnant women with chronic hypertension tend to be older, fatter, and slightly taller. Frequently they have clear family histories of hypertension. Owing to the physiological changes of pregnancy their hypertension may be ameliorated or masked by the beginning of the second trimester, so that the diagnosis is missed unless prepregnancy blood pressure readings are available. As explained above, the blood pressure tends to revert to the levels that characterize the nonpregnant state towards the end of the third trimester. If these are high, this normal change can be misinterpreted as pre-eclampsia or PIH. The difference is that the blood pressure fails to settle after delivery.

Pre-eclampsia superimposed on chronic hypertension tends to be more severe, to occur at earlier stages of pregnancy, to cause more fetal growth retardation, and to be recurrent in later pregnancies. Pre-eclampsia occurring in normotensive women tends not to recur. If a blood pressure of 140/90 mmHg in the first half of pregnancy is taken as evidence of chronic hypertension, then the affected woman has an approximately fivefold increased risk of later pre-eclampsia compared to normotensive women. This close link between the two conditions led earlier clinicians to conclude that chronic hypertension is itself extremely dangerous in pregnancy. In fact the risks are almost entirely attributable to the increased chance of developing superimposed pre-eclampsia. Most chronically hypertensive women who do not get pre-eclampsia can expect normal pregnancies.

Chronic hypertension can only be diagnosed with certainty during pregnancy on the basis of readings taken in the first half, preferably before 16 weeks of gestation. Without the benefit of such readings, hypertension in the second half of pregnancy cannot be interpreted because the possibility that it may represent pre-eclampsia cannot be excluded. The signs of pre-eclampsia in chronically hypertensive women are the same as in other women, except that the blood pressure increases from a higher baseline. There may be progressive hyperuricaemia, abnormal activation of the clotting system, or new proteinuria.

Treatment of chronic hypertension in pregnancy

If antihypertensive treatment has been started before conception, the patient may seek advice about the possible effects of her medication on the growth and development of her fetus. Of the commonly used antihypertensive drugs only ACE inhibitors and the related angiotensin II receptor inhibitors are teratogenic, and ACE inhibitors are also fetotoxic (causing growth restriction, oligohydramnios, intrauterine, and postnatal renal failure in the second and third trimester). But this does not preclude the possibility of subtle problems which are as yet unknown, and for this reason it is appropriate that women with no more than moderate hypertension stop treatment before conception. By the 12th week of pregnancy the normal fall in blood pressure is such that treatment may no longer be needed, at least until the beginning of the third trimester. In the unlikely event that diuretics are essential for good blood pressure control they can be continued throughout pregnancy, but their use carries disadvantages if pre-eclampsia supervenes, as already discussed.

If chronic hypertension is diagnosed for the first time in pregnancy, it is necessary to treat only those in whom it presents an immediate (as opposed to a long-term) hazard to the woman. It needs to be re-emphasized that the indications for antihypertensive treatment in general medical practice are to prevent long-term complications such as coronary and cerebral vascular disease, which are not relevant concerns for the brief period of pregnancy. Thus moderate hypertension *per se* carries no intrinsic maternal risk over the short time of 9 months, except insofar as it may be the precursor of more severe hypertension. It is true that the higher the arterial pressure, the greater is the eventual perinatal mortality. Among this group are those in whom the mild hypertension indicates early pre-eclampsia, in which case the risks evolve through simple progression. But if the mild hypertension indicates a pre-existing problem then the risk is of later superimposition of pre-eclampsia which is, as stated above, several times more likely in chronically hypertensive women. Antihypertensive treatment would only be useful if either it halts the progression of mild

---

Box 14.4.6 Eclampsia

- Rare: 1/2000 of all pregnancies
- Characterized by grand-mal convulsions, PIH, and new proteinuria
- May occur before during or after labour
- May be heralded by signs of pre-eclampsia or unheralded
- Maternal mortality 1/50

pre-eclampsia or prevents the superimposition of pre-eclampsia in women with long-term hypertension, but there is no evidence for either possibility, indeed there is good evidence that control of moderate long-term hypertension does not prevent superimposed pre-eclampsia but does cause mild fetal growth retention. Thus there are neither clear fetal nor maternal indications for treating moderate hypertension in pregnancy.

Secondary hypertension (Box 14.4.7)

Women with secondary hypertension in pregnancy are rare but important to detect (Box 14.4.7)

Phaechromocytoma is a very rare but dangerous disease in pregnancy. Maternal mortality is higher if it is not diagnosed before the peripartum period. Presentation is variable but includes extreme hypertension, severe pre-eclampsia, cardiomyopathy with heart failure, cardiovascular collapse, or diabetes mellitus. Diagnosis depends primarily on the appropriate level of clinical suspicion and investigations as are used in nonpregnant patients, including biochemical measures of catecholamine secretion and examination of the adrenals by MRI or CT. If the condition is identified and treated before delivery the maternal mortality is reduced, especially if α-adrenergic blockade has been used. Treatment with α-adrenergic blockade with or without addition of β-adrenergic blockade is compatible with normal fetal survival. Given adequate medical treatment, tumour resection (preferably laparoscopically) can be successfully accomplished early in pregnancy, at delivery or at a later elective date. Both malignant and ectopic tumours have been reported in pregnancy.

Coarctation of the aorta may present for the first time in pregnancy, and patients with previous surgical correction may become pregnant. A previous successful resection is not a contraindication to undertaking pregnancy, but consideration of the possible long-term complications following repair need to be borne in mind. These include recurrent hypertension, recoarctation, repair site aneurysms, and aortic root problems, which are best reassessed before pregnancy. However, the advisability of a pregnancy in a woman with a coarctation frequently depends more on related factors such as associated cardiac malformation than on the presence of the coarctation itself. Surgical resection during pregnancy is not advisable, but has been reported.

Cushing's syndrome is associated with amenorrhoea and therefore rarely seen in pregnancy. It usually presents in pregnant women with hypertension, often associated with diabetes and other clinical features discussed elsewhere. Diagnosis should take account of the increased urinary free cortisol of normal pregnancy associated with some blunting of its diurnal variation. Suppression of cortisol production by dexamethasone is the appropriate diagnostic test, although normally this is less complete than in

Table 14.4.4 Antihypertensive drugs and breastfeeding

Drug	Secretion in breast milk
Methyldopa	Minimal secretion; too small to be harmful
Labetalol	Secreted in breast milk in small amounts
Atenolol	Secreted in breast milk in small amounts
Nifedipine	Secreted in breast milk
ACE inhibitors	Secreted in breast milk but in small amounts that are unlikely to be harmful

nonpregnant women. There is a relatively high incidence of primary adrenal tumours, including carcinoma in rare instances. For these reasons surgical exploration and removal should be considered once the diagnosis is made.

Conn's syndrome is also rare in pregnancy. It has usually been diagnosed on the basis of hypokalaemia combined with hypertension. During pregnancy both plasma concentration and urinary excretion of aldosterone are increased, which makes diagnosis difficult. Remission of the disorder may occur during pregnancy, possibly due to progesterone antagonizing the renal action of aldosterone, which then reasserts its action postpartum. Successful pregnancies with and without medical treatment have been reported.

Renovascular hypertension in pregnancy may be due to stenosis, thrombosis, or embolism. The diagnosis needs to be considered when there is atypical severe hypertension. Renal ultrasonography may reveal one or two small kidneys. Renal artery magnetic resonance angiograms may be helpful and avoid the risks of irradiation of the fetus. Percutaneous renal artery angioplasty has been safely completed during pregnancy.

Hypertension in the puerperium

In relation to both chronic hypertension and pre-eclampsia the highest blood pressures are often recorded in the puerperium, typically peaking at about 5–7 days after delivery. Antihypertensive treatment has to be continued, in some women for 3–6 weeks or even longer after delivery. It is preferable to stop methyl dopa which causes depression and substitute other preparations which may include ACE inhibitors. There is no clear evidence that treatment interferes with breastfeeding (Table 14.4.4).

Long-term sequelae of hypertension in pregnancy

Women who have had pre-eclampsia have an increased risk in later life of sustained hypertension, ischaemic heart disease, and stroke. Although it is inappropriate to immediately place this burden of knowledge on women who already have had the troubled experience of pre-eclampsia, organization of low-key community follow-up is likely to be helpful.

Further reading

Altman D, et al. (2002). Do women with pre-eclampsia, and their babies, benefit from magnesium sulphate? The Magpie Trial: a randomised placebo-controlled trial. Lancet, **359**, 1877–90.

Higgins JR, De Swiet M (2001). Blood-pressure measurement and classification in pregnancy. Lancet, **357**, 131–5.

Box 14.4.7 Secondary hypertension in pregnancy

- Phaechromocytoma
- Cushing's syndrome
- Primary hyperaldosteronism (Conn's syndrome)
- Coarctation of the aorta
- Renovascular hypetension

Lain KY, Roberts JM (2002). Contemporary concepts of the pathogenesis and management of preeclampsia. *JAMA*, **287**, 3183–6.

Redman, CWG, Sargent IL (2004). Preeclampsia and the systemic inflammatory response. *Semin Nephrol*, **24**, 565–70.

Redman CWG, Sargent IL (2005). Latest advances in understanding preeclampsia. *Science*, **308**, 1592–4.

Sibai BM, *et al.* (1993). Maternal morbidity and mortality in 442 pregnancies with hemolysis, elevated liver enzymes, and low platelets (HELLP syndrome). *Am J Obstet Gynecol*, **169**, 1000–1006.

von Dadelzsen P, *et al.* (2000). Fall in mean arterial pressure and fetal growth restriction in pregnancy hypertension: a meta-analysis. *Lancet*, **355**, 87–92.

Renal disease in pregnancy

John D. Firth

Essentials

Renal complications that can occur during pregnancy

Urinary tract infection—2 to 10% of pregnancies are complicated by asymptomatic bacteriuria, which progresses to symptomatic infection in 40% of cases and is associated with adverse fetal outcome. Antibiotic treatment reduces the chances of developing symptomatic infection and of infants being born with low birth weight.

Acute kidney injury—causes of particular note in pregnancy include (1) haemolytic uraemic syndrome (HUS, idiopathic postpartum renal failure)—typically presents 1 day to several weeks after delivery with rising creatinine and microangiopathic haemolytic anaemia, often in association with cardiac failure and neurological dysfunction; treatment is with supportive care and infusion of fresh plasma or plasma exchange. (2) Obstetric acute renal failure—responsible for about 1% of cases of acute renal failure in the developed world, but up to 30% in some countries; often caused by septic abortions and/or poor perinatal care; may be due to acute cortical necrosis with risk of permanent renal failure.

Pregnancy in women with known renal disease

Immediate effects of pregnancy include increase in proteinuria (50% of cases), development of or deterioration in hypertension (25%), and marked worsening of oedema.

Outcome in relation to baseline GFR—(1) GFR normal or mildly reduced (serum creatinine <125 μmol/litre, eGFR >45; CKD stages 1, 2 and 3A)—pregnancy is most unlikely to be associated with permanent decline in renal function and there is a greater than 90% chance of a successful obstetric outcome. (2) GFR is moderately reduced (serum creatinine 125–250 μmol/litre, eGFR 20–45; CKD stages 3B and 4)—about 40% will have a rise in creatinine during pregnancy (instead of the usual fall), up to one-third will have a greater than expected irreversible decline in GFR, and around 10% will progress fairly rapidly to endstage renal failure. Preterm delivery will be required in 60% of pregnancies because of pre-eclampsia and/or intrauterine growth retardation, but overall there is an approximately 90% chance of a successful obstetric outcome as long as blood pressure is well controlled. (3) Serum creatinine >250 μmol/litre (eGFR <20; CKD stages 4 and 5)—women with such gross impairment of renal function are rarely fertile. Pregnancies are not common in women receiving dialysis treatment, but with intensive management (including haemodialysis six times per week) about 50% result in (premature) live births. Successful renal transplantation restores fertility.

Changes in the kidneys and urinary tract during normal pregnancy

Anatomical

The most obvious anatomical change in the urinary tract during pregnancy is dilatation of the calyces, renal pelvis, and ureter. Contrary to popular belief, the ureters are not floppy and toneless, indeed tone is increased, but urinary stasis within the ureters may nevertheless contribute to the risk of asymptomatic bacteriuria developing into acute pyelonephritis. Ureteric dilatation can persist for 3 or 4 months after pregnancy, and long term in about 10% of women who have had children. The kidney enlarges by about 1 cm in length during pregnancy.

Functional

Renal blood flow increases by 70 to 80% between conception and mid pregnancy, falling to a value 50 to 60% above the nonpregnant level during the third trimester. Between conception and 16 weeks of pregnancy the glomerular filtration rate increases about 50% above baseline and remains at this elevated level until delivery. Plasma creatinine decreases from a mean nonpregnant value of 73 μmol/litre to 65, 51, and 47 μmol/litre in successive trimesters.

Urinary excretion of glucose increases soon after conception and may rise 10-fold above nonpregnant values, hence glycosuria is common during pregnancy. This occurs because of decreased tubular reabsorption of glucose, the reason for which is not known. Glucose excretion returns to normal nonpregnant levels within a week of delivery.

Plasma uric acid concentration decreases by about 25% during normal pregnancy because of increased urinary excretion (the precise mechanism is unknown). In pregnancies complicated by preeclampsia or intrauterine growth retardation, the plasma uric acid concentration is higher than normal and serial measurements can be used to monitor progress. (See Chapter 14.4 for further discussion.)

The mean albumin excretion rate in pregnancy is 12 mg/day, with 29 mg/day the upper limit of normal (no different from that in the nonpregnant state). However, slightly increased urinary protein excretion is normal in pregnancy, such that proteinuria in pregnancy should not be considered abnormal until it exceeds 500 mg/day, which is over twice the upper limit of normal outside of pregnancy.

Renal complications that can occur in pregnancy

Urinary tract infection

Asymptomatic bacteriuria

The incidence of asymptomatic bacteriuria is 2 to 10% in pregnant and nonpregnant young women, but it is two to three times more common in pregnant diabetic women. It is associated with increased risks of pre-term birth, low birth weight, and perinatal mortality, and—if not treated—40% of women with asymptomatic bacteriuria will develop acute symptomatic infection during pregnancy, including many with acute pyelonephritis. A recent Cochrane review of 14 studies found that antibiotic treatment (compared to placebo or no treatment) is effective at clearing asymptomatic bacteriuria (risk ratio [RR] 0.25, 95% CI 0.14–0.48), reducing the risk of pyelonephritis (RR 0.23, 95% CI 0.13–0.41), and reducing the incidence of low birth weight (RR 0.66, 95% CI 0.49–0.89), but had no effect on the risk of preterm delivery.

Screening for asymptomatic bacteriuria should be performed at 12 to 16 weeks gestation or at the first prenatal visit (if later). If this is negative, then no further screening is required, excepting in women thought to be at high risk of infection, e.g. urinary tract abnormalities, preterm labour.

Escherichia coli is responsible for over 75% of cases of bacteriuria in pregnancy. If treatment is to be given, then the choice of drug should be determined by the sensitivity of the organism isolated. Amoxicillin and cephalosporins are safe in pregnancy, as is nitrofurantoin, except in the last few weeks (it can rarely produce neonatal haemolysis if used at term). Trimethoprim is contraindicated in the first trimester (folate antagonist) and quinolones should not be used at all in pregnancy (they cause arthropathy in animal studies). There is no good evidence to determine the first choice of antibiotic (pending culture results) or the duration of treatment. The United Kingdom Health Protection Agency guidelines recommend a 1-week course of antibiotic, but there is wide variability in practice as is common when high quality evidence is scarce: fosfomycin 3 g orally as a single dose has been shown to be effective, as have 3-day courses of a variety of antibiotics. Urinary culture should be performed 1 week after treatment is stopped and monthly thereafter until delivery. About 25% of patients will suffer recurrent infection and require a second course of treatment,

with 15% continuing to have positive cultures thereafter, for which suppressive therapy with a nocturnal dose of nitrofurantoin or cephalexin is recommended.

After delivery, most physicians would not pursue urinary/renal investigation of women with asymptomatic bacteriuria during pregnancy unless there were other reasons to do so.

Symptomatic infection

Acute cystitis affects about 1% of pregnant women. Treatment is as for asymptomatic bacteriuria, with the aim of abolishing symptoms and preventing acute pyelonephritis. A Cochrane review that included nine studies of antibiotic treatment of symptomatic urinary infection in pregnancy concluded that there were no significant differences between any of the treatments studied (excepting that cefuroxime was better than cephradine) and was unable to recommend any particular regimen.

Acute pyelonephritis presents with the same symptoms as it does in patients who are not pregnant, i.e. flank pain, nausea/vomiting, fever ($>38\,°C$), tenderness in the renal angle, with or without symptoms of cystitis (see Chapter 21.13), but the differential diagnosis in pregnancy includes uterine fibroid degeneration and placental abruption, and distinction from appendicitis can be particularly difficult. Complications include anaemia (23% of cases, mechanism not known), bacteraemia (17%), and respiratory failure due to adult respiratory distress syndrome (7%, higher in severe cases). Preterm labour occurs in about 4% of mild cases and 20% of severe cases. Treatment is usually with intravenous antibiotics (choice as determined by likely local resistance patterns, typically co-amoxiclav (amoxicillin–clavulanate) or a third-generation cephalosporin) in the first instance, switching to oral therapy after the patient has improved and been afebrile for 24 h, continuing to complete a 10- to 14-day course. Pyelonephritis recurs in 5 to 10% of women during pregnancy, hence it is important to continue close monitoring for evidence of recurrent urinary infection, with or without instigating prophylactic treatment with a bedtime dose of nitrofurantoin or cephalexin.

Causes of acute renal failure specific to pregnancy

Acute renal failure in pregnancy can be caused by any of the conditions that affect those who are not pregnant, but there are some causes of acute renal failure that are specific to pregnancy. The priorities in dealing with acute renal failure in a pregnant woman are no different from those that apply to any other patient: treatment of life-threatening complications, fluid resuscitation (if necessary), establishing a precise diagnosis, treatment of any underlying condition (if possible), and timely provision of renal replacement therapy (if indicated).

Acute renal failure with thrombotic microangiopathy

Acute renal failure associated with microangiopathic haemolytic anaemia and thrombocytopaenia in late pregnancy can be caused by thrombotic thrombocytopaenic purpura/haemolytic uraemic syndrome (TTP/HUS) or severe pre-eclampsia, the latter often in association with the HELLP (haemolysis associated with elevated liver enzymes and low platelets) syndrome.

TTP/HUS is a spectrum of disease, with presentations dominated by fever and neurological symptoms at one extreme (TTP) and with renal failure at the other (HUS). In the context of pregnancy TTP-like presentations are more likely to occur antepartum, and HUS-like presentations postpartum. The cause(s) is (are) unknown.

Regarding HUS-like presentations, these most typically occur one day to several weeks after delivery, leading to the term 'idiopathic postpartum renal failure'. Aside from oliguria (sometimes anuria), other manifestations include evidence of cardiac failure (pulmonary oedema, with clinical and imaging features of dilated cardiomyopathy) and neurological dysfunction (lethargy, convulsions, coma) that is out of proportion to the physiological and metabolic disturbance. Blood pressure can vary from low to very high. The blood film shows a microangiopathic haemolytic anaemia, sometimes with a consumptive coagulopathy in addition, although the latter is not typical and should lead to consideration of other diagnoses (e.g. placental abruption, hepatic rupture, or liver failure as a complication of pre-eclampsia). Renal biopsy is rarely performed because the risks are high and histological information is not likely to alter diagnosis or management in most cases, but changes in glomerular capillaries similar to those of HUS in the nonpregnant patient (see Chapter 21.10.5) and/or arteriolar changes similar to those seen in malignant hypertension or scleroderma are seen.

The main differential diagnosis, as stated above, is severe pre-eclampsia, which is much commoner than TTP/HUS, typically develops late in the third trimester (with only a few cases postpartum), and is usually preceded by the characteristic features of hypertension, proteinuria and oedema. Distinction of TTP/HUS from HELLP can be difficult: see Chapter 14.9 for further discussion.

In addition to supportive care, standard treatment of HUS in pregnancy or the puerperium is with infusion of fresh plasma or plasma exchange. In this rare condition there are no randomized controlled trials to justify this approach, but mortality was about 90% in series before the widespread use of these treatments, compared to around 20% in recent series. Renal function rarely, if ever, recovers completely, and many remain dependent on dialysis (see Chapter 20.10.5 for further discussion). Fetal mortality is high in cases developing antepartum.

Acute fatty liver of pregnancy

Acute fatty liver of pregnancy is a disease of the third trimester or puerperium in which there is jaundice and severe hepatic dysfunction. In early series the incidence of acute renal failure was over 50%, but this is now much reduced, both as a consequence of the recognition of milder cases and through improved management of severe cases, which require supportive care for disseminated intravascular coagulation and immediate delivery of the fetus. The explanation for acute renal failure is unknown but usually presumed to be 'haemodynamic'. Renal biopsy shows nonspecific changes. (See Chapter 14.9 for further discussion.)

Obstetric acute renal failure

In the developed world, the incidence of obstetric acute renal failure has fallen dramatically over the last 40 years. In Leeds (United Kingdom), obstetric causes accounted for 26% of cases of acute renal failure between 1956 and 1959, compared to 1.3% between 1980 and 1988. A significant fall, although not so dramatic, has also been seen in some parts of the developing world, where in Chandigarh (north India) obstetric causes were responsible for 25% of cases of acute renal failure 30 years ago, compared with less than 10% today. But this is not universal: studies from Argentina and Nigeria show that obstetric causes continued to account for 26 to 32% of cases of acute renal failure reported in series

Table 14.5.1 Some obstetric causes of acute renal failure

Pathogenesis	Clinical condition
Volume depletion + hypotension	Antepartum haemorrhage
	Postpartum haemorrhage
	Abortion
	Hyperemesis gravidarum
Volume depletion + hypotension + coagulopathy	Antepartum haemorrhage
	Pre-eclampsia/eclampsia
	Amniotic fluid embolism
	Acute fatty liver of pregnancy
	HELLP syndrome
	Haemolytic uraemic syndrome (idiopathic postpartum renal failure)
Volume depletion + hypotension + coagulopathy + infection	Septic abortion
	Chorioamnionitis
	Puerperal sepsis
	Pyelonephritis[a]
Urinary tract obstruction	Damage to ureters during caesarean section
	Haematoma in the pelvis

[a] Can cause acute renal failure outside of pregnancy, but pregnant women are at particular risk.

published in the 1990s. Where a decline in the incidence of obstetric acute renal failure has been seen, this is almost certainly attributable to improvements in perinatal care and a reduction in the numbers of septic abortions. Should acute renal failure develop in pregnancy or the puerperium, then obstetric causes listed in Table 14.5.1 should be considered in addition to the conditions that can present in any patient (see Chapter 21.5).

In most cases of acute renal failure in pregnancy the clinical progress of the condition is typical of acute tubular necrosis, with full recovery of renal function if the patient survives. However, for reasons that are not known, pregnant women are particularly susceptible to acute cortical necrosis, which is most often a complication of placental abruption. The incidence of this has fallen in the developed world, from 1 in 10 000 in the decade from 1960 to less than 1 in 80 000 pregnancies in the decade from 1970 in one large study, but it still carries the risk of permanent renal failure, although delayed and partial recovery is not uncommon. (See Chapter 21.5 for further discussion.)

Miscellaneous conditions

Acute hydroureter and hydronephrosis and the overdistension syndrome

The anatomical changes associated with pregnancy can very occasionally be exaggerated, with massive distension of the ureters and renal pelvis. This is usually asymptomatic, but can rarely have clinical consequences. The 'overdistension syndrome' varies from transient, mild loin pain to recurrent attacks of severe loin or lower abdominal pain radiating to the groin. Variation in symptoms with posture and position are typical. Urine specimens are sterile, but can show microscopic haematuria. Diagnosis is confirmed by ultrasonography. Nursing in the knee–chest position often provides relief, but very uncommonly nephrostomy and/or ureteral stenting are required.

Rupture of the urinary tract

The development of severe, persistent pain or haematuria in a pregnant patient with acute pyelonephritis or the overdistension syndrome suggests the very rare complication of rupture of the urinary tract. This can be retroperitoneal or intraperitoneal and is more likely to occur in those with pre-existing disease of the kidneys or urinary tract, perhaps because mild weaknesses are exposed by the physiological changes of pregnancy. Distinction from other obstetric or abdominal catastrophes can be very difficult.

Pregnancy in women with known renal disease

Women with renal disease who are considering pregnancy or who are already pregnant will often ask their physicians one or more of the following questions: 'Is pregnancy advisable?; Will pregnancy do me any harm?; Will pregnancy be straightforward?; Will the baby be normal and healthy?' It is never possible to give any woman a guarantee that pregnancy will be straightforward and culminate in a healthy normal baby, but based on the nature and severity of their renal disease it is possible to make a clear statement of risks for the woman to consider.

Effects of pregnancy on renal disease

The immediate effects of pregnancy in patients with renal disease include increase in proteinuria (50% of cases), development of or deterioration in hypertension (25%, with severe hypertension sometimes leading to maternal complications and poor fetal outcome), and marked worsening of oedema in those who are nephrotic. However, these changes usually resolve after delivery and most women contemplating pregnancy are willing to tolerate short-term problems, hence of much greater concern are possible long-term effects of pregnancy on renal function.

When the GFR is normal or mildly reduced (creatinine <125 μmol/litre, eGFR >45) pregnancy is associated with little chance of permanent decline in renal function. In one study of 360 such women with chronic glomerulonephritis followed for 30 years, there was no difference in renal survival between the 171 who became pregnant and the others who did not. By contrast, if GFR is moderately reduced (creatinine 125–250 μmol/litre, eGFR 20–45), the situation is different: about 40% of such women will have a rise in serum creatinine during pregnancy (instead of the usual fall), and as many as one third will have an irreversible decline in GFR that is greater than would be expected on the basis of their previous renal behaviour, including around 10% who will progress fairly rapidly to end stage renal failure. The higher the initial serum creatinine and the worse the control of blood pressure, the greater the chance of such irreversible decline.

Women with a baseline creatinine creatinine >250 μmol/litre (eGFR <20) are rarely fertile and the chances of conception, a normal pregnancy, and a healthy child are extremely low; the risks to maternal health are high; and pregnancy should be strongly discouraged. Women in this situation who are desperate to conceive should be told that their best chance of becoming pregnant and having a child is 1 year after successful renal transplantation.

Effects of pregnancy on specific renal conditions

It has been suggested that some renal conditions are more likely than others to deteriorate under the stress of pregnancy, and that more guarded advice than that described above should be given to patients with lupus nephropathy, mesangiocapillary glomerulonephritis, focal segmental glomerulosclerosis, and (perhaps) IgA nephropathy and reflux nephropathy. It would be generally agreed that women with systemic lupus erythematosus should be discouraged from pregnancy until their disease has been inactive for at least 6 months, but the evidence that women with the other conditions listed should be specifically discouraged from pregnancy is not strong.

Effects of renal disease on pregnancy

Women with a serum creatinine of less than 125 μmol/litre (eGFR >45) have a greater than 90% chance of a successful obstetric outcome, and the chances are only slightly lower in patients with moderate depression of GFR (creatinine 125–250 μmol/litre, eGFR 20–45) as long as blood pressure is well controlled.

The presence of hypertension during pregnancy in women with renal disease has a substantial influence on pregnancy outcome: the overall risk of fetal death for women with renal disease of any severity that is complicated by hypertension in pregnancy (compared to pregnancies in women with renal disease that are not complicated by hypertension) is 12% (vs 6%), of intrauterine growth retardation is 16% (vs 2%), and of preterm delivery is 20% (vs 11%).

Women with kidney disease are at much greater risk for pre-eclampsia than those without. This can be difficult to diagnose as distinct from the deterioration of renal function that is commonly seen during pregnancy in women with moderately impaired renal function, but typically presents in the third trimester (much less commonly in the second) with significant worsening of hypertension and proteinuria in association with a falling platelet count and/or increased liver enzymes. Preterm delivery is required in 60% of pregnancies in women with moderately impaired renal function because of pre-eclampsia and/or intrauterine growth retardation.

Monitoring and management of pregnancy in women with renal disease

Patients with renal disease who are pregnant require close attention, with prenatal monitoring every 2 weeks until 32 weeks gestation and every week thereafter. This monitoring should include measurement of blood pressure, testing of urine for proteinuria (by dipstick, with quantitation if positive), urinary culture for bacteriuria (which should be treated promptly, as discussed above), estimation of serum creatinine (at least monthly), and (as appropriate) ultrasonography to check fetal growth and fetal heart rate monitoring to check fetal well-being.

The management of hypertension in pregnancy is discussed in Chapter 14.4. In routine obstetric practice, blood pressure above 170/110 mmHg in the third trimester is certainly an indication for starting antihypertensive treatment, and many obstetricians will have a lower threshold of 160/100 mmHg. Whether or not the threshold should be reduced below this in women with renal disease is a contentious issue, but many renal physicians recommend more aggressive treatment in the belief (but without proof) that this may preserve renal function.

As described previously, it is common for proteinuria to develop or to increase substantially during pregnancy in women with renal disease. Pregnancy can be allowed to continue as long as blood pressure is normal and renal function does not deteriorate. Reversible causes, such as volume depletion or urinary infection, should be sought if renal function does decline, but significant and otherwise unexplained deterioration in renal function is reason to recommend elective delivery. Management of difficult cases requires achieving an acceptable balance between maternal and fetal interests, which is not always easy, but if in doubt the mother's interests should come first.

Women on dialysis

The rate of pregnancy amongst women of childbearing age on dialysis is 0.3 to 1.5% per year. With intensive management, including increased dialysis (six sessions of haemodialysis per week instead of the usual three) and higher doses of erythropoietin to maintain haemoglobin levels, about 50% of pregnancies can result in a live birth, but there is high risk that the mother will develop severe hypertension and most infants are premature, with mean gestational age 30.5 weeks in one large series.

Women with renal transplants

Fertility returns in women of child-bearing age after renal transplantation and over 90% of pregnancies that survive the first trimester end successfully. It is generally recommended that women should not attempt to conceive for the first year after transplantation. Thereafter the risks are similar to those indicated above for a woman with disease of her native kidneys, being low in the patient with good renal function, no proteinuria, and no hypertension, but high in the presence of hypertension, heavy proteinuria, and with a poorly functioning graft. Prednisolone, azathioprine, ciclosporin, and tacrolimus seem to be safe in pregnancy, but doses of ciclosporin and tacrolimus may need to be modified to ensure maintenance of stable therapeutic levels in the blood. Mycophenolate mofetil and sirolimus are strongly contraindicated

in pregnancy: women taking mycophenolate mofetil who wish to conceive should be switched onto azathioprine at least 6 weeks before they attempt to do so, and women taking sirolimus should be switched on to ciclosporin or tacrolimus at least 12 weeks beforehand. The presence of a renal transplant is not a contraindication to normal vaginal delivery and is not an indication for caesarean section. There is no increase in the incidence of congenital abnormalities in the infants of mothers with renal transplants. Pregnancy does not have an adverse long term effect on transplant kidney function.

Further reading

George JN (2003). The association of pregnancy with thrombotic thrombocytopenic purpura-hemolytic uremic syndrome. *Curr Opin Hematol*, **10**, 339–44.

Hill JB, *at al.* (2005). Acute pyelonephritis in pregnancy. *Obstet Gynecol*, **105**, 18–23.

Hou S (2003). Pregnancy in dialysis patients: where do we go from here? *Semin Dial*, **16**, 376–8.

Jones DC, Hayslett JP (1996). Outcome of pregnancy in women with moderate or severe renal insufficiency. *N Engl J Med*, **335**, 226–32.

Jungers P, *et al.* (1995). Influence of pregnancy on the course of primary chronic glomerulonephritis. *Lancet*, **346**, 1122–4.

McKay DB, Josephson MA. (2006). Pregnancy in recipients of solid organs—effects on mother and child. *N Engl J Med*, **354**, 1281–93.

Meyers SJ, *et al.* (1985). Dilatation and nontraumatic rupture of the urinary tract during pregnancy: a review. *Obstet Gynecol*, **66**, 809–15.

Pertuiset N, Grünfeld JP (1994). Acute renal failure in pregnancy. *Baillière's Clin Obstet Gynaecol*, **8**, 333–51.

Selcuk NY, *et al.* (1998). Changes in frequency and etiology of acute renal failure in pregnancy (1980–1997). *Ren Fail*, **20**, 513–7.

Smaill F, Vazquez JC (2007). Antibiotics for asymptomatic bacteriuria in pregnancy. *Cochrane Database Syst Rev*, **2**, CD000490.

Vazquez JC, Villar J (2003). Treatments for symptomatic urinary tract infections during pregnancy. *Cochrane Database Syst Rev*, **4**, CD002256.

Heart disease in pregnancy

Catherine E.G. Head

Essentials

Pregnancy is a vasodilator state in which plasma volume and cardiac output increase such that many symptoms and signs of cardiac disease can occur physiologically. Disproportionate symptoms or abnormal signs such as a diastolic murmur require investigation as usual; necessary radiological investigations should not be withheld as the risks to the fetus are generally low.

Prepregnancy risk assessment—this is ideally based on data related to the specific cardiac abnormality, with prepregnancy functional status an important predictor of outcome. Issues of particular note are (1) pregnancy is high risk in pulmonary hypertension or severe left ventricular dysfunction—effective contraception and termination should be offered; (2) women at risk of aortic dissection are at increased risk during pregnancy—prepregnancy elective replacement of the aortic root should be considered if its diameter at its widest point is greater than 4.5 cm; β-blockers and regular echo monitoring should continue through pregnancy.

Delivery of the baby—vaginal delivery is recommended, other than in the presence of a dilated aortic root, aneurysm or dissection, or if the fetal INR is elevated. Low dose infusions of epidural anaesthesia and oxytoxic drugs are safe.

Heart conditions arising in pregnancy

Peripartum cardiomyopathy—this should be considered in any woman presenting peripartum with dyspnoea or tachycardia.

Myocardial infarction—when occurring in pregnancy this may be due to coronary dissection: immediate angiography with percutaneous coronary intervention is the management of choice, but thrombolysis is not contraindicated.

Pregnancy in women with known cardiac disorders

Valve diseases and cardiomyopathies—(1) Symptomatic mitral stenosis—may be managed medically with diuretics, β-blockade and maintenance of sinus rhythm; failing this, balloon valvuloplasty is usually successful. (2) Aortic stenosis—women with satisfactory prepregnancy haemodynamics are at low risk of problems in pregnancy. (3) Hypertrophic cardiomyopathy—patients generally tolerate pregnancy well.

Congenital cardiac lesions—low-risk conditions include atrial septal defect, restrictive ventricular septal defect and corrected tetralogy of Fallot in the absence of severe pulmonary regurgitation. All cases other than those at low risk should be managed by a multidisciplinary team in a specialist centre.

Anticoagulation—the optimal anticoagulation management of a pregnant patient with a mechanical prosthetic valve is not known. Continued warfarin therapy carries the risk of warfarin embryopathy for the fetus, but switching to heparin increases the maternal risk of thromboembolism, although newer regimens using LMW heparin with monitoring of anti-Xa levels almost certainly perform better than historical regimens using unfractionated heparin.

Introduction

Cardiac disease is the commonest cause of maternal death in the United Kingdom. Historically most of these women had rheumatic mitral stenosis, but in the developed world today the most important causes are pulmonary vascular disease, cardiomyopathy, aortic dissection, and myocardial infarction. Maternal death is fortunately rare, but the proportion of pregnant women who have cardiac disease is increasing, reflecting both the improved survival of adults with congenital heart disease and changes in pregnancy demographics.

Cardiovascular changes in pregnancy

Early in gestation the up-regulation of nitric oxide synthesis by oestradiol causes arterial vasodilatation and a reduction in both systemic and pulmonary vascular resistance. Simultaneously the normal fall in heart rate at the end of the menstrual cycle fails to occur, and the heart rate increases by 10 to 20 beats/min for the duration of the pregnancy. The reduction in afterload and blood pressure stimulates an increase in plasma volume and hence preload by activation of the renin–angiotensin–aldosterone system. End diastolic volume, stroke volume and contractility increase such that cardiac output reaches about 140% of prepregnancy level by mid gestation. These changes combined with the development of the low resistance uteroplacental circulation cause blood pressure (systolic and diastolic) to decline by around 10 mmHg to a nadir at about 20 weeks, before returning to prepregnancy levels by term (see Chapters 14.1 and 14.4). Although central venous pressure and pulmonary capillary wedge pressure remain unchanged, serum colloid osmotic pressure is reduced by plasma expansion and the pregnant woman is therefore at increased risk of pulmonary oedema. The 50% increase in plasma volume combined with the 25% increase in red cell mass accounts for a haemoglobin level of around 11 g/dl—the physiological anaemia of pregnancy.

Labour, particularly the second stage, is associated with a further increase in cardiac output as pain increases heart rate via the sympathetic response and stroke volume is augmented by autotransfusion during contractions and postpartum. This means that the later stages of labour are a period of high risk for pulmonary oedema.

Structural changes to the heart and great vessels occur. Orifice areas of all four valves increase, causing a higher incidence of valvular regurgitation. Changes in the extracellular matrix of the aortic media increase compliance but also, in combination with the increased cardiac output, the risk of dissection.

Cardiac clinical features of normal pregnancy

Fatigue, dizziness, palpitation, oedema, dyspnoea, and reduced exercise tolerance may occur in a normal pregnancy. Pressure of the uterus on the inferior vena cava when supine can significantly reduce preload and therefore cardiac output, causing presyncope. Symptoms are rapidly relieved by turning on one side. The increased cardiac output of pregnancy, together with the relative sinus tachycardia and the increased tendency to ectopy, may be experienced as palpitation, often particularly when at rest lying down. Physiological hyperventilation of pregnancy is perceived as breathlessness, particularly when speaking, by most women at some point during a normal pregnancy.

Normal cardiovascular examination findings in pregnancy are

- increased volume 'bounding' peripheral pulses
- third heart sound
- soft ejection systolic murmur at the left sternal edge
- peripheral oedema

  Abnormal findings that require further assessment include:
- fourth heart sound
- diastolic murmur

Cardiovascular investigation in pregnancy

Electrocardiogram

The rotated position of the heart causes left axis deviation. Changes in autonomic control and ion channel expression result in an increase in corrected QT interval and QT dispersion.

Exercise testing

Maximal exercise testing is safe for both mother and fetus in a normal pregnancy, with maximal oxygen uptake the same as that of non-pregnant matched controls in non-weight-bearing (static cycle) protocols. There is no data on the use of exercise testing to diagnose ischaemic heart disease during pregnancy and so sensible extrapolation from the nonpregnant data should be used, remembering that nonspecific T wave changes can be normal in pregnancy. Prepregnancy testing is useful in risk stratification.

Chest radiograph/CT

The fetal absorbed dose of ionizing radiation is <0.01 mGy from a chest radiograph and <1 mGy (mean 0.06 mGy) from a chest CT. Maximum recommended total occupational exposure during pregnancy is 1 mGy, the mean annual dose received from background radiation. The threshold dose for fetal malformation is 100 mGy, and while there is no threshold associated with an increased rate of later malignancy, the relative risk is modest at ×1.4 for a dose of >10 mGy. Thus a chest radiograph or CT necessary to make a diagnosis should not be withheld from a pregnant woman.

Echocardiogram

Echocardiography is safe and useful. Views are standard other than for the absence of a subcostal view in later pregnancy. Normal findings include a small increase in the size of all cardiac chambers, mild regurgitation of all four valves, and the presence of a small pericardial effusion.

Cardiac catheterization

Diagnostic cardiac catheterization is rarely indicated in pregnancy, but percutaneous intervention may be required for valvular or coronary disease. Most interventional cardiac procedures are associated with a total exposure of <50 mGy (usually 1–10 mGy). External shielding of the pelvis and abdomen is of limited protective value as most fetal exposure is caused by internally scattered radiation. However, fetal doses can be reduced by use of adjunctive imaging modalities such as transoesophageal echo, use of the transradial route for coronary intervention, and imaging of the woman in the first trimester with an empty bladder. A wedge should be placed under one hip during the procedure to prevent aortocaval compression.

MRI

MRI avoids ionizing radiation and yields very high-quality diagnostic information but is associated with theoretical fetal risk from heat, noise, and electromagnetic fields. If MRI is necessary in pregnancy, often for imaging of the aorta, the first trimester and gadolinium contrast are avoided if possible.

Prepregnancy assessment and risk stratification

In all but the most straightforward cases a planned pregnancy is preferable to one that is unplanned. Prior to pregnancy a full clinical assessment should be made, including measurement of oxygen saturation, ECG, chest radiography, and echocardiogram. Prepregnancy functional capacity is an important predictor of a woman's ability to tolerate pregnancy, with those in

> **Box 14.6.1** High-risk lesions—advise against pregnancy
>
> ◆ Pulmonary hypertension
> ◆ Aortopathy with root >4.5 cm or aneurysm, advise surgery first
> ◆ Severe aortic stenosis (peak gradient > 80 mmHg or symptoms), advise surgery first
> ◆ Systemic ventricular dysfunction NYHA III or IV symptoms

NYHA classes I and II generally having a good outcome. Treadmill exercise testing can be useful to define this: achievement of a level of above 7 METS (multiples of resting oxygen consumption) being used empirically by some centres to predict a good outcome. Invasive investigation may also be necessary. An estimate of maternal and fetal risk can then be given, together with recommendations for any medical, interventional, or surgical treatment before conception (Box 14.6.1). Although it is a difficult issue to discuss, it is also important that the prospective mother is fully aware of her expected lifespan and capacity.

Maternal

In parallel with the known lesion-specific risks, a generic scoring system can be used to predict the risk of an adverse maternal event by awarding a point for each of:

◆ cyanosis (oxygen saturation <90%) or NYHA functional class >II

◆ left heart obstruction (mitral valve area <2 cm^2, aortic valve area <1.5 cm^2 or left ventricular outflow tract gradient >30 mmHg by echocardiography)

◆ left ventricular dysfunction (ejection fraction <40%)

◆ prior cardiac event (pulmonary oedema, arrhythmia, stroke or transient ischaemic attack)

Adverse event rates are approximately 5%, 30%, and 70% for 0, 1, and >1 points.

Fetal

In addition to the factors above, smoking, anticoagulation, and multiple pregnancy are adverse predictors of fetal and neonatal outcome, especially prematurity and low birth weight. Recurrence risk of any non-monogenic congenital heart disease is 3 to 6%, which is up to a 10-fold increase over the general population. Affected women should be offered fetal echocardiography and families with multiple cases of congenital heart disease should be offered referral to a clinical geneticist.

Management—general principles

Antenatal care

Women with a risk score of 0 (as defined above) and no additional lesion-specific risk factors can generally be managed locally, but in all other cases antenatal care should be multidisciplinary in a specialist centre. Many cardiac drugs are relatively or absolutely contraindicated in pregnancy (see Chapter 14.18), and therapy should be reviewed before conception. In general warfarin should be changed to subcutaneous low molecular weight heparin

(with anti-Xa level monitoring) for the duration of pregnancy, except in the case of mechanical valve replacements discussed below.

Cardiac surgery during pregnancy

Maternal mortality rates are similar to those reported for emergency procedures in nonpregnant patients, but rates of fetal loss associated with cardiopulmonary bypass are high at 15 to 33%. Modifications to standard cardiopulmonary bypass may improve fetal outcome, but consideration should also be given to early delivery, balancing the risk of fetal loss against those of prematurity.

Labour and delivery

In all but low-risk cases, delivery should occur at the tertiary centre with a written management plan in place. In most United Kingdom units antibiotic prophylaxis was until recently given to all women at risk of endocarditis at the onset of active labour, reflecting a pragmatic approach to the emergency nature of instrumented delivery and reports of bacteraemia rates of 14% after labour or rupture of membranes. Current NICE guidelines do not recommend antibiotic prophylaxis for delivery.

Vaginal delivery is generally recommended, cardiac indications for caesarean section being:

◆ aortopathy with aortic root >4.5 cm or rapidly dilating

◆ aortic dissection

◆ warfarin therapy within the preceding 2 weeks (although the maternal INR may be normal, the fetus clears warfarin more slowly and may still be at risk of cerebral haemorrhage)

Low dose epidural anaesthesia does not cause excessive vasodilatation, and with adequate volume expansion is the analgesia of choice. Invasive blood pressure monitoring is advisable in women with obstructive lesions (e.g. aortic stenosis), in whom large fluid shifts may be poorly tolerated. Observation and monitoring on a high-dependency unit may be required for up to 1 week postpartum.

Specific cardiac conditions in pregnancy

Cardiomyopathy

Peripartum cardiomyopathy

This is defined as the development of left ventricular (LV) systolic dysfunction that occurs between the last month of pregnancy and 5 months postpartum in the absence of an identifiable cause or previous cardiac disease. Incidence in Western countries is 1 in 4000. Although risk factors—multiple pregnancy, multiparity, hypertension, increased maternal age, and black ethnicity—have been identified, the aetiology is unknown. There is evidence for infective, inflammatory, and autoimmune mechanisms, in addition to a genetic predisposition. Clinical features are those of LV failure; the diagnosis should be suspected in any peripartum woman with dyspnoea, orthopnoea, paroxysmal nocturnal dyspnoea, or tachycardia. Echocardiography is key in the diagnosis, both to establish LV systolic dysfunction and to exclude other cardiac causes (Fig. 14.6.1). Management is as standard for LV failure, with oxygen, diuretics, vasodilators (angiotensin-converting enzyme (ACE) inhibitors postpartum only), β-blockers, and occasionally digoxin. There is a high risk of thromboembolism,

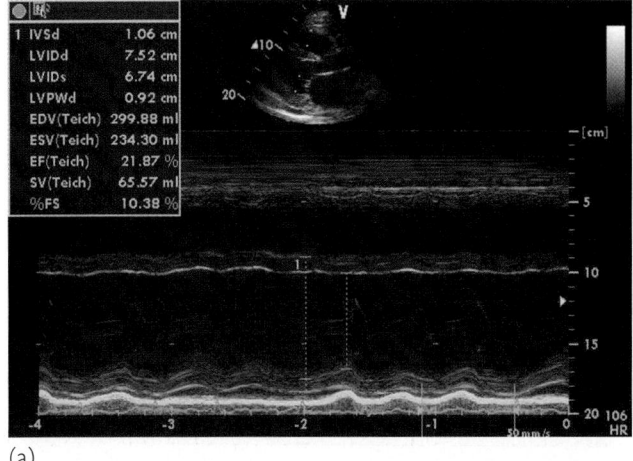

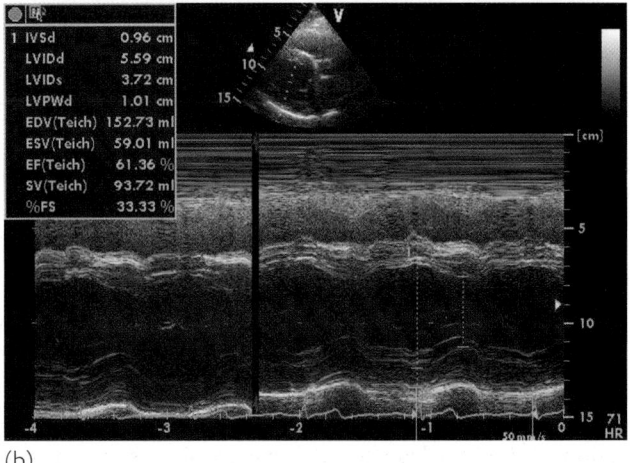

Fig. 14.6.1 Left ventricular dimensions on M mode echocardiogram. (a) Dilated impaired ventricle in peripartum cardiomyopathy. (b) Normal ventricle.

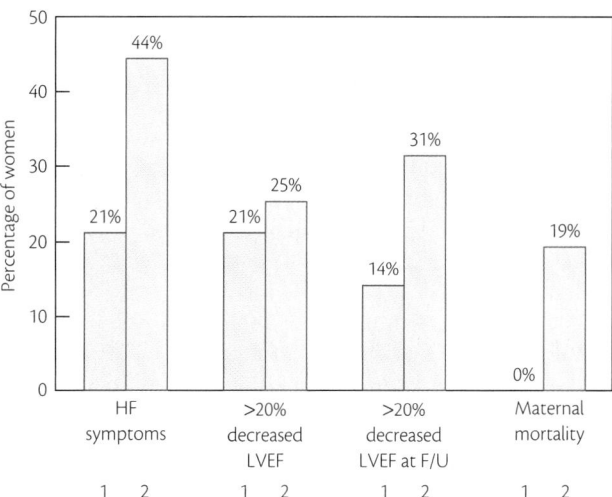

Fig. 14.6.2 Maternal complications in subsequent pregnancy in patients with previous peripartum cardiomyopathy. Group 1, LVEF >50% prior to subsequent pregnancy; group 2, LVEF <50%. HF, heart failure.
(From Elkayam U. (2002). Pregnant again after peripartum cardiomyopathy: to be or not to be? *European Heart J*, **23**, 753–6, with permission.)

necessitating the addition of a prophylactic or, in high risk cases, treatment dose of low molecular weight heparin.

Mortality is 9 to 15%, usually occurring within 3 months and predicted by poor NYHA class at presentation, larger LV dimensions, lower ejection fraction (LVEF), and lack of contractile reserve on dobutamine stress echocardiography. Cases refractory to standard medical therapy may require intensive care with inotropic support and consideration of a ventricular assist device or cardiac transplantation.

Up to 60% of patients recover normal resting LV function, which is crucial to the outcome of a future pregnancy (Fig. 14.6.2). We counsel against subsequent pregnancy in women whose LV function has not recovered and offer termination of unplanned pregnancy. In those who are NYHA I with a normal resting echocardiogram we attempt to refine their risk by dobutamine stress echocardiography, judging empirically that women with a normal contractile reserve are less likely to deteriorate during a pregnancy. This, however, will not predict cases of recurrence of the original pathological process and thus a further pregnancy will always involve a degree of risk.

Dilated cardiomyopathy

As in peripartum cardiomyopathy the diagnosis depends on the identification of left ventricular dilatation and dysfunction in the absence of an identifiable cause. Women may present with a pre-existing diagnosis or *de novo* in pregnancy. LVEF <40% is a predictor of adverse events in pregnancy and <30% or NYHA III/IV clinical status is a contraindication. Management is as discussed for peripartum cardiomyopathy, with the important addition of consideration of termination of pregnancy for women with worsening symptoms or ventricular function prior to fetal viability.

Hypertrophic cardiomyopathy

Women with hypertrophic cardiomyopathy generally tolerate pregnancy well, with outcome predicted by prepregnancy functional status. An asymptomatic woman has a better than 90% chance of remaining so throughout her pregnancy. Reported mortality rates are 0 to 1%, with the two deaths in a recent series both being high-risk cases who had been advised against pregnancy. Prepregnancy assessment should include exercise testing, echocardiography, and standard assessment of sudden cardiac death risk. Women with severe systolic or diastolic dysfunction should be advised against pregnancy; those with moderate diastolic dysfunction may require diuretic treatment if they do not cope with volume expansion. Pre-existing β-blockers should be continued and atrial fibrillation treated if it occurs. An implantable cardioverter-defibrillator is no bar to pregnancy. During labour cardiac filling pressures should be maintained by fluid infusion, especially in the event of postpartum haemorrhage, and any epidural analgesia/anaesthesia should be low dose to avoid vasodilatation.

Ischaemic heart disease

In the 10 years from 1994 a small decrease in the female prevalence of hypertension and smoking, combined with an increase in diabetes and obesity, resulted in an unchanged prevalence of cardiovascular disease in women. However, the proportion of live births occurring to women in their thirties or older has more than doubled over the last 30 years, such that the prevalence of coronary atheroma in pregnant women is increasing.

Known ischaemic heart disease prepregnancy is rare and should be assessed as if risk-stratifying for noncardiac surgery. Previous percutaneous coronary intervention (PCI) or coronary artery bypass grafting (CABG) is no bar to pregnancy if functional status is good and ventricular function normal. Angina presenting in pregnancy should be managed with standard medical therapy, other than a statin as these are teratogenic. PCI is feasible, as described above. Troponin I is unaffected by normal pregnancy and delivery.

In the United States myocardial infarction occurs in 3 to 6 in 100 000 deliveries, with mortality 5 to 7%. Most cases occur in the third trimester, largely peripartum. Risk factors include thrombophilia, infection, and transfusion in addition to standard coronary risk factors. Coronary atheroma is present in less than half of cases (43%), with the remainder caused by spontaneous dissection, thrombosis or embolus. In 29% of cases angiography is entirely normal and coronary spasm the presumed diagnosis; this has been reported following administration of the vasoconstrictor ergometrine to prevent postpartum haemorrhage (transfusion, listed above as a risk factor, may be a surrogate marker for this). Immediate angiography is the management of choice as it allows percutaneous intervention and appropriate targeting of secondary coronary prevention. Thrombolysis is not contraindicated, but best avoided 2 weeks peripartum because of the risk of postpartum haemorrhage. Aspirin is safe, but there is only case report evidence about other antiplatelet drugs.

Aortopathy

Dilated aortic root

Aortic root dilatation secondary to cystic medial necrosis occurs in association with Marfan syndrome and related disorders, Turner syndrome, familial thoracic aneurysm, bicuspid aortic valve, and repaired tetralogy of Fallot, but has also been reported in healthy pregnant women. Together with hypertension, atherosclerosis, and infection it confers a risk of type A dissection, most commonly in the third trimester or peripartum—the time of greatest haemodynamic shear stress to the aortic wall. Most of the literature concerns Marfan syndrome, with an overall pregnancy mortality of 1%. It is important to note that although prepregnancy aortic root dimensions less than 4 cm tend to remain stable during pregnancy, dissection can occur in a nondilated root, especially if there is a family history. Although the number of reported cases is small the risk appears to increase significantly if the aortic root diameter is greater than 4 to 4.5 cm, in which case elective aortic root replacement before conception should be considered. The aortic root should be screened by echocardiography before conception and every 4 to 10 weeks during pregnancy and the puerperium (Fig. 14.6.3). It is recommended that regardless of root diameter all at risk women are fully β-blocked throughout pregnancy. If despite these measures the root dilates rapidly or dissects, the management of choice is caesarean delivery of a viable fetus followed by root replacement. If the fetus is nonviable, surgery should proceed, accepting the risk of fetal loss. Low-risk cases may have a normal delivery with an assisted second stage but most specialist units recommend caesarean section for higher-risk women, although there are no randomized data to support this. Obstetric complications of Marfan syndrome include recurrent miscarriage, preterm rupture of membranes, and postpartum haemorrhage.

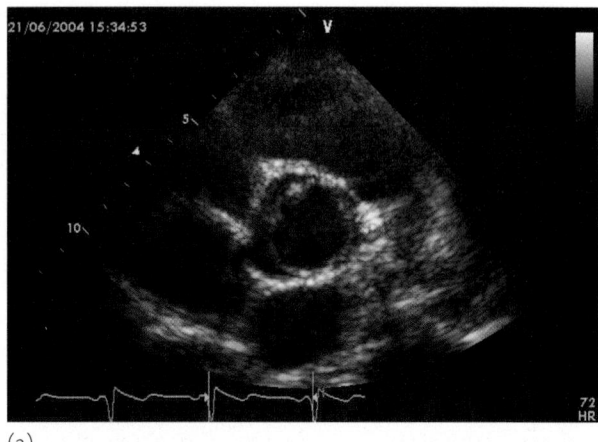

(a)

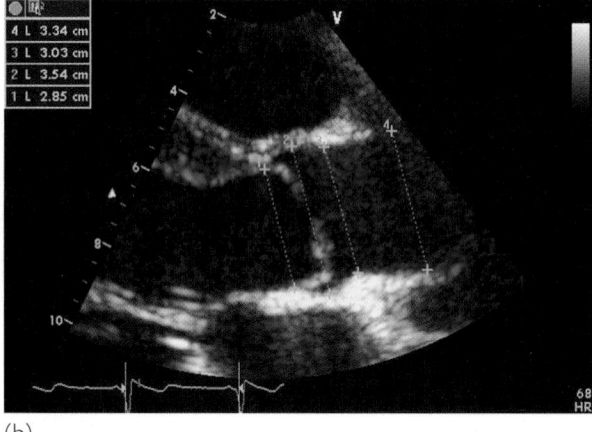

(b)

Fig. 14.6.3 Bicuspid aortic valve (a) in short axis, (b) showing the aortic root measurements used in monitoring.

Coarctation of the aorta

Pregnancy is low risk in repaired coarctation as long as there is no aneurysm at the site of repair: MRI or CT should be performed before conception to exclude this if the patient has undergone patch graft repair. Two recent series reported a single death, by type A dissection, in 104 women (20 unrepaired) undergoing 244 pregnancies. The incidence of hypertension is fourfold higher than in the general pregnant population, particularly in those women with a residual or native gradient higher than 20 mmHg. In the presence of a significant gradient the concerns are dual: maternal hypertension, with risk of aortic dissection and stroke, and hypotension of the fetoplacental unit. Blood pressure should therefore be measured in the right arm and either leg, using β-blockers as the first line antihypertensive agent to achieve systolic pressures of less than 140 mmHg in the arm and more than 70 mmHg in the leg. Delivery should usually be vaginal, with consideration of assisted second stage in the presence of a significant gradient or hypertension, and by caesarean section if there is an aneurysm. Angioplasty and stenting of coarctation during pregnancy and the puerperium is not recommended because of the increased predisposition to dissection during this period, although there are no series from which to estimate risk.

Pulmonary hypertension

Pulmonary hypertension (mPAP >25 mmHg at rest or 30 mmHg on exercise) of any cause is high risk for pregnancy, with maternal mortality around 40%. Effective contraception or termination should be advised. Women who elect to continue should be monitored closely and advised strongly to reconsider termination should they deteriorate in the first or second trimester.

Suggested treatments include bed rest, oxygen, anticoagulation, and targeted pulmonary vascular therapies such as sildenafil, nitric oxide, and prostacyclin analogues, but the evidence is scant. Bosentan is not recommended as it has been associated with animal teratogenesis. One small series reported an improved maternal mortality with a regimen of oxygen, heparin before delivery, and warfarin after 48 h; 60% of infants were liveborn, with most premature. Early reports of the use of nebulized iloprost, intravenous prostacyclin, and oral sildenafil are optimistic, but numbers are small and deaths still occur.

Admission for bed rest and timing of delivery are determined by the clinical status of the woman. There is no evidence to support the choice of either vaginal or caesarean delivery for cardiac reasons: vaginal delivery is associated with a lower average blood loss but also increased maternal effort. In practice early caesarean delivery is often required because of intrauterine growth retardation. In either case regional is preferable to general anaesthesia, as positive pressure ventilation reduces preload. Invasive blood pressure monitoring is required, and oxytocic drugs should be given as a low dose infusion, rather than a bolus dose. Monitoring should continue for at least a week after delivery because the risk of sudden death postpartum is high.

Valvular lesions

Mitral stenosis

This is generally rheumatic in aetiology, occurring predominantly in those born outside the developed world. The volume expansion and tachycardia of pregnancy can unmask a previously clinically silent lesion. Death rates are low but pulmonary oedema or arrhythmia occur in one-third, particularly those with valve area less than $1.5\,cm^2$ or a history of cardiac events. Medical therapy includes β-blockade to increase time for diastolic filling, diuretics, and consideration of anticoagulation, as left atrial thrombus has been reported in pregnancy even in sinus rhythm. New atrial fibrillation should be cardioverted promptly. If NYHA III/IV symptoms develop despite medical therapy, and the valve is morphologically suitable, balloon mitral valvuloplasty is the treatment of choice, being clinically successful in more than 95% with significantly lower rates of fetal loss than surgery.

Aortic stenosis and bicuspid aortic valve

Bicuspid aortic valve (Fig. 14.6.3) in the absence of any stenosis or root dilatation can be managed as a normal pregnancy.

Aortic stenosis is well tolerated if before pregnancy the patient is asymptomatic, has a normal resting ECG, echocardiography shows normal LV function with peak aortic valve gradient less than 80 mmHg and mean less than 50 mmHg, and a treadmill exercise test to target heart rate (220 minus age) reveals no ST segment change or arrhythmia and a normal haemodynamic response. Otherwise aortic stenosis should be relieved before conception using balloon dilatation or a tissue valve if feasible, to avoid mechanical valve replacement. A recent series reported a 10% complication rate in pregnant women with peak gradient more than 64 mmHg or valve area less than $1\,cm^2$ and no complications in those with less severe stenosis. The valve gradient will increase

as pregnancy progresses and failure to do so is a warning sign of ventricular dysfunction. There is benefit in bed rest and β-blockade if a pregnant woman presents or becomes severely symptomatic with dyspnoea, angina or syncope, but balloon valvuloplasty may need to be considered. Valve replacement during pregnancy carries a maternal mortality of 1.5 to 6% and fetal of 30%. Delivery should be vaginal, avoiding vasodilatation and fluid shifts. It is unknown whether pregnancy accelerates the progression of congenital aortic stenosis.

Pulmonary stenosis

This is generally well tolerated, although in severe cases may precipitate right heart failure, tricuspid regurgitation, or atrial arrhythmia. Women with a prepregnancy peak-to-peak catheter gradient of more than 50 mmHg or symptoms should be considered for balloon valvuloplasty or surgery before conception. Balloon valvuloplasty is also possible during pregnancy if symptoms develop. It has been suggested that women with pulmonary stenosis are at increased risk of hypertensive disorders and preterm delivery, but this requires confirmation.

Mitral and aortic regurgitation

Left-sided valve regurgitation is generally very well tolerated in pregnancy if ventricular function is normal. The offloading of the left ventricle caused by systemic vasodilatation is beneficial, but diuretics and vasodilators such as nitrates may be necessary in addition. ACE inhibitors are contraindicated in pregnancy.

Small left-to-right shunts

Atrial septal defect

In the presence of a normal pulmonary vascular resistance an unrepaired atrial septal defect should be well tolerated. The pre-existing tendency to atrial arrhythmia may increase with the increase in cardiac output. The potential to shunt right to left in combination with the hypercoagulable state of pregnancy increases the risk of paradoxical embolism, especially with increases in intrathoracic pressure during labour. There should therefore be a low threshold for the use of compression stockings and prophylactic heparin in the presence of immobility or additional risk factors for venous thrombosis. This also applies to patients known to have a patent foramen ovale. Surgical or device closure of the atrial septal defect removes this risk and if planned should therefore be carried out before pregnancy, although there is no evidence to support the same recommendation for patent foramen ovale.

Ventricular septal defect or patent ductus arteriosus

A small defect with normal right-sided pressures confers no added risk in pregnancy. Because of the large pressure gradient across the defect paradoxical embolism is extremely unlikely. Large defects causing pulmonary vascular disease (Eisenmenger's syndrome) are high risk as discussed above.

Complex congenital heart disease

For full descriptions of these lesions and their sequelae see Chapter 16.12.

Transposition of the great arteries—post Mustard or Senning atrial repair

Successful tolerance of pregnancy depends largely on good function of the systemic right ventricle and its atrioventricular valve. In a total of 195 pregnancies reported in 104 women there were 2 deaths, 1 heart transplant, and 7 women with a permanent reduction in ventricular function or functional class. Atrial arrhythmia occurs in 10 to 20%, those with a previous history being at higher risk. There is an increased incidence of miscarriage, prematurity, and low birth weight. More recently, repair has been by the arterial switch operation, following which pregnancy should in theory be well tolerated—but this remains to be seen.

Congenitally corrected transposition of the great arteries

Outcome of this rare condition (where the circulation is physiologically 'corrected', with blood passing from the pulmonary veins to the left atrium, to the right ventricle, to the aorta) depends on systemic right ventricular function and the presence of associated lesions such as complete heart block, ventricular septal defect, or pulmonary stenosis.

Fontan operation for univentricular circulation

These patients have two separate circulations in series and are therefore usually not cyanosed, but they experience a chronic low-output state and are at risk of ventricular failure, atrial arrhythmia, and thrombosis. They are generally anticoagulated with warfarin, which should be converted to full dose low molecular weight heparin for the duration of pregnancy. Maternal outcome again depends on functional capacity and ventricular function. If these are satisfactory and the woman accepts the two to threefold increase in the rate of first trimester fetal loss, then there is no reason to advise against pregnancy, as any deterioration appears to be reversible.

Surgically corrected tetralogy of Fallot

Women with good functional capacity and no significant haemodynamic abnormality tolerate pregnancy well, although the presence of severe pulmonary regurgitation confers a 20 to 30% risk of symptomatic heart failure. If the mother carries del22q11 the recurrence risk is 50%.

Cyanotic heart disease without pulmonary hypertension

Cyanosis is associated with a poorer outcome for both mother and fetus. The risk of paradoxical embolism should be reduced by appropriate hydration, mobilization, and use of compression stockings. Because cyanosis also confers an increased bleeding tendency anticoagulants are not used routinely, but only if there is an additional indication. Increased right-to-left shunting can occur with the systemic vasodilatation of pregnancy, causing worsening cyanosis. Fetal outcome is dependent on maternal saturation—the chance of a live birth decreases from 92% with prepregnancy maternal saturation over 90%, to 12% if maternal saturation is less

than 85%, and many of these infants are premature or of low birth weight.

Prosthetic valves

Bioprosthetic valves do not confer increased risk if haemodynamics are normal, and they do not degenerate more rapidly in pregnancy as previously feared. The management of a mechanical prosthesis is far less straightforward and represents a conflict of interest between the mother and fetus. Complication rates associated with the alternative anticoagulation regimens are shown in Table 14.6.1. The increased rate of fetal loss associated with all effective anticoagulation may reflect placental haemorrhage.

A relatively safe option for the mother is to remain on warfarin for the duration of the pregnancy, stopping only for elective caesarean delivery at 38 weeks with intravenous heparin perioperatively. If vaginal delivery is planned this change should occur at 36 weeks to allow the fetus to clear the warfarin. This strategy is associated with a risk of warfarin embryopathy, which is significantly reduced if the dose required to achieve target INR is <6 mg daily.

Heparin does not cross the placenta, hence a strategy of substituting heparin for warfarin during the period of organogenesis (6–12 weeks) abolishes the risk of warfarin embryopathy, but it doubles the maternal thromboembolism rate. Heparin throughout pregnancy has historically been associated with a high risk of thromboembolism, but has not always been appropriately dose-adjusted. With twice daily dosing of low molecular weight heparin and antiXa levels monitored fortnightly, achieving a level of 1 to 1.2 IU/ml 4 to 6 h post dose, the thromboembolism rate in a recent meta-analysis was only 2%.

Arrhythmia

Ectopy occurs in most pregnancies, but sustained arrhythmia in less than 1%. A pre-existing tachyarrhythmia confers a 50% chance of a recurrence of supraventricular tachycardia and 25% of ventricular tachycardia. The principles of diagnosis and management are the same as in the nonpregnant state—only recurrent symptomatic or life-threatening arrhythmia should be treated and underlying causes such as thyroid disease should be sought and corrected. Vagal manoeuvres are useful as a first line to diagnose or terminate a narrow complex tachycardia. Adenosine is safe in pregnancy, as is DC cardioversion with fetal monitoring. The risk/benefit ratio of all drugs should be assessed: no drug is absolutely contraindicated, as maternal haemodynamic instability may result in worse fetal outcome. Bradyarrhythmia is rare; the presence of a permanent pacemaker or implantable cardioverter-defibrillator is no problem,

Table 14.6.1 Complication rates (%) of anticoagulation regimens in pregnant women with mechanical heart valves

Regimen	Maternal thromboembolism	Maternal death	Fetal abnormality	Fetal loss[a]	Source
Warfarin to 38/40, then heparin	4	2	6	34	Chan *et al.* (2000)
Heparin 6–12/40, warfarin otherwise	9	4	0[b]	16	Chan *et al.* (2000)
Heparin throughout	25	7	0	44	Chan *et al.* (2000)
Heparin anti-Xa adjusted throughout	2	0	0	12[c]	Oran *et al.* (2004)

[a] Refers to abortion, stillbirth, or neonatal death.
[b] If heparin instituted at or before 6/40.
[c] Abortion and stillbirth only.

but the permanent pacemaker may need to be reprogrammed for delivery. Equipment for temporary pacing during labour is recommended, though not usually needed, for nonpaced women with complete heart block.

Contraception

Barrier methods

These are safe for all cardiac patients and have the added benefit of protection against sexually transmitted diseases, but reported failure rates are 2 to 26 per 100 woman years.

Hormonal methods

The oestrogen component of the combined oral contraceptive, whether oral or transdermal, confers an increased risk of thrombosis that is not completely abolished by warfarin. These preparations are therefore contraindicated in women who already have a high thrombotic risk, i.e. pulmonary hypertension, the Fontan circulation, older mechanical valves, dilated cardiac chambers with the risk of atrial fibrillation, or in cyanosed patients in whom paradoxical embolism may occur. The standard progesterone-only 'minipill' is safe, but is less reliable than the combined oral contraceptive pill and therefore not the method of choice for women in whom avoidance of pregnancy is critical. Recommended progesterone only preparations, more reliable as they act by suppression of ovulation, include daily oral desogestrel, 3-monthly depot medroxyprogesterone, and a subcutaneous etonogestrel implant (Implanon), which is the method of choice for complex congenital heart disease. Women concurrently taking the endothelin antagonist bosentan require additional protection.

Intrauterine devices

These are not contraindicated, but insertion of the device can be associated with bacteraemia and a vasovagal response. Antibiotic prophylaxis protects against endocarditis, a vasovagal response associated with which can be life-threatening in a haemodynamically unstable patient such as those with a Fontan circulation or Eisenmenger's syndrome.

Sterilization

Sterilization by tubal ligation may be appropriate for women in whom pregnancy would be high risk. However, failure may result in ectopic pregnancy and the surgery is not trivial, especially in women at risk of paradoxical embolism, as it includes a head-down tilt and distension of the abdomen with CO_2. Sterilization of the male partner is not generally advised if he has a much longer potential lifespan than his partner and may therefore wish to father children in a subsequent relationship.

Further reading

Bates SM, et al. (2008). Venous thromboembolism, thrombophilia, antithrombotic therapy, and Pregnancy. ACCP Clinical Practice Guideline. *Chest*, **133**, 844S–66S.

Beauchesne LM, et al. (2001). Coarctation of the aorta: outcome of pregnancy. *J Am Coll Cardiol*, **38**, 1728–33.

Chan WS, Anand S, Ginsberg JS (2000). Anticoagulation of pregnant women with mechanical heart valves: a systematic review of the literature. *Arch Intern Med*, **160**, 191–6.

Gowda RM, et al. (2003). Cardiac arrhythmias in pregnancy: clinical and therapeutic considerations. *Int J Cardiol*, **88**, 129–33.

James AH, et al. (2006). Acute myocardial infarction in pregnancy: a United States population-based study. *Circulation*, **113**, 1564–71.

Meijboom LJ, et al. (2005). Pregnancy and aortic root growth in the Marfan syndrome: a prospective study. *Eur Heart J*, **26**, 914–20.

Oran B, Lee-Parritz A, Ansell J (2004). Low molecular weight heparin for the prophylaxis of thromboembolism in women with prosthetic mechanical heart valves during pregnancy. *Thromb Haemost*, **92**, 747–51.

Presbitero P, et al. (1994). Pregnancy in cyanotic congenital heart disease. Outcome of mother and fetus. *Circulation*, **89**, 2673–6.

Silversides CK, et al. (2003). Cardiac risk in pregnant women with rheumatic mitral stenosis. *Am J Cardiol*, **91**, 1382–5.

Silversides CK, et al. (2003). Early and intermediate-term outcomes of pregnancy with congenital aortic stenosis. *Am J Cardiol*, **91**, 1386–9.

Siu SC, et al. (2001). Prospective multicenter study of pregnancy outcomes in women with heart disease. *Circulation*, **104**, 515–21.

Sliwa K, Fett J, Elkayam U (2006). Peripartum cardiomyopathy. *Lancet*, **368**, 687–93.

Steer PJ, Gatzoulis MA, Baker P (eds) (2006). *Heart disease and pregnancy*, RCOG Press, London.

Task Force on the Management of Cardiovascular Diseases During Pregnancy of the European Society of Cardiology (2003). Expert consensus document on management of cardiovascular diseases during pregnancy. *Eur Heart J*, **24**, 761–81.

Thaman R, et al. (2003). Pregnancy associated complications in women with hypertrophic cardiomyopathy. *Heart*, **89**, 752–6.

Thorne SA, et al. (2006). Pregnancy and contraception in heart disease and pulmonary arterial hypertension. *J Fam Plann Reprod Health Care*, **32**, 75–81.

Veldtman GR, et al. (2004). Outcomes of pregnancy in women with tetralogy of Fallot. *J Am Coll Cardiol*, **44**, 174–80.

Vitale N, et al. (1999). Dose-dependent fetal complications of warfarin in pregnant women with mechanical heart valves. *J Am Coll Cardiol*, **33**, 1637–41.

Vriend JWJ, et al. (2005). Outcome of pregnancy in patients after repair of aortic coarctation. *Eur Heart J*, **26**, 2173–8.

Walker F (2007). Pregnancy and the various forms of the Fontan circulation. *Heart*, **93**, 152–4.

Weiss BM, Hess OM. (2000). Pulmonary vascular disease and pregnancy: current controversies, management strategies, and perspectives. *Eur Heart J*, **21**, 104–15.

14.7

Thrombosis in pregnancy

I.A. Greer

Essentials

Aetiology—features that predispose to venous thromboembolism include (1) pregnancy is a thrombophilic state; (2) there is relative venous stasis during pregnancy; and (3) some endothelial damage to the pelvic vessels occurs during delivery.

Epidemiology— venous thromboembolism complicates around 1 in 1000 pregnancies, with highest risk just after delivery. Deep venous thromboses usually occur on the left side, and a much higher proportion are ileofemoral than in patients who are not pregnant.

Screening—there is no evidence to support universal screening for thrombophilia in pregnancy, but such screening is appropriate for women with a personal or well-proven family history of venous thromboembolism, also in patients who might reasonably be suspected of having antiphospholipid antibody syndrome.

Diagnosis—ultrasound venography is the first line diagnostic test for deep venous thrombosis in pregnancy. If pulmonary thromboembolism is suspected, ultrasound venography of the leg veins can also be performed: if positive anticoagulation can be given; if negative a chest radiograph and ventilation–perfusion scan or CT pulmonary angiogram are required.

Management—low molecular weight heparin (LMWH) is the anticoagulant of choice in pregnancy because of a better side-effect profile than warfarin or unfractionated heparin, good safety record for mother and fetus, and convenient once-daily dosing for prophylaxis. Typical recommendations are as follows: (1) prophylaxis for women at low but still probably increased risk, e.g. history of previous venous thromboembolism that was not pregnancy-related, associated with a risk factor that is no longer present, and with no additional risk factor or underlying thrombophilia can be offered surveillance antenatally, with postpartum anticoagulation therapy (usually with LMWH) for at least 6 weeks; antenatal LMWH would not be routinely given. (2) Prophylaxis for women at higher risk of recurrent venous thromboembolism in pregnancy—these should usually be prescribed prophylactic LMWH, which should be started as soon as possible following the diagnosis of pregnancy and continued for at least 6 weeks after delivery. (3) Treatment of proven venous thromboembolism in pregnancy—in most cases a twice-daily regimen (because of increased renal excretion) of LMWH is the treatment of choice, but intravenous unfractionated heparin remains the preferred treatment in massive pulmonary thromboembolism.

Introduction

Pulmonary thromboembolism remains a major direct cause of maternal mortality. Venous thromboembolism complicates around 1/1000 pregnancies, with the greatest risk after delivery. Almost half antenatal venous thromboembolism occurs before 15 weeks gestation, emphasizing the need for risk assessment before pregnancy and prophylaxis in early pregnancy. Almost 90% of pregnancy-associated deep venous thromboses occur on the left side, compared with 55% in nonpregnant women, possibly reflecting some compression of the left common iliac vein by the right iliac artery. Over 70% of gestational deep venous thromboses are ileofemoral, compared with around 9% in nonpregnant women, where calf vein thromboses predominate. This is important because ileofemoral thromboses are more likely to embolize than calf vein thromboses.

Venous thromboembolism causes long-term problems as well as acute problems. Deep venous thrombosis is associated with a significant risk of recurrent venous thromboembolism and deep venous insufficiency. Mild to moderate post-thrombotic syndrome can be found in over 60% of cases within 5 years, and about 5% of patients with deep venous thromboses develop venous ulcers within 10 to 20 years of the primary event. The risk of pulmonary hypertension after pulmonary thromboembolism is probably 3 to 4%.

The physiological changes in the haemostatic system in pregnancy (see Chapter 14.16) result in an acquired thrombophilic state due to increased concentrations of coagulation factors such as factor VIII and fibrinogen, reduced endogenous anticoagulants, and suppression of fibrinolysis. Relative venous stasis also occurs, with a 50% reduction in venous flow velocity by 25 to 29 weeks gestation, reaching a nadir at 36 weeks. In addition, some degree of endothelial damage to pelvic vessels is inevitable during vaginal or abdominal delivery. Thus the components of Virchow's triad are all present in the course of normal pregnancy and delivery.

Risk factors for gestational venous thromboembolism and thrombophilia screening

Thromboprophylaxis in pregnancy depends on identifying the level of risk for individual women. The common risk factors for venous thromboembolism are set out in Box 14.7.1.

With regard to thrombophilia, the likelihood of thrombosis depends on the thrombophilia (Table 14.7.1), whether more than one thrombophilia is present or the woman is homozygous for factor V Leiden or prothrombin G20210A, whether previous venous thromboembolism have occurred, and additional risk factors, such as obesity. At present there is no evidence to support universal screening for thrombophilia in pregnancy. The natural

---

Box 14.7.1 Common risk factors for venous thromboembolism in pregnancy

Patient related factors

- Age over 35 years
- Obesity (BMI $\geq$30 kg/m^2) in early pregnancy
- Thrombophilia
- Past history of venous thromboembolism (especially if idiopathic pregnancy or thrombophilia associated)
- Gross varicose veins
- Significant current medical problem (e.g. nephrotic syndrome, heart failure)
- Current infection or inflammatory process (e.g. active inflammatory bowel disease or urinary tract infection)
- Immobility (e.g. bed rest or lower limb fracture)
- Paraplegia
- Recent long-distance travel
- Dehydration
- Intravenous drug abuse
- Ovarian hyperstimulation (NB associated with internal jugular vein thrombosis presenting with neck pain and swelling; subclavian, axillary and brachiocephalic veins thrombosis can also occur, with slight preponderance in the right-sided vessels)

Pregnancy/obstetric related factors

- Caesarean section, particularly as an emergency in labour
- Major obstetric haemorrhage with blood/blood product transfusion
- Hyperemesis gravidarum
- Pre-eclampsia

---

history of many of these thrombophilias—particularly in asymptomatic kindred—is not yet established, appropriate intervention is unclear, and screening is not cost effective. Selective screening (after appropriate counselling) of women with venous thromboembolism in pregnancy or who have a personal or family history of venous thromboembolism (preferably objectively confirmed) may be of value, with around 50% of such women having a heritable thrombophilia. Screening for thrombophilia in patients with problems such as recurrent miscarriage or severe pre-eclampsia, which may be associated with an underlying thrombophilia and therefore risk of venous thromboembolism, should also be considered. However, apart from recurrent miscarriage associated with antiphosphlipid antibody syndrome (see Chapter 14.14), effective intervention for these pregnancy complications is not established.

Antithrombotic therapy in pregnancy

Antithrombotic therapy in pregnancy is limited essentially to warfarin and heparin. There are insufficient data on newer antiocoagulants such as recombinant hirudin and fondaparinux to allow recommendations in pregnancy. Low dose aspirin is not associated with adverse pregnancy outcome in the second and third trimesters and may be useful in some situations, either alone or combined with low molecular weight heparin (LMWH) such as in antiphospholipid syndrome.

Warfarin

The use of warfarin in pregnancy is restricted to only a few situations where heparin is considered unsuitable. Although warfarin is not secreted in breast milk in significant amounts and is safe to use during lactation, it crosses the placenta and is teratogenic with around 6% of pregnancies exposed being associated with congenital abnormalities. With exposure between 6 and 9 weeks' gestation warfarin embryopathy (midface hypoplasia, stippled chondral calcification, scoliosis, short proximal limbs, and short phalanges) may occurs with estimates varying from 0.6 to 5%. This problem is potentially preventable by substitution of heparin for warfarin during the first trimester. Prenatal exposure to coumarins is also associated with an increased risk of neurodevelopmental problems. Warfarin should be avoided around the time of delivery because of maternal and fetal bleeding risk, and hence if used in pregnancy is usually stopped at around 36 weeks gestation (see Chapter 14.6).

Heparin

Neither unfractionated heparin (UFH) nor LMWH appears to cross the placenta and there is no evidence of teratogenesis or risk of fetal haemorrhage. Heparins are not secreted in breast milk and can be used during breastfeeding.

Prolonged use of UFH is associated with symptomatic osteoporosis, with a 2% incidence of osteoporotic fractures. Allergy and heparin-induced thrombocytopenia, an antibody-mediated effect that leads to arterial and venous thrombosis due to platelet activation, may occur.

LMWHs appear safe for the mother and fetus, with a substantially lower risk of osteoporosis and a negligible risk of heparin-induced thrombocytopenia compared to UFH, but local allergic reactions (itchy, erythematous lesions at the injection sites) can occur as with UFH. Changing the heparin preparation may be

Table 14.7.1 Typical prevalence of particular causes of thrombophilia and association with gestational venous thromboembolism in European populations

Thrombophilia	Population prevalence (%)	Approximate prevalence in women with gestational venous thromboembolism (%)	Typical estimate of odds ratio of venous thromboembolism in woman with specific thrombophilias
Factor V Leiden heterozygous	2–7	20–40	8 (homozygote OR 34)
Prothrombin G20210A heterozygous	2	6 (increasing to 20% with strong family history)	2–7 (homozygote OR 26)
Antithrombin deficiency	0.25–0.55	<10	Type 1 280 Type 2 28
Protein C deficiency	0.20–0.33		4–5
Protein S deficiency	0.03–0.13		3

NB: combined defects substantially increase risk, with an odds ratio estimated at 107 for factor V Leiden and prothrombin G20210A compound heterozygotes.

helpful, but cross-reactivity is common. Skin reactions can be associated with heparin-induced thrombocytopenia, hence the platelet count should be checked if these develop. The risk of recurrent venous thrombosis with LMWH used for thromboprophylaxis in pregnancy is less than 1%. LMWHs are not associated with an increased risk of severe peripartum bleeding, hence LMWH is now the anticoagulant of choice in pregnancy because of a better side effect profile, good safety record for mother and fetus, and convenient once-daily dosing for prophylaxis.

Graduated elastic compression stockings

In view of the pregnancy-related changes in the venous system, graduated elastic compression stockings should be of value in pregnancy and postpartum. Full-length stockings are usually used in pregnancy where ileofemoral thrombosis is more common, and indeed they are recommended in high-risk situations for prophylaxis, but most data on efficacy in nonpregnant women come from below-knee stockings, which patients may be more likely to wear. Antiembolism stockings for prophylaxis have a pressure of around 20 mmHg at the ankle, but graduated elastic compression stocking with an ankle pressure of 30 to 40 mmHg should be used after a deep venous thromboses. Long-term use after deep venous thromboses may reduce the risk of post-thrombotic syndrome.

Thromboprophylaxis in pregnancy

The woman with a previous venous thromboembolism that was not pregnancy-related, associated with a risk factor that is no longer present, and with no additional risk factor or underlying thrombophilia, should not routinely receive antenatal LMWH as her risk of recurrence is considered relatively low, but this strategy must be discussed with the woman and her views taken into account because of the relatively limited data available. Surveillance can be offered antenatally to such women, with postpartum anticoagulant therapy, usually with LMWH, for at least 6 weeks (Table 14.7.2).

In women with a single previous venous thromboembolism and an underlying thrombophilia, or where the venous thromboembolism was idiopathic or pregnancy-related (or related to the oral contraceptive 'pill'), or where there are additional risk factors such as obesity or nephrotic syndrome, there is a stronger case for LMWH prophylaxis. Antenatally, these women should usually be prescribed prophylactic LMWH, which should be started as soon as possible following the diagnosis of pregnancy. More intense LMWH therapy may be indicated in the presence of antithrombin deficiency. Postpartum anticoagulant therapy for at least 6 weeks is recommended (Table 14.7.2).

Women with more than one previous venous thromboembolism or on long-term anticoagulant therapy usually require LMWH prophylaxis. Following delivery, particularly if by caesarean section, a risk assessment should be made and those at increased risk prescribed thromboprophylaxis.

Use of LMWH in pregnancy

The prophylactic dose of LMWH may need adjustment in women with very low or very high body weight, with lower doses (e.g. 20 mg enoxaparin daily or 2500 IU dalteparin daily) at low body weight (<50 kg or BMI less than 20 kg/m^2), and higher doses in obese women. There are no data to guide practice on this issue: clinical judgement of risk is required after individual assessment. In women with morbid obesity the author uses 40 mg enoxaparin or 5000 IU dalteparin twice daily; or for those considered at greater risk but with a lower level of obesity 60 mg enoxaparin or 7500 IU dalteparin once daily.

Traditionally the platelet count was checked before and 1 week after the introduction of LMWH, then on around a monthly basis to detect heparin-induced thrombocytopenia. However, where a woman has not previously received UFH the risk of heparin-induced thrombocytopenia with exclusive use of LMWH is so low that current guidelines do not recommend routine monitoring of the platelet count in this situation.

There has been concern with regard to LMWH and epidural haematoma. As a general rule, neuraxial anaesthesia is not used until at least 12 h after the previous prophylactic dose of LMWH, and regional techniques should not be employed for at least 24 h after the last dose when a woman presents while on a therapeutic regimen of LMWH. LMWH should not be given for at least 3 h after an epidural catheter has been removed, and the cannula should not be removed within 10 to 12 h of the most recent injection. Planning management of anticoagulation around delivery requires prior involvement and discussion with obstetric anaesthetists. LMWH may preclude urgent regional analgesia and anaesthesia and assessment of general anaesthetic risk may influence timing and route of delivery.

Table 14.7.2 Suggested management strategies for various clinical situations (NB: specialist advice for individualized management of patients is advisable in many of these situations)

Clinical situation	Suggested management
Single previous venous thromboembolism (not related to pregnancy or oral contraceptive) associated with a transient risk factor and no additional current risk factors, such as obesity.	Antenatal—surveillance or prophylactic doses of LMWH (e.g. 40 mg enoxaparin or 5000 IU dalteparin daily). Discuss decision regarding antenatal LMWH with the woman Postpartum—anticoagulant therapy for at least 6 weeks (e.g. 40 mg enoxaparin or 5000 IU dalteparin daily or warfarin (target INR 2–3) with LMWH overlap until the INR is ≥2.0) ± graduated elastic compression stockings
Single previous idiopathic venous thromboembolism or single previous venous thromboembolism with underlying thrombophilia or positive family history and not on long-term anticoagulant therapy, or single previous venous thromboembolism and additional current risk factor(s) (e.g. morbid obesity, nephrotic syndrome)	Antenatal—prophylactic doses of LMWH (e.g. 40 mg enoxaparin or 5000 IU dalteparin daily) ± graduated elastic compression stockings. NB: there is a strong case for more intense LMWH therapy in antithrombin deficiency, homozygotes or compound heterozygotes for FV Leiden and prothrombin 20210A (e.g. enoxaparin 0.5–1 mg/kg 12 hourly or dalteparin 50–100 IU/kg 12 hourly) Postpartum—anticoagulant therapy for at least 6 weeks (e.g. 40 mg enoxaparin or 5000 IU dalteparin daily or warfarin (target INR 2–3) with LMWH overlap until the INR is > 2.0.) ± graduated elastic compression stockings
More than one previous episode of venous thromboembolism, with no thrombophilia and not on long-term anticoagulant therapy	Antenatal—prophylactic doses of LMWH (eg 40 mg enoxaparin or 5000 IU dalteparin daily) + graduated elastic compression stockings. Postpartum—anticoagulant therapy for at least 6 weeks (e.g. 40 mg enoxaparin or 5000 IU dalteparin daily or warfarin (target INR 2–3) with LMWH overlap until the INR is ≥2.0.) + graduated elastic compression stockings
Previous episode(s) of venous thromboembolism in women receiving long-term anticoagulants (e.g. with underlying thrombophilia)	Antenatal—switch from oral anticoagulants to LMWH therapy (e.g. enoxaparin 0.5–1 mg/kg 12 hourly or dalteparin 50–100 IU/kg 12 hourly) by 6 weeks gestation + graduated elastic compression stockings Postpartum—resume long-term anticoagulants with LMWH overlap until INR in prepregnancy therapeutic range + graduated elastic compression stockings
Thrombophilia (confirmed laboratory abnormality) but no prior venous thromboembolism	Antenatal—surveillance or prophylactic LMWH ± graduated elastic compression stockings. An individual risk assessment is required. The indication for pharmacological prophylaxis in the antenatal period is stronger in AT-deficient women, homozygotes, or compound heterozygotes for FV Leiden and prothrombin 20210A than the other thrombophilias, in symptomatic kindred compared to asymptomatic kindred, and also where additional risk factors are present Postpartum—anticoagulant therapy for at least 6 weeks (e.g. 40 mg enoxaparin or 5000 IU dalteparin daily or warfarin (target INR 2–3) with LMWH overlap until the INR is ≥2.0) ± graduated elastic compression stockings
Following caesarean section or vaginal delivery	Carry out risk assessment for venous thromboembolism. If additional risk factors such as emergency caesarean section in labour, age >35 years, high BMI, etc. present, then consider LMWH thromboprophylaxis (e.g. 40 mg enoxaparin or 5000 IU dalteparin) ± graduated elastic compression stockings

Diagnosis of venous thromboembolism in pregnancy

The clinical diagnosis of deep venous thromboses and pulmonary thromboembolism is unreliable and objective testing is required if there is substantial clinical suspicion. Anticoagulant treatment should be employed in women with clinical features consistent with venous thromboembolism until an objective diagnosis is made.

Ultrasound venography is the first line diagnostic test for deep venous thromboses in pregnancy. If ultrasonography is negative but there is a high level of clinical suspicion, then the patient should be anticoagulated and ultrasonography repeated in one week, or an alternative test such as radiological venography should be considered. If repeat testing is negative, anticoagulant treatment should be discontinued.

If pulmonary thromboembolism is suspected, ultrasound venography of the leg veins can also be performed: if positive anticoagulation can be given; if negative a chest radiograph and ventilation–perfusion scan or CT pulmonary angiogram should

be performed. None of these investigations is considered to pose a significant radiation risk to the fetus in the context of the diagnosis of pulmonary thromboembolism, and they should not be withheld in pregnancy because of fetal considerations when pulmonary thromboembolism is suspected. The average fetal radiation dose with CT pulmonary angiogram is less than that with ventilation–perfusion lung scanning during all trimesters of pregnancy. However, this is offset by the relatively high radiation dose (≥0.02 Gy) to the mother's thorax and in particular breast tissue, which may be especially sensitive to radiation exposure during pregnancy. The delivery of 0.01 Gy to a woman's breast has been calculated to increase her lifetime risk of developing breast cancer by up to 14%. This emphasizes the continued role for ventilation–perfusion scans in pregnancy.

In an appropriate clinical context outside pregnancy an increased level of D-dimer suggests that thrombosis may be present and an objective diagnostic test for deep venous thromboses and/or pulmonary thromboembolism should be performed. In pregnancy, D-dimer can be elevated due to the physiological changes in the coagulation system, and levels become 'abnormal' at term and in the post-natal period in most healthy pregnant women. Furthermore, D-dimer levels are increased if there is a concomitant problem such as pre-eclampsia. Thus a 'positive' D-dimer test in pregnancy does not indicate the presence of venous thromboembolism and objective testing is required, but a low level of D-dimer in pregnancy is likely—as in the nonpregnant—to suggest that there is no venous thromboembolism. However, it is important to note that in the nonpregnant, even with a high pretest probability and a highly sensitive D-dimer assay, around 4% of DVTs will not be identified by a D-dimer test. Hence in patients with a moderate or high pretest probability—which accounts for most pregnant patients—it would be inappropriate to rely on D-dimer to exclude venous thromboembolism in pregnancy.

Treatment of venous thromboembolism in pregnancy

LMWH is the treatment of choice for venous thromboembolism in pregnancy in most cases. With massive pulmonary thromboembolism causing haemodynamic compromise there may be a place for management with intravenous UFH and thrombolysis. In women at risk of thrombosis and with concurrent high risk of haemorrhage, such as those with major antepartum haemorrhage, coagulopathy, progressive wound haematoma, suspected intra-abdominal bleeding, or postpartum haemorrhage, UFH is often preferred as it has a shorter half-life than LMWH and its activity is more completely reversed with protamine sulphate.

A large systematic review demonstrated a risk of recurrent venous thromboembolism of 1.15% when treatment doses of LMWH were used to manage venous thromboembolism in pregnancy, which compares favourably with recurrence rates of 5 to 8% reported in trials carried out in nonpregnant patients treated with LMWH or UFH followed by coumarin therapy who were followed up for 3 to 6 months.

In view of the increased renal excretion of dalteparin and enoxaparin during pregnancy, a twice daily dosage regimen for these LMWHs in the treatment of venous thromboembolism in pregnancy is currently recommended (enoxaparin 1 mg/kg twice daily; dalteparin 100 units/kg twice daily) for initial treatment (Table 14.7.3). Experience indicates that satisfactory anticoagulant effects are obtained using this weight-based regimen. Monitoring of anti-Xa to assess the effect of LMWH is not routinely required, particularly as there are concerns over the accuracy of such monitoring, but there is a case doing so at extremes of body weight or in the presence of renal impairment: the target therapeutic range is 0.5 to 1.2 units/ml for peak levels (around 3 h post injection).

As warfarin is generally avoided for maintenance therapy in pregnancy, women with antenatal venous thromboembolism are usually managed with therapeutic subcutaneous LMWH for the remainder of the pregnancy. They should be taught to self-inject, appropriate arrangements should be made to allow safe disposal of needles and syringes, and they can then be managed as outpatients until delivery.

In order to avoid an unwanted anticoagulant effect during delivery, it is suggested that heparin be discontinued 24 h before elective induction of labour or caesarean section.

Anticoagulant therapy should be continued for at least 6 weeks postpartum, and longer if required to allow a total duration of

Table 14.7.3 Typical initial doses of LMWH used for treatment of acute venous thromboembolism in pregnancy.

Early pregnancy weight (kg)	Initial dose of enoxaparin (mg, twice daily)
<50	40
50–69 kg	60
70–89 kg	80
≥90 kg[a]	100

[a] In obese patients it is recommended that dose capping is not used.

treatment of 6 months. If the woman chooses to commence warfarin postpartum, this can usually be initiated on the third postnatal day. Switching from LMWH to warfarin can be associated with secondary postpartum haemmorrhage, hence warfarin administration should be delayed further in women with risk of postpartum haemmorrhage.

Massive pulmonary thromboembolism

Intravenous UFH remains the preferred treatment in massive pulmonary thromboembolism because of its rapid effect and extensive experience of its use in this situation. A loading dose of 5000 IU followed by continuous intravenous infusion of 1000 to 2000 IU/h adjusted by the activated partial thromboplastin time (APTT) (target APTT ratio usually 1.5–2.5) monitoring 6 h after the loading dose and then at least daily. However, the APTT is unreliable in pregnancy and an apparent heparin resistance occurs due to the coagulation changes in pregnancy. Anti-Xa monitoring can be used in this situation (target 0.35–0.70 IU/ml—note that this is different for the target used with LMWH due to differences in action of UFH). Thrombolysis can be considered in severe cases.

Women receiving therapeutic-dose UFH should have their platelet count monitored (see above). Pregnant women who develop HIT and require ongoing anticoagulant therapy should be managed with the heparinoid danaparoid sodium, or possibly fondaparinux. Warfarin may also be justified in this situation.

Further reading

Bates SM, et al. (2008). Thromboembolism, thrombophilia, antithrombotic therapy, and Pregnancy, *Chest*, **133**, 844S–886S.

Confidential Enquiry into Maternal and Child Health. *Saving Mothers' Lives: Reviewing Maternal Deaths to Make Motherhood Safer, 2003–2005. The Seventh Report of the Confidential Enquiries into Maternal Deaths in the United Kingdom*. London: CEMACH; 2007 [www.cmace.org.uk/Publications/CEMACHPublications/Maternal-and-Perinatal-Health.aspx].

Gherman RB, et al. (1999). Incidence, clinical characteristics, and timing of objectively diagnosed venous thromboembolism during pregnancy. *Obstet Gynecol*, **94**, 730–4.

Greer IA, Nelson-Piercy C (2005). Low-molecular-weight heparins for thromboprophylaxis and treatment of venous thromboembolism in pregnancy: a systematic review of safety and efficacy. *Blood*, **106**, 401–7.

Greer IA, Thomson AJ (2001). Management of venous thromboembolism in pregnancy. *Best Pract Res Clin Obstet Gynaecol*, **15**, 583–603.

Robertson L, et al. (2006). Thrombophilia in pregnancy: a systematic review. *Br J Haematol*, **132**, 171–96.

Scarsbrook AF, et al. (2006). Diagnosis of suspected venous thromboembolic disease in pregnancy. *Clin Radiol*, **61**, 1–12.

Chest diseases in pregnancy

Minerva Covarrubias and Tina Hartert

Essentials

Respiratory changes in pregnancy include an increase in tidal volume and minute ventilation, leading to a primary respiratory alkalosis. During a normal and uncomplicated pregnancy many women experience the sensation of dyspnea, hence it is important—but sometimes difficult—for the clinician to distinguish breathlessness resulting from normal physiological changes from that caused by underlying medical diseases.

Chest conditions arising in pregnancy—these include (1) amniotic fluid embolism—unique to pregnancy; (2) venous air embolism—a rare condition that can occur in pregnancy; (3) venous and pulmonary thromboembolism—pregnancy is a risk factor (see Chapter 14.7); (4) pulmonary oedema—this can be caused by heart disease, as in the nonpregnant state, but it can also be associated with

pre-eclampsia or HELPP syndrome and be induced by tocolysis; (5) varicella pneumonia—the risk of this potentially devastating complication of primary varicella zoster virus infection (50% require mechanical ventilation, of whom 25% die) occurs particularly in the second or third trimester; (6) influenza—associated with high maternal morbidity.

Pregnancy in women with known chest disorders—(1) asthma—patients with a history of admission to an intensive care unit for asthma, prior mechanical ventilation, or frequent health care visits, are at risk of developing severe or life-threatening asthma exacerbations during pregnancy. The treatment of chronic asthma and acute asthma exacerbations during pregnancy is largely the same as in the nonpregnant state.

Respiratory changes in pregnancy

The respiratory system undergoes many changes during pregnancy, in part as a result of elevated oestrogen and progesterone levels (Fig. 14.8.1).

Chest wall and diaphragm

Changes to the chest wall and diaphragm occur early in pregnancy in response to changing hormone levels and before the uterus is large enough to exert any mechanical effects. The diameter of the chest wall increases, the diaphragm rises up to 4 cm into the chest, and the ligaments of the ribs relax and cause the subcostal angle of the rib cage to increase.

Ventilation and gas exchange

Very early in pregnancy, changes in respiratory drive, ventilation, and gas exchange occur secondary to the stimulatory response from increased progesterone levels. The mechanism by which progesterone affects respiratory drive and ventilation is explained by alterations in the sensitivity of chemoreceptors in the medulla to CO_2: even slight increases in arterial P_{CO_2} will cause an increase in tidal volume. Tidal volume increases up to 40% during pregnancy, resulting in increased minute ventilation. The arterial P_{CO_2} falls

from 40 mmHg (5.3 kPa) in the nongravid patient to approximately 30 mmHg (4.0 kPa) in the pregnant patient, resulting in a primary respiratory alkalosis. In response the kidney excretes bicarbonate to normalize the pH, hence it is usual to see bicarbonate levels of approximately 20 mEq/litre during pregnancy. A second effect of increased minute ventilation is a rise in alveolar and arterial oxygenation that produces arterial P_{O_2} levels ranging from 100 to 110 mmHg (13.3–14.6 kPa).

Lung volumes

As tidal volume increases during pregnancy, the functional residual capacity (FRC) decreases because the diaphragm rises up into the chest, resulting in lower residual and expiratory reserve volumes. The forced expiratory volume in 1 s (FEV_1), FEV_1/forced vital capacity (FVC) ratio, and peak expiratory flow rates (PEFR) are unchanged during pregnancy. Hence a reduction in FEV_1 or FVC should prompt the clinician to seek out underlying pulmonary disease pathology to explain the spirometric changes.

Cardiovascular

As outlined in Fig. 14.8.1, the cardiovascular changes that impact on pulmonary physiology are observed as early as 6 to

The authors wish to acknowledge the editorial assistance of Mr Adam S Morgan.

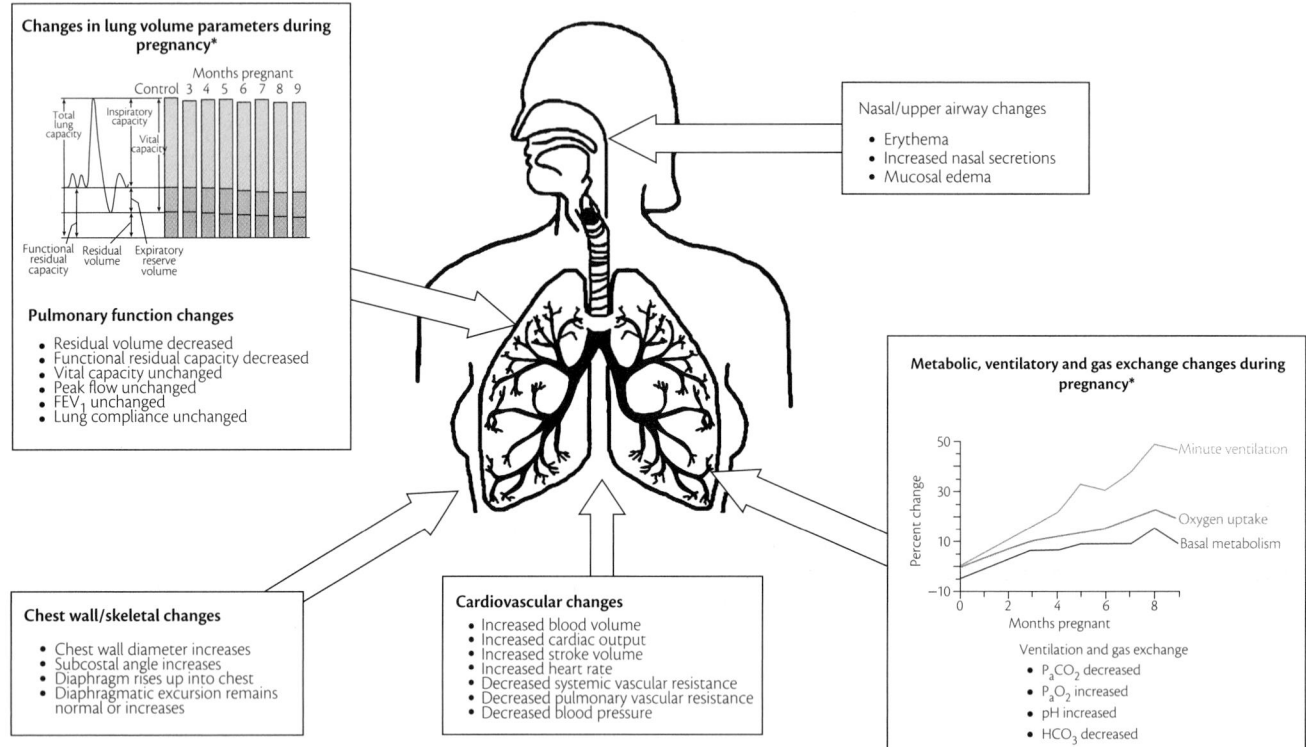

Fig. 14.8.1 Physiological changes of the upper airway, lung, and cardiovascular system during pregnancy that impact signs and symptoms of lung diseases.
*(From Prowse CM, Gaensler EA (1965). Respiratory and acid-base changes during pregnancy. *Anesthesiology*, **26**, 381–92. Top left inset redrawn, with permission.)

8 weeks gestation. There is a 50% increase in blood volume to meet the increased metabolic demands of pregnancy and an increase in cardiac output by 1 to 2 litre/min. Systemic and pulmonary vascular resistances are also reduced.

Respiratory conditions in pregnancy

Up to 70% of women experience the sensation of dyspnoea during a normal and uncomplicated pregnancy, hence it is important for the clinician to distinguish dyspnoea resulting from normal physiological changes of pregnancy from that caused by underlying medical diseases. The obstetric patient presenting with acute onset of shortness of breath requires a careful assessment to exclude life threatening conditions detrimental to the mother or the fetus.

Pregnancy-associated rhinitis

Among the several causes of dyspnoea, an underappreciated condition that may have significant impact on a patient's ability to breathe comfortably is nasal congestion, known as pregnancy-associated rhinitis. Treatment includes raising the head of the bed 30 to 45°, saline nasal spray washings to help clear secretions, and nasal corticosteroids. Nasal sprays containing phenylephrine or oxymetazoline should be used with caution.

Embolic disease

Venous thromboembolism (VTE)

VTE is a significant cause of morbidity and mortality during pregnancy and complicates approximately 1 to 2 out of every 1000 pregnancies. Diagnosing VTE during pregnancy may be challenging since many of the symptoms of VTE in the nongravid patient

can be a part of the normal physiologic changes observed in pregnancy (e.g. tachycardia, dyspnoea, lower extremity oedema). The diagnostic evaluation of VTE in pregnant patients is similar to nonpregnant patients. The PIOPED II recommendations published in December 2006 for suspected pulmonary embolus during pregnancy include D-dimer testing, and if the D-dimer is positive, then venous ultrasonography is the next step before considering imaging tests using radiation. If venous ultrasonography is negative and a significant clinical suspicion for pulmonary embolism exists, then either ventilation–perfusion scan or CT angiogram should be performed. Low molecular weight heparin is the agent of choice for prophylaxis or treatment in most cases. See Chapter 14.7 for further discussion.

Venous air embolism

The postulated mechanism for venous air embolism is air travelling through the placental venous sinuses into the venous circulation, then passing through the right ventricle, and ultimately causing obstruction of the right ventricular outflow tract. The presenting symptoms and signs are dyspnoea, hypotension, tachycardia, tachypnea, a characteristic 'millwheel murmur', or sudden cardiac arrest. Treatment is supportive.

Amniotic fluid embolism (AFE)

AFE is a rare disorder unique to pregnancy. It is thought to occur due to amniotic fluid components entering the maternal circulation, most commonly during labour and delivery or in the immediate postpartum period. The characteristic presentation is rapid onset of severe hypoxic respiratory and/or cardiogenic shock. It may present with a coagulopathy resembling disseminated intravascular coagulation. Diagnosis is clinical, although amniotic fluid elements may be found in sputum or alveolar spaces. Treatment is supportive, focusing on rapid cardiorespiratory stabilization and delivery of the fetus if necessary. Maternal mortality is very high (60–90%).

Acute pulmonary oedema

The incidence of acute pulmonary oedema during pregnancy is about 0.08% (based on the results of a large retrospective study from a single medical centre). In this series, half of all patients developed pulmonary oedema as a result of either cardiac disease or tocolytic therapy: the remaining causes included pre-eclampsia and iatrogenic volume overload.

Cardiogenic pulmonary oedema

Cardiogenic pulmonary oedema can result from established or newly diagnosed cardiac disease. In one large series the development of cardiogenic pulmonary oedema preceded the diagnosis of valvular or myocardial dysfunction in 6 of 13 patients (46%); the 7 cases of acute decompensation in patients with known heart disease occurred in those with aortic valve disease (stenosis or regurgitation), idiopathic subaortic stenosis, and dilated cardiomyopathy. An additional cause of pulmonary oedema is peripartum cardiomyopathy, defined as the development of heart failure in the last month of pregnancy or up to 5 months postpartum in the absence of other causes. See Chapter 14.6 for further discussion.

Pre-eclampsia

The risk of developing pulmonary oedema is highest after delivery when plasma oncotic pressures drop to their lowest values and the distal air spaces of the lung fill with fluid. HELLP syndrome (haemolysis, elevated liver enzymes, and low platelets) can also result in pulmonary oedema. See Chapters 14.4 and 14.9 for further discussion.

Tocolytic-induced pulmonary oedema

Tocolytic-induced pulmonary oedema accounts for about 25% of all cases of pulmonary oedema during pregnancy. Most cases occur in the setting of prolonged systemic β-agonist use for refractory preterm labour. The mechanism is unclear, but it is suspected that changes in haemodynamics as a secondary effect of β-receptor stimulation (i.e. tachycardia and increased stroke volume) accompanied by increased hydrostatic pressures lead to pulmonary oedema. Treatment consists of discontinuing tocolytic agents, oxygen, and diuretics.

Aspiration

During normal pregnancy, decreased oesophageal sphincter tone, delayed gastric emptying, and increased gastric pressures are seen as consequences of the hormonal changes and enlarging uterus. These normal physiological changes place pregnant patients at risk for aspiration. Preventive measures that can be instituted to reduce the risk of aspiration include using regional anaesthesia, gastric acid suppression, and limiting oral intake around the time of labour and delivery.

Asthma

As mentioned previously, FEV_1 is unchanged during pregnancy and should be compared to normal or personal best values, but a recent longitudinal study has suggested that PEFR declines with increasing gestational age and is position dependent. Health surveys from 1997 and 2001 determined that asthma affected up to 8.4% of pregnant women in the United States of America. Potential adverse outcomes of poorly controlled or severe asthma during pregnancy are increased risk of pre eclampsia, low birth weight infants, preterm delivery and perinatal mortality. Patients with a history of admission to an intensive care unit for asthma, prior mechanical ventilation, and frequent health care visits are at risk of developing severe or life-threatening asthma exacerbations during pregnancy. Several studies have demonstrated that optimal management of asthma is associated with improved outcomes.

The principles of managing asthma during pregnancy are not different from those in nongravid women, and management goals focus on controlling symptoms, optimizing pulmonary function, and preventing and appropriately treating exacerbations. The treatment of chronic asthma and acute asthma exacerbations during pregnancy is largely the same as in the nonpregnant state.

Limited information is available regarding the safety and efficacy of asthma medications in pregnant women, primarily because pregnant women are generally excluded from clinical studies. Schatz and colleagues evaluated more than 2000 pregnant women to determine the relationship between asthma medications and adverse outcomes. No significant relationship between adverse outcomes and the use of chronic asthma medications was identified.

Pulmonary infections during pregnancy

Despite new antibiotics and advances in respiratory support, pneumonia during pregnancy is still a significant cause of maternal and fetal morbidity and mortality, even though the incidence is similar to the general population. Respiratory failure due to pneumonia is the third leading indication for intubation during pregnancy. Adverse fetal outcomes include preterm labour, increased need for tocolytics, and lower birth weights.

Community acquired pneumonia (CAP)

The presentation and management of CAP during pregnancy is similar to that in the nonpregnant state. Pneumococcal vaccine has been shown to be effective in decreasing the prevalence of pneumococcal pneumonia in patient populations considered at high risk for mortality from pneumonia: it is recommended for patients considered immunosuppressed (e.g. diabetes mellitus, asthma, chronic obstructive pulmonary disease) and may be given during pregnancy.

Varicella pneumonia

Varicella-zoster virus (VZV) infection in pregnancy is serious for both mother and fetus (see Chapter 14.15). Signs and symptoms of VZV include vesicular rash, dyspnoea, cough, fever, malaise, and pleuritic chest pain. The risk of varicella pneumonia complicating primary VZV infection during pregnancy occurs particularly in the second or third trimester. The diagnosis is usually made clinically; radiographic findings are nonspecific. Samples from vesicular lesions can be sent for polymerase chain reaction or viral culture. IgM antibody may be detected as soon as 3 days, and IgG may be detected as early as 7 days after symptoms appear. The pregnant patient with VZV pneumonia should be treated with aciclovir 10 mg/kg every 8 h intravenously for a minimum of 5 days. Mechanical ventilation may be required in about 50% of patients with varicella pneumonia (25% mortality).

The best method for preventing maternal and fetal complications of VZV infection is preconception counselling and documentation of a history of varicella or presence of serum varicella antibodies (IgG). If either of these conditions is not met, then varicella vaccination is recommended before pregnancy, preferably 1 to 3 months before conception. Varicella vaccination is not recommended for use during pregnancy. Pregnant women without evidence of immunity to VZV who are at high risk for severe disease and who have been exposed to VZV are eligible to receive varicella zoster immune globulin, which is recommended by the United States Advisory Committee on Immunization Practices.

Influenza

Influenza A and B are common causes of respiratory illness, with influenza A being the most virulent strain in humans. During the influenza season pregnant women have over fivefold higher influenza-related morbidity compared to nongravid women, and also increased mortality during pandemic years.

Vaccination against influenza is able to prevent illness in 70 to 90% of healthy adults less than 65 years of age during the influenza season, and no adverse fetal outcomes have been identified in women who received the inactivated vaccine during pregnancy. Influenza vaccine is recommended for all women pregnant during the influenza season, regardless of trimester.

Antiviral medications are effective in preventing and treating the two most common types of influenza illness. Administered within the first 48 h from the onset of symptoms, the neuraminidase inhibitors (zanamivir, oseltamivir) are effective in shortening the course of symptoms and decreasing viral load. These antiviral medications are classified as category C, US FDA (Food and Drug Administration) pregnancy risk category, indicating that risks of using them in pregnancy cannot be excluded since human studies are lacking. The benefits of therapy may outweigh the risks depending on the clinical scenario.

Coccidioidomycosis pneumonia

Fungal pneumonias during pregnancy are rare, but in the setting of disseminated disease carry an increased risk of maternal mortality, preterm births, and perinatal mortality. Coccidioidomycosis is primarily found in semiarid areas in the western hemisphere, such as the south-western portion of the United States, central and northern areas of Mexico, and endemic pockets in Central and South America. Coccidioidomycosis pneumonia tends to occur in the third trimester of pregnancy. For patients with severe pneumonia or disseminated disease, amphotericin B is recommended, followed by oral antifungals such as fluconazole after delivery. In pregnant women without pre-existing medical diseases, coccidioidomycosis pneumonia usually resolves on its own regardless of whether or not treatment is given.

Mechanical ventilation during pregnancy

The physiological changes of pregnancy need to be considered when optimizing pulmonary mechanics and gas exchange during mechanical ventilation. Pregnant women normally exhibit a respiratory alkalosis with a mean baseline arterial pH of 7.44 and an arterial CO_2 of approximately 32 mmHg (4.3 kPa), and this level of CO_2 should be considered the target during mechanical ventilation. Animal studies suggest that overventilation to an arterial partial pressure of CO_2 significantly below this level may compromise uterine blood flow and should be avoided. The strategy of permissive hypercapnoea, which may be necessary when ventilation is difficult, does not appear to have adverse effects on the fetus, at least to a CO_2 level of 60 mmHg (8 kPa). Adequate fetal oxygenation requires an arterial oxygen tension of at least 70 mmHg (9.3 kPa), which corresponds to a maternal oxygen saturation of 95%.

Further reading

Physiology of pregnancy

Gilroy RJ, Mangura BT, Lavietes MH (1988). Rib cage and abdominal volume displacements during breathing in pregnancy. *Am Rev Resp Dis*, **137**, 668–72.

Lim VS, Katz AI, Lindheimer MD (1976). Acid-base regulation in pregnancy. *Am J Physiol*, **231**, 1764–9.

Pernoll ML, *et al.* (1975). Ventilation during rest and exercise in pregnancy and postpartum. *Resp Physiol*, **25**, 295–310.

Prowse CM, Gaensler EA (1965). Respiratory and acid-base changes during pregnancy. *Anesthesiology*, **26**, 381–92.

Embolic disease

Clark SL, *et al.* (1995). Amniotic fluid embolism: analysis of the national registry. *Am Jo Obstet Gynecol*, **172**, 1158–67.

James AH, *et al.* (2006). Venous thromboembolism during pregnancy and the postpartum period: incidence, risk factors, and mortality. *Am J Obstet Gynecol*, **194**, 1311–15.

Acute pulmonary oedema

Pisani RJ, Rosenow EC, III (1989). Pulmonary edema associated with tocolytic therapy. *Ann Inter Med*, **110**, 714–18.

Asthma

National Asthma and Education Prevention Program (NAEPP) working group report on managing asthma during pregnancy: recommendations for pharmacologic treatment. NIH Publication No. 05-5236. http://www.nhlbi.nih.gov/health/prof/lung/asthma/astpreg/astpreg_full.pdf

Schatz M, *et al.* (2004). The relationship of asthma medication use to perinatal outcomes. *J Allergy Clin Immunol*, **113**, 1040–5.

Pulmonary infections during pregnancy

Harger JH, *et al.* (2002). Risk factors and outcome of varicella-zoster virus pneumonia in pregnant women. *J Infect Dis*, **185**, 422–7.

Hartert TV, *et al.* (2003). Maternal morbidity and perinatal outcomes among pregnant women with respiratory hospitalizations during influenza season. *Am J Obstet Gynecol*, **189**, 1705–12.

Martin SR, Foley MR (2006). Intensive care in obstetrics: an evidence-based review. *Am J Obstet Gynecol*, **195**, 673–89.

Pastuszak AL, *et al.* (1994). Outcome after maternal varicella infection in the first 20 weeks of pregnancy. *N Engl J Med*, **330**, 901–5.

Liver and gastrointestinal diseases in pregnancy

Alexander Gimson

Essentials

Liver and gastrointestinal diseases unique to pregnancy

Hyperemesis gravidarum—a condition of unknown cause where severe vomiting can lead to volume depletion, ketonuria, electrolyte disturbances, and nutritional deficiency. Management is supportive.

Intrahepatic cholestasis of pregnancy—a common cause of jaundice in pregnancy, presenting in the second or third trimester, usually with pruritus. Serum bilirubin and aminotransferases may be elevated, with no significant rise in alkaline phosphatase (beyond the normal elevation expected in pregnancy) or γ-glutamyl transpeptidase. Serum bile acids increase 3- to 100-fold. The cause is unknown, but there is marked geographical variation. Treatment is symptomatic with the bile salt ursodeoxycholic acid, and most obstetric physicians recommend delivery at 38 weeks to prevent late fetal complications.

Acute fatty liver of pregnancy—a rare complication that usually arises between 34 and 36 weeks of gestation. Often associated with features of pre-eclampsia, with peripheral oedema, hypertension and proteinuria, and occasionally the HELLP syndrome (haemolysis, elevated liver enzymes and low platelet count). Some cases may be due to abnormalities of mitochondrial fatty acid oxidation. The most important component of management is early delivery of the fetus.

In association with hypertension—abnormalities of liver blood tests have been described in three clinical syndromes associated with high blood pressure in pregnancy: (1) pre-eclampsia/eclampsia—see Chapter 14.4. (2) HELLP syndrome—diagnosis requires haemolysis with a characteristic peripheral blood smear, serum lactate dehydrogenase 600 U/litre or more, serum aspartate aminotransferase 70 U/litre or more, and platelet count less than 100×10^9/litre. Usually presents in the second or third trimester. Maternal complications and perinatal mortality are common. Management of the coexisting pre-eclampsia is crucial, with seizure prophylaxis using magnesium sulphate and blood pressure control. Aside from signs of significant fetal distress, indications for urgent delivery include persistent severe right upper quadrant or shoulder tip pain, often associated with hypotension and thrombocytopenia, which indicate possible liver haematoma or impending rupture. (3) Spontaneous hepatic rupture.

Differential diagnosis of liver diseases associated with pregnancy—it can be difficult to distinguish acute fatty liver of pregnancy, pre-eclampsia, and HELLP syndrome. The size of the liver, degree of hyperbilirubinaemia, abnormalities on peripheral blood film, presence of hypoglycaemia, and disseminated intravascular coagulation are the most discriminatory features.

Other liver and gastrointestinal diseases in pregnancy

When dealing with a pregnant woman with liver disease it is important to remember that pregnancy does not protect against conditions that are common in those who are not pregnant. Acute viral hepatitis is the most common cause of jaundice during pregnancy: the outcome is the same as in patients who are not pregnant, with the notable exception of hepatitis E (20% mortality in pregnancy).

Introduction

This chapter discusses gastrointestinal and liver diseases specific to pregnancy, those occurring with increased frequency during pregnancy, and those already present at conception or arising coincidentally during the course of pregnancy (Table 14.9.1). Liver or gastrointestinal dysfunction is present in fewer than 5% of pregnancies in Europe and the United States of America, but their recognition and management is important because increased maternal and fetal morbidity and mortality may result without prompt intervention.

There are significant physiological changes in hepatic function during pregnancy. The increased circulating blood volume and cardiac output are not associated with any changes in hepatic blood flow, but there is increased azygous flow that results rarely in

Table 14.9.1 Liver diseases during pregnancy

Diseases specific to pregnancy	Hyperemesis gravidarum
	Intrahepatic cholestasis of pregnancy
	Acute fatty liver of pregnancy
	Hypertension-associated liver diseases of pregnancy
Diseases where pregnancy increases frequency or severity of presentation	Budd–Chiari syndrome—increased frequency, possibly related to low antithrombin III levels
	Acute cholecystitis—increased risk of gallstones/complications
	Acute viral hepatitis E—increased frequency of acute liver failure in the third trimester
	Hepatic tumours—vascular hepatic tumours may enlarge and rupture
	Variceal haemorrhage—more common in non-cirrhotic portal hypertension
Liver diseases manifesting during but unrelated to pregnancy	Acute viral hepatitis A, B, cytomegalovirus, Epstein–Barr virus
	Chronic liver diseases
	Drug hepatotoxicity

the formation of small oesophageal varices. Gallbladder motility is reduced and bile lithogenicity increased due to increased hepatic cholesterol synthesis and excretion into bile. Minor but important changes in laboratory blood tests occur due to haemodilution or alteration in hepatic synthesis (Table 14.9.2).

Increased gastric myoelectric activity may be manifest as nausea and vomiting, but there are few other significant changes in gastrointestinal function during normal pregnancy.

Table 14.9.2 Effects of pregnancy on laboratory blood tests

Parameter	Effect	Trimester with maximum change	Mechanism
Bilirubin	Nil	–	–
AST/ALT	Nil	–	–
Bile salts	Nil	–	–
5-Nucleotidase	Nil	–	–
γ-Glutamyl transpeptidase	Nil	–	–
Alkaline phosphatase	+100–300%	3rd	Increased bone/placental isoenzyme
Albumin	−10–60%	2nd	Dilution, reduced synthesis
Gammaglobulin	−10%	2nd	Dilution
Fibrinogen	+50%	2nd	Increased hepatic synthesis
Cholesterol	+100%	3rd	Increased hepatic synthesis

Liver diseases specific to pregnancy

Hyperemesis gravidarum

Although nausea and vomiting may occur in up to 75% of pregnancies, severe vomiting leading to dehydration, ketonuria, electrolyte disturbances, and nutritional deficiency is rare, developing in 2 to 16 of every 1000 pregnancies. Nutritional deficiency has been so severe as to progress to Wernicke's encephalopathy and changes in serum sodium may precipitate osmotic demyelination (central pontine myelinolysis). This is more common in younger women, in obesity, and in those with pre-existing diabetes or gastrointestinal disorders; recent surveys do not suggest any relationship with parity or gravidity. Elevated transaminases, by two- to threefold, occur in 50% of cases, with a minor rise in alkaline phosphatase and bilirubin in 10%. Liver histology shows few abnormalities or hepatic steatosis only. The aetiology is unclear and may be multifactorial: positive helicobacter serology has been reported in up to 90% of cases, and changes in thyroid function are present in 50%. An elevated free thyroxin (T_4) with suppressed thyroid-stimulating hormone (TSH) correlates with elevated human chorionic gonadotrophin (hCG) levels in these patients, raising the possibility that gestational thyrotoxicosis may also have role in pathogenesis. In some cases psychological factors are also important.

Management, which may require hospitalization, is symptomatic and includes rehydration and correction of nutritional deficiencies. Psychological support is crucial. Treatment of symptomatic gastro-oesophageal reflux is important and antiemetics are required, with metoclopramide and promethazine as effective as newer 5-HT_3 antagonists. There are uncontrolled reports and a single controlled trial demonstrating benefit with corticosteroids. In rare cases there may be recurrence in subsequent pregnancies.

Intrahepatic cholestasis of pregnancy

This cholestatic disorder of the second and third trimesters is the most common cause of jaundice during pregnancy, after acute viral hepatitis. Initially starting with pruritus, jaundice follows after 1 to 4 weeks in 20 to 60% of cases, associated with pale stools and dark urine. Diagnosis is by history and the classic biochemical features of an elevated bilirubin (<100 µmol/litre) and increased aminotransferases (rarely >250 IU/litre), with no significant rise in alkaline phosphatase (beyond the normal elevation expected in pregnancy) or γ-glutamyl transpeptidase. Serum bile acids increase 3- to 100-fold, those factors with the highest predictive diagnostic value being total bile acid concentration of more than 11.0 µmol/litre and a cholic/chenodeoxycholic acid ratio of more than 1.5 with a cholic acid percentage over 42. In a large cohort study fetal complications were most common in those cases with bile acid level greater than 40 µmol/l. An ultrasound scan is necessary to exclude choledocholithiasis, and further imaging of the bile duct with magnetic resonance cholangiopancreatography will occasionally be needed. A liver biopsy is not required for diagnosis, but shows a canalicular cholestasis with no hepatocellular necrosis.

The epidemiology of intrahepatic cholestasis of pregnancy is interesting, with marked geographical variation. The highest incidence, over 10%, has been recorded in Arauncanian Indians in Chile, with 2 to 3% in Sweden and 0.1% in Canada. It is rare in Afro-Caribbeans. It is more common in women with a history of contraceptive pill induced jaundice (50%) and those with benign recurrent intrahepatic cholestasis who have multiple gestations, and it may be more common in women who are positive for hepatitis C virus antibodies. In France it has been associated with use of progesterone in early pregnancy.

The aetiology is unknown, but one hypothesis suggests enhanced sensitivity of components of the bile salt excretion apparatus to oestrogen: pregnancy impairs sulphation of both monohydroxy bile salts and oestrogen, which may enhance the cholestatic potential of both compounds. Family studies have suggested a dominant mode of transmission in a few kindreds. Mutations in the *MDR3* gene (*ABCB4*) that encodes an ATP-dependent transporter of phosphatidylcholine across the canalicular membrane occur more commonly in those with the severe form of the disease.

Intrahepatic cholestasis of pregnancy is associated with an increased incidence of fetal prematurity (fivefold increase), fetal distress, stillbirths, and meconium staining of amniotic fluid (1.5-fold increase), but perinatal mortality is normal with modern management. Reports of maternal morbidity from postpartum haemorrhage relate to vitamin K deficiency and are not a feature of recent series.

Treatment is symptomatic, with the bile salt ursodeoxycholic acid (10–15 mg/kg per day) the treatment of choice and better than *S*-adenosylmethionine. Ursodeoxycholic acid relieves pruritus, reduces bile salt levels in maternal serum, and may reduce the frequency of fetal complications. Both bile salt sequestration with cholestyramine and dexamethasone have given variable results. Vitamin K should be given before delivery.

Most authors recommend elective delivery at 38 weeks to prevent late fetal complications, and this has been shown to improve fetal outcome. More recently there have been suggestions that a policy of careful observation and induction of labour only for fetal distress may be used in those with lower bile acid levels, but there is anxiety that classical markers of fetal distress may not be adequate in this setting.

Intrahepatic cholestasis of pregnancy recurs in up to 60 to 80% of subsequent pregnancies and is associated with a late increased incidence of gallstones. Oral contraceptives should be used with caution, although early reports of liver abnormalities were predominantly with high-dose pills and combined low-dose preparations may cause fewer problems.

Acute fatty liver of pregnancy

Acute fatty liver of pregnancy, a microvesicular steatosis during the last trimester of pregnancy, was first adequately described by Sheehan in 1940. Occurring in 1 in 14 000 pregnancies between the 34th and 36th weeks, it is more common in primigravidae, with male fetuses, and with twin pregnancies. Up to 40% may have associated features of pre-eclampsia, with peripheral oedema, hypertension, and proteinuria, and occasionally the HELLP syndrome (haemolysis, elevated liver enzymes and low platelet count; see below). Acute fatty liver of pregnancy occurs only rarely before the third trimester, but postpartum presentations are well recorded. Initial symptoms are of headache, fatigue, nausea, and vomiting with abdominal discomfort. In severe cases jaundice develops within 14 days. This may progress to manifest all the features of acute liver failure, including coma, renal failure and death. However, less severe cases are now described more commonly, with recent series reporting a 10 to 20% fetal and maternal mortality.

The cause of many cases of acute fatty liver of pregnancy may be a fetal–maternal interaction resulting from abnormalities of mitochondrial fatty acid oxidation, more commonly with long than medium or short chain defects. A mutation involving substitution of glutamine for glutamic acid at amino acid residue 474 of the α subunit of long-chain 3-hydroxyacyl-CoA dehydrogenase, an enzyme that forms one component of a trifunctional protein catalysing the last three steps in the β-oxidation of fatty acids within mitochondria, has been found in up to 20% of pregnancies in this condition. Up to 80% of heterozygote mothers carrying fetuses with long-chain 3-hydroxyacyl-CoA dehydrogenase deficiency may develop either acute fatty liver of pregnancy or HELLP syndrome. Mitochondrial oxidation of fatty acids is already impaired during pregnancy, mediated by oestrogen and progesterone, and long-chain 3-hydroxyacyl metabolites produced by the fetus can accumulate and be toxic to the liver. Because presentation of children with long-chain 3-hydroxyacyl-CoA dehydrogenase deficiency may occur late after birth, with nonketotic hypoglycaemia and sudden infant death, the early identification and treatment of such cases is important. For this reason diagnostic molecular testing is recommended on all mothers and offspring of acute fatty liver of pregnancy and HELLP pregnancies.

The important differential diagnosis is between acute viral hepatitis with liver failure, acute fatty liver of pregnancy, and hypertension-associated liver dysfunction of pregnancy. The presence of features of pre-eclampsia in up to 40% may make this distinction difficult. In acute fatty liver of pregnancy transaminases are elevated to less than 500 IU/litre, in contrast to viral hepatitis where values are usually higher. Hypoglycaemia is more common in acute fatty liver of pregnancy than in pre-eclampsia, and a blood film commonly showing neutrophilia, normoblasts, thrombocytopenia, target cells and giant platelets may also help to make the diagnosis of acute fatty liver of pregnancy. Prothrombin and partial thromboplastin times are prolonged with low antithrombin III levels. Although hepatic steatosis in acute fatty liver of pregnancy may be detected by ultrasonography, CT scanning is more sensitive with attenuation values less than half normal and less than spleen, the reverse of normal. Hyperuricaemia is present in 80%, but is not pathognomonic as this may also be found in pre-eclampsia.

Despite all these biochemical and radiological tests, and because differentiation of acute fatty liver of pregnancy from acute viral hepatitis and hypertension-associated liver diseases is important in assessing the prognosis for future pregnancies, a liver biopsy may be necessary to distinguish between these three diagnoses. Histology demonstrates a microvesicular fat deposition with rare hepatocyte necrosis and minimal inflammation, a pattern similar to that seen in Reye's syndrome, tetracycline and sodium valproate hepatotoxicity, Jamaican vomiting sickness due to a toxin in unripe ackee fruit, some urea cycle enzyme deficiencies, and defects in mitochondrial fatty acid oxidation.

Other obstetric causes of renal failure that are associated with minor changes in liver blood tests rarely need to be considered. These include thrombotic thrombocytopenic purpura and haemolytic uraemic syndrome. The former is particularly associated with neurological signs, including epileptic fits, without evidence of disseminated intravascular coagulation, whereas haemolytic uraemic syndrome may occur postpartum and with microangiopathic anaemia.

After the diagnosis of acute fatty liver of pregnancy has been established, the most important component of management is early delivery of the fetus. A policy of careful monitoring has been proposed for the mildest cases, but extreme caution is required as deterioration can be sudden and unpredictable. Vaginal delivery can be tried first, but caesarean section will usually require general anaesthesia as a spinal anaesthetic in the presence of coagulation deficits is dangerous. Hypoglycaemia is prevented by intravenous dextrose infusion; aggressive correction of coagulation abnormalities with fresh frozen plasma, cryoprecipitate, and antithrombin III has also been recommended. Liver transplantation has been used (very rarely) for cases failing to respond to early delivery and intensive care.

The risk of recurrence of acute fatty liver of pregnancy is very low, the few recorded cases most probably being due to associated recurrent metabolic defects in the fetus.

Hypertension-associated liver diseases of pregnancy

Hypertension occurs in up to 8% of pregnancies and is the most common cause of maternal mortality in developed countries. Abnormalities of liver blood tests have been described in three clinical syndromes associated with hypertension in pregnancy: pre-eclampsia/eclampsia, spontaneous hepatic rupture, and the HELLP syndrome.

Pre-eclampsia/eclampsia

Pre-eclampsia is discussed in detail in Chapter 14.4. There are abnormalities of liver biochemistry in up to 25% of mild cases and up to 80% of those with severe disease, i.e. those with renal impairment, visual disturbance, headache, fits, and the onset of eclampsia. The usual abnormality is a rise in transaminases, with jaundice occurring only in the most severe cases. The alanine aminotransferase levels are usually less than 150 IU/litre, lower than in acute fatty liver of pregnancy, and bilirubin is less than 100 μmol/litre. Changes in coagulation parameters, with elevated d-dimers, reflect the intravascular activation and consumption of clotting factors. Antithrombin III levels are low. Liver histology in the early stages shows few changes except for deposition of fibrinogen within sinusoids and the space of Disse. Blockage of sinusoids by fibrin may progress to frank infarction of hepatic parenchyma, when the low levels of coagulation factors may then predispose to haemorrhage into these infarcted areas. This combination of infarcts and associated haemorrhage, often covert and without apparent clinical consequence, may be demonstrated on ultrasound or CT scan of the liver.

The management of liver dysfunction in this context is that for pre-eclampsia, with correction of hypertension and coagulation defects, early delivery being the most important aspect. Anticonvulsant prophylaxis must be considered. Very close fetal monitoring is important. Liver biochemistry improves after delivery, but a late cholestatic phase with rise in alkaline phosphatase and γ-glutamyl transpeptidase is common.

Spontaneous hepatic rupture

Spontaneous rupture of the liver is fortunately rare, occurring in 1 in 100 000 deliveries. In 80% of cases liver haematomas, segmental or larger infarcts, and rupture occur in patients with severe pre-eclampsia and eclampsia: the remainder occur in association with acute fatty liver of pregnancy, or underlying hepatic adenomata, hepatocellular carcinoma, haemangioma, choriocarcinoma, or liver abscess.

The classical presentation is with right upper quadrant pain, nausea, vomiting and hypotension in an older woman with severe pre-eclampsia during the third trimester. Right upper quadrant tenderness may be associated with frank peritonism where rupture into the peritoneum has occurred. The diagnosis can be confirmed by ultrasonography or CT scanning. Treatment is conservative if possible, starting with angiography and hepatic artery embolization, proceeding to laparotomy, use of collagen meshes, and hepatic artery ligation if necessary. Successful orthotopic liver transplantation has been performed, but associated coagulation abnormalities are difficult to manage. The baby should be delivered by caesarean section. Successful subsequent pregnancies are recorded, as is recurrent haemorrhage, hence careful monitoring of any future pregnancy is necessary.

Haemolysis, elevated liver enzymes, and low platelet count (HELLP syndrome)

Weinstein first described a syndrome of haemolysis, elevated liver enzymes, and a low platelet count in patients with severe pre-eclampsia or eclampsia. HELLP syndrome occurs in 10% of pregnancies with severe pre-eclampsia. Strict criteria should be used for the diagnosis: haemolysis with a characteristic peripheral blood smear, serum lactate dehydrogenase 600 U/litre or more, serum aspartate aminotransferase 70 U/litre or more, and platelet count less than 100×10^9/litre. An abnormal peripheral blood smear with fractured red blood cells (schistocytes, echinocytes, spherostomatocytes) is sensitive but not specific for HELLP, and the elevated serum lactate dehydrogenase is simply another indicator of haemolysis. Some cases display only one or two of the above criteria and have been labelled as having partial HELLP: these have been shown to follow a less severe clinical course. HELLP syndrome has also been classified (by Martin and colleagues) according to platelet count: in class 1 the platelet count is 50×10^9/litre or less, in class 2 it is 50 to 100×10^9/litre, and in class 3 more than 100×10^9/litre, which is equivalent to partial HELLP.

The reason why some cases with severe pre-eclampsia progress to HELLP syndrome is not clear. The haemolysis is clearly related to intravascular deposition of thrombin and mechanical fracture of red cells, and there is fibrin deposition obstructing hepatic sinusoids, but the factors causing particular damage to the hepatic microcirculation are unknown. Overt disseminated intravascular coagulation is not usually a major component: when defined as hypofibrinogenaemia (<300 mg/dl) and elevated d-dimers (>40 μg/ml) it occurred in 21% of a series of 442 cases. Compared with other cases with severe pre-eclampsia, those with HELLP syndrome tend to be older, white, and multiparous. HELLP may be more common in mothers heterozygous for thrombophilic states.

Symptoms usually start in the second or third trimester, with 15% starting prior to 26 weeks and 30% only developing symptoms after delivery. HELLP syndrome has protean manifestations but universal early symptoms include malaise and fatigue, followed by nausea, vomiting, and headache shortly thereafter (Table 14.9.3). Epigastric and right upper quadrant pain are ominous signs, particularly when accompanied by right shoulder tip pain. Weight gain and peripheral oedema are found in 50%, with diastolic blood pressure 90 mmHg or more in all but a small minority.

Table 14.9.3 Clinical features and complications of hypertension-associated liver diseases

	HELLP syndrome		Pre-eclampsia	
	Martin et al. (1999)	Sibai et al. (1993)	Audibert et al. (1996)	Martin et al. (1999)
Symptoms (%)				
Nausea/vomiting	35	36	5	15
Headache	61	31	40	68
Epigastric/abdominal pain	50	65	5	13
Maternal complications (%)				
None	51		91	89
Haematological/DIC	32	21	0	1
Cardiopulmonary	22	6	1	10
Renal	3	8	0	0
Neurological/Ophthalmic	4.5	2	0	1
Hepatic	1.5	1	0	0
Obstetric complications (%)				
Eclampsia	13	8	9	5
Placental abruption	3	16	5	1
Perinatal mortality/1000 births	119	–	–	57

DIC, disseminated intravascular coagulation.

The fall in platelet count and rise in transaminases usually reach their nadir in the first 2 days postpartum. Aspartate aminotransferase and lactate dehydrogenase are elevated in unison, along with other markers of hepatocellular or sinusoidal cell dysfunction, glutathione-S-transferase and hyaluronic acid.

Maternal complications associated with HELLP syndrome occur in up to 50% of cases. Blood transfusion to correct hypovolaemia, anaemia, or coagulopathy is required in 50%, with features of disseminated intravascular coagulation in 25%, and pleural effusions or pulmonary oedema in 15 to 20%. Renal failure due to acute tubular necrosis may occur in 3 to 8%. Obstetric complications are also associated with the degree of fall in platelet counts, with placental abruption (16%) and wound haematomas after caesarean section the most prevalent. Eclampsia is approximately two to three times more common in patients with class 1 HELLP than in those with milder varieties, and consistent with this the maternal mortality was 1.5% in a large series, with a perinatal mortality in Martin et al.'s tertiary referral practice of 119/1000 infants. Overall perinatal mortality is strongly related to time of delivery, with rates as high as 30% in some series, although this may be due to case selection. Mortality was 9.5% in a large series assessing class 1, 2, and 3 cases. Preterm infants born before 32 weeks from mothers with HELLP syndrome had a higher frequency of severe intraventricular haemorrhage than other preterm infants.

Birth weights tend to be lower in severe HELLP than in pre-eclampsia alone.

Preterm patients with HELLP syndrome should be treated at a referral centre with appropriate obstetric, anaesthetic, and haematological support. Management of the coexisting pre-eclampsia is crucial, with seizure prophylaxis using magnesium sulphate and blood pressure control with labetolol, ketanserin, or hydrallazine if blood pressure is more than 160/105 mmHg. Antenatal corticosteroids enhance fetal lung maturity if the pregnancy is of less than 32 weeks gestation. Careful fluid resuscitation is required to prevent volume overload, particularly in the presence of renal impairment, as is very close fetal monitoring.

Aside from signs of significant fetal distress, indications for urgent delivery include persistent severe right upper quadrant or shoulder tip pain, often associated with hypotension and thrombocytopenia, which indicate possible liver haematoma or impending rupture. Early delivery, at the safest time for mother and fetus, is strongly recommended in the absence of treatment that unequivocally improves the haematological abnormalities and both maternal and fetal outcome. Although arguments have been put forward for a more conservative approach in patients with mild disease—with careful monitoring of coagulation profiles, fetal growth and well-being, and with the timing of delivery depending on clinical judgement—this management strategy is not without risk and has not been examined in a randomized controlled trial.

Attempts have been made to improve the outcome of HELLP with medical management alone in an effort to buy time to enhance fetal maturity and to improve the mother's clinical condition prior to delivery. Although plasma volume expansion, antithrombotic agents, plasma exchange and corticosteroids have all been advocated, no therapies have been shown to allow safe deferral of delivery and improve outcome. In one study dexamethasone given before delivery resulted in a modest prolongation of pregnancy, whereas two other trials showed significant improvements in haematological and biochemical parameters when this was given postpartum. In a trial of invasive haemodynamic monitoring, plasma volume expansion and afterload reduction, laboratory parameters improved with prolongation of gestation by 21 days, but no significant change in perinatal mortality.

Recurrence of HELLP syndrome in subsequent pregnancies is uncommon: it recurred in only 5% of a series of 139 normotensive women after an index pregnancy with HELLP syndrome, despite 25% developing pre-eclampsia. In hypertensive cases a further pregnancy was associated with pre-eclampsia in 70% and HELLP syndrome in 8%.

Differential diagnosis of jaundice during pregnancy

Many patients with acute fatty liver of pregnancy have signs of pre-eclampsia and such cases may be part of a clinical syndrome that includes hypertension-associated liver diseases. Evidence for this possibility includes the finding of microvesicular hepatic steatosis in cases with pre-eclampsia; indeed one study found fat deposition by special staining in all 41 cases examined. Histological evidence of both pre-eclampsia and acute fatty liver of pregnancy has also been demonstrated in some cases, and pregnancies associated with pre-eclampsia have been followed in the next by HELLP syndrome.

Table 14.9.4 Clinical features and laboratory variables in acute fatty liver of pregnancy, HELLP syndrome, and pre-eclampsia

	Acute fatty liver of pregnancy	HELLP	Severe pre-eclampsia
Frequency	1/13 000	4/1000	7/100
Clinical features	Nausea/vomiting (70%)	Malaise/lethargy (90%)	Oedema (80%)
Examination	RUQ pain (65%)	Nausea/vomiting (35%)	Weight gain (75%)
	Small liver	Oedema/weight gain (60%)	RUQ tenderness
	Jaundice	RUQ tenderness (80%)	Mental status changes
	Encephalopathy later	Hypertension (80%)	
	Hypertension 40%	Liver normal size	
Investigations	Leucocytosis	Bilirubin <100 μmol/litre	Bilirubin variable
	Bilirubin >100 μmol/litre	ALT 150 IU/litre	ALT 150–200 IU/litre (unless infarction)
	ALT 300 IU/litre	Hypoglycaemia rare	DIC 7%
	Hypoglycaemia	DIC 25%	
	DIC 75%		
Maternal mortality	<20%	1.5%	<1%
Fetal mortality	15%	35%	–
Recurrence	Very rare	4–8%	25%

ALT, serum alanine aminotransferase; DIC, disseminated intravascular coagulation; RUQ, right upper quadrant.

Despite this there are usually features in the clinical history or laboratory findings (Table 14.9.4) that allow discrimination between these diagnoses. The size of the liver, degree of hyperbilirubinaemia, abnormalities on peripheral blood film, presence of hypoglycaemia, and disseminated intravascular coagulation are the most discriminatory tests. The differential diagnosis of jaundice and abnormal liver blood tests differs in the three trimesters of pregnancy (Table 14.9.5).

Liver diseases that are commoner in pregnancy

Budd–Chiari syndrome

Thrombosis in one or more hepatic veins has an increased prevalence during pregnancy and in those on the oral contraceptive pill. This relates to low antithrombin III levels and may be more common in those with an underlying procoagulant state or presence of antiphospholipid antibodies. Right upper quadrant pain, hepatomegaly and maternal ascites should suggest the diagnosis, with confirmation by ultrasonography or hepatic venous angiography. Although hepatic venous balloon dilatation or insertion of a transjugular intrahepatic stent shunt has been recommended for Budd–Chiari syndrome, there are few data on their use during pregnancy. Maternal mortality remains very high.

Cholelithiasis

Gallbladder sludge and gallstones develop in 31% and 9% of pregnancies respectively, although most resolve thereafter. Prior use of oral contraceptives, increased cholesterol synthesis, reduced cholesterol carriage in bile, and impaired gallbladder motility all account for the increased lithogenicity of bile. Symptomatic gallstone disease should be managed in the usual way. Magnetic resonance cholangiopancreatography (MRCP) can accurately

detect common bile duct stones without exposing the fetus to radiation, with endoscopic sphincterotomy and/or stent placement reserved for those in whom they are detected. In most cases surgery can be deferred until after delivery.

Other hepatological conditions in pregnancy

Viral hepatitis

Acute viral hepatitis is the most common cause of jaundice during pregnancy (Table 14.9.5), with no specific change to presentation, clinical course or outcome for acute hepatitis A, B, cytomegalovirus, or Epstein–Barr virus infection.

Transmission of virus from a mother with acute hepatitis B to her child occurs in 50% of cases, rising to 70% when hepatitis starts in the third trimester. Transmission of virus from mothers with chronic hepatitis B carriage is less common, but depends on the level of viral replication. The rate is at least 90% in those who are hepatitis B virus DNA positive, and who are usually hepatitis B e antigen positive, as is most common in East Asians. Following vertical transmission up to 80% of offspring become chronic HBsAg carriers. Transmission of hepatitis B can be effectively interrupted by use of hepatitis B immunoglobulin at birth, with hepatitis B virus vaccination within 7 days and at 1, 2, and 12 months.

Transmission of hepatitis C from chronic carriers occurs in up to 8% of cases, being higher in those with high maternal viral load. Hepatitis C virus antibody seroconversion of infants following transmission may take 6 to 12 months to appear, but detection of hepatitis C virus RNA by polymerase chaine reaction allows detection of transmission sooner.

Acute hepatitis E is due to an RNA virus and occurs, often in waterborne epidemics, predominantly in the Middle East and East Asia. In pregnancy it is associated with a mortality of up to 20%

Table 14.9.5 Differential diagnosis of abnormal liver blood tests during pregnancy

Diagnosis	Frequency	Clinical features, diagnostic criteria, and investigations
First trimester		
Acute viral hepatitis	As general population	IgM anti-HAV, IgM anti-HBc, IgM anti-HEV CMV PCR, EBV serology, IgM anti-herpes simplex
Cholelithiasis	Unknown	RUQ pain, fever, gallstones/dilated common bile duct on USS/MRCP for choledocholithiasis
Drug-induced hepatotoxicity	Unknown	Drug history
Hyperemesis gravidarum	0.3–1%	Young, overweight, multiple births. ALT <200 IU/litre. Low TSH in 50%
Intrahepatic cholestasis of pregnancy	0.1%	Pruritus. ALT <300 IU/l, bilirubin <100 μmol/litre, bile acids × 30–100
Second trimester		
Acute viral hepatitis	As general population	As for first trimester
Cholelithiasis	Unknown	As for first trimester
Drug hepatotoxicity	Unknown	As for first trimester
Intrahepatic cholestasis of pregnancy	0.1%	As for first trimester
Pre-eclampsia–eclampsia[a]	5–10%	Lethargy (90%), weight gain, hypertension. Bilirubin <100 μmol/litre, ALT 150–300 IU/litre unless infarction. Hypoglycaemia rare, DIC 7%
HELLP syndrome[a]	0.1%	RUQ pain, vomiting, haemolysis (LDH >600 IU/litre, blood film), ALT >70 IU/litre, platelets <100, bilirubin <100 μmol/litre, ALT 150–300 IU/litre unless infarction. Hypoglycaemia rare, DIC 25%
Third trimester		
Intrahepatic cholestasis of pregnancy	0.1%	As for first trimester
Pre-eclampsia–eclampsia	5–10%	As for second trimester
Hepatic rupture	0.0001%	RUQ/shoulder tip pain, low blood pressure/peritonism. CT, angiography
HELLP syndrome	0.1%	As for second trimester
Acute fatty liver of pregnancy	0.008%	Nausea/vomiting (70%), RUQ pain (65%), small liver, hypertension (40%), encephalopathy later, leucocytosis. Bilirubin >100 μmol/litre, ALT 300 IU/litre. Hypoglycaemia, DIC 75%. USS
Acute viral hepatitis	As general population	As for first trimester
Cholelithiasis	Unknown	As for first trimester
Drug hepatotoxicity	Unknown	As for first trimester

[a] Rare in this trimester.

ALT, serum alanine aminotransferase; CMV, cytomegalovirus; DIC, disseminated intravascular coagulation; EBV, Epstein–Barr virus; HAV, hepatitis A virus; HEV, hepatitis E virus; LDH, serum lactate dehydrogenase; MCRP, magnetic resonance cholangiopancreatography; PCR, polymerase chain reaction; RUQ, right upper quadrant; TSH, thyroid-stimulating hormone; USS, ultrasound scan.

due to development of acute liver failure during the third trimester, but transmission to offspring has not been recorded.

Liver tumour during pregnancy

The first presentations of focal nodular hyperplasia, hepatic adenoma, hepatocellular carcinoma, and cholangiocarcinoma have all been reported during pregnancy. Adenomas, in some cases related to prior oral contraceptive use, may undergo vascular engorgement during pregnancy and rupture has been reported. Secondary tumours, including hepatic choriocarcinoma and ovarian teratomas, may also rupture.

Pregnancy during chronic liver disease

Most patients with established cirrhosis are infertile, but a few remain fertile, although with a high rate of prematurity, low-birthweight babies, and stillbirths. There is little evidence that pregnancy results in deterioration in liver dysfunction in patients with cirrhosis, and improvement of inflammatory activity occurs in some cases of autoimmune chronic active liver disease. There is no increased rate of relapse after delivery. Patients with treated Wilson's disease are able to conceive and successful pregnancies whilst taking d-penicillamine or trientine have been reported.

Variceal haemorrhage

Changes in splanchnic haemodynamics, increased cardiac output and azygous blood flow, and an increase in circulating blood volume have all been suggested as risk factors for variceal bleeding during pregnancy. Evidence for this remains controversial, although recent large series of patients with noncirrhotic portal hypertension report a haemorrhage rate of 13%. Treatment of variceal bleeding during pregnancy should be by conventional endoscopic techniques, with use of transjugular intrahepatic stent shunts or surgical shunts reserved for rescue therapy.

Pregnancy following orthotopic liver transplantation

Fertility returns quickly following liver transplantation. Pregnancy does not alter the risks of cellular rejection, but immunosuppressive drug toxicity needs to be carefully monitored. Azathioprine may cause neonatal pancytopenia, and ciclosporin A is associated with a 40% incidence of hypertension, which may be lower with tacrolimus.

Pregnancy during gastrointestinal disease

Only a few gastrointestinal diseases occur with altered frequency during pregnancy.

Gastro-oesophageal reflux

Symptomatic gastro-oesophageal reflux is present at some stage in up to 80% of pregnancies. It is mainly due to a reduced lower oesophageal sphincter pressure rather than elevated intra-abdominal pressure from a gravid uterus. Treatment with antacid is recommended, with avoidance of H_2 antagonists or proton pump inhibitors unless symptoms and complications of gastro-oesophageal reflux outweigh potential drug toxicity. Acid–pepsin reflux combined with vomiting in early pregnancy may precipitate haematemesis, occasionally with a Mallory–Weiss tear, for which management should be as in the nonpregnant state. Upper gastrointestinal endoscopy is a safe procedure during pregnancy.

Inflammatory bowel disease

Stable inactive ulcerative colitis and Crohn's disease do not affect fertility and are not associated with increased fetal risk; disease control is not impeded by pregnancy. There are few data on the effect of drug therapy on fertility, although sperm counts may be reduced in men on salazopyrine. The risk of relapse of inflammatory bowel disease during pregnancy has been assessed at between 30 and 50%, but this is no higher than comparable nonpregnant control groups. Folate and iron supplementation are recommended, with regular monitoring of nutritional status.

Active inflammatory bowel disease is associated with involuntary infertility, and when very severe it is prudent to recommend deferring any attempt to conceive. Increased fetal loss may occur when active inflammatory bowel disease is first manifest during pregnancy, with recent reports suggesting that the site of disease activity (colonic or small bowel) does not affect outcome. Most studies have demonstrated that corticosteroids, sulphasalazine, and 5-aminosalicylic acid preparations are safe to use during pregnancy. Colonoscopy, in expert hands, can be performed during pregnancy without risk, although it is often possible to defer this procedure.

Acute appendicitis

Acute appendicitis, the most common nonobstetric emergency requiring surgery, occurs in 1 in 2500 to 1 in 3500 pregnancies. It is not clear if reports of a more aggressive clinical course reflect delays in diagnosis or reporting bias. Clinical management is similar to that of the nonpregnant case: surgery must not be deferred, as the frequency of prematurity and perinatal mortality may be increased if perforation occurs.

Coeliac disease

Women with untreated coeliac disease have a markedly increased risk of abortion and low birthweight babies, which can be reversed following institution of a gluten-free diet. Screening for coeliac disease should be considered in women with a previous history of abortion or unfavourable pregnancy outcomes.

Further reading

Audibert F, *et al.* (1996). Clinical utility of strict criteria for the HELLP syndrome. *Am J Obstet Gynecol*, **175**, 460–4.

Geenes V, Williamson C (2009). Intrahepatic cholestasis of pregnancy. *World J of Gastroenterol*, **15**(17), 2049–66.

Hay JE (2008). Liver Disease in pregnancy. *Hepatology*, **47**, 1067–76.

Ibdah JA, *et al.* (1999). A fetal fatty-acid oxidation disorder as a cause of liver disease in pregnant women. *N Engl J Med*, **340**, 1723–31.

Knox T, Olans L (1996). Liver disease in pregnancy. *N Engl J Med*, **335**, 569–76.

Kochhar R, *et al.* (1999). Pregnancy and its outcome in patients with noncirrhotic portal hypertension. *Digest Dis Sci*, **44**, 1356–61.

Korelitz BI (1992). Inflammatory bowel disease and pregnancy. *Gastroenterol Clin North Am*, **27**, 213–24.

Martin JN, *et al.* (1999). The spectrum of severe preeclampsia: comparative analysis by HELLP (hemolysis, elevated liver enzyme levels, and low platelet count) syndrome classification. *Am J Obstet Gynecol*, **180**, 1373–84.

Martinelli P, *et al.* (2000). Coeliac disease and unfavourable outcome of pregnancy. *Gut*, **46**, 332–5.

Mayberry J, Weterman IT (1986). European survey of fertility and pregnancy in women with Crohn's disease; a case control study by the European Collaborative group. *Gut*, **27**, 821–5.

Modigliani R, (1997). Drug therapy for ulcerative colitis during pregnancy. *Eur J Gastroenterol Hepatol*, **9**, 854–7.

Nicastri P, *et al.* (1998). A randomised placebo-controlled trial of ursodeoxycholic acid and S-adenosylmethionine in the treatment of intrahepatic cholestasis of pregnancy. *Br J Obstet Gynaecol*, **105**, 1205–7.

Palma J, *et al.* (1997). Ursodeoxycholic acid in the treatment of cholestasis of pregnancy: a randomized, double-blind study controlled with placebo. *J Hepatol*, **27**, 1022–8.

Sibai BM, *et al.* (1993). Maternal morbidity and mortality in 442 pregnancies with hemolysis, elevated liver enzymes, and low platelets (HELLP syndrome). *Am J Obstet Gynecol*, **169**, 1000–1006.

14.10

Diabetes in pregnancy

Moshe Hod and Yariv Yogev

Essentials

Diabetes is one of the most common medical complications in pregnancy: 0.4 to 2% of all births are complicated by pregestational diabetes; about 3% of pregnancies are complicated by gestational diabetes mellitus, with substantially more in some populations.

Pregestational diabetes

Preconceptional evaluation—this should include evaluation of glycaemic control, blood pressure, retinal disease, renal status, thyroid function, peripheral and autonomic neuropathy, peripheral vascular disease, and hypoglycaemic symptoms.

Pregnancy outcome—(1) Pregnancy complicated by diabetes is associated with increased perinatal mortality. (2) Early growth delay, major congenital malformations, and abortions are related to poor glycaemic control around the time of conception and in the first trimester. (3) Macrosomia may be associated with significant obstetrical morbidity such as shoulder dystocia, which may result in severe birth trauma.

Gestational diabetes mellitus

Screening and diagnosis—selective or universal screening for gestational diabetes mellitus should be determined by population characteristics. The most commonly accepted method of diagnosis of gestational diabetes mellitus is the 100-g oral glucose tolerance test, using either the National Diabetes Data Group criteria or Carpenter and Coustan criteria.

Medical management—the key to improving pregnancy outcome in women with diabetes is strict glycaemic control. Proper diet has a very important function unique to maternal diabetes: it must assure adequate nourishment to the developing fetus without risking significant and prolonged hyperglycemia. Medical therapy with pharmacological agents should be reserved for those who fail to achieve desired level of glycaemic control despite diet therapy, and for those who are not appropriate candidates for diet therapy alone. Glibenclamide is safe and effective for the treatment of gestational diabetes mellitus.

Obstetric management—important aspects include: (1) Measurement of the fetal abdominal circumference early in the third trimester may identify infants at risk for macrosomia in the absence of maternal pharmacological therapy. (2) The timing of delivery of the patient with diabetes is a balancing act between potential intrauterine death, shoulder dystocia and the consequences of premature delivery—expectant management beyond the estimated due date is not recommended generally, although an ultrasound estimate of fetal weight may help to rule out macrosomia. Cesarean delivery to prevent traumatic birth injury may be considered if the estimated fetal weight is greater than 4000 to 4500 g. (3) Poor glycaemic control in late pregnancy is a significant risk factor for fetal distress and neonatal asphyxia—a team of professionals (physicians, neonatal nurse practitioners, midwives, and/or respiratory therapists) trained in the paediatric management of complicated deliveries should be present in the delivery room.

Postpartum management—at 6 to 8 weeks a 75-g oral glucose tolerance test should be administered to all women with gestational diabetes mellitus. The test should be repeated on a regular basis every 1 to 3 years, depending upon the patient's risk factors for developing type 2 diabetes.

Introduction

Diabetes is one of the most common medical complications in pregnancy, affecting 4 to 10% of women worldwide and even more highly prevalent in specific geographic regions and ethnic populations. In the United States of America and Europe, about 135 000 to 200 000 women are diagnosed annually with gestational diabetes (GDM), adding to the number of women who have diabetes (type 1 or type 2) before pregnancy. The increasing prevalence of type 2 diabetes in general, and in younger people in particular, has led to an increasing number of pregnancies with this complication.

During normal pregnancy, a marked reduction of insulin sensitivity is compensated by a reciprocal increase in β-cell secretion, hence pregnancy is characterized as a state of hyperinsulinaemia and insulin resistance in response to diabetogenic effects of normal carbohydrate metabolism. The increased risk for maternal hyperglycaemia and the resultant fetal hyperinsulinaemia are central to the pathophysiology of diabetic complications. All types of diabetes have increased risk for stillbirth, deviant fetal growth (macrosomia, growth restriction), metabolic (e.g. hypoglycaaemia, hypocalcaemia), haematological (e.g. hyperbilirubinaemia, polycythaemia) and respiratory complications that increase neonatal intensive care unit admission rates; also a greater incidence of birth trauma (e.g. shoulder dystocia). The most significant fetal complications in type 1 and type 2 diabetes are congenital anomalies; there is also a high risk of spontaneous abortion.

Historical perspective

Before the discovery of insulin, diabetes was an affliction with a dismal prognosis. A successful pregnancy was virtually impossible when compromised by untreated diabetes. Pregnancy worsened the disease and shortened the lives of these women, many of whom died either during or shortly after the pregnancy. Poor interventional obstetric care with increased risk of puerperal sepsis further compromised the pregnancies. The link between congenital malformations and maternal diabetes in pregnancy is of more recent concern.

With the discovery and use of insulin, a new hope arose for diabetic women and their reproductive potential. With the introduction of insulin, maternal mortality fell dramatically, and perinatal mortality decreased over time. However, the introduction of insulin did not ameliorate the problems of macrosomia and associated traumatic injury to mother and fetus, as well as continuing complications such as neonatal hypoglycaemia, congenital malformations, pre-eclampsia, and infection. By the 1940s insulin had made pregnancy relatively safe for the diabetic mother, but it also complicated the problem because physicians saw patients with severe diabetes who in the pre-insulin era would never have become pregnant. During this period, several attempts were made to ameliorate fetal death due to diabetes. It was observed that there was a significant stillbirth rate beyond 36 weeks of gestation, hence diabetic patients were routinely delivered at or before 36 weeks by caesarean section or by induction of labour if fetal death had not already occurred, or if maternal complications had not mandated an earlier delivery. At the Joslin Clinic in Boston, under the leadership of Priscilla White, new clinical recommendations for the care of pregnant diabetic women consisted of strict glycaemic control, long-term hospitalization, and sound obstetrical management.

Gestational diabetes (GDM)—a term first used by O'Sullivan in 1961—is defined as 'carbohydrate intolerance of varying severity with onset or first recognition during pregnancy'. At about the same time, others reported increased perinatal mortality associated with abnormal oral glucose tolerance during pregnancy, but gestational diabetes as a clinical entity was slow to win converts, partly because of the relatively short phase of hyperglycaemia during the latter part of pregnancy and partly on account of its disappearance after the delivery. However, it has become increasingly accepted as a disease, not only for its implications on the immediate outcome of pregnancy, but also for long-term effects on child and mother (maternal development in later life of type 2 diabetes).

Classification

Patients with pregestational diabetes are categorized according to length of disease and the presence of microvascular or other end-organ complications (Table 14.10.1). GDM—defined as stated above as carbohydrate intolerance of varying severity with onset or first recognition during pregnancy—is further stratified by fasting plasma glucose and treatment modality to A1 and A2 (Table 14.10.1).

Epidemiology

GDM is a problem with major public health implications and one that is growing in magnitude as its incidence climbs. The principal sources of epidemiological information are national and local statistics, hospital and ambulatory medical records, and research studies and specialized registries. These epidemiological data vary as to their specificity, population size, criteria for ascertainment, and definition of disease. Estimates that diabetes (type 1, type 2, and GDM) occurs annually in 1% to 14% of all pregnancies are based on both national birth statistics and small community studies.

Since the prevalence of type 1 and type 2 diabetes varies by both race and age, it is difficult to differentiate the number of births complicated by type 1 diabetes from those complicated by type 2 diabetes in the population as a whole or in any of its components. However, it is estimated that between 0.4% and 2% of all births are complicated by pregestational diabetes. Moreover, it is assumed that the prevalence of pregnancies complicated by pregestational diabetes will increase. This is based on several factors that have emerged in recent years: (1) increased incidence in type 2 diabetes among adolescents and women less than 25 years of age; (2) increased birth rate among adolescents; (3) population growth (due to immigration and higher birth rate) among groups with higher risk of diabetes (specifically Hispanic and Asian-American); (4) increased incidence of obesity in women of childbearing age.

The epidemiology of GDM is subject to substantial limitations due to disagreement over: (1) who should be screened; (2) when screening should occur; (3) screening test criteria; and, (4) diagnostic test criteria. Screening recommendations for GDM range from

Table 14.10.1 Classification of diabetes in pregnancy

Class	Onset	Fasting plasma glucose	Therapy
A1	Gestational	<105 mg/dl (5.8 mmol/litre)	Diet
A2	Gestational	>105 mg/dl (5.8 mmol/litre)	Pharmacological

Class	Age of onset (years)	Duration (years)	Vascular complication	Insulin
B	>20	<10	None	Insulin
C	10–19	10–19	None	Insulin
D	<10	>20	Benign retinopathy	Insulin
F	Any	Any	Nephropathy	Insulin
R	Any	Any	Proliferative retinopathy	Insulin
H	Any	Any	Heart	Insulin

the inclusion of all pregnant women (universal) to the exclusion of all women except those with very specific risk factors (selective), the latter being estimated to omit more than 5% of women with the condition. Based on the United States Vital Statistics database in 2002, GDM occurred in the pregnancies resulting in live births of 3.4% Hispanic women, 2.7% African-American women, and 2.8% white women. However, the situation is still complicated by disagreement as to diagnostic criteria for GDM. For example, there is a controversy as to whether the 75-g 2-h oral glucose tolerance test (OGTT) should be considered in place of the 100 g 3-h OGTT, and the interpretation of OGTT criteria is also subject to debate. Some advocate that one abnormal value on the OGTT has the same risk of adverse perinatal outcome as does two abnormal values, hence the true prevalence of GDM in a studied population is still a matter of definition and classification.

Aetiology, genetics, pathogenesis, and pathology

GDM is characterized by carbohydrate intolerance of variable severity, with onset or first recognition during pregnancy. This definition applies whether or not there is a need for insulin and whether or not it disappears after pregnancy: it does not apply to gravid patients with previously diagnosed diabetes. Pregnancy can be viewed as a progressive condition of insulin resistance, hyperinsulinaemia, and postprandial hyperglycaemia. Glucose is transferred through the placenta by facilitated diffusion, with postprandial elevation increasing nutrient availability (glucose) to the fetus. In addition, peripheral insulin resistance is more pronounced in skeletal muscle than in the adipose tissue, resulting in ingested nutrients being shunted towards the adipose tissue. This promotes maternal anabolism and energy storage needed in late pregnancy when fetal growth is maximal.

As pregnancy advances the increasing tissue resistance to insulin creates a demand for more insulin, which is readily met in most women such that normoglycaaemia is maintained. Hyperglycaemia develops if insulin secretion is inadequate to overcome insulin resistance: in most cases this happens in the last half of pregnancy, with insulin resistance increasing progressively until delivery, when in most cases it rapidly disappears.

The physiological changes responsible for insulin resistance in pregnancy appear to be related to the metabolic effects of several hormones and other factors that are elevated in the maternal circulation during gestation. The development of insulin resistance and GDM during pregnancy tends to parallel the growth of the fetomaternal unit and the levels of hormones secreted by the placenta. Progesterone signalling may play a vital role in insulin release and pancreatic function and may affect susceptibility to diabetes; moreover progesterone prohibits normal adaptation of the pancreatic β-cell reserve during pregnancy and is a major contributor to increased insulin resistance. Human placental lactogen (hPL) levels increase at the onset of the second trimester, causing a decrease in phosphorylation of insulin receptor substrate-1 and intense insulin resistance. In addition cortisol and prolactin increase insulin resistance and alter insulin function.

Leptin is a 16-kDa protein encoded by the ob/ob (obesity) gene, secreted by adipocyte tissue, and also produced by a number of other tissues including the stomach, intestine, and placenta in humans. It acts on hypothalamic receptors to decrease food intake and increase energy expenditure. Fasting insulin and leptin concentrations correlate closely with body fat, making leptin a good marker of obesity and insulin resistance. The serum leptin levels in women with GDM are significantly higher than in women whose pregnancies are not compromised by this condition.

Adiponectin is an adipose tissue hormone secreted by adipocytes that may facilitate the regulation of glucose and lipid metabolism. It decreases hepatic glucose production and insulin resistance by up-regulating fatty acid oxidation. Adiponectin may emerge as a significant factor in carbohydrate-fat metabolism and in the development of insulin resistance during pregnancy because of data suggesting that there are decreased adiponectin levels in women with GDM compared with healthy control subjects.

Risk factors for the development of GDM are specified in Table 14.10.2.

Screening

There is considerable controversy concerning who should be screened for GDM. The American Diabetes Association proposed that all pregnant women undergo risk assessment for GDM at the first office visit as early as possible, with the recommendation that they need not be screened for GDM if they have none of the risk factors described in Table 14.10.2, but they should be screened if any risk factors are present. If they are found to not have GDM on the initial screening (negative screening results), they should be retested between 24 to 28 weeks of gestation. By contrast, the American College of Obstetricians and Gynecologists recommends that all pregnant women be screened for GDM between 24 and 28 weeks of gestation, except women who meet all the low risk criteria.

The 4th Workshop Conferences on GDM recommended screening with a 50-g oral glucose load followed 1 h later with a blood glucose determination, with those found to have a value of 130 mg/dl (7.2 mmol/litre) followed up with a 100-g OGTT. Using their data, this approach had a sensitivity of 79% and specificity of 87% for the diagnosis of GDM by the OGTT. To account for plasma determination, the cut-off was modified to 140 mg/dl (7.8 mmol/litre) and this threshold has been widely applied as the indication for a follow-up OGTT. Coustan et al. studied 6000 women using a 50-g oral glucose challenge test: using an abnormal threshold designated as 130 mg/dl (7.2 mmol/litre) had a sensitivity of nearly 100%, with 23% requiring a 3-h OGTT; by contrast, the use of a threshold of 140 mg/dl (7.8 mmol/litre) resulted in sensitivity of 80 to 90%, with 15% requiring a 3-h OGTT. Hence, lowering the threshold

Table 14.10.2 Risk factors for GDM

Risk factor	Description
Age	>25 years
Obesity	Prepregnancy BMI> 30 kg/m^2
Ethnicity	Hispanic, Native American, Asian American, African-American
Family history	First degree relative with type 2 diabetes
Previous GDM	
Previous infant large for gestational age	

from 140 mg/dl (7.8 mmol/litre) to 130 mg/dl (7.2 mmol/litre) resulted in an 11% increase in test sensitivity, but there was a significant increase in the numbers of women requiring an OGTT. About 10% of individuals with screening results between 130 and 139 mg/dl (7.2–7.8 mmol/litre) will manifest GDM if tested with a 3-h OGTT. Because the precise cost–benefit ratio for diagnosing GDM remains unresolved, either threshold is acceptable, hence the selection should be decided mainly by demographic/geographic considerations. In regions with a high prevalence of GDM/type 2 diabetes, it is reasonable to use the lower threshold (130 mg/dl or 7.2 mmol/litre—increasing sensitivity); in an area of lower prevalence, cost-effectiveness may dictate the choice of a higher threshold (140 mg/dl or 7.8 mmol/litre).

Diagnosis

The ideal diagnostic test for gestational diabetes has not yet been developed. The limitations of the OGTT include test duration, time of performance (morning only, after nocturnal fast), patient discomfort, especially during the first trimester with potential nausea and vomiting, as well as the supraphysiological glucose load unrelated to body weight. Finally, the issue of reproducibility remains a limitation. The most commonly accepted method of diagnosis of GDM is the 100-g 3-h OGTT, using either the National Diabetes Data Group or the Carpenter and Coustan criteria. Both diagnostic criteria require two or more abnormal values for the diagnosis of GDM (Table 14.10.3). Despite repeated reports of the association between one abnormal value on the OGTT results and adverse outcome in pregnancy, the use of one abnormal value for the diagnosis of GDM remains controversial.

There is no consensus on the glucose load concentration that should be used for the glucose test. Several clinical studies have attempted to test if the 75-g load (recommended by the World Health Organization and by the American Diabetes Association) will be more convenient and provide greater accuracy than the 100-g load, while others have suggested that some GDM women will not be identified with the lower load. Some advocate that the 75-g load be used in the diagnosis of GDM using the threshold suggested by the Carpenter–Coustan criteria, i.e. fasting 95 mg/dl (5.3 mmol/litre), 1 h 180 mg/dl (10 mmol/litre), 2 h 155 mg/dl (8.6 mmol/litre). This recommendation eliminated the 3-h sample and used two or more abnormal values for diagnosis. The result was a one-step approach in which the OGTT is performed without prior plasma or serum glucose screening, which may be cost-effective for high-risk patients.

Recently, the Hyperglycemia & Adverse Pregnancy Outcome (HAPO) study has collected data from around 25 000 pregnancies to examine the relationships between maternal glycaemia and pregnancy outcome in a setting where both caregivers and subjects were masked or blinded to glucose tolerance test results. It is anticipated that the results of the HAPO study will provide data that lead to criteria for the diagnosis of GDM that are linked to risk of adverse outcome.

Towards new diagnostic criteria for diagnosing GDM-The HAPO Study

The HAPO Study was an investigator initiated project, planned as a prospective, observational, multicentre, blinded study. The study was held in a multinational, multi cultural, ethnically diverse population, from various countries. It was designed to find if, and what is the correlation between adverse pregnancy outcomes to maternal glucose intolerance, that fall short of overt diabetes values. Also, it was meant to set the evidence-based criteria for diagnosis and classification of GDM, to be based upon the correlation between glycaemic levels and perinatal outcome. The preliminary hypothesis of the study was that gestational hyperglycaemia, even below the threshold for diabetes, will be associated with increased maternal, fetal and neonatal morbidities

A total of 23 316 women completed the course of the study, not being lost to follow-up, and remaining with their data blinded. The results of the HAPO study demonstrate an association between increasing levels of fasting, 1-h and 2-h plasma glucose post a 75 g OGTT, to the four primary endpoints of the study: birth weight above the 90th percentile, cord blood serum C-peptide level above the 90th percentile, primary caesarean delivery and clinical neonatal hypoglycaemia. Although significant correlations were present for the two latter outcomes, they were not as strong as those with the two former endpoints. Positive correlations were also found between increasing plasma glucose levels to the five secondary outcomes: premature delivery, shoulder dystocia or birth injury, intensive neonatal care admission, hyperbilirubinaemia, and pre-eclampsia. Adjustments were made for field centre, maternal BMI, blood pressure, height, parity, baby gender, and ethnic group—these reduced the observed associations, but they generally remained valid. This validates the results for all age groups, countries, and ethnic origin—thus, eliminating the proposed impacts of some speculated confounders .

Additional analyses examined the issue of neonatal adiposity. Out of the total HAPO participants, cord serum C-peptide results were available for 19 885 newborns and skin-fold measurements for 19 389. These measurements were used to determine the relationship between neonatal adiposity (defined as the sum of skin folds higher than 90th percentile or body fat percentage over 90th percentile) to maternal glucose levels. There is a statistically significant correlation between increasing values of maternal glycemia, on all OGTT values, and cord serum C-peptide to neonatal adiposity. The pattern is similar to the correlation between maternal glucose values and birth weight above the 90th percentile, and was held true also for fat free mass (derived by subtracting fat mass from total body weight) .

The HAPO study therefore demonstrates that fasting glucose levels and post 75 g OGTT are correlated to maternal, perinatal, and neonatal outcomes and this is essentially in a linear manner. Glucose has an impact on pregnancy outcome, even at levels below the current, commonly accepted range. There seems to be no apparent threshold, but rather a continuum of glucose levels. These results now provide the evidence base for developing perinatal outcome-based standards to diagnose and classify GDM, that

Table 14.10.3 Diagnostic criteria for GDM

Status	Carpenter and Coustan	NDDG
Fasting	95 mg/dl (5.3 mmol/litre)	105 mg/dl (5.8 mmol/litre)
1 h after GTT	180 mg/dl (10 mmol/litre)	190 mg/dl (10.6 mmol/litre)
2 h after GTT	155 mg/dl (8.6 mmol/litre)	185 mg/dl (10.3 mmol/litre)
3 h after GTT	140 mg/dl (7.8 mmol/litre)	145 mg/dl (8.0 mmol/litre)

NDDG, National Diabetes Data Group.

are valid and therefore applicable worldwide Furthermore, these associations between adverse outcomes and 'nondiabetic' hyperglycaemia, suggest the need to lower current diagnostic thresholds for GDM. It is anticipated that the International Association of Diabetes and Pregnancy Study Groups (IADPSG) will shortly publish its recommended criteria for GDM which are based on the findings from the HAPO study.

Effects of diabetes in pregnancy

All types of diabetes have increased risk for stillbirth, deviant fetal growth (macrosomia, growth restriction), metabolic complications (e.g. hypoglycaemia, hypocalcaemia), haematological complications (e.g. hyperbilirubinaemia, polycythaemia), respiratory complications that increase neonatal intensive care unit admission, and birth trauma (e.g. shoulder dystocia). It has been demonstrated in both randomized and cohort studies that lack of treatment for GDM is associated with increased risk of these serious perinatal morbidities.

Treatment

Preconception care for pregestational diabetes

About 50% of all pregnancies are unplanned and do not have the advantages of preconception care. Congenital anomalies and spontaneous abortions are more serious complications in pregestational diabetes than in GDM. Preconception counselling for women with pregestational diabetes mellitus has been reported to be beneficial and cost-effective and should be encouraged. A search for underlying vasculopathy is advisable and, in selected patients, may include a retinal examination, estimation of urinary protein excretion (albumin creatinine ratio or protein creatinine ratio or 24-h urinary collection) and renal function (eGFR or creatinine clearance), and electrocardiography. Due to comorbidity with type 1 diabetes mellitus, thyroid function studies also should be obtained. Folic acid should be prescribed to all women contemplating pregnancy, which is particularly important in women with diabetes given their increased risk of neural tube defects.

Intensified therapy in pregnancy

Intensified therapy in the management of GDM and pregestational diabetes is aimed at achieving best possible levels of glycaemic control. It involves frequent self-monitoring of blood glucose (SMBG), diet, oral hypoglycaemic drugs, multiple injections of insulin or its equivalent, and a multidisciplinary team effort. This approach often makes the difference between success and failure in diabetes management. Regardless of the treatment modality used, the purpose is to achieve glycaemic control that diminishes the rate of hypoglycaemia and ketosis and maximizes perinatal outcome. Although there is ample evidence that there is an association between glycaemic control and the occurrence of maternal/fetal complications, this association does not prove cause and effect. It does, however, provide the rationale to attempt to control blood glucose levels, the accepted glycaemic metabolic goals being specified in Table 14.10.4.

Diet and exercise

For all types of diabetes, the underlying foundation of treatment is diet. Two approaches are currently recommended: decreasing the proportion of carbohydrates to 35 to 40% in a daily regimen of three meals and three or four snacks, and lowering glycaemic index carbohydrates for approximately 60% of daily intake. The assignment of daily caloric intake is similar for gestational and pregestational diabetes and is calculated based on prepregnancy body mass index (20–25 kcal/kg for obese women and 35 kcal/kg for nonobese women, of actual pregnancy weight). An appropriate exercise programme may improve postprandial blood glucose levels and insulin sensitivity for pregnant diabetic women who are not only willing but also able (socioeconomic limitations, obesity, multiparity) to participate. Patients with GDM who fail to achieve the desired level of glycaemic control should be treated with pharmacological agents.

Oral hypoglycaemic agents

Historically, oral antidiabetic agents were contraindicated in pregnancy. The early-generation sulfonylureas crossed the placenta and had the potential to stimulate the fetal pancreas, leading to fetal hyperinsulinaemia, and they were potentially associated with fetal malformations. Of the sulfonylurea family of drugs, only glibenclamide has been shown to have minimal (4%) transfer across the human placenta and has not been associated with excess neonatal hypoglycaemia in clinical studies. Moreover, it has been demonstrated to be safe and as efficient as insulin for the treatment of GDM in both randomized and prospective studies. Dosing must be carefully balanced with meals and snacks to prevent maternal hypoglycaemia (as with insulin therapy).

Metformin does cross the placenta and should not be used for treatment of GDM except in clinical trials, which should include long-term follow-up of infants. Patients with pregestational diabetes that requires pharmacological treatment should be treated exclusively with insulin.

Insulin treatment

There is a gradual increase in insulin requirement throughout pregnancy: 0.7 units/kg per day in the first trimester; 0.8 units/kg per day at week 18, 0.9 units/kg per day at week 26, and 1.0 units/kg per day from week 36 until delivery. Women with pregestational diabetes need adjustment of insulin dose for each trimester in addition to frequent assessment and individualization of dosage. Mounting evidence of the beneficial effects of insulin lispro in type 1 and type 2 nonpregnant diabetic women includes decreased frequency of severe hypoglycaemic episodes, limited postprandial glucose excursions, and a possible decrease in glycosylated haemoglobin when the drug is administered by continuous subcutaneous infusion. Insulin lispro also provides greater convenience in the timing of administration (analogues administered up to 15 min after the start of a meal, compared to soluble insulin taken 30 min

Table 14.10.4 Recommended glycaemic metabolic goals in the treatment of diabetes in pregnancy

	Plasma glucose
Fasting	60–95 mg/dl (3.3–5.3 mmol/litre)
Before a meal	<95 mg/dl (<5.3 mmol/litre)
1 h after a meal	<140 mg/dl (<7.8 mmol/litre)
2 h after a meal	<120 mg/dl (<6.7 mmol/litre)
Mean blood glucose	<95 mg/dl (<5.3 mmol/litre)

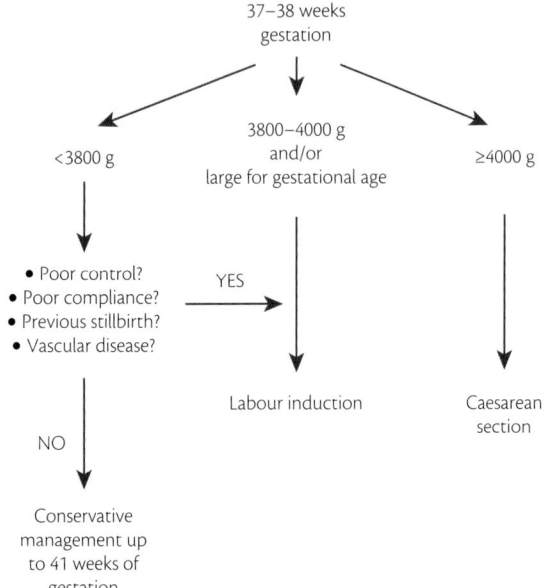

Fig. 14.10.1 Decision analysis for timing and mode of delivery depending on fetal size in pregnancies complicated by diabetes.

before a meal). Insulin Aspart has been shown to be superior to human insulin for postprandial glycaemic control. As far as is known, maternal safety profile and fetal/perinatal outcomes with respect to fetal loss, perinatal mortality, congenital malformation, and child health are not affected by choice of insulin.

Experience of the use of insulin pumps in pregnancy has been limited. For patients treated with an insulin pump or intensified conventional therapy, comparable maternal/fetal outcomes and metabolic control have been achieved. However, improvement in patient lifestyle and success after difficulties achieving acceptable levels of metabolic control with conventional therapy may justify the use of a pump.

When should treatment be intensified?

Measurement of the fetal abdominal circumference above the 70 to 75th percentile early in the third trimester may identify infants at risk for macrosomia in the absence of maternal insulin therapy. Studies primarily in pregnancies with maternal fasting glucose levels of <105 mg/dl (<5.8 mmol/litre) have evaluated this approach. The measurement of both maternal and fetal factors may eventually enhance fetal outcome in a subset of patients with GDM.

Fetal assessment

The main contributor to perinatal mortality and morbidity for the offspring of the patient with pregestational diabetes is congenital malformations of the fetus. Abnormalities commonly affect the central nervous system, heart, and genitourinary and gastrointestinal systems. Detection of congenital anomalies should be initiated as early as the first trimester of pregnancy and repeated in the second trimester. If possible, early anomaly scan using transvaginal ultrasonography may be helpful (14–16 weeks); a basic examination is mandatory in the second trimester of pregnancy.

Antepartum fetal monitoring—including fetal movement counting, the nonstress test, the biophysical profile, and the contraction stress test—can be used to monitor women with pregnancy complicated by diabetes. Initiation of testing is appropriate for most patients at 32 to 34 weeks of gestation, but testing at earlier gestational ages may be warranted in some pregnancies complicated by additional high-risk conditions. The primary clinical value of current antepartum fetal monitoring tests is their low false-negative rate and ability to reassure the clinician that the fetus with normal test results is unlikely to die in utero. In a metabolically stable patient such testing therefore allows prolongation of pregnancy with continued fetal maturation.

Timing and mode of delivery

The care provider's decision on the optimum time to deliver the infant in the pregnancy complicated by diabetes needs to balance between the perceived risk of late intrauterine death and shoulder dystocia and the consequences of unnecessary prematurity and caesarean section delivery. The indications for planned delivery of a patient with diabetes include macrosomia or fetus large for gestational age, previous stillbirth, prevention of fetal demise, and reduction in potential shoulder dystocia. Maternal indications for planned delivery include hypertension, diabetic vasculopathy, and poor compliance to the diabetic management resulting in adverse glycaemic control.

Rouse *et al.* calculated the probability of shoulder dystocia based on birth weight in diabetic and nondiabetic pregnancies. For birth weights of 4500 g or more there was a 52% probability in diabetic compared to 14% in nondiabetic pregnancies, and the mean probability that a neonatal brachial plexus injury would persist was 6.7% (range 0–19%). Thus, to prevent one case of permanent brachial plexus injury in babies weighting 4500 g or more would necessitate performing 153 caesarean deliveries in diabetic mothers and 419 in nondiabetic mothers. If a cut-off of 4000 g is used, then 169 caesarean sections would be required in diabetic women compared to 654 in nondiabetic women. However, Erb's palsy should not be the only consideration in evaluation of morbidity prevention by caesarean delivery. Although Erb's palsy is a severe complication, bone fractures, asphyxia, respiratory complications requiring neonatal intensive care admission, and neonatal and fetal demise should be considered when calculating the cost of caesarean sections performed to prevent shoulder dystocia and adverse outcome.

When diabetes is well controlled and gestational age is well documented, respiratory distress syndrome at or beyond 39 weeks of gestation is rare enough that routine amniocentesis for pulmonary maturity is not necessary. At earlier gestational ages, or when control is poor or undocumented, pulmonary maturity should be assessed before induction. However, when early delivery is planned because of maternal or fetal compromise, the urgency of the indication should be considered in the decision to perform amniocentesis. Figure 14.10.1 summarizes a decision analysis for timing and mode of delivery in pregnancies complicated by diabetes.

Postpartum considerations

Immediate postpartum management for patients with pregestational diabetes should include adjustment of insulin dosage. Usually, due to substantial decrease in insulin resistance shortly after delivery, insulin dose should be reduced by 50%.

In women with GDM, diabetes will be diagnosed in some women soon after pregnancy, suggesting they had pre-existing diabetes that was not diagnosed before pregnancy. The estimate of long-term risk for developing diabetes among women who have had GDM depends on the diagnostic test used, the duration of follow-up, age, and other characteristics of the population studied. It is recommended that all women with GDM should be screened for type 2 diabetes 6 weeks postpartum using a 75-g OGTT. Factors identifiable during or shortly after pregnancy that increase the risk for subsequent diabetes include the degree of abnormality of the diagnostic OGTT, the presence or absence of obesity, the gestational age at diagnosis of GDM, and the degree of abnormality of the postpartum OGTT. Individuals at increased risk should be counselled regarding diet, exercise, and weight reduction or maintenance to forestall or prevent the onset of type 2 diabetes.

Further reading

American College of Obstetricians and Gynecologists Committee on Practice Bulletins. Obstetrics (2001). American College of Obstetricians and Gynecologists Practice Bulletin: Gestational diabetes. *Obstet Gynecol*, **98**, 525–38.

American Diabetes Association (2003). Gestational diabetes mellitus. *Diabetes Care*, **26** Suppl 1, S103–5.

Buchanan TA, *et al.* (1994). Use of fetal ultrasound to select metabolic therapy for pregnancies complicated by mild gestational diabetes. *Diabetes Care*, **17**, 275–83.

Carpenter MW, Coustan DR (1982). Criteria for screening tests for gestational diabetes. *Am J Obstet Gynecol*, **144**, 768–73.

Coustan DR, *et al.* (1989). Maternal age and screening for gestational diabetes: a population based study. *Obstet Gynecol*, **73**, 557.

Crowther CA, *et al.* (2005). Australian Carbohydrate Intolerance Study in Pregnant Women (ACHOIS) Trial Group. *N Engl J Med*, **352**, 2477–86.

Downs B (2003). *Fertility of American women in current population reports*. US Department of Commerce, US Census Bureau, Washington, DC.

HAPO Study Cooperative Research Group (2002). The Hyperglycemia & Adverse Pregnancy Outcome study. *Int J Gynecol Obstet*, **78**, 69.

HAPO Study Cooperative Research Group. Metzger BE, Lowe LP, Dyer AR, *et al.* (2008). Hyperglycemia and adverse pregnancy outcomes. *N Engl J Med*. **358**, 1991–2002.

The HAPO Study Cooperative Research Group (2009). Hyperglycemia and Adverse Pregnancy Outcome (HAPO) Study: associations with neonatal anthropometrics. *Diabetes*, **58**, 453–9.

Langer O, *et al.* (1994). Intensified vs. conventional management of gestational diabetes. *Am J Obstet Gynecol*, **170**, 1036–47.

Langer O, *et al.* (2000). A comparison of glyburide vs. insulin in women with gestational diabetes mellitus. *N Engl J Med*, **343**, 1134–8.

Langer O, *et al.* (2005). Gestational diabetes: the consequences of not treating. *Am J Obstet Gynecol*, **192**, 989–97.

Metzger BE, Coustan DR (1998). Summary and recommendations of the Fourth International Workshop-Conference on Gestational Diabetes Mellitus. The Organizing Committee. *Diabetes Care*, **21** Suppl 2, B161–7.

National Diabetes Data Group (1979). Classification and diagnosis of diabetes mellitus and other categories of glucose intolerance. *Diabetes*, **28**, 1039–57.

O'Sullivan JB, Mahan C (1964). Criteria for the oral glucose tolerance test in pregnancy. *Diabetes*, **13**, 278–85.

Rouse DJ, Owen J (1999). Prophylactic cesarean delivery for fetal macrosomia diagnosed by means of ultrasonography—a Faustian bargain? *Am J Obstet Gynecol*, **181**, 332–8.

White P (1949). Pregnancy complicating diabetes. *Am J Med*, **7**, 609–16.

Yogev Y, *et al.* (2004). Glucose screening in Mexican-American women. *Obstet Gynecol*, **103**, 1241–5.

14.11

Endocrine disease in pregnancy

John H. Lazarus

Essentials

Endocrine function in the developing fetus is initially almost entirely dependent on the mother, with the fetus becoming less reliant on maternal hormones as the fetal glands develop and mature from the second trimester onwards.

Endocrine diseases particular to pregnancy

Lymphocytic hypophysitis—typically presents with symptoms of an expanding pituitary tumour; increasingly recognized as a cause of hypopituitarism occurring late in pregnancy and in the postpartum period.

Sheehan's syndrome (postpartum hypopituitarism)—caused by pituitary infarction following significant hypotension occurring at the time of delivery.

Postpartum thyroiditis—characterized by transient hyperthyroidism followed by hypothyroidism; occurs in 50% of anti-thyroid peroxidase (anti-TPO) positive women and only rarely in antibody negative women.

Pregnancy in women with endocrine disorders

Hyperprolactinaemia—this must be corrected to allow ovulation and fertility. Prolactinomas may enlarge during pregnancy and cause visual impairment: the risk is 2% for a microprolactinoma and >15% for a macroprolactinoma.

Acromegaly—fertility is impaired in women with acromegaly, and management of pregnancy is difficult because there is a risk that the responsible pituitary adenoma may enlarge and cause visual impairment. Very close monitoring by testing of visual fields and pituitary MRI scanning is required.

Cushing's syndrome—difficult to diagnose in pregnancy, and there is a high risk of maternal and fetal complications.

Hyperthyroidism—occurs in 0.2% of pregnancies, usually due to Graves' disease, and is best diagnosed on the basis of an elevated serum free tri-iodothyronine (T_3) in association with a suppressed TSH. The baby is at risk of hyperthyroidism due to the transplacental passage of thyroid stimulating antibodies. Treatment can be by antithyroid drugs or surgery, but not by radio-iodine.

Hypothyroidism—associated with a number of complications in pregnancy, including fetal neurological problems ranging from cretinism to impaired child development. Pregnant patients with hypothyroidism should always be treated with thyroxine, with increased dose requirements during gestation.

Introduction

During pregnancy the endocrine physiology of the mother and fetus changes constantly. Endocrine function in the fetus is initially dependent on maternal function as most endocrine glands do not produce hormones until the second trimester. Thereafter the fetus is less reliant on maternal function, but the fetal glands are continually developing and maturing throughout pregnancy. This section will indicate the important therapeutic aspects of endocrine disease in pregnancy.

Pituitary disease

Prolactinoma

Pituitary adenomas are the most common pituitary disorder affecting pregnancy and prolactinomas are the most common of the hormone-secreting adenomas. Prolactinomas are a common cause of reproductive and sexual dysfunction and hyperprolactinaemia must be corrected to allow ovulation and fertility. The main concern during pregnancy is of symptomatic enlargement leading to visual impairment: there is less than a 2% risk of this happening with a microprolactinoma, but a greater than 15% risk with a macroprolactinoma. Bromocriptine is safe for use during gestation, but a macroadenoma may require debulking prior to pregnancy. Cabergoline has also been used during pregnancy with no deleterious effects. It is safe for patients to become pregnant following dopamine agonist treatment, when prolactinomas may decrease in size, show no change, or achieve complete resolution.

Acromegaly

Fertility is impaired in acromegaly due to concomitant hyperprolactinaemia and decreased gonadotropin reserve due to the

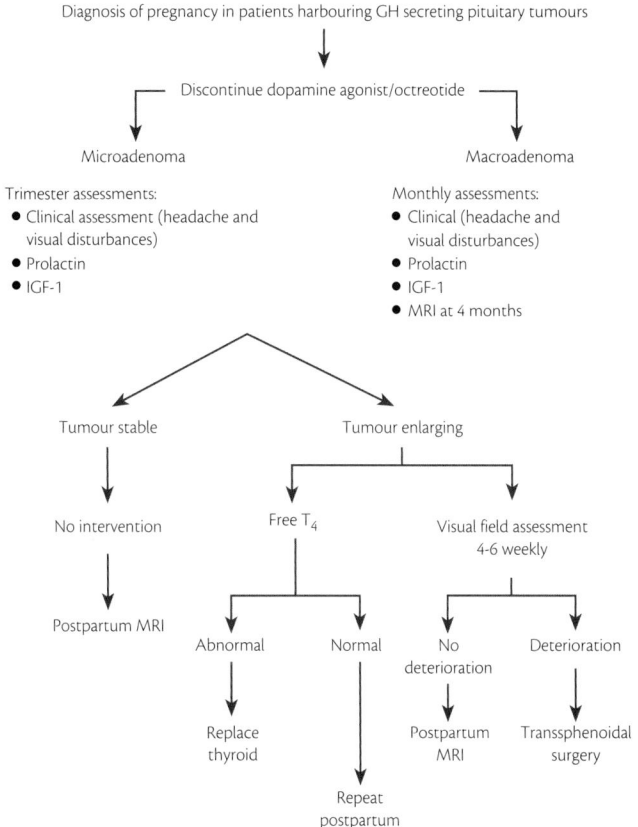

Diagnosis of pregnancy in patients harbouring GH secreting pituitary tumours

↓

Discontinue dopamine agonist/octreotide

Microadenoma

Trimester assessments:
• Clinical assessment (headache and visual disturbances)
• Prolactin
• IGF-1

Macroadenoma

Monthly assessments:
• Clinical (headache and visual disturbances)
• Prolactin
• IGF-1
• MRI at 4 months

Tumour stable

No intervention

↓

Postpartum MRI

Tumour enlarging

Free T$_4$

Abnormal

Replace thyroid

Normal

Repeat postpartum

Visual field assessment 4-6 weekly

No deterioration

Postpartum MRI

Deterioration

Transsphenoidal surgery

Fig. 14.11.1 Scheme for the management of growth hormone secreting pituitary tumours in pregnancy.
(From Herman-Bonert V, Seliverstov M, Melmed S. (1998) Pregnancy in acromegaly: successful therapeutic outcome. *J Clin Endocrinol Metab*, **83**, 727–31, with permission from The Endocrine Society.)

expanding tumour. In an acromegalic woman wishing to conceive, prolactin (PRL) and growth hormone (GH) levels must be normalized to promote fertility (Fig. 14.11.1). Patients with microadenomas should discontinue medical therapy (bromocriptine or somatostatin analogues) during pregnancy and be assessed at each trimester. In patients with macroadenomas removal before pregnancy leads to a greater risk of infertility, but if they are not resected there is a greater risk of pituitary enlargement and visual impairment during gestation.

Pregnancy may influence the size of the adenoma, particularly as the pituitary gland enlarges during normal gestation and may increase by 45% during the first trimester. Pregnancy exacerbates acromegaly in about 17% of cases, and patients with adenomas larger than 1.2 cm are at greater risk of visual loss during pregnancy. Regular visual field checks and MRI examinations are required in such cases.

Cushing's syndrome

Cushing's syndrome during pregnancy has a high incidence of maternal and fetal complications; only one-quarter of patients have an uncomplicated pregnancy. Diagnosis is difficult because many biochemical features such as elevated cortisol levels and loss of the normal glucocorticoid feedback are present during normal pregnancy. Corticotropin-releasing hormone (CRH) and dexamethasone testing is helpful, as is MRI. Transphenoidal surgery is indicated following the enlargement of any pituitary tumour in

pregnancy, especially when there is evidence of increasing visual field impairment.

Diabetes insipidus

Central diabetes insipidus may present during pregnancy. It is seen in women with Sheehan's syndrome, partial postpartum hypopituitarism, and is associated with infiltrative disorders such as histiocytosis X. Synthetic 1-deamino-8-D-arginine-vasopressin (DDAVP) is normally used in the management of diabetes insipidus, with a therapeutic dose of about 30 μg (range 7.5–100 μg) given intranasally. Use during pregnancy seems to be safe for both mother and baby: DDAVP does not affect delivery and has no adverse effects on the neonate.

Postpartum hypopituitarism

Postpartum hypopituitarism due to Sheehan's syndrome is now uncommon because of improved obstetric care. The syndrome is caused by pituitary infarction consequent on significant hypotension occurring at the time of delivery, the diagnosis typically being made when a woman who has survived such an insult fails to establish lactation or menstruation afterwards.

Lymphocytic hypophysitis is increasingly recognized as a cause of hypopituitarism occurring late in pregnancy and in the postpartum period, and around 60% of cases of women found to have adenohypophysitis are pregnant or have recently been delivered. Women may present with symptoms of an expanding pituitary tumour, with headaches and visual symptoms. Inability to lactate and amenorrhoea have been noted. Hyperprolactinaemia and elevated GH levels are also observed. Imaging (CT or MRI) reveals a pituitary mass mimicking an adenoma in about four-fifths of patients. Evaluation of pituitary function shows isolated or multiple anterior pituitary deficiency. ACTH secretion is impaired most frequently, followed by TSH, gonadotropins, GH, and PRL. Histology shows lymphocytic infiltration, which may extend up to the pituitary stalk to the infundibulum. Antibodies to pituitary tissue may be present but are often absent. Other autoimmune diseases, particularly postpartum thyroiditis, may be associated. In addition to the pituitary symptoms described, patients are at risk of adrenal failure and death has been reported, hence adrenal function should be assessed in all cases. Surgery may be required for diagnosis, but should be avoided if the condition is suspected beforehand and corticosteroids given, since these can reduce the size of the pituitary mass.

Thyroid disease
Maternal thyroid function during pregnancy

Thyroid volume increases in iodine-deficient areas but not in iodine-sufficient ones. Thyroxine binding globulin synthesis increases during pregnancy; free thyroxine increases during the first trimester and falls thereafter. Placental human chorionic gonadotropin(hCG), a weak thyroid activator, stimulates maternal thyroid function in the first trimester and results in TSH suppression.

Hyperthyroidism

Hyperthyroidism, usually due to Graves' disease, occurs in 0.2% of pregnancies and is associated with impaired fertility. Other causes include gestational thyrotoxicosis due to high hCG concentrations and hydatidiform molar disease. The diagnosis is made by

---

Box 14.11.1 Management of Graves' hyperthyroidism in pregnancy

- Confirm diagnosis
- Start propylthiouracil
  - Render patient euthyroid—aiming to continue with low-dose antithyroid drug up to and during labour
- Monitor thyroid function regularly throughout gestation (4–6-weekly)
  - Adjust antithyroid drug if necessary
- Check thyroid-stimulating antibodies at 36 weeks gestation
- Discuss treatment with patient
  - Effect on patient
  - Effect on fetus
  - Breastfeeding
- Inform obstetrician and paediatrician
- Review postpartum
  - Check for exacerbation

---

noting an elevated serum free tri-iodothyronine (FT_3) in association with a suppressed TSH, the free thyroxine (FT_4) being elevated or at the upper limit of normal. Ideally each laboratory should establish pregnancy-related normal thyroid reference ranges. Untreated hyperthyroidism is associated with an increased risk of abortion, and if the pregnancy is completed the baby may be of low birth weight and be neonatally transiently hyperthyroid due to the transplacental passage of thyroid-stimulating antibodies. High concentration of TSH receptor antibodies at 28 to 36 weeks gestation suggests the possibility of neonatal thyrotoxicosis. This can also occur in infants whose mothers are currently being treated for Graves' disease or who have received treatment in the past.

Management of hyperthyroidism in pregnancy is either with antithyroid drugs (Box 14.11.1) or surgery, the latter being optimally performed in the second trimester. Radio-iodine therapy is completely contraindicated during pregnancy, and nonpregnant women receiving radioiodine should be advised not to conceive for at least 6 months. There may be a case for therapeutic abortion if radio-iodine has been administered after 12 weeks gestation (i.e. after the fetal thyroid is functional). Propylthiouracil (PTU) is the preferred antithyroid drug as rare but significant side effects due to carbimazole (or methimazole) have been reported: these include aplasia cutis and a methimazole embryopathy characterized by choanal atresia and other defects.

Exacerbation of Graves' disease often occurs postpartum, hence thyroid function tests should be checked routinely at this time. PTU does cross into breast milk, but in lower concentrations than carbimazole or methimazole, hence breastfeeding may normally be permitted, but thyroid function should be monitored in the neonate if breastfeeding is prolonged.

Hypothyroidism

Hypothyroidism is associated with relative infertility because of anovulation and menorrhagia, and the presence of thyroid antibodies is a marker for miscarriage and recurrent abortion even in euthyroid patients. There is an increased incidence of stillbirths and congenital malformations as well as maternal obstetric complications if the condition is untreated. In iodine-deficient areas the risk of neonatal brain damage is increased, resulting in cretinism in severe cases. This is due to maternal hypothyroxinaemia, particularly in the first trimester when the developing fetal nervous system is entirely dependent on maternal T_4. Even in iodine-sufficient areas mild gestational hypothyroidism (seen in 2.5% of pregnancies) is associated with impaired child development, hence there is a case for screening for thyroid function—including for thyroid antibodies—in early pregnancy. Patients with hypothyroidism of any degree should be treated with thyroxine and those already receiving T_4 when found to be pregnant should increase the dose by at least 50 μg per day, and more if necessary.

Fetal and neonatal thyroid dysfunction

Fetal hyperthyroidism is diagnosed by noting a high fetal heart rate and may be confirmed if necessary by fetal blood sampling. Treatment is by maternal administration of high-dose PTU (300–450 mg/day) together with thyroxine during gestation to prevent maternal hypothyroidism. Neonatal hypothyroidism may also occur at birth due to maternal TSH receptor blocking antibodies, maternal antithyroid drug administration, iodine deficiency and maternal goitrogen ingestion. All these conditions are transient and the mother can be reassured.

Postpartum thyroid disease

Anti-thyroid peroxidase (anti-TPO) antibodies, found in 10% of euthyroid pregnant women in early gestation, are a marker for development of postpartum thyroid dysfunction. Postpartum thyroiditis, a destructive process characterized by transient hyperthyroidism followed by hypothyroidism, occurs in 50% of anti-TPO positive women and only rarely in antibody negative women. The hyperthyroidism is relatively asymptomatic but may require treatment with β-adrenoreceptor blocking agents in some cases. By contrast, the hypothyroidism is often symptomatic and thyroxine therapy is required. Mild depressive symptomatology is more common in postpartum women with anti-TPO antibodies than those without. Following recovery from transient postpartum thyroid dysfunction nearly 50% will develop permanent hypothyroidism after 7 years, and recurrent disease follows future pregnancies up to 75% who have experienced a previous episode. Screening for TPO antibodies should be included in the suggested routine antenatal thyroid screening (see above).

Thyroid nodules

Thyroid nodules occur in up to 10% of pregnant women and are usually benign, but 5 to 20% are either benign follicular adenomas or carcinomas of follicular or parafollicular (C-) cell origin. Fine-needle aspiration biopsy (ultrasound-guided if necessary) is the investigation of choice. Surgery should be performed during the second trimester to avoid abortion in the first trimester and premature labour in the third. Pregnancy does not adversely affect the rate of recurrence or distant metastases. A goitre found early in gestation should be evaluated, but the investigation of nodules presenting after 5 to 6 months gestation should occur postpartum.

Differentiated thyroid cancer should not be a contraindication to pregnancy or an indication for abortion.

Parathyroid disease

Diseases of the parathyroid glands are uncommon in women of childbearing age, but hyperparathyroidism during pregnancy can lead to acute pancreatitis, hypercalcaemic crisis, and toxaemia. There is an increased incidence of prematurity and neonatal hypercalcaemia if maternal calcium levels are high. Surgical management can be undertaken safely in the second trimester. Hypoparathyroidism is treated with vitamin D analogues, with dosage often needing to be increased during pregnancy to maintain normocalcaemia, hence calcium levels should be monitored regularly throughout pregnancy, at least in each trimester.

Adrenal disease

The diagnosis of adrenal disease in pregnancy is often delayed. Adrenal tumours are very rare, but their pathophysiological consequences for the mother and fetus are dire. Hypertension is a major feature in patients with phaeochromocytoma and may be initially mistaken for pregnancy-associated hypertension. Such uncommon cases should be managed medically during pregnancy, with surgical resection in the postpartum period, and a similar approach should be taken to the exceptionally rare problem of primary aldosteronism (Conn's syndrome) presenting during pregnancy.

Addison's disease

Addison's disease is only rarely diagnosed during pregnancy but may present as an addisonian crisis in the postpartum. The diagnosis may be missed, with symptoms erroneously attributed to those of pregnancy or its complications. The condition is readily confirmed with measurement of plasma cortisol, the short Synacthen test, and ACTH levels. Antibodies to 21-hydroxylase should be measured to confirm the autoimmune nature of the disease, and the patient screened for other autoimmune conditions.

Congenital adrenal hyperplasia (CAH)

Women with severe CAH have decreased fertility because of oligo-ovulation due to elevated androgen levels. Successful conception requires careful endocrine monitoring and sometimes induction of ovulation. During pregnancy problems are seen in those women with 21-hydroxylase deficiency (P450c21 deficiency, OMIM 201910), 11-hydroxylase deficiency (P450c11, OMIM 610613), and 3-β-hydroxysteroid dehydrogenase deficiency (OMIM 201810). Gestational management must involve adequate adrenal steroid replacement and adrenal androgen suppression. Clinical status, serum electrolytes, and androgen levels should be measured regularly and glucocorticoid and mineralocorticoid therapy adjusted or increased as necessary. As many of the genes for the described enzymes have been isolated, accurate prenatal diagnosis of 21- and 11-hydroxylase deficiency is now possible. The infant should be evaluated clinically and, in most cases, biochemically.

Miscellaneous endocrine conditions

Bartter's syndrome (OMIM 241200, 601678) is a rare renal tubular autosomal recessive disorder in which hypokalaemia, hyperaldosteronism, and sodium wasting occur. The main concern in pregnancy is to maintain normal serum potassium levels which, if done, results in a normal gestation. Gestational hypomagnasaemia may require replacement therapy.

Gonadal dysgenesis (Turner's syndrome) is characterized by streak ovaries and infertility. However, advances in *in vitro* fertilization and embryo transplantation have made pregnancy possible for some women with this condition.

Further reading

Bronstein MD (2005). Protactinomas and pregnancy. *Pituitary*, **8**, 31–8.

Gillam MP, *et al.* (2006). Advances in the treatment of prolactinomas. *Endocr Rev*, **27**, 485–534.

Glinoer D (1997). The regulation of thyroid function in pregnancy: Pathways of endocrine adaptation from physiology to pathology. *Endocr Rev*, **18**, 404–33.

Gutenberg A, *et al.* (2006). Primary hypophysitis: clinical–pathological correlations. *Eur J Endocrinol*, **155**, 101–7.

Gyamfi C, Wapner RJ, D'Alton ME. (2009). Thyroid dysfunction in pregnancy: the basic science and clinical evidence surrounding the controversy in management. *Obstet Gynecol*, **113**, 702–7.

Herman-Bonert V, Seliverstov M, Melmed S. (1998). Pregnancy in acromegaly: successful therapeutic outcome. *J Clin Endocrinol Metab*, **83**, 727–31.

Kelestimur F (2003). Sheehan's syndrome. *Pituitary*, **6**, 181–8.

Lazarus JH (2005). Thyroid disorders associated with pregnancy: etiology, diagnosis and management. *Treat Endocrinol*, **4**, 31–41.

Lindsay JR, Neiman LK. (2005). The hypothalamic-pituitary-adrenal axis in pregnancy: challenges in disease detection and treatment. *Endocr Rev*, **26**, 775–99.

Mestman JH. (1998). Parathyroid disorders of pregnancy. *Semin Perinatol*, **22**, 485–96.

Ogilvie CM, *et al.* (2006) Congenital adrenal hyperplasia in adults: a review of medical, surgical and psychological issues. *Clin Endocrinol (Oxf)*, **64**, 2–11.

14.12

Neurological disease in pregnancy

G.G. Lennox and John D. Firth

Essentials

Neurological conditions of particular note in pregnancy

Thiamine deficiency—caused by the combination of the nutritional demands of pregnancy and hyperemesis gravidarum, presenting as a subacute sensory neuropathy or (less commonly) acute Wernicke's encephalopathy.

Chorea—all types are exacerbated in pregnancy, an effect termed chorea gravidarum.

Malignancies—choriocarcinoma (see Chapter 14.17) can cause brain or spine metastases, the former giving rise to strokes through infarction or haemorrhage, and the latter to cord or cauda equina compression.

Obstetric nerve palsies—seen in cases of prolonged or complicated labour; pressure on the lower lumbosacral plexus leads to foot drop, and on the upper lumbosacral plexus to weakness of iliopsoas and quadriceps; obturator neuropathy leads to weakness of hip adduction and rotation; pudendal nerve damage may be asymptomatic initially, but probably contributes to later stress incontinence.

Cerebrovascular disorders—'postpartum angiopathy' is a rare syndrome of segmental cerebral vasoconstriction in the puerperium, which usually presents with headaches, seizures, or focal deficits (especially visual field defects).

Pregnancy in other common neurological conditions

Epilepsy—most women with pre-existing epilepsy have no change in the frequency of their seizures during pregnancy, but

in 30% they become more frequent. Sodium valproate used as part of polytherapy for epilepsy, or as a single agent, is clearly associated with increased risk of major congenital malformations, but other antiepileptic drugs probably are not. Carbamazepine is probably the safest antiepileptic drug in pregnancy, but use of valproate at doses less than 1 g daily should not be discounted for the treatment of women with conditions for which it is particularly effective. Anticonvulsant plasma levels tend to fall in the later stages of pregnancy: close monitoring and adjustment of dosing are required.

Multiple sclerosis—the incidence of relapses falls during pregnancy itself, but 20 to 40% of women report exacerbation of symptoms in the puerperium. Relapses in pregnancy are treated in the normal way, with rest supplemented by a short course of oral or intravenous steroid if there is serious new disability. Patients with impaired bladder emptying are predisposed to urinary tract infection, and severe spinal cord disease may mask the usual symptoms of such infection; regular urine culture is a sensible precaution.

Muscle diseases—most congenital myopathies and muscular dystrophies cause no special problems in pregnancy unless they are severe enough to compromise ventilation, either because of respiratory muscle weakness or associated scoliosis. Mothers with myotonic dystrophy may have prolonged labour, increased risk of postpartum haemorrhage, and may develop symptoms of cardiomyopathy during labour, and their infants are high risk of perinatal death.

Neurological conditions particular to pregnancy or of particular note in pregnancy

Thiamine deficiency

The combination of the nutritional demands of pregnancy and hyperemesis gravidarum can lead to thiamine deficiency. This most commonly causes a subacute sensory neuropathy, but cases of

acute Wernicke's encephalopathy (with any combination of altered consciousness, ataxia, and ophthalmoplegia, leading if untreated to death) have been described. Both conditions respond promptly to parenteral thiamine, 100 mg daily.

Movement disorders

Pregnancy aggravates any tendency to chorea, an effect termed chorea gravidarum. This should not be regarded as a specific diagnosis, and unless there is a definite history of previous Sydenham's chorea it should prompt a search for all the usual causes of the condition, including thyrotoxicosis and systemic lupus erythematosus. Chorea can be florid and exhausting, such that treatment with a small dose of a neuroleptic such as haloperidol may be required. Recurrence in subsequent pregnancies (or with the combined oral contraceptive) is common, perhaps because of the effects of oestrogens on the sensitivity of dopamine receptors.

Obstetric nerve palsies

Obstetric nerve palsies are becoming less common with improvements in obstetric care, but still occur in cases of prolonged or complicated labour (e.g. due to cephalopelvic disproportion, dystocia, and primiparity), in difficult forceps deliveries, and as a result of traction or haematoma formation in caesarean section. Damage to the common peroneal nerve from incorrectly positioned leg holders is now rare.

The baby may compress the lower parts of the lumbosacral plexus during labour, which will typically give rise to focal neurological deficits that depend on which parts of the plexus have borne the brunt of the pressure. Most commonly there is a unilateral foot drop, which may only become apparent when the mother starts to mobilize. Examination reveals sensory loss that characteristically involves the dorsolateral foot and leg, distinguishing plexus damage from a common peroneal palsy where the sensory loss is confined to the dorsum of the foot. Compression of the upper lumbosacral plexus leads to weakness of iliopsoas as well as the quadriceps muscles, which distinguishes it from more distal damage to the femoral nerve. Both may give rise to sensory loss in the anteromedial thigh and loss or depression of the knee jerk. In most cases the prognosis is good, with spontaneous recovery over a couple of months. Particular care must be taken in subsequent deliveries to avoid further damage to the same nerve, as recovery after repeated injury tends to be less complete.

Long, complicated, or instrumental deliveries may also damage the obturator or pudendal nerves. Obturator neuropathy leads to weakness of hip adduction and rotation, together with some sensory loss in the upper medial thigh. Pudendal nerve damage may be asymptomatic initially, but probably contributes to the subsequent development of perineal descent and stress incontinence.

Malignancies

Choriocarcinoma is a tumour peculiar to pregnancy and the most common form of malignancy associated with pregnancy. It usually presents after molar pregnancy or abortion, but 15% of cases occur during or after normal pregnancy. Neurological manifestations due to brain or spine metastases are common. The brain metastases have a tendency to invade blood vessels, giving rise to strokes through infarction or haemorrhage. Spinal metastases cause cord or cauda equina compression that may be rapid in onset. There are usually multiple pulmonary metastases on chest radiography and the serum chorionic gonadotrophin is greatly elevated. Early diagnosis and treatment (with chemotherapy and radiotherapy) improves survival, but the mortality rate of cases with neurological manifestations remains high. See Chapter 14.17 for further discussion.

Cerebrovascular disorders

There is a rare syndrome of segmental cerebral vasoconstriction in the puerperium, which usually presents with headaches, seizures, or focal deficits (especially visual field defects). It has a predilection for the posterior cerebral circulation and can give rise to multiple infarcts or haemorrhages. The condition, generally termed postpartum angiopathy, can occur spontaneously but has also been described in women taking bromocriptine. There are reports of successful treatment with corticosteroids and vasodilators, but there have been no prospective studies. The condition can recur in subsequent pregnancies.

Effects of pregnancy on neurological diseases and their treatment

Disorders of muscle and neuromuscular transmission

Muscle disorders

Muscle cramps, particularly on waking, are extremely common in the third trimester. They are almost never a symptom of serious neurological disease and often respond to calcium supplements. Restless legs syndrome, in which there is a feeling of discomfort in the legs that is relieved by movement, is also common, especially on retiring to bed. It may respond to correction of underlying anaemia (particularly if this is due to folate or iron deficiency); otherwise management in pregnancy is aimed at promoting the rapid onset of sleep, e.g. by reducing caffeine intake. Drug treatment (with levodopa, clonazepam, or codeine) is best avoided. Polymyositis, although rare in young women, can deteriorate during pregnancy. Treatment with corticosteroids is thought to be safe, as is azathioprine if another immunosuppressive agent is necessary.

Most of the congenital myopathies and muscular dystrophies, apart from myotonic dystrophy, cause no special problems in pregnancy unless they are of sufficient severity to compromise ventilation, either because of respiratory muscle weakness or associated scoliosis. Such cases should ideally be assessed in a specialist unit prior to pregnancy because the cardiorespiratory demands of pregnancy, combined with the splinting effect of the fetus on the diaphragm, can lead to ventilatory failure and a temporary need for mechanical ventilation.

Myotonic dystrophy

Myotonic dystrophy is an autosomal dominant disorder due to an expanded triplet repeat in the myotonin protein kinase gene (OMIM 160900). The expansion tends to increase during transmission from mother to child, so that a mildly affected or asymptomatic mother may have a severely affected fetus. This probably accounts for the excess of polyhydramnios and perinatal death. The myotonia affects the smooth muscle of the uterus, prolonging labour and increasing the risk of postpartum haemorrhage because of uterine inertia. Moderately affected mothers may also develop symptoms of cardiomyopathy during labour (see Chapter 24.24.2 for further discussion).

Myasthenia gravis

Myasthenia gravis deteriorates, improves, and remains stable during pregnancy in roughly equal proportions of patients, but the response is neither predictable nor reproducible in subsequent pregnancies. It deteriorates during the puerperium in about half of all patients, an effect that may also occur after abortion. The mechanism of these changes is not clear. Corticosteroids, oral anticholinesterases, and plasmapheresis can all be employed in the usual manner during pregnancy. It is reasonable to continue azathioprine where this has been prescribed before pregnancy for severe myasthenia, bearing in mind the risk of inducing neonatal leucopenia. Thymectomy can be performed during pregnancy (e.g. where a malignant thymoma is suspected), but may take up to a year to have a therapeutic effect and ideally should be performed well before any planned pregnancy.

Myasthenia does not usually influence labour, although the second stage may be prolonged by fatigue, and obstetric anaesthesia is complicated by the need to avoid drugs with adverse effects on neuromuscular transmission—regional anaesthesia being preferable when possible.

Acetylcholine receptor antibodies can cross into the fetal circulation, giving rise to transient neonatal myasthenia in up to 20% of the babies from affected mothers. Expert paediatric support must therefore be available at delivery (see Chapter 24.23 for further discussion).

Disorders of nerves and nerve roots

Facial palsy

The incidence of facial nerve palsy (Bell's palsy) is substantially increased during pregnancy and the puerperium (as Bell himself described). The reason for this is not known. There have been no studies of treatment in this specific context, but it is reasonable to treat promptly with prednisolone, beginning at 40 mg daily and reducing over a 2-week course.

Mononeuropathies

Carpal tunnel syndrome, due to compression of the median nerve in the wrist, is very common in pregnancy, characteristically causing pain and tingling in the hands at night and after use. Most cases can be managed with nocturnal wrist splints, although steroid injections into the carpal tunnel may tide the patient over into the puerperium, when symptoms usually remit. Diuretics are of little value. Surgical decompression during pregnancy should be reserved for cases with severe pain, weakness, or wasting, when usually there have been symptoms either before pregnancy or early in the first trimester. In troublesome cases it is worth considering delayed surgery to prevent recurrence in subsequent pregnancies, which is common.

The lateral cutaneous nerve of the thigh can be compressed as it crosses the inguinal ligament. This is particularly common in the third trimester and causes tingling, hypersensitivity, or numbness in the midlateral thigh, which may be bilateral. Usually no treatment is required, but troublesome cases may respond to transcutaneous nerve stimulation or a local nerve block. Remission after delivery is the rule.

Lumbosacral root and plexus problems

Backache is very common in pregnancy, particularly in women with a past history of back pain or occupations that involve bending and lifting. It is traditionally blamed on changes in posture and hormonally mediated relaxation of spinal and sacroiliac joints. The pain is usually confined to the lumbar region, but may radiate into the buttock or thigh. There may be tenderness over one or other sacroiliac joints. Radiological investigations are not needed if there are no abnormal neurological signs. Management is conservative.

Abrupt onset of pain that radiates below the knee with focal weakness, numbness, or reflex loss is most likely to be due to a prolapsed intervertebral disc. Provided that the signs are unilateral with no sphincter impairment, conservative management is again appropriate, with analgesia and advice to keep mobile. If this fails then MRI is thought to be a safe method of investigation prior to consideration of lumbar microdiscectomy.

Generalized neuropathies

Chronic inflammatory demyelinating polyradiculoneuropathy can present or relapse during pregnancy, and can be treated with corticosteroids or (if necessary) intravenous immunoglobulin. The incidence of acute Guillain–Barré syndrome is increased in the puerperium, when it is managed in the usual ways. Pregnancy can precipitate relapse in acute intermittent porphyria: abdominal pain typically precedes autonomic and sensory neuropathy, sometimes with seizures and psychiatric disturbance. Lepromatous neuropathies may present or deteriorate during pregnancy, making careful clinical supervision advisable.

Disorders of the central nervous system

Headache

The most common form of headache during pregnancy (as at other times) is chronic daily headache of the tension type. This may be a continuation of pre-existing headaches or a new phenomenon, compounded by anxiety, depression, or poor sleep. Neurological examination is normal in such cases, and treatment should concentrate on explanation and reassurance, coupled if necessary with advice about relaxation techniques. Occasional paracetamol may be helpful; aspirin should be avoided in the third trimester.

Migraine usually improves during pregnancy, but about 20% of sufferers get worse, and occasionally migraine actually begins in pregnancy. No single hormonal change has been convincingly linked to these divergent responses. Although migraine can generally be identified accurately on clinical grounds, diagnosis is more difficult when the condition presents for the first time in pregnancy, particularly if accompanied by the transient focal deficits of migraine aura such visual disturbances or hemiplegia. Other potential causes of headache in pregnancy, such as eclampsia (Chapter 14.4), subarachnoid haemorrhage, cerebral venous thrombosis, cerebral infarction, intracranial tumour, and intracranial infection must be considered and excluded by careful neurological and general examination, supplemented if necessary by brain imaging (see below). Some women present in pregnancy with migraine aura without headache, which can also give rise to diagnostic difficulty: it may be necessary to exclude causes of transient ischaemic attack.

Acute migraine attacks should be treated promptly with rest and paracetamol; prochlorperazine is probably a safe treatment for vomiting. Ergot derivatives must be avoided in pregnancy (and breastfeeding), and the triptan drugs have not yet been shown to be safe. If attacks are frequent then attention should be paid to relevant lifestyle factors such as irregular sleep or meals, and to worry. Prophylactic drug treatment is occasionally necessary, for which the greatest experience lies with propranolol that in doses of 20–80 mg three times a day appears to be both effective and safe, despite its effect on placental blood flow. Women with migraine commonly develop a dull, nonspecific headache of variable severity in the first few days after delivery: this usually responds to simple analgesia, particularly if the woman has been warned about the phenomenon.

Tumours

Although the incidence of cerebral and spinal tumours is probably no greater than at other times, some tumours expand during pregnancy and may present unusually rapidly. This probably reflects a mixture of hormonal and vascular factors; most meningiomas, also some neurofibromas and gliomas, express oestrogen and progesterone receptors and placental growth factor.

Neurofibromatosis type 1 presents particular problems in pregnancy. Women with this condition experience an increased rate of spontaneous first-trimester abortions, perhaps also intrauterine fetal growth retardation and stillbirths, and have a high rate of caesarean section. Most women notice that cutaneous neurofibromas grow or appear *de novo* during pregnancy.

Meningiomas are particularly liable to expand in the third trimester, causing local mass effects such as headache, cranial nerve palsies, hemiparesis, or paraparesis, which may remit after delivery. Corticosteroids can be given to reduce surrounding oedema, and surgery can often be delayed until after delivery. Gliomas tend to present earlier in pregnancy and have a reputation for following an aggressive course. They may require early surgical intervention, and it is sometimes also appropriate to consider termination of the pregnancy. Women with known intracranial mass lesions require careful assessment prior to delivery: prolonged Valsalva manoeuvres can increase intracranial pressure, hence elective caesarean section may be necessary.

The normal pituitary gland and some pituitary tumours such as prolactinomas expand during pregnancy. Their management, the possibility of pituitary apoplexy, and the postpartum differential diagnosis of lymphocytic hypophysitis are discussed in Chapter 14.11.

Stroke

There is probably an increased incidence of stroke during pregnancy and the puerperium, although it remains rare. There are some causes of stroke which seem to be more common in pregnancy, but most cases are due to one of the usual causes of stroke in nonpregnant young women. Cerebral infarction due to large cerebral artery occlusion may be slightly more common. Possible explanations for this include the mild hypercoagulable state that develops in the later stages of pregnancy and persists for a few weeks afterwards, also the phenomenon of paradoxical embolism from the leg or pelvic veins. Cerebral infarction may occur as a result of hypoxia–ischaemia or disseminated intravascular coagulation in the context of major obstetric emergencies such as amniotic fluid embolism. Unless the cause is obvious, ischaemic stroke in pregnancy should be investigated comprehensively in the same way that it would in a young nonpregnant woman.

Cerebral venous thrombosis, like deep vein thrombosis of the legs, is commoner in the puerperium, and the two conditions may coexist. Classically it gives rise to headache and neurological deficit that evolves over several hours and may become bilateral, with seizures and papilloedema; other cases present with the syndrome of benign intracranial hypertension. The diagnosis can usually be made with MRI, including MR venography. Although venous infarcts frequently undergo haemorrhagic transformation, the currently available evidence favours treatment with heparin. Recovery may be surprisingly complete if the patient survives.

The incidence of aneurysmal subarachnoid haemorrhage is not increased during pregnancy, but its management is difficult.

In general, neurosurgical considerations take precedence over obstetric ones, and the aneurysm is treated in the usual way. If it is not technically possible to deal with the aneurysm surgically or radiologically, then conventional wisdom is to deliver the baby (once it is mature) by caesarean section, although there is no definite evidence to suggest an increased risk of rebleeding during vaginal delivery. Intracranial and subarachnoid haemorrhage from arteriovenous malformations is much less common, but the same principles of management apply. Women with untreatable vascular malformations (including cavernomas) should be counselled about the increased risk of bleeding (perhaps due to a mixture of hormonal and vascular factors) throughout pregnancy.

Epilepsy

Most women with pre-existing epilepsy have no change in the frequency of their seizures during pregnancy, but some 30% have more frequent seizures. These are often women whose epilepsy has been hard to control at other times. Anticonvulsant plasma levels (particularly of lamotrigine) tend to fall in the later stages of pregnancy through increased volumes of distribution and rates of elimination: consensus guidelines recommend that plasma levels are monitored routinely and dosage adjusted to keep these steady. This approach is not entirely foolproof because most laboratories are unable to measure the changes in protein binding that also occur during pregnancy, increasing the availability of free drug. If the dosage is increased prophylactically during pregnancy then it is important to remember to reduce the dosage again in the postpartum period.

An equally important reason for deteriorating control of seizures is lack of adherence to anticonvulsant therapy because of fear of teratogenic effects. This is best addressed by counselling well before pregnancy, which should include a discussion of the risks of uncontrolled epilepsy to both mother and fetus, although it must be admitted that this is made difficult by the lack of quantitative data. As always, the aim of treatment is to control the epilepsy using a single anticonvulsant in the lowest effective dosage, and it is reasonable to try to reduce or withdraw anticonvulsants prior to pregnancy if there is a chance that the epilepsy may have remitted, but it is unwise to attempt this during pregnancy itself.

It is routinely stated that many anticonvulsant drugs are known teratogens, and that the safety of others cannot be guaranteed in pregnancy, with facial clefts, cardiac septal defects, and a pattern of craniofacial and digital dysmorphism known as the fetal anticonvulsant syndrome being described. However, recent data suggests that sodium valproate used as part of polytherapy, or as a single agent, is clearly associated with increased risk, but other agents probably are not. In the best available study the absolute risks of major congenital malformations were carbamazepine 2.2%, lamotrigine 3.2%, phenytoin 3.7%, compared to untreated women with epilepsy 3.5% and valproate 6.2%. Limited information is available for many of the newer anticonvulsants (e.g. gabapentin, vigabatrin, topiramate, tiagabine, etc.), and of those that have been used for a long time, carbamazepine is traditionally regarded (and supported by recent data) as the safest. However, it is worth noting that the teratogenic effects of sodium valproate appear to be dose dependent and dosages of less than 1 g daily may be equally safe. This is important when treating women with conditions such as juvenile myoclonic epilepsy which respond much better to valproate than to carbamazepine.

Sodium valproate and (to a lesser extent) carbamazepine appear to be associated with neural tube defects, some of which may be secondary to drug-induced folate deficiency, hence it is good practice to offer folate supplements (5 mg daily) routinely to all potentially fertile women who are taking anticonvulsants, especially in the 3 months prior to and the first trimester of any planned pregnancy.

In addition to worries about teratogenic effects (which arise in the first 8 weeks of gestation), there are concerns about the potential for anticonvulsants to produce more subtle adverse effects on brain development and the subsequent behaviour and intelligence of the child. *In utero* exposure to valproate is associated with children having a verbal IQ approximately 10 points lower than controls; polytherapy is associated with poorer cognitive outcome, and monotherapy with phenytoin or phenobarbital may be, whereas carbamazepine appears to pose no risk.

Carbamazepine, phenytoin, and the barbiturates accelerate vitamin K metabolism and increase haemorrhagic risks, hence it is good practice to offer the mother vitamin K supplements during the last month of pregnancy and to give the baby vitamin K at birth.

Epilepsy presenting for the first time in pregnancy requires investigation in the same way as adult-onset epilepsy in general. Idiopathic epilepsy that occurs only in pregnancy (so-called gestational epilepsy) is rare. Women presenting with serial seizures or status epilepticus are particularly likely to have an underlying secondary cause such as eclampsia, stroke, tumour, or encephalitis. Epilepsy during labour is usually either iatrogenic (for example, omission of normal anticonvulsant therapy) or again symptomatic of serious intracranial disease. Eclampsia (see Chapter 14.4) is clearly the first consideration, but other possibilities include amniotic fluid embolism and cerebral venous thrombosis.

All anticonvulsants pass into breast milk to some extent, but this need not prevent breastfeeding. Only the barbiturates occasionally cause problems with excessive sedation, but this small risk must be balanced against the problems of effectively withdrawing barbiturates by not breastfeeding. This can lead to the baby becoming irritable and jittery; impaired suckling and withdrawal seizures have also been reported.

Multiple sclerosis

Pregnancy raises complex issues for women with multiple sclerosis. Preconceptual considerations include the small risk (*c*.3%) of their child inheriting the disease, and the practical burdens that child care imposes upon a mother with existing and potentially progressive disability. Several epidemiological studies have shown that the incidence of relapses of multiple sclerosis falls during pregnancy itself, with a compensatory rise in the puerperium (with between 20 and 40% of women reporting an exacerbation of symptoms.) It has been suggested that this reflects the production of pregnancy-associated proteins with immunosuppressive properties, such as α-fetoprotein, and changes in T-lymphocyte subsets. There is no evidence of any long-term detrimental effect on disability, and no evidence of any adverse effect from epidural anaesthesia or breastfeeding.

Relapses in pregnancy are treated in the normal way, with rest supplemented by a short course of oral or intravenous steroid if there is serious new disability. High-dose steroids given late in

pregnancy can cause neonatal adrenal suppression. The manufacturers of interferon-β advise women taking it to avoid pregnancy and discontinue it during pregnancy and breastfeeding unless there are compelling reasons to continue with therapy.

Many women with multiple sclerosis have impaired bladder emptying, which predisposes to urinary tract infection. Severe spinal cord disease is a particular risk because it may mask the usual symptoms of urinary infection; regular urine culture is a sensible precaution. Paraplegia (from any cause) otherwise has little effect on pregnancy, but can lead to premature and unheralded labour, hence regular monitoring is needed in the third trimester. High spinal cord lesions can cause autonomic instability during labour; this can be blocked by careful regional anaesthesia.

Movement disorders

Parkinsonism is rare in women of childbearing age, but tends to worsen slightly during pregnancy. Preconceptual counselling is difficult because there are no useful data in relation to the teratogenicity of the drugs used in young patients; levodopa has teratogenic effects in animals. Dystonic disorders also sometimes worsen in pregnancy, the effect being especially marked in dopa-responsive dystonia where an increase in levodopa therapy may be required. Wilson's disease is an exception and sometimes improves in pregnancy. Concerns about the potential teratogenic effects of therapy with penicillamine must be balanced against the risks of catastrophic neurological deterioration if therapy is abruptly withdrawn, although in the future treatments such as zinc may turn out to be a safe alternative.

Further reading

Aube M (1999). Migraine in pregnancy (review). *Neurology* **53** Suppl. 1, 26–8.

Batocchi AP, *et al.* (1999). Course and treatment of myasthenia gravis during pregnancy. *Neurology*, **52**, 447–52.

Battino D, Tomson T. (2007). Management of epilepsy during pregnancy. *Drugs*, **67**, 2727–46.

Ferrero S, *et al.* (2005). Myasthenia gravis: management issues during pregnancy. *Eur J Obstet Gynecol Reprod Biol*, **121**, 129–38.

Grosset DG, *et al.* (1995). Stroke in pregnancy and the puerperium: what magnitude of risk? *J Neurol Neurosurg Psychiatr*, **58**, 129–31.

Harden CL. (2007). Antiepileptic drug teratogenesis: what are the risks for congenital malformations and adverse cognitive outcomes? *Int Rev Neurobiol*, **83**, 205–13.

Harden CL, Sethi NK (2008). Epileptic disorders in pregnancy: an overview. *Curr Opin Obstet Gynecol*, **20**, 557–62.

Isla A, *et al.* (1997). Brain tumour and pregnancy. *Obstet Gynecol*, **89**, 19–23.

Liang CC, *et al.* (2006). Stroke complicating pregnancy and the puerperium. *Eur J Neurol*, **13**, 1256–60.

Lee M, O'Brien P. (2008). Pregnancy and multiple sclerosis. *J Neurol Neurosurg Psychiatr*, **79**, 1308–11.

Pennell PB (2004). Pregnancy in women who have epilepsy. *Neurol Clin*, **22**, 799–820.

Rudnick-Schoneborn S, *et al.* (1998). Different patterns of obstetric complications in myotonic dystrophy in relation to the disease status of the fetus. *Am J Med Genet*, **80**, 314–21.

Sax TW, Rosenbaum RB. (2006). Neuromuscular disorders in pregnancy. *Muscle Nerve*, **34**, 559–71.

Shneerson JM (1994). Pregnancy in neuromuscular and skeletal disorders. *Arch Chest Dis*, **49**, 227–30.

The skin in pregnancy

Fenella Wojnarowska

Essentials

Pregnancy dermatoses are common, and because they are usually very itchy may ruin the life of the pregnant woman. It is particularly important to recognize when itch is due to intrahepatic cholestasis of pregnancy, which has important implications for the health of both mother and fetus (see Chapter 14.9).

Atopic eruption of pregnancy—affects 1/300 pregnancies, typically with an eczematous eruption over abdomen and limbs. Treatment is difficult: there is a dilemma in balancing the need for treatment with the wish to minimize the use of potent topical steroids that will be absorbed and may affect the fetus.

Polymorphic eruption of pregnancy—affects about 1 in 240 pregnancies, usually beginning with red papules and plaques on the abdomen and thighs before spreading more widely. Treatment is with reassurance and emollients, with steroids avoided if possible.

Pemphigoid gestationis—the most severe of the pregnancy dermatoses. It occurs in 1 in 50 000 pregnancies and is due to circulating antibodies against the skin basement membrane zone. The eruption begins around the umbilicus and spreads to the whole trunk, limbs, hands and feet. Systemic steroids are usually required. Transplacental transmission to the fetus may occur. Recurrence in future pregnancies is to be expected.

Introduction

The skin undergoes profound alterations during pregnancy as a result of endocrine, metabolic, and physiological changes. Some of these are trivial and chiefly cosmetic, producing no or minor symptoms; others can be distressing and/or of major medical importance. Pregnancy will profoundly modify expression of pre-existing skin disease, and there are dermatoses that are specific to pregnancy.

Common skin changes in pregnancy

Vascular changes and lesions

There is increased skin blood flow during pregnancy, making the skin more prone to itch and to oedema, manifest as tightening of rings and shoes. Spider naevi and palmar erythema are common, and there maybe erythema of the gums (with gingivitis) and vulvovaginal area. Unilateral telangiectasia may appear for the first time, as may haemangiomas.

Pyogenic granuloma, a benign tumour with a tendency ulcerate and to bleed, may develop on the skin or oral cavity, where they are known as pregnancy tumours (Fig. 14.13.1). They are sometimes confused with melanoma and often recur after local destruction.

Pigmentary changes and pigmented lesions

Increased skin pigmentation is common, particularly in dark-skinned women, up to 90% of whom may be affected. There is darkening of the nipples, genitalia, and linea alba. In some women recent scars will darken. The unsightly and sometimes psychologically distressing facial pigmentation of melasma (chloasma, formerly known as the 'mask of pregnancy') affects many women, is worse with sunlight, and can be reduced by the use of high protection factor (SPF 50) UVB and UVA sun screens (Fig. 14.13.2).

Pigmented naevi can increase in number, size and pigmentation. Melanoma may occur and is not associated with a poorer prognosis in pregnant women. Any rapidly changing, irregularly shaped, or irregularly pigmented mole should be biopsied to exclude a dysplastic naevus or melanoma.

Hair changes

There is diminished shedding of hair due to prolongation of anagen. This is perceived as thickening of the hair, which increased sebum secretion makes appear more lustrous. The synchronized shedding after parturition gives rise to the distressing postpartum telogen effluvium. Hirsutism may begin or worsen in pregnancy, as there is an associated increase in androgens.

Pilosebaceous changes

The increased oestrogens of pregnancy usually improve acne, but there may be worsening of acne in some unfortunate patients, and the entire skin is usually greasier.

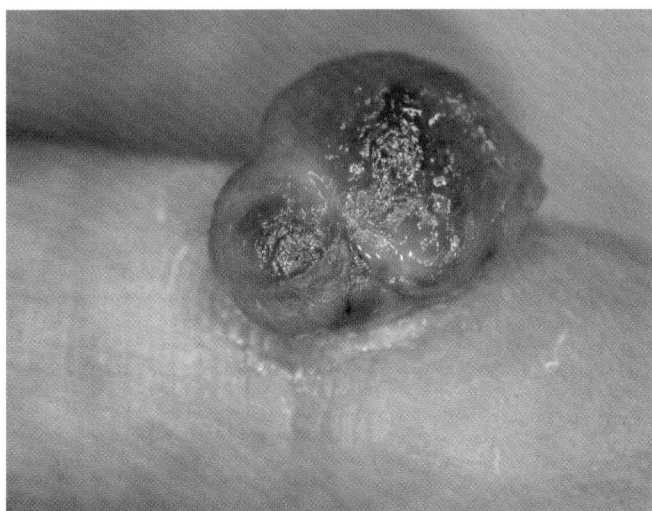

Fig. 14.13.1 Pyogenic granuloma on the finger.
(Courtesy of Dr Jonathan Bowling, Oxford Radcliffe Hospital NHS Trust, UK.)

Striae gravidarum

Striae gravidarum (stretch marks) are common in pregnancy. They affect about half of white women, are more frequent in dark-skinned women, and are familial in about 50% of cases. They are commoner and more severe in young women and teenagers, who are a group already at risk for striae, and they are more likely if a woman has had them previously. They are associated with a raised maternal body mass index and large babies.

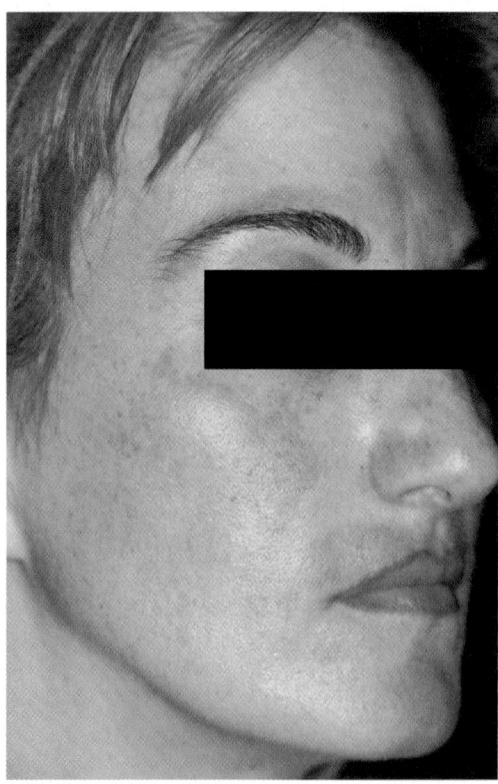

Fig. 14.13.2 Melasma
(Courtesy of Dr Christina Ambros-Rudolph, University of Graz, Austria.)

The breasts and sides and lower areas of the abdomen are the typical sites, but thighs and arms can be affected. They start as linear depressed purple lesions and fade to pale, atrophic, scar-like lesions. They may be itchy. There is an association with subsequent tendency to prolapse.

Cutaneous infections

Candida of the vulva as well as the vagina is common and occurs in about 15% of pregnant women, causing itching, burning, and discharge.

Cutaneous and genital warts thrive in pregnancy, often commencing, proliferating, or enlarging. Treatment of genital warts is by physical destruction: podophyllin must not be used in pregnancy. Genital herpes simplex infections can pose problems with delivery during active infections.

The pregnancy dermatoses

Historical perspective

The striking blistering eruption known as 'pemphigoid gestationis' was described in 1867 by Wilson and named by Milton in 1872 as 'herpes gestationis'. During the 1980s it was characterized as an autoimmune blistering disease by Black, Charles-Holmes, and Shornick, and renamed as 'pemphigoid gestationis' to emphasize the close relationship to the commoner autoimmune blistering disease bullous pemphigoid and to prevent confusion with viral herpes disease.

The other skin diseases that arise in pregnancy have been confusing in their nomenclature and clinical descriptions, but recently Ambros-Rudolph and colleagues proposed a new and much simpler classification (Table 14.13.1).

Pruritus of pregnancy and intrahepatic cholestatis of pregnancy

Itching occurs in about 20% of pregnancies, frequently in association with an inflammatory dermatosis. Often pruritus occurs without physical signs, other than scratch marks. The most serious cause is intrahepatic cholostasis of pregnancy, which is the cause in about 3% of itchy pregnant women (see Chapter 14.9). The itching

Table 14.13.1 Major pregnancy dermatoses

Pregnancy dermatosis	Frequency (%)	Effect on fetus	Effect on mother
Intrahepatic cholestatis of pregnancy	3	Can be major (see Chapter 14.9)	Can be major (see Chapter 14.9)
Atopic eruption of pregnancy	50		
Polymorphic eruption of pregnancy	22		
Urticaria	2		
Pemphigoid gestationis	4[a]	Small for dates	

Numbers based on 505 pregnant patients with skin problems (Ambros-Rudolph *et al.* 2006).
[a] Raised frequency as tertiary referral centre.

begins in the third trimester and affects the abdomen, palms, and soles. Liver function tests are abnormal and bile salts are raised; iron deficiency should be excluded. The condition resolves postpartum but will recur in subsequent pregnancies. Management is with emollients and sometimes antihistamines, chlorpheniramine usually being recommended in pregnancy. The nonsedating antihistamines are probably ineffective.

Atopic eruption of pregnancy

This condition includes entities formerly known as prurigo of pregnancy and pruritic folliculitis. It may affect 1 in 300 pregnancies. It occurs in women with an atopic background (personal or family history), of whom about 20% have had previous eczema. The immunological changes of pregnancy and the tendency to pruritus may both contribute to the worsening of atopic eczema or its first occurrence with pregnancy.

Atopic eruption of pregnancy commences early, in three-quarters of women before the beginning of the third trimester. There is intense pruritus. The eruption is scattered over the abdomen and limbs (Fig. 14.13.3). The lesions can be chiefly eczematous. The skin is red, dry, and scaly, with areas of excoriation and thickening or lichenification. Pre-existing atopic eczema often deteriorates becoming more widespread and may result in erythroderma in the most severe cases. Another presentation is with excoriated papules and nodules (prurigo of pregnancy). The least common form is follicular pruritic papules and pustules (pruritic folliculitis), which may present in the third trimester and in a

Table 14.13.2 Examples of topical steroids

Group	Generic name	Trade names
Mild	Hydrocortisone 1%	Numerous
Moderately potent	Hydrocortisone 1% with urea	Alphaderm, Calmurid HC
	Clobetasone butyrate	Eumovate
	Flurandrolone	Haelan
Potent	Betamethasone valerate	Betnovate RD, Betnovate
	Betamethasone dipropionate	Propaderm, Diprosalic, Diprosone
	Hydrocortisone 17-butyrate	Locoid
	Fluticasone propionate	Cutivate[a]
	Mometasone furoate	Elocon[a]
Very potent	Clobetasol propionate	Dermovate

[a] Newer topical steroids.

small series was associated with male infants and low birth weight. Secondary infection with *Staphylococcus aureus* and streptococci is a frequent complication.

Histopathology is usually nonspecific, but may show a perivascular infiltrate with thickened epidermis. Direct and indirect immunofluorescence are negative.

Treatment is difficult: there is a dilemma in balancing the need for treatment with the wish to minimize the use of potent topical steroids that will be absorbed and may affect the fetus. The use of emollients may lessen the requirements for topical steroids, and steroids should be used in the minimum quantities and strengths necessary to control the disease (see Table 14.13.2). Many topical steroids contain antiseptics and antibiotics which will be absorbed and may be contraindicated in pregnancy. The sedating antihistamine chlorpheniramine may help with sleep. Secondary infection often requires systemic antibiotics such as erythromycin or flucloxacillin.

The condition resolves in days to weeks after delivery. It may recur in one-third of pregnancies.

Polymorphic eruption of pregnancy

This condition was formerly known as 'pruritic urticated papules and plaques of pregnancy' or 'toxic erythema of pregnancy'. Its aetiology is unknown, but there is an association with a low serum cortisol. It affects 1 in 240 singleton pregnancies, being most common in first pregnancies, with multiple births (and hence following *in vitro* fertilization)—perhaps related to the mechanical effect of the abdominal stretching or to an increased immune complex load—and with a male fetus.

The dermatosis usually begins in the third trimester and occasionally postpartum. The lesions typically begin in the striae on the abdomen and thighs and then spread to the whole trunk and limbs, including the hands and feet. They are very itchy, and the itching can be so severe as to prevent sleep. Initially the lesions are raised red papules (Fig. 14.13.4) and plaques; with time they become more diverse in morphology, occasionally polycyclic or blistering.

The histopathology shows oedema, perivascular lymphocytes, and eosinophils. Immunofluorescence does not demonstrate any circulating or bound immunoreactants.

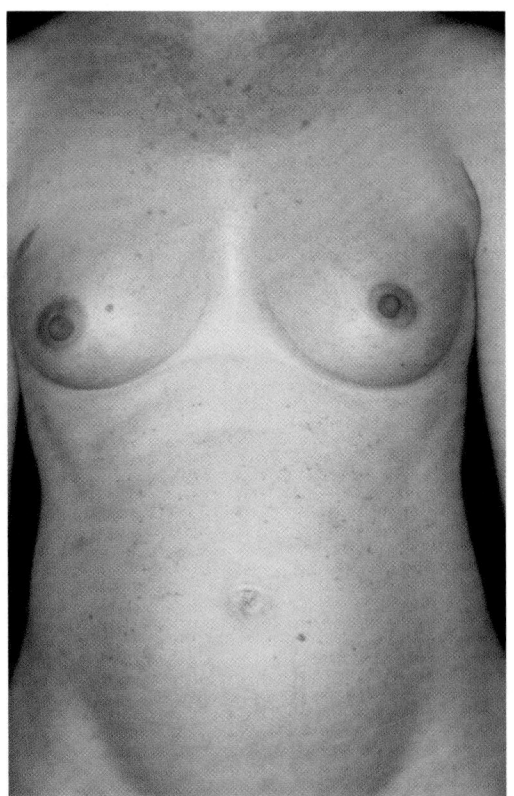

Fig. 14.13.3 Atopic eruption of pregnancy in a 24-year-old gravida 2 at 19 weeks gestation: small red pruritic papules and eczematous features on the trunk (and limbs).
(Courtesy of Dr Christina Ambros-Rudolph, University of Graz, Austria.)

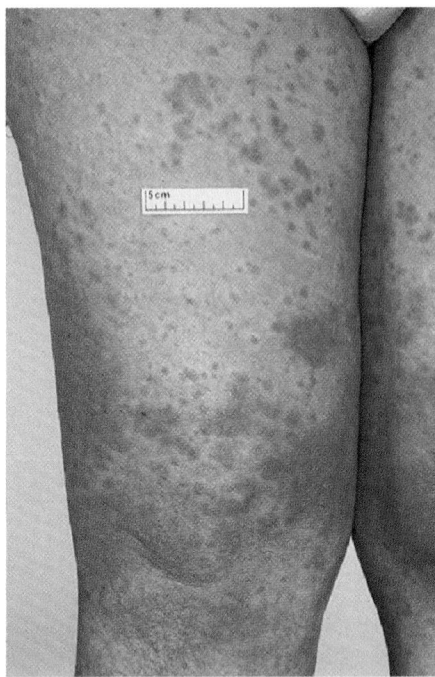

Fig. 14.13.4 Polymorphic eruption of pregnancy: urticated papules and plaques on the thigh.

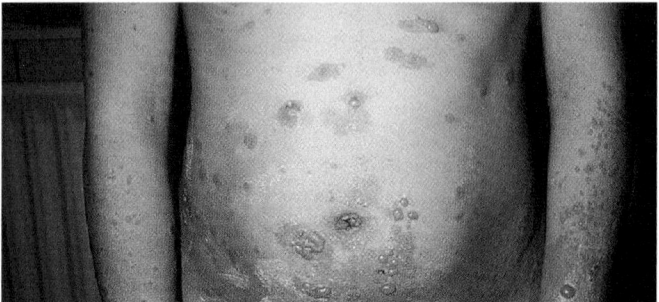

Fig. 14.13.5 Pemphigoid gestationis: urticated papules and plaques and blisters. (From Charles-Holmes R, Black MM (1990). Herpes gestationis. In: Wojnarowska F, Briggaman RA (eds) *Management of blistering disease*, pp. 93–104. Chapman & Hall, London, with permission.)

Treatment is with reassurance and emollients, e.g. aqueous cream and 1 to 2% menthol. This is helpful, but not always sufficient. Antihistamines and moderate to very potent topical steroids, which will have significant absorption (see Table 14.13.2), may be required, and occasionally systemic steroids for induction.

The condition resolves over days to weeks after delivery. It does not usually recur. The outcome of the pregnancy is not adversely affected.

Pemphigoid gestationis (herpes gestationis)

Pemphigoid gestationis is the most severe of the pregnancy dermatoses. The name 'herpes gestationis' is best abandoned as the herpes refers to the herpetiform grouping of the blisters rather than herpes infection.

The aetiology is only partially understood. The pathogenicity of the circulating basement membrane zone antibodies is demonstrated by transplacental transmission of the disease. The major target antigen is BP180/collagen XVII (chief epitope being the transmembrane NC16A domain); BP230 is a less common antigen. Both antigens are present in skin, mucosa, and amnion, associated with the hemidesmosome and adhesion complex linking epithelium to dermis/mesenchyme, which are targets in other autoimmune blistering diseases. The placenta shows increased expression of antigen-presenting cells, but it is unclear why breakdown of tolerance occurs, and why normal components of amnion and stratified squamous epithelium become antigenic. The mothers have the HLA DR 3, 4, haplotype and are C4 null, and there is an association with thyroid and less commonly other autoimmune disease.

Pemphigoid gestationis occurs in 1 in 50 000 pregnancies. It commences from the second trimester onwards and quite often in the first week postpartum (range from 5 weeks of gestation to 4 weeks postpartum). It usually occurs in the first and subsequent pregnancies, although 8% of pregnancies are skipped.

The eruption begins around the umbilicus and spreads to the whole trunk, limbs, hands and feet, including the palms and soles, and rarely the face. The mouth and vulva may be involved. It usually commences as an annular red raised plaque around the umbilicus. The lesions comprise annular lesions, papules and plaques. Vesicles and blisters are seen (Fig. 14.13.5). The mucosal lesions may be blisters or erosions. Pruritus is severe and sleep often impossible. Transplacental transmission to the fetus occurs in about 3% of affected pregnancies, the neonate developing transient self-limiting blisters (Fig. 14.13.6).

Histopathology demonstrates eosinophilia, subepidermal blisters, and teardrop vesicles within the epidermis, continuous with the subepidermal blisters. Direct immunofluorescence demonstrates that C3 component of complement and IgG1 are bound at the basement membrane zone of the dermoepidermal junction. The patient's serum has circulating IgG1 basement membrane zone antibodies that bind C3. These immunoreactants are also found at the basement membrane zone of the amnion (Fig. 14.13.7).

Treatment with potent or very potent topical steroids and chlorpheniramine is sometimes successful, but usually systemic steroids (e.g. prednisolone 20–80 mg daily) are required, with

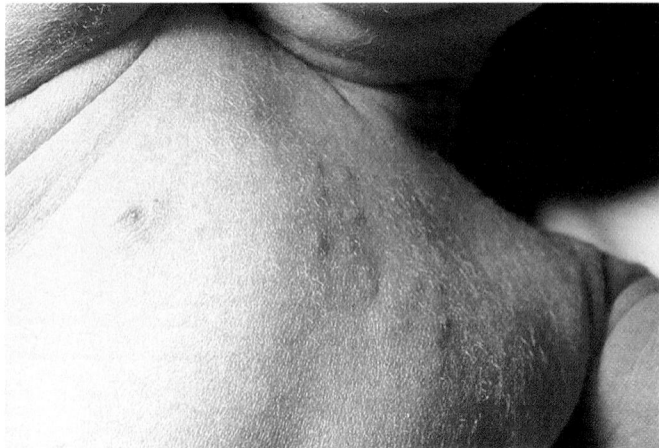

Fig. 14.13.6 Pemphigoid gestationis: urticated papules in the neonate. (From Charles-Holmes R, Black MM (1990). Herpes gestationis. In: Wojnarowska F, Briggaman RA (eds) *Management of blistering disease*, pp. 93–104. Chapman & Hall, London, with permission.)

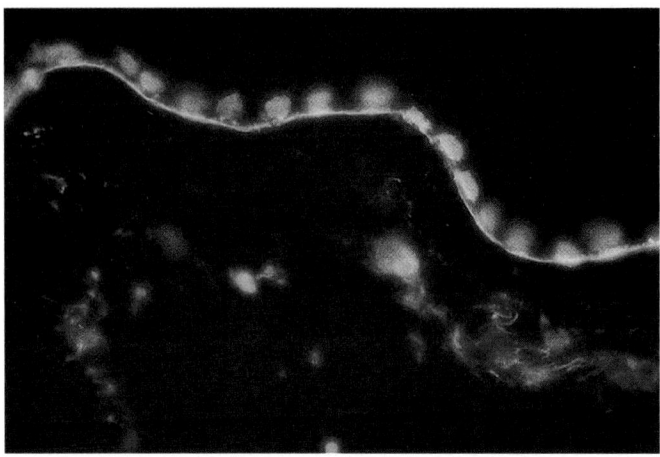

Fig. 14.13.7 Pemphigoid gestationis: linear deposition of C3 at the amnion basement membrane zone as demonstrated by immunofluorescence. The nuclei are counter-stained with propidium iodide.
(Courtesy of B S Bhogal and M M Black, St John's Institute of Dermatology, St Thomas's Hospital, London.)

the dose adjusted according to disease activity. There is usually a postpartum flare, necessitating increased steroids.

The disease slowly resolves postpartum, but persists for several months. Recurrence in subsequent pregnancies is usual, only about 8% being spared. The classical teaching is that it recurs earlier and is more severe in subsequent pregnancies, but this has not always been our experience. There is an increased incidence of premature births and small-for-dates babies.

Urticaria

Urticaria (hives) and dermographism (wealing in response to pressure, e.g. scratching) may be precipitated by pregnancy. This has been attributed by some authors to physiological changes in vascular reactivity. Physical factors such as pressure and heat may evoke it. Drugs may be the cause in some patients. Treatment is with chlopheniramine or a nonsedating antihistamine such as loratidine.

Dermatoses and the effect of pregnancy

Atopic eczema

Atopic eczema commonly worsens in pregnancy (see above). It can be severe and life ruining, and life threatening if secondary infection with herpes simplex (eczema herpeticum) or streptococci occurs.

Psoriasis

Psoriasis improves in most women during pregnancy, but can deteriorate. Therapy poses special problems as all the systemic treatments are contraindicated: methotrexate is a folic acid

antagonist; acitretin is teratogenic; psoralens with UVA are still not proven to be safe. Topical therapy with steroids should be avoided if possible. Coal tars and dithranol have been widely used in pregnancy but are not proven to be safe, and the new vitamin D analogues are not licensed for use in pregnancy. The ideal is minimum treatment, with emollients and if necessary UVB. A severe form of pustular psoriasis, impetigo herpetiformis, may occur in pregnancy and is best managed with bed rest and emollients.

Autoimmune dermatoses in pregnancy

Cutaneous lupus erythematosus

Cutaneous lupus erythematosus may be adversely affected or improved or unchanged by pregnancy. However such patients should be screened for anti-Ro and anticardiolipin antibodies etc., preferably prior to conception, to identify at-risk pregnancies (see Chapter 14.14).

Autoimmune bullous diseases

Linear IgA disease, an autoimmune blistering disease with IgA basement membrane zone antibodies, usually improves with pregnancy, such that some patients can discontinue their dapsone therapy. Despite the deposition of immunoreactants in the amnion basement membrane zone the fetus is not adversely affected. There is usually an exacerbation 3 months postpartum.

Pemphigus vulgaris is an autoimmune blistering disease with widespread mucosal an/or cutaneous erosions caused by antibodies to desmosomal components. The desmosomal antibodies are directed at desmoglein 3, a major adhesion molecule in mucosa and neonatal skin, and can be transmitted across the placenta, causing severe neonatal pemphigus with devastating results to the fetus. This does not occur in the related pemphigus foliaceus, which is endemic in Brazil, characterized by superficial cutaneous erosions and mediated by desmoglein 1 antibodies that do not cause oral lesions or affect neonatal skin. Both forms of pemiphigus often worsen in pregnancy.

Further reading

Ambros-Rudolph CM, *et al.* (2006) The specific dermatoses of pregnancy revisited and reclassified: results of a retrospective two-center study on 505 pregnant patients. *J Am Acad Dermatol*, **54**, 395–404.

Collier P, Kelly SE, Wojnarowska F (1993). Linear IgA disease and pregnancy. *J Am Acad Dermatol*, **30**, 407–12.

Holmes RC, *et al.* (1982). A comparative study of toxic erythema of pregnancy and herpes gestationis. *Br J Dermatol*, **106**, 499–510.

Jenkins RE, Hern S, Black MM (1999). Clinical features and management of 87 patients with pemphigoid gestationis. *Clin Exp Dermatol*, **24**, 255–9.

Muller S, Stanley JR (1990). Pemphigus: pemphigus vulgaris and pemphigus foliaceus. In: Wojnarowska F and Briggaman RA (eds) *Management of blistering disease*, Chapman & Hall, London, pp. 43–62.

Vaughan Jones SA, *et al.* (1999). A prospective study of 200 women with dermatoses of pregnancy correlating clinical findings with hormonal and immunopathological profiles. *Br J Dermatol*, **141**, 71–81.

Autoimmune rheumatic disorders and vasculitis in pregnancy

Sarah Germain and Catherine Nelson-Piercy

Essentials

Autoimmune diseases affect 5 to 7% of people, are commoner in women of childbearing age, and are frequently encountered in pregnancy. They may remit or improve during pregnancy, but can flare or present in pregnancy with disastrous consequences. The postpartum period is a time of susceptibility to autoimmune disorders, and women who already have an autoimmune disorder may suffer disease exacerbation following pregnancy.

Systemic lupus erythematosus (SLE)

The mother—pregnancy probably exacerbates SLE and increases the likelihood of a flare, which can be difficult to diagnose since many features (e.g. hair loss, oedema, facial erythema, fatigue, musculoskeletal pain) also occur in normal pregnancy. Differentiation of active renal lupus from pre-eclampsia is notoriously difficult, and the two conditions may be superimposed: renal flares are more common if disease is active within 6 months of conception, in particular in women with hypertension, heavy proteinuria, or high baseline serum creatinine. There is an increased risk of maternal thrombosis and premature atherosclerosis.

The fetus—SLE is associated with increased risks of adverse pregnancy outcome including fetal death and IUGR. Most fetal losses occur in association with secondary antiphospholipid syndrome or active disease, particularly renal. For women with SLE in remission and without hypertension, renal involvement, or the antiphospholipid syndrome, the risk of problems in pregnancy is similar to that of the general population.

Management—flares of SLE must be actively managed, pre-pregnancy counselling should be encouraged with treatment depending on both organ involvement and severity. Mild cases can be managed with analgesics alone (paracetamol); rash and arthritis will usually respond to NSAIDs, low dose prednisolone and/or hydroxycholorquine; more severe disease may require introduction of a disease modifying agent e.g. azathioprine or higher steroid dose. Steroids remain first-line treatment for severe lupus flares in pregnancy (and treatment of other autoimmune conditions), with the benefits of rapid disease control outweighing the risks.

The baby—neonatal lupus syndromes are caused by transplacental passage of autoantibodies directed against cytoplasmic ribonucleoproteins Ro and La. Cutaneous neonatal lupus is the most common manifestation (5%) and congenital heart block the most serious (20% mortality).

Antiphospholipid syndrome

Clinical features—antiphospholipid antibodies include anticardiolipin antibodies (IgG and/or IgM), lupus anticoagulant and anti-β_2-glycoprotein-I antibody. Antiphospholipid syndrome (APS) is the combination of any of these with one or more of the characteristic clinical features: (1) thrombosis—arterial, venous or capillary; (2) recurrent or late pregnancy loss—typically in the second trimester; and (3) adverse pregnancy outcome.

Management— aim is to improve pregnancy outcome and prevent maternal thrombosis. This will require aspirin and/or LMWH, and close fetal and maternal surveillance.

Rheumatoid arthritis

Rheumatoid arthritis has no adverse effect on fertility or pregnancy and often improves during pregnancy. The main concerns relate to the safety during pregnancy and lactation of the medications used in treatment—although most women can be managed on analgesics and low dose prednisolone.

Introduction

Autoimmune diseases affect 5 to 7% of the population, are commoner in women of childbearing age, and are frequently encountered in pregnancy.

Pregnancy is associated with suppressed cell-mediated immunity (Th1) and enhancement of humoral immunity (Th2), but these changes revert postpartum accompanied by sudden reductions of oestrogen, progesterone, and cortisol levels. The postpartum period is therefore a time of susceptibility to autoimmune disorders and women who already have an autoimmune disorder may suffer disease exacerbation following pregnancy. Conversely, autoimmune diseases may remit or improve during pregnancy, but this is not a universal rule, and autoimmune rheumatic diseases can flare or present in pregnancy with disastrous consequences.

This chapter considers the relationship between pregnancy and systemic lupus erythematosus (SLE), antiphospholipid syndrome (APS), rheumatoid arthritis (RA), vasculitides, and scleroderma, and how pregnancy affects treatment of these conditions. The management of these conditions during pregnancy provides the obstetrician and physician with particular challenges and concerns related to not only the mother but also the fetus.

Systemic lupus erythematosus (SLE)

SLE is a multisystem autoimmune rheumatic disorder of unknown aetiology, although genetic and environmental factors have been identified, including sunlight and various drugs. It is much more common in women than men (ratio 9:1), with peak onset during the childbearing years. A recent extensive review of published epidemiological studies demonstrated that the prevalence ranges from 0.07/1000 in white Americans to 1.59/1000 in British Afro-Caribbeans.

Effect of pregnancy on SLE

SLE flares may be difficult to diagnose during pregnancy since many features such as hair loss, oedema, facial erythema, fatigue, musculoskeletal pain, anaemia, and raised ESR also occur in normal pregnancy. Disease activity scores have now been validated for use in pregnancy.

Pregnancy probably exacerbates SLE and increases the likelihood of a flare. A number of case–control studies have addressed this issue, but differ in patient ethnicity, criteria for flare and SLE activity scales employed. Some found no increased risk of deterioration in pregnancy, but most suggest that SLE was more likely to flare during pregnancy and the puerperium. In one prospective case–control study, 65% of women flared during pregnancy, compared to 42% nonpregnant women during the same time period. The type of flare usually follows previous disease pattern. Steroids do not prevent flares, and therefore it is not appropriate to prescribe or increase the dose of steroids prophylactically during pregnancy or postpartum.

Renal flares are more common if disease is active within 6 months of conception. As with all types of renal disease there is a risk of deterioration of renal function in pregnancy, in particular in patients with hypertension, heavy proteinuria, or high baseline serum creatinine. As a general rule, if serum creatinine is greater than 2 mg/dl (177 μmol/litre) then deterioration is often irreversible, whereas it is usually transient if creatinine is less than 2 mg/dl.

However, lupus nephritis may have a more favourable outcome: a recent meta-analysis reported that the incidence of renal lupus flares during pregnancy was 11 to 69% and renal impairment occurred in 3 to 27%, which was irreversible in 0 to 10%. SLE nephritis may also present for the first time during pregnancy. Worsening proteinuria in pregnancy can provide a diagnostic challenge, as in addition to nephritic flare, it may be due to physiological change, discontinuation of angiotensin-converting enzyme (ACE) inhibitor, or pre-eclampsia.

Women with SLE have an increased risk of maternal thrombosis, especially in the puerperium, and this is usually associated with antiphospholipid antibodies. They are also at risk of premature atherosclerosis, and myocardial infarction should be considered if presenting with chest pain or shortness of breath. Pulmonary hypertension, present in up to 14% of patients, carries a significant risk of maternal death.

Effect of SLE on pregnancy

Fertility is not usually affected by SLE, except for cyclophosphamide-induced ovarian failure, but SLE is associated with increased risks of adverse pregnancy outcome. These include early miscarriage, intrauterine fetal death, pre-eclampsia, intrauterine growth restriction (IUGR), and preterm delivery. The main factors influencing the effect of SLE on pregnancy are disease activity (especially at time of conception), hypertension, renal involvement, antiphospholipid antibodies, and anti-Ro/La antibodies (see below).

In a prospective study of 267 pregnancies in 203 lupus patients, live birth rate was 86%, with incidence of prematurity 31% and small for gestational age 23%. Most of the fetal losses were in association with secondary APS or active disease.

Pregnancy outcome is particularly affected by renal disease, with active nephritis an independent risk factor for fetal loss. In the meta-analysis discussed above, fetal loss ranged from 25 to 50% in patients with active disease at conception to 8 to 12% if disease was inactive. Similar to the risk of renal deterioration during pregnancy, the risk of adverse pregnancy outcome is increased with higher baseline creatinine. Even quiescent renal lupus is associated with increased risk of the adverse outcomes above, particularly if there is hypertension or proteinuria. One case–control study showed that 28% of patients with class III or IV lupus nephritis developed pre-eclampsia, 35% had a preterm delivery, and average birthweight was 2.21 kg, compared to 4.6%, 18.6%, and 2.87 kg respectively for women with SLE but no nephritis, 21.4% having active disease in the former group, compared to 11.1% in the latter.

For women with SLE in remission, and without hypertension, renal involvement, or APS, the risk of problems in pregnancy is similar to that of the general population.

Management of SLE in pregnancy
Preconception counselling

When possible, management should begin with preconception counselling. Knowledge of renal function, blood pressure, and the antiphospholipid and anti-Ro/La antibody status allows prediction of the risks to the woman and her baby (see below). Appropriate baseline investigations are listed in Box 14.14.1. A decision should be made as to whether to start aspirin and/or heparin if the woman is antiphospholipid antibody positive (see later).

The outlook is better if conception occurs during remission, and women should be advised to avoid pregnancy until 6 months post-flare, especially if there is renal involvement. Current drug treatments should be reviewed and adjusted if necessary, as discussed below, preferably at least 3 to 6 months preconception to allow stabilization.

Maternal surveillance

Pregnancy care is best undertaken in multidisciplinary, combined clinics where physicians and obstetricians can monitor disease activity, fetal growth, and uterine and umbilical artery Doppler blood flow regularly.

Diagnosis of flare

Differentiation of active renal lupus from pre-eclampsia is notoriously difficult, and the two conditions may be superimposed. Table 14.14.1 lists features to help to distinguish them. The only definitive investigation to reliably differentiate a renal lupus flare from pre-eclampsia is renal biopsy, but this is rarely undertaken in pregnancy.

Management of flare

Disease flares must be actively managed. Treatment will depend on the organ involvement and severity. Mild cases can be managed with analgesics alone (paracetamol). Rash and arthritis will usually respond to nonsteroidal anti-inflammatory drugs (NSAIDs), low-dose prednisolone, and/or hydroxycholorquine. More severe disease may require introduction of a disease-modifying agent or

Table 14.14.1 Features to help distinguish lupus nephritis flare and pre-eclampsia

Both	Lupus nephritis flare	Pre-eclampsia
Hypertension	Symptoms of lupus flare in other systems	Raised uric acid
Thrombocytopenia	Rising dsDNA titre	Raised liver function tests
Renal impairment	Fall in C3 and C4	
Proteinuria	Active urinary sediment (red blood cells or cellular casts)	

higher steroid dose, and azathioprine is often used as a steroid-sparing drug.

Paracetamol, which has no known adverse effects in pregnancy, should be the first-line analgesic. Aspirin and NSAIDs are not teratogenic, but both aspirin (in analgesic doses) and NSAIDs may increase the risk of neonatal haemorrhage via inhibition of platelet function. Low-dose aspirin has not been shown to have adverse effects on neonatal renal function, pulmonary hypertension, or clotting ability. NSAIDs may also lead to oligohydramnios via effects on the fetal kidney, and as they are prostaglandin synthetase inhibitors may cause premature closure of the ductus arteriosus (because prostaglandin E_2 relaxation of pulmonary vessels is inhibited) with neonatal primary pulmonary hypertension. They are usually avoided in pregnancy, especially in the last trimester, but the risk to the ductus arteriosus may have been exaggerated since premature closure has not been encountered when indomethacin is used for the treatment of premature labour. Impairment of ductal flow is rare before 27 weeks and resolves within 24 to 48 h of NSAID discontinuation. Oligohydramios is also reversible. In occasional circumstances, and especially before 28 weeks gestation, NSAIDs may be used for control of arthritic pain if there are relative contraindications to steroids, e.g. in patients with severe osteoporosis. They should be discontinued at least 6 to 8 weeks before delivery. Preparations in combination with misoprostol are contraindicated because of the latter's abortifacient effect.

The newer cyclo-oxygenase type 2 selective (COX-2) NSAIDs, currently contraindicated in pregnancy, also appear to have significant, but reversible, effects on fetal renal function and the ductus arteriosus, but these may be less than with nonselective COX inhibitors.

Prednisolone is metabolized by the placenta and very little (10%) active drug reaches the fetus, unlike dexamethasone and betamethasone which cross the placenta more readily. In animal studies, large doses of prednisolone or hydrocortisone are associated with an increased incidence of cleft palate. Clinical experience varies, with some studies—including a meta-analysis—showing an increased risk of oral clefts following first-trimester exposure. There are many other studies supporting no increased risk of congenital malformations, miscarriage, adverse fetal effects, stillbirth, or neonatal death attributable to maternal steroid therapy. However, in women with APS treated with high doses of prednisolone throughout pregnancy, an increased frequency of premature rupture of the membranes has been reported, and some studies suggest an increased incidence of IUGR, although this is controversial. Betamethasone and dexamethasone are used to reduce respiratory distress syndrome in those at risk of preterm delivery, but there is increasing evidence that repeated courses—particularly of dexamethasone—can adversely affect the child's later neuropsychological development. Other potential fetal or neonatal adverse effects are limited to rare case reports, including suppression of the fetal hypothalamic–pituitary–adrenal axis, infections, and neonatal cataract. Corticosteroid usage in pregnancy does increase the maternal risk of gestational diabetes, hypertension, infection and osteoporosis. Women on long-term maintenance steroids (>7.5 mg/day for >2 weeks) require parenteral steroids to cover the stress of labour and delivery. Prednisolone is safe in breastfeeding mothers since less than 10% of active drug is secreted into breast milk. Notwithstanding the above risks, steroids remain first-line treatment for severe lupus flares in pregnancy (and treatment of other autoimmune conditions), as the benefits of rapid disease control outweigh the risks.

Disease-modifying antirheumatic drugs (DMARDs) are discussed in Table 14.14.2.

Treatment of systemic and pulmonary hypertension

For control of hypertension, the drug of choice in pregnancy is methyldopa, with calcium channel blockers (e.g. nifedipine) or hydralazine as second-line agents. β-Blockers are avoided if possible because of the increase in IUGR when high-dose atenolol was used long-term throughout pregnancy, although this adverse effect has not been seen with labetalol despite extensive experience in pregnancy. ACE inhibitors and angiotensin-2 receptor blockers should be stopped before pregnancy. Until recently some have advocated their continued until the first trimester, as only after that time is their use associated with renal tract abnormalities, oligohydramnios, hypotension, and decreased skull ossification in the fetus. However, there is now evidence that even exposure periconceptually is associated with a 2.7-fold increased risk of overall congenital abnormalities, especially cardiovascular (3.7-fold) and neurological (4.4-fold).

Since maternal mortality is so high with pulmonary hypertension, continued use of sildenafil, bosentan, and epoprostenol analogues may be appropriate. There is little experience regarding potential adverse effects of these drugs on the human fetus, but bosentan is teratogenic in animals.

Postpartum

Drugs used during pregnancy are generally safe when breast-feeding, but a risk–benefit assessment should always be made (see Table 14.14.2).

When considering postnatal contraception, the combined oral contraceptive pill should probably be avoided because of the increased risk of thrombosis in SLE, especially if antiphospholipid antibodies are present. It had been suggested that exogenous oestrogens also increase the risk of disease flare, but two recent studies have not confirmed this.

Neonatal lupus syndromes

These conditions are models of passively acquired autoimmunity. Autoantibodies, known as extractable nuclear antibodies (eNA), directed against cytoplasmic ribonucleoproteins Ro and La, cross the placenta and cause immune damage in the fetus. Several clinical syndromes have been described, of which cutaneous neonatal lupus is the most common and congenital heart block is the most serious. Anti-Ro/La antibodies do not appear to increase the risk of other adverse pregnancy outcomes. In the mother they tend to be associated with photosensitivity, subacute lupus erythematosus, Sjögren's syndrome, Raynaud's syndrome, and ANA-negative SLE. Assay of eNAs does not need to be repeated in pregnancy if the mother's status is already known.

About 30% of patients with SLE are anti-Ro positive. In such women the risk of transient cutaneous lupus is about 5% and the risk of congenital heart block about 2%, with the two conditions rarely coexisting. Anti-Ro antibodies are present in 90 to 100% of mothers of affected offspring, and 68 to 91% have anti-La antibodies. The risk of neonatal lupus is increased if a previous child has been affected, at 15 to 25% if one and 50% if two previous children are affected. Not all anti-Ro/La-positive mothers of

neonates with congenital heart block have SLE: most are asymptomatic, but 48% of these developed symptoms of connective tissue disease in a median 3.7 years follow-up in one study. In mothers who do have SLE there is no correlation between the severity of maternal disease and the incidence of neonatal lupus.

Cutaneous neonatal lupus usually manifests in the first 2 weeks of life. The infant develops typical annular skin lesions similar to those of adult subacute cutaneous lupus, usually of the face and scalp, which appear after sun or UV light exposure. The rash disappears spontaneously within 6 months, suggesting a direct antibody-mediated mechanism as this correlates with the half-life of maternal IgG in the neonatal circulation. Residual hypopigmentation or telangiectasia may persist for up to 2 years, but scarring is unusual and parents can be reassured. No specific treatment is required, except topical steroids in severe cases.

Congenital heart block usually appears in utero, around 18 to 20 weeks, but may not present until the neonatal period or later. It is typically associated with a structurally normal heart, but there may be associated cardiac abnormalities. Any degree of heart block can be present, but complete heart block is the most serious, and can be fatal. The mechanism of damage is not fully understood, but appears to involve binding of the anti-Ro/La antibodies to antigens on the fetal cardiocytes, inducing an inflammatory process which leads to tissue damage and fibrosis of the conducting system. One hypothesis is that the maternal autoantibodies prevent physiological clearance of apoptotic cardiocytes, promoting an inflammatory cascade involving macrophages and release of transforming growth factor beta (TGFβ). Anti-idiotypic antibodies to anti-La antibodies may be protective by blocking the pathogenic maternal antibodies. In women known to be anti-Ro/La positive, the fetal heart rate should be monitored at each visit, and fetal cardiology scans offered at approximately 18 weeks gestation and again in the third trimester. Complete heart block causes bradycardia which can be detected on auscultation, but lesser degrees of heart block require Doppler echocardiography. Incomplete heart block can be reversible, but can also progress to complete heart block. There is no treatment that reverses complete heart block, but there are reports of second-degree heart block reverting to first-degree heart block after treatment with betamethasone or dexamethasone. Fluorinated glucocorticosteroids, plasmapheresis, salbutamol, and digoxin have all been used if hydrops fetalis or pleuropericardial effusion develop, but benefit has to be balanced against maternal side effects. Small studies have examined the benefit of prophylactic corticosteroids in preventing recurrence of congenital heart block in mothers with a previously affected child, and show some benefit, but this approach exposes women and babies to the risks of corticosteroids when most would not have developed the disease. Prophylactic intravenous immunoglobulin is also being investigated. Overall mortality is around 20%, with deaths usually occurring in utero or the neonatal period, but can be up to 3 years of age. Most infants who survive the neonatal period do well, although two-thirds require pacemakers.

Antiphospholipid syndrome (APS)

Antiphospholipid antibodies include anticardiolipin antibodies (IgG and/or IgM), lupus anticoagulant (LA), and more recently anti-β_2-glycoprotein I antibody. The combination of any of these with one or more of the characteristic clinical features of

Table 14.14.2 Use of disease-modifying drugs in rheumatic disorders in pregnancy and breastfeeding

Drug	Evidence	Can drug be used?	
		Pregnancy	**Breast-feeding**
Hydroxychloroquine and chloroquine	At high doses concentration in melanin-containing structures in fetal uveal tract and inner ear can cause retinopathy and ear malformations. No increased risk of miscarriage, congenital malformation, or stillbirth at doses used in rheumatic diseases. Cessation increases risk of flare and long half-life means stopping does not prevent fetal exposure.	Yes	Yes
Azathioprine	Fetus lacks enzyme to convert to active form. Fetal and neonatal immunosuppression minimal if dose <2 mg/kg and normal maternal WCC	Yes	Yes
Ciclosporin	No increase in congenital malformations. Trend towards prematurity and IUGR not significant and probably related to more severe maternal disease. Small amounts in breast milk, but no adverse effects reported	Yes	If benefits outweigh potential risks
Tacrolimus	No increase in congenital malformations. Increased rates of prematurity related to severity of maternal disease. In one case report baby received maximum of 0.02% of maternal dose via breast milk	Yes	Yes, with caution
Intravenous immunoglobulin	Cross placenta after 32 weeks but no adverse fetal effects	Yes	Yes
Mycophenolate (MMF)	Increased risk of congenital abnormalities. Enterohepatic recirculation and long half-life	No (stop 6 weeks prior to conception)	No
Cyclophosphamide	Alkylating agent. Teratogenic and fetotoxic. Risk of neonatal haematopoiesis suppression	No (stop 3 months prior to conception)	No
Chlorambucil	Alkylating agent. Teratogenic and fetotoxic	No (stop 3 months prior to conception)	No
Methotrexate	Folate antagonist Teratogenic and fetotoxic	No (stop 3 months prior to conception, and folic acid peri-conceptually and throughout pregnancy)	No
Leflunomide	Congenital abnormalities in animal studies; human studies are limited. Long half-life of active metabolites	No (chole-styramine to increase clearance pre-conception)	No
D-Penicillamine	Chelating agent. Teratogenic in humans, with 5% risk of congenital cutis laxa and associated collagen disorders. Is crucial for successful pregnancy in Wilson's disease and often used in cystinuria	No in rheumatic disorders (stop pre-conception)	No
Sulphasalazine	Used extensively in treatment of IBD during pregnancy and appears safe. Keep doses <2 g/day to avoid neonatal neutropenia or aplastic anaemia. May displace bilirubin from albumin and induce neonatal pathological jaundice	Yes (with folate supplementation pre-conception and throughout pregnancy)	Yes (unless premature or other increased risk of hyperbilirubinaemia)
Gold salts	Teratogenic in animals, but limited data in humans	Can continue if controlling disease, but usually avoid initiation	Yes (with monitoring for toxicity)
Biological agents (e.g. etanercept, infliximab, adalimumab, rituximab)	Limited experience in human pregnancies and breastfeeding, but no adverse fetal or neonatal outcomes to date	Limit to severe disease	Probably avoid

IBD, inflammatory bowel disease; IUGR, intrauterine growth retardation; WCC, white cell count.

Table 14.14.3 Revised classification criteria for the antiphospholipid syndrome

Diagnostic criteria	Other clinical features include
◆ Antiphospholipid antibody positive (at least one of following, on two or more occasions, at least 12 weeks apart) • lupus anticoagulant • anticardiolipin antibody (medium or high titre) • anti-β_2-glycoprotein-I antibody (titre >99th centile) plus at least one of: ◆ Vascular thrombosis—arterial, venous, or capillary ◆ Pregnancy morbidity (with normal fetal morphology, parental chromosomes and maternal hormones): • recurrent 1st trimester miscarriage (at least three consecutively, <10 weeks gestation) • late fetal loss (2nd or 3rd trimester, >10 weeks gestation) • premature delivery <34 weeks because of severe pre-eclampsia/ eclampsia or other features of placental insufficiency	Thrombocytopenia Haemolytic anaemia Livedo reticularis Neurological manifestations e.g. epilepsy, cerebral infarction, chorea, migraine Heart valve disease (especially mitral valve) Systemic and pulmonary hypertension Nephropathy (including thrombotic microangiopathy) Metatarsal fractures, avascular necrosis Leg ulcers

Adapted from Miyakis S, et al. (2006). International consensus statement on an update of the classification criteria for definite antiphopholipid syndrome (APS). J Thromb Haemost, **4**, 295–306.

thrombosis, recurrent pregnancy loss, or adverse pregnancy outcome (as detailed in Table 14.14.3) is known as the antiphospholipid syndrome (APS).

APS was first described in patients with SLE (secondary APS), but it is now recognized both that most patients with APS do not fulfil the diagnostic criteria for SLE, and that those with primary APS do not usually progress to SLE. In one prospective study following 128 patients with primary APS for a mean duration of 9 years, only 8% developed SLE and 5% a lupus-like disease. Those patients with SLE who have APS (up to 35%) have a higher morbidity and mortality. Although the clinical features of primary and SLE-associated APS are similar, and the antibody specificity is the same, the distinction is important: patients with primary APS should not be labelled as having 'lupus'.

Antiphospholipid antibodies can be measured in pregnancy as levels are not altered, but their prevalence in the general obstetric population is low (up to 5% depending on assay), hence universal screening is not warranted. However, the prevalence of antiphospholipid antibodies is increased in women with pregnancy complications including severe early-onset pre-eclampsia, abruption, intrauterine fetal death, or IUGR without hypertension. The role of antiphospholipid antibodies in the broader spectrum of pre-eclampsia is more controversial. Many studies have shown an increased incidence of antiphospholipid antibodies in cases of severe early-onset pre-eclampsia, such as one in which 20.9% of these women were found to have anticardiolipin antibodies compared with 7.5% of controls. By contrast, studies looking at women

with anticardiolipin antibodies have not consistently shown an increased risk of pre-eclampsia, but that may be because the incidence of the more severe form of the disease is relatively rare.

Fetal loss represents one end of a spectrum of fetal compromise and a wide range of pregnancy morbidity has been reported in APS, including recurrent first-trimester miscarriage, second- and third-trimester loss, severe early-onset pre-eclampsia, IUGR, placental abruption, and prematurity. Recurrent pregnancy loss, typically in the second trimester, is one of the most consistent features of APS, but is not necessary for diagnosis of the condition (Table 14.14.3). Fetal death is typically preceded by IUGR, oligohydramnios, and features of pre-eclampsia. The risk of fetal loss is directly related to antibody titre, particularly the IgG anticardiolipin antibodies, although many women with a history of recurrent loss have only IgM antibodies. Quantifying the risk is difficult, and the presence of antiphospholipid antibodies does not preclude successful pregnancy. The antibodies should be regarded as markers for a high-risk pregnancy, but previous poor obstetric history remains the most important predictor of fetal loss in these women.

The pathogenesis of fetal loss in these patients is not fully understood, although a variety of mechanisms have been suggested and there appear to be both thrombotic and inflammatory components. Early pregnancy losses are probably related to a failure in placentation itself, whereas later losses are related to thrombosis in the uteroplacental vessels, with evidence of placental infarction and spiral artery vasculopathy. One hypothesis is that anticardiolipin antibodies cause thrombosis by binding to molecules involved in the regulation of coagulation, such as β_2-glycoprotein, an endogenous coagulation inhibitor. This interaction may also affect earlier placentation since β_2-glycoprotein is present on trophoblasts. Other postulated mechanisms include oxidant-mediated injury of the vascular endothelium due to anticardiolipin antibodies binding oxidized cardiolipin, and displacement of annexin V (another endogenous anticoagulant).

APS is the most frequent cause of acquired thrombophilia. However, unlike the inherited thrombophilias, thrombosis can be arterial or venous, and affects vessels of all sizes. The risk of recurrent thrombosis in patients with APS may reach 70%, and women with APS and previous thromboembolism are at extremely high risk in pregnancy and the puerperium.

Studies on pregnancy outcome in women known to have APS show differing rates of obstetric complications depending on their presentation: those found to have APS as a result of recurrent miscarriage have lower rates of complications than those discovered because of late fetal losses, thrombosis or other systemic manifestations (Table 14.14.4). Rates are even lower in studies that have

Table 14.14.4 Pregnancy complications in different populations of women with antiphospholipid antibodies or APS

	Pre-eclampsia	Preterm delivery
APS with predominantly recurrent miscarriage	Mean 10.5% Range 0–15%	Mean 10.5% Range 5–40%
APS with predominantly late loss/thrombosis/SLE	Median 32% Range up to 50%	Range 32–65%

Adapted from Ware Branch D, Khamashta MA (2003). Antiphospholipid syndrome: obstetric diagnosis, management, and controversies. Obstet Gynecol, **101**, 1333–44.

measured the presence of antiphospholipid antibodies in the general obstetric population with no history of thrombosis or pregnancy morbidity.

Management of APS in pregnancy

The management of pregnancy in women with APS, in particular the use of anticoagulation, is the subject of much debate. The main aims are to improve pregnancy outcome and prevent maternal thrombosis.

Maternal and fetal surveillance

Pregnancy complicated by APS requires expert care and a team approach by obstetricians, physicians, and haematologists. Close monitoring of both mother and fetus is essential. Ultrasound monitoring of fetal growth and uteroplacental blood flow is crucial, allowing for timely delivery. Uterine artery waveforms are assessed between 20 and 24 weeks gestation, and those pregnancies with evidence of early diastolic notch(es) or other abnormalities are monitored very closely with 4-weekly growth scans because of the high risk of IUGR. Where there are no abnormalities, scans are only performed for the usual obstetric indications. Doppler flow studies of the umbilical artery may be used, as in other pregnancies at high risk of fetal compromise through uteroplacental insufficiency.

Anticoagulation

The main therapeutic options are low-dose aspirin (75–100 mg/day) or heparin—low molecular weight (LMWH) or unfractionated (UFH)—neither, or both. Neither LMWH nor UFH crosses the placenta.

The most controversial areas are the treatment of those who are antiphospholipid antibody positive with either no previous thrombosis or adverse obstetric event, or with recurrent first-trimester miscarriage. There have been few randomized controlled trials. In the former group, which has a very low risk of an adverse pregnancy outcome, the use of single-agent aspirin showed no benefit. However, there are several nonrandomized studies in women with fetal loss suggesting that the drug is effective, and it can prevent pregnancy loss in experimental APS mice. Many clinicians would advocate using aspirin throughout pregnancy as it may benefit some and has low toxicity. Some would even start before conception, in the belief that the placental damage occurs early in gestation, and that aspirin prevents failure of placentation. Heparin is added only if there are other risk factors for thrombosis.

The evidence in those with recurrent miscarriage is also the subject of much debate. Two prospective trials have shown that adding heparin to aspirin is more effective than aspirin alone, with live birth rates of 71% and 80% with additional heparin, compared to 42% and 44% with aspirin alone. However, this was not confirmed by a subsequent randomized controlled trial, when a live birth rate of 78% with heparin and aspirin was not significantly different from that of 72% with single-agent aspirin. Another recent randomized controlled trial from Canada did not show any difference in the live birth rate with aspirin and low molecular weight heparin (78%) compared to that with aspirin alone (79%). Interestingly, the benefit of heparin in the first study was only in preventing miscarriages up to 13 weeks, and there was no difference in the treatment arms in pregnancies that advanced beyond this gestation. In addition, a double-blind randomized placebo-controlled trial of 50 women with at least 3 recurrent miscarriages failed to show any benefit of aspirin alone, with live birth rates of 85% in the placebo group and 80% in the aspirin-treated group, suggesting some patients may not require any treatment at all.

Table 14.14.5 Anticoagulation during pregnancy in women who are antiphospholipid antibody positive

Antiphospholipid antibody positiveplus		Antenatal management	
Previous obstetric adverse events	Previous thrombosis	Aspirin (75 mg)	Low molecular weight heparin (LMWH)
None	None	Yes, but controversial (see text)	No (unless other risk factors for thrombosis e.g. family history of thrombosis, raised BMI)
Recurrent 1st-trimester miscarriage (at least 3 consecutively)	None	Yes	Controversial (see text). Low prophylactic dose from beginning of pregnancy (e.g. enoxaparin 40 mg once daily), but stop either after 1st trimester, or after 20–24 weeks if uterine artery Dopplers normal (if no history of thrombosis or late fetal loss)
Late fetal loss (2nd or 3rd trimester) or Premature delivery <34 weeks because of severe pre-eclampsia/eclampsia or other features of placental insufficiency	None	Yes	Low prophylactic dose throughout pregnancy.
Any of above	Yes	Yes	Swap warfarin to LMWH before 6 weeks gestation. High prophylactic dose, e.g. enoxaparin 40 mg twice daily (once daily until 16–20 weeks).
Any of above	Yes, and continued TIAs in pregnancy despite high prophylactic LMWH dose	Yes	Full anticoagulant dose, e.g. enoxaparin 1 mg/kg twice daily. May also consider re-warfarinizing between 14 and 34 weeks gestation (INR 2–3).

BMI, body mass index; LMWH, low molecular weight heparin; TIA, transient ischaemic attack.

Management is less controversial in women with previous thrombosis or adverse pregnancy outcome, when aspirin and heparin are required, as detailed in Table 14.14.5. One prospective study using this regimen in 33 pregnant women with primary APS achieved a 91% live birth rate. Warfarin should be stopped and heparin started before 6 weeks gestation to avoid warfarin embryopathy. LMWH appears to be as effective as UFH, with fewer side effects and without the need for monitoring of APTT or (usually) anti-Xa levels.

Other agents

Treatment with high-dose corticosteroids (in the absence of active lupus) to suppress lupus anticoagulant and anticardiolipin antibodies has previously been recommended (in combination with aspirin) because of improved fetal survival compared to historical controls. However, high doses of prednisolone caused considerable maternal morbidity and subsequent studies have failed to demonstrate better fetal outcome compared to aspirin and heparin, and suggest that steroids may even worsen outcome because of an increased risk of preterm labour.

Immunosuppression with intravenous immunoglobulin has been used, particularly for recurrent miscarriage, and case series have shown improvement in pregnancy outcome. However, more recent studies have shown no benefit either compared to, or in addition to, aspirin and heparin. In the comparison study in recurrent miscarriage there was a higher rate of live births (84%) with aspirin and heparin than with immunoglobulin (57%): the study in which intravenous immunoglobulin was added showed no significant difference in live birth rate. Intravenous immunoglobulin is best reserved for 'refractory' cases of women with APS who continue to have pregnancy losses despite aspirin and heparin. Other immunosuppressive agents have also been used, including azathioprine and plasmapheresis, but the numbers treated do not allow firm conclusions regarding efficacy.

Postpartum

The postpartum period continues to pose an increased thrombotic risk. Those on heparin for previous maternal thrombosis should be converted back to warfarin. Those on heparin for previous adverse fetal outcome or obstetric history should continue heparin for 6 weeks, although there is little evidence as to the exact length of time needed. For those with recurrent miscarriage heparin is usually given postpartum for 1 week, especially if there are other risk factors such as increased body mass index or caesarean section, although again there is little evidence for this. Aspirin is usually continued long-term in all. All these agents can be used while breastfeeding.

As mentioned previously, the combined oral contraceptive pill should be avoided as contraception, but alternative methods should be discussed.

Rheumatoid arthritis (RA)

The adult form of the disease is more common in women (female to male ratio 3:1), and approximately 1 in every 1000 to 2000 pregnancies are affected.

Effect of pregnancy on RA

Up to 75% of women with RA experience improvement during pregnancy. There have been a number of hypotheses to explain this, but data for most are conflicting. They include the shift in pregnancy from a predominantly Th1 to Th2 immune response

and cytokine repertoire; raised levels of circulating hormones (including cortisol, progesterone, and oestrogen); the maternal immune response to fetal paternally inherited HLA class II gene products, with maternal–fetal mismatch for certain HLA alleles being beneficial; pregnancy-specific proteins such as α_2-glycoprotein; and removal of immune complexes by the placenta.

Improvement usually begins during the first trimester, when rheumatoid nodules may also disappear, but 90% of those who experience remission suffer postpartum exacerbations. A large study of disease activity in pregnancy in 140 women with RA confirmed improvement in joint swelling and pain in two-thirds of subjects by the third trimester. However, only a minority had no joints with active disease, disability as assessed by the Health Assessment Questionnaire changed little compared to prepregnancy, and only 16% went into complete remission. Disease response in a previous pregnancy was predictive of response in the index pregnancy. An increase in the mean number of inflamed joints was seen postpartum, but this could not be predicted from previous puerperal relapse. In women without RA there is an increased incidence of developing the condition in the postpartum period. Studies looking at the effect of breastfeeding on disease have shown conflicting results, with some suggesting it is protective against disease development and others that it increases postpartum flare. Overall the evidence of an adverse effect is not strong enough to advise women against.

Effect of rheumatoid arthritis on pregnancy

Unlike SLE, RA seems to have no adverse effect of on pregnancy, and neither fertility rate nor spontaneous abortion rate is significantly altered. Most women with RA have no increased risk of pregnancy complications compared to the background population, although there are some reports of an increased risk of lower birth weight, prematurity, pre-eclampsia, and caesarean section, which may be related to medications used and/or disease activity.

Atlantoaxial subluxation is a rare complication of a general anaesthetic for a caesarean section, and very rarely limitation of hip abduction is severe enough to impede vaginal delivery. The main concerns relate to the safety during pregnancy and lactation of the medications used to treat RA, although only 20 to 30% of pregnant women with RA will require medications to control flares or systemic disease. The infants of women who have Ro or La antibodies are at risk of neonatal lupus (see above).

Management of rheumatoid arthritis in pregnancy

As with SLE, women should ideally be reviewed before conception to optimize medication for pregnancy. They can often reduce their medication in pregnancy, but usually require some maintenance therapy. Most women can be managed on analgesics and low-dose prednisolone, with azathioprine or ciclosporin added in for more severe cases. Many of the drugs used in RA overlap with those used in SLE, but additional agents include D-penicillamine, sulphasalazine and gold (Table 14.14.2). They may be used if high doses of steroids are being required, but their delayed onset of action means benefit is often not fully seen for several months.

Women should be reviewed by an obstetric anaesthetist to assess cervical spine involvement and degree of jaw movement, and to anticipate any problems if she was to require a general anaesthetic. Ro and La antibodies should be measured, as discussed for SLE.

Vasculitides

Wegener's granulomatosis, polyarteritis nodosa (PAN), and Churg–Strauss syndrome occur principally in the post-childbearing years and more often in men, so pregnancy is very uncommon in these conditions. Henoch–Schönlein purpura (HSP) tends to affect the paediatric population, but there have been a few case reports of presentation in pregnancy, or pregnancy after previous HSP. Pregnancy is more likely in Takayasu's arteritis and Behçet's disease, as they usually occur in the reproductive years.

In general, maternal and fetal outcome are dependent on disease activity and pre-existing complications. Numbers of reported cases are generally too small to determine definitively if disease onset or flare is more likely during pregnancy or postpartum, but the trend suggests this is so.

A recent literature review showed that pregnancy outcome in Wegener's is worse with active disease at conception or disease onset during pregnancy. Even if disease is in remission at the beginning of pregnancy there are significant risks of preeclampsia (25%) and prematurity (41%), and there were 2 maternal deaths out of 30 women with 36 pregnancies. Pre-eclampsia was more common with renal involvement. PAN carries a high risk of maternal mortality (up to 100%) if diagnosed during pregnancy or immediately postpartum, whereas the maternal and fetal outcome is much better if diagnosed prepregnancy and disease is in remission. There are some reports of neonatal cutaneous vasculitis, resolving with treatment, in infants of mothers with PAN. Churg–Strauss syndrome tends to be less aggressive than Wegener's syndrome or PAN, especially if women conceive during remission. Maternal and fetal outcomes are significantly worse if Churg–Strauss syndrome presents during pregnancy, and cardiac disease is an important cause of maternal death. Issues with Takayasu's arteritis include hypertension and involvement of the aortic valve and abdominal aorta, and superimposed pre-eclampsia and IUGR are common. Pulmonary hypertension should be excluded before pregnancy. Behçet's disease may relapse or remit in pregnancy, with relapses tending to be mucocutaneous rather than thrombotic or ocular. Most case series have not reported an adverse affect on maternal or fetal outcome. The main concern regarding HSP in pregnancy is renal involvement, which is usually mild and resolves spontaneously, but may lead to nephrotic syndrome or acute renal failure and needs to be distinguished from pre-eclampsia.

In view of the significant maternal and fetal morbidity and mortality associated with active disease, women should be advised to delay pregnancy until disease is in remission, and in the case of flare or onset of disease during pregnancy it is important to adopt an aggressive approach to treatment with immunosuppression. Corticosteroids are usually first-line, followed by azathioprine. Life-threatening disease may necessitate the use of pulsed cyclophosphamide (especially in Wegener's syndrome) or methotrexate despite the risks, although more recent case reports have successfully used intravenous immunoglobulin or plasmapheresis in refractory disease, thus minimizing the fetal risk.

Scleroderma

Scleroderma (or systemic sclerosis) is more common in women (female to male ratio 3:1), with peak age of onset 30 to 50 years old. Although it is a rare disease, more cases are being reported in pregnancy as maternal age increases.

Effect of pregnancy on scleroderma

In general, women with limited scleroderma without organ involvement do better than those with diffuse disease. The extent of diffuse disease and systemic involvement (particularly lung, cardiac, and renal) influences prognosis, but there are no absolute rules. Those with early (<4 years) or diffuse disease, or with anti-topoisomerase (anti-ScL-70) antibodies, are at greater risk of having more active aggressive disease than those with long-standing disease and anticentromere antibodies.

One of the main concerns is the risk of renal crisis, although it is still debatable whether this occurs more commonly in pregnancy. Women with renal involvement often have associated hypertension and rapid deterioration is possible. Progressive cutaneous disease is unusual during or immediately after pregnancy. Raynaud's phenomenon usually improves as a result of vasodilation, but reflux and oesophagitis are often exacerbated due to reduced lower oesophageal tone, and arthralgia also worsens. There is no evidence that pregnancy worsens cardiac or respiratory disease, although those with severe pulmonary fibrosis and pulmonary hypertension are at extremely high risk of postpartum deterioration, as with pulmonary hypertension from any cause.

It has been suggested that pregnancy, including miscarriage, may have an aetiological role in scleroderma, with some studies showing persistent fetal microchimerism and HLA-DR compatibility between mother and fetus are more common in women with scleroderma than controls. Hypotheses implicating the persistence of these fetal cells in the pathogenesis of scleroderma include the development of a fetal antimaternal graft vs host reaction and/or the maternal response to fetal cells becoming redirected against the mother herself.

Effect of scleroderma on pregnancy

Some studies suggest no effect on fertility, whereas others show increased incidence of infertility even before disease onset. The rate of spontaneous miscarriage is probably increased in those who become pregnant before the diagnosis of scleroderma, but data are inconclusive regarding the miscarriage rate in pregnancies after diagnosis.

If pregnancy is well timed and carefully monitored then the outcome is usually good, and overall pregnancy success rate is now 70 to 80%. There is some evidence of an increased risk of IUGR and prematurity, but no increased risk of pre-eclampsia in the absence of hypertension or renal involvement. The risks of adverse outcome are highest for women with early diffuse disease.

Management of scleroderma in pregnancy

Women should be assessed before conception for the extent of organ involvement. Those with significant renal impairment, severe restrictive lung disease, pulmonary hypertension, or severe cardiomyopathy should be advised against pregnancy. Those with early diffuse disease should delay pregnancy until the disease stabilizes. Disease-remitting drugs such as D-penicillamine and ciclosporin should preferably be discontinued before conception if disease is stable.

High-level joint obstetric and medical care is appropriate, with frequent and regular multidisciplinary monitoring of disease activity and fetal growth.

Management of scleroderma during pregnancy is largely symptomatic, including calcium antagonists for Raynaud's phenomenon, and histamine antagonists and proton pump inhibitors for reflux. NSAIDs are best avoided, as previously discussed, and corticosteroids (>15 mg/day) must also be avoided in early diffuse scleroderma since they can precipitate a renal crisis.

Features indicating the development of a renal crisis include hypertension, rapidly rising creatinine, thrombocytopenia and microangiopathic haemolytic anaemia, with pre-eclampsia the main differential to be considered. Prompt initiation of an ACE inhibitor is required in a renal crisis. This class of drug is usually contraindicated in pregnancy, as discussed previously, but the benefits in renal scleroderma in treating uncontrolled hypertension and preventing maternal mortality usually far outweigh the fetal risks.

Venepuncture, venous access, oxygen saturation, and blood pressure measurements may be difficult because of skin, nail, or blood vessel involvement. General anaesthesia may be complicated by difficult endotracheal intubation, and regional anaesthesia may also be problematic. Early assessment by an obstetric anaesthetist is advisable, and epidural anaesthesia and analgesia are encouraged as vasodilation improves skin perfusion of the extremities. Other measures to reduce problems related to Raynaud's phenomenon include warming of the delivery room and any intravenous fluids as well as socks and gloves.

Close observation must continue in the immediate postnatal period, particularly in those with cardiac, pulmonary or renal involvement.

Further reading

General

Ostensen M, Forger F, Villiger PM (2006). Cytokines and pregnancy in rheumatic disease. *Ann N Y Acad Sci.* 1069, 353–63. [Review of the involvement of pregnancy-related immune changes in the pathophysiology of rheumatic diseases].

Pregnancy and rheumatic disease (2007). *Rheum Dis Clin N Am*, 33, 227–364. [Recent edition dedicated to rheumatic disease in pregnancy.]

Antirheumatic drugs and immunosuppressive agents in pregnancy

Chambers CD, et al. (2006). Human pregnancy safety for agents used to treat rheumatoid arthritis: adequacy of available information and strategies for developing post-marketing data. *Arthritis Res Ther*, 8, 215–24. [Comprehensive review.]

Ostensen M (2006). Anti-inflammatory and immunosuppressive drugs and reproduction. *Arthritis Res Ther*, 8, 209–27. [Excellent in-depth review.]

Systemic lupus erythematosus

Clark CA, Spitzer KA, Laskin CA (2005). Decrease in pregnancy loss rates in patients with systemic lupus erythematosus over a 40-year period. *J Rheumatol*, 32, 1709–12. [Meta-analysis of published pregnancy loss rates for SLE over past 40 years, showing prognosis is now more encouraging]

Clowse MEB, et al. (2005). The impact of increased lupus activity on obstetric outcomes. *Arthritis Rheum*, 52, 514–21. [Large cohort study of pregnancy outcomes related to disease activity.]

Cortes-Hernandez J, et al. (2002). Clinical predictors of fetal and maternal outcome in systemic lupus erythematosus: a prospective study of 103 pregnancies. *Br J Rheumatol*, 35, 133–8. [Study identifying predictors of adverse outcome in SLE pregnancies.]

D'Cruz DP, Khamashta MA, Hughes GRV (2007). Systemic lupus erythematosus. *Lancet*, 369, 587–96. [Review of recent developments in SLE including pregnancy-related issues.]

Germain S, Nelson-Piercy C (2006). Lupus nephritis and renal disease in pregnancy. *Lupus*, 15, 1–8. [Review of features and management of renal disease in pregnancy.]

Khamashta MA, Ruiz-Irastoza G, Hughes GRV (1997). Systemic lupus erythematosus flares during pregnancy. *Rheum Dis Clin N Am*, 23, 15–30. [Review of studies examining frequency of lupus flares in pregnancy.]

Moroni G, Ponticelli C (2003). The risk of pregnancy in patients with lupus nephritis. *J Nephrol*, 16, 161–7. [Important meta-analysis of fetal and maternal outcomes with lupus nephritis, and factors associated with adverse outcomes.]

Neonatal lupus

Buyon JP, et al. (1998). Autoimmune-associated congenital heart block: demographics, mortality, morbidity and recurrence rates obtained from a national neonatal lupus registry. *J Am Coll Cardiol*, 31, 1658–66. [Large series of long-term outcome with auto-immune associated congenital heart block.]

Brucato A, et al. (2002). Pregnancy outcome in 100 women with autoimmune diseases and anti-Ro/SSA antibodies: a prospective controlled study. *Lupus*, 11, 716–21. [Large cohort study demonstrating incidence of congential heart block.]

Cimaz R, et al. (2003). Incidence and spectrum of neonatal lupus erythematosus: a prospective study of infants born to mothers with anti-Ro autoantibodies. *J Pediatr*, 142, 678–83. [Prospective study showing incidence of anti-Ro associated cutaneous neonatal lupus and congenital heart block.]

Clancy RM, et al. (2006). Impaired clearance of apoptotic cardiocytes is linked to anti-SSA/Ro and -SSB/La antibodies in the pathogenesis of congenital heart block. *J Clin Invest*, 116, 2413–22. [Recent experimental evidence regarding pathogenesis of congenital heart block.]

Friedman DM, Rupel A, Buyon JP (2007). Epidemiology, etiology, detection and treatment of autoantibody-associated congenital heart block in neonatal lupus. *Curr Rheumatol Rep*, 9, 101–8. [Up-to-date comprehensive review.]

Antiphospholipid syndrome

Backos M, et al. (1999). Pregnancy complications in women with recurrent miscarriage associated with antiphospholipid antibodies treated with low dose aspirin and heparin. *Br J Obstet Gynaecol*, 106, 102–7. [A study describing obstetric outcome in treated APS pregnancies with history of recurrent miscarriage.]

Clark EA, Silver RM, Branch DW (2007). Do antiphospholipid antibodies cause preeclampsia and HELLP syndrome? *Curr Rheumatol Rep*, 9, 219–25. [Review of evidence for an association between APS, antiphospholipid antibodies, and preeclampsia.]

Cowchock FS, et al. (1992). Repeated fetal losses associated with antiphospholipid antibodies: a collaborative randomized trial comparing prednisone with low-dose heparin treatment. *Am J Obstet Gynecol*, 166, 1318–23. [Important trial showing aspirin and heparin is better than aspirin and prednisolone.]

Derksen RHWM, Khamashta MA, Ware Branch D (2004). Management of the obstetric antiphospholipid syndrome. *Arthritis Rheum*, 50, 1028–39. [Comprehensive review of management of APS in pregnancy.]

Farquharson RG, Quenby S, Greaves M (2002). Antiphospholipid syndrome in pregnancy: a randomized, controlled trial of treatment.

Obstet Gynecol, **100**, 408–13. [A study suggesting no benefit of adding heparin to aspirin alone in improving pregnancy outcome.]

Gomez-Puerta JA, *et al.* (2005). Long-term follow-up in 128 patients with primary antiphospholipid syndrome: do they develop lupus? *Medicine (Baltimore)*, **84**, 225–30. [Study following women with primary APS to determine how many develop SLE.]

Laskin CA *et al.* (2009). Low Molecular Weight Heparin and Aspirin for Recurrent Pregnancy Loss: Results from the Randomized, Controlled HepASA Trial. *J Rheumatol*. 2009 Feb 4. [Epub ahead of print]

Laskin CA, *et al.* (1997). Prednisone and aspirin in women with autoantibodies and unexplained recurrent fetal loss. *N Engl J Med*, **337**, 148–53. [Study showing no benefit of adding prednisolone to aspirin in APS with recurrent miscarriage, and the increased risk of prematurity.]

Lim W, Crowther MA, Eikelboom JW (2006). Management of antiphospholipid antibody syndrome: a systemic review. *JAMA*, **295**, 1050–7. [Recent review of thrombosis risk and management in APS.]

Lima F, *et al.* (1996). A study of sixty pregnancies in patients with the antiphospholipid syndrome. *Clin Exp Rheumatol*, **14**, 131–6. [A study describing obstetric outcome in different populations of treated APS pregnancies.]

Lynch A, *et al.* (1994). Antiphospholipid antibodies in predicting adverse pregnancy outcome: a prospective study. *Ann Intern Med*, **120**, 470–5. [Study showing increased fetal loss rate but not other pregnancy adverse outcomes in healthy pregnant women with antiphospholipid antibodies.]

Miyakis S, *et al.* (2006). International consensus statement on an update of the classification criteria for definite antiphopholipid syndrome (APS). *J Thromb Haemost*, **4**, 295–306. [Most recent consensus update on criteria for definition of APS.]

Noble LS, *et al.* (2005). Antiphospholipid antibodies associated with recurrent pregnancy loss: prospective, multicenter, controlled pilot study comparing treatment with low-molecular-weight heparin versus unfractionated heparin. *Fertil Steril*, **83**, 684–90. [Study showing low molecular weight heparin is as effective as unfractionated heparin in preventing recurrent miscarriage.]

Pattison NS, *et al.* (2000). Does aspirin have a role in improving pregnancy outcome for women with the antiphospholipid syndrome? A randomized controlled trial. *Am J Obstet Gynecol*, **183**, 1008–12. [Study showing aspirin had no benefit over placebo in APS pregnancies with recurrent miscarriages.]

Rai R, *et al.* (1997). Randomized controlled trial of aspirin and aspirin plus heparin in pregnant women with recurrent miscarriage associated with phospholipid antibodies (or antiphospholipid antibodies). *BMJ*, **314**, 253–7. [A study suggesting aspirin and heparin superior to aspirin alone for first trimester miscarriage in APS.]

Stone S, *et al.* (2005). Primary antiphospholipid syndrome in pregnancy: an analysis of outcome in a cohort of 33 women treated with a rigorous protocol. *J Thromb Haemost*, **3**, 243–5. [Study showing successful outcome can be achieved in APS pregnancies with a rigorous anticoagulation regime.]

Tincani A, *et al.* (2006). Pregnancy, lupus and antiphospholipid syndrome (Hughes syndrome). *Lupus*, **15**, 156–60. [Succinct review.]

Triolo G, *et al.* (2003). Randomized study of subcutaneous low molecular weight heparin plus aspirin versus intravenous immunoglobulin in the treatment of recurrent fetal loss associated with antiphospholipid antibodies. *Arthritis Rheum*, **48**, 728–31. [Study demonstrating that heparin is more effective than intravenous immunoglobulins when added to aspirin in APS-associated recurrent miscarriage.]

Ware Branch D, Khamashta MA (2003). Antiphospholipid syndrome: obstetric diagnosis, management, and controversies. *Obstet Gynecol*, **101**, 1333–44. [Excellent review of controversies in management.]

Ware Branch D, *et al.* (2000). A multi-center, placebo-controlled pilot study of intravenous immune globulin treatment of antiphospholipid syndrome during pregnancy. *Am J Obstet Gynecol*, **182**, 122–7. [A pilot study using intravenous immunoglobulin in APS pregnancies.]

Wilson WA, *et al.* (1999). International consensus statement on preliminary classification criteria for definite antiphospholipid syndrome: Report of an international workshop. *Arthritis Rheum*, **42**, 1309–11. [Paper discussing previously updated criteria for APS.]

Rheumatoid arthritis

Barrett JH, *et al.* (1999). Does rheumatoid arthriitis remit during pregnancy and relapse postpartum? Results from a nationwide study in the United Kingdom performed prospectively from late pregnancy. *Arthritis Rheum*, **42**, 1219–27. [Excellent report and review of effect of pregnancy on RA.]

Golding A, Haque UJ, Giles JT (2007). Rheumatoid arthritis and reproduction. *Rheum Dis Clin North Am*, **33**, 319–43. [Comprehensive review].

Vasculitides

Hot A, *et al.* (2007). Marked improvement of Churg-Strauss vasculitis with intravenous gamma globulins during pregnancy. *Clin Rheumatol*, **26**, 2149–151. [Encouraging report of use of intravenous immunoglobulins to treat Churg–Strauss in pregnancy].

Jadaon J, *et al.* (2005). Behçet's disease and pregnancy. *Acta Obstet Gynecol Scand*, **84**, 939–44. [Most recent case–control study and literature review.]

Koizumi M, *et al.* (2004). Schönlein–Henoch purpura during pregnancy: Case report and review of the literature. *J Obstet Gynecol Res*, **30**, 37–41. [Case report and literature review.]

Langford CA, Kerr GS (2002). Pregnancy in vasculitis. *Curr Opin Rheumatol*, **14**, 36–41. [Excellent review of literature.]

Seo P (2007). Pregnancy and vasculitis. *Rheum Dis Clin North Am*, **33**, 299–317. [Up-to-date review.]

Soh MC *et al* (2009). Pregnancy complicating Wegener's Granulomatosis. *Obstet Med*, **2**, 77–80.

Scleroderma

Chung L, *et al.* (2006). Outcome of pregnancies complicated by systemic sclerosis and mixed connective tissue disease. *Lupus*, **15**, 595–9. [Most recent study of pregnancy outcome with scleroderma.]

Steen VD (2007). Pregnancy in scleroderma. *Rheum Dis Clin North Am*, **33**, 345–58. [Up-to-date review.]

Infections in pregnancy

Lawrence Impey

Essentials

The mother

Maternal illness is often more severe in pregnancy, e.g. varicella, malaria, and the treatment of infections in pregnancy is complicated by potential effects of drugs on the fetus. Peri- and postpartum maternal infection is a major cause of maternal mortality.

The fetus

The effects of infection in pregnancy can be broadly categorized as follows (these are not mutually exclusive): (1) transplacental infection causing fetal malformation, e.g. treponema pallidum, rubella; (2) transplacental infection causing severe in utero illness, e.g. parvovirus; (3) neonatal infection / carrier status as a result of transplacental or intrapartum infection, e.g. HIV, herpes zoster; such neonatal infection may be severe; (4) preterm delivery, late miscarriage, perinatal death and cerebral palsy at term delivery are more common in the presence of in utero and placental infection (chorioamnionitis), e.g. Group B streptococcus.

The baby

Viral—(1) HIV—transmission of carrier status occurs most frequently at vaginal delivery. Prevention is achieved by caesarean delivery, antiretroviral and avoidance of breastfeeding.

(2) Parvovirus—transplacental infection can cause fetal anaemia and cardiac failure. (3) CMV—transplacental infection is variable, but severe neurological damage, impaired growth and deafness may follow. (4) Herpes simplex—intrapartum infection can cause severe neonatal illness following a primary attack. (5) Herpes zoster—chickenpox in early pregnancy is occasionally teratogenic, but severe neonatal illness can follow late pregnancy disease; maternal disease is often severe. (6) Hepatitis B—vertical transmission usually causes chronic carrier status and is reduced by neonatal immunization.

Other—(1) Bacterial vaginosis—associated with preterm delivery. (2) Streptococcal infection—Group A causes puerperal sepsis, a major cause of maternal mortality; Group B can cause severe neonatal illness following intrapartum infection. (3) Chlamydia—associated with preterm delivery and neonatal conjunctivitis. (4) Syphilis—although rare in the West, syphilis is endemic in many countries, with transplacental infection causing congenital syphilis and perinatal death. (5) Toxoplasmosis—transplacental infection can cause severe fetal disease; treatment may prevent transmission and reduce disease severity. (6) Malaria—a major cause of neonatal mortality in parts of Africa; prevention is with nets and chemoprophylaxis.

Introduction

Immunity is mildly suppressed in pregnancy and the fetal immune system is developmentally immature. Infections in pregnancy can therefore be devastating both for the mother, as is occasionally seen with varicella, and for the fetus, as exemplified by congenital infections such as those caused by rubella, cytomegalovirus (CMV), syphilis, and toxoplasmosis.

Preterm delivery accounts for 80% of neonatal unit cot days, is the single most important contributor to long-term handicap, and is a major cause of perinatal mortality. In addition to the specific effects of individual infections, infection in pregnancy is an important risk factor for these adverse outcomes. Infection is implicated in over 50% of preterm deliveries and considerably worsens the prognosis for the neonate at any given preterm gestation.

The vaginal pathogens, including bacterial vaginosis and Group B streptococcus, (GBS) are varied and only intermittently associated with adverse outcomes: it is likely that cervical integrity is both affected by bacteria and affects the access of bacteria to the uterus. Non-'ascending' infection may also be important, with periodontal disease recently associated with an increased risk of preterm delivery.

At term, clinical or histological chorioamnionitis are associated with a large increase in the risk of neonatal death, neonatal encephalopathy, and cerebral palsy. The relative contributions of infection and an inflammatory response associated with other risk factors (e.g. pre-eclampsia) are not known, although the limited but potentially devastating role played by bacteria such as GBS is clearly understood. Currently, with the exception of GBS, it remains unknown whether the use of antibiotics or antipyretics reduces the associated risks.

The most important infective organisms in pregnancy are described in this chapter: detailed discussion of their pathology and features in adults are described in Section 7.

Viral infections

HIV

The HIV1 and 2 retroviruses are the cause of AIDS. In some parts of sub-Saharan Africa 20% of pregnant women are affected; in the United Kingdom more than 50 000 people are infected, over half of whom acquired their infection abroad. The predominant mode of infection is heterosexual sexual contact, and almost as many women as men are now infected. The risk of infection is 0.03 to 1% per episode of sexual intercourse, and it is estimated that about one-half of all partners of known HIV-positive women in the United Kingdom are unaware of the diagnosis. HIV in pregnancy is associated with an increased risk of complications, notably pre-eclampsia, intrauterine growth restriction (IUGR), and still-birth. It appears that women taking highly active antiretroviral therapy (HAART) are at greater risk of developing pre-eclampsia. In the United Kingdom, viral antigen enzyme-linked immuno-sorbent assay (ELISA) screening for HIV is offered to all pregnant women.

Vertical transmission occurs largely but not exclusively during delivery or breastfeeding. Its prevalence is highest in developing countries, if there are concomitant sexually transmitted diseases, in preterm delivery, and where the CD4 count is low and the viral load is high, as in early and late disease. Transmission rates are 15 to 20% in Europe and North America if preventative measures are not taken, and 25 to 35% in Africa, India, and Thailand. Women with HIV are at greater risk of other sexually transmitted infections and other coexisting disease: these increase vertical transmission rates and lead to poorer obstetric outcomes. HIV infection in the neonate leads to over one-third dying in infancy; 25% will develop AIDS within 1 year.

Practical prevention of vertical transmission needs to vary according to resources and availability of health care. Interdisciplinary cooperation is required, with screening and treatment for other sexually transmitted infections early in gestation and again at 28 weeks. Under ideal circumstances, combination therapy using HAART is advised; zidovudine alone is probably less effective and allows the emergence of resistant strains. A woman with HIV already receiving treatment should continue to do so during pregnancy, and treatment is usually started at 28 weeks in a patient who has not previously met criteria for doing so. With advanced disease, viral loads should be checked, and the regimen changed if viraemia is not suppressed.

Delivery should be by caesarean section after 38 weeks: this definitely reduces vertical transmission if antiretroviral therapy is not taken, or if there is a detectable viral load. The effect of caesarean section in women on treatment and with an undetectable viral load is uncertain, but most women are nevertheless delivered this way. In women who do labour, vertical transmission is higher the longer the rupture of the membranes. Antiretroviral therapy should be given to the neonate for 6 weeks and breastfeeding should be avoided. Overall, these manoeuvres can reduce the vertical transmission rate to less than 1%.

A different strategy is required in developing countries where resources are scarce, caesarean section is less readily available and with higher operative and future obstetric risks, and the avoidance of breastfeeding has more serious implications (while reducing neonatal infection rates it is associated with a higher mortality). Nevirapine is given both in labour and to the neonate. Amniotomy is avoided. Breastfeeding is exclusive, limited to 6 months, and combined with antiretroviral therapy.

Rubella

Up to 20% of women in North America and more in developing countries are nonimmune, hence small outbreaks of rubella still occur. Most women in the United Kingdom are immune as a result of widespread immunization programmes, and fewer than 10 affected neonates are born each year.

The incubation period is 14 to 21 days, with infectivity 7 days before and 7 days after the appearance of the characteristic rash, which is preceded by a short prodrome of low-grade fever, headache, malaise, and lymphadenopathy. Arthritis and arthralgia occur in up to 70% of adult women, and rare maternal complications are thrombocytopenia, acute postinfectious encephalitis, myocarditis, Guillain–Barré syndrome, relapsing encephalitis, optic neuritis, bone marrow aplasia, and progressive panencephalitis.

The fetus is at greatest risk during the first trimester, when 90% will be affected. Embryo resorption may occur in very early gestation, or abortion, or the congenital rubella syndrome. This consists of congenital heart disease—especially pulmonary arterial hypoplasia, patent ductus arteriosus, and coarctation of the aorta—learning difficulties, ocular defects such as cataracts, glaucoma, and microphthalmia, and sensorineural deafness. Between 12 and 16 weeks the sequelae are less severe, with sensorineural deafness predominating. At 25 weeks vertical transmission is approximately 25%, rising to 100% at term, but the fetus is almost invariably unaffected.

Congenital rubella can only be prevented by immunization; termination of pregnancy may be offered where infection has occurred in the first trimester. Immunization programmes vary worldwide, but in the United Kingdom rubella forms part of the MMR vaccination in early childhood. Immunity is routinely checked in early pregnancy, and postnatal vaccination is offered if a mother is nonimmune or has low immunity. The vaccine is live attenuated and therefore contraindicated in pregnancy, although inadvertent administration has not led to recorded problems.

Parvovirus

The parvovirus B19 is the only pathogenic parvovirus in humans. Infectivity is high and via respiratory secretions, often from children. More than 50% of adults in Western countries are immune; 0.25% of women are infected in pregnancy, but infection can be epidemic. Viraemia appears about 7 days after infection and has disappeared within a few days, before symptoms occur. The classic 'slapped cheek' rash is not invariable and most have an arthralgia; 20% of adults have no symptoms. Pregnancy does not alter these symptoms.

Infection in pregnancy leads to a 9% excess risk of fetal loss, with an approximately 30% rate of fetal infection, largely with exposure before 20 weeks gestation. A characteristic effect is due to the parvovirus binding to the P antigen present on erythrocytes,

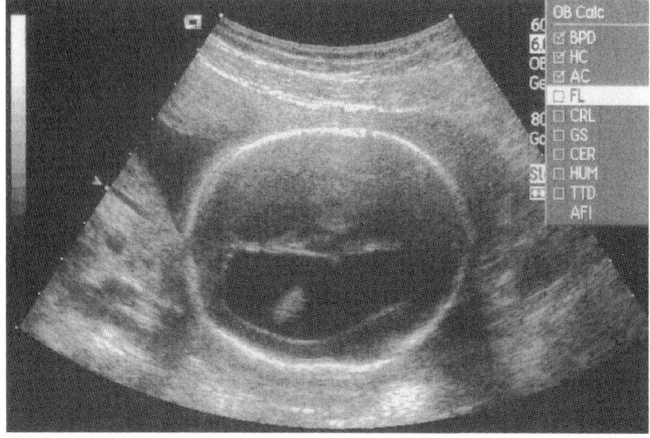

(a)

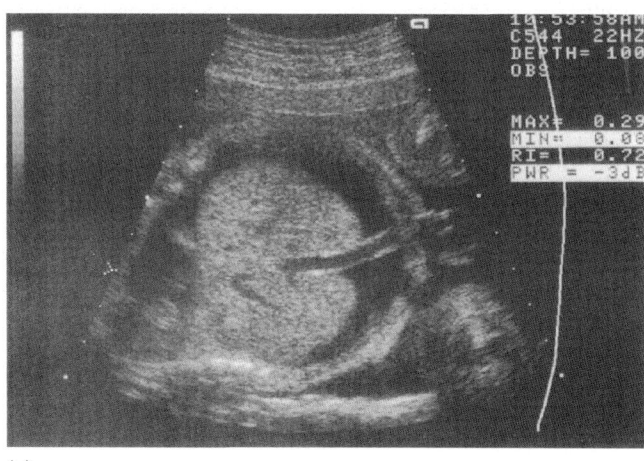

(b)

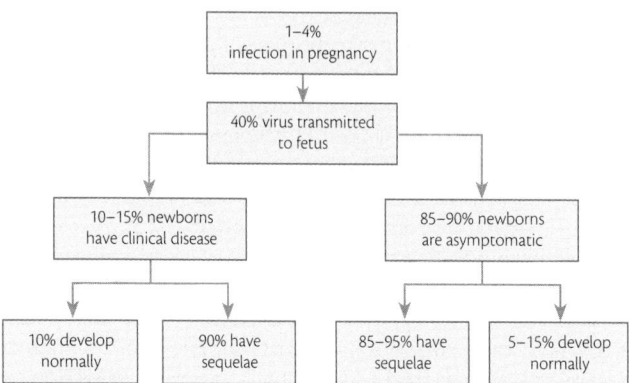

(c)

Fig. 14.15.1 Antenatal ultrasound scans: (a) fetal head showing ventriculomegaly secondary to congenital toxoplasmosis; (b) fetal abdomen showing intrahepatic calcification seen in congenital varicella infection; (c) fetal abdomen showing ascites in parvovirus infection.

erythroblasts, and myocardium. This can cause a predominantly aplastic anaemia that is of minimal significance in healthy children or adults. By contrast, the fetus is vulnerable, largely because of the short half-life of fetal red blood cells and the need for erythropoiesis, and it may develop a severe aplastic anaemia with a variable but occasionally severe thrombocytopenia. This is a cause of nonimmune hydrops (Fig. 14.15.1), exacerbated in some cases by cardiac dysfunction, which is self-limiting in more than 50% of cases but fatal in the rest. Fetal death typically occurs 3–6 weeks after infection and is very unusual more than after 18 weeks afterwards.

Parvovirus in pregnancy is encountered either during investigation of fetal hydrops, or where there has been maternal infection or contact with an infected individual. For the former, the diagnosis is made when the hydropic fetus is established to be anaemic, usually by the finding of a raised peak systolic velocity in the fetal middle cerebral artery, and by exclusion of other causes of hydrops. Maternal blood will usually show IgM; if IgG is present, a stored early-pregnancy booking sample can be checked for comparison. Viral identification by PCR of a fetal blood sample is more reliable. An *in utero* transfusion is given if the degree of anaemia appears to be increasing and the fetal state worsens. This involves injection of high haematocrit blood into the umbilical vein at the cord insertion. When the disease appears to be severe, an *in utero* platelet transfusion is recommended by some because of the potential for thrombocytopenia and reports of severe and fatal fetal bleeding during *in utero* transfusion.

Management of the woman infected by parvovirus involves close follow-up of the fetus, usually with ultrasound scans assessing the middle cerebral artery, at least every 2 weeks and up until 4 months after infection, when the mother can be reassured that her risk of fetal loss is low.

Long-term follow-up of babies affected *in utero* by parvovirus are reassuring, but there are reports both of fetal loss at transfusion and of severe cerebral damage following very severe fetal anaemia.

Cytomegalovirus (CMV)

CMV is the commonest congenital infection in developed countries. Immunity is present in up to 75% of women; less in higher socioeconomic classes or in developing countries. Infection in pregnancy occurs in about 1%. Maternal infection is usually asymptomatic but can cause an infectious mononucleosis-like illness.

Vertical transmission occurs during pregnancy following 40% of primary infections and less than 1% of secondary recurrences. After primary infection, 5 to 15% of neonates are symptomatic, and of these more than 80% develop severe neurological sequelae

Fig. 14.15.2 The outcome of CMV infection in pregnancy.

including mental impairment and sensorineural hearing loss. Even asymptomatic infants have a 5 to 15% risk of hearing impairment. Overall, the chance of normal childhood development without evidence of fetal damage is approximately 75%. The outcomes of CMV infection in pregnancy are shown in Fig. 14.15.2. Ultrasound abnormalities, particularly intracranial or hepatic calcifications, cerebral ventriculomegaly, oligohydramnios, and IUGR are detected in only 20%.

CMV is encountered in pregnancy usually because IgM is found incidentally, although it may be detected as part of the investigation of a fetus with abnormalities. CMV IgM is long lasting and its identification in pregnancy may predate the pregnancy, hence a negative retrospectively tested booking sample, or low IgG avidity, or rising IgG or IgM titres are required to confirm maternal infection. Vertical transmission is detected using amniocentesis and PCR, which needs to be performed no earlier than 20 weeks gestation and 6 weeks after maternal infection, or in the presence of ultrasound abnormalities (which have multiple causes), to exclude fetal infection. Ultrasound abnormalities, high viral load, and thrombocytopenia are associated with more severe sequelae, and fetal blood sampling later in the pregnancy may help determine the prognosis where ultrasound abnormalities are not detected. There is no effective therapy and termination of pregnancy may be offered: currently in the United Kingdom this can be performed late in the pregnancy. Intravenous ganciclovir given to the infant reduces hearing loss in the most severely affected. CMV screening is currently not recommended.

Herpes simplex (HSV)

HSV-2 is the predominant cause of genital herpes, but in up to 30% of cases it is HSV-1 that is responsible. In the United States of America the seroprevalence of HSV-1 and HSV-2 is 63% and 23% respectively, with about 90% of those seropositive to HSV-2 giving no history of infection. Primary infection in pregnancy occurs in 2% of susceptible women. This is usually asymptomatic, but primary herpes may be characterized by genital pain and ulceration, discharge, dysuria, lymphoedema, and systemic symptoms. The development of vesicles may occur for the first time in a woman previously infected: it does not necessarily imply recent transmission. A rare but severe manifestation of HSV infection in pregnancy is disseminated disease, with necrotizing hepatitis, thrombocytopenia, leucopenia, disseminated intravascular coagulopathy, and more than 50% mortality.

Herpes simplex is transmitted vertically at delivery, but very rarely during pregnancy. Transmission is almost 50% in active primary infection, with the greatest risk in late pregnancy, but nearer 1% with active recurrent herpes because of passive fetal immunity. Nevertheless, most neonatal herpes occurs in women without a history. It is rare (1.65/100 000 live births in the United Kingdom), although less so in the United States, but causes severe illness including encephalitis and death, particularly in preterm neonates.

Caesarean delivery is recommended when genital lesions from primary infection are evident at the time of delivery, and usually also where primary infection has occurred in the 6 weeks prior to delivery. This should be performed before, or as soon as possible after the membranes have ruptured. If vaginal delivery is unavoidable or the membranes have been ruptured for more than 4 h, then the neonate should be treated with aciclovir. Caesarean delivery is not advised if primary infection has occurred earlier in the pregnancy

or where there is asymptomatic recurrent herpes. Where recurrent herpes is symptomatic at delivery the neonatal risk is extremely small and probably not an indication for caesarean section. Oral aciclovir may be safely used in pregnancy for all women with a primary episode and may prevent recurrences at term. Screening and searching for asymptomatic viral shedding is not advised.

Herpes zoster

In Western countries, more than 90% of adults are immune to varicella zoster virus (VZV), with infection only occurring in 3 per 1000 pregnancies. In developing countries, many more are nonimmune. Transmission is by respiratory droplets and personal contact with the vesicles. Primary infection causes chickenpox; reactivation of the virus that has lain dormant in sensory nerve root ganglia causes shingles. The incubation period is 10 to 21 days, infectivity being from 48 h before the rash appears to when all the vesicles are covered. Primary infection in pregnancy may be severe, with pneumonia in 10% and occasional maternal death. Maternal shingles is not associated with neonatal risk.

The principal risk to the fetus is with primary infection in late pregnancy, when varicella infection of the newborn occurs in 50% and is associated with a neonatal mortality approaching 30%. Infection between 20 and 36 weeks gestation, in the absence of preterm delivery, does not have sequelae. Before 20 weeks, however, 1 to 2% of fetuses develop the congenital varicella syndrome, characterized by neurological, optical, and limb anomalies. Ultrasound findings 5 weeks after infection include polyhydramnios and echogenic foci in the fetal liver (Fig. 14.15.1).

Maternal infection is confirmed by the presence of IgM; maternal IgG indicates immunity. A nonimmune mother with significant exposure should be given varicella zoster immune globulin (VZIG) within 10 days, and if chickenpox develops oral aciclovir is recommended within 24 h of the rash if the gestation exceeds 20 weeks. Careful fetal ultrasound evaluation is required when the mother is infected before 20 weeks. In late pregnancy, VZIG is given to the neonate if delivery occurs 5 days after or 2 days before maternal infection. Vigilance for neonatal infection is required: this has a mortality of up to 30% and is treated with aciclovir.

Hepatitis B

Less than 1% of pregnant women in Western countries are HepBsAg positive, although the incidence is rising; in parts of Africa and Asia the rate is 25%. Vertical transmission can occur throughout pregnancy and is particularly important because 90% of infected neonates become chronic carriers (in contrast to adults, 10% of whom become chronic carriers) that are both infectious and at risk of liver disease. The risk of transmission relates to maternal viral antigen status: in HepBsAg positive/HepBeAg negative mothers the risk is 5 to 20%; in HepBsAg positive/HepBeAg positive it is 70 to 90%.

Vertical transmission can be reduced by more than 90% by active neonatal immunization, using 0.5 ml hepatitis B vaccine. This is recommended to all infants born to HepBsAg positive mothers; additional passive immunization (200 IU of hepatitis B immunoglobulin within 12 h of birth) for infants born to HepBeAg positive or HepBsAb negative mothers is also advised. Targeted screening only identifies about half of chronic carriers, so universal screening has been advocated in developed countries, with the World Health Organization recommending universal vaccination in countries with high prevalence.

Hepatitis C

Worldwide, 3% of pregnant women have been infected with hepatitis C virus (HCV), but the figure is 30% in HIV-positive women. The principal risk factor in the United Kingdom, where about 0.5% of women have been infected, is intravenous drug abuse, and sexual transmission is unusual. Hepatitis C leads to chronic hepatitis in about 80%; progression is insidious and most pregnant women are asymptomatic. Liver transaminases may be normal, but tend to reduce during pregnancy if elevated. Antibody levels are usually detectable within 3 months after infection; the persistence of HCV antibody implies persistent infection and infectivity.

Interferon-α with ribavirin reduces disease activity, but ribavirin may be teratogenic, hence interferon is used (rarely) for treatment of severe cases in pregnancy and (more commonly) postpartum. Vertical transmission of HCV occurs in approximately 6% if HCV is detectable by polymerase chain reaction (PCR) in the mother; otherwise the risk is very low. Coexisting HIV infection increases the rate of vertical transmission to 23%. Transmission is not thought to be significantly affected by mode of delivery. Transmission by breast feeding is unlikely. Elective caesarean section, formula feeding, and administration of immune globulin do not reduce vertical transmission to the neonate.

Maternal antibodies may persistent for months, hence PCR is used to confirm infection in infants. Infected infants usually remain viraemic and prone to chronic hepatitis.

Bacterial diseases

Bacterial vaginosis

This occurs when there is an overgrowth of anaerobic organisms such as *Gardnerella vaginalis* and *Mycoplasma hominis*, and characterized by excessive Gram-negative bacilli and cocco-bacillary organisms compared to lactobacilli on Gram staining. The prevalence varies from 5 to 20%, depending much on the diligence with which the diagnosis is sought. Bacterial vaginosis is not sexually transmitted, but is associated with sexually transmitted diseases and is rare before the onset of sexual activity. Three of four Amsel's criteria are required for diagnosis: a thin white homogeneous discharge, clue cells, raised vaginal pH (>4.5), and a positive 'whiff test' (fishy odour when 10% KOH is added to the discharge). At least 50% of women with bacterial vaginosis have no symptoms, but an offensive, thin white discharge is often found.

Bacterial vaginosis is associated with late miscarriage and preterm birth. Prematurity is a major cause of neonatal mortality and morbidity in developed countries.

Symptomatic bacterial vaginosis is treated with oral clindamycin. In women with risk factors for preterm birth, particularly a prior history of this or late miscarriage, treatment of asymptomatic infection is indicated as it reduces the risk of recurrence. It is not known whether screening and treatment in low-risk women has the same effect. Vaginal clindamycin is not effective and metronidazole has paradoxically been associated with an increased risk of preterm delivery.

Streptococci

Group A streptococci (*Streptococcus pyogenes*) remain an important cause of puerperal sepsis worldwide, but this is now rare in developed countries. Group B streptococci (GBS, *Streptococcus agalactiae*) are an important cause of neonatal disease but cause less severe maternal disease. Up to 25% of pregnant women are colonized by GBS, usually without symptoms, although maternal urinary tract infection is not uncommon.

GBS is associated with preterm delivery but it is ascending infection at the time of delivery that is best understood. Although 70% of neonates born to carriers are colonized, only 1 to 2% will develop disease of chorioamnionitis and fetal infection leading to early-onset neonatal streptococcal sepsis. The incidence of this is 0.5 to 3.7 per 1000 live births with a mortality of 6%. Intrauterine infection may also cause antepartum stillbirth. Infection usually occurs following rupture of the membranes: risk factors are prematurity, prolonged rupture of the membranes, intrapartum maternal fever, heavy colonization, low maternal antibody levels, and a previously affected infant.

Intrapartum high-dose intravenous penicillin greatly reduces early-onset neonatal disease. Preventive strategies are based on risk factors, either alone or in conjunction with screening. With the former approach, women are treated if they have a previous history, intrapartum fever, are in preterm labour, or where the membranes have been ruptured for more than 18 h: at least 70% of neonatal sepsis is prevented by treating approximately 18% of women. In the latter approach, a combined screening and risk-based strategy, third-trimester vaginal and anal swabs are taken. Women identified as carriers are then also treated intrapartum. This leads to approximately 25% of all pregnant women being treated, with 86% of cases of sepsis prevented. The former is the currently preferred approach because of implications of cost and allergy to penicillin. Vaccines for GBS are under development.

Listeria

Infection is from salads contaminated with animal faeces, undercooked meats, unpasteurized milk, soft cheeses, some fruit, hummus, and patés. In the United Kingdom the incidence is up to 5 per 100 000 live births. Worldwide the incidence has fallen as a result of public health campaigns about the likely source of infection. Maternal disease manifests as bacteraemia, with fever, sore throat, headache, and chills: diarrhoea, pyelitis, and backache may also occur. It is treated with ampicillin with an aminoglycoside for synergy.

Infection of the fetus occurs transplacentally. Before 24 weeks gestation this usually results in miscarriage; after 24 weeks neonatal mortality is approximately 20%.

Chlamydia

Chlamydia trachomatis is the most common sexually transmitted infection, with up to 7% of pregnant women being infected, depending on age, marital status, and socioeconomic class. Infection is mostly asymptomatic. Pelvic infection is very rare during pregnancy, but after delivery endometritis and salpingitis may lead to tubal damage and infertility, and 12% of induced abortions are followed by pelvic infection.

Maternal infection, particularly if recently acquired, is associated with preterm delivery and a significant cause of neonatal handicap. Treatment reduces but does not eradicate these risks. Neonatal conjunctivitis occurs in up to 50% of neonates exposed to chlamydia, with a smaller proportion developing pneumonia.

The identification of maternal infection warrants referral to a genitourinary medicine clinic, with contact tracing for treatment of sexual partners. Erythromycin is effective, and a single dose of azithromycin (1 g) ensures compliance and is also known to be safe. Tetracyclines are contraindicated in pregnancy as they cause tooth discoloration in the child. Reinfection rates are high and repeat testing is advised after at least 3 weeks to ensure a cure has been achieved. Screening or even prophylaxis of all mothers following abortion is cost-effective, but routine screening in pregnancy should currently be limited to those at risk of infection who are also at increased risk of preterm delivery.

Gonorrhoea

Neisseria gonorrhoea is endemic in many developing countries, and having fallen to low rates in many areas of the developed world in the late 1980s and early 1990s is now gradually increasing again. Pharyngeal and disseminated systemic infection with fever, rash, and septic arthritis are more common in pregnancy, but salpingitis is rare. Cervical culture detects most infections; PCR testing is expensive and does not enable antibiotic sensitivity testing. As with nonpregnant women, 80% are asymptomatic.

Gonococcal cervicitis is associated with a fourfold increase in prematurity and chorioamnionitis. Further, 40% of neonates exposed to gonorrhoea at delivery will develop ophthalmia neonatorum. Gonococci have also been implicated in postpartum and postabortion endometritis and salpingitis.

Treatment is best with a single intramuscular dose of ceftriaxone (250 mg). Disseminated infection warrants intravenous therapy. Penicillinase-producing strains are common. The patient should be screened for other sexually transmitted infections and antichlamydia therapy is often given at the same time. A test of cure should be taken at least 3 days after antibiotics. Because of the frequency of infection and the serious risks, screening is warranted in high-risk groups such as those undergoing first-trimester termination.

Syphilis

The incidence of infection in pregnancy is 0.02% in the United Kingdom, but in Africa, South-East Asia, and Russia it is endemic. Pregnancy does not alter the clinical manifestations. Screening with nontreponemal tests (e.g. VDRL) is routine in many countries, including the United Kingdom. Sensitivity is highest in secondary syphilis and lowest early in the infection, and false-positive results occur with concomitant infections or autoimmune disease.

Vertical transmission is predominantly transplacental, occurring in up to 90% of untreated women, particularly those with early disease. Most affected pregnancies result in congenital syphilis, miscarriage, preterm delivery or perinatal death. Ultrasound examination of the infected fetus may be normal or show hepatomegaly and other abnormalities. At birth, babies exhibit rhinitis, osteitis, and skin bullae. Hutchinson's triad of abnormal teeth, interstitial keratitis, and sensorineural deafness arise later in the untreated child.

Syphilis is usually diagnosed in pregnancy after the development of suggestive symptoms or a positive screen. A positive VDRL should be confirmed with a specific treponemal test (e.g. FTA-ABS). Treatment is with two intramuscular doses of benzyl penicillin (2.4 MU, 1 week apart). In true penicillin allergy, a 5- to 10-day regimen of high-dose oral ceftriaxone is recommended. VDRL titres should fall until undetectable or less than 1 in 4, otherwise retreatment is necessary. Treatment will prevent congenital infection in 98% of cases. The rare Jarisch–Herxheimer reaction to treatment

may precipitate preterm labour. Screening in pregnancy is cost-effective, even where the disease is rare: 121 women were identified by antenatal screening in the United Kingdom from 1994 to 1997, with 18 600 tests needing to be performed to detect 1 case.

Tuberculosis

Mycobacterium tuberculosis infection (TB) is extremely common in the developing world. The proportion of younger people infected—including women of reproductive age—is rising, in part due to HIV infection. Pregnancy has little effect on the course of either symptomatic or latent TB, but the diagnosis may be delayed in pregnancy because of the nonspecific symptoms.

Congenital tuberculosis is acquired transplacentally and is potentially fatal but extremely rare; treatment is advised principally for maternal health. Coinfection with HIV should be considered. Isoniazid, ethambutol, pyrazinamide, and probably rifampicin are safe in pregnancy; streptomycin can cause ototoxicity. Vitamin B_6 and vitamin K supplementation are indicated. Breastfeeding is not contraindicated. Infectivity is greatly reduced after 2 weeks of therapy, hence separation of mother and child is inappropriate.

Protozoal infections

Toxoplasmosis

In the United Kingdom and North America 15 to 20% of adults have antibodies to *Toxoplasma gondii*; infection in pregnancy occurs in 0.2%. It is more common in mainland Europe and in developing countries. Infection is acquired from contact with soil, uncooked meat, or contaminated salad, and is more common in women with HIV. The condition is frequently asymptomatic, but 10 to 20% of mothers have lymphadenopathy or a flu-like episode.

Vertical transmission occurs during pregnancy in about 30%. Transmission is lower (<10%) in early gestation, but has greater impact: over 75% will have clinically apparent disease. This includes the classic neonatal triad of chorioretinitis, cerebral calcification, and microcephaly. Ultrasound findings include intracranial calcification, cerebral ventriculomegaly (Fig. 14.15.3), ascites, and hepatomegaly. With increasing gestation, vertical transmission increases to about 75% by term, but the risks of severe

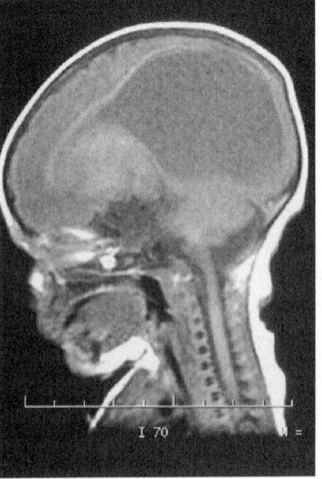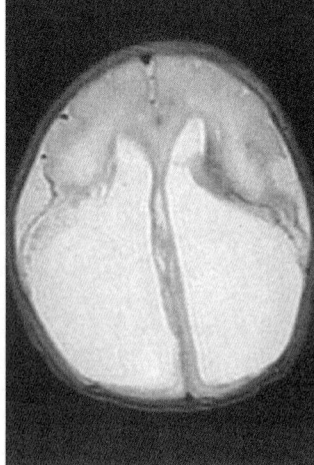

Fig. 14.15.3 MRI head of a 20-day-old baby with congenital toxoplasmosis, showing severe ventriculomegaly from hydrocephalus.

Table 14.15.1 Notes on other infections in pregnancy

Infection	Notes
HHV6	Transplacental transfer occurs, probably without any effect on the fetus
HPV	Vertical transmission has been reported rarely; if vaginal warts are massive they may obstruct delivery
Enteroviruses	50% have a mild respiratory or gastrointestinal illness; some have severe cramping abdominal pains simulating placental abruption that can lead to unnecessary emergency caesarean section; newborns with vertically acquired echoviral infections may have fulminant hepatic necrosis, severe coagulopathy from disseminated intravascular coagulopathy, and meningitis or myocarditis
Japanese B encephalitis virus	Particularly high mortality rates with fetal death have been reported in pregnancy
Lassa fever	Increased mortality for women in pregnancy, survival is improved by abortion and ribavirin (see Table 14.15.1)
Trichomonas vaginalis	Infections are common in pregnancy, can be transmitted to the newborn around birth, but there are no adverse effects on the fetus
Mycoplasma hominis	A commensal of the lower female genital tract; controversial disease role in newborns
Ureaplasma urealyticum	As for *M. hominis*
Lyme disease	*Borrelia burgdorferi* in gestation has a good prognosis if recognized early and treated aggressively; fetal death or disease, including meningoencephalitis, occurs without maternal treatment
Schistosomiasis	Placental infection occurs in up to 25% in bilharzia infested areas, but there is no effect on gestational age or birth weight
Candida	The incidence of vaginal thrush increases with each trimester; rarely, vaginal thrush in pregnancy predisposes to congenital candidiasis

sequelae are less. The highest risk for congenital toxoplasmosis with a poor outcome is therefore when maternal infection occurs around 20 to 24 weeks' gestation. At this stage the risk of severe handicap is approximately 10%.

Toxoplasmosis is encountered in pregnancy either as part of investigations for abnormal fetal ultrasound appearances, or as a result of screening. Toxoplasmosis screening is imprecise: IgM may not be detected with proven disease, and it may also persist for months after infection. Infection is nevertheless unlikely in the previous 3 months if IgM is negative, or there is high-avidity IgG. Maternal infection is confirmed by a change from negative to positive IgG, or low to high levels of IgM. Mothers infected in pregnancy are treated with spiramycin with the aim of reducing vertical transmission, this being diagnosed or excluded using PCR on amniotic fluid taken after 18 weeks. Combination therapy of pyrimethamine and sulfadiazine with folinic acid is used if fetal infection is detected. Although reversal of ultrasound abnormalities has been recorded after therapy, there is no consistent evidence that treatment is effective when vertical transmission has occurred. In the neonate, diagnosis requires IgA or IgM testing because maternal IgG will persist for up to 1 year. Neonatal infection is treated for 1 year. Because of the perceived effectiveness of therapy in preventing vertical transmission, screening is widely practised in Europe.

Malaria

In sub-Saharan Africa up to 8% of infant mortality is attributable to malaria in pregnancy. Pregnant women are more susceptible to malaria and complications such as cerebral malaria, pulmonary oedema, and renal failure occur more commonly.

Severe malarial anaemia of pregnancy causes spontaneous abortion, premature birth, IUGR, and stillbirth. Congenital malaria from transplacental spread occurs in approximately 1% of infected pregnancies. The newborns have fever, respiratory distress, pallor, anaemia, hepatomegaly, jaundice, and diarrhoea.

Prevention of malaria infection advocated by the World Health Organization involves insecticide-treated mosquito nets, intermittent preventive treatment with antimalarial drugs, and febrile malaria case management. Antimalarial drugs reduce parasitaemia, placental malaria, low birth weight, and—depending on their timing—perinatal death. Drugs used depend on the sensitivity of the relevant plasmodium locally and include proguanil, chloroquine, mefloquine, and artemisinin compounds. Most falciparum malaria is now resistant to mefloquine and chloroquine. Sulfadoxine–pyrimethamine is most commonly used as intermittent preventive treatment, this chemoprophylaxis involving two doses at least 1 month apart to all pregnant women in stable transmission areas. A third dose is recommended where HIV infection is common. Artemisinin combination therapy is increasingly used for febrile malaria because of resistance to other drugs and lower frequency of few side effects, although there are less safety data, particularly for the first trimester.

Trypanosomiasis

Infection in pregnancy can cause miscarriage, IUGR, and preterm delivery. Congenital infection occurs in about 10% and may be initially asymptomatic, but jaundice, anaemia, hepatosplenomegaly, encephalitis and pneumonitis can then develop. Diagnosis is through placental histology, blood smear examination for parasitaemia, and ELISA. There is no safe and reliable treatment in pregnancy.

Other conditions

Notes on other infections in pregnancy are given in Table 14.15.1.

Antimicrobial agents in pregnancy

A guide to the safety of antimicrobial agents in pregnancy is given in Table

Table 14.15.2 A guide to the safety of antimicrobial agents in pregnancy

Drugs	Probably safe but limited human studies	Potential or proven risk in pregnancy, but benefits may outweigh risk	Fetal abnormalities, risk greater than benefit
β-Lactams	+		
Aminoglycosides		+	
Macrolides	+		
Sulfonamides		+	
Tetracycline			+
Antiparasitic agents, except quinine		+	
Quinine			+
Antimycobacterial agents: INH, pyrazinamide, rifampicin, dapsone, ethambutol		+	
Antimycobacterial agents: ethionamide, thalidomide, clofazimine/cycloserine			+
Aciclovir, valaciclovir, famciclovir	+		
Ribavirin			+

Adapted from: Gilbert DN, Moellering RC, Sande MA (2000). *The Sandford guide to antimicrobial therapy*, 13th edirionn. Antimicrobial Therapy, Inc, Sandford, USA.

Further reading

De Santis M, *et al.* (2006). Rubella infection in pregnancy. *Reprod Toxicol*, **21**, 390–8.

Doroshenko A, Sherrard J, Pollard AJ (2006). Syphilis in pregnancy and the neonatal period. *Int J STD AIDS*, **17**, 221–7.

Gibbs RS, Schrag S, Schuchat A (2004). Perinatal infections due to group B streptococci. *Obstet Gynecol*, **104**, 1062–76.

Grether JK, Nelson KB (1997). Maternal infection and cerebral palsy in infants of normal birth weight. *JAMA*, **278**, 207–11.

Levy R, *et al.* (1997). Infection by parvovirus B19 during pregnancy: a review. *Obstet Gynecol Surv*, **55**, 254–9.

RCOG (2004). *Management of HIV in pregnancy*. Green Top Guideline 39. Royal College of Obstetricians and Gynaecologists, London.

Ormerod P (2001). Tuberculosis in pregnancy and the puerperium. *Thorax*, **56**, 494–9.

Ornoy A, Diav-Citrin O (2006). Fetal effects of primary and secondary cytomegalovirus infection in pregnancy. *Reprod Toxicol*, **21**, 399–409.

Rorman E, *et al.* (2006). Congenital toxoplasmosis—prenatal aspects of *Toxoplasma gondii* infection. *Reprod Toxicol*, **21**, 458–72.

Steer P (2005). The epidemiology of preterm labor—a global perspective. *J Perinat Med*, **33**, 273–6.

Useful websites

Centers for Disease Control. *Malaria during pregnancy*. http://www.cdc.gov/malaria/pregnancy.htm

NAM. *Reproductive health*. http://www.aidsmap.com/cms1044917.asp

Royal College of Obstetricians and Gynaecologists. *Infection and pregnancy—study group statement*. http://www.rcog.org.uk/womens-health/clinical-guidance/infection-and-pregnancy-study-group-statement

Blood disorders specific to pregnancy

David J. Perry and Katharine Lowndes

Essentials

Plasma volume increases by more during pregnancy than does red cell mass, leading to haemodilution and a fall in the haematocrit from about 40% to 33%, with the nadir usually reached at 24 to 32 weeks gestation. Anaemia during pregnancy is defined as a haemoglobin concentration of <10.5 g/dl during the second and third trimesters.

Anaemias and haemoglobinopathies

The commonest haematological problem encountered in pregnancy is iron deficiency anaemia. Routine iron supplementation in all pregnant women is probably not justified in developed countries, but if iron deficiency is detected it is advisable to treat as early as possible.

Folic acid—the requirement for folic acid doubles in pregnancy and dietary folate deficiency is the most frequent cause of gestational megaloblastic anaemia. This can be prevented by supplementation with 300 μg folic acid daily, although higher doses of folate (up to 5 mg daily) are recommended to prevent neural tube defects.

Haemoglobinopathies—the diagnosis of variant haemoglobins and the thalassaemia syndromes before pregnancy or early in gestation is important. Screening is usually performed on a blood sample taken at booking. If a haemoglobin variant or thalassaemic indices are detected, then the partner should be tested to determine the risk of having an affected fetus and allowing informed prenatal counselling.

Haemostatic disorders

Normal pregnancy is associated with marked changes in all aspects of haemostasis, the overall effect of which is to generate a state of hypercoagulability. These changes in haemostasis, whilst reducing the risks of excessive blood loss at delivery, significantly increase the risk of venous thromboembolic disease in pregnancy (see Chapter 14.7).

Gestational thrombocytopenia—seen in about 8% of all pregnancies and accounts for more than 70% of cases of thrombocytopenia in pregnancy: its main differential diagnosis is immune thrombocytopenic purpura.

Disseminated intravascular coagulation—can be caused by intrauterine death with a retained fetus, severe pre-eclampsia, premature separation of the placenta (placental abruption), retained placenta, amniotic fluid embolism, haemorrhagic shock and transfusion reaction.

Inherited haemostatic disorders, e.g. haemophilia, von Willebrands disease—women with these conditions require specialist management during pregnancy.

Anaemia

Plasma volume will increase by about 1250 ml in a singleton pregnancy, approximately 45% of the average nonpregnant female plasma volume. This increase occurs mainly after the first trimester and peaks at 34 to 36 weeks gestation. The increase is greater in multiparous women with larger babies and in multiple pregnancies. The total red cell mass increases after the first trimester by about 250 ml, approximately 20% of the average nonpregnant female value. This can increase to 400 ml in women taking iron supplementation.

The consequence of the greater relative increase in the plasma volume leads to haemodilution and a fall in the haematocrit from about 40% to 33%. The nadir is usually reached at 24 to 32 weeks gestation, with the haemoglobin then starting to rise again towards term. The degree of haemodilution shows considerable variation between women, meaning that haemoglobin alone is not a valid marker of iron status. The normal range of haemoglobin in pregnancy can lie between 10.0 and 14.5 g/dl, but anaemia during pregnancy is usually defined as a haemoglobin concentration of less than 10.5 g/dl during the second and third trimesters and requires further investigation. The World Health Organization, however, recommends that it should not fall below 11 g/dl at any time during pregnancy. There is a gradual increase in erythropoietin levels with increasing gestation, although this increase is blunted by the use of iron supplementation.

Iron deficiency anaemia

During pregnancy the daily requirements for iron increase from 0.8 to 7.5 mg/day between the first and third trimesters. Iron is needed to expand the maternal erythrocyte mass, fulfil fetal requirements, and prepare the mother for any iron loss at delivery. This increased requirement is met by increased absorption, which is most pronounced after 20 weeks gestation.

Iron deficiency anaemia is the commonest haematological problem encountered in pregnancy. In nonpregnant women this is often seen as a hypochromic, microcytic anaemia, but in the pregnant woman, owing to a relative increase in the number of larger immature red cells, the mean cell volume (MCV) may remain unchanged, but the red cell distribution width (RDW) increases. A serum ferritin level of less than 30 μg/L reflects a loss of storage iron and indicates iron deficiency. It occurs before the haemoglobin falls, which is a relatively late manifestation. Mothers who enter pregnancy iron deficient will have no stores remaining at term.

Transferrin levels double during the course of pregnancy, leading to a fall in percentage saturation. Transferrin receptors are present on the surface of young erythrocytes and also circulate within the blood as soluble transferrin receptors (sTfR). These increase in number during iron deficiency and are independent of total body iron stores. They can, therefore, be a helpful measure of iron deficiency in women with a raised ferritin for other reasons.

Mild iron deficiency anaemia is unlikely to have any harmful effects on the mother, but if it is more severe the symptoms of anaemia can make the last few weeks of pregnancy difficult to tolerate. Women that are iron deficient are unlikely to tolerate significant blood loss at delivery and may indeed have increased blood loss due to impaired neuromuscular transmission. An uncorrected anaemia may be associated with placental enlargement, which in turn leads to a higher incidence of fetal abnormalities, low birth weight, and increased preterm births. However, a similar outcome has been associated with high haemoglobin concentrations as this is related to inadequate haemodilution which is a characteristic of pre-eclampsia.

Iron replacement

Routine iron supplementation in all pregnant women is probably not justified in developed countries, but if iron deficiency is detected it is advisable to treat as early as possible as the demands for iron will increase as the pregnancy progresses. There is no advantage in giving parenteral rather than oral iron. The maximal increase in haemoglobin that can be expected is approximately 0.8 g/week.

Pregnancy leaves a lasting impression on a woman's iron stores, with nulliparous women having higher serum ferritin levels than multiparous women. These differences can persist even into menopause. However, if iron supplementation is given the haemoglobin will reach prepregnancy levels within 5 to 7 days of delivery assuming there has not been excessive blood loss.

Vitamin B$_{12}$ and folate deficiency

Vitamin B$_{12}$ and folate are required in pregnancy for the growing uterus, fetus and the expanding red cell mass. The requirement for folic acid doubles in pregnancy, and dietary folate deficiency is the most frequent cause of gestational megaloblastic anaemia. Megaloblastic anaemia secondary to a deficiency of either vitamin B$_{12}$ and/or folate is most common in countries with inadequate nutrition. Folate deficiency is more frequent in multiple pregnancies and multiparous women, with most cases presenting in the third trimester and postpartum. It is known to be associated with an increase in neural tube defects and can also lead to an increased incidence of prematurity and low birth weight infants.

In most women the diagnosis of folate deficiency is made in the last 4 weeks of pregnancy, usually without symptoms excepting failure to respond to iron supplementation. An earlier presentation, in the second trimester, should prompt a search for another cause of folate deficiency such as chronic haemolysis or anticonvulsant therapy.

Folate supplementation is recommended before conception and during the first trimester to prevent neural tube defects. The current recommendation is 400 μg/day, which will reduce the risk of neural tube defects by 36%, but there is a linear dose response, and a dose of 5 mg daily improves this reduction to 85%. Megaloblastic anaemia due to poor dietary folate intake is prevented by 300 μg daily, but if the folate deficiency is due to malabsorption it will need to be given parenterally.

Initial concerns that folate supplementation would mask an underlying B$_{12}$ deficiency, allowing continued neurological deterioration, have not been borne out. This is probably because severe B$_{12}$ deficiency due to Addisonian pernicious anaemia and of sufficient severity to cause megaloblastosis is likely to be associated with infertility. Vitamin B$_{12}$ stores are large (c.3000 μg) and therefore more or less unaffected by pregnancy. The daily requirements for vitamin B$_{12}$ are increased in pregnancy (1.4 μg/day in pregnancy vs 1.0 μg/day in the nonpregnant female), but this is easily met by a diet containing animal products. Dietary deficiency of vitamin B$_{12}$ is rare in pregnancy, but can occur and was previously termed 'pernicious anaemia of pregnancy'. It responds to oral vitamin B$_{12}$ supplementation and is not associated with an autoimmune aetiology.

Haemoglobinopathies

Genetic defects in the structure, function, and production of haemoglobin can be divided into two clinically significant groups: variant haemoglobins and the thalassaemia syndromes. Diagnosis prior to, or early in, pregnancy is important so that obstetric management can be tailored appropriately. It is also now possible to offer prenatal diagnosis, which can shape parental decisions with regards to termination of the pregnancy or can direct maternal and fetal management prior to delivery.

Screening is usually performed on the blood sample taken at booking. This can be directed at high-risk populations, although with the increased migration of people from varied racial backgrounds it can be difficult to isolate this population accurately and therefore it is prudent to offer the screening to all mothers. An algorithm for screening blood tests is outlined in Fig. 14.16.1. If a haemoglobin variant or thalassaemic indices are detected, then the

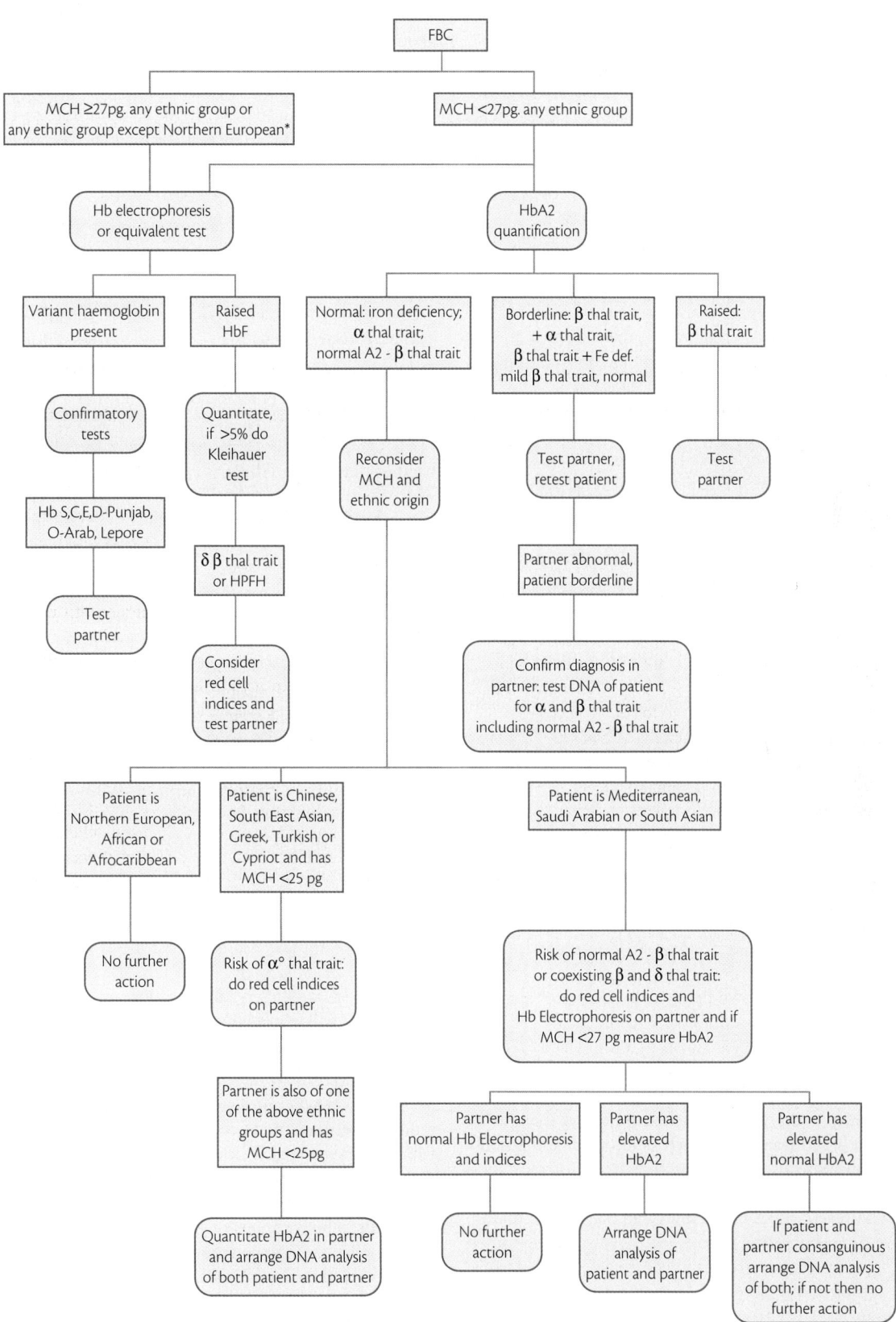

Fig. 14.16.1 An algorithm for screening for haemoglobinopathies in pregnant women.

partner should be tested to determine the risk of having an affected fetus and allowing informed prenatal counselling.

Variant haemoglobins and sickle cell syndromes

Clinically the important haemoglobin variants are those that are associated with red cell sickling. The sickle cell syndromes with major clinical symptoms include sickle cell anaemia (HbSS), sickle cell haemoglobin C (HbSC) disease, and sickle cell β-thalassaemia (HbS β-Thal). Other haemoglobin variants in combination with HbS, e.g. HbSE and HbSD, are in general associated with a milder disorder, but vasocclusive crises may occur in pregnancy.

Mothers with sickle cell trait, i.e. heterozygotes for haemoglobin A and S (HbAS), have no increased risk of sickle cell crises during normal pregnancy, but they do have an increased incidence of some infections, e.g. pyelonephritis. Caution should also be exercised if a general anaesthetic is required in these women as they have an increased risk of placental infarction and pre-eclampsia if they develop severe dehydration or become shocked.

Outcome data in pregnancy for women with sickle cell disease (SCD), i.e. HbSS, HbSC, and HbS β-thal, is based upon retrospective case series; overall maternal mortality is less than 2% and neonatal mortality is less than 5%. There is an increased tendency to pre-eclampsia, preterm labour, and low birth weight babies. The main medical problems facing a pregnant woman with SCD are those of increased sickle cell crises causing tissue infarction, severe anaemia, and an increased risk of infection. The crises are predominantly vaso-occlusive in nature and can be triggered by infection or by the pregnancy alone. If associated with a parvovirus infection the crisis can become aplastic, resulting in a rapid drop in haemoglobin. Painful vaso-occlusive crises can occur in any organ, leading to infarction and dysfunction, but the lungs are particularly susceptible and can progress to a life-threatening chest crisis.

Treatment of a sickle crisis in pregnancy is the same as for the nonpregnant woman, i.e. oxygen, fluids, and analgesia, with the addition of antibiotics if an infective trigger is suspected. There should be a low threshold for proceeding to red cell exchange transfusion if the mother is not improving. It is particularly important that pregnant women with SCD are on continuous folic acid supplementation because of the high erythrocyte turnover rate. In addition, as most adults with SCD have functional hyposplenism, they should receive pneumococcal vaccination and twice daily penicillin prophylaxis.

No correlation has been shown between the degree of anaemia and obstetric or perinatal complications in the sickle cell syndromes, and no benefit has been shown by prophylactic red cell transfusion to keep the haemoglobin at 10 to 11 g/dl, rather than transfusing when indications arise. In addition to the issues of cost and availability, prophylactic transfusion exposes the mother to the hazards of blood transfusion such as infection and notably the risk of alloimmunization of the mother to minor red blood cell antigens. This can lead to severe, delayed, and sometimes fatal haemolytic reactions in the mother and haemolytic disease of the fetus and newborn. Indications for transfusion in women with SCD during pregnancy are anaemia associated with cardiac or respiratory compromise, severe SCD-related complications (e.g. acute chest syndrome), preparation for caesarean section or refractory pre-eclampsia. More controversial indications are increasing frequency of painful crises, SCD-related complications during a previous pregnancy, and multiple-gestation pregnancy.

The increased risk of intrauterine growth retardation (IUGR) is probably due to a combination of decreased oxygen supply from the maternal anaemia and some placental infarction. Fetal growth should therefore be monitored with regular ultrasound scans. The method of delivery is based on the obstetric considerations.

For an infant with SCD, the first 2 years of life are particularly hazardous, with an increased risk of death due to infection and splenic sequestration. Hence, if the diagnosis is not made antenatally, it needs to be made as soon as possible after birth so that the parents can be aware of the need for early investigation and treatment of any possible symptoms.

Thalassaemias

α-Thalassaemia

The clinical syndromes are dependant on the number of α genes that have been deleted.

Four-gene deletion α-thalassaemia

A complete absence of all four α-globin genes results in a fetus that cannot make any α chains and therefore no fetal or adult haemoglobin can be synthesized. The remaining γ chains form tetramers known as haemoglobin Barts (Hb Barts (γ_4)). This has a high oxygen affinity, which restricts oxygen delivery to the tissues and results in a hydropic fetus which usually dies *in utero* or shortly after birth. Pregnancy with an α-thalassaemia hydrops fetus is associated with severe hypertension and proteinuria early in pregnancy, along with a high risk of antepartum and postpartum haemorrhage, in addition to other obstetric complications secondary to a large fetus and bulky placenta.

Routine antenatal screening can detect women at risk of carrying an affected fetus. Parents should be referred for counselling and offered prenatal diagnosis, as termination of pregnancy may be required to avoid serious obstetric complications. Most cases of Hb Barts hydrops fetalis are seen in eastern Asia. However, with increased immigration this disorder will become more prevalent in Western countries. Transfusion *in utero* has been performed and has been successful in a few cases.

Haemoglobin H (β_4)

This is the result of the deletion of three α-globin genes. The fetus can make some α chains, so there will be some fetal Hb (HbF ($\alpha_2\gamma_2$)) production, but most of the haemoglobin will be Hb Barts. The neonate appears healthy at birth but soon develops a severe haemolytic anaemia as HbF levels fall. The Hb Barts (γ_4) is replaced with HbH (β_4), which results in a lifelong anaemia. This varies in severity and will worsen during pregnancy.

One- or two-gene deletion α-thalassaemia

Mothers with one- (– α/αα) or two-gene deletion α-thalassaemia (– –/αα or –α/–α) can range from being asymptomatic to having a mild hypochromic microcytic anaemia. The partners of all women with suspected two-gene deletion α-thalassaemia should be screened, and if necessary the couple should be referred for genetic counselling. Two-gene deletion α-thalassaemia does not affect the pregnancy, but if both parents posses two-gene deletion α-thalassaemia and the deletion occurs on the same allele (i.e. – –/αα), then there is a 1:4 chance of having a Hb Barts hydropic fetus.

β-Thalassaemia

The β-thalassaemias are due to point mutations in the β-globin genes that cause varying degrees of reduction in the amount of β-chains produced.

β-Thalassaemia major

In β-thalassaemia major the production of β-globin chains is severely impaired because both β-globin genes are mutated. The severe imbalance of globin chain synthesis results in ineffective erythropoiesis and a severe microcytic hypochromic anaemia. The excess unpaired α-globin chains aggregate to form precipitates that damage red cell membranes, resulting in intravascular haemolysis. Premature destruction of erythroid precursors results in intramedullary death and ineffective erythropoiesis. This is not apparent in the fetus until the HbF production switches to HbA, when the infant will become anaemic.

Women with transfusion-dependent β-thalassaemia major have historically been infertile, but with improving iron chelation therapy the number of successful pregnancies is increasing. There are also an increasing number of women with thalassaemia intermedia proceeding to pregnancy. Both groups of women have an increased incidence of antepartum and postpartum complications with IUGR, recurrent infections, and hypersplenism. They need to continue with regular transfusions throughout pregnancy, with the incumbent risks and complications. Iron chelation therapy is teratogenic, hence consideration should be given to aggressive chelation therapy before planned conception.

β-Thalassaemia minor (β-thalassaemia trait)

In β-thalassaemia minor (β-thalassaemia trait) one of the two β-globin genes is defective. The defect can be a complete absence or a reduced synthesis of the β-globin protein. Women with β-thalassaemia minor are either asymptomatic or have a mild hypochromic microcytic anaemia, with a raised proportion of HbA_2 which does not affect the pregnancy. However, it is important to identify such women and screen their partners to see if they are similarly affected, and if necessary to offer prenatal diagnosis. If both partners have β-thalassaemia minor, there is a 1:4 chance of having a child with severe β-thalassaemia major.

Other anaemias

Aplastic anaemia

Coincidental aplastic anaemia can occur in pregnancy in the same way as acute leukaemia, but there does appear to be a rare form of aplasia that develops due to the hormonal influences of pregnancy and may resolve following delivery. Diagnosis is often made in the second and third trimesters, and treatment depends on the severity of the aplasia.

Haemolytic anaemia

Pregnancy-related haemolytic anaemia is a rare disorder which occurs in the third trimester of pregnancy and remits spontaneously following delivery. The cause remains unknown. Treatment with steroids and intravenous immunoglobulin (IVIG) is often unhelpful and red cell transfusions may be required.

Disorders of haemostasis in pregnancy

Normal pregnancy is associated with marked changes in all aspects of haemostasis, the overall effect of which is to generate a state of hypercoagulability (Table 14.16.1). The evolutionary benefit of this is clear when one considers that at the time of delivery placental separation provokes an acute massive blood loss in the region of 700 ml/min, which must be stopped immediately. Three weeks

Table 14.16.1 Haemostatic changes in normal pregnancy

Haemostatic factor	Effect of pregnancy
Platelet count	Decreases during pregnancy
Factor XIII, V	Increase in early pregnancy but returns to the prepregnancy state by the 3rd trimester
Factors XII, X, VIII, VII, VWF, and fibrinogen	Increase throughout pregnancy
Factor IX	No change
Factor XI	Either no change or a slight fall
Protein C and antithrombin	No change
Protein S	Progressive decrease during pregnancy
Activated protein C resistance	Gradual fall during pregnancy
PAI-1, TAFI	Increases throughout pregnancy
PAI-2	Appears during pregnancy

after delivery most of the changes in clotting factors have returned to normal.

These changes in haemostasis, while reducing the risks of excessive blood loss at delivery, significantly increase the risk of venous thromboembolic disease in pregnancy. Increasingly it is recognized that disordered haemostasis has a role in IUGR, pre-eclampsia, early and late pregnancy loss, and placental abruption.

Thrombocytopenia in pregnancy

Thrombocytopenia is a common finding in pregnancy and may be due to a variety of causes (Table 14.16.2).

Gestational thrombocytopenia

Gestational thrombocytopenia is seen in about 8% of all pregnancies and accounts for more than 70% of cases of thrombocytopenia in pregnancy. The aetiology is unknown, but probably represents increased peripheral destruction. The platelet count is, in general, only mildly reduced, and in 95% of women is between 100 and 150×10^9/litre. Rarely does the count fall below 80×10^9/litre. The major differential diagnosis is between gestational thrombocytopenia and immune thrombocytopenic purpura (ITP).

Table 14.16.2 Causes of thrombocytopenia in pregnancy

Increased destruction or utilization	
Immunological	ITP, SLE
Consumption	DIC
Microangiopathies	+ HELLP + TTP + HUS
Gestational thrombocytopenia	
Decreased production	Leukaemia, aplastic anaemia, folate deficiency, medications, viral infections
Sequestration	E.g. secondary to portal hypertension

DIC, disseminated intravascular coagulation; HELLP, haemolysis, elevated liver enzymes, low platelets; HUS, haemolytic uraemic syndrome; ITP, immune thrombocytopenic purpura; SLE, systemic lupus erythematosus; TTP, thrombotic thrombocytopenic purpura.

Immune thrombocytopenic purpura (ITP)

ITP has a prevalence of 1 to 5 cases per 10 000 pregnancies, i.e. it is approximately 100 times less common than gestational thrombocytopenia. The diagnosis is largely one of exclusion as there is no confirmatory laboratory test. In pregnancy ITP has implications for both the mother and the fetus.

All women with platelet counts $<100 \times 10^9$/litre should be screened for clinical or laboratory evidence of pre-eclampsia, a coagulopathy, or autoimmune disease. A screen for antinuclear antibodies (ANA) should be performed and if positive it is essential to screen for anti-Ro and anti-La antibodies. Anti-Ro/La antibodies can result in congenital heart block in approximately 2 to 5% of infants born to mothers with such antibodies (see Chapter 14.14).

Asymptomatic women with platelet count higher than 20×10^9/litre do not require treatment until delivery is imminent, but they should be carefully monitored, both clinically and haematologically. Platelet counts higher than 50×10^9/litre are regarded as safe for normal vaginal delivery and for caesarean section, but would preclude the use of spinal or epidural anaesthesia for which the platelet count should be higher than 80×10^9/litre because of the theoretical risk of haematoma formation and neurological damage.

Therapies aimed at increasing the platelet count during pregnancy or before delivery include the use of oral prednisolone, IVIG, and—in rhesus-negative women—anti-D. Splenectomy is rarely performed during pregnancy. The mode of delivery for women with ITP is dictated by obstetric reasons rather than the platelet count, there being no good evidence that caesarean section is less traumatic than an uncomplicated vaginal delivery.

The main risk to the fetus is of neonatal thrombocytopenia. The platelet count may be low at birth but reaches a nadir on the third day following delivery. The risk of neonatal thrombocytopenia does not correlate with the maternal platelet count, although a previous splenectomy for ITP or a previously affected infant with significant thrombocytopenia may increase the risk of significant fetal thrombocytopenia in subsequent pregnancies.

Alloimmune thrombocytopenia

In this disorder the maternal platelet count is normal but the mother is sensitized to paternally derived fetal platelet antigens, the most common of which is HPA-1. This can result in severe fetal and neonatal thrombocytopenia, beginning early in pregnancy. Women at risk can be tested for the presence of platelet alloantibodies during gestation. In neonates with severe thrombocytopenia, the most common presentations are petechiae, purpura or cephalohaematoma at birth, associated with major risk of intracranial haemorrhage (up to 20% of reported cases) leading to death or neurological sequelae. The treatment of affected infants involves the transfusion of compatible platelets: washed maternal platelets are often used. Antenatal management is controversial but can include a combination of maternal IVIG administration, intrauterine platelet transfusions, and corticosteroid therapy, while monitoring fetal platelet counts closely throughout the pregnancy.

HELLP

The HELLP syndrome (haemolytic anaemia, elevated liver enzymes, and a low platelet count) occurs in approximately 10% of pregnant women with pre-eclampsia or eclampsia (see Chapters 14.4 and 14.9). The haemolysis in the HELLP syndrome is a microangiopathic haemolytic anaemia. Red blood cells become fragmented as they pass through small blood vessels with endothelial damage and fibrin deposits. The elevated liver enzyme levels in the syndrome are thought to be secondary to obstruction of hepatic blood flow by fibrin deposits in the sinusoids. The thrombocytopenia has been attributed to increased consumption and/or destruction of platelets.

Thrombotic thrombocytopenic purpura (TTP)

TTP is a life-threatening multisystem disorder characterized by a pentad comprising microangiopathic haemolytic anaemia, thrombocytopenia, neurological abnormalities, fever, and renal dysfunction.

In most cases of acquired TTP in pregnancy, women develop an autoantibody directed against ADAMTS13 and as a consequence cannot break down the ultra-large Von Willebrand factor multimers that are secreted from endothelial cells. The absence of this cleavage and the presence of ultra-large Von Willebrand factor multimers in the circulation is believed to lead to platelet activation and the generation of platelet microthrombi.

Congenital TTP is a rare disorder, due to a mutation within the gene encoding ADAMTS13 that results in a deficiency or functional abnormality of the protein. Although congenital TTP usually presents in childhood there are cases in which the presentation is in adulthood.

The diagnosis of TTP is a clinical one. Although assays of ADAMTS13 may be of value, they are not widely available and are time consuming to perform. The mainstay of treatment for TTP is early plasma exchange to remove the autoantibody and to increase ADAMTS13 levels. With the introduction of plasma exchange, the survival rate has improved from approximately 3% before the 1960s to 82% now.

Disseminated intravascular coagulation (DIC)

DIC is an acquired syndrome characterized by the intravascular activation of coagulation. It can originate from and cause damage to the microvasculature, which if sufficiently severe can produce organ dysfunction. DIC can arise for a variety of reasons, including sepsis, major trauma and an incompatible blood transfusion. In pregnancy it may occur secondary to:

- intrauterine death with a retained fetus
- severe pre-eclampsia
- premature separation of the placenta (placental abruption)
- retained placenta
- amniotic fluid embolism
- haemorrhagic shock
- transfusion reaction

Systemic activation of the clotting cascade leads to depletion of procoagulant clotting factors, consumption of the natural anticoagulants that regulate the activity of clotting cascade (antithrombin, protein C, and protein S), activation of the fibrinolytic system leading to hyperfibrinolysis, and consumption of platelets leading to thrombocytopenia.

The major clinical manifestation of DIC is haemorrhage secondary to the consumption of clotting factors and platelets. Treatment involves identifying and removing the trigger and replacing the missing clotting factors with fresh frozen plasma, restoring fibrinogen with cryoprecipitate or fibrinogen concentrate, and correcting the thrombocytopenia with platelet transfusions.

Other disorders of haemostasis

Haemophilia A and B in pregnancy

Haemophilia A and B are uncommon X-linked disorders due to mutations within the genes for factor VIII (*F8*) and factor IX (*F9*) respectively. Female carriers of haemophilia A or B may have low levels of factor VIII or factor IX as a consequence of Lyonization. Rarely women who are carriers may have severe haemophilia either because of extreme Lyonization or because they have a second mutation in the other *F8* or *F9* gene.

Counselling should be offered to all potential carriers of haemophilia to discuss prenatal diagnosis and other aspects of pregnancy management, with carrier status established by DNA analysis. Women who may require blood product therapy should be immunized against hepatitis B.

Prenatal diagnosis by chorionic villus sampling or amniocentesis can now be readily performed to allow identification of an affected male fetus. Initial fetal sexing is performed, followed—if a male fetus is confirmed—by a search for the disease-specific mutation. Direct mutation analysis has now almost entirely replaced the use of linkage analysis in both carrier detection and prenatal diagnosis. For couples who do not wish to have prenatal diagnosis, fetal sexing either by free fetal DNA [ffDNA] analysis of maternal blood at 7–8 weeks gestation or by ultrasonography at 16 weeks of gestation is recommended when an anomaly scan is performed: if this shows a male fetus, then it should be assumed that this is an affected male.

Factor VIII levels increase significantly during pregnancy, but this rise is unpredictable and a small proportion of women may still have low levels at the time of delivery. Levels of factor VIII and factor IX should be checked at booking, at 28 weeks, and again at 34 weeks: levels that are low (<50 IU/dl) at 34 weeks are unlikely to rise into the normal range by delivery, and treatment to prevent haemorrhage will be required. Factor IX levels do not rise during pregnancy. Women who undergo any form of invasive prenatal diagnostic procedure or who have a spontaneous abortion or a termination of pregnancy will require prophylactic replacement therapy if their factor levels are less than 50 IU/dl. Women who require clotting factor replacement should receive recombinant products.

Epidural anaesthesia may be safely used in haemophilia carriers providing a coagulation screen (including the platelet count) is normal and the factor level is at least 50 IU/dl.

Von Willebrand's disease (VWD)

VWD is due to a deficiency or functional abnormality of Von Willebrand factor (VWF). VWF has two main functions: firstly as a carrier protein for factor VIII; secondly as an adhesive protein involved in vessel wall–platelet interaction. Inherited defects in VWF may, therefore, cause bleeding by impairing either platelet adhesion or fibrin clot formation. VWD is the most common of the inherited disorders of coagulation and is classified into types 1, 2, and 3: type 1 accounts for 80% of cases and is a partial quantitative defect; type 3 is rare and represents a complete absence of VWF in plasma; type 2 (subclassified into types 2A, 2B, 2M, and 2N) represents qualitative defects in VWF.

In women with type 1 VWD, the levels of VWF increase during pregnancy and usually normalize by delivery. In type 2 VWD, although levels may increase, this increase is of a functionally abnormal protein and replacement therapy may be required at

delivery. In women with type 1 or 2 VWD, VWF levels should be checked at 34 to 36 weeks. Vaginal delivery is generally regarded as safe in types 1 and 3 if VWF activity (VWF:RCo) is more than 40 IU/dL. For caesarean section VWF activity should be more than 50 IU/dL. In type 3 VWD the levels will remain low and replacement therapy with a VWF-containing concentrate will be needed at the time of delivery.

In women with type 1 VWD, VWF levels may fall rapidly following delivery although the rate of fall is unpredictable. In some cases a rapid fall in VWF levels may lead to a delayed postpartum haemorrhage and women should be made aware of this possibility.

DDAVP is widely used in the treatment of Type 1 VWD but it tends to be avoided in pregnancy because of concerns that it may cause vasoconstriction with subsequent placental insufficiency, or increase the risk of premature labour due to its potential oxytocic effect, and increase the risk of maternal and neonatal hyponatraemia. However, DDAVP increases the levels of factor VIII and VWF via its action on V2 receptors and its potential for vasoconstriction and stimulation of uterine contraction is negligible because it is practically devoid of these biologic activities that are mediated by V1 vasopressin receptors.

Factor XI deficiency

Factor XI deficiency is a recessively inherited disorder that is rare except in Ashkenazi Jews where the frequency of heterozygosity may approach 10%. There is a poor correlation between absolute factor XI levels and the risk of bleeding, but individuals with levels below 30 U/dl tend to have a positive bleeding history. Observations of factor XI levels in pregnancy are contradictory, but changes are generally not clinically significant. Women with factor XI levels in the heterozygous range may bleed at delivery. A policy of 'watch and wait' is justified in those with factor XI levels between about 15 and 70 U/dl and no bleeding history despite previous haemostatic challenges. For women with the same levels of factor XI but with a significant bleeding history, or without previous haemostatic challenges, tranexamic acid is often used for 3 days, with the first dose being administered during labour. Factor XI concentrate should be given during labour to women with severe factor XI deficiency (FXI:C <10–20 U/dl).

Rarer clotting factor deficiencies

Inherited deficiencies of all of the clotting factors have been reported and these may result in haemorrhage at the time of delivery. These rare inherited coagulation disorders affect between 1 in 500 000 and 1 in 2 million of the population, although because they are recessively inherited they are significantly more common in countries where consanguineous relationships are found. Readers wanting information on the management of these conditions in pregnancy should consult specialist references and guidelines.

Acquired factor VIII inhibitors

Acquired haemophilia is a rare disorder with an incidence of 1.5 per million per year. It is due to the formation of an autoantibody ('inhibitor') that results in the depletion or inhibition of a coagulation factor, most commonly factor VIII, but antibodies to all of the coagulation factors have been described.

Acquired haemophilia A leads to a potentially severe bleeding diathesis, often of sudden onset, and although the condition is most common in older people, with a median age of 70 to 80 years, it can present earlier and pregnancy is a recognized risk factor for the development of the disorder.

In women who are actively bleeding secondary to an autoantibody to factor VIII, options for treatment include recombinant factor VIIa and activated prothrombin complex concentrates. Elimination of the inhibitor should be attempted using immunosuppression, which is initiated as soon as the diagnosis has been established. Where successful, this restores haemostasis to normal.

Relapse of pregnancy-related acquired haemophilia is relatively rare, but it may occur and women should be warned of this possibility. The antibody may affect the factor VIII level of the fetus and this must be considered at the time of delivery.

Miscellaneous haematological conditions

Myeloproliferative diseases

Pregnant patients with essential thrombocythemia and polycythemia vera may be difficult to manage and the disorder is associated with a high fetal mortality. The live birth rate is approximately 60% in both thrombocythemia and polycythemia vera, with spontaneous abortion during the first trimester being the most common complication and occurring in about 20 to 30% of all pregnancies. Major maternal complications are more frequent in polycythemia vera than in thrombocythemia, but are reduced with low-dose aspirin treatment. In high-risk pregnancies, the additional use of low molecular weight heparin and/or interferon-α has also been beneficial.

Further reading

Bolton-Maggs PH, *et al.* (2004). The rare coagulation disorders—review with guidelines for management from the United Kingdom Haemophilia Centre Doctors' Organisation. *Haemophilia*, **10**, 593–628.

Franchini M (2006). Haemostasis and pregnancy. *Thromb Haemost*, **95**, 401–13.

Frenkel EP, Yardley DA (2000). Clinical and laboratory features and sequelae of deficiency of folic acid (folate) and vitamin B_{12} (cobalamin) in pregnancy and gynecology. *Hematol Oncol Clin N Am*, **14**, 1079–100, viii.

Griesshammer M, Struve S, Harrison CM (2006). Essential thrombocythemia/polycythemia vera and pregnancy: the need for an observational study in Europe. *Semin Thromb Hemost*, **32**, 422–9.

Guidelines for the investigation and management of idiopathic thrombocytopenic purpura in adults, children and in pregnancy (2003). *Br J Haematol*, **120**, 574–96.

Hay CR, *et al.* (2006). The diagnosis and management of factor VIII and IX inhibitors: a guideline from the United Kingdom Haemophilia Centre Doctors' Organisation. *Br J Haematol*, **133**, 591–605.

Kadir RA, *et al.* (2006). Screening for factor XI deficiency amongst pregnant women of Ashkenazi Jewish origin. *Haemophilia*, **12**, 625–8.

Lapido OA (2000). Nutrition in pregnancy: mineral and vitamin supplements. *Am J Clin Nutr*, **72** Suppl, 280–90S.

Lee CA, *et al.* (2006). The obstetric and gynaecological management of women with inherited bleeding disorders—review with guidelines produced by a taskforce of UK Haemophilia Centre Doctors' Organisation. *Haemophilia*, **12**, 301–36.

Letsky EA (1985). Haematological disorders in pregnancy. In: Letsky EA (ed.) *Clinics in Haematology*, **14**(3).

Lottenberg R, Hassell KL (2005). An evidence-based approach to the treatment of adults with sickle cell disease. *Hematology Am Soc Hematol Educ Program*, 2005, 58–65.

Milman N (2006). Iron and pregnancy—a delicate balance. *Ann Hematol*, **85**, 559–65.

Nassar AH, *et al.* (2006). Pregnancy in patients with beta-thalassemia intermedia: outcome of mothers and newborns. *Am J Hematol*, **81**, 499–502.

Nugent DJ (2006). Immune thrombocytopenic purpura of childhood. *Hematology Am Soc Hematol Educ Program*, 2006, 97–103.

Pasi KJ, *et al.* (2004). Management of von Willebrand disease: a guideline from the UK Haemophilia Centre Doctors' Organization. *Haemophilia*, **10**, 218–31.

Scully M, *et al.* (2006). Successful management of pregnancy in women with a history of thrombotic thrombocytopaenic purpura. *Blood Coagul Fibrinolysis*, **17**, 459–63.

World Health Organization. *Standards for maternal and neonatal care.* http://www.who.int/making_pregnancy_safer/publications/standards/en/index.html

Malignant disease in pregnancy

Robin A.F. Crawford

Essentials

Cancer in pregnancy is rare, affecting less than 1 in 1000 live births. It may be specific to pregnancy (gestational trophoblastic disease) or incidental to it, the less infrequent conditions being melanoma, lymphoma, and cervical malignancy.

Malignant disease particular to pregnancy

Gestational trophoblastic disease—a group of conditions that arise in the fetal chorion during various types of pregnancy: histologically they are categorized as (1) partial or complete hydatidiform mole, (2) gestational choriocarcinoma, or (3) placental site trophoblastic tumour. The most common of these conditions is molar pregnancy, when villi are present in association with malignant trophoblast in gestational choriocarcinoma.

Any woman of reproductive age who has an undiagnosed tumour or unexplained bleeding from any organ other than the uterus should have a human chorionic gonadotrophin estimation to exclude highly treatable gestational trophoblastic disease.

General aspects of management during pregnancy

Consideration must be given both to the mother who is affected and the unborn fetus, with the balance of care favouring the mother's well-being.

Anaesthesia and extra-abdominal surgery—these rarely carry any risks to the fetus, and intra-abdominal surgery may be safely carried out in the second trimester.

Exposure to ionizing radiation—during the first trimester this can increase the risk of fetal abnormalities and childhood cancers. The dose of radiation, the gestational age of the fetus, and the practicability of shielding the fetus from radiation must be balanced against potential benefits to the mother.

Chemotherapy—administration during the first trimester carries risks that include abortion or congenital abnormalities. Treatment after the first trimester, when structural development is largely complete, is reasonably safe in many diseases and more appropriate than postponement of treatment.

Introduction

Cancer is rare during pregnancy, occurring in only about 1 per 1000 live births. Most malignancies affecting this age group have been seen during pregnancy. Tumours of the uterine cervix, ovary, breast, or thyroid can metastasize to the placenta, but not to the fetus. Gestational trophoblastic disease arises from fetal chorion and is a malignant transformation of the placenta. Melanoma and haematological tumours, which also can invade the placenta, may cross into the fetal circulation. Pregnancy may cause enlargement of a pituitary tumour and a previously silent tumour may present with symptoms in pregnancy. Rare cases of colonic and neurological cancers developing in pregnancy have been reported.

Concurrence of pregnancy and cancer raises complex therapeutic and ethical dilemmas because the most appropriate and timely treatment for the mother may not be in the best interests of the fetus. Anaesthesia and extra-abdominal surgery during pregnancy rarely carry any risks to the fetus, and intra-abdominal surgery may be safely carried out in the second trimester. However, fetal cells divide and differentiate rapidly during the first trimester, hence radiation and chemotherapy carry well-recognized risks to the fetus, including the risk of abortion, congenital abnormalities, or preterm birth. As a result, physicians may be reluctant to treat the mother aggressively at the time of initial diagnosis, preferring to defer treatment for several weeks or months until the fetal lungs have matured, a delay which may substantially reduce the mother's chance of surviving the disease.

It is impossible to establish a threshold dose of ionizing radiation below which such treatment is safe for the fetus, inasmuch as exposure during the first trimester to a dose as low as 10 cGy appears to increase the risk of fetal abnormalities and exposure to 3 to 5 cGy increases the risk of childhood cancers. The risk is negligible if exposure to the fetus is less than 1 cGy. The dose of radiation, the gestational age of the fetus, and the practicability of shielding the fetus from radiation must be balanced against potential benefits to the mother.

Chemotherapy administered to the mother during the first trimester carries well-recognized risks that include abortion or congenital abnormalities. Drugs that preferentially interfere with rapidly growing tissues, e.g. methotrexate, can harm the fetus. Use of antagonists of folate, purine, or pyrimidine synthesis during organogenesis result in congenital malformations in up to 25% of fetuses, although this figure is much lower if the mother only receives therapy with a single agent. Treatment after the first trimester, when structural development is largely complete, is reasonably safe in many diseases and more appropriate than postponement of treatment. Chemotherapy after the first trimester has been associated with slight increases in the incidence of preterm birth and fetal growth retardation and, when administered shortly before delivery, with transient neonatal myelosuppression. Nevertheless, the long-term outcomes of the children of women who received chemotherapy during the second or third trimester are generally good.

In practical terms, acute leukaemia is virtually the only condition requiring immediate chemotherapy in a pregnant woman. When faced with cancer in the first trimester, the available information should be explained to the woman and her partner, who should give informed, unhurried consent before treatment starts. In most situations a consensus decision to proceed with chemotherapy can be reached between the woman, her partner, and the responsible physician, but the ethical issues are very complex and decisions have to be made on an individual basis.

Increasing success with the treatment of childhood cancers means that more women are entering the reproductive age group having survived cancer treatment. An increased incidence of spontaneous abortions, low birth weight babies, and neonatal deaths has been described in women with Wilms' tumour who had received at least 20 Gy abdominal radiation. Survivors of Hodgkin's disease treated with both radiation and chemotherapy (but not either alone) also appear to be at increased risk of spontaneous abortions. However, based on series of several thousand children there appears to be no overall increased risk of either congenital malformations or childhood cancers in the offspring of cancer survivors.

Malignant diseases specific to pregnancy

Gestational trophoblastic disease

Gestational trophoblastic disease is a group of diseases that arise in the fetal chorion during various types of pregnancy. Histologically they are categorized as one of two types of hydatidiform mole (partial or complete), gestational choriocarcinoma, or placental site trophoblastic tumour.

Gestational trophoblastic disease is notable for several reasons. First, the tumours are genetically different from the host, having antigens derived from the male partner. Secondly, apart from placental site tumour, they secrete human chorionic gonadotrophin (hCG) in amounts proportional to the viable tumour volume, allowing hCG to be used as an ideal tumour marker. Thirdly, even metastatic disease can be cured with chemotherapy, the use of methotrexate in the early 1950s having shown reproducible results.

Complete and partial hydatidiform moles present as abnormal pregnancies ending in first or second trimester abortions.

The complete mole is diploid (of paternal origin), is commonly diagnosed on ultrasound scan, and has no fetal elements present. The partial mole is triploid with paternal and maternal origin, has fetal elements present, and is usually diagnosed after the products of conception are examined pathologically. Gestational choriocarcinoma is a highly malignant tumour derived from syncytial and cytotrophoblastic cells. When villi are present in association with malignant trophoblasts, it is classified as a molar pregnancy. If there is diagnostic doubt about the possibility of combined molar pregnancy with a viable fetus, then ultrasound scanning should be repeated before intervention. If a twin pregnancy is associated with a partial mole, it should be allowed to proceed; if a twin pregnancy is associated with a complete mole, it may proceed after appropriate counselling. These pregnancies are associated with a reduced live birth rate of 25% and are at risk of pre-eclampsia and haemorrhage. The subsequent need for chemotherapy in these rare cases is about 20% and is the same whether the pregnancy is terminated spontaneously or therapeutically, or allowed to proceed to term.

Gestational trophoblastic disease arises in various types of pregnancy, most of which are clinically recognized as abnormal. The incidence is 1.54 per 1000 live births. The most common are molar pregnancies, but gestational trophoblastic disease can also arise following abortions, ectopic pregnancies, or even normal full-term pregnancies. Clinical surveillance of patients who have had a molar pregnancy is the only practical method of detecting and preventing gestational trophoblastic disease. In the United Kingdom all patients with a histological diagnosis of a molar pregnancy are registered and followed up at one of three screening centres (Charing Cross Hospital in London, Sheffield, and Dundee). Only 7.5% of women with hydatidiform mole require chemotherapy, and more than half of the patients who require chemotherapy for gestational trophoblastic disease have a preceding molar pregnancy.

Patients who develop gestational trophoblastic disease after an abortion or full-term pregnancy are more difficult to detect. They present with symptoms attributable to metastases, the sites of initial metastasis being (in order of frequency) lung, vagina, brain, liver, gastrointestinal tract, and kidney. The interval between pregnancy and the development of metastatic gestational trophoblastic disease may be years. Because these tumours are rare, many clinicians are unfamiliar with them and do not consider gestational trophoblastic disease as part of any differential diagnosis. Any woman of reproductive age who has an undiagnosed tumour or unexplained bleeding from any organ other than the uterus should have an hCG estimation to exclude highly treatable gestational trophoblastic disease.

Patients with gestational trophoblastic disease are classified as having a low or high risk depending on a scoring system devised at Charing Cross Hospital and now modified by the World Health Organization. The score relies on factors such as age, the antecedent pregnancy, the interval between presentation and the previous pregnancy, the hCG level, the blood group, the size of the largest tumour, site and number of metastases, and whether the patient had previously received chemotherapy. In the United Kingdom the low-risk group will be offered methotrexate with folinic acid rescue. The high-risk group and those low-risk patients who have resistant or persistent disease will be offered combination chemotherapy. The initial diagnosis may be made by surgical excision or biopsy of a suspicious lesion, but surgery otherwise has little role, excepting rarely to remove a cerebral metastasis to prevent a cerebral bleed.

The overall survival for patients with gestational trophoblastic disease is now about 94%. Women should be advised not to conceive for 6 months after a negative hCG reading. The risk of further molar pregnancy is low (1 in 74).

Malignant diseases not specific to pregnancy

Gynaecological cancers

Cancer of the cervix

Carcinoma of the cervix is diagnosed during approximately 1 in 2200 pregnancies. In the United Kingdom, with the recent success of the cervical screening programme, the incidence is probably lower. Pregnant women with cervical cancer generally present with early stage disease, their prognosis being similar to that of patients who are not pregnant.

The presenting symptom is usually vaginal bleeding, hence it is important to check the cervix with a visual examination when pregnant women present with irregular vaginal bleeding. There is a tendency to assume that vaginal bleeding in early pregnancy is related to miscarriage, organize an ultrasound scan to check for fetal viability, and forget vaginal examination. In the case of an obvious cancer, a wedge biopsy under general anaesthetic is appropriate for diagnosis and staging. If there is any doubt, colposcopy can be used to assess the cervix. There is an increased risk of bleeding when taking a biopsy from the pregnant cervix, but there is no increased rate of fetal loss.

Patients with cervical intraepithelial neoplasia can be managed expectantly until after delivery. There is no contraindication to a vaginal delivery for women with cervical intraepithelial neoplasia; indeed, there are several series which suggest that vaginal delivery is associated with a higher rate of regression of severe dysplasia than is usually seen. Standard practice would be to review with colposcopy at about 3 months after delivery. Management of women with microinvasion of the cervix is usually via cone biopsy under a general anaesthetic, allowing the pregnancy to continue.

When cervical cancer is diagnosed in early pregnancy, treatment options include immediate radical hysterectomy or delaying treatment until the fetus is viable, followed by classical caesarean section (scar in the upper segment of the uterus) and radical hysterectomy. This is appropriate for stage 1B cases, where the tumour is confined to the cervix and is less than 4 cm in diameter. In one series there was no difference in survival between the two modes of treatment. Typically, women diagnosed in the first trimester will be offered immediate surgery. Women diagnosed after 24 to 28 weeks gestation are usually managed expectantly until after 32 weeks gestation and then delivered by caesarean radical hysterectomy. Steroids are usually given to accelerate fetal lung maturity. The outlook may be worse for patients who deliver vaginally across a cervical cancer, but this has not been substantiated.

Cancer of the ovary

The incidence of adnexal masses occurring in pregnant women has been reported as being as rare as 1 in 2500 to as frequent as 1 in 81 live births. With the use of routine early ultrasound the true incidence of adnexal masses is closer to the latter figure. Most of these

(>95%) are benign. Complications of a benign adnexal mass include pain due to torsion, rupture, or haemorrhage; obstruction of the pelvic outlet; and infection. Most cysts are managed conservatively, avoiding surgery, but when necessary surgery to remove cysts is usually performed in the second trimester. The advantage of waiting until the second trimester is that most cysts resolve spontaneously and that the rate of fetal loss is reduced.

The rationale for removing a persistent adnexal mass is to exclude malignancy. Ovarian cancer in pregnancy is rare, with a reported incidence of 1 case in 17 000 to 38 000, because the usual age of childbirth is greater than the peak incidence of germ cell tumours and substantially less than the usual age of those with epithelial cancer. In addition, pregnancy protects against ovarian cancer. Two-thirds of the cancers detected are epithelial and the remaining are germ cell (usually dysgerminoma) and stromal cell types. Cysts that are simple on ultrasound scan and less than 5 cm in diameter have almost no malignant potential: larger cysts with nodules, septa, or rapid growth are more likely to be malignant. Tumour markers are not helpful in pregnancy: CA-125 can be raised by pregnancy, as can α-fetoprotein and hCG.

The management of the ovarian cancer is similar to that in the nonpregnant woman. Appropriate surgical staging is required, the author's preference being removal of the cyst, taking of peritoneal washings for cytology, biopsy of the contralateral ovary, and biopsies of any abnormal areas are sufficient at the primary operation. It is also preferable to wait 48 h for a definitive diagnosis from paraffin sections, rather than expect the pathologist to give an immediate result from frozen section. This delay also allows the woman and her partner to consider the implications of the diagnosis. Most of the women seen with a malignant diagnosis in pregnancy will have early stage epithelial cancer: FIGO stage 1A or B, meaning well or moderately differentiated tumour confined to one or both ovaries, or will have borderline histology. No further therapy would then be necessary. Therapeutic termination is not required and pregnancy per se does not worsen outcome. Fuller staging may be considered 6 to 12 weeks after delivery. The decision to use chemotherapy postoperatively depends on the stage and differentiation of the tumour, the gestational age of the fetus, and the wishes of the mother. The treatment of malignant germ cell tumours can be carried out without affecting the pregnancy in the second two trimesters, especially if alkylating agents are avoided.

Other gynaecological cancers

Other gynaecological cancers are rarely seen. Cancer of the endometrium is associated with infertility in the reproductive age group and cancer of the vulva is predominantly a disease of older women.

Cancer of the breast

Gestational breast cancer is defined as a breast cancer presenting either during pregnancy or up to 1 year postpartum. It was originally thought that pregnancy-related cancer carried a worse prognosis, but this has not been substantiated. Although breast cancer is regarded as a hormone-dependent tumour, termination of pregnancy and oophorectomy do not provide a better outcome for the woman. Women becoming pregnant after treatment for breast cancer have a similar or better survival when controlled for age and stage.

Breast cancer is often diagnosed at a late stage as breast lumps may be difficult to detect against a background of pregnancy-related hypertrophy. Consequently, investigation of masses is often delayed. Mammography is not harmful to the fetus with appropriate shielding. When a breast mass is found, the most important step is to make a histological diagnosis. If the diagnosis of breast cancer is made, treatment is the same as for the nonpregnant woman. Obviously, chemotherapy in the first trimester is associated with risks for the developing fetus.

Suppression of lactation as a therapeutic manoeuvre is not necessary, with two exceptions. Firstly, if breast surgery is required during the puerperium, suppression of lactation can decrease the size and vascularity of the breast and allow a safer surgical procedure. Secondly, suppression of lactation is recommended in women receiving chemotherapy as some of the drugs can reach the breast milk and cause neonatal neutropenia.

Melanoma

The incidence of melanoma in pregnancy is between 0.14 and 2.8 cases per 1000 deliveries. Melanoma in pregnancy is unusual in that it can metastasize to the placenta and to the fetus. As this is a rare phenomenon, therapeutic abortion is not indicated, but careful examination and follow-up of the baby is warranted. Current evidence suggests that the clinical outcome for pregnant patients is similar to that of those who are not pregnant. Early detection and biopsy are performed as usual, and the surgical management is the same. Since most recurrences of melanoma occur in the first 3 years following initial diagnosis, it may be appropriate to delay further pregnancies until this time period has elapsed.

Thyroid and other endocrine cancers

It is not uncommon to find thyroid nodules that require further investigation during pregnancy. Most cancers are well differentiated, with a very good prognosis. When a diagnosis is made, treatment proceeds as normal, with the exception that radio-iodine is contraindicated. Cancers discovered early in the pregnancy can be treated surgically in the second trimester. Tumours discovered in later pregnancy can be investigated and treated after delivery. Thyroxine is given to reduce the level of thyroid-stimulating hormone. There is no evidence to suggest that pregnancy alters the outcome for thyroid cancer. Thyroid cancer is not an indication for termination of pregnancy.

Phaeochromocytoma is rare in pregnancy but has been described. It is difficult to diagnose because elevation of blood pressure is almost invariably attributed to pregnancy-induced hypertension, which is very much more common.

Lymphoma

Hodgkin's disease is a disease of young adults (mean age 32 years), hence it is not surprising that there are more cases diagnosed in pregnancy than there are of non-Hodgkin's lymphoma (mean age of diagnosis 42 years). The reported incidence of Hodgkin's disease in pregnancy is between 1 in 1000 and 1 in 6000 deliveries.

Although it was historically believed to be exacerbated by pregnancy, there does not seem to be any influence of pregnancy on the outcome for Hodgkin's disease. If treatment is required, most patients can be managed without compromise to mother or fetus. Patients presenting with localized Hodgkin's disease relatively late in pregnancy may be observed with limited staging and not treated until after delivery.

By contrast, in non-Hodgkin's lymphoma, patients with Burkitt's lymphoma in pregnancy appear to have a highly aggressive disease involving the breast or ovary. The outlook for pregnant women with non-Hodgkin's lymphoma is bleak, some dying before delivery.

Leukaemia

Leukaemia in pregnancy is rare, with an incidence of 1 per 100 000 pregnancies. This may be because most cases of acute lymphoblastic leukaemia occur before reproductive age and most cases of acute myeloid leukaemia occur afterwards. Chronic lymphocytic leukaemia is a disease of older people, hence chronic myeloid leukaemia constitutes 90% of the cases of chronic leukaemia seen in pregnancy.

Since the introduction of intensive chemotherapy, the survival of pregnant women with leukaemia is similar to that of nonpregnant women. It does not appear that intrauterine exposure to antileukaemic chemotherapy produces detrimental late effects on the resulting children. Women treated with nonalkylating agents have no apparent decrease in fertility, although this is reduced by one-third when alkylating agents are used.

Cancer of the colon

The reported incidence of colorectal cancer in pregnancy of 1 per 50 000 pregnancies may now be an underestimate as a reflection of the trend for women to delay pregnancy until later in life; a more recent study has reported an incidence of 1 per 13 000 live births. By contrast, with increased awareness of inherited genetic traits and the availability of genetic testing, more and more patients at risk (for example those with familial adenomatous polyposis and hereditary nonpolyposis coli) are undergoing screening, which may reduce the numbers of pregnant women diagnosed with colon cancer.

Colorectal cancer in pregnancy is particularly common in the rectal region, below the peritoneal reflection. The importance of this is that 88% of tumours are within reach of the flexible sigmoidoscope, allowing detection with a minimum of inconvenience to the patient and no risk to the fetus.

Presenting symptoms are similar to those in nonpregnant women. However, the combination of altered bowel habit, abdominal pain/swelling, and anaemia is common in pregnancy, such that these symptoms are frequently ascribed to the pregnancy itself. Assessment of the pregnant patient with colorectal cancer is similar to that of the nonpregnant patient. Radiological imaging is avoided in the first trimester. Carcinoembryonic antigen is not affected significantly by pregnancy and so can be used as a marker.

Patients younger than 40 years generally have a poorer prognosis because of delayed diagnosis and advanced stage at presentation. Pregnant women are no different in this respect. The overall fetal prognosis is relatively favourable as the diagnosis is usually made close to term and the fetus can be delivered coincident with the surgery for the colon cancer.

Further reading

Barnea ER, Jauniaux E, Schwartz PE (eds) (2001). *Cancer and pregnancy.* Springer, London.

Charing Cross Hospital Trophoblast Disease Service. *Hydatidiform mole and choriocarcinoma UK information and support service.* http://www.hmole-chorio.org.uk. [Information website with up-to-date recommendations about management.]

Ngan S, Seckl MJ (2007). Gestational trophoblastic neoplasia management: an update. *Curr Opin Oncol*, **19**, 486–91.

Wright TC Jr, *et al.* (2007). 2006 consensus guidelines for the management of women with cervical intraepithelial neoplasia or adenocarcinoma in situ. *Am J Obstet Gynecol*, **197**, 340–5.

14.18

Prescribing in pregnancy

Peter Rubin

Essentials

Only prescribe if it is essential to do so—the guiding principle when prescribing in pregnancy, or in a woman who may become pregnant, is to use no drug at all if possible. If it is necessary to prescribe, then use the smallest number of drugs in the lowest possible doses, balancing the benefits of treatment for the mother against what (if anything) is known about its risks to the developing baby. Prepregnancy evaluation is invaluable for chronic conditions.

Stage of pregnancy—the period of organogenesis, which extends for about 2 months following the last period, is the critical time for major structural abnormalities, but growth and development can be affected by some drugs in the remainder of pregnancy.

Handling of drugs by the body—the distribution and elimination of some drugs is affected to a clinically significant extent by pregnancy.

Breastfeeding—many commonly used drugs, including some that are unsafe in pregnancy, can safely be used by mothers who are breastfeeding.

Introduction

Prescribing in pregnancy is essentially about balancing risks. The damage that a drug may cause to the fetus must be weighed against the harm that may befall the mother and her unborn child if a disease goes unchecked.

While knowledge in most therapeutic areas has grown rapidly in recent decades, information on the use of drugs in pregnancy has developed sporadically, with case reports being more usual than large, prospective clinical trials. The reasons are not surprising and largely relate to concern about teratogenesis.

Thalidomide is a name inescapably associated with prescribing in pregnancy. Drug-induced fetal abnormality did not begin with thalidomide: there is an Old Testament exhortation to have 'no strong drink, neither eat any unclean thing' during pregnancy. However, the scale of the thalidomide tragedy brought to the general public for the first time the realization that drugs could harm the developing baby. Thalidomide was marketed in Germany in 1956 and subsequently in other countries as a sedative and hypnotic which had the particular attraction of being safe in overdose. Indeed, the drug was considered so safe that in some countries it was available without prescription. Then between 1960 and 1961 Germany experienced what amounted to an epidemic of phocomelia, a birth defect involving absence of the long bones with hands and feet being attached directly to the trunk. What had previously been an extremely rare condition (no cases had been reported in the 10 years to 1959) was being seen almost commonly. Various causes—viral, radioactivity, food preservatives—were considered as culprits, until one doctor retrospectively questioned his patients and found that 20% had taken thalidomide in early pregnancy. On repeat questioning, asking specifically about the drug, 50% admitted taking thalidomide, many having not mentioned it before since the drug was so obviously innocent. In fact, around 80% of women who took thalidomide in the first trimester had a deformed baby. More than 10 000 such babies had been born before the drug was removed from the market.

The thalidomide experience had far-reaching ramifications. Drug regulation as we know it stems largely from this disaster. Doctors and their patients recognized that there is no such thing as a safe drug. In addition, the pharmaceutical industry has largely avoided obtaining systematic information on drug use in pregnancy. The reasons are obvious and understandable, but for the prescribing doctor the statement that 'the safety of this drug in pregnancy has not been established' is not helpful when faced with a woman who is, or may become, pregnant.

Identifying teratogenic drugs

Information on drug-induced fetal abnormality comes from case reports, case studies, and epidemiological studies. Case reports are a two-edged sword. Describing a single association between a drug and a fetal abnormality can be very useful in first identifying a real problem: warfarin was first linked to teratogenesis in this way. However, the problem with case reports is that they may be showing nothing more than a chance association, because fetal abnormalities occur in around 2% of pregnancies, and caution must be exercised in their interpretation. This is well demonstrated by the Debendox saga.

Most cases of morning sickness do not require treatment. However, some do, and the drug for which most information is available was withdrawn from the market in 1983 in view of mounting public concern about its safety. This drug was a mixture of doxylamine succinate and pyridoxine hydrochloride and was marketed as Debendox or Bendectin. Despite having been used by over 30 million pregnant women over a quarter of a century, and notwithstanding carefully designed clinical trials suggesting that the drug was not teratogenic, individual case reports linking the use of the drug to fetal abnormality were given considerable publicity and led to its withdrawal. In view of the extremely high number of exposures, many chance associations between drug use and fetal abnormality were inevitable. This episode illustrated that in an emotional area such as the use of drugs during pregnancy, well-chosen and carefully presented anecdotes can be more powerful than a substantial body of scientific data carefully accumulated over many years.

Case studies are more secure in that they describe several patients where the same drug and malformation were linked: phenytoin and the retinoids were found to be teratogenic in this way. Epidemiological studies are of two major types: cohort studies, which prospectively study exposed and unexposed groups, and case–control studies, which retrospectively compare the pregnancies of abnormal and normal offspring. So far as teratogenesis is concerned, case–control studies are the norm because of the size and expense of cohort studies. The relationship between use of diethylstilbestrol in the first trimester and vaginal adenocarcinoma in teenage offspring was found in a case–control study.

Effects of drugs on the fetus

A drug can harm the fetus only if it crosses the placenta, but most drugs do. The placenta offers a lipid barrier to the transfer of drugs, and the rate at which a drug crosses from mother to baby will depend on its lipophilicity and polarity. However, with the exception of drugs administered acutely around the time of delivery, the rate of transfer is of little importance, and for any course of drug treatment it should be assumed that transfer will occur. The only notable exceptions are heparin—including low molecular weight preparations—and insulin.

Drugs can adversely affect the developing fetus in different ways depending on the gestation at which exposure occurs. For this reason it is appropriate to consider organogenesis, fetal growth and development, the breastfed infant, and childhood growth and development separately.

Prescribing in the first trimester

Teratogenesis

Organogenesis occurs between 18 and 55 days of gestation and it is during this time that drugs can cause anatomical defects. A drug can cause a teratogenic effect only if it is present in the embryo during organogenesis, and even a definite teratogen will not cause a structural defect if it is given following this period. These seemingly obvious statements become relevant in prepregnancy counselling and in providing advice when exposure to a possible teratogen has occurred during pregnancy. Being present in the embryo during organogenesis is not necessarily synonymous with being prescribed during this period. The retinoids are stored in adipose tissue and released slowly, so a teratogenic effect can occur long after the course of treatment has been completed. It is important to recognize that teratogenic effects are not seen in all cases: on the contrary, most first-trimester exposures to teratogenic drugs will not harm the baby. Clearly there is more to drug-induced fetal abnormality than simply the drug: the genetic make-up of the baby is important too. Some drugs that are definitely teratogenic in humans, together with approximate risks, are listed in Table 14.18.1.

Anticonvulsants, and the difficulties of establishing good data on drug toxicity in pregnancy

Anticonvulsants have been extensively studied over the last 40 years and illustrate well some of the principles and pitfalls associated with producing robust information. Many of the studies have serious weaknesses, involving design, ascertainment, classification, and statistical power. However, the advent of epilepsy-pregnancy registers from the mid 1990s has improved the quality of data available. Some themes are remarkably consistent. Polytherapy is accompanied by a greater risk of fetal abnormality. The United Kingdom Epilepsy and Pregnancy Register found that 6% of babies whose mothers had taken more than one anticonvulsant had a major abnormality, compared to 3.7% following monotherapy (except for valproate, which carried a risk of 6.2%) and 1 to 2% in the unaffected population. However, women taking several drugs are likely to have more severe disease, hence cause and effect is hard to establish, and interestingly the abnormality rate in epileptic women who had not taken any drugs was 3.5%, still higher than the general population. This finding is consistent and has generated much debate about the relative roles of drug, disease and inheritance. Several studies have suggested that the teratogenic effects of valproate increase above 800 to 1000 mg daily, and lamotrigine may also show dose-dependent teratogenicity.

A further very important theme that runs through the consideration of anticonvulsant teratogenicity is that new drugs are often welcomed as being safer, until experience demands otherwise. Valproate was heralded as the drug of choice for women of child-bearing age

Table 14.18.1 Some commonly used drugs that are known to be teratogenic

Drug	Main abnormality	Approximate risk (%)
Phenytoin	Craniofacial; cardiac	4
Carbamazepine	Craniofacial, limb	2
Sodium valproate	Neural tube; possible neurodevelopmental	6
Lamotrigine	Oral cleft; possibly others	3
Warfarin	Chondrodysplasia punctata	Up to 25
	Facial anomalies	
	CNS anomalies	
Lithium	Cardiac (Ebstein complex)	2
Danazol	Virilization of female fetus	Uncertain
Retinoids	Multiple	High

CNS, central nervous system.

in the early 1980s. Lamotrigine enjoyed similar claims but is now known to increase the risk of oral clefts.

Another aspect to the consideration of anticonvulsants in pregnancy is the extent to which a 'fetal anticonvulsant syndrome' exists. The term was first coined many years ago to describe a constellation of features including major malformations, microcephaly, hypoplasia of the midface and fingers, and growth retardation. More recently there have been several reports of dysmorphic features, particularly with valproate. There is, however, considerable overlap between the appearances claimed for individual drugs and indeed with those seen in the children of epileptic women who have not had *in utero* drug exposure.

Preventing drug-induced teratogenesis

It is difficult to prevent drug-induced teratogenesis, short of the obvious solution of not taking the drug. Where there is a risk of neural tube defect, folic acid 5 mg daily should be prescribed from the time that pregnancy is planned. There is no direct evidence to support this approach, but it is logical: folic acid is known to be effective in the secondary prevention of naturally occurring neural tube defect, and anticonvulsants lower folate levels.

The overall message—not just for anticonvulsants but for any drug treatment in pregnancy—is to use no drug if you can, but if you must then use the smallest number of drugs in the lowest possible doses.

Many of the abnormalities caused by drugs can be detected by detailed ultrasound scanning at 18 to 20 weeks gestation, but the defects caused by warfarin involve mainly soft tissue and do not fall into this category.

Table 14.18.1 is not comprehensive and includes only those drugs commonly encountered in general medical practice. Some drugs used in specialist areas are teratogenic, e.g. several agents used in cancer chemotherapy. Many more drugs may be teratogenic in a small percentage of exposures, but definitive information is not available because both prediction and detection of human teratogens is difficult. Predicting the effect of a drug in humans usually depends on studying its pharmacology in experimental animals. However, this is not fruitful in the area of teratogenesis because species variation is so great: e.g. thalidomide causes phocomelia only in primates, while lithium causes cardiac abnormalities in humans at doses that produce no effect in the rat. Detecting teratogenic effects is complicated by the normal occurrence of fetal abnormalities, hence if a drug is teratogenic very occasionally it can be exceedingly difficult to distinguish its effects from those arising naturally.

Balance of benefits and risks

Even if a drug is a teratogen, the balance of benefits and risks may still be in favour of its use. For example, chloroquine and proguanil are indicated for malarial prophylaxis in areas where *Plasmodium falciparum* remains sensitive. Currently available evidence suggests that chloroquine may cause a very small increase in birth defects: in one study 169 infants whose mothers took chloroquine base 300 mg once weekly were compared with 454 children whose mothers took no drug. Abnormal babies were born to 1.2% of the treated group, compared to 0.9% of the controls: not a significant difference, but the study was too small to detect anything less than a fivefold increase in abnormality rate. By contrast to the possibility of this small increase in risk, malaria presents a major risk to the health and life of both mother and baby, particularly when an

expatriate woman is travelling in an endemic area. The argument in favour of using prophylaxis is therefore overwhelming—but not so overwhelming as the advice for pregnant travellers to avoid malarial areas!

Similar arguments apply to corticosteroids, which have acquired a reputation for causing oral cleft defects. The evidence in support of this effect is at best conflicting and is easily outweighed by the benefits of steroids in conditions such as severe asthma, inflammatory bowel disease, systemic lupus erythematosus, or organ transplantation. The placenta inactivates around 90% of prednisolone, but corticosteroids such as betamethasone, which are used to accelerate fetal lung maturity, have much greater penetration to the fetus.

Prescribing later in pregnancy

Beyond organogenesis, the fetus undergoes growth and development. The scope for producing anatomical defects has largely passed, exceptions being premature closure of the ductus arteriosus caused by indometacin and bleeding into the fetal brain produced by warfarin. Growth and function tend to be the targets of drug adverse effects for the remainder of the pregnancy.

The possible effects of some commonly used drugs later in pregnancy are shown in Table 14.18.2.

Drugs and breastfeeding

Most women who breastfeed their babies will take a drug during this time. Iron, mild analgesics, antibiotics, laxatives, and hypnotics

Table 14.18.2 Some drugs that can cause harm later in the pregnancy

ACE inhibitors	First trimester exposure fairly common and low risk Avoid in remainder of pregnancy because of fetal and neonatal renal damage
Antithyroid drugs	Fetal hypothyroidism if used in excessive dose
Aspirin	Analgesic doses associated with neonatal bleeding; not seen with low-dose aspirin
β-Agonists	Pulmonary oedema can occur in management of preterm labour, particularly when combined with excessive fluids and/or corticosteroids
β-Blockers	Use throughout pregnancy associated with around 25% risk of intrauterine growth retardation; not seen with short-term use in third trimester
Benzodiazepines	Drug dependence in the fetus
Corticosteroids	Claims that these drugs cause intrauterine growth retardation, or suppress the fetal adrenal, are not supported by the available evidence
Heparin	Maternal osteoporosis: risk increases with dose and duration of exposure
Indomethacin	Multiple neonatal morbidity; premature closure of ductus
Phenytoin	Neonatal haemorrhage accompanied by low levels of vitamin K-dependent clotting factors
Tetracyclines	Tooth discoloration. No evidence of harm following limited exposure in first trimester
Warfarin	Fetal cerebral haemorrhage—can occur with therapeutic INR in the mother

ACE, angiotensin-converting enzyme.

are the most commonly used. Much work has been performed on the pharmacokinetic aspects of breastfeeding, but systematic studies on the effect of drug ingestion by the mother on her breastfed baby are lacking.

Milk consists of fat globules suspended in an aqueous solution of protein and nutrients. Drugs move from plasma to milk by passive diffusion of the unionized and non-protein-bound fraction. Since breast milk has a slightly lower pH than plasma, drugs that cross most extensively into breast milk are lipid-soluble, poorly protein-bound, weak bases. However, even for drugs that cross readily into breast milk, considerable dilution has already occurred in the mother. Thus, when the concentration of a drug in breast milk and the volume of the milk consumed by the baby are translated into a dose, it is often the case that the baby receives too little drug to have any detectable pharmacological effect.

Some of the more commonly used drugs that, on the basis of experience, have a good safety record in breastfeeding mothers are listed in Table 14.18.3. It will be seen from this that many of the drugs that would be indicated for common medical problems in this context are safe to use. However, some qualification is needed about two of the drugs listed in Table 14.18.3. Oestrogen-containing oral contraceptives may suppress lactation if they are taken before the milk supply is well established, and in some women may do so even after this time: progestogen-only contraceptives do not influence lactation at any stage. Metronidazole is not harmful to the baby but is said to make the milk taste bitter and may therefore interfere with feeding.

Some drugs have been shown to affect the baby when ingested in breast milk: these are listed in Table 14.18.4. There are several other drugs for which theoretical risks exist, or for which isolated reports of serious adverse consequences have appeared. For example, aspirin is contraindicated in young children because of the possible association with Reye's syndrome, and some authorities consider that the drug should therefore be avoided in women who are breastfeeding. No evidence is available to support this view, but unless the use of aspirin is considered essential in a breastfeeding woman (and such an eventuality must be rare), then it is probably best avoided. Similarly, indometacin has been associated with one case of neonatal convulsion when used during lactation: a decision with regard to its appropriateness in any given patient would depend on the likelihood of real benefit accruing from its use.

Behavioural teratology

The most obvious consequences of a drug-induced fetal abnormality occur at or shortly after birth in the form of anatomical defects, and studies in teratology have largely concentrated on immediate pregnancy outcome. However, drugs can, on occasion, cause problems that become manifest only after several years. The most striking example is diethylstilbestrol which, when given during early pregnancy, can lead to adenocarcinoma of the vagina in teenage offspring. In addition to late morphological effects, concern has been expressed that drugs given during pregnancy can influence behavioural development.

Anticonvulsants

Several studies have claimed that the use of anticonvulsants during pregnancy is associated with impaired intellectual development of the children, but findings have been conflicting. It is difficult to carry out studies in this area and the choice of control group is crucially important. In general, all studies have suffered from small size and many from possible selection bias. When all children of treated epileptic mothers in a single hospital in Finland were studied prospectively, using the offspring of untreated epileptic women and age-matched children of the same social class as controls, no difference was found in intellectual development at the age of 5.5 years. Similarly, children exposed to carbamazepine *in utero* have been found in two studies to be of normal intelligence. In contrast, there have been several reports suggesting that valproate causes neurodevelopmental delay. The absence of methodologically sound research makes it difficult to draw reliable conclusions.

Table 14.18.3 Some drugs that have been used in breastfeeding women without evidence of harm to the baby

Drug	Notes
β-Blockers	
Bronchodilators	Inhaled
Carbamazepine	
Carbimazole	High doses may suppress the neonatal thyroid
Codeine	
Corticosteroids	
Digoxin	
Heparin	
H₂-antagonists	
Methyldopa	
Metronidazole	
Opioids	Therapeutic administration
Oral contraceptives	
Paracetamol	
Penicillins	
Phenytoin	
Propylthiouracil	High dose may suppress neonatal thyroid
Sodium valproate	
Tricyclic antidepressants	
Warfarin	

Table 14.18.4 Some drugs that may be harmful to the baby when used in breast-feeding women

Drug	Possible effects
Amiodarone	Neonatal hypothyroidism
Barbiturates	Drowsiness
Benzodiazepines	Lethargy and weight loss
Iodine	Risk of neonatal hypothyroidism
Laxatives	Diarrhoea
Lithium	Hypotonia, lethargy, cyanosis
Phenobarbital	Drowsiness
Sulphonamides	Risk of kernicterus in preterm, ill, or stressed babies, but safe in healthy term infants

Antihypertensive drugs

One of the earliest trials on the treatment of hypertension during pregnancy involved a comparison of methyldopa with no treatment. The children underwent physical and psychomotor assessment at 4 and 7.5 years. The 4-year-old children from the treatment group had a slightly smaller head circumference than their untreated controls, but there were no other physical or psychomotor differences. The evaluation at 7.5 years revealed no differences between the two groups. The reputation of methyldopa as a safe drug in pregnancy is largely based on this very well-conducted study.

The effects on childhood development of atenolol vs placebo have similarly shown no detrimental effects, a wide range of physical and psychomotor tests being performed on the children at the age of 1 year.

Effects of pregnancy on drugs

Influence of pregnancy on dose requirements

While the emphasis on what drugs can do to a pregnancy is both understandable and appropriate, the physiological changes of pregnancy can have a clinically important influence on drug disposition and effect. The plasma concentrations of some drugs fall to an extent that is clinically important during pregnancy.

Changes in drug clearance in pregnancy

Among the many physiological changes in pregnancy, the most important from the standpoint of drugs are those that influence clearance. By the third trimester renal blood flow has nearly doubled and the activity of some, but not all, liver metabolic pathways is increased during pregnancy. A further factor tending to reduce drug concentrations is an increase in body water, with around an additional 7 litres being retained by the end of pregnancy.

The importance of these changes is well illustrated by the influence of pregnancy on anticonvulsant dose requirements. The plasma concentrations of phenytoin and carbamazepine decrease as pregnancy progresses. An increase in systemic clearance is the main reason—e.g. the clearance of phenytoin increases by over 100% by the third trimester—with an increased volume of distribution making a further contribution. An example of the influence of pregnancy on the concentration of phenytoin is shown in

Fig. 14.18.1. The reduction in anticonvulsant concentration can be substantial and, if the dose is not increased, then seizure control may be lost. The physiological changes of pregnancy resolve in the 6 weeks following delivery, and there is a progressive return to prepregnancy dose requirements during this time.

Not all drugs metabolized in the liver show reductions in plasma concentration during pregnancy. For example, the clearance of propranolol is unchanged, presumably because this is determined by liver blood flow, which is not altered by pregnancy.

Since renal blood flow increases during pregnancy, the clearance of drugs eliminated by this route can also be expected to increase. Lithium clearance doubles during pregnancy, so that dose increases, guided by drug-level monitoring, are likely to be needed. Dose requirements fall rapidly following delivery and care must be taken to avoid the development of toxicity. The clearance of ampicillin nearly doubles during pregnancy. Formal pharmacokinetic studies have not been performed with cephalosporins, but plasma levels of around 50% of those found in nonpregnant women have been reported. By contrast to drugs with a reasonably well-defined therapeutic range, the falling plasma levels of penicillin or cephalosporin antibiotics are of less obvious significance. However, it seems prudent to give doses at the higher end of the recommended range when using these agents to treat systemic infections during pregnancy.

Drug protein binding in pregnancy

The protein binding of drugs is also altered by pregnancy. The mechanism is not fully understood: although the concentration of albumin falls substantially in a normal pregnancy, there is no correlation between the concentration of albumin and the free fraction of the drug, at least not for all drugs. The free and pharmacologically active concentration of anticonvulsants is increased in pregnancy by 30 to 50%, which has consequences for the interpretation of plasma drug levels.

Therapeutic drug monitoring during pregnancy

Epilepsy is the commonest condition for which therapeutic drug monitoring during pregnancy should be performed. This area is controversial because in nonobstetric practice therapeutic drug monitoring is considered of less value than seizure control as a guide to drug management. However, during pregnancy there is a high likelihood that drug levels will fall because of pharmacokinetic changes. In addition, measuring levels is a useful guide to poor compliance with treatment, which is a feature of pregnant epileptic women. Waiting for a seizure to occur is not without risk: women die from poorly controlled epilepsy in pregnancy. Since the free fraction of anticonvulsants increases during pregnancy, it is the unbound level that should preferably be recorded. Alternatively, saliva samples can be used to guide treatment, since these have been shown to correlate well with the plasma concentration of unbound drug.

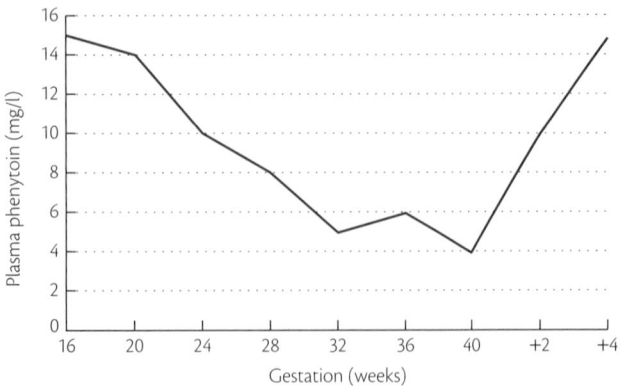

Fig. 14.18.1 Plasma phenytoin concentration during and following pregnancy in a woman who remained on a constant dose of 300 mg/day throughout. She had a seizure at 38 weeks gestation and delivered at 40 weeks. The dose should have been increased when the phenytoin concentration began to fall.

Further reading

Briggs GG, Freeman RK, Yaffe SJ (2005). *Drugs in pregnancy and lactation*, 7th edition. Lippincott, Williams & Wilkins, Baltimore, MD.

Rubin PC (2007). *Prescribing in pregnancy*, 4th edition. Blackwell Publishing, Oxford.

Benefits and risks of oral contraception

John Guillebaud

Essentials

Efficacy of the 'pill' as an oral contraceptive—users of combined oral contraceptives (COC) must understand the importance of not lengthening the pill-free (contraception-deficient) time, and be appropriately advised if prescribed enzyme-inducing drugs.

Noncontraceptive benefits of COC use—these include fewer disorders of the menstrual cycle and less risk of colorectal cancer and cancers of the ovary and endometrium, which may sometimes provide the principal indication for prescription.

Risks of COC use—these include (1) cancer of the breast (possible cofactor) and of the cervix (probable cofactor, with impact reducible through cervical screening); (2) venous thromboembolism—the attributable risk with any formulation of COC is very small without a hereditary or acquired predisposition, including obesity

and immobility; (3) vascular diseases—the attributable risk of both acute myocardial infarction and haemorrhagic stroke is negligible without an added arterial risk factor; migraine with aura is a specific thrombotic stroke risk factor and contraindicates use of any oestrogen-containing method of contraception. By 10 years all-cause mortality in past-users is indistinguishable from that in never-users of the COC.

Progestogen-only pills—these have fewer contraindications than COC. Desogestrel 75 µg (Cerazette) blocks ovulation in 97% of cycles, hence it relies less than other progestogen-only pills on the cervical mucus effect and is a more effective option if COC is contraindicated.

Introduction

Combined oral contraceptives (COCs) contain an oestrogen (ethinylestradiol 20–35 µg in the majority of products in the United Kingdom) combined with one of eight progestogens. Progestogen-only pills (POP) have far fewer contraindications than COCs, since these are mainly oestrogen-related. Desogestrel 75 µg (Cerazette) is a useful new POP since it blocks ovulation in 97% of cycles, whereas other POPs do this only half the time, hence Cerazette relies less on the (weaker) contraceptive effect on the cervical mucus. This makes Cerazette, like all the COCs, highly effective in 'perfect' use (see Box 8.6.2 on p. 1263).

The COC replaces normal cycling with a 21-day cycle that is user-produced and caused directly at the end organ, i.e. the endometrium, during the (usually) 7 days of taking placebo or no pill. The withdrawal bleeding has minimal medical significance, can be deliberately postponed or made infrequent, and if it fails to occur poses no problem—once pregnancy is excluded. However, users must be advised never to lengthen the pill-free (contraception-deficient) time (Fig. 14.19.1), and to act appropriately if tablets are missed (Box 14.19.1)

All medical treatments are a matter of balancing benefits and risks. In relation to the COC there are numerous reviews,

chapters, systematic reviews, and guidance documents based on a vast literature since it was first marketed in 1960, comprising three main prospective studies (the Royal College of General Practitioners and Oxford/Family Planning Association in the United Kingdom and the Nurses Study in the United States of America) supplemented by numerous case–control studies and a few randomized controlled trials conducted by the World Health Organization (WHO) and other bodies.

Benefits of COC use

Contraceptive

The COC is extremely effective: failures are less than 1 per 100 woman-years with 'perfect use', but this is rare and in the real world failure rates of 8 per 100 woman-years are common (see Box 8.6.2, p. 1263). Furthermore, the COC is convenient to use, not being related to intercourse, and its effects are reversible.

Noncontraceptive

There are often times when the COC pill is principally indicated for noncontraceptive purposes, e.g. in the treatment of dysmenorrhoea in a teenager who is not yet sexually active, or of menorrhagia

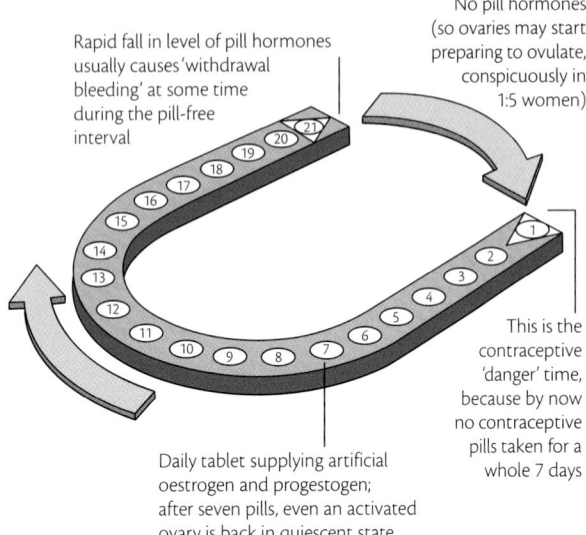

Rapid fall in level of pill hormones usually causes 'withdrawal bleeding' at some time during the pill-free interval

No pill hormones (so ovaries may start preparing to ovulate, conspicuously in 1:5 women)

This is the contraceptive 'danger' time, because by now no contraceptive pills taken for a whole 7 days

Daily tablet supplying artificial oestrogen and progestogen; after seven pills, even an activated ovary is back in quiescent state

Fig. 14.19.1 'Horseshoe' analogy to explain the 21-day cycle. Omission of tablets on either side of the gap in the horseshoe lengthens the 'contraceptive-losing interval'.

in nulliparae unwilling to use an intrauterine system such as Mirena.

In the treatment of menstrual cycle disorders the COC pill can offer the following advantages:

- less heavy bleeding, and hence less anaemia
- less dysmenorrhoea; regular bleeding, the timing of which can be controlled—no COC-taker need ever have 'periods' at weekends, indeed continuous pill-taking with or without infrequent breaks reduces the number of days of (inconvenient) bleeding per year, increases efficacy, e.g. during enzyme-inducing drug therapy, avoids hormone-withdrawal headaches, and has become an option marketed in some countries
- less premenstrual tension
- usually no ovulation pain and fewer functional ovarian cysts

Other advantages of the COC include:

- reduced risk of cancers of ovary and endometrium, and very probably also colorectal cancer
- fewer extrauterine pregnancies because ovulation is inhibited
- reduction in pelvic inflammatory disease

Box 14.19.1 Appropriate action if tablets are missed

- In the final active-pill week, omit the oncoming placebo week
- In the first week, take emergency contraception if any more than two of pills 1 to 7 are missed and unprotected intercourse has occurred since the last active tablet
- 7 days of condom use whenever any pill is more than 24 hours late (though this is less important in contraceptive terms)

- fewer sebaceous disorders, especially acne and mild hirsutism (with oestrogen-dominant COCs such as Marvelon and Yasmin)—with or without the diagnosis of polycystic ovarian syndrome (PCOS)
- beneficial social effects (facilitating women's higher education and careers).

Disadvantages of COC use

Tumours

The COC is a possible cofactor for cancer of the breast, but risk relates to recency, i.e. it occurs during use but diminishes to nil thereafter over 10 years. COC use for any duration ceasing at age 35 years appears to add one case to the background 10 per 1000 by age 45 years, with no subsequent added risk.

COC is a probable cofactor for cancer of the cervix, weaker than cigarette smoking, but with both increasing the rate of progression of (human papilloma virus-induced) cervical intraepithelial neoplasia. However, invasive cervical cancer should be an avoidable risk for COC users (with/without smoking), so long as there is 3-yearly cervical cytology from age 25 years, plus colposcopy as indicated, and eventually through earlier vaccination against causative human papilloma virus.

Malignant and benign tumours of liver have been said to be associated with the COC, but their rarity has led to imprecise but always very small relative risk estimations. However, the attributable death rate of this rapidly fatal cancer has not changed detectably in the United States or in Sweden, where the COC has been very widely used since the 1960s, moreover, there is no evidence of synergism with either cirrhosis or hepatitis B infection.

No other cancers have beneficial or adverse associations in the causation of with COCs or POPs (Fig. 14.19.2).

Circulatory disease

Venous thromboembolism (VTE)

The main outcome of the 1995 'pill scare' was an understanding that ethinylestradiol is the prothrombotic hormone, but for a given ethinylestradiol dose second-generation levonorgestrel (LNG) and norethisterone (NET) progestogens reduce VTE risk. Using absolute rates from the Committee on Safety of Medicines in 1999, the risk amounts to around 100 extra cases per million users per year, and assuming 2% mortality for VTE, gives 2 per million difference in annual VTE mortality between third-generation

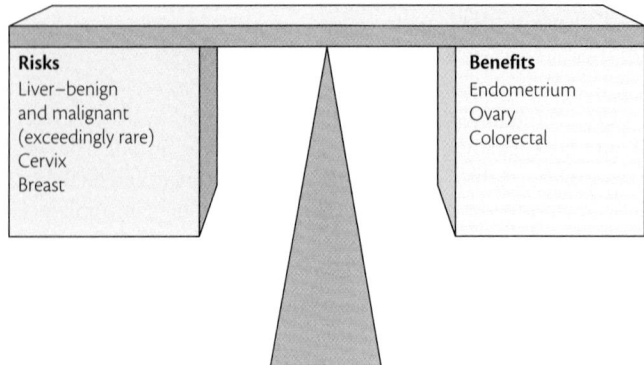

Risks
Liver—benign and malignant (exceedingly rare)
Cervix
Breast

Benefits
Endometrium
Ovary
Colorectal

Fig. 14.19.2 Cancer and COC: a balance.

desogestrel (DSG)/gestodene (GSD) products and second-genera-tion LNG/NET products. To put this into context (Fig. 14.19.3), 1 h of driving gives a 1 per million mortality risk, hence if a pill-taker chooses to control any minor side effect by switching—as she sensibly may—from Microgynon 30 (the usual first-line COC) to (say) Marvelon or Femodene, then if she avoids one 2-h drive in a whole year, she will have the same overall VTE risk next year as she would otherwise have if she did not change brands. It is important to recognize that the risk factors for VTE (Table 14.19.1), obesity and immobility above all, affect risk far more than the differences between formulations of contraceptive pill.

Arterial disease

Although the relative risk is increased, the attributable risk of acute myocardial infarction and of haemorrhagic stroke from the COC is negligible unless there is an added risk factor such as those listed in Table 14.19.2, the commonest of these being smoking. Thrombotic stroke risk can be minimized by using an ethinylestradiol-free method (e.g. a POP such as Cerazette) for all women with the

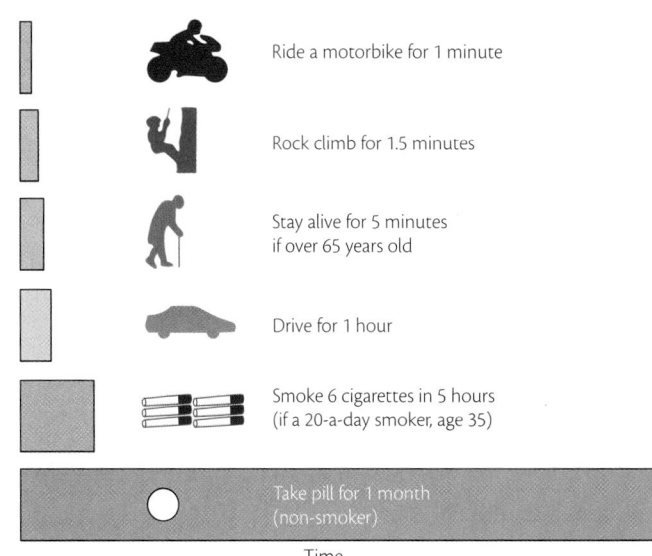

Ride a motorbike for 1 minute

Rock climb for 1.5 minutes

Stay alive for 5 minutes if over 65 years old

Drive for 1 hour

Smoke 6 cigarettes in 5 hours (if a 20-a-day smoker, age 35)

Take pill for 1 month (non-smoker)

Time

Fig. 14.19.3 The time required to have a one-in-a-million chance of dying.

Table 14.19.1 Risk factors for venous thromboembolism and their relation to use of oral contraceptives

Risk factor	Absolute contraindication	Relative contraindication		Remarks
	WHO 4	WHO 3	WHO 2	
Personal or FH of thrombophilias, or of venous thrombosis in sibling or parent	Past VTE event; or identified clotting abnormality whether hereditary or acquired FH of a defined thrombophilia or idiopathic thrombotic event in parent or sibling <45 and thrombophilia screen not (yet) available	FH of thrombosis in parent or sibling <45 with recognized precipitating factor (e.g. major surgery, postpartum) and thrombophilia screen not available	FH of thrombotic event in parent or sibling <45 with or without a recognized precipitating factor and normal thrombophilia screen FH in parent or sibling ≥45 or FH in second-degree relative (classified WHO 2 but tests not indicated)	Idiopathic VTE in a parent or sibling <45 is an indication for a thrombophilia screen if available. The decision to undertake screening in other situations (including where there was a recognized precipitating factor), will be unusual because very cost-ineffective—might be done on clinical grounds, in discussion with the woman. Even a normal thrombophilia screen cannot be entirely reassuring, as some predispositions not yet known
Overweight—high BMI	BMI ≥40	BMI 30–39	BMI 25–29	
Immobility	Bed-bound, with or without major surgery; or leg fractured and immobilized	Wheelchair life, debilitating illness	Reduced mobility for other reason	Minor surgery such as laparoscopic sterilization is WHO 1
VVs	Current superficial vein thrombosis in the upper thigh Current sclerotherapy for VVs (or imminent VV surgery)		History of superficial vein thrombosis (SVT) in the lower limbs, no deep vein thrombosis	SVT does not result in pulmonary embolism, although this past history means some caution (WHO 2) in case it might be a marker of future VTE risk Uncomplicated VVs are irrelevant to VTE risk (WHO 1)
Cigarette smoking		≥15 cigarettes/day	<15 cigarettes/day	On balance the literature suggests a VTE risk from smoking, though less than the arterial disease risk
Age >35	>51		35–51 if age is sole risk factor	VTE risk like arterial diseases risk goes up with increasing age

BMI, body mass index; FH, family history; VTE, venous thromboembolism; VV, varicose veins(s).

Notes

1. A single risk factor in the relative contraindication columns indicates use of LNG/NET pill if any COC used (as in *BNF*).

2. Beware of synergism: more than one factor in either of relative contraindication columns. As a working rule, two WHO 2 conditions makes WHO 3; and if WHO 3 applies (eg BMI 30–39) addition of either a WHO 3 or WHO 2 (eg reduced mobility) condition normally means WHO 4 (do not use).

3. Nonhereditary predispositions include antiphospholipid syndrome

4. There are also important acute VTE risk factors, which need to be considered in individual cases, notably major surgery, all leg surgery, long-haul flights, and dehydration through any cause.

5. There are minor differences in above table from the Faculty of Family Planning and Reproductive Health Care UK Medical Eligibility Criteria (see 'Further reading'), notably the author's more cautious categorization of BMI above 25.

Table 14.19.2 Risk factors for arterial disease and their relation to use of oral contraceptives

Risk factor	Absolute contraindication	Relative contraindication		Remarks
	WHO 4	WHO 3	WHO 2	
FH of atherogenic lipid disorder or of arterial CVS event in sibling or parent	Identified familial hyperlipidaemia, persisting despite treatment	FH of known familial lipid disorder or idiopathic arterial event in parent or sibling <45 and client's lipid screening result not available or confirmed and responding to treatment	Client has the less problematic common hyper-lipidaemia and well treated FH of arterial event with risk factor (e.g. smoking), in parent or sibling < 45, and lipid screen not available	FH of premature arterial CVS disease without other risk factors, or a known atherogenic lipid disorder in a parent or sibling <45 indicate fasting lipid screen, if available. Despite any FH, normal lipid screen in client is reassuring, means WHO 1 (in contrast to thrombophilia screening)
Cigarette smoking	≥40 cigarettes/day	15–39 cigarettes/day	<15 cigarettes/day	Cut-offs here are somewhat arbitrary
DM	Severe, longstanding or diabetic complications present (e.g. retinopathy, renal damage)	Not severe/labile and no complications, young patient with short duration of DM		DM is always at least WHO 3 (safer options available)
Hypertension (consistently elevated BP, with properly taken measurements)	Systolic BP ≥160 mmHg Diastolic BP > 95 mmHg	Systolic BP ≥140–159 mmHg Diastolic BP > 95 mmHg or: On treatment for essential hypertension, with good control	Past history of pre-eclampsia (WHO 3 if also a smoker)	Levels for WHO 4 and WHO 3 consistent with UKMEC
Overweight, high BMI	BMI >40	BMI 30–39	BMI 25–29	High BMI increases arterial as well as VTE risk
Migraine	Migraine with aura Migraine without aura if severe + prolonged attacks (>72 h)	Migraine without aura plus a strong added arterial risk factor	Migraine without aura	Relates to thrombotic stroke risk Triptan treatment does not affect the category
Age > 35	Age >51 (safer options available)		Age 35–51 if no other risk factors	In persistent smokers, age >35 remains best classified as WHO 4 In ex-smokers, UKMEC permits WHO 2 category after one year of not smoking

BMI, body mass index; BP, blood pressure; CVS, cardiovascular system; DM, diabetes mellitus; FH, family history; VTE, venous thromboembolism.
Notes

1. Beware of synergism: more than one factor in either of relative contraindication columns. As a working rule, two WHO 2 conditions makes WHO 3; and if WHO 3 applies, (e.g. smoking >15 cigarettes/day) addition of either a WHO 3 or WHO 2 (eg. age >35) condition normally means WHO 4 (as in table).
2. The pill seems to have negligible adverse effect in arterial disease unless there is a risk factor. In continuing smokers the COC is generally stopped at age 35 years in the UK.
3. WHO numbers also relate to use for contraception: use of COCs for medical indications such as PCOS often entails a different risk/benefit analysis, i.e. the extra therapeutic benefits might outweigh expected extra risks, such as a high BMI-common in PCOS.
4. There are minor differences in above Table from UK Medical Eligibility Criteria of Faculty Family Planning and Reproductive Health Care (see references), notably the author's more cautious categorization with respect to smoking, hyperlipidaemia and DM.

specific risk factor of migraine with aura, but migraine without aura adds minimal extra risk.

Reassuringly, COCs have their main (small) effect on every known associated cause of mortality during current use and the excess thrombotic risk has vanished by 4 weeks. By 10 years all-cause mortality in past users is indistinguishable from that in never-users.

Prescribing oral contraceptives

Current scientific evidence suggests only two prerequisites for the safe provision of COCs: a careful personal and family history with particular attention to cardiovascular risk factors, and a well-taken blood pressure at baseline and follow-up. The WHO has introduced an invaluable 1 to 4 scale for risks and many, though not all, relevant conditions are now usefully categorized on this scale by the United Kingdom Medical Eligibility Criteria of Faculty Family

Planning and Reproductive Health Care (see Tables 14.19.1 and 14.19.2).

Principles for establishing contraindications

A careful personal and family history excludes absolute (WHO 4) and relative (WHO 3 or 2) contraindications to COC use (Tables 14.19.1 and 14.19.2). It is impossible to list them all here; indeed. for many diseases the relevant data do not exist. The working rules therefore require prescribers to ascertain whether or not any condition might lead to summation with a known major adverse effect of COCs, particularly relating to arterial or venous circulatory disease (see Box 14.19.2), or a current hormone-sensitive tumour (breast, liver, or trophoblastic), or might affect COC metabolism in the liver, e.g. severe hepatocellular disease or enzyme-inducing drug use. All these usually mean WHO 4 (Do Not Use), or sometimes—as with enzyme-inducing drug use—WHO 3. The use of enzyme-inducing drugs always means that

Box 14.19.2 Important examples of circulatory conditions to be considered with respect to COC use

- A personal history of definite VTE, acute myocardial infarction, any kind of stroke or transient ischaemic attack, or of migraine with aura are all WHO 4 contraindications.

- Structural (uncorrected) heart disease such as valvular heart disease or shunts/septal defects are WHO 4, but if there is little or no direct or indirect risk of thrombo-embolism—this being the crucial point to check with the cardiologist—the COC is usable (WHO 3 or even 2), especially if patient is on lifetime warfarin.

- Important WHO 4 heart conditions are pulmonary hypertension, cyanotic heart disease, atrial fibrillation or flutter whether sustained or paroxysmal—or not current but high risk (e.g. mitral stenosis), dilated left atrium (>4 cm), any dilated cardiomyopathy (but this is classified only as WHO 2 with a past history of any type in full remission, including pregnancy cardiomyopathy).

another method (specifically an injectable or intrauterine method) would be preferable, but if these are not acceptable oral contraceptive use requires special conditions (i.e. double dose with elimination and/or shortening of the contraception-deficient intervals).

It is important to emphasize that WHO 4 means 'do not use' any hormonal method containing ethinylestradiol (including the patch Evra or vaginal ring NuvaRing) combined with any progestogen, but all progestogen-only methods are usable. Indeed, Cerazette and Mirena are most valuable options, the former especially in adolescents with treated congenital heart disease. More generally, Cerazette is a realistic alternative if the COC is WHO 4 or 3 in any young woman, although the cheaper old-type POPs suffice in low-fertility states such as lactation or above age 40 years.

In all other medical conditions the use of COCs is generally graded as WHO 2, though always with alertness for the onset of new risk factors. Reliable protection from pregnancy is often particularly important in chronic disease states.

Further reading

Amy, J-J,Tripathi V (2009). Clinical Review. Contraception for women:an evidence-based overview. *BMJ* **339**, 563–8.

Beral V, *et al.* (1999). Mortality associated with oral contraceptive use: 25 year follow up of cohort of 46 000 women from RCGP OC study. *BMJ*, **318**, 96–100.

Cochrane Collaboration. *Cochrane systematic reviews in fertility regulation.* http://www.cochrane.org/reviews/en/topics/64.html

Collaborative Group on Hormonal Factors in Breast Cancer (1996). Breast cancer and hormonal contraceptives: collaborative reanalysis of individual data of 53,297 women with breast cancer and 100,239 women without breast cancer from 54 epidemiological studies. *Lancet*, **347**, 1713–27.

Edelman AB, *et al.* (2005). Continuous or extended cycle versus cyclic use of combined oral contraceptives for contraception. *Cochrane Database Syst Rev*, **3**, CD004695.

Faculty of Family Planning and Reproductive Health Care (2006). *First prescription of combined oral contraception*, pp. 1–18. FFPRHC Guidance from Clinical Effectiveness Unit, London.

Faculty of Family Planning and Reproductive Health Care (2006). *UK medical eligibility criteria (UKMEC 2005/2006).* http://www.ffprhc.org. uk/admin/uploads/298_UKMEC_200506.pdf Also UK selected practice recommendations http://www.ffprhc.org.uk/admin/uploads/Final%20 UK%20recommendations1.pdf

Guillebaud J (2009). The combined oral contraceptive—selection and eligibility; follow-up. The progestogen-only pill. In: *Contraception—your questions answered*, 5th edition, pp. 97–326. Churchill-Livingstone, Edinburgh.

Hannaford P, Webb A (1996). Evidence-guided prescribing of combined oral contraceptives: consensus statement. *Contraception*, **54**, 125–9.

Lidegaard O, *et al.* (2009). Hormonal contraception and risk of venous thromboembolism. *BMJ*, **339**, 557–560.

Miller L, Hughes JP (2003). Continuous combination oral contraceptive pills to eliminate withdrawal bleeding: a randomized trial. *Obstet Gynecol*, **101**, 653–61.

O'Brien MD, Guillebaud J (2006). Critical review: contraception for women with epilepsy. *Epilepsia*, **47**, 1419–22.

Smith J, *et al.* (2003). Cervical cancer and use of hormonal contraceptives, a systematic review. *Lancet*, **361**, 1159–67.

Thorne S, *et al.* (2006). Pregnancy and contraception in heart disease and pulmonary arterial hypertension. *J Fam Plann Reprod Health Care*, **32**, 75–81.

Benefits and risks of hormone replacement therapy

J.C. Stevenson

Essentials

Hormone replacement therapy (HRT) comprises oestrogen with or without progestogen.

Benefits—HRT is the most effective treatment for the relief of menopausal symptoms and for the primary prevention of postmenopausal osteoporosis. There are also possible benefits for coronary heart disease, colorectal cancer, and neurocognitive function, but these are yet to be established.

Risks—the main risk of HRT is perhaps a small increase in incidence of breast cancer, but this risk may be confined to women with a long exposure to certain oestrogen–progestogen combinations.

There is a small increased risk of stroke if HRT is initiated in older women and a small increased risk of venous thromboembolism with oral therapy.

Balance of benefits and risks—given appropriately, the benefits of HRT outweigh the risks. The choice and dose of therapeutic agents should be tailored to suit the individual case, but usually the therapy used should be the one that the patient finds most acceptable. Risks and benefits should be reviewed annually, but no limit on duration of treatment need be set.

Introduction

The menopause, the time of a woman's last spontaneous menstrual period, is a useful marker for ovarian failure and occurs naturally at an average age of around 51 years, although it may occur at any time after puberty. Symptoms arising around the time of the menopause include hot flushes and night sweats, and psychological symptoms such as mood swings, depression, anxiety and irritability, and difficulties with memory and concentration. Later there may be genitourinary problems such as vaginal dryness and dyspareunia, and increased urinary frequency and urge incontinence. However, it is the long-term consequences of hormone deficiency, particularly osteoporosis and cardiovascular disease, which pose a major health problem.

Benefits of hormone replacement therapy (HRT)

The main indications for use of HRT are relief of menopausal symptoms and prevention of osteoporosis.

Vasomotor symptoms

HRT will abolish vasomotor symptoms, often within days of starting treatment, but psychological and genitourinary symptoms may take weeks or even months to respond. It is therefore worthwhile persisting with therapy for several months in the absence of rapid symptomatic response, and treatment should be continued for at least several months after symptomatic relief has been obtained.

Osteoporosis

HRT is well established for both the prevention and treatment of osteoporosis, and is as effective as any other agent currently available. It conserves—and to some extent increases—bone density, and results in a reduction in fracture risk. Therapy should be offered to any woman considered at increased risk of osteoporosis, and particularly those with an early menopause. When risk of osteoporosis is uncertain, bone density measurement can aid clinical decision making.

Hormone replacement may need to be given for several years when started in the early postmenopause. Benefits in reducing risk of osteoporotic fracture may persist into old age. Cessation of HRT leads to a loss of bone density, but only at the usual postmenopausal rate.

Older women are less tolerant of treatment side effects, particularly cyclical bleeding and mastalgia, hence for this age group regimens that avoid bleeding are to be preferred, and much lower doses of oestrogen than are used early after the menopause appear effective for bone conservation.

Cardiovascular disease

Observational studies have shown prevention of cardiovascular disease with HRT. There are many mechanisms, both established and potential, whereby HRT might benefit the cardiovascular system: these are summarized in Box 14.20.1. The effects vary depending on the dose and type of oestrogen or progestogen and the route of administration. In general, hormone replacement produces favourable metabolic effects for lipids, and glucose and insulin metabolism, thus reversing the changes brought about by the menopause. There are also direct effects of oestrogen on arteries, which improve their function by endothelium-dependent and non-endothelium-dependent mechanisms.

In contrast to the observational studies, randomized prospective studies of HRT for both primary and secondary prevention of coronary heart disease have failed to show any overall benefit in clinical events. Although eventual reductions in events by 20 to 30% were observed by the end of the trials, these were counterbalanced by early increases in events with hormone replacement. The doses of oestrogens used were inappropriately high for the older women in the study groups, which could result in transient increases in thrombogenesis and adverse vascular remodelling. Indeed, in these trials younger women appeared to show some benefit while older women did not. Further studies are necessary to clarify the position.

Colorectal cancer

There is some epidemiological evidence that oestrogen–progestogen therapy may result in a decrease in the incidence of colorectal cancer, also seen in a large randomized trial.

Side effects and risks of HRT

Oestrogenic side effects such as breast tenderness and nausea are sometimes experienced on commencing therapy, but these are transient and usually resolve by about 3 months of therapy. More commonly side effects are due to the progestogen and can include breast tenderness, abdominal and pelvic pain, backache, depression, irritability, and migraine.

Breast cancer

The main concern about HRT is the risk of breast cancer. Epidemiological evidence remains conflicting: some studies show no overall increased risk of breast cancer, whereas others show an increase with prolonged usage. The largest randomized trial showed a small increase in risk of developing breast cancer with one oestrogen–progestogen regimen, but a small decreased risk with oestrogen alone. It seems prudent to avoid HRT where possible in women with breast cancer, but previous disease need not be considered a total contraindication in all cases.

Other risks

Previous endometrial hyperplasia or neoplasia is not a contraindication, provided the disease has been eradicated. Similarly, endometriosis and uterine fibroids rarely cause a problem, although they may occasionally worsen.

HRT does not usually cause hypertension and some regimens may reduce blood pressure. There is a small but transient dose-dependent increase in venous thromboembolism risk, but this is not seen with nonoral therapy. It is prudent to exclude a preexisting thrombophilia in patients with a relevant past or family history, and avoid oral therapy in such women. There is also a small increased risk of stroke, which may also be dose dependent.

Many women gain weight after the menopause, most commonly due to excessive calorie intake. Weight gain may occasionally occur due to fluid retention, although antimineralocorticoid progestogens prevent this. Increases in body fat are not caused by HRT.

Therapeutic regimens

HRT consists of oestrogen, which should be given continuously, with the addition of cyclical progestogen in women who have not had a hysterectomy. Low starting doses of oestrogen are now recommended. Progestogens are necessary to prevent endometrial hyperplasia and neoplasia, and to regulate any uterine bleeding that may occur.

The choice and dose of therapeutic agents should be tailored to suit the individual case. There are advantages and disadvantages of certain preparations and combinations, but usually the therapy used should be the one that the patient finds most acceptable.

Box 14.20.1 Hormone replacement therapy and the cardiovascular system: possible mechanisms of action

- Decreased total cholesterol
- Decreased triglycerides
- Decreased LDL cholesterol
- Decreased LDL cholesterol oxidation
- Increased HDL and HDL_2 cholesterol
- Increased small dense LDL particle clearance
- Increased postprandial lipid clearance
- Decreased insulin resistance
- Decreased circulating insulin concentrations
- Decreased proportion of insulin propeptides
- Improved glucose tolerance
- Decreased proportion of android fat
- Decreased NEFA flux
- Decreased fibrinogen
- Decreased plasminogen activator inhibitor-1
- Increased tissue plasminogen activator
- Decreased homocysteine
- Increased arterial NO production
- Decreased endothelin-1 release
- Reduced calcium channel ion flux
- Enhanced potassium channel ion flux
- Decreased ACE activity
- Decreased blood pressure
- Increased arterial blood flow
- Improved arterial remodelling

ACE, angiotensin-1 converting enzyme; HDL, high density lipoprotein; LDL, low density lipoprotein; NEFA, nonesterified fatty acids; NO, nitric oxide.

Annual review of risks and benefits should be undertaken, but no time limit on duration of treatment need be set.

Various types of natural oestrogens and various routes of administration can be used. The synthetic alkylated oestrogens, such as ethinyloestradiol, are not used in HRT because of their potency and unwanted side effects. The progestogens currently used are either derivatives of 19-nor-testosterone, C-21 steroids, or a spironolactone analogue. Progestogens are usually given in the minimal dose necessary for endometrial protection for 12 or more days per month, and result in a regular uterine bleed. Commonly used hormones are shown in Box 14.20.2.

A major drawback to cyclical HRT regimens is the necessity of uterine withdrawal bleeding, although this is often fairly light, particularly in older women, and tends to diminish with time. With a satisfactory and regular bleeding pattern, there is usually no need for endometrial screening. However, cyclical bleeding becomes less acceptable as women get older and regimens that avoid such bleeding become preferable. Preparations giving continuous progestogen with continuous oestrogen are used to prevent endometrial stimulation and hence abolish uterine bleeding, resulting in amenorrhoea in up to 70 to 80% of women. These therapies are less successful in women close to menopause, where transient episodes of spontaneous ovarian activity may result in irregular bleeding.

Tibolone, a synthetic compound with oestrogenic, progestogenic, and androgenic properties, is an alternative that avoids cyclical bleeding. It relieves vasomotor symptoms and appears as effective as HRT for the prevention and treatment of osteoporosis, but it is not established whether it has other benefits associated with HRT, such as desirable cardiovascular effects or effects on the central nervous system. However, it has the same potential risks, for the breast and for stroke.

Raloxifene, a selective oestradiol receptor modulator (SERM), is a synthetic compound which binds to the oestrogen receptor but causes conformational changes that result in different tissue-specific actions. Thus it can act similarly to an oestrogen in the skeleton, preventing osteoporotic vertebral fractures although not hip fractures, but like an antioestrogen in the breast, causing a reduction in breast cancer incidence. It does not cause uterine bleeding, but does not relieve vasomotor or genitourinary symptoms. Its cardiovascular effects may be favourable if initiated in postmenopausal woman below age 60 years.

Box 14.20.2 Oestrogens and progestogens used in HRT

Oral preparations

Oestrogens

- Micronized oestradiol-17β
- Oestradiol valerate
- Oestrone sulphate
- Conjugated equine oestrogens

Progestogens

- *dl*-Norgestrel
- Norethisterone acetate
- Dydrogesterone
- Medroxyprogesterone acetate
- Micronized progesterone
- Drospirenone

Others

- Tibolone
- Raloxifene

Nonoral preparations

Oestrogens

- Transdermal oestradiol-17β patch
- Percutaneous oestradiol-17β gel
- Oestradiol-17β implant

Progestogens

- Transdermal norethisterone acetate (combination patch)
- Transdermal levonorgestrel (combination patch)

The lowest doses are often sufficient for older women; higher doses may be needed for young or acutely postmenopausal women.

Further reading

Bush TL, Whiteman M, Flaws JA (2001). Hormone replacement therapy and breast cancer: a qualitative review. *Obstet Gynecol*, **98**, 498–508.

Cauley JA, *et al.* (2003). Effects of estrogen plus progestin on risk of fracture and bone mineral density. The Women's Health Initiative randomized trial. *JAMA*, **290**, 1729–38.

Hulley S, *et al.* (1998). Randomized trial of estrogen plus progestin for secondary prevention of coronary heart disease in postmenopausal women. *JAMA*, **280**, 605–13.

Manson JE, et al (2003). Estrogen plus progestin and the risk of coronary heart disease. *N Engl J Med*, **349**, 523–34.

Scarabin P-Y, Oger E, Plu-Bureau G (2003). Differential association of oral and transdermal oestrogen-replacement therapy with venous thromboembolism risk. *Lancet*, **362**, 428–32.

Stefanick ML, *et al.* (2006). Effect of conjugated equine estrogens on breast cancer and mammography screening in postmenopausal women with hysterectomy. *JAMA*, **295**, 1647–57.

Stevenson JC (2005). Menopausal hormone therapy. In: Wenger NK, Collins P (eds) *Women and heart disease*, pp. 375–90. Taylor & Francis, London.

Stevenson JC on behalf of the International Consensus Group on HRT and Regulatory Issues (2006). Hormone replacement therapy, osteoporosis and regulatory authorities. Quis custodiet ipsos custodes? *Hum Reprod*, **21**, 1668–71.

Stevenson JC, *et al.* (2009). Coronary heart disease and menopause management: The swinging pendulum of HRT. Atherosclerosis, In press, Available online.

Women's Health Initiative Steering Committee (2004). Effects of conjugated equine estrogen in postmenopausal women with hysterectomy. *JAMA*, **291**, 1701–12.

Writing Group for the Women's Health Initiative Investigators (2002). Risks and benefits of estrogen plus progestin in healthy postmenopausal women. *JAMA*, **288**, 321–23.

SECTION 15

Gastroenterological disorders

Structure and function of the gut

D.G. Thompson

Essentials

The gastrointestinal tract is a hollow tube stretching from the oral cavity through the oesophagus, stomach, small intestine, colon, and rectum to the anal sphincter. Its function is the transport, digestion, and elimination of ingested material to supply nutrients, vitamins, minerals, and electrolytes that are essential for life, together with the protection of the rest of the body from injurious or allergenic material. The stomach acts as a storage, sterilizing, and digestive tank; the small intestine is the major site of digestion and absorption; the colon's function is to salvage water and electrolyte from the small intestinal effluent; and the rectum provides a storage function, enabling the elimination of colonic residue (defecation) to be restricted to times of personal convenience.

Introduction

This chapter provides a brief overview of the structure and function of the gastrointestinal tract (excluding the liver and pancreas). Emphasis has been placed on those aspects of gastrointestinal anatomy and physiology which illuminate understanding of the nature of gastrointestinal symptoms and inform treatment.

Anatomy

Gross anatomy

The gastrointestinal tract is a hollow tube of approximately 5 to 6 m in length, stretching from the oral cavity to the anal sphincter (Fig. 15.1.1). It is arbitrarily divided into a series of organs which serve different functions, and is joined to the liver and pancreas, the major organs of digestion.

Anatomical structure

The gastrointestinal tract possess a broadly similar structure throughout its length (Fig. 15.1.2) with an innermost epithelium, a subepithelial lamina propria, and two muscle layers, an inner circular and an outer longitudinal layer, between which lies the myenteric plexus, the intrinsic neural control system of the musculature. While this description most accurately describes the small intestine, the other organs of the gastrointestinal tract differ only subtly from this stereotype.

Oesophagus

In the oesophagus, the innermost layer is a squamous rather than columnar epithelium. The musculature in the upper one-third is striated and controlled directly via extrinsic neural pathways, unlike the lower two-thirds which has smooth muscle and a myenteric plexus.

Stomach

The anatomy of the stomach differs from that of the intestine, possessing an additional oblique muscular layer and at either end, a sphincter—specialized musculature designed to act as a unidirectional valve to control the flow of luminal contents. The sphincter between the oesophagus and stomach (the lower oesophageal sphincter) lies at the level of the diaphragm. The sphincter between the stomach and small intestine is known as the pylorus.

Small intestine

The small intestine is arbitrarily divided into duodenum, jejunum, and ileum. The duodenum (so named because it is 12 fingers' breadth in length) is retroperitoneal, and possess on its medial aspect the ampulla of Vater which connects the pancreatic and common bile ducts to the duodenal lumen. The jejunum (Latin, empty, after death) is mobile and free on a mesentery. The ileum (Greek, twisted) begins indistinctly from the jejunum and ends at the caecum.

Colon and rectum

The colon differs from the small intestine in its muscular structure—the inner circular layer is similar but the outer longitudinal layer is condensed into three 'wormlike' structures, the taeniae coli. At the proximal end of the colon, the caecum (Latin, blind ending) arises the vermiform appendix, named because of its worm-like appearance. The ascending and descending colon are retroperitoneal whereas the transverse and sigmoid colon are freely mobile on a mesentery, extending to the pelvic floor, after which it expands into the rectum.

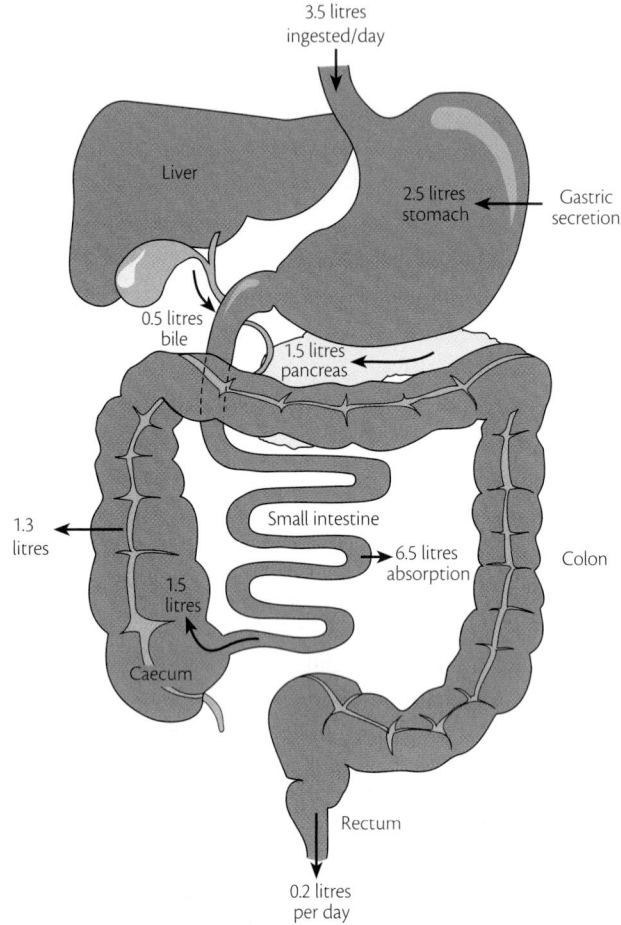

Fig. 15.1.1 Schematic diagram of the gastrointestinal tract showing the major organs of the tract and their connections. The figure also shows the average daily fluid flux across the intestinal mucosae to indicate sites and volumes of absorption and secretion in the various organs.

Anal sphincter

The anal sphincter provides an important continence mechanism and has two parts, an internal sphincter of smooth muscle and an external sphincter of striated muscle.

Functional anatomy

The function of the gastrointestinal tract is closely associated with its structure.

Epithelial layer

The epithelium lies in contact with the luminal contents and ranges in permeability from being largely impermeable (oesophageal squamous epithelium) to highly permeable (intestinal epithelium). The absorptive function of the epithelial layer is modulated by a network of neurons, the submucous plexus, which receive input from the central nervous system. In addition, the neurons of the submucous plexus and the nerve terminals of extrinsic afferent nerves, particularly those running in the vagus trunk, are modulated by signals arising from the epithelium.

Neuromusculature of the gut

The striated muscle in the gastrointestinal tract (upper oesophagus and anus) is directly innervated by second-order (lower motor)

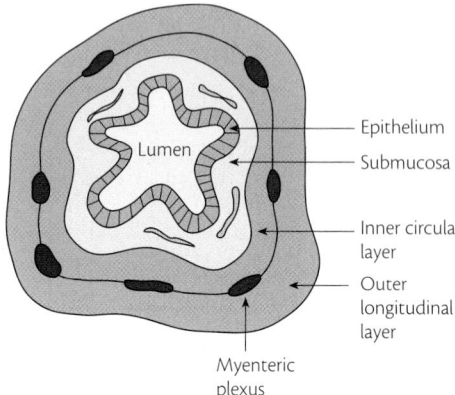

Fig. 15.1.2 Generalized structure of the intestine in cross section. A central lumen is bounded by an epithelial layer, which in turn is surrounded by a submucosal layer containing neural and vascular connections to the epithelium. Outside the submucosae lie circumferential and longitudinal muscular layers with the controlling neuronal myenteric plexus lying between.

neurons (arising from the brainstem and spinal cord respectively) and therefore under direct central nervous system control, whereas smooth muscle is largely autonomous, being controlled 'locally' by the enteric nervous system without direct innervation from the central nervous system. The central nervous system can, however, indirectly influence the muscular function of the gastrointestinal tract via its innervation of the myenteric plexus.

Immune system of the gastrointestinal tract

Throughout the gastrointestinal tract lie discreet clusters of immune cells which provide immunosurveillance and immune protection. These immune cell clusters form the so-called Peyer's patches in the small intestine and the appendix (see Chapter 15.5).

Function of the gastrointestinal tract

The function of the gastrointestinal tract is the transport, digestion, and elimination of ingested material to supply nutrients, vitamins, minerals, and electrolytes which are essential for life, together with the protection of the rest of the body from injurious or allergenic material.

Secretion/absorption

The gastrointestinal tract is responsible for movement of very large volumes across its lumen (Fig. 15.1.1). Overall, more than 8 litres enter the lumen per day. In contrast, only 200 to 300 ml is expelled per day as stool, the remainder being efficiently absorbed by the small intestine and proximal colon. The major digestive/absorptive organ of the gastrointestinal tract is the small intestine. Without the small intestine life is impossible, whereas possession of the small intestine without oesophagus, stomach, or colon is still compatible with reasonable nutrition. The various organs of the gastrointestinal tract subserve different functions to ensure that ingested nutrients are adequately digested or eliminated.

Oesophageal function

The oesophagus functions as a conduit to transport ingested food masticated by the mouth and salivary glands, through the thoracic cavity and into the proximal stomach.

Gastric function

The stomach acts as a storage, a sterilizing, and a digestive tank. Its receptive function enables large quantities of food to be eaten rapidly and stored and processed until adequately prepared for delivery to the small intestine. The presence of pathogens in food is reduced by the secretion of hydrochloric acid upon meal ingestion while the production of peptidases and lipase capable of operating in a low pH commence the process of digestion.

Small intestinal function

The small intestine is the major site of digestion and absorption. It regulates the speed of delivery of gastric contents via a sensing mechanism located in the epithelium, comprising endocrine cells sensitive to the pH, osmolarity, and chemical composition of the luminal contents, and signals both to intrinsic neurons and to extrinsic neurons of the vagus to delay gastric emptying. This sensory signal also stimulates the delivery of bile and the production of pancreatic secretion ensuring that these major digestive materials are delivered to the intestine in the presence of nutrients.

The absorption of digested material is achieved through the intestinal mucosa. While some passes between the intestinal cells, most is actively transported through the epithelial cells via specific transporters (e.g. peptide and hexose transporters). The small intestinal is also a major fluid absorptive organ, retrieving more than 6 litres of fluid per day from the lumen (Fig. 15.1.1), the end result of which is the delivery of a small quantity of unabsorbed food (1.5 litres) into the caecum.

Regional variation in intestinal absorption

The intestine shows regional differences in its absorptive function. The jejunum is responsible for the majority of nutrient and fluid absorption, whereas the ileum has additional, specific absorptive functions, in particular the absorption of vitamin B_{12} and the absorption of bile salts. Surgical resection of the ileum may thus be associated with development of vitamin B_{12} deficiency and of diarrhoea resulting from passage of bile salts into the colon where they induce secretion.

Colon

The colon's function is to salvage water and electrolyte from the small-intestinal effluent, converting over 1 litre of material arriving from the intestine into small pellets for elimination via the anus. In addition to its water and electrolyte absorptive function, the colon also salvages unabsorbed calories from the lumen, particularly undigested carbohydrate, e.g. starch polysaccharides. These are incompletely digested in the small intestine and pass to the colon where the anaerobic bacteria of the lumen ferment the carbohydrate to short chain fatty acids, which are absorbed to provide a secondary energy source.

Rectum

The rectum provides a storage function, enabling the elimination of colonic residue (defecation) to be restricted to times of personal convenience.

Neural control of gastrointestinal function

For the greater part of the time, the gastrointestinal tract is controlled by its own nervous system—the enteric nervous system.

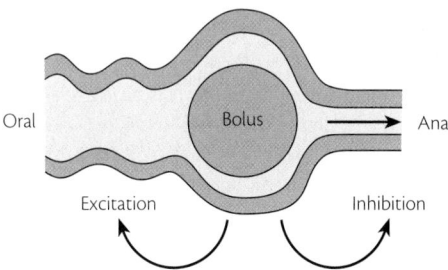

Fig. 15.1.3 Peristaltic reflex. The peristaltic reflex is the mechanical response of the intestine to the intraluminal distension. Note the presence of proximal motor excitation and distal inhibition which together propel the distending bolus from mouth to anus.

The enteric nervous system is not entirely autonomous, however, and requires some local and central nervous system 'reflexes' for adequate coordination of functions along its length. For example, the coordination of the passage of luminal contents into the small intestine from the stomach requires sophisticated control, which is provided by a vagally mediated reflex operating via the brainstem. This circuitry alters the function of the gut from its fasted state to the fed state, initiating gastric relaxation and the induction of gallbladder emptying and pancreatic secretion, thus ensuring the provision of digestive enzymes at the appropriate time. An additional relay function is provided by prevertebral ganglia where visceral afferent neurons synapse with efferent relay neurons to integrate contractile patterns and control contraction force.

Intrinsic nervous system

The intrinsic nervous system acts as a local control system with its own 'programmes', examples of which are the peristaltic reflex and the migrating motor complex.

Peristaltic reflex

This basic programme responds to local luminal distension by inducing a pattern of ascending muscular excitation and descending inhibition (Fig. 15.1.3) which ensures aboral propulsion of luminal contents. This reflex is best seen in the oesophagus where it is known as secondary or non-swallow-related peristalsis. Although the reflex can be induced in the small intestine or colon, it is not a major factor for luminal transit.

Migrating motor complex

This comprises a triphasic pattern of aborally propagating contractions in the distal stomach and small intestine during the fasted state which probably serve to maintain an empty lumen and reduce bacterial growth. Periods of quiescence are followed by irregular contractile activity, which then terminates in a aboral migrating burst of regular contractions that migrate slowly from the distal stomach down to the terminal ileum. This pattern, which characterizes the fasted state, is interrupted on food ingestion by a vagally mediated reflex that converts the pattern into a fed one.

Immune function of the gut

Being the major route of nutrient absorption, the gastrointestinal tract is also a potential portal for pathogen entry. The gastrointestinal tract therefore requires a sophisticated immune surveillance system together with a process for eliminating intestinal pathogens and the ability to either tolerate or eliminate ingested antigens. Details of this process are more fully dealt with in Chapter 15.5.

Disturbances of local physiological control mechanisms and origins of symptoms

Disturbances of local neuromuscular function are associated by the disturbances in transit and elimination or secretion and absorption. Example of disturbed transit resulting from disturbed neuromuscular function are achalasia or slow transit constipation. Examples of disturbance of secretion and absorption are secretory diarrhoeas or the hyperacidity associated with *Helicobacter pylori* infection. Examples of symptoms which follow damage to extrinsic neural control are exemplified by the symptoms of truncal vagotomy, i.e. rapid transit and impaired nutrient–enzyme mixing, result in poor digestion and an osmotic diarrhoea.

The relationships between gastrointestinal symptoms and the central nervous system are relevant to the understanding of functional gastrointestinal disorders. It is well recognized that psychological disturbances, e.g. anxiety or depression, combined with local disturbances of gastrointestinal physiology produce pain, nausea and vomiting, and altered bowel habit.

Further reading

Schultz SG (ed.) (1991). The gastrointestinal system. In: *Handbook of physiology*, Section 6, Vols I–IV. American Physiological Society, Oxford University Press, New York.

Symptomatology of gastrointestinal disease

Graham Neale

Essentials

The skilful analysis of symptoms indicating disorders of the digestive system is an integral part of the practice of internal medicine. Many patients with abdominal symptoms do not have easily defined organic conditions. The traditional skills of taking a careful history and examining the patient thoroughly are invaluable in managing patients who have functional disorders such as 'irritable bowel', nonulcer dyspepsia, nonspecific diarrhoea, recurrent abdominal pain, and somatization disorder.

The enormous advances in endoscopy, scanning, and other investigative techniques have not made clinical diagnosis less important. Most gastrointestinal disorders are minor self-limited conditions of uncertain cause or are functional in nature, thereby often eluding definition even if extensive diagnostic procedures are (unnecessarily) employed. At the other extreme, the early suspicion of life-threatening disease and prompt referral of patients for investigation depends on clinical judgement.

Oesophageal symptoms

Dysphagia

Difficulty in swallowing (dysphagia) is an important symptom that requires prompt resolution. Oropharyngeal disorders cause difficulty in initiating swallowing, regurgitation through the nasopharynx, a sensation of sticking in the throat, or the feeling of a lump in the throat on or after swallowing. Coughing and choking on swallowing is usually a symptom of pharyngeal disease and indicates failure to close the larynx. More rarely it is a sign of an obstructive lesion in the lower gullet that allows food and secretions to accumulate and spill into the larynx, especially at night. This symptom needs urgent attention to reduce the risk of aspiration pneumonia. Painful lesions of the oropharynx are usually demonstrated quite easily by simple inspection.

Patients with neurological disorders such as Parkinson's disease, motor neurone disease, myaesthenia gravis, and dermatomyositis rarely present with disorders of swallowing and the clinician has only to be aware of the way in which known illnesses may affect the swallowing process. Oropharyngeal dyskinesia is common in the early phase of recovery after a stroke and may be persistently troublesome in patients with brainstem lesions.

Dysphagia due to pharyngeal disease usually presents as a sensation of a lump in the throat on or after swallowing. An imaging technique is necessary to look for a pharyngeal pouch, a post-cricoid web or carcinoma, and rarely extrinsic compression caused by a large osteophyte as a result of cervical spondylosis. It is unwise to submit patients with suspected pharyngeal lesions to conventional fibre-optic oesophagoscopy as a first examination because of the risks of perforation. Patients with a persistent feeling of 'a lump in the throat' without any demonstrable disease ('globus hystericus') usually respond well to the taking of a careful history, a single scanning procedure, and firm reassurance. They are more often women than men and they nearly always show signs of an anxiety state.

Dysphagia caused by oesophageal disorders gives a sensation of food sticking in the gullet, and this symptom is nearly always due to organic disease. The symptoms vary from discomfort to severe pain and the patient is rarely able to localize the site of the obstruction accurately. Associated symptoms such as regurgitation, vomiting, and coughing or choking are common. Oesophageal dysphagia is caused either by an obstructive lesion or more rarely by a neuromuscular disorder. The common obstructive lesions are tumours or inflammatory strictures secondary to gastric acid reflux. Extrinsic compression may occur as a result of mediastinal lesions or vascular disorders (e.g. an aortic aneurysm). Neuromuscular disorders such as achalasia, Schatzki ring, diffuse oesophageal spasm, and dystrophia myotonica may cause dysphagia for both solids and fluids, usually with an insidious onset. In achalasia there are no other clues as to the nature of the problem. In its early stages the disease is often attributed to a functional disorder especially as the symptoms may be episodic. The duration, progression, and frequency of symptoms help determine the likely nature of the pathology. Steady progression of dysphagia over a few weeks suggests malignant obstruction whereas association with a long history of heartburn suggests an inflammatory stricture.

Heartburn

Heartburn is an extremely common symptom. It is an episodic lower retrosternal or epigastric burning that radiates upwards. It is caused by gastro-oesophageal reflux and commonly occurs an hour or two after meals (especially if these are fatty or spicy); it may be precipitated by heavy physical work and bending. Symptoms often occur on lying down and are characteristically relieved by the ingestion of antacids. Most pregnant women suffer heartburn.

Oesophageal pain

Odynophagia is oesophageal pain felt within 15 s of swallowing and may be associated with the impaction of a lump of food at a site of mechanical blockage or a hold-up with oesophageal spasm. Odynophagia without hold-up occurs with intrinsic inflammatory disorders (such as reflux or candidal oesophagitis) and extrinsic disorders (such as mediastinitis). Hot liquids and alcohol may cause odynophagia in a normal gullet (the so-called 'tender oesophagus').

Oesophageal pain not clearly related to swallowing is characteristically retrosternal, often has a crushing quality, and may radiate to the jaw thereby mimicking cardiac pain. Patients with such symptoms are usually investigated for angina before being referred to a gastroenterologist: some will be shown to have reflux-associated chest pain or a primary disorder of motility (e.g. diffuse oesophageal spasm). High-amplitude contractions of the distal oesophagus are often discovered in patients with attacks of chest pain of uncertain cause; these are believed to be related to psychological stress.

Dyspepsia, nausea, and vomiting

Dyspepsia, nausea, and vomiting are extremely common linked symptoms that can be produced by a wide range of conditions from the most serious (such as endstage neoplastic disease) to the most trivial (such as overindulgence in food or alcohol). Patients may speak of 'indigestion' (to describe any low-grade upper abdominal discomfort) and 'sickness' (to describe either nausea or vomiting).

Dyspepsia

Dyspepsia is upper abdominal or lower chest discomfort or pain related to eating. It may be described by the patient as a burning, a heaviness, or an aching and is often accompanied by other symptoms such as nausea, fullness in the upper abdomen, or belching. Although the symptoms of upper gastrointestinal disease are imprecise and nonspecific, care in taking the clinical history will often facilitate making the correct diagnosis quickly and limit unnecessary investigation. All too often, an over-stretched, relatively inexperienced clinician will spend a few minutes talking to the patient and then arrange a battery of blood tests, gastrointestinal endoscopy (and biopsy), ultrasound examination of the abdomen, and some conventional radiology before telling the patient that he can find nothing wrong (and possibly implying that the patient is too ready to complain). Certain aspects of history-taking yield important clues:

◆ How clear cut is the patient's description of symptoms? Peptic ulcer often gives well-localized pain in the epigastrium. For many patients with dyspepsia this comes on after a meal and wakes the patient at night. Attacks of central abdominal pain which cause the patient to double up may indicate gallstones although, if there

is associated severe cholecystitis, the pain is more likely to be in the right upper quadrant (often radiating to the right shoulder).

◆ For how long has the patient had symptoms and how constant are they? A short history makes organic disease likely.

◆ Has the patient any associated diseases and what drugs are being taken? Many drugs cause upper abdominal symptoms, especially aspirin and nonsteroidal anti-inflammatory drugs.

◆ Has the patient lost significant weight? Are there associated symptoms? Vomiting suggests organic disease, alcoholism, or pregnancy.

◆ Has the patient any worries or anxieties that may be related to dyspepsia of recent onset (especially in women and young people)? Sometimes patients will deliberately conceal their worries for fear that the clinician will too readily accept them as the cause of their symptoms.

◆ Details about dietary habits, smoking, and intake of alcohol should be obtained and it may be necessary not to take what the patient says at face value.

Functional dyspepsia (sometimes termed nonulcer dyspepsia) is a common condition. Localized tenderness in the abdominal wall that increases with contraction of abdominal muscles may be helpful in excluding intra-abdominal pathology (Carnett's sign). Unfortunately symptoms and signs rarely distinguish organic disease from functional dyspepsia with certainty. In the older patient (>45 years), with dyspepsia of recent onset, gastroscopy is indicated in order to identify early gastric cancer. By the time the patient has the classical triad of symptoms of this disease—loss of appetite, loss of weight, and loss of strength—it is usually too late to achieve a surgical cure. Regrettably, the early symptoms of gastric cancer are usually mild and nonspecific. The symptoms of patients shown to have infection with *Helicobacter pylori* by serological testing are difficult to assess. Most infected patients are symptomless and most of those who have dyspeptic symptoms without ulceration are not cured by treatment with appropriate antibiotics. In unravelling the pathogenesis of nonulcer dyspepsia the place of newer tests of upper gastrointestinal physiology such as gastric emptying and impaired fundic accommodation remain uncertain.

Nausea

This term should be restricted to the feeling of being about to vomit. Acute nausea is usually accompanied by hypersalivation. Nausea is caused by labyrinthine stimulation (as in motion sickness); distension of hollow viscera, or any severe somatic pain and by some drugs, especially opiates and those used in chemotherapy for malignant conditions.

Again the clinician has to define carefully what the patient means by nausea. It may be used to describe anorexia, an aversion to food, abdominal fullness, or a sinking feeling in the abdomen. In the absence of a recognizable cause, persistent or frequent nausea without vomiting often proves to be psychologically determined.

Vomiting

Vomiting is the forceful ejection of gastric contents through the mouth by the coordinated contraction of abdominal and gastric muscles with relaxation of the lower oesophageal sphincter. Nonproductive vomiting is called retching. Gastroenteritis is the commonest cause of self-limited vomiting. The small round structured (SRSV) family of viruses (especially Norwalk) causing 'winter vomiting syndrome' or 'gastric flu' are highly infectious and may be spread by nasopharyngeal droplets as well as by the orofaecal route. Symptoms usually last 12–48 h.

Repeated vomiting occurs with peptic ulceration, especially when there is delayed gastric emptying (pyloric stenosis) and with advanced gastric cancer. It occurs with disorders of the biliary tree (especially as a result of gallstones) and with acute pancreatitis (in which it is a prime symptom). It is an important symptom of intestinal obstruction, especially with lesions above the ileocaecal valve, and it may occur with any cause of peritoneal inflammation such as appendicitis. Metabolic causes of vomiting include diabetic ketoacidosis, hypoadrenalism, and uraemia. Drugs which cause vomiting include opiates, some antibiotics (e.g. erythromycin), and chemotherapeutic agents. Alcoholism, raised intracranial pressure, and pregnancy are important causes of early morning vomiting.

Effortless vomiting without a definable cause may be psychogenic. This is usually a disorder of young women, many of whom have suffered psychological trauma (such as sexual abuse). It is not related to the vomiting of bulimia, a condition that is part of the anorexia nervosa syndrome (see Chapter 26.5.6).

Rumination has to be distinguished from vomiting. It is the repetitive regurgitation of gastric contents into the mouth after meals, the regurgitated material then being re-swallowed. It is not associated with nausea, heartburn, or discomfort and often appears to be simply an acquired habit.

Cyclical vomiting is a rare condition usually described in children. It is characterized by repeated episodes of vomiting/retching perhaps 5 to 10 times an hour for several hours (occasionally for days). Investigation fails to reveal organic pathology and emotional stress may appear to be a trigger factor. The condition is sometimes called 'abdominal migraine'.

Abdominal pain

Pain in the 'acute abdomen'

Most patients with acute abdominal pain are promptly referred to a surgeon. However, this does not always happen and delay in diagnosis may be disastrous. Thus all clinicians should be able to assess a patient with acute abdominal pain. The site of the pain is usually helpful, but it is diffuse or atypical in at least 25% of patients with acute gastrointestinal pathology. It is useful to determine whether movement or coughing aggravate the pain as occurs in appendicitis and generalized peritonitis (including perforated peptic ulcer and pancreatitis). Pain exacerbated by inspiration points to pathology in the upper abdomen (especially cholecystitis) or adjacent to the diaphragm. A detailed analysis of the type of pain is usually unhelpful but it is useful to know if it is intermittent, colicky, or constant. Some pain radiates in a characteristic manner—urological (loin-to-groin), gynaecological (to the back or thigh), and cholecystitis (to the shoulder tip). In contrast, the pain of appendicitis and diverticulitis does not radiate. The pain of intestinal obstruction is colicky and often associated with vomiting. Severe pain without physical signs and with normal routine tests (laboratory and simple radiological) raises the possibility of mesenteric vascular occlusion, especially in patients over the age of 50 years or those known to be at risk of thromboembolic disease.

First attacks of conditions causing recurrent abdominal pain such as acute porphyria and familial Mediterranean fever very occasionally enter the diagnostic spectrum of an 'acute' abdomen. In exacerbations of porphyria the pain is diffuse and severe and occur most frequently in the third decade with females being much more frequently affected than males. Tenderness is almost always absent but tachycardia and anxiety are prominent. During the attack the urine will contain excess δ-aminolaevulinic acid and, usually, porphobilinogen.

Upper abdominal pain

Pain in the upper abdomen has been considered under the heading dyspepsia. Upper abdominal discomfort is so common that its presence alone is of no value in distinguishing between those patients with organic disease and those with a functional disorder. Moreover patients with an irritable bowel, diverticular disease, and occasionally with other colonic pathology may have discomfort in the centre of the abdomen which they may describe as indigestion. In such circumstances there is usually also a history of some change in bowel habit that will indicate the true nature of the condition. Disease in the small intestine is proportionately rather uncommon and is frequently misdiagnosed as an irritable bowel. Symptoms are rarely specific but should be reinterpreted in the light of screening investigations (such as the blood count, a straight radiograph of the abdomen, and assessment of serum markers of inflammatory disease).

Lower abdominal pain

With lower abdominal pain analysis of symptoms often does not help to determine the cause. Indeed, inflammatory and neoplastic colonic disorders often may not give rise to pain and when pain does occur, it is usually diffuse and central. However, focal pain and tenderness in the left iliac fossa often indicates diverticulitis and, more rarely, colonic cancer. Focal pain in the right iliac fossa may be a marker of Crohn's ileocaecal disease. The passage of stool or flatus will often relieve the pain of colonic disease and an irritable bowel; in contrast, it tends to exacerbate the pain of local rectal conditions. A history of recent-onset lower abdominal pain in patients over the age of 40 years is an indication for prompt investigation.

The pelvis should be examined in patients with deep-seated lower abdominal pain. If pathology is present it is usually gynaecological, but it may be in the intestine, especially the appendix and distal colon.

Proctalgia fugax is a very painful paroxysmal perineal pain occurring unexpectedly often at night and may last for up to half an hour. The pathogenesis is uncertain and it is unassociated with any signs of disease. The condition is often recurrent but is self-limiting.

Irritable bowel

'Irritable bowel' is a common diagnosis in young adult patients, especially women. The symptoms are variable but usually comprise nonspecific abdominal discomfort especially cramping pain eased by the passing of wind, abdominal 'bloating', an irregular bowel habit and perhaps a sensation of incomplete defecation. There are often nonspecific associated symptoms such as headache and tiredness.

Altered bowel habit

The general public knows well what is meant by 'an attack of diarrhoea' or 'being constipated' but these conditions are not easy to define in medical terms. First, one must recognize that to a lay person, constipation means passing a stool less often than normal and usually with difficulty. But 'normal' may be anything from two or three times a day to two or three times a week. Moreover the mass and consistency of a normal stool varies considerably, depending on diet, gender, and individual factors. Subjects eating a Western diet pass 80 to 200 g of stool each day, with more women at the lower end of this range. To add to the difficulty of assessing bowel function, the frequency of bowel habit may bear no relation to the volume of faecal material passed nor to the amount of stool in the colon. Thus care must be taken to define exactly what is happening and it is advisable to take the commonsense view that a change in normal bowel habit is the significant issue. Two warnings are appropriate: first, most people are loath to mention incontinence (they will usually say that they have diarrhoea and will have to be asked specifically about soiling); secondly in those with persistent unexplained diarrhoea, it is best to examine the stool because patients' descriptions of their faeces are rarely informative.

Diarrhoea

The clinician needs to understand some basic gastrointestinal physiology in order to understand the mechanisms of diarrhoea and to make sense of a patient's symptoms (Table 15.2.1). Most cases of diarrhoea can be diagnosed quite simply from the history,

an examination of the stools, and, when appropriate, direct examination of the rectal mucosa. Acute infective diarrhoea is recognized by its recent onset, sometimes preceded by nausea or vomiting and a general systemic upset. Abdominal pain often occurs with *Campylobacter* infection, and although passage of blood and mucus can occur with any severe infection, it is more common with *Shigellosis* and infection with *E. coli* 0157.

In assessing chronic or recurrent diarrhoea, it is worth trying to distinguish diarrhoea of large bowel origin from that of the small intestine. Large-bowel diarrhoea characteristically occurs on rising, may be associated with pain which is relieved by defecation, and often contains mucus and sometimes red blood. The differential diagnosis usually rests between inflammation and neoplasm. Small-bowel diarrhoea occurs at any time, and although often watery, the stool may also contain excess fat. Steatorrhoea occurs in coeliac disease, pancreatic insufficiency, stagnant loop syndromes, and massive intestinal resection. Drugs (such as β-blockers, diuretics, antacids, and antibiotics) as well as excess intake of beer may also cause diarrhoea.

In assessing diarrhoea, that otherwise remains unexplained, a sensible first step is to test the effect of fasting. If the diarrhoea ceases, a dietary nutrient is like to be the cause—usually carbohydrate or fat—and the patient needs to be investigated for causes of malabsorption. If the diarrhoea persists one may assume that there is malabsorption of fluid secreted into the gut. This may be mediated by infection, gastrointestinal hormones, and bile salts. The astute physician must also be aware of the possibility of purgative abuse. Theoretically it is worth distinguishing between osmotic and secretory mechanisms. This is done by measuring the concentration of the major cations (sodium and potassium) and stool osmolality. If the measured osmolality is little more than the sum of the cations multiplied by two (to allow for the unmeasured anions), then the patient has a secretory diarrhoea. In contrast, if there is a significant osmolar gap then there must be another solute in the stool. However, in practice this not often used. The normal osmolar gap is difficult to define and diarrhoea in some of the more common conditions such as coeliac disease have both absorptive and secretory mechanisms.

Table 15.2.1 Salt and water absorption by the gastrointestinal tract

Site	Passage of fluid in 24 h	Concentration of Na⁺ in the lumen (mM)	Total Na⁺ received in 24 h (mmol)	Mucosal characteristics with respect to salt/water
Duodenum/ jejunum	7–8 litres	150	1000	Acts as semi-permeable membrane. Salt and water follows absorption of nutrients and bicarbonate
Ileum	? 2–3 litres	100–110		Active absorption of salt/water (chloride/ bicarbonate exchange)
Proximal colon	1.5 litres	100	160	Decreasing permeability. Active absorption of salt and water
Distal colon/ rectum	50–100 ml	40–50	3–5	Low permeability. Na/K exchange

Salt and water absorption is disturbed by: osmotic pressure from the gut (e.g. malabsorbed sugars/peptides; purgative salts); reduced mucosal permeability (mucosal enteropathies as in coeliac disease); reduced active absorption (e.g. by the small intestine in coeliac disease and by the large intestine in colitis); increased mucosal secretion (in response to bacterial toxins (e.g. cholera), inflammatory mediators (e.g. cytokines/leukotrienes), or neurohormonal mediators (as in a patient with aVIPoma); abnormal motility (e.g. diabetic autonomic neuropathy).

Box 15.2.1 Causes of constipation

- Poor diet (inadequate intake of poorly absorbed carbohydrate)
- Functional disorders (slow transit constipation, 'outlet obstruction' constipation—see Fig. 15.2.1)
- Failure to respond to rectal distension (bed-bound patients, some psychiatric patients)
- Extrinsic disorders of colonic innervation especially to sacral outflow
- Intrinsic neurological pathology: Hirschsprung's, diabetic neuropathy
- Chronic pseudo-obstruction (neuromuscular)
- Metabolic disorders, e.g. myxoedema, hypercalcaemia
- Drugs: opiates, anticholinergics
- Obstructive: neoplasm, inflammatory (e.g. Crohn's disease)

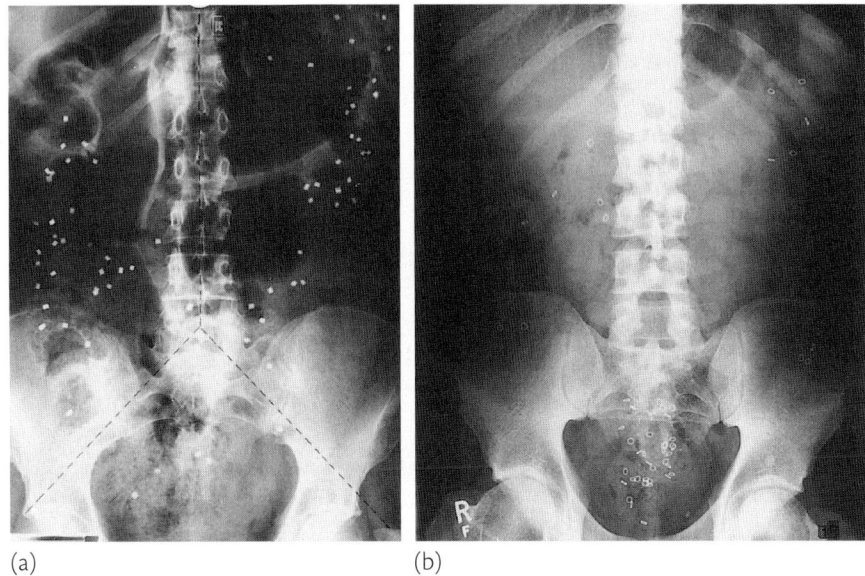

(a)   (b)

Fig. 15.2.1 Functional constipation illustrated by the use of markers (patient takes one marker capsule daily for 14 days, each capsule containing 10 radio-opaque pellets). (a) Abdominal radiograph of a 58-year-old woman with 'slow transit' constipation (colonic inertia). Seventy-three pellets were retained after 14 days, equally distributed between right and left colons (mean transit time 7.3 days, median normal for women 3.0 days). (b) Abdominal radiograph of a 30-year-old man who, a year previously, had an emergency laminectomy for an acute prolapsed disc. He complained of constipation since the operation and was shown to have 'outlet obstruction' presumably due to impaired rectoanal reflexes. Fifty-seven pellets were retained with 9 in the right colon, 9 in the left colon, and 39 in the rectosigmoid segment (mean transit time 5.7 days, median normal for men 2.3 days).
(Courtesy of Dr J H Cummings, MRC Microbiology and Gut Biology Group, University of Dundee. Figure 15.2.1a has been published previously in Misiewicz JJ, Pounder RE, Venables CW (eds) *Diseases of the gut and pancreas*, and is reprinted with permission of Blackwell Scientific Publications.)

The very rare cases of watery diarrhoea from birth indicate the need to investigate enzymes and transporters needed for nutrient absorption and ion exchange, and the presence and activity of enteroendocrine cells.

Constipation

Each year about 1% of the population consult their family doctor complaining of constipation. The mode of presentation ranges from the acute onset of colonic obstruction to a lifelong disability. The most common causes of constipation are shown in Box 15.2.1. In taking a clinical history it is important to determine exactly what the patient means by constipation. A relatively sudden change in bowel habit without any significant change in dietary habit or medication suggests an organic disorder. A desire to defecate, especially if associated with colicky discomfort, suggests organic obstruction. Constipation from a young age, increasing slowly with time, indicates a disorder of normal colonic function, a condition that is much more common in women than men. Colon physiologists distinguish between 'slow transit' and 'outlet obstruction' constipation (Fig. 15.2.1) but this distinction is of limited value in management. 'Low fibre' diets (as ingested by many young people living away from the family home for the first time), some drugs (especially opiates and drugs with anticholinergic activity such as antidepressants), metabolic disorders, and neurological disease must be considered—although in most cases no cause can be established. In women it is also necessary to consider the obstetric history and to consider the possibility of pelvic floor dysfunction. Straining at stool over a prolonged period may lead to rectal prolapse and incontinence and it may be necessary to ask the patient specifically about such symptoms.

Further reading

Binder HJ (2006). Causes of chronic diarrhea. *N Engl J Med*, **355**, 236–9.

Feldman M, Friedman LS, Brandt LJ (eds) (2006). *Sleisenger and Fordtran's gastrointestinal and liver disease*, 8th edition, Vol. 1 Chapter 2. WB Saunders/Elsevier, Philadelphia, PA. [Latest version of this leading textbook.]

Longstreth GF (2006). Functional dyspepsia—managing the conundrum. *N Engl J Med*, **354**, 701–3. [A well-balanced paper, with useful references, on a condition that depends on the careful assessment of symptomatology.]

Yamada T, *et al.* (2005). *Handbook of gastroenterology*. Lippincott, Williams and Wilkins, Philadelphia, PA. [Contains the essential information from Yamada's exceptionally comprehensive textbook.]

Methods for investigation of gastrointestinal disease

Contents

15.3.1 Colonoscopy and flexible sigmoidoscopy

Christopher B. Williams and Brian P. Saunders

Essentials

Colonoscopy and flexible sigmoidoscopy are techniques for visualizing the lumen of the large bowel. In expert hands, after appropriate explanation to the patient (which increases the chances of the procedure being well tolerated), bowel preparation, and (usually) some form of 'conscious sedation', then total colonoscopy is possible in 98 to 99% of cases in the absence of obstruction, a severely ulcerated colon, or other contraindication.

The indications for colonoscopy are wide and constantly expanding, and are likely to continue to do so until alternative less invasive techniques ('virtual colonoscopy' or genetic tests) are perfected. Common indications include patients with or requiring: (1) bleeding, anaemia, or occult blood loss; (2) chronic diarrhoea or known inflammatory bowel disease, which is accurately and easily assessed by endoscopy and biopsy; (3) polyps that can be removed endoscopically; (4) surveillance for cancer prevention. Abnormalities found by other diagnostic methods frequently turn out to be spurious when checked colonoscopically. Findings such as anastomotic strictures, typically after Crohn's resection, are usually easily and effectively dilated by the endoscopist using a 'through the scope' balloon.

Flexible sigmoidoscopy is the best means of examining the bowel proximal to the rectosigmoid junction (the distal rectum and anal canal are well seen with a rigid instrument).

Introduction

Colonoscopes range from 60 to 70 cm flexible sigmoidoscopes or thin, very flexible paediatric instruments also used in adults with fixation or stricturing, up to 165 cm colonoscopes with different flexibility characteristics and instrumentation channel sizes. Further technical improvements include higher resolution, zoom magnification, better control ergonomics, adjustable shaft flexibility, image enhancement, and magnetic imaging of shaft loops without fluoroscopy. Ultrasound colonoscopes, thin ultrasound probes for use with conventional instruments, and other more advanced technologies are available in specialist centres. Experimental efforts continue in the quest to develop self-propelled colonoscopes.

A large range of accessories can be introduced through the suction/instrumentation channel of a colonoscope, including biopsy or grasping forceps; washing, spraying or deflation tubes; cytology brushes; and injection needles. Therapeutic accessories include insulated forceps, polypectomy snares and retrieval devices, cutting wires, coagulating probes and argon plasma coagulating catheters, laser light guides, haemostatic clip and nylon loop applicators, dilating balloons, and metal stent introducers. Experimentation continues on the long-established principle of having an external 'overtube' in place beforehand which can be slid inwards to control problematic shaft looping. CO_2 insufflation apparatus is also available which, since the gas is exhaled within 10 to 15 min, ensures that patients are not left distended after the procedure.

Cleaning and disinfection

As for all flexible endoscopes, skilled maintenance, regular checks, and meticulous cleaning are essential. All parts, including air, water, and instrumentation channels must be accessed during cleaning. It is not possible to sterilize a colonoscope but scrupulous mechanical cleaning and 'high-level disinfection' rapidly inactivate viral agents (including HIV and hepatitis B) and bacteria. However, mycobacterial spores require prolonged disinfection agents and may be present in AIDS patients, thus mandating invariably high standards of disinfection. Even with purpose-built washing machines, designed to perfuse the various channels of an endoscope, it can take up to an hour to clean and disinfect an instrument, so multiple colonoscopes are required to provide a routine service. Most accessories such as biopsy forceps or polypectomy snares are 'single use' disposables but any others require equally rigorous cleaning and autoclave sterilization or high-level disinfection.

Patient preparation

Psychological preparation of the patient should not be forgotten, since most of those scheduled for colonoscopy are apprehensive, whether through embarrassment, expected discomfort, or fear of colorectal cancer. Explanatory literature and a friendly telephone manner at the time of booking the exam can help a great deal. Equally, a warm and reassuring atmosphere on reception, while obtaining 'informed consent', and also during the procedure, can help transform colonoscopy from an ordeal into a reasonable and well-tolerated experience.

Flexible sigmoidoscopy preparation is normally by disposable enema (hypertonic phosphate or similar) given or self-administered 10 to 15 min before the procedure. Some patients prefer to avoid the indignity of an enema by taking full oral preparation and this is also advisable in any patient with a colon narrowed by pronounced diverticulosis or stricturing.

Full bowel preparation is usually the most unpleasant part of colonoscopy. Oral preparation must be preceded by dietary restrictions, which include stopping iron or constipating agents in the preceding days and a low-fibre diet (with no nuts, mushrooms, or iron-containing red wine) for at least 24 h.

Fluid overload is the commonest approach, usually achieved by ingestion of 3 to 4 litres of isotonic polyethylene glycol (PEG)–electrolyte solution, which avoids electrolyte losses. Various commercial PEG–electrolyte combinations exist, flavoured and packaged for posting. However, up to 10% of patients become nauseated, vomit, or become distended and stop drinking, which can result in poor preparation, especially in the proximal colon. A hypertonic phosphate solution is available, easier to drink and generally preferred, but with a bitter taste disliked by some patients.

Purgative preparation is a very cheap and well-tolerated alternative, although a few individuals can suffer cramping, incontinence, or vasovagal reaction. After the dietary restrictions described above and senna or bisacodyl tablets on the afternoon before examination, a litre of isotonic osmotic laxative (commonly magnesium citrate) is drunk followed by other clear fluids to taste (including alcohol in moderation). Drinking continues up to the time of the procedure to avoid solidification in the proximal colon, which can result in adherent residue, difficult to flush or aspirate.

If there is any possibility that the patient is obstructed, full oral preparation is contraindicated because of the possibility of perforation; a smaller volume should be given, supplemented by enemas. In the presence of massive bleeding it may be preferable to proceed directly to colonoscopy, relying on the purgative effect of blood rather than wasting time on preparation. Nasal-tube lavage is an alternative compromise before emergency colonoscopy (with the angiography team alerted in case adequate views prove impossible).

Medication

There is surprisingly wide variation around the world in attitudes to colonoscopy. In certain countries with enough anaesthetists available (France, Australia) propofol anaesthesia is routinely employed. In others (Japan, China) and many institutions in Scandinavia, Germany or northern Italy, unsedated colonoscopy is the norm. Fashions and opinions change and the trend is to some form of medication.

'Conscious sedation' is offered to most patients in the United Kingdom, unless they are likely to be easy to examine (flexible sigmoidoscopy, previously easy examination, male gender, sigmoid resection, or stoma) or are motivated to manage without medication in order to leave rapidly afterwards or to drive home. To generalize, women have longer colons and are more likely to suffer without sedation. The unpleasant gnawing quality of 'visceral pain' caused by the inevitable stretching of colon or attachments during insertion is, in a tolerant patient, quite manageable for a few spells of 20 to 30 s. However, prolonged examinations or the sensitivity of patients with irritable bowel syndrome can be much helped by a minimal dose of a sedative–analgesic combination. Combining a low dose of benzodiazepine (typically, midazolam 2–3 mg, intravenously), with an opiate analgesic (pethidine 25–50 mg, intravenously) reduces discomfort and anxiety and gives the patient a well-deserved feeling of euphoria. Low-level sedation of this kind does not inhibit conversation or the ability to complain of pain or to change position when necessary. Smaller doses should be given in older or sick patients but incremental larger doses (especially opiates) can be needed in apprehensive younger ones. Pulse oximetry monitoring and nasal oxygen is routine, resuscitation equipment, and reversal agents (flumazenil, naloxone) should be immediately accessible. Sedated patients should be accompanied home.

General anaesthesia is rarely needed and, we believe, generally best avoided. An unconscious patient cannot change position spontaneously and removal of the warning given by pain may tend to more aggressive technique. However, physician-administered 'propofol sedation' is increasingly advocated in the United States of America and Germany and undoubtedly, in patients with particular reasons for anaesthesia, propofol gives excellent results with rapid recovery compared to high doses of conventional sedation.

Antispasmodics are decried by many on the basis that they are thought to elongate the colon and make insertion more difficult. Randomized trial shows this to be untrue and we routinely use hysocine-N-butyl bromide to speed insertion and optimize the view.

Antibiotics are only given to those with immunosuppression or immunodepression, previous endocarditis, heart valve prosthesis, septal defects, recent vascular prosthesis, or ascites.

Flexible sigmoidoscopy

Flexible sigmoidoscopy is the kindest and most logical means of examining proximal to the rectosigmoid junction (15 cm), whereas the distal rectum and anal canal are well, and in skilled hands often better, seen with a rigid instrument. In the presence of severe diverticular disease it may be impossible to reach even mid-sigmoid without expertise and a thin endoscope. After hysterectomy it may be cruel to examine without sedation. For this reason, although flexible sigmoidoscopy is both better tolerated and more accurate and effective than aggressive, rigid proctosigmoidoscopy, depth of insertion should be limited to what is tolerable by the individual patient. Some endoscopists mistakenly attempt to 'reach the splenic flexure' routinely. Without fluoroscopy or magnetic endoscope imaging, even expert endoscopists can be completely mistaken between sigmoid-descending junction and splenic flexure. At 60 cm of insertion the tip of the instrument can be anywhere between mid-sigmoid and hepatic flexure, and there are no positive localizing landmarks.

Insertion usually follows digital lubrication with jelly, the blunt tip of the instrument being inserted as the sphincters relax. Thereafter the instrument is coaxed in, as gently as possible, without haste or force, steering and 'corkscrewing' around bends with twisting movements. Forceful insertion with 'red-out', guesswork, or blind 'push through' are all avoided as far as possible. Any small polyps (up to 5 mm) that may be adenomas are normally snared or destroyed at once, as they may be difficult to see on withdrawal (when the colon has been shortened and convoluted) or if left for subsequent colonoscopy. Because of the remote possibility of explosive gas concentrations after limited preparation, either repeated suction with air reinflation or use of CO_2 should precede electrosurgery; alternatively, 'cold snaring' with physical removal of the polyp can be employed. If in doubt a biopsy can be taken, both to give some idea of the size of any lesion against the open forceps and to give partial histology.

Total colonoscopy

In expert hands, and in the absence of obstruction, a severely ulcerated colon, or other contraindication, total colonoscopy is possible in 98 to 99% of cases, with little sedation or suffering and virtually no complications. In less expert hands 'total colonoscopy' or 'completion' rates as low as 75% have been reported. The principal difference in technique between expert and inexpert is the ability, while keeping sufficient orientation for steering purposes, to pull back and crumple the segment of colon already traversed, and simultaneously straighten the way or bend ahead. The ideal is to keep the colonoscope as straight as possible and to pleat or 'concertina' the colon over it, avoiding the unnecessary loops and pain caused by pushing too hard or too long. The ideal is not always immediately achievable, so patience and determination—tempered by humanity—are essential qualities for the colonoscopist.

Paradoxically, a freely mobile colon, without the conventionally fixed segments in the descending and ascending parts, can be as difficult to traverse as one with adhesions. This is principally because atypical loops may form, sometimes uncontrollable until the instrument tip eventually reaches a fixed point, which gives a 'hold' and allows the shaft to be straightened back. Happily, this type of long and mobile colon, although a nightmare for the endoscopist, typically also has long attachments so that the patient experiences little discomfort.

From the point of view of the patient, colonoscope stretch discomfort is felt as 'wind pain', rapidly relieved as soon as the causative loop can be straightened. True overdistension is easily removed by aspiration. Further distress may be produced by the unpleasant illusion of incontinence when the body-warmed and lubricated shaft is withdrawn through the sensitive anal canal; it is kind to warn the patient of this phenomenon in advance, and to preserve decorum by aspirating any fluid found during insertion through the rectosigmoid.

Once the colonoscope has successfully passed into the descending colon and has been straightened back to remove sigmoid colon looping, it is likely that the rest of the insertion phase will be considerably easier. When the colonoscope shaft is straight it feels responsive and free, as do the angling controls: the more looped the colonoscope is, the more 'snarled up' everything becomes, and the more the patient suffers. Avoiding looping and responding to pain are the basis for successful, kind, and safe insertion. Good technique also minimizes instrument repair bills and maximizes accuracy and ease of targeting lesions, since a straight instrument handles better.

This practical philosophy underlies the reason for simple but effective 'tricks of the trade' such as position change. It is obvious that in left lateral position there will be pooling of any fluid in the left colon; the transverse colon will also tend to sag down and so make the splenic flexure more acute. It therefore follows that, where there is a poor view or difficulty in insertion, position change may improve matters (to supine or right lateral at the splenic, but back to left lateral again for the hepatic flexure). Adding only the simple principles of pulling back as often as possible to straighten each loop before tackling the next, avoiding overdistension to keep the bowel reasonably deflated and supple, and trying hand pressure from an assistant whenever an unavoidable loop may be accessible (sigmoid and transverse colon), the art of colonoscopy is explained. Insensitivity, impatience, or aggression results in the endoscopist being too muscular and tense to handle the shaft and controls sensitively, and so more likely to cause needless looping, pain, failure, and complications.

Contraindications, risks, and limitations

There are few contraindications to colonoscopy. It is, however, a relatively strong vasovagal assault with potential for arrhythmias and so is contraindicated for 2 to 3 months after myocardial infarction. The tip, shaft, and air pressure involved in insertion have potential to exacerbate any existing risk of perforation. Colonoscopy is thus contraindicated in the acute phase and 2 weeks after an episode of diverticulitis and in severe acute or deeply ulcerated colitis of any variety (ulcerative, Crohn's, ischaemic or infective). Patients with acute localized or rebound tenderness of the abdomen, free air, or dilated colon on radiograph should not be submitted to colonoscopy without special reason, due consultation, and by an expert endoscopist—who may decide to abandon the procedure.

The risks of diagnostic colonoscopy, as implied above, are to a great extent related to the training, personality, and manual skills of the endoscopist. Regrettably, large-scale audit shows figures of around 1 perforation in 1500 examinations, whereas in specialist centres complications are exceedingly rare. The overall figures can be justified by the avoidance of the morbidity and mortality of surgery. Therapy inevitably increases the likelihood of complications, principally bleeding but occasionally perforation after polypectomy or dilatation. Perforation may be actual (perhaps needing surgery) or threatened as the 'postpolypectomy syndrome' (managed conservatively with rest and antibiotics). Immediate bleeding can occur in around 1% of polypectomies but is usually easily stopped by submucosal adrenaline injection (5–20 ml of 1/10 000 dilution, which is safe because of portal drainage) or by local electrocoagulation, clipping, or nylon loop application. Delayed haemorrhage can occur up to 10 to 14 days after removal or local coagulation of even small polyps; it is usually self-limiting, but can be substantial and require admission to hospital and transfusion. Aspirin is no longer considered a risk factor but antiplatelet agents such as clopidogrel should be stopped for a week before and after polypectomy. Anticoagulants should similarly be discontinued or special measures instituted.

The greatest causes of colonoscopy-related mortality (1 in 10 000 examinations) are patients referred (not always correctly) for surgery following endoscopic complications and deaths directly due to oversedation, usually in older people. There have been unnecessary deaths when an physician has persisted in conservative management without involving a surgeon in management of suspected perforation. Surgical fatalities or major morbidity have resulted in others found at operation to have sustained only a point perforation, which would clearly have sealed spontaneously. In managing suspected perforation, due consultation between endoscopist and an endoscopically aware, preferably laparoscopy oriented, surgeon is essential. The endoscopist should not be too proud to abandon an examination which is proving unreasonable, rather than to 'flatten' the patient with extra sedation; it is safer and kinder to change to CT colography ('virtual colonoscopy') to image the unexamined proximal colon during the same visit.

The major limitations of colonoscopy relate to the fact that it is dependent on manual skills and that tortuous, angulated, and haustrated colonic anatomy results in some blind spots for the endoscopist. Areas that the endoscopist sees are extremely accurately evaluated, with a resolution of less than 1 mm. The percentage of mucosa unseen is uncertain but is probably around 10 to 15% overall. The likelihood of larger and 'significant' lesions being missed is much lower than this because colonic neoplasms are usually protuberant. Paradoxically, pathology can be missed in the capacious distal rectum or the anal canal, which can be avoided by retroverting the endoscope and/or examining with a rigid proctoscope as well.

Indications

The indications for colonoscopy are wide and constantly expanding, and are likely to continue to do so until alternative less invasive techniques (virtual colonoscopy or genetic tests) are perfected. Where there is a shortage of endoscopic personnel, skill, or facilities it is possible to reduce the load of total colonoscopy by cross-referring for CT imaging. It is also possible to combine CT with prior flexible sigmoidoscopy on the same visit, on the basis that limited colonoscopy covers the highest yield area, which is also the most prone to missed diagnosis or overdiagnosis.

High-yield indications include patients with bleeding, anaemia, or occult blood loss. Persistent bleeding, especially if dark or mixed in with the stool, is of sinister import, although it may be due only to local mucosal traumatization in diverticular disease. Good clinicians may select out for sigmoidoscopy patients with obviously fresh bleeding on defecation or with spotting on toilet paper. However, the presence of blood in a patient aged 50 years or more (so at risk for colorectal neoplasia) is increasingly used as an excuse for the reassurance of a whole-colon screening examination. Of all patients with blood loss referred for colonoscopy, around 10% will have a 'significant' lesion, either a neoplastic polyp of 1 cm diameter or greater or malignancy. Colonoscopy is considered the investigation of choice for major bleeding, being readily available and offering immediate therapy and a high degree of diagnostic accuracy. Angiodysplasia, small ectatic vascular lesions in the proximal colon of older people with bleeding or anaemia, is relatively rare but is an example of a condition easily diagnosed and treated by colonoscopy.

Chronic diarrhoea or known inflammatory disease is accurately and easily assessed by endoscopy and biopsy. The terminal ileum can be accessed in more than 80% of cases by an experienced endoscopist. Endoscopic differential diagnosis between the focal or aphthoid ulcers with intervening normal mucosa in Crohn's disease and the generally reddened surface of ulcerative colitis is easy and definitive in around 90% of cases. A few remain as 'indeterminate colitis' and differential diagnosis can be more difficult in severe or chronic cases. The possibility of infective colitis, including tuberculous or amoebic, must be borne in mind and extra specimens taken for microscopy and culture if in doubt. Biopsies typically show somewhat greater extent of inflammation than is visible to the eye, and so must be taken at intervals around the colon in any patient with bowel frequency to exclude 'microscopic colitis' or the related phenomenon of 'collagenous colitis'. Chronic inflammatory disease affecting more than one-half of the colon carries an increased long-term risk of cancer or mucosal dysplastic (precancerous) change, and so indicates intermittent surveillance from 8 to 10 years after onset of symptoms. Ischaemic colitis, typically affecting a short segment around the splenic flexure, can show changes ranging from mild reddening to marked ulceration or even near gangrene.

There are low-yield indications for colonoscopy, where alternative investigations such as flexible sigmoidoscopy or 'virtual colonoscopy' may be justified. These include patients with simple constipation of long standing, bloating, left iliac fossa discomfort, or combinations of these symptoms suggesting 'irritable bowel syndrome'. In many patients the extra accuracy and therapeutic potential of one-off colonoscopy may be justified. In older patients, however, the greater likelihood of diverticular disease and difficult (so more hazardous) colonoscopy is a disincentive compared to the rapidity and safety of scanning.

Polyps of almost any size can be removed endoscopically. Removal of very large sessile polyps in the distal rectum, for which transanal proctological management has been indicated, was traditionally not attempted by endoscopists but these are now manageable by endoscopic submucosal dissection (ESD), with superior view and greater safety. The place of laparoscopic removal or a combined approach for large sessile polyps in the proximal colon is in evolution. Otherwise even overtly malignant polyps or polypoid cancers with no adenoma present can be managed by endoscopy alone if complete removal is confirmed histologically (a margin of 1 mm between the limit of invasion and the plane of excision, and the tumour well or moderately differentiated). Around 5 to 10% of polyps will contain focal, high-grade dysplasia or invasive carcinoma but are endoscopically removable. Placing one or more Indian ink tattoos near a polypectomy site gives a permanent marker for endoscopic follow-up, or localizes it if surgery or laparoscopy become indicated by the histology results. Lasers were previously used for ablation of postpolypectomy remnants, but the alternative of argon plasma coagulation (APC) is cheaper, easier and safer.

Cancer prevention or surveillance colonoscopy gives a good guarantee to the patient, even when negative, both because of the accuracy of colonoscopy and the generally slow time-course of development of colonic neoplasms. Follow-up at 3 to 5-year intervals after polypectomy yields further (usually small) adenomas in 30 to 50% of patients, especially those with three or more, or large, polyps on the initial examination. There is reasonable evidence to suggest that the incidence of colorectal cancer is significantly reduced by polypectomy and follow-up, but occasional breakthrough cancers occur and any bleeding or suggestive symptoms should be reported. Patients at genetic risk merit colonoscopic surveillance, especially those with a first-degree relative with colorectal cancer under 45 years of age, two or more affected first-degree relatives, or those assessed genetically as belonging to a hereditary non-polyposis colon cancer (HNPCC) family with autosomal dominant risk (see Chapter 14.15). Follow-up, ablating minute or 'flat' adenomas, is scheduled at intervals of 1 to 5 years according to perceived individual risk.

Abnormalities found on other diagnostic methods, when checked colonoscopically, frequently turn out to be spurious—presumably faecal. The majority of positive occult blood tests prove to be false positive for neoplasm. Other findings, such as anastomotic strictures, typically after Crohn's resection, are usually easily and effectively dilated by the endoscopist using a 'through the scope' balloon. Even patients with typical malignant 'applecore' strictures should ideally have preoperative total colonoscopy to exclude other synchronous neoplasms, if necessary using a small-diameter instrument (sometimes a paediatric gastroscope). If this proves impossible, endoscopy should be rescheduled within 6 months after resection. Colonoscopy has effectively supplanted diagnostic laparotomy and avoids the numerous resections previously performed for diverticular disease when the radiologist 'could not exclude the possibility of malignancy'—which the endoscopist can achieve in a few minutes.

Cost-effectiveness and relationship to other techniques

Flexible endoscopy seems superficially expensive and is demanding of professional time. However, modern colonoscopes are surprisingly robust and, properly handled and maintained, will perform thousands of examinations without expensive repairs.

Newer teaching methods, including use of computer simulation and imaging techniques that do not use X-rays, should help to improve manual skills and instrument handling and speed up the training and assessment of doctors or nurse practitioners performing colonoscopy or flexible sigmoidoscopy. There has been shown to be considerable variation between endoscopists in picking up adenomas, so quality control is desirable.

Flexible endoscopy leaves only gas (air or CO_2) in the colon, and can immediately be followed by scanning if incomplete. Total colonoscopy, its accuracy increasing to near microscopic levels with newer and more agile instruments, is likely to remain the diagnostic 'gold standard' for the foreseeable future. However, evolving newer methods such as virtual colonoscopy by scanning will be more acceptable to some patients and so have an invaluable role in screening and selection, in spite of their lack of tissue diagnosis or therapy. Since endoscopy can check an abnormal scan immediately, it is quite likely that colonoscopy will lose some of its present front-line diagnostic role. Nonetheless it is equally likely that requirements for colonoscopy will increase overall as population screening for colorectal cancer prevention becomes an accepted routine.

Further reading

Waye, Rex, Williams (eds) (2009). Colonosopy–principles and practice. Wiley-Blackwell.

15.3.2 **Upper gastrointestinal endoscopy**

Adrian R.W. Hatfield

Essentials

Flexible fibre optic endoscopes were developed in the mid-1960s, leading to the growth of gastrointestinal endoscopy as we now know it. The recent availability of cheaper, miniaturized colour chips has led to the development of video endoscopes, providing an excellent clear view that does not deteriorate with age (as it does with fibre optic devices). With improvements in software, the endoscopic video image can be magnified: modern instruments will zoom up to 25 × magnification, and mucosal detail can also be enhanced electronically so that small lesions a few millimetres in size can be seen quite clearly. The modern video endoscope image can be instantly printed out and archived digitally on a computer system.

Endoscopy has now become the investigation of choice in patients with retrosternal or upper abdominal symptoms where barium radiology would previously have been employed. The advantages of detecting grades of inflammation and erosive change, rather than radiologically obvious ulceration, are obvious. Equally, the ability to take samples from the gastrointestinal tract with brush cytology or biopsy greatly enhances the diagnostic accuracy, not just in differentiating between benign and malignant ulcers and strictures, but also in assessing degrees of inflammatory change and in detecting dysplasia, e.g. in Barrett's oesophagus.

Endoscopy is essential in significant gastrointestinal bleeding to identify and—in many cases—treat the cause, with various therapeutic methods possible for erosions, ulcers, and oesophageal varices.

More recent developments in the practice of upper gastrointestinal endoscopy include the use of enteroscopy for direct vision of the jejunum, video capsule endoscopy for diagnosis of obscure bleeding lesions, and an impressively useful range of therapeutic techniques including laser therapy. Endoscopic retrograde cholangiopancreatography (ERCP) is useful for the diagnosis and noninvasive removal of gallstones from the common bile duct.

In a wider perspective, upper gastrointestinal endoscopy has had a driving role in the development of the specialty of gastroenterology as a result of the imaginative application of techniques and applied physics to common medical conditions affecting hitherto inaccessible regions of the abdomen and its hollow viscera.

Development

The external specifications and handling of the new video endoscopes are similar to their earlier fibre optic counterparts and thus the techniques for disinfection and endoscopy are similar for both ranges of equipment. The disadvantage of the modern equipment is that the video endoscopy system needs considerable hardware. In most instances a video monitor, light source, and processor are located in an endoscopy unit and are not so easily moved to a different location such as the intensive therapy unit or operating theatre for emergency endoscopy. In the acutely bleeding patient, the presence of excessive blood in the lumen of the gastrointestinal tract diminishes the efficiency of the video processing so that the image obtained may be unsatisfactory.

The latest type of high-definition endoscope, processor, and monitor can be used for two new techniques, narrow band imaging (NBI) and autofluorescent imaging (AFI). NBI uses the properties of short-wavelength light of two different wavelengths to enhance the visualization of capillaries in the superficial mucosa and vessels deeper in the mucosa. These are seen as two different colours, which enhances the visualization and diagnosis of otherwise poorly identifiable lesions. AFI utilizes the property of short-wave light in the blue area of the spectrum to elicit a green fluorescence from normal mucosa. Thickening of the mucosa by malignant infiltration tends to inhibit this and abnormal tissue may fluoresce less, allowing for endoscopic detection of submucosal abnormality.

Endoscopy units and disinfection techniques

It is now well recognized that the care of the instruments and other equipment, together with the important aspects of patient safety, are greatly improved by having a purpose-built endoscopy unit staffed by experienced endoscopic nursing staff who are trained in handling and disinfecting endoscopes and in patient safety during and after intravenous sedation.

Most endoscopy units have a purpose-built disinfecting machine which can take single or multiple instruments. After suitable mechanical cleaning, a disinfecting agent will be automatically pumped through the channels of the instrument for a given period of time and flushed out afterwards. The choice of disinfecting agent varies between units but the trend has been away from hazardous agents such as glutaraldehyde (Cidex) to less harmful agents, such as Nu-Cidex or Tristel, that do not need sophisticated extraction and ventilation.

For routine, simple diagnostic upper gastrointestinal endoscopy many patients are now routinely endoscoped without sedation, after local anaesthesia to the throat only. 'No sedation endoscopy' is suitable for busy units with long lists of day cases. However, large numbers of endoscopies, particularly in apprehensive or sick inpatients and those needing more complicated procedures, are still performed under intravenous sedation.

There are now clear guidelines, such as those drawn up by the British Society of Gastroenterology, for the practice of administering intravenous sedation for endoscopic procedures. Patients are now monitored with pulse oximetry and oxygen is given routinely to ill or elderly patients, and to other patients if oxygen saturation falls during the procedure. The precise choice of sedation varies between units and will depend on the patient and the type of procedure performed; however, diazempam and midazolam remain the two most common sedative agents used, often combined with pethidine for more lengthy or invasive procedures. It is not uncommon to reverse the effect of the benzodiazepine sedation with flumazenil and any opiate sedation with naloxone. On rare occasions general anaesthesia will need to be used for endoscopy, usually for children or adults with ventilatory problems. There is an increasing trend in some countries, but not yet to any major extent in the UK, for complex procedures to be performed under propofol anaesthesia. Specially trained anaesthetic nurses can be trained to administer this.

Specific risk of infection with endoscopy

In the past patients with heart murmurs were routinely given antibiotics to cover endoscopic procedures. It is now recommended that only patients with prosthetic valves need be given routine prophylactic antibiotic cover, with a single parenteral dose of a broad-spectrum penicillin before the procedure.

Current disinfecting agents and schedules will cope with hepatitis B and C and HIV infection. All endoscopic staff wear disposable gloves and the nurse nearest the patient's mouth will usually wear a visor to cover eyes, nose, and mouth, particularly with a patient of known infective risk. As there is no effective way of sterilizing an endoscope against prions (at present thought to be the transmissible agent in Creutzfeldt–Jakob disease), the current United Kingdom Department of Health guidelines make it clear that all equipment used on patients with suspected Creutzfeldt–Jakob disease should be quarantined afterwards and if the diagnosis were proven at a later date, only used thereafter on patients with Creutzfeldt–Jakob disease. Patients with suspected Creutzfeldt–Jakob disease should therefore not be endoscoped and alternative ways of diagnosis or treatment should be sought.

Diagnostic endoscopy in the gastrointestinal tract

In recent years, it has become routine to take gastric biopsies in patients with peptic problems to detect the presence of *Helicobacter pylori*. The routine use of a simple CLO test, where mucosal biopsies are inserted into a gelatin well containing a colouring agent that turns yellow to red in the presence of helicobacter urease, will be satisfactory. In some patients with infection resistant to multiple eradication therapies, gastric biopsies are necessary in this situation for culturing the bacteria to ascertain sensitivity. In younger patients where malignant disease is less of a concern, serum, faecal, or breath test analysis is an acceptable alternative to establishing helicobacter infection and thus such patients could be treated initially without endoscopy and gastric biopsy.

Most gastric cancers in the United Kingdom are diagnosed when the patient is symptomatic and thus the finding of a mucosal cancer is rare. Most lesions are straightforward to diagnose endoscopically and biopsies are usually confirmatory. Cancers that infiltrate the wall of the stomach below the mucosa are difficult to diagnose endoscopically as endoscopic biopsies are usually quite superficial. In this situation a 'double punch' type technique is useful, where a second biopsy is taken from the deeper submucosa through the small defect of the first biopsy. Linitis plastica is difficult to assess endoscopically, particularly where anticholinergic and other agents may have been used routinely to inhibit peristalsis at the start of the endoscopy. In such patients, a barium meal may help in the diagnosis by showing the lack of gastric motility.

Small bowel endoscopy (enteroscopy)

For many years, routine upper gastrointestinal endoscopes were not of sufficient length to pass beyond the duodenojejunal flexure into the small bowel. Enteroscopes are now made that can be advanced under direct vision down the upper small intestine or, alternatively, a thinner endoscope is allowed to pass down the small bowel spontaneously with the help of an inflated balloon and then the bowel lumen is visualized on withdrawal. Such endoscopic procedures are lengthy and difficult and will not necessarily view the entire small bowel. A more comprehensive view is sometimes obtained, particularly in the hunt for obscure bleeding lesions, by passing a standard upper gastrointestinal endoscope up and down the small intestine through small enterotomies at the time of laparotomy, with a surgeon concertina-ing the small bowel over the shaft of the endoscope.

The rather lengthy, tedious, and unpredictable techniques of small bowel biopsy using a Crosby capsule have been completely superseded by routine upper gastrointestinal endoscopy with biopsies from the distal duodenum. Such biopsies have been shown to be very representative of the upper jejunal mucosa. This technique is now used routinely in the diagnosis of coeliac disease.

Video capsule endoscopy of the small bowel

Over the last few years a new technique of visualizing the small intestine has been developed and, although expensive, is readily available. A small capsule containing a minute camera and transmitter can be swallowed by the patient or released at the time of endoscopy. Providing the small intestine has been cleared with a colonoscopy-type bowel preparation, the capsule transmits individual images of amazing clarity every 0.5 s to a receiver strapped on the abdomen. The capsule takes about 4 h to pass down the small intestine.

This technique is particularly useful in the detection of superficial mucosal lesions, such as angiodysplasia in difficult gastrointestinal bleeding or early Crohn's disease, that might otherwise be undetected by x-ray examination using barium contrast.

Therapeutic endoscopy in the upper gastrointestinal tract

Over the last 20 years, a wide range of therapeutic manoeuvres have been developed for use in various situations in the upper gastrointestinal tract.

Gastrointestinal bleeding

Oesophageal varices can be injected through the mucosa with ethanolamine oleate under direct vision. Paravasal injection is best avoided as it can lead to secondary bleeding from mucosal ulceration and sometimes later oesophageal stricture formation. Endoscopic sclerotherapy can be repeated at weekly or monthly intervals until the varices have been obliterated. Bleeding gastric varices can also be injected, but these are more difficult to obliterate. More recently, endoscopic banding techniques have been employed, both in the acutely bleeding patient and the chronic

situation. Single or multiple bands could be put on varices in the oesophagus or, sometimes, in the fundus of the stomach. The addition of thrombin into gastric varices after banding may enhance successful eradication and reduce the risk of bleeding if the bands slip off too early.

Bleeding erosions and ulcers can be injected with dilute adrenaline (1:10 000). This may be satisfactorily in reducing bleeding in the short term and can always be repeated if necessary. A similar effect can be obtained by the use of multicontact diathermy probes or heater probes. Bleeding vascular abnormalities, such as angiodysplasia, can be treated with thermal probes but more satisfactorily with noncontact laser which does not pull off a coagulum and has the extra benefit of destroying vessels just below the mucosa.

More recently argon photocoagulation (APC) has become available. A diathermy current in a beam of argon gas provides a safe and predictable way of coagulation without direct contact with the mucosa. Although more costly, it is more effective than simple touch diathermy devices and a very reasonable alternative to thermal laser coagulation.

Benign oesophageal strictures

Commonly, a peptic stricture above a hiatus hernia secondary to reflux will produce dysphagia but benign strictures due to other causes, such the swallowing of corrosive substances and postsurgical anastomotic strictures, can be treated by the same endoscopic techniques. In the past, bougies of increasing size were passed over a previously endoscopically placed guide wire and the stricture slowly dilated. More recently, high-pressure dilating balloon catheters, passed over the wire under radiological screening or directly through the scope under direct endoscopic vision, have been used. These are useful for short strictures, but there is still a place for over the wire bougies in very long strictures.

Achalasia of the cardia can be treated with balloon dilatation using a larger balloon of 30 to 40 mm diameter, where the aim is to rupture muscle fibres to weaken the circular muscle sphincter. Alternatively, botulinum toxin can be injected through the mucosa into the muscle sphincter circumferentially at the time of endoscopy. The improvement in swallowing after this procedure is limited and may need to be repeated every 6 months.

Malignant gastro-oesophageal strictures

Most patients with nonoperable tumours of the stomach or oesophagus producing dysphagia are palliated by the insertion of some sort of oesophageal stent. The older silicon rubber prostheses have been replaced by self-expanding metal stents which can be very easily and safely placed through a malignant stricture, often without the need for prior dilatation, thus reducing the risk of perforation. Most of these stents now have a membrane to prevent tumour ingrowth through the mesh but this will sometimes occur at one or either end. Such tumour overgrowth can be treated with endoscopic laser therapy. Brachytherapy can be given via an endoscopically sited tube through the stricture before or after stenting.

Postoperative anastomotic strictures after oesophagogastric resection, sometimes associated with a leak, can now be managed with membrane-covered self-expanding metal stents. The newer stents are potentially removable a few months later when the stricture and leak have sealed.

Removal of foreign objects

Most solid objects such as marbles, rings, and coins should pass spontaneously. The need for removing foreign bodies is usually because they are sharp and may cause damage if left *in situ*. Most objects can be snared or trapped in a basket and removed intact. Sharp objects can be pulled into a endoscopic overtube to protect the oesophagus from damage during removal.

Polyps and mucosal cancers

Most gastric polyps are entirely benign and do not need removing. Leiomyomas of the stomach or duodenum can be watched if small, but if ore than 5 cm in size should probably be removed.

Endoscopic mucosal resection (EMR)

Patients with larger mucosal tumours usually used to undergo open surgery but newer endoscopic techniques using submucosal resection can tackle lesions that do not infiltrate beyond the submucosa. Careful prior assessment with endoscopic ultrasound is usually needed to make sure that a small tumour can be technically removed in this way. Lesions can be elevated by the submucosal injection of saline and then removed intact or piecemeal, like polyps in the colon. This can be done for small mucosal cancers or dysplasic lesions in Barrett's oesophagus or similar lesions of the stomach, duodenum, or ampulla of Vater. Newer accessories with a suction cap and banding device, similar to that used with varices, allow the mucosal lesion to be trapped and removed with a snare without damage to the muscle layer and therefore without risk of perforation.

Laser therapy

Thermal coagulation with a YAG laser via a fibre under direct endoscopic vision has been used for many years as a complex but highly effective way of recanalizing tumour obstruction in the oesophagus, stomach, and colon. It is used less now with the widespread development of self-expanding metal stents to relieve luminal tumour obstruction.

Photodynamic laser therapy (PDT) has gained increasing popularity as the lasers used are considerably smaller and cheaper than those used for thermal coagulation. It is also easier to use and safer, and the fibre can be in contact with tissue. The technique is currently used in head and neck, oesophageal, and biliary tumours. After the administration of a photosensitizing drug, such as porfimer sodium, a low-power laser light can be passed down a diffuser fibre which can be endoscopically and radiologically positioned, sometimes inside a balloon to keep it centralized, particularly in the oesophagus, where it is also used for treating high-grade dysplasia in Barrett's oesophagus. An alternative to PDT in the latter situation is a radiofrequency (RF) probe that can be placed on the surface of an oesophageal balloon or clipped on the end of an endoscope.

Assisted nutrition

There are now many types of enteral feeding tube that can be sited in the upper gastrointestinal tract. Although most fine-bore feeding tubes can be passed on the ward or under radiological control, the prior passage into the stomach of an endoscopic guide wire that is then rerouted through the nose can allow feeding tubes to be positioned accurately, often through an oesophageal stricture or difficult anastomosis, or positioned in the duodenum in patients with gastric stasis. The endoscopic positioning of a nasojejunal feeding tube, beyond the duodenojejunal flexure, is now becoming a common alternative to intravenous feeding in patients with complicated pancreatitis where 'pancreatic rest' is needed.

Techniques for placing a gastrostomy tube endoscopically (percutaneous endoscopic gastrostomy, PEG) are now simple and straightforward. After transabdominal puncture into a distended stomach under direct endoscopic vision, a PEG tube with diameter from 8FG to 24FG can be pulled back down the oesophagus through the stomach and a flange, balloon, or button will allow the tube to be anchored firmly up against the gastric mucosa. In patients where there is gastric stasis or in pancreatitis a small jejunal extension tube can be inserted through the PEG tube and positioned endoscopically into the distal duodenum or beyond the duodenojejunal flexure (PEJ).

Endoscopic ultrasound

Special endoscopes are available with a dual capability of endoscopic and ultrasound imaging. Either a rotating or a fixed linear array transducer will provide an ultrasound image at a point where the endoscopist can accurately direct the probe in the lumen of the oesophagus, stomach, or duodenum. Although CT scanning will stage most larger tumours of the upper gastrointestinal tract, pancreas, and bile duct, endoscopic ultrasonography is particularly useful in staging small tumours and particularly mucosal tumours. The linear array ultrasound endoscope can be used for needle biopsy of tumours in the wall of the gastrointestinal tract or head of pancreas and sometimes lymph nodes, either adjacent to stomach, duodenum and increasingly in the mediastinum, through the oesophagus.

There is an increasing use of endoscopic ultrasonography in therapeutic procedures such as coeliac plexus block and endoscopic drainage of pancreatic pseudocysts.

Endoscopy and disorders of the pancreas and biliary tree

Diagnostic endoscopic retrograde cholangiopancreatography (ERCP)

The development of side-viewing duodenoscopes in the 1970s allowed endoscopic visualization of the papilla of Vater and cannulation of the pancreatic and biliary duct systems, endoscopic retrograde cholangiopancreatography (ERCP). For many years ERCP was the gold standard for investigating pancreatic and biliary disorders but, with the advent of CT and MRI scanning, the need for diagnostic ERCP has diminished. ERCP is still extremely useful in the diagnosis of patients with gallstones, sclerosing cholangitis, and biliary tumours where scanning is normal or equivocal, in the absence of overt jaundice. A tissue diagnosis can be obtained with brush cytology and endoscopic biopsy within the bile duct, avoiding the need for percutaneous biopsy.

Diagnostic ERCP is still useful in the assessment of patients with pancreatitis, congenital abnormalities, such as pancreas divisum, and in some patients with a pancreatic mass on scanning where the diagnosis is not clear. Most patients with a carcinoma of the pancreas will present with obstructive jaundice and will need a therapeutic procedure; others without jaundice will usually be diagnosed on ultrasound or CT scanning.

In specialized centres, biliary and pancreatic manometry is performed to assess patients with pancreatobiliary pain with no apparent structural abnormalities. At ERCP, a perfused catheter can be inserted into the bile duct and into the pancreatic duct and pull-through manometry performed. This will show whether elevated basal and peak pressures indicate dysfunction of the sphincter of Oddi.

Therapeutic ERCP
Gallstones
The endoscopic removal of common bile duct stones at the time of ERCP is the treatment of choice for patients presenting with pain, abnormal liver function tests, jaundice, or cholangitis. Following previous cholecystectomy, about 10% of patients will ultimately represent with bile duct stones and endoscopic management is far safer than further surgical exploration of the bile duct. Before laparoscopic cholecystectomy, it is particularly important to investigate and to endoscopically clear the bile duct of stones, if suspected. Failure to do so may increase the likelihood of postoperative bile duct leaks. At the time of ERCP if stones are located in the biliary tree, a small diathermy cut is made into the bile duct through the papilla and, through the sphincterotomy, stones can be extracted with a balloon or basket. If the stones are too numerous or too large to extract at the first procedure, small pigtail stents are inserted into the bile duct to guarantee good drainage without stone impaction and therefore reduce the incidence of postprocedure cholangitis.

Most large stones can ultimately be removed using a mechanical crushing basket (lithotripter) or sometimes with the help of extracorporeal shock wave lithotripsy, following which fragments can be removed from the bile duct at follow-up ERCP. In experienced hands, the technical failure rate is low and thus the need for surgical reintervention is uncommon. Only in patients with very large bile duct stones, intrahepatic stones, or stones above biliary strictures is there a need for further procedures, such as intraduct choledochoscopy, using small endoscopes passed directly into the bile duct, with direct contact lithotripsy using a pulse dye laser or an electrohydraulic probe. Very elderly or frail patients with large bile duct stones can be managed long-term by simple placement of an endoscopic stent beside the stones for drainage to prevent jaundice and/or cholangitis. Such stents can be changed over the years as necessary.

Benign strictures
Postoperative anastamotic strictures or those following bile duct damage at the time of cholecystectomy can initially be managed with intermittent biliary balloon dilatation at the time of ERCP or simple endoscopic stent placement. In the young patient, after a trial of dilatation or stenting for a reasonable length of time, surgical reconstruction of the bile duct might be needed if it is clear that endoscopic treatment is not leading to resolution of the stricture. In patients with primary sclerosing cholangitis, there may be single or multiple strictures in the intrahepatic and extrahepatic biliary tree, often in association with pigment stones, which can be difficult to dilate or stent. A variable proportion (5–20%) of patients with primary sclerosing cholangitis develop a cholangiocarcinoma and this can be very difficult to prove even with good ERCP, biliary cytology, CT, and MR scanning.

Malignant bile duct obstruction
Pancreatic and bile duct cancer and carcinoma of the ampulla of Vater can all produce stricturing of the biliary tree at different levels. At ERCP the stricture can be dilated and then an endoscopic 10FG polyethylene stent placed to relieve jaundice. These stents are cheap and usually stay patent for 4 to 5 months. In pancreatic cancer, about one-third of patients will survive long enough to occlude their stent, in which case a further procedure is performed to remove the blocked stent and replace it with a new one. Self-expanding metal stents offer a way of palliating patients for longer as they have a lumen of 10 mm which gives excellent long-term drainage. At present, biliary metal stents have an open mesh and tumour infiltration may occur, causing recurrent jaundice and/or sepsis. In that situation, a plastic stent can be inserted through the blocked metal stent to achieve drainage. Membrane-covered metal stents are now available which should result in long term patency and, hopefully, avoid the problem of tumour ingrowth.

In some patients with cholangiocarcinoma at the hilum of the liver, separate obstruction to right and left main ducts or subsegments may be found. In such a situation, more than one stent may be necessary to relieve jaundice or sepsis. Brachytherapy for cholangiocarcinoma can be administered endoscopically using an iridium wire source inserted down an endoscopically placed catheter inside the stent within the cholangiocarcinoma. Photodynamic therapy can also be administered using a diffuser laser fibre, endoscopically sited within the malignant biliary stricture(s).

Pancreatitis
In patients with acute, relapsing, and chronic pancreatitis a variety of endoscopic therapies can be performed. After pancreatic sphincterotomy, stones can be removed from the pancreatic duct, strictures can be stented, and drainage of the dorsal duct in pancreas divisum can be achieved. Peripancreatic fluid collections and pseudocysts can also be managed by pancreatic duct drainage or direct endoscopic cyst puncture and stenting techniques. Pancreatic endotherapy is difficult and can be associated with complications. Nevertheless, in selected patients it may be very valuable and could avoid difficult and complex pancreatic surgery.

Gastric outlet obstruction
About 10% of patients with pancreatobiliary tumours will develop gastric outlet obstruction as a late complication as tumour infiltrates the duodenum. Conventionally, a surgical gastric bypass has been unavoidable and this has carried a substantial morbidity/mortality as these patients are often very frail in the latter stages of their malignant disease. A large-diameter self-expanding metal 'enteral' stent can now be placed in the stomach and duodenum at the time of endoscopy. This rapidly relieves symptoms of gastric outlet obstruction and allows the patients to eat a reasonable diet without vomiting, thus avoiding the need for bypass surgery.

Hazards and complications
Diagnostic endoscopy carries very few risks. With careful attention to nursing techniques and sedation protocol, cardiovascular problems during endoscopy and aspiration pneumonia after it are extremely rare. Direct damage to the upper gastrointestinal tract during insertion and subsequent inspection down to the duodenum is extremely unusual but rarely the cricopharynx, lower oesophagus above the cardia, and duodenal cap are sites of direct

perforation with the endoscope, more commonly with inexperienced endoscopists. An unrecognized pharyngeal pouch represents a real hazard during insertion of the endoscope and might lead to a perforation if undue force is applied.

Most complications of endoscopy occur during therapeutic procedures and are specific to the type of procedure being performed.

◆ The perforation rate following oesophageal dilatation is extremely low now that techniques and equipment have improved. The development of self-expanding stents in the oesophagus avoids the need for forceful dilatation of malignant strictures and this has radically lowered the postprocedure complication rate of perforation. Due to the size of the balloon used in dilating achalasia of the cardia, perforations can be seen. Anyone who develops pain or discomfort after oesophageal dilatation should be assumed to have developed perforation, a chest radiograph should be obtained and if there is evidence of mediastinal air or surgical emphysema, conservative management with nil by mouth, parenteral antibiotics, and intravenous feeding is advocated. Many patients will settle conservatively without the need for surgical intervention.

◆ The complications of ERCP are well known and more frequent than those of other endoscopic manoeuvres in the upper gastrointestinal tract. Even with diagnostic ERCP, up to 2% of patients may develop postprocedure pancreatitis after either manipulation at the papilla or the injection of contrast into the pancreas. Such pancreatitis is usually self-limiting and mild. Some patients may have a very elevated amylase in the absence of pancreatitis or pain. After endoscopic sphincterotomy and any therapeutic manoeuvre in the pancreatic or biliary tree, pancreatitis and bleeding can occur. Between 2 and 5% of patients may have some degree of bleeding, but only a small proportion of these will need a blood transfusion or, rarely, surgical intervention. There is also a small risk of retroperitoneal leakage and perforation after sphincterotomy. With the use of periprocedure antibiotics and the routine use of biliary stents after incomplete gallstone clearance within the bile duct, the incidence of postprocedure cholangitis is minimal.

15.3.3 Radiology of the gastrointestinal tract

A.H. Freeman

Essentials

The widespread introduction of endoscopic techniques has lessened the need for radiological examination of the intestinal tract, and has almost completely replaced it in the examination of the stomach. There remains, however, a major radiological role in the investigation of the small and large bowel; and clinically useful information can be obtained from thoughtful use of radiology in the diagnosis of abdominal and gastrointestinal disease in those regions of the world where facilities for endoscopy are not available.

The small intestine may be examined by a number of radiological means, including plain films, barium contrast studies, ultrasonography, CT, MRI, and nuclear medicine. Barium studies (follow-through or small-bowel enema) can provide good morphological detail of the mucosal surface of the bowel; cross-sectional imaging (usually CT or MRI) is required for disease in the wall of the bowel or outside it. CT is increasingly used as the primary investigation in suspected bowel obstruction. Nuclear medicine studies have two major roles in the examination of the small bowel: imaging with labelled white blood cells for the demonstration of inflammatory conditions, and with labelled red blood cells for the demonstration of potential bleeding sources.

Colonoscopy has revolutionized imaging approaches to the colon because of its therapeutic as well as diagnostic role, but it is not without risk and barium enema examination remains a much used alternative. CT is an increasingly used technique, particularly since the advent of multidetector CT (MDCT) allows three-dimensional reconstruction and thus so-called virtual colonoscopy.

The small intestine

The small intestine may be examined by a number of radiological means which include plain radiographs, barium contrast studies, ultrasonography, CT, MRI, and nuclear medicine. Plain film radiography is performed in cases of suspected small-bowel obstruction and typically includes films taken with both vertical and horizontal beam, the object being to demonstrate dilated loops and air–fluid levels. CT, however, is increasingly used as the primary investigation in this situation and therefore there is now little role for plain film examinations.

Barium studies of the small bowel have been the mainstay examination for almost a century and, if correctly performed, provide good morphological detail of the bowel. There are two types of examination: the first is the so-called barium follow-through wherein the patient drinks a quantity of barium sulphate and then sequential films are taken of its passage through the small bowel. The second is the small-bowel enema or enteroclysis and in this technique a tube is passed into the third part of the duodenum and barium sulphate is continuously infused, thus outlining the small intestine. This latter technique can also be used to provide a double contrast effect by infusing methyl cellulose, which provides a negative contrast against the positive contrast of barium sulphate. Both techniques have advantages and disadvantages. The follow-through is simple to perform and of course is more comfortable for the patient. However, it is imperative that fluoroscopy is performed at regular intervals together with abdominal compression so that all loops of small bowel are outlined. Enteroclysis by its very nature means that the barium column is observed in a continuous fashion and any minor obstruction or abnormality is thus more likely to be observed. Proponents of enteroclysis therefore argue that it is a more accurate test, but it is difficult to make a direct comparison as it is obviously difficult to perform both techniques on a cohort of patients. Given the relatively low incidence of disease of the small intestine, it seems reasonable in most scenarios to perform a follow-through study in the first instance and to reserve enteroclysis for unresolved problems, subacute obstruction, etc.

Both types of contrast study suffer from the fact they only demonstrate the mucosal surface of the bowel and disease in the wall of the bowel or outside it may be easily overlooked. In this situation, some form of cross-sectional imaging, typically ultrasound, CT, or MRI, may well give more information.

Ultrasonography, to date, has not found a huge role because it is highly operator dependent and results are variable. Its advantage, of course, is that it is radiation free—a major consideration in the paediatric population. Usually, a high-frequency ultrasound probe, of the order of 5 mHz, is used and the whole abdomen is carefully covered quadrant by quadrant with graded compression. Dilated, fluid-filled loops of bowel are relatively easy to examine, but the presence of excess gas within bowel loops, deep pelvic loops, and patient obesity all provide major impediments to full examination by ultrasound.

These factors, however, provide no problem for CT which, despite its use of ionizing radiation, is finding an increasing role in the investigation of small-bowel disease. This particularly applies to acute small-bowel obstruction where it provides not only confirmation of the diagnosis but often demonstrates the site and the nature of the obstructing lesion. As the images are usually enhanced by means of intravenous contrast agents, they can provide useful information as to the viability or otherwise of the obstructed loops. Thickening and infiltration of the bowel wall is readily appreciated on CT, as is the demonstration of exophytic tumours such as leiomyomas and lymphoma.

MRI of the small bowel holds huge promise and is likely to become the most important technique in the future, subject to availability. It has major advantages in that it involves no radiation and image reconstruction can be performed in almost any plane. Indeed, image reconstruction is so fast that in effect, MR fluoroscopy of the bowel can produce images similar to those obtained at barium enteroclysis. Because of the lack of ionizing radiation, areas of interest or difficulty can be 'revisited' time and again until fully evaluated. To obtain these images, the bowel needs to be distended which usually involves passing a nasoduodenal tube and utilizing water or methyl cellulose as distension agents. However, reasonable results can be obtained by simple oral preparation.

Nuclear medicine studies, which involve the injection of a radiolabelled substance, have two major roles in the examination of the small bowel: first in the demonstration of inflammatory conditions, and secondly in the demonstration of potential bleeding sources. In the former, the patient's white blood cells are extracted and then labelled with [99]Tcm pertechnetate. These white cells are then re-injected into the patient. The cells concentrate at the site of inflammation and this activity is demonstrated on a gamma camera. The technique is known as labelled white cell scanning. Alternatively, indium may be used as the isotope when a longer half-life is required and this particularly applies in the diagnosis of possible intra-abdominal abscess. However, this does involve a higher radiation dose to the patient.

If bleeding from the small bowel is the clinical problem, then the patient's red blood cells are extracted and again labelled with [99]Tcm pertechnetate. The labelled cells are re-injected into the patient and the abdomen is again scanned under a gamma camera. A bleeding source of more than approximately 0.5 ml/min, can be identified as a hot spot, indicating the probable site. A more specific bleeding source is a Meckel's diverticulum and if this is symptomatic it is likely to contain ectopic gastric cells which may be demonstrated by the simple injection of pertechnetate by itself.

The emerging role of capsule enteroscopy should also be noted. This investigation involves the ingestion of a small capsule which continuously views the mucosa of the small bowel during its passage through it. Images are transmitted to a detector worn by the patient and are then downloaded to a work station at the end of the procedure. Excellent detail can be obtained of those areas of the small bowel not accessible to conventional endoscopes. This technique is replacing a number of the indirect methods of imaging of the small bowel such as those used to identify occult bleeding lesions, etc.

Anatomy of the small bowel

Strictly speaking, the small bowel commences at the pylorus and includes duodenum, jejunum, and ileum. However, the first part of duodenum, proximal to the superior duodenal flexure, is related more closely to the stomach in both diseases and investigations. Therefore, for practical purposes, this chapter will discuss small bowel from mid-descending duodenum onwards. The third part of the duodenum commences at the inferior duodenum flexure and passes across the midline at roughly the level of L3 to ascend to the duodenal–jejunal junction. This is marked by the peritoneal ligament of Treitz. At this point, the small bowel emerges from the retroperitoneum to become an intraperitoneal structure. It is then divided roughly into equal lengths of jejunum and ileum, with jejunal loops occupying the left upper quadrant and ileal loops the right lower quadrant. The ileum terminates at the ileocaecal junction where it again becomes a retroperitoneal structure. Morphologically, jejunum can be distinguished from ileum both by its size (it is usually c.1 cm larger in diameter) and by the presence of valvulae connivente or plicae semilunaris. The latter gives it its characteristic fold pattern on contrast studies, as opposed to the relatively featureless ileum.

Pathology of the small bowel

Coeliac disease and malabsorption states

Coeliac disease, caused by a sensitivity to gluten, is characterized by atrophy of the small intestinal villous pattern. The definitive diagnosis thus rests with duodenal or jejunal biopsy, but radiology retains a role in evaluating complications as well as excluding other causes of malabsorption.

Barium follow-through studies demonstrate changes which include dilatation of jejunal loops (to >3.5 cm), flocculation of the barium suspension, thickening of the fold pattern (particularly if there is associated hypoproteinaemia), and delayed transit. Many of these features are very subjective and thus radiology cannot be used as a test to exclude coeliac disease. Marked mucosal effacement typically involving the duodenum, but sometimes the whole of the jejunum, may be a prominent feature leading to the so-called 'moulage' appearance (Fig. 15.3.3.1). This is specific for two conditions- coeliac disease and for the rarer graft-versus-host syndrome. In addition, transient intussusceptions may be observed during the examination and these are only seen with coeliac disease.

Complications, such as the development of lymphoma, may be demonstrated by both barium studies and CT, whereas stricture formation following ulcerative jejunitis, often regarded as a pre-lymphomatous condition, is best assessed by barium studies.

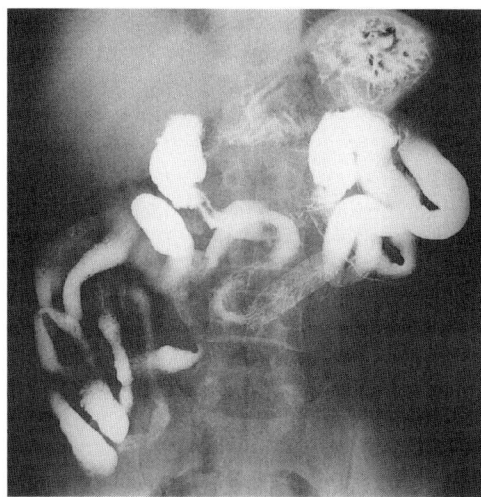

Fig. 15.3.3.1 Severe coeliac disease showing moulage phenomena. There has been complete obliteration of the small-bowel fold pattern such that the barium follow-through appearances resemble toothpaste squeezed from a tube, leading to the alternative term of 'tube of toothpaste' sign. This particular study was performed because the patient was thought to have a carcinoma of the stomach and thus illustrates one of the very varied ways in which coeliac disease can manifest itself.

Other causes of malabsorption include jejunal diverticulosis and short bowel syndrome, plus infiltrative causes such as intestinal lymphangectasia, Whipple's disease, eosinophilic gastroenteritis, amyloidosis, and mastocytosis:

- Jejunal diverticulosis causes malabsorption because of intestinal stasis and subsequent bacterial overgrowth. The diverticula usually protrude through the mesenteric border of the jejunum and can be demonstrated on small-bowel series as a number of sac-like structures containing barium.

- Short-bowel syndrome results if extensive lengths of small bowel have been resected, often either as a result of vascular accidents or following complications of Crohn's disease. The bowel will adapt by increasing its diameter, but an overall length of less than 50 cm is usually incompatible with life. The malabsorption situation is compounded if the terminal ileum has

been resected because of its specialized function in the absorption of vitamin B_{12}, and its role in the enterohepatic circulation of bile salts.

The various small-bowel infiltrations are rare:

- Intestinal lymphangiectasia is characterized by the presence of dilated lymph vessels in the mucosa which cause protein and lymphocytic loss into the small bowel. It may be primary or secondary. The secondary form is caused by conditions which obstruct the bowel lymphatics, such as lymphoma, carcinoma, postradiation changes, and occasionally in association with heart failure and constrictive pericarditis. High-quality barium studies may demonstrate the dilated lymphatics as very fine, millimetre-size nodules, mainly in the jejunum.

- Whipple's disease is caused by a bacillus resulting in a syndrome of steatorrhoea, abdominal pain, and arthralgia. It has a male predominance. Barium studies show thickened folds together with slight dilatation of the bowel lumen. In addition, CT may demonstrate bowel wall thickening together with mesenteric lymphadenopathy, the lymph nodes usually being of low attenuation.

- Eosinophilic gastroenteritis. In this condition, the wall of the bowel is infiltrated with eosinophils and there is usually a peripheral eosinophilia as well. Often, there is a history of atopy and the triad of eosinophilic gastroenteritis, asthma, and mononeuritis multiplex comprise the Churg–Strauss syndrome. Symptoms resulting from small-bowel involvement depend on the major site of location of eosinophilic infiltration, which may be either mucosal or serosal. With the former diarrhoea, malabsorption, and protein loss are dominant, whereas the latter is characterized by ascites. Barium studies in cases of mainly mucosal involvement show fold thickening together with nodular filling defects, whereas serosal involvement is better assessed by CT, which shows both the bowel wall thickening and ascites.

- Amyloidosis and mastocytosis are very rare causes of malabsorption with infiltration in both cases, causing thickening of the valvulae conniventae. Amyloidosis is characterized by the deposition of amyloid fibres in the small bowel and may be primary or secondary (Fig. 15.3.3.2).

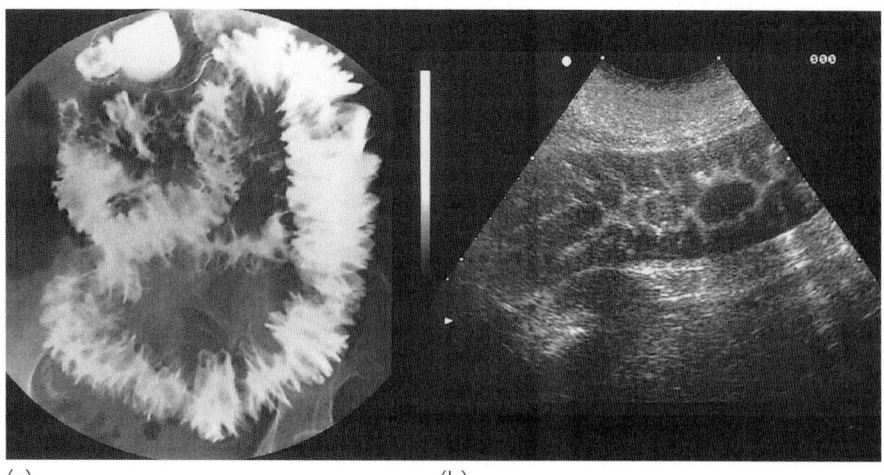

(a) (b)

Fig. 15.3.3.2 Amyloidosis of the small bowel shown on barium follow through (a) and ultrasound examination (b). There is complete disorganization of the normal small-bowel fold pattern (a) and the degree of thickening of the small-bowel wall is best appreciated on the ultrasound scan (b).

Tumours of the small intestine

These may be benign or malignant and are relatively uncommon.

Benign tumours

These include leiomyomas, haemangiomas, and adenomas. Bleeding and intussusception are the commonest presentations, particularly from leiomyomas. These tumours may grow into the bowel lumen, but often have a significant exoenteric mass, in which case they can grow to a very large size without causing clinical symptoms. They may, therefore, be demonstrated on barium studies as a filling defect, sometimes with a central ulcer which results from necrosis, whereas CT is the best method for demonstrating the exocentric component. A number of syndromes include small bowel polyps as part of their features and these include Peutz–Jegher's with small-bowel hamartomas, Gardener's with adenomas, and Cronkhite Canada with retention polyps. Many of these have an association with periampullary carcinoma.

Malignant tumours

These include carcinoid, carcinoma, lymphoma, and metastases.

◆ Carcinoid typically arises in the distal ileum and presents as a smooth, submucosal mass. At this stage, it behaves like a benign tumour. Later, local infiltration occurs causing extensive tissue thickening and a desmoplastic reaction. This may be severe enough to cause bowel obstruction. Once the tumour has reached a size of 2 cm or more, it is likely to display true invasiveness, metastasizing via the portal vein to the liver. Radiological assessment is best by CT, which may show evidence of local infiltration into the mesentery typically with a central spiculated mass, and later very vascular liver metastases.

◆ Adenocarcinoma of the small bowel is rare, with an approximate incidence of 1 in 100 000. These tumours are most commonly found in the jejunum. The usual macroscopic appearance is that of an annular, concentric tumour which gives rise to an apple-core appearance on barium studies or sometimes a large mass (Fig. 15.3.3.3). Prognosis is poor, as the majority of tumours have metastasized at the time of surgery.

◆ Lymphoma may involve the gastrointestinal tract and indeed is the most common location for extranodal disease. In contradistinction to carcinoma, the ileum is more frequently involved than the jejunum. A number of macroscopic forms are seen including: (1) multiple nodular defects; (2) diffuse infiltration (Fig. 15.3.3.4); (3) the infiltration may destroy the muscularis propria leading to the so-called aneurysmal form with bowel dilatation; (4) large endoexoenteric masses with excavation; (5) large extraluminal masses. The latter is a particular feature of HIV-associated Burkitt's lymphoma.

◆ Metastatic disease to the small bowel may arrive by either transcoelomic spread or via the haematogenous route. Common tumours to seed across the peritoneal cavity are from the colon, pancreas, and stomach with the addition of the ovary in women. The commonest source for haematogenous metastases to the small bowel is malignant melanoma which produces characteristic submucosal masses with a central umbilical-type ulcer. Carcinoma of the bronchus and breast are also major causes of haematogenous metastases.

Crohn's disease and inflammatory small-bowel conditions

Crohn's disease is the commonest inflammatory condition to affect the small bowel in Western populations and is characterized by a chronic course of progression with spontaneous remission. The cause remains unknown and despite the presence of noncaseating granulomas on biopsy, extensive investigation into infectious agents has so far proved inconclusive. It may involve any part of the gastrointestinal tract, but in the great majority of cases the small bowel demonstrates most macroscopic change, and when involved the terminal ileum is the usual site.

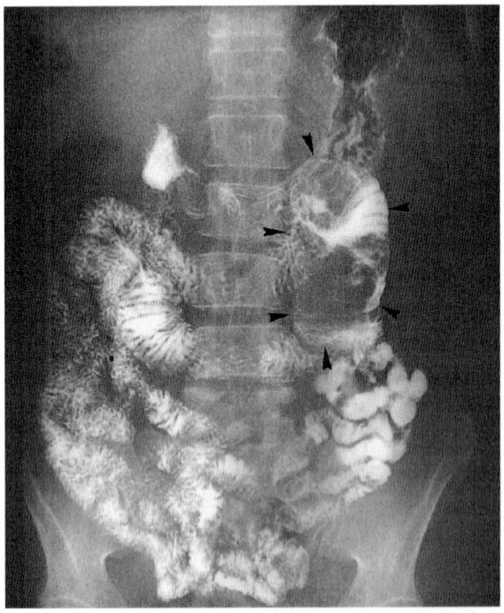

Fig. 15.3.3.3 Adenocarcinoma of the jejunum. This follow-through examination in an anaemic patient demonstrates the large mass (arrowheads) arising from the proximal jejunum at a site just distal to the ligament of Treitz—a common position. Note also the normal small bowel pattern distal to this tumour when compared to the abnormal patterns shown on Figs. 15.3.3.1 and 15.3.3.2.

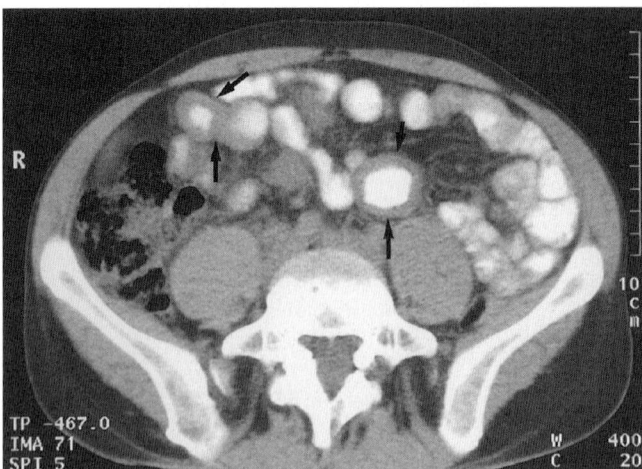

Fig. 15.3.3.4 Lymphoma of the small bowel as demonstrated by CT. Several loops are involved demonstrating marked thickening of the bowel wall to a width of 5 to 6 mm (arrows).

The disease starts with mucosal ulceration which then becomes transmural with fissure ulcers. Healing is accompanied by fibrosis and stricture formation and there is considerable thickening of the bowel wall. Skip lesions may occur affecting considerable lengths of small bowel. Fistula formation is a characteristic of the disease and these may be enteric, enterocutaneous, or extend into the muscles of the abdominal wall and pelvis. Intra-abdominal abscesses also characterize severe disease. Radiological assessment is by means of [99]Tcm white blood cell scanning, barium follow-through studies, CT, and MR. White cell scanning is used as the initial test for a patient with symptoms and signs of possible Crohn's disease (Fig. 15.3.3.5). It is also used to document disease activity and response to therapeutic measures. It is highly sensitive but may produce false-positive results from other conditions which cause terminal ileal inflammation. Barium studies demonstrate morphological detail. These may show the earliest change of Crohn's disease which is an aphthoid ulcer resulting from ulceration on the tip of a lymphoid follicle. Next, distortion and thickening of the fold pattern occurs which in some instances becomes completely effaced. Finally, development of deep, interlacing, linear ulcers give rise to the characteristic cobblestone pattern due to oedema of mucosal islands between the ulcers. If stricture formation occurs, it sometimes results in a long segment of stenosis across the terminal ileum, referred to as the string sign. Fistula formation may be demonstrated by barium studies, CT, and MRI. CT in particular shows other complications such as the formation of intra-abdominal abscesses and communications outside of the abdomen. The role of MRI in Crohn's disease is also evolving rapidly because it can define both morphological detail with function. Thus not only can it demonstrate thickened bowel wall (Fig. 15.3.3.6), inflammatory changes in the mesentery, and the presence of fistulae, but it can also assess physiological action in the small bowel.

Other inflammatory conditions of the small bowel include infection, such as *Yersinia enterocolitica* and tuberculosis. The former is

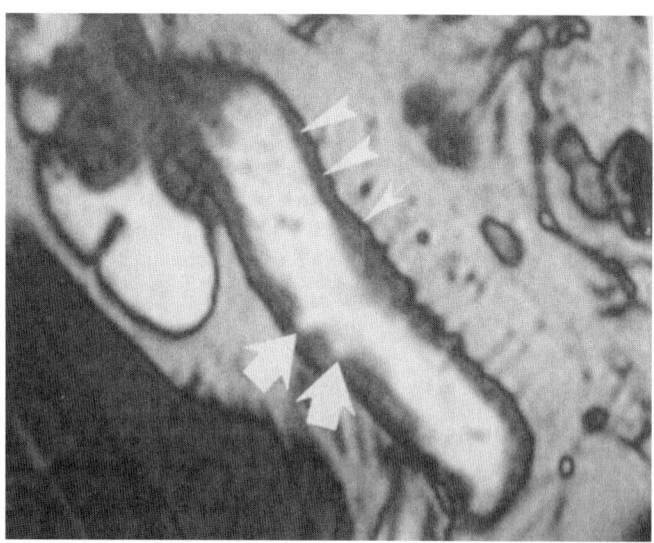

Fig. 15.3.3.6 Crohn's disease of the small bowel as demonstrated at MRI. Note the discrete ulcers (arrows) and the thickened bowel wall (arrowheads). (Courtesy of Professor N Gourtsoyiannis and Springer-Verlag, the publishers of *Radiological imaging of the small intestine*)

associated with changes of terminal ileitis and is usually self limiting. The latter may affect any part of the gastrointestinal tract, but typically the ileocaecal region. Now that bovine tuberculosis has largely disappeared, the bacillus in most cases has arrived from swallowing infected sputum. Barium studies usually demonstrate changes in both the terminal ileum and caecum, a helpful point in distinguishing this from Crohn's disease, although the appearances can be very similar. There may be two type of appearance—the ulcerative form and the hypertrophic form. The latter is characterized by thickened and matted loops of bowel in the right iliac fossa. In addition, tuberculous enteritis may present as ascites from tuberculous peritonitis.

Postradiation enteritis and bowel ischaemia

Postradiation enteritis is considered here because the pathophysiology is that of endarteritis obliterans. This may follow any form of radiotherapy, either external beam or cavity therapy, and is most commonly encountered in female patients who have had therapy for carcinoma of the cervix. Thus, it typically involves small-bowel loops which lie deep in the pelvis and these are made more susceptible if there is adhesive disease which fixes them in this position. Initial changes are of mucosal oedema but major problems from fibrosis and stricture formation occur later, in some instances after a latent period as long as 25 years. Sinuses and fistulae can be particularly problematic if there has been previous surgery to the radiation-damaged bowel. These changes are well appreciated at barium follow-through studies.

Bowel ischaemia and infarction may result from both arterial and venous occlusion. Arterial thrombosis of the superior mesenteric artery results in catastrophic infarction of most of the small bowel and carries a dismal prognosis. On the other hand, multiple, small emboli may cause episodes of nonocclusive ischaemia from which the bowel makes a good recovery. These typically are shown as areas of narrowing due to oedema with an abrupt transition to normal small bowel between the involved segments. Venous occlusion may

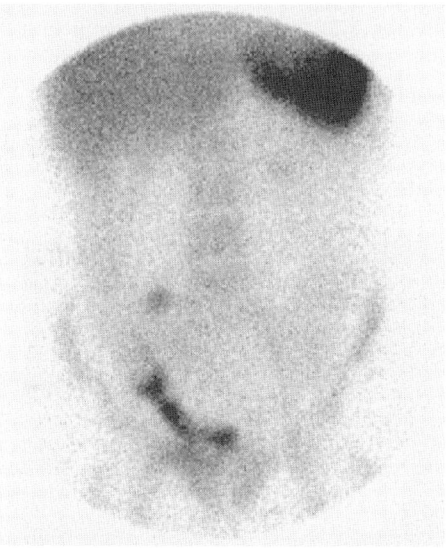

Fig. 15.3.3.5 Crohn's disease of the small bowel as demonstrated by a [99]Tcm-labelled white cell scan. There is grade III activity in the right iliac fossa indicative of highly active Crohn's disease in the terminal ileum. Note the normal accumulation of isotope in the spleen. (Courtesy of Dr Jane Dutton)

result from volvulus of the bowel, blood dyscrasias, and malignant infiltration in the mesentery.

The colon

Colonoscopy has revolutionized imaging approaches to the colon because of its therapeutic as well as diagnostic role. However, it is not without risk, and barium enema examination still remains a much used alternative. CT is an increasingly used technique, particularly since the advent of multidetector CT (MDCT) allows three-dimensional reconstruction and thus so-called virtual colonoscopy.

For all three techniques a completely clean and empty colon is a prerequisite. This is achieved by colonic lavage, usually using an oral preparation the day before the examination, such as Picolax or Klean prep. For barium enema examination, the patient is placed on a fluoroscopic table and barium sulphate is run into the colon up to the level of the transverse colon. The excess is then drained out and air or carbon dioxide is insufflated into the colon to achieve a so-called double contrast effect, i.e. luminal distension with air and mucosal coating by barium sulphate. Up to 12 to 15 images are then taken of the colon with the patient in different positions so that the entire bowel is demonstrated in double contrast.

For CT examination, the colon is simply distended with air, usually after the administration of a spasmolytic drug such as butylscopolamine and an intravenous contrast agent. So-called volume rendering of the data following MDCT examination permits a three-dimensional reconstruction of the lumen of the colon, thus allowing the operator to apparently 'fly' through the colon in a manner similar to colonoscopy, hence the term virtual colonoscopy.

CT without bowel preparation has also been used in the detection of gross colonic abnormalities in elderly patients, thus sparing them the discomfort of bowel preparation and a barium enema, both of which are likely to be less than optimal in this group.

Anatomy of the large bowel

The colon commences with the caecum and appendix in the right iliac fossa and these structures lead into the ascending colon which is a retroperitoneal structure. The hepatic flexure then leads into the transverse colon which is intraperitoneal, suspended by the transverse mesocolon. The splenic flexure marks the transition to descending colon, which is again retroperitoneal. Finally, the sigmoid and proximal rectum are intraperitoneal structures as the peritoneal reflection is sited at the junction of the mid and lower third of rectum.

Pathology of the colon

Diverticular disease and irritable bowel syndrome

Diverticular disease and its complications are among the commonest conditions to affect the colon. It results from raised intraluminal pressure causing a bleb of mucosa to herniate through the bowel wall at points of potential weakness, where the nutrient artery pierces the wall to supply the colon. This is accompanied by hypertrophy of the circular muscle fibres in the bowel wall, which is the first sign of this condition. Diverticula by themselves may not cause symptoms, and indeed they are said to be present in one-third of the population over the age of 60. They may, however, become inflamed, resulting in a number of complications which include local and segmental abscesses, perforation and fistula formation, strictures, and colonic bleeding. The usual location is the sigmoid colon which, with severe diverticular change, may become extremely distorted. A barium enema is the best technique for demonstrating the presence and extent of diverticulosis and these are shown as small barium-filled outpouchings from the bowel wall. Most of the complications of diverticular disease, however, are best appreciated on CT. This demonstrates the marked thickening of the bowel wall as well as the presence of fistulae and abscesses. The latter are shown as soft tissue areas of fluid density either within or immediately adjacent to the wall of the bowel (Fig. 15.3.3.7). Stricture formation, however, is best assessed by barium enema and will usually require colonoscopy for biopsy purposes as the distinction between benign diverticular stricture and one secondary to malignancy is often difficult.

The diagnosis of irritable bowel syndrome is not radiological but clinical. However, in many instances the distinction from diverticular disease and colonic carcinoma is impossible and therefore a further examination, usually a barium enema, is indicated to exclude these diseases.

Fig. 15.3.3.7 Diverticular disease and its complication as shown at CT examination (a) demonstrating the marked thickening of the sigmoid wall and to the right of this is a fluid collection demonstrated by a low attenuation mass. This has been drained under CT control with the drainage catheter shown in position (b).

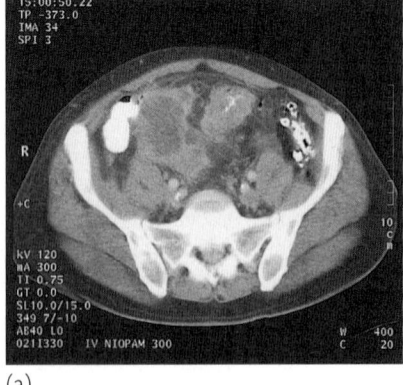

(a)

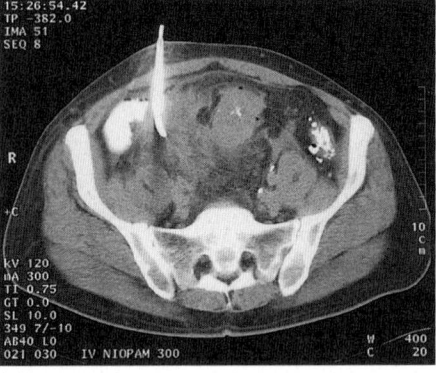

(b)

Colorectal cancer and polyp formation

Colorectal cancer is the second most common cause of death from cancer in the Western world and early detection can have a profound effect on prognosis. It is now clear that colorectal cancer arises as a result of a number of mutations resulting in a chromosome instability pathway. The first macroscopic change is the formation of an adenomatous polyp which over time, often two or three decades, will eventually become a frank carcinoma. The percentage of polyps, which if left alone will become a carcinoma is unknown, but any attempt to reduce the mortality from colorectal cancer starts with their detection and subsequent removal. Polyp detection is achieved by both barium enema and CT colonography.

At barium enema, a polyp may be demonstrated as a filling defect in the barium column or as a ring of increased density on the air-contrast views. They may be sessile or pedunculated (Fig. 15.3.3.8). The size of the polyp is significant, as lesions under 5 mm in size have little or no statistical association with an increased risk of cancer. Any polyp larger than 10 mm should be removed and once they reach 20 mm they will almost certainly be malignant. For obvious reasons, their detection requires a colon that is completely clean as residual faecal material can readily be misinterpreted as polyp.

Carcinoma of the colon has several macroscopic appearances including annular stricture, a proliferative type, a large polypoid type, and schirrous. Both barium enema (Fig. 15.3.3.9) and CT examinations detect of all of these.

CT colonography has two major advantages. First, if a tumour is demonstrated, then it can be formally staged at the same examination, i.e. by looking for involvement of the lymph nodes or the presence of liver metastases. Second, as only air has been insufflated an optical colonoscopy may be performed immediately after the CT, for further diagnostic or therapeutic indications.

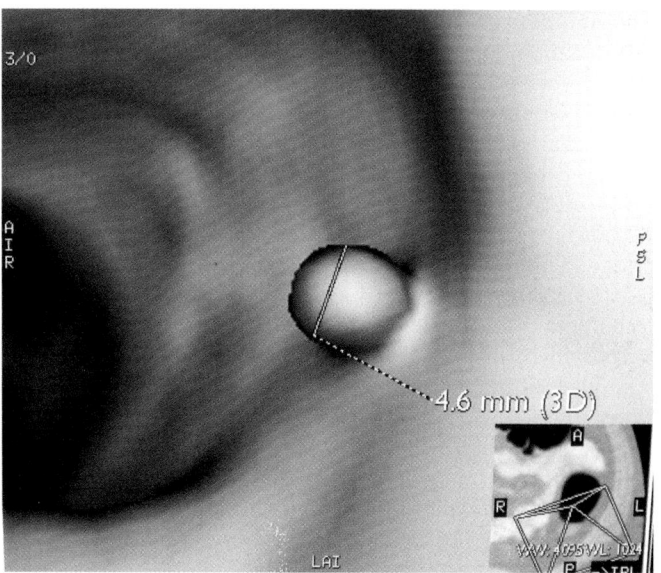

Fig. 15.3.3.8 Colorectal polyp in the mid sigmoid demonstrated at virtual colonoscopy. This small (4 mm) polyp is almost certainly benign in nature.

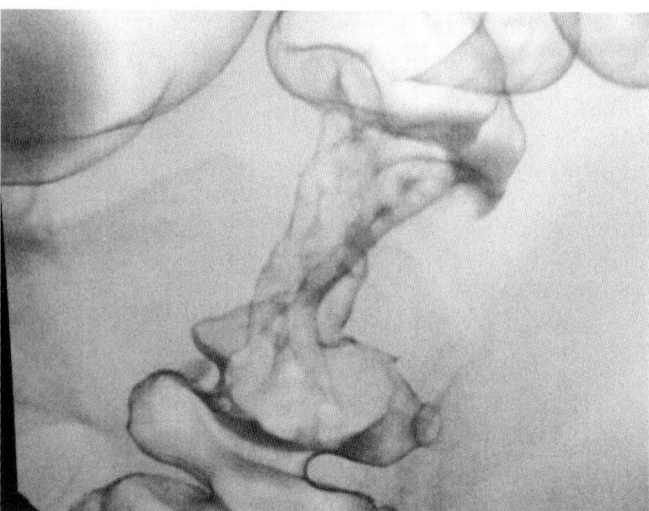

Fig. 15.3.3.9 Colorectal cancer as demonstrated on a barium enema. Note the typical apple-core deformity caused by an annular carcinoma.

Inflammatory bowel disease

The two main causes of idiopathic inflammatory bowel disease are ulcerative colitis and Crohn's disease, with the former approximately three times more common than the latter. Ulcerative colitis invariably starts in the rectum and spreads proximally, whereas Crohn's disease more commonly involves the right colon. Both conditions are readily appreciated at barium enema, though the complications of Crohn's disease, i.e. fistulae and abscess formation, are best demonstrated by CT. The radiological appearances reflect the pathophysiology. Ulcerative colitis results in fine mucosal ulceration which always involves the rectum and then may spread proximally to involve the entire colon. There is loss of the haustral pattern and the mucosa demonstrates a fine granular appearance. Crohn's disease in contradistinction demonstrates more discreet and deep ulcers. The latter represent fissure ulcers, which may extend throughout the whole thickness of the bowel wall. There is discontinuity and asymmetry of involvement. The picture is completed by terminal ileal involvement. An unusual feature of Crohn's disease is its earliest appearance, which is that of aphthous ulceration caused by ulcers appearing on the surface of hypertrophied lymphoid aggregates.

Other causes of colitis include pseudomembranous (caused by an overgrowth of *Clostridium difficile* often following antibiotic usage) as well as the various infective colitides, e.g. shigella, campylobacter, or cytomegalovirus. The last-named is usually only a problem in the immunocompromised patient. Postradiation colitis typically affects the sigmoid colon, for example after treatment for carcinoma of the cervix.

Further reading

Chapman AH (ed.) (2004) *Radiology and imaging of the colon*. Springer-Verlag, Heidelberg.

Freeman AH (2001). CT and bowel disease. *Br J Radiol*, **74**, 4–14.

Gourtsoyiannis NC (ed.) (2002) *Radiological imaging of the small intestine*. Springer-Verlag, Heidelberg.

15.3.4 Investigation of gastrointestinal function

Julian R.F. Walters

Essentials

Many blood measurements of absorbed dietary components (such as iron, folate, vitamin B_{12}, cholesterol, and triglycerides) or their metabolic products (such as haemoglobin or albumin) can be abnormal when gastrointestinal function is impaired, and their serial changes can be used to follow progress of disease. Specific assessment of the function of the gastrointestinal tract complements the findings of imaging, endoscopy, and histology in the diagnosis of digestive diseases.

Measures of nutritional status (e.g. body mass index, anthropometry, body density), nutrient intake (e.g. dietary history) and faecal output (e.g. stool weight and volume, faecal fat) provide indications of the net effects of absorption.

In patients with possible malabsorption an important clinical decision is whether digestion is at fault (such as pancreatic exocrine insufficiency) or whether absorption is the problem (as in coeliac disease). Often this is rapidly established by employing tests with high positive predictive values for common individual diseases, such as tissue transglutaminase serology for coeliac disease, or imaging studies for chronic pancreatitis.

When a more systematic approach is required to reach a diagnosis, there are many tests that indirectly measure digestion and absorption and can help to differentiate between disorders affecting the two processes, e.g. reduced levels of faecal elastase in pancreatic insufficiency. Increased excretion of breath hydrogen after administration of lactose is found in lactase deficiency, and rapid excretion of hydrogen occurs after administration of glucose or lactulose when there is small-bowel bacterial overgrowth.

Evidence for infection, structural damage, or loss of barrier functions of the gut can also be obtained, e.g. (1) *Helicobacter pylori* infection of the stomach can be detected by the urea breath test—^{13}C-labelled urea is given by mouth; the urease activity of *H. pylori* in the stomach metabolizes this to CO_2, which is then exhaled; a standard amount of CO_2 is collected in a breath sample and the activity of ^{13}C determined by mass spectrometry.

Introduction

Digestion and absorption of food by the gastrointestinal tract is achieved by the integration of multiple steps. The complex foods taken in through the mouth are digested into simpler molecules which can be transported across mucosal epithelial cells into the metabolic pool of the body. The contents of the gastrointestinal tract also need to be moved to regions where specialized digestive and absorptive functions can take place, and physical and immunological

barriers must be maintained to prevent injury from toxic or immunologically active substances and bacteria.

These functions are assessed clinically in a variety of ways. Much can be learnt indirectly from techniques not principally aimed at defining gastrointestinal function. Patients will describe appetite, dietary intake, weight changes, and the frequency and nature of their bowel movements. Clinical examination may reveal malnutrition, either generalized or specific. Many blood measurements of absorbed dietary components (such as iron, folate, vitamin B_{12}, cholesterol, and triglycerides), or their metabolic products (such as haemoglobin or albumin) can be abnormal when gastrointestinal function is impaired, and their serial changes can be used to follow improvements with treatment. Radiological studies (see Chapter 15.3.3) can demonstrate functional changes as well as anatomy, and physiological measurements are central to studies of motility disorders. Tests aimed at giving specific measurements of gastrointestinal function are described below.

Intake and output

Nutritional assessment

The dietary history is a critical part of the investigation of gastrointestinal function. For instance, a high intake of milk in a patient of African ethnicity will suggest that diarrhoea may be due to nonpersistence of lactase. Vitamin B_{12} deficiency in a vegan is more likely to be due to dietary deficiency than to malabsorption.

Patients may not accurately recall what they eat. Assessment can be improved by keeping a detailed diary with formal recording of the diet over a week, which will enable the usual intakes of a full range of nutrients to be calculated. Total calories, fat, protein and nitrogen, water, electrolytes, individual vitamins, minerals, and trace elements can all be assessed in this way.

Assessment of nutritional status can indirectly provide evidence of gastrointestinal dysfunction. Calculation of the body mass index (kg/m^2) gives a measure of obesity, and hence fat stores. More detailed estimates of body composition can be made by anthropometry, measuring skin-fold thickness, or body density. Dual-energy X-ray absorptiometry (DEXA) will assess the percentage of fat, and bone mineral density as a measure of calcium stores.

These estimates of nutritional status can change over time. If the intake of any particular nutrient exceeds the losses, the body is in positive balance, as occurs during growth. If the losses are greater, the result is a negative balance. Losses from all sources must be included. Urinary loss is obvious for water, electrolytes, and minerals, and nitrogenous compounds. Carbon dioxide and heat losses reflect metabolism and energy consumption: research calorimetric techniques can estimate these accurately. Absorption by the gastrointestinal tract is a major factor in determining overall balance, with unabsorbed nutrients and excreted matter being egested in faeces.

Faecal output

Stool weight and volume can vary in the healthy individual, but averages about 200 g/24 h. This volume increases in diarrhoea or other forms of malabsorption, and may be as high as several litres in 24 h in patients with secretory diarrhoea, such as that due to cholera. Accurate measurements of faecal volume and electrolyte composition are then helpful in maintaining an accurate fluid balance.

Patients may complain of diarrhoea when they mean urgent, frequent, or unformed stools, rather than an increase in volume. Stool charts, recording frequency and volume, help to define the change in the nature of the stools. Changes in frequency and volume with simple changes such as fasting help to differentiate osmotic diarrhoea from secretory or inflammatory causes. Stool electrolytes and osmolarity are also helpful here: a large osmotic gap suggests an unabsorbed ion e.g. from magnesium salts taken as laxatives, or the products of unabsorbed carbohydrate fermentation. Stool pH is low after carbohydrate malabsorption, as in lactase deficiency (nonpersistence) or sucrase–isomaltase deficiency.

Faecal fat output is increased in most forms of generalized malabsorption and results in steatorrhoea. Patients frequently describe stools that float or are foul-smelling, but to be sure that this is due to fat, qualitative and quantitative estimations need to be performed. Fat droplets in the stool can be detected microscopically after staining with lipid-soluble dyes. Accurate estimation of the loss of fat in the faeces requires a 3-day collection of stools while the patient is on a defined fat-intake diet. An average output of more than 5 g/24 h for a 70 to 100 g daily fat intake is abnormal. Patients and clinical and laboratory staff dislike this test for obvious reasons.

Gas, wind, explosive stools, and foul odours are frequent complaints. Although volumes of flatus and the presence of various gases have been measured in research studies, these have not been adopted as routine clinical investigations.

Stool microscopy for faecal leucocytes can be helpful in diagnosing inflammatory diarrhoea. Detection of bacterial pathogens, parasites, ova, or toxins may show the cause.

Digestive secretions

In patients with possible malabsorption, who have an adequate dietary intake but large volume stools, an important clinical decision is whether digestion is at fault (such as pancreatic exocrine insufficiency) or whether absorption is the problem (as in coeliac disease). Often this is rapidly established by employing tests with high positive predictive values for common individual diseases, such as tissue transglutaminase or endomysial IgA serology for coeliac disease, or imaging studies for chronic pancreatitis.

Intubation of the lumen to collect the contents for measurements of secretory rates and composition is the definitive way to study digestive juices produced by the stomach, pancreas, liver, and intestine. Though necessary for basic physiological and pharmacological studies, tube tests are now rarely performed in a clinical setting. Endoscopy is generally now used, which enables direct vision and biopsy of anatomical lesions, and can, on occasions, also provide functional information (see Chapter 15.3.2).

A large number of tubeless tests have been developed to indirectly measure digestion and absorption, or to help differentiate between the two types of disorder. Many involve small doses of radionuclides. Other tests use markers of breath hydrogen or urinary excretion (Table 15.3.4.1). Selection of these tests in clinical practice depends on their predictive values, reliability, cost, and ease of use.

Gastric secretion

The gastric mucosa secretes acid, pepsin, and some other products such as intrinsic factor. Measurements of acid output

Table 15.3.4.1 Breath tests in general use for gastrointestinal diseases

Type of test	Substrate	Clinical use
Hydrogen	Lactose	For lactase deficiency
	Lactulose	For orocaecal transit
	Glucose	For small intestinal bacterial overgrowth
Carbon dioxide (^{13}C)	Urea	Urease activity from gastric *Helicobacter pylori* infection

have historically been important in diagnosing the cause and response to treatment of acid-related diseases such as duodenal ulceration. This has become less relevant with the discovery of *Helicobacter pylori* and potent acid suppression with histamine H_2-receptor antagonists and proton-pump inhibitors.

Intubation of the stomach with a nasogastric tube allows the gastric contents to be sampled. Tube positioning is important. Swallowed salivary secretion will raise the pH and so will refluxing duodenal contents, common after retching. The yellow colour of bile will indicate duodenal reflux into the stomach. After an overnight fast, gastric aspiration allows the volume of resting secretions to be measured and the pH determined. Normal resting volumes are less than 50 ml. pH values above 4 suggest impaired acid secretion, as in the gastric atrophy and achlorhydria found in pernicious anaemia, or as the result of acid-suppressant drugs. Gastric pH can also easily be measured at endoscopy.

Estimation of basal and peak acid output requires continuous sampling and titration of the aspirate with sodium hydroxide. A marker can be infused to correct for loss of gastric contents into the duodenum. A basal acid output of about 5 mmol over 1 h is normal. Low values are found in achlorhydria. The detection of a high basal output is important in making the diagnosis of Zollinger–Ellison syndrome. However, this clinical decision is now usually made after finding a high serum gastrin level in a patient treated with a proton-pump inhibitor, who because of symptoms is unable to discontinue therapy.

Peak acid output following pentagastrin stimulation quantifies the ability of the stomach to maximally produce acid. There was considerable interest in the use of this test for research purposes before the aetiology of duodenal ulcer became clear but it is of little clinical use now that our understanding of pathophysiology and therapeutics has advanced.

Biliary secretions

Bile samples, mixed with pancreatic secretions and other duodenal contents, can be collected from the duodenum at upper endoscopy (or after intubation). Endoscopic retrograde cholangiopancreatography (ERCP) allows bile to be collected from the bile ducts. Microscopy of bile can detect cholesterol crystals. The proportions of bile acids, phospholipids, and cholesterol are relevant in the study of biliary cholesterol saturation and gallstone formation, but have little clinical use.

Bile secretion by the liver is not easily measured directly. Clearance from the circulation can be determined for a number of compounds normally secreted into the bile. Apart from measurements of bilirubin, such tests have found little clinical use. The nuclear medicine HIDA (hepatoiminodiacetic acid; lidofenin) scan gives a measure of biliary secretion as well as helping define functional anatomy. The gallbladder function of contraction in response to a meal, or cholecystokinin, can be measured by imaging techniques, of which ultrasonography is the most convenient.

Pancreatic secretions

Pancreatic secretion of a large number of digestive enzymes and bicarbonate is crucial for the digestive process. Duodenal intubation allows their collection for assay of the activities of some of the key enzymes such as trypsin, lipase, and amylase; however, these duodenal contents will be mixed with bile and duodenal secretions, or with those from the stomach. Pure pancreatic juice can be collected at ERCP.

Although a number of stimulation tests have been used to diagnose pancreatic exocrine insufficiency, their clinical usage is very limited: virtually all patients can be managed without the need to resort to these function tests. The duodenum is intubated, under fluoroscopic control or endoscopically. Secretin, which stimulates bicarbonate secretion, or cholecystokinin, which stimulates enzyme secretion, is given intravenously, either alone or in combination. The contents of the duodenum are then aspirated for assay of bicarbonate and enzyme concentrations.

Several indirect, tubeless pancreatic tests have been developed and are much simpler and more convenient to perform. The pancreolauryl test relies on the hydrolysis of fluorescein dilaurate by pancreatic esterases. The fluorescein is absorbed and excreted in the urine where it can be assayed easily. The test is administered on 2 days, each time with a standard breakfast and similar urine collections. On the first day, a test capsule containing fluorescein dilaurate is given, and on the second, a control capsule of non-esterified fluorescein. To diagnose pancreatic insufficiency, the ratio of fluorescein recovered in the urine with the dilaurate test substance will be less than 20% of that with the control. Another test uses *N*-benzoyl-l-tyrosyl-*p*-aminobenzoic acid as an alternative substrate. Following a similar principle, pancreatic chymotrypsin activity releases *p*-aminobenzoic acid, which is assayed in the urine. This test seems to be less reliable than that with pancreolauryl.

A different type of indirect test for pancreatic exocrine dysfunction involves the determination of proteolytic enzymes in the faeces. These enzymes are produced by the pancreas and are stable during passage through the intestine. Chymotrypsin activity has been used as a test for many years, but an improved method using an immunological assay for human-specific elastase I has been developed and is now more commonly employed.

All of these indirect tests are generally reliable in patients with severe exocrine pancreatic insufficiency causing steatorrhoea, where they can have adequate specificity for pancreatic disease if borderline test results are repeated or ignored. Many patients with severe intestinal disease will have somewhat abnormal results. The sensitivity of the tests is such that patients with lesser degrees of pancreatic functional impairment will be missed and considerable pancreatic damage may have occurred before the tests become abnormal.

Intestine

The role of brush-border enzymes in digestion is clearly important. Individual enzyme activities (e.g. sucrase–isomaltase) can be measured directly in small-bowel biopsies, now usually obtained at endoscopy. Indirect tests of intestinal digestive enzyme function

are closely linked with those of absorption and are described below. Intestinal secretions, such as those from the Brunner's glands in the duodenum or from the crypts in secretory diarrhoea, are not directly measured.

Absorption

Carbohydrates

The xylose absorption test was used as a simple measure of absorption and malabsorption. Xylose does not need to be digested, is absorbed by the jejunum, does not undergo significant metabolism, is excreted efficiently by the kidney, and is measured in the urine. The test measures the area of functioning mucosa and has reasonably good sensitivity for intestinal mucosal abnormalities such as coeliac disease. The measurement of blood levels is said to improve accuracy. False-positive low levels of xylose excretion can occur with delayed gastric emptying, ascites, or insufficient urinary output. As described elsewhere, serological tests are now available that are simpler, more specific, and more sensitive in screening for coeliac disease.

Lactose tolerance testing can be performed to diagnose lactase deficiency. This is similar to the glucose tolerance test, except that 50 g of lactose is given instead of glucose. Blood glucose levels are measured, and should increase if brush-border lactase is present to split the lactose into glucose and galactose. In subjects without brush-border lactase, the lactose is not digested or absorbed and the blood glucose level does not rise. The lactose passes through the small bowel to the large intestine where it is then broken down by bacteria, thereby causing symptoms of gaseousness and diarrhoea.

The breath-hydrogen test for lactose intolerance is based on this principle (Fig. 15.3.4.1). Hydrogen is only produced in the body from the bacterial fermentation of carbohydrates in the gut. It diffuses into the blood and is excreted in the breath. Breath hydrogen can be measured simply and relatively cheaply to an accuracy of a few parts per million. Colonic bacteria produce a background level of breath hydrogen from the fermentation of unabsorbed colonic contents. After taking oral lactose, breath hydrogen is measured every 30 min. An increase greater than 20 parts per million implies that, rather than being absorbed in the small intestine, the sugar has been broken down by bacteria in the colon. As described below, bacterial overgrowth in the small intestine elevates breath

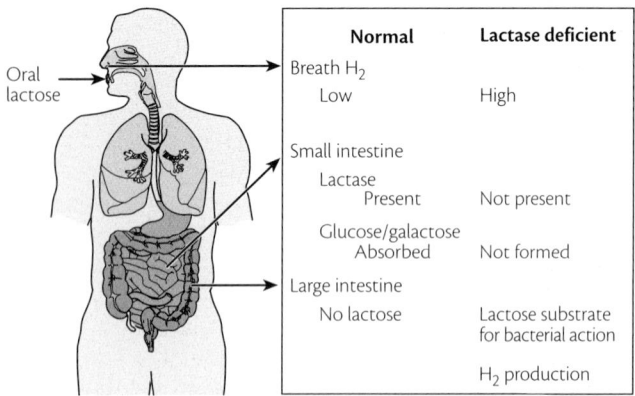

Fig. 15.3.4.1 Lactose-hydrogen breath test for lactase deficiency.

hydrogen after glucose administration, and can also do this when lactose is given. Similar breath-hydrogen tests can be performed with other sugars when fructose or sucrose malabsorption is suspected.

Fat

The estimation of nonabsorbed fat, i.e. faecal fat, is discussed above. A tubeless test, which does not require faecal collection, is the triolein test. This has been advocated as a simple method to determine lipid absorption. After digestion and absorption of the ^{13}C- or ^{14}C-labelled triglyceride, metabolism in the liver produces labelled CO_2 which is detected in the breath. This test is not widely used and is only sensitive to large changes in fat absorption.

Bile salts

Bile salts, critical for lipid absorption, undergo an enterohepatic circulation where the conjugated salts (such as glycocholate and taurocholate) are reabsorbed in the ileum. Failure to reabsorb these salts increases their concentrations in the colon, where they produce a secretory diarrhoea. Tests have been developed to look for evidence of bile salt malabsorption.

The SeHCAT test uses radiolabelled selenohomocholic acid as the taurine conjugate. This is given orally and whole-body retention is measured with a gamma camera after 7 days. Low values result from an excessive loss of bile salts. Bile acid malabsorption, often producing SeHCAT retention values of less than 5%, is found after ileal resection, with ileal disease such as Crohn's, and in idiopathic bile acid malabsorption. Small-intestinal bacterial overgrowth results in deconjugation of the bile salts, which will also impair absorption and retention.

Vitamin B_{12}

Absorption of vitamin B_{12} (the cobalamins) is particularly complex. Vitamin B_{12} deficiency is common, and, if not nutritional, is due to one of several gastrointestinal disorders. Intrinsic factor, produced by the stomach, binds cobalamins in the intestine. The intrinsic factor–vitamin B_{12} complex interacts with a receptor in the brush-border membrane of the terminal ileum and is taken up by the cell. Vitamin B_{12} is stored in the liver. Pancreatic enzyme activity is necessary to release dietary vitamin B_{12} from R-proteins in the diet so that it can bind to intrinsic factor. Bacterial overgrowth in the small intestine can split the intrinsic factor–vitamin B_{12} complex before it can be absorbed.

The Schilling test uses radioisotopes of cobalt to label cobalamin. A two-part test is usually performed, with two isotopes, ^{57}Co and ^{58}Co, simultaneously. One isotope is used to label free vitamin B_{12} and the other to label a complex of intrinsic factor and vitamin B_{12}. After an overnight fast, both are given together by mouth, and unlabelled cobalamin is given by intramuscular injection to ensure that binding sites are occupied. Absorbed radiolabelled vitamin B_{12} is excreted in the urine. This is collected for 24 h and should normally contain more than 10% of the ingested dose, with an equal ratio of the two isotopes. In gastric disease, such as pernicious anaemia, or after gastrectomy, absorption is reduced when vitamin B_{12} is given alone but not when it is given with intrinsic factor. In terminal ileal disease, or after resection, absorption of both forms is low. Small-bowel bacterial overgrowth mimics ileal disease, but antibiotic treatment restores vitamin B_{12} absorption to normal.

Gastrointestinal transit

Physiological function tests have been developed to measure the motility of the gut in propelling the contents of the diet through the areas involved in digestion and absorption.

Oesophageal function

Peristalsis in the oesophagus, with appropriately timed relaxation of the upper and lower oesophageal sphincters, is necessary for efficient and comfortable swallowing, without symptoms of dysphagia. Gastrooesophageal reflux through the lower sphincter will produce heartburn. Oesophageal manometry, with multiple fine tubes passed through the nose and connected to sensors, will measure the pressures in the oesophagus and at the sphincters at rest and during swallowing. Disordered peristalsis, spasm, achalasia, nutcracker oesophagus, and conditions associated with reflux can be diagnosed.

Monitoring gastrooesophageal acid reflux with pH-sensitive electrodes over 24 h is useful in diagnosing the severity of gastrooesophageal reflux disease, and in relating atypical symptoms to episodes of reflux. A small, portable recording device allows the times of symptoms, meals, and sleeping to be recorded, so they can be analysed together with episodes of low pH. A composite score can be calculated, reflecting the severity of reflux. A bile-sensitive electrode is also available, and may be of use in patients with adequate acid suppression but who still suffer symptoms from duodenogastric and gastrooesophageal reflux.

Gastric emptying

This can be measured by a range of imaging tests, of which radionuclide labelling of liquid and solid food is probably the most effective technique. Tracer quantities of technetium and/or indium are incorporated into simple foods. Gamma scanning over the stomach allows the time course of gastric emptying to be determined. These measurements are useful in conditions such as diabetic gastroparesis or after gastric surgery where bloating, nausea, or vomiting are problems. Radiological measurements of barium emptying, although widely available, are less reliable unless the contrast is incorporated into food. Ultrasonography and MRI have also been used.

Intestinal transit

- Radionuclide techniques, as used to measure gastric emptying, can also determine small-bowel transit by timing the appearance of counts over the caecum. Estimates of transit times through the large intestine can be obtained with further imaging.

- Mouth-to-caecum transit times can be estimated simply with breath-hydrogen testing. As described above, breath hydrogen is derived from the bacterial metabolism of unabsorbed carbohydrates. Lactulose, a non-absorbed sugar, is given by mouth and breath hydrogen sampled every 15 to 30 min. A rise in breath-hydrogen values indicates that the lactulose has reached the caecum. A rapid rise will occur if there is bacterial overgrowth in the small intestine.

- Dye markers taken by mouth will give an estimate of the whole-gut transit time when they are detected in the stool.

◆ Radiological markers, small differently shaped pieces of radio-opaque plastic, can be useful in determining transit through the large intestine. These are taken daily for several days. A plain abdominal radiograph shows the number remaining and their distribution in the parts of the colon.

◆ Defecation and anorectal physiology can be measured with manometry in response to balloon inflation in the rectum.

Tests of gastrointestinal integrity and barrier functions

Several tests examine other aspects of gastrointestinal physiology not discussed above. Evidence for infection, structural damage, or loss of barrier functions can be obtained.

Infection

Helicobacter pylori infection of the stomach is common and can be detected at endoscopy by microscopy, culture, or the biopsy urease test. The urea breath test, an indirect test, is now one of the commonest breath tests performed to look at gastric pathophysiology. Urea labelled with the stable isotope ^{13}C is given by mouth to fasting subjects (Fig. 15.3.4.2). The urease activity of *H. pylori* in the stomach metabolizes this to CO_2, which is then exhaled. A standard amount of CO_2 is collected in a breath sample and the activity of ^{13}C determined by mass spectrometry. As there are no other sources of urease activity in the body, this is a very specific test. Low-level *H. pylori* infection, as can occur when acid production is suppressed with histamine H_2-receptor antagonists or proton-pump inhibitors, can give negative results, reducing the sensitivity of this test. Hence it should only be performed several weeks after treatment aimed at eradication of *H. pylori*, and after discontinuing acid suppressants.

Bacterial overgrowth in the small intestine can be detected by the glucose–hydrogen breath test (Fig. 15.3.4.3). Glucose given by mouth is normally fully absorbed, but some metabolism to hydrogen will occur if bacteria are present in the small intestine. This will be measurable in the exhaled breath, which is collected every 30 min for 2 h. A positive test produces a diagnostic rise of 20 parts per million above a low baseline. It may be necessary to give a diet low in nonabsorbable polysaccharides to reduce baseline hydrogen production. This test has a sensitivity of about 80%. Lactulose will also detect small-bowel bacterial overgrowth, where an early rise in

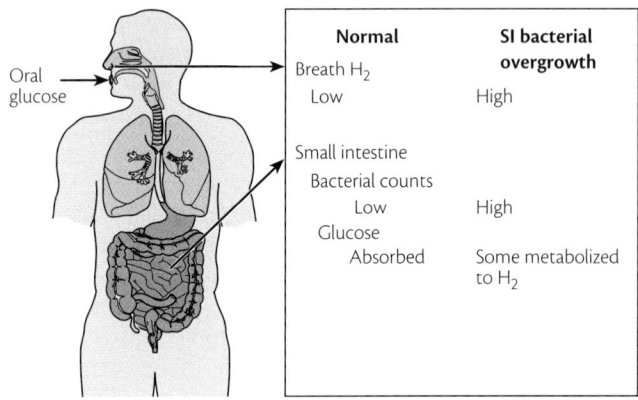

Fig. 15.3.4.3 Glucose-hydrogen breath test for small-bowel bacterial overgrowth.

breath hydrogen will occur before this nonabsorbed sugar reaches the caecum.

Mucosal damage

Several tests will give abnormal results if the gastrointestinal mucosa is damaged. The faecal occult blood test becomes positive with a relatively small loss of blood per day. Dietary components containing blood or peroxidase can give positive tests. The presence of leucocytes in faeces suggest inflammatory causes of diarrhoea.

White-cell scanning has a role in diagnosing and assessing the activity of inflammatory bowel disease. Autologous white cells, labelled with indium or technetium, are reinjected intravenously and collect in areas of inflammation. Imaging with a gamma camera, at multiple time points, indicate white-cell accumulation at sites of diseased bowel and chemokine production. The complexity and the radiation dosage involved limits the use of this test.

Calprotectin is a calcium-binding protein found in leucocytes. It is stable in the gut lumen and so can be quantified in the stool. It can be detected in faeces in a variety of inflammatory conditions and its simplicity may make it suitable as a first-line screening test. Lactoferrin can also be used.

In patients with small intestinal lymphangiectasia, lymphocytes are lost into the lumen of the gut. The full blood count may then show a lymphopenia. Protein loss also occurs in this disorder. Many other inflammatory and ulcerative conditions can produce a protein-losing enteropathy, and several tests have been employed in attempts to quantify this loss. Since α_1-antitrypsin is resistant to breakdown in the intestine, faecal measurements can provide an indication of the loss of serum proteins into the lumen. *In vivo*-labelled $[^{51}Cr]$albumin is also used to estimate gastrointestinal protein loss.

The permeability of the intestine can be investigated using a number of different probes: usually sugars, which normally have little uptake in the gut but can enter the body in disease states. These probe substances will then be excreted and measured in the urine. Lactulose is one such sugar that is normally excluded. When administered together with another molecule that is taken up and excreted readily, such as rhamnose or mannitol, the ratio can correct for individual differences in gastric emptying or urine collection. Although the results of these tests are usually abnormal in coeliac disease, specific serological tests (tissue transglutaminase IgA antibodies) are much more specific and sensitive for use

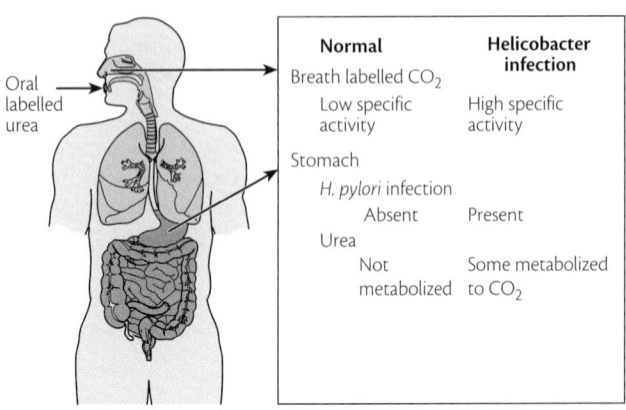

Fig. 15.3.4.2 Urea breath test for *H. pylori* infection.

in screening. Intestinal permeability changes have been described in other diseases but roles in their pathogenesis are uncertain.

Further reading

Luth S, *et al.* (2001). Fecal elastase-1 determination: 'gold standard' of indirect pancreatic function tests? *Scand J Gastroenterol*, **36**, 1092–9.

Schibli S, *et al.* (2006). Towards the ideal quantitative pancreatic function test: analysis of test variables that influence validity. *Clin Gastroenterol Hepatol*, **4**, 90–7.

Simren M, Stotzer PO (2006). Use and abuse of hydrogen breath tests. *Gut.* **55**. 297–303.

Yamada T, *et al.* (eds) (2003). *Textbook of gastroenterology*, 4th edition, Lippincott, Philadelphia, PA.

15.4

Common acute abdominal presentations

Contents

15.4.1 The acute abdomen

Chris Watson

Essentials

The term 'acute abdomen' is commonly used to describe abdominal pain of recent onset requiring urgent surgical assessment. Most cases of acute abdominal pain present in the community and are managed by family practitioners, with only a few presenting to a hospital. Those cases that do present to hospital are usually referred to the general surgeons. In a third of cases, no specific diagnosis is made, although many will subsequently re-present with identifiable pathology.

Only a few patients with an acute abdomen present directly to medical specialities or occur in patients already on a medical ward. These patients are often older, and the acute abdomen may present on a background of other comorbidities; hence a patient with known ischaemic heart disease who presents with upper abdominal pain from biliary colic or reflux may be misdiagnosed with cardiac chest pain. In addition, the disorders most commonly causing an acute abdomen in a medical patient differ from those occurring in the community and referred to surgeons, since the more obvious causes are likely to have been identified and referred appropriately. In elderly medical patients vascular events and intestinal obstruction due to malignancy are much more common than the appendicitis seen in the typical 'surgical' patient.

Management of the acute abdomen in medical patients can be extremely difficult: there is no substitute for an experienced and vigilant physician working together with a thoughtful surgeon and radiologist. The key question is, 'Does this patient need an operation?', a decision which depends on (1) symptoms, e.g. severe pain; (2) findings on examination, e.g. a rigid abdomen; (3) findings on investigation, e.g. subdiaphragmatic air; (4) excluding nonoperative diagnoses, e.g. pancreatitis; and (5) the presumed diagnosis, e.g. appendicitis as opposed to Crohn's ileitis. But it must be remembered that in very sick patients it may be necessary to proceed straight to surgery without any supportive imaging.

Assessment

Principles of management

Unlike the management of a medical condition, where achieving a precise diagnosis is often essential before treatment can be initiated, the management of the acute abdomen is more generic but no less imperative. The principle of management is to answer the question: 'Does this patient need an operation?' If the answer is yes, then the surgeon must decide the optimal timing of surgical intervention.

The surgical assessment of any patient with abdominal pain should be undertaken with this point in mind, and the decision to undertake surgical intervention is generally based upon the following:

- Symptoms, e.g. severe pain
- Findings on examination, e.g. a rigid abdomen
- Findings on investigation, e.g. subdiaphragmatic air
- Excluding nonoperative diagnoses, e.g. pancreatitis
- The presumed diagnosis, e.g. appendicitis as opposed to Crohn's ileitis

In very sick patients it may be necessary to proceed straight to surgery without any supportive imaging. The best place for a patient with acute abdominal pain radiating into the back, a palpable abdominal aortic aneurysm and an unrecordable blood pressure is in an operating theatre and not a CT scanner. Nevertheless, in most patients urgent imaging and laboratory investigations can be undertaken and a definitive diagnosis made.

There are two further management principles that are worthy of discussion at this stage:

♦ In a patient with an acute abdomen, administration of analgesia may affect the findings on clinical examination, but there is good evidence to suggest that it does not prevent the appropriate management being undertaken. There is therefore no justification in withholding analgesia from patients in pain with an acute abdomen. However, repeated administration of opiate analgesia without appropriate surgical review is unwise.

♦ Antimicrobial treatment can influence the course of an acute abdomen and may confuse the clinical findings. It should be withheld until a diagnosis is made, at which point appropriately targeted therapy may be commenced.

History

The common causes of the acute abdomen can usually be diagnosed by careful history taking, the principles which are enunciated in Chapter 15.2. See Table 15.4.1.1.

Pain

The hallmark of the acute abdomen is abdominal pain, and ascertaining the tempo of onset is important. Pain of sudden onset (coming on in seconds) suggests rupture of an abdominal viscus or sudden intra-abdominal bleeding (and occasionally torsion of an ovary or testis). Rapid onset pain, reaching maximum intensity within an hour, is typical of acute pancreatitis whereas other inflammatory conditions have a slower onset pain. Loss of consciousness when the pain starts is suggestive of abrupt blood loss as in a ruptured aneurysm.

Colicky pain, described as gripes or cramping by patients, comes and goes in waves and originates from a muscular-walled hollow viscus, such as the intestine or ureter. It also occurs during parturition, with a tubal ectopic pregnancy, and in acute urinary retention. Colicky pain typically makes patients restless; the pain of peritonitis is exacerbated by movement so the patient lies still.

Biliary colic typically is a sustained pain lasting 2 to 3 h coming on a couple of hours after a fatty meal; unless a stone is stuck in the sphincter of Oddi, colicky pain is not a feature. The marked intensity of this pain, lack of fever, and minimal abdominal tenderness may result in such patients being misdiagnosed with cardiac pain. The true diagnosis is suggested by pain radiating round to the inferior angle of the right scapula.

Other symptoms

Nausea and vomiting often occur in patients with an acute abdomen, and are typical of appendicitis and obstruction. Retching is suggestive of pancreatitis and typically the patient sits forward to relieve pain. Changes in bowel habit, particularly absence of flatus and faeces, distension ('bloating'), and a history of previous abdominal surgery should be sought. Similarly urinary symptoms, such as haematuria, dysuria, and frequency are important in indicating the cause of pain.

Examination

A thorough clinical examination should confirm the diagnosis, and will go a long way to indicating whether immediate surgery is required. A patient who is walking about or eating food is unlikely to be in need of urgent operative intervention. In contrast, the

Table 15.4.1.1 Common causes of an acute abdomen

Cause	Approximate incidence (%)
Nonspecific abdominal pain	35
Infection, e.g. viral or bacterial gastroenteritis	
Irritable bowel syndrome	
Psychosomatic pain	
Abdominal wall pain, e.g. herpes zoster, rectus sheath haematoma	
Acute appendicitis	20
Intestinal obstruction	15
Adhesions from previous surgery (60%)	
Hernia (20%)	
Cancer—colon/small intestine	
Volvulus ± malrotation	
Intussusception	
Crohn's disease	
Congenital bands	
Gallstone ileus	
Biliary pain	10
Acute cholecystitis	
Biliary colic	
Urological causes	6
Renal colic	
Testicular torsion	
Acute pyelonephritis	
Acute colonic diverticulitis	3
Perforation	2
Peptic ulcer	
Colonic diverticulum	
Carcinoma of colon	
Ulcerative colitis	
Pancreatitis	2
Ruptured abdominal aneurysm	<1
Aortic, iliac, mesenteric arteries	
Mesenteric ischaemia	<1
Arterial embolus or thrombosis	
Venous thrombosis	
Aortic dissection	
Gynaecological emergencies	<1
Salpingitis	
Ovarian torsion	
Ruptured ectopic pregnancy	

(Continued)

Table 15.4.1.1 (cont'd) Common causes of an acute abdomen

Cause	Approximate incidence (%)
Miscellaneous examples	
Primary peritonitis (streptococcal infection)	
Torted appendix epiploica	
Omental torsion	
Meckel's diverticulitis	
Jejunal diverticulitis	

patient who lies still for fear of exacerbating the pain, is dehydrated from vomiting, and has a foetor is much more likely to have serious abdominal mischief. Adequate exposure for a thorough clinical examination is important. The common missed diagnoses are in the groins (e.g. femoral hernia) and scrotum (e.g. testicular torsion) and these must be exposed, as should the upper abdomen up to the nipples. Not infrequently breast cancer is diagnosed on clinical examination, and may explain jaundice, lymphadenopathy, and back pain (all a result of secondary deposits).

Asking the patient to cough, upon which the patient experiences severe pain, indicates peritonitis. Palpation should seek features of peritonitis, such as guarding (increased resistance to increased palpation) and rigidity; eliciting rebound tenderness is unnecessary and cruel where coughing has been demonstrated to cause pain and other features are present—gentle percussion usually suffices. In more equivocal cases, the absence of rebound tenderness is reassuring. Abdominal aortic aneurysms are palpated by placing the flat of the hand just above the umbilicus (which is where the aorta bifurcates); once ruptured, the presence of a large retroperitoneal haematoma and hypotension will make them difficult to palpate. The hernial orifices (inguinal and femoral canals) should always be examined carefully—obstructed hernias are one of the first things a surgeon looks for on a patient on a medical ward, and it is surprising how often a previously unnoticed hernia is identified. Similarly, remember that testicular torsion may present with abdominal pain and vomiting, and unless the testes are palpated the diagnosis is missed, as is the opportunity to avoid the need for an orchidectomy.

Auscultation may confirm absence of bowel sounds, indicating generalized peritonitis; but their presence does not exclude a localized peritoneal reaction as is present in appendicitis, for example.

Finally, the value of a digital rectal examination should not be underestimated. In the jaundiced patient it could reveal the abscess that caused the portal pyaemia or the primary tumour that has metastasized to the liver; in the patient with diarrhoea and vomiting, or dysuria and pyuria, it may reveal peritoneal irritation due to a pelvic appendicitis.

Investigations

The laboratory investigation of patients with an acute abdomen usually contributes little to diagnosis, with the exception of serum amylase, which can be diagnostic and could avoid an inappropriate laparotomy. Raised concentrations of inflammatory markers such as C-reactive protein, or a moderate leucocytosis (up to 20×10^9/litre)

are nonspecific, although a very high leucocyte count ($>30 \times 10^9$/litre) is suggestive of mesenteric ischaemia.

Imaging

The contribution of radiology in the assessment of the acute abdomen has changed in recent years, particularly with the enhanced resolution of modern helical CT, and it is now common for patients with undiagnosed pain to have an emergency CT. Table 15.4.1.2 details the appropriate investigations and their limitations.

Initial management

Patients with an acute abdomen are usually volume depleted and require fluid resuscitation. The fluid losses in vomiting and third space losses in intestinal obstruction are usually underestimated, and regular review of volume status is required to ensure adequate replacement. Since many patients will require urgent surgery they should be kept nil by mouth. Nasogastric suction is indicated in the presence of continued vomiting and suspected intestinal obstruction. Decompressing the stomach with a wide-bore tube may later prevent aspiration on induction of anaesthesia.

Common causes of an acute abdomen

Acute appendicitis

Appendicitis, the most common surgical cause of the acute abdomen, typically starts with a central periumbilical pain which migrates to the right iliac fossa over the course of 3 to 12 h, during which nausea and vomiting are common. Although common in children and young adults it can occur at any age, and is usually missed in older people in whom the mortality is around 3%. Laparoscopic appendicectomy has become standard practice, permitting confirmation of the diagnosis (particularly in young women in whom gynaecological pathology is common), as well as facilitating rapid recovery after surgery.

Intestinal obstruction

This is suggested by a history of colicky pain and distension, with vomiting or constipation. Any patient presenting with a history of vomiting should be examined to exclude an occult hernia, and obstruction considered as a possibility. Conservative treatment with nasogastric aspiration and intravenous fluid replacement is only indicated in patients with a history of previous abdominal surgery, when adhesive small-bowel obstruction is a likely diagnosis and surgery is withheld; for other causes of small-bowel obstruction, surgery is usually inevitable. The timing of surgery depends whether there is evidence that the blood supply of the bowel is compromised, so called strangulating obstruction. Features suggestive of strangulation include colicky pain that becomes constant, a pyrexia ($>37.5°C$) and a tachycardia, together with features of peritonitis and leucocytosis. Strangulation is an indication for urgent surgery.

Perforated viscus

Acute perforation is usually associated with a sudden onset of severe abdominal pain. When a peptic ulcer perforates the patient suffers a chemical irritative peritonitis, and is seldom septic. In contrast, faecal peritonitis that follows perforation of a colonic diverticulum is associated with profound sepsis, in addition to pain. The mortality from faecal peritonitis is high, and increases with increasing age.

Table 15.4.1.2 Preferred investigations for the acute abdomen

Condition	Investigation	Comments
Right lower quadrant pain	CT	Reasonably sensitive in confirming appendicitis or other causes of right iliac fossa pain
Intestinal obstruction	Supine abdominal radiograph	Shows dilated small or large bowel, but seldom indicates cause
	CT	Demonstrates obstruction and may indicate cause, particularly if it is a hernia missed on clinical examination or in an unusual place (e.g. obturator hernia). In cases of malignancy CT may also reveal liver metastases that could alter surgical approach
Acute gallbladder disease	Ultrasonography	Identifies gallstones, thickened gallbladder wall (suggesting inflammation), dilated bile duct (suggesting biliary obstruction/stones in bile duct). Does not reliably detect stones in bile duct. Also identifies liver metastases which may present with right upper quadrant pain. Murphy's sign elicited by the ultrasound probe when the abdominal wall is indented into the gallbladder is diagnostic of acute cholecystitis.
	CT	Better to detect complications of cholecystitis, (e.g. emphysematous cholecystitis and gallbladder perforation). Not so sensitive for gallstones
Pancreatitis	Amylase	Typically very high (>1000 units) in pancreatitis, but goes down within a few days. Nonspecific—also very high in inflammation of salivary glands, perforation of peptic ulcer, ruptured aortic aneurysm, and in patients with macroamylasaemia. Moderately raised (300 to 1000 units) in many other causes of acute abdomen including biliary colic, cholecystitis, mesenteric ischaemia. Also said to be raised in renal failure
	CT	Best for detecting pancreatitis in patients presenting late where amylase not very high, as well as assessing severity and complications of pancreatitis
Perforated viscus	Erect chest radiograph	The patient needs to have been sitting up for some time to optimize the chances of picking up subdiaphragmatic air. Misses 10% of perforations
	CT	Most sensitive in detection of free air, and may also indicate what has perforated
Mesenteric ischaemia	CT	Readily available and noninvasive compared to angiography, but reported sensitivity varying from 40 to 80%. Nonspecific features include bowel dilatation, bowel wall thickening, and abnormal wall enhancement. Occlusion of mesenteric vessels may be seen after contrast. In addition infarction (nonperfusion) of other abdominal organs suggests multiple emboli. In many cases imaging is not diagnostic, and if suspicion is high laparotomy is indicated, although the chances of successful outcome are limited
Left iliac fossa pain (presumed diverticulitis)	CT	Barium enema and colonoscopy are contraindicated due to risk of converting inflammation into perforation. CT is sensitive in confirming diverticulitis, and will confirm complications such as abscess and perforation. It also detects other causes of left iliac fossa pain, including ruptured aneurysms. It is underused in patients thought to have diverticulitis, in whom left iliac fossa peritonitis is too frequently assumed to be diagnostic of uncomplicated colonic diverticulitis
Renal colic	Supine abdominal radiograph	Traditionally the investigation of choice, it is now been superseded by CT
	CT	Thin slice CT reliably detects stones. Will exclude abdominal aortic aneurysm where confusion exists
Gynaecological	Transvaginal ultrasonography	Not advisable if a high suspicion of a ruptured ectopic pregnancy due to risk of precipitating further haemorrhage. Should detect ovarian abnormalities

Diverticulitis

Often a label given to any left iliac fossa pain, acute colonic diverticulitis is a gradual onset lower abdominal pain that locates to the left iliac fossa, although it may cause suprapubic or right iliac fossa pain if the sigmoid colon is very mobile. It is similar to a left-sided appendicitis, and like appendicitis can result in abscess formation or perforation. Following initial cultures, antimicrobial therapy is commenced; if the pain does not improve over the next 24h, or if there are other features suggesting that this is a complicated diverticulitis, an urgent CT should be performed.

The acute abdomen on the medical ward

Acute pseudo-obstruction (adynamic ileus)

Originally described by Ogilivie in two patients with retroperitoneal malignancy, colonic pseudo-obstruction is common in hospitalized patients with acute infections, metabolic disorders (including electrolyte disorders), and following orthopaedic and pelvic surgery; drugs, particularly anticholinergics, are also associated. It is believed to arise from an imbalance in autonomic innervation of the colon, with a relative excess of sympathetic stimulation and reduction in parasympathetic activity. This results in an atonic distal colon, while the small bowel continues normal peristalsis. The ensuing features are typical of large-bowel obstruction, with vague central colicky abdominal pain, distension, and vomiting. Rectal examination reveals a capacious rectum, and imaging confirms a dilated large bowel with no obstructing cause seen on contrast enema. Left untreated the colon, in particular the caecum, distends and becomes ischaemic leading to necrosis and perforation. Treatment involves correcting any identifiable cause, such as electrolyte imbalances. Infusion of neostigmine (a cholinesterase inhibitor) or colonoscopic decompression are effective treatments. Surgery is indicated when perforation has occurred. Laxatives should be avoided since they worsen the distension and precipitate perforation. Prokinetic agents, such as erythromycin which stimulates the motilin receptor, have been reported to be effective.

The acute abdomen in older patients

Acute abdominal pain is common in older people, but tends to present less dramatically, such that severe mesenteric ischaemia or diverticular perforation might be associated with surprisingly few physical signs. The pain may be nonspecific, and pyrexia maybe absent in spite of intra-abdominal sepsis. On occasion the acute abdomen may precipitate an acute confusional state, so a thorough abdominal examination is important in all such patients. The pattern of disease also changes in older people. Diverticular disease and colonic cancer are common, as is biliary disease, alcohol use and, in consequence, acute pancreatitis. Obstruction due to adhesions and hernias is also more common, the hernias often being overlooked by patient and physician alike. Comorbidity is routine, so the morbidity and mortality from the acute abdomen are higher.

The acute abdomen in immunosuppressed patients

In immunosuppressed patients, as in older people, the typical presentation and course of an acute abdomen may alter. In addition the presence of immunosuppression might make other diagnoses more likely, particularly lymphoma and viral diseases such as cytomegalovirus. Immunosuppression often reduces the inflammatory response to the abdominal pathology, so signs of peritonitis might be much less impressive than in the nonimmunosuppressed; but such patients tolerate the untreated acute abdomen badly. For this reason urgent imaging and early surgery are appropriate. Likewise a less ambitious surgical approach is required, such that exteriorization of the bowel should be considered routine rather than risking a primary anastomosis. An early leak from an anastomotic disruption could be fatal in an immunosuppressed patient, but is obviated if the bowel is defunctioned.

The acute abdomen with peritoneal dialysis

The peritonitis that occurs in patients on peritoneal dialysis is commonly due to skin organisms such as *Staphylococcus epidermidis* and *Staph. aureus*. In addition to abdominal pain and tenderness the peritoneal dialysis fluid is cloudy with a high cell count. Culture of the fluid usually confirms the causative organism, and systemic and intraperitoneal antibiotics usually treat the infection completely. The presence of gut organisms in the fluid, particularly where more than one organism is identified, suggests a bowel perforation, as does the presence of free intraperitoneal air (best seen on CT). Although peritoneal dialysis exchanges can result in free intraperitoneal air, in the context of abdominal pain a perforation is more likely. Perforations are usually of diverticular origin, and can be very difficult to find at laparotomy because of the effective irrigation that the peritoneal dialysis provides and the small size of an early perforation. A negative laparotomy should therefore not be taken as eliminating perforation as a diagnosis, and continued pain is an indication for a second look, even within 48 h of the original laparotomy.

The acute abdomen in chronic liver disease

In cirrhotic patients with ascites, translocation of gut flora, or haematogenous seeding of bacteria, can result in bacterial infection of the fluid, a condition referred to as spontaneous bacterial peritonitis.

This is diagnosed by a high white cell count (>250 cells/mm^3) on aspiration, and is treated by systemic antibiotics even where culture is negative. Culture is negative in over one-half of the cases, although sensitivity of culture can be increased by direct inoculation into culture bottles at the bedside. Where the liver disease is advanced it often precipitates encephalopathy or renal failure and there is some evidence to suggest it may precipitate variceal haemorrhage. Surgery is not usually necessary, and if undertaken in this setting is associated with a high mortality due to decompensated liver disease.

The iatrogenic acute abdomen

Modern investigation and minimally invasive treatments carry risks, including the precipitation of an acute abdomen. These should be borne in mind by anyone reviewing a patient in pain in the following circumstances.

- Angiography/angioplasty—dislodged plaque fragments may result in mesenteric or renal ischaemia. Angioplasty to a branch of the aorta, such as a renal artery or mesenteric artery may cause *in situ* thrombosis. Since mesenteric ischaemia is difficult to diagnose, a high index of suspicion is necessary.

- Percutaneous drainage, be it under radiological guidance or unguided drainage of ascites, runs the risk of bowel perforation. Typical presentation as following a perforation of any aetiology, with the added diagnostic aid being the colour and nature of the fluid being drained.

- Liver procedures, such as transjugular portosystemic shunt formation, percutaneous transhepatic cholangiography, or endoscopic retrograde cholangiopancreatography may result in a bile leak and biliary peritonitis. Liver biopsy and percutaneous transhepatic cholangiography may also result in intraperitoneal haemorrhage.

- Endoscopic retrograde cholangiopancreatography is occasionally associated with acute pancreatitis. It may also cause a retroperitoneal perforation.

- Endoscopic investigation and treatment, whether upper or lower gastrointestinal tract—perforation of the bowel is recognized. Typically patients present with acute abdominal pain if the perforation is intraperitoneal; occasional retroperitoneal perforations may result in local abscess formation and be difficult to diagnose without cross-sectional imaging.

Medical causes of an acute abdomen

While the keen student will recount the acute abdomen that results from porphyria or sickle crisis, or in association with tabetic crises, it should be borne in mind that common things are common and that applies particularly to the acute abdomen. Nevertheless some nonsurgical causes are important to note:

- Diabetic ketoacidosis is associated with abdominal pain; it might also be precipitated by intra-abdominal pathology such as appendicitis and ectopic pregnancy.

- Herpes zoster often presents with a prodromal pain a few days before the rash appears. Its unilateral nature may result in diagnoses of diverticulitis or cholecystitis being made.

- Pneumonia—particularly in young people and older people, lower lobe pneumonia can present with upper abdominal pain.

A careful history, chest examination, and radiology should provide the correct diagnosis. Occasionally the pneumonia is secondary to upper abdominal pathology which has resulted in reduced respiratory effort.

◆ Gastroenteritis can present with colicky pain followed by diarrhoea and/or vomiting. The history of exposure to a potential infective source, as well as contacts with similar symptoms is usually helpful. Stool cultures should be taken, and the patient nursed appropriately.

◆ Constipation can often cause concern, particularly in patients with Parkinson's disease where both disease and treatment contribute. Constipation may present with colicky pain and distension, and may be the first manifestation of a colonic carcinoma. Occasionally chronic constipation might result in sigmoid volvulus, diagnosed radiologically and treated sigmoidoscopically.

◆ Acute porphyria causes abdominal pain and other features of neurovisceral manifestations. It is a disease that is worthy of consideration since specific treatment with haem arginate and avoidance of precipitating factors such as drugs, starvation, surgical procedures, and anaesthetics is often life-saving. A characteristic feature of acute porphyria is the distress that accompanies the pain and the associated hypertension and tachycardia: a notable aspect is the lack of tenderness. The diagnosis is based on history, family history, and specific urinary tests (see Chapter 12.5).

Further reading

Burnand KG *et al.* (eds) (2005). The acute abdomen, Chapter 25 in *The new Aird's companion in surgical studies*, 3rd edition. Churchill Livingstone, Edinburgh.

Flasar MH, Goldberg E (2006). Acute abdominal pain. *Med Clin N Am*, **90**, 481–503. [Acute abdominal pain for physicians, with an American flavour.]

Ranji SR *et al.* (2006). Do opiates affect the clinical evaluation of patients with acute abdominal pain? *JAMA*, **296**, 1764–74. [Evidence that opiates do not alter the outcome in acute abdominal pain, although they may increase the time to diagnosis.]

Saunders MD, Kimmey MB (2005). Systematic review: acute colonic pseudo-obstruction. *Aliment Pharmacol Ther*, **22**, 917–25. [A review of the aetiology and treatment of pseudo-obstruction.]

15.4.2 Gastrointestinal bleeding

T.A. Rockall and H.M.P. Dowson

Essentials

Gastrointestinal bleeding is a common emergency, with an incidence in the United Kingdom of about 1 per 1000 adults/year. It is subdivided into upper and lower, and acute or chronic, with acute upper gastrointestinal haemorrhage further subdivided into variceal and nonvariceal bleeding. Risk stratification in acute upper gastrointestinal haemorrhage can be performed using simple clinical and endoscopic criteria that can be used to estimate the risk

of mortality, which overall is about 10% for both upper and lower gastrointestinal bleeds.

The immediate management of the hypovolaemic patient is first directed towards resuscitation (see Chapter 17.3) and then to identification of the site and cause of bleeding.

Most patients (80% in upper and 85–90% in lower gastrointestinal bleeding) will stop bleeding spontaneously and should then be investigated with either endoscopy or colonoscopy as appropriate. Patients with acute ongoing haemorrhage require urgent investigation (following fluid resuscitation) by oesophagogastroduodenoscopy with a view to applying endoscopic haemostatic therapy. Therapeutic techniques include injection of adrenaline, application of heat energy, and clipping, with data from randomized controlled trials demonstrating that such endoscopic therapy is efficacious in up to 95% of patients with upper gastrointestinal bleeding. In patients with major ulcer bleeding, treatment with a high dose proton pump inhibitor following successful endoscopic therapy has been shown to reduce the risk of rebleeding (but not overall mortality). If these techniques fail to arrest bleeding, then either selective mesenteric angiography with embolization or surgery is indicated.

Uncontrolled variceal haemorrhage may be controlled with a Sengstaken–Blakemore tube as a temporary measure before more definitive treatment. Where endoscopic therapies subsequently fail, transjugular intrahepatic portosystemic shunt is a minimally invasive method of creating a portosystemic shunt, and oesophageal transection is occasionally life saving where all other attempts at haemostasis have failed.

Definition

Acute gastrointestinal haemorrhage is classified by its origin, from either the upper or the lower gastrointestinal tract, anatomically demarcated by the ligament of Treitz (at the junction of the duodenum and jejunum). It is further subdivided into nonvariceal and variceal haemorrhage. Only when gastrointestinal bleeding is acute does it constitute an emergency. Chronic, low-volume blood loss is usually subclinical until such time as it presents with iron deficient anaemia.

Acute upper gastrointestinal haemorrhage (AUGIH)

Aetiology and pathogenesis

Many gastrointestinal lesions may result in haemorrhage but peptic ulcer is the most frequent cause in the United Kingdom (Table 15.4.2.1). Each diagnostic group has its own aetiological factors.

Peptic ulcer disease

Helicobacter pylori infection and ingestion of aspirin and nonsteroidal anti-inflammatory drugs (NSAIDs) are important for ulcer disease and erosions of the upper gastrointestinal tract. Ulceration may also occur at the site of surgical enterostomies (stomal ulcers) and in association with the Zollinger–Ellison syndrome. Peptic ulceration at specific sites is associated with major haemorrhage due to the anatomical relation of major arteries—the posterior wall of the first part of the duodenum (gastroduodenal artery), the

Table 15.4.2.1 Diagnoses following acute upper gastrointestinal haemorrhage

Diagnosis	%
Peptic ulcer	35–50
Erosive disease	10–15
Oesophagitis	10
Mallory–Weiss tear	5–10
Oesophageal varices	5–10
Upper gastrointestinal malignancy	<5
Vascular malformations	5
Other/not established	5–15

lesser curve of the stomach (left gastric artery), and posterior wall of stomach (splenic artery).

Varices

Liver disease due to alcohol and hepatitis are the principal causes in Western countries of portal hypertension, which leads to oesophageal varices; variceal bleeding may rarely affect the stomach and the remaining gastrointestinal tract.

Mallory–Weiss tears

These are mucosal lesions at the oesophagogastric junction associated with profuse vomiting; the haematemesis that occurs follows a normal vomit, and is usually minor and nearly always self-limiting.

Rare causes

The most common malignant causes of upper gastrointestinal haemorrhage are adenocarcinoma of the stomach and gastric lymphoma, but acute bleeding is an unusual presentation. Other causes include gastrointestinal stromal tumours which may bleed when the mucosal surface ulcerates, angiodysplasia (and other vascular lesions), aortoduodenal fistula, haemobilia, and trauma.

Epidemiology

The incidence of AUGIH in the United Kingdom is approximately 1 per 1000 adults/year, of which 15% of cases occur in patients already in hospital. The male incidence is twice that of the female in all age groups except older people, where they are similar. The annual incidence increases dramatically with age, rising to nearly 5 per 1000/year in the over-75 age group. In the United Kingdom in 1993, about one-quarter of cases occurred in patients over the age of 80 years.

Prevention

All patients with a peptic ulcer should be tested for *Helicobacter pylori* infection, and if positive, eradication therapy should be prescribed. This significantly reduces the risk of ulcer recurrence.

Patients in hospital, particularly old people and those who have had surgery, are at higher risk of AUGIH. For this group in whom use of NSAIDs is being considered, it is prudent to consider cover with a proton pump inhibitor.

Variceal haemorrhage can be prevented through programmes of variceal eradication by injection or banding and also by transjugular intrahepatic portosystemic shunt, or ultimately liver transplantation where indicated.

Box 15.4.2.1 Melaena

This is a clinical diagnosis made on the observation of black, tarry, offensive stool on rectal examination (or passed spontaneously). It occurs as the result of digestive enzymes and bacteria acting on haemoglobin. Although melaena is usually due to AUGIH, bleeding from the right side of the colon may also present in this way.

Clinical features

History

- Upper gastrointestinal haemorrhage usually presents with haematemesis or 'coffee-ground' vomiting and melaena (see Box 15.4.2.1). Frank haematemesis indicates a severe bleed. It is not always a feature, but melaena will always follow a significant bleed. The absence of blood in the first vomit suggests a Mallory–Weiss tear.

- In rapid bleeding, symptoms of hypovolaemia may precede haematemesis or melaena. These include postural hypotension, syncope, shock, and even death.

- Past medical history—liver disease (alcohol, risk factors for hepatitis).

- Drug history—the patient should be asked about ingestion of aspirin and other NSAIDs, and anticoagulants.

Examination

- Airway, breathing, circulation—the patient must be assessed rapidly for signs of shock.

- Gastrointestinal—signs of liver disease may be present in patients with oesophageal varices but this does not confirm the cause of blood loss since peptic ulcer is a common synchronous lesion.

- Rectal examination—looking for fresh blood or evidence of melaena.

Differential diagnosis

In patients with rapid haemorrhage, usually accompanied by shock, fresh blood may be passed per rectum (haemochezia) and may thus be difficult to distinguish from lower gastrointestinal haemorrhage. A large nasopharyngeal bleed, resulting in a significant volume of swallowed blood, can also present with haematemesis.

Investigations

AUGIH is mainly a clinical diagnosis.

- Full blood count and coagulation tests. The initial haemoglobin estimation is not a useful indicator of the volume of blood lost until time for haemodilution has passed. The haemoglobin level may be normal in a patient with a large, acute haemorrhage. Equally, it may be low in a patient with iron deficiency anaemia resulting from chronic haemorrhage who presents with a small, acute bleed. The haemoglobin and haematocrit after volume resuscitation are more useful. Platelet count and coagulation studies are important to exclude a bleeding disorder and are of particular relevance in patients receiving therapeutic anticoagulants and in those with liver disease.

Table 15.4.2.2 The Rockall score: acute upper gastrointestinal haemorrhage scoring system

Variable	Score			
	0	1	2	3
Age (years)	<60	60–79	≥80	
Shock	'No shock'	'Tachycardia'	'Hypotension'	
Systolic BP	≥100	≥100	<100	
Pulse	<100	≥100		
Comorbidity	No major comorbidity		Cardiac failure	Renal failure
			Ischaemic heart disease	Liver failure
			Any major comorbidity	Disseminated malignancy
Diagnosis	Mallory–Weiss tear	All other diagnoses	Malignancy of upper gastrointestinal tract	
	No lesion identified and no stigmata of recent haemorrhage			
Major stigmata of recent haemorrhage	None or dark spot only		Blood in upper gastrointestinal tract	
			Adherent clot	
			Visible or spurting vessel	

- Urea, creatinine, and electrolytes. The blood urea may rise as the absorbed products of luminal blood are metabolized by the liver. It is also important to have a baseline renal function.

- Serum liver-related tests—liver disease.

- Group and save, or cross-match, depending on clinical severity.

- Endoscopy. See below.

Treatment

The management of acute upper gastrointestinal haemorrhage falls into four principal stages.

1 Assessment, resuscitation, and monitoring

Important aspects of assessment are confirmation that a bleed has occurred and the degree of hypovolaemic shock that has resulted.

- Resuscitation is as for any hypovolaemic patient with the immediate aim of rapidly replenishing blood. Tachycardia, vasoconstriction, sweating, hypotension (including a postural drop), tachypnoea, and a low central venous pressure all indicate hypovolaemia. Large-bore peripheral venous access, central venous access, and placement of a urinary catheter will help in the resuscitation and monitoring of the more severe cases and those with major cardiovascular and respiratory comorbidity.

- Monitoring—once circulating blood volume has been restored, management should be aimed at monitoring the patient for continued or recurrent bleeding, replacing blood, making a diagnosis, and instituting therapy. Regular pulse, blood pressure, central venous pressure, and urine output will give a good guide. High risk patients should be monitored in an high-dependency unit or intensive therapy unit. Fresh haematemesis obviously indicates further acute haemorrhage. The passage of further fresh melaena has to be interpreted in the light of the cardiovascular signs and repeated estimations of blood haemoglobin concentration.

- Assessment of bleeding severity. It is essential to categorize patients at the time of admission into high or low risk of death.

Independent risk factors that accurately predict mortality have been identified (see 'Prognosis' below, and Tables 15.4.2.2 and 15.4.2.3). These include:

- increasing age
- comorbidity
- shock
- endoscopic findings

2 Diagnosis and haemostasis

In most instances, the diagnosis is obscure until upper gastrointestinal endoscopy is undertaken (see Chapter 15.3.2). This diagnostic, and potentially therapeutic, procedure should be undertaken as soon as possible after resuscitation is complete. Haemostasis occurs spontaneously in most cases. When bleeding continues, haemostasis can be achieved by endoscopic, surgical, or radiological means.

Endoscopy

The aim of endoscopy is fourfold:

- To make a diagnosis

- To assess the risk of further haemorrhage based upon the site, size, and nature of the lesion (including stigmata of recent haemorrhage)

Table 15.4.2.3 Observed rebleeding and mortality by risk score

Score	0	1	2	3	4	5	6	7	8+
Rebleed (%)	4.9	3.4	5.3	11.2	14.1	24.1	32.9	43.8	41.8
Deaths No rebleed (%)	0	0	0.3	2.0	3.5	8.1	9.5	14.9	28.1
Deaths Rebleed (%)	0	0	0	10.0	15.8	22.9	33.3	43.4	52.5
Deaths Total (%)	0	0	0.2	2.9	5.3	10.8	17.3	27.0	41.1

- To apply haemostatic therapy where appropriate

- To inform the surgeon as to the site of the lesion in cases requiring urgent surgery due to rapid, ongoing blood loss and to exclude varices in these cases.

Endoscopic haemostatic therapy may be given in the form of:

- Injection of adrenaline. This is performed in quadrants around the bleeding point, and then into the bleeding vessel, using a total of 4 to 16 ml of a 1:10000 adrenaline solution in normal saline. Haemostasis is achieved in 95% of cases, although bleeding can recur in 15 to 20%.

  - Injection of other agents such as sclerosants (e.g. polidocanol) or alcohol does not confer additional advantage, but does increase the risk of perforation

  - Fibrin glue, by encouraging clot formation, has been shown to be effective, but is not widely available.

- The application of heat energy in the form of a heater probe or diathermy is also effective. The heater probe is useful because it includes a powerful water jet which aids clot removal. Laser therapy is no longer used.

- Mechanical clips can be applied to bleeding points, and are particularly useful for actively bleeding large vessels.

- Combination therapy. The combination of two endoscopic therapeutic measures (the injection of adrenaline, and application of heat or haemoclipping) has been shown in randomized controlled trials and a meta-analysis to be more efficacious than single-modality therapy in preventing rebleeding.

- Endoscopic therapy can be repeated if a patient rebleeds.

There is good trial evidence that endoscopic therapy reduces the rate of rebleeding and mortality. There is no evidence from randomized controlled trials that planned, repeated endoscopic therapy further reduces rebleeding in peptic ulcer. Repeated injection or banding have been shown to reduce rebleeding and mortality from oesophageal varices.

Surgery

This is indicated in massive, acute bleeding not amenable to endoscopic therapy or where endoscopic therapy fails to control active bleeding. However, a second attempt at endoscopic therapy should be made (especially in young patients) before resorting to surgery, although there is rarely any place for a third attempt. There is some evidence that early surgical intervention in those over 60 is appropriate. It is important to inform an experienced surgeon about the possible need for surgery at an early stage. In cases where endoscopic therapy has failed and surgery is deemed to be exceptionally high risk, visceral angiography may allow for embolization (e.g. the gastroduodenal artery in duodenal ulcer).

Drug therapy

In patients with major ulcer bleeding, following successful endoscopic therapy, treatment with a high dose proton pump inhibitor is recommended, such as omeprazole 80 mg immediately followed by an infusion of 8 mg hourly for 72 h. This has been shown to reduce the risk of rebleeding, although studies have not demonstrated a significant reduction in overall mortality.

Uncontrolled variceal haemorrhage

This may be controlled with a Sengstaken–Blakemore tube as a temporary measure before more definitive treatment. Where endoscopic therapies subsequently fail, transjugular intrahepatic portosystemic shunt is a minimally invasive method of creating a portosystemic shunt. Finally, oesophageal transection is occasionally life saving where all other attempts at haemostasis have failed.

3 Treatment of causative lesion

Treatment of the causative lesion should be started as soon as possible after diagnosis. Proton pump inhibitors are effective in healing peptic ulcers, and have been shown to reduce rebleeding rates in patients with a nonbleeding visible vessel, and also in patients with active bleeding when used in combination with endoscopic therapies. Where the causative lesion is a tumour (benign or malignant) then elective surgery may be indicated. Angiodysplasia can be treated with laser or argon beam. Specific treatments may be required for rarer causes such as Crohn's disease or tuberculosis.

4 Prevention of recurrence

Recurrent episodes of bleeding from peptic ulcers can be prevented by eradicating *H. pylori* infection and through the avoidance of ulcerogenic drugs. Persistent ulceration despite these measures may require long-term acid suppressive therapy and Zollinger–Ellison syndrome should be excluded.

Prognosis

Prognosis depends on many factors including the severity of the bleed, the age of the patient, the associated comorbidity of the patient, the diagnostic category, the endoscopic features (stigmata of recent haemorrhage), and whether continued or recurrent bleeding is a feature.

Overall, the crude mortality for patients presenting to emergency departments with acute upper gastrointestinal haemorrhage is about 10%, but is significantly higher (up to 33%) among inpatients who develop gastrointestinal bleeding while hospitalized for other reasons. Most deaths occur in older people and those with severe comorbidity.

Death in those under the age of 60 with no comorbidity is very low (0.1%) regardless of the severity of the haemorrhage. The factors that contribute to mortality have been combined in a prognostic risk score which is represented in Table 15.4.2.2. The mortality associated with each risk score is represented in Table 15.4.2.3.

Acute lower gastrointestinal haemorrhage
Epidemiology

The incidence of lower gastrointestinal haemorrhage has not been well defined but it is common, and accounts for approximately 1% of acute hospital admissions. Most (85–90%) of acute lower gastrointestinal bleeds will stop spontaneously although 35% will require blood transfusion, and 5 to 10% will require urgent surgical intervention.

Aetiology

As in upper gastrointestinal haemorrhage, several pathological causes are responsible. Most causative lesions are colonic or anorectal with only 5 to 10% originating in the small bowel (Table 15.4.2.4). In developed countries, diverticular disease represents

Table 15.4.2.4 Source of lower gastrointestinal haemorrhage

Diagnosis	%
Diverticulosis	35
Colonic polyp or cancer	15
Benign anorectal conditions (including haemorrhoids)	10
Inflammatory bowel disease (including UC, Crohn's, infective colitis)	15
Ischaemic colitis	5
Angiodysplasia (including angiomas and AV malfunctions)	10
Small bowel (including Meckel's diverticulum)	1–2
Others (including rectal ulcer, postpolypectomy, radiation colitis, rectal varices)	10

AV, arteriovenous; UC, ulcerative colitis.

the largest proportion of cases. Bleeding is not uncommonly associated with coagulopathy but studies have shown the distribution of causative lesions in these cases to be the same. In severe cases, however, generalized mucosal bleeding may occur.

Diverticular disease
Acute colonic diverticular bleeding is common. The estimated risk of bleeding with this disease is about 15%. After a single bleed, the risk of recurrence is 25% and after two bleeds it is 50%. Eighty per cent of all bleeds stop spontaneously and no therapy is indicated. Operative intervention should be considered after two major bleeds because the risk of further recurrence is high. However, many of these patients are frail and elderly, and continuation of conservative treatment for multiple, self-limiting episodes may be appropriate.

Inflammatory bowel disease
This often manifests itself as bloody diarrhoea but more rarely may present with profuse haemorrhage. This is more common in Crohn's disease than in ulcerative colitis because the inflammation involves the whole thickness of the bowel wall. Up to 6% of patients with this disease may sustain a major haemorrhage. About 50% stop bleeding spontaneously but of these 35% will rebleed. For this reason, urgent surgery is usually indicated for patients with a life-threatening haemorrhage as a result of inflammatory colitis. The operation usually required is a subtotal colectomy, with the rectum usually being preserved at this stage unless this is the site of major haemorrhage. Ischaemic colitis rarely causes severe haemorrhage. Bloody diarrhoea is more usual and may be accompanied by pain.

Colonic tumours
Benign and malignant colonic tumours may present as profuse bleeding although occult blood loss and minor fresh bleeding is more common. Rarely is urgent surgical intervention required.

Angiodysplasia
Vascular anomalies occur with increasing frequency with age. They may originate from chronic, partial venous obstruction of submucosal veins due to incompetence of the precapillary sphincters and arteriovenous malformations. These lesions are usually multiple and are most frequent in the caecum and ascending colon. Bleeding is usually slow, intermittent, and recurrent although once again it is occasionally massive (2–15%). Most (90%) stop spontaneously but 25 to 85% will recur. The treatment of choice is endoscopic

coagulation if the lesions can be identified. Colectomy is reserved for those with repeated major haemorrhage.

Benign anorectal disease
Benign anorectal disease does present as lower gastrointestinal haemorrhage and a careful examination of the anorectum (with proctosigmoidoscopy) is imperative before initiating more invasive examinations. However, anorectal lesions are common and complete colonic evaluation is usually required even after identifying an anorectal source such as haemorrhoids.

Iatrogenic haemorrhage
The risk of haemorrhage after polypectomy is estimated to be between 0.2 and 3%. Haemorrhage is usually immediate but may be delayed. When identified, endoscopic haemostatic techniques are usually successful (injection of adrenaline, resnaring, recoagulating, placement of a ligature or clip).

Clinical features
History
A good history from the patient may give clues as to the cause of colorectal haemorrhage. Important points include:

- A prior history of bleeding
- The exact nature of the bleeding—specifically the duration, the colour of the blood, the relationship to defecation, whether the blood is mixed with or separate from the stool, an associated change in bowel habit, or mucus discharge. Bright red blood separate from the stool suggests an anorectal cause. Diarrhoea and mucous associated with darker blood mixed in with the stool suggests colitis or neoplasm. None of these clinical features, however, is absolutely diagnostic.
- Co-morbidities
- Drug usage (aspirin, NSAIDs, and warfarin)

Examination
A full clinical examination should be performed, with particular focus on examination of the abdomen and rectum. Proctosigmoidoscopy is mandatory to identify anorectal causes of bleeding.

Treatment
Resuscitation
Immediate resuscitation is as for bleeding from the upper gastrointestinal tract. In a patient with significant bleeding, it is essential that good intravenous access is established, even in the stable patient. The patient should be catheterized, closely monitored, and if necessary transferred to a high-dependency setting.

Subsequent management
Since most lower gastrointestinal bleeds stop spontaneously, initial management should be conservative with transfusion and correction of clotting abnormalities. Once haemorrhage has ceased, bowel preparation and colonoscopy can be undertaken in a stable patient and with a much higher chance of detecting the pathological lesion (>90%).

In the small proportion of patients in whom active colonic bleeding continues, investigation to localize the source of the haemorrhage is indicated so that directed treatment can be administered in the form of endoscopic therapy, interventional radiology, or surgery.

Clinical investigation and further treatment

In a patient with significant haemorrhage, it may be necessary to delineate the location of the gastrointestinal bleed, prior to evaluation of the colon. This is because massive upper gastrointestinal bleeding can masquerade as lower gastrointestinal bleeding, with up to 15% of those patients presenting with haematochezia having an upper gastrointestinal source. An oesophagogastroduodenoscopy will exclude an upper gastrointestinal cause, although historically, passing a nasogastric tube and the aspirate checked for blood was used.

Colonoscopy

Colonoscopy is favoured by many clinicians as both an investigative and a therapeutic measure, although the use of bowel preparation is still debated. In studies, some using bowel preparation and some without, the causative lesion was identified in approximately three-quarters of patients. Colonoscopy should be abandoned if massive haemorrhage obscures the diagnosis or severe mucosal or ischaemic colitis is encountered, as the risk of perforation in these cases is high.

Control of active bleeding is an important therapeutic indication for colonoscopy, with haemostasis achievable in many cases such as diverticular haemorrhage, angiodysplasia, and postpolypectomy bleeding. Control of bleeding can be accomplished with monopolar or bipolar coagulation, heater probe, injection of various agents (such as epinephrine), use of Nd:YAG laser, and clipping.

Endoscopic treatment of focal bleeding lesions in the colon is highly effective and safe, diminishing the need for surgical intervention. However, rebleeding rates have been reported of between 13 and 53%, and many patients require further treatments.

Radiology

Nuclear scintigraphy can be used to detect active haemorrhage. It is very sensitive and can detect bleeding rates of 0.1 ml/min, and has been reported to detect bleeding rates as low as 0.02 ml/min. Technetium-99 (^{99}Tcm) labelled sulphur colloid can be used, which has the advantage of no preparation but the half-life is very short. If there is no active bleeding at the moment it is given, the test may be nondiagnostic, and its rapid enhancement of the liver and spleen can also obscure the diagnosis.

A better method is the use of ^{99}Tcm labelled red cells. Unfortunately, although sensitive, it is also very nonspecific and localizes the lesion very poorly. Its half-life of up to 12–24 h means that, even if the bleeding is intermittent, the labelled blood cells can accumulate at the site of bleeding up to 24 h after injection.

There is still controversy over the role of nuclear scintigraphy, and many surgeons are reluctant to proceed to a colectomy based solely on its results. It may be useful immediately before angiography (as scintigraphy can detect lower bleeding rates) to confirm active haemorrhage before undertaking the more invasive procedure. Whenever there is massive, active haemorrhage, however, this is unnecessary and the patient should proceed directly to visceral angiography.

Sensitivity for scintigraphy is over 90%, although specificity is lower (76–95%), and overall accuracy reported in the literature is between 41 and 94%.

Selective mesenteric angiography can detect a rate of bleeding of 0.5 to 1.0 ml/min. The sensitivity of angiography reported in various studies ranges from 40 to 86%, although this may be increased by the use of so-called provocative measures, such as vasodilators, heparin, or thrombolytic agents.

Once the site of haemorrhage is identified, there is the therapeutic possibility of arterial infusion of vasopressin or selective embolization, or the patient can proceed directly to surgery. Vasopressin infusion (via a catheter positioned in the artery supplying the site of bleeding) has considerable side effects including mesenteric thrombosis, intestinal infarction, myocardial ischaemia, hypertension, arrythmias, and death. Nitroglycerine may be infused simultaneously to counteract the systemic effects of the drug. Vasopressin infusion is successful in stopping bleeding in about 80% of patients, but the rebleeding rate is high (30%), giving an overall success rate of approximately 50%.

Selective embolization using coil springs, polyvinyl alcohol foam, or gel foam into the most distal vessel results in high initial rates of haemostasis and the rate of intestinal infarction is low. It is a good technique for patients with a very high predicted operative mortality.

Surgical options

An emergency operation for lower gastrointestinal haemorrhage is required in 10 to 25% of patients. Indications for surgery include:

- Haemodynamic instability
- Clinical deterioration
- Transfusion requirements >6 units
- Persistent or recurrent haemorrhage

Surgery consists of a segmental resection, or a subtotal colectomy in nonlocalized gastrointestinal haemorrhage. Whilst the mortality rates following a segmental resection are lower, the rebleeding rate is much higher: between 14% (with a positive angiogram) and 42% (with a negative angiogram).

Obscure bleeding

In about 5% of cases the source of bleeding remains obscure, despite multiple attempts at localization. In many of these cases the bleeding source is found to be in the small bowel, with the commonest causes being angiodysplasia (accounting for 75% of episodes), Meckel's diverticula, neoplasia, and Crohn's disease. Wireless capsule endoscopy has been shown to be useful in such cases. The videocapsule is a self-contained unit, approximately 1×3 cm in size, and contains a miniature image-capturing system, battery, light source, and transmitter. Additional investigations may include small-bowel enteroscopy or laparotomy with on-table enteroscopy.

Likely future developments

Improved diagnostic capabilities

- Identifying feeding vessels and collaterals by endoscopic ultrasonography may be beneficial in AUGIH.

- Capsule endoscopy is the most sensitive modality for identifying lesions in the small bowel, and this investigative technique needs to be more widely available. It is also useful in the investigation of recurrent obscure gastrointestinal bleeds.

Improved therapeutic capabilities

◆ Rebleeding still occurs in 20% of upper gastrointestinal bleeds. New therapeutic endoscopic techniques such as endoscopic suturing devices may reduce the need for salvage surgery.

Further reading

British Society of Gastroenterology Endoscopy Committee (2005). Non-variceal upper gastrointestinal haemorrhage: guidelines. *Gut*, **51** Suppl IV, iv1–6.

Calvet X, *et al.* (2004). ddition of a second endoscopic treatment following epinephrine injection improves outcome in high-risk bleeding ulcers. *Gastroenterology*, **126**, 41–50.

Hoedema RE, Luchtefeld MA (2005). The management of lower gastrointestinal hemorrhage. *Dis Colon Rectum*, **48**, 2010–24.

Jensen DM, *et al.* (1999). Prospective effectiveness study of an urgent endoscopic approach to diagnosis and treatment of patients hospitalized with recurrent hematochezia. *Gastrointest Endosc*, **49**, 331.

Jensen DM, Machicado GA (2005). Endoscopic hemostasis of ulcer hemorrhage with injection, thermal, and combination methods. *Tech Gastroint Endosc*, **7**, 124–31.

Kahi CJ, *et al.* (2005). Endoscopic therapy versus medical therapy for bleeding peptic ulcer with adherent clot: a meta-analysis. *Gastroenterology*, **129**, 855–62.

Khorrani GJP, *et al.* (2004). *H. pylori* eradication therapy vs. Antisecretory non-eradication therapy (with or without long-term maintenance antisecretory therapy) for the prevention of recurrent bleeding from peptic ulcer. *Cochrane Database Syst Rev*, **2**, CD004062.

Martins NB, Wassef W (2006). Upper gastrointestinal bleeding. *Curr Opin Gastroenterol*, **22**, 612–19.

Palmer KR, Church NI (1999). Therapeutic endoscopy for upper gastrointestinal bleeding. *Cont Med Ed J Gastroenterol Hepatol Nutr*, **2**, 75–8.

Rockall TA, *et al.* (1995). Incidence of and mortality from acute upper gastrointestinal haemorrhage in the United Kingdom. *BMJ*, **311**, 222–6.

Rockall TA, *et al.* (1996). Risk assessment following acute upper gastrointestinal haemorrhage. *Gut*, **38**, 316–21.

Vernava AM, *et al.* (1997). Lower gastrointestinal bleeding. *Dis Colon Rectum*, **40**, 846–58.

Williams SG, Westaby D (1994). Management of variceal haemorrhage. *BMJ*, **308**, 1213–17.

Immune disorders of the gastrointestinal tract

M.R. Haeney

Essentials

The gastrointestinal tract is protected by gut-associated lymphoid tissue that provides an environment where interaction occurs between luminal antigen and specially adapted immune tissue in Peyer's patches. T lymphocytes (cytotoxic effector cells) and B lymphocytes primed in Peyer's patches migrate into the systemic circulation via the thoracic duct but home preferentially to the lamina propria of the intestine. Plasma cells of the lamina propria secrete immunoglobulin A as a dimer linked by a joining peptide.

Ingestion of antigen can lead to local immunity, systemic immunity, or a state of specific immune unresponsiveness (tolerance). Normally, the intestinal immune system steers a course between immunological incompetence on the one hand, with vulnerability to ingested pathogens, as in primary and secondary immunodeficiencies, and hypersensitivity to dietary antigens on the other, with immunologically mediated adverse reactions each time that antigen is eaten.

Immunodeficiency disorders

Common variable immunodeficiency provides an example of the intestinal complications of primary antibody deficiency syndromes, with 30% to 50% of patients having gastrointestinal problems at some time: achlorhydria is common; there is an increased risk of gastric cancer and B cell lymphoma; infestation with *Giardia lamblia* and infection with cryptosporidium or campylobacter are common causes of diarrhoea and/or malabsorption; nodular lymphoid hyperplasia is frequently asymptomatic.

Secondary immunodeficiency disorders, e.g. AIDS, are far more common than primary immunodeficiencies. The gastrointestinal tract is a major target organ in HIV infection, with intestinal consequences arising from (1) direct infection of enterocytes by HIV; (2) opportunistic and other infections; and (3) opportunistic tumours.

Food allergy and intolerance

Food allergy refers to a form of exaggerated reactivity (hypersensitivity) of the immune system to an ingested antigen, and is mostly synonymous with reactions involving IgE antibodies. The term 'food intolerance' should be used to describe all abnormal, reproducible reactions to food when the causative mechanism is unknown or is not immunological. These are controversial topics—public perception is that a wide variety of symptoms are due to food 'allergy', but this is rarely supported by objective scientific evidence. It is highly debatable whether food intolerance plays any part in symptoms remote from the gut—e.g. attention-deficit hyperactivity disorder or intractable epilepsy in children, or arthritis in adults—but food allergy and intolerance remain particularly susceptible to those advocating unorthodox diagnostic tests or treatments, the main hazard of which is that potentially serious problems can be misdiagnosed or mistreated.

Most cases of IgE-mediated food allergic reactions occur in infants and children: these are caused by cow's milk (in infants), peanuts, tree nuts, eggs, fish, and shellfish, and relatively easy to diagnose because of the clear relationship between typical symptoms (e.g. angioedema, vomiting, diarrhoea) and exposure. Food allergy should not be diagnosed without good clinical indications, and no laboratory test can replace a careful clinical history. Skin prick tests and tests for circulating antigen-specific IgE antibodies are positive in about 75% of patients with IgE-mediated acute reactions to foods. Recognition of the offending food and its elimination from the diet is the cornerstone of treatment. Some patients require a preloaded syringe of adrenaline (epinephrine) for self-injection, together with clear instruction and training in its use (see Chapter 17.2).

Elimination diets and food challenges form the basis of diagnosis of food intolerance, the gold standard being a double-blind, placebo-controlled challenge under medical supervision (there is danger of precipitating an anaphylactic reaction, particularly in children), although this is difficult to undertake in practice. Laboratory tests are of little diagnostic help for most patients with food intolerance.

Introduction

The gut is protected by several mechanisms. The intercellular tight junctions of the epithelial cells form an important physical barrier; these cells turn over every 24 to 96 h. Any injury to the epithelial barrier results in rapid migration of adjacent viable epithelial cells to cover the denuded area, a process called 'restitution', while lymphocytes and macrophages migrate through pores in the basement membrane to provide temporary protection. The acid pH of the stomach and the proteolytic enzyme content of the intestine are formidable chemical barriers to many organisms. A change in the normal microflora of the intestine or impaired gut motility may allow pathogenic bacteria to flourish. Microbial antigens that resist these defences and penetrate the epithelial surface encounter the mucosal immune system.

Functional morphology of the gut-associated lymphoid tissue

Lymphocytes are found at three sites within the mucosa (Fig. 15.5.1):

♦ Organized lymphoid aggregates (Peyer's patches) beneath the epithelium of the terminal small intestine

♦ Lymphocytes within the epithelial cell layer (intraepithelial lymphocytes)

♦ Lymphocytes scattered among other immunocompetent cells within the lamina propria

Gut-associated lymphoid tissue (GALT) is divided into two functional compartments: an afferent arm—Peyer's patches—where interaction occurs between luminal antigens and the immune system; and an effector arm—the diffusely distributed intraepithelial and lamina propria lymphocytes.

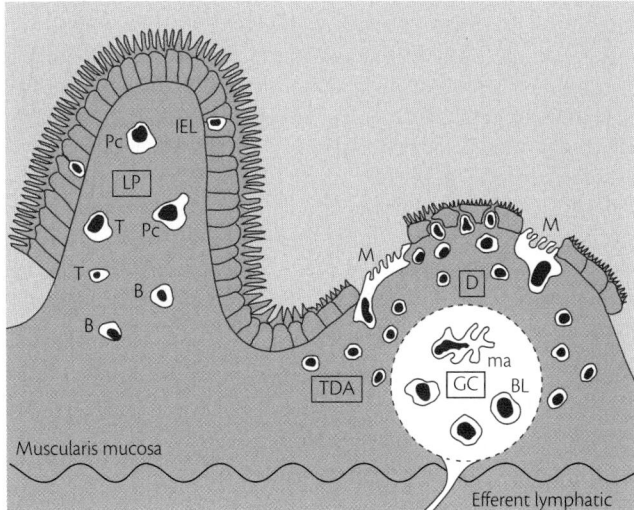

Fig. 15.5.1 Organization and structure of gut-associated lymphoid tissue. On the left, T and B lymphocytes and plasma cells (PC) can be seen in the lamina propria, with intraepithelial lymphocytes (IEL) between the columnar epithelial cells. On the right, there is a Peyer's patch covered by cuboidal epithelium with occasional 'M' cells. The Peyer's patch comprises three areas: the dome (D) of T and B lymphocytes; the thymus-dependent area (TDA); and the germinal centre (GC) containing macrophages (Ma) and B lymphoblasts (BL).

Peyer's patches

These are covered by a specialized epithelium (follicle-associated epithelium) that has no microvilli but whose surface seems wrinkled or folded under the scanning electron microscope (Fig. 15.5.1). These microfold, or M, cells sample and transport particulate antigens from the lumen into the 'dome' area, where T and B cells mix freely with the microfolds of the M cells and priming of both types of lymphocyte occurs. Within Peyer's patches are specialized T cells that induce immature IgM-bearing B lymphocytes to switch isotype to IgA.

Lymphocytes are mobile: an array of cell surface receptors permits adhesion to endothelial cells and to components of the extracellular matrix. Primed B lymphoblasts, committed mainly to producing IgA antibody, migrate from Peyer's patches, via the lymphatics and mesenteric lymph nodes, to the thoracic duct and hence into the circulation. These cells return preferentially to the lamina propria, a process known as 'homing'. Once back in the gut, they mature into IgA plasma cells and are responsible for local and secretory antibody defences. The number of IgA-containing cells in the lamina propria far exceeds the numbers containing IgM, IgG, or IgE.

Homing appears to depend on three factors: (1) retinoic acid produced by dendritic cells in GALT; (2) upregulated expression of the chemokine receptor CCR9; and (3) expression of the integrin $\alpha_4\beta_7$. Retinoic acid increases the gut homing receptors $\alpha_4\beta_7$ and chemokine receptor 9 on antigen-primed IgA committed B cells which direct them into the lamina propria in response to mucosal adressin cell adhesion molecule 1 (MAdCAM1) expressed on the microvascular endothelium and to the chemokine CCL25 selectively produced by gut epithelial cells.

Intraepithelial lymphocytes

There is a similar migration pathway for T lymphocytes whereby T blasts from mesenteric nodes 'home' both to the epithelium and to the lamina propria. Intraepithelial lymphocytes are phenotypically and functionally distinct from peripheral blood lymphocytes. Intraepithelial lymphocytes express both innate and adaptive immune receptors and have been conserved throughout vertebrate evolution. Peripheral T cells rarely express the human mucosal lymphocyte antigen (CD103) but nearly all intraepithelial lymphocytes do. CD103 is an adhesion molecule of the β_7 integrin family and important in the homing of IEL, allowing these cells to bind via CD103 to its ligand, E-cadherin, expressed on epithelial cells. Intraepithelial lymphocytes are not a homogeneous population: about 70% are CD8+ and show increased expression of the γ/δ form of the T-cell receptor compared with peripheral blood lymphocytes (see Chapter 5.1). Another population expresses the α/β form of the T-cell receptor, while a third subset expresses both CD4 and CD8 and is not found elsewhere in lymphoid tissue. In rodents and probably in humans also, intraepithelial lymphocytes are cytotoxic effector cells: upon activation *in vitro*, cytotoxicity is mediated by perforin released from granules in their cytoplasm. Activated intraepithelial lymphocytes also express FasL and following interaction with Fas on target cells induce programmed cell death, a function important in the control of enterovirus infection. Intraepithelial lymphocytes also seem to have a role in controlling the cell barrier function of epithelial cells, i.e. restitution.

Lamina propria lymphocytes

Large numbers of lymphocytes, natural killer cells, mast cells, macrophages, and plasma cells occur in the lamina propria. T and B lymphocytes are both found, but T cells predominate in a ratio of about 4:1. They do not proliferate well after stimulation of the T-cell receptor, yet produce large amounts of cytokines (interleukin 2, interleukin 4, interferon-γ, and tumour necrosis factor α). T-cell homing to the lamina propria is determined mainly by the integrin $\alpha_4\beta_7$ on primed cells interacting preferentially with MAdCAM 1 expressed on the microvascular endothelium in the lamina propria and by chemokine receptor 9 which attracts them to the chemokine CCL25 secreted by gut epithelium. Interleukins 5 and 6 produced by CD4 + Th2 cells induce terminal differentiation of IgA+ B cells to IgA-producing plasma cells secreting dimeric IgA (see below).

Secretory immunoglobulins

The plasma cells of the lamina propria secrete mainly IgA, which is specially adapted for its function. IgA is synthesized as a dimer with two IgA molecules linked by a smaller 'joining' peptide (the J chain), also produced by the plasma cells. The secretory component is a 70 kDa fragment of the polymeric immunoglobulin receptor synthesized by epithelial cells and is essential for transport of secretory IgA into the gut lumen. The polymeric Ig receptor binds the dimeric IgA; the complex is endocytosed and transported through the cytoplasm to the luminal surface of the cell where proteolysis of the receptor occurs. The IgA dimer is released into the gut attached to the proteolytic fragment of the receptor now called secretory component. Secretory component protects the IgA molecule from degradation by proteolytic enzymes.

Secretory IgA predominates in the saliva and in gastric and intestinal secretions, where it tends to be concentrated in the mucous layer overlying epithelial cells. Secretory IgA neutralizes viruses, bacteria, and toxins and prevents the adherence of pathogenic microorganisms to gut epithelium and so blocks the uptake of antigen into the systemic immune system—a role termed 'immune exclusion'.

Spectrum of intestinal immune responses

Ingestion of antigens can lead to local immunity, a systemic immune response, or a state of specific immune unresponsiveness (tolerance).

Local immune responses

These can occur independently of a systemic response. For example, immunization against poliomyelitis with oral Sabin vaccine gives better protection than the injected Salk vaccine, even though both induce serum antibodies. Local IgA antibody, produced in response to the oral vaccine partly blocks uptake of pathogenic virus into the circulation. Unfortunately, the oral vaccine contains attenuated but still living virus that can cause poliomyelitis in immunocompromised recipients.

Systemic immune responses

Macromolecules are absorbed by the intestine into the portal or systemic circulations, via either the glandular epithelium covering the villus or the M cells. Up to 2% of a dietary protein load appears antigenically intact in the circulation. Sinusoidal phagocytes (Kupffer cells) of the liver destroy much of the antigen but enough passes through the liver to stimulate systemic antibody production, particularly in the spleen. Antibody formed in the spleen enters the portal circulation to complex with incoming antigen. Circulating immune complexes of IgA and dietary antigens are regularly found in normal people after meals.

Systemic tolerance

A unique feature of the mucosal immune system is its ability to down-regulate immune responses to dietary antigens (oral tolerance). In animal models, oral feeding of antigen makes them immunologically unresponsive (tolerant) to subsequent parenteral injections of that antigen. Oral tolerance is an active process mediated by multiple mechanisms and can affect all aspects of the systemic immune response: a single feed of protein antigen suppresses systemic, humoral responses as well as down-modulating T cell receptors and inducing apotosis of Th1-like lymphocytes. This has led to attempts to treat autoimmune diseases by feeding autoantigens to patients.

Immunological disorders of the gastrointestinal tract

Normally, the intestinal immune system steers a delicate course between the undesirable extremes of immunological incompetence, with resulting vulnerability to ingested pathogens (for instance, the gastrointestinal consequences of primary and secondary immunodeficiencies), and hypersensitivity to dietary antigens, with immunologically mediated reactions each time that antigen is eaten.

Primary immunodeficiency diseases

Immunocompromised patients are at risk from two sources of infection: common pathogens, which invade even the immunologically healthy, and opportunistic agents that can invade and infect only those with weakened defences. In the compromised host, most infections are due to common pathogens that are readily identified and controlled. The difficult problems arise from opportunistic infections because these often elude isolation, may not respond to available drugs, and carry a high fatality. Indeed, the identification of certain opportunistic infections implies an underlying immunodeficiency that demands further investigation.

It is beyond the scope of this section to deal with all the gastrointestinal complications of every known form of primary and secondary immunodeficiency. Instead, attention will be focused on representative disorders.

Common variable immunodeficiency

Common variable immunodeficiency is an example of one of the primary antibody deficiency syndromes described in Section 5.

Definition

Common variable immunodeficiency is a heterogeneous group of disorders characterized by low serum immunoglobulin levels, a normal or low proportion of circulating B lymphocytes, and, in about one-third of patients, impaired cell-mediated immunity. It can present at any age and, in the United States and western Europe, the prevalence is about 40 per million of the population. Although most cases appear sporadic, about 20% have a genetic background and mutations in four genes have been documented which imply that impaired T–B cell collaboration within the germinal centre and intrinsic B-cell defects are key aetiological factors in this group of conditions.

Clinical features

Patients present typically with recurrent sinopulmonary infections, most frequently caused by pneumococci, streptoccoci, and *Haemophilus influenzae*. Less commonly, they present with arthropathy, skin sepsis, meningitis, osteomyelitis, or other severe systemic bacterial infections (see Section 7).

With the exception of chronic echovirus infection, these patients are not unduly susceptible to viral or fungal infections, because cell-mediated immunity is usually preserved. There are rarely any diagnostic physical signs of antibody deficiency, although examination often shows evidence of the consequences of previous infections, particularly bronchiectasis.

Between 30 and 50% of patients with common variable immunodeficiency have gastrointestinal problems at some time. Virtually any part of the gastrointestinal tract may be affected (Table 15.5.1) but the most common symptoms are diarrhoea (intermittent or chronic) and weight loss. An approach to the diagnosis of these complications is shown in Fig. 15.5.2.

Stomach Achlorhydria is found in about 30% of patients and the associated atrophic gastritis occasionally leads to a syndrome resembling pernicious anaemia except that the atrophic gastritis involves the whole stomach without antral sparing, the serum gastrin concentrations remain normal, and autoantibodies to gastric parietal cells and intrinsic factor are absent.

Patients with common variable immunodeficiency have been reported to have an almost 50-fold increase in the incidence of carcinoma of the stomach, although a report from Scandinavia has suggested that this extra risk is less than previously thought (standardized incidence ratio 10.3, 95% confidence interval 2.1–30.2). There was no increase in risk of cancer in relatives, suggesting that

the increased risk in common variable immunodeficiency patients is related to the immune deficiency rather than any specific genetic trait. *Helicobacter pylori* infection is found in more than 40% of gastric biopsies from common variable immunodeficiency patients, suggesting that chronic active gastritis induced by *H. pylori* and overexpression of p53 may play a role in gastric carcinogenesis.

Small intestine

Infections Although infestation with *Giardia lamblia* is the most common identifiable cause of malabsorption, in many patients the cause is never found. Giardiasis is virtually confined to adults and is rarely seen in boys with X-linked agammaglobulinaemia. Giardiasis may also cause diarrhoea, villous abnormalities, vitamin B_{12} and folate malabsorption, steatorrhoea, disaccharidase deficiency, and protein-losing enteropathy, but the pathogenetic mechanisms are poorly understood.

Examination of at least three consecutive fresh stool specimens is essential to detect the cysts of *G. lamblia* (Fig. 15.5.2). If this fails, duodenal aspiration and jejunal biopsy are needed to establish the diagnosis. In particularly difficult cases, a therapeutic trial of metronidazole can be useful, although infestation frequently recurs. Most patients show symptomatic improvement after treatment with either a 7-day course of metronidazole (2 g daily as a single dose) or a single dose of tinidazole (2 g immediately). Other parasitic infestations occur. Cryptosporidium infection occasionally causes self-limiting diarrhoea but has a much more sinister outcome in boys with CD40 ligand deficiency (hyper-IgM syndrome) and in patients with HIV infection.

Bacterial infections also cause diarrhoea in patients with common variable immunodeficiency and *Campylobacter jejuni* is frequently responsible. Rarely, campylobacter causes an ascending cholangitis and hepatitis. Treatment is a 2-week course of erythromycin (500 mg, four times daily) with follow-up stool culture to ensure that treatment has been effective.

Shigella or salmonella diarrhoea does not occur more commonly than normal. Similarly, while overgrowth of commensal bacteria is common, bacterial counts rarely exceed 10^5 organisms/ml, compared with counts of more than 10^6/ml in the blind-loop syndrome. Nevertheless, it is common practice to treat these patients empirically with tetracycline and metronidazole, often with symptomatic improvement.

Nodular lymphoid hyperplasia Nodular lymphoid hyperplasia describes the presence of lymphoid nodules in the lamina propria of the gut. Although described in many disorders and occasionally in healthy individuals, finding nodular lymphoid hyperplasia should make the clinician suspect common variable immunodeficiency. It occurs in 20% to 50% of patients but is not necessarily symptomatic. The nodules, which are 1 to 3 mm in diameter, appear as protrusions on fibreoptic endoscopy (Fig. 15.5.3) and as multiple filling defects on barium studies (Fig. 15.5.4). Nodular lymphoid hyperplasia restricted to the rectum or colon can present with rectal bleeding, abdominal pain and features of intestinal obstruction, but rarely with diarrhoea.

The ultrastructure of these nodules is similar to Peyer's patches, and lymphoblasts containing IgM are found in the centres of the follicles. The condition probably represents hypertrophy of the gut-associated lymphoid tissue in response to antigens in the gut lumen. In one series of nodular lymphoid hyperplasia in individuals with normal serum immunoglobulins, every patient had

Table 15.5.1 Gastrointestinal disorders associated with common variable immunodeficiency and other forms of primary antibody deficiency

Infective	Giardiasis
	Campylobacter enteritis
	Cryptosporidiosis
	Strongyloides stercoralis
	Salmonella/shigella infection
	Viral enteritis
	Bacterial overgrowth
Other	Pernicious anaemia-like syndrome
	Hypogammaglobulinaemic sprue
	Coeliac disease
	Carcinoma of the stomach
	Nodular lymphoid hyperplasia
	Inflammatory bowel disease
	Non-granulomatous jejunoileitis

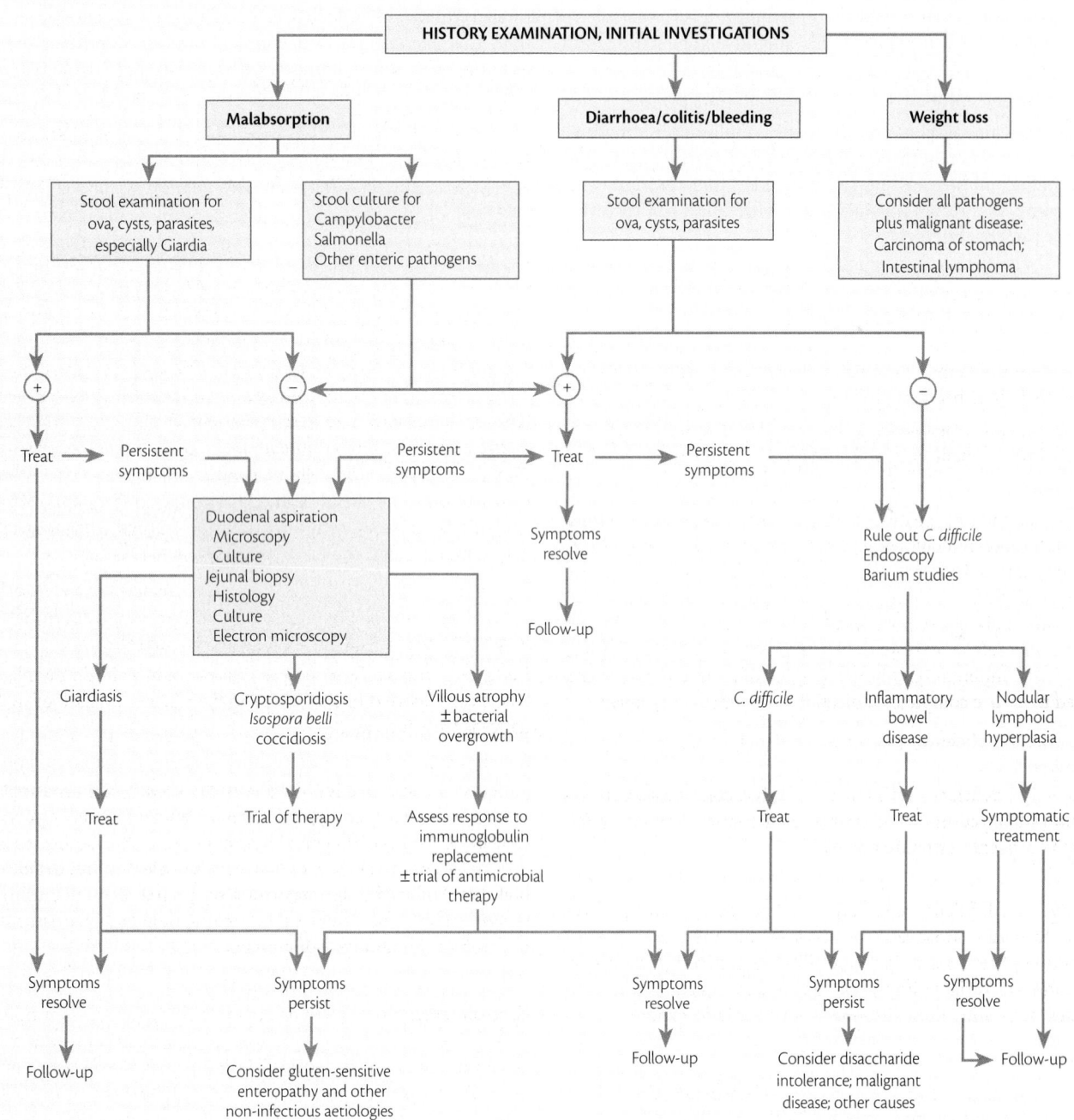

Fig. 15.5.2 A scheme for the investigation of gastrointestinal complications in patients with common variable immunodeficiency.
(Reproduced from Haeney MR (1989). Gastrointestinal disease in the immunocompromised host. In: Turnberg LA, ed. *Clinical gastroenterology* by permission of Blackwell Science, Oxford.)

intestinal giardiasis, suggesting an aetiological link with persistent infestation. Intestinal lymphoma has been reported in apparently immunocompetent subjects with extensive small-bowel nodular lymphoid hyperplasia.

Hypogammaglobulinaemic sprue In a few patients with unexplained diarrhoea, the mucosal lesion resembles coeliac disease or tropical sprue but with reduced or undetectable plasma cells within the lamina propria. In tropical regions, about 1% of patients with 'sprue' may be suffering from a primary humoral immunodeficiency syndrome. Malabsorption in patients with

hypogammaglobulinaemic sprue can improve rapidly after replacement immunoglobulin therapy.

Although extremely rare, patients with common variable immunodeficiency may have concomitant gluten-sensitive coeliac disease.

Inflammatory bowel disease About 5% of patients with common variable immunodeficiency have features of inflammatory bowel disease with radiological and histological findings of Crohn's disease. Others have proposed a specific common variable immunodeficiency enteropathy characterized by low-grade microscopic colitis, increased intraepithelial lymphocytes, and an intact crypt

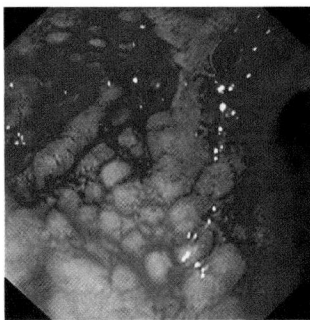

Fig. 15.5.3 The appearance of nodular lymphoid hyperplasia on upper gastrointestinal endoscopy.

architecture which may respond to an elemental diet or treatment with anti-tumour necrosis factor-α.

Nongranulomatous jejunoileitis This is a rare feature of common variable immunodeficiency and has a poor prognosis.

Management

The cornerstone of treatment of antibody deficiency is immunoglobulin replacement; enough must be given to prevent further infections and reduce the incidence of complications. Intravenous or subcutaneous immunoglobulin therapy is the treatment of choice and is discussed more fully in Section 5.

Antibody-deficient patients respond as promptly as others to appropriate antibiotics but longer courses of treatment are usually needed to ensure complete eradication of the micro-organism.

Selective IgA deficiency (see also Section 5)
Definition

Selective IgA deficiency refers to a serum IgA concentration below the limit of detection (<0.01 g/litre). By definition, the serum IgG and IgM concentrations are normal.

Aetiology

Selective IgA deficiency is common and occurs in about 1 in 700 of healthy adults. Most cases are sporadic, but there is an association with deficiencies of IgG2 and IgG4. Selective IgA deficiency and common variable immunodeficiency can occur in the same families, suggesting these disorders reflect variable expression of a

common genetic defect(s). Selective IgA deficiency may also be due to treatment with drugs such as phenytoin or penicillamine.

Clinical features

Although selective IgA deficiency is associated with a range of disorders, most IgA-deficient individuals are asymptomatic, possibly because IgM-producing cells provide high local concentrations of IgM antibody or because symptomatic individuals are those who also have deficiency of IgG2 antibodies to polysaccharide antigens.

Gastrointestinal complications (Table 15.5.2)

Pernicious anaemia Selective IgA deficiency is associated with pernicious anaemia. Unlike common variable immunodeficiency, the anaemia conforms to the classical addisonian type in that atrophic gastritis and raised serum gastrin levels occur.

Malabsorption and steatorrhoea IgA deficiency occurs in about 1 in 40 of patients with coeliac disease, over 15 times more frequently than in the general population. Patients with selective IgA deficiency and a flat jejunal mucosa respond to dietary gluten withdrawal in a way typical of classical coeliac disease.

Gastrointestinal infection With the exception of *G. lamblia* infestation, other infections rarely persist. Even giardiasis is far less frequent than in common variable immunodeficiency.

Inflammatory bowel disease Crohn's disease and ulcerative colitis occur in patients with IgA deficiency but their frequency is difficult to judge from the widely varying published reports.

Malignant disease Oesophageal, gastric, and colonic neoplasms have been reported but it is not certain whether the risk of malignancy is truly increased.

Management

Patients with selective IgA deficiency rarely warrant immunoglobulin replacement therapy, unless IgG2 deficiency and/or polysaccharide antibody deficiency is also present. Antibodies to IgA develop in about one-fifth of patients with selective IgA deficiency: high titres of antibodies may cause severe reactions to plasma or blood transfusions or even the trace amounts of IgA present in intravenous immunoglobulin preparations.

Other types of primary immunodeficiency

Gastrointestinal problems occur in other types of immunodeficiency (Table 15.5.3) (see Section 5). These conditions are much rarer than primary antibody deficiency. Most defects involving cell-mediated immunity present within the first 6 months of life. Infants with severe combined immunodeficiency, for example, grow and develop normally for a few months but then fail to thrive, frequently with a clinical triad of pneumonia, mucocutaneous

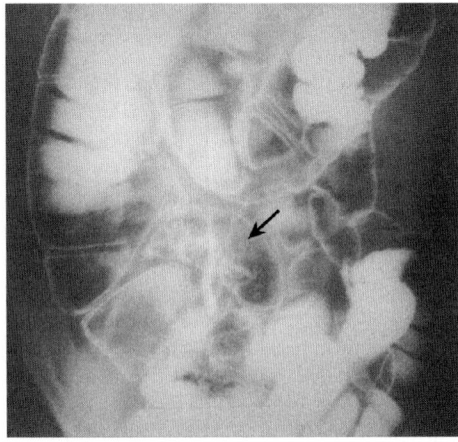

Fig. 15.5.4 A double-contrast barium enema showing nodular lymphoid hyperplasia in the terminal ileum (arrowed).

Table 15.5.2 Gastrointestinal disorders sometimes associated with selective IgA deficiency

Infections	Giardiasis, bacterial overgrowth
Autoimmune disease	Pernicious anaemia, antiepithelial cell antibody
Hypersensitivity disorders:	Coeliac disease, cows' milk protein intolerance, inflammatory bowel disease
Neoplasia	Carcinoma of the oesophagus, stomach, colon
Other	Nodular lymphoid hyperplasia, disaccharidase deficiency.

Table 15.5.3 Gastrointestinal disease in selected types of primary immunodeficiency. (Reproduced from Haeney MR (1989). Gastrointestinal disease in the immunocompromised host. In: Turnberg LA, ed, *Clinical gastroenterology*, Ch.16, pp. 371–55, by permission of Blackwell Scientific Publications, Oxford)

Condition	Functional defect	Typical age at presentation	Major clinical features	Gastrointestinal complications
X-linked lymphoprolif-erative syndrome	Inherited vulnerability to infection with Epstein–Barr virus	Childhood	Fatal or chronic infectious mononucleosis. Aplastic anaemia. Hypogammaglobulinaemia. Malignant B-cell lymphoma	As for antibody deficiency. Malignant lymphoma of the terminal ileum
Severe combined immunodeficiency	Impairment of cell-mediated immuni-ty and antibody production. Multiple pathogenic mechanisms resulting from genetic defects in cell surface receptors or intracellular signalling enzymes.	Infancy	Wide spectrum of severe infection. Nonimmunological features in subtypes	Chronic oral and intestinal candidiasis. Persistent diarrhoea due to rotavirus, cytomegalovirus, other viruses, crypt-osporidium, *Campylobacter*, *Salmonella*
CD40 ligand deficiency (hyper IgM syndrome)	Defective interaction between T and B lymphocytes: failure to switch from IgM to IgG production. Defective interaction between T cells and mac-rophages	Infancy	Impaired antibody production. Neutropenia. Suspectibility to *Pneumocystis carinii* pneumonia and cryptosporidiosis	Persistent cryptosporidiosis. Ascending cholangitis and cirrhosis
Di George anomaly (a catch 22 syndrome with Chromosome 22q 11 deletions)	Impairment of cell-mediated immu-nity and antibody production (non-familial)	From birth	Hypoparathyroidism: tetany and convulsions. Cardiovascular defects. Immunodeficiency (Mild). Abnormal facies	Oesophageal atresia. Chronic intestinal candidiasis. Diarrhoea of uncertain aeti-ology
Wiskott–Aldrich syn-drome	Progressive impairment of antibody production and cell-mediated immunity	Infancy or early childhood	Thrombocytopenia: bleeding. Eczema. Immunodeficiency. Malignant disease	Bloody diarrhoea. Food allergic disease. Intestinal lymphoma
Chronic granulomatous disease	Defective neutrophil killing of catala-se-producing organisms (X linked or autosomal recessive)	Infancy	Severe skin sepsis due to *Staphylococcus aureus*, fungi, Gram-negative bacilli. Lymphadenopathy. Hepatosplenomegaly. Deep abscesses	Diarrhoea and steatorrhoea with PAS-positive histiocytes in the lamina propria Granuloma formation
Autoimmune polyendocrinopathy, candidiasis, ectodermal dysplasia (APECED)	Imparied cell-mediated immunity to *Candida albicans* caused by mutations in Autoimmune regulator (AIRE) gene on chromosome 21	Childhood	Chronic *Candida* infection of mucous membranes, nails, skin. Associated endo-crinopathy: Addison's disease, hypopar-athyroidism, diabetes mellitus, thyroiditis, skin and tooth changes	Chronic oral and intestinal candidiasis

candidiasis, and intractable diarrhoea caused by one or more of a range of microorganisms. Some disorders are associated with unusual gastrointestinal features (Table 15.5.3).

Secondary immunodeficiency

Secondary immunodeficiency describes conditions in which the immune defect results from underlying disease, and is far more common than primary immunodeficiency. In many cases, the secondary immunodeficiency is of minor relevance to the clinical picture but occasionally its severity may mask the underlying condition. AIDS is a florid example of the gastrointestinal compli-cations seen in patients with secondary defects predominantly involving cell-mediated immunity.

HIV and the gastrointestinal tract

The gastrointestinal tract is a major target organ in HIV infection and AIDS, irrespective of the route of acquisition of the infection. The enhanced susceptibility of intestinal lymphoid tissue to HIV-1 is related to the large population of memory CD4+ T lymphocytes expressing chemokine receptor 5 resident in the gut. In simian models, and in human studies, severe depletion of CD4+ lym-phocytes in the lamina propria and of intraepithelial lymphocytes occurs during primary infection and persists throughout the course of the infection. These dynamic changes in intestinal T lymphocytes occur much earlier and are more severe than those seen in blood or peripheral lymph nodes.

About one-half of patients with HIV infection will have sympto-matic gastrointestinal involvement at some time, and any level of the tract, from mouth to anus, can be involved (see also Section 7). There are three main pathogenic mechanisms: direct infection of enterocytes by HIV, opportunistic and other infections, and oppor-tunistic tumours (Figs. 15.5.5 and 15.5.6). A major change in the small intestine is a partial villous atrophy, detectable early in the natural history of HIV infection. Enteropathogens causing intesti-nal infections are of the same types as in immunocompetent sub-jects but the infections are much more aggressive and invasive, and elicit little host immune response, so familiar symptoms and signs may be absent. A systematic and thorough search for likely patho-gens is essential (Fig. 15.5.6). Multiple infections and tumours may coexist, so the organism isolated is not necessarily the cause

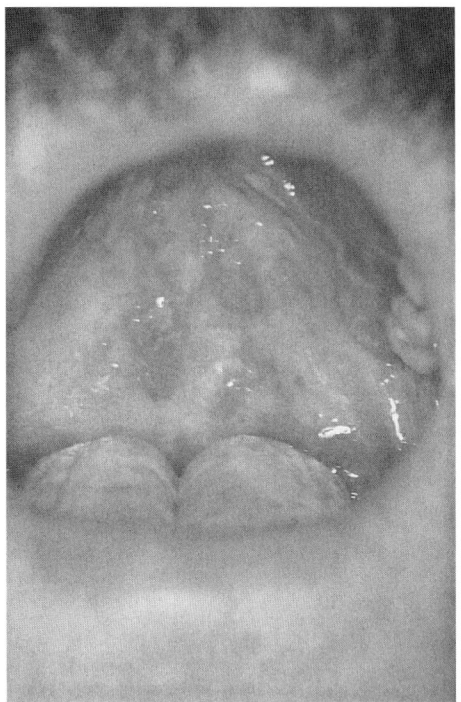

Fig. 15.5.5 Kaposi's sarcoma of the oral cavity in a patient with AIDS.

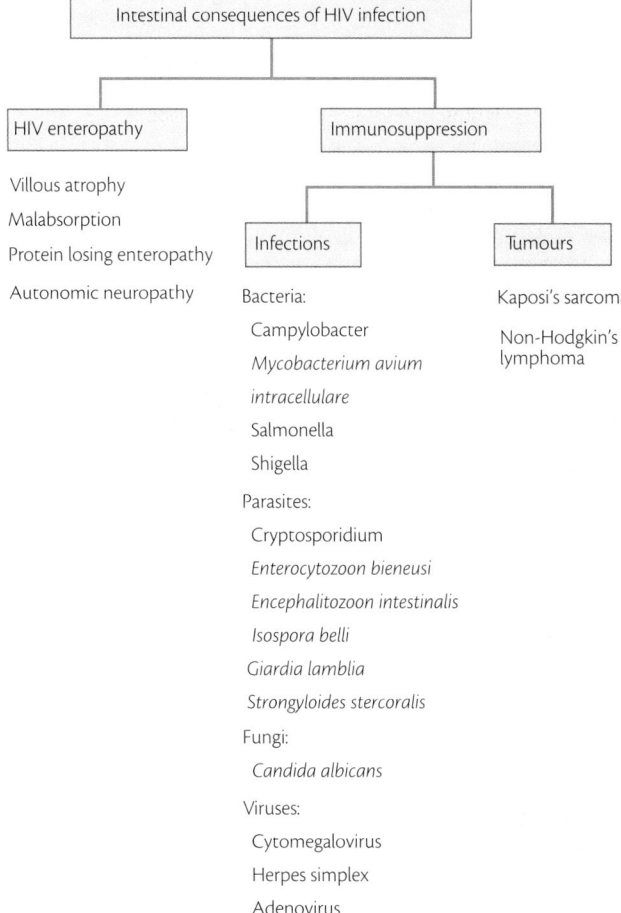

Fig 15.5.6. Gastrointestinal consequences of HIV infection.
(Redrawn from Chapel HM *et al.* (2006). *Essentials of clinical immunology*, 5th edn, by permission of the authors and Blackwell Science, Oxford.)

of the symptoms. Colonic complications increase in frequency as immunodeficiency worsens. Clinically, patients experience diarrhoea, intestinal bleeding, and abdominal pain. Toxic megacolon, intussusception, idiopathic colonic ulceration, and pneumatosis intestinalis have also been described.

The clinical features of HIV infection and AIDS are discussed in detail in Chapter 7.5.23.

Immunodeficiency secondary to gastrointestinal disease

A low serum IgG concentration may be due to increased intestinal loss of immunoglobulin. A useful clue is a low serum albumin because there are no known conditions where immunoglobulin is selectively lost from the gut. The major causes of protein-losing enteropathy are discussed in Chapter 15.26.

Intestinal lymphangiectasia (see also Chapter 15.16)

This immunodeficiency results from increased loss of lymphatic fluid containing immunoglobulins and lymphocytes. There is a selective loss of naive T lymphocytes expressing CD4/CD45RA. The basic defect is an abnormal dilatation of the lymphatic vessels in the intestine. There is a primary familial form in children, who present with diarrhoea, malabsorption, and growth retardation. Such children may have abnormal lymphatics elsewhere in the body causing chylous ascites, pleural effusions, and localized areas of oedema. The condition may also occur secondarily to lymphatic obstruction, for example due to intestinal lymphoma or constrictive pericarditis (see Sections 15 and 22). The diagnosis should be suspected when there is T-cell lymphopenia, hypoalbuminaemia, and hypogammaglobulinaemia. On endoscopy, white villi or white submucosal nodules may be seen. The diagnosis is confirmed by finding dilated lymphatics in a jejunal biopsy (Fig. 15.5.7). The primary form of the disease responds to a low-fat diet with additional medium-chain triglycerides. Octreotide has produced symptomatic improvement and reduced intestinal protein loss in some case reports. In secondary forms, correction of the underlying disease process is needed.

Food allergy and intolerance

Food allergy is one of the most controversial topics in medicine. It undoubtedly exists, but extravagant claims that a staggering array

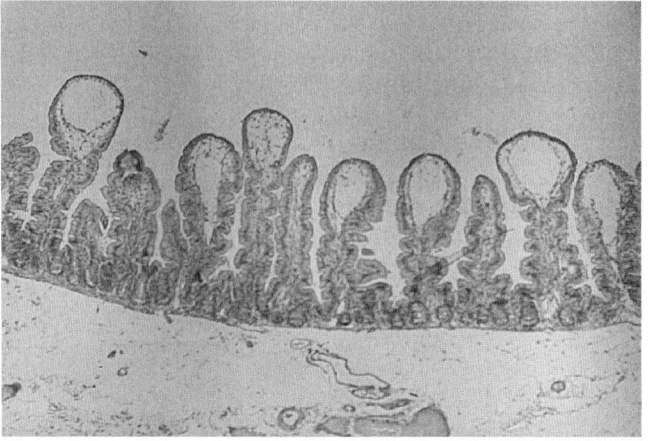

Fig 15.5.7. A jejunal biopsy from a patient with intestinal lymphangiectasia showing dilated central lacteals.

Table 15.5.4 Classification of adverse reactions to foods

Reproducible adverse reaction on food challenge		Immune mechanism		Non-immune mechanism	Examples
Open	Blind	IgE	Other		
Food allergy					
+	+	+	–	–	Immediate reactions to nuts, eggs, milk shellfish, fish
+	+	–	+	–	Coeliac disease, cows' milk protein intolerance
Food intolerance					
+	+	–	–	?	Irritable bowel syndrome (some), food induced migraine, reactions to sulphites, nitrites, food additives
Food aversion					
+	–	–	–	–	

of symptoms are due to food 'allergy' have confused the subject. Such claims are too rarely supported by objective, scientific observations and have provoked a sceptical response from many doctors. The major cause of confusion lies in the lack of agreement on definitions and diagnostic criteria.

Definition

Food allergy refers to a form of exaggerated reactivity (hypersensitivity) of the immune system to an ingested antigen. The term should be used only when the abnormal reaction is proved to be immunologically mediated, and is mostly synonymous with reactions involving IgE antibodies (Table 15.5.4). The term 'food intolerance' should be used to describe all abnormal, reproducible reactions to food when the causative mechanism is unknown or is nonimmunological. Food allergy and intolerance must be distinguished from food fads and psychological aversion to foods.

Aetiology

Food allergy

Although the gut provides a physical barrier to the antigen load in the lumen, up to 2% of a protein meal can appear antigenically intact in the circulation. This was shown by injecting serum from a patient with known sensitivity to fish into the skin of a normal subject. A wheal and flare response at the skin test site (positive Prausnitz–Kustner reaction) was observed shortly after the normal subject ate the appropriate antigen, showing that this must have crossed the gut and triggered IgE-sensitized mast cells at the skin test site.

The vast majority of food allergic reactions present in the first year of life and atopic individuals have a higher prevalence of food allergy. The allergic components of foods are mainly glycoproteins with molecular weights between 10 and 70 kDa and most are heat stable and resistant to proteolysis, with the exception of those causing the oral allergy syndrome (see below).

Sometimes, gut damage involves immune mechanisms other than IgE. For instance, in coeliac disease there is strong evidence that exaggerated local T-cell mediated reactivity to dietary gluten causes the villous atrophy.

Food intolerance

Nonimmunological mechanisms of reproducible, adverse reactions to food are much more common and include irritant, toxic, pharmacological, or metabolic effects of foods, enzyme deficiencies, or even the release of substances produced by fermentation of food residues in the bowel. Some foods contain pharmacologically active substances (such as tyramine or phenylethylamine) that act directly on blood vessels in sensitive subjects to produce migraine. Traces of drugs, food additives (e.g. monosodium glutamate), colouring agents (e.g. tartrazine), or preservatives (for example benzoic acid) can also cause symptoms in susceptible people by mechanisms which are ill understood, but are probably due to direct effects on mast cells.

Prevalence

The general public perceives food allergy to be a major health problem but epidemiological studies do not support this view. Food allergy affects 2 to 5% of children under 5 years but only 1% of adults. In one survey of 7500 households in the United Kingdom, about 20% of the sample reported a food intolerance but this was confirmed by double-blind, placebo-controlled food challenge in only 1.4%. However, the prevalence of peanut allergy appears to have increased significantly over the last 20 years.

Reactions to food additives, while they exist, are also not as common as most people believe. In a second population study in the United Kingdom, 7.4% had symptoms suggestive of intolerance to food additives; further clinical assessment and additive challenge showed a true prevalence of 0.01 to 0.23%.

Clinical features

Food reactions can be early or late, confined to the gastrointestinal tract or occur at sites remote from the gut (Fig. 15.5.8).

Gut-related symptoms

About 75% of young children, but only 10% of adults, present with local gastrointestinal symptoms of food intolerance.

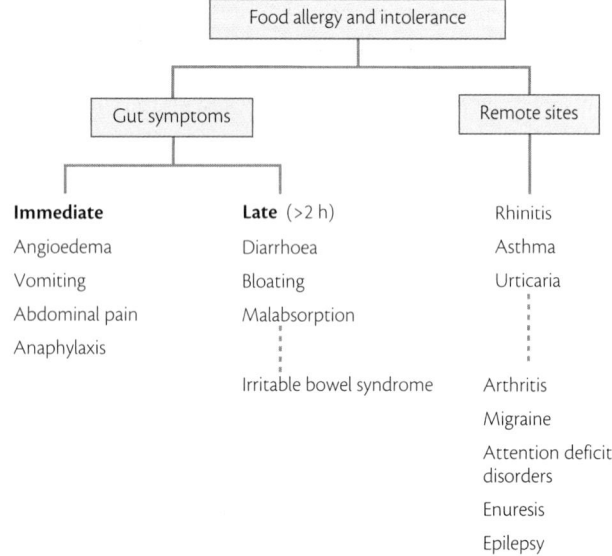

Fig 15.5.8. Clinical spectrum of food allergy and intolerance.
(Redrawn from Chapel HM *et al.* (2006). *Essentials of clinical immunology*, 5th edn, by permission of the authors and Blackwell Science, Oxford.)

Early reactions

These are often 'immediate' in onset, occurring within minutes or rarely up to 2 h after ingestion. They recur on challenge testing, and include, apart from gastrointestinal disturbances, such features as perioral rash, angioedema of the lips or tongue, tingling of the throat, urticaria, asthma, or even anaphylaxis. Such acute and severe allergic reactions are mostly due to IgE antibodies to foods and are the least controversial form of food allergy. They are fairly easy to diagnose and the offending food is readily identified, usually by the patient or parent: although any food may be responsible, 90% of reactions are caused by cows' milk (in infants), peanuts, tree nuts, eggs, fish, and shellfish. Peanut is the most allergenic food known and peanut allergy is usually regarded as lifelong.

In some cases, anaphylaxis only occurs when the food is eaten 2 to 4 h before exercise, so-called food-dependent exercise-induced anaphylaxis.

Allergy to latex rubber is increasingly common and several high-risk groups are recognized, notably patients with spina bifida or multiple urological procedures, rubber-industry workers and health care workers. Latex allergy may cross-react with plant defence proteins, called chitinases, in foods, typically kiwi fruit, melon, banana, avocado, chestnut, celery, or passion fruit.

Oral allergy syndrome, also called pollen–fruit allergy syndrome, describes itching and lip swelling without involvement of other target organs. It is a form of contact urticaria and occurs in patients with tree pollen allergy and is due to cross-reactivity with epitopes in fresh (but not cooked) fruits and vegetables such as apples, peaches, pears, plums, carrots, hazelnuts, or raw potatoes. Commercially available skin prick testing solutions may not contain the fresh allergenic epitopes and it is essential to use the fresh fruit itself to undertake 'prick-prick' testing whereby the skin test lancet is pricked into the fruit and then immediately into the patient's skin. Allergic eosinophilic gastroenteritis is characterized by intolerance to multiple foods, eosinophilic infiltration of the stomach and small intestine, peripheral eosinophilia, and positive skin prick tests and radioallergosorbent tests (see below) to foods.

Late reactions

Symptoms occurring more than 2 h after food ingestion, such as diarrhoea, bloating, or a fatty stool, may be suggestive of food intolerance, if not allergy. Features of the irritable bowel syndrome (see below) may be accompanied by allergic symptoms elsewhere but usually occur in isolation and without any evidence of an immunological reaction.

Remote symptoms

Some patients with acute, IgE-mediated reactions to foods also experience rhinitis, asthma, urticaria, angioedema, or eczema. However, eating the implicated foods does not always cause these remote symptoms. Sneezing bouts, blocked nose, or asthma can also occur after taking wine or other alcoholic drinks because of the irritant effect of sulphite preservatives or other components. This is not an immunological reaction. Many patients with atopic eczema find that certain foods provoke a transient red and blotchy rash but it is mainly in children that food makes eczema worse. Elimination diets rarely improve atopic eczema in adults.

What is more debatable is whether food intolerance plays any part in remote symptoms such as hyperactivity/attention deficit disorder, enuresis, or arthritis.

Specific syndromes of food allergy

Food allergy contributes to a number of common intestinal disorders where the immunological mechanisms are not IgE mediated.

Coeliac disease

The characteristic histological lesion in untreated cases of coeliac disease (see Chapter 15.10.3) is loss of normal villi and a marked increase in the numbers of CD8+ intraepithelial lymphocytes, particularly those expressing the γ/δ T-cell receptor. Two factors are important in pathogenesis: exposure to gluten and a genetic predisposition to react to it. A unique 33-amino-acid gluten peptide (33-mer) is thought to initiate the disease because it encloses several, partly overlapping HLA-DQ2 binding and T cell-stimulating epitopes that are resistant to intestinal proteases. This peptide undergoes deamidation by the enzyme tissue transglutamidase in the small intestine and is then endocytosed and processed by antigen-presenting cells to three epitopes that preferentially bind to HLA-DQ2 or -DQ8 and are subsequently recognized by T cell receptors on CD4+ T cells. These activated T cells generate interferon-γ and other cytokines and are believed to cause the villous atrophy and crypt hyperplasia characteristic of coeliac disease. Gliadin-specific HLA-DQ2-restricted T cells have been isolated from small-intestinal biopsies of coeliac patients. T-cell infiltration of the small-bowel epithelium is seen within hours of gluten exposure and resolves on treatment with a gluten-free diet—supportive evidence that intestinal damage is due to a T-cell mediated reaction to gluten.

Cows' milk protein enteropathy

Milk proteins can cause a malabsorption syndrome similar to coeliac disease. Cows' milk protein enteropathy in babies causes failure to thrive, diarrhoea, malabsorption, and even intestinal bleeding and colitis. Jejunal biopsies show villous atrophy and lymphocytic infiltration.

Symptoms disappear when cows' milk is removed from the diet. Reintroduction of cows' milk causes a recurrence of symptoms. After a viral gastrointestinal infection, cows' milk may also be poorly tolerated for a while because of a temporary inability to digest lactose. Thus, in babies and small children with chronic gastrointestinal symptoms and failure to gain weight, trials (under medical supervision) of milk exclusion are justified and the diagnosis can usually be confirmed by food challenge. Recovery often occurs within a few months.

Recognized syndromes of food intolerance

In some conditions, a relationship to foods can be convincingly demonstrated in a proportion of patients. Sometimes symptoms are provoked by the known irritant, pharmacological, or metabolic effects of food.

Irritable bowel syndrome

Irritable bowel syndrome is a descriptive term for several conditions that produce a similar range of abdominal symptoms (see Chapter 15.13). Irritable bowel syndrome is characterized by alternating constipation and diarrhoea, abdominal bloating, and colicky pain. In a variant of this disorder, however, constipation predominates and gastrointestinal transit times are greatly increased. Most cases are unrelated to food intolerance but in a minority of patients—usually those with predominant diarrhoea, with some bloating and pain—a relationship to specific foods can be demonstrated. Some patients who improve on a restricted diet identify certain foods, notably cereals and dairy products, that provoke symptoms when reintroduced. However, not all gastroenterologists are convinced of a causal relationship between food and irritable bowel syndrome. It has also been claimed that the removal of foods based on the presence of IgG antibodies to foods in an ELISA assay decreases symptoms of irritable bowel. However, IgG antibodies to foods reflect exposure, not disease, and are common and nonspecific findings in asymptomatic people, and the diagnostic value of this test is highly questionable.

Lactose intolerance

Many adults cannot digest lactose because of a deficiency of the enzyme lactase (see Chapter 12.3.3). In them, undigested sugar is fermented in the lower bowel, causing diarrhoea and wind. Lactose intolerance is not common in Europeans but affects up to 90% of adult Africans and Asians. It can also occur as a transient result of gastroenteritis and even as a secondary effect of cows' milk protein intolerance. This can cause confusion in diagnosis unless a lactose challenge is performed separately from a cows' milk protein challenge.

Fructose intolerance

This is discussed in Chapter 12.3.2.

Miscellaneous syndromes
Migraine and headache

Coffee and coffee withdrawal can provoke migraine in susceptible people. Certain cheeses cause headaches in many people, probably due to their tyramine or phenylethylamine content. Red wines, especially port, cause headaches in susceptible people because of their content of congeners.

Asthma

Foods preserved by sulphites, particularly white wine, dried fruit, and fruit salads in supermarkets and restaurants, sometimes provoke asthma by the release of sulphur dioxide.

Urticaria

While IgE-mediated food allergy can cause acute urticaria and angioedema, allergy rarely induces chronic urticaria. However, food dyes and preservatives often trigger chronic urticaria in sensitive subjects.

Chinese restaurant syndrome

Monosodium glutamate, used to enhance flavour in food and found in large amounts in Chinese food, may cause a syndrome of chest pain, sweating, nausea, dizziness, and fainting in susceptible individuals. However, double-blind studies have not convincingly demonstrated that monosodium glutamate is the culprit.

Controversial issues
Behavioural problems in children

The belief that foods and food additives can induce behavioural problems, particularly attention deficit hyperactivity disorder, is a controversial one. A diet free of preservatives, salicylates, and artificial flavours has been claimed to benefit up to 70% of such children but most well-designed, double-blind, placebo-controlled challenges have failed to support a causal link. Children with behavioural disorders may improve temporarily for a few weeks when given a diet avoiding food additives but this appears to be a placebo effect. Parents who suspect food additive intolerance in

their child may insist on maintaining the child on a restrictive or nutritionally deficient diet, even when dietary challenges prove negative.

Psychological distress in adults

Some patients with a multiplicity of vague and variable symptoms, such as unexplained fatigue and malaise, and disturbances of sleep, appetite, or libido turn to the diagnosis of food allergy as an explanation. Only a few have clear cut psychiatric illness, others inadvertently cause symptoms by overbreathing or by somatizing their psychological distress. Having made their own diagnosis of food allergy, they have difficulty in accepting they are not allergic to foods, even though their food aversions may have resulted in a dangerously inadequate diet. They will frequently seek out practitioners who are prepared to endorse their views, whether valid or not. Early diagnosis and sympathetic management are essential if unnecessary consultations and inappropriate allergy tests are to be avoided.

Diagnosis

Food allergy should not be diagnosed without clear indications, as needless dietary restrictions can seriously disrupt not only the patient's life but also the whole family and may occasionally cause malnutrition. No test can replace a careful clinical history and thorough examination to exclude other, sometimes more likely, causes of the patient's symptoms.

Skin tests and radioallergosorbent tests

Skin prick tests and radioallergosorbent tests for detecting serum IgE antibodies are positive in about 75% of patients who have IgE-mediated, acute, early reactions to foods such as nuts, egg, or fish. Usually, the offending antigen is obvious from the clinical history and confirmatory tests are needed only if there is clinical doubt. In patients with late symptoms at sites remote from the gut (see Fig. 15.5.6), skin and blood tests are notoriously unreliable for many reasons:

- Foods, as antigen sources, are poorly standardized and contain multiple, ill-defined antigens.
- The antigen content of the food will depend on whether it is raw or cooked.
- Some foods cause nonspecific ('irritant'), positive skin reactions.
- Patients may have IgE antibodies but no symptoms.
- Food reactions can be mediated by mechanisms other than IgE antibodies.

For most patients with suspected food intolerance, laboratory tests are of little diagnostic value.

Elimination diets and challenge tests

In the absence of reliable laboratory tests, elimination diets and food challenge form the basis of diagnosis. To minimize bias and suggestion, the relationship between food and symptoms should be established by a placebo-controlled, double-blind challenge under medical supervision. In some cases, e.g. in chronic urticaria or when the symptoms are mild and largely subjective, it may be necessary to repeat the challenge before accepting that the association is not simply coincidental. In several series, only a quarter of reported 'adverse reactions' can be confirmed by double-blind challenge. Although these rules are simple to state, they are difficult to carry out in practice. However, the alternative is that of prolonged, unsupervised, dietary manipulation, usually self-imposed or inflicted by parents on their children, with the attendant risks.

Food challenges are not without risk: there is a danger of precipitating an anaphylactic reaction. This is well recognized in children with relatively mild symptoms of food intolerance, who develop anaphylaxis when the food, often cows' milk, is reintroduced after a period of avoidance.

Bogus or unproven laboratory tests

The absence of reliable laboratory tests has led to the promotion of controversial 'alternative' tests: these are at best misleading and at worst dangerous. New diagnostic procedures, like new drugs, require scientific validation: they must be reliable and reproducible. When presented with coded, duplicate samples, some 'alternative' laboratories in the United Kingdom were unable reliably to identify food allergies in patients known to have them; they gave inconsistent results for paired samples from the same patient; they reported many allergies in nonallergic subjects; and they often gave dubious and risky dietary advice.

Provocation–neutralization testing

This has been critically evaluated by the Royal College of Physicians of London, the American College of Physicians, and the California Medical Association. These bodies concluded that reported studies were seriously flawed and that the method lacked scientific validity. Under double-blind conditions, the response of patients to active and control injections appeared to be due to suggestion and chance.

Leucocytotoxic testing

This involves incubating a patient's leucocytes with various food extracts and inspecting the cells for damage. The high number of false positive and false negative results led the American Academy of Allergy to conclude that there was no evidence that the test was effective in diagnosis of food allergy.

Other tests

Electrodermal (Vega) testing, whereby skin electrical resistance is measured with food extracts present in the same circuit, has been assessed in a double-blind, randomized block design study: it was unable to distinguish between healthy and allergic individuals or between control and allergen extracts, and yielded results that did not correlate with conventional test results.

Hair analysis, applied kinesiology, radionics, radiaesthesia, psionic medicine, and auriculocardiac reflex testing have never been objectively evaluated and are more a matter of gullibility and faith than science.

Treatment

Dietary management

Recognition of the offending food and its elimination from the diet is the cornerstone of treatment. In patients with acute IgE-mediated reactions to a single food, such as shellfish, this is usually straightforward. Patients with anaphylactic reactions to foods need to be careful to avoid accidental exposure. A problem for such patients is the use of a food, most notably nuts, as an undeclared or 'hidden' ingredient in manufactured foods or restaurant meals. Where there remains a risk of accidental ingestion it may be appropriate for some patients to carry a preloaded syringe of adrenaline (epinephrine) for self-injection.

In less clear cut situations, certain foods or food additives are eliminated empirically because they are frequently implicated in that form of food intolerance. For example, a diet free of cereal grains and dairy products may sometimes be beneficial in certain patients with irritable bowel syndrome, while a diet free of azo dyes, preservatives, and salicylates helps a proportion of patients with chronic intractable urticaria.

Patients who seem intolerant of a wide range of foods may need a very restricted diet, sometimes called a 'few food' diet. If symptoms are improved, then foods can be reintroduced one at a time. This is both diagnostic and therapeutic, but care is essential as anaphylaxis can occur on reintroduction, especially in children. Expert advice from specially trained dietitians is essential to avoid nutritional deficiency.

Sodium cromoglicate

Oral sodium cromoglicate has been used as an adjunct to diet in selected patients with food allergy, especially those with accompanying allergic reactions in the eyes, nose, and skin. Its effectiveness is minimal.

Immunotherapy

Although immunotherapy (hyposensitization) is effective in wasp or bee venom anaphylaxis and in some forms of allergy to inhaled allergens, it has never been evaluated scientifically in food intolerance. There is considerable interest in future vaccines for immunotherapy for food-induced anaphylaxis.

'Alternative' therapies

Provocation–neutralization therapy and enzyme-potentiated desensitization are two treatments used by 'alternative' practitioners: neither is of proven value, although both induce significant placebo responses.

Food allergy seems particularly vulnerable to unorthodox treatments which have not been scientifically validated by double-blind, placebo-controlled trials or confirmed by independent investigators. The hazard of the unconventional approach to therapy is that potentially serious problems can be misdiagnosed and mistreated.

Further reading

Agace WW (2006). Tissue-tropic effector T cells: generation and targeting opportunities. *Nat Rev Immunol*, **6**, 682–92.

Ament ME, Ochs HD, Davis SD (1973). Structure and function of the gastrointestinal tract in primary immunodeficiency syndromes. A study of 39 patients. *Medicine (Baltimore)*, **52**, 227–48.

Australian Society of Clinical Immunology and Allergy (2007). *ASCIA position statement: unorthodox techniques for the diagnosis and treatment of allergy, asthma and immune disorders.* http://www.allergy.org.au/pospapers/unorthodox.htm

Barrett S (2007). *Quackwatch*. http://www.quackwatch.com

Burks W, Ballmer-Weber HL (2006). Food allergy. *Mol Nutr Food Res*, **50**, 595–603.

Cunningham-Rundles C (1999). Common variable immunodeficiency: clinical and immunological features of 248 patients. *Clin Immunol*, **92**, 34–48.

David TJ (1993). *Food and food additive intolerance in childhood.* Blackwell Scientific, Oxford.

Lewith GT, *et al.* (2001). Is electrodermal testing as efficient as skin prick tests for diagnosing allergies? A double blind, randomised block design study. *BMJ*, **322**, 131–4.

McCabe RP (2002). Gastrointestinal manifestations of non-AIDS immunodeficiency. *Curr Treat Opt Gastroenterol*, **5**, 17–25.

Martin A (2007). *Intestinal lymphangiectasia*. http://www.emedicine.com/med/topic1178.htm

Mehandru S, *et al.* (2005). The gastrointestinal tract is critical to the pathogenesis of acute HIV-1 infection. *J Allergy Clin Immunol*, **116**, 419–22.

Mellemkjaer L, *et al.* (2002). Cancer risk among patients with IgA deficiency or common variable immunodeficiency and their relatives: a combined Danish and Swedish study. *Clin Exp Immunol*, **130**, 495–500.

Neutra MR and Kozlowski PA (2006). Mucosal vaccines: the promise and the challenge. *Nat Rev Immunol*, **6**, 148–58.

Nowak-Wegrzyn A, Sampson HA (2006). Adverse reactions to food. *Med Clin N Am*, **90**, 97–127.

Pribila JT, *et al.* (2004). Integrins and T cell-mediated immunity. *Annu Rev Immunol*, **22**, 157–80.

Salzer U, Grimbacher B (2006). Common variable immunodeficiency: the power of stimulation. *Semin Immunol*, **18**, 337–46.

Schwartz R (2007). *Common variable immunodeficiency*. http://www.emedicine.com/derm/topic870.htm

Weiner HL (2004). Current issues in the treatment of human diseases by mucosal tolerance. *Ann N Y Acad Sci*, **1029**, 211–24.

Young E, *et al.* (1994). A population study of food intolerance. *Lancet*, **343**, 1127–30.

The mouth and salivary glands

T. Lehner and S.J. Challacombe

Essentials

Stomatology is the branch of medicine that deals with oral diseases of both hard and soft tissues. For historical reasons and due to the rather technical aspects of treatment of teeth, dentistry has been separated from the main body of teaching medicine. This has created a curious anomaly in the training of doctors, namely that oral diseases receive low priority in teaching, and yet many systemic diseases are associated with oral symptoms and signs.

Dental caries, caused by bacterial action, is one of the most common human diseases and causes considerable misery: it results from the interaction of dietary sugars with cariogenic bacteria. Chronic gingivitis and periodontal disease are also very common diseases of the oral cavity which are related to accumulation of dental plaque; host factors related to immunological responses to mixed organisms or specific microbes, e.g. *Porphyromonas gingivalis*, may be involved. Chronic periodontal disease is the most important cause of dental loss in adults. Host factors, including smoking, diabetes mellitus, and genetic determinants increase susceptibility to periodontitis.

Acute oral infections include fusospirochaetal gingivitis (Vincent's gingivitis or necrotizing ulcerative gingivitis), a bacterial infection responsive to antimicrobial therapy that requires differentiation from herpetic gingivostomatitis, caused by herpes simplex virus type 1, which may respond to early treatment with aciclovir. However, the most common oral lesion is recurrent aphthous stomatitis, the treatment of which is fraught with difficulties.

Immunodeficiency (e.g. related to iatrogenic immunosuppression) can be associated with many oral infections, e.g. HIV recurrent herpetic lesions, or oropharyngeal candidiasis. Early manifestations of HIV infection are often found in the mouth, with oral candidiasis, Kaposi sarcoma or periodontal disease.

The oral cavity is affected in diverse diseases of the skin such as pemphigus vulgaris, benign pemphigoid, lichen palnus, erythema multiforme and Stevens–Johnson syndrome, in autoimmune rheumatic or vasculitic disorders (e.g Sjögren's syndrome, Behçet's disease, Wegener's granulomatosis), in various internal conditions (e.g. Crohn's disease, ulcerative colitis, coeliac disease). Oral cancer may involve the lips, cheeks, tongue, gums and oropharynx and a variety of tumours affect the salivary gland.

Dental caries

Aetiology

Dental caries (decay) may be defined as the localized destruction of tooth tissue by bacterial action. Dissolution of the hydroxyapatite crystals seems to precede the loss of organic components of both enamel and dentine, and thus demineralization is thought to be caused by acids resulting from the bacterial fermentation of dietary carbohydrates. Dental caries comprises one of the most common diseases of humankind. In spite of recent reductions in the rate of decay in Western societies, the prevalence of caries in developed countries remains at more than 95% of the population. Caries is still increasing in the developing countries with the increased consumption of refined sugars. The prevalence of caries is greatest in children and young adults where it affects the pits and fissures of the occlusal surfaces, and the enamel of the approximal surfaces of teeth. However, an increasing prevalence of root caries (at the neck of the tooth) occurs later in life, especially as teeth are now increasingly retained to old age.

Caries is an infection caused by aggregation of bacteria on the tooth surface, usually referred to as dental plaque. The development of dental caries requires (1) the presence of cariogenic bacteria that are capable of rapidly producing acid below the critical pH required for dissolving enamel; and (2) sugar in the diet that favours colonization of these bacteria and that can be metabolized by the bacteria to form acid. Cariogenic bacteria can be defined by their ability to colonize teeth, to reduce the pH to about 4.1 in the presence of a suitable sugar substrate, and to induce caries in germ-free animals. *Streptococcus mutans*, *Streptococcus sanguis*, *Lactobacillus acidophilus* and *casei*, and *Actinomyces viscosus* fulfil most of these criteria. However, *Strep. mutans* appears to be the most efficient cariogenic organism. Germ-free studies have clearly shown that *Strep. mutans* can induce caries rapidly in the absence of other organisms, even though in humans plaque is always a mix of many bacterial species. *S. mutans* is a facultative anaerobic, non-haemolytic, acidogenic Gram-positive coccus, producing extracellular and intracellular polysaccharides. The organism fulfils Koch's postulates as a cause of dental caries.

In addition to microorganisms, a sugar substrate is essential for caries formation. The most common carbohydrates in our diet are starch and sucrose, with smaller amounts of glucose, fructose, and lactose. Quantitatively and functionally the most important substrate in the human diet is sucrose. Addition of glucose to the diet makes little difference. Sucrose gives rise to heavy plaque formation, with considerable amounts of extracellular polysaccharide. The most important polysaccharide is dextran (glucan), which is synthesized in large amounts by the constitutive enzyme glucosyltransferase. Dextran may give plaque the necessary quality of stickiness to the enamel surface.

Streptococci do not possess a cytochrome system but contain the Embden–Meyerhof glycolytic enzymes, which will convert glucose to lactic and other organic acids. The pH inside the plaque may fall within 2 to 3 min of rinsing the mouth with glucose or sucrose from a level of about 6.5 to 4.5; the critical pH below which decalcification of enamel occurs is thought to be about 5.5. Caries is thus the end result of a complex sequence of microbial and biochemical processes terminating in acid formation.

Pathology

Caries develops as a result of acid produced from sugar fermentation by bacteria present in plaque. The enamel becomes demineralized and plaque bacteria penetrate along the enamel prisms. Dissolution of the hydroxyapatite crystals seems to precede the loss of organic components of both enamel and dentine; it proceeds slowly through the enamel layer, but once the dentine is reached, destruction by decalcification and proteolysis of the dentine is rapid. The pulp reacts by an acute inflammatory response that results in necrosis and pain, as the pulp is enclosed within the rigid walls of the tooth and the exudate cannot expand to adjacent tissues. Eventually, infection and toxic materials spread from the root-canal opening to the tissues around the apex of the tooth and induce periapical inflammatory changes, which may terminate in an acute or chronic abscess, or a chronic granuloma. If epithelial proliferation takes place within the granuloma or abscess, then a cyst may develop, which will increase in size over many years before it may be revealed clinically. A dental abscess shows a mixed bacterial infection with a variety of streptococci, enterococci and other organisms including *Prevotella* and *Bacteroides*.

The tooth sits in a unique position between the secretory immune system and the systemic immune system. Both systemic and secretory systems have been examined for natural immunity in humans, and for the protective effects in vaccination experiments in animal models. Most of the tooth surface would seem to be accessible to saliva and the secretory immune system, although the most caries-susceptible sites around the gingival margin and between the teeth (where the systemic immune system might be expected to play a larger role) are bathed in crevicular fluid and thus antibodies derived from serum. Serum IgG, IgA, and IgM antibodies, as well as cell-mediated immunity to *Strep. mutans*, can be correlated with the DMF (decayed, missing, and filled teeth) index of caries. Salivary IgA antibodies are also found. Although

there is evidence that natural immunity against dental caries can be found in humans, the immunity achieved is commonly ineffective. This might be associated with the immune responsiveness linked with the HLA class 2 gene products.

Theoretically either local immunization giving rise to salivary antibodies, or systemic immunization via serum antibodies and the gingival crevice, might lead to protection against dental caries. Mucosal immunization has been studied in several animal models, particularly the rat, and several groups have shown that the induction of salivary IgA antibodies may be related to a reduction in dental caries. Such salivary IgA antibodies can be induced by direct immunization of the minor salivary glands or by immunization of the gut-associated lymphoid tissue or nasal-associated lymphoid tissue, from where sensitized B cells may home to the salivary glands. Systemic immunization experiments with *Strep. mutans* have been repeatedly performed in the rhesus monkey model, and have demonstrated unequivocally that caries can be reduced by immunization and the induction of serum IgG antibodies. Salivary or serum-derived antibodies may prevent *Strep. mutans* from adhering to the tooth surface or inhibit glucosyltransferase activity and thereby prevent caries. Systemic immunization elicits antibodies, complement, polymorphonuclear leucocytes, lymphocytes, and macrophages which pass from the gingival blood vessels to the gingival domain of the tooth. Bacterial colonization of the tooth can therefore be influenced by the systemic immunity and an important mechanism is probably that of IgG-induced opsonization, binding, phagocytosis, and killing of *Strep. mutans* by phagocytes.

Clinical features (Fig. 15.6.1)

Toothache that is made worse by any hot or cold drinks or food is characteristic: the throbbing pain becomes progressively worse, affects the patient especially at night time, and may radiate to the face and ear. The pain becomes excruciating, and the tooth tender followed by death of the dental pulp and the development of swelling due to an abscess or cellulitis. With an acute abscess the inflammatory exudate may penetrate through the bone to the soft tissues. Whilst the pain is reduced, facial oedema increases, and if the upper canine is involved the swelling spreads to the eyelid—with sometimes an alarming appearance. The regional lymph nodes are tender and enlarged; there may be fever and malaise.

Occasionally, a cellulitis derived from the infected periapical tissues gives rise to a spreading infection along the fascial planes, especially of the submaxillary and sublingual spaces. This can also occur with intraoral infection by β-haemolytic streptococci. The inflammatory exudate may spread along the parapharyngeal spaces into the loose connective tissue of the glottis causing oedema of the glottis and respiratory obstruction. The attendant brawny swelling of the neck and floor and the mouth, difficulty in swallowing, trismus, fever, and malaise is referred to as Ludwig's angina.

An alternative and more common chronic course is the insidious development of a chronic pulpitis, granuloma, abscess, and eventually cyst around the apex of the offending tooth. There may be few symptoms. Although the patient may indicate a painful tooth, this can be misleading, because the pain often radiates to adjacent teeth. The offending tooth is located by finding the caries. The tooth responds with pain on application of a hot or cold stimulus, and later is tender to percussion; it may be discoloured. Dental radiographs may confirm or localize the carious tooth and, at a later stage, any periapical pathological changes.

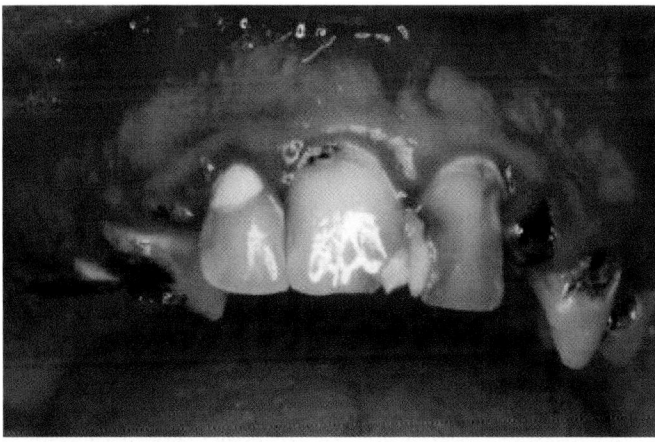

(a)

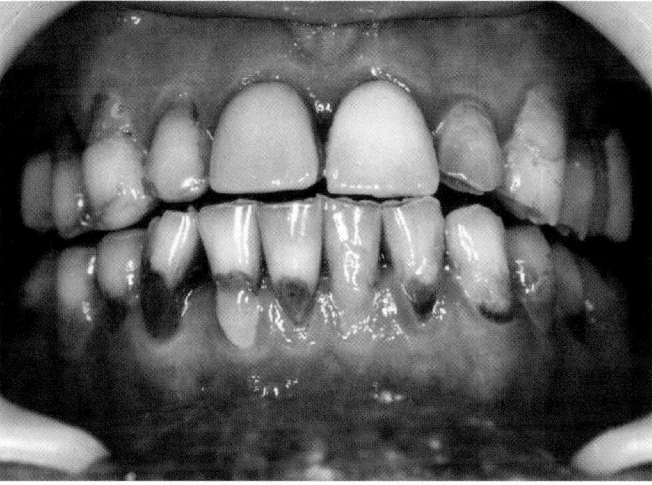

(b)

Fig. 15.6.1 Dental caries: (a) extensive destruction of the enamel and dentine; (b) cervical caries secondary to xerostomia.

Treatment

The principles of treatment are to remove the caries, apply a nonirritant material such as zinc oxide and eugenol dressing to protect the pulp, and then restore the tooth with a filling. If the pulp is damaged irreversibly it will have to be extirpated and root canal therapy instituted. The alternative to conservative treatment is extraction. A dental abscess is effectively dealt with by extraction of the diseased tooth, for this removes the source of infection and drains the pus.

If the tooth is to be saved, the pus is drained by an intraoral incision and/or establishing drainage through the root canal. Antibiotics are usually given in acute abscesses: amoxicillin or ampicillin 250 mg four times a day for about 7 days, or metronidazole 400 mg three times daily for up to 7 days is adequate. Cellulitis may be treated by amoxicillin 500 mg 3 times a day or intramuscular benzylpenicillin, 1 megaunit (MU) four times a day. The swelling should then be incised, to relieve the pressure and provide drainage; extraction of the tooth under general anaesthesia should take place as soon as the patient's condition permits it.

Prevention of dental caries is best practised by careful plaque removal by the individual, and by limiting the intake of sugar, especially the frequent consumption of sweets and sweetened drinks. Fluoride in toothpaste decreases the incidence of caries

in children by up to 40% but effective tooth brushing is essential. Water fluoridation, however, is the most effective public health preventive measure. One part per million of fluoride in the drinking water will decrease the incidence of caries in children by up to 60%. There is no evidence of toxicity from water fluoridation. The ethical and scientific issues of water fluoridation are complex and have been the subject of a number of reports, including one by the Royal College of Physicians of London.

Differential diagnosis

Toothache has a characteristic quality but occasionally needs to be carefully differentiated from sinusitis and neuralgia. Throbbing pain exacerbated by thermal stimuli and more severe at night is an important diagnostic feature. An abscess or cellulitis caused by dental caries has been, on a few occasions, confused with mumps, although mumps is confined predominantly to the parotid fascia. Earache may be a prominent feature, and pain is elicited by pulling on the earlobe. A chronic granuloma or a dental cyst is usually diagnosed radiologically, unless the cyst becomes large and a swelling becomes clinically evident.

Course and prognosis

The acute sequence of events from dental caries is acute pulpitis, apical periodontitis, resulting in an abscess or cellulitis. If treated promptly the sequelae can be prevented, but if not treated the patient will lose the tooth and may also develop facial scarring due to a discharging sinus. With slow progression of caries or incomplete removal of decay, a chronic pulpitis may supervene, which may result in a periapical granuloma, abscess, or cyst. Dental caries is in most instances a progressive condition and can be halted only by the dental surgeon.

Gingival and periodontal diseases

Aetiology

Many diseases affect the gingivae and periodontium but the two most common conditions, chronic gingivitis (Fig. 15.6.2) and chronic inflammatory periodontal disease (Fig. 15.6.3), are both related to accumulation of plaque on the interface between teeth and gingivae. Chronic gingival inflammation may persist for many years; it is followed by breakdown of the periodontal membrane, with loss of the supporting bone, and then teeth over the years. Progression of chronic inflammatory periodontal disease (Box 15.6.1) may be related to genetically controlled immune responses. Associations have been described between chronic inflammatory periodontal disease and atherosclerosis, and between maternal chronic inflammatory periodontal disease and low infant birth weights. Mild inflammation of the gingivae (gums) (chronic marginal gingivitis) and/or slight destruction of the collagen fibres of the periodontal membrane (early periodontitis) are found in most adults. Advanced destruction of the periodontal membrane, including the supporting bone, is found in about one-half of the middle-aged or older population. Gingivitis is an inflammatory response to plaque bacteria, is thought to be reversible, and does not necessarily proceed to periodontitis; but chronic inflammatory periodontal disease is preceded by gingivitis and is irreversible. Plaque begins as a Gram-positive biofilm but changes to a complex population of filamentous organisms, spirochaetes, vibrios, and

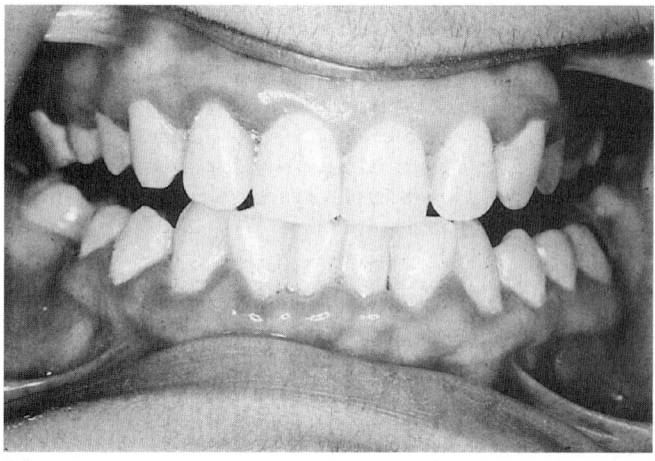

(a)

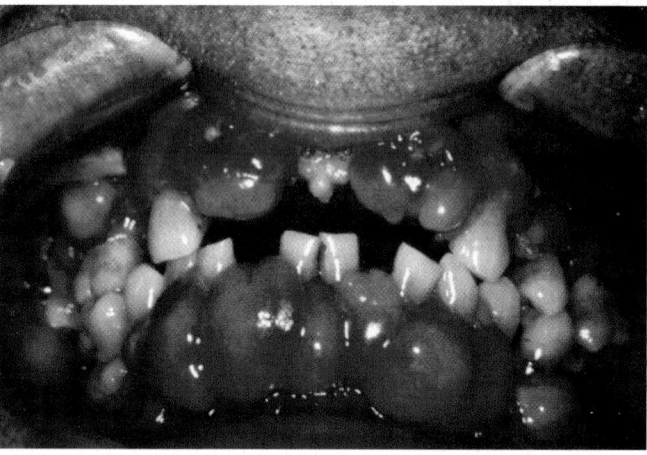

(b)

Fig. 15.6.2 (a) Chronic gingivitis, with erythema and oedema of the gingival margin of the lower teeth and especially the upper right lateral incisor. (b) Drug-induced gingival hyperplasia (ciclosporin).

Gram-negative cocci. Of the Gram-positive organisms, *Actinomyces viscosus* appears to be involved in the development of gingivitis. Gram-negative organisms are thought to be essential in the development of periodontal disease. *Porphyromonas gingivalis*, *Actinobacillus actinomycetemcomitans*, *Capnocytophaga* spp., and spirochaetes have all been implicated.

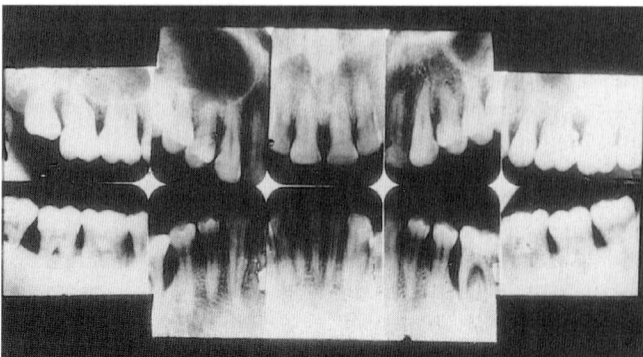

Fig. 15.6.3 Radiograph of teeth showing advanced periodontitis with loss of supporting bone of the teeth.

Plaque is a prerequisite for both gingivitis and for chronic inflammatory periodontal disease, but there are two main views concerning the microbial aetiology for periodontal disease: (1) that it mainly an immunological response to nonspecific mixed organisms in dental plaque or (2) that specific organisms are responsible for the development of periodontal disease. The specific microbial aetiology hypothesis has recently received support from the observations that *P. gingivalis* is the predominant organism isolated from periodontal disease and produces powerful extracellular toxins. Invasiveness of these microorganisms probably plays an important part in their virulence. Periodontitis is the most important cause of loss of teeth after the age of 40, when the incidence of dental caries has greatly diminished. An important feature of periodontitis is that it usually affects many teeth, resulting in a complete loss of the dentition.

A rare type of rapid destruction of the supporting dental tissues is found in children or young adults and is referred to as aggressive (or juvenile) periodontitis; one or more teeth may become mobile and may be lost before 21 years of age. Both this juvenile form and rapidly progressing adult periodontitis are associated with *Actinobacillus actinomycetemcomitans*.

If left undisturbed, bacterial plaque calcifies to form dental calculus. Calculus is often found on the lingual surface of the lower incisors and the buccal surface of the upper molars, i.e. opposite the orifices of the major salivary glands. Dental calculus above and

---

Box 15.6.1 Classification of periodontal diseases

Gingivitis

Acute

- Acute necrotizing gingivitis (ANUG)
- Acute gingivostomatitis
- Traumatic gingivitis

  Physical (toothbrushing)
  Chemical (aspirin burn)

- Leukemia

Chronic

- Chronic marginal gingivitis
- Plasma cell gingivitis
- Desquamative gingivitis (dermatomes)
- Necrotizing ulcerative gingivitis
- Drug-induced gingivitis (phenytoin)

Periodontal diseases

- Adult periodontitis
- Early-onset periodontitis
- Rapidly progressing periodontitis
- Periodontitis with systemic disease

  Diabetes, Down's syndrome, Papillon–Lefevre syndrome, HIV infection

- Necrotizing periodontitis

below the gum line must be removed completely by the dental hygienist or dentist to treat gingivitis and periodontitis. Although the primary causes of gingivitis and periodontitis are the bacteria that adhere to the tooth surface, there are many other modifying factors. One of the strongest of these is tobacco use. Another very strong factor is one's inherited or genetic susceptibility. Several diseases including diabetes, Down syndrome and diseases that affect resistance to infection also increase susceptibility to periodontitis.

Pathology

There are four immunopathological stages of periodontal disease:

1 The initial lesion is found in the normal clinical state, with a localized inflammatory response of polymorphonuclear leucocytes; complement activation and chemotaxis generated by plaque antigens and possibly immune complexes may account for this stage.

2 The early lesion shows a localized infiltration of predominantly T with a few B lymphocytes. In the circulation, lymphocytes are sensitized at this stage to plaque antigens.

3 The established lesion is characterized by a localized plasma-cell infiltration and peripheral blood lymphocytes can be stimulated to proliferate by plaque antigens. This stage can persist for years, with early pocket formation.

4 The advanced lesion marks the transition to a destructive immunopathological mechanism, with ulceration of the pocket epithelium and localized destruction of collagen and bone.

The immunological processes of periodontitis are complex, and may involve type I, II, III, and IV reactions, with the protective–destructive mechanisms of lymphocyte and macrophage functions, antibodies, and complement activation. Repair, with collagen formation and destruction of the tissues, eventually leads to loss of support of the teeth.

An attractive hypothesis for the destructive phase of periodontal disease is that bacterial toxins or the reactions to them inhibit normal healing and repair and that this inhibition leads to progressive damage to the periodontium. Macrophages are important for tissue repair; when activated macrophages produce fibroblast-activating factors that stimulate the fibroblasts into active proliferation. Fibroblast function is also affected by lymphocytes in inflammatory lesions since the latter produce a chemotactic factor for fibroblasts. Both macrophages and lymphocytes therefore produce factors that recruit fibroblasts to the area of inflammation, stimulate their proliferation, and thus indirectly stimulate collagen production. Bacterial factors that interfere with this repair could have profound effects on the effects of disease.

Clinical features (Figs. 15.6.2 and 15.6.3)

The symptoms of chronic gingivitis or periodontitis are usually so mild that they go unnoticed by the patient. Symptoms may include:

◆ occasional redness or bleeding of gums while brushing teeth, using dental floss or biting into hard food (e.g. apples)

◆ occasional gum swellings that recur, halitosis or bad breath

◆ persistent bad taste in the mouth, recession of gums resulting in apparent lengthening of teeth (which may also be caused by heavy-handed brushing)

◆ periodontal pockets between the teeth and the gums

◆ loose, shaky teeth in later stages

Differential diagnosis

Chronic gingivitis is relatively painless. It can be differentiated from acute ulcerative gingivitis (see below) by the sudden onset, malaise, characteristic halitosis, pain, and ulceration of the gingiva in the latter. Herpetic gingivostomatitis occurs predominantly in children and again the onset is acute, with fever, malaise, pain, and ulceration of the gingiva and oral mucosa (see below). Desquamative gingivitis usually involves the full thickness of the gingivae, is caused either by lichen planus or mucous membrane pemphigoid (see below) but may cause difficulties in differential diagnosis. The points to bear in mind are that the attached gingiva shows diffuse erosive areas and there may be evidence of lesions elsewhere in the oral mucosa.

Treatment

The general principles are control of bacterial plaque, establishment of healthy gingiva accessible to plaque control, the use of local antibiotics in selected cases, and mucogingival surgery in selected cases. The aims in the management of gingivitis and mild periodontitis are to remove dental plaque and calculus by scaling the teeth, and this can be done only by the dentist or, where available, by a dental hygienist. Prevention is, however, much more effective by plaque control, which involves careful tooth brushing, with the aid of plaque-disclosing solutions and regular use of dental floss and wood points. However, once deep periodontal pockets have been formed, these can be treated by root planing, gingival curettage, or surgically. It should be appreciated that the success of treatment of periodontal disease is in the hands of the patient: any type of treatment is dependent on meticulous plaque control.

Course and prognosis

If the bacterial plaque is not removed, the gingivitis may progress to periodontitis and after many years will progress to loss of the periodontium with loosening and loss of teeth. This process may, however, be arrested by plaque control and, if necessary, eradication of pockets, as long as there is sufficient bone to support the teeth.

Acute (necrotizing) ulcerative gingivitis

Synonyms

This is also called Vincent's gingivitis or acute fusospirochaetal gingivitis.

Aetiology

The bacteria responsible for acute necrotizing ulcerative gingivitis are a complex mixture of spirochaetes and fusiforms aided by other Gram-negative species. *Fusobacterium nucleatum* and *Treponema vincenti* have been favoured on account of their presence in large numbers in direct examination of smears from the lesions. *Prevotella intermedia* and *Porphyromonas gingivalis* have also been implicated as causative organisms, but *Leptotrichia* and *Selenomonas* species can commonly be found.

Whatever role microorganisms may play, a number of predisposing factors are recognized. Of the local factors, poor oral hygiene, with accumulation of dental bacterial plaque, defective restorations, and pericoronitis are most important. Acute ulcerative gingivitis is seen more commonly in young adults and particularly in smokers. A lowered general resistance may also predispose to the disease, as was commonly seen in trench warfare during the First World War. A chronic form of necrotizing ulcerative gingivitis is seen in HIV-induced immunodeficiency.

Pathology

The gum undergoes an acute inflammatory reaction, with an intense polymorphonuclear response and fibrinous exudate. This leads soon to necrosis of the epithelium and thrombosis of the small blood vessels.

Clinical features (Fig. 15.6.4)

Acute necrotizing ulcerative gingivitis is readily recognized by the sudden onset of painful, bleeding gums and a characteristic foul breath. Except for primary herpetic stomatitis, this is the only other oral mucosal infection in which there is a rise in temperature, which may reach 39 °C, regional lymphadenitis, anorexia, and significant malaise. Oral examination reveals necrotic, punched-out ulcers, affecting predominantly the interdental gingiva. At times there are shallow necrotic ulcers affecting the oropharyngeal mucosa, which shows diffuse erythema; this has been referred to as Vincent's angina. In the presence of erupting wisdom teeth, the overlying gum can show ulceration and oedema causing partial trismus of the jaws.

Diagnosis

This disease is often confused with primary herpetic stomatitis, because of the acute onset. However, these patients are usually younger, their breath is stale but lacks the distinct foul quality of that found in ulcerative gingivitis. First vesicles and then numerous well-defined ulcers are scattered over the oral mucosa unlike the tendency to localization of necrotic sites to the gingiva in ulcerative gingivitis. Direct examination of a smear from the lesion reveals a large number of spirochaetal and fusiform organisms, with a decrease in the mixed bacterial flora.

Treatment

Metronidazole is very effective and should be taken 200 mg by mouth three times daily for 3 to 4 days. Phenoxymethyl penicillin, 250 mg taken four times daily for a week, is equally effective in

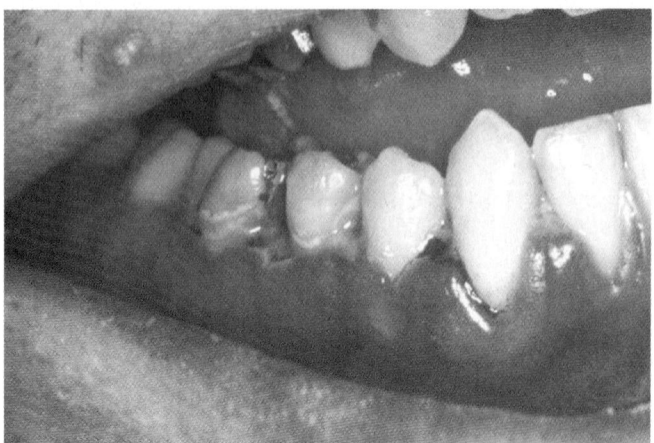

Fig. 15.6.4 Acute necrotizing ulcerative gingivitis.

clearing the symptoms. Oxidizing agents, hydrogen peroxide mouthwash, and a variety of peroxyborate preparations are also useful. During the acute phase, patients are advised to use a soft toothbrush or a soft cloth to clean their teeth, and they are encouraged to rinse their mouths forcibly with warm saline every 3 h.

Although treatment by drugs is effective in clearing the acute phase, recurrences can be prevented only by careful oral hygiene. The teeth have to be scaled and polished, and the patient is instructed as to the best method of tooth brushing and dental plaque control. Frequent review by the dental surgeon is advisable.

Course and prognosis

In the absence of treatment, the acute phase resolves gradually leaving a partially necrosed gingiva and chronic inflammation. Inadequate treatment commonly leads to recurrent ulcerative gingivitis over many years, with halitosis, gingival bleeding, and recession.

Herpes simplex and other viral infections

Herpes simplex virus type 1 is responsible for certain orofacial infections (see also Section 7).

Primary herpetic gingivostomatitis

Aetiology

Primary infection is caused by herpes simplex virus, usually type 1 which can present as an acute vesiculating stomatitis. Clinical or subclinical primary infections by herpes simplex virus type 1 are usually acquired in early childhood,. Primary herpetic infection in the first year is rare, because most mothers have neutralizing IgG antibodies to the virus that are transferred through the placenta to the fetus. Serum virus neutralizing antibodies are found in about 50% of children at 5 years of age and in 70% by age 20. Transmission is by close contact. Thus primary infection is common in children, but seen less frequently in adults.

Pathology

Herpes simplex virus is a DNA virus and there are two types: type 1 is found predominantly in the orofacial region and type 2 in the genital region. There are three genes (α, β, γ) and the β-gene codes for viral glycoproteins gB, gC, gD, and gE. These viral glycoproteins have been well characterized: gB is involved in viral penetration of the cell membrane, gC constitutes the C3b receptor (binding activated C3b), and gE is the Fc receptor for IgG. Antibodies against gD neutralize herpes simplex virus and block its penetration. Hence, this viral infection generates a number of significant immunological molecules in the host cell, in addition to expressing a viral antigen on the cell surface.

Infection starts with the herpesvirus gaining entry into epithelial cells. Virus replication takes place inside the nucleus, and this is associated with formation of intranuclear inclusion bodies and giant cells. As more epithelial cells become infected, degenerative and oedematous changes give rise to vesicle formation. The intraepithelial vesicles contain oedematous fluid, with giant cells and degenerating cells with intranuclear inclusion bodies. The vesicles rupture early, resulting in ulcers that heal rapidly.

Clinical features

The disease is recognized by an acute onset of a sore mouth and often sore throat, fever, and extensive inflammation of the gum, followed by formation of vesicles and ulcers of the oral mucosa, and regional lymphadenitis. Infants display considerable fretfulness, sleeplessness, and refusal to eat. Initially there are crops of small ulcers but these coalesce to produce large, shallow, irregular ulcers with surrounding inflammation. Herpetic keratitis is not often associated with herpetic stomatitis, and herpetic encephalitis is extremely rare but may occasionally complicate herpetic stomatitis.

Diagnosis

The clinical picture is usually distinctive but the early phase of infection can be confused with a cold, though the development of vesicles and ulcers makes that diagnosis unlikely. In the adult, herpetic infection may be confused with recurrent aphthous stomatitis, though the important differentiating points are the acute onset, sore throat, fever, and lymphadenitis in herpetic infection. A smear from the lesion showing virally damaged cells, intranuclear inclusion bodies or giant cells is helpful. Culture of the virus may assist in the diagnosis, but the herpesvirus is also found in carriers. A rise in antibody titre to the virus reaching a peak 2 to 3 weeks after an infection gives a retrospective confirmation of diagnosis.

Treatment

Aciclovir tablets (200 mg), four times daily for 7 days can be helpful if started at an early stage of infection; or in children aciclovir elixir used as a rinse and then swallowed. However, in late onset of primary herpetic infection, tetracycline mouthwash can speed up recovery. Patients are advised to rest for 2 to 4 days; a soft diet is indicated and an adequate fluid intake is emphasized. The mouth is cleansed by thorough rinsing with hot salt water six times daily and the teeth are cleaned with a wet flannel. In infants, special attention must be paid to the fluid intake and sleep. A useful sedative to use is promethazine elixir, given in doses of 1 teaspoonful (5 mg/5 ml) at night time.

Course and prognosis

The natural course of this infection is 7 to 14 days, during the initial days of which eating is usually difficult, but healing of the ulcers occurs spontaneously. Unusually prolonged infection or failure to respond to aciclovir suggests immunodeficiency. Recurrence of herpetic lesions intraorally is rare in otherwise healthy subjects, but is found commonly in patients with cellular immunodeficiencies.

Recurrent herpetic infection

Synonyms

This is also called recurrent herpes labialis or cold sore.

Aetiology

Recurrent herpes labialis is a reactivation of latent virus in those who have had a primary infection. It is caused by herpes simplex virus type 1; it is commonly found from childhood to past middle age and affects both sexes. It may be present in up to 15% of the population. Fever, exposure to sunlight, local trauma, emotional stress, menstruation, and section of the sensory root of the trigeminal ganglion are among the most common precipitating factors. Severe herpetic infections, affecting the lips, perioral skin, and mouth, are seen in patients receiving immunosuppressive drugs.

Pathology

Primary herpes simplex infection is followed by latency of the virus in the trigeminal ganglion. The relation between primary infection, latency, and recurrent infection by herpes simplex virus has not been completely elucidated, but it seems that after primary infection the virus ascends sensory axons via retrograde axonal flow, replicates, and establishes latency within the trigeminal ganglion. The entire herpes simplex virus genome can be found in the trigeminal ganglion, though the DNA is qualitatively different. During latency, there is down-regulation of the replicative process, infectious virus and viral antigens are not detectable, and the virus evades immune surveillance. When an appropriate trigger occurs (such as illness, sunlight, trauma, emotional stress, or menses), the virus reactivates, replicates in the ganglion, and travels centrifugally along the axon to the skin or mucosal site to be shed at the nerve endings. These may include intraoral sites where shedding can be detected but where probably the powerful antiviral factors in saliva usually prevent lesions. The virus may also establish latency in nonneuronal sites such as within the epithelium of the primary infection, although this concept is controversial. Primary infection induces immune responses to the virus, and antibody and cell-mediated cytotoxic mechanisms kill most of the virus and virus-infected cells that are accessible to killer cells. After latency is established, it is possible that re-activation occurs in the presence of some local defect in cell-mediated immunity, acting at the neuroepithelial junction. Cytokine production, especially interferon-γ and interleukin-2, may be impaired, and a decrease in cytotoxic CD8T cells is involved in recurrent herpetic infection. However, antibodies to herpes simplex virus are not impaired.

Clinical features (Fig. 15.6.5)

The lesions are usually limited to the vermilion border of the lips and adjacent skin. A single blister or a crop of blisters may develop a day after the prodromal phase of a burning sensation. The duration of the lesion varies usually between 3 and 10 days, but secondary infection by *Staph. aureus* occurs commonly. The lesion recurs at various intervals, often at the same site for many years, and the rate of recurrence may be related to the type of precipitating factor involved. The significance of cellular immunity is highlighted by herpes simplex virus infections found in cell-mediated immunodeficiency states, such as AIDS, and in patients receiving immunosuppressive therapy. Both primary and secondary herpetic lesions

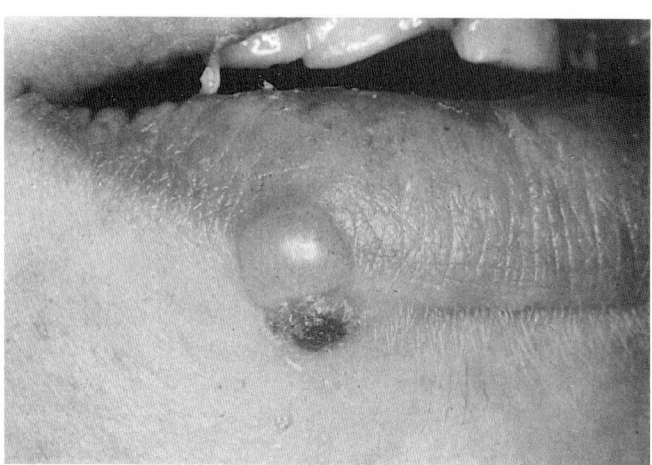

Fig. 15.6.5 Recurrent herpes labialis vesicle on the vermilion border of the lower lip.

are contagious, and herpetic whitlows on digits in contact with lesions are a hazard to the patient and others.

Diagnosis

Localization to the vermilion border of the lips and the history of recurrences make this a readily recognizable condition. Laboratory assistance is rarely required but the findings are similar to those described for primary herpetic infection, except that there is usually already a detectable antibody titre which shows little change following recurrent infection. Staphylococcal infection from the anterior nares should be excluded.

Treatment

Aciclovir (5% in the cream base)may reduce the duration of lesions if applied early. Recurrent herpetic infection (and recurrent intraoral herpes simplex virus infections) can be effectively treated with aciclovir 400 mg three times a day or valaciclovir 500 to 1000 mg twice a day. There is sound evidence that recurrent herpetic infection in the immunocompetent host can also be effectively prevented with sunscreen alone (SPF 15 or above). Valaciclovir 500 mg twice a day is also effective in suppressing erythema multiforme triggered by herpes simplex virus. Staphylococcal infection responds readily to mupirocin or fucidin ointment, applied three times daily. In the severe type of mucocutaneous herpetic infection in immunosuppressed patients, aciclovir tablets (200 mg) are administered two to four times daily.

Course and prognosis

The lesions heal usually within a week, but recurrences are difficult to prevent. If the precipitating factors are known, some preventive measures can be taken, as by applying a barrier cream to the lips before exposure to the sun.

Herpes zoster infection

Herpes zoster infection of the skin of the face, innervated by the second or third branches of the trigeminal nerve, may be associated with unilateral distribution of oral vesicles (Fig. 15.6.6). It is caused by varicella zoster virus and characterized by pain, a vesicular rash on the face, and vesicles in the oral cavity in the related

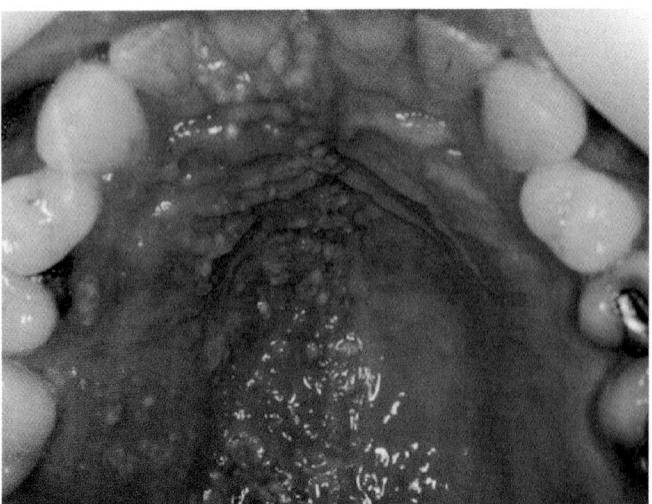

Fig. 15.6.6 Herpes zoster of the maxillary branch of the trigeminal nerve showing vesicular ulceration of half of the palate.

dermatome. These break down early to produce ulcers along the oral distribution of the maxillary or mandibular branches. Patients are sometimes unable to distinguish the pain of trigeminal zoster from severe toothache. Unlike herpes labialis, recurrences are rare.

Treatment is by oral aciclovir, 200 to 800 mg five times daily for 7 days, given at the earliest time possible, together with analgesics. In immunocompromised patients, intravenous aciclovir may be required.

Herpangina

This is a rare infection by the group A coxsackieviruses, usually affecting the soft palate and the oropharyngeal region. Children tend to be affected more often than adults and the mode of presentation of the disease is similar to that in primary herpetic stomatitis. The diagnosis can be firmly established only by isolating the virus from a lesion or by showing an increase in antibody titre. The disease appears to be self-limiting and specific treatment is not necessary.

Hand, foot, and mouth disease

This is another virus infection caused by coxsackievirus A5, 10 and 16 (see Section 7). It is a common mild infection, sometimes causing mild epidemics among schoolchildren. The mouth is sore due to multiple small vesicles or ulcers, which affect most commonly the hard palate, tongue, and buccal mucosa. There are associated deep-seated vesicular lesions on the hands and feet. The diagnosis is confirmed by isolating the virus from the lesion. The disease is self-limiting within about 2 weeks and no specific treatment is necessary.

Measles

This is an acute exanthematous virus infection of children (see Chapter 7.5.6). Whitish macules on the buccal mucosa, known as Koplik's spots, may precede the development of the red macular rash by 2 to 3 days.

Oral manifestations of HIV infection and AIDS (see Chapter 7.5.23)

Aetiology

AIDS is an HIV infection affecting primarily CD4+ cells. The resulting immunodeficiency allows coinfection with a number of viruses, bacteria, and fungi. There is also evidence that the virus may have a direct effect on epithelial cells, altering their cytokine responses.

Pathology

Entry of HIV into the host is primarily by the interaction between gp120 and the CD4 glycoprotein on the cell membrane, which acts as a receptor and enables the viral particle to enter the cell by fusion between viral and cell membranes or receptor-mediated endocytosis. Hence, the primary target of HIV is the CD4 subset of T cells (helper-inducer cells), but macrophages, dendritic, and Langerhans cells may also express CD4 and become infected. CD4 cells decrease in number as the cells become infected and killed, but the CD8 subset is not affected, resulting in a decrease in the CD4:CD8 cell ratio. It is not clear how the virus kills CD4 cells; it might be mediated by interaction between CD4 protein and the HIV envelope protein that results in lethal cell-to-cell fusion (syncytium formation), or by the induction of apoptosis.

Clinical features

The disease affects five at-risk populations:

1 Heterosexual transmission during sexual intercourse with HIV-positive partners is numerically the greatest number, especially in Africa and parts of Asia where more than one-third of the adult population may be HIV positive; female prostitutes may carry the virus in their genital secretions.

2 Homosexual men, especially those with multiple sex partners, and the anal-receptive partner in anogenital intercourse, are at greatest risk.

3 Intravenous drug users spread the virus by infected needles from one person to another, directly by the vascular route.

4 Blood transfusion with HIV-infected blood, especially in haemophiliacs treated with factor VIII.

5 Perinatal HIV infection of babies from infected mothers.

Oral transmission of HIV by orogenital intercourse, with ejaculation of infected semen into the mouth, is very uncommon but there is some epidemiological evidence that oral sex might enable HIV transmission. However, doubt remains, as anal sex is practised more frequently than the participants are prepared to admit. The potential of salivary transmission of HIV is of immense significance to the public, as saliva is encountered during daily social interchanges—talking, coughing, sneezing, and particularly kissing. Oral fluid consists of saliva and gingival fluid and the latter contains high numbers of white cells. Although about 90% of the gingival fluid cells are neutrophils, the rest consists of T and B cells and macrophages. Oral fluid may then contain CD4+ cells, thereby creating the essential conditions for HIV transmission. Nevertheless, there is little evidence that salivary transmission of HIV can occur. Saliva contains a number of powerful anti-HIV factors including salivary leucocyte protease inhibitor, lactoferrin, mucins, and proline-rich peptides. In addition, comparative isolation studies of HIV from body fluids have been made and their results suggest that the quantity of HIV isolated from saliva is usually low though hypersecretors may exist.

The special significance to dentists of oral transmission of HIV is self-evident, as they work in a pool of saliva and often gingival bleeding. However, the prevalence of transmission of HIV to dentists from patients is extremely low and in studies from the United States and Germany involving more than 2000 dentists, only one occupationally acquired seroconversion was found in spite of a high rate of admitted needlestick injuries. The possibility of HIV transmission during dental procedures remains a possibility, especially as documented by the case of the Californian dentist passing HIV to his patients. However, the details of this case are most perplexing and the route of transmission was never established.

Oral manifestations of HIV disease

Over the last 20 years a body of literature has chronicled the frequency and type of oral disease in HIV infection around the world. These have been classified into three groups according to their relative frequency (Box 15.6.2). There is a group of seven lesions which are strongly associated with HIV infection and these include hairy leukoplakia, pseudomembranous and erythematous candidiasis, Kaposi's sarcoma, necrotizing ulcerative periodontal disease and non-Hodgkin's lymphoma. Hairy leukoplakia (Fig. 15.6.7)

Box 15.6.2 Oral manifestations of HIV infection

Group I: Lesions strongly associated with HIV infection

- Candidiasis

  Erythematous
  Pseudomembranous

- Hairy leukoplakia (Epstein–Barr virus)
- Kaposi's sarcoma
- Linear gingival erythema
- Necrotizing (ulcerative) gingivitis
- Necrotizing (ulcerative) periodontitis
- Non-Hodgkin's lymphoma

Group II: Lesions less commonly associated with HIV infection

- Bacterial infections
- Melanotic hyperpigmentation
- Necrotizing (ulcerative) stomatitis)
- Salivary gland disease

  Dry mouth due to deceased salivary flow rate
  Unilateral or bilateral swelling of major salivary glands

- Thrombocytopenic purpura
- Ulceration NOS (not otherwise specified)

Viral infections

- Herpes simplex virus
- Human papillomavirus

  Condyloma acuminatum
  Focal epithelial hyperplasia
  Verruca vulgaris

- Varicella-zoster virus

  Herpes zoster
  Varicella

Group III: Lesions seen in HIV infection

A variety of other lesions have been reported in HIV positive individuals but their association with HIV induced immunodeficiency is unclear

---

most commonly bilateral white lesions on the lateral borders of the tongue, and pseudomembranous candidiasis (Fig. 15.6.8) are the most frequently seen lesions in HIV infection and AIDS. The prevalence of these two lesions increases with time from seroconversion and their increasing prevalence and incidence rates correlate with falling CD4 counts and disease progression. Kaposi's sarcoma (Fig. 15.6.9) can frequently be the presenting sign of AIDS. This group of oral lesions not only indicates the presence of HIV infection but often constitutes early clinical features of HIV disease and predicts progression from asymptomatic HIV to AIDS. They can

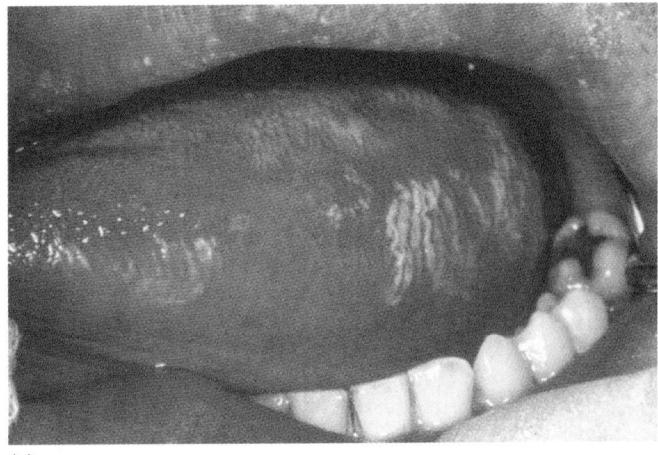

(a)

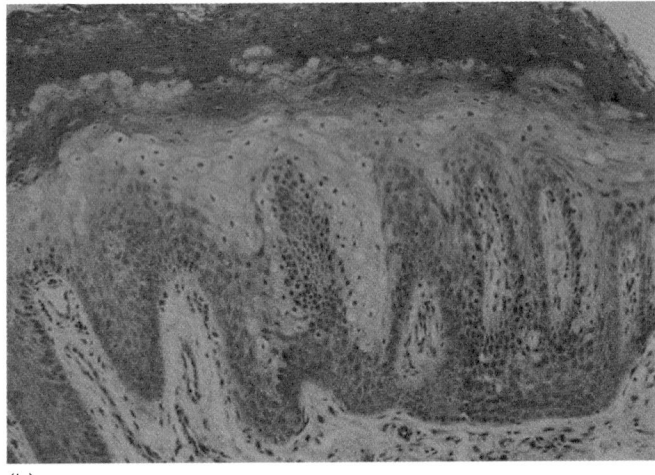

(b)

Fig. 15.6.7 (a) Oral hairy leukoplakia. Note the vertical lines of keratosis on the sides of the tongue. These are characteristically bilateral. (b) Histologically, in addition to acanthosis, frequent koilocyte-like cells (swollen epithelial cells) are seen indicating infection by Epstein–Barr virus.

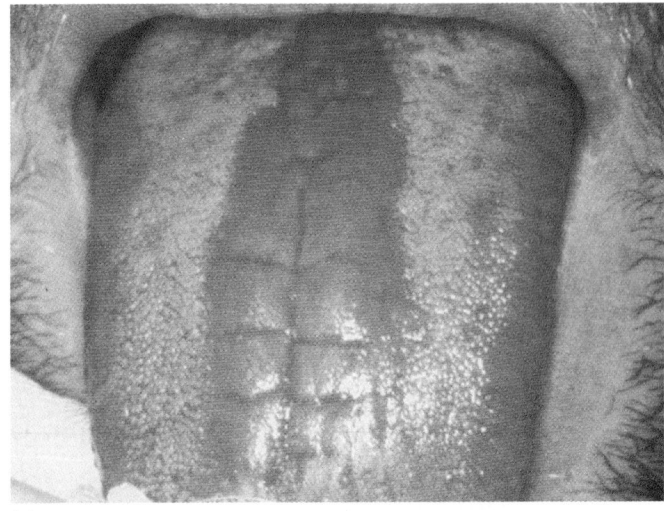

(a)

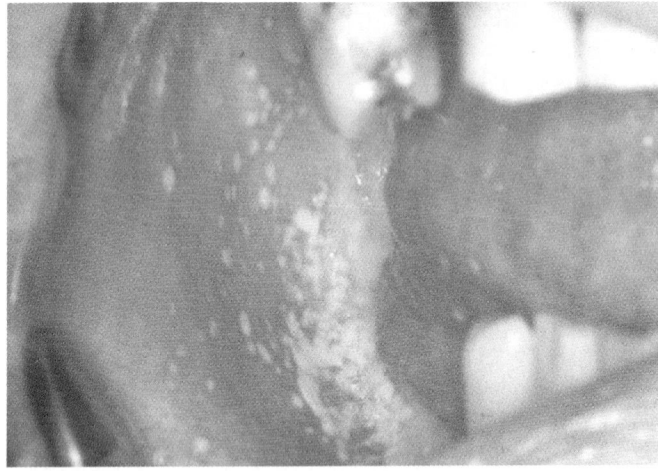

(b)

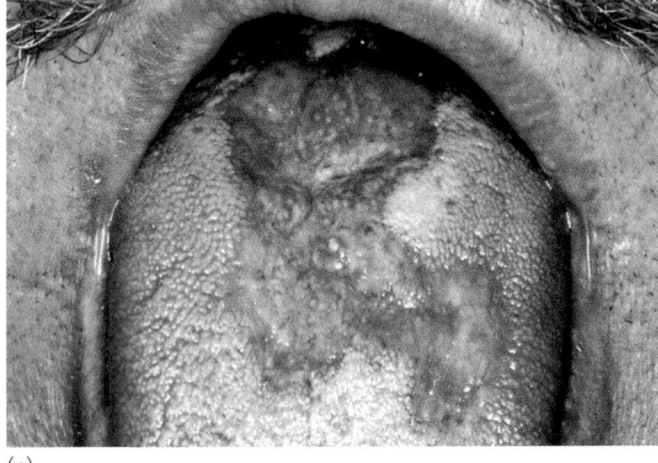

(c)

Fig. 15.6.8 Candidiasis in HIV-positive patients: (a) Erythematous candidiasis of the dorsum of the tongue; (b) pseudomembranous candidiasis of lower alveolus; (c) Chronic hyperplastic candidiasis of the dorsum of the tongue.

be used as entry or end points in therapy and vaccine trials or as determinants of anti-opportunistic infection therapy and anti-HIV therapy and can be utilized in staging and classification systems.

The most common types of candidiasis in HIV-infected individuals are pseudomembranous and erythematous, with both types occurring simultaneously in some patients. Hairy leukoplakia is the name given to the corrugated white patches occurring on the lateral borders of the tongue. The lesion has a characteristic histopathological appearance characterized by high-level Epstein–Barr virus replication, multiple Epstein–Barr virus strains, and extensive inter- and intrastrain recombination. Treatment with the antiviral aciclovir leads to a resolution of the lesion, which then reappears after medication stops.

Kaposi's sarcoma is a neoplasm of the vascular endothelial cells. Oral lesions present as red or purple macules or papules, often affecting the palate and tongue (Fig. 15.6.9). Other neoplasias are less common, but non-Hodgkin's lymphomas and carcinomas have been recorded.

Viral infections in HIV are common. Infection with herpes simplex virus gives rise to recurrent oral herpetic lesions affecting the palate or gum and presenting as painful vesicles that ulcerate.

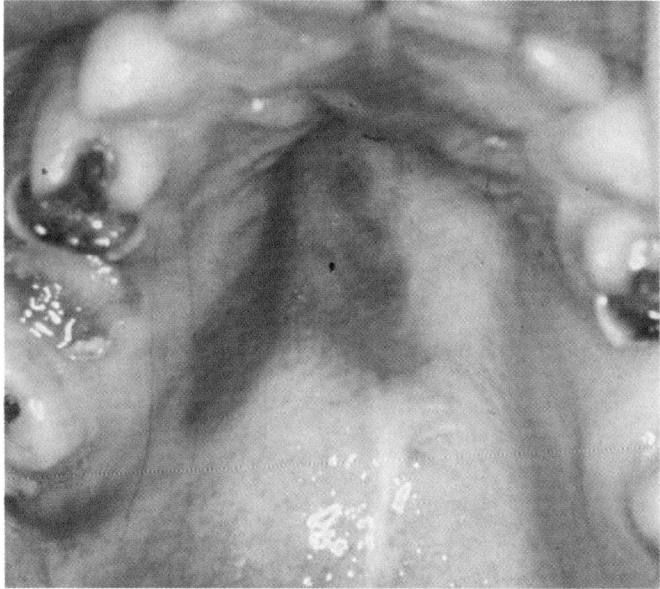

(a)

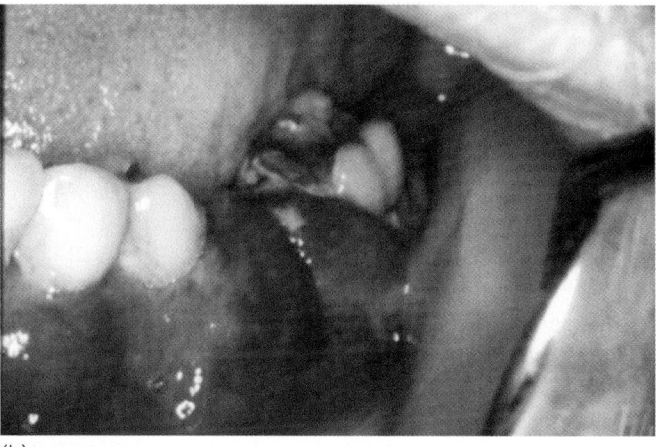

(b)

Fig. 15.6.9 Early Kaposi's sarcoma in the palate (a) and established in the gingiva (b).

Orofacial lesions due to herpes zoster have also been recorded but are rather rare. Human papillomavirus may induce single or multiple warts in the mouths of AIDS patients. Salivary gland enlargement as part of diffuse infiltrative leucocytosis syndrome, especially of the parotid glands, is often seen, particularly in children and may well be caused by a viral infection.

Chronic necrotizing ulcerative gingivitis and chronic necrotizing periodontitis are frequently found in HIV immunocompromised patients, often superimposed on the more common chronic inflammatory periodontal disease. The conditions can be painful and can be associated with rapid loss of soft tissue and bone support, leading to loss of teeth.

Differential diagnosis

As oral manifestations of AIDS may occur early in the disease, oral candidiasis, herpetic infections, leukoplakia, oral or gingival ulcers, salivary gland swellings, and oral tumours should be suspected, especially in young men (and women) falling into the HIV risk populations.

Treatment

In addition to the general management of AIDS, the teeth and gums should receive a great deal of attention, so as to maintain a high standard of oral hygiene. Otherwise, the oral lesions should be treated topically as for any other oral condition. Most routine dental treatment in HIV-positive patients can be performed in a dental practice setting, but many hospitals have made special arrangements for AIDS patients.

Fungal infections (see Section 7)

Candidiasis

Synonyms

This is also called moniliasis or thrush.

Aetiology

Candida species can be found as commensals in the mouths of some 40% of normal subjects in amounts up to approximately 800/ml. There is usually some underlying precipitating factor for oral candidiasis, often an immunodeficiency and in patients with various forms of candidiasis, salivary counts of more than 20 000/ml may be found. Oral candidiasis is a common condition, especially in patients with xerostomia, those taking immunosuppressive drugs, those with other oral diseases, and in patients with HIV infection where some 40% may have oral candidiasis. All forms of oral candidiasis are strongly associated with smoking. Although most species of candida can become pathogenic, *Candida albicans* is most frequently found in oral infections.

Pathology

The different varieties of candidiasis have in common a superficial invasion of epithelium by hyphae of candida and it is unusual for the hyphae to penetrate the basement membrane. However, occasionally candida may spread by the vascular route to the heart, kidneys, and brain, especially where there may be breaches of the mucosa such as in leukaemia or cytotoxic therapy. Pseudomembranous plaques are a mixture of desquamated epithelial cells, polymorphonuclear leucocytes, and candida hyphae, whereas fewer hyphae are present with the erythematous forms of candida. In chronic hyperplastic candidiasis, hyphae characteristically penetrate the epithelium. Antibodies and complement are necessary for optimal phagocytosis of candida by polymorphonuclear leucocytes or macrophages, though epithelial cells themselves secrete defensins especially in the presence of CD4+ lymphocytes.

Clinical features

Oral candidiasis develops in a variety of conditions predisposing to candidal proliferation: xerostomia, diabetes mellitus, anaemias, cell-mediated immunodeficiencies (such as AIDS or thymic defects), broad-spectrum antibiotics, immunosuppressive drugs, and leukaemias. Local factors commonly predisposing to oral candidiasis are dry mouth due to Sjögren's or sicca syndrome, irradiation, dentures, or steroid sprays used for asthma.

There are four main varieties of oral candidiasis:

Acute pseudomembranous candidiasis (thrush) (Fig. 15.6.10)

This disease is commonly seen in infants as well as in debilitated adults, particularly in diabetes mellitus and malignant diseases, especially leukaemia and lymphoma. Iatrogenic agents are also important predisposing factors; systemic antibiotics, corticosteroids, and

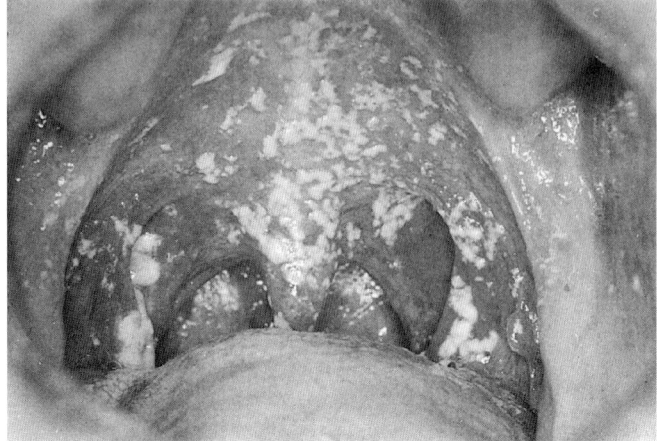

Fig. 15.6.10 Pseudomembranous candidiasis (thrush) showing white removable plaques on the hard and soft palate. Similar appearances can be seen following the application of a steroid spray in a patient with asthma.

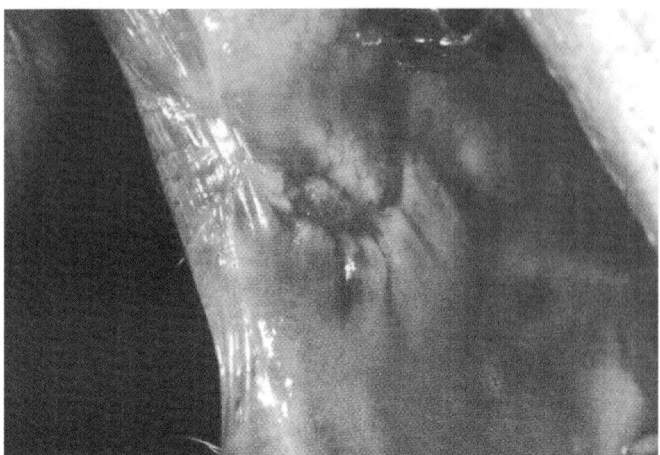

Fig. 15.6.12 Chronic hyperplastic candidiasis inside the mouth at the buccal mucosa.

immunosuppressive drugs seem to enhance candida infection. Local antibiotic and corticosteroid treatment can enhance oral candidiasis. Clinical manifestations of thrush are usually symptomless white papules or cotton-wool-like exudates that can be rubbed off leaving an erythematous mucosa.

Acute atrophic candidiasis

This may follow acute pseudomembranous candidiasis and is usually associated with broad-spectrum antibiotic therapy, hence referred to as 'antibiotic sore tongue'. It is the only type of oral candidiasis that is consistently painful, showing a smooth erythematous tongue, with angular cheilitis and (less often) inflamed lips and cheeks.

Chronic atrophic candidiasis

This type of candida infection is better known as 'denture stomatitis', for it presents as a diffuse erythema of the palate, limited to the denture-bearing mucosa. The denture covering the palatal mucosa predisposes to proliferation of candida. The lesion is usually symptomless but is often associated with angular cheilitis (Fig. 15.6.11).

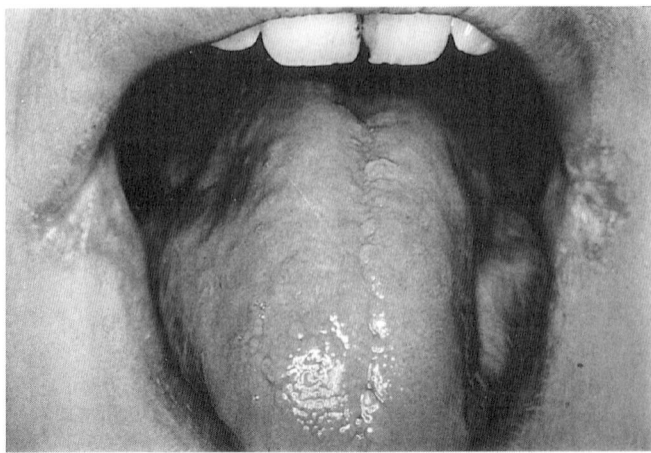

Fig. 15.6.11 Angular cheilitis caused by candidal infection.

Chronic hyperplastic candidiasis (Fig. 15.6.12)

This lesion presents as a firm, diffuse, white patch, or as numerous white papules with intervening erythema on the tongue, cheeks, or lips. The lesion may persist for many years or for life and should be distinguished from leukoplakia. This variety of candidiasis can be associated with skin lesions in mucocutaneous candidiasis.

Erythematous candidiasis (Fig. 15.6.8) These lesions are associated with HIV and are found predominantly on the dorsum of the tongue where the appearance is of bilateral depapillation and on the palate where 'thumb print erythema' in the absence of any white plaques is characteristic.

Chronic mucocutaneous candidiasis This starts in childhood as an intractable oral candida infection, with involvement of nails and sometimes the adjacent skin of hands and feet. A number of other skin sites may show persistent candida infection. Alopecia secondary to dermal candida may be present. In the granulomatous type, masses on the scalp and skin may be seen. Recurrent respiratory tract infection has been recorded in one-quarter of these children.

Chronic localized mucocutaneous candidiasis with endocrine disorder This can be found in children and young adults. A strong familial incidence is often found and candidiasis commonly precedes the endocrine abnormalities. The clinical features of candida infection are similar to those seen in the localized mucocutaneous variety. The association with hypoparathyroidism and Addison's disease, and less often pernicious anaemia and hypothyroidism, illustrates the relationship between cell-mediated immunodeficiencies and autoimmune endocrine disorders.

Differential diagnosis

Chronic hyperplastic candidiasis can cause some difficulties in differential diagnosis from leukoplakia and the laboratory tests are useful in this, as well as in the other types of candidiasis, in establishing the diagnosis. AIDS must be considered, particularly in homosexual men. A culture from the lesion yields candida, usually *C. albicans*, and direct examination of scrapings shows Gram-positive hyphae and yeast cells of candida. Biopsy of the lesion in chronic mucocutaneous candidiasis is helpful, as in addition to the superficial invasion of epithelium by candida hyphae, there is usually extensive epithelial hyperplasia. The dermis shows an intense mononuclear cell infiltration with a large proportion of plasma cells.

A rise in convalescent serum antibody titre to candida may assist in the diagnosis of the acute types of candidiasis, but there may be an impaired antibody titre in the chronic type of candidiasis. Chronic mucocutaneous candidiasis is usually associated with some defects in cell-mediated immunity and this should be determined by investigating delayed hypersensitivity *in vivo* and lymphocyte proliferative and cytokine responses to candida antigens. It is essential that the endocrine function should be tested in children with chronic candidiasis of the mouth and nails.

Treatment

Oral candidiasis responds readily to topical oral treatment with antifungal drugs, either polyenes or azoles; sucking tablets of nystatin 500 000 units four times a day, or amphotericin 10 mg four times a day, for 1 to 2 weeks is very effective. For chronic hyperplastic candidiasis, systemic therapy is needed and fluconazole 100 mg tablets or itraconazole is usually effective. Topical antifungal agents, such as miconazole, are effective when applied to the denture in chronic atrophic candidiasis or to the lips in angular cheilitis provided in the latter that the intraoral reservoir is also treated. Chronic mucocutaneous candidiasis usually does not respond to topical oral treatment, however, and necessitates systemic azoles such as voriconazole or in severe cases intravenous administration of amphotericin. Although almost complete eradication of the lesions can be accomplished, amphotericin is nephrotoxic and the disease tends to return after the drug is discontinued. This is comprehensible on the basis of an underlying immunological defect, which, if it is not rectified, will lead to reinfection with candida.

Bacterial infections

Tuberculosis

Oral tuberculosis is rare and usually secondary to pulmonary tuberculosis. Commonly the presenting feature is a painful ulcer or a firm, small swelling. Ulcers may be single or multiple, but they are usually large, with a depressed and granulomatous floor and some induration of the base. The tongue, lips, and cheeks may be affected. Diagnosis is based on microscopical and cultural demonstration of *Mycobacterium tuberculosis* and a biopsy of the lesion, which will show a tuberculous granuloma. Oral tuberculosis responds readily to specific chemotherapy.

Syphilis

Treponema pallidum may affect the mouth in all stages of syphilis (see also Section 7).

Primary stage

A chancre appears within 2 to 4 weeks of infection. The lesion that presents on the lip or tongue as a painless, small, firm nodule about 6 mm across that breaks down and forms an ulcer with raised indurated edges. This can resemble a carcinoma, especially if on the lips. A chancre is typically painless and the regional lymph nodes show discrete, rubbery enlargement. The diagnosis depends on direct observation of *T. pallidum* by dark-ground illumination. This stage is highly infective, but serological tests are usually negative during the initial 3 to 4 weeks and the chancre heals after 8 to 9 weeks.

Secondary stage

This develops 1 to 4 months after infection and presents as a generalized maculopapular rash and lymphadenitis. Oral lesions rarely appear without the rash and are usually flat ulcers covered by a fibrinous membrane (snail-track ulcers) affecting the tonsils, tongue, or lips, and the saliva is highly infective. The serological tests for syphilis are positive. It typically causes mild fever with malaise, headache and sore throat accompanied by a generalized lymphadenopathy. The rash consists of asymptomatic macules, symmetrically distributed and beginning on the trunk.

Tertiary stage

This is delayed by 3 to 15 years after infection. The onset is insidious and during the latent period (since secondary syphilis) the patient may appear well. Gumma and leukoplakia are the typical oral manifestations at this stage. A gumma starts as a swelling of the palate, tongue, or tonsils; it undergoes necrosis and results in a painless, punched-out, deep ulcer, with a 'wash leather' floor. Gummas vary from one to several centimetres in diameter. The lesion may heal by scarring, or give rise to perforation. Leucoplakia usually affects the dorsum of the tongue as an irregular, diffuse white patch that cannot be rubbed off. Histological appearances are often nonspecific, so confirmation of the diagnosis depends on serology. The treatment of oral syphilis is the same as that used in other sites, but the response in the tertiary stage is rather poor.

Cancrum oris (noma)

This is a rapidly spreading gangrene of the lips and cheeks, mostly confined to children in parts of tropical Africa. It is thought to be an extension of acute ulcerative gingivitis (see above) when associated with other diseases, especially measles. Cancrum oris is very rare in the United Kingdom, but can be seen during the terminal stages in patients with leukaemia, especially when treated by a variety of cytotoxic, antiinflammatory, and immunosuppressive drugs. It is more commonly seen in Africa, usually associated with malnutrition.

Oral ulceration

In view of the great variety of oral ulcers a classification will be given first (Box 15.6.3). Only recurrent oral ulcers will be dealt with fully and the other types of ulcers will be considered predominantly under differential diagnosis.

Recurrent aphthous stomatitis

Synonyms

Three types of ulcers will be described: minor aphthous ulcers, also known as aphthae; major aphthous ulcers, often referred to in the literature as periadenitis mucosa necrotica recurrens; and herpetiform ulcers.

Aetiology

Recurrent aphthous stomatitis or recurrent oral ulceration is characterized by oral ulcers, occurring singly or in crops that usually last for 7 to 21 days before healing spontaneously. These ulcers recur after a variable period, which may be a few days or several weeks. Recurrent aphthous stomatitis can be separated clinically into three types: minor aphthous ulcers (Fig. 15.6.13), major aphthous ulcers

Box 15.6.3 Classification of oral ulcers related to cause

Recurrent ulceration

◆ Recurrent aphthous ulcers

  Minor
  Major
  Herpetiform

◆ Recurrent aphthous ulcers associated with Behçet's disease

◆ Smoking-related aphthous ulcers

◆ Atypical recurrent oral ulceration

◆ Recurrent erythema multiforme

Recurrent/persistent oral ulceration

◆ Secondary to haematological deficiency state/anaemia

  B$_{12}$/folate/iron

◆ Secondary to a gastrointestinal enteropathy

  Ulcerative colitis
  Crohn's disease
  Coeliac disease

◆ Secondary to a dermatological condition

  Benign mucous membrane/bullous pemphigoid
  Pemphigus
  Erosive lichen planus
  Dermatitis herpetiformis and linear IgA disease

◆ Secondary to connective tissue disease

  Systemic/discoid lupus erythematosus
  Oral ulcers as part of Reiter's syndrome

Single episode of ulceration

◆ Infective

  Viral (may also be recurrent)
  Syphilitic
  Tuberculous

◆ Traumatic

  Physical/mechanical
  Chemical

◆ Drug reaction

Single persistent ulcer

◆ Neoplastic

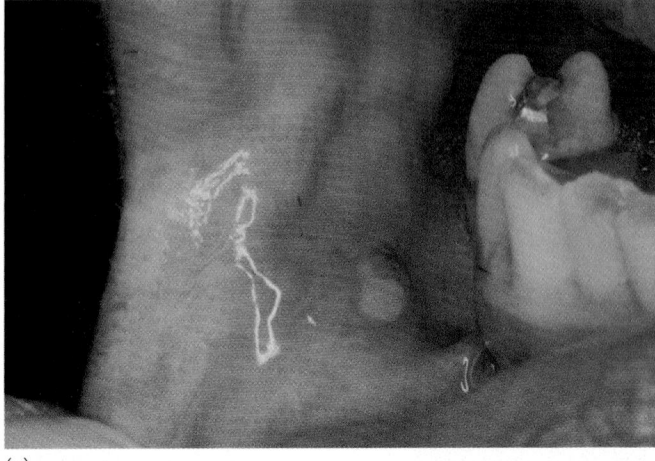

(a)

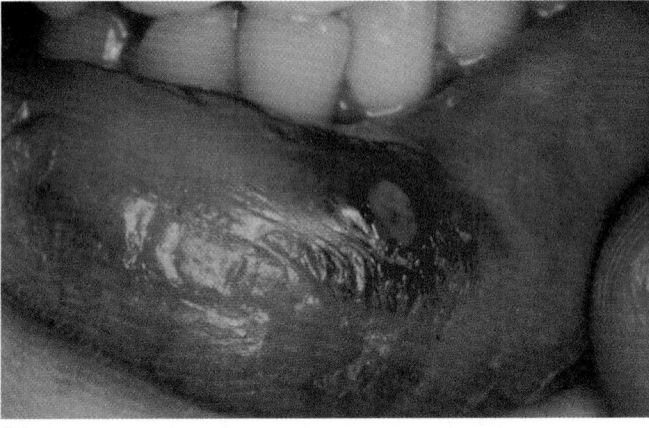

(b)

Fig. 15.6.13 Minor aphthous ulceration of (a) the buccal mucosa and (b) the lower lip. Note normal appearance of mucosa away from ulcers. One of the three types of recurrent aphthous stomatitis.

aetiology of recurrent aphthous stomatitis has not been fully established. Trauma is unlikely to play an essential role, though it might precipitate ulceration. There is no evidence that vitamin deficiency or food allergy are involved. Infection by the herpes simplex virus has been excluded as a cause of this type of ulceration. Although emotional stress may often influence the pattern of the disease, it is unlikely to be the direct cause. A family history of recurrent aphthous ulcers is often present and the highest incidence of ulcers is recorded in siblings in whom both parents have recurrent aphthous ulcers. A hormonal disturbance may play a part, as in some female patients there is a relationship between the ulcers and menstrual period; the onset of ulceration may coincide with puberty, or the ulcers may develop only after the menopause and the ulcers often disappear during pregnancy. The part that autoimmunity may play in the pathogenesis of this disease has not been fully elucidated, but the *in vitro* response of lymphocytes to epithelial antigens has been related to the clinical features, and lymphocytes are cytotoxic to oral epithelium. Oral mucosa shares common antigens with the 65-kDa heat shock protein that is found in Gram-positive organisms and human cells. A specific peptide of 15 amino acid residues (91–105) derived from the sequence of

(Fig. 15.6.14), and herpetiform ulcers (Fig. 15.6.15). There has been a tendency for clinicians to describe any ulcer occurring in the mouth as aphthous. However, aphthous ulcers have been carefully defined to allow differentiation from the many other types of ulcers occurring in the oral cavity (see Table 15.6.1). Recurrent aphthous ulcers are the most common lesions affecting the oral mucosa with a prevalence of about 10%, with a wide range reported in the literature. Although a large variety of causes has been suggested, the

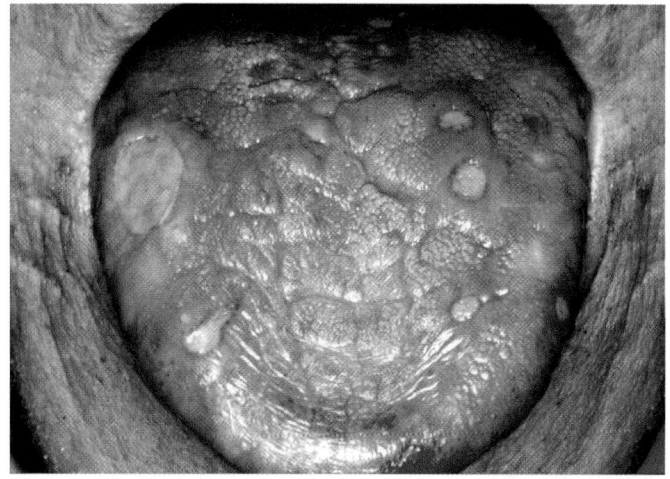

(a)

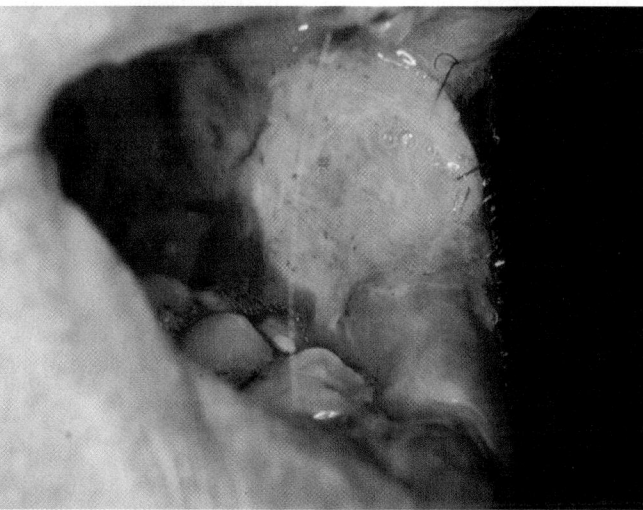

(b)

Fig. 15.6.14 Major aphthous ulcers. Note ulcers more than 10 mm in diameter on (a) the tongue with several smaller ulcers and (b) the left buccal mucosa. One of three types of recurrent aphthous stomatitis.

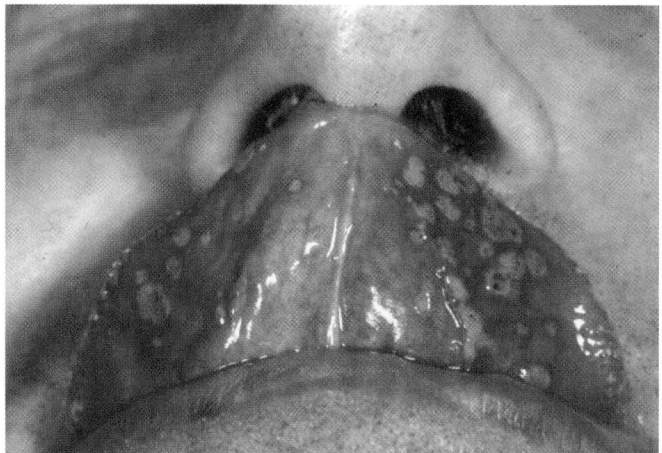

Fig. 15.6.15 Herpetiform ulceration: multiple coalescing ulcers characteristically on the ventral surface of the tongue or floor of the mouth. One of three types of recurrent aphthous stomatitis.

Table 15.6.1 Differentiating features of the three varieties of recurrent aphthous stomatitis

	Minor aphthous ulcers	Major aphthous ulcers	Herpetiform ulcers
Sex ratio F:M	1.5:1	1:1	3:1
Age of onset (peak incidence) (years)	10–19	10–19	20–29
Number of ulcers	1–5	2–10	10–100
Size of ulcers	<10 mm	>10 mm (some)	1–2 mm but coalesce
Duration (days)	4–14	10–30	7–10
Healing with scars (%)	8	64	32
Recurrence	1–4 months	<monthly	<monthly
Sites	Lips, cheeks, sides of tongue	Lips, cheeks, tongue (dorsum), pharynx, palate, gums	Lips, cheeks, tongue (ventral), pharynx, floor of mouth,
Associated oral lesions	None	Erythema migrans	None
Treatment	Corticosteroids (local)	Corticosteroids, immunosuppressives	Tetracycline as mouthwash

the 65-kDa heat shock protein has recently been found to stimulate lymphocytes from patients with recurrent oral ulcers. The role of this peptide in the pathogenesis of oral ulceration is under investigation.

Pathology

An early intense lymphomonocytic infiltration, especially with a perivascular distribution, is a constant histological finding, suggesting a delayed hypersensitivity reaction. This is followed by a polymorphonuclear infiltration. Immunohistological investigations suggest an enhanced immune response, with a significant increase in the number of CD4 and CD8 subsets of T cells, Langerhans cells, and macrophages and the expression of HLA-DR in the epithelial cells.

Clinical features

Minor aphthous ulcers (Fig. 15.6.13)

About 80% of recurrent oral ulcers are of this type; they are very common, especially in the 10 to 40 year age group, and they are found more frequently in females than males.

A prodromal phase is recognized by most patients, 1 to 2 days before the onset of ulceration, as a soreness or burning sensation. With the breakdown of epithelium and associated inflammatory reaction the pain increases in severity, particularly on eating. The ulcers are round or oval, up to five in number, and enlarge in size, although they remain well under 1 cm. They have a yellow floor with a slightly raised margin and often marked surrounding erythema and oedema. The most common sites of involvement are the mucosa of the lips and cheeks and margin of the tongue, and the ulcers last 4 to 14 days. The rate of recurrences varies from 1 to 4 months and is usually irregular, though in some females ulcers may precede the menstrual period. Enlargement of lymph nodes is uncommon and the patients do not have a raised temperature.

Major aphthous ulcers (Fig. 15.6.14)

These are severe variants of minor aphthous ulcers and less than 10% of patients with recurrent aphthous stomatitis have this type of ulcers. The pain that develops after the prodromal symptoms can be severe and persistent, so that patients find it difficult to eat and swallow food and often lose weight. Examination may reveal up to 10 ulcers at a time and some of these may enlarge to about 3 cm. The ulcers are necrotic with a raised margin and inflammation of the adjacent tissue, so they occasionally mimic a carcinomatous ulcer. In addition to the lips, cheeks, and tongue, the soft palate and tonsillar region are commonly involved. Healing of an ulcer may take 10 to 40 days and recurrences are so frequent that the patient suffers from continuous ulceration. Multiple, small scars may result from the large ulcers and these may assist in the diagnosis of major aphthous ulcers. The prevalence of major aphthous ulcers is raised in ulcerative colitis. A striking association has been found in smokers who give up the habit and develop recurrent aphthous ulcers.

Herpetiform ulcers (Fig. 15.6.15)

These are recurrent crops of small ulcers, up to 100 in number, affecting any part of the mouth including the gum, palate, and dorsum of the tongue. They account for less than 10% of recurrent oral ulcers and are much more common in females than males. Patients present with pain on eating and talking, and often with dysphagia; malaise and loss of weight can be prominent features. The lesions persist for 7 to 14 days and commonly new ulcers appear before the previous crop has healed, so that ulceration becomes continuous.

Diagnosis

The differential diagnosis of the three types of recurrent oral ulcers is given in Table 15.6.1. It is important to differentiate these ulcers from those found in patients with iron, folate, or vitamin B_{12} deficiency, which constitutes less than 5% of patients with recurrent oral ulcers. About 2% may suffer from coeliac disease, due to gluten enteropathy, and these ulcers respond readily to a gluten-free diet.

Agranulocytosis or neutropenia may manifest themselves as shallow necrotic ulcers, affecting predominantly the oropharyngeal region. The ulcers tend to persist, unlike major aphthous ulcers, which recur at different sites. However, cyclical neutropenia can mimic minor aphthous ulcers and the diagnosis depends on serial weekly white blood-cell counts.

One of the most common diagnostic errors is to confuse the effects of denture trauma with aphthous ulcers, although the former are usually localized to the mucosa covering the mandibular and maxillary alveolus and the buccal and lingual sulci. The relation between denture trauma and ulceration is usually simple to find and requires the attention of a dentist.

The differential diagnosis from pemphigus, benign mucous membrane pemphigoid, and erythema multiforme will be described below. Not infrequently, patients with major aphthous ulcers are suspected of having a carcinoma, though a careful history will make it evident that these ulcers have been recurring at different sites in the mouth. Although major aphthous ulcers may have a raised margin, this is due to inflammation and not invasion, so that palpation fails to elicit the induration usually detected in carcinomatous ulcers.

Treatment

Topical corticosteroids are at present the most helpful agents in alleviating minor and major aphthous ulcers. They are most effective if application is started during the prodromal phase, when the mucosa has not yet ulcerated, and the intensity of lymphocyte transformation has not reached peak values. If steroids are applied early, ulceration may be prevented, but application at a later stage may reduce the severity and duration of ulceration. The most useful preparations are triamcinolone in orabase, containing 0.1 mg triamcinolone per 100 g of an adhesive base; hydrocortisone sodium succinate, having 2.5 mg of the steroid per tablet; and betamethasone, containing 0.5 mg steroid per tablet and used as a mouthwash The hydrocortisone tablets are kept in the mouth, or the ointment is applied to the ulcers, three to four times daily until the ulcer disappears. Systemic prednisolone or azathioprine has to be resorted to occasionally in patients with major aphthous ulcers, when topical corticosteroids fail to control the ulcers.

Topical tetracycline is the drug of choice in suppressing herpetiform ulcers, but is also useful in controlling some major aphthous ulcers, particularly when there is excessive amount of inflammation. Its mode of action is not clear and an effective preparation is to use capsules containing 250 mg tetracycline; the powder from a capsule is dissolved in 10 ml of water and kept in the mouth four times daily. Chlorhexidine solution (0.2%) can be used as a mouthwash, which keeps the teeth free of dental plaque, and may facilitate remission of ulceration.

Course and prognosis

Minor aphthous ulcers may recur from early childhood for many years, and often these ulcers may cause only transient discomfort to which the patient becomes accustomed. However, major aphthous and herpetiform ulcers usually cause a great deal of discomfort, difficulty in eating, and loss of weight. In children, major aphthous ulcers are particularly troublesome and need careful management. In the majority of patients with recurrent oral ulceration the disease burns itself out but this may take many years.

Behçet's syndrome

In a very small proportion of patients, extraoral sites may become involved, of which the vulvovaginal region is most common, to form part of Behçet's syndrome. There is no way of predicting the development of Behçet's syndrome in patients with recurrent oral ulcers apart from the increased association with HLA-B51 in Behçet's (see Chapter 19.11.5).

Recurrent aphthous stomatitis, genital ulcers, and uveitis are the major features of Behçet's syndrome. Cutaneous, vascular, arthritic, neurological, and gastrointestinal manifestations may also occur. The condition is uncommon in the United Kingdom and United States, but it is probably underdiagnosed. A high prevalence has been reported in Japan and the eastern Mediterranean countries. Patients may suffer a variety of manifestations, and, as only some may have the classical triad of recurrent aphthous stomatitis, genital ulcers, and iridocyclitis, it has suggested that involvement of a minimum of two of the major sites is sufficient for diagnosis (see Chapter 19.11.5).

Oral manifestations of dermatological conditions

Common oral manifestations of dermatological conditions include lichen planus, pemphigus, mucous membrane pemphigoid, and erythema multiforme.

Lichen planus

This is a disease that may affect the skin, or the mouth or both mucocutaneous surfaces (see Section 23).

Aetiology

Oral lichen planus is a common and distinctive mucocutaneous disease that usually presents in the mouth as bilateral symmetrical white patches or striae on the mucosa, but may present as a bullous, ulcerative, or atrophic condition, or even as desquamation of the gingivae. It is thought to affect between 1% and 2% of the adult population with a peak incidence in middle age, and the lesions of the mucosa may persist for several years. The lesions of the mucosa may persist for many years. Oral lichen planus is classified as a potentially malignant condition since there is an increased rate of malignant transformation.

Lichen planus is regarded as a cell-mediated autoimmune disease targeted against hitherto unidentified antigens in the basement membrane zone. A similar condition can develop in graft-vs-host reaction after bone marrow transplantation, and a variety of drugs are capable of inducing lichenoid changes in the mouth (e.g. penicillinase, colloidal gold). It seems to be exacerbated by emotional or psychiatric stress. However, in most patients no obvious initiating factors or cause can be determined.

Pathology

The pathological changes are hyperkeratosis, hyperplasia, and a characteristic degeneration of the basal cell layers of epithelium due to the induction of apoptosis of these cells. The lamina propria shows a well-defined lympho-monocytic infiltration.

Clinical features

There are three main clinical presentations of oral lichen planus: hypertrophic/papular, atrophic, and ulcerative (Fig. 15.6.16). In all three types the lesions are bilateral and frequently symmetrical. About 10% of patients presenting with oral lesions have cutaneous manifestations, which appear as a papular rash, predominantly affecting the flexor surfaces of the arms.

In the mouth the milder lesions may remain symptomless for years and not infrequently they are first noticed by the dentist during routine examination. Some patients complain of a furry thickening of the mucosa and others of pain or bleeding from the gums on eating. The hypertrophic variety is most common. There are white striae and minute papules, most commonly affecting the posterior part of the buccal mucosa, lips, and dorsum of tongue, though the palate, gum, and floor of the mouth are also involved. The striae criss-cross, giving rise to a fine lacy pattern. At times the striae may fuse together and result in a diffuse, somewhat smooth, shiny white plaque which may be difficult to differentiate from leukoplakia. Indeed, the dorsum of the tongue usually manifests diffuse white patches instead of the striated pattern.

Ulcerative lichen planus is common, however, and patients complain of pain and discomfort on eating. There may be large shallow ulcers up to 3 cm in size surrounded by white striae and

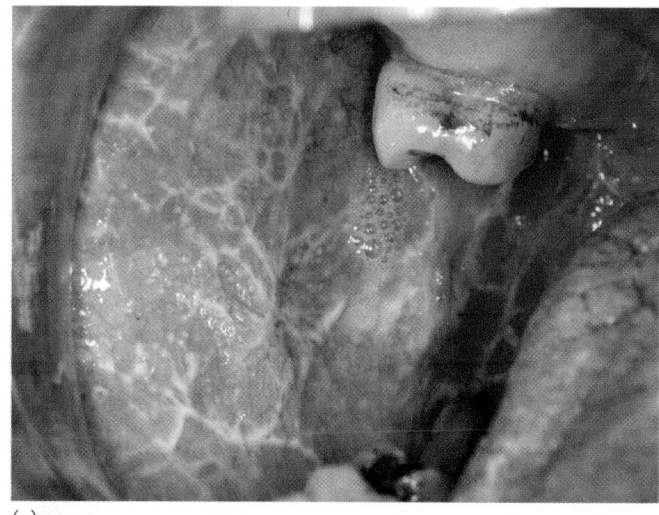

(a)

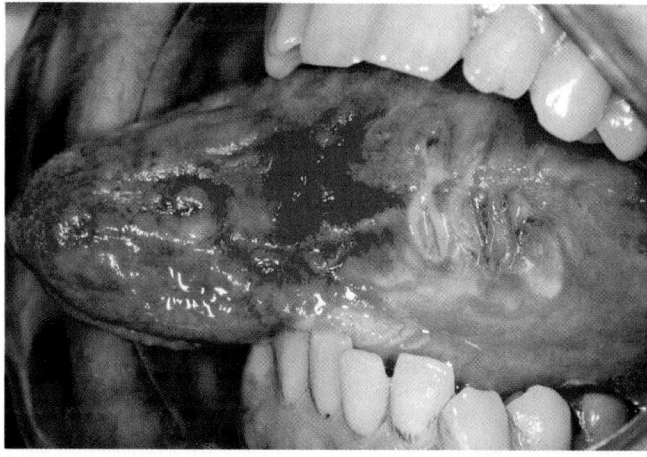

(b)

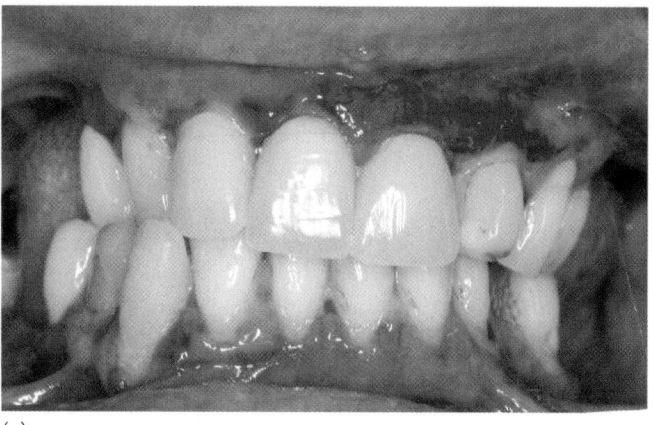

(c)

Fig. 15.6.16 Oral lichen planus: (a) reticular pattern in buccal mucosa; (b) ulcerative and (c) atrophic forms.

papules (Fig. 15.6.16). The sites of predilection are the same as in the hypertrophic variety, and whilst the latter may break down to result in ulcerative lichen planus, it is remarkable how often the hypertrophic variety remains unchanged. Except for discomfort, difficulties with eating, and occasionally loss of weight, there are no general manifestations and the regional lymph nodes are not enlarged, except with secondary infection. Not infrequently lichen planus may affect only the gum, inducing a diffuse, fiery-red gingivitis and scattered erosions. Desquamative gingivitis is essentially an atrophic form of lichen planus. This is a particularly troublesome type of lichen planus, with pain and bleeding, and tends to be quite resistant to treatment.

Differential diagnosis

The striae and papules of lichen planus are sufficiently distinctive features in the mouth to differentiate it from other lesions, without the necessity of a biopsy examination. However, the diffuse hypertrophic variety can be confused with leukoplakia and then a biopsy is helpful. Ulcerative lichen planus may very occasionally lack the distinctive striae, and then erythema multiforme and benign mucous membrane pemphigoid should be excluded. Both systemic and discoid lupus erythematosus can present in the mouth as central erosions, surrounded by a keratinized margin.

Treatment

In the absence of symptoms, hypertrophic lichen planus does not require any treatment but the patient needs to be informed of the nature of the disease. Topical corticosteroids are usually effective in the treatment of ulcerative lichen planus but also suppress the striae and papules of the hypertrophic variety. Triamcinolone in orabase ointment applied four times a day is useful in localized lesions, but betamethasone (as sodium phosphate) is more effective and is usually used in the form of 0.5 mg tablets used as a mouthwash three times daily. For these drugs to be helpful, they must be applied for one to several months. The lesions recur almost invariably, though the length of remissions varies greatly and corticosteroids may have to be applied with every remission. Systemic therapy may be needed to control the more severe ulcerative presentations, usually prednisolone and/or azathioprine.

Cleaning the teeth tends to be painful and the accumulation of a large amount of dental plaque aggravates the gingivitis. The patient should use a very soft toothbrush and needs to have the teeth scaled every 3 to 6 months. Chlorhexidine mouthwash can be helpful in controlling dental plaque.

Course and prognosis

The disease is chronic and tends to persist for years, with natural remissions and exacerbations. Topical corticosteroids prolong the remissions, and the erosions and discomfort are kept under control. In a very small number of patients, carcinomatous transformation, especially of the erosive type of lichen planus, can take place. In view of this possibility patients should be followed up regularly at an oral medicine clinic.

Leukoplakia

White patches of the oral mucosa that cannot be removed by scraping are referred to as leukoplakia. By convention, lichen planus and lupus erythematosus are excluded from this group. They are regarded as potentially malignant with a transformation rate of about 0.4% per year. High risk sites include the floor of the mouth and sides of the tongue.

Aetiology

The prevalence of leukoplakia is not known, but it seems that during the past two decades it has become less frequent. There are many causes of leukoplakia and as these may have distinctive features they will be classified below. It should be noted, however, that in about half the leukoplakias a cause cannot be found. Syphilitic, candidal, and AIDS leukoplakias have been discussed elsewhere. Causes include:

- physical and chemical agents: frictional keratosis, smoker's keratosis
- microbial infection: chronic hyperplastic candidiasis, tertiary syphilis, and AIDS
- congenital and hereditary leukokeratosis
- idiopathic.

Pathology

The microscopical features of leukoplakia show a spectrum of changes; at the benign end is epithelial keratosis alone, followed by hyperplasia and then epithelial atypia at the premalignant end. The lamina propria shows in parallel an increase in mononuclear cells, especially plasma cells. Carcinoma *in situ* is the least common histological finding.

Clinical features

The white patches vary from a soft, slightly thickened mucosa, involving a small or very large mucosal surface, to hard, irregular white plaques with intervening normal, erosive, or ulcerated sites. The latter is often referred to as 'speckled leukoplakia' and must be recognized clinically because of its greater propensity to carcinomatous transformation. Any part of the oral mucosa or gum may be involved but the cheeks and tongue are most often affected.

Frictional keratosis is usually found along the occlusal line of buccal mucosa and presents as a linear white patch of even consistency.

Smoker's keratosis (see Fig. 15.6.26) shows a characteristic distribution of the soft and adjacent hard palate, as keratinized papules with central red dots. The distribution is due to involvement of the palatal mucous glands and the red dots are the openings of the ducts. It is usually caused by pipe smoking, but cigarette smoking may also lead to keratosis of a diffuse type, affecting most commonly the cheeks.

Congenital and hereditary leukokeratosis can be distinguished by the presence of diffuse, soft, white plaques, often with a folded surface. The lesions tend to be symmetrical; they affect the floor of the mouth. Members of the family may have similar lesions.

Differential diagnosis

All leukoplakias should be biopsied, except smoker's keratosis of the palate, as even small white patches have at times proved to be early carcinomas (see Fig. 15.6.27). It is, furthermore, essential to find out the degree, if any, of epithelial atypia as this affects the prognosis of leukoplakia. Cytological examination can be helpful in the presence of hyphae of candida; cultures should also be set up for candida. Serological tests can further aid in the diagnosis of candidiasis but are essential in the diagnosis of syphilitic leukoplakia.

Treatment

Smoker's keratosis is reversible in many instances, if the patient gives up smoking. Frictional keratosis can also be cleared, if some local cause of irritation is removed. Candidal leukoplakia (chronic hyperplastic candidiasis) should be treated with systemic antifungal drugs, though this rarely results in permanent clearance of the lesion.

Syphilis should be managed by a course of penicillin and stringent follow-up, so as to detect early any carcinomatous transformation. Leucoplakia showing evidence of epithelial atypia should be excised and if the lesion is large a skin graft may be required. However, in many cases the lesion recurs, even after repeated excision. There is no satisfactory treatment of leukoplakia and the most important point is long-term follow-up, so as to detect in time the development of an incipient carcinoma.

Course and prognosis

Leucoplakia may persist for life, without any discomfort or change. However, about 0.5% of all leukoplakias undergo malignant changes per year and this figure increases to about 3.0% per year in leukoplakias showing histological evidence of epithelial atypia. Epithelial atypia is more commonly associated with speckled leukoplakia. In contrast, smoker's keratosis and frictional keratosis have a very good prognosis if the offending cause is removed. Congenital or hereditary leukokeratosis were thought to be free of malignant changes, though recently a few cases with carcinomatous transformation have been reported.

Bullous lesions

These are diseases that often affect the skin and oral mucosa, but sometimes involve only one type of epithelium. Three conditions will be discussed in this section: pemphigus vulgaris, benign mucous membrane pemphigoid, and erythema multiforme (see Section 23).

Pemphigus vulgaris

Aetiology

Pemphigus is a potentially lethal chronic bullous disease of the stratified squamous mucosa and skin, occurring mainly in adults over the age of 60 but sometimes in young adults. It commonly affects the oral mucosa and may present orally. Histologically there is acantholysis with intraepithelial bulla formation. Serum IgG, IgM, or sometimes IgA autoantibodies to desmogleins (Dsg) in skin and mucosa are found in nearly all cases of pemphigus. Desmoglein 1 predominates in skin and Dsg 3 in mucosa. Thus antibodies against Dsg1 will result in skin lesions, those against Dsg3 oral lesions, and if antibodies against both Dsg1 and 3 are present, the patient may have a combination of skin and mucosal lesions. The autoantibody titre is correlated with the severity of pemphigus, and antibody disappears as the lesions heal. Antibodies to pemphigus antigens may be present in saliva and may be of both IgG and IgA isotypes. HLA class II allele associations in pemphigus vulgaris are found with HLA-DR4 (DRB1*0402), DRw14 (DRB1*1041) and DQB1*0503. These HLA class II alleles appear critical to T-lymphocyte recognition of Dsg 3 peptides.

Pathology

This shows loss of interepithelial adhesion, intraepithelial bullae, and acantholytic cells, with a diffuse leucocytic infiltration of the lamina propria.

Clinical features

The disease affects males and females, usually over the age of 50 years. Painful, fluid-filled blisters or bullae may appear in the mouth and burst within a few hours, resulting in shallow ulcers (Fig. 15.6.17). These persist for weeks or months, but new lesions

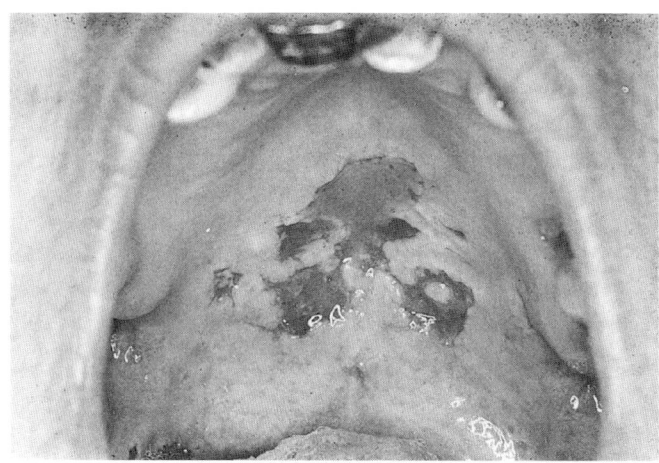

(a)

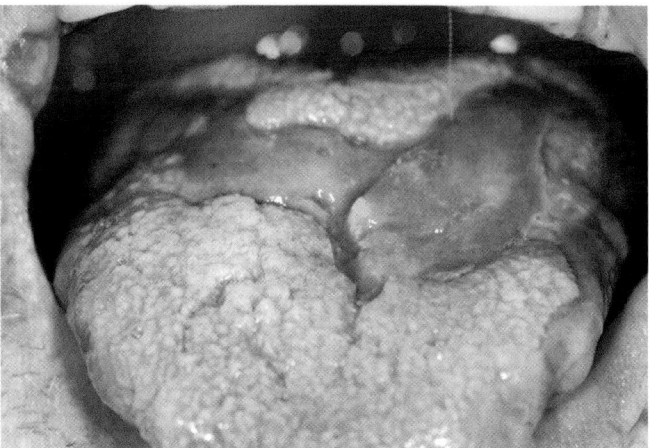

(b)

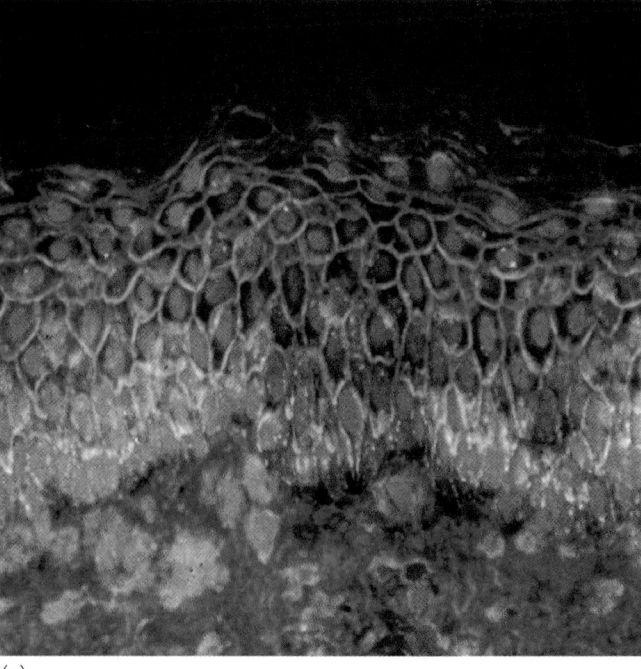

(c)

Fig. 15.6.17 Pemphigus vulgaris: erosions involving (a) the soft palate and buccal mucosa; (b) the lower lip; (c) direct immunofluoresence on human oral mucosa showing intercellular IgG autoantibodies (to desmoglein 3).

recur throughout the disease process. Oral manifestations of the disease may persist for many months, without overt ill-health but skin lesions, malaise, and loss of weight may occur at a later stage.

Differential diagnosis

Clinically the lesions can be differentiated from recurrent aphthous ulcers by the presence of bullae and when these ulcerate the edges lack the well-defined character of aphthous ulcers. Only occasionally is the Nikolsky sign helpful, by rubbing the mucosa to induce a bulla. The most important diagnostic test is the presence of acantholytic cells on microscopic examination of direct scrapings from the lesion and a biopsy must always be taken. Both direct and indirect immunoflourescence are usually positive (see Fig. 15.6.17) and specific antibodies to Dsg1 and Dsg 3 may also assist in the diagnosis. Pemphigus must be differentiated from pemphigoid and dermatitis herpetiformis (see below).

Other types of pemphigus such as pemphigus foliaceus and erythematosus and pemphigus vegetans only rarely affect the oral mucosae. In vegetans, vegetation-type lesions may be found on the oral mucosa and lips, and histological examination shows intraepithelial abscesses containing numerous eosinophils. Apart from pemphigus vulgaris, the other important form affecting the oral mucosa is paraneoplastic pemphigus, usually associated with lymphoproliferative disease. Oral lesions have also been seen in all reported cases of paraneoplastic pemphigus and may be the sole manifestation. Failure to respond to therapy may give an indication.

Treatment

Systemic corticosteroids such as prednisolone are given initially in doses of 40 to 60 mg/day and this is gradually reduced to the minimal dose that will prevent formation of new lesions. In order to keep the steroid dose to a minimum, azathioprine can also be used, with a dose of up to 2 mg/kg per day.

Course and prognosis

Treatment with corticosteroids has completely changed the prognosis of the disease. Steroids may need to be maintained for life, but clinical improvement along with reduction in circulating antibody titre allows the dose to be reduced to minimal levels. Patients rarely die now from the disease but they may develop the side effects of steroid therapy.

Mucous membrane pemphigoid

Aetiology

Mucous membrane pemphigoid comprises a heterogeneous group of disorders characterized by subepithelial separation and deposition of autoantibodies and complement along the basement membrane zone. Mucous membrane pemphigoid is distinguished from bullous pemphigoid by its predilection for mucosal sites and the tendency to form scars, leading to oesophageal strictures, laryngeal stenosis, and blindness in extreme cases of conjunctival cicatrization. Most cases are detected in the fourth and fifth decade, and the disease is more frequent in women than in men.

Pathology

This shows subepithelial bullae, and the epithelium tends to detach itself from the underlying lamina propria. Antibodies (IgG, IgA or IgM, with or without complement) to the basement membrane are found. More than 90% of patients with mucosal disease alone have

IgG antibodies to basement membrane zone in their sera whereas previously it was thought that few patients with mucosal disease had these circulating autoantibodies. In addition, IgA antibodies are associated with a more persistent and severe form of the disease. Recent immunopathological and immunochemical techniques have revealed that are found to the basement membrane consists of several distinct subgroups based on the specificity of antibodies. The largest subgroup target bullous pemphigoid antigen 180 (BP180). A further group has circulating IgG antibodies that bind to the dermal side of salt split skin and recognize laminin 5 (previously known as epiligrin). This group may also have antibodies directed against laminin 6. Among the clinical subgroup with pure ocular disease, IgA antibodies may target an uncharacterized keratinocyte-derived 45 kD antigen and IgG antibodies may target epitopes on β_4-integrin.

Clinical features

Intraorally, two variants of benign mucus membrane pemphigoid are seen. The most common is bullous lesions involving much of the nonkeratinized and occasionally the keratinized mucosa (Fig. 15.6.18). The other type is a form of desquamative gingivitis and involves only the gingivae around the teeth. The gingivae are

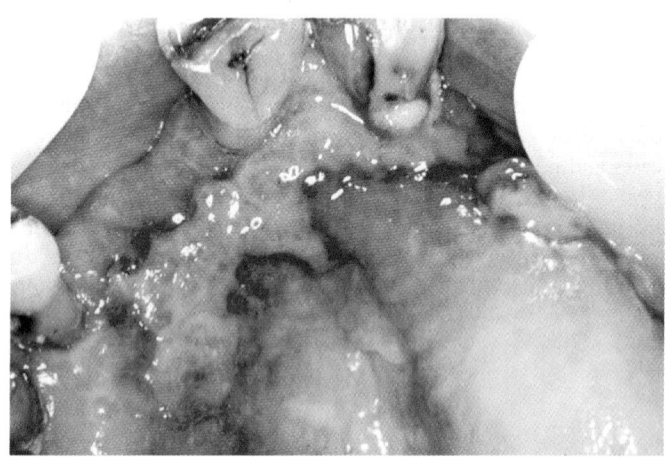

(a)

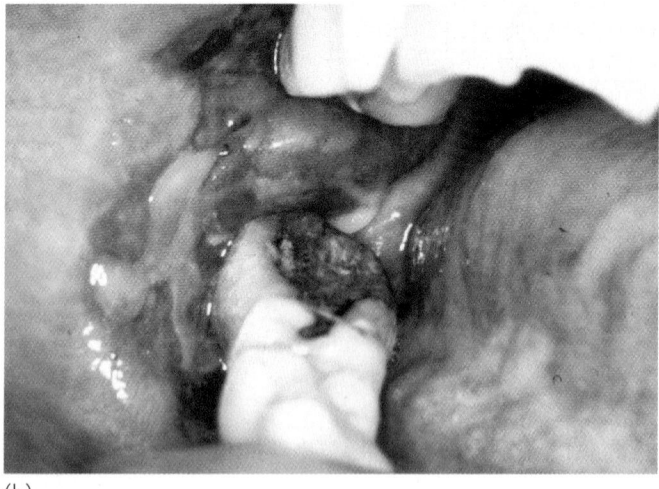

(b)

Fig. 15.6.18 Mucous membrane pemphigoid showing irregular and persistent ulceration (a) of the palate and (b) of the buccal mucosa.

highly erythematous and hyperaemic. Small bullae may be formed in protected areas around the teeth. It is not clear whether the molecular heterogeneity of bullous pemphigoid antigens (see previous discussion) or whether their recognition by IgG and IgA isotypes is responsible for the varied clinical presentations. Bullous lesions involve the oral mucosa, conjunctiva, and skin around the genitals and orifices, but in some patients only the mouth is involved. The bullae rupture within a day or two leaving erosions and ulcers. The gingiva is commonly involved, giving rise to persistent pain, bleeding, and a diffuse, raw, fiery red lesion. Other mucous membranes can be involved, such as the nose, larynx, pharynx, oesophagus, vulva, vagina, penis, and anus. The oral lesions usually heal without scarring, unlike those of the conjunctiva.

Differential diagnosis

Benign mucous membrane pemphigoid can often be differentiated from pemphigus vulgaris on clinical grounds but a biopsy is needed to establish the diagnosis. There are no acantholytic cells and the bullae are subepithelial and not suprabasilar. Direct immunofluorescence shows, autoantibodies, binding to the basement membrane of epithelium and not to the interepithelial substance as in pemphigus. In linear IgA disease there is linear deposition of IgA along the basement membrane without IgG, and in dermatitis herpetiformis IgA deposits are found in the papillae.

Treatment

If the disease is confined to the mouth, topical corticosteroids are often adequate to control the lesions. However, in the more severe cases and if there is involvement of other sites, systemic corticosteroids, azathioprine, dapsone and other immunosuppressive medications may be needed to control the ulceration.

Course and prognosis

This is a chronic disease, which persists, often with exacerbations and remissions, over many years. The conjunctivitis may result in adhesions, corneal opacity and blindness.

Erythema multiforme

Aetiology

Erythema multiforme is a mucocutaneous disease characterized by typical target skin lesions, with oral or ocular involvement in some cases, and a marked tendency to recur. Erythema multiforme may develop at any age but often occurs in young males. Many agents have been associated with this disease: drugs, such as sulphonamides and barbiturates, microbial infections, especially with herpes simplex virus, but a large proportion appear to be idiopathic.

Pathology

There is intracellular oedema with a zone of liquefaction degeneration of the upper layers of epithelium. Often subepithelial bullae are present and the lamina propria is infiltrated with leucocytes, especially lymphomonocytic cells, neutrophils, and eosinophils.

Clinical features

The disease most commonly involves the skin, and oral manifestations may not be a significant feature. However, the mouth can be affected without skin involvement and the diagnosis then is more difficult. The patient develops painful, extensive erosions and ulcers with a predilection for the palate, tongue, and cheeks. The gum

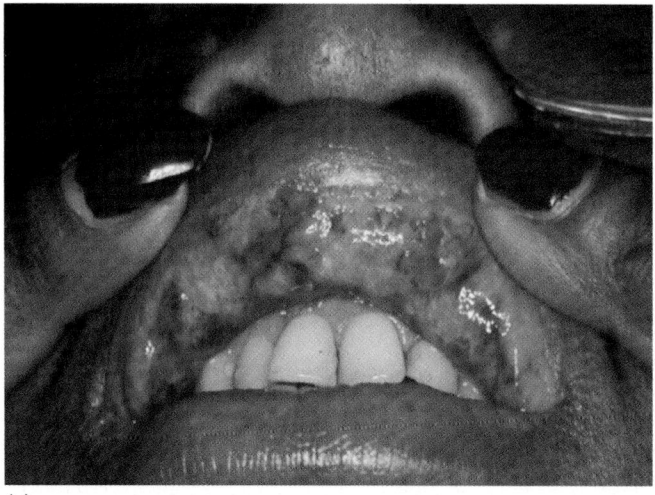

(a)

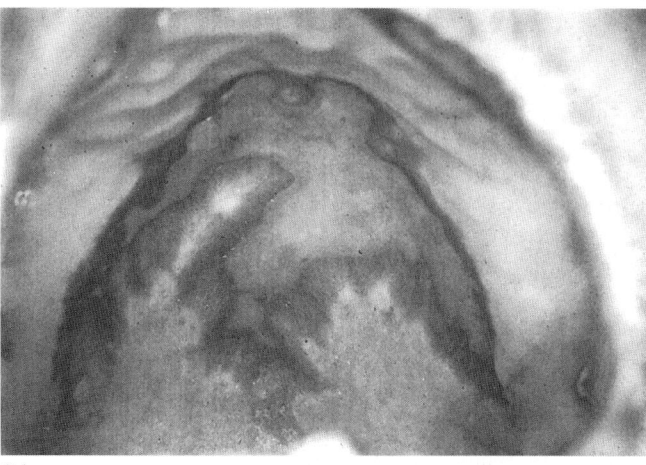

(b)

Fig. 15.6.19 Erythema multiforme: (a) haemorrhagic crusted upper lip; (b) diffuse erosion of the palate.

may show extensive erosions, which tend to bleed. Haemorrhagic crusting of the lips is often seen (Fig. 15.6.19). A severe variant of erythema multiforme, which affects the eyes and genitalia in addition to the skin and mouth, is referred to as Stevens–Johnson syndrome.

Differential diagnosis

The diagnosis of oral lesions without the typical skin manifestation can be very difficult. The clinical features to note are the very extensive erosions affecting the palate, tongue, cheeks, and gingiva and the haemorrhagic crusting of the lips. These features should avoid confusion with aphthous ulcers. An association with drugs or microbial infection is helpful. The age and sex prevalence differs from those in benign mucous membrane pemphigoid. A biopsy examination can definitely exclude pemphigus and erosive lichen planus.

Treatment

Whenever possible the offending drug or infection should be eliminated. The oral lesions often respond to topical tetracycline. With extraoral manifestations, treatment with systemic corticosteroids may be indicated.

Course and prognosis

If the offending agent is not found, the lesions may recur over many years and cause a great deal of discomfort. In Stevens–Johnson syndrome, blindness may result from intercurrent bacterial infection.

Discoid lupus erythematosus

Traditionally lupus erythematosus is classified into a chronic discoid type and a systemic type. Both types may give rise to lesions within the oral mucosa. The buccal mucosa is most frequently involved and bilateral lesions are common. Classically the lesions appear as an atrophic erythematous area surrounded by a keratotic border. Sometimes the lesions are more plaque-like and may resemble lichen planus or leukoplakia. Skin lesions are found in about half the patients. Histologically the epithelium always shows orthokeratosis and parakeratosis, and areas of moderate epithelial hyperplasia alternate with areas of epithelial atrophy. There is a rather deep-seated focal or perivascular accumulation of lymphocytes. Although there is a genetic susceptibility in systemic lupus erythematosus. with an increased frequency of HLA-DR2 and DR3 in white populations, no such relationship has been established with discoid lupus erythematosus.

Oral manifestations of gastrointestinal diseases

Coeliac disease, ulcerative colitis, and Crohn's disease can all appear in the oral cavity. Frequently, the oral cavity can be the presenting site, and Crohn's disease may be limited to the oral cavity. Each of these gastroenteropathies can give rise to oral ulceration, but is a feature of ulcerative colitis and coeliac disease.

Crohn's disease and orofacial granulomatosis

The term orofacial granulomatosis describes a group of conditions characterized by typical features of noncaseating granulomata, lymphocytic infiltration, and oedema at various sites in the oral cavity. Orofacial granulomatosis is a chronic inflammatory disorder presenting characteristically with lip swelling but also affecting gingivae, buccal mucosa, floor of mouth, and a number of other sites in the oral cavity. Most cases of orofacial granulomatosis occur as a separate clinical entity but a proportion present in association with established Crohn's disease of the small or large intestine. A smaller number of cases of orofacial granulomatosis may be a manifestation of dietary intolerance or sarcoidosis, or occur as part of the Melkersson–Rosenthal syndrome.

Aetiology

Although Crohn's disease and orofacial granulomatosis share a number of clinical and histological features, the exact relationship between the two conditions is unknown. Non-specific oral lesions are common in Crohn's disease usually reflecting periods of nutritional deficit or active disease. Conversely, changes like those of orofacial granulomatosis, usually lip swelling or buccal involvement, are uncommon in established gut Crohn's disease.

Clinical features

Crohn's disease in the oral cavity or orofacial granulomatosis usually presents as thickened rubbery lips (Fig. 15.6.20) and thickened

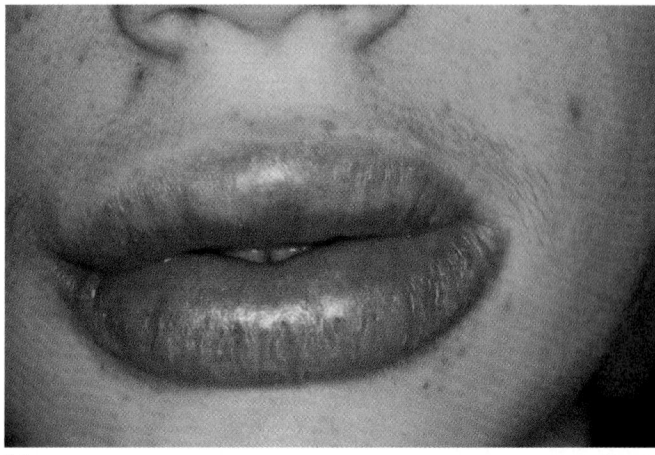

(a)

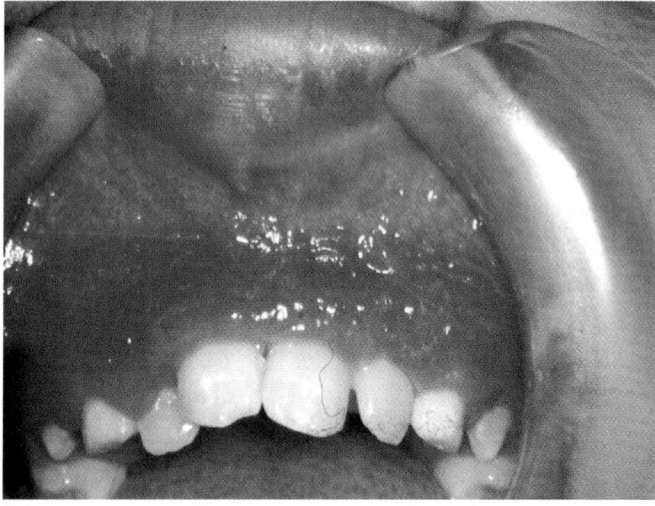

(b)

Fig. 15.6.20 Orofacial granulomatosis in a 15-year-old boy showing (a) enlarged lips and (b) hyperplastic gingivae.

'lumpy' cheeks (cobblestone appearance) with deep fissures of the tongue and hyperplastic enlarged gingiva. More severe cases may have linear type ulcers and epithelial tags in the buccal sulci. In both these clinical manifestations, biopsy of the affected areas will show granulomata. The clinical appearance is similar to the oral signs in patients with systemic Crohn's disease. A number of cases present with swollen lips without any other intraoral signs, and these have also been classified as oral Crohn's disease by some workers, although the term cheilitis granulomatosa is be more appropriate.

A significant proportion of patient with orofacial granulomatosis have chronic inflammation of the gut detected by endoscopy or subsequently develop Crohn's disease despite the absence of gastrointestinal symptoms at presentation. Although the cellular and humoral immunology of Crohn's disease has been extensively studied, few studies have addressed the immunological aspects of orofacial granulomatosis. The demonstration of raised SIgA and IgA2 subclasses in orofacial granulomatosis and increased serum IgA responses to *S. cerevisiae* antigens in Crohn's disease suggests that the two diseases can be distinguished.

Aetiology

The aetiology remains unknown, although claims that Crohn's disease is associated with altered immune responses to microbes persist; there is no conclusive evidence of an infective origin. Associations with measles virus, *Mycobacterium paratuberculosis*, and *Saccharomyces* have been reported with Crohn's disease, but it is not clear whether any of these hypotheses apply to orofacial granulomatosis. The role of allergy to food or other substances has not been fully investigated, although some patients have been reported to be sensitive to cinnamon or sodium benzoate and clinical responses to cinnamon- and benzoate-free diets suggest that hypersensitivity to some dietary components may play a role.

Management

Diagnosis is by a combination of clinical features and the demonstration of granulomata histologically. Treatment is challenging and systemic immunosuppression using azathioprine at 1 to 3 mg/kg has become a standard, but may need to be continued for 2 years. Topical steroids and tacrolimus have met with limited success, and systemic steroids mostly lead to short-term improvement. Exclusion diets appear to be useful in more than 50% of patients.

Coeliac disease

It is reported that some 25% of patients with coeliac disease may give a history of oral ulceration. The oral ulcers of patients with coeliac disease often respond extremely well to correction of underlying haematological deficiencies, particularly folate and iron. It seems that the oral ulceration is often due to the associated deficiencies rather than a direct response of the oral mucosa to the allergen.

Some reports have described adult female patients suffering from abdominal pain and chronic diarrhoea who responded immediately to a gluten-free diet and in whom symptoms returned on gluten challenge. Oral ulceration and macroglossia were described in several of these patients, but jejunal biopsies were normal. This suggests that oral signs and symptoms can be associated with gluten in the absence of coeliac disease and that such oral symptoms are accompanied by varying abdominal problems.

Screening patients for the presence of endomysial autoantibody and antigliaden antibody is worthwhile in patients in whom the ulceration is atypical and similar in appearance to herpetiform recurrent aphthous stomatitis; however, there are wide variations in the incidence within populations.

Ulcerative colitis

Oral ulceration is frequently associated with ulcerative colitis and may be one of at least four types: (1) aphthous, (2) pyostomatitis necrotica, (3) pyostomatitis vegetans, or (4) hemorrhagic. The incidence of oral lesions in patients with ulcerative colitis is approximately 20%. The oral ulcers of groups 2, 3, and 4 are readily distinguishable from the more common types of recurrent aphthous ulceration. Unlike Crohn's disease, these lesions do not appear to occur in the oral cavity in the absence of any bowel symptoms.

Benign neoplasms, cysts, and developmental and inflammatory lesions of the soft tissues

There are numerous benign neoplasms and soft-tissue lesions of the mouth. The section will be restricted to some essential features of the following lesions: papilloma, fibroma, lipoma, neurofibroma, hamartoma, pigmented naevus, lymphangioma, denture granuloma, giant-cell reparative granuloma, fibrous polyp, pregnancy tumour, mucous retention, and extravasation cysts.

Aetiology

The cause of benign neoplasms is unknown and the parts that physical or chemical irritation and microbial infection may play are ill understood. Mucous retention or extravasation cysts are caused by trauma or obstruction of the duct orifice of the minor salivary glands. Whereas true benign neoplasms are rare, inflammatory lesions and cysts are commonly found in the mouth.

Clinical features

The soft-tissue tumours present as painless, slow-growing swellings affecting any part of the mouth, but if they originate from the gum they are referred to as epulides. Fibrous polyps are the most common inflammatory lesions of the oral mucosa and result from trauma or irritation from rough edges of carious teeth. Most of the tumours are sessile, some are pedunculated as with some fibromas, and others are flat and pigmented as with the naevi. They are usually symptomless except for bleeding from hamartomas and giant-cell reparative granulomas.

Differential diagnosis

There are some distinguishing clinical features but the definitive diagnosis will depend on the histological examination of the excised specimen.

- A papilloma can be recognized by its firm, small, keratinized, finger-like processes.
- Lymphangiomas are soft swellings, which may cause considerable enlargement of the lip or tongue.
- Hamartomas are flat or nodular red lesions that may blanch when compressed; they are occasionally confused with pregnancy tumours, which are rather vascular granulomatous swellings of the gingiva found during pregnancy.
- Giant-cell reparative granulomas are also very vascular, maroon-coloured lesions originating from the gingiva.
- Denture granulomas can be readily recognized from their relation to the flange of a denture; the lesion is often elongated, can be indented or ulcerated by the denture.
- Mucous retention or extravasation cysts are small, often bluish swellings affecting the lips or cheeks.

Treatment

Surgical excision, with a margin of normal tissue at the base of the lesion, is usually indicated. Pregnancy tumours, however, commonly regress spontaneously.

Course and prognosis

The soft-tissue neoplasms will enlarge over the years and interfere with the normal functions of the mouth. Bleeding from any of the lesions is rarely profuse. Only the giant-cell reparative granuloma has a tendency to recur after excision.

Oral carcinoma

Aetiology

Carcinoma of the mouth accounts for about 2% of all cancers in the United Kingdom but in some parts of the world, such as India, may account for 40%. The prevalence increases significantly after the age of 45 years and more than twice as many men as women are affected. The incidence of oral cancer has been decreasing over the last four decades, unlike that of lung cancer. As in other carcinomas the cause is unknown, but smoking and alcohol have been implicated. There is some epidemiological evidence to support this, but unlike lung cancer it is the smoking of pipes or cigars, rather than cigarettes, that has been associated with oral cancer. The association with chronic oral sepsis and irritation has not been critically examined. There is some evidence that microbial agents, particularly *Treponema pallidum, Candida albicans,* human papilloma virus, and HIV, may directly or indirectly influence the development of carcinoma.

Among the predisposing lesions, leukoplakia is the best-known one; in 5% of all patients and in about 30% of those showing evidence of epithelial atypia the leukoplakia may eventually undergo carcinomatous transformation. This is especially true in the presence of smoking (Fig. 15.6.21). Submucous fibrosis is another precancerous condition and is found predominantly in India and Sri Lanka. It seems to be related to eating chillis and possibly chewing betel nut, and affects the palate, buccal mucosa, and tongue.

Pathology

Squamous-cell carcinoma in the mouth is usually a well-differentiated keratinizing neoplasm invading the surrounding tissue. Poorly differentiated and anaplastic oral carcinomas are much less frequent and especially rare with carcinoma of the lip. Spread occurs by local invasion; lymph node metastasis is less common than is generally thought, and occurs at a late stage.

Clinical features

The presenting features of carcinoma vary with the site of involvement but there are two types, a lump or an ulcer. The patient complains of a swelling or ulcer that is resistant to healing and gradually

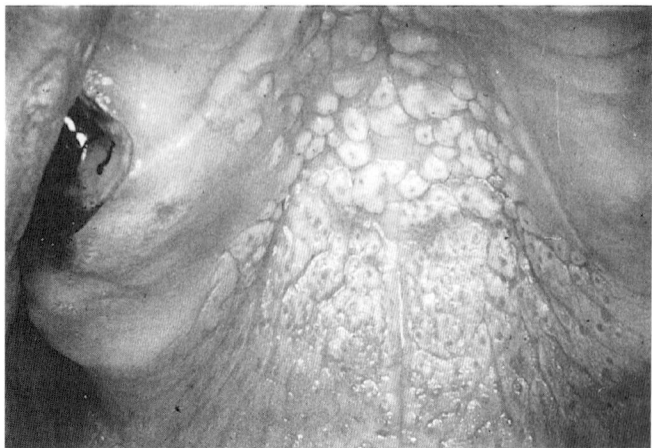

Fig. 15.6.21 Smoker's keratosis (leukoplasia) of the palate.

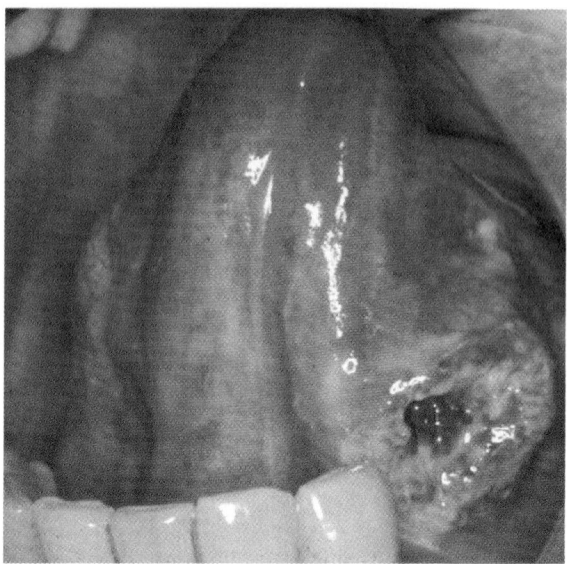

Fig. 15.6.22 Squamous cell carcinoma on the ventral surface of the tongue showing necrotic centre and rolled indurated margins.

enlarging in size. There may be little pain initially, but at a later stage discomfort and occasional bleeding may occur. Cancer of the tongue may give rise to local pain and earache. Whereas some patients complain of excess of saliva, especially with the larger tumours, a dry mouth may be found during the early stages of malignant change and should be noted as another feature favouring malignancy. A small lump may enlarge to a hard swelling before the covering mucosa breaks down. A malignant ulcer shows a raised and often everted edge, and the most important feature is induration at the base of the lesion. Any part of the mouth can be involved but the lips (usually the lower lip) and tongue are most common, each accounting for about 25% of oral carcinomas (Fig. 15.6.22). The floor of the mouth, gingiva, cheek, hard and soft palate, and oropharynx may account for about 10% of the carcinomas. In most patients there is only one lesion but some patients may have two or even multiple carcinomas. Metastasis may occur at a late stage to the submandibular or upper cervical lymph nodes, and occasionally to the submental nodes.

Differential diagnosis

Any long-standing or indurated lesion in the mouth, especially of elderly or middle-aged patients, should be queried for malignancy and biopsy examination is essential. A traumatic ulcer caused by a denture can be confused with a malignant ulcer, but it may lack induration, the offending part of the denture may fit into the ulcer, and removing the denture for about a week may bring about healing of the lesion. Major aphthous ulcers have been mentioned elsewhere (see above), but the salient differentiating features are a history of recurrent ulcers at different sites of the mouth, over many years.

Adenocarcinoma of the small salivary glands may present as a lump of the soft palate, lips, or cheeks and only a biopsy will establish the diagnosis firmly. Carcinoma *in situ* is rare in the mouth, but it may present as a diffuse, erythematous, somewhat velvety lesion, affecting the mucosa of one half of the soft palate or cheek. Again a biopsy examination must be carried out for diagnosis.

Treatment

The principles of treatment of oral carcinomas are those applied to other carcinomas of the body. Surgical excision of the lesion and a margin of adjacent tissue is the most common practice, and this may be extended if necessary to block dissection of the regional lymph nodes. Radiotherapy is an alternative approach and is commonly used in primary treatment of cancer of the lip, in inoperable cases, or with recurrent carcinoma following surgery. Cytotoxic drugs have also been used in the management of cancer of the mouth with variable results. Management of oral cancer is a complex subject outside the scope of this section. It should be emphasized that oral hygiene is particularly important with any treatment so as to avoid ascending parotitis. A dry mouth usually follows radiotherapy and again meticulous oral hygiene should be advised, so as to prevent rampant caries and candida infection.

Course and prognosis

The 5-year survival rates differ considerably with the anatomical site of the cancer. Carcinoma of the lip has by far the best prognosis, irrespective of whether treatment is by surgery or radiotherapy, and the 5-year survival rate is about 80%. In contrast, the figures for carcinoma of the tongue range from 25 to 35%, floor of the mouth 20 to 40%, cheek 30 to 50%, and oropharynx, palate, and gingiva about 25%. The prognosis is significantly better in the absence of lymph node involvement.

Salivary gland diseases

Xerostomia

Xerostomia is a term describing dryness of the mouth either as a symptom or sign, though the latter is best termed salivary hypofunction. It is very prevalent and is a major side effect of much drug therapy.

Aetiology

Dry mouth is a common symptom, and can be caused by anxiety or emotional and mental stress. Iatrogenic xerostomia is secondary to a large number of drugs, the most common of which are antihistamines, tranquilizers (phenothiazine), anxiolytics, antihypertensive agents, and diuretics.

Pathology

Pathology of the glands is seen in Sjögren's and SNOX syndromes, but not usually in drug induced hyposalivation. In Sjögren's syndrome there is an intense focal lymphocytic infiltrate of lymphocytes with ensuing loss of acinar function and an increased propensity of developing B-cell lymphomas (maltomas). In SNOX syndrome there is a nonspecific (nonfocal) sialadentitis of chronic inflammatory cells, mainly lymphocytes, and the disease is associated with nodal osteoarthritis with the xerostomia.

Clinical features (Fig. 15.6.23)

The patient complains of dryness of the mouth and sometimes the eyes, soreness of the mouth, especially the tongue and throat, and discomfort on swallowing of solids and at times difficulty in speaking. The best clinical evidence of xerostomia is an atrophic, dry oral mucosa, often fiery red, due to secondary infection by candida. Inspection of the duct orifices of the major salivary glands will fail to reveal salivary flow and in severe cases stimulation by lemon

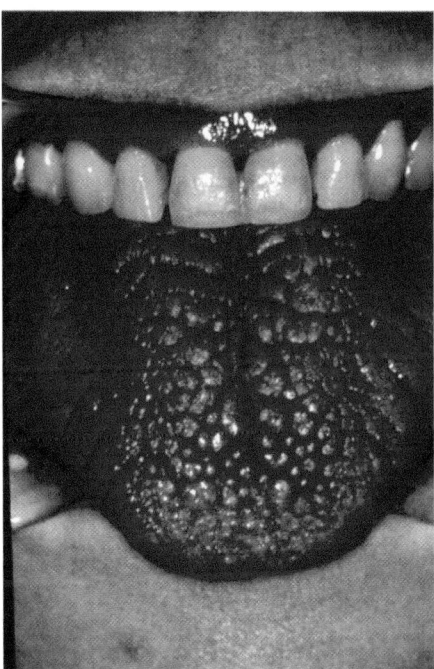

Fig. 15.6.23 Lobulated tongue in a female patient with Sjögren's syndrome. Note also glassy gingivae secondary to persistent dryness.

juice applied to the tongue may not induce a flow of saliva. Patients may develop rampant cervical caries, and for denture wearers there may be difficulties with retention.

Differential diagnosis

A thorough history may establish psychogenic or iatrogenic causes, and diseases affecting fluid balance. Sjögren's syndrome is diagnosed by sialography showing sialectasis (Fig. 15.6.24) and labial minor salivary gland biopsy showing focal lymphocytic infiltrates as well as demonstration of reduced lachrymal and salivary flows. Extractable nuclear antigens are present in the majority of Sjögren's syndrome patients. Other findings useful in making the diagnosis include a raised erythrocyte sedimentation rate, rheumatoid factor,

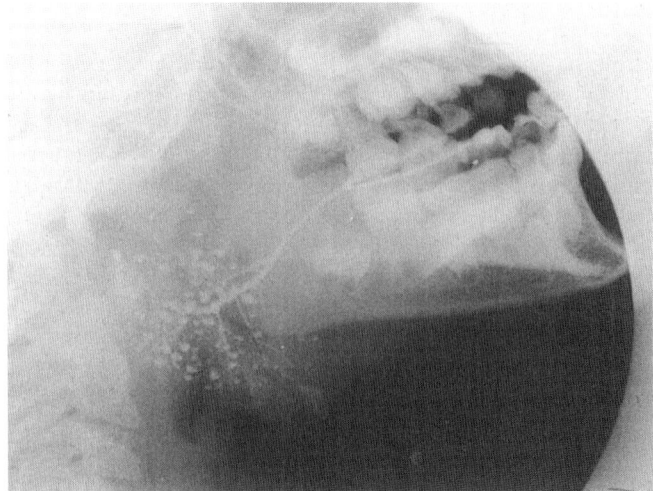

Fig. 15.6.24 Sialography of parotid gland in a patient with Sjögrens syndrome showing marked sialectasis ('snowstorm' appearance).

antinuclear factor, autoantibodies, and HLA typing. Nevertheless there will be a large proportion of patients in whom a specific cause cannot be found. The high prevalence of nonspecific symptoms (dryness, fatigue, and myalgia) and antinuclear antibodies in the general population makes the distinction of Sjögren's syndrome from other connective tissue diseases difficult (e.g. fibromyalgia patients with low levels of antinuclear antibodies). A further complication is the presence of rheumatoid factor in 70% of primary Sjögren's syndrome patients.

Treatment

Management of the patient involves elimination of the cause of xerostomia where this is possible or alleviation of symptoms where it is not. In such cases, palliative measures are helpful and these include frequent sips of water, meticulous oral hygiene, early treatment or preferably prevention of candidiasis by regular topical nystatin or amphotericin. Useful salivary substitutes include glycerine-type gels, carboxymethylcellulose as a solution or aerosol (e.g. Glandosane) or a mucin preparation as a spray (e.g. Saliva Orthana).

Sialadenitis

Bacterial or viral infections and rarely allergic reactions may cause inflammation of the salivary glands. These agents may give rise to acute, chronic, and allergic sialadenitis, and recurrent parotitis.

Aetiology

Ascending infection of the parotid gland used to be a common complication in older postoperative patients who were predisposed by dehydration, reduced salivary flow, and lack of oral hygiene. Acute parotitis may also follow the use of drugs causing xerostomia. The most common microorganisms involved are *Staphylococcus aureus, Streptococcus milleri group*, and other members of the oral flora. The most common acute parotitis is mumps (see Chapter 7.5.5). Salivary glands are sometimes affected by HIV infection, with an enlargement of the parotid glands. Chronic sialadenitis is usually associated with duct obstruction and therefore affects usually the submandibular gland. Recurrent sialadenitis is a disease of unknown aetiology and may be associated with a decreased salivary flow causing retrograde infection. The disease may affect both adults and children.

Pathology

Acute sialadenitis shows an acute inflammatory reaction of the salivary tissue, with a predominantly neutrophil infiltration, except in mumps, which shows an infiltration by mononuclear cells. In both chronic and recurrent sialadenitis there is a marked periductal and acinar infiltration by mononuclear cells, with some duct epithelial hyperplasia, accompanied by acinar atrophy and fibrosis.

Clinical features

The presenting symptom of acute sialadenitis is a painful swelling in one of the parotid glands of an elderly patient. Commonly the patient has a low-grade fever, oedema of the cheek and some trismus, and a purulent discharge may be expressed from the duct opening. In contrast, mumps affects healthy children and young adults.

In chronic sialadenitis there are usually clinical features of duct obstruction of one of the submandibular glands. There is pain and swelling in the submandibular or retromandibular region, with a reddened duct orifice discharging pus. Recurrent parotitis presents as an acute pain and swelling of one or both parotid glands, with erythema of the duct orifices and pus discharging from them. There may be an associated fever and malaise. Recurrences vary from weeks to months and after repeated attacks the affected gland may remain enlarged.

Differential diagnosis

There is little clinical difficulty in the differential diagnosis between acute sialadenitis of the parotid gland in older patients due to ascending infection and mumps in healthy young subjects. Any discharging pus should be cultured for organisms and its antibiotic sensitivity should be determined. Recurrent parotitis can, however, cause difficulties; in addition to a history of recurrent painful swelling and discharging pus, sialography may help and show sialectasis and duct dilatation. In chronic sialadenitis there is usually clinical or radiological evidence of calculus and sialography may show duct dilatation.

A variety of granulomatous diseases may very occasionally affect the salivary glands, such as sarcoidosis, tuberculosis, syphilis, and actinomycosis. When there is bilateral salivary and lachrymal enlargement this is often referred to as Mikulicz's syndrome. Allergic sialadenitis is also rare and to determine the allergic agent can be difficult as drugs, foods, pollen, and other agents have been implicated.

Treatment

In acute, chronic, or recurrent sialadenitis the relevant antibiotics should be used to control the infection, but occasionally surgical drainage may also be necessary. Careful oral hygiene measures are important in all types of sialadenitis. There is no special treatment for mumps, but rest and isolation for about a week are indicated. In chronic sialadenitis the cause of obstruction, such as a calculus, should be removed. The treatment of recurrent parotitis is more difficult and if antibiotics do not control the disease, surgical intervention should be considered.

Course and prognosis

Acute sialadenitis will resolve with the aid of antibiotics and general management of the patient. Mumps will resolve spontaneously and second attacks are very rare. Chronic sialadenitis may persist for many years and may lead to destruction of the gland, unless the cause of duct obstruction is removed early. Recurrent parotitis in childhood may show spontaneous recovery after puberty.

Salivary duct obstruction due to calculus

Aetiology

The submandibular salivary ducts and, to a less extent, glands are the most common sites for the development of stones. Calcium phosphates and carbonates are deposited from the saliva round a nidus of desquamated cells or microorganisms.

Clinical features

Salivary calculus is usually found in adults and the presenting symptoms are a sudden unilateral swelling and pain of the gland related to eating. The swelling may take minutes to appear and hours to subside. Examination reveals a soft swelling of the affected gland and careful digital palpation along the course of the salivary duct will localize the calculus. This may vary in size from a small grain to a concretion 10 to 20 mm in length. The presence and localization of a stone in a duct should be confirmed by radiographs and the presence of calculi in the gland can be diagnosed only by radiography.

Differential diagnosis

Recurrent unilateral swelling associated with eating is characteristic of salivary gland obstruction but occasionally this may be caused by external agents. Trauma from a denture or sharp tooth may cause obstruction of the orifice of the parotid duct.

Treatment

If the calculus is near the orifice of the duct it can occasionally be teased out, otherwise surgical removal is indicated.

Course and prognosis

Single calculi do not tend to recur, but if treatment has been delayed numerous calculi may have formed inside the gland, which may occasionally have to be excised.

Salivary gland tumours

A variety of epithelial tumours affects the major and minor salivary glands of which the most common is the pleomorphic adenoma, or mixed salivary tumour (74%), followed by adenocarcinoma (12%), adenoma (8%), mucoepidermoid tumour (3%), and acinic cell tumour (2%); the percentages give the prevalence in the parotid glands. Only pleomorphic adenoma will be considered in any detail and the further reading list should be consulted for other tumours.

Pleomorphic adenoma

Aetiology

The cause of this tumour is unknown, though salivary gland tumours can be produced in animals by carcinogenic hydrocarbons, polyomavirus, and other agents. The tumour originates from epithelial cells of the ducts, acini, or myoepithelial cells; the last are thought to be capable of producing the stromal mucins of this tumour.

Pathology

The epithelial cells proliferate in duct-like structures, sheets, and cords, within a connective tissue stroma, which may show mucous, cartilaginous, or hyaline appearance. The tumour is encapsulated, though satellite tumours are often found outside the capsule.

Clinical features

The tumour is usually found in adults and the parotid salivary gland is most commonly affected, followed by the submandibular gland and rarely the sublingual gland. The minor salivary glands, however, are also affected, and the most frequent sites are the glands of the palate, lips, and cheeks. The tumour presents as a small, painless swelling, which may take years to enlarge and is not attached to the overlying skin or mucosa.

Differential diagnosis

As the tumour is slow growing it needs to be differentiated only from other tumours. Adenocarcinoma, mucoepidermoid carcinoma, and adenoid cystic carcinoma may mimic pleomorphic adenoma in its slow growth, but some may grow more rapidly, invade the adjacent skin or mucosa, and metastasize. These tumours can often be differentiated only on histopathological examination, and wherever possible an excision biopsy should be done.

Treatment

Surgical excision with a margin of normal tissue is always practised, as the tumour is radio resistant.

Course and prognosis

If left untreated the tumour may enlarge to a grotesque size. A small proportion of pleomorphic adenomas may undergo carcinomatous transformation. The tumour has a bad record for recurrences after excision and this is thought to be due to leaving behind satellite tumours outside the capsule.

Neoplasms, cysts, developmental lesions, and dystrophies of the bones and teeth

This section covers a very large number of lesions found in the jaws. Only essential features, especially of differential diagnosis, will be covered in the following disorders: (1) benign neoplasms: osteoma, chondroma, fibroma, ossifying fibroma, and giant-cell tumour; (2) malignant neoplasms: osteosarcoma, and chondrosarcoma; (3) cysts and tumours of dental origin: periodontal and dentigenous cysts, keratocysts, and ameloblastoma; (4) dental malformations or odontomes; (5) osteodystrophies: giant-cell reparative granuloma, brown tumour of hyperparathyroidism, fibrous dysplasia, and Paget's disease.

Aetiology

The cause of the neoplasms and osteodystrophies is not known. Periodontal cysts, which are the most common lesions in this group, develop as a consequence of chronic periapical infection.

Clinical features

Bony tumours and cysts are commonly symptomless, unless they have reached a large size and the patient notices a swelling, or a denture ceases to fit. Often pathological changes are noticed by the dentist through movement of teeth or on routine radiographic examination of the teeth. Hyperparathyroidism should be excluded, in cases when a giant-cell granuloma is suspected. Cysts can be found at any age, but giant-cell reparative granulomas, ossifying fibroma, and fibrous dysplasia are often seen in young people, unlike Paget's disease of bone, which is seen only in old people. There is a predilection for the mandible to be involved more commonly with ossifying fibroma and giant-cell reparative granuloma. Odontomes are developmental malformations of dental tissue that become calcified. This is a diverse group of disorders and varies from a simple enamel pearl, consisting of a nodule of ectopic enamel attached to a tooth, to a complex composite odontome, which is an irregular mass of calcified dental tissues. Ameloblastoma is a rare but important epithelial neoplasm of the jaws. Young adults are most often affected; the tumour is slow-growing and affects the mandible more often than the maxilla. The neoplasm is locally invasive but does not metastasize. Osteosarcoma and chondrosarcoma are found in children or young adults but may develop in older people with Paget's disease. They present as fast-growing, painful, and firm swellings and they may metastasize to the lungs early.

Differential diagnosis

The diagnosis of bony lesions of the jaws is made on the basis of a characteristic radiological picture, coupled with the histological features of the biopsy. Periodontal cysts are very frequent and show a radiolucent rounded area with a sharply defined outline. If the crown of a tooth is enclosed within the cyst, it is referred to as a dentigerous cyst. The latter and keratocysts are usually found in the young, but with some keratocysts a tooth may be missing. Dental cysts must be differentiated from ameloblastomas, which tend to show multilocular and sometimes a honeycomb pattern on radiographs. These radiolucent lesions should also be differentiated from secondary carcinoma and myelomatosis. Giant-cell reparative granuloma and tumour (osteoclastoma) show a radiolucent area, sometimes loculated, and the outline is not as well defined as a dental cyst. Hyperparathyroidism can be excluded by radiographic appearance of other bones and by the calcium and phosphate levels in the blood. Ossifying fibromas are more common than fibromas and the radiographs show a well-defined radiolucent area with speckled calcification. This can usually be distinguished from the 'ground glass' appearance, without a distinct border, found in fibrous dysplasia. In Paget's disease there is a distinctive 'cotton wool' appearance on radiographic examination and the alkaline phosphatase levels are high. Odontomes can be readily recognized on clinical examination, but those that are unerupted, particularly the compound and complex composite odontomes, show on radiographs a mass of overlapping denticles and an irregular radio-opaque mass, respectively. Osteosarcoma and chrondrosarcoma show patchy areas of bone resorption and deposition.

Treatment

The treatment of dental cysts is by enucleation of the cyst lining and usually extracting the involved tooth. The tumours and malformations are usually excised but some, such as giant-cell reparative granuloma, can be curettaged. Brown tumours will recur unless the underlying hyperparathyroidism has been dealt with. Fibrous dysplasia may require removal of excessive tissue for cosmetic or functional reasons, but this should be delayed until normal bone growth has ceased. Bony changes in Paget's disease are best not interfered with, except if there are functional reasons, such as inability to fit a denture. Composite odontomes should be removed surgically. The treatment of ameloblastoma is by local excision, with a generous margin of normal bone, or by hemimandibulectomy. Sarcoma of the jaw must be dealt with by early radical excision.

Course and prognosis

If the cysts and benign tumours are removed surgically, they do not recur, except with keratocysts and the reparative granulomas. Ameloblastomas may recur after several excisions, without metastases, and this is why some surgeons prefer to do a hemimandibulectomy. The prognosis of the jaw sarcomas is very poor and the 5-year survival rate is between 25 and 40%. Fibrous dysplasia tends to be self-limiting, but in Paget's disease there may be progressive enlargement, especially of the maxilla.

Miscellaneous disorders

In this section a brief discussion will be given of the following three topics: (1) oral manifestations of blood disorders, (2) halitosis, and (3) disorders of the temporomandibular joint.

Oral manifestations of blood disorders

The main oral manifestations of blood dyscrasias are glossitis, oral ulceration, erythematous patches, and nonspecific stomatitis. Mild anaemias or deficiencies of iron, folate, or vitamin B$_{12}$ may manifest themselves as glossitis (Fig. 15.6.25) with a sore tongue or mouth, angular cheilitis, or recurrent ulceration (see Section 22). The tongue is commonly depapillated, the corners of the mouth may be inflamed and fissured, and occasionally there may be small shallow ulcers affecting the lips, tongue, and cheeks. The cause of any haematological deficiency should be investigated and, especially with folate deficiency, coeliac disease should be excluded. Replacement therapy usually deals effectively with the clinical features. It should, however, be emphasized that the complaint of a sore tongue can be associated with many other causes, such as erythema migrans, candidiasis, lichen planus, recurrent aphthous ulceration, and black hairy tongue. Erythema migrans (geographical tongue, or best known as benign migratory glossitis) is particularly common and is characterized by oval, depapillated areas

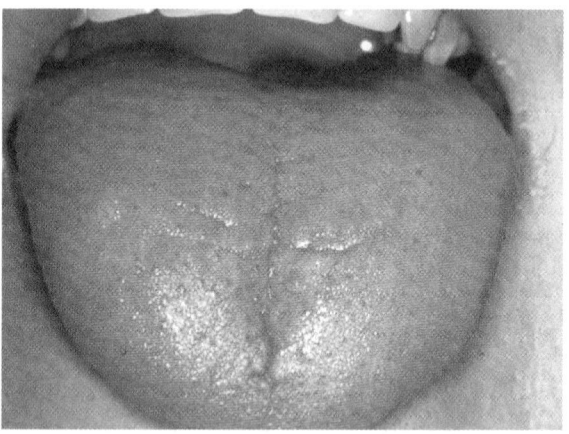

(a)

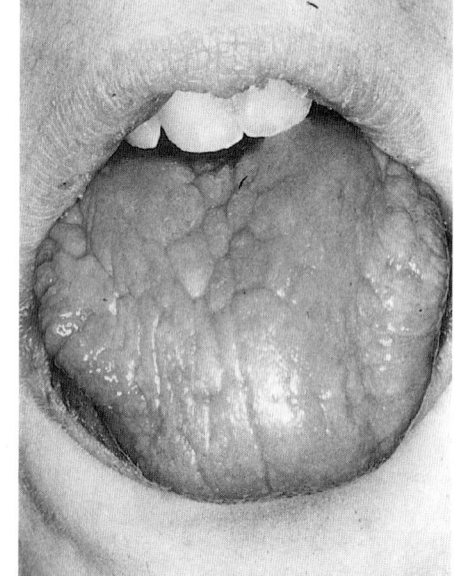

(b)

Fig. 15.6.25 Tongue showing depapillation secondary to iron deficiency: (a) early (b) late.

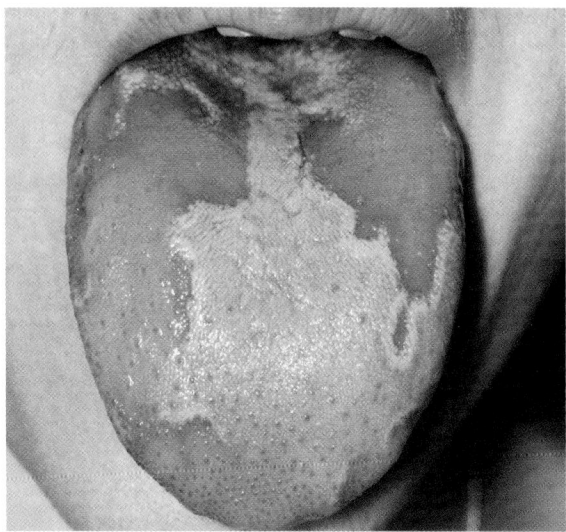

Fig. 15.6.26 Benign migratory glossitis (erythema migrans or geographical tongue). A common benign lesion frequently misdiagnosed as candida infection or anaemia.

with a well-defined edge affecting the dorsum of the tongue (Fig. 15.6.26). The lesions move from one site to another. The aetiology of erythema migrans is unknown and treatment is rather unsatisfactory. A sore tongue is a frequent complaint in middle-aged women, often without any demonstrable aetiological factor.

Acute leukaemia, particularly the myelomonocytic form, may occasionally present in young people in the form of sore, bleeding gums (Fig. 15.6.27). This may vary from slight inflammation to that showing bulbous enlargement of the gingiva. There are usually inadequate local causes for such a gingivitis and anaemia may be evident; blood tests should be requested to exclude leukaemia.

Leucopenia and agranulocytosis, especially those due to drugs, may become clinically evident by ulceration of the throat or the mouth. Purpura may be associated with a deficiency of platelets, so that bleeding from the gum may also be a feature.

Many haemorrhagic disorders may become evident after extraction of a tooth, because bleeding does not stop. Less commonly, gingival bleeding may attract attention to the blood disorder.

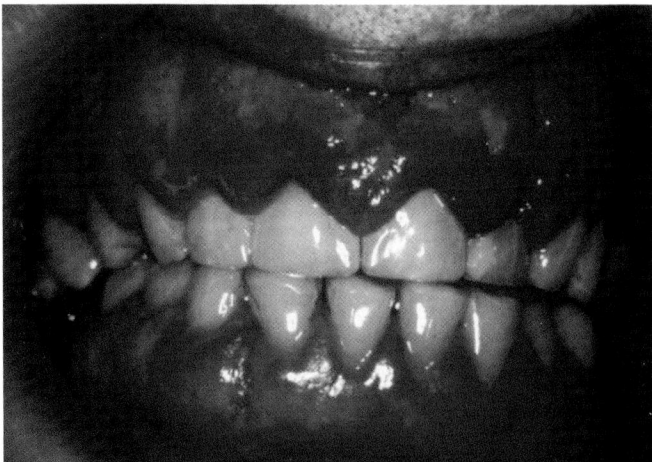

Fig. 15.6.27 Chronic myeloid leukaemia presenting as a hyperaemic swollen gingivitis.

Halitosis

Bad breath is usually a trivial complaint, though it seems to be heightened by the attention drawn to it by advertising. There are four possible sources of halitosis: the mouth, nasopharynx, lungs, and gastrointestinal tract. Altered blood round the gum may be the most important oral cause, and this may be associated with debris or pus from gingivitis and periodontal pockets. A characteristic halitosis is found in acute ulcerative gingivitis. It should be noted that bad taste and bad breath are subjective sensations which are often confused. Excessive bacterial plaque on the teeth is not a principal cause of halitosis; nevertheless, meticulous oral care should be advised.

Chronic tonsillitis may be responsible for halitosis but atrophic rhinitis causing ozena is probably the most important cause to be excluded. Occasionally, respiratory tract infections may cause halitosis, and a variety of gastrointestinal disorders have been associated with bad breath but there is little evidence to substantiate this. Frequently all these sources of halitosis may be excluded without finding a cause and these patients may have a fixation about bad breath related to emotional or sexual problems.

Temporomandibular joint disorders

Temporomandibular arthrosis is the most common disorder of this joint and the patient complains of pain, clicking, or limitation of movement. It is found in young women more often than men. Examination may reveal limitations in jaw movement, tenderness of the joint, and crepitus on movement, discovered by palpating the head of the condyle through the overlying skin. The cause is difficult to establish but malocclusion might be one of several factors. The condition may clear spontaneously, but in some patients the occlusion should be checked and a bite-raising appliance is often helpful. Rheumatoid arthritis and osteoarthritis of this joint are occasionally seen clinically. Dislocation of the joint, which becomes fixed in the open position, may be caused by a blow on the jaw or during dental extractions under general anaesthesia. Ankylosis of the joint is nowadays extremely rare and used to be secondary to osteomyelitis.

Further reading

Atkinson JC, *et al.* (1990). Major salivary gland function in primary Sjögren's syndrome and its relationship to clinical features. *J Rheumatol*, **17**, 318–22.

Azarpazhooh A, Leake JL (2006). Systematic review of the association between respiratory diseases and oral health. *J Periodontol*, **77**, 1465–82. [Review.]

Bouquot JE, Weiland LH, Kurland LT (1988). Leukoplakia and carcinoma *in situ* synchronously associated with invasive oral/oropharyngeal carcinoma in Rochester Minn., 1935–1984. *Oral Surg Oral Med Oral Pathol*, **65**, 199–207.

Carlos JP, *et al.* (1988). Periodontal disease in adolescents: some clinical and microbiological correlates of attachment loss. *J Dent Res*, **67**, 1510–14.

Carlsson J (1989). Microbial aspects of frequent intake of products with high sugar concentrations. *Scand J Dent Res*, **97**, 110–14.

Chau MN, Radden BG (1989). A clinical-pathological study of 53 intra-oral pleomorphic adenomas. *Int J Oral Maxillofac Surg*, **18**, 158–62.

Dummer PMH, *et al.* (1990). Factors influencing the caries experience of a group of children at the ages of 11–12 and 15–16 years: results from an ongoing study. *J Dent*, **18**, 37–48.

Dzink JL, Socransky SS, Haffajee AD (1988). The predominant cultivable flora of active and inactive lesions of destructive periodontal diseases. *J Clin Periodontol*, **15**, 316–23.

Eisen D, *et al.* (2005) Oral lichen planus: clinical features and management. *Oral Dis*, **11**, 338–49. [Review.]

Farah CS, Ashman RB, Challacombe SJ (2000) Oral candidosis. [Review.] *Clin Dermatol*, **18**, 553–62.

Fox PC, Busch KA, Baum BJ (1987). Subjective reports of xerostomia and objective measures of salivary gland performance. *J Am Dent Assoc*, **115**, 581–4.

Genco RJ, Christersson LA, Zambon JJ (1986). Juvenile periodontitis. *Int Dent J*, **36**, 168–76.

Gibbons RJ (1989). Bacterial adhesion to oral tissues: a model for infectious diseases. *J Dent Res*, **68**, 750–60.

Greenspan JS, Greenspan D (2002) The epidemiology of the oral lesions of HIV infection in the developed world. *Oral Dis*, **8** Suppl 2, 34–9. [Review.]

Greenspan JS, Greenspan D, Winkler JR (1988). Diagnosis and management of the oral manifestations of HIV infection and AIDS. *Infect Dis Clin N Am*, **2**, 373–85.

Hasan A, *et al.* (2005). The immune responses to human and microbial heat shock proteins in periodontal disease with and without coronary heart disease. *Clin Exp Immunol*, **142**, 585–94.

Herrod HG (1990). Chronic mucocutaneous candidiasis in childhood and complications of non-Candida infection. *J Pediatr*, **116**, 377–82.

Hogewind WF, *et al.* (1989). The association of white lesions with oral squamous cell carcinoma: a retrospective study of 212 patients. *Int J Oral Maxillofac Surg*, **18**, 163–4.

Holmstrup P, *et al.* (1988). Malignant development of lichen planus-affected oral mucosa. *J Oral Pathol*, **17**, 219–25.

Kashima HK, *et al.* (1990). Human papilloma virus in squamous cell carcinoma, leukoplakia, lichen planus, and clinically normal epithelium of the oral cavity. *Ann Ontol Rhinol Laryngol*, **99**, 55–61.

Lehner T (1992). *Immunology of oral diseases.* Blackwell, Oxford.

Lindhe J, *et al.* (1989). Longitudinal changes in periodontal disease in untreated subjects. *J Clin Periodont Res*, **16**, 662–70.

Lloyd RE, Ho KH (1988). Combined CT scanning and sialography in the management of parotid tumors. *Oral Surg Oral Med Oral Pathol*, **65**, 142–4.

Lozada-Nur F, Gorsky M, Silverman S (1989). Oral erythema multiforme: clinical observations and treatment of 95 patients. *Oral Surg Oral Med Oral Pathol*, **67**, 36–40.

Mitchell TJ (2003) The pathogenesis of streptococcal infections: from tooth decay to meningitis. *Nat Rev Microbiol*, **3**, 219–30. [Review.]

Mithani SK, *et al.* (2007) Molecular genetics of premalignant oral lesions. *Oral Dis*, **13**, 126–33. [Review.]

Moller H (1989). Changing incidence of cancer of the tongue, oral cavity and pharynx in Denmark. *J Oral Pathol Med*, **18**, 224–9.

Newbrun E (1989). Frequent sugar intake—then and now: interpretation of main results. *Scand J Dent Res*, **97**, 103–9.

Renehan A, *et al.* (1996) Long-term follow-up of over 1000 patients with salivary gland tumours treated in a single centre. *Br J Surg*, **83**, 1750–4.

Sciubba JJ (2001) Oral cancer. The importance of early diagnosis and treatment. *Am J Clin Dermatol*, **2**, 239–51. [Review.]

Seaman S, Thomas FD, Walker WA (1989). Differences between caries levels in 5 year old children from fluoridated Anglesey and non-fluoridated mainland Gwynedd in 1987. *Commun Dent Health*, **6**, 215–21.

Silva TA, *et al.* (2007) Chemokines in oral inflammatory diseases: apical periodontitis and periodontal disease. *J Dent Res*, **86**, 306–19. [Review.]

Slots, J (1986). Bacterial specificity in adult periodontitis. *J ClinPeriodontol*, **13**, 912–17.

Stanford M, *et al.* (2004). Oral tolerization with peptide 336–351 linked to cholera toxin B subunit in preventing relapses of uveitis in Behcet's disease. *Clin Exp Immunol*, **137**, 201–8.

von Bultzingslowen I, *et al.* (2007). Salivary dysfunction associated with systemic diseases: systematic review and clinical management recommendations. *Oral Surg Oral Med Oral Pathol Oral Radiol Endod*, **103** Suppl 57, e1–15.

Williams DM (1989). Vesiculobullous mucocutaneous disease: pemphigus vulgaris. *J Oral Pathol Med*, **18**, 544–53.

Williams RC (1990). Periodontal disease. *N Engl J Med*, **322**, 373–82.

Zakrzewska JM, Chan ES, Thornhill MH (2005). A systematic review of placebo-controlled randomized clinical trials of treatments used in oral lichen planus. *Br J Dermatol*, **153**, 336–41. [Review.]

15.7

Diseases of the oesophagus

Rebecca Fitzgerald

Essentials

Defective conduit function of the oesophagus readily induces clinical symptoms and may have serious effects on nutrition and the lungs, the latter resulting from aspiration of gastro-oeophageal contents. Oesophageal pain and dysphagia caused by benign or malignant diseases of the muscular layer or epithelium are often disabling.

The oesophagus is exposed to numerous hostile environments including carcinogens in food or those derived from tobacco, betel nuts, and other ingested sources and hence carcinomas can occur. Chronic reflux disease from exposure to corrosive upper gastrointestinal secretions are also associated with malignant disease—adenocarcinoma—as well as benign stricture formation related to the action of pepsin.

Introduction

The oesophagus is responsible for transporting food to the stomach without compromising the safety of the airway. Imprecise muscle coordination of the oropharynx and the oesophageal body can have serious consequences such as aspiration pneumonia and malnutrition. Diseases of the oesophagus generally present with symptoms of pain or dysphagia either alone or in combination (odynophagia). True oesophageal dysphagia should be distinguished from oropharyngeal dysphagia, an abnormality of transfer of food from the mouth to the oeosphagus, by a careful history. Other symptoms and signs of oesophageal disease include weight loss, anaemia, cough, hoarse voice, and breathlessness secondary to aspiration pneumonia. The most common oesophageal disorder is gastro-oesophageal reflux disease which should be taken seriously because of its profound impact on quality of life in some people and since it can be a precursor to oesophageal adenocarcinoma. The diagnosis of oesophageal disease may generally be determined by a thorough history and a small number of focused investigations outlined below.

Investigation

Diagnosis and treatment of suspected oesophageal disease has been enhanced by the introduction of endoscopic techniques, but in some circumstances radiological investigations and dynamic studies of oesophageal motor function using manometry provide essential guidance for diagnosis of achalasia, oesophageal spasm, and motor disorders related to systemic diseases such as scleroderma.

Endoscopy

An oesophagogastroduodenoscopy is usually the first investigation of choice to determine whether there is a mechanical cause for the symptoms and whether there is any evidence of inflammation or mucosal damage. Direct visualization of the oesophagus combined with biopsy as appropriate, offers immediate benefit for the diagnosis of mucosal diseases such as: (1) infections due to candida and herpes simplex virus; (2) benign and malignant strictures; (3) bleeding lesions, including varices. Although the endoscopic appearances may be suggestive of a motility disorder this is not the investigation of choice for assessing oesophageal function. Endoscopic technology is advancing rapidly and enhanced magnification coupled with permutations in the parts of the light spectrum used for image processing (e.g. narrow band imaging) permit a more detailed analysis of the mucosa in real time. It is hoped that these technologies will aid diagnosis, e.g. of dysplasia.

Endoscopic ultrasound is an important staging investigation for oesophageal cancer (see below) and also has a role in characterizing submucosal lesions.

Radiology

A plain cervical and chest radiograph should be taken in cases where oesophageal perforation is suspected. The barium or gastrograffin swallow has largely been superseded by endoscopy for the diagnosis of structural abnormalities; however, it can be a useful guide prior to interventions such as endoscopic stent insertion and to evaluate conduit functioning postoperatively. Useful information can also be obtained about the motor function of the pharynx and oesophagus by videotaping the images and analysing, in slow-motion replay, repeated tests of standardized stimuli such as bread or barium tablets. Optimal results from radiology are achieved when there is a partnership between a clinician and a radiologist who both have a special interest in oesophageal motor disorders, so that the examination technique can then be tailored accordingly. CT scanning and positron emission tomography, increasingly as part of a combined procedure (CT-PET), are part of the staging investigations for oesophageal cancer (see below). MRI has a limited role for oesophageal disease.

Oesophageal function testing

Techniques are now available for the precise measurement of oesophageal motor function. These include oesophageal manometry, intraluminal impedance monitoring, video fluoroscopy, and high-resolution oesophageal manometry with isocontour mapping. Together these techniques build a dynamic picture of the physiological sequence of events and the effectiveness of contraction which can be compared with resultant functional outcome. These tests may also have a clinical role for explaining symptoms to patients even in the absence of therapy.

Oesophageal manometry provides the most direct indication of patterns of oesophageal motor function. It is most helpful in the diagnosis of dysphagia, after exclusion of fixed, structural defects. Manometry may also be useful to confirm the placement of intraluminal devices such as pH probes and to assess pre- and postoperative results following surgery for achalasia or reflux. It may be performed as a stationary test with a liquid swallow or as a prolonged, ambulatory 24-h manometry. This is conventionally performed with a transnasal catheter although, more recently, wireless devices have become available. To determine the association between reflux episodes and symptoms pH catheters can be used to provide either a stationary or ambulatory recording. Again wireless devices are increasingly used. Ambulatory monitoring is particularly useful to determine the association between symptoms and episodes of acid reflux in a minority of patients in whom the origin of troublesome symptoms is unclear. This test is generally performed off medication but may occasionally be useful to assess response to therapy.

Radionuclide measurement of oesophageal transit

Computerized scintigraphic analysis of the movement of swallowed radiolabelled boluses can give quantitative information about the patterns of movement of material down the oesophagus. However, its poor spatial resolution makes it an inadequate method for the display of oesophageal anatomy. If structural abnormalities have been adequately excluded, slow or interrupted transit suggests abnormal motility, although patterns of transit are usually nonspecific.

Gastro-oesophageal reflux disease

This is by far the most common oesophageal disorder and management should be tailored to the severity, which may vary considerably.

Definition

Some reflux of gastric and duodenal contents into the oesophagus occurs in everybody due to vagally mediated transient lower oeophageal sphincter relaxations. It should only be considered a disease when it gives rise to symptoms or complications sufficient to impair quality of life. Pathogenic reflux may occur without causing mucosal damage. The terms reflux or peptic oesophagitis should be reserved for circumstances when endoscopy demonstrates that the oesophageal mucosa is clearly breached by the action of the refluxed gastric contents. Minor changes such as erythema, oedema, or friability have been shown to be very unreliable indicators of the presence of oesophagitis. The disease can be further classified into oesophageal and extra-oesophageal syndromes using the Montreal classification.

Aetiology

In most patients reflux disease arises from the excessive exposure of the distal oesophagus to gastric contents which are primarily acid and/or bile. This is usually because of an abnormal frequency or duration of reflux episodes. In a few patients, however, symptoms arise with relatively normal levels of acid exposure, presumably because of sensitization of the oesophageal mucosa. In normal individuals excessive reflux is prevented by the lower oesophageal sphincter and an external sphincter formed by the crural diaphragm. Pathological reflux generally occurs as a result of defective neural control of the lower oesophageal sphincter. Hiatus hernia is common in patients with reflux disease and causes displacement of the sphincter from the hiatus formed by the diaphragmatic crura. Most reflux occurs during the day, usually after food, but lying down will ameliorate the antireflux effect of gravity and nocturnal reflux can be a disabling symptom. Refluxate is cleared from the oesophagus by peristalsis and swallowed saliva. Slow clearance of oesophageal acidification contributes significantly to prolonged acid exposure in about 50% of patients. This can be an important contributor to severe gastro-oesophageal reflux disease in systemic disorders such as scleroderma which affect gut motility.

Risk factors for gastro-oesophageal reflux disease include heritability (up to 30% of the risk), obesity, and age but not gender. Alcohol and smoking may play a role. Asthma increases the risk as do medications which relax the lower oesophageal sphincter such as calcium channel antagonists, nitrates, anticholinergics, and methyl xanthines.

Consequences of excessive reflux
Symptoms

These are an important source of disability. Evidence suggests that heartburn occurring on more than 2 days a week causes significant impairment of quality of life. However, presentation may be with the less specific symptom of dyspepsia (or epigastric discomfort), belching, nausea or with regurgitation, and dysphagia due to either stricture or motor dysfunction of the oesophageal body. There are a number of extra-oesophageal manifestations of reflux including respiratory symptoms such as hoarseness, persistent cough, and asthma. Chronic sinusitis, otalgia, and glue ear may also be associated with reflux.

Complications of reflux disease

The chemical insult from excessive exposure of the mucosa to gastro-duodenal contents leads to distal oesophageal erosion or ulceration in between 40 and 60% of patients with troublesome reflux symptoms and columnar-lined (Barrett's) oesophagus in between 5 and 10% of individuals, as discussed in detail below. The extent of ulceration varies greatly, from tiny patches of erosion to extensive circumferential ulceration in a small minority. Peptic stricture

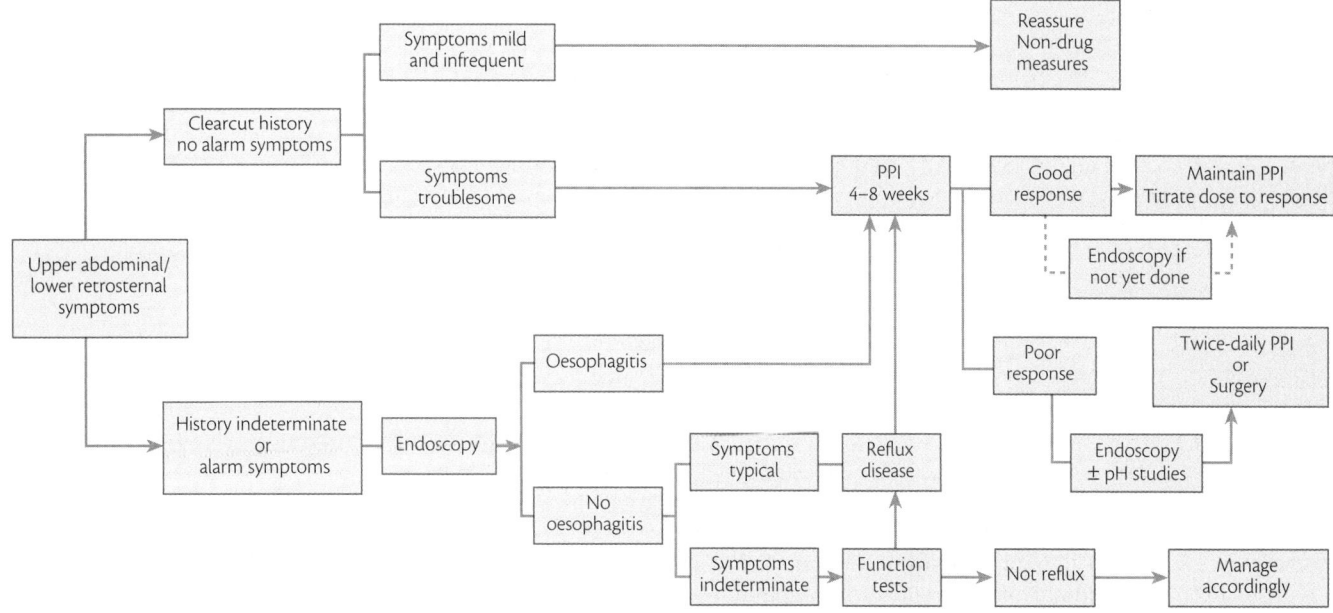

Fig. 15.7.1 Principal decision paths for management of reflux disease.

sufficient to cause dysphagia is typically only associated with severe oesophagitis. When strictures are severe this may lead to malnutrition. Bleeding from oesophagitis may occur but is rarely life-threatening except when it occurs from a deep ulcer associated with columnar metaplasia.

Diagnosis and assessment of severity

History

The history is pivotal for diagnosis because of the extremely high prevalence of reflux-induced symptoms and the lack of a definitive, inexpensive diagnostic test for reflux disease. A trial of acid-suppression therapy can be used as an aid to diagnosis.

Endoscopy

When investigation is required, endoscopy is the first choice as it is the only test that can give sensitive recognition and grading of oesophagitis (e.g. Los Angeles classification system) and reliable diagnosis of oesophageal columnar metaplasia (Barrett's oesophagus). Endoscopy also allows for the effective identification of significant peptic strictures, other types of oesophagitis (discussed below), and peptic ulcer disease as well as malignancies. The value of endoscopy as the initial investigation is greatly enhanced by the accurate diagnosis of endoscopic biopsy and, where indicated, cytology brushings. As discussed above, however, most patients with reflux disease do not have endoscopically visible mucosal damage, so a negative endoscopy does not exclude the diagnosis of reflux disease (so-called nonerosive reflux disease).

Oesophageal function tests

The place of these is summarized in Fig. 15.7.1. Oesophageal manometry and ambulatory 24-h pH monitoring have a limited but important role in the diagnosis of reflux disease (Fig. 15.7.2). Oesophageal pH monitoring is most useful in patients with troublesome symptoms but without endoscopic signs of oesophagitis in whom a trial of therapy has failed, and patients with atypical symptoms that cannot be clearly related to reflux. Patients with suspected reflux symptoms but with no endoscopic evidence of

oesophagitis who are being considered for antireflux surgery should also undergo oesophageal pH monitoring.

Recently, multichannel oesophageal impedance monitoring (Fig. 15.7.3) has been shown to distinguish between swallowed or refluxed fluid and gas, although at present its use is mainly confined to the research setting. Combined with pH monitoring, it may identify individuals with 'nonacid' who fail to respond to treatment. Bile reflux can be assessed using Bilitec probes, but these are not routinely available anywhere.

Barium swallow and meal

This is an inappropriate primary diagnostic test; it is of no value for the detection of abnormal reflux, and is insensitive for the diagnosis of oesophagitis and cannot grade it. Other pathologies such as gastric ulcer and oesophageal stricture are demonstrated with reasonable sensitivity, but adequate evaluation of these findings requires endoscopic biopsy. However, barium swallow is the best method for recognizing extrinsic oesophageal compression which may be producing symptoms that could be interpreted as being due to reflux, and in the assessment of an anatomically complex hiatus hernia. The mere demonstration of hiatus hernia, however, does not necessarily indicate the presence of reflux disease.

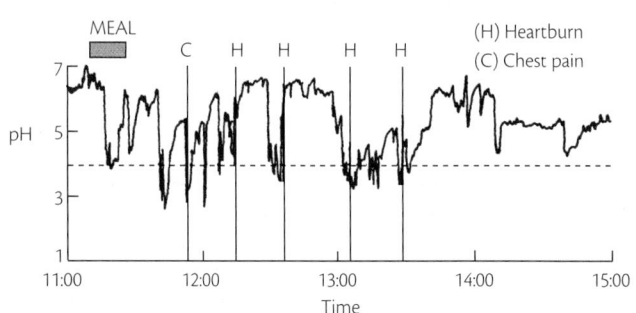

Fig. 15.7.2 Section of a 24-h oesophageal pH monitoring study showing the association of heartburn with episodes of acid reflux after a meal.

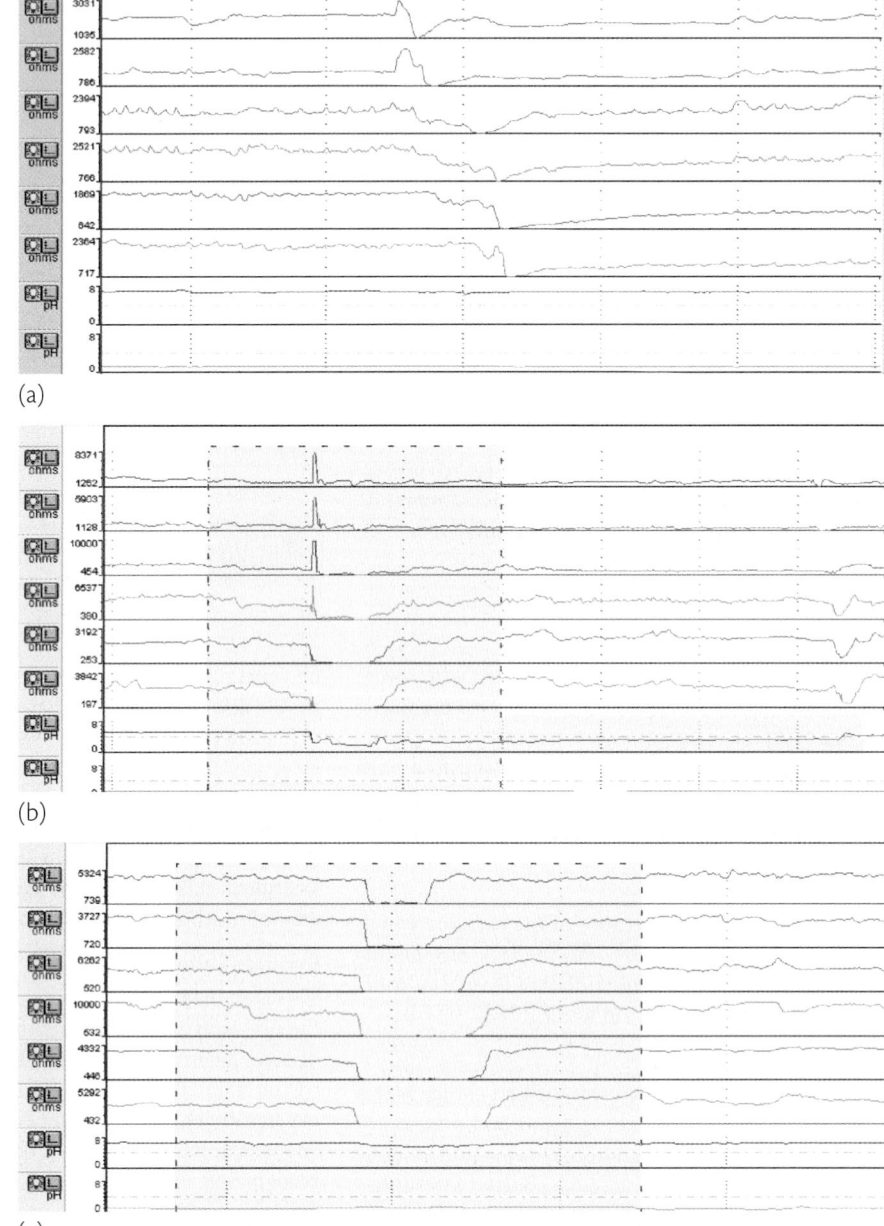

Fig. 15.7.3 Example impedance images obtained from six impedance and two pH channels placed in the oesophagus. (a) Impedance changes for normal liquid swallow. Usually air is ahead of liquid bolus. (b) Mixed (gas and liquid) acid reflux episode. Mixed reflux is more frequent than liquid only reflux. Gas (belch) reflux is evidenced by short rise in impedance migrating rapidly into the proximal oesophagus. (c) Nonacid reflux. Oesophageal pH is unchanged, while impedance channels are showing a liquid reflux episode migrating into the proximal oesophagus.
(Courtesy of Qasim Aziz, Professor of Physiology, Barts and the London School of Medicine and Dentistry.)

Principles of management

The major aims of treatment are to provide adequate symptomatic relief and control of oesophagitis. Reduction of oesophagitis to minor patchy erosions is probably sufficient to prevent the complications of oesophagitis, although adequate symptomatic relief is usually achieved only when oesophagitis is completely healed.

Tailoring and titration of therapy

The severity and frequency of symptoms and the endoscopic findings should be used to choose an appropriate level of initial therapy (Fig. 15.7.1). There is some debate about whether to treat patients with a high or low dose of acid-suppressant drugs initially. An initial trial of low- to medium-dose empirical therapy has the disadvantage of giving less precise diagnostic information, and often gives only slow relief of symptoms. Patients with severe oesophagitis will usually not respond adequately to low dose acid-suppression. Initial high-dose proton pump inhibitor therapy is likely to give more immediate confirmation of the diagnosis and prompt relief of symptoms. For optimum cost-effectiveness and to reduce complications high dose treatment should be followed by a step-down approach to long-term therapy as outlined in Fig. 15.7.1.

Nondrug measures and antacids

The efficacy of these traditional approaches is often overrated. The most useful measures are avoidance of large meals and provocative foods, drinks, and physical activities. The benefits to reflux disease of stopping smoking, weight loss, and elevation of the bed head are uncertain. Antacids will not usually prevent symptoms, but may be effective in aborting episodes of heartburn. These low-cost measures are worth a trial in patients with mild intermittent symptoms and should be used as maintenance therapy if they prove effective, provided that their impact on lifestyle is acceptable to the patient.

Acid suppression

Inhibition of secretion of gastric acid makes gastric juice less injurious but does not stop reflux. This has deservedly become the most widely used drug therapy because of its high efficacy and adjustability. Proton pump inhibitors are the mainstay of treatment because of their effectiveness in reduction of food-stimulated acid secretion and their greater overall efficacy in control of acid secretion compared with histamine-2 receptor antagonists. However, histamine-2 receptor antagonists can be a useful adjunct to proton pump inhibitors for controlling nocturnal reflux.

Long-term treatment with acid suppressants maintains patients free of symptoms and oesophagitis indefinitely, but withdrawal is usually associated with prompt relapse. The maintenance dose appears to be the same as the lowest effective healing dose. There have been concerns about the safety of long-term acid suppression ever since the introduction of istamine-2 receptor antagonists. To date, follow-up of patients treated continuously for 10 years or more with acid suppression has shown no evidence of any effects of significance, but in the context of patients who may require treatment with these agents for decades, more extensive follow-up is still needed. Given these theoretical safety considerations and also drug cost, long-term treatment of reflux disease with these agents should use the lowest effective dose. In some patients use of proton pump inhibitors is limited by side effects such as diarrhoea and patients on long-term therapy may be prone to increased gastrointestinal infections due to loss of the antimicrobial effects of low gastric pH.

Motility stimulants

The best researched, most efficacious motility stimulant is cisapride, which is a parasympathomimetic that acts as a serotonin 5-HT$_4$ receptor agonist. It mainly acts through enhancing oesophageal acid clearance as well as increasing muscle tone in the lower oesophageal sphincter. Unfortunately, cisapride can have effects on cardiac conductance that may rarely lead to sudden death at peak serum levels, especially when various drugs are co-administered. Cisparide has therefore been withdrawn from the market in many countries and should only be used cautiously in severe cases. Alternative prokinetics such as metoclopramide and domperidone may be useful adjuncts, again when used in combination with acid-suppression therapy.

Endoscopic antireflux procedures

Techniques include endoscopic suturing, radiofrequency energy delivery to the lower oesophageal sphincter, and submucosal prosthetic implants. Effectiveness has mainly been assessed in uncontrolled trials without long-term follow-up data. There is no place for such therapies outside clinical trials at present.

Antireflux surgery

In skilled hands, antireflux surgery is a very effective long-term therapy. Negative factors are the dependence of the results on the expertise of the surgeon and the morbidity and small (approximately 0.5%) mortality associated with the surgery itself. Laparoscopic antireflux surgery (usually a Nissen fundoplication) is a major advance, as it achieves good control of reflux with a major reduction in the morbidity inherent in the more traditional approach.

Choice between medical and surgical therapies

Selection of a medical or surgical therapy should take account of the severity of disease and the risks of antireflux surgery specific to the patient. It should also take account of the patient's age, both from the point of view of operative risk and the time over which the patient will need treatment for reflux disease, the cost of effective medical therapy, and, naturally, the preferences of the patient. The choice between medical therapies should be largely governed by the local cost of the alternatives that give the necessary level of treatment, as all of the first-line options are effective, safe, and well tolerated.

Management of complications of reflux disease

The important complication of oesophageal columnar metaplasia is discussed in a separate section below.

Peptic stricture

Dysphagia secondary to stricture formation needs to be distinguished from the more common dysphagia seen in patients with reflux disease which is due to defective triggering and control of oesophageal body peristalsis (see the section on nonspecific oesophageal motor disorders, below). Peptic stricture is managed by a combination of peroral dilatation and healing of oesophagitis by either medical or surgical means. All strictures should be treated as malignant until proven otherwise by repeated biopsy. Provided oesophagitis is healed, stricture is usually not an ongoing problem.

Respiratory complications

Respiratory disease may occur either as a result of direct aspiration of refluxed gastric contents or from the reflex effects of gastro-oesophageal reflux. It is difficult to prove that reflux disease which coexists with respiratory disease is actually the cause of the respiratory problem. The best investigative approach is probably a trial of high-level acid inhibition with at least a double dose of proton pump inhibitor and prokinetics for at least 2 months. Management of respiratory disease by antireflux surgery is not guaranteed to be successful.

Regurgitation

Voluminous regurgitation is the main symptom in a small subgroup of patients with reflux disease. They may present complaining of vomiting, but a detailed history reveals that there is no prior nausea, and no effort involved in the appearance of the gastric content in the mouth. The determinants of high-volume reflux and regurgitation have not been defined. Treatment with proton pump inhibitors and prokinetics can have substantial benefits, but in more severe cases antireflux surgery is usually the only effective management.

Noncardiac chest pain

Reflux is also an important cause of noncardiac chest pain (see below).

Oesophageal columnar metaplasia (Barrett's oesophagus)

Definition and nomenclature

Oesophageal columnar metaplasia (Barrett's oesophagus) is defined as the conversion of the normal stratified squamous epithelium with a columnar-lined mucosa which may have characteristics of gastric or intestinal epithelium. The lack of international consensus on the definition of this disease has led to confusion in the literature. However, it is widely accepted that it is the subtype characterized by intestinal metaplasia with goblet cells which has the highest risk for malignant progression and in many countries the term Barrett's oesophagus has been restricted to this subtype. The extent of the metaplasia may vary from 1 cm to the entire oeosophageal length and there appears to be a correlation between the length of the segment and the proximal extent of reflux exposure. The metaplasia generally starts in the distal oesophagus although discrete columnar islands may occur. The accepted nomenclature for describing the endoscopic features is the Prague classification in which C indicates circumferential involvement in centimetres and M is the maximal disease extent in centimetres (e.g. C2,M5 for a 5 cm segment with 3 cm of metaplastic tongues).

Aetiopathogenesis

Columnar metaplasia occurs in the context of chronic gastro-oesopageal reflux, predominantly in white males. Its incidence appears to have increased, even taking into account the more frequent use of endoscopy, and the reasons for this are still under intense scrutiny. Possible explanations include an increase in obesity leading to an increased susceptibility to reflux and the reduced prevalence of *Helicobacter pylori* infection with a consequent increase in gastric acid secretion. Columnar metaplasia carries a 40-fold increased risk for the development of oesophageal adenocarcinoma compared with the general population, which equates to an annual incidence of 0.5 to 1%. Occurrence of adenocarcinoma is very strongly associated with prior development of high-grade dysplasia in the metaplastic segment and therefore endoscopic surveillance is generally advocated.

Management

Surveillance hinges on the subjective interpretation of dysplasia in multiple, random biopsies (usually quadrantic biopsies every 2 cm according to the Seattle protocol). The frequency of surveillance depends on the degree of dysplasia (Table 15.7.1). This arduous protocol has not been uniformly accepted since no data from randomized controlled trials support a reduction in population mortality from oesophageal adenocarcinoma using this approach. On the other hand, the outcome for individuals with symptomatic invasive adenocarcinoma is universally poor compared with surveillance-detected disease. Failure to discuss the risk for adenocarcinoma and the option of endoscopic surveillance with a patient who has oesophageal columnar metaplasia could well be viewed as an indefensible lapse of practice, despite the uncertainties about cost-effectiveness.

The treatment of high-grade intraepithelial neoplasia (dysplasia) in oesophageal columnar metaplasia is controversial. First, the diagnosis should be corroborated by two independent pathologists, preferably on biopsies taken at two separate endoscopies (Table 15.7.1). Increasingly, endoscopic mucosal resection can be used as a diagnostic adjunct to determine depth of invasion. This will inform management decisions and in some cases will turn out to be a therapeutic local excision. Endoscopic ultrasound may be useful but there is a danger of overestimating the depth of invasion. The management options will be determined by the extent of dysplasia and the fitness of the individual as well as local expertise. Oesophagectomy (which may be performed as a transhiatal or even a laparsocopic procedure with a limited lymph node resection) is still considered to be the gold standard management option although increasingly endoscopic ablation using photodynamic therapy, argon plasma coagulation, or more recently radiofrequency ablation are being offered. Some centres favour frequent continued surveillance until there is clear evidence of invasion. Lack of detailed knowledge about the natural history of high-grade dysplasia makes the decision-making process especially difficult. Discussion with a multidisciplinary team with expertise in oesophageal cancer is recommended as well as full consultation with the patient.

Barrett's oesophagus may also be associated with deep benign oesophageal ulceration within the columnar-lined segment and strictures usually at the squamocolumnar junction. Occasionally ulcers can erode into mediastinal structures or the pleural space although this is encountered much less frequently with the ready availability of acid suppressants.

The diagnosis and management of invasive oeosphageal adenocarcinoma is discussed in the malignancy section.

Nonreflux causes of oesophagitis

Infective oesophagitis

Infective oesophagitis has become more prevalent with the increasing number of people who are immunosuppressed through HIV infection or chemotherapy. The more important causes of infective oesophagitis are summarized in Table 15.7.2. Immune status is a major determinant of the pattern of infection and simultaneous infection with two or more infective agents is not unusual (Table 15.7.2).

Table 15.7.1 Surveillance protocol for columnar lined (Barrett's) oesophagus for patients willing and fit to undergo regular endoscopy

Histopathological diagnosis	Endoscopy frequency	Clinical management
Intestinal metaplasia No dysplasia	2 years	Treat heartburn symptoms with PPI
Intestinal metaplasia Indefinite intraepithelial neoplasia/dysplasia	6 months after index finding. Annual if changes persist. Revert 2 yearly when 2 consecutive endoscopies no dysplasia	Ensure adequate acid suppression to prevent inflammation confounding diagnosis
Intestinal metaplasia Low grade intraepithelial neoplasia	6 months after index finding. Annual if changes persist. Revert 2 yearly when 2 consecutive endoscopies no dysplasia (caution if multifocal change)	Ensure adequate acid suppression to prevent inflammation confounding diagnosis
Intestinal metaplasia High grade intraepithelial neoplasia	Confirm diagnosis on second endoscopy with 1 cm 4-quadrant biopsy and assessment by two independent pathologists	Consider endoscopic or surgical intervention—method depending on comorbidity and focality of lesion

Table 15.7.2 Major causes of infective oesophagitis

Pathogen	Management	Remarks
Immunocompetent patients		
Candida albicans	Topical/oral antifungals	By far the most common
Herpes simplex	Aciclovir if severe	Unusual, may denude mucosa
Varicella zoster	Aciclovir if severe	In association with chickenpox/herpes zoster
Bacteria		Rare in well individuals
Immunocompromised patients		
Candida albicans	Systemic antifungals	Most common; oral disease almost diagnostic
Cytomegalovirus	Prophylaxis and treatment with ganciclovir or foscarnet	Serpiginous to giant ulcers in distal half
Herpes simplex	Prophylaxis and treatment with aciclovir or foscarnet	Circumscribed ulcers, raised edges to coalescence. Oral lesions
Tuberculosis	Conventional	From miliary and local spread
Gram-positive cocci, Gram-negative bacilli	Intravenous antibiotics	Often with systemic infection
Syphilis	Conventional	Associated with tertiary syphilis elsewhere. Inflammatory stricture

Helicobacter pylori does not appear to be of any primary significance in the pathogenesis of oesophageal mucosal disease.

Patients may present with pain or dysphagia. Viral oesophagitis can sometimes cause major haemorrhage. The dysphagia is generally secondary to superficial mucosal damage and inflammation, but some disorders damage the full thickness of the oesophageal wall and so lead to stricturing.

A full history to determine the setting in which the oesophageal problem occurs is often very helpful. Cutaneous or oral disease can inform the oesophageal diagnosis. Endoscopy is the investigation of choice since the mucosal appearance and the distribution of oesophageal lesions can be virtually diagnostic. In addition, biopsies and brushings allow for histological diagnosis and identification of fungal elements, viral inclusions, or rarely, pathogenic bacteria.

Although infective oesophagitis may be severe in immunocompetent patients it is characteristically self-limiting and topical therapy is normally all that is needed. Immunocompromised patients usually need aggressive, systemic therapy to resolve the infection (Table 15.7.2). Some infections tend to recur, which can cause major disability.

Eosiniphilic oesophagitis

Eosinophilic oesophagitis (sometimes referred to as allergic oesophagitis) affects children and adults worldwide, with a male preponderance. The incidence appears to be increasing in line with other associated allergic conditions such as asthma, hay fever, allergic rhinitis, and atopic dermatitis. Although the exact aetiology is not understood there does seem to be an aberrant immune-mediated response and activated eosinophils may cause activation of acetyl choline via histamine. Food impaction and dysphagia are the common presenting symptoms. Heartburn is often present but refractory to standard treatments for gastro-oesophageal reflux disease. Approximately 50% of patients will have other allergic symptoms. Endoscopy is the investigation of choice and the findings range from grossly abnormal to normal. Findings include a small-calibre oesophagus, proximal strictures, white exduates, oeosphageal rings, and fragile mucosa. The diagnosis is made on oesophageal biopsy in which there is a dense eosiniphilic infiltration within the epithelium (Fig. 15.7.4). If the eosinophilic infiltration is more generalized this suggests eosinophilic gastroenteritis. There is a lack of randomized controlled trial evidence to guide treatment. Strategies include dietary elimination in consultation with an allergy assessment and steroids given topically or systemically in severe cases. Endoscopic food disimpaction and dilatation may be necessary. There is some data on leukotriene inhibitors and anti-interleukin-5 antibody therapy. There is limited data on the long-term outcome for these patients.

Medication-induced oesophagitis

This entity was only recognized in 1970. The chemical properties of medications pose hazards to the oesophageal mucosa because of its relative susceptibility to injury through pH-dependent mechanisms. This susceptibility arises in part from the high local concentrations of medications that occur in the oesophageal lumen, since pills

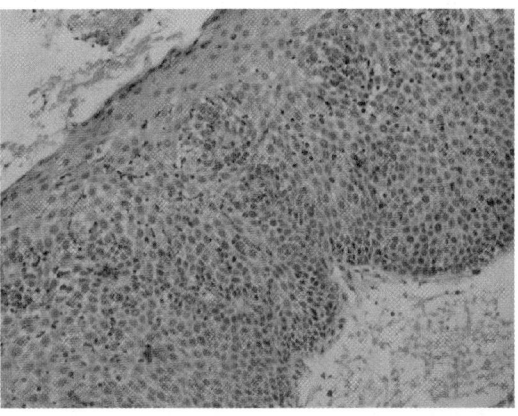

(a)

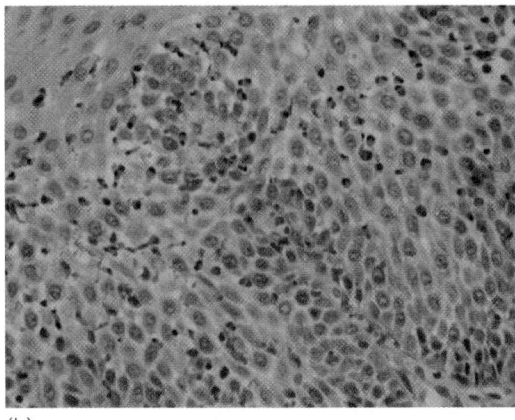

(b)

Fig. 15.7.4 Histopathological appearance of eosinophilic oesophagitis: Low power (a) and high power (b).
(Courtesy of Vicki Save, Lothian University Hospital, NHS Trust.)

Table 15.7.3 Common causes of medication-induced oesophagitis

Severe injury—high risk	Slow-release potassium chloride
	Aspirin and nonsteroidal anti-inflammatory drugs
	Doxycycline/tetracycline
	Quinidine
	Alendronate
	Potassium chloride
Less severe injury—high risk	Many antibiotics
	Iron supplements
Occasional injury	Ascorbic acid
	Mexiletine
	Slow-release theophylline
	Captopril
	Phenytoin
	Zidovudin
	Corticosteroids

move surprisingly slowly through the normal oesophagus especially at the level of the aortic arch. Defective oesophageal transport, poor pill design, increased mucosal susceptibility to injury, and poor pill-taking technique contribute to the problem. Medications known to have an especially high risk for oesophageal damage are listed in Table 15.7.3.

Symptoms are those for any form of stricture associated oesophagitis, and much pill-induced injury probably goes unrecognized. Injury at the distal oesophagus, the other common site of hold-up, may be commonly misdiagnosed as being due to reflux disease.

Medications and formulations with a high risk of injury should be identified and avoided if possible, especially in older patients with reflux disease or abnormal oesophageal transit. Pill transit is facilitated if medications are taken in the erect position with plenty of water. Pharmaceutical companies need to pay more attention to the use of shapes, sizes, and coatings that can assist transit of pills through the oesophagus. Stricturing may occasionally require surgery.

Caustic injury
See 'Caustic ingestion', below.

Primary oesophageal motor disorders
Idiopathic achalasia and achalasia-like states
Definition
These disorders are characterized by increased lower oesophageal sphincter tone, absence of lower oesophageal sphincter relaxation with swallowing, and impairment of peristalsis of the oesophageal body. Idiopathic achalasia, which was first described over 300 years ago, accounts for more than 95% of cases and has an annual incidence of approximately 1 to 2 per 100 000. It affects all ages, but is diagnosed most often in early to mid adult life. Primary familial achalasia, which is genetically transmitted accounts for less than 1% of cases.

There are a number of causes of secondary or pseudoachalasia. The most common are due to malignant infiltration of the gastro-oesophageal junction which has been reported with carcinoma of

the stomach, oesophagus, lung, pancreas, and prostate, and with lymphoma. It may also be a manifestation of paraneoplastic neural dysfunction. Chagas' disease is an important cause worldwide and can sometimes accompany the intestinal pseudoobstructive syndrome. There are a number of other secondary causes including oesophageal amyloidosis and sarcoidosis. Achalasia can also occur in associated with neurodegenerative diseases including Parkinson's disease and cerebellar ataxia.

Aetiology
Impairment of inhibitory neural control of the distal oesophagus is the universal abnormality. The clearest evidence is degeneration of myenteric inhibitory neurons which, in the early stages, is associated with an inflammatory response. There is increasing evidence that the resulting nitric oxide deficiency may be causative.

Symptoms
Dysphagia with solids is almost universal, but the symptoms may extend to include liquids and regurgitation is also prominent. The regurgitated material tastes bland because it never enters the stomach. Cramping chest pain occurs in some patients during an early hypercontracting phase of the disorder. Weight loss is seen in patients with disabling dysphagia. The course of symptoms over time is variable in contrast to the progressive symptoms in patients with a malignant cause. Over a prolonged period of a hypertonic lower oesophageal sphincter, continuing oesophageal dilatation may result with increasing regurgitation. When this occurs, respiratory problems secondary to aspiration can become a major feature.

Diagnosis
Idiopathic achalasia is diagnosed on average 2 years after its first presentation. Oesophageal manometry is the only sensitive method for demonstration of the characteristic motor dysfunction. It is not unusual for manometry to be diagnostic of achalasia even though barium studies have been judged to be normal. In advanced disease a barium swallow may reveal gross oesophageal dilatation with a gastro-oesophageal junction that tapers smoothly to a closed sphincter, with occasional spurts of flow into the stomach (Fig. 15.7.5).

As noted above, idiopathic achalasia and achalasia-like states should be distinguished from constriction of the gastro-oesophageal junction by an infiltrating or encasing malignancy at the cardia. This can be difficult to ascertain with certainty. If there are any grounds to suspect malignancy then an endoscopy should be performed including multiple biopsies from the gastro-oesophageal junction. CT scanning may also be helpful in these circumstances.

Treatment
There are three potential approaches to treatment: drug therapy with agents that relax the lower oesophageal sphincter, mechanical disruption of the sphincter by either pneumatic dilatation or surgical myotomy, and pharmacological poisoning of the remaining excitatory nerves to the sphincter with botulinum toxin. The results of reduction of lower oesophageal sphincter pressure with drugs such as calcium antagonists and β-adrenergic agonists compare poorly with mechanical techniques.

Oesophagomyotomy can now be performed as a laparoscopic or thoracoscopic procedure. It is highly effective but is associated with a 5 to 10% risk of troublesome gastro-oesophageal reflux. This risk can be minimized by the incorporation of an antireflux procedure.

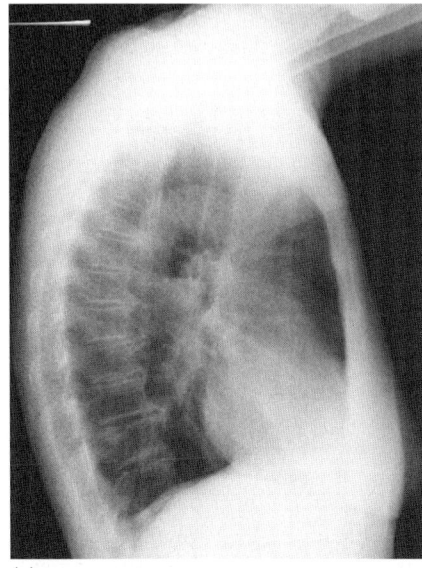

(a)

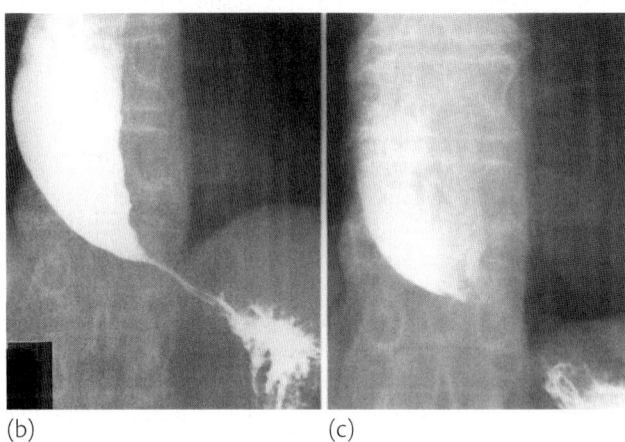

(b)   (c)

Fig. 15.7.5 Chest radiograph and barium studies from a case of advanced achalasia.

Balloon dilatation is an attractive approach because of its simplicity and low cost, but it often needs to be repeated and may fail in up to 40% of patients, especially those who are young. It also carries a risk of perforation of about 5%. With the development of minimally invasive surgery for oesophagomyotomy, balloon dilatation is generally reserved for older patients who have other medical problems that increase the risks of surgery.

Endoscopic injection of the sphincter with botulinum toxin acts on residual excitatory nerves, thereby lowering sphincter pressure. Short-term results are comparable to those of pneumatic dilatation but the procedure usually has to be repeated within 1 to 2 years. The toxin is also relatively expensive. It is a simple, low-risk procedure and most applicable to patients with significant coexisting morbidity which renders them unfit for dilatation or myotomy.

When oesophageal dilatation is present, prompt treatment is indicated because of the morbidity and poor therapeutic outcome associated with gross oesophageal dilatation.

Prognosis

Results are excellent if effective treatment is applied before the development of major dilatation, despite the persistence of major physiological abnormalities. Achalasia carries a significantly increased risk for oesophageal malignancy (squamous cell and, more recently appreciated, adenocarinoma) up to three decades later. The prevalence ranges from 2 to 7% (or a standardized incidence ratio of around 10) in the most comprehensive reports. There is no apparent reduction of this risk with treatment. It is not usual practice to undertake surveillance for this condition.

Diffuse oesophageal spasm

Definition

Episodic chest pain and/or dysphagia resulting from abnormal contractions of the distal half of the oesophageal body in the absence of any precipitating structural stenosis. There are no generally agreed criteria for diagnosis.

Aetiology

The aetiology of this disorder is poorly understood. Stress is an unlikely primary precipitant but may exacerbate the problem. Good prevalence data are lacking but it affects all age groups.

Symptoms

Virtually all patients have episodic, crushing central retrosternal pain which can be excruciating and may be misinterpreted as cardiac ischaemia. Intermittent dysphagia occurs in about two-thirds of patients and leads to temporary abandonment of eating until symptoms abate. Episodes of oesophageal obstruction usually last for approximately 30 min but can last for several hours. In most patients, symptomatic episodes occur less than once a month but in severe cases these may occur several times a week, or each time food intake is attempted.

Diagnosis

Due to the intermittent nature of the problem investigations may be normal. Most frequently the diagnosis is made on the basis of the history and the exclusion of other problems that may mimic diffuse oesophageal spasm such as myocardial ischaemia and a Schatzki ring (see below). Oesophageal manometry may show intermittent, simultaneous, prolonged, and vigorous oesophageal contractions interspersed with normal swallow-induced peristalsis. Relaxation of the lower oesophageal sphincter is normal thus excluding achalasia as a cause. 24-h ambulatory manometry may improve diagnostic accuracy by increasing the likelihood of capturing symptomatic episodes.

Barium swallow may show trapping of contrast beads in the distal oesophagus—the 'corkscrew oesophagus'—or sustained obliteration of the distal oesophageal lumen. This is not the investigation of choice.

Treatment

There is no specific therapy. Smooth muscle relaxants such as nitrites, nitrates (given as sublingual spray), and calcium antagonists may reduce symptoms but their use is often limited by side effects. In many patients, reassurance is the most important management since the intensity and nature of symptoms gives rise to great concern. Opiate therapy is sometimes necessary. In the rare case of frequent, disabling spasm oesophagomyotomy can give good relief.

Prognosis

The major significance is impairment of quality of life and concern about life-threatening cardiac disease. There is no consistent progression over time. There are several reports of progression of diffuse oesophageal spasm to achalasia but in most of these it seems likely that achalasia was initially misdiagnosed as diffuse oesophageal spasm.

Hypertensive peristalsis or nutcracker oesophagus

Definition

This is defined purely by the manometric demonstration of primary peristaltic pressure waves in the oesophageal body that have peaks in excess of 250 mmHg in a symptomatic patient (Fig. 15.7.6). There is preservation of the normal peristaltic pattern with a broad progression of the time of onset of the contraction wave in the oesophageal body.

Aetiology

It is not clear if this is a true motor disorder or whether it represents the upper end of a continuum of peristaltic wave amplitudes. It has been shown to vary over time within individuals. There are indications that psychological factors can influence peristaltic amplitude. A minority of patients with hypertensive peristalsis also experience episodes of diffuse oesophageal spasm, suggesting that their underlying dysfunction may be related and involve neural control mechanisms.

Symptoms

The only clinical significance of hypertensive peristalsis is its relationship to noncardiac chest pain. Hypertensive peristalsis alone does not produce dysphagia or derangement of oesophageal transit, because, by definition, peristalsis is preserved.

Treatment and prognosis

These are discussed in the section on noncardiac chest pain.

Nonspecific oesophageal motor disorders

Definition

These are departures from normal patterns of oesophageal motor function which do not actually define specific diseases, but which are of clinical significance. These are separate from oeosphageal dysmotility arising in association with diseases such as gastro-oesophageal reflux disease, diabetes, and other autonomic neuropathies. Nonspecific oesophageal motor disorder is the commonest single functional diagnosis made in most oesophageal manometric laboratories.

Aetiology

There are likely to be several mechanisms involved. The intermittent occurrence of dysfunctions suggests that they are due to defective neural control.

Symptoms

Swallow-induced distal oesophageal body contraction waves with multiple peaks stand out from the other patterns not only functionally but also symptomatically. This pattern is loosely associated with the hypercontraction disorders of diffuse oesophageal spasm and hypertensive peristalsis, but sometimes does not appear to have any clinical significance. Hypocontraction dysfunctions, recently termed 'ineffective' peristalsis, are associated with defective triggering and progression of both primary and secondary peristalsis. Failure to develop a propagated pressure wave of sufficient strength to maintain closure of the oesophageal lumen leads to deranged oesophageal transit. This probably explains the association of these disorders with mild intermittent dysphagia which occurs characteristically with solids. The nonobstructive dysphagia and slow oesophageal acid clearance seen in gastro-oesophageal reflux disease are due to such dysfunction. Secondary oesophageal body peristalsis has not yet been widely evaluated, but it is probably an important cause of intermittent dysphagia, since, at least in patients with nonobstructive dysphagia and reflux disease, dysfunction of secondary peristalsis is substantially more common than primary peristaltic dysfunction. Oesophageal manometry with an adequate number of recording points in the oesophageal body is the only sensitive means for diagnosis.

Treatment

In most cases patients seek reassurance and an explanation about the origin of their symptoms. Prokinetic agents may improve triggering and amplitude of peristaltic contractions and so, theoretically, of transit. Secondary peristaltic dysfunction may be more troublesome, but there is no good information on the effect of prokinetic or other drugs on this.

Prognosis

These dysfunctions do not remit spontaneously. Patients are often helped by the measures outlined in the section on general management of oesophageal dysphagia, which minimize the demands on oesophageal transport mechanisms and provide propulsive forces that substitute for oesophageal contractions.

Noncardiac chest pain

Definition

Implicit in this rather circuitous and negative label is the view that this pain has a cardiac-like quality, but there is no evidence for a cardiac origin. The oesophagus is the next most likely origin, but it is unlikely that all such pain arises from the oesophagus.

Aetiology

Evidence for triggering of pain by reflux or oesophageal motor dysfunction has been found in between one-fifth and one-half of patients evaluated. Oesophageal mucosal pain due to gastro-oesophageal reflux is the most common and helpful diagnosis.

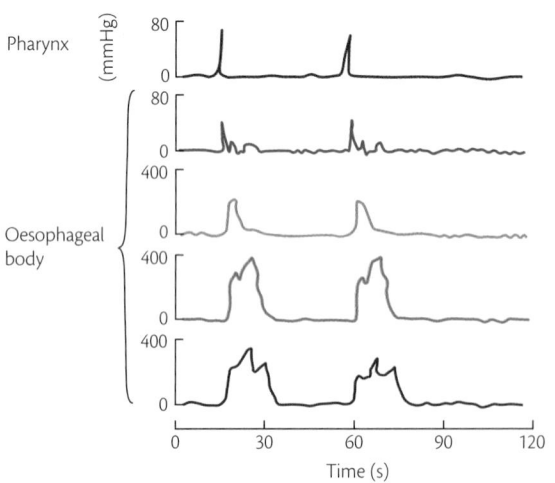

Fig. 15.7.6 Oesophageal manometric tracing in a patient with hypertensive peristalsis.

Frank oesophageal spasm associated with achalasia and diffuse oesophageal spasm is an unusual but convincing cause of noncardiac chest pain. In the majority of patients, most episodes of pain occur independently of reflux and any motor abnormality, although many of these patients have nonspecific oesophageal motor disorders or hypertensive peristalsis (see above). Sustained contraction of the longitudinal muscle has been identified by prolonged intraluminal ultrasonography in association with a high proportion of episodes of pain. Nevertheless, in many patients noncardiac chest pain appears to be a primary oesophageal hypersensitivity disorder and any motor disorder may be an epiphenomenon. Recent work to understand the neurophysiological basis for the hypersensitivity suggests that there may be distinct phenotypic subclasses of disease based on enhanced afferent transmission defects vs heightened secondary cortical processing.

Symptoms

By definition, the pain resembles cardiac pain in its sensation and distribution. It can be very intense and distressing, can disturb sleep, and may be worse during periods of emotional stress. Postprandial occurrence, in association with heartburn, suggests that it may be caused by reflux. When pain is associated with dysphagia, vigorous achalasia or oesophageal spasm are very possible.

Diagnosis

Myocardial ischaemia should first be excluded as the cause. Endoscopy should then be performed followed by oesophageal pH and motility studies when symptoms are disabling. Investigation can be unrewarding.

Treatment

Reassurance is essential to prevent repeated hospital admissions for fear of a cardiac cause. If the pain is triggered by gastro-oesophageal reflux, high-level acid-suppression therapy should be tried (see section on gastro-oesophageal reflux disease). Achalasia and diffuse oesophageal spasm should be treated on their own merits. In patients with no clear cut diagnosis, treatment with anxiolytics and antidepressants has been found to be moderately effective. Agents that reduce the strength of oesophageal contraction, such as calcium antagonists, appear ineffective in hypertensive peristalsis.

Oesophageal motor disorders secondary to systemic disease

Oesophageal motility may be affected by a number of systemic diseases (Table 15.7.4). These diseases may affect the striated or smooth muscle itself or the neural control.

The division of the oesophageal musculature into striated and smooth muscle components is revealed clearly by the myopathic diseases that affect the oesophageal musculature. In patients with peripheral myopathy this would normally have already been diagnosed. Weak or absent oesophageal contraction in the affected segment has the expected adverse impact on oesophageal transit, with a pattern of symptoms similar to the hypocontraction states of nonspecific oesophageal motor disorders (see above). The management of these dysfunctions is along general lines (see section on general management of oesophageal dysphagia).

Table 15.7.4 Systemic diseases associated with disturbance to oesophageal symptoms

Systemic diagnosis	Oesophageal symptom(s)	Pathophysiology
Rheumatological disorders		
Systemic sclerosis (limited and diffuse types)	Dysphagia, heartburn, regurgitation, weight loss	Oesophageal dysmotility, lower oesophageal sphincter incompetence, oesophagitis, columnar lined oesophagus
Mixed connective tissue disease	Dysphagia	Oropharyngeal and body dysmotility
Sjögren's syndrome	Dysphagia	Xerostomia, oesophageal mucosal dryness
Polymyositis/dermatomyositis	Dysphagia, nasal regurgitation, aspiration	Oropharyngeal and body dysmotility
Systemic lupus erythematosus	Dysphagia, odynophagia	
Seronegative spondyloarthropathies	Dysphagia	
Rheumatoid arthritis	Dysphagia, odynophagia	Oesophageal body dysmotility, oesophageal vasculitis, atlantoaxial subluxation
Paget's disease		Atlantoaxial subluxation, oesophageal vasculitis, secondary amyloid, micrognathia
Neuromuscular disorders	Dysphagia, chronic aspiration, disordered phonation	
Myotonic dystrophy	Dysphagia	Oropharyngeal and oesophageal dysmotility
Myasthenia gravis	Dysphagia	Oropharyngeal and oesophageal dysmotility
Chronic intestinal pseudoobstruction	Dysphagia	Oesophageal dysmotility
Other disorders		
Vasculitic syndromes	Dysphagia, odynophagia, chest pain, haematemesis	Oesophageal vasculitis, ulcers, pharyngeal stenosis
Diabetes mellitus	Dysphagia	Oesophageal dysmotility
Alcohol abuse	Dsyphagia, odynophagia, heartburn	Oesophageal dysmotility, oesophagitis, varices and haematemesis
Infiltrative disorders (amyloidosis, sarcoidosis)	Dysphagia	Oesophageal dysmotility

Diseases of oesophageal smooth muscle

Systemic sclerosis (scleroderma)

Definition and aetiology

60% of cases are limited cutaneous scleroderma, previously called CREST (**c**alcinosis, **R**aynaud's syndrome, (o)**e**sophageal dysphagia, **s**clerodactyly, **t**elangiectasia) syndrome. The remaining 40% of cases are now termed diffuse cutaneous scleroderma, with widespread involvement of other organs apart from the skin. The timing of onset of symptoms from oesophageal involvement are very variable in relation to other manifestations but are sometimes the presenting complaint. Oesophageal muscle atrophy and fibrosis are the cardinal features, but neuropathic abnormalities may also contribute to dysfunction. Smooth muscle peristalsis and the tone of the lower oesophageal sphincter is feeble or absent (Table 15.7.4).

Symptoms

Troublesome reflux symptoms are the most common consequence of loss of function. The pattern of dysphagia resembles that seen in nonspecific oesophageal motor disorder (see above). If dysphagia is severe, peptic stricture should be excluded, as complete loss of oesophageal smooth muscle peristalsis rarely leads to disabling dysphagia.

Treatment

Reflux disease is frequently severe and should be managed by high-level medical therapy in order to prevent complications such as stricture (see above). Antireflux surgery is relatively contraindicated because of the poor propulsive function of the oesophageal body.

Other rheumatological disorders

A scleroderma-like picture of oesophageal dysfunction is sometimes seen in other connective tissue disorders such as mixed connective tissue disease. The smooth muscle segment is also involved in systemic myopathies including polymyositis–dermatomyositis and myotonic dystrophy. It should be remembered that in addition to effects on motility rheumatological disorders may also lead to oesophageal symptoms via a combination of effects including mucosal dryness and associated reflux disease (Table 15.7.4).

Other disorders

Abnormal oesophageal motility is common in diabetes mellitus, and may be a feature of amyloidosis, chronic alcoholism, and the pseudoobstructive syndrome. In these disorders, the disturbance is believed to be primarily due to dysfunction of neural control mechanisms.

Disorders of striated muscle

Involvement of the striated muscle segment of the oesophagus is rare and patients usually present with high dysphagia, often in association with oropharyngeal dysfunction (see Chapter 15.6). The inflammatory myopathies (dermatomyositis, polymyositis, and inclusion body myositis), the muscular dystrophies (myotonia dystrophica and oculopharyngeal dystrophy), and myasthenia gravis are the most common causes.

General management of oesophageal dysphagia

Symptomatic treatment of dysphagia is frequently necessary because of the limited options and efficacy of specific treatments for oesophageal disorders. Although these measures may appear obvious, this aspect of management is commonly neglected by both patient and physician.

Optimization of bolus consistency

Large particles of solid food may impact on strictures. Large boluses require greater propulsive force even in the absence of stricture, and may trigger oesophageal spasm. Boluses should therefore be small and, in some circumstances, reduced to semiliquid or liquid form. Poor dentition should be treated. In some patients, defects of oesophageal function may be so severe that the diet should be puréed. Consultation with a dietitian will assist patients in identifying and preparing suitable food and in maintaining nutrition.

Assistance with oesophageal transit

Liquids assist transit by reducing the viscosity of food and providing a pressure head in the oesophagus. Gas generated within the oesophageal body from effervescent drinks can act as a piston which displaces oesophageal contents into the stomach in the erect position and may be sufficient to overcome an achalasic sphincter. The value of gravity in assisting transit should never be forgotten. Patients with severely impaired oesophageal transit should be advised to swallow medications in the upright position and with plenty of water so as to avoid injurious contact of the oesophagus with potentially corrosive tablets.

Alternative/supplementary approaches to feeding

Rarely, the above measures fail to maintain nutrition. Percutaneous endoscopic gastrostomy should then be used.

Oesophageal neoplasms

The two most frequently occurring malignancies of the oesophagus are adenocarcinoma and squamous cell carcinoma, defined according to the histopathological characteristics. Occasionally mixed cell types are seen. Cure is only possible in the small minority (10–20%) of patients whose disease presents early. Several approaches are possible for palliation, although data are somewhat conflicting about the relative merits of each.

Oesophageal adenocarcinoma and tumours of the gastro-oesophageal junction

Definition

Over 80% of adenocarcinomas arising in the oesophagus occur in association with oesophageal columnar metaplasia, or Barrett's oesophagus (Fig. 15.7.7). In the cases with no co-incident Barrett's the oesophageal mucous glands or the adjacent gastric cardia mucosa are presumably the source of malignant change.

Aetiology

As discussed above, columnar oesophageal metaplasia occurs in the context of chronic gastro-oesophageal reflux disease usually manifest as heartburn symptoms. The incidence of oesophageal adenocarcinoma has increased rapidly in Western countries over the past 20 to 30 years, surpassing the incidence of squamous cell carcinoma in these populations. The disease has a male preponderance. An increase in the prevalence of reflux disease related to the rise in obesity and reduced prevalence of *Helicobacter pylori* infection, with consequent increase in gastric acid secretion, are plausible explanations.

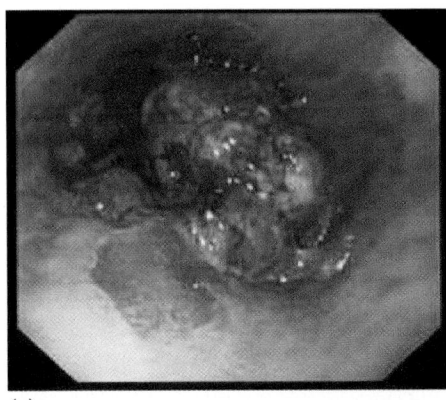

(a)

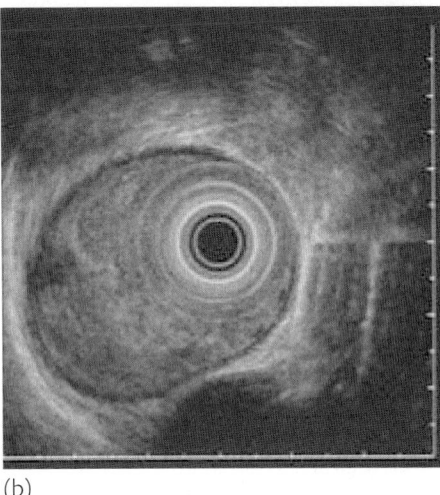

(b)

Fig. 15.7.7 Barrett's associated adenocarcinoma. (a) demonstrates the endoscopic view in which tongues of salmon pink columnar lined mucosa are seen extending beyond the exophytic tumour mass. (b) is the corresponding endoscopic ultrasound image of this case in which the tumour is seen to invade through the muscularis (T3).

Symptoms

Dysplasia and carcinoma *in situ* are asymptomatic. Inexorable progression of dysphagia to solids, and eventually to liquids, over several weeks is the almost universal presentation. Dysphagia usually occurs only when the tumour has become circumferential or bulky. Sometimes, malignant mucosal ulceration presents with pain. Substantial weight loss has often occurred by the time of presentation.

Endoscopy and biopsy is the first investigation of choice. The lesion may be stricturing or exophytic. Multiple biopsies should be taken to avoid a missed diagnosis due to sampling bias. In stricturing lesions, dilatation for diagnostic purposes should be avoided if possible due to the risk of perforation. Biopsies can usually be taken from the proximal portion of the stricture even if intubation is limited. Brush cytology may be a useful adjunct to diagnosis but biopsies are preferable to confirm invasion. If performed, a barium swallow typically reveals a stricture with an irregular, lobulated mucosal outline. However, it is important to note that occasionally the barium appearance mimics a benign peptic stricture.

Occasionally, an asymptomatic oesophageal carcinoma is diagnosed when endoscopy is done for some other reason. Early lesions arising in Barrett's mucosa may be inconspicuous endoscopically or be associated with a nodule or ulcer.

Staging

Staging using the TNM system is essential for all patients fit for radical therapy in order to optimize management. The staging criteria of gastro-oesophageal junction tumours will depend on whether the cancer is thought to arise primarily in the oesophagus or proximal stomach. CT scanning is very useful to determine nodal status and the presence of any distant metastases which most commonly affect the liver, lungs, adrenal glands and peritoneum. In order to obtain the best views the stomach should be distended with water before scanning (Fig. 15.7.8). In the absence of metastatic disease on the CT scan, endoscopic ultrasound should be performed to determine the degree of invasion through the oesophageal wall (T stage) (see Fig. 15.7.7). Paraoesophageal lymph

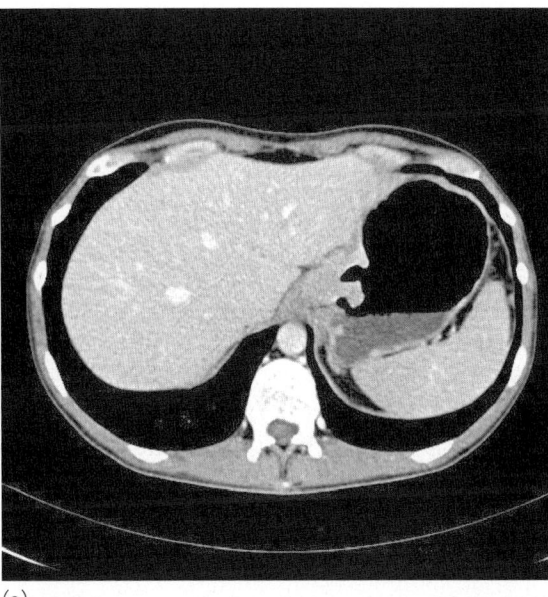

(a)

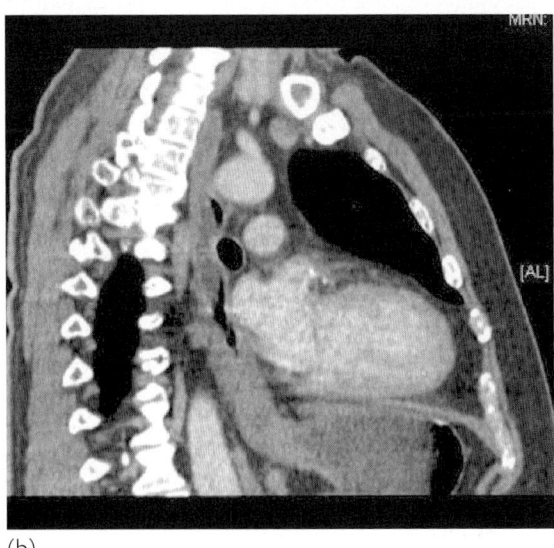

(b)

Fig. 15.7.8 (a) Transaxial CT staging of a type 3 tumour of the gastro-oesophageal junction (primarily within the proximal stomach and extending into the oesophagus). (b) Reformatted view of a gastro-oesophageal junction tumour with extensive involvement of lower oesophagus extending into the proximal stomach with proximal oesophageal dilatation.
(Courtesy of Dr Nicholas Carroll, Consultant Radiologist, Addenbrooke's Hospital Cambridge.)

nodes can also be assessed and sampled if necessary using fine needle aspiration. Positron emission tomography can provide further information on whether lymph nodes are involved and to characterize distant spread. Ideally this is now increasingly performed in combination with CT (CT-PET). Bronchoscopy or thoracoscopy can be useful to look for signs of airway infiltration in proximal disease.

Treatment

For disease limited to the mucosa, endoscopic therapy may be sufficient. In early stage disease extending into the submucosa and beyond surgery is the treatment of choice as it achieves high rates of cure. The surgical approach depends on the location of the tumour. A transthoracic approach is standard (Ivor Lewis) but other options such as a transhiatal operation have a lower morbidity if a less radical lymph node resection is required. If lymph nodes are involved (N1) or if the cancer is invading through the muscularis and into the adventitia (T3) then multimodal therapy is usually required. By the time the disease is stage T2, it is usually associated with lymph node involvement. Multimodal therapy generally involves neo-adjuvant chemotherapy which in some cases is combined with radiotherapy prior to surgery. The precise algorithm will depend on the details of the individual case and the local expertise. Combined modality therapies have significant morbidity and mortality and an expert multidisciplinary approach, which takes into account quality of life issues for the patient, is required to achieve the best results.

When curative treatment is not possible, palliation of dysphagia poses many challenges and the field is hampered by a lack of critical comparisons. Surgery is not a good palliative option because of its morbidity and mortality. Radiotherapy applied as external beam or internal brachytherapy can provide useful relief from dysphagia. There may, however, be a temporary worsening of symptoms due to mucositis and nasogastric feeding may be required over this period. Peroral dilatation of malignant strictures, except prior to stent insertion, should be avoided due to the risk of perforation. Peroral placement of stenting tubes (usually covered, to prevent tumour ingrowth), laser photocoagulation, argon plasma coagulation, injection of sclerosants and radiotherapy (external beam or brachytherapy) are all options for the management of dysphagia which have potential for improving the quality of life. Laser and injection therapies are most useful when there is an exophytic tumour component. Stent insertion has the advantage of being a once-only treatment with immediate effect, although pain after insertion can sometimes be a problem. Alternative endoscopic therapies can provide more physiological improvements in swallowing.

Oesophagopulmonary fistula is a distressing development which usually causes pneumonia and persistent cough and which can sometimes be controlled by stenting. Bleeding can be managed with radiotherapy, argon plasma coagulation, or laser.

Palliative chemotherapy can increase survival and help symptoms in carefully selected patients fit enough to withstand the treatment. Other critical aspects of palliative care include pain control as well as nutritional advice and support (e.g. oral supplements) which are best done within the context of an expert multidisciplinary team.

Prognosis

This remains dismal except where screening programmes identify early, asymptomatic cases. In patients presenting with symptomatic disease only about one-quarter of patients are deemed to be potentially curable by surgery, and the overall 5-year survival rate is approximately 13%.

Squamous cell carcinoma

Squamous cell carcinoma has marked geographical variation. It is common in the developing world with an annual incidence of 6 in 100 000 men and 1.6 in 100 000 women. There are areas of especially high incidence (northern China, northern Iran, Kazakhstan, and the Transkei region of South Africa with >35/100 000 cases per year). Its incidence is stable in Western countries where it is six times more common in black men than in white men.

Aetiology

The striking geographical variation in incidence suggests a major aetiological contribution from environmental factors. The risk factors include heavy alcohol use, tobacco, and dietary factors including high rates of consumption of nitrosamines and aflatoxins. Other factors implicated are previous treatment for head and neck cancers, Plummer Vinson syndrome, human papilloma virus infection, vitamin A deficiency, chronic candida infection, injury to the oesophageal mucosa due to ingestion of a corrosive substance years previously, and chronic irritation from oesophageal retention in achalasia. Invasive carcinoma is preceded by mucosal dysplasia and carcinoma *in situ* and there may be a lag phase of many years which affords the possibility for screening in high-risk regions. Some patients may be genetically predisposed to this cancer. The best-documented example is tylosis, which is an autosomal dominant condition with associated palmar and plantar hyperkeratosis. Linkage studies suggest that the causative gene resides on chromosome 17q25.

Symptoms and staging

The presentation and investigation algorithms for squamous cell carcinoma are essentially as described for adenocarcinoma. Patients may present to the ear, nose and throat department if the dysphagia is very high or if hoarseness is a key symptom. Orolaryngsocopy may reveal the cause but flexible oesophagoscopy is usually required.

In very high-risk areas screening programmes have been set up which generally hinge on cytological sampling methods using either standard endoscopy or nonendoscopic balloons and mesh catheters. Lugol's iodine spray can be very useful to highlight dysplastic mucosa and newer endoscopic techniques such as narrow band imaging can be a useful aid to diagnosis (Fig. 15.7.9).

Treatment

The treatment is essentially similar for all oesphageal malignancies. Squamous carcinomas are generally more radiosensitive than adenocarcinomas and radiotherapy can be given as definitive treatment either alone or combined with chemotherapy. The standard multimodal therapy generally involves neo-adjuvant chemotherapy, with or without radiotherapy, before surgery. Again the precise algorithm will depend on the details of the individual case and the local expertise. Unfortunately, for many patients palliative therapy is all that can be offered. Critical aspects of palliative care include pain control as well as nutritional advice and support (e.g. oral supplements) which are again best done within the context of an expert multidisciplinary team.

Prognosis

As for adenocarcinoma this remains dismal except where screening programmes identify early, asymptomatic cases. The overall 5-year survival rate is less than 20%.

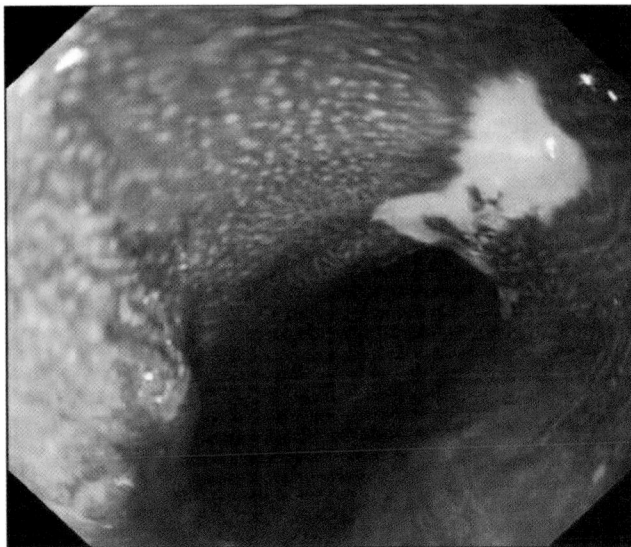

(a)

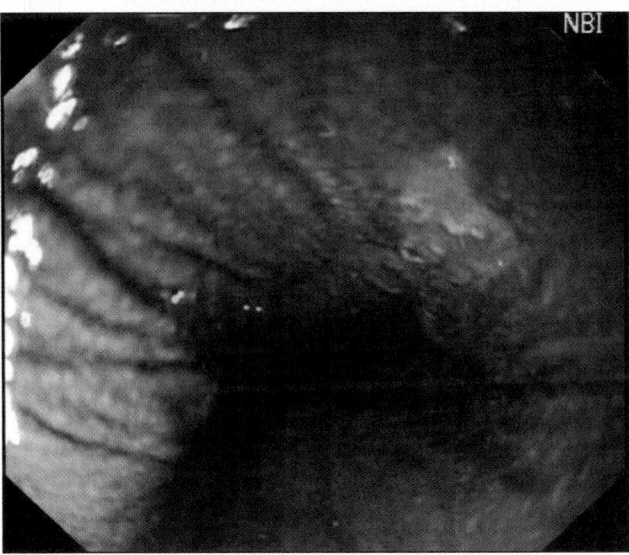

NBI

(b)

Fig. 15.7.9 Lugol's iodine spray reveals early squamous cell carcinoma as seen by white light (a) and with narrow-band imaging (b).
(Courtesy of Mr Peter Safranek, Consultant Upper Gastrointestinal Surgeon, Addenbrooke's Hospital, Cambridge.)

Other primary oesophageal tumours

Other primary malignant tumours are rare and all have a poor prognosis. These include malignant melanoma, lymphoma, carcinoid, leiomyosarcoma, neuroendocrine carcinoma (small-cell carcinoma), adenoid cystic carcinoma, and pseudosarcoma reflecting the cell types present within the oesophagus. These tumours show a mixture of polypoid and infiltrating features and are usually only clearly distinguished from the more common malignancies by histology.

Although rare in the oesophagus, gastrointestinal stromal tumours (which were previously classified as smooth muscle tumours) are the most common benign oesophageal tumour although they may have malignant potential. Approximately one-half of patients are asymptomatic and the remainder exhibit symptoms which may include dysphagia, retrosternal chest pain, pyrosis, cough, odynophagia, and weight loss. Bleeding is unusual,

in contrast to gastric gastrointestinal stromal tumours. They are usually intramural but can become pedunculated and they usually only cause symptoms if they are very large, or on a long pedicle. On endoscopy the mucosa is intact but there may be central umbilication or ulceration. Because of the submucosal nature of the lesion biopsy is often negative and endoscopic ultrasonography is a useful diagnostic tool which can be combined with fine needle aspiration. The majority have a gain of function mutation of the protooncogene growth factor receptor c-kit. The malignant potential is determined by the size and mitotic index. Most small lesions do not require treatment. Surgery should be considered in symptomatic patients or when the risk of malignant transformation is high. Treatment with a tyrosine kinase inhibitor can be useful for metastatic disease.

Other benign intramural tumours of the oesophagus include lipomas and granular cell tumours. The main risk of these is that they are mistaken for malignant tumours and operated on inappropriately.

Squamous cell papillomas of the mucosa can mimic a polypoid squamous carcinoma and so should be removed endoscopically for histological diagnosis.

Abnormalities of oesophageal anatomy

Non-neoplastic abnormalities which distort oesophageal anatomy may interfere with normal function or may merely pose difficulties in the interpretation of findings.

Sliding hiatus hernia

Definition

Around 90% of hiatus hernias are of this type, in which the gastro-oesophageal junction is displaced upwards into the thorax, giving a simple shaped pouch of intrathoracic stomach. This can be mistaken for a columnar-lined oesophagus unless the anatomical landmarks are clearly defined. These landmarks include the proximal extent of the gastric folds and the pallisading of vessels in the squamous oesophagus.

Aetiology

The phreno-oesophageal ligament is effaced in sliding hiatus hernia, but it is not clear whether this is a primary defect of gastric anchorage.

Symptoms

Many patients with hiatus hernia are asymptomatic. Despite this, physiological studies indicate that herniation of the gastro-oesophageal junction impairs its function as an antireflux barrier by removing the normal diaphragmatic crural compression from the lower oesophageal sphincter. Thus, hiatus hernia can be taken as a risk factor for reflux disease, but not an abnormality that makes the diagnosis.

Treatment

Symptoms of gastro-oesophageal reflux are the only ones of major significance. These should be treated along conventional lines (see gastro-oesophageal reflux disease).

Prognosis

This is essentially that of any associated reflux disease.

Rolling or para-oesophageal hiatus hernia

Definition

A variable part of the stomach herniates through the hiatus alongside a normally situated gastro-oesophageal junction. This pattern of herniation may produce a gross disturbance of gastric anatomy, usually with a narrow exit from the herniated pouch into the main stomach cavity. Some rolling hernias are also associated with displacement of the gastro-oesophageal junction above the hiatus, in which case these are known as mixed hernias.

Symptoms

Obstruction and distension of the pouch causes upper abdominal discomfort and can progress to strangulation. Gastric volvulus can occur because of the laxity of the gastric anchorage and may obstruct the gastro-oesophageal junction. Both of these problems have a very high mortality and demand urgent surgery. It is controversial whether elective surgery should be performed to reduce and anchor rolling hiatus hernias in order to remove these risks.

Prognosis

Unfortunately, there are no adequate data on the degree of risk associated with rolling hiatus hernia.

Schatzki ring (B ring)

Definition

This is a characteristic short luminal stenosis which occurs at the gastro-oesophageal junction. It is made up only of mucosa and submucosa, and may narrow the lumen to a few millimetres or cause a clinically insignificant minor indentation.

Aetiology

This is unknown. They have been postulated to be congenital although evidence now suggests that they can occur in later life. Reflux and pill oesophagitis have been implicated.

Symptoms

With mechanically significant rings, intermittent dysphagia occurs on eating solids. Meat is often the culprit, leading to the common term of 'steakhouse syndrome'. Episodes of bolus obstruction are not unusual, with associated chest pain caused by powerful oesophageal contractions. Failure to recognize a Schatzki ring frequently leads to the incorrect diagnosis of primary diffuse oesophageal spasm. Endoscopy is the investigation of choice (Fig. 15.7.10). If barium studies are performed adequate distal oesophageal distension during the barium swallow is essential for detection and this is best achieved by prone-oblique views.

Treatment

No treatment may be necessary. Disruption of the ring by simple peroral dilatation or endoscopic diathermy or laser is very rewarding, as the dysphagia and chest pain are cured, sometimes after many years of symptoms. However, there is a significant incidence of recurrence and repeated dilatations at intervals are often needed.

Other rings and webs

Other short oesophageal stenoses may develop because of peptic stricture, muscular rings, and cervical webs with iron-deficiency anaemia (Plummer–Vinson syndrome) or without.

Oesophageal diverticula and pseudodiverticula

Wide-mouthed multiple diverticula are characteristic of scleroderma oesophagus. In the nonsclerodermatous oesophagus diverticula occur in the mid and distal oesophagus, both types probably being 'blow-outs' secondary to hypercontraction motor disorders. These can become very large. It is rare for them to cause symptoms,

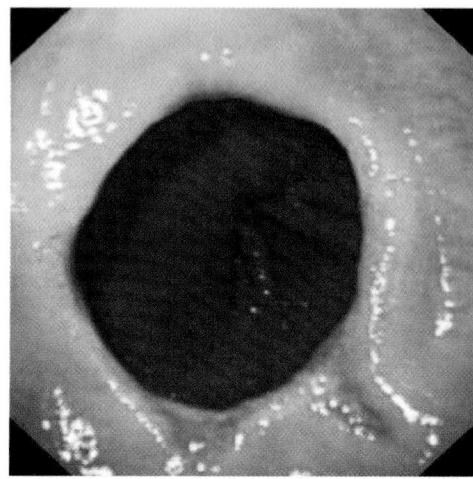

Fig. 15.7.10 Endoscopic appearance of a Schatzki ring.
(Courtesy of Dr Ewen Cameron, Consultant Gastroenterologist, Addenbrooke's Hospital, Cambridge.)

but they may be associated with dysphagia and regurgitation of retained contents. Unless symptoms are disabling, they are best left undisturbed because leakage is common following surgical removal.

Multiple intramural outpouchings of barium are characteristic of intramural pseudodiverticulosis which appears to be due to dilatation of the ducts of submucosal glands by an unknown process.

Extrinsic oesophageal compression

This is a relatively common cause of dysphagia, and is most often a result of malignant mediastinal lymphadenopathy. Barium swallow or endoscopy usually shows a relatively long constriction of the oesophageal lumen of variable calibre, associated with a normal mucosal appearance. Dilatation of such a compression is usually unrewarding because of its elastic recoil. Mechanically significant extrinsic compression may also result from an enlarged heart, a dilated or unfolded aorta, or an aortic aneurysm. Kyphosis may accentuate the mechanical impact of these abnormalities. Mechanical changes along the cervical spine can also interfere with swallowing such as atlantoaxial spurs, osteophytes associated with osteoarthritis, and Forestier's disease. In patients with rheumatoid arthritis atlantoaxial joint subluxation can lead to dysphagia and other signs of spinal cord compression (Table 15.7.4). Congenital vascular abnormalities can also compress the oesophagus in adults, an aberrant right subclavian artery being by far the most common.

Mechanical, chemical, and radiation trauma

Mallory–Weiss tear

These mucosal tears extend across the gastro-oesophageal junction and are normally induced by vigorous straining associated with vomiting. Bleeding is the only consequence of significance. In 10% of cases bleeding is severe enough to cause hypovolaemia. The history is usually quite characteristic, but definitive diagnosis requires endoscopy. Continued bleeding usually responds to endoscopic injection, electrocoagulation, vascular embolization, or vasopressin infusion. Very rarely, surgery is needed to under-run a persistently bleeding artery at the base of the tear.

Barogenic oesophageal rupture (Boerhaave's syndrome)

In this uncommon condition, straining and vomiting cause oesophageal rupture, most often in the left lower third of the oesophagus. High-volume spillage of the gastric contents into the pleural space causes shock and pain in the chest and upper abdomen with radiation to the back, left chest, or shoulder. The chest radiograph becomes abnormal only some hours after rupture. Surgical repair and drainage are usually necessary, and if this is delayed beyond 24 h the mortality is very high. Unfortunately, diagnostic delay is not unusual.

Iatrogenic oesophageal perforation

Physicians encounter this problem most often as a result of their involvement in dilatation of oesophageal strictures, pneumatic bag dilatation for achalasia, or through problems with the management of oesophageal varices by balloon tamponade. Even with meticulous technique and appropriate equipment, oesophageal perforation can occur. Perforation is strongly suggested by development of chest or epigastric pain directly after instrumentation, sometimes with dyspnoea. Pneumothorax and surgical emphysema are diagnostic. Any suspicion of perforation should be acted upon by taking a chest radiograph which should be repeated in several hours if it is negative. Broad-spectrum antibiotics should be given on suspicion, as they are most effective in minimizing the risks of mediastinitis when given from the outset. Surgical consultation should occur promptly; the choice between conservative and surgical management needs to be individualized. Increasingly, instrumental perforation is being managed nonsurgically with nasogastric suction, antibiotics, and intravenous nutrition with good results, primarily because instrumental injury usually occurs when the stomach is empty.

Caustic ingestion

Definition and aetiology

Strong acids and alkalis are both very damaging to the oesophagus and are found in high concentrations in many agents commonly used in the household for cleaning and maintenance. Laryngeal and gastric injuries may overshadow oesophageal injury. Because of their relative lack of taste, alkaline solutions are more likely to be swallowed accidentally in large amounts. Alkaline injury is especially deep; acid tends to form a superficial coagulant, which limits penetration.

Symptoms

The severity and extent of injury are immensely variable and cannot be predicted accurately from estimates of the volume ingested. Around one-half of patients with a history of caustic ingestion have no significant injury. Oropharyngeal and laryngeal injury confirm caustic ingestion and can be a major threat to the airway, but do not predict the existence and severity of oesophageal injury which causes odynophagia, dysphagia, or haematemesis. Prompt fibreoptic panendoscopy appears to be safe. This may be normal or show only patchy mucosal oedema, erythema, and small haemorrhagic ulcers, indicative of superficial damage with a good prognosis. Extensive and circumferential ulceration, and grey or brown/black ulceration suggest transmural injury.

Treatment

Patients with severe injury must be observed closely for signs of perforation. Nasogastric suction should be used with the administration of broad-spectrum antibiotics as these appear to reduce the severity of infective complications. The use of steroids is controversial, the balance of evidence tending to oppose their use. Oesophageal stricture is to be expected with severe injury and appears not to be prevented by routine dilatation in the first 2 weeks after injury. A barium study should be done at 2 to 3 weeks to screen for stricturing, and then subsequently at about 3-monthly intervals thereafter for a year, so that the development of stricturing is recognized at a stage when dilatation may have some impact.

Prognosis

The main short- to medium-term risk is the development of stricture. Caustic strictures are difficult and hazardous to treat by peroral dilatation so that about half of patients require oesophageal resection. In the long term (average onset 40 years after injury) carcinoma of the oesophagus is a major hazard, the risk being 1000 to 3000 times the expected risk.

Chemotherapy-induced oesophageal problems

Chemotherapy causes oesophageal problems in several ways. Therapy may impair mucosal defences by affecting cell turnover leading to 'mucositis'. This in turn may reduce resistance of the mucosa to damage from other agents, and increase susceptibility to infective oesophagitis from immune suppression. Oesophageal transit and acid clearance may be impaired through the neurotoxic effects of some agents. Fistulation or perforation may occur through cytotoxic effects on a malignancy in the oesophageal wall. It has been reported that combination chemotherapy is associated with the development of oesophageal columnar metaplasia in women being treated for breast cancer.

Other non-neoplastic mucosal diseases

Skin and systemic diseases associated with lesions of the oropharynx may also involve the oesophagus. These include epidermolysis bullosa, Behçet's disease, lichen planus, pemphigus vulgaris, bullous pemphigoid, benign mucous membrane (cicatrial) pemphigoid, and drug-induced disease (Stevens–Johnson syndrome and toxic epidermal necrolysis).

Chronic, and less frequently acute, graft vs host disease may cause severe oesophageal problems through mucosal desquamation or mural damage. Resultant stricturing shows considerable variation in appearance. Rarely, Crohn's disease can cause indolent, craggy ulceration and/or stricturing. Oesophageal sarcoidosis can mimic Crohn's disease.

Further reading

Armstrong D, *et al.* (2005). Canadian Consensus Conference on the management of gastroesophageal reflux disease in adults—update 2004. *Can J Gastroenterol*, **19**, 15–35.

Boeckxstaens GE (2007). Achalasia. *Best Pract Res Clin Gastroenterol*, **21**, 595–608.

Clouse R, Diamant N (2006). Motor function of the esophagus. In: Johnson L (ed.) *Physiology of the gastrointestinal tract*, 4th edition. Elsevier, Boston, MA.

Cowgill SM, *et al.* (2007). Ten-year follow up after laparoscopic Nissen fundoplication for gastroesophageal reflux disease. *Am Surg*, **73**, 748–52; discussion 752–3.

Curvers WL, *et al.* (2008). Endoscopic tri-modal imaging for detection of early neoplasia in Barrett's oesophagus; a multi-centre feasibility study using high-resolution endoscopy, autofluorescence imaging and narrow band imaging incorporated in one endoscopy system. *Gut*, **57**, 167–72.

Ellis FH Jr. (1998). Long esophagomyotomy for diffuse esophageal spasm and related disorders: an historical overview. *Dis Esophagus*, **11**, 210–14.

Enzinger PC, Mayer RJ (2003). Esophageal cancer. *N Engl J Med*, **349**, 2241–52.

Falk GWM, Fennerty B, Rothstein RI (2006). AGA Institute technical review on the use of endoscopic therapy for gastroesophageal reflux disease. *Gastroenterology*, **131**, 1315–36.

Fitzgerald RC (2006). Molecular basis of Barrett's oesophagus and oesophageal adenocarcinoma. *Gut*, **55** (12), 1810–20.

Fitzgerald RC, Triadafilopoulos G (1997). Esophageal manifestations of rheumatic disorders. *Semin Arthritis Rheum*, **26**, 641–66.

Furuta GT, *et al.* (2007). Eosinophilic esophagitis in children and adults: a systematic review and consensus recommendations for diagnosis and treatment. *Gastroenterology*, **133**, 1342–63.

Galmiche JP, *et al.* (2006). Functional esophageal disorders. *Gastroenterology*, **130**, 1459–65.

Hobson AR, *et al.* (2006). Neurophysiologic assessment of esophageal sensory processing in noncardiac chest pain. *Gastroenterology*, **130**, 80–8.

Jones R, Bytzer P (2001). Review article: acid suppression in the management of gastro-oesophageal reflux disease—an appraisal of treatment options in primary care. *Aliment Pharmacol Ther*, **15**, 765–72.

Kahrilas PJ, Ghosh SK, Pandolfino JE (2008). Challenging the limits of esophageal manometry. *Gastroenterology*, **134**, 16–18.

Lagergren J, *et al.* (1999). Symptomatic gastroesophageal reflux as a risk factor for esophageal adenocarcinoma. *N Engl J Med*, **340**, 825–31.

Mainie I, *et al.* (2006). Acid and non-acid reflux in patients with persistent symptoms despite acid suppressive therapy: a multicentre study using combined ambulatory impedance-pH monitoring. *Gut*, **55**, 1398–402.

Malfertheiner P, *et al.* (2005). Prognostic influence of Barrett's oesophagus and Helicobacter pylori infection on healing of erosive gastro-oesophageal reflux disease (GORD) and symptom resolution in non-erosive GORD: report from the ProGORD study. *Gut*, **54**, 746–51.

Matthews PJ, Aziz Q (2005). How useful are proton-pump inhibitors for diagnosis and therapy of patients with noncardiac chest pain? *Nat Clin Pract Gastroenterol Hepatol*, **2**, 506–7.

Mulhall BP, Wong RK (2003). Infectious Esophagitis. *Curr Treat Options Gastroenterol* **6** (1), 55–70.

Pandolfino JE, *et al.* (2006). Obesity: a challenge to esophagogastric junction integrity. *Gastroenterology*, **130**, 639–49.

Pandolfino JE, *et al.* (2006). Transient lower esophageal sphincter relaxations and reflux: mechanistic analysis using concurrent fluoroscopy and high-resolution manometry. *Gastroenterology*, **131**, 1725–33.

Pech O, *et al.* (2007). Endoscopic resection of early oesophageal cancer. *Gut*, **56**, 1625–34.

Rastogi A, *et al.* (2007). Incidence of esophageal adenocarcinoma in patients with Barrett's esophagus and high-grade dysplasia: a meta-analysis. *Gastrointest Endosc*, **67**, 394–8.

Ross WA, *et al.* (2007). Evolving role of self-expanding metal stents in the treatment of malignant dysphagia and fistulas. *Gastrointest Endosc*, **65**, 70–6.

Ruigómez A, *et al.* (2007). Endoscopic findings in a cohort of newly diagnosed gastroesophageal reflux disease patients registered in a UK primary care database. *Dis Esophagus*, **20**, 504–9.

Shaheen NJ, *et al.* (2009). Radiofrequency ablation in Barrett's esophagus with dysplasia. *N Engl J Med*, **360**, 2277–88.

Sharma P, *et al.* (2006). The development and validation of an endoscopic grading system for Barrett's esophagus: the Prague C & M criteria. *Gastroenterology*, **131**, 1392–9.

SIGN (Scottish Intercollegiate Guidelines network) (n.d.) *Management of oeosphageal and gastric cancer*. June 2006. http://www.sign.ac.uk

Spechler SJ (2007). Screening and surveillance for Barrett's esophagus—an unresolved dilemma. *Nat Clin Pract Gastroenterol Hepatol*, **4**, 470–1.

Vakil N, *et al.* (2006). The Montreal definition and classification of gastroesophageal reflux disease: a global evidence-based consensus. *Am J Gastroenterol*, **101**, 1900–20.

Zendehdel K, *et al.* (2007). Risk of esophageal adenocarcinoma in achalasia patients, a retrospective cohort study in Sweden. *Am J Gastroenterol*, **102**, 1–5.

Peptic ulcer disease

Joseph Sung

Essentials

Helicobacter pylori infection and the use of nonsteroidal anti-inflammatory drugs (NSAIDs) including aspirin are the most important causes of peptic ulcer disease. Cigarette smoking also increases the risk, but—although often alleged—there is little evidence to implicate psychological stress. Zollinger–Ellison syndrome, which consists of a gastrin-secreting islet cell tumour (gastrinoma) leading to marked hypergastrinemia, is a rare cause of recurrent peptic ulceration.

Peptic ulcer disease is characterized by a history of waxing and waning symptoms of localized, dull, aching pain in the upper abdomen. Bleeding is the most common complication. Free perforation of the stomach or duodenum into the peritoneal cavity is an uncommon but serious complication.

The diagnosis of peptic ulcer disease is made by endoscopy, which can (1) confirm the diagnosis of peptic ulcer; (2) offer an opportunity for biopsy of gastric ulcers, which may be malignant; and (3) reveal important prognostic indicators in patients with bleeding ulcers (Forrest classification: grade I ulcers are those with active bleeding; grade II have signs of recent bleeding; grade III have a clean base).

A single daily dose of a proton pump inhibitor gives quick relief of symptom and effective healing of peptic ulcers in 4 to 6 weeks. These drugs are more effective than misoprostol and H_2-receptor antagonists in healing ulcers, as well as in preventing further peptic ulcerations and erosions.

The management of patients with upper gastrointestinal haemorrhage requires a multidisciplinary medical and surgical approach.

Upper gastrointestinal bleeding stops spontaneously in about 80 to 85% of patients, but the remaining 15 to 20% continue to bleed or develop recurrent bleeding, and these patients constitute a high-risk group with substantially increased morbidity and mortality. Early risk stratification based on clinical and endoscopic criteria allows delivery of appropriate care, with endoscopic intervention (endoscopic injection, thermal coagulation, or mechanical haemostasis, i.e. clipping or banding) now widely accepted as the first line of therapy. This should be applied to actively bleeding ulcers or ulcers covered with an adherent clot to reduce both recurrent bleeding and the need for surgical intervention, and be followed by administration of a high dose of intravenous proton pump inhibitor to further reduce recurrent bleeding.

Treatment of *H. pylori* is a cure for peptic ulcer disease in most patients with the condition. Many antimicrobials can be effective, but successful cure usually requires at least two antimicrobial agents, with the most popular triple therapy combining a proton pump inhibitor with any two of amoxicillin, metronidazole, and clarithromycin for 7 to 14 days. Eradication of *H. pylori* can be confirmed by either urea breath test, stool antigen test, or biopsy urease test, which should be done at least 4 weeks after finishing the anti-helicobacter regimen and discontinuation of the proton pump inhibitor for at least 2 weeks.

Eradication of *H. pylori* infection, avoidance of high-dose NSAIDs or aspirin, and the maintenance use of proton pump inhibitors in high-risk individuals are the best ways to prevent recurrence of ulcer and ulcer complications.

Introduction

Peptic ulcer is defined as a distinct breach in the mucosa of the gastrointestinal tract as a result of caustic effects of acid and pepsin in the lumen. The term 'peptic ulcer disease' usually refers to ulceration of the stomach, duodenum, or both but it can also occur in the oesophagus in gastro-oesophageal reflux disease and in the distal ileum as a result of a Meckel's diverticulum lined with an acid-secreting gastric epithelium. Histologically, peptic ulcer is identified as necrosis of the mucosa extending through the muscularis

mucosae into the submucosa. In the endoscopic or radiological view, there is an appreciable depth of the lesion. When the break of epithelial lining is confined to the mucosa without penetrating through the muscularis mucosae, the superficial lesion is called 'erosion'.

For more than a century, peptic ulcer disease has been a major cause of morbidity and mortality. The Schwarz dictum introduced in 1910 says 'no acid, no ulcer', indicating that the presence of acid is essential for peptic ulceration. Indeed, peptic ulcers rarely develop in patients with achlorhydria. Thus the therapy has always been focused on acid neutralization or suppression of acid secretion. The discovery of *Helicobacter pylori* in the highly acidic environment by Marshall and Warren in 1984 has revolutionized the concept of ulcerogenesis. In many cases, peptic ulcer disease is an infectious disease which can be cured by a single course of antimicrobial therapy. In recent decades, however, there has been a rapid change in the epidemiology of peptic ulcer disease. With the improvement in sanitary conditions in many countries, there has been a dramatic decline in *H. pylori* infection and hence the associated peptic disease in the stomach and duodenum. On the other hand, with the increasing use of aspirin and nonsteroidal anti-inflammatory drugs (NSAIDs), a new epidemic of peptic ulcer disease and complications has arisen. Our understanding of peptic ulcer disease is not complete. With the decline of *H. pylori* infection, peptic ulcers emerge that are not related either to *H. pylori* or to NSAIDs.

Aetiology, pathogenesis, and pathology

Gastric acid and pepsin

Despite the importance of *H. pylori* infection and ulcerogenic drugs such as NSAIDs and aspirin as the initiating events in the development of peptic ulcer disease, gastric acid and pepsin remain the ultimate injurious factors in the development of peptic ulcers. Ulceration is a result of an imbalance between the damaging effects of acid and pepsin and the defensive effects of bicarbonate and mucin on the mucosal surface. Factors that may account for increased secretion of acid and pepsin include increased parietal cell mass, increased stimulation of acid secretion (e.g. gastrin), increased parietal cell sensitivity to stimuli, and attenuated inhibition of acid secretion (e.g. somatomedin). Patients with peptic ulcer disease often have higher parietal cell mass, leading to increased basal and nocturnal unstimulated acid output as well as peak acid output under stimulation by food and gastrin. Several of these abnormal physiological responses are probably related to *H. pylori* infection (hypersecretion of gastrin, raised basal and gastrin-releasing peptide-stimulated acid output, decreased inhibitory drive mediated by somatostatin and hypersecretion of pepsinogen) as they disappear after successful cure of *H. pylori* infection. It is known that even peptic ulcer disease induced by NSAIDs or aspirin is an acid-dependent process. In the low secretory state, NSAID and aspirin exposure are less likely to induce peptic ulcer in the upper gastrointestinal tract.

With high exposure to gastric acid, epithelium of the duodenal bulb develops gastric metaplasia. Wyatt and colleagues postulated that gastric metaplasia is essential for the colonization of *H. pylori* in the duodenum and subsequent development of duodenal ulceration. *H. pylori* is found colonizing only part of the duodenum with gastric metaplasia, setting off duodenitis and eventually duodenal ulcer. However, the data for the correlation of intragastric pH with occurrence of gastric metaplasia in the duodenum are inconsistent.

Duodenal bicarbonate secretion

Patients with duodenal ulcer are found to have impaired bicarbonate secretion in the proximal duodenum in face of influx of gastric acid. This impaired response is reversed by the eradication of *H. pylori*. The mechanism by which *H. pylori* hampers duodenal bicarbonate secretion is not understood. One proposed mechanism is that nitric oxide synthase activity in the duodenum interferes with bicarbonate secretion.

Helicobacter pylori

Since the discovery of *H. pylori* in the stomach of patients with gastritis and peptic ulcer, this bacteria has been reported in approximately 90% of cases of duodenal ulcer and 60% of cases of gastric ulcer. *H. pylori* is a slow-growing, microaerophilic, highly motile, Gram-negative spiral organism aetiologically linked to gastritis, peptic ulcer disease, gastric lymphoma, and adenocarcinoma of the stomach. *H. pylori* infection has a long latent period before symptomatic disease appears. *H. pylori* is tropic for gastric epithelium (i.e. stomach and areas of gastric metaplasia outside the stomach) and is found either attaching to the surface epithelium through a pedestal or dwelling within the mucous coating on the surface of gastric epithelium. A very small proportion of organisms can be found intracellularly, but the significance of this in relation to the inflammatory response and evasion of antimicrobial therapy is still under investigation. *H. pylori* infection elicits robust chronic active inflammatory and immune responses that continue throughout life. *H. pylori* produces abundant amount of urease, which is important for its colonization and survival in the stomach.

H. pylori infection is primarily acquired in childhood, such that the prevalence at the age of 20 approximates the prevalence of that birth cohort throughout life. Acquisition during adulthood is rare, with estimates ranging from 0.3 to 0.5% per year, and recurrence of infection after successful eradication is therefore uncommon. The primary mode of transmission is person to person, probably via a gastro-oral route (through vomitus) or oro-oral route (through contamination of saliva). There are links between the bacterial genotype, its virulence factor, and the development of gastroduodenal disease. CagA, a 120- to 140-kDa highly antigenic protein, is encoded by the *cagA* gene as part of the *cag* pathogenicity island. In Western countries 60 to 80% of *H. pylori* express CagA, compared to 90% of isolates from Asian patients. The presence of the *cag* pathogenicity island is associated with a more prominent inflammatory tissue response than is seen with strains lacking this virulence factor. This increase in inflammation is associated with an increased risk of developing of peptic ulcer disease and adenocarcinoma of the stomach. The *cag* pathogenicity island encodes a type IV secretory apparatus that injects CagA and possibly other bacterial proteins into mammalian cells. CagA undergoes phosphorylation in the cell and is responsible for the changes in actin polymerization seen in the infected cell, resulting in conformational change. Besides cytoskeletal changes, CagA also enhances inflammatory response which is mediated through NF-κB. Attachment of *H. pylori* to the cell is required for *cagA*-positive *H. pylori* to elicit an interleukin-8 (IL-8) response in the gastrointestinal epithelium triggering gastritis. Beside CagA, approximately 50% of *H. pylori* strains produce a protein that induces vacuole formation in eukaryotic cells. This protein, which is called VacA, has been purified and the gene *vacA* has bee cloned. The *vacA* gene has two families of alleles of the middle region (m1, m2) and at least three families of alleles of the signal sequence (s1a, s1b, s2). The *vacA* genotype s1 is strongly, but not exclusively, associated with the *cagA* gene. So far, studies have not found an important role for VacA in relation to histological findings, or risk of *H. pylori*-related disease. The function of VacA remains unclear.

Despite the establishment of a strong association between *H. pylori* infection and peptic ulcer disease, it is still unclear why

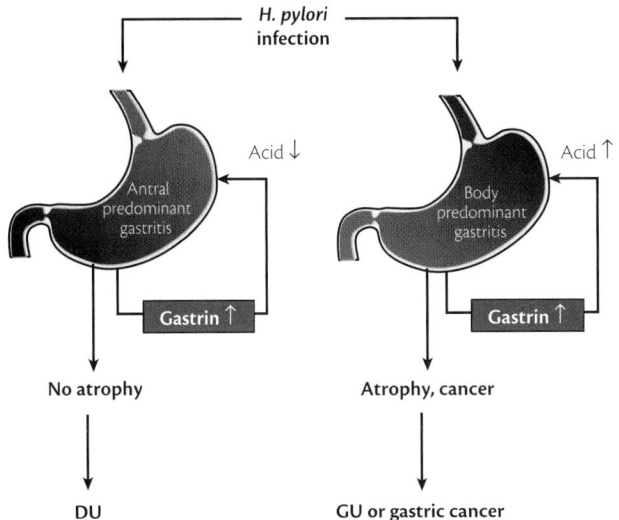

Fig. 15.8.1 Association between pattern of *H. pylori* gastritis and disturbance in gastric physiology. Antral-predominant gastritis is associated with duodenal ulcer (DU), body-predominant gastritis with gastric ulcer (GU) or cancer.
(Modified from McColl KEL, El-Omar E (2000). Mechanism involved in the development of hypochlorhydria and pangastritis in *Helicobacter pylori* infection. In: Hunt RH, Tytgat GNJ (ed) *Helicobacter pylori: basic mechanisms to clinical cure.* Kluwer, Dordrecht.)

some patients develop duodenal ulcer and others gastric ulcer. McColl and El-Omar proposed an intriguing paradigm (Fig. 15.8.1). In patients with duodenal ulcer, *H. pylori* colonizes mainly the antrum. The antral-predominant gastritis stimulates production of gastrin-releasing peptide, triggering secretion of gastrin leading to excessive output of gastric acid. Profuse amount of acid flooding in the duodenum leads to gastric metaplasia, which allows colonization of *H. pylori* in the duodenum. This sets up an intense inflammation in the duodenum, further weakening mucosal protection and eventually developing into duodenal ulcer. On the other hand, in patients with gastric ulcer, *H. pylori* is often found throughout the entire body of the stomach, leading to diffuse gastritis. The intense inflammation in the body of stomach tends to reduce gastric acid secretion as a result of glandular atrophy. In these patients other bacterial virulence factors come into play, leading to development of either gastric ulcer or adenocarcinoma in the distal stomach. Although this schema is probably oversimplified, it provides a broad-brush picture explaining how an infection can induce two distinctly different diseases.

The ultimate proof of causal relationship between *H. pylori* and peptic ulcer disease comes from interventional studies. If peptic ulcer disease is merely a result of altered gastric physiology in bacterial infection, eradication of *H. pylori* in the stomach and duodenum should rectify the physiological change and cure the disease. And, if re-infection with *H. pylori* is rare, peptic ulcer disease should not recur. Indeed, this has been proved in clinical trials. In a study that randomized duodenal ulcer patients to receive either 1-week bismuth triple therapy or bismuth triple therapy plus 4-week therapy with proton pump inhibitor, ulcers healed in 90 to 95% of cases with or without acid suppressive therapy. Similarly, when non-NSAID-related gastric ulcer was treated by 1-week bismuth triple therapy or 4-weeks proton pump inhibitor therapy, ulcer healing was higher with anti-*Helicobacter* therapy. More importantly, ulcer recurrence was much lower after patients

received anti-*Helicobacter* therapy with successful eradication than with a full course of proton pump inhibitor. Studies have also shown that peptic ulcer bleeding and bowel perforation does not recur, obviating the need for acid-reduction surgery.

Ulcerogenic drugs

In the last three decades, NSAIDs and antiplatelet agents have become increasingly important as a cause of peptic ulcer disease. It has been estimated that NSAIDs and aspirin increase the risk of gastric ulcer fourfold and the risk of gastrointestinal bleeding threefold. The risk of drug-induced peptic ulcer is substantially higher in older people and those with previous history of peptic ulcer disease. Patients who are taking concomitant NSAIDs, aspirin, anticoagulants and corticosteroids are also exposed to a higher risk of peptic ulcer disease. *H. pylori* infection further increases the risk of peptic ulcer and ulcer complication in users of NSAIDs and aspirin.

Aspirin and acidic NSAIDs were initially believed to have only a topical injurious effect by direct damage to the gastric epithelium as a result of intracellular accumulation of these drugs in an ionized state. However, the fact that enteric-coated formulations, prodrugs, and systemic administration of NSAIDs fail to reduce the frequency of gastroduodenal ulceration implies that the chief mechanism of injury might not be a local action. NSAIDs reduce the hydrophobicity of mucous gel on the intestinal epithelium and this may hamper the defensive mechanism of the gut. The most important mechanism of drug-induced peptic ulcer disease is inhibition of prostaglandin synthesis by NSAIDs. Prostaglandins regulate mucosal blood flow, epithelial cell proliferation, and basal acid secretion as well as mucus and bicarbonate secretion. The rate-limiting enzyme in prostaglandin synthesis is cyclooxygenase (COX). Most NSAIDs are found to suppress prostaglandin synthesis via reversible inhibition of COX, but aspirin acetylates COX and inhibits its enzyme activity irreversibly in a dose-dependent manner. In the early 1990s two structurally related COX isoforms, COX-1 and COX-2, were identified. COX-1 is found in most of the body's tissues, including the gastrointestinal tract and the kidney, and COX-2 is an inducible enzyme produced principally in inflammation. The discovery of these isoforms has prompted the development of COX-2 selective inhibitors as anti-inflammatory analgesics, with the aim of protecting against gastrointestinal damage. Yet this approach is an oversimplification, as evidence indicates that both COX-1 and COX-2 must be inhibited for gastric ulceration to occur. Selective suppression of COX-1 does not cause gastric damage. Clinical trials have shown that COX-2 selective inhibitors cause less peptic ulcer and ulcer bleeding than nonselective NSAIDs. Yet, in high-risk patients with a history of peptic ulcer disease, ulcer complication as a result of using COX-2 selective inhibitors is still a possibility.

Gastric acid exacerbates NSAID injury by disrupting the basement membrane to produce deep injury, impairing platelet aggregation and potentiating enzymatic erosion of pepsin. It is therefore logical that suppression of acid secretion by potent agents such as proton pump inhibitors can confer at least partially protection against injury induced by NSAIDs and aspirin.

More recently, attention has been focused on the role of nitric oxide in maintenance of intestinal mucosal blood flow. Like prostaglandins, nitric oxide has been shown to increase blood flow, stimulate mucin secretion, and inhibit neutrophil adherence.

It may thus protect the gastroduodenal tract against injury by aspirin and NSAIDs. Nitric oxide-releasing NSAIDs have been developed and found to produce less gastric damage than their parent drugs.

Tobacco, alcohol, and stress

Cigarette smoking increases the risk of peptic ulcer diseases and their complications. As with NSAID usage, tobacco decreases prostaglandin production and inhibits acid-stimulated bicarbonate secretion in the duodenum. Increase in gastric acidity, reduction in epithelial cell proliferation, and impairment of mucosal blood flow have also been demonstrated with consumption of tobacco. Cigarette smokers are found to have slower healing of peptic ulcers and higher relapse rate of the disease. However, when *H. pylori* is eradicated, the effects of tobacco appear to be mitigated.

It is a misconception that alcohol as such increases the risk of peptic ulcer disease. There are no convincing data in the literature supporting this notion. Although high concentrations of alcohol can cause damage to mucosa in animal studies, normal drinks such as wine and beer do not contain a high enough concentration of alcohol to cause ulceration in the stomach and duodenum. However, peptic ulcer disease is more common in liver cirrhosis and alcohol consumption is certainly one of the most important underlying causes of this condition. The mechanism of peptic ulcer development in cirrhosis remains to be elusive.

Psychological stress has always been implicated in peptic ulcer disease but there is little scientific evidence to confirm the correlation. After all, stress is difficult to measure and its effects are hard to assess. Historical records during natural disasters (e.g. earthquakes and tsunami) and wars report an upsurge of peptic ulcer disease. During peacetime, however, stress seldom reaches high enough levels to lead to peptic ulcers. However, hospitalized patients with multiple illnesses and critical medical conditions can develop peptic ulcer and complications such as bleeding. Stress related to serious medical conditions and multiorgan failure is likely to produce peptic ulcer bleeding and the mortality of these patients has been estimated to be 10 times higher than for those without comorbid illnesses.

Other causes

Zollinger–Ellison syndrome consists of a gastrin-secreting islet cell tumour (gastrinoma) leading to marked hypergastrinemia, outpouring of gastric acid, and recurrent peptic ulceration. Most cases of Zollinger–Ellison syndrome are sporadic but some are associated with multiple endocrine neoplasia syndrome type I (MEN-1). As well as peptic ulcer disease, these patients may complain of diarrhoea, steatorrhoea, symptoms of gastro-oesophageal reflux, weight loss, and other presentations of MEN-1 (e.g. hypercalcaemia and renal stones). The diagnosis is confirmed by finding a markedly raised serum gastrin level stimulated by secretin and radiological identification of tumour in the pancreas.

Beside *H. pylori*, other infections such as cytomegalovirus or *Helicobacter heilmannii* may lead to peptic ulcer disease. *H. heilmannii* has been found to cause intense inflammation in the stomach and occasionally peptic ulcers, especially in children. *Helicobacter felis*, a species that usually infects dogs and cats, has also been reported to cause peptic ulcer in pet owners.

Crohn's disease affects the whole gastrointestinal tract and may be a cause of peptic ulcer disease in the stomach, duodenum or even the oesophagus. With the rising incidence of Crohn's disease in Asia, peptic ulcers related to it are more commonly seen.

Epidemiology

It is hard to follow the temporal trend and geographical variation of peptic ulcer disease as the condition may not manifest itself in clinical settings. From records of peptic ulcer perforation, it has been suggested that this disease was uncommon before the 19th century. Over the ensuing decades, the incidence of peptic ulcer disease escalated. By the end of the 19th century, duodenal ulcer frequency had surpassed gastric ulcer disease in frequency. The incidence of peptic ulceration rose dramatically throughout the first half of the 20th century, and then started to decline again in the second half of the century. Thus peptic ulcer disease appears to follow the trend of urbanization. The temporal trends of frequency of peptic ulcer disease are best studied by following birth cohorts. In Western countries and in Japan, the risk of developing peptic ulcer disease rose in birth cohorts born before the turn of 20th century and then declined in subsequent generations.

In addition to changes in the prevalence of peptic ulcer disease over time, there is also evidence that it shows geographical variations. For example, it is more common in Scotland and northern England than in southern England. Similarly, ulcers are more common in the south of India than in the north. Environmental factors are likely to play an important role in the development of peptic ulcer disease. Human-to-human transmission of *H. pylori* in urban dwellers, improvement of sanitation in recent decades, and increased consumption of tobacco and analgesics might be important factors affecting the changing epidemiology of the disease.

The incidence of bleeding resulting from peptic ulcer disease is much better documented than uncomplicated peptic ulcers. Based on the American Society of Gastrointestinal Endoscopy survey and two large United Kingdom audits made available in the 1990s, the reported incidence of gastrointestinal bleeding is approximately 100 per 100 000 population. The national United Kingdom audit was a population-based, prospective collection of data on 4185 cases in 74 acute hospitals over a 4-month period. Acute upper gastrointestinal bleeding is a disease primarily affecting the older age groups. In this audit, 68% of patients were older than 60 years and 27% were more than 80 years of age. In comparison with historic British series, a steady rise in the incidence over the last few decades was observed. The crude mortality rate increased from 9.9% in the 1940s to 11% in the 1990s. It is often argued that advances in the care of patients with upper gastrointestinal bleeding have been offset by an ageing population. There has also been a trend towards increasing hospital admissions among older subjects and a corresponding decline for younger patients, resulting in little change in the overall admission rate. Hospital statistics from the United Kingdom Office of National Statistics revealed that from 1989 to 1999, admission rates for peptic ulcer haemorrhage increased among older people. Over this period, admissions increased by one-third among older women and by almost 50% among older men.

The epidemiology of peptic ulcer disease has changed in the last two decades. With the declining prevalence of *H. pylori* infection in the developed countries, the proportion of patients with ulcers attributed to the use of aspirin and NSAIDs as well as *H. pylori*-negative 'idiopathic' ulcers is on the rise. However, there is evidence suggesting that between 20% and 40% of peptic ulcers in North America are not associated with *H. pylori* infection or the use of NSAIDs. Is there truly a rise in non-*H. pylori*, non-NSAID ulcer, or does this merely reflects the declining trend of the disease and therefore a proportionate rise in idiopathic ulcers? The existing evidence suggests that the prevalence of these idiopathic ulcers is probably increasing. Two prospective cohort studies in Hong Kong, each lasting 1 year, looked at idiopathic ulcers in 1997–1998 and 2000–2001. The total number of bleeding peptic ulcers was more than 1500. Comparing the two time periods, the total number of bleeding ulcers per year had decreased by 33.1% and the number of *H. pylori*-associated ulcers by over 30%. On the other hand, the absolute number of idiopathic ulcers increased 4.5-fold. Patients suffering from idiopathic ulcers are older and sicker, and the ulcers more frequently developed after patients had been admitted to hospital for other medical conditions. Up to one-half of idiopathic ulcer patients have major medical conditions such as advanced cardiopulmonary or liver disease. Ulcer recurrence is higher in patients with idiopathic ulcers than for *H. pylori*-associated ulcers treated with eradication therapy. Future studies should focus on unveiling the underlying cause of these ulcers.

Clinical features

Dyspepsia

Peptic ulcer disease is characterized by a history of waxing and waning symptoms of localized, dull, aching pain in the upper abdomen, which is called dyspepsia. Many patients notice that symptoms often worsen in winter. Eating spicy food and drinking coffee and tea may aggravate the symptoms, but these dietary habits do not lead directly to ulcer formation. Pain may occur sooner after meals in gastric ulcers than in duodenal ulcers, and is not necessarily relieved by food and antacids. The relationship between symptoms and eating is an unreliable predictor of peptic ulcer disease. Gastric ulcers are more often found in older patients, especially those taking NSAIDs or aspirin. Approximately 20% of complicated ulcers presents without dyspeptic symptoms. These 'silent' ulcers are more common in individuals consuming NSAIDs, owing to their analgesic effects. The lack of warning signs in these ulcers make them more dangerous.

Haemorrhage

Gastrointestinal bleeding is the most common complication associated with peptic ulcer disease (Fig. 15.8.2). Vomiting of fresh blood, or haematemesis, indicates that bleeding originates from a site proximal to the suspensory muscle of the duodenum (ligament of Treitz). A history of fresh haematemesis usually implies a significant bleed and the patients may go into haemodynamic instability due to hypovolaemia. 'Coffee ground' vomiting, usually arising from altered black blood, often indicates that active bleeding may have ceased. Melaena is the passage of black tarry stool. It occurs when haemoglobin in the gut is converted to haematin by bacterial degradation. As little as 200 ml of bleeding inside the digestive tract can produce melaena. Although melaena generally connotes bleeding proximal to the suspensory muscle of the duodenum, bleeding from small bowel or proximal colon may also cause it, especially when colonic transit is slow. Haematochezia, passage of pure red blood or blood admixed with stool, occurs when bleeding comes from the lower gastrointestinal tract. It can also present in a massive upper gastrointestinal bleeding. When a substantial amount of blood is lost into the gastrointestinal lumen, pulses start to rise and blood pressure drops. The haemoglobin levels at this stage may not reflect the actual amount of blood loss before haemodilution sets in. A close monitoring of vital signs and estimation of volume of vomitus offer a better prognostic indicator of the severity of the illness.

Perforation

Free perforation of the stomach or duodenum into the peritoneal cavity is a rare but serious complication. It is more commonly found in older patients using aspirin or NSAIDs, leading to life-threatening catastrophe. The use of cocaine has also been related to peptic ulcer perforation. The classic presentation is a sudden onset of intense abdominal pain at the onset with gastric juice pouring into peritoneal cavity. This is followed a period of stabilization and amelioration of symptoms. Ulcer perforation may be concealed by the omentum. However, signs of peritonitis such as guarding and

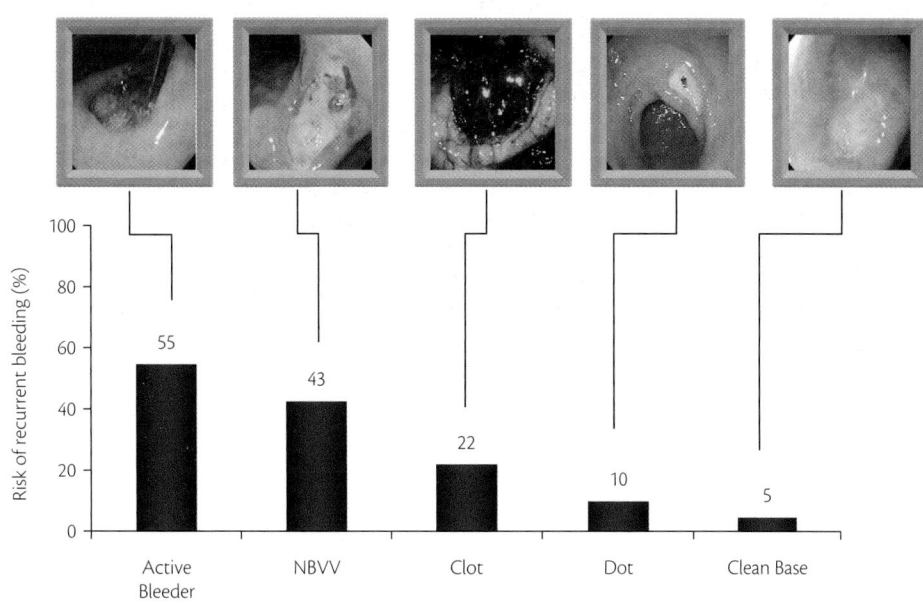

Fig. 15.8.2 Features of bleeding ulcers and the risk of recurrent bleeding. NBVV, nonbleeding visible vessel.
(From Lau JY, et al. (1998). The evolution of stigmata of hemorrhage in bleeding peptic ulcers: a sequential endoscopic study. *Endoscopy*, **30**, 513–18.)

rebound tenderness persist. Bowel sounds are silent and liver dullness to percussion diminishes. A plain abdominal radiograph may demonstrate free gas between the upper border of the liver and the diaphragm and may also outline the serosal surfaces of the bowel wall. If prompt treatment is not provided, the patient will develop frank peritonitis and severe sepsis. Body temperature will rise and breathing becomes shallow. Leucocytosis and acidosis may appear at this stage.

Besides free perforation, peptic ulcer may also penetrate into adjacent organs such as the pancreas, the bile duct, or even the colon, resulting in pancreatitis or gastrobiliary or gastroenteric fistula. With prompt medical attention, these complications are rarely seen nowadays.

Obstruction

In patients with recurrent peptic ulceration at the prepyloric antrum, pylorus, and duodenal bulb, oedema and/or scarring of the tissue may lead to obstruction of the gastric outlet. Pyloric obstruction usually presents with bloating, early satiety, and vomiting. The patient may recognize food ingested several days ago in their vomitus. Weight loss may be profound and dehydration with electrolyte disturbance (metabolic alkalosis with acidic urine) is common. On examination of the abdomen, an audible splash of the gastric content can be demonstrated by shaking the patient's abdomen (succussion splash). Aspiration of gastric content through a nasogastric tube will empty litres of fluid and undigested food from the stomach, giving quick relief for the patient. Obstruction due to acute peptic ulcer and tissue oedema usually resolve in a few weeks as the ulcer heals. On the other hand, severe scarring of the pylorus and duodenum leads to permanent gastric outflow obstruction and requires endoscopic or surgical treatment.

Differential diagnosis

Symptoms are neither sensitive nor specific for the diagnosis of peptic ulcer disease. A wide range of conditions ranging from functional dyspepsia to malignancy of the gastrointestinal tract can produce symptoms mimicking peptic ulcer disease. Pancreatitis and cholecystitis often produce more severe pain than peptic ulcer, so the differentiation may not be difficult. On the other hand, it is a disaster to miss a diagnosis of malignancy of the stomach, pancreas, or hepatobiliary tract. A high index of suspicion, especially in older patients with anorexia and weight loss, is needed to minimize the possibility of missing the diagnosis. In countries where the prevalence of gastric cancer is high, symptom of dyspepsia should be managed carefully.

Clinical investigation

With the advent of endoscopy, barium studies are less frequently used in the diagnosis of dyspepsia. Endoscopy serves three purposes in diagnosis and evaluation of the patients. First, it confirms the diagnosis of peptic ulcer disease by its morphology, location and, in case of gastric ulcer, offering an opportunity for biopsy. Endoscopic features of bleeding ulcers are important prognostic indicators. The presence of signs of recent bleeding in an ulcer confirms the source of bleeding.

The Forrest classification categorizes ulcers into those that are actively bleeding, show signs of recent bleeding, or simply have a clean base:

- Forrest class I ulcers are actively bleeding, either spurting (Forrest class IA) or oozing (Forrest class IB).

- Forrest class II ulcers show signs of recent bleeding including nonbleeding visible vessel (Forrest class IIA), adherent clots (Forrest class IIB), or flat pigmented spots (Forrest IIC).

- Forrest III ulcers have a clean base. The risk of continuous or recurrent bleeding of these ulcers is related to their appearance (Fig. 15.8.3).

An evolutionary scheme for the natural history of signs of haemorrhage for peptic ulcers has been proposed. Major bleeding from a peptic ulcer is arterial in origin. A sentinel clot (a term used synonymously with 'visible vessel') plugs the bleeding point. This can initially be contiguous with a larger overlying clot, which resolves in time. The clot may be variable in colour: initially it is red, but it darkens in time and subsequently the colour disappears leaving a plug of fibrin and platelets. Eventually the plug disappears, as the healing process is complete (see Fig. 15.8.3). Ulcers with an adherent clot or protuberant vessels have a 20 to 40% chance of recurrent bleeding without proper endoscopic or pharmacologic therapy. Endoscopic features, including the size and the site of bleeding ulcers, should be interpreted along with clinical factors. Ulcers at the lesser curve of the stomach or posterior duodenal bulb are a high risk because of their proximity to the left gastric artery and the gastroduodenal artery respectively.

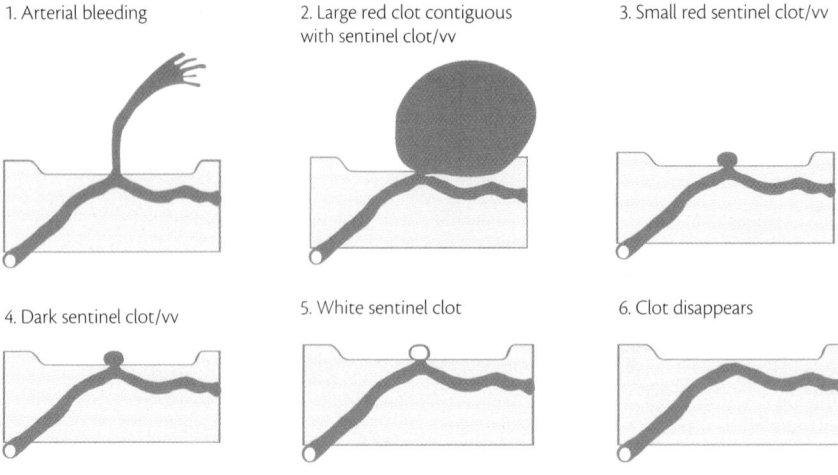

1. Arterial bleeding   2. Large red clot contiguous with sentinel clot/vv   3. Small red sentinel clot/vv

4. Dark sentinel clot/vv   5. White sentinel clot   6. Clot disappears

Fig. 15.8.3 Evolution of signs of recent haemorrhage. vv, visible vessel. (From Johnston JH (1990). Endoscopic risk factors for bleeding peptic ulcer. *Gastrointest Endosc*, **36** Suppl, S16–20.)

Gastric outlet obstruction due to recurrent peptic ulcer disease may produce a pinhole pylorus and dilated stomach. The endoscope may not be able to pass through the area of obstruction, leading to difficulty in assessment. Radiological imaging such as contrast studies is useful in this situation.

Treatment

Treatment of peptic ulcer disease can be divided into two stages: (1) treatment of acute symptoms and complications such as pain and bleeding, and (2) treatment of the underlying cause to prevent ulcer recurrence.

Treatment of acute symptoms and complications

Relief of symptoms and healing of peptic ulcer

Before the 1970s treatment of peptic ulcer relied on antacids, anticholinergics, a bland diet, and bed rest. The therapeutic efficacy was low and many patients resorted to surgery such as partial gastrectomy and vagotomy.

In 1977, the first H_2-receptor antagonist, cimetidine, was introduced. Subsequently, ranitidine, famotidine, and nizatidine became available. These are effective acid-suppressive agents, easy to use with an excellent safety profile. H_2-Receptor antagonists quickly became the treatment of choice for peptic ulcer disease, but they have several disadvantages. Cimetidine has mild antiandrogenic effects, leading to gynaecomastia and impotence in some patients. The ability of cimetidine to bind to hepatic enzyme cytochrome P450 has also led to many interactions with other drugs, altering the pharmacokinetics of medications. Cimetidine is reported to interact with theophylline, phenytoin, lidocaine, warfarin, β-blockers, tricyclic antidepressants, benzodiazepines, and many others. A variety of neurological reactions have also been reported such as headache, lethargy, depression, memory impairment, and confusion, especially in older patients. Furthermore, the reversible competitive inhibition of histamine-stimulated acid secretion provides only a modest suppression of acid secretion. The postprandial acidity of the stomach is still relatively high.

In addition to the acid-suppressive agents, drugs claimed to have 'cytoprotective' activities were developed in the 1980s. Sucralfate is a complex salt of sucrose in which the eight hydroxyl groups of sucrose are replaced by sulfate and aluminium hydroxide. It is insoluble in water, forming a thick, tenacious paste that covers the surface of gastrointestinal mucosa. Sucralfate has no acid-suppressing effects and is believed to work by coating the luminal surface of the ulcer, absorbing bile salts and pepsin and protecting the injured mucosa from further insult by erosive substances in the stomach. However, its ulcer healing effect is slow. Because of its aluminium content, it is considered unsafe in patients with chronic renal insufficiency. Acute aluminium toxicity has been reported in patients with end-stage renal failure. Sucralfate is now rarely used in the clinical management of peptic ulcers.

Bismuth salts have been used for many years for the treatment of diarrhoea, dyspepsia, and abdominal pain. As in case of sucralfate, bismuth has no effect on acid secretion in the stomach. The mechanism of action is unknown but it is found to preferentially cover the ulcer crater. In the early 1980s bismuth was found to inhibit the growth of *H. pylori*, which may partially explain its ulcer healing activity. Colloidal bismuth subcitrate and bismuth subsalicylate (BSS) are available for clinical use. The use of bismuth subcitrate will blacken stool. which might be confusing for patients suffering from gastrointestinal bleeding. There are isolated reports of neurotoxicity related to the use of bismuth subcitrate and bismuth subsalicylate when used in large doses in older patients. Otherwise, bismuth is a fairly safe drug. Its use is now mainly confined to the treatment of *H. pylori* infection in combination with other antimicrobial agents.

Prostaglandins are derivatives of unsaturated fatty acid known as eiconsanoids. The human gastrointestinal tract synthesizes several prostaglandins such as PGE_2 and PGF_2. Prostaglandins have been found to have a modest effect in inhibiting acid secretion in the stomach as well as stimulating the production of bicarbonate and mucin. Misoprostol has been developed as a prostaglandin analogue for human use. The standard dose of the drug is 800 μg/day taken in four divided doses. The ulcer-healing effect is not as potent as other acid-suppressive agent and the regimen is inconvenient, but because of the nature of its action misoprostol offers one of the best treatments for NSAID-related ulcers and prevention of this condition. Diarrhoea is the most common side effects and limits the use of misoprostol in daily practice. It is also contraindicated in pregnancy as it may induce abortion. Uterine bleeding has been reported in a substantial proportion of patients.

Proton pump inhibitors represents a major advancement in the treatment of acid-related gastrointestinal disorders. The final step of hydrogen ion secretion by the parietal cells is accomplished by H^+,K^+-APTase, an acid pump that exchanges hydrogen for potassium. These pumps are located at the apical membrane of tubulovesicular apparatus of the parietal cells. Proton pump inhibitors such as omeprazole, lansoprazole, pantoprazole, and rabeprazole are substituted benzimidazoles that bind to the acid pump irreversibly. These drugs turn off acid secretion stimulated by any kind of stimulants. Recovery of acid secretion requires synthesis of new enzyme in the acid pump. The most effective way of administering a proton pump inhibitor is to take the drug before meals, i.e. before acid secretion is triggered by food. Usually, a single daily dose gives quick relief of symptoms and effective healing of peptic ulcers in 4 to 6 weeks. Compared to misoprostol and H_2-receptor antagonists, a proton pump inhibitor such as omeprazole is more effective in healing the ulcer as well as preventing further peptic ulcerations and erosions. As the most potent inhibitors of acid secretion, proton pump inhibitors are also the treatment of choice for Zollinger–Ellison syndrome. They have also been found to suppress the growth of *H. pylori* and forms an integral part in combination therapy to eradicate *H. pylori* in the stomach ('proton pump inhibitor triple therapy'). Initial suspicion that prolonged suppression of the proton pump leads to enterochromaffin-like cell hyperplasia has not been proved in humans. Patients who have received proton pump inhibitors for more than 10 years have not reported significant side effects.

Treatment of ulcer bleeding

The management of patients with upper gastrointestinal haemorrhage requires a multidisciplinary approach mandating cooperation among medical and surgical gastroenterologists with access to skills in endoscopic and surgical haemostasis. Endoscopic therapy is often the first treatment in the management algorithm. Approximately 80 to 85% of upper gastrointestinal bleeding stops spontaneously. The remaining 15 to 20% continue to bleed or develop recurrent bleeding and these patients constitute the high-risk group with substantial increased morbidity and mortality. Early risk stratification of patients with upper gastrointestinal bleeding based on clinical and endoscopic criteria allows delivery of an appropriate level of care to patients. Endoscopic therapy is now widely accepted as the first line of therapy for upper gastrointestinal bleeding. It should be applied to actively bleeding ulcers or ulcers covered with an adherent clot (Forrest class IIB). Many clinical trials and at least two meta-analyses have confirmed the efficacy of endoscopic haemostasis with dual therapy. Endoscopic therapy reduces recurrent bleeding and the need for surgical intervention.

Endoscopic therapy can be broadly categorized into endoscopic injection, thermal coagulation, and mechanical haemostasis:

◆ Epinephrine, polidocanol, sodium tetradectyl sulphate, absolute alcohol, and even saline solution have been used for injection. No single agent for endoscopic injection is superior to another for achieving haemostasis. The mechanism of action is mostly related to a tamponade effect produced by the solution injected. The haemostatic effect of endoscopic injection is only transient, as the solution will be absorbed by the tissue. Injection is therefore not recommended as the sole therapy for peptic ulcer bleeding. Combination with other modalities is required.

◆ Thermal devices include heated probes; electrocoagulation is required to secure haemostasis. Thermal devices seal blood vessels underneath the ulcer base by pressure and heat energy. This combined pressure–thermal energy effect is called 'coaptive coagulation'. Like endoscopic injection, no single method of endoscopic coaptive therapy is superior to the others.

◆ Mechanical haemostasis can be achieved by endoscopic clipping or, in some cases, banding ligation. Various kinds of endoscopic clips have been developed and they are useful device to deal with protruding vessels at the ulcer base. Mechanical haemostasis is found to be as effective as thermal device in controlling peptic ulcer bleeding.

Combining endoscopic injection with either thermal coagulation or mechanical haemostasis represents the best endoscopic therapy, with an overall success rate of around 90%.

As an acidic environment in the stomach and duodenum inhibits platelet aggregation and activates enzymatic activity of pepcinogen, suppression of acid, especially in the early phase of peptic ulcer bleeding, is useful as an adjuvant therapy. Randomized studies and a subsequent systematic review have confirmed that high-dose intravenous proton pump inhibitor offers an effective inhibition of gastric acid secretion and reduces recurrent bleeding. Patients receiving these intravenous infusions require less blood transfusion, fewer repeated endoscopic treatments, and fewer surgical operations. Recent data suggest that the use of intravenous proton pump inhibitor in the early phase of bleeding, before endoscopy, may reduce the requirement for endoscopic therapy and shorten hospital stay. An algorithm for the management of peptic ulcer bleeding is proposed in Fig. 15.8.4.

Prevention of ulcer recurrence

Treatment of H. pylori infection

Treatment of *H. pylori* is a cure for peptic ulcer disease in most patients. *H. pylori* is susceptible to many different antimicrobials and a variety of combinations have been used successfully. Antimicrobials that have proved effective include amoxicillin, metronidazole, tetracycline, clarithromycin, and furazolidone.

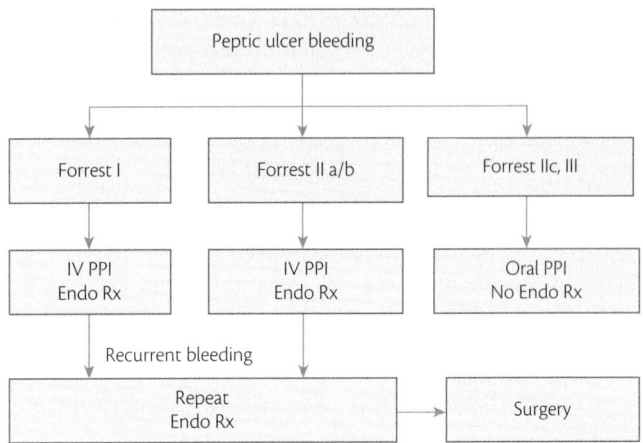

Fig. 15.8.4 Management strategy for peptic ulcer bleeding.
(From Sung J (2006). Current management of peptic ulcer bleeding. *Nat Clin Pract Gastroenterol Hepatol*, **3**, 24–32.)
IVPPI = intravenous proton pump inhibitor.
Ento Rx = endoscopic treatment.

Other less commonly used antimicrobials include rifabutin and several fluoroquinolones. Successful cure of infection usually requires two antimicrobial agents. Cure rates with single antimicrobial agents are poor, ranging from 0 to 35%, and monotherapy is also associated with the rapid development of antibiotic resistance. It is therefore not recommended for *H. pylori* infections. In principle, only those regimens that give high cure rates (>90%) should be used as first line therapy. Generally, higher doses and longer durations provide better results. Antibiotic resistance leads to reduced efficacy of therapy. The antimicrobial resistance pattern of *H. pylori* should be monitored and made known in each locality. The patient's compliance with therapy is very important for successful cure of the infection, so regimens should be simple and with few side effects that might affect compliance.

Treatment regimens for *H. pylori* infection are classified by the number of antibiotics and adjunctive agents employed. Dual therapies were the first therapies to be introduced for *H. pylori*. Because of low cure rates and a high frequency of clarithromycin resistance among the treatment failures, dual therapies with a proton pump inhibitor and clarithromycin or amoxicillin, or ranitidine and bismuth citrate with clarithromycin, are no longer recommended. Triple therapy with either bismuth or a proton pump inhibitor combined with two antibiotics is now the most widely used regimen. Ranitidine bismuth citrate may be substituted for bismuth or a proton pump inhibitor, but in many countries this drug is not available. Therapy with metronidazole, tetracycline, and bismuth ('traditional' triple therapy) produces very good cure rates, especially with organisms sensitive to metronidazole. However, the side effects of metronidazole may be prohibitive in some patients. Substitution of clarithromycin for metronidazole gives similar results. Amoxicillin should be substituted for tetracycline in children to avoid staining of teeth. The most popular triple therapy combines a proton pump inhibitor with any two of these three antimicrobials: amoxicillin, metronidazole, and clarithromycin. The triple therapy described above is often enough unless the organism being treated is resistant to clarithromycin or metronidazole.

The most effective regimens to cure *H. pylori* infection are combinations of two antibiotics and adjunctive agents taken for 7 to 14 days (Table 15.8.1). Although regimens composed of two antibiotics with a proton pump inhibitor are expensive, they are

Table 15.8.1 Recommended first-line regimens to treat *Helicobacter pylori*

Adjuvant	Antimicrobial 1	Antimicrobial 2	Duration of therapy (days)
Proton pump inhibitor twice daily	Clarithromycin twice daily	Amoxicillin twice daily or metronidazole twice daily	7–14
Ranitidine bismuth citrate twice daily	Clarithromycin twice daily	Amoxicillin twice daily or metronidazole twice daily	7–14
Bismuth four times daily	Tetracycline four times daily	Metronidazole three times daily	7–14

easy to take and have few major side effects. Unless a patient has taken clarithromycin previously, one of the two regimens containing this antibiotic, with an additional antimicrobial plus a proton pump inhibitor, is recommended. The most effective and best-tolerated combination seems to be a twice daily combination of a proton pump inhibitor with clarithromycin 500 mg twice daily plus 1000 mg of amoxicillin (PPI +AC) or 500 mg of metronidazole (PPI +MC). The choice of antibiotic should be determined by the local antibiotic resistance pattern and the history of treatment received by the patient.

Eradication of *H. pylori* can be confirmed by urea breath test, stool antigen test, or biopsy urease test. In order to differentiate temporary suppression of *H. pylori* from successful eradication, these tests should be done at least 4 weeks after finishing the anti-*Helicobacter* regimens and discontinuation of proton pump inhibitor for at least 2 weeks.

Patients who fail to respond to these first line therapies should be considered for repeat proton pump inhibitor-based therapy switching between clarithromycin and metronidazole. As clarithromycin resistance readily developed after exposure, repeating the same regimen with clarithromycin is usually futile. A longer treatment duration such as 2 to 4 weeks is desirable to ensure optimal antimicrobial activity. The other option is to use a quadruple therapy combining proton pump inhibitors twice daily, bismuth salt four times daily, tetracycline 500 mg four times daily and metronidzole 500 mg three times daily. This is a more complicated regimen, with significant side effects. Patient compliance is a main determining factor for the success of therapy. In recent years, levofloxacin 250 mg twice daily and rifabutin 150 to 300 mg daily in combination with a proton pump inhibitor and amoxicillin has been advocated for multidrug resistant *H. pylori*.

Prevention of NSAID-associated ulcer

NSAID-associated ulcer and ulcer complications are more commonly reported in high-risk individuals, i.e. older people and those with history of peptic ulcer disease or chronic medical illness. Concomitant use of NSAIDs with aspirin, anticoagulants or corticosteroid also increases the risk of bleeding from peptic ulcers. Special caution has to be exercised before prescribing NSAIDs to these patients.

Various prophylactic strategies to reduce gastroduodenal injury by NSIADs have been investigated. These include concurrent treatment with H_2-receptor antagonist, misoprostol, proton pump inhibitor, and substitution of conventional NSAIDs by COX-2 selective inhibitors. Systematic review pooling over 30 randomized controlled clinical trials of misoprostol, H_2-receptor antagonist, or proton pump inhibitor for the prevention of gastroduodenal ulcer showed that these drugs have different efficacy. H_2-Receptor antagonists reduce the risk of duodenal ulcer, but not not of gastric ulcer, except at very high dose. Misoprostol at 80 μg per day can reduce ulcer and ulcer complication but its side effects are significant. Proton pump inhibitors can reduce the risk of both duodenal and gastric ulcers associated with NSAIDs and they are much better tolerated than misoprostol.

The interaction between *H. pylori* and NSAIDs in the development of peptic ulcer disease is a complex. Clinical studies reported by different investigators have yielded conflicting results. Part of the confusion stems from the recruitment of different patient groups and use of different outcome measurement. Meta-analysis of 16 studies showed that *H. pylori* infection and NSAID use increase the risk of ulcer bleeding by 1.8-fold and 4.8-fold respectively. The risk of ulcer bleeding increases to around sixfold when both factors are present. This implies that NSAIDs and *H. pylori* are independent but additive risk factors for ulcer development. *H. pylori*-infected individuals taking NSAIDs will have an increased risk of peptic ulcer and ulcer complications. If a patient known to have *H. pylori* infection requires an NSAIDs, eradicating *H. pylori* before using the NSAID may substantially reduce the risk of peptic ulcer disease. However, simply curing *H. pylori* infection may not be sufficient to protect the stomach and duodenum from ulcer formation in high-risk individuals. In elderly patients with history of ulcer complication, concomitant use of a proton pump inhibitor is warranted. In these patients, even the use of COX-2 selective inhibitors is not entirely safe. The risk of recurrent bleeding with celecoxib is comparable to the use of diclofenac combined with omeprazole, according to one study. In patients with a history of ulcer bleeding, a combination of COX-2 selective inhibitors with a proton pump inhibitor offers the best safety profile for the gastrointestinal tract (Table 15.8.2).

Prevention of ulcer associated with antiplatelet agents

Aspirin and clopidogrel are increasing used in the prevention of cardiovascular and cerebrovascular diseases. Aspirin-induced peptic ulcer disease is dose dependent, so the lowest dose of aspirin should be prescribed. Aspirin is often used in elderly patients who require NSAID or COX-2 selective inhibitors for musculoskeletal pain. Combinations of aspirin with NSAIDs and COX-2 selective

Table 15.8.2 Recommendations for reducing the risk of ulcer and ulcer complications in high-risk patients (NSAID and aspirin users)

Strategies	NSAID users	Aspirin users
Choice of medication	Choose less ulcerogenic NSIAD (e.g. ibuprofen) or short-term COX-2 selective inhibitors	Use low-dose aspirin (80–100 mg/day)
H. pylori infection	Eradicate *H. pylori* infection with proton pump inhibitor triple therapy	Eradicate *H. pylori* infection with proton pump inhibitor triple therapy
Concomitant medication	Avoid combining with aspirin, anticoagulants, and steroid	Avoid combining with NSAID, clopidogrel, COX-2 selective inhibitors, anticoagulant, and steroid
Ulcer-preventing drugs	Proton pump inhibitor or high-dose H_2-receptor antagonist in high-risk individuals	Proton pump inhibitors in high-risk individuals

inhibitors have been shown to increase the risk of ulcer bleeding substantially. The gastric sparing effect of COX-2 inhibitors is off-set by the concomitant use of low-dose aspirin, so this combination should be avoided if possible. Eradication of *H. pylori* infection has been shown to reduce the risk of peptic ulcer bleeding in high-risk individuals (Table 15.8.2). Recent study shows that if aspirin is discontinued for a prolonged period after peptic ulcer bleeding, patient survival may be jeopardized as a result of cardiovascular or cerebrovascular conditions. Clinicians are advised to exercise discretion and balance the risk and benefit of discontinuing antiplatelet agents in these patients.

Clopidogrel has an improved gastrintestinal safety profile compare to aspirin in general use. However, in high-risk individuals, e.g. elderly patients with a history of ulcer or ulcer complication, the risk of peptic ulcer with clopidogrel should not be underestimated. In a head-to-head comparison between clopidogrel and low-dose aspirin combined with proton pump inhibitors, the risks of peptic ulcer bleeding were shown to be similar for both strategies. In recent years, there has been a trend to combine aspirin and clopidogrel in the management of patients with myocardial infarction, especially after percutaneous coronary interventions with stenting. A combined use of two antiplatelet agents is recommended for at least 6 months after the procedures. The combination of clopidogrel and aspirin is expected to further increase the gastrointestinal risk, so the benefit of using these antiplatelet agents must be balanced against the risk of causing gastrointestinal toxicity in these patients. This could be a difficult decision in elderly patients with life-threatening cardiovascular disease and a history of ulcer complication in the past. Future studies should be directed towards prevention of ulcer bleeding in patients requiring double antiplatelet agents.

Surgery and peptic ulcer complications

With the improvement of ulcer treatment using proton pump inhibitors and anti-*Helicobacter* therapy, the role of ulcer surgery has diminished. Classical operative procedures such as partial gastrectomy (Billroth I and Billroth II gastrectomy) and vagotomy are now rarely performed except for unhealed or recurrent peptic ulcers in the stomach or duodenum. As a result, postgastrectomy complications such as afferent loop syndrome, dumping syndrome, postvagotomy diarrhoea, and bile reflux gastropathy are disappearing in clinical practice.

Surgery is still the most effective method of treating peptic ulcer bleeding arising from ulcers at difficult positions or large submucosal vessels, e.g. the gastroduodenal artery. Plication of the bleeding vessels and/or removal of part of the stomach or duodenum remain the definitive method of controlling bleeding that cannot be stopped by pharmacological and endoscopic measures. Often, this is a life-saving procedure. The decision to operate is best made by a team of experienced gastroenterologists and gastrointestinal surgeons with a close working relationship. Repeated, unsuccessful attempts at endoscopic haemostasis leads to undue delay in surgery, massive blood transfusion, and multiorgan failure, jeopardizing the patient's survival. In a study comparing second-attempt endoscopic therapy vs surgery, ulcer surgery showed a superior haemostasis result although postoperative complications were frequent. An individual-based decision and the exercise of clinical discretion are therefore required.

Despite initial enthusiasm for endoscopic dilatation of pyloric stenosis, the long-term result is disappointing. Gastric outlet obstruction often recurs months or years after endoscopic balloon dilatation. Partial gastrectomy and vagotomy may solve the problem of obstruction once and for all, saving the patient repeated admissions to hospital. Free perforation of the ulcer into the peritoneum is another indication for ulcer surgery. Repair of perforation and vagotomy is usually adequate to control the disaster. Treatment of *H. pylori* infection and a maintenance dose of proton pump inhibitor are indicated as follow-up therapy.

Areas of uncertainty and future development

We have come a long way in the last two decades in the understanding of pathogenesis of peptic ulcer disease and its management. Substantial improvements have been made in preventing recurrent disease and in the treatment of its associated complications. There are, however, areas of uncertainty and room for future improvement.

Although *H. pylori* has been identified as the major cause of peptic ulcer disease in individuals who do note use NSAIDs or aspirin, it is still not clear why only a relatively small proportion of infected subjects develop peptic ulcer disease. Bacterial factors (other than the *cag* pathogenesity island) and host factors (other than IL-1b polymorphism) need further studies to elucidate the difference in outcome. With rapid emergence of antimicrobial resistance in *H. pylori*, cure cannot be assumed without confirmation. An effective second-line therapy is still much needed.

The best strategy for high-risk individuals requiring antiplatelet, NSAIDs, or COX-2 inhibitors needs further studies. There are, at present, very few data on the effective protection of the gastrointestinal tract when patients are prescribed double antiplatelet agents. Scepticism still persists about the safety of eradicating *H. pylori* as the only prophylaxis for aspirin users. In view of the complicated interaction between NSAIDs, COX-2 inhibitors, and antiplatelet agents in vascular and gastrointestinal safety, a matrix for choice of therapy under different circumstances is much desired. Guidelines need to be developed for primary care physicians, cardiologists, and gastroenterologists looking after these patients.

The role of nitric oxide is receiving more attention in understanding the gastrointestinal toxicity of NSAIDs and analgesics. The development of NSAIDs and aspirin coupled with a molecule of nitric oxide is an exciting area that opens up a new horizon in the management of peptic ulcer disease in those who requires anti-inflammatory medication and antiplatelet therapy. The efficacy and safety of these drugs can only be confirmed by carefully designed clinical studies.

Despite the advances in pharmacological and endoscopic therapy, the mortality of ulcer bleeding remains at 7 to 10%. Especially in the elderly patients, death is often related to non-bleeding causes such as cardio-pulmonary conditions, multi-organ failure and terminal malignancy. Clinicians are reminded to manage the comorbid illness instead of focusing on bleeding lesions alone. In difficult cases of ulcer bleeding, endoscopy and surgery are the two common approaches available at this stage. The role of radiological intervention, i.e. embolization of the feeding artery at the ulcer base, deserves a more careful investigation.

Further reading

Blaser MJ (1996). Role of *vac A* and the *cag A* locus of *Helicobacter pylori* in human disease. *Aliment Pharmacol Ther*, **10**, 73–77.

Calvet X, et al. (2004). Addition of a second endoscopic treatment following epinephrine injection improve outcome in high-risk bleeding ulcers. Gastroenterology, 126, 441–50.

Chan FKL, et al. (2001). A randomised comparison of Helicobacter pylori eradication and omeprazole for the prevention of recurrent upper gastrointestinal bleeding in chronic users of low-dose aspirin and non-aspirin non-steroidal anti-inflammatory drugs. N Engl J Med, 344, 967–73.

Chan FKL, et al. (2002). Celecoxib versus diclofenac and omeprazole in preventing recurrent ulcer bleeding in patients with arthritis. N Engl J Med, 347, 2104–10.

Chan FKL, et al. (2002). Screen-and-treat Helicobacter pylori to reduce the risk of peptic ulcers for patients starting long-term non-steroidal anti-inflammatory drug treatment: a double blind randomised placebo-controlled trial. Lancet, 359, 9–13.

Chan FKL, et al. (2005). Clopidogrel versus aspirin and esomeprazole to prevent recurrent ulcer bleeding. N Engl J Med, 352, 238–44.

Chan HLY, et al. (2001). Is non-Helicobacter non-NSAID peptic ulcer a common cause of upper gastrointestinal bleeding? A prospective study of 977 patients. Gastroint Endosc, 53, 438–42.

Cook DJ, et al. (1992). Endsocopic therapy for acute non-variceal upper gastrointestinal haemorrhage: a meta-analysis. Gastroenterology, 102, 139–48.

Dorward S, et al. (2006). Proton pump inhibitor treatment initiated prior to endoscopic diagnosis in upper gastrointestinal bleeding. Cochrane Database Syst Rev, CD005415.

El-Omar EM, et al. (1995). Helicobacter pylori infection and abnormalities of acid secretion in patients with duodenal ulcer disease. Gastroenterology, 109, 681–91.

El-Omar EM, et al. (1997). Helicobacter pylori infection and chronic gastric acid hypo-secretion. Gastroenterology, 113, 15–24.

European Helicobacter pylori Study Group. (1997). Current European concepts in the management of Helicobacter pylori infection. The Maastricht Consensus Report. Gut, 41, 8–13.

Forrest JA, Finlayson ND, Shearman DJ. (1974). Endoscopy in gastrointestinal bleeding. Lancet, 2, 392–7.

Graham DY, Yamaoka Y (2000). Disease-specific Helicobacter pylori virulence factors—the unfulfilled promise. Helicobacter, 5, 3–9.

Hawkey CJ. (1990). Non-steroidal anti-inflammatory drugs and peptic ulcers. BMJ, 300, 764.

Hawkey CJ, et al. (1998). Omeprazole compared with misoprostol for ulcer associated with non-steroidal anti-inflammatory drugs. Omeprazole versus misoprostol for NSAID-induced ulcer management (OMNIUM) study group. N Engl J Med, 338, 727–34.

Hosking SW, et al. (1994). Duodenal ulcer healing by eradication of Helicobacter pylori without anti-acid treatment: randomized controlled trial. Lancet, 343, 508–10.

Huang JQ, Sridhar S, Hunt RH. (2002). Role of Helicobacter pylori infection and non-steroidal anti-inflammatory drugs in peptic ulcer disease: a meta-analysis. Lancet, 359, 12–22.

Hung LCT, et al. (2005). Long-term outcome of H. pylori-negative bleeding ulcers: A prospective cohort study. Gastroenterology, 128, 1845–50.

Lanas A, et al. (2006). Risk of upper gastrointestinal ulcer bleeding associated with selective cyclo-oxygenase 2 inhibitors, traditional non-aspirin non-steroidal anti-inflammatory drugs, aspirin and combinations. Gut, 55, 1731–8.

Lau JYW, et al. (1999). Endoscopic re-treatment versus surgery in patients rebleeding after initial endoscopic ulcer hemostasis: a prospective randomized controlled trial. N Engl J Med, 340, 751–6.

Lau JYW, et al. (2000). A comparison of high-dose omeprazole infusion to placebo after endoscopic hemostasis to bleeding peptic ulcer. N Engl J Med, 343, 310–316.

Lau JYW, et al. (2007). Omeprazole before endoscopy in patients with gastrointestinal bleeding. N Engl J Med, 356, 1631–40.

Leontiadis G, Sharma VK, Howden CW (2006). Proton pump inhibitor treatment for acute peptic ulcer bleeding. Cochrane Database Syst Rev, CD002094.

Malfertheiner P, et al. (2002). Current concepts in management of Helicobacter pylori infection. The Maastricht 2–2000 Consensus Report. Aliment Pharmacol Ther, 16, 167–80.

Marmo R, et al. (2007). Dual therapy versus monotherapy in the endoscopic treatment of high-risk bleeding ulcers: a meta-analysis of controlled trials. Am J Gastroenterol, 102, 270–89.

Marshall BJ, Warren JR (1984). Unidentified curved bacilli in the stomach of patients with gastritis and peptic ulceration. Lancet, 1, 1311–15.

Masferrer JL, et al. (1994). Selective inhibition of inducible cyclooxygenase-2 in vivo is anti-inflammatory and non-ulcerogenic. Proc Natl Acad Sci U S A, 91, 3228–32.

McColl KE, El-Omar E (1996). Helicobacter pylori and distrubance of gastric function associated with duodenal ulcer disease and gastric cancer. Scand J Gastroenterol (suppl), 215, 32–7.

Patrono C, et al. (2005). Low dose aspirin for the prevention of atherothrombosis. N Engl J Med, 353, 2373–83.

Rockall TA, et al. (1995). Incidence of and mortality from acute upper gastrointestinal haemorrhage in the United Kingdom. Steering Committee and members of the National Audit of Acute Upper Gastrointestinal Haemorrhage, BMJ, 311, 222–6.

Rostom A, et al. (2002). Prevention of NSAID-induced gastroduodenal ulcers. Cochrane Database Syst Rev, 4, CD002296.

Sacks HS, et al. (1990). Endoscopic haemostasis: an effective therapy for bleeding peptic ulcers. JAMA, 264, 494–9.

Silverstein FE, et al. (1981). National ASGE survey on upper gastrointestinal bleeding: study design and baseline data. Gastrointest Endosc, 27, 73–9.

Silverstein FE, et al. (1995). Misoprostol reduces serious gastrointestinal complications in patients with rheumatoid arthritis receiving non-steroidal anti-inflammatory drugs. A randomized double-blind placebo-controlled trial. Ann Intern Med, 123, 241–9.

Sonnenberg A. (1995). Temporal trends and geographical variations of peptic ulcer disease. Aliment Pharmacol Ther, 9 Suppl 2, 3.

Sung JJY, et al. (1995). Antibacterial treatment of gastric ulcers associated with Helicobacter pylori. N Engl J Med, 332, 139–42.

Sung JJY, et al. (2007). Endoscopic clipping versus injection and thermo-coagulation in the treatment of non-variceal upper gastrointestinal bleeding: a meta-analysis. Gut, 56, 1364–73.

Sung JJY, et al. (2009). Intravenous esomeprazole for prevention of recurrent peptic ulcer bleeding: a randomized trial. Ann Intern Med, 150(7), 455–64.

Sung JJY, et al. (2010). Causes of mortality in patients with peptic ulcer bleeding: a prospective cohort study of 10,428 cases. Am J Gastroenterol, 105(1), 84–9.

Sung JJY, et al. (2010). Continuation of low-dose aspirin therapy in peptic ulcer bleeding: a randomized trial. Ann Intern Med, 152(1), 1–9.

Taha AS, et al. (1996). Famotidine for the prevention of gastric and duodenal ulcers caused by non-steroidal anti-inflammatory drugs. N Engl J Med, 334, 1435–9.

Vane JR (1971). Inhibition of prostaglandin synthesis as a mechanism of action for aspirin-like drugs. Nat New Biol, 231, 232–5.

Walan A, et al. (1989). Effect of omeprazole and ranitidine on ulcer healing and relapse rates in patients with benign gastric ulcer. N Engl J Med, 320, 69–75.

Wallace JL, et al. (2000). NSAID-induced gastric damage in rats: requirement for inhibition of both cyclooxygenase 1 and 2. Gastroenterology, 119, 706.

Wyatt JI, et al. (1987). Campylobacter pyloridis and acid induced gastric metaplasia in the pathogenesis of duodenitis. J Clin Pathol, 40, 841–8.

Yeomans ND, et al. (1998). A comparison of omeprazole with ranitidine for ulcers associated with nonsteroidal anti-inflammatory drugs. Acid suppression trial: Ranitidine versus omeprazole for NSAID-associated ulcer treatment (ASTRONAUT) study group. N Engl J Med, 338, 719–26.

Hormones and the gastrointestinal tract

A.E. Bishop, P.J. Hammond, J.M. Polak, and S.R. Bloom

Essentials

The gastrointestinal tract is the largest endocrine organ in the body, with its component cells dispersed along its length rather than being clustered in glands. Gut peptides integrate gastrointestinal function by regulating the actions of the epithelium, muscles, and nerves, affect the growth and development of the gut and—as has emerged comparatively recently—they also have a major role in appetite control. There is little evidence that many gut peptides act as hormones in a classical endocrine fashion: many are autocrine, regulating the function of the cell secreting them, or paracrine, influencing the behaviour of neighbouring cells of different types.

Many gut peptides have been described, including the following.

The gastrin–cholecystokinin family—gastrin, which stimulates gastric acid secretion and has a trophic effect on the gastric mucosa, and cholecystokinin, a postprandial satiety signal.

The secretin family—secretin, which stimulates production of watery, alkaline pancreatic juices; glucose-dependent insulinotropic peptide, which stimulates insulin release in response to a mixed meal; vasoactive intestinal peptide (VIP), a stimulator of small-intestinal and colonic enterocyte secretion of water and electrolytes.

Peptide products of preproglucagon—enteroglucagon, which may be important in gut adaptation; glucagon-like peptides 1 and 2 and oxyntomodulin, which induce satiety.

Peptide products of preproghrelin—ghrelin, which is the only hormone known to stimulate food intake; obestatin, whose physiological function is uncertain; and motilin, which accelerates intestinal transit.

Peptide tyrosine tyrosine (PYY), which slows intestinal transit, and neuropeptide Y, which is a potent vasoconstrictor, inhibits intestinal secretion, and depresses colonic motility.

Others—bombesin and the gastrin-releasing peptides; opioids; tachykinins; other gut peptides—neurotensin; somatostatin; chromogranin-derived peptides; and other peptide neurotransmitters.

Gastrointestinal disease may cause abnormalities of these gut peptides, e.g. (1) achlorhydria (from atrophic gastritis or drug-induced) causes elevation of circulating gastrin; (2) malabsorptive conditions are associated with a decrease in the amount of peptides produced in the affected region, and a compensatory elevation of other peptides.

Carcinoid syndrome

Carcinoid tumours are capable of producing serotonin (5-hydroxytryptamine; 5-HT). Carcinoid syndrome occurs in about 10% of patients with carcinoid tumours, usually midgut tumours that have metastasized to the liver. The cardinal feature is the carcinoid flush; other characteristic symptoms are secretory diarrhoea, cramping abdominal pain, nausea, and vomiting; and about 50% of patients have cardiac valve abnormalities. The diagnosis is made on the basis of elevated concentrations of 5-hydroxyindoleacetic acid in a 24-h urine collection, with localization by octreoscan (using radiolabelled octreotide), ultrasonography/CT, or endoscopy. Treatment is with simple antidiarrhoeal agents and octreotide, a long-acting, subcutaneously administered, somatostatin analogue. The 5-year survival rates for carcinoids (depending on location) are 33 to 98%.

Introduction

The discovery of secretin, the first recognized hormone, by Bayliss and Starling in 1902 marked the birth not only of gastrointestinal endocrinology, but of endocrinology itself. This first discovery was followed in 1905 by the identification of gastrin, but the technique of identifying hormones was, thereafter, more successfully applied to the study of secretions from the ductless glands, and gastrointestinal endocrinology languished for the next six decades. The determination of the amino acid structure of gastrin following its extraction from a solid tumour in 1964 marked a renewed interest in the field, and the introduction of techniques for large-scale chemical extraction and purification of hormones resulted in the discovery of further gut peptides. Many of these proved to be neuropeptides and have been identified within the central and peripheral nervous systems.

This section describes gut peptide hormones and neurotransmitters, classifying them by common structure or precursor peptides, and then outlines abnormalities in gastrointestinal disease. The roles

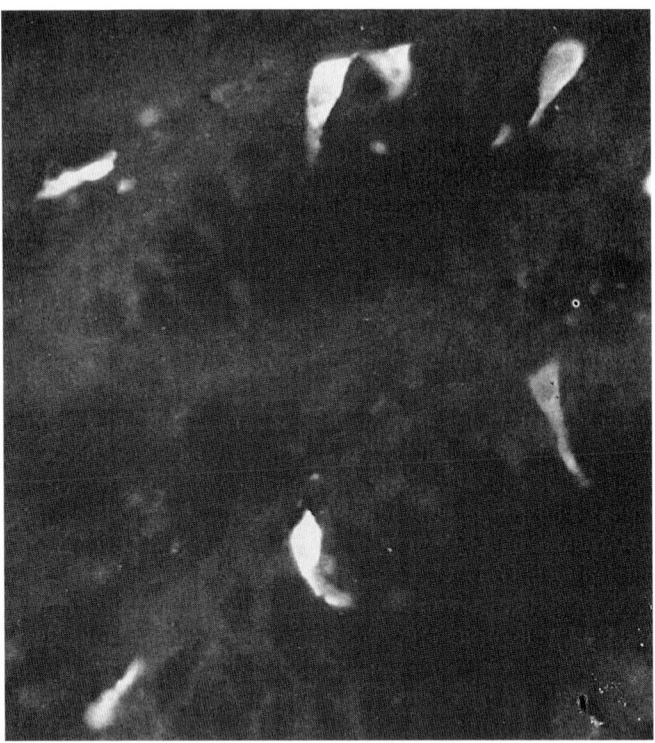

Fig. 15.9.1 Somatostatin cells in the mucosa of human colon, immunostained using the technique of indirect immunofluorescence (×300).

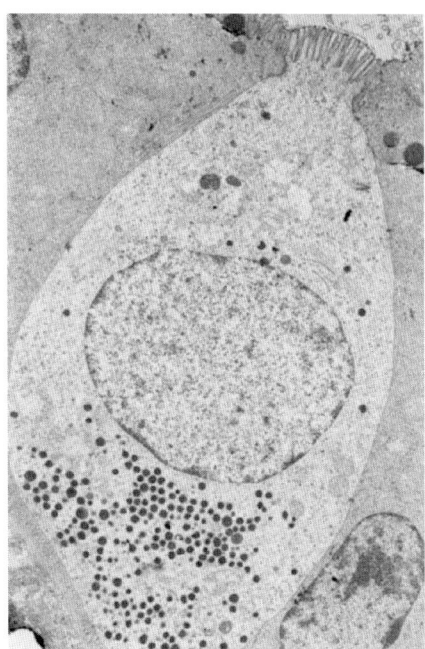

Fig. 15.9.2 Electron micrograph showing the typical morphology of an endocrine cell of the gut mucosa, with well-developed microvilli at the luminal border and secretory granules grouped towards the basal membrane (×5500).

of gut peptides in the syndromes associated with gastroenteropancreatic tumours are considered in detail elsewhere, while the carcinoid syndrome is described at the end of this chapter.

Techniques that have contributed to our understanding of gastrointestinal endocrinology include molecular biology, which has helped identify members of peptide families by molecular cloning techniques and has provided information about peptide processing that, in turn, has shown that different peptides may originate from a single common precursor. Sensitive peptide radioimmunoassay has allowed detection of gut peptides, which often have very low concentrations in plasma and tissues. Furthermore, specific peptide antibodies can be used for immunocytochemistry to demonstrate the cellular localization of peptide-producing cells (Fig. 15.9.1), and for immunoneutralization studies to elucidate the pathophysiological functions of gut peptides. Peptide localization can be further defined by electron microscopy, which demonstrates specific peptide storage granules (Figs. 15.9.2, 15.9.3), and *in situ* hybridization, which allows the sites of peptide synthesis to be identified by revealing the cellular distribution of specific mRNA species. A major advance in gastrointestinal endocrinology has been the molecular characterization of hormone receptors by cloning techniques. This has demonstrated different receptors for the same ligand and provides an explanation for the diverse biological actions of many gut peptides in the same tissues.

Gut peptides

Gastrin–cholecystokinin family

Gastrin

Gastrin occurs in various molecular forms, but all the biological activity resides in the four C-terminal amino acids. The major

molecular forms contain 17 (G17; 2098 Da), 14 (G14; pentagastrin), and 34 (G34; big gastrin) amino acids. Larger molecular forms have been described but may be artefacts. In humans, gastrin is mainly in the gastric antrum, where G17 predominates, but is also found in the upper small intestine, mainly as G34. These two are

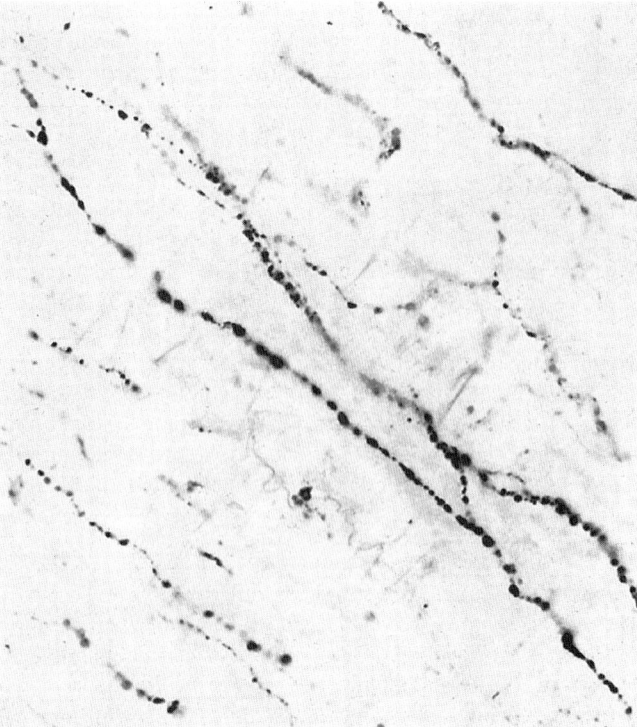

Fig. 15.9.3 Vasoactive intestinal polypeptide (VIP) fibres, immunostained using the unlabelled antibody enzyme (PAP) method, in the submucosa of human colon (×500).

the predominant circulating forms. Gastrin is synthesized in G cells where it is stored in large electron-lucent granules.

Gastrin release, following protein ingestion and gastric distension, stimulates gastric acid secretion and has a trophic effect on the gastric mucosa. Infusion of gastrin stimulates gastric motor activity and contraction of the lower oesophageal sphincter, although the physiological significance of this action is unclear.

Cholecystokinin

Cholecystokinin has a C-terminal sequence of five amino acids identical to gastrin, but its specificity is conferred by the adjacent three amino acids, and this octapeptide confers its biological activity. It is found in the gut predominantly in molecular forms with 33, 39, or 58 amino acids, and is produced by the I cells of the duodenal and jejunal mucosa. The octapeptide cholecystokinin is a neurotransmitter in the central and enteric nervous systems.

Cholecystokinin is a postprandial satiety signal. The development of antagonists specific for the two cholecystokinin receptor subtypes (CCK1R/CCK-A, which is cholecystokinin-specific, and CCK2R/CCK-B, which appears to be also the only gastrin receptor) has allowed the important physiological roles of cholecystokinin to be characterized. The CCK-A receptor appears to be involved in stimulation of gallbladder contraction and trophic effects on the duodenum and pancreas. The ability of CCK1R receptor antagonists potently to inhibit meal-stimulated gallbladder contraction may be of therapeutic value in biliary colic.

Secretin family

In addition to secretin itself the secretin family includes glucose-dependent insulinotropic peptide, glucagon, enteroglucagon, vasoactive intestinal peptide (VIP), peptide histidine methionine, and growth hormone (GH) releasing factor. The latter is released from the hypothalamus, mainly as a peptide of 44 amino acids, to stimulate release of GH, but is also found in significant concentrations, mainly in a 40 amino acid form, in the small intestinal mucosa, where its function is unknown.

Secretin

Secretin is a 3056-Da peptide of 27 amino acids, which appears to occur in only one molecular form, the whole molecule being needed for full biological activity. It is produced by S cells sparsely scattered throughout the duodenal and jejunal mucosa. The main stimulus to secretin release is a duodenal pH of less than 4.5, although this occurs rarely. It is probably also secreted late after a meal, but the timing and quantities of this secretion are uncertain. The main physiological role of secretin is stimulating the production of watery, alkaline pancreatic juices in response to acid in the duodenum. It may play an important part in the developing gastrointestinal tract, concentrations of secretin being particularly high in the early postnatal period.

Glucose-dependent insulinotropic peptide

Glucose-dependent insulinotropic peptide is a 5105-Da peptide of 42 amino acids produced by K cells, predominantly in the upper small intestinal mucosa, but also in the gastric antrum and ileum, and is stored in large granules.

At pharmacological doses, glucose-dependent insulinotropic peptide inhibits gastric secretions, hence its original name of gastric inhibitory peptide (GIP). However, its physiological role appears to be as a component of the enteroinsular axis, being released in response to a mixed meal, particularly carbohydrates and long-chain fatty acids, and stimulating insulin release. This incretin effect, also exerted by GLP1 (see later), has been shown to be accompanied by increased levels of cAMP in islet β cells with consequent increased cell mass and resistance to apoptosis.

Vasoactive intestinal peptide (VIP)

VIP is a 3326-Da peptide neurotransmitter of 28 amino acids widely distributed throughout the central and peripheral nervous systems. Its highest concentrations occur in the submucosa of the intestinal tract, where it is found in postganglionic intrinsic nerves (Fig. 15.9.4). It is a potent stimulator of small-intestinal and colonic enterocyte secretion of water and electrolytes, acting via elevation of cAMP. Other important actions include smooth-muscle relaxation, both in the alimentary tract and in the systemic vasculature; stimulation of insulin release, counteracted by a direct glucagon-like effect of VIP in stimulating hepatic gluconeogenesis and glycogenolysis; stimulation of pancreatic bicarbonate secretion; and relaxation of the gallbladder, pyloric sphincter, and circular muscle of the small intestine with contraction of the longitudinal muscle.

Peptide histidine methionine, a neuropeptide of 27 amino acids with considerable sequence homology to VIP, is derived from the adjacent exon of the prepro-VIP gene. It mimics the actions of VIP, probably acting via the same receptor, but is less potent.

Another peptide with considerable sequence homology to VIP is pituitary adenylate cyclase-activating peptide, which occurs in forms with 27 and 38 amino acids. It has a similar tissue distribution to VIP, sharing the same receptor outside the central nervous system and pituitary gland, and similar actions on intestinal secretion and motility.

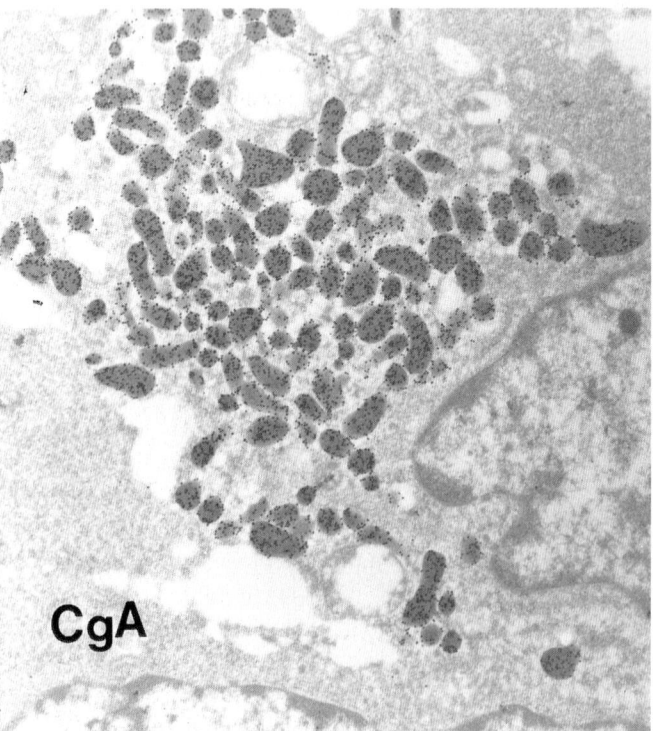

Fig. 15.9.4 Electron micrograph of secretory granules within an endocrine cell of the gut mucosa immunostained for chromogranin A using antibodies labelled with colloidal gold particles (small black dots) (×6500).

Peptide products of preproglucagon

In the pancreas the major product of the preproglucagon molecule is pancreatic glucagon, but in the intestinal L cells preproglucagon is cleaved into enteroglucagon, a peptide of 69 amino acids containing the entire sequence of pancreatic glucagon, two glucagon-like peptides (GLP-1$_{7-36}$ NH$_2$ and GLP-2), and oxyntomodulin.

Enteroglucagon

Enteroglucagon (sometimes called glicentin) is found in high concentrations in the mucosa of the ileum, colon, and rectum. It is released after a mixed meal, particularly of carbohydrate and long-chain fatty acids. The amount of enteroglucagon secreted is proportional to the amount of unabsorbed food entering the colon, and high enteroglucagon concentrations are found in conditions associated with loss of the small-intestinal absorptive capacity. Thus, it has been postulated that enteroglucagon has a trophic effect on the small intestinal mucosa and may be important in gut adaptation.

Glucagon-like peptide 1

The most common circulating form of glucagon-like peptide 1 is as GLP-1$_{7-36}$ NH$_2$. It is released after a meal and, in humans, is the most potent incretin. It induces satiety, inhibiting secretion of glucagon and potentiating the release of somatostatin.

Glucagon-like peptide 2

This appears to stimulate motility and absorption and has trophic effects on the intestine.

Oxyntomodulin

Enteroglucagon is further cleaved by the L cells to produce oxyntomodulin, a peptide of 37 amino acids which is released into the circulation and is a potent inhibitor of gastric motility and secretion. Like glucagon-like peptide 1, it is released postprandially and appears to induce satiety; chronic administration has been shown to reduce weight. Oxyntomodulin appears to act via the receptor for glucagon-like peptide 1 and reduces food intake with similar potency, despite having a 50-fold lower affinity.

Peptide products of preproghrelin

Ghrelin

Studies on growth hormone (GH) secretagogues led to the identification of a specific G-protein-coupled receptor termed the GH secretagogue receptor (GHSR). Subsequently, the endogenous ligand for this receptor was identified as an acylated peptide of 28 amino acids, called ghrelin, cleaved from a 117 amino acid precursor, preproghrelin. Ghrelin and motilin (see below), along with their precursors and receptors, are structurally related, leading to suggestions that they form a new family of peptides. Ghrelin is a circulating hormone secreted predominantly from the oxyntic mucosa of the stomach but is found in other areas of the gut. Its major action is to stimulate food intake. It is, to date, the only known orexigenic hormone and, as such, it opposes the satiety signal leptin.

Obestatin

The only other product of preproghrelin described so far is the 23 amino acid amidated peptide obestatin. It was reported that its administration, peripherally or centrally, to obese rats suppresses food intake and decreases body weight. However, this suggestion that the two known cleavage products of preproghrelin play antagonistic roles in the control of food intake has not been substantiated by subsequent studies.

Motilin

Motilin, a 2700-Da peptide of 22 amino acids, secreted by small intestinal M cells, was first characterized in 1971. Peaks in motilin secretion coincide with initiation of the duodenal myoelectric complex, and so motilin appears to control the reflex motor activity of the small intestine, keeping the small intestine free of debris. Circulating amounts of motilin rise after a meal or drinking water and it may have a physiological role in accelerating gastric emptying and colonic transit. Macrolide antibiotics, e.g. erythromycin, are motilin receptor agonists, hence their side effects of diarrhoea and abdominal cramps.

Peptide tyrosine tyrosine (PYY) and neuropeptide Y

The pancreatic polypeptide-fold (PP-fold) family includes the gut hormone peptide tyrosine tyrosine, the neurotransmitter neuropeptide Y, and, in the pancreatic islets, pancreatic polypeptide. All are 36 amino acid peptides that require C-terminal amidation for bioactivity and share the PP-fold structural motif. They interact with the Y family of receptors that couple to inhibitory G proteins and are probably derived from a common ancestral gene.

Peptide tyrosine tyrosine

Peptide tyrosine tyrosine (PYY) is a 36 amino acid peptide found in the L cells of the distal gut. It is released into the circulation following a meal, mostly as PYY$_{3-36}$, and its levels are reduced during fasting. Its main function appears to be to slow intestinal transit, allowing more time for absorption. Other actions include delaying gastric emptying, decreasing intestinal motility, and inhibiting gastric acid secretion. Clinical trials are testing the efficacy of PYY$_{3-36}$ as an antiobesity agent.

Neuropeptide Y

Neuropeptide Y is a 36 amino acid peptide neurotransmitter, which is often colocalized with noradrenaline. It is found in both extrinsic adrenergic nerves to the myenteric plexus and in intrinsic nerves in the myenteric and submucosal plexi, and highest concentrations occur in the upper intestine and distal colon. It is a potent vasoconstrictor, inhibits intestinal secretion, and depresses colonic motility.

Bombesin and the gastrin-releasing peptides

Bombesin is a 1620-Da peptide of 14 amino acids initially isolated from amphibian skin. It was found to be a potent stimulator of gastrin, and hence of gastric acid secretion. Its mammalian counterparts have similar properties and so were named gastrin-releasing peptides. In humans, gastrin-releasing peptide is a 27 amino acid peptide found in the gut in the intrinsic neurons of the myenteric and submucosal plexuses, particularly in the stomach and pancreas. In addition to its effect on gastrin, it stimulates release of motilin and cholecystokinin, and pancreatic enzyme secretion. Gastrin-releasing peptide is mitogenic and has been reported to have trophic effects on the developing gut. It is also a potent chemoattractant of macrophages and lymphocytes and enhances the phagocytic process in macrophages.

Opioids

The opioid peptides leu-enkephalin, met-enkephalin, and dynorphin are widespread throughout the nerves of the myenteric and submucosal plexuses of the gastrointestinal tract. Their principal actions appear to be inhibition of gastrointestinal secretion and increased smooth muscle contractility. In addition, observations of the activity of μ opioid receptors in inflammatory bowel diseases indicate that endogenous opiates may confer a measure of protection against inflammation.

Tachykinins

The existence of substance P, a 1345-Da peptide of 11 amino acids, was demonstrated in 1931 through its ability to cause smooth-muscle contraction and vasodilatation. Several homologous peptides have since been characterized and are collectively known as tachykinins, because of their rapid action. In humans, there are two tachykinin genes; preprotachykinin A (*TAC1*) encoding substance P and neurokinin-α, and preprotachykinin B (*TAC3*) encoding neurokinin-β. These three tachykinins are localized to neurons in the myenteric and submucosal plexuses throughout the gastrointestinal tract and their principal effects are smooth-muscle contraction, vasodilatation, and inhibition of intestinal absorption.

Other gut peptides

Neurotensin

Neurotensin is a 1673-Da peptide of 13 amino acids present throughout the central nervous system, and in enteric neurons and N cells of the ileal mucosa. It was originally isolated from bovine hypothalamus. Plasma neurotensin concentrations rise postprandially, particularly after fatty food. At physiological doses, neurotensin inhibits gastric acid secretion and gastric emptying, and stimulates pancreatic exocrine and intestinal secretion.

Somatostatin

Somatostatin was initially isolated from the hypothalamus as a 1640-Da peptide of 14 amino acids that inhibited the release of GH. It is widely distributed throughout the central and peripheral nervous systems and is found in a variety of endocrine tissues. In the gastrointestinal tract, it occurs in 14 and 28 amino acid forms secreted by specialized (D) cells distributed throughout the gut mucosa (Fig. 15.9.1) and on the inner rim of the pancreatic islets. D cells have all the characteristics of endocrine cells, but also possess axon-like basal elongations along which the peptide can be transported and secreted directly on to local cells. Somatostatin inhibits hormone release, blocks the response of the effector tissue and inhibits a wide range of gastrointestinal functions (Table 15.9.1). Five human somatostatin receptors have been identified and cloned, the type 1 receptor predominating in the gastrointestinal tract. As gastrointestinal and other neuroendocrine tumours often possess high-density somatostatin receptors, scintigraphy with radiolabelled somatostatin analogues has been used for tumour localization (see 'Carcinoid syndrome', below).

Chromogranin-derived peptides

These structurally related acidic proteins are present in the secretory granule matrix of neuroendocrine cells (see Fig. 15.9.3) and are useful markers of normal and neoplastic neuroendocrine cells. To date, this family of proteins has been shown to consist of three molecules: chromogranin A, the first to be identified and also known as (parathyroid) secretory protein I; chromogranin B, or secretogranin I; and chromogranin C, or secretogranin II. It appears that the chromogranins have dual physiological roles: they may act in the processing of some regulatory peptides and prohormones. Their latter property was suspected when the primary structures of

Table 15.9.1 Inhibitory actions of somatostatin

Hormone release	Physiological function
Growth hormone	Lower oesophageal sphincter contraction
Thyroid-stimulating hormone	Gastric acid secretion
Insulin	Gastric emptying and secretions
Glucagon	Absorption of nutriments
Pancreatic polypeptide	Splanchnic blood flow
Gastrin	Gallbladder contraction and secretions
Secretin	Pancreatic enzyme and bicarbonate secretion
Gastric inhibitory polypeptide	
Motilin	
Enteroglucagon	

the three proteins were determined. All were found to contain multiple pairs of basic amino acids, forming sites for potential proteolytic cleavage. Chromogranin A gives rise to several peptides, including catestatin, chromostatin, vasostatin, and parastatin. Another derived peptide, pancreastatin, was first characterized as a potent inhibitor of insulin release and later found in mucosal cells throughout the gut, where it is often co-stored with other peptides. It is released by gastrin from enterochromaffin-like cells of the gastric fundus, fitting with its action of enhancing meal-stimulated gastric acid secretion. The chromogranin B molecule yields, among other peptides, GAWK (named from its first four amino acids: glycine, alanine, tryptophan, and lysine), a peptide distributed abundantly throughout the gut in both mucosal endocrine cells and intramural nerves. Chromogranins are proving to be of relevance to clinical medicine as plasma concentrations of chromogranins A and B can be used to determine the presence of a neuroendocrine tumour and as a means to monitor the efficacy of treatment.

Other peptide neurotransmitters

Calcitonin gene-related peptide (CGRP) is a peptide of 37 amino acids produced by alternative splicing of the calcitonin gene transcript. It is a widespread neurotransmitter and in the gut occurs in both extrinsic sensory nerves and intrinsic neurons. It inhibits gastric acid and pancreatic secretion, and causes relaxation of vascular smooth muscle.

Galanin is a peptide neurotransmitter of 29 amino acids isolated from porcine intestine. It is widely distributed in enteric nerve terminals and in nerves supplying the liver and pancreatic islets. Its main actions are inhibition of intestinal smooth-muscle contraction and inhibition of postprandial insulin release.

The potent vasoconstricting peptide endothelin has been demonstrated in the plexuses of the gastrointestinal tract and in mucosal epithelial cells. However, its role in the regulation of gastrointestinal function is unknown.

Gut peptides in gastrointestinal disease

Gastric pathology

The commonest cause of elevated levels of circulating gastrin is achlorhydria, which may result from atrophic gastritis, pernicious anaemia, or uraemia, or from iatrogenic causes such as the use of H$_2$-receptor antagonists or proton pump inhibitors such as omeprazole, or following vagotomy. The elevation is a consequence of the loss of negative feedback on gastrin secretion by the low stomach pH. If the antrum is mistakenly retained after gastric surgery, this similarly removes the antral G cells from exposure to gastric acid and is associated with high gastrin concentrations. Achlorhydria-related hypergastrinaemia results in hyperplasia of the gastric histamine-producing enterochromaffin-like cells (Fig. 15.9.5). Long-term increases in gastrin levels are associated with gastric carcinoid tumours that are thought to develop as a result of the direct trophic effect of gastrin on enterochromaffin-like cells. Antisecretory therapy in humans has not been associated with the development of these tumours, but recommended therapeutic doses should not be exceeded and hypergastrinaemia should be avoided in patients on long-term therapy.

Peptic ulcer disease is not usually associated with abnormalities in gut peptide secretion, although a decrease in somatostatin release in patients infected with *Helicobacter pylori* may influence the paracrine regulation of gastric function.

After gastrectomy or truncal vagotomy, patients may develop the dumping syndrome due to accelerated gastric emptying. In these individuals there is a marked increase in the postprandial rise of VIP, neurotensin, PYY, and enteroglucagon, and a decrease in the release of motilin. VIP and neurotensin may both contribute to the postprandial hypotension associated with dumping, but neurotensin may have a beneficial effect in slowing gastric transit. The long-acting somatostatin analogue octreotide is often a very effective treatment for this condition.

Malabsorption

Malabsorptive conditions are associated with a decrease in the amount of peptides produced in the affected region, and a compensatory elevation of other peptides, particularly those trophic peptides implicated in the bowel's adaptation to loss of absorptive surface, such as enteroglucagon.

The postprandial peptide response in patients with untreated coeliac disease shows greatly reduced secretion of glucose-dependent insulinotropic peptide and secretin, which originate from the affected region of bowel. In contrast, there is marked elevation of enteroglucagon, neurotensin, and PYY (Fig. 15.9.6). The decrease in secretin and increase in PYY may be responsible for the reduced pancreatic exocrine and biliary secretion found in this condition. Enteroglucagon stimulates enterocyte turnover in the affected segment, despite the villous atrophy. It may have a trophic effect on the remaining small-intestinal mucosa and delay gut transit time, and neurotensin may help to improve absorption by delaying gastric emptying. In tropical sprue, a postinfective malabsorptive state, a different profile of postprandial peptide release is seen with marked elevation in enteroglucagon and PYY, as in coeliac disease, but also in motilin secretion, while other peptides behave normally. Successful treatment of coeliac disease or tropical sprue returns peptide responses to normal.

The malabsorption associated with pancreatic exocrine insufficiency of any cause leads to an excess of nutriments in the colon, and as a result the concentrations of enteroglucagon, PYY, and neurotensin are raised. The gut adaptation resulting from the effects of these peptides may contribute to the improvement in absorptive function with age in patients with cystic fibrosis.

Intestinal resection

Intestinal resection has profound effects on gut peptide concentrations. A jejunoileal bypass used to be constructed in patients with gross obesity. Peptide concentrations were normal preoperatively, but patients were hyperinsulinaemic and glucose intolerant. After the procedure there was an almost complete absence of the prandial glucose-dependent insulinotropic peptide response and consequently a much reduced first-phase insulin response. The initial beneficial effects of the operation were ultimately negated by massive hypertrophy of the remaining bowel.

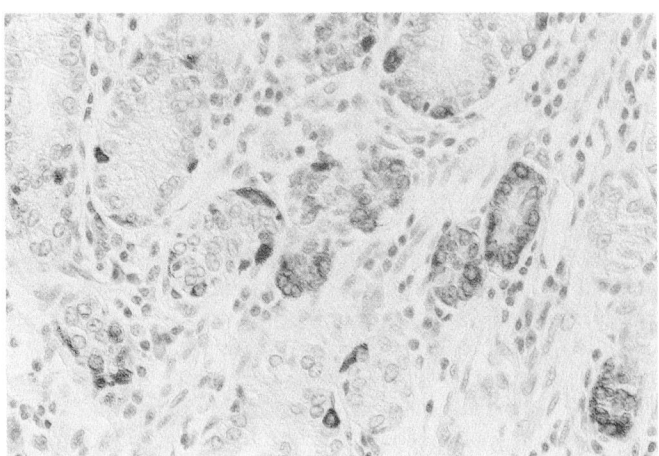

Fig. 15.9.5 Histological section of gastric fundus (oxyntic mucosa) from a patient with pernicious anaemia. Long-standing achlorhydria has led to hyperplasia of enterochromaffin-like (ECL) cells, demonstrated by immunostaining of the general endocrine cell marker chromogranin. In addition to the abnormally high number of cells in the mucosa, small nodules (microcarcinoids) have formed in the submucosa (×180).

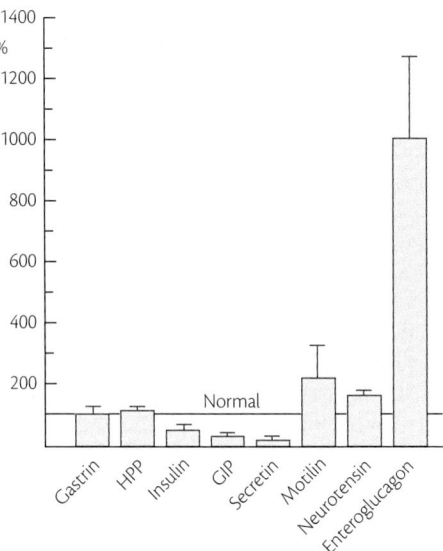

Fig. 15.9.6 The percentage incremental rise in gut hormones following a standard test breakfast in patients with coeliac disease compared with normal controls.

The appearance of large volumes of undigested nutrients in the distal ileum is associated with a 16-fold increase in enteroglucagon responses and an 8-fold increase in neurotensin secretion, and this may provide an explanation for the hypertrophy. After partial ileal resection, the concentrations of gastrin, enteroglucagon, pancreatic polypeptide, motilin, and PYY are elevated, but after colonic resection only gastrin and pancreatic polypeptide are raised, as there is a decrease in production of the other predominantly colonic peptides.

Diarrhoea

In acute infective diarrhoea, the concentrations of enteroglucagon, PYY, and motilin are increased, probably contributing to the altered gut motility and aiding mucosal repair. Patients with Crohn's disease have an elevated pancreatic polypeptide, glucose-dependent insulinotropic peptide, motilin, and enteroglucagon, while in ulcerative colitis there is a modest elevation in pancreatic polypeptide, glucose-dependent insulinotropic peptide, motilin, and gastrin, the last in response to the hypochlorhydria associated with the disease. Elevated levels of endothelin have been reported in ulcerative colitis and Crohn's disease and oral administration of an endothelin receptor antagonist in a model of colitis was found to ameliorate diarrhoea and tissue damage. No demonstrable abnormalities in gut peptides account for disordered motility in the irritable bowel syndrome.

Intestinal tumours

The trophic effects of gut peptides may contribute to proliferation of malignant gut tumours. In particular, colon carcinoma cells have receptors for a number of potentially mitogenic peptides, including gastrin, gastrin-releasing peptides, and VIP.

Neuropathic disease

In conditions associated with destruction of intrinsic enteric nerves there is loss of the neurocrine peptides found in the affected region. Chagas' disease (see Chapter 7.8.11) results from chronic infection with *Trypanosoma cruzi* and in the gastrointestinal tract can result in mega-oesophagus and megacolon. Concentrations of VIP and substance P and of their nerve fibres are greatly reduced in biopsies from affected segments. Similar changes are seen in the affected bowel from children with Hirschsprung's disease, which results from an aganglionic colonic segment. In contrast, neuropeptide Y-containing, mostly adrenergic, nerves are not reduced. Also, patients with the Shy–Drager syndrome, who have chronic autonomic failure with loss of preganglionic extrinsic nerves, have no abnormalities in neurocrine peptides or peptidergic nerve fibres on rectal biopsies (Fig. 15.9.7). AIDS is frequently accompanied by diarrhoea without evidence of secondary infection, and reduced immunostaining for substance P, VIP, and somatostatin in biopsies suggests a neuropathic process may be responsible. Alterations in neuroactive peptides have been observed in a number of inflammatory diseases. Increased density of VIP innervation has been reported in several gut diseases including reflux oesophagitis, radiation colitis, ulcerative colitis, and Crohn's disease. CGRP has been shown to mediate the protective effect of sensory nerves in experimental colitis. It was recently reported that upregulation of the galanin-1 receptor is a mechanism for the increased colonic fluid secretion in infectious diarrhoea resulting from various pathogens.

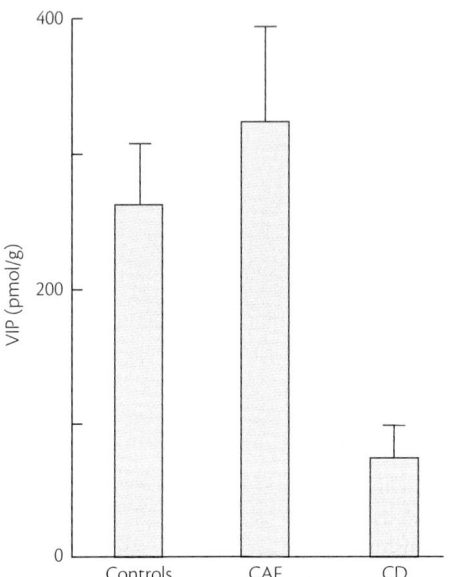

Fig. 15.9.7 Rectal vasoactive intestinal polypeptide (VIP) concentrations (pmol/g wet tissue) in controls and patients with chronic autonomic failure (CAF) and Chagas' disease (CD) with gastrointestinal involvement. Reduced concentrations were seen in Chagas' specimens
(From Long RG, *et al.* (1980). Neural and hormonal peptides in rectal biopsy specimens from patients with Chagas' disease and chronic autonomic failure. *Lancet*, **i**, 559–62, with permission).

Carcinoid syndrome

Introduction

The term *Karzinoide* was originally used by Obendorfer in 1907 to describe a carcinoma-like lesion without malignant qualities. It has now come to refer to tumours capable of producing serotonin (5-hydroxytryptamine, 5-HT). However, several different cell types either synthesize or take up 5-HT and so the term carcinoid is applied to a variety of malignant tumours with different biological behaviour grouped by their similar histological appearances. This section focuses primarily on those tumours associated with the classic carcinoid syndrome.

Primary gastrointestinal carcinoid tumours are derived from the embryonic foregut (thyroid, bronchus, stomach, common bile duct, and pancreas), midgut or hindgut. The most common sites for carcinoid tumours are the appendix and rectum, but these tumours, often found incidentally on histological examinations of appendicectomy and rectal biopsy specimens, are almost always benign. Rectal neuroendocrine tumours generally produce glucagon-like peptides and PYY rather than 5-HT and are not usually associated with a clinical syndrome, even when they metastasize.

The carcinoid syndrome occurs in about 10% of patients with carcinoid tumours. It does not develop when the tumour drains through a normal liver, and so midgut tumours have almost always metastasized, usually to the liver, before symptoms develop. The carcinoid syndrome is most commonly due to a metastatic midgut tumour, about 50% of which metastasize to the liver. Primary carcinoid tumours are bronchial in origin in about 10% of cases, and rarely occur in the ovary and testis. Tumours in these sites may be associated with the syndrome in the absence of metastases. The annual incidence of the carcinoid syndrome is about 1 in 500 000.

Clinical manifestations

The cardinal feature of the classic carcinoid syndrome is the flush. The carcinoid flush predominantly involves the head and upper thorax, and is usually associated with tachycardia, hypotension, increased skin temperature and, sometimes, wheezing. Rarely, flushing extends to the trunk and limbs, and may be associated with lacrimation, facial oedema, and great distress. Attacks are paroxysmal and usually unprovoked, although precipitating factors include alcohol or food ingestion, stress, emotion, or exertion. Flushing initially lasts for only a few minutes, but as the disease progresses may become almost continuous, and such patients often develop a chronically reddened and cyanotic facial hue, with widespread telangiectasia, the 'leonine facies'. This fixed flush is more commonly seen with bronchial carcinoids, which are often metabolically inactive, but when associated with flushing can cause severe attacks lasting for hours or days, occasionally with profound hypotension and even anuria. Gastric carcinoids are often associated with raised, localized, wheal-like areas of flushing, which are usually pruritic and may migrate.

The other characteristic feature of the syndrome is secretory diarrhoea, which may be profuse and accompanied by electrolyte disturbance, cramping abdominal pain, nausea, and vomiting. Rarely these symptoms may result from small-bowel obstruction by a large ileal carcinoid tumour, but the majority of primary tumours are small, usually being less than 1% of total body tumour weight. Hepatic metastases may cause right hypochondrial pain, particularly if the liver capsule is involved or stretched, and acute exacerbations may occur if metastases become ischaemic and undergo autonecrosis. Weight loss and, in the later stages, cachexia are common as a result of poor dietary intake, malabsorption, and increased catabolism. Pellagra with dermatitis of sun-exposed areas may occur, the increased conversion of 5-hydroxytryptophan into 5-HT causing nicotinamide deficiency.

Cardiac valve abnormalities affect about 50% of patients. They occur as a result of endocardial fibrosis, with plaques of smooth muscle in a collagenous stroma deposited on the valves. Lesions are almost always on the right-hand side, left-sided valve damage occurring only in association with bronchial carcinoids, which drain into the left atrium, or atrioseptal defects with right to left shunting. The most common lesions are tricuspid incompetence and pulmonary stenosis, and the usual clinical outcome is oedema and breathlessness due to right ventricular failure, which can be fatal. The other causes of breathlessness in association with the carcinoid syndrome are bronchospasm, which affects a small number of patients, often occurring with flushing attacks, and metastatic involvement of the lung and pleura. Arthritis occurs in a small number of patients, and sclerotic bone metastases may be seen, usually in association with foregut tumours.

Carcinoid tumours, in common with other gastroenteropancreatic tumours, have the potential to produce a variety of peptide products and may be associated with other syndromes, with or without the carcinoid syndrome. The most common of these associated syndromes is Cushing's, due to an ectopic ACTH-secreting, bronchial or pancreatic carcinoid. Carcinoid tumours may also be a feature of multiple endocrine neoplasia type 1.

Biochemistry

The biologically active metabolite characteristically produced by metastatic carcinoid tumours is 5-HT, synthesized from the amino acid tryptophan (Fig. 15.9.8). 5-HT probably plays a part in the pathogenesis of some of the symptoms of the carcinoid syndrome, particularly the diarrhoea and bronchoconstriction. It is metabolized to 5-hydroxyindoleacetic acid (5-HIAA), which accounts for 95% of the urinary excretion of 5-HT.

A variety of vasoactive substances may be secreted by carcinoid tumours and have been implicated in the pathogenesis of the flush. Flushing can be provoked by intravenous noradrenaline, which has been shown to activate kallikrein in the tumour, leading to synthesis and release of bradykinin. Other possible mediators of the flush include histamine, the tachykinins substance P and neurokinin A, and prostaglandins, although the flush is rarely affected by inhibitors of prostaglandin synthesis, such as indomethacin. Gastric carcinoids are derived from histamine-producing enterochromaffin-like cells and histamine is possibly the cause of the characteristic wheal-like flush seen with gastric tumours.

Investigations

The diagnosis of carcinoid syndrome is made on the basis of elevated concentrations of 5-HIAA in a 24-h urine collection, and urinary 5-HIAA acts as a marker of disease progression. Various foods, including avocados, bananas, aubergines, pineapples, plums, and walnuts, should be avoided while collecting specimens, to prevent false-positive results. A number of drugs and other substances interfere with the spectrophotometric assay: paracetamol, fluorouracil, methysergide, and caffeine give false-positive results, and ACTH, phenothiazines, methyldopa, monoamine oxidase inhibitors, and tricyclic antidepressants false negatives. The other products of carcinoid tumours are not routinely assayed.

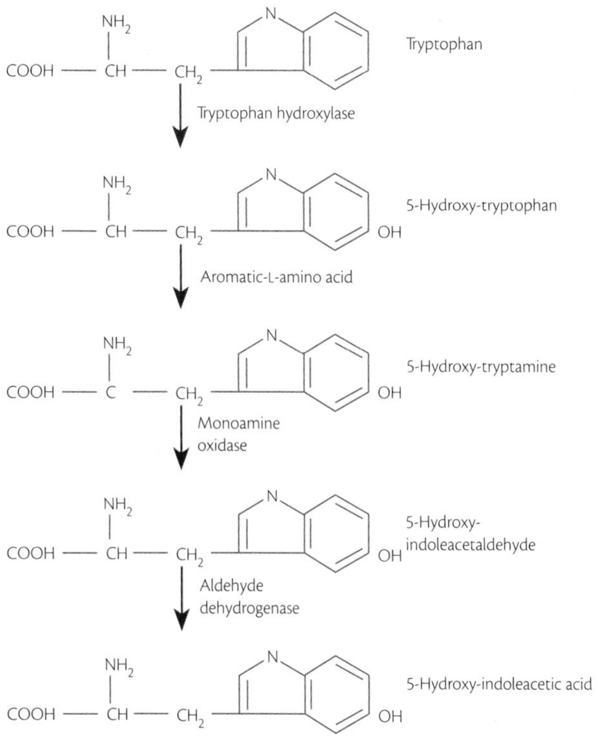

Fig. 15.9.8 Biochemical pathway for the synthesis and degradation of 5-hydroxytryptamine.

Topographic localization of carcinoid tumours can be done by Octreoscan (Fig. 15.9.9), CT scan, or endoscopy/ultrasound and is rarely a problem, as most have gross hepatic metastases, visible on CT scan or abdominal ultrasonography, at the time of diagnosis. In those rare cases where the syndrome occurs in the absence of metastases, tumour localization may offer the prospect of cure. These tumours are unlikely to be in the gastrointestinal tract and so chest radiographs and CT scans of the chest and pelvis should be taken. Angiography may be of value in assessing suitability for hepatic embolization. Carcinoid tumours have characteristic histological features being composed of regular polygonal cells arranged in nests. The capacity of 5-HT to reduce silver salts (so-called argentaffinity) led to the development of a classical diagnostic histochemical stain (Fig. 15.9.10), although immunostaining for 5-HT is also used to identify the tumours.

Treatment

The realistic aim of therapy in patients with the carcinoid syndrome is to relieve the symptoms. Simple treatments such as codeine phosphate, diphenoxylate, and loperamide may help to control the diarrhoea. Many of the symptoms can be controlled with the peripheral 5-HT antagonists: cyproheptadine, a 5-HT type 2 receptor blocker, often helps the diarrhoea; ketanserin may be effective in reducing flushing; and the 5-HT type 3 receptor antagonist ondansetron can alleviate nausea and anorexia. Parachlorphenylalanine, an inhibitor of tryptophan hydroxylase, and chlorpromazine block synthesis of 5-HT, but are rarely used. Histamine may mediate some of the features of the syndrome, especially in patients with gastric carcinoids, and in these cases H_1- and H_2-receptor blockade may be useful. With the exception of simple antidiarrhoeal agents, these treatments have been largely superseded by the long-acting, subcutaneously administered, somatostatin analogue octreotide. This inhibits the release of the mediators of the syndrome by the tumour and antagonizes their peripheral effects. Octreotide is effective in alleviating symptoms in more than 90% of patients. It is rarely associated with significant side effects: the acidic solution can cause pain at the injection site; gallstones often develop, but are rarely of clinical significance; and a few patients develop steatorrhoea, which can be prevented by giving pancreatic enzyme supplements. Octreotide is now the first-line treatment for most patients and may be life-saving in the carcinoid crisis, when symptoms become severe and continuous. In addition to octreotide, during crises patients usually need close monitoring of fluid and electrolytes, often by measurement of

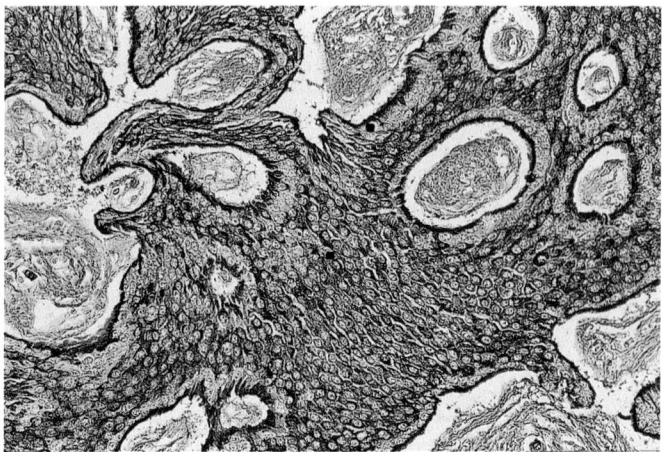

Fig. 15.9.10 Histological section of ileum from a patient with carcinoid syndrome showing a malignant carcinoid tumour stained with silver salts (Masson's argentaffin stain) (×120).

central venous pressure, and appropriate replacement therapy. Minor injury, including overenthusiastic clinical examination of large carcinoid masses in the liver, may induce a life-threatening state akin to the tumour lysis syndrome characterized by pain, fever, shock, and renal failure compounded by hyperuricaemia and hyperphosphataemia. Allopurinol, and the judicious use of infusions of sodium bicarbonate to make the urine more alkaline, as well as antimicrobials, may reduce the threat of renal failure in this condition. Corticosteroids may improve shock.

The principal disadvantage of octreotide is that patients develop resistance with time, and most become refractory to any form of treatment after about 4 years. Vitamin supplements containing nicotinamide are necessary when patients have pellagra, and these can be given prophylactically. The treatment of cardiac manifestations is the same as for valve disease and cardiac failure of other causes. Patients with painful bony metastases may benefit from palliative radiotherapy.

In patients who fail to respond to octreotide or are intolerant to it, tumour debulking may provide palliative relief. Surgery is rarely indicated, although enucleation of large metastases may give some benefit. Carcinoid tumours rarely respond to any form of chemotherapy. The most effective means of debulking is hepatic embolization, which devascularizes the tumour while the blood supply to the normal liver is maintained by the portal vein. Octreotide should be given in high dose during this intervention, as the necrotic metastases release large quantities of vasoactive mediators that can cause a severe carcinoid crisis with profound hypotension, leading to acute renal failure (see tumour lysis syndrome, above).

Prognosis

Carcinoid tumours behave like other gastroenteropancreatic tumours, with the majority following an indolent course. Estimates given for 5-year survival rates for carcinoids are; appendiceal 98%, gastric (types I/II) 81%, rectal 87%, small intestinal 60%, colonic carcinoids 62%, and gastric type III/IV 33%. Palliation is very worthwhile in these patients, allowing them to lead a normal life until the terminal stages of the disease.

Multiple endocrine neoplasia and nondiabetic pancreatic endocrine disorders are described elsewhere.

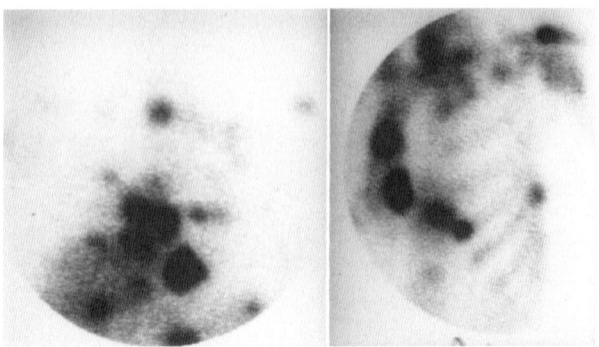

Fig. 15.9.9 ¹¹¹In-labelled somatostatin analogue scan (left) in a patient with carcinoid syndrome showing metastases to liver, bone, and intrathoracic lymph nodes compared with a conventional base scan (right).

Further reading

Besterman HS, *et al.* (1978). Gut hormone profile in coeliac disease. *Lancet*, **i**, 785–8.

Bishop AE, Polak JM (1997). Classification of neuroendocrine tumours. In: Sheaves R, Jenkins P, Wass JAH (eds). *Clinical endocrine oncology*, pp. 369–376. Blackwell Scientific Publications, Oxford.

Bishop AE, Polak JM (1999). The gut and the autonomic nervous system. In: Bannister R, Mathias C (eds) *Autonomic failure*, pp. 117–25. Oxford University Press, Oxford.

Bloom SR, Long RG (eds) (1982). *Radioimmunoassay of gut regulatory peptides*. Saunders, London.

Coll AP, Farooqi IS, O'Rahilly S (2007). The hormonal control of food intake. *Cell*, **129**, 252–62.

Cook GC, *et al.* (1979). Gut hormone responses in tropical malabsorption. *Br Med J*, **i**, 1252–5.

Cummings DE, Overduin J (2007). Gastrointestinal regulation of food intake. *J Clin Invest*, **117**, 13–23.

Drucker DJ (2007). The role of gut hormones in glucose homeostasis. *J Clin Invest*, **117**, 24–32.

Gorden P, *et al.* (1989). NIH conference. Somatostatin and somatostatin analogue (SMS 201–995) in treatment of hormone-secreting tumors of the pituitary and gastrointestinal tract and non-neoplastic diseases of the gut. *Ann Intern Med*, **110**, 35–50.

Gutniak M, *et al.* (1992). Antidiabetogenic effect of glucagon-like peptide-1 (7–36) amide in normal subjects and patients with diabetes mellitus. *N Engl J Med*, **326**, 1316–22.

Hodgson HJ, Maton PN (1987). Carcinoid and neuroendocrine tumours of the liver. *Baillière's Clin Gastroenterol*, **1**, 35–61.

Jensen RT (ed.) (1989). Gastrointestinal endocrinology. *Gastroenterol Clin N Am*, **18**, 671–931.

Kvols LK (1989). Therapy of the malignant carcinoid syndrome. *Endocrinol Metabol Clin N Am*, **18**, 557–68.

Lacroix A, *et al.* (1992). Gastric inhibitory polypeptide-dependent cortisol hypersecretion—a new cause of Cushing's syndrome. *N Engl J Med*, **327**, 974–80.

Long RG, *et al.* (1980). Neural and hormonal peptides in rectal biopsy specimens from patients with Chagas' disease and chronic autonomic failure. *Lancet*, **i**, 559–62.

Long RG, Adrian TE, Bloom SR (1981). Gastrointestinal hormones in pancreatic disease. In: Mitchell CJ, Kelleher J, eds. *Pancreatic diseases in clinical medicine*, pp. 223–39. Pitman Medical, Tunbridge Wells.

Maton PN, Jensen RT (1992). Use of gut peptide receptor agonists and antagonists in gastrointestinal diseases. *Gastroenterol Clin N Am*, **21**, 551–664.

Merchant JL (2007). Tales from the crypts: regulatory peptides and cytokines in gastrointestinal homeostasis and disease. *J Clin Invest*, **117**, 6–12.

Modlin IM, *et al.* (2006). Gastrointestinal carcinoids: the evolution of diagnostic strategies. *J Clin Gastroenterol*, **40**, 572–82.

Moss SF, *et al.* (1992). Effect of *Helicobacter pylori* on gastric somatostatin in duodenal ulcer disease. *Lancet*, **ii**, 930–2.

Murphy KG, Bloom SR (2006). Gut hormones and the regulation of energy homeostasis. *Nature*, **444**, 854–9.

Reznik Y, *et al.* (1992). Food-dependent Cushing's syndrome mediated by aberrant adrenal sensitivity to gastric inhibitory polypeptide. *N Engl J Med*, **327**, 981–6.

Thompson JC (1991). Humoral control of gut function. *Am J Surg*, **161**, 6–18.

Winkler H, Fischer-Colbrie R (1992). The chromogranins A and B: the first 25 years and future perspectives. *Neuroscience*, **49**, 497–528.

15.10

Malabsorption

Contents

15.10.1 Differential diagnosis and investigation of malabsorption

Julian R.F. Walters

Essentials

Malabsorption by the gastrointestinal tract results in excess loss of dietary nutrients in the faeces and, if dietary intake does not increase to compensate, nutritional deficiency in the body. Digestion and absorption involve multiple processes in the entire gastrointestinal tract and hence a large number of different conditions can result in specific or generalized patterns of malabsorption.

The diagnosis of malabsorption is often missed until it is advanced. There may be nonspecific symptoms such as loss of weight, lassitude, and weakness; changes in the nature of the stool or frequency of bowel habit are not invariable. Examination may reveal poor general nutritional status and features of specific deficiencies, e.g. anaemia.

Commonly obtained haematological and biochemical investigations can show abnormalities—e.g. anaemia; low serum iron, transferrin saturation, vitamin B_{12}, and folate—but deficiency can be due to malnutrition, maldigestion (usually from pancreatic insufficiency), or malabsorption.

Coeliac disease, one of the commonest causes of malabsorption, is now easily screened for by specific serology for tissue transglutaminase (tTG) antibodies. Endoscopy to obtain intestinal histology, imaging, and certain function tests (see Chapter 15.3.4) are necessary to make alternative diagnoses.

Principles of normal absorption

The normal physiology of nutrient absorption is complex—specific molecular mechanisms have evolved for each of the various types of nutrient. Understanding the principles involved in normal absorption enables different causes of malabsorption to be appreciated, appropriate differential diagnoses to be made, and investigations planned accordingly.

Absorptive capacity

For each of the classes of nutrients, the overall efficiency of intestinal absorption varies. Some compounds, such as components of dietary fibre, are not absorbed even in health. Others are normally almost completely absorbed, but in disease, absorption is insufficient to cope with the load, giving symptoms of diarrhoea from excess faecal water, or steatorrhoea from excess faecal fat.

The principal determinants of the maximum absorptive capacity are the area of the intestinal mucosa, increased by surface folding, villi, and microvilli to about 200 m^2, and the function of the individual cellular transporting mechanisms. As part of the total absorptive process, the intestine also has to reabsorb endogenous secretions produced to aid digestion. Approximately 7 litres of digestive fluids from salivary, gastric, biliary, pancreatic, and intestinal sources add significantly to the absorptive requirements for water, electrolytes, protein, and fat. Secretory diarrhoea and protein-losing enteropathy are conditions where endogenous output exceeds the absorptive capacity of the bowel.

Sites of absorption

Gastrointestinal motility mixes food with digestive secretions and propels them from the mouth to the anus. During this passage, nutrients are exposed to specialized areas of the gut with specific digestive or absorptive functions. The duodenum and proximal jejunum are mostly involved with digestion and fluid secretion. However, the more acidic pH in this area means the solubility and hence the absorption of polyvalent cations such as iron and calcium is high. The bulk of nutrient absorption takes place in the more distal jejunum and ileum. The terminal ileum is specialized for absorption of cobalamin (vitamin B_{12}) and bile salt. The colon salvages fluid and electrolytes not absorbed by the small intestine and absorbs short-chain fatty acids produced by colonic bacteria from poorly digested carbohydrates. Loss of specialized areas by surgical resection or disease activity can produce specific patterns of malabsorption.

The intestinal epithelial cells differentiate as they move from crypt to villus tip. The older villus-tip enterocytes perform most of the absorptive functions, though some digestive enzymes are found in less mature cells. Fluid secretion probably occurs from the crypts. Goblet cells secrete mucus, trapping an unstirred water layer which is a relative barrier to the diffusion of large molecules but allows the smaller products of digestion to reach the surface of the epithelium. Other epithelial cells secrete various hormones or have immunological functions.

Mechanisms of absorption

Absorption occurs by transcellular and paracellular pathways. The paracellular pathway is through the tight junctions which link the epithelial cells. By this pathway, passive absorption of small molecules occurs by diffusion down electrical and concentration gradients. 'Solvent drag' is the term used to describe movement down concentration gradients, which are themselves created by the movement of water. Active transport takes place through the epithelial cell against these gradients and necessitates the expenditure of energy generated within the cell.

Three steps are involved in transcellular absorption: entry to the cell at the apical (brush border) membrane; passage through the cytoplasm; and exit from the cell at the basolateral membrane. Polarization of the enterocyte produces differences in structure and function of the apical and basolateral membranes. Specific carrier molecules are present in one of these membranes but not the other; this asymmetry generates vectorial flow in a single direction through the cell. The molecular basis for absorption of most types of nutrients has now been defined.

Diagnosis of malabsorption

The diagnosis of malabsorption is often missed until it is advanced. Diseases of the small intestine, colon, pancreas, liver, and stomach can all produce malabsorption; these may be obvious (such as the result of previous surgery) or may not be suspected until malabsorption is diagnosed.

History

Delayed growth and development, loss of weight, lassitude, and weakness may be described, but can be due to many other conditions. Changes in the nature of the stool or frequency of bowel habit suggest gastrointestinal disease but are not invariable, as apparently normal stools or constipation can also be found. In describing their faeces, patients may indicate the features of steatorrhoea, rather than watery diarrhoea. Careful questioning is needed to differentiate descriptions of changes in stool frequency or volume, and the passage of gas, liquid, oil, or grease. Bloating, borborygmi, and abdominal discomfort are often reported and seepage of oil from the anus may be described.

A previous history of abdominal surgery, radiation, and alcohol or drug usage may immediately make obvious the likely cause of malabsorption. A family history of coeliac disease or dermatitis herpetiformis makes gluten sensitivity more likely. Malabsorption of nutrients such as iron, folate and vitamin B_{12}, calcium, or vitamin K can give specific histories of anaemia, bone disease, and fractures, or bleeding and bruising.

Examination

General nutritional status can be assessed by height, weight, body mass index, and by anthropomorphic measurements such as skin fold thickness. Anaemia, bruising, petechiae, ascites, oedema, glossitis, mucosal changes, and neuromuscular irritability (including positive Trousseau's or Chvosteck's signs) may be found and indicate specific deficiencies. Pigmentation and clubbing can occur. Abdominal distension, scars from previous surgery, masses, or fistulas can suggest specific diagnoses. The nature of the stools must be examined.

Evidence from routine investigations

Commonly obtained haematological and biochemical investigations can show a reduced haemoglobin concentration, microcytosis or macrocytosis, raised red cell distribution width, thrombocytopenia, and low serum iron, transferrin saturation, vitamin B_{12}, and folate. The prothrombin time or international normalized ratio (INR) may be raised. Albumin, calcium, phosphate, 25-hydroxyvitamin D (calcidiol), zinc, and other nutrients may be reduced. Elevated alkaline phosphatase and parathyroid hormone can suggest metabolic bone disease secondary to malabsorption.

Differential diagnosis

When malabsorption is suspected, two parallel diagnostic pathways need to be followed: first, to define the extent of the nutritional deficiency, and second, to define the cause of the malabsorption.

Generalized or isolated nutrient malabsorption?

When an isolated nutritional deficiency, such as that of B_{12} or iron, is identified, it must be remembered that this may be due to a more generalized process and evidence for malabsorption of other nutrients may be found if looked for. However, abnormalities in specific transport pathways, either genetic or acquired, account for some common types of malabsorption (Table 15.10.1.1).

Malnutrition, maldigestion, or malabsorption?

Evidence of deficiency of a nutrient does not necessarily imply malabsorption. In many cases, nutritional intake is impaired, or insufficient to meet increased demands. Pregnancy places additional

Table 15.10.1.1 Common forms of malabsorption of specific nutrients

Nutrient	Condition
Lactose	Lactase nonpersistence
Vitamin B_{12}	Pernicious anaemia (loss of intrinsic factor)
Bile salts	Bile acid diarrhoea

demands on iron, calcium, and many other nutrients. Menorrhagia requires extra iron intake. Excessive loss of protein, electrolytes, and water may require increased intake, and additional calories are required in catabolic states such as infection, surgery, and critical care. Assessment of intake and requirements may determine that poor nutrition is the principal factor and dietary supplementation is required.

Impaired digestion, usually from pancreatic insufficiency, will produce a clinical state similar to malabsorption resulting from intestinal disease. Absorption of simple nutrients, as in an elemental diet, will be normal, but complex foods, particularly fats, will not be hydrolysed to forms that can be absorbed. Evidence of pancreatic disease should be looked for with imaging and function tests.

Conditions that cause malabsorption are listed in Table 15.10.1.2. Some, such as coeliac disease, are common; others such as the short bowel syndrome in patients with extensive surgery, may be obvious, but other diagnoses may not be made unless specifically sought.

Investigation of malabsorption

Function tests

Tests to investigate absorptive functions are described in Chapter 15.3.4. These may be necessary to define the extent of nutrient malabsorption, but in most cases are not needed in routine clinical practice, where the emphasis is usually on defining the precise pathological cause of the malabsorption.

Faecal fat measurements may have to be performed occasionally to confirm that malabsorption (or maldigestion) is present and needs further investigation. The absorption of fat depends on a large number of different steps making it a sensitive indicator of malabsorption. Faecal collections are made over several days on a defined fat intake. However, the unpleasantness of these collections and assays has resulted in a number of other tests being developed in attempts to circumvent these problems.

Measurement of faecal pancreatic elastase-1 immunoreactivity is widely used to predict significant pancreatic insufficiency. This test is easy to perform although it is not sensitive enough to detect less severe degrees of functional impairment. Other indirect tests for pancreatic function, such as the pancreolauryl test, have now been made unnecessary.

The Schilling test has been useful in differentiating vitamin B_{12} malabsorption caused by ileal disease from autoimmune gastritis (pernicious anaemia), but with good tests for autoantibodies to intrinsic factor and gastric parietal cells is usually unnecessary. The xylose absorption test has largely been superseded by tests aimed at detecting specific pathologies.

Testing stools or urine for laxative abuse may be necessary, and endocrine causes of diarrhoea and malabsorption, although rare, should not be forgotten. The SeHCAT test is necessary to make a definitive diagnosis of bile acid malabsorption.

Table 15.10.1.2 Causes of malabsorption

Common	
Coeliac disease	Gluten-sensitive enteropathy
Small-bowel bacterial overgrowth	Gastric surgery and achlorhydria
	Intestinal blind loops postsurgery
	Jejunal diverticula
	Intestinal strictures
	Fistulas (as in Crohn's disease)
	Impaired peristalsis (fibrosis)
Pancreatic insufficiency	Chronic pancreatitis
	Cystic fibrosis
Less common	
Short bowel syndrome	Intestinal resection for Crohn's disease, mesenteric vascular disease, or injury
Chronic infections	Tropical sprue
	Giardiasis
	Other parasites (e.g. *Strongyloides* sp.)
	Tuberculosis
	AIDS
Lymphoma	Immunoproliferative small-intestinal disease
	Enteropathy-associated T-cell lymphoma
	Refractory sprue and ulcerative jejunoileitis
Radiation enteritis	Fibrosis
	Atrophy
	Strictures
	Lymphangiectasia
Intestinal lymphangiectasia	Congenital
	Infective
	Fibrotic
	Malignant
	Cardiac
Drugs	Orlistat
	Laxatives
	Neomycin (and many others rarely)
	Cholestyramine (and certain others with specific interactions)
Allergic	Eosinophilic enteritis
	Milk and soya enteropathy
Immunodeficiency	Autoimmune enteropathy
Rare	Whipple's disease
	Amyloidosis
	Abetalipoproteinaemia
	Most specific transporter defects

Serological tests for coeliac disease

IgA-class antibodies to tissue transglutaminase or endomysium are highly sensitive and specific, and have simplified screening for coeliac disease in patients with any suggestion of possible malabsorption. Endomysial antibodies are detected by immunofluorescence and are a subclass of the previously used reticulin antibodies.

Tissue transglutaminase (tTG) is the antigen recognized by endomysial antibodies. The presence of tTG antibodies is detected more conveniently than endomysial antibodies, being an enzyme-linked immunoassay (ELISA). This is now the usual screening test, with endomysial antibodies being used for confirmation. Test employing human recombinant tTG have the best sensitivity. False-negative results to both antibodies in coeliac disease occur in the presence of selective IgA deficiency (approximately 1 in 50 of the population), but IgG-class antibodies are then detected. With effective treatment of coeliac disease on a gluten-free diet, tTG and endomysial antibodies become negative. Gliadin antibodies have much lower specificity and are not valuable in screening.

The availability of these simple blood tests for tTG antibodies, with high positive and negative predictive values for coeliac disease, means that this condition can now be strongly suspected before intestinal biopsy is performed.

HLA class II typing (now usually done by polymerase chain reaction rather than by serology) has a limited role in clarifying whether coeliac disease is likely in atypical cases. As essentially all proven coeliac subjects are either HLA DQ2 or DQ8, the diagnosis is improbable with alternative types.

Endoscopy and small bowel histology

Endoscopy is widely available and enables tissue to be taken from the small intestine to make a histological diagnosis of the pathology causing malabsorption. Oesophagogastroduodenoscopy allows biopsies from the upper duodenum. At colonoscopy, biopsies can be taken from the terminal ileum. Fortunately, common intestinal diseases such as coeliac disease are diffuse and diagnosis can usually be made from duodenal biopsies taken at routine upper endoscopy. Multiple biopsies reduce the likelihood of sampling error.

Mucosal appearances at endoscopy may be abnormal, suggesting histological diagnoses. With modern endoscopes, the resolution and magnification is such that villi can be detected. A smooth mucosa, with reduced folds of Kerckring, scalloped valvulae conniventes, pallor, and a mosaic appearance suggest villous atrophy, as in coeliac disease. Small white spots can indicate areas of intestinal lymphangiectasia. In the terminal ileum, ulceration can indicate Crohn's disease. Biopsies can be directed to abnormal areas.

Push enteroscopy or double balloon enteroscopy allows much more of the small bowel to be inspected and biopsies taken. Wireless capsule endoscopy has been recently developed to allow simple and relatively noninvasive visualization of the entire small intestine. The early changes of small-intestinal Crohn's disease (aphthoid ulcers) are best detected by this method, but advanced stricturing may result in capsule retention. Coeliac disease also has characteristic appearances. It is not possible to obtain biopsies with the wireless capsule.

Other systems such as the Crosby capsule, designed to take biopsies remotely, are used infrequently now that coeliac disease is usually diagnosed by endoscopic duodenal biopsies. These methods do not allow reliable targeting to specific areas of small intestine

seen on radiology. Laparotomy (or laparoscopy) may be needed to take full-thickness biopsies from jejunal and ileal lesions.

Histology will be definitive in most small-bowel diseases. Villous atrophy with crypt hyperplasia is most frequently caused by coeliac disease. Tropical sprue, allergy to cows' milk protein in children, and a range of other conditions occasionally cause a similar picture. Intestinal lymphangiectasia, lymphoma, eosinophilic enteritis, Whipple's disease, amyloid, and abetalipoproteinaemia have characteristic appearances. Parasites including *Giardia* sp. may be seen.

Radiology

Plain abdominal radiographs may show calcification in chronic pancreatitis, faecal loading, or abnormal gas-filled loops of bowel.

Contrast studies of the small intestine will define abnormal anatomy. Small-bowel enema (enteroclysis) is preferred for showing mucosal detail, although barium follow-through studies are more easily tolerated and can give better images of proximal duodenum and terminal ileum. Mass lesions or strictures from Crohn's disease, tuberculosis, lymphoma, other tumours, fibrosis, radiation, ischaemia, or drug-induced injury will be demonstrated. Enteric fistulas and diverticula are diagnosed. Postsurgical anatomy can be defined and the length of remaining intestine in the short bowel syndrome estimated.

Endoscopic retrograde cholangiopancreatography (ERCP) and magnetic resonance cholangiopancreatography (MRCP) show pancreatic abnormalities that can cause pancreatic exocrine insufficiency.

CT, ultrasonography, and angiography have roles in further defining conditions associated with malabsorption. Magnetic resonance enteroclysis is increasingly being used to diagnose small-intestinal Crohn's disease.

Microbiology

Small-bowel bacterial overgrowth is a common and frequently undiagnosed cause of malabsorption. Absolute bacterial counts in proximal small-intestinal fluid are hard to obtain without contamination, so diagnosis tends to be on clinical suspicion confirmed indirectly via glucose hydrogen breath testing (see Chapter 15.3.4).

Infestations causing malabsorption (including *Giardia* and *Strongyloides* spp.) will be diagnosed by demonstrating parasites in fresh stool, or duodenal aspirates.

Response to treatment

Confirmation of the diagnosis of malabsorption is often made by assessing the response to treatment. Symptomatic patients with typical villous atrophy and positive antibody tests, who respond clinically and serologically to a gluten-free diet, can be confirmed to have coeliac disease and do not routinely need further biopsies. In small-intestinal bacterial overgrowth, the diagnosis is often only finally made by the response to broad-spectrum antibiotics. Pancreatic exocrine insufficiency can be confirmed with a satisfactory response to enzyme replacements.

Further reading

American Gastroenterological Association (1999). American Gastroenterological Association medical position statement: guidelines for the evaluation and management of chronic diarrhea. *Gastroenterology*, **116**, 1461–3.

Hill ID, *et al.* (2005). Guideline for the diagnosis and treatment of celiac disease in children: recommendations of the North American Society for Pediatric Gastroenterology, Hepatology and Nutrition. *J Pediatr Gastroenterol Nutr*, **40**, 1–19.

Lewis NR, Scott BB. (2006). Systematic review: the use of serology to exclude or diagnose coeliac disease (a comparison of the endomysial and tissue transglutaminase antibody tests). *Aliment Pharmacol Ther*, **24**, 47–54.

Thomas PD, *et al.* (2003). Guidelines for the investigation of chronic diarrhoea, 2nd edition. *Gut*, **52** Suppl 5, v1–15.

Walker-Smith J, *et al.* (2002). Chronic diarrhea and malabsorption (including short gut syndrome): Working Group Report of the First World Congress of Pediatric Gastroenterology, Hepatology, and Nutrition. *J Pediatr Gastroenterol Nutr*, **35** Suppl 2, S98–105.

15.10.2 Small-bowel bacterial overgrowth

P.P. Toskes

Essentials

Malabsorption in a patient with overgrowth of bacteria in the small intestine is known as small-bowel bacterial overgrowth (SBBO). Predisposing causes include sustained hypochlorhydria induced by proton pump inhibitors, small-intestinal stagnation due to anatomical (e.g. diverticulosis, postsurgical) or motor (e.g. scleroderma) abnormalities, and chronic pancreatitis.

Presenting symptoms include diarrhoea, steatorrhoea, weight loss, and flatulence. Investigation may reveal low levels of cobalamin (metabolized by Gram-negative anaerobes), increased serum folate (synthesized by overgrowth flora), and decreased urinary excretion of xylose (intraluminal degradation of the sugar by overgrowth flora).

Definitive diagnosis is time-consuming and expensive, requiring a properly collected and appropriately cultured aspirate from the proximal small intestine revealing a total concentration of bacteria generally greater than 10^5 organisms/ml, with *Bacteroides*, anaerobic lactobacilli, coliforms, and enterococci all likely to be present. Alternative investigations are frequently employed, of which the most reliable is the ^{14}C-xylose breath test, with elevated levels of $^{14}CO_2$ found in the breath after 30 min in SBBO.

Aside from supportive care, specific treatment is with an antimicrobial that is effective against both aerobic and anaerobic enteric bacteria, e.g. tetracycline (but resistance is an increasing problem), amoxicillin-clavulanic acid, or norfloxacin.

Introduction

The occurrence of malabsorption in a patient with overgrowth of bacteria in the small intestine is known as small-bowel bacterial overgrowth (SBBO). This occurs in a range of conditions associated with abnormal motility, including gastroparesis, irritable bowel syndrome, and chronic pancreatitis—three conditions that

---

Box 15.10.2.1 Characteristic clinical features of SBBO

- Diarrhoea
- Steatorrhoea
- Cobalamin (vitamin B_{12}) malabsorption
- Decreased urinary xylose excretion
- Hypoalbuminaemia

---

now account for most patients in whom bacterial overgrowth is documented. Thus SBBO should be suspected in patients with these conditions whose symptoms prove resistant to conventional treatment or in whom steatorrhoea, weight loss, flatulence or other problems (Box 15.10.2.1) develop unexpectedly. SBBO is now also recognized as the most important cause of malabsorption in older people, in whom a structurally intact small intestine becomes inhabited by colonic flora. Establishing a diagnosis of suspected SBBO by rigorous investigation is of key importance to its proper treatment.

Indigenous bacterial populations of the normal gastrointestinal tract

An understanding of SBBO is based upon a thorough knowledge of the indigenous bacterial populations of the normal gastrointestinal tract (Table 15.10.2.1). The proximal small intestine is normally inhabited by a few bacteria. Qualitative and quantitative changes appear at the ileum and become quite striking in the colon. Box 15.10.2.2 indicates the endogenous factors that prevent SBBO in humans, by far the two most important of which are the normal intestinal motility and an appropriate amount of gastric acid secretion: SBBO may ensue when either or both of these mechanisms are inhibited.

The relatively few bacteria normally present in the stomach and proximal small intestine are usually lactobacilli, entercocci, Gram-positive aerobes, or facultative anaerobes, which are present in concentrations of up to 10^4 viable organisms per gram of jejunal contents. Coliforms are rarely found in the healthy proximal small intestine, and anaerobic bacteroides are not found in the proximal small intestine of a healthy gastrointestinal tract. The ileum is a zone of transition from the sparse populations of the proximal small intestine to the very dense bacterial populations of the colon. In the colon the bacterial population increases up to 10^6 times and reaches 10^9 to 10^{12} bacteria per gram of colonic content. The nature of the bacteria also change remarkably in the colon, where there are fastidious anaerobic bacteria such as bacteroides,

Table 15.10.2.1 Indigenous bacterial population of the normal human gastrointestinal tract

Feature	Stomach	Jejunum	Ileum	Colon
Total bacterial counts[a]	0–3	0–4	5–8	10–12
Aerobes/facultative anaerobes[a]	0–3	0–4	2–5	2–9
Anaerobes[a]	0	0	3–7	9–12

[a] Log_{10} colony-forming units (CFU) per gram of contents.

anaerobic lactobacilli, and clostridia. These anaerobes outnumber the aerobic bacteria by as much as 10 000 to 1. The complexity of the colonic flora is such that more than 400 different species may be present in the colon of a single individual.

Bacteria normally metabolize bile acids, androgens and oestrogens, exogenous and endogenous cholesterol, unabsorbed dietary lipids, proteins, and carbohydrates as well as fibre, protein, urea, and other substances. The by-products of this metabolism may be of benefit or harm to the normal host. An exaggeration of this metabolism occurs in the presence of SBBO. It is noteworthy that the normal bacterial flora is also important in the metabolism of some drugs and other xenobiotics (Box 15.10.2.3), although the importance of the excessive metabolism of medications that may occur in SBBO is yet to be defined. Perhaps the relatively frequent occurrence of SBBO in older people may lead to ineffective medication of this age group.

Mechanisms of the metabolic abnormalities

The malabsorption of nutrients associated with SBBO can largely be attributed to the abnormal intraluminal effects of the overgrowth flora, combined with enterocyte injury induced by the overgrowth flora. A patchy small-intestinal mucosal lesion has been identified in experimental animals with SBBO and in people with the condition.

Steatorrhoea associated with SBBO results from bacterial alteration or bile salts, which leads to an impairment of micelle formation. Accumulation of toxic concentrations of free bile acids may also contribute to the steatorrhoea by inducing a patchy intestinal mucosal lesion, thereby impairing the transport of fat.

The predominant cause of the anaemia associated with SBBO is cobalamin deficiency. The anaemia is megaloblastic and serum cobalamin levels are low. Neurological changes indistinguishable from those of pernicious anaemia may ensue. The anaemia can be

corrected by physiological doses of cobalamin. Cobalamin malabsorption that cannot be corrected by exogenous intrinsic factor is a characteristic of clinically significant SBBO, with competitive uptake of cobalamin, particularly by Gram-negative anaerobes, appearing to be the mechanism responsible. Iron deficiency may also occur in association with SBBO due to blood loss through the gastrointestinal tract, perhaps resulting from patchy ulceration. These patients may have blood detected on examination of their stools, together with a microcytic and hypochromic anaemia. In some patients there may be two populations of red blood cells, microcytic and macrocytic. Folate deficiency is not a common occurrence in SBBO because the overgrowth flora synthesize folate which is available for the host to utilize, indeed serum folate levels may be elevated.

Hypoproteinaemia is frequent in SBBO and is occasionally severe enough to lead to oedema. Its causes are multifactorial but include decreased uptake of amino acids by a damaged small intestine, intraluminal breakdown of protein and protein precursors by bacteria, and protein-losing enteropathy.

A decrease in urinary xylose excretion is frequently seen in patients with SBBO, the primary reason for which is intraluminal degradation of the sugar by the overgrowth flora.

Diarrhoea has many potential causes: the overgrowth flora may produce organic acids that increase osmolarity of the small intestine and decrease intraluminal pH. Furthermore, bacterial metabolites such as free bile acids, hydroxy fatty acids, and organic acids stimulate secretion of water and electrolytes into the lumen.

Clinical manifestations

SBBO may present with nonspecific symptoms of nausea, bloating, abdominal distension and abdominal pain, or—no matter what the underlying clinical condition leading to SBBO may be—with one or more of the typical features listed in Table 15.10.2.1.

Thorough evaluation of suspected cases is warranted. Many of these patients may have had small-bowel diverticula for years before suddenly developing marked symptoms as a result of SBBO, possibly because they needed to have a significant reduction in their gastric acid secretion before the structural abnormality could precipitate the condition. It is important to realize that SBBO may be superimposed on several clinical conditions whose initial symptoms are exactly those of SBBO, e.g. Crohn's disease, radiation enteritis, short bowel syndrome, or lymphoma. To what extent the malabsorption is the result of the primary intestinal disease or the consequence of SBBO is often difficult to determine. Weight loss associated with clinically apparent steatorrhoea has been observed in about one-third of patients with SBBO severe enough to cause cobalamin deficiency. Osteomalacia, vitamin K deficiency, night blindness, and even hypocalcaemic tetany as well as the vitamin E deficiency syndromes (neuropathy, retinopathy, T-cell abnormalities) may result.

Associated clinical conditions

The clinical conditions associated with SBBO are listed in Table 15.10.2.2. In the past, when gastrointestinal surgery was more frequently performed, the common causes of clinically significant bacterial overgrowth were structural abnormalities (e.g. Billroth II anastomosis, surgery for Crohn's disease). Stagnant loops of intestine resulting from fistulas or surgical enterostomies and leading to

Table 15.10.2.2 Clinical conditions associated with SBBO

Site	Associated clinical condition
Gastric proliferation	Hypochlorhydria or achlorhydria, especially when combined with motor or anatomical disturbances
	Sustained hypochlorhydria induced by proton pump inhibitor
Small intestinal stagnation:	Afferent loop of Billroth II partial gastrectomy
Anatomical	Duodenal–jejunal diverticulosis
	Surgical blind loop (end-to-side anastomosis)
	Surgical recirculating loop (end-to-side anastomosis)
	Ileal anal pouch
	Obstruction (stricture, adhesion, inflammation, neoplasm)
Motor	Scleroderma
	Idiopathic intestinal pseudoobstruction
	Absent or disordered migrating motor complex
	Diabetic autonomic neuropathy
Abnormal communication between proximal and distal gastrointestinal tract	Gastrocolic or jejunocolic fistula
	Resection of diseased ileocaecal valve
Miscellaneous	Chronic pancreatitis
	Immunodeficiency syndromes
	Cirrhosis

SBBO were also common. Duodenal and jejunal diverticula can lead to SBBO, particularly if there is an associated hypo- or achlorhydria (Fig. 15.10.2.1). Obstruction of the small intestine caused by Crohn's disease, adhesions, radiation damage, lymphoma, or tuberculosis may cause SBBO. Devastating malabsorption may occur secondary to SBBO associated with a gastrocolic or gastrojejunocolic fistula, with colonic contents passing into the stomach or upper small intestine. SBBO may result from the ileal anal pouch procedure used to treat ulcerative colitis and adenomatous polyposis. The dysmotility syndrome, especially if combined with hypo- or achlorhydria, may lead to SBBO. Such motility disturbances include scleroderma (Fig. 15.10.2.2), intestinal pseudoobstruction, and diabetic autonomic neuropathy. Subjects with an absent or disordered migrating motor complex may develop SBBO. Such patients have no radiographic abnormalities and present with unexplained malabsorption. Elderly patients may develop malabsorption secondary to SBBO, and indeed it has been suggested that bacterial overgrowth may be the most common cause of clinically important malabsorption in older people. Also, older people often have motor disorders (sometimes induced by previous gastrointestinal tract surgery) and decreased acid secretion.

The importance of both normal intestinal motility and normal gastric acid secretion in the prevention of clinically significant SBBO cannot be overemphasized. For example, patients with scleroderma and reflux oesophagitis who are well while receiving H_2-receptor antagonists may develop marked malabsorption

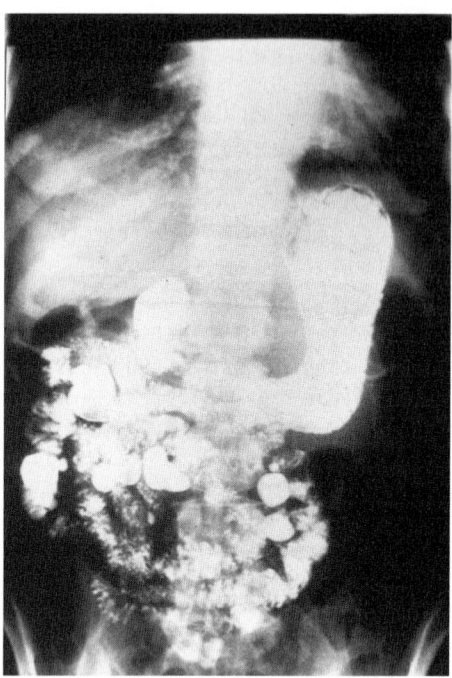

Fig. 15.10.2.1 Multiple duodenal and jejunal diverticula in a patient with cobalamin malabsorption and deficiency and steatorrhoea associated with SBBO.

manifested by diarrhoea and steatorrhoea after introduction of a proton pump inhibitor.

Up to 40% of patients with chronic pancreatitis may have concomitant SBBO because of a decrease in intestinal motility resulting from pain, use of narcotics, inflammatory changes or obstruction from the large inflamed pancreas, or previous pancreatic surgery. Management is problematic unless the clinician recognizes the need to treat both the pancreatic insufficiency and the SBBO.

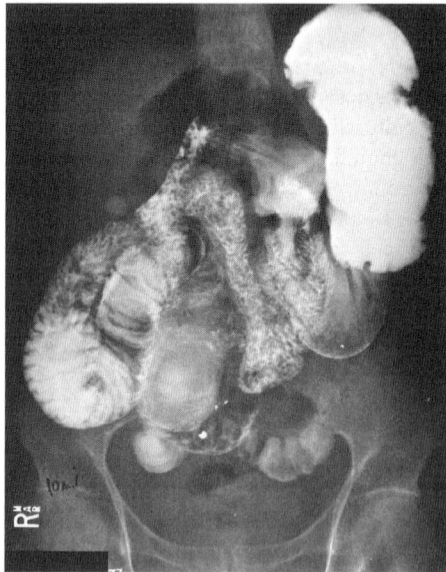

Fig. 15.10.2.2 An upper gastrointestinal and small-bowel series in a woman with scleroderma who presented with severe weight loss, cobalamin (vitamin B$_{12}$) deficiency and marked steatorrhoea. These abnormalities were corrected by broad spectrum antibiotics. Note the marked dilatation of intestinal segment was seen throughout the entire small bowel.

Several other clinical entities are associated with SBBO, but the pathogenesis is ill understood. These include end-stage renal disease, cirrhosis, myotonic muscular dystrophy, fibromyalgia, chronic fatigue syndrome, and various immunodeficiency syndromes such as chronic lymphocytic leukaemia, immunoglobulin deficiencies, and selected T-cell deficiency.

Data coming primarily from one laboratory have suggested that bacterial overgrowth is found in most (84%) patients with irritable bowel syndrome. However, this is based on findings of lactulose hydrogen breath testing, which is well known to be associated with a high degree of false positives and false negatives, and has not been confirmed in many other laboratories when intestinal cultures have been performed in patients with irritable bowel syndrome.

Diagnosis

The general approach to the patient with malabsorption is discussed in Chapter 15.10.1, but it is essential that SBBO should be considered in the differential diagnosis of any patient who presents with diarrhoea, steatorrhoea, weight loss, or macrocytic anaemia, particularly if the patient is elderly and has had previous abdominal surgery. A history of previous surgery for small-intestinal obstruction should raise the question of whether the obstruction was bypassed by an end-to-side anastomosis, leaving a blind pouch, or side-to-side anastomosis, resulting in recirculation of the contents of the small intestine. The presence of dysphagia in a patient with malabsorption should suggest the diagnosis of scleroderma, and repeated bouts of intestinal obstruction without obvious organic cause should suggest intestinal pseudoobstruction.

If a patient has clinically significant bacterial overgrowth, cobalamin absorption is frequently impaired, even though they may not yet have developed low levels of serum cobalamin. Intrinsic factor will not improve cobalamin absorption in these patients. As stated above, the urinary excretion of xylose may be decreased, and the serum folate level may be increased in some—but not all—patients with SBBO.

Bacterial culture and other investigations

The definitive diagnosis of SBBO requires a properly collected and appropriately cultured aspirate from the proximal small intestine. The specimen should be obtained under anaerobic conditions, serially diluted, and cultured on several selected media. In patients with SBBO, the total concentration of bacteria generally exceeds 10^5 organisms per millilitre of jejunal secretions. Bacteroides, anaerobic lactobacilli, coliforms, and enterococci are all likely to be present in varying numbers. Although in most patients the intraluminal microbial proliferation can be documented in the proximal jejunum, it is important to recognize that pockets of overgrowth may be missed by a single culture and that bacterial overgrowth may occur in the more distal parts of the small intestine.

A properly collected and analysed quantitative intestinal culture requires intubation of the small intestine and is both time-consuming and expensive, hence this is often simply not performed. A variety of surrogate tests for detecting SBBO have been devised, based on the varied metabolic actions of the bacteria within the overgrowth flora. Table 15.10.2.3 lists these various tests and compares them in respect to sensitivity, specificity, and simplicity. Measurement of urinary excretion of indican, phenols, drug metabolites, and deconjugated para-amino benzoic acid

Table 15.10.2.3 Tests for SBBO

Tests	Simplicity	Sensitivity	Specificity	Safety
Culture	Poor	Excellent	Excellent	Good
Urinary indican	Good	Poor	Poor	Excellent
Jejunal fatty acids	Poor	Fair	Excellent	Good
Jejunal bile acids	Poor	Fair	Excellent	Good
Fasting breath H_2	Excellent	Poor	Excellent	Excellent
^{14}C-bile acid breath test	Excellent	Fair	Fair	Good
^{14}C-xylose breath test	Excellent	Excellent	Excellent	Good
Lactulose-H_2 breath test	Excellent	Fair	Fair	Excellent
Glucose-H_2 breath test	Excellent	Good	Fair	Excellent

suffer from a lack of sensitivity and specificity in distinguishing SBBO from other causes of malabsorption. The quantification of deconjugated bile acids and short-chain fatty acids in jejunal secretions requires an intubation of the intestine and thus is resisted by clinicians and patients for the same reasons that cultures of the intestine are not popular.

Breath tests

Another approach to diagnosing SBBO is the timed analysis of breath excretion of volatile metabolites produced by intraluminal bacteria. Both the measurement of expired, labelled CO_2 after oral administration of ^{14}C- or ^{13}C-labelled substrates, and breath hydrogen after administration of nonlabelled fermentable substrate, have been utilized.

The first breath test to be utilized clinically to detect SBBO was the bile acid or ^{14}C-cholylglycine breath test, which unfortunately suffered from significant false-negative and false-positive results. It does not distinguish SBBO from ileal damage or resection with excessive breath $^{14}CO_2$ production resulting from bacterial deconjugation within the colon of the unabsorbed labelled bile salt, which is particularly problematic because SBBO may be superimposed on ileal damage in conditions such as Crohn's disease, lymphoma, and radiation enteritis. False-negative results have also been described with this test in 30 to 40% of patients with culture-proven SBBO.

Studies in experimentally induced SBBO demonstrated that the overgrowth flora had the capacity to metabolize significant quantities of xylose and produce CO_2. A 1-g ^{14}C-xylose breath test was developed and found to be sensitive and specific for detecting the presence of SBBO in patients with culture-proven SBBO. Xylose was chosen as a substrate because: (1) it is catabolized by Gram-negative aerobes which are always part of the overgrowth flora; (2) it is predominantly absorbed in the proximal small intestine in contrast to the predominant ileal absorption of bile salts, leading to virtually no 'dumping' of xylose into the colon; and (3) it is metabolized substantially less than other proximally absorbed substrates such as glucose. Elevated $^{14}CO_2$ levels appear in the breath of 85% of patients with culture-proven SBBO within the first 60 min of the test, with the 30-min sample being the most reliable. Laboratories throughout the world have demonstrated the reliability of the ^{14}C-xylose breath test when compared with intestinal culture. In those studies that utilized intestinal culture as the gold standard and evaluated shorter sampling intervals, particularly the 30-min time point, the sensitivity and specificity approximated 90%. However, some studies have raised doubts about the reliability of the ^{14}C-xylose breath test, but these evaluated patients with severe disorders of motility and it is quite possible that the xylose never left the stomach appropriately to come in contact with the overgrowth flora in the proximal small intestine. In addition, there must be an overgrowth of Gram-negative coliforms for the xylose test to be positive, and in at least one of the studies failing to confirm the reliability of the ^{14}C-xylose breath test, the cultures also lacked Gram-negative coliforms. Others have suggested refinement of the ^{14}C-xylose breath test to include a transit marker for intestinal motility, which may enhance its specificity.

It is not recommended that ^{14}C-labelled xylose be used as a substrate in the diagnosis of SBBO in children or fertile women, hence ^{13}C-labelled xylose has been developed and demonstrated to be effective, but this is not in general use in clinical practice.

Breath hydrogen analysis allows a distinct separation of metabolic activities of the overgrowth flora from that of the human host because hydrogen is not produced to any significant extent in mammalian tissue. Excessive breath hydrogen production has been noted in patients with bacterial overgrowth after the administration of 50 to 80 g of glucose or 10 to 12 g of lactulose. A fasting elevation of breath hydrogen is an excellent test for detecting SBBO, but only about one-third of subjects with culture-proven SBBO will have elevated fasting levels of breath hydrogen.

Rigorous attention must be paid to methodological details when utilizing a hydrogen breath test. Certain foods that cause prolonged excretion of hydrogen must be avoided the night before the test, and 2 h must elapse after cigarette smoking or physical exercise sufficient to produce hyperventilation before taking the test. It is also recommended that a mouthwash be performed before testing to eliminate the possibility of an early hydrogen peak resulting from oral bacteria. Finally, strict interpretation criteria must be adopted, but even with careful attention to these details the sensitivity and specificity of the hydrogen breath test is disappointing when it is used to detect SBBO, and many studies indicate that this test is too unreliable for clinical use.

Management

The aim of therapy for SBBO is to correct when feasible the cause of the stasis, but surgery is often impractical (scleroderma, multiple diverticula, diabetes, intestinal pseudoobstruction) and unacceptable to the patient. Thus, management of patients with SBBO is lifelong. Antibiotic therapy is the cornerstone of treatment and remarkable improvement in symptoms can be achieved in most cases. It is important to emphasize once again that SBBO may be a treatable component of the malabsorption seen in those with conditions such as Crohn's disease, intestinal lymphoma, or radiation enteritis, and deterioration in absorption in such patients may not be caused by their primary disease process but by the associated overgrowth. Clinicians also must be aware that bacterial overgrowth may be present without causing any disease. Not all patients who have a pathological flora in the proximal small intestine develop clinically important symptoms. An abnormal breath test or a pathological culture must be put into proper clinical perspective before therapeutic decisions are made.

Antimicrobials

It would seem attractive to select the appropriate antibiotic by evaluation of the sensitivity of the bacteria present in the small bowel lumen. However, this approach is very problematic because there are many different bacterial species present, often with very different antimicrobial sensitivities. Under such conditions it may be extremely difficult to select the most appropriate agent on the basis of the sensitivity results. It is important to select an antibiotic that is effective against both aerobic and anaerobic enteric bacteria. Although most patients with clinically significant malabsorption secondary to SBBO have a flora that is largely overgrown with anaerobes, malabsorption associated predominantly with the overgrowth of Gram-negative aerobes also occurs.

Table 15.10.2.4 lists antimicrobial agents that have been effective in treating SBBO, whether in controlled clinical trials or extensive clinical practice. Antibiotics whose activities are largely limited to anaerobes, such as metronidazole or clindamycin, are not usually effective as monotherapy. Antibiotics that are known to have poor activity against anaerobes should not be used in treating SBBO; such antibiotics include penicillin, ampicillin, the oral aminoglycosides, kanamycin, and neomycin. Historically, the treatment of first choice has been tetracycline, but experience in the United States suggests that up to 60% of patients with SBBO do not respond to tetracycline largely because of bacteroides resistance to this drug.

In most patients, a single course of therapy (7 to 10 days) markedly improves symptoms and the patient may remain symptom-free for months; in others, symptoms recur quickly and acceptable results can only be obtained with cyclic therapy (1 week out of every 4); and in still others, continuous therapy may be needed for 1 to 2 months. If the antimicrobial agent is effective there will be a resolution or marked diminution of symptoms within 1 week: diarrhoea and steatorrhoea will decrease and cobalamin malabsorption will be corrected.

Table 15.10.2.4 Effective antimicrobial agents for treating SBBO

Agent	Dose/day (10-day course)
Tetracycline	250 mg four times
Doxycycline	100 mg twice
Minocycline	100 mg twice
Amoxycillin–clavulanic acid	850 mg twice
Cephalexin +	250 mg four times
metronidazole	250 mg three times
Colistin +	250 000 IU/kg
metronidazole	250 mg three times
Trimethoprim–sulphamethoxazole	One double-strength tablet twice
Chloramphenicol	250 mg four times
Ciprofloxacin	500 mg twice
Norfloxacin	400 mg twice
Rifaximin	400 mg three times
Nitazoxanide	500 mg twice

Other treatments

Prolonged antibiotic therapy poses potential clinical problems including diarrhoea, enterocolitis, patient intolerance, and bacterial resistance. A prokinetic agent that could help clear the small intestine of the overgrowth flora would be an attractive therapy, and experimental animal studies suggest that this might be helpful. There have been two small studies of these agents in patients with SBBO, one utilizing cisapride and one using octreotide, both leading to positive results. Another study utilizing octreotide and erythromycin in patients with scleroderma and SBBO attained positive responses. Large controlled trials of prokinetic therapy in patients with SBBO have yet to be completed.

Since the days of Metchkinoff, it has been thought that one could manipulate the intestinal flora by giving live 'probiotic' microbial supplements that would change the balance in the intestinal flora. Studies to date with probiotic therapy in subjects with SBBO have been disappointing. A placebo-controlled, randomized crossover trial compared norfloxacin, amoxicillin–clavulanic acid, and *Saccharomyces boulardii* in 10 symptomatic patients with SBBO. Both antibiotic treatments led to significant decreases in symptoms and a substantial improvement in the results of hydrogen breath testing, but the probiotic treatment did not result in any improvement in these parameters.

Nutritional support is an important part of treatment of SBBO and may be needed despite attempts to control the bacterial overgrowth by antimicrobial agents because of irreversible damage to the enterocytes. A lactose-free diet and substitution of a large proportion of dietary fat by medium-chain triglycerides may be necessary. Patients with cobalamin malabsorption should receive monthly injections of cobalamin ($1000\,\mu g$). Deficiencies of other nutrients such as calcium and vitamin K should also be corrected.

Further reading

Attar A, *et al.* (1999). Antibiotic efficacy in small intestinal overgrowth-related chronic diarrhea: a cross-over, randomized trial. *Gastroenterology*, **117**, 794–7.

Bishop WP (1997). Breath hydrogen testing for small bowel bacterial overgrowth—a lot of hot air? *J Pediatr Gastroenterol Nutr*, **25**, 245–9.

Bouhnik Y, *et al.* (1999). Bacterial populations contaminating the upper gut in patients with small intestinal bacterial overgrowth syndrome. *Am J Gastroenterol*, **94**, 1327–9.

Bratten JR, Spanier J, Jones MP. (2008). Lactulose breath testing does not discriminate patients with irritable bowel syndrome from healthy controls. *Am J Gastroenterol*, **103**, 958–63.

Corazza GR, *et al.* (1990). The diagnosis of small bowel bacterial overgrowth. *Gastroenterology*, **98**, 302–5.

Fried M, *et al.* (1996). Duodenal bacterial overgrowth during treatment with omeprazole in outpatients. *Gut*, **35**, 23–7.

King CE, Toskes PP (1986). Comparison of the 1-gram [^{14}C]xylose, 10-gram lactulose-H$_2$, and 80-gram glucose-H$_2$ breath tests in patients with small intestine bacterial overgrowth. *Gastroenterology*, **91**, 1447–51.

Lin HC (2004). Small intestinal bacterial overgrowth; a framework for understanding irritable bowel syndrome. *JAMA*, **292**, 852–8.

Postsserud I, *et al.* (2007) Small intestinal bacterial overgrowth in patients with irritable bowel syndrome. *Gut*, **56**, 802–8.

Rana SV, Bhardwaj B (2008). Small intestinal bacterial overgrowth. *Scand J Gastroenterol*, **43**, 1030–7.

Saltsman J, *et al.* (1994). Bacterial overgrowth without clinical malabsorption in elderly hypochlorhydric subjects. *Gastroenterology*, **106**, 615–18.

Singh VV, Toskes PP. (2003). Small bowel bacterial overgrowth: Presentation, diagnosis and treatment. *Curr Gastroenterol Rep*, **5**, 365–72.

Soudah H, Hasler W, Owyang C (1991). Effect of octreotide on intestinal motility and bacterial overgrowth in scleroderma. *N Engl J Med*, **325**, 1461–7.

Walters B, Vanner JS. (2005).Detection of bacterial overgrowth in IBS using the lactulose H$_2$ breath test: Comparison with ^{14}C D-xylose and healthy controls. *Am J Gastroenterol*, **100**, 1566–70.

15.10.3 **Coeliac disease**

Patrick C.A. Dubois and David A. van Heel

Essentials

Coeliac disease is a common disorder of the small intestine in which storage proteins in dietary wheat, rye, and barley (gliadin, secalins, hordeins, usually referred to as 'gluten') induce T-cell responses restricted by HLA DQ2 or DQ8. This immune response drives intestinal inflammation and loss of villous architecture and can lead to a wide spectrum of clinical manifestations.

The condition presents most commonly either in early childhood or in the third or fourth decade of life. A 'classical' malabsorption syndrome characterized by diarrhoea, steatorrhoea, weight loss, fatigue, and anaemia may occur in severe cases, but is now rare: most patients have a milder constellation of symptoms such as abdominal discomfort, bloating, indigestion or nongastrointestinal symptoms (e.g. dermatitis herpetiformis), and many have no symptoms at all.

Diagnosis is made by serological testing for antitissue transglutaminase/antiendomysial antibodies, which have excellent sensitivity and specificity. About 1% of the (white European origin) population have positive coeliac serology, but many are undiagnosed. Positive serological tests should be followed by small intestinal biopsy, whilst a normal (gluten containing) diet is continued, looking for histological features of intraepithelial lymphocytosis, chronic immune cell infiltration of the lamina propria, loss of villous height (villous atrophy), and crypt hyperplasia.

Treatment is by strict avoidance of dietary wheat, rye, and barley (a gluten-free diet), which is safe and usually effective, but constitutes a major challenge for some people. Most patients (but not all) can eat pure oats. Screening for osteoporosis, vitamin D deficiency, and osteomalacia is advised, with treatment if indicated.

Intestinal complications include enteropathy-associated T-cell lymphoma, which should be considered particularly in older patients experiencing a clinical relapse in symptoms, despite effective gluten exclusion, after a prolonged period of clinical response. The overall prognosis of coeliac disease is excellent, but requires lifelong commitment to a gluten-free diet to reduce the risk of complications.

Introduction

Coeliac disease is a common (*c.*1% prevalence) inflammatory disorder of the small intestine occurring in both children and adults. Specific proteins in dietary wheat, rye, and barley (gliadin, secalins, hordeins, usually referred to as 'gluten') induce T cell responses restricted by HLA DQ2 or DQ8. These responses are central to the subsequent intestinal inflammation and loss of villous architecture that characterizes the disease (Fig. 15.10.3.1). Now that serological testing is widespread, symptoms observed in diagnosed individuals vary greatly and are often absent. Classical malabsorption is now infrequent, and only the most florid of the spectrum of presentations seen in coeliac disease. Strict avoidance of dietary wheat, rye, and barley (a gluten-free diet) usually induces remission. Disease reappears on re-challenge and dietary treatment is lifelong.

Historical perspective

Aretaeus (2nd century AD) gave the first recognizable account of coeliac disease (Greek: *koiliakos*, abdominal) describing steatorrhoea, that disease occurred in both children and adults, and that it was more common in women than men. Samuel Gee presented the first clear modern description of coeliac disease in 1888. Willem Dicke (1950) in his doctoral thesis entitled 'Investigation of the harmful effects of certain types of cereal on patients suffering from coeliac disease' outlined the modern treatment of a gluten-free diet. Dicke came to these observations in part by noticing that when wheat flour (i.e. bread) became scarce in the wartime Netherlands, children with coeliac disease paradoxically improved. John Paulley (1954) demonstrated using surgical operative specimens that villous atrophy occurs in the small-intestinal mucosa in coeliac patients. A technique enabling small-bowel biopsy by the oral route was first developed by Margot Shiner (1956), refined as the 'Crosby capsule' (1957), and subsequently replaced in the 1980s by fibre optic endoscopy. Shiner and Doniach (1960) were then able to show using light and electron microscopy the identical histology of adult idiopathic steatorrhoea and childhood coeliac disease. Marsh described the sequence of changes in small-intestinal histology, and a classification system. Duhring (1884) was the first to describe dermatitis herpetiformis, and the often coexisting coeliac small bowel changes were described by Marks and Watson (1966).

The cultivation of wheat in Europe began about 5000 years ago, and (with rye) it became more common in the diet with the introduction of crop rotation in the Middle Ages. Serological diagnostic tests became available in the 1960s (antigliadin antibodies) and 1970s (antireticulin antibodies), although they lacked specificity until the development of the antiendomysial antibody test (1984). The HLA association was recognized in 1972. Dieterich and colleagues (1997) identified tissue transglutaminase as the endogenous target of antiendomysial antibodies and the key autoantigen in coeliac disease.

Aetiology

Many of the immunological mechanisms by which dietary wheat (and to a lesser extent rye and barley) induce coeliac disease are now understood. Wheat gluten is partially digested, but key toxic protein sequences are resistant to intestinal proteases—in part due to high proline (P) and glutamine (Q) content. Tissue transglutaminase in the intestinal epithelium deamidates critical peptide sequences such as the dominant HLA DQ2 restricted wheat epitope sequence PQPQLPY to PQPELPY, and (cross-linked to critical wheat peptides during the deamidation step) is the antigen detected by current diagnostic serological tests such as the antiendomysial or tissue transglutaminase antibody assays. It is unclear if these antibodies have a pathological role in coeliac disease. Work using intestinal T cell clones, intestinal biopsy culture, and peripheral blood T cells in wheat antigen challenged coeliac patients, has shown that wheat peptides are presented by HLA DQ2 (or in a few patients DQ8) to CD4+ helper T cells. Immunodominant wheat (and rye, barley) epitopes that are capable of inducing T cell responses in almost all coeliac patients have been defined, and the crystal structure of these epitopes bound to HLA DQ2 or DQ8 has been elucidated. Activated T cells secrete interferon-γ, and other cytokines. Interleukin-15, expressed by intestinal epithelial cells and lamina propria macrophages, appears to activate intraepithelial lymphocytes and leads to epithelial cell killing. Multiple pathways lead to intestinal inflammation, villous atrophy and subsequent malabsorption.

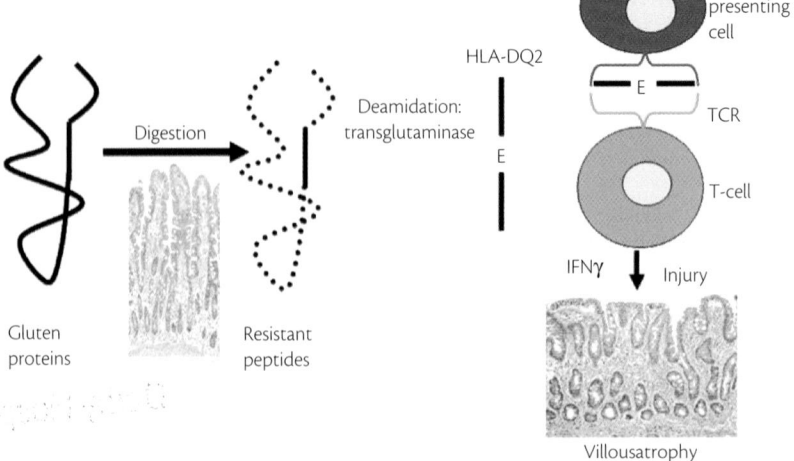

Fig. 15.10.3.1 Model of gluten toxicity in coeliac disease. Toxic peptides in gluten are resistant to human digestive enzymes. Deamidation of key glutamine residues by mucosal tissue transglutaminase creates gluten epitopes with enhanced affinity for the peptide-binding groove of HLA DQ2. These gluten peptides are taken up by antigen presenting cells and presented by HLA DQ2 heterodimers to CD4+ T cells. Upon activation CD4+ T cells secrete interferon-γ and other cytokines and drive the intestinal inflammatory response.

Gluten proteins

Digestion

Resistant peptides

Deamidation: transglutaminase

HLA-DQ2

Antigen presenting cell

TCR

T-cell

IFNγ   Injury

Villousatrophy

The full HLA DQ2 heterodimer (encoded at the DNA level by the combination of HLA DQA1*0501 and DQB1*0201) is found in around 90% of coeliac disease patients, compared to around 30% of white European population controls. The remaining 10% of coeliac disease individuals either carry HLA DQ8, or part of the HLA DQ2 heterodimer. Carriage of one of these HLA types is therefore necessary but not sufficient to develop coeliac disease.

The HLA only explains around 30% of the heritable risk of coeliac disease; other genetic and environmental risk factors play a major role. Genetic risk variants on chromosome 4 (in a region containing the genes for the T-cell cytokines interleukin-2 and interleukin-21) as well as variants in other immune system genes have recently been identified. Several of these have independently been shown to influence risk to other autoimmune diseases, especially type 1 diabetes mellitus. The timing of the introduction of wheat during infant feeding is probably important, some studies suggesting that continued breastfeeding while weaning is protective. Whether gastrointestinal infections (e.g. rotavirus) in infancy are important triggers remains unclear.

Epidemiology

Prevalence estimates of clinically diagnosed coeliac disease (i.e. where symptoms lead to diagnostic testing) should be distinguished from population prevalence studies that employ serological screening. Most studies have been performed in populations of mainly white European origin, and used combined serological and intestinal biopsy testing. In these studies the prevalence of clinically diagnosed disease is around 0.1% (range 0.05 to 0.3%), whereas seroprevalence (including previously undiagnosed cases) in the general population is around 0.5 to 1% in both children and adults. Prevalence is even higher in close relatives of affected individuals; about 10% in first degree relatives. A large proportion of coeliacs in most populations remain undiagnosed—recently estimated at four out of five affected individuals in the United Kingdom. The highest population prevalence of 5% was found in Saharawi refugees living in Algeria. Coeliac disease occurs in Asians, but is extremely rare in individuals of tropical African, Japanese, and Chinese descent.

The similar United Kingdom population seroprevalence found in studies of children (1.0% in 5470 7-year-olds) and adults (1.2% in 7550 over-45-year-olds), suggests the coeliac trait is present from childhood in all cases, even those subsequently diagnosed as adults. Environmental trigger factors resulting in breakdown of oral tolerance to wheat, rye, and barley are therefore likely to occur in the first few years of life. The clinical observation that some adults suddenly develop symptoms in later life remains unexplained, but may reflect a later event in the control of immunological tolerance.

Clinical features

Although coeliac disease can be diagnosed at any age, it presents most commonly either in early childhood (between 9 and 24 months) or in the third or fourth decade of life. Coeliac disease is more common in females, with an approximately 2:1 sex ratio. Although the 'classical' gastrointestinal malabsorption syndrome characterized by diarrhoea, steatorrhoea, weight loss, fatigue, and anaemia may occur in severe cases, most patients nowadays have a milder constellation of symptoms such as abdominal discomfort, bloating, indigestion, or nongastrointestinal symptoms

---

Box 15.10.3.1 Clinical presentations in coeliac disease

With the advent of highly sensitive serological tests, coeliac disease is diagnosed in several settings.

- Classical: symptoms and clinical features of intestinal malabsorption—a relatively infrequent presentation in the developed world

- Atypical: minimal or no gastrointestinal symptoms. Coeliac disease suspected due to presence of associated features or conditions. Examples include iron and folate deficiencies, raised hepatic transaminases, osteoporosis, infertility, or short stature

- Silent: asymptomatic with no clinical manifestations of coeliac disease, diagnosed by serological screening or intestinal biopsy performed for another reason

- Latent: patients who may later develop coeliac disease, but who currently have normal intestinal mucosa on a gluten-containing diet. These include individuals with positive coeliac serology but normal intestinal biopsies

---

(or no symptoms at all). The clinical manifestation appears to be changing, with increasing numbers being diagnosed as a result of the investigation of iron deficiency (anaemia), fatigue and/or 'nonclassical' symptoms (Box 15.10.3.1).

Although the natural history of the disease may be changing (possibly due to environmental factors), a more likely explanation for the current clinical manifestations is that the ability to make the diagnosis has improved (both better tests, and greater test accessibility) throughout the last 20 years with the development of accurate serological markers of the disease and increasing use of endoscopic biopsy techniques. Therefore a much broader spectrum of individuals are being investigated for coeliac disease and consequently being diagnosed (Fig. 15.10.3.2).

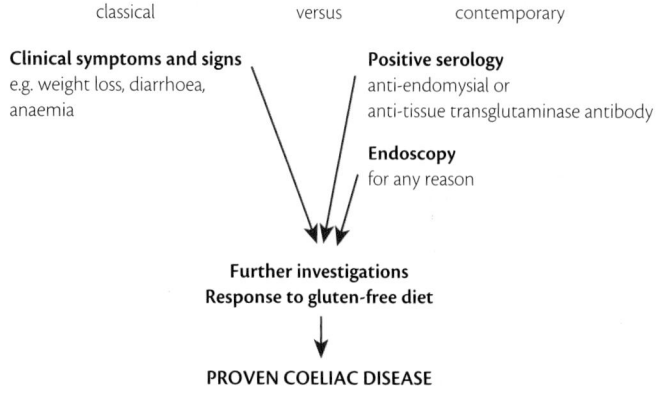

Fig. 15.10.3.2 Contemporary and classical diagnosis of coeliac disease. In the past, coeliac disease was mainly diagnosed after clinical presentation. Nowadays, many more patients are referred on the basis of positive serological tests. Endoscopy and 'routine' duodenal biopsy (without prior suspicion of coeliac disease) may also lead to diagnosis.
Adapted from Green PHR, Jabri N (2005). Diagnosis of coeliac disease. *Best Pract Res Clin Gastroenterol* **19**, 389–400, and van Heel DA, West J (2006) Recent advances in coeliac disease. *Gut*, **55**, 1037–46.

Intestinal complications

Refractory coeliac disease

This term is used for the small minority of patients (<5%) who show persistent histological features of coeliac disease with villous atrophy, despite apparently strict exclusion of gluten. In some individuals, this occurs due to the development of an aberrant, premalignant intraepithelial lymphocyte population. Immunohistochemistry is helpful in distinguishing these patients (see below) from those with persistent villous atrophy without aberrant lymphocytes, who have a very low risk of progression to lymphoma.

Enteropathy-associated T cell lymphoma (EATL)

This is a rare complication of coeliac disease but should be considered particularly in older patients experiencing a clinical relapse in symptoms, despite effective gluten exclusion, after a prolonged period of clinical response. Symptoms may include anorexia, weight loss, abdominal pain, fever, night sweats, and diarrhoea.

Ulcerative jejunitis

This presents with small intestinal ulcerations and stricturing—a high index of suspicion should be maintained for the presence of an EATL, as lymphoma may also cause similar appearances, including benign-appearing ulcerations.

Small-bowel adenocarcinoma

The risk of small-bowel adenocarcinoma is increased in coeliac disease, but the absolute risk of this rare cancer is still very small.

Extraintestinal manifestations and associated conditions

Coeliac disease shares similarities with autoimmune diseases, even though the trigger for inflammation in the intestine is not an autoantigen, but dietary gluten. Coeliac disease may have multisystemic effects, thought to be immune-mediated phenomena, although the pathophysiology is unproven in most cases.

Skin

Dermatitis herpetiformis is an inflammatory skin condition characterized by pruritic papules and vesicles over extensor surfaces and IgA deposition in the dermal papillae adjacent to lesions. Histological features of coeliac disease are present on intestinal biopsy in nearly all patients, but only 20% have intestinal symptoms. Dermatitis herpetiformis responds to gluten exclusion, but this may take months to years. Dapsone provides relief of the intense pruritus associated with dermatitis herpetiformis within 2 or 3 days and can lead to healing of the skin lesions, but not cure, as lesions recur rapidly on discontinuation of therapy.

Liver

Mild elevations of hepatic transaminases are common in untreated coeliac disease, which resolve in most cases within 6–12 months of starting a strict gluten-free diet. Separately, there are also associations between coeliac disease and autoimmune liver disorders including autoimmune hepatitis and primary biliary cirrhosis. The progression of these autoimmune disorders in the presence of coeliac disease is unaffected by subsequent gluten exclusion. Although accounting for a small minority of coeliac patients with abnormal liver function tests, these diagnoses should be considered in patients whose abnormal liver function tests do not improve despite prolonged gluten exclusion.

Neurological

Malabsorption may rarely lead to neurological sequelae from vitamin deficiency: vitamin B_{12} deficiency may cause peripheral neuropathy and myelopathy; vitamin E deficiency can cause cerebellar ataxia or myopathy. Tetany may be seen with severe hypocalcaemia or hypomagnesaemia. Associations with coeliac disease have also been reported for several neurological disorders, notably cerebellar ataxia, peripheral neuropathy, and epilepsy, although most studies have been small or inconsistent. A large Swedish study that retrospectively compared the frequency of several neurological diseases in 14 000 coeliac cases and population controls, found an increased risk of polyneuropathy, but not of other neurological diseases including ataxia.

Other immune-mediated diseases

There is an approximately fivefold increased risk of autoimmune disorders in coeliac disease. Definite associations include type 1 diabetes mellitus, autoimmune thyroid disease, Sjögren's syndrome, and Addison's disease.

Miscellaneous

Several cross-sectional studies have shown that the prevalence of coeliac disease is increased (approximately fivefold) in individuals with Down's syndrome. In untreated coeliac disease, rates of miscarriage and infertility are increased, possibly due to undernutrition, but rates return to near normal following diagnosis and institution of a gluten-free diet.

Differential diagnosis

Several other small-intestinal diseases can cause villous atrophy (Box 15.10.3.2). However, most conditions bear only partial resemblance to coeliac disease and can usually be distinguished either through the clinical history or histologically on careful review. Response to treatment (gluten exclusion) plays an important part in confirming the diagnosis of coeliac disease and excluding other causes. Patients who do not show a clinical or histological response to a strict gluten-free diet warrant consideration of alternative diagnoses and complications of coeliac disease. As well as other causes of villous atrophy, many comorbid conditions may mimic symptoms of coeliac disease and other causes of malabsorption should be excluded. Conditions occurring more frequently in coeliac disease, that may have similar symptoms, include small intestinal bacterial overgrowth, secondary lactase deficiency, microscopic colitis, Crohn's disease, and ulcerative colitis.

Clinical investigation

Pathology

The coeliac lesion occurs predominantly in the proximal small intestine, reflecting the distribution of gluten encounter. Changes may be mild and patchy and for this reason it is recommended that multiple (>4) biopsies are taken from separate sites, usually by

Box 15.10.3.2 Non-coeliac-related causes of villous atrophy

- Autoimmune enteropathy
- Common variable immunodeficiency
- Crohn's disease
- Eosinophilic gastroenteritis
- Giardiasis
- Graft-vs-host disease
- HIV enteropathy
- Ischaemic enteritis
- Nonsteroidal anti-inflammatory drug enteropathy
- Peptic duodenitis
- Post-chemotherapy intestinal mucositis
- Radiation enteritis
- Tropical sprue

upper gastrointestinal endoscopy from the second part of the duodenum. The classic histological features are intraepithelial lymphocytosis, chronic immune cell infiltration of the lamina propria, loss of villous height (villous atrophy), and crypt hyperplasia. These features may be graded according to a commonly used classification proposed by Marsh. Intraepithelial lymphocytosis is the earliest change, but specificity for the diagnosis of coeliac disease increases with the presence of the other accompanying features, particularly villous atrophy.

Immunohistochemistry for T-cell markers (CD3, CD8) and the epithelial integrin CD103 are of value in refractory coeliac disease in detecting an aberrant intraepithelial T cell population that can precede the development of overt lymphoma.

Haematological abnormalities

A variety of haematological abnormalities may occur, arising from haematinic deficiencies, hyposplenism, and autoimmune phenomena. IgA deficiency (2–3%) and non-Hodgkin's lymphoma (see below) are also more common in coeliac disease.

Anaemia occurs frequently with microcytosis due to iron deficiency, but folate deficiency is also common and may cause macrocytosis. Vitamin B_{12} levels are usually preserved, except in severe, long-standing disease with involvement of the whole small intestine. Pancytopenia may occur in these cases as a result of folate or vitamin B_{12} deficiency.

Leucopenia and thrombocytopenia may also occur rarely as an autoimmune phenomenon.

Thrombocytosis is common in coeliac disease and can occur as a result of iron deficiency or hyposplenism, but usually resolves with gluten exclusion.

Morphological red cell changes characteristic of functional hyposplenism (Howell–Jolly bodies, target cells, acanthocytosis) may be apparent on blood film. Hyposplenism (based on sensitive research techniques, such as pitted red cell counting) is common in adult coeliac disease, but is rare in children and may be more frequent in patients with associated autoimmune disorders. The cause of hyposplenism in coeliac disease is unknown. Most studies suggest

hyposplenism does not revert after treatment with a gluten-free diet. The risk of infection due to hyposplenism in coeliac disease is likely to be increased, but to date there have been only a few studies. A modest increased risk of infections in all patients with coeliac disease has been suggested by a large Swedish cohort study examining hospital inpatient episodes. The increased risk is partly accounted for by a 2.5-fold increase in the rate of pneumococcal infections. Immunization against the encapsulated organisms *Haemophilus influenza* type b, *Streptococcus pneumonia*, and *Neisseria meningitidis* should be considered in those with blood film evidence of hyposplenism. However, as yet no studies evaluating the effectiveness of this approach in coeliac disease have been performed. Immunization against influenza should also be considered in older patients because of the risk of secondary bacterial infections.

IgA deficiency

This occurs more commonly in coeliac disease, affecting 2 to 3% of patients. Conversely, the prevalence of coeliac disease in IgA deficiency is also increased and may be as high as 8%. IgA deficiency is important in coeliac disease as it may be a cause of false negative IgA endomysial or tissue transglutaminase tests.

Biochemistry

Fat malabsorption occurs in classical coeliac disease, leading to steatorhoea and malabsorption of vitamins A, D, E, and K. Hypocalcaemia and hypomagnesaemia may occur due to vitamin D deficiency. Rarely coagulopathy with prolonged prothrombin time is seen due to vitamin K malabsorption. Serum albumin can be low in the setting of intestinal inflammation, but systemic inflammatory markers such as C-reactive protein or ESR are not usually raised.

Antibody tests

Antiendomysial antibody (EMA) and human recombinant tissue transglutaminase (TTG) antibody tests have about 95% sensitivity and specificity in untreated coeliac disease. These tests have superseded both antigliadin and antireticulin antibody tests which have much lower diagnostic accuracy. The sensitivity and specificity estimates for EMA and TTG antibody tests were obtained in studies with patients with classical histological changes on biopsy including villous atrophy. Diagnostic difficulties therefore may arise in patients with mild disease, who may have negative serology and only mild inflammatory (infiltrative) changes on biopsy. Such patients may still have clinical manifestations that respond to gluten exclusion. Intestinal biopsy should therefore be obtained in all patients with unexplained features consistent with coeliac disease even if antibody tests are negative. EMA is assayed by indirect immunofluorescence (most commonly against monkey oesophagus) whereas TTG antibody titres are measured by ELISA and provide a quantitative measure that may be useful in assessing patients' compliance with a gluten-free diet.

Radiology

Barium radiology (barium follow-through, enteroclysis) lacks sensitivity in coeliac disease and is rarely used in diagnosis, but is of value when complications are suspected (lymphoma, ulcerative jejunitis) or alternative diagnoses such as Crohn's disease need to be excluded. Intestinal lymphoma usually has a diffuse pattern of bowel involvement and can be particularly difficult to diagnose. Barium studies in uncomplicated disease may show thickening of mucosal folds and flocculation, segmentation or clumping of barium. CT or MR cross-sectional imaging with enteroclysis is superior when complications are suspected, enabling assessment of the intestinal wall but also regional lymphadenopathy and extra-intestinal disease.

Wireless capsule enteroscopy

This technique has good sensitivity and specificity for the diagnosis of coeliac disease and may be considered where upper gastrointestinal endoscopy and duodenal biopsies are nondiagnostic, but suspicion of small-bowel pathology remains (e.g. iron deficiency). Wireless capsule enteroscopy also has a role in investigation of patients with refractory sprue to help exclude complications such as lymphoma, small-bowel adenocarcinoma, and ulcerative jejunitis. This may lead on to targeted biopsies of suspicious areas by laparoscopy or double balloon enteroscopy.

HLA DQ typing

Genetic testing for HLA DQ2/8 is valuable, but only as an exclusionary test. The absence of genes encoding subunits of the HLA DQ2 or DQ8 heterodimers has almost 100% negative predictive value. However, local laboratories vary greatly in the format in which results are reported, making this a confusing area, and clinicians without experience are advised to refer back to the laboratory to ensure correct interpretation. The test is particularly useful in those in whom the diagnosis remains uncertain after serological testing and intestinal biopsy.

Criteria for diagnosis

Definitive diagnosis is based on intestinal biopsy and the finding of characteristic histological features of coeliac disease, together with clinical improvement on a gluten-free diet. Published guidelines on diagnosis (including NICE guidance) and treatment are listed below (see 'Further reading'). Upper gastrointestinal endoscopy and distal duodenal biopsy can be undertaken as an outpatient with local throat anaesthetic spray or intravenous sedation. An improvement in symptoms and nutritional parameters, including micronutrient deficiencies, occurs in most patients within months after commencing a gluten-free diet and provides important confirmatory support for the diagnosis. Repeat intestinal biopsy after gluten exclusion to observe recovery of the intestinal mucosa is no longer considered necessary for diagnosis in adults, provided other objective indicators of response to gluten exclusion are observed (e.g. disappearance of positive coeliac antibody titres).

In patients with suspected coeliac disease who have commenced a gluten-free diet before a small-intestinal biopsy has been obtained and in whom serological tests and biopsies are nondiagnostic, biopsy after prolonged gluten challenge (equivalent to 4 slices of bread per day for at least 2 weeks) is helpful to confirm the diagnosis.

Treatment

Strict, lifelong gluten exclusion is the cornerstone of therapy and is effective in most individuals. The gluten-free diet is safe and

---

> **Box 15.10.3.3** Action after diagnosis of coeliac disease
>
> **Initiate gluten-free diet**
> - Referral to a dietitian with suitable expertise
> - Membership of a coeliac support society
> - (In the United Kingdom: prescription of gluten-free foods)
>
> **Possible investigations for comorbid conditions**
> - Full blood count
> - Iron studies, vitamin B_{12}, and folate
> - Calcium, phosphate, patathyroid hormone, vitamin D
> - Liver function tests
> - Thyroid function tests
> - Bone densitometry scan
>
> **Additional therapy**
> - Correct iron, vitamin B_{12}, folate deficiency
> - Calcium and vitamin D supplements
> - Pneumococcal, meningococcal, and *Haemophilus influenza* type b immunization in patients with hyposplenism

usually effective, but constitutes a major challenge for some people because of the pervasiveness of these grains in modern diets and the paucity of palatable alternatives. Resolution of symptoms and nutrient deficiencies are the earliest markers of response. Bone density and other nutritional parameters such as body mass index and fat mass also increase, predominantly in the first year after starting a gluten-free diet. Subjective indices of well-being, such as self-reported vitality, may also improve. In children histological recovery is usually complete within a few months, but recovery in adults may be slower. Box 15.10.3.3 summarizes a typical course of treatment and additional investigation after diagnosis of coeliac disease.

Resolution of positive EMA and TTG antibody titres provides a useful objective marker of response to gluten exclusion and usually occurs within 6 to 12 months. However, it should be remembered that these antibodies are commonly negative in the presence of low-grade histological abnormalities and are therefore insensitive markers of the extent of disease response. Monitoring of antibody tests, particularly quantitative TTG antibodies, is useful in patient follow-up to assess compliance. Major dietary indiscretions can lead to a rise in antibody levels, and can be helpful to reinforce efforts to improve compliance.

Compliance is also aided by joining a local coeliac society and by review with a dietitian with coeliac expertise. In the United Kingdom, Coeliac UK provides direct patient support and a comprehensive directory of gluten-free and gluten-containing food products. In general, wheat, rye, and barley should be avoided entirely. Feeding studies have established that pure oats are safe for most patients, but contamination of oat products with wheat gluten during harvesting or production is a common problem. A small number of patients appear to have a true coeliac intolerance to gluten-related avenins in oats. T-cell lines reactive to avenins in oats can be generated from the intestinal mucosa of some of these patients.

It is unclear whether there is a safe amount of gluten that may be consumed without adverse effects, although for the majority even small amounts of gluten (50 mg/day) appear sufficient to cause ongoing intestinal inflammation. Individuals appear to vary considerably in their sensitivity to gluten. A few are exquisitely sensitive and even minimal amounts of gluten may provoke gastrointestinal symptoms and histological abnormalities. At the opposite end of the spectrum, some patients have no symptoms despite a normal gluten-containing diet.

Patients with coeliac disease show a modestly increased risk of osteoporosis and fractures. Hip fractures are increased nearly twofold, a significant concern given the high incidence of these fractures in ageing populations. The most effective intervention is the gluten-free diet, which improves bone density in coeliac disease, predominantly in the first year. Patients should be encouraged to undertake regular weight-bearing exercise, and advised on consuming adequate dietary calcium (c.1000 mg/day). Calcium supplements may be prescribed to meet these targets. Screening for osteoporosis with bone densitometry scanning should be considered, particularly in older patients who have the greatest risk of fractures and in those with other risk factors (low body mass index, weight loss, poor adherence to gluten-free diet). Patients at high risk of fractures, with osteoporosis determined by bone densitometry scanning, should receive appropriate supplementary therapies for osteoporosis including bisphosphonates.

Patients should be screened for vitamin D deficiency and osteomalacia. This may be suggested by hypocalcaemia, hypophosphataemia and raised alkaline phosphatase and is confirmed by serum 25-hydroxyvitamin D (calcidiol) assay. The British Society of Gastroenterology have produced guidelines on the management of low bone mineral density in coeliac disease. These guidelines recommend screening for secondary hyperparathyroidism as a surrogate marker of vitamin D deficiency, by measuring serum calcium and parathyroid hormone. Patients with a high parathyroid hormone level and normal calcium should receive supplementation with calcium and vitamin D (800–1000 units/day).

Persistent clinical symptoms

The commonest reason for recurrent or persistent clinical manifestations in coeliac disease is inadequate adherence to a gluten-free diet. This may be inadvertent, and a careful dietary review should be undertaken to assess presence of gluten in the diet. Symptoms may also commonly persist or recur due to the presence of comorbidities, which should be carefully sought and treated (see above).

Rarely patients have true refractory coeliac disease, if symptoms and histological features persist despite strict gluten exclusion over several months. Intestinal complications of coeliac disease, including enteropathy-associated T-cell lymphoma, should be considered and excluded in these patients (see above). It is worth remembering that the incidence of several gastrointestinal conditions that are not connected to coeliac disease, e.g. sporadic colorectal carcinoma greatly exceeds that of enteropathy-associated T-cell lymphoma and should also be excluded in patients with persisting symptoms.

Table 15.10.3.1 Estimates of relative and absolute risks in coeliac disease

	Relative risk	Absolute risk (incidence per 100 000 person-years)	
		General population	Coeliac
Any sepsis	2.6	58	139
Hip fracture	2.2	128	197
Any fracture	1.5	444	600
Lymphoma	5.9	8	45

Comparisons of events in the cohort of coeliacs (>10 000 cases) in the Swedish inpatient register with the general population. Includes first year after diagnosis.
Adapted from the analysis of Walters JRF, et al. (2008). Coeliac disease and the risk of infections. Gut, **57**, 1034–5.

Prognosis

Prognosis in coeliac disease is excellent, provided a prompt diagnosis is made and treatment instituted with strict adherence to a gluten-free diet. In long-term treated coeliac disease mortality is comparable to that of population controls.

The largest cohort studies point to an increased risk (c.twofold) of malignancy and mortality occurring within the first 2 or 3 years after diagnosis, although there is evidence for a sustained (c.sixfold) increased risk of lymphoproliferative disorders beyond this. It should be noted that absolute risks (i.e. at an individual patient level) of malignancy are small (Table 15.10.3.1). The increased risk appears to correlate with disease severity as it is highest in those with overt malabsorption but not detected in studies of patients with asymptomatic disease.

Screening

Screening for coeliac disease in asymptomatic individuals (including those at higher risk, e.g. with a family history or coexisting type 1 diabetes) remains controversial. The natural history of disease (especially risk of complications) in asymptomatic screening-detected cases is currently unknown, hence clear guidance on whether such individuals should commence a gluten-free diet cannot be given.

Likely developments over the next 5 to 10 years

Understanding of the heritable genetic risk factors predisposing to coeliac disease is rapidly increasing, driven by advances in genetics. Several new approaches to therapy are currently being developed or in early clinical trials. These include oral peptidase supplements designed to breakdown toxic cereal peptides, small molecules to inhibit various steps in pathogenesis (e.g. directed against transglutaminase, HLA DQ2, zonulin), and cereals genetically modified to reduce antigenicity.

Further reading

Halfdanarson TR, Litzow MR, Murray JA (2007). Hematologic manifestations of celiac disease. *Blood*, **109**, 412–21.

Hill ID, et al. (2005). Guideline for the diagnosis and treatment of celiac disease in children: recommendations of the North American Society for Pediatric Gastroenterology, Hepatology and Nutrition. *J Pediatr Gastroenterol Nutr*, **40**, 1–19. [Provides paediatric guidance including information on presentation of disease in infancy and childhood, diagnostic and therapeutic approaches in children.]

Hunt KA, *et al*. (2008). Newly identified genetic risk variants for celiac disease related to the immune response. *Nat Genet*, **40**, 395–402.

Kagnoff, MF (2006). AGA Institute Medical Position Statement on the Diagnosis and Management of Celiac Disease. *Gastroenterology*, **131**, 1977–80. [Provides practical clinical guidance for management of adults and children including internationally oriented dietary advice and list of useful websites.]

Ludvigsson JF, *et al*. (2008). Coeliac disease and risk of sepsis. *Gut*, **57**, 1074–80.

National Institute for Health and Clinical Excellence (2009). *NICE clinical guideline 86 – Coeliac Disease. Recognition and assessment of coeliac disease.* (http://www.nice.org.uk/CG86)

Rostom A, Murray JA, Kagnoff MF (2006). American Gastroenterological Association (AGA) Institute technical review on the diagnosis and management of celiac disease. *Gastroenterology*, **131**, 1981–2002. [Provides guidance in adults with coeliac disease. Strong focus on diagnosis, including difficulties encountered by physicians and use of serological tests.]

Scott, BB, Lewis NR (2007). *Guidelines for osteoporosis in inflammatory bowel disease and coeliac disease.* British Society of Gastroenterology (http://www.bsg.org.uk). [Provides practical guidance on targeted screening and treatment of osteoporosis in coeliac disease.]

Sollid LM (2002). Coeliac disease: dissecting a complex inflammatory disorder. *Nat Rev Immunol*, **2**, 647–55.

van Heel DA, West J (2006). Recent advances in coeliac disease. *Gut*, **55**, 1037–46.

WGO Celiac Disease Review Team (2007). *World Gastroenterology Organization Practice Guideline: celiac disease.* http://www.worldgastroenterology.org/assets/downloads/en/pdf/guidelines/04_celiac_disease.pdf

15.10.4 **Gastrointestinal lymphoma**

P.G. Isaacson

Essentials

Primary gastrointestinal lymphoma, which is the commonest extranodal lymphoma and almost exclusively of non-Hodgkin's type, is defined as lymphoma that has presented with the main bulk of disease in the gastrointestinal tract, with or without involvement of contiguous lymph nodes, and necessitating direction of treatment to that site.

MALT lymphoma describes a group of low-grade B-cell lymphomas whose histology recapitulates the features of mucosa-associated lymphoid tissue (MALT). It most commonly affects the stomach, presenting with nonspecific dyspepsia. Endoscopy typically shows inflamed or eroded mucosa rather than tumour mass. Many if not all cases appear to be driven by *Helicobacter pylori*, with 75% regressing following eradication of the organism with appropriate antibiotics. Deeply invasive lymphomas and those with adverse histological or cytogenetic features are unlikely to respond.

Enteropathy-associated T-cell lymphoma (EATL) is an intestinal tumour of intraepithelial T lymphocytes that occurs most commonly in the jejunum or ileum and is sometimes associated with coeliac disease. It presents with abdominal pain, often due to intestinal perforation, and in some cases there is a prodromal period of refractory coeliac disease (sometimes accompanied by ulcerative jejunitis). The prognosis is usually poor, with death frequently resulting from abdominal complications in patients already weakened by uncontrolled malabsorption.

Burkitt's lymphoma is the most frequent childhood gastrointestinal lymphoma and is particularly common in the Middle East. B-cell lymphoproliferative conditions associated with immunodeficiency commonly present in the gastrointestinal tract and are increasingly important.

Introduction

The lymphomas that may arise in the gastrointestinal tract are listed in Box 15.10.4.1. Two of these, namely B-cell lymphoma of mucosa-associated lymphoid tissue (MALT) and enteropathy-associated T-cell lymphoma (EATL), do not arise in peripheral lymph nodes and will be discussed in more detail in this section. Any of the lymphomas that normally arise in lymph nodes may present as a primary gastrointestinal tumour, the most frequent being diffuse large B-cell lymphoma which, in fact accounts for the majority of primary gastrointestinal lymphomas, and mantle-cell lymphoma, which typically manifests in the gut as lymphomatous polyposis. Burkitt's lymphoma, is the commonest childhood gastrointestinal lymphoma, and is an especially common primary small intestinal lymphoma in the Middle East. The increasingly important group of B-cell lymphoproliferative conditions

---

Box 15.10.4.1 Primary gastrointestinal non-Hodgkin's lymphoma

B cell

- MALT lymphoma (including IPSID) with or without evidence of high-grade transformation
- Mantle-cell lymphoma (lymphomatous polyposis)
- Burkitt's lymphoma
- Other types corresponding to lymph node equivalents:

  follicular lymphoma
  lymphocytic lymphoma
  diffuse large B-cell lymphoma

- Immunodeficiency-related lymphomas:

  post-transplant
  acquired (AIDS)
  congenital

T cell

- EATL
- Other types not associated with enteropathy

Rare types
(including conditions that may simulate lymphoma)

associated with immunodeficiency commonly present in the gastrointestinal tract, but they are more properly considered in the context of immunodeficiency-related lymphoproliferative conditions as a whole.

MALT lymphomas

The term MALT lymphoma is used to designate a group of low-grade B-cell lymphomas whose histology recapitulates the features of mucosa-associated lymphoid tissue (MALT) as exemplified by the Peyer's patch. Another term for these lymphomas that reflects their normal cell counterpart is 'extranodal marginal zone B-cell lymphoma'. Paradoxically, there is usually no lymphoid tissue in the sites where MALT lymphomas occur, but lymphoid tissue of MALT type accumulates prior to the development of lymphoma. In the stomach this is usually the result of chronic inflammation in response to *Helicobacter pylori* infection. Intestinal MALT lymphomas are less frequent but include the entity known as immuno-proliferative small intestine disease (IPSID) that has interesting parallels with gastric MALT lymphoma.

Gastric MALT lymphoma

Clinical presentation

Gastric MALT lymphoma typically occurs in patients over 40 years of age but can occur at any age. The sex incidence is equal. The presenting symptoms are usually those of nonspecific dyspepsia and more suggestive of gastritis or peptic ulcer than a neoplastic lesion. Likewise, endoscopy more often shows inflamed, sometimes eroded mucosa than a tumour mass.

Pathology

Most MALT lymphomas of the stomach arise in the antrum, and macroscopically are characterized by an ill-defined thickened, inflamed, and ulcerated mucosa. The histological features closely simulate those of MALT as exemplified by Peyer's patches (Fig. 15.10.4.1a). Reactive non-neoplastic follicles are surrounded by the lymphomatous infiltrate in the region corresponding to the Peyer's patch marginal zone (Fig. 15.10.4.1b). The infiltrate extends into the surrounding tissue and invades individual gastric glands to form characteristic lymphoepithelial lesions (Fig. 15.10.4.2). The cytological appearances of the cells of MALT lymphomas are typically heterogeneous. They may resemble centrocytes, small lymphocytes, or monocytoid B-cells and are collectively referred to as 'marginal zone B-cells'. Scattered transformed blasts are usually present and plasma-cell differentiation, characteristically maximal beneath the surface epithelium, is present in one-third of cases. The lymphoma cells may specifically colonize the reactive follicle centres in a way that may lead to an appearance closely resembling follicular lymphoma. Gastric MALT lymphoma is characteristically multifocal.

Biopsy appearances of gastric MALT lymphoma

There are many pitfalls in making the diagnosis of MALT lymphoma in small endoscopic biopsies. Amongst these are the retrieval of inadequate tissue, the presence of predominantly sub-mucosal lymphoma, and the presence of cryptic foci of high-grade lymphoma or an associated adenocarcinoma. The differential diagnosis between MALT lymphoma and florid *H. pylori*-associated chronic gastritis (follicular gastritis) can be especially difficult. Molecular evidence of B-cell monoclonality is also helpful, but a

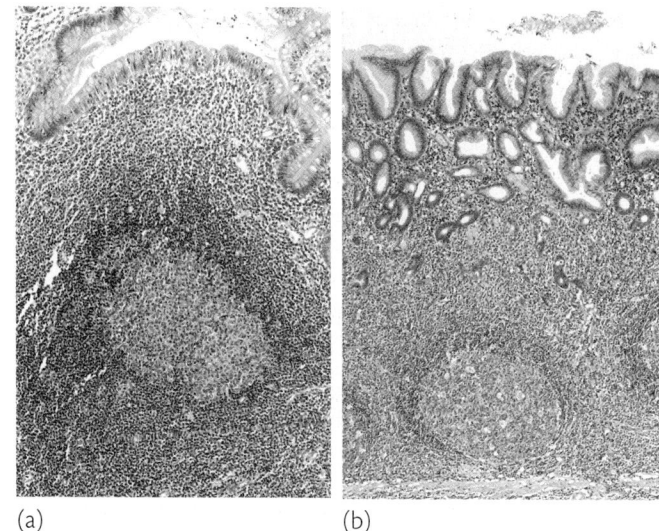

(a)   (b)

Fig. 15.10.4.1 (a) Peyer's patch comprising a B-cell follicle surrounded by a mantle zone external to which is the marginal zone. There are collections of small B lymphocytes within the dome epithelium. (b) Gastric MALT lymphoma. The tumour cells surround the reactive B-cell follicle in the marginal zone and invade gastric glands to form lymphoepithelial lesions. The overall structure is similar to the Peyer's patch.

diagnosis of lymphoma should never be made unless the histological criteria are fulfilled.

Dissemination to lymph nodes and other sites

Most gastric MALT lymphomas are at clinical stage 1_E at the time of diagnosis, but approximately 20% have spread to the gastric lymph nodes or beyond. The more common distal sites include the small intestine, spleen, and bone marrow. In both lymph nodes

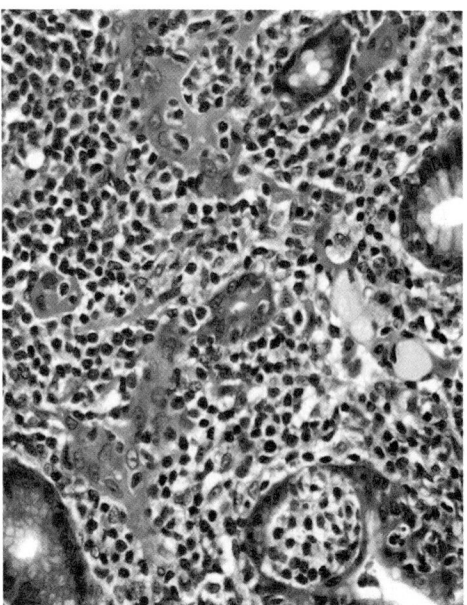

Fig. 15.10.4.2 Detail of the neoplastic infiltrate in a gastric MALT lymphoma showing 'centrocyte-like' cells invading gastric glands to form lymphoepithelial lesions (bottom right) and eosinophilic change in gastric gland epithelium (centre).

and spleen the lymphomatous infiltrate tends to concentrate in the marginal zone.

Phenotype and genotype of gastric MALT lymphoma

The B cells of MALT lymphoma express surface and, to a lesser extent, cytoplasmic immunoglobulin (usually IgM), which shows light-chain restriction. The cells express mature B-cell antigens including CD21 and CD35. They are CD5- and CD10-negative. This phenotype is homologous with that of marginal zone B cells, which are acknowledged as the normal-cell counterpart. The immunoglobulin (Ig) genes are mutated with ongoing mutations. Detection of monoclonal Ig gene rearrangement, usually by polymerase chain reaction (PCR), can assist in making the diagnosis of lymphoma in gastric biopsies, but caution is required since PCR evidence of monoclonality has been reported in biopsies from cases of florid *H. pylori*-associated gastritis. A number of translocations have been described in MALT lymphomas, including t(1;14)(p22;q32), t(11;18)(q21;q21), t(14;18)(q21;q21) and others. These have the common effect of activating the nuclear factor kappa B (NF-κB) pathway.

High-grade transformation of gastric MALT lymphoma

Transformation of MALT lymphoma to diffuse large B-cell lymphoma is heralded by the emergence of increased numbers of transformed blast cells, which eventually form sheets or clusters (Fig. 15.10.4.3) and finally grow to confluence effacing any trace of the preceding low-grade tumour. This gives rise to difficulty both in grading some MALT lymphomas and in classifying diffuse large B-cell lymphomas of the stomach and other parts of the gastrointestinal tract. Those large-cell lymphomas in which no MALT component is evident are best classified as diffuse large B-cell lymphoma without reference to MALT.

Clinical behaviour

In comparison with nodal low-grade B-cell lymphomas, such as follicular lymphoma, which, at the time of diagnosis are characteristically at an advanced stage, MALT lymphoma is usually at stage I_E or II_E when diagnosed and is slow to disseminate. Hence low-grade MALT lymphomas respond favourably to therapy and

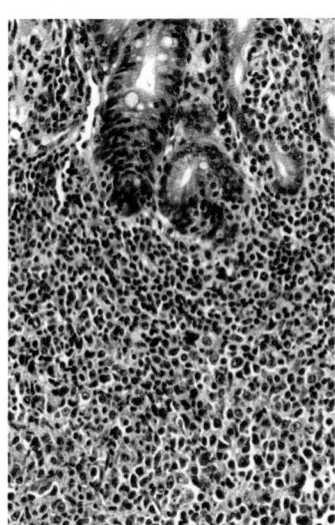

Fig. 15.10.4.3 MALT lymphoma showing transformation from low-grade (small cell) histology (upper half of figure) to high-grade (large cell) lymphoma (bottom half of figure).

there is an excellent overall survival approximating 90% at 10 years. The survival for cases in which there is evidence of high-grade transformation is significantly worse: 45% at 10 years.

H. pylori and gastric MALT lymphoma

There are several lines of evidence that implicate *H. pylori* in the pathogenesis of gastric MALT lymphoma. These include the fact that normal gastric mucosa is devoid of organized lymphoid tissue which, however, accumulates as a consequence of *H. pylori* infection, and the observation that the organism can be detected in most cases. This association has been supported by epidemiological studies which have shown that there is a significantly higher frequency of preceding *H. pylori* infection in patients with gastric lymphoma compared to matched controls with nongastric lymphoma. The evidence became even more compelling following *in vitro* studies, which showed that the cells of low-grade gastric MALT lymphoma respond to *H. pylori* antigens via a T-cell mediated mechanism. The clinical significance of these findings is that 75% of gastric MALT lymphoma regress following eradication of *H. pylori* using appropriate antibiotics. Deeply invasive lymphomas, those in which there are foci of high-grade transformation, and cases with t(11;18) are unlikely to respond.

Immunoproliferative small intestinal disease (IPSID)

This condition is a subtype of MALT lymphoma, which occurs most commonly in the Middle East, although small numbers of cases have been reported from elsewhere. It is a disease of young adults and usually presents with severe malabsorption. The histology of IPSID is similar to that of gastric MALT lymphoma, except that plasma-cell differentiation is much more prominent both in the intestine and mesenteric lymph nodes. These plasma cells synthesize large amounts of α heavy chain without light chain, which can be detected in the serum, hence the term 'α-chain disease' that was first used for this condition. IPSID remains localized to the small intestine for prolonged periods and patients usually die from the severe malabsorption. High-grade transformation may also occur.

In its early stages, IPSID may be responsive to broad-spectrum antibiotics, which presumably eradicate bacterial species from the intestinal lumen. There is some evidence that *Campylobacter jejuni* may be implicated in IPSID in parallel with the relationship between *H. pylori* and gastric lymphoma.

Enteropathy-associated T-cell lymphoma (EATL)

This is an intestinal tumour of intraepithelial T-lymphocytes, showing varying degrees of transformation but usually presenting as a tumour composed of large lymphoid cells. Two subtypes are described. In type 1 EATL, which accounts for 80 to 90% of cases, the lymphoma comprises large, often polymorphic cells and in type 2, which accounts for the remaining 10 to 20%, the lymphoma comprises small round cells. Adjacent small intestinal mucosa shows villous atrophy with crypt hyperplasia. The disease is uncommon in most parts of the world, but is seen with increasing frequency in those areas with a high prevalence of coeliac disease. The lymphoma occurs most commonly in the jejunum or ileum. Presentation in the duodenum, stomach, colon, or outside the gastrointestinal tract may occur but is rare.

Clinical features

In type 1 EATL, a small proportion of the patients have a history of childhood onset coeliac disease. Most show adult onset disease or are diagnosed as having coeliac disease in the same clinical episode in which the lymphoma is diagnosed. In type 2 EATL there is no clear link with coeliac disease. Both groups of patients present with abdominal pain, often associated with intestinal perforation. In a proportion of patients there is a prodromal period of refractory coeliac disease that is sometimes accompanied by intestinal ulceration (ulcerative jejunitis). In type 1 EATL the association with coeliac disease is borne out by positive serological tests, HLA DQ2 or DQ8 expression and associated clinical findings such as dermatitis herpetiformis and hyposplenism. In type 2 there is no such evidence for this association.

Pathology

The tumour usually presents as multiple ulcerating raised mucosal masses but may present as one or more ulcers or as a large exophytic mass. There are two distinct tumour types. In type 1 (Fig. 15.10.4.4) there is a wide range of cytology. Most commonly, the tumour cells are relatively monomorphic medium-sized to large cells with round or angulated vesicular nuclei, prominent nucleoli, and moderate to abundant, pale-staining cytoplasm. Less commonly, the tumour exhibits marked pleomorphism with multinucleated cells bearing a resemblance to anaplastic large cell lymphoma. Most tumours show infiltration by inflammatory cells, including large numbers of histiocytes and eosinophils, and in some cases these may be so abundant as to obscure the relatively small number of tumour cells present. Infiltration of the epithelium of individual crypts is present in many cases. The intestinal mucosa adjacent to the tumours, especially those in the jejunum, usually shows enteropathy comprising villous atrophy, crypt hyperplasia, increased lamina propria

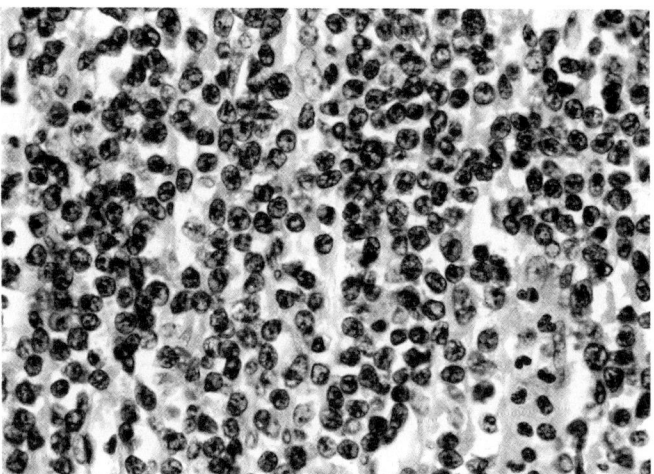

Fig. 15.10.4.5 Type 2 EATL. The lymphoma is composed of monomorphic small lymphocytes.

lymphocytes and plasma cells, and intraepithelial lymphocytosis. The degree of enteropathy is highly variable, however, and may consist only of an increase in intraepithelial lymphocytes.

In type 2 (Fig. 15.10.4.5) the neoplastic cells are small, round and monomorphic with darkly staining nuclei and a narrow rim of cytoplasm. There is usually florid infiltration of intestinal crypt epithelium. The adjacent intestinal mucosa shows villous atrophy and crypt hyperplasia with striking intraepithelial lymphocytosis involving both crypt and surface epithelium.

The histology of the small intestine remote from the site of the tumour is an important consideration in the diagnosis of EATL. In most cases the changes are identical with those of coeliac disease and consist of villous atrophy with crypt hyperplasia, plasmacytosis of the lamina propria, and an increase in intraepithelial lymphocytes.

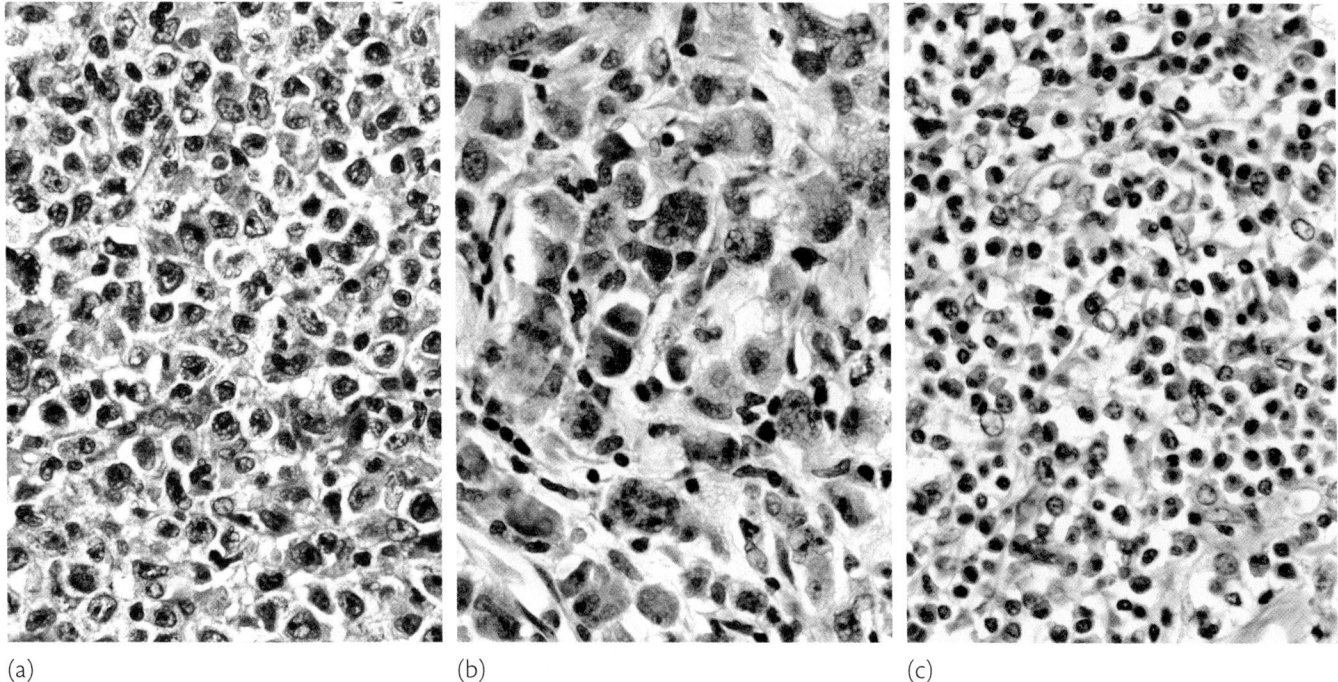

(a)   (b)   (c)

Fig. 15.10.4.4 Type 1 EATL. Three different cases showing the cytological variability. In (a) the tumour is composed of large polymorphic lymphocytes; in (b) the tumour shows striking pleomorphism and in (c) tumour cells are overrun by inflammatory cells, principally eosinophils.

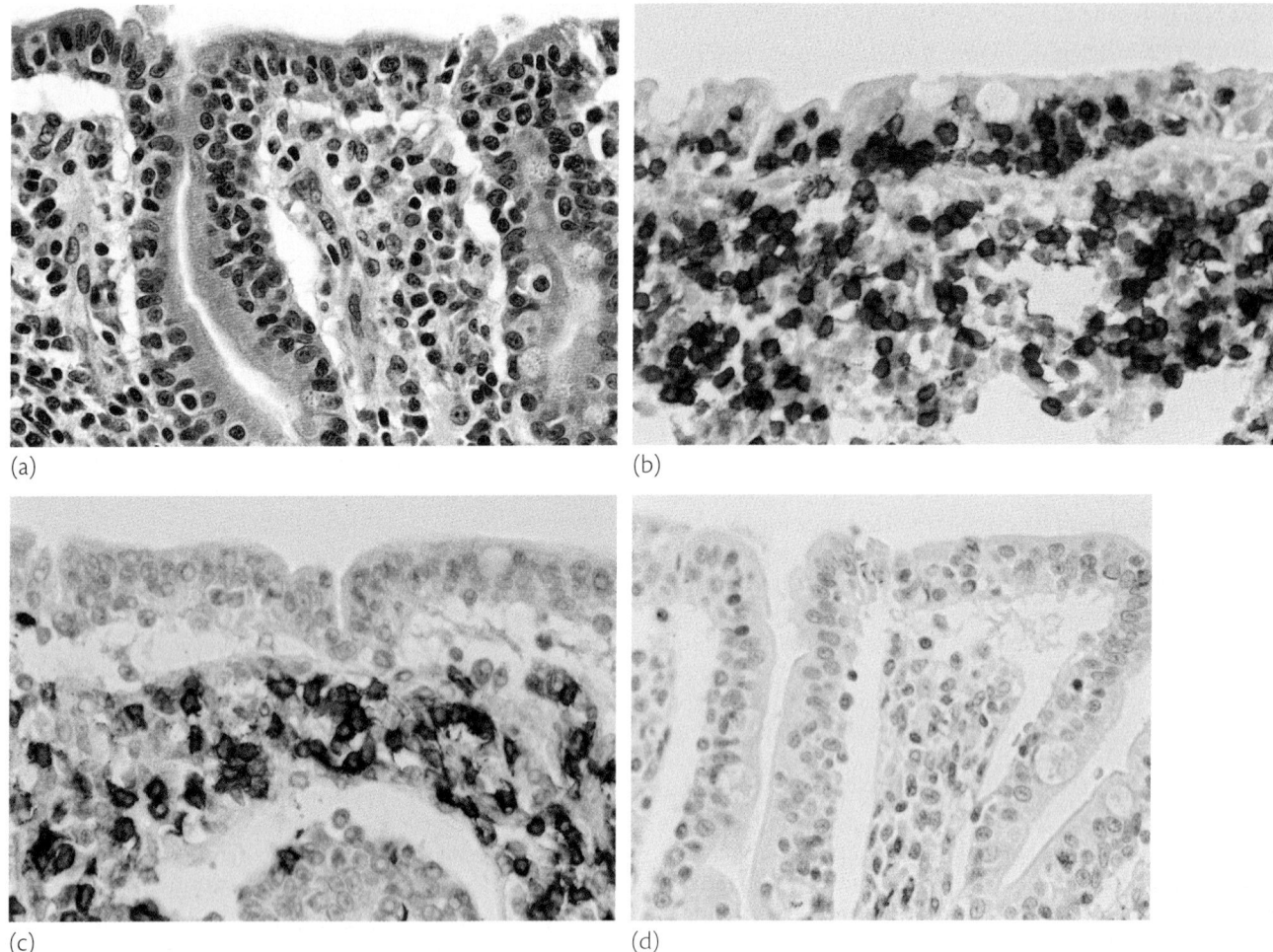

Fig. 15.10.4.6 Uninvolved mucosa adjacent to type 1 EATL showing (a) increased intraepithelial lymphocytes that are (b) CD3 positive, (c) CD8 negative, and (d) CD56 negative.

In type 2 EATL, the degree of intraepithelial lymphocytosis may be spectacular and so extreme as to virtually obscure the epithelial cells. The lymphocytes are small, without neoplastic features, and in these extreme cases spill into the lamina propria where they may merge with the lymphomatous infiltrate.

Immunophenotype

In type 1 EATL the tumour cells are CD3+, CD5–, CD7+, CD8–/+, CD4–, CD103+, TCRβ +/– and contain cytotoxic granule associated proteins. In almost all cases, a varying proportion of the tumour cells express CD30. The intraepithelial lymphocytes in the adjacent enteropathic mucosa (Fig. 15.10.4.6) may show an abnormal immunophenotype, usually CD3+, CD5–, CD8–, CD4–, identical to that of the lymphoma. In type 2 cases the tumour cells are CD3+, CD4–, CD8+ CD56+ and TCRβ+ and the intraepithelial lymphocytes in the adjacent mucosa share the identical immunophenotype. The postulated cell of origin is the intestinal intraepithelial T cell.

Genetics

The TCR β and γ genes (*TCRB* and *TCRG*) are clonally rearranged in both types of EATL and also frequently in the 'uninvolved' mucosa adjacent to the lymphoma. Type 1 EATL frequently homozygously expresses HLA DQA1*0501, DQB1*0201 genes that

characterize coeliac disease, while patients with type 2 EATL do not differ in their genetic HLA DQB1 constitution from the average population of white European origin. In contrast to primary nodal peripheral T-cell lymphomas, most EATL cases (58–70%) harbour complex segmental amplifications of the 9q31.3-qter chromosome region or, alternatively, show deletions in 16q12.1. These features are prevalent in both type 1 and 2 EATL and form a common genetic link between the two types. Type 1 EATL, however, frequently displays chromosomal gains in 1q and 5q, while type 2 EATL is more often characterized by 8q24 (*MYC*) amplifications.

Precursor lesions

As indicated above, type 1 EATL may be preceded by refractory coeliac disease with or without ulceration In some cases of refractory coeliac disease the intraepithelial lymphocytes are phenotypically aberrant, showing down-regulation of CD8 similar to the intraepithelial lymphocytes in mucosa adjacent to EATL (see Fig. 15.10.4.6). These cases also show monoclonal T-cell rearrangement of the intraepithelial lymphocytes similar to the clonal rearrangements that may be found in the enteropathic mucosa adjacent to EATL, suggesting that the immunophenotypically aberrant intraepithelial lymphocytes constitute a neoplastic population. In those cases of refractory coeliac disease where EATL subsequently develops, the intraepithelial lymphocytes share the same monoclonal TCR gene rearrangement with the subsequent T-cell lymphomas. Furthermore, the intraepithelial lymphocytes in these cases of refractory coeliac disease carry gains of chromosome 1q in common with type I EATL. Thus, refractory coeliac disease in which the intraepithelial lymphocytes show these immunopheno-typic and genetic features can be considered as examples of intraepithelial T-cell lymphoma or, alternatively EATL *in situ*. Type 2 EATL may also be preceded by refractory coeliac disease in which the immunophenotype of the intraepithelial lymphocytes is similar to that of the neoplastic cells in the subsequent lymphoma, namely CD8+ and CD56+. This type of refractory coeliac disease has not been well characterized. In a second group of patients with refractory coeliac disease the intraepithelial lymphocytes express a normal immunophenotype and are polyclonal. These cases probably do not progress to EATL.

Prognosis

The prognosis is usually poor, with death frequently resulting from abdominal complications in patients already weakened by uncontrolled malabsorption. Long-term survivals are recorded, typically in cases presenting with a localized tumour that can be surgically excised. Recurrences are most frequent in the small intestine.

Further reading

Cellier C, *et al.* (2000). Refractory sprue, coeliac disease, and enteropathy-associated T-cell lymphoma. *Lancet*, **356**, 203–8.

De Leeuw RJ, *et al.* (2007). Whole genome analysis and HLA genotyping of enteropathy-type intestinal T-cell lymphoma reveals two distinct lymphoma subtypes. *Gastroenterology*, **132**, 1902–11.

Isaacson PG, Du M-Q (2004). Malt lymphoma: from morphology to molecules. *Nat Rev Cancer*, **4**, 6644–653.

Isaacson PG, Du M-Q (2005). Gastrointestinal lymphoma: where morphology meets molecular biology. *J Pathol*, **205**, 255–74.

15.10.5 Disaccharidase deficiency

Timothy M. Cox

Essentials

Disaccharidases occur in the microvilli of the small intestine and are required for the complete assimilation of nearly all carbohydrate present in food and drinks, apart from free glucose and fructose. The enzymes cleave disaccharides such as sucrose, maltose, and lactose, as well as dextrins derived from starch, into their component monosaccharides, and their activity is reduced in hereditary conditions or in generalized intestinal diseases.

Disaccharidase deficiency causes carbohydrate intolerance induced by bacterial fermentation of undigested sugars which are delivered to the colon. Abdominal symptoms (e.g. nausea, bloating, distension, colicky pain, watery diarrhoea) are usually noticed within an hour of the ingestion of foods containing the offending sugars.

By far the most common cause of disaccharidase deficiency is lactose intolerance. During infancy, when milk is the principal food, lactase activity is high, but in most humans it declines after weaning and remains low (lactase nonpersistence), with such individuals having a low capacity to breakdown lactose. By contrast, in other healthy subjects a mendelian dominant trait means that intestinal lactase expression remains high throughout life (lactase persistence), and these can digest large quantities (loading doses >50 g). The global distribution of lactase activity in adult populations is subject to wide variation: nonpersistence of lactase expression predominates in nearly every population in East Asia, whereas in populations of northern and central European origin, and in Afro-Arabian nomads who have developed or maintained pastoralist dairy cultures, lifelong lactase expression in the intestine is sustained by most individuals.

Intestinal lactase phenotypes can be identified by assay of mucosal biopsy samples or appropriate sugar-tolerance tests, as can other (much rarer) genetically determined disaccharidase variants. Disaccharide intolerance is readily treated by institution of a strict exclusion diet; enzymatic supplementation may benefit patients with severe enzymatic deficiency.

Physiology of carbohydrate digestion (Fig. 15.10.5.1)

Luminal phase

Free disaccharides occur in the diet or originate from luminal hydrolysis of starch and glycogen by salivary and pancreatic α-amylase. Since amylase cannot hydrolyse the α-1,6 branching linkages that contribute to the complex arborized structure of starch and glycogen, and has little action on the linear α-1,4 bonds adjacent to these points, the initial products of starch digestion are branched oligosaccharides containing at least one α-1,6 bond. Maltase–glucoamylase is a mucosal α-glucosidase that removes glucose moieties sequentially from the nonreducing terminus of linear oligosaccharides to generate limit α-dextrins within the lumen; these are branched, short-chain carbohydrate molecules.

Mucosal phase

Isomaltase (α-dextrinase) promotes the further digestion of starch at the intestinal brush border by cleaving the α-1,6 glycosidic bonds of the limit dextrins. Isomaltase is a component of the bifunctional complex sucrase–isomaltase, the sucrase moiety of which hydrolyses sucrose into fructose and glucose.

The disaccharides sucrose, lactose, and trehalose, like the α-dextrins, are poorly absorbed: to be assimilated, they are also split into monosaccharides by glycosidases located on the brush-border (microvillus) membrane (sucrase, lactase, and trehalase). Mucosal disaccharidases are optimally active at pH 6.0 and are present principally in the duodenum and jejunum; some activity persists in the ileum but is absent in the colon. Lactase is the familiar name for lactase–phlorizin hydrolase, a membrane-bound microvillous enzyme with β-galactosidsase activity responsible for the cleavage of lactose into its component glucose and galactose moieties.

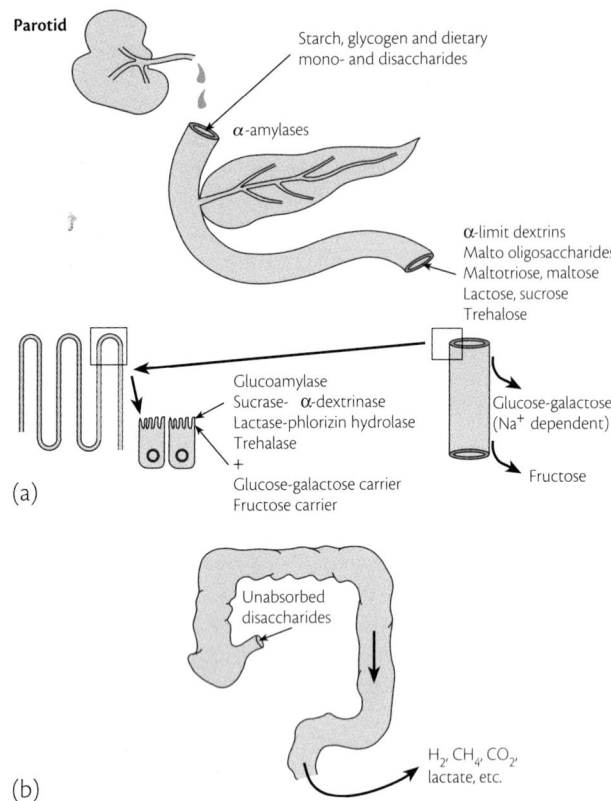

Fig. 15.10.5.1 Carbohydrate digestion and absorption.

Specific carriers in the microvilli for the transport of glucose and galactose, as well as fructose, mediate the uptake of monosaccharides released by the mucosal disaccharidases—and absorption occurs rapidly. Active transport by the sodium-dependent glucose–galactose carrier is accompanied by the passive flux of water from the lumen. Unabsorbed disaccharides are fermented by bacteria in the colon to short-chain organic acids, hydrogen, and methane. Maldigestion of osmotically active sugars thus leads to retention of fluid in the gut. When digestion of disaccharides is incomplete, ingestion of carbohydrate induces pain caused by distension of the bowel with fluid and gas, accompanied by watery diarrhoea.

For most carbohydrates, hydrolysis in the lumen and at the mucosal surface is sufficiently rapid to saturate the pathways for glucose and fructose transport. For lactose, however, the rate of mucosal hydrolysis, rather than glucose and galactose uptake, may easily become limiting. Hence the functional reserve of lactase in the human intestine is restricted and assimilation of lactose is often noticeably impaired in the early stages of mucosal disease.

Although the biosynthesis of surface disaccharidases continues throughout the life of the epithelium, the enzymes are only active in mature cells on the upper reaches of small-intestinal villi. Complete turnover of the enzyme molecules occurs several times during the lifespan of the mature enterocyte. Brush-border disaccharidases are complex glycoproteins that undergo proteolytic processing; extensive glycan modification in the Golgi apparatus occurs before insertion into the membrane. The mature enzymes are derived from large, single-chain polypeptides. The genetically determined mechanism by which lactase expression decreases after infancy is not fully understood but influences transcription of the lactase gene.

Carbohydrate intolerance syndrome (Table 15.10.5.1)

Abdominal symptoms are usually noticed within an hour of the ingestion of foods containing the offending sugars. There is nausea, bloating, and distension of the abdomen accompanied by borborygmi and flatulence. Colicky pain precedes watery diarrhoea, usually associated with flatus, and it may be explosive; the anal region is often sore as a result of stool acidity. Diarrhoea due to the maldigestion of carbohydrate can occur several hours after ingestion of the noxious food or drink. These symptoms may be induced by only a few grams of the offending sugar. Intestinal hurry aggravates fat malabsorption and may obscure the underlying cause of the diarrhoea. Deficiency of particular disaccharidases is responsible for the dietary intolerance of specific foods and drinks: milk-containing products in the case of lactase deficiency; table sugar and starch in asucrasia; mushrooms (and probably shellfish) in the rare trehalase deficiency. Identification of a cause-and-effect relationship between particular items and the intolerance syndrome is often impossible, given the ubiquity of sucrose and lactose in commercial foods.

Lactose intolerance

Most patients suffering from intolerance of lactose in the diet suffer either from lactase deficiency acquired as a result of intestinal disease, especially postinfective gastroenteritis in children, or as a result of genetically determined restriction of lactase expression.

Congenital lactase deficiency

A few infants have been reported in whom diarrhoea occurred after the first feed with breast milk and who responded completely to a lactose-free formula feed. This disorder is distinct from congenital glucose–galactose malabsorption, in which lactose exclusion alone is ineffective. Congenital lactose intolerance is associated with a severe inherited deficiency of mucosal lactase activity and, unlike the intolerance of lactose associated with prematurity or secondary to diffuse intestinal disease, remains lifelong. This syndrome leads to lactosuria due to the abnormal absorption of intact lactose, principally in the stomach; renal tubular acidosis and aminoaciduria have been recorded in this autosomal recessive disease that leads to vomiting, failure to thrive, and dehydration.

Table 15.10.5.1 Carbohydrate intolerance syndromes due to deficiency of disaccharidases

Lactose intolerance
Congenital (inherited) lactase deficiency
Lactase restriction (genetically determined)
Lactase deficiency secondary to intestinal disease
Sucrose intolerance*
Congenital asucrasia (inherited)
Sucrase deficiency secondary to intestinal disease
Trehalose intolerance
Congenital atrehalasia

* Accompanied by reduced tolerance of starch.

Table 15.10.5.2 Foods containing lactose

Fresh, dried, skimmed, non-fat, and condensed milks
Cream
Yoghurt
Cheese
Processed meats and sausages
Sauces, stuffings, salad dressings
Custard powder
Canned and dried soups
Biscuits, cakes, cookies, pancakes, waffles, dried cereals
Confectionery
Frozen and canned fruits
Instant coffee
Lactose is also frequently used as a filler in powdered medicines and tablets

Lactase deficiency of prematurity

Unlike the other mucosal glycosidases, which appear early during fetal development, intestinal lactase activity is not fully expressed until after the 28th week of gestation and transient intolerance of milk feeds is common before this age. Abdominal distress due to gaseous distension and diarrhoea requires careful attention to the diet and fluid balance in premature infants.

Lactase restriction in children and adults

The capacity of the intestine to digest lactose is a mendelian dominant trait which is retained into adult life. Persistence of high intestinal lactase activity is unusual in adult mammals, and in humans is believed to have been maintained by selection in populations that adopted dairy culture about 10 000 years ago. Thus, tolerance of lactose in milk, dairy products (and many processed and ready-to-eat foods; see Table 15.10.5.2), is found mainly in peoples of northern and central European descent. Lactose tolerance is also prevalent in the nomadic Tuareg and Bedouin, as well as the Peuhl of Senegal and Nigerian Fulani peoples, all of whom retain strong dairy-based pastoral traditions. In about 5% of northern European adults, compared with more than 90% in most of Africa and Asia, the genetically determined decline in mucosal lactase activity occurs after weaning. Reduction of mucosal lactose activity is associated with reduced synthesis of the precursor protein in the epithelial cells with apparently normal processing to the mature enzyme. The physiological decline in activity occurs between 3 and 5 years of age.

Low lactase activity, considered in the clinical context as lactase deficiency, is thus a frequent genetic variant among healthy adults. Extensive family studies demonstrate transmission as a simple mendelian factor: healthy adults with low lactase activity are homozygous for an autosomal recessive allele that causes the physiological decline of lactase activity after weaning (lactase nonpersistence or restriction, also referred to as adult-type hypolactasia), whereas those in whom high lactase activity persists in adult life are either heterozygous or homozygous for a dominant allele, the persistence allele, which prevents 'physiological' decline of lactase activity. Globally, lactase persistence is thus the minor, low-frequency variant, and its high prevalence in specific populations

was probably maintained by natural selection in groups that settled to invest in dairy culture from Neolithic times. The development of cheese manufacture, as well as yogurt and other milk fermentation products such as kvass in which the sugar content is markedly reduced, would allow individuals with diminished capacity to digest lactose to thrive.

The element which determines lactase activity in adults acts in *cis* with the human lactase gene on chromosome 2q21; however, the molecular mechanism which regulates transcriptional and developmental expression of the enzyme in the intestine has yet to be unravelled. A C/T polymorphism approximately 14 kb upstream of the gene is tightly linked to the deficient/persistent lactase phenotype in several populations and constitutes part of a haplotype extended over more than 500 kb of genomic DNA. Homozygosity for the *C* allele at nucleotide position −13910 is associated with nonpersistence of lactase expression in adults. This polymorphic site might itself determine lactase expression, at least in part, since studies have shown that the presence of the −13910*T* allele enhances binding of the transcription factor Oct1, and thereby promotes lactase gene expression *in vitro*. Additional sequence variants in the vicinity of the locus at position −13910 are strongly associated with determinants that lead to persistence of lactase expression in populations of sub-Saharan African and Afro-Arabian origin.

Symptoms develop on exposure to excessive milk-and lactose-containing foods or medicines in late childhood or early adult life. The selective pressures that maintain this physiological reduction in mucosal lactase deficiency in childhood are unknown but the concept of 'lactase deficiency' in adults is difficult to justify, since lactase persistence is the least frequent state. Nonetheless, with the increasing migration of peoples and the widespread adoption of Western-style diets, physiological loss of lactase activity is a prevalent cause of abdominal distress. A significant proportion of patients with spastic colon, irritable bowel disease, or other 'functional' abdominal disturbances may prove to have lactase deficiency.

The speculative possibility arises that lactase-deficient subjects are at risk from osteoporosis in countries at high latitudes because of a dietary deficiency of calcium or vitamin D. There is a higher frequency of lactase nonpersistence in osteoporotic women when compared with appropriate control subjects; this extends in some studies to reduced bone mineralization density with increased fractures. It is presumed, but not proven, that reduced calcium intake is responsible. In contrast, in lactase-persistent subjects, increased milk consumption may contribute to hyperlipidaemia and coronary heart disease. Moreover, by analogy with the role of galactitol in galactokinase deficiency, a disorder of galactose metabolism associated with cataract ('galactose diabetes'), sustained consumption of large amounts of milk and lactose-containing foods has been implicated in the development of premature cataract. There have been several European reports that adults with idiopathic and diabetic senile and presenile cataracts have a higher frequency of lactase persistence than population controls without cataract and at least one other study has shown that high intake of milk correlated with cortical cataracts. Similar surveys in populations with a higher general prevalence of lactose persistence showed no correlation; but a high risk of cataract formation has been reported in subjects with high lactose intake and low activities of galactokinase.

Diagnosis of lactose malabsorption

Intolerance of dietary carbohydrate caused by the maldigestion of lactose may be suspected from the dietary history of a patient typically complaining of abdominal pain, flatulence, and diarrhoea. Symptoms are often related to changes in social circumstances and are frequently reported by Asian immigrants to Western countries; they may also become manifest when lactose-rich foods are administered inappropriately to children and adults by Western agencies in famine relief programmes. In this respect, the promotion by large multinational corporations of commercial infant feeds heavily based on milk products has attracted adverse international criticism. The relative lack of functional reserve of mucosal lactase activity also explains the frequency with which lactose malabsorption becomes manifest after partial gastrectomy and related procedures that accelerate delivery of dietary carbohydrate to the jejunum.

The stool has an acidic pH (<6) and the osmolality of stool water is generally greater than 350 mosmol/kg because of the presence of lactate and other organic anions; in infants and children with complete lactase deficiency, reducing substances may be abundant in the stool water. Breath-hydrogen analysis is a useful confirmatory test. Hydrogen excretion, determined by rebreathing 2 h after the ingestion of 50 g of lactose, identifies patients with lactase deficiency diagnosed by enzymatic assay of jejunal mucosa obtained by biopsy. This latter procedure is difficult to standardize and is now rarely justified outside the research setting. Other investigations, such as the lactose barium-meal examination and determination of blood glucose profile after oral challenge with lactose, are cumbersome and, because they give false-positive results, are now obsolete. Several initiatives are under way to promote the diagnosis of lactose persistence/nonpersistence by molecular analysis of the lactase–phlorizin hydrolase gene, with particular emphasis on the polymorphic variants at position −13910. However, without a complete molecular understanding of the mechanisms by which lactase activity is controlled and the appearance of different lactase haplotypes in different population groups, in all but selected groups, genetic diagnosis should at present be regarded as premature.

Secondary lactase deficiency

Lactase activity may be depressed by mucosal disease of the small intestine and often occurs transiently after infective gastroenteritis. It is particularly frequent in infants suffering from gastroenteritis due to enterocytopathic viruses, and continuing symptoms provoked by milk feeds can persist for days or some weeks. Dehydration may develop rapidly in infants and is accompanied by prominent bloating; disacchariduria is found and acid, sour-smelling stools may be obvious. These symptoms usually resolve rapidly when dairy products are excluded. Decreased lactase activity also accompanies extensive and longstanding mucosal disease so that a milk intolerance syndrome due to maldigestion may complicate coeliac disease, intestinal giardiasis, and Crohn's disease.

In secondary deficiencies of disaccharidases, because of the critical relationship between lactase activity and the rate at which this sugar is digested, intolerance of lactose predominates. However, the use of high-calorie preparations containing large amounts disaccharides and short-chain carbohydrates other than lactose (especially maltose, sucrose, and dextrins) to supplement the nutrition of patients with intestinal disease, may exacerbate their symptoms and induce a florid carbohydrate intolerance syndrome.

Sucrase–isomaltase (α-dextrinase) deficiency

This recessively inherited enzyme deficiency of the mucosal brush border is rare in all populations except the Inuit of Greenland, in whom the frequency of homozygotes is up to 10%. Cetacean mammals also lack sucrase–isomaltase. Several defects of the human gene on chromosome 3q appear to be responsible; in some, there is aberrant glycosylation and the enzyme is inefficiently transported to the brush border. Substantial degradation of the abnormal polypeptide occurs within the epithelial cell.

Intolerance of sucrose is responsible for most of the symptoms, which develop as table sugar and sugar-containing foods are introduced during weaning. Intolerance of starch is less prominent because the osmotic contribution of the larger α-dextrin molecules that remain unsplit in the gut lumen is less. However, ingestion of large, starchy meals may induce cramping discomfort, flatulence, and diarrhoea. While taking a normal diet, patients with deficiency of sucrase–isomaltase have persistent diarrhoea with the passage of acid and frothy stools containing increased concentrations of lactate and other short-chain acids.

The diagnosis may be suspected on the basis of the history of diarrhoea at weaning and on the character of the stools. Differentiation from coeliac disease, cow's milk allergy, infective or postinfective gastroenteritis, pancreatic failure, and other disaccharide intolerance syndromes (particularly lactose intolerance, caused by inflammatory bowel disease) is important, and biopsy of the jejunal mucosa for enzymatic assay and histological examination should be considered. In inherited sucrase–isomaltase deficiency, these activities are selectively reduced to less than 10% of control values in histologically normal mucosa. Hydrogen breath tests after ingestion of sucrose and isomaltose may also prove to be useful in diagnosis, but experience is limited.

Trehalase deficiency

A few patients have been reported with mushroom intolerance due to the absence of mucosal trehalase. Trehalase is a brush-border α-glycosidase that cleaves the unusual 1α–1α bond of trehalase into its component glucose moieties. Trehalose is found in the haemolymph of arthropods and in fungi, so that intolerance of crustacean shellfish as well as mushrooms in the diet might be expected. Given that intolerance of edible fungi is not uncommon, trehalase deficiency may prove to be more frequent than previously supposed. Trehalase deficiency has also been reported to occur in 10 to 15% of Greenland Inuit (and in cetacean mammals from the same environment) but the functional significance of this is unknown.

Treatment

Dietary exclusion of the offending sugar is the best method of preventing symptoms in individuals with primary or acquired disaccharidase deficiency. Symptoms recur as soon as excessive lactose or sucrose is reintroduced and advice from a professional dietitian may be needed to avoid indiscretions. This is especially important in the case of young infants and children with marked deficiency of particular disaccharidases, where special food supplements may be required (see below). In hypolactasia, complete elimination is not usually required, as lactase deficiency is rarely absolute; nevertheless, if symptoms persist there are many potential sources of lactose that warrant investigation (see Table 15.10.5.2).

An early, alternative, method for preventing symptoms in patients with lactose intolerance was the use of β-galactosidases obtained from yeast or other microorganisms. These enzymes were added to dairy products before consumption and often changed the taste.

In the United States of America, β-galactosidase is obtained from yeast (LactAid) and has been shown to reduce symptoms as well as breath-hydrogen excretion in subjects with maldigestion of lactose. In the United Kingdom, a concentrated liquid lactase preparation (Colief, 50 000 units/g) is licensed and for use in infants and children with symptomatic lactose intolerance. β-Galactosidase derived from *Aspergillus oryzae* (Lactrase), taken in tablet form immediately before challenge with lactose, is effective in children with late-onset intolerance of lactose. Its cost, compared with dietary exclusion, may not be justified. More recently there has been a resurgence of the avid 19th-century interest in the use of so-called 'prebiotic agents' for a wide diversity of abdominal and other complaints; there have been claims of benefit in rotavirus infection and in the control of symptomatic lactose intolerance. At present, it is too early to decide whether these highly commercialized agents have any useful role in lactose intolerance but, despite their high cost, on balance some preparations may have a modest benefit in symptomatic control.

In infants and young children with proven lactose intolerance, Farley's Soya formula, Galactomin Formula 17, Isomil, SMA FF, Enfamil Lactofree, and other preparations provide protein and suitable carbohydrate in a powdered form so that adequate nutrition can be maintained. For older children and severely ill adults with disaccharide intolerance, other preparations may be required (see below). In the future, microbial β-galactosidases might be justified for food supplementation programmes in countries where lactose intolerance and nutritional deprivation in the adult population are widespread.

Complete absence of sucrase–isomaltase activity in most patients with sucrose intolerance, together with the ubiquity of sucrose in modern diets, complicates symptom management. Modest reduction of amylopectin-rich foods usually suffices to improve symptoms of starch intolerance, but complete avoidance of sucrose-containing foods can be difficult especially in infants and young children. Powdered and liquid preparations such as Caloreen, Maxijul LE, Polycal liquid and powder, amongst others, may be needed for sucrase–isomaltase deficiency. Glucose (or fructose) can be used as a sweetener. It has been reported that ingestion of dried brewer's yeast (containing invertase or sucrase but little lactase activity) after food is effective in patients with sucrase–isomaltase deficiency. However, dried yeast is rather unpalatable and not readily accepted by children. A high-potency liquid preparation of invertase used in the industrial manufacture of fructose from unrefined sugar cane juice (Sacrosidase), has been approved by the Food and Drug Administration in the United States. In a double-blind randomized controlled trial in patients with sucrase–isomaltase deficiency, the agent was found to be safe, acceptable, and effective for the symptomatic treatment of this disease in patients receiving a low-starch diet.

Further reading

Arola H, et al. (1999). Low trehalase activity is associated with abdominal symptoms caused by edible mushrooms. *Scand J Gastroenterol*, **34**, 898–903.

Baudon JJ, et al. (1996). Sucrase-isomaltase deficiency: changing pattern over two decades. *J Pediatr Gastroenterol Nutr*, **22**, 284–8.

Bodé S, Gudmand-H yer E (1988). Incidence and clinical significance of lactose malabsorption in adult celiac disease. *Scand J Gastroenterol*, **23**, 484–8. [Provides an important clinical perspective in common diseases presenting to gastroenterologists and other practitioners.]

Bolin TD, Davis AE, Duncombe VM (1982). A prospective study of persistent diarrhoea. *Austral N Z J Med*, **12**, 22–6. [Careful study of operational importance for practitioners.]

Clare H, Ruth M (1997). Phylogenetic analysis of the evolution of lactose digestion in adults. *Hum Biol*, **69**, 605–28.

Corazza GR, et al. (1992). Beta-Galactosidase from *Aspergillus niger* in adult lactose malabsorption: a double blind crossover study. *Aliment Pharmacol Therapeut*, **6**, 61–6.

Di Stefano M, et al. (2002). Lactose malabsorption and intolerance and peak bone mass. *Gastroenterology*, **122**, 1793–99.

Ennatah NS, et al. (2002). Identification of a variant associated with adult-type hypolactasia. *Nat Genet*, **30**, 233–7.

Farnworth ER (2008). The evidence to support health claims for probiotics. *J Nutr*, **138**, 1250S–54S.

Gray GM (1975). Carbohydrate digestion and absorption. Rôle of the small intestine. *N Engl J Med*, **292**, 1225–30. [An informative and accessible biochemical review.]

Heyman MB (2006). Committee on Nutrition. Lactose intolerance in infants, children, and adolescents. *Pediatrics*, **118**, 1279–86.

Hoskova A, et al. (1980). Severe lactose intolerance with lactosuria and vomiting. *Arch Dis Child*, **55**, 304–16.

King CE, Toskes PP (1983). The use of breath tests in the study of malabsorption. *Clin Gastroenterol*, **12**, 591–610.

Kuokkanen M, et al. (2006). Mutations in the translated region of the lactase gene (LCT) underlie congenital lactase deficiency. *Am J Hum Genet*, **78**, 339–44.

Lewinsky, RH et al. (2005). T-13910 DNA variant associated with lactase persistence interacts with Oct-1 and stimulates lactase promoter activity in vitro. *Hum Mol Genet*, **15**, 3945–53.

Madzarovova-Nohejlova J (1973). Trehalase deficiency in a family. *Gastroenterology*, **65**, 130–3.

Medow MS, et al. (1990). β-Galactosidase tablets in the treatment of lactose intolerance in pediatrics. *Am J Dis Child*, **144**, 1261–4. [Promising results with enzyme replacement therapy.]

Montalto M, et al. (2005). Effect of exogenous beta-galactosidase in patients with lactose malabsorption and intolerance: a crossover double-blind placebo-controlled study. *Eur J Clin Nutr*, **59**, 489–93.

Sibley E (2004). Carbohydrate intolerance. *Curr Opin Gastroenterol*, **20**, 162–7.

Simoons FJ (1978). The geographic hypothesis and lactose malabsorption. *Am J Digest Dis*, **23**, 963–80.

Swallow DM (2003). Genetics of lactase persistence and lactose intolerance. *Annu Rev Genet*, **37**, 197–219. [A first-rate comprehensive essay on the biochemical genetics and evolutionary significance of intestinal lactase polymorphisms in humans.]

Swallow DM (2006). DNA test for hypolactasia premature. *Gut*, **55**, 131.

Treem WR (1995). Congenital sucrase–isomaltase deficiency. *J Pediatr Gastroenterol Nutr*, **21**, 1–14.

Treem WR, et al. (1999). Sacrosidase therapy for congenital sucrase–isomaltase deficiency. *J Pediatr Gastroenterol Nutr*, **28**, 137–42.

Wang Y, et al. (1998). The genetically programmed down-regulation of lactase in children. *Gastroenterology*, **114**, 1230–6.

15.10.6 Whipple's disease

H.J.F. Hodgson

Essentials

Whipple's disease is an uncommon infection caused by the actinomycete *Tropheryma whipplei*. It is most commonly diagnosed when overt small-intestinal disease leads to malabsorption, but before this there are often several years of nonspecific prodromal manifestations such as fever and arthralgia/arthritis, and the disease can present in many other ways, e.g neurological manifestations (of many forms, including movement disorders, ocular manifestations and meningitis) or endocarditis.

Diagnosis usually depends upon (1) demonstration of classical histological features in the small intestine, which is thick and oedematous, with stubby or absent villi and dilated lacteals, and with the lamina propria stuffed with macrophages containing foamy material which stains brilliant magenta with periodic acid–Schiff reagent (diastase resistant); and (2) positive identification of *Tropheryma whipplei* DNA by polymerase chain reaction. Molecular techniques have increased the frequency with which individuals with minimal or absent gastrointestinal disease are diagnosed.

Treatment is with antibiotics (initially a bactericidal agent with CSF penetration, followed by long-term therapy with e.g. trimethoprine-sulphamethiazole). Clinical improvement occurs within a few weeks, but prolonged treatment for at least a year is recommended. Relapse can occur, even after many years, especially when progressive central nervous system disease occurs in the absence of other systemic manifestations.

Pathology and aetiology

Advanced or fatal cases of Whipple's disease predominantly show severe intestinal and intraabdominal pathology. Fatty deposits in the small intestine and mesenteric lymph nodes prompted Whipple to call the disease 'intestinal lipodystrophy'. The small intestine is thick and oedematous, with stubby or absent villi and dilated lacteals (secondary lymphangiectasia reflecting obstructed lymph flow). The absorptive enterocyte layer is virtually normal, but the lamina propria is stuffed with macrophages containing foamy material which stains brilliant magenta with periodic acid–Schiff reagent (diastase resistant) (Fig. 15.10.6.1). There is little inflammation otherwise. There are fatty deposits, and occasionally granulomas, in the mesenteric nodes as well as the characteristic macrophages. Other organs are involved to a varying degree, with foamy macrophages in spleen, lymph nodes, central nervous system, liver, lung, heart, and joints. Valvular endocarditis and localized brain deposits account for two of the most severe forms of the disease. The rod-shaped bacteria, the source of the periodic acid–Schiff-positive material, are identifiable at light and electron microscope level in affected tissues. The presence of the organism in sewage-exposed water suggests that infection occurs by invasion of the alimentary tract, and may explain the preponderance of small-intestinal disease, with subsequent haematogenous or lymphatic dissemination. It remains unclear whether those who become infected have an

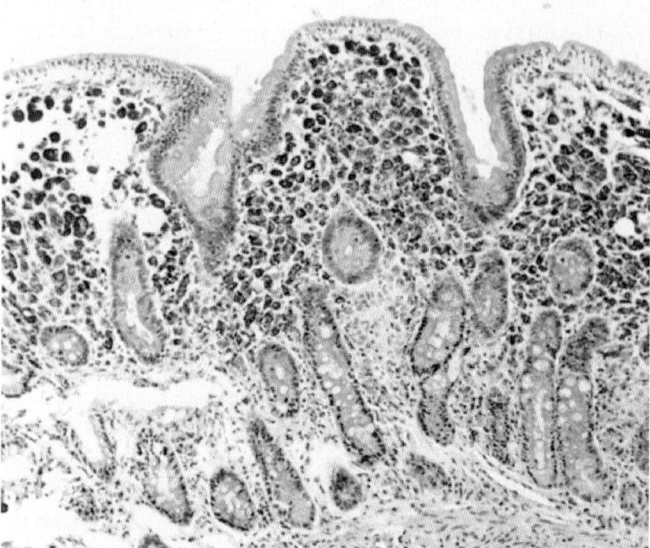

Fig. 15.10.6.1 Jejunal biopsy specimen from a 50-year-old man with Whipple's disease showing stunted villi and infiltration of the lamina propria with densely staining macrophages (periodic acid–Schiff stained, ×150).

underlying immunodeficiency, but host factors are certainly relevant as immunosuppressive drugs have hastened disease progression. Abnormal monocyte function may persist after successful treatment, and a weak HLA B27 association has also been reported.

Clinical features and diagnosis

The condition is most frequently diagnosed in middle-aged or older men, but women and children may be affected. The classical patient is a white man diagnosed with relatively advanced disease with malaise, weight loss, diarrhoea, and arthralgias; on examination there may be marked pigmentation, lymphadenopathy, anaemia, finger clubbing, hypotension, and oedema. Rarely, gastrointestinal bleeding may also occur. In such cases, investigation of an obvious gastrointestinal complaint should quickly establish the diagnosis. Recognition is far more difficult if symptoms are limited to fever or arthritis, or another systemic manifestation, which may be present transiently or intermittently for many years before the disease is diagnosed. The arthritis is migratory, nondeforming, and seronegative, predominantly affecting peripheral joints and in some series affects up to 90% of patients. Other early features include respiratory symptoms with pleurisy and pulmonary infiltrates, and pericarditis. Chylous or serous ascites, endocarditis, cardiac conduction defects, coronary arteritis, and neurological abnormalities may occur with progression of the condition, but in particular endocarditis (predominantly aortic and mitral) or neurological manifestations may occur in isolation. In recent surveys more than 80% of patients had gut disease at diagnosis but 15% had no gastrointestinal disorder at any time. Joint symptoms were present at some time in 75% of patients, 33% had neurological disease, 17% cardiovascular disease, and 15% mucocutaneous manifestations (pigmentation or sarcoid-like plaques). The central nervous system manifestations are diverse and include depression, apathy, fits, and myoclonus, and a variety of ocular manifestations including supranuclear ophthalmoplegia, papilloedema, scotomata, pseudotumour, and uveitis. Meningitis and a hypothalamic syndrome with insomnia, hyperphagia, and polydipsia also occur. Oculomastatory myorhythmia is said to be diagnostic.

Diagnosis usually depends upon demonstration of classical histological features in the small intestine, reflecting the ease with which tissues can be obtained at routine upper gastrointestinal endoscopy, and a positive identification of *Tropheryma whipplei* DNA by molecular amplification in the polymerase chain reaction (PCR). The combination of histological and molecular identification avoids pitfalls. For example, *Mycobacterium avium* infection may be histologically similar, and some reports on saliva suggest the organism may reside as a commensal, emphasizing the need for clinical interpretation. PCR positivity in patients has been reported on peripheral blood, lymph nodes, synovial tissue, bone marrow, and even faeces, and may yield positive results on small-intestinal and other tissues in which characteristic histology cannot be identified. Use of the technique in patients with arthritis, pyrexia of unknown origin, and other chronic undiagnosed conditions can, however, identify cases in which small-intestinal disease is not apparent. Its use has suggested that intractable idiopathic thrombocytopenia, quadriparesis, isolated muscle weakness, and juvenile chronic arthritis may form part of the clinical spectrum of Whipple's disease.

Supplementary investigations are of value in confirming the involvement of different organs, but are not diagnostic of the disease. Radiographs of the small intestine characteristically show dilatation. Ultrasonography and CT of the abdomen may show lymphatic masses, and CT or MRI of the brain may show multiple lesions in the white matter and grey–white junction with characteristic appearances. The sedimentation rate is generally but not inevitably elevated, and anaemia due to folate or iron deficiency may be present. Eosinophilia and thrombocytosis may be apparent on blood films. Steatorrhoea, hypocalcaemia, vitamin deficiencies, and an elevated alkaline phosphatase occur with advanced gut disease, which may also give rise to hypoproteinaemia and protein-losing enteropathy.

Differential diagnosis

The differential diagnosis clinically includes chronic rheumatological conditions, connective tissue disorders, other causes of malabsorption, Addison's disease, bacterial endocarditis, and a wide variety of neurological diseases. Histological appearances suggestive of Whipple's disease have been reported in AIDS patients affected with atypical mycobacteria and rhodococci.

Treatment and prognosis

Whipple's disease progresses slowly, but unrecognized disease is eventually fatal. Antibiotic therapy is effective, although short-term corticosteroid therapy may occasionally be required in malnourished individuals to correct the metabolic and nutritional state. Administration of many different oral and parenteral antibiotics has been successful. Parenteral high-dose penicillin, third-generation cephalosporins, or carbapenems, for induction therapy, followed by prolonged therapy with oral co-trimoxazole, is recommended. Clinical improvement occurs within a few weeks, but prolonged treatment for at least a year is recommended. Relapse some years after treatment is common (up to 30%), often with central nervous system manifestations, particularly if the initial regime involved drugs with poor blood–brain barrier penetrance. Current regimens include 2 weeks' therapy with either parenteral Ceftriaxone 2 g daily, or meropenem 3 g daily, or penicillin G 1.2 million units daily, or streptomycin 1 g daily in penicillins sensitive patients, followed by 1–2 years therapy with trimethoprine 160 mg and sulphamethoxazole 800 mg daily. The use of mammalian cell cultures may shortly define bactericidal strategies (e.g. doxycycline/hydroxychloroquine) which will need prospective assessment.

A Herxheimer-like syndrome with fever and vasculitic manifestations has been reported at the start of treatment. The histological appearance of the gut mucosa returns to normal within a few months, although scattered periodic acid–Schiff-positive macrophages may persist for longer. Serial studies show that analysis of affected tissues by the polymerase chain reaction becomes negative in advance of histological improvement, and patients with clearance of tissues, documented by the polymerase chain reaction, appear to have a low risk of subsequent relapse. However, it is important to be aware of the possibility of relapse even after many years, especially when progressive central nervous system disease occurs in the absence of other systemic manifestations.

Further reading

Durand DV, et al. (1997). Whipple disease. Clinical review of 52 cases. *Medicine (Baltimore)*, **76**, 170–84.

Dutly F, et al. (2000). *Tropheryma whippelii* DNA in saliva of patients without Whipple's disease. *Infection*, **28**, 219–22.

Ectors NL, et al. (1994). Whipple's disease: a histological, immunocytochemical, and electron microscopic study of the small intestinal epithelium. *J Pathol*, **172**, 73–9.

Fenollar F, Puechal X, Raou D (2007). Whipple's disease. *N Engl J Med*, **356**, 55–66.

Feurle GE, Junga NS, Marth T. (2009). Efficacy of Ceftriaxone or Meropenem as initial therapies in Whipple's Disease. *Gastroenterology*. Oct 28. [Epub ahead of print]

Finzi G, et al. (2007). Ultrastructural evidence of *Tropheryma whippelii* in PAS-negative granulomatous lymph nodes. *Ultrastruct Pathol*, **31**, 169–72.

Gubler J, et al. (1999). Whipple endocarditis without overt gastrointestinal disease. *Ann Intern Med*, **131**, 112–16.

Knaapen HK, Barrera P (2007). Therapy for Whipple's disease. *J Antimicrob Chemother*, **60**, 457–8.

Maizel H, Ruffin J, Dobbins W (1993). Whipple's disease: a review of 19 patients from one hospital and a review of the literature since 1950. *Medicine (Baltimore)*, **72**, 343–55.

Marín M, et al (2007). *Tropheryma whipplei* infective endocarditis as the only manifestation of Whipple's disease. *J Clin Microbiol*, **45**, 2078–81.

Marth T, et al. (1997). Defects of monocyte interleukin 12 production and humoral immunity in Whipple's disease. *Gastroenterology*, **113**, 442–8.

O'Duffy JD, et al. (1999). Whipple's arthritis: direct detection of *Tropheryma whippelii* in synovial fluid and tissue. *Arthritis Rheum*, **42**, 812–17.

Playford RJ, et al. (1992). Whipple's disease complicated by a retinal Jarisch–Herxheimer reaction. *Gut*, **33**, 132–4.

Pron B, et al. (1999). Diagnosis and follow-up of Whipple's disease by amplification of the 16S rRNA gene of *Tropheryma whippelii*. *Eur J Clin Microbiol Infect Dis*, **18**, 62–5.

Puéchal X, Fenollar F, Raoult D (2007). Cultivation of *Tropheryma whipplei* from the synovial fluid in Whipple's arthritis. *Arthritis Rheum*, **56**, 1713–18.

Schneider T, et al. (2008). Whipple's disease: new aspects of pathogenesis and treatment. *Lancet Infect Dis*, **8**(3), 179–90.

Wilson K, et al. (1991). Phylogeny of the Whipple's-disease-associated bacterium. *Lancet*, **338**, 474–5.

15.10.7 Effects of massive small bowel resection

R.J. Playford

Essentials

Major vascular events involving the superior mesenteric artery and Crohn's disease are the two main reasons for adults requiring massive intestinal resection. The ability of the residual bowel to adapt after resection varies greatly between patients, with factors influencing the ability to absorb nutrients being (1) the extent and site of resection, (2) the condition of the remaining intestine, (3) the presence of the ileocaecal valve, and (4) the function of other digestive organs.

Clinical problems are more likely to occur following large resections that include most of the ileum and include diarrhoea, malnourishment (protein–energy malnutrition, mineral and vitamin deficiencies), gallstones, and renal stones.

In the initial postoperative period management requires assiduous fluid and electrolyte replacement, with many patients requiring parenteral nutritional supplements while the residual bowel adapts. Oral nutrition, initially consisting of elemental or polymeric diets administered by nasogastric or enteral tube feeding, should ideally be started within the first few days of surgery. Subsequently, small-volume, frequent, solid or semisolid meals with low fat and oxalate content should be introduced. Oral multivitamin and mineral supplements are needed; vitamin B_{12} injections are required following terminal ileum resection; regular long-term monitoring of fat-soluble vitamins (A, K, and D), vitamin B_{12}, folate, magnesium, zinc, and bone status is required. Long-term total parenteral nutrition is sometimes needed, and small-bowel transplantation is considered for some patients.

Aetiology and prevention

The two main reasons why adults require massive intestinal resection are major vascular events involving the superior mesenteric artery, usually thrombosis or embolus, or multiple surgical resections of the small bowel in patients with Crohn's disease (regional ileitis). Surgical intervention for vascular catastrophes is usually unavoidable. In regards to Crohn's disease, the use of biological therapies such as antitumour necrosis factor alpha (anti-TNFα) antibodies has had a major impact in inducing remission in severe cases and reduced the number of surgical procedures required. Nevertheless, operative interventions may still be required and as this is a lifelong recurrent disease, it is imperative that the minimum amount of bowel is resected. Stricturoplasty, rather than resection, may be possible and multiple small segments of relatively normal intestine should be retained *in situ* and joined in series, rather than removed. Preservation of only a few additional centimetres of gut may be enough to allow the patient to be maintained on oral rather than parenteral nutrition.

The principal conditions requiring massive resection in children include segmental volvulus in the prenatal period and necrotizing enterocolitis postnatally. Rarer causes affecting all ages include trauma, retroperitoneal tumours, radiation enteritis, and strangulation, mainly resulting from adhesions.

Physiology

Although digestion and absorption of water, electrolytes, and nutrients occurs throughout the small intestine, there are regional differences. Regional functions of the jejunum include iron and folate absorption and disaccharide digestion and, in combination with the duodenum, the production of cholecystokinin and secretin.

The ileum is the principal site for absorption of vitamin B_{12} and bile salts and, in contrast to the jejunum, is capable of absorbing sodium against a steep gradient. It also plays a key role, in combination with the proximal colon, in mediating the 'ileal brake', in which intestinal transit and secretions are reduced when nutrients reach the terminal small bowel. Hormones, particularly peptide tyrosine tyrosine, probably mediate this phenomenon.

Factors, including adaptation, that influence the metabolic consequences of massive resection

The ability of the residual bowel to adapt after resection varies greatly between patients; it influences the development of symptoms and may determine the long-term requirement for parenteral nutrition. Four main factors influence the patient's ability to absorb nutrients:

◆ Extent and site resected. The length of the small intestine varies between individuals. In general, patients with an intact duodenum but less than 50 cm of additional small bowel if the colon is *in situ*, or less than 100 cm if the colon has been removed, will require long-term total parenteral nutrition. Conversely, a requirement for parenteral nutrition is unlikely if more than 25% of the small bowel remains.

◆ Condition of the remaining intestine. The capacity of the residual bowel to adapt postoperatively is influenced by any underlying condition. Patients in which the residual bowel is damaged or abnormal due to conditions such as Crohn's disease or radiation enterocolitis are more likely to have metabolic disturbances.

◆ Presence of the ileocaecal valve. Removal of the ileocaecal valve has a major impact on subsequent clinical progress and troublesome watery diarrhoea that compounds malabsorption is frequent. Factors contributing to this include faster intestinal transit, possibly related to loss of the ileal brake mechanism, and a much higher likelihood of bacterial overgrowth.

◆ Function of other digestive organs. Pancreatic hypofunction, resulting from malnutrition and reduced hormonal stimulation, may exacerbate fat malabsorption; this is sometimes compounded by gastric hypersecretion that inactivates pancreatic enzymes in the lumen.

Pathophysiology

Because regional differences in the function of the small intestine exist, the clinical sequelae of resection vary according to the site removed. Resection of most of the jejunum can usually be compensated for by the distal bowel, and the consequences of proximal resections are usually slight. Patients may experience iron and folic acid deficiency as well as lactose intolerance, resulting in abdominal bloating and watery diarrhoea.

Clinical problems are more likely to occur following large resections that include most of the ileum. Intractable (cholerheic) diarrhoea, often with steatorrhoea, and consequential metabolic abnormalities including vitamin B_{12} deficiency occur.

Diarrhoea

This is probably the most troubling symptom. Multiple factors are involved in its aetiology (Table 15.10.7.1):

♦ Decreased transit time due to the reduced length of bowel and alteration in the control of its motility.

♦ Increased luminal osmolality, partly due to reduced absorption of lactose and other carbohydrates, which are then metabolized by colonic bacteria. Severe metabolic (lactic) acidosis may develop—the increased anion gap being due to the microbial generation of D-lactate.

♦ Disruption of the enterohepatic circulation of bile salts reduces the total body pool of bile salts. This is initially compensated for by a homeostatic up-regulation of bile salt production by the liver. Increased delivery of bile salts into the colon, however, stimulates colonic adenylate cyclase activity, increasing colonic secretion of water and electrolytes, resulting in watery diarrhoea sometimes termed cholerheic diarrhoea.

♦ If most of the ileum has been removed, the compensatory up-regulation of bile salt production may be insufficient to balance losses. This leads to decreased micelle formation in the lumen of the small bowel with a resultant reduction in absorption of water-insoluble fatty acids, causing the patient to have steatorrheic diarrhoea. Resection of the terminal 100 cm of ileum is typically associated with clinically significant malabsorption of bile salts. The presence of excess α-hydroxy fatty acids derived from bacterial metabolism in the colonic lumen stimulates adenylate cyclase, further increasing secretion of fluids and electrolytes.

Table 15.10.7.1 Aetiology and therapy of diarrhoeal symptoms

Condition	Mechanism, effect	Potential therapy
Shortened bowel	Reduced time and surface for absorption	Antiperistaltic drugs
Lactose intolerance	Reduced mucosal surface area and lactase, increases luminal osmolality	Reduce dietary dairy products
Bile salt diarrhoea	Increased bile salts in colon stimulates fluid secretion	Bile salt sequestrants
Steatorrhoea	Bile salt deficiency, fatty acids stimulate colonic secretion and contractility, reducing transit time	Reduce fat intake, pancreatic supplements
Pancreatic hyposecretion	Malnutrition, exacerbates steatorrhea	Maintain nutritional support
Gastric hypersecretion	Increases gastric fluid secretion and inactivates pancreatic enzymes	Acid suppressants

♦ In massive intestinal resections, the reduced micellar solubilization of fat and consequential impairment of lipolysis is compounded by the loss of absorptive mucosa, thus aggravating the effects of maldigestion and fluid loss.

Stones

Gallstone formation is two to three times more common after ileal resection and the stones may be of the cholesterol-rich or pigment type. Reduced concentrations of bile salts within the bile due to depletion of the body pool of bile salts, in combination with gallbladder hypomotility, facilitate the formation of cholesterol crystals.

Renal stones (usually calcium oxalate) commonly result from increased absorption of oxalate and hyperoxaluria. The availability of free oxalate within the colon is increased by excessive complexation of calcium by fatty acids which normally promote formation of insoluble (nonabsorbable) calcium oxalate. Although concentrations of bile salts in the small intestine may be reduced, the failure to reabsorb bile salts in the ileum increases luminal bile salts in the colon; this increases colonic permeability and further promotes oxalate absorption.

Gastric hypersecretion

This phenomenon occurs in some patients, although its severity tends to lessen over time. Hyperacidity may inactivate pancreatic enzymes by precipitating bile salts and lowering intraduodenal pH as in Zollinger–Ellison syndrome.

Nutritional status

Many patients undergoing resections will be malnourished preoperatively and energy consumption increases in the immediate postoperative period. If not appropriately managed, long-term protein–energy malnutrition as well as life-threatening mineral and vitamin deficiencies develop.

Adaptation

Morphological and functional adaptive changes follow resection of the small intestine. The residual bowel undergoes mucosal hyperplasia and its capacity to absorb fluids and nutrients increases over a period of weeks or months. The molecular events that underlie these changes are unclear but may include circulating trophic factors and growth factors present in pancreatic juice or secreted into the intestinal lumen. Early intervention is required to achieve maximal adaptation, and maintenance of a supply of luminal nutrients is a prerequisite for the adaptive changes. It is therefore important that luminal feeding is started as early as possible after surgery even if the patient also requires parenteral nutrition.

Management

Initial therapy

In the initial postoperative period, vigorous intravenous fluid and electrolyte replacement is required to prevent dehydration and to compensate for intestinal losses. Many patients will also require parenteral nutritional supplements while the residual bowel adapts. Ingestion of water may exacerbate diarrhoea and be counterproductive. The use of an oral isoosmolar saline–glucose solution containing bicarbonate, similar to that used for the treatment of cholera, may often assist in reducing intravenous requirements without increasing intestinal fluid loss.

Nutrition

Oral nutrition, initially consisting of elemental or polymeric diets administered by nasogastric or enteral tube feeding, should ideally be started within the first few days of surgery. The introduction of luminal nutrition tends, however, to exacerbate the diarrhoea. Many high-calorie enteral supplements for use in malnourished patients who have little or no impairment of small intestinal function have a very high osmolality, thereby inducing catastrophic egress of luminal fluid and diarrhoea in patients with large resections. These preparations must be used with great caution or avoided altogether in patients suffering the effects of massive bowel resections. Subsequently, small-volume, frequent, solid or semi-solid meals with low fat and oxalate content should be introduced. Low-fat meals and supplements containing large quantities of medium-chain fatty acids tend to be unpalatable. Compliance of patients with dietary advice is therefore best if symptoms are used as a guide to the amount of fat that is included in the diet. Since much of the energy content of the ingested diet may well be lost in the stool, the daily intake of calories often has to be greater than expected. This is best provided in a complex form, including glucose polymers and starch, which have little osmotic effect in the lumen and are hydrolysed rapidly by brush-border hydrolases at the site of absorption. Lactose intolerance, seen particularly in patients following significant jejunal resections, may induce bloating and exacerbation of diarrhoea but usually responds to reduction in lactose-containing dairy products. Low-fibre diets are helpful in some patients although they may aggravate symptoms in others; treatment must be tailored to the individual. Patients should be encouraged to take multivitamin and mineral supplementation at levels two to five times the normal recommended daily requirements; vitamin B_{12} injections are required following terminal ileum resection. In all patients, regular long-term monitoring of fat-soluble vitamins (A, K, and D), vitamin B_{12}, folate, magnesium, zinc, and bone status is required.

In some patients, adequate fluid and nutritional balance cannot be maintained by the oral route alone and long-term total parenteral nutrition is needed. These patients should be encouraged to continue oral nutrition, for social and psychological reasons as well as to minimize the amount of parental nutrition required.

Drugs

Most patients will require antiperistaltic drugs to increase the time of contact between luminal contents and residual bowel. A stepwise approach should be used, starting with agents such as loperamide or codeine phosphate. Long-term administration of the more potent constipating, but potentially addictive, opiates should be used only in intractable cases. Since diarrhoea may be particularly troublesome in the initial postoperative period, liquid or occasionally intravenous formulations may be needed.

Administration of H_2-receptor antagonists or proton pump inhibitors may reduce diarrhoea and promote digestion, as well as prevent peptic ulceration, by decreasing gastric secretions and preventing inactivation of pancreatic enzymes. Cholerheic diarrhoeas may respond well to bile acid sequestrants such as cholestyramine, but its use can worsen the fatty component of diarrhoea by exacerbating the deficiency of bile salts. Similarly, the use of long-acting somatostatin analogues can reduce gastrointestinal secretions and fluid loss but may exacerbate steatorrhea and formation of gallstones. In patients with marked steatorrhea who do not respond to restriction of fat intake, the addition of oral pancreatic enzyme supplements to food may assist lipolysis and improve digestion.

Bacterial overgrowth

Colonization of the small bowel by colonic or pathogenic bacteria results in exacerbation of diarrhoea, malabsorption, and nutritional deficiencies. Culture and analysis of small-bowel aspirates is required for definitive diagnosis but is a moderately invasive procedure. Because results from many of the usual noninvasive tests, e.g. glucose or lactulose hydrogen breath tests, are abnormal in all patients after significant resection, empirical trials of antibiotics may be justified.

Surgical options

In patients with severe intractable diarrhoea further surgery should be considered, although it is usually of limited benefit. Although not in general clinical use, reversal of a small segment of small bowel can delay gut transit; however, if too long a segment is used, obstruction may occur. Longitudinal lengthening may also be of value, particularly in paediatric patients.

Small-bowel transplantation is now available in a limited number of centres. Because of the high morbidity and mortality associated with transplantation, it is usually only offered to those patients who cannot be maintained on total parenteral nutrition. Patients who have undergone intestinal transplantation are particularly prone to infections and lymphoma. Problems with acute and chronic rejection are also common. Patients therefore require detailed counselling about the risks of any such procedure.

Future directions

Administration of gut trophic factors, such as glucagon-like peptide 2, hepatocyte growth factor, epidermal growth factor, and growth hormone (possibly in combination with glutamine supplements) during the early postoperative period may increase the rate and extent of mucosal adaptation that occurs in the intestine. These are, however, unlikely to be a panacea: side effects, such as fluid retention, are not uncommon and adaptive changes seem to rapidly disappear when treatment is stopped, meaning that such therapies may be required lifelong. In patients who prove not to adapt adequately, continuing advances in techniques for small-bowel transplantation and in antirejection therapy offers future hope. In the longer term, advances in tissue engineering technology may allow intestinal mucosa to be obtained from humanized animal gut or to be reconstituted in culture from the patient's own residual bowel, thereby removing the problems of rejection and immunosuppression.

Further reading

Gupta A, *et al.* (2006). Tissue engineering of small intestine—current status. *Biomacromolecules*, **7**, 2701–9. [A useful review of the state of play in this area.]

Pereira PM, Bines JE (2006). New growth factor therapies aimed at improving intestinal adaptation in short bowel syndrome. *J Gastroenterol Hepatol*, **21**, 932–40. [Overview of potential value of growth factors to stimulate small-bowel function.]

Ruiz P, Kato T, Tzakis A (2007). Current status of transplantation of the small intestine. *Transplantation*, **83**, 1–6. [Useful overview of the successes and challenges of this approach.]

15.10.8 Malabsorption syndromes in the tropics

V.I. Mathan

Essentials

Causes of secondary malabsorption that are mainly prevalent in the tropics include (1) progressive wasting in people infected with HIV, which is known as 'slim disease'; (2) various infections—protozoal (e.g. *Gardia lamblia*, *Cryptosporidium parvum*), helminthic (e.g *Capillaria philippinensis*, *Strongyloides stercoralis*), bacterial (*Mycobacterium tuberculosis*); (3) immunoproliferative small intestinal disease; (4) hypolactasia (see Chapter 15.10.5).

When patients with conditions that can cause secondary malabsorption are excluded, a group remains who have chronic diarrhoea, malabsorption, and its nutritional sequelae. This primary or idiopathic malabsorption syndrome is called 'tropical sprue', and it occurs against the background of tropical enteropathy (which describes the fact that the morphology of the mucosa of normal gut is different in tropical preindustrialized countries from that in temperate-zone industrialized countries).

The aetiology of tropical sprue is not known: epidemiological data suggests an infective cause, but no causal agent has been identified. Presentation is typically with loose or watery stools lasting for several weeks or months, and with symptoms and signs of nutritional deficiency. Management involves symptomatic relief from diarrhoea, correction of fluid and electrolyte abnormalities and nutritional deficiencies, and attempts at specific curative measures—vitamin B$_{12}$, folic acid, and tetracyclines—are usually given for up to 6 months.

Introduction

Patients, in whom the 'digestive fire is weakened and food is expelled from the body without contributing to growth' were described in *Charaka-Samhita*, an ancient Indian treatise on medicine compiled some time between the 6th and 12th centuries BCE. The clinical description in the section on 'Grahani Vyadhi' or diseases of the organ of assimilation, clearly describes patients gradually wasting with chronic diarrhoea and loud borborygmi. Malabsorption of nutrients with its sequelae has therefore long been recognized as a clinical entity in some tropical regions.

Even in the globalized context of the third millennium, there are defined tropical malabsorption syndromes. All the diseases with malabsorption of nutrients that are prevalent in temperate climates also occur in the tropics, but there are certain conditions, the majority being chronic enteric infections or infestations, that are geographically primarily limited to the tropics. Expatriates from other parts of the world visiting the tropics may have a higher susceptibility to some of these conditions.

Causes of malabsorption primarily prevalent in the tropics

Malabsorption in the tropics, as elsewhere, may have an identifiable underlying aetiology, when it is classified as secondary malabsorption. When no primary cause has yet been identified it is considered primary or idiopathic malabsorption (Table 15.10.8.1).

The importance of a variety of protozoal infections, especially intracellular protozoans, was recognized in temperate-zone countries at the beginning of the AIDS epidemic, these organisms having been identified as opportunistic infections. In tropical countries these protozoa have been identified in symptomatic and asymptomatic immunocompetent subjects.

Capillaria philippinensis infection has been reported in epidemics from the Philippines and as sporadic cases from other tropical countries including India. Hyperinfection with *Strongyloides stercoralis* can occur rarely. Both these helminths burrow into the mucosa and form tunnels.

Abdominal tuberculosis occurs much less frequently than pulmonary tuberculosis and is often secondary. Malabsorption in abdominal tuberculosis is the result of bacterial colonization of the small intestinal lumen secondary to strictures and extensive ulceration, or due to obstruction of the lymphatic outflow (tabes mesenterica).

Progressive wasting in people infected with HIV is known as 'slim disease', especially in Africa. This is usually considered a consequence of malabsorption secondary to enteric opportunistic infections. However there is some evidence to suggest that a primary HIV enteropathy can also contribute to malabsorption.

Calcific pancreatitis affecting young adults, particularly in economically disadvantaged sections of society, is another cause of

Table 15.10.8.1 Classification of tropical malabsorption syndromes

Secondary malabsorption	
Protozoal infections	*Giardia lamblia*
	Cryptosporidium parvum
	Isospora belli
	Enterocytozoon bieneusi
	Septata intestinalis
Helminthic infections	*Capillaria philippinensis*
	Strongyloides stercoralis
Bacterial infections	*Mycobacterium tuberculosis*
Viral infections	Human immunodeficiency virus
	Tropical (calcific) pancreatitis
	Immunoproliferative small intestinal disease (IPSID)
	Late-onset hypolactasia
Primary malabsorption	
Tropical sprue (idiopathic tropical malabsorption syndrome)	

malabsorption unique to the tropics. The aetiology may be related to malabsorption and dietary 'toxins'.

Immunoproliferative small intestinal disease (IPSID; see Chapter 15.10.4) is due to the clonal expansion of immunocytes producing altered α heavy-chain immunoglobulin. This is also known as Mediterranean lymphoma and has been reported from several tropical countries. The characteristic histology in the premalignant stage is diagnostic and can be reversed by prolonged antibiotic therapy at this stage, suggesting a trigger that may be related to enteric infection. Once malignant transformation has occurred the treatment is as for other lymphomas, but the prognosis is guarded.

In many tropical regions, particularly south and south-east Asia, the high lactase activity in the intestinal epithelium in neonates declines rapidly after weaning. Since most adults in such countries do not regularly consume milk or lactose in their diets, this abnormality is of relatively small significance. The use of fermented milk and milk products (e.g. yoghurt) can ensure that milk-based nutritional supplementation is still possible in such populations (see Chapter 15.10.5).

Malabsorption, or increased secretion, is an invariable part of all acute diarrhoeal infections. These episodes, most frequent in children, are of short duration, usually a few days. A small proportion of infants and young children have diarrhoea that persists for longer than 2 weeks following an acute episode. This persistent diarrhoea syndrome, seldom if ever seen in adolescents and adults, is not usually considered as one of the malabsorption syndromes.

The concept of a 'postinfective malabsorption state' associated with the presence of a mixed bacterial flora in the small intestine has been postulated to explain, in particular, the persistent diarrhoea and malabsorption reported in many European travellers to the Indian subcontinent. By extension, it has been suggested that the syndrome of primary malabsorption in the tropics, tropical sprue, is only another form of postinfective malabsorption. Several facts are against this assumption. Significant bacterial colonization of the small intestine has been found in apparently healthy asymptomatic adults resident in the tropics. Detailed investigation of many overland travellers from Europe to the Indian subcontinent identified several of the infections described earlier as the cause of persistent malabsorption, along with an altered luminal bacterial flora. The epidemiology of tropical sprue is distinctly different from that of acute infectious diarrhoea. Detailed clinical and laboratory investigations of adults and children in more than 20 epidemics of acute diarrhoea, studied in south India, identified no single case of persistent malabsorption, other than the background prevalence of tropical enteropathy. There are also well-documented instances of expatriates from Europe who developed a primary malabsorption syndrome many years after their return to temperate climes. A careful analysis of the available literature therefore suggests that significant persistent and symptomatic malabsorption following acute enteric infectious diarrhoea is a rare event in the tropics.

When patients with conditions that can give rise to secondary malabsorption unique to the tropics or elsewhere are excluded, a group remain who have chronic diarrhoea, malabsorption, and its nutritional sequelae. Such patients are relatively rare in temperate climates, but frequently encountered in regions such as southern India and the Caribbean islands. This primary or idiopathic malabsorption syndrome has been called 'tropical sprue'. Tropical sprue occurs against the background of tropical enteropathy in the indigenous population of these regions.

Tropical enteropathy

The intestinal mucosal morphology of germ-free rats differs from that of their conventionally reared litter-mates; the latter have shorter villi, higher crypts, and increased mononuclear cells infiltrating the lamina propria and epithelium. These differences are attributed to the modulating effect of the microbial flora in the intestinal lumen of the conventionally reared litter-mates.

Similar morphological differences are found between the jejunal mucosa of apparently healthy asymptomatic individuals living in temperate-zone industrialized countries and those in tropical preindustrialized countries. The morphological features of this tropical enteropathy are characterized by the replacement of finger- and tongue-shaped villi by broader structures in the upper small intestine, reduction in the height of villi with an increase in crypt thickness, and increased infiltration by mononuclear cells of the lamina propria and the epithelium. Similar mucosal morphological changes have also been shown to occur in the large intestine.

The morphology of fetal intestinal mucosa is identical in both geographical regions, the earliest differences appearing shortly after birth. The morphological changes are not apparent in biopsies from residents of Singapore—although this is a tropical country, it has standards of environmental hygiene and nutrition that equal those in temperate-zone industrialized countries. People expatriated from temperate countries to tropical countries develop these mucosal morphological changes over time. Expatriates from tropical countries living in a temperate zone, even if they continue to ingest a diet similar to that in their original home, eventually revert to having temperate-zone morphology. The evidence therefore suggests that the morphological alteration in the small intestine of residents of tropical countries is not a result of climatic differences, but is probably a reflection of an adaptation to environmental factors. *In vitro* organ culture studies have shown slightly accelerated cell turnover in the jejunal mucosa of people living in the tropics, further supporting an adaptive response as the basis for the change.

Extensive bacterial colonization of the upper small-intestinal lumen and mucosa by aerobes and anaerobes, in apparently healthy adults, has been documented in studies from southern India. Enteric pathogens can be cultivated from the stools of asymptomatic individuals resident in many tropical countries. It is also known that the first dose of oral immunization agents to enteric pathogens usually results in a secondary response, even in children as young as 2 years old living in the tropics. There is no evidence that the macronutrient deficiency widely prevalent in many tropical countries influences intestinal structure or function. All of this suggests that the enteropathy of tropical regions is an adaptation to environmental contamination resulting from poor sanitation practices. Conceptually, it may be useful to categorize 'specific pathogen-free' populations (temperate zone) and 'conventional' populations (tropical)! Whether these changes in the enteric mucosa, a primary barrier between the internal and external environment, would disappear with improving socio-economic status as a result of industrialization, is an intriguing question.

Minor abnormalities in absorption can also be demonstrated in these healthy subjects, with xylose malabsorption in 40%, mild steatorrhoea in 10%, and vitamin B_{12} malabsorption in 3%. The overall absorption of calories is reduced by about 5%, while the colonic bacterial mass is increased. Colonic salvage of unabsorbed calories is thereby reduced. There is no evidence that these changes in the lining epithelium of the intestinal tract significantly affect the health of these 'conventional' populations. However, the reduction in overall caloric absorption can raise the question as to whether the absence of tropical enteropathy can increase the effective availability of food without an increase in supply.

Tropical sprue

Definition

Tropical sprue is defined as a primary (idiopathic) malabsorption syndrome affecting residents of, or visitors to, certain tropical regions. It is characterized by enterocyte damage, usually associated with chronic diarrhoea and the nutritional sequelae of persisting malabsorption. The underlying aetiology (or aetiologies) is not yet understood. There are differences in the presentation, epidemiology, and clinical course in different geographical regions and between expatriates to endemic regions and indigenous residents affected by the syndrome.

History

William Hillary described a chronic wasting diarrhoea in European expatriates in Barbados in 1759, probably the first description of the syndrome in the English literature. The disease apparently attained epidemic proportions 3 years after he arrived in Barbados. With expanding colonization, the syndrome was well recognized in expatriates by British and Dutch physicians in south and south-east Asia. However, no cases were described from tropical Africa. Tropical sprue assumed epidemic proportions during the Second World War and was a major factor for repatriation from the Assam and Burma theatres of war. Indian troops were also affected. It was only in the postcolonial era, with the work of Baker and colleagues in southern India and of Klipstein in Puerto Rico and Haiti, that the extent of the problem of tropical sprue in indigenous populations was defined.

Epidemiology

Endemic cases in indigenous and expatriate residents in the tropics and epidemics in troops and indigenous populations have been documented. Endemic tropical sprue is apparently geographically restricted to south and south-east Asia and the Caribbean islands other than Jamaica, with a few case reports from Central and South America and sub-Saharan Africa. In fact, much of the literature up to the 1960s is limited to expatriate populations. In India, only two large medical institutions, with well-developed laboratory facilities, have reported detailed studies, suggesting that in marginally nourished indigenous populations many cases may be missed because of the poor availability of diagnostic facilities.

Apart from the reports during the Second World War, large epidemics have only been described from southern India. The first such reported epidemic in 1960–61 affected approximately 100 000 patients, with a 40% case fatality. This was reflected in the unusual death rates in the North and South Arcot Districts of Madras state in the 1961 census of India. The last epidemic was detected in 1978. In all the epidemics, patients initially developed an apparent episode of acute diarrhoea accompanied by vomiting in about 30% and fever in 25% of cases. Significant malabsorption of fat, carbohydrate, and vitamin B_{12} was present even during the first week of illness and 50% of those affected had diarrhoea for longer than 1 month. The epidemics evolved with new cases occurring over a period of months to years, in contrast to epidemics of acute infectious diarrhoea which are usually over in a few weeks. Adults had a significantly higher attack rate and were affected earlier during the course of the epidemic. The epidemiological data suggested an infective aetiology, but no causal viral, bacterial, or parasitic agent has been identified.

Clinical features

The patient with tropical sprue is usually an adult with a history of loose or watery stools lasting for several weeks or months and with symptoms and signs of nutritional deficiency. There is usually anorexia, a feeling of abdominal distension, and loud, abnormal borborygmi. The signs of nutritional deficiency include pallor due to anaemia, angular stomatitis, glossitis, oedema, and the skin and hair changes of severe hypoproteinaemia. The prevalence of nutritional deficiency, measured by clinical or laboratory parameters, is higher in those patients with a longer duration of symptoms. In the epidemic situation the prevalence of nutritional deficiency in patients during the first month of illness was no different from that in the unaffected people in the same village. However, in patients affected in the epidemics persistent malabsorption begins during the first few days of illness. The diarrhoea can be severe enough to produce life-threatening dehydration. In the epidemics the early deaths were mainly due to fluid and electrolyte imbalance, which can be prevented by maintenance of hydration. As the disease progresses the sequelae of severe malnutrition and consequential acute infections, especially of the respiratory tract, contribute to mortality. The natural history of the illness shows periods of remission, relapses, and spontaneous recovery, which make an evaluation of specific therapy difficult. Although patients have been followed for up to 25 years in southern India, intestinal neoplasms have not developed.

Investigation

Investigation of these patients should confirm the presence of intestinal malabsorption, exclude conditions that can give rise to secondary malabsorption, and evaluate the nutritional sequelae of malabsorption (Table 15.10.8.2).

A simple faecal smear stained with a fat stain such as Sudan 3 can often detect fat globules and fatty acid crystals associated with steatorrhoea. The extent of tests for confirming the presence of malabsorption is determined by the availability of facilities, which in many tropical areas is still limited. Tests of xylose absorption should be interpreted in the light of xylose malabsorption as a part of tropical enteropathy in the particular community.

The exclusion of conditions that can give rise to secondary malabsorption is of importance since many of these conditions are amenable to therapy. The diagnosis of the syndrome of primary malabsorption is one of exclusion.

Evaluation of the nutritional sequelae of malabsorption, especially the presence of megaloblastic anaemia, provides useful benchmarks for appropriate nutritional rehabilitation.

Table 15.10.8.2 Investigation of a patient with tropical malabsorption syndrome

1. Confirmation of the presence and extent of malabsorption
Steatorrhoea
D-Xylose absorption
Vitamin B$_{12}$ absorption
Breath hydrogen or CO$_2$ estimation with stable isotopes and other tests of absorption, depending on availability
2. Exclusion of conditions leading to secondary malabsorption
Faecal examination for parasites
Small intestinal luminal fluid cultures to exclude bacterial overgrowth
Careful radiological examination of the small and large bowel including small bowel enema
Duodenal or jejunal mucosal biopsy
Serum protein electrophoresis for heavy-chain abnormality
3. Evaluation of the sequelae of malabsorption
Haemoglobin, haematocrit, reticulocyte count
Bone marrow morphology, when indicated
Serum protein and albumin
Serum electrolytes
Vitamin B$_{12}$ and folate
Estimation of other micronutrients based on availability

Pathology and pathogenesis

The wide availability of peroral mucosal biopsies confirmed the report, as early as 1924, that the primary lesion in tropical sprue was in the small-intestinal mucosa. Electron microscopic examination of jejunal mucosal biopsies confirmed the presence of damage to enterocytes in the crypt (regenerative) and villous (functional) compartments. This damage can be demonstrated in the first weeks of illness in patients affected during epidemics. Accelerated cell turnover in the regenerative compartment and increased loss of enterocytes from the functional compartment was demonstrated by *in vitro* culture of jejunal mucosal biopsies labelled with tritiated thymidine. In fact these changes in the enterocyte lifecycle explain the observed mucosal architecture, which has often been called partial villous atrophy. In contrast to the situation in coeliac disease, where the initial damage to enterocytes occurs in the functional compartment and the crypts are hypertrophied with morphologically normal enterocytes, in tropical sprue the primary lesion appears to affect the regenerative compartment. These findings have only been confirmed in patients studied in southern India.

The mucosal lesion in tropical sprue is not confined to the small intestine, since functional and structural abnormalities have also been demonstrated in the stomach and the colon. Significant water malabsorption in the colon may contribute to the severity of diarrhoea.

An appreciation of regional differences in the patient profile is essential for understanding the pathology and pathogenesis.

All patients have malabsorption, but vitamin B$_{12}$ malabsorption is only found in about 70% of patients in southern India, while it is almost invariable in expatriates from the temperate zones and in the Caribbean. In Haiti and Puerto Rico the observed seasonal incidence is ascribed to small-intestinal colonization by toxin-producing coliforms, probably secondary to the consumption of rancid pork fat. In southern India, the extent and severity of small-bowel colonization by enterotoxin-producing coliforms is no higher than in matched controls. Identification of one or more 'agents' that can damage the mucosal epithelial cells will enable a clearer understanding of these differences.

Treatment

Provision of symptomatic relief from diarrhoea, correction of fluid and electrolyte abnormalities and nutritional deficiencies, and attempts at specific curative measures are the cornerstone of treatment. Diarrhoea and abdominal distension can be helped by the judicious use of loperamide and dimethyl polysiloxane. Increasing the nutrient intake and providing therapeutic supplements such as vitamin B$_{12}$ and folic acid, as indicated, is beneficial. However, specific therapy to cure the condition awaits understanding of its aetiology.

Empirical evidence from patients in the Caribbean and European expatriate community indicates that folic acid can alleviate symptoms in cases of less than 2 months duration. In patients with a longer duration of symptoms, the addition of oral tetracycline for up to 6 months leads to the restoration of normal intestinal absorption. In southern India, the results of therapy with vitamin B$_{12}$, folic acid, and tetracyclines were not so clear cut and a few patients were resistant to all therapy. Nevertheless, the recommended management includes the use of all three of these therapeutic agents for up to 6 months.

Further reading

Baker SJ (1973). Geographical variation in the morphology of the small intestinal mucosa in apparently healthy individuals. *Pathol Microbiol*, **294**, 222–37.

Baker SJ, Mathan VI (1972). Tropical enteropathy and tropical sprue. *Am J Clin Nutr*, **25**, 1047–55.

Humphrey JH (2009). Child undernutrition, tropical enteropathy, toilets, and handwashing. *Lancet*, **374**, 1032–5.

Manson-Bahr PH (1924). The morbid anatomy and pathology of sprue and their bearing upon aetiology. *Lancet*, **i**, 1148–51.

Mathan M, Mathan VI, Baker SJ (1975). An electron-microscopic study of jejunal mucosal morphology in control subjects and patients with tropical sprue in southern India. *Gastroenterology*, **68**, 17–32.

Mathan M, Ponniah J, Mathan VI (1986). Epithelial cell renewal and turnover and its relationship to the morphological abnormalities in the jejunal mucosa in tropical sprue. *Dig Dis Sci*, **31**, 586–93.

Mathan M, *et al.* (1990). Ultrastructure of the jejunal mucosa in human immuno deficiency virus infection. *J Pathol*, **16**, 119–27.

Mathan VI (1988). Tropical sprue in southern India. *Trans R Soc Trop Med Hyg*, **82**, 10–14.

Owens SR, Greenson JK (2007). The pathology of malabsorption: current concepts. *Histopathology*, **50**, 64–82.

Ramakrishna BS, Mathan VI (1982). Water and electrolyte absorption by the colon in tropical sprue. *Gut*, **23**, 843–6.

Wellcome Trust (1971). *Tropical sprue and megaloblastic anaemia*. Churchill Livingstone, London.

15.11

Crohn's disease

Miles Parkes

Essentials

Crohn's disease is a common form of chronic inflammatory bowel disease. Typically involving the terminal ileum, colon, and perineum, it causes patchy transmural inflammation characterized microscopically by granulomata. Common complications include fibrotic strictures, fistulas, and abscesses.

The trigger is unknown but an unregulated mucosal immune response to commensal bacteria drives the chronic inflammation. Variants in several genes involved in innate immunity are strongly associated, with NOD2, interleukin-23, and autophagy pathways all recently implicated. Smoking also increases the risk.

With a pattern of episodic flares, Crohn's disease has significant morbidity but low mortality. Treatment of acute inflammatory disease is usually with corticosteroids or therapeutic diets; for steroid-dependence or frequent relapse immunosuppression with azathioprine, 6-mercaptopurine or methotrexate is indicated.

Antitumour necrosis factor (anti-TNFα) antibody therapy can induce rapid remission of resistant disease and can be used as maintenance therapy.

Despite increased use of immunosuppressants 80% of patients require surgery in the long term, most commonly for ileal stricturing. Timely, conservative surgery is the key, minimizing the length of small-bowel resected and using laparoscopic approaches where possible. For colonic disease requiring surgery, segmental colectomy or subtotal colectomy with ileorectal anastomosis are preferred, but significant rectal or perianal involvement may require proctocolectomy and ileostomy.

Perianal Crohn's disease is treated medically with antibiotics, azathioprine, and anti-TNF antibody therapy; and surgically with abscess drainage and placement of seton sutures through fistulas where possible, rather than more radical options.

Introduction and history

Crohn's disease is a form of chronic, relapsing inflammatory bowel disease characterized by discontinuous segments of transmural inflammation. It can affect any part of the gastrointestinal tract but most commonly involves the terminal ileum, colon, and perineum. The eponymous term 'Crohn's disease' derives from the index description of chronic ileal inflammation in young people in 1932 by Crohn, Ginzburg, and Oppenheimer. However, many much earlier reports describe what would now be called Crohn's disease. Colonic Crohn's disease was formally differentiated from ulcerative colitis by Lockhart-Mummery and Morson in 1960, although recent genetic studies suggest, perhaps unsurprisingly, that they are closely related.

Aetiology

Precise pathogenic mechanisms are unknown, but Crohn's disease evidently results from a complex interplay of genetic and environmental factors producing an excessive, unregulated inflammatory response to luminal microflora in susceptible individuals. The trigger has not been identified.

Susceptibility to the initial trigger may result from a defective mucosal barrier: either increased intestinal permeability, allowing luminal antigens to access the mucosal immune system, or aberrant innate immunity, which would increase risk of microbial invasion. Evidence from genetic studies increasingly implicates the latter in Crohn's disease, the former perhaps being more relevant in ulcerative colitis. Early failure to control microbial ingress may lead to activation of alternative, adaptive immune pathways mediated by CD4+ T cells. In Crohn's disease these are predominantly Th1 cells, secreting cytokines interferon (IFN)-γ and interleukin (IL)-2, with TNFα and IL-23 also being critical mediators.

Environmental factors

The clearest environmental association is with smoking which more than doubles the risk of developing Crohn's disease, while being protective against ulcerative colitis. The mechanism is unclear. Use of nonsteroidal anti-inflammatory drugs (NSAIDs) and the oral contraceptive pill are also associated, the former perhaps by increasing intestinal permeability—well recognized to precede flares of Crohn's disease. Interestingly, 10% of healthy first-degree relatives of Crohn's disease patients have increased intestinal permeability, suggesting a heritable basis.

Many patients are concerned about dietary precipitants for Crohn's disease. Excess refined sugar and lack of fibre have been noted in retrospective studies, but may reflect dietary accommodation to early symptoms. Response to therapeutic diets also suggests food antigens are important but no single foodstuff is consistently associated.

Microbiological determinants represent obvious potential triggers, and self-limiting infections such as yersinia do precede Crohn's disease in some instances. More contentiously, specific chronic infections might cause the persisting inflammation. Advocates of *Mycobacteria paratuberculosis*, which causes the granulomatous intestinal inflammation of Johne's disease in cattle, highlight its common presence in pasteurized milk and detection of its DNA in Crohn's ulceration. However epidemiological evidence shows no clustering of Crohn's disease in livestock farmers, antituberculous therapy is not effective in Crohn's disease, and the molecular findings could reflect predilection of *M. paratuberculosis* for intestinal ulceration. Its contribution thus remains speculative.

A role for commensal bacteria appears more secure, particularly in perpetuating intestinal inflammation after the initial trigger. Clinical evidence comes from attenuation of Crohn's disease inflammation following diversion of the faecal stream with ileostomy; while experimentally, intestinal inflammation in animal models of inflammatory bowel disease is markedly reduced in 'germ-free' conditions. Some commensals are particularly implicated, including bacteroides and adherent invasive *Escherichia coli*, while others confer protection, including *Faecalibacterium prausnitzii* and 'probiotic' strains of lactobacilli and bifidobacter.

Genetic determinants

Although environmental influences are clearly important, it is genetic studies that have made most progress in recent years. The effect sizes for most confirmed susceptibility genes are modest but they highlight critical molecular pathways predisposing to Crohn's disease. The major theme emerging is the importance of the early host immune response to bacterial ingress—particularly innate immunity.

NOD2, the first Crohn's disease gene identified, encodes an intracellular receptor for bacterial muramyl dipeptide and (by poorly understood mechanisms) modulates toll-like receptor signaling and activation of NF-κB, a transcription factor for several proinflammatory mediators. For *NOD2* heterozygotes the risk of Crohn's disease is doubled compared to wild type, while homozygotes have 17-fold increased risk. Interestingly there is significant heterogeneity, both for disease (*NOD2* variants are specifically associated with ileal Crohn's disease) and ethnicity (no *NOD2* mutations are found in Japanese patients).

Signals identified by genome-wide association scans in Crohn's disease converge on two other key immune pathways. One is the activation of naive CD4+ T cells by IL-23. Confirmed association with variants in genes for the IL-23 receptor and IL-12B (which encodes a subunit common to IL-12 and IL-23) among other components of this pathway strongly corroborates functional experiments in mouse models, which also implicate IL-23 in chronic intestinal inflammation.

Another key components is autophagy. Replicated association in two separate autophagy genes, *ATG16L1* and *IRGM*, has highlighted this previously unsuspected pathway. Autophagy is the mechanism by which cells engulf, compartmentalize, and digest cytoplasmic debris and intracellular bacteria. Its disruption permits prolonged survival of several intracellular microorganisms—perhaps important for the intracellular bacteria postulated to play a role in Crohn's disease pathogenesis, including adherent invasive *E. coli* and *M. paratuberculosis*.

In which cell the primary genetic abnormalities impact remains unknown (prime candidates being intestinal macrophages, dendritic cells, T cells, and epithelial cells) but already the idea that Crohn's disease results from an 'overactive' immune system appears simplistic. Increasing laboratory and clinical evidence suggests that at least some elements of the immune response are defective. Whether intestinal inflammation is driven by failure to eliminate intracellular infection, inappropriate activation of adaptive immune pathways, failure of immune regulation, or some other mechanism entirely must await further investigation.

Pathology

Crohn's disease can affect any part of the gastrointestinal tract but most commonly causes ileocaecal (40%), exclusively ileal (30%), or exclusively colonic (25%) inflammation with or without perianal involvement (25%). Diffuse small-bowel, upper gut, or oral Crohn's disease are less frequent. Colonic disease often spares the rectum. These patterns typically remain stable in any given patient over time. Ulcers are usually present, with appearances varying from small aphthous lesions overlying lymphoid aggregates to scattered punched-out, serpiginous, longitudinal or pleomorphic ulcers (see Fig. 15.11.2). Inflammation is patchy, giving rise to 'skip lesions', and transmural—manifest as deep ulceration and cobblestoning endoscopically, and fat wrapping at surgery. The bowel wall is usually thickened, often producing luminal stenosis, and the mesentry oedematous with regional lymph node enlargement.

Histologically Crohn's disease is characterized by a patchy chronic transmural inflammatory infiltrate, maximal in the submucosa and lamina propria. This consists of lymphocytes, characteristically organized as lymphoid aggregates, macrophages and plasma cells. Acutely, neutrophils infiltrate around crypts producing cryptitis. Fissuring ulcers can penetrate deeply, sometimes to the serosal surface to produce fistulas, and noncaseating epithelioid granulomata formed from macrophages and giant cells may be found at any level—present in up to 60% of cases (Fig. 15.11.1). Typically in the colon there is preservation of goblet cell numbers and crypt architecture compared to ulcerative colitis.

Epidemiology

Crohn's disease can affect people of any age but peak incidence occurs in early adulthood, with a smaller peak in the seventh decade. There is a marginal predominance in women and 15% of patients have an affected relative. Crude annual incidence in Western countries ranges from 1.8 to 10 per 100 000, with a north–south gradient (higher in the north) across Europe and North America. Incidence is highest in Ashkenazi Jews and low in Japan (0.25 per 100 000).

Longitudinal studies from the United States of America and Denmark showed that Crohn's disease incidence increased significantly (2.7-and 6-fold respectively) between 1960 and 1980 but has since stabilized. This contrasts with the currently increasing incidence

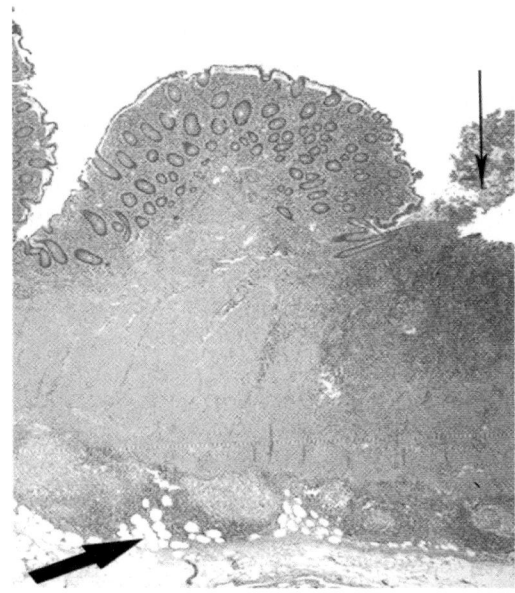

Fig. 15.11.1. Crohn's disease affecting large bowel, showing fissuring ulceration (narrow arrow) and transmural inflammation with a 'Crohn's rosary'—lymphoid aggregates studded along the outer border of the muscularis propria (broad arrow). (Courtesy of Dr Vicki Save, Addenbrooke's Hospital, Cambridge.)

in paediatric populations and non-Western societies, perhaps reflecting adoption of 'Western' lifestyles. Increased awareness and improved diagnostics have undoubtedly also contributed.

Estimates of Crohn's disease prevalence also vary significantly, in part according to ascertainment method. Thus population- and primary-care-based surveys in the United Kingdom put the prevalence as high as 140 to 210 per 100 000, while studies in secondary/tertiary care are lower at 70 to 100 per 100 000. Either figure indicates that the burden of disease is substantial in terms of both morbidity and cost. Best estimates of direct health care costs suggest an average figure of £3300/patient-year for Crohn's disease (2004 data), but with large variation and much higher costs with severe disease or complications requiring hospitalization.

Clinical features

The clinical presentation of Crohn's disease varies from 'classical' to diagnostically challenging and nonspecific. With severe disease patients may have systemic upset, with fever, tachycardia, and anaemia. More often, however, a modestly raised C-reactive protein (CRP) and vague or irritable-bowel-like symptoms may be the only clues mandating further investigation. Many patients report remitting and relapsing symptoms for years before the diagnosis is made. A family history of inflammatory bowel disease and smoking history should be sought.

For patients with established disease the Harvey–Bradshaw index provides a simple objective assessment of activity, while the Crohn's disease activity index requires symptom diaries plus laboratory data, limiting it to clinical trials. The Inflammatory Bowel Disease Questionnaire (IBDQ) is the best validated quality of life tool.

Symptoms

Symptoms are significantly determined by site of intestinal inflammation and typically include lower abdominal pain, diarrhoea,

anorexia, and weight loss. Tiredness, malaise, sweats, and extraintestinal manifestations can be prominent.

Abdominal pain reflects gut wall ulceration and mesenteric oedema, and often localizes to the right iliac fossa with ileocaecal disease. It may be constant or colicky, exacerbated by eating and associated with other obstructive features such as vomiting or bloating. The absence of tenderness suggests a fibrotic stricture—usually the small bowel. Abdominal pain due to coincident gallstones or renal stones, both associated with Crohn's disease, can cause confusion.

Weight loss is common with active Crohn's disease, particularly involving the small bowel, so patients should be weighed at each clinic visit. Contributory factors include food avoidance due to abdominal pain or mouth ulceration, intestinal protein loss, catabolism induced by inflammation or sepsis, and malabsorption reflecting the combination of diffuse small-bowel disease, resection, and bacterial overgrowth.

Diarrhoea occurs in 80% of patients. Bowel frequency correlates with inflammatory activity, particularly in the colon, with bacterial overgrowth and ileal resection potentially contributing. Bleeding is less common than in ulcerative colitis, as is urgency—unless the rectum is involved or the anal sphincter damaged. An important point: many Crohn's disease patients consider three to four semisolid bowel evacuations per day to be 'normal' and it is the change from baseline, including nocturnal frequency, which is important in assessing disease activity.

Perianal symptoms are often mild, even with apparently severe involvement: pain usually indicates an abscess; fistula discharge is common; and anal stricture may produce constipation or tenesmus.

Signs

Many patients with even severely active Crohn's disease appear deceptively well. A minority are anaemic or malnourished. A persisting tachycardia may point to dehydration, severe inflammation, or sepsis. The oral cavity should be inspected for ulceration and glossitis, and nails for clubbing.

The commonest abnormal examination finding is right iliac fossa tenderness, often with associated fullness or a mass due to thickened and matted bowel loops. Equivalent findings may be found over any affected bowel segment.

Anorectal examination may reveal various signs from violaceous fleshy skin tags to anal fissure, ulcer, abscess, and fistulas. Anal stenosis may be detected.

Signs related to specific complications may be evident—e.g. fever and tachycardia with intraabdominal collection, distension and high-pitched bowel sounds with obstruction, and so on.

Extraintestinal manifestations

Extraintestinal manifestations of Crohn's disease commonly affect the mouth, joints, skin, and eyes and less commonly the liver and lungs. These are more frequent with colonic involvement and may precede intestinal symptoms.

Aphthous mouth ulcers are usually associated with active intestinal inflammation. These should be distinguished from haematinic deficiency (glossitis, angular cheilitis), oral candida, and particularly oropharyngeal Crohn's disease—which usually causes fissuring and thickening of the lips but can present with deep sulcal ulceration and buccal cobblestoning. There is overlap with orofacial granulomatosis where 60% have asymptomatic intestinal lesions of Crohn's disease. Both oral Crohn's disease and orofacial granulomatosis can be successfully treated with a low-benzoate, low-cinnamon diet or topical steroids.

Joint involvement is seen in up to 30% of Crohn's disease patients. It ranges from arthralgia to inflammatory arthritis and includes ankylosing spondylitis. The inflammatory arthritis can be an asymmetric large-joint arthropathy with pain and effusions prominent with active intestinal inflammation, or a symmetrical small-joint arthropathy. Each has distinct genetic associations. Where possible NSAIDs should be avoided as they increase gut permeability and can trigger a Crohn's disease flare.

Eczema and psoriasis often flare with active Crohn's disease, but the most common specific dermatological manifestation is erythema nodosum. Usually found at initial presentation, it settles with resolution of bowel inflammation rarely to recur.

Ocular inflammation usually presents as uveitis, episcleritis, or conjunctivitis. Crohn's disease patients developing red eye, eye pain, and/or visual disturbance should receive emergency ophthalmic assessment. Persistently abnormal, particularly cholestatic liver function tests should prompt investigation including magnetic resonance cholangiography for primary sclerosing cholangitis.

Differential diagnosis

The differential diagnosis of Crohn's disease depends on its specific presentation.

Ileitis in young patients closely mimics appendicitis, while chronic symptoms are often diagnosed as irritable bowel syndrome. In older patients colonic, particularly caecal, carcinoma must be considered. Clinicians often rely on a raised CRP or faecal calprotectin to identify patients with irritable-bowel-like symptoms needing further investigation. However, strong clinical suspicion (e.g. family history of Crohn's disease) may warrant further investigation despite normal screening tests.

With demonstrated intestinal inflammation, distinguishing inflammatory bowel disease from infection is the commonest challenge. Occasionally the diagnosis of Crohn's disease cannot be confirmed until the second flare. In known Crohn's disease patients, when abdominal symptoms recur the challenge is distinguishing active inflammation from other causes. Most of the latter are discussed below (see 'Complications') but it is noteworthy that a history of inflammatory bowel disease increases susceptibility to infectious enterocolitis, and that irritable bowel syndrome is as common in individuals with Crohn's disease as in the general population. Failure to appreciate these points can cause both diagnostic confusion and inappropriate treatment choices such as over-use of corticosteroids.

Yersinia enterocolitica and *M. tuberculosis* can mimic Crohn's disease, sharing an ileocaecal predilection and causing acute and chronic inflammation respectively. However, the cause of most cases of acute ileitis is never determined and only a minority develop Crohn's disease. Campylobacter, shigella, and salmonella cause an acute colitis usually with fever and sometimes with a reactive arthritis and *Clostridium difficile* is increasingly found outside conventional risk groups. *E. coli* can cause colitis, the 0157 serotype triggering haemolytic uraemic syndrome. Rarer causes of enterocolitis include amoebae, schistosomiasis, and cytomegalovirus, emphasizing the need for careful microbiological and histopathological assessment. Rectal and perianal ulceration can be caused by sexually transmitted infections such as gonorrhoea, syphilis, and lymphogranuloma venerium.

Noninfectious mimics of Crohn's disease include drugs, ischaemia, Behçet's disease, lymphoma, small-bowel carcinoma, solitary rectal ulcer, and radiotherapy. NSAIDs can produce intestinal inflammation and rarely 'diaphragm' strictures, and Fleet phospho-soda colonoscopy bowel preparation commonly causes rectal aphthoid ulceration with focal active colitis on histopathology. Nicorandil can produce oral and deep perianal ulceration, and mycophenolate mofetil occasionally causes right colonic ulceration. Ischaemic colitis can mimic Crohn's disease with segmental involvement and solitary rectal ulcers can be large and pleiomorphic but histopathology discriminates. Diverticulitis can mimic Crohn's disease clinically and histopathologically: colonoscopic biopsies from a diverticular segment must be labelled as such.

For colonic inflammation the major differential diagnosis for Crohn's disease is ulcerative colitis. Differentiation is possible for about 95% of cases (Table 15.11.1), leaving 5% as indeterminate or, more accurately, unclassified due to equivocal appearances. Ulcerative colitis can mimic Crohn's disease with a prominent caecal patch of inflammation well recognized in distal ulcerative colitis, or where inflammation becomes patchy on treatment.

Clinical investigation

With any significant acute enterocolitis excluding infection is critical. Three stool samples should be sent for microscopy, culture and *C. difficile* toxin assay. Serological tests for yersinia and polymerase chain reaction for cytomegalovirus should also be requested where appropriate.

For chronic symptoms a few baseline tests provide important diagnostic indicators. Faecal calprotectin, although not widely available, is highly sensitive for intestinal inflammation. On blood tests an even modestly elevated CRP or ESR is consistent with

Table 15.11.1 Features distinguishing Crohn's disease from ulcerative colitis

	Crohn's disease	**Ulcerative colitis**
Clinical features		
Bloody diarrhoea	Uncommon	Common
Perianal disease	Common	Uncommon
Abdominal mass	Common	Rare
Endoscopy/radiology		
Rectal inflammation	Uncommon	Defining feature
Distribution	Patchy	Continuous
Ulceration	Pleomorphic, deep	Superficial, fine
Strictures/fistulas	Characteristic	Rare
Histology		
Depth	Transmural	Superficial
Infiltrate	Lymphocytes, macrophages, plasma cells	Neutrophils, plasma cells, eosinophils
Granulomas	Characteristic	Confined to ruptured crypts

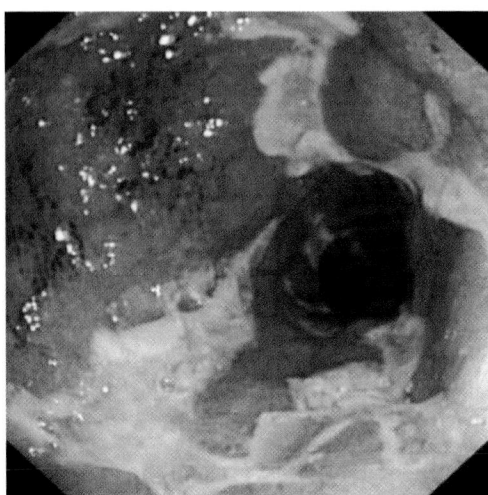

Fig. 15.11.2 Colonoscopic appearance of linear and pleomorphic ulceration of Crohn's disease.

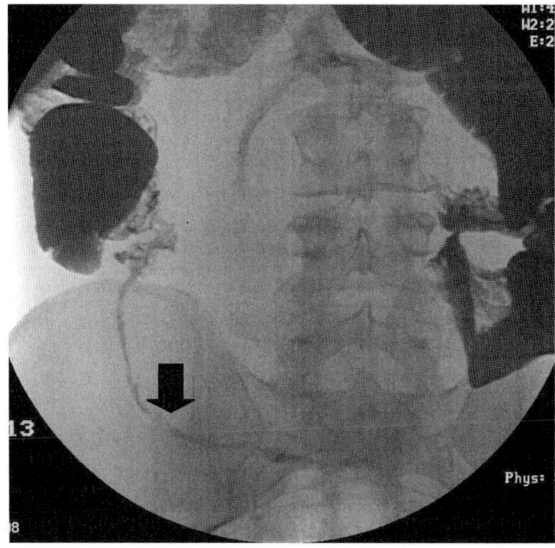

Fig. 15.11.3 A long ileal stricture shown on barium small-bowel radiology. (Courtesy of Dr Nicholas Carroll, Addenbrooke's Hospital, Cambridge.)

active Crohn's disease, sometimes accompanied by elevated platelet and neutrophil counts and a low serum albumin. The latter reflects cytokine-mediated down-regulation of hepatic synthesis and intestinal protein loss. Anaemia is common, and multifactorial in origin; ferritin, vitamin B_{12}, and folate should be checked. Liver and renal function tests and coeliac serology are advisable. Anti-*Saccharomyces cerevisiae* antibody assays are positive in 50 to 75% of cases but not widely used. Plain abdominal radiography helps assessment of severe diarrhoea or possible obstruction, although increasingly CT is the investigation of choice for the latter.

Where baseline tests indicate possible Crohn's disease, choice of next investigation depends on clinical context. Ileocolonoscopy with biopsies is highly sensitive for Crohn's disease presenting with diarrhoea. Appearances vary, but Crohn's disease hallmarks are segmental inflammation with pleomorphic ulceration and cobblestoning, most commonly ileocaecal (Fig. 15.11.2). Endoscopists should biopsy the rectum and intervening normal colon where inflammation is patchy to aid histopathological interpretation.

Where abdominal pain predominates, the choice usually lies between CT scan and barium small bowel radiology (enteroclysis having higher sensitivity for subtle mucosal change than follow-through)—with abdominal ultrasound scanning or MR/CT enteroclysis alternatives in some centres (see Chapter 15.3.3). The goal is to identify small-bowel ulceration, oedema and luminal stenosis (Fig. 15.11.3). Cross-sectional modalities also show wall thickening and inflammatory change in the mesentry, while dynamic studies (ultrasound, enteroclysis) are particularly helpful in assessing obstruction.

Special tests

- MRI perineum—detailed anatomical assessment of perianal fistulas
- Sinograms—to delineate enterocutaneous fistulas
- ^{99}Tc HMPAO-labelled white cell scans—detect and localize intestinal inflammation
- Capsule endoscopy—highly sensitive for subtle small-bowel ulceration; avoid in stricturing disease

Criteria for diagnosis

No single feature is sufficient or necessary to diagnose Crohn's disease. Instead, diagnosis is based on cumulative clinical, laboratory, radiological, endoscopic, and histopathological evidence. This is usually straightforward, but where uncertainty exists the multidisciplinary team should carefully review the evidence.

Treatment
Overview

Treatment of Crohn's disease must be tailored to the individual. Patients need a consistent medical approach underpinned by information and support, e.g. from specialist nurses and national patient organizations (see 'Useful websites'). Nutritional deficits must be corrected, with medical therapy for active disease and timely surgery for refractory inflammation or complications. Treatment should be escalated according to disease severity and clinical progress. Mucosal healing is the goal and probably reduces risk of complications. Those with severe disease should be admitted to hospital for intravenous corticosteroids, fluids and electrolytes, and close monitoring. Most improve within 5 to 7 days. Site of disease affects treatment choice, as does the patient's previous experience and views regarding tolerability and risks vs benefits. Prognostic markers are lacking, but Crohn's disease often behaves more aggressively in those with early age of onset, diffuse disease, marked perianal involvement, early requirement for steroids, and prominent extraintestinal manifestations. In such patients, and those with recurrent relapse, maintenance immunosuppressive therapy must be considered early. The clinician must synthesize all these strands in formulating an appropriate, individualized treatment plan.

Smoking

All Crohn's disease patients who smoke should be advised to stop. This halves risk of relapse.

Diet and nutrition

Dietetic assessment and advice is critical, particularly in patients who have lost weight. The large majority should be fed or supplemented enterally. Parenteral nutrition is reserved for those with intestinal failure due to obstruction, high output fistula, or short bowel syndrome.

For Crohn's disease affecting the upper gastrointestinal tract and small bowel, therapeutic diets can—by poorly understood effects on mucosal immunity and gut flora—suppress inflammation. Amino acid ('elemental'), peptide, and protein-based liquid feeds are equally effective, being nutritionally replete and used exclusive of all other foods for 2 to 4 weeks. Disease remission occurs in 40 to 80% of patients able to tolerate them.

Advantages of therapeutic diets include rapid nutritional restitution and avoidance of corticosteroids—limiting their adverse impact on growth (in children), osteoporosis, and superadded sepsis. Limitations mainly relate to palatability and frequency of early relapse. Specialist dietetic supervision, offering choice of flavour or preparation, and building gradually towards calculated nutritional requirements greatly increases adherence. Nasogastric or gastrostomy tube feeding are occasionally required. Successful transition to eating should start with a basic low fat, low fibre exclusion diet with phased reintroduction of normal foods over several weeks to identify specific dietary intolerances. This in itself can produce prolonged remission, although addition of immunomodulatory therapy may be required.

Patients with a stricture should have a low-residue diet to avoid bolus obstruction (avoiding sweetcorn, apple skins, etc.); and lactose intolerance is common in Crohn's disease requiring a lactose-free diet with calcium supplementation. Oral Crohn's disease often responds to a low-benzoate, low-cinnamon diet.

Medical therapy

5-Aminosalicylates

Early randomized controlled trials of sulphasalazine in active Crohn's disease showed nonsignificant advantage over placebo, but subgroup analysis suggested possible benefit in colonic Crohn's disease. Mesalazine also lacks efficacy in Crohn's disease. Of six methodologically rigorous trials, some indicated modest benefit but this was not significant on metaanalysis. There is a strong case for dropping mesalazine from the treatment algorithm of mild to moderately active Crohn's disease.

Mesalazine should also be abandoned as maintenance therapy following medically induced remission, because of its demonstrated lack of efficacy. After many years on treatment many patients may be resistant to the idea of stopping (indeed, may report symptom recurrence). A pragmatic approach is to try a slow wean.

After surgical resection maintenance mesalazine may confer some benefit, although the effect size is small (number needed to treat (NNT) = 11 to prevent one relapse at 12 months) and appears restricted to exclusively small-bowel disease. Given the cost and inconvenience it should be reserved for selected cases, and only after more effective measures such smoking cessation.

Antibiotics

Antibiotics can successfully treat perianal abscesses, discharging fistulas, and small-bowel bacterial overgrowth complicating Crohn's disease. Metronidazole with or without ciprofloxacin is best and may be required for several weeks. Some clinicians recommend antibiotics for active Crohn's colitis but supporting trials evidence is modest. A randomized controlled trial of antimycobacterial therapy for Crohn's disease showed no benefit over placebo.

Corticosteroids

For most gastroenterologists, corticosteroids constitute the therapeutic mainstay for active Crohn's disease. They induce symptomatic remission or satisfactory clinical response in 80% of patients with active disease. Typically given as a course of oral treatment reducing over 6 to 8 weeks, the conventional starting dose is prednisolone 40 mg/day. Smaller starting doses appear less effective. Severe disease mandates hospital admission for intravenous therapy with hydrocortisone (100 mg four times daily) or methyl prednisone (40 mg twice daily).

Corticosteroid side effects can be mitigated by using oral budesonide, formulated for ileocaecal release. High first-pass hepatic metabolism ensures low systemic availability. Trials data and clinical experience suggest that budesonide's efficacy approaches that of prednisolone. Where the latter is required, e.g. for more severe and extensive disease, calcium and vitamin D with or without oral bisphosphonate should be co-prescribed to limit osteoporosis.

Long-term corticosteroid therapy is ineffective and should be avoided in Crohn's disease. For the 35 to 40% of patients relapsing frequently off steroids (e.g. at least two relapses a year) or unable to wean without relapse, immunosuppressive or biological therapies are mandated.

Immunosuppressants

Azathioprine and 6-mercaptopurine are the most commonly used immunosuppressants, with methotrexate second-line and alternatives such as tacrolimus and thalidomide used less frequently. Where remission is maintained the vogue is towards increased duration of therapy—driven by evidence of increased risk of relapse on stopping even after many years in remission.

Azathioprine and 6-mercaptopurine

The thiopurines azathioprine (2–2.5 mg/kg) and 6-mercaptopurine (1.5 mg/kg) are steroid-sparing and effective in maintaining remission in Crohn's disease (NNT = 3). They inhibit purine synthesis via 6-thioguanine triphosphate to prevent leucocyte proliferation. Azathioprine or mercaptopurine take up to 16 weeks to work and should be considered early for aggressive disease, severe perianal disease, steroid-dependence or patients requiring two or more courses of corticosteroids per year. Treatment should continue for at least 4 years when effective and well tolerated.

Some 10 to 20% of patients will be intolerant of thiopurines due to myalgias, nausea, rash, mild hepatitis, or cytopenias, and occasionally pancreatitis (2%). Risk of lymphoma appears slightly increased but it remains extremely rare. Patients should be warned of possible profound neutropenia and need regular monitoring of blood count and liver function, particularly following commencement or dose increase. Minor elevations of liver enzymes, lymphopenia, and macrocytosis are not significant.

Variation in the thiopurine methyltransferase (TPMT) gene affects efficacy and safety of thiopurines. 1 in 300 Europeans have negligible enzyme activity and risk severe neutropenia—preventable by measuring TPMT activity or genotype before starting therapy. However subsequent blood test monitoring is still required. TPMT heterozygotes are predisposed to thiopurine side effects, and may respond to lower doses.

Where toxicity develops, switching from one thiopurine to the other often helps, despite their chemical similarity. For patients seemingly unresponsive or intolerant, doses should be pushed to the limit of the dosing range or tolerability for 16 weeks before trying alternatives.

Methotrexate

Methotrexate is also effective for inducing and maintaining steroid-free remission in Crohn's disease. The index randomized controlled trial used an induction dose of 25 mg/week and 15 mg/week maintenance given intramuscularly. Most centres now use oral methotrexate at these doses—supported by retrospective evidence of efficacy. Blood test monitoring is again advised. Methotrexate is teratogenic and should be avoided in women of child-bearing potential.

Other immunosuppressants

Randomized trial evidence is lacking for other immunosuppressants. From available data tacrolimus appears promising for refractory inflammatory disease and closing fistulas, and thalidomide may have a short-term role but is limited by toxicity. Oral ciclosporin is not effective.

Biological therapies

Infliximab is an effective treatment for severe, refractory Crohn's disease whether acute or chronic. A chimeric human/mouse monoclonal antibody targeting TNFα, it neutralizes circulating TNFα, mediates antibody-dependent cellular cytotoxicity, and induces T-cell apoptosis. The ACCENT 1 study showed 60% of patients with active luminal Crohn's disease experienced rapid improvement of symptoms following one intravenous infusion (5 mg/kg). Subsequent data demonstrated benefit in closing fistulas, healing ulcerated mucosa, and maintaining steroid-free remission in 30 to 50% of patients responding to initial induction and then given 8 weekly infusions of infliximab. Improved quality of life and reduced hospitalization significantly offset the high treatment costs. Newer, subcutaneously administered anti-TNF antibody therapies such as adalimumab and certolizumab appear equally effective.

Anti-TNF therapies are generally well tolerated but major side effects include life-threatening infection (sepsis must be excluded and abscesses drained before treatment), reactivation of tuberculosis (mandating screening), infusion reactions including anaphylaxis, and increased risk of lymphoma. Recent data from the SONIC study showed the combination of infliximab and azathioprine to be more effective than either alone at inducing and maintaining remission. Questions relate to treatment duration. For steroid-refractory or -dependent Crohn's disease where thiopurines have not been tried, doses not maximized, or insufficient time allowed, infliximab provides a therapeutic 'bridge' to an optimized thiopurine regime. It should then be withdrawn. Where Crohn's disease has flared in spite of such an optimized regime, or patients are intolerant of immunosuppressants, regular anti-TNF antibody therapy may be required long term.

Anti-TNF antibody therapies appear less effective in smokers, patients with small-bowel disease, and those without raised CRP. Concerns regarding infliximab efficacy dwindling over time have been reduced by the arrival of the alternatives adalimumab and certolizumab.

Other therapies

Several novel therapies are currently being evaluated. These include antibodies targeted at adhesion molecules (natalizumab demonstrated efficacy but causes demyelination) and proinflammatory cytokines, antisense intercellular adhesion molecule-1, inhibitors of chemotactic factors, and a variety of small molecules. Less conventional approaches include trials of *Trichuris suis*, a helminth from pigs, and probiotics. Given recent data highlighting the central role of IL-23 and autophagy in Crohn's disease, these represent exciting potential therapeutic targets.

Surgery

Despite the substantially increased use of immunosuppression since 1980, surgery is still required in 80% of patients with Crohn's disease long term. The two main indications are refractory inflammation and complications of disease (the latter are discussed in the next section). Close collaboration between experienced supervising physicians and surgeons, and open discussion with the patient regarding treatment options, facilitates joined-up clinical management.

Surgery for refractory Crohn's disease should be timely and conservative. Increasingly, laparoscopic approaches are used. Timeliness means patients not enduring medical therapies when it is clear they are not working, nor being propelled toward surgery before it is warranted (e.g. for radiologically severe but minimally symptomatic strictures). Patients should be involved in discussions regarding long-term efficacy and safety of second-line medical therapies vs risks, benefits, and expected outcomes of surgery.

Conservative surgery minimizes risk of long-term harm, particularly short-bowel syndrome. Thus strictureplasties (incising longitudinally and suturing vertically) effectively open short strictures and are favoured over small-bowel resections where possible, while for resections only macroscopically involved bowel is removed. For colonic disease panproctocolectomy carries the lowest risk of relapse but at the cost of permanent ileostomy. Segmental colectomy or sub-total colectomy with ileorectal anastomosis are usually preferred where possible. Surgery for perianal sepsis and fistulas usually involves drainage and placement of seton sutures, together with medical management, rather than more aggressive interventions which carry high risk of nonhealing wounds or faecal incontinence.

Optimization for surgery includes dietitian-supervised correction of any malnutrition. Oral supplements are preferred but parenteral nutrition may be required. Corticosteroids should be minimized to limit adverse impact on wound healing—but evidence indicates continued azathioprine/mercaptopurine therapy perioperatively reduces complications, including sepsis. For severe coloanal Crohn's disease a defunctioning ileostomy should be considered. Technically straightforward, diverting the faecal stream usually settles coloanal inflammation, relieving symptoms and permitting subsequent elective panproctocolectomy on a clinically fit patient. Whether some patients might avoid colectomy and be maintained in remission on stoma reversal if started on thiopurine or biological therapy is unclear.

Approximately one-half of patients requiring surgery for small-bowel Crohn's disease require a repeat operation within 10 years, especially smokers. For patients deemed at high risk of early postoperative relapse, e.g. those requiring resections in quick succession or with residual diffuse disease, azathioprine should be considered. Increasingly clinicians recommend colonoscopy for all patients 6 months post-ileal resection, with institution of azathioprine in those with perianastomotic ulceration. This is a sensible strategy but its long-term benefit has yet to be established in prospective trials.

Complications and their management

The complications of Crohn's disease confer significant morbidity and some mortality.

Acute complications of Crohn's disease

◆ Venous thromboembolism is common and potentially life-threatening, requiring vigilance and low-molecular-weight heparin during all hospital admissions.

◆ Intestinal obstruction manifesting as colicky pain, vomiting, distension, and absolute constipation presents acutely or subacutely and is due variably to food bolus, active inflammation (with mural oedema), adhesions, and fibrotic stenosis. Strictures usually affect the terminal ileum but can occur anywhere from oesophagus to anal canal. Inflammatory markers and abdominal CT constitute key investigations. Episodes usually resolve with conservative management: nil by mouth, intravenous fluids, corticosteroids, and nasogastric tube for pronounced vomiting. Recurrent episodes refractory to low-residue diet (exclusion of mushrooms, sweetcorn, vegetable skins, etc.) and increased immunosuppression (if evidence of inflammation) require endoscopic dilatation or surgical resection/strictureplasty.

◆ Intestinal perforation, caused by deep fissuring ulcers characteristic of Crohn's disease, presents acutely as peritonitis but symptoms may be considerably masked by corticosteroid therapy. Following diagnostic confirmation, usually on CT, urgent surgical resection is mandated. Fortunately, free perforation is rare as fibrotic serosal reaction and fat wrapping contain most leaks.

◆ Toxic megacolon is rare in Crohn's disease, but those with acute severe colitis and systemic upset (fever, tachycardia, etc.) require close monitoring and serial abdominal radiographs. Where transverse colonic diameter is more than 6 cm at presentation and this persists despite 24 to 48 h maximal medical therapy, or develops during such treatment, colectomy is mandated to prevent perforation.

◆ Severe bleeding is rare. After resuscitation, therapeutic options include endoscopic haemostasis (adrenaline injection and clipping), angiographic occlusion, or surgical resection.

Subacute/chronic complications

◆ Intraabdominal or pelvic abscesses can result from localized perforation or internal fistulation. Symptoms include abdominal pain and marked weight loss but can be surprisingly nonspecific and frequently mistaken for active luminal inflammation. Markedly elevated inflammatory markers indicate sepsis and mandate abdominal CT. Treatment options, decided by multidisciplinary review and depending on the patient's clinical status, include antibiotics (metronidazole and ciprofloxacin) with radiological drainage and elemental diet or corticosteroids to suppress Crohn's inflammation. Surgical drainage/resection is usually best deferred while sepsis is thus controlled. Parenteral nutrition and intensive care may be required in severe cases.

◆ Perianal abscesses and fistulas present with pain, swelling, and discharge. This can be cyclical. Fistulas may be simple (single intra- or trans-sphincteric track) or complex (including extension above levators, 'horseshoeing' contralaterally, or secondary tracks). Management includes defining the anatomy (using pelvic MRI), drainage of abscesses, control of infection with metronidazole ± ciprofloxacin and suppression of disease activity. Insertion of seton sutures keeps fistula tracks open, preventing repeated blockage and abscess formation. For recurrent perianal Crohn's disease, azathioprine or infliximab reduces inflammation and fistula activity. Severe, refractory disease may require defunctioning ileostomy or panproctocolectomy.

◆ Symptomatic anal strictures should be dilated under anaesthetic, with benefit prolonged by using a dilator at home.

◆ Internal fistulas. Rectovaginal fistulas cause faeculent vaginal discharge; colovesical fistulas cause pneumaturia / recurrent urinary infections; and enterocolic fistulas present with diarrhoea, 'malabsorption', and weight loss. Enterocutaneous fistulas are postoperative complications, mostly closing spontaneously by 6 weeks unless communicating with inflamed or obstructed bowel. Resectional surgery for fistulas should be preceded by control of sepsis and inflammatory disease, optimization of nutrition and delineation of fistula anatomy by appropriate imaging.

◆ Short-bowel syndrome following extensive resection is likely if there is less than 120 cm of small bowel ending in ileostomy or 80 cm with colon *in situ* (colonic bacteria 'scavenge' calories by fermentation, producing volatile fatty acids which are absorbed).

◆ Other patterns of malabsorption in Crohn's disease include:
  • Vitamin B12 deficiency—following ileal resection levels should be monitored yearly and replaced parenterally where deficient.
  • Choleretic diarrhoea—ileal resection prevents resorption of bile acids in the enterohepatic circulation. In the colon they can stimulate marked watery diarrhoea. Treat with cholestyramine.
  • Bacterial overgrowth of the small bowel results from stasis produced by scarring and stricturing. Symptoms include diarrhoea, nausea, bloating and flatulence. Treat with antibiotics (e.g. metronidazole, doxycycline, coamoxiclav); often prolonged or rotating courses required.
  • Iron deficiency. Oral iron preparations frequently poorly tolerated or ineffective—intravenous iron sucrose/iron dextran often required.
  • Zinc, magnesium, and selenium deficiency should be ascertained and treated.

◆ Growth failure is a major risk in adolescents, particularly with disease activity around puberty. Height and weight must be monitored on growth charts. Acute relapse should be managed with dietary therapy (elemental/polymeric) where possible. The priority is rapid induction of remission to restore growth, and infliximab or surgery may be required to achieve this. Long-term corticosteroids must be avoided: azathioprine or infliximab are frequently used to maintain remission.

◆ Osteoporosis occurs in approximately 12% of Crohn's disease patients, with increased fracture risk. Corticosteroid therapy, low body mass, poor dietary intake of calcium, smoking, hypogonadism, and uncontrolled inflammation all contribute. Regular bone densitometry is indicated, with calcium/vitamin D supplements and bisphosphonates given as required.

◆ Gallstones and renal stones are more common, and symptoms may be confused with active Crohn's disease. Conventional management is indicated.

◆ Colon cancer is increased in Crohn's disease. As with ulcerative colitis, risk correlates with disease extent, activity and duration. In one study neoplasia was detected in 16% of patients over 20 years. Regular surveillance colonoscopy is warranted after 10 years extensive Crohn's colitis, with biopsy series including any mucosal irregularities. Risk of small bowel carcinoma increases 40-fold compared to the general population, usually within chronic strictures, but remains very rare.

Prognosis

To a patient newly diagnosed with Crohn's disease the lack of a cure and uncertain future is understandably concerning. However, an aggressive or refractory course is unusual, and although morbidity during flares is substantial these are mostly short-lived and usually interspersed with long periods of remission with near-normal quality of life. Although prognostic markers are lacking, population-based data from Denmark indicate 55% of patients to be in remission and 15% with mild disease only 1 year after diagnosis. Some 10 to 30% of patients relapse each year, less if immunomodulatory drugs are used.

Up to 80% of Crohn's disease patients require surgery long-term, a figure unchanged over 30 years despite substantially increased azathioprine use. For ileal/small-bowel Crohn's disease, surgery is required on average 8 years after diagnosis. Some 30 to 40% of patients experience symptomatic relapse by 5 years postoperatively, with 30% requiring further surgery within 10 years. Smoking more than doubles this risk. Surgery is required less frequently for exclusively colonic disease. Risk of relapse following panproctocolectomy is low in such individuals.

Despite the imperfections of current therapies Crohn's disease does not dramatically increase mortality. In a large United Kingdom-based cohort study, Crohn's disease was associated with an overall hazard ratio of 1.73. The effect was greatest in 20- to 39-year-olds, reflecting the large impact of a small number of deaths in this age bracket, usually due to acute complications such as sepsis, pulmonary embolism, bowel perforation, and postoperative complications.

Heredity, fertility, and pregnancy

Each child of a Crohn's disease-affected individual has a 2 to 4% risk of developing Crohn's disease, rising to approximately 30% where both parents are affected. Fertility is reduced in women with Crohn's disease, and miscarriage rate is higher particularly with active disease during pregnancy. Most Crohn's disease therapies are safe in pregnancy but risks and benefits should be carefully discussed with patients. Acute flares should be treated with corticosteroids or dietary therapy (elemental or polymeric); and maintenance treatment with azathioprine or infliximab (the latter until the third trimester) should usually be continued. Methotrexate,

however, is contraindicated in pregnancy, and thiopurines should not be used by breastfeeding mothers.

Areas of controversy

◆ The precise role of commensal gut flora (and the possible contribution of one or a small number of pathogens) in triggering and sustaining the intestinal inflammation of Crohn's disease

◆ Use of systemic corticosteroids for Crohn's disease in view of side effects and possibly the increased risk of fistulas

◆ For patients in remission on azathioprine, 6-mercaptopurine, methotrexate, or anti-TNF antibody therapy, how long to continue these treatments and when risks of long-term immunosuppression outweigh benefits of controlling active Crohn's disease

◆ Whether anti-TNF antibody therapy provides more effective and safer control of Crohn's disease than thiopurines long term

◆ Whether surgical resection (especially laparoscopic) is preferable to long-term immunosuppression for corticosteroid-refractory terminal ileal Crohn's disease

◆ For protection against osteoporosis, optimal use and timing of calcium supplementation and/or bisphosphonates with respect to corticosteroids

Likely future developments

◆ Increasing use of specialist nurses and patient self-management

◆ Use of the internet rather than the physician as primary information source

◆ More widespread use of biological therapies

◆ Use of genetic data to delineate heterogeneity within the Crohn's disease population; value for prognosis, stratification for drug trials, and possibly 'personalized' therapy

◆ Progress in characterizing environmental trigger(s) facilitated by genetic knowledge

◆ Increased knowledge regarding pathogenic mechanisms feeding development of rational new therapies and possibly vaccines for those identified as genetically at risk

Further reading

Barrett JC et al (2008). Genome-wide association defines more than 30 distinct susceptibility loci for Crohn's disease. *Nature Genetics*, **40**(8), 955–62.

Colombel JF, et al. (2004). The safety profile of infliximab in patients with Crohn's disease: the Mayo clinic experience in 500 patients. *Gastroenterology*, **126**, 19–31.

Cosnes J, et al. (2001). Smoking cessation and the course of Crohn's disease: an intervention study. *Gastroenterology*, **120**, 1093–9.

Cosnes J, et al. (2005). Impact of the increasing use of immunosuppressants in Crohn's disease on the need for intestinal surgery. *Gut*, **54**, 237–41.

ECCO (2006). Consensus guidelines for Crohn's disease. *Gut*, **55** Suppl 1.

Hanauer SB, et al. (2002). Maintenance infliximab for Crohn's disease: the ACCENT I randomised trial. *Lancet*, **359**, 1541–9.

Heetun ZS, et al. (2007). Review article: Reproduction in the patient with inflammatory bowel disease. *Aliment Pharmacol Ther*, **26**, 513–33.

Irving P, Rampton D, Shanahan F (eds) (2006). *Clinical dilemmas in inflammatory bowel disease*. Blackwell, Oxford.

Lemann M, *et al.* (2006). Infliximab plus azathioprine for steroid-dependent Crohn's disease patients: a randomized placebo-controlled trial. *Gastroenterology*, **130**, 1054–61.

Loftus EV (2004). Clinical epidemiology of inflammatory bowel disease: Incidence, prevalence, and environmental influences. *Gastroenterology*, **126**, 1504–17.

Pearson DC, *et al.* (1995). Azathioprine and 6-mercaptopurine in Crohn disease. A meta-analysis. *Ann Intern Med*, **123**, 132–42.

Sandborn W, *et al.* (2000). Azathioprine or 6-mercaptopurine for inducing remission of Crohn's disease. *Cochrane Database Syst Rev*, **2**, CD000545.

Sandborn WJ, Feagan BG, Lichtenstein GR (2007). Medical management of mild to moderate Crohn's disease: evidence-based treatment algorithms for induction and maintenance of remission. *Aliment Pharmacol Ther*, **26**, 987–1003.

Sartor RB (2006). Mechanisms of disease: pathogenesis of Crohn's disease and ulcerative colitis. *Nat Clin Pract Gastroenterol Hepatol*, **3**, 390–407.

Satsangi J, Sutherland L (eds) (2003). *Inflammatory bowel diseases*. Churchill Livingstone, Edinburgh.

Targan S, Shanahan F, Karp L (eds) (2003). *Inflammatory bowel disease—from bench to bedside*, 2nd edition. Kluwer, London.

Useful websites

Crohn's and Colitis Foundation of America, http://www.ccfa.org

National Association for Colitis and Crohn's Disease, http://www.nacc.org.uk

Ulcerative colitis

D.P. Jewell

Essentials

Ulcerative colitis is a chronic inflammatory disease of the colon that always affects the rectum, extends proximally to a variable extent, and is characterized by a relapsing and remitting course. In mild disease the mucosa is hyperaemic and granular; punctate ulcers appear in more severe disease, and these may then enlarge and extend deeply. Infiltration with acute and chronic inflammatory cells is largely confined to the mucosa, with histological features of chronicity, e.g. distorted crypt architecture, important in clinical distinction from other causes of colitis, e.g. infective.

The cause of ulcerative colitis is unknown: genetic factors are involved although not all the relevant genes are yet identified. A dysregulated immune response to luminal antigen may be important.

Clinical features and investigation

Typical presentation of mild or moderate disease is with a gradual onset of symptoms including diarrhoea, rectal bleeding, the passage of mucus, and—less frequently—abdominal pain; such patients usually look well and exhibit few abnormal physical signs.

Severe disease is characterized by anorexia, nausea, weight loss, and severe diarrhoea (>6 motions daily) that becomes a slurry of faecal material, pus, and blood. The patient is likely to look unwell with fever, tachycardia, and other signs of volume depletion, and the abdomen is often distended and tympanitic, with reduced bowel sounds and marked colonic tenderness.

Extraintestinal manifestations may be related to activity of the colitis (e.g. aphthous ulceration of the mouth, erythema nodosum, peripheral arthropathy, pyoderma gangrenosum) or not (e.g. anterior uveitis, sacroiliitis, primary sclerosing cholangitis). Local colonic complications of acute disease include acute dilatation and perforation, and complications of longstanding disease include carcinoma (7–15% risk after 20 years).

Diagnosis is usually made of the basis of exclusion of infective colitis by stool culture and the finding of typical diffuse sigmoidoscopic appearances in the rectum. All patients with a severe attack require a plain abdominal radiograph, primarily to exclude acute dilatation. Active disease is often accompanied by a neutrophil leucocytosis, thrombocytosis, and a rise in inflammatory markers.

Management

For active disease treatment depends on severity, but initial therapy is usually as follows: (1) proctitis—a 5-aminosalicylic acid drug, given by mouth and concurrently as a suppository; (2) mildly active disease ($\leq$4 motions/day)—oral prednisolone (20 mg daily), together with topical steroids or 5-aminosalicylic acid (or both); (3) moderately active disease (>4 motions/day, but not systemically ill) – as for mild disease, but with prednisolone 40 mg daily; (4) severe disease (>6 bowel motions/day, with blood; systemically ill) – resuscitation/ intravenous fluids; hydrocortisone, 100 mg intravenously every 6 h and 100 mg as a rectal drip twice daily; those who deteriorate during the first few days of intravenous treatment, or who have not made a substantial improvement after 3–4 days, need either 'rescue' therapy with ciclosporin or infliximab, or colectomy. Patients with chronic active disease that prevents steroid withdrawal are treated with immunosuppressants, azathioprine and ciclosporin being most widely used.

In the long term, drugs containing 5-aminosalicylic acid (e.g. sulphasalazine, mesalazine) reduce the relapse rate and are able to maintain remission over many years. Patients with extensive longstanding disease require regular colonoscopic surveillance, with prophylactic colectomy usually advised if biopsies reveal dysplasia.

Indications for surgery include (1) severe inflammation unresponsive to medical therapy; (2) acute complications (perforation, dilatation); (3) chronic active disease; and (4) prevention of cancer. Restorative proctocolectomy with ileoanal reservoir/pouch is the procedure of choice in specialist centres, provided the anal sphincter is intact.

Introduction

Ulcerative colitis is a chronic inflammatory disease of the colon, of unknown cause. It always affects the rectum and extends proximally to involve the colon to a variable extent. It is characterized by a relapsing and remitting course.

The disease was first described in 1859 by Samuel Wilks, a physician at Guy's Hospital, who recognized that 'simple, idiopathic colitis' could be distinguished from other forms of colitis, mainly bacterial dysentery. It took many years for the concept to be accepted, but finally, in 1931, Sir Arthur Hurst was able to give a complete description of the disease including the sigmoidoscopic appearances. Nevertheless, he still considered the disease to be primarily infective, even though its chronic nature might be induced secondarily by other factors.

Epidemiology

Ulcerative colitis is a worldwide disease, although it may be difficult to diagnose in areas where infective colitis is prevalent. Accurate figures for incidence and prevalence are not universally available, but the disease is now recognized in most countries. Table 15.12.1 lists data for high-incidence areas and also shows that there have been no trends to suggest the disease is becoming more common, which is in contrast to Crohn's disease. Low-incidence areas include Asia, Japan and South America, where the incidence rates are at least tenfold less than in those Western countries with a high prevalence, although this is increasing, which may to some extent reflect better diagnostic awareness.

The age of onset peaks between 20 and 40 years, but the disease may present at all ages from the first few months of life to the eighties. Some series show a secondary peak of onset in the 60- to 70-year-old age group, but this has not been a universal finding. Earlier series suggested a predominance of the disease in women,

but more recently there has been little difference between the sexes.

Both in the United States of America and South Africa (Cape Town), Jews are more prone to ulcerative colitis than non-Jews by a factor of 3 or 4. Within Israel, Ashkenazi Jews have a higher incidence than Sephardim, but it is still less than the incidence in Jews in the United States of America or, indeed, than the European incidence. This suggests that environmental factors may be involved in addition to genetic factors. However, the differences in incidence between urban as opposed to rural communities or between different socio-economic groups have been slight and inconstant.

Aetiology

The cause(s) of ulcerative colitis remains unknown. The main hypotheses that have been proposed include genetic predisposition, infection, allergy to dietary components, immune responses to bacterial or self-antigens, an abnormality in epithelial cell integrity, and the psychosomatic theory. There are virtually no data to support a primary role for psychosomatic factors in the aetiology of the disease, although they may play a secondary role in determining the pattern of symptoms and must always be considered when managing individual patients.

Genetic factors

The familial incidence of ulcerative colitis has long been recognized, with 10 to 20% of patients likely to have at least one other family member affected either with ulcerative colitis or with Crohn's disease. Most of the familial association is within first-degree relatives. Within a multiply affected family there is a high degree of concordance for disease characteristics (e.g. extent, severity, presence of extraintestinal manifestations). Familial incidence may, of course, reflect that family members are often exposed to common environmental factors. However, the higher concordance in monozygotic twins than in dizygotic twins provides strong evidence that genetic factors play a role in determining disease susceptibility. Nevertheless, the concordance rates for ulcerative colitis in monozygotic twins is still quite low at 6 to 12%, suggesting that the genetic component of an individuals risk of developing the disease is much less than it is for Crohn's disease, where concordance rates for identical twins is 35 to 45%.

The mode of inheritance is unknown, but as with Crohn's disease, multiple genes are probably involved in determining disease susceptibility and its behaviour. Studies of multiply affected families, using microsatellite technology, have demonstrated linkage to chromosome 12 and, less strongly, to chromosomes 3 and 7. These susceptibility loci are shared by patients with Crohn's disease, although some evidence suggests that the locus on chromosome 12 contains two separate genes, one for ulcerative colitis and a second for Crohn's disease. Large genome-wide association studies are defining genomic regions of interest more accurately and hence aid the detection of the relevant genes. In most studies, ulcerative colitis is more strongly linked to chromosome 6p (the HLA region) than is Crohn's disease. Study of individual HLA alleles has shown that possession of HLA DRI03 is likely to be associated with severe disease. In Japan and in the Jewish population of California the disease is associated with HLA DRI502 (an allele of DR2 common in these populations but very uncommon in Europeans).

Table 15.12.1 Incidence of ulcerative colitis

	Period of study	Incidence (per 10^5)
USA		
Minnesota	1935–64	7.2
Baltimore	1960–63	4.6
UK		
Oxford	1951–60	6.5
Wales	1968–77	7.2
Aberdeen	1967–76	11.3
Denmark		
Copenhagen	1962–78	8.1
	1981–88	9.5
Netherlands		
Leiden	1979–83	6.8
Sweden		
Stockholm County	1975–79	4.3
Israel		
Tel-Aviv	1961–70	3.6

The occurrence of extraintestinal manifestations also appears to be related to genetic make-up. For example, patients who develop a reactive, large-joint arthropathy in association with active disease are likely to possess the HLA DR103 allele (35%), compared with patients who do not (8%) or healthy controls (3%). In contrast, the small-joint, seronegative arthropathy is associated with HLA B44 (77%) and MICA-8 (98%). Nevertheless, it is not possible to be sure on the basis of present knowledge whether these associations are biologically meaningful, or whether they represent linkage disequilibrium with a nearby gene.

Infection

No specific infective organism has been consistently isolated from patients with ulcerative colitis. However, the recognition that the strains of *Escherichia coli* in the normal colon are continually changing has led to the concept that patients may carry strains which, by releasing enzymes or other toxic products, might damage the mucosa. The demonstration that, even in remission, patients with ulcerative colitis are more likely than control subjects to harbour *E. coli* expressing adhesins is a particularly interesting observation, as these may allow the bacteria to adhere readily to the epithelium. The role of sulphate-reducing bacteria is also of interest as these organisms are found more commonly in those with colitis. They reduce sulphate to sulphide which, in turn, inhibits butyrate oxidation in epithelial cells. Several investigators have demonstrated reduced activity of butyrate dehydrogenase within colitic epithelium, even in remission, raising the possibility that luminal bacteria may have a deleterious effect on epithelial cell metabolism and, hence, integrity. Studies of the luminal microbiota using ribosomal RNA analysis have not only shown that the human colon contains at least 500 species of bacteria, less than one-half having been identified by culture, but that changes occur in patients with ulcerative colitis, although these do not appear to be consistent from one patient to another. Evidence is accumulating that disease susceptibility may be mediated by host genetic factors affecting adaptive immunity, innate immunity, and autophagy (a normal intracellular process for degrading organelles but also involved in antigen presentation and bacterial degradation), although this is admittedly stronger for Crohn's disease than for ulcerative colitis.

Food allergy

The early suggestions of allergic responses to milk proteins, eggs, and other dietary proteins have not been substantiated as an aetiological factor. Milk-free diets may be beneficial in a few patients, but it is not clear whether this results from an associated hypolactasia, an immunological response, or some other mechanism. The failure of ulcerative colitis to respond either to avoidance of oral food by intravenous nutrition, or to colonic isolation by means of a split ileostomy, are further pointers that dietary factors play little part.

Other environmental factors

As well as infection and diet, smoking and the use of oral contraceptives may influence disease. Many studies have now shown that ulcerative colitis is more common in non-smokers than smokers, with a relative risk of 2 to 6. Ex-smokers have a particularly high incidence, and this is highest for former heavy smokers compared with light smokers. Women taking oral contraceptives may have a slightly increased risk of the disease, but this association is weak and loses significance when the data are corrected for smoking habits and social class. Minor infections, paracetamol, and nonsteroidal anti-inflammatory drugs (NSAIDs) have been implicated, especially as triggers for a relapse, but the data are inconclusive, which largely reflects small sample sizes.

Immunopathogenesis

The intense infiltration of the inflamed mucosa with plasma cells, B and T lymphocytes, and macrophages suggests immunological activity. It is not known whether activation of both humoral and cellular immune mechanisms merely reflects increased antigenic absorption through an abnormal epithelium, a response to a specific aetiological agent, or an underlying defect in mucosal immunoregulation. The inability to down-regulate an immune response to luminal antigen is a hypothesis that is supported by some of the genetic data, as well as by experiments using animal models of colitis. A wide variety of immune-manipulated mouse models have shown that these animals develop colitis when grown in a specific pathogen-free environment, but that colitis does not develop in animals reared in germ-free environments until they are given oral bacteria. Interestingly, some strains of mice are more susceptible than others, which clearly indicates a genetic susceptibility to exogenous antigen, hence a dysregulated response to luminal antigen may underlie much of the pathogenesis of ulcerative colitis.

There is an increase in plasma cells synthesizing all three of the major immunoglobulin isotypes: IgA, IgG, and IgM. However, the largest proportional increase is in IgG-producing cells, and this is predominantly of the IgG1 and IgG3 subclasses, in contrast to Crohn's disease where an IgG2 response is predominant. IgG1 and IgG3 are synthesized in response to protein antigen and are effective in fixing complement. Complement activation is known to occur in active colitis, probably as a result of the formation of antigen–antibody complexes, and is likely to be one of the principal effector mechanisms in establishing the inflammatory lesion. Some of the increased mucosal IgG synthesized is known to have antibody specificity for bacterial and epithelial antigens. As antibody to epithelial antigens, especially a 40-kDa protein, is a feature of ulcerative colitis, rather than Crohn's disease, it is possible that autoimmunity plays a part in ulcerative colitis. This concept is strengthened by the association with other autoimmune disorders and with circulating antibodies to neutrophils (pANCA), neither of which is associated with Crohn's disease. Nevertheless, whether anticolon antibodies or pANCA have a pathogenetic role is still uncertain.

The main subsets of T cells (CD4+, CD8+) are present in increased numbers in the inflamed mucosa, but their proportions do not change significantly. Several lines of evidence suggest that the T cells are activated and release a variety of cytokines. Whether there is a failure of T cells to either up-regulate or down-regulate the mucosal immune response has not been clearly shown. However, data suggest that there may indeed be a failure to induce suppression to specific antigens, which could lead to some of the immunological overactivity that is observed in this disease. Intraepithelial T lymphocytes isolated from colons resected for severe ulcerative colitis also fail to suppress T-cell proliferative responses to specific antigens, a property that is not due to the increased numbers of intraepithelial T lymphocytes using γδ T-cell receptors.

As well as T-cell activation, there is also a marked increase in the population of activated macrophages, which not only release inflammatory mediators (reactive oxygen metabolites, leukotrienes, platelet-activating factor) but serine proteases, metalloproteinases, and cytokines. The release of interleukin 1 (IL-1), IL-6, and tumour necrosis factor (TNF) will not only lead to tissue damage but will initiate an acute-phase response, down-regulate albumin synthesis, and induce fever. Release of interferon-γ from activated T cells induces HLA class II molecules on colonic epithelial cells, which are then able to present antigen to the adjacent CD4+ lymphocytes and activate CD8+ intraepithelial T lymphocytes. Changes in epithelial permeability induced by interferon-γ and inflammatory mediators, endothelial damage by a wide variety of cytokines and mediators leading to local ischaemia, and stimulation of collagen synthesis by transforming growth factor β (TGFβ), IL-1 and IL-6, may all contribute to the inflammatory process.

Pathology

Macroscopic features

Ulcerative colitis always involves the rectum, but in about 40% of patients the disease is limited to the rectum and sigmoid. In adults, only about 20% will have the whole colon involved, although this proportion rises to about 50% in children. In mild disease, the mucosa is hyperaemic and granular, but small punctate ulcers appear as the disease becomes more severe, which may then enlarge and extend deeply into the lamina propria. The ulceration may be linear along the line of the taeniae coli, and the mucosa can become intensely haemorrhagic. Inflammatory polyps (pseudopolyps) may develop in patients with longstanding disease: these are usually found in the colon and rarely in the rectum, are of no significance, and have no malignant potential. In some patients they may regress over time.

When the disease goes into remission, the colonic appearances may return to normal, but—especially in patients who have had recurrent attacks—the mucosa becomes atrophic and featureless. There is often narrowing and shortening of the bowel. Fibrous strictures complicating long-standing chronic disease are extremely rare.

If an acute dilatation occurs in a patient with severe disease, the bowel becomes thin and congested. There is usually severe ulceration, with only small islands of mucosa remaining, and the bowel may perforate.

Microscopic features

The inflammation of ulcerative colitis is largely confined to the mucosa. The lamina propria becomes oedematous, with dilated and congested capillaries, and extravasation of red blood cells. There is a cellular infiltrate of acute and chronic inflammatory cells: neutrophils, lymphocytes, plasma cells, macrophages, mast cells, and eosinophils.

The neutrophils invade the epithelium, usually in the crypts, giving rise to a cryptitis and eventually to a crypt abscess. The triggers for this migration of neutrophils are unknown, but chemotactic peptides of colonic bacteria (e.g. formyl methionyl leucyl phenylalanine) as well as IL-8, leukotriene B4, platelet-activating factor, and activated complement are potential candidates.

Damage to the crypts leads to increased epithelial cell turnover and discharge of mucus from goblet cells. With increasing inflammation, the surface epithelial cells become flattened and irregular, and eventually ulcerate. Deep ulcers may extend into the lamina propria, leading to inflammatory changes in the submucosa that may be accompanied by an acute dilatation or perforation.

Many of the acute changes of ulcerative colitis are nonspecific and may also be seen in infective colitis. However, the diagnosis of ulcerative colitis can be made with some accuracy (>80% probability) if features of a chronic inflammatory process are present. These include distorted crypt architecture, crypt atrophy, basal lymphoid aggregates, and a chronic inflammatory infiltrate.

Histological appearances may return to normal once the disease has gone into remission, but there is frequently evidence of bifid or shortened crypts, hyperplasia of the muscularis mucosae, neuronal hypertrophy, and Paneth-cell metaplasia at the base of the crypts.

Clinical features

Patients usually present with a gradual onset of symptoms, often intermittent, but becoming progressively more severe. Occasionally, ulcerative colitis can present much more rapidly and may mimic an infective colitis. Indeed, some patients begin with a documented infection such as campylobacter or salmonella colitis, but continue to have symptoms that ultimately lead to the correct diagnosis.

The principal symptoms include diarrhoea, rectal bleeding, the passage of mucus, and—less frequently—abdominal pain. When the inflammation is confined to the rectum (proctitis), patients often pass fresh blood, which is usually mixed with the stool but can be streaked on the surface. These patients often complain of constipation rather than diarrhoea and, on clinical symptoms alone, may be mistakenly diagnosed as suffering from haemorrhoids. When the inflammation extends beyond the rectum, there is usually diarrhoea with the passage of partly altered blood. The diarrhoea is often accompanied by urgency and tenesmus, and patients can be incontinent. Nocturnal diarrhoea is a common symptom in the presence of severe inflammation. When severe ulcerative colitis affects most or all of the colon, patients are usually anorexic, nauseated, and have lost weight. They usually have severe diarrhoea (>6 motions daily) that becomes a slurry of faecal material, pus, and blood that resembles anchovy sauce—indeed, some patients may fail to recognize that they are passing blood. Patients may also complain of malaise, lassitude, and symptoms referable to chronic iron deficiency or to some of the extraintestinal manifestations, especially recurrent aphthous ulcers of the mouth.

On examination, patients with mild or moderate attacks usually look well and exhibit few abnormal physical signs. Weight should always be recorded and, for children and adolescents, both height and weight should be noted on growth charts. Abdominal examination may reveal a tender colon but is often normal. Bowel sounds are normal and rectal examination is also normal, apart from revealing blood in some cases.

Patients with a severe attack may also look deceptively well, with tachycardia or a tender colon sometimes the only abnormal signs. However, many of these patients are obviously ill, with fever, salt and water depletion, anaemia, and evidence of weight loss. There may be oral candidiasis, aphthous ulceration, signs of iron deficiency, and finger clubbing. The skin changes of hypoalbuminaemia and dependent oedema may occur. The abdomen is often distended and tympanitic, with reduced bowel sounds and marked colonic tenderness.

Minor perianal disease, such as a fissure, may occur in patients with an active ulcerative colitis, but this is never as severe as is seen in patients with Crohn's disease.

Assessment of disease severity

This can be done clinically, by grading the degree of inflammation seen endoscopically or histologically, and by using laboratory tests of inflammatory activity. Many activity indices have been devised for the purpose of clinical trials, but these are rarely used in day-to-day practice apart from the following simple guide.

Clinical grading

1 Mild—there are fewer than four stools daily, with or without blood, with no systemic disturbance and a normal erythrocyte sedimentation rate

2 Moderate—this is between mild and severe

3 Severe—there are at least six stools daily, with bleeding, and evidence of systemic illness as shown by fever, tachycardia, a falling haemoglobin, hypoalbuminaemia, and raised erythrocyte sedimentation rate and C-reactive protein (CRP).

Laboratory markers of inflammation

Active disease is often accompanied by a neutrophil leucocytosis, thrombocytosis, and a rise in acute-phase proteins (e.g. CRP) and in erythrocyte sedimentation rate (ESR). There may also be a fall in haemoglobin and albumin levels. These inflammatory markers are useful when measured serially during the course of treatment as an indicator of disease activity. However, if corticosteroids are used, the white cell count can no longer be used as a marker of disease activity because it will often rise in response to the steroids. Patients with a proctitis rarely have a rise in CRP unless the inflammation is particularly severe.

Faecal calprotectin, which is released from neutrophils and therefore a marker of acute inflammation even in the absence of symptoms, has recently been identified as a sensitive marker of disease activity. It may be useful in differential diagnosis (e.g. an elevated faecal calprotectin value in a patient previously diagnosed as having an irritable bowel syndrome indicates the need to reconsider the diagnosis), and it may also be useful to monitor the response to therapy and to screen asymptomatic relatives who are concerned about familial risk.

Investigation and diagnosis

The diagnosis of ulcerative colitis is made on the basis of the history, the absence of faecal pathogens, and the endoscopic and histological appearances of the colon.

Stool cultures

Stool cultures should be set up for all patients presenting for the first time and, ideally, for all those presenting with a relapse of established disease. Special culture conditions are required for campylobacter, yersinia, gonococci, and *Clostridium difficile*. The possibility of an infection with *E. coli* 0157 must also be considered, especially in patients in whom bleeding and abdominal pain are predominant symptoms. An infective colitis with opportunistic organisms in patients with immunodeficiency syndromes has become much more common and has to be remembered in the differential diagnosis.

Sigmoidoscopy and colonoscopy

Sigmoidoscopy is safe, even in patients with a severe attack, and not only confirms rectal inflammation but also allows a biopsy specimen to be taken and an assessment of severity to be obtained. Although some centres use colonoscopy in severe attacks, this is rarely necessary for diagnosis, for assessment of severity, or for determining management. It is best avoided in the acute stage. The earliest signs of colitis on sigmoidoscopy are blurring of the vascular pattern associated with hyperaemia and oedema, leading to blunting of the valves of Houston. With increasing severity, the mucosa becomes granular and then friable. With severe inflammation, the mucosa shows spontaneous bleeding and ulceration (Fig. 15.12.1). These changes begin in the rectum, they are diffuse, and extend proximally to affect a variable length of the colon. Severe attacks of the disease can be associated with relative rectal sparing. The reason for this is not known, but the finding can be wrongly used to diagnose Crohn's disease of the colon. Pseudopolyps (inflammatory polyps) often occur in patients with long-standing disease, but tend to be in the colon rather than the rectum: they have no malignant potential and may even regress over many years if the disease remains in remission.

Colonoscopy with multiple biopsies is useful for assessing the extent of disease and is mandatory for patients with a colonic stricture. It is also required for cancer surveillance (see later). Preparation of the colon should follow the normal methods, with osmotic purgation being the most satisfactory. However, a more gentle approach is needed if colonoscopy is done in the presence of severe inflammation, but this is rarely indicated.

Biopsy specimens must be taken at sigmoidoscopy or colonoscopy, preferably with small, cupped forceps. Histological assessment contributes to grading severity as well as the differential diagnosis.

Imaging

All patients with a severe attack must have a plain abdominal radiograph. Not only does this exclude a dilated colon, but it may

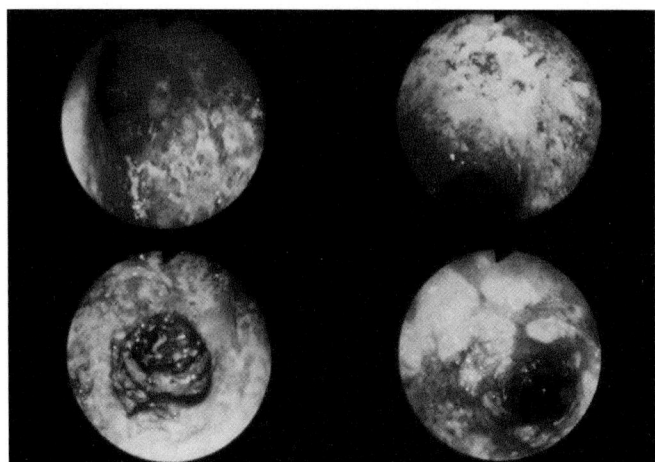

Fig. 15.12.1 Sigmoidoscopic appearances of severe ulcerative colitis showing spontaneous bleeding and ulceration.

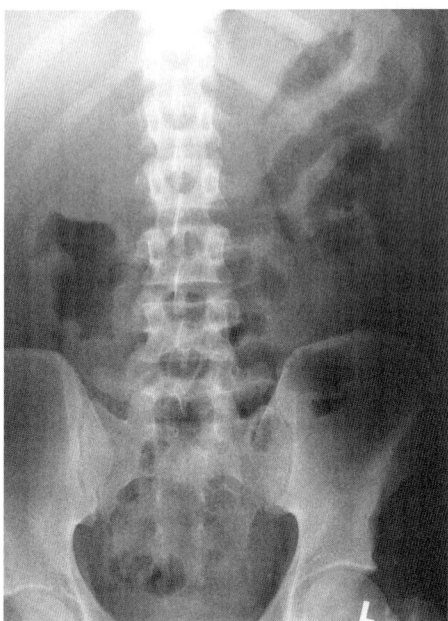

Fig. 15.12.2 Plain abdominal radiograph of a 24-year-old man with severe ulcerative colitis. The ascending and transverse colon arc grossly oedematous and diseased with loss of the normal haustral pattern. In addition, there are multiple loops of distended small intestine.

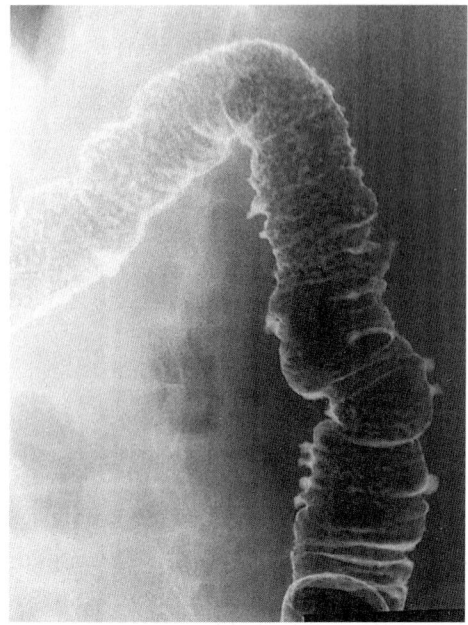

Fig. 15.12.3 A double-contrast barium enema in a patient with active ulcerative colitis. The figure is a close-up view of the splenic flexure to show extensive mucosal ulceration, loss of haustration, and narrowing of the colon. The patient also has diverticula in the descending colon.

provide prognostic information (mucosal islands, distended small-bowel loops) and demonstrate the extent of the disease. An abnormal haustral pattern, thickening of the bowel wall, and mucosal oedema can be detected on a plain film (Fig. 15.12.2). As an inflamed colon does not hold faecal material, the presence of faecal matter in the ascending or transverse colon will indicate that the inflammation is distal.

Barium radiography has largely been superseded by colonoscopy and is virtually never indicated in a severe attack, but—if required—a single-contrast study in an unprepared colon with barium entering the colon at low pressure should be used. In less severe disease, a double-contrast barium enema can be safely given (Fig. 15.12.3), but the colon must not be overdistended and the procedure must be stopped if the patient complains of pain.

Other laboratory data

These are required for assessing severity, as discussed above, and to document haematological or biochemical complications.

Iron deficiency is common as a result of chronic iron loss; this can be exacerbated by a severe attack, in which 0.5 g of elemental iron can be lost. Thus, a hypochromic, microcytic anaemia is frequently present. A neutrophil leucocytosis, thrombocytosis, eosinophilia, or monocytosis may also be present and are indicators of active inflammation.

Biochemical abnormalities are rare in mild or moderate attacks, but hypokalaemia, hypoalbuminaemia, and a rise in gammaglobulin frequently accompany a severe attack. Minor elevations of the aspartate transaminase or alkaline phosphatase are also frequently seen in patients with a severe attack, but they return to normal when the disease goes into remission. They probably reflect a fatty liver, together with the effects of toxaemia or poor nutrition. Persistent elevation, especially of alkaline phosphatase, may indicate underlying chronic liver disease and needs further investigation

(see below). Serum immunoglobulins rarely exceed the upper limit of normal during a relapse, but usually fall as remission occurs.

Differential diagnosis

Symptoms of gradual onset

If the patient has a history of slow onset of symptoms, including blood and mucus, and has diffuse inflammation on sigmoidoscopy, the diagnosis of ulcerative colitis is highly probable. The major differential diagnosis is Crohn's disease (see Chapter 15.11). If clinical, radiological, endoscopic, and histological information is considered together, less than 10% of patients fall into the category of indeterminate colitis, a term originally used to describe an uncertain colitis based on the examination of a colectomy specimen and therefore inappropriate when only biopsy specimens are available, hence the recommended term is 'colitis, not yet classified'.

Collagenous colitis usually has only a mild inflammation on colonoscopy and is diagnosed on the basis of a thickened subepithelial collagen band (wider than 15 μm) seen in a rectal biopsy specimen. Microscopic or lymphocytic colitis has a normal endoscopic appearance but shows a diffuse infiltration of the lamina propria with lymphocytes and eosinophils on histological examination. Although ischaemic colitis classically occurs around the splenic flexure, it may occur in the rectum, especially in older people, and can be diagnosed histologically. Radiation damage to the rectum may occur, especially in men who have had radiotherapy to the prostate.

Rarely, a drug-induced colitis may occur. The drugs that have been implicated include NSAIDs, gold, penicillamine, and 5-aminosalicylic acid. This last drug may cause considerable diagnostic confusion in patients who already have ulcerative colitis. An antibiotic history must be taken, but a pseudomembranous colitis secondary to *C. difficile* can occur in the absence of antibiotic usage, especially in older people.

Symptoms of acute onset

For those patients presenting with a much more acute history, infective forms of colitis must be excluded by stool culture. A sudden onset of symptoms, the predominance of abdominal pain, the ingestion of potentially infected food (chicken, shellfish), and evidence of diarrhoeal disease in contacts are obvious pointers to an infection. Sigmoidoscopic appearances are usually very similar to ulcerative colitis, but a rectal biopsy can be very useful in distinguishing an infective from a more chronic ulcerative colitis. The presence of a chronic inflammatory infiltrate, architectural disturbances of the glands, and basal lymphoid aggregates favour ulcerative colitis. The common organisms causing an infective colitis are salmonella, shigella, and campylobacter. Yersinial infections may also cause colitis and can pursue a chronic course over many months before resolving. Special culture conditions may isolate the organism from stool, but a rising titre of serum antibody is often the more reliable method of identifying the infection. *E. coli* 0157 is a recognized cause of an acute colitis, especially in institutions, and massive bleeding is often a characteristic feature. Children may develop a haemolytic uraemic syndrome. Diagnosis is difficult because most laboratories are not equipped either to detect this strain of *E. coli* or to measure specific antibody. For patients who have travelled in endemic areas, amoebic and schistosomal colitis must be considered; stool examination and histological demonstration of amoebas or schistosomal ova in rectal biopsy specimens make the diagnosis.

Other causes of infective colitis can occur in immunosuppressed patients and include cytomegalovirus, herpes simplex, and *Mycobacterium avium intracellulare*. Although these organisms usually cause fairly characteristic sigmoidoscopic appearances, they can be associated with a more diffuse pattern of inflammation. Other sexually transmitted causes of proctitis (gonorrhoea, chlamydia, lymphogranuloma) do not usually cause diarrhoea and, especially with gonorrhoea, are associated with the passage of watery pus.

Other considerations

Ulcerative colitis also has to be differentiated from irritable bowel syndrome, colonic polyps or carcinoma, diverticular disease, solitary rectal ulcer syndrome, and factitious diarrhoea. Sigmoidoscopy usually clarifies the diagnosis, but if the ulceration of the solitary rectal ulcer syndrome becomes circumferential, this can be mistaken for ulcerative colitis. A biopsy specimen showing strands of smooth muscle radiating up into the lamina propria between the glands is characteristic of the solitary ulcer syndrome.

Extraintestinal manifestations

The extraintestinal manifestations of ulcerative colitis are listed in Box 15.12.1.

Skin

An erythematous, macular skin rash, sometimes photosensitive, that used to be common in patients with ulcerative colitis was a hypersensitivity rash to sulphasalazine (related to the sulphapyridine moiety). However, this is now rarely seen because most patients are maintained on other formulations of 5-aminosalicylic acid

---

Box 15.12.1 Extraintestinal manifestations of ulcerative colitis

Related to activity of colitis
- Aphthous ulceration of the mouth
- Fatty liver
- Erythema nodosum
- Peripheral arthropathy
- Episleritis
- Pyoderma gangrenosum

Usually unrelated to activity of colitis
- Anterior uveitis
- Unrelated to colitis
- Sacroiliitis
- Ankylosing spondylitis
- Primary sclerosing cholangitis
- Cholangiocarcinoma

---

which do not contain the sulphonamide. Urticaria can rarely occur in association with mesalazine.

Erythema nodosum occurs in about 2 to 4% of patients and is mostly associated with active disease. The lesions occur most commonly on the anterior aspect of the lower legs. Pyoderma gangrenosum is rare (1–2%) and is usually seen in patients with active disease, but occasionally persists despite inactive colitis. The lesions usually begin as sterile pustules, usually on the limbs, which break down as they enlarge and finally coalesce. Ulceration leads to necrosis and the lesions become surrounded by black, necrotic tissue. Treatment of the colitis is usually followed by regression of the skin lesions, but pyoderma can be very resistant to therapy and may only respond following colectomy, but it can persist even then. Recently, anti-TNF monoclonal antibodies (e.g. infliximab, adalimumab, certolizumab) have been shown to be very useful in treating refractory pyoderma, including peristomal lesions in patients who have an ileostomy: following an induction regimen, maintenance administration is usually necessary to keep the pyoderma in remission.

Mouth

Crops of aphthous ulcers are common in patients with active disease. A sore tongue and angular stomatitis often accompany chronic iron deficiency.

Eyes

Episcleritis or anterior uveitis occur in 5 to 8% of patients. Local corticosteroids and treatment of active colitis usually lead to resolution.

Joints

An acute arthropathy occurs in 10 to 15% of patients with active disease. It affects the larger joints (knees, hips, ankles, wrists, elbows) and is usually asymmetrical. It is a non-erosive condition and settles as the colitis goes into remission. A less common joint complication is a symmetrical small-joint polyarthropathy, which is seronegative and is unrelated to the activity of the colitis.

Low back pain is a common symptom and usually due to sacroiliitis, which can be seen by plain radiology in 12 to 15% of patients and in 30 to 35% by MRI. It is unrelated to the activity of the colitis, is not strongly associated with HLA B27, and rarely progresses to ankylosing spondylitis. The latter disease occurs in only 1 to 2% of patients, with 60% of these having the HLA B27 phenotype. There is a 2:1 ratio in favour of males with this complication. The spondylitis may present before the colitis becomes apparent or may follow the intestinal symptoms. Its natural history is independent to that of the colitis and should be treated with physiotherapy, hydrotherapy, and—if necessary—NSAIDs. However, these drugs can occasionally worsen the colitis and should therefore be used cautiously. Anti-TNF antibodies are highly effective in relieving the pain of either sacroiliitis or ankylosing spondylitis.

Liver disease

Patients with severe attacks of ulcerative colitis often have minor elevations of alkaline phosphatase or transaminases. The cause of these enzyme rises is probably multifactorial, including malnutrition, sepsis, and a fatty liver, which occurs in up to 60% of patients undergoing urgent colectomy. The liver enzymes return to normal when remission is achieved, but there may be persistent abnormalities in liver enzymes in about 3% of patients, usually a rise in alkaline phosphatase. The overwhelming majority of these patients will have primary sclerosing cholangitis when the bile duct is visualized by endoscopic cholangiography (see Chapter 15.21.4). Histologically, liver biopsy specimens show evidence of chronic liver disease, but the spectrum of appearances ranges from those of an autoimmune hepatitis to the classic picture of concentric periductular fibrosis with obliteration of bile ducts.

Many patients with ulcerative colitis and sclerosing cholangitis remain well for many years. The colitis is often very mild, though frequently affecting the whole colon, but the liver disease is progressive and ultimately leads to portal hypertension and liver failure. Sclerosing cholangitis is a premalignant condition and explains the well-recognized association between ulcerative colitis and cholangiocarcinoma. Furthermore, there is a high incidence of colorectal cancer, especially of the right colon, in these patients. Colonoscopic surveillance is mandatory. The pathogenesis and treatment of the liver disease are discussed in Chapter 15.21.4. The mild nature of the colonic inflammation despite extensive disease, the frequently observed rectal sparing, and the right-sided cancers have called into question whether the colonic disease is really the same as ulcerative colitis. At the present time there is no clear answer, but the possibility that primary sclerosing cholangitis (PSC)-colitis might be a distinct entity should be remembered when posing questions about pathogenesis.

Rare associations

Pericarditis with or without an effusion has been described in association with an acute attack of colitis, but a true association is not yet proven. Autoimmune haemolytic anaemia has been reported in ulcerative colitis and may recur when the colonic disease becomes active. Amyloid rarely occurs in ulcerative colitis; it is much more likely to be associated with Crohn's disease. A rapidly progressing bronchiectasis has also been described in some patients with ulcerative colitis.

Medical management

The main principles of therapy for the treatment of ulcerative colitis are to control active disease rapidly, to maintain remission, to select patients for whom surgery is appropriate, and to ensure as good a quality of life as possible. Patient education about their disease is essential, and all patients should be given the opportunity to subscribe to patient self-help groups such as the National Association for Colitis and Crohn's Disease (in the United Kingdom) or the Crohn's and Colitis Foundation of America.

Treatment of active disease

The most effective drugs for controlling active disease are the corticosteroids, which may be given systemically, topically, or in combination. Drugs containing 5-aminosalicylic acid (sulphasalazine, olsalazine, balsalazide, mesalazine) are often used to treat a mild colitis, but prednisolone has been shown to be more effective and to control symptoms more rapidly, which make it the drug of choice. The dosage and route of administration are largely governed by disease severity. Once active inflammation has been controlled and remission obtained, the corticosteroids should be tailed off because they are ineffective as maintenance therapy and prolonged use puts the patient at risk of long-term side effects such as osteoporosis.

Proctitis

Proctitis refers to disease limited to the rectum: in practice it refers to inflammation that does not extend beyond the limits of a rigid sigmoidoscope. It can be remarkably difficult to treat. Initial therapy is usually a 5-aminosalicylic acid drug by mouth in combination with topical therapy. The latter can be a corticosteroid or 5-aminosalicylic acid in the form of a suppository, with the latter shown by metaanalysis of clinical trials to be more effective and therefore the drug of choice. If a good response is not obtained, then a 5-aminosalicylic acid suppository in the morning and a steroid one in the evening can produce a better response than either alone. For patients who do not respond, oral prednisolone may be given. Some have sufficiently severe proctitis to warrant intravenous steroids, and occasionally colectomy may be necessary.

Many patients with refractory proctitis develop a severe proximal constipation, which can cause considerable abdominal discomfort, bloating, and nausea. Relief of the constipation, usually by gentle osmotic purgation, will often give considerable symptomatic benefit, and it may also be associated with a marked improvement in the inflammation. Some patients appear to be refractory because foam or enema preparations are used: changing to a suppository allows a much higher concentration of drug in the rectum and is frequently associated with improvement in symptoms.

Mildly active disease

Patients who have no more than four motions daily on average, with inflammation extending beyond the limits of the rigid sigmoidoscope, should be given 20 mg of oral prednisolone daily, together with topical steroids or 5-aminosalicylic acid (or both). Treatment should be given for at least 4 weeks, before being tailed off over the subsequent 3 to 4 weeks. Clinical trials have shown that oral 5-aminosalicylic acid formulations are more effective than placebo in treating active disease, especially in high doses. However, corticosteroids achieve remission more quickly and in a higher proportion than 5-aminosalicylic acid drugs.

Moderately active disease

Patients who have, on average, more than four bowel motions daily but who are not systemically ill should be given 40 mg of prednisolone by mouth daily. Giving larger doses (such as 60 mg daily) provides only a marginally better effect but increases the frequency of side effects quite considerably. The dose is reduced to 20 mg daily over 2 to 3 weeks and the regimen then follows that described for mild disease.

Severe disease

This is defined as an attack in which the patient has more than six bowel motions daily, with blood, and who is systemically ill as shown by tachycardia, fever, and anaemia. The colon is usually tender on palpation. These patients should be admitted to hospital and assessed by both physician and surgeon. Fluid and electrolyte losses are replaced intravenously, and blood transfusion should be given if the haemoglobin is less than 10 g/dl. Patients are given intravenous corticosteroids (such as 100 mg of hydrocortisone, 6-hourly) together with a twice daily rectal drip of hydrocortisone (100 mg in 100 ml water).

Parenteral nutrition is indicated for those who are malnourished, but intravenous saline and dextrose–saline are sufficient for most, together with potassium supplements. Most patients with a severe attack prefer to have only clear fluids by mouth during the first 24 h. Thereafter, there is no evidence that a light diet has any adverse effect on the disease, but many clinicians will leave the patient on only clear fluids for the first few days. Prophylactic heparin should be given, either unfractionated or low molecular weight, since thomboembolism is still a cause of death in these patients: this is safe and only very rarely associated with massive haemorrhage.

Provided the patient is improving, treatment is continued for 5 to 7 days. At this time, a good response is one in which the patient feels well, there is no fever or tachycardia, the colon is not tender on abdominal palpation, and the diarrhoea has largely settled, usually to less than four motions daily, with the stools rarely formed, but without macroscopic bleeding. These patients can then go on to oral prednisolone (e.g. 40 mg daily), a retention enema, an oral 5-aminosalicylic acid drug, and a light diet. By contrast, those who deteriorate during the first few days of intravenous treatment, or who have not made a substantial improvement after 3 to 4 days, need further treatment: simply continuing intravenous therapy for more than 7 to 10 days is rarely beneficial, and surgery is usually required. Indeed, it is now clear that patients who, after 3 days of intravenous steroid therapy, still have marked diarrhoea (>8 stools/24 h) or 4 to 6 stools daily with a CRP of more than 45 mg/litre, have a very high chance (85%) of requiring urgent surgery. For this group of patients, proceeding directly to urgent surgery may be appropriate if they have had difficult, refractory colitis prior to the current admission, but 'rescue' therapy with either ciclosporin or infliximab should be considered for those having their first attack of colitis, or for patients whose previous history of colitis has always been associated with good quality of life.

Rescue therapies

Ciclosporin will induce remission in 60 to 80% of patients not responding to intravenous steroids. This should be added after 3 to 5 days of steroid therapy. It is usually given intravenously, a dose of 2 mg/kg being as effective as 4 mg/kg (although an oral formulation may be just as effective), and most patients respond very quickly (3 to 4 days), hence—for those in whom surgery becomes necessary—a decision about colectomy can be made after a week or so of treatment. Those who do respond to drug therapy can be converted to oral treatment with decreasing doses of prednisolone. Practice varies between continuing oral ciclosporin for some months, changing to azathioprine, or using the two in combination. No controlled trial data are yet available to provide evidence-based guidelines. However, it is important to recognize that ciclosporin is not a cure, and 50% of those responding will have further relapses of their ulcerative colitis and require colectomy within 5 years. For those who do ultimately come to surgery, the initial response to ciclosporin provides time for educating patients about their disease, the implications of life with a colectomy (with or without an ileoanal pouch), and the long-term prognosis. This is particularly important for young patients, especially if it is their first attack. The use of ciclosporin in the manner and dosage (low with respect to its usage in organ transplantation) described above has not been associated with major side effects, although prolonged use of high-dose steroids and ciclosporin can be associated with pneumocystis pneumonia. Blood pressure and renal function need to be closely monitored.

A small trial of intravenous infliximab has recently been published from Sweden, in which patients not responding to intravenous steroids after 5 to 10 days were randomized to receive infliximab (5 mg/kg) or placebo while continuing the steroid. The colectomy rate in the infliximab group was significantly less than in the placebo group. This trial, together with a number of small open-label studies, have shown that 65 to 80% of patients not responding to steroid therapy can be saved from colectomy during the index admission by infliximab. This is a very similar proportion to that achieved with ciclosporin, and the long-term outlook is similar, with about 50% coming to colectomy during subsequent follow-up. Whether maintenance infusions every 8 weeks will reduce the long-term colectomy rate remains to be established.

Whether ciclosporin or infliximab is used as rescue therapy is largely a matter for physician preference. In the absence of a direct comparison in the setting of a formal randomized, double-dummy trial, both drugs seem to be associated with very similar outcomes. Side-effect profiles are clearly different, but whether in the long-term infliximab is safer than ciclsporin is not known. What should be avoided is using these drugs sequentially if there is no response to one: a small series from Mount Sinai Hospital in New York showed that no therapeutic benefit is gained by so doing, whether ciclosporin was given first followed by infliximab, or vice versa, and there was high morbidity and even mortality in those who had both drugs in addition to prolonged intravenous corticosteroids.

Approximately 15–25% of patients with a severe attack will require an urgent colectomy regardless of medical therapy given. These patients can often be identified early on, using clinical and radiological features that have been shown to have prognostic significance, namely the passage of more than nine stools daily, a pulse rate greater than 100/min, or a temperature greater than 38 °C during the first 24 h of treatment. A serum albumin level of less than 30 g/litre during the first few days or the failure of acute-phase proteins such as the serum CRP to fall are also poor prognostic signs. Seventy-five per cent of patients showing mucosal islands in the colon or having more than three loops of distended small bowel on a plain abdominal radiograph will come to urgent surgery. These findings, based on retrospective studies, have been confirmed by prospective series. If rescue therapy is to be used, it should be introduced (as discussed above) on day 4 of steroid therapy so that a decision about the need for surgery can still be made within 10 days of admission. This approach minimizes the risks of patients developing opportunistic infections (e.g. pneumocystis, cytomegalovirus), of becoming malnourished, and of postoperative complications.

Chronic active disease

Some patients repeatedly relapse when they come off corticosteroids or receive a daily dose of less than 10 to 15 mg of prednisolone. Immunosuppression therapy with azathioprine or 6-mercaptopurine is often beneficial in this group. In the United Kingdom, azathioprine is the drug that is most used, in doses of 2.0 or 2.5 mg/kg, and may allow the prednisolone to be withdrawn. It usually takes 4 to 6 weeks before an effect is seen, and the drug is then continued for several months. Although few long-term sequelae have been encountered, most clinicians do not usually continue therapy for more than 18 to 24 months.

Oral ciclosporin (5 mg/kg) has also been used for chronic active disease, but no formal clinical trials have been made. High-dose prednisolone (40 mg) given on alternate days is another approach that may be useful. However, if the patient's lifestyle is impaired by chronic disabling symptoms or by the side effects of treatment, surgical management should be considered. Recently, two trials have reported favourably on the use of infliximab in patients refractory to medical therapy: following infusions at 0, 2, and 6 weeks about 60% had a response, but only about 20% went into prolonged remission.

Maintenance of remission

Salicylate drugs

Sulphasalazine and its active moiety, 5-aminosalicylic acid, reduce the relapse rate by about fourfold and are able to maintain the disease in remission when given over many years. Thus, provided they are well tolerated, they should be given indefinitely. For sulphasalazine, the optimal dose to obtain good therapeutic efficacy with the least side effects is 2 g daily. Common side effects are nausea, anorexia, and headache: these are dose related and caused by the sulphapyridine component. Other side effects, which are also usually due to the sulphonamide but are not dose related, include hypersensitivity skin rashes, male infertility, agranulocytosis, and Heinz-body haemolytic anaemia. Overall, 10 to 15% of patients are unable to take the drug, although the nausea and headache can often be overcome by starting at a low dose and gradually increasing.

Sulphasalazine is an unusual drug in that it is poorly absorbed in the stomach and small intestine. When it reaches the colon, the azobond linking the 5-aminosalicylic acid and sulphapyridine moieties is split by bacterial azoreductases. The sulphapyridine is absorbed, metabolized in the liver, and excreted in the urine. The majority of the 5-aminosalicylic acid (c.70%) is poorly absorbed and excreted in the faeces. As it is the 5-aminosalicylic acid that is the active compound, several drugs are now available that present 5-aminosalicylic acid to the colon without the sulphapyridine that causes most of the side effects of sulphasalazine. The 5-aminosalicylic acid cannot simply be given by mouth as it is rapidly absorbed. Thus, it is either given as a delayed-release formulation (the mesalazine group) or as a prodrug (olsalazine, balsalazide). Table 15.12.2 lists these and details their characteristics.

Table 15.12.2 The salicylate drugs

	Characteristics
Mesalazine preparations	
Enteric coated	
Asacol	Coated with Eudragit, S 5-ASA released at pH 7.0
Claversal, Salofalk	Coated with Eudragit, L 5-ASA released at pH 6.5
Controlled release	
Pentasa	Tablets comprise 5-ASA granules coated with ethyl cellulose; released with time at pH >6.5
Mezavant (Lialda in USA)	Mesalazine in multimatrix formulation
Prodrugs	
Sulphasalazine	5-ASA linked to sulphapyridine by an azo bond which is split by colonic bacteria
Olsalazine	Two molecules of 5-ASA linked with an azo bond
Balsalazide	5-ASA lined to an amino acid by an azo bond

5-ASA, 5-aminosalicylic acid.

Which drug containing 5-aminosalicylic acid should be prescribed as maintenance therapy for ulcerative colitis? Sulphasalazine is well tolerated by 85% or so of patients, is cheap, and serious side effects (such as Stevens–Johnson syndrome, agranulocytosis, and pancreatitis) are very rare. The newer drugs are more expensive than sulphasalazine, but they have equal therapeutic efficacy and are now the drugs of choice. In general they are associated with fewer side effects, but occasional patients develop typical salicylate reactions (rhinitis, urticaria, and colitis). About 10 to 12% of patients will develop loose stools when given olsalazine: this gradually settles if treatment is continued, but about 5% will develop severe watery diarrhoea that usually necessitates stopping the drug. The risk of diarrhoea can be minimized by taking the drug with food. Progressive renal failure due to chronic interstitial nephritis is a recognized complication, mostly associated with the delayed-release forms of mesalazine, and all patients taking this require regular monitoring of their serum creatinine (eGFR), with renal consultation in the event that this deteriorates. Sulphasalazine is still a useful drug for those patients with joint symptoms as it often benefits those while maintaining the colonic disease in remission.

Diet

Patients with recurrent, severe disease are slightly prone to hypolactasia, and a lactose-free diet may be beneficial. Individual patients may be intolerant of dairy products, wheat, eggs, and other dietary constituents, but most patients should have a normal, well-balanced diet.

Surgical management

The indications for surgery are:

1 severe inflammation unresponsive to medical therapy

2 acute complications-perforation, dilatation

3 for chronic active disease

4 to prevent cancer

The choice of operation is partly determined by the expertise available and the activity of the disease. When surgery is performed for a severe attack, a one-stage proctocolectomy with a Brooke ileostomy has been shown to be a safe and effective procedure. The major problems with the operation are poor healing of the perineal wound, adhesion obstruction, and ileostomy dysfunction. Sexual dysfunction in males rarely occurs if a perimuscular excision of the rectum is made. However, with the advent of restorative proctocolectomy with the formation of an ileoanal reservoir or pouch, many surgeons will do only a colectomy in the acute stage. The rectal stump is either oversewn (which is not recommended as it often leaks, with abscess formation), or brought out as a mucous fistula either in the lower end of the wound or in the left iliac fossa. This allows histological examination of the whole colon to exclude Crohn's disease. The rectum is excised and the pouch formed some months later when nutrition has been restored and the patient is not taking corticosteroids or immunosuppressive drugs.

Restorative proctocolectomy with ileoanal reservoir/pouch

Restorative proctocolectomy has become the procedure of choice in specialist centres, provided the anal sphincter is intact, hence this operation is not advised over the age of 65 years. The two-limb (J) pouch is now the favoured design, with most surgeons preserving the anal transitional zone by anastomosing the pouch 1 to 2 cm above the dentate line. This allows for a stapled anastomosis, which shortens the operation and is associated with better continence than a mucosectomy that inevitably requires anal dilatation by retractors. If the operation is being carried out for high-grade dysplasia or cancer, most surgeons will perform a mucosectomy and hand-sew the pouch to the dentate line.

Most patients who undergo a pouch operation have excellent function, with less than 10% having any leakage, which is usually limited to night-time soiling. Nevertheless, all patients should be advised to wear a pad at first after a pouch procedure. The pouch usually requires emptying 6 to 12 times daily within the first few weeks of functioning, and loperamide is usually needed. Adaptation occurs during the first few months, and by the end of a year the emptying frequency is around four to six times daily, but without urgency. Good function persists in the long term (>10 years). Complications of the pouch, once the immediate surgery is over, include anal stenosis, adhesion obstruction and pouchitis, at least one attack of which occurs in 40 to 50% of patients during the first 5 years, consisting of diarrhoea with blood and evidence of inflammation on endoscopy. It usually responds to antibiotics such as metronidazole or ciprofloxacin, but occasionally requires topical treatment with corticosteroids or 5-aminosalicylic acid. Refractory pouchitis can be a severe management problem: the use of probiotic preparations can maintain some of these patients in remission, but others may require immunosuppressives, infliximab or even removal of the pouch.

The causes of pouchitis are heterogeneous and include ischaemia, infection with a recognized pathogen (such as campylobacter), and poor emptying, but most pouchitis attacks are unexplained. Poor emptying can be recognized by isotopic scanning using a radiolabelled artificial stool and usually responds to regular catheterization of the pouch. Idiopathic pouchitis is particularly interesting in so far as it is only seen in patients who have previously had ulcerative colitis, and rarely if ever in patients who have a pouch for other reasons. After the formation of a pouch, for whatever indication, the ileal mucosa undergoes colonic metaplasia. The triggers for this are unknown but almost certainly involve luminal stasis. Thus, whatever factors first render individuals susceptible to developing ulcerative colitis also seem to render them susceptible to developing acute inflammation in ileal mucosa that has undergone colonic metaplasia.

With increasing use of restorative proctocolectomy, there is increasing recognition that there is often a reduced fecundability in female patients. This problem should be discussed with the patient before the procedure is performed and, in some centres, ova are harvested and frozen in case of subsequent infertility. Male patients should also be counselled with regard to subsequent impotence, although this is a rare occurrence given good surgical technique.

Some patients have poor pouch function which is not due to pouchitis. Some will have cuffitis or prepouch ileitis to account for symptoms, but others have poor function due to noninflammatory causes. These include dietary intolerance, motility disorders, bacterial overgrowth in the small intestine, and a concomitant irritable bowel syndrome.

Local complications and their treatments
Perianal lesions

Minor lesions such as fissures, perianal abscesses, or haemorrhoids may occur in patients with ulcerative colitis, but extensive lesions such as fistulas are exceptional and suggest Crohn's disease. Treatment of fissures involves treatment of active inflammation. Surgical treatment should be avoided wherever possible and, if necessary, should be conservative.

Massive haemorrhage

This rarely occurs in association with severe attacks. Intravenous corticosteroids and blood transfusion usually allow the bleeding to stop. However, urgent colectomy must be considered if patients have already received six or more units of blood and are still bleeding.

Perforation

This is the most dangerous of the local complications and carries appreciable mortality. In patients receiving corticosteroids, the physical signs of peritonitis may not be obvious, and malaise, tachycardia, and reduced or absent bowel sounds may be the only clinical features. Plain abdominal films usually show free intraabdominal gas. It may complicate an acute dilatation but can occur in its absence. Management consists of immediate intravenous fluid, electrolytes, antibiotics and hydrocortisone, with urgent colectomy performed within 24 h as soon as the patient has been resuscitated. The mortality of a perforation is as high as 16%, even in specialist centres.

Acute dilatation

This is defined as a transverse colon with a diameter of greater than 5.0 to 6.0 cm, with loss of haustration seen on a plain radiograph in a patient with a severe attack of ulcerative colitis. It occurs in about 5% of severe attacks and can be precipitated by hypokalaemia or the administration of opiates. Abdominal signs are often minimal, but the patient is usually obtunded, the bowel sounds are reduced, and the abdomen may become distended. Medical therapy with intravenous steroids is given as usual if the colon is already dilated on presentation of a severe attack: about 50% will settle on medical therapy alone, but urgent surgery is required for those who continue to deteriorate or do not improve within 24 h. Colectomy should be performed if the colon dilates during the course of treating a severe attack.

Strictures

These occur very rarely in patients with long-standing ulcerative colitis with a shortened, narrow colon. Colonoscopy with multiple biopsies must be performed as there should be a high index of suspicion for carcinoma.

Pseudopolyps

These are common and may be filiform, sessile, or may form bridges. They can occur throughout the colon but often spare the rectum. They are not premalignant and may occasionally regress.

Colonic carcinoma

The risk of cancer is mainly in patients who have had extensive disease for more than 10 years, especially if they have had recurrent attacks. The most recent series studying primary cohorts suggest that the cumulative risk for patients with extensive disease is about 7 to 15% at 20 years, with very little risk up to 15 years of disease.

Carcinoma is usually, but not always, preceded by dysplasia. This can be detected histologically and has led to colonoscopic surveillance programmes for patients with longstanding ulcerative colitis affecting most or all of the colon. Provided no dysplasia is found (at least 30 biopsies around the colon are recommended), the examination is repeated every 1 to 3 years. If high-grade dysplasia is present, prophylactic colectomy is usually considered. For low-grade dysplasia, repeat colonoscopy within a few months is usually advised, but there are increasing reports of cancers occurring in association with low-grade dysplasia, hence colectomy is increasingly being recommended whenever dysplasia is recognized, regardless of grade. As large numbers of colonoscopies are involved in a surveillance programme, the question of cost benefit has been raised. However, two recent studies have shown that patients have a worse outcome with respect to cancer if they are not in a surveillance programme. The recent introduction of chromoendoscopy has allowed targeted biopsy of suspicious areas, which not only allows a high pick-up rate of dysplasia but also reduces the number of biopsies that need to be taken, a saving that partly offsets the increased time of the procedure. In a few specialist centres, confocal laser endoscopy provides an even more sensitive way of detecting epithelial dysplasia.

Course and prognosis

Most patients with ulcerative colitis have intermittent attacks of the disease, but the duration of remission between attacks can vary from a few weeks to many years. About 10 to 15% of patients will have a chronic continuous course and rarely achieve a full remission for any appreciable time. A few (5–10%) will have a severe first attack requiring urgent surgery, but fewer—if any—have one attack only and never relapse.

Patients with extensive or total disease are much more likely to have a severe attack within 1 year of diagnosis than patients with distal disease and are therefore at greater risk of colectomy. However, a year from diagnosis the risk of colectomy is similar in all groups, with a cumulative rate of about 1% per year. Patients with disease limited to the rectum are a special group in so far as most of them continue to have very limited involvement, with only about 30% developing more extensive disease in the 20 years after diagnosis.

Despite having a chronic relapsing disease, 90% or so of patients are able to work, with very few days of sick leave each year. Nevertheless, quality of life can be impaired in many patients. During active inflammation, lassitude, discomfort, and urgency of defecation are the major symptoms that limit everyday activities. Sexual and marital problems are not uncommon, but may be no more frequent than that seen in other populations of patients with acute-on-chronic illnesses. Most of these problems disappear during remission, although fear of relapse and the need for continuing treatment and medical supervision can cause considerable anxiety. Many patients will alter their lifestyle with respect to daily activity, travel, and diet, but with prompt treatment of active disease and supportive medical care, most are able to have a normal life for most of the time. The development of patient self-help groups (such as the National Association for Colitis and Crohn's Disease in the United Kingdom) has been of tremendous value in providing education and an environment in which patients can regain their confidence and overcome the problem of isolation, an important and common factor in patients with an uncommon and socially unpleasant disease.

There has been a dramatic fall in the mortality rates for ulcerative colitis since the introduction of corticosteroids in the 1950s and improvement in the management of severe attacks. The mortality rate for a severe attack, including urgent surgery, should now be less than 2%. In the longer term, mortality differs hardly at all from that expected in a matched healthy population, a fact which the majority of life assurance companies fail to recognize.

Ulcerative colitis in particular groups of patients

Pregnancy

Women with ulcerative colitis have normal fertility and are not at increased risk of having a spontaneous abortion, and there is no evidence that pregnancy is a risk factor for relapse. If they do become pregnant, the chance of having a normal baby is the same as for healthy women. Furthermore, there is no good evidence that corticosteroids, drugs containing 5-aminosalicylic acid, or azathioprine are harmful. Maintenance treatment should be continued throughout pregnancy and, if a relapse does occur, it should be treated aggressively with corticosteroids to obtain a rapid remission. There is now a cohort of women who have conceived while receiving infliximab, and no adverse outcomes have been seen although the drug is not recommended either during pregnancy or in women wanting to conceive. Methotrexate is totally contraindicated if conception is possible, as it is known to be teratogenic.

Childhood

Ulcerative colitis is less common in children than in adults and, for the United Kingdom, the prevalence is about 6 to 7 per 100 000.

Nevertheless, it can present within the first few weeks of life, although the mean age of presentation is about 10 years. The symptoms are those of diarrhoea, rectal bleeding, abdominal pain, and failure to thrive. There may be delayed growth, but this is more commonly a feature of childhood Crohn's disease. The proportion of children with a total colitis is about 50%, which is higher than in adults, and probably accounts for the higher rate of colectomy reported in most series.

Treatment follows the same principles as for adults, although dosages are adjusted for the child's weight. In addition, great attention must be made to nutrition to allow for adequate growth. For children requiring repeated courses of corticosteroids, an alternate-day regimen usually controls the disease activity but prevents growth retardation. If colectomy becomes necessary, a restorative proctocolectomy should be done.

Further reading

Allan RN, *et al.* (eds) (1996). *Inflammatory bowel diseases*, 3rd edition. Churchill Livingstone, Edinburgh.

Anderson CA, *et al.* (2009). Investigation of Crohn's disease risk loci in ulcerative colitis further defines their molecular relationships. *Gastroenterology*, **136**, 523–9.

Jewell DP, *et al.* (ed) (2006). *Challenges in inflammatory bowel disease*, 2nd editon. WileyBlackwell, Oxford.

Sartor RB, Sandborn WJ (2004). *Kirsner's inflammatory bowel disease*, 6th edition. WB Saunders, Philadelphia, PA.

Irritable bowel syndrome and functional bowel disorders

D.G. Thompson

Essentials

Symptoms suggestive of disturbed lower gastrointestinal function without adequate explanation are very common in adults in the Western world, up to 15% of whom experience such symptoms at any one time, although most do not seek medical advice. It is not clear whether the symptoms of those individuals who do seek medical help have a different pathophysiological basis from those who do not, and whether the seeking of medical advice is more an indication of a worried individual than of disturbed gut function.

The currently used terms are best viewed as an attempt to provide some clinically useful rather than pathophysiologically accurate categorization of patients and their symptoms. The 'Rome criteria' recognize (1) irritable bowel syndrome, characterized by abdominal pain that is relieved by defecation with associated change in frequency in defecation and/or stool consistency; (2) functional bloating; (3) functional constipation; (4) functional diarrhoea; and (5) functional abdominal pain.

Routine haematological and biochemical screening is usually done on the assumption that they will be normal. Features that raise the suspicion of organic disease and indicate a need for further investigation include the onset of symptoms in middle-aged or older individuals, weight loss, or blood in the stool.

Management remains empirical: no single pharmacological agent or group of agents has ever been found to be consistently effective. The principal task of the physician is to give explanation and reassurance (sometimes supplemented by psychological treatments), but particular symptoms are often treated as follows: (1) constipation—defecation may be eased by supplementary dietary fibre and poorly absorbed fermentable carbohydrates which increase faecal bulk and soften the stool; osmotic laxatives and enemas are used for the severely constipated patient with slow transit; (2) diarrhoea—attention to diet is often helpful, as are simple antidiarrhoeal agents; (3) abdominal pain—antispasmodics (e.g. hyoscine butyl bromide) are frequently employed, as are low doses of antidepressants.

Introduction and definition of terms

Over the last century many attempts have been made to categorize functional bowel disorders. It is not surprising that most have failed to stand the test of time, as the symptoms suffered by the patient (although genuine and troublesome) are often difficult to define, variable in their expression, and defy pathophysiological explanation. The latest and perhaps most comprehensive attempt has been made by a working group whose recommendations, known as the 'Rome criteria', are now accepted as a consensus view and provide a useful research tool. Whether these criteria will be better than previous attempts will, however, depend upon whether they turn out to provide a better understanding of the pathogenic mechanisms of the disease or to aid its therapy. The Rome Working Group (who are now in their third iteration of their classification) has suggested the division of functional bowel disease into a number of symptom-based categories (Box 15.13.1). Because they do seem to have some practical value in guiding approaches to management, this chapter is based on some of the Rome categories, with emphasis on those

previously encompassed by the term 'irritable bowel syndrome'. However, it must be recognized that the Rome criteria do not necessarily include all symptoms presented by patients with abnormal bowel function. Failure to allocate a patient into one or other category should therefore not be taken to mean that the patient does not have a functional bowel disorder.

Irritable bowel syndrome

Definition

This syndrome is characterized by the presence of abdominal pain associated with defecation, or a change in bowel habit, together with disordered defecation and the sensation of abdominal distension. For practical purposes, its recognition relies upon the presence of abdominal pain that is relieved by defecation and of an associated change in frequency in defecation and/or stool consistency.

Box 15.13.1 Categorization of functional bowel disease according to the 'Rome criteria'

Functional bowel disorders
Irritable bowel syndrome
Functional abdominal bloating
Functional constipation
Functional diarrhoea
Functional abdominal pain

These criteria are themselves based on the studies of Manning and of Kruis, which identified that the above features were reported most frequently in patients with bowel problems but were very unusual in patients with structural disease of the colon.

Recognition

The recognition of irritable bowel syndrome is clinically based, and relies on a carefully taken history and examination, there being no specific endoscopic, radiological, or laboratory investigation that is yet capable of providing a positive diagnosis. Despite the absence of a specific pathological indicator, the identification of irritable bowel syndrome is usually not difficult, and in most cases it is unnecessary to investigate the patient extensively in an attempt to exclude other, more serious disease.

Clinical features

History

In addition to the careful elicitation of the above specific symptoms, other features may be found that serve to increase clinical confidence. For example, many patients have upper-gut symptoms, e.g. food-related abdominal distension. Women may also complain of menstrual and bladder symptoms, and there is also an increased prevalence of psychosexual problems.

Examination

Clinical examination is important. Although there is no physical abnormality that is diagnostic of irritable bowel syndrome, a number of features occur commonly. Palpation over the site of the lower colon, particularly in the left iliac fossa, may produce discomfort, and a sigmoid colon containing faeces is often palpable. Similar tenderness may be present under the rib margins and in the right iliac fossa.

Rectal examination and sigmoidoscopy should be conducted as part of the initial clinical assessment. Characteristic findings are the presence of pellety stools in the rectum and a mucosa of normal appearance, evidence of mucosal inflammation is incompatible with the diagnosis. A further helpful pointer is the response to air insufflation during the sigmoidoscopy; abdominal discomfort is often reproduced and relieved by air expulsion. Evidence of a pigmented rectal mucosa (melanosis coli) may be found in patients who have been taking stimulant laxatives and is a useful indicator of the chronicity of the problem.

Further laboratory investigations remain at the discretion of the clinician, depending upon the confidence with which a clinical diagnosis is made. Routine haematological and biochemical screening is usually done on the assumption that they will be normal, and thus to provide reassurance both to the patient and the doctor. Radiological and endoscopic examination of the colon is not mandatory unless a clinical suspicion of a structural colonic disorder, particularly neoplasia, remains after the history and examination have been completed.

Features that raise the suspicion of organic disease and indicate a need for further investigation include the onset of symptoms in middle-aged or older individuals, weight loss, or blood in the stool. The development of new colonic symptoms in a patient with a long history of irritable bowel syndrome should also be taken seriously, as there is no evidence that the syndrome protects against the development of other disease and the incidence of colonic neoplasia increases with age.

Pathophysiology

Despite much interest and many painstaking clinical studies, our understanding of the pathophysiology of irritable bowel syndrome remains limited and the following hypotheses are discussed solely as a guide to current thinking.

Neuromuscular dysfunction

The most popular hypothesis is that these patients have a disorder of neuromuscular function of the gastrointestinal tract. However, although this seems eminently plausible, evidence is lacking. Manometric studies of the colon do show an increased contractile activity in patients with this syndrome, particularly after food, but the neurophysiological basis of this finding and its relationship to symptoms remains to be determined.

Visceral hypersensitivity

Another currently popular hypothesis is that visceral sensation from the gastrointestinal tract is somehow enhanced in these patients. This idea is based on the observation that distension of the rectum and colon produces greater discomfort than in people with normal bowel function. This increased sensory awareness appears to be viscerally specific, as cutaneous responsiveness is normal. However, it remains to be determined whether the mechanism for this hypersensitivity is peripheral (abnormal mechanoreceptor responsiveness in the gut) or central (abnormal sensory processing by the brain and spinal cord) or even both.

Psychiatric disease

There is convincing evidence that psychiatric disease and abnormal illness behaviour are more prevalent in patients with irritable bowel syndrome. The relationship between the psychological problem and any neuromuscular abnormality remains uncertain, although it is recognized that a heightened awareness of visceral sensation is a feature of affective disorders, particularly depression.

Diet

It is customary to regard diet as being a pathogenic factor and to attribute constipation symptoms to fibre deficiency, on the basis that irritable bowel syndrome is uncommon in those parts of the world where a high-fibre diet is consumed. While it is true that faecal bulk can be increased by ingesting more fibre and that constipation is improved, careful studies of fibre intake and symptom development do not show a clear causal relationship. Food 'allergy' or 'sensitivity' is occasionally confused with irritable bowel syndrome because abdominal pain and diarrhoea can accompany both problems (see Chapter 15.5). Classic food allergy with measurable immunological alterations in response to a particular food (e.g. eggs, shellfish) is readily distinguishable from irritable bowel syndrome by a clear relationship between ingestion of the implicated food and symptom development. More subtle forms of food intolerance (e.g. lactose intolerance, fructose intolerance; see Chapter 15.10.5) that produce gut symptoms without an accompanying immune response are much more difficult to recognize because the nutrient in question is often present throughout the diet. Recognition requires a painstaking dietary history and the clear demonstration of a relationship between symptoms and food intake. In most patients such a relationship is not found.

Functional bloating

Recognition

This is characterized by symptoms of abdominal fullness or distension, awareness of audible bowel sounds, and excessive flatus with no evidence of either maldigestion and malabsorption or excessive consumption of poorly absorbed fermentable carbohydrate.

Pathophysiology

Distension of the colon at sigmoidoscopy characteristically produces greater discomfort than normal, suggesting increased gut sensitivity. However, there is no evidence that intestinal gas production is increased. As in irritable bowel syndrome, the prevalence of psychological disorders is high.

Clinical features

The clinical assessment of such patients is identical to that for irritable bowel syndrome and features will be identical.

Functional constipation

Recognition

This is arbitrarily defined as either persistently difficult, infrequent defecation or the sensation of incomplete defecation. Usually, two or more of the following are present: straining at defecation; lumpy or hard stools; the sensation of incomplete evacuation; and two or fewer bowel movements per week.

Clinical evaluation

As with the other categories of functional bowel disorders, its recognition is based on a carefully conducted history and examination designed to exclude the possibility of more serious colonic disease, particularly cancer. When considering the problem, it is important to enquire about immobility, concomitant drug therapy (particularly opiate analgesia), and a low-roughage diet, all of which are well recognized as contributing to constipation, particularly in infirm individuals.

An abnormality of pelvic-floor function on attempted defecation is an unusual cause of constipation that should be suspected in individuals who feel the need to defecate but cannot expel faeces despite severe straining. Such a problem should be considered when symptoms develop following pelvic trauma or difficult childbirth. Clinical evidence of diabetes, hypothyroidism, and hypercalcaemia must also be sought, as these may also lead to altered colonic function and constipation.

Physical examination should include a rectal and vaginal examination. The absence of perineal descent on straining is a simple indicator of impaired pelvic-floor relaxation, while descent below the level of the ischial tuberosities indicates pelvic-floor weakness. Sigmoidoscopy is required to identify the presence of formed faeces, and to exclude faecal impaction and organic obstruction of the lower colon and rectum.

Laboratory examination

Extensive laboratory investigation is usually unnecessary in the absence of clinical indicators of systemic disease and in the presence of the above criteria. A plain abdominal radiograph is often helpful to confirm the presence of faecal material throughout the colon and to allow estimation of the diameter of the small intestine and colon, which helps to exclude the rare cases of intestinal pseudoobstruction and megacolon caused by intestinal myopathies and neuropathies.

Transit studies using radio-opaque markers are commonly performed as part of the investigation of constipated patients to determine the severity of transit delay, and to distinguish those with a pancolonic abnormality from a more localized problem of pelvic relaxation. However, measurement of whole-gut transit should not be regarded as necessary for the diagnosis—documented infrequent defecation is usually sufficient. The electrophysiological and radiological assessment of anorectal function is only indicated if there is evidence of abnormal perineal descent or rectal prolapse, as the accurate recognition of pelvic-floor dysfunction can influence the choice of therapy. Such investigations are indicated when Hirschsprung's disease is suspected.

Pathophysiology

The cause of functional constipation is uncertain. Factors likely to be of relevance are similar to those proposed for irritable bowel syndrome, in particular enteric neural dysfunction.

In the mildest cases, dietary fibre deficiency may be relevant; however, in the more severely affected patients, fibre supplementation does not abolish the problem and may even worsen symptoms, making a causal role for fibre untenable in such individuals. By contrast, a histological abnormality of the enteric nerves of the colon or muscle of the colon may be found in the most severe cases; for the great majority of constipated patients, however, no structural abnormality has been identified.

In a proportion of patients, almost invariably female, defecatory dysfunction appears to be the major factor. A failure of the pelvic-floor muscles to relax on attempted stool expulsion is identifiable in these patients; this appears to be a 'learned' phenomenon with a psychophysiological aetiology rather than peripheral nerve dysfunction. In other patients, low tone in the pelvic floor and rectal prolapse appear to be the result of damage to the pudendal nerve from straining at stool or parturition and thus may be a consequence of the constipation rather than its cause.

In some severely affected women there is a relationship between symptom severity and the luteal phase of the menstrual cycle, which has led to the suggestion of a sex-hormonal aetiology. In support of this hypothesis is the fact that colonic muscle tone is reduced by progesterone and that constipation is a frequent accompaniment of normal pregnancies. Against the hypothesis, however, is the failure to demonstrate abnormal colonic sensitivity to progesterone in constipated women, leaving the possibility that the menstrual cycle-related events are merely the expression of a normal cyclical progesterone effect on a malfunctioning colon.

Functional diarrhoea

Recognition

This is defined as the frequent passage of unformed stool without the presence of other features of irritable bowel syndrome. Neither abdominal pain nor the frequent passage of formed stools is included in the symptoms.

The diagnosis of functional diarrhoea depends on the presence of two or more of the following: unformed stool; three or more bowel movements per day; and increased stool weight, more than 200 g/day.

Clinical features

This disorder is recognized only after excluding other, more medically serious conditions, in particular inflammatory bowel disease and secretory diarrhoeas. The possibility of surreptitious laxative use should always be borne in mind. Some patients identify the time of onset of the problem to a specific life event, particularly a bout of severe gastroenteritis. The possibility of a chronic intestinal infection needs to be considered carefully in such patients, although evidence of an infective agent will be lacking in most and the label 'postinfective diarrhoea' is usually applied.

Physical examination should determine the extent of nutritional deficiency, exclude metabolic disorders such as hyperthyroidism, and rule out intraabdominal structural abnormalities. Careful examination of stool samples for pathogens and laxatives is required.

Laboratory investigations

Unlike the other functional diseases, it is important to make a careful search for a structural mucosal disease in such patients. Key diagnoses that must be excluded are chronic malabsorption due to pancreatic insufficiency or gluten sensitivity, inflammatory bowel disease, infections, and infestations of the gastrointestinal tract.

Pathophysiology

In the absence of any definable structural abnormality, functional diarrhoea is generally assumed to be a disorder of neuroenteric control of intestinal epithelial transport.

In some patients, there is a clear relationship between psychological state and symptoms, with diarrhoea worsening whenever anxiety occurs. However, whether the relationship is truly causal is unknown.

Functional abdominal pain

Recognition

While this symptom category is commonly included amongst the functional bowel disorders, the relationship between the abdominal pain and a disturbance of gastrointestinal tract function is difficult to ascertain. Abdominal pain is frequent, recurrent, or continuous, and characteristically persists for many months. The relationship between pain and recognizable physiological events such as eating, defecation, or menstruation is lacking, and evidence of organic disease in the abdomen is absent. Most of these patients show a major loss of daily functioning capacity and exhibit chronic illness behaviour.

Management of functional bowel disorders

The management of patients with functional bowel disorders remains empirical. Perhaps it should not be surprising that in an area of human suffering with such symptom diversity and in which the pathophysiological mechanisms remain obscure, no single pharmacological agent or group of agents have ever been found to be consistently effective.

A review of randomized, double-blind, placebo-controlled trials for the treatment of irritable bowel syndrome examined 43 trials and concluded that none offered convincing evidence that any therapy was effective, a conclusion which is perhaps as much a reflection of the difficulty of trial design as the efficacy of the drug therapy. Furthermore, in a condition in which the patient's mental state plays such an important part in defining symptom severity, it is not surprising that in most clinical trials placebo responses have been very high, usually up to 50%. Also, short-term trials of therapeutic agents in diseases where symptoms are intermittent may be unable to distinguish a true drug effect from a placebo response.

So what can the clinician do to help patients with functional bowel disease? As in all chronic problems without a cure, a principal task is to give an explanation and reassurance. Therapy must be patient-centred and designed to provide a solution for the patient's personal needs and expectations. The clinician should give a full explanation of the likely nature of the problem and firm reassurance that organic disease is not likely to be present. Attention to the patient's psychological state is very important, as it is clear that mood is a powerful modulator of symptoms.

In more severe cases of irritable bowel syndrome, psychological treatment using a variety of techniques has been found to provide greater improvement in a patient's sense of well being than drug therapy alone. Good prognostic factors for improvement seem to be overt psychiatric symptoms, particularly anxiety or depression, together with intermittent pain exacerbated by stress. In contrast, patients in whom the abdominal pain is constant, and who exhibit evidence of chronic illness behaviour, do not seem to be helped by a psychotherapeutic approach although they may respond to antidepressants.

In mild cases, attention to the individual and his/her symptoms is usually the approach taken. In patients with predominant constipation, supplementary dietary fibre and poorly absorbed fermentable carbohydrates increase faecal bulk, soften the stool, and may ease defecation. On occasion, however, this approach can exacerbate symptoms of abdominal distension, probably as a result of increased colonic gas produced by the fermentation of the unabsorbed carbohydrate. Wherever possible, long-term use of stimulant laxatives is best avoided because of the concern that such drugs may themselves damage the colonic enteric-neural function and eventually make the problem worse. Osmotic laxatives and enemas are the mainstay of therapy of the severely constipated patient with slow transit.

For the patient who appears unable to relax the pelvic floor musculature on attempted defecation, a variety of biofeedback techniques are now available that help the individual to 'relearn' the process. Patient satisfaction is high in those able to engage closely with the therapist in the process.

For patients with diarrhoea-predominant symptoms, attention to diet is also often helpful, as the size of and timing of meals is likely to influence the frequency and social inconvenience of the diarrhoea. Fermentable carbohydrates are best taken in moderation because they can exacerbate symptoms. In the more persistent cases of diarrhoea, symptoms can be improved by simple antidiarrhoeal agents, the dose being adjusted according to the symptoms and administered before a meal.

In the management of patients with unexplained abdominal pain it is tempting to prescribe opiate-derivative analgesics. These are unlikely to be of benefit in the long term, however, and may even exacerbate symptoms because of their constipating effect. Antidepressants are often prescribed empirically in low doses, with evidence of benefit at least in mood elevation. Antispasmodics (e.g. hyoscine butyl bromide) are frequently employed. Although there are undoubtedly a number of patients and doctors who are convinced of their value, a beneficial effect has yet to be proven beyond doubt by clinical trial. Outside Europe, 5-HT$_3$ antagonists are becoming increasingly used for severe diarrhoea-predominant irritable bowel symptoms.

Relaxation therapy, in particular hypnosis, seems to benefit those individuals who are prepared to participate. In the right conditions, programmes of self-delivered 'autohypnosis' may offer a satisfactory approach for some sufferers.

Surgical intervention for symptoms of functional bowel disorders is usually best avoided, as benefit is unlikely. On occasions, however, subtotal colectomy and ileorectal anastomosis will provide symptomatic benefit in carefully selected patients with severe constipation.

Further reading

Afzalpurkar RG, *et al.* (1992). The self-limited nature of chronic idiopathic diarrhoea. *N Engl J Med*, **327**, 1849–52.

Christensen J (1992). Pathophysiology of the irritable bowel syndrome. *Lancet*, **ii**, 1444–7.

Creed F, *et al.* (2003). The cost-effectiveness of psychotherapy and paroxetine for severe irritable bowel syndrome. *Gastroenterology*, **124**, 303–17.

Creed F, *et al.* (2005). Outcome in severe irritable bowel syndrome with and without accompanying depressive, panic and neurasthenic disorders. *Br J Psychiatry*, **186**, 507–15.

Drossman D (2006). The functional gastrointestinal disorders and the Rome III process. *Gastroenterology*, **130**, 1377–91.

Klein KB (1988). Controlled treatment trials in the irritable bowel syndrome: a critique. *Gastroenterology*, **95**, 232–41.

Kruis W, *et al.* (1984). A diagnostic score for the irritable bowel syndrome: its value in the exclusion of organic disease. *Gastroenterology*, **87**, 1–7.

Longstreth GF, *et al.* (2006). Functional bowel disorders. *Gastroenterology*, **130**, 1480–92.

Manning AP, *et al.* (1978). Towards a positive diagnosis of the irritable bowel. *Br Med J*, **2**, 653–4.

Read NW, Timms JM, Barfield LJ (1986). Impairment of defecation in young women with severe constipation. *Gastroenterology*, **90**, 53–61.

Wexner SD, *et al.* (1992). Prospective assessment of biofeedback for the treatment of paradoxical puborectalis contraction. *Dis Colon Rect*, **35**, 145–50.

Whorwell PJ, Prior A, Faragher EB (1984). Controlled trial of hypnotherapy in the treatment of severe refractory irritable bowel syndrome. *Lancet*, **ii**, 1232–4.

Colonic diverticular disease

S.Q. Ashraf, M.G.W. Kettlewell, and
N.J. McC. Mortensen

Essentials

Diverticula, which are herniations of mucosa through the bowel musculature, are seen most often in the sigmoid and descending colon, with prevalence <5% at age 40 years rising to 65% by age 85 in European populations, but around 0.2% in African and Asian countries. They are ascribed to a lifelong diet deficient in dietary fibre, but it is not known why some diverticula become symptomatic, although rises in intradiverticular pressure are thought to play a role in perforation.

Diverticula are usually discovered incidentally, but symptoms which are attributable to diverticular disease include colicky abdominal pain and bloating, often accompanied by a change in bowel habit with the passage of broken, pellety stools after considerable straining. All patients with such presentation should have a rigid or flexible sigmoidoscopy in addition to a barium enema or colonoscopy to exclude a rectal or sigmoid carcinoma. Treatment is with reassurance that there is no serious underlying disease, a high-fibre diet, and—for patients with pain—antispasmodics such as mebeverine. Elective resection is indicated in the few patients who have repeated severe attacks.

Complications of diverticular disease include diverticultis, pericolic abscess formation, peritonitis, intestinal obstruction, haemorrhage, and fistula formation. Acute diverticulitis typically presents with pain and tenderness over the left lower abdomen, and the patient may have pyrexia, malaise, anorexia and nausea. Treatment is with rest, antibiotics (usually cefuroxime 750 mg and metronidazole 500 mg 8-hourly) and analgesia. Resection of the sigmoid colon may be necessary if symptoms fail to resolve or recur.

Epidemiology

The term diverticular disease was first described in the medical literature at the turn of the20th century. The first case of resection for a complication of diverticular disease was documented by Mayo in 1907. Autopsy studies in the United Kingdom and Australia have shown that the prevalence of colonic diverticula increases with age. It is less than 5% at the age of 40 years; at the age of 60 it is 30% and rises to 65% by the age of 85. Subtle gender differences have also been observed. In Edinburgh, 23% of all barium enemas demonstrated diverticula. The annual incidence increased from 0.17 in 1000 in those under 45 years to 5.7 in 1000 in those over 75 years of age. Women were affected more than men. A study in eastern England measured the incidence of perforation secondary to diverticular disease. They observed that there was increase in perforation with age and after adjusting for age there was a higher incidence in males (5.1 in 100 000 per year male and 3.6 in 100 000 per year female). In spite of the introduction of high-fibre diets, there is no evidence that the incidence of diverticular disease is declining. A recent review has observed a slight rise in the prevalence of perforated diverticular disease in Western countries from 2.4 in 100 000 in 1986 to 3.8 in 100 000 in 2000.

On the other hand, colonic diverticulosis is very rare in African and Asian countries where the prevalence is 0.2%. Interestingly, in a review of 600 Japanese patients with diverticular disease, right-sided colonic disease was demonstrated in 70%. This geographical distribution is not simply due to genetic factors and race, as Asian and African migrants moving to the United Kingdom or the United States of America have acquired the prevalence of disease seen in the native white population, which suggests an environmental risk factor, thought to be dietary. This is in agreement with the observation that patients presenting with complicated diverticular disease have a low intake of dietary fibre, and vegetarians have a low incidence of the disease.

Aetiology

Diverticular disease is said to be a disease of the 20th century and in the United Kingdom there is a correlation between the rising incidence at the beginning of the 20th century and an increased consumption of refined flour and sugar. Sugar consumption has trebled since 1860, and in the late 1870s the stone grinding of flour was replaced by roller milling, which removes more fibre. Modern white bread and some brown breads contain little fibre compared with the amount in wholemeal bread, which was previously a staple part of the diet.

The development of diverticula can therefore be ascribed to a lifelong diet deficient in dietary fibre. A high-fibre diet is related to reduced gut transit times, with less strain on the colon. Modern, fibre-deficient diets on the other hand give rise to stiff, viscous stools that need high intracolonic pressures to propel them. High luminal pressures cause a protrusion of the mucosa through vulnerable points in the sigmoid and descending colon. They usually occur at the site where colonic blood vessels penetrate the wall. This hypothesis is supported by the observation that, although basal intracolonic pressures are similar in health and diverticular disease, when the diseased colon is activated by emotion, eating, mechanical stimuli, or drugs such as morphine or prostigmine, high pressures are generated in those segments that have diverticula. This is due to hypersegmentation by the colonic smooth muscle, and the difference has been recorded in the earliest stage of disease and may explain its progressive nature. In symptomatic patients an increase in dietary fibre causes a relief of symptoms in many cases.

Changes in the colon wall also play a part. With age, and following episodes of diverticulitis, the colonic wall becomes stiff and less distensible, aggravating the effects of raised intracolonic pressure. An increase in elastin and changes in collagen have been reported. Diabetic patients are prone to diverticular disease at an earlier stage, suggesting a defect in glycolysation of colonic collagen with advancing age. In those with connective tissue disorders such as Ehlers–Danlos syndrome or Marfan's disease, diverticula are also seen at an unusually early age.

Pathogenesis of diverticular complications

The distinction between symptomatic and asymptomatic diverticular disease is important, for although something is known about the formation of diverticula it is not known why some diverticula become symptomatic.

A large American cohort study has shown that high red meat intake and a diet deficient in fruit and vegetables multiplied the risk of developing symptomatic diverticular disease threefold. The benefits of fibre are thought to be secondary to their effect in reducing gut transit times and colonic segmentation. Secondly, there may be a symbiotic effect related to the formation of short-chain fatty acids, which are released after bacterial action on fibre. On the other hand, certain chemicals in cooked meat such as hetrocyclic amines are thought to trigger cytotoxicity of colonocytes.

The pathogenesis of diverticular perforation is not clear. However, rises in intradiverticular pressure are thought to play a role. This may be secondary to a blockage of the mouth with faecal material or colonic segmentation. Once the pressure rises over a critical threshold, focal ischaemia leading to necrosis occurs. This would then allow the passage of luminal bacteria into the local pericolic tissue. With time this would mature into a local abscess. In cases of failure of local tissue to contain the infection, there may be a progression to a faecal peritonitis. This spectrum of diverticular complications can be classified into the four stages as proposed by Hinchey (see Table 15.14.1).

The sigmoid colon, which is less compliant than other colonic segments, is where intraluminal colonic pressures are highest. This reflects the observation that the sigmoid colon is the commonest area in the colon to develop diverticular disease and also secondary complications such as perforation. It has also been noted that diverticula are very distensible and other factors are thought to play a role in whether complications such as perforation occur. Pathology reveals that diverticula consists mainly of a mucosal layer and any factor that results in changes of the integrity of the mucosal barrier

Table 15.14.1 Hinchey classification of sepsis/contamination in diverticulitis

Stage	Characteristics
1	Pericolic abscess
2	Contained pelvic, retroperitoneal or distant intraperitoneal abscess
3	Generalized purulent peritonitis, no communication with bowel lumen
4	Generalized purulent peritonitis, communication with bowel lumen

will result in alteration of the ability microbial population to pass into the local tissues. This can be divided into factors affecting the microbial flora (antibiotics and fibre deficiency), mucin secretion (nonsteroidal anti-inflammatory drugs (NSAIDs) and fibre), epithelial cell insult (NSAIDs) and immune activity in the colonic wall (age, drugs such as corticosteroids and immunosuppressants).

There is growing body of evidence that NSAIDs have a role to play in complicated diverticular disease. Two prospective case–control studies have shown patients with complications of diverticular disease were more likely to be taking NSAIDs than age-matched controls. Another study compared 115 cases with complicated diverticular disease with 77 with uncomplicated disease. NSAIDS and corticosteroids were found to be associated with development of peritonitis and abscess formation. Also, a large American cohort study following over 35 000 male health professional showed that individuals on NSAIDS had a relative risk of 2.2 of developing symptoms of abdominal pain, bleeding, or change in bowel habit secondary to diverticular disease. The action of NSAIDs may be secondary to a reduction in mucosal blood flow as a result of modulation of prostaglandin levels.

Pathology

A diverticulum consists of a herniation of mucosa through the colonic musculature. As it enlarges its muscular covering atrophies, so that the fully developed diverticulum consists of mucosa, connective tissue, and peritoneum. The striking abnormality is in the thickening of the circular and longitudinal muscle, which both narrows the colonic lumen and shortens the sigmoid like a concertina to give a sawtooth appearance on barium enema. The diverticula occur as slit-like apertures between the muscle clefts.

Inflammation in diverticular disease is the result of infection around diverticula, which spreads within the pericolic fat to form a dissecting abscess. Usually a single diverticulum is the cause of a pericolic abscess, perhaps initiated by the presence of a faecolith. Involvement of the peritoneum results in local peritonitis, which may become generalized in the event of a perforation. This may also give rise to intraabdominal abscesses or fistulas to the bladder, small bowel, vagina, or uterus. Repeated episodes of diverticulitis lead to a contracted, narrowed sigmoid colon surrounded by fibrous tissue. Bleeding in diverticular disease can often be traced to an infected diverticulum. This may cause either the erosion of a vessel in its wall or the formation of granulation tissue inside the diverticulum, which then bleeds.

Clinical features

Only 10 to 15% of cases of diverticular disease result in symptoms, of which 75% develop diverticultis. They are usually discovered incidentally. The symptoms usually result from disordered motility rather than secondary complications of the disease.

Uncomplicated diverticular disease

Symptoms which are attributable to diverticular disease include colicky abdominal pain and bloating. Pain can be felt along the course of the colon, particularly over the sigmoid, and is often accompanied by a change in bowel habit with the passage of broken, pelletty stools after considerable straining. Examination may reveal some tenderness over the sigmoid colon without guarding or evidence of systemic upset. These symptoms may be indistinguishable from those of the irritable bowel syndrome. The passage of blood with an unformed stool needs to be investigated thoroughly to exclude more sinister pathology.

Management

All patients should have a rigid or flexible sigmoidoscopy in addition to a barium enema to exclude a rectal or sigmoid carcinoma (Fig. 15.14.1). They should be reassured that there is no serious underlying disease and a high-fibre diet should be recommended. Exercise and high dietary fibre have been shown to be prevent the development of diverticular disease in prospective studies. However, evidence for the efficacy of dietary fibre for treatment of established diverticular disease is not conclusive, as shown by two randomized controlled trials where only one showed improved symptoms. Current dietary recommendations include wholemeal bread, wholewheat breakfast cereals, rough porridge or muesli, and fresh fruit and vegetables daily. Fibre increases stool bulk in three ways—by holding water, by proliferation of bacteria, and from the by-products of bacterial fermentation. The coarser the fibre the greater is the faecal bulk, but also the greater the unpalatability. Although cooking bran improves its taste, it reduces its water-holding capacity. A good clinical response is usually achieved by including two tablespoons of bran with the morning cereal, but about one-half of patients will experience gaseous distension or cramps on starting the high-fibre diet. It is worth warning them that this is likely to happen and that it will resolve within a month or so if they persist with the diet.

More recent studies looking at pharmacological agents have shown some benefit with rifamaxin (a derivative of rifamycin) and fibre. Mesalazine has also been associated with a decreased recurrence of symptoms over placebo. However this study also showed that abdominal pain was more common in the treatment group. A case–control study has shown that mesalazine is associated with reduced intracolonic pressure and a reduction in the perforation rate. A reduction in perforation rate was also observed with the use of calcium channel blockers. This is thought to act via the mechanism of reducing intracolonic pressure. Long term use of opioids may be detrimental in such patients, resulting in an increased the risk of developing perforation. More research needs to be done in this field.

In patients with pain, antispasmodics such as mebeverine may be useful, and in a minority with repeated severe attacks an elective resection is then indicated (Table 15.14.2). This is probably more effective than sigmoid myotomy, an operation that became popular in the mid-1960s. In this procedure the circular muscle is divided with a longitudinal incision to widen the colonic lumen. The incision is made through the taenia so as to avoid opening diverticula, and is deepened until the mucosa is just seen. The operation lowers the sigmoid intraluminal pressures and improves symptoms but, after 3 years, pressures return to their former levels. The need for myotomy has declined but it may still be useful in some elderly or obese patients.

Complicated diverticular disease

Complications of diverticular disease include diverticultis, percolic abscess formation, peritonitis, intestinal obstruction, haemorrhage, and fistula formation. This results in the significant morbidity and mortality in this subgroup of patients. This has obvious cost implications in terms of expenditure in health services across the Western world. It is important to distinguish the minority of patients who suffer from a febrile attack with left iliac fossa peritonism, sometimes called left-sided appendicitis, from those with chronic pain and diarrhoea. The inflammation may settle with minimal symptoms or develop into a pericolic abscess or peritonitis.

Acute diverticulitis

Pain is felt over the left lower abdomen, and the patient may have pyrexia, malaise, anorexia, and nausea which evidence of systemic upset. The neutrophil count is raised. This is as a result of localized

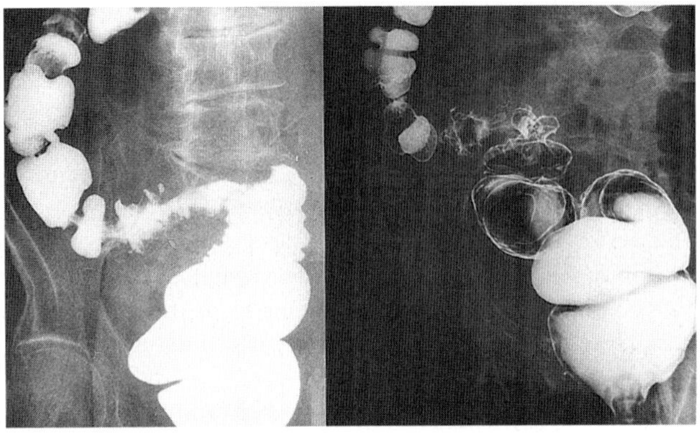

Fig. 15.14.1 Barium enema showing a narrowed sigmoid colon with a few diverticula. This appearance can be confused with those of a carcinoma and colonoscopy would be indicated to clarify the diagnosis.

Table 15.14.2 Indications for surgery

Sepsis
Recurrent diverticulitis
Perforated diverticulitis
Purulent peritonitis
Faecal peritonitis
Pelvic or paracolic abscess

Colonic obstruction
Inflammatory stricture
Fibrotic stricture
Suspected malignancy

Fistulae
Colovesical
Colovaginal
Ileocolic
Major haemorrhage

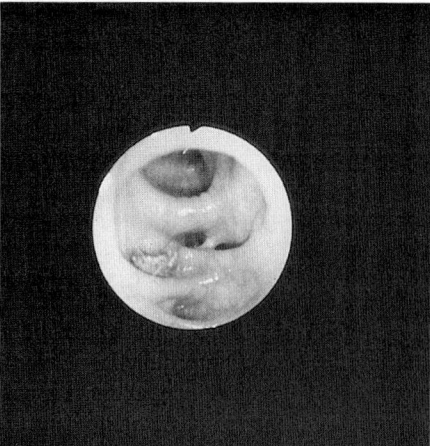

Fig. 15.14.2 The typical appearance of diverticula seen at colonoscopy. Note the muscular haustra and the mouths of diverticula—one with a faecolith. (From the *Slide atlas of gastroenterology*, Gower Medical Publishing, London, with permission.)

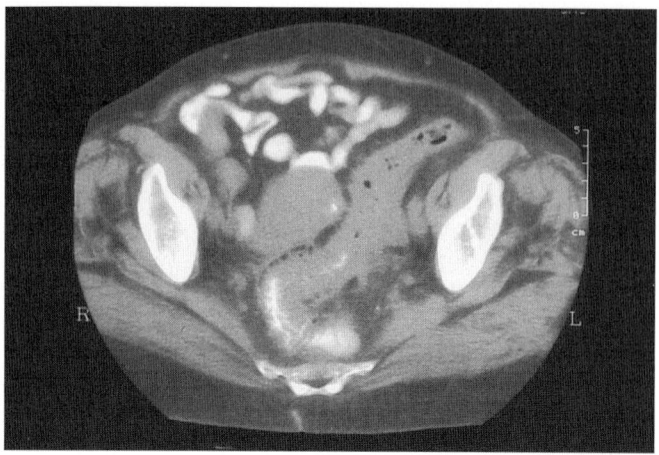

Fig. 15.14.3 CT of the pelvis in a patient with acute diverticulitis. The sigmoid colon is grossly thickened, the lumen narrowed, and pockets of air are seen in the diverticular disease.

bacterial infection in the colonic wall causing an inflammatory infiltrate thus resulting in systemic manifestations. In certain cases, right iliac fossa tenderness may be present due to sigmoid colon looping to the right side of the abdomen. This may be diagnosed at laparoscopy for right iliac pain.

Treatment is with rest, antibiotics, usually coamoxiclav 1.2 g and metronidazole 500 mg 8-hourly (effective against Gram-negative bacteria and anaerobes), and analgesia. Most cases settle within a few days and the diagnosis can be confirmed after 2 to 3 weeks by barium enema. A narrow segment can sometimes be difficult to distinguish from a carcinoma and any doubtful cases can be clarified by subsequent colonoscopy (Fig. 15.14.2).

If symptoms fail to resolve, or recur, resection of the sigmoid colon may be necessary. When it is necessary to resect an acutely inflamed and unprepared colon, a Hartmann's operation may be safer than a primary anastomosis.

However complications will normally develop during the primary episode with further episodes having less inflammatory sequelae. Risk of recurrence after the first episode ranges from 7 to 45%. For recurrent diverticulitis operated electively, a primary anastomosis would be ideal. The accepted management policy for recurrent diverticulitis is elective surgery after two episodes of uncomplicated diverticulitis in order to reduce the morbidity and mortality risk associated with admission for complicated diverticulitis. However this needs to be tempered by the observation from a population-based study that only 25% of patients with perforated diverticulitis actually had a previous history of diverticular disease. This is in agreement with other studies which puts the range at 3 to 30%. Furthermore following elective operation, 10% develop recurrent diverticulitis. Patients being consented for elective operations therefore need to be fully informed of risk and benefits.

Diverticular abscess

Acute diverticulitis can lead to a local peritonitis with abscess formation, either in the paracolic or pelvic area. There may be a palpable mass and a swinging fever. When in doubt the diagnosis can be confirmed by CT scanning with rectal contrast (Fig. 15.14.3). The latter investigation is excellent at demonstrating bowel wall thickening, abscess formation, and extraluminal disease. The specificity is high. The size of the abscess can be measured. Small abscesses

less than 5 cm in size can be treated with antibiotics with good outcome. Those less than 2 cm in size can be treated with antibiotics in the community.

It is wise to let an abscess localize whilst treating the patient with rest, antibiotics, and analgesia. Some abscesses will be amenable to drainage by direct incision, either over them or via the rectum or vagina. More complicated collections are best drained by CT-guided aspiration or drain placement. There is rarely any need to do a proximal transverse colostomy. If drainage persists, an elective sigmoid colectomy with primary anastomosis can be done at a later time. Even when an abscess is localized, however, the condition remains potentially dangerous as it may rupture into the peritoneal cavity giving rise to peritonitis.

Perforated diverticulitis

Acute diverticulitis can be complicated by generalized purulent peritonitis, either by direct spread from the inflamed colon or by rupture of a peridiverticular abscess. The clinical picture is of severe intraperitoneal sepsis with toxaemia, ileus, and abdominal pain, and septicaemia will often follow. Before surgery such patients need to be intensively resuscitated with intravenous colloids together with administration of systemic antibiotics. Once stabilized, they require emergency laparotomy.

Other causes of the acute abdomen that may not require surgery should be excluded, including pelvic inflammatory disease, ureteric calculus, and even pulmonary embolus. In these circumstances a CT scan is invaluable.

Surgical options include a defunctioning transverse colostomy, Hartmann's procedure—removing the diseased sigmoid, over-sewing the distal rectum, and bringing out an end colostomy—or colonic resection and primary anastomosis. The first option tends to be performed by more junior surgeons in the middle of the night; however, this is associated with complications of ongoing sepsis secondary to the ongoing faecal stream through the septic colon. Historically, complicated diverticular disease was managed in three stages in which initially the sepsis was drained together with the formation of transverse loop colostomy. This was then followed by resection of the diseased segment and end colostomy followed by reversal. However, this required three hospital admissions and resulted in considerable morbidity. The reduction to two-stage (Hartmann's) resulted in a drop in mortality rates. More recent studies suggest that in a selected case group a one-stage process involving primary anastomosis is not associated with increased mortality rates. This has the added advantages of reducing hospital re-admissions, although there is a risk of potential leak. There has been a shift away from the more conservative procedures in this situation due to the residual 'septic colon' and the further problem of the unsuspected carcinoma within the inflammatory mass. For these reasons more radical measures are favoured by experienced surgeons. Hartmann's operation is the procedure most frequently used (Fig. 15.14.4).

Hartmann's procedure is safe and effective and removes the postoperative risk of anastomotic leak, although subsequent reconnection may involve a major operation in older patients. Purulent peritonitis carries a mortality of around 15%.

Faecal peritonitis

This is a catastrophic complication with a mortality of around 50%, particularly in older patients. A diverticulum ruptures, often with little or no inflammation, liberating quantities of faeces into

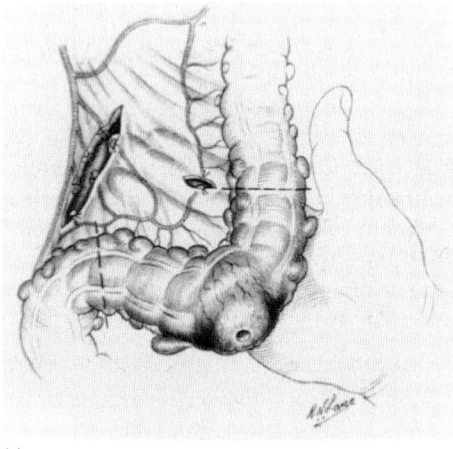

(a)

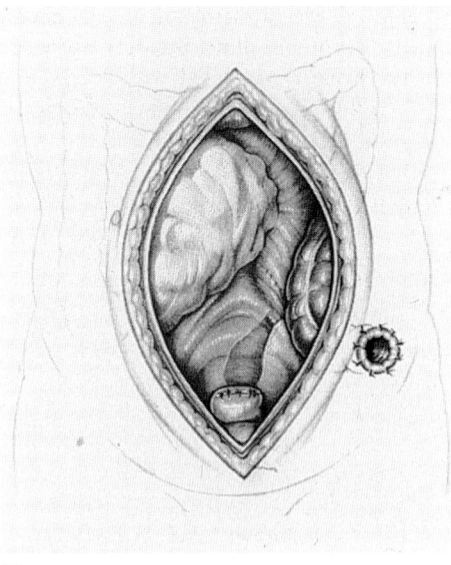

(b)

Fig. 15.14.4 (a) The area of sigmoid colon resected for perforated diverticular disease. (b) Hartmann's operation—the sigmoid colon has been resected, the rectum oversewn, and a left iliac fossa colostomy fashioned.

the peritoneal cavity. Rapid and severe shock with septicaemia ensues. Energetic resuscitation is necessary, followed promptly by surgery and a Hartmann's operation. These patients often need to be stabilized in an intensive care unit postoperatively.

Intestinal obstruction

Recurrent inflammation with fibrosis and muscular hypertrophy can lead to progressive stenosis and colonic obstruction, which is usually chronic but may present acutely. Conservative treatment is worth trying at first, provided a carcinoma has been excluded. With the aid of a stool softener the symptoms may resolve and the stricture gradually dilate. If these measures fail, the bowel should be prepared for a resection, with care taken not to aggravate the obstruction.

Small-bowel obstruction is sometimes a complication of acute diverticulitis, as the bowel may adhere to the inflammatory mass. It usually resolves as the inflammation subsides but on occasion a laparotomy and division of adhesions or even a small-bowel resection may be necessary.

Colonic fistulas

A colovesical fistula usually presents with recurrent urinary tract infections, together with pneumaturia or faecuria. The fistula arises in the sigmoid, which has often folded over into the pouch of Douglas, and adheres to the apex of the bladder. This is the most frequent cause of colovesical fistula but carcinoma and Crohn's disease should be excluded.

Fistulas may also occur between the sigmoid and vagina, uterus, ureter, and ileum. They seldom heal spontaneously but do not always give rise to disabling symptoms and so represent a relative indication for surgery. Sigmoid colectomy as a one-stage procedure is the best option, and colostomy is rarely required. A fistula into the bladder is simply closed and urethral catheter drainage continued for a week.

Haemorrhage

Major haemorrhage is an uncommon but well-recognized complication. Bleeding from the colon only accounts for 20% of gastrointestinal haemorrhages, of which 50% are diverticular in origin. It is important that other more common causes for bleeding such as polyps and angiodysplasia are excluded by angiographic studies and colonoscopy. Most patients who present tend to be elderly. Massive bleeding is defined when over 40% of blood volume is lost. This can be catastrophic in older patients who have a reduced physiological capacity to maintain vital organ perfusions.

Massive bleeds tend to present as fresh rectal bleeding. Up to 80% will settle down spontaneously and require only transfusion and supportive measures. The initial management of these patients includes oxygen therapy with adequate venous access. Disorders of coagulation need to be identified and corrected during the ongoing resuscitation process. It is important to exclude upper gastrointestinal bleeding by way of endoscopy. Colonoscopy in the immediate aftermath of a bleed can be difficult but in experienced hands the diagnostic yield can be high as 70%. The endoscope needs to have a wide-bore suction channel and excessive insufflation needs to be avoided due to the risk of causing a re-bleed. In units with access to vascular services, mesenteric angiography can be performed. Localization of the bleeding point needs to be at least 1 to 1.5 ml/h. Therapeutic interventions that are available include vasopressin injection and selective embolization. Radiolabelling is usually reserved for patients who are haemodynamically stable, with no access to vascular radiology and failure to establish a diagnosis during endoscopy. However, in circumstances where there is accelerated transit if blood, localization can be poor. As the haemorrhage can be from any part of the colon, good localization is an essential prelude to any operation. Blind colonic resections have a particularly poor record and if the site of bleeding has still not been located, on-table colonic lavage via the appendix stump and intraoperative colonoscopy will usually target the bleeding segment.

A study published in the *New England Journal of Medicine* reported the results of urgent colonoscopy in bleeding diverticular disease. Instead of the traditional conservative measures patients were given bowel preparation and colonoscoped within 12 h. Bleeding sites thus identified were treated by colonoscopic diathermy and the number of major bleeds, blood transfusions, and operations was reduced together with length of hospital stay. It remains to be seen whether this will result in a major shift of emphasis in management.

Further reading

Boulos BP, *et al.* (1984). Is colonoscopy necessary in diverticular disease? *Lancet*, **i**, 95–6.

Brodribb AJ (1977). Treatment of symptomatic diverticular disease with a high fibre diet. *Lancet*, **i**, 644–66.

Campbell K, Steele RJ (1991). Non-steroidal anti-inflammatory drugs, and complicated diverticular disease: a case-control study. *Br J Surg*, **78**, 190–1.

Eastwood MA, *et al.* (1977). Variation in the incidence of diverticular disease within the city of Edinburgh. *Gut*, **18**, 571–4.

Eastwood MA, *et al.* (1978). Comparison of bran, ispaghula and lactulose on colon function in diverticular disease. *Gut*, **19**, 1144–7.

Gear JSS, *et al.* (1979). Symptomless diverticular disease and intake of dietary fibre. *Lancet*, **i**, 511–14.

Gianfranco JA, Abcarian H (1982). Pitfalls in the treatment of gastrointestinal bleeding with blind subtotal colectomy. *Dis Colon Rect*, **25**, 441–5.

Grief JM, Fried DO, McSherry CK (1980). Surgical treatment of perforated diverticulitis of the sigmoid colon. *Dis Colon Rect*, **23**, 483–7.

Heaton KW (1985). Diet and diverticulosis—new leads. *Gut*, **26**, 541–3.

Hughes LE (1969). Postmortem survey of diverticular disease of the colon. *Gut*, **10**, 336–51.

Hyland JMP, Taylor I (1980). Does a high fibre diet prevent the complications of diverticular disease? *Br J Surg*, **67**, 77–9.

Janes SEJ, Meagher A, Frizelle FA (2006). Management of diverticulitis. *BMJ*, **332**, 271–5.

Jensen DM, *et al.* (2000). Urgent colonoscopy for the diagnosis and treatment of severe diverticular haemorrhage. *N Engl J Med*, **342**, 78–82.

Kettlewell MGW, Moloney GE (1977). Combined horizontal and longitudinal colomyotomy for diverticular disease: preliminary report. *Dis Colon Rect*, **20**, 24–8.

Krukowski ZH, Mattheson NA (1985). Emergency surgery for diverticular disease complicated by generalised and faecal peritonitis: a review. *Br J Surg*, **71**, 921–7.

Krukowski ZH, Koruth NM, Mattheson NA (1985). Evolving practice in acute diverticulitis. *Br J Surg*, **72**, 684–6.

Morris CR, *et al.* (2002). Epidemiolgy of perforated colonic diverticular disease. *Postgrad Med J*, **78**, 654–9.

Ornstein MH, *et al.* (1981). Are fibre supplements really necessary in diverticular disease of the colon? A controlled clinical trial. *BMJ*, **282**, 1353–6.

Painter NS (1975). *Diverticular disease of the colon*. Heinemann Medical, London.

Papi C, *et al.* (1995). Efficacy of rifaximin in the treatment of symptomatic diverticular disease of the colon: a multi-centre double-blind placebo-controlled trial. *Aliment Pharmacol Ther*, **9**, 33–9.

Reilly M (1966). Sigmoid myotomy. *Br J Surg*, **53**, 859–63.

Smith AN, Attisha RP, Balfour T (1969). Clinical and manometric results one year after sigmoid myotomy for diverticular disease. *Br J Surg*, **56**, 895–9.

Whiteway J, Morson BC (1985). Elastosis in diverticular disease of the sigmoid colon. *Gut*, **26**, 258–66.

Wilson RG, Smith AN, Macintyre IM (1990). Complications of diverticular disease and non-steroidal anti-inflammatory drugs: a prospective study. *Br J Surg*, **77**, 1103–4.

Congenital abnormalities of the gastrointestinal tract

V.M. Wright and J.A. Walker-Smith

Essentials

Congenital abnormalities of the gastrointestinal tract usually manifest shortly after birth, but on occasion symptoms may be delayed for months or even years. Any part of the gut can be affected, with problems including oesophageal atresia and tracheo-oesophageal fistula, anterior abdominal wall defects, congenital pyloric stenosis, atresia and stenosis of the small intestine, duplication of the gastrointestinal tract, small-intestinal malrotation with or without volvulus, small-intestinal lymphangiectasia, Meckel's diverticulum, meconium ileus, congenital short intestine, colonic atresia, Hirschprung's disease, and imperforate anus.

The widespread use of ultrasonography to assess the fetus allows many of these abnormalities to be recognized prenatally, and associated anomalies (e.g. cardiac lesions) may indicate a major chromosomal abnormality. This allows parental choice to continue with or terminate the pregnancy.

Presentation of congenital abnormalities of the gastrointestinal tract in adult life is uncommon, but small intestinal lymphangiectasia can present in adults with a picture mimicking coeliac disease, and Meckel's diverticulum—a vestigial remnant of the vitellointestinal duct on the antimesenteric surface of the distal ileum—can cause rectal bleeding or small-intestinal obstruction in young adults.

Embryology of congenital gastrointestinal tract abnormalities

The primitive gut is initially a simple tube of endoderm, the muscle and connective tissue developing from the splanchnopleuric mesoderm. Cranially, the gut terminates at the buccopharyngeal membrane and caudally at the cloacal membrane. Both membranes disappear; failure of the cloacal membrane to do so results in one of the rarer forms of imperforate anus. The primitive foregut diverticulum gives rise to the respiratory system, oesophagus, stomach, duodenum to the level of the ampulla of Vater, liver, and pancreas. The primitive oesophagus lengthens rapidly, becomes narrow, and frequently the lumen is transiently obliterated. A longitudinal, ventral diverticulum of the foregut forms the trachea with ridges on either side that fuse, initially caudally with progression cranially, until the primitive respiratory system is separated from the oesophagus. Failure of this complex process results in the various forms of oesophageal atresia and tracheo-oesophageal fistula. Dilatation of the foregut distal to the oesophagus produces the stomach, initially slung from the dorsal body wall by the dorsal mesentery and from the septum transversum by the ventral mesentery. Rapid differential growth results in the stomach rotating through 90° on its long axis, the dorsal border becoming the greater curvature and the ventral border the lesser curvature.

The dorsal mesentery forms the greater omentum. The ventral mesentery, into which the liver bud grows, forms the falciform ligament and coronary ligaments attaching the liver to the diaphragm, and the lesser omentum. Congenital abnormalities of the stomach are excessively rare. The liver arises as a shallow groove on the ventral aspect of the duodenum. The groove becomes tubular and invades the septum transversum and the ventral mesentery. Bile is secreted from the fifth month, and gives meconium its characteristic dark-green appearance. The mesoderm of the septum transversum forms the fibrous tissue of the liver.

The pancreas develops as two outgrowths of the duodenum. One comes from the dorsal aspect, the other from the ventral. The dorsal bud grows into the dorsal mesentery and the ventral bud is swept around dorsally into the mesentery when the duodenum rotates to the right. These two primordia fuse, the ducts fuse, and the main pancreatic duct joins the bile duct to enter the duodenum at the ampulla of Vater. If the ducts do not fuse, an accessory pancreatic duct persists. Annular pancreas is a congenital anomaly where the pancreas surrounds the duodenum, which may be atretic or intrinsically stenosed. Annular pancreas is not the primary cause of the duodenal obstruction in these cases.

The duodenum is derived partly from foregut and partly from the midgut. The loop of primitive duodenum is fixed at the pyloric end, and by the ligament of Treitz at the duodenojejunal flexure to the left of the first lumbar vertebra. By rotating to the right, the entire duodenum comes to lie retroperitoneally in a curve around the head of the pancreas. Failure of the duodenum to fix in this position is a fundamental reason for the gut failing to rotate correctly. During rapid growth the duodenal lumen is obliterated and partial or total failure of recanalization will result in the anomalies of duodenal atresia or stenosis. The small intestine and colon, suspended on the dorsal mesentery, rapidly lengthen and outgrow the primitive peritoneal cavity, and herniation occurs into the umbilical sac during the fifth week of development. Growth in length continues, the loop of bowel rotating through 90° anticlockwise, the cranial limb lengthening more than the caudal limb. About the tenth week the loops of bowel return to the peritoneal cavity, undergoing a further 180° anticlockwise rotation. The small intestine goes first, the large intestine subsequently. Thus the large intestine lies in front of the small. The caecum is initially subhepatic, the large liver occupying the right side of the abdomen, eventually retreating to the right upper quadrant and allowing growth in the length of the ascending colon. The caecum, ascending colon, and descending colon become fixed to the posterior abdominal wall; thus the small bowel is suspended from a mesentery that runs from the left side of the first lumbar vertebra to the right iliac fossa. Failure of the duodenum to rotate and fix, coupled with a failure of normal rotation of the bowel with consequent lack of normal fixation, gives rise to malrotation of the intestine. Abnormal bands run from the caecum, which lies to the left of the midline, to the region of the gallbladder and may compress the duodenum. The narrow mesentery of the small intestine predisposes to a volvulus of the entire midgut.

At the apex of the midgut loop, the primitive gut is in continuity with the extraembryonic yolk sac via the vitellointestinal duct, which runs in the umbilical cord. Obliteration and disappearance of this duct occurs, allowing the bowel to return from the umbilical sac to the enlarged peritoneal cavity. Failure of the duct to disappear may result in a Meckel's diverticulum, a band connecting the ileum to the umbilicus, a communication between the lumen of the ileum and the umbilicus, or failure of the gut to return completely to the peritoneal cavity, resulting in a small umbilical hernia.

Persistence of the umbilical sac will result in an exomphalos, with the sac containing a variable amount of gut and much of the liver. The embryology of gastroschisis is disputed. It may be due to early rupture of the umbilical sac allowing the primitive gut to extrude into the extraembryonic coelom, or failure of fusion of the lateral body folds producing a defect in the anterior abdominal wall adjacent to the umbilicus.

The midgut comprises the duodenum distal to the ampulla of Vater, jejunum, ileum, caecum, and colon as far as the left transverse colon. Atresia affecting the midgut may occur at single or multiple sites. The cause is probably intrauterine interference with the blood supply to that part of the gut which is affected, with consequent resorption of the ischaemic bowel.

The hindgut gives origin to the left third of the transverse colon, the descending colon, sigmoid, rectum, and upper part of the anal canal, and a considerable part of the urogenital system. The hindgut terminates in the primitive cloaca, which is separated from the proctodaeum (a shallow ectodermal depression) by the cloacal membrane. The primitive cloaca communicates with the hindgut and the allantois. Early in development the cloaca is joined by the pronephric ducts. A coronal septum (the urorectal septum) arises in the angle between the allantois and hindgut, grows caudally,

fuses with the cloacal membrane, and divides the cloaca into a dorsal primitive rectum and a ventral primitive urogenital sinus. The cloacal membrane breaks down, establishing continuity between the endodermal hindgut and the ectodermal part of the anal canal. There are many varieties of imperforate anus. Absence of a variable length of rectum and anal canal, known as the 'high' anomaly, is frequently associated with the bowel terminating via a rectourethral or rectovaginal fistula. Ten per cent of babies with an imperforate anus will have oesophageal atresia, with or without a fistula, suggesting that the division of trachea and oesophagus and urogenital system and rectum must be occurring at a similar time in gestation, with possibly a similar mechanism producing the division. Anomalies of the urogenital system occur in a very high proportion of affected infants. Abnormalities of the ectodermal component of the anal canal result in 'low' imperforate anus.

The ganglion cells of the gut lie in the submucosa and intermyenteric plane. Ectodermal in origin, they migrate caudally along the length of the gut. Failure of migration down to the internal sphincter of the anal canal results in an aganglionic segment extending for a variable distance proximally, and is the underlying abnormality in Hirschsprung's disease.

Mucosal differentiation occurs in the early months. The inner circular muscle differentiates earlier than the outer longitudinal. Thus the fetal intestinal tract is prepared for digestion, absorption, and propulsion at a comparatively early stage in development.

Intestinal histology in neonates with congenital gastrointestinal tract abnormalities

Histological architecture of the intestines in neonates with abnormalities of the gastrointestinal tract when compared to normal fetuses, is abnormal. The villi may be blunted, the crypts disorganized, and crypt depth significantly decreased, yet enterocyte height may be increased. These findings may be relevant to malabsorption which may complicate such disorders.

Oesophageal atresia and tracheo-oesophageal fistula

The incidence of this condition is approximately 1 in 3500 live births.

The upper oesophagus ends in a blind pouch. In the majority of cases, the lower oesophagus communicates at its upper end with the trachea, that is there is a tracheo-oesophageal fistula. Although much less common, there are a number of well recognized anatomical variations illustrated in Fig. 15.15.1.

Clinical features

Frequently the infant with oesophageal atresia is premature or small for gestational age. In 50% there is a history of polyhydramnios. Shortly after birth, because swallowing is impossible, copious amounts of frothy saliva dribble from the mouth, associated with choking, dyspnoea, and cyanotic episodes. Frequent suction is required to keep the airway clear. The infant with a tracheo-oesophageal fistula without associated oesophageal atresia coughs, chokes, and becomes cyanosed during feeds. Because air escapes through the fistula into the oesophagus, gaseous distension of the

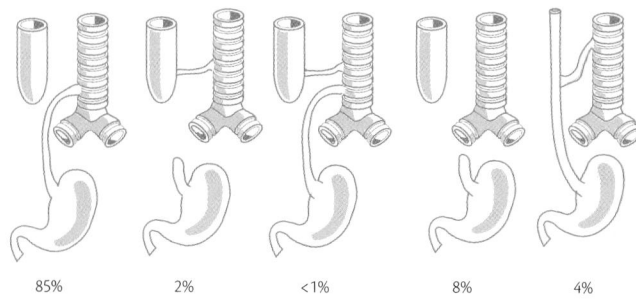

85%   2%   <1%   8%   4%

Fig. 15.15.1 Anatomical variations of oesophageal atresia and tracheo-oesophageal fistula, indicating the relative frequency.

abdomen is frequently present. Aspiration of feed into the airway results in pulmonary collapse and consolidation.

Over 50% of infants with oesophageal atresia have significant associated anomalies. Of particular importance are cardiac, anorectal, urogenital, and skeletal anomalies. The premature infant or the infant who is small for gestational age is more likely to have multiple anomalies than is the full-term infant.

Survival of infants with oesophageal atresia depends on birth weight and associated abnormalities. All infants with a birth weight greater than 1.8 kg and no associated abnormalities or pneumonia should survive; this is also true of larger infants with a moderately severe associated abnormality or pneumonia. The mortality for infants with birth weight less than 1.5 kg, or with multiple severe congenital abnormalities, remains in the region of 20 to 30%.

Diagnosis

When oesophageal atresia is suspected, a size 10 or 12 FG catheter is passed through the mouth and into the oesophagus. If the oesophagus is obstructed, the catheter meets a resistance 9 to 11 cm from the gum margin. A smaller catheter may curl up in the obstructed oesophagus. Contrast studies of the oesophagus are rarely necessary. A chest and abdominal radiograph will show the position of a radio-opaque tube in the upper oesophagus, and the presence of gas in the bowel if a tracheo-oesophageal fistula is present. Complete absence of gas in the abdomen is diagnostic of an oesophageal atresia without a distal tracheo-oesophageal fistula. The radiograph will also reveal any abnormalities of ribs or vertebrae, signs of pneumonia, and may provide evidence of an associated cardiac abnormality.

In isolated tracheo-oesophageal fistula, very careful contrast studies of the oesophagus are required to demonstrate the fistula. Endoscopic examination of trachea and oesophagus is usually diagnostic.

Management

Early division of the tracheo-oesophageal fistula and anastomosis of the oesophagus are possible in the majority of cases. Postoperatively, mechanical ventilation may be necessary, but usually the full-term infant with no preoperative complications only needs careful suction of the nasopharynx to maintain a clear airway. A gastrostomy or a transanastomotic nasogastric tube is usually used to enable the infant to be fed within 48 h of operation. A primary anastomosis may not be feasible in pure oesophageal atresia, extreme prematurity, or where the infant's general condition is poor. In such cases a tracheo-oesophageal fistula, if present, would be divided and a feeding gastrostomy established. Subsequently, an oesophageal anastomosis, after a delay of 4 to 6 weeks, having left

the upper oesophageal pouch intact and kept empty of saliva by continuous suction, may be feasible. Alternatively, a cervical oesophagostomy is done with the intention, when the infant's condition permits, of establishing continuity between mouth and stomach, using a length of colon, a tube of stomach, or the whole stomach. The choice depends on the surgeon's preference.

Anterior abdominal wall defects

The incidence of exomphalos and gastroschisis is approximately 1 in 3000 births. An exomphalos occurs because the abdominal contents herniate through the umbilical ring into the base of the umbilical cord and are covered by a translucent membrane composed of peritoneum and amnion. Exomphalos major indicates that the diameter of the defect is greater than 5 cm, exomphalos minor that the defect is less than 5 cm. The contents of the exomphalos almost always include liver and a variable amount of bowel. On occasion, a very small amount of bowel alone herniates into the base of the cord. The diagnosis is frequently made on a prenatal ultrasonographic scan and prompts a search for associated major abnormalities, particularly anencephaly, chromosomal trisomies, major cardiac anomalies, and the Beckwith–Wiedemann syndrome. Associated abnormalities occur in 40%.

The Beckwith–Wiedemann syndrome, also termed the exomphalos macroglossia gigantism (EMG) syndrome, usually presents as a large-for-dates infant with a small exomphalos. The tongue is strikingly large, there are frequently ridges in the earlobes, and a prominent naevus flammeus on the forehead. Hypoglycaemia as a result of hyperinsulinism produced by islet-cell hyperplasia is a common early problem, which may require steroids, glucagon, and rarely subtotal pancreatectomy to effect control. In the long term, children with this syndrome have an increased incidence of solid tumours, particularly nephroblastoma and hepatoblastoma.

In gastroschisis there is a full-thickness defect in the anterior abdominal wall, usually to the right of the umbilical cord. The defect is small but most of the gastrointestinal tract may be extruded through it. In contrast to exomphalos, other abdominal organs are rarely eviscerated and abnormalities outside the gastrointestinal are unusual. Again, prenatal diagnosis on ultrasound scan is common.

Exomphalos

Clinical features

The lesion will be obvious at birth. Occasionally the membrane will rupture during, or shortly after, delivery. Careful examination for associated defects is essential.

Management

A nasogastric tube is passed to decompress the bowel. The sac can be very satisfactorily covered and supported by wrapping clingfilm around the exomphalos and the baby's trunk. Plain radiographs of chest and abdomen are taken preoperatively in order to study the cardiac contour and the intestinal gas pattern, and to look for evidence of an associated diaphragmatic hernia. If the contents of the sac can be reduced into the peritoneal cavity, the abdominal wall can be closed in layers. If closure of all layers of the abdominal wall is impossible, skin closure alone may be used, or a synthetic material such as Silastic sheeting or Prolene mesh is used to enclose the sac after suturing it to the margins of the defect. Gradual reduction of the contents into the peritoneal cavity is then possible, with delayed closure of the abdominal wall. An alternative is to paint the sac with an antiseptic solution such as 70% alcohol or one of the iodine-based preparations. This results in the formation of a dry eschar that separates after some weeks, leaving a granulating surface, which gradually epithelializes. Any method that does not achieve muscle closure will leave a ventral hernia, which requires surgery at a later date.

Postoperatively, ventilatory support may be necessary. Antibiotics commenced preoperatively are continued postoperatively, particularly if an artificial material is used. Parenteral nutrition will be necessary if oral feeds cannot be given. Survival is related to the size of the lesion and the severity of any associated abnormalities.

Gastroschisis

Clinical features

Babies with this abnormality are frequently small for gestational age. After delivery, heat loss from the exposed bowel rapidly causes hypothermia. Hypoproteinaemia is very common. The small size of the defect in the anterior abdominal wall and the often narrow pedicle from which the bowel is suspended may impair the blood supply and result in infarction of much of the extruded intestine. Atresia may have occurred because of intrauterine impairment of the blood supply.

Management

A nasogastric tube is passed and the bowel decompressed. The bowel can be enclosed in clingfilm (plastic wrap) wrapped around the baby's trunk, or the baby can be placed in a large polythene bag taped around the chest. This keeps the bowel moist and prevents excessive heat loss. Antibiotics are commenced preoperatively and colloid is given to counteract the existing hypoproteinaemia and hypovolaemia. At operation the anterior abdominal wall is stretched and any meconium washed out *per rectum* to reduce bulk. Reduction of the extruded bowel is attempted and abdominal wall closure achieved where possible.

In about 10% of cases, primary closure is not possible and a Silastic sheet or Prolene mesh is used to form an artificial sac to enclose the intestine. The material is sutured to the margins of the defect and the size of the sac gradually reduced over some days, squeezing the bowel back into the peritoneal cavity until closure of the abdominal wall becomes feasible—usually after 10 to 14 days. Ventilatory support postoperatively is often necessary. Parenteral nutrition is essential and may need to continue for many weeks until gastrointestinal motility and absorption are adequate. Sepsis is a considerable hazard. The mortality is now 5 to 10% compared with 80% 10 years ago. Improved postoperative management is largely responsible for this.

Congenital pyloric stenosis

Congenital hypertrophic pyloric stenosis is a disorder characterized by hypertrophy of the circular muscle of the pylorus and so obstruction to the gastric outlet. The incidence is 2 per 1000 live births. The aetiology is unknown. Theories include primary muscle hypertrophy, abnormalities of the maturation of ganglion cells, absence of a certain type of ganglion cell, or a response to abnormally high concentrations of circulating gastrin. Genetic and environmental factors play an important part. There is an increased incidence of pyloric stenosis in siblings of an affected child and in the offspring of a woman who has had the condition. Environmental factors include social class, type of feeding, and a seasonal variation with an increase in the winter months. In any large series the male:female ratio is 3 or 4:1 and half the cases will be first-born children.

Clinical features

The onset of symptoms is usually between 3 and 6 weeks of age, but may present shortly after birth. Vomiting of increasing severity is the cardinal symptom, eventually occurring after most feeds and becoming projectile. The vomitus is milk and mucus, and may contain altered blood suggesting an oesophagitis or gastritis; bile is never present. The baby stops gaining weight and becomes constipated. Characteristically the baby is alert, anxious, and hungry. If diagnosis is delayed, severe malnutrition may develop.

Examination reveals evidence of weight loss and in advanced cases signs of dehydration will be evident. When the stomach is full, waves of peristalsis travelling from left to right in the epigastrium will be seen (visible peristalsis). The thickened pylorus is felt as an olive-sized tumour lying deep to the edge of the right rectus and is often most easily felt when the stomach is empty. The diagnosis of pyloric stenosis is made on clinical grounds in the majority of cases. A plain radiograph of the abdomen may be very helpful in revealing a large stomach with a paucity of distal gas. A barium meal is diagnostic when the 'string' sign of the elongated pylorus is demonstrated. The barium study may also reveal gastro-oesophageal reflux, which is commonly associated with pyloric stenosis. Ultrasonography is now widely used—pyloric length more than 1.2 cm and wall width more than 3 mm supporting the diagnosis.

Management

In the child presenting early, electrolyte disturbance and dehydration are minimal. In the later case, dehydration with hypochloraemic alkalosis and marked potassium depletion occurs. Preoperative correction of water and electrolyte deficits is essential. The operation of pyloromyotomy, described by Ramstedt in 1912, splits the hypertrophied muscle longitudinally allowing the mucosa to bulge through the defect, thus enlarging the pyloric canal. Postoperatively, various feeding regimens are advocated; all aim to have the baby on a normal feeds by 48 to 72 h postoperatively. The prognosis is excellent.

Atresia and stenosis of the small intestine

An intrinsic obstruction may produce either complete or partial obliteration of the bowel lumen. Complete obliteration may be due to a gap between the two ends of the small intestine, with or without a connecting band between these ends, or a complete mucosal diaphragm. Such complete obstruction is known as atresia. When obstruction is incomplete it may be due to a narrowing of the lumen—a stenosis—or a mucosal diaphragm with a hole. Small-intestinal atresia is a more common finding than is stenosis. The duodenum is most often affected, followed by jejunum, and least often ileum.

Associated abnormalities of the gastrointestinal tract, including malrotation, oesophageal atresia, imperforate anus, biliary atresia, and annular pancreas are a feature of duodenal atresia/stenosis. Localized volvulus and meconium ileus are associated with jejunoileal atresias.

Intrinsic obstruction of the small intestine of congenital origin presents most often in the neonatal period but when the obstruction is partial it may first present much later, in infancy and childhood.

Congenital intrinsic duodenal obstruction

When duodenal obstruction is complete, vomiting usually occurs within a few hours of birth and is bile stained unless the obstruction is proximal to the ampulla of Vater, when the vomiting is persistent and copious but not bile stained. Meconium may be passed normally and there may be obvious epigastric distension. In view of the association with other abnormalities, these should be sought carefully. In particular, the infant should be examined for evidence of Down's syndrome. Duodenal lesions are an association of this syndrome and occur in 10% of cases. When obstruction is incomplete the symptoms may be intermittent and the diagnosis delayed.

Congenital intrinsic duodenal obstruction may be accompanied by an annular pancreas; this is a sign of failure of duodenal development rather than an obstructive lesion *per se*. In infants with duodenal atresia, at operation, it often looks as if there is an annular pancreas because there is interposition of the pancreas between the two ends of the duodenal atresia.

Congenital intrinsic duodenal obstruction is not, in general, associated with multiple atresias in the remainder of the small intestine, but there may be obstruction at two levels in the duodenum.

Jejunoileal obstruction

Symptoms, typically bile-stained vomiting and abdominal distension, usually occur within the first 2 days of life. Meconium may or may not be passed. When obstruction is incomplete the diagnosis may again be long delayed and the child may present with intermittent vomiting, abdominal distension, and even with features of malabsorption—a clinical picture that may resemble coeliac disease.

Diagnosis

Plain radiographs of the abdomen are usually diagnostic in infants who present with a complete obstruction. In duodenal atresia there is the characteristic 'double bubble' (Fig. 15.15.2). When duodenal obstruction is incomplete there may be small amounts of air in the lower bowel. A barium meal may be necessary to demonstrate the obstruction and may suggest an associated malrotation. When there is complete jejunoileal obstruction there are usually multiple dilated loops of intestine. A barium enema may reveal an unused microcolon. When obstruction is incomplete a barium follow-through may be needed to establish the diagnosis. Rarely, laparotomy may be the final court of appeal.

Management

A nasogastric tube is passed to empty the stomach and allow accurate measurement of gastric losses. Correction of fluid and electrolyte disturbances, if present, should precede surgery, provided that gangrenous or ischaemic bowel is not suspected. At laparotomy, care should be taken to exclude any other gastrointestinal abnormality. In duodenal obstruction, the operation of choice is duodenoduodenostomy. In jejunoileal lesions, adequate resection of the proximal dilated gut reduces the great discrepancy in size between the two blind ends and so facilitates end-to-end anastomosis, although an oblique-to-end anastomosis is sometimes necessary. Leaving the dilated gut immediately proximal to the anastomosis results in ineffective peristalsis and delay in establishing enteral feeds.

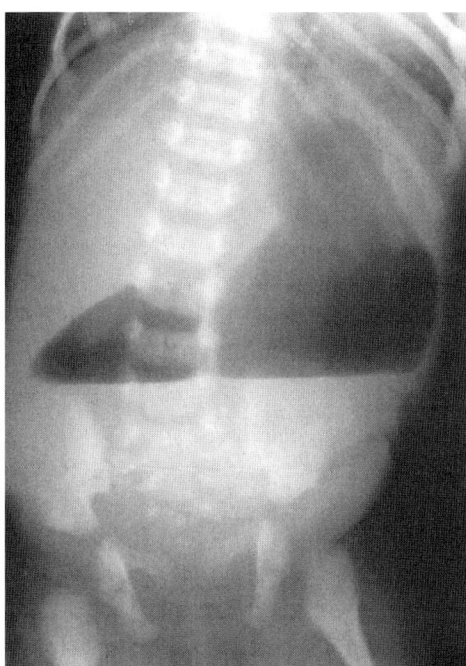

Fig. 15.15.2 Plain radiograph of the abdomen of an infant with duodenal atresia showing characteristic 'double bubble'.

Considerable loss of intestinal length may occur as a result of the intrauterine process producing the atresia; surgical correction, particularly of multiple atresias, will result in further loss. Every effort is made to preserve some ileum and the ileocaecal valve. Loss of considerable lengths of jejunum is well tolerated. Loss of ileum, particularly if the ileocaecal valve is also lost, presents management problems throughout childhood because malabsorption of a variety of important nutrients occurs. The enterohepatic circulation may be impaired. Early liver damage is a consequence of prolonged parenteral nutrition and episodes of sepsis.

Duplication of gastrointestinal tract

Definition

Duplications are cystic or tubular structures whose lumen is lined by a mucous membrane, usually supported by smooth muscle. They occur most often within the dorsal mesentery of the gut. They are also sometimes described as enteric cysts, neurenteric cysts, and reduplications. Duplications may occur anywhere along the alimentary tract but they are found most often in relation to the small intestine, particularly the ileum. They may not communicate with the lumen of the gastrointestinal tract. Duplications may be found in association with intestinal atresias. Sometimes those associated with the small intestine are lined by gastric mucosa and peptic ulceration of the adjacent small-intestinal mucosa, with bleeding, may occur. Those associated with the colon never contain ectopic gastric mucosa.

Clinical features

These are congenital malformations that present most often in early infancy. Later presentation, even into adult life, is well recognized. Duplications may present in infancy as a small-bowel obstruction, or a small cystic duplication may form the lead point of an intussusception. A palpable abdominal mass in infancy, as well as rectal bleeding and volvulus, may also be modes of presentation of this disorder. The clinical diagnosis is often difficult and the diagnosis may sometimes be made only at laparotomy. A technetium scan may be helpful by demonstrating ectopic gastric mucosa. Initial presentation may be a posterior mediastinal cystic mass, possibly associated with cervical or upper thoracic vertebral abnormalities. The mass is likely to communicate through the diaphragm with an intestinal duplication.

Management

Excision of a cystic duplication with or without the adjacent intestine is usually straightforward. Any associated thoracic cyst will also need excision. Short tubular duplications can be excised with the adjacent intestine; very extensive tubular duplications can be opened longitudinally and the mucosa stripped out, leaving the common muscle wall.

Small-intestinal malrotation with or without volvulus

Malrotation of the small intestine is due to disordered movement of the intestine around the superior mesenteric artery during the course of development of the embryo.

Two main abnormalities that produce symptoms may occur. First, there is a gross narrowing of the base of the mesentery, which may allow the midgut to twist around and cause a volvulus. This may occur acutely, causing complete obstruction, or it may occur intermittently, producing bouts of partial or complete obstruction that release themselves spontaneously. Secondly, there may be partial duodenal obstruction from extrinsic compression of the small intestine by peritoneal bands (Ladd's bands) that extend from the caecum to the subhepatic region.

Malrotation may be associated with duodenal atresia or stenosis. It is also found in association with diaphragmatic hernia, omphalocele, and gastroschisis. However, malrotation may be asymptomatic and is sometimes discovered only as an incidental finding on a barium study. The majority of children who develop symptoms related to malrotation do so within the neonatal period, presenting with features of intestinal obstruction, complete or incomplete. When there is a volvulus there may also be obstruction to the blood supply to the bowel, which if complete will lead to extensive gangrene of the small bowel. The passage of bloody stools may be an early sign of this complication.

Those children with malrotation who present later in childhood may do so with features of intermittent obstruction such as episodes of vomiting, often bile stained, and abdominal pain, but sometimes they may manifest with features of malabsorption and many clinical features suggestive of coeliac disease. This is due to intestinal stasis with bacterial overgrowth in the lumen of the small intestine. Steatorrhoea may be accompanied at times by protein-losing enteropathy from obstruction of the mesenteric lymphatics, and chylous ascites may also occur.

Diagnosis

The diagnosis needs to be considered in the differential diagnosis of small-intestinal obstruction in infancy.

Plain radiographs of the abdomen may be very useful, typically revealing an air-filled stomach with some gas scattered through the lower part of the abdomen. However, a malrotation may not be accompanied by any abnormality on the plain radiograph of the abdomen and a barium meal will then be necessary to reveal the presence of malrotation by outlining the failure of the duodenum to cross to the left of the vertebral bodies with the fourth part lying adjacent to the first lumbar vertebra. A barium enema may be useful if it demonstrates the abnormal position of the caecum, but a barium meal is more reliable.

Management

Surgical intervention is indicated when a firm diagnosis is established. Ladd's operation is usually the procedure of choice. This involves, in general, the placement of the colon on the left and the small intestine on the right, having divided any bands and adhesions between the duodenum and large bowel, and, by dissection, broadened the base of the mesentery as much as possible. After a volvulus, total bowel necrosis is untreatable, but severe bowel ischaemia can be reversible and a 'second look' laparotomy may be necessary.

Small-intestinal lymphangiectasia

Small-intestinal lymphangiectasia has been described as a primary, i.e. a congenital, abnormality or as a secondary manifestation of some other disease process such as constrictive pericarditis. The primary abnormality may be accompanied by generalized lymphatic abnormalities including lymphoedema, chylous ascites, and hypoplasia of the peripheral lymphatic system, but the lymphatic abnormality may be confined to the small bowel and its mesentery. It is usually, but not invariably, accompanied by hypoproteinaemic oedema. Radioisotope studies have demonstrated that the hypoproteinaemia is due to abnormal protein loss into the gut. The pathogenesis of the hypoproteinaemia has been attributed to the rupture of dilated lymphatic channels or to protein exudation from intestinal capillaries via an intact epithelium, where there is obstruction of lymphatic flow.

Clinical features

It is a rare condition, which may present throughout life but most often in the first 2 years with diarrhoea and failure to thrive and, later, generalized oedema with hypoproteinaemia. The clinical picture may resemble coeliac disease. There is lymphopenia in the presence of a normal bone marrow and reduction of serum albumin, serum IgG, and carrier proteins such as protein-bound iodine. The severe protein loss may be accompanied by enteric calcium loss, leading to hypocalcaemia. Steatorrhoea is often found in this disorder.

Diagnosis

Diagnosis is made by showing the characteristic lymphatic abnormality on small intestinal biopsy, that is dilated lacteals, but the lesion is patchy. One negative biopsy does not exclude the diagnosis. Radioisotope demonstration of abnormal enteric protein loss using a technique such as intravenous chromium trichloride ($CrCl_3$) is helpful in diagnosis but is not specific. Barium studies in most cases show coarse mucosal folds.

Pathology

Autopsy studies reveal a considerable variation in the distribution of the lymphatic abnormality along the length of the small intestine. Dilated lacteals may occur irregularly along the small bowel and there may be gross dilatation of lymphatics projecting into the lumen. Lymphatic proliferation and dilation may also occur within the mesentery, as well as the serosal, muscular, and submucosal layers of the small-intestinal wall, and extend into the lymph nodes and occupy part of the nodal tissue.

Treatment

This is usually dietetic, as the lymphangiectasia is rarely localized enough to allow surgical excision to effect a permanent cure. The amount of long-chain fat in the diet, which is normally absorbed via the intestinal lymphatics, should be limited. This leads to a reduction in the volume of intestinal lymph and in the pressure in the dilated lymphatics. It is best done by placing the child on a low-fat diet (5–10 g/day) and adding medium-chain triglycerides, instead of the usual long-chain dietary fats, in unrestricted amounts. A milk containing medium-chain triglyceride such as Pregestimil may be used, with medium-chain triglyceride oil for cooking. Some children may be resistant to this therapy when the abnormality is very extensive and, on occasion, death may result despite therapy. Albumin infusions are of little value in management as their benefit is so transitory. Steroids have been advocated but there is little evidence to justify their use. In a follow-up study of children, although there was a continuing chyle leak, as shown by persistent lymphopenia and hypoalbuminaemia, there was a rapid and sustained improvement in dependent oedema following the use of the diet recommended above, although asymmetrical oedema from peripheral lymphatic abnormalities was unaffected. Their growth rate improved on the diet. Clinical relapse occurred quickly when the diet was relaxed. Continued adherence to a strict diet, at least through puberty, is therefore recommended. Indeed it seems probable that this is a lifelong disorder and that some dietetic management may usually need to be permanent.

Meckel's diverticulum

This diverticulum is the vestigial remnant of the vitellointestinal duct. Although most people who have such a diverticulum are asymptomatic, complications may arise, which may present in a variety of ways. In children, these complications chiefly arise in association with the presence of ectopic gastric mucosa in the diverticulum. Other ectopic tissue, for example pancreatic tissue and colonic mucosa, may be found in some cases.

The diverticulum is located in the distal ileum within 100 cm of the ileocaecal valve. It is always antemesenteric.

Clinical features

Rectal bleeding is the main symptom. This is usually the passage of bright blood rather than tarry melaena stools. Typically the stool is at first dark in colour but later bright red. Bleeding may be acute, with shock requiring urgent blood transfusion, or it may be chronic. From a practical viewpoint any child who has a massive, painless, rectal bleed should be regarded as having a Meckel's diverticulum until proved otherwise. Most often bleeding from a Meckel's diverticulum is associated with ulceration of the small bowel adjacent to ectopic gastric or pancreatic mucosa but this is not always the case as bleeding may occur in the absence of ectopic mucosa.

Small-intestinal obstruction may also be a mode of presentation. This may be as a volvulus associated with a band, or an intussusception with the diverticulum as the lead point. Acute diverticulitis occurs and may produce a picture indistinguishable from acute appendicitis.

Diagnosis and management

This depends upon the mode of presentation. When rectal bleeding occurs, other causes need to be excluded. Investigation may include colonoscopy to exclude colonic causes and upper endoscopy to exclude peptic ulceration or oesophagitis.

Barium follow-through is usually an unrewarding investigation. a technetium scan is usually the most important investigation. The radionuclide ^{99}Tcm concentrates in the gastric mucosa. When it is given intravenously, ectopic gastric mucosa appears as an abnormal localization on abdominal imaging with a gamma-camera. In this way a Meckel's diverticulum with ectopic gastric mucosa or indeed a duplication with such ectopic tissue may be diagnosed. A negative scan may prompt angiography. However, negative investigations in a child with severe bleeding should not deter a surgeon from proceeding with a diagnostic laparotomy, or laparoscopy if appropriately skilled. Indeed, when considering the other modes of presentation of Meckel's diverticulum it is often only at laparotomy that the role of a Meckel's diverticulum in the child's intestinal pathology is appreciated.

Meconium ileus

This is a manifestation of cystic fibrosis, the disorder sometimes known as fibrocystic disease of the pancreas. Meconium ileus is the earliest mode of presentation of this disorder during the neonatal period. A similar syndrome in older children and young adults who have cystic fibrosis may occur—the meconium ileus equivalent. The abnormally viscid consistency of the meconium produces an intraluminal obstruction. It may result from several factors including the lack of pancreatic enzymes during fetal life, which may account for the high protein content of the meconium. There is also evidence of reduced secretion of water and electrolytes in such infants, which may further render the meconium more viscid. The meconium, because of its high viscosity and tendency to adhere to the mucosa, cannot be propelled along the bowel and so small-intestinal obstruction results. This occurs most often in the distal ileum.

Clinical features

The neonate with this disorder usually develops signs of intestinal obstruction within the first 24 to 48 h of life, with the classical signs of bile-stained vomiting, progressive abdominal distension, and failure to pass meconium. In simple meconium ileus, the meconium is the sole source of the obstruction, but meconium ileus may be complicated by perforation of the gut and, when this occurs *in utero*, intraperitoneal calcification may be observed on a plain radiograph of the abdomen, providing evidence of meconium peritonitis. Perforation may also occur in the neonatal period. Volvulus and atresia may also complicate meconium ileus.

In simple meconium ileus, the plain radiograph of the abdomen may show dilated bowel but few fluid levels. Sometimes there is the appearance of bubbly meconium in the right lower quadrant. Bowel loops may be palpable. If a contrast enema is performed a microcolon, a consequence of disuse, will be demonstrated. Atresia associated with meconium ileus is frequently indistinguishable radiologically from an atresia of ischaemic origin.

Management

When meconium ileus is complicated by atresia or perforation, gangrene, peritonitis, or associated volvulus, surgical intervention is essential. Surgical options include the formation of a double-barrelled stoma with subsequent irrigation of the meconium from the distal bowel over a week or so, or intraoperative irrigation of the bowel with an immediate end-to-end anastomosis. In both options, an associated atresia or necrotic bowel are resected. The treatment of uncomplicated meconium ileus using enemas containing pancreatic enzymes, mucolytic agents such as acetylcysteine, and the detergent Tween 80 had been advocated for some time: Noblett in Melbourne, in 1969, used a Gastrografin enema to relieve intraluminal obstruction. Gastrografin is a radio-opaque, hyperosmolar solution that is effective because of its hypertonicity. This technique should not be used until a plain radiograph of the abdomen has excluded the possibility of complicated meconium ileus. An initial barium enema should exclude Hirschsprung's disease and demonstrate a microcolon extending to the proximal colon. The retrograde passage of contrast medium through the ileocaecal valve should demonstrate intraluminal meconium with passage into proximal dilated ileum, thus excluding an ileal atresia. After a successful Gastrografin enema, large amounts of meconium will be passed.

Although there may be no signs clinically or radiologically of pulmonary complications in the neonatal period, physiotherapy should be started and any chest infections treated with antibiotics when they occur (as for older children with cystic fibrosis). A pancreatic enzyme preparation should also be started, at first in small dosage when milk feeds have begun. The diagnosis should be confirmed by sweat electrolyte estimations; concentrations of sweat sodium above 60 mmol/litre are abnormal. In the majority of infants with cystic fibrosis, the finding of the abnormal gene ΔF508 or one of the other recognized mutations confirms the diagnosis. In a minority the abnormal gene is not identifiable.

Congenital short intestine

There is a syndrome of congenital short intestine in association with malrotation with clinical features similar to those that follow massive intestinal resection. There is also another syndrome of congenital short intestine in association with pyloric hypertrophy and malrotation. This latter syndrome is due to an absence or diminution of argyrophil ganglion cells in the small-intestinal wall. These cells normally organize peristalsis and ensure that the bolus moves forward at the correct speed. In the absence of such innervation, smooth muscle of the small-intestinal wall contracts spontaneously and rhythmically, but segmentation is not coordinated and the food bolus does not move forward, and there is work hypertrophy of smooth muscle. Both syndromes are rare and often only diagnosed at laparotomy.

Colonic atresia

Atresia of the large intestine is rare. In any series of cases of intestinal atresias, fewer than 10% will have isolated colonic atresia.

Clinical features

The baby presents in the first 24 to 48 h with marked abdominal distension, vomiting, and failure to pass meconium.

Diagnosis

Abdominal radiographs reveal multiple dilated loops of bowel with fluid levels; the position of the loops may suggest a large bowel obstruction. Confirmation of the level of the atresia is obtained by barium enema.

Management

Nasogastric suction and intravenous fluids are commenced preoperatively. At laparotomy the lesion may be an isolated atresia or associated with multiple atresias of small and large bowel. If the atresia is solitary, it may be possible to perform an anastomosis after resection of the atresia and a length of the grossly dilated proximal bowel. Frequently a colostomy is fashioned to allow the dilated proximal bowel to contract before an end-to-end anastomosis some weeks later.

Hirschsprung's disease

In this condition, ganglion cells are absent in the bowel wall. The distal rectum is always aganglionic and the aganglionosis extends proximally for a variable distance. In 70% the rectosigmoid is involved, in 20% the aganglionosis extends proximal to the sigmoid for a variable distance up the colon, and in 10% the aganglionosis extends into the small intestine. The aganglionic bowel is incapable of coordinated peristalsis and passively constricts, resulting in a mechanical obstruction. The incidence is approximately 1 in 5000 births.

Clinical features

Hirschsprung's disease is not associated with a high incidence of prematurity, and most of the babies have a birth weight appropriate for gestational age. This contrasts sharply with most of the other congenital obstructions of the alimentary tract. Associated abnormalities are rare. The most important association is with Down's syndrome.

Symptoms of Hirschsprung's disease are present in the first few days of life in almost all cases. Exceptionally, a baby will have no symptoms during the early neonatal period. The major symptoms are failure to pass meconium within 36 h of birth, abdominal distension, vomiting, and poor feeding. These may occur singly or in combination. Frequently, a rectal examination will relieve the obstruction by passively dilating the aganglionic segment. Twenty to 50% of patients with Hirschsprung's disease are not diagnosed in the early weeks of life. Later presentation is with constipation that dates back to the neonatal period. It is not accompanied by soiling and is frequently associated with failure to thrive. Presentation may be delayed for months or years.

Hirschsprung's enterocolitis may be the mode of presentation in the infant of a few weeks of age. This condition, the precise cause of which is unknown, presents with abdominal distension, profuse diarrhoea, and circulatory collapse. The infant is gravely ill and the mortality is 20%. The child with this complication, successfully treated initially, may have absorptive problems for some time, suffer recurrent episodes of enterocolitis despite successful surgery, and the surgery is attended by a higher rate of complications. The incidence of enterocolitis can be greatly reduced if the diagnosis of Hirschsprung's disease is made in the first week of life.

Diagnosis

In the neonatal period a plain abdominal radiograph will reveal distension of small and large bowel. A barium enema may show the

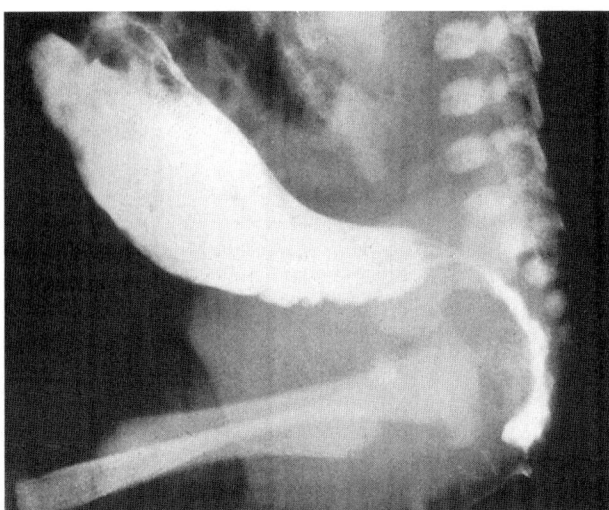

Fig. 15.15.3 Barium enema in Hirschsprung's disease illustrating a narrow aganglionic rectum with dilation proximally.

narrow aganglionic bowel with dilated proximal bowel (Fig. 15.15.3) but a normal barium enema does not exclude Hirschsprung's disease. A 24-h film showing retained barium in the colon is often more helpful than the actual enema in confirming the clinical suspicion of Hirschsprung's disease. The definitive diagnostic procedure is a rectal biopsy. Suction biopsy enables the pathologist to look for ganglion cells in the submucosal plexus; full-thickness biopsy provides the intermyenteric plexus as well but this is usually unnecessary. In Hirschsprung's disease, ganglion cells are absent, hypertrophic nerve trunks are present, and if a histochemical stain for acetylcholinesterase is used, this reveals excessive amounts of this enzyme in the bowel wall. Anorectal manometry in Hirschsprung's disease typically shows failure of relaxation of the internal sphincter in response to rectal distension but this reflex is frequently absent in normal term babies until after the second week of life. This method of diagnosis is therefore unreliable in the neonatal period, requires considerable expertise to obtain reliable results, and cannot be regarded as suitable for the routine diagnosis of Hirschsprung's disease.

Management

Following diagnosis, either definitive surgery is carried out or a colostomy is fashioned in ganglionic bowel and definitive surgery deferred for a period of time. Definitive surgery consists of excision of aganglionic bowel with a 'pull through' procedure, enabling an anastomosis to be made between the anus and ganglionic colon. The three operations most often performed are those described by Swenson, Duhamel, and Soave. Provided that the surgery is uncomplicated, the long-term complications, which include faecal and urinary incontinence, and impotence, should be minimal. Bowel control is likely to be imperfect for a number of years, with soiling as a major problem, but good bowel control will be achieved in the majority of patients treated by experienced surgeons.

Imperforate anus

The exact incidence of this abnormality is not known but the usual incidence quoted is 1 in 5000 births. The basic classification differentiates between the high anomalies, where the bowel terminates above the pelvic floor, the bowel narrowing down to communicate with the urethra in the male (a rectourethral fistula) and the vagina or vestibule in the female (a rectovaginal/vestibular fistula) in the majority of cases. In the low anomalies, the bowel passes through the pelvic floor and either opens on to the perineum in an ectopic position, or lies just beneath the skin-covered anus. The high anomaly is more likely to occur in boys, the low in girls. Overall, more boys than girls present with an imperforate anus. Associated anomalies of the urogenital tract, oesophagus, heart, and skeletal system are common.

Clinical features

Early examination of the perineum will establish the presence of an anorectal anomaly. In boys, the presence of meconium on the perineum usually indicates a low anomaly. In girls, careful inspection is necessary to differentiate meconium being passed *per vaginum*, indicating a high anomaly, from meconium emerging from a perineal site, suggesting a low anomaly. Careful probing of any opening will enable the direction in which the bowel is running to be established. In girls, doubt about the precise anatomy of the anomaly may be resolved by contrast studies. In boys, differentiating a completely covered anus from a high anomaly may be difficult in the early hours after birth. Examination of the urine microscopically may reveal the presence of squamous cells or debris, suggesting a fistula between bowel and urethra. Occasionally, meconium is passed *per urethra*.

A lateral film of the pelvis taken after the infant has lain 'bottom up' over a foam wedge for some minutes will often reveal the level at which the rectum terminates, but this film cannot be reliably interpreted in the first few hours after birth because air may not have reached the distal bowel. In boys, a micturating cystourethrogram will demonstrate a rectourethral fistula in a high proportion of cases, but is rarely necessary as an initial diagnostic procedure. Having defined the nature of the anorectal anomaly, evidence of any associated abnormality should be sought by careful clinical examination and radiographs of chest, abdomen, and the vertebral column.

Management

A low anomaly usually requires a perineal procedure to enlarge the opening. Dilatation alone may suffice, but in the majority of cases a simple anoplasty produces a more satisfactory result. In the long term, the functional results for the low anomalies should be very good. A high anomaly necessitates a defunctioning colostomy in the neonatal period. Definitive surgery involves division of any fistula and positioning the bowel accurately within the pelvic floor and sphincter muscles. Delay in achieving bowel control is common and a number of secondary operations designed to improve control have been advocated. However, if the initial surgery is meticulous, acceptable continence should be achieved in over 80% of children within the first 10 years. A permanent colostomy should rarely be necessary. The high incidence of associated genitourinary abnormalities makes it mandatory to investigate carefully the urinary tract at an early stage. The mortality for anorectal anomalies is largely dictated by the presence of other serious abnormalities.

Further reading

Brown RL, Azizkhan RG (1999). Gastrointestinal bleeding in infants and children: Meckel's diverticulum and intestinal duplication. *Semin Pediatr Surg*, **34**, 202–9.

Condino AA, *et al.* (2004). Abnromal intestinal histology in neonates with congenital anomalies of the gastrointestinal tract. *Biol Neonate*, **85**, 145–50.

Dalla Vecchia LK, *et al.* (1998). Intestinal atresia and stenosis: a 25 year experience with 277 cases. *Arch Surg* **133**, 490–6.

De Backer AI, *et al.* (1997). A patient with congenital short small bowel associated with malrotation. *J Belge Radiol*, **80**, 71–2.

Freeman NV, *et al.* (eds) (1994). *Surgery of the newborn*. Churchill Livingstone, London.

Gupta AK, Cuglani B (2005). Imaging of congenital anomalies of the gastrointestinal tract. *Ind J Pediatr*, 72, 403–14.

Khong PL, *et al.* (2003). Ultrasonography of Intra-abdominal cystic lesions in the newborn. *Clin Radiol*, **58**, 449–54.

Langer JC (1996). Gastroschisis and omphalocele. *Semin Pediatr Surg*, **5**, 124–8.

Larsen WJ (1997). *Human embryology*. Churchill Livingstone, New York.

Pierro, A *et al.* (1997). Staged pull-through for rectosigmoid Hirschsprung's disease is not safer than primary pull-through. *J Pediatr Surg*, **32**, 505–9.

Roberts HE, *et al.* (1998). Increased frequency of cystic fibrosis among infants with jejunoileal atresia. *Am J Med Genet*, **78**, 446–9.

Shaul DB, Harrison EA (1997). Classification of anorectal malformations—initial approach, diagnostic tests, and colostomy. *Semin Pediatr Surg*, **6**, 187–95.

Swaniker F, Soldes O, Hirschl RB (1999). The utility of technetium 99 m pertechnetate scintigraphy in the evaluation of patients Meckel's diverticulum. *J Pediatr Surg*, **34**, 760–4.

Veereman-Wauters G (1996). Normal gut development and postnatal adaptation. *Eur J Pediatr*, **155**, 627–32.

Cancers of the gastrointestinal tract

J.A. Bridgewater and S.P. Pereira

Essentials

Cancers of the gastrointestinal tract are one of the most rewarding interfaces in translational medicine, with recent work—particularly on colorectal cancer—leading to greater understanding of the genetic mechanisms leading to cancer and the development of novel targeted therapies.

Diagnosis of gastrointestinal tract cancers is usually made or suspected at endoscopy, confirmed by biopsy.

Oesophageal cancer

A common cancer, usually of squamous cell histology, that is particularly prevalent in China (male incidence 28/100 000), southern and eastern Africa, and Japan. Typical presentation is with dysphagia, initially to solids and then to liquids. Staging investigations include contrast-enhanced CT, 2-[^{18}F] fluoro-2-deoxy-D-glucose positron emission tomography (FDG-PET scan), and endoscopic ultrasonography. In patients who are fit and suitable for surgery, neoadjuvant chemotherapy is commonly given, but most patients are elderly with comorbid disease and unsuitable for curative surgery, and many others present with advanced disease such that palliation with or without systemic therapy is the only option. For locally advanced inoperable patients, chemoradiation in preference to radiation alone may confer a survival benefit. Specific palliation for dysphagia can include laser, brachytherapy, external beam therapy or stenting. Overall survival is less than 40% at 2 years.

Stomach cancer

A common cancer, usually adenocarcinoma, that is particularly prevalent in eastern Asia (male incidence 46/100 000), eastern Europe, Polynesia and South America. Predisposing factors include deprivation, *Helicobacter pylori* infection, tobacco, alcohol, and diet. Dysphagia, early satiety, and anaemia are common presenting features, with weight loss being an indication of advanced disease. Tumour staging is by CT and, in some centres, endoscopic ultrasonography. Best treatment, when appropriate and when possible, is by surgery with extensive nodal resection with postoperative chemoradiation, neoadjuvant chemotherapy or adjuvant chemotherapy. Palliation in advanced disease is as for oesophageal cancer. Overall survival is 40 to 50% at 5 years.

Colorectal cancer

A common cancer, predisposed to by a Westernized diet (male incidence in the United Kingdom is 56/100 000). It arises in many cases by transformation of adenoma to carcinoma by sequential inherited and acquired mutations: some cases are associated with well-characterized polyposis syndromes (e.g. familial adenomatous polyposis, hereditary nonpolyposis colorectal cancer). Typical presentation of left sided tumours is with alteration of bowel habit, obstruction or overt bleeding, and of right sided tumours is with iron-deficiency anaemia. Staged by Dukes' classification: stage A, confined to the bowel wall; stage B, full thickness involvement of the bowel wall with extension through to the serosa; stage C, spread to lymph nodes; stage D, distant spread, usually to the liver. Surgical resection is the primary treatment and potentially curative in all except Dukes' stage D, with adjuvant fluorouracil or fluoropyrimidine providing benefit. Fluoropyrimidine, in combination with both oxaliplatin and irinotecan, can improve survival in patients with advanced disease. Colonic stenting is an effective technique for symptoms from bowel obstruction. Overall survival is 83% at 5 years for Dukes' stage A, declining to 3% for Dukes' stage D.

Introduction

Cancers of the gastrointestinal tract provide a paradigm for the investigation and treatment of cancer. The relationship between basic research and clinical management has generated one of the most rewarding interfaces in translational medicine, particularly with respect to novel targeted therapies. This has occurred on the background of an increasing understanding of the genetic predisposition to cancer, in particular the influence of common, low-penetrance susceptibility alleles in conferring predisposition to neoplasia. Examples of this include sporadic colorectal carcinoma as well as the better understood genetic syndromes listed in Table 15.16.1.

There is increasing interest in the influence of genetic polymorphisms on treatment toxicity. For instance, *UGT1A1* promoter polymorphisms have been demonstrated to predict early haematologic toxicity following treatment with irinotecan and fluorouracil. The microsatellite instability pathway, which involves failure of the

Table 15.16.1 Gastrointestinal cancer syndromes and their molecular defects

Clinical syndrome	OMIM	Gene	Gene function
Familial adenomatous polyposis	175100	*APC*	Antagonist in WNT signalling pathway
Peutz–Jeghers syndrome	175200	*STK11*	Probable involvement in p53, TGFβ and VEGF signalling pathways
Cowden's syndrome	158350	*PTEN, MMAC1*	Protein acts in late nuclear division and may play a role in preparation for DNA replication; interacts with BMP pathway
Juvenile polyposis	174900	*BMPR1A*	Interacts with PTEN; interacts with WNT signalling pathway
Biallelic mismatch repair	604933	*MUTYH*	Corrects A/G and A/C mismatches
Hereditary nonpolyposis colorectal cancer	609310	*MLH1/ MSH2*	Involved in DNA mismatch repair

nucleotide mismatch recognition and repair system, has been proposed as a form of genomic instability that can predict for survival and response. The consequent loss of DNA repair signals for apoptosis may confer resistance to specific chemotherapy drugs. More recently, the development of a molecular classification for gastrointestinal malignancy using genome-wide screens using C DNA or by microRNA have increased the potential for predicting prognosis and response in parallel with standard molecular techniques.

Although much of the translational work and trials using novel targeted agents have been in colorectal cancer, they are of potential relevance to all types of gastrointestinal malignancy.

Oesophageal cancer

There are approximately 12 000 new cases of oesophageal cancer in the United Kingdom per year (see http://info.cancerresearchuk. org/cancerstats/types/oesophagus/ and Fig. 15.1.6.1). Mortality rates closely resemble incidence and, despite some progress in diagnosis and treatment, there has been little overall impact on the disease. The incidence of oesophagogastric carcinoma is increasing, with the male European age-standardized rate per 100 000 population rising from 7.8 to 13.4 between 1971 and 2005. The corresponding rates for women were 4.2 to 4.9. Worldwide, there is an 18-fold variation in male incidence rates between different regions and an almost 40 fold variation in female rates. There is also ethnic variation, with a six times higher rate in black men than in white men. Most cases (80–85%) of oesophageal cancer are diagnosed in developing countries, where it is the fourth most common cancer in men. The usual histology is squamous cell carcinoma, although the incidence of adenocarcinoma is increasing. This increase is likely to be environmental, although no single agent has been identified and it is uncertain whether or not it is related to the increase in Barrett's oesophagus.

Predisposing factors

It has been proposed that the family of Napoleon Bonaparte had a predisposition to stomach cancer, although epidemiological and genetic aetiologies are somewhat wrong-footed by the conclusion

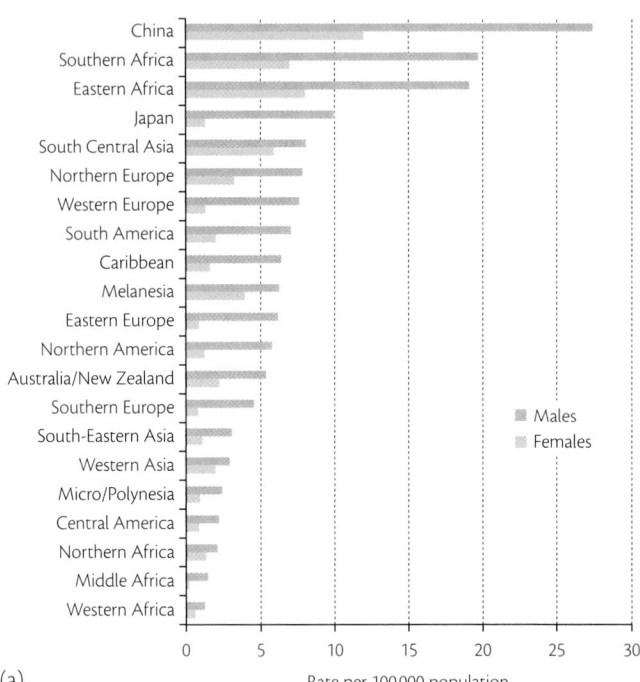

(a)

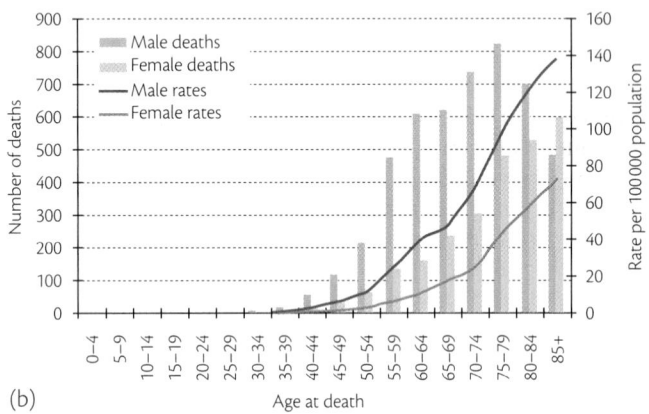

(b)

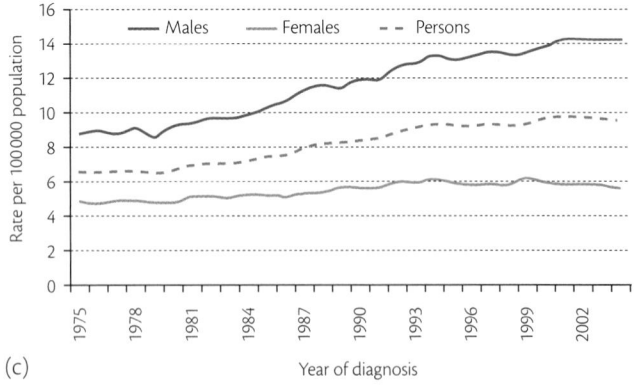

(c)

Fig. 15.16.1 (a) World age-standardized incidence rates for oesophageal cancer, 2002 estimates (http://www.cancer.org.uk). (b) Number of deaths and age-specific mortality rates for oesophageal cancer, by sex, United Kingdom, 2005 (http://www.cancer.org.uk). (c) Age-standardized incidence rates for oesophageal cancer in Europe, 1975–2004 (http://www.cancer.org.uk).

that 'An analysis of Bonaparte's case may convince one that human predisposition to cancer is a phenomenon of an unstable, variable nature, which is easily broken by marriage'. More classically described is tylosis, a syndrome of familial oesophageal cancer and hyperkeratosis of the palms and soles, as well as thickening of the oral mucosa. For an affected family member, the estimated lifetime risk of cancer is 92% by age 70. The linkage has been localized to chromosome 17q25 and associated with down-regulation of the cytoglobin gene.

Environmental factors that may be incriminated in oesophageal cancer include smoking and high alcohol intake, also achalasia, oesophageal strictures due to ingestion of corrosives, radiotherapy, and coeliac disease. The Paterson–Kelly (Plummer–Vinson) syndrome, characterized by iron deficiency anaemia, glossitis, postcricoid webs, and dysphagia has been associated with squamous carcinoma in up to 20% of cases, most commonly in Scandinavian populations.

Clinical features

Approximately 55% of patients have cancers in the lower section of the oesophagus, 30% in the upper section, and 15% in the middle section. Middle and upper oesophageal cancers are more likely to be squamous cell carcinomas, whereas those in the lower oesophagus are commonly adenocarcinoma, potentially arising from a Barrett's oesophagus.

Patients classically present with dysphagia, initially to solids and then to liquids. Other late symptoms such as dyspnoea, a hoarse voice, constant pain and weight loss suggest advanced disease and confer a poor prognosis. Initial diagnosis is made at upper gastrointestinal endoscopy (Fig. 15.16.2a) or occasionally contrast radiology (Fig. 15.16.3), and confirmed by endoscopic biopsy. Standard staging investigations include contrast-enhanced CT, 2-[^{18}F] fluoro-2-deoxy-D-glucose positron emission tomography (the FDG-PET scan), and endoscopic ultrasonography (EUS, Fig. 15.16.2b).

Management

In patients who are fit and suitable for surgery, neoadjuvant chemotherapy is commonly given and confers an improvement in survival from 34% after oesophagectomy alone to 43% at 2 years. For locally advanced inoperable patients, or patients unfit for surgery

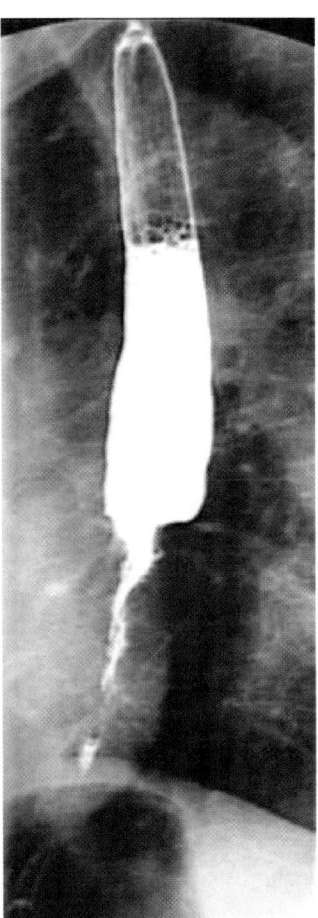

Fig. 15.16.3 Barium swallow demonstrating an obstructing lesion in the mid-oesophagus with proximal dilatation and minimal passage of contrast distally.

chemoradiation in preference to radiation alone may confer a survival of 38% vs 10% at 2 years, although these data come from a small unrepeated study. Attempts to combine surgery and chemoradiation or neoadjuvant chemotherapy and chemoradiation have failed to demonstrate a survival advantage and there is still debate as to the best approach.

Surgery

Surgery is performed using a transhiatal or thoracic approach. There is increasing evidence to suggest that a two-phase oesophagectomy (abdomen and right or left chest approach) with a two-field lymphadenectomy (abdomen and thorax) is oncologically favoured, but this remains controversial.

Palliative approaches

Most patients with oesophageal cancer are elderly with comorbid disease and are unsuitable for curative surgery and 40% of patients present with advanced disease in whom palliation is the only option. Specific palliation for dysphagia can include laser, brachytherapy, external beam therapy, or stenting.

Laser endoscopic therapy vaporizes exophytic tumour under direct vision without mechanical stress on the oesophageal wall so that stenting is usually not required. Successful tumour recanalization can be achieved in more than 90% of appropriately selected patients, and a return to eating solids is seen in most patients after treatment. However, laser therapy needs to be repeated every

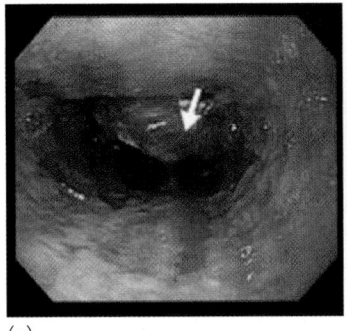 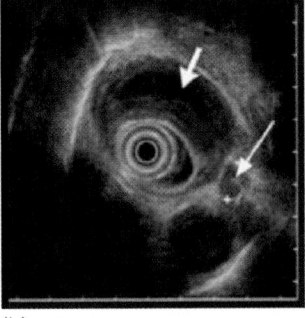

(a)   (b)

Fig. 15.16.2 (A) Mass arising from a Barrett's oesophagus segment at endoscopy. Note the abnormal epithelium which lies distally and around the mass. (B) Endoscopic ultrasound demonstrating the mass that has not penetrated the wall of the oesophagus (short arrow) and an associated enlarged lymph node (long arrow).

4–6 weeks as the tumour regrows. The palliation can be improved with radiation, either external beam or brachtherapy.

Palliative chemotherapy improves survival, although this remains poor with a 1 year survival of 40%. It is likely that three drug combinations offer the best results. Survival and prognosis can be predicted using microRNA arrays, but these methodologies have yet to be prospectively validated.

Stomach cancer

As for oesophageal cancer, stomach cancer occurs mainly in older people and has a striking variation in worldwide incidence (Fig. 15.16.4a, b). Unlike oesophageal cancer, however, the age-standardized incidence rates for males have halved from 31.0 per 100 000 in 1975 to 14.3 in 2004.

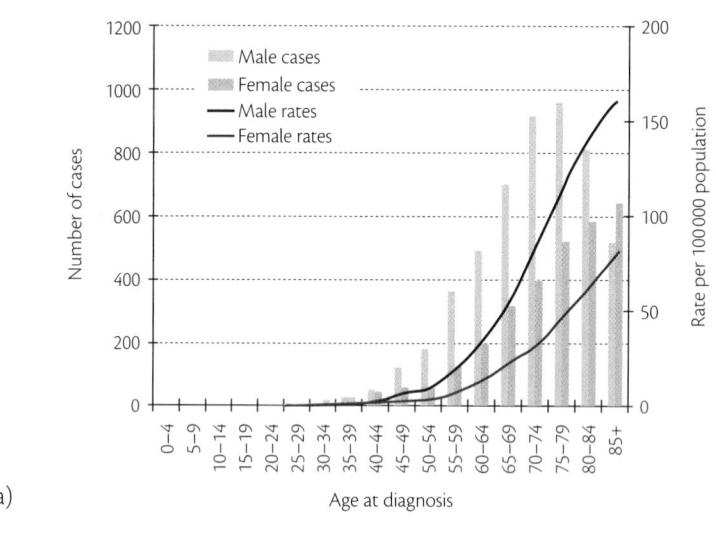

(a)

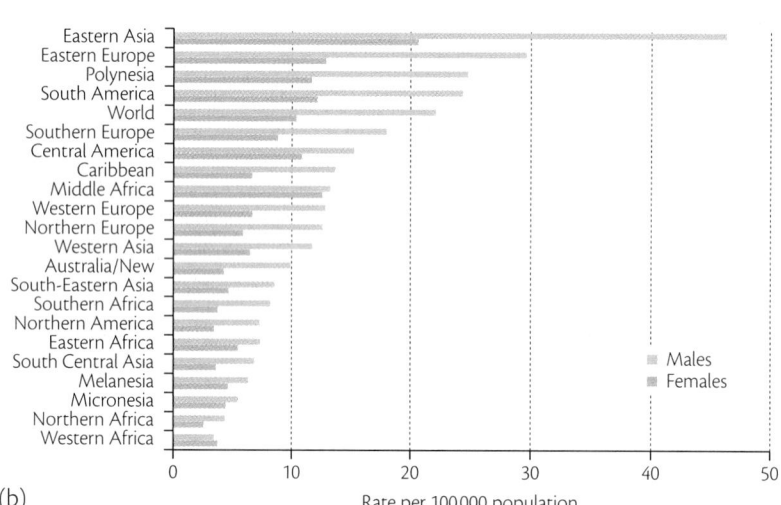

(b)

Fig. 15.16.4 (a) Numbers of new cases and age specific incidence rates, by sex, for stomach cancer, United Kingdom 2004 (http://www.cancer.org.uk). (b) Age-standardized incidence rates for stomach cancer, by sex and region of world (2002 estimates), showing extensive variation in the incidence of stomach cancer (http://www.cancer.org.uk). (c) Age-standardized incidence and mortality, cause-specific 5-year survival by deprivation quintile for stomach cancer in Scotland, 1991–1995, showing a strong link between incidence and deprivation (http://www.cancer.org.uk).

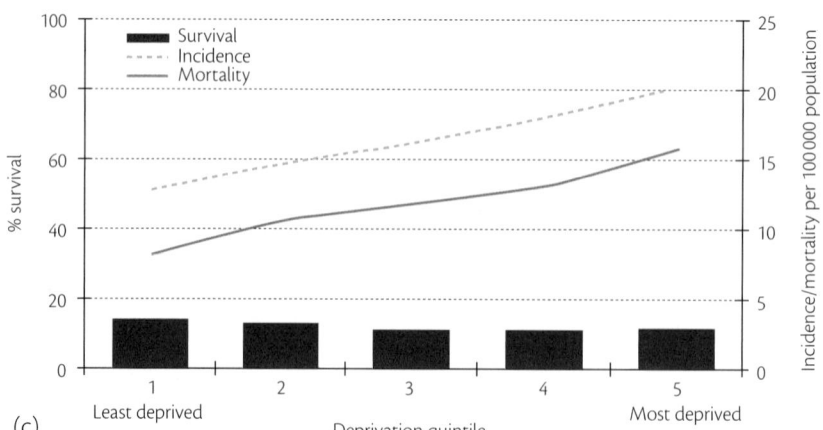

(c)

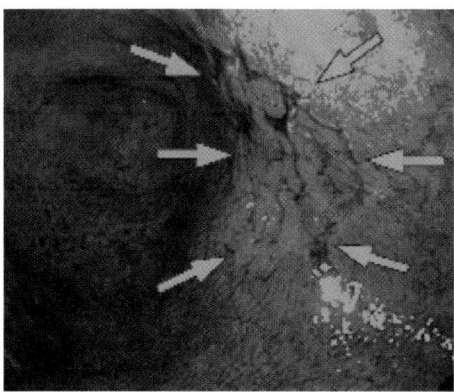

Fig. 15.16.5 Abnormal gastric mucosa suggesting malignancy at the cardia.

Predisposing factors

There are clear links to deprivation (Fig. 15.16.4c), *Helicobacter pylori* infection, tobacco, alcohol and diet. The compelling relationship between *H. pylori* infection and gastric neoplasia (also gastric lymphoma, see Chapter 15.10.4) has led to proposals for national screening programmes, but few countries have implemented these in preference to investigation of symptomatic individuals. Diffuse adenocarcinoma is associated with an E-Cadherin mutation, conferring almost 100% penetrance in the inherited form of this gastric cancer, and leading to recommendations for 'curative' prophylactic gastrectomy in affected families.

Pathology

Most stomach cancers (around 95%) are adenocarcinomas, which may be further classified into 'intestinal' and 'diffuse' types. Intestinal-type adenocarcinomas are found in older patients, are associated with a history of atrophic gastritis, and have better survival. The incidence is falling, probably as a result of decreasing levels of *H. pylori*-associated gastritis.

'Diffuse' adenocarcinomas (also known as linitis plastica or signet cell cancers of the stomach) are more common than intestinal-type

tumours, are associated with a poorer survival, and occur more frequently in women and people with blood group A.

Clinical features

Dysphagia, early satiety, and anaemia are common presenting features, with weight loss being an indication of advanced disease. Gross haematemesis is unusual. An epigastric mass is palpable in about 30% of patients, and palpable lymphadenopathy in the left supraclavicular fossa (Virchow's node; Troisier's sign) may be present. Metastasis occurs to the peritoneum (with ascites and sometimes ovarian involvement—Krukenberg's tumour), to the liver, and in later stages to the lung and other sites. Gastric cancer is the most common malignancy to be associated with dermatomyositis or acanthosis nigricans.

Diagnosis is usually made by upper gastrointestinal endoscopy (Fig. 15.16.5) and biopsy. Tumour staging is by CT and, in some centres, endoscopic ultrasonography, together with careful preoperative assessment to determine fitness for surgery.

Management

Outcome is critically dependent on the success of surgery, although other significant risk factors include comorbidity and nodal status. Most authorities agree that an extensive nodal resection—meaning resection of all perigastric lymph nodes and some coeliac, splenic or splenic–hilar, hepatic artery, and cardia lymph nodes, depending on the location of the tumour in the stomach (a D2 resection)—confers an improved survival over a limited resection (Fig. 15.16.6).

Neo-adjuvant and adjuvant treatment

In patients with resectable gastric cancer, a survival benefit has been demonstrated in large well-designed clinical trials for postoperative chemoradiation, neoadjuvant chemotherapy, and adjuvant chemotherapy. However, these studies have not escaped criticism: one was criticized for suboptimal surgery (only 10% of patients had undergone a formal D2 dissection), and the benefit of chemoradiation may not have been seen with optimal surgery; another was criticized for the inclusion of patients with oesophagogastric tumours (11%), although there was a clear overall benefit of adjuvant treatment for both oesophagogastric and gastric cancers.

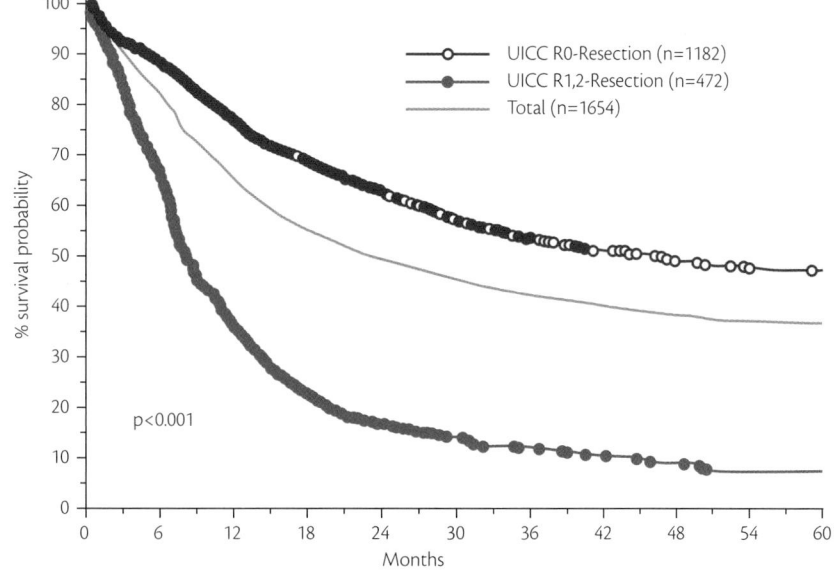

p<0.001

UICC R0-Resection (n=1182)
UICC R1,2-Resection (n=472)
Total (n=1654)

Fig. 15.16.6 5-year survival is critically dependent upon a complete resection (R0) compared to microscopic (R1) or macroscopic (R2) residual disease at resection.
(From Roder (1993), with permission.)

Advanced disease

Palliation of proximal gastric obstruction and palliative chemo-therapy is similar to that for oesophageal cancers. Malignant gastric outlet obstruction can be palliated with stenting, although this is less successful (up to a 25% migration or fracture rate) than for stents placed more proximally. Surgical bypass is an option for patients who are sufficiently fit, but postsurgical gastroparesis may be a problem, particularly in those with metastatic disease.

Small-bowel cancers

Small-bowel adenocarcinoma is rare, accounting for 0.2 to 0.3% of all malignant tumours but associated with a poor 5-year survival of around 25%. The incidence is increased in coeliac and Crohn's disease, and there is some evidence that the incidence is increasing, particularly in black men.

Duodenal polyps are associated with several gastrointestinal polyposis syndromes, but most commonly with familial adenomatous polyposis, with transformation to duodenal carcinoma (resembling adenoma–carcinoma progression in the large bowel) the leading cause of death amongst familial adenomatous polyposis patients who have had a total colectomy. Endoscopic surveillance and prophylactic duodenal resection is recommended in this high risk group.

Hamartomatous polyps are common in the jejunum in Peutz–Jeghers syndrome: these can undergo malignant change, leading to a 500-fold relative risk of small-bowel carcinoma. Carcinoid tumours are usually found in the ileum (see Chapter 15.9).

The most common histological findings are of adenocarcinoma in 40%, with other histologies being lymphoma and gastrointestinal stromal tumours (GIST).

Clinical features

Presentation is with nonspecific symptoms of abdominal pain, change in bowel habit, weight loss, and anaemia. Appearances on noninvasive imaging may be nondiagnostic, hence the diagnosis is usually made at upper gastrointestinal endoscopy or laparotomy.

Management

Surgical resection offers the only opportunity of long-term survival. There is no evidence to support the use of adjuvant or palliative therapy, although this may reflect the paucity of data rather than a true lack of effect.

Colorectal cancer

Incidence and epidemiology

In the United Kingdom, approximately 36000 people are diagnosed with colorectal cancer every year, of which 16000 die of their disease. The incidence had been rising until 1999, since which time it has fallen slightly, and overall mortality has been falling steadily since 1975 (Fig. 15.16.7). The peak incidence of the disease is between the ages of 70 to 80, with less than 5% of cases under the age of 50 years.

There is a clear link between diet and relative risk of colorectal cancer, with subjects consuming more than one portion of red or processed meat a week having a relative risk of 1.63, and there is a strong protective influence of fish, fibre, calcium and dietary folate (Fig. 15.16.8). This effect of a Westernized diet is supported by data demonstrating an increase in incidence of colorectal cancer in first-generation Japanese immigrants to the United States of

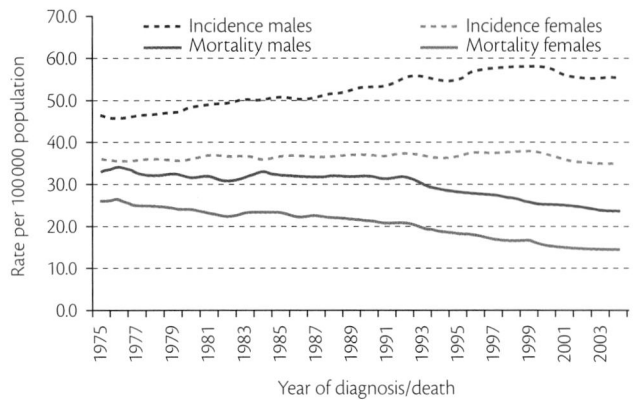

Fig. 15.16.7 Age-standardized incidence and mortality rates by sex for colorectal cancer, United Kingdom, 1975–2004 (http://www.cruk.co.uk).

America compared to their parents. Recent improvements in the diet of Western nations is likely to contribute to a continued decline in incidence. Other factors, but with lesser effects, may include hormone replacement therapy and oral contraceptives, obesity, alcohol intake, tobacco, aspirin, and statins.

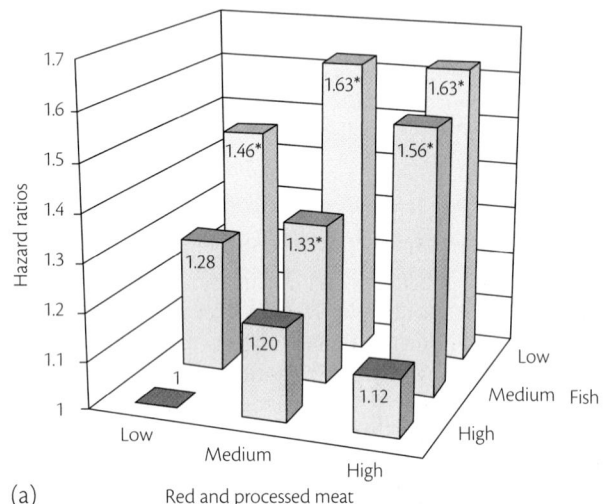

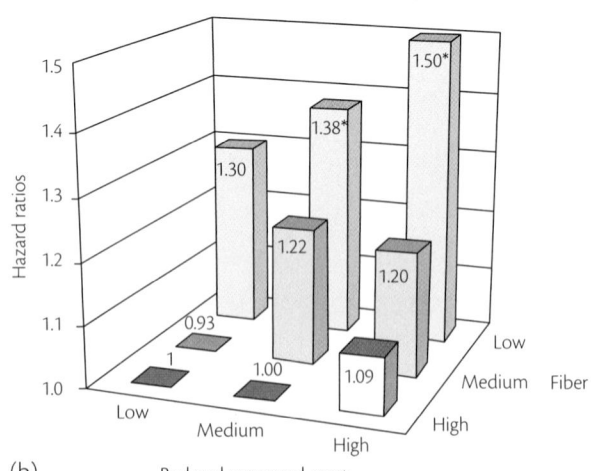

Fig. 15.16.8 Relative risk of developing colorectal cancer increases with diets high in processed meat, low in fibre, and low in fish.
(from Norat 2005.)

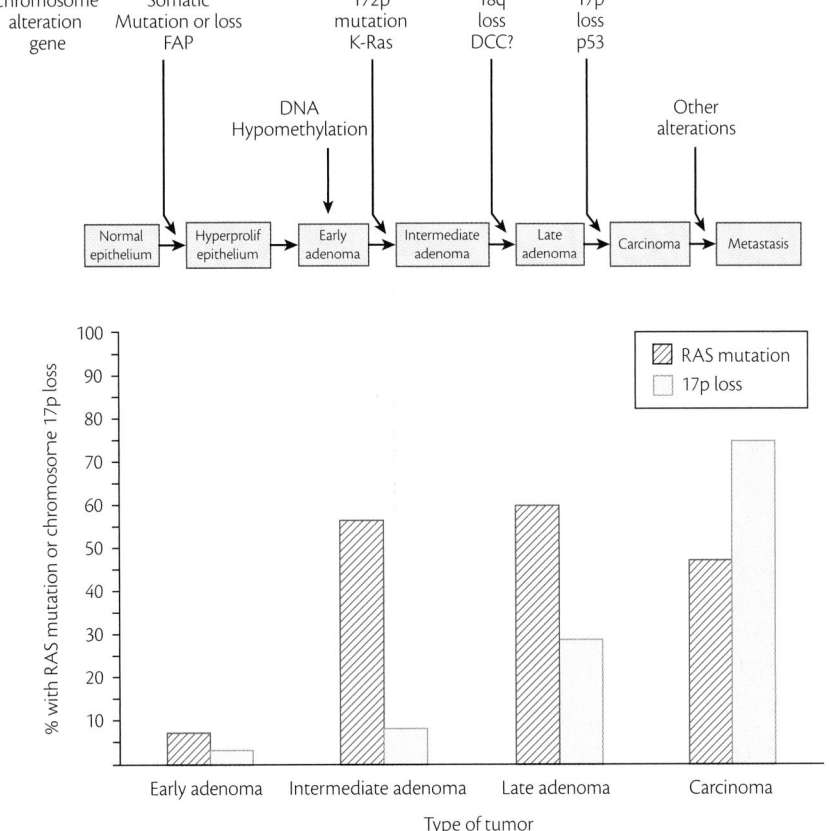

Fig. 15.16.9 Sequential mutation is mirrored by histopathological change and clinical behaviour. (From Fearon ER, Vogelstein B (1990). A genetic model for colorectal tumorigenesis. *Cell*, **61**, 759–767.)

Genetic processes and pathology

Vogelstein and colleagues described the adenoma–carcinoma pathway in which sequential inherited and acquired mutations lead to the development of colorectal cancer following waves of clonal expansion involving *APC/β-catenin*, *KRAS/BRAF*, *TGF-β*, *PIK3CA*, and *TP53* (Fig. 15.16.9). However, this is clearly not the malignant process for all cancers, over 50% of which retain wild-type RAS and over 20% wild-type p53. Similarly, tumour response to agents targeted at the RAS and phosphatidylinositol 3-kinase pathways (cetuximab and panutumumab, see below) are effective only in patients with wild-type RAS and not in patients with mutated RAS.

The Dukes' classification remains the mainstay of staging of colorectal carcinoma: stage A is confined to the bowel wall with no extension to the serosal fat; in stage B there is full thickness involvement of the bowel wall with extension through to the serosa; in stage C there is spread to local nodes (C1) or to more proximal mesenteric nodes (C2); and in stage D there is distant spread, usually to the liver (Fig. 15.16.10). The frequency of the different Dukes' stages, and the impact of staging on survival, are shown in Table 15.16.2

Colorectal cancers can arise in any part of the large bowel or rectum, but are most frequent in the rectum, sigmoid colon, and caecum (Fig. 15.16.11).

The polyposis syndromes

The known polyposis syndromes, all of which have some predisposition to malignancy, are listed in Table 15.16.3

Familial adenomatous polyposis

Familial adenomatous polyposis (FAP) is responsible for 1% of all colorectal cancers, with a reported incidence of 1 in 7000 to 1 in 22 000 live births. The principal feature of the condition is the

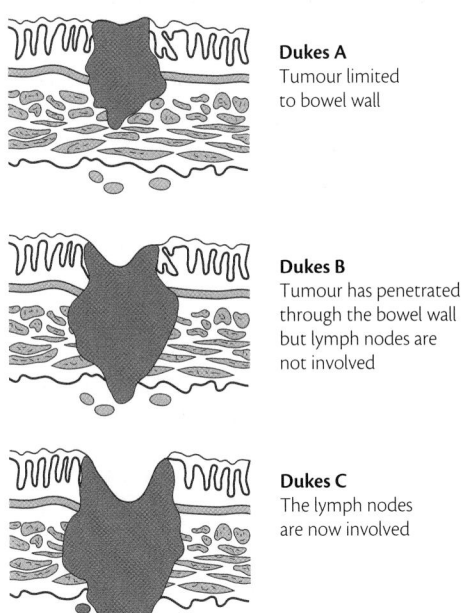

Dukes A
Tumour limited to bowel wall

Dukes B
Tumour has penetrated through the bowel wall but lymph nodes are not involved

Dukes C
The lymph nodes are now involved

Fig. 15.16.10 Dukes' classification of colorectal carcinoma.

Table 15.16.2 Staging and prognosis of colorectal cancer

Dukes'	Cancer	Frequency (%)	5-year survival (%)
A	Localized in bowel wall	11	83
B	Beyond lamina propria	35	64
C	Nodal involvement	26	38
D	Distant metastases	28	3

presence of hundreds to thousands of adenomatous polyps throughout the colon. It is inherited as an autosomal dominant condition, although about one-quarter of cases arise without a family history, thus implying a high rate of new mutations. The gene responsible for FAP—the adenomatous polyposis coli (*APC*) gene—is located on chromosome 5. Most mutations are nonsense mutations, resulting in a truncated protein of less than the predicted 310-kDa (2843 amino acids) wild-type APC protein. Some of these germ-line mutations correlate with phenotypic manifestations, such as retinal pigmentation, desmoids, the severity of polyposis, upper gastrointestinal malignancies, and attenuated FAP (Fig. 15.16.12). As well as colonic polyps, adenomas are found in the duodenum in most patients, and also in the stomach and elsewhere in the small intestine.

There is a 10- to 20-year period between the appearance of an adenoma and its progression to colorectal carcinoma, but the risk of colorectal cancer developing in one of the adenomas is essentially 100% by the age of 40 years, so that this condition is fully penetrant. Adenomas usually begin to develop during the second decade, hence screening by flexible sigmoidoscopy is commenced between 12 and 14 years of age (Fig. 15.16.13, Table 15.16.4). Biopsy of polyps detected at screening for histological diagnosis confirms the condition and allows surgery before the age of 20. Screening family members by flexible sigmoidoscopy confirms or eliminates the diagnosis.

Colectomy with ileorectal or ileoanal anastomosis, or total proctocolectomy with ileostomy, are the recommended surgical procedures. If the rectal stump is left, this will require continued surveillance as the likelihood of malignant change in high.

Table 15.16.3 Colonic polyps and polyposis: a classification

Pathogenesis	Polyps	Polyposis
Metaplastic	Hyperplastic	Hyperplastic polyposis
Inflammatory	Inflammatory	Inflammatory polyposis
Lymphatic	Benign lymphoid	Malignant lymphomatous polyposis
Traumatic	Mucosal prolapse syndrome	Inflammatory cap polyp polyposis
Neoplastic	Adenoma	Familial adenomatous polyposis, if >100
Hamartomatous	Juvenile	Juvenile polyposis
	Peutz–Jeghers syndrome	Peutz–Jeghers syndrome
		Cronkhite–Canada syndrome
Stromal origin		
Neoplastic	Leiomyomatous polyp	Cowden's syndrome
	Lipomatous polyp	
Hamartomatous	Vascular hamartoma	
	Neurofibroma	
	Ganglioneuroma	

Surveillance programmes (Table 15.16.4) have reduced the incidence of colorectal cancer due to FAP, but the prolonged survival of patients post colectomy has highlighted other features of the condition, primarily desmoids and adenomas in the duodenum and stomach. Guidelines have been published for continued clinical management, including suggested surveillance of the duodenum, and also the management of duodenal polyposis and desmoid tumours.

Hereditary nonpolyposis colorectal cancer

Hereditary nonpolyposis colorectal cancer (HNPCC) accounts for 5% of colorectal cancer. Cancer occurs at a mean age of 45 years, with primarily right-sided colorectal cancer and an excess of synchronous colorectal cancer. There is also an excess of extracolonic cancers (endometrium, small bowel, pancreas, hepatobiliary tract, brain, and upper uroepithelial tract). Patients with HNPCC may also have sebaceous adenomas, sebaceous carcinomas, and multiple keratoacanthomas.

At-risk patients are identified using the Amsterdam criteria (Box 15.16.1)

HNPCC arises as a result of the germ-line transmission of mutations and polymorphisms in six genes encoding components of the DNA mismatch repair enzyme system and the TGFβ receptor II gene. The encoded proteins repair DNA mismatches arising as a result of replication errors and are described as RER+ (positive replication error), mostly the *MLH1*, *MSH2*, and *MSH6* genes. Replication of DNA is particularly prone to error in those regions of DNA known as microsatellites, where multiple short nucleotide repeat sequences occur. Loss of DNA repair function leads to the so-called 'microsatellite instability' of these regions, such that the allele sizes of microsatellites are different in tumours than in normal cells from the same individual. PCR-based methods are readily

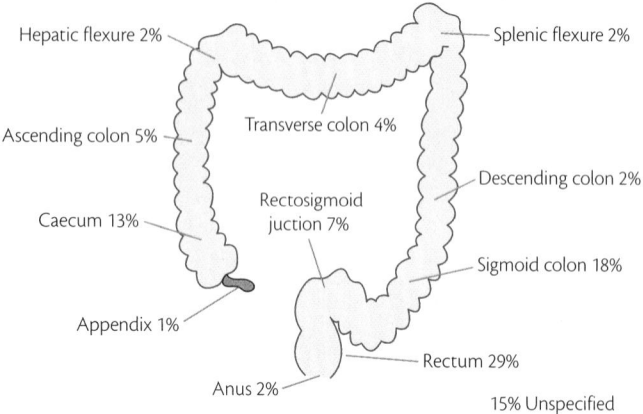

Fig. 15.16.11 Anatomical distribution of adenocarcinoma within the large bowel.

Hepatic flexure 2%
Splenic flexure 2%
Ascending colon 5%
Transverse colon 4%
Descending colon 2%
Caecum 13%
Rectosigmoid juction 7%
Sigmoid colon 18%
Appendix 1%
Rectum 29%
Anus 2%
15% Unspecified

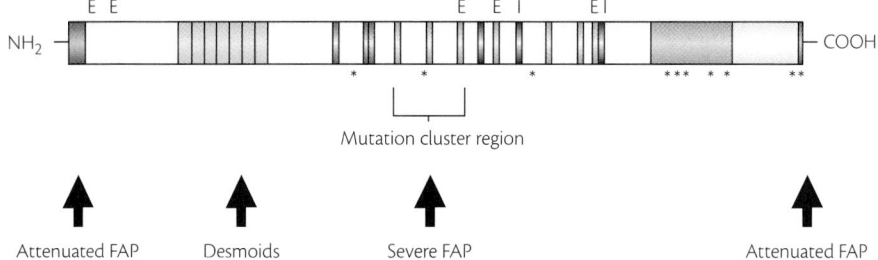

Fig. 15.16.12 Phenotypes can be predicted form the site of mutation on the APC gene. FAP, familial adenomatous polyposis. (Adapted from Fodde R, Smits R, Clevers H (2001). APC, Signal transduction and genetic instability in colorectal cancer. *Nat Rev Cancer*, **1**, 55–67.)

able to detect this to establish that a given tumour has an RER+ phenotype. The extent of microsatellite instability varies between tumours and there is some disagreement as to how many loci need to be modified before a tumour can be classified as RER+. In addition to patients with HNPCC, between 10 and 15% of sporadic colorectal cancers are also RER+.

Screening and prevention

Three randomized studies have demonstrated the potential improvement in survival of screening for colorectal cancer using guaiac faecal occult blood testing in the 50- to74-year-old population, which is now being piloted throughout the United Kingdom and Europe. The results of a trial in Nottingham (United Kingdom) showed a reduction in mortality from colorectal cancer in the intervention group of 15% at a median follow-up of 7.8 years, and there are early data to suggest a decrease in the incidence of new cancers in the general population as a result of faecal occult blood testing.

Clinical features

The site of a colorectal cancer influences the symptoms that it is likely to produce. The stool becomes more solid as it passes through the colon, hence obstruction and overt bleeding are increasingly likely with distal lesions. Blood is typically dark and mixed in with the stool, in contrast to the fresh or dripping bleeding that is caused by haemorrhoids. Alteration of bowel habit may be in terms of frequency or increased constipation where the flow of solid stool is obstructed, which is particularly likely with left-sided lesions. Tumours can grow to considerable size in the right colon without affecting faecal flow, often leading to presentation with iron-deficiency anaemia as a consequence of long-standing but occult blood loss. Pain in a patient with colorectal cancer suggests obstructive disease or invasion, and weight loss is a late symptom suggesting advanced disease and poor prognosis.

Digital rectal examination is an essential part of the physical examination of any patient with symptoms that might be attributable to colorectal cancer. The finding of an enlarged, irregular, hard liver clearly suggests metastatic disease.

Routine laboratory investigation may reveal iron-deficiency anaemia and abnormal liver blood tests, but specific investigations obviously focus on the bowel. Patients with new symptoms require endoscopy (flexible sigmoidoscopy or colonoscopy, Box 15.16.2) or other imaging (barium enema or CT, including CT colonography). For rectal cancers, MRI and endoanal ultrasonography improve staging (http://www.nice.org.uk/nicemedia/pdf/CSGCCfullguidance.pdf).

Management

Surgery

Surgical resection is the primary treatment and potentially curative. There are no differences between open and laparoscopic-assisted surgery with respect to tumour and nodal status, short-term endpoints, and quality of life, hence surgery for resectable colon cancer is increasingly a laparoscopic procedure. However, although almost three-quarters of patients have no evidence of metastases at diagnosis (Table 15.16.2), about one-third of these relapse, mostly with incurable disease.

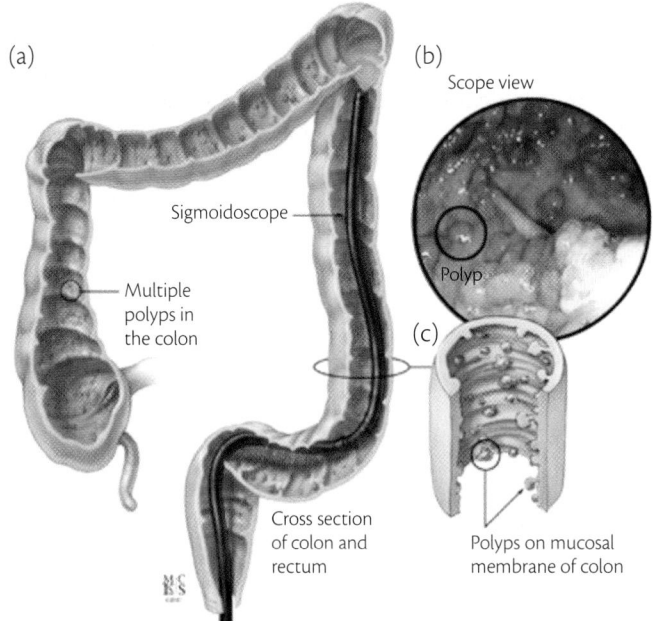

Fig. 15.16.13 Familial adenomatous polyposis. Sigmoidoscopy reveals carpeting of the colon by hundreds of adenomas.

Table 15.16.4 Colorectal surveillance protocol in family members at risk for FAP

	Type of investigation	Lower age limit	Interval
Classical FAP	Sigmoidoscopy*	10–12 years	2 years[a]
AFAP	Colonoscopy	18–20 years	2 years[a]

[a] Once adenomas are detected, annual colonoscopy should be performed until colectomy is planned.

AFAP, attenuated familial adenomatous polyposis.

(Adapted from Vasen 2008.)

Box 15.16.1 Amsterdam criteria for hereditary nonpolyposis colorectal cancer (HNPCC)

Amsterdam I criteria

At least three relatives must have histologically verified colorectal cancer, with one being a first-degree relative of the other two:

1 At least two successive generations must be affected.

2 At least one of the relatives with colorectal cancer must have received the diagnosis before the age of 50 years.

3 FAP must have been excluded.

Amsterdam II criteria

At least three relatives must have a cancer associated with hereditary nonpolyposis colorectal cancer (colorectal, endometrial, stomach, ovary, ureter or renal–pelvis, brain, small-bowel, hepatobiliary tract, or skin (sebaceous tumours)):

1 One must be a first-degree relative of the other two.

2 At least two successive generations must be affected.

3 At least one of the relatives with cancer associated with HNPCC should have received the diagnosis before the age of 50 years.

4 FAP should have been excluded in any relative with colorectal cancer.

5 Tumours should be verified whenever possible.

FAP, familial adenomatous polyposis.

Adjuvant and neo-adjuvant therapy

In 1990, Moertel and colleauges described a reduction in death of 33% following 12 months of adjuvant fluorouracil. Oral fluoropyrimidine is more convenient, as effective, and can obviate complications associated with central venous catheters although toxicity may be greater. There is a further improvement in survival of 4.4% with the addition of oxaliplatin, although this is accompanied by significant neurotoxicity.

Advanced disease

Fluoropyrimidine, in combination with both oxaliplatin and irinotecan, can improve survival in patients with advanced disease. Oral fluoropyrimidines have been shown to be as effective as 5-fluorouracil but incur more toxicity. Targeted agents such as the anti-vascular endothelial growth factor antibody bevacizumab and

---

Box 15.16.2 Common indications for colonoscopy

♦ Rectal bleeding and or change in bowel habit to a looser stool in patients >50 years

♦ History of ulcerative colitis, previous polyps, previous colorectal cancer, family history in patients >45 years.

♦ Iron-deficiency anaemia without an obvious cause

♦ Palpable right-sided abdominal or rectal mass

National Institute for Health and Clinical Excellence (2005). *Referral guidelines for lower gastrointestinal cancer.*

---

the anti-epidermal growth factor receptor cetuximab have further increased survival. Neo-adjuvant therapy and surgery for liver metastases has been shown to improve disease-free survival, and the resection of lung metastases as well as locally ablative techniques such as radioactive yttrium and radiofrequency ablation are having an impact on the long-term survival of patients once thought to have incurable disease.

The molecular genotyping of patients is likely to play an increasing role in treatment decisions, e.g. patients with a mutant kRAS are unlikely to benefit from epidermal growth factor receptor inhibition.

Palliation

Colonic stenting is an effective technique for symptoms from bowel obstruction, and in some cases can be used as a precursor to resection, allowing the performance status of the patient to improve and permit definitive surgery. Octreotide may improve symptoms in those with disease at multiple sites precluding stenting or surgery.

Rectal cancer

If the mesorectal margin is threatened or breached, chemoradiation with fluoropyrimidine as a radiosensitizer can render cancers operable. Patients in whom complete microscopic resection (R0) cannot be obtained have a universally poor prognosis. In operable cancers, a total mesorectal excison preceded by short course irradiation has been shown to reduce local relapse, although survival benefit is disputed (Fig. 15.16.14).

Tumours that occur throughout the gastrointestinal tract

Several types of malignancy can occur throughout the gastrointestinal tract. Initial symptoms may be related to the mass effect that occurs within that site, e.g. a caecal B-cell lymphoma may present with obstruction, in which case initial management should be as for all obstructing tumours of the caecum, but subsequent treatment should be based on pathology rather than anatomy, i.e. of curative intent with lymphoma-specific combination chemotherapy rather than as the much more common adenocarcinoma of the caecum. Exceptions are the neuroendocrine malignancies that have specific management determined by primary site.

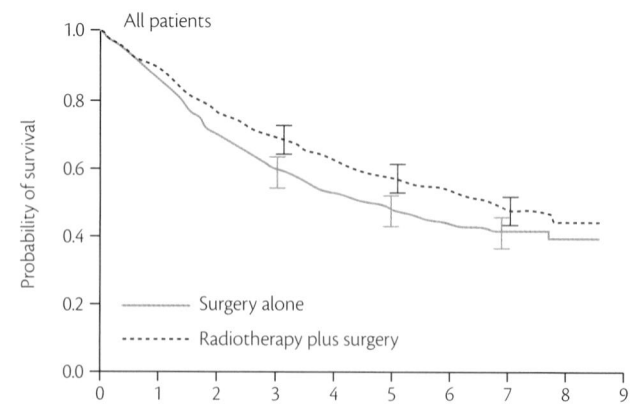

Fig. 15.16.14 A short course of irradiation before surgery for operable rectal cancer improves survival.
(From Swedish Rectal Cancer Consortium 1999.)

Non-Hodgkin's lymphoma

There are two commonly occurring lymphomas of the gastrointestinal tract, mucosa-associated lymphoid tissue (MALT) and a high-grade B-cell lymphoma, the latter being managed with chemotherapy without surgery and without significant risk of perforation. See Chapter 15.10.4 for further discussion.

Gastrointestinal stromal tumour

Gastrointestinal stromal tumours (GISTs) arise from the interstitial cells of Cajal, thought to be the pacemaker cells for gastric contraction. They occur throughout the gastrointestinal tract, and the most common stomach GIST frequently grows to a significant size before there are any local symptoms. They are associated with mutations within the cKIT domain, leading to constitutive activation and oncogenic development, with median survival approaching 5 years. Treatment options were limited to surgery and the prognosis was poor before the introduction of imatinib, a small molecule that inhibits tyrosine kinase domains of the cKIT and platelet derived growth factor (PDGF) receptors. Unlike chemotherapy, responses can occur many months into treatment. Patients with *KIT* exon 11 mutations have a higher rate of objective response (86%) than patients with exon 9 mutation (48%) or no mutations in *KIT* or *PDGFRA* (0%). GISTs are typically responsive before the development of novel mutations in further cKIT domains, responsible also for primary nonresponsiveness. Salvage therapies include other kinase inhibitors or surgery.

Melanoma

Primary melanoma occurs throughout the gastrointestinal tract, most commonly in the nasopharynx, rectum, and anus, but care must be taken to exclude metastasis from cutaneous melanoma whenever a lesion is found in the bowel. Surgery is often the first treatment, but there is no evidence-based management algorithm. Staging and treatment is usually based on that for cutaneous melanoma.

Linitis plastica

Although linitis plastica (signet cell carcinoma) occurs most frequently in the stomach, in can also occur in the colon and rectum, gallbladder, and pancreas. Such cases must be carefully differentiated from the more common scenario of a linitis plastica of the stomach with peritoneal spread.

Neuroendocrine tumours

Neuroendocrine tumors are a group of neoplasms arising from neuroendocrine cells of the diffuse endocrine system. They comprise approximately 2% of all malignant tumors of the gastrointestinal tract, and are usually sporadic, but they may occur as part of multiple endocrine neoplasia 1 syndrome (MEN1), von Hippel–Lindau syndrome, neurofibromatosis, and tuberous sclerosis. Most have relatively slow tumor growth, but malignant potential, and most are diagnosed when distant (mainly liver) metastases have developed. Gastrointestinal neuroendocrine tumors (carcinoids) and neuroendocrine pancreatic tumours (islet cell tumours) make up the majority. Surgery of the primary and metastasis, where possible, remains the only chance of cure. Somatostatin analogues control symptoms in cases of functional tumors, and peptide receptor treatment, transarterial hepatic embolization (or chemoembolization), chemotherapy are options for palliative therapy. See Chapters 15.9 and 15.24.3 for further information.

Sarcoma

Sarcomas of the gastrointestinal tract are exceedingly rare, with angiosarcomas of the large bowel and liposarcomas of the oesophagus being the least uncommon, and should be treated like all other sarcomas.

Small-cell carcinoma

Small-cell carcinomas have been described in all parts of the gastrointestinal tract. Treatment is as for primary small cell carcinoma of the lung, but prognosis is poor.

Metastasis

Metastasis in the gastrointestinal occurs commonly in the liver (see Chapter 15.22.6) and following intracoelomic dissemination, but has been described uncommonly in pancreas. The liver is the most common site of metastatic presentation for carcinoma of unknown primary. Metastasis must be suspected in patients with a history of prior malignancy. Biopsy and comparison with prior histopathology is essential to confirm the diagnosis where there is clinical doubt and the overall condition of the patient makes this appropriate.

Further reading

Clarke CA, McConnell RB (1954). Six cases of carcinoma of the oesophagus occurring in one family. *Br Med J*, **2**, 1137–8.

Cunningham D, Allum WH, Stenning SP, et al. (2006). Perioperative Chemotherapy versus Surgery Alone for Resectable Gastroesophageal Cancer. In, 11–20.

Fearon ER, Vogelstein B (1990). A genetic model for colorectal tumorigenesis. *Cell*, **61**, 759–67.

Fishman PN, et al. (2006). Natural history and chemotherapy effectiveness for advanced adenocarcinoma of the small bowel: a retrospective review of 113 cases. *Am J Clin Oncol*, **29**, 225–31.

Fodde R, Smits R, Clevers H (2001). APC, Signal transduction and genetic instability in colorectal cancer. *Nat Rev Cancer*, **1**, 55–67.

Gebski V., et al. (2007). Survival benefits from neoadjuvant chemoradiotherapy or chemotherapy in oesophageal carcinoma: a meta-analysis. *Lancet Oncol*, **8**, 226–34.

Haselkorn T, Whittemore AS, Lilienfeld DE (2005). Incidence of small bowel cancer in the United States and worldwide: geographic, temporal, and racial differences. *Cancer Causes Control*, **16**, 781–7.

Hermans J, et al. (1993). Adjuvant therapy after curative resection for gastric cancer: meta- analysis of randomized trials. *J Clin Oncol*, **11**, 1441–7.

Herskovic A, et al. (1992). Combined chemotherapy and radiotherapy compared with radiotherapy alone in patients with cancer of the esophagus. *N Engl J Med*, **326**, 1593–8.

Hurwitz H, et al. (2004). Bevacizumab plus irinotecan, fluorouracil, and leucovorin for metastatic colorectal cancer. *N Engl J Med*, **350**, 2335–42.

Kapiteijn E, et al. (2001). Preoperative radiotherapy combined with total mesorectal excision for resectable rectal cancer. *N Engl J Med*, **345**, 638–46.

Kim GP, et al. (2007). Prognostic and predictive roles of high-degree microsatellite instability in colon cancer: A National Cancer Institute-National Surgical Adjuvant Breast and Bowel Project Collaborative Study. *J Clin Oncol*, **25**, 767–72.

Kronborg O, et al. (1996). Randomised study of screening for colorectal cancer with faecal-occult-blood test. *Lancet*, **348**, 1467–71.

Law W, Choi HK, Chu KW (2003). Comparison of stenting with emergency surgery as palliative treatment for obstructing primary left-sided colorectal cancer. *Br J Surg*, **90**, 1429–33.

Leung WK, *et al.* (2008). Screening for gastric cancer in Asia: current evidence and practice. *Lancet Oncol*, **9**, 279–87.

Lynch HT, de la Chapelle A (2003). Hereditary colorectal cancer. *N Engl J Med*, **348**, 919–32.

Macdonald JS, Smalley SR, Benedetti J, *et al.* (2001). Chemoradiotherapy after Surgery Compared with Surgery Alone for Adenocarcinoma of the Stomach or Gastroesophageal Junction. *N Engl J Med*, **345**, 725–30.

Massacesi C, Galeazzi G (2006). Sustained release octreotide may have a role in the treatment of malignant bowel obstruction. *Palliat Med*, **20**, 715–16.

McRonald FE, Liloglou T, Xinarianos G, *et al.* (2006). Down-regulation of the cytoglobin gene, located on 17q25, in tylosis with oesophageal cancer (TOC): evidence for trans-allele repression. *Hum Mol Genet*, **15**, 1271–7.

Modlin IM, *et al.* (2008). Gastroenteropancreatic neuroendocrine tumours. *Lancet Oncol*, **9**, 61–72.

MRC Working Party for Oesophageal Cancer (2002). Surgical resection with or without preoperative chemotherapy in oesophageal cancer: a randomised controlled trial. *Lancet*, **359**, 1727–3.

Pashayan N, *et al.* (2006). Survival trends for small intestinal cancer in England and Wales, 1971–1990: national population-based study. *Br J Cancer*, **95**, 1296–300.

Sakuramoto S, Sasako M, Yamaguchi T, *et al.* (2007). Adjuvant Chemotherapy for Gastric Cancer with S-1, an Oral Fluoropyrimidine. *N Engl J Med*, **357**, 1810–20.

Schlabach MR, *et al.* (2008). Cancer proliferation gene discovery through functional genomics. *Science*, **319**, 620–4.

Scholefield JH, *et al.* (2002). Effect of faecal occult blood screening on mortality from colorectal cancer: results from a randomised controlled trial. *Gut*, **50**, 840–4.

Sokoloff B (1938). Predisposition to cancer in the Bonaparte family. *The American Journal of Surgery*, **40**, 673–8.

Spirio L, *et al.* (1993). Alleles of the *APC* gene: an attenuated form of familial polyposis. *Cell*, **75**, 951–7.

Swedish Rectal Cancer Trial (1997). Improved survival with preoperative radiotherapy in resectable rectal cancer. *N Engl J Med*, **336**, 980–7.

Toumpanakis CG, Caplin ME. (2008). Molecular genetics of gastroenteropancreatic neuroendocrine tumors. *Am J Gastroenterol*, **103**, 729–32.

Vasen HF, *et al.* (1999). New clinical criteria for hereditary nonpolyposis colorectal cancer (HNPCC, Lynch syndrome) proposed by the International Collaborative group on HNPCC. *Gastroenterology*, **116**, 1453–6.

Wagner AD, *et al.* (2006). Chemotherapy in advanced gastric cancer: a systematic review and meta-analysis based on aggregate data. *J Clin Oncol*, **24**, 2903–9.

Wild CP, Hardie LJ (2003). Reflux, Barrett's oesophagus and adenocarcinoma: burning questions. *Nat Rev Cancer*, **3**, 676–84.

15.17

Vascular and collagen disorders

Graham Neale

Essentials

A wide range of vascular and collagen disorders may affect the gastro-intestinal tract. Most are quite uncommon but presentations are often dramatic with intestinal bleeding or gangrene.

Vascular insufficiency leading to ischaemic damage of the gut may be caused by occlusion of mesenteric vessels by either arterial thrombosis (usually with atheromatous pathology); or venous thrombosis (in thrombophilic conditions); or arterial emboli (as occurs with atrial fibrillation); or diffuse small vessel occlusion. There are four primary syndromes. (1) Acute mesenteric ischaemia—typically manifest as the sudden onset of abdominal pain, initially without marked tenderness or localizing signs. Diagnosis requires a high index of suspicion and is often delayed. Imaging serves primarily to exclude other causes of an apparent abdominal catastrophe but prompt laparotomy for embolectomy and/or arterial re-construction and/or bowel resection is required to minimize damage to the gut. (2) Chronic mesenteric ischaemia—usually due to atheroma, presents with severe cramping abdominal pain 20 to 60 min, after eating. Diagnosis requires vascular imaging and usually the condition can be relieved only by revascularization. (3) Ischaemic colitis—presents with pain and tenderness in the left iliac fossa, nausea and vomiting, followed by the passage of a loose motion containing dark blood. Contrast enema examination characteristically shows 'thumbprinting' of the colonic mucosa. Most cases resolve spontaneously so supportive management is usually sufficient. (4) Ischaemia–reperfusion injury—diminishes the barrier function of the gut and may lead to septicaemia in those who are already critically ill.

Vascular malformations in the intestine may present with acute bleeding or an iron deficient anaemia. Conditions include (1) Dieufaloy's disease—an arterial malformation in the upper stomach that usually presents with recurrent massive bleeding; (2) hereditary telangiectasia—with skin lesions and low grade gastrointestinal bleeding; and (3) angiodysplasia—occurs most commonly in the caecum and ascending colon of older patients and is difficult to diagnose. Discrete vascular malformations may be treated endoscopically, although surgical resection is required in some cases.

Collagen-vascular disorders (systemic sclerosis, systemic lupus erythematosus (SLE), and primary vasculitides) may be associated with damage to the intestine. Abdominal symptoms may occur when the pathological process affects the gut but these rarely dominate the clinical picture.

Causes of segmental mesenteric ischaemia

The blood supply to the gut may be impaired by compression, by intraluminal occlusion of vessels, or by intrinsic vascular pathology, including vasospasm (Box 15.17.1).

Compression of mesenteric vessels

The mesenteric vessels may be compressed by torsion or strangulation of the mesentery, retroperitoneal haematomas, neoplastic infiltration, and rarely by proliferating fibrous tissue such as occurs in retroperitoneal fibrosis or occasionally around carcinoid or desmoid tumours. Venous occlusion with thrombosis is a rare complication of excessive gaseous pressure during laparoscopy.

Intraluminal occlusion of mesenteric vessels

Thrombosis

Thrombosis may occur in arteries or veins. In arteries thrombosis usually occurs on an ulcerated atheromatous plaque but it may occur spontaneously in polycythaemia, sickle cell disease, cryoglobulinaemia, and amyloidosis. Thromboangiitis obliterans (Buerger's disease) is a rare condition which does not usually affect mesenteric vessels, but intestinal infarction has been described as a first manifestation of the disorder in women who smoke. Mesenteric arterial thrombosis has also been described in cocaine addicts.

Mesenteric venous thrombosis is less common than arterial occlusion. An inherited thombophilia (such as deficiency of

Box 15.17.1 Causes of ischaemia of the gut

Mechanical occlusion of vessels

+ Torsion of the mesentery

+ Strangulation of a loop of intestine

+ Extraluminal compression

Intraluminal vascular occlusion

+ Thrombosis—arterial or venous

+ Emboli

+ Diffuse microthrombosis

Intrinsic vascular pathology

+ Atheromatous occlusion

+ Inflammation of blood vessels

Nonocclusive mesenteric ischaemia (severe constriction of splanchnic vessels)

+ Profound hypotension as a result of cardiac decompensation, sepsis, acute pancreatitis

+ Post major procedures including dialysis

+ Intestinal reperfusion injury

protein C, protein S, or antithrombin III) is the most likely cause. It may also occur in the primary antiphospholipid antibody syndrome and with dysfibrinogenaemia and has been described in women taking oral contraceptives (especially those who smoke), after splenectomy and in association with pancreatitis.

Arterial embolism

Emboli cause up to one-third of cases of mesenteric vascular occlusion. They arise from the heart, especially in patients with mitral stenosis and atrial fibrillation, with myocardial infarction and endomyocardial thrombosis, and with bacterial endocarditis. Paradoxical embolism through a patent foramen ovale and embolism from aortic mural thrombi are uncommon causes.

Diffuse microthrombosis

Diffuse thrombosis of small vessels may occur as a result of disseminated intravascular coagulation. The haemolytic–uraemic syndrome and thrombotic thrombocytopenic purpura are related conditions in which platelet aggregation occurs in small vessels (see Section 22). Renal failure usually dominates the clinical picture, but in most patients there is evidence of widespread involvement of the intestine and related organs. The haemostatic abnormalities and their relationship to microvascular injury are complex and give rise to diverse and often confusing clinical and laboratory findings. Infusions of platelets and fresh plasma are usually beneficial, but therapy must be individualized depending on the nature of the underlying pathology and the site and severity of haemorrhage or thrombosis.

Intrinsic vascular pathology

Atheromatous occlusion

Atheroma is the most common cause of mesenteric vascular insufficiency. It often remains undiagnosed in life, probably because the

slowness of the pathological process allows for the development of a compensatory collateral circulation. Intestinal infarction secondary to atheromatous occlusion of one major mesenteric vessel is uncommon. Indeed, rarely, all three vessels may be occluded without visceral damage.

Inflammation of blood vessels

Vasculitis is primarily a disorder of small vessels and affects many organs (Box 15.17.2). Involvement of the mesenteric circulation rarely causes infarction of long segments of the gut but may cause a wide spectrum of gastrointestinal disorders that are described later in this chapter.

Damage to the arterial wall in the splanchnic circulation sometimes occurs a few days after surgical correction of coarctation of the aorta. There is necrotizing arteritis with fibrinoid necrosis which is most marked at arterial bifurcations and appears to be related to the sudden sustained increase in blood pressure. It usually resolves spontaneously but may occasionally lead to intestinal infarction requiring operative intervention.

The walls of the mesenteric arteries may be involved in fibroelastic hyperplasia and in Takayasu's disease. In malignant hypertension, intimal hyperplasia and fibrinoid necrosis of arteriolar walls may lead to patchy ischaemia of the intestines. Irradiation of the

Box 15.17.2 Vasculitides that may affect the gut

Involving vessels of all sizes

+ Polyartertis nodosa

+ Churg–Strauss disease

+ Giant cell arteritis

+ Takayasu's arteritis

+ Transplant rejection

Involving predominantly medium and small vessels

+ Wegener's granulomatosis

+ Kawasaki disease

+ Buerger's disease

Vasculitis of collagen–vascular disorders[a]

+ Rheumatoid disease

+ SLE

+ Progressive systemic sclerosis

+ Dermatomyositis

Involving predominantly small vessels

+ Hypersensitivity angiitis (microscopic polyarteritis)

+ Henoch–Schönlein purpura

+ Serum sickness

+ Infective angiitis (e.g. typhoid, tuberculosis)

[a] The vasculitides of these disorders often involve only small vessels and the histological features may be indistinguishable from hypersensitivity angiitis. However, significant gastrointestinal pathology rarely occurs without the involvement of medium-sized vessels.

abdomen leads to vascular necrosis and thrombosis, which in turn may cause ischaemic ulceration that, on healing, leaves a fibrosed intima and a poorly perfused segment of intestine.

Mesenteric veno-occlusive disease (previously described as idiopathic venous thrombosis) has been described as a discrete entity that may affect adults of any age.

Nonocclusive mesenteric ischaemia (Box 15.17.3)

Sporadic and epidemic cases of necrotizing enteritis occurring without evidence of vascular occlusion have been described from many parts of the world and in all age groups. Neonatal necrotizing enterocolitis occurs in the first week of life of premature and low-birth-weight infants. Artificial hyperosmolar feeds may promote damage, whereas breast milk appears to be protective, possibly by providing passive enteric immunity. Lesions occur most frequently in the stomach, the distal ileum, and the colon; as mucosal integrity disintegrates bacterial invasion enhances the damage. The condition may also occur in infants of normal birth weight who have a hyperviscosity syndrome or who have been exposed to cocaine *in utero*.

In adults, infarction of the gastrointestinal tract without vascular occlusion is seen mainly in older people with severe low-output cardiac failure; in hypotensive patients requiring intensive care; and in patients undergoing haemodialysis, especially when overtreated with erythropoietin. Curiously, it has also rarely been described in women in middle life without obvious risk factors. In tropical and subtropical areas the condition is more common and may be related to environmental factors including diet, infection, and infestation.

Nonocclusive focal ischaemia appears to underlie the pathogenesis of uraemic colitis, radiation enteritis, potassium-induced ulcers, and multiple stress ulcers of the upper gastrointestinal tract. The verotoxin of *Escherichia coli* 0157:H7, which causes haemorrhagic colitis, is another aetiological agent. This is a particularly potent cause of disseminated intravascular coagulation, which may occur as a result of the absorption of bacterial endotoxin and thromboplastins from damaged tissues. It is associated with the development of the haemolytic–uraemic syndrome in children and more rarely with thrombotic thrombocytopenic purpura in adults (Box 15.17.2).

Intestinal ischaemia: the clinical syndromes

The clinical effects of mesenteric vascular insufficiency will be considered under four headings: acute mesenteric ischaemia, chronic mesenteric ischaemia, ischaemic colitis, and ischaemia–reperfusion injury. Focal ischaemia of the intestine will be considered in the section on collagen disorders.

Acute mesenteric ischaemia

Despite increasing knowledge of the causation of acute mesenteric ischaemia and improved methods of diagnosis, this is a condition that still carries a high mortality rate (probably >50%).

Clinical features

Necrosis, incipient or complete, of that part of the gut supplied by the superior mesenteric artery is life-threatening. The onset is usually abrupt. Abdominal pain is the key symptom and at the onset it is usually colicky in nature. As the condition progresses the pain becomes constant and unremitting. Initially it is felt in the right iliac fossa and then spreads over the entire abdomen. Diarrhoea is usual and the motions may contain blood. Vomiting occurs in some cases but haematemesis is rare. There may be slight tenderness in the right iliac fossa and some exaggeration of bowel sounds. Over the course of hours (or a day or two at most) the abdomen becomes distended and silent with increasing tenderness and a positive rebound sign. At this stage there are usually signs of peripheral circulatory failure. The patient is pale, anxious, sweating, and tachypnoeic. Later the blood pressure falls and the patient becomes cyanosed and anuric; by then, damage to the intestine is irrecoverable.

Diagnosis is often delayed because there are no clinical signs apart from overwhelming patient distress which itself indicates the need for urgent specialist attention. Duplex Doppler ultrasonography and contrast-enhanced MRI are probably the best means of confirming impaired blood flow. For practical purposes, the diagnosis still depends on the efficiency with which other causes of an apparent abdominal catastrophe can be excluded. Plain radiographs of the abdomen may show nonspecific dilatation of loops of intestine with multiple fluid levels. The presence of gas bubbles in the portal vein is diagnostic of intestinal necrosis at a stage when the patient is beyond recovery. Needle aspiration of the peritoneal cavity may be a helpful procedure because necrotic intestine usually seeps blood-stained fluid.

Management

Early laparotomy is essential. First the clinician has to combat the effects of loss of water, electrolytes, and protein leading to hypovolaemia and impaired tissue perfusion; and then combat bacterial invasion and disseminated intravascular coagulation. The value of pharmacological agents (such as phenoxybenzamine, glucagon, or dopamine) for improving the mesenteric circulation remains uncertain.

As soon as the patient is sufficiently fit, the abdomen must be opened. If a large vessel is occluded, the surgeon may be able to undertake embolectomy or arterial reconstruction. In both occlusive and nonocclusive vascular disease it is necessary to decide how much intestine to resect. If there is doubt about the viability of the residual intestine the abdomen may be closed and re-explored 24h later.

Box 15.17.3 Intestinal infarction without acute vascular occlusion

Neonatal
- Necrotizing enterocolitis

Haemorrhagic enteritis or colitis
- Bacterial toxins (e.g. *E. coli* 0157:H7, *Clostridium perfringens*)

Focal ulceration
- Stress ulcers (especially stomach and duodenum)
- Drug-induced ulcers (e.g. potassium, nonsteroidal anti-inflammatory drugs)
- Radiation enteritis
- Uraemic ulceration (especially in the colon)

After prolonged period of poor perfusion
- Low-output cardiac failure (?digitalis predisposed)
- Hyperviscosity syndromes
- Polycythaemia and haemoconcentration

Infiltrating the coeliac and mesenteric plexuses with local anaesthetic may help relieve vascular spasm and should be used if there is no evidence of vascular occlusion. Treatment with anticoagulants may also be indicated.

Chronic intestinal ischaemia

Chronic intestinal ischaemia is usually due to atheroma. The coeliac axis and superior mesenteric artery are commonly affected and the inferior mesenteric artery to a much lesser extent. Stenotic lesions occur at the aortic origins of the vessels. Diffuse, severe atheroma throughout the intestinal arterial tree is uncommon and therefore arterial reconstruction may be very rewarding.

Clinical features

Patients with chronic ischaemia of the gut suffer poorly localized severe cramping abdominal pain. This occurs every day and is usually worse 20 to 60 min after eating. The pain may be relieved by simple analgesics or by vasodilator drugs. As the condition progresses the patient becomes afraid to eat and loses weight. There are no diagnostic physical signs and in particular the finding of a vascular bruit is not clinically helpful. Diagnosis may be made by one of several noninvasive methods including CT angiography, MR angiography, and duplex ultrasonography as well as invasive catheter angiography.

Compression of the coeliac axis

Occasionally, relatively young patients, with pain after eating, will be found to have an abdominal bruit in the epigastrium increased by inspiration. Aortography may show constriction of the coeliac axis by the median arcuate ligament. It has been claimed that the arteries in the territory of the coeliac axis 'steal' blood from that of the superior mesenteric artery, thereby causing an intestinal angina that may be relieved by dividing the median arcuate ligament and possibly by reconstructing the coeliac axis. The validity of this syndrome is regarded as uncertain but ischaemia detected by gastric exercise tonography appears to be a useful method of diagnosing patients who may benefit from surgical intervention.

Ischaemic colitis

The colon is more prone to ischaemic damage than the small intestine. The transverse and descending segments of the colon are supplied by marginal branches of the middle colic (superior mesenteric territory) and left colic (inferior mesenteric territory) arteries. An arterial and lymphatic watershed exists close to the splenic flexure, which is supported to a variable extent by an additional vascular arcade. This segment of the colon is at risk when the mesenteric circulation is compromised. In addition, distension of the colon may impair blood flow. Thus ischaemic colitis may occur in the segment of intestine immediately proximal to an obstructing lesion (stercoral ulceration) or with colonic pseudo-obstruction. Venous occlusion may also cause ischaemic colitis.

Clinical features

In the acute phase of ischaemic colitis the clinician has to differentiate between mild injury, that responds quickly and effectively to supportive measures and treatment with appropriate antibiotics, and severe injury, in which gangrene may develop. Typically the affected person complains of pain in the left iliac fossa, nausea, and vomiting followed by the passage of a loose motion containing dark blood.

Marked tenderness in the left iliac fossa is the most constant physical sign. At colonoscopy the mucosa may be blue and swollen without contact bleeding. The rectum is invariably spared. Plain radiographs of the abdomen may show an abnormal segment of large intestine outlined with gas.

Contrast enema examination of the colon is a most useful way of demonstrating ischaemic damage. In the early phase 'thumb-printing' is the characteristic sign. This may persist for several days (Fig. 15.17.1). Subsequently the mucosal appearance may return to normal or progress to mucosal ulceration, giving an appearance that may be indistinguishable from segmental ulcerative colitis or Crohn's disease. These changes may resolve spontaneously or progress to tubular narrowing of the intestine with or without sacculation on the anti-mesenteric border.

Ischaemic colitis may be confused with dysenteric conditions, acute diverticular disease of the colon, acute inflammatory bowel disease, perforation of a hollow viscus, or left-sided peritonitis caused by pancreatitis. The most important distinguishing features are the association with degenerative cardiovascular disease and the distinctive, although not pathognomonic, radiographic and colonoscopic appearances.

Management

On establishing the diagnosis of ischaemic colitis the treatment is initially expectant. The patient should be given intravenous fluid as necessary, together with systemic broad-spectrum antibiotics. Well over 90% of recognized cases resolve spontaneously. A stricture may develop in up to one-third of patients but this is usually asymptomatic and only rarely needs to be resected. Surgery is indicated if there is evidence of peritonitis, persistent bleeding, or an underlying colonic disorder (such as carcinoma).

Intestinal reperfusion injury

The gut mucosa may be transiently but seriously damaged after a period of ischaemia which is followed by apparently

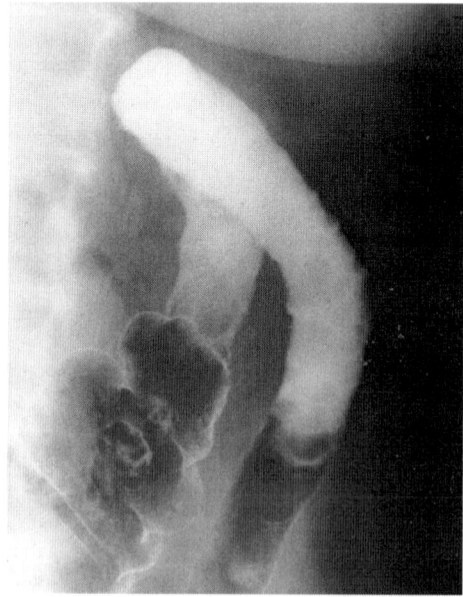

Fig. 15.17.1 Ischaemic colitis: barium enema showing thumbprinting at the splenic flexure.
(Courtesy of Dr A Freeman, Addenbrooke's Hospital.)

adequate reperfusion. The damage appears to be caused by the generation of reactive oxygen metabolites (including superoxide, hydrogen peroxide, and hydroxyl radicals). These alter the vascular permeability of endothelial cells and damage epithelial cells by peroxidation of cell membranes. The injured tissues are strongly chemotactic for neutrophils and this leads to an acute inflammatory response. Such damage diminishes the barrier function of the gut, increasing intestinal permeability and allowing the translocation of bacteria. Injury of the intestinal mucosa is now recognized as an important factor in the prognosis of critically ill patients in intensive care.

Vasculitis and the collagen disorders: effects on the gut

The gut may be involved in any of the systemic collagen–vascular disorders. Vasculitis may cause focal ischaemic damage of the intestine (Box 15.17.2) but this is a feature of many conditions other than the collagen disorders, such as drug-induced ulceration (e.g. by potassium salts), the after-effects of blunt trauma to the abdomen, irradiation, and rarely infective disease (e.g. typhoid or leprosy) (Box 15.17.3).

In the collagen disorders, the visceral muscle may be damaged and the resulting dysmotility may cause dysphagia, delayed gastric emptying, small intestinal stasis with bacterial overgrowth, or colonic inertia. Gas may infiltrate the tissues, giving rise to pneumatosis intestinalis.

The specific pathological diagnosis is usually based on the systemic features of the illness and the laboratory findings rather than on the mostly nonspecific abdominal complications. But the inquisitive physician may also recognize curious associations in patients with multisystem disorders. Thus, intestinal malabsorption and protein-losing enteropathy have been described in association with systemic lupus erythematosus (SLE) and rheumatoid arthritis; pancreatic insufficiency with systemic sclerosis; acute pancreatitis during the course of Behçet's disease; and apparently classical inflammatory bowel disease with SLE.

Systemic sclerosis

In primary systemic sclerosis (see Chapter 19.11.3), fibrous connective tissue proliferates. In the gastrointestinal tract it may replace smooth muscle, especially in the oesophagus (which is involved in 80% of cases), to a lesser extent in the small intestine (although duodenal involvement is quite common), and rather rarely in the colon.

Overt vasculitis is a less common feature but occasionally causes intestinal infarction. Pneumatosis cystoides intestinalis is also described, especially in association with intestinal pseudo-obstruction or a pneumoperitoneum.

Clinical features

In systemic sclerosis progressive dysphagia is the most frequent gastrointestinal symptom. Initially there is a decrease in the incidence and amplitude of contractions of the lower oesophagus and incomplete relaxation of the lower oesophageal sphincter. In addition, the resting tone of the sphincter is reduced, allowing reflux of gastric juices, oesophagitis, shortening of the oesophagus, and occasionally stricture formation. Associated hiatal herniation is common.

More rarely the stomach is involved, causing delayed emptying that on occasion is exacerbated by associated stenosis of the pyloric canal. Changes lower down the gastrointestinal tract also occur. Characteristically the duodenum is dilated, the valvulae of the small intestine are thickened, and pseudodiverticula may form. These changes are associated with abdominal discomfort, distension, and borborygmi, especially after the taking of meals. The impaired motility of the small intestine leads to stasis of its contents and bacterial overgrowth causing malabsorption, especially of fat and vitamin B_{12} (see Chapter 15.10.2) (Fig. 15.17.2). Progressive constipation due to impaired colonic motility is uncommon.

Management

There is no specific treatment of primary systemic sclerosis. Lesions in the gastrointestinal tract need to be managed on their merits. It is important to recognize early the patient with gastro-oesophageal reflux. A proton pump inhibitor should be given to prevent the ravages of acid-peptic digestion of the oesophageal mucosa. When strictures occur these should be dilated by bouginage. Surgical intervention is occasionally necessary.

A breath test (see Chapters 15.3.3 and 15.10.2) is a useful screening test for delayed passage of contents and bacterial proliferation in the small intestine. Patients with a positive breath test should be assessed for evidence of malabsorption, and if this is found intermittent therapy with antibiotics for an indefinite period may be of clinical value.

Systemic lupus erythematosus (SLE)

SLE (see Chapter 19.11.2) may cause abdominal symptoms arising from any part of the gastrointestinal tract. Clinical manifestations are nonspecific and can be difficult to differentiate from infective (especially with cytomegalovirus), thrombotic and therapy-related aetiologies. Anorexia, weight loss, nausea, vomiting, and diarrhoea are relatively common. Dysphagia, abdominal pain, distension due to ascites, and gastrointestinal bleeding are less frequent symptoms. Occasionally a patient with SLE develops an acute abdomen, which may be due to localized or widespread lupus vasculitis causing ischaemic damage to the gut or its related organs, including the gallbladder and pancreas. Arteriography may be helpful in diagnosis by revealing diffuse irregularities in the branches of mesenteric vessels.

Treatment with oral corticosteroids usually relieves minor SLE-related abdominal symptoms and will lead to rapid resolution

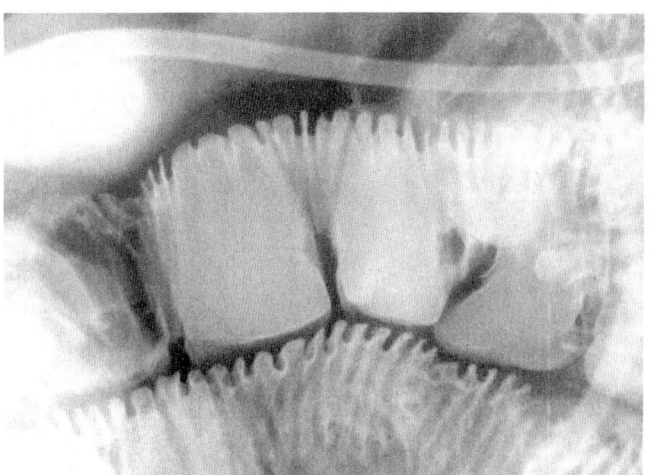

Fig. 15.17.2 Systemic sclerosis. Typical 'sacculation' appearance of the bowel.

of simple ascites. In the acute stage of the disease, however, surgery may be necessary to deal with infarcted intestine, serious bleeding, or intestinal obstruction.

Other systemic disorders

In rheumatoid arthritis, vasculitis is associated with long-standing disease, seropositivity, and florid subcutaneous nodule formation (see Section 19.11). Occasionally, a severe diffuse and necrotizing angiitis causes infarction in the gallbladder, pancreas, or intestine. Symptoms vary from vague abdominal pain, with or without diarrhoea, to the development of an acute abdomen.

Dermatomyositis rarely causes damage to the viscera although thrombosis of small vessels occasionally causes gastrointestinal ulceration.

In Behçet's syndrome the triad of relapsing iritis, painful ulcers of the mouth, and genital ulceration is only part of the spectrum of disease (see Chapter 19.11.5). Again, vasculitis appears to be the underlying histopathological lesion. In the gastrointestinal tract this may lead to ulceration of the colon, malabsorption (sometimes with lymphangiectasia), and pancreatitis.

Primary vasculitis

Henoch–Schönlein purpura (anaphylactic purpura)

This is a self-limiting disorder of unknown cause characterized by small-vessel vasculitis (see Chapter 19.11). Gastrointestinal disease occurs in at least two-thirds of cases and is manifest as abdominal pain and gastrointestinal bleeding. Intramural haematomas are common and rarely may be complicated by intussusception, perforation, or an infarcted segment of gut.

Polyarteritis nodosa

Abdominal pain and other gastrointestinal symptoms are common in patients with polyarteritis nodosa. The underlying cause is usually recognized by evidence of systemic disease such as skin lesions, renal involvement, hypertension, and eosinophilia. Mesenteric angiography is useful as a diagnostic tool because up to two-thirds of cases have recognizable aneurysms of mesenteric and renal vessels. A small proportion of patients with polyarteritis have acute abdominal episodes including ulceration, haemorrhage, perforation and segmental necrosis of intestine, cholecystitis, pancreatitis, and hepatic infarction. Kawasaki disease (infantile acute febrile mucocutaneous lymph node syndrome; see Chapter 19.11.8) proceeds to a disorder indistinguishable histopathologically from infantile periarteritis nodosa. Cardiac involvement is most common, but the gastrointestinal tract is affected in up to one-third of cases.

Antineutrophilic cytoplasmic antibody-positive vasculitides

Wegener's granulomatosis, Churg–Strauss syndrome, and microscopic polyarteritis are conditions frequently associated with the finding of antineutrophilic cytoplasmic antibodies. Gastrointestinal symptoms are common in these conditions, although the intra-abdominal pathology has not been well characterized except when angiitis has led to a life-threatening condition such as visceral perforation or infarction.

Giant cell arteritis

This characteristically affects the larger cranial arteries including the ciliary and central retinal arteries (see Chapter 19.11.4) and

rarely limb arteries. Very occasionally a similar pathology affects mesenteric arteries and causes bowel infarction.

Localized arteritis

Arteritis has been described causing pathology solely in the appendix, the gallbladder, and the pancreas. The relationship of a localized arteritis to systemic polyarteritis is uncertain. Similarly, localized leucocytoclastic (hypersensitivity) vasculitis has been described in the abdominal cavities.

Other vascular disorders that may affect the gut

Aneurysms of the aorta and its major branches

Rarely, aneurysms fistulate into the stomach or duodenum. This usually causes catastrophic bleeding and rapid death. Even more rarely there is intermittent bleeding (e.g. from the splenic artery into the stomach), which may be difficult to diagnose.

Superior mesenteric artery syndrome

A syndrome of postprandial epigastric pain, distension, and vomiting may occur in asthenic young people, especially those who have lost weight or who are fixed in a position of hyperextension after spinal injury. Barium studies show a distended proximal duodenum with a sharp cut-off at the line where the superior mesenteric artery crosses the duodenum. Symptoms may be relieved if the patient adopts the prone position after meals and usually disappear as the patient gains weight. Surgery is occasionally necessary. The condition must be distinguished from duodenal ileus caused by mesenteric bands, a condition that is associated with partial malrotation of the midgut.

Vascular malformations

Vascular malformations in the gastrointestinal tract are not uncommon and may be diagnosed at any age. They may present with acute bleeding, anaemia or even a mass lesion leading to intussusception. They include Dieufaloy's disease, an arterial malformation in the upper stomach, usually presenting, in older men, with recurrent massive bleeding; haemangiomas especially in the jejunum; and telangiectases occurring especially with Osler–Weber–Rendu disease (see Chapter 22.4.4).

Vascular dysplasia is a more recently recognized and not uncommon disorder causing occult bleeding from the gut in older people. The lesions occur as small arteriovenous malformations or as foci

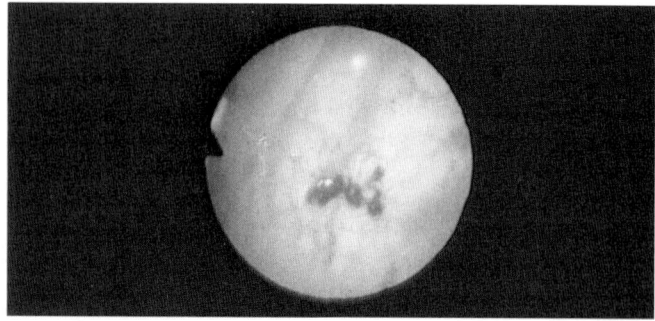

Fig. 15.17.3 Angiodysplastic lesion in the caecum, photographed through a colonoscope.
(Courtesy of Dr R Hunt, RN Hospital, Haslar.)

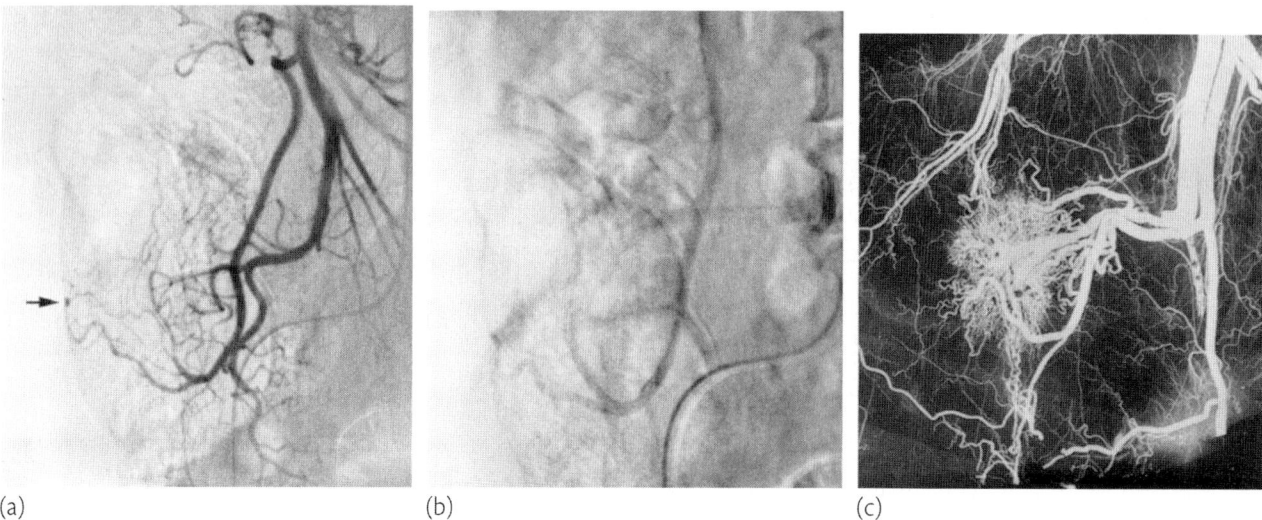

(a)   (b)   (c)

Fig. 15.17.4 (a) Angiodysplastic lesion in the caecum: superior mesenteric angiogram in a 53-year-old man with anaemia for 20 years (no lesion found at previous operations). Vascular lake in caecum (arrowed). (b) Angiodysplastic lesion in the caecum: superior mesenteric angiogram in a 53-year-old man with anaemia for 20 years (no lesion found at previous operations). Capillary phase, showing early filling vein arising from lesion. (c) Angiodysplastic lesion in the caecum: superior mesenteric angiogram in a 53-year-old man with anaemia for 20 years (no lesion found at previous operations). Injected specimen magnified ×30.
(Courtesy of Dr D J Allison, Royal Postgraduate Medical School; previously published in *Br J Hosp Med* (1980), **23**, 358.)

of ectatic capillaries or veins with little supporting stroma. They are found predominantly in the caecum and ascending colon. There may be an association with aortic stenosis but none with cutaneous telangiectases and no familial aggregations have yet been described. Patients give a history of recurrent anaemia or episodes of bleeding from the gut, have usually been investigated repeatedly without getting a firm diagnosis, and sometimes have had one or more operations (including resection of a segment of the gastrointestinal tract) without relief of symptoms. The diagnosis of vascular dysplasia should be considered in all cases of obscure gastrointestinal haemorrhage and may be made by direct visualization of the intestinal mucosa (Fig. 15.17.3) or by selective mesenteric arteriography (Fig. 15.17.4). The lesions may be multiple, in which case resection of the affected segment of gut may be indicated. Many patients, however, can be treated successfully by fulguration of the lesion through an endoscope. If the lesion(s) cannot be obliterated, a trial of treatment with an oestrogen–progesterone preparation is often effective in women.

More generalized genetic disorders affecting blood vessels include vascular Ehlers–Danlos syndrome and pseudoxanthoma elasticum. Spontaneous rupture of arteries in the abdomen in these conditions is life-threatening. Delayed diagnosis is common and great care is necessary with arterial catheterization and surgical intervention.

Intramural bleeding

Bleeding into the wall of the bowel may occur as a result of treatment with anticoagulants or from the inflammation of small vessels (as occurs classically in Henoch–Schönlein purpura). The usual presentation is with colicky abdominal pain, with bleeding into the lumen of the gut. Appropriate radiological examination with barium contrast may show the classical sign of 'thumbprinting'. The condition usually resolves spontaneously providing that the underlying disorder can be treated. A blood transfusion may be needed.

Further reading

Garcia-Porrua C, *et al.* (2006). Localised vasculitis of the gastro-intestinal tract. *Semin Arth Rheum*, **35**, 403–6.

Lock G (2001). Acute intestinal ischaemia: global review. *Best Pract Res Clin Gastroenterol*, **15**, 83–98.

Marshall SE (2004). Behcet's disease. *Best Pract Res Clin Gastroenterol*, **18**, 291–311.

Mensink PB, *et al.* (2006). Gastric exercise tonometry: the key investigation in patients with suspected celiac artery compression syndrome. *J Vasc Surg*, **44**, 277–81.

Mok CC (2005). Investigation and management of gastrointestinal and hepatic manifestations of systemic lupus erythematosus. *Best Pract Res Clin Gastroenterol*, **19**, 741–66.

Schneider A, Merikhi A, Frank BB (2006). Auto-immune disorders: gastrointestinal manifestations and endoscopic findings. *Gastrointest Endosc Clin N Am*, **16**, 133–51.

Steenarasimhaiah J (2005). Chronic mesenteric ischaemia. *Best Pract Res Clin Gastroenterol*, **19**, 283–95.

15.18

Gastrointestinal infections

Davidson H. Hamer and Sherwood L. Gorbach

Essentials

Gastrointestinal infections, especially diarrhoea, are responsible for substantial morbidity, mortality, and socioeconomic penalties worldwide. In poor countries, the greatest burden of disease is borne by infants and young children, although older people and immunocompromised patients are also at great risk of severe and complicated disease. Poor sanitation, inadequate water supplies, and globalization of food marketing increase the risk of large epidemics of food- and water-borne outbreaks of gastrointestinal disease.

Clinical syndromes

Enteric pathogens can cause intestinal disease by means of enterotoxins, adherence to gut mucosa, or invasion of enterocytes. Acute diarrhoea can be caused by pathogens ranging from toxin-producing strains of *Escherichia coli* to rotavirus and *Giardia* spp. Gastrointestinal pathogens usually cause three principal syndromes: noninflammatory diarrhoea, inflammatory diarrhoea, and systemic disease. Noninflammatory diarrhoea targets the small intestine and inflammatory diarrhoea the colon, the site of infection influencing the clinical and diagnostic features. Organisms affecting the small intestine tend to produce watery, potentially dehydrating diarrhoea, whereas those infecting the large intestine cause bloody, mucoid diarrhoea.

Patients who do not have high fever (>38.5°C), systemic illness, tenesmus, bloody diarrhoea, a prolonged course (>2 weeks), or dehydration require neither investigation nor treatment. Investigation is required in patients with any of these features, with faecal specimens subjected to microscopy (ova and parasites), direct electron microscopy (viruses), bacteriological and viral culture, and identification of microbial antigens (viruses, bacteria, parasites, or toxins). A specific laboratory diagnosis is useful epidemiologically and therapeutically, especially for invasive pathogens and diarrhoea in high-risk patients such as the very young, elderly, or immunocompromised.

Treatment and prevention

Oral rehydration therapy is the priority in management of children and adults with mild to moderate diarrhoea as long as vomiting is not a major feature, and it can also follow initial parenteral rehydration in severely dehydrated patients. Empirical antimicrobial therapy is necessary in more severe cases, pending the results of stool and blood cultures. Antibiotic treatment benefits cholera, giardiasis, cyclosporiasis, shigellosis, *E. coli* diarrhoea in infants, symptomatic traveller's diarrhoea, *Clostridium difficile* diarrhoea, and typhoid. Fluoroquinolones were the ideal choice for empirical therapy because of their broad spectrum of activity against common gastrointestinal bacterial pathogens, but increasing resistance and clinical treatment failures in South East Asia and the Indian subcontinent have forced a switch to azithromycin for acute traveller's diarrhoea and other forms of diarrhoea in this region. Antimotility drugs are useful in controlling moderate to severe diarrhoea.

Strict attention to food and water precautions and hand washing helps reduce the risk of gastrointestinal infections in poor countries. Although immunization offers an ideal way to prevent certain bacterial and viral diseases, it has not yet proved successful for combating many gastrointestinal pathogens, with the notable exception of rotavirus.

Introduction

Diarrhoea, the most common manifestation of intestinal tract infections, is a leading cause of death in most developing countries where its greatest impact is seen in infants and children. Infectious diarrhoea may be accompanied by numerous complications (Table 15.18.1). The financial burden associated with medical care and lost productivity due to infectious diarrhoea amounts to more than $20 billion/year in the United States of America alone.

The aetiology and severity of gastrointestinal infections are determined by several epidemiological factors. Young children and elderly people are at greatest risk for more severe disease and complications. The presence of underlying medical conditions, especially those that compromise immunity, greatly enhances the risk of acquiring an infection and its ultimate severity. Poor sanitation, inadequate water supplies, and increasing globalization of food transport systems all predispose to the development of large

Table 15.18.1 Complications of gastrointestinal infections

Complication	Causative pathogens
Dehydration	*Vibrio cholerae, Cryptosporidium parvum* (especially in immunocompromised hosts), enterotoxigenic *Escherichia coli* (ETEC), rotavirus
Severe vomiting	Staphylococcal food poisoning, norovirus, rotavirus
Haemorrhagic colitis	*Campylobacter jejuni*, enterohemorrhagic *E. coli* (EHEC), salmonella, shigella, *V. parahaemolyticus*
Toxic megacolon, intestinal perforation	EHEC, shigella, *C. jejuni* (rare), *Clostridium difficile* (rare), salmonella (rare), yersinia (rare)
Haemolytic uraemic syndrome (HUS), thrombotic thrombocytopenic purpura (TTP)	EHEC, shigella, *C. jejuni* (rare)
Reactive arthritis	*C. jejuni*, shigella, salmonella, yersinia
Malabsorption/malnutrition	*Cyclospora cayetanensis, Giardia lamblia, C. parvum* (especially immunocompromised hosts)
Distant metastatic infection	Salmonella, *C. jejuni* (rare), yersinia (rare)
Guillain–Barré syndrome	*C. jejuni* (rare)

epidemics of food- and water-borne outbreaks of gastrointestinal disease. Seasonal or cyclic weather variations also influence the epidemiology of diarrhoeal disease and food poisoning.

A wide array of bacterial, protozoal, and viral pathogens is responsible for gastrointestinal tract infections. The characteristics of specific organisms are described in detail in Section 7 of this book: here are presented the pathophysiology, common clinical syndromes, diagnosis, management, and prevention of gastrointestinal diseases.

Pathophysiology

Host factors

Normal intestinal flora
The proximal small bowel, including the stomach, duodenum, jejunum, and upper ileum, has a relatively sparse microflora, mainly derived from the oropharynx. Colonization of the upper intestine by Gram-negative bacilli is an abnormal event, characteristic of illness due to pathogens such as *Vibrio cholerae* and *Escherichia coli*. The large bowel has an abundant microflora, with total concentrations of 10^{11} bacteria per gram of content. Anaerobes including bacteroides, clostridium, and anaerobic streptococci outnumber aerobic bacteria, such as coliforms, by 1000-fold. During an episode of acute diarrhoea, regardless of the aetiology, the colonic flora becomes less anaerobic because of the rapid transit of intestinal contents. As a consequence, strictly anaerobic bacteria decrease in number while there is an increase in coliforms, which are often aberrant types such as enterobacter, klebsiella, and proteus. The pathogen itself assumes a dominant position in the flora, so that the major faecal isolate may be salmonella or *V. cholerae*.

In addition to the longitudinal distribution of bacteria in the gastrointestinal tract, the bowel microflora is found both within the lumen and adherent to the mucous layer overlying epithelial cells. Invasive pathogens such as campylobacter, shigella, salmonella, and yersinia can penetrate the mucosal surface and infect epithelial cells, or translocate into the mesenteric lymph nodes and bloodstream.

Control mechanisms
At the portal of entry, gastric acid suppresses most organisms that are ingested. When gastric acid is reduced or absent, there is a higher incidence of bacterial colonization of the upper small intestine. Consequently, people with hypochlorhydria, achlorhydria, or those using drugs such as proton pump inhibitors that inhibit gastric acid secretion are susceptible to diarrhoeal diseases. A critical element in maintaining the sparse flora of the upper bowel is propulsive motility. The antibacterial properties of biliary fluid may control the intestinal flora. The glycocalyx and intestinal mucins secreted by epithelial cells provide a mechanical barrier to invasion by gut pathogens and antibacterial substances produced by the normal intestinal microflora help to maintain the stability of normal populations of organisms and to prevent the implantation of pathogens.

Intestinal immunity (see Chapter 15.5)
The intestinal immune system plays a major role in the host's response to enteric pathogens. The human gut contains a large amount of lymphoid tissue in the form of intraepithelial lymphocytes, lamina propria lymphoid cells, and Peyer's patches. Peyer's patches are lymphoid aggregates in the mucosa and submucosa of the distal small intestine where antigens are presented to B and T lymphocytes. After activation by antigens, bacteria, or viruses in the Peyer's patches, the lymphocytes migrate to the lamina propria and the intraepithelial portion of the intestinal lining where, along with macrophages and other types of white blood cells, they protect the host from specific pathogens. Plasma cells in the lamina propria produce secretory immunoglobulin A, which is released into the intestinal lumen. When the mechanical barrier of the gut fails, the intraepithelial and lamina propria lymphocytes provide the next level of protection against pathogenic enteric organisms.

Microbial factors
The number of organisms that need to be ingested to establish a gastrointestinal tract infection varies from as few as 10 to 100 in the case of shigella to as many as 10^8 for *V. cholerae*. In the presence of reduced gastric acidity or underlying immunosuppression, the inoculum needed to establish infection is reduced.

Enteric pathogens can cause intestinal disease by means of enterotoxins, adherence to gut mucosa, or invasion of enterocytes.

Toxins
Bacterial enteric pathogens can elaborate enterotoxins that act directly on intestinal epithelial cells (e.g. cholera toxin) or preformed toxins that are ingested in contaminated food (e.g. *Bacillus cereus* toxin). Invasive bacteria penetrate the mucosal surface of the gut as the primary event, and they may also secrete enterotoxins. Production of enterotoxin can be demonstrated in the laboratory by *in vivo* tests, such as the rabbit ileal loop model and the suckling mouse model, or by *in vitro* tests involving a tissue culture line, such as Y-1 adrenal cells or Chinese hamster ovary cells. Polymerase chain reaction (PCR) with specific molecular probes can also be used to detect enterotoxins and other bacterial virulence factors.

Many organisms elaborate enterotoxins that cause fluid and electrolyte secretion in the gut. Diarrhoeal toxins can be grouped into two categories: cytotonic, which produce fluid secretion by activation of intracellular enzymes such as adenylate cyclase, without causing any damage to the epithelial surface; and cytotoxic, which cause injury to the mucosal cell while also inducing fluid secretion, but not primarily by activation of cyclic nucleotides. V. cholerae and enterotoxigenic Escherichia coli (ETEC) are examples of pathogens that cause dehydrating diarrhoea by producing enterotoxins of the cytotonic type (see Chapter 7.6.7.1).

Intestinal fluid loss is the primary manifestation of cholera (Chapter 7.6.11). It results from the action of enterotoxin on the epithelial cells of the small bowel. These organisms colonize the small intestine, adhering to epithelial cells and then elaborating enterotoxin. There is no invasion of the mucosal surface, so there is no evidence of damage to the mucosal architecture and bacteraemia is not a complication. The faecal effluent is watery, often voluminous, and produces the clinical features of dehydration. The most sensitive areas are the upper bowel, particularly the duodenum and upper jejunum; the ileum is less affected, and the colon is usually in a state of absorption since it is relatively insensitive to the toxin. This is a form of 'overflow' diarrhoea, with a large volume of fluid produced in the upper intestine that overwhelms the capacity of the lower bowel to absorb.

ETEC produces two types of enterotoxins: a heat-labile (LT) and a heat-stable toxin (ST). LT is a protein that is destroyed by heat and acid. Like cholera toxin, it activates adenylate cyclase, causing secretion of fluids and electrolytes into the lumen. In contrast, ST can withstand heating to $100\,^{\circ}\text{C}$ and acts by activating guanylate cyclase. Despite the differences between them, the ultimate effect of both enterotoxins is a noninflammatory secretory diarrhoea.

Invasion

Whereas toxigenic organisms usually involve the upper intestine, invasive pathogens target the lower intestine, particularly the distal ileum and colon. Histological findings include evidence of mucosal ulceration with acute inflammation in the lamina propria. Principal pathogens in this group are salmonella, shigella, enterohaemorrhagic E. coli (EHEC), enteroinvasive E. coli (EIEC), campylobacter, and yersinia. Although there are important differences between these organisms, they all have in common the property of mucosal invasion as the initiating event. To date, three theories have been invoked to explain the mechanism of fluid production in invasive diarrhoea. First, fluid production may result from an enterotoxin, at least in the initial phase of the illness. Most shigella strains elaborate an enterotoxin that differs substantially from cholera toxin, but which does result in fluid and electrolyte secretion by the intestine. A similar toxin has been proposed for salmonella, and there is suggestive evidence that campylobacter and yersinia elaborate enterotoxins. Second, invasive organisms lead to an increased local synthesis of prostaglandins at the site of the intense inflammatory reaction that may be responsible for fluid secretion and diarrhoea. Third, damage to the epithelial surface may prevent reabsorption of fluids from the lumen and thereby result in a net accumulation of fluid in the bowel lumen, resulting in diarrhoea.

A series of pathogenic factors, each controlled by plasmids or chromosomal loci, are used by pathogenic strains of salmonella. Specific plasmids encode for bacterial spread from Peyer's patches to other sites in the body, for the ability of certain strains to survive within macrophages following phagocytosis, and for the ability of salmonellae to elicit transepithelial signalling to neutrophils (see Chapter 7.6.8). Invasion by shigella is also associated with diverse virulence factors related to various stages of invasion. The end result is the death of the intestinal epithelial cell, focal ulcers, and inflammation of the lamina propria. The shigella virulence factors are encoded by chromosomal and plasmid genes, all of which are needed for the full expression of virulence. Various genetic loci encode for an invasion plasmid antigen (ipa), which seems to determine recognition of the epithelial cell, inv invasion factors, and a series of vir loci that are involved in regulation within the infected cell. After penetrating the mucosal surface of the gut, shigella multiply within epithelial cells and extend the infected area by direct cell-to-cell migration of bacilli. Shigella rarely penetrate beyond the intestinal mucosa and therefore do not usually invade the bloodstream (Chapter 7.6.7).

Adherence

Specific fimbriae or adhesins mediate the attachment of pathogenic bacteria to gut mucosal cells. For example, the attachment of V. cholerae is mediated by a fimbrial colonization factor, known as the toxin-coregulated pilus. Some enteric pathogens such as enteropathogenic E. coli (EPEC) attach to the intestinal mucosa in a characteristic manner, producing ultrastructural changes known as attachment–effacement lesions; this leads to the elongation and destruction of microvilli. Protozoal parasites such as Giardia lamblia use a ventral adhesive disc to attach to the mucosal surface of the small intestine. Thus, enteropathogens have devised a number of different ways to adhere to the surface of the gut.

Clinical syndromes of gastrointestinal infections

Gastrointestinal infections usually result in three principal syndromes: noninflammatory diarrhoea, inflammatory diarrhoea, and systemic disease. Noninflammatory diarrhoea primarily involves the small intestine, whereas inflammatory diarrhoea predominantly affects the colon. The location of infection influences the clinical characteristics and certain diagnostic features of the diarrhoeal disease (Table 15.18.2). Thus, the organisms that target the small intestine tend to produce watery, potentially dehydrating diarrhoea, whereas those infecting the large intestine cause bloody mucoid diarrhoea associated with tenesmus.

Noninflammatory diarrhoea

Bacteria

Cholera, the prototypic noninflammatory diarrhoea, can cause dehydration and death within 3 to 4 h of onset. As in many other infectious diseases, there is a spectrum of clinical manifestations, from an asymptomatic carrier state to severe dehydration with shock. Initial symptoms of vomiting and abdominal distension are rapidly followed by diarrhoea, which accelerates over the next few hours to frequent purging of large volumes of 'ricewater' stools. The acutely ill patient has marked dehydration manifested by poor skin turgor, 'washerwoman's hands', feeble to absent pulses, reduced renal function, and hypovolaemic shock.

Non-01 cholera vibrios have also been associated with severe, dehydrating diarrhoea as well as wound infections and septicaemia. V. vulnificus is one of the most important noncholera vibrios,

Table 15.18.2 Clinical features of diarrhoeal diseases

Feature	Site of infection	
	Small intestine	**Large intestine**
Pathogens	*Escherichia coli* (EPEC, ETEC)	*E. coli* (EIEC, EHEC)
	Cryptosporidium parvum	*Entamoeba histolytica*
	Giardia lamblia	Shigella
	Norovirus	
	Rotavirus	
	Vibrio cholerae	
Location of pain	Mid abdomen	Lower abdomen, rectum
Volume of stool	Large	Small
Blood in stool	Rare	Common
Faecal leucocytes	Rare	Common (except in amoebiasis)
Sigmoidoscopy	Normal	Mucosal ulcers, haemorrhagic foci, friable mucosa

judging by the severity of illness that it causes, especially in patients with underlying liver disease and especially iron-storage disease. This infection can be acquired by direct consumption of seafood, usually raw oysters, or as a wound infection in people who have direct contact with salt water. Susceptible people may contract fatal infections and so should be warned not to eat raw seafood, especially oysters. *V. parahaemolyticus* is an important cause of sporadic outbreaks of gastroenteritis associated with the consumption of contaminated seafood.

ETEC infections are one of the most common causes of diarrhoea in travellers to less developed countries and children living in these regions. The incubation period of this infection is usually between 24 and 48 h, after which the disease often begins with upper intestinal distress, followed soon thereafter by watery diarrhoea. The infection can be extremely mild, with only a few loose movements, or it can be quite severe, mimicking cholera with profuse watery diarrhoea leading to severe dehydration. Other strains of *E. coli* such as enteroaggregative (EAEC), diffusely adhering, and EPEC, may also be associated with watery diarrhoea.

Viruses (see also Chapter 7.5.9)

Numerous viruses are responsible for as many as 30 to 40% of self-limited episodes of noninflammatory diarrhoea, especially in children. Rotavirus causes a range of clinical manifestations from asymptomatic carriage to severe, potentially fatal dehydration. The disease occurs primarily in children aged between 3 and 15 months; infections continue into the second year of life, but after this age are less common. Adults can develop mild infections with group A rotaviruses, especially if there is a sick child in the household. The disease process often begins with vomiting, followed shortly thereafter by watery diarrhoea. The incubation period is between 1 and 3 days, with an average duration of illness of 5 to 7 days, although some instances of chronic diarrhoea have been described.

Caliciviruses are single-stranded RNA viruses that are responsible for human and animal infections. Recent molecular studies have shown that noroviruses (formerly known as Norwalk and Norwalk-like viruses) have a genetic composition that places them in the taxonomic family of Caliciviridae. This family of viruses typically causes disease mainly in infants and young children, especially in daycare centres. The illness is generally mild and indistinguishable from that due to rotavirus or even epidemic noroviral disease. Noroviruses cause explosive epidemics of diarrhoea that sweep through communities with a high attack rate. These agents have become notorious in recent years as causes of diarrhoea outbreaks associated with cruise ships. Noroviruses show no respect for age, as they can affect virtually all age groups except infants. Infections caused by noroviruses tend to be relatively mild and short-lived, with common symptoms including diarrhoea, nausea, abdominal pain, vomiting, and myalgias. Generally, the clinical illness lasts no longer than 24 to 48 h.

Astroviruses are responsible for outbreaks of diarrhoea in day-care centres and in communities with infants. The disease is characterized by watery or mucoid stools, nausea, vomiting, and occasionally fever, but it tends to be milder than rotavirus diarrhoea as there is less dehydration. Adenovirus serotypes 40 and 41 are responsible for day-care centre and nosocomial outbreaks of gastroenteritis in children under 2 years of age. As opposed to rotavirus or norovirus, infection with enteric adenovirus has a long incubation period lasting approximately 8 to 10 days, and the illness can be prolonged for as long as 2 weeks.

Other infections (see also Section 7)

Giardia are responsible for clinical syndromes ranging from asymptomatic cyst passage, to self-limited diarrhoea, to chronic diarrhoea with malabsorption and weight loss. After an incubation period between 1 and 2 weeks, patients experience the onset of frequent, loose to watery bowel movements associated with abdominal cramps, bloating, belching, nausea, anorexia, and flatulence (Chapter 7.8.8).

Patients with cryptosporidiosis present with watery diarrhoea associated with abdominal pain, nausea, vomiting, low-grade fever, malaise, and anorexia. Faecal output may be voluminous and dehydrating in immunocompromised patients, particularly those with underlying HIV infection. Symptoms usually resolve by 5 to 10 days (Chapter 7.8.5). Infection with *Cyclospora cayetanensis* is manifested by anorexia, intermittent diarrhoea, and nausea. Diarrhoea is usually self-limiting, but it can last for several weeks in immunocompetent patients and result in significant weight loss (Chapter 7.8.6). *Cytoisospora (Isospora) belli* also causes a self-limited illness characterized by watery, non-bloody diarrhoea, abdominal cramping, anorexia, weight loss, and, less commonly, fever (Chapter 7.8.8). Any of the parasitic infections is more severe and longer lasting in immunocompromised patients, such as those with HIV or organ transplants.

Food poisoning

Food poisoning is most commonly caused by the consumption of food contaminated with bacteria or bacterial toxins. Food poisoning can also be due to parasites (e.g. trichinosis), viruses (e.g. hepatitis A), and other toxins (e.g. of aquatic animals—Chapter 9.2, and mushrooms—Chapter 9.3). The best-recognized causes of bacterial food poisoning are the following: *Clostridium perfringens*, *Staphylococcus aureus*, vibrios (including *V. cholerae* and *V. parahaemolyticus*), *Bacillus cereus*, salmonella, *C. botulinum*, shigella, toxigenic *E. coli* (ETEC and EHEC), and certain species of campylobacter, yersinia, listeria, and aeromonas.

An enterotoxin elaborated by type A strains of *C. perfringens* is responsible for food-borne outbreaks with high attack rates but of short duration. *C. perfringens* food poisoning is characterized by severe, crampy abdominal pain and watery diarrhoea, usually without vomiting, beginning 8 to 24 h after the incriminating meal. Fever, chills, headache, or other signs of infection are usually absent. Strains of *C. perfringens* type C elaborate a similar enterotoxin that has been implicated in outbreaks of enteritis necroticans secondary to the consumption of rancid meat in Europe, also known as 'pigbel' in Papua New Guinea. This is a much more severe necrotizing disease of the small intestine and carries a high mortality rate (Chapter 7.6.24).

Staphylococcal food poisoning presents with severe vomiting, nausea, and abdominal cramps, often followed by diarrhoea. *B. cereus* is an aerobic, spore-forming, Gram-positive rod that has been associated with two clinical types of food poisoning—a diarrhoea syndrome and a vomiting syndrome. The latter has a short incubation period of about 2 h, after which nearly all affected persons experience vomiting and abdominal cramps. In contrast, the diarrhoea syndrome has a median incubation period of 9 h; clinical illness is characterized by diarrhoea, abdominal cramps, and vomiting. *B. cereus* is particularly associated with the ingestion of contaminated rice that has been kept for a long time in a warm or partially cooked state in takeaway food outlets. Fevers are uncommon with all three of these bacterial toxin-mediated syndromes. Episodes of staphylococcal and *B. cereus* food poisoning are short-lived, usually resolving within 24 h. The staphylococcus has often been introduced by contamination from a small abscess, whitlow, or other discharging lesion present during preparation of food, which is allowed to remain warm and not fully cooked before serving.

Traveller's diarrhoea (see Chapter 7.4)

People who travel from industrialized countries to less developed areas of the world are at risk of contracting traveller's diarrhoea. As many as 25 to 50% or more of them suffer from one or more episodes of diarrhoea. The greatest frequency of diarrhoea occurs in students or low-budget tourists. Business travellers are at intermediate risk, while travellers who are visiting relatives have the lowest risk. Young travellers, particularly those 20 to 29 years old, have the highest risk, whereas the lowest rates of traveller's diarrhoea are noted in those over 55 years of age. The disease does not begin immediately but generally starts 2 to 3 days after the traveller's arrival. While most people have 3 to 5 watery, loose stools daily, about 20% can have as many as 6 to 15. A minority of patients, approximately 2 to 10%, have fever, bloody stools, or both. These people are more likely to have shigellosis. Diarrhoea is frequently associated with gas, cramps, fatigue, nausea, abdominal pain, fever, and anorexia. The illness usually resolves without specific therapy within 3 to 5 days, although a few unfortunate travellers will have persistent diarrhoea.

Infectious microorganisms in contaminated food and drink are the main source of traveller's diarrhoea. Especially risky foods include uncooked vegetables, salsa, meat, and seafood. Tap water, ice, unpasteurized milk and dairy products, salads, and unpeeled fruits are also associated with an increased risk. Although an array of pathogens has been found, the leading culprits are various forms of *E. coli*, particularly ETEC and EAEC. *Campylobacter jejuni* is common, particularly during cooler seasons. Viruses, shigella, salmonella, giardia, cryptosporidium, and cyclospora are responsible for a minority of cases.

Prudent selection of beverages and foods can help reduce the risk of developing traveller's diarrhoea. Bottled carbonated beverages, hot coffee or tea, beer, and boiled water are generally safe choices for fluids. Avoiding salads, unpeeled fruit, ice, and undercooked or raw meat, poultry, and seafood can help lower the risk. Travellers should avoid eating food from street vendors. Although studies have shown high protection rates when prophylactic antimicrobial agents such as ciprofloxacin or rifaximin are taken, this approach is generally not recommended because of the risk of side effects and emergence of antibiotic-resistant enteric flora.

Chronic noninflammatory diarrhoea

Certain pathogens cause chronic diarrhoea of small-intestinal origin. Some patients with giardiasis develop chronic diarrhoea associated with fatigue, steatorrhoea, weight loss, and intermittent constipation, along with malabsorption of fat, vitamins A and B$_{12}$, protein, and D-xylose. Acquired lactose intolerance is common, but a lactose-free diet should be recommended in such cases. Cryptosporidiosis can result in chronic, dehydrating diarrhoea in immunocompromised patients, especially in those with AIDS. Complications of chronic cryptosporidiosis include malabsorption, wasting, and biliary tract disease. Patients with AIDS are also at risk of chronic noninflammatory diarrhoea due to diffusely adherent *E. coli*, microsporidia, cytoisospora, and cyclospora.

About 1 to 3% of travellers returning from a developing country will have persistent diarrhoea that may last for 1 month or more. Some suffer from a prolonged irritable bowel-like syndrome. Giardia, cyclospora, and, rarely, shigella, salmonella, or *C. jejuni* may be responsible but in many cases, the cause is not found. Some of these unfortunate people will respond to empirical therapy with broad-spectrum antibiotics since they have 'tropical jejunitis' or a mild form of tropical sprue. Returning travellers with irritable bowel symptoms may experience these symptoms for many months.

Bacterial overgrowth in the small intestine can result in chronic diarrhoea, steatorrhoea, bloating, abdominal pain, and wasting. Contributing factors include achlorhydria, decreased motility (as in diabetes mellitus or scleroderma), and stasis due to diverticula or blind loops of bowel. Treatment with amoxicillin/clavulanic acid, erythromycin, or tetracycline in conjunction with a lactose-free diet will often lead to resolution of the diarrhoea.

Inflammatory diarrhoea

Acute inflammatory diarrhoea is the result of infection with bacterial enteropathogens such as shigella, campylobacter, salmonella, EHEC, *V. parahaemolyticus*, and *C. difficile*. Among the parasites, *Entamoeba histolytica* is the most common cause of dysenteric illness although *Balantidium coli*, *Schistosoma mansoni*, *S. japonicum*, *Trichuris trichiura*, hookworms, and *Trichinella spiralis* can all cause bloody, mucoid diarrhoea (see Section 7).

Dysentery is a commonly used term referring to a diarrhoeal stool that contains an inflammatory exudate composed of blood and polymorphonuclear leucocytes. Patients with bacillary dysentery classically present with crampy abdominal pain, rectal burning (or 'rectal tenesmus'—painful and ineffectual straining to pass a stool), and fever, associated with multiple small-volume, bloody mucoid, bowel movements. The most constant findings are lower abdominal pain and diarrhoea. Fever is present in less than one-half of patients and the typical dysentery stool, consisting of blood and mucus, in only one-third. Sigmoidoscopy reveals acute mucosal inflammation with ulcerations and focal haemorrhage.

Bacteria

The shiga bacillus *Shiga dysenteriae* type 1 produces the most severe form of dysentery, while *S. sonnei* produces the mildest disease. *S. flexneri* is the most commonly encountered serogroup in tropical regions, whereas *S. sonnei* is the most common in industrialized countries. Many patients with shigellosis manifest a biphasic illness. The initial symptoms of fever, abdominal pain, and watery, nonbloody diarrhoea result from the action of enterotoxin. The second phase, starting 3 to 5 days after the onset of symptoms, is notable for tenesmus and small-volume bloody stools. This period corresponds to invasion of the colonic epithelium and acute colitis. Infection with *S. dysenteriae* type 1 and malnutrition, especially in young children, are factors associated with a more severe course. Complications of shigellosis include intestinal perforation, protein-losing enteropathy, hypoglycaemia, seizures, thrombocytopenia, and haemolytic–uraemic syndrome—the latter three being particularly common in children.

Campylobacter species, especially *C. jejuni*, have gained in prominence as invasive diarrhoeal pathogens. Clinically, disease manifestations range from frank dysentery, to watery diarrhoea, to asymptomatic excretion. Most patients have diarrhoea, fever, and abdominal pain—about 50% will note bloody stools. Constitutional symptoms such as headache, myalgias, backache, malaise, anorexia, and vomiting are often present. The illness usually resolves in less than 1 week, although symptoms can persist for 2 weeks or more, and relapses occur in as many as one-quarter of patients. Rare complications include gastrointestinal haemorrhage, toxic megacolon, pancreatitis, cholecystitis, haemolytic uraemic syndrome, bacteraemia, meningitis, and reactive arthritis, and Guillain–Barré syndrome.

Recent years have seen an increasing frequency of outbreaks of *Salmonella enterica* serovar Enteritidis associated with the consumption of uncooked or raw eggs. Salmonella gastroenteritis is characterized by initial symptoms of nausea and vomiting, followed by abdominal cramps and diarrhoea which is accompanied by fever in about 50% of persons. The diarrhoea varies from a few loose stools, to dysentery with grossly bloody, purulent faeces, to a cholera-like syndrome.

Yersinia enterocolitica can cause illness ranging from acute nonbloody diarrhoea to invasive colitis and ileitis. Fever, abdominal cramps, and haem-positive diarrhoea that may persist for several weeks characterize yersinia enterocolitis (Chapter 7.6.17). *V. parahaemolyticus* outbreaks have been associated with the consumption of raw fish or shellfish. Illness is generally characterized by explosive, watery diarrhoea, abdominal cramps, nausea, vomiting, and headaches. In some cases a bloody dysenteric syndrome is observed.

EIEC strains are capable of invading epithelial cells and producing a shiga-like toxin. Patients with EIEC present with diarrhoea, tenesmus, fever, and abdominal cramps. EHEC strains possess at least two virulence factors that produce intestinal damage: an adherence mechanism causing attachment-effacement lesions similar to those seen with EPEC; and the production of two shiga-like cytotoxins (SLT I and II). Some EHEC strains produce only SLT I or II, whereas others produce both toxins. After a mean incubation of 3 to 4 days, illness begins with watery, nonbloody diarrhoea associated with severe abdominal cramping, nausea,

vomiting, chills, and low-grade fever. The diarrhoea then often progresses to visibly bloody stools. Leucocytosis with a shift to the left is usually present, but anaemia is uncommon unless infection is complicated by the development of the haemolytic–uraemic syndrome (HUS) or thrombotic thrombocytopenic purpura (TTP). The median duration of diarrhoea is 3 to 8 days, but longer durations have been described in children and persons with bloody diarrhoea.

Parasites (see Section 7)

While infection with a number of different intestinal nematodes and trematodes can be associated with an inflammatory diarrhoea, *E. histolytica* is by far the most common parasitic cause of dysenteric illness (see Chapter 7.8.1). Approximately 50 million cases of invasive colitis due to *E. histolytica* occur worldwide each year, primarily in developing countries. In industrialized countries, populations at high risk of infection include institutionalized persons, especially the mentally impaired, recent immigrants, returning travellers, and sexually active male homosexuals. Malnutrition, malignancy, glucocorticoid use, pregnancy, and young age are risk factors for greater severity of infection.

There are two distinct species of entamoeba that can be differentiated on the basis of antigenic structure, isoenzyme analysis, host specificity, *in vitro* growth characteristics, *in vivo* virulence, and DNA characterization. The two species, *E. histolytica* and *E. dispar*, have the same life cycle and are morphologically identical. However, *E. dispar* is associated with an asymptomatic carrier state, whereas *E. histolytica* is capable of invading tissue and causing symptomatic infection.

A spectrum of clinical illness occurs with *E. histolytica* infections including asymptomatic carriage, nonbloody diarrhoea, acute dysenteric colitis, fulminant colitis with perforation, chronic nondysenteric colitis, and the formation of an amoeboma, an annular lesion of the colon that can be confused with colon cancer. Patients with acute amoebic dysentery usually present with a 1- to 3-week history of bloody diarrhoea, tenesmus, and abdominal pain. Fever and dehydration are present in a minority of patients. Complications of amoebic colitis include intestinal perforation and toxic megacolon. Although nearly all patients have blood in the stool, faecal leucocytes are usually absent, probably as a result of the lysis of inflammatory cells by trophozoites. Amoebic liver abscess can occur with or independent of acute colitis. The fulminant variant of amoebic colitis is characterized by the rapid onset of fever, bloody mucoid diarrhoea, diffuse abdominal pain with peritoneal signs, and leucocytosis. Chronic nondysenteric amoebiasis is a syndrome usually lasting more than 1 year with intermittent diarrhoea, mucus, abdominal pain, flatulence, and weight loss.

Antibiotic-associated colitis (see Chapter 7.6.23)

Although the mechanism has not been fully elucidated, it appears that the normal bowel flora inhibits overgrowth by *C. difficile* in the large intestine. Factors such as antibiotic use or chemotherapy disrupt the suppressive effects of the microflora and allow *C. difficile* to propagate and to secrete its toxins. This organism produces two cytotoxins, one of which, cytotoxin A, appears to be responsible for damaging the colonic mucosa, while the other, cytotoxin B, is used for diagnosis based on its cytotoxic effects in tissue culture.

Although classically acquired in hospitals and chronic-care facilities, toxin-producing strains of *C. difficile* have been increasingly recognized as a cause of community-acquired diarrhoea.

Recent treatment with antibiotics, especially cephalosporins and clindamycin, or chemotherapeutic agents such as methotrexate, usually precedes the development of illness. Clinical findings range from asymptomatic carriage to fulminant colitis with perforation. Symptomatic patients have frequent, malodorous bowel movements that are not grossly bloody. Associated signs and symptoms include crampy abdominal pain, fever, and abdominal tenderness. Leucocytosis with an increase of immature neutrophil forms is often present. Complications of *C. difficile* colitis include toxic megacolon, perforation, electrolyte disturbances, and hypoalbuminaemia.

Invasive infections

There are many infections of the gastrointestinal tract that do not present with diarrhoea, but instead are manifested by a systemic illness in which constitutional symptoms and signs predominate. Enteric fever, particularly when caused by *Salmonella enterica* serovar Typhi, may be the most common bacterial infection worldwide.

Typhoid fever (see Chapter 7.6.8)

After ingestion in contaminated food or water, *S.* Typhi penetrates the small-bowel mucosa and makes its way rapidly to the lymphatics, the mesenteric nodes, and finally the bloodstream. Following an initial bacteraemia, the organism is sequestered in cells of the reticuloendothelial system where it multiplies and re-emerges several days later in recurrent waves of bacteraemia, an event that initiates the symptomatic phase of infection.

Typhoid fever is a febrile illness of prolonged duration, characterized by hectic fever, delirium, persistent bacteraemia, splenomegaly, abdominal pain, and a variety of systemic manifestations. Pulse–temperature dissociation is present in some patients. In approximately 50% of patients, there is no change in bowel habits; in fact, constipation is more common than diarrhoea in children with typhoid fever. As a result of recurrent waves of bacteraemia, patients with typhoid fever can develop pneumonia, pyelonephritis, osteomyelitis, septic arthritis, and meningitis. Intestinal haemorrhage and perforation, the most common complications, often occur in the third week of infection or during convalescence.

While *S.* Typhi is the main cause of typhoid fever, other serotypes of salmonella occasionally produce a similar clinical picture, known as enteric or paratyphoid fever. These serotypes include *S.* Paratyphi, *S.* Schottmülleri (formerly *S.* Paratyphi B), and *S.* Hirschfeldii (formerly *S.* Paratyphi C), as well as others such as *S.* Typhimurium.

Parasitic infections (see Section 7)

Certain gastrointestinal parasites are associated with systemic signs and symptoms during the extraintestinal stages of their life cycles. Gut infections with *Strongyloides stercoralis* manifest with vague symptoms such as abdominal pain, bloating, and diarrhoea, frequently associated with eosinophilia. During the migration of this parasite through the skin and lung, specific symptoms attributable to the local inflammatory response in these tissues may occur. Hyperinfection or disseminated strongyloidiasis develops in immunocompromised patients, especially those with HIV infection, haematological malignancies, or those treated with systemic steroids or other immunosuppressive agents. Individuals with the hyperinfection syndrome have heavy worm burdens that can lead to intestinal obstruction, respiratory failure, Gram-negative bacteraemia, or meningitis.

Other intestinal parasites such as hookworm, *T. trichiura*, and *Schistosoma* species can cause gradual blood loss from the intestine that, in prolonged infections, can lead to clubbing, severe malnutrition, pica, stunting of growth, and congestive heart failure secondary to severe anaemia. Chronic infections with all schistosoma species with the exception of *S. haematobium* can cause significant morbidity and mortality as a result of granuloma formation in the intestine and liver. The resulting hepatic fibrosis leads to portal hypertension that can eventually be complicated by splenomegaly, oesophageal varices, haematemesis, and death.

Intestinal tuberculosis (see Chapter 7.6.25)

Mycobacterium tuberculosis is responsible for most cases of intestinal tuberculosis. In some developing countries, however, cases caused by *M. bovis*, an organism found in unpasteurized dairy products, still occur. The most frequent sites of intestinal involvement are the distal ileum and caecum, although any region of the gastrointestinal tract can be involved. Most patients with intestinal tuberculosis are asymptomatic. The most common complaint is chronic, nonspecific abdominal pain. Weight loss, fever, diarrhoea or constipation, and blood in the stool may be present. An abdominal mass, commonly located in the right lower quadrant of the abdomen, is appreciated in about two-thirds of patients. Complications include haemorrhage, obstruction, perforation, fistula formation, and malabsorption.

Peritoneal tuberculosis results from the haematogenous spread of *M. tuberculosis* to mesenteric lymph nodes. Ascites is the most common presenting feature and is often associated with fever, lethargy, and weight loss. The ascitic fluid is notable for an elevated white blood cell count with a lymphocytic predominance, and a high albumin concentration.

Diagnosis and management of gastrointestinal infections

Diagnosis

Although there is considerable overlap in presenting signs and symptoms, a pathophysiological approach can be used to make a presumptive aetiological diagnosis in patients with infectious diarrhoea (Table 15.18.2). By separating microorganisms that target the upper small intestine from those that attack the large bowel, the clinician can categorize the general type of pathogen based on the initial symptoms and the type of diarrhoea. In the case of the non-inflammatory bowel pathogens, microscopy of the stool reveals no leucocytes or erythrocytes, whereas these are often abundant in the faeces of patients with invasive diarrhoeal pathogens. Several organisms including salmonella, yersinia, *V. parahaemolyticus*, and *C. difficile* produce variable findings on microscopic examination of stools. Depending on the invasiveness of the strain and the extent of colonic involvement, there can be few to many red blood cells and/or polymorphonuclear leucocytes in the stool.

A diagnostic algorithm can be used to help decide which patients should be treated symptomatically and which require further diagnostic studies and treatment (Fig. 15.18.1). Approximately 90% of cases of acute diarrhoea fall into the 'no studies–no treatment' category. Because of the significant morbidity and cost associated with infectious diarrhoea, making a specific laboratory diagnosis can be useful epidemiologically, diagnostically, and therapeutically. A definitive diagnosis is achieved mainly through study of faecal specimens, using bacteriological culture, viral culture, or direct

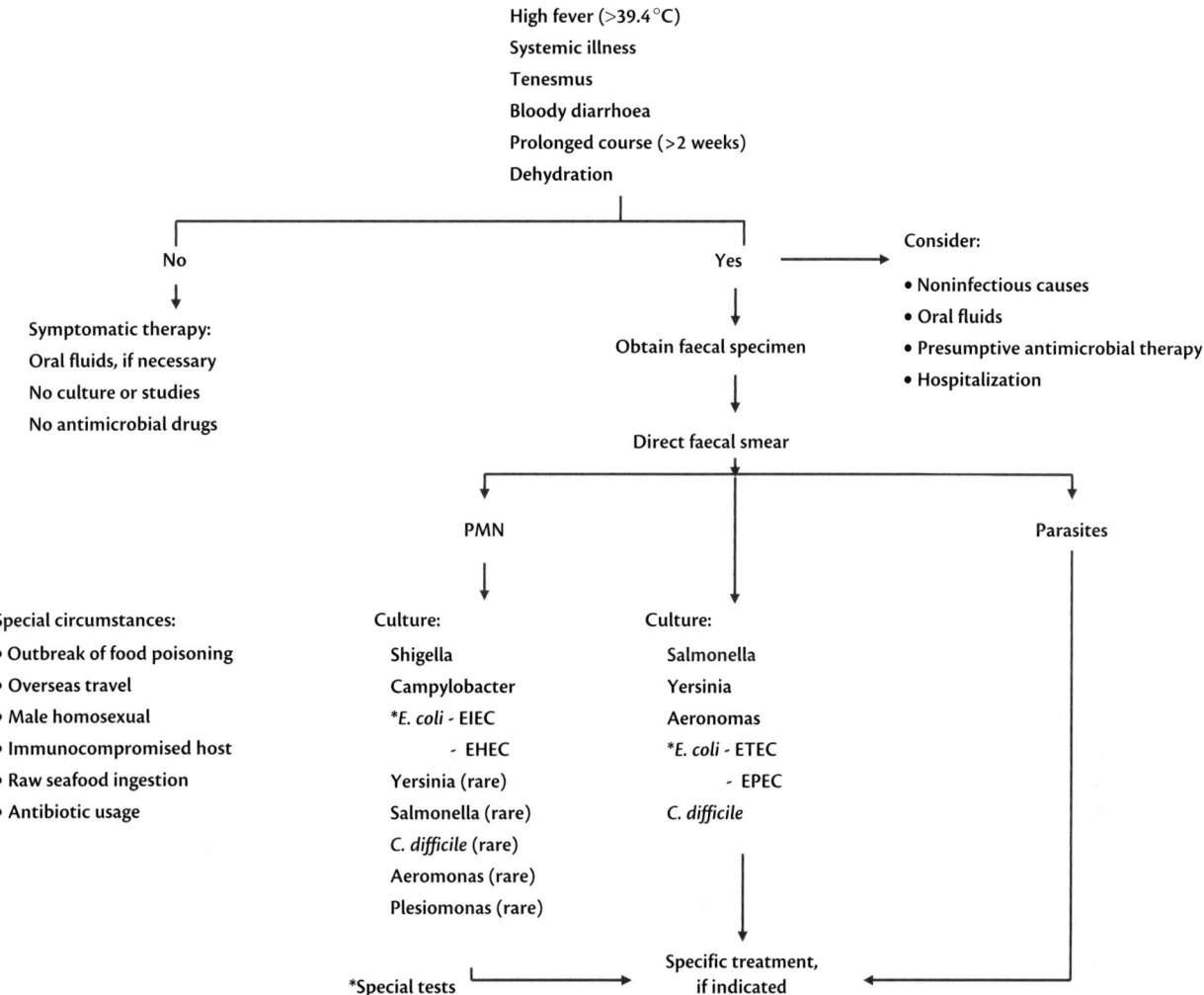

Fig. 15.18.1 Algorithm for the diagnosis and treatment of diarrhoea.

electron microscopy for viral particles, and identification of microbial antigens (viruses, bacteria, parasites, or toxins). DNA probes, PCR, and immunodiagnostic tests can now be used to identify several pathogens in stool specimens. Although some diseases can be diagnosed by elevations of serum antibody titres, this method is usually retrospective and often inaccurate.

Invasive procedures such as sigmoidoscopy or upper endoscopy generally play a limited role in the diagnosis of bacterial infections of the gastrointestinal tract. Proctoscopy or sigmoidoscopy of patients with colitis due to shigella, salmonella, and other invasive pathogens will show a diffusely ulcerated, haemorrhagic, and friable colonic mucosa. Large-bowel involvement with *C. difficile* manifests as an acute inflammatory colitis with or without pseudomembranes. Although the demonstration of pseudomembranes by colonoscopy can provide a rapid diagnosis, this method is relatively insensitive. Sigmoidoscopy with biopsy of the rectal mucosa is often helpful in identifying parasitic infections such as *E. histolytica* or *S. mansoni*. Endoscopy with duodenal aspirates or biopsies may help to establish the diagnosis of giardiasis, cryptosporidiosis, microsporidiosis, or strongyloidiasis. These procedures should be carried out during the evaluation of patients with chronic diarrhoea if stool cultures and examinations for ova and parasites have failed to elucidate the aetiology.

Differential diagnosis

Noninflammatory diarrhoea

A large number of noninfectious causes of food poisoning such as heavy metals (e.g. arsenic or cadmium), mushrooms (e.g. *Amanita phalloides*), and other chemical substances can result in acute diarrhoea, nausea, and vomiting. Various toxin-mediated forms of shellfish or seafood poisoning, including ciguatera, scombroid, and toxic encephalopathic shellfish poisoning, can all present with nausea, vomiting, and diarrhoea as part of a constellation of symptoms. A history of recent seafood consumption and the presence of other characteristic symptoms or signs should alert the clinician to the cause.

Endocrine disorders associated with diarrhoea include thyrotoxicosis and Addison's disease. Some secretory tumours such as carcinoid, medullary tumour of the thyroid, and vasoactive intestinal peptide-secreting adenomas have watery diarrhoea as a prominent symptom. Chronic, nonbloody diarrhoea is seen in patients with coeliac disease, laxative abuse, Whipple's disease, short-gut syndrome, and pancreatic insufficiency.

Inflammatory diarrhoea

Bloody diarrhoea due to invasive enteropathogens is difficult to distinguish from that caused by inflammatory bowel disease.

Two features help to distinguish dysentery from an acute attack of idiopathic ulcerative colitis: a positive culture for a pathogen and a self-limited course without relapse. However, positive cultures are encountered in only 40 to 60% of reported dysentery cases. Biopsy of colonic mucosa from patients with both bacterial dysentery and ulcerative colitis show oedema, neutrophils in the lamina propria, and superficial cryptitis with preservation of the normal crypt pattern. Yet, biopsy from idiopathic ulcerative colitis also reveals signs of chronicity such as crypt distortion and plasmacytosis in the lamina propria. In clinical practice, the main diagnostic quandary is the patient with severe, acute colitis who has failed to respond to antimicrobial therapy. Presumptive treatment should include a fluoroquinolone for bacterial pathogens and metronidazole for protozoa. The decision to use other treatments, such as corticosteroids and antimetabolites, rests on the distinction between these diseases, although it may be difficult to make this decision based on culture or histopathological findings. In addition to inflammatory bowel disease, often noninfectious causes such as ischaemic colitis, acute diverticulitis, and, rarely, colon cancer can present with bloody diarrhoea.

Enteric fever

Because the initial presentation of typhoid and paratyphoid fever is pyrexia, there is a large differential diagnosis during the early stages of enteric fever. Depending on epidemiological and clinical factors, a range of infectious (e.g. malaria, Gram-positive sepsis, brucellosis, occult abscess) and noninfectious (e.g. rheumatological diseases and malignancy) aetiologies need to be considered. Blood cultures are an essential part of the diagnostic evaluation for enteric fever.

Management

Rehydration

Since the most devastating consequences of acute infectious diarrhoea result from fluid losses, the major goal of treatment is the replacement of fluid and electrolytes. While the intravenous route of administration has been traditionally used, oral rehydration solutions (ORS) have been shown to be equally effective physiologically and logistically more practical and less costly to administer, especially in developing countries. ORS is the treatment of choice for mild to moderate diarrhoea in both children and adults, provided that vomiting is not a major feature of the gastrointestinal infection. ORS can also be used in severely dehydrated patients after initial parenteral rehydration.

Although there is no doubt about the value of ORS in treating dehydrating diarrhoea, the optimal concentration of sodium that should be used remains in dispute, particularly in regard to the treatment of mild to moderate diarrhoea in well-nourished children in industrialized countries. The high concentration of sodium (90 mmol) in the World Health Organization's standard ORS formulation may cause hypernatraemia and even seizures in children with noncholera watery diarrhoea. Consequently, lower concentrations of sodium and a reduced osmolarity solution have been found to be effective for rehydration and not to be associated with any serious adverse clinical events. The substitution of starch derived from rice or cereals for glucose in ORS has been another approach. Rice-based salt solutions produce lower stool losses, a shorter duration of diarrhoea, and greater fluid and electrolyte absorption than do glucose-based solutions in treating childhood and adult diarrhoea.

The provision of zinc supplements in conjunction with oral rehydration therapy serves to shorten the duration of diarrhoea and reduce the risk of subsequent episodes among children in resource-poor settings. This approach is now advocated by the World Health Organization for the routine treatment of childhood diarrhoea in developing countries.

Diet

The traditional approach to an acute diarrhoeal illness—dietary abstinence—restricts the intake of necessary calories, fluids, and electrolytes. During an acute attack, the patient often finds it more comfortable to avoid spicy, high-fat, and high-fibre foods, all of which can increase stool volume and intestinal motility. Although giving the bowel a rest provides symptomatic relief, continued oral intake of fluids and foods is critical for both rehydration and the prevention of malnutrition. In children, it is particularly important to restart feeding as soon as the child is willing to accept oral intake.

Because certain foods and fluids can increase intestinal motility, it is wise to avoid fluids such as coffee, tea, cocoa, and alcoholic beverages. Ingestion of milk and dairy products can potentiate fluid secretion and increase stool volume. Besides the oral rehydration therapy outlined above, acceptable beverages for mildly dehydrated adults include fruit juices and various bottled soft drinks. Carbonated drinks should be allowed to 'de-fizz' by letting them stand in a glass before ingestion. Soft, easily digestible foods are generally acceptable to the patient with acute diarrhoea.

Antimicrobial therapy

Since most patients with infectious diarrhoea, even those with a recognized pathogen, have a mild, self-limited course, neither a stool culture nor specific treatment is required for such cases (Fig. 15.18.1). For more severe cases, however, empirical antimicrobial therapy should be instituted, pending the results of stool and blood cultures. Gastrointestinal infections likely to respond to antibiotic treatment include cholera, giardiasis, cyclosporiasis, shigellosis, *E. coli* diarrhoea in infants, symptomatic traveller's diarrhoea, *C. difficile* diarrhoea, and typhoid fever. The choice of antimicrobial drug should be based on *in vitro* sensitivity patterns, which vary from region to region. A fluoroquinolone antibiotic is a good choice for empirical therapy, since these agents have broad-spectrum activity against virtually all bacterial pathogens responsible for acute infectious diarrhoea (except *C. difficile*). Resistance to fluoroquinolones in South and South East Asia is an increasing problem. The presence of nalidixic acid resistance among gastrointestinal pathogens such as *S.* Typhi is associated with clinical treatment failures with fluoroquinolones. Alternative therapies including azithromycin or third-generation cephalosporins are recommended in these circumstances.

In patients with severe community-acquired diarrhoea—characterized by more than four stools per day lasting for at least 3 days or more with at least one associated symptom such as fever, abdominal pain, or vomiting—there is a high likelihood of isolating a bacterial pathogen. In this setting, a short course of a fluoroquinolone (duration 1–3 days) will generally provide prompt relief with a low risk of adverse effects. Fluoroquinolones will not be effective for parasitic infections—specific antiparasitic drugs should be prescribed after identification of the offending pathogen in stool smears.

Self-treatment with an effective antimicrobial agent is advised for traveller's diarrhoea. While a fluoroquinolone is the treatment of choice, travellers to parts of Asia where resistance has become widespread should be provided with azithromycin for standby therapy. Rifaximin may also be used, but this nonabsorbable antibiotic is not recommended for treatment of invasive diarrhoea, which is common among travellers to Asia, especially Thailand.

There are conflicting reports regarding the efficacy of antimicrobial drugs in several important infections, such as those caused by campylobacter, and insufficient data for infections caused by yersinia and aeromonas, vibrios, and several forms of *E. coli*. In cases of EHEC, there is evidence that antibiotics are not helpful and may even be harmful.

The duration of antimicrobial therapy has not been clearly defined. Courses of anywhere from 3 to 10 days of treatment have been recommended, but several studies that included severe forms of diarrhoea have suggested that a single dose is as effective as more prolonged therapy. For example, single-dose fluoroquinolone therapy is highly effective for infections due to *V. cholerae*, *V. parahaemolyticus*, and most shigella species. On the other hand, short-course treatment of salmonella gastroenteritis with fleroxacin has not been found to be clinically beneficial. When treatment is indicated, a number of studies have shown that the combination of an antimicrobial drug and an antimotility drug provides the most rapid relief of diarrhoea.

Antidiarrhoeal agents (Table 15.18.3)

Antimotility drugs are particularly useful in controlling moderate to severe diarrhoea. These agents disrupt propulsive motility by decreasing jejunal motor activity. Opiates may decrease fluid secretion, enhance mucosal absorption, and increase rectal sphincter tone. The overall effect is to normalize fluid transport, slow transit time, reduce fluid losses, and ameliorate abdominal cramping.

Loperamide is the best agent because it does not carry a risk of habituation or depression of the respiratory centre. Treatment with loperamide produces rapid improvement, often within the first day of therapy. Although there has been a long-standing concern

Table 15.18.3 Nonspecific treatments for diarrhoeal disease

Effective	Not effective
Fluids	Anticholinergics
Intravenous	Cholestyramine
Oral rehydration therapy	Kaolin, pectin, charcoal
Food	Lactobacilli
Continue food intake	Hydroxyquinolones (may be harmful)
Avoid caffeine, lactose, and methylxanthines	
Antimotility drugs	
Diphenoxylate	
Loperamide	
Codeine, paregoric, tincture of opium	
Bismuth subsalicylate	
Antisecretory drugs (e.g. zaldaride maleate)	
Lactobacillus GG (may be effective in rotavirus diarrhoea)	

that antimotility agents might exacerbate cases of dysentery, this has largely been dispelled by clinical experience. Patients with shigellosis, even *S. dysenteriae* type 1, have been treated with loperamide alone and have had a normal resolution of symptoms without evidence of prolonging the illness or delaying excretion of the pathogen. However, as a general rule, antimotility drugs should not be used in patients with acute severe colitis, whether infectious or noninfectious in origin.

Bismuth subsalicylate (BSS), an insoluble complex of trivalent bismuth and salicylate, is effective in treating mild to moderate forms of diarrhoea. Bismuth possesses antimicrobial properties, whereas the salicylate moiety has antisecretory properties. In trials of diarrhoea among travellers in Mexico and West Africa, BSS reduced the frequency of diarrhoea significantly relative to placebo, but results were generally better when a high dose (e.g. 4.2 g/day) was used. A number of studies have shown that the combination of an antimicrobial drug and an antimotility drug provides the most rapid relief of diarrhoea.

Prevention

Strict adherence to food and water precautions as outlined above will help travellers to less developed areas of the world to decrease their risk of acquiring gastrointestinal infections. Parasitic infections, such as strongyloidiasis and hookworms, can be avoided by the use of footwear. Avoiding contact with fresh water such as rivers and lakes in endemic areas serves to prevent schistosomiasis. In developing countries, interventions promoting hand washing have successfully reduced the incidence of diarrhoeal disease in young children.

Probiotics, especially *Lactobacillus rhamnosus* GG, effectively reduce the frequency and duration of diarrhoea in children and adults. Probiotics are also useful for the prevention of antibiotic-associated diarrhoea.

Immunization represents an ideal way to prevent certain bacterial and viral diseases, but has not yet proved successful for combating many gastrointestinal pathogens. The cholera vaccine that has been available for decades suffers from low efficacy, a moderate risk of side effects, and a short duration of action. Newer oral cholera vaccines, such as the inactivated B subunit vaccine, are highly effective for prevention of severe cholera. New rotavirus vaccines, now available for the prevention of rotaviral diarrhoea in children, have not been associated with intussusception. Immunization has been partially effective for the prevention of typhoid fever, especially in endemic areas. Although the efficacy of the currently available typhoid vaccines has not been determined in persons from industrialized regions, these vaccines are widely used for the prevention of typhoid fever in travellers to developing countries.

Further reading

Brooks JT, *et al.* (2006). Surveillance for bacterial diarrhea and antimicrobial resistance in rural western Kenya, 1997–2003. *Clin Infect Dis*, **43**, 393–401.

Bhutta ZA (2006). Current concepts in the diagnosis and treatment of typhoid fever. *BMJ*, **333**, 78–82.

DuPont HL (2006). Travellers' diarrhoea: contemporary approaches to therapy and prevention. *Drugs*, **66**, 303–14.

Hamer DH (2003). Treatment of bacterial and viral diarrhea and food poisoning. In: Baddour L, Gorbach SL (eds). *Therapy of infectious diseases*. Elsevier Science, Philadelphia, PA.

Hamer DH, Snydman DR (2004). Food poisoning. In: Gorbach SL, Bartlett JG, Blacklow NR (eds) *Infectious diseases*, 3rd edition. Lippincott Williams & Wilkins, Philadelphia, PA.

Kaper JB, Nataro JP, Mobley HL (2004). Pathogenic *Escherichia coli*. *Nat Rev Microbiol*, **2**, 123–40.

McFarland LV (2006). Meta-analysis of probiotics for the prevention of antibiotic associated diarrhea and the treatment of *Clostridium difficile* disease. *Am J Gastroenterol*, **101**, 812–22.

Niyogi SK (2005) Shigellosis. *J Microbiol*, **43**, 133–43.

Qadri F, *et al.* (2005). Enterotoxigenic *Escherichia coli* in developing countries: epidemiology, microbiology, clinical features, treatment, and prevention. *Clin Microbiol Rev*, **18**, 465–83.

Sack DA, *et al.* (2004) Cholera. *Lancet*, **363**, 223–33.

Thapar N, Sanderson IR (2004). Diarrhoea in children: an interface between developing and developed countries. *Lancet*, **363**, 641–53.

Thielman NM, Guerrant RL (2004). Acute infectious diarrhea. *N Engl J Med*, **350**, 38–47.

Structure and function of the liver, biliary tract, and pancreas

Alexander Gimson and Simon M. Rushbrook

Essentials

Liver and biliary tract

The liver, sited in the right upper quadrant of the abdomen, comprises eight segments, each of which is a complete functional unit with a single portal pedicle and a hepatic vein. Within the functional segments, the structural unit is the hepatic lobule, a polyhedron surrounded by four to six portal tracts containing hepatic arterial and portal venous branches from which blood perfuses through sinusoids, surrounded by walls of hepatocytes that are a single cell thick and lined by specialized endothelial cells with 'windows' (fenestrae), to the centrilobular region and the central hepatic veins. Bile secreted through the canalicular membrane of the hepatocyte collects in biliary canaliculi, from which it passes through the biliary tract into the gut.

The liver secretes bile, which aids digestion by emulsifying lipids, and has a central role in metabolism of (1) bilirubin, from haem; (2) bile salts, the principal mechanism for clearance of cholesterol; (3) carbohydrates, e.g. maintenance of blood glucose within a narrow range; (4) amino acids and ammonia, e.g. control of the plasma concentration of amino acids, and clearing portal venous ammonia generated within the gut lumen; (5) proteins, most circulating plasma proteins being produced by hepatocytes; and (6) lipid and lipoproteins.

Pancreas

The pancreas lies in the retroperitoneum and is composed of (1) an exocrine portion centred on acini, producing an alkaline secretion containing digestive enzymes including serine proteases (e.g. trypsinogen, chymotrypsin, which act at various cleavage points), exopeptidases (e.g. carboxypeptidases A and B, which cleave C-terminal amino acids) and lipolytic enzymes, draining through a ductal system into the duodenum; and (2) the islets of Langerhans, which secrete insulin (also glucagon, somatostatin, and pancreatic polypeptide).

Liver and biliary tract

The liver weighs 1.2 to 1.5 kg and has a highly vascular architecture. The classic descriptions of liver anatomy demonstrating the complexity of different parenchymal and nonparenchymal elements have a long history, but only recently have they been united with an increasing understanding of the intricate functional organization and physiological compartmentalization of liver structure. This has had a profound effect on our understanding of the control of physiological processes and the development of liver surgery. A grasp of the hepatic anatomy is key to an appreciation of these complex functional arrangements.

Morphological anatomy

This describes the classic structure of the liver into two lobes, right and left, and the accompanying vascular structures, lymphatics, and biliary tract.

The liver, situated in the right upper quadrant of the abdomen, is covered by Glisson's capsule, a visceral continuation of the peritoneum. Three ligaments attach to surrounding structures—the falciform ligament anterior and superiorly, and the two posterior triangular ligaments which enclose the retrohepatic vena cava and the small bare area of the liver. Inferiorly Glisson's capsule attaches to the lesser curve of the stomach and at the hepatic hilus encases the hepatic pedicle consisting of hepatic artery, portal vein, and common hepatic bile duct.

Hepatic lobes

The two major lobes, right and left, and two accessory lobes, quadrate and caudate, are defined by points of surface anatomy (Fig. 15.19.1a). The larger right lobe comprises the dome of the liver under the diaphragm and is limited anteriorly and medially by the falciform ligament and posteriorly by the right border of the inferior vena cava. The quadrate lobe inferiorly abuts on to the antrum of the stomach and first part of the duodenum and is bordered by the posterior transverse hilar fissure, the gallbladder fossa laterally, and the umbilical fissure medially. The caudate lobe lies posterior and superior to the quadrate lobe limited by the vena cava and the ligamentum venosum. Finally, the left lobe has the umbilical fissure medially and the falciform ligament anteriorly.

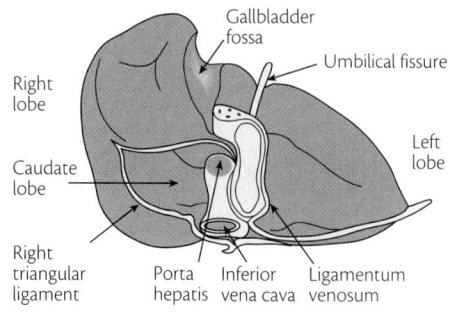

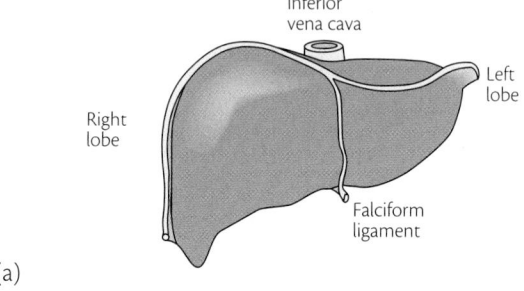

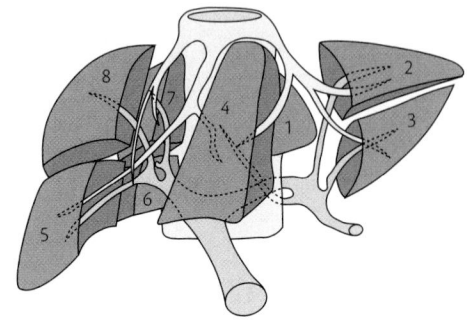

Fig. 15.19.2 Functional anatomy of the liver with Couinaud's segments.

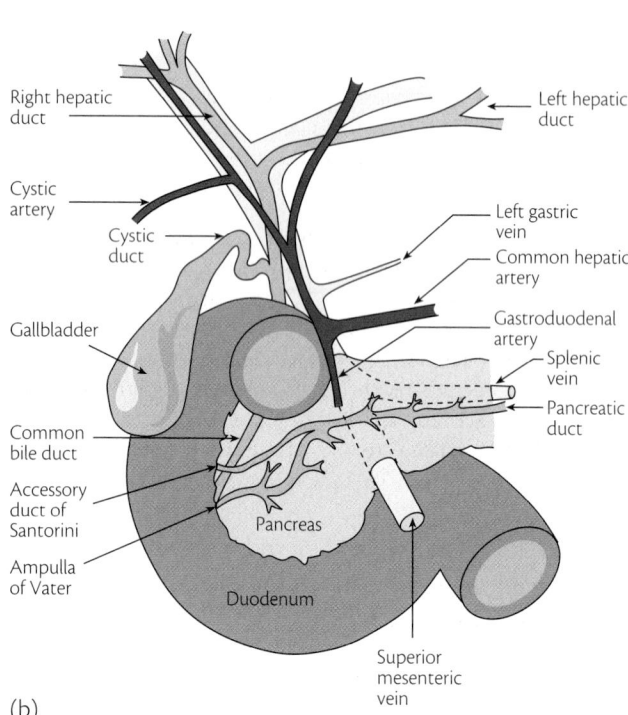

Fig. 15.19.1 (a) Lobar anatomy and relations. (b) Hilar, portal biliary tract, and pancreatic anatomy.

Vascular anatomy

The portal vein, hepatic duct, and hepatic artery form the hepatic pedicle with the bile duct anterior in the free edge of the lesser omentum and the portal vein posteriorly (Fig. 15.19.1b). The latter is formed by the confluence of the superior mesenteric vein and the splenic veins running posteriorly in the pedicle, dividing into left and right branches to supply each lobe. The left gastric vein also drains into the portal vein and may, in the presence of portal hypertension, be a major feeding vessel for gastro-oesophageal varices.

The hepatic artery arises from the coeliac axis as the common hepatic artery before dividing into a gastroduodenal and the main hepatic artery. There are several common anatomical variants of the arterial supply of the liver, which are of no functional significance but which are of importance in liver transplantation and during surgical resection. The standard division into single left and right hepatic arteries is present in approximately 70% of cases (Fig. 15.19.1b), but common variants include a separate second right hepatic artery (10%), separate right and left hepatic arteries (8%), and origin of the main hepatic artery off the superior mesenteric artery (2.5%). Variants of the left hepatic arterial supply also occur, with a separate left hepatic artery arising from the left gastric artery in 10% of cases.

Venous drainage of the liver is through the three main hepatic veins, right, left, and middle, the latter two coalescing before joining the inferior vena cava. The caudate lobe drains separately through an array of small spigelian veins directly into the inferior vena cava. The functional anatomy of the liver (see below) describes the relationship between the main divisions of the portal vein and their draining hepatic veins running in the right, left, and main scissures (Fig. 15.19.2).

Biliary anatomy

Biliary canaliculi drain into left and right hepatic bile ducts forming the common hepatic duct until entry of the cystic duct, after which it is designated the common bile duct and has a diameter of less than 8 mm. The left hepatic duct follows a nearly horizontal course, partially extrahepatic. Anatomical variants are again quite frequent, and are surgically important, the most common being drainage of the cystic duct directly into the right hepatic duct. The common bile duct passes behind the first part of the duodenum, through pancreatic tissue to the ampulla of Vater joining drainage of the pancreatic duct (Fig. 15.19.1b). The gallbladder lies in a shallow depression in the underside of the liver, may contain up to 50 ml of bile, and is connected to the cystic duct with a spiral valve.

Lymphatics

The liver has a high blood flow and a highly permeable microcirculation. The consequent production of interstitial fluid, intrahepatic lymph, is formed in the perisinusoidal space of Disse between the hepatocytes and sinusoidal lining endothelium. Lymphatic vessels drain via the portal tracts, closely applied to the hepatic arterial branches, to the hilum and thence to the thoracic duct. A smaller proportion drains with the hepatic veins and some interstitial fluid drains through Glisson's capsule into the peritoneum. Lymph flow acts to drain from the liver that interstitial fluid and protein that forms inevitably through microvascular filtration. The lymph flow rate in mammalian liver is approximately 0.5 ml/kg of liver per minute, making up 25 to 50% of thoracic duct lymph flow, and may be increased either by elevated microvascular pressure (hydrostatic pressure) through increased hepatic venous pressure or increased inflow pressure, or by reduced transcapillary oncotic pressure.

Nervous system

Both sympathetic and parasympathetic efferent innervation of the liver are described, an anterior plexus around the hepatic artery and posterior around the portal vein. Sympathetic stimulation increases glucose release and glycogenolysis, and reduces oxygen consumption, ammonia uptake, and bile formation. Hepatic vascular resistance also rises as does portal pressure and there is rapid expulsion of blood out of the liver into the systemic circulation. An intrinsic nervous system with a wide variety of neurotransmitters, including noradrenaline, prostanoids, neuropeptide Y, substance P, and vasoactive intestinal peptide, is closely located to smooth muscle cells, fibroblasts, endothelial lining cells, and biliary epithelium within the liver and may be involved in chemoreception and osmoreception.

Extrinsic nervous regulation of hepatic physiological processes seems to be of minor importance as there is no apparent impairment of liver metabolism or bile formation following orthotopic liver transplantation. It may be more relevant during pathophysiological stress: the existence of a hepatorenal reflex is patients with cirrhosis has been postulated whereby an increase in sinusoidal pressure is associated with increased efferent renal sympathetic activity and reduced renal blood flow. In animal models of chronic liver disease, the metabolic consequences of sympathetic nerve stimulation are impaired but the haemodynamic responses exaggerated.

Functional anatomy

Following the initial descriptions by Cantlie in 1898, there has been an increasing appreciation of the importance of the functional anatomy of the liver, the culmination of which was the description by Couinaud of the present eight liver segments that underpins all modern hepatic surgery. Each segment is a complete functional unit with a single portal pedicle and a hepatic vein (Fig. 15.19.2). There are four portal pedicles, two for each lobe, each supplying a sector of the liver, divided from each other by the three hepatic veins lying in a right, middle, and left scissure. This separates the liver into a right and left liver, different from lobes, with independent vascular supply and biliary drainage. Within each sector of the liver there are further subdivisions into segments. The caudate lobe (segment 1) has its own venous drainage, manifest during the Budd–Chiari syndrome with thrombosis of hepatic veins when all venous drainage attempts to pass through this segment with consequent lobar hypertrophy.

The left liver consists of the left posterior sector of segment 2 alone, and a left anterior sector of segment 3 medially and segment 4 laterally separated by the umbilical fissure. The right liver comprises a posterior sector of segment 7 superiorly and segment 6 inferiorly and an anterior sector of segment 5 inferiorly and segment 8, being most of the dome of the liver, superiorly (Fig. 15.19.2).

Structural organization

Within the functional segments of the liver the structural unit is the hepatic lobule, a polyhedron (2 mm × 0.7 mm) surrounded by four

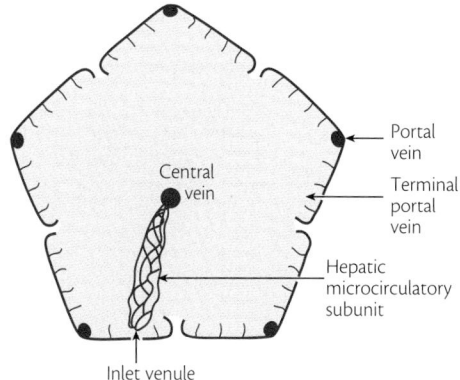

Fig. 15.19.3 Hexagonal lobule with portal venous branches and hepatic microcirculatory subunit—sinusoids.

to six portal tracts containing hepatic arterial and portal venous branches from which blood perfuses through sinusoids, surrounded by walls of hepatocytes that are a single cell thick and lined by specialized endothelial cells with 'windows' (fenestrae), to the centrilobular region and the central hepatic veins (Fig. 15.19.3).

The portal vein branches give off numerous terminal portal venules that run around the lobules in the interlobular septa accompanied by arterioles and bile ductules, and subsequently branch into inlet venules which each supply a hepatic microcirculatory subunit consisting at the base of numerous interconnected sinusoids and, at the apex, the central vein (Fig. 15.19.3).

Sinusoids

Sinusoids are specialized capillaries without a basement membrane and lined with endothelial lining cells through which proteins of low molecular weight may percolate into the space of Disse. The sinusoidal membrane of the surrounding hepatocytes is covered by microvilli that increase the surface area sixfold (Fig. 15.19.4). Within the sinusoids, Kupffer cells and liver-associated lymphocytes may be found, and within the space of Disse, the hepatic stellate cells (also called Ito, fat storage, or perisinusoidal cells), which respectively make up 2%, 0.2%, and 1.4% of the lobular parenchyma (Table 15.19.1).

Biliary canaliculi

Bile secreted through the canalicular membrane of the hepatocyte collects in biliary canaliculi, which pass around hepatocytes until

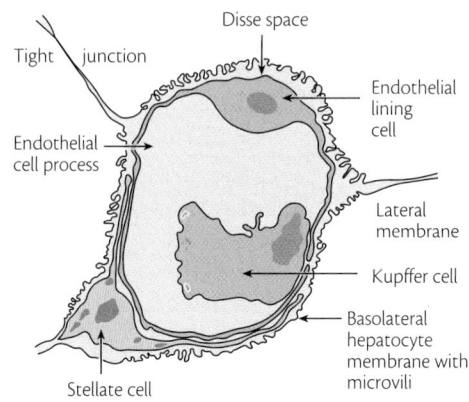

Fig. 15.19.4 Hepatic sinusoid, sinusoidal cells, and functional spaces.

Table 15.19.1 Hepatic parenchymal cellular elements and physiological functions

Cell type	Percentage of parenchyma	Surface receptors	Cellular functions
Hepatocytes	94	Asialoglycoprotein receptors, IL-6, cytokine receptors, albumin, transferrin, mannose, annexin, MHC class 1, Fas ligand	Maintain glucose, amino acid, ammonia, and bicarbonate homeostasis. Bile acid synthesis and transport. Synthesis of most plasma proteins. Processing of absorbed nutrient fuels and xenobiotics. Lipoprotein metabolism. Processing of hormones and signal mediators
Endothelial lining cells	2.5	Scavenger receptor, Fc IgM, MHC class II (CD4), CD58, thrombospondin receptor	Acts as physical barrier lining to sinusoids allowing passage of molecules via fenestrations up to 100 nm or numerous pinocytotic vesicles. Receptor-mediated uptake of HDL, LDL by scavenger receptor. May express numerous adhesion molecules marginating leucocytes and lymphocytes to sites of inflammation
Kupffer cells	2	KP-1, (CD68), Fc and complement receptors, VCAM, ICAM-1	Phagocytosis of numerous particles including cellular debris, denatured albumin, bacteria, complement. After stimulation, release inflammatory mediators: oxygen radical species, nitric oxide, proteases, TNF-α, IL-1, -6, -10, TGF-β, prostanoids, interferons
Stellate, fat storage, or Ito cells	1.4	Retinoid, cytokine receptors, platelet-derived growth factor, TGF-β, endothelin receptor	Vitamin A storage. Under a wide range of stimuli, including TNF-α, TGF-β, acetaldehyde, CCL$_4$, prostanoids, cytokines, and oxygen species, transform into myofibroblasts. Secrete extracellular matrix proteins after activation (collagen, fibronectin, laminin, chondroitin sulphate, hyaluronic acid) resulting in fibrogenesis. Activated transformed stellate cells control sinusoidal blood flow
Pit cells	0.1	CD2, CD18	Natural killer cell activity that may be directed against tumour cells and virus-infected cells and occurs without prior activation

draining through the short canal of Hering into the bile ductule. Cholangioles are lined by three or four cells that eventually become cuboidal epithelium.

The volume and flow rate of bile are low; secretion into the duodenum is controlled by gallbladder contraction and sphincter of Oddi tone. Agents that cause gallbladder contraction, including cholecystokinin, secretin, and motilin, also relax the sphincter of Oddi (Table 15.19.2). Factors modulating biliary motility have received increased attention recently with the realization that the syndrome of biliary dysmotility may be the cause of biliary-type pain in some cases. Changes in gallbladder motility may also be important in gallstone pathogenesis.

Table 15.19.2 Physiological effects of neurotransmitters and hormones on biliary function

Contraction	Relaxation
Gallbladder motility	
Acetylcholine	Secretin
Cholecystokinin	Glucagon
Motilin	Vasoactive intestinal peptide
β-Adrenergic agents	Pancreatic polypeptide
Endorphins	
Sphincter of Oddi	
Secretin	Cholecystokinin
Motilin	Vasoactive intestinal peptide
β-Adrenergic agents	Pancreatic polypeptide

Cellular elements

Hepatocytes are arranged in unicellular plates (Remak's plates) that branch and divide around sinusoids, and are covered by specific membranes at each surface: sinusoidal (70% of surface area) for exchange of material between the Disse space and intracellular compartment (endo- and exocytosis); canalicular membrane (15%) for exchange with the smallest of biliary canaliculi or hemi-canals; and lateral membrane (15%) separated from the former by tight junctions and involved in intercellular transport between hepatocytes. There is abundant smooth and rough endoplasmic reticulum, numerous mitochondria, and glycogen. There is an extensive cytoskeleton. Other cells making up 6% of all parenchyma include sinusoidal-lining endothelial cells, Kupffer cells, hepatic stellate cells (Ito cells, fat-storing cells), and pit cells (intrahepatic lymphocytes) (Table 15.19.1). These cells each differ in morphology, patterns of function, reactions to stimuli and disease, and expression of surface molecules and receptors. Interplay between these cells is critical, with communication via tight junctions allowing complex modulation of hepatocyte growth and function by sinusoidal lining cells. Parenchymal cells may clear mediators, including cytokines, secreted by endothelial lining and Kupffer cells. Waves of cellular activity may pass down the length of sinusoids. Importantly some cells show heterogeneity of function relative to their zonal location. Periportal hepatocytes differ from perivenous cells in both the direction of carbohydrate metabolism and ammonia/glutamine synthesis. Ito cells show zonal differences in desmin and cytokeratin staining, vitamin A storage, and α-smooth muscle actin.

Endothelial lining cells

These cells are central to the processes that control entry and exit trafficking of molecules from the sinusoidal flow into the Disse space.

Fenestrae with a diameter of 100 nm, occupying up to 8% of the sinusoidal surface, act as a physical barrier to access of parenchymal cells by large molecules including lipids, cholesterol, vitamin A, and possibly some viruses. Endothelial cells also possess numerous specialized endocytotic mechanisms, some linked to specific receptors including mannose, transferrin, caeruloplasmin, modified high-density lipoprotein (HDL), low-density lipoprotein (LDL), glucosaminoglycans, and hyaluronic acid. Nonspecific endocytosis of molecules and small particles up to 0.1 µm also occurs. Endothelial cells are also capable of expressing a range of surface adhesion molecules including E- and P-selectins, intercellular adhesion molecule 1 (ICAM-1), and lymphocyte function-associated antigen-4 (LFA-4) that enhance polymorphonuclear leucocyte and lymphocyte adherence, activation, and migration towards sites of inflammation.

Kupffer cells

These cells represent part of the mononuclear phagocyte system and are adherent to the sinusoidal surface of endothelial lining cells, predominantly in a periportal distribution. Covered with numerous microvilli and with a number of intracytoplasmic vesicles, their main function is to phagocytose a range of particulate material including cellular debris, senescent red blood cells, parasites, bacteria, endotoxin, and tumour cells. Phagocytosis is via a range of mechanisms including coated pits, macropinocytotic vesicles, and phagosomes aided by opsonization of particles by fibronectin or opsonin. Kupffer cells may be activated by molecules including *Escherichia coli* endotoxin, interferon-γ, tumour necrosis factor α (TNFα), and arachidonic acid as well as zymosan and phorbol myristate to release a range of inflammatory mediators that include oxygen radical species, nitric oxide, proteases, TNFα, interleukins 1, 6, and 10 (IL-1, -6, -10), transforming growth factor β (TGFβ), prostanoids, and interferon-α and -γ. Some of these may act in an autocrine or paracrine loop to further activate other Kupffer cells. These inflammatory products have a range of effects including significant modulation of parenchymal cell function (down-regulation of albumin synthesis and up-regulation of acute-phase protein gene expression), and induction of adherence of polymorphonuclear leucocytes and lymphocytes to endothelial lining cells due to enhanced expression of endothelial adhesion molecules.

Hepatic stellate cells

Stellate cells (Ito cells, fat-storing cells) have a similar morphology to fibroblasts with the addition of fat droplets, and are located within the Disse space. A fine branching array of cytoplasmic processes circle sinusoids under the endothelial cells. Stellate cells contain most of the body's stores of vitamin A. Retinoids are taken up from chylomicrons by specific receptors on hepatocytes and stellate cells and stored within the latter. These cells are central to the process of hepatic fibrogenesis, responding to mediators released by parenchymal and Kupffer cells, causing transformation into myofibroblasts. TGFβ initiates this process, stimulating production by the transformed stellate cell of extracellular matrix products (collagen types I, III, and IV, fibronectin, laminin, chondroitin sulphate, and hyaluronic acid) in addition to products for matrix degradation (collagenase, metalloproteinase, and its inhibitor TIMP-1). Activation of stellate cells is also an important mechanism for control of sinusoidal perfusion, through cytoskeletal actin within branching cellular processes beneath the endothelium.

Pit cells

Similar to large granular lymphocytes and located in clefts within endothelial lining cells, pit cells have natural killer cell properties with spontaneous activity against tumour cells in the absence of prior activation. They may also play a role in hepatic regeneration.

Physiological processes

Hepatic blood flow

The liver receives approximately 25% of cardiac output, one-third from the hepatic artery and two-thirds from the portal vein with a plasma flow at rest of 1600 ml/min in women and 1800 ml/min in men. Hepatic blood flow increases after feeding and with expiration and decreases with standing, inspiration, and sleep. In contrast to other organs, metabolic autoregulation of blood flow is not observed. Changes in hepatic oxygen consumption do not seem to control hepatic blood flow. Vascular autoregulation of hepatic arterial blood flow mediated by adenosine is present, but may not be of great physiological importance. Hepatic arterial resistance increases with increasing hepatic venous pressure due to a stepwise myogenic response in the hepatic artery to increased pressure. There is an important reciprocity between portal venous and hepatic arterial flow with a reduction in portal venous input being associated with significant compensatory decrease in hepatic arterial resistance and rise in arterial flow. The mechanism for this relationship is unproven but may be due to adenosine-mediated arterial vasodilatation.

The portal venous system is passive, without pressure-dependent autoregulation, and the major physiological factors controlling flow are those modulating supply to the intestines and spleen. The sites of portal venous resistance are not fully defined in humans but may be at sinusoidal or postsinusoidal levels. The significant capacitance of the hepatic circulation, with blood comprising up to 20% of liver volume, is reflected in the important role of the liver and splanchnic circulation in acting as a blood reservoir. Sympathetic nerve stimulation may reduce hepatic blood volume by up to 50%.

Sinusoidal perfusion

Blood pressure in sinusoids ranges from 4.8 to 1.7 mmHg, with flows of 270 to 410 ml/s. There is likely to be considerable heterogeneity of the unidirectional sinusoidal flow, control for which can be considered as either passive (haemodynamic) or active. Passive control mechanisms include: (1) the arterial input pressure and flow at the level of the arteriosinous twig at the origin of the sinusoid; and (2) changes in right atrial pressure, central venous pressure, and hepatic venous pressure that are transmitted to the sinusoid from the centrilobular veins. Active control mechanisms include: (1) the presence of 'functional' sphincters at the inlet and outlet of the sinusoid due to indentations by the cell bodies of sinusoidal lining cells, which under different physiological stimuli may change dimension and alter sinusoidal perfusion; (2) plugging by leucocytes, which are less compressible than erythrocytes and may under physiological stimuli adhere to endothelial lining cells; (3) activation of Kupffer cells within sinusoids and release of other vasoactive mediators including nitric oxide, cytokines, and prostanoids; and (4) transformation of hepatic stellate cells into activated contractile myofibroblasts that constrict the sinusoidal lumen. Sinusoidal flow will also affect the transendothelial traffic into and out of the Disse space by the processes of forced sieving and

Table 15.19.3 Physiological functions of bile

Digestion
Neutralization of duodenal pH
Bile salt activation of lipase, formation of micelles
Emulsification, lipolysis, and solubilization of fat
Absorption of fat-soluble substances
Excretion, including xenobiotics
Cholesterol
Bilirubin
Drugs
Environmental toxins
Heavy metals
Mucosal immunity
Secretory IgA

endothelial massage that may affect, respectively, the passage of lipoprotein particles and the appropriate mixing of the interstitial fluid. Therefore, sinusoidal flow is likely to have a profound effect on numerous hepatic metabolic functions and clearance of xenobiotics.

Bile formation

The formation of bile by hepatocytes and its modification by bile ductular epithelium serves many functions (Table 15.19.3). In humans the daily production of 600 ml of bile is made up of 75% of canalicular origin and 25% from ductules. Bile is formed by osmotic filtration, with the secretion of the two primary bile salt anions, taurine and glycine conjugates of cholic acid and chenodeoxycholic acid, across the canalicular membrane by an active transport mechanism against a concentration gradient of 5000:1 (Fig. 15.19.5). Negatively charged intercellular tight junctions prevent back diffusion of these anions, allowing the selective passage of cations, predominantly sodium, and to a smaller extent potassium, calcium, and magnesium, followed by the passive transit of water, transcellularly or between cells. The resulting bile salt-dependent bile flow makes up 50% of canalicular bile flow, with the remaining bile salt-independent flow resulting from the active secretion of bicarbonate and glutathione.

Bile in biliary ductules is further modified by reabsorption of glucose, amino acids, and bile salts, as well as active secretion. Reabsorption of bile salts, the cholehepatic shunt pathway, occurs after their protonation in bile with the generation of further bicarbonate into bile stimulating bile flow. Active secretion of bicarbonate and chloride within ductules is mediated by the secretin receptor and the cystic fibrosis transmembrane receptor. Gallbladder epithelium further modifies and concentrates bile by an active anion transport process.

Bile salt conjugates secreted from hepatocytes into bile are deconjugated in the jejunum and ileum with reabsorption and reuptake by the liver—this enterohepatic circulation conserves bile acids and maintains their high concentration within bile. The 5% of bile acids passing through the ileocaecal valve are fully deconjugated by colonic bacteria and reabsorbed as the secondary bile acids deoxycholic acid and lithocolic acid, which are in turn secreted as taurine and glycine conjugates.

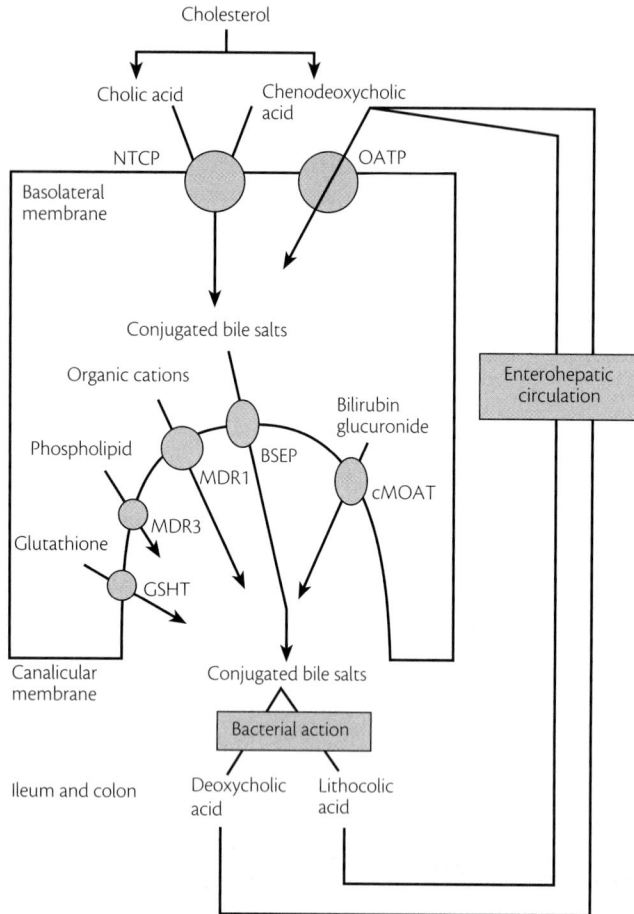

Fig. 15.19.5 Bile salt metabolism and enterohepatic pathway. NTCP, Na-taurocholate cotransporters; conjugated bile salt uptake from portal blood. OATP, organic anion transporter; bile salt, organic anion, and amphipathic solutes uptake. BSEP, bile salt export pump; ATP-dependent bile export—bile salt-dependent bile flow. MDR1, multidrug resistance; organic cation, xenobiotic export. MDR2, bilirubin glucuronide export; bile salt-independent bile flow. MDR3, multidrug resistance; translocation of phosphatidylcholine. GSHT, glutathione transporter; gluthathione transport independent of bile flow.

Metabolic processes

Hepatic metabolic processes have a central role in protein, carbohydrate, and lipid metabolism and fuel economy, orchestrating a diverse interplay between central splanchnic and peripheral organs. Interruption to these processes results in the major metabolic consequences of acute and chronic liver disease. Modulation of these metabolic processes can occur at a number of levels. Transport of molecules across membranes and through cells is an important control mechanism as are rate-limiting enzyme levels, controlled at a number of transcriptional and translational points. There is important zonal heterogeneity of hepatocyte function, with periportal zone 1 cells with a higher oxidative capacity and larger mitochondria involved in gluconeogenesis, β-oxidation of fatty acids, amino acid catabolism, ureagenesis, cholesterol synthesis, and bile secretion, whereas perivenular cells are more involved with glycolysis, lipogenesis, ammonia clearance with glutamine synthesis, detoxification, and biotransformation.

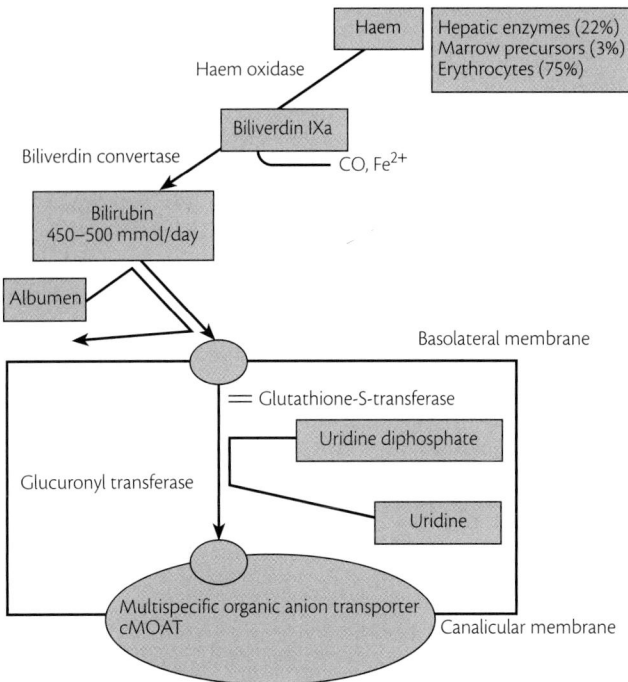

Fig. 15.19.6 Metabolism of haem and bilirubin with clearance through canalicular membrane to bile.

Bilirubin metabolism (see Chapter 15.20)

The first step in the production of bilirubin is the formation of biliverdin IXa by the action of haem oxidase on haem-containing proteins including catalases, cytochromes as well as haemoglobin in senescent red cells, with the release of carbon monoxide and Fe^{2+}. Biliverdin convertase within the cytosol reduces biliverdin to unconjugated bilirubin (Fig. 15.19.6). Both biliverdin convertase and haem oxidase are predominantly found within reticuloendothelial cells.

Bilirubin is transported within plasma bound with high affinity to albumin. A few substances may displace bilirubin from albumin, including sulphonamides and fatty acids. Unbound bilirubin, which is insoluble in water, is present only in nanogram quantities but may cause significant cellular toxicity in neonates and in the Crigler–Najjar syndrome.

Bilirubin uptake by hepatocytes occurs via an organic anion-binding protein receptor. Within the hepatocyte the unbound bilirubin is transported by organelles and a number of transport proteins including glutathione-*S*-transferase (ligandin) to the endoplasmic reticulum. This reduces back diffusion into sinusoids of the lipid-soluble unbound bilirubin. Glucuronidation to the mono- and diglucuronides renders bilirubin water soluble. Secretion across the canalicular membrane occurs at the canalicular multispecific membrane organic anion transporter.

Bile salt metabolism

In addition to their role in digestion, bile acids are the principal mechanism for clearance and metabolism of cholesterol, which acts as a substrate for their synthesis and in turn promotes biliary cholesterol secretion as lamellar vesicles. The first step in bile acid synthesis is rate limiting and involves cholesterol 7α-hydroxylase. Transcriptional control of the cholesterol 7α-hydroxylase gene has been demonstrated with thyroxine and glucocorticoids increasing,

and glucagon decreasing, gene expression. Preformed (nondietary) cholesterol and bile acids may also control this enzyme. The close association between bile acid and cholesterol metabolism is reflected in the often parallel activation of 7α-hydroxylase and HMG-CoA reductase, which is of critical importance in bile acid synthesis. The two major bile acids, cholic acid (60% of bile acid pool) and chenodeoxycholic acid are secreted into bile as taurine and glycine conjugates. The transport receptors for both uptake into hepatocyte and transport across the canalicular membrane are controlled at both transcriptional and post transcriptional levels by multiple factors including bile acids, cytokines and hormones. Nuclear receptors such as the farnesoid X and liver X receptor also regulate transcription.

Carbohydrate metabolism (Fig. 15.19.7)

The liver has a central role in maintaining blood glucose within a narrow margin. During fasting, hepatic glucose release is contributed to by both glycogenolysis (33%) and gluconeogenesis (67%) from lactate, pyruvate, glycerol, and the glucogenic amino acids alanine and glutamine (Fig. 15.19.7). This process is regulated by at least four levels: (i) hormonal control, with glucagon accounting for up to two-thirds of basal fasted glucose output, and cortisol, growth hormone, and catecholamines also contributing; (ii) the supply of substrates, fatty acids, lactate, pyruvate, and amino acids for hepatic gluconeogenesis; (iii) metabolic regulation of hepatic enzyme activity; and (iv) the degree of hepatocellular hydration. The direction of gluconeogenesis or glycogenolysis is controlled at the level of three paired enzyme cycles—glucose/glucose 6-phosphate, fructose 6-phosphate/fructose 1,6-bisphosphate, and pyruvate/phosphoenolpyruvate. In contrast, after a glucose load, insulin suppresses

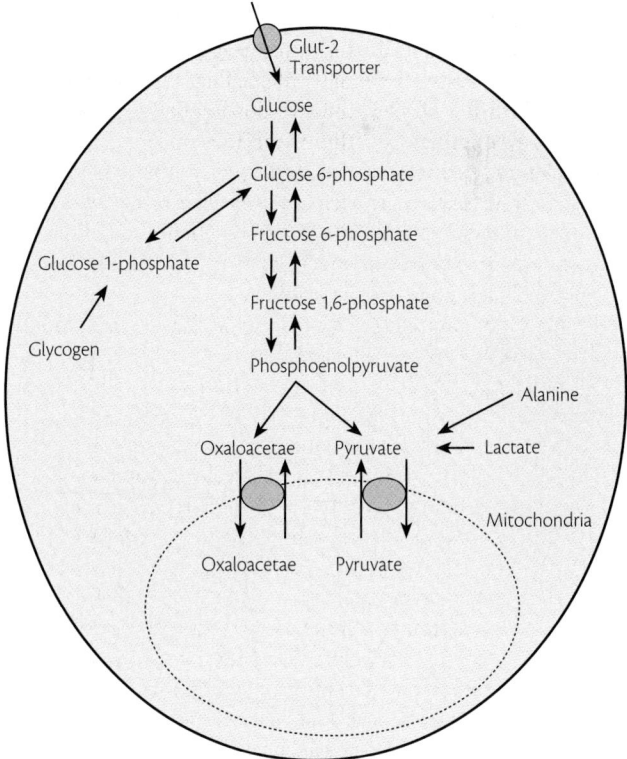

Fig. 15.19.7 Carbohydrate metabolism and pathways for glycolysis and glycogenesis.

hepatic glucose release and activates glucose synthetase, while autoregulation of hepatic glucose extraction by glucose itself within the portal venous circulation is an important factor in controlling the distribution of the load between liver and peripheral tissues.

Amino acid and ammonia metabolism

The liver is the most important organ in controlling the plasma concentration of amino acids. During prolonged starvation, hepatic proteolysis stimulated by glucagon increases splanchnic export of amino acids, whereas during the postprandial absorptive state, amino acid uptake is significantly increased. The gluconeogenic amino acids are preferentially extracted and metabolized, whereas the branched chain amino acids valine, leucine, and isoleucine are only cleared in the liver for protein synthesis and are catabolized in the muscle. During sepsis and under the influence of cytokines IL-1, IL-6, and TNFα, the liver may significantly enhance gluconeogenesis and protein synthesis of acute-phase reactants (C-reactive protein, serum amyloid A).

The liver has a critical role in clearing portal venous ammonia generated within the gut lumen, by both formation of carbamoyl phosphate and entry into the urea cycle in periportal hepatocytes, and glutamine synthetase-driven glutamine synthesis in perivenous hepatocytes.

Protein synthesis

Most circulating plasma proteins with the exception of immunoglobulins and von Willebrand factor are produced by hepatocytes. The major controlling factors for this constitutive protein secretion are substrate delivery and the degree of hydration of hepatocytes. Acute-phase protein secretion is also specifically controlled by cytokines with a reciprocal relationship to albumin and other carrier protein synthesis.

Lipid and lipoprotein metabolism (Fig. 15.19.8) (see Chapter 12.6)

Plasma lipoproteins are particles with an outer layer of cholesterol, phospholipids, and apoproteins and an inner core of cholesterol

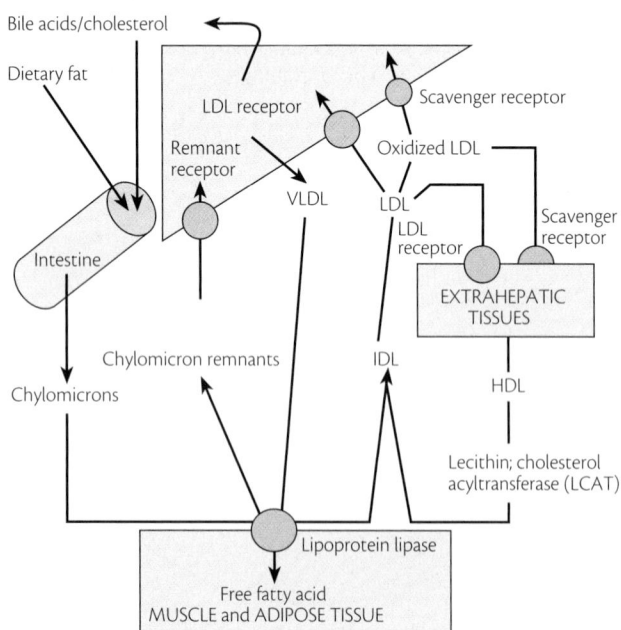

Fig. 15.19.8 Lipoprotein metabolism.

esters and triglycerides. The various lipoproteins differ in the relative proportions of these elements. Dietary derived chylomicrons, consisting of more than 90% triglyceride, are processed within muscle and adipose tissue by lipoprotein lipase, extracting free fatty acids and the remnant, enriched in cholesterol, are extracted by the liver—an exogenous lipid pathway. During carbohydrate feeding, free fatty acids formed within the liver are exported as very-low-density lipoprotein (VLDL) and taken up by muscle and adipose tissue with extraction of free fatty acids, leaving intermediate-density lipoprotein and subsequently LDL. Specific LDL receptors on hepatocytes or scavenger receptors on Kupffer cells remove LDL where cholesterol may be utilized for bile salt metabolism or excreted into bile. Peripheral LDL receptors in extrahepatic tissues also extract cholesterol. Export of cholesterol from peripheral tissues in high-density lipoprotein is modified in plasma by lecithin; cholesterol acyltransferase (LCAT) and LDL is formed for further recirculation.

Pancreas

Structure and function

A retroperitoneal organ receiving arterial supply from splenic, superior mesenteric, and gastroduodenal arteries, the pancreas is composed of an exocrine portion centred on acini producing digestive enzymes draining through a ductal system into the duodenum, and the islets of Langerhans which make up 1 to 2% of the whole volume and are predominantly located along arterioles.

Development and congenital anomalies

The pancreas develops from ventral and dorsal buds of the primitive duodenum. With rotation around the duodenum the two portions fuse together and the duct originating from the dorsal portion (duct of Santorini) forms the accessory duct whilst the main drainage of the gland is through the duct of Wirsung to the ampulla of Vater. Failure of ductal fusion, pancreas divisum, in which most of the gland drains through the duct of Santorini to the minor papilla, occurs in approximately 8% of the population, and in a small proportion may lead to recurrent acute pancreatitis. Annular pancreas results from pancreatic tissue remaining wrapped around the duodenum during rotation of the ventral portion. Ectopic pancreatic tissue may occur in a submucosal location within the stomach and duodenum.

Exocrine pancreas

The pancreas secretes up to 2 litres of fluid per day although resting secretion rates are very low (0.3 ml/min). Acini are located in lobules draining into extralobular ducts. Cells lining the ducts secrete bicarbonate, the major anion within pancreatic juice. The acinar cells are pyramidal with the nucleus and endoplasmic reticulum towards the base and zymogen storage granules towards the apex and draining duct. Two classes of proteolytic enzymes are secreted—the serine proteases and the exopeptidases. Serine proteases all require activation either by intestinal endopeptidase in the case of trypsinogen or by trypsin itself in the case of chymotrypsin, elastase, and protease E. Serine protease act at various cleavage points whereas the carboxypeptidases A and B (exopeptidases) cleave C-terminal amino acids. The lipolytic enzymes include phospholipase A$_2$, lipase, and carboxylesterase. Other proteins found in

Table 15.19.4 Source and metabolic control of pancreatic endocrine function

	Source	Stimuli for release	Inhibitors of release	Physiological role
Insulin	B cells	Glucose, leucine, inosine, sulphonylureas Secondary stimuli: free fatty acids, arginine, alanine, acetylcholine, glucagon, GIP	Hypoglycaemia, adrenaline, noradrenaline, somatostatin, insulin-like growth factor	Increases rate of transport of glucose across cell membrane Enhances glycogen synthesis and inhibits gluconeogenesis; increases protein, triglyceride, and VLDL synthesis in hepatocytes Enhances protein and glycogen synthesis in muscle cells Enhances triglyceride deposition and inhibits lipolysis in adipocytes.
Glucagon	A cells	Glucose, catecholamines Secondary stimuli: glutamine, alanine, arginine, vasoactive intestinal peptide	Insulin, somatostatin	Stimulates glycogenolysis. Promotes gluconeogenesis from amino acids Increases lipolysis in adipose tissue
Somatostatin	D cells	Glucose, arginine, GIP, glucagon, sulphonylureas	Sympathetic nerve stimulation	Suppresses pancreatic exocrine release of insulin and glucagon Reduces gastric motility Inhibits growth hormone-releasing hormone
Pancreatic polypeptide	PP cells	Protein intake, sympathetic nerve stimulation	?	Probable inhibition of pancreatic acinar and ductal secretion

GIP, glucose-dependent insulinotropic polypeptide.

pancreatic secretions include lysosomal proteins, ribonucleases, and amylase.

Control of the secretory process involves hormones as well as sympathetic and parasympathetic nerve fibres. Secretin is the main stimulus to ductal bicarbonate secretion, whereas cholecystokinin, acetylcholine, and to a lesser extent gastrin and neurotensin stimulate zymogen release of digestive enzymes at the apical membrane. Although often described as having cephalic, gastric, and intestinal phases to indicate the origin of the pancreatic stimulus, this distinction is physiologically artificial since the phases run concurrently. Somatostatin and glucagon inhibit pancreatic proenzyme secretion.

Endocrine pancreas

The islets of Langerhans represent an endocrine organ consisting of four cell types: α cells secreting glucagon, β cells secreting insulin, δ cells secreting somatostatin, and PP cells secreting pancreatic polypeptide. The β cells constitute 80% of islet volume and form the central core around which the others cells form a mantle. The principal physiological function of these cells is to maintain stable glucose concentration irrespective of substrate delivery.

The β cells act as a sensor of glucose concentration over a wide range, with rapid equilibration of glucose levels across the cell membrane by the GLUT-2 transporter. The molecular basis for this sensor is considered to be glucokinase, the activity of which closely follows glucose levels. Enhanced glucose metabolism increases ATP/ADP ratios, which in turn blocks potassium ion channels, and the subsequent change in membrane potential allows an influx of calcium that promotes exocytosis of insulin-containing granules. Many other hormones, neuropeptides, and neurotransmitters also modulate glucose-dependent insulin secretion (Table 15.19.4).

Further reading

Balabaud C, *et al.* (1988). Light and transmission electron microscopy of sinusoids in human liver. In: Bioulac Sage P, Balabaud C (eds) *Sinusoids in human liver; health and disease*, pp. 87–110. Kupffer Cell Foundation, Rijswik.

Erlinger S (1993). Intracellular events in bile acid transport by the liver. In: Tavoloni N, Berk PD (eds) *Hepatic transport and bile secretion. Physiology and pathophysiology*, pp. 467–75. Raven Press, New York.

Gumucio JJ (1999). Functional organisation of the liver. In: Bircher J, *et al. Oxford textbook of clinical hepatology*, pp. 437–46. Oxford University Press, Oxford.

Kang S, Davis RA (2000). Cholesterol and hepatic lipoprotein assembly and secretion. *Biochim Biophys Acta*, **1529**, 223–30.

Knook DI, Wisse E (eds) (1982). *Sinusoidal liver cells*. Elsevier, Amsterdam.

Tukey RH, Strassburg CP (2000). Human UDP-glucuronosyltransferases: metabolism, expression, and disease. *Ann Rev Pharmacol Toxicol*, **40**, 581–616.

Jaundice

R.P.H. Thompson

Essentials

Physiology of bilirubin

All haem molecules are degraded in macrophages by haem oxygenase to biliverdin, and then by biliverdin reductase to bilirubin, which is selectively removed by hepatocytes from sinusoidal blood and then conjugated, mainly by one of the two specific isoforms of the microsomal enzyme UDP-glucuronyl (glucuronate-glucuronosyl) transferase, chiefly with two glucuronic acid moieties. Conjugated bilirubin is excreted into the bile by the anionic conjugate transporter protein (MRP2), but in many liver diseases it readily refluxes back into blood and—since it is water soluble and less firmly bound to albumin than unconjugated bilirubin—about 1% is filtered across the glomerular membrane and darkens the urine (choluria). In the distal intestine conjugated bilirubin is deconjugated and reduced to a series of uro- and stercobilinogens that give the normal colour to faeces. Some colourless urobilinogen is normally absorbed from the colon and undergoes an enterohepatic circulation, with a small amount being excreted in urine. If this biliary excretion is impaired in liver disease, or increased in haemolysis, then excess urobilinogen is excreted in urine, where it is easily detected by routine clinical 'stix'.

Clinical approach

Jaundice is the clinical sign of hyperbilirubinaemia and usually indicates disease of the liver or biliary tree. Dark urine and, less commonly, pale stools indicate cholestasis. Stigmata of chronic liver disease are important, but do not define the cause of jaundice.

Unconjugated hyperbilirubinaemia—should be sought for by testing if serum bilirubin levels are raised, while other liver-related blood tests are normal. Causes include (1) haemolysis, which if severe enough to raise bilirubin levels is likely to cause an elevated reticulocyte count and reduction in plasma haptoglobin; (2) benign constitutional unconjugated hyperbilirubinaemia (Gilbert's syndrome)—a common recessive condition (affecting at least 3% of the normal adult population) due to homozygous polymorphisms in the promoter region of the specific glucuronyl transferase gene; recognized by a fluctuating, elevated serum bilirubin concentration that rises excessively on fasting; patients require reassurance that the results do not indicate liver disease.

Conjugated hyperbilirubinaemia—routine liver-related blood tests cannot differentiate between intra- or extrahepatic causes of jaundice, unless the transferases are very high, in which case hepatitis (e.g. viral, alcoholic) is certain. Cholestasis should be sought by abdominal ultrasonography to detect a dilated intra- and/or extrahepatic biliary tree (and often also reveal its cause, e.g. gallstones, tumour). Further investigation depends on clinical context: (1) likely biliary disease—endoscopic retrograde cholangiopancreatography (ECRP), magnetic resonance cholangiography (MRC); (2) likely intrahepatic cholestasis—hepatitis A, B, and C serology, autoantibodies, serum caeruloplasmin/copper, plasma α_1-antitrypsin concentration; liver biopsy.

Introduction

Jaundice is the clinical sign of hyperbilirubinaemia, and hence usually indicates disease of the liver or biliary tree. The pigment in the tissues in best seen as yellowing of the sclera; eventually the skin and soft palate become tinted, but not saliva nor sputum. The urine usually becomes dark. Rarely, carotenaemia, from eating carrots or vitamin A in excess, can mimic jaundice, but then the colour is more prominent in the palms than the sclera.

Physiology of bilirubin

All haem molecules in haemoglobin or cytochrome enzymes are stoichiometrically (1:1) degraded in macrophages via biliverdin to bilirubin, especially in the spleen and liver, but also macrophages in other tissues, including skin, and renal tubular cells. Haem oxygenase breaks open the asymmetric tetrapyrrole haem molecule specifically at the α-methene bridge, releasing carbon monoxide and iron, and forming biliverdin (Fig. 15.20.1). One principal

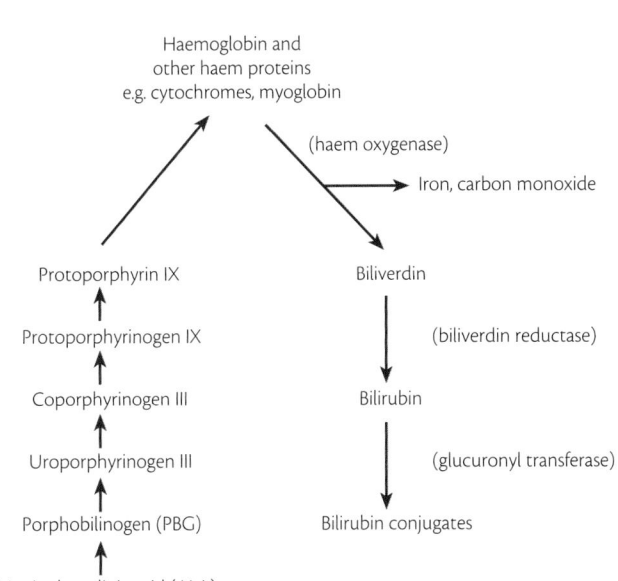

HAEM

Haemoglobin and
other haem proteins
e.g. cytochromes, myoglobin

(haem oxygenase)

Iron, carbon monoxide

Protoporphyrin IX

Biliverdin

Protoporphyrinogen IX

(biliverdin reductase)

Coporphyrinogen III

Bilirubin

Uroporphyrinogen III

(glucuronyl transferase)

Porphobilinogen (PBG)

Bilirubin conjugates

δ-Aminolaevulinic acid (ALA)

Glycine + succinyl CoA

Fig. 15.20.1 The porphyrin–bilirubin pathway.

isomer of biliverdin, namely IXα, is formed, although small amounts of the other three possible isomers (β, γ, and δ) can be detected in bile. The excretion of carbon monoxide in breath can be used quantitatively to determine the breakdown of haem to bilirubin, of which 200 to 350 mg (340–600 μmol) is produced daily. About 85% of biliverdin, and therefore bilirubin, is derived from the delayed breakdown of the haemoglobin in ageing red blood cells, while the remainder is either from the breakdown of haem proteins, chiefly in the liver, or from ineffective erythropoiesis in the bone marrow; these constitute the so-called 'early labelled' bilirubin, defined by isotopic studies *in vivo*.

Biliverdin is green and is directly excreted in bile by birds, amphibians, and reptiles, but not by mammals in whom biliverdin is reduced by the macrophage cytosolic enzyme biliverdin reductase chiefly to the yellow bilirubin IXα, which has then to be excreted. The reason for this species difference was obscure, for bilirubin is lipid soluble and potentially toxic, and has to be conjugated before it is excreted in bile, whereas biliverdin is water soluble and can be readily excreted in urine and bile by mammals. However, bilirubin is an antioxidant or free radical scavenger in plasma and bile, particularly when bound to copper, and this may be particularly important in the neonate, especially when levels of the antioxidant ascorbate are low. Hence bilirubin probably has a function and is not just a waste product. Bilirubin is surprisingly lipid soluble; this is due to internal hydrogen bonding in the molecule so that it forms a tight, nonpolar, nonlinear, three-dimensional structure. After its release from macrophages, it is firmly bound to plasma albumin, so that none enters the urine. At high concentrations in the blood it slowly diffuses into tissues, where it can be toxic, particularly in the neonatal brain (kernicterus), or the kidney. Jaundice is less obvious in unconjugated, than in conjugated, hyperbilirubinaemia since its diffusion into the tissues is more limited. Bilirubin is readily

oxidized back to biliverdin; hence the green vomit of intestinal obstruction.

The circulating pool of bilirubin in the plasma (c.100 μmol) is almost all unconjugated. Routine measurements still rely on the Van den Bergh diazo reaction, which yields either an indirect (unconjugated bilirubin) or direct (conjugated) reaction and, although this overestimates the true level of conjugated bilirubin, the results indicate whether or not circulating bilirubin is chiefly unconjugated. The direct and indirect reactions depend on the slow reaction of the unconjugated bilirubin with the reagent; this is accelerated when solvents, such as methanol, which break the internal hydrogen bonding of bilirubin, are added. The normal range of plasma bilirubin is wide (c.5–19 μmol/litre), reflecting wide variation in the rate of conjugation in the liver, and is higher than in most other mammals in which hepatic clearance and excretion are more efficient. The distribution of values is Gaussian, so that the true upper limit of normal is arbitrary (see 'Familial unconjugated hyperbilirubinaemia', below). Hepatic enzyme-inducing drugs reduce the plasma level by increasing hepatic conjugation and hence the plasma clearance of bilirubin.

Bilirubin is selectively removed by hepatocytes from sinusoidal blood, although its plasma clearance (c.50 ml/min) is low compared e.g. with that of bile acids, and so its extraction (1.5% of plasma pool/min) is dependent more upon hepatocyte distribution and function than on hepatic blood flow. It is initially surprising that bilirubin can be displaced from its plasma binding sites and enter hepatocytes. Specific hepatic cytoplasmic binding proteins have been described, but binding to the active site of the microsomal conjugating enzyme would be sufficient to maintain a low level of free bilirubin in the cytoplasm, which, without the need for specific transfer proteins, should alone produce a gradient sufficient to allow bilirubin slowly to enter the hepatocyte. This uptake of bilirubin is facilitated by the direct contact of plasma with the hepatocyte in the interstitial space of Disse through fenestrations in the endothelium of hepatic blood capillaries. Although uptake predominates, dynamic studies show that there is also considerable reflux of bilirubin out of the cell back into the plasma.

Within the hepatocyte bilirubin is principally conjugated by one of the two specific isoforms of the microsomal enzyme UDP-glucuronyl (glucuronate-glucuronosyl) transferase, chiefly with two glucuronic acid moieties. Minor quantities of bilirubin are conjugated with one glucuronic acid molecule (monoglucuronide) or with combinations of related sugars (xylose, glucose); a small amount of unconjugated bilirubin also appears in bile. The chemical properties of the conjugated molecules are quite different from those of unconjugated bilirubin, for there is no internal hydrogen bonding of bilirubin—they now become more linear, fully water-soluble molecules and are efficiently excreted in bile. In many liver diseases conjugated bilirubin readily refluxes back into blood and, since it is water soluble and less firmly bound to albumin than unconjugated bilirubin, about 1% is filtered across the glomerular membrane and darkens the urine (choluria). Hepatocytes have at least six specific active transporters for the canalicular excretion of the major components of bile, although not for cholesterol, and isolated autosomal recessive defects in them have now been identified. Conjugated bilirubin is excreted out of the endoplasmic reticulum and then across the microvillous intercellular canalicular membrane by the anionic conjugate transporter protein (MRP2).

There is a specific canalicular bile acid export pump protein (BSEP) and one for phospholipid (MDR3). MRP2 also transports other multivalent anions, such as conjugated bromsulphthalein.

The urinary excretion of conjugated bilirubin is increased by the bile acids that also accumulate in liver disease. If renal function is normal, this renal excretion of bilirubin eventually matches its normal rate of production when conjugated bilirubin levels in the plasma reach about 600 µmol/litre. With renal failure, or haemolysis, plasma levels rise higher. Little bilirubin, even if conjugated, diffuses through renal dialysis membranes.

Recently it has been shown that deconjugated bilirubin can undergo a substantial enterohepatic circulation; it is absorbed from the colon, particularly when there is bile acid malabsorption and hence the concentration of bile acids in the colon is increased, for example as a result of disease or resection of the ileum. This reabsorption then increases the concentration of bilirubin re-excreted in bile, and may in part explain the increased incidence of pigment gallstones in patients with ileal disease. Oral ursodeoxycholic acid also increases the enterohepatic recycling of bilirubin perhaps by solubilizing bilirubin in the intestinal lumen, or by impairing the reabsorption of other bile acids in the ileum. This may explain the rim of calcification in an outer pigment layer of cholesterol gallstones during their treatment with ursodeoxycholic acid, and thus the frequent resistance to such dissolution therapy. Similarly, fasting increases unconjugated bilirubin levels in the plasma by increasing the reabsorption of bilirubin, because it reduces intestinal motility and improves absorption.

In the distal intestine conjugated bilirubin is deconjugated and reduced to a series of uro- and stercobilinogens that give the normal colour to faeces. Some colourless urobilinogen is normally absorbed from the colon and undergoes an enterohepatic circulation, with a small amount being excreted in urine. If this biliary excretion is impaired in liver disease, or increased in haemolysis, then excess urobilinogen is excreted in urine, where it can oxidize on standing to dark brown urobilins. Urobilinogen is easily detected by routine clinical 'stix'. Ehrlich's aldehyde reagent was at one time used; urine containing excess urobilinogen turns red with this reagent and the urobilinogen pigment can then be extracted into an organic solvent, such as chloroform. This is unlike the similar pigment formed from the more polar porphobilinogen adduct in acute porphyria, which remains in the upper aqueous phase.

Management of jaundice

Complex algorithms for the management of the patient with hyperbilirubinaemia or jaundice have been published, but a simple pragmatic approach is proposed here (Fig. 15.20.2).

Raised plasma bilirubin levels, and eventually frank jaundice, are due to excessive unconjugated or conjugated bilirubin levels in blood, depending respectively on whether the abnormality in bilirubin metabolism is either in its production and/or conjugation, or in the subsequent hepatic excretion of conjugated bilirubin. Impaired excretion is almost always combined with impaired bile flow and is best termed cholestasis, when other liver-related blood tests are abnormal, especially the biliary enzymes alkaline phosphatase and γ-glutamyl transpeptidase, serum bile acids are also raised, there is often itching, and the microvilli lining the biliary canaliculi are injured. Examination of a liver biopsy specimen taken

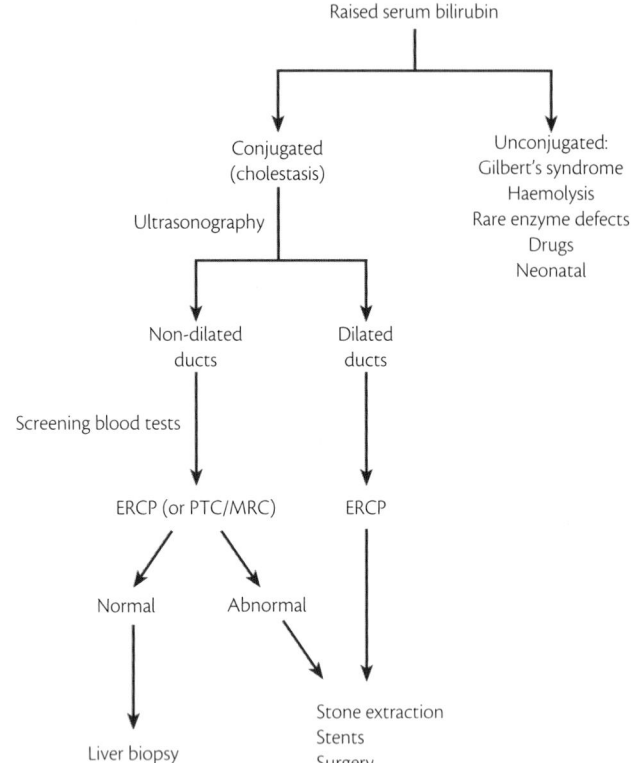

Fig. 15.20.2 Investigation of jaundice.

from a patient with cholestasis may show bile plugs under light microscopy. These findings, however, are often termed 'obstructive jaundice'—an unfortunate term, since it implies extrahepatic obstruction of the biliary tree. Prolonged cholestasis, as from bile duct obstruction, down regulates the MRP2 exporter transporter that is also found in enterocytes, so that the oral bioavailability of many drugs is increased. The molecular events underlying some forms of intrahepatic cholestasis are now being unravelled (see below).

History

Dark urine and, less commonly, pale stools indicate cholestasis. Many drugs, including alcohol, can cause unconjugated and conjugated hyperbilirubinaemia and should be rigorously sought. Fever (hepatitis, cholangitis, abscesses), travel (hepatitis, amoebiasis), sexual history (hepatitis A, B, or C), surgery and anaesthesia (postoperative jaundice, see below; biliary tract disease), herbal medicines (e.g. West Indian teas, Chinese herbs), and transfusions or blood products (hepatitis B or C) can be important clues.

Clinical examination

Stigmata of chronic liver disease (e.g. spider naevi, facial telangiectases, parotid enlargement, Dupuytren's contractures, muscle wasting, hepatosplenomegaly, dilated abdominal wall veins and ascites) are important, but do not define the cause of jaundice.

Testing for unconjugated hyperbilirubinaemia

If serum bilirubin levels are raised but other liver-related blood tests are normal, unconjugated hyperbilirubinaemia should be excluded by testing whether the bilirubin in blood is predominantly conjugated or unconjugated. An abnormal reticulocyte count will suggest haemolysis severe enough to raise bilirubin levels and blood film examination may be informative. Suspected haemolysis is investigated as described elsewhere in chapter.

If no cause of unconjugated hyperbilirubinaemia is identified, then benign constitutional unconjugated hyperbilirubinaemia (Gilbert's syndrome) is diagnosed (see below).

Conjugated hyperbilirubinaemia

The familial syndromes without cholestasis (Dubin–Johnson and Rotor) are rare (see below).

Routine liver-related blood tests cannot differentiate between intra- or extrahepatic causes of jaundice, unless the transferases are very high (e.g. >1000 IU/litre), in which case hepatitis (e.g. viral, alcoholic) is certain. A greatly raised alkaline phosphatase level does not necessarily imply an extrahepatic lesion; intrahepatic causes are common (Table 15.20.1). Research methods for assessing liver function (e.g. galactose tolerance test, aminopyrine breath test) are of no value in the management of the patient with jaundice.

Cholestasis should be investigated first with abdominal ultrasonography, which will accurately detect a dilated intra- and/or extrahepatic biliary tree and often also reveal its cause (e.g. gallstones, tumour). Oral cholecystography, or the now little used intravenous cholangiography, will fail in the presence of jaundice. If biliary disease is thus suspected, an endoscopic retrograde

Table 15.20.1 Intrahepatic cholestasis

Infection	Viral hepatitis A, B, C, or E
	Bacterial: sepsis, miliary tuberculosis, leptospirosis
	Neonatal hepatitis syndrome
Toxins	Alcohol
	Drugs: hepatotoxic, idiosyncratic
	Oestrogens: pregnancy, contraceptive pill
	α_1-Antitrypsin deficiency
	Parenteral nutrition
Infiltration	Carcinoma: metastases
	Lymphoma
	Adenocarcinoma of kidney (non-metastatic)
	Sarcoidosis
Familial	Benign recurrent
	Neonatal cholestatic syndromes
Reduced blood flow	Perioperative hypoperfusion/shock
	Sickle-cell anaemia
Intrahepatic ducts	Biliary atresia
	Malignant infiltration of ducts
Autoimmune	Chronic active hepatitis
	Primary biliary cirrhosis
	Sclerosing cholangitis
	Rejection of liver graft

cholangiogram (ERCP) or, failing that, a fine-needle percutaneous transhepatic cholangiogram (PTC), will define the anatomy more accurately and often provide definitive therapy (removal of biliary stones, stenting), thus avoiding surgery. Magnetic resonance cholangiography (MRC) is increasing in sensitivity and availability and can now produce high-quality noninvasive images of the biliary tree and pancreas; it is useful even for intrahepatic biliary disease. It cannot, of course, be therapeutic. Endoscopic ultrasonography (EUS) can show accurately the presence of stones, biliary or pancreatic tumours and sclerosing cholangitis, while gamma-camera scans with technetium-labelled hydroxyiminodiacetic acid (HIDA) can be used to indicate biliary obstruction, particularly in the neonate, if ultrasonography is normal.

If intrahepatic cholestasis is suspected because of a normal sized biliary tree on ultrasonography, the following tests should be considered: hepatitis A, B, and C serology, autoantibodies (antimitochondrial for primary biliary cirrhosis, antinuclear, smooth muscle and liver–kidney microsomal for autoimmune chronic hepatitis) and immunoglobulins, serum caeruloplasmin and copper for Wilson's disease if less than 40 years of age, or plasma α_1-antitrypsin concentrations for homozygous deficiency of this enzyme. Intrahepatic masses seen by ultrasonography will prompt measurement of α-fetoprotein for primary hepatoma, and other tumour markers. A percutaneous needle liver biopsy (or aspiration of an abscess) may then be indicated, provided that blood coagulation and the platelet count are normal. Guidelines for liver biopsy have been published. A transjugular venous approach for the biopsy is appropriate if the risks of bleeding are increased.

Unconjugated hyperbilirubinaemia

Plasma bilirubin levels are exponentially and positively related to the half-life of circulating red blood cells, which determines bilirubin load, and negatively to the hepatic clearance rate of bilirubin. This relationship is analogous to that of muscle breakdown, plasma creatinine, and glomerular filtration rate. Hence, if the rate of haemolysis rises or clearance falls, bilirubin levels may rise rapidly in response to small changes of the load or removal rate from plasma, or both.

Haemolytic jaundice is most commonly encountered in the haemoglobinopathies of sickle-cell anaemia (homozygous SS or heterozygous SC disease) or homozygous thalassaemia major, although dark skin may render it difficult to detect. The 'acholuric jaundice' of hereditary spherocytosis is rare. Mildly elevated bilirubin levels are described in ineffective erythropoiesis of the bone marrow in vitamin B_{12} deficiency (pernicious anaemia), or in thalassaemia minor.

Drugs may cause haemolysis (e.g. methyldopa, sulphasalazine), or impair hepatic bilirubin clearance (e.g. rifampicin). Infections (e.g. malaria) or mismatched blood transfusions can produce massive haemolysis, but this overshadows the raised bilirubin levels. Autoimmune haemolytic anaemia, such as in lupus erythematosus, or haemolysis due to glucose-6-phosphate dehydrogenase deficiency, or to leaking prosthetic cardiac valves, can cause clinical jaundice.

Familial unconjugated hyperbilirubinaemia

A series of defects of the hepatic bilirubin conjugating enzyme UDP-glucuronyl transferase produce various degrees of unconjugated hyperbilirubinaemia due to impaired bilirubin clearance; they have long fascinated physiologists and more recently molecular biologists.

At least 3% of the normal adult population have mildly raised unconjugated bilirubin levels in blood that rise excessively on fasting. This 'phenomenon' is commonly termed 'Gilbert's syndrome' (OMIM 143500), although it is unclear whether the eponym is justified. The raised concentrations of bilirubin develop in early adult life and are often associated with mild degrees of haemolysis. Any combination of an increased bilirubin load from the haemolysis and a mildly impaired clearance will increase plasma bilirubin concentrations more than would either alone, and hence together they bring the underlying condition to notice. Various associated defects of hepatic drug metabolism have also been described and these are probably linked genetic abnormalities. The syndrome is not a discrete entity, but rather different defects of conjugation and haemolysis that elevate bilirubin levels above an arbitrary upper limit of normal. Determination of the bilirubin-conjugating capacity of liver biopsy tissue has shown that the activity of glucuronyl transferase is reduced by 60 to 70%, and this impairs bilirubin clearance.

Gilbert's syndrome is recognized by a fluctuating, raised serum bilirubin concentration with the other routine liver-related blood tests remaining normal, and a normal reticulocyte count to exclude overt haemolysis. It can be confirmed by measuring the unconjugated fraction of the bilirubin, which should be greater than 90%. Measuring the pronounced increase of plasma bilirubin that occurs after a 48-h fast on 400 kcal/day or provocation with intravenous nicotinic acid are research procedures. A liver biopsy is not needed. Reassurance that the results do not indicate liver disease and will not affect life insurance is important. Plasma bilirubin concentrations rise in patients with Gilbert's syndrome during intercurrent illness and jaundice may then be observed.

It is said that Gilbert's syndrome can follow an attack of viral hepatitis, although this may be due to ascertainment bias.

The genetic basis of Gilbert's syndrome remains controversial but it appears that it is a recessive condition in which there are homozygous polymorphisms in the promoter region affecting expression of the specific glucuronyl transferase gene. Heterozygotes have normal bilirubin levels. There must be another factor responsible for the increased bilirubin concentrations as the heterozygote abnormality occurs in 40% of normal individuals. The variable bilirubin load from red cell breakdown is one factor that will influence the underlying prevalence of the anomaly in the population.

Crigler–Najjar syndromes

Two syndromes of more severe unconjugated hyperbilirubinaemia have been described, namely the rare type I Crigler–Najjar (OMIM 218800; 100 cases reported), which without treatment causes neonatal death, and the more common, and benign type II (OMIM 606785). Both are due to severe deficiency in the UDP-glucuronyl transferase enzymes.

In type I, first reported in 1952, with a recessive inheritance, neonates rapidly become progressively jaundiced in the first days of life (bilirubin levels reach 350–950 µmol/litre) and, if untreated, develop kernicterus or brain damage. Death usually occurs within a year but delayed kernicterus has been reported.

There is no conjugated bilirubin in bile, but small quantities of unconjugated bilirubin can be found in bile and also cross the intestinal wall.

The inheritance of type II is complex, and is reported both to be dominant with incomplete penetrance or recessive. Bilirubin levels are lower (<350 µmol/litre), and persistent mild jaundice is only noticed in childhood. Brain damage does not occur, and the only problem is cosmetic. One-third of the conjugated bilirubin in bile is present as the monogluronide (normally <10%). In the Gunn strain of laboratory rat severe unconjugated hyperbilirubinaemia occurs and glucuronyl transferase activity is absent in the liver, as it is in Crigler–Najjar type I. In type II, enzyme activity is less than 10% of normal, but measurable.

It has long been known that there is a spectrum of bilirubin levels in type II Crigler–Najjar and Gilbert's syndromes and indeed both conditions have been observed within the same families, suggesting different degrees of enzyme activity. Phenobarbitone or other hepatic microsomal enzyme-inducing agents markedly reduce bilirubin levels in Gilbert's and Crigler–Najjar type II syndromes, although unfortunately not in Crigler–Najjar type I, and increase the activity of glucuronyl transferase. Such treatment, however, is not needed.

Molecular analysis of the genes encoding human UDP-glucuronyl transferases has both clarified and complicated our understanding of the genetic basis of these disorders. The complementary DNAs for the two human isoforms of the enzyme have been sequenced; they differ from those that encode the other glucuronyl transferases, which conjugate e.g. steroids. The UDP-glucuronyl transferases map to human chromosome 2, where at least five exons encode the specific mRNAs of the isoenzymes. Analysis of DNA from patients with type I Crigler–Najjar syndrome has identified homozygous or heterozygous defects in the exons encoding particularly the most active of the two bilirubin transferase isoforms. Similar defects occur in the Gunn rat.

In Crigler–Najjar type II syndrome, mutations have been described in the gene encoding the more active bilirubin glucuronyl transferase isoform. Phenobarbitone induces the expression of the abnormal enzyme, explaining its efficacy in this condition. Probably a heterozygous combination of an abnormality of the promoter region (Gilbert's defect) and a Crigler–Najjar I defect is responsible for the phenotype of type II Crigler–Najjar syndrome. This explains the presence of patients with Gilbert's syndrome within families with type II Crigler–Najjar.

It seems likely that a series of rare abnormalities in the gene for bilirubin glucuronyl transferases will be found in each of the three arbitrary phenotypes, which are clinically defined by the degree of impairment of conjugation and hence plasma bilirubin levels.

Crigler–Najjar type I syndrome can now be successfully treated by whole-body blue-light phototherapy for 16 h daily or by plasmapheresis until liver transplantation can be carried out as a definitive treatment. Severe kernicterus is a contraindication to transplantation as it is not reversible. Some patients have received successful transplants. Hepatocyte transplantation, in which donor hepatocytes are infused into the portal vein, has been partially successful. Drugs that displace unconjugated bilirubin from albumin (sulphonamides, salicylates, penicillin) increase brain damage in type I Crigler–Najjar syndrome and must be avoided.

Neonatal jaundice

Unconjugated hyperbilirubinaemia, often with mild clinical jaundice, occurs in all full-term newborn infants, and is harmless and probably beneficial. Bilirubin concentrations are maximal at 2 to 5 days after birth, but the plasma bilirubin rarely exceeds 90 µmol/litre; neonatal jaundice is more severe in premature infants. It is attributed to a combination of immaturity of hepatic glucuronyl transferase and the added load of bilirubin from rapid haemolysis of surplus fetal red blood cells in the neonatal period. Before birth, fetal bilirubin is excreted by the mother, and meconium and stools are pale because of the limited excretion of bilirubin by the fetus.

If haemolysis is increased, as in rhesus or other fetomaternal incompatibility of red cell antigens when transplacental maternal antibodies cause intravascular haemolysis of fetal red blood cells, severe jaundice and kernicterus can occur. Acidosis and some drugs (sulphonamides, salicylates, penicillin) may increase kernicterus by displacing unconjugated bilirubin from albumin. Glucose 6-phosphate deficiency can also cause jaundice and anaemia in the neonatal period, usually in infants of Mediterranean, African, or Chinese ancestry.

Treatment with phenobarbitone induces hepatic glucuronyl transferase and lowers bilirubin levels, but its effect is slow unless it is given to the mother before birth. Exchange transfusion or plasmapheresis are more effective. Phototherapy, namely exposure of the near-naked infant to blue light in an incubator, is also effective. Being yellow, bilirubin absorbs light at approximately 450 nm, which oxidizes it to water-soluble, nontoxic products. Hence, exposure of the bilirubin in skin capillaries to light reduces its plasma concentration and the breakdown products are excreted safely in urine and bile. Reabsorption of bilirubin from the intestine can also be reduced by giving agar by mouth, thus interrupting its enterohepatic circulation. Nevertheless, it seems that moderate hyperbilirubinaemia does not adversely affect development.

Breastfeeding slightly increases serum bilirubin levels and about 1 in 40 breast-fed infants develop jaundice, which remits on transfer to cow's milk within 24 h; this jaundice does not always recur when breast milk is reintroduced. Breastfeeding increases the enterohepatic cycling of bilirubin from the intestine, since stool weights and frequency are less than when taking formula feeds, and hence intestinal motility is decreased. Steroid molecules in breast milk may also inhibit glucuronyl transferase activity in the neonatal liver.

Hypothyroidism increases jaundice and should be sought in neonates with unexplained hyperbilirubinaemia since it may not be associated with obvious cretinism. The rare Crigler–Najjar type I syndrome (see above) presents with florid jaundice in the first few days of life.

Sickle-cell anaemia and β-thalassaemia

Jaundice is common in homozygous sickle-cell anaemia due to the unconjugated hyperbilirubinaemia from persistent haemolysis. During crises jaundice often deepens in association with increasing anaemia, suggesting accelerated haemolysis, although transient bone marrow failure may also occur. Occasionally, conjugated hyperbilirubinaemia with dark urine occurs during these episodes, and hepatic histology may show areas of necrosis due to thrombosis and bile thrombi. Patients with sickle-cell anaemia are also prone to pigment gallstones, due to the excessive bilirubin constantly being excreted, and these can cause extrahepatic biliary obstruction; conjugated hyperbilirubinaemia and dark urine may then be clues. Unconjugated hyperbilirubinaemia occurs in homozygous thalassaemia as a result of increased red cell destruction and the intramedullary haemolysis associated with ineffective erythropoiesis; there may also be unexplained episodes of intrahepatic cholestasis.

Cholestasis

There are many causes of intrahepatic cholestasis (Table 15.20.1).

Neonatal cholestasis

Conjugated hyperbilirubinaemia and cholestasis in the neonate, with dark urine and pale stools, is always pathological and if it continues beyond 2 weeks of age requires urgent investigation. There are many causes.

In many instances the cause is never established and then, although it was once called neonatal hepatitis, it is better termed the hepatitis syndrome; hepatic histology shows hepatitis, sometimes with giant cells. Some babies recover, while perhaps half progress to hypoplasia of the intrahepatic bile ducts, which then overlaps with intrahepatic biliary atresia.

Infections, particularly urinary, can cause transient cholestasis. Syphilis is now rare, as is toxoplasmosis. Various viral infections (rubella, cytomegalovirus) can cause neonatal jaundice. The hepatotropic hepatitis B virus contracted from an HBe antigen-positive mother rarely causes jaundice. Metabolic diseases that may cause neonatal jaundice include galactosaemia, hereditary fructose intolerance (fructosaemia), and tyrosinosis—all of which need to be diagnosed quickly so as to start dietary treatment early—as well as homozygous α_1-antitrypsin deficiency, and intravenous feeding per se. Other genetic diseases include trisomy 13 and trisomy 18 (one-quarter of babies developing the hepatitis syndrome) and cystic fibrosis.

Several familial syndromes presenting with neonatal cholestasis have been described, some with other congenital abnormalities, such as arteriohepatic dysplasia (Alagille's syndrome), and others solely with cholestasis featuring persistent jaundice, raised serum bile acids, hepatosplenomegaly, steatorrhoea and failure to thrive, such as Byler's syndrome in Amish families, which is genetically related to benign recurrent cholestasis. Bile duct hypoplasia, cirrhosis, and liver failure often follow unless liver transplantation is carried out. There are several different mutations of the genes described in the various syndromes of progressive familial intrahepatic cholestasis (PFIC), namely those encoding the canalicular transport proteins for bile acids (BSEP), phospholipid (MDR3), or bilirubin and other anions (MRP2), or for bile acid synthesis. Canalicular excretion of bile acids and conjugated bilirubin are severely impaired, and cholestasis develops early in life. Some are more common in infants born to mothers with obstetric cholestasis. Surprisingly, external biliary drainage may be beneficial.

Extrahepatic cholestasis in the neonate is most commonly due to biliary atresia, but a choledochal cyst or bile duct perforation can also cause jaundice at this age. Biliary atresia appears to represent a form of sclerosing cholangitis with progressive loss of intra- and extrahepatic ducts. HIDA scans, percutaneous liver biopsy, and retrograde cholangiography can establish the diagnosis without laparotomy.

Benign recurrent intrahepatic cholestasis (BRIC)

In this rare syndrome, recurrent reversible episodes of cholestasis start in childhood or adult life. Each attack is characterized by jaundice, anorexia, and itching for several months, which then subsides with no residual effects. Hepatic histology only shows cholestasis. Phenobarbitone or ursodeoxycholic acid may shorten and attenuate attacks. So far two mutations have been identified in patients with BRIC, one of which is similar to that in Byler's disease.

Postoperative jaundice

Jaundice due to halothane hepatitis, post-transfusion viral hepatitis, incompatible blood transfusion, drugs, and bile duct damage is described elsewhere.

Prolonged intrahepatic cholestasis used to be common after cardiac surgery. It is related to the length of surgery and intraoperative cardiac function, and may be due to reduced hepatic blood flow during surgery. Improvements in intra- and postoperative care seem to have improved hepatic function and rendered the syndrome uncommon. Transfused red blood cells are prone to rapid haemolysis and this increases the bilirubin load, while impaired renal function reduces the urinary excretion of conjugated bilirubin. Drug-induced liver injury should be considered.

Prolonged parenteral nutrition is sometimes associated with cholestasis, fatty liver, and eventually fibrosis, especially in the neonate. The mechanism is unclear.

Cholestasis after liver transplantation has multiple causes, including rejection.

Drug cholestasis

This is described in Chapter 15.22.8, but it is increasingly likely that the sensitivity of many examples of idiosyncratic drug-induced cholestasis is due to genetic abnormalities of the bile acid, phospholipid, or bilirubin excretion systems.

Cholestasis of pregnancy (obstetric cholestasis)

Slight impairment of the hepatic excretion of bilirubin can be demonstrated during normal pregnancy or after the administration of oestrogens, but in less than 1% of pregnancies bilirubin and alkaline phosphatase levels rise during the third trimester and intolerable itching and frank jaundice develop, all of which rapidly remit after delivery (see Chapter 14.9). The severity of obstetric cholestasis increases in successive pregnancies. There is an increased incidence of premature births, fetal distress, and intrauterine death, and so premature induction of labour may be needed. The incidence is higher in South America than Europe, and it is commoner in mothers of babies with familial intrahepatic cholestasis. This is not surprising because the syndrome is caused by mutational dysfunction of the biliary canalicular transporter proteins MRP3 and BSEP, which is exacerbated by the high levels of oestrogens and progesterone in pregnancy. Thus the contraceptive pill frequently causes a milder syndrome in the same susceptible women. Ursodeoxycholic acid is reported to ameliorate the condition and is safe, at least during late pregnancy. Phenobarbitone may help the

itching, although there is a small risk of impairing neonatal respiration. Cholestyramine has also been used.

Other causes of jaundice in late pregnancy should be remembered, including acute fatty liver, extrahepatic biliary obstruction, such as from gallstones, and toxaemia.

Pregnancy, by affecting bilirubin excretion, may bring to notice the jaundice of primary biliary cirrhosis or the Dubin–Johnson/Rotor syndromes.

Sepsis

Abnormal liver-related blood tests, and occasionally cholestatic jaundice, often develop during bacterial/viral infections, unrelated to the administration of drugs. In animals this has been shown to be due to endotoxins and cytokines that rapidly down-regulate and translocate the canalicular transport protein MRP2, which excretes conjugated bilirubin into the canaliculus. At the same time other pump proteins are up-regulated, a complex rearrangement that may protect the hepatocyte against oxidative damage. Jaundice is especially common in patients with glucose-6-phosphatase deficiency when they develop sepsis, such as pneumonia, since the haemolysis exacerbates the jaundice. This combination of high conjugated bilirubin levels and sepsis is particularly damaging to the kidney.

Dubin–Johnson and Rotor syndromes

These are two rare, familial forms of nonhaemolytic, conjugated hyperbilirubinaemia without cholestasis.

The Dubin–Johnson syndrome (OMIM 237500), first described in 1954, is a chronic, relapsing jaundice, without itching or raised serum bile acids. Other liver-related blood tests are normal, but there are associated defects in the excretion of other anions, such as bromsulphthalein, radiographic dyes, and urobilinogen. Hence cholecystography fails, there is excess urobilinogen in the urine, and a delayed rise of the plasma levels of bromsulphthalein after an injection of the dye due to reflux of the conjugated anion from hepatocytes. Jaundice increases during pregnancy or when taking the contraceptive pill because oestrogens further impair bilirubin excretion. A black pigment accumulates in the liver so that at laparoscopy the liver appears strikingly black, as do needle biopsy specimens. Urinary coproporphyrin excretion is abnormal. Some at least seem to be due to abnormality of the MRP2 canalicular bilirubin transporter. The inheritance seems to differ between families, and a similar condition occurs in a mutant strain of Corriedale sheep, although then photosensitivity also occurs, and in a laboratory rat model. Other families have been described in which there are similar findings but no hepatic pigment, the so-called Rotor syndrome (OMIM 237450). No treatment of either syndrome is required apart from reassurance, and support when seeking life insurance.

Further reading

Chowdury JR, Chowdury NR (1993). Unveiling the mysteries of inherited disorders of bilirubin glucuronidation. *Gastroenterology*, **105**, 288–93.

Elferink RPJO, van Berge Henegouwen GP (1998). Cracking the genetic code for benign recurrent and progressive familial intrahepatic cholestasis. *J Hepatol*, **29**, 317–20.

Elferink RO (2003). Cholestasis. *Gut*, **52** Suppl 2, ii42–48.

Grant A, Neuberger J (1999). Guidelines on the use of liver biopsy in clinical practice. *Gut*, **45** Suppl IV, 1–11.

Jansen PLM (1996). Genetic diseases of bilirubin metabolism: the inherited unconjugated hyperbilirubinemias. *J Hepatol*, **25**, 398–404.

Jansen PLM, Müller M (1998). Early events in sepsis-associated cholestasis. *Gastroenterology*, **116**, 486–8.

Jansen PLM, Muller M (2000). The molecular genetics of familial intrahepatic cholestasis. *Gut*, **47**, 1–5.

Jansen PLM, Sturm E (2003). Genetic cholestasis, causes and consequences for hepatobiliay transport. *Liver Int*, **23**, 315–22.

Milkiewicz P, *et al.* (2002). Obstetric cholestasis. *BMJ*, **324**, 123–4.

Pauli-Magnus C, Meier PJ (2006). Hepatobillary transporters and drug-induced cholestasis. *Hepatology*, **44**, 778–87.

Sherlock S, Dooley J (2002). *Diseases of the Liver and Biliary System*. (11th edition). Blackwell.

Soloway RD (1996). The increasingly complex molecular life cycle of bilirubin. *Gastroenterology*, **110**, 2013–14.

Strassburg CP, Manns MP (2000). Jaundice, genes and promoters. *J Hepatol*, **33**, 476–9.

Watchko JF (2006). Neonatal hyperbilirubinemia–what are the risks? *New Engl J Med*, **354**, 1947–9.

15.21

Hepatitis and autoimmune liver disease

Contents

15.21.1 Viral hepatitis—clinical aspects

H.J.F. Hodgson

Essentials

There are five major hepatitis viruses—A, B, C, D, and E—with the clinical picture depending on the severity of the inflammation induced in the liver, and on whether the virus is cleared from the liver or persists long-term.

Acute icteric hepatitis, characterized by jaundice and right upper quadrant abdominal tenderness, is the commonest clinically recognized consequence of infection. This is generally a self-limited condition with low mortality and complete recovery: only hepatitis B and C have the propensity to cause chronic viral hepatitis. Typically, hepatocellular enzyme levels in blood are prominently raised at the time of the onset of symptoms, whilst the serum alkaline phosphatase level is only slightly increased. Specific diagnosis is made by serological testing for particular viruses. Uncomplicated

cases recover spontaneously; there is no proven therapy to enhance recovery, but alcohol and potentially hepatotoxic drugs should be withdrawn. Fulminant hepatic failure caused by viral hepatitis has 80% mortality and should be treated (if possible) by orthotopic liver transplantation.

Protection against hepatitis A and B is available, both passive (gammaglobulin preparations) and active (vaccinations). Vaccines are not yet available for hepatitis C or E, but vaccination against hepatitis B also protects against hepatitis D.

Features of particular hepatitis viruses

Hepatitis A virus (HAV)—faecal–oral transmission; incubation 2–6 weeks; acute self-limited hepatitis; no specific treatment.

Hepatitis B virus (HBV)—parenteral transmission; incubation 4–24 weeks; may present with acute hepatitis, with prodrome sometimes including prominent arthritis, fever, and urticarial rash, but anicteric attacks are common; most (>90%) patients clear HBV after acute infection, but failure to clear HBsAg (hepatitis B surface antigen) within 6 months defines 'chronic carriage', which is associated with a spectrum of histological damage and clinical manifestations ranging from being clinically silent to producing cirrhosis and hepatocellular cancer. Some patients with chronic infection will benefit from treatment with α-interferons and/or inhibitors of viral replication (nucleotide and nucleoside analogues).

Hepatitis C virus (HCV)—parenteral transmission; incubation 2 to 26 weeks; acute episode most often subclinical; 70% of patients fail to clear the virus and become chronic carriers, which often leads to cirrhosis after 15 to 25 years and then predisposes to hepatocellular cancer; treatment is with the combination of IFN-α2a or IFN-α2b plus ribavirin, and the use of pegylated interferon preparations.

Hepatitis D virus (HDV)—an RNA virus 'parasitic' on HBV, with dual infection tending to produce more severe liver disease; treatment is as for hepatitis B.

Hepatitis E virus (HEV)—faecal–oral transmission; incubation about 6 weeks; high risk of fulminant hepatitis if acquired during midtrimester pregnancy; no specific treatment.

Table 15.21.1.1 Viruses affecting the liver

Major hepatotrophic viruses	A, B, C, D, E
Minor hepatotrophic viruses	G, transfusion-transmitted virus (TTV)
Systemic viruses capable of causing hepatitis[a]	Herpesviruses, Epstein–Barr virus, cytomegalovirus, varicella virus, adenovirus
Tropical viruses	Yellow fever, dengue, haemorrhagic viruses

[a] More frequently in immunosuppressed patients.

Introduction

Viral hepatitis is a major clinical problem worldwide, particularly in developing countries, though no society is exempt. There are five major hepatitis viruses—A, B, C, D, and E. These have tropism for the liver, and the liver bears the brunt of the disease. Other viruses can infect the liver (Table 15.21.1.1), but with many of these (e.g. Epstein–Barr virus, cytomegalovirus), hepatic involvement is merely one facet of a systemic infection, and the liver involvement is usually trivial, although occasionally it may dominate. Other hepatitis viruses are being described and their clinical relevance is under investigation. This chapter will describe the clinical and pathological consequences of viral hepatitis in general, identify virus-specific clinical patterns, and discuss the investigation, management, and prophylaxis of viral hepatitis.

Clinical outcome of hepatitis virus infection

The clinical picture in viral hepatitis depends on the severity of the inflammation induced in the liver, and on whether the virus is cleared from the liver or persists long-term. These in turn reflect characteristics both of the virus and of the host immune response, so the clinical patterns are very varied. They range from a short-lived episode that may not even be clinically apparent, to chronic infection leading to cirrhosis and predisposing to hepatocellular carcinoma.

Acute icteric hepatitis is the commonest clinically recognized consequence of infection with a hepatitis virus. It is generally a self-limited condition with a low mortality and complete recovery. Typically, after an initial prodrome lasting from several days to a couple of weeks, comprising malaise, anorexia, mild fever, and upper abdominal discomfort, the patient becomes jaundiced (icteric). The icteric period lasts for a few days to a few weeks, after which jaundice slowly subsides. Pruritus may occur, generally after the onset of jaundice. Development of ascites or oedema is uncommon but may occur in more severe cases. Return to normality after an attack of hepatitis may take several weeks to a few months and residual fatigue is common.

There are a number of variations on the clinical course of acute hepatitis:

- In anicteric hepatitis jaundice does not occur, and the episode is asymptomatic or dismissed as 'flu-like'. This may in fact be a more frequent pattern than a clinically recognized episode, as evidenced by serological surveys for immunity to hepatitis viruses in populations.

- In cholestatic hepatitis, jaundice with pruritus, pale stools, and dark urine persists for up to 2 or 3 months before recovery.

- In relapsing hepatitis there is a transient worsening of jaundice after an initial improvement before recovery eventually occurs.

- Acute hepatitis is only rarely fatal. If it is, patients usually rapidly develop hepatic encephalopathy, and the timing of onset of this has been used to define subtypes of acute severe hepatitis.

- In 'fulminant hepatitis' encephalopathy develops within 2 weeks of jaundice.

- In 'subfulminant hepatitis' encephalopathy develops later.

Hepatitis A, B, C, and E can all initiate an acute self-limited hepatitis, although hepatitis C is particularly unlikely to give rise to the fulminant form. Only hepatitis B and C have the propensity to cause chronic viral hepatitis: this is generally an indolent disease, in which viral carriage in the liver persists over years or decades, with inflammation that varies in intensity. Hepatitis D, which coinfects patients infected with hepatitis B, can contribute to either acute or chronic inflammation.

Features of acute hepatitis caused by different viruses

Hepatitis A virus (HAV)

This causes acute self-limited hepatitis, but not chronic viral carriage or chronic liver disease. The RNA virus is acquired orally. The incubation period is between 2 and 6 weeks. Transmission generally follows the ingestion of food or water contaminated with faeces from an HAV-infected individual. Viral shedding in the faeces ceases at approximately the onset of clinical symptoms. Transmission may occur in epidemics, following floods, or after sewage contamination of shellfish beds. The disease is also endemic in all parts of the world. In developing countries, infection is frequent; there is serological evidence of past infection in up to 100% of 10-year-olds in some countries. In Western countries, evidence of prior infection varies, typically ranging from 5 to 40% dependent on age, social class, and other factors. Promiscuous homosexual males have a high incidence of infection. Very rarely, pooled blood products have transmitted the disease parenterally. Clinically the disease is often anicteric or mild, particularly in young children. About 10% of patients have a relapse before recovery. The mortality rate is low, about 0.3%. Deaths occur predominantly in older people, among whom mortality rates may exceed 2%, and pre-existing chronic viral hepatitis B or C may predispose to a fatal outcome. A rare sequel is aplastic anaemia some months after recovery from hepatitis.

Hepatitis B virus (HBV)

Hepatitis B viral infection was recognized by its parenteral transmission route, classically as serum- and then transfusion-associated hepatitis. The incubation period of this DNA virus varies from 4 to 24 weeks. In between 90 and 95% of adult cases the infection is self-limited and the HBV is cleared. In infants, clearance rates are as low as 5 to 10%. The incidence of acute hepatitis B varies widely, and is very high in east Asia and Africa. Transmission may be vertical—i.e. infection of a newborn or infant child usually by a chronically infected mother, either at the time of birth or during close family contact. Horizontal transmission routes include blood transfusion and blood products, the use of contaminated needles medically or by drug addicts, exposure in dialysis units, tattooing, and sexual contact. Promiscuous homosexuals and heterosexuals are at risk.

Anicteric attacks of acute HBV are common. If the acute infection is recognized clinically, in addition to the typical clinical

SECTION 15 GASTROENTEROLOGICAL DISORDERS

features of any acute hepatitis, the preicteric prodrome may include prominent arthritis, fever, and an urticarial rash, due to immune complex deposition. Hepatitis B is fulminant in about 0.3% of cases, and both the strain of HBV and a very active host immune response may contribute. In the great majority of cases, in which HBV is cleared after acute infection, hepatitis B surface antigen (HBsAg) disappears from the blood within weeks to a few months. Failure to clear within 6 months defines 'chronic carriage'.

Hepatitis C virus (HCV)

This was recognized as a cause of transfusion-associated hepatitis. The incubation period ranges from 2 to 26 weeks, usually between 5 and 12 weeks. Apart from blood transfusion and blood product administration, drug addiction and renal dialysis are strong epidemiological associations. Sexual transmission and horizontal transmission are uncommon, but not unknown. Fulminant hepatitis due to HCV is rare. Indeed, the initial acute episode is most often subclinical, but after acquiring the infection about 70% of individuals fail to clear the virus. HCV infection is therefore usually not recognized until the chronic phase.

Hepatitis D virus (HDV)

The unique position of hepatitis D virus, an RNA virus 'parasitic' on HBV, is discussed in Chapter 7.5.21. If HBV and HDV coinfect simultaneously, either unremarkable acute hepatitis, or on occasion fulminant disease, result. If HBV is cleared, HDV must be so also. Acute HDV infection can superinfect a chronic HBV carrier, and result in worsening of liver function, particularly if the HBV has previously caused significant liver disease. In such a carrier, the superinfection with HDV may be transient, or chronic hepatitis D carriage may persist. Both coinfection and superinfection are recognized initiators of fulminant hepatitis. In Westernized countries, intravenous drug abuse is a prominent epidemiological association, but all parenteral modes demonstrated by HBV occur, including sexual transmission. The southern Mediterranean, eastern Asia, and South America are areas of high or moderate incidence.

Hepatitis E virus (HEV)

Like HAV, this enterally acquired RNA virus causes acute hepatitis without chronic carriage. Most major epidemics of acute hepatitis in the Indian subcontinent and east Asia are due to HEV. Such epidemics affect adults as well as children, indicating that immunity in those areas is not regularly acquired in childhood. Flooding and sewage contamination often precede epidemics. The incubation period is about 6 weeks, and faecal excretion of the virus may persist for nearly 2 months after the onset of hepatitis. A striking feature of HEV infection, and the main clinical difference from HAV, is the propensity to induce fulminant hepatitis if acquired during mid-trimester pregnancy, and mortality rates of 10 to 40% are recorded amongst pregnant women. In Western countires, HEV cases may be imported, or be a zoonosis from infected pigs.

Other hepatotrophic viruses

Other hepatotrophic viruses remain to be described, in particular to explain non-A/B/C/D/E fulminant and transfusion hepatitis. Although the hepatitis G virus and transfusion-transmitted virus (TTV) have been well characterized, they do not appear to give rise to significant disease.

Clinical examination

Jaundice and right upper quadrant abdominal tenderness characterize acute hepatitis. Skin manifestations include spider naevi (which often disappear after recovery), scratch marks in the pruritic phase, and rarely a vasculitic or urticarial rash. Mild hepatomegaly is common, but a rapid shrinkage in hepatic size may occur in severe or fulminant hepatitis. Splenomegaly is uncommon, and suggests alternative viral causes such as Epstein–Barr virus or cytomegalovirus, or pre-existing liver disease. Marked nausea and persistent vomiting indicate a severe hepatitis and increase the chance of developing hypoglycaemia. Stools become pale and urine darkens as jaundice is established. Ascites and peripheral oedema may occur in prolonged or severe episodes. The most significant clinical indicator of deterioration is the development of hepatic encephalopathy, indicating the onset of hepatic failure. In fulminant viral hepatitis deterioration can be very rapid, and indeed rarely encephalopathy may occur before obvious jaundice has had time to develop.

Laboratory investigations

Virological investigations depend on serological testing as outlined in Table 15.21.1.2. The initial 'screen' for the cause of suspected acute viral hepatitis is for anti-HAV IgM antibodies, for HBsAg, and for anti-HCV antibodies. Figures 15.21.1.1 to 15.21.1.3 indicate the typical serological evolution of self-limited episodes of A, B, and C viral hepatitis.

Typically, hepatocellular enzyme levels in blood (AST, aspartate aminotransferase; ALT, alanine aminotransferase) are prominently raised at the time of the onset of symptoms, often more than 10-fold above normal, whilst the serum alkaline phosphatase level is only slightly increased, less than 2.5-fold As an episode evolves, transaminase levels fall and alkaline phosphatase may rise, notably if there is prolonged intrahepatic cholestasis. Urinary analysis shows excess urobilinogen in early and late phases of an episode, with excess bilirubin at the height of jaundice. The severity of the attack is best reflected in the synthetic parameters of albumin and clotting factors: in particular, progressive prolongation of the prothrombin time mirrors the onset of liver failure. A low factor V ($<c.30\%$ of normal) level has been used as an indicator of irreversible failure.

Hepatic imaging techniques such as ultrasonography contribute to diagnosis primarily by excluding other causes. Patients with uncomplicated hepatitis do not require a liver biopsy, but hepatic histology is very helpful if there is diagnostic uncertainty or an unusual course in severity or duration (Fig. 15.21.1.4). In such cases, biopsy may require correction of clotting factors and use of the transjugular route or 'plugged' biopsy techniques.

Differential diagnosis

Drug-induced jaundice is the most common differential diagnosis, and its course may be very similar. Drug history and drug screening should particularly enquire about the use of acetaminophen and nonsteroidal anti-inflammatory drugs. Other potential drugs and toxins include halothane, antituberculous drugs, carbon tetrachloride, and mushroom poisoning. Alcoholic hepatitis often presents with less marked elevations of serum transaminases and a high circulating leucocyte count. About one-third of patients with

Table 15.21.1.2 Serological tests used in the assessment of acute hepatitis

Test	Interpretation	Timing in relation to jaundice
HAVAg	Not tested in routine practice	Disappears at time of onset
HAVAb-Ig^M	Acute or recent infection	From onset for approximately 4 months
HAVAb-Ig^G	Acute, recent, or past infection	Persists till old age
HBeAg	Viral protein in blood	Cleared by 6 months in >90% of cases; persistence beyond 6 months confirms chronicity
HBsAb	Viral clearance occurring	Few weeks after jaundice—persists lifelong
HBeAg	Infectious phase, high-titre HBV DNA	Cleared by 1 month in >90% of cases
HBeAb	Immune response to infectious virus indicates that the virus will be cleared	Appears as HbeAg cleared
HBcAb-Ig^M	Acute infection	Present at onset, persists for *c.* 4 months
HBcAb-Ig^G	Acute, recent, or past infection	Persists for 2–5 years if virus cleared
HBV-DNA	Infectious virus in blood	Cleared in 2 months in >90% of cases
HCV-RNA	Active viral replication	Present at onset
HCVAb	Acute, recent, or past infection	May not appear until a few weeks after onset
HDVAg	Presence of viral protein in blood	Present at onset
HDVAb-Ig^M	Acute or chronic infection	Present at onset, persists in chronic carriage
HEVAb-Ig^M	Acute or recent infection	From onset for 4–6 months
HEVAb-Ig^G	Acute, recent, or past infection	From onset for several years

Ab, antibody; Ag, antigen; HBs, hepatitis B surface; HBc, hepatitis B core.

autoimmune hepatitis present with a clinical picture of acute hepatitis. Autoantibody testing is generally helpful: the majority of patients with autoimmune disease having high levels of circulating autoantibodies. However, there are often low- or moderate-titre antinuclear and anti-smooth muscle antibodies in uncomplicated viral hepatitis. Similarly, there may be some increase of immunoglobulin levels in acute hepatitis, though not the doubling characteristic of autoimmune hepatitis. Although uncommon,

acute Wilson's disease is an important diagnosis to make, because of the high incidence of acute liver failure and the rapid necessity for transplantation. 'Surgical' obstructive jaundice tends not to raise transaminase levels markedly, but serum alkaline phosphatase levels are high. Obstruction is generally confirmed by imaging techniques, notably ultrasound. Individual causes may be suspected from features in the history such as nausea and biliary colic in cholelithiasis, and painless jaundice without systemic upset in an elderly patient with pancreatic cancer. Pregnancy-associated syndromes—acute fatty liver and HELLP (haemolysis, elevated liver function tests, low platelets)—are in fact less common in pregnancy than acute hepatitis. Occasionally ischaemia, generally after profound hypotension over many hours, and rapidly progressive malignant infiltration may mimic acute viral hepatitis.

Management

Uncomplicated cases of hepatitis recover spontaneously. Classical studies in military personnel demonstrated no benefit from bed rest, though whether the same applies to older people is unknown. In any case malaise and nausea often enforce rest. Clinicians must

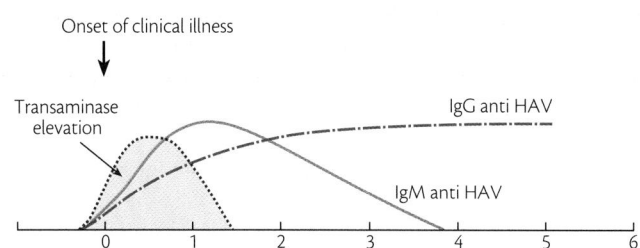

Fig. 15.21.1.1 Typical serology of hepatitis A infection.

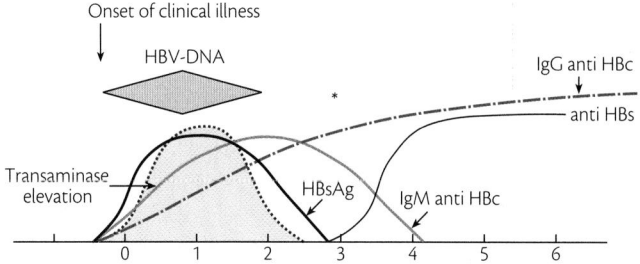

Fig. 15.21.1.2 Serological changes during acute hepatitis B with viral clearance. *, 'Window phase' after elimination of HBsAg and before the emergence of anti-HBs, during which anti-HBc may be the sole indicator of infection.

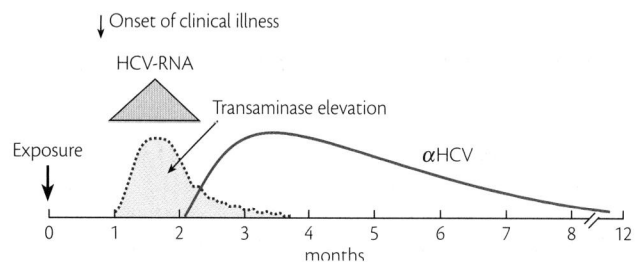

Fig. 15.21.1.3 Serological changes during acute hepatitis C with viral clearance.

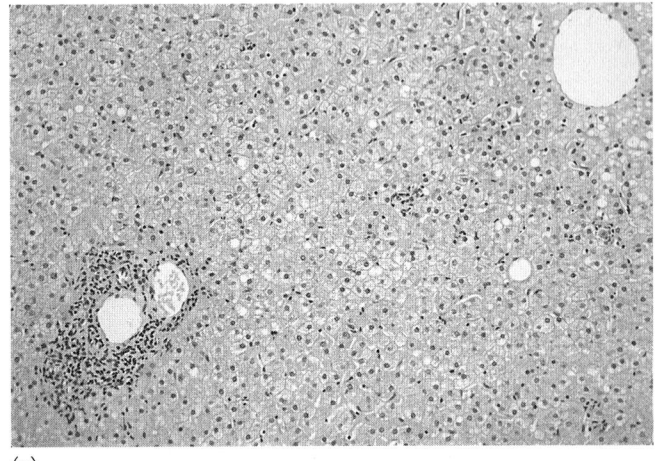

(a)

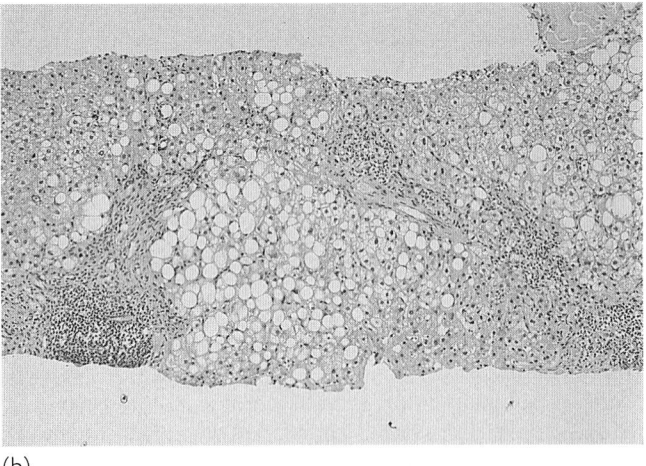

(b)

Fig. 15.21.1.4 Haematoxylin and eosin staining of liver biopsies from (a) mild hepatitis with inflammation restricted to the portal tracts and minimal fibrosis, and (b) severely active but still precirrhotic liver with bridging necrosis. (Courtesy of Professor P. Dhillon.)

be alert to signs of impending liver failure and ensure that hypoglycaemia is avoided, if necessary by parenteral administration of glucose. No diets are of established benefit, but dietary fat is often poorly tolerated. There is no rationale for protein restriction unless evidence of hepatic encephalopathy has emerged. Alcohol and potentially hepatotoxic drugs should be withdrawn. Troublesome pruritus can be treated with colestyramine, which is preferable to antihistamines because of their potential hepatotoxicity. There is no proven therapy to enhance recovery. Corticosteroids do not speed recovery or improve survival, although they do lower serum bilirubin levels. In hepatitis B, and particularly hepatitis C, the use of interferon has been advocated to enhance the chance of elimination of the virus. There is little evidence of its efficacy with HBV. Hepatitis C is rarely recognized during the stage of acute infection, but if it is, the use of interferon-α is associated with a very high rate of clearance of HCV (>95% with 6 months therapy) and thus should be used in patients with acute infection who have not cleared the virus within 12 weeks.

In fulminant hepatic failure, which in the setting of viral hepatitis carries a mortality risk of 80%, patients should, if possible, undergo orthotopic liver transplantation. Criteria for listing differ in different centres, but include a marked abnormality of clotting parameters (e.g. prolongation of the prothrombin time to >50 s or a factor V level <20–30%) and the development of significant encephalopathy. Patients awaiting transplantation require glucose supplementation, full intensive care monitoring, and prophylaxis of infection. Some patients require renal support, such as haemofiltration, and ventilation. Some units invasively monitor intracerebral pressure, which may rise dangerously, so that cerebral oedema may be treated with intravenous mannitol or other manoeuvres.

Prevention of viral hepatitis

Sanitation and hygiene reduce the frequency of the enteric-borne infections HAV and HEV. Passive protection against hepatitis A (to close family contacts) and hepatitis B (after exposure to risk factors such as sexual contact with an individual incubating acute hepatitis B, or a needlestick injury) are available using gammaglobulin preparations (standard preparations for protection against HAV, specific high-titre preparations for HBV). Active immunization to HAV, using formalin-inactivated viral preparations, provides a high level of protective immunity within a few days—suitable, for example, for use prior to travel from Western countries to highly endemic areas, and also advisable in patients with established chronic liver disease, particularly chronic viral hepatitis. Active immunization to HBV is discussed below, which also protects against HDV. Vaccines are not yet available for HCV or HEV.

Features of chronic viral hepatitis caused by different viruses

Chronic hepatitis B

Up to 10% of adults and more than 90% of infants become chronic B carriers after infection, defined by the persistence of HBsAg in the blood for more than 6 months. Subsequently, a low proportion of patients will clear the virus spontaneously each year, but most are infected long-term. Failure to clear the virus is more common in neonates or those infected as infants, in males, and those with natural or iatrogenic immunosuppression. Carriage rates in the population vary widely geographically, and are notably high in east Asia and southern Africa (10–20%), and low in northern Europe and North America (<1%).

The consequences of long-term carriage are varied, reflecting the strength of the immune response mounted by the host, the duration of infection, and alteration in the mechanisms of viral replication with time (Fig. 15.21.1.5). Viral mutation may also contribute to modulation of the host response and viral replication. During the early years, the 'replicative' phase, HBeAg (hepatitis B e antigen)-expressing virus replicates independently of the host chromosomes, resulting in the production of fully infectious viral particles in the blood with high levels of HBV DNA (Table 15.21.1.3). The early replicative phase is associated with a state of relative immune tolerance by the host, and may be very prolonged if infection is acquired as an infant. In the later replicative phase there is expression of immune responses associated with inflammation. Thereafter, HBeAg expression is often lost, HBeAb is expressed ('seroconversion'), and HBsAg production may be driven by viral sequences integrated into the genome

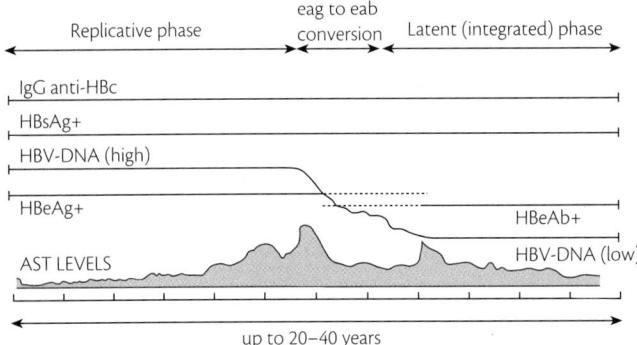

Fig. 15.21.1.5 Serological markers during chronic hepatitis B. Note that HBV mutants not expressing HBeAg may emerge and that HBV DNA quantitation is required to assess their replicative phase.

(integrative phase). In many patients this is associated with low or undetectable levels of HBV DNA in the blood, but in others HBV DNA levels may rise, particularly if HBV mutants not expressing HBeAg emerge.

Chronic hepatitis B infection is associated with a spectrum of histological damage and clinical manifestations. The inflammatory response to the virus may sometimes be so slight that the histological appearances of the liver are virtually normal, with the exception of evidence of virally infected hepatocytes seen as 'ground-glass' cells on routine eosin staining or by histochemistry. More commonly, the immune response is adequate to inflame the liver but

Table 15.21.1.3 Serological tests in chronic HBV carriage

First few months	
HBsA g+	HBsAb–
HBeAg+	HBeAb–
HBcAb IgM+[a]	
HBcAb IgG+	
HBV DNA+	
Replicative phase (several years but variable)	
HBsAg+	HBsAb–
HBeAg+	HBeAb–
HBcAb IgM–[a]	
HBcAb IgG+	
HBV DNA+	
Late phase (variable duration)	
HBsAg+	HBsAb–
HBeAg–	HBeAb+[b]
HBcAb IgM–[a]	
HBcAb IgG+	
HBV DNA–, or minimal	

+, Positive; –, negative; see Table 15.21.1.2 for other abbreviations.

[a] HbcAb-IgM tests are set to be positive only at high titre and thus detect acute infections. Lower titres of IgM antibody persist long-term and the test may again become positive during flares.

[b] Infection with the pre-core mutant of HBV does not lead to HbeAg expression but is associated with HBV DNA in blood and with active disease. Patients with this mutant form are often HbeAb+.

inadequate to clear the virus. The resulting chronic inflammation may be confined to the portal tracts, with a chronic lymphocytic infiltration, associated to varying extent with periportal and/or lobular inflammation, a tendency to develop fibrosis spreading from the portal tracts, and in some cases eventually cirrhosis. These appearances can be categorized in terms of inflammatory activity and fibrosis (Table 15.21.1.4). In general, the replicative phase of HBV infection with HBeAg-positivity, particularly in its later phase, is associated with more marked inflammation than the subsequent HBeAb-positive stage.

Chronic hepatitis B infection may be clinically silent for years, or give rise only to nonspecific symptoms of fatigue. The condition may be recognized on screening (e.g. during pregnancy) or the investigation of coincidentally detected abnormal liver function tests. Some patients present with nonspecific indications of chronic liver disease (malaise or hepatomegaly), or at a late stage with a complication of established cirrhosis. Episodes of enhanced inflammation ('flares') may give rise to transient worsening of liver function tests, particularly transaminase elevations and jaundice at any stage of the disease; precipitating events may include a reduction of prior immunosuppression, or the time of conversion from HBeAg- to HBeAb-positivity. Usually the progression to cirrhosis takes many years, but the rate varies. The incidence of hepatocellular cancer in chronic hepatitis B is high, probably increased 100-fold over noninfected controls. Most, but not all, patients with hepatocellular cancer will have cirrhosis.

Chronic HBV infection may also give rise to a number of extrahepatic manifestations. These include membranous glomerulonephritis, polyarteritis nodosa, and cryoglobulinaemia.

After establishing the diagnosis of chronic HBV infection, it is necessary to define the virological status of the patient with respect to infectivity and viral replication (see Table 15.21.1.3), and the hepatic status with respect to the presence of inflammation and liver damage. Interpretation of viral status may be complicated by the emergence of viral mutants, particularly the 'precore' mutant that results in absent HBeAg expression, but which, none the less, is associated with active inflammation and circulating HBV DNA levels.

Treatment

The general measures relevant to chronic liver disease of any aetiology are discussed elsewhere.

Table 15.21.1.4 Grading of chronic hepatitis

Grade	Activity	Staging
I	Minimal inflammation in portal tracts; scanty piecemeal necrosis; no lobular necrosis	Mild fibrous expansion of portal tracts
II	Mild portal inflammation; piecemeal necrosis; scanty lobular necrosis	Periportal fibrosis, only fine strands of fibrosis into parenchyma
III	Moderate portal inflammation; piecemeal necrosis; lobular necrosis	Bridging of fibrosis with confluent portal tracts or portocentral vein bridging
IV	Marked portal inflammation; prominent piecemeal necrosis; lobular necrosis including confluent bridging necrosis between portal tracts	Cirrhosis–bridging fibrosis and nodular regeneration

With respect to HBV infection, the prospects for inducing viral clearance in an individual patient are relatively low, but the viral load, infectivity, and intensity of hepatic inflammation can often be reduced. The two current approaches are the use of α-interferons, which combine immunomodulatory and antiviral properties, and the use of inhibitors of viral replication, nucleotide and nucleoside analogues.

Patient selection is important. Those with active inflammation, viral replication independent of host DNA, but low levels of HBV DNA have the greatest potential to benefit. Most such patients will have circulating HBeAg present. Whilst some patients will clear HBsAg from the blood in response to treatment, loss of HBeAg is a more common event. In the absence of elevated transaminases the response to treatment is very poor.

α-Interferons (IFN-α) act predominantly by enhancing T-cell-mediated viral clearance, by processes including the enhancement of hepatocyte class I HLA expression. Treatment involves parenteral IFN-α—best administered weekly in pegylated form (long-acting, conjugated to polyethylene glycol) for 6 to 12 months. If viral clearance or HBeAg to HBeAb conversion occurs, there is generally an inflammatory flare during the second or third month. Side effects include malaise, fever (particularly in the first weeks of treatment), anaemia, alopecia, and depression. HBeAg to HBeAb conversion or loss of HBV DNA occurs in 30 to 40% of cases, HBsAg clearance in about 10%. Women, those with a shorter duration of carriage, Westerners, and those without an additional immunosuppressed background (such as HIV infection) respond more favourably. Relapse after the clearance or sustained loss of HBV replication is rare (5–10%). Successful treatment slows histological progression and reduces liver-related mortality (including hepatocellular cancer).

Nucleoside and nucleotide analogues can inhibit viral reverse transcriptase and inhibit replication, and have the advantage of oral bioavailablity. They have the disadvantage of a tendency to induce viral mutation, and their effect is suppressive rather than curative, so once treatment has been initiated logic suggests long-term therapy is indicated, particularly as occasionally cessation of therapy can be followed by a disease flare. The first drug in use, lamivudine (100 mg daily), markedly reduced HBV DNA during treatment, lead to HBeAg to HBeAb conversion in one-third of patients after 12 months, and reduced serological and histological parameters of inflammation. Loss of HBsAg was infrequent. However, lamivudine-esistant strains predictably emerged at the rate of around 20% of treated patients per year, so after 3 to 4 years most patients carried viruses with mutations in the DNA polymerase (YMDD mutants). Newer agents used in combination (adefovir 10 mg daily plus lamivudine) and more powerful single agents (e.g. tenofovir 245 mg daily, entecavir 0.5–1mg daily) have much lesser tendencies to induce mutations. Monitoring of HBV DNA levels is now a key part of effective management of antiviral therapy. A particular use of antivirals is prior to chemotherapy or immunosupression in chronic carriers.

Prevention of hepatitis B

Active immunization for the prevention of HBV infection initially involved a vaccine derived from viral proteins in infected blood, but now uses recombinant HBsAg proteins. Vaccination strategies range from universal vaccination in infancy to the vaccination of only high-risk individuals. In areas of high carriage in east Asia, universal vaccine programmes have already reduced the national incidence of infection, carriage, and hepatocellular cancer. Conventional three-dose immunization in adults leads to protective immunity, as judged by anti-HBsAg, in 90% of individuals.

Passive immunization with anti-HBsAg hyperimmune globulin provides rapid protection after exposure (e.g. after needlestick injury). A combination of passive and active immunization is recommended immediately after birth for children born to infected mothers. In some infants, chronic infection with a mutant 'escape' virus has subsequently occurred.

Chronic hepatitis C

Around 70% of patients who become infected with HCV fail to clear the virus and become chronic carriers. In the majority of cases the initial presentation will have been asymptomatic, and HCV infection is generally recognized in the chronic phase. An asymptomatic indolent necroinflammatory response to the persistent virus in the liver tends to persist long term, and often, but not inevitably, leads to cirrhosis after 15 to 25 years and predispose to hepatocellular cancer thereafter.

Mechanisms of transmission and prevalence rates vary geographically from around 0.5% in the United Kingdom to greater than 20% in some parts of Asia, perhaps 2 to 2.5% of the world's population. In Western countries, blood transfusion and treatment of clotting disorders with plasma concentrates (prior to the early 1990s) and intravenous drug abuse constitute the main routes of transmission. Medical use of unsterilized needles, including in vaccination programmes, tattooing, dentistry, and communal shaving practices, may all contribute worldwide. Vertical transmission is uncommon and has been estimated at around 3%. Sexual transmission is low (<5% in stable heterosexual relationships).

As with HBV, the severity of liver damage reflects host–virus responses. Severe inflammation is less common if the virus is acquired in childhood and progression to cirrhosis less frequent and probably slower. HBV coinfection and alcoholism worsen disease and increase the likelihood and rate of developing cirrhosis. The histological response of the liver shows a similar variety of response to that seen in HBV infection, from minimal to severe portal inflammation, periportal hepatocyte necrosis, and progressive fibrosis leading to cirrhosis. The presence of lymphoid follicles in portal tracts and parenchymal steatosis are characteristic of the response to HCV.

Patients may be diagnosed coincidentally during the investigation of fatigue or abnormal liver function tests, or with manifestations of chronic liver disease. In addition, there are a variety of extrahepatic manifestations thought to reflect either antigen–antibody complex formation or the induction of crossreacting autoimmunity. These include a vasculitic rash associated with cryoglobulinaemia (type 2, polyclonal immunoglobulin plus rheumatoid factor), glomerulonephritis, abnormal thyroid function, thrombocytopenia, and porphyria cutanea tarda. As in HBV, assessment of a patient with HCV involves both the virological and the hepatic status.

The initial screening test for HCV is detection of circulating anti-HCV antibody. If present, confirmation is required using polymerase chain reaction (PCR) for viral RNA (Fig. 15.21.1.6). Viral genotyping (types 1–6) is important as response to treatment varies between genotypes, and quantitative PCR is valuable in judging treatment response.

The severity of inflammation in the liver is poorly judged from routine liver function tests such as aminotransferase level measurements.

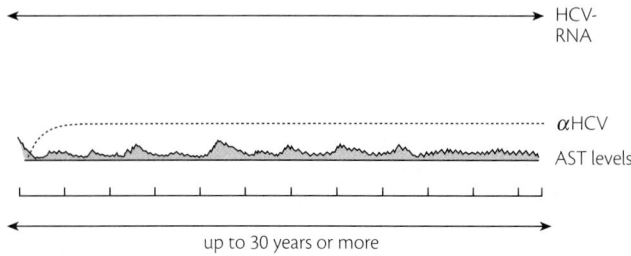

Fig. 15.21.1.6 Serological changes during chronic hepatitis C.

Histological assessment may reveal both significant inflammation and progressive fibrosis despite normal serum enzyme levels.

Treatment of chronic HCV

The main aim of treatment in chronic HCV infection is to clear the virus, which has been established to be associated with a reduction in necroinflammation and slowing in the rate of accumulation of fibrosis in the liver. There is general agreement that patients with the full spectrum from mild to severe precirrhotic disease as judged by activity grading, and with well-compensated cirrhosis, should be considered for treatment, but in decompensated cirrhosis current treatment may induce deterioration.

Treatment results have improved markedly over the last decade, with the introduction of combination therapy with IFN-α2a and IFN-α2b plus ribavirin, and the use of pegylated interferon preparations. Successful treatment produces a sustained virological response, which combines end-of-treatment suppression of viral RNA with persistent negativity 6 months after cessation of treatment. Sustained virological response rates to IFN-α of as low as 10 to 12% reported in the 1990s have been transformed by the coadministration of ribavirin (ineffective alone) and the longer-acting pegylated interferons. Genotypes 2 and 3 respond well to 6 months treatment with IFN-α (pegylated, weekly) plus ribavirin orally, with clearance rates of around 80%. For genotypes 1 and 4, treatment for 12 months is recommended, and clearance rates are 40 to 50%. Older people respond less well. Interferon dosage varies with the preparation, and both IFN-α2a and IFN-α2b are effective; dosage may require to be decreased in response to lowering of platelet and white cell counts. Ribavirin dose varies between 800 and 1200 mg/day; the drug is teratogenic and can induce haemolysis. Use of serial and quantitative RNA analysis can define nonresponders to IFN-α plus ribavirin—in whom therapy can be abandoned after 3 months—and also identify rapid responders who may have sustained remission with shorter duration therapy.

IFN-α regimens have side-effects as discussed under HBV treatment, and in particular may induce thyroiditis and some other auto-immune phenomena. Thrombocytopenia, leucopenian, and anaemia may limit the ability to sustain IFN therapy, though the use of growth factors for this may help. Ribavirin induces cough, rash, dyspnoea, and insomnia in about 25% of patients, and there is predictably a dose-dependent haemolytic anaemia. The drug is contraindicated in renal failure as it accumulates and then causes severe haemolysis. Both pregnancy and fathering children need to be avoided whilst taking ribavirin. The full role of interferon therapy in established cirrhosis, and possible long-term benefits (less fibrosis, lower incidence of hepatocellular cancer) in patients in whom viral clearance is not been achieved, are currently under investigation; in decompensated cirrhosis, however, it is contraindicated.

The next few years are likely to see the emergence into clinical practice of other antiviral strategies currently under clinical trial, such as the use of HCV protease and polymerase inhibitors, analogous to those use for the treatment of HIV. Genetic approaches such as the initiation of expression of inhibitors of RNA expression (RNAis) may also enter the clinical arena.

Treatment of HIV–HCV coinfected patients is a growing practice; there is a greater risk of metabolic complications of highly active retroviral therapy and of decompensation in cirrhosis.

Prevention of hepatitis C

There is no vaccine available for HCV; the major difficulty is the rapid evolution of changes in the composition of the HCV structural proteins as the virus mutates rapidly and many quasi-species develop. Passive immunization with gammaglobulin containing antibodies to HCV is not protective. For similar reasons, patients successfully treated with a sustained virological response do remain susceptible to re-infection.

Chronic hepatitis D

Chronic HDV generally follows superinfection of a chronic HBV carrier in whom ample HBsAg to permit HDV encapsulation is already present. The spectrum of chronic liver disease associated with the double chronic infection is as variable as with HBV alone. Overall, however, the liver tends to be more severely affected, and in 10 to 15% of chronic carriers there may be a rapid (1–2 year) evolution to cirrhosis. HDV acts to suppress HBV infection, so that markers of HBV activity, such as HBV DNA, in the serum may become suppressed. Many patients with HDV may therefore be HBeAb positive.

The treatment of HDV mirrors that for HBV. Prolonged courses of IFN-α (≥6 months) may transiently clear HDV in some patients in whom HBsAg persists. In general, HBsAg clearance is required to cause sustained HDV clearance.

Liver transplantation for viral hepatitis

Liver transplantation is indicated both in fulminant hepatic failure due to acute hepatitis and in advanced chronic hepatitis with cirrhosis. Recurrence of viral hepatitis after transplantation is a major concern. The use of hyperimmune globulin, interferon, and nucleoside analogues allows control in HBV, but severe recurrence remains a significant problem after transplantation for HCV.

Further reading

Coiffier B (2006). Hepatitis B virus reactivation in patients receiving chemotherapy for cancer treatment: role of lamivudine prophylaxis. *Cancer Invest*, **24**, 548–52.

Cooksley WG (2004). The role of interferon therapy in hepatitis B. *Med Gen Med*, **6**, 16.

European Association for the Study of the Liver (2009). EASL Clinical Practice Guidelines: management of chronic hepatitis B. *J Hepatol*, **50**, 227–42.

Heathcote J, Main J (2005). Treatment of hepatitis C. *J Viral Hepat*, **12**, 223–35.

Hoofnagle JH, Seeff LB (2006). Peginterferon and ribavirin for chronic hepatitis C. *N Engl J Med*, **355**, 2444–51.

Martin A, Lemon SM (2006). Hepatitis A virus: from discovery to vaccines. *Hepatology*, **43**(2) Suppl 1, S164–72.

NIH consensus development statement on management of hepatitis B. (2008). *NIH Consens State Sci Statements*. **25**, 1–29.

Poland GA, Jacobson RM (2004). Clinical practice: prevention of hepatitis B with the hepatitis B vaccine. *N Engl J Med*, **351**, 2832–8.

Rehermann B, Nascimbeni M (2005). Immunology of hepatitis B virus and hepatitis C virus infection. *Nat Rev Immunol*, **5**, 215–29.

Sharma P, Lok A (2006). Viral hepatitis and liver transplantation. *Semin Liver Dis*, **26**, 285–97.

Taylor JM (2006). Hepatitis delta virus. *Virology*, **344**, 71–6.

Villeneuve JP (2005). The natural history of chronic hepatitis B virus infection. *J Clin Virol*, **34** Suppl 1, S139–42.

Wang L, Zhuang H (2004). Hepatitis E: an overview and recent advances in vaccine research. *World J Gastroenterol*, **10**, 2157–62.

15.21.2 Autoimmune hepatitis

H.J.F. Hodgson

Essentials

Autoimmune hepatitis describes chronic inflammation in the liver attributed to immune responses against self-antigens in the liver, typically in the form of a marked portal tract infiltrate containing both plasma cells and T cells. It usually affects women (female:male, 8:1), is often familial, and 60% of patients have other autoimmune diseases (e.g. thyroiditis, type 1 diabetes) in addition.

Presentation may be with anorexia, nausea, hepatic discomfort, and the development of jaundice, but other patients present just with malaise, or with extrahepatic manifestations such as arthralgia, arthritis, or fever. Clinical signs vary greatly: there may be jaundice and tender hepatomegaly; or evidence of fulminant hepatic failure such as encephalopathy; or splenomegaly that indicates that cirrhosis has already developed.

Characteristic laboratory findings include high transaminase levels, marked hyperglobulinaemia (particularly IgG), and circulating autoantibodies (antinuclear antibodies (ANA), titre 1:40 or greater; anti-smooth muscle antibodies (SMA), titre 1:80 or greater; anti-liver–kidney microsomal (LKM-1) antibodies). There are no critical symptoms, signs, biochemical, immunological, or liver biopsy abnormalities that are sufficiently specific to provide diagnostic criteria: diagnosis depends on the constellation of features.

Autoimmune hepatitis tends to progress with the development of hepatic fibrosis and cirrhosis. Severe cases should be treated with an immunosuppressive regimen for 1 to 2 years, typically prednisolone with or without azathioprine in the first instance. The 10-year survival rate is 65% for those presenting with cirrhosis and >95% for those presenting without. Endstage cirrhosis and acute nonresponsive autoimmune hepatitis leading to acute or subacute liver failure are indications for orthotopic liver transplantation.

Introduction

Autoimmune hepatitis describes chronic inflammation in the liver attributed to immune responses against self-antigens in the liver. Patients generally have circulating autoantibodies, and 60% have other autoimmune diseases in addition. In severe cases autoimmune hepatitis can lead to acute liver failure, and untreated there is often progression to cirrhosis. There is generally a good response to corticosteroid therapy.

The term 'autoimmune hepatitis' should be reserved for patients with clinically significant liver disease, and not used to describe the very mild chronic inflammation often seen in the livers of patients with systemic autoimmune conditions. Previous terms for autoimmune hepatitis include 'autoimmune chronic active hepatitis' and 'lupoid hepatitis'.

Aetiology

Autoimmune hepatitis is often familial, and a constellation of autoimmune diseases (e.g. thyroiditis, type 1 diabetes) may occur in affected families. Some of the predisposing genetic factors have been characterized. There are strong HLA associations. In the United Kingdom and the United States of America the strongest association is with HLA DR haplotype B1*030 (50% of patients vs 20% of controls), and a secondary association with *0401, but in other geographical areas there are different associations. The DR4 association is strongest in Japan. Deficiency of the C4 component of complement also predisposes to the disease. In Western countries DR3 is associated with more severe disease and a younger onset, and DR4 with an older onset and better treatment response. In most cases there is no clear initiating event for the development of autoimmune hepatitis, but occasionally drugs (α-methyldopa, oxyphenisatine, nitrofurantoin, isoniazid, minocycline, dihydralazine, diclofenac, pemoline, and atorvastatin) and herbal remedies (e.g. black cohosh) can precipitate the condition. As discussed below, in some patients with chronic hepatitis C, autoimmune manifestations develop and may contribute to the inflammatory processes in that chronic viral condition.

Histological appearances and immunopathogenesis

The histological appearances used to be referred to as 'chronic active hepatitis', but pathologists now grade chronic hepatitis in respect of aetiology, disease activity (grading), and progression (staging). There is a marked portal tract infiltrate containing both plasma cells and T cells. Cytotoxic T cells spread out across the limiting plate of the portal tract, associated with piecemeal necrosis of periportal hepatocytes, and lymphocytes are often present diffusely within the parenchyma (Fig. 15.21.2.1). Compared with the inflammation seen in chronic hepatitis B and C, the plasma-cell component of the portal tract infiltrate is more prominent, as is regenerative 'rosette' formation by the hepatocytes. The portal tract lymphoid aggregates and steatosis common in hepatitis C are less frequent in autoimmune hepatitis. With progression, periportal fibrosis, bridging necrosis linking portal tracts to central veins, and hyperplasia of regenerating hepatocytes all occur leading to cirrhosis.

Antibody and T-cell reactivity to a panel of hepatic antigens, both intracellular and on the cell surface, are described. Some of these may be the primary mechanism of liver damage, and others a secondary response to tissue injury. Cell-surface targets such as the hepatocyte-specific asialoglycoprotein receptor may be particularly relevant to the development of tissue damage.

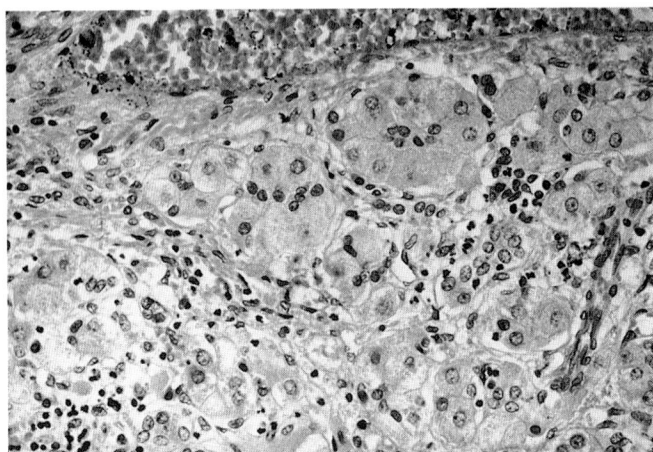

Fig. 15.21.2.1 Haematoxylin and eosin stained liver histology showing 'rosettes' of regenerated hepatocytes, surrounded by lymphocytes that have spread into the hepatic parenchyma.

Table 15.21.2.1 Associated conditions

Arthropathy[a]	Skin rashes[a]
Keratoconjunctivitis sicca[a]	
Autoimmune thyroiditis[b]	Diabetes[b]
Renal tubular acidosis[b]	
Peripheral neuropathy[c]	
Fibrosing alveolitis[d]	Ulcerative colitis[d]
Coeliac disease[d]	Immune thrombocytopenia[d]
Rheumatoid arthritis[d]	Glomerulonephritis[d]
Autoimmune haemolytic anaemia[d]	

Approximate relative frequency of finding in patients with autoimmune hepatitis:
[a] 20–40%; [b] 10–20%; [c] 5–10%; [d] 1–5%.
In the rare autoimmune polyendocrine syndrome type 1 (adrenal insufficiency, mucocutaneous candidiasis, hypoparathyroidism) c.20% of patients have hepatic involvement.

Epidemiology

Most reported cases are of European ancestry, although cases occur worldwide. Most patients are female, with female:male ratios of up to 8:1 reported in some series. Northern European prevalence figures are about 20 per 100 000, similar to those for primary biliary cirrhosis and primary sclerosing cholangitis. The age of onset varies widely, but young adults and children are most commonly affected. Perhaps 20% of cases occur after the age of 65.

Clinical manifestations

In about 30% of cases the onset is indistinguishable clinically from acute viral hepatitis, with anorexia, nausea, hepatic discomfort, and the development of jaundice. Other patients present just with malaise, or with extrahepatic manifestations such as arthralgia, arthritis, or fever, or right upper quadrant abdominal discomfort, and subsequent investigation demonstrates high circulating transaminase levels. Despite an acute onset, many patients have cirrhosis at the time of presentation.

Clinical signs may therefore vary greatly. Cutaneous manifestations of palmar erythema and prominent spider naevi, a maculopapular or acneiform rash, and occasionally abdominal striae (without corticosteroid therapy) may be found both in acute and insidious presentations. In an acute presentation, jaundice and tender hepatomegaly may be prominent, with severe cases demonstrating ascites and most sinisterly the development of encephalopathy. Acute severe autoimmune hepatitis may progress to fulminant hepatic failure. Splenomegaly, which is often marked, indicates that cirrhosis has already developed. There may also be evidence of other autoimmune conditions (Table 15.21.2.1).

Investigations

High transaminase levels, marked hyperglobulinaemia (particularly IgG), and circulating autoantibodies characterize the condition. Transaminase levels are often five or ten times the upper normal limit. Hyperglobulinaemia may include IgG levels of more than 30 g/litre when the condition is active. The major serological diagnostic markers are the presence of autoantibodies demonstrated by tissue immunofluorescence, prominently antinuclear antibodies (ANA), titre 1:40 or greater, and an anti-smooth muscle (SMA) titre 1:80 or greater. In addition, other autoantibodies may be present, in particular to liver–kidney microsomes (liver and proximal renal tubule, LKM-1). However, the antibody profiles in the disease are variable and may alter over time: some cases identified on clinical and histological grounds may lack circulating antibodies on routine testing. Other autoimmune associations of the disease may be manifest with antithyroid, parietal cell, and intrinsic factor antibodies, or antibodies leading to immune thrombocytopenia or haemolysis. Other positive immune tests include a moderate frequency of antibodies to double-stranded and single-stranded DNA. The positive lupus erythematosus cells described in early reports of the condition led to the designation of 'lupoid hepatitis'.

Diagnostic criteria

There are no critical signs, symptoms, or liver test abnormalities that are sufficiently specific to provide diagnostic criteria. The diagnosis is therefore made on a constellation of features, each of which may also occur in other conditions. Diagnosis during the active phase of the disease generally reflects the presence of elevated serum transaminase levels without marked elevation of alkaline phosphatase, elevated globulins, positive antibodies to ANA, SMA, or LKM-1, seronegativity for hepatitis viruses (although the overlap with hepatitis C is discussed below), and characteristic or compatible liver histology. A 'scoring system' to identify definite or probable autoimmune hepatitis from a combination of clinical and histological features has been proposed by an international group.

Differential diagnosis

The differential diagnosis during investigation includes not only viral and drug-induced hepatitis, but the metabolic conditions of Wilson's disease and α_1-antitrypsin deficiency. Some alcoholic patients may manifest histological appearances overlapping with autoimmune hepatitis. The immune biliary diseases primary biliary cirrhosis (PBC) and primary sclerosing cholangitis (PSC) are generally easy to differentiate by the predominant elevation of serum alkaline phosphatase and the antimitochondrial antibody in

PBC, and antineutrophil cytoplasmic antibodies (ANCA) and cholangiography in PSC. However, as already mentioned, each of the suggestive indicators for autoimmune hepatitis may be absent in particular cases, and in some series up to 20% of cases lack any ANA, SMA, and anti-LKM-1 antibodies. Furthermore, there is overlap in the autoimmune profiles of various immunological liver diseases, e.g. with low titres of ANCA often found in autoimmune hepatitis, and SMA in both PBS and PSC. Autoimmune hepatitis is not part of the spectrum of systemic lupus erythematosus.

Autoimmune hepatitis subtypes

A subclassification of autoimmune hepatitis into according to a combination of autoantibody profiles and clinical features has also been suggested (Table 15.21.2.2):

- Type I—classical autoimmune hepatitis with high-titre ANA and SMA. The SMA antibody has anti-F-actin specificity, as can be demonstrated using cell lines as immunofluorescent substrates.
- Type II—anti-LKM-1 antibodies are present, with specificity for a cytochrome P450 antigen, CYP4502D. The disease may be particularly severe, and tends to affect children, and responds less well to immunosuppression. However, anti-LKM-1 may also be found in sera from patients with chronic hepatitis C infection, which can itself also predispose to a variety of autoimmune manifestations. It has therefore been suggested that type II autoimmune hepatitis should be further subdivided to separate those with a primary autoimmune condition (IIa) from those in whom hepatitis C has triggered an autoimmune response (IIb). This, however, introduces further confusion as some patients with hepatitis C have ANA and SMA but not anti-LKM.

Other autoantibodies that may be detected include antibodies to liver cytosol (usually in type II but sometimes type I) and antibodies to soluble liver antigen (in either type).

The issue of autoautoantibodies is complex. Antibodies identified by immunofluorescence are often relatively nonspecific, and reactions to different epitopes may give similar staining patterns. Many of the more recently described antibodies are found in more than one type of autoimmune hepatitis and in other immune conditions affecting the liver. Also, as described below, there are well-described 'overlap' cases, with patients with autoimmune hepatitis also showing manifestations of another immune liver disease. Subtyping on autoantibody criteria alone is therefore unlikely to be definitive. Importantly, there are some patients—perhaps 10%—who otherwise fit criteria, including treatment response, for a diagnosis of autoimmune hepatitis but have no detectable autoantibodies, emphasizing that sometimes a trial of corticosteroids may be worthwhile even if autoantibodies have not been identified.

Associated liver diseases and overlap conditions

Up to 10% of cases may show mixed autoimmune hepatitis and immune biliary disease, generally PBC and less frequently PSC. The disease may also coexist with autoimmune cholangitis (which resembles PBC but is antimitochondrial antibody-negative). In children the overlap with autoimmune primary sclerosing cholangitis is marked, and patients frequently evolve for hepatitis to sclerosing cholangitis over time.

Natural history

Untreated, autoimmune hepatitis may occasionally spontaneously remit, but there is a marked tendency for progression with the development of hepatic fibrosis and cirrhosis, and subsequently the complications thereof. Childhood-onset and type II autoimmune hepatitis have a bad prognosis. Over one-half of the patients with severe disease die within 5 years if untreated. Epidemiological features suggest that inapparent autoimmune hepatitis is the cause of a significant number of cases of cryptogenic cirrhosis. Cirrhosis arising as a consequence of autoimmune hepatitis only rarely leads to hepatocellular carcinoma.

Treatment regimens

Specific therapy for autoimmune hepatitis is aimed at reducing or abolishing inflammation. Patients, particularly those with cirrhosis,

Table 15.21.2.2 Subtypes of autoimmune hepatitis based on autoantibody profiles

Disease	Antibody profile	Descriptive features	Treatment
Autoimmune hepatitis			
Type I	ANA++ SMA++	Classical AIH 70–80% of cases	Corticosteroids
Type II	LKM-1++	Often childhood or adolescent 5% of cases. Overlap with hepatitis C	Corticosteroids (except hepatitis C)
Autoantibody –ve	ANA– SMA–: LKM–	15% of cases	Corticosteroids
Drug-induced	Variable—includes LM+	Drug withdrawal and corticosteroids	
Hepatitis C	ANA± SMA± LKM-1±	c.30% hepatitis C. Less female preponderance	IFNα/ribavirin

AIH, autoimmune hepatitis; ANA, antinuclear antibody; IFN-α, interferon-α; LKM, liver–kidney microsomal antibody: LKM-1, anti-CYP450II; LM, liver microsomal antibodies; SLA, anti-soluble liver antigen (specificity contentious—includes glutathione S-transferase); SMA, anti-smooth muscle (F-actin specificity).
++, highly positive; +, positive; ±, variable; –, negative.

may require treatment for the complications of portal hypertension and liver failure discussed in Chapter 15.21.2.

There is consensus that severe cases of autoimmune hepatitis should be treated with an immunosuppressive regimen for 1 to 2 years. Evidence of benefit is firm in patients with transaminase levels more than five times normal, and those with histological evidence of bridging necrosis on biopsy. Whether patients with mild disease (minor elevations of transaminase, minor inflammation on biopsy without developing fibrosis) benefit from immunosuppressive therapy is unclear, and in such patients a period of observation followed by repeat biopsy to gauge progression may be helpful. The finding of established cirrhosis should not be taken as a reason to prevent treatment, provided there is active inflammation.

Corticosteroid treatment of patients with severe disease reduces inflammation in 80 to 90% of cases, reduces the chance of progression to cirrhosis if it has not already occurred, and prolongs survival. In assessing the short-term effects of corticosteroid or other therapy, responses are characterized as 'complete' if transaminase levels normalize and remain so for a year or more, or if repeat histology shows only minimal activity. A 'partial response' describes improvement but the persistence of transaminase abnormalities at more than twice the upper limit of normal, or persistent histological activity despite the normalization of transaminase levels. In the most successful cases, complete responses with regression of fibrosis and normalization of architecture have been reported.

A variety of corticosteroid-based regimens are in use. Comparative studies demonstrate equivalent anti-inflammatory efficacy of a solely corticosteroid regimen of prednisolone 20 mg/day, and a steroid-sparing combination of 75 mg azathioprine plus 10 mg prednisolone, but a lesser incidence of side effects over 2 years with the latter. Many physicians use higher doses of prednisolone initially (30–45 mg), until there is a definite improvement in liver function tests. Amongst those who respond, corticosteroid treatment will significantly reduce or normalize transaminase levels within a few weeks to a few months. Symptoms tend to resolve over a similar period, but corticosteroids may not abolish inflammation, as judged histologically, for a year or more. Therefore, if a complete clinical and biochemical remission is established, generally within a few months, most physicians advocate treatment for between 1 and 2 years and a repeat liver biopsy after that to see if there is still histological evidence of inflammation. A biopsy at this interval may also demonstrate that cirrhosis has supervened, despite clinical and biochemical control of the disease. If there is no active inflammation, or only mild inflammation, on the follow-up biopsy, cautious withdrawal of corticosteroids—e.g. reducing the dose at a rate of 1 mg/month—may allow their discontinuation. However, the chances of relapse are high (perhaps 70%) either during withdrawal or later, in which case immunosuppressive therapy will again be required and should then be continued long-term. When this is required, azathioprine alone may be all that is required. For patients who have only partially responded to corticosteroids—judged by the failure to reduce transaminase levels significantly or by persisting inflammation on follow-up biopsy—long-term immunosuppression is advocated, and increased corticosteroid or azathioprine dosage may be required to achieve remission.

Minimizing the incidence and severity of corticosteroid side effects is very important. Glucose intolerance and hypertension should be screened for, and the enhanced risk of infection warrants increased vigilance. Strategies to reduce bone loss include oral supplementation with calcium and vitamin D, or the use of bisphosphonates to restore lost bone mass. The orally administered halogenated corticosteroid budesonide is rapidly metabolized by the liver, and reports indicate that it may be effective in treating autoimmune liver disease with less effect on the pituitary–adrenal axis than prednisolone. Theoretically, lesser effects on bone would also be anticipated.

For patients who fail to respond to corticosteroid-based immunosuppression there is anecdotal evidence of a reasonable response rate to each of mycophenylate, ciclosporin, tacrolimus, methotrexate, and rapamycin, Failure to respond should also prompt reconsideration of the diagnosis, in particular exclusion of previously unrecognized Wilson's disease.

In the overlap syndrome of primary biliary cirrhosis-autoimmune hepatitis, the periportal inflammatory element of the condition and the serum transaminase elevations generally respond to corticosteroid therapy, but the biliary component is not improved. Conversely, bile acid therapy with ursodeoxycholic acid can improve the biliary manifestations whilst leaving the transaminase levels and periportal inflammation unaffected. Combination of the two therapeutic approaches may be necessary to restore normal biochemical markers of liver disease. Patients with the autoimmune hepatitis–PSC overlap syndrome respond poorly to treatment.

Prognosis after treatment

Amongst patients presenting without cirrhosis, long-term survival is excellent (>95% at 10 years), and the 10-year survival rate is about 65% if cirrhosis is present initially. Corticosteroid therapy increases the survival of both cirrhotic and noncirrhotic patients.

Transplantation

Endstage cirrhosis due to autoimmune hepatitis, and acute nonresponsive autoimmune hepatitis leading to acute or subacute liver failure, provide firm indications for orthotopic liver transplantation. Failure to achieve an early response in acute disease, with a shrinking liver volume, should prompt consideration of transplantation. Overall, the prognosis after transplantation is good, with 5-year survival rates in excess of 80%, and a similar incidence of acute rejection episodes (50–60%) to that seen in other immunological liver diseases. Autoantibodies persist after transplantation, though at lower titre. There is a tendency for the disease to recur in the transplanted liver, with a frequency of up to 50% at 5 years, sometimes necessitating retransplantation. Interestingly, de novo autoimmune hepatitis can occur after liver transplantation performed for other indications. Whether more aggressive immunosuppressive antirejection regimens will prevent this remains to be established.

Further reading

Czaja AJ, Carpenter HA (1993). Sensitivity, specificity, and predictability of biopsy interpretations in chronic hepatitis. *Gastroenterology*, **105**, 1824–32.
Czaja AJ, Freese DK (2002). Diagnosis and treatment of autoimmune hepatitis. *Hepatology*, **36**, 479–97.
De Silva S, Neuberger J (2006). HLA and autoimmune hepatitis. *Liver Int*, **26**, 509–11.
Dufour JF, DeLellis R, Kaplan MM (1997). Reversibility of hepatic fibrosis in autoimmune hepatitis. *Ann Intern Med*, **127**, 981–5.
Gautam M, Cheruvattath R, Balan V. (2006). Recurrence of autoimmune liver disease after liver transplantation: a systematic review. *Liver Transpl*, **12**, 1813–24.

Ichiki Y, *et al.* (2005). T cell immunity in autoimmune hepatitis. *Autoimmun Rev*, **4**, 315–21.

Krawitt EL. (2006). Autoimmune hepatitis. *N Engl J Med*, **354**, 54–66.

Manns MP, Vogel A. (2006). Autoimmune hepatitis, from mechanisms to therapy. *Hepatology*, **43** Suppl 1, S132–44.

Poupon R (2003). Autoimmune overlapping syndromes. *Clin Liver Dis*, **7**, 865–78.

Ratziu V, *et al.* (1999). Long term follow up after liver transplantation for autoimmune hepatitis, evidence of recurrence of primary disease. *J Hepatol*, **30**, 131–4　1.

Vergani D, Mieli-Vergani G (2004). Autoimmune hepatitis and sclerosing cholangitis. *Autoimmunity*, **37**, 29–32.

Vergani D, *et al.* (2004) Liver autoimmune serology: a consensus statement from the committee for autoimmune serology of the International Autoimmune Hepatitis Group. *J Hepatol*, **41**, 677–83.

Yeoman AD, Westbrook *et al.* (2009). Diagnostic value and utility of the simplified International Autoimmune Hepatitis Group (IAIHG) criteria in acute and chronic liver disease. *Hepatology*, **50**, 538–45.

15.21.3 **Primary biliary cirrhosis**

M.F. Bassendine

Essentials

Primary biliary cirrhosis is a chronic, cholestatic liver disease in which the biliary epithelial cells lining the small intrahepatic bile ducts are the target for immune-mediated damage leading to progressive ductopenia. The cause is unknown, but presumed to be autoimmune.

The disorder affects women (>90% of cases) and usually has an insidious onset in middle age. Fatigue and pruritus are the most common presenting symptoms. Findings on examination vary widely, ranging from no abnormality to jaundice with hyperpigmentation, scratch marks, and signs of long-standing cholestasis.

Diagnosis of primary biliary cirrhosis is based on three criteria: (1) cholestatic liver function tests, with increases in serum alkaline phosphatase and γ-glutamyl transferase, but only modest changes in transaminases; (2) presence of serum antimitochondrial antibodies (AMA), which are found in more than 95% of cases; and (3) compatible liver histology. Many asymptomatic patients are recognized following the incidental discovery of AMA or elevated levels of serum alkaline phosphatase.

Treatment with ursodeoxycholic acid can lead to significant improvement in liver biochemical values and is recommended for some patients. Cholestyramine is used to treat pruritus. No immunosuppressive drug regimen has been proven to be effective. Progression may be slow, but eventually patients can develop cirrhosis, and death may occur from liver failure or complications of cirrhosis such as bleeding oesophageal varices. The disease at one time was a leading indication for liver transplantation, but earlier diagnosis and treatment has now improved the prognosis for many patients.

Historical perspective

In 1851 Addison and Gull described six patients with jaundice and xanthomas, the dominant presenting features of disease for over a century. In 1965 the clear association between antimitochondrial antibodies (AMA) and primary biliary cirrhosis (PBC) was recognized and in 1988 the major mitochondrial autoantigen was identified as an enzyme component of pyruvate dehydrogenase complex. Routine use of laboratory tests for AMA and liver function have changed the clinical presentation of the disease and over half of patients are now asymptomatic at diagnosis. The term 'primary biliary cirrhosis' was first used in 1950 but is a misnomer as cirrhosis is not often present. The first randomized controlled trial of therapy was initiated in 1968 and many treatments have since been evaluated but none have been shown to cure the disease; only liver transplantation is curative.

Aetiology

Genetics

In common with most autoimmune disorders, genetic factors play a role in determining susceptibility to PBC, but the pattern of inheritance is complex. Familial clustering is well documented, and the sibling relative risk is 10.5, similar to values seen in other autoimmune disorders where it is thought that genetic factors may contribute up to 50% of the total risk. The concordance rate of PBC in identical twins is among the highest reported in autoimmunity at 63%. There is no association of the disorder with major histocompatibility complex (MHC) class I antigens. An immunogenetic predisposition has been confirmed by a genomewide association study identifying HLA class II genes (DQB1, DPB1, DRB1, and DRA), IL12A, and IL12RB2 as susceptibility loci. Genetic factors may also impact on the severity of PBC.

Pathogenesis

Over 95% of patients have antibodies to mitochondria, with the dominant autoantibody response being directed against two components (dihydrolipoamide acetyltransferase (E2) and E3-binding protein) of pyruvate dehydrogenase complex (PDC) (Table 15.21.3.1). The loss of tolerance to these autoantigens is an early event in this progressive disease, with AMA being detectable in serum before abnormalities in liver function and long before the onset of symptoms. One hypothesis is that the development of these AMA marks the exposure of a genetically susceptible individual to an initiating environmental factor. Autoreactive T cells play a central role in the development of various autoimmune diseases and an immunodominant T-cell epitope within PDC-E2 (peptide 163–176) has been identified in patients with PBC. This epitope is within the lipoyl domain of PDC-E2 and in the same region where AMA bind. T-cell clones reactive to this peptide can also be activated by mimicry peptides derived from several xenobiotics and microbial proteins, supporting the hypothesis that autoreactive T-cells present in the peripheral blood and liver can be activated and clonally expanded by antigenic stimulation by mimicry peptides derived from environmental nonself antigen.

Antinuclear antibodies are found in a minority of patients with PBC (Table 15.21.3.1) and display unique immunofluorescence patterns such as nuclear dots or a nuclear ring-like pattern.

Table 15.21.3.1 Reactivity of disease-specific autoantibodies in PBC

	Molecular mass (×10³)	Occurrence (%)
Mitochondrial antigens		
Pyruvate dehydrogenase complex (PDC): lipoyl domain of E2 acetyltransferase	74	95
PDC: lipoyl domain of E3-binding protein	52	95
PDC E1α decarboxylase	41	40–66
PDC E1β decarboxylase	36	2–10
2-oxoglutarate dehydrogenase complex: lipoyl domain of E2 succinyl transferase	48	39–88
Branched chain 2-oxo-acid dehydrogenase complex: lipoyl domain of E2 acyltransferase	50	53–89
Nuclear antigens		
Glycoprotein of the nuclear-pore membrane	210	10–47
Nucleoporin p62	62	32
Sp100	100	20

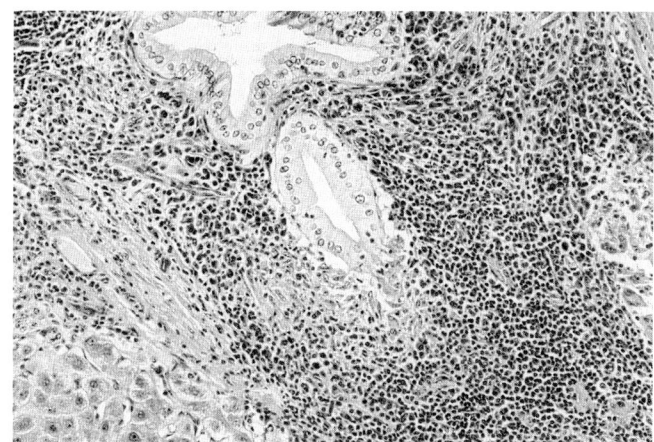

Fig. 15.21.3.1 Bile duct lesion in PBC. There is granulomatous destruction of a medium-sized bile duct radicle in which the epithelium appears hyperplastic. Epithelioid macrophages are surrounded by a chronic inflammatory cell infiltrate. Haematoxylin and eosin.
(Courtesy of A D Burt.)

Disease-specific nuclear antigens include a 210-kDa glycoprotein of the nuclear-pore membrane (gp 210), nucleoporin p62, and Sp100, an interferon-inducible 100-kDa nucleoprotein.

Despite progress in characterizing the reactivity of the disease-specific autoantibodies and autoreactive T-cell responses in PBC, the elucidation of early events in the pathogenesis of bile duct damage remains elusive. Progress has been hampered by the practical limitations in accessing human liver tissue and the lack of a suitable animal model. There is a controversial report that PBC is associated with a retroviral infection; however, the balance of evidence in PBC remains strongly in favour of an autoimmune process in which autoreactive effector mechanisms are directed at epitopes within self-PDC-E2 expressed normally or aberrantly by biliary epithelial cells.

Pathology

The characteristic early lesion of PBC is inflammatory duct destruction. Later there is fibrosis, often patchy, and eventually a frank cirrhotic picture. Histologically this disease appears to evolve from a florid duct lesion to cirrhosis. This has led to a morphological classification into four stages. It must be recognized, however, that overlaps between stages is common in different parts of the liver. In stage 1, the duct lesion is florid (Fig. 15.21.3.1) with the epithelium irregular, hyperplastic, or ulcerated. There is a heavy infiltrate of lymphocytes, plasma cells, and neutrophils, with occasional eosinophils. Aggregates of histocytes with granulomas ranging from foci of epithelioid cells to rounded lesions with multinucleated giant cells are present. In stage 2 there is established duct destruction and the bile ducts may be replaced by lymphoid aggregates with fibrosis. In stage 3 there is relatively little inflammation, though lymphoid aggregates may be present and fibrous septa extend from the portal tract. In stage 4 there is an established cirrhosis, paucity of bile ducts, and lymphoid infiltration (Fig. 15.21.3.2). Mallory bodies similar to those seen in alcoholic liver disease may be present adjacent to the areas of inflammation

and there is excess stainable copper-binding protein, a reflection of the cholestasis.

Epidemiology

There is a marked geographical variation in the prevalence of the disease; it is commonest in northern Europe but rare in the Indian subcontinent and Africa. It was previously considered to be rare and account for fewer than 5% of patients dying of cirrhosis in Western communities, but appears to be becoming commoner. In the north-east of England the prevalence rose from 202 per million adults and 541 per million women over 40 in 1987 to 335 per million adults and 940 per million women over 40 in 1994. In Finland a similar increase in prevalence has been documented, from 161 per million women in 1988 to 292 per million in 1999. It remains unclear whether this represents better diagnosis or a true increase in prevalence. In Victoria, Australia the prevalence in British-born immigrant women is 344 cases per million, compared to 160 per million in Australian-born women, suggesting that environmental

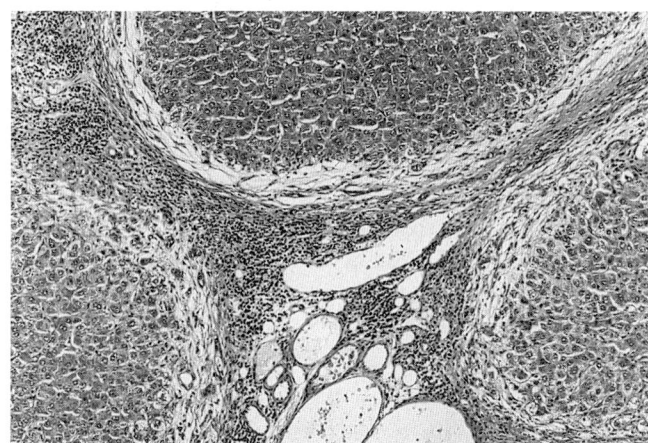

Fig. 15.21.3.2 Stage 4 PBC: an established micronodular cirrhosis; the halo effect seen around the nodules is a characteristic feature of biliary cirrhosis. Haematoxylin and eosin.
(Courtesy of A D Burt.)

factors may play a role in the aetiology of PBC. A significant role for environmental factors in the triggering of PBC is also suggested by the demonstration, using formal cluster analysis, of disease 'hot spots' in the north-east of England.

Clinical features

Patients with early disease may be asymptomatic or complain of fatigue or symptoms of coexisting autoimmune disease. Profound fatigue affects 50% of patients and can be a significant cause of disability. It is not related to the severity of underlying liver disease or itch. Pruritus can be local or diffuse, is worse at night, and usually precedes the onset of jaundice by months to years. Those with more advanced disease have evidence of cholestasis, with jaundice, light stools, easy bruising, and weight loss; itch may become the most distressing symptom. Rarely patients present with ascites, gastrointestinal bleeding from oesophageal varices, or associated peptic ulcer.

Findings on examination vary widely. At one extreme, there may be no abnormality, whereas at the other the patient is jaundiced, with hyperpigmentation, scratch marks, and signs of long-standing cholestasis. The planus form of xanthoma occurs characteristically as xanthelasmas around the eyes and in the palmar creases.

The liver is often enlarged and firm, and splenomegaly may be present, with or without portal hypertension. Spider naevi and palmar erythema are less frequent than in patients with alcoholic cirrhosis. Fluid retention with ascites and oedema is usually a late complication, as is bleeding from oesophageal varices. Steatorrhoea occurs primarily in patients who have advanced cholestasis, leading to malabsorption of fat-soluble vitamins, especially vitamin D. Deficiency of vitamin K sometimes results in easy bruising or other haemorrhagic phenomena. Bone pain due to osteomalacia can occur, as can liver failure with encephalopathy. However, such late manifestations of disease are now rarely seen in Western countries as liver transplantation is performed in most patients before their development. Osteoporosis in PBC is related to advancing age and disease severity; there is a twofold increase in both the absolute and relative fracture risk in people with PBC compared with the general population.

Hepatocellular carcinoma (HCC) is a recognized complication of cirrhosis from any cause. Men are afflicted at least twice as often as women, and PBC is no exception to this rule. HCC is a relatively common cause of death in male PBC patients with cirrhosis and surveillance with regular liver ultrasound is recommended.

PBC is associated with past smoking and a number of other autoimmune diseases. These include Sjögren's syndrome, seropositive and seronegative arthropathy, thyroiditis, scleroderma, and renal tubular acidosis. The CRST syndrome (calcinosis, Raynaud's phenomenon, sclerodactyly, and telangiectasia), pulmonary fibrosis, psoriasis, and coeliac disease have also been reported.

Differential diagnosis

The main differential diagnosis is from other causes of cholestasis. Good ultrasound examination of the liver and biliary tree is mandatory to exclude extrahepatic biliary obstruction or gallstones. CT, magnetic resonance cholangiopancreatography (MRCP), or endoscopic retrograde cholangiopancreatography (ERCP) may be necessary for patients without detectable antimitochondrial antibody, many of whom have a positive antinuclear antibody and

may be thought to have 'autoimmune cholangitis'. There is an overlap with autoimmune hepatitis, which can be diagnosed on liver histology, whilst primary sclerosing cholangitis will be evident on MRCP or ERCP.

Clinical investigation

The serological hallmark of PBC is a positive AMA, which may antedate all other abnormalities. The presence of AMA is not sufficient by itself to allow the diagnosis of PBC but indicates a substantial risk of onset of PBC over the next decade. Liver function tests reflect cholestasis, with increases in serum alkaline phosphatase and γ-glutamyl transferase, but only modest changes in transaminases. At presentation total serum bilirubin is usually normal or only modestly increased. The serum globulins are usually raised, particularly the IgM, but the serum albumin is usually maintained until late in the disease. Other tests such as erythrocyte sedimentation rate and autoantibodies other than antimitochondrial antibodies are less specific. Serum lipid levels may be strikingly elevated in PBC but it is not clear if this is associated with atherosclerotic risk. The increased cholesterol levels found in PBC are primarily due to LP-X, an abnormal low-density lipoprotein (LDL) particle with antiatherogenic properties.

The use of liver biopsy has diminished in recent years in the setting of 'typical' PBC, i.e. a patient with symptoms of fatigue or itch, cholestatic LFTs, and a strongly positive AMA. However the histological features are very specific, and although several different histological stages may be found in one biopsy, the presence of fibrosis or cirrhosis indicates a worse prognosis. Liver stiffness measurement (transient elastography) is a promising new noninvasive test for assessment of liver fibrosis and monitoring its progression over time. In patients with more advanced disease, surveillance for osteopenia and hepatocellular cancer should be undertaken.

Criteria for diagnosis

As many patients are asymptomatic at presentation, diagnosis is currently based on three criteria: cholestatic liver function tests, presence of serum AMA, and liver histology that is compatible with PBC. A definite diagnosis requires the presence of all three criteria and a probable diagnosis requires two of these three.

Treatment

This consists of therapy aimed at modifying the disease process and progression to cirrhosis, and treatment of symptoms and late complications.

Numerous trials of specific therapy have been undertaken in the last 40 years; the main agents that have been assessed are shown in Table 15.21.3.2. Over recent years the naturally occurring bile acid, ursodeoxycholic acid (UDCA), which is safe and well tolerated, has become an established treatment of PBC. The mechanism of action of UDCA is uncertain and is probably multifactorial. Many randomized controlled trials comparing ursodeoxycholic acid with placebo have been published. All the trials reported an improvement in biochemical liver indices. However, a recent updated systematic review to evaluate the benefits and harms of UDCA in patients with PBC did not demonstrate any benefit of UDCA on mortality or liver transplantation in patients with PBC. Another meta-analysis that was confined to trials using an appropriate dose

Table 15.21.3.2 Therapeutic agents evaluated in PBC

Agent	Dosage	Comment
UDCA	13–15 mg/kg per day	Improvement in biochemistry. May delay progression to cirrhosis and normalize survival rate when given in early stages of disease. Approved by FDA for use in PBC. Well tolerated
UDCA + budesonide	6 mg/day	Improvement in liver histology and biochemistry. May worsen osteopenia
UDCA + fibrate	Not determined	Small studies show improvement in biochemistry compared to UDCA monotherapy
Ciclosporin	2.5–4mg/kg per day	Limited efficacy; renal toxicity and hypertension
Methotrexate	15 mg/week	Some benefit but toxicity possible. Use not recommended outside randomized trials
Prednisolone	30 mg/day reducing to 10 mg/day	Improved hepatic function in one small study
Azathioprine	1–2 mg/kg per day	Limited efficacy
Mycophenolate mofetil	1 g/dy	Pilot study showed limited efficacy
Chlorambucil	0.5–4 mg/day	Potentially toxic
Colchicine	0.6–1.2 mg/day	Minor benefits but insufficient evidence to support use
D-Penicillamine	250–100 mg/day	No convincing benefit. Excessive toxicity

UDCA, ursodeoxycholic acid.

of ursodeoxycholic acid (>10 mg/kg body weight per day) and with sufficient follow-up (at least 2 years) found that treatment with UDCA resulted in significant improvement in liver biochemical values. In addition subjects without evidence of fibrosis (histological stages I and II) who were treated with UDCA had slower disease progression than did subjects in the control group. UDCA therapy does not seem to benefit the symptom of fatigue and has a variable effect on pruritus. The practice guidelines of the American Association for the Study of Liver Diseases state that appropriately selected patients with PBC and abnormal liver biochemical values should be advised to take UDCA at a dose of 13 to 15 mg/kg daily either in divided doses or as a single daily dose. If cholestyramine is used to treat pruritus, 4 h should elapse between the administration of cholestyramine and that of UDCA.

There is a continued need for new therapeutic options in patients with advanced disease.

Immunosuppressive agents

As PBC appears to be a classic autoimmune disease, a number of immunosuppressive agents have been assessed. There is currently insufficient evidence to support or reject the use of glucocorticosteroids. Budesonide combined with UDCA improves liver histology and the results of biochemical tests of liver function, but may worsen osteopenia in patients with more advanced disease; monitoring of bone mass density is recommended. Other immunosuppressive drugs that have been evaluated but found to be either ineffective or toxic include azathiabrine, chlorambucil, cyclosporin, methotrexate, and mycophenolate mofetil.

Other agents

D-Penicillamine was used for patients with PBC because of its ability to decrease hepatic copper and modulate the immune response, but did not reduce the risk of mortality or morbidity, and led to more adverse events. Colchicine has been evaluated because of its immunomodulatory and antifibrotic potential, but there is insufficient evidence to support its use outside clinical trials. Statins effectively reduce cholesterol levels but do not improve cholestasis in PBC. Fibrates have been used in nonicteric patients who have not shown a complete response to UDCA; combination of bezafibrate or fenofibrate with UDCA appears promising in preliminary studies, with significant improvement in serum alkaline phosphatase and IgM, compared with UDCA monotherapy.

Treatment of symptoms

Fatigue in PBC may be associated with the presence of daytime somnolence, and modafinil has been used with good effect in a pilot study. Itching can be an intolerable symptom and the first line of treatment is with cholestyramine. Improvement in itching has also been reported with rifampicin and opioid antagonists (naloxone and naltrexone). A prolonged prothrombin time is treated with intramuscular vitamin K, 10 mg monthly. Injections of vitamin A (100 000 IU) and vitamin D (100 000 IU) are usually given every 2 to 3 months in jaundiced patients and vitamin E supplements may also be required. Osteomalacia is now rare, given such treatment. The principles developed for monitoring and treating postmenopausal osteoporosis can be followed for patients with PBC. The complications of portal hypertension and of liver failure are treated appropriately.

Liver transplantation

This has greatly improved survival in patients with PBC, and it is the only effective treatment for those with liver failure. The requirement for liver transplantation for endstage PBC is falling in both Europe and North America. Referral to a transplant centre should be considered as the bilirubin approaches 100 μmol/litre, though patients with particular problems such as intractable itching may need to be considered individually. Current data suggest that the survival benefit from transplantation occurs when the MELD score exceeds 15. Survival rates at 5 and 10 years are in excess of 80% and 50% respectively. Recurrence of PBC may occur but graft loss from PBC recurrence is rare. The main risk factor for recurrence is the use of tacrolimus compared with ciclosporin for immunosuppression.

Prognosis

People with PBC have a threefold mortality increase when compared with the general population, which is somewhat reduced by regular treatment with UDCA. The clinical and biochemical response to UDCA can be used to predict outcome. Patients with a decrease in serum alkaline phosphatase of at least 40% or a decrease to the normal range at 1 year have a prognosis similar to that of an age-matched healthy population. The most reliable determinant of prognosis is the level of the serum bilirubin; other factors associated with poor prognosis include weight loss, hepatomegaly, splenomegaly, histological stage, patient age, and impaired liver synthetic function. Several similar prognostic models have been validated in clinical studies; the most widely used is the Mayo Risk Score (an online tool for calculating this is available at http://www.mayoclinic.org/gi-rst/mayomodel1.html).

Future developments

Progress in understanding the aetiopathogenesis of PBC has been hampered by the absence of a suitable model, but three spontaneous autoimmune biliary disease mouse models have recently been reported. These will help in the study of genetics and immunoregulation in early PBC and may suggest new therapeutic approaches to reverse the disease process. The role of combination regimens of UDCA with other agents should become clearer in the next 5 to 10 years after assessment in appropriately designed trials.

Further reading

Corpechot C, et al. (2005). The effect of ursodeoxycholic acid therapy on the natural course of primary biliary cirrhosis. *Gastroenterology*, **128**, 297–303. [Study using multistate modelling approach to assess the effect of UDCA on the natural history of PBC, showing that UDCA alone normalizes the survival rate of patients when given at early stages.]

EASL and collaborators (2009). EASL Clinical Practice Guidelines: management of cholestatic liver diseases. *J Hepatol*, **51**, 237–67. [Guidelines developed under the auspices and approved by the European Association for the Study of the Liver.]

Gershwin ME, et al. (2005). USA PBC Epidemiology Group. Risk factors and comorbidities in primary biliary cirrhosis: a controlled interview-based study of 1032 patients. *Hepatology*, **42**, 1194–202. [Multicentre study evaluating factors associated with increased risk of PBC.]

Gong Y, Christensen E, Gluud C (2007). Azathioprine for primary biliary cirrhosis. *Cochrane Database Syst Rev* **3**, CD006000. [Review; 63 references.]

Gong Y, Christensen E, Gluud C (2007) Cyclosporin A for primary biliary cirrhosis. *Cochrane Database Syst Rev* **3**, CD005526 [Review; 55 references.]

Gong Y, Gluud C (2005). Colchicine for primary biliary cirrhosis: a Cochrane Hepato-Biliary Group systematic review of randomized clinical trials. *Am J Gastroenterol*, **100**, 1876–85. [Systematic review of 10 trials involving 631 PBC patients, 4 of which were high-quality trials, concluding that there is insufficient evidence to support the use of colchicine.]

Gong Y, Klingenberg SL, Gluud C (2006). Systematic review and meta-analysis: D-penicillamine vs. placebo/no intervention in patients with primary biliary cirrhosis—Cochrane Hepato-Biliary Group. *Aliment Pharmacol Therapeut*, **24**, 1535–44. [Systematic review with meta-analysis of seven trials including 706 PBC patients, showing D-penicillamine did not reduce the risk of mortality or morbidity and led to more adverse events.]

Gong Y, et al. (2007). Ursodeoxycholic acid for patients with primary biliary cirrhosis: an updated systematic review and meta-analysis of randomized clinical trials using Bayesian approach as sensitivity analyses. *Am J Gastroenterol*, **102**, 1799–807. [Meta-analysis of all placebo-controlled trials of UDCA in PBC.]

Hirschfield GM, et al. (2009). Primary biliary cirrhosis associated with HLA, IL12A, and IL12RB2 variants. *N Eng J Med*, **360**, 2544–55. [A genomewide association study identifying susceptibility loci in primary biliary cirrhosis.]

Jones DE (2007). Pathogenesis of primary biliary cirrhosis. *Gut*, **56**, 1615–24. [Review of evidence supporting autoimmune aetiology of PBC.]

Kaplan MM, Gershwin ME (2005). Medical progress: primary biliary cirrhosis. *N Eng Med*, **353**, 1261–73. [Comprehensive review of the condition.]

Lindor K (2007). Ursodeoxycholic acid for the treatment of primary biliary cirrhosis. *N Engl J Med*, **357**, 1524–9. [Review of major clinical studies using UDCA based around a 'typical' case vignette and explaining areas of uncertainty.]

Lindor KD, et al. (2009). Primary biliary cirrhosis. *Hepatology*, **50**, 291–308.

McNally RJ, et al. (2009). Are transient environmental agents involved in the cause of primary biliary cirrhosis? Evidence from space-time clustering analysis. *Hepatology*, **50**, 1169–74. [Analysis of >1000 PBC cases indicates that transient environmental agents may play a role in the aetiology of PBC.]

Prince MI, et al. (2004). Asymptomatic primary biliary cirrhosis: clinical features, prognosis, and symptom progression in a large population based cohort. *Gut*, **53**, 865–70. [Follow-up study of 770 patients with PBC, 61% asymptomatic at diagnosis.]

Prince M, Christensen E, Gluud C (2005). Glucocorticosteroids for primary biliary cirrhosis. *Cochrane Database Syst Rev* **2**, CD003778. [Review with 59 references.]

Prince MI, James OFW (2003). The epidemiology of primary biliary cirrhosis. *Clin Liver Dis*, **7**, 795–819. [Comprehensive review of epidemiology.]

Rautiainen H, et al. (2005). Budesonide combined with UDCA to improve liver histology in primary biliary cirrhosis: a three-year randomized trial. *Hepatology*, **41**, 747–52. [Trial in 77 patients with precirrhotic PBC showing budesonide combined with UDCA improved liver histology.]

Rieger R, Gershwin ME (2007). The X and why of xenobiotics in primary biliary cirrhosis. *J Autoimmunity*, **28**, 76–84. [Review of data supporting an environmental trigger for PBC.]

Shi J, et al. (2006). Long-term effects of mid-dose ursodeoxycholic acid in primary biliary cirrhosis: a meta-analysis of randomized controlled trials. *Am J Gastroenterol*, **101**, 1529–38. [Meta-analysis confined to placebo-controlled trials using an appropriate dose of UDCA and with sufficient follow-up.]

Yeaman SY, et al. (1988). Primary biliary cirrhosis: Identification of two major M2 mitochondrial autoantigens. *Lancet* i, 1067–70. [Landmark paper characterizing reactivity of AMA.]

15.21.4 Primary sclerosing cholangitis

R.W. Chapman

Essentials

Primary sclerosing cholangitis is a chronic cholestatic liver disease caused by diffuse inflammation and fibrosis that can involve the entire biliary tree. The cause is unknown, but presumed to be immune mediated, and there is a very close association with inflammatory bowel disease, particularly ulcerative colitis.

The disorder tends to affect men (male:female 2:1), some presenting with fatigue, intermittent jaundice, weight loss, right upper quadrant pain, and pruritus, but many are asymptomatic at diagnosis, which is made incidentally when a persistently raised serum alkaline phosphatase is discovered, usually in the setting of ulcerative colitis.

Serum biochemical tests usually indicate cholestasis, but diagnosis is based on three criteria: (1) generalized beading and stenosis of the biliary system on cholangiography; (2) absence of choledocholithiasis or a history of bile duct surgery; and (3) exclusion of bile duct cancer, usually by prolonged follow-up.

There is no curative treatment. Pruritus is initially managed with cholestyramine, with second-line treatments including rifampicin and naltrexone. Orthotopic liver transplantation is the only option available for young patients with advanced liver disease.

Introduction

Primary sclerosing cholangitis (PSC) is a chronic cholestatic liver disease caused by diffuse inflammation and fibrosis that can involve the entire biliary tree. The progressive pathological process obliterates intrahepatic and extrahepatic bile ducts, ultimately leading to biliary cirrhosis, portal hypertension hepatic failure. Cholangiocarcinoma develops in about 10 to 30% of patients during the course of the disease. PSC was initially considered to be a rare disease; however, the advent of endoscopic retrograde cholangiopancreatography (ERCP) in the early 1970s established the diagnosis in a progressively larger number of patients. This led to the realization that PSC has a much wider clinical and pathological spectrum than was previously recognized.

The generally accepted diagnostic criteria of PSC are: (1) generalized beading and stenosis of the biliary system on cholangiography (Fig. 15.21.4.1); (2) absence of choledocholithiasis or a history of bile duct surgery; and (3) exclusion of bile duct cancer, usually by prolonged follow-up.

The term 'secondary sclerosing cholangitis' is used to describe the typical bile duct changes when a clear predisposing factor to duct fibrosis, such as previous bile duct surgery, can be identified. The causes of secondary sclerosing cholangitis are shown in Box 15.21.4.1.

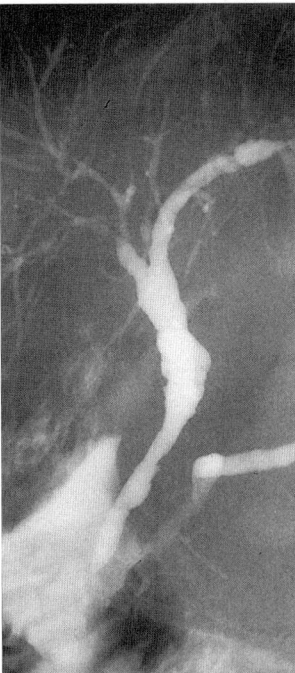

Fig. 15.21.4.1 Endoscopic retrograde cholangiogram (ERCP) showing the typical features of PSC with stricturing and dilatation of the intra- and extrahepatic biliary tree.

> **Box 15.21.4.1** Causes of secondary sclerosing cholangitis
>
> - Previous bile duct surgery with stricturing and cholangitis
> - Bile duct stones causing cholangitis
> - Intrahepatic infusion of 5-fluorodeoxyuridine
> - Formalin insertion into hepatic hydatid cysts
> - Alcohol insertion into hepatic tumours
> - AIDS/immunodeficiency states—probably infective (chronic cytomegalovirus or cryptosporidial infection)
> - IgG4-associated sclerosing cholangitis

Aetiology

The cause of PSC remains unknown. There is a very close association, however, between PSC and inflammatory bowel disease, particularly ulcerative colitis. Approximately two-thirds of northern European patients with PSC have coexisting ulcerative colitis, and PSC is the most common form of chronic liver disease found in ulcerative colitis. In southern Europeans about one-half of patients with PSC will have ulcerative colitis. However in Japan only 20% of patients will also have inflammatory bowel disease. This difference in populations may be real or may represent differences in case finding as not all the patients studied had had colonoscopy and colonic biopsies performed.

Some 3 to 10% of patients with ulcerative colitis will develop PSC, and the prevalence is greater in patients with substantial or total colitis than in those with distal colitis only. In a Swedish study, the prevalence of ulcerative colitis was 171 per 100 000 population and that of PSC 6.3 per 100 000 population. Recent studies from North America and South Wales have demonstrated a prevalence of 20 per 100 000 population in male patients.

Any proposed aetiopathogenic factor must explain this close association with inflammatory bowel disease. Current evidence suggests that PSC is an immunologically mediated disease, probably triggered in genetically susceptible by acquired toxic or infectious agents, which may gain access through the 'leaky' diseased colon.

Immunogenetic factors

Case reports of families in whom members developed ulcerative colitis and PSC led to the search for an HLA association. A close link with the HLA *A1-B8-DR3* haplotype has been found, in common with other organ-specific autoimmune diseases such as autoimmune chronic active hepatitis. Independent associations with HLA *DR2* and *DR6* have also been documented. HLA *A1-B8-DR3*, *DR2*, and *DR6* are equally distributed in patients with PSC, with or without ulcerative colitis. It has been suggested that *DR3*, *DR6*, and *DR2* encode for amino acids in the HLA β-chain that may enhance antigen presentation by the HLA molecule to the T-cell receptor. Further evidence of an immune-mediated basis for this condition has been provided by many studies that have shown humoral and cellular immune abnormalities.

Humoral immune abnormalities

Like primary biliary cirrhosis, a disease with which it shares many features (see Chapter 15.21.3), symptomatic PSC is characterized by hypergammaglobulinaemia; high concentrations of serum IgM are found in patients with advanced disease, and high levels of IgG are found in all children with PSC. Smooth-muscle antibody and antinuclear factor are also found in approximately one-third of patients with PSC, usually in low titres.

A cytoplasmic antineutrophil antibody is found in the serum of 80% of patients with PSC and approximately 30 to 40% of patients with ulcerative colitis. However, the antibody is not specific for PSC and is found in 50% of patients with autoimmune chronic active hepatitis (type 1). The antigen(s) are distinct from those found in Wegener's granulomatosis, which have been shown to be proteinase 3 and myeloperoxidase. Current evidence suggests that the antigen may be a nuclear envelope protein. The pathogenetic significance of the circulating antibody is not clear, but it may prove to be useful in a diagnostic test. Titres of the antibody do not change after hepatic transplantation.

Cellular immune abnormalities

Elevated circulating immune complexes associated with activation of complement via the classic pathway have been found in the serum and bile of patients with PSC. In common with other autoimmune diseases, there are reduced levels of T-suppressor cells circulating in the serum of these patients, leading to an increased ratio of T-helper to T-suppressor cells. Infiltration of portal tracts by increased numbers of mononuclear cells is seen in liver biopsies from patients with PSC. The majority of these cells are activated T lymphocytes.

Current evidence suggests that PSC is an immunologically mediated disease, perhaps triggered in genetically susceptible subjects by acquired toxic or infectious agents, which are presented through antigen-presenting cells to activated T lymphocytes. Unlike normal biliary cells, the biliary epithelial cells in PSC express HLA class II molecules and also intercellular adhesion molecules (ICAM) such as ICAM-1. It has been suggested that the biliary disease is mediated by long-lived memory T cells derived from the inflamed gut which enter the enterohepatic circulation,hence gaining access to the liver. Aberrant expression of chemokines and adhesion molecules on biliary cells cause recruitment of these gut-derived T cells, to the liver which in turn leads to biliary inflammation and damage. However, the reason ('trigger factor') for the aberrant expression is unknown.

Alternative hypothesis—exposure to bacterial components

An alternative hypothesis has been proposed in which the initial event is the reaction of an immunologically susceptible host to bacterial cell wall products. This reaction would result in hepatic macrophages producing tumour necrosis factor-α (TNFα) and endotoxin. The exposure to bacterial components and increased gut permeability would be increased by the presence of inflammatory bowel disease, but could also, in theory, occur during episodes of gut infection. The resulting increase in peribiliary cytokine and chemokine secretion would attract activated neutrophils, monocyte/macrophages, T cells, and fibroblasts. The deposition of concentric fibrosis could result in atrophy of the biliary epithelial cells secondary to ischaemia. The resulting bile duct loss would lead to progressive cholestasis, fibrosis, and secondary biliary cirrhosis. This hypothesis does not explain the relative scarcity of patients with Crohn's colitis and does not take into account the strong circumstantial evidence of immune mediation and autoimmunity, previously described.

Clinical features

There is a clear male predominance, with a male:female ratio of 2:1. The majority of patients present between the ages of 25 and 40 years, although PSC may be diagnosed at any age. Indeed, it has recently become recognized as an important cause of chronic liver disease in children.

The clinical presentation is variable: some patients may present with fatigue, intermittent jaundice, weight loss, right upper quadrant pain, and pruritus. Attacks of acute cholangitis are surprisingly rare and usually follow instrumental biliary intervention, such as ERCP. Physical examination is abnormal in approximately one-half of symptomatic patients; the most common findings are jaundice and hepatosplenomegaly. The majority of patients with PSC are asymptomatic at diagnosis, which is made incidentally when a persistently raised serum alkaline phosphatase is discovered, usually in the setting of ulcerative colitis.

Serum biochemical tests usually indicate cholestasis, but PSC may cause no abnormalities of serum biochemistry. The serum alkaline phosphatase is often raised to more than three times normal, and mild elevations in liver transaminases are seen in the majority of patients. Serum bilirubin is not usually elevated until later stages of the disease. Levels of bilirubin and alkaline phosphatase may fluctuate widely in an individual patient during the course of the disease. Hypoalbuminaemia is unusual until the disease becomes advanced. As mentioned above, increased serum IgM concentrations are seen in about one-half of the symptomatic adult patients, but high concentrations of IgG are always found in children with PSC.

In addition to the serum antineutrophil antibodies, low levels of antinuclear antibody and smooth-muscle antibody may be found in approximately one-third of patients, but serum mitochondrial antibodies are absent.

Diagnosis
Radiological features

The cholangiographic appearances on ERCP are usually diagnostic and consist of multiple, irregular stricturing and dilatation (beading of the intrahepatic and extrahepatic biliary ducts) (Fig. 15.21.4.1). Occasionally, involvement is localized to the intrahepatic system, and even more rarely, only the extrahepatic bile ducts may be involved. Small diverticula are found along the common bile duct in about 20% of patients and are pathognomonic (Fig. 15.21.4.2). Magnetic resonance cholangiopancreatography (MRCP) provides a noninvasive method of imaging the biliary tree, and has become established as the standard technique for the diagnosis of PSC (Fig. 15.21.4.3) as there is a significant risk of cholangitis or acute pancreatitis after diagnostic ERCP. Approximately 20% of patients have stricturing of the main pancreatic duct, although exocrine pancreatic insufficiency is rare.

Pathological features

The histological appearances of liver are not usually diagnostic for PSC, although some form of biliary disease can usually be identified. The characteristic early features of PSC are periductal 'onion skin' fibrosis and inflammation, portal oedema, and bile ductular proliferation resulting in the expansion of the portal tracts (Fig. 15.21.4.4). Later, fibrosis spreads into the liver parenchyma to form

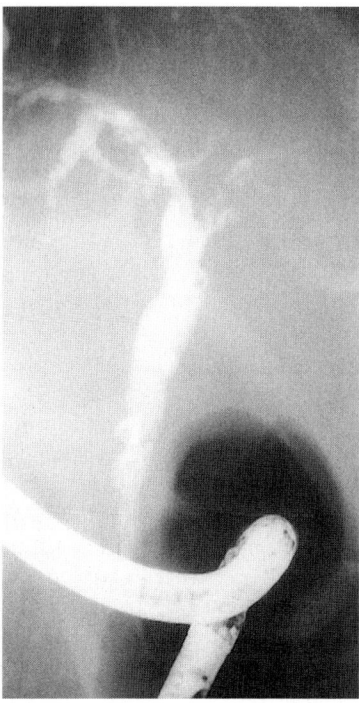

Fig. 15.21.4.2 ERCP from a patient with PSC showing a diverticular appearance of the common bile duct.

fibrous septa, leading inevitably to biliary cirrhosis. As in primary biliary cirrhosis, with disease progression an obliterative cholangitis occurs, leading to complete replacement of the intralobular bile ducts by connective tissue—the so-called 'vanishing bile duct' syndrome. In addition, piecemeal necrosis, copper-binding protein, cholestasis, and occasional portal phlebitis may be present.

Small duct PSC

A variant of the disease called 'small duct PSC' is applied to the small percentage (approximately 10%) of patients with characteristic clinical and histological findings but who have normal cholangiography. These patients usually present with abnormal cholestatic

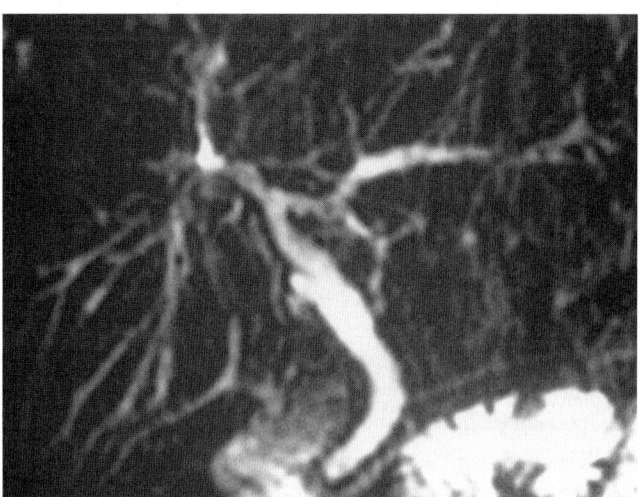

Fig. 15.21.4.3 MRCP demonstrating hilar stricture and intrahepatic involvement of the biliary tree.

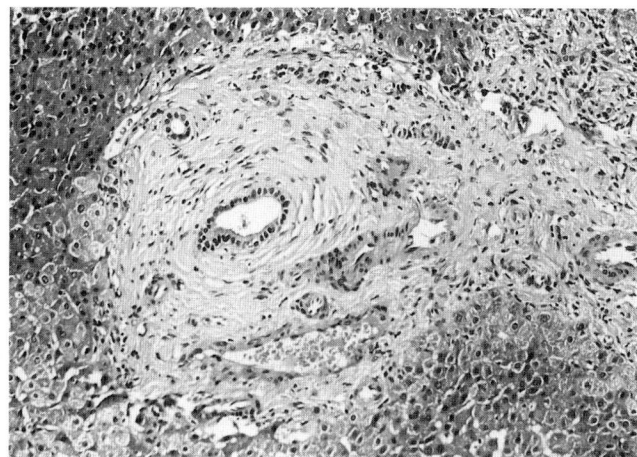

Fig. 15.21.4.4 The hepatic histological changes of early PSC showing a concentric (onion skin) fibrosis around the bile ducts.

biochemical tests in the context of inflammatory bowel disease. The absence of macroscopic cholangiographic abnormalities necessitates liver biopsy for the diagnosis of small duct PSC.

Small duct PSC appears to have a more favourable prognosis, with a median survival of 29.5 years compared to 17 years for classical PSC. Only around 25% of patients with small duct PSC progress to large duct disease and no cases of cholangiocarcinoma have been reported.

Association with other diseases

A large number of diseases have been associated with PSC (Box 15.21.4.2). The most important association, as discussed above, is with inflammatory bowel disease, particularly ulcerative colitis. The extent of the colitis is usually total but symptomatically, and paradoxically, mild, often with no rectal bleeding and characterized by prolonged remission. Rectal sparing is found in 20% of patients with ulcerative colitis and PSC compared with 5% of patients with ulcerative colitis alone. These differences have led to the suggestion that the colitis associated with PSC may represent a distinct form of colitis viz PSC/IBD with a distinct genetic background.

Box 15.21.4.2 Diseases associated with primary sclerosing cholangitis
◆ Ulcerative colitis
◆ Crohn's colitis
◆ Chronic pancreatitis
◆ Retroperitoneal fibrosis
◆ Riedel's struma
◆ Autoimmune pancreatitis
◆ Retroorbital tumours
◆ Sjögren's syndrome
◆ Angioimmunoblastic lymphadenopathy
◆ Histiocytosis X
◆ Autoimmune haemolytic anaemia

Although the symptoms of ulcerative colitis usually develop before those of PSC, the onset of the latter may precede the symptoms of colitis by some years. The outcome of PSC is completely unrelated to the activity, severity, or clinical course of the colitis, and colectomy has no effect on the progression of the cholangitis. PSC is less common in Crohn's disease, occurring in less than 1% of patients and only in those with Crohn's colitis. Patients with PSC and ulcerative colitis are at greater risk of developing colorectal dysplasia and colonic cancer than those with ulcerative colitis alone. In a Swedish study, the absolute accumulative risk of developing colorectal dysplasia/cancer in the PSC/ulcerative colitis group was 9, 31, and 50%, respectively, after 10, 20, and 25 years of disease duration. In the group with ulcerative colitis alone, the corresponding risk was 2, 5, and 10%, respectively.

Some patients with autoimmune pancreatitis develop biliary strictures similar to PSC viz IgG4-associated sclerosing cholangitis. Serum IgG4 levels are increased in patients with autoimmune pancreatitis and the disease is highly responsive to corticosteroids with improvement in the biliary stricturing (unlike PSC). Elevated IgG4 levels have been found in around 10% of a primary sclerosing population, and further studies are required to clarify the relationship between the two conditions. It is recommended that all patients with presumed PSC should be screened for IgG4-associated sclerosing cholangitis.

Natural history and prognosis

The course of PSC is highly variable and unpredictable. The median survival from presentation to death or liver transplantation in symptomatic patients is approximately 10 to 12 years, and approximately 75% of asymptomatic patients survive 15 years or more. In the past, the majority of patients died of hepatic failure following deepening cholestatic jaundice. However, with the advent of successful liver transplantation the majority of patients die of malignancy, either hepatobiliary or colonic. Approximately 10 to 30% of patients with long-standing PSC die from the development of bile duct carcinoma, which often follows a very aggressive course. The mean survival after the diagnosis of cholangiocarcinoma is only 9 months. Unfortunately, there are no factors that will predict which patients will develop this cancer. Tumour markers such as CEA and CA 19-9 have been investigated as potential serum markers of the development of bile duct cancer in PSC. Although some centres have found elevations in serum CA 19-9 a useful predictor, these results have not been confirmed in other units. Attempts to model factors that will predict the risk of progression to liver failure and death have yielded conflicting data from different centres. It is probable that the majority of asymptomatic patients will progress insidiously to symptomatic liver disease, liver failure, and death.

Treatment

Symptomatic measures

There is no curative treatment for PSC. This is indicated by the plethora of medical, endoscopic, and surgical approaches that has been advocated. Treatment of cholestasis, complications, and specific disease processes may all be required in the management of an individual patient.

Management of cholestasis

Symptomatic patients are frequently troubled by pruritus. This is best managed initially by cholestyramine and the dose should be increased until relief is obtained. Second-line treatments include rifampicin and the opioid antagonist naltrexone. In addition, replacement of fat-soluble vitamins is necessary when patients become jaundiced. Metabolic bone disease (usually osteoporosis) is a common complication of advanced PSC. Calcium supplementation with vitamin D_3 should be given prophylactically in jaundiced patients and bisphosphonates considered in patients with osteoporosis.

Management of complications

Broad-spectrum antibiotics such as ciprofloxacin should be given for acute attacks of cholangitis. If cholangiography shows a well-defined obstruction to the main extrahepatic bile ducts, then mechanical relief must be considered. Balloon dilatation of the strictures may prove useful in a minority of patients with well-defined localized particularly main duct strictures and can lead to a striking improvement in symptoms and serum biochemistry.

In a minority of patients the best approach is to introduce a temporary prosthesis (stent) through the obstruction. This may be placed nonoperatively by the percutaneous transhepatic route or at ERCP.

Another common complication is the development of small biliary stones (brown pigment) and biliary sludge, which can lead to a rapid clinical or biochemical deterioration. In these patients, endoscopic sphincterotomy with extraction of the biliary debris can be beneficial.

Specific treatment

Medical

The medical treatment of PSC has included trials of corticosteroids, immunosuppressive drugs, cholecystogogues, and antibiotics, either alone or in combination. The results have been universally disappointing, although assessment of treatment of this uncommon disease is difficult because the clinical course fluctuates, survival is variable, and some patients may remain asymptomatic for long periods of time. The role of corticosteroid therapy is unclear. There have been no large controlled trials, but corticosteroids have been used topically and systemically in small and generally uncontrolled studies. However, there is evidence that, even in male patients, metabolic bone disease may be accelerated by corticosteroids and in general they should not be used in this condition. They should be reserved for the minority of patients who also exhibit features of autoimmune hepatitis (PSC/autoimmune overlap) or in those patients with IgG4-associated biliary disease.

A number of immunosuppressant agents have been tried, either alone or in combination, including azathioprine, methotrexate, and ciclosporin. Overall, the results have been disappointing.

Ursodeoxycholic acid (UDCA) is a nonhepatotoxic hydrophilic bile acid which has been used widely for the treatment of cholestasis—it reduces levels of cholestatic liver enzymes. Controlled trials in PSC have shown no effect on symptoms, histology, or survival. However, UDCA has been shown to lower the prevalence of colonic dysplasia and possibly cholangiocarcinoma.

Surgical

The role of hepatobiliary surgery in the treatment of PSC remains controversial. Good results have been claimed for the resection of the extrahepatic biliary tree followed by biliary reconstruction with silastic transhepatic stents. However, controlled trials are needed to confirm the efficacy of these and other surgical techniques, as previous biliary surgery will increase perioperative mortality from hepatic transplantation.

Transplantation

Orthotopic liver transplantation is the only option available in young patients with PSC and advanced liver disease. PSC is now the second most common indication for liver transplantation in the United Kingdom. Recent results have been very encouraging, with 5-year survival rates of 75 to 90% being obtained in most centres. These rates compare favourably with those for other forms of chronic liver disease. It has become clear that PSC recurs in the transplanted liver in 30% of patients at 5 years post-transplant. In a minority of patients recurrence has led to problems with liver decompensation, requiring retransplantation. Recurrence is commoner in male patients with an intact colon. Proven cholangiocarcinoma is a contradiction to transplantation because the tumour recurs rapidly after transplantation with immunosuppression. As patients suffering from PSC in combination with ulcerative colitis have an increased risk for the development of colon cancer after transplantation, yearly colonoscopy has been recommended in this group. Several centres have noted a worsening in the symptoms of ulcerative colitis after transplantation; the explanation for this phenomenon remains unclear.

Further reading

Bambha K, *et al.* (2003). Incidence, clinical spectrum, and outcomes of primary sclerosing cholangitis in a United States community. *Gastroenterology*, **125**, 1364–9.

Bergquist A, *et al.* (2002). Hepatic and extra hepatic malignancies in primary sclerosing cholangitis. *J Hepatol*, **36**, 321–7.

Broome U, *et al.* (1995). Primary sclerosing cholangitis and ulcerative colitis: evidence for increased neoplastic potential. *Hepatology*, **22**, 1404–8.

Broome U, Olsson RK, Loof L (1996). Natural history and prognostic factors in 305 Swedish patients with primary sclerosing cholangitis. *Gut*, **38**, 610–15.

Burak K, *et al.* (2004). Incidence and risk factors for cholangiocarcinoma in primary sclerosing cholangitis. *Am J Gastroenterol*, **99**, 523–6.

Chalasami N, *et al.* (2000). Cholangiocarcinoma in patients with primary sclerosing cholangitis: a multicentre case–control study. *Hepatology*, **31**, 7–11.

Chapman RW (2006). Primary sclerosing cholangitis. *Semin Liver Dis*, **26**, 1–88.

Chapman RW, *et al.* (1980). Primary sclerosing cholangitis—a review of its clinical features, cholangiography and hepatic histology. *Gut*, **21**, 870–7.

Donaldson PT, *et al.* (1991). Dual association of HLA DR2 and DR3 with primary sclerosing cholangitis. *Hepatology*, **13**, 129–33.

Gow PJ, Chapman RW. (2000). Liver transplantation for primary sclerosing cholangitis. *Liver*, **20**, 97–103.

Graziadei IW, *et al.* (1999). Recurrence of Primary sclerosing cholangitis following liver transplantation. *Hepatology*, **29**, 1050–6.

Kingham JG, Kochar N, Gravenor MB (2004). Incidence, clinical patterns, and outcomes of Primary sclerosing cholangitis in South Wales, United Kingdom. *Gastroenterology*, **126**, 1929–30.

Levy C, *et al.* (2005). The value of serum CA 19-9 in predicting cholangiocarcinomas in patients with primary sclerosing cholangitis. *Digest Dis Sci*, **50**, 1734–40.

Lindor KD, *et al.* (2009). High-dose ursodeoxycholic acid for the treatment of primary sclerosing cholangitis. *Hepatology*, **50**, 808–14.

Lo SK, Fleming KA, Chapman RW (1992). Prevalence of antineutrophil antibody in Primary sclerosing cholangitis and ulcerative colitis using an alkaline phosphatase method. *Gut*, **33**, 1370–5.

Loftus EV Jr, *et al.* (2005). PSC_IBD:a unique form of inflammatory bowel disease associated with primary sclerosing cholangitis. *Gut*, **54**, 91–6.

Ludwig J, *et al.* (1981). Morphological features of chronic hepatitis associated with Primary sclerosing cholangitis and ulcerative colitis. *Hepatology*, **1**, 632–40.

Mitchell SA, *et al.* (2001). A preliminary trial of high dose ursodeoxycholic acid in primary sclerosing cholangitis. *Gastroenterology*, **122**, 900–7.

Olsson R, *et al.* (2005). Five year treatment with high dose UDCA in PSC. *Gastroenterology*, **129**, 1464–72.

Pardi DS, Lindor KD (2003). Ursodeoxycholic acid as a chemopreventitive agent in patients with ulcerative colitis and primary sclerosing cholangitis. *Gastroenterology*, **124**, 889–93.

Stiehl A, *et al.* (2002). Development of dominant bile duct stenoses in patients with Primary sclerosing cholangitis treated with ursodeoxycholic acid:outcome after endoscopic treatment. *J Hepatol*, **36**, 151–6.

Terjung B, *et al.* (1998). Atypical antinuclear cytoplasmic antibodies with perinuclear fluorescence in chronic inflammatory bowel diseases and hepatobiliary disorders colocalise with nuclear lamina proteins. *Hepatology*, **28**, 332–40.

15.22

Other disorders of the liver

Contents

titis and/or cirrhosis. It is not clear how alcohol causes liver disease, but likely mechanisms include (1) oxidative stress and acetaldehyde produced during ethanol metabolism, and (2) innate and adaptive immune responses. Factors determining the variable susceptibility to liver disease in heavy drinkers include a variety of host and environmental factors which affect these mechanisms.

Clinical manifestations can be extremely variable, ranging from completely asymptomatic to severe hepatic failure. Although patients can present with a life-threatening complication, most often they do so with symptoms unrelated to the liver, typically nonspecific digestive symptoms or vague psychiatric complaints. The key to the early recognition of alcohol-related disease is having a high index of suspicion, with confirmation by (1) direct questioning for alcohol history and alcohol-related symptoms; (2) clinical examination for signs of chronic liver disease; (3) supportive investigations, including elevation of serum γ-glutamyl transferase (γGT) and aspartate transaminase (AST); and (4) liver biopsy, which is often required for accurate prognostication, revealing alcoholic fatty liver, alcoholic hepatitis, or cirrhosis.

Management is governed by the stage and severity of the liver disease, but always includes abstinence and adequate nutritional support. Corticosteroids and pentoxifylline can reduce mortality in selected patients with severe acute alcoholic hepatitis. Transplantation remains the only effective treatment for alcoholic cirrhosis, although this remains controversial, principally due to concerns over the risk of post-transplant recidivism.

15.22.1 **Alcoholic liver disease**

Stephen F. Stewart and Chris P. Day

Essentials

The incidence of alcoholic liver disease (ALD) follows the trend of *per capita* alcohol consumption, with the spectrum of hepatic injury ranging from the preliminary stage of fatty liver to alcoholic hepa-

Introduction

It is likely that humans have been consuming alcohol in excess since the Stone Age, and the ancient Greeks made the link between alcohol and liver damage. In spite of this association, the consumption of potentially hazardous quantities of alcohol persists and alcoholic liver disease (ALD) is currently the most common cause of liver disease in the Western world. In some countries consumption is increasing. The magnitude and range of the health and socioeconomic problems attributable to alcohol abuse are enormous, but this chapter will primarily focus on pathogenesis, epidemiology, and treatment.

Pathogenesis

There are several pathogenetic mechanisms through which ethanol can cause liver injury. These include the direct effect of ethanol metabolism on liver biochemistry and hepatocyte functioning, the release of cytokines as a result of portal endotoxinemia, and liver-directed adaptive immune responses generated towards new antigens formed through these first two mechanisms.

Ethanol metabolism and pathogenesis

Ethanol metabolism

Over 90% of circulating alcohol is oxidatively metabolized, primarily in the liver, and excreted as CO_2 and water.

Alcohol oxidation in the liver takes place via three steps. First alcohol is oxidized, principally within the cytosol, to acetaldehyde. Then acetaldehyde is further oxidized to acetate, primarily within the mitochondria, and finally, acetate is released into the blood and oxidized to CO_2 and water in peripheral tissues. At least three enzyme systems with the capacity to oxidize alcohol to acetaldehyde are present within the liver (Fig. 15.22.1.1), although in normal individuals only the alcohol dehydrogenase enzymes are important.

ADHs catalyse the oxidation of a variety of alcohols to aldehydes and ketones. This includes catalysing the oxidation of ethanol to acetaldehyde and transferring hydrogen to the cofactor nicotinamide adenine dinucleotide (NAD) which is converted to its reduced form, NADH. In addition to ADH, alcohol is metabolized by the microsomal ethanol oxidizing system (MEOS), an accessory pathway that principally involves a specific alcohol-inducible form of cytochrome P450 designated CYP2E1. Its K_m for alcohol

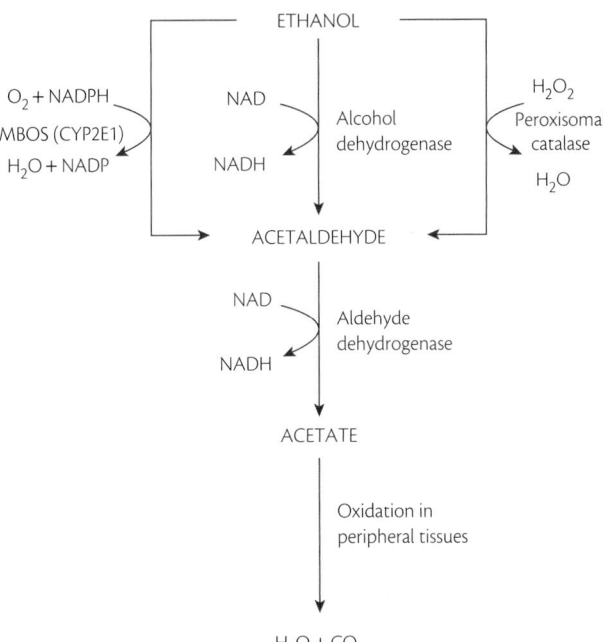

Fig. 15.22.1.1 The three common pathways of ethanol metabolism: alcohol dehydrogenase (ADH), the microsomal ethanol oxidizing system (MEOS) and catalase. NAD(H), nicotinamide adenine dinucleotide and its reduced form; NADP(H), nicotinamide adenine dinucleotide phosphate and its reduced form.

is in the order of 50 to 80 mg/100 ml, so in view of its inducibility it appears to play an important role at high blood alcohol levels or following chronic alcohol abuse.

The third pathway for alcohol oxidation is catalysed by the enzyme catalase. This enzyme is located in the peroxisomes of most tissues and the pathway accounts for less than 2% of overall *in vivo* alcohol oxidation.

Acetaldehyde is further oxidized in the liver to acetate by aldehyde dehydrogenases (ALDHs). ALDH, like ADH, uses NAD as a cofactor and further increases the NADH/NAD ratio. ALDH2 is responsible for the majority of acetaldehyde oxidation and exists in at least two allelic forms, *ALDH2*1* and *ALDH2*2*, with the gene product of the *ALDH2*2* allele (found in 50% of east Asians) having little or no catalytic activity. Homozygotes for the *ALDH2*2* allele develop an unpleasant 'flushing' reaction after alcohol that is thought to be due to acetaldehyde. ALDH inhibitors such as disulfiram (Antabuse) use this mechanism in the treatment of alcoholism.

Ethanol metabolism may result in the generation of fatty liver (steatosis), oxidative stress/lipid peroxidation, and acetaldehyde, all of which are thought to be important in disease pathogenesis.

Pathogenesis of fatty liver

Accumulation of triacylglycerol is the consequence of increased substrate (free fatty acids and glycerol 3-phosphate) supply, increased esterification, and decreased export from the liver. Alcohol intake increases availability of free fatty acids through the lipolysis of adipose tissue, impairment of gluconeogenesis, increased fatty acid synthesis, and reduced oxidation. The altered NADH/NAD ratio generated during ethanol metabolism also increases the production of glycerol 3-phosphate, thereby again promoting triacylglycerol synthesis. The decrease in export of triacylglycerol from the liver appears to be primarily due to ethanol-induced down-regulation of microsomal triglyceride transfer protein (MTP), the principal enzyme responsible for packaging triacylglycerol and apolipoprotein B (apoB) into very low-density lipoprotein (VLDL) particles.

Oxidative stress and lipid peroxidation

An accumulating body of evidence now supports a role for oxidative stress and lipid peroxidation in the pathogenesis of ethanol-induced liver injury, though considerable controversy remains regarding the most important source of reactive oxygen species in ALD. The most likely candidates are microsomal CYP2E1 (the only source of hydroxyethyl radicals), the mitochondrial electron transport chain, inducible nitric oxide synthase, and Kupffer cells (Fig. 15.22.1.2). Any liver injury due to oxidative stress is compounded by the depletion in antioxidant defences found after chronic alcohol consumption.

Acetaldehyde

It has been known for some time that acetaldehyde can form Schiff bases with the valine, lysine, and tyrosine residues on cellular proteins, resulting in both stable and unstable adduct formation. This may disrupt protein function and can result in the production of immunodominant antigenic determinants. In addition, acetaldehyde mediates the ethanol-induced susceptibility of hepatocytes to cytotoxicity induced by tumour necrosis factor-α (TNFα).

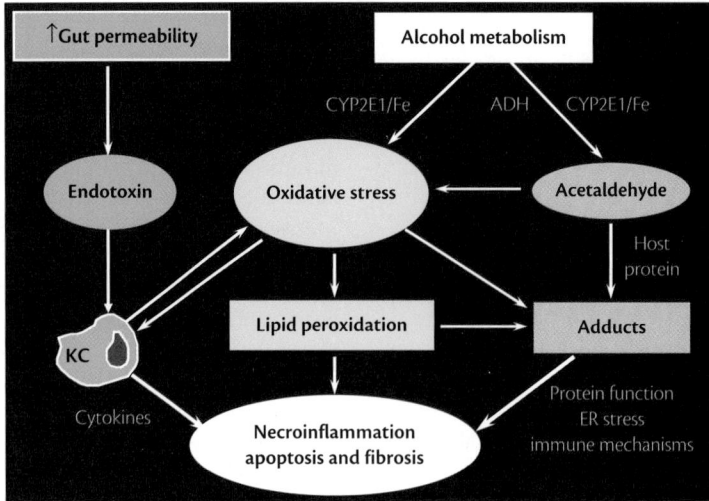

Fig. 15.22.1.2 Mechanisms of hepatocyte injury in alcoholic steatohepatitis. The metabolism of ethanol through the cytochrome P450 2E1 pathway results in oxidative stress and lipid peroxidation. Ethanol metabolism produces acetaldehyde which is directly, through disturbing protein function and generating endoplasmic reticular stress, and indirectly, through the generation of immunogenic adducts, hepatotoxic. Ethanol consumption also increases gut permeability, resulting in portal endotoxinaemia and cytokine production from Kupffer cells. ADH, alcohol dehydrogenase; CYP2E1, cytochrome P450 2E1; ER, endoplasmic reticular; Fe, iron; KC, Kupffer cell.

Innate immune system

Endotoxin, which refers collectively to the lipopolysaccharide components of the cell wall of all Gram-negative bacteria, appears to play a central role in the development of ALD. Ethanol ingestion increases the translocation of endotoxin from the gut lumen to the portal circulation where it induces macrophages (Kupffer cells) to produce cytokines and Reactive oxygen species. These Kupffer cells are the primary intrahepatic source of TNFα, a cytokine believed to be central to disease pathogenesis.

Adaptive immune system

Several clinical features imply that adaptive immune mechanisms may have a role in disease pathogenesis. Patients often display hypergammaglobulinemia, and lymphocyte infiltration is a well-recognized histological feature of advanced disease. Studies to date have revealed that there are specific antibody and cellular responses to proteins formed during ethanol metabolism and in some patients there is also autoantibody formation. Further work is required to determine whether these specific immune responses are an important part of disease progression or an epiphenomenon.

Susceptibility

It is still not clear why only around one-third of heavy drinkers develop alcoholic hepatitis and fewer progress to cirrhosis. The risk of developing ALD appears to begin at around 30 g/day of ethanol, but only around 5% of the individuals drinking this much show signs of liver disease. There is evidence to suggest that risk is higher in women and among individuals over 50 if alcohol is drunk outside mealtimes or consumed in a variety of different beverages. The highest risk is seen in drinkers who do not include wine in their drinking repertoire. No dose of alcohol confers a guarantee of developing cirrhosis, regardless of the length of time over which it is consumed, and relatively low doses can cause problems.

It is now clear that obesity and associated hyperglycaemia increase the incidence of all stages of ALD in heavy drinkers. Animal studies coupled with epidemiological data point to the fact that dietary fats, particularly polyunsaturated fats, may have a role in disease progression.

Evidence for the importance of genetic factors comes from a study showing that concordance rates for alcoholic cirrhosis are three times higher in monozygotic than in dizygotic twin pairs. This is not entirely explained by the difference in concordance rates for alcoholism *per se* and associations have been found between disease and polymorphisms in genes influencing the severity of steatosis (microsomal triglyceride transfer protein), ethanol metabolism (ADH2 and ALDH2), and cytokine production (TNFα and IL-10 promoters).

Epidemiology

During a period of wine rationing in France during the Second World War, cirrhosis deaths reduced by 80%. A similar effect was observed during the Prohibition era in the United States of America (1919–1933). These and other studies have highlighted the close correlation between deaths from cirrhosis and *per capita* alcohol consumption. The worldwide increase in mortality from cirrhosis observed during the 1950s and 1960s was associated with a similar rise in alcohol consumption, attributed largely to the falling price of alcohol relative to income. This reduction in real price, the increased availability of alcohol, and heavy promotion by the drinks industry have lead to a doubling of alcohol consumption in the United Kingdom since 1960. This increase in consumption has been followed by a dramatic increase in cirrhosis mortality in the United Kingdom between the late 1980s and 2000. This contrasts sharply with a reduction in mortality in most other European countries and the United States of America. These latest data closely link cirrhosis mortality with a rise in alcohol consumption.

Clinical features

Diagnosis

Alcohol-related liver damage is a spectrum, with the various lesions (fatty liver (steatosis), alcoholic hepatitis, and cirrhosis) occurring more commonly in combination than in isolation. The clinical manifestations can be extremely variable, ranging from completely asymptomatic to severe hepatic failure.

Initially, patients most commonly present with symptoms unrelated to the liver, typically nonspecific digestive symptoms or vague psychiatric complaints. The key to the early recognition of patients with alcohol-related disease is a high index of suspicion. Once the diagnosis is suspected it is usually easy to confirm by direct questioning for alcohol history and alcohol-related symptoms, careful clinical examination, and supportive laboratory investigations.

Important features to note on examination are the signs of chronic liver disease including hepatomegaly and signs indicative of alcohol-related pathology in other organs such as hypertension, atrial fibrillation, and a cushingoid appearance. Many of the classical signs of chronic liver disease, including spider nevi, Dupuytren's contractures, palmar erythema, and parotid swelling, can occur in alcoholics in the absence of cirrhosis. Clinical signs and history cannot be relied upon to distinguish the various histological subtypes of ALD, since patients with cirrhosis can be asymptomatic while patients with hepatocellular failure may have only severe fatty change.

Biochemical and haematological tests can suggest the presence of alcohol abuse and indicate the presence of liver damage, but are not useful in determining the severity of the histological lesion. Elevation of γ-glutamyl transferase (γGT) has been reported in up to 90% of patients abusing alcohol but is not specific for alcohol abuse. Its main clinical use is probably in monitoring a period of supposed abstinence, since it falls within a week of cessation of drinking. A raised mean corpuscular volume (MCV) occurs in 80 to 100% of alcoholics with and without liver disease and is due to a direct toxic effect of alcohol on the marrow.

With regard to biochemical markers of alcohol-related liver damage, a rise in serum aspartate transaminase activity (AST) of up to five times normal is common in patients abusing alcohol and reflects the presence, but not the severity, of liver damage. Alanine transaminase (ALT) activity is raised less often than AST, and the AST/ALT ratio is usually greater than 1.

Liver biopsy is useful to accurately stage alcohol-related liver disease. Although many clinicians withhold biopsy, it is often required for accurate prognostication.

Alcoholic fatty liver

Alcoholic fatty liver is indistinguishable histologically from nonalcoholic fatty liver (NAFLD) associated with the metabolic syndrome. Patients with fatty liver are usually asymptomatic or present with nonspecific digestive symptoms. Rarely fatty liver may be associated with hyperlipidaemia, haemolytic anaemia and jaundice (Zieve's syndrome, discussed below) or hepatic failure. Smooth, nontender hepatomegaly is usually the only clinical finding and the γGT, AST, and MCV are often mildly raised.

A growing body of evidence suggests that, rather than being an epiphenomenon of excessive alcohol intake, steatosis may play a direct role in progression to more advanced disease. In several prospective studies of heavy drinkers the severity and pattern of steatosis on index biopsy predicts the subsequent risk of fibrosis and cirrhosis.

Alcoholic hepatitis

Alcoholic hepatitis consists of a constellation of histological abnormalities including ballooning degeneration of hepatocytes, Mallory bodies, and a neutrophil inflammatory cell infiltrate. In addition there is pericellular and perivenular fibrosis, producing a 'chicken-wire' appearance. Progression to cirrhosis is associated with the extent and degree of fibrosis, a panlobular distribution, and widespread Mallory body formation.

There is no good correlation between the severity of the histological lesion and the clinical presentation, although patients with severe histology usually present with symptoms specifically related to hepatocellular failure such as jaundice, ascites and encephalopathy, or variceal bleeding. Clinical decompensation may be precipitated by vomiting, diarrhoea, anorexia, increased alcohol intake, or intercurrent infection. The majority of patients have tender, smooth, hepatomegaly and signs of chronic liver disease may be present.

Blood abnormalities include decreased albumin and increased γGT, AST, bilirubin, alkaline phosphatase, and prothrombin time (PT). Blood urea and serum sodium and potassium are all low, unless hepatorenal syndrome supervenes, and hypoglycaemia may be present. Macrocytic anaemia, neutrophil leucocytosis, and thrombocytopenia are present in all but the mildest cases. Patients with severe alcoholic hepatitis often rapidly deteriorate in the days immediately following hospital admission. The pathophysiological basis of this is not clear.

Clinical and laboratory variables have been used to derive scores to predict short-term mortality in alcoholic hepatitis. The most widely used is the discriminant function which is based on PT and bilirubin only. This has been confirmed as a useful predictor of mortality prospectively. The recently derived Glasgow Alcoholic Hepatitis Score (GAHS) incorporates INR, bilirubin, age, creatinine, and white cell count. Although this scoring system needs validation in large numbers prospectively, initial work suggests that it is more sensitive and specific than the discriminant function at determining prognosis. If the patient survives to hospital discharge, then the long-term prognosis is determined by the initial histology, the progression to cirrhosis, and subsequent drinking behaviour.

Cirrhosis

With progressive injury, fibrous septa link hepatic and portal veins, and regenerative nodules eventually appear. This cirrhosis is usually micronodular and frequently reverts to a macronodular cirrhosis with abstention. Clinical presentation can range from asymptomatic hepatomegaly to hepatic failure and the complications of portal hypertension such as ascites or variceal bleeding. Presentation with severe hepatic decompensation usually implies the presence of continued drinking or the development of hepatocellular carcinoma or portal vein thrombosis. The clinical findings will depend on the presence of portal hypertension or encephalopathy and do not differ significantly from those observed in other forms of cirrhosis. Patients with compensated cirrhosis, particularly if abstinent from alcohol, can have completely normal laboratory investigations, while patients with continued intake will have a similar range of abnormal laboratory investigations to those seen in patients with alcoholic hepatitis. A raised α-fetoprotein suggests the presence of hepatocellular carcinoma and indicates the need for further investigations.

The survival of patients with alcoholic cirrhosis is determined by the clinical and histological severity of the disease at presentation and their subsequent drinking behaviour. In patients with alcoholic cirrhosis hepatocellular carcinoma occurs at a rate of 1 to 2%/year. It is most common in abstaining men.

Treatment

Achieving abstinence

Measures aimed at establishing and maintaining abstinence are critical in the management of patients with ALD. This is best achieved by close liaison between liver physicians and addiction psychiatrists with support from specialist alcohol nurses and trained counsellors. Available treatments for alcohol-dependent patients can be divided into psychological and pharmacological (Table 15.22.1.1). 'Brief intervention' involves educating patients about the nature of their problem and providing then with advice on how to change their behaviour. In spite of the apparent simplicity of this form of management, brief interventions have been shown to significantly increase the chances of heavy drinkers moderating their drinking at 6 and 12 months in an outpatient setting. Cognitive-behavioural therapy and motivational enhancement therapy have also both been shown to reduce drinking in dependent patients in a randomized controlled trial.

Both acamprosate and naltrexone aim to reduce alcohol craving and have been shown to reduce drinking days and increase abstinence rates. Disulfiram, an inhibitor of acetaldehyde dehydrogenase, has been used for many years with conflicting results. The only treatment to undergo assessment in drinkers with liver disease has been the $GABA_B$-receptor antagonist baclofen, which has shown promise in small numbers with short follow-up.

Up to 50% of patients will either abstain completely or achieve a significant reduction in intake after being given simple advice by physicians during their initial presentation, with a significant improvement in survival compared to continued heavy drinkers.

Alcoholic hepatitis

Almost all treatment trials in patients with alcoholic hepatitis have been short-term (usually 1 month) and restricted to patients with a discriminant function greater than 32 and/or encephalopathy. Many treatment modalities have been tried in patients with alcoholic hepatitis, but none has achieved consensus status among practising hepatologists.

Corticosteroids

Steroids are aimed at suppressing the hepatic inflammatory response seen in liver biopsies from patients with severe alcoholic hepatitis. Concern over adverse effects coupled with a continued uncertainty over efficacy has contributed to the reluctance of many clinicians to prescribe steroids for patients with alcoholic hepatitis. This uncertainty may be due to the fact that initial studies were often poorly designed and included patients with a variety of disease severities. The most recent meta-analysis pooled the individual patient data from the three large randomized controlled trials, only including patients with encephalopathy and/or a discriminant function greater than 32. This study showed that steroids improved survival vs placebo (85% vs 65%), with increasing age and creatinine independent predictors of mortality on multivariate analysis. For these patients 40 mg prednisolone for 28 days with a 2-week taper is recommended. If the bilirubin has not fallen by the seventh day of steroid treatment the prognosis is very poor and alternative treatments should be considered. Steroid treatment is still relatively contraindicated in the large number of patients with concomitant infection and gastrointestinal bleeding.

Pentoxifylline is a nonselective phosphodiesterase inhibitor that is approved for use in claudication due to its effect on red blood cell deformability, but also has an anticytokine effect attributed to a reduction in TNFα gene transcription. In the only randomized controlled trial of pentoxifylline, the effective claudication dose (400 mg three times a day) led to a 40% reduction in 28-day mortality in patients with a discriminant function greater than 32. Importantly, almost all of the improvement in survival was due to a fall in mortality from hepatorenal syndrome, suggesting that pentoxifylline may have a specific beneficial effect in

Table 15.22.1.1 Therapeutic options in patients with alcoholic liver disease

Target	Treatment
Addiction	Nonpharmacological
	Brief intervention
	Cognitive therapy
	Motivational enhancement therapy
	Psychotherapy
	Pharmacological
	Baclofen
	Acamprosate
Alcoholic hepatitis	Probable benefit
	Corticosteroids
	Pentoxifylline (one RCT only)
	Possible benefit
	Infliximab
	MARS
Alcoholic cirrhosis	Confirmed benefit
	Liver transplantation
	Possible benefit
	Propylthiouracil
	S-Adenosylmethionine
	Phosphatidylcholine

alcoholic hepatitis patients developing this ominous complication. Clearly, further trials are needed.

Protein–calorie malnutrition is seen in patients presenting with acute severe alcoholic hepatitis and there is a correlation between the severity of malnutrition and mortality. Enteral tube feeding with an energy-dense formula can reduce this mortality and is advised for all these patients.

In spite of the likely role of oxidative stress in disease pathogenesis there is evidence that antioxidants are ineffective in acute alcoholic hepatitis. Likewise, insulin and glucagon, anabolic steroids, and propylthiouracil have no proven role in treatment.

The anti-TNFα drugs infliximab and etanercept have been trialled in acute severe alcoholic hepatitis because of the putative role of TNFα in disease pathogenesis. Although the only large randomized trial using high-dose infliximab in combination with steroids was stopped as a result of a higher mortality in the treatment arm, these drugs may yet prove to have some role. Likewise, the molecular adsorbents recycling system (MARS) has shown promise in preliminary studies and further data is awaited.

A major improvement in survival in patient with severe disease has been seen with the use of glypressin and albumin for hepatorenal syndrome.

Alcoholic cirrhosis

At present the management of patients with advanced fibrotic liver disease is directed at preventing and treating the complications of portal hypertension, liver failure and hepatocellular carcinoma and deciding if and when to consider patients for orthotopic liver transplantation.

No medical therapy for alcoholic cirrhosis has yet reached clinical practice, but some agents have shown initial promise. These will need further trials before general use. Cirrhotic patients who continue to drink moderately may benefit from propylthiouracil, an antithyroid drug that targets the hypermetabolic state seen in ALD. A second agent, S-adenosylmethionine, acts both as an antioxidant by replenishing glutathione and as a methyl donor maintaining cell membrane fluidity. In one trial, a significant beneficial effect of treatment has been found in patients with Child's A and B cirrhosis. Clearly further trials with this agent are awaited with interest. After promising results in baboons, a large, long-term study of phosphatidylcholine in humans with cirrhosis was negative, possibly due to the number of drinkers who dramatically reduced their consumption while under observation.

Liver transplantation

Transplantation for ALD remains controversial, principally due to concerns over the risk of post-transplant recidivism. In spite of initial concerns with regard to comorbidities, patients transplanted for cirrhosis have 5- and 10-year survival rates somewhere between those of patients transplanted for cholestatic and viral hepatitis-related liver disease. In general, transplantation should be restricted to patients with Child's C cirrhosis or a MELD score of greater than 14. The potential effect of abstinence on the severity of disease has lead most units to adopt a policy of offering transplantation only to those patients who continue to have severe liver disease after a period of abstinence.

Around 10% of patients transplanted for ALD will return to problem drinking. This has no impact on early mortality, but mortality in recidivists is significantly higher than in abstainers 10 years post transplant. Efforts to minimize the risk of post-transplant recidivism are important, to avoid the likely adverse effect on the organ-donating public.

Many units have previously insisted on a 6-month period of abstinence. Although this can allow recovery, there is conflicting evidence about whether it can predict recidivism. The chance of recovery in patients with decompensated liver disease can be predicted as early as 3 months.

Transplantation for acute alcoholic hepatitis is very controversial. Although many of these patients undoubtedly have a poor prognosis, and there have been isolated reports of survival following transplantation, most clinical centres do not consider this therapeutic alternative.

Conclusions

Alcohol use and abuse is widespread and endstage liver disease is the result of prolonged heavy alcohol intake in only a small proportion of users. Nevertheless, these patients make up a significant proportion of the workload of most liver units in the Western world. The complex pathogenesis makes it an intriguing disease to study and the overlap of physical and psychological problems make this patient population a fascinating group. Unfortunately, improvements in management of alcoholic hepatitis are slow considering the high mortality of the condition. Liver transplantation remains the mainstay of treatment for advanced cirrhosis. Further research to understand the basics of hepatocyte injury is required to inform further clinical trials and improve mortality in this widespread disease.

Further reading

Akriviadis E, et al. (2000). Pentoxifylline improves short-term survival in severe acute alcoholic hepatitis: a double-blind, placebo-controlled trial. Gastroenterology, 119, 1637–48. [The first trial of pentoxifylline in alcoholic hepatitis.]

Becker U, et al. (2002). Lower risk for alcohol-induced cirrhosis in wine drinkers. Hepatology, 35, 868–75. [A very large epidemiological study into pattern of drinking and susceptibility.]

Bellentani S, et al. (1997). Drinking habits as cofactors of risk for alcohol induced liver damage. The Dionysos Study Group. Gut, 41, 845–50. [A landmark study of liver disease in a given population.]

Cabre E, et al. (2000) Short- and long-term outcome of severe alcohol-induced hepatitis treated with steroids or enteral nutrition: a multicenter randomized trial. Hepatology, 32, 36–42. [RCT of enteral nutrition vs steroids.]

Carithers RL, et al. (1989) Methylprednisolone therapy in patients with severe alcoholic hepatitis. A randomized multicenter trial. Ann Intern Med, 110, 685–90. [RCT of steroids in alcoholic hepatitis noted for the introduction of the discriminant function.]

Day CP (2006). Genes or environment to determine alcoholic liver disease and non-alcoholic fatty liver disease. Liver Int, 26, 1021–8. [Review of susceptibility to alcoholic liver disease.]

Day CP, James OF (1998). Hepatic steatosis: innocent bystander or guilty party? Hepatology, 27, 1463–6. [Review of the role of fat in alcoholic liver disease.]

Hrubec Z, Omenn GS (1981). Evidence of genetic predisposition to alcoholic cirrhosis and psychosis: twin concordances for alcoholism and its biological end points by zygosity among male veterans. Alcohol Clin Exp Res, 5, 207–15. [Only large twin study defining host factors that determine susceptibility.]

Leon DA, McCambridge J (2006). Liver cirrhosis mortality rates in Britain from 1950 to 2002: an analysis of routine data. *Lancet*, **367**, 52–6. [Study of cirrhosis mortality rates showing recent rises in UK.]

Lelbach WK (1975). Cirrhosis in the alcoholic and its relation to the volume of alcohol abuse. *Ann N Y Acad Sci*, **252**, 85–105. [Classic study of alcohol consumption and risk of cirrhosis.]

Lieber CS (2004). The discovery of the microsomal ethanol oxidizing system and its physiologic and pathologic role. *Drug Metab Rev*, **36**, 511–29. [Review of the characteristics of this important pathogenic pathway.]

Mathurin P, *et al.* (2002) Corticosteroids improve short-term survival in patients with severe alcoholic hepatitis (AH): individual data analysis of the last three randomized placebo controlled double blind trials of corticosteroids in severe AH. *J Hepatol*, **36**, 480–7. [Landmark 'super' meta-analysis showing benefit of corticosteroids in well selected patients.]

Mathurin P, *et al.* (2003) Early change in bilirubin levels is an important prognostic factor in severe alcoholic hepatitis treated with prednisolone. *Hepatology*, **38**, 1363–9. [Development of a criterion that allows early detection of patients not responding to steroids.]

Mato JM, *et al.* (1999). S-Adenosylmethionine in alcoholic liver cirrhosis: a randomized, placebo-controlled, double-blind, multicenter clinical trial. *J Hepatol*, **30**, 1081–9. [A rare positive RCT in alcoholic cirrhosis.]

Neuberger J, *et al.* (2002). Transplantation for alcoholic liver disease. *J Hepatol*, **36**, 130–7. [Thorough review of transplantation.]

Sorensen TI, *et al.* (1984) Prospective evaluation of alcohol abuse and alcoholic liver injury in men as predictors of development of cirrhosis. *Lancet*, **ii**, 241–4. [Biopsy predictors of progression.]

Stewart SF, Day CP (2003). The management of alcoholic liver disease. *J Hepatol*, **38** Suppl 1, S2–13. [Review of current treatment for alcoholic liver disease.]

Stewart SF, Day CP (2006). Alcoholic liver disease. In: Boyer T, Manns M, Wright T (eds) *Zakim and Boyer's hepatology*, 5th edition, Chapter 30. Elsevier, Edinburgh.

Stewart SF, Day CP (2007). Ethanol metabolism and pathogenesis of alcoholic liver injury. In: Benhamou JP, *et al.* (eds) *Textbook of hepatology; from basic science to clinical practice*, 3rd edition, Chapter 12.2. Blackwell Publishing, Oxford.

Wilfred de Alwis NM, Day CP (2007). Genetics of alcoholic liver disease and nonalcoholic fatty liver disease. *Semin Liver Dis*, **27**, 44–54. [Thorough review of the genetics of alcoholic liver disease.]

15.22.2 Nonalcoholic steatohepatitis

Stephen F. Stewart and Chris P. Day

Essentials

Nonalcoholic fatty liver disease (NAFLD) is the commonest liver disorder in the developed world, affecting 20 to 30% of Western adults. It comprises a spectrum of disease ranging from simple steatosis through nonalcoholic steatohepatitis (NASH) to fatty fibrosis and ultimately cirrhosis. It is a manifestation of the metabolic syndrome, strongly associated with obesity, insulin resistance, and dyslipidaemia, with dietary and genetic factors determining susceptibility to the disease and its progression.

Most patients present with incidentally found abnormal liver blood tests. Diagnosis is usually one of exclusion: liver biopsy is not required for diagnosis in a typical patient, but is required for disease staging. Treatment is directed at components of the metabolic syndrome: diet and exercise have been shown to reduce steatosis; metformin and pioglitazone can have beneficial effects on steatosis, inflammation and fibrosis in patients with type 2 diabetes; pharmacological antiobesity agents and other treatments are under evaluation.

Introduction

Nonalcoholic fatty liver disease (NAFLD) is considered to be the commonest liver disorder in Western countries. It comprises a disease spectrum ranging from simple steatosis through nonalcoholic steatohepatitis (NASH) to fatty fibrosis and ultimately cirrhosis. It is strongly associated with obesity, insulin resistance, and dyslipidaemia and is now regarded as the liver manifestation of the metabolic syndrome (Fig. 15.22.2.1).

Epidemiology

The prevalence of NAFLD appears to be around 20 to 30% in Western adults, with around 1 in 10 of NAFLD patients having NASH. The prevalence of NAFLD is much higher in obesity and type 2 diabetes, with recently reported prevalences of 90% and 70% respectively. There are no accurate data regarding temporal changes in the prevalence of NAFLD; however, the rising prevalence of obesity, diabetes, and the metabolic syndrome seems likely to be reflected in an increasing prevalence of NAFLD. This trend is of particular concern in the paediatric population where the prevalence of NAFLD has been reported to be as high as 50% in obese children, and primary school children with NAFLD-related cirrhosis have already been reported.

Natural history of NAFLD

The long-term hepatic prognosis of patients with NAFLD depends on the histological stage of disease at presentation. Among patients with simple steatosis 12–40% will develop NASH with early fibrosis after 8–13 years follow-up. Of patients presenting with NASH and early fibrosis, around 15% will develop cirrhosis and/or evidence of hepatic decompensation over the same time period. About 7% of subjects with compensated cirrhosis associated with NAFLD will develop a hepatocellular carcinoma (HCC) within 10 years, while 50% will require a transplant or die from a liver-related cause. NAFLD is becoming one of the most common indications for liver transplantation in the United Kingdom and the United States of America. The overall survival of patients with NAFLD is less than that of an age- and sex-matched population with liver disease the third leading cause of death in NAFLD patients compared to the thirteenth leading cause in a general population.

Clinical presentation

NAFLD is a largely asymptomatic condition. Right upper quadrant discomfort, fatigue, and lethargy have been reported in up to

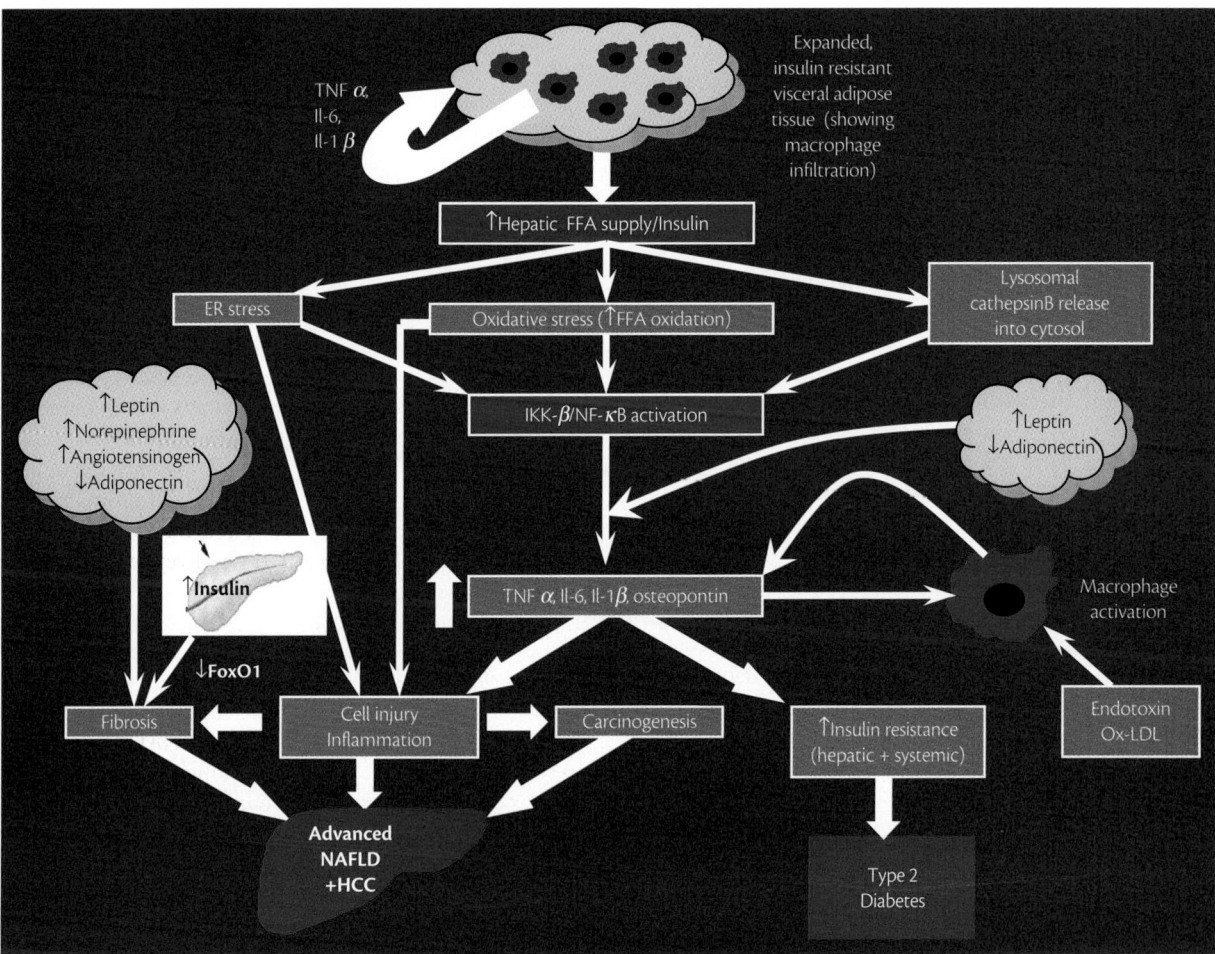

Fig. 15.22.2.1 Potential links between obesity. NAFLD, and type 2 diabetes. FFA, free fatty acids; HCC, hepatocellular carcinoma; Ox-LDL, oxidized low-density lipoprotein.

50% of patients but are uncommon modes of presentation. Most patients with NAFLD are diagnosed after they are found to have hepatomegaly, or more commonly, unexplained abnormalities of liver blood tests performed as part of routine health checks or during drug monitoring (e.g. statin therapy). NAFLD is the commonest cause of incidental abnormal liver blood tests, accounting for between 60 and 90% of such cases. Importantly, the vast majority (c.80%) of patients with NAFLD have normal liver blood tests. NAFLD should therefore be suspected and sought in all patients with established risk factors, regardless of liver blood tests. These risk factors include the presence of polycystic ovary syndrome and obstructive sleep apnoea, both of which have been associated with NAFLD. History is based on determining the presence/absence of conditions associated with NAFLD and excluding alternative causes of steatosis including excess alcohol intake, previous abdominal surgery, and drugs such as amiodarone and tamoxifen.

Investigation

Blood tests are aimed at detecting associated conditions and excluding alternative causes of abnormal liver blood tests.

Serum ferritin is often raised in NAFLD patients and has been associated with advanced fibrosis. HFE genotyping should be carried out when hyperferritemia is associated with raised transferrin saturation. Currently available imaging modalities, including ultrasound, CT, and MRI, are all excellent at detecting steatosis but none can reliably detect NASH or fibrosis. Newer imaging techniques, including proton magnetic resonance spectroscopy and transient elastography, show promise but require further study prior to routine use for disease staging. Liver biopsy is not required for diagnosis in a typical patient with classical risk factors and compatible imaging although may be required when other blood tests suggest an alternative or coexistent diagnosis. The main indication to perform a biopsy is accurate disease staging since (1) different stages have different prognoses and therefore require different management strategies, and (2) no currently available imaging techniques can perform this role. Clinical or laboratory features associated with advanced disease include advanced age (>45 years), body mass index more than $30\,\mathrm{kg/m^2}$, type 2 diabetes, serum aspartate aminotransferase/alanine aminotransferase (AST/ALT) ratio greater than 1, hyperferritinaemia, and positive autoantibodies At present, it would therefore seem reasonable to restrict liver biopsy to patients with at least some, if not all, of these risk factors. Some of these factors have recently been combined together with platelet count and serum albumin into a NAFLD fibrosis 'score' which accurately predicts the presence or absence of advanced disease in the majority of patients, and a recent serum test capable of accurately identifying the presence of NASH has also been described.

Management strategy for NAFLD

Almost no large randomized controlled trials (RCTs) have been published on which to establish evidence-based treatment recommendations for NAFLD. Accordingly, current management strategies are directed at treating, where present, the individual components of the metabolic syndrome since this will reduce risk of cardiovascular disease and may also be beneficial for the liver. This is particularly important in light of recent evidence that NAFLD may be an independent risk factor for cardiovascular disease in patients with obesity and type 2 diabetes. Alcohol intake should not exceed 'sensible' limits. In view of their largely benign prognosis, these strategies are all that is required for patients with simple steatosis who can be managed by general or primary care physicians. In contrast, patients with more advanced NAFLD require long-term follow-up by gastroenterologists/hepatologists in light of their increased propensity for disease progression. These patients will also be candidates for emerging second-line therapies currently being evaluated in large RCTs. The rationale for NAFLD therapies is based on a growing understanding of disease pathogenesis with a particular focus on reducing insulin resistance, hepatic free fatty acid levels, and oxidative, endoplasmic reticulum and cytokine-mediated stress; and also influencing the balance and effects of profibrotic, proinflammatory and antifibrotic, anti-inflammatory adipokines released from adipose tissue.

Treatment of obesity with diet and exercise is the first-line therapy and has been shown to reduce steatosis with less effect on inflammation and fibrosis. Encouraging results have been reported for gastric bypass and banding surgery with studies with longer follow-up reporting improvements in necroinflammation and fibrosis as well as steatosis. Pharmacological antiobesity agents are currently under evaluation. For patients with associated type 2 diabetes, insulin-sensitizing agents including metformin and glitazones would be the rational choice given their mode of action. Small RCTs of metformin and pioglitazone have recently reported beneficial effects on steatosis, inflammation, and fibrosis. There is, as yet, no evidence that any particular lipid-lowering agents are beneficial for NAFLD although there is considerable evidence that statin therapy is safe.

With respect to treatments directed primarily at the liver rather than the associated metabolic syndrome, there have been encouraging pilot studies with antioxidants and anticytokine agents, including pentoxifylline, though as yet no RCT-based evidence. Liver transplantation is successful for patients with NAFLD but the high risk of disease recurrence makes management of the metabolic syndrome a priority both prior to and following transplantation.

Further reading

Angulo P, et al. (2007). The NAFLD fibrosis score: a noninvasive system that identifies liver fibrosis in patients with NAFLD. *Hepatology*, **45**, 846–54. [Derivation of a simple scoring system based on routine laboratory and clinical variables that accurately predicts the presence of advanced fibrosis in NAFLD.]

Belfort R, et al. (2006) A placebo-controlled trial of pioglitazone in subjects with nonalcoholic steatohepatitis. *N Engl J Med*, **355**, 2297–307. [First RCT demonstrating that a glitazone improves liver histology in NASH patients.]

Day CP (2006). From fat to inflammation. *Gastroenterology*, **130**, 207–10. [Review of pathogenesis of progressive NAFLD.]

De Alwis NMW, Day CP (2007). Genetics of alcoholic liver disease and nonalcoholic fatty liver disease. *Semin Liver Dis*, **27**, 44–54.

De Alwis NMW, Day CP (2008). NAFLD: the mist gradually clears. *J Hepatol*, **48** Suppl 1, S104–12.

Dixon JB, et al. (2004). Nonalcoholic fatty liver disease: Improvement in liver histological analysis with weight loss. *Hepatology*, **39**, 1647–54. [First evidence that weight reducing surgery improves fibrosis in NAFLD.]

Ekstedt M, et al. (2006) Long-term follow-up of patients with NAFLD and elevated liver enzymes. *Hepatology*, **44**, 865–73. [Longest natural history study with histological follow-up.]

Harrison SA, Day CP (2007). Benefits of lifestyle modification in NAFLD. *Gut*, **56**, 1760–9. [Review of role of diet and exercise in the pathogenesis and treatment of NAFLD.]

Neuschwander-Tetri BA, Caldwell SH. (2003). Nonalcoholic steatohepatitis: summary of an AASLD Single Topic Conference. *Hepatology*, **37**, 1202–19. [Excellent summary of a state-of-the-art conference.]

Saadeh S, et al. (2002). The utility of radiological imaging in nonalcoholic fatty liver disease. *Gastroenterology*, **123**, 745–50. [Provides evidence that neither CT, ultrasound not MRI can detect NASH or fibrosis short of cirrhosis in NAFLD.]

Skelly MM, James PD, Ryder SD (2001). Findings on liver biopsy to investigate abnormal liver function tests in the absence of diagnostic serology. *J Hepatol*, **35**, 195–9. [Largest study demonstrating that NAFLD is the commonest diagnosis in patients presenting with incidental abnormal LFTs.]

Targher G, et al. (2007). Prevalence of non-alcoholic fatty liver disease and its association with cardiovascular disease among type 2 diabetic patients. *Diabetes Care*, **30**, 1212–18. [Largest study on the prevalence of NAFLD in type 2 diabetes demonstrating a strong association between the presence of NAFLD and cardiovascular disease in this patient group.]

Wieckowska A, et al. (2006) In vivo assessment of liver cell apoptosis as a novel biomarker of disease severity in nonalcoholic fatty liver disease. *Hepatology*, **44**, 27–33. [Identification of new serum marker of NASH based on the presence of apoptosis.]

15.22.3 **Cirrhosis and ascites**

Kevin Moore

Essentials

Ascites is the accumulation of fluid in the peritoneal cavity: 75% of cases are associated with cirrhosis, but there are many other causes, of which the commonest are malignancy and cardiac failure. The occurrence of ascites in patients with cirrhosis is associated with a poor prognosis, with survival around 50% at 1 to 2 years.

In cirrhosis, the presence of portal hypertension (>8 mmHg) is necessary but not sufficient for the development of ascites: other factors involved include hyperaldosteronism, activation of the sympathetic nervous system, and reduction in renal blood flow, perhaps stimulated by reduction in actual or perceived central blood volume ('vasodilatation hypothesis').

Clinical presentation is with abdominal distension and/or abdominal pain, and many patients complain of back ache. Three grades of severity are recognized: grade 1 is only detectable by ultrasound examination; grade 2 is moderate, detected by a shifting dullness; grade 3 is gross, with tense abdominal distension and fluid thrill on palpation.

Investigation

Essential tests are (1) serum electrolytes and renal function tests; patients with ascites due to cirrhosis are prone to hyponatraemia and/or renal impairment; (2) ascitic tap, with fluid sent for (a) microscopy and culture to exclude bacterial peritonitis, (b) protein/albumin concentration to determine whether the fluid is an exudate (protein >25 g/litre; serum-ascites albumin gradient <11 g/litre) or transudate (protein <25 g/litre; serum–ascites albumin gradient >11 g/litre)—exudates are most likely to be due to malignancy and transudates to cirrhosis, but the distinction is unreliable and not of great clinical utility, (c) cytology for malignant cells, (d) amylase for pancreatic cause; (3) ultrasonography of liver for evidence of cirrhosis, congestion or metastases, and of portal vein to exclude thrombosis.

Management

First-line manoeuvres include (1) dietary salt restriction (<90 mmol/day); (2) diuretics—initially spironolactone, with addition of furosemide if required; (3) therapeutic paracentesis—all ascitic fluid should be drained in a single session as rapidly as possible, with the cannula removed immediately afterwards to reduce the risks of infection and colloid replacement given to prevent circulatory disturbance. Water restriction and (in a few centres) an oral vasopressin receptor antagonist is recommended if there is significant hyponatraemia. Refractory ascites is managed by repeated paracentesis or insertion of a transjugular intrahepatic portosystemic shunt (TIPS).

Complications

The most important complication is spontaneous bacterial peritonitis (SBP), which within 3 years will affect 15% of patients presenting with ascites. Typical symptoms are abdominal pain and fever, but there may be none. The gut and urine are the most frequent source of organisms, but treatment with appropriate antibiotics (e.g. cefotaxime; ciprofloxacin with amoxicillin; piperacillin with tazlocillin) should be started as soon as a presumptive diagnosis is made following microscopy of ascitic fluid (neutrophil count >250/mm^3). Prophylactic ciprofloxacin can reduce the risk of recurrent attacks. Mortality is around 30% for the acute episode and 75% at 1 year, hence (unless contraindicated) all patients with SBP should be considered for orthotopic liver transplantation. Other complications of ascites include (1) pleural effusion; (2) paraumbilical hernia; (3) hepatorenal syndrome (see Chapter 21.5); and (4) respiratory compromise from diaphragmatic splinting.

Introduction

Ascites is the accumulation of fluid in the peritoneal cavity. Studies on its pathogenesis began in the 17th century when Richard Lower (1631–1691), a physician based in Oxford, demonstrated that ascites developed in dogs following ligation of the inferior vena cava. Ernest Henry Starling (1866–1927), a physiologist based at University College London, made a major contribution to the study of oedema formation with the demonstration that both hydrostatic forces and oncotic forces were involved, and that the increase in thoracic lymph flow following obstruction of the inferior vena cava is mainly derived from the liver.

Aetiology

Ascites is a common complication of cirrhosis and indicates the presence of portal hypertension and hepatic decompensation. It occurs in at least 50% of patients within 10 years of the diagnosis of cirrhosis, which accounts for over 75% of cases presenting with ascites.

Ascites may also be caused by malignancy, pancreatitis, tuberculosis, cardiac failure, myxoedema, or other rarer causes, each of which may also occur in patients with cirrhosis (Table 15.22.3.1). Ascites does not occur in patients with portal vein thrombosis or other forms of noncirrhotic portal hypertension such as congenital hepatic fibrosis, except as a transient finding following a gastrointestinal haemorrhage. It frequently occurs in patients with the Budd–Chiari syndrome or late-onset hepatic failure (subfulminant hepatic failure), and—to a lesser extent—where small amounts of peritoneal fluid accumulate in cases of acute liver failure.

Other (rare) causes of ascites include constrictive pericarditis, malnutrition, stromal tumours and Meigs' syndrome, hypothyroidism, Budd–Chiari syndrome, veno-occlusive disease, or lymphatic leak (chylous ascites). Rare infections include candidiasis and filariasis. Granulomatous liver disease such as sarcoidosis may cause severe portal hypertension and (occasionally) ascites. Although ascites commonly occurs in patients with cardiac failure, it is not usually a presenting feature. Ascites may also occur in the ovarian hyperstimulation syndrome in women undergoing fertility treatment.

Epidemiology

Cirrhosis is the fifth leading cause of death in the United Kingdom. It heralds the beginning of a usually rapid decline of liver function, with about half of patients dying within 2 years of the onset of ascites.

Pathogenesis of ascites due to cirrhosis

The presence of portal hypertension is essential for the development of ascites: fluid accumulation does not occur at a portal pressure below 8 mmHg. However, factors other than portal pressure are important, since ascites does not develop spontaneously in patients with portal vein thrombosis. Ascites develops as a consequence of sodium and water retention, which in the presence of portal hypertension causes transudation of fluid into the peritoneal cavity, and together with an increased production of hepatic

Table 15.22.3.1 Underlying causes of patients presenting with ascites in the United States of America

Cause	% Total
Cirrhosis (ALD)	65
Cirrhosis (viral)	10
Cirrhosis (other)	6
Malignancy	10
Heart failure	3
Tuberculosis	2
Pancreatic disease	1
Other causes	3

ALD, alcoholic liver disease

lymph may cause a massive accumulation of fluid—a moderate to marked ascites will comprise about 5 to 25 litres of fluid. It is well recognized that abnormal sodium handling occurs in patients with advanced cirrhosis, but less well known that sodium handling is abnormal even in the preascitic stage. Experiments by Dudley and colleagues have shown that the proximal tubular reabsorption of sodium is enhanced in early cirrhosis, and that some patients exhibit glomerular hyperfiltration.

Sodium retention does not occur solely as a result of hyperaldosteronism, for approximately 60% of patients with ascites have normal aldosterone levels at initial presentation. There is no doubt, however, that aldosterone is involved: it increases sodium retention in the distal tubules, and the administration of high doses of spironolactone increases natriuresis in patients with cirrhosis and ascites, despite apparently normal plasma aldosterone levels, which has given rise to the concept that renal sensitivity to aldosterone may be enhanced in cirrhosis.

Other factors involved in sodium homeostasis include the sympathetic nervous system, which is activated in decompensated liver disease and which enhances sodium reabsorption along the proximal tubules. Another important factor is the rate of sodium delivery to the tubules: renal blood flow is decreased in cirrhosis, and decreases further with decompensation, and sodium reabsorption is enhanced during decreased sodium delivery. Other factors such as atrial natriuretic peptide, endothelin-1, or urodilatin may be involved, but their role is as yet undefined.

The underlying cause of the activation of sodium-retaining pathways is still disputed, with data to support both the 'underfill' and 'overfill' hypotheses. Thus, the same patient may exhibit signs of both an expanded and a contracted central blood volume at different stages of disease development. A unifying hypothesis, known as the 'vasodilatation hypothesis', was put forward to explain the observations regarding the development of salt-retaining states (Fig. 15.22.3.1). In this, the central stimulus for activation of neurohumoral pathways is a decrease in the central blood volume, which differs in severity depending on the intensity of liver disease. Whilst superficially attractive, this hypothesis fails to explain why many patients develop salt retention in the presence of normal aldosterone concentrations, and why systemic vasodilatation is only observed in the supine state.

Clinical features

Ascites is graded 1 to 3 depending on its severity. Grade 1 ascites is mild, and only detectable by ultrasound examination; grade 2 ascites is moderate, and is manifest by moderate symmetrical distension of the abdomen; grade 3 ascites is large or gross, with marked abdominal distension. A grade 2 ascites is most easily detected by a shifting dullness. Grade 3 ascites is usually tense and easily detected by the presence of a fluid thrill on palpation. Aside from an unpleasant feeling of abdominal distension and/or abdominal pain, many patients will complain of backache. There is often divarification of the rectus abdomini muscles, and prominent veins may be evident on the abdominal wall (Fig. 15.22.3.2). Paraumbilical hernias develop in about 20% of patients with ascites, an incidence that increases to up to 70% in those with long-standing recurrent tense ascites, with the main risks being rupture and strangulation.

Pleural effusions (hepatic hydrothorax) develop in about 5% of patients with cirrhosis and may develop in patients with no discernible ascites. The pleural effusions are right-sided in 85% of cases, left-sided in 13%, and bilateral in 2%.

Laboratory diagnosis

The cause of ascites or its precipitation is often obvious. Where there are no obvious clues to its aetiology, tests must be directed both at diagnosing the presumed cause of liver disease and at excluding other causes of ascites such as malignancy or tuberculosis. Other causes of abdominal distension such as huge masses, Meigs' syndrome, or pregnancy should be considered. The essential investigations on admission of a patient to hospital include the following.

- Serum electrolytes and renal function tests—patients with ascites due to cirrhosis are prone to hyponatraemia or renal impairment, either spontaneously or following diuretic therapy.

- Ascitic aspiration with microscopy, determination of albumin or protein content, culture, cytology, and amylase measurement should be performed to confirm or exclude spontaneous bacterial

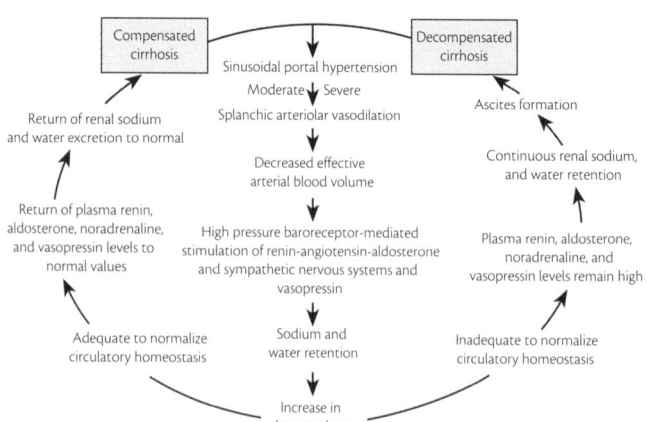

Fig. 15.22.3.1 Outline of peripheral vasodilation hypothesis. (From Schrier RW *et al.* (1988). Peripheral arterial vasodilation hypothesis: a proposal for the initiation of renal sodium and water retention in cirrhosis. *Hepatology*, **8**, 115–17).

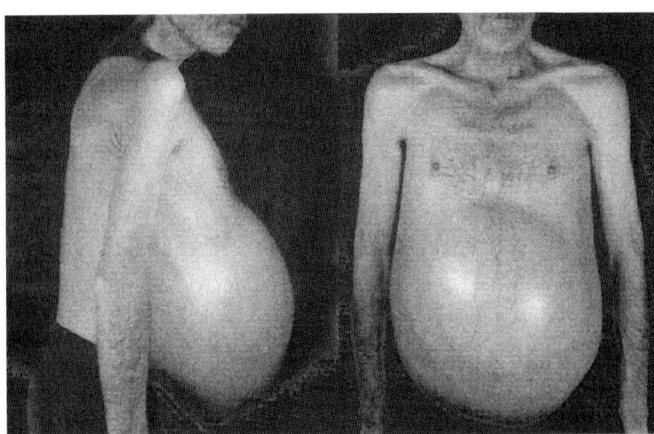

Fig. 15.22.3.2 Alcoholic cirrhosis with ascites is often associated with marked anorexia.

peritonitis, tuberculosis, malignancy, or pancreatic disease. A Gram stain is usually uninformative.

♦ Ultrasound scans are needed to evaluate liver appearance (nodular and cirrhotic) or congested (e.g. congestive cardiac failure (CCF)), as well as blood flow in the portal vein (to exclude the portal vein thrombosis that occurs in 8% of patients with cirrhosis, and which may precipitate hepatic decompensation), a semi-quantitation of the amount of ascites, and the presence of tumour in the liver or other masses.

Paracentesis

An ascitic tap is used for either diagnostic purposes or for the therapeutic removal of large volumes of ascites. The most common site for aspirating ascites is about 15 cm lateral to the umbilicus, with care being taken to avoid an enlarged liver or spleen. The epigastric arteries run just lateral to the umbilicus towards the midinguinal point and should also be avoided.

For diagnostic purposes, between 20 and 50 ml of ascitic fluid should be withdrawn, and 3 to 5 ml placed under aseptic conditions (i.e. the needle changed) into each of two blood culture bottles (cultures for tuberculosis have to be requested specifically). A 5-ml aliquot of fluid should also be sent in a plastic container (containing ethylenediaminetetraacetic acid (EDTA) if the sample has a tendency to clot) to the microbiology department for a polymorphonuclear neutrophil (PMN) or lymphocyte count. The microbiologist should report a neutrophil count (e.g. <250 PMNs/mm^3) together with a limited differential (i.e. PMN or lymphocytes). Coulter counter estimations of ascitic neutrophil numbers are probably unreliable at the lower end of a pathologically increased white blood cell count. A 5-ml aliquot should be also sent for measurement of ascitic protein content or, ideally, ascitic albumin. Cytological examination requires 20 to 50 ml of ascitic fluid and the attention of a cytopathologist. There is little diagnostic value in an analysis of ascitic fluid pH or of lactate or glucose concentrations.

Ascitic fluid investigations

A diagnostic paracentesis should be performed in all patients with new onset grade 2 or 3 ascites, and in all patients hospitalized for worsening of ascites or any complications of cirrhosis, with the most important investigations being polymorphonuclear leucocyte count by microscopy and culture to exclude bacterial peritonitis. The next most important investigation is the measurement of ascitic total protein concentration, since patients with low ascitic protein concentration (<15 g/litre) have an increased risk of developing spontaneous bacterial peritonitis and may benefit from antibiotic prophylaxis.

Ascitic protein concentration

The main purpose of measuring ascitic protein concentration is to identify patients at risk of developing spontaneous bacterial peritonitis (SBP). However, ascitic protein is often measured to try and determine the cause of ascites, and is much over-rated, and misinterpreted in this respect. Conventionally, ascites is described as being an exudate or a transudate depending on whether ascitic protein concentration is respectively more or less than 25 g/litre. The purpose of this subdivision is to narrow the differential diagnosis of its cause, but many physicians erroneously assume that cardiac ascites will have a low level of ascitic protein, when this is rarely the case, and that patients with tuberculous peritonitis have a high ascitic protein content, when in fact it is low in 30% of patients. Moreover, about 15% of cases of cirrhotic ascites have an ascitic protein level of more than 25 g/litre, and 20% of patients with a malignancy have a low ascitic protein level. The causes of transudative and exudative ascites are given in Table 15.22.3.2.

For patients with cirrhosis, a very low ascitic protein level (<10 g/litre) is associated with an increased risk of SBP at the time of hospital admission, and SBP is present in about 15% of all patients admitted with cirrhotic ascites. The use of ascitic protein estimations to subdivide exudative or transudative causes of ascites is considerably enhanced by measuring the difference between ascitic and serum albumin levels (see below).

Serum–ascites albumin gradient

The measurement of serum–ascites albumin gradient may be useful in patients in whom the diagnosis of the cause of ascites is unclear. Several studies have compared the value of ascitic protein concentration with that of serum-ascitic albumin gradient measurements in patients with ascites resulting from cirrhosis and other causes. In one study comprising 44 patients, it was reported that 5/29 (17%) patients with cirrhotic ascites had an ascitic protein level above 25 g/litre, whereas 3/15 (20%) with malignant ascites had an ascitic protein level below 25 g/litre. In contrast, the overlap in each group was reduced to 1/29 and 1/15 respectively when a serum–ascites albumin gradient above 11 g/litre was used, hence it is clearly preferable to measure the serum–ascites albumin gradient in patients presenting with ascites. This method, which involves subtraction of the ascitic albumin concentration from that observed in ascites, divides patients into two groups: those with a high gradient (>11 g/litre) and those with a low gradient (<11 g/litre). The overall accuracy of this method is high, although its actual impact in day to day clinical practice is small (Table 15.22.3.3).

Ascitic amylase

The ascitic fluid amylase level should always be measured in patients with an exudative or unexplained ascites, since it is cheap

Table 15.22.3.2 Subdivision into exudative and transudative ascites

Exudative ascites (protein>25 g/l)	Transudative ascites (protein <25 g/l)
Malignancy (80%)	Cirrhosis (85%)
Tuberculosis (70%)	Malignancy (20%)
Congestive cardiac failure	Protein-losing enteropathy
Cirrhosis (15% of cases)	Tuberculosis (30%)
Pancreatitis	
Budd–Chiari syndrome	
Myxoedema	
Constrictive pericarditis	
Nephrotic syndrome	

and quick to measure and may yield a rapid diagnosis. A very high value is obtained when ascitic fluid results from a pancreatic pseudocyst or mass.

Ascitic fluid microscopy

An ascitic neutrophil count of more than 250 PMNs/mm³ is diagnostic of spontaneous bacterial peritonitis. An elevated lymphocyte count should raise the possibility of tuberculous peritonitis. Excess red blood cells are most commonly due to a traumatic tap, but should raise the possibility of malignancy.

Ascitic fluid culture

If aspirated fluid is placed in a sterile container and sent to the microbiology department for microscopy and culture, then a positive culture will be obtained in only about 40% of (truly infected) samples. However, if—as described above—ascitic fluid is treated in the same way as blood cultures, and fluid inoculated directly into blood culture bottles at the bedside, the positive culture rate is double that observed when fluid is sent in a sterile pot. A single study has evaluated the effectiveness of cytospin with cell lysis to improve the efficacy of culturing ascitic fluid, and again found that direct inoculation of ascitic fluid into blood culture bottles was far superior (79% positivity) compared with the cell-lysis method (46% culture-positive).

If an ascitic microscopy is reported as showing less than 250 PMNs/mm³ but subsequent culture grows an organism (monomicrobial bacterascites), then the ascitic tap should be repeated since the patient may have resolved the incipient infection (now

Table 15.22.3.3 Subdivision of patients into high and low ascitic albumin gradient

Serum-ascites albumin gradient <11 g/l (Low gradient)	Serum-ascites albumin gradient >11 g/l (High gradient)
Malignancy	Cirrhosis
Tuberculosis	Cardiac failure
Pancreatic	Budd–Chiari syndrome
Biliary	Myxoedema
Nephrotic syndrome	
Connective tissue disease	

culture-negative and low ascitic white cell count), or may have developed spontaneous bacterial peritonitis (high white cell count and culture-positive) and thus require treatment with antibiotics and albumin.

Ascitic fluid cytology

Ascitic cytology should involve liaison with the cytopathologist so that the index of suspicion and type of potential tumour are discussed. A 20- to 50-ml sample of ascitic fluid is required to produce a cell concentrate for cytology—obtained by centrifuging the ascites fluid, removing supernatant, and resuspending the cells. A sample of the concentrate then undergoes a cytospin to deposit cells on to microscope slides, following which the cells are stained. Typical stains include the Papanicolaou and May-Grünwald–Giemsa stain.

Ascitic volume

Ascitic volume is not usually determined in clinical practice. It can, however, be quantified radiologically or by indicator-dilution. As a rough guide, patients with barely detectable ascites usually harbour between 1 and 4 litres, those with moderate ascites 4 to 8 litres, and those with marked ascites more than 8 litres of fluid. Ultrasonographic determination of ascitic volume involves measurement of the abdominal circumference and the deepest vertical depth of the fluid, with subsequent modelling as a segment of a sphere. Isotopic determination of ascitic volume involves the injection of radiolabelled 99Tc- macroalbumin.

Treatment

Patients with ascites can be divided into those who are easy to treat and those who are difficult. In general, patients with their first presentation of ascites and normal renal function, who have a spot urine sodium concentration of more than 20 mmol/litre, or an identifiable source of dietary sodium excess, respond well to simple measures. Likewise, when ascites has developed as a consequence of bleeding or infection, it usually resolves more readily. The treatment of ascites is summarized in Box 15.22.3.1.

Bed rest

Bed rest is of no benefit in patients with reasonably preserved renal function, as indicated by a serum creatinine concentration of less than 125 μmol/litre, and a good initial response to diuretics.

Dietary salt restriction

There is a consensus that dietary salt restriction is important in the management of patients with cirrhosis and ascites, but it is important to maintain an adequate level of nutrition. Standard practice is to restrict sodium intake to less than 90 mmol/day, which in effect amounts to a 'no added salt' diet with avoidance of preprepared meals. It is generally agreed that salt restriction should be an adjunct to diuretic therapy, and that it is rarely effective alone.

Water restriction

As a general recommendation

There are no studies evaluating the role of water restriction on the resolution of ascites, although in many studies from the United States of America and Europe it has been customary to restrict

Box 15.22.3.1 Summary of treatment of ascites

♦ Bed rest is of little value

♦ Sodium restriction to 90 mmol/day

♦ Water restriction should only be used in severely hyponatraemic patients with caution

♦ Diuretic therapy should employ spironolactone as the first-line drug

♦ Total paracentesis should initially be carried out on patients with moderate or marked ascites

♦ Shunts may be used in those with refractory ascites in whom recurrent paracentesis is too frequent or poorly tolerated, or in those with a hepatic hydrothorax

water intake to between 1 and 1.5 litres/day, a recommendation that has appeared in many major texts for the last 20 to 30 years. This treatment has thus crept into current dogma without clinical or scientific basis to support its use. It is well known that water follows salt, and thus fluid loss will occur if a patient achieves negative sodium balance with dietary salt restriction and/or natriuresis.

In patients with hyponatraemia

In a study of 55 patients with ascites, none of whom had taken any diuretics for 2 weeks, 21 had spontaneous hyponatraemia and 34 were normonatraemic. In all patients with normonatraemia, the free-water clearance (see Chapter 21.2.1) was normal. Of those with hyponatraemia, 13 had a marked reduction in free-water clearance and glomerular filtration rate, with the remaining 8 having a relatively normal free-water clearance. The patients with hyponatraemia and poor renal function did not respond to diuretic therapy, and had a poor prognosis with 60% inpatient mortality, compared to 15% in the other patients.

Hyponatraemia is caused by excessive water retention, primarily as a result of increased circulating vasopressin levels, hence patients with significant hyponatraemia are usually subject to a water restriction of less than 500 ml/day. However, not least because of difficulty ensuring compliance, this is often ineffective, and the response—if any—is slow. It is sometimes more prudent to try to improve renal function with volume expansion, in the first instance with colloid.

A more recent approach has been to use vasopressin receptor antagonists with the aim of improving serum sodium concentration by increasing solute-free water excretion. The effect of satavaptan, a highly selective vasopressin V2 receptor antagonist, on ascites management and serum sodium in hyponatremic patients with cirrhosis has been studied in a multicentre double-blind randomized controlled study of 110 patients. Patients were treated for 14 days, with all continuing to receive spironolactone at 100 mg/day. Satavaptan led to improved control of ascites, as indicated by a reduction in body weight (1.5–1.7 kg for those treated at the higher dose of drug), compared to no mean change for placebo, and serum sodium increased by 5 to 7 mmol/litre in those treated. Thirst was significantly more common in patients treated with satavaptan compared to those on placebo, but the frequency of other adverse events was similar among groups.

Diuretics

The goal of treatment is to maintain patients free of ascites with the minimum dose of diuretics. Thus, once the ascites has largely resolved the dose of diuretics should be reduced to the minimum or discontinued if possible.

Many diuretic agents have been evaluated over the years, but in the United Kingdom and Europe this has been mainly confined to spironolactone, amiloride, frusemide, and bumetanide. Patients who develop ascites for the first time should receive spironolactone, starting at 100 mg/day, increasing to maximum of 400 mg/day. In patients who do not respond to spironolactone, as defined by a reduction of body weight of less than 2 kg per week, or in patients who develop hyperkalaemia, frusemide should be added at an increasing dose from 40 mg/day to a maximum of 160 mg/day.

The safe upper limit of the rate of weight loss is contentious, but most experts agree that the diuretic dose should be adjusted to achieve a rate of weight loss below an average of 500 g per day in patients without peripheral oedema, or 1 kg per day in those with peripheral oedema.

Diuretic agents
Spironolactone
Spironolactone is an aldosterone antagonist, acting mainly on the distal tubules to increase natriuresis and conserve potassium. In a controlled study comparing the efficacy of spironolactone in 40 nonazotaemic patients with ascites who were excreting less than 12 mmol of sodium/day, 18 of 19 patients responded to spironolactone alone, whereas only 11 of 21 patients responded to frusemide alone. Most patients responding to spironolactone required 150 mg/day, and a few required 300 mg/day. In all cases diuresis occurred by the third day. For those given frusemide, most responders required 80 mg/day, but a few required 160 mg/day. Frusemide was associated with a decrease in the serum potassium concentration, which necessitated potassium supplementation. In those given spironolactone, serum potassium concentrations increased appreciably, and the main problem with clinical use in men is the development of gynaecomastia, which is often painful. Other side effects of spironolactone include hyponatraemia, impotence, menstrual disturbance (although most ascitic patients are amenorrhoeic), and osteomalacia.

Amiloride
Amiloride combined with either frusemide or ethacrynic acid results in a satisfactory diuresis in most cirrhotic subjects with ascites. In one study of amiloride in patients with cirrhosis and ascites resistant to bed rest and a very low salt diet (<20 mmol Na/day), it induced a satisfactory response in 80% of patients at doses of 15 to 30 mg/day when used alone.

Frusemide
Frusemide is a loop diuretic that causes a marked natriuresis and diuresis in normal subjects. Its efficacy compared with spironolactone is discussed above. In normal subjects it has a half-life of about 75 min, increasing to about 130 min in patients with cirrhosis. It is generally used as an adjunct to spironolactone treatment and has poor efficacy when used alone in cirrhosis, probably because there is salt retention in the distal tubules in the subset of patients with high plasma aldosterone concentrations. Frusemide should be used in a dose not exceeding 160 mg/day; its use is associated with severe electrolyte disturbance, and therefore requires close monitoring.

Complications and benefits of diuretic therapy

Diuretic therapy generally improves morbidity and well-being, since it causes resolution of ascites, allows a more liberal diet, decreases portal pressure, and increases the opsonic activity of ascitic fluid, thereby decreasing the risk of spontaneous bacterial peritonitis. However, diuretic use is associated with complications in many patients (Box 15.22.3.2), although these are less frequent with usage as described above than in some historical series.

Therapeutic paracentesis

Paracentesis has been in use for at least 2000 years, and was widely used in the earlier part of the last century. When diuretics first became available in the 1940s the practice declined, but it was still used as an adjunct to therapy until the early 1960s, when it gradually fell into disrepute with the recognition that repeated paracentesis resulted in salt depletion and oliguria, and became virtually banned as a treatment. However, it re-emerged in the mid 1980s when several controlled clinical studies demonstrated that paracentesis with colloid replacement was safe and associated with fewer complications than diuretic therapy. In a large controlled study, patients with tense ascites were randomized to receive either paracentesis with intravenous albumin (40 g after each paracentesis) or diuretics (spironolactone 200–400 mg/day plus frusemide (40–240 mg/day). Patients with significant renal impairment (serum creatinine concentration >250 μmol/litre) were excluded. Paracentesis (4–6 litres/day) was effective in all patients, and no significant change in electrolytes or renal function was observed. Diuretics were effective in 28 out of 34 patients. There was, however, a significant increase in serum creatinine and decrease in sodium levels in the diuretic-treated group, and the duration of inpatient treatment was considerably longer. Total paracentesis does, however, lead to a modest decrease in blood pressure (Fig. 15.22.3.3) by 7 to 10 mmHg. This research was followed by many other studies evaluating the speed of paracentesis, the haemodynamic changes following paracentesis, and the need for colloid replacement therapy.

Practical aspects

The most important feature of a paracentesis cannula is that it should have multiple side perforations to avoid obstruction by omentum. All ascitic fluid should be drained in a single session as rapidly as possible over 1 to 4 h: if 25 litres of ascites can be drained within 2 to 4 h it is quite safe to do so. The old dogma that rapid paracentesis causes marked hypotension is false, and the haemodynamic changes

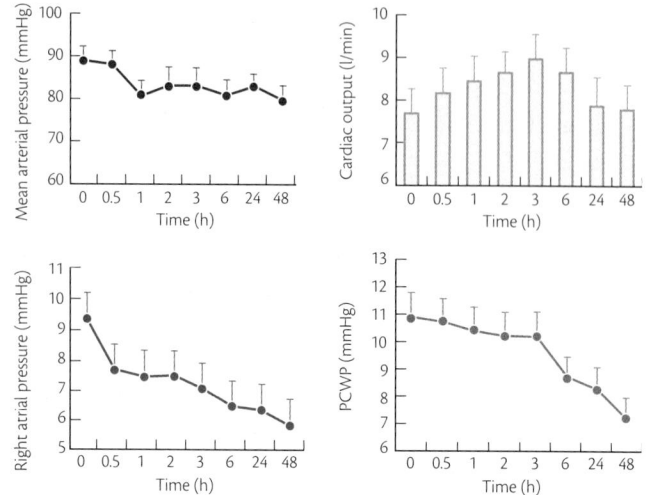

Fig. 15.22.3.3 Haemodynamic changes following acute total paracentesis of approximately 10 litres of ascites over 1 h. Paracentesis was commenced at time 0 h and sequential changes were monitored by a Swan–Ganz catheter, without albumin replacement.
(Modified from Panos MZ, *et al.* (1990). Single, total paracentesis for tense ascites: sequential haemodynamic changes and right atrial size. *Hepatology*, **11**, 662–7.)

that occur do so after the removal of as little as 1 litre of fluid. There is an immediate fall in right atrial pressure (within 30 min), due to a decrease in intra-abdominal pressure and a decrease in compression of the right atrium. There is a rapid decrease in systemic vascular resistance and increase in cardiac output that peaks at 3 h. Pulmonary capillary wedge pressure remains constant for 6 h (in the absence of colloid), and decreases after this interval in the absence of colloid replacement. Mean arterial pressure decreases by about 8 mmHg. These changes are shown in Fig. 15.22.3.3. The drainage system should never be left in place overnight since this carries a high risk of infection.

Colloid replacement

It is very important that colloid replacement is given following paracentesis to prevent circulatory disturbances. After total paracentesis, synthetic plasma substitutes may be used if the volume of ascites removed is less than 5 litres, but albumin should be used when more than 5 litres is removed, and based on studies of the haemodynamic changes that follow paracentesis this should be given after paracentesis has been completed. All or most trials have used albumin at a dose of 8 g/litre of ascites removed: there are no data on whether smaller or larger amounts of albumin have differing degrees of efficacy.

Benefits

Paracentesis most obviously provides immediate relief from ascites and a tense abdomen, but also a number of other benefits, including (1) relief of respiratory muscles—tense ascites clearly restricts breathing, and increases both the workload of respiration and energy expenditure, with paracentesis providing immediate relief; (2) reduction in resting energy expenditure, which is increased by ascites; (3) enhanced salt and water excretion—due to acute reduction of renal venous pressure and consequent increase in renal perfusion, also acute decrease in plasma arginine vasopressin levels, which are directly related to intrathoracic or intra-abdominal pressure, with

---

Box 15.22.3.2 Complications of diuretics in the management of ascites

- Hyponatraemia (50%)
- Hyperkalaemia (spironolactone) or hypokalaemia (loop diuretics)
- Hepatic encephalopathy (secondary to electrolyte disturbance)
- Hyperuricaemia (30%)
- Renal impairment
- Gynaecomastia, osteomalacia, and mild metabolic acidosis with spironolactone

both of these perhaps making patients more responsive to diuretic therapy.

Contraindications

It is generally agreed that there are no contraindications to paracentesis, although studies to date have excluded several subsets of patients, primarily because of inadequate data. In practice, some clinicians have concerns about carrying out paracentesis in patients who have a severe coagulopathy or marked thrombocytopenia in case localized bleeding complications arise, but there are no data to support this view.

Intravenous albumin infusion

There is a persistent belief that the infusion of albumin is beneficial to patients with cirrhosis. It does have a useful role in relation to paracentesis (see above), and it also has a role in the treatment of spontaneous bacterial peritonitis (see below). Several studies in the 1940s evaluated the effect of fractionated human albumin solution in patients with cirrhosis, demonstrating that this could correct the low plasma levels of albumin observed and result in a modest diuresis in some patients, but overall the results were disappointing. The identification of new hepatitis viruses, HIV, and the advent of new variant Creutzfeldt–Jakob disease should make all clinicians cautious in the administration of human products.

Angiotensin-converting enzyme (ACE) inhibitors

The therapeutic effect of ACE inhibitors is attractive since they directly target the system involved most intimately with salt and water retention. However, the acute administration of either captopril or enalapril may cause an acute fall in blood pressure. Some studies have suggested that in patients with ascites the chronic administration of enalapril suppressed plasma aldosterone levels and increased urinary sodium excretion and GFR, as well as increasing urinary prostaglandin E_2 and 6-oxo-prostaglandin $F_1\alpha$. More studies on the efficacy of these drugs and of angiotensin antagonists on portal pressure and the treatment of ascites are expected. Recent studies have suggested that low doses of ACE inhibitors may enhance salt excretion, but they should be used very carefully and they have not been widely adopted in clinical practice.

Patients with severe liver dysfunction and ascites

Patients with endstage liver disease often have subclinical renal impairment, with a typical GFR of around 60 ml/min, and up to 90% of patients dying from alcoholic hepatitis develop renal failure. For patients with alcoholic liver disease, with or without alcoholic hepatitis, the presence of ascites does not generally affect the clinical outcome, unless the ascites becomes a focus for infection. For those with alcoholic hepatitis that resolves spontaneously or with treatment, the ascites usually improves as salt and water excretion increase with improvement of the liver disease. Most patients with severe liver failure have been excluded from clinical studies assessing the efficacy of diuretics or paracentesis. However, it is recommended that extreme caution is exerted when trying to induce diuresis in patients with endstage liver disease, and it is probably safer to use paracentesis rather than give potentially nephrotoxic drugs, although few relevant studies have been conducted. Such patients also have lower cardiac reserve due to the presence of cirrhotic cardiomyopathy, hence particular caution should be exerted in fluid replacement.

Refractory ascites

Refractory ascites is defined as ascites that cannot be mobilized, or the early recurrence of which (post paracentesis) cannot be prevented because of lack of response to maximal diuretic therapy and salt restriction (<80–120 mmol salt/day), or who cannot reach an effective diuretic dose because of side effects. The assessment of the response of patients with ascites to diuretic therapy and salt restriction should only be performed in stable patients without associated complications such as bleeding or infection, but 5 to 10% do not respond adequately. This may be because the diuretics induce an electrolyte disturbance or encephalopathy, necessitating a temporary and recurrent withdrawal of medication, or alternatively the patient may be genuinely resistant. In both these groups, there is invariably significant renal dysfunction when assessed by creatinine clearance or other techniques measuring GFR. The mainstay of treatment for these patients is repeated paracentesis or insertion of a shunt.

Shunts

Transjugular intrahepatic portosystemic shunts (TIPS)

TIPS may improve natriuresis in patients with diuretic-resistant ascites. In one study, 50 patients with refractory ascites were treated by TIPS, sufficient to decrease the portal pressure gradient by over 60%. Some 75% of all patients showed complete resolution of their ascites by 3 months, and 20% achieved a partial response, but new onset of hepatic encephalopathy occurred in 10%. However, several other studies have reported a 45% incidence of hepatic encephalopathy post-TIPS, which was severe and disabling in 15% of all treated patients.

TIPS is associated with deterioration of liver function, improvement in renal function (at 6 months), and some patients develop severe haemolysis. Overall the mean 1-year survival post-TIPS is less than 50%.

Peritoneovenous shunts (Le Veen shunts or Denver shunts)

Peritoneovenous shunting became very popular in the 1970s, with numerous publications on its benefits to renal function and resolution of ascites. However, it soon became apparent that many shunts became blocked or infected and caused scarring of the peritoneum, which can make liver transplantation difficult. There have been three clinical trials evaluating the efficacy of the peritoneovenous shunt, showing that the technique offers no survival advantage over medical therapy or repeated paracenteses. With respect to its effects on renal function, it has been shown that shunting had no overall effect on mortality in patients with the hepatorenal syndrome.

Prognosis

The occurrence of ascites in patients with cirrhosis is associated with a poor prognosis, and patients with ascites may have a much worse prognosis than currently reflected in the MELD or UKELD score system, commonly used in organ allocation for liver transplantation.

Survival rates are around 50% at 1 to 2 years, but somewhat better in alcoholic patients with ascites who stop drinking. The development of bacterial peritonitis in patients with ascites is associated with a mortality of 75% at 1 year, hence the development of this complication is associated with an overall poor prognosis and, unless contraindicated, all patients should be considered for orthotopic liver transplantation.

Complications

The complications of ascites are shown in Box 15.22.3.3 and discussed below.

Pleural effusion

Pleural effusions (hepatic hydrothorax) develop in about 5% of patients with cirrhosis. Fluid tracks up into the pleural cavity via defects in the diaphragm (e.g. holes or blebs), which occasionally close spontaneously. Hepatic hydrothorax may develop in patients with no discernible ascites. The pleural effusions are right-sided in 85% of cases and bilateral in 2% of cases. To confirm the diagnosis, if doubt exists, a radiotracer should be injected under aseptic conditions into the abdomen and its appearance followed in the pleural fluid. A pleural effusion should be managed as for conventional ascites unless it is unresponsive and causing severe dyspnoea, in which case a TIPS should be inserted.

Paraumbilical hernia

Paraumbilical hernias develop in about 20% of patients with ascites, an incidence that increases up to 70% in those with long-standing recurrent tense ascites. The main risks are rupture and strangulation.

Hepatorenal syndrome

Hepatorenal syndrome is the development of renal failure in patients with advanced liver disease (acute or chronic) in the absence of any pathological cause of renal failure. It is due to a reduction of renal blood flow, an increased renal sympathetic drive, and increased circulating or increased renal production of various vasoactive mediators such as endothelin-1, cysteinyl-leukotrienes, thromboxane A_2, or F(2)-isoprostanes. See Chapter 21.5 for further discussion.

Hypercatabolic state

Many patients with ascites present in a hypercatabolic state, which may be secondary to low-grade endotoxaemia, together with their general state of malnutrition. This can be reversed, particularly in alcoholic patients who stop drinking and improve their nutritional lifestyle, and successful TIPS can also improve matters, although this may of course be secondary to cessation of alcohol intake.

Respiratory difficulties

Increasing abdominal distension due to the accumulation of peritoneal fluid increases the effort required for breathing. Occasionally, this may precipitate extreme difficulty in breathing that should be treated by rapid paracentesis.

Spontaneous bacterial peritonitis (SBP)

The spectrum of bacterial peritonitis includes spontaneous bacterial peritonitis, monomicrobial bacterascites, culture-negative neutroascites, and secondary bacterial peritonitis. SBP is defined as the combination of a positive ascitic fluid culture, an ascitic fluid neutrophil count of more than 250 cells/mm^3, and no evident intra-abdominal source of infection. Secondary bacterial peritonitis is identical, excepting that an intra-abdominal source is apparent and the culture is frequently polymicrobial.

About 11% of patients presenting with ascites will develop SBP within 1 year and 15% within 3 years. For those with an ascitic protein level less than 10 g/litre the risk is 24% within 3 years. For patients admitted to hospital with ascites, with or without other complications (e.g. bleeding), the incidence of SBP on admission, based on a review of several reports, is about 10%.

The symptoms of SBP are shown in Box 15.22.3.4 and the pathogenesis in Fig. 15.22.3.4. It is apparent that a source for bacteraemia gives rise to organisms in the hepatic lymph and thence the ascitic fluid. Before an inflammatory reaction occurs, an ascitic tap will yield a positive culture, but a low neutrophil count. This is termed 'monomicrobial bacterascites', and in the absence of any intervention it is estimated that two-thirds of these cases will resolve as a consequence of complement-mediated bacterial lysis: that is to say, they will not develop into SBP but will be resolved by the normal antimicrobial defences of the body. If the organisms multiply and neutrophils are mobilized, the ascitic neutrophil count increases, and an ascitic tap at this stage yields a positive culture and an elevated white blood cell count. By contrast, if the infection of monomicrobial bacterascites resolves (that is, the organisms are lysed) and an ascitic tap is then performed, the ascitic neutrophil count will be increased but the ascitic fluid will be sterile. This is termed 'culture-negative neutrocytic ascites' (CNNA), but it should be remembered that the most common cause of this finding is poor culture technique.

The organisms isolated are shown in Table 15.22.3.4. If there is a polymicrobial growth with a low ascitic neutrophil count, which occurs in 0.6% of all ascitic taps, then the tap is likely to have been traumatic.

Risk factors

The risk factors for the development of SBP are summarized in Table 15.22.3.5 and discussed below.

Decreased opsonic activity

The protein concentration of ascitic fluid does not change with the advent of SBP. Patients with a low protein content (<15 g/litre)

Box 15.22.3.3 Complications of ascites
◆ Pleural effusion
◆ Paraumbilical hernia
◆ Hepatorenal syndrome
◆ Respiratory difficulties
◆ Hypercatabolic state
◆ Spontaneous bacterial peritonitis

Box 15.22.3.4 Symptoms of spontaneous bacterial peritonitis
◆ Asymptomatic 25%
◆ Abdominal pain 60%
◆ Abdominal tenderness 10%
◆ Fever 50%
◆ Encephalopathy 10%
◆ Shock <5%

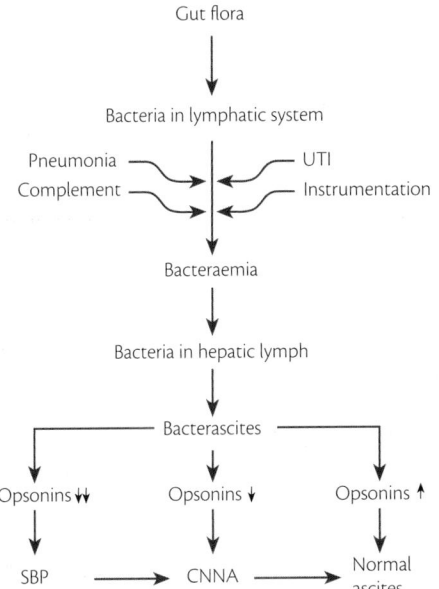

Fig. 15.22.3.4 Pathogenesis of spontaneous bacterial peritonitis. Bacteria can enter ascites through the lymphatic system. In many cases this is resolved through complement mediated bacterial lysis. When opsonins are decreased (e.g. low ascitic protein) or host defence is poor, bacteria multiply and cause SBP. CNNA, culture negative neutrocytic ascites; SBP, spontaneous bacterial peritonitis.

have an increased risk of developing SBP, compared to those with a high ascitic protein content. Patients with cirrhotic and nephrotic ascites are prone to infection, whereas those with malignant ascites or cardiac ascites are not. The risk of SBP is increased sixfold for those with an ascitic protein of less than 10 g/litre. When bacteria enter ascitic fluid they may be lysed by the activity of complement if they are serum-sensitive, or they may be coated with opsonins such as IgG or the third component of the complement pathway (C3). Complement deficiency also predisposes to infection. The opsonic activity of ascitic fluid correlates with the total protein, as well as that of CH100 (total haemolytic complement), C3, and C4 concentration. These concentrations may be increased by diuresis, thus decreasing the risk of SBP, and (for reasons that are not

Table 15.22.3.4 Organisms causing spontaneous bacterial peritonitis

The gut and urine are the most frequent source of organisms
Enteric organisms (75%)
Enterobacteria (mainly *E. coli* (60%)
Other Gram-negative bacilli, e.g. *Klebsiella* spp. (8%)
Enterococcus faecalis (6%)
Anaerobes (1–5%)
Non-enteric organisms (25%)
Gram-positive cocci
Streptococcus pneumoniae (12%)
Other *Streptococcus* spp. (7%)
Staphylococcus spp. (4%)
Others (2%)

Table 15.22.3.5 Risk factors for spontaneous bacterial peritonitis (SBP)

- Instrumentation procedures (endoscopy, sigmoidoscopy, balloon tamponade)
- Gastrointestinal haemorrhage
- Bacterial infections (e.g. chest, urinary tract infections, bacteraemia)
- Previous episodes of SBP
- Decreased opsonic activity
    - Low ascitic protein (<10 g/l)
    - Low ascitic C3 concentration
    - Complement deficiency

understood) diuretics may also increase the neutrophil count in ascitic fluid.

Recent instrumentation
Recent instrumentation such as endoscopy or sigmoidoscopy increases the risk of SBP, but the risk is not increased by paracentesis. A study compared the risk of SBP in two groups of patients and found that it was slightly less, if anything, in those treated with paracentesis rather than with diuretics.

Gastrointestinal haemorrhage
There is a 21% incidence of SBP in patients admitted to hospital with a gastrointestinal haemorrhage. While it is assumed that bleeding predisposes to infection, there is data to suggest that infection may predispose to bleeding. Since the incidence of SBP immediately following a gastrointestinal bleed is high, many clinicians now advocate the prophylactic use of broad-spectrum antibiotics in such situations.

Previous spontaneous bacterial peritonitis
The recurrence rate for SBP is 47% at 6 months and 69% at 1 year.

Treatment
The mortality associated with SBP is approximately 30% in most series, hence it must be treated as soon as a presumptive diagnosis is made following microscopy of ascitic fluid. For patients with bacterascites but no rise in the neutrophil count, the ascitic tap should be repeated, while those with an increased neutrophil count should be treated.

The treatment of SBP is summarized in Box 15.22.3.5. Appropriate antibiotics—based on the types of organism most frequently encountered—include cefotaxime, ciprofloxacin with amoxicillin, and piperacillin with tazlocillin (PIP/TAZ). Treatment is continued until complete resolution of all signs of infection and the ascitic neutrophil count decreases to within the normal range, which is generally achieved within week of treatment. The administration of albumin at a dose of 1.5 g/kg at the time of diagnosis and 1 g/kg at 48 h decreases the incidence of renal dysfunction and decreases mortality from 30% to 18%.

Prophylaxis
Many clinicians in the United Kingdom now use ciprofloxacin. A French study has evaluated the efficacy of this antibiotic in patients with cirrhosis who have an ascitic protein level of less than 15 g/litre, showing that the administration of 750 mg ciprofloxacin given in a single dose per week decreased the incidence of SBP from

> **Box 15.22.3.5**   Treatment of spontaneous bacterial peritonitis (SBP)
>
> 1   Diagnosis of SBP on ascitic microscopy (>250 PMNs/mm^3)
>
> 2   Commence third-generation cephalosporin or ciprofloxacin with amoxicillin
>
> 3   Infuse albumin at 1.5 g/kg at diagnosis and 1g/kg at 48 h
>
> 4   Treat until resolution (~1 week, mortality up to 30%)
>
> 5   Commence prophylaxis against future SBP
>
> 6   Consider liver transplantation as 1-year mortality is 75%

22% to 4% at 6 months, with a corresponding decrease in hospital admission over this period (18 days to 9 days). These authors concluded that prophylaxis with ciprofloxacin was effective, and cost-analysis studies have shown such antimicrobial prophylaxis to be cost-effective.

Other issues

Drug prescribing

When prescribing a drug for any patient with liver disease it is always sensible for the physician to check the product literature or some source such as the British National Formulary (BNF), but in patients with ascites the following are worthy of particular comment:

* Nonsteroidal anti-inflammatory drugs are contraindicated in patients because of the high risk of developing renal failure.

* Drugs that can cause a reduction in arterial pressure or decrease renal blood flow—e.g. ACE inhibitors, angiotensin II and α_1-adrenergic receptor blockers—should be used with caution because of an increased risk of renal impairment.

* Aminoglycosides are associated with an increased risk of nephrotoxicity and renal failure, hence their use should be reserved for patients with bacterial infections that cannot be treated with less toxic antibiotics.

* Contrast media for radiological investigations should be used with care, particularly if the patient has significant renal impairment (beware the patient whose serum creatinine is 'not too bad' as a consequence of low muscle mass or body mass index).

Fertility

Women with cirrhosis and ascites rarely, if ever, become pregnant, since ovulation has usually ceased before the onset of ascites.

Areas of controversy and for further research

Current areas of controversy include the use of albumin or plasma substitutes following paracentesis. Although albumin has been shown to be superior to plasma substitutes in preventing the activation of hormonal systems that indicate hypovolaemia, there is no hard data to show that albumin is more effective than colloid substitutes in terms of overall patient survival or duration of hospital stay. There is also controversy over the issue of central blood volume, with two groups reporting diametrically opposite findings. This is a crucial argument since the current peripheral vasodilatation hypothesis is based on the premise of a decreased central blood volume. Studies by Mauro Bernardi's group have shown that vasodilatation disappears during upright posture, and it appears that patients may exhibit features of both underfill and overfill depending on their posture and severity of liver disease.

Ideally, longitudinal studies conducted over many years need to be performed in newly diagnosed patients with cirrhosis, including baseline clinical, hormonal, and sodium-balance studies, as well as long-term (10 years or more) investigations of systemic haemodynamics and portal pressure. Why do patients develop vasodilatation? Although current ideas favour a role for nitric oxide, the evidence to support this is unclear. What is the role of hydrogen sulphide or carbon monoxide? Why do patients develop ascites after liver transplantation? This complication is unusual but can be very striking and disruptive to management. Finally, controlled studies are needed to determine whether it is beneficial to employ paracentesis in patients with spontaneous bacterial peritonitis.

Further reading

Arroyo V, Ginés P (1992). Arteriolar vasodilatation and the pathogenesis of the hyperdynamic circulation and renal sodium and water retention in cirrhosis. *Gastroenterology*, **102**, 1077–8.

Bernard B, *et al.* (1995). Prognostic significance of bacterial infection in bleeding cirrhotic patients a prospective study. *Gastroenterology*, **108**, 1828–34.

Bernardi M, *et al.* (1995). Hyperdynamic circulation of advanced cirrhosis: a re-appraisal based on posture-induced changes in haemodynamics. *J Hepatol*, **22**, 309–18.

Campra JL, Reynolds TB (1978). Effectiveness of high-dose spironolactone therapy in patients with chronic liver disease and relatively refractory ascites. *Digest Dis*, **23**, 1025–30.

Chavez-Tapia NC, *et al.* (2009). Antibiotics for spontaneous bacterial peritonitis in cirrhotic patients. *Cochrane Database Syst Rev*, **21**, CD002232.

Dolz C, *et al.* (1991). Ascites increases the resting energy expenditure in liver cirrhosis. *Gastroenterology*, **100**, 738–44.

Ginés P, *et al.* (2008). Effects of satavaptan, a selective vasopressin V(2) receptor antagonist, on ascites and serum sodium in cirrhosis with hyponatremia: a randomized trial. *Hepatology*, **48**, 2041–3.

Ginés P, Cardenas A. (2008). The management of ascites and hyponatremia in cirrhosis. *Semin Liver Dis*, **28**, 435–8.

Henriksen JH, *et al.* (1989). Reduced central blood volume in cirrhosis. *Gastroenterology*, **97**, 1506–13.

Heuman DM, *et al.* (2004). Persistent ascites and low serum sodium identify patients with cirrhosis and low MELD scores who are at high risk for early death. *Hepatology*, **40**, 802–10.

Iwakiri Y (2007). The molecules: mechanisms of arterial vasodilatation observed in the splanchnic and systemic circulation in portal hypertension. *J Clin Gastroenterol*, **41**, S288–94.

Luca A, *et al.* (1994). Favorable effects of total paracentesis on splanchnic haemodynamics in cirrhotic patients with tense ascites. *Hepatology*, **20**, 30–3.

Nevens F, *et al.* (1996). The effect of long-term treatment with spironolactone on variceal pressure in patients with portal hypertension without ascites. *Hepatology*, **23**, 1047–52.

Panos MZ, *et al.* (1990). Single, total paracentesis for tense ascites: sequential haemodynamic changes and right atrial size. *Hepatology*, **11**, 662–7.

Pare P, Talbot J, Hoefs JC (1983). Serum-ascites albumin concentration gradient: a physiologic approach to the differential diagnosis of ascites. *Gastroenterology*, **85**, 245–53.

Perez-Ayuso RM, et al. (1983). Randomized comparative study of efficacy of furosemide versus spironolactone in non-azotemic cirrhosis with ascites. *Gastroenterology*, **84**, 961–8.

Runyon BA (1986). Low-protein-concentration ascitic fluid is predisposed to spontaneous bacterial peritonitis. *Gastroenterology*, **91**, 1343–6.

Runyon BA, Hoefs JC (1984). Culture-negative neutrocytic ascites a variant of spontaneous bacterial peritonitis. *Hepatology*, **4**, 1209–11.

Runyon BA, et al. (1990). Bedside inoculation of blood culture bottles with ascitic fluid is superior to delayed inoculation in the detection of spontaneous bacterial peritonitis. *J Clin Microbiol*, **28**, 2811–12.

Saab S, et al. (2009). Oral antibiotic prophylaxis reduces spontaneous bacterial peritonitis occurrence and improves short-term survival in cirrhosis: a meta-analysis. *Am J Gastroenterol*, **104**, 993–1001.

Salerno F, et al. (1991). Randomized comparative study of hemaccel vs. albumin infusion after total paracentesis in cirrhotic patients with refractory ascites. *Hepatology*, **13**, 707–13.

Simón M-A, Díez J, Prieto J (1991). Abnormal sympathetic and renal response to sodium restriction in compensated cirrhosis. *Gastroenterology*, **101**, 1354–60.

Solà R, et al. (1995). Spontaneous bacterial peritonitis in cirrhotic patients treated using paracentesis or diuretics results of a randomized study. *Hepatology*, **21**, 340–4.

Sort P, et al. (1999). Effect of intravenous albumin on renal impairment and mortality in patients with cirrhosis and spontaneous bacterial peritonitis. *N Engl J Med*, **341**, 403–9.

Stanley MM, et al. (1989). Peritoneovenous shunting as compared with medical treatment in patients with alcoholic cirrhosis and massive ascites. *N Engl J Med*, **321**, 1632–8.

Strauss RM, Boyer TD (1997). Hepatic hydrothorax. *Semin Liver Dis*, **17**, 227–32.

15.22.4 Hepatocellular failure

E. Anthony Jones

Essentials

Hepatocellular failure occurs when loss of liver parenchymal cell function exceeds the capacity of hepatocytes to regenerate or repair liver injury. Acute hepatocellular failure is characterized by hepatocellular jaundice, elevated serum aminotransferase levels, and prolongation of the prothrombin time associated with an acute liver disease/insult. Fulminant hepatic failure is the syndrome of acute hepatocellular failure complicated by hepatic encephalopathy, occurring within 8 weeks of the onset of clinical liver disease. Chronic hepatocellular failure is characterized by a chronic hepatocellular disease and one or more features of hepatocellular failure.

The most common causes of fulminant hepatic failure are acute viral hepatitis and drugs. Prevention may be achieved by vaccination against hepatitis B, avoidance of re-exposure to drugs that have previously induced hepatitis, avoidance of poisons (e.g. *Amanita* mushrooms), and—after exposure to a relevant toxin—the use of antidotes, e.g. *N*-acetylcysteine after paracetamol (acetaminophen) overdose. Chronic hepatocellular failure may complicate any progressive chronic hepatocellular process, such as cirrhosis.

There are four main manifestations of hepatocellular failure. (1) Hepatic encephalopathy. This complex neuropsychiatric syndrome is divided into four stages of increasing severity: stage I—psychiatric and behavioural changes; stage II—drowsiness and lethargy; stage III—reversible somnolence; and stage IV—coma. Clinical signs are non-specific. Asterixis ('liver flap') can often be elicited. Raised brain concentrations of ammonia and increased GABA-mediated inhibitory neurotransmission may be important in pathogenesis. (2) Haemorrhagic diathesis. The responsible factors include impaired synthesis of hepatocyte-derived blood clotting factors and thrombocytopenia. (3) Ascites. see Chapter 15.22.3. (4) Hepatocellular jaundice—see Chapter 15.20. Other features of particular importance include increased susceptibility to infection, cerebral oedema and raised intracranial pressure, hypoglycaemia, hepatorenal syndrome, portopulmonary hypertension, and hepatopulmonary syndrome. Patients with hepatocellular failure complicating chronic liver disease may manifest peripheral stigmata, such as spider naevi or clubbing.

In patients with chronic liver disease hepatic encephalopathy can be precipitated by a wide range of factors. These include: (1) gastrointestinal disturbance—e.g. bleeding oesophageal varices, constipation; (2) fluid/electrolyte imbalance—e.g. diuretics-induced; (3) metabolic disturbance—e.g. hypoglycaemia, hypoxia; (4) drugs—particularly sedatives and hypnotics; (5) infection.

Management

Specific and effective therapy for the underlying liver disease is administered when available, but this is not possible for most causes of hepatocellular failure. Treatment is therefore predominantly supportive, with particular emphasis on: (1) correction or removal of precipitating factors; (2) if encephalopathy is present minimizing absorption of nitrogenous substances from the gut by administration of a nonhydrolysed disaccharide laxative (e.g. lactulose, lactitol) with or without an oral poorly absorbed broad-spectrum antibiotic (e.g neomycin); and (3) very careful monitoring of clinical status and laboratory data to facilitate early detection and prompt treatment of complications, such as hypoglycaemia, hypokalaemia, cerebral oedema, and bleeding.

All patients with fulminant (or subfulminant) hepatic failure should be considered to have potentially reversible disease. Nevertherless, when a patient develops stage II encephalopathy intensive supportive care should be instituted and transfer of the patient to a unit with the potential for undertaking orthotopic liver transplantation is recommended.

Course and prognosis

Patients with acute liver failure who do not develop encephalopathy can be expected to recover completely. The mortality of fulminant hepatic failure (without liver transplantation) is about 40%; there are no reliable criteria that enable prediction of whether an individual patient will die or regain consciousness and ultimately survive. The most important determinant of mortality in chronic liver disease is the severity of hepatocellular failure.

Introduction

Hepatocellular failure is the syndrome that occurs when loss of liver parenchymal cell function exceeds the capacity of hepatocytes to regenerate or repair liver injury. Its clinical manifestations include hepatic encephalopathy, a haemorrhagic diathesis, ascites, and hepatocellular jaundice. The syndrome may complicate any disease in which the pathophysiology includes hepatocellular necrosis or apoptosis, or hypofunction of hepatocellular organelles. The onset of overt hepatocellular failure is variable, ranging from a few days to many years after the onset of liver disease.

The term hepatocellular failure does not necessarily imply impaired function of hepatic cells other than hepatocytes: the function of Kupffer cells, sinusoidal cells or stellate (fat-storing) cells may remain intact. Although many biochemical lesions induced by specific chemical, immunological or cytopathic hepatotoxic factors have been associated with hepatocellular failure, the mechanisms by which such factors induce hepatocellular failure—with the notable exception of hypoxia—are poorly understood. Factors that may contribute to hepatocellular injury include immunological damage mediated by T lymphocytes, macrophage activation, direct cytopathic effects of viruses, cytokine-induced activation of cellular functions, and oxidative stress. An influx of calcium ions into hepatocytes appears to be a late phenomenon in the sequence of biochemical events that culminates in hepatocellular death.

Definitions

Acute hepatocellular failure

Acute hepatocellular failure is the syndrome of hepatocellular jaundice, elevated serum aminotransferase levels, and prolongation of the prothrombin time associated with an acute liver disease/insult.

Fulminant hepatic failure

Fulminant hepatic failure is classically defined as the syndrome of acute hepatocellular failure complicated by hepatic encephalopathy occurring within 8 weeks of the onset of clinical liver disease. The King's College Hospital (London) group has introduced the terms 'hyperacute liver failure' for the occurrence of encephalopathy within 7 days of the onset of jaundice and 'late-onset liver failure' for the syndrome in which hepatic encephalopathy occurs 8 to 24 weeks after the onset of clinical evidence of liver disease. In addition, the Beaujon Hospital (Paris) group has proposed that the term 'fulminant hepatic failure' be applied to acute liver failure associated with a plasma factor V level less than 50% of normal and hepatic encephalopathy occurring less than 2 weeks after the onset of jaundice, and that the term 'subfulminant hepatic failure' be used for acute liver failure with a plasma factor V concentration less than half of normal and hepatic encephalopathy occurring 2 weeks to 3 months after the onset of jaundice.

Chronic hepatocellular failure

Chronic hepatocellular failure is the syndrome of decompensated chronic liver disease, which is characterized by a chronic hepatocellular disease and one or more features of hepatocellular failure.

Hepatic encephalopathy (portosystemic encephalopathy)

Hepatic encephalopathy is a complex neuropsychiatric syndrome attributable to impaired hepatocellular function and increased portosystemic shunting. The terms hepatic encephalopathy and portosystemic encephalopathy are often used interchangeably. However, whereas the term portosystemic encephalopathy may be appropriate for encephalopathy complicating increased portosystemic shunting in the absence of overt hepatocellular failure, it may be inappropriate to use the term hepatic encephalopathy in this context. Portosystemic encephalopathy appears to be the preferred term for chronic or recurrent encephalopathy associated with chronic hepatocellular disease.

Aetiology

Acute hepatocellular failure

The most common causes of fulminant hepatic failure are acute viral hepatitis and drugs. About one-third of cases appear to be due to non-A, non-B, non-C (i.e. seronegative) hepatitis of undetermined aetiology. Markers of acute infection with specific hepatitis viruses (such as IgM anti-HAV, IgM anti-HBc, IgM anti-HDV) may be useful in suggesting a specific aetiology. A syndrome similar to acute liver failure with encephalopathy may be associated with infection with other viruses (such as herpes, varicella, cytomegalovirus), particularly in immunocompromised patients.

Only drugs that can induce acute hepatocellular injury (rather than cholestasis alone) have the potential of inducing fulminant hepatic failure. Examples can be classified into two groups according to the characteristics of associated hepatic histology, one of which includes paracetamol (acetaminophen), halothane and ecstasy, and the other includes tetracycline, valproate and certain antiretroviral drugs (see 'Pathology', below). Fulminant hepatic failure due to poisoning may be caused by *Amanita* mushrooms or industrial solvents, particularly chlorinated hydrocarbons.

Hypoxic hepatocellular injury may be attributable to reduced hepatic perfusion, but rarely leads to fulminant hepatic failure (for example following cardiac arrest). Important vascular causes of fulminant hepatic failure include the Budd–Chiari syndrome and veno-occlusive disease. The latter may be induced by pyrolizidine alkaloids, chemotherapy, or irradiation.

Rare causes of fulminant hepatic failure include heat stroke and fatty liver of pregnancy. Acute liver failure associated with intravascular haemolysis suggests Wilson's disease. Autoimmune chronic active hepatitis may present with a syndrome similar to subfulminant hepatic failure; type I antibodies to liver and kidney microsomes may be present.

Fulminant hepatic failure may be precipitated by partial hepatectomy (removal of more than 80% of a normal liver or a smaller proportion of a cirrhotic liver). Fulminant hepatic failure soon after orthotropic liver transplantation may be due to hyperacute allograft rejection or hepatic arterial thrombosis. In carriers of the hepatitis B or C viruses, fulminant hepatic failure may be precipitated by modulation of the host's immune response to the virus as a consequence of immunosuppressive chemotherapy or its withdrawal. In Reye's syndrome a fulminant hepatic failure-like syndrome may occur, but there are additional mitochondrial changes in the brain which are not features of liver failure.

Chronic hepatocellular failure

Chronic hepatocellular failure may complicate any progressive chronic hepatocellular process, or any lesion causing chronic hepatic central venous congestion.

Prevention

The incidence of fulminant hepatitis B should be substantially reduced by widespread vaccination. Fulminant hepatic failure can be prevented by avoiding poisons, such as *Amanita* mushrooms, and avoiding re-exposure to an agent that has induced an idiosyncratic acute hepatitis, such as halothane. Abstinence from alcohol for a period of 6 months is recommended after recovery from an episode of acute liver failure not precipitated by alcohol. If alcohol was implicated in such an episode, lifelong abstinence is advocated.

In some circumstances the use of specific antidotes may prevent liver failure. *N*-acetylcysteine, preceded by activated charcoal, is routinely given after paracetamol overdose. Silibinin, the active constituent of silymarin from milk thistle, is used in Europe as an antidote after *Amanita* poisoning: it may prevent transport of amatoxin into hepatocytes and has other potential actions. Difficulties in designing prospective trials in this rare but important cause of acute liver failure render licensing and proof of efficacy difficult, but evidence from animal studies and retrospective analyses of data on patients exposed to lethal quantities of mushrooms give support to its use.

Common clinical features and their pathophysiology

Hepatic encephalopathy

Impaired mental function due to liver failure may lead to many psychiatric and neurological abnormalities. Impaired psychometric and/or brain electrophysiological function in a patient with chronic liver disease, in whom a routine neurological examination is normal, may imply subclinical or minimal hepatic encephalopathy. The earliest clinical signs are psychiatric and behavioural changes that are primarily due to subtle impairment of intellectual function that reflect predominantly bilateral forebrain dysfunction.

Conventionally, four clinical stages of overt hepatic encephalopathy of increasing severity are recognized (Table 15.22.4.1). Both clinical and electrophysiological manifestations of hepatic encephalopathy are nonspecific and potentially reversible. Advanced hepatic encephalopathy is characterized by loss of consciousness and coma. Myoclonal twitching with increased muscle tone and cogwheel and neck rigidity may occur. Asterixis ('liver flap') can often be elicited (Table 15.22.4.1, Fig. 15.22.4.1). The mouth may be difficult to open. With progression, deep tendon reflexes may be increased and subsequently decreased. One or both plantar responses may become extensor. With progression, the frequency of the electroencephalogram decreases and its amplitude increases, and in later stages the amplitude decreases and triphasic waves may occur.

Hepatic encephalopathy complicating chronic liver disease may be acute or chronic. When acute it is usually associated with one or more recognized precipitating factors (Table 15.22.4.2), but, with the notable exception of sedative–hypnotic drugs, the mechanisms by which these exacerbate hepatic encephalopathy are poorly understood. Failure to identify a precipitating factor may imply deterioration of overall hepatocellular function.

Pathogenesis is multifactorial. Traditionally, factors arising from the intestine have been considered to play an important role. In liver failure, decreased hepatic extraction and metabolism of substances derived from the gut, as a consequence of their passage through intrahepatic and extrahepatic collateral channels and hepatocellular hypofunction, lead to their accumulation in the systemic circulation. Some of these substances have the potential to cross the blood–brain barrier and modulate brain function. The blood–brain barrier is normally highly permeable to nonpolar substances, such as nonionic ammonia and benzodiazepines, but has a low permeability to polar compounds. However, in liver failure the permeability of the barrier to polar compounds, such as the inhibitory neurotransmitter γ-aminobutyric acid (GABA), may increase. Most of the manifestations of hepatic encephalopathy appear to be consistent with a global suppression of central nervous system function, which could be due predominantly to a net increase in inhibitory neurotransmission, as a consequence of increased

Table 15.22.4.1 Clinical stages of hepatic encephalopathy

Stage	Mental status	Asterixis	Electroencephalographic changes
I (prodrome, often diagnosed in retrospect)	Mild confusion, euphoria or depression, decreased attention, slowing of ability to perform mental tasks, untidiness, slurred speech, irritability, reversal of sleep rhythm	Usually absent	Often lacking
II (impending coma)	Drowsiness, lethargy, gross deficits in ability to perform mental tasks, obvious personality changes, inappropriate behaviour, intermittent disorientation (usually for time), lack of sphincter control	Present (with or without incoordination)	Generalized slowing
III	Somnolent but rousable, unable to perform mental tasks, persistent disorientation with respect to time and/or place, amnesia, occasional fits of rage, speech present but incoherent, pronounced confusion	Usually present (if patient can cooperate)	Always present
IV	Coma; with (IV-A) or without (IV-B) response to painful stimuli	Usually absent	Always present

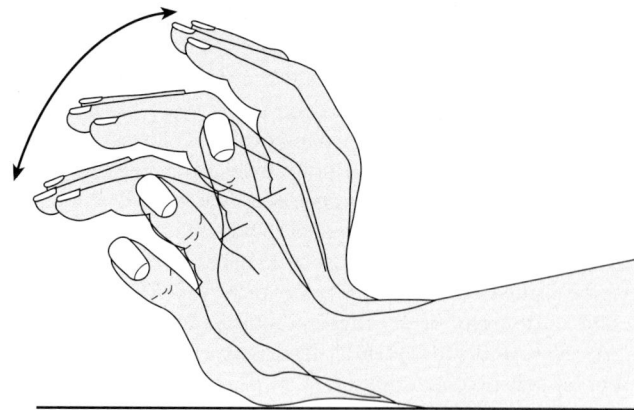

Fig. 15.22.4.1 The 'liver flap' is a slow, flapping tremor (one flap every 1–2 s), which can be elicited by asking the patient to dorsiflex the hands with the arms outstretched and the fingers extended and parted. It is due to neuromuscular incoordination between flexor and extensor muscles: the hands tend to fall forward, but this involuntary movement is rapidly corrected by readoption of the dorsiflexed position, thereby creating a 'flap'. The same phenomenon may be elicited by asking the patient to squeeze the physician's extended finger: neuromuscular incoordination is indicated by repeated augmentation and relaxation of the intensity of the squeeze ('milkmaid's grip').

neurotransmission mediated by inhibitory neurotransmitters such as GABA, and/or possibly decreased neurotransmission mediated by excitatory neurotransmitters, such as glutamate. Currently, the two factors considered to be most important in pathogenesis are raised brain concentrations of ammonia and increased GABA-mediated inhibitory neurotransmission.

Increased GABAergic neurotransmission is associated with impaired motor function and decreased consciousness, two of the cardinal manifestations of hepatic encephalopathy.

Table 15.22.4.2 Factors that may precipitate encephalopathy in a patient with cirrhosis

Precipitating factor	Comments
Constipation Oral protein load Upper gastrointestinal bleed	Gut factors contribute to hepatic encephalopathy
Diuretic therapy Paracentesis Diarrhoea and vomiting	Dehydration, electrolyte and acid–base imbalance
Hypoglycaemia Hypoxia Hypotension Anaemia	Factors with adverse effects on both liver and brain function
Sedative/hypnotic drugs[1]	Benzodiazepines and barbiturates enhance the action of GABA
Azotaemia[2] Infection[3] Induction of a portosystemic shunt[4] General surgery	

[1] Includes drugs acting on the GABA$_A$/benzodiazepine receptor complex.
[2] Blood urea is a source of intestinal ammonia.
[3] May cause dehydration and increased release of nitrogenous substances.
[4] For example, a transjugular intrahepatic portosystemic shunt.

Potential mechanisms for increased GABAergic tone in liver failure include: (1) increased availability of GABA at GABA$_A$ receptors in synaptic clefts; (2) increased astrocytic synthesis and release of neurosteroids that are potent agonists of the GABA$_A$ receptor complex; and (3) increased brain concentrations of naturally occurring ligands that act as central, benzodiazepine receptor agonists.

Ammonia was originally implicated in pathogenesis because it was recognized to be neurotoxic, plasma concentrations tend to be raised in liver failure, and plasma ammonia readily enters the brain. Plasma ammonia concentrations higher than those usually found in liver failure (>1 mmol/litre) are associated with increased neuronal excitation and seizures. By contrast, plasma ammonia concentrations typically found in patients with precoma stages (I–III) of hepatic encephalopathy (100–400 μmol/litre) may enhance neural inhibition by: (1) directly facilitating GABA-gated chloride conductance; (2) selectively increasing the binding of agonist ligands of the GABA$_A$/benzodiazepine receptor complex, and (3) up-regulating peripheral-type benzodiazepine receptors on astrocytic mitochondria, thereby stimulating astrocytic synthesis and release of neurosteroid agonists of the GABA$_A$ complex. An increasing understanding of interorgan ammonia metabolism, which includes its production by small intestine and kidney and its removal by skeletal muscle, may facilitate the development of novel therapies.

Possible roles for neurotransmitter systems other than the GABA system have been postulated. Some of the features of hepatic encephalopathy can be explained by disturbances in functional loops of basal ganglia, which could arise as a consequence of an imbalance between glutamatergic and GABAergic neurotransmission.

Haemorrhagic diathesis

The basis of the haemorrhagic diathesis is multifactorial. Of major importance is impaired synthesis of hepatocyte-derived blood clotting factors, which leads to prolongation of the prothrombin time that cannot be corrected by vitamin K. Thrombocytopenia is often present and may be secondary to the hypersplenism of portal hypertension. However, in fulminant hepatic failure, platelet structure and function are abnormal and the capillary bleeding time is greater than that predicted from the platelet count. Mild disseminated intravascular coagulation is often detectable, but is rarely clinically significant. Upper gastrointestinal haemorrhage frequently occurs, for example from gastritis, gastro-oesophageal varices, or ulcers. A common clinical manifestation of the bleeding tendency is bruising around venepuncture sites.

Ascites

Ascites due to hepatocellular failure complicates lesions that cause sinusoidal portal hypertension, such as cirrhosis, or impaired hepatic venous drainage. However, hepatocellular failure is not invariable when ascites is associated with hepatic venous congestion. See Chapter 15.22.3 for further discussion.

Hepatocellular jaundice

The jaundice of hepatocellular failure has an orange tint and is attributable to conjugated hyperbilirubinaemia due to impaired secretion of conjugated bilirubin into the bile canaliculus because the transport maximum for conjugated bilirubin across the bile canaliculus is reduced relative to bilirubin production and conjugation (see Chapter 15.20).

In acute hepatitis the degree of conjugated hyperbilirubinaemia reflects the extent of hepatocellular necrosis, but even when jaundice is deep, other features of hepatocellular failure, such as a prolonged prothrombin time, may be absent, reflecting the large normal hepatic reserve. By contrast, in chronic noncholestatic liver disease, hepatocellular jaundice usually reflects severe hepatocellular failure.

Other clinical features

Increased susceptibility to infection

About 80% of infections are bacterial, but about one-third are complicated by tissue invasion by fungi (e.g. aspergillosis, candidiasis), which is suggested by antibiotic-resistant fever. However, infection may occur without fever or leucocytosis, and mortality is high.

The increased frequency of infections may be related to a decrease in levels of complement components and opsonins, impairment of the phagocytic and bacteriocidal properties of polymorphonuclear leucocytes, and reduced clearance function of Kupffer cells. Spontaneous bacterial peritonitis is a common complication of ascites due to hepatocellular failure (see Chapter 15.22.3). Sepsis may precipitate acute-on-chronic liver failure.

Foetor hepaticus

Foetor hepaticus is the term applied to the particular smell of the breath that commonly occurs in patients with cirrhosis and extensive portosystemic shunts or fulminant hepatic failure. It has been attributed to gut-derived sulphur-containing products of methionine metabolism. Descriptions vary and include a sweetish, slightly pungent, or faecal smell, similar to that of a rotten apple, mice, or a freshly opened corpse; such subjectivity leads to considerable variation in the recognition of foetor hepaticus.

Acid–base and electrolyte changes

A wide range of abnormalities occur, particularly in fulminant hepatic failure, and may contribute to altered neurological and cardiac function. Hyponatraemia may be due to impaired free-water clearance, failure of the sodium pump, or diuretics. Hypernatraemia is usually iatrogenic, such as when precipitated by lactulose or lactitol therapy. Hyponatraemia or its rapid correction may precipitate central pontine myelinolysis. Respiratory alkalosis, secondary to hyperventilation of central origin, is common in fulminant hepatic failure. Loop diuretics often precipitate a hypokalaemic metabolic alkalosis. Metabolic acidosis may be associated with extensive tissue damage, hypoxia and lactic acidosis. Respiratory acidosis may be associated with hypercapnia and respiratory infection.

Cerebral oedema and raised intracranial pressure

Hepatic encephalopathy in fulminant hepatic failure may be compounded by cerebral oedema and raised intracranial pressure, hypoglycaemia, hypoxia, renal failure, and acid–base/electrolyte changes. Cerebral oedema and raised intracranial pressure occur in about 80% of patients with fulminant hepatic failure with stage IV encephalopathy; they are rarely diagnosed in patients with chronic hepatocellular failure. The relationship, if any, between these complications and hepatic encephalopathy is uncertain, and they are usually classified separately.

Herniation of the cingulate, uncus, or cerebellar tonsil secondary to raised intracranial pressures is a frequent cause of death in fulminant hepatic failure. Antemortem diagnosis of cerebral oedema and raised intracranial pressure is suggested by sudden deterioration of consciousness, increased muscle tone, unequal pupils, abnormally reacting pupils, myoclonus, focal seizures, decerebrate posturing, fixed pupils with spontaneous respiration and/or absent ciliospinal reflexes; such signs become apparent when intracranial pressure exceeds 30 mmHg. Sudden changes in pulse and blood pressure unrelated to haemorrhage, rapid deterioration of the electroencephalogram, sweating, tachycardia, arrhythmias, intermittent systemic hypertension, sudden severe hypotension, bursts of hyperventilation, and fever may all be manifestations of raised intracranial pressure. Papilloedema is rare.

A failure of cellular osmoregulation, with intracellular accumulation of osmolytes, such as glutamine, appears to be a pathogenic mechanism (cytotoxic). Compensatory loss of other intracellular osmolytes, such as inositol, may be more effective in chronic liver disease than in fulminant hepatic failure. Increased blood-to-brain transfer of fluid across the blood–brain barrier (vasogenic), and expansion of the extravascular space (interstitial or hydrocephalic) may also contribute to pathogenesis. The systemic response to inflammation may play a synergistic role through its effect on cerebral blood flow.

Hypoglycaemia

Severe hypoglycaemia (blood glucose <2.2 mmol/litre, i.e. <40 mg/dl) occurs in about 40% of patients with fulminant hepatic failure, particularly children, and may exacerbate encephalopathy. The clinical and electroencephalographic features of hepatic and hypoglycaemic encephalopathies are similar. In acute liver failure, hypoglycaemia may occur in the absence of hepatic encephalopathy. Hypoglycaemia may develop rapidly and may be associated with sepsis. It is due primarily to impaired hepatic glucose release secondary to glycogen depletion. In contrast to hepatic encephalopathy, hypoglycaemic coma may cause irreversible brain damage.

Cardiovascular changes

Hepatocellular failure is associated with systemic vasodilatation and a hyperdynamic circulation. Cardiac output is increased, peripheral vascular resistance decreased, blood pressure reduced, and splanchnic and capillary flow increased, but perfusion of the renal cortex is decreased (see below). Features of a hyperdynamic circulation include a bounding pulse, capillary pulsation, vasodilated extremities, a precordial heave, and an ejection systolic murmur. The increased cardiac output has been attributed to an increased vascular capacitance and hence relative hypovolaemia with low jugular venous pressure. Endogenous cannabinoids acting at vascular CB1 receptors have been implicated in this state of vasodilation.

Arrhythmias, other than sinus tachycardia, frequently occur with hypoxia and stage IV encephalopathy due to fulminant hepatic failure. Cardiac arrest, unrelated to respiratory arrest, may occur.

Hepatorenal syndrome

In many cases renal impairment is attributable to concurrent hypovolaemia (e.g. following gastrointestinal haemorrhage or use of diuretics) and/or sepsis, but in the absence of such factors, renal failure may be due to the hepatorenal syndrome. This syndrome which may be rapidly progressive, occurs in the setting of decreased cardiac output associated with a decrease in effective arterial blood volume due to severe splanchnic arterial vasodilatation and a reduction in venous return; the renal failure is functional and associated with intense renal arterial vasoconstriction, a reduced glomerular filtration rate and oliguria. Two patterns of the syndrome have been recognized: in the first (type 1), impairment in circulatory and renal function is rapidly progressive and usually associated with a major precipitating factor; in the second (type 2), there is a steady impairment of circulatory and renal function associated with refractory ascites. The kidneys in this syndrome function normally when transplanted into subjects without liver disease. Several humoral systems have been implicated in pathogenesis. Acute tubular necrosis, usually precipitated by an ischaemic insult, may supervene. See Chapter 21.5 for further discussion.

Portopulmonary hypertension and hepatopulmonary syndrome

Portopulmonary hypertension, which is common in cirrhotic patients with portal hypertension, is due to pulmonary vasoconstriction and vascular remodelling; it may lead to hypoxaemia, dyspnoea and right ventricular failure. The hepatopulmonary syndrome is characterized by the triad of liver disease, intrapulmonary microvascular dilatation with deceased pulmonary vascular resistance (right to left shunt), and an increased alveolar–arterial oxygen gradient, leading to hypoxaemia. Ventilation perfusion ratios are abnormal and diffusion capacity is impaired. Cyanosis may occur. The mechanism of the pulmonary vasoconstriction and/or vasodilatation in these syndromes is unknown, but factors such as endothelin, that modulate the pulmonary circulation may be involved.

Rarely, in patients with cirrhosis, intractable hypoxaemia may be due to large pulmonary arteriovenous shunts. Pulmonary oedema, not attributable to left ventricular failure, and respiratory arrest of central origin may occur in fulminant hepatic failure.

Skin changes

Recognition of certain skin changes in a patient with chronic liver disease alerts the clinician to the possibility of incipient or overt chronic hepatocellular failure, but no skin changes are specific for hepatocellular failure.

Spider naevi are often present in patients with cirrhosis. They consist of a central protuberant arteriole from which small vessels radiate in a manner that has been likened to the appearance of a spider's legs (Fig. 15.22.4.2). Their diameter is usually less than 0.5 cm. They occur in the area of drainage of the superior vena cava and should be distinguished from telangiectasia, corkscrew sclera vessels, and purpura. Development of new spider naevi suggests progressive hepatocellular disease.

Palmar erythema occurs less frequently than spider naevi. It is characterized by an exaggeration of the normal mottling of palmar surfaces of the hands, resulting in well-demarcated redness of the thenar and hypothenar eminences, and of the pulps of the fingers (Fig. 15.22.4.3). Dilated, thread-like blood vessels in the skin, having an apparently random distribution, may occur, and may resemble a United States dollar note ('paper money skin'). White nails with loss of demarcation of the lunulae (leuconychia, Terry's nails) (Fig. 15.22.4.4) and finger clubbing (Fig. 15.22.4.5) may also occur.

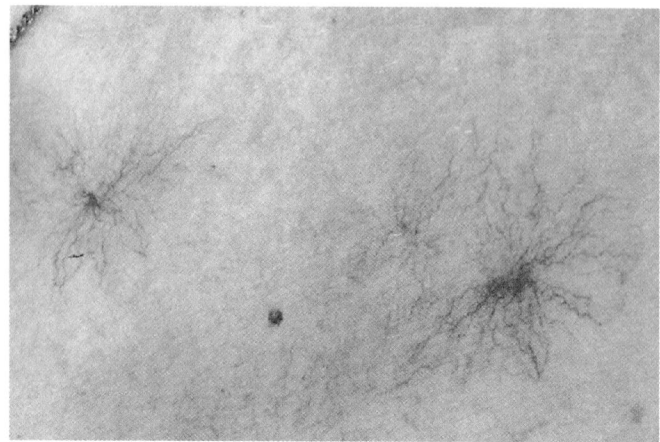

Fig. 15.22.4.2 Spider naevi in a patient with cirrhosis.

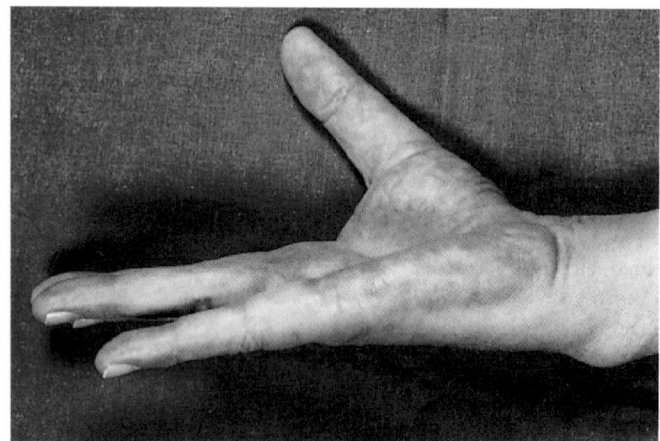

Fig. 15.22.4.3 Palmar erythema in a patient with cirrhosis.

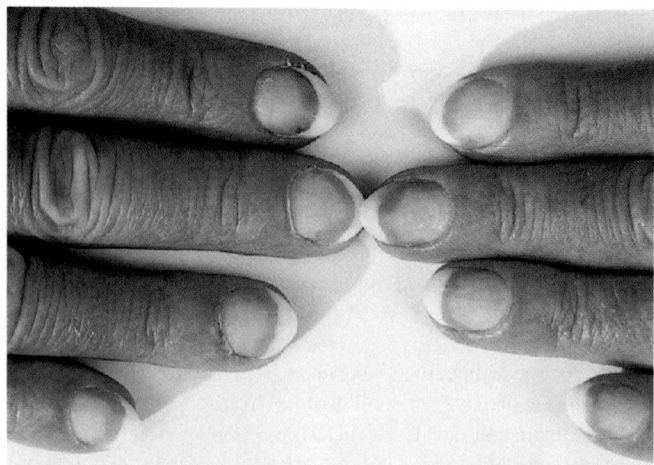

Fig. 15.22.4.4 White nails in a patient with cirrhosis.

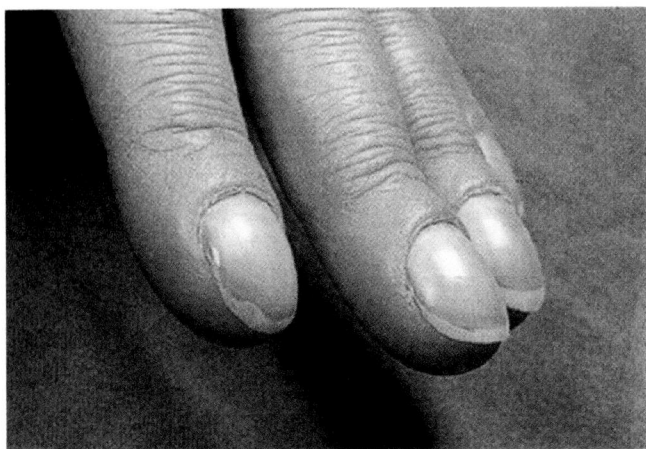

Fig. 15.22.4.5 Finger clubbing in a patient with cirrhosis.

Endocrine changes

Chronic liver disease may be associated with reduced concentrations of testosterone. Some male patients with cirrhosis develop hypogonadism and feminization. The former is characterized by testicular atrophy, decreased potency and libido, and a reduced need to shave; the latter is characterized by gynaecomastia and female hair distribution and body habitus. Some female patients with cirrhosis develop infertility, scanty irregular menstruation, and an asexual appearance due to loss of female characteristics. Unilateral or bilateral (tender) gynaecomastia may be a complication of cirrhosis (Fig. 15.22.4.6) or spironolactone therapy.

Fatigue

Severe disabling fatigue that seems to be out of proportion to a patient's general condition may occur in patients with chronic liver disease, such as those with primary biliary cirrhosis and chronic hepatitis C, before the onset of overt hepatocellular failure.

Abnormal protein metabolism

In cirrhosis the degree of hypoalbuminaemia reflects both decreased hepatocellular synthesis and an increase in plasma volume. Because of albumin's long plasma half-life, hypoalbuminaemia may not be present early in the course of fulminant hepatic failure. Chronic hepatocellular failure is associated with increased protein catabolism and a loss of skeletal muscle mass.

Other features

A low-grade fever may accompany severe active hepatocellular disease, such as acute alcoholic hepatitis, in the absence of infection. A normochromic normocytic anaemia is a feature of chronic hepatocellular disease. Osteopenia is common in patients with decompensated cirrhosis.

Diagnosis

The syndrome of hepatocellular failure constitutes a clinical spectrum from acute liver failure at one extreme to decompensated chronic hepatocellular disease at the other. A patient dying from hepatocellular failure usually exhibits all four of the cardinal manifestations, with or without complicating sepsis.

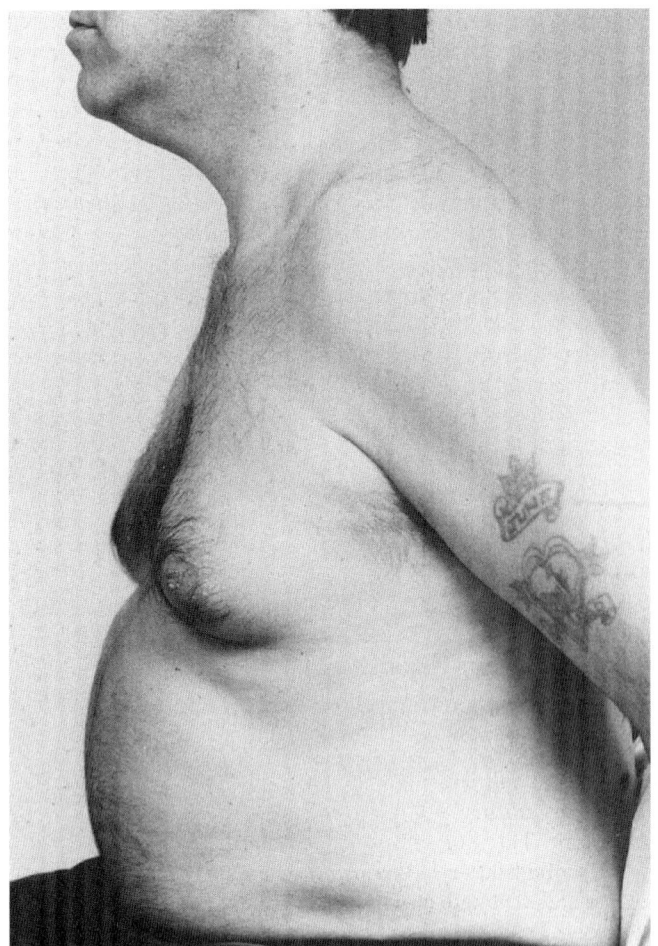

Fig. 15.22.4.6 Gynaecomastia in a male alcoholic patient with cirrhosis.

Hepatic encephalopathy

Hepatic encephalopathy is a clinical diagnosis that is usually made by recognizing the presence of encephalopathy and excluding nonhepatic causes. No individual clinical or laboratory abnormality is specific for hepatic encephalopathy. In the early stages of presentation special attention is paid to changes in personality, hypersomnia, and deterioration of performance at work or school. Asterixis (liver flap) is commonly present, but is not pathognomonic. Signs of portal hypertension, nonspecific cutaneous stigmata of liver disease, and/or foetor hepaticus may be present. It is necessary to recognize and distinguish disorders with neurological manifestations that may mimic those of hepatic encephalopathy, and to which many of the same patients are prone, such as alcohol intoxication, subdural haematoma, and Wernicke's and Korsakoff's syndromes. More than one type of encephalopathy may coexist.

Psychometric tests are useful in detecting and monitoring subtle mental dysfunction in patients with minimal or early stages of hepatic encephalopathy. The quantitative number connection test is often applied, but allowance must be made for the effects of learning and age on test scores. EEG abnormalities are nonspecific, but there is usually a fairly good correlation between the clinical stage of encephalopathy and the degree of abnormality of the EEG. The EEG is of value in differential diagnosis, sometimes revealing focal lesions in the brain, seizure activity, and other findings that might suggest an alternative diagnosis. Visual evoked potentials that depend on cognitive function are sensitive in the detection of mild mental changes in patients with cirrhosis who do not have overt encephalopathy.

Routine laboratory tests aid in the differential diagnosis of encephalopathies, and in the detection of factors that may precipitate hepatic encephalopathy (Table 15.22.4.2). An elevated plasma ammonia concentration may be helpful in suggesting a hepatic origin for an undiagnosed encephalopathy and is consistent with increased portosystemic shunting. Plasma ammonia concentrations are modestly increased in most patients with hepatic encephalopathy, but correlate poorly with the clinical stage and are not useful in management.

Haemorrhagic diathesis

The most important and readily obtainable markers of the diathesis are the prothrombin time and the platelet count. Plasma activities of individual clotting factors that are synthesized by hepatocytes, such as factor V, are reduced.

Ascites

When the presence of ascites on physical examination is in doubt, the issue may be resolved by ultrasonography, which can detect as little as 100 to 200 ml of intraperitoneal fluid. Careful examination of the jugular veins is necessary in the exclusion of cardiac causes. On ultrasonography, diffuse inhomogeneity of the liver suggests cirrhosis, and difficulty in visualizing major hepatic veins suggests the Budd–Chiari syndrome. See Chapter 15.22.3 for further discussion.

Hepatocellular jaundice

The conjugated hyperbilirubinaemia of hepatocellular failure has to be distinguished from: (1) acquired intrahepatic cholestatic disease, e.g. primary biliary cirrhosis, before decompensation; (2) cholestasis due to large duct biliary obstruction, e.g. due to stones or tumours; and (3) rare congenital conjugated hyperbilirubinaemia, in which results of other routine serum biochemical liver tests are normal, e.g. the Rotor and Dubin Johnson syndromes.

Recognition that conjugated hyperbilirubinaemia is attributable to hepatocellular failure is usually possible from clinical and routine haematological and serum biochemical findings and an ultrasound showing no evidence of dilated bile ducts. Unconjugated hyperbilirubinaemia is not a feature of hepatocellular failure.

Acute hepatocellular failure

Acute hepatocellular disease associated with conjugated hyperbilirubinaemia may be classified as acute liver failure when the prothrombin time is prolonged. If acute liver failure is due to hypoxia, a cause is usually obvious, such as a hypotensive episode during surgery.

A diagnosis of fulminant hepatic failure requires the presence of encephalopathy, elevated serum alanine aminotransferase (ALT) activities early in the course, and marked prolongation of the prothrombin time (see 'Definitions', above). ALT concentrations exceeding 50 times the upper limit of normal are common in massive hepatocellular necrosis, but may be less than three times the upper limit of normal with minimal hyperbilirubinaemia when fulminant hepatic failure is associated with microvsicular hepatic

steatosis (see 'Pathology', below). Abdominal pain may occur with poisoning. Rarely, hepatic encephalopathy precedes jaundice and abnormal behaviour may have to be distinguished from non-hepatogenous acute psychiatric disease. However, patients with fulminant hepatic failure due to massive hepatocellular necrosis who survive more than a few days develop deep jaundice. Lumbar puncture should usually be avoided, because of the coagulopathy and possible raised intracranial pressure. However, a baseline CT scan of the brain is prudent. Evidence for the presence of other types of encephalopathy is routinely sought. Severe sepsis or falciparum malaria may occasionally mimic the syndrome of fulminant hepatic failure. A very large liver or a history of malignancy suggests neoplastic infiltration of the liver. In subfulminant hepatic failure, ultrasonography may reveal inhomogeneity of the liver due to nodular transformation.

Chronic hepatocellular failure

The diagnosis of chronic hepatocellular failure requires the demonstration of an appropriate chronic liver disease and evidence of hepatocellular failure. Mild conjugated hyperbilirubinaemia and a modest prolongation of the prothrombin time tend to occur before the onset of overt hepatic encephalopathy or ascites. By contrast with diseases that lead to sinusoidal portal hypertension, such as cirrhosis, those that cause presinusoidal portal hypertension, such as schistosomiasis, do not usually progress to hepatocellular failure. Diagnosis of the hepatorenal syndrome requires exclusion of other causes of renal failure.

Pathology

There is no single hepatic histological change that is pathognomonic of hepatocellular failure. Fulminant hepatic failure is usually associated with massive or confluent hepatocellular necrosis. However, occasionally, e.g. when fulminant hepatic failure is due to acute fatty liver of pregnancy, valproic acid, tetracycline, or antiretroviral drugs, liver histology reveals microvesicular hepatocellular steatosis in which the nucleus retains its central position within hepatocytes.

In many autopsies on patients who succumb to fulminant hepatic failure, there is evidence of cerebral oedema and raised intracranial pressure, such as increased brain weight, tense dura, flattened cortical gyri, dilated ventricles, and cingulate, uncal, or cerebellar herniation. The histology of the brain is essentially normal, whereas that of patients who died from chronic liver failure typically reveals an increase in the number and size of Alzheimer type 2 astrocytes (astrocytosis), which may reflect toxic effects of ammonia on astrocytes. Functional renal failure, in the absence of complicating acute tubular necrosis, is associated with no gross pathological changes in the kidney.

Course and prognosis
Acute hepatocellular failure

In patients with acute liver failure who do not develop encephalopathy, as in most cases of acute icteric viral hepatitis, complete recovery is the rule.

The course of fulminant hepatic failure is variable, and there are no reliable criteria that enable prediction of whether an individual patient will die or regain consciousness and ultimately survive.

Overall survival appears to have improved with advances in intensive supportive care, and currently may be about 40% without liver transplantation. Mortality tends to be greater when encephalopathy is severe and prolonged, and when coagulopathy is profound (prothrombin time >100 s). Mortality is particularly high (>80%) in cases caused by halothane, or drugs other than paracetamol, but is about 50% when paracetamol is implicated. Major complications, such as gastrointestinal haemorrhage, renal failure, cerebral oedema, and raised intracranial pressure, increase mortality. Indeed, fulminant hepatic failure may be characterized by multiorgan failure. Small or decreasing liver size, convulsions, cardiac arrhythmias other than sinus tachycardia, and marked foetor hepaticus are ominous signs. Serum concentrations of aminotransferases may decrease abruptly, but have no prognostic value. Factor VII levels are favoured as a prognostic marker early in the course, and factor V levels later with progression. No available prognostic scoring system adequately predicts outcome or candidacy for liver transplantation. The course of fulminant hepatic failure can be divided into five phases.

1 Preencephalopathy

In acute liver failure a progressive increase in prothrombin time is ominous and often precedes the onset of hepatic encephalopathy. After paracetamol overdosage the onset of encephalopathy may be predicted from plasma concentrations of the drug.

2 Encephalopathy

About one-third of patients die within 2 days of the onset of stage IV encephalopathy. About 20% of deaths appear to be due to progressive liver failure. In other cases, death can be attributed to one or more complications of the syndrome, such as upper gastrointestinal haemorrhage, cerebral oedema and raised intracranial pressure, sepsis, and renal failure. In subfulminant hepatic failure, death due to raised intracranial pressure and/or sepsis is more common than in fulminant hepatic failure.

3 Hepatic regeneration

The key factor in determining the outcome of fulminant hepatic failure, in the absence of liver transplantation, is the ability of the liver to regenerate. Nodules of hyperplastic regenerating liver tissue may be found at autopsy in patients who survive more than 10 days after the onset of encephalopathy. In general, such patients have usually died of a complication of fulminant hepatic failure at a time when indices of hepatocellular function were improving. Serum concentrations of α-fetoprotein, which are regarded as an index of hepatic regeneration, do not usually become elevated until at least 10 days after the onset of encephalopathy, and the concentration tends to correlate fairly well with the amount of hepatic regeneration found at autopsy. Recovery is usually heralded by clinical improvement in encephalopathy, which may be preceded by a decreasing prothrombin time. The EEG may remain abnormal for several days after consciousness is regained.

4 Cholestasis

A phase of profound cholestasis often develops 2 to 3 weeks after patients regain consciousness. When death has occurred during this phase, large regenerative nodules and intense cholestasis in hepatocytes have been found at autopsy.

5 Long-term sequelae

Complete restoration of normal hepatic function and structure usually occurs in survivors of fulminant hepatic failure, even after

cerebral oedema, decerebrate rigidity, and episodes of flattening of the EEG. Serum biochemical liver tests and hepatic histology typically return to normal 45 to 75 days after the onset of hepatic encephalopathy. Permanent neurological sequelae have been reported when recovery has occurred after respiratory arrest.

Chronic hepatocellular failure

In patients with chronic hepatocellular disease, hepatic encephalopathy is often reversible, particularly if a precipitating factor is identified. An MRI scan of the brain typically reveals symmetrical pallidal hyperintensities, possibly due to increased deposition of manganese in the basal ganglia. These hyperintensities appear to correlate with the degree of impairment of hepatocellular function, but not with hepatic encephalopathy. Elevated serum conjugated bilirubin in cirrhosis or precirrhotic chronic alcoholic liver disease is associated with a poor prognosis. An increasing serum conjugated bilirubin concentration in a patient with a chronic cholestatic liver disease, such as primary biliary cirrhosis, may reflect progression of the liver disease and/or the development of hepatocellular failure. The serum total bilirubin is regarded as a good index of prognosis in primary biliary cirrhosis. When ascites first develops in a patient with cirrhosis, 1-year survival is about 50% and 5-year survival about 20%. Survival after the onset of the hepatorenal syndrome is usually no more than a few weeks for type 1 cases or a few months for type 2 cases.

Management

The first concern is whether there is any effective therapy for the underlying liver disease. A treatment that suppresses the pathological process responsible for impairing hepatocellular function may decrease or reverse manifestations of hepatocellular failure. For most patients with acute liver failure, corticosteroids appear to be harmful, with exceptions being the few patients in whom the underlying lesion is an autoimmune hepatitis, and carriers of the hepatitis B or C virus in whom acute liver failure has been precipitated by withdrawal of immunosuppressive chemotherapy. Nucleoside analogues may have a place in preventing a reactivation/acute flare of hepatitis in HBsAg carriers, but antiviral therapy has not been shown to be efficacious in preventing acute liver failure in patients with acute viral hepatitis. N-Acetylcysteine, preferably preceded by activated charcoal, has been shown to improve survival in patients who have taken an overdose of paracetamol, and may do so even if given after the onset of hepatic encephalopathy. Viral infections other than viral hepatitis, such as those due to herpes simplex, herpes zoster or cytomegalovirus, may be treated with appropriate antiviral therapy, e.g. aciclovir or ganciclovir. Induced early delivery may be advocated to improve survival in patients with fulminant hepatic failure due to acute fatty liver of pregnancy or the HELLP syndrome (haemolysis, elevated liver enzymes, low platelets).

In addition to discontinuing drugs that may have contributed to the clinical condition, especially neuroactive, hepatotoxic, and nephrotoxic drugs, it is necessary to take into account hepatocellular disease-associated alterations in drug pharmacokinetics and pharmacodynamics when prescribing for the patient in hepatocellular failure. For example, in hepatocellular failure the plasma half-life of benzodiazepines is prolonged (altered pharmacokinetics), and the sensitivity of the brain to the neuroinhibitory effects of benzodiazepines is increased (altered pharmacodynamics) (see Section 10).

It is useful to consider management of acute and chronic hepatocellular failure separately. The chronic syndrome accounts for the great majority of cases of hepatocellular failure, whereas the acute syndrome, when severe, is one of the most challenging in clinical medicine, presenting the physician with a unique constellation of difficult problems. Whether liver transplantation is an appropriate option must be considered in all patients with hepatocellular failure (see Chapter 15.22.5).

Hepatic encephalopathy

The following general principles underlie the management of hepatic encephalopathy (Table 15.22.4.3): (1) removal or correction of any precipitating factor; (2) reduction of absorption of nitrogenous substances from the gut; (3) in some (rare) cases, reduction of increased portal systemic shunting (if practical) and, although still experimental, (4) reversal of contributing neuropathophysiology with drugs that act directly on the brain.

Acute hepatic encephalopathy

All drugs that might contribute to encephalopathy, including diuretics, should be stopped, and consideration given to administering an antidote, such as naloxone or flumazenil. Meticulous attention is required to maintain fluid and electrolyte balance, and ensure adequate urine flow. Dietary protein intake is restricted, and enemas, such as magnesium sulphate or phosphate, are administered.

A nonhydrolysed disaccharide, such as lactulose or lactitol, is given by mouth routinely: their metabolism by colonic bacteria leads to production of lactic acid and other organic acids, a fall in colonic pH, increased ionization, and, hence, reduced absorption of nitrogenous compounds, including ammonia. Lactulose is widely believed to be effective in the management of hepatic encephalopathy, but its efficacy has not been confirmed by rigorously designed randomized controlled trials. However, its cathartic effect should be useful in correcting one of the precipitating factors, constipation (Table 15.22.4.2), although it must also be recognized that lactulose may induce hypernatraemia due to increased faecal fluid loss.

Table 15.22.4.3 Treatment of hepatic encephalopathy

Treatment	Comments
1. Correction or removal of precipitating factors	Mandatory
2. Institution of manoeuvres to minimize absorption of nitrogenous substances: Dietary protein restriction Evacuation of the bowel Non-hydrolysed disaccharide (lactulose or lactitol) and/or oral poorly absorbed broad-spectrum antibiotic (such as neomycin)	Routine
3. Reduction of portosystemic shunting	Rarely practical
4. Drugs that directly reverse brain pathophysiology, such as flumazenil	Experimental

In addition to lactulose, a poorly absorbed broad-spectrum antibiotic may be administered enterally to reduce the enteric bacterial flora and hence gut production of nitrogenous substances, such as ammonia, but the efficacy of such antibiotics has not been definitively demonstrated. Neomycin, up to 6 g daily, has been most extensively used; potent alternatives include kanamycin and paramomycin. Metronidzaole, which is effective against anaerobes, may also be given.

Chronic hepatic encephalopathy

Precipitating factors should be carefully avoided. In the absence of protein intolerance, a nutritious diet that includes a high protein content (80–100 g/day) is encouraged to maintain a positive nitrogen balance and optimize liver function. Vegetable protein diets seem to be better tolerated than animal protein diets, possibly due to the cathartic effect of the former caused by their high fibre content. If protein intolerance develops, dietary protein intake is reduced to as low as 40 g per day; lower intakes are associated with negative nitrogen balance.

Vitamins are given empirically. Thiamine replacement may be indicated in malnourished patients who are alcoholic. Oral branched chain amino acids may decrease protein catabolism and facilitate maintenance of a positive nitrogen balance, but are not efficacious in ameliorating the encephalopathy. Lactulose or lactitol is given orally in doses that produce two or three semiformed bowel actions daily, but may be associated with bowel distension at liver transplantation. If disaccharide intolerance develops, a broad-spectrum antibiotic may be given orally. However, long-term neomycin should be avoided because of the risk of ototoxicity and nephrotoxicity, and metronidazole may induce a peripheral neuropathy.

If intractable portosystemic encephalopathy occurs in a patient with a large spontaneous or surgically induced portosystemic shunt, the technique of balloon occlusion, coupled with embolization of collateral veins, may reverse portal blood flow from hepatofugal to hepatopetal, improve hepatocellular function, and ameliorate the encephalopathy. Similarly, in a patient with chronic portosystemic encephalopathy and a patent transjugular intrahepatic portosystemic shunt (TIPS), the shunt can be narrowed or closed.

Drugs acting directly on the brain

A novel experimental therapeutic approach is to administer a drug that acts on the target organ of hepatic encephalopathy, the brain, by reversing a major contributing neurophysiological mechanism. The benzodiazepine receptor antagonist, flumazenil, is the first promising drug of this type. It competes with high specificity with other benzodiazepine receptor ligands for binding to central benzodiazepine receptors, and rapidly and completely reverses the sedative and other neurological effects of benzodiazepine agonists, such as diazepam. When given as a bolus intravenously, flumazenil induces transient, incomplete, clinical and electrophysiological ameliorations of overt hepatic encephalopathy in an appreciable proportion of patients with acute or chronic liver failure. That flumazenil is currently not widely used in the management of hepatic encephalopathy does not imply that benzodiazepine antagonists lack efficacy, but rather that the properties of flumazenil are not optimal. Other benzodiazepine antagonists with superior properties to those of flumazenil, such as a longer plasma half-life and less partial agonist effects, may well be more efficacious: sarmazenil shows such promise.

Acute hepatocellular failure

Acute liver failure

Treatment of acute liver failure in the absence of encephalopathy is expectant, but frequent monitoring is necessary when the prothrombin time is prolonged and prompt admission to hospital is indicated at the first sign of encephalopathy. Referral to a specialized liver unit has been recommended before encephalopathy develops if levels of factor V fall to less than 50% of normal.

Fulminant and subfulminant hepatic failure

Routine management for acute hepatic encephalopathy is instituted (by extrapolation from the management of acute hepatic encephalopathy complicating chronic liver disease). With the onset of stage 2 hepatic encephalopathy, intensive supportive care should be instituted, and transfer of the patient to a unit with the potential for undertaking orthotopic liver transplantation is recommended. All patients should be considered to have potentially reversible disease.

Treatment is designed to buy time to allow hepatic regeneration to take place and to avoid iatrogenic deterioration. No factor reported to stimulate hepatic regeneration experimentally is of proven clinical benefit. Conventional intensive care for the unconscious patient is provided. A fluid intake of 1 to 2 litres daily is usually adequate; in the presence of haemodynamic instability, pulmonary artery catheterization may facilitate monitoring fluid replacement. Caloric intake is maintained by infusing hypertonic dextrose (10–50%), usually 200 to 300 g per day, into a central vein. Intravenous lipids and amino acids may also be given. Vitamins may be given empirically. A nasogastric tube is used to decompress the stomach and detect upper gastrointestinal haemorrhage. Despite the coagulopathy, an arterial catheter is useful for monitoring blood pressure, sampling blood, and measuring blood gases. Unless the aetiology is known to be noninfectious, blood and all secretions are considered to be infectious. Hence, attending personnel should wear gowns, gloves, and masks, enteric isolation procedures should be enforced, and all specimens from the patient should be labelled as infectious.

Frequent semiquantitative assessment of neurological status, such as the Glasgow Coma Score, and continuous monitoring of the electroencephalogram and electrocardiogram are undertaken. Blood is withdrawn at the outset for serological markers, such as those of hepatitis viruses and cytomegalovirus, screening for common drugs, and estimation of serum copper.

Regular monitoring

Blood glucose is checked as frequently as every 1 to 2 h. The following investigations are carried out every 12 h—haemoglobin, total and differential leucocyte count, platelet count, urea, creatinine, potassium, sodium, chloride, and bicarbonate. Daily investigations include prothrombin time, total and direct bilirubin, alkaline phosphatase, alanine and aspartate aminotransferases, albumin, amylase, calcium, phosphate, magnesium, fibrinogen, and fibrinogen split products. Regular careful review of the results of these tests, with appropriate response to abnormalities or trends detected, facilitate maintenance of metabolic homeostasis, which may be important in encouraging hepatic regeneration.

Chest radiographs should be obtained daily, and may show a high diaphragm, basal pulmonary infiltrates, or pulmonary oedema. Serial ultrasonographic determination of liver size may be useful in predicting the course: a massive liver or a history of cancer suggests extensive neoplastic replacement of the liver. In general, needle biopsy of the liver is contraindicated, but this procedure may occasionally be considered if the outcome is likely to influence management, e.g. to confirm a diagnosis of autoimmune hepatitis; a transjugular approach may be preferred if fresh frozen plasma fails to correct the coagulopathy.

Patients should be monitored frequently for complications, which must be treated promptly and vigorously. A major goal is the prevention of brain damage: if agitation, piercing cries, delirium, or seizures occur, then the patient should be restrained in a dark, quiet room. Administration of sedatives or tranquillizers should, if possible, be avoided. Phenytoin is not given prophylactically, but may be preferable to a short-acting benzodiazepine for seizures.

Specific problems

Susceptibility to infections

Extensive and frequent microbiological monitoring is necessary. In fulminant hepatic failure, daily cultures of blood, urine, sputum, and swabs of intravenous cannulas are recommended. Although not of proven benefit, prophylactic antimicrobial therapy has been advocated for patients admitted to a liver unit, such as intravenous broad-spectrum antibiotics, oral or nasogastric amphotericin B suspension, and (in women) vaginal clotrimazole cream. Nephrotoxic amino glycosides are avoided. Antibiotics are recommended to cover invasive procedures. Potential sources of infection, such as intrauterine devices, are removed.

Acid–base and electrolyte disturbances

Alkalosis does not require treatment. Acidosis should be managed by specific treatment of the cause; intravenous sodium bicarbonate increases body sodium. Hypokalaemia (potassium <3.5 mmol/litre) is corrected by adding potassium chloride to intravenous fluids, but the serum potassium is not increased above 4.0 mmol/litre if liver transplantation is an option, as graft reperfusion may precipitate hyperkalaemia. Addition of sodium chloride to intravenous fluids is not indicated in the presence of hyponatraemia unless there is clear evidence of excessive loss of sodium. Sudden changes in sodium concentration should be avoided, because of the risk of precipitating central pontine myelinolysis.

Cerebral oedema and raised intracranial pressure

Cerebral oedema precedes raised intracranial pressure; it is not always demonstrable on CT scan, but may be indicated by a loss of demarcation between grey and white matter. To avoid precipitating an increase in intracranial pressure, patients are nursed in a quiet room with the trunk and head elevated 30 to 40°; jugular venous compression is avoided.

Intracranial pressure can only be measured by direct monitoring, for which a parietal or temporal burr hole is required to place an extramural or subdural pressure transducer, a procedure which should be undertaken by a neurosurgeon in an operating theatre. This procedure is controversial because it is hazardous. Complications include cerebral haemorrhage precipitated by coagulopathy. Epidural monitoring is safer, but less accurate, than subdural monitoring. The appropriate time to instigate intracranial pressure monitoring is uncertain, but may be when there is progression to stage III encephalopathy or when the patient becomes a candidate for liver transplantation. Cerebral perfusion pressure (mean arterial pressure minus intracranial pressure) is maintained at a minimum of 60 mmHg. However, it is uncertain whether such monitoring is associated with improved survival. If intracranial pressure monitoring is not undertaken, frequent clinical examination to detect complications of intracranial hypertension is necessary.

Mannitol has been shown to reduce elevated intracranial pressure that is not greater than 60 mmHg. It is given as an intravenous bolus of a 20% solution (1 g/kg); further infusions (0.5 g/kg) can be administered every 4 h if the previous infusion induced a diuresis, plasma osmolarity does not exceed 315 mosmol/litre, and azotaemia is not present. However, mannitol has variable and potentially dangerous effects on intracranial pressure when the initial pressure exceeds 60 mm Hg. and should probably not be given without prior measurement of intracranial pressure. Mechanical hyperventilation may be tried, but not prophylactically. For refractory intracranial hypertension other options include thiopentone (185–500 mg intravenously over 15 min) and indomethacin. Induction of mild hypothermia is safe, may successfully prevent increases in intracranial pressure, and may attenuate upregulation of peripheral-type benzodiazepine receptors and thereby prevent an augmentation of GABAergic tone. Infusion of hypertonic saline (145–155 mmol/litre) has been reported to decrease the incidence and severity of intracranial hypertension. Corticosteroids have been tried, but not been shown to be effective.

Haemorrhagic diathesis

Skin puncture sites may require protracted pressure to achieve haemostasis. Administration of an H_2-antagonist or a proton pump inhibitor to maintain gastric pH above 5.0 decreases transfusion requirements due to bleeding from stress ulcers in fulminant hepatic failure; in the presence of renal failure dose reduction may be necessary or sulcralfate may be considered. A substantial increase in intracranial pressure may be due to an intracranial haemorrhage and is an indication for a CT scan of the head.

The haemorrhagic diathesis requires no specific treatment in the absence of overt bleeding. Vitamin K (10 mg/day) is usually given intravenously, in spite of the low risk of inducing anaphylaxis. Fresh frozen plasma is not given routinely so that plasma levels of clotting factors, some of which, such as factor VII, have short half-lives, can be used as prognostic indicators. Infusion of platelets and fresh frozen plasma may be indicated to cover invasive procedures, but tends to increase further an expanded plasma volume and may increase intracranial pressure. Clotting factor concentrates, which may exacerbate disseminated intravascular coagulation, are contraindicated. Heparin is not indicated for mild disseminated intravascular coagulation. A haematocrit of at least 30 or 35% should be maintained.

Hypoglycaemia

Hypoglycaemia must be prevented. Dextrose is administered intravenously to maintain a plasma glucose of 60 to 200 mg/dl (3.3–10.2 mmol/litre). Occasionally, massive amounts of dextrose amounting to 1 kg/day or more are required.

Cardiovascular changes

Maintenance of a normal blood pressure may reduce the risk of cerebral oedema or lessen its severity. Cardiovascular support is the principal intervention for shock liver. Ionotropes, e.g. adrenalin and noradrenalin, may be administered if there is failure to maintain a mean arterial blood pressure of 50 to 60 mmHg, but tissue hypoxia may increase and their efficacy has not been conclusively demonstrated. If hypertension occurs, hypotensive or vasodilator drugs may not be indicated as they may adversely affect intracranial pressure. Arrhythmias may subside with correction of hypoxia, or acid–base or electrolyte disturbances.

Hepatorenal syndrome

Prerenal failure is corrected by promoting renal blood flow. In particular, cautiously infusing 20% albumin tends to improve renal function by correcting relevant haemodynamic disturbances. Care must be taken not to overload the circulation to avoid an adverse affect on intracranial pressure. Any therapeutic agents that may contribute to impaired renal function, including diuretics, are avoided.

Development of acute hepatorenal syndrome may be prevented in patients with cirrhosis and spontaneous bacterial peritonitis by administering intravenous albumin and antibiotics, and in patients with severe alcoholic hepatitis by administering pentoxifylline.

An improvement in circulatory function, normalization of serum creatinine, and prolongation of survival may be achieved in patients with acute hepatorenal syndrome by administering intravenous albumin and arterial vasoconstrictors, such as a vasopressin analogue (e.g. terlipressin) or an α_1-adrenergic agonist (e.g. midodrine or noradrenalin). Fashioning a TIPS may also be tried, but there is a risk of precipitating encephalopathy. A molecular absorbent recirculating system has also been applied in this context, but without clear evidence of benefit in all studies, and the technique is not in routine clinical use.

Severe acid–base/electrolyte disturbances, fluid overload, and (rarely) azotaemia may be indications for renal replacement therapy, which may also be necessary to optimize a patient's condition before liver transplantation, but should not be expected to alter the course of hepatic or renal dysfunction. This approach must be undertaken carefully because of cardiovascular instability and coagulopathy. Hence, continuous (e.g. haemofiltration) rather than intermittent (e.g. dialysis) treatments are often preferred, particularly in the presence of raised intracranial pressure. Use of vasopressin analogues is still experimental.

Portopulmonary hypertension and hepatopulmonary syndrome

No attempt should be made to correct hyperventilation. Hypoxaemia is usually reversed by 100% oxygen by face mask. Endotracheal intubation, with a tube large enough to permit bronchoscopy, is recommended at the onset of stage III encephalopathy, and assisted mechanical ventilation is indicated for patients with stage IV encephalopathy, respiratory failure (increasing P_{CO_2}) or pulmonary oedema. Positive end-expiratory pressure, which may reduce hepatic blood flow and increase intracranial pressure, should be avoided. Right heart catheterization may be necessary to confirm the presence of portopulmonary hypertension. The heptopulmonary syndrome may be identified in up to 20% of patients evaluated for liver transplantation.

Ascites

Treatment of ascites is discussed in Chapter 15.22.3.

Future developments

Temporary hepatic support

The original rationale for providing temporary hepatic support was based on the assumption that the hepatic lesion in fulminant hepatic failure is potentially reversible, provided that the patient can be kept alive sufficiently long for hepatic regeneration to take place. Theoretically, the patient selected for temporary hepatic support would die if treated by conventional intensive supportive care alone, but might survive if the functions of the liver could be provided artificially over a finite period (Fig. 15.22.4.7). Temporary hepatic support should not only maintain the general condition of the patient, but also prevent life-threatening complications of fulminant hepatic failure.

As there is a lack of detailed understanding of the biochemical disturbances that need to be corrected in fulminant hepatic failure, the design of temporary liver support systems has been largely empirical. Attempts have been made to: (1) remove substances that accumulate in the body as a consequence of impaired hepatocellular function using a nonbiological system, such as charcoal haemoperfusion (artificial system); (2) provide deficient factors synthesized by the normal liver as well as remove accumulated substances using biological systems, for example, haemoperfusion through devices containing hepatocyte preparations (bioartificial system); and (3) combine both of these approaches (hybrid system).

Logistical and ethical issues make it a formidable undertaking to conduct randomized controlled trials to assess the risk/benefit ratio associated with the clinical application of temporary hepatic support systems. Thus far, no temporary hepatic support system to treat fulminant hepatic failure has been shown to benefit the patient unequivocally. Many authorities consider that clinical application of any temporary hepatic support system should not be undertaken outside the context of controlled, ethically approved clinical trials. The potential of temporary hepatic support in the management of chronic irreversible liver disease, such as cirrhosis, is limited to bridging the patient to liver transplantation (buying time). When a patient with fulminant hepatic failure or cirrhosis is a candidate for liver transplantation, effective temporary hepatic support would nonetheless have the potential not only of extending the waiting time for a donor liver, but also, perhaps, of reducing operative or perioperative mortality.

Further reading

Als-Neilsen B, Gludd LL, Gludd C (2004). Non-absorbable disaccharides for hepatic encephalopathy; systematic review of randomised trials. *BMJ*, **328**, 1046–50.

Basile AS, Jones EA, Skolnick P (1991). The pathogenesis and treatment of hepatic encephalopathy; evidence for the involvement of benzodiazepine receptor ligands. *Pharmacol Rev*, **43**, 27–71.

Batkal S, *et al.* (2001). Endocannabinoids acting at vascular CB1 receptors mediate the vasodilator state in advanced liver cirrhosis. *Nat Med*, **7**, 827–32.

Bernal W, *et al.* (2008). Intensive care management of acute liver failure. *Semin Liver Dis*, **28**, 188–200.

Blei AT (2005). The pathophysiology of brain edema in acute liver failure. *Neurochem Int*, **47**, 71–7.

Gines P, *et al.* (2003). Hepatorenal syndrome. *Lancet*, **362**, 1819–27.

Hoeper MM, Krowka MJ, Strassburn CP (2004). Portopulmonary hypertension and hepatopulmonary syndrome. *Lancet*, **363**, 1461–8.

Larsen FS (2004). Optimal management of patients with fulminant hepatic failure: Targeting the brain. *Hepatology*, **39**, 229–301.

McKenzie TJ, Lillegard JB, Nyberg SL (2008). Artificial and bioartificial liver support. *Semin Liver Dis*, **28**, 210–17.

Moreau R, Lebrec D (2006). The use of vasoconstrictors in patients with cirrhosis: Type 1HRS and beyond. *Hepatology* **43**, 385–94.

Munoz SJ, Stravitz RT, Gabriel DA (2009). Coagulopathy of acute liver failure. *Clin Liver Dis*, **13**, 95–107.

Polson J (2008). Assessment of prognosis in acute liver failure. *Semin Liver Dis*, **28**, 218–25.

Riordan SM, Williams R (2008). Perspectives on liver failure: past and future. *Semin Liver Dis*, **28**, 137–41.

Schafer DF, Sorrell MF (1997). Power failure, liver failure. *New Engl J Med*, **336**, 1173–4.

Stravitz RT, Kramer DJ (2009). Management of acute liver failure. *Nat Rev Gastroenterol Hepatol*, **6**, 542–53

Vaquero J, Rose C, Butterworth RF (2005). Keeping cool in acute liver failure: Rationale for the use of mild hypothermia. *J Hepatol*, **43**, 1067–77.

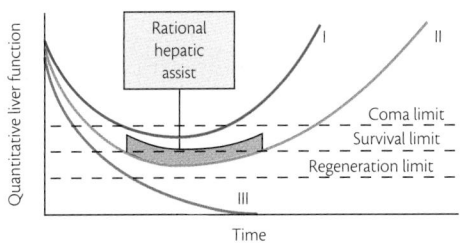

Fig. 15.22.4.7 Three hypothetical courses of fulminant hepatic failure (as envisaged by N Tygstrup).

In patients in group I, liver function deteriorates below the coma limit, but does not fall below the survival limit; these patients should survive with intensive medical supportive care alone.

In patients in group II, liver function deteriorates below the survival limit, but—if it can be maintained above this limit for a sufficient time by providing effective temporary hepatic support—liver function would not fall below the regeneration limit; these patients should also survive.

In patients in group III, liver function deteriorates below the survival and regeneration limits, irrespective of whether temporary hepatic support is provided; liver transplantation offers the only hope of survival for these patients. To facilitate optimal selection of patients for temporary hepatic support and liver transplantation it is necessary to develop reliable criteria for predicting which course an individual patient will follow: this goal has not yet been achieved.

15.22.5 Liver transplantation

Gideon M. Hirschfield, Michael E.D. Allison, and Graeme J.M. Alexander

Essentials

Liver transplantation is considered for patients with liver disease that is predicted to shorten life or causes symptoms that preclude an acceptable quality of life, and for individuals with life-shortening genetic disease that can be cured by transplantation. One-year survival is 90%, 5-year survival approaches 80%, and individual median survival exceeds 20 years.

The selection of patients and timing of transplantation is difficult, since both premature transplantation and delayed grafting can shorten life. Manifestations of chronic liver disease that should prompt referral to a transplant centre include hepatic encephalopathy, ascites, spontaneous bacterial peritonitis, jaundice, malnutrition, hepatic osteodystrophy, hepatorenal syndrome, reversed portal vein blood flow, portal vein thrombosis, and hepatocellular carcinoma. Super-urgent liver transplantation is often life saving for those with acute liver failure (encephalopathy, coagulopathy, liver disease of <6 months duration).

Liver transplantation usually involves a whole liver graft from a deceased donor, but innovations include the use of split livers, auxiliary grafts, and living related transplantation. Size matching between donor and recipient is important, but transplantation across the ABO barrier can be performed, and HLA matching and pre-existing donor sensitization are not important. Therapeutic immunosuppression is most commonly with triple therapy: calcineurin inhibitor (tacrolimus, ciclosporin), azathioprine, and prednisolone.

In the immediate postoperative period most complications relate to bleeding or poor graft function. Early postoperative complications include infection (bacterial, viral (cytomegalovirus), fungal), problems with vascular and biliary anastomoses, and acute rejection. In the longer term the consequences of immune suppression (impaired renal function, increased cardiovascular risk, malignancy) remain important, alongside chronic vascular rejection and disease recurrence.

Introduction

Liver transplantation is an established procedure with 90% 1-year survival, 5-year survival approaching 80% and individual median survival exceeding 20 years. Improvements in quality of life are such that a return to normal personal, professional and family life is expected. The current challenge is to ensure equity of access in the context of a limited donor pool.

Indications for liver transplantation

Liver transplantation is considered for patients with liver disease that is predicted to shorten life, subjects in whom symptoms of liver disease preclude an acceptable quality of life and individuals in whom life shortening genetic disease can be cured by transplantation. The most common indications are shown in Box 15.22.5.1.

Assessment and waiting for transplantation

The selection of patients and timing of transplantation is difficult, since both premature transplantation and delayed grafting can shorten life. Organ transplantation should occur when there is clear evidence of benefit; a composite assessment of medical, surgical, and psychological factors that may preclude transplantation is essential. All individuals who may benefit from liver transplantation should be referred for early assessment. Manifestations of chronic liver disease prompting referral include hepatic encephalopathy, ascites, spontaneous bacterial peritonitis, jaundice, malnutrition, hepatic osteodystrophy, hepatorenal syndrome, reversed portal vein blood flow, portal vein thrombosis, and hepatocellular carcinoma.

Box 15.22.5.1 Accepted indications for liver transplantation

Liver failure

Acute/subacute

◆ Drug induced:

  direct toxicity, e.g. paracetamol and herbal remedies
  idiosyncratic, e.g. isoniazid and nitrofurantoin

◆ Viral hepatitis, e.g. hepatitis A, B, D, E, non-A, non-B

◆ Acute onset autoimmune hepatitis

◆ Budd–Chiari syndrome

◆ Metabolic disease, e.g. Wilson's disease, neonatal haemochromatosis

Chronic

◆ Alcohol-related liver disease

◆ Chronic hepatitis B or C virus infection

◆ Malignancy, e.g. hepatocellular carcinoma, very rarely neuroendocrine tumours, haemangioendothelioma and AL amyloidosis

◆ Nonalcoholic steatohepatitis

◆ Autoimmune hepatitis

◆ Biliary cirrhosis, usually primary, but secondary causes include cystic fibrosis

◆ Sclerosing cholangitis, usually primary, but secondary causes include histiocytosis X

◆ Haemochromatosis/Wilson's disease/α_1-antitypsin deficiency

◆ Gaucher's disease, glycogen storage disease, Crigler–Najar syndrome, familial intrahepatic cholestasis syndromes

Surgical gene therapy

◆ Primary oxalosis

◆ Familial amyloidosis (transthyretin and fibrinogen-α)

◆ Familial hypercholesterolaemia

Miscellaneous (with or without significant chronic liver disease)

◆ Polycystic liver disease/Caroli's disease

◆ Portopulmonary hypertension/hepatopulmonary syndrome

The concept of minimum listing criteria for transplantation is being evaluated and implemented currently in an attempt to ensure equity of access to, and maximal benefit from, a limited donor pool. Increasing age, renal dysfunction, poor nutritional status and jaundice are associated with poor outcome. Liver disease severity algorithms such as MELD (bilirubin, creatinine, INR) and UKELD (bilirubin, creatinine, INR and Na$^+$) will be used increasingly as a basis for listing as well as for prioritization and removal from the list. Patients with diseases in which a synthetic-based algorithm would put them at a disadvantage (e.g. hepatocellular carcinoma) need to be managed in a modified way.

The basis for many presumed contraindications is the likelihood that 5-year survival will fall beneath 50% as a result of operative risk, pre-existing medical conditions, or both.

Extrahepatic and metastatic malignancy is still considered a contraindication with rare exceptions (certain neuroendocrine tumours and haemangioendothelioma). Many other factors may contribute to a decision not to proceed including continued injecting drug or substance abuse, severe cardiorespiratory disease (hepatopulmonary syndrome or portopulmonary hypertension are anaesthetic risk factors but not necessarily contraindications), malnutrition, and (increasingly) obesity. Surgical factors such as portal vein thrombosis and previous laparotomy need to be considered. Factors such as age, HIV coinfection, previous ischaemic heart disease, diabetes, and severe psychiatric illness are not in themselves contraindications to transplantation.

Individuals who are turned down should be re-assessed if circumstances change, as well as having a second opinion if wanted.

Listed patients need close management. Vaccination against hepatitis B virus (HBV) is recommended if the patient has not been exposed previously, as donor organs positive for anti-HBc carry a risk of subsequent HBV infection. Factors that may require temporary or permanent suspension from the list include sepsis, hyponatraemia (risk of central pontine myelinolysis), renal impairment, new portal vein thrombosis, new or further growth of hepatocellular carcinoma, and substance abuse.

Specific disorders

Acute and subacute liver failure

Super urgent liver transplantation is often life saving for those with acute liver failure (encephalopathy, coagulopathy, liver disease of <6 months duration). The chance of spontaneous recovery is least in those with subacute liver failure, whose clinical course may mimic chronic liver disease. Various criteria based on outcome allow selection of patients with acute liver failure for transplantation. Most use a combination of aetiology, age, coagulopathy, renal failure, acidosis, and bilirubin to identify those with poor survival without transplantation at 1 year. When compared to other aetiologies the 1-year survival is lower, but these patients are often cured by transplantation and many are young; the longer-term outcome is excellent. Psychiatric follow-up may be indicated for some.

Chronic liver disease

Alcohol

The outcome of transplantation for alcohol-related liver disease is equivalent to that following transplantation for other liver disorders. Abstinence is an absolute requirement because clinical status may improve substantially such that patients may not need transplantation. Most units look for a 6- to 12-month alcohol-free period, with a clear commitment to lifelong abstinence because disease may recur in the graft. Factors that predict recidivism include alcohol consumption in the year prior to transplantation, the duration of abstinence, and the extent of social support. Severe acute alcoholic hepatitis is not an accepted indication for transplantation because of continued alcohol consumption until presentation and because survival post-transplant is poor.

Chronic viral hepatitis

Chronic infection with hepatitis B, C, or D are all indications for transplantation if patients have complications. Results improve if viraemia is controlled or eradicated pretransplant.

Hepatobiliary malignancy

Surgery, where possible, is the best treatment for hepatocellular carcinoma (HCC). In patients with a normal background liver or in those with compensated cirrhosis, resection may be possible. In others with more advanced liver disease transplantation is beneficial with a low risk of recurrence if tumour bulk is limited. According to the Milan criteria transplantation is indicated if there is a single tumour of less than 5 cm diameter or three tumours all less than 3 cm in size, in the absence of portal vein involvement or extrahepatic spread. Imaging modalities include ultrasound, contrast CT, MRI, and hepatic angiography.

The fibrolamellar variant of HCC is more common in young patients without cirrhosis and is slower growing. Resection is performed more commonly than transplantation. Outside clinical trials, transplantation cannot be recommended for cholangiocarcinoma because of unacceptable recurrence rates. Occasionally transplantation has a role in the management of neuroendocrine tumours (particularly if the primary can be resected), hepatic haemangioendothelioma and large biliary cystadenoma.

Nonalcoholic steatohepatitis

As a component of the metabolic syndrome, nonalcoholic steatohepatitis leads to chronic liver disease, cirrhosis, and HCC. Fibrosis progression may be ameliorated by aggressive management of modifiable risk factors but, as an indication for transplantation, this disease is increasingly important. Patients need careful assessment of their cardiovascular risk profile pretransplant and continued aggressive management of diabetes, hyperlipidaemia, hypertension, and weight is needed post-transplant. Disease recurrence is common.

Primary biliary cirrhosis

Most patients with primary biliary cirrhosis (PBC) do not need liver transplantation, and most clinicians accept that ursodeoxycholic acid at appropriate doses has improved transplant free survival. However those with decompensated liver disease, HCC, or severe unremitting symptoms benefit from transplantation. A bilirubin in excess of 100 µmol/litre predicts a high mortality without transplantation in the absence of other indications.

Primary sclerosing cholangitis

The timing of transplantation for primary sclerosing cholangitis (PSC) is difficult. The disease has a fluctuating course, previous bowel surgery often raises the perioperative risk, and patients face a 10 to 20% lifetime risk of inoperable cholangiocarcinoma. Transplantation is not indicated as prophylaxis against malignancy. Frequent episodes of jaundice (often unremitting) or cholangitis should prompt assessment. Endoscopic retrograde cholangiopancreatography (ERCP) (with biliary cytology) and endoscopic ultrasonography may help the assessment of a superimposed cholangiocarcinoma; CA19-9, a tumour marker associated with cholangiocarcinoma, is not wholly reliable (marked elevations are seen with biliary disease and sepsis). Careful surveillance and management of inflammatory bowel disease are essential.

Autoimmune hepatitis

Transplantation can be avoided in many patients with autoimmune hepatitis, even in those who present with chronic liver failure. Transplants are performed for those with complications of endstage liver disease and, less often, poor control despite appropriate therapy.

Budd–Chiari syndrome

The presentation of hepatic vein thrombosis can be acute or chronic. In those with acute liver failure, transplantation is accepted first-line therapy. In those with a less dramatic presentation, radiological intervention (hepatic vein angioplasty and/or transjugular intrahepatic portosystemic shunting) or surgical shunts can be effective, followed by long-term anticoagulation. Transplantation remains an option. The majority of patients with Budd–Chiari syndrome have an underlying coagulopathy; appropriate investigation (e.g. thrombophilia screen and Jak-2 mutation analysis) and treatment of haematological disease is essential. Most patients require anticoagulation from the early postoperative period.

Metabolic/genetic disease

Transplantation is successful where metabolic/genetic disorders lead to liver failure. These include Wilson's disease, α_1-antitrypsin deficiency (increasingly recognized as a cofactor in many other liver diseases), Gaucher's disease, glycogen storage disease, Crigler–Najar syndrome, and familial intrahepatic cholestasis syndromes. Patients with haemochromatosis may avoid transplantation with early diagnosis and venesection, but may present with complications of chronic liver disease, including HCC. This group has an increased post-transplant morbidity related to cardiovascular disease, diabetes and an increased susceptibility to postoperative bacterial infection.

Polycystic liver disease, unlike polycystic kidney disease, causes hepatic failure rarely, but patients may suffer pain and abdominal distension such that transplantation is considered. Those with associated renal failure may benefit from combined liver–kidney transplantation. Hereditary haemorrhagic telangiectasia may be associated with massive hepatic haemangioma that leads to portal hypertension, secondary biliary disease (ischaemic bile duct injury due to shunting), or HCC; in these rare cases transplantation may be indicated.

Patients with cystic fibrosis (CF) may develop a secondary biliary cirrhosis and significant portal hypertension in addition to cardiorespiratory disease. Empirically it appears that ursodeoxycholic acid slows down the progression of CF-associated liver disease; occasional well-selected patients benefit from transplantation. Nutritional gains from transplantation may aid longer-term cardiorespiratory function. Realistically, because of donor organ shortages, most centres do not offer multivisceral transplantation at present.

Surgical gene therapy

This term describes the practice of liver transplantation to treat life-threatening inherited disorders in which the genetic abnormality is cured by giving the recipient a healthy donor liver. Examples include primary oxalosis (unless performed in childhood, concurrent renal transplantation is usually performed), hypercholesterolaemia, and familial amyloidosis. Unique features of individual diseases require modifications to standard transplant management, e.g. risk of heart block in transthyretin amyloidosis and risk of acute oxalate nephropathy following liver–kidney transplantation in oxalosis.

Transplant procedure

Liver transplantation usually involves a whole liver graft from a deceased donor, but innovations continue in the use of split livers, auxiliary grafts, and living related transplantation. Early morbidity and mortality continue to improve with increased surgical and anaesthetic expertise; massive transfusion is now the exception.

Donor organ

Extended criteria have been introduced to widen the pool of donors because of increasing disparity between the number of available organs and possible recipients, albeit with the potential for greater recipient morbidity and mortality. Livers may now be used with mild or moderate steatosis, from individuals with previous exposure to HBV, from individuals with HCV, from donors over the age of 65 and from non-heart-beating donors. Extrahepatic malignancy in the donor is assessed on an individual basis.

Size matching between donor and recipient is important. Transplantation across the ABO barrier can be performed, but it is routine to match for blood group, except in acute liver failure. HLA matching and pre-existing donor sensitization is not important. The intention is to implant the new liver so that the cold ischaemic time is less than 12 h. *In situ* perfusion with cold University of Wisconsin solution has permitted prolongation of the cold ischaemic time.

Surgical aspects

The transplantation procedure consists of three operations. Hepatectomy, which can be difficult with portal hypertension or previous abdominal surgery, is followed by the anhepatic phase with liver implantation. Reperfusion and abdominal closure follow. Variations in techniques exist for caval anastomosis. In up to 20% of patients the donor hepatic arteries have anomalous anatomy requiring adjustments to the nature of the hepatic artery anastomosis. Veno-venous bypass with extracorporeal circulation of blood via the portal vein back into the systemic circulation is used on occasion and reduces subsequent rates of renal failure and sepsis. The biliary anastomosis can be carried out as duct-to-duct or as duct-to-small bowel (Roux-en-Y-hepatico-jejunostomy). Primary Roux loop formation is carried out where there are doubts about the vascular supply to the biliary tree, with retransplantation, and often in patients with PSC, who have a risk of cholangiocarcinoma in residual recipient biliary tissue. Previous techniques using the gallbladder as a biliary conduit were unsuccessful and the use of an externally draining T-tube over a duct-to-duct anastomosis has lost favour. Donor cholecystectomy removes the potential for a denervated, atonic gallbladder to act as a nidus for stone formation and sepsis.

Recent innovations in transplantation have focused on using split liver grafts, in which the donor liver is divided and offered to two recipients. This carries greater procedural risk but utilizes the donor organ more effectively. Auxiliary transplantation, where the recipient liver remains in place and another whole or partial (reduced size) liver is transplanted adjacently, may have a role in acute liver failure and the treatment of genetic liver disease. Problems with the vascular anastomosis and the lack of a reliable method of proportionally dividing the portal vein blood flow between two livers causes significant morbidity. Living related transplantation is likely to increase in frequency and is well established in many countries. The advantages are those of an elective procedure with excellent donor liver function, minimal cold/warm ischaemia, and lower rates of rejection. There are increased vascular and biliary complication rates for the recipient, along with the potential for 'small-for-size syndrome'. The donor operation has a defined morbidity and mortality.

Anaesthetic aspects

Close attention to donor haemodynamics are important to avoid organ injury during retrieval. During the transplant itself the anaesthetist has the task of maintaining adequate cardiorespiratory function, in the face of significant swings in cardiac output, cardiac filling, and systemic vascular resistance. Particularly critical moments can occur on mobilization of the recipient liver, on manipulation of the inferior vena cava, and during the anhepatic and reperfusion phases. Bleeding complications have been reduced by the use of aprotinin and by monitoring coagulation closely, e.g. thromboelastography.

Post-transplant course

Surgical, medical, and immunological factors account for morbidity and mortality. In the immediate postoperative period most complications relate to bleeding or poor graft function. Early postoperative complications include sepsis, problems with vascular and biliary anastomosis, and acute rejection. In the late postoperative period the consequences of immune suppression (renal function, cardiovascular risk, malignancy) are more important, alongside chronic vascular rejection and disease recurrence.

Immediate

Bleeding varies from inconsequential to life threatening, with the associated complications of haemodynamic instability and massive transfusion. Very early graft failure is suggested by coma following withdrawal of sedation, a rapidly rising prothrombin time, acidosis, high insulin requirements, thrombocytopenia, and hyperkalaemia. The differential diagnosis is primary nonfunction, nonthrombotic graft infarction, or hepatic artery thrombosis. The patient develops acute liver (and multiorgan) failure and imaging by ultrasound and/or angiography of the graft vascular supply is important. Super-urgent retransplantation can be life saving. The blood supply to the liver can also be affected catastrophically by inappropriate use of inotropes, and marginal graft function can be made critical by inappropriate vasoconstriction. Hyperacute rejection (antibody mediated) is extremely rare; thus a positive cross-match is not a contraindication.

Early

The combination of a demanding procedure in immunocompromised, chronically ill individuals can make diagnosis of complications challenging, with a low specificity for routine symptoms and signs. In addition to blood tests, investigations such as ultrasonography, CT, MRI, and liver biopsy are often sufficient for diagnosis, although more invasive investigations (e.g. ERCP, angiography, exploratory surgery) are sometimes needed.

Sepsis

All patients are at risk of sepsis, but those transplanted for acute liver failure and/or with renal failure face additional risk. The sites of infection are commonly chest, urine, blood, abdomen (wound, haematomas, bilomas) and indwelling cannulae, although other locations of sepsis to consider include frontal sinuses, teeth, and heart valves. The risk of sepsis is increased with a second transplant.

Most units give 48 h of antibiotic prophylaxis; the choice is dependent on local microbiology advice, methicillin-resistant *Staphylococcus aureus* (MRSA) status, and antimicrobial allergy. Subsequent courses of antibiotics are where possible guided by culture.

Cytomegalovirus (CMV) can cause disease early post-transplant. The advent of valganciclovir (an oral prodrug of ganciclovir) has simplified prophylaxis, which is indicated if the donor has serological evidence of past CMV, but the recipient is negative. Clinical disease with CMV is diminished by 3 months prophylaxis; if disease occurs after completing prophylaxis it is usually less severe. Primary or secondary CMV viraemia can be identified early by surveillance with PCR of plasma for CMV DNA. Active disease (cytopenia, pneumonitis, colitis, hepatitis, retinitis, wound infection) can be treated by reduced immune suppression and with intravenous ganciclovir; oral valganciclovir may not be reliable in this setting. Reduced immune suppression alone may be sufficient in secondary reactivation. HSV DNA detection suggests that herpes simplex is reactivated commonly early after transplant; symptomatic infection is less common but warrants topical or systemic treatment with aciclovir. Varicella zoster recrudescence should always be treated. Occasionally marked hepatitis from donor-derived herpesviruses such as herpes simplex or Epstein–Barr virus occur and a low threshold for virological testing is needed to make the diagnosis. Infections with human herpesvirus 6 and 8 are now documented.

Fungal infection can be devastating, especially if associated with vascular anastomoses. High-risk groups include individuals transplanted for acute liver failure, patients with renal failure, and individuals with an ischaemic graft. Prophylaxis with fluconazole is recommended and is effective against the commonly isolated candida species. Tacrolimus metabolism is modified by fluconazole. Most patients are discharged with topical prophylaxis in the form of nystatin or amphotericin lozenges. Systemic disease may require treatment with higher doses of fluconazole, or where appropriate amphotericin B or caspofungin, and should be guided by culture.

Lymphopenia is a risk factor for infection with *Pneumocystis jirovecii* but prophylaxis with co-trimoxazole (or dapsone if allergic) is usually effective. Toxoplasmosis is rare but prophylaxis is recommended if the donor is seropositive and the recipient naive.

Anastomotic complications

Each surgical anastomosis is subject to complications. Hepatic artery thrombosis (1–2% incidence except in paediatric practice) may be suspected by worsening liver function tests, by zone 3 centrilobular ischaemia on a biopsy, by the occurrence of a biliary leak or the development of nonanastomotic biliary strictures. Bacterial or fungal sepsis may be associated. Diagnosis usually requires ultrasonography or angiography (CT, MR, or classical) and management usually entails retransplantation. Patients transplanted for PSC seem to be more prone to arterial thrombosis. Hepatic artery stenosis may be amenable to vascular reconstruction. Portal vein thrombosis or stenosis is less common and maybe suspected by the development of ascites. Caval anastomotic strictures are infrequent, but may present as rapid weight gain, recurrent pleural effusions, ascites, peripheral oedema, protein-losing enteropathy, or pulmonary emboli. Angioplasty with or without stenting can be successful. Biliary complications relate to either leaks or strictures. Anastomotic strictures are usually technical, whereas non-anastomotic strictures often relate to hepatic ischaemia, although recurrent PSC and Roux loop reflux cholangiopathy are in the differential. The use of non-heart-beating donors is particularly associated with nonanastomotic biliary complications. Treatment options include therapeutic ERCP, external biliary drainage, biliary reconstruction, and retransplantation.

Acute rejection and graft-vs-host disease

Acute cellular rejection of the graft is common and occurs to some degree in most subjects. The target tissues include bile ducts and endothelial cells (hepatic artery, portal vein, and less frequently, central vein). Symptoms are nonspecific, including fever, jaundice, and pain. More often acute rejection is suspected on the basis of deterioration in liver function, especially the bilirubin accompanied by eosinophilia; rejection needing treatment is less likely if the patient is not jaundiced. In most cases biopsy confirmation is required in order that the severity of the rejection can be graded and pulsed doses of methylprednisolone given only where appropriate (moderate or severe rejection). Steroid-resistant rejection and multiple episodes of acute rejection, although uncommon, carry a poor prognosis for the longer term.

Very rarely donor-derived lymphocytes generate graft-vs-host disease (GVHD). The patient (often underweight and previously alcoholic with lymphopenia) presents within a few months with systemic disease: rash (cutaneous), diarrhoea (gastrointestinal tract), and pancytopenia (bone marrow). In contrast to classical GVHD seen in bone marrow transplantation the liver is 'immune' to attack and liver function tests are classically normal. The diagnosis of acute GVHD can be difficult, since many of its features are similar to drug reactions or viral infection; the demonstration by molecular testing for donor lymphoid chimaerism is diagnostic. Outcome is almost universally fatal, with progressive malnutrition and intractable sepsis. No treatment modality is proven.

Late

Although late presentations of technical complications do occur, such as delayed hepatic artery thrombosis, intrahepatic biliary strictures, and recurrent cholangitis, these are less important than medical complications.

Renal failure and cardiovascular disease

It is estimated that by 5 years post-transplant 10 to 20% of patients develop chronic renal failure, usually related to calcineurin inhibitor toxicity but also secondary to diabetes and vascular disease. The day 30 creatinine is a good predictor of long-term renal function. Care with calcineurin dosing is essential in the early postoperative period, when patients often have marginal renal function. Patients are also at heightened risk from hypertension, hypercholesterolaemia, obesity, metabolic syndrome, and diabetes. Ambulatory post-transplant care focuses on these issues to reduce the probability of cardiovascular events.

Malignancy

A spectrum of predominantly Epstein–Barr virus (EBV)-driven B-cell lymphomas occurs with an incidence of 2 to 4%. It is more common in paediatric practice, especially where the recipient is EBV naive. Although disease in or around the liver is most common, widespread disease is not infrequent. Management is focused on minimizing (or even stopping) immunosuppression, along with systemic chemo- and biological therapies. Prognosis may be guarded and disease resolution can be tempered by development of chronic rejection. There is a substantial increased incidence of almost all carcinomas, some of which relates to pretransplant risk factors, and others to the consequence of long-term immunosuppression. Sun protection, appropriate breast and cervical screening, and smoking cessation are recommended.

Osteodystrophy

Osteoporosis, and more rarely osteomalacia, are important complications of chronic liver disease and both conditions are associated with significant morbidity through fractures resulting in pain, deformity, and immobility. The increasing trend to rapidly wean steroids has reduced post-transplant fracture rates. Patients should have their bone density measured, in addition to vitamin D and testosterone levels, and appropriate treatment initiated (e.g. calcium/vitamin D and bisphosphonates).

Chronic rejection

Chronic rejection is a vasculopathy with characteristic obliteration by foamy macrophages of the main branches of the hepatic artery and bile duct loss ('vanishing bile ducts') probably secondary to ischaemia. Chronic rejection is more common in those with severe acute rejection, steroid-resistant acute rejection, or multiple episodes of acute rejection. It can also occur after a switch in immunosuppression. Presentation can be acute, with an initial cellular component, or more insidious. The switch from cyclosporin to tacrolimus and the aggressive prevention and treatment of CMV disease has probably reduced its incidence. Retransplantation is often needed and carries a high risk of chronic rejection in the second graft.

Immune suppression

To achieve tolerance, which is an active immunological process between the transplant recipient and the graft, the donor's antigens must imprint their pattern of specificity on the recipient's immune system. Ironically immunosuppressive agents, such as tacrolimus, while reducing rejection probably prevent true tolerance. Liver allografts have immunologic advantages over other organs and liver transplantation in patients appears to protect against rejection of other organs transplanted from the same donor. Currently used immunosuppressive drugs are outlined in Table 15.22.5.1.

A wider range of alternative immune suppressive agents has improved outcome and allowed protocols to be tailored to the aetiology of the original disease, the risk of disease recurrence and renal function. Most start with triple therapy: calcineurin inhibitor (we favour tacrolimus over ciclosporin), azathioprine, and prednisolone. Corticosteroids (we favour 20 mg prednisolone daily) are weaned over 6 weeks, but azathioprine (approximately 1 mg/kg) is continued for 6 to 12 months.

Calcineurin inhibitors form the backbone of treatment but side effects are substantial, including hypertension, hyperlipidaemia, weight gain, nephrotoxicity, and neurotoxicity. Tacrolimus is diabetogenic; ciclosporin causes hirsutism and gum hypertrophy.

Different scenarios demand different approaches. Where there is concern about renal function some centres delay introduction of calcineurin inhibitors, using monoclonal antibodies against the interleukin-2 receptor instead (e.g. basiliximab). When calcineurin inhibitors cause renal toxicity, rapamycin is an effective alternative. Many centres favour mycophenolate mofetil rather

Table 15.22.5.1 Currently used immunosuppressive agents

Drug	Mechanism	Side effects	Comments
Prednisolone	Synthetic corticosteroid with broad anti-inflammatory effects	Weight gain Hyperglycaemia Osteoporosis	Enhances HBV and HCV replication
Azathioprine	Purine synthesis inhibitor that inhibits cell proliferation	Marrow suppression Pancreatitis Veno-occlusive disease	Harmful interaction with allopurinol
Mycophenolate mofetil	Mycophenolic acid inhibits *de novo* purine synthesis by inhibiting inosine monophosphate dehydrogenase	Diarrhoea Marrow suppression	
Tacrolimus	Calcineurin inhibitor: macrolide antibiotic that inhibits both T-lymphocyte signal transduction and IL-2 transcription	Nephrotoxicity Neurotoxicity Hypertension Diabetes	Reduces the rate of chronic rejection as compared to cyclosporin and more reliably absorbed
Cyclosporin	Calcineurin inhibitor: inhibition of T-lymphocyte signal transduction and IL-2 transcription	Nephrotoxicity Neurotoxicity Hypertension	
Rapamycin	Inhibition of IL-2 receptor signalling (mTOR inhibitor)	Pneumonitis Atypical infection Impaired wound healing	Antitumour and antifibrotic effects may be of value in HCC and HCV
Antilymphocyte and antithymocyte globulin	Lymphocyte depletion	Infection Serum sickness Lymphoma	Retains a role in steroid-resistant acute rejection
Anti-CD25 monoclonal antibodies	IL-2 receptor blockade	Hypersensitivity reactions	May allow delayed tacrolimus use in those with renal impairment

than azathioprine as it is perceived to be more lymphocyte specific. Comparative data are lacking and cost is an important factor.

Antilymphocyte and antithymocyte globulin are often effective following failed treatment for acute rejection; there are concerns about sustained lymphopenia.

Recurrent disease

Disease 'recurrence' in the graft is a significant concern.

Hepatitis B (HBV)

Accelerated, devastating graft infection by HBV can occur in those transplanted for HBV (particularly if HBV DNA positive at transplant) or in recipients who receive a donor organ positive for anti-HBc. Graft infection can be prevented by the combination of pooled HBV immunoglobulin (HBIg) and antiviral chemotherapy. HBIg revolutionized treatment of this group of patients. With the dual use of an antiviral agent the duration of prophylaxis with HBIg can be shortened. Lifelong antiviral therapy with lamivudine has inevitably driven resistant strains and alternative antiviral agents such as adefovir, tenofovir, and entecavir now also play a role to prevent disease recurrence. Prednisolone enhances HBV replication *in vivo* and *in vitro* and has led to early steroid withdrawal.

Hepatitis C (HCV)

Liver transplantation for HCV does not cure the disease and infection of the graft, with the potential for accelerated disease, is nearly inevitable. A significant proportion of patients have cirrhosis by 5 to 10 years and a small proportion lose the graft within 1 to 2 years. Factors associated with graft damage include the age and

quality of the donor (older, more marginal livers are more prone to recurrence) and the cumulative dose of immune suppression. Many transplant units avoid using marginal donors in HCV-positive recipients where possible and some use a steroid-free regime. Rapamycin has *in vitro* antifibrogenic properties and trials are under way of its use in the context of HCV-related fibrosis post-transplant. Adoption of antiviral therapy post-transplant has not been widespread because of overall poor response rates, but selected patients, e.g. genotype 3, may benefit. Passive specific antibody-based therapy is ineffective.

Autoimmune hepatitis

Autoimmune hepatitis can 'recur' causing graft damage and loss. Patients transplanted for autoimmune hepatitis appear to have an increased risk of acute rejection; many centres use long-term dual or triple immunosuppression. A smaller group of individuals, particularly those transplanted as children, develop a *de novo* 'alloimmune hepatitis' which responds to enhanced immunosuppression. This may be a variant of rejection; mismatch between donor and recipient for expression of the enzyme glutathione *S*-transferase T1 is one recognized risk factor.

Primary sclerosing cholangitis (PSC)

PSC is likely to 'recur' in the graft of perhaps 20% of individuals within 5 years of transplantation and may cause graft dysfunction and cholangitis. Immune suppression does not prevent disease recurrence. Risk factors for recurrence include male sex and having an intact colon before transplantation. Despite immune suppression inflammatory bowel disease can be more severe after transplantation. Furthermore, colon cancer appears within the first few years after transplantation in approximately 7% of patients with IBD who are transplanted for PSC. Annual colonoscopy in this population is therefore essential.

Primary biliary cirrhosis (PBC)

Recurrent PBC is well recognized and although cirrhosis with portal hypertension has been reported by 2 years, it is more commonly a histopathological diagnosis than a major clinical problem affecting graft function or patient survival. Interestingly there is a suggestion that ciclosporin (as opposed to tacrolimus) prolongs the median time to recurrence. There is, however, insufficient evidence to suggest adjusting immunosuppression regimes at present.

Alcohol

Recidivism for alcoholism and the development of alcohol-related liver disease after transplantation are well recognized. Approximately 20% of patients who undergo transplantation for alcoholic liver disease use alcohol post-transplant; one-third of these individuals exhibit repetitive or heavy drinking. Liver damage can lead to graft loss within 1 year if consumption is heavy.

The future of transplantation

Long-term survival following transplantation is a testament to the refinement of the entire procedure from assessment to post-transplant care. Future strategies must focus on avoiding transplantation. Surgical advances are needed to increase the donor pool, along with ongoing efforts to improve deceased donation rates. Safer, individualized, immune suppression will need major advances in the understanding and targeting of the immune system.

Further reading

Burroughs AK, *et al.* (2006). 3-month and 12-month mortality after first liver transplant in adults in Europe: predictive models for outcome. *Lancet*, **367**, 225–32.

Muiesan P, Vergani D, Mieli-Vergani G (2007). Liver transplantation in children. *J Hepatol*, **46**, 340–8.

Neuberger J (2004). Developments in liver transplantation. *Gut*, **53**, 759–68.

O'Grady JG, *et al.* (2007). Randomized controlled trial of tacrolimus versus microemulsified cyclosporin (TMC) in liver transplantation: poststudy surveillance to 3 years. *Am J Transplant*, **7**, 137–41.

Wiesner R, *et al.* (2003). Model for end-stage liver disease (MELD) and allocation of donor livers. *Gastroenterology*, **124**, 91–6.

15.22.6 Liver tumours—primary and secondary

William J.H. Griffiths and Simon M. Rushbrook

Essentials

A number of benign and malignant tumours may arise in the liver, the most important of which are:

Hepatocellular carcinoma (HCC)

HCC is the fifth most common cancer worldwide, but with great geographical variation in incidence, ranging from around 2 per 100 000 population in western Europe to 100 per 100 000 population in some parts of Africa. Most tumours arise on the background of cirrhosis, commonly due to hepatitis B, hepatitis C, or alcohol.

Symptoms may not be apparent until the cancer is already advanced, patients typically presenting with a triad of pain in the right upper quadrant, hepatomegaly, and weight loss. Decompensation in patients with cirrhosis may be precipitated by tumour and is signified by worsening ascites, variceal bleeding, jaundice, and/or encephalopathy.

The diagnosis of HCC is made primarily on contrast imaging (CT or MRI) where arterial enhancement and portal venous washout are characteristically seen. The tumour marker α-fetoprotein (AFP) is elevated in 80% of cases and is diagnostic when greater than 200 ng/ml in the presence of cirrhosis and a suspicious mass. Biopsy is reserved for indeterminate cases and immunohistochemical staining may help distinguish from adenocarcinoma.

Symptomatic presentation carries a poor prognosis, with less than 10% of patients surviving 3 years. However, ultrasound surveillance programmes of patients at risk (for example, those with cirrhosis or active hepatitis B infection) enable one-third of patients to be diagnosed at an early stage, when curative treatments are possible including (1) surgical resection, (2) ethanol/radiofrequency ablation, or (3) liver transplantation. Transarterial chemoembolization is an established palliative treatment. Cytotoxic drugs are generally not effective though new multikinase inhibitors appear promising.

Cholangiocarcinoma

Cholangiocarcinoma is an epithelial malignancy of the biliary tree that accounts for 7 to 10% of primary liver malignancies. Bile duct cancer is thought to be induced by chronic inflammation within the biliary tree, with risk factors including biliary infection by particular endemic trematodes and flukes, and primary sclerosing cholangitis.

Patients with peripheral intrahepatic masses typically present with upper abdominal pain, anorexia, malaise, and weight loss: jaundice is an early feature of those with hilar or extrahepatic tumours.

It can be difficult to establish the diagnosis of cholangiocarcinoma. Blood concentrations of CA19-9, a glycoprotein secreted by bile duct cells, are often elevated. Depending on tumour location, cross-sectional imaging or magnetic resonance cholangiopancreatography (MRCP) may be suggestive but not diagnostic. Options for obtaining tissue include (1) percutaneous biopsy if peripheral; (2) biliary brushings and/or intraductal biopsy at ERCP; (3) endoscopic ultrasound fine needle aspiration of hilar lesions where the differential includes inflammatory pseudotumour and metastasis.

Surgical resection can offer cure for a few patients, but results are generally disappointing. Useful palliation may be offered by photodynamic therapy, conventional radiotherapy and high-dose local irradiation, and biliary stenting.

Benign liver tumours

Haemangiomas are usually discovered incidentally during abdominal imaging and have a prevalence of 2 to 5% in the general population. Large symptomatic haemangiomas can be managed by surgical enucleation or embolization, but most do not require treatment and patients can be reassured.

Focal nodular hyperplasia (FNH) has a prevalence of 0.4 to 0.8% in the general population. FNH is usually found in women (female:male 9:1) and is typically discovered as an incidental solitary lesion during abdominal imaging. Appearances on MRI may be diagnostic, but biopsy is required if there is uncertainty particularly to differentiate from adenoma. The importance of diagnosing FNH is that it is a truly benign lesion.

Hepatic adenomas are associated with long-term use of the oral contraceptive pill, often incidental, but can present with abdominal pain. Lesions more than 5 cm in size should be considered for resection because of the risk of bleeding and malignant transformation. A conservative approach involves discontinuation of the oral contraceptive pill and surveillance imaging. Adenomas are currently being subclassified according to histopathological features and presence of somatic mutations (HNF1alpha, gp130, beta-catenin) with associated distinct prognosis.

Secondary liver tumours

Secondaries are commonly discovered as part of the staging process for primary malignancy (synchronous) or during follow-up (metachronous), or indeed may be the initial presentation. Symptoms and signs include abdominal pain and hepatomegaly; jaundice and ascites may occur with extensive infiltration. If the primary is not apparent, a targeted liver biopsy under ultrasound guidance usually confirms malignancy, with immunohistochemical assessment helpful in determining type.

For most primary cancers with liver involvement the prognosis is poor and treatment palliative. Surgical resection and other treatments have been shown to improve survival in the setting of colorectal liver metastases, neuroendocrine malignancies, and gastrointestinal stromal tumours (GISTs).

Introduction

A number of benign and malignant tumours may arise in the liver, given the proliferative nature of its component tissues which include hepatocytes, biliary epithelium, and vascular endothelium. Benign tumours are relatively common and often incidental; distinction is occasionally challenging and some may harbour malignant potential. Hepatocellular carcinoma (HCC) is the most common primary hepatic malignancy, almost always arising on a background of liver damage. Early diagnosis and careful patient selection can lead to cure with treatment such as liver transplantation. Furthermore, advances in our understanding of molecular mechanisms involved in hepatocarcinogenesis are yielding novel therapeutic agents for this disease. The prognosis of cholangiocarcinoma remains poor although prospects for earlier diagnosis and curative treatment are improving; intrahepatic cholangiocarcinoma and intermediate hepatocellular-cholangiocarcinoma are increasingly recognized subtypes. Other primary liver malignancies are rare and thus optimal management, including the role of transplantation, is evolving. Secondary liver tumours are common and treatment is palliative save for colorectal metastases, for which surgical resection can achieve cure, and neuroendocrine tumour where liver-directed therapies and transplantation can be of benefit.

Hepatocellular carcinoma (HCC)

HCC is the fifth most common cancer worldwide as well as the third most common cause of cancer-related death. Most tumours arise on the background of cirrhosis and typically grow slowly with late spread to extrahepatic sites. Symptoms may not be apparent until the cancer is already advanced and most deaths occur within one year of diagnosis. Selected at-risk patients benefit from enrolment into surveillance programmes with the prospect of early detection and potentially curative therapy, principally surgical.

Epidemiology

The geographical distribution of HCC worldwide is uneven, with more than 80% of cases occurring in sub-Saharan Africa and eastern Asia. Indeed, half of global cases occur in China alone (incidence 35 per 100 000 males). The incidence is much lower in western Europe and North and South America—around 2 per 100 000 population vs up to 100 per 100 000 population in some parts of Africa. Certain Asian populations are now experiencing a decline in incidence, following the introduction of hepatitis B vaccination programmes. In the West, however, the incidence of HCC is rising partly due to a rise in cirrhosis due to hepatitis C and also because the usage and sensitivity of liver radiology has increased. In the United States of America HCC is the fastest-growing cause of cancer-related death in men, with marked ethnic variation and highest rates particularly in Asian Americans.

Men have higher primary liver cancer rates than women, approximately three-fold. As well as greater exposure to hepatitis viruses, alcohol, and cigarettes, the higher levels of androgenic hormones in males may be an important aetiological factor. In most populations the highest rates of HCC occur in those aged 75 and over. In Africa, where hepatitis B is often acquired very young, male rates peak between 60 and 65 years. In all regions female rates peak 5 years later than those for men. For tumours arising in noncirrhotic liver the sex incidence is equal and patients usually present younger. In Asia approximately 40% of HCC arises in noncirrhotic livers, mainly hepatitis B-related; in the West the proportion is closer to 5% but incidence may be increasing.

Aetiology and prevention

HCC usually occurs in the context of chronic liver disease: worldwide, 80% of patients with HCC are cirrhotic and 80% can be attributed to hepatitis B, C, or alcohol. Prevention of HCC on a global scale is therefore linked to ameliorating these factors in particular. HCC is long established as the commonest cause of death in haemochromatosis, and HCC complicating cirrhosis due to nonalcoholic steatohepatitis is increasingly recognized. HCC is seen less commonly in cirrhosis due to α_1-antitrypsin deficiency and autoimmune hepatitis. Often several factors may contribute to cirrhosis and subsequent tumour development. In addition, acute intermittent porphyria is a rare hepatic condition prone to complication by HCC.

Hepatitis B virus (HBV) is the most common cause for HCC worldwide, with an estimated 380 million infected individuals harbouring a 100-fold relative risk of developing HCC compared with noncarriers. HCC can arise in chronic HBV infection without cirrhosis—integration of viral DNA into the hepatocyte genome appears to be a prerequisite for oncogenic transformation of these cells. In HBV endemic areas vertical transmission results in high rates of chronic infection, whereas in low-risk areas the virus is acquired horizontally and 90% will clear the acute infection. Risk factors for HCC among HBV carriers include male sex, cirrhosis, older age, family history of HCC, Asian or African ethnicity, and coinfection with hepatitis C or D. Aflatoxin B1, a hepatocarcinogen produced by the *Aspergillus* fungus and present on stored foods in HBV-endemic areas, has been implicated in susceptibility to HCC via a direct disruption of the *TP53* tumour-suppressor gene. Higher circulating viral DNA levels are associated with greater risk of HCC and treatment which suppresses viral load appears to partly protect against HCC development. In Taiwan, following the introduction of routine infant hepatitis B immunization, the incidence of HCC is expected to fall by 80% over the next three decades and with other countries following suit global mortality from HBV-related HCC should reduce.

Hepatitis C virus (HCV) is a leading cause for cirrhosis and HCC development in Western countries and in Japan where HBV is not endemic. HCV-infected individuals have a 17-fold relative risk of developing HCC compared with the general population. Approximately 25% of HCV-infected individuals will develop cirrhosis over a period of 25 years with an annual incidence of HCC thereafter of 1 to 4%. Although most tumours will arise following the lag period to cirrhosis, HCC can occur in noncirrhotic hepatitis C. In the West the peak incidence of HCC in hepatitis C may not have been reached, particularly as many individuals remain undetected. Although no vaccine is currently available, successful antiviral therapy has been shown to reduce cancer risk and continuing advances in treatment together with improvements in prevention and screening are the mainstay for lessening the future burden of HCV-related HCC.

Alcohol is a well-established risk factor for HCC and acts synergistically with hepatitis B and C in causing cirrhosis. Attempts to reduce *per capita* alcohol consumption may impact favourably on HCC prevalence. Patients with haemochromatosis and cirrhosis have up to a 200-fold relative risk of HCC, which persists despite iron removal. Iron has a direct mitogenic effect through stimulation of hepatocyte proliferation. Early recognition and venesection treatment before the onset of significant fibrosis should reduce deaths from HCC in this condition. Importantly, obesity is associated with a two- to threefold increased risk of HCC, most likely via its association with cirrhosis due to nonalcoholic steatohepatitis. Obesity rates are increasing in the West and this may adversely influence future incidences of HCC. Diabetes mellitus, associated with nonalcoholic fatty liver disease, has been similarly identified as an independent risk factor for HCC. For both obesity and type 2 diabetes a direct effect of hyperinsulinaemia on hepatocyte mitogenesis has been proposed.

Pathogenetic mechanisms

Important strides have been made in understanding the molecular biology of HCC development and progression. Alterations of proteins involved in cell cycle regulation, such as p53 and cyclin/CDK complex, and several intracellular signalling pathways undergoing oncogenic activation (specifically Ras/Raf/Mek/Erk, Wnt/β-catenin and PI3k/Akt/mTOR) appear key. Moreover. the role of several growth factors and angiogenic factors in the tissue microenvironment such as epidermal growth factor (EGF) and vascular EGF has been confirmed. Increasing evidence supports the notion that HCCs are monoclonal tumours with different oncogenic pathways and distinct biological phenotypes.

Cirrhosis is characterized by decreasing hepatocyte proliferation as regenerative capacity becomes exhausted. A hypothesis for HCC development in the context of hepatocyte senescence involves critical telomere shortening which then triggers DNA repair mechanisms and chromosomal instability as the first step. Some tumours may originate from a particular subpopulation of stem cells which persist in the adult liver and are found in portal triads. These 'oval' cells retain the potential to proliferate and differentiate into either hepatocytes or biliary epithelial cells; they have been implicated in the development of HCC as well as intermediate hepatocellular-cholangiocarcinoma.

Clinical presentation

HCC may present with a triad of pain in the right upper quadrant, hepatomegaly, and weight loss. In high-incidence areas the presentation is usually shorter, over a period of weeks, whereas in low-incidence areas patients tend to present more insidiously over several months. Diarrhoea is also a common feature. Patients presenting with these symptoms usually have significant-sized tumours which may be palpable; a bruit may be auscultated. Decompensation in cirrhotic individuals may be a sign of tumour and is signified by worsening ascites, variceal bleeding (particularly if the portal vein is directly invaded by tumour), jaundice, encephalopathy, or a combination of these. Occasionally patients present with sudden abdominal pain and swelling associated with haemoperitoneum due to tumour rupture. The latter diagnosis is usually confirmed by imaging and ascitic fluid sampling. Other presentations include secondary Budd–Chiari syndrome, obstructive jaundice, haemobilia, and pyrexia of unknown origin. Paraneoplastic manifestations include polycythaemia, hyperthyroidism, hypercalcaemia, and hypoglycaemia. Asymptomatic tumours are increasingly being detected through surveillance imaging, typically 1 to 2 cm in size.

Investigations

The diagnosis of HCC may be confirmed following a combination of blood tests, various imaging techniques and histology if necessary (Fig. 15.22.6.1).

Serum markers

α-Fetoprotein (AFP) is the only commonly used laboratory test for the diagnosis of HCC. AFP is a glycoprotein synthesized by the fetal liver and its plasma concentrations reach their maximum at the end of the first trimester, declining rapidly after birth to adult levels (0–10 ng/ml). Elevated levels are found in about 80% of patients with HCC and tend to be higher in African and east Asian populations (median 10 000 ng/ml) than in those from low-incidence areas (median 1000 ng/ml). Concentrations of AFP above 500 ng/ml in patients with a liver mass suggest HCC, the differential diagnosis including nonseminomatous germ cell tumours, hepatoblastoma (in infants), and hepatic metastases usually from pancreas or stomach. In patients with cirrhosis and a suspicious liver mass on imaging, an AFP level above 200 ng/ml can be considered diagnostic. Serum AFP increases with tumour growth, and serial measurements showing a steady rise are strongly indicative of HCC. Note that 50% of noncirrhotic patients with HCC have a normal AFP level. A modestly raised and fluctuating AFP level is common in patients with chronic HCV infection.

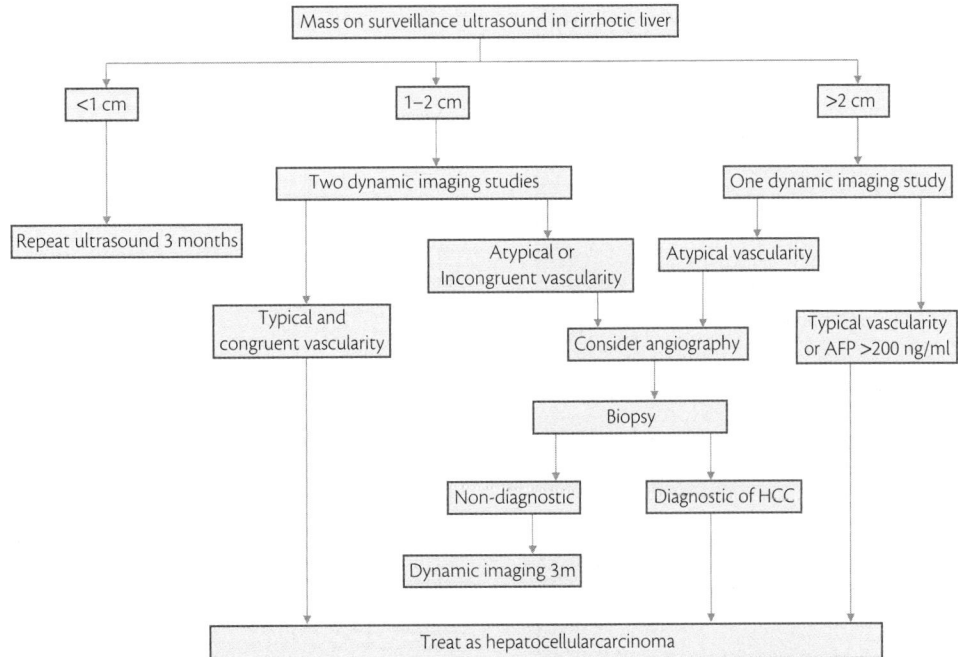

Fig. 15.22.6.1 Suggested pathway of investigation for suspected hepatocellular carcinoma.

Liver imaging

Ultrasound is relatively inexpensive, safe, and can detect an HCC as small as 1 cm in size. Such tumours typically appear hypoechoic. Further imaging is usually required for confirmation of diagnosis, although ultrasound remains a useful screening modality. Sensitivity depends on operator experience, however, and tumours within an irregular and heterogeneous liver may be easily missed. Use of microbubble contrast enhancement improves sensitivity. Visibility on ultrasound may inform subsequent attempts at biopsy or ablation, and use of Doppler can confirm forward portal vein flow prior to hepatic arterial embolization.

Multislice CT is an established imaging modality for diagnosis and staging of HCC, as well as for planning surgical resection. Use of intravenous contrast allows more detailed characterization: a combination of arterial enhancement and portal venous 'washout' is virtually diagnostic for HCC in lesions over 2 cm with known cirrhosis. Smaller lesions and those with a less typical vascular profile require additional dynamic imaging which may improve diagnostic certainty. Sensitivity of CT remains imperfect with 30% of tumours under 2 cm undetected when compared with subsequent explant histology. CT may be helpful in demonstrating hepatic features consistent with cirrhosis and the presence of portal hypertension. Portal venous invasion and extrahepatic disease, both signifying poor prognosis, can be evaluated using this technique.

The sensitivity and specificity of MRI for detection of HCC is similar to that of CT, but without the radiation exposure (Fig. 15.22.6.2). For 1 to 2 cm tumours MRI is slightly more sensitive than CT and can be used for follow-up of indeterminate lesions particularly where the background liver is difficult to assess by ultrasound. For such lesions a low signal on T2-weighted imaging and lack of arterial enhancement are example features which would suggest a regenerative nodule rather than HCC. Excellent visualization of the hepatic arterial supply can be

obtained by selective catheterization at angiography; as the vascular supply for HCC is predominantly arterial, a diagnostic 'tumour blush' is seen in a high proportion of cases. An absent blush or indeterminate appearance may point towards an alternative explanation such as dysplastic or regenerative nodule or a region of fibrosis.

If uncertainty remains, the clinician must weigh up the pros and cons of obtaining liver tissue to establish a firm diagnosis. Where biopsy is not possible or is nondiagnostic, close surveillance with dynamic imaging to look for temporal changes in characteristics, number and size of lesions is the preferred option.

Liver biopsy

Histology is the gold standard for diagnosis, although interpretation of core biopsies may be challenging, e.g. distinguishing well-differentiated HCC from severe dysplasia. On microscopic examination, HCC is typically composed of large eosinophilic or clear cells, arranged in trabeculae; intercellular bile is diagnostic when present (Fig. 15.22.6.3). Immunohistochemical markers for hepatocytes, such as HepPar-1 and AFP, may help where morphology is not characteristic. Biopsy of the background liver to confirm cirrhosis greatly increases the probability of a focal lesion being HCC where this is uncertain.

Percutaneous biopsy carries a small risk (<2%) of tumour seeding along the tract and historically has been avoided prior to potentially curative surgical treatment. Coagulopathy and ascites are additional hazards. For inaccessible lesions of sufficient concern, and where imaging is not diagnostic, laparoscopic biopsy or wedge resection is an alternative. Furthermore histological examination and staging of surgical specimens are important for prognosis in HCC—poor differentiation and vascular invasion are strongly associated with tumour recurrence following resection or transplantation. Determining prognosis based on needle-derived specimens is more challenging due to variation of differentiation

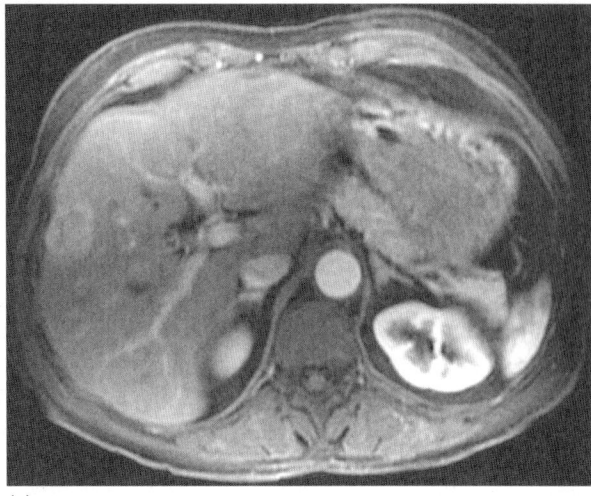

(a)

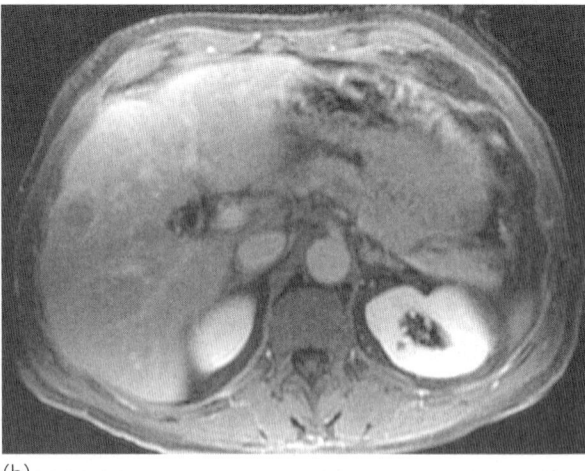

(b)

Fig. 15.22.6.2 T_1-weighted MRI scan of a cirrhotic liver with an irregular lesion in the right lobe which demonstrates contrast enhancement on arterial phase imaging (panel A). Delayed portal phase imaging shows 'washout' consistent with hepatocellular carcinoma (panel B).

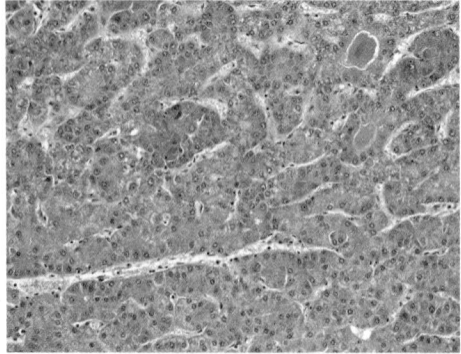

Fig. 15.22.6.3 Targeted biopsy of a liver lesion showing eosinophilic cells arranged in a trabecular pattern with pseudoglandular formation—bile plugs are noted. The morphology is typical for a well-differentiated hepatocellular carcinoma (haematoxylin and eosin, ×20).

and vessel involvement across the tumour. However, identification of prognostically accurate biological markers may change practice in favour of always obtaining tissue prior to radical therapies.

Surveillance

Ultrasound surveillance has been shown to be cost-effective in cirrhosis where the annual risk of HCC exceeds 1.5%. Fulfilling this criterion includes cirrhosis due to HBV, HCV, alcohol, and haemochromatosis as well as stage 4 primary biliary cirrhosis. Incidence data for HCC in cirrhosis due to nonalcoholic steatohepatitis, autoimmune hepatitis, and α_1-antitrypsin deficiency are less robust. At-risk HBV carriers who should be surveyed include Asians (men >40 years, women >50 years), Africans from adulthood, and older white men with active disease. With HCV infection the risk rises following the onset of severe fibrosis and noninvasive fibrosis markers appear promising for determining this time-point. Ultrasound has 65 to 80% sensitivity and greater than 90% specificity for HCC when used as a surveillance tool and the standard 6-month interval is based on average tumour doubling times. AFP alone is inadequate as a screening test, as it lacks sensitivity, though is typically used in addition to ultrasound. Proteomic profiling may in future yield useful serum biomarkers for detection of HCC.

Treatment

Several treatment options may be available but selecting the one with the highest benefit/risk ratio is key. Importantly, survival may be limited by liver disease as well as by tumour. Transplantation, resection, and ablation are potentially curative and surgery in particular should be considered if at all eligible. Chemoembolization is an established palliative treatment with associated survival benefit. Cytotoxic drugs are generally nonefficacious but novel agents against specific molecular targets are showing promise.

Surgical resection

Nowadays operative mortality is low, following careful patient selection, and laparoscopic approaches may be feasible. The best candidates are noncirrhotic with a single tumour or cirrhotic but with well-preserved liver function, i.e. Child–Pugh A. Survival in those with normal bilirubin and absence of portal hypertension (hepatic venous pressure gradient <10 mmHg) reaches 70% at 5 years. However, this falls to 50% in the presence of portal hypertension and 30% if the bilirubin is also raised. In cirrhosis, therefore, transplantation would usually be the preferred option if feasible. Apart from liver decompensation, the principal problem with resection is tumour recurrence, which reaches 70% at 5 years. Early recurrence is usually due to previous dissemination whereas later recurrence is a result of *de novo* tumour development. Recurrence is associated with microvascular invasion and presence of satellite nodules, rather than size of lesion *per se*, although larger lesions are more likely to have adverse features. Surgery for recurrence can only be justified if thought to be a *de novo* tumour. Surgical resection for spontaneously ruptured tumours appears to offer satisfactory outcomes despite the expectation of intraperitoneal seeding at time of rupture.

Liver transplantation

This confers significant long-term survival benefit for patients with cirrhosis curing both the tumour and the liver disease, but not without risk. Donor shortages have restricted selection to those with predicted survival comparable to non-HCC indications.

When adhering to the Milan criteria (single tumour ≤5 cm or up to 3 tumours ≤3 cm) a 70% 5-year survival and 10% recurrence rate are anticipated. Long waiting times result in dropout due to tumour growth, approximately 25% after 12 months. Patients awaiting transplantation therefore commonly receive embolization or ablative therapy with a view to staying within criteria—the benefit of this on an intention-to-treat basis is unproven, however. Compared with non-HCC patients, those with HCC have a typically lower severity of liver disease so should be afforded greater priority on the list and may tolerate a marginal donor liver with less chance of early graft dysfunction.

Expansion of the Milan criteria is currently being debated, the risk being that of listing a greater number of patients who would be subject to dropout or recurrence post-transplant. Better methods to predict tumour behaviour, independently of size, are required. With recurrent HCC, 50% is extrahepatic; treatment options have to be individualized, and surgery or indeed radiotherapy may be useful for isolated secondary deposits. Recent observations suggest that post-transplant immunosuppression using the mTOR inhibitor sirolimus reduces risk of tumour recurrence—a strategy perhaps for those with adverse prognostic features on explant histology.

Ablative therapies

Local ablation involves destruction of tumour cells by chemical substances (alcohol or acetic acid) or temperature (radiofrequency, microwave, laser, high-intensity focused ultrasound, or cryoablation) with the aim of creating a 1 cm 'ablation ring' around the tumour. Ablation is potentially curative but usually reserved for those where surgery is contraindicated. The procedure is most commonly performed using ultrasound guidance and carries a small risk (c.1%) of needle-track seeding. Follow-up arterial-phase imaging is required to ensure the tumour has been adequately treated and to identify local recurrence due to incomplete therapy.

Percutaneous ethanol injection is well tolerated, inexpensive, and highly efficacious for solitary tumours under 3 cm. Survival figures are similar to those for surgical resection in this group. For larger tumours mortality and recurrence rates increase exponentially with size. Radiofrequency ablation (RFA) has comparable efficacy to ethanol for small tumours, with 75% survival at 3 years. Furthermore, fewer treatments are required and RFA can be used intraoperatively. RFA is superior to ethanol for larger tumours although beyond 5 cm local recurrence is common. This technique works less well if the tumour is adjacent to a major blood vessel, as the latter removes heat. Subcapsular tumours are more likely to result in pain and risk of neoplastic seeding. Morbidity is generally higher than with ethanol but RFA has become the established method in most centres. Data on the remaining thermal techniques is limited although these are showing promise as adjuncts to embolization therapy for prolonging survival in a palliative setting.

Transarterial chemoembolization (TACE)

This has been the most widely used primary treatment for unresectable HCC. TACE involves injection of chemotherapeutic agent (typically doxorubicin or cisplatin) into hepatic arterial branches supplying the tumour, followed by embolic occlusion. Infarction and necrosis ensue, since tumours derive 95% of their blood supply from the hepatic artery. To avoid infarction of neighbouring liver tissue, adequate portal vein flow is required. Up to 60% of patients respond and tumour progression is delayed with a 20 to 60% improvement in 2-year survival. A postembolization syndrome of abdominal pain and fever is common, indicating tumour necrosis. Complications include liver failure and abscess formation, hence prophylactic antibiotics are advised. The best candidates have preserved liver function and no vessel involvement or extrahepatic spread. Although transarterial embolization (TAE) achieves similar objective responses, only TACE has shown survival benefit on recent meta-analysis. New embolic agents incorporating a radio-isotope or gene vector are under study.

Chemotherapy

HCC is a highly chemoresistant cancer with little benefit from systemic therapy. Responses to cytotoxic drugs, typically doxorubicin, are limited and hampered by side effects. Tamoxifen, octreotide, pravastatin, and gemcitabine have not shown any impact on survival. Agents targeting molecular abnormalities have shown promise and are being studied in patients with advanced HCC. Sorafenib is a multikinase inhibitor against Ras kinase, involved in proliferative signalling, and VEGF receptors which stimulate angiogenesis. In a recent randomized placebo-controlled trial in patients with advanced HCC and Child–Pugh A cirrhosis this agent demonstrated a significant survival advantage (median 10.7 vs 7.9 months). Targeted drug therapies may become useful in preventing progression while awaiting liver transplantation and as adjuvant treatment after resection or transplantation, particularly where there is histological evidence of aggressive tumour biology.

Prognosis

Symptomatic presentation carries a poor prognosis with less than 10% of patients surviving 3 years. Surveillance programmes, however, enable one-third of patients to be diagnosed at the early stages when curative treatments are possible. Accurate prognostic modelling requires not only tumour stage but other tightly-related aspects such as liver reserve and general condition. Several staging systems have been proposed though none is universally accepted. The Barcelona Clinic Liver Cancer system usefully links tumour stage and Child–Pugh status with treatment strategy to optimize prognosis. Molecular profiling of tumours will be incorporated undoubtedly into staging systems of the future.

Fibrolamellar HCC

This rare variant presents in younger individuals with median age of presentation around 20 years. Risk factors are not apparent, cirrhosis is typically absent and AFP levels normal. The tumour is generally slow growing, although regional lymph node metastases are common. Histology reveals dense fibrotic bands surrounding eosinophilic tumour cells. The prognosis is better than for HCC although recurrence is common following surgical resection.

Hepatoblastoma

This primary hepatic malignancy occurs in children, mostly under 3 years of age. The optimal treatment approach of resection combined with chemotherapy may achieve a 5-year survival of 80%. Transplantation has proved to be an effective rescue therapy.

Cholangiocarcinoma

This is an epithelial malignancy of the biliary tree which on anatomical grounds can be separated into intrahepatic or extrahepatic, the latter divided into hilar and lower duct tumours. Cholangiocarcinoma is less common than HCC and comprises around 7 to 10% of primary liver malignancies. Prognosis is generally poor unless detected very early or a more favourable subtype.

Epidemiology and aetiology

Cholangiocarcinoma occurs most commonly in the sixth and seventh decades, is 50% more common in men and twice as common in Asians. Furthermore the incidence of intrahepatic cholangiocarcinoma worldwide appears to be increasing. The highest incidence is in northern Thailand, due to endemic biliary infection by the trematode *Opisthorchis viverrini*. High incidence is also seen in Korea where similar infection by the fluke *Clonorchis sinensis* is prevalent. Other risk factors for the intrahepatic variant include oriental fibrocholestatic hepatitis, primary sclerosing cholangitis (PSC), EBV, HCV infection, and exposure to thorotrast. The developmental abnormalities Caroli's disease, congenital hepatic fibrosis, and von Meyenburg complexes are also associated with intrahepatic cholangiocarcinoma. Extrahepatic cholangiocarcinoma is associated with PSC, abnormal choledochopancreatic junction, choledochal cysts, and infection by *Clonorchis sinensis* and *Opisthorchis viverrini*.

Pathogenesis

Most of the aetiological factors associated with cholangiocarcinoma induce chronic inflammation within the biliary tree. Chronic inflammation stimulates inducible nitric oxide and free radical production in bile duct epithelial cells. These processes in turn induce oxidative DNA damage and telomere shortening with resultant loss or gain of critical genes involved in cellular control. Methylation of tumour suppressor promoters and cholangiocyte resistance to apoptosis are thought to be relevant mechanisms in oncogenesis.

Pathology

Cholangiocarcinoma is an adenocarcinoma with a prominent stromal reaction. Histological variants include adenosquamous, signet cell, sarcomatous, clear cell, and lymphoepithelial. Three contrasting growth patterns have been applied to both intrahepatic and extrahepatic cholangiocarcinoma: mass-forming, periductal-infiltrating, and intraductal-growing.

- Mass-forming is the commonest mode of presentation of intrahepatic cholangiocarcinoma and these tumours are often large, up to 15 cm in diameter. The margin is typically well circumscribed and lobulated and central necrosis may be present. Multicentricity is common, probably because of the propensity of the tumour to invade the adjacent peripheral branches of the portal vein. Mass-forming tumours arising from the extrahepatic ducts tend to be smaller, typically less than 2 cm.

- Periductal-infiltrating cholangiocarcinoma is most common at the hilum, growing along the bile ducts and therefore elongated, spiculated, or branchlike. These tumours tend to be difficult to detect radiologically.

- Most intraductal-growing cholangiocarcinomas are papillary adenocarcinomas comprising innumerable frond like infoldings of proliferated columnar epithelial cells with slender fibrovascular cores. The tumours are usually small, sessile, or polypoid, often spreading superficially along the mucosal surface and resulting in multiple tumours (papillomatosis) along various

regions of the biliary tree. Occasionally a large mass occludes the bile duct and some tumours produce profuse amounts of mucin akin to pancreatic intraductal papillary mucinous tumours.

Signs and symptoms

With peripheral intrahepatic masses, patients present with upper abdominal pain, anorexia, malaise, and weight loss. Jaundice is an early feature of hilar tumours. Hepatomegaly is usual and splenomegaly may occur in the context of a secondary biliary cirrhosis due to prolonged obstruction.

Diagnosis

Liver function tests are typically cholestatic with elevation of plasma bilirubin and alkaline phosphatase concentrations. AFP concentrations are usually normal or only slightly raised. CA19-9, a glycoprotein secreted by bile duct cells, is a commonly used tumour marker. In patients with PSC a CA19-9 level over 100 U/mL is 80% specific for the presence of complicating cholangiocarcinoma.

Mass-forming intrahepatic cholangiocarcinomas may show persistent peripheral enhancement on contrast-enhanced CT imaging. For extrahepatic hilar tumours MR cholangiopancreatography (MRCP) demonstrates first- and second-order duct involvement and a mass may be evident which is hypointense on T1-weighted imaging and hyperintense on T2-weighted imaging. Differential diagnosis of hilar lesions includes inflammatory pseudotumour and metastasis. A periductal-infiltrating tumour appears on MRCP as a concentric irregular thickening of the bile duct with an abrupt transition. An intraductal-growing neoplasm may be visualized as an enhancing mass confined to the lumen of the bile duct. In all three types, the ducts peripheral to the tumour may appear dilated with associated atrophy of the liver.

Percutaneous transhepatic cholangiography (PTC) may be used if the proximal involvement of the biliary tree cannot be determined adequately by MRCP and to drain segments prior to surgery. Endoscopic retrograde cholangiopancreatography (ERCP) with brush cytology and biopsy or with newer choledochoscopy may assist in the diagnosis of a malignant biliary stricture. Analysis on cytological specimens of aneuploidy by digital image analysis or of chromosomal alterations using fluorescence *in situ* hybridization improves diagnostic accuracy but is not routinely available. Endoscopic ultrasound-guided fine-needle aspiration of hilar masses can achieve a sensitivity and specificity for malignancy of 89% and 100%, respectively, in expert hands. This technique can also be used to identify neighbouring malignant lymph nodes. Positron emission tomography (PET) imaging may be a useful adjunct for diagnosis and laparoscopy can detect occult peritoneal spread.

Treatment and prognosis

For peripheral tumours the main treatment approach is resection with prospect of cure, although results are generally disappointing. Poor prognostic factors include a preoperative CA19-9 more than 1000 U/mL, multifocal disease, liver capsule invasion, R1 resection, regional lymph node metastases, and mass-forming or periductal infiltrating type.

Extrahepatic tumors of the distal duct may be treated by pancreaticoduodenectomy (Whipple's operation). Hilar tumours may be suitable for curative resection with extended hemihepatectomy and anastomosis of a Roux loop of jejunum to a hilar bile duct. Contraindications to surgery include bilateral involvement of the second-order radicles and portal vein or hepatic artery encasement contralateral to the side being resected. Despite surgical advances, the median 5-year survival for hilar tumours following resection is around 20% and controlled trials of adjuvant chemotherapy are needed. More commonly curative excision is not possible, and the aim is to establish biliary drainage. A stent can be placed through the growth endoscopically or via a percutaneous transhepatic route. Unilateral self-expanding metal stent placement has been shown to be as efficacious as bilateral and cost-effective compared with plastic if survival more than 6 months is expected. MRCP may assist in optimum stent positioning and method. A recent palliative advance is photodynamic therapy which has been shown to prolong survival. Conventional radiotherapy and high-dose local irradiation within the biliary tree, by means of iridium-192 wire, may produce useful symptomatic relief. If biliary drainage can be achieved by these procedures, survival for 1 to 2 years is not unusual.

Within the UK, liver transplantation is not an accepted treatment option for cholangiocarcinoma as historical data indicates an unacceptably high level of recurrence and mortality. However, long-term survival has been achieved in highly selected cases with unresectable hilar cholangiocarcinoma. A regimen involving high-dose neoadjuvant radiotherapy (external and internal) with chemosensitization and operative staging, to exclude patients with regional lymph node metastases, has recently been associated with a 5-year post-transplant survival of greater than 80%. In one-quarter of explants no tumour was identified and—of note—pretransplant histological confirmation of the diagnosis was not a prerequisite. Furthermore, a high rate of arterial and venous complications in the post-operative period has been reported. These results are nonetheless impressive and await validation in other centres before transplantation can be universally accepted as a treatment for cholangiocarcinoma.

Malignant vascular tumours

Angiosarcoma

Angiosarcoma of the liver is a rare and aggressive primary tumour, often multifocal, which may arise in a cirrhotic liver. Worldwide, 200 new cases are reported annually. Peak incidence is in the sixth and seventh decades of life and men are three times more commonly affected than women. In 75% of cases there is no recognized cause. Previous research has outlined the associations with specific carcinogens such as arsenic, vinyl chloride, and thorotrast. Thorotrast (thorium dioxide) was used as a radiological contrast dye during angiographic procedures between the 1930s and 1950s. More recently the tumour has been found in workers in the vinyl chloride industry and, though strict safety regulations have been introduced, new cases continue to present due to the long latent period. Long-term androgen use, haemochromatosis, and von Recklinghausen's disease are known associations. The genetics associated with angiosarcoma vary according to the aetiological agent. For vinyl chloride-associated tumours, TP53 mutations with A:T→T:A transversions have been identified, generally uncommon in other carcinomas. K-ras-2 mutations have been associated with thorotrast-related and sporadic angiosarcoma.

Patients may present with an hepatic venous outflow syndrome of abdominal pain and ascites, mimicking primary Budd–Chiari syndrome; 15% present with an acute intrabdominal crisis due to tumour rupture and 15% present with splenomegaly and pancytopenia.

A small number present with distant metastases, especially to lung, spleen, and bone marrow. An hepatic bruit and signs of high-output cardiac failure may be present, and ascites may be bloodstained due to spontaneous haemoperitoneum. Disseminated intravascular coagulation may be associated (Kasabach–Merritt syndrome). On CT and MRI these tumours demonstrate a variety of appearances although the majority have focal hypodense areas, often haemorrhagic, which demonstrate arterial enhancement with intravenous contrast. A typical reticular pattern due to thorotrast accumulation may be evident on CT and vascular lakes may be observed on angiography. Diffuse infiltration may give rise to a nonspecific heterogeneous appearance of the liver.

Liver biopsy is diagnostic in 25% of percutaneous and 65% of open procedures, the latter preferred because of bleeding risk. Histology shows typical spindle or pleomorphic tumour cells with eosinophilic cytoplasm growing along the lumina of previous vascular structures. The growth and blockage of sinusoids is associated with sinusoidal

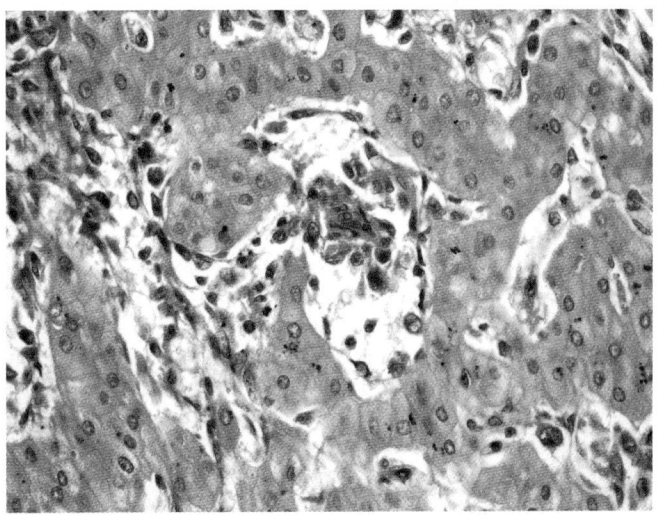

(a)

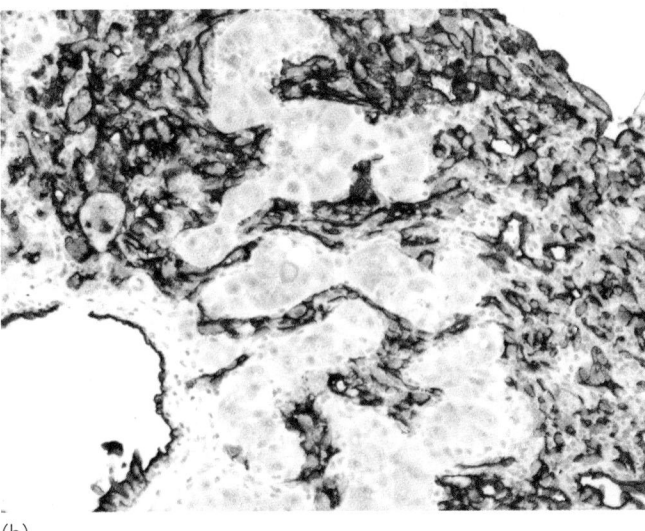

(b)

Fig. 15.22.6.4 Irregular cells with pleomorphic and hyperchromatic nuclei are seen infiltrating sinusoids and terminal hepatic vein branches (haematoxylin and eosin, ×40—panel A). These cells are strongly positive for CD34 and consistent with angiosarcoma (×20—panel B).

congestion and liver cell atrophy. As these cells are derived from vascular structures they stain positive with antibody markers to CD34 (Fig. 15.22.6.4). If thorotrast or vinyl chlorides are the cause there may be considerable periportal and subcapsular fibrosis. Four growth patterns are typically recognized: nodular, large dominant nodule, mixed features, and a rarer diffusely infiltrating type. Curative resection is rarely possible and chemotherapy may increase survival for what is an otherwise poor prognosis.

Hepatic epithelioid haemangioendothelioma

This rare malignant tumour of vascular endothelial origin runs a clinical course akin to a low-grade angiosarcoma. It is usually multifocal and slow growing, with a slight female preponderance. Patients present typically around 40 to 45 years with right upper quadrant pain. Histological appearances are fairly characteristic, with a spindle lesion infiltrating hepatocyte plates and hepatic veins. Immunohistochemistry for vascular markers, such as CD34, can aid diagnosis. Resection is associated with a 5-year survival of 75% but this approach is usually not feasible and aggressive recurrence has been reported. Transplantation is an acceptable therapy even with limited extrahepatic disease—again unpredictable and rapid recurrence can occur. The role of chemotherapy is unclear.

Benign liver tumours

Haemangioma

This is the most common benign tumour of the liver with a prevalence of 2 to 5% in the general population and a reported female preponderance. Although thought to be congenital, growth can occur, and in 50% of cases more than one lesion is present. Histology reveals multiple large blood-filled spaces, lined by endothelial cells, with varying degrees of hyalinization and fibrosis. The term 'cavernous' haemangioma is used for larger lesions over 4 cm. These are fed by hepatic artery branches and have a slow internal circulation.

Haemangiomas are usually discovered incidentally during abdominal imaging. Larger tumours can cause abdominal symptoms from mass affect and have been reported to cause portal hypertension, haemobilia, caval thrombosis, and a consumptive coagulopathy (Kasabach–Merritt syndrome). Spontaneous and traumatic rupture have also been reported. The typical appearance on ultrasound is a well-circumscribed and uniform hyperechoic mass. MRI is a more sensitive and specific modality demonstrating a lesion which is hypointense on T1-weighted imaging and hyperintense on T2-weighted views. Dynamic imaging characteristically shows nodular peripheral enhancement with progressive centripetal 'fill-in' and retention of contrast in the portal phase (Fig. 15.22.6.5). Occasionally biopsy is required to confirm diagnosis in larger lesions where typical features are not present. Usually no treatment is required and patients can be given reassurance. Large symptomatic haemangiomas can be managed by surgical enucleation or embolization. Liver transplantation has rarely been performed when unresectable and causing intractable symptoms.

Focal nodular hyperplasia (FNH)

FNH is the second most common benign tumour of the liver, with a prevalence of 0.4 to 0.8% in the general population. It is nine times more prevalent in women than men and usually presents in the third or fourth decade. Typically a solitary lesion is present which may be over 5 cm in size. The oral contraceptive pill is not

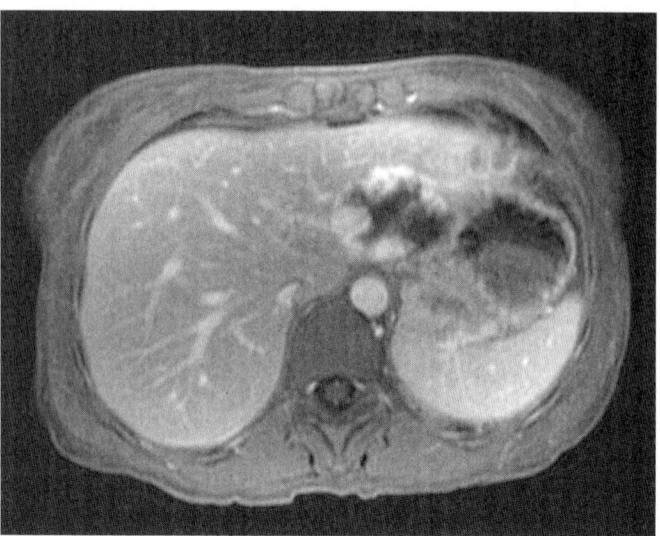

Fig. 15.22.6.5 Delayed MRI during the portal phase demonstrates the characteristic centripetal filling of a left liver lobe cavernous haemangioma in an otherwise normal liver.

thought to induce FNH formation, but studies have suggested that oestrogens can promote FNH growth and vascularity.

Histology typically shows a central large fibrous septum containing a branch of hepatic artery which divides in a star-shaped manner and is not accompanied by either portal vein or bile duct. Within this central 'stellate scar' there is bile ductular proliferation and surrounding it is polyclonal nodular hyperplasia of the hepatic parenchyma giving a pseudobiliary cirrhotic pattern. The hyperplastic response of the hepatic parenchyma may be driven by angiopoietins released from the hepatic artery branch, or in response to a hyperperfusion injury. The less common, recently recognized 'telangiectatic' variant is thought to be better classified as an adenoma (see below).

FNH is usually detected on ultrasonography but requires further characterization. On MRI the lesion demonstrates homogenous signal intensity with the central scar appearing hypointense on T1-weighted imaging and usually hyperintense on T2-weighted imaging. With administration of contrast, dense enhancement occurs and the lesion then becomes isointense in the portal phase (Fig. 15.22.6.6). With delayed imaging the central scar may become hyperintense. It is noteworthy that in 80% of lesions under 3 cm in size, a central scar may not be visible. If the imaging techniques are nondiagnostic, targeted biopsy usually confirms the diagnosis. The prognosis is excellent and malignant change has not been recorded. For women on the oral contraceptive pill where FNH appears likely, but biopsy is not straightforward, a surveillance approach with cessation of oestrogen use may provide reassurance.

Hepatic adenoma

Hepatic adenoma is 10 times less common than FNH and rare in men, with a female to male ratio of 4:1. The incidence of adenomas among long-term users of the oral contraceptive pill is approximately 4 per 100 000 and increases with length of contraceptive use. In women who do not use oral contraceptives, or have used them for less than 2 years, the incidence is 1 per million. In addition, the incidence of adenoma is increased in patients with type 1 glycogen storage disease, diabetes mellitus, haemochromatosis, acromegaly, and in men using anabolic steroids. The presence of

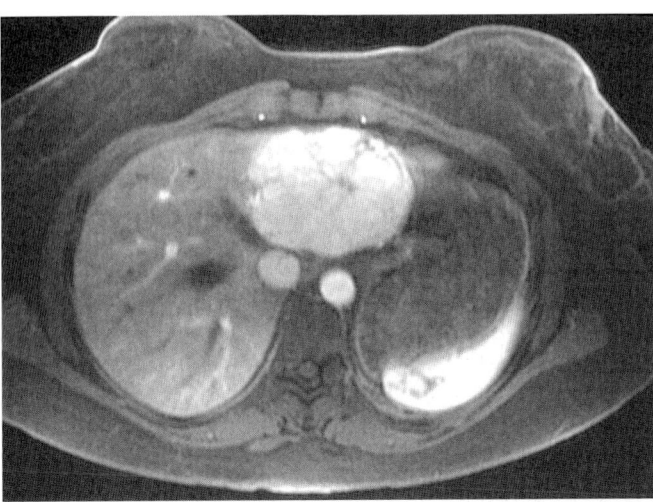

(a)

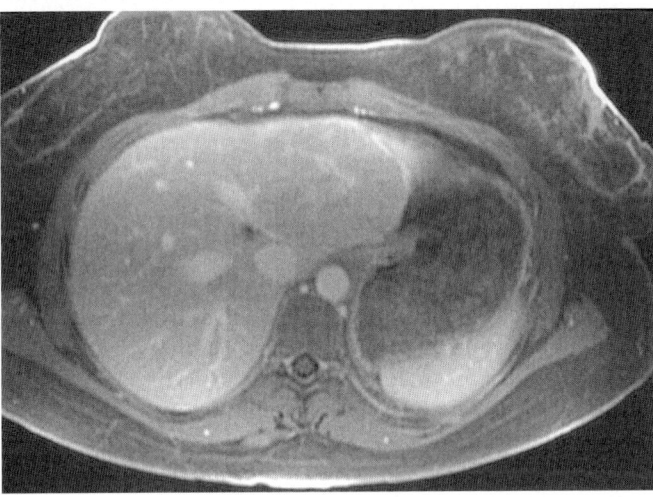

(b)

Fig. 15.22.6.6 A large lesion in the left lobe of the liver avidly enhances with Gadolinium on arterial phase MRI (panel A). The lesion becomes isointense during the portal phase and a central scar is evident (panel B). This lesion was confirmed as an FNH on histology.

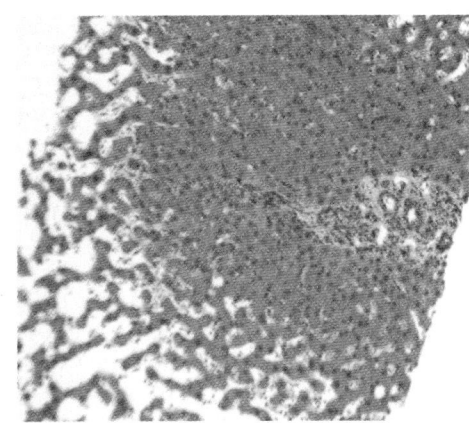

Fig. 15.22.6.7 Targeted biopsy of a liver lesion which shows a portal tract-like area, containing multiple atypical blood vessels, and a region of prominent sinusoidal ectasia. These findings are in keeping with the telangiectatic adenoma variant (haematoxylin and eosin, ×10).

more than 10 adenomas defines hepatic adenomatosis. Adenomas may increase in size in pregnancy and shrink with suspension of oestrogen use. Abdominal pain is relatively common and, rarely, spontaneous rupture and bleeding can occur.

On microscopic examination, adenomas consist of trabeculae of mature-appearing hepatocytes with absent portal tracts and Kupffer cells, though arterial branches are present. Recently genetic mutations have been identified which correlate with distinct biological phenotypes. Biallelic *HNF1A* mutations define adenomas with marked steatosis, a lack of both cytological abnormalities and inflammatory infiltrates, and a very low risk of malignant transformation. Mutations resulting in β-catenin (*CTNNB1*) activation are present in 15% of cases and are associated with a high risk of transformation into hepatocellular carcinoma. A third group of adenomas has been defined by the absence of known mutations but presence of inflammatory infiltrates and features such as sinusoidal dilatation, ductular reaction and cytological abnormalities. These 'telangiectatic' adenomas, originally called telangiectatic FNH, are thought to have a higher risk of bleeding and may harbour malignant potential

(Fig. 15.22.6.7). Mutations in the *IL6ST* gene encoding gp130, activating the interleukin-6 pathway, have been associated with the majority of these inflammatory lesions. A fourth group comprises adenomas without known mutations or inflammatory infiltrates.

CT imaging of adenomas may demonstrate an area of haemorrhage and occasionally internal fat or calcification. After intravenous contrast homogeneous enhancement in the hepatic arterial phase is characteristic with lesions becoming isoattenuating in the portal venous phase (Fig. 15.22.6.8). With MRI adenomas are hyperintense or isointense lesion on T1-weighted imaging and often slightly hyperintense to liver tissue on T2-weighted imaging. It is suggested that lesions over 5 cm should be considered for resection because of risk of bleeding and malignant transformation. A conservative approach involves discontinuation of the oral contraceptive pill and surveillance imaging with AFP monitoring. Predicting subsequent behaviour is key and inhibitors of β-catenin are being sought for targeted therapy.

Lymphangioma

Lymphangiomas are made up of dilated lymphatic channels that compress the normal liver parenchyma. Often these occur as part of a multisystem disease affecting bone, brain, soft tissues, and lung. Typically with MRI multiple cystic areas in the liver are seen that do not enhance with contrast.

Angiomyolipoma

While common in the adrenals and kidneys, these lesions can be found in the liver and are associated in 6 to 10% of cases with tuberous sclerosis.

Mesenchymal hamartoma

This lesion is more common in males and usually manifests within the first 2 years of life. Patients usually present with progressive abdominal swelling. Structurally the tumour is composed of mixed endodermal and mesodermal components in a connective tissue stroma. Surgical resection is the treatment of choice.

Biliary cystadenoma

This cystic lesion usually occurs in middle-aged women. Papillary infoldings are a characteristic finding on ultrasound or CT.

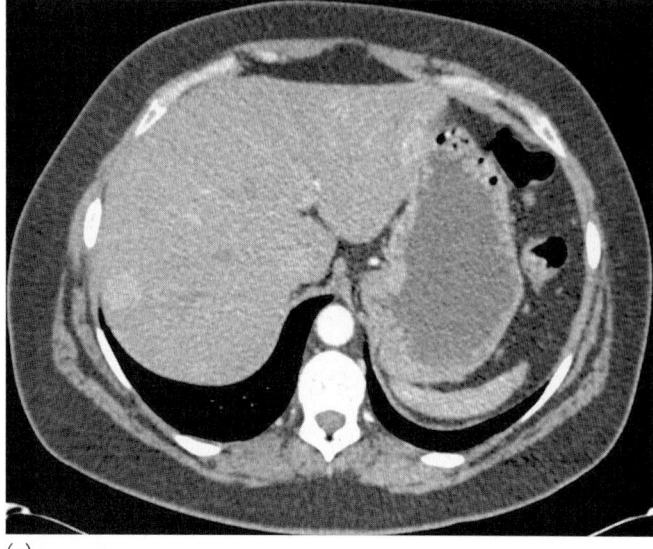

(a)

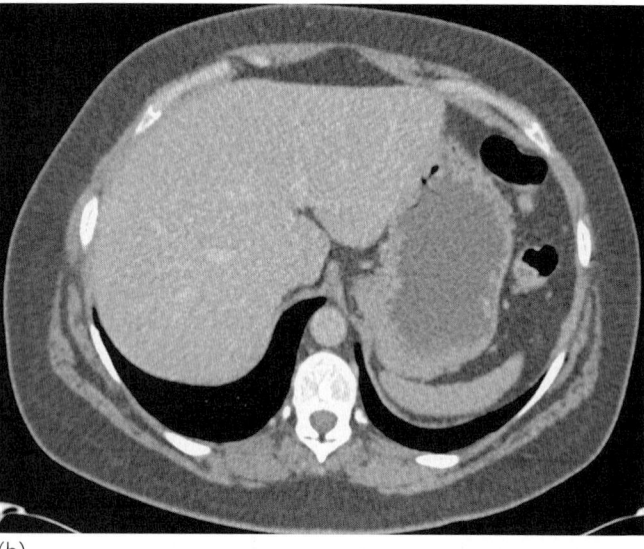

(b)

Fig. 15.22.6.8 A well-circumscribed liver lesion in the right lobe is demonstrated on CT. This lesion enhances in the arterial phase (panel A) and becomes isoattenuating in the portal phase (panel B). Subsequent histology confirmed this to be an adenoma.

Malignant potential is recognized and distinguishing from cystadenocarcinoma on radiology alone is difficult. Cystic aspiration for diagnosis is unhelpful and complete excision is required to avoid recurrence.

Secondary liver tumours

The liver is a common site for metastases which thrive on a rich blood supply and favourable milieu for tumour growth. Secondaries are commonly discovered as part of the staging process for primary malignancy (synchronous) or during follow-up (metachronous) or indeed may be the initial presentation. Liver function tests may be normal but the alkaline phosphatase level usually rises as the tumour mass enlarges. Symptoms include abdominal pain and, with extensive infiltration, jaundice and ascites may occur. If a primary tumour is not apparent a targeted liver biopsy under

ultrasound usually confirms malignancy and an immunohisto-chemical panel for antigens may point to the origin.

For most primary cancers with liver involvement the prognosis is poor and treatment palliative. However, there are notable exceptions such as colorectal and neuroendocrine. A quarter of patients with colorectal cancer have liver metastases at presentation with a median survival untreated of between 6 and 9 months. Hepatic resection in appropriate candidates, where the primary has been removed, can achieve a 30 to 40% 5-year survival with cure in some patients. The liver remnant must be adequate and disease should be preferably unilobar. The role of adjuvant chemotherapy is unclear, as is whether there is any benefit in synchronous resection of primary and secondary disease. Portal vein embolization of the tumour-affected lobe has become a standard method for increasing the size of the liver remnant to reduce the risk of decompensation. Innovative approaches include down-staging tumour using systemic chemotherapy to within criteria for resection, hepatic arterial infusion of chemotherapy, targeted therapies against EGF receptors, and combining RFA with surgery to preserve liver volume. None of these modalities has been subject to randomized study.

Neuroendocrine tumours typically grow slowly and are therefore amenable to therapy even when multifocal within the liver. Directed therapies such as surgical debulking, embolization, TACE, and ablation have been shown to improve symptoms and slow progression although survival benefit is unproven. Sirolimus, somatostatin analogues, and targeted agents against VEGF activity also appear efficacious. For carcinoid tumour, where the primary has been removed and there is no evidence of extrahepatic disease, survival after liver transplantation approaches 70% at 5 years with recurrence-free survival nearer 50%. Gastrointestinal stromal tumours (GISTs) are also slow-growing and metastasize to the liver—good control can be achieved using a combination of surgical resection and tyrosine kinase inhibitors.

Further reading

Bioulac-Sage P, *et al.* (2009). Hepatocellular adenoma management and phenotypic classification: the Bordeaux experience. *Hepatology*, **50**, 48–9.

Chan JA, Kulke MH (2007). Emerging therapies for the treatment of patients with advanced neuroendocrine tumors. *Expert Opin Emer Drugs*, **12**, 253–70.

El-Serag HB, Rudolph KL (2007). Hepatocellular carcinoma: epidemiology and molecular carcinogenesis. *Gastroenterology*, **132**, 2557–76.

Garrot C, Stuart K (2007). Liver-directed therapies for metastatic neuroendocrine tumours. *Hematol Oncol Clin North Am*, **21**, 545–60.

Ito F, *et al.* (2009). Hilar cholangiocarcinoma: current management. *Ann Surg*, **250**, 210–18.

Khatri VP, *et al.* (2007). Modern multimodality approach to hepatic colorectal metastases: Solutions and controversies. *Surg Oncol*, **16**, 71–83.

Lizardi-Cervera J, *et al.* (2006). Focal nodular hyperplasia and hepatic adenoma: a review. *Ann Hepatol*, **5**, 206–11.

Llovet JM, Bruix J (2003). Systematic review of randomized trials for unresectable hepatocellular carcinoma: Chemoembolization improves survival. *Hepatology*, **37**, 429–42.

Llovet JM, *et al.* (1999). Prognosis of hepatocellular carcinoma: the BCLC staging classification. *Semin Liver Dis*, **19**, 329–38.

Malhi H, Gores GJ (2006). Review article: the modern diagnosis and therapy of cholangiocarcinoma. *Aliment Pharmacol Therapeut*, **23**, 1287–96.

Maluf D, *et al.* (2005). Hepatic angiosarcoma and liver transplantation: case report and literature review. *Transplant Proc*, **37**, 2195–9.

Mazzaferro V, *et al.* (1996). Liver transplantation for treatment of small hepatocellular carcinomas in patients with cirrhosis. *N Engl J Med*, **334**, 693–9.

Mehrabi A, *et al.* (2006). Primary malignant hepatic epithelioid hemangioendothelioma: a comprehensive review of the literature with emphasis on the surgical therapy. *Cancer*, **107**, 2108–21.

Nissen NN, *et al.* (2004). Emerging role of transplantation for primary liver cancers. *Cancer J*, **10**, 88–96.

Pang RW, Poon RT (2007). From molecular biology to targeted therapies for hepatocellular carcinoma: the future is now. *Oncology*, **72**, 30–44.

15.22.7 **Hepatic granulomas**

C.W.N. Spearman, Pauline de la Motte Hall[‡], M.W. Sonderup, and S.J. Saunders

Essentials

Granuloma formation occurs when persistent antigenaemia or poorly degradable antigens, such as chemicals or toxins, provide an ongoing stimulus that results in the focal accumulation of activated lymphocytes and macrophages, with the macrophages undergoing epithelioid transformation.

The diagnosis of granulomatous hepatitis is usually made during the investigation of a systemic illness, often presenting as a pyrexia of unknown origin. Serum liver enzymes are frequently normal, but alkaline phosphatase activity may be elevated. The histomorphology of the granuloma, their distribution in the liver and special stains, e.g. Ziehl–Neelsen for mycobacteria and methenamine silver for fungi, may yield a definite diagnosis.

The causes of hepatic granulomas vary depending on the patient population and country studied. In the developed world most cases are due to sarcoidosis, primary biliary cirrhosis or are drug-induced, whilst infectious causes such as mycobacterial infections, schistosomiasis and AIDS-related infections predominate in the developing world.

Introduction

Granulomas are localized collections of modified macrophages, known as 'epithelioid'cells that have become transformed from a predominantly phagocytic cell to a more secretory cell in response to ingested antigens. The epithelioid cells, which are derived from blood monocytes, have abundant amounts of eosinophilic cytoplasm. Langhans' or foreign body-type giant cells, which form by fusion of the epithelioid cells, are often seen in granulomas. Granulomas are usually surrounded by a rim of mononuclear cells predominantly lymphocytes. Granulomas may be progressively replaced by collagen.

The aetiology of hepatic granulomas varies depending on the patient population and country studied. In the developed world, sarcoidosis, primary biliary cirrhosis, and drug-induced hepatic granulomas probably account for the majority, while infectious causes such as mycobacterial infections, schistosomiasis, and AIDS-related infections predominate in the developing world.

The diagnosis of granulomatous hepatitis is usually made during the investigation of a systemic illness, frequently presenting as pyrexia of unknown origin. However, granulomas are found in 10 to 15% of all liver biopsies and may be an unexpected finding. The histomorphology of the granuloma, their distribution in the liver and special stains, e.g. Ziehl–Neelsen for mycobacteria and a methenamine silver for fungi, may yield a definite diagnosis.

Pathogenesis

Granuloma formation represents a specialized cellular immune-mediated response involving presentation of antigen, either endogenous or exogenous, by activated macrophages to CD4 lymphocytes, which are in turn activated by the secretion of macrophage derived interleukin (IL)-1. The activated CD4 lymphocytes secrete interferon, resulting in the up-regulation of MHC class II molecules on the surface of the activated macrophages. Up-regulation of the HLA DR-positive macrophage and the resulting increased interaction with stimulated CD4 lymphocytes, is accompanied by the increase in IL-2 receptor expression and IL-2 secretion. This results in a clonal increase in the CD4 lymphocytes, leading to the recruitment of B cells which are activated and produce immunoglobulins, antibodies and autoantibodies. Persistent antigenaemia or poorly degradable antigens, such as chemicals or toxins, provide an ongoing stimulus for the cytokine cascade which results in the focal accumulation of activated lymphocytes and macrophages, with the macrophages undergoing epithelioid transformation.

In infections, the microorganisms, together with their by-products, are the sensitizing exogenous antigens, whereas in malignancy or immune complex disease sensitizing endogenous antigens may trigger an interaction between the activated macrophages and lymphocytes.

The characteristic immune response is dependent on whether the foreign particle is intra- or extracellular in origin. Intracellular pathogens generally provoke a Th1 response with the secretion of IFN-γ, IL-2, and IL-12. A Th2 response with the secretion of IL-4, IL-6, and IL-10 is usually associated with extracellular pathogens. The Th1 responses are usually associated with larger and more active granulomas. The cytokines produced by Th1 or Th2 immune responses are responsible for the formation and maintenance of liver granulomas.

Depending on the aetiology of the hepatic granuloma, differences are seen in the above described structural/functional arrangement of the granuloma. The well-studied sarcoid granuloma has a central core of HLA DR-positive macrophages, epithelioid cells, and giant cells with a peripheral rim of CD4 lymphocytes. The macrophages surrounding the central core are distinguishable from those in the centre by their reactivity with the macrophage monoclonal antibody RFD-1 as opposed to RFD-2. CD8 suppressor cells and some CD4 cells may be found at the periphery, but not in the centre of the granuloma. The epithelioid cells in sarcoid granuloma secrete a number of compounds including angiotensin-converting enzyme, lysozyme, glucuronidase, collagenase, elastase, and calcitriol. In AIDS patients with *Mycobacterium avium intracellulare* (MAI) infection, there is a paucity of CD4 lymphocytes in the granulomas, while in the granulomas in *Schistosoma mansoni*, the CD4 cells show increased Th2 cooperation. The granulomas in tuberculoid leprosy contain very few bacilli, whereas bacilli are profuse in lepromatous leprosy.

[‡] It is with regret that we report the death of Professor Pauline de la Motte Hall during the preparation of this edition of the textbook.

Aetiology

The many causes of hepatic granulomas are shown in Table 15.22.7.1. Granulomas are frequently nonspecific in appearance and a clinicopathological correlation is essential for diagnosis. In 10 to 30% of hepatic granulomas, the aetiology remains unknown. However, caseating granulomas are characteristic of mycobacterium tuberculosis; the presence of ova and noncaseating granulomas permit the diagnosis of schistosomiasis; fat droplets are seen in the granuloma (lipogranuloma) that accompanies mineral oil ingestion and fibrin-ring granulomas are highly suggestive of Q fever.

Clinical presentation

Fever (pyrexia of unknown origin) is the most common presenting symptom. The diverse clinical features, which include weight loss, anorexia, fatigue, hepatosplenomegaly, and abdominal pain, depend on the underlying aetiologies. Serum liver enzymes are frequently normal but alkaline phosphatase activity may be elevated. Jaundice is uncommon unless there is bile duct injury e.g. primary biliary cirrhosis (PBC), sarcoidosis or drug-induced bile duct injury.

Infectious causes

Mycobacterium tuberculosis

Tuberculosis is a common cause of hepatic granulomas in the developing world. There may be evidence of pulmonary tuberculosis or of tuberculosis elsewhere, or the patient may present with a pyrexia of unknown origin. Hepatic granulomas are commonly found in miliary tuberculosis, more often than in bone marrow biopsies. Caseation occurs in about one-third of cases and, although characteristic of tuberculosis, is not unique to it, occurring also in candidiasis, histoplasmosis and cryptococcosis. Acid-fast bacilli are seen in 10 to 15% of cases, in 31% of autopsy specimens and therefore the biopsy must always be cultured. More recently, the use of the polymerase chain reaction (PCR), based on amplification of IS6110 insertion sequences, was shown to have a sensitivity of 58% in the diagnosis of hepatic granulomas of definitive tuberculosis origin and a specificity of 96% and is a useful test as it can be performed on paraffin-embedded tissue. BCG vaccination may also cause hepatic granulomas.

HIV/AIDS

The presence of hepatic granulomas is a common finding in a number of biopsy or autopsy series. Most series from North America predate the era of effective antiretroviral therapy. Granulomatous change was the finding in 14 to 40% of HIV-positive patients biopsied for abnormal liver enzymes, hepatomegaly or fever. The most prevalent aetiology was *Mycobacterium avium-intracellulare* followed by *Mycobacterium tuberculosis*, *Histoplasma capsulatum*, and occasionally drugs.

Similarly, biopsy and autopsy series from Thailand, India, and sub-Saharan Africa have demonstrated granulomas in 21 to 41% of HIV-positive patients. The major difference from the developed world is that invariably the aetiology is *Mycobacterium tuberculosis*. The organism can be cultured from liver tissue in approximately one-third of patients and liver biopsy is a useful diagnostic technique.

Table 15.22.7.1 Causes of hepatic granulomas

Infections	
Mycobacteria	Tuberculosis
	Leprosy
Atypical bacteria	Brucella
	Francisella tularense
	Yersinia
	Burkholderia pseudomallei (melioidosis)
Spirochaetes	Treponema
Fungi	Blastomyces
	Candida
	Coccidioides
	Histoplasma
	Cryptococcus
Protozoa	Leishmania
	Toxoplasma
Metazoa	Schistosoma
	Toxocara
	Rickettsia
	Q fever
	Boutonneuse fever
Viruses	Epstein–Barr virus
	Cytomegalovirus
	Hepatitis C virus
Helminths	
Chemicals	Copper
	Talc
	Silica
Immunological or systemic disease	Sarcoidosis
	Inflammatory bowel disease
	Primary biliary cirrhosis
	Immune complexes
	Hepatic granulomatous disease
	AIDS
Enzyme defect	Chronic granulomatous disease of children
Neoplasia	Lymphoma—Hodgkin's disease
	Carcinoma
	Melanoma
Miscellaneous	BCG vaccine
	Cholestasis
	Polymyalgia rheumatica
Drugs	(see Table 15.22.7.2)

All HIV-positive patients who have a liver biopsy should have tissue sent for tuberculosis testing and fungal culture.

A notable histological feature is that tuberculous granulomas in HIV-positive patients may be poorly formed or non-necrotizing. This is not surprising, as HIV-positive patients with tuberculous liver disease often have advanced HIV/AIDS with significant immunosuppression. Acid-fast bacilli may be sparse and careful histological review following appropriate staining is warranted. In addition, up to 20% of HIV-positive patients with granulomatous disease have coexisting liver pathology with steatosis, the most prevalent concomitant pathology observed.

Histoplasmosis, cryptococcosis, toxoplasmosis, and cytomegalovirus may also cause granulomas in AIDS patients. However, an infectious cause is not always found; presumably there are as yet unidentifiable infections.

Drugs, Hodgkin's disease, and non-Hodgkin's lymphoma may also cause hepatic granulomas in AIDS patients.

Leprosy

Millions of people living in the Indian subcontinent have leprosy and it is also common in Africa. Hepatic granulomas are more common in lepromatous leprosy. The diagnosis is usually made from the characteristic skin and peripheral nerve lesions; only occasionally is the physician alerted to the diagnosis by the finding of an otherwise unexplained hepatic granuloma.

Histoplasmosis

Histoplasmosis is an important cause of hepatic granulomas in the United States of America. The fungus may be seen in the granulomas and may be cultured from liver biopsies, blood or bone marrow. The chest radiograph is usually abnormal and diagnosis is confirmed serologically.

Q fever

The patients usually present with a pyrexia of unknown origin or an illness resembling viral hepatitis. The typical granuloma contains inflammatory cells and fat droplets and has a fibrin ring within or at its margin. However, fibrin-ring granulomas may also be seen in cytomegalovirus infection, Hodgkin's disease, leishmaniasis, and drug reactions. e.g. allopurinol.

Schistosomiasis

Schistosoma japonicum and *S. mansoni* infestation occurs commonly in Africa, South America, and eastern Asia. Ova are usually deposited in the portal tracts within the portal vein radicles where a Th2-based granulomatous reaction occurs around the ova. Patients who develop a predominant Th1 cytokine profile eventually develop an obliterative portal venular fibrosis and presinusoidal portal hypertension results with the characteristic 'pipestem' cirrhosis. Common presenting features are hepatomegaly and portal hypertension. Eosinphlilia also occurs.

Hepatitis C virus (HCV)

Sparse noncaseating hepatic granulomas have been described in chronic hepatitis C and in recurrent HCV post-liver transplant. There is controversy whether the presence of hepatic granulomas is predictive of a favourable response to interferon therapy. Interferon-α therapy maybe associated with granuloma formation and may trigger the development of sarcoidosis in susceptible individuals.

Noninfective causes

Sarcoidosis

This is the most common noninfectious cause of hepatic granuloma formation. Although it is thought to be immunologically mediated, the triggering precipitant remains unknown. Hepatic granulomas are found in 60% of liver biopsies performed on patients with sarcoidosis. The granulomas are thought to result from a Th1 response to unknown retained antigens.

Well-formed noncaseating granulomas occur in clusters in the parenchyma and the portal tracts. There may be associated portal fibrosis, which in some patients, progresses though bridging fibrosis to cirrhosis. Other features that are sometimes seen include bile duct damage and loss, which needs to be differentiated from PBC, other causes of ductopaenia, and acute cholangitis associated with bile duct obstruction. Damage to large bile ducts may lead to a clinical picture that resembles primary sclerosing cholangitis. A lobular hepatitis, portal inflammation with interface hepatitis, may also occur. The development of nodular regenerative hyperplasia as well as fibrosis and cirrhosis may be associated with granulomatous phlebitis of the portal and hepatic veins.

Hepatic sarcoidosis is frequently asymptomatic. Although significant hepatomegaly is uncommon, splenomegaly is often present. The liver enzymes may be normal, or there may be elevated alkaline phosphatase and aminotransaminases. Portal hypertension and cholestasis are rare complications occurring in only 1 in 300 European patients, but appear to be more common in the United States of America, and particularly in African American males. Patients may present with intrahepatic cholestasis and later cirrhosis. Differentiation from primary biliary cirrhosis is often difficult. The portal hypertension is presinusoidal and is thought to be due to granulomatous involvement of the portal venous radicals. These patients may present with variceal bleeds in the absence of cirrhosis.

Treatment with steroids often results in the reduction of size of the hepatosplenomegaly and in improvement in liver enzymes. Steroids have little effect on portal hypertension, but together with ursodeoxycholic acid may have some beneficial effects in those patients with intrahepatic cholestasis.

Primary biliary cirrhosis (PBC)

Hepatic granulomas are found in approximately 25 to 50% of patients with PBC. The granulomas are noncaseating and are in close proximity to the septal and interlobular bile ducts. This granulomatous cholangitis leads to bile duct injury and loss and increasing cholestasis. Occasionally, granulomas are seen in the parenchyma. The granulomas are seen in the early stages of PBC. PBC has a female to male ratio of 8:1, tends to present in the fifth decade of life and does not usually have extrahepatic systemic manifestations. Pruritus tends to be marked; clubbing and hepatomegaly are frequent. These clinical features help to differentiate PBC from sarcoidosis. The latter has an equal female to male ratio, occurs in the third and fourth decades of life and frequently has extrahepatic manifestations such as erythema nodosa, uveitis, pulmonary involvement, hilar adenopathy, and abnormalities of calcium metabolism with hypercalcaemia and hypercalciuria. Antimitochondrial antibodies are positive in over 95% of patients with PBC. The serum angiotensin-converting enzyme activity test may be elevated in both conditions. Treatment with long-term ursodeoxycholic acid is associated with histological improvement and reduces the need for liver transplantation.

Neoplasia

Noncaseating hepatic granulomas occur with a variety of neoplasms, including lymphoma and carcinoma. These granulomas may occur in the absence of tumour deposits and may represent an immune response to tumour antigens.

Lymphoma

Hepatic granulomas may occur in both Hodgkin's and non-Hodgkin's lymphoma. Granulomas may mask the infiltrates of malignant lymphoma and in Hodgkin's disease. Immunohistochemistry may demonstrate a clonal lymphocytic population in or around the granulomas associated with lymphoma.

Chronic granulomatous disease of childhood

This is a classical X-linked disorder, presenting usually at about 5 years of age with hepatosplenomegaly, generalized lymphadenopathy, granulomatous skin lesions and diffuse miliary lung infiltration. The neutrophils of children with chronic granulomatous disease are unable to kill ingested bacteria, as they are deficient in those enzymes required for the superoxide respiratory burst. The diagnostic test for this condition is the inability of neutrophils to reduce nitroblue tetrazolium from colourless to blue-black formazan granules in the cytoplasm in the presence of a bacterial infection.

Crohn's disease

Noncaseating granulomas are found in the intestine, perineum and occasionally in the liver. The clinical manifestations are typical of Crohn's disease and diagnosis is not usually problematic.

Hepatic granulomatous disease

Hepatic granulomatous disease is a diagnosis of exclusion. The granulomas are seen in the portal tracts and lobules but there is no evidence of hepatitis. There appear to be two variants: one an acute febrile illness characterized by respiratory symptoms, a high white cell count, and splenomegaly, and the other a more chronic condition presenting more frequently in middle-aged men with recurrent fevers, rigors, sweating, general malaise, and loss of weight. Neuralgia and arthralgia are common and there may be a mild, tender hepatomegaly and liver enzyme abnormalities are nonspecific, including bilirubinaemia, mild elevation of transaminases, and elevated alkaline phosphatase. There is usually a good response to steroid therapy with pyrexia resolving and liver enzymes improving. Aetiology remains uncertain.

Drugs and chemicals

Many drugs can cause granulomatous hepatitis (Table 15.22.7.2). Drug-induced liver injury is frequently due to a hypersensitivity reaction. Although drug reactions may result in eosinophil-rich granulomas, in most cases the granulomas are nonspecific.

Drug-induced hepatic granulomas may be completely asymptomatic or present with features suggestive of a drug allergy with a swinging fever, skin rash, eosinophilia and abnormal liver enzymes. Although the diagnosis of drug-induced granulomatous hepatitis is one of exclusion, drugs should always be considered when granulomas are found in the liver.

Table 15.22.7.2 Drugs and chemicals causing hepatic granulomas

Allopurinol	Glibenclamide	Penicillin
Amiodarone	Gold	Perhexiline
Amoxicillin–clavulinic acid (co-amoxiclav)		Phenylbutazone
Amoxycillin	Halothane	Phenytoin
Ampicillin	Hydralazine	Procainamide
Aspirin		Procarbazine
	Isoniazid	Pyrazinamide
Beryllium		
	Mebendazole	Quinidine
Carbamazepine	Mesalamine	
Carbutamide	Methyldopa	Ranitidine
Cephalexin	Metolazone	Rosiglitazone
Chlorpromazine	Mineral oil	
Chlorpropamide		Salicylazosulphapyridine
Copper salts	Nitrofurantoin	Silica
	Nomifensine	Steroids
Dapsone	Norfloxacin	Sulphonamides
Diazepam		
Diltiazem	Oral contraceptive	Tetrahydroaminoacridine
	Oxacillin	Tocainide
Fenfluramine		Tolbutamide
Flucloxacillin	Papaverine	Trichlormethiazide

Exposure to various chemicals such as beryllium, silica, starch, talc, and suture material has also been associated with the development of hepatic granulomas.

Granulomatous liver disease after liver transplantation

Granulomas are seen in 3 to 9% of biopsies performed in liver transplant patients. The most common causes include cytomegalovirus, hepatitis B virus, HCV, preservation injury, and acute cellular rejection. A granulomatous cholangitis may represent the recurrence of the original disease such as PBC or sarcoidosis. Except for acute rejection or PBC, post liver transplant granulomas are usually seen in the parenchyma. Up to 30% of post liver transplant granulomas are idiopathic, but infectious causes must always be excluded.

Investigation and management

A detailed history including travel and drug/chemical exposure and physical examination is important. The presence of portal hypertension raises the suspicion of schistosomiasis, sarcoidosis, or PBC. In order to obtain the correct diagnosis and determine the appropriate therapy, it is important to always consider the epidemiological background of the patient. In developed countries, the common causes of granulomas in the liver are sarcoidosis, PBC, drugs and neoplasms. In developing countries infectious causes must be considered first, and excluded before considering other causes. However, the global problem of HIV/AIDS may well place mycobacterial and other infections at the forefront of causes of granulomatous hepatitis.

Further reading

Barceno R, et al. (1998). Post-transplant liver granulomatosis associated with hepatitis C. Transplantation, 65, 1494–5.

Denk H, et al. (1994). Guidelines for the diagnosis and interpretation of hepatic granulomas. Histopathology, 25, 209–18.

Devaney K, et al. (1993). Hepatic sarcoidosis. Clinicopathologic features in 100 patients. Am J Surg Pathol, 17, 1272–80.

Diaz ML, et al. (1996). Polymerase chain reaction for the detection of Mycobacterium tuberculosis DNA in tissue and assessment of its utility in the diagnosis of hepatic granulomas. J Lab Clin Med, 127, 359–63.

Emile JF, et al. (1993). The presence of epithelioid granulomas in hepatitis C virus-related cirrhosis. Hum Pathol, 24, 1095–7.

Farrell GC (1995). Drug-induced granulomatous hepatitis. In: Drug-induced liver disease, Chapter 13, pp. 301–17. Churchill Livingstone, Edinburgh.

Goldin RD, et al. (1996). Granulomas and hepatitis C. Histopathology, 28, 265–7.

Ishak KG (1998). Sarcoidosis of the liver and bile ducts. Mayo Clin Proc, 73, 467–72.

Lanjewar DN, et al. (2004). Hepatic pathology in AIDS: a pathological study from Mumbai, India. HIV Med, 5, 253–7.

Lee RG, et al. (1981). Granulomas in primary biliary cirrhosis: a prognostic feature. Gastroenterology, 81, 983–6.

Lefkowitch JH (1999). Hepatic granulomas. J Hepatol, 30, 40–5.

Matheus T, Muñoz S (2004). Granulomatous liver disease and cholestasis. Clin Liver Dis, 8, 229–46.

O'Connell MJ, et al. (1975). Epithelioid granulomas in Hodgkin's disease: a favorable prognostic sign. JAMA, 233, 886–9.

Poles MA, et al. (1996). Liver biopsy findings in 501 patients infected with HIV. J AIDS Hum Retrovirol, 11, 170–7.

Simon HB, Wolff SM (1973). Granulomatous hepatitis and prolonged fever of unknown origin: a study of 13 patients. Medicine (Baltimore), 52, 1–20.

15.22.8 Drugs and liver damage

J. Neuberger

Essentials

Drug-induced liver injury is relatively uncommon but can very rarely be fatal. Almost all patterns of liver disease can be induced by drugs, and some drugs may be associated with more than one type of reaction. Most cases present with jaundice and hepatitis.

Good data on incidence are hard to find. The diagnosis of drug-induced liver damage is largely circumstantial and by exclusion of other causes of liver disease, and many cases are not reported to regulatory or monitoring bodies. The more common culprits are antibiotics (especially amoxicillin/clavulanate, flucloxacillin) and nonsteroidal anti-inflammatory drugs (especially diclofenac);

chlorpromazine and isoniazid are both associated with a high incidence of liver injury; recognized causes of fatal liver injury are halothane, perhexiline and erythromycin.

Withdrawal of the drug will usually lead to resolution of the liver damage, but liver damage sometimes progresses despite this, particularly if there is cholestatic hepatitis and with amoxicillin/clavulanate, atorvastatin, captopril, and bentazepam.

Introduction

Drug-induced liver injury (DILI) is relatively uncommon, but unless it is recognized early and the drug discontinued it may cause death. Adverse drug reactions are responsible for up to 3% of all hospital admissions. Reliable data are difficult to come by: a relatively recent study has shown that in 1986 to 1987 about 1600 cases/year of adverse drug reactions were reported in England. Hepatic reactions accounted for 3.5% of which 7% were fatal. Similar figures were found in New Zealand. A total of 205 drugs were associated with 943 reports of adverse liver injury between 1974 and 1994: 20 drugs accounted for nearly 60% of reports. Most reactions are of jaundice and hepatitis; the more common are due to antibiotics and nonsteroidal anti-inflammatory drugs. Halothane, perhexiline, and erythromycin were common causes of death and diclofenac, augmentin, and flucloxacillin were the most important causes of liver damage. In Denmark, it was estimated that drug-induced liver injury accounts for between 1 in 600 and 1 in 3500 hospital admissions, amounting to 2 to 3% of all hospital admissions due to adverse reactions and about 3% of all jaundiced patients. In general practice, the spectrum of liver damage is slightly different: drugs associated with a high incidence of acute liver injury (>100/100 000 users) were chlorpromazine and isoniazid; drugs with intermediate incidence of acute liver damage (>10/100 000 users) were amoxicillin/clavulanic acid and cimetidine. More recently, the top 10 drugs or classes of drugs associated with either jaundice or hepatitis referred to the West Midlands Committee for Safety of Medicine in the United Kingdom were amiodarone, terbinafine, atorvastatin, paroxetine, lansoprazole, simvastatin, hepatitis A vaccine, minocycline, omeprazole, and carbamazepine. Currently, interest has focused on DILI associated with antiretroviral agents, some herbal remedies, statins, and thiazolidinediones.

It is important to put drug-induced liver damage into appropriate context and toxicity has to be balanced against efficacy: many potentially hepatotoxic drugs are withdrawn before coming to market and only a few (such as troglitazone) are withdrawn afterwards: indeed, to detect reliably an adverse drug reaction affecting the liver at a rate of 1:10 000, 30 000 patients would need to be studied. With the advent of transcriptomics and proteomics, the understanding of the mechanisms of toxicity is becoming increasingly better understood and so the risk of hepatotoxicity may be reduced.

Drug-induced liver damage may be caused by agents not considered as conventional drugs, such as herbal remedies (e.g. kava kava and celandine), and by 'recreational drugs' such as ecstasy (methylene dioxymethamphetamine, MDMA) and cocaine (see Box 15.22.8.1). The wide regional and individual variation in reporting rates and failure to report reactions after deliberate overdose combine to underestimate the frequency and severity of

Box 15.22.8.1   The 'rules' of drug-induced liver disease

- Assume that all drugs may cause liver damage
- All patterns of liver damage have been associated with drug toxicity
- Some drugs may cause more than one pattern of liver damage
- Always take a full drug history
- Ask about other drugs—including herbal remedies, recreational drugs, vitamins
- The diagnosis of an adverse drug reaction is one of exclusion and temporal relationship
- Drug withdrawal is not always associated with improvement in liver function
- Reports of drug-associated liver damage do not necessarily mean causality
- Clinical challenge is rarely justified, may be fatal, and may be misleading

Table 15.22.8.1 Patterns of adverse hepatic drug reactions

Adverse reaction	Drug
Hepatitis	
Fulminant	Paracetamol
Acute	Amoxycillin/clavinulate, NSAIDs
Subacute	
Chronic	Methyldopa, nitrofurantoin
Cholestatic	Phenothiazines
Granulomatous	Phenytoin
Autoimmune	Minocycline, terbinafine
Cirrhosis	
Cholestasis	
Bland	Anabolic steroids, oestrogens
Vanishing bile duct syndrome	Chlorpromazine, penicillins
Sclerosing cholangitis	Floxuridine
Granulomas	Sulphonamides
Steatosis	
Macrovesicular	Amiodarone
Microvesicular	Valproic acid
Tumours	
Adenoma	Oestrogens
Carcinoma	Oestrogens, androgens
Angiosarcoma	Arsenicals, thorium dioxide
Cholangiocarcinoma	Thorium dioxide
Vascular lesions	
Peliosis	Oestrogens
Budd–Chiari syndrome	Oestrogens
Veno-occlusive disease	Azathioprine
Fibrosis	Vitamin A, arsenicals

adverse drug reactions. Most adverse drug reactions are not fatal, and withdrawal of the drug will usually lead to resolution of the liver damage. However, sometimes liver damage progresses despite withdrawal of the drug: those with cholestatic hepatitis and those with hepatotoxicity associated with drugs for cardiovascular disease and those affecting the central nervous system seem to be implicated most commonly (especially amoxicillin/clavulanate, atorvastatin, captopril, and bentazepam)

Almost all patterns of liver disease can be induced by drugs (Table 15.22.8.1) and some drugs may be associated with more than one type of reaction. For example, oral contraceptives are associated not only with the development of cholestasis but also with adenoma, hepatocellular carcinoma, peliosis hepatis, and Budd–Chiari syndrome. It is important therefore to consider the possible contribution of drugs in a patient with any type of hepatic abnormality.

The diagnosis of drug-induced liver damage is largely circumstantial and by exclusion of other causes of liver disease. It must be remembered that the reporting of an associated drug reaction does not prove causality. The temporal association between the onset of damage and timing of drug exposure, and the response to drug withdrawal (Table 15.22.8.2) and the known patterns of drug reaction all help in establishing a drug as the cause of liver damage. Rarely, the presence of specific serological markers may help confirm the association between the drug and liver damage. For example, an antibody to tifluoroaceylated proteins is found in halothane-associated hepatitis, and anti liver–kidney microsomal antibodies occur in tienilic acid-associated hepatitis. Use of a clinical challenge is rarely justified, may be misleading, and may prove fatal.

Acute hepatitis

The severity of liver cell necrosis associated with drugs varies from a mild elevation of serum transaminases without symptoms to fulminant hepatic failure. Many drugs have been associated with acute liver failure (Table 15.22.8.3). Clinically, the picture may be indistinguishable from that of viral hepatitis. Occasionally, right upper quadrant pain may be so severe as to lead to the mistaken diagnosis of acute cholecystitis. The serological changes are those of acute hepatitis with initial elevations of serum aminotransferases. Prolongation of the prothrombin time and jaundice may occur in more severe cases. Histologically, the appearances vary from a mild focal necrosis to massive liver cell damage. In some cases, e.g. paracetamol, the damage is predominantly centrilobular, whereas in others, e.g. α-methyldopa, the whole lobule is affected. Steatosis, granulomas, and eosinophilia are variable features. The most common causes of drug-associated fulminant hepatic failure are paracetamol overdose and halothane hepatitis. Liver failure may also be associated with 'recreational' drugs.

The development of abnormalities of liver tests during prolonged drug use poses particular problems, e.g. with antituberculous therapy. Derangement of serum aminotransferases occurs in approximately 10% of patients and, if the noxious drug is continued, up to l0% of these develop severe hepatic necrosis. Identification of those patients who will develop severe hepatic failure is difficult, and the clinician has to decide whether the risks of continuing therapy outweigh the potential benefits. Drugs such

Table 15.22.8.2 Criteria for defining adverse drug reactions

Drug reaction	Suggestive compatible		Incompatible		From cessation
	From onset	From onset	From cessation	From onset	
Hepatitis					
Initial exposure	5–90 days	<5 or >90 days	<15 days	Drug started after onset	>15 days
Subsequent exposure	1–15 days	>15 days	<15 days	Drug started after onset	>15 days
Cholestasis					
Initial exposure	5–90 days	>5 days	<1 month	Drug started after onset	>1 month
Subsequent exposure	1–90 days	>90 days	<1 month	Drug started after onset	

(From Danan O (1990). Consensus meeting. Criteria of drug induced liver disorders. *J Hepatol*, **11**, 272–6.)

Table 15.22.8.3 Drugs associated with hepatocellular necrosis

Area of drug use	Drug
Anaesthesia	Chloroform
	Cyclopropane
	Desflurane
	Enflurane
	Ethyl ether
	Fluroxene
	Halothane
	Isoflurane
	Methoxyflurane
	Trichloroethylene
	Vinyl ether
Antineoplastic disorders	Carmustine
	Chlorozotocin
	Cyclophosphamide
	Cytarabine
	Dacarbazine
	Flutamide
	Hydroxycarbamide
	Mithramycin
	Procarbazine
	Streptozotocin
	Vincristine
Cardiovascular disease	Captopril
	Coumarins
	Enalapril
	Ezetimibe
	Frusemide
	HMG Co-A reductase

Table 15.22.8.3 (*Cont'd*) Drugs associated with hepatocellular necrosis

Area of drug use	Drug
	Hydralazine
	Lisinopril
	Methyldopa
	Metoprolol
	Nicotinic acid
	Nifedepine
	Papavarine
	Quinidine
	Verapamil
Endocrine disorders	Acetohexamide
	Carbutamide
	Flutamide
	Metahexamide
	Propylthiouracil
	Troglitazone
Gastroenterological disorders	Chenodeoxycholic acid
	Ebrotidine
	Omeprazole
	Salazopyrine
Herbal remedies	Chinese herbal tea
	Germander
	Mistletoe
	Pennyroyal oil
Infectious disorders	Amiodaquine
	p-Aminosalicylic acid
	Carbenicillin
	Ciprofloxacillin
	Clindamycin

(Continued)

Table 15.22.8.3 (*Cont'd*) Drugs associated with hepatocellular necrosis

Area of drug use	Drug
	Cotrimoxazole
	Dapsone
	Dideoxyinosine
	Erythromycin
	Fluconazole
	Fusidic acid
	Hycanthone
	Isoniazid
	Ketoconazole
	Levamisole
	Mebendazole
	Mepacrine
	Minocycline
	Nevirapine
	Oxacillin
	Piperazine
	Ritonavir
	Sulphonamides
	Telithromycin
	Zidovudine
Neuropsychiatric disorders	Amitriptyline
	Bromocryptine
	Carbamazepine
	Dantrolene
	Desipramine
	Disulphiram
	Ferpexide
	Feltamate
	Imipramine
	Iproniazid
	Isaxonine
	Lergotrile
	Levodopa
	Loxapine
	Methylphenidate
	Nomifensine
	Oxapozin

Table 15.22.8.3 (*Cont'd*) Drugs associated with hepatocellular necrosis

Area of drug use	Drug
	Pemoline
	Pergomide
	Phenacetamide
	Phenelzine
	Pheniprazine
	Phenoxyproperazine
	Phenytoin
	Phethenylate
	Valproate
	Viloxazine
Nutritional and metabolic diseases	Clofibrate
	Fenofibrate
	Gemfibrozil
	Nicotinamide
Others	Ampfetamine
	Cocaine
	MDMA ('ecstasy')a
Radiological examinations	Iodapamide
	Iopanoic acid
Rheumatic and musculoskeletal disorders	Allopurinol
	Aspirin
	Baclofen
	Benorylate
	Benoxaprofen
	Clomacetin
	Dantrolene
	Glafenine
	Nimesulide
	Paracetamol
	Piroxicates
	Salicylates
Skin diseases	Elretinate
	Methoxsalen
	Povidone-iodine
	Tannic acid

a Methylenedioxymethamphetamine.

Table 15.22.8.4 Patterns of acute hepatitis associated with drugs

Type	Onset	Reaction on re-exposure	Dose dependent	Reproducible in animals	Hypersensitivity features
Predictable	Rapid	Rapid	++	+	−
Idiosyncratic					
Metabolic	Variable	Delayed	±	−	−
Immune mediated	Variable	Rapid	−	−	+

as heparin are commonly associated with abnormal liver enzymes but very rarely with liver disease. The reason is not known but it may be due to loss of a few sensitive hepatocytes or to adaptation.

Conventionally, hepatic drug reactions are classified into predictable and idiosyncratic (Table 15.22.8.4). Predictable reactions are dose dependent, i.e. the greater the amount of drug ingested, the greater the probability of developing liver damage. Because animal models can usually be developed, screening will detect many of these drug reactions and the drug withdrawn before reaching the market. Hence this type of drug reaction is relatively uncommon, except in overdose. The classic example is paracetamol toxicity, which is described in detail in Chapter 9.1. None the less, there may exist great variability between individuals in the probability of developing predictable drug reactions.

With very few exceptions, drugs require metabolism before cytotoxicity develops. Variations in susceptibility may, therefore, be a consequence of genetic variations in drug metabolism. Well-recognized genetic polymorphisms include variations in the cytochrome P450 isoenzymes, drug oxidation, acetylation, and hydroxylation. Adverse drug reactions have been associated with genetic polymorphisms in a variety of enzymes, including manganese superoxide dismutase, glutathione S-transferase, and quinone oxireductase. Thus deficiency of CYP2D6 is associated with perhexiliene hepatotoxicity and CYP2C19 with troglitazone; slow acetylation of N-acetyl-transferase (NAT2) is associated with isoniazid and sulphonamide DILI. HLA status may also be associated with heptatotoxicty (DRB*1501 with amoxicillin and DR3, DR4, DR7 with statin toxicity).

Age, too, is associated with differences in susceptibility to toxicity. In general, younger children metabolize drugs differently from adults. Those taking enzyme inducers such as alcohol, rifampicin, or phenobarbital are at a greater risk of increased metabolism of the drug and hence of forming toxic metabolites. Those with reduced glutathione stores, e.g. due to fasting, malnutrition, or associated disease, may be at greater risk of developing paracetamol toxicity because detoxification mechanisms are impaired. Other factors determining susceptibility include ethnicity, smoking, and coexisting diseases; e.g. methotrexate toxicity is more common in individuals with diabetes. Finally, liver disease itself may alter susceptibilities to drug toxicity. However, because of potential alterations in absorption, volume of distribution, protein binding, detoxification, and excretion it is difficult to predict the effect of disease on susceptibility to drug toxicity. Many drugs induce hepatitis by apoptosis which may be accompanied by simultaneous or secondary necrosis.

In contrast, idiosyncratic drug reactions are dose independent and may be due either to metabolic idiosyncrasy or to the involvement of immune mechanisms. Immune involvement rather than metabolic idiosyncrasy is suggested by a rapid onset after subsequent exposure and the appearance of markers such as peripheral and intrahepatic eosinophilia, granulomas, circulating immune complexes, autoantibodies, and other autoimmune phenomena, e.g. haemolytic anaemia. Two drugs in particular have been well studied with respect to immune-mediated hepatitis—halothane (no longer in common use) and tienilic acid (now withdrawn from the market). Halothane hepatitis occurs rarely and after multiple exposures. Risk factors include female sex, obesity, and repeated or subsequent exposure within 3 months. Immune involvement is suggested by an increased incidence of organ non-specific autoantibodies, peripheral eosinophilia, and circulating immune complexes, and the presence of antibodies reacting with a variety of halothane-associated liver cell macromolecules. In other examples, antibodies to drug-metabolizing enzymes are present in serum. Tienilic acid-associated hepatitis is associated with a circulating liver–kidney microsomal antibody that reacts with the cytochrome P450 enzyme CYP 2C9, associated with metabolism of the drug; antibodies to CYP 1A2 are associated with hydralazine and disulfiram hepatitis; alcohol and halothane hepatitis are associated with antibodies to CYP 2E1. Iproniazid hepatitis is associated with antibodies to MAO-B. Whether these antibodies are involved in the pathogenesis of the disease remains uncertain.

Cross-reaction between two drugs may occur. Thus, halothane sensitization may predispose to toxicity from other halogenated hydrocarbon anaesthetic agents such as isoflurane. This may be due to the two drugs inducing similar antigenic determinants, leading to cross-sensitization, or to a different mechanism of toxicity, as suggested for captopril and enalapril hepatotoxicity, where a similar metabolic pathway of toxicity has been postulated.

Statins

Mild and asymptomatic elevation of serum aminotransferase concentration is often seen in patients taking statins, especially during the first 3 months. Levels often settle despite continuation of therapy. Greater elevations can occur in about 0.5%. Acute liver failure and autoimmune hepatitis have both been described in patients receiving statins but are rare. There is no significant differences between the different statins with respect to DILI. Whether patients receiving statin therapy need monitoring of liver tests is uncertain.

Thiazolidinediones

Troglitazone was withdrawn from use because of cases of acute liver failure. There have been isolated reports of hepatitis associated with both rosiglitazone and pioglitazone.

Antiretroviral agents

Hepatitis and acute liver failure are associated with all three classes of antiretroviral agents: protease inhibitors, nucleoside and non-nucleoside reverse transcriptase inhibitors (NRI and NNRI). Of the protease inhibitors, ritonavir is most commonly associated with hepatitis and may be more common in those with concurrent infection with either hepatitis B or C virus. Of the NNRIs, nevirapine is most frequently associated with hepatitis.

Acute cholestatic hepatitis

Acute cholestatic hepatitis is characterized by jaundice, pruritus, pale stools, and dark urine. There are usually few clinical findings, although the liver may be enlarged. Serologically, in the early stages there is elevation of the serum alkaline phosphatase and γ-glutamyl transpeptidase; as the disease progresses, hepatocellular enzymes start to rise. Histologically, the liver shows dilated sinusoids with cholestasis often predominating in the centrilobular region. There may be an associated portal inflammation and liver cell necrosis. In the majority of cases there is rapid resolution following withdrawal of the drug, although with chlorpromazine and other phenothiazines the cholestasis may take up to 1 to 2 years to resolve. Many drugs cause a mixed hepatitis, where there are features of both cholestasis and liver cell damage (Table 15.22.8.5).

Table 15.22.8.5 Drugs associated with cholestatic hepatitis

Area of drug use	Drug
Cancer	Aminoglutethimide
	Arabinoside
	Azathioprine
	Chlorambucil
	Chlorotozotocin
	Cisplatin
	Cytosin
	Mitomycin
	Streptozotocin
Cardiovascular disease	Ajmaline
	Captopril
	Diltiazem
	Disopyramide
	Flecanide
	Hydrallazine
	Methyldopa
	Mexilitine
	Nifedepine
	Phenindione
	Prajmaline
	Procaineamide
	Propafenone
	Quinine

Table 15.22.8.5 (*Cont'd*) Drugs associated with cholestatic hepatitis

Area of drug use	Drug
	Spironolactone
	Ticlopidine
	Verapamil
	Warfarin
Endocrine disease	Acetohexamide
	Carbimazole
	Chlorpropamide
	Glibenclamide
	Metahexamide
	Methimazole
	Propylthiouracil
	Tamoxifen
	Thiouracil
	Tolbutamide
Gastroenterological disorders	Cimetidine
	Ranitidine
Infectious and parasitic disease	p-Aminosalacylic acid
	Arsphenamine
	Cefalexin
	Chloramphenicol
	Claxacillin
	Clindamycin
	Cotrimoxazole
	Erythromycin
	Griseofulvin
	Nalidixic acid
	Nitrofurantoin
	Quinine
	Rifampicin
	Sulphadiazine
	Sulphonamides
	Tiabendazole
	Troleandomycin
	Tryparsamide
Neuropsychiatric disease	Amitryptaline
	Bromocryptine
	Carbamazepine
	Chlordiazepoxide
	Chlorpromazine

(Continued)

Table 15.22.8.5 (*Cont'd*) Drugs associated with cholestatic hepatitis

Area of drug use	Drug
	Desipramine
	Diazepam
	Fluphenazine
	Flurazepam
	Haloperidol
	Imipramine
	Iprindole
	Mianserin
	Phenobarbital
	Phenytoin
	Prochlorperazine
	Promazine
	Thioridizine
	Triazolam
	Trifluoperazine
	Zimeldine
Rheumatic and musculoskeletal diseases	Allopurinol
	Baclofen
	Colchicine
	Diclofenac
	Diflunisal
	Fenbrufen
	Feprazon
	Flurbiprofen
	Gold salts
	Ibfenac
	Ibuprofen
	Indomethacin
	Kebuzone
	Naproxen
	Oxyphenbutazone
	Penicillamine
	Phenopyrazone
	Phenylbutazone
	Piroxicam
	Probenacid

Table 15.22.8.5 (*Cont'd*) Drugs associated with cholestatic hepatitis

Area of drug use	Drug
	Propoxyphene
	Proquazone
	Sulindac
	Zoxazolamine
Skin disease	Isoretanoin

Bland cholestasis

Bland cholestasis is characterized by cholestasis in the absence of hepatitis and is due to specific interference with bile secretion. The two main groups of drugs associated with this condition are oral contraceptives and oestrogens, and anabolic steroids. Cholestasis occurs in women taking oral contraceptives and in pregnancy. Prevalence varies, being low in southern Europe and North America (1 in 10 000) and high (1 in 4000) in parts of Chile and Scandinavia. Cholestasis associated with anabolic and contraceptive steroids is well recognized and may occur in association with virtually all the anabolic steroids with a C17 group; these drugs include norethandrolone, oxymethalone, danazol, stanozalol, and methyltestosterone. Indinavir and atazanabir are also associated with cholestasis, especially in those who are homozygous for UGT1A1*28 (associated with Gilbert's syndrome). Other drugs are listed in Table 15.22.8.6. In some cases, drug-induced cholestasis leads to a progressive 'vanishing bile duct' syndrome.

Treatment is symptomatic: the itching may be intense and sometimes responds to colestyramine or colestipol; other therapies include antihistamines, ursodeoxycholic acid, rifampicin, androgenic anabolic steroids, and opiate receptor antagonists.

Table 15.22.8.6 Drugs associated with acute cholestasis

Class of drug/area of drug use	Drug
Anticancer drugs	Azathioprine
	Busulfan
	Chlorambucil
	Cytarabine
Anticonvulsants	Carbamazepine
	Phenobarbitone
	Phenytoin
Anti-inflammatory and analgesic agent	Benoxaprofen
	Dextropropoxyphene
	Diflunisal
	Gold
	Naproxen
	Nimesulide

(Continued)

Table 15.22.8.6 (*Cont'd*) Drugs associated with acute cholestasis

Class of drug/area of drug use	Drug
	Penicillamine
	Phenylbutazone
	Piroxicam
Antimicrobials	Amoxicillin/clavulinic acid
	Cephalosporins
	Co-trimoxazole
	Erythromycin
	Flucloxacillin
	Griseofulvin
	Ketoconazole
	Nitrofurantoin
	Penicillins
	Rifampicin
	Sulphones
	Thiobendazole
	Trimethoprim
Antithyroid drugs	Carbimazole
	Methimazole
	Thiouracil
Cardiovascular drugs	Ajmaline
	Captopril
	Chlorthalidone
	Disopyramide
	Hydralazine
	Nifedepine
	Thiazides
	Verapamil
Cytokines	Interleukin-2
	Tumour necrosis factor
Other	Ciclosporin A
	Warfarin
Psychiatric disease	Amitryptiline
	Chlordiazepoxide
	Chlorpromazine
	Flurazepam
	Haloperidol
	Imipramine
	Nomifensine
	Thioridizine
	Prochlorperazine
	Resperidone

Table 15.22.8.6 (*Cont'd*) Drugs associated with acute cholestasis

Class of drug/area of drug use	Drug
	Quetiapine
	Zemeldene
Steroids	Aminoglutethemide
	Anabolic steroids (C17)
	Danazol
	Stanozolol
	Tamoxifen

Steatosis

Steatosis may be micro- or macrovesicular. Differentiation is important because the clinical features and outcomes are different. (Table 15.22.8.7).

Microvesicular steatosis

In microvesicular steatosis, the fat is distributed in small lipid droplets and the hepatocellular nucleus is not displaced. There may be an associated hepatitis. Extensive microvesicular steatosis, even in the absence of liver cell necrosis, may lead to a serious clinical syndrome with haemorrhage, syncope, hypotension, lethargy, coma, and hypoglycaemia. In some cases, renal failure and pancreatic inflammation may occur. Biochemically, serum aminotransferases and bilirubin are not greatly increased, although the prothrombin time may be greatly prolonged. Microvesicular steatosis is thought to be related to drug inhibition of mitochondrial oxidation of fatty acids.

Macrovesicular steatosis

In contrast, macrovesicular steatosis is usually far less serious. The hepatocyte contains a large droplet of fat, which displaces the nucleus to the periphery. Liver tests are usually only minimally

Table 15.22.8.7 Drugs associated with steatosis

Type of steatosis	Drug
Microvesicular	Amineptine
	Aureomycin
	Bleomycin
	Cisplatin
	Mitomycin C
	Pirprofen
	Tetracycline
	Valproate
Macrovesicular	Asparaginase
	Glucocorticosteroids
	Methotrexate
	6-Mercaptopurine

deranged. Damage is thought to be related to impaired release of lipids from liver cells.

Granulomatous hepatitis

The spectrum of granulomatous hepatitis varies from an asymptomatic finding to a systemic illness characterized by generalized aches and pains, pruritus, jaundice, and hepatomegaly. Serologically. the main abnormality is an increase in serum alkaline phosphatase. Histologically the liver is infiltrated by granulomas— small, rounded foci of epithelioid cells with multinucleated giant cells. Drugs associated with granulomatous hepatitis are listed in Table 15.22.8.8.

Table 15.22.8.8 Drugs associated with hepatic granulomas

Area of drug use	Drug
Antineoplastic	Procarbazine
Cardiovascular	Amiodarone
	Diltiazem
	Hydralazine
	Methyldopa
	Procaineamide
	Quinidine
	Quinine
	Tocainade
Endocrine	Chlorpropamide
	Glibenclamide
	Tolbutamide
Gastroenterological	Ranitine
	Sulphasalazine
Infectious disease	Amoxicillin/clavulinic acid
	Cephalexin
	Dapsone
	Isoniazid
	Nitrofurantoin
	Oxacillin
	Penicillin
	Sulphonamides
Neuropsychiatric disease	Carbamazepine
	Chlorpromazine
	Diazepam
	Nomifensine
Rheumatological	Allopurinol
	Aspirin
	Gold
	Oxyphenbutazone
	Phenylbutazone

Phospholipidosis

Phospholipidosis is characterized by the accumulation of phospholipids in liver cell lysosomes. The major drugs associated with this form of liver damage, perhexiline and amiodarone, are cationic, amphiphilic compounds that accumulate within the liver cell lysosomes where they form complexes with phospholipids. Accumulation can be detected by immunohistochemistry or electron microscopy. The compounds are stored in these complexes and may be released very slowly, even after ingestion has stopped. The extent to which these complexes accumulate in patients without toxicity remains uncertain.

Nonalcohol steatotic hepatitis

Long-term treatment with perhexiline and amiodarone may be associated with a syndrome that is clinically and histologically identical to alcoholic hepatitis. The disease develops insidiously and is characterized by hepatomegaly, jaundice, ascites, and encephalopathy. Other drugs implicated in this syndrome include diltiazem and nifedipine.

Fibrotic and vascular disease (Table 15.22.8.9)

Perisinusoidal fibrosis

Perisinusoidal fibrosis is characterized by accumulation of collagen within the space of Disse. This may be asymptomatic or lead to hepatomegaly and portal hypertension. The most common causes of perisinusoidal fibrosis due to drugs are large doses of vitamin A given for prolonged periods, or methotrexate. Liver damage may be associated with alopecia. Characteristically the liver shows hyperplasia of the Ito cell as a consequence of vitamin A accumulation. Serum concentrations of vitamin A may he normal, even in the presence of marked liver damage. Patients with a high intake of alcohol are at greater risk of fibrosis.

Peliosis hepatis

Peliosis hepatis is a histological diagnosis and is characterized by blood-filled cavities, bordered by hepatocytes, which may be distributed throughout the liver. Originally described in association with tuberculosis, it is now appreciated that peliosis hepatis may be drug induced and is often asymptomatic. The major drugs involved are the anabolic steroids, androgenic steroids, azathioprine, vinyl chloride, and pyrizolide derivatives.

Hepatic venous damage

Obstruction of the large hepatic veins results in the Budd–Chiari syndrome, characterized by the onset of abdominal pain and ascites, often with diarrhoea. In the acute form the patient may develop liver failure. Most cases of Budd–Chiari syndrome are due to myeloproliferative disorders, either clinically apparent or latent, but it may be associated with the use of oral contraceptives and some antineoplastic drugs such as dacarbazine, doxorubicin, and cyclophosphamide.

Obstruction of the small veins leads to hepatic veno-occlusive disease, characterized by nonthrombotic, concentric narrowing of the small centrilobular veins. Clinical presentation is often chronic but rarely may be acute. Veno-occlusive disease was initially described

Table 15.22.8.9 Drug-related vascular diseases of the liver

Vascular disorder	Drug
Budd–Chiari syndrome	Actinomycin
	Dacarbazine
	Oral contraceptives
Nodular regenerative hyperplasia	Azathioprine
	Busulfan
Perisinusoidal fibrosis	Arsenicals
	Azathioprine
	Mercaptopurine
	Methotrexate
	Vitamin A excess
Veno-occlusive disease	Actinomycin D
	Azathioprine
	Busulfan
	Cyclophosphamide
	Mercaptopurine
	Herbal remedies comfrey, ilex plants, Chinese medicinal teasa
	Mitomycin
	Pyrrolizidine alkaloids
	Thioguanine
	Vincristine

a May be due to pyrrolizidine alkaloids.

in association with ingestion of the pyrrolizidine alkaloids present in plants of the genus *Senecio*, but may be seen in patients treated with immunosuppressives, especially with organ transplantation.

Hepatic tumours

Hepatic tumours may be benign or malignant (Table 15.22.8.10). Hepatocellular adenoma has been associated with the use of oral contraceptives and anabolic steroids. These tumours have a potential for malignant transformation. Usually withdrawal of the steroid results in a reduction in the size of the tumour.

In contrast, hepatocellular carcinoma is also associated with the anabolic and androgenic steroids, oral contraceptives, and thorium dioxide. Although the risk of malignancy increases with

Table 15.22.8.10 Malignant liver tumours associated with drugs

Type of tumour	Drug
Angiosarcoma	Anabolic/androgenic steroids
	Arsenicals
	Thorium dioxide
Cholangiocarcinoma	Thorium dioxide
Hepatocellular carcinoma	Anabolic/androgenic steroids
	Oral contraceptives
	Thorium dioxide

the prolonged use of oral contraceptives, up to eightfold after 8 years, it must be emphasized that the overall risk of developing hepatocellular carcinoma with oral contraceptives is extremely small, and must be balanced against their beneficial, therapeutic effects. Angiosarcomas and cholangiosarcomas may also be related to drugs, although the association is less clear-cut.

Chronic disease

Cirrhosis and chronic hepatitis

Some drugs are associated with chronic liver disease. It may be that the initial lesions develop subclinically and that only prolonged use of the drug will result in cirrhosis. Rarely, a short-term exposure to a drug results in chronic liver disease. In some instances, there is a syndrome resembling autoimmune hepatitis: although corticosteroids may be given, withdrawal of the drug usually leads to resolution of the hepatic inflammation. Some of the drugs associated with the development of cirrhosis and chronic hepatitis are listed in Table 15.22.8.11.

Intrahepatic chronic cholestasis

In some instances of drug-related cholestasis, jaundice or cholestatic liver tests persist for 6 months or more (Table 15.22.8.12). In these cases it is important to exclude other causes of cholestatic disease, such as primary biliary cirrhosis or primary sclerosing cholangitis, which may have been brought to light by drug-induced disorders. However, some drugs may be associated with a chronic vanishing bile duct syndrome, which may be indistinguishable from primary biliary cirrhosis. A syndrome virtually identical to primary sclerosing cholangitis can be induced by infusion into the hepatic artery of floxuridine for the treatment of intrahepatic malignancy. Sclerosing cholangitis may develop several months after starting chemotherapy. The outcome is variable. A vanishing bile duct syndrome has been associated with carbamazepine, thiobendazole, flucloxacillin, haloperidol, ajmaline, cyproheptidine,

Table 15.22.8.11 Commoner drugs associated with subacute and chronic hepatitis and cirrhosis

Acetohexamide	Isoniazid[a]
Amiodarone	Methotrexate
Amodiaquine	Methyldopa[a]
Aspirin	Minocycline[a]
Benzarone	Nicotinic acid
Busulfan	Nitrofurantoin[a]
Chlorambucil	Oxyphenisatin[a]
Cimetidine	Perhexiline
Clometacin[a]	Propylthiouracil
Dantrolene	Sulphonamides[a]
Doxorubicin[a]	Tienilic acid[a]
Diclofenac[a]	Urethane
Etridonate[a]	Valproate
Iproniazid	Vitamin A (excess)

a May also be associated with autoimmune hepatitis.

Table 15.22.8.12 Drugs associated with chronic cholestasis

Phenothiazines	
Tricyclic antidepressants	
Sex steroids	
Sulphonylureas	
Penicillins	
Others	Arsenicals
	Cyproheptidine
	Haloperidol
	Thiobendazole
	Troleandomycin
	Piroxicam

and chlorpromazine. There has been a suggestion that primary biliary cirrhosis is associated with the use of benoxaprofen. The cause of the chronic cholestasis is uncertain; both immune mechanisms and the recirculation of toxic metabolites have been implicated.

Further reading

Abboud G, Kaplowitz N (2007). Drug-induced liver injury. *Drug Safety*, **30**, 277–94.

Aithal PG, Day CP (1999). The natural history of histologically proved drug induced liver disease. *Gut*, **44**, 731–5.

Andrade RJ, et al (2006). Outcome of acute idiosyncratic drug-induced liver injury: long-term follow-up in a hepatotoxicity registry. *Hepatology*, **44**, 1581–8.

Bem JL, Msann R, Rawlins MO (1988). Review of yellow cards. *Br Med J*, **296**, 1319.

Chang CY, Schiano TD (2007). Drug hepatotoxicity. *Aliment Pharmacol Therapeut*, **25**, 1135–51.

Danan O (1990). Consensus meeting. Criteria of drug induced liver disorders. *J Hepatol*, **11**, 272–6.

Dossing M, Sonne J (1993). Drug-induced hepatic disorders. *Drug Safety*, **9**, 441–9.

Friis H, Andreason P (1991). Drug induced hepatic injury: an analysis of 1100 cases reported to the Danish Committee on Adverse Drug Reactions between 1978 and 1987. *Intern Med*, **232**, 133–42.

Garcia Rodriguez LA, Ruigomez A, Jick H (1997). A review of epidemiologic research on drug-induced acute liver injury using the general practice research data base in the United Kingdom. *Pharmacotherapy*, **17**, 721–8.

Merrick BA, Bruno M (2004). Genomic and proteomic profiling for biomarkers and signature profiles of toxicity. *Curr Opin Mol Therapeut*, **6**, 600–7.

Neuberger J (1989). Drug induced jaundice. *Clin Gastroenterol*, **3**, 447–66.

Pessayre D, et al. (1999). Withdrawal of life support, altruistic suicide, fratricidal killing and euthanasia by lymphocytes: different forms of drug-induced hepatic apoptosis. *J Hepatol*, **31**, 760–70.

Pillans PI (1996). Drug associated hepatic reactions in New Zealand: 21 years experience *N Z Med J*, **109**, 315–19.

Seminars in Liver Disease (2009), **29** (4).

Shaw D, et al. (1997). Traditional remedies and food supplements. A 5 year toxicological study (1991–1995). *Drug Safety* **17**, 342–56.

15.22.9 The liver in systemic disease

J. Neuberger

Essentials

The liver is affected in many systemic diseases, with important examples being:

Cardiovascular diseases—raised venous pressure, e.g. cardiac failure, constrictive pericarditis, can lead to hepatic congestion, which sometimes causes nausea, vomiting, and right upper quadrant pain. Hepatomegaly is frequent in moderately severe heart failure. Cardiac cirrhosis is a rare complication.

Pulmonary diseases—conditions that involve the liver as well as the lungs include cystic fibrosis, sarcoidosis, and α_1-antitrypsin deficiency.

Gastrointestinal diseases—inflammatory bowel disease is associated with a range of hepatic pathology including fatty change, pericholangitis, sclerosing cholangitis, chronic active hepatitis, cirrhosis, and amyloidosis. Hepatobiliary disease associated with total parenteral nutrition varies from a mild, asymptomatic disease to jaundice, cirrhosis, and liver failure. Coeliac disease may rarely present with abnormal liver tests.

Endocrine diseases—autoimmune hepatitis may be associated with autoimmune endocrine disorders. Both hypothyroidism and hyperthyroidism can cause abnormalities of liver function, which are usually mild.

Haematological diseases—conditions associated with abnormal blood clotting, such as protein C or S deficiency and paroxysmal nocturnal haemoglobulinuria, may lead to Budd–Chiari syndrome (hepatic vein thrombosis). The liver may be involved in both non-Hodgkin's lymphoma and leukaemia.

Infectious diseases—agents that particularly affect the liver, e.g. viral hepatitis, are discussed in other chapters. Abnormal liver function may occur during many systemic infections, but it is rare for patients with sepsis to present primarily with liver symptoms, although jaundice, abnormal liver function tests or (very rarely) fulminant hepatic failure may be the principal presenting feature.

Rheumatological diseases—hepatic disease may either be a consequence of treatment or occur in association with other autoimmune diseases.

Introduction

The liver is affected in many systemic diseases. It most instances, disturbance of liver structure and/or function is a relatively minor component of the illness, but in some cases abnormalities of liver function may be the presenting symptom. This chapter describes abnormalities of liver function that occur in some systemic diseases.

Cardiovascular disease

Congestive cardiac failure

Most patients with congestive cardiac failure have few symptoms related to hepatic congestion, although nausea, vomiting, and right upper quadrant pain may occasionally occur. Hepatomegaly is frequent in moderately severe heart failure. Rarely, cardiac cirrhosis develops and may be associated with splenomegaly and ascites. Jaundice occurs in about one-quarter of patients with persistent hepatic venous congestion.

The standard serum liver-related tests may show a rise in bilirubin, which rarely exceeds 50 µmol/litre. The level of unconjugated bilirubin usually exceeds that of conjugated bilirubin. The serum aminotransferases may also be elevated but rarely exceed twice the upper limit of normal. However, in severe, acute heart failure, concentrations in excess of 1000 IU/litre may be found. Serum alkaline phosphatase is rarely elevated. The prothrombin time is often prolonged by a few seconds. The liver is usually enlarged and ultrasound examination may show dilated hepatic veins and a congested liver. Macroscopically, the liver shows the classical nutmeg appearance, with the pale periportal zones alternating with darker centrilobular zones. Microscopically there is congestion, with dilatation of the terminal hepatic venules and adjacent sinusoids, and areas of centrilobular necrosis due to hypoperfusion injury. With chronic heart failure centrilobular necrosis may be associated with fibrosis.

Constrictive pericarditis

Hepatic complications of constrictive pericarditis occur late in the course of the illness. Cardiovascular features of constrictive pericarditis are described elsewhere (see Section 15). The liver is enlarged and there may be associated splenomegaly. Jaundice and ascites may develop. Ultrasonography will show enlargement of the liver with dilated hepatic veins.

Tricuspid incompetence

Tricuspid incompetence most commonly occurs as a result of failure of right heart dilatation but may also result from congenital or acquired disease of the tricuspid valve. The liver is enlarged and pulsatile.

Tumours of the heart

Tumours of the right atrium, including myxoma and myosarcoma, may infiltrate the hepatic veins resulting in Budd–Chiari syndrome (a syndrome of hepatic venous thrombosis, characterized by abdominal pain, progressive ascites, and diarrhoea). Cardiac myxoma may be associated with abnormalities of liver function tests, including increased serum bilirubin and alkaline phosphatase and a reduction in serum albumin and total protein.

Drug reactions

As described in Chapter 15.22.8, many drugs used for the treatment of heart disease may be associated with adverse reactions that involve the liver. The pattern of hepatotoxicity associated with drug toxicity is wide and, in any person with unexplained liver abnormalities, a drug aetiology should be considered. The diagnosis of an adverse drug reaction is one of exclusion and based on the temporal association between the onset of liver abnormalities and the taking of the medication, the effect of withdrawal of the drug, and its known pattern toxicity.

Hypoxia

Hypoxic episodes, especially during surgery, may lead to an acute liver injury resulting from an ischaemic hepatitis. The clinical severity ranges from an asymptomatic elevation of serum aminotransferases to fulminant hepatic failure. The syndrome may be followed by a period of cholestasis. The aminotransferases may become greatly elevated (in excess of 10 000 IU/litre); histologically there is hepatocellular necrosis in the absence of inflammation, most marked in acinar zone 3 (the perivenular area). Similar changes occur in patients with heat stroke. Fulminant hepatic failure may rarely develop but the prognosis is usually dependent on the cause of the ischaemia rather than the effects on the liver.

Syndromes affecting both the heart and the liver

Several conditions affect both the heart and the liver; these include Alagille's syndrome (a multisystemic disorder, associated with a paucity of intrahepatic bile ducts, leading to a biliary cirrhosis with pulmonary stenosis and other cardiac abnormalities), biliary atresia (where up to 10% of patients may have congenital heart disease), and cardiomyopathy which may be associated with a variety of inherited and acquired conditions affecting both organs, these include alcohol toxicity, haemochromatosis, tyrosinaemia, and mitochondrial cytopathy. Drugs such as the immunosuppressive agent tacrolimus may also cause cardiomyopathy.

Pulmonary disease

Cirrhosis

Lung disease may complicate cirrhosis; the hepatopulmonary syndrome, discussed elsewhere, may resolve after treatment of the underlying liver disease or after liver transplantation. In contrast, abnormalities of liver function in patients with pulmonary disease arise either as a consequence of that disease or of diseases affecting both lung and liver. In most patients with chronic lung disease, abnormalities of liver function are mild. In more advanced disease, associated with hypoxia, there may be more widespread disturbances of liver function, with elevation of serum aminotransferase, bilirubin, alkaline phosphatase, and γ-glutamyltransferase. However, abnormality of liver function in patients with pulmonary disease is associated mainly with pulmonary hypertension rather than lung disease or hypoxia as such.

Pneumonia

Some patients with pneumococcal pneumonia may have jaundice. It usually occurs on the fourth or fifth day of the illness and is seen particularly in patients with consolidation of the right lower lobe. The serum bilirubin rarely exceeds 100 µmol/litre, and abnormalities of other liver tests are unusual. The cause of the jaundice is not known: factors that have been implicated are glucose-6-phosphatase deficiency, associated acute haemolysis, hypoxia, fever, and direct toxicity. The increased amounts of inflammatory cytokines seen in such patients may also contribute to the jaundice.

Abnormal liver function tests are also seen in patients with Legionnaire's disease and are characterized by elevation of aspartate aminotransferase and alkaline phosphatase. Jaundice is less common and tends to occur only in patients who are severely ill.

Diseases that involve lung and liver

α₁-Antitrypsin deficiency (see Chapter 11.13)

α_1-Antitrypsin deficiency was initially described in relation to pulmonary emphysema but it is now known that the liver, kidney, and pancreas can also be diseased. In children, α_1-antitrypsin deficiency often presents as neonatal hepatitis: in one-third it resolves, one-third develop fibrosis, and the remainder develop progressive cirrhosis, often requiring transplantation. In adults the disease often presents with cirrhosis or its complications. The liver shows the characteristic histological features of periodic acid–Schiff-positive, diastase-resistant globules in the liver. These globules are not diagnostic of the disease. Patients usually express the Pi zz phenotypic α_1-antitrypsin variant; other isoforms of α_1-antitrypsin are usually not associated with liver disease. Histological features of granules of α_1-antitrypsin may be seen in conditions other than α_1-antitrypsin deficiency.

The course is unpredictable, but many patients develop progressive disease that requires liver transplantation. There is no other proven effective treatment. The onset of cholestasis often heralds liver failure. In cases where lung and liver disease coexist, the only effective therapy is transplantation of the lungs and liver.

Cystic fibrosis

The increasing success in treating respiratory complications in children with cystic fibrosis has resulted in a greater number surviving to develop liver disease. Abnormal liver tests are found in up to one-half of these children, and in adults up to one-quarter of patients with cystic fibrosis develop a biliary cirrhosis. These patients present with cholestasis and jaundice. The pathogenesis and aetiology of this cholestasis are poorly understood. In most cases, liver disease is characterized by the development of a focal biliary cirrhosis that increases with time with cirrhosis usually being evident by the age of 10 years. Early involvement of the liver is characterized by the presence of eosinophilic granular material in the portal ducts. There is proliferation of bile ducts and portal fibrosis. This progresses to a focal biliary cirrhosis, which then develops into a multilobular cirrhosis with the onset of symptoms of cholestasis and jaundice. However, many patients have evidence of biliary obstruction shown by imaging the biliary tree by magnetic resonance cholepancreatography (MRCP) or endoscopic retrograde cholepancreatography (ERCP). There is some evidence that infusion of *N*-acetylcysteine into the biliary tree may relieve the obstruction in the extrahepatic biliary tree. The onset of jaundice and ascites is associated with a poor prognosis. Standard liver tests may underestimate the severity of the liver disease. Treatment with ursodeoxycholic acid will improve the liver tests and may improve liver function.

Other causes of cholestasis in patients with cystic fibrosis include gallstones and pancreatic insufficiency associated with increased loss of faecal bile salts, a consequent decrease in the size of the bile salt pool, and the development of lithogenic bile.

Treatment is uncertain. Open studies have suggested that ursodeoxycholic acid, 10 mg/kg per day, may result in biochemical improvement, weight gain, and improved nutrition. However, whether this agent has any long-term effect remains to be established.

Sarcoidosis

Sarcoidosis is a systemic granulomatous disease of unknown aetiology. The liver is commonly affected, with evidence of infiltration in up to 70% of cases. However, symptoms and signs of hepatic disease are uncommon. Hepatomegaly and splenomegaly occur in about one-quarter of patients. While jaundice is rare, elevation of the serum alkaline phosphatase is frequently observed. Complications of granulomatous infiltration of the liver are unusual. Liver failure may supervene, but portal hypertension occurs more frequently and causes bleeding varices or ascites. Sarcoidosis of the liver has been reported in association with other conditions, such as the Budd–Chiari syndrome.

As with sarcoid elsewhere, the diagnosis is usually made by the finding of noncaseating granulomas around the portal tracts. These granulomas are usually large and consist of multinuclear giant cells with T lymphocytes. Most patients respond to corticosteroids, although the portal hypertension may persist, possibly due to established presinusoidal fibrosis.

Overlap syndromes with primary biliary cirrhosis are well recognized: in patients with typical sarcoid infiltration in lungs and liver in the presence of bile duct damage consistent with primary biliary cirrhosis (PBC) and with positive antimitochondrial antibody tests, treatment should be directed against the sarcoid because, as yet, there is no treatment that improves survival in primary biliary cirrhosis. Other causes of granulomatous hepatitis are discussed elsewhere.

Drugs

As indicated elsewhere, many drugs used for the treatment of lung diseases may be associated with abnormal liver function. Inhaled disodium chromoglicate reportedly causes a syndrome that transiently resembles primary biliary cirrhosis. However, inhaled medications otherwise rarely cause significant abnormalities of liver-related tests.

Disorders of the gastrointestinal tract

Inflammatory bowel disease

The range of liver abnormality associated with inflammatory bowel disease includes fatty change, pericholangitis, sclerosing cholangitis, chronic active hepatitis, cirrhosis, and amyloidosis. The reported incidence of serum liver test abnormalities in inflammatory bowel disease varies from 3 to 10%. In general, abnormalities of liver tests correlate poorly with the severity of liver disease determined histologically. Ulcerative colitis is more commonly associated with abnormal serum liver-related tests than is Crohn's disease.

There is no clear relation between the onset of symptoms of inflammatory bowel disease and liver abnormalities. In general, symptoms of ulcerative colitis precede changes in liver function tests by about 8 years, but liver disease may precede the onset of clinically apparent inflammatory bowel disease by many years. Conversely, liver disease may become manifest several years after colectomy. Furthermore, there is little correlation between the severity of inflammatory bowel disease and the incidence or severity of liver disease. Indeed, in many patients with sclerosing cholangitis the colitis tends to be a pancolitis but is often quiescent (Table 15.22.9.1). Fatty change is relatively common on histological examination of the liver in patients with inflammatory

Table 15.22.9.1 Liver and biliary disorders associated with inflammatory bowel disease

	Disorder
Parenchymal	Granuloma
	Pericholangitis
	Autoimmune hepatitis
	Primary biliary cirrhosis
	Liver abscess
	Amyloid
Biliary	Gallstones
	Primary sclerosing cholangitis
	Cholangiocarcinoma

bowel disease and is probably multifactorial in origin, relating to the degree of ill health, poor nutrition, and use of corticosteroids. As a patient's condition improves, the fatty infiltration resolves. Primary sclerosing cholangitis (PSC) is associated with inflammatory bowel disease in about 10% of cases, whereas nearly 90% of patients with sclerosing cholangitis have inflammatory bowel disease. PSC is a premalignant condition, associated with bile duct carcinoma in 5 to 20% of cases. In patients with PSC and ulcerative colitis, there is an increased risk of colon cancer.

Cirrhosis occurs in up to 10% of patients who die with ulcerative colitis. The cause of the cirrhosis is not known, but in some cases it may be caused by chronic hepatitis C infection from drug transfusions or by drug toxicity, rather than primary sclerosing cholangitis.

Although chronic active hepatitis in association with inflammatory bowel disease is rare, its recognition is important because it resembles autoimmune chronic active hepatitis and may respond well to corticosteroid treatment. Other hepatic complications of inflammatory bowel disease include granulomatous hepatitis, amyloid infiltration of the liver, bile duct carcinoma, gallbladder cancer, and gallstones.

Coeliac disease

In patients with coeliac disease there may be minor abnormalities of liver function tests, characterized by elevation of serum aminotransferases; they usually resolve within 6 months of institution of a gluten-free diet. Rarely, both cirrhosis and acute liver failure has been attributed to coeliac disease. Coeliac disease may also be associated with autoimmune diseases affecting the liver, including PBC, cryptogenic cirrhosis, PSC, and autoimmune hepatitis. Up to 4% of patients with PBC may have coeliac disease and up to 3% of patients with coeliac disease may have PBC (see Chapter 15.10.3).

Gastrointestinal bypass surgery

Jejunoileal bypass surgery may be associated with liver disease; the changes in the liver range from simple fatty infiltration to cirrhosis. In a few cases there may be features identical to those of alcoholic hepatitis. In those in whom liver function tests are deranged, progressive injury is likely; although treatment with metronidazole has been advocated, restoration of normal anatomy appears to be the only effective measure.

Total parenteral nutrition

The association of hepatobiliary disorders with total parenteral nutrition has been recognized over the last two decades. Although the pathogenesis remains obscure, most studies suggest that the incidence is now less than 5%. Hepatobiliary disease associated with total parenteral nutrition varies from a mild, asymptomatic disease with acalculous cholecystitis, biliary sludge, or hepatomegaly to jaundice, cirrhosis, and liver failure. Biochemically, the severity of abnormalities will reflect the severity of the disease but elevations of serum liver enzymes such as aspartate and alanine transferases, lactate dehydrogenase, and alkaline phosphatase, and serum bilirubin, are common. The histological features vary from a mild fatty infiltrate or cholestasis to a more severe picture resembling alcoholic fatty liver. Cirrhosis will develop in chronic cases. The mechanism is uncertain but hypoxic enterocytes, nutritional depletion, sepsis, toxicity of certain unidentified amino acids, and even carnitine deficiency have been implicated (Table 15.22.9.2). Once a patient develops abnormal liver function, and provided that other causes have been excluded, there is little alternative other than to reduce or stop parenteral nutrition and find other ways of providing adequate nutrition. It has been suggested that substitution of a fish-oil based fat emulsion for the soya bean-based emulsion may be beneficial.

Obesity

Obesity, especially when associated with the metabolic syndrome, may be associated with abnormalities of serum liver tests, which may vary from minor and asymptomatic elevation of the serum aminotransferases to decompensated liver disease. Nonalcoholic fatty liver disease is becoming an increasing problem and is discussed in greater detail in Chapter 15.22.2. Cutaneous manifestations of chronic liver disease may develop. The liver ultrasound scan will show a fatty liver and liver histology a macrovesicular fatty infiltration, which may be associated with a hepatitic picture. There is considerable serological and histological overlap between fatty liver disease from alcohol and nonalcohol related factors (such as obesity, diabetes mellitus, drugs, and gastric bypass surgery)

Table 15.22.9.2 Factors contributing to liver dysfunction in patients receiving total parenteral nutrition

Underlying sepsis:	Systemic
	Local
	Small-bowel colonization
Underlying disease	
Duration of TPN	
Pre-existing liver disease	
Underlying condition	
Nutritional factors:	Excess nonprotein calories
	Essential fatty acid deficiency
	Amino acid toxicity
	Carnitine deficiency
	Bile acid abnormalities
Drug toxicity	

TPN, total parenteral nutrition.

Liver in endocrine disease

Autoimmune hepatitis may be associated with autoimmune endocrine disorders, such as thyroid disease, vitiligo, and diabetes mellitus.

In haemochromatosis, where both liver and pancreas are affected, diabetes itself is associated with liver abnormalities. The liver may be enlarged due to excess stores of fat and glycogen. In severe cases there may be a non-alcoholic steatohepatitis syndrome which can lead to hepatic fibrosis and cirrhosis. Liver abnormalities are seen much more commonly in type 2 diabetes (20–75% of patients) compared with well-controlled type I diabetes (<1% of patients).

Hypothyroidism may be associated with a mild hyperbilirubinaemia and elevated serum transaminases (which may be of muscular origin). Ascites occurs very rarely. Hyperthyroidism is also associated with mild abnormalities of liver function which resolve on treatment of the thyroid disorder; severe uncontrolled thyrotoxicosis is associated with cardiac failure, atrial fibrillation, and jaundice (Habershon's jaundice) in which hypoperfusion and the toxic effects of thyroid hormone lead to hepatocellular dysfunction. This syndrome carries a poor prognosis and requires urgent treatment for thyroid stores.

Liver in haematological diseases

In general, diseases of the blood do not affect the liver. However, diseases associated with abnormal blood clotting, such as protein C or S deficiency and paroxysmal nocturnal haemoglobulinuria, may lead to Budd–Chiari syndrome (hepatic vein thrombosis).

Haemolysis

Jaundice may accompany haemolysis and is principally associated with an increase in unconjugated bilirubin. In patients with underlying liver disease both conjugated and unconjugated bilirubin are elevated out of proportion to the degree of haemolysis. Patients with chronic haemolytic anaemia are at risk of developing haemosiderosis. Iron is deposited initially in the Kupffer cells, but spread to the parenchyma will subsequently occur. The identification of the gene for hereditary haemochromatosis has assisted in the distinction between primary and secondary iron overload. The haemolytic anaemias are associated with an increased risk of pigment gallstones, which may lead to liver and biliary tract disease.

Sickle cell disease

Most of the abnormalities of liver function in sickle cell disease are due to haemolysis or infections transmitted by blood transfusion. Kupffer cell hyperplasia, haemosiderosis, fibrosis, or cirrhosis may be due to iron overload following multiple transfusions. Sometimes, patients present with severe pain in the right upper quadrant and rapid enlargement of the liver is part of the hepatic sequestration syndrome. Liver histology may show clumps of sickled red cells in the sunusoids, erythrophagocytosis, and sinusoidal dilatation. There is an increased risk of gallstones.

Thalassaemia

As with sickle cell disease, there is an increase in haemolysis and the complications of blood transfusions. Gallstones are common.

Multiple transfusions

Patients who receive regular blood transfusions or blood products, e.g. those with thalassaemia or haemophilia, are at risk of developing viral hepatitis B or C. It is now clear that such patients are at an increased risk of hepatitis C which may lead to cirrhosis and liver cell cancer. With screening, the incidence of hepatitis C virus infection through this cause will fall. Blood transfusion is also associated with secondary haemochromatosis since each unit of blood provides the equivalent of 225 mg of iron which may ultimately causes iron storage disease in the liver and in other organs.

Lymphomatous disease

In patients with Hodgkin's disease, liver function tests are of limited value in predicting liver involvement, although jaundice is a recognized feature and may be due to a number of different causes. For example, haemolysis may complicate Hodgkin's disease, and occasionally there is a bland cholestasis in the absence of infiltration, which resolves when the disease is treated. The clinical manifestations of liver involvement in Hodgkin's disease relate to the degree of infiltration. In rare cases, patients with Hodgkin's disease develop fulminant hepatic failure: the clue to infiltration is a large liver, as most cases of viral or drug-related fulminant hepatic failure are associated with small livers. Liver biopsy may be diagnostic. Primary lymphoma of the liver has been described, but is rare. The liver may be involved in both non-Hodgkin's lymphoma and leukaemia and the diagnosis is usually made by biopsy. Some patients with non-Hodgkin's lymphoma have chronic hepatitis preceding diagnosis or treatment. A causal effect cannot be excluded. Hodgkin's disease and non-Hodgkin's lymphoma may be associated with obstructive jaundice due to invasion of the bile duct by invasive nodal disease in the hilum.

Liver and infections

Abnormal liver function may occur during systemic infections but it is rare for patients with sepsis to present primarily with liver symptoms (Table 15.22.9.3). However, jaundice, abnormal liver function tests, or even, occasionally, fulminant hepatic failure may be the principal presenting feature.

Bacterial infections

Pneumococcal infections are discussed above. Meningococcal infections are occasionally associated with features suggestive of viral hepatitis. Jaundice may be associated with the toxic shock syndrome associated with *Staphyloccus aureus*. Gonococcal infection is a well-recognized cause of liver disease. The classical Fitzhugh–Curtis syndrome, perihepatitis, is characterized by sudden onset of severe pain in the right upper quadrant, occurring classically in a woman with a previous history of pelvic inflammatory disease. On examination there may be little to find, although tender hepatomegaly and a hepatic rub may be present. Where laparotomy has been performed in the mistaken diagnosis of cholecystitis, perihepatitis with adhesions and pus around the liver may give the clue to the diagnosis. In chronic infection, adhesions develop between the surface of the liver and the anterior abdominal wall. The condition usually resolves without treatment, although the use of penicillin promotes more rapid resolution. Abnormalities of liver function may occur in gonococcal bacteraemia, peritonitis, and endocarditis. Perihepatitis is also reported in association with syphilis

Table 15.22.9.3 Systemic infections affecting the liver

Bacterial	Actinomycoses
	Brucellosis
	Chlamydia
	Clostridium welchii
	Escherichia coli
	Gonorrhoea
	Granuloma inguinale
	Listeriosis
	Legionella pneumophila
	Meliodosis
	Meningococcus
	Nocardia
	Shigella
	Staphyloccus
	Streptococcus
	Typhoid and paratyphoid
	Tularaemia
	Yersinia
Fungal	Aspergillosis
	Blastomycosis
	Candidosis
	Coccidiodomycosis
	Cryptococcus
	Histoplasmosis
Mycobacterial	Leprosy
	Others
	Tuberculosis
Protozoal	Giardiasis
	Kala-azar
	Malaria
	Toxoplasmosis
Rickettsial	Q fever
	Rocky Mountain spotted fever
Spirochaetal	Leptospirosis
	Lyme disease
	Relapsing fever
	Syphilis

and chlamydial infections. Chlamydial infection is today the most frequent cause of chronic perihepatic adhesions.

In childhood, some infections with *Escherichia coli* may be associated with hepatitis and jaundice. Jaundice is rare in older patients, although pregnant women seem more susceptible. Abnormalities of liver function occur in systemic streptococcal and staphylococcal infection and in enteric fevers, paratyphoid, and typhoid.

Hepatomegaly is common in typhoid infection and jaundice occurs in about 10% of patients, although up to one-third have abnormal liver function tests with increased levels of aminotransferase and normal values for alkaline phosphatase. The hepatomegaly rapidly responds with treatment. In gas gangrene, deep jaundice may occur may occur in up to one-fifth of patients. The liver may be infected and a plain radiograph of the abdomen may show gas within the liver. Liver damage and jaundice are associated with *Listeria monocytogenes* and *Legionella pneumophila* infections.

Brucellosis may also be associated with jaundice and abnormal liver function tests. All three species of brucella have been associated with abnormal liver function. Characteristically, the liver biopsy shows a marked inflammatory infiltrate and fibrosis with multiple large or small granulomas scattered throughout the parenchyma. Some reports have suggested that granulomatous hepatitis due to brucella may cause cirrhosis, but this is questionable. The common causes of liver granulomas, including infections, are listed in Table 15.22.9.4. The liver damage asociated with leptospirosis (Weil's disease) is described elsewhere (Section 7).

Actinomyces spp. are commensal organisms that rarely cause disease. Actinomycotic infection of the liver may occur, the patient presenting with abdominal pain, anorexia, and fever. In one case report the liver was found to have small, multilocular abscesses.

Tuberculosis may present with granulomatous hepatitis, biliary tuberculosis, a solitary tuberculoma, or tuberculosis of the biliary tract. The liver is involved in up to 85% of patients with tuberculosis, especially in those with miliary disease. The presence of multiple granulomas in the liver should raise the possibility of tuberculosis, although the differential diagnosis of granulomatous hepatitis is long (see Table 15.22.9.4). With the increasing incidence of atypical mycobacterial infections, lesions similar to tuberculosis can be found. In those infected with *Mycobacterium avium intracellulare* there are numerous acid-fast bacilli, often in the absence of granulomas.

Leptospirosis

Leptospiral infections are described in Section 7. Acute leptospirosis is frequently accompanied by jaundice, although frank liver failure is uncommon. The jaundice is mainly cholestatic, although there may be liver cell injury.

Rickettsial infection

Liver injury in Q fever (*Coxiella burnetti*) is recognized, although symptoms of liver disease are uncommon. Hepatomegaly is frequent and liver function tests may show an elevation of serum alkaline phosphatase and, rarely, a picture resembling viral hepatitis. Histologically, the liver has areas of focal necrosis, Kupffer cell proliferation, lipogranuloma formation, and mononuclear cell infiltration in the portal tracts. The characteristic histological feature of Q fever is eosinophiliic fibrinoid necrosis but this is not specific. Treatment is with chloramphenicol or tetracycline. Liver disease is much more frequent in Rocky Mountain spotted fever (*Rickettsia rickettsia*).

Fungal infections

The liver may be involved in fungal infection, often in patients with immunodeficiency such as with AIDS, following chemotherapy, and after organ transplantation. Histoplasmosis, cryptococcosis,

Table 15.22.9.4 Common causes of hepatic granulomas

Drugs	Allopurinol
	Phenylbutazone
	Sulphonamides
Infective	Bacterial
	Brucellosis
	Mycobacteria
	Rickettsial
	Spirochaetal
	Fungal
	Parasitic
	Amoebiasis
	Ascariasis
	Giardiasis
	Schistosomiasis
	Toxocara
	Yersinia
	Viral
	Cytomegalovirus
	Epstein–Barr virus
Malignancy	Hodgkin's disease
Other	Collagen disease
	Crohn's disease
	Erythema nodosum
	Sarcoid
	Systemic lupus erythematosus
	Toxins: beryllium and silicon
	Whipple's disease
Parenchymal disease	Primary biliary cirrhosis
	Primary sclerosing cholangitis

aspergillosis, blastomycosis, and candidiasis are all causes of liver damage. The liver is usually involved in disseminated fungal infections. Cryptococcal infection has also been associated with a PBC-like condition.

Protozoal infections

Protozoal infections are described in detail in Chapter 7.13. Many of them involve the liver. In toxoplasmosis, while most patients are asymptomatic and liver involvement is mild, hepatitis may occur and *Toxoplasma gondii* may be found in liver biopsy samples. In malaria, due to either *Plasmodium falcipartun* or *P. vivax*, abnormalities of liver tests may be observed. Hepatomegaly is common and is often associated with jaundice. The jaundice is in part due to haemolysis but liver tests may provide a picture suggestive of viral hepatitis. Histological examination may show characteristic features of Kupffer cell proliferation with black malarial pigment and mononuclear cell infiltrate. Frank hepatic failure is extremely rare.

Schistosomiasis is one of the most common causes of liver disease worldwide. A heavy infection of fertile schistosomes in the portal system results in deposition of eggs that induce an immune response, leading to portal fibrosis and granuloma formation, portal hypertension with consequent splenomegaly, ascites, and variceal haemorrhage. Hepatocyte function is well preserved. There is a complex interaction between schistosomal eggs and the immune system; the degree of fibrosis is directly related to the number of eggs and the duration of infection. The diagnosis is made on stool examination or finding schistosomes in the liver. Serological tests are unreliable at present. Treatment is described in Chapter 7.16.1. Successful treatment is associated with a significant but variable improvement in the degree of portal hypertension. Treatment of the portal hypertension is dependent on the medical facilities available. As parenchymal function is well preserved, these patients usually tolerate a portosystemic shunt.

Coinfection of patients with schistosomiasis and hepatitis B or C virus is associated with an aggressive progression.

Viral infections

Hepatitis may be a significant feature of viral infection other than with the classical hepatitis viruses. Thus, infection with cytomegalovirus, Epstein–Barr virus, herpesviruses, measles, rubella, coxsackievirus, adenoviruses, and echoviruses may all cause a significant hepatitis. Such viral infections (especially cytomegalovirus) are more common in immunosuppressed patients. The diagnosis is made serologically, but in some cases, such as with cytomegalovirus, herpes, and adenoviral infections, the liver histology may show characteristic features.

Pyogenic liver abscess

Pyogenic liver abscesses may occur as part of a systemic illness, or as a consequence of portal phlebitis. Abscesses are often associated with bowel sepsis, biliary tract disease, direct trauma, septicaemia, and in association with carcinoma of the colon or bacterial endocarditis. Abscesses most commonly arise out of portal phlebitis, with the primary focus being the appendix, colon, diverticular disease, or in the pelvis (Table 15.22.9.5). Although abscesses may occur in patients with inflammatory bowel disease, this is relatively rare. The patient presents with abdominal pain, pyrexia, nausea, and weight loss. However, fever is less common in children. Hepatomegaly may be present and the liver is sometimes tender. The serum albumin is often reduced and alkaline phosphatase elevated. There is usually marked neutrophil leucocytosis, but this is not invariable. The diagnosis is made on imaging of the liver. A chest radiograph may show elevation of the right hemidiaphragm with an associated pleural effusion or even lung consolidation. Ultrasonography, CT, or MRI may define a hepatic abscess.

Table 15.22.9.5 Sources of a pyogenic abscess

Source	Percentage of cases
Obstructive biliary tree	30–40
Intra-abdominal infection	15–25
Systemic infection	15–20

Treatment of a solitary abscess is usually by percutaneous drainage in the first instance. Under the guidance of ultrasonography or CT, a percutaneous drain should be established for single abscesses, and even in some cases of multiple abscesses. The abscesses should be drained to dryness, and antibiotics should be given according to the sensitivities of the organisms isolated. Pathogens are usually anaerobic or aerobic gut coliforms, especially *Streptococcus milleri*, but in children *Staphylococcus aureus* is common. The success rate of treatment with drainage and systemic antibiotics is 80 to 90%. Fatality is high in children and older people, in those with coexisting disease such as diabetes mellitus, and in those with delayed diagnosis. Once the abscess has been drained, the primary source of infection must be sought and appropriate management instituted. Surgery may be required for patients with multiple abscesses or for those with abscesses that do not respond to simple drainage and antibiotic therapy. Liver abscess due to hydatid and amoebal infection is discussed elsewhere.

AIDS and liver disease

Liver disease in patients with HIV infection may be due to pre-existing hepatitis virus, opportunistic infections, or neoplasms. In some cases the abnormality of liver function may be due to virus itself. Such patients have nontender hepatomegaly with anorexia, weight loss, and low-grade fever. Liver function tests show slight derangement with cholestasis. The liver biopsy shows non-specific features including Kupffer cell hyperplasia, fat infiltration, noncaseating granulomas, and portal tract inflammation; Mallory hyaline bodies may occasionally be present.

Other causes of hepatobiliary abnormality in patients with HIV include primary hepatic infection due to viral hepatitis.

Other causes of liver damage in AIDS

Many patients with AIDS are also at risk from hepatitis B, C, and D. As discussed elsewhere, these patients respond less well to interferon than do those who are HIV negative. Other infections that are more common in HIV-positive patients include cytomegalovirus, herpesvirus, cryptosporidiosis, and mycobacterial infections including tuberculosis and *Mycobacterium avium intracellurare*. Drug-induced liver damage must always be considered in HIV patients with abnormal liver tests, and it has been suggested that such patients are more susceptible to drug hepatotoxicity. Thus, many of the anticonvulsants, analgesics, and antimicrobials are associated with hepatocellular damage, and antibiotics may also be associated with cholestasis. Other abnormalities that may be of less significance clinically include peliosis hepatis and fatty infiltration.

The biliary tree may also be affected in HIV infection inducing a syndrome superficially resembling primary sclerosing cholangitis. This is characterized by a rapid elevation of the serum alkaline phosphatase, which may be associated with pain in the right upper quadrant and, later, jaundice. Ultrasonography may be unhelpful, although dilated and thickened walls of the bile duct may be seen. Otherwise, ERCP will show the characteristic changes of sclerosing cholangitis with bleeding, dilatation, and stricture. Both cryptosporidial and cytomegaloviral infections have been associated with this form of sclerosing cholangitis.

The liver may be affected by HIV in other ways. There is an association between AIDS and lymphomas, be they Burkitt's, large cell, or immunoblastic lymphomas. The liver and/or spleen may be the site of these tumours and hepatic infiltration may be present in up to one-third of those with gastrointestinal lymphomas. Tumours may be microscopic or macroscopic. The hepatic masses are often asymptomatic but if large they may cause pain in the right upper quadrant, fever, jaundice, and abnormalities of serum liver tests, especially of the serum alkaline phosphatase. Kaposi's sarcoma may affect the liver and biliary tree but is often asymptomatic.

Liver and rheumatological disease

Liver abnormalities occur in patients with rheumatological disorders, although they rarely prove to be clinically significant. Hepatic disease may either be a consequence of treatment or occur in association with other autoimmune diseases. For example, those diseases assumed to have an autoimmune basis, such as autoimmune hepatitis or primary biliary cirrhosis, may be associated with extrahepatic rheumatological diseases such as the sicca syndrome.

Rheumatoid arthritis

Abnormalities of liver structure and function are uncommon in patients with rheumatoid arthritis, although minor abnormalities of liver function tests occur in 20 to 50% of cases. Nodular regenerative hyperplasia may cause complications of portal hypertension.

Felty's syndrome

Felty's syndrome is characterized by the triad of splenomegaly, hypersplenism, and seropositive rheumatoid arthritis. Liver function tests tend to be more commonly deranged than in uncomplicated rheumatoid arthritis. Anti-inflammatory therapy may contribute to the abnormal liver tests. Histological examination of the liver shows lymphocytic infiltration and, rarely, an established cirrhosis. Nodular regenerative hyperplasia occurs in patients with Felty's syndrome, as with rheumatoid arthritis. Although portal hypertension and variceal haemorrhage may occur, jaundice is unusual.

Connective tissue disease

Systemic lupus erythematosus

Usually only minor abnormalities of liver function occur in patients with systemic lupus erythematosus, although spontaneous rupture of the liver has been described. The pattern of liver disease in patients with systemic lupus erythematosus varies from minimal change to chronic persistent hepatitis, chronic active hepatitis, and cirrhosis. The inflammation and necrosis may affect portal and lobular areas. In others, a granulomatous hepatitis has been identified. There is usually a good response to corticosteroids.

Polyarteritis nodosa

In contrast to rheumatoid arthritis, liver injury in polyarteritis nodosa is relatively uncommon, although a hepatic arteritis may occur, leading to aneurysm. Rupture of an aneurysm is rare and is characterized by fever, pain in the right upper quadrant, and jaundice. In most cases, abnormalities of liver function are due to an associated hepatitis C virus infection.

Polymyalgia rheumatica

Abnormalities of liver function are well recognized in patients with polymyalgia rheumatica. These abnormalities (of elevation of serum alkaline phosphatase and aminotransferase activity) usually resolve with effective treatment. Histologically, the liver shows mild portal inflammation with occasional liver cell necrosis. Granulomas and steatosis may also be seen.

Sjögren's syndrome

Symptoms of sicca syndrome are common in patients with liver disease, particularly primary biliary cirrhosis, and abnormalities of salivary gland function have been described in all patients in some series. Sicca syndrome is also found in patients with cryptogenic cirrhosis and autoimmune chronic active hepatitis. In patients with Sjögren's syndrome there is often hepatomegaly and minor derangement of liver function tests, particularly serum alkaline phosphatase, in 25% of cases. The liver may show nonspecific inflammatory infiltration.

Amyloid (see Chapter 11.12.4)

The liver is infiltrated in both primary and secondary amyloidosis; liver disease is found in over 80% of patients with either form. In general, however, liver amyloidosis has few significant clinical consequences, although jaundice, hepatitis, portal hypertension, and spontaneous hepatic rupture occur. Clinically, the liver is enlarged; the serum alkaline phosphatase is usually greatly elevated and jaundice is uncommon. It is believed that liver biopsy may be particularly hazardous in patients with amyloid because there may be an increased risk of bleeding after biopsy. There is no treatment other than that which addresses the underlying cause.

Cryoglobulinaemia

The reported incidence of liver disease in essential, mixed cryoglobulinaemia varies greatly. In 20 to 50% of patients there is an association with hepatitis C viral infection. Up to half of patients have evidence of infection with hepatitis B virus, and up to 10% have an active hepatitis or cirrhosis with jaundice.

Liver in malignancy

Although the liver may become infiltrated by metastatic cancer, abnormalities of liver tests can be seen in the absence of infiltration. This may be due to a systemic effect of tumour-derived cytokines, to the hepatotoxic effects of drugs, or to the effects of irradiation.

Liver in the sick patient

Abnormalities of serum liver tests are frequent in patients who are critically sick, and are associated with a poor prognosis. There are many causes of abnormal liver tests in this situation (Table 15.22.9.6). 'Intensive therapy unit' jaundice occurs in up to 10%

Table 15.22.9.6 Abnormal liver tests in the critically ill

Patient
Underlying, pre-existing liver disease
Drug reactions
Trauma
Sepsis
Ischaemia
Haemolysis
Parenteral nutrition
Acalculous cholecystitis

of patients so treated, usually in the context of sepsis or abdominal trauma. Hepatomegaly is often present, but the cutaneous features of chronic liver disease are absent. Encephalopathy is uncommon. The liver tests show a rise in serum bilirubin with a smaller and less consistent rise in serum alkaline phosphatase and aminotransferase levels. Blood coagulation tests are mildly deranged and blood sugar levels tend to be high rather than low. The cause of intensive therapy unit jaundice is unclear but factors such as ischaemia, hypoxia, and hepatocyte necrosis may occur.

Liver disease in pregnancy

This is discussed in Chapter 14.9.

Further reading

Birrer MJ, Young RC (1987). Differential diagnosis of jaundice in lymphoma patients. *Semin Liver Dis*, **7**, 269–77.

Drebber U, *et al.* (2008). Hepatic granulomas: histological and molecular pathological approach. *Liver Int*, **28**, 828–34.

Fuchs M, Sanyal AJ (2008). Sepsis and cholestasis. *Clin Liver Dis*, **12**, 151–72.

Geier A, Fickert P, Trauner M (2996). Mechanisms of disease: mechanisms and clinical implications of cholestasis in sepsis. *Nat Clin Pract Gastroenterol Hepatol*, **3**, 574–85.

Guglielmi FW, *et al.* (2006). Total parenteral nutrition-related gastroenterological complications. *Digest Liver Dis*, **38**, 623–42.

Krowka MJ (2000). Hepatopulmonary syndromes. *Gut*, **46**, l–4.

Matsumoto T, *et al.* (2000). The liver in collagen diseases: pathologic study of 160 cases with particular reference to hepatic arteritis, primary biliary cirrhosis, autoimmune hepatitis and nodular regenerative hyperplasia of the liver. *Liver*, **20**, 366–73.

Valla DC, Benhamou JP (2000). Hepatic granulomas and hepatic sarcoidosis. *Clin Liver Dis*, **4**, 269–85.

Volta U (2009). Pathogenesis and clinical significance of liver injury in celiac disease. *Clini Rev Allergy Immunol*, **36**, 62–70.

Diseases of the gallbladder and biliary tree

J.A. Summerfield

Essentials

Diseases of the gallbladder and bile ducts are common, with gallstones and their complications being most frequent. Less common are biliary strictures, usually malignant, which are caused by adenocarcinomas of the pancreas, bile ducts, ampulla of Vater, and gallbladder. Rarely encountered are sclerosing cholangitis and a variety of congenital disorders.

Disorders of the biliary system usually give rise to the symptoms and signs of biliary obstruction (cholestasis), including pain (ranging from 'dyspepsia' to severe right hypochondrial colic), jaundice, itching, nausea and vomiting (which may be prominent in sudden obstruction of the bile duct, usually by a gallstone), fevers, and rigors (indicating bacterial infection of the biliary tract, which frequently accompanies partial obstruction). Jaundice, dark urine, and pale stools indicate obstruction of the bile duct. Weight loss may be due to fat malabsorption, but can also be caused by malignancy. Prolonged biliary obstruction leads to skin changes of increased pigmentation (due to melanin) and cholesterol deposition (xanthelasma and xanthoma). Biliary cirrhosis can cause portal venous hypertension and liver cell failure.

Disorders of the biliary system generally give rise to the biochemical picture of cholestasis: the serum (conjugated) bilirubin concentration may be normal or raised; serum alkaline phosphatase, γ-glutamyl transferase and bile acids are elevated; serum transaminases show only modest elevation. Bilirubinuria is present, with the disappearance of urobilinogen from the urine indicating complete biliary obstruction.

Imaging is critical in the diagnosis of biliary disease, initially by ultrasonography, with CT scanning and MRI then employed in more complicated cases. However, these investigations sometimes provide insufficient anatomical detail for diagnosis or planning of treatment, in which cases further imaging with the cholangiographic techniques of magnetic resonance cholangiography (MRC), endoscopic retrograde cholangiopancreatography (ERCP) or percutaneous transhepatic cholangiography (PTC) are required. ERCP and PRC can be used to place biliary stents.

Gallstones

Cholesterol gallstones account for 75% of gallstones in Europe and the United States of America. They result from the secretion of cholesterol-saturated bile by the liver, the cause of which is unclear. Pure cholesterol stones are usually solitary; mixed stones—which contain cholesterol in a matrix of calcium bilirubinate, calcium phosphate, and protein—are usually multiple and faceted.

Bile pigment stones consist of mucoprotein matrix, calcium bilirubinate, cholesterol, and calcium compounds: in east Asia they tend to be soft, friable, and brown and are associated with biliary infection; in the West they tend to be hard, brittle, and black and are found in patients with cirrhosis, chronic bile duct obstruction and chronic haemolytic anaemias.

Some 10 to 20% of the population have gallstones, most of which remain in the gallbladder (cholelithiasis) and give rise to no symptoms, but clinical presentations include (1) acute or chronic cholecystitis—due to impaction of a gallstone in the neck of the gallbladder; (2) choledocholithiasis—when gallstones pass through the cystic duct into the bile duct resulting in biliary obstruction and jaundice, and which may be complicated by bacterial infection (cholangitis); and less commonly, (3) perforation—through the inflamed gallbladder wall to form an internal fistula, usually to the small intestine or colon, and (4) gallstone ileus—a large gallstone passing into the small intestine may impact in the ileum and cause intestinal obstruction.

The usual treatment for symptomatic gallstones is cholecystectomy, performed (when available) laparoscopically. It is also appropriate to offer this to young patients with asymptomatic gallstones (who, with many years ahead of them, will have a greater likelihood of developing complications), but to advise against treatment in older people with other major medical problems. Chemical agents that dissolve gallstones (e.g. oral bile acid therapy, contact dissolution after transhepatic catheterization of the gallbladder) and physical methods (e.g. extracorporeal shock-wave lithotripsy) have a role to play in a very few patients. Endoscopic sphincterotomy is used to remove gallstones from the common bile duct.

Anatomy

The biliary system comprises the collection of ducts extending from the biliary canaliculus of each hepatocyte to the ampulla of Vater opening into the duodenum. The biliary canaliculi drain into interlobular and then septal bile ducts. These further ramify to form the intrahepatic bile ducts which are visible on cholangiography (Fig. 15.23.1). They eventually form the right and left hepatic ducts draining bile from the right and left lobes of the liver, respectively. The junction of the hepatic ducts at the porta hepatis forms the common hepatic duct. The cystic duct, linking the gallbladder to the bile duct, arises from the lower end of the common hepatic duct. The gallbladder rests in a fossa under the right lobe of the liver. Anatomical variations in the size and position of the gallbladder and the insertion of the cystic duct into the bile duct are of major surgical importance. The common hepatic duct becomes the common bile duct below the insertion of the cystic duct. The common bile duct passes through the head of the pancreas and the sphincter of Oddi to drain into the duodenum via the ampulla of Vater. The bile duct usually exits through a common channel with the pancreatic duct in the ampulla of Vater, although anatomical variations are frequent.

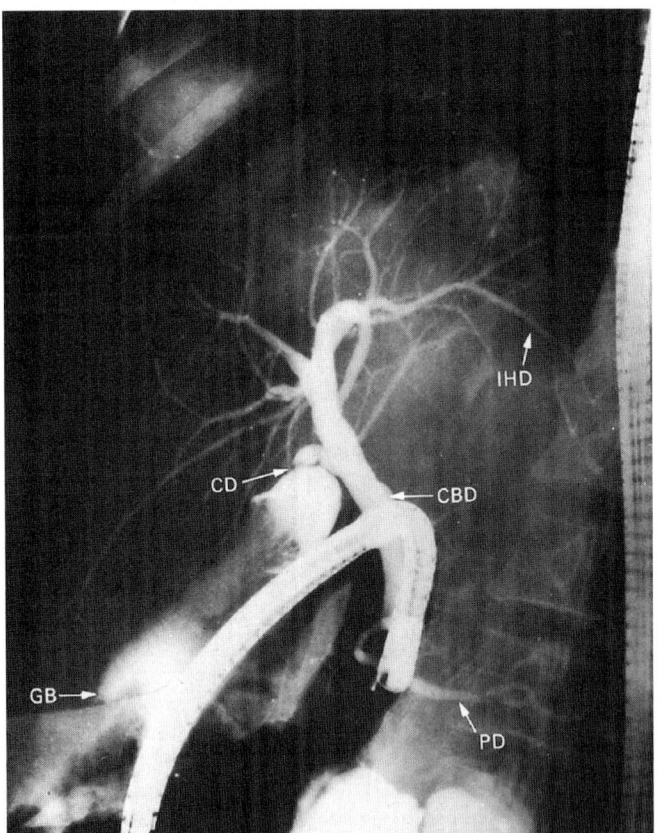

Fig. 15.23.1 The normal biliary tree. The intrahepatic bile ducts (IHD) taper smoothly and extend deep into the liver. The gallbladder (GB) drains via the cystic duct (CD) into the common bile duct (CBD). The pancreatic duct (PD) has also been opacified in this endoscopic retrograde cholangiogram.

The investigation of biliary disease

Objectives

The clinical and laboratory features of biliary disease may also be caused by hepatic disorders. Consequently, the primary objective of investigations is to establish that the cause is due to biliary and not hepatic disease. The secondary objective is to define the anatomy of the lesion to permit a rational choice of the many surgical and nonsurgical therapeutic options which are now available. To achieve these objectives requires not only a careful history and physical examination, but also the use of various imaging techniques and sometimes aspiration liver biopsy.

Symptoms and signs

Disorders of the biliary system usually give rise to the symptoms and signs of biliary obstruction (cholestasis). The repertoire is rather limited: pain, jaundice, itching, nausea and vomiting, fevers, and rigors. The pain can range from abdominal discomfort described as 'dyspepsia' to severe right hypochondrial colic caused by a sudden rise in biliary pressure. Jaundice, dark urine, and pale stools indicate obstruction of the bile duct. Itching is an important sign of biliary obstruction. Nausea and vomiting may be prominent in sudden obstruction of the bile duct, usually by a gallstone. The milder symptoms of flatulence and intolerance of fatty food are more common. Fever and rigors indicate bacterial infection of the biliary tract, which frequently accompanies partial obstruction. In jaundiced patients weight loss is usual and results from fat malabsorption due to the lack of bile acids reaching the gut; it may also indicate a malignant tumour. Prolonged biliary obstruction leads to skin changes: increased pigmentation (due to melanin) and cholesterol deposits (xanthelasma and xanthoma). Finally, biliary cirrhosis may develop causing the signs of portal venous hypertension and liver cell failure.

Laboratory investigations

In general, disorders of the biliary system give rise to the biochemical picture of biliary obstruction (cholestasis). A notable exception is gallstones in the gallbladder (cholelithiasis) where the liver function tests are usually normal. In cholestasis, the serum bilirubin concentration may be normal or raised and most of the bilirubin is esterified (conjugated). Bilirubinuria is present. The disappearance of urobilinogen from the urine indicates complete biliary obstruction. Elevation of the serum alkaline phosphatase is an important but not invariable sign of biliary obstruction; the rise is usually greater than three times normal. Other biliary canalicular enzymes accumulate in the blood, including γ-glutamyl transpeptidase. This enzyme is only found in the liver and is estimated if there is doubt as to whether the alkaline phosphatase is of bony or hepatic origin. This may be required in children and patients with malignancy. Serum transaminases, such as aspartate aminotransferase, show only modest elevation in contrast to the rises which occur in hepatitis. The serum cholesterol concentration rises and may cause abnormalities of red cell shape (target cells) (see Section 22). A raised concentration of serum bile acids is a sensitive index of biliary disease. A prolonged prothrombin time reflects intestinal malabsorption of fat-soluble vitamin K owing to a lack of bile acids. Vitamin A and D deficiency may also develop. The serum albumin and gammaglobulin levels are normal until biliary cirrhosis develops.

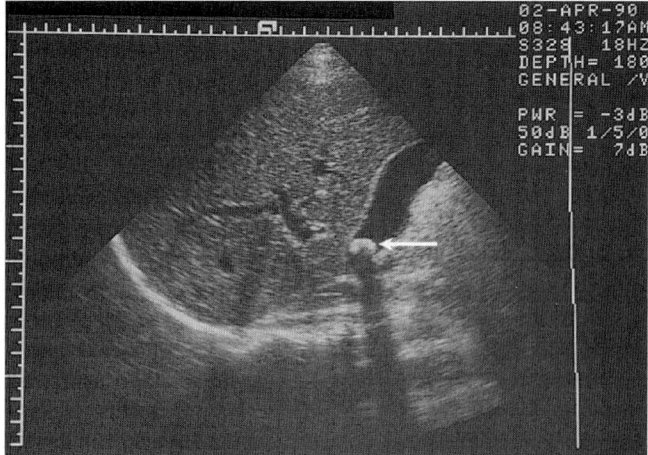

Fig. 15.23.2 Ultrasound scan of the gallbladder shows gallstones (arrowed) as bright round objects which cast acoustic shadows.

A polymorphonuclear leucocytosis accompanies bacterial infections of the biliary system.

Imaging techniques

A plain radiograph of the abdomen may reveal an enlarged liver, calcified gallstones, or air in the biliary tree. Plain radiographs of the abdomen are now rarely done. The preferred first investigation is ultrasonography (Fig. 15.23.2). CT and MRI are used in complicated diagnostic problems. These tests reveal dilated bile ducts and may also indicate the position of the obstruction in the biliary tree and dense structures such as gallstones. Hepatic scintiscanning with 99Tcm-labelled HIDA (dimethyl acetanilide iminodiacetic acid) is an alternative and is of value in the diagnosis of acute cholecystitis. Oral cholecystograms are rarely done nowadays but are useful to determine whether the gallbladder is functioning in patients with gallstones being assessed for oral bile acid dissolution therapy (see below). Intravenous cholangiography is obsolete. However, these noninvasive investigations usually provide insufficient anatomical detail for diagnosis or planning of treatment. A further cholangiographic technique such as magnetic resonance cholangiography (MRC), percutaneous transhepatic cholangiography (PTC), or endoscopic retrograde cholangiopancreatography (ERCP) is necessary. MRC is now the preferred investigation in the first instance. The quality of MRC images now approaches that of ERCP and PTC (Fig. 15.23.3). ERCP and PTC are usually reserved for patients in whom MRC fails and for therapeutic interventions. ERCP and PTC carry small risks including haemorrhage, biliary peritonitis, and cholangitis (with PTC), and bowel perforation, cholangitis, and pancreatitis (with ERCP). Should cholangiography reveal a normal biliary system in a jaundiced patient, a liver biopsy is indicated. Endoscopic ultrasound (EUS) is a new technique which appears to have promise in biliary disease.

This diagnostic approach is ideal but expensive both in terms of human and material resources. The apparatus required is costly and procedures such as ERCP require considerable expertise. Obviously local factors will determine the diagnostic pathway that is adopted. Nevertheless, these techniques have revolutionized the management of patients with biliary disease. It is now a routine matter to achieve a precise diagnosis rapidly. In addition, a series of nonoperative therapeutic options with ERCP ranging from the introduction of endoprostheses for the management of benign and

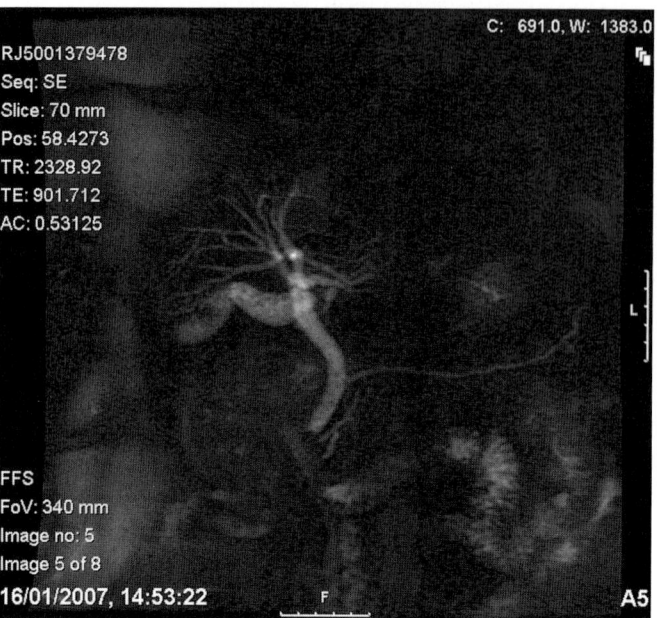

Fig. 15.23.3 Magnetic resonance cholangiogram (MRC) shows gallstones in the gallbladder and common bile duct.
(Courtesy of Professor W Gedroyc.)

malignant biliary structures to endoscopic sphincterotomy for the removal of the biliary calculi are direct consequences of these diagnostic approaches.

Bile composition and gallstone formation

Bile composition

Bile is secreted by the hepatocytes and its water and electrolyte composition altered during its passage down the biliary system. Between meals much of the bile is diverted to the gallbladder where it is concentrated by the removal of sodium, chloride, bicarbonate, and water. In response to food, the gallbladder contracts, emptying bile into the duodenum. Apart from water (97%) the major components of bile are bile acids, phospholipids, and cholesterol. Bile is also the major excretory route of other compounds including bilirubin and certain drugs and their metabolites. Cholesterol is insoluble in water but is held in solution by the detergent action of bile acids with the aid of phospholipids.

Cholesterol is synthesized primarily in the liver and small intestine. The rate-limiting enzyme for cholesterol production is hydroxymethylglutaryl-CoA reductase (EC 1.1.1.34), which catalyses the first step, the conversion of acetate to mevalonate. Subsequently, nonesterified (free) cholesterol is secreted into bile. Dietary cholesterol also contributes to biliary cholesterol secretion. The control of cholesterol metabolism is complex. It is not yet clear what proportion of biliary cholesterol is derived from circulating lipoproteins and what proportion is newly synthesized by the liver.

The primary bile acids, cholic and chenodeoxycholic acid, are synthesized in the liver from cholesterol. The economy of the bile acid pool is preserved by efficient reabsorption, principally in the terminal ileum. About 95% of the bile acids are reabsorbed and pass back to the liver in the portal venous system (enterohepatic circulation). The remainder enters the colon where bacteria form the secondary bile acids, deoxycholic and lithocholic acid, from cholic and chenodeoxycholic acid, respectively. Some of the secondary bile acids are absorbed from the colon but most are excreted in the faeces. The normal bile acid pool is about 3 to 5 g and circulates 6 to 10 times each day. Synthesis is controlled by the negative feedback of bile acids returning in the portal venous blood which act on the rate-limiting hepatic enzyme, cholesterol-7α-hydroxylase (EC 1.14.13.17). The principal phospholipid in bile is lecithin. It is produced in the liver and secreted into the bile. In the intestine lecithin is hydrolysed to lysolecithin by pancreatic phospholipase and is subsequently reabsorbed.

Above a certain level (the critical micellar concentration) bile acids coalesce to form micelles that have a hydrophilic external surface and hydrophobic internal surface. Cholesterol is incorporated into the hydrophobic interior. Phospholipids are inserted into the micellar wall so that the micelles are enlarged; these 'mixed micelles' are thus able to hold more cholesterol.

Consequently, the solubility of cholesterol in bile depends on the concentrations of bile acid and phospholipid. In the presence of a relative excess of bile acids and phospholipid (on a molar basis) the cholesterol-holding capacity of bile is increased and it is said to be unsaturated. However, if there are insufficient micelles of bile acid and phospholipid to hold the cholesterol, the solution is referred to as saturated and the excess cholesterol tends to precipitate. With a knowledge of the molar concentration of cholesterol, phospholipid, and bile acids, the cholesterol saturation of bile can be predicted using triangular coordinate diagrams.

Gallstone formation

Gallstone disease is common and afflicts between 10 and 20% of the world's population. Gallstones are classified according to their composition into two main groups: cholesterol stones and bile pigment stones. Cholesterol stones are composed mainly of cholesterol (>70%) and can be subdivided into pure cholesterol stones (usually solitary) and mixed stones which contain cholesterol in a matrix of calcium bilirubinate, calcium phosphate, and protein (Figs. 15.23.4 and 15.23.5). Mixed stones are usually multiple and faceted. Bile pigment stones can also be divided into two main groups. Brown pigment stones are soft and friable and consist of calcium bilirubinate, cholesterol, and calcium soaps. Pure pigment stones ('black stones') are black, hard, and brittle and contain an insoluble black pigment, calcium bilirubinate, calcium carbonate and phosphate, calcium salts of fatty acids, and bile acids. All pigment stones contain a large amount of mucoprotein matrix (up to 70%). Gallstones are rare before the age of 10 years. The incidence increases progressively with age. Cholesterol gallstones account for about 75% of the gallstones in Europe and the United States of America.

Cholesterol gallstones

Cholesterol gallstones result from the secretion of cholesterol-saturated bile by the liver. The cause of the saturation is unclear. Patients with gallstones usually have a smaller bile acid pool than controls and it circulates more frequently. The rapid recycling of bile acids may be responsible for the smaller bile acid pool by excessive inhibition of the enzyme that controls bile acid synthesis, cholesterol-7α-hydroxylase. However, diminished bile acid synthesis is probably not the most important factor in the production of saturated bile. This appears to be an elevated biliary cholesterol secretion rate, due either to increased hepatic cholesterol synthesis or to increased transfer of plasma lipoprotein cholesterol into bile. Nevertheless, saturated bile may be encountered in

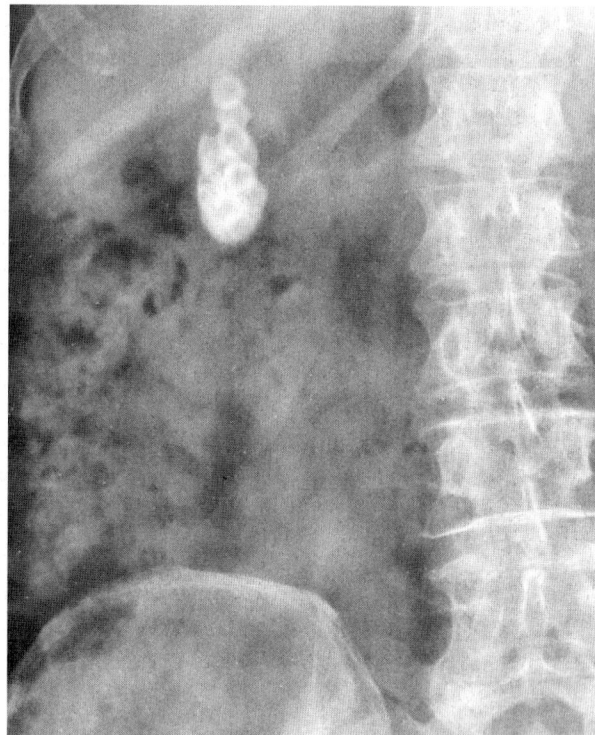

Fig. 15.23.4 Calcified gallstones. Gallstones contain sufficient calcium to be visible on a plain abdominal radiograph in about 10% of patients. The gallbladder stones are surrounded by a ring of calcium salts.
(From Sherlock S, Summerfield JA (1979). *A colour atlas of liver disease*, Wolfe Medical Publications, London, with permission.)

normal subjects, especially during fasting. It is therefore likely that other factors such as the condition of the gallbladder, the mechanism of seeding (nucleation) of gallstones, and the control of gallstone growth are important. Furthermore, racial differences, advancing age, female sex, obesity, diet, drugs (such as the

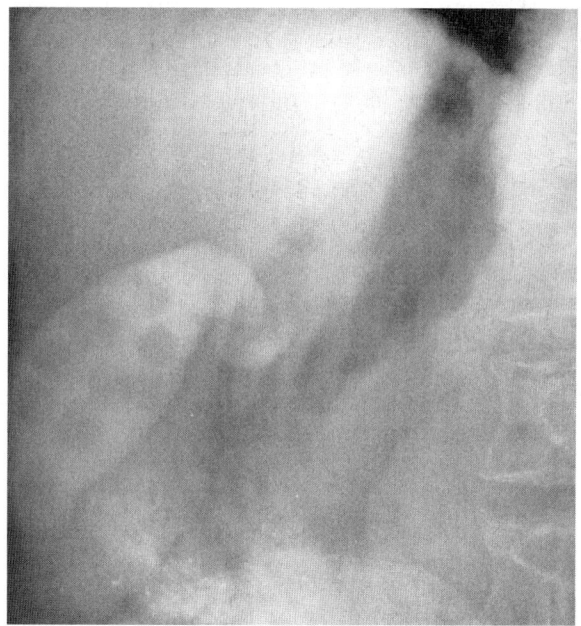

Fig. 15.23.5 Cholesterol gallstones. An intravenous cholangiogram has opacified the gallbladder showing multiple faceted radiolucent gallstones. These are typical features of cholesterol stones.

contraceptive pill and clofibrate), and gastrointestinal disease (such as Crohn's disease) are known to have a significant influence on the development of gallstones.

Bile pigment gallstones

In contrast to cholesterol stones, little is known of the aetiology of bile pigment stones. The soft, friable, brown-pigmented stones are especially common in the east Asia and are associated with *Escherichia coli*, bacteroides, and clostridium infection of the biliary tract. It is probable that these bacteria contribute to stone formation by producing β-glucuronidase that deconjugates bilirubin diglucuronide to form free unconjugated bilirubin. This combines with calcium to form sparingly soluble calcium bilirubinate that precipitates.

The black, hard, and brittle pure-pigment stones are the type commonly encountered in the West. The incidence of pure pigment stones increases with age and they are found in patients with cirrhosis, chronic bile duct obstruction (such as biliary strictures), chronic haemolytic anaemias including haemolysis induced by prosthetic heart valves, and malaria. Pure pigment stones affect both sexes equally. The mechanism of stone production is unclear, but does not appear to be due to cholesterol saturation of hepatic or gallbladder bile. About 50% of all pigment stones are radio-opaque and they account for about 70% of all opaque stones.

Natural history of gallstones

The majority of gallstones remain in the gallbladder (cholelithiasis) and may give rise to no symptoms ('silent' gallstones), being discovered incidentally during investigation or at autopsy. Impaction of a gallstone in the neck of the gallbladder results in gallbladder inflammation and the symptoms and signs of acute or chronic cholecystitis. Acute cholecystitis will subside if the stone spontaneously disempacts, or may progress to gangrene and perforation of the gallbladder or empyema of the gallbladder. Gallstones may pass through the cystic duct into the bile duct (choledocholithiasis), resulting in biliary obstruction and jaundice. Bacterial infection (cholangitis) commonly accompanies choledocholithiasis and can lead to a liver abscess. Gallstones may perforate through the inflamed gallbladder wall to form an internal fistula, usually to the small intestine or colon. A large gallstone passing into the small intestine may impact in the ileum resulting in intestinal obstruction (gallstone ileus). Finally, surgical treatment for gallstones, while usually curative, may result in a postcholecystectomy syndrome or a benign stricture of the bile duct.

Treatment

The usual treatment for gallstones remains cholecystectomy although medical treatments may be employed in selected patients (see below). The advent of laparoscopic cholecystectomy has swung the balance in favour of surgery since this technique carries so little morbidity and a very short hospital stay. Treatment is obviously indicated for symptomatic gallstones and for their complications. However, in patients in whom 'silent' gallstones are discovered incidentally and in patients with minimal symptoms it is by no means clear that treatment is always the best solution. The problem revolves around the probability of serious complications in the future. It is appropriate to offer treatment to young patients (who, with many years ahead of them, will have a greater likelihood of developing the complications of gallstones) and to advise against

treatment in older people with other major medical problems. However, in fit middle-aged patients with no or minimal symptoms it is reasonable to tell the patient of the finding and to withhold surgery until it is warranted by symptoms or complications.

Gallstone dissolution and disruption

Cholesterol gallstones can be removed from the gallbladder and bile ducts in a proportion of patients by medical treatments. These techniques avoid the discomfort, disability, and risks of general anaesthesia and surgical exploration of the abdomen and bile ducts. However, with the widespread availability of laparoscopic cholecystectomy these techniques are now used rarely. There are two types of medical method: chemical agents that dissolve gallstones, and physical methods such as endoscopic sphincterotomy and extracorporeal shock-wave lithotripsy (ESWL). Judicious combinations of chemical and physical methods yield the best results.

Chemical methods

Oral bile acid therapy

Oral treatment with chenodeoxycholic acid or ursodeoxycholic acid can dissolve cholesterol gallstones. These bile acids, normal constituents of bile, reduce the cholesterol saturation of bile and result in the leaching of cholesterol from gallstones. They act by reducing the hepatic synthesis and biliary excretion of cholesterol. Ursodeoxycholic acid has advantages over chenodeoxycholic acid in that it does not cause diarrhoea or elevations of serum transaminases. These bile acids differ in the way that they remove cholesterol from gallstones and have been shown to dissolve gallstones better in combination than singly. Combination therapy is the preferred treatment.

Contact dissolution of gallstones

Cholesterol stones in the gallbladder can be dissolved by the direct instillation of methyl tertbutyl ether (MTBE) into the gallbladder via a percutaneous catheter. MTBE is a foul-smelling, volatile, inflammable colourless substance that remains liquid at body temperature. The gallbladder is catheterized by the transhepatic route, entering it through the area of attachment of the gallbladder to the liver and MTBE is continually infused and aspirated with vigour until the stones have disappeared (which typically takes 5–7 h).

Physical methods

Extracorporeal shock-wave lithotripsy (EWSL)

This is a noninvasive and safe but expensive way of rapidly shattering gallstones into a coarse powder. The gallbladder must contain no more than three stones to allow accurate focusing of the shock waves.

Endoscopic sphincterotomy

Endoscopic sphincterotomy can remove gallstones from the bile duct. The bile duct is entered by a cannula passed via a duodenoscope and the bile duct is opened by diathermy cutting of the ampulla of Vater. Stones are removed by balloon or wire catheters.

Patient selection and results

Medical treatment with oral bile acid therapy, ESWL, or contact dissolution is suitable for patients with cholesterol gallstones in a functioning gallbladder (as judged by an oral cholecystogram). Calcified gallstones do not dissolve. Radiolucent gallstones are usually, but not always, composed of cholesterol. CT scans are useful for detecting low levels of gallstone calcification. These treatments should be reserved for patients with mild or no symptoms in whom the risk of cholecystectomy is high, including those with pre-existing disease, older people, and very obese individuals. They are also of value in patients who refuse surgery. Drugs which increase the cholesterol saturation of bile should be avoided; these include oestrogens, the oral contraceptive pill, and clofibrate.

Oral bile acid therapy is protracted but safe. It dissolves gallstones in about 25% of patients fulfilling the selection criteria by 6 months. It should not be taken during pregnancy. The preferred treatment is combination therapy with chenodeoxycholic acid (7 mg/kg) and ursodeoxycholic acid (7 mg/kg). Proprietary combination tablets are available. Gallstone dissolution usually requires 6 to 24 months of therapy depending on stone size. Oral cholecystograms are performed every 6 months to assess progress. Combining oral bile acid therapy with ESWL speeds up the process greatly: gallstones will be cleared in more than 90% of patients within 18 months. Furthermore, slightly calcified gallstones can be treated in this way. MTBE therapy is invasive and the ether is unpleasant to use, but dissolution is rapid. Endoscopic sphincterotomy removes gallstones from the common bile duct. Any type of stone can be removed up to about 20 mm in diameter.

Side effects and toxicity

The most frequent side effect of oral bile acid therapy is diarrhoea. It is dose related and usually mild and transient. It can be minimized by slowly increasing the dose to the required level. Transient elevations of serum transaminase activity are also common; liver function tests should be monitored. Ursodeoxycholic acid may cause calcification of gallstones. Gallstone recurrence remains a major problem with oral bile acid therapy. About 30% of patients will have had a recurrence 1 year after gallstone dissolution. Unwanted effects of ESWL include biliary colic, skin petechias, and haematuria. The principal unwanted side effects of MTBE are sedation, burning upper abdominal pain, nausea, and vomiting. Endoscopic sphincterotomy can cause gastrointestinal haemorrhage and acute pancreatitis.

Acute cholecystitis

Aetiology

Acute cholecystitis is associated with gallstones in over 90% of patients. It follows the impaction of a gallstone in the cystic duct. Continued secretion by the gallbladder leads to a rise in pressure. Inflammation of the gallbladder wall results from the toxic effects of the retained bile and bacterial infection. The gallbladder bile is usually turbid but may become frank pus (empyema of the gallbladder). Intestinal organisms, especially anaerobes, are commonly cultured from the gallbladder. Ischaemia in the distended gallbladder wall may lead to infarction and perforation. Generalized peritonitis may follow, but the leak is usually localized to form a chronic abscess cavity. Some patients have repeated attacks of acute cholecystitis which are probably exacerbations of chronic cholecystitis. Acute cholecystitis in the absence of gallstones (acalculous cholecystitis) is very rare. However, acalculous cholecystitis is a particular problem in patients with AIDS. Cytomegalovirus and cryptosporidium are the most commonly associated organisms in acalculous cholecystitis in AIDS.

Symptoms and signs

The typical patient is an obese middle-aged woman, and the acute attack is often precipitated by a large or fatty meal. However, there are many exceptions to this pattern. The principal symptom is pain, of fairly sudden onset, which is severe, continuous or minimally fluctuating, and localized to the epigastrium or right hypochondrium. The pain often radiates to the back. The constancy of the pain is in contrast to the repeated short bouts of biliary colic. In uncomplicated cases the pain gradually subsides over 12 to 18 h. Flatulence and nausea are common, but persistent vomiting suggests the presence of a stone in the common bile duct. Examination reveals an ill, sweating patient with shallow, jerky respiration. Fever indicates a complicating bacterial cholangitis. Jaundice may accompany acute cholecystitis but is usually a sign of a stone in the bile duct. The abdomen moves poorly with respiration. Right hypochondrial tenderness is present and is exacerbated by inspiration (Murphy's sign). Muscle guarding and rebound tenderness are common. The gallbladder is usually impalpable but occasionally a tender mass of omentum and gallbladder may be felt under the liver.

Laboratory investigations

The white cell count is usually moderately elevated ($12–15 \times 10^9$/litre) as a result of a polymorphonuclear leucocytosis. Serum bilirubin concentrations between 17 and 68 μmol/litre (1–4 mg/dl) may be seen in uncomplicated acute cholecystitis, but should raise the suspicion of a stone in the bile duct. Modest rises in the serum alkaline phosphatase, aspartate transaminase, and amylase may also be seen. An abdominal radiograph will show gallstones in about 10% of patients. Ultrasound scanning of the gallbladder is the preferred first investigation. Scintiscanning with ^{99}Tcm-labelled HIDA provides similar information. It is important to establish the correct diagnosis before starting surgery.

Differential diagnosis

Acute cholecystitis may be confused with other abdominal emergencies including perforated peptic ulcer, acute pancreatitis, retrocaecal appendicitis, perforated carcinoma or diverticulum of the hepatic flexure of the colon, and liver abscess. Cardiac infarction and pneumonia with right-sided pleurisy should also be considered.

Complications

Gangrene of the gallbladder

Pain, tenderness, and fever progressively increasing or persisting for longer than 24 to 48 h are indications of gangrene of the gallbladder. The prognosis is poor if necrosis and perforation occur. In patients who are elderly and obese, perforation of the gallbladder can occur without definite signs. Perforation into an adjacent viscus may produce a cholecystenteric fistula and may lead to gallstone ileus.

Cholangitis

Intermittent high temperatures often accompanied by rigors indicate bacterial infection of the bile duct and usually follow the passage of a stone into the bile duct.

Treatment

In most patients acute cholecystitis subsides in a few days with conservative treatment. Cholecystectomy is performed either a few days after the symptoms have settled or 2 to 3 months later. In the latter event, if the symptoms recur during the interval, cholecystectomy is performed without delay. Immediate surgery is mandatory if signs of gangrene or perforation develop.

Conservative treatment

Oral feeding is stopped. Intravenous fluids, and analgesia with nalbuphine or pethidine (demerol) and atropine are administered. Antibiotics are given to all but the most mild cases; tetracycline, amoxicillin, or a cephalosporin are satisfactory for general use. The patient should be observed frequently with abdominal examination and sequential leucocyte counts to detect signs of gangrene of the gallbladder or cholangitis.

Surgical treatment

Cholecystectomy is the operation of choice. Laparoscopic cholecystectomy is the preferred approach. About 10% of patients with acute cholecystitis will have stones in the common bile duct. The bile ducts should be assessed by MRC or ERCP and bile duct stones removed by endoscopic sphincterotomy. If an open cholecystectomy is performed, intraoperative cholangiography may be performed to determine whether bile duct stones are present. In high-risk patients and when technical difficulties are encountered a cholecystotomy may be performed.

Chronic cholecystitis

This is the most common form of gallbladder disease that results from gallstones. Pathologically it is characterized by chronic inflammation and thickening of the gallbladder wall. In addition to stones the gallbladder may contain brown sediment ('biliary mud'). A proportion of these patients have cholesterolosis of the gallbladder ('strawberry gallbladder'). This describes the deposition of yellow specks of cholesterol in the pink gallbladder wall and is a consequence of cholesterol-saturated bile. Cholesterolosis of the gallbladder is asymptomatic but about one-half of the patients develop gallstones. Chronic cholecystitis usually develops insidiously but may follow an attack of acute cholecystitis.

Symptoms and signs

Some patients complain of bouts of constant right hypochondrial or epigastric pain. If it is intermittent, that is, biliary colic, the height of the pain is separated by 15- to 60-min intervals. The pain may last several hours or be as brief as 15 to 20 min. It may radiate to the right shoulder or the back. More commonly the symptoms are vague and ill-defined and include abdominal discomfort and distension, nausea, flatulence, and intolerance of fatty foods. Unfortunately, many patients who do not have chronic cholecystitis complain of these symptoms. Examination of the abdomen may reveal tenderness over the gallbladder and a positive Murphy's sign. Laboratory investigations are usually unhelpful.

Imaging techniques

An ultrasound scan is used to detect gallstones. A plain radiograph of the abdomen may reveal calcified stones or opacification of the gallbladder caused by high concentrations of calcium carbonate ('limey bile') but is not often used now. If these investigations fail to show stones, but stones are still suspected on clinical grounds, an MRC or ERCP should be performed before surgery is undertaken.

Differential diagnosis

Dyspepsia and fat intolerance are common symptoms that may be caused by many conditions including peptic ulcers, hiatus hernia, irritable bowel syndrome, chronic relapsing pancreatitis, and tumours of the stomach, pancreas, colon, or gallbladder. Other functional disorders may also mimic chronic cholecystitis.

Complications

The complications of chronic cholecystitis include acute exacerbations (acute cholecystitis), passage of stones into the bile duct (choledocholithiasis or Mirizzi's syndrome), pancreatitis, cholecystenteric fistula formation and gallstone ileus, and rarely carcinoma of the gallbladder. Occasionally the accumulation of mucus and gallstones produces hydrops of the gallbladder, which is characterized by a tender mass without the symptoms of acute cholecystitis.

Treatment

In established cases of chronic cholecystitis the treatment of choice is cholecystectomy. When the diagnosis is in doubt, especially when vague symptoms are associated with a well-functioning gallbladder containing stones, a conservative approach is worth trying. This includes weight reduction and a low-fat diet, especially if fatty food is associated with the symptoms. Oral bile acid therapy may also be considered (see above).

Prognosis

Chronic cholecystitis carries a good prognosis. Cholecystectomy is curative and should have a mortality below 1%. However, if cholecystectomy is performed indiscriminately on patients with 'dyspeptic' symptoms who happen to have incidental gallstones, the results will be unpredictable and often unsatisfactory.

Choledocholithiasis

Most stones in the common bile duct originate in the gallbladder. About 15% of patients with cholelithiasis have common duct stones. This proportion rises with age so that nearly 50% of elderly patients with cholelithiasis may have common duct stones. Stones may develop in the bile duct in diseases causing chronic biliary obstruction such as benign bile duct strictures and sclerosing cholangitis.

Clinical features

The classic triad of symptoms is right upper abdominal pain, jaundice, and fever. The abdominal pain is typically colicky, severe, and persists for hours. It is often associated with vomiting. Fever and rigors indicate cholangitis, which commonly accompanies bile duct stones. Jaundice is variable; it may be mild or deep and is often intermittent. The urine is dark due to conjugated bilirubin and the faeces are pale. Frequently, the amount of pigment in the faeces varies. Itching may be prominent. However, common bile duct stones may also be silent, especially in older people. Alternatively, only one of the triad of symptoms may be present; the patient presenting with jaundice, abdominal pain, or cholangitis. The liver is moderately enlarged and there may be tenderness in the right upper quadrant. Prolonged biliary obstruction lasting months or years eventually leads to biliary cirrhosis with portal venous hypertension and liver cell failure.

Laboratory investigations

Liver function tests show a cholestatic (biliary obstructive) pattern. The prothrombin time may be prolonged due to inadequate absorption of vitamin K. A polymorphonuclear leucocytosis is common and indicates biliary infection. Blood cultures should be performed repeatedly during the fevers to isolate the organism and determine sensitivities.

Imaging techniques

A plain radiograph of the abdomen will show calcified gallstones in 10% of patients, but is rarely performed now. Ultrasonography is useful for demonstrating the dilated biliary tree that results from obstruction and may reveal biliary gallstones. Unfortunately, an ultrasound scan frequently fails to detect common duct stones obstructing the lower end of the bile duct. Cholangiography by MRC or ERCP is required in these patients (Fig. 15.23.6). Common bile duct stones should be removed by endoscopic sphincterotomy before the patient is submitted to cholecystectomy.

Differential diagnosis

Common duct stones are the most common cause of cholestatic (biliary obstructive) jaundice. Next in frequency are carcinomas of the head of the pancreas, bile duct, and ampulla of Vater (Box 15.23.1). Intrahepatic diseases may also cause a cholestatic jaundice; the causes include viral and alcoholic hepatitis, drugs, and pregnancy.

Treatment

Common bile duct stones must be removed. The optimal treatment is endoscopic sphincterotomy to remove bile duct stones

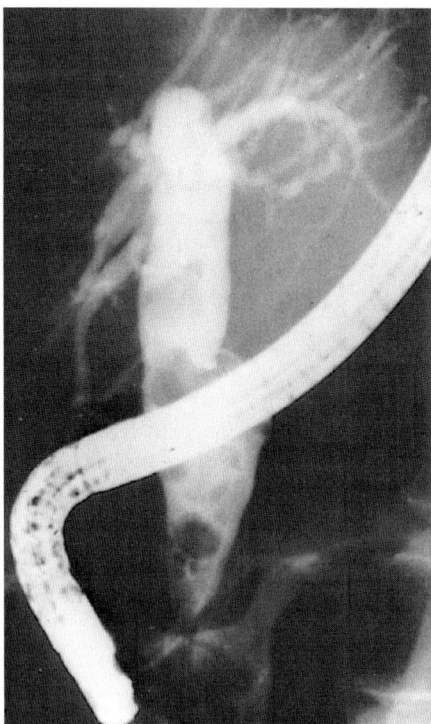

Fig. 15.23.6 Choledocholithiasis. An endoscopic retrograde cholangiogram shows multiple faceted radiolucent stones in a dilated bile duct. The gallbladder has not been opacified.

Box 15.23.1 Causes of bile duct obstruction

Intrinsic causes
- Common bile duct gallstones
- Cholangitis
- Carcinoma of the bile duct
- Carcinoma of the gallbladder
- Benign post-traumatic stricture
- Sclerosing cholangitis (primary and secondary)
- Haemobilia

Extrinsic causes
- Carcinoma of the pancreas
- Carcinoma of the ampulla of Vater
- Metastatic carcinoma
- Lymphoma
- Pancreatitis (acute and chronic)
- Pancreatic cysts

Congenital causes
- Biliary atresia
- Choledochal cyst
- Congenital intrahepatic biliary dilatation (Caroli's disease)

---

followed by laparoscopic cholecystectomy. This approach avoids the hazards of open exploration of the common bile duct. Endoscopic removal of common duct gallstones without cholecystectomy is appropriate in patients unfit for surgery. Few patients will have further problems from the gallbladder that remains. Stones overlooked at surgery (residual calculi) are best treated by endoscopic sphincterotomy or, if a T-tube is in place, removed by a steerable basket catheter manipulated down the T-tube track. Open exploration of the common bile duct is required if gallstones are too large to be removed endoscopically (>2 cm). Preoperative preparation includes appropriate antibiotics for cholangitis, the correction of fluid and electrolyte balance, nutrition, and anaemia, and if the prothrombin time is prolonged, parenteral vitamin K.

Postcholecystectomy syndromes

After cholecystectomy a proportion of patients continue to complain of symptoms such as right upper quadrant pain, flatulence, and fatty food intolerance. However, the vast majority of patients with gallstones are improved by surgery. The persistence of symptoms in many is probably a consequence of the wrong diagnosis being made before surgery, and other diseases such as oesophagitis, pancreatitis, or functional bowel disease should be sought. In others, technical problems during surgery may have resulted in a benign post-traumatic biliary stricture or residual calculi. However, there remains a group of patients where the cause appears to be due to less common biliary disorders such as long, dilated cystic duct remnants, amputation neuromas of the cystic duct, and spasm or stenosis of the sphincter of Oddi. The biliary tract must be carefully investigated in these patients, especially if colicky pain, fever, jaundice, or cholestatic liver function tests persist. Biliary tract manometry is of value when spasm or stenosis of the sphincter of Oddi is suspected.

Biliary infections

Bacterial cholangitis (suppurative cholangitis)

This is usually associated with common bile duct calculi and benign biliary structures. Malignant strictures produce complete obstruction and the bile remains sterile. Other conditions associated with cholangitis are biliary enteric fistulas—both spontaneous and surgical—sclerosing cholangitis, and congenital intrahepatic biliary dilation (Caroli's disease). Organisms of the gut flora are usually cultured in these infections, including aerobes such as *E. coli*, *Streptococcus faecalis*, *Proteus vulgaris* and staphylococci, and anaerobes such as bacteroides, aerobacter, and anaerobic steptrococci.

Clinical features and treatment

The onset of malaise, fever, and rigors is followed by pain, vomiting, jaundice, and itching. The urine turns dark and the faeces pale. The biliary obstructive features are probably due to oedema of the bile duct wall. Recurrent attacks are common. Hepatic abscesses may result. Repeated blood cultures are performed during the fever to isolate the organisms. Culture of a liver biopsy fragment may also yield the organism. The main element of treatment is drainage of the biliary tract, which is best achieved by emergency endoscopic sphincterotomy. Additionally, appropriate antibiotics such as cefuroxime and metronidazole are given. For recurrent attacks of cholangitis, tetracycline, amoxicillin, or cephalexin are usually effective.

Infestations

Infestations (see Section 7) with the roundworm *Ascaris lumbricoides* and the liver fluke *Clonorchis sinensis* are particular problems of East Asia. Both lead to cholangitis. *C. sinensis* infestation predisposes to bile duct carcinoma and primary liver cancer. The common sheep fluke *Fasciola hepatica* may be encountered as a cause of cholangitis in Europe during wet summers.

Benign biliary strictures

In about 95% of patients these are a consequence of biliary tract surgery. The remainder are caused by gallstones eroding the bile duct and, rarely, blunt injury to the abdomen. Signs of biliary stricture may be detected in the immediate postoperative period but are often delayed. Disasters such as ligation or section of the bile duct present early with jaundice and drainage of bile from the wound drains. With lesser damage to the duct the patient presents after an interval with cholangitis and jaundice. Liver function tests reveal a cholestatic pattern and blood cultures may yield an organism. The precise delineation of the stricture requires MRC, ERCP or PTC. Biliary stricture is not a benign condition; untreated, it will usually progress to biliary cirrhosis with portal venous hypertension and liver failure. Treatment is surgical and should be performed by a surgeon skilled in this difficult repair.

Malignant biliary stricture

This is most commonly due to adenocarcinoma of the head of the pancreas but may also be caused by adenocarcinomas of the bile

ducts, of the ampulla of Vater, and rarely of the gallbladder. Occasionally the cause is lymph node enlargement at the porta hepatis due to malignant metastases or lymphoma.

Symptoms and signs

Cancers of the pancreas and biliary tree (Figs. 15.23.7 and 15.23.8) usually affect middle-aged and elderly individuals. The onset is insidious, with deepening jaundice, itching, and weight loss. A dull, nagging upper abdominal pain which radiates to the back is common. In contrast to choledocholithiasis and benign strictures, cholangitis is unusual. Examination reveals a deeply jaundiced patient often excoriated from scratching. The liver is enlarged but not tender. If the malignant obstruction is below the level of the cystic duct, the gallbladder is distended and may be palpable (Courvoisier's law). The urine is dark and the stools pale. In cancer of the ampulla of Vater, a film of blood on the pale stool may give it a silvery colour ('silver stools').

Laboratory investigation

Liver function tests reveal a cholestatic pattern. The serum bilirubin may be very high (600 µmol/litre; 35 mg/dl). A microcytic hypochromic anaemia indicates blood loss from the tumour.

Imaging techniques

An ultrasound or CT scan examination will reveal dilatation of the biliary tree and may demonstrate the level of the obstruction. Ultrasound-guided percutaneous needle biopsy may be employed

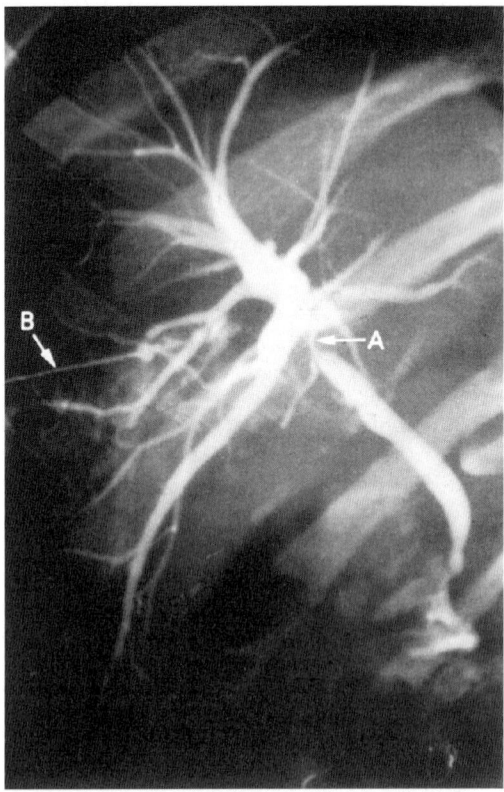

Fig. 15.23.7 Carcinoma of the bile duct. A percutaneous transhepatic cholangiogram (PTC) shows a stricture (a) high in the bile duct at the porta hepatis intrahepatic bile ducts are moderately dilated. The transhepatic track of the 'skinny' needle used for the PTC is also visible (b).

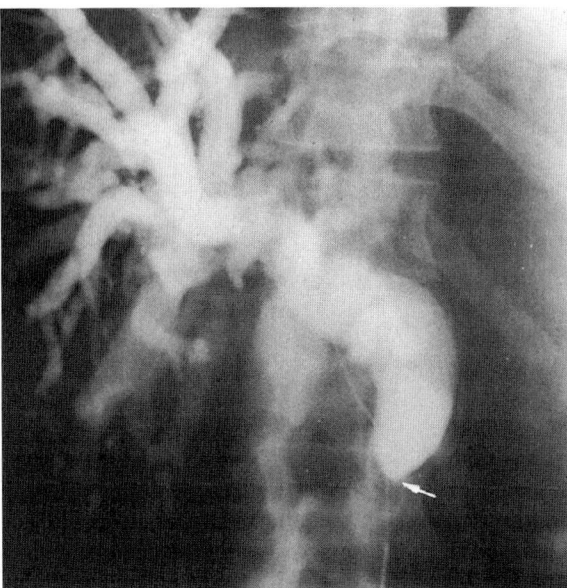

Fig. 15.23.8 Carcinoma of the pancreas. The percutaneous transhepatic cholangiogram shows a very dilated biliary tree which terminates in a blunt 'nipple-like' obstruction (arrow) at the lower end of the common bile duct. This is the usual finding in the cancers of the head of the pancreas which obstruct the bilary system.

to provide a histological diagnosis. Bile duct carcinoma frequently causes obstruction at the porta hepatis and, consequently, at laparotomy the extrahepatic biliary tract appears nondilated. Even if operative cholangiography is performed, the constrast medium frequently fails to pass the obstruction and fill the dilated intrahepatic biliary tree. Therefore it is important to establish the diagnosis precisely before surgery is contemplated by performing an MRC, ERCP or PTC. This is particularly important because most of these patients are best treated by endoscopic or percutaneous biliary stents rather than surgery (see below).

Treatment

Occasionally, small tumours confined to the head of the pancreas and ampulla of Vater may be treated curatively by a Whipple's operation. Unfortunately the great majority of pancreatic and bile duct cancers can only be treated palliatively with a bypass procedure such as a cholecystojejunostomy. The prognosis for these patients is poor. An alternative treatment is endoscopic or percutaneous transhepatic introduction of prostheses (stents) through the biliary stricture. Patients with endoscopic prostheses have the same median survival as those with surgical bypass procedures, but the operative mortality and morbidity rate is much lower for endoscopic prostheses. Endoscopic prostheses are the preferred treatment for unresectable biliary and pancreatic cancers. The prostheses may block after about 3 months and need to be replaced.

Other causes of bile duct obstruction

Pancreatitis may obstruct the common bile duct during its passage through the head of the pancreas. Transient jaundice is common in acute pancreatitis due to compression by pancreatic oedema.

In chronic pancreatitis, especially alcoholic, persistent jaundice can develop requiring a surgical bypass procedure such as a cholecysto-jejunostomy. This biliary obstruction is probably a consequence of pancreatic fibrosis. Pancreatic cysts may rarely cause extrinsic compression of the bile duct. Haemobilia or haemorrhage into the biliary tract is uncommon but may follow trauma, liver biopsy, biliary tumours, and gallstones. In addition to jaundice, the blood clots cause biliary pain. Massive gastrointestinal haemorrhage may occur. The diagnosis of these conditions relies on accurate cholangiography (usually MRC or ERCP).

Sclerosing cholangitis

Sclerosing cholangitis is the description applied to multiple strictures and bead-like dilatations of the intrahepatic and extrahepatic biliary tree.

Primary sclerosing cholangitis (Fig. 15.23.9)

This should only be diagnosed if the following criteria are satisfied: (1) absence of gallstones; (2) absence of previous biliary surgery; and (3) sufficiently long follow-up to exclude carcinoma of the bile duct. Primary sclerosing cholangitis affects men more than women (2:1) and about 70% of patients have ulcerative colitis. The usual clinical presentation is cholestatic jaundice and cholangitis. However, a significant proportion of patients are asymptomatic or present with cirrhosis and portal venous hypertension. There is associated retroperitoneal fibrosis or Riedel's thyroiditis in some cases. Serum biochemistry shows cholestatic liver function tests. A raised serum alkaline phosphatase is almost invariable. Consequently the diagnosis should be considered in patients with cirrhosis whose liver function tests show cholestatic features. The IgM concentration is commonly elevated. Liver biopsy may be

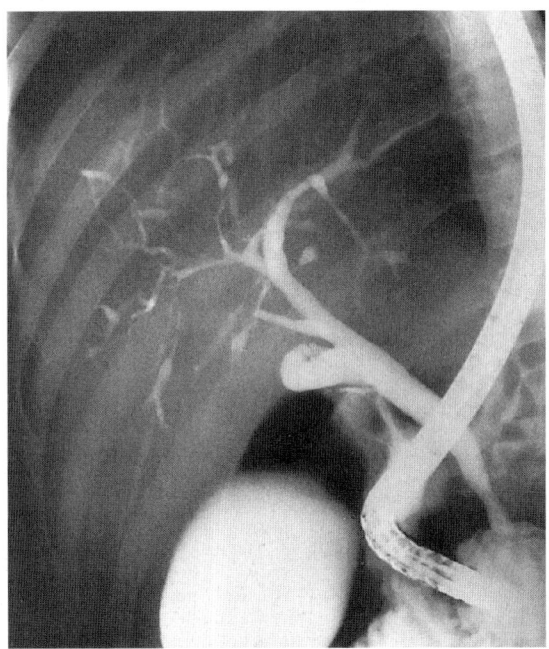

Fig. 15.23.9 Primary sclerosing cholangitis. The intrahepatic bile ducts show alternate strictures and dilatations ('beading'). The common bile duct, cystic duct, and gallbladder appear normal in this study but may also be involved.

helpful and usually indicates large bile duct obstruction. The diagnosis is established by cholangiography with ERCP or PTC. Laparotomy should not be performed. Lone tight strictures and stones can be treated by endoscopic techniques. Primary sclerosing cholangitis is being recognized more frequently as a result of the widespread use of ERCP and PTC. It may be confused with primary biliary cirrhosis, but the serum mitochondrial antibody is always negative in primary sclerosing cholangitis. Treatment is unsatisfactory, neither corticosteroids nor azathioprine are of proven value. Ursodeoxycholic acid improves liver function tests but has not been shown to prolong survival. Pruritus may be helped by cholestyramine. The prognosis is variable but most patients eventually develop cirrhosis and liver failure. Liver transplantation yields excellent results in these patients. Bile duct adenocarcinoma is a late complication.

Secondary sclerosing cholangitis

Several causes of secondary sclerosing cholangitis are now recognized. These include recurrent bacterial cholangitis due to gallstones or benign biliary strictures. Children with primary immunodeficiency syndromes and patients with AIDS also develop sclerosing cholangitis. Cytomegalovirus and cryptosporidium are the organisms most commonly associated with AIDS-related sclerosing cholangitis. Sclerosing cholangitis may also develop in patients treated by hepatic arterial infusion of cytotoxic drugs and after the introduction of caustics into hydatid cysts.

Congenital disorders of the gallbladder and biliary tract

This subject is discussed in Chapter 15.25.

Further reading

Angulo P, Lindor KD (1999). Primary sclerosing cholangitis. *Hepatology*, **30**, 325–32.

Donovan JM (1999). Physical and metabolic factors in gallstone pathogenesis. *Gastroenterol Clin North Am*, **28**, 75–97.

Ko CW, Lee SP (1999). Gallstone formation. Local factors. *Gastroenterol Clin North Am*, **28**, 99–115.

Martin DJ, Vernon DR, Toouli J (2006). Surgical versus endoscopic treatment of bile duct stones. *Cochrane Database Syst Rev*, **19**, CD003327.

Schiff L, Schiff ER (1993). *Diseases of the liver*, 7th edn. Lippincott, Philadelphia, PA.

Sherlock S, Dooley JS (1997). *Diseases of the liver and biliary system*, 10th edition. Blackwell Scientific Publications, Oxford.

Sherlock S, Summerfield JA (1991). *A colour atlas of liver disease*, 2nd edition. Wolfe Medical Publications, London.

Diseases of the pancreas

Contents

15.24.1 **Acute pancreatitis**

C.W. Imrie and R. Carter

Essentials

Acute pancreatitis affects 300 to 600 new patients per million population per year and is most commonly caused by gallstones or alcohol, but there are many other causes and associations. Careful imaging reveals that most so-called idiopathic acute pancreatitis is due to small (1–3 mm diameter) gallstones.

Typical presentation is with sudden onset of severe upper abdominal pain and vomiting. Diagnosis is made by exclusion of other causes of an acute abdomen and by finding of raised serum amylase (over three times upper limit of normal) and/or lipase (over twice upper limit of normal). CT scanning may reveal pancreatic swelling, fluid collection, and change in density of the gland.

Initial management is with (1) analgesia, with morphine or buprenorphine; (2) ensuring adequate oxygenation, with supplemental oxygen and/or ventilatory support as required; (3) restoration of circulating volume; and (4) grading of severity, for which several scoring systems have been developed, e.g. (a) Glasgow Prognostic Score, (b) modified Marshall critical illness scoring system, which takes account of five elements—blood pressure, arterial oxygenation, neurological function (Glasgow Coma Score), haematological function (platelet count), and renal function (serum creatinine)—to allow early referral of serious cases to high-dependency or intensive care facilities.

Mild acute pancreatitis responds to analgesia and intravenous fluids, and patients rarely need to be in hospital beyond 7 to 10 days. If gallstones have been identified by ultrasound scanning, then laparoscopic or open cholecystectomy (or ERCP sphincterotomy in very frail individuals) should be performed in the same admission to prevent recurrence.

Severe acute pancreatitis is a devastating condition with high mortality (35–55%). Management requires support for respiratory, circulatory, and renal failure, with consideration of the following: (1) ERCP—biliary decompression is of proven benefit in patients with pancreatitis associated with cholangitis (jaundice and pyrexia); (2) antibiotics—should not be given until and unless a specific indication arises; there is no benefit to early initiation of prophylactic antibiotics; (3) nutrition support—the mode does not appear to affect the disease process, but enteral feeding is associated with fewer risks and side effects than total parenteral nutrition; (4) surgical intervention—the indications for this are (a) to establish the diagnosis when this is uncertain, rare nowadays (b) to eradicate gallstones, (c) removal of pus and infected necrotic tissue, and (d) drainage of pseudocysts with solid or semi-solid content (those that are mainly composed of fluid and be drained by endoscopic ultrasound guided endoscopic transmural procedures).

Epidemiology

In different countries incidence figures vary from 40 to 500 new cases of acute pancreatitis per million of the population each year. Data usually derives from hospital record systems and it is important to identify new patients separately from those with recurrent disease. In large population studies from Scotland and Finland the incidence of the disease has risen steadily to the current 400 patients/million per year. A study including data on 84713 patients from 470 Californian hospitals collected from 1992 to 2000 indicated approximately 300 new patients/million per year. A recent epidemiological study utilizing biochemical factors in diagnosis in north-east England, with individual accurate case verification, yielded just over 600 new patients/million per year, probably a more reliable incidence. The disease was most prevalent in those with poorer socioeconomic status, especially associated with alcohol abuse as the cause.

Overall mortality is from 4.0 to 7.5%, highest in those who are over 70 years, obese individuals, and those with comorbidity at the time of onset. In all parts of the world both prospective and retrospective studies record 45 to 50% of deaths as occurring in the initial 2 weeks of illness, with some studies identifying a peak of deaths in the initial 48 h. Death is usually due to multiple organ failure in which respiratory failure predominates.

Aetiology

Aetiological factors and rare associations of acute pancreatitis are listed in Boxes 15.24.1.1 and 15.24.1.2.

Major factors

Biliary disease and alcohol abuse together account for over 80% of patients with acute pancreatitis in most prospective studies.

Gallstones

The increased early use of endoscopic retrograde cholangiopancreatography (ERCP) and endoscopic ultrasound (EUS) results in most so-called idiopathic acute pancreatitis being identified as due to small (1–3 mm diameter) stones, which account for nearly all female

---

Box 15.24.1.2 Rare associations with acute pancreatitis

- Hypothermia
- Sclerosing cholangitis
- α_1-Antitrypsin deficiency
- Pancreatic cancer
- Cancers metastatic to pancreas:
  Renal
  Stomach
  Breast
  Ovarian
  Lung
- Virus infection:
  Hepatitis
  ECHO
- Duodenal reduplication
- Autoimmune pancreatitis

Box 15.24.1.1 Aetiological factors in acute pancreatitis (according to frequency)

Major
- Biliary disease
- Alcohol abuse

Minor
- Post-ERCP
- Blunt trauma
- Coxsackie B virus
- Mumps virus
- Hyperlipoproteinaemia
- Ampullary tumour
- Hyperparathyroidism
- Worm infestation[a]
- Scorpion bites[b]
- Drugs
- Hereditary (trypsinogen gene defects)
- Sphincter of Oddi dysfunction

[a] In South-East Asia.
[b] In Trinidad.
ECRP, endoscopic retrograde cholangiopancreatography

---

patients as well as older males. EUS is both less interventional and more sensitive at detecting these smaller stones than ERCP, but each approach is contingent on the skill of the operator.

Prospective studies in the United Kingdom, without EUS, have revealed that 40 to 65% of patients with pancreatitis have gallstones. In Ohio (United States of America) a similar incidence was reported, and in Argentina over 80% were found to have small gallstones when faecal sieving was employed. Such studies link the passage of small stones migrating from the gallbladder down the common bile duct and into the gut, after usually transient impaction in the ampulla of Vater, with acute pancreatitis. Increased back pressure in the pancreatic duct is likely to be an important element, but other factors are probably also involved.

Eradication of stones nearly always frees the patient from further episodes of acute pancreatitis.

Alcohol

Pancreatitis due to alcohol abuse occurs in over 80% of patients from downtown New York (United States of America), and around 70% in Helsinki (Finland). This association is usually found in young males who drink in excess of 80 g alcohol per day, but anyone having a heavy regular alcohol intake is at risk. Careful investigation of the possibility of small gallstones in these patients is necessary. Some patients have both the most common aetiologies. Alcohol may provoke acute pancreatitis by intracellular lysosomal release modulated through elevations in cytosolic and mitochondrial ionized Ca^{2+} concentration.

Minor factors

Drugs

The drugs most commonly implicated in causing acute pancreatitis are valproic acid, azathioprine, L-asparaginase, and corticosteroids. There is equivocal evidence regarding thiazide and other diuretics. However, unless viral titres have been determined, together with adequate biliary investigations including endoscopic examination of the ampulla of Vater, it is unwise to ascribe acute pancreatitis to a particular drug. Repeat exposure to the same drug again causing acute pancreatitis is the strongest evidence of a direct association.

Viral infection

Viral infection, particularly mumps, Coxsackie B, and viral hepatitis, can cause acute pancreatitis. One clinical feature that may prove useful is prodromal diarrhoea, which is rare in all other types of acute pancreatitis. Of increasing importance in endemic areas are the effects of HIV infection. There are also concerns that some antiretroviral therapy may cause acute pancreatitis.

Pancreatic duct stricture

Benign

A focal area of pancreatic necrosis in a primary attack of acute pancreatitis can cause secondary fibrosis with main duct stricture formation, with segmental 'upstream' recurrent attacks of pancreatitis as a consequence. Stricture dilatation or occasionally surgical decompression or distal pancreatectomy may be required.

Congenital or developmental anatomical abnormalities can present with pancreatitis (choledochal cyst, duodenal duplication, anomalous pancreaticobiliary junction). Pancreas divisum (non-union of main and accessory ducts) occurs in 3 to 5% of people and is not usually a primary cause of pancreatitis.

Tumours

Periampullary adenoma or carcinoma is an important association, best diagnosed by endoscopic biopsy. With the increase in this approach to diagnosis, tumours at or close to the ampulla have been shown to have a greater association (0.4%) with acute pancreatitis than hyperparathyroidism. Effective treatment of the tumour abolishes recurrent attacks. This usually involves surgical resection, but endoscopic laser therapy or endoscopic papillectomy can be effective in older and less fit patients.

Carcinoma of pancreas can occasionally present with clinical acute pancreatitis and other primary tumours metastasizing to the pancreas may present in this way.

Hyperparathyroidism

This is now recognized to be an uncommon accompaniment of acute pancreatitis. Indeed, many of the reported patients have also had gallstones. The association is calculated at 0.1%. Removal of a parathyroid adenoma usually prevents further acute pancreatitis since persistent hypercalcaemia appears to be the provoking factor.

Hyperlipoproteinaemia

Patients with type I and V hyperlipoproteinaemia may develop acute pancreatitis. The significance of this association can be difficult to validate where alcohol ingestion compounds the problem. Those patients with primary hyperlipoproteinaemia with chylomicronaemia and hypertriglyceridaemia are prone to attacks of acute pancreatitis in the absence of alcohol ingestion. Dietary restriction of lipids and various lipid-lowering drugs are valuable in therapy.

Hypothermia

This is an important association in the elderly, when pancreatitis may be associated with myxoedema coma. In younger patients, alcohol abuse may be linked, particularly if patients fall asleep out of doors or in a cold, unheated house. Management is directed at gradual warming and supportive measures for organ compromise (see Chapter 9.5.2).

Hereditary

This condition is increasingly being studied since the 1996 discovery of genetic mutations of the cationic trypsinogen gene (*PRSS1*), which shed light on the mechanism of acute pancreatitis. A Europe-wide study (EUROPAC) has tracked multiple families in the United Kingdom, Germany, and France, and similar work in Japan and the United States of America is ongoing. Somewhat confusingly, the numbering of the two most common defects has altered in the intervening years, with R117H changing to R122H and N211 to N291.

An autosomal dominant family history of pancreatic disease is customary. Severe acute inflammatory changes are rare and diagnosis is often delayed. Patients usually have a long history of recurrent abdominal pain from childhood or adolescence. Changes of chronic fibrosis may be present at diagnosis. Typically chronic pancreatitis is evident by the age of 20 to 40 years, and the risk of pancreatic carcinoma over 60 years is significantly increased.

Mutations in the cystic fibrosis transmembrane conductance regulator gene (*CTFR*) and the pancreatic secretory trypsinogen inhibitor gene (*SPINK1*) are also linked to pancreatitis.

Trauma

Hyperamylasaemia may occur after blunt abdominal trauma, usually from a crush injury to the body of the pancreas against the vertebral column (Fig. 15.24.1.1). The risk of associated injuries to surrounding organs must be considered, and assessment by CT scan is important. When there is transaction of the main pancreatic, therapeutic options include endoscopic transpapillary stenting and distal pancreatectomy. Late presentation is associated with pseudocyst formation due to leakage from the damaged pancreatic duct.

Iatrogenic

Surgical or endoscopic procedures involving the ampulla of Vater can induce pancreatitis. The large decrease in diagnostic ERCP (1% risk of acute pancreatitis) as a result of noninvasive imaging modalities of EUS and magnetic resonance cholangio-pancreatography (MRCP) has reduced the overall incidence of post-procedural acute pancreatitis. The risk of acute pancreatitis increases to 3% where a therapeutic endoscopic sphincterotomy has been performed, and in such patients the potential of iatrogenic duodenal perforation should be explored by CT.

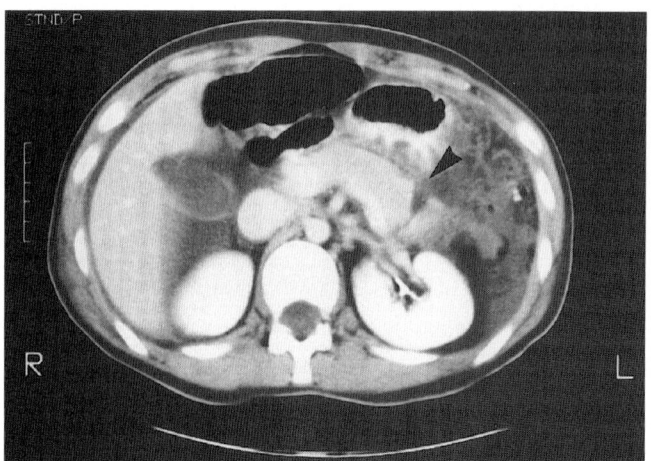

Fig. 15.24.1.1 Blunt trauma causing pancreatitis by transection at the arrowpoint on the CT scan.

Autoimmune pancreatitis

This is a rare condition, which is considered part of the IgG4-related autoimmune disease spectrum and associated with other autoimmune diseases (polyarteritis nodosa, systemic lupus erythematosus, other vasculitides) and inflammatory bowel disease (Crohn's disease and ulcerative colitis). It may present as abdominal pain with obstructive jaundice more typical of chronic than acute pancreatitis. Other features may include: (1) an increased IgG4/IgG ratio in serum; (2) homogeneous gland enlargement with a well-defined edge on CT; (3) periductal lymphoplasmocytic infiltrate on biopsy, which may also be associated with abnormalities in the extrahepatic biliary tree resembling sclerosing cholangitis. Focal autoimmune pancreatitis may prove difficult to differentiate from carcinoma. A good response to steroids is diagnostic.

Worm infestation

Ascaris lumbricoidis within the ampullary area may manifest as acute pancreatitis clinically, and other worms stuck in this area can produce the same effect.

Scorpion bites

Bartholomew showed elegantly that the Trinidad scorpion bite was associated with the production of a clinical episode of acute pancreatitis soon after the victim was bitten. Patients customarily brought the dead scorpion to show the doctor.

Sphincter of Oddi dyskinesia

A few patients present with recurrent abdominal pain associated with raised pressures on sphincter manometry. If this is part of a global gut dysmotility spectrum in an individual patient, then symptoms may originate from motility abnormalities in more than one area of the gastrointestinal tract and division of the sphincter of Oddi may only partly resolve such a person's symptoms. The benefit of intervention is more likely in patients with type 1 Geenan and Hogan sphincter of Oddi dyskinesia (Table 15.24.1.1). Traditional treatment involves endoscopic sphincterotomy, but the risk of post-ERCP pancreatitis in these patients is high (30%). The use of preliminary sphincter paralysis by the injection of botulinum toxin can provide temporary symptom relief at minimal risk, and helpful information on whether more prolonged response may be achieved by sphincterotomy.

Table 15.24.1.1 Geenan and Hogan classification of sphincter of Oddi dysfunction

Biliary SOD	Pancreatic SOD
Type 1	**Type 1**
Biliary type pain	Pancreatic-type pain
Elevated liver enzymes	Amylase/lipase elevation
CBD dilatation	MPD dilatation
Delayed contrast drainage from the CBD > 45 min	Delayed contrast drainage from the MPD >8 min
Type 2	**Type 2**
Biliary type pain	Pancreatic-type pain
One or two of the above criteria	One or two of the above criteria
Type 3	**Type 3**
Biliary type pain only	Pancreatic-type pain only

CBD, common bile duct; MPD, main pancreas duct; SOD, sphincter of Oddi dysfunction.

Pathology

All patients with acute pancreatitis have microscopic evidence of necrosis, but macroscopic changes, particularly black discoloration of necrosis of the pancreas, are confined to the most severe cases. It is more frequent for this gross degree of necrosis to occur in the peripancreatic fatty tissue than in the pancreas itself. When it is present in the pancreas there is usually a panlobular necrosis, and it is impossible to delineate where the disease initiated. In a classical paper, Foulis claimed that the most common microscopic abnormality seen in humans, periductal necrosis, is typical of biliary and alcohol causation. Less commonly a perilobular necrosis is found, usually in patients with hypothermia or gross hypotension. In experimental acute pancreatitis the initial lesion is now considered to be intracellular, featuring coalescence of lysozymes and zymogen granules. Acinar cell disruption is found with many of the hyperstimulation models such as caerulein-induced acute pancreatitis. It is now believed that this initial event may be associated with oxidative stress.

Clinical features

Sudden onset of severe upper abdominal pain with vomiting is the most common manner of presentation. The pain may focus in the epigastrium or right or left upper quadrant, with penetration through to the back, and occasionally it encircles the upper abdomen. Patients who have experienced both a myocardial infarct and acute pancreatitis usually describe the latter pain as being much more severe. However, it tends to lessen in severity progressively over the first 72 h, and it is not usually a significant factor beyond this time. There may be upper abdominal tenderness and guarding, but these signs are often less marked than might be suspected from the severity of the pain, and bowel sounds are usually absent in the early stages.

Up to 90% of patients with acute pancreatitis have troublesome vomiting in the first 12 h of illness, and this contributes to hypovolaemia and hypotension. Clinical jaundice and pyrexia are rare on admission, although abnormalities of biochemical liver blood tests occur in 80% of patients with a biliary aetiology. Occasionally pancreatitis occurs in association with cholangitis, which is of importance in that organ failure may be driven by the cholangitis, not pancreatitis, such that urgent ERCP and biliary decompression is required.

Biochemical abnormalities

A multitude of biochemical phenomena are found in acute pancreatitis. Various pancreatic enzymes are released that are useful as diagnostic markers. Acinar cell disruption leads to high serum levels of amylase, lipase, trypsin, chymotrypsin, phospholipase, elastase, trypsinogen activation peptide, and phospholipase activation peptide, and these are also elevated in peritoneal and retroperitoneal tissues as well as lymph. The cheapest and most durable of these measurements as a diagnostic marker has been the total activity of serum amylase, and levels over three times the upper limit of normal in blood are now usually taken as diagnostic of acute pancreatitis in an appropriate clinical context. The serum lipase activity is a more specific measure and is almost as cheap to measure; levels of twice the upper limit of normal are significant.

C-reactive protein (CRP) is an acute phase reactant, which 36–48 h after onset of acute pancreatitis can be used for both assessment of severity (>150 mg/litre) and longitudinal monitoring of progress (see below).

Very high concentrations of circulating cytokines occur in the blood at an early stage in the disease, including tumour necrosis factor α (TNFα), platelet activating factor (PAF), and interleukin 6 (IL-6) with maximal levels in those with severe pancreatitis.

Diagnosis

The diagnosis is usually made from the clinical presentation, particularly the rapid onset of upper abdominal pain and vomiting, associated with an elevation of serum amylase and lipase. Where doubt exits, CT will reveal pancreatic swelling, fluid collection, and change in density of the gland. Contrast-enhanced CT is mandatory to identify areas of pancreatic ischaemia and infarction. MRI may ultimately replace contrast-enhanced CT in this area, but currently difficulties in access or with the availability of MRI-compatible equipment in the intensive care unit often limit its applicability in patients with organ failure. Occasionally the diagnosis may be made at laparotomy, when cholecystectomy plus cholangiography is good treatment, otherwise simple washout and closure is all that should be done.

Differential diagnosis

The differential diagnosis is that of an acute abdomen (Box 15.24.1.3). Perforated peptic ulcer may be associated with a raised amylase (although it is unusual for blood amylase to be elevated in <5 h of pain onset), but plain abdominal radiograph or CT usually confirms the diagnosis (most typically by demonstrating free intraperitoneal air). A dissecting aortic aneurysm usually presents with an initial history of chest pain in a known hypertensive; abdominal pain and loss of arterial pulses occur later. High amylase activity in ectopic pregnancy derives from the fallopian tubes, but the clinical presentation should not be mistaken for acute pancreatitis. Mesenteric ischaemia or infarction are important to consider: CT of abdomen and the associated metabolic acidosis help the differentiation.

Elevated amylase activities are frequently present in patients with renal failure, while a lifetime of high amylase occurs in those with macroamylasaemia, when failure to filter the amylase complex molecule results in very low urine levels. Occasionally a presentation of diabetic ketoacidosis exhibits exocrine involvement by elevated amylase/lipase.

Grading disease severity

The importance of objective grading of disease severity is that less experienced clinicians can direct the more serious cases to high-dependency or intensive care facilities at an early stage of their illness, or instigate contrast enhanced CT scanning and early ERCP for patients who will derive most benefit. Grading is also useful for trials of different forms of therapy. The original Ranson grading system of 11 prognostic factors was developed for patients with acute pancreatitis due to alcohol abuse, but later an alternative system was introduced by him for those with gallstones. A single system, validated for both the common causes, is the modified Glasgow scoring system of eight prognostic factors (Box 15.24.1.4). Validation came from a multicentre randomized British study by Corfield that assessed the place of peritoneal lavage in the management of severe acute pancreatitis.

Atlanta criteria

In 1992 in Atlanta a group of 40 multidisciplinary experts decided that severe acute pancreatitis was defined by the presence of failure of one or more organs, or the development of a major later complication (infected necrosis, abscess, or pseudocyst).

It is now recognized that neither transient hypoxaemia nor pseudocyst development is a good criterion for severe acute pancreatitis.

CT scanning

This can be very useful in confirming the diagnosis and also in grading severity of disease. It is very helpful in assessing an individual patient by demarcating location and extent of pancreatic damage (Fig. 15.24.1.2). The area of nonperfused pancreas corresponds to the extent of necrosis. More than 50% necrosis (especially if the head of the pancreas is involved) is associated with the most severe disease.

The APACHE II system

This can be used to grade the severity of many diseases and has been shown to be useful in acute pancreatitis (Fig. 15.24.1.3).

Box 15.24.1.3 Differential diagnosis of acute pancreatitis

- Perforated duodenal ulcer
- Acute cholangitis[a]
- Acute cholecystitis[a]
- Mesenteric ischaemia/infarction
- Small bowel obstruction/perforation
- Atypical myocardial infarction[a]
- Ectopic pregnancy
- Renal failure
- Macroamylasaemia
- Dissecting aortic aneurysm
- Diabetic ketoacidosis

[a] Amylase is usually normal.

Box 15.24.1.4 Glasgow Prognostic Score—three or more prognostic factors indicates severe acute pancreatitis

- WBC >15 000/mm^3
- Glucose >10 mmol/litre (no diabetic history)
- Urea >16 mmol/litre (despite intravenous infusion)
- Po_2 < 8 kPa (60 mmHg)
- Albumin <32 g/litre
- Calcium <2.0 mmol/litre
- LDH >600 IU/litre
- AST/ALT >200 units/litre

ALT, serum alanine aminotransferase; AST, serum aspartate aminotransferase; LDH, lactate dehydrogenase; WBC, white blood count.

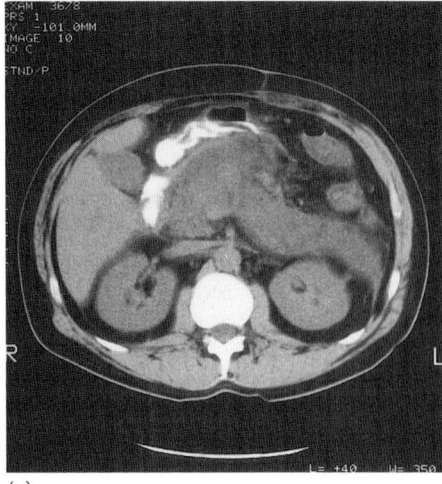

(a)

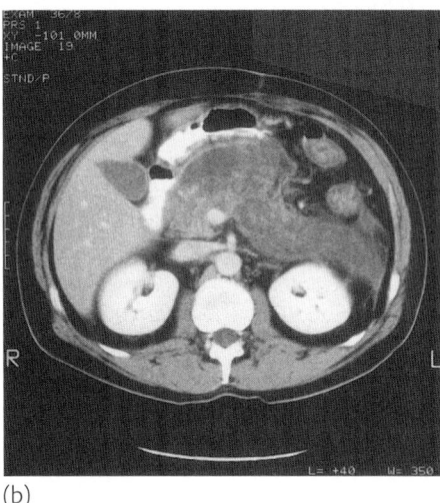

(b)

Fig. 15.24.1.2 (a) Severe acute pancreatitis with diffuse pancreatic swelling (CT scan). (b) Same scale level as in (a) with angiogram enhancement, revealing hypodense areas of poor perfusion.

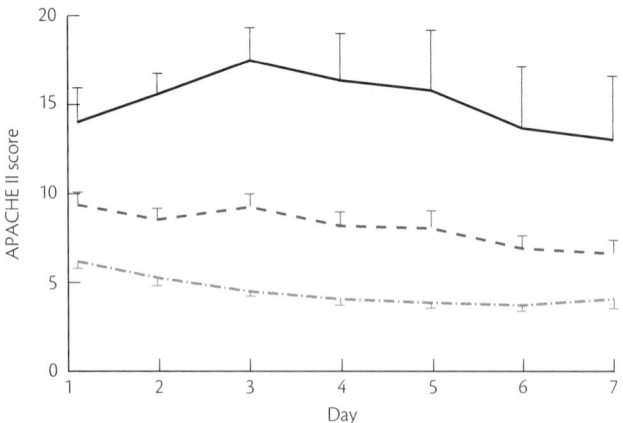

Fig. 15.24.1.3 Mean daily APACHE II scores by outcome in 119 patients with an uncomplicated course (·—·—·), 26 patients with a complicated course (– –), and 12 patients with a fatal outcome (——). The differences between fatal and uncomplicated and between complicated and uncomplicated were highly significant (p < 0.001) for each day (Mann–Whitney U test).
(From the *British Journal of Surgery*, with permission).

It takes time for an individual clinician to learn to use the system, but it has the advantage that it can be applied throughout the first week of illness. The higher the score the worse the prognosis, and patients with the most severe acute pancreatitis have scores in excess of 10. A recent large (>1500 patients) clinical study assessing the potential role of a PAF antagonist in the management of higher-risk patients revealed major concerns about an admission entry criterion of APACHE II score of 6 or more to select patients, as the mortality rate in each of three groups of approximately 500 patients was less than 10%. Admission APACHE II scores of 8 or above are now recommended to identify severe disease.

Organ failure scoring

Clinical assessment by an expert is probably better than any of the other systems described to identify the most ill patients. Quantification of the clinical assessment by scoring 0 to 4 points for each of several organ systems using the modified Marshall Critical Illness Scoring System (Table 15.24.1.2) has revealed that 44% of patients with an APACHE II score of 6 or more will show an organ failure score of 2 or more at admission (Table 15.24.1.3). The hepatic index in the Marshall score is excluded in acute pancreatitis assessment as the presence of stones in the bile duct is so common. Many patients improve fairly rapidly with intensive supportive intravenous fluids and oxygen: they are regarded having low risk transient organ failure with mortality of less than 1%. By contrast, those who continue with a minimum modified Marshall score of 2 have persistent organ failure and high mortality (35–55%). It is this dynamic aspect of organ failure that is not recognized by the Atlanta criteria.

Other predictors

Age

Many studies indicate that those over 70 years have a higher mortality, with one study finding 18.8% risk of death for this group. Any form of chronic cardiorespiratory or similar impairment is most common in this age group and further increases the risk of death.

Obesity

Acute pancreatitis carries a significantly higher mortality and morbidity in patients with a body mass index of more than 30 kg/m²,

Table 15.24.1.2 Modified Marshall Critical Illness Scoring System (excludes hepatic index)

Score	0	1	2	3	4
Systolic BP (mm Hg)	>90	<90 responds to fluid	<90 poor response to fluid	<90 (pH<7.3)	<90 (pH<7.2)
	>400	301–400	201–300	101–200	<101
Glasgow Coma Score	15	13–14	10–12	6–9	<6
Platelet count × 10⁹/litre	>120	81–120	51–80	21–50	<21
Creatinine (μmol/litre)	<134	134–169	170–310	311–439	>439

FiO₂, fraction of inspired oxygen; PO₂, partial pressure of oxygen.

Table 15.24.1.3 Importance of the dynamics of organ failure in acute pancreatitis

	Patient nos.	Deaths
Transient organ failure	104 (25.3%)	1 (1.0%)
Persistent organ failure	123 (29.9%)	47 (38.2%)
No organ failure	184 (44.8%)	5 (2.7%)

Outcome derived from combined data from Buter *et al.* (2002) and Johnson and Abu Hilal (2004). All patients had a minimum APACHE II score of 6 at admission.

mainly because of increased risk of hypoxaemia, but also from other associated factors.

CRP

The main value of this acute phase reactant is at around 36 to 48 h of illness, when values between 200 and 600 mg/litre are found in the most severely ill patients (Fig. 15.24.1.4).

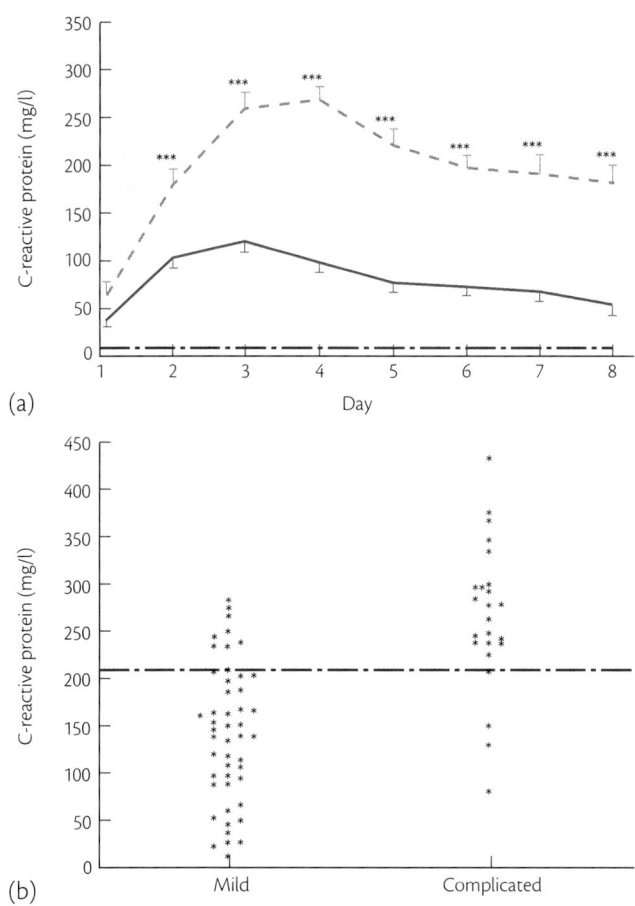

Fig. 15.24.1.4 (a) Sequential C-reactive protein concentrations in 47 patients with mild pancreatitis (—) and 25 with complicated attacks (– – –). Results are expressed as mean ± standard error of the mean: *$p < 0.05$; **$p < 0.01$; ***$p < 0.01$ (mild vs complicated); (–·– –·-), upper limit of normal for C-reactive protein. (b) Scattergram showing discrimination between mild and complicated attacks of pancreatitis based on the peak C-reactive protein concentration recorded on days 2 to 4 (–·– –·-). The peak concentration providing the best discrimination was greater than or equal to 210 mg/litre.
(From the *British Journal of Surgery*, with permission).

Serum amyloid A

Preliminary studies measuring this substance hold considerable promise that it may be the most useful single marker of disease severity, but additional clinical studies are needed and its measurement is not routine clinical practice.

Trypsinogen activation peptide

The activation of trypsinogen releases trypsin and a small peptide (trypsinogen activation peptide), which passes unchanged in the urine, where its level can be used as a marker of severity. It has now been employed in two clinical studies with the promise of this being a valuable step forward in assessment of severity, but its measurement is not routine clinical practice.

Clinical progress and outcome

Mild acute pancreatitis

Those patients who fail to meet objective criteria of severe acute pancreatitis tend to have a low mortality (maximum 2%) and rarely need to be in hospital beyond 7 to 10 days. Simple therapeutic measures normally suffice through the first 24 to 48 h, after which time monitoring and support can usually be discontinued, but it is best to assume at presentation that a patient may develop severe disease and to provide monitoring within a high dependency environment when possible.

Good prospective studies of analgesia in acute pancreatitis are notable for their absence. Pain is usually treated with morphine or buprenorphine. Care is required if nonsteroidal anti-inflammatories are used because they may exacerbate renal compromise. Epidural analgesia is employed in some German hospitals. Agitation is common, particularly with alcoholic pancreatitis, and intravenous benzodiazepines or haloperidol may also be required.

Even in patients with mild disease it may occasionally be necessary to provide 4 to 5 litres of intravenous fluid in the first 24 h of the illness.

When the acute attack has resolved, it is important to consider prevention of further episodes of pancreatitis. If gallstones have been identified by ultrasound scanning, then laparoscopic or open cholecystectomy should be performed in the same admission, with ERCP sphincterotomy alone considered a satisfactory alternative in patients who are infirm.

Severe acute pancreatitis

The mainstays of treatment are reversing hypoxaemia, restoration of circulating volume, maintaining tissue perfusion, and organ support. Patients who meet objective criteria of severe acute pancreatitis are often tachypnoeic, tachycardic, and hypotensive. They should be managed within a high-dependency environment, with facilities for invasive monitoring. Successful resuscitation and prevention of secondary organ dysfunction is key to improving outcome, especially as 40 to 50% of deaths result from multiple organ failure within the first week of illness rather than the late infective complications.

Body wall staining at the umbilical area (Cullen's sign) or in the flanks (Grey Turner's sign) can occur, usually appearing around the fourth day of illness. This results from transudation of blood stained retroperitoneal fluid.

Respiratory failure

Hypoxaemia reflects disease severity in acute pancreatitis, and all systems of grading severity include hypoxaemia. Basal atelectasis and respiratory compromise are very common and must be expected. Early pleural effusions (more commonly on left side) indicate severe disease. The onset of respiratory failure may be insidious, with an initial compensatory tachypnoea easily overlooked, although this can be highlighted by the routine use of Modified Early Warning Score (MEWS) systems that mandate recording of respiratory rate and request for patient review if the MEWS score increases beyond an agreed level. Pulse oximetry is valuable in monitoring, but arterial gas analysis may be needed three or four times in the first 24 h to make sensible decisions about humidified oxygen therapy and possible ventilator support. Most patients can be managed with supplemental humidified oxygen, but assisted ventilation may be required in more severe cases for several weeks.

Circulatory failure

The initial therapy of hypovolaemia is of great importance in maintaining cardiac and renal function. Intravascular fluid deficits in the more severe cases are considerable, often underestimated, and intravascular fluid monitoring is required where tissue perfusion is not easily restored. The combination of fluid lost from vomiting and loss of capillary integrity can be very substantial. The use of catecholamines should only be considered after it is established that adequate fluid restoration has been achieved. In the most severe cases of acute pancreatitis the cardiovascular changes are very similar to those encountered in septic shock, with a high cardiac output and low peripheral vascular resistance. Stress on the heart may cause arrhythmias and ischaemic changes.

Renal failure

After immediate resuscitation, intravenous fluid should be given at sufficient rate to produce 0.5 ml/kg of urine per hour, but oliguric acute tubular necrosis is not uncommon in patients presenting with hypovolaemia and poor tissue perfusion, in which case fluid challenges should not be pursued to the point of inducing pulmonary oedema. The use of mannitol or furosemide is without proven benefit. Renal replacement therapy by haemodialysis or haemofiltration may be required if renal failure becomes established.

Pyrexia

This reflects cell damage and necrosis, as with any condition associated with tissue destruction. High fever within the first 24 h is rare and, if associated with jaundice, is suspicious of ascending cholangitis; consideration should be given to biliary decompression. In the more severe cases of acute pancreatitis the first week is characterized by the development and persistence of a systemic inflammatory response syndrome, one aspect being the development of a swinging pyrexia. This is often inappropriately taken as evidence of infection but is a reflection of the inflammatory cascade and the presence of devitalized tissue in the retroperitoneum.

Specific aspects of management of severe acute pancreatitis

Initial management

Analgesia (with pethidine or buprenorphine) and restoration of circulating volume is the mainstay of early treatment. Although nasogastric decompression has no effect on outcome, it can sometimes alleviate vomiting. In all but the mildest cases, careful monitoring of organ function is required with pulse oximetry, urinary catheterization, and noninvasive blood pressure measurement in addition to biochemical, haematological, and blood gas analysis. Treatment is directed towards support and restoration of lung, renal, and cardiac function.

As stated above, those who have severe acute pancreatitis are usually very ill at the time of admission or within 24 h and warrant high-dependency or intensive care therapy. Close routine monitoring for system failures as well as biochemical and haematological abnormalities is required. An algorithm for suggested steps in the management of severe acute pancreatitis (Fig. 15.24.1.5) is based on the United Kingdom National Guidelines published in 1998 and revised in 2005. Particular interventions are discussed below.

ERCP

The one group of patients with proven benefit from ERCP and biliary decompression are those with pancreatitis associated with cholangitis (jaundice and pyrexia), where the cholangitis, rather than any pancreatic inflammation, is driving organ dysfunction. The role of ERCP is more debatable in other circumstances. There is no role for early ERCP in mild disease. For severe acute pancreatitis there are four randomized trials of early ERCP, three reported in peer-reviewed journals and one in abstract form. The evidence is equivocal, and ERCP is probably difficult to justify in patients who are not jaundiced. No study has addressed the question of whether sphincter decompression in the absence of a common bile duct stone affects disease progression.

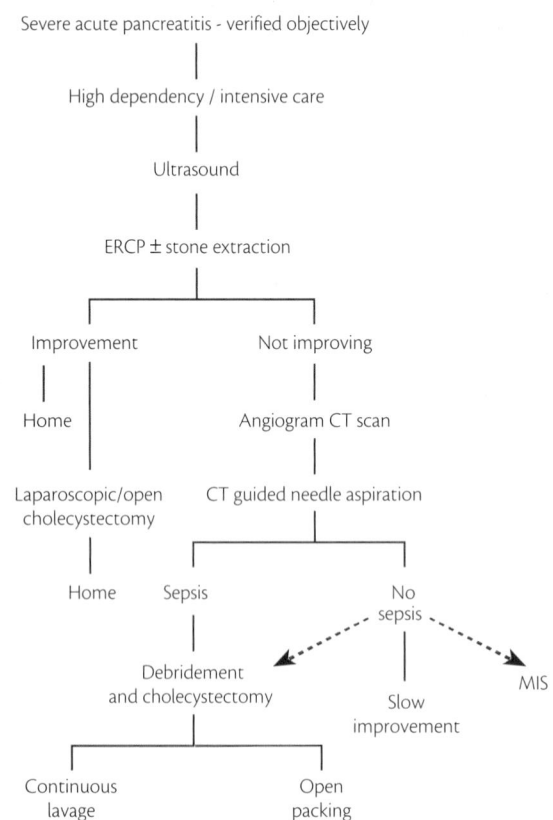

Fig. 15.24.1.5 Summary of management of acute pancreatitis. MIS=minimally invasive surgery

Antibiotics

Several studies in the 1990s advocated the early initiation of prophylactic antibiotics such as imipenem for 10 to 14 days in patients with predicted severe disease, and most clinicians adopted this policy. However, the quality of these clinical trials was not to the accepted standard for randomized double-blind studies, and two larger higher-quality multicentre studies—both mainly including patients with CT-proven necrosis—have more recently failed to demonstrate benefit in terms of either the primary endpoint of pancreatic infection, or the secondary one of mortality (Table 15.24.1.4). One of these employed ciprofloxacin and metronidazole vs placebo in 114 patients, and meropenem vs placebo was used in 100 patients in the other study. Although it could be argued that neither of these trials was adequately powered, the clinical effort and expense of mounting even larger antibiotic studies of only the most severely ill patients, with poor prospects of a positive outcome, means such a future trial is highly improbable. It seems appropriate to recommend that antibiotic therapy should not be given until and unless a specific indication arises.

Nutrition support

Before the 1960s, gut rest was not considered an issue, but intake was often limited because of gastric stasis. The development of modern parenteral support in the late 1960s, along with laboratory studies investigating the stimulation of pancreatic exocrine function, led to the avoidance of enteral intake during the acute phase of disease. However, randomized studies have since shown that early nasojejunal nutritional support is cheaper and associated with fewer side effects than total parenteral nutrition, also that there is no difference in outcome with nasogastric compared to nasojejunal feeding. In clinical practice, therefore, the mode of nutrition support does not appear to affect the disease process, and the choice of delivery relates to tolerance and minimizing morbidity associated with the delivery system.

Small studies indicated potential benefit from adding probiotics to nasoenteral feeds, but surprising and disturbing adverse effects were found when the large Dutch PROPATRIA randomized study of 298 patients was reported in 2008: infective complications occurred in approximately 30% of each group of patients, but the mortality in the probiotic group was 16% vs 6% in the placebo group, and bowel ischaemia or infarction was found in eight fatal cases in the treatment group but none of the placebo group. Probiotics should not be used.

Other approaches

In the 1990s, there was considerable interest in the potential of manipulating the inflammatory response to prevent cytokine cascade modulated multiorgan failure, but the initial promise of the PAF antagonist studies proved unfounded after a multinational study of >1500 patients failed to show benefit. In a similar way, high dose intravenous antiprotease and antioxidant therapy as well as the somatostatin analogue octreotide showed no benefit in randomized double-blind studies. There is no clinically available specific intervention that can be recommended in addition to respiratory, fluid, and circulating volume support in the early phase of disease.

Surgical intervention

The roles of surgery in acute pancreatitis are shown in Box 15.24.1.5. There is no place for early intervention, other than occasionally to establish the diagnosis where diagnostic doubt remains despite clinical, biochemical, and radiological assessment, but surgery does have an important role in the management of complications.

In patients with mild attacks, gallstones (when relevant) should be eradicated, ideally within the same hospital admission. In those with severe disease, the role of surgery is aimed at the control of sepsis, usually several weeks after disease onset. Most sterile collections can be managed conservatively and drainage achieved with low morbidity as a delayed procedure once the acute phase has passed.

The indication for surgical intervention is the development of infection within an acute fluid collection, which is normally heralded by deterioration in biochemical and haematological markers, and deterioration in organ function. Traditional management demanded complete debridement of any devitalized tissue at the earliest opportunity, but it is now clear that maintaining adequate drainage is more important than eradication of necrosis, and options for intervention include open surgical drainage, percutaneous, or endoscopic minimally invasive approaches, with choice of procedure determined by local expertise and preference.

In open surgical debridement, the necrotic tissue is removed by a combination of gentle finger and forceps dissection, after which there are two options: (1) to establish a postoperative lavage system, which may necessitate up to three inflow and three outflow drains because of the tendency for retroperitoneal extension of the infected necrosis down the paracolic gutters and upwards towards the diaphragm; or (2)—if venous ooze of blood is a particular problem—packing of the abdominal cavity with large cotton packs wrapped in nonadhesive paraffin gauze, together with limited closure or nonclosure of the abdominal wall. Such patients are invariably in intensive care and receiving mechanical ventilation. The packs should be changed at intervals of 48 to 72 h, with removal of any extension of infection or necrosis. Abdominal wall closure and postoperative lavage may be established after the second or subsequent operations.

Table 15.24.1.4 Deaths in early antibiotic randomized double-blind studies in severe acute pancreatitis

Study	Antibiotic	Placebo
Isenmann *et al.* (2004)	3/58	4/56
Dellinger *et al.* (2007)	10/50	9/50
Totals	13/108	13/106

Box 15.24.1.5 Role of surgery in acute pancreatitis

- ◆ To establish diagnosis when this is uncertain (rare)
- ◆ Eradication of gallstone risk in primary admission, if possible
- ◆ Removal of pus and infected necrotic tissue
- ◆ Drainage of pseudocysts with solid/semi-solid content

Minimally invasive surgical approaches have been developed to achieve adequate drainage of sepsis whilst minimizing the surgical insult. The first of these was developed in Glasgow, utilizing either a left flank retroperitoneal approach (80%) or right anterior drainage (20%), and is now our standard surgical approach. Other variations, including endoscopic drainage methods, have been described, but our own experience of these has highlighted the difficulties in maintaining drainage in collections with a large solid component, and we find this method more useful in fluid-predominant collections being drained several months after an acute attack. However, to emphasize the point again, in practical terms achieving continued sepsis control is probably more important than the method used.

Specific complications of acute pancreatitis

Acute pancreatic pseudocyst

This is probably a misnomer in that acute fluid collections requiring intervention rarely contain little or no debris (as required by the Atlanta definitions). Unfortunately, necrosis is poorly demonstrated by CT (MRI is much more sensitive), and an acute fluid collection on CT may appear homogeneous and invite radiological intervention. This leads to inadequate drainage and persistent infection. We prefer the terms 'fluid-predominant' or 'solid-predominant' acute fluid collection or pseudocyst, as this defines subsequent treatment.

Pancreatic pseudocyst most commonly occurs in the lesser sac and often represents a closed pancreatic fistula, as a breach in the main or major pancreatic duct can frequently be demonstrated at ERCP. Transpapillary duct stenting and ERCP should be avoided if possible, as this leads to the introduction of infection in more than 10% of patients. Percutaneous aspiration alone invariably results in recollection of the fluid quite rapidly, while infection is potentially associated with long-term percutaneous drainage. In the absence of sepsis, fluid-predominant acute fluid collections may be adequately drained as a one-step procedure by EUS-guided endoscopic transmural procedures, although repeated tract dilatation is often required. By contrast, solid-predominant acute fluid collections, especially in younger, fit patients, may be best dealt with by internal surgical drainage to the stomach or to a defunctioned Roux loop of jejunum. This procedure can be done either laparoscopically or at open surgery, depending on local expertise, and can also be combined with a cholecystectomy.

Pancreatic ascites

This condition rarely occurs in association with acute pancreatitis, but when it does it is due to spontaneous decompression of a pancreatic pseudocyst, with escape of pancreatic juice into the peritoneal cavity. Amylase-rich fistula fluid is common after surgical drainage and can often be successfully managed by endoscopic transpapillary drainage.

Rare complications

These include splenic vein thrombosis and subcutaneous fat necrosis. Increased availability and use of high-quality imaging techniques mean that splenic and segmental portal vein thrombosis are increasingly detected. Painful subcutaneous bright red nodules (mimicking erythema nodosum) may occasionally occur on upper and lower limbs when spontaneous decompression of a pseudocyst takes place: skin biopsy makes the diagnosis. Cranial areas of fat necrosis have also been noted at autopsy.

Further reading

Acosta JM, Ledesma CL (1974). Gallstone migration as a cause for acute pancreatitis. *N Engl J Med*, **290**, 480–7.

Balthazar EJ, *et al.* (1990). Acute pancreatitis: value of CT in establishing diagnosis. *Radiology*, **156**, 767–72.

Besselink MGH, *et al.* (2008). Probiotic prophylaxis in predicted severe acute pancreatitis: a randomised, double-blind, placebo-controlled trial. *Lancet*, **371**, 651–9.

Bradley EL (1993). A clinically based classification system for Acute Pancreatitis: Atlanta International Symposium Summary. *Arch Surg*, **128**, 586–90.

Blamey SL, *et al.* (1984). Prognostic factors in acute pancreatitis. *Gut*, **25**, 1340–46.

Buter A, *et al.* (2002). Dynamic nature of early organ dysfunction determines outcome in acute pancreatitis. *Br J Surg*, **89**, 298–302.

Carter CR, *et al.* (2000). Percutaneous necrosectomy and sinus tract endoscopy in the management of infected pancreatic necrosis: an initial experience. *Ann Surg*, **232**, 175–80.

Connor S, *et al.* (2005). Early and late complications after pancreatic necrosectomy. *Surgery*, **137**, 499–505.

Corfield AP, *et al.* (1985). Prediction of severity in acute pancreatitis: prospective comparison of three prognostic indices. *Lancet*, **ii**, 403–7.

Dellinger EP, *et al.* (2007). Early antibiotic treatment for severe acute necrotising pancreatitis: a randomised, double blind placebo controlled study. *Ann Surg*, **245**, 674–83.

Eatock FC, *et al.* (2005). A randomized study of early nasogastric versus nasojejunal feeding in severe acute pancreatitis. *Am J Gastroenterol*, **100**, 432–9.

Frey C, *et al.* (2007). Co-morbidity is a strong predictor of early death and multi-organ system failure among patients with acute pancreatitis. *J Gastrointest Surg*, **11**, 733–42.

Foulis AK (1982). Morphological study of the relation between accidental hypothermia and acute pancreatitis. *J Clin Pathol*, **35**, 1244–8.

Heath Dl, *et al.* (1993). Role of interleukin-6 in mediating the acute phase protein response and potential as an early means of severity assessment in acute pancreatitis. *Gut*, **34**, 41–5.

Imrie CW, *et al.* (1977). Arterial hypoxia in acute pancreatitis. *Br J Surg*, **64**, 185–8.

Imrie CW, *et al.* (1978). A single centre double blind trial of Trasylol therapy in primary acute pancreatitis. *Br J Surg*, **65**, 337–41.

Isenmann R, *et al.* (2004). Prophylactic antibiotic treatment in patients with predicted severe acute pancreatitis: a placebo controlled double blind trial. *Gastroenterology*, **126**, 997–1004.

Johnson CD, Abu Hilal M (2004). Persistent organ failure during the first week as a marker of fatal outcome in acute pancreatitis. *Gut*, **53**, 1340–44.

Larvin M, McMahon MJ (1989). APACHE II score for assessment and monitoring of AP. *Lancet*, **ii**, 201–4.

Luiten EJ (1995). Controlled clinical trial of selective decontamination for the treatment of severe acute pancreatitis. *Ann Surg*, **222**, 57–65.

Marshall JC, *et al.* (1995). Multiple organ dysfunction score; a reliable descriptor of a complex clinical outcome. *Crit Care Med*, **23**, 1638–52.

McKay, CJ *et al.* (1999). High early mortality rate from acute pancreatitis in Scotland. 1984–1995. *Br J Surg*, **86**, 1302–6.

Mofidi R, *et al.* (2007). An audit of the management of patients with acute pancreatitis against national standards of practice. *Br J Surg*, **94**, 844–8.

Neoptolemos JP, *et al.* (1987). Acute cholangitis in association with acute pancreatitis: incidence, clinical features, outcome and the role of ERCP and endoscopic sphincterotomy. *Br J Surg*, **74**, 1103–6.

Olah A, *et al.* (2002). Early nasojejunal feeding in acute pancreatitis is associated with a lower complication rate. *Nutrition*, **18**, 259–62.

Pandol SJ, *et al.* (2007). Acute pancreatitis: bench to the bedside. *Gastroenterology*, **132**, 1127–51.

Ranson JHC, *et al.* (1974). Prognostic signs and the role of operative management in acute pancreatitis. *Surg Gynecol Obstet*, **139**, 69–81.

Siriwardena AK, *et al.* (2008). Randomised,double blind, placebo controlled trial of intravenous antioxidant(*N*-acetyl cysteine, selenium, vitamin C) therapy in severe acute pancreatitis. *Gut*, **56**, 1439–44.

Wilson C, *et al.* (1989). C-reactive protein, antiproteases and complement factors as objective markers of severity of AP. *Br J Surg*, **76**, 177–81.

Wilson C, *et al.* (1990). Prediction of outcome in acute pancreatitis: a comparative study of APACHE II, clinical assessment, and multiple scoring systems. *Br J Surg*, **77**, 1260–4.

Windsor AC, *et al.* (1998). Compared with parenteral nutrition, enteral feeding attenuates the acute phase response and improves disease severity in acute pancreatitis. *Gut*, **42**, 431–5.

15.24.2 Chronic pancreatitis

P.P. Toskes

Essentials

Chronic pancreatitis is most commonly due to chronic alcoholism in adults and cystic fibrosis in children, but there are many other causes/associations. Typical presentation is with (1) abdominal pain—but this is not always a feature and when present can vary from being mild to extremely severe; and/or (2) maldigestion—diarrhoea/steatorrhoea and weight loss.

Accurate diagnosis requires a combination of a hormone stimulation test (e.g. secretin–cholecystokinin stimulation of bicarbonate and enzyme secretion) and a structural test, e.g. endoscopic ultrasonography or endoscopic retrograde cholangiopancreatography ERCP). In routine clinical practice common strategy is to evaluate patients suspected of having chronic pancreatitis with a noninvasive test, e.g. faecal elastase (reduced), and initiate treatment if the result is abnormal, reserving invasive tests for cases where diagnostic doubt remains or clinical progress is unsatisfactory.

Management requires use of (1) potent enzyme formulations—protease for pain, lipase for steatorrhoea; given before meals and (if pain is a symptom) before bedtime, (2) acid suppressive therapy—H$_2$ antagonist or proton pump inhibitor; (3) abstinence from alcohol; (4) diet that is moderate in fat (30%), high in protein (24%), and low in carbohydrate (40%); (5) pain control—if required, (a) non-narcotic analgesics are the pain-relieving medications of choice, and (b) lateral pancreaticojejunostomy (Peustow procedure) should be considered if there is dilatation of the main pancreatic duct.

Introduction

Patients with chronic pancreatitis usually come to medical attention with abdominal pain or maldigestion (diarrhoea, steatorrhoea, weight loss), but the frequency of chronic pancreatitis is underestimated because of inadequate investigation of these symptoms. The realization that impaired pancreatic exocrine function can occur

without obvious dilatation of the main duct, i.e. 'small-duct disease', has greatly influenced management. Symptomatic variability and the many causes of this disease have made its classification difficult.

Three forms of chronic pancreatitis are now recognized: (1) chronic calcifying, (2) chronic obstructive, and (3) chronic inflammatory. Alcohol abuse and/or malnutrition are the most common causes of the calcifying type. Obstruction of the main pancreatic duct with secondary fibrosis in that part of the pancreas proximal to the obstruction leads to the obstructive type. Chronic inflammatory pancreatitis is not well characterized, and many patients with chronic pancreatitis of unknown cause fall into this group. Irreversible changes often occur in the gland, making a cure improbable. Nevertheless, the chief complaints of pain and/or maldigestion can be effectively treated.

Inflammation and sclerosis with progressive damage to the acini and ducts are the histological hallmarks of chronic pancreatitis. In advanced stages the gland may be fibrotic and calcified and the main duct may be dilated. Islet cells are usually lost more slowly than the exocrine part, hence diabetes is a late feature.

Aetiology

Table 15.24.2.1 classifies chronic pancreatitis into a number of different conditions associated with this disease. Chronic alcoholism and cystic fibrosis are the most frequent causes in adults and children, respectively. Gallstones rarely cause chronic pancreatitis because a cholecystectomy is almost always performed after the first or second attack of acute pancreatitis related to gallstones, after which the pancreas recovers. Hypertriglyceridaemia may cause chronic as well as acute pancreatitis. Some patients with chronic pancreatitis may have suffered autoimmune pancreatitis: they have had enlargement of the pancreas, strictures of the pancreatic duct, autoantibodies in the serum, elevated plasma immunoglobulins, and histology showing a dense lymphocytic infiltrate. Some respond to steroid therapy. Tropical pancreatitis (Africa and Asia) is characterized by calcific disease, glucose intolerance, and infrequent pain. Pancreatic exocrine impairment occurs in patients with haemochromatosis and α_1-antitrypsin deficiency, but the pancreatic disease is usually asymptomatic. Secondary pancreatic exocrine insufficiency may occur after gastric surgery, leading to postprandial asynchrony; usually the maldigestion is not very severe. Similarly, the acid hypersecretion associated with gastrinoma may irreversibly inactivate lipase, causing steatorrhoea. Hereditary pancreatitis and developmental anomalies leading to pancreatitis are discussed later.

Idiopathic chronic pancreatitis remains controversial and may account for up to 30% of cases, depending on the population. Many patients with this condition present solely with unexplained abdominal pain, with no evidence of maldigestion, and they have small-duct disease, often without overt radiographic abnormalities by CT or magneric resonance cholangiopancreatography (MRCP). It may be necessary to perform endoscopic ultrasonography or direct intubation (hormone stimulation) to identify this condition. Endoscopic retrograde cholangiopancreatography (ERCP), which is often used to diagnose chronic pancreatitis, may miss up to 30% of patients with chronic pancreatitis who have abnormal hormone stimulation tests. It is not know how many patients with unexplained abdominal pain may indeed suffer from small-duct chronic pancreatitis: some will be thought to have nonulcer

Table 15.24.2.1 Causes of chronic pancreatitis and pancreatic insufficiency

Toxic–metabolic	Alcohol
	Tobacco smoking
	Hypercalcaemia
	Hyperlipidaemia
	Chronic renal failure
	Medications—phenacetin abuse
	Toxic organic compounds
Idiopathic	Early onset
	Late onset
	Tropical
Genetic	Hereditary pancreatitis—mutations in CFTR, SPINK1, PRSS1
Autoimmune	Isolated autoimmune chronic pancreatitis
	Syndromic autoimmune chronic pancreatitis – associated with Sjögren's syndrome, inflammatory bowel disease, primary biliary cirrhosis
Recurrent and severe acute pancreatitis	Postnecrotic (severe acute pancreatitis)
	Recurrent acute pancreatitis
	Vascular diseases/ischaemia
	Postirradiation
Obstructive	Pancreas divisum
	Duct obstruction (e.g. tumour)
	Preampullary duodenal wall cysts
	Post-traumatic pancreatic duct scars
	Sphincter of Oddie disorders (controversial)

Causes can be remembered by the mnemonic 'TIGAR-O': Toxic-metabolic, Idiopathic, Genetic, Autoimmune, Recurrent and severe acute pancreatitis, Obstructive.

dyspepsia, and others with idiopathic pancreatitis may present at an older age with painless diarrhoea, steatorrhoea, and secondary diabetes mellitus, and they often have pancreatic calcification.

Several investigators have documented mutations of the cystic fibrosis, transmembrane-conductance regulator gene (CFTR), which functions as a cAMP-regulated chloride channel, in idiopathic chronic pancreatitis. More than 1000 mutant alleles of the CFTR gene have been identified, which has hampered attempts to elucidate the relationship between the genotype and pancreatic manifestations. Two reports have shown cystic fibrosis gene mutations in 13 to 40% of patients with idiopathic chronic pancreatitis (the observed frequency of a single CFTR mutation was 11 times greater than expected); moreover, the frequency of two mutant alleles was increased 80-fold. Most of these patients were adults with chronic pancreatitis, none of whom had any clinical evidence of pulmonary disease, and the results of sweat chloride measurements were not diagnostic of cystic fibrosis. A further study examining all known CFTR mutations noted abnormalities in 55% of 16 patients, 14 of whom had idiopathic chronic pancreatitis. Some of these patients

with either one or two mutations had evidence of defective CFTR-mediated ion transport in nasal epithelium. It is not yet clear whether these CFTR abnormalities are primarily responsible for chronic pancreatitis or whether they are, at least in some cases, unrelated.

Pathophysiology

Although alcohol-induced chronic pancreatitis has been studied extensively, it remains uncertain as to whether the biochemical and histological lesions are caused by a reduced secretion of pancreatic-stone protein or alcohol toxicity. Ingestion of alcohol may decrease stone protein secretion below a critical level, allowing calcium and other secretory components to precipitate and obstruct pancreatic ductules. Alcohol may also cause abnormalities in acinar cells, leading to an imbalance of proteases and their cognate inhibitors, resulting in the initiation of a necroinflammatory process. In tropical pancreatitis, a combination of protein deficiency and a dietary toxin that occurs in cassava or sorghum may be responsible. A primary defect in the permeability of the ductal epithelium to electrolytes in patients with cystic fibrosis reduces secretory fluxes such that the hyperconcentrated proteinaceous fluid precipitates and obstructs the pancreatic ducts. The pathophysiology of the other causes of chronic pancreatitis is not understood.

Although it is widely believed that when a patient develops their first attack of acute alcoholic pancreatitis they have already sustained chronic damage to the pancreas, some individuals who do not abuse alcohol regularly develop acute pancreatitis after ingesting uncommonly large quantities of alcohol (binge drinking).

Incidence

The exact prevalence and incidence of chronic pancreatitis is unknown. The prevalence in autopsy studies varies from 0.04 to 5.0%. The only prospective study (Copenhagen Pancreatic Study), which mainly reflected alcohol-induced pancreatitis, found a prevalence of 26.4 cases per 100 000 population and an incidence of 8.2 new cases per 100 000 per year.

Clinical features

Abdominal pain is the cardinal symptom of chronic pancreatitis, but its pattern, severity, and frequency vary considerably. Whereas the pain of acute pancreatitis is often located in the epigastrium and bores through to the back, the pain of chronic pancreatitis has no characteristic features and may be constant or intermittent. Eating often increases the severity of the pain, resulting in the avoidance of food and subsequent weight loss. The pain may be mild, requiring no therapy, or severe, leading to the frequent use of analgesics and narcotic addiction.

Patients with abdominal pain may develop steatorrhoea and/or diarrhoea, but this is not inevitable. Approximately 15% of patients never suffer with abdominal pain but present with steatorrhoea, diarrhoea, and weight loss. In those who only have abdominal pain, there are few physical findings except for abdominal tenderness and mild pyrexia. There is a marked disparity between the severity of the abdominal pain and the physical findings.

Signs and symptoms of liver disease may be present in patients with maldigestion and weight loss due to alcohol-induced pancreatitis. Clinically apparent deficiencies of fat-soluble vitamins or vitamin B_{12} are uncommon.

Investigation and diagnosis

Table 15.24.2.2 lists selected tests of pancreatic function and structure, with abnormalities of function generally preceding abnormalities in structure.

Blood tests rarely contribute to a diagnosis of chronic pancreatitis. The plasma activities of pancreatic enzymes (amylase, lipase, trypsin) are usually normal, except in patients who have a pseudocyst of the pancreas. There may be evidence of cholestasis (elevated alkaline phosphatase, elevated bilirubin) caused by inflammatory reactions around the common bile duct. Some patients with severe disease may have raised fasting blood-glucose levels.

Calcification may be seen on a plain abdominal radiograph (Fig. 15.24.2.1) and by ultrasonography, with the latter also sometimes revealing dilatation of the pancreatic duct (Fig. 15.24.2.2). CT scans may reveal diffuse enlargement of the pancreas and, occasionally, a pseudocyst (Figs. 15.24.2.3 and 15.24.2.4). ERCP may reveal more subtle changes (Figs. 15.24.2.5 and 15.24.2.6). Newer techniques for imaging the pancreas include MRCP and endoscopic ultrasonography (EUS). MRCP provides a satisfactory morphological assessment of the main pancreatic duct but does not provide detailed imaging of the secondary ducts, or even the main pancreatic duct if it is small. EUS provides detailed assessment of both the pancreatic duct and parenchyma. A total of nine abnormal features have been defined, with more than five of these criteria being required in most studies for a diagnosis of chronic pancreatitis. EUS may find abnormalities that are not depicted by CT or ERCP (Figs. 15.24.2.7 and 15.24.2.8), and has replaced ERCP as a diagnostic modality in selected patients with suspected chronic pancreatitis. What is not yet clear is how sensitive and specific EUS is in defining abnormalities in patients considered to have early or mild chronic pancreatitis, or in those in whom only hormone stimulation testing has been found to be abnormal.

Currently, the most accurate means of detecting chronic pancreatitis is a combination of a hormone stimulation test and a structural test such as endoscopic ultrasonography or ERCP, but as many as 30% of patients with chronic pancreatitis may have a normal ERCP in combination with an abnormal hormone stimulation test, and occasionally the converse will be true. Two significant causes of a false-positive (abnormal) ERCP are normal ageing and recent acute

Table 15.24.2.2 Selected pancreatic diagnostic tests

	Principle/main utility	Comment
Functional tests		
Hormone stimulation	Secretin stimulates bicarbonate; CCK stimulates enzyme output	Reduced bicarbonate and enzyme output in pancreatic exocrine dysfunction. Sensitive and specific, requires intubation
Pancreolauryl test	Fluorescein diaurate cleaved to release fluorescein which appears in urine	Reduced urinary excretion of fluorescein in pancreatic exocrine dysfunction. Will detect severe disease
Bentiromide test	Synthetic peptide cleaved to release PABA which is excreted	Similar to pancreolauryl
Faecal chymotrypsin	Residual secretion	Reduced level in pancreatic exocrine dysfunction. Insensitive, frequent false- positive/ negative tests
Serum trypsinogen	Blood spillover	Highly specific; insensitive, inexpensive, and simple
Faecal elastase	Residual secretion	Reduced level in pancreatic exocrine dysfunction. Unknown sensitivity, excellent specificity; inexpensive and simple
Quantitative faecal fat	Maldigestion of exogenous fat	Elevated level in pancreatic exocrine dysfunction—the 'gold standard'. Does not distinguish pancreatic from intestinal causes of fat maldigestion/malabsorption. Laborious; requires 3-day collection; expensive
Structural tests		
Plain abdominal radiographs (Fig. 15.24.2.1)	Detection of pancreatic calcification	Simple, inexpensive; diffuse calcification indicates severe damage and is hallmark of alcoholic pancreatitis; focal calcification seen in trauma, islet- cell tumours, hereditary pancreatitis, malnutrition, hypercalcaemia, idiopathic pancreatitis
Ultrasonography (Fig. 15.24.2.2)		Simple, cheap, no radiation. Can provide information on cysts, phlegmon, calcification, abscesses
CT (Fig. 15.24.2.3)	Detailed visualization of pancreas	Early detection of masses. Expensive; high-dose radiation; may not distinguish inflammation from cancer
ERCP (Figs. 15.24.2.4 and 15.24.2.5)	Direct imaging of pancreatic ducts	Sensitivity 70%; specificity 90%. Differentiation of cancer may be difficult. Expensive, invasive—3% risk of acute pancreatitis
MRCP	Visualization of pancreatic and biliary ducts	Cannot offer therapeutic intervention
EUS (Figs. 15.24.2.6 and 15.24.2.7)	Assessment of intraductal system and pancreatic parenchyma	Highly skilled operator needed. May be combined with FNA

CCK, cholecystokinin; ERCP, endoscopic retrograde cholangiopancreatography; EUS, endoscopic ultrasonography; FNA, fine needle aspiration; MRCP, magnetic resonance cholangiopancreatography; PABA, *para*-aminobenzoic acid.

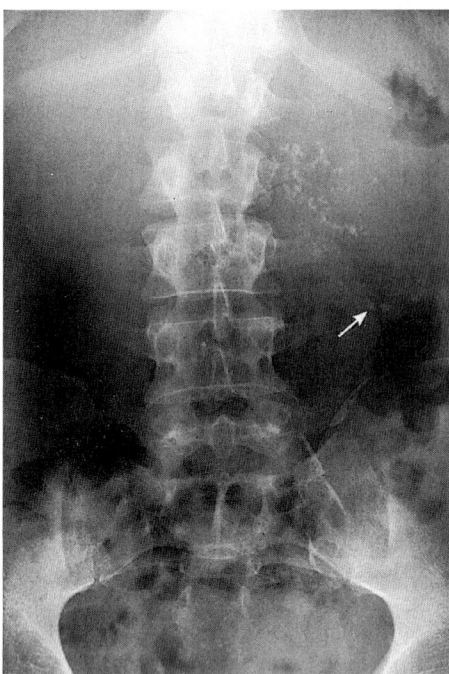

Fig. 15.24.2.1 Plain film of the abdomen showing diffuse pancreatic calcification; the arrow points to one of the calcified areas.

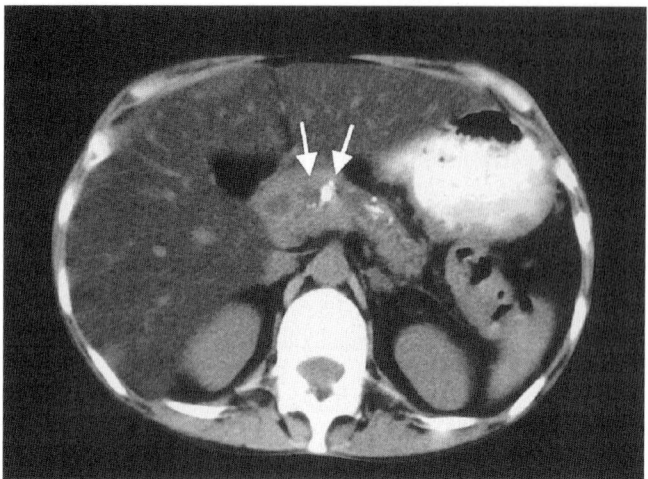

Fig 15.24.2.3 CT scan showing a fatty liver and chronic pancreatitis. Note the dilated pancreatic duct (left arrow) and calcification in the body of the pancreas (right arrow), also the very low attenuation of the liver (the normal density relationship of unenhanced hepatic vessels and liver is reversed) due to diffuse fatty infiltration (steatosis) that is most commonly caused by alcohol excess. (From the 4th edition of *Oxford Textbook of Medicine*, with acknowledgements to C S Ng, D J Lomas, and A K Dixon.)

pancreatitis, but ageing does not appear to affect the hormone stimulation test. Simple, noninvasive tests (bentiromide, pancreolauryl, serum trypsinogen, fecal elastase) are not sensitive and are used to confirm the clinical impression, and the same can be said for radiography other than endoscopic ultrasonography or ERCP.

Almost any test listed in Table 15.24.2.2 will identify patients with severe disease, but a hormone stimulation test is often needed to diagnose those with abdominal pain only. In comparison with the true 'gold standard'—histological examination of the pancreas—the most discriminatory function after hormone stimulation testing is the maximum bicarbonate concentration, followed by volume and amylase output. In one study of 29 patients with

histologically confirmed pancreatitis, the cholecystokinin–secretin test had a sensitivity of 79%, compared with 66% for ERCP. A simple, inexpensive test that has a sensitivity and specificity approaching that of hormone stimulation is needed but is not yet available. A cost-effective approach to the evaluation of patients suspected of having chronic pancreatitis would first be to use a simple noninvasive test like serum trypsinogen, bentiromide or fecal elastase, and initiate pancreatic enzyme therapy if the result is abnormal.

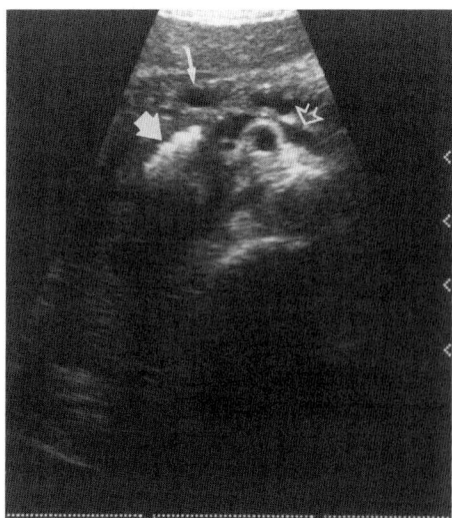

Fig. 15.24.2.2 Ultrasonogram of chronic pancreatitis. The large closed arrow points to pancreatic calcification; the small closed arrow shows a dilated pancreatic duct; and the open arrow identifies the splenic vein.

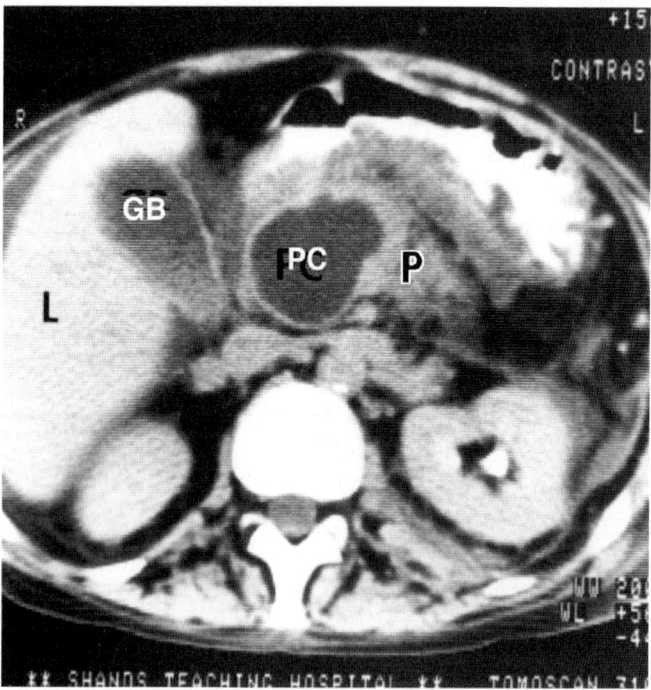

Fig. 15.24.2.4 CT scan demonstrating a pseudocyst (PC) in the head of the pancreas, diffuse enlargement of the pancreas (P), a normal liver (L), and normal gallbladder (GB).

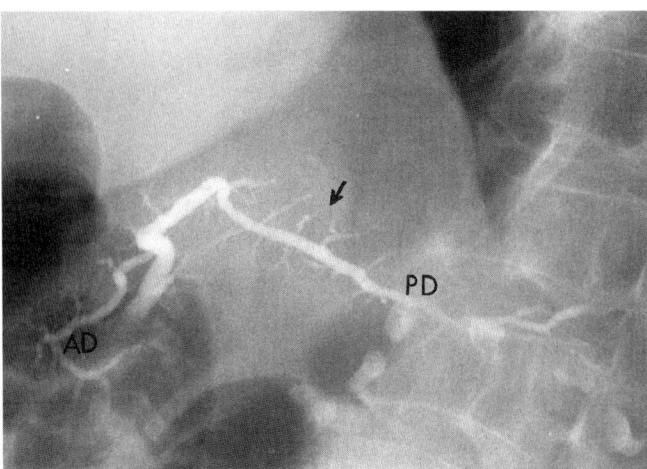

Fig. 15.24.2.5 ERCP showing early changes of chronic pancreatitis. A non-dilated main pancreatic duct with mild dilatation and clubbing of the side branches are seen.

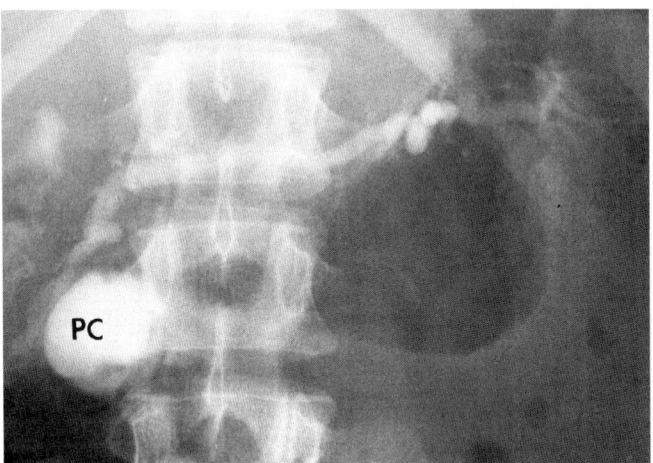

Fig. 15.24.2.6 ERCP showing a dilated main pancreatic duct (compare with that demonstrated in Fig. 15.24.2.4) with a communicating pseudocyst (PC).

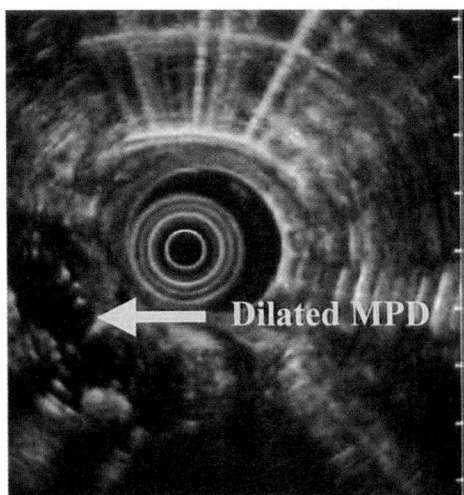

Fig. 15.24.2.7 Endoscopic ultrasonogram showing a dilated main pancreatic duct (MPD).

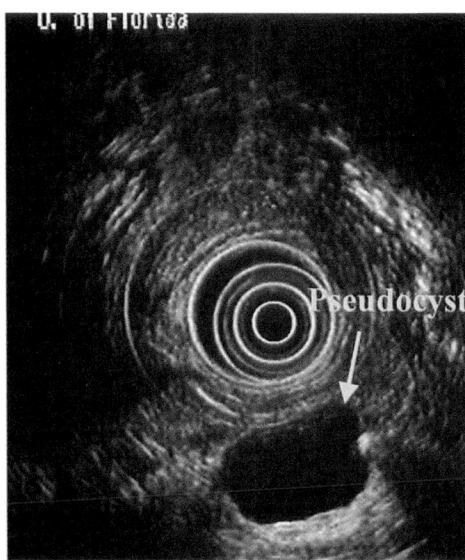

Fig. 15.24.2.8 Endoscopic ultrasonogram showing a pseudocyst.

However, if this first-ordered test is normal, the next step would be EUS or a hormone stimulation test, as further discussed below.

Management

The most important aspect of the medical management of chronic pancreatitis is the use of pancreatic enzyme formulations, which can be effective in treating both pain and steatorrhoea. A potent enzyme formulation must be used to ensure that the relevant enzymes (protease for pain, lipase for steatorrhoea) escape destruction by gastric acid and reach the duodenum.

Abstinence from alcohol is recommended. The diet should be moderate in fat (30%), high in protein (24%), and low in carbohydrate (40%). When required, non-narcotic analgesics are the pain-relieving medications of choice.

To date, three controlled trials have shown that pancreatic enzymes decrease abdominal pain in 75% of patients with chronic pancreatitis. Those most likely to respond have small-duct disease, i.e. a minimal to moderate impairment of exocrine function (normal fat absorption, abnormal hormone stimulation test, minimal abnormalities on ERCP; see Fig. 15.24.2.5). By contrast, patients with severe (large-duct) disease (steatorrhoea, abnormal hormone stimulation test, marked abnormalities on ERCP; see Fig. 15.24.2.6) do not respond well to enzyme therapy for pain. These clinical observations fit well with findings in experimental animals and humans, which demonstrate the negative-feedback regulation of pancreatic secretion controlled by the amount of proteases within the proximal small intestine. Treatment comprising eight tablets or capsules of a potent, non-enteric-coated enzyme preparation should be given at mealtimes and at bedtime, with appropriate adjuvant therapy (Box 15.24.2.1). Enteric-coated preparations are not the preparations of choice because they often release their proteases in the jejunum or ileum rather than the duodenum, thus failing to deliver to the feedback-sensitive segment of the intestine; these preparations may also cause acute colonic disease and rupture.

Figure 15.24.2.9 outlines an approach to patients with abdominal pain thought to be caused by chronic pancreatitis. After other causes of abdominal pain have been excluded, ultrasonography should be performed. If no pseudocyst or mass is found, a

Box 15.24.2.1 Frequently used pancreatic enzyme therapy

Pancrelipase

- Viokase 8 (C), 8 tablets each time
- Viokase 16 (C), 4 tablets each time

Pancreatin

- Creon (E), 3 capsules each time
- Pancrease MT (E), 3 capsules each time
- Ultrase (E), 3 capsules each time

Adjuvant

- H$_2$-receptor antagonist in usual acid-suppressive dose twice a day
- Proton pump inhibitor in usual acid-suppressive dose once a day

The enzymes should be administered before meals; a bedtime dosage should be given if the enzymes are being used to treat pain.

hormone stimulation test should be performed; this will invariably be abnormal in patients with abdominal pain secondary to chronic pancreatitis. A 4-week trial of pancreatic enzymes (with adjuvant) is indicated, as described above. If pain is not relieved, ERCP is appropriate to characterize the pancreatitis as small- or large-duct disease, and possibly to define the surgical approach.

If there is large-duct disease (diameter of the main pancreatic duct >7 mm), a lateral pancreaticojejunostomy (Peustow

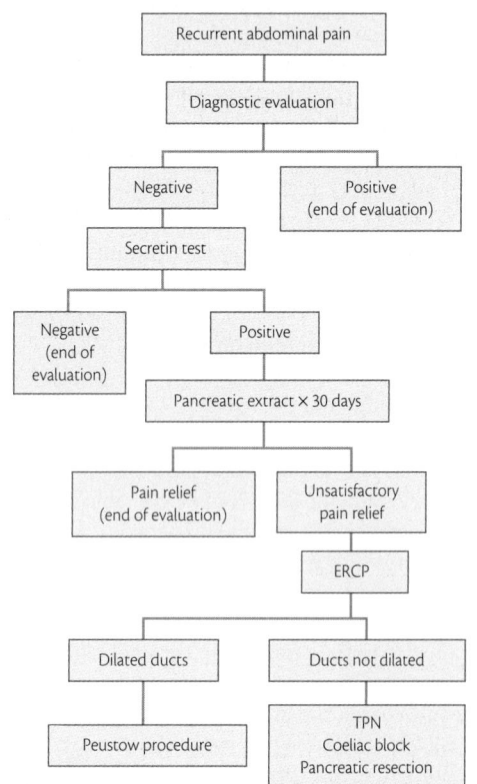

Fig. 15.24.2.9 Approach to the management of chronic pancreatitis and abdominal pain.

procedure) should be performed. Immediate pain relief occurs in 80% of patients, with satisfactory pain relief sustained in about 50% at 1 to 3 years follow-up. If the ducts are not significantly dilated, most patients can eventually have their pain controlled by adjusting their enzyme and adjuvant therapy, e.g. substitution of a proton pump inhibitor for an H$_2$ receptor antagonist, total parenteral nutrition with no food orally for several weeks, or by performing a nerve block. It is now rare for a major pancreatic resection to be undertaken to control pain, but whether ductal decompression or major resection are performed, enzyme therapy for enhancing digestion should still be given. In some preliminary controlled trials, octreotide given subcutaneously in doses up to 200 µg three times daily has been effective in reducing pain in patients with severe chronic pancreatitis.

Endoscopic therapy for the pain of chronic pancreatitis—which has included dilatation or stenting of duct strictures, removal of calculi, and treatment of biliary obstruction—has been disappointing. With the exception of acute biliary decompression, none of these therapies has been shown to be effective. Complications such as bleeding, sepsis, pancreatitis, and perforation have occurred after stent placement; moreover, stents can induce progressive ductal changes similar to the abnormalities seen in chronic pancreatitis.

Steatorrhoea in chronic pancreatitis is a late finding and does not occur until lipase secretion is reduced by 90%. With eight conventional or three enteric-coated enzyme tablets or capsules (see Table 15.24.2.3), control of steatorrhoea and diarrhoea, and weight gain, can be readily achieved, even though some steatorrhoea persists. Formulations containing 25 000 units or more of lipase have recently been associated with the occurrence of colonic strictures in patients with cystic fibrosis who were taking large doses of these high-potency preparations. In the United States of America, all pancreatic enzyme preparations with more than 20 000 units of lipase per capsule have been taken out of clinical use.

Decreasing the amount of long-chain triglycerides in the diet and/or adding medium-chain triglycerides (which do not require pancreatic lipase for absorption) should decrease the steatorrhoea and enhance weight gain and energy.

Complications

Table 15.24.2.3 lists the structural and other complications of chronic pancreatitis. Inflammatory masses are common. Ultrasonography and CT greatly assist in discriminating phlegmon from a pseudocyst and from an abscess. The management of

Table 15.24.2.3 Complications of chronic pancreatitis

Structural	Other
Phlegmon	Narcotic addiction
Pseudocyst	Diabetes mellitus
Abscess	Cobalamin (vitamin B$_{12}$) malabsorption (deficiency rare)
Ascites	Subcutaneous fat necrosis
Common bile duct obstruction	Bone pain (osteomalacia)
Duodenal obstruction	Nondiabetic retinopathy
Splenic vein thrombosis	Pancreatic cancer
Gastrointestinal bleeding	

pseudocysts is currently being re-evaluated: most clinicians have hitherto recommended drainage if they persist for longer than 7 weeks, but the ability of pseudocysts to undergo late resolution may have been underestimated and the incidence of serious complications exaggerated. A mature pseudocyst that has benign radiological appearances should be observed in a patient who has minimal symptoms and is not actively abusing alcohol: nine out of ten such pseudocysts will resolve without complications.

Pancreatic ascites occurs when there is a rent in the pancreatic duct or a leaking pseudocyst. The amylase content in the ascitic fluid is extraordinarily high, averaging 20 000 IU/litre, which distinguishes this true pancreatic ascites from 'reactive ascites' in patients with pancreatitis. In reactive ascites the amylase content of the fluid is increased, but is not nearly as high as in the pancreatic ascites. Pancreatic stimulation should be avoided in patients with pancreatic ascites: they should receive total parenteral nutrition and no food by mouth; proton pump inhibitors or H_2 antagonists will reduce pancreatic stimulation resulting from gastric acid release into the duodenum. Surgery may be needed if the ascites persists after several weeks of conservative therapy, with ERCP sometimes required to determine the site of duct leakage.

Obstruction of the common bile duct is common, but may be temporary owing to the resolution of inflammation. Biliary obstruction due to fibrosis of the pancreas rarely leads to cholangitis. Conservative management is justified unless the alkaline phosphatase level remains very high or cholangitis develops. In a few patients obstruction may require surgical relief by anastomosis of the dilated common bile duct to the duodenum or jejunum.

Gastrointestinal bleeding may arise from portal hypertension associated with splenic vein thrombosis caused by inflammation of the tail of the pancreas. Bleeding may also occur if a pseudocyst erodes into the duodenum, or from a pseudoaneurysm within the wall of a pseudocyst. However, the most common cause of bleeding in chronic pancreatitis is a related duodenal ulcer or alcohol-induced gastritis.

Up to 30% of patients with chronic pancreatitis have impaired glucose tolerance. Although pancreatic diabetes is usually manageable, destruction of glucagon-containing cells may render hypoglycaemia more likely. Diabetic retinopathy occurs as often in pancreatic diabetes as in other types of diabetes mellitus, and retinopathy due to a zinc or vitamin A deficiency may also occur.

Cobalamin (vitamin B_{12}) malabsorption is common in chronic pancreatitis, but clinical vitamin B_{12} deficiency is rare. It is caused by the failure to release free cobalamin by proteolysis of transcobalamin complexes. The exogenous administration of pancreatic enzymes corrects the maldigestion.

Familial and congenital diseases

Hereditary pancreatitis (OMIM 167800)

Familial or hereditary pancreatitis is an autosomal dominant disorder with approximately 80% penetrance that is responsible for about 1% of all cases of chronic pancreatitis. These patients often present in childhood with recurrent acute pancreatitis which causes chronic pancreatitis and often pancreatic insufficiency. The lifetime risk of developing pancreatic cancer is quite high. The genetic abnormality is a defect in the cationic trypsinogen gene (*PRSS1*), which appears to interfere with the inactivation of trypsin after it is cleaved. Mutations in the cystic fibrosis transmembrane conductance regulator gene (*CTFR*) and the pancreatic secretory trypsinogen inhibitor gene (*SPINK1*) are also linked to pancreatitis. See Chapter 15.24.1 for further discussion.

Shwachman–Diamond syndrome (OMIM 260400)

This familial disorder is caused by homozygous or compound heterozygous mutations of the Shwachman–Bodian–Diamond syndrome gene (*SBDS*), whose function is not known. The condition affects the pancreas, bone marrow and skeletal system, and is second only to cystic fibrosis as a cause of pancreatic insufficiency in infants. Neonates present with severe steatorrhoea that can be well treated by pancreatic enzymes. The associated neutropenia leads to frequent infections, and there is a high lifetime risk of transformation into acute myeloid leukaemia. Severe skeletal defects result in dwarfism.

Isolated pancreatic enzyme deficiencies

Protease deficiencies result from a lack of enterokinase (proximal small-intestine mucosal enzyme) or trypsinogen. The addition of exogenous enterokinase to duodenal secretions will differentiate these two deficiencies; it will not activate duodenal secretions lacking trypsinogen. Both conditions respond to pancreatic enzyme therapy. Lipase and colipase deficiencies are also rare isolated deficiencies that cause steatorrhoea. Patients with these pancreatic lipase deficiencies retain a residual fat-absorbing capacity, presumably from the action of other lipases such as gastric lipase.

Developmental anomalies

Annular pancreas

A failure of the ventral and dorsal embryonic elements of the pancreas to unite produces a ring of pancreatic tissue encircling the duodenum. This may lead to intestinal obstruction in the neonate or the adult. Nonspecific symptoms of postprandial fullness, nausea, abdominal pain, and vomiting may be present for years before the diagnosis is made. Radiographs show fixed symmetrical dilatation of the proximal duodenum, with bulging of the recesses on either side of the annular band, effacement of the duodenal mucosa without obstruction of the mucosa, and accentuation of the findings in the right anterior oblique position. The differential diagnosis should include duodenal webs, tumours of the pancreas or duodenum, postbulbar peptic ulcer, Crohn's disease of the proximal intestine, and adhesions. Patients with an annular pancreas have an increased incidence of pancreatitis and peptic ulcer. Surgery may be necessary because of these and other intestinal complications. Retrocolic duodenojejunostomy is the procedure of choice, although some surgeons prefer a Billroth II gastrectomy with gastroenterostomy and vagotomy.

Pancreas divisum

Pancreas divisum is the most common congenital anatomical abnormality of the human pancreas. It occurs when the ventral and dorsal parts of the pancreas fail to fuse, so that pancreatic drainage is accomplished mainly through the accessory papilla. Current evidence indicates that this anomaly predisposes, albeit infrequently, to the development of pancreatitis. The combination of a pancreas divisum and a small accessory orifice could result in dorsal-duct obstruction. The challenge is to identify this subset of patients. Cannulation of the dorsal duct by ERCP is not as easy as cannulation of the ventral duct. Patients with pancreatitis and pancreas divisum demonstrated by ERCP should be treated conservatively, including with pancreatic enzyme therapy. Many of them have idiopathic pancreatitis unrelated to the pancreas divisum and will respond well to pancreatic enzymes. Endoscopic or surgical intervention is indicated only when these methods fail. Surgical ductal decompression is indicated if marked dilatation of the dorsal duct can be demonstrated. However, the appropriate therapy for those patients without dilatation of the dorsal duct is not yet defined. It should be emphasized that the ERCP appearance of pancreas divisum (i.e. a small-calibre ventral duct with an arborizing pattern) may be confused with an obstructed main pancreatic duct caused by a pancreatic tumour.

Further reading

Amann ST, Toskes PP (1998). Hyperlipidemia and pancreatitis. In: Berger HG, *et al.* (eds) *The pancreas*, pp. 311–16. Blackwell Science, Oxford.

Cahen DL, *et al* (2007). Endoscopic versus surgical drainage of the pancreatic duct in chronic pancreatitis. *N Engl J Med*, **356**, 676–84.

Chowdhury R, *et al.* (2003). Prevalence of gastroparesis in patients with small duct chronic pancreatitis. *Pancreas*, **26**, 235–8.

Chowdhury R, *et al* (2005). Comparative analysis of direct pancreatic function testing versus morphological assessment by endoscopic ultrasonography for the evaluation of chronic unexplained abdominal pain of presumed pancreatic origin. *Pancreas*, **31**, 63–8.

Fazel A, Draganov P (2004). EUS in the evaluation and management of chronic pancreatitis. *Tech Gastrointest Endosc*, **6**, 107–44.

Gupta V, Toskes PP. (2005). Diagnosis and management of chronic pancreatitis. *Postgrad Med J*, **81**, 491–7.

Milmerowicz H, *et al.* (2007). Dysfunction of the pancreas in healthy smoking persons and patients with chronic pancreatitis. *Pancreas*, **34**, 46–54.

Pannala R, Chavist ST (2008). Autoimmune pancreatitis. *Curr Opin Gastroenterol*, **24**, 591–6.

Somogyi L, *et al.* (2000). Synthetic porcine secretin is highly accurate in pancreatic function testing in individuals with chronic pancreatitis. *Pancreas*, **21**, 262–5.

Vitab GJ, Sarr MG (1992). Selected management of pancreatic pseudocysts: operative versus expectant management. *Surgery*, **111**, 124–30.

Walsh TN, *et al.* (1992). Minimal change chronic pancreatitis. *Gut*, **33**, 1566–71.

Whitcomb DC, *et al.* (1996). Hereditary pancreatitis is caused by a mutation in the cationic trypsinogen gene. *Nat Genet*, **14**, 141–5.

15.24.3 **Tumours of the pancreas**

Martin Lombard and Ian Gilmore

Essentials

Pancreatic cancer, most commonly in the form of a solid ductal adenocarcinoma, accounts for 3% of all cancers but ranks in the top five leading causes of cancer deaths in most developed coun-

tries, reflecting the fact that it has a very poor prognosis (median survival 6 to 9 months). It is a disease of old age (85% of patients >65 years), and commoner in smokers.

Most patients present with locally advanced or metastatic disease, often with obstructive jaundice. Pain is unusual in early disease, but when present is characteristically described as 'gnawing', ever present, and frequently radiating into the back. Weight loss is commonly due to anorexia as a result of jaundice or pain, but can occasionally be the only presenting symptom. Increased use of abdominal imaging means that incidental discovery of pancreatic cancer is becoming more common.

Serum biochemistry will typically show elevated bilirubin and a cholestatic picture of liver enzymes, with particular elevation of alkaline phosphatase and γ-glutamyl transferase. Transabdominal ultrasonography is usually the primary investigation in a patient with jaundice and can detect pancreatic tumours >2 cm in size or hepatic metastases with a diagnostic accuracy of 75%, but identifies smaller tumours much less reliably. The essential investigations for the diagnosis and staging of pancreatic cancer are contrast-phased CT scan or MRI.

The only curative treatment for pancreatic cancer is surgical excision. This is technically feasible in up to 40% patients at presentation, but even after careful selection almost 40% of these will have positive microsopic resection margins, and overall postoperative survival is only around 10% at 5 years, the remainder experiencing metastatic disease in the peritoneum, liver, or lungs. Adjuvant chemotherapy with 5-fluorouracil or gemcitabine can double the 5-year survival rate.

Palliative management may require biliary stenting for jaundice, duodenal stenting (or surgical bypass) for gastric outlet obstruction, and pain control.

Introduction

Pancreatic cancer is a devastating illness with an incidence in the United Kingdom of about 12.4/100 000 population per year. Thus there are 7500 new cases each year in the United Kingdom and this incidence is mirrored elsewhere: 32 000 in the United States of America and an estimated 232 000 worldwide. Eighty-five per cent of pancreatic cancer presents in patients >65 years and incidence rates are almost equivalent in both genders with a declining trend in males and an increasing occurrence in females during the past 30 years. It accounts for only 3% of all cancers but ranks in the top five leading causes of cancer deaths in most developed countries. Annual mortality statistics are almost identical to incidence, underscoring the fact that this disease has a very poor prognosis (see below). This is in part because of the late presentation of the disease, most tumours being already surgically unresectable, and in part because of the aggressive tumour biology.

Aetiology, genetics, pathogenesis, and pathology

The vast majority of pancreatic cancers arise from the ductular cells of the exocrine acini, usually as a solid ductal adenocarcinoma. Rarely (3%), they are mucin-producing neoplasms which can be cystic or intraductal; other rare primary tumours of the pancreas include lymphomas and endocrine tumours. These less common types are worth diagnosing because of their substantially better outlook.

Cigarette smoking is the only consistently reported risk factor and may contribute to up to 30% of pancreatic cancers. The risk appears to be dose- and possibly duration- dependent. For a man smoking more than 25 cigarettes/day the relative risk is 3.2; it is 1.8 for a man smoking less than 25 cigarettes/day, and 1.4 for an ex-smoker compared to nonsmokers. Smokers tend to develop cancer on average 10 years younger than nonsmokers.

Chronic pancreatitis is thought to double the risk of developing cancer, particularly when long-standing and calcific in nature, but there is some shared aetiological background that is difficult to untangle. In hereditary pancreatitis, a rare autosomal dominant condition where there is a defect in the *PRSS1* gene that regulates trypsin activation, there is a greatly increased risk of malignant change.

Overall up to 10% of cases may have a genetic cause, and sometimes clustering of pancreatic cancer is seen in families with breast and other cancers. No single gene has been identified in familial pancreatic cancer, but germ-line mutations in the *BRCA2* gene appear to be involved in a significant number. Patients with Peutz–Jeghers syndrome have a more than 100-fold increased lifetime risk and patients with cystic fibrosis living into adulthood are also at increased cancer risk, but there is currently no case for screening as effective protocols and tests have not been devised.

Diabetes mellitus has an association with pancreatic cancer and a significant number of patients with cancer have had type 2 diabetes diagnosed within 2 years previous to presentation. This is not just because the cancer may be the cause of the diabetes through pancreatic destruction, as the association holds good with long-standing pre-existing glucose intolerance and possibly with type 1 diabetes too. There is also an association with increased body weight, but this does not necessarily hold true if physical activity is also increased. There are a few industries, such as paint and textile manufacturing, that appear to have increased risk, possibly related to hydrocarbon exposure, and nickel and insecticides have also been implicated. The effects of diet or alcohol on risk of pancreatic cancer has been studied extensively but the results are inconsistent. Similarly, suggestions that gallbladder disease, previous cholecystectomy, peptic ulcer disease, or hypertension are linked remain unproven.

Prevention

At present, there is no effective population-based strategy for the prevention of pancreatic cancer. The only consistent aetiological factor is cigarette smoking and it may be expected that in those countries that have legislated against smoking in public, and adopted other strategies to reduce cigarette consumption overall, the incidence may decline. Otherwise, health policies are currently best directed at early diagnosis and devising effective screening protocols in populations identified to be at risk.

Clinical features

Almost 80% of patients with pancreatic cancer present with locally advanced or metastatic disease with a median survival of 6 to 9 months. Two-thirds of pancreatic cancers occur in the head or uncinate parts of the organ and their growth beyond 1 cm will usually cause obstruction of the common bile duct as it passes through the head. Most patients therefore present with jaundice and frequently give a history of pale stools and dark urine consistent with cholestatic jaundice. Although cancer at this site all too often presents at a stage where there is local invasion, it may be an earlier and more visible presentation than when the cancer arises more peripherally in the gland. Pain is unusual as a feature of early pancreatic cancer but is more common if the cancer arises in the body, possibly because of invasion of a rich neural plexus. The pain is characteristically described as 'gnawing' and ever present, and frequently radiates into the back.

Weight loss is commonly due to anorexia as a result of jaundice or pain but can occasionally be the only presenting symptom. It can be due to pancreatic enzyme deficiency and this is an important consideration in managing the patient. A tendency to looser bowel motions is frequent, but diarrhoea is unusual. Steatorrhoea is sometimes seen. Very occasionally the patient will present with abdominal swelling due to ascites but it is unusual for this to be the sole presenting feature.

A common presentation of pancreas cancer now (and many other cancers) is as an incidental finding picked up on abdominal imaging done for other reasons or a presentation unrelated to the cancer itself. This is particularly so for cystic pancreatic tumours, which make up about 15% of pancreatic cysts and can be a chance finding at abdominal ultrasound examination.

Differential diagnosis

The alternative possible diagnoses depend on the patient's clinical presentation. The commonest presentation, with jaundice and dilated bile ducts on ultrasound scan, is more often due to choledocholithiasis especially in younger patients, and particularly those who have had a cholecystectomy, more often women. Older women (>80 years) with stones in the common bile duct can often present with minimal jaundice, abnormal liver enzymes, dilated ducts, and/or abdominal pain but men older than 60 years presenting in this way are more likely to have pancreatic tumours.

It is important to distinguish cancer of the ampulla of Vater as this has a better prognosis and this should be suspected in patients presenting with jaundice associated with dilated bile ducts and microcytic anaemia—these intraluminal tumours usually bleed.

Patients with tumours of the common bile duct (cholangiocarcinoma) or gallbladder cancer can present in exactly the same way as those with pancreas cancer and occasionally can be difficult to distinguish. They are less common tumours, the work-up for diagnosis is similar, and their management is usually by the same multidisciplinary team of clinicians involved with pancreas cancer.

Patients with previous abdominal surgery can present with jaundice and dilated bile ducts. A recent cholecystectomy or surgery involving the bile duct suggests the possibility of a bile duct injury, but stones in the common bile duct following cholecystectomy are much more common. Occasionally patients who have had a gastrectomy or vagotomy previously for ulcer disease can present many years later with dilated bile ducts or jaundice, and this scenario also is more usually due to common bile duct stones.

Clinical investigation, diagnosis, and staging

Clinical presentation will be most commonly with jaundice of a cholestatic nature (pale stools and dark urine). Serum biochemistry confirms an elevated bilirubin level, often at levels up to 10 times normal, and abnormal liver enzymes, particularly alkaline phosphatase (AlkP) and γ-glutamyl transferase (GGT). In situations where the patient is not jaundiced, liver enzymes can be normal or only very slightly elevated. Full blood count is usually normal. Occasionally tumours are found incidentally in patients presenting with recent-onset diabetes mellitus or who are under investigation for other reasons. Tumours are detected and staged by a variety of imaging techniques.

Ultrasonography

Transabdominal ultrasound scan is usually the primary investigation in a patient with jaundice and can detect dilatation of bile ducts with a sensitivity of 90%. It can detect pancreatic tumours >2 cm in size or hepatic metastases with a diagnostic accuracy of 75% but detects smaller tumours much less reliably. Ultrasonography identifies the cause of biliary obstruction in only 60% of cases, but the clinical presentation and context together with the age and gender of the patient frequently lead to the diagnosis. A dilated bile duct in the absence of jaundice is rarely due to pancreatic tumour but requires further investigation to exclude this possibility.

Transabdominal ultrasonography is often used for the investigation of abdominal pain in patients without jaundice and may identify a tumour in the body of pancreas, but this is not a common presentation; experience and expertise of the operator and the patient's body habitus are important determinants of its usefulness in this situation.

Contrast-enhanced ultrasonography using an intravenous microbubble infusion is useful in detecting or characterizing liver metastases but is no more sensitive than noncontrast techniques for detecting small primary tumours of the pancreas and is probably not practical in routine practice.

CT

Contrast-phased CT is essential for the diagnosis and staging of pancreatic cancer. It is more accurate than ultrasonography at identifying the level and cause of obstructed bile ducts. Published sensitivity and specificity rates are determined by the quality of the scan (e.g. multislice using a pancreas protocol and 1 mm images), the size of the tumour, and expert interpretation. Tumours of 1 cm and sometimes less can be detected with a diagnostic accuracy of 90%. Prediction of unresectability is also greater than 90% but prediction of curative resection is slightly less accurate, often because of peritoneal seeding or small metastases. CT is good at detecting lymph node enlargement but much less accurate at determining, without the aid of a biopsy, whether or not these contain metastatic tumour.

MRI and positron-emission tomography (PET)

MRI can produce results similar to contrast CT and the choice between them depends on local facilities, expertise, and protocols. It has advantages in patients who have difficult venous access, renal insufficiency, or allergy to contrast, but the claustrophophic environment is not tolerated by all patients. It is very useful in the differential diagnosis of biliary obstruction, for identifying stones in the bile duct and is recommended in preference to ERCP in nonjaundiced patients (i.e. where endoscopic therapy is not required) to avoid the risk of pancreatitis. Magnetic resonance spectroscopy to examine tumour metabolism is being explored as a

diagnostic tool. PET and PET-CT have been assessed for the diagnosis of pancreatic tumours but are much less accurate than MRI or contrast CT and cannot reliably distinguish tumour from inflammatory mass in the pancreas. Angiography has been superseded by CT and MR and does not usually provide additional useful information.

Endoscopic ultrasound (EUS)

EUS is ultrasonography undertaken from the lumen of the stomach and duodenum via a fibreoptic endoscope. It has a similar accuracy to contrast CT and MRI for diagnosis and local staging but its disadvantage is that it is more invasive. It has a superior sensitivity for smaller tumours (2–10 mm) and can more reliably identify neuroendocrine tumours in the pancreas. It is equally effective at assessing local invasion or lymph node involvement but less accurate at predicting resectability overall as it cannot reliably detect metastases or involvement of the coeliac axis. It is at least as effective as ERCP and MRCP at identifying stones as the cause of jaundice or dilated bile ducts in patients being investigated for obstructed bile ducts.

Used in conjunction with fine needle aspiration or biopsy (FNAB), it has a diagnostic accuracy of greater than 90% which is particularly useful for assessing nodal disease and is thought to pose less risk of seeding peritoneum or adjacent organs than transabdominal FNAB. EUS–FNAB should be reserved for patients who are deemed to have an unresectable tumour but for whom a tissue diagnosis is required to enable other treatments or trials to take place.

Endoscopic retrograde cholangiopancreatography (ERCP)

ERCP is best reserved for jaundiced patients whose imaging has been completed and have a working diagnosis of pancreas tumour. It is essential that patients suspected to have pancreatic cancer have had staging CT or MRI prior to ERCP, as the complication of post-ERCP pancreatitis may make subsequent staging difficult or impossible.

The objective of ERCP should be to acquire tissue samples for diagnosis and to place an endoprosthesis across the stricture to relieve jaundice. Contrast imaging of the bile ducts (cholangiography) can confirm tumour obstruction of the common bile duct but usually adds little to previous imaging. Brush cytology to confirm the nature of the obstruction is mandatory. Specificity is almost 100% and sensitivity is reported to be 40 to 80% depending on the technique used. A combination of sonicating the cellular sample from the brush and subsequent cytospin preparation has yielded the most accurate results. Brush cytology at ERCP is preferable to FNAB as it avoids risk of tumour seeding.

Relief of obstruction and jaundice can be achieved in 90% of patients by insertion of an endoprosthesis, but the goals of this manoeuvre should be defined. It does not affect the outcome of resectional surgery but is effective in relieving jaundice and pruritus while improving appetite and morale. For patients with unresectable disease, there are advantages in inserting wide-bore self-expanding metal endoprosthesis as these are less likely than smaller-bore plastic stents to occlude and usually provide very effective palliation.

For patients in whom therapeutic ERCP is unsuccessful, a percutaneous transhepatic cholangiogram (PTC) can achieve similar rates of cytological diagnosis and relief of obstruction by insertion of endoprosthesis although the morbidity is higher.

Laparoscopy

For patients deemed to have resectable disease on noninvasive imaging, laparoscopy—particularly combined with intraoperative ultrasonography—can be very effective in detecting small hepatic or peritoneal seeding, and may avoid unnecessary and ineffective radical surgery in 15% of patients otherwise thought operable. Selection of less than 50% of patients for laparoscopic staging by using the level of serum CA19.9 (see below) has been shown to promote efficient use of this modality and improves the yield of metastatic disease to 25%.

Tumour markers

Serum tumour markers are usually based on immune assays exploiting antibodies to mucoproteins expressed on or released by mucinous cells in pancreatic adenocarcinoma. The most commonly used serum marker is CA19-9, which can have a sensitivity of more than 70%. Its specificity is less than 90%, but as it can be elevated in the presence of jaundice or ascites, which are common with pancreatic cancer, caution is advised in its interpretation. Extremely high levels (>20 000 IU/litre) can be present in acute cholangitis. It should not be used as a screening test for patients in patients with abnormal liver enzymes or abdominal pain in the absence of jaundice as it has a very poor specificity in this context. A variety of other tumour markers (DU-PAN-2, CA50, CAM17.1) have been reported but have not proved as useful as CA19-9. Proteomic techniques to identify tumour associated proteins, or gene expression and mutation profiling, in samples of serum, pancreatic or duodenal juice, or bile (e.g. k-ras, p-53 m DPC-4) are being evaluated and may help in tailoring specific treatments to predictable tumour behaviour in the future.

Histopathology

Adenocarcinoma accounts for 95% of pancreatic tumours. It is usually well differentiated and can be identified in small cytology samples following cytospin, or in more substantial samples obtained by Tru-cut biopsy.

Cystic tumours are increasingly identified incidentally as a result of imaging rather than because of any specific clinical presentation. Seventy per cent of these are serous cystic neoplasms affecting the head or mucinous cystic neoplasms of the body or tail, both more commonly occurring in middle-aged women. By contrast, intraductal papillary mucinous neoplasms arise from the main pancreatic duct or its side branches and tend to affect older patients, predominantly men, and often cause pancreatic duct dilatation. All of these tend to be slow-growing neoplasms; the serous variety is often considered benign but the mucinous cystic and papillary types can undergo aggressive transformation and are also associated with other tumours of the pancreas or colon.

Endocrine tumours can be found as incidental lesions in the pancreas as part of an abdominal scan for other reasons but otherwise come to light only if they are secretory tumours that have hormonal effects. The two commonest endocrine tumours are insulinoma and gastrinoma. Recurrent bouts of hypoglycaemia with episodic hyperinsulaemia are characteristic of insulinoma, while gastrinomas can present with a history of recurrent abdominal pain, recalcitrant peptic ulcers, upper gastrointestinal haemorrhage, or duodenal perforation. In the initial investigation, serum levels of gut hormones should be measured but are often normal. Serum chromogranin-A has been shown to have a high sensitivity (80%) for neuroendocrine

tumours and its level reflects tumour burden, but it is not specific. Portal venous sampling for hormone levels can be useful but localizing these tumours precisely is difficult. Contrast CT or MRI scan should be undertaken but EUS is much more sensitive and specific for these tumours. Radiolabelled octreotide and/or ^{131}I-MIBG (*meta*-iodobenzylguanidine) can be used to locate tumours and to assess the possibility of using this modality for treatment. Surgical excision is usually curative. Endocrine syndromes require palliation and may occasionally respond to ^{131}I-MIBG or ^{90}Y-DOTOTOC, a somatostatin analogue.

Treatment

Surgery

The only curative treatment for pancreatic cancer is surgical excision. This is technically feasible in up to 40% of patients at presentation but, even after careful selection, almost 40% of these will have positive microsopic resection margins. The traditional operation is a Kausch–Whipples subtotal pancreatoduodenectomy, but a more commonly used approach is a pylorus-preserving partial pancreatoduoenectomy. Surgical-related mortality for this major operation is <4% but postoperative morbidity can be as high as 40%.

Resection margins are important in predicting recurrence. Also, comorbidity but not age has a significant effect on surgical outcomes. Radical resection in carefully selected patients is usually followed by a reported survival of only 10% at 5 years, the remainder experiencing metastatic disease in the peritoneum, liver, or lungs. Adjuvant chemotherapy with 5-fluorouracil or probably gemcitabine can double the 5-year survival rate. Adjuvant chemoradiotherapy is not beneficial unless the chemotherapy is continued long term and confers no advantage over chemotherapy alone. Evidence for effective neoadjuvant treatment is not available at present.

Surgical palliation is reserved for relief of gastric outlet obstruction by providing a gastroenterostomy but this can also now be achieved by endoscopic placement of wide-bore transduodenal self-expanding endoprosthesis.

Endoscopic therapy

This can provide effective palliation for relief of jaundice with consequent improvement in appetite, quality of life and pruritus. Usually a 2 to 3 mm diameter Teflon or plastic endoprosthesis is inserted into the common bile duct across the stenosing tumour at the time of ERCP. Complications of this procedure are rare but include pancreatitis, or bleeding if ampullary sphincterotomy is required to gain access to the duct. Silting and occlusion of the endoprosthesis is common at 3 to 4 months but replacement is straightforward. As overall survival improves with better palliation, a wider-bore 10 mm diameter self-expanding nitinol stent is now frequently inserted either at the first ERCP or at the time of replacement for stent occlusion. These tend to have a longer lifespan of 6 to 12 months, but tumour ingrowth is a problem for longer-surviving patients. Preoperative stenting for patients with resectable disease is probably unnecessary but is often undertaken if operation is delayed.

Medical treatment

This is used for symptom control or in an attempt to modify the natural history.

Pain is commonly a feature of cancer of the body of pancreas, possibly because of involvement of the neural plexus. Escalating doses of opioid analgesia with appropriate measures to avoid constipation are usually required. Coeliac plexus neurolysis by either an endoscopic posterior gastric route or a transcutaneous lumbar approach, or bilateral transthoracic sympathectomy, is a useful alternative in some patients.

Weight loss is often due to anorexia, and relief of jaundice can be helpful. Occasionally pancreatic supplements can produce impressive reversal of previous weight loss. They can also help if diarrhoea due to malabsorption becomes a problem.

The common type of pancreatic cancer is intrinsically drug-resistant. However, palliative improvement in survival has been demonstrated with infusions of 5-fluorouracil, which interferes with cell proliferation by incorporation of metabolites into RNA and DNA and inhibition of thymidylate synthase. This is still considered superior to best supportive care but within the last 10 years has been replaced by gemcitabine which is less toxic and confers significant advantages to the longer-term survivors (e.g. 18% vs 2% at 12 months). Gemcitabine is a fluorinated pyrimidine nucleoside analogue that interferes with cell division. Recently, a combination of gemcitabine with capecitabine has been shown to confer additional benefit and other combinations with oxalipaltin or irinotecan are being assessed. Median survival for most unresected patients is still around 6 months, however, and the improved survival for most patients with these regimens, although statistically significant, amounts only to a few weeks.

Radiotherapy for pancreatic tumours is limited by the proximity of adjacent radiosensitive structures and the inherent insensitivity of pancreatic adenocarcinoma. To improve potential for resectability, radiosensitizers such as gemcitabine, capecitabine or bevacizumab have demonstrated some promise in preliminary trials but these await confirmation. However, the specific role of radiation as opposed to the drugs remains unclear.

Prognosis

Although 1-year survival statistics in the United Kingdom have improved from 6% in 1971 to 13% in 2002, overall 5-year survival rates remain dismal at less than 3%. Better 1-year survival can be attained in certain groups, e.g. 25% of patients under 50 years of age will survive 1 year, but the 5-year survival is still poor. Ninety-five per cent of pancreatic cancers are adenocarcinomas of ductal origin, but better survival rates can be attained in some of the less common types of cancer.

Likely future developments

Understanding of tumour biology has increased greatly in the past 10 years. For pancreatic cancer, up-regulation or activation of many growth factors and receptors has been identified and the characterization of their role in development of cancer has suggested many candidate targets for therapy and also for more specific diagnosis. For example, vascular endothelial growth factor (VEGF) enhances peritumour angiogenesis and is present in 90% cases of pancreatic cancer. Bevazizumab and sunitimib are VEGF inhibitors that have shown promise in trials when combined with gemcitabine. Inhibition of other tumour-expressed molecules such as k-ras, the ErbB family of receptor tyrosine kinases, and downstream signals have also been targeted.

Another important development has been the collaborative approach undertaken by groups capable of recruiting larger numbers of patients into clinic trials. Thus the European Study Group for Pancreatic Cancer (ESPAC) and the Gastrointestinal Tumour Study Group (GITSG) have devised prospective randomized trials to assess adjuvant chemotherapy or chemoradiotherapy to improve resectability outcomes and this approach is more likely to give clear clinical guidance in the future for this challenging disease.

Further reading

Ghaneh P, Costello E, Neoptolemos JP. (2007). Biology and management of pancreatic cancer. *Gut*, **56**, 1134–52.

Kleef J, *et al.* (2006). Pancreatic cancer from bench to 5-year survival. Pancreas, **33**, 111–18.

Mancuso A, Calabro F, Sternberg CN (2006). Current therapies and advances in the treatment of pancreatic cancer. *Crit Rev Oncol Hematol*, **58**, 231–41.

Schima W, *et al.* (2007). Pancreatic adenocarcinoma. *Eur Radiol*, **17**, 638–49.

Website

Cancer Research UK. *Pancreatic cancer.* http://www.cancerhelp.org.uk/help/default.asp?page=2795

Congenital disorders of the liver, biliary tract, and pancreas

J.A. Summerfield

Essentials

Congenital disorders of the liver, biliary tract, and pancreas are rare or very rare.

Biliary atresias present with cholestatic jaundice starting after the first 2 weeks of life and may eventually cause biliary cirrhosis and liver failure. Prognosis depends on the type of atresia: (1) intrahepatic—both nonsyndromic (with cirrhosis usually developing in late childhood, and fatal without liver transplantation) and syndromic (e.g. Alagille's syndrome, due to mutation in the *JAG1* gene, with dysmorphic and other features, and a tendency for recovery of liver function in adolescence), or (2) extrahepatic—which is usually fatal within 6 months of birth unless treated by hepatic portoenterostomy and/or liver transplantation.

Fibropolycystic diseases include polycystic liver, congenital hepatic fibrosis, congenital intrahepatic biliary dilatation (Caroli's disease), choledochal cysts, and microhamartomas (von Meyenberg complexes). Patients may have more than one of these diseases, some of which may be complicated by biliary malignancy. Associated renal diseases can be severe.

Congenital pancreatic diseases comprise a heterogeneous group of conditions of varying severity, ranging from annular pancreas (where pancreatic tissue encircles the duodenum) that may be discovered incidentally, to pancreatic agenesis, which is usually fatal soon after birth.

Pathogenesis of congenital disorders of the biliary tract

During the 4th week of gestation the liver arises as a bud of cells (the hepatic diverticulum) from the ventral wall of the foregut. At about the 8th week of gestation a layer of liver precursor cells around the portal vein branches differentiate to form a sleeve, termed the ductal plate. This sleeve duplicates to form a double layer of cells which by 12 weeks is remodelled by dilatation of segments of the double-layered ductal plate to form tubules that become the intrahepatic bile ducts. Nontubular parts of the plate disappear and the bile ducts form part of the portal tracts.

Congenital disorders of the biliary tract are classified into two main groups: diseases characterized by inflammatory destruction of the bile ducts (the biliary atresias) and diseases marked by ectasia of the bile ducts with varying degrees of fibrosis (the fibropolycystic diseases). Both of these groups of disorders are related to the persistence or lack of remodeling of the embryonic ductal plate. They are termed 'ductal plate malformations'.

Ductal plate malformations can be seen on ultrasound or CT scans as a circular lumen containing a fibrovascular cord. Figure 15.25.1 shows ductal plate malformations in a CT scan of a patient with Caroli's disease (a fibropolycystic disease).

Biliary atresia

Classification

Biliary atresias are classified into extrahepatic biliary atresia and intrahepatic biliary atresia (paucity of intrahepatic bile ducts). Biliary atresia does not represent agenesis of the bile ducts but is the result of progressive bile duct destruction from an inflammatory disease of unknown cause. In extrahepatic biliary atresia the destructive cholangitis affects not only part or the whole of the extrahepatic bile duct but also intrahepatic bile ducts and leads to paucity of intrahepatic bile ducts. In intrahepatic biliary atresia the destructive cholangitis is restricted to the intrahepatic bile ducts. Intrahepatic biliary atresia can be classified further into a nonsyndromatic or a syndromatic type (Alagille's syndrome or arteriohepatic dysplasia). About one-quarter of patients with extrahepatic biliary atresia have evidence of ductal plate malformation indicating that the destructive cholangitis started early in fetal life.

Symptoms and signs

Biliary atresia presents as cholestatic jaundice starting after the first 2 weeks of life. The infant develops jaundice with pale stools, dark urine, and hepatomegaly. Itching is often prominent. Bile pigments may stain the growing teeth greenish. The jaundice steadily

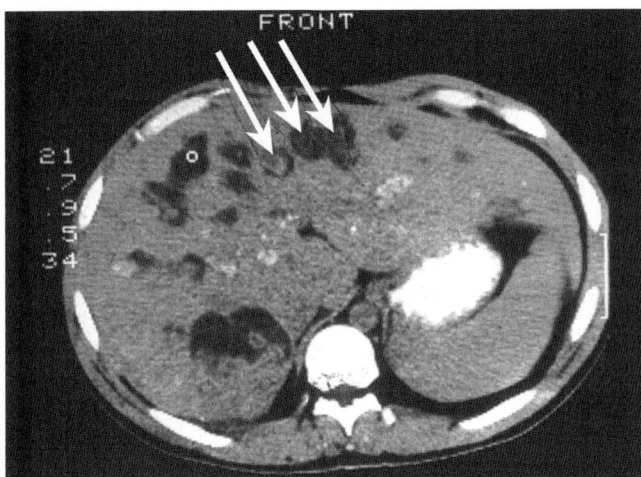

Fig. 15.25.1 Caroli's disease. Intravenous contrast enhanced CT scan of the liver shows dilated intrahepatic bile ducts containing filling defects which are portal vein branches (arrowed). This is an example of a ductal plate malformation. (From Sherlock S, Summerfield JA (1991). *A colour atlas of liver disease*, 2nd edition. Wolfe Medical Publications, London, with permission.)

deepens and xanthomas of the palm and knees, rickets, a bleeding tendency, and growth failure may develop. Biliary atresia may eventually cause biliary cirrhosis with pigmentation (due to melanin), portal hypertension, ascites, and liver failure.

The progress of biliary atresia depends on the type. Infants with extrahepatic biliary atresia (usually girls) have a steadily deepening jaundice and biliary cirrhosis soon develops. Untreated, these children usually die by 6 months of age. The fate of infants with intrahepatic biliary atresia depends on whether they have a syndromatic or nonsyndromatic atresia. Children with nonsyndromatic intrahepatic biliary atresia survive longer than those with extrahepatic biliary atresia, but biliary cirrhosis eventually develops in later childhood. In contrast, patients with syndromic intrahepatic biliary atresia (Alagille's syndrome) tend to recover normal liver function as they become adolescent. Infants with Alagille's syndrome can be recognized by the associated features, which include a characteristic facies (a flattened and triangular-shaped face), pulmonary stenosis, vertebral abnormalities, and a change in the eyes (embryotoxon). Some patients have growth and mental retardation. Alagille's syndrome is a dominantly inherited disorder associated with mutations in the Jagged 1 (*JAG1*) gene. *JAG1* encodes a ligand in the Notch intercellular signaling pathway.

Differential diagnosis

Jaundice is common in early infancy. In the early neonatal period jaundice is usually due to haemolysis and impaired bilirubin conjugation. After 2 weeks, jaundice is usually cholestatic. There are many causes of cholestasis in infancy and childhood. The most common are extrahepatic and intrahepatic biliary atresias, neonatal hepatitis (such as hepatitis A, B, and C, rubella, and cytomegalovirus infection), metabolic causes (such as galactosaemia, α_1-antitrypsin deficiency, and tyrosinaemia), and the 'inspissated bile syndrome' (congenital spherocytosis).

Laboratory investigations

Liver function tests show a cholestatic (biliary obstructive) pattern. Serum bilirubin and alkaline phosphatase levels are markedly raised with only modest elevations of serum transaminases. Later, very high levels of serum cholesterol may develop.

Histological examination of the liver cannot distinguish between intrahepatic and extrahepatic biliary atresia. Liver biopsy shows severe centrizonal cholestasis and a prominent giant-cell reaction. In the portal tracts bile ducts are reduced. Later in the course of the disease the portal tracts are devoid of bile ducts and biliary cirrhosis is present.

Imaging

The initial step in the management of infants with cholestasis is to differentiate between intrahepatic and extrahepatic biliary atresia. Since the clinical and laboratory findings are similar, this distinction requires imaging techniques. In extrahepatic biliary atresia, scintiscanning with ^{99}Tcm-labelled HIDA (dimethyl acetanilide iminodiacetic acid) shows accumulation of the label in the liver but none enters the biliary tree. Percutaneous and endoscopic cholangiography provides more precise anatomical detail.

Treatment and prognosis

General supportive measures include parenteral administration of fat-soluble vitamins A, D, K, and E. Medium-chain triglycerides as a source of fat, cholestyramine to relieve itching, and ursodeoxycholic acid as a choleretic help some patients.

Extrahepatic biliary atresia

Hepatic portoenterostomy (Kasai's operation) has been the treatment of choice for extrahepatic biliary atresia and is still widely performed. Approximately 25 to 35% of patients who undergo a Kasai portoenterostomy will survive more than 10 years without liver transplantation. One-third of the patients drain bile but develop complications of cirrhosis and require liver transplantation before the age of 10. For the remaining one-third of patients, bile flow is inadequate following portoenterostomy and the children develop progressive fibrosis and cirrhosis. The portoenterostomy should be done before there is irreversible sclerosis of the intrahepatic bile ducts. Consequently, a prompt evaluation for conjugated hyperbilirubinaemia is indicated for any infant older than 14 days with jaundice.

Intrahepatic biliary atresia

All infants should receive general supportive measures. Definitive treatment depends on the type of intrahepatic biliary atresia. Nonsyndromic intrahepatic biliary atresia eventually progresses to biliary cirrhosis and liver failure. Liver transplantation should be performed before the onset of liver failure. Syndromic intrahepatic biliary atresia (Alagille's syndrome) has a good prognosis in most children and few develop biliary cirrhosis. General supportive measures are usually sufficient until the cholestasis disappears.

Fibropolycystic disease

Fibropolycystic disease encompasses a family of rare congenital hepatobiliary diseases that arise due to malformations of the embryonic ductal plate. These diseases include polycystic liver, congenital hepatic fibrosis, congenital intrahepatic biliary dilatation (Caroli's disease, Fig. 15.25.1), choledochal cysts, and microhamartomas (von Meyenberg complexes). Many patients will have more than one disease. The combination of congenital hepatic fibrosis and Caroli's disease is characteristic as these patients develop first variceal haemorrhage (due to congenital hepatic fibrosis) and later recurrent cholangitis (due to Caroli's disease). Associated kidney defects are common. Malignant change may complicate congenital hepatic fibrosis, Caroli's disease, choledochal cysts, and microhamartomas. These diseases are of widely differing severity and the prognosis in an individual patient is determined by the fibropolycystic diseases present.

Polycystic liver disease

The infantile type is inherited as an autosomal recessive disease and is usually rapidly fatal due to the associated renal disease. Adult polycystic liver disease is more common and has a dominant inheritance. Two separate genes, *PRKCSH* and *SEC63*, have been identified to cause familial adult polycystic liver disease. The patient is usually a woman presenting in the fourth or fifth decade. The liver contains many thin-walled cysts filled with a clear or brownish liquid (due to altered blood). The cysts vary in size from a pinhead to about 10 cm in diameter. The remainder of the liver is normal. Patients present with right upper quadrant pain and increasing girth. Examination reveals an enlarged liver as the cause of the upper abdominal swelling. Liver function tests are normal. Provided no other fibropolycystic diseases are present, polycystic liver disease is benign. Some patients with polycystic liver disease also have polycystic kidneys or nephrocalcinosis. The associated renal disease may cause serious complications including renal failure. The diagnosis can be confirmed by ultrasound or CT scanning, which show numerous thin-walled cysts of low density (Fig. 15.25.2). The enlarged polycystic liver causes some patients considerable discomfort. It is best treated by percutaneous aspiration of the larger cysts using ultrasound guidance in order to reduce liver size. Percutaneous aspiration treatment can be performed repeatedly.

Congenital hepatic fibrosis

This is a rare autosomal recessive condition which is usually diagnosed before 10 years of age. The main complication is portal hypertension. Children present with a large, very hard liver and splenomegaly or bleeding from oesophageal varices. Congenital hepatic fibrosis may be misdiagnosed as cirrhosis. Liver function tests are normal or only slightly deranged. Ultrasound scans show the liver contains many bright areas due to the dense bands of fibrous tissue. The diagnosis is made by liver biopsy which shows normal liver parenchyma surrounded by fibrous septa containing structures resembling bile ducts.

Patients with congenital hepatic fibrosis bleed repeatedly from oesophageal varices, but because liver function is well preserved they do not develop portosystemic encephalopathy. Portocaval shunts will stop the variceal bleeding and are well tolerated. Liver transplantation has also been used successfully.

The long-term prognosis in congenital hepatic fibrosis is usually determined by the associated renal disease. Renal lesions include renal dysplasia, medullary cystic disease, and infantile or adult-type polycystic kidneys. The kidneys are rarely normal and renal failure eventually develops in many patients. However, renal transplants have been successful.

Congenital intrahepatic biliary dilatation (Caroli's syndrome)

In Caroli's syndrome the common bile duct is normal but the intrahepatic ducts have bulbous dilatations with normal ducts between (Fig. 15.25.3). The mode of inheritance is unknown. While the cystic dilatations of the bile ducts remain uninfected the patient is symptom free. Eventually, ascending infection leads to cholangitis, which can be intractable with the formation of gallstones and liver abscesses. Caroli's syndrome usually presents in early adulthood as cholangitis. Most patients are male. Liver function tests show cholestasis with elevations of serum bilirubin and alkaline phosphatase and modest elevations of the transaminases. The diagnosis is made by endoscopic cholangiography. Magnetic resonance cholangiography (MRC) and CT scans can also demonstrate the syndrome (see Fig. 15.25.1). The natural history of Caroli's disease is of recurrent cholangitis which is very resistant to antibiotics. Biliary cirrhosis eventually develops. Bile duct cancer develops in about 10% of cases. Treatment is difficult; antibiotics are usually only partially effective, and liver transplantation is compromised by the extensive sepsis.

About one-half of the patients with congenital hepatic fibrosis or Caroli's disease will also have the other disease. The clinical

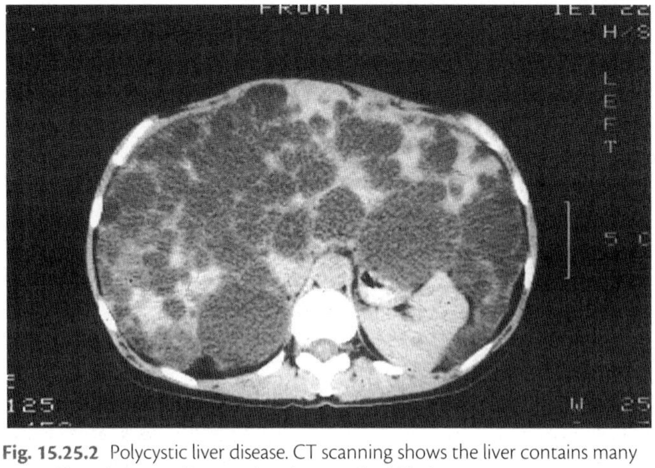

Fig. 15.25.2 Polycystic liver disease. CT scanning shows the liver contains many cysts of low density, indicating that they are fluid filled.
(From Sherlock S, Summerfield JA (1991). *A colour atlas of liver disease*, 2nd edition. Wolfe Medical Publications, London, with permission.)

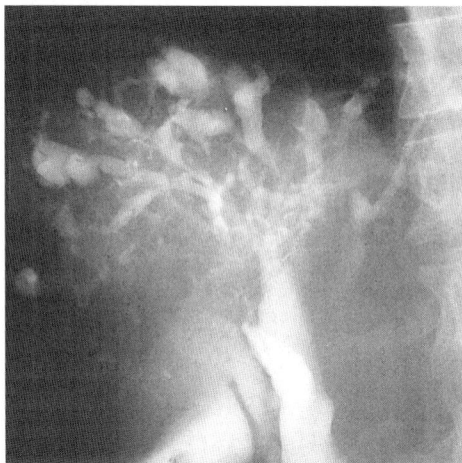

Fig. 15.25.3 Caroli's disease. An endoscopic cholangiogram shows bulbous dilatations of the intrahepatic bile ducts. The rest of the biliary tree is normal.
(From Sherlock S, Summerfield JA (1991). *A colour atlas of liver disease*, 2nd edition. Wolfe Medical Publications, London, with permission.)

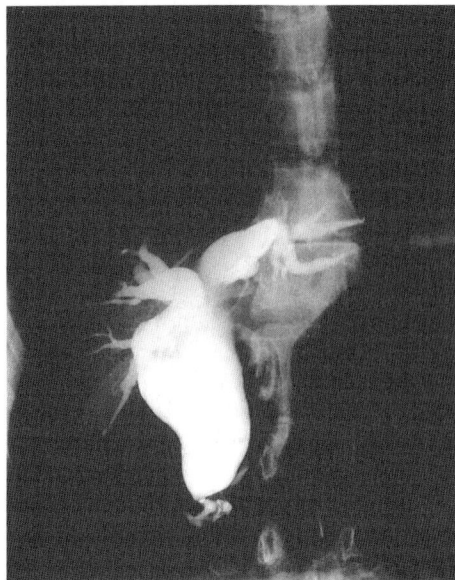

Fig. 15.25.4 Choledochal cyst in a 20-year-old woman. The endoscopic cholangiogram shows a massively dilated common bile duct. The gallbladder was normal but obscured by the dilated bile duct.
(From Sherlock S, Summerfield JA (1991). *A colour atlas of liver disease*, 2nd edition. Wolfe Medical Publications, London, with permission.)

presentation in these patients is distinctive. As in Caroli's disease, males predominate. The first complication is variceal haemorrhage followed about 10 years later by recurrent cholangitis.

Choledochal cyst

Choledochal cyst is a congenital dilatation of part or the whole of the common bile duct (Fig. 15.25.4). It is more common in girls and usually presents in childhood but may appear in early adulthood. Choledochal cysts classically cause a triad of intermittent pain, jaundice, and a right hypochondrial mass. Choledochal cysts are particularly common in Japanese and Chinese individuals. Liver function tests show cholestasis, similar to Caroli's disease. Ultrasound and MRC or CT scans show cystic dilatation of the bile duct. The diagnosis is made by endoscopic or percutaneous cholangiography. Choledochal cysts should be treated by surgical excision because of the risk of bile duct malignancy. Caroli's disease is a common associated disease.

Microhamartomas (von Meyenberg complexes)

Microhamartomas are groups of rounded biliary channels embedded in a collagen stroma located around portal tracts. The appearances are of localized islands of congenital hepatic fibrosis. Microhamartomas are usually asymptomatic and discovered incidentally on liver biopsy. They may be associated with other fibropolycystic diseases and are a rare cause of portal hypertension. Bile duct and pancreatic cancers are commoner in these patients.

Congenital disorders of the pancreas

Agenesis of the pancreas

Pancreatic agenesis is rare and may occur as an isolated anomaly or be associated with other defects. These children usually die soon after birth. Agenesis of either the dorsal or ventral pancreas may occur, although agenesis usually involves the dorsal segment.

Annular pancreas

This is a rare condition where pancreatic tissue encircles the descending duodenum. It results from persistence of part of the ventral pancreas during embryonic development. Annular pancreas is the most common cause of duodenal obstruction in infancy and often involves growth of pancreatic tissue into the duodenal wall. However, the clinical presentation is variable and annular pancreas may first present as an incidental finding at surgery or autopsy.

Pancreas divisum

Pancreas divisum results from failure of fusion of the ducts of the dorsal and ventral portions of the pancreas. The body and tail of the pancreas drain through the narrow duct of Santorini into the accessory papilla. Only the head of the pancreas drains into the ampulla of Vater (Fig. 15.25.5). This is the commonest congenital abnormality of the pancreas, occurring in about 5% of patients. Pancreas divisum appears to be associated with an increased incidence of pancreatitis affecting the body and tail of the pancreas which drains into the accessory papilla. Endoscopic sphincterotomy of the accessory papilla is reported to lead to clinical improvement in this type of pancreatitis.

Hereditary pancreatitis

This rare form of pancreatitis is inherited as an autosomal dominant disorder. Recurrent attacks of abdominal pain start in childhood or the second decade. Hereditary pancreatitis tends to be troublesome rather than life-threatening and attacks become less severe as the patient gets older. They often disappear by middle age. Hereditary pancreatitis is associated with mutations in the cationic trypsinogen gene, which probably render the protease more resistant to autocatalytic trypsinogen breakdown.

Other rare abnormalities causing pancreatic disease

Congenital abnormalities adjacent to the pancreas are rare causes of pancreatitis. These include duodenal diverticulum, duplication of the duodenum, stenosis of the sphincter of Oddi, and choledochal cyst. These abnormalities seem to cause pancreatitis by obstructing the pancreatic duct.

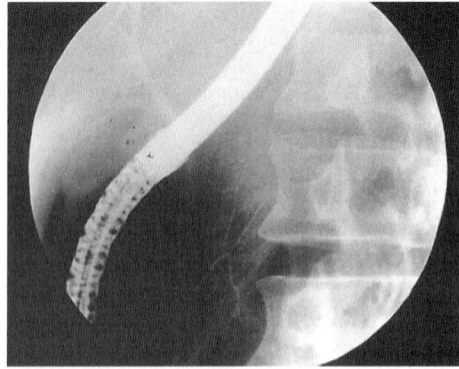

Fig. 15.25.5 Pancreas divisum. An endoscopic pancreatogram following injection of contrast medium into the ampulla of Vater shows only the ducts of the head of the pancreas, characterized by a trefoil pattern. The body and tail of the pancreas drain via the accessory ampulla.

Further reading

Chardot C, *et al.* (1999). Prognosis of biliary atresia in the era of liver transplantation: French national study from 1986 to 1996. *Hepatology*, **30**, 606–11.

Desmet VJ (1992). Congenital diseases of intrahepatic bile ducts: variations on the theme 'ductal plate malformation'. *Hepatology*, **16**, 1069–83.

Sherlock S, Dooley JS (1997). *Diseases of the liver and biliary system*, 10th edition. Blackwell Scientific Publications, Oxford.

Sherlock S, Summerfield JA (1991). *A colour atlas of liver disease*, 2nd edition. Wolfe Medical Publications, London.

Summerfield JA *et al.* (1986). Hepatobiliary fibropolycystic diseases; a clinical and histological review of 51 patients. *J Hepatol*, **2**, 141–56.

Miscellaneous disorders of the bowel and liver

Alexander Gimson

Essentials

A wide range of miscellaneous disorders can affect the bowel and liver: some that are relatively common and of particular note are:

Microscopic colitis—characterized by the triad of watery diarrhoea, a normal macroscopic colonoscopy, and specific histology showing either a lymphocytic colitis or collagenous colitis. May resolve spontaneously, but treated with budesonide if it does not.

Intestinal pseudo-obstruction—acute massive dilatation of the caecum and colon can occur following intra-abdominal surgery or in any critically ill patient. Most patients have constant dull pain with marked abdominal distension and vomiting. The diagnosis is made on plain abdominal radiography. After exclusion of other causes of colonic dilatation, treatment is with nasogastric suction, intravenous fluids and electrolytes, and cessation of drugs that impair bowel motility.

Solitary rectal ulcer syndrome—caused in most cases by mucosal ischaemia and infarction and usually presents with bleeding per rectum, often leading to anaemia. Biopsy is required to rule out malignancy. Treatment is often difficult but requires correction of constipation with bulking agents and avoidance of straining at stool.

Ischaemic hepatopathy—diffuse hepatic injury can occur with acute reduction in hepatic blood flow, e.g. following shock. Blood tests demonstrate marked elevation of transaminases and prolongation of prothrombin time. There is no specific treatment.

Portal vein thrombosis—can be associated with a range of conditions, e.g. pancreatitis, abdominal surgery/malignancy, thrombophilic states. Often asymptomatic, but may present as haemorrhage from oesophageal or gastric varices. Diagnosis is made by Doppler ultrasonography, CT, or magnetic resonance angiography. Variceal band ligation or injection sclerotherapy may be required. Anticoagulation with warfarin reduces the risk of further thrombotic events in the splanchnic circulation and does not increase the risk of variceal haemorrhage.

Microscopic colitis

This syndrome is characterized by the triad of watery diarrhoea, a normal macroscopic colonoscopy, and specific histology showing either a lymphocytic colitis or collagenous colitis. Although usually considered together as microscopic colitis there are some distinct epidemiological, histological, and therapeutic differences between the two types. There is an annual incidence rate of 10/100 000 with lymphocytic colitis being marginally the most common. It is five times more common over the age of 65 years and in women. There have been associations with coeliac disease, hypothyroidism, and a family history of inflammatory bowel disease.

Collagenous colitis

This was first recognized by Linstrom in 1976. Patients, mostly women, usually present in the fifth and sixth decade but the disease can occur in young adults as well as in older people. Watery diarrhoea accompanied by occasional abdominal cramps, wind, distension, and some nausea are usual. Diarrhoea can be severe and may seem secretory in nature. There may be some mucus, but bleeding per rectum does not occur. Despite such severe symptoms the patients look well, with a good appetite, and they do not lose weight. There are no abnormal physical signs and on colonoscopy the mucosa looks normal although it may seem somewhat granular and hyperaemic. Such endoscopic changes can occur throughout the colon but are usually patchy and never severe. The diagnosis is made on the appearance of the biopsy where there is a thickened band of subepithelial collagen extending 15 μm compared with a normal thickness of 2 to 6 μm. The collagen band is widest in the right colon and tends to become thinner more distally. Immunohistochemical studies have shown that the abnormal tissue consists predominantly of collagen type 3 and there is a patchy variable inflammatory infiltrate in the lamina propria consisting of lymphocytes, plasma cells, and some neutrophils. The disease is confined to the colon and is distinct from collagenous sprue.

Lymphocytic colitis

The clinical symptoms are similar to collagenous colitis but the mucosa always looks normal at colonoscopy. Histological examination shows a diffuse inflammatory cell infiltrate throughout the lamina propria with no architectural changes to the glands. The infiltrate is predominantly lymphocytes but there may also been eosinophils and a characteristic feature is the marked increase in intraepithelial lymphocytes, which clearly distinguishes it from ulcerative colitis where they are normal or reduced.

In some cases of microscopic colitis there may be spontaneous remissions and symptoms may have been preceded by some infectious trigger, including *Campylobacter jejeuni*, *Clostridium difficile*, or yersinia infection. In cases that do not resolve, treatment is now more rational as recent meta-analyses have demonstrated significant improvement with budesonide although there are also reports of improvements with mesalazine, cholestyramine, bismuth, or just simply with loperamide.

Complications of parenteral nutrition and intestinal failure

A number of complications of parenteral nutrition have been described relating to vascular thrombosis and catheter-related sepsis, but metabolic complications and the development of a cholestatic liver disease are the most important. Metabolic dysfunction includes hyperglycaemia, dyslipidaemia, manganese toxicity, oxalate renal stones, osteoporosis, and a refeeding syndrome which includes hypophosphataemia, hypernatraemia, and hypokalaemia shortly after starting nutrition in a malnourished patient. Hepatobiliary disease includes cholelithiasis and a progressive cholestasis resulting in liver failure. This progressive liver disease is more common in children with intestinal failure (due for instance to necrotizing enterocolitis) but may also occur in adults. In larger cohort studies about 25% of cases receiving total parenteral nutrition (TPN) will have significantly abnormal liver blood tests with up to 5% showing evidence of fibrosis leading to cirrhosis. The liver disease may be driven by the TPN itself and result from nutrient excess, deficiency, or toxicity, and is suggested by the dramatic improvements in liver function that can occur with manipulation of the contents of the nutrition support. On the other hand, it may also be related to the accompanying bowel resection. Bacterial overgrowth, increased permeability of the bowel wall due to intestinal atrophy, gut-derived endotoxins, and lithocolic acid with a reduced circulating bile salt pool and bile flow promoting cholestasis have all been suggested. The development of a similar liver disease in patients following a jejeuno-ileal bypass and other forms of bariatric surgery and the fact that liver dysfunction is less common in patients with an intact colon or who can maintain small amounts of enteral feeding are evidence in favour of the gut being a major driver of the liver pathology.

Management of these cases should be centralized in intestinal failure units experienced in the complex management of nutrition support and scrupulous catheter care. A careful balance in lipid composition, where both too much and too little must be avoided as well as too much carbohydrate, is important. Cyclical feeding and wherever possible maintaining at least some enteral nutrition are recommended. Ursodeoxycholic acid, as a choleretic, has been shown to prevent liver dysfunction and antibiotics to prevent bacterial overgrowth in children but there is less evidence of their efficacy in adults. Supplementation with choline and taurine are also important. Bowel-lengthening surgical techniques in children are still unproven but there is increasing evidence of the benefit of transplantation of the small bowel (with or without a liver) and 50% 5-year survival is now being recorded.

Miscellaneous vascular disorders of the intestine
Spontaneous intramural haemorrhage

Spontaneous bleeding into the bowel wall may occur following trauma; during excessive anticoagulation with warfarin; in patients with coagulation disorders, particularly haemophilia; and in vasculitis. It may present as pain, symptoms of partial intestinal obstruction, intussusception, and rarely intestinal haemorrhage. Diagnosis is best made by abdominal CT scan or barium radiology and treatment is usually conservative with correction of the coagulation deficit and transfusion.

Aorto-enteric fistulas

Aorto-enteric fistulas are rare but serious conditions that may arise as a complication following abdominal aortic surgery or rarely spontaneously. Clinical symptoms range from occult recurrent gastrointestinal bleeding and intermittent unexplained fever attacks to dramatic massive intestinal blood loss with shock. The fistula is usually in the second or third part of the duodenum and may be diagnosed by CT, angiography, or occasionally red cell scintigraphy. Treatment is by surgery although recently endoluminal aortic stents have been successfully used. Overall mortality remains high.

Vascular malformations; haemangiomas of the bowel

Angiodysplasia of the bowel is described in Chapter 15.4.2. Cavernous haemangiomas of the bowel are rare occurring most commonly in the rectosigmoid region. Some are found as a component of the blue rubber bleb nevus syndrome (Bean syndrome) associated with cutaneous haemangiomas. They present in young patients with iron deficiency anaemia. Diagnosis may be made by endoscopic examination, CT or MRI, and surgical resection of the lesions is necessary if the haemangiomas are associated with significant symptoms.

Miscellaneous vascular disorders of the liver
Congestive hepatopathy

The liver's complex blood supply and high metabolic activity may be affected in a number of clinical situations when there is reduced splanchnic inflow and impaired hepatic venous outflow. Hepatic venous outflow obstruction and Budd–Chiari syndrome are dealt with in Chapter 15.22.3. Congestive hepatopathy may occur in the context of reduced cardiac output and high right-sided venous pressure, due to constrictive pericarditis, mitral stenosis, tricuspid regurgitation, and cardiomyopathy. The hepatic congestion and reduced liver sinusoidal perfusion is usually asymptomatic as the heart failure dominates the clinical scenario. There is an elevated jugular venous pressure, with 'v' waves in the presence of tricuspid regurgitation, hepatomegaly, and a positive hepatojugular reflex. The liver may be pulsatile when tricuspid regurgitation is severe. The consequent reduced sinusoidal blood flow can lead to ischaemia in zone 3 of the hepatic lobule and histological changes are characterized by centrilobular congestion with surrounding fatty change, initially described as the 'nutmeg liver'. If the disorder is long-standing there may be progressive fibrosis extending peripherally from the centrilobular to the periportal areas although regenerative nodules are usually not present. A modestly elevated serum bilirubin level may be the only abnormality, with a normal serum alkaline phosphatase and elevated aminotransferases. Although minor changes in liver biochemistry are observed in cases with chronic biventricular heart failure, true cases of cardiac cirrhosis are very uncommon as are major complications from portal hypertension. Occasionally this situation is complicated by the presence together of an alcohol-induced liver injury and an alcoholic cardiomyopathy. In these circumstances it may be necessary to undertake histological examination of the liver as well as measuring right-sided cardiac pressures and free and wedged hepatic venous pressure gradients. The treatment for congestive hepatopathy centres on improving cardiac function with standard therapies.

Ischaemic hepatopathy

This refers to the diffuse hepatic injury that follows an acute reduction in hepatic blood flow. It may be due to any of the causes of sudden shock (haemorrhage, cardiac arrest, severe septic shock) but a similar syndrome has also been described in hepatic sickle cell crisis, following liver transplantation with hepatic artery thrombosis, and in severe respiratory failure and hypoxaemia. Histology shows a centrizonal necrosis and blood tests demonstrate marked elevation of transaminases, prolonged prothrombin time, and jaundice. The differential diagnosis includes other cause of sudden hepatocyte necrosis including drug hepatotoxicity and viral hepatitis. Rarely, acute liver failure with encephalopathy may develop in the most severe cases of ischaemic hepatopathy. There is no specific treatment for the liver dysfunction in this context, management being directed at the cause of the impaired hepatic perfusion.

Hepatic artery aneurysm

Hepatic artery aneurysms have been found in a number of conditions but are most common after surgery. They may also be found in the Osler–Weber–Rendu syndrome, Behçet's syndrome, polyarteritis nodosa, and as part of systemic sepsis with fungal infection. It may be an incidental finding on an angiogram or present with pain, sometimes in the back and rarely after cholecystectomy with jaundice and biliary obstruction. Spontaneous rupture has been associated with haemobilia and is a major medical emergency presenting with severe abdominal pain and shock followed by jaundice. Treatment is with either hepatic artery embolization or surgery.

Portal vein thrombosis

Spontaneous thrombosis of the portal vein, although often asymptomatic, may cause a range of serious medical complications. A thrombosis may develop in one or more of the intrahepatic portal vein branches, or within the main portal vein itself and may involve the superior mesenteric or splenic veins which join to form the main trunk of the portal vein. Thrombosis may result from infection after birth arising in the umbilical vein, following acute pancreatitis (occasionally isolated to the splenic vein alone), surgery or abdominal trauma, as a complication of cirrhosis with or without an additional hepatocellular carcinoma, pancreatic and other intrabdominal malignancy, retroperitoneal fibrosis and a

number of thrombophilic states. These include polycythaemia rubra vera, any cause of thrombocytosis, factor V Leiden and factor II (G20210A) deficiency, antithrombin III, protein C and S deficiency, paroxysmal nocturnal haemoglobinuria, and the lupus anticoagulant. Septic thrombosis of the portal vein may also occur associated with another infective focus within the abdomen such as acute appendicitis or diverticular disease. Often asymptomatic, it may present as haemorrhage from oesophageal or gastric varices and rarely with biliary obstruction from choledochal varices. The diagnosis can be made at Doppler ultrasound examination of the liver, CT or magnetic resonance angiography. When portal vein thrombosis presents with variceal haemorrhage endoscopic therapy with variceal band ligation or injection sclerotherapy is required. Occasionally surgical shunts can decompress the portal venous system, but this is often not possible due to the extensive nature of the thrombosis. Clot lysis is not possible as the thrombosis is usually long-standing. Anticoagulation with warfarin has been shown to reduce the risk of further thrombotic events in the splanchnic circulation and does not increase the risk of variceal haemorrhage.

Cystic disorders of the bowel

Colitis cystica profunda

First described by Stark in 1766 and then by Virchow as colitis cystica polyposa in 1863, the disorder is characterized by submucosal mucin-filled cysts. They may be single or multiple, within 12 cm of the anal verge, and are more common in younger men. It may represent a subgroup of the solitary rectal ulcer/rectal prolapse syndrome but has also been associated with Crohn's disease. The cysts are seen at colonoscopy as a submucosal mass covered by normal rectal mucosa that may be occasionally hyperaemic, polypoid, or ulcerated. Diagnosis can be made with transrectal ultrasound, MRI, or colonoscopy, as it is important to exclude malignancy. Treatment is with bulking agents and laxative, re-education to avoid straining at stool, and surgery only if there is associated rectal prolapse.

Pneumatosis cystoides intestinalis

Gas-filled cysts within the small or large bowel are rare and can develop in a wide range of conditions. Some are primary, asymptomatic, often in the left colon and with no apparent cause. Others are secondary, involve the ileum and right colon, and can be associated with chronic obstructive pulmonary disease, intestinal obstruction, severe colonic inflammation (pseudomembranous colitis, necrotizing enterocolitis), connective tissue disease (systemic sclerosis, mixed connective tissue disease), amyloidosis, endoscopy, or CT colography. Pneumatosis cystoides intestinalis has recently been described in patients receiving α-glucosidase inhibitors. The submucosal or subserosal cysts are lined by histiocytes and giant cells and, although easy to diagnose on resection, specimens can be difficult with biopsies. Symptoms, where present, may include diarrhoea, vague abdominal discomfort, blood per rectum, and weight loss. The air-filled spaces may be seen on abdominal films but CT is best to diagnose them. They appear as submucosal masses on colonoscopy. Rarely portal venous gas can also be visualized, which implies associated bowel infarction. In some primary cases a conservative approach is possible but when symptomatic treatment is with high flow oxygen therapy 55 to 75% O_2 aiming for a PaO_2 greater than 200 mmHg for 4 to 10 days or, avoiding oxygen toxicity, with hyperbaric oxygen. If colonic integrity is compromised, or there is evidence of systemic sepsis or bowel perforation, broad spectrum antibiotics and surgery are required.

Disorders of the peritoneum

A number of rare disorders can specifically affect the peritoneum and serosal surfaces of the large and small bowel (Box 15.26.1). Their importance is firstly as a differential diagnosis for diffuse malignant infiltration of the peritoneum, by far the commonest cause of widespread peritoneal deposits seen on cross-sectional imaging, but also because they may require specific therapy.

Disseminated malignancy is common, with ovarian and adenocarcinoma most prevalent. Patients present with abdominal swelling, ascites, pain, and weight loss. CT scanning will reveal peritoneal deposits and biopsy is mandatory in order to tailor chemotherapy to specific cancers. Primary peritoneal mesothelioma presents in a similar manner with a slightly better prognosis. Peritoneal carcinomatosis is associated with poor survival and reduced quality of life, but a significant improvement in survival has recently been associated with cytoreductive surgery and hyperthermic intraperitoneal chemotherapy (HIPEC) in patients with disseminated ovarian and gastric cancer and peritoneal mesothelioma.

Desmoid tumours (aggressive fibromatosis) are rare benign neoplasms of fibroblastic origin, that can be either extra- or intra-abdominal (mesenteric fibromatosis). They are locally invasive, with high recurrence rates. It occurs as a sporadic form and associated with familial neoplastic syndromes including Gardner's syndrome and familial adenomatous polyposis (FAP). Sporadic cases may have mutations in the adenomatous polyposis coli (*APC*) or β-catenin (*CTNNB1*) genes. In FAP, tumours carry biallelic APC mutations. Overall desmoids can occur in up to 15% of FAP cases rising to 65% after abdominal surgery in those with 3′ APC mutations. They are a leading cause of death after colectomy. Symptoms include pain, features of intestinal obstruction, and often a palpable mass. Treatment remains unsatisfactory and includes surgery, nonsteroidal anti-inflammatory drugs, and tamoxifen.

Pseudomyxoma peritonei has been linked to peritoneal spread of appendiceal and ovarian mucinous tumours.

Erdheim–Chester disease is a multisystem xanthomatosis with histiocytic proliferation similar to Langerhans cell histiocytosis but with a different immunohistochemical profile. Sheets of foamy histiocytes can involve lung, skin, brain, adrenals, renal tract, liver and peritoneum. Treatment is with corticosteroids.

The syndrome of retractile mesenteritis (sometimes referred to as sclerosing mesenteritis or mesenteric panniculitis) may present with abdominal discomfort, pain, diarrhoea and weight loss. Chronic fibrosing inflammation involves the root of the mesentery and small bowel. In some cases it has been associated with retroperitoneal fibrosis a desmoid or carcinoid tumour of the small bowel. It is more common in males and may have a prolonged debilitating course. Treatment is with tamoxifen and corticosteroids.

Leiomyomatosis peritonealis disseminata is an uncommon condition characterized by subperitoneal proliferation of benign nodules composed of smooth muscle cells. It is most common in premenopausal women and hormonal influences may play a role in its pathogenesis. The macroscopic appearance mimics peritoneal carcinomatosis but the clinical course is usually benign.

Endometriosis

Endometriosis is defined as the presence of endometrium and stroma outside the uterine cavity and myometrium was first described by von Rokitansky in 1860. It is commonly asymptomatic and occurs in up to 15% of menstruating women. Involvement of the bowel is much less common and only rarely causes symptoms, but when they occur they are often debilitating and may take years to be diagnosed. The pathogenesis is considered to be retrograde passage of endometrial tissue into the pelvic organs and subsequent spread by haematogenous or lymphatic dissemination. When implanted, the tissue continues to be hormonally modulated. It is most commonly left-sided within the abdomen in the rectosigmoid region (80%) followed by ileum, caecum, and appendix. Small serosal endometriotic nodules rarely cause symptoms, but large collections and those in a subserosal location may result in vague abdominal and back pain, diarrhoea, constipation, and abdominal bloating, symptoms that closely mimic the irritable bowel syndrome. Rectal bleeding may occur, but symptoms are not often cyclical. Symptomatic endometriosis is found in women of childbearing age and is uncommon before age of 20 years. It is important to consider the diagnosis in any women with prolonged symptoms suggestive of the irritable bowel syndrome who does not respond to initial therapies and in those whose pain is not relieved by defecation. Nevertheless, diagnosis may be difficult as symptoms can be multiple and diffuse especially if the lesions are widespread. Imaging is the mainstay of diagnosis and includes transvaginal ultrasonography, double contrast barium enemas, and colonoscopy, but endometriosis is increasingly being identified with MRI. The presence of methaemoglobin from recurrent haemorrhage within the lesion causes hyper-intense T_1 weighted images and hypo-intensity on T_2. Old endometriotic lesions with significant fibrosis are less well identified on MRI, and CT scans may be necessary. Some cases are only diagnosed at laparotomy or laparoscopic examination of the bowel. Management must be individualized and can include in some a solely expectant and conservative approach or medical therapy. Few trials have been performed. Inducing a pseudo-pregnancy state with low-dose oestrogen–progestogen is not recommended for intestinal disease,

---

Box 15.26.1 Diffuse disorders of the peritoneum

- Malignancy

  Primary: mesothelioma, leiomyosarcoma, solitary fibrous tumour

  Secondary: ovary, stomach, colon, kidney

  Pseudomyxoma peritonei

  Desmoid tumours

- Erdheim–Chester disease
- Sarcoidosis
- Amyloidosis
- Tuberculosis
- Retractile mesenteritis
- Leiomyomatosis peritonealis disseminata

and agents that are effective in pelvic endometriosis including the synthetic androgen danazol or gonadotrophin-releasing hormone agonists may not be appropriate in bowel endometriosis as they may promote fibrosis. A cautious trial of therapy as a first line may be indicated but laparoscopy or surgery will be needed in those with severe symptoms or partial bowel obstruction.

Isolated ulcers of the intestine

Solitary rectal ulcer syndrome

The solitary rectal ulcer syndrome is somewhat misnamed as it may occasionally occur above the rectum and be multiple or circumferential. It occurs across the age spectrum and is seen into the ninth decade. The ulcer may be at one end of the spectrum of clinical disorders associated with rectal mucosal prolapse and caused in most cases by mucosal ischaemia and infarction. It presents with blood per rectum in 90% of cases and less frequently with abdominal pain, mucus per rectum, straining at defecation, diarrhoea, and constipation. The cases are commonly anaemic and the symptoms have serious impact on the quality of life. The ulcers may be located anteriorly (70%), posteriorly or circumferentially, and are multiple in one-third of cases. At colonoscopy the ulcer may be surrounded by a minimal area of inflamed mucosa or it may be at the end of a polypoid lesion simulating a carcinoma. Biopsy is crucial to rule out that diagnosis. Histology usually shows evidence of ischaemia but the characteristic feature is hypertrophy of the muscularis mucosae with smooth muscle fibres extending between the crypts and down into the epithelium. Treatment is commonly difficult but should be centred on correction of constipation with bulking agents (with or without lactulose) and patients should be warned not to strain at stool. Topical treatments with 5-aminosalicylic acid or corticosteroids have been helpful in small series. As these ulcers can remit spontaneously, it is difficult to be sure whether treatment has been effective in an individual patient. For patients with continuing disabling symptoms, anorectal physiological measurements should be considered because there may be evidence of impaired pelvic floor muscle innovation. A defecating proctogram may determine whether the anorectal angle changes when the patient attempts to empty the rectum and record the degree of mucosal prolapse. Surgical therapy with a rectopexy may be helpful in some cases.

Stercoral ulcers

These occur in association with faecal impaction and are most commonly found in the recto sigmoid area. The patients are usually elderly, but these ulcers can occur at any age in severely constipated individuals, including patients with a neurological cause for constipation. The common symptoms are those associated with constipation—nausea, abdominal distension, pain, and anorexia. The ulcers are frequently asymptomatic but may be the cause of anaemia from chronic bowel loss. The differential diagnosis includes other ulcers within the colon, particularly those with an infectious cause (tuberculosis and amoebiasis) as well as malignancy.

Isolated ulcers of the large intestine not associated with underlying colitis are rare but may be an incidental finding on screening colonoscopy or present with abdominal pain, acute blood per rectum bleeding, or chronic gastrointestinal blood loss. A common cause, particularly when the ulcers are caecal or right sided, is the use of nonsteroidal anti-inflammatory drugs.

Protein-losing enteropathy

This is a syndrome due to excessive loss of protein from the gastrointestinal tract. It should be considered in any case where hypoproteinaemia or a low albumin cannot be explained by renal loss (nephritic syndrome) or reduced hepatic synthesis. The cardinal features are peripheral oedema, occasionally diarrhoea and weight loss. There is a low albumin (occasional falling to very low levels, <15 g/dl), reduced immunoglobulins, caeruloplasmin, and fibrinogen.

Gastrointestinal protein loss may be due to a wide range of cause (Box 15.26.2). Increased interstitial pressure within the intestine can lead to protein loss due to lymphangiectasia (Waldmann's disease, lymphedema–lymphangiectasia–mental retardation, Hennekam syndrome), chronic lymphatic obstruction due to tuberculosis, sarcoidosis, lymphoma, retroperitoneal fibrosis, or in association with an elevated right-sided heart pressure (constrictive pericarditis, following Fontan's procedure). Various ulcerative disorders of the gastrointestinal tract include severe erosive gastritis, Crohns disease, pseudomembranous colitis, and acute graft vs host disease. Finally, it has been associated with Menetrier's disease, bacterial overgrowth of the small bowel, Whipple's disease, eosinophilic gastroenteritis, coeliac disease, and tropical sprue. A number of radio-isotopes have been used for diagnosis, with ^{51}Cr-labelled chromium chloride being most commonly used. Stool α_1-antitrypsin levels are also used, as this protein is not broken

---

Box 15.26.2 Causes of a protein-losing enteropathy

Inflammatory conditions
- Inflammatory bowel disease—Crohn's disease
- Gastric cancer
- Intestinal lymphoma
- α-Chain disease

Lymphatic obstruction
- Intestinal lymphangiectasia
- Right-sided heart failure
- Congestive cardiac failure
- Constrictive pericarditis
- Fontan procedure for single ventricle
- Hepatic venous outflow obstruction
- Mesenteric TB, sarcoidosis
- Intestinal lymphoma

Increased permeability without ulceration
- Coeliac disease
- Tropical sprue
- Menetrier's disease
- Amyloidosis
- Bacterial overgrowth of small bowel
- Connective tissue diseases
- Allergic gastroenteropathy
- Eosinophilic gastroenteropathy

down within the gut. Treatment should be aimed at raising the serum albumin level and management for each specific cause of the protein loss.

Malakoplakia

This is a rare chronic granulomatous condition, most commonly affecting the genitourinary tract, skin, lung, bone, or brain; within the gastrointestinal tract it is most common in the sigmoid colon or rectum. It is observed in two clusters: in children and older people. It is more common in diabetic, immunosuppressed, or immunocompromised patients including those with hypogammaglobulinaemia, HIV infection, or after organ transplantation. Yellowish soft plaques 1 to 20 mm diameter show a histiocytic infiltrate with eosinophils and characteristic basophilic laminated calcium containing Michaelis–Guttman bodies. It may occur with isolated rectosigmoid involvement, as diffuse colonic involvement or as a focal lesion associated with a polyp or cancer. It is usually considered to be a granulomatous reaction to a chronic infection: *Escherichia coli*, klebsiella and proteus have been implicated. Treatment has revolved around antibiotic therapy (quinolone and co-trimoxazole–trimethoprim) and minimizing immunosuppression.

Intestinal pseudo-obstruction

Acute colonic pseudo-obstruction

Acute massive dilatation of the caecum and right colon, sometimes extending into the transverse and left side of the colon, can occur following intra-abdominal surgery for any cause as well as in any critically ill patient with severe sepsis, respiratory, or cardiac disease. In Ogilvie's original report two patients had retroperitoneal malignancy, currently an exceptionally rare cause for this syndrome. Most patients have constant dull pain with marked abdominal distension associated with vomiting. There is constipation, but many patients continue to pass wind and some occasionally have diarrhoea despite the colonic dilatation. Bowel sounds are variable in pitch and frequency but are absent only rarely. The diagnosis is

---

Box 15.26.3 Causes of chronic intestinal pseudo-obstruction

- Familial visceral myopathy
- Familial visceral neuropathy
- Paraneoplastic neuropathy
- Scleroderma
- Dermatomyositis/polymyositis
- Mixed connective tissue disease
- Diabetic neuropathy
- Spinal cord injury
- Neurofibromatosis
- Myotonic dystrophy
- Amyloidosis
- Hypothyroidism
- Hypoparathyroidism

---

made on a plain radiograph of the abdomen which can be undertaken to monitor the risk of colonic perforation—the main risk from this disorder. The differential diagnosis includes toxic megacolon (a complication of inflammatory bowel disease or *C. difficile* infection) and mechanical colonic obstruction. Intravenous fluids and electrolytes are given, together with nasogastric suction, and any drugs that might be implicated in reduced colonic motility, e.g. opioids, tricyclic antidepressants, or anticholinergic agents, should be stopped. Pharmacological stimulation has been recommended with neostigmine (an acetylcholinesterase inhibitor), and small controlled trials have been positive. There are some reports of success with other prokinetic agents such as erythromycin or cisapride. Decompression of the colon with a rectal tube or with colonoscopy is occasionally needed although the long-term value has been contested. Equally it has previously been recommended that the patient is turned from side to side at regular intervals or nursed prone with elevated hips, although the benefit of this is not proven. Very rarely surgical decompression with a caecostomy may be needed if the colon is more than 12 cm diameter, which may be accompanied by resection if there is evidence of obvious colonic ischaemia.

Chronic intestinal pseudo-obstruction

This is a rare syndrome associated with symptoms and signs suggesting mechanical obstruction of the large or small bowel in the absence of any obstructive lesion. A similar disorder of the intestinal but without features of obstruction or bowel dilatation has been termed 'chronic intestinal dysmotility'. The main features are of nausea, repeated vomiting, and abdominal pain. There may be significant bowel distension and constipation or occasionally diarrhoea. Bowel sounds are usually hyperactive. There are a number of causes (Box 15.26.3) which include familial visceral neuropathies and myopathies, which may present in infancy or adulthood; collagen vascular disorders; neuromuscular disorders and endocrinopathies; infections; and with some drugs. The diagnosis requires features of colonic or small-bowel dilatation and may require specific electrophysiological studies or full-thickness bowel biopsy at laparotomy. Treatment is directed at the underlying disease or the use of prokinetic agents. Rarely surgery may be needed for isolated sections of affected bowel or substantial sections if symptoms are severe and chronic. Some cases have done well following small-bowel transplantation.

Further reading

Cameron IC, *et al.* (1995). Intestinal endometriosis: Presentation, investigation, and surgical management. *Int J Colorectal Dis*, **10**, 83–6.
Cipolletta L, *et al.* (1995). Malakoplakia of the colon. *Gastrointest Endosc*, **41**, 225–8.
Gagliardi G, *et al.* (1996). Pneumatosis coli: A proposed pathogenesis based on study of 25 cases and review of the literature. *Int J Colorectal Dis*, **11**, 111–18.
Giallourakis CC, Rosenberg PM, Friedman LS (2002). The liver in heart failure. *Clin Liver Dis*, **6**, 947–67.
Kelly D (2006). Intestinal failure associated liver disease—what do we know today? *Gastroenterology*, **130**, 870–7.
Nyhlin N, *et al.* (2006). Systematic review: microscopic colitis. *Aliment Pharmacol Ther*, **23**, 1525–34.
Webster G, Buroughs A, Riordan S (2005). Portal vein thrombosis—new insights into aetiology and management. *Aliment Pharmacol Ther*, **21**, 1–9.

SECTION 16

Cardiovascular disorders

16.1

Structure and function

Contents

16.1.1 Blood vessels and the endothelium

Patrick Vallance

Essentials

Anatomy of blood vessels

There are three basic layers to blood vessels—the intima, the media, and the adventitia. Not all vessels have each layer, and the layers vary in size and structure between vessels. (1) The intima comprises a single layer of endothelial cells on a basement membrane, beneath which—depending on vessel size—there may be a layer of fibro-elastic connective tissue and an internal elastic lamina that provides both structure and flexibility. Embedded in the intima are pericytes. (2) The media is made up predominantly of smooth muscle cells, but also has elastic fibres and contains the external elastic lamina. (3) The adventitia is the outermost part of the vessel, composed mainly of fibroelastic tissue but also containing nerves, small feeding blood vessels (the vasa vasorum), and lymph vessels.

Function of particular constituents of blood vessels

Endothelial cells are metabolically very active and exert a profound influence on vascular reactivity, thrombogenesis, and the behaviour of circulating cells. They produce at least three key vasodilator mediators: nitric oxide, prostanoids, and hyperpolarizing factor. Although the predominant background influence of the endothelium is as dilator, it also produces important vasoconstrictor factors, including endothelin, angiotensin-converting enzyme, certain prostanoids, and the superoxide anion.

The endothelium synthesizes and releases prothrombotic and antithrombotic factors, with antithrombotic factors predominating under basal conditions. It also prevents cells from adhering fully to the vessel wall, but allows leucocytes to roll along its surface.

Vascular smooth muscle cells—these are remarkably plastic and may adopt a range of phenotypes: they can leave the contractile state and enter a replicative state, migrate into the intima, adopt a secretory phenotype that results in matrix deposition (including developing bone-like features and calcification), and under some conditions, can contribute to inflammation within the vessel wall.

Vascular resistance—there is a fourth power relationship between resistance to flow and the radius of a blood vessel, which means that relatively small changes in the thickness or contractile state of smooth muscle in small arteries and arterioles have big effects on systemic vascular resistance.

Integrated responses of blood vessels

Basal endothelium-dependent dilator tone is due to the production of nitric oxide and seems to provide a physiological counterbalance to the continuous constrictor tone of the sympathetic nervous system. Veins differ from arteries and arterioles, and do not seem to be actively dilated by continuous release of nitric oxide.

Flow-mediated dilatation is an autoregulatory property of blood vessels that tends to oppose classical myogenic autoregulation—the process by which a blood vessel constricts in response to an increase in intraluminal pressure.

There are important interactions between the sympathetic nervous, the renin–angiotensin, and the endothelin systems, with these acting in concert to control constrictor tone, and with the endothelin system providing a slowly modulating, background constrictor tone.

Pathophysiology

Several clinical conditions—including atherosclerosis, hypertension, hypercholesterolaemia, and diabetes—are associated with a functional loss of nitric oxide-mediated effects. Overproduction of nitric oxide may also contribute to disease, with induction of inducible nitric oxide synthase by sepsis leading to production of large amounts of nitric oxide and resulting in vascular paresis. Expression of adhesion molecules by the vascular endothelium is an important mechanism of cellular adhesion during inflammation and is also important in recruitment of T cells and monocytes in atherosclerosis.

Introduction

Blood vessels range in size from microscopic capillaries to large vessels, such as the aorta and vena cava, and vary in specialized function from tissue to tissue. They deliver oxygen and nutrients, remove waste, control the passage of cells and macromolecules from the blood into the tissues, and are equipped to sense and respond to physical and chemical signals. There are three basic layers to blood vessels—the intima, the media, and the adventitia.

The intima comprises a single layer of endothelial cells on a basement membrane, beneath which—depending on vessel size—there may be a layer of fibroelastic connective tissue and an internal elastic lamina that provides both structure and flexibility. Embedded in the intima are pericytes—intriguing cells of smooth muscle cell lineage that make contact with multiple endothelial cells. The media is made up predominantly of smooth muscle cells, but also has elastic fibres and contains the external elastic lamina. The outermost part of the vessel is the adventitia, a less well-defined layer composed mainly of fibroelastic tissue but also containing nerves, small feeding blood vessels (the vasa vasorum), and lymph vessels. In simple terms, the intima may be considered as the layer that transduces signals from the lumen of the vessel to the rest of the vessel wall and controls the interface with the blood; the media is the mechanical workhorse of the vessel, and the adventitia houses links to the wider environment beyond the circulation. Not all vessels have each layer, and the layers vary in size and structure between vessels. For example, capillaries are essentially endothelial cell tubes surrounded by pericytes, resistance vessels have a relatively thick media, and the large conduit arteries have a high proportion of elastic tissue and a rich vasa vasorum. In disease states, particularly atherosclerosis (see Chapter 16.13.1), the vessel wall may have a high content of inflammatory cells.

It can also be convenient to consider the many vessel types that make up the vascular tree in simplified groups. Large arteries perform the function of mass transport, smaller arteries and arterioles provide the predominate resistance to flow, and therefore, are key determinants of blood pressure, capillaries are thin-walled and contribute most to passage of nutrients, gases, and cells through to tissues, venules provide postcapillary resistance and help determine capillary pressure, and larger venules and veins dynamically regulate the total capacitance of the circulatory system.

Cellular constituents of blood vessels

Endothelium

A monolayer of endothelial cells lines the intimal surface of the entire vascular tree (Fig. 16.1.1) to form the largest endocrine/paracrine organ in the body. Endothelial cells are metabolically very active and exert a profound influence on vascular reactivity, thrombogenesis, and the behaviour of circulating cells. Abnormalities of endothelial function have been implicated in a wide variety of diseases ranging from atheroma and hypertension to acute inflammation and septic shock.

During early development, the endothelium forms the first layer of the circulatory system and extends to produce a network of interconnecting tubes, and this ability of endothelial cells to form tube-like structures is retained even when they are grown *in vitro*. *In vivo* the endothelial tubes differentiate into arteries, arterioles, capillaries, veins, and lymph vessels, and regional differences in function and structure evolve such that the properties of endothelial cells vary between arterial and venous beds, between micro- and macrovasculature, between organs, and between different parts of individual organs—perhaps the most striking example being the specialized layer of endothelial cells and pericytes that forms the blood–brain barrier. Heterogeneity of endothelial cell function undoubtedly has implications for physiology, pathophysiology, and therapeutics. However, endothelial cells from different vessels also have many features in common and a number of pathologies, including those causing premature vascular disease, are associated with widespread changes in the behaviour of endothelial cells.

Anatomy of the endothelium

Each endothelial cell is between 25 and 50 μm long, 10 and 15 μm wide, and up to 5 μm deep, and lies with its long axis aligned in the direction of the blood flow (Fig. 16.1.1). The underlying smooth muscle cells lie radially, are about 5 to 10 μm wide, and taper at either end so that a single endothelial cell can communicate with many smooth muscle cells, and vice versa. The endothelium also comes into intimate contact with circulating cells, and the total area of the luminal surface of the endothelium is in excess of

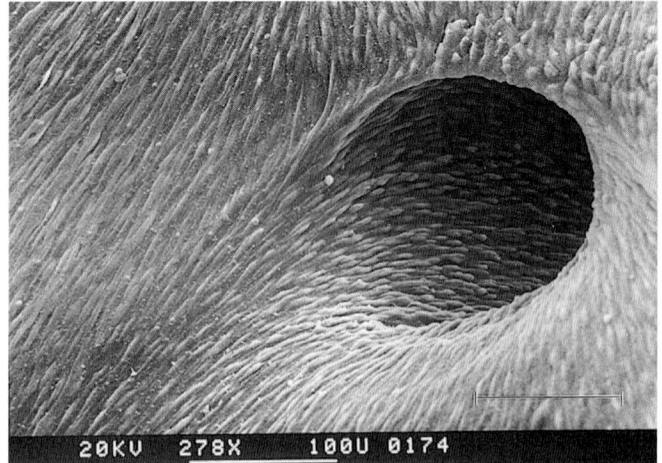

Fig. 16.1.1.1 Scanning electron micrograph showing endothelial lining to a human coronary artery. Note that the endothelial cells are aligned in the direction of blood flow.
Supplied by P. M. Rowles.

$500 \, m^2$. This thin layer of cells is particularly susceptible to injury, and changes in endothelial cell morphology and turnover occur in experimental hypertension, diabetes, and atheroma.

Signal detection by endothelial cells

The endothelial cell membrane expresses a large number of receptors for circulating hormones, local mediators, and vasoactive factors released from blood cells. It can also sense changes in pressure and flow. Although the precise nature of endothelial flow, stretch, and pressure sensors is not clear, stretch of the cell membrane leads directly to the opening of a cation channel that is permeable to calcium, and flow across the cell surface leads to the opening of a potassium channel, which hyperpolarizes the cell. The intracellular signalling mechanisms linking agonist occupation of receptors or physical activation of the cell surface to mediator release is outside the scope of this chapter, but changes in the concentration of intracellular free calcium, and the temporal and spatial profile of calcium change, influences which endothelial functions are activated, and therefore, which message is produced by the cell. The endothelial cell also adjusts the expression and localization of certain key enzymes in response to physical or chemical stimuli. For example, changes in shear stress across the endothelial cell surface lead to alterations in gene activation and can produce longer-term phenotypic alterations in the cell. Translocation of enzymes from cytosol to the cell surface or to specialized invaginations in the cell surface (caveolae) in response to stimuli can greatly alter the signalling capacity of the endothelial cell.

The mobile endothelial cell and vascular repair

Endothelial cells are not static: they can and do move (Fig. 16.1.1.2), and are renewed. Endothelial cells move in response to specific chemical signals and can migrate to recover areas of endothelial

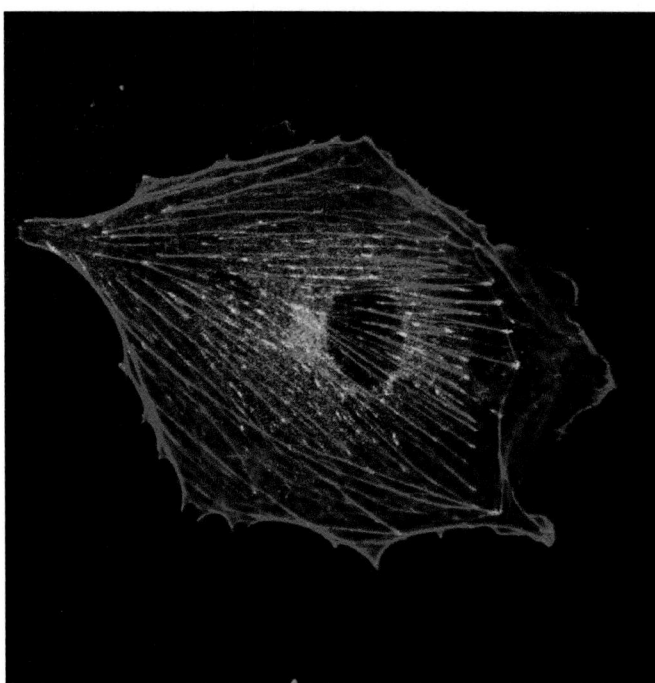

Fig. 16.1.1.2 An endothelial cell moving. The front end of the cell with leading lamella is on the right, stress fibres of contractile elements are seen in the centre and these end in focal adhesions. The retracting rear end of the cell is on the left. Courtesy of Dr B. Wojciak-Stothard.

damage or denudation. The basic mechanisms of movement are probably the same as those required to form vessels during development or during the process of formation of new vessels in adults, e.g. in tumour angiogenesis. There is also evidence that endothelial cells may circulate. This apparent paradox of a cell of the vessel wall circulating is explained in two ways. The first is that the circulating endothelial cells are cells that have become damaged and detached and are undergoing a terminal process. The second is that circulating cells represent a progenitor population (or populations) that arises largely from the bone marrow and may be instrumental in the process of vascular repair. These progenitor cells are characterized by the expression of specific cell-surface markers (CD34 and CD133) and can form colonies when cultured *in vitro*.

The literature on the relationship between circulating endothelial cells and cardiovascular disease is confused. The most straightforward interpretation at the moment is that there is an increase in the number of circulating mature (dying?) endothelial cells in the presence of a wide variety of vascular diseases, and that there is a positive relationship between the number of these circulating cells and the degree of impairment of endothelial function measured *in vivo* (see below). By contrast, the number of endothelial progenitor cells (EPCs) is thought to represent the restorative capacity of the vessel wall, with low numbers being indicative of disease progression and increased cardiovascular risk. Perhaps the ability to increase EPCs in response to vascular damage is a key feature of a healthy cardiovascular system able to repair itself. Despite the intense interest in circulating endothelial cells and their potential use as markers of disease or restorative capacity, there is also evidence that the repair process is dependent on resident stem cells—cells that have the properties of clonality, self-renewal, and multipotentiality.

Pericytes

Pericytes are about $70 \, \mu m$ in length and extend long cytoplasmic processes over endothelial cells in order to make multiple contacts (Fig. 16.1.1.3). In small capillaries, it also seems that pericytes may extend connections to more than one vessel, possibly exerting some sort of coordinating influence. The overall coverage of the endothelium by pericytes varies between vascular beds from 10 to 50%. The junctions between pericytes and endothelial cells appear to be rich in growth factors (particularly epidermal growth factor) that are important in regulating endothelial cell growth and may be vital for angiogenesis. Of particular importance in this interaction may be a signalling molecule known as angiopoietin and its receptor Tie2.

The nature of the junction between pericytes and endothelial cells may be important for regulating permeability at specialized sites such as the blood–brain barrier. In other areas, the contractile function of pericytes may predominate. In the retina, where pericytes are particularly prevalent, their loss is associated with impaired hierarchical organization of vessels or even vessel regression, and this might contribute to diabetic retinopathy. The only genetic disease to date in which pericyte loss has been implicated is Adams–Oliver syndrome, a rare developmental disorder characterized by scalp and limb malformations, telangiectasia, and vascular problems.

The potential roles of pericytes are listed in Box 16.1.1.1. These rather under-investigated cells seem to retain a plasticity that enables them to differentiate into smooth muscle cells.

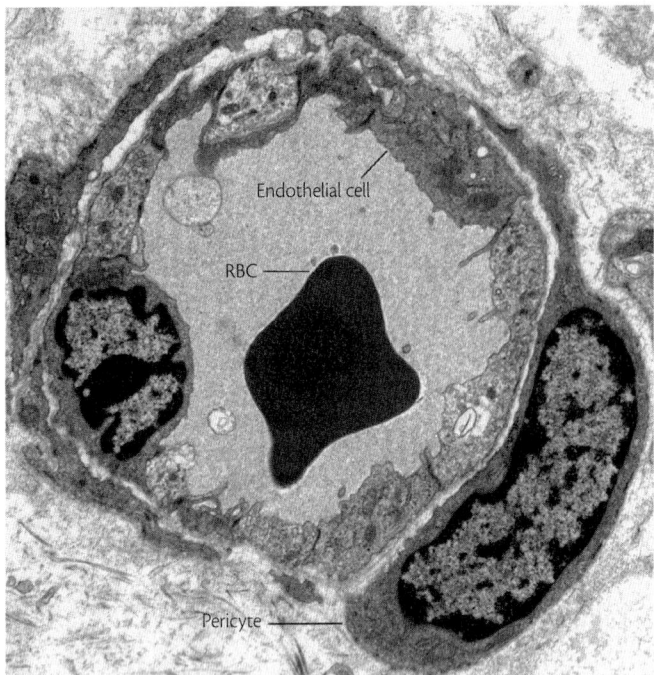

Fig. 16.1.1.3 Pericytes are observed outside small blood vessels in close association with endothelial cells.
Reproduced with kind permission from the Department of Pathology and Laboratory Medicine, University of Pennsylvania.

Vascular smooth muscle cells

Smooth muscle cells largely lie radially around the vessel to provide contractile function. Their state of contractility is influenced by hormonal, endothelial, neuronal, and intrinsic influences, and contraction is triggered by a wave of calcium release. In some vessels, smooth muscle cells show rhythmic contraction and it may be that this, rather than a static degree of contraction, is a ubiquitous feature. The complex determinants of vascular smooth muscle cell contraction, the signalling pathways and ion channels that determine smooth muscle cell membrane potential and calcium entry, are outside the scope of this chapter, but there are many good review articles that cover this topic.

It is worth considering briefly the relationship between smooth muscle contraction and resistance to flow, there being a fourth-power relationship between resistance to flow and the radius of the vessel, which means that relatively small changes in the contractile state of smooth muscle can produce large changes in the resistance offered by the vessel. This is particularly important for small arteries and arterioles that are the major determinants of systemic vascular resistance. The relative thickness of the vessel wall

---

Box 16.1.1.1 Roles of pericytes

- Contractility
- Barrier function and regulation of permeability
- Signalling to control endothelial growth and angiogenesis
- Vascular stabilization
- Sensors of hypoxia and hypoglycaemia
- Trans-differentiation into fibroblasts for wound healing

---

compared to the size of the lumen is also an important determinant of resistance. As the wall:lumen ratio increases, there is a comparatively larger reduction in lumen size for every incremental shortening of the smooth muscle. In this way, smooth muscle hypertrophy or hyperplasia can lead to a functional hyper-reactivity of the vessel wall, exemplifying the intimate connection between structure and function (Fig. 16.1.1.4).

Vascular smooth muscle cells are remarkably plastic and may adopt a range of phenotypes in response to local environmental changes. They may leave the contractile state and enter a replicative state, migrate into the intima, adopt a secretory phenotype that results in matrix deposition (including the development of bone-like features and calcification), and may, under certain conditions, contribute to inflammation within the vessel wall. Smooth muscle cells that replicate and secrete matrix contribute to the process of thickening of the vessel wall. Signalling through the so-called Notch pathway seems to be particularly important in some of the phenotypic plasticity of smooth muscle cells and defects in Notch signalling have been implicated in cerebro- and renovascular disorders as well as vascular calcification.

Control of vascular tone

Endothelium extracts and inactivates circulating hormones, converts inactive precursors to active products, and synthesizes and releases a variety of vasoactive mediators (Fig. 16.1.1.5). Vasoconstrictor and vasodilator mediators allow the vessel to respond to changes in the local milieu, but the predominant background influence of the endothelium is dilator, with the removal of the endothelium leading to vasoconstriction. A basal endothelium-dependent dilator tone seems to provide a physiological counterbalance to the continuous constrictor tone of the sympathetic nervous system.

Vasodilators

The endothelium produces at least three key vasodilation mediators (Fig. 16.1.1.5): nitric oxide, prostanoids, and hyperpolarizing factor.

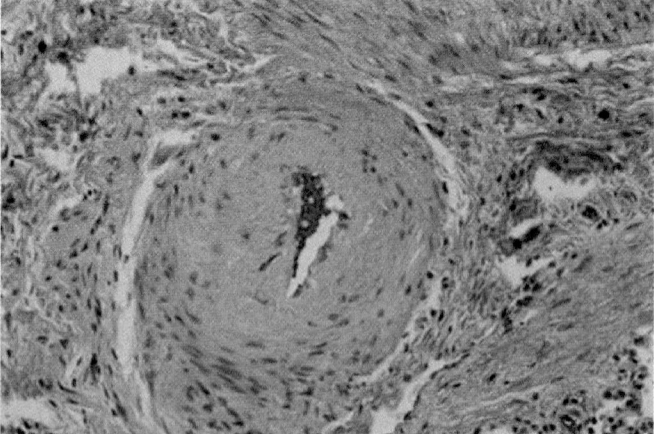

Fig. 16.1.1.4 Resistance vessels showing substantial medial hypertrophy. The increase in wall thickness will cause an exaggerated response to vasoconstrictors and is seen in patients with hypertension, in this case pulmonary hypertension.
http://www.lumen.luc.edu/lumen/MedEd/medicine/pulmonar/images/path/sld40.jpg.

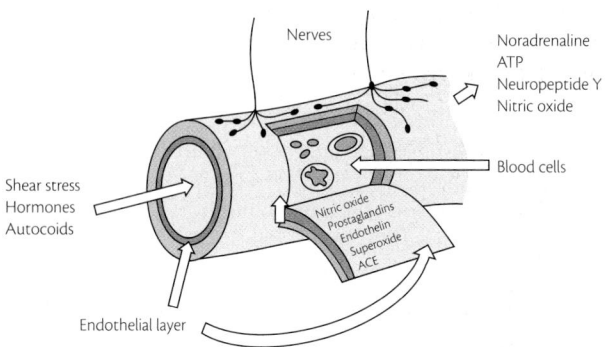

Fig. 16.1.1.5 Vascular endothelial cells lie at the interface between blood and the smooth muscle cells. They detect chemical and physical signals in the lumen of the blood vessel and adjust their output of biologically active mediators accordingly. This provides a mechanism of local regulation of vascular function. Rapid adjustment of vascular tone is probably achieved through a balance of endothelium-derived nitric oxide and neuronally derived noradrenaline. Endothelin provides a slowly modulating constrictor tone and angiotensin II has the capacity to fine-tune neuronal, endothelial, and smooth muscle function. ACE, angiotensin converting enzyme.

Nitric oxide

Physiology

The production of nitric oxide is responsible for basal endothelium-dependent dilator tone. This simple compound is a potent vasodilator: its synthesis is described in Fig. 16.1.1.6. Many of its actions are mediated through the second messenger cGMP, but in addition to signalling through activation of guanylyl cyclase, nitric oxide inhibits cytochrome *c* oxidase, initially in a reversible manner, but irreversibly under certain conditions. Inhibition of this enzyme decreases oxygen utilization, and the release of nitric oxide by endothelial cells appears to be an important determinant of oxygen consumption in the vasculature. Nitric oxide is also able to modify protein function through the chemical reactions of nitrosation of cysteine residues and nitration of tyrosines. It is possible that there are additional important targets for nitric oxide, including ion channels and various enzymes. Nitric oxide modifies the adhesiveness of the endothelial cell for circulating white cells, but rapid inactivation by haemoglobin prevents any significant downstream effect.

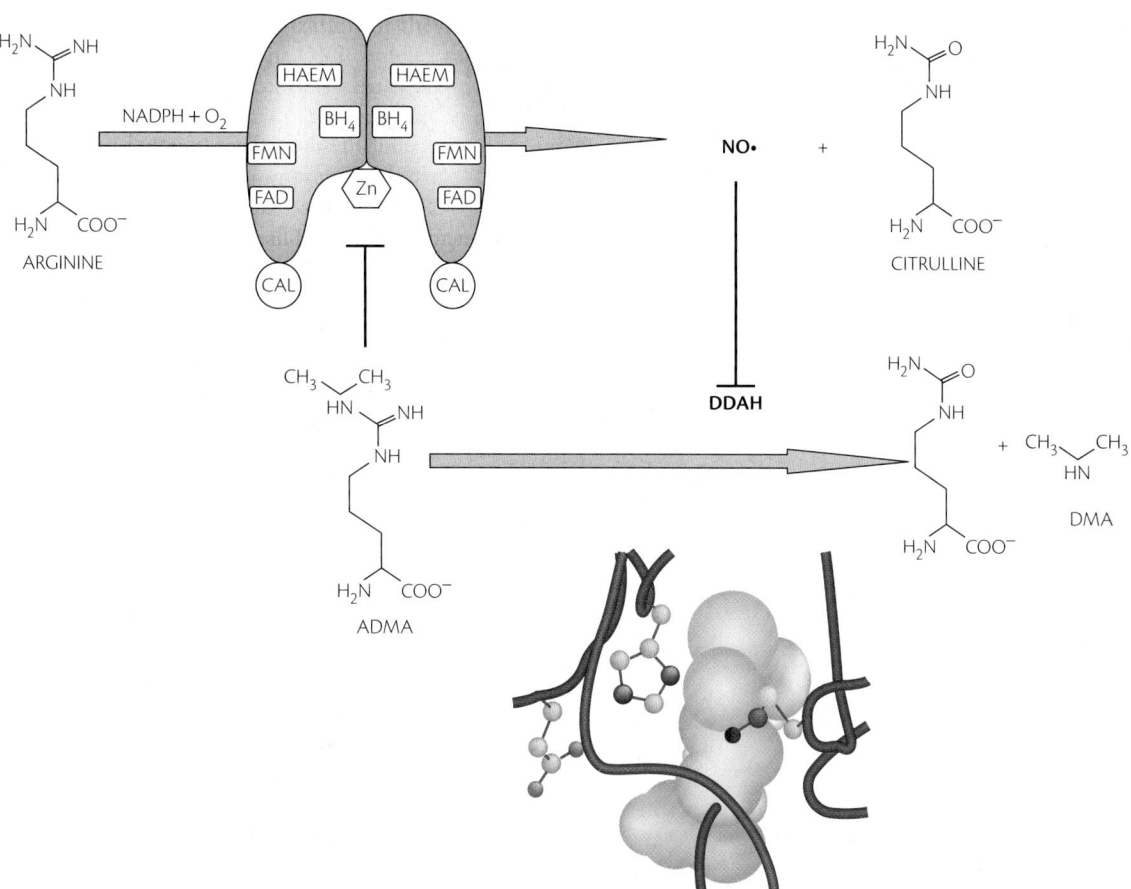

Fig. 16.1.1.6 Nitric oxide synthase (NOS) catalyses the conversion of L-arginine and molecular oxygen to citrulline and NO. NOS enzymes are catalytically active as homodimers and require the binding of cofactors (flavin adenine dinucleotide (FAD), flavin mononucleotide (FMN), haem, and tetrahydrobiopterin (BH$_4$)) and calmodulin for optimal activity. Each NOS dimer coordinates a single atom of zinc. NO directly inhibits DDAH by S-nitrosation of the active site cysteine residue. Inhibition of dimethylarginine dimethylaminohydrolase (DDAH) results in accumulation of asymmetric dimethylarginine (ADMA) and inhibition of NOS. Inset: a structural model of the active site of DDAH containing ADMA. The catalytic triad of glutamine, histidine, and cysteine residues is shown. S-nitrosation of the sulfur atom (green) of the active site cysteine deactivates this residue and might also sterically hinder the binding of ADMA.
From Arteriosclerosis Thrombosis and Vascular Biology 2004;24:1023-1030 (Vallance P and Leiper J).

Nitric oxide is a free radical (it has an unpaired electron in its outer orbit), and as such, reacts readily with other free radicals and reactive oxygen species. The reaction between nitric oxide and the superoxide anion (O^-_2) is extremely rapid and can result in the formation of either the toxic product peroxynitrite ($ONOO^-$) or the inactive breakdown product nitrate (NO_3^-). Such interactions between radicals can greatly influence the overall behaviour of the wall of the blood vessel and lead to an apparent defect in endothelial function even when the output of endothelial mediators is normal.

The arterial circulation of animals and humans is vasodilated continuously and actively by endothelium-derived nitric oxide, and inhibition of the synthesis of nitric oxide with certain guanidino-substituted analogues of L-arginine, including *N*-G-monomethyl-L-arginine, leads to vasoconstriction, hypertension, and sodium retention. Shear stress—the force caused by the viscous drag of flowing blood—is probably an important physiological stimulus for the continuous production of nitric oxide. As shear stress increases more nitric oxide is produced and the blood vessel relaxes, reducing the stress. This process of flow-mediated dilatation appears to be a homeostatic mechanism to prevent shear stress from increasing to levels that might initiate activation of platelets or other cells and may also help coordinate tissue perfusion. Flow-mediated dilatation is an autoregulatory property of blood vessels that tends to oppose classical myogenic autoregulation—the process by which a blood vessel constricts in response to an increase in intraluminal pressure.

Synthesis of nitric oxide is stimulated by acetylcholine, bradykinin, and substance P, and in many vessels the release of nitric oxide accounts for the vasodilator actions of these mediators, which are known as 'endothelium-dependent vasodilators'. Circulating hormones, including insulin and oestrogens, may also act on receptors on or within the endothelial cell to stimulate the release of nitric oxide acutely or to alter the expression of endothelial nitric oxide synthase chronically.

Veins differ from arteries and arterioles in that they do not seem to be actively dilated by the continuous release of nitric oxide. The venous endothelium releases nitric oxide when it is stimulated by acetylcholine or bradykinin, but not under basal conditions. Furthermore, human veins do not release much nitric oxide in response to platelet-derived mediators. Indeed, aggregating platelets constrict veins, due to the unopposed action of the platelet-derived mediators on the vascular smooth muscle. The reasons for the arteriovenous difference in nitric oxide production are not fully understood, but one consequence is that the guanylyl cyclase in venous smooth muscle is relatively up-regulated and veins respond to smaller amounts of nitric oxide than do arteries or arterioles. This is of therapeutic relevance; nitric oxide is the active moiety of glyceryl trinitrate and other nitrovasodilators, and the low basal synthesis of endogenous nitric oxide by venous endothelium accounts, in part, for the venoselective action of these drugs.

Pathophysiology

Loss of nitric oxide leads to arterial vasoconstriction, has the potential to enhance platelet and white cell adhesion, and, in experimental models, may enhance atherogenesis. Several clinical conditions—including atherosclerosis, hypertension, hypercholesterolaemia, and diabetes—are associated with a functional loss of nitric oxide-mediated effects.

Box 16.1.1.2 Sildenafil and ADMA

The pulmonary vasculature seems to be particularly sensitive to nitric oxide and the inhibition of nitric oxide synthesis causes pulmonary hypertension. These observations have been utilized therapeutically in the form of inhaled nitric oxide treatment, and amplification of nitric oxide signalling by inhibition of cGMP phosphodiesterase with sildenafil (see Chapter 16.15.2). Recently, it has become clear that a naturally occurring amino acid, asymmetric dimethylarginine (ADMA), acts as an important endogenous inhibitor of nitric oxide synthesis and that the concentration of ADMA in blood is a predictor of cardiovascular risk. Accumulation of ADMA may be important in renal failure, providing a possible mechanism to link failing renal function with increased risk of atherothrombotic complications.

In the coronary vasculature, loss of nitric oxide predisposes to vasospasm and may contribute to the onset of anginal symptoms. Atherosclerotic coronary arteries constrict in response to the platelet-derived mediator serotonin (5-hydroxytryptamine), whereas healthy vessels are stimulated to produce more nitric oxide and dilate. Flow-dependent dilatation is also lost in such vessels, and the response to sympathetic stimulation is converted from dilatation to unopposed constriction. Endothelial dysfunction precedes the development of overt atheroma, and there is a relationship between risk factors for ischaemic heart disease and impaired responsiveness of coronary arteries to endothelium-dependent vasodilators. Furthermore, hypercholesterolaemia, even in the absence of angiographic evidence of atheroma in large vessels, is associated with abnormal endothelium-dependent vasodilatation in coronary and peripheral arterioles. Modified low-density lipoproteins appear to inhibit nitric oxide synthesis or speed its destruction, possibly by enhancing production of the superoxide anion.

Basal endothelium-dependent dilatation is also impaired in patients with essential hypertension and the degree of impairment increases with increasing blood pressure. It is not known whether the defect is a consequence or a cause of the raised pressure, but the fact that endothelial function appears to be restored by antihypertensive therapy argues in favour of such dysfunction being a response to raised pressure. Patients with diabetes show diminished endothelium-dependent dilatation, and this defect does not reverse with treatment. Thus, patients with uncontrolled hypertension, diabetes, and hypercholesterolaemia all display defects of nitric-oxide-mediated vasodilatation and this could provide a common mechanism of vascular dysfunction in these diseases.

Overproduction of nitric oxide may also contribute to disease. Bacterial endotoxin and some cytokines, including interleukin (IL)-1 and interferon-γ, induce expression of a second nitric oxide synthesizing enzyme that appears in the endothelium, vascular smooth muscle, and inflammatory cells invading the vessel wall. Unlike the constitutive enzyme present in healthy endothelium (endothelial nitric oxide synthase), this inducible isoform of nitric oxide synthase is not regulated by calcium and produces large amounts of nitric oxide. In these quantities nitric oxide, either alone or in combination with superoxide, may contribute to tissue damage in addition to causing profound vasodilatation and hypotension such as that seen in septic shock. This essentially results in vascular paresis. Excess production of nitric oxide from endothelial nitric oxide synthase due to stimulation of certain essential cofactors including tetrahydrobiopterin may also contribute to these effects.

Prostanoids

Nitric oxide appears to be the dominant vasoactive factor released from endothelial cells under basal conditions, but it is by no means the only mediator produced. The endothelium is a rich source of prostanoids, including the vasodilators prostacyclin and prostaglandins E_2 and D_2 (PGE_2 and PGD_2). However, whereas inhibition of nitric oxide leads to profound and widespread changes in vascular tone, inhibition of prostanoid synthesis with aspirin (or other nonsteroidal anti-inflammatory drugs, NSAIDs) does not, excepting in the renal vasculature where dilator prostanoids do appear to be important in the regulation of basal renal blood flow: aspirin and other NSAIDs lead to vasoconstriction in the kidney, indicating tonic release of vasodilator prostanoids in this vascular bed. Furthermore, in the fetus and newborn, indomethacin leads to the closure of the ductus arteriosus and a fall in cerebral blood flow suggesting a significant contribution of endothelium-derived prostanoids to tonic vasodilatation in these beds, at least during development. The cerebral blood flow in adults also falls in response to indomethacin, but not to aspirin and other cyclo-oxygenase (COX) inhibitors, and so the role of prostanoids is unclear. Vasodilator prostanoids are important in the vascular changes of inflammation, although whether these prostanoids derive exclusively from the endothelium is not known. The finding that the inhibition of COX-II appears to be associated with increased cardiovascular risk is important and suggests that the balance of prostanoids in the vessel wall, and between endothelium and platelets, is a key determinant of the 'stickiness' of the endothelium to platelets and other circulating cells.

Hyperpolarizing factor

An endothelium-derived hyperpolarizing factor has been identified in some animal and human blood vessels. Hyperpolarization of vascular smooth muscle cells leads to a fall in calcium entry and vascular relaxation. Increasing evidence suggests that endothelium-dependent hyperpolarization may be particularly important in small arteries and arterioles. The chemical identity of endothelium-derived hyperpolarizing factor has not been clearly established, but products of activity of cytochrome P450, the cannabinoid anandamide, and the potassium ion have all been suggested as possible candidates. Recent data also suggests that the C-type natriuretic peptide accounts for this activity in some vessels. A picture is emerging that endothelium-derived hyperpolarizing factor is not a single entity, but rather that hyperpolarization is a mechanism utilized by different mediators that vary between vessels. In addition, direct contact through gap junctions also provides a means for endothelial cells to hyperpolarize smooth muscle cells. Without specific inhibitors, it is not yet clear what role the variations in endothelial cell hyperpolarization of smooth muscle cells plays in human disease.

Vasoconstrictors

Although the predominant background influence of the endothelium is dilator, important vasoconstrictor factors are also synthesized and released (See Box 16.1.1.2).

Endothelin

The endothelins are a family of potent vasoconstrictor peptides of 21 amino acids, which are closely related to the snake-venom toxin of the Israeli burrowing asp. Three types of endothelin have been described—endothelin 1, 2, and 3—and there are at least two endothelin receptors in human blood vessels, the endothelin A and endothelin B receptors. Endothelins vasoconstrict and can promote the growth of vascular smooth muscle cells. Effects are mediated in part through the stimulation of increases in calcium and in part through calcium-independent mechanisms, including activation of protein kinases.

Endothelin 1 is synthesized from 'big endothelin' within human endothelial cells (Fig. 16.1.1.7). It is a potent and long-lasting constrictor of human blood vessels, and causes widespread vasoconstriction, hypertension, and sodium retention when infused into healthy volunteers. Antagonists of the endothelin A receptor cause vasodilatation and can lower blood pressure, indicating that there is a tonic synthesis and release of endothelin A. A number of studies suggest that there may be important interactions between the sympathetic nervous system, the renin–angiotensin system, and the endothelin system, and that these may act in concert to control constrictor tone, with the endothelin system providing a slowly

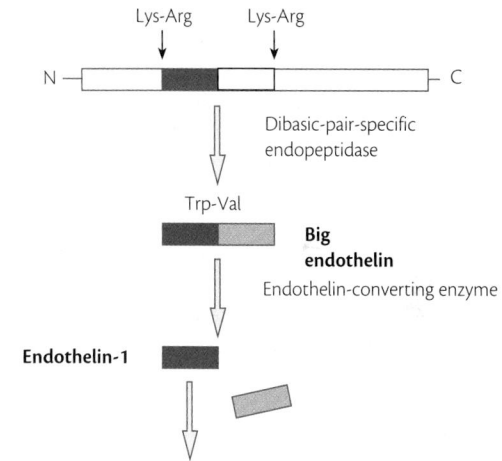

Activation of endothelin A and endothelin B receptors

Fig. 16.1.1.7 Endothelin-1 (ET-1), a cyclic (Cys^1–Cys^{15} and Cys^3–Cys^{11}) 21-amino acid peptide, is synthesized within the vascular endothelium as the product of an 'inactive' 39-amino acid precursor known as 'big ET-1', a conversion catalysed by a specific membrane-bound zinc metalloproteinase endothelin-converting enzyme. Big ET-1, in turn, is the catalytic product of a larger (203 amino acids) precursor polypeptide termed 'preproET-1' (a conversion that is believed to be mediated by a 'furin-like' protease). The ECE-mediated conversion of big ET-1 to mature ET-1 is an essential step in the expression of full biological activity. Upon release from the vascular endothelium, ET-1 interacts with the underlying smooth muscle cells resulting in vasoconstriction. This action is mediated by two distinct G-protein-coupled receptors, ET_A and ET_B. Whilst the predominant action of ET-1 is that of a vasoconstrictor, this effect is regulated by the concomitant release of vasodilatory factors (e.g. PGI_2, NO) by the action of ET-1 on endothelial ET_B-receptors. Although such an action tempers the contractile actions of ET-1, it is postulated that endothelial dysfunction (e.g. diminished ability to synthesize and/or release NO such as is seen in hypertension, atherosclerosis) results in aberrant ET-mediated vasoconstrictor tone due to a loss in concomitant endothelial regulation.

modulating, background constrictor tone. Endothelins also exert an important influence on sodium reabsorption in the kidney.

Although activation of endothelin B receptors on vascular smooth muscle causes constriction, activation of endothelial endothelin B receptors leads to the generation of vasodilator prostanoids and/or nitric oxide, hence endothelin can also produce transient vasodilatation in some circumstances. Binding of endothelin to endothelin B receptors also seems to be important to clear the peptide from the circulation. Stimuli for endothelin production include thrombin, insulin, cyclosporine, adrenaline, angiotensin II, cortisol, various proinflammatory cytokines, hypoxia, and shear stress.

The concentrations of endothelins circulating in plasma are low and may not reflect local concentrations achieved within the vessel wall. It is difficult to interpret the elevated values reported in many conditions. A role for endothelin in the pathogenesis of vasospasm associated with subarachnoid haemorrhage and some types of renal ischaemia is suggested by experiments in animals, and endothelin A/B antagonists produce short-term changes in haemodynamics in patients with heart failure that suggest a possible beneficial therapeutic effect.

Once again, the pulmonary vasculature seems to be of particular interest. Endothelin antagonists lower pulmonary pressures and exert beneficial effects in resistant pulmonary hypertension. The increased production of endothelin has also been clearly implicated in the pathogenesis of a very rare form of secondary systemic hypertension caused by malignant haemangioendothelioma, a vascular tumour characterized by intravascular proliferation of atypical endothelial cells. In this condition, the degree of hypertension correlates with plasma levels of endothelin, and when the tumour is removed blood pressure and plasma endothelin levels fall.

Angiotensin converting enzyme (ACE)

ACE is located primarily on the luminal surface of the endothelium. This enzyme converts angiotensin I to angiotensin II and also metabolizes bradykinin to inactive products. The pulmonary vasculature provides the largest area of endothelium and is important in the regulation of circulating levels of angiotensin II, but the activity of endothelial ACE in systemic vessels may be more important in determining the final concentrations of angiotensin II and bradykinin that reach the blood vessel wall. Furthermore, endothelial cells also have the ability to synthesize renin and its substrate. It seems, therefore, as though the enzymatic machinery for a complete renin–angiotensin system is present within the vessel wall.

The activity of the renin–angiotensin system is clearly important in cardiovascular diseases including hypertension and heart failure, but the relative importance of local, compared with systemic, regulation of angiotensin II production is not yet clear. Furthermore, the full clinical significance of bradykinin metabolism by endothelial ACE (see Fig. 16.1.1.5) has yet to be determined. It has been demonstrated that at least part of the vasodilator action of ACE inhibitors in certain isolated blood vessels is due to accumulation of bradykinin, which stimulates nitric oxide synthesis.

Prostanoids

The endothelium synthesizes thromboxane and the unstable prostaglandin endoperoxides PGG_2 and PGH_2. Overproduction of constrictor prostanoids by the endothelium has been implicated in

animal models of diabetes and hypertension, but the significance of these findings for human disease remains uncertain.

Superoxide

The superoxide anion (O^-_2) is synthesized within endothelial cells. There are several possible enzymatic sources, including cofactors that deplete nitric oxide synthase and cyclo-oxygenase. In neutrophils, NADH/NADPH oxidase is the major source of superoxide. Components of this system have been detected in endothelial cells and appear to be the major site of superoxide generation in the vessel wall, but it is important to note that generation of superoxide is not limited to the endothelium and may also occur in smooth muscle cells. Stimulation by angiotensin increases superoxide generation within the endothelium and elevated superoxide production is emerging as a key feature of pathophysiology, at least in animal models. Individuals with deficiency in NADH/NADPH oxidase suffer from chronic granulomatous disease: they may also have abnormal vascular reactivity.

Regulation of platelet function and haemostasis

The endothelium synthesizes and releases prothrombotic and antithrombotic factors. However, healthy endothelium presents a thromboresistant surface, indicating that the antithrombotic factors predominate under basal conditions.

Platelets

Endothelial cells inhibit the aggregation and adhesion of platelets, and disaggregate aggregating platelets. Two mediators are of particular importance: nitric oxide and prostacyclin (or PGE_2 in the microvascular endothelium), which act synergistically through different second messenger systems: cGMP for nitric oxide and cAMP for prostacyclin.

Thiols and sulphydryl-containing molecules react with nitric oxide to produce more stable adducts, including nitrosocysteine, nitrosoglutathione, nitrosoalbumin, and even nitrosohaemoglobin. Some of these compounds are formed *in vivo* and may enhance the antiplatelet effects of endothelium-derived nitric oxide. Furthermore, interaction between nitric oxide and tissue plasminogen activator leads to the formation of nitroso-tissue plasminogen activator, a molecule with fibrinolytic, antiplatelet, and vasorelaxant properties. It is not yet clear how important these nitric oxide adducts are in human physiology or pathophysiology.

Deficient production of nitric oxide has been implicated in a wide variety of cardiovascular diseases (see above), and abnormalities of prostanoid synthesis occur in experimental models of atherosclerosis and diabetes. In the presence of a quiescent healthy endothelium, loss of basal nitric oxide alone does not lead to significant systemic platelet activation. However, loss of nitric oxide and prostacyclin at sites of endothelial damage, dysfunction, or activation promotes the formation of platelet aggregates and may contribute to thrombosis and vessel occlusion. In animals, stenosed endothelium-denuded vessels lead to cyclical variations in flow as platelets stick to the vessel wall and release vasoactive and proaggregant mediators. If this also occurs in human vessels *in vivo*, it might be an important mechanism of vasospasm and thrombosis.

Under basal conditions the endothelium inhibits platelet activation, but in response to certain stimuli, proaggregant, proadhesive mediators may be synthesized and released. Unstable prostaglandin endoperoxides activate platelets, platelet activating factor may be produced, and von Willebrand factor—which is synthesized and stored within endothelial cells—increases platelet adhesion. These changes occur in response to inflammatory mediators and may also result from repeated endothelial 'injury'.

Coagulation

Heparan sulphate is a glycosaminoglycan closely related to heparin, but less potent, which is found on the surface of endothelial cells. Antithrombin III is also expressed on the endothelial cell surface and, together with heparan sulphate, provides a mechanism for binding and inactivating thrombin. In addition, endothelial cells participate in the activation of the anticoagulant protein C, and secretion of protein S and thrombomodulin that is found on the cell surface.

In the quiescent state, expression of anticoagulant factors predominates, but when activated the endothelium may promote coagulation. Receptors for clotting factors appear on the endothelial surface, von Willebrand factor is secreted, and tissue factor—the principal cellular initiator of coagulation—is expressed. Bacterial endotoxin, inflammatory cytokines, and glycosylated proteins activate the endothelium and shift the balance in favour of coagulation. This may occur in response to infection, inflammation, or endothelial injury. Circulating levels of von Willebrand factor are increased in some patients with diabetes or hypertension.

Fibrinolysis

The endothelial cell surface has a fibrinolytic pathway. Urokinase and tissue plasminogen activator are secreted and there are specific binding sites for plasminogen activators and plasminogen. Thrombin, adrenaline, vasopressin, and stasis of blood may be physiological stimuli for the release of tissue plasminogen activator from human endothelium.

Plasminogen activator inhibitor 1 is also synthesized and bound by endothelium, providing a pathway for local inhibition of the fibrinolytic system. Under basal conditions fibrinolysis is dominant, but the balance may be altered by a variety of local and circulating factors, including inflammatory cytokines and the atherogenic particle lipoprotein(a), which inhibits plasminogen binding and hence plasmin generation. In the presence of atherosclerosis, the fibrinolytic properties of the endothelium are diminished.

Other important aspects of vascular and endothelial biology

Cellular adhesion

The resting endothelium prevents cells from adhering fully to the vessel wall, but allows leucocytes to roll along its surface. The regulation of 'rolling', adhesion, and migration is governed largely by specialized glycoproteins known as cell adhesion molecules, which are expressed in varying amounts on the endothelial cell surface and interact with complementary adhesion molecules on circulating cells. Endothelial-leucocyte adhesion molecule 1 (ELAM-1, also known as E-selectin), vascular adhesion molecule 1 (VCAM-1),

intercellular adhesion molecule 1 (ICAM-1), and P-selectin (also known as GMP-140) are all expressed on cytokine-activated endothelium. The degree of expression and the type of adhesion molecules expressed determines the 'stickiness' of the endothelium for different cell types.

Expression of adhesion molecules is an important mechanism of cellular adhesion during inflammation and is also important in recruitment of T cells and monocytes in atherosclerosis. Increased expression of E-selectin is seen in the coronary arteries of transplanted hearts, and has been implicated in the rapid development of atherosclerosis in these vessels. Nitric oxide and prostacyclin inhibit the adhesion of white cells to the endothelium and this effect may be mediated by changes in the expression or configuration of adhesion molecules. Certain endothelial cell-adhesion molecules are shed into the plasma: changes in their concentration have been detected in a variety of cardiovascular diseases, but the significance of this is uncertain.

Proinflammatory cytokines

Cytokines are released from activated leucocytes in response to infection and immunological stimulation and are also produced by the vessel wall itself; IL-1, IL-6, and IL-8, and colony-stimulating factors (CSF) are synthesized by endotoxin-stimulated endothelial cells, and tumour necrosis factor (TNF) by human smooth muscle cells. A large number of cytokines and chemokines alter endothelial functions, upsetting the balance of vasoactive mediators, altering thrombotic activity and the expression of adhesion molecules, or initiating apoptosis (programmed cell death). IL-1 and some other proinflammatory cytokines alter the synthesis of nitric oxide (see above) and a variety of prostaglandins; enhance the generation of thrombin, platelet-activating factor, von Willebrand factor, and plasminogen activator inhibitor; alter endothelial permeability; increase expression of ICAM-1 and VCAM-1; and may also cause endothelial cell damage and death. These findings are of direct relevance to the vascular changes occurring in inflammation and sepsis, and might also provide a link between acute or chronic immunological stimulation (e.g. infection) and the development of cardiovascular disease, including atherosclerosis or acute cardiovascular events.

Cell growth and angiogenesis

The endothelium of healthy differentiated vessels inhibits proliferation of the underlying smooth muscle. Endothelium-derived vasodilator, antiplatelet, and antithrombotic mediators (e.g. nitric oxide, prostacyclin) tend to inhibit the growth of vascular smooth muscle cells, whereas vasoconstrictor and prothrombotic mediators (e.g. endothelin, angiotensin) tend to promote it. Thus the basal state of the endothelium, in which dilatation and thromboresistance predominates, also prevents the growth of smooth muscle. The heparin-like molecules prevent cell growth and molecules similar or identical to platelet-derived growth factor (PDGF) and fibroblast growth factor (FGF) are endothelium-derived growth promoters. Others such as transforming growth factor β (TGFβ), produced by endothelial cells, may either inhibit or promote cell growth, and the precise role of this molecule in vivo is unclear. The basal antiproliferative effects of the endothelium may retard the development of atherosclerosis and intimal proliferation.

Fig. 16.1.1.8 Formation of new blood vessels. Endothelial cells grown in a matrix (Matrigel) form tube-like structures. The right-hand panel shows the effect of inhibiting angiogenic signals such as vascular endothelial growth factor (VEGF). Reprinted from *Biochemical and Biophysical Research Communications*, Vol 308, Issue 4, Smith, C L et al, *Dimethylarginine dimethylaminohydrolase activity modulates ADMA levels, VEGF expression, and cell phenotype*, pp984–89. Copyright (2003), with permission from Elsevier.)

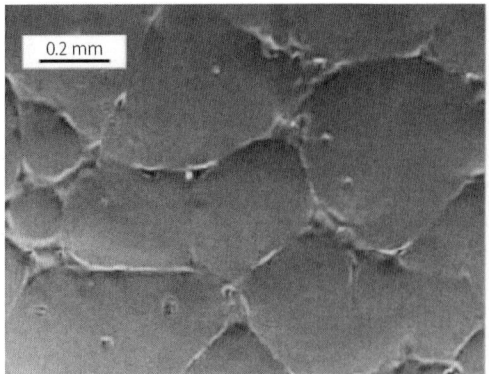
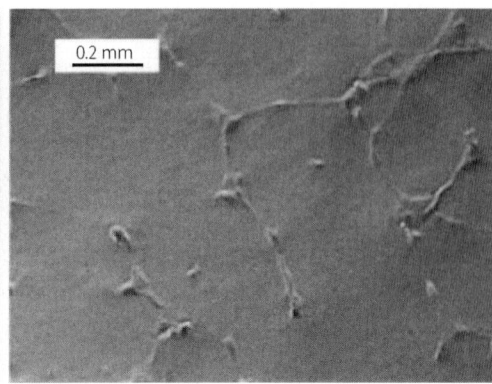

In addition to affecting the growth of underlying smooth muscle, endothelial cells are essential for the formation of new blood vessels. The ability of endothelial cells to initiate the formation of new vessels (angiogenesis and vasculogenesis; Fig. 16.1.1.8) is retained in adults, but the only place this occurs physiologically to any great extent is in the female reproductive tract. However, angiogenesis occurs in a wide range of disease states including atherosclerosis, rheumatoid arthritis, and tumour growth, and during wound healing or in response to ischaemia. Positive and negative regulators of angiogenesis have been identified and a wide variety of cytokines, growth factors, and local autacoids can act alone or in concert to promote endothelial cell growth, migration, and tube formation. Of particular interest is vascular endothelial growth factor (VEGF), a growth factor produced by smooth muscle cells in response to hypoxia, inflammatory cytokines, and certain other growth factors. There is good evidence that VEGF can promote angiogenesis in a variety of animal models and in humans. Intriguingly, it appears as though VEGF can increase the production of nitric oxide by endothelial cells, and this may be one of the effector molecules mediating some of the actions of this growth factor. In order to form tubes through tissues, endothelial cells must degrade matrix and they are capable of synthesizing and releasing a variety of matrix metalloproteinases. Some of these matrix metalloproteinases may, in turn, affect endothelial function by regulating cell attachment, proliferation, and migration. Failure of endothelial cells to initiate appropriate angiogenesis in response to ischaemia may lead to tissue hypoxia, whilst excessive or inappropriate angiogenesis may contribute to a sustained inflammatory response in the vessel wall, disrupt vessel wall architecture, or lead to haemorrhage into atherosclerotic plaques.

Transport and metabolism

The endothelium presents a permeability barrier for molecules in the bloodstream. Transfer of molecules from the bloodstream into the vessel wall across the endothelium can occur by transport through the endothelial cells or between them. The junctions between endothelial cells are maintained by specialized molecules, including cadherins, and are actively regulated. Transport between cells occurs when endothelial cells contract to leave intercellular gaps. This is an important mechanism for formation of localized oedema. Transport through cells occurs by transcytosis and is an important mechanism for the passage of some macromolecules, including insulin. In addition, specialized channels for transport of water have been identified—the aquaporins.

The endothelium is intimately involved in lipid metabolism. Lipoprotein lipase is located on the endothelial cell surface, and receptors for low-density lipoproteins are present in varying amounts. In quiescent endothelium, lipoprotein lipase is active, but there are few low-density lipoprotein receptors, indicating that healthy endothelium provides a barrier for the entry of low-density lipoproteins into the vessel wall. However, under conditions in which a low-density lipoprotein is taken into the endothelium, modification by oxidation occurs and this step may stimulate atherogenesis.

Adventitial function

Nerves supplying the vessel wall enter through the adventitia into the media to provide a key influence on the contraction of vascular smooth muscle cells. The sympathetic nervous system is, of course, of prime importance in determining the contractile state of the vessel. In addition, cholinergic innervation influences some vascular beds, as do purinergic nerves. Pharmacological observation suggests that not all vessels are equally affected by denervation or interruption of specific neuronal influences. Resistance vessels and capacitance veins seem to be particularly regulated by sympathetic tone, and blockade of the sympathetic system causes not only a fall in arterial pressure but also major venous dilatation that leads to postural hypotension. In the brain, local neuronal projections have been implicated in providing a link between cerebral activation and the consequent increase in blood flow.

Lymph vessels also permeate the adventitia of large vessels and are important to remove fluid. Finally, a network of small blood vessels, the vasa vasorum, is found in the adventitia of larger blood vessels. Vasa vasorum are found mainly in vessels that have relatively thick walls with many layers of vascular smooth muscle cells. An increase in vasa vasorum may be taken as an indication of vessel-wall hypoxia. Stripping the vasa vasorum in large veins leads ultimately to both smooth muscle and endothelial dysfunction and damage, and, in the arterial system, can stimulate smooth muscle-cell replication and promote an atherogenic type of lesion. The vasa vasorum responds to vasoactive agents, but the pharmacology of these vessels is relatively poorly understood. Infiltration of the adventitia with inflammatory cells may be an important feature of atherogenesis (see Chapter 16.13.1), and perivascular fat may interfere with vascular function through the generation of adipokines and inflammatory cytokines. It is worth noting that obese individuals have more perivascular fat.

Further reading

Allt G, Lawrenson JG (2001). Pericytes: Cell biology and pathology. *Cells Tissues Organs*, **69**, 1–11.

Armulik A, Abramsson A, Betsholtz C (2005). Endothelial/pericyte interactions. *Circ Res*, **97**, 512–23.

Boos CJ, Lip GY, Blann AD (2006). Circulating endothelial cells in cardiovascular disease. *J Amer Coll Cardiol*, **8**, 1538–47.

Dhaun N, Goddard J, Webb DJ (2006). The endothelin system and its antagonism in chronic kidney disease. *J Am Soc Nephrol*, **17**, 943–55.

Feletou M, Vanhoutte PM (1999). The alternative: EDHF. *J Mol Cell Cardiol*, **31**, 15–22.

Folkman J. (2003). Fundamental concepts of the angiogenic process. *Curr Mol Med*, **3**, 643–51.

Furchgott RF, Zawadzki JV (1980). The obligatory role of endothelial cells in the relaxation of arterial smooth muscle. *Nature*, **288**, 373–6.

Garry DJ, Olson EN (2006). A common progenitor at the heart of development. *Cell*, **127**, 1101–4.

Hayden MR, Reidy M (1995). Many roads lead to atheroma. *Nat Med*, **1**, 22–3.

Isner JM, Asahara T (1999). Angiogenesis and vasculogenesis as therapeutic strategies for postnatal neovascularization. *J Clin Invest*, **103**, 1232–6.

Kinlay S, Libby P, Ganz P (2001). Endothelial function and coronary artery disease. *Curr Opin Lipid*, **12**, 383–9.

Mason JC, Haskard DO (1994). The clinical importance of leucocyte and endothelial cell adhesion molecules in inflammation. *Vasc Med Rev*, **5**, 249–75.

Panes J, Perry M, Granger DN (1999). Leukocyte-endothelial cell adhesion: avenues for therapeutic intervention. *Br J Pharmacol*, **126**, 537–50.

Ross R (1999). Atherosclerosis—an inflammatory disease. *N Engl J Med*, **340**, 115–26.

Vallance P, Collier J, Bhagat K (1997). Infection, inflammation and infarction: does acute endothelial dysfunction provide a link? *Lancet*, **349**, 1391–2.

Vallance P, Leiper J (2004). Cardiovascular biology of the asymmetric dimethylarginine:dimethylarginine dimethylaminohydrolase pathway. *Arterioscler Thromb Vasc Biol*, **24**, 1023–30.

Vane JR, Bakhle YS, Botting RM (1998). Cyclooxygenases 1 and 2. *Annu Rev Pharmacol Toxicol*, **38**, 97–120.

16.1.2 Cardiac myocytes and the cardiac action potential

Kenneth T. MacLeod, Steven B. Marston, Philip A. Poole-Wilson[†], Nicholas J. Severs, and Peter H. Sugden

Essentials

Functional anatomy of the cardiac myocyte

Cardiac myocytes are the contractile cells of the heart and constitute the bulk of heart mass. There are differences between the myocytes of the ventricles, the atria, and the conduction system: ventricular myocytes are elongated cells and packed with myofibrils (the contractile apparatus) and mitochondria (for ATP production).

The myofibrils are repeating units (sarcomeres) made up of thin actin filaments anchored at the Z discs at either end of the sarcomere, and thick myosin filaments which interdigitate and interact with the thin filaments. Contraction results from sarcomere shortening produced by the ATP-dependent movement of the thin and thick filaments relative to one another. Atrial myocytes are long and slender, and differ in some of the features of ventricular myocytes. For example, transverse tubules (T-tubules) which are involved in entry of Ca^{2+} into the ventricular myocyte are essentially absent but there are more caveolae. Myocytes of the conduction system are small cells that possess only a rudimentary myofibrillar structure.

Myocytes are attached to their neighbours and to the extracellular matrix to allow transmission of force. At some regions of contact (the intercalated discs), specialized structures (the gap junctions) contain channels which form contiguous electrical connections between a myocyte and its neighbours, and allow passage of ions and small molecules.

Cardiac action potential

There is a potential difference (the membrane potential) across the plasma membrane such that the inside of the cell is negative compared to the outside by about 80 mV. This is caused largely by the efflux of K^+ from the cell through K^+ channels and down its concentration gradient until the electronegative force retaining K^+ in the cell balances the tendency for efflux.

The sarcoplasmic reticulum (SR) is a lace-like membranous structure that surrounds the myofibrils and is a reservoir of the Ca^{2+} which participates in myofibrillar contraction. The plasma membrane of the ventricular myocyte contains deep, finger-like indentations (the T-tubules) that abut with the SR at junctional regions in register with the Z discs of the superficial sarcomeres.

When a myocyte is electrically excited, Na^+ channels open and Na^+ enters the cell down its own concentration gradient, thus producing an inward current and depolarizing the cell towards its equilibrium potential. This represents the initial phase (phase 0) of the action potential. As the myocyte depolarizes, the L-type Ca^{2+} channels in the T-tubules and plasma membrane open and Ca^{2+} enters the cell down its concentration gradient. The Na^+ channels close rapidly, but the L-type Ca^{2+} channels remain open for longer and produce further depolarization. This is followed by phases 1 and 2 of the action potential where the tendency to depolarize is balanced by repolarizing outward current flow carried by a variety of K^+ channels. The membrane potential in phase 2 is relatively stable and hence this phase is also known as the plateau phase.

The entry of Ca^{2+} in close apposition to the junctional SR causes the SR Ca^{2+}-release channels to open, discharging about half of the SR Ca^{2+} reservoir into the cytoplasm in a process known as Ca^{2+}-induced Ca^{2+}-release. This increase in Ca^{2+} concentration (the Ca^{2+} transient) is sensed by a Ca^{2+}-binding protein (troponin C) that is a component of the thin filament regulatory complex (the troponin–tropomyosin complex). This initiates myofibrillar contraction, which starts about halfway though phase 2.

As the L-type Ca^{2+} channels close, outward current flow though K^+ channels predominates and the myocyte repolarizes towards the K^+ equilibrium potential (phase 3). Ca^{2+} is removed from the cytoplasm and returned to the SR in an ATP-requiring process

---

[†] It is with regret that we report the death of Professor Philip A. Poole-Wilson during the preparation of this edition of the textbook.

mediated by the sarcoplasmic/endoplasmic Ca^{2+} ATPase (SERCA2). Ca^{2+} is also expelled from the cell by the plasma membrane Na^+,Ca^{2+} exchanger, which is electrogenic (three Na^+ exchanged for one Ca^{2+}) and tends to prolong the plateau phase. The behaviour of the Na^+,Ca^{2+} exchanger is complex because—depending on the Na^+ and Ca^{2+} concentrations and the membrane potential—it can reverse, thus mediating Ca^{2+} entry and repolarization. This occurs at depolarized potentials, and more so when intracellular Na^+ is increased. In phase 4, repolarization is complete and the myocyte is electrically quiescent until the next depolarization.

Cardiac pacemaker and regulation of contractility

The 'pacemaker' or sinoatrial node contains myocytes that exhibit a different form of action potential from the ventricular myocytes because of differences in the expression of ion channels. The Na^+ channel is essentially absent and depolarization is mediated by Ca^{2+} channels. The cell depolarizes spontaneously and gradually during phase 4 until the Ca^{2+} channels open and an action potential is produced. This partly results from the presence of hyperpolarization-activated cyclic nucleotide-gated (HCN) channels which are absent from ventricular myocytes and which carry an inward-depolarizing Na^+ current. The stimulus is then transmitted in a controlled manner via the conduction system to all regions of the heart.

Cardiac contractility is controlled largely by the sympathoadrenal system and the parasympathetic nervous system. β-Adrenergic stimulation increases the tendency of the L-type Ca^{2+} channel to open (positive inotropism). β-Stimulation also increases relaxation (positive lusitropism) by stimulation of SERCA2 and an increased rate of release of Ca^{2+} from the troponin complex. The positive chronotropic effects of β-stimulation result from increased HCN channel opening, causing an increased frequency of pacemaker depolarization. These effects are all opposed by the (cholinergic) muscarinic receptors of the parasympathetic nervous system.

Introduction

Cardiac myocytes are the contractile cells of the heart, though some have evolved to fulfil other specialized roles, e.g. the myocytes that constitute the electrical conduction system. The aims of this chapter are threefold: (1) to describe the functional anatomy of the cardiac myocyte, (2) to describe the origins of the cardiac action potential, and (3) to describe the mechanism of contraction. We will focus largely on the ventricular rather than the atrial myocyte, though the specialized characteristics of the latter will be described. In the ventricle, the myocytes constitute the bulk of the cellular volume and protein although, because they are large cells, they are in the minority with respect to cell number, being outnumbered by endothelial cells, smooth muscle cells of the vasculature, fibroblasts, and others. It remains controversial, but the overall view is that ventricular myocytes are terminally differentiated cells that withdraw from the cell cycle during the perinatal period in mammals, and thus are incapable of further complete cycles of replication. This is less clear for the atrial myocyte. Terminal differentiation has important consequences for the heart in terms of its limited ability to survive haemodynamic insults or stresses, but also means that the myocardium is essentially resistant to malignant transformation.

Functional anatomy of the cardiac myocyte

Overall morphology of the ventricular myocyte and its contractile machinery

The ventricular myocyte is an elongated cell (100–150 μm long and 20–35 μm wide) and is packed with striated myofibrils (the contractile elements) that alternate with rows of mitochondria (Figs. 16.1.2.1 and 16.1.2.2). Each myofibril is roughly cylindrical (2–3 μm in diameter), stretches the length of the cell and is anchored at each end in a fascia adherens junction. The myofibril is made up of sarcomeres arranged in series. Sarcomeres consist of two arrays of filaments: the thin filaments, and the thick filaments which interdigitate with the thin filaments (Fig. 16.1.2.2). The thin filaments are comprised predominantly of the protein actin and the thick

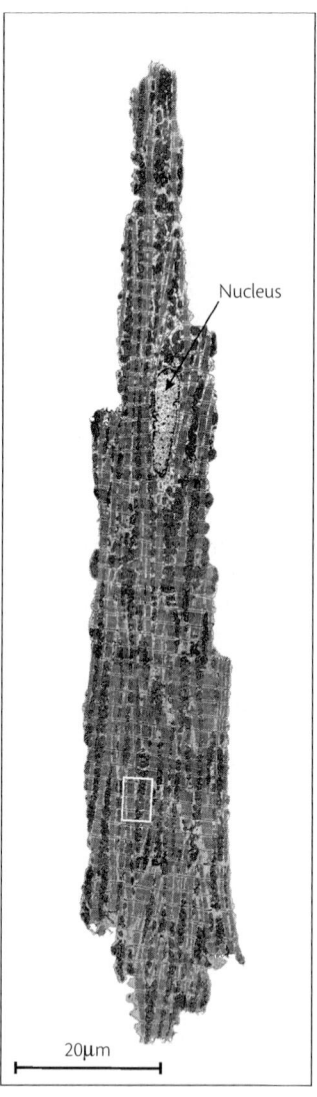

Nucleus

20μm

Fig. 16.1.2.1 Low-magnification thin-section electron micrograph of an isolated ventricular cardiac muscle cell. This cell is from a rat, though the human cell is essentially indistinguishable. Note that the cell is packed full of striated myofibrils, with rows of mitochondria—just visible as darker bodies—lying between. An electron micrograph of an area equivalent to the white rectangle in the lower part of the image is shown in Fig. 16.1.2.2.
Reprinted from Journal of Ultrastructure Research, 81:, N.J. Severs et al, Correlation of ultrastructure and function in calcium-tolerant myocytes isolated from the adult rat heart, 222–239. Copyright (1982) with permission from Elsevier.

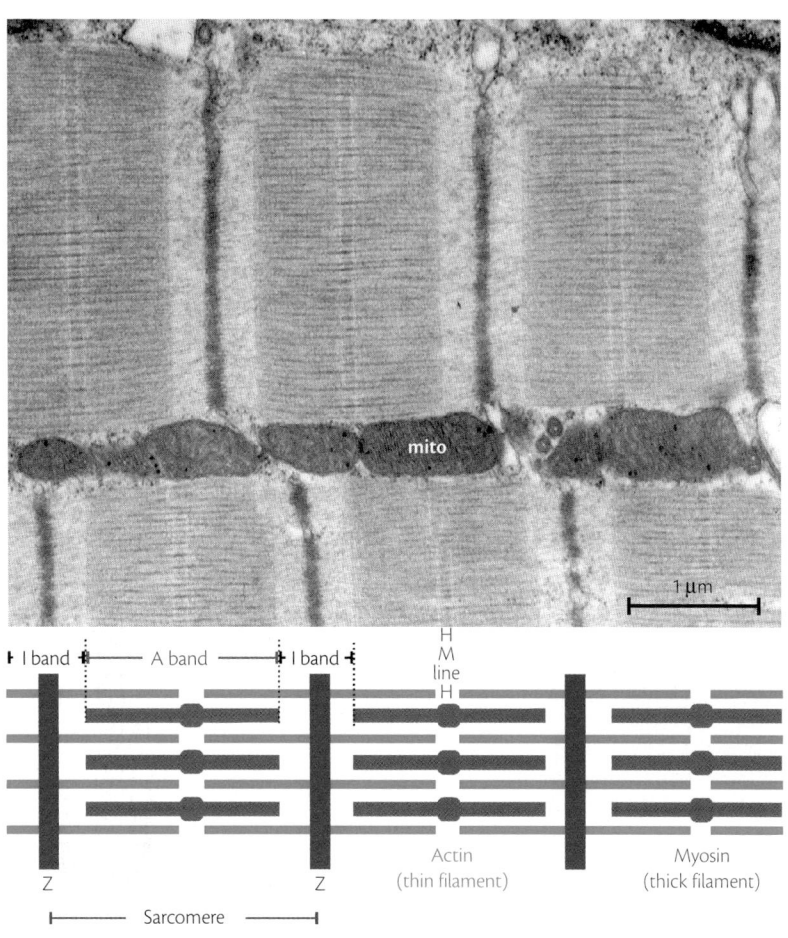

Fig. 16.1.2.2 Upper panel: Thin-section electron micrograph of an area equivalent to that in the rectangle in Fig. 16.1.2.1, showing the structure of the myofibrils. Portions of two myofibrils are shown in the field, with a row of mitochondria between (mito). Lower panel: Diagrammatic representation of the arrangement of the thick and thin filaments in relation to the striated pattern shown in the upper panel.

filaments of myosin. The characteristic striated appearance arises from the organization of the myofibril and the associated proteins within it (Fig. 16.1.2.2). The thick filaments are confined to the A band at the centre of the sarcomere. The thin filaments extend out from either side of the Z-band, crossing the I-band, and penetrate partially into the A-band, where they overlap and interact with the thick filaments. Each Z- to Z-band repeat constitutes a sarcomere, and the distance between consecutive Z-bands (the sarcomere length) is a measure of the contractile state of the myofibril. At the centre of the sarcomere lies the M-line. At the maximum longitudinal dimension of the myocyte, each myofibril contains 70-80 sarcomeres (Fig. 16.1.2.3). Myocytes have an irregular 'branched' morphology, readily appreciated in confocal microscopical reconstructions of the cell (Fig. 16.1.2.3). Through these branches, each ventricular myocyte typically connects to 10 or more of its neighbours to form the three-dimensional branching structure of the myofibre.

Structure of the contractile apparatus

Thick filaments

The myosin molecule is made up of two heavy chains (molecular mass 200 kDa) and two pairs of light chains (mass 18–28 kDa). The myosin heavy chains form a dimer, which consists of a long tail and two roughly globular heads (Fig. 16.1.2.4). The myosin tails are packed side by side to form the shaft of the thick filament, while the heads protrude from the filament and lie close to the thin actin

filaments. The myosin heads in the two halves of the thick filament either side of the M-line (Fig. 16.1.2.2) have opposite polarities, whilst the shaft at the centre of the filament is bare. The myosin heads are the motor units of muscle: they bind and hydrolyse ATP to ADP and convert the free energy of hydrolysis into mechanical work through their interaction with actin in the thin filaments (described in detail below).

Thin filaments

Each thin filament extending from the Z-line is made up of a double helical polymer (Fig. 16.1.2.4) of about 300 globular actin subunits (mass 42 kDa). The actin monomers have sites for interaction with the myosin heads involved in contraction and with a regulatory protein complex that confers Ca^{2+} sensitivity. The latter consists of the troponin complex and the elongated protein, α-tropomyosin (Fig. 16.1.2.4). Troponin complexes are located at intervals along the actin filament. Tropomyosin forms two continuous strands along the thin filament and is responsible for cooperative propagation of regulatory signals.

Other structural components of the sarcomere

The thin filaments are attached to the Z-discs in a regular array with filaments on each side in opposite orientations. The main structural component of the Z-disc is the actin cross-linking protein, α-actinin (Fig. 16.1.2.2). Z-discs are also associated with the T-tubules and costameres (see below), and contain a number of additional proteins believed to be associated with cell signalling. At the centre of

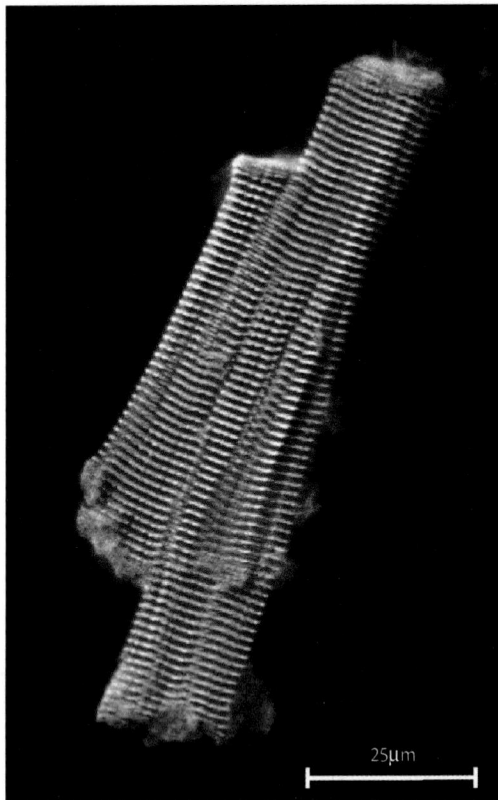

Fig. 16.1.2.3 A rat ventricular myocyte viewed by confocal microscopy. The myofibrils have been visualized by immunolabelling α-actinin, a component of the Z-discs. The blunted ends of the cell are the sites of the intercalated discs, through which individual myocytes are linked together.

Reprinted from Severs NJ (2000). The cardiac muscle cell. Bioessays, 22:188–199 (Fig. 2A). With permission from Wiley-Blackwell.

the sarcomere lies the M-line (Fig. 16.1.2.2) containing the protein myomesin that cross-links the thick filaments to maintain them in a regular array and to keep them in register. In addition, the giant protein titin extends from the M-line to the Z-disc. Titin contains hundreds of binding sites for myosin, myosin-binding protein-C (MyBP-C), other M-line proteins, and several Z-disc and I-band proteins that have not yet been identified. It contributes to elasticity, passive tension, and thick filament positioning in the sarcomere. MyBP-C is associated with myosin tails in the overlap zone, and nebulin extends along, and may control, the length of the thin filament. Familial hypertrophic cardiomyopathy is caused by mutations in sarcomeric proteins (principally myosin heavy chain and MyBP-C) (see Chapter 16.7.2).

Intermediate filaments, costameres, and the plasma membrane skeleton

The myofibrils are held in position by scaffold-like webs of intermediate filaments made from the (non-contractile) protein, desmin. Desmin filaments are anchored to costameres, vinculin-rich rib-like plaques that circumscribe the lateral plasma membrane in discontinuous fashion (Fig. 16.1.2.5). Apart from maintaining the spatial organization of the contractile apparatus, the costameres mechanically couple the cells laterally to the extracellular matrix. Associated with the costameres, but closely applied to the entire cytoplasmic aspect of the lateral plasma membrane, is the membrane skeleton, a peripheral membrane protein network of dystrophin and spectrin (Fig. 16.1.2.5). The membrane skeleton strengthens the plasma membrane against the rigours of contraction, and further contributes to lateral force transmission. The costameres, membrane skeleton, and intermediate filaments are linked to the glycocalyx (a glycoprotein-rich coating of the

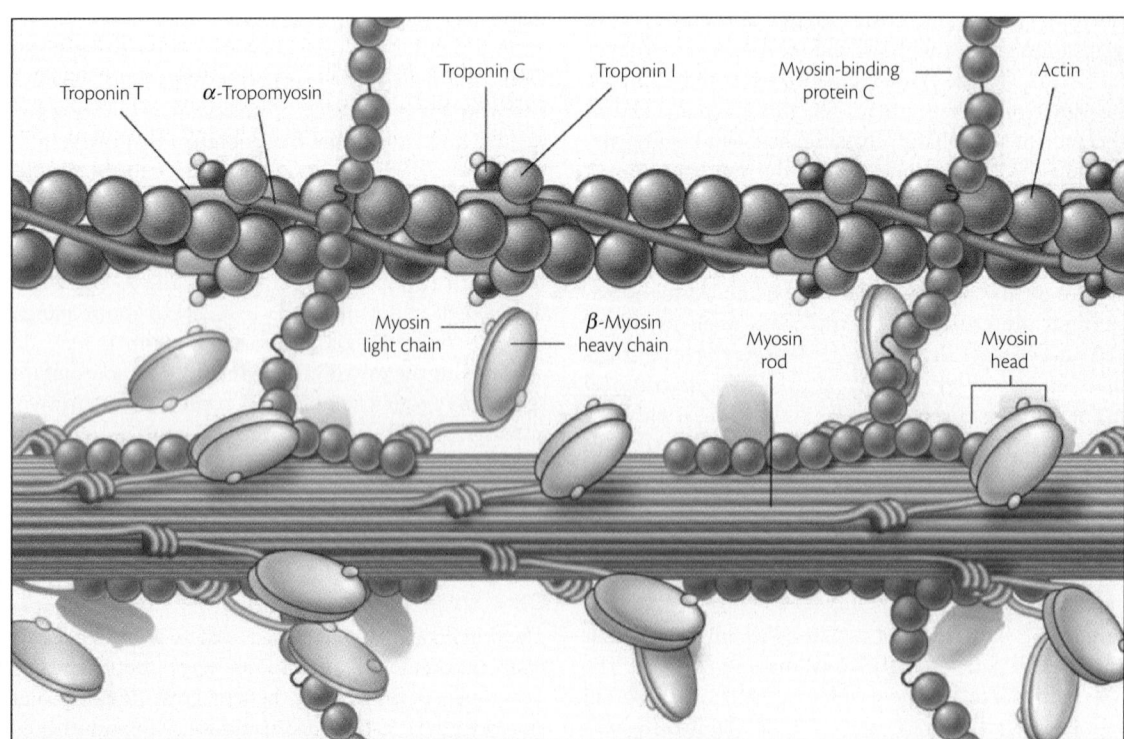

Fig. 16.1.2.4 Structural arrangement of contractile proteins in the filament overlap zone of the sarcomere.

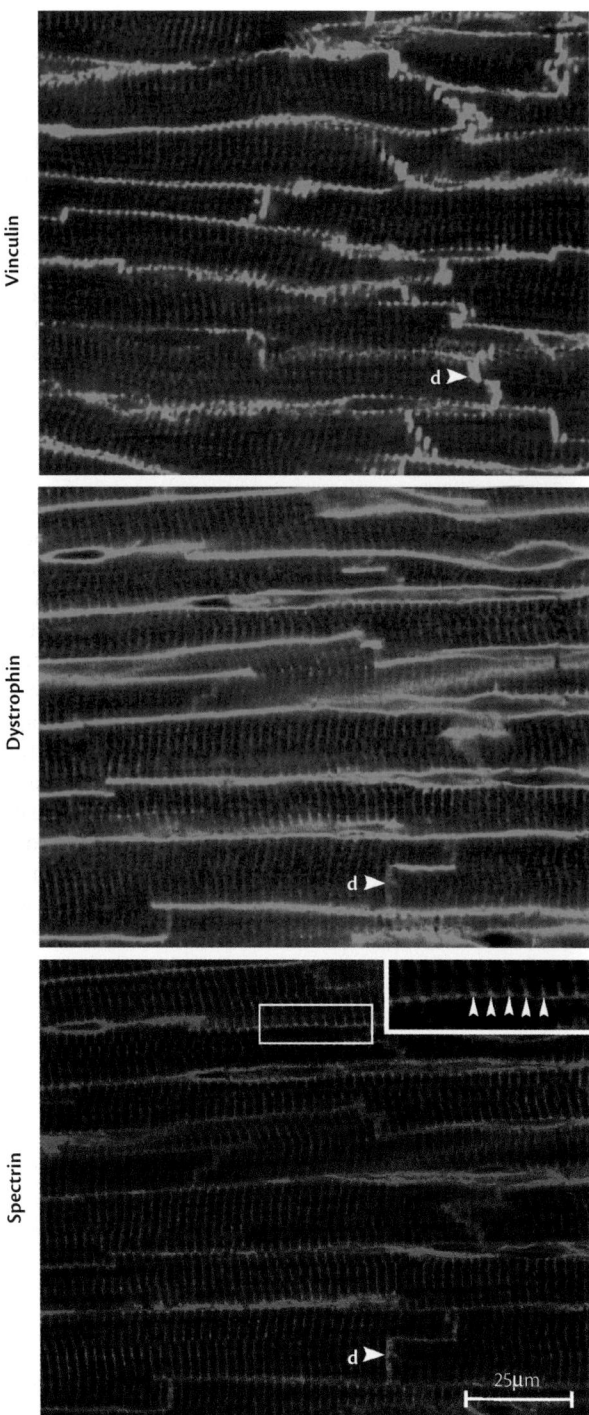

Fig. 16.1.2.5 Immunolocalization of vinculin (upper panel), dystrophin (centre panel) and spectrin (lower panel) by confocal microscopy. Vinculin localization reveals the classic punctate pattern at the cell periphery representing the costameres, with prominent immunolabelling of the fasciae adherentes of the intercalated discs (d). Weaker transverse (T)-tubule immunolabelling seen as interior striations is also apparent. Dystrophin and spectrin show a continuous distribution at the peripheral plasma membrane, and regularly spaced foci of higher-intensity spectrin labelling are present at the costameres (arrowheads, inset). Regular striations (T-tubules) penetrating deep within the cells are also seen for both proteins. Spectrin, but not dystrophin, is present at the intercalated discs.

Reprinted from Eur J Cell Biology, Vol 84: Issue 12, Stevenson et al, High-resolution en-face visualization of the cardiomyocyte plasma membrane reveals distinctive distributions of spectrin and dystrophin, pp. 961–971. Copyright (2005), with permission from Elsevier.

plasma membrane) and extracellular matrix by sets of integral plasma membrane proteins, notably the integrins and the components of the dystrophin–glycoprotein complex.

The coupling of the plasma membrane to the SR

The surface structure of the plasma membrane is shown in Fig. 16.1.2.6. Important features are the transverse (T)-tubule openings and the caveolae, which are cholesterol-enriched membrane invaginations in which signal-transducing and water-channel proteins are concentrated (Fig. 16.1.2.6a). T-tubules are the long, finger-like extensions of the plasma membrane that lie adjacent to the costameres and the Z-bands of the superficial myofibrils and which penetrate deeply into the cell (see Fig. 16.1.2.7, represented diagrammatically in Fig. 16.1.2.8a). These are stabilized by the coat of vinculin and dystrophin continuous with that at the lateral surface of the cell shown in Fig. 16.1.2.5. As described below, the T-tubules mediate the entry of extracellular Ca^{2+} (Ca^{2+}_o) into the cell through the L-type Ca^{2+} channels. Each myofibril is surrounded by a network of interconnecting membranous tubules and cisternae known as the sarcoplasmic reticulum (SR) (Fig. 16.1.2.7a, represented diagrammatically in Fig. 16.1.2.8a). At multiple sites within this network, the membranes broaden out to form flattened sacs, the junctional SR (JSR) cisternae, which press tightly against the peripheral plasma membrane and T-tubules (Figs. 16.1.2.7b and c). The plasma membrane (including T-tubule) domains facing the JSR membrane contain clusters of L-type Ca^{2+} channels (Fig. 16.1.2.6d), whilst the apposing domains of the JSR are packed with Ca^{2+}-release channels (Fig. 16.1.1.7c), also known as 'ryanodine receptors' because of their sensitivity to interference by the plant alkaloid ryanodine. The JSR contains high concentrations of the Ca^{2+}-binding protein calsequestrin and is the major reservoir of the cytoplasmic Ca^{2+} of the Ca^{2+} transient. The close spatial apposition of the two-channel clusters and calsequestrin is an important facet of the machinery controlling the Ca^{2+} transient required for myofibrillar contraction. Following contraction, the sarcoplasmic/endoplasmic reticulum Ca^{2+}ATPase 2 (SERCA2) pumps Ca^{2+} back into the SR lumen, causing myofibrillar relaxation. SERCA2 can be visualized as prominent particles by freeze-fracture electron microscopy (Fig. 16.1.2.7a) in the network of nonjunctional SR surrounding the myofibrils.

Connections between cardiac myocytes

The microanatomical machinery we have seen so far allows each myocyte to function as an autonomous contractile unit. To produce a heart beat, the contractile capabilities of the 3 billion myocytes that make up the human heart have to be mustered in a synchronous fashion. This requires both an orderly spread of the wave of electrical activation and the effective transmission of contractile force from one cell to the next, throughout the heart. These functions are fulfilled by the intercalated discs, formed from specialized regions of the plasma membrane where adjacent cells interact.

Intercalated discs are situated at the blunted ends of myocytes, both at ends of the main body of the cell and its side branches (Figs. 16.1.2.1 and 16.1.2.3). Three types of cell junction—the gap junction, the fascia adherens, and the desmosome—physically connect the adjacent membranes at the disc, acting in concert to integrate cardiac myocyte electromechanical function (Fig. 16.1.2.9).

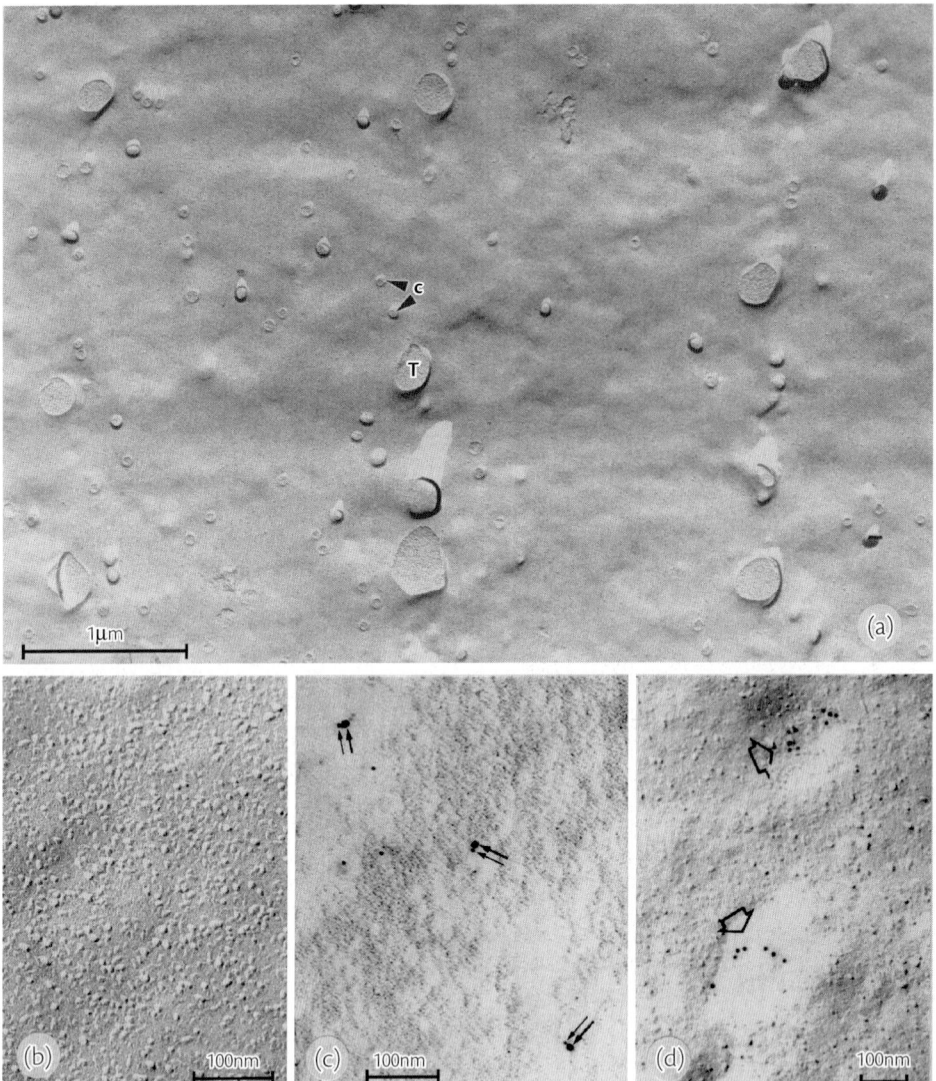

Fig. 16.1.2.6 Details of plasma membrane architecture. Freeze-fracture electron microscopy images reveal membrane structure at a macromolecular resolution in *en face* view. Panel a: Planar freeze-fracture view of part of the lateral plasma membrane of a ventricular myocyte. The portion of membrane viewed is equivalent to the length of two, side-by-side sarcomeres. T-tubule openings (T) are present in a regular array in this portion of the membrane. Caveolae (c) are seen as smaller, scattered vesicular structures. Panel b: Higher-magnification freeze-fracture views of the plasma membrane disclose a heterogeneous collection of intramembrane particles, 3–10 nm in diameter, embedded in a smooth background matrix (the hydrophobic lipid interior of the membrane). These particles represent the integral membrane proteins, including the channels, transporters, pumps, receptors, and matrix-linking proteins that endow the plasma membrane of the myocyte with its unique properties. Freeze-fracture cytochemistry enables identification of these proteins and analysis of their spatial organization (panels c and d). Panel c: By combining freeze-fracture with double immunogold-labelling at the plasma membrane interface, it is possible to demonstrate a direct molecular interaction between the C-terminal domains of dystrophin (a peripheral membrane protein of the membrane skeleton) and β-dystroglycan, an integral membrane protein which in turn binds to the extracellular matrix protein laminin via α-dystroglycan on the extracellular side of the membrane (arrows: large gold particles, β-dystroglycan; small gold particles, dystrophin). Panel d: L-type Ca^{2+} channels are demonstrated by freeze-fracture immunogold labelling to be clustered in the plasma membrane (arrows). Reprinted from: Severs NJ (2000). The cardiac muscle cell. BioEssays. 22:188–199 (Fig. 3). With permission from Wiley-Blackwell.

The fascia adherens and desmosome are forms of anchoring junction, responsible respectively for attachment of the myofibrils and the desmin cytoskeleton to sites of cadherin-mediated adhesion between the adjacent plasma membranes. Gap junctions contain clusters of connexons (described in detail in Fig. 16.1.2.9). These junctions are essentially clusters of intercellular channels which span two closely apposed plasma membranes and directly link adjacent cytoplasmic compartments of neighbouring cells. They form the sites of electrical coupling between individual cardiac myocytes that mediate the orderly spread of electrical excitation throughout the heart. They also allow direct cell-to-cell transmission of chemical signals (ions and small molecules of <1 kDa). The combination of connexin isoforms constituting a gap-junction channel is a major determinant of the functional properties of the gap-junction channel. Three connexins (connexins 43, 40, and 45) are differentially expressed in various combinations and relative quantities in different, functionally specialized subsets of cardiac myocytes. Ventricular myocytes express predominantly

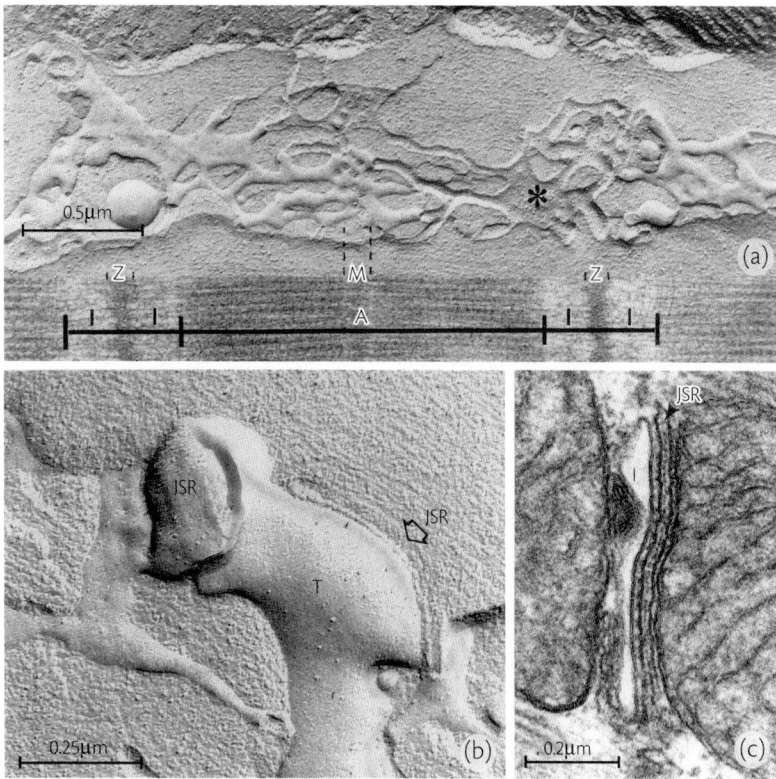

Fig. 16.1.2.7 SR, and its relationships to T-tubules and sarcomeres. Panel a: Freeze-fracture electron microscopic view of the SR network that surrounds each myofibril (the thin-section image below shows alignment of the SR with respect to the sarcomere bands). The numerous particles visible on the protoplasmic fracture face of the SR membrane (*) represent SERCA2. Panel b: Organization of the junctional sarcoplasmic reticulum (JSR) as revealed by freeze-fracture. The JSR is continuous with the free SR network. Two cisternae of JSR are illustrated, making intimate contact with a T-tubule (T). The cisterna to the right of the field has been cross-fractured, while that to the left has been fractured to reveal its membrane *en face*. Panel c: Thin-section electron-microscopic view of JSR. The JSR cisterna contains the Ca^{2+}-binding protein, calsequestrin, which is seen as conspicuous electron-dense material in the lumen. Projecting from the JSR membrane towards the T-tubule (T) is a series of electron-dense structures which represent the SR Ca^{2+}-release channels.
Reprinted from Severs NJ (2000). The cardiac muscle cell. BioEssays. 22:188–199, (Fig 4). With permission from Wiley-Blackwell.

connexin43 with small quantities of connexin45, atrial myocytes express connexins 43 and 40 with some connexin45, and myocytes of the impulse generation and conduction system express principally connexins 45 and 40.

Cardiac myocyte subtypes

The type of myocyte on which we have focused so far, the working ventricular cell, is the archetypal cardiac myocyte that is responsible for the powerful contractions that pump blood through the vascular system. Their counterparts in the atria, whose action facilitates filling of the ventricles, are modelled on a similar plan, although atrial cells are long and slender, and have few or no T-tubules but more abundant caveolae. By producing the peptide hormone atrial natriuretic factor (ANF), also known as atrial natriuretic peptide, they also function as secretory cells. Natriuretic peptides participate in the control of sodium and water balance and are hence important in the control of blood pressure.

A third, somewhat heterogeneous, group of myocytes makes up the impulse generation and conduction system. Although these cells show some resemblance to ventricular and atrial cells, their primary function is the generation of the impulse and its precisely timed distribution to the working cells of the chambers at the appropriate point in the cardiac cycle. This is reflected in quite distinctive morphological features. The cardiac impulse is generated in the sinoatrial node (the 'pacemaker') from where it crosses and activates the atria, before converging on the atrioventricular node for distribution to the ventricles via the specialized conduction system (His bundle, main bundle branches to each ventricle, and Purkinje fibre network).

Myocytes of the sinoatrial and atrioventricular nodes are typically small ($c.5\,\mu m$ diameter), containing just a few rudimentary, haphazardly distributed myofibrils, and small, sparse, dispersed gap junctions composed of connexin45. These features contribute to poor coupling, which in the atrioventricular node is essential to slowing of conduction to ensure sequential contraction of atria and ventricles. It should be emphasized, however, that even within the nodes, the cell population is not of uniform morphology and exhibits differences in protein expression. For example, cells of the compact atrioventricular node—and those of the surrounding areas (the transitional cells and posterior nodal extension)—are quite distinctive, and detailed three-dimensional models of the node are required to relate cell morphology to function. Similarly, myocytes of the bundle branches and Purkinje system show a range of morphologies according to their location, progressively increasing in size, myofibril content, and showing more developed intercalated discs distally, towards the working ventricular myocardium.

(a)

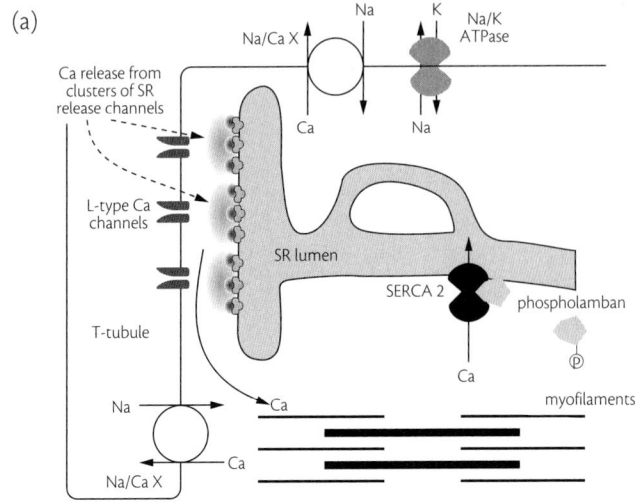

(b)

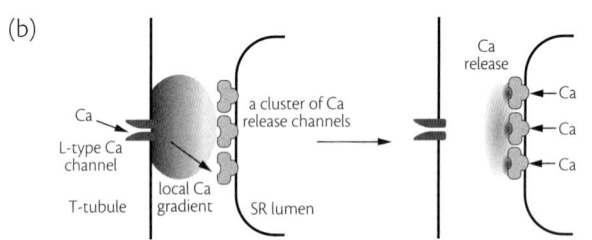

Fig. 16.1.2.8 EC coupling in the heart. Panel a. L-type Ca^{2+} channels allow Ca^{2+} influx across the plasma membrane and this creates I_{Ca}. This influx increases the local Ca^{2+} concentration around a cluster of SR Ca^{2+}-release channels in sufficient amounts to open them (Ca^{2+}-induced Ca^{2+}-release). Panel b. The opening of clusters of SR Ca^{2+}-release channels allows SR Ca^{2+} reservoir to be discharged into the cytoplasm. The fluxes of Ca^{2+} combine to initiate contraction. The contraction process is terminated (1) by SERCA2 (regulated by phospholamban and dependent on phospholamban phosphorylation state), which removes Ca^{2+} from the cytoplasm and pumps it into the SR, and (2) by the plasma membrane Na/CaX which expels Ca^{2+} from the cell. In steady-state conditions, the amount of Ca^{2+} leaving the cell (via the Na/CaX) balances the amount entering (via the L-type Ca^{2+} channel).

Apart from high glycogen content, one notable feature that marks out distal Purkinje fibre myocytes from working ventricular cells is the presence of high levels of connexin40—a connexin that gives high conductance channels and may contribute to rapid distribution of the impulse to all parts of the working ventricular myocardium.

The cardiac action potential

The membrane potential

Ion channels

The incremental excitation of the heart, from its initiation in the sinoatrial node through its passage across the atrium and along the atrioventricular node, His bundle, and Purkinje fibres into the ventricular myocardium provides a means of coordinating the contractile activities of the four chambers and is the basis for the ECG (see Chapter 16.3.1). Electrical excitation of each myocyte involves the movement of ions through ion channels. These are 'excitable' proteins embedded in the plasma (or other) membranes that contain pores capable of opening or closing in response to a stimulus, which could be a change in membrane potential, a

neurotransmitter or hormone, an intracellular second messenger or ion, or mechanical stretch of the membrane. When a channel opens, it becomes selectively permeable to a restricted series of ions, selectivity being determined by the interaction of the various ions with the channel pore. There are a large number of different types of channel, often named after the most important permeant ion they pass, e.g. Na^+, Ca^{2+}, and K^+ channels. The groups of channels are functionally distinct and can be further divided into subgroups on the basis of primary (i.e. amino acid) sequence and higher-order structure, and their electrical behaviour. Ions move down their electrochemical gradients through each channel at high rates (>10^6 ions/s), which distinguishes them from other ion-transport proteins (e.g. the Na^+,K^+-ATPase or pump, and the Na^+,Ca^{2+} exchanger (Na/CaX), see below) which move ions across plasma membranes several orders of magnitude more slowly.

The origin of the membrane potential

When a ventricular myocyte is at rest (diastole), there is a potential difference of about −80 mV across the plasma membrane, the inside of the cell being negative with respect to the outside. This is caused by K^+ channels being open, making the plasma membrane more permeable to K^+ than any other ion. The extracellular concentration of K^+ (K^+_o) is about 4 mmol/litre, and the intracellular (cytoplasmic) concentration (K^+_i) is about 140 mmol/litre, so K^+ tends to leave the cell by diffusing down its concentration gradient, resulting in the interior becoming negatively charged. Although there is some movement of Cl^- across the plasma membrane, there is not sufficient net movement to balance the K^+ loss. An equilibrium is thus established where the electronegative force retaining K^+ inside the cell balances its tendency to diffuse out of the cell down its concentration gradient. This is termed the equilibrium potential (E) and can be calculated from the Nernst equation (see Table 16.1.2.1 for E values of relevant ions). At this potential, there will be no net flux of K^+ ions through K^+ channels and, if the membrane is only permeable to K^+, then the membrane potential will be equal to E_K.

The membrane potential at any moment is dependent upon the equilibrium potentials for all permeant species and their relative permeabilities. The actual transmembrane potential difference at rest and the calculated E_K are rarely the same owing to a small leakage, mainly of Na^+ into the cell down its concentration gradient (Na^+_o = 140 mmol/litre, Na^+_i = 7–10 mmol/litre). To counteract this leak and to maintain the concentration gradients of Na^+ and K^+ upon which the generation of the membrane potential depends, the plasma membrane Na^+,K^+-ATPase uses free energy derived from the hydrolysis of ATP to pump these ions against their concentration gradients. This process is electrogenic (three Na^+ are extruded for two K^+ entering) and generates 3 to 10 mV of the membrane potential.

The action potential

The action potential is divided into five phases (Fig. 16.1.2.10). The currents that flow are described in Table 16.1.2.2 and Fig. 16.1.2.10. Depolarization from the resting potential is said to be mediated by inward current flow.

Phase 0 of the action potential

When a myocyte is electrically excited, Na^+ channels open and allow Na^+ ions to enter the cell. The channels open by sensing the

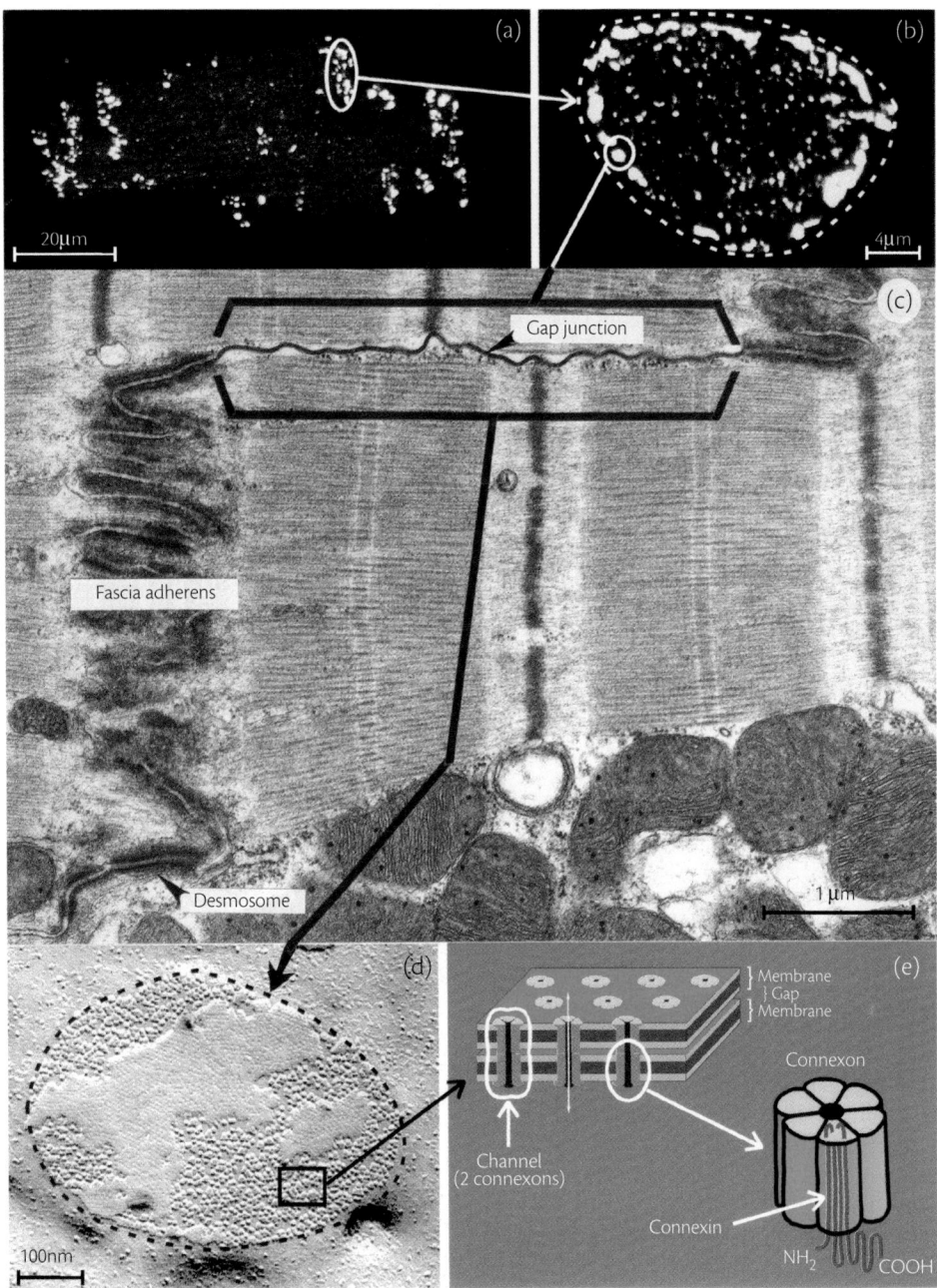

Fig. 16.1.2.9 The intercalated disc and cardiac gap junction organization and structure. Panel a Clusters of gap junctions at the intercalated discs revealed in a single ventricular cardiac myocyte by immunoconfocal microscopy with connexin43 labelling. Panel b One disc-cluster of gap junctions viewed *en face* (reconstruction from a stack of serial optical sections). One of these immunolabelled spots corresponds to a single gap junction, as seen by electron microscopy in panels c and d. Panel c: Thin-section electron micrograph illustrating the three types of cell junction of the intercalated disc. Gap junctions are recognized where the adjacent plasma membrane profiles run in close contact, separated by a gap of 2 nm. The fascia adherens and the desmosome are characterized by a much wider intermembrane space (*c.*25 nm) and by prominent electron-dense membrane-associated proteins. The mature intercalated disc appears as a set of irregular steps, with the fasciae adherentes occupying interdigitating transverse regions, and the gap-junctional membrane and most of the desmosomes in the intervening 'horizontal' membrane zones. Panel d: Viewing the membrane *en face* by freeze-fracture reveals the gap junction as a cluster of particles (connexons). Panel e: The gap junction channel is comprised of a pair of connexons (hemichannels), one contributed by each of the adjacent plasma membranes. The connexon spans the full depth of the membrane and is coaxially aligned across the narrow extracellular gap with its partner in the adjacent membrane. Each connexon is itself formed from six connexin molecules. The connexins are a family of conserved proteins encoded by about 20 genes in humans. The specific connexin type or types within the connexon is a major determinant of the functional properties of the gap junction channel.
Reprinted from Severs NJ (2000). The cardiac muscle cell. BioEssays. 22:188–199, (Fig 5). With permission from Wiley-Blackwell.

potential difference across the cell membrane (Fig. 16.1.2.10). Excitation depolarizes the cell membrane slightly and this increases the probability of Na$^+$ channels opening. A cardiac myocyte contains many thousands of Na$^+$ channels, hence the current (I) generated by the movement of Na$^+$ ions into the cell (I_{Na}) is the

sum of the small currents that flow though each individual channel. Positive charge is taken into the cell, the membrane potential increases towards the equilibrium potential for Na$^+$ (E_{Na} = +70 mV, Table 16.1.2.1), and the cell depolarizes (Fig. 16.1.2.10). The Na$^+$ current causes the rapid upstroke (phase 0) of the action

Table 16.1.2.1 Intracellular and extracellular concentrations of pertinent ions in the quiescent myocyte, and their calculated equilibrium potentials (*E*). *E* is calculated from the Nernst equation, $E = (RT/zF) \ln(a_o/a_i)$, where *E* is in volts, *T* is the absolute temperature, *R* is the gas constant, *F* is the Faraday constant, *z* is the valency, and a_o and a_i are the extracellular and intracellular activities of the ion in question

Ion	Intracellular concentration (mmol/litre)	Plasma concentration (mmol/litre)	Calculated E (mV)
Na^+	10	140	+70
K^+	140	4.5	−91
Ca^{2+}	0.0001	2.3	+131
Cl^-	20	110	+45

potential and, like a similar current in nerve tissue, is inhibited by procaine, quinidine, and tetrodotoxin (a toxin found particularly in some species of *fugu*, the Japanese puffer fish). The propagation velocity of the action potential across the whole heart is related to the rate of change of the rapid upstroke. Some antiarrhythmic therapies are directed towards inhibiting a proportion of Na^+ channels to decrease the upstroke velocity and, therefore, to slow conduction. Following opening (or activation), the channels close very rapidly, even though the myocyte remains depolarized. This process is termed 'inactivation'. Channels that have inactivated cannot open again until the cell repolarizes. This is the mechanism responsible for the existence of the refractory period during which a further stimulus cannot evoke another action potential (Fig. 16.1.2.10).

The inactivation of each channel decreases the total number of Na^+ channels that are conducting such that I_{Na} almost entirely inactivates within the first 5 ms of the action potential (the overall action potential in humans at rest lasts *c.*350 ms). Some Na^+ channels do not inactivate quite so rapidly and this allows a small inward current to persist during the plateau phase of the action potential (phase 2, see below). Some mutations in Na^+ channels interfere with the inactivation process and the inward current persists, thus prolonging the action potential and increasing the QT interval on the ECG. The clinical manifestation of this mutation is a form of long-QT syndrome (LQT3). Other mutations reduce the number of functional Na^+ channels or accelerate their inactivation and these lead to the Brugada syndrome phenotype. See Chapter 16.4 for further discussion.

Phase 1 of the action potential

The characteristic notch observed in phase 1 of the action potential in ventricular myocytes (Fig. 16.1.2.10) (the notch is also particularly apparent in the Purkinje cell action potential; see Fig. 16.1.2.11) is caused by a transient outward current (I_{TO}), carried mainly by K^+ ions flowing out of the cell, that activates rapidly and partially repolarizes the membrane. The current inactivates within 30–40 ms (hence the term 'transient'), but plays a large role in governing action potential duration. For example, in the failing heart, channels associated with I_{TO} are poorly expressed and this is a major cause of the prolonged action potential in cells isolated from such hearts. A component of I_{TO} appears to be dependent upon intracellular Ca^{2+} concentration (raised Ca^{2+}_o increases I_{TO}).

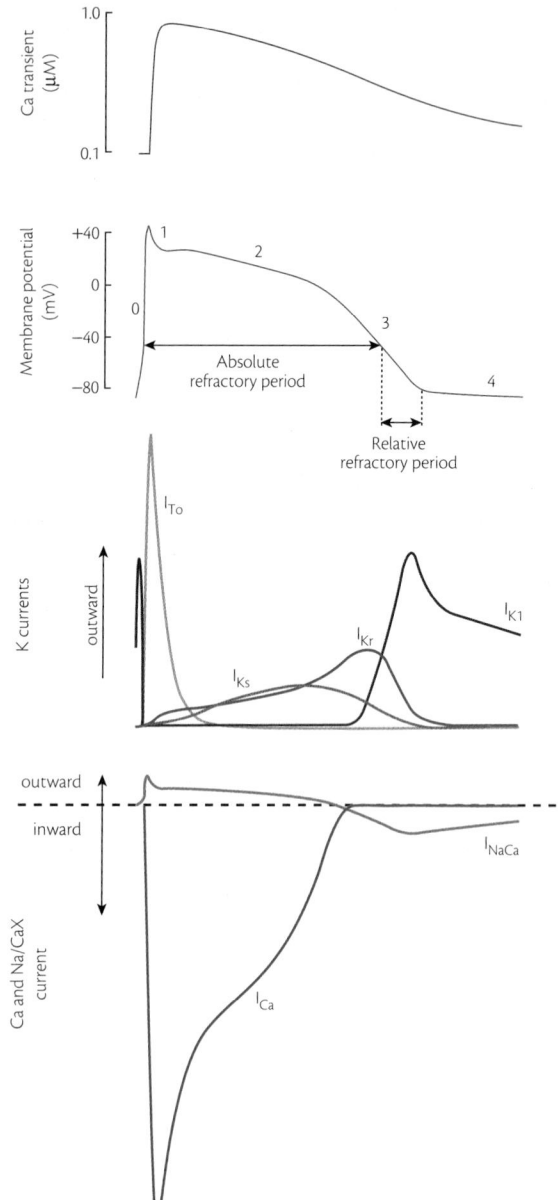

Fig. 16.1.2.10 Ca^{2+} transient, membrane potential, K^+ currents and Ca^{2+}-related currents flowing during a ventricular myocyte action potential. The inward Na^+ current that produces the rapid upstroke of the action potential is not shown Top panel: Changes in cytoplasmic Ca^{2+} concentration during the action potential (Ca^{2+} transient). Upper middle panel: The phases of the ventricular myocyte action potential. For a period between phase 0 and about halfway through phase 3, cardiac muscle cannot be excited with another stimulus—no matter how strong—and the muscle is in its absolute refractory period (thus tetanic contraction of the type seen in skeletal muscle cannot occur). From about halfway through phase 3 until just the end of phase 3, cardiac muscle is in its relative refractory period when it is possible for a stronger stimulus than normal to initiate an action potential. The states of refractoriness are related to the ability of ion channels to recover from a stimulus. This recovery is both voltage- and time-dependent. Lower middle panel: Time courses and relative sizes and directions of K^+ currents during one action potential. All K^+ currents (I_{TO}, I_{Ks}, I_{Kr} and I_{K1}) repolarize the myocyte because of outward K^+ movement. Bottom panel: Time courses and relative sizes and directions of Ca^{2+}-related currents during one action potential. Because of the inward movement of Ca^{2+}, Ca^{2+} current (I_{Ca}) is depolarizing. The Na/CaX produces both outward and inward current ($I_{Na,Ca}$) depending the phase of the action potential. Note that the inward Na^+ current is roughly 8 to 10 times the size of the Ca^{2+} current and has largely inactivated by the time the peak of the Ca^{2+} current is reached.

Table 16.1.2.2 Plasma membrane currents in the cardiac myocyte

Current	Name	Activated by	Blocked by	Gene	Protein	Function
Inward currents						
I_{Na}	(Fast) Na^+ current	Depolarization	Tetrodotoxin, local anaesthetics	SCN5A	Nav1.5	Rapid upstroke of action potential
$I_{Ca,L}$	L-type Ca^{2+} current	Depolarization	Verapamil, Cd^{2+}, dihydropyridines	CACNA1C	Cav1.2	Ca^{2+} influx that activates CICR, provides some Ca^{2+} for contraction
$I_{Ca,T}$	T-type Ca^{2+} current	Activates on depolarization but at more negative potentials than L-type current	Ni^{2+}, mibefradil	CACNA1G CACNA1H	Cav3.1 Cav3.2	Channel density high in pacemaker and conducting tissue so may contribute to pacemaker activity. Role in ventricular cells unclear.
I_f	Hyperpolarization-activated, cyclic nucleotide-gated cation channel	Hyperpolarization, noradrenaline, cyclic AMP	Cs^+, ZD7288, ivabradine, zatebradine, cilobradine	HCN2 HCN4		Exists in sinoatrial node and Purkinje fibres bringing membrane potential slowly to threshold
Inward and outward current						
$I_{Na/Ca}$	Na/CaX current	Ca^{2+}_i	Ni^{2+}, KB-R7943	NCX1		Expels Ca^{2+} from the cell, maintains inward current flow near end of action potential, at positive potentials may reverse and mediate Ca^{2+} influx
Outward currents						
I_{TO}	Transient outward current	Depolarization	4-Aminopyridine	KCNA4 KCND2 KCND3	Kv1.4 Kv4.2 Kv4.3	Early repolarization (notch)
I_{Cl}	Chloride current	Cyclic AMP		CFTR		Early repolarization
$I_{Cl,Ca}$	Ca^{2+}-activated chloride current	Ca^{2+}		CLCA1		Early repolarization
I_{Kur}	Ultra-rapid delayed rectifier	Depolarization	Tetraethylammonium, Cs^+, Ba^{2+}, 4-aminopyridine, flecainide, nifedipine, diltiazem, bupivacaine, propafenone, quinidine	KCNA5	Kv1.5	Repolarization of cell
I_{Kr}	Rapid delayed rectifier	Depolarization	Tetraethylammonium, Cs^+, Ba^{2+}, E-4031, dofetilide, D-sotolol, cisapride, BRL32872	KCNH2	herg, Kv11.1	Repolarization of cell
I_{Ks}	Slow delayed rectifier	Depolarization	Chromanol 293B	KCNQ1	KvLQT1	Repolarization of cell
I_{K1}	Inward (anomalous) rectifier	Depolarization from E_K Conductance of channel increases then decreases to zero at 0 mV	Cs^+, Rb^+, Ba^{2+}, intracellular Mg^{2+}, spermidine, spermine	KCNJ2 KCNJ12	Kir2.1 Kir2.2	Prolongs action potential duration, background K^+ conductance,
I_p	Na^+/K^+ pump current	Na^+_i, K^+_o	Cardiac glycosides			Maintains low $[Na^+]_i$
$I_{K,ACh}$	Acetylcholine-activated K^+ current (inward rectifier)	ACh	Ba^{2+}	KCNJ3 KCNJ5	Kir3.1 Kir3.4	Muscarinic receptor-coupled. Activates additional K^+ channels so slowing pacemaker potential

This is the probable mechanism underlying the shortening of action potential duration during tachycardia. When cells are paced rapidly, the resting (diastolic) intracellular Ca^{2+} concentration will increase and this augments I_{TO} so more outward current flows, repolarizing the cell more quickly.

Phase 2 of the action potential

A number of different currents flow during phase 2 (the action potential plateau), the most important—from the point of view of the generation of contraction—being I_{Ca} (Fig. 16.1.2.10). L-type Ca^{2+} channels, which take longer to activate and inactivate than Na^+ channels, open within 3–5 ms of the start of the upstroke and allow Ca^{2+} to flow into the cell. L-type Ca^{2+} channels activate at more positive voltages than Na^+ channels, hence the cardiac cell must be depolarized to potentials around −35 mV before the L-type Ca^{2+} channels open, whereas Na^+ channels begin to open at potentials more positive than −65mV. The inward flow of Ca^{2+} maintains depolarization (Fig. 16.1.2.10, Tables 16.1.2.1 and 16.1.2.2)

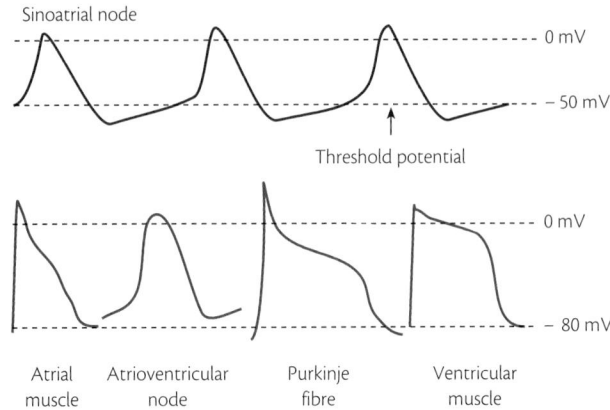

Threshold potential

Fig. 16.1.2.11 Regional configurations of the action potential. In the sinoatrial (SA) and atrioventricular (AV) nodes, the cells spontaneously depolarize during diastole (phase 4 depolarization). When the membrane potential reaches a threshold value, the complete action potential is initiated. Because the SA nodal cells have the fastest phase 4 depolarization, they act as the cardiac pacemaker.

and can be inhibited by 'Ca^{2+} antagonists' such as verapamil and the dihydropyridines. The influx of Ca^{2+} initiates Ca^{2+}-induced Ca^{2+}-release (CICR) from the SR through the SR Ca^{2+}-release channels, and the increase in cytoplasmic Ca^{2+} concentration causes the myocyte to contract (see below).

The plateau phase (phase 2) of the action potential (Fig. 16.1.2.10) is prolonged in ventricular myocytes because of the properties of several types of K$^+$ channel that give rise to several different K$^+$ currents. The main repolarizing current, I_K, is composed of two pharmacologically and kinetically distinct currents, one activating more rapidly (I_{Kr}) than the other (I_{Ks}) (see Table 16.1.2.2). Both channels open at positive membrane potentials and close (deactivate) at negative potentials, akin to K$^+$ channels in nerve. However, the activation kinetics of these channels are much slower than in nerve so that the repolarization process takes longer. This is one of the reasons that a cardiac myocyte action potential is so much longer than a nerve action potential. The plateau of the action potential is, therefore, the result of a delicate balance of inward (Ca^{2+}) and outward (K$^+$) current flow.

Mutations in the genes encoding the K$^+$ channels through which I_{Kr} and I_{Ks} flow are associated with the most common forms of inherited long-QT syndrome (LQT1 and LQT2). The mutations reduce the amount of repolarizing current, leading to a prolongation of action potential duration. Drug-induced long-QT syndrome is becoming a more widely recognized problem: drugs that can cause this condition (e.g. erythromycin, terfenadine, and ketoconazole) inhibit I_{Kr}, which seems more sensitive to drugs in comparison to other K$^+$ currents.

Phase 3 of the action potential

The final phase of repolarization begins with the termination of I_{Ca} and progressively increasing K$^+$ current (I_{Kr} and I_{Ks}) (Fig. 16.1.2.10). As repolarization proceeds, the Na/CaX responds to the increase in cytoplasmic Ca^{2+} concentration and produces an inward current ($I_{Na,Ca}$) through the exchange of three Na$^+$ entering the cell for one Ca^{2+} expelled. By producing an inward current, the Na/CaX helps to prolong the plateau and slows repolarization.

In ventricular myocytes, complete repolarization and a return to a negative resting membrane potential is eventually achieved by I_{K1}, which is larger than other K$^+$ currents (Fig. 16.1.2.10). The channel through which this current flows possesses peculiar characteristics. Normally, because of the relative concentrations of K$^+$ inside and outside the cell, there is outward movement of K$^+$ ions that becomes larger the more positive the displacement from E_K. However, the current I_{K1} flows through a channel that first increases its conductance but then decreases it as the cell depolarizes away from E_K (anomalous rectification). Thus, there is outward flow of repolarizing current only over a narrow voltage range (around –30 to –80 mV), which is another reason for the prolonged cardiac action potential because a large, rapid, outward K$^+$ current does not flow despite the membrane potential approaching 0 mV during the plateau phase.

I_{K1} underlies the main flow of K$^+$ that gives rise to the membrane potential. The channels through which I_{K1} flows are numerous in ventricular cells, fewer in atrial cells, and absent in pacemaker cells. The current is therefore large in ventricular cells and this is the reason that the resting membrane potential of ventricular myocytes lies near E_K, whereas atrial cells have a more positive resting membrane potential and SA nodal cells do not have a stable resting potential. The clinical consequences of the presence of I_{K1} are profound and result from this channel being acutely sensitive to the extracellular concentration of K$^+$. For example, shortly after myocardial infarction, there is a loss of K$^+$ from cells and local K^+_o concentrations increase. Since extracellular K^+_o increases I_{K1}, the outward movement of K$^+$ is increased. Thus, more outward current flows, larger depolarizing currents are required to induce excitation, and conduction problems occur.

Phase 4 of the action potential

This phase relates to the membrane potential during the electrically silent period between excitatory events in ventricular myocytes (Fig. 16.1.2.10). For the reasons outlined above, phase 4 is stable in these cells.

Regional variations in action potential

The configuration of the cardiac action potential differs regionally (Fig. 16.1.2.11) because ion-channel expression varies between cells. In the sinoatrial node, I_{Na} is very small and the main current responsible for the depolarizing upstroke is I_{Ca}, carried mainly by L-type Ca^{2+} channels. The only repolarizing current is I_K. I_{K1} is absent and, as mentioned above, this partially explains why sinoatrial node cells have a more depolarized 'diastolic' potential than ventricular myocytes. Sinoatrial node cells depolarize spontaneously during phase 4 (Fig. 16.1.2.11), owing to the absence of I_{K1}, the presence of a current activated on hyperpolarization called the 'funny' current (I_f) which is carried mainly by Na$^+$ through hyperpolarization-activated cyclic nucleotide-gated (HCN) channels, and current ($I_{Ca,T}$) resulting from an influx of Ca^{2+} through T-type Ca^{2+} channels (which are more abundant in these cells than in ventricular myocytes). Phase 4 is often termed the 'pre- or pacemaker potential' in nodal cells and is caused by the gradual decrease in I_K and increase in I_f and $I_{Ca,T}$ (Fig. 16.1.2.11). Once the cell has depolarized to a voltage at which L-type Ca^{2+} channels open (the threshold), a more rapid depolarization (caused by $I_{Ca,L}$) takes place, forming the upstroke of the sinoatrial node action potential. When the cholinergic drive from autonomic neurons to the nodal cells is increased, the slope of the pacemaker potential is decreased

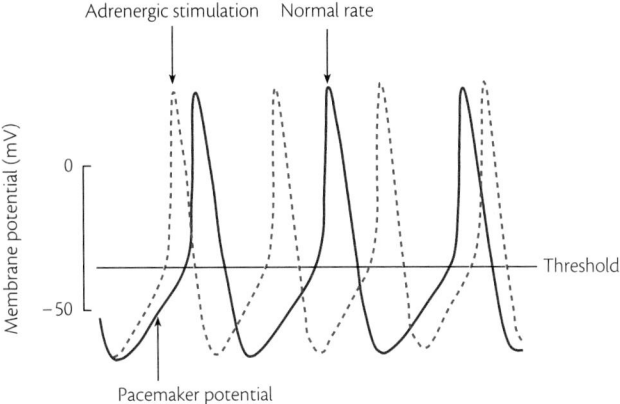

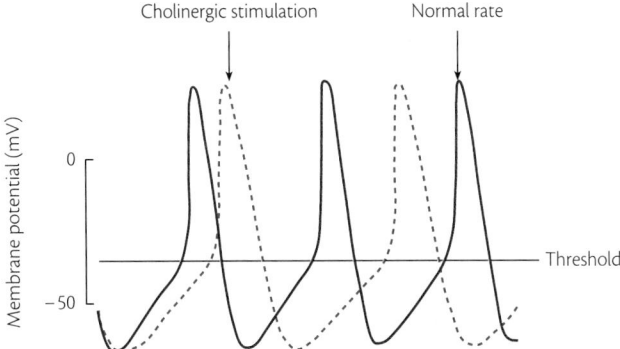

Fig. 16.1.2.12 Change in heart rate produced by altering the phase 4 slope of the pacemaker potential in the sinoatrial (SA) node. β-Adrenergic stimulation increases, and cholinergic stimulation decreases, the slope of the pacemaker potential, affecting the time taken to reach threshold.

and heart rate slows (Fig. 16.1.2.12). Acetylcholine (ACh) opens another group of K^+ channels and activates $I_{K,ACh}$, which helps drive the membrane potential towards E_K and slows the rate of depolarization. I_f and I_{Ca} are also reduced and the overall effect is a reduction in the rate of production of action potentials. As described below, β-adrenergic stimulation increases the slope of the pacemaker potential and heart rate through an effect on I_f.

Atrial and ventricular myocytes do not have pacemaker potentials and spontaneously discharge only when injured or when there is abnormal intracellular Ca^{2+} balance. The longest action potential is in Purkinje fibres (Fig. 16.1.2.11) and this acts as a 'gate' preventing retrograde activation by depolarization of adjacent ventricular myocytes. The action potential is longer in the endocardium than in the epicardium and longer still in the mid-myocardial layer of cells. This also is the result of differential expression of ion channels. For example, there is more I_{TO} in epicardium than in endocardium, so repolarization is more rapid in the former. The expression of channels producing I_{Ks} in mid-myocardium is about half that in epi- and endocardium and so the action potential is more prolonged in this region.

The mechanism of myocyte contraction

Excitation–contraction coupling

As outlined so far, the electrical events throughout the heart initiate and regulate contraction (Fig. 16.1.2.10). The coupling of the electrical excitation of the heart to the production of contraction (called excitation–contraction coupling or EC coupling) by Ca^{2+} ions involves the interaction of a number of proteins involved in Ca^{2+} homeostasis (Fig. 16.1.2.8). The T-tubules allow the wave of depolarization of the action potential to reach deeply into the cell. As described earlier, the SR is an intracellular membranous lace-like structure surrounding the myofibrils, with JSR 'swellings' where the membrane of the SR comes close to the T-tubules (Figs. 16.1.2.7 and 16.1.2.8). During diastole, when cytoplasmic Ca^{2+} concentrations are low (c.0.1 µmol/litre), Ca^{2+} is sequestered by the Ca^{2+}-buffering protein calsequestrin within the JSR. Depolarization then opens the L-type Ca^{2+} channels in the T-tubule and plasma membrane allowing influx of Ca^{2+} (Figs. 16.1.2.8a and b, and 16.1.2.10) and producing I_{Ca} (Fig. 16.1.2.10). This influx of Ca^{2+} increases the local Ca^{2+} concentration around clusters of SR Ca^{2+}-release channels sufficiently to open them (i.e. CICR), the number of channels activated in this way being mainly, though not exclusively, determined by the size of the Ca^{2+} current. Ca^{2+} in the SR Ca^{2+} reservoir is thus discharged into the cytoplasm. Two features of CICR are important. First, it provides an amplification step as the small 'trigger' Ca^{2+} influx through the L-type Ca^{2+} channels evokes a much larger release of Ca^{2+} from the SR. Secondly, the release of Ca^{2+} from the SR is under precise control as it is closely matched to the amount of Ca^{2+} influx. The fluxes of Ca^{2+} combine to raise the cytoplasmic concentration of Ca^{2+} to between 1 and 3 µmol/litre (Fig. 16.1.2.10). The release of Ca^{2+} ceases because the L-type Ca channels inactivate so the trigger influx declines and, via a complex series of events, this leads to the closing of SR Ca^{2+} release channels.

The mechanism of myofibrillar contraction

The release of Ca^{2+} from the SR activates the contractile apparatus of the sarcomere (Figs. 16.1.2.4 and 16.1.2.13). The temporal relationship between the action potential, the Ca^{2+} transient, and the subsequent development of tension is shown in Fig. 16.1.2.14. Sarcomere shortening is caused by the interaction of motor protein myosin in the thick filaments with actin in the thin filaments (Fig. 16.1.2.13). Myosin heads bind and hydrolyse ATP, retaining bound ADP and phosphate and trapping the free energy of hydrolysis within the myosin molecule. The myosin–ADP–phosphate complex then binds to actin, leading to the release of the stored energy by a conformational change that moves the actin filament by about 10 nm relative to the thick filament. This is known as the cross-bridge cycle (Fig.16.1.2.13).

The summation of many cross-bridge cycles results in the sliding of the thin filament past the thick filaments and sarcomere shortening. If the muscle is under load, the cross-bridge cycle generates force and work is done (the maximum efficiency is more than 60% in intact muscle). The mechanical characteristics of contracting muscle can be described in terms of the relationship between shortening speed and force, and between sarcomere length and force (Fig. 16.1.2.15a). Maximum force is produced under isometric conditions, while maximum shortening speed is observed in unloaded muscle. In the (left ventricular) cardiac cycle, the myocardium first contracts isometrically, until pressure inside the heart exceeds the pressure in the aorta (termed afterload), and then contracts isotonically as the aortic valve opens. Power output is the product of force and velocity and is optimal at about 30% of maximum shortening speed (Fig. 16.1.2.15a).

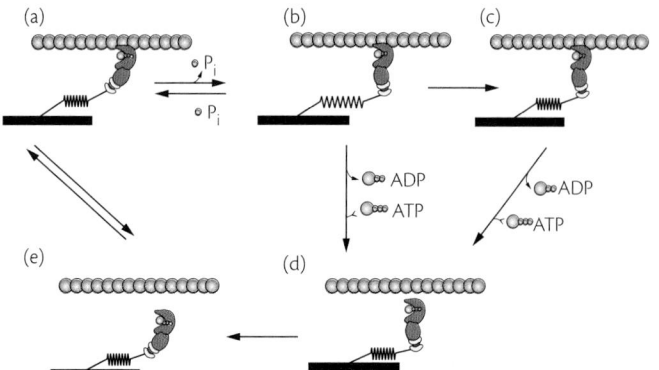

Fig. 16.1.2.13 The cross-bridge cycle. Exchange of ATP with ADP on either a load-bearing (b) or a resting-length myosin head (c) results in a conformational change in the myosin head, causing a rapid, almost irreversible dissociation of the myosin head from actin ((b) to (d) and (c) to (d), respectively). Following detachment from actin, the ATP is hydrolysed to ADP and Pi, both of which remain very tightly bound to the myosin head (e). The hydrolysis is relatively rapid (taking about 10 ms). The small value of K_{eq} (c.10) suggests that the reaction is reversible. Because the free energy of ATP hydrolysis is much greater than that for this reaction, this indicates that the free energy of ATP hydrolysis is not released but remains within the structure of the myosin–ADP–phosphate complex. Hydrolysis is accompanied by a major conformational change which represents the reversal or a repriming of the power stroke. If an actin site is within reach of the myosin head, it will bind rapidly and reversibly to the actin site (a). When the myosin head binds actin, the interaction can promote a major change in conformation (the power stroke) which is accompanied by the dissociation of Pi ((a) to (b)). This step approximates to isometric contraction (no relative movement of actin and myosin) whereas the (a) to (c) steps approximate to an isotonic contraction (relative movement, with a release of the myosin 'spring'). This power stroke consists of a reorientation of part of the myosin head that results in the displacement of the tip by up to 10 nm. In isometric contraction, ADP is released slowly from the strained cross-bridges ((b)–(d)). If the muscle can shorten ((b)–(c)), ADP release is accelerated ((c)–(d)).
Reproduced with permission from S. Weiss and M.A Geeves.

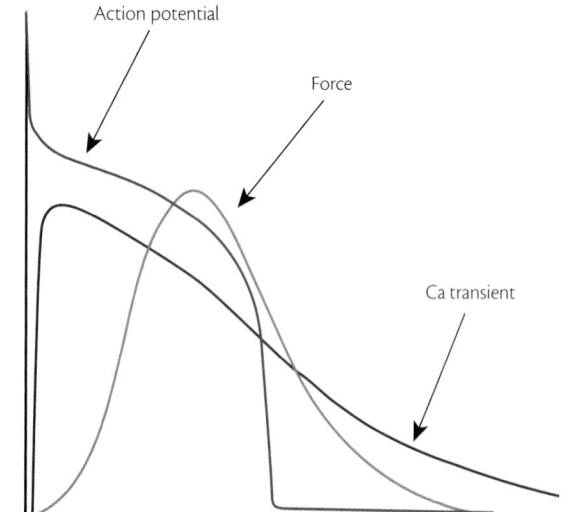

Fig. 16.1.2.14 The relationship between the action potential, the Ca^{2+}-transient and the generation of force. The peak of force production is not achieved until near the end of the plateau phase of the action potential and lags behind the peak of the Ca^{2+}-transient. This reflects the time required for Ca^{2+}-induced Ca^{2+}-release and cross-bridge cycling.

The isometric force produced by a muscle depends on the sarcomere length, being optimal at 2.00–2.25 μm where the overlap of thick and thin filaments is such that all the myosin cross-bridges can interact with actin (Fig. 16.1.2.15b). In the heart, the sarcomere length is generally less than optimal, with 'preload' stretching the sarcomere to 2.1 μm at the end of diastole and the sarcomere shortening to 1.6 μm during systole. In this length range, stretching the cardiac muscle when it is relaxed leads to increased force in the subsequent contraction. This characteristic is responsible in part for Starling's law of the heart. In dilated cardiomyopathy, sarcomeres may be stretched beyond 2.3 μm, leading to reduced force that is reduced still further by stretching.

Control of contraction by Ca^{2+}

As explained, muscle contraction is initiated by an increase in cytoplasmic Ca^{2+}, which binds to the troponin complex of the thin filament. Troponin is made up of three subunits (Fig. 16.1.2.16). Troponin C is the Ca^{2+}-binding protein. In cardiac myocytes, the thin filament is activated when a single Ca^{2+} ion binds to the N-terminal domain of troponin C. The second component is troponin I, which is the inhibitory subunit. In relaxed muscle, the Ca^{2+} concentration is low and the troponin I C-terminal region binds to a site on actin, which blocks the binding of myosin cross-bridges, thus preventing cross-bridge cycling. In the presence of activating Ca^{2+} concentrations, Ca^{2+} binds to troponin C, and the C-terminus of troponin I becomes bound to the N-terminus of troponin C and is not able to interact with actin, thus allowing the actin–myosin interaction. The third component, troponin T, binds to troponin C and troponin I and also to tropomyosin, independently of the Ca^{2+} concentration, thereby anchoring the regulatory complex on the thin filament. The inhibitory effect of troponin I binding to actin is propagated along the actin filament by a concerted cooperative conformational change that involves all the proteins of the thin filament. This results in the movement of the tropomyosin strand to a position that prevents cross-bridge binding to all actins, thus switching off contraction (Fig. 16.1.2.16).

The Ca^{2+}-sensitivity of cardiac myocytes is increased by stretch. In a chemically skinned muscle preparation, EC_{50} for Ca^{2+} decreases from 4.9 μmol/litre at a sarcomere length of 1.9 μm to 3.0 μmol/litre at a length of 2.4 μm. This phenomenon promotes relaxation at the start of diastole (short sarcomere lengths) and activates contraction at start of systole (long sarcomere lengths). Moreover, this 'stretch activation' is delayed so that the enhanced contractility is synchronized with systole, thus contributing to the Starling effect. Recent research using mice in which the MyBP-C gene is homozygously deleted indicates that the timing of stretch activation is determined by MyBP-C, and it is also modulated by cAMP-dependent protein kinase (PKA)-mediated phosphorylation of MyBP-C.

Termination of contraction

Sarcoplasmic/endoplasmic reticulum ATPase type 2 (SERCA 2)

Contraction is terminated predominantly by reuptake of Ca^{2+} into the SR by activation of SERCA2, an ATP-requiring Ca^{2+} pump present in the network of non-junctional SR surrounding the myofibrils (Figs. 16.1.2.7 and 16.1.2.8a). The activity of SERCA2 is regulated by the extent of phosphorylation of the SERCA2-associated protein phospholamban. Hypophosphorylated phospholamban

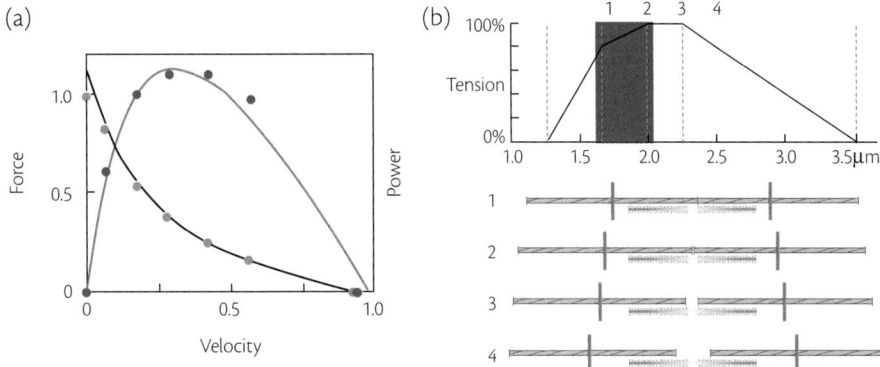

Fig. 16.1.2.15 Force–velocity–power relationship in cardiac muscle. The force–velocity relationship is described by the Hill equation $(P + a)(V + b) = (P_o + a)b$, where P is force during shortening at velocity V, P_o is the isometric force and a and b are constants (red symbols, black line). Maximum force is produced under isometric conditions ($V = 0$), whilst maximum shortening speed is observed in unloaded muscle ($P = 0$). Power output is the product of P and V. The force–power relationship (blue symbols, green line) is a parabola with maximum power being produced at an intermediate force and velocity. Panel B: Length–tension relationship in cardiac muscle. At sarcomere length greater than 2.0 μm, isometric tension depends on the amount of overlap between myosin cross-bridges and actin filaments. At shorter sarcomere lengths (down to 1.6 μm), tension is reduced because of interference of thin filaments from opposite ends of the sarcomere. Below 1.6 μm sarcomere length, myosin filaments interfere with the Z-line and tension falls rapidly. The relative positions of the thick and thin filaments corresponding to stages 1 to 4 of the length–tension relationship are shown below. The range of sarcomere lengths during a normal cardiac cycle is shown in blue.

tonically inhibits SERCA2. As phosphorylation increases, the inhibition is removed and more Ca^{2+} is pumped into the SR (Fig. 16.1.2.8a).

The Na^+,Ca^{2+} exchanger (Na/CaX) and the Na^+,K^+-ATPase

The plasma membrane Na/CaX additionally contributes to the lowering of cytoplasmic Ca^{2+} during the later part of the action potential and during diastole (Fig. 16.1.2.10 and Table 16.1.2.2). The Na/CaX utilizes the energy associated with the concentration and electrical gradients for Na^+ to expel Ca^{2+} from the cell.

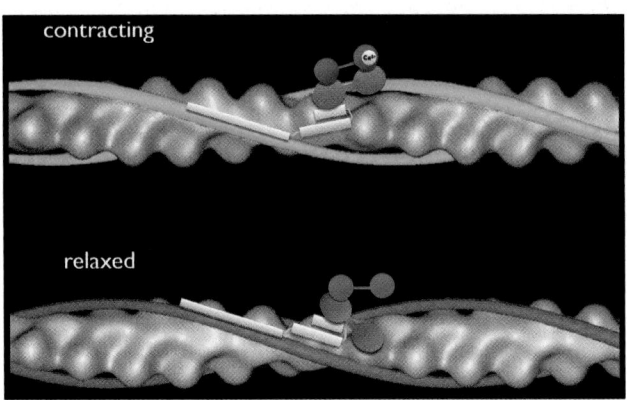

Fig. 16.1.2.16 Regulation of the thin filament by Ca^{2+}. The thin filament is composed of actin, tropomyosin, and troponin. Actin is rendered in orange, tropomyosin in green for activated filaments and red for the 'switched off' filament. Troponin T is grey, troponin I is magenta, and troponin C is blue. In contracting muscle, troponin I is bound to troponin C and the myosin-binding sites on actin are accessible. In relaxed muscle, the C-terminus of troponin I is bound to actin and the tropomyosin strand has moved to a position that blocks the access of myosin heads.

(The structure of the actin–tropomyosin complex is based on helical reconstructions of electron micrographs of thin filaments by Xu C, et al. (1999). Tropomyosin positions in regulated thin filaments revealed by cryoelectron microscopy. *Biophys. J*, **177**, 985–992, with permission from the Biophysical Journal. The structure of the troponin complex is shown diagrammatically and is based on the model of Malnic B, et al. (1998). Regulatory properties of the NH_2- and COOH-terminal domains of troponin T. ATPase activation and binding to troponin I and troponin C. *J Biol Chem*, **273**, 10594–10601.)

As mentioned, it is electrogenic, promoting depolarization under these conditions. However, a thermodynamic prediction is that the direction of ion movement mediated by the Na/CaX will vary according to the membrane potential and the intracellular and extracellular concentrations of Na^+ and Ca^{2+}. The exchange is sensitive to Na^+_i concentration. When membrane potential is near its diastolic level and Na^+_i at normal physiological concentration, the Na/CaX will eject Ca^{2+} from the cell. If Na^+_i increases by a few mmol/litre and the membrane potential becomes depolarized, the exchanger can reverse and mediate Ca^{2+} entry.

The (plasma membrane) Na^+,K^+-ATPase is responsible for the extrusion of Na^+. Cardiac glycosides (e.g. digoxin) inhibit the Na^+,K^+-ATPase, preventing the extrusion of Na^+_i. This, in turn, causes the Na/CaX to spend less time extruding Ca^{2+}_i during the cardiac cycle and more time in 'reverse' Ca^{2+}_o uptake mode. Under these conditions, Ca^{2+} uptake by the SR may be increased, thereby augmenting the cardiac Ca^{2+} pool and facilitating CICR. The net effect of the cardiac glycosides is to increase the cytoplasmic concentration and availability of Ca^{2+} resulting in an increased force of contraction.

Although ventricular myocytes possess other systems to decrease cytoplasmic Ca^{2+} concentrations (namely the plasma membrane Ca^{2+} ATPase and mitochondrial Ca^{2+} uptake), these contribute less than 5% towards relaxation of a normal twitch. SERCA2 and Na/CaX contribute about 70% and 25%, respectively, towards relaxation, though these figures vary greatly between species. In steady-state conditions, the amount of Ca^{2+} leaving the cell via the Na/CaX is the same as the amount entering (via I_{Ca} carried by the L-type Ca^{2+} channel) to evoke CICR, hence precise Ca^{2+} homeostasis is achieved.

Control of myocardial contractility

The contractility of heart muscle is determined by three factors: the initial sarcomere length (preload), the force against which the muscle must shorten (afterload), and the speed and force of contraction. Speed and force of contraction can be modulated independently of preload and afterload by changing the inotropic state.

This is controlled largely, but not exclusively, by stimuli from the sympathoadrenal system and the parasympathetic nervous system. β-Adrenergic agonists (e.g. adrenaline, noradrenaline, and the synthetic pharmacological agonist isoprenaline (isoproterenol)) or β-blockers/β-antagonists (which compete with β-agonists) bind to the extracellular domain of transmembrane β_1-adrenergic receptors. In the case of β-agonists, this binding increases the activity of the membrane-bound adenylyl cyclases, leading to an increase in the intracellular concentrations of cyclic adenosine monophosphate (cyclic AMP). Cyclic AMP dissociates the regulatory and catalytic subunits of the protein kinase A (PKA) heterotetramer. The catalytic subunits, now freed from the repression of their activity by the regulatory subunits, covalently phosphorylate a number of intracellular proteins including those concerned with the regulation of Ca^{2+} movements and contractility. To terminate these events when plasma concentrations of β-agonists fall, cyclic AMP is hydrolysed by the cyclic nucleotide phosphodiesterases, and protein phosphatases hydrolyse the protein-bound phosphate. Conversely, acetylcholine, when bound to certain subclasses of muscarinic receptors, inhibits adenylyl cyclases and decreases inotropic drive.

Positive inotropism, lusitropism, and chronotropism

Positive inotropism

The major influence of catecholamines on the speed and force of contraction is mediated by a PKA-mediated phosphorylation of the L-type Ca^{2+} channel, which increases the probability of channels opening when the cell is depolarized, thus increasing I_{Ca}.

Positive lusitropism

Catecholamines are also positively lusitropic (i.e. they increase the rate of relaxation). Positive lusitropism is achieved by a PKA catalytic subunit-mediated phosphorylation of phospholamban which inhibits SERCA2 in its hypophosphorylated state (Fig. 16.1.2.8a). Phosphorylated phospholamban does not inhibit SERCA2. The effect of phospholamban phosphorylation is thus to activate SERCA2 and stimulate Ca^{2+} reuptake into the SR. In addition, protein kinase-A phosphorylates cardiac troponin I, and this increases the rate of dissociation of Ca^{2+} from troponin C, increasing the rate of dissociation of myosin cross-bridges from actin (i.e. stimulating relaxation).

Positive chronotropism

Positive chronotropism is achieved by increasing the frequency of depolarization in the sinoatrial node. Upon stimulation of the sympathoadrenal system, I_f (generated by HCN channels) is activated to depolarize the membrane to the threshold level more quickly and increase the rate of production of action potentials. The positive chronotropism of the sympathoadrenal system is in part mediated by the binding of cyclic AMP to these HCN channels. This shifts their voltage dependence of activation to more depolarized potentials and increases both the rate of channel opening and the maximal current level. The net result is an increased frequency of depolarization and the heart rate increases.

The sympathoadrenal system and heart failure

In heart failure, the myocyte becomes unresponsive to β-adrenergic agonists, and consequently phosphorylation of the proteins responsible for the control of contractility is diminished. The β_1-adrenergic receptor abundance is decreased and the expression of proteins which antagonize β_1-receptor signalling is increased, thus the efficacy of β-agonism is diminished. Many drugs that mitigate heart failure are targeted at the proteins that regulate the inotropic state. There is evidence also that SERCA2 expression is decreased and this may contribute to the elevated cytoplasmic Ca^{2+} concentrations sometimes seen in diastole during heart failure and the poorer contraction of the heart in this condition.

Further reading

Bagshaw CR (1993). *Muscle contraction*, 2nd edition. Chapman & Hall, New York.

Bers DM (2001). *Excitation-contraction coupling and cardiac contractile force*, 2nd edition. Kluwer, Dordrecht.

Houser SR, Margulies KB (2003). Is depressed myocytes contractility centrally involved in heart failure? *Circ Res*, **92**, 350–8.

Katz AM (2006). *Physiology of the heart*, 4th edition. Lippincott Williams and Wilkins, Philadelphia.

Ko Y-S, *et al.* (2004). Three-dimensional reconstruction of the rabbit atrioventricular conduction axis by combining histological, desmin, and connexin mapping data. *Circulation*, **109**, 1172–9.

Opie LH (2004). 4th edition. Lippincott Williams and Wilkins, Philadelphia.

Rüegg JC (1992). *Calcium in muscle contraction*, 2nd edition. Springer-Verlag, Berlin.

Severs NJ (2000). The cardiac muscle cell. *BioEssays*, **22**, 188–99.

Severs NJ, *et al.* (2004). Gap junction alterations in human cardiac disease. *Cardiovasc Res*, **62**, 368–77.

Stevenson S, *et al.* (1998). Spatial relationship of the C-terminal domains of dystrophin and β-dystroglycan in cardiac muscle supports a direct molecular interaction at the plasma membrane interface. *Circ Res*, **82**, 82–93.

16.1.3 **Clinical physiology of the normal heart**

David E.L. Wilcken

Essentials

The function of the heart is to provide the tissues of the body with sufficient oxygenated blood and metabolites to meet the moment-to-moment needs as dictated by physical activity and postural and emotional changes.

The energy requirements of the heart during rest and exertion are influenced by ventricular volume, outflow resistance (blood pressure), venous return, and the activity of the autonomic nervous system. An increase in ventricular volume increases wall tension during contraction, and an augmented myocardial oxygen supply is then required to maintain the same systemic blood pressure and stroke volume.

The normal integration of the venous return, heart rate, stroke volume, and arterial blood pressure ensures that there is an adequate supply of oxygen and nutrients to the tissues. The activities of the sympathetic and parasympathetic nervous systems contribute to the adjustment of cardiac performance to immediate needs—the former by increasing heart rate and myocardial contractility during exertion and emotion, the latter by maintaining a relatively slow heart rate at rest. Vagal fibres in the heart are distributed mainly to the sinoatrial node and the atria; sympathetic innervation is to both the atria and the ventricles. There is a normal diurnal variation in autonomic function, with an increased sympathetic outflow in the mornings, soon after wakening.

Coronary flow occurs largely in diastole. It is finely adjusted to meet metabolic requirements and may increase five- or sixfold during strenuous exercise. The inner layers of the ventricular muscle normally receive a slightly greater blood flow than the outer layers. Haemodynamic and ventilatory responses during exercise take 2 to 3 min to equilibrate and adjust to an increased workload and reach a new steady state. Regular exercise to least 60% of maximal heart rate about three times a week improves effort tolerance. Measurement of the cardiovascular response to exercise provides an objective assessment of cardiac function.

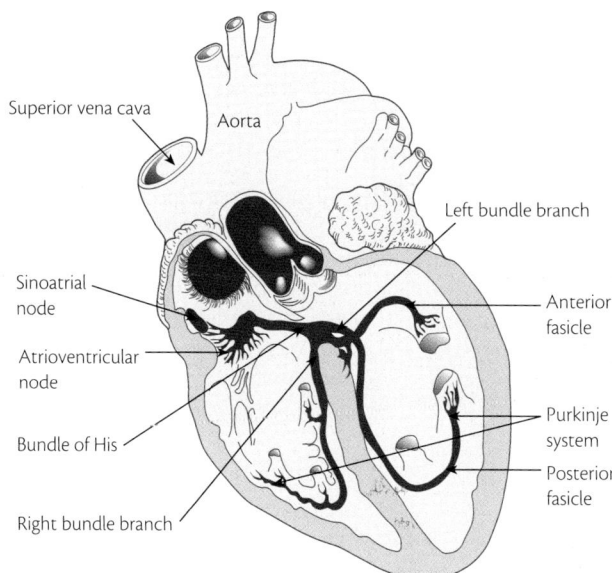

Fig. 16.1.3.1 Diagram of the heart showing the impulse-generating and impulse-conducting system.
From Junqueira LC, Carneiro J, (2005). Basic histology,11th edn. McCgraw-Hill, New York.

Introduction

The function of the heart is to pump sufficient oxygenated blood containing nutrients, metabolites, and hormones to meet moment-to-moment metabolic needs and preserve a constant internal environment. The heart has two essential characteristics—contractility and rhythmicity. The nervous system and neurohumoral agents modulate relationships between the venous return to the heart, the outflow resistance against which it contracts, the frequency of contraction, and its inotropic state; there are also intrinsic cardiac autoregulatory mechanisms. This chapter describes normal cardiac function and discusses the principal mechanisms contributing to its regulation.

The cardiac cycle

Electrical events initiate the cardiac cycle with depolarization of the sinoatrial (SA) node in the upper right atrium (Fig. 16.1.3.1). Cardiac muscle acts as a functional syncytium. Communication between neighbouring cells is mediated by 'gap junctions' which form arrays of cell-to-cell channels. The generated action potential spreads from the sinoatrial node across the functional syncytium at a speed of 1.0 to 1.2 M/s. The first mechanical response is atrial systole.

The cell-to-cell conduction of the electrical impulse from atrium to ventricle normally occurs only through the atrioventricular (AV) node (Fig. 16.1.3.1), a region of slow conductance at 0.02 to 0.1 m/s. This delays activation of the cells of the bundle of His and allows time for completion of ventricular filling. The conduction velocity in the bundle of His is from 1.2 to 2.0 m/s. The impulse passes via the right bundle branch and the two branches of the left bundle, and spreads rapidly (2.0–4.0 m/s) through the Purkinje fibres and each muscle cell to produce an orderly sequence of ventricular contraction (Fig. 16.1.3.1). Atrial and ventricular depolarization (P wave and QRS complex) and repolarization (T wave) can be recorded on the ECG (Fig. 16.1.3.2)—see Chapter 16.3.1 for further details.

The specialized cells of pacemaker tissue have an inherent rhythmicity that is shared by the sinoatrial node, the atrioventricular node, and Purkinje tissue. Unlike other myocardial cells, these cells do not maintain a diastolic intracellular potential of about −90 mV, but tend to depolarize spontaneously. Because the sinoatrial node has the fastest inherent discharge (depolarization) rate, and because there is a brief period after depolarization of the whole heart during which a further stimulus is ineffective—the absolute refractory period—the sinoatrial node is normally the pacesetter for the heart. However, if this does not occur, pacemaker tissue in

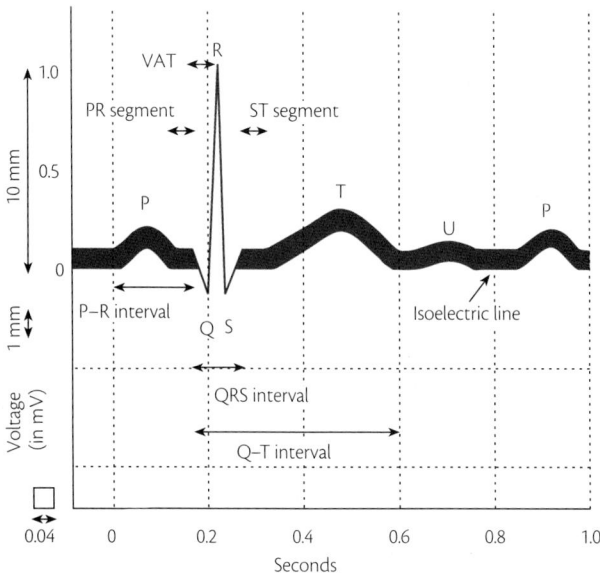

Fig. 16.1.3.2 Diagram of electrocardiographic complexes, intervals, and segments. VAT, ventricular activation time.
From Goldschlager N, Goldman MJ (1989). Principles of clinical electrocardiography, 13th edn. Appleton and Lange, East Norwalk, Connecticut.

the atrioventricular node, the bundle of His, or the Purkinje system will assume this role, in which case the heart rate is then considerably slower.

Mechanical events

The mechanical events following depolarization of the atrial and ventricular muscle and their timing in relation to the ECG, to pressure and flow changes, and to heart sounds are shown in five phases in Fig. 16.1.3.3. After the P wave, and coinciding with atrial systole, 'a' waves appear in left atrial and right atrial pressure tracings due to atrial contraction, and an 'a' wave can be seen in the jugular venous pulse. Atrial contraction increases ventricular filling by about 10% (phase 1).

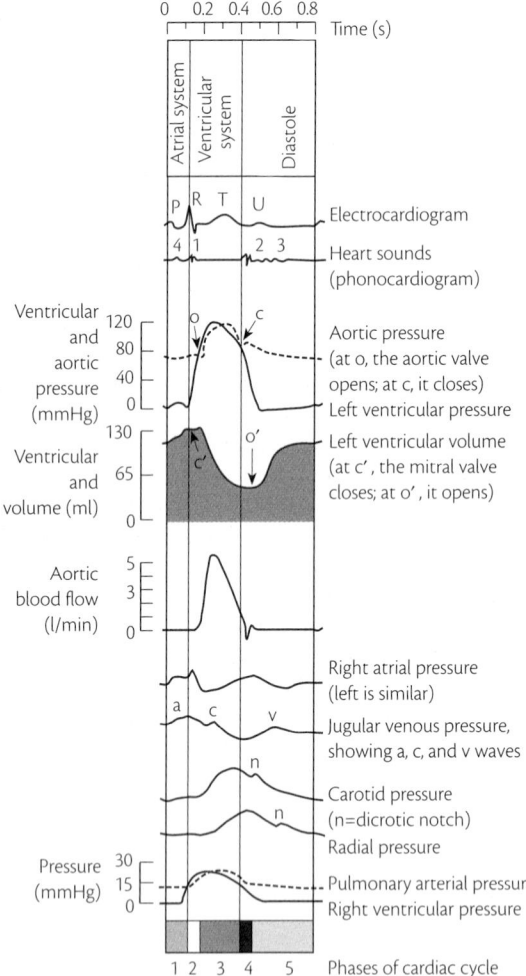

Fig. 16.1.3.3 Events of the cardiac cycle at a heart rate of 75 beats/min. The phases of the cardiac cycle identified by the numbers at the bottom are: (1) atrial systole; (2) isovolumetric ventricular contraction; (3) ventricular ejection; (4) isovolumetric ventricular relaxation; and (5) ventricular filling. Note that late in systole, aortic pressure actually exceeds left ventricular pressure. However, the momentum of the blood keeps it flowing out of the ventricle for a short time. The pressure relationships in the right ventricle and pulmonary artery are similar. The jugular venous pulse is similar in form to that seen in the right atrial pressure tracing. The 'c' wave interrupts the 'x' descent of the 'a' wave. The decline in pressure from the peak of the 'v' is the 'y' descent; the rate of decline reflects speed of ventricular filling. Atr. syst, atrial systole; ventric. syst, ventricular systole. Modified with permission from Ganong WF (2005). Review of medical physiology, 22nd edn. McGraw-Hill, New York.

The onset of ventricular contraction coincides with the peak of the R wave of the ECG; a rapid rise in intraventricular pressure closes the mitral and tricuspid valves, causing the first heart sound. During this short isovolumetric period (phase 2 of Fig. 16.1.3.3), the pressure rises rapidly in the ventricles. When ventricular pressures exceed those in the pulmonary artery and aorta, the outflow valves open and ventricular ejection follows. The highest flow rate is in early systole, and pressures in the aorta and pulmonary artery rise. Normally, between 50 and 70% of the ventricular volume is ejected during systole, and this can be seen in the volume curve included in Fig. 16.1.3.3 (phase 3).

The jugular venous pulse, during ventricular contraction, has a positive deflection in early systole, the 'c' wave, due to right ventricular contraction and bulging of the tricuspid valve into the right atrium. Descent of the tricuspid ring caused by ventricular contraction then produces a negative 'x' descent, but as atrial inflow continues the pressure rises in the atria and great veins, producing the 'v' wave. This reaches its peak just before the opening of the tricuspid valve, declining during early ventricular filling as the negative 'y' descent. The changes in the pulmonary veins and left atrium are similar.

As the strength of ventricular contraction declines, coinciding with the end of the T wave, the aortic and pulmonary valves close, producing the dicrotic notch seen on both, aortic and pulmonary, artery pressure tracings in Fig. 16.1.3.3. Aortic closure slightly precedes pulmonary closure, and together these are responsible for the two components of the second heart sound. A short period of further rapid decline in ventricular pressure ensues without change in the ventricular volume (the period of isovolumetric ventricular relaxation, phase 4), and at the end of this the mitral and tricuspid valves open. There is a pressure gradient from atrium to ventricle so that a period of rapid ventricular filling follows, which coincides with the timing of the third heart sound. The rapid ventricular filling is reflected in the shape of the ventricular volume curve, and is followed by a period of slower filling (phase 5) with a final sudden small increment from the next atrial contraction as diastole ends (phase 1).

Third heart sounds are normally audible in children and young adults, but over the age of about 40 years this usually indicates elevation of ventricular end-diastolic pressure (most frequently in the left ventricle). The myocardium and valvular structures become stiffer with ageing, and large increases in ventricular end-diastolic pressure are then required to tense valvular structures and generate audible vibrations. A fourth heart sound almost always indicates abnormal ventricular function, with increased end-diastolic pressure. A fourth heart sound precedes the Q wave of the ECG, and must be distinguished from a normal splitting of the two components of the first heart sound. The latter occurs after the Q wave (Figs. 16.1.3.2 and 16.1.3.3).

Normal volumes, pressures, and flows

The blood volume in normal adults is about 5 litres (haematocrit 45%), and, of this, about 1.5 litres are in the heart and lungs—the central blood volume. The pulmonary arteries, capillaries, and veins contain about 0.9 litres, with only about 75 ml being in the pulmonary capillaries at any one instant. The volume of blood in the heart is about 0.6 litres. Left ventricular end-diastolic volume is about 140 ml, stroke volume about 90 ml, and end-systolic volume around 50 ml, reflecting an ejection fraction (stroke volume/end-diastolic volume) of between 50 and 70%. The right ventricular ejection fraction is similar.

Of the 3.5 litres in the systemic circulation, most—at least 60% of the total blood volume—is in the veins. The systemic veins containing most of the blood volume are easily distensible, and input of blood into the contracting heart is associated with only small changes in venous pressure. By contrast, ejection of blood into the much less distensible arterial tree produces large pressure changes.

The normal values for pressures generated in the heart and great vessels during the cardiac cycle are shown in Table 16.1.3.1. Pressures are measured with reference to a zero pressure arbitrarily set at 5 cm below the sternal angle with the patient recumbent. 'Normal' arterial blood pressure is considered later (see below).

Cardiac output is the product of stroke volume and heart rate. It is related to body size and is best expressed as litre/min per m² of body surface area: the 'cardiac index'. The mean cardiac index under resting and relaxed conditions is 3.5 litre/min per m², and values below 2 and above 5 are abnormal. The cardiac index declines with age. In persons of average size, resting oxygen consumption is about 240 ml/min, and the difference in oxygen content between arterial and mixed venous blood is about 40 ml/litre (arteriovenous oxygen difference), giving a basal cardiac output of 6 litre/min. In normal subjects, the arteriovenous difference in oxygen content at rest is maintained within narrow limits, from 35 to 45 ml/litre; values of 55 ml/litre and above are always abnormal.

Pulmonary or systemic vascular resistance is estimated by dividing the difference between mean inflow pressure (pulmonary artery or aortic) and mean outflow pressure (left atrial or right atrial) in mmHg by the flow in litre/min through the respective circulations. In normal subjects and patients without intracardiac shunts, this flow is the cardiac output. Normal pulmonary vascular resistance is less than 2 mmHg/litre per min (16 MPa•s/m³, 160 dyn s⁻¹cm⁻⁵). Arterial blood pressure is the product of cardiac output and total peripheral resistance.

Stroke work is the integral of instantaneous ventricular pressure with respect to stroke volume, but is usually estimated as the product of stroke volume and mean ejection pressure. The orderly sequence of contraction in the normal cardiac cycle coordinates changes in instantaneous pressure and flow, so maximizing the transfer of energy to the circulation. Normal left ventricular work output at rest is about 6 kg/m² per min.

Myocardial mechanics

When a muscle is activated to contract, it develops a potential for doing work. In isolated skeletal and heart muscle preparations, the stretching force applied to the muscle—and therefore the length of the muscle—can be varied before contraction; this is the preload. The activated muscle will begin to shorten when it has generated a force sufficient to overcome that exerted by the attached weight or load against which it contracts. When the force exerted by the load is so arranged that it is not applied to the relaxed muscle and is applied only after the muscle has begun to develop tension, it is termed the afterload. If this load is so large that the activated muscle is unable to overcome it, and so cannot shorten, the contraction produces tension only, and the contraction is isometric. When shortening does occur, external work is done. If the load is constant during the shortening, the contraction is said to be isotonic; if it changes, it is auxotonic.

The tension produced by both skeletal and cardiac muscle during contraction depends on initial fibre length; during afterloaded isotonic contractions from a particular length, the amount and the speed of fibre shortening and the tension developed all depend upon the afterload. Over a range of loads the initial velocity of muscle shortening is most rapid and the most extensive shortening occurs when the load is smallest.

The inverse relationship between initial velocity of fibre shortening and load in an isotonic contraction is a fundamental one for both skeletal and cardiac muscle. There is, however, a major difference between the two types of muscle in that the relationship at any one length is constant in a skeletal muscle, whereas in cardiac muscle there are variations in inotropic state that are accompanied by considerable changes in the relationship between force and velocity. A positive inotropic effect produces a more extensive contraction from the same initial length and afterload, and a faster maximum velocity of shortening (V_{max}). An increase in initial fibre length with no increase in inotropic state increases the force of contraction but does not, however, change the maximum velocity of shortening. This is illustrated in Fig. 16.1.3.4.

The contraction of the intact heart can be visualized as being similar mechanically to the afterloaded contraction of an isolated muscle strip. For the left ventricle, the preload is the distending force which stretches the muscle fibres in end-diastole, and the initial afterload is the force the ventricle must generate in order to open the aortic valve and eject blood. At the end of ejection, the ventricular muscle is isolated from the peripheral circulation, with the afterload then supported by the competent aortic valve, and the muscle relaxes against a comparatively small force. Relaxation of the heart is an active process due to withdrawal of calcium ions from the cytoplasm surrounding the myofibrils. 'Active' relaxation is still proceeding in the ventricular wall when the atrioventricular valves open, and, if it is delayed—as in the hypoxic heart—the slower relaxation increases the stiffness of the ventricular wall and reduces filling. Wall thickness is also a determinant of relaxation rate and compliance. For this reason, filling pressures are higher for the thicker and stiffer left ventricle than for the thinner and

Table 16.1.3.1 Normal resting values for pressures in the heart and great vessels

Site	Systolic pressure (mmHg)	Diastolic pressure (mmHg)	Mean pressure (mmHg)
Right atrium	'a' up to 7, 'v' up to 5	'y' up to 3, 'x' up to 3	Less than 5
Right ventricle	Up to 25	End pressure before 'a' up to 3; end pressure on 'a' up to 7	Not applicable
Pulmonary artery	Up to 25	Up to 15	Up to 18
Left atrium (direct or indirect pulmonary capillary wedge)	'a' up to 12, 'v' up to 10	'x' up to 7, 'y' up to 7	Up to 10
Left ventricle	120	End pressure before 'a' up to 7; end pressure on 'a' up to 12	Not applicable

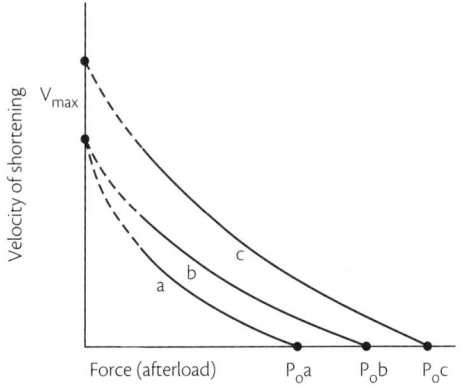

Fig. 16.1.3.4 Idealized relationships between velocity of fibre shortening and afterload or force developed during contraction of a strip of cardiac muscle under three different conditions. Curves a and b were obtained with the muscle in the same inotropic state but with a longer initial fibre length (greater preload) for curve b. Curves b and c were obtained with initial fibre length the same but with contractility increased in c by the addition of a drug producing a positive inotropic effect. The terms V_{max} and P_0 describe, respectively, a hypothetical maximum shortening velocity in the absence of any load (hence the broken lines), and the force developed in an isometric contraction. An increase in initial fibre length increases P_0 but not V_{max}; a positive inotropic change increases both P_0 and V_{max}.

more distensible right ventricle (Table 16.1.3.1). When the left ventricle is hypertrophied due to chronic pressure overload, as in systemic hypertension or aortic stenosis, it becomes stiffer and filling pressures may then be abnormally high.

Regulation of cardiac function

Four essential factors determine the performance of the heart: (1) venous return, (2) outflow resistance (afterload), (3) inotropic state or contractility, and (4) heart rate. Changes in cardiac performance are accomplished by mechanisms that alter these four determinants.

Venous return, preload, and the Frank–Starling relationship

The relationship described independently by Frank and Starling between end-diastolic fibre length and force of contraction is shown in Fig. 16.1.3.5. When the ventricle ejects against a constant pressure, variations in venous return alter the degree of stretch of the muscle fibres in diastole, and this determines contraction strength and work output. The number of active force-generating sites in each fibre increases as it lengthens so that, within limits, the force of contraction and stroke work are positively related to end-diastolic fibre length. The relationship is curvilinear when stroke work is plotted against end-diastolic pressure as an index of preload, reflecting the exponential relationship between end-diastolic pressure and end-diastolic volume. When stroke work is plotted against end-diastolic volume, the relationship between stroke work and preload is linear.

The response of the heart at any particular time depends upon: (1) the intrinsic state of the muscle, i.e. the biochemistry and contractile machinery; (2) the prevailing neurohumoral state, e.g. increased sympathetic outflow produces a more forceful contraction at any end-diastolic fibre length; (3) extrinsic inotropic influences—drugs which have either positive or negative inotropic effects.

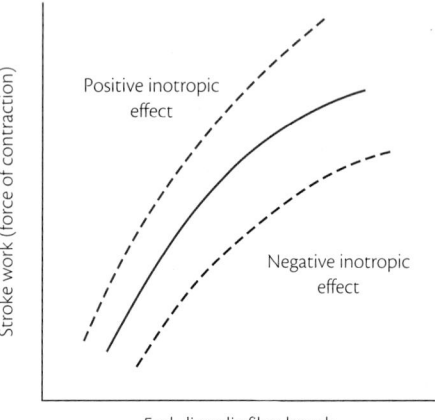

Fig. 16.1.3.5 The relation between left ventricular end-diastolic fibre length and left ventricular stroke work showing displacement upward and to the left with an increase in contractility and downward and to the right with a reduction in contractility. Similar but not identical curves are obtained by plotting left ventricular stroke work as one measure of the force of contraction against ventricular end-diastolic pressure or volume (see text). Similar function curves may be obtained from both ventricles and both atria.

End-diastolic fibre length is determined by the force distending the ventricle at end-diastole, and end-diastolic pressure provides a reasonable indication of this force when the ventricle has normal distensibility or compliance; this is the preload. The systemic venous return and the elastic properties of the myocardium produce the end-diastolic distending pressure for the right ventricle, and the pulmonary venous return and myocardial elasticity that for the left ventricle. For clinical purposes, it is convenient to equate venous return with preload because, as it changes from beat to beat, it adjusts the strength of the subsequent ventricular (and atrial) contraction by varying the force stretching the relaxed cardiac muscle and changing end-diastolic fibre length.

Outflow resistance or afterload

Pulmonary and aortic valve opening pressures are determined largely by the pulmonary and systemic vascular resistances, as shown for the latter in Fig. 16.1.3.6. These resistances, together with an inertial component dependent upon the mass of blood within the vessels, the compliance (stiffness) of the vessels, and the physical characteristics of each vascular tree combined with the pulsatile nature of the flow, constitute the impedance to ventricular outflow. This is the load against which the ventricle must contract and shorten. As this load is not applied in diastole to the relaxed muscle, it then being supported by competent aortic and pulmonary valves, it is described clinically as the afterload: it becomes applied to the muscle only after the ventricle has begun to develop tension.

Regulation of systemic arterial blood pressure

The regulation of the systemic circulation is well adapted to the vital function of maintaining constant, adequate cerebral perfusion. There is a need to maintain a relatively constant arterial blood pressure when there are changes in posture and circulating blood volume. The baroreceptors mediate rapid responses to alterations in aortic pressure, whilst a variety of hormonal and physical factors regulate the circulating blood volume.

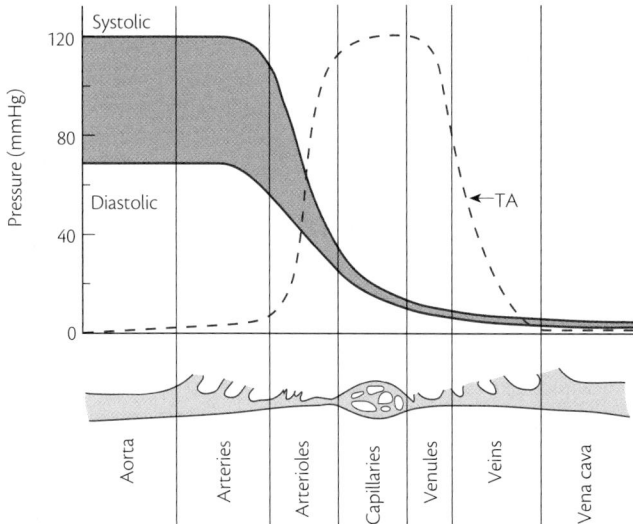

Fig. 16.1.3.6 Diagram of the changes in pressure as blood flows through the systemic circulation. The total cross-sectional area of the vessels (TA) increases from 4.5 cm² to 4500 cm² in the capillaries. The major resistance to flow is at the arteriolar level.

Modified and reproduced with permission from Ganong WF (2005). *Review of medical physiology*, 22nd edn. McGraw-Hill, New York.

Baroreceptors

The baroreceptor regulatory system comprises two groups of stretch receptors: one group in the carotid sinuses near the bifurcations of the common carotid arteries in the neck and a second group in the arch of the aorta. These respond to an increase in central arterial pressure by the firing of impulses, which pass by the glossopharyngeal and vagus nerves to the solitary tract nucleus in the medulla and inhibit sympathetic outflow. Efferent impulses from these central connections pass via the right vagus nerve mainly to the sinoatrial node, and via the left vagus mainly to the atrioventricular node. The effect is to decrease the heart rate and the force of atrial contraction. There is also attenuation of sympathetic discharge to arteriolar smooth muscle in the limbs and visceral circulation, resulting in a release of peripheral arteriolar constriction and, therefore, peripheral vasodilatation. Thus the immediate response to a rise in arterial pressure is slowing of the heart rate, reduced force of atrial contraction, and reduced vascular resistance. The net effect of this negative feedback system is to offset the elevation in blood pressure. Conversely, a lowering of blood pressure diminishes stimulation of the stretch receptors and reduces afferent traffic to the solitary tract nucleus, resulting in reduced inhibition of sympathetic outflow. There is, then, a quickening of the heart rate and peripheral vasoconstriction so that the blood pressure increases. The changes in heart rate take place within 1 to 2 s and changes in vasomotor control within 5 or 6 s.

Baroreceptor mechanisms effectively modulate the responses of blood pressure to postural change. Additionally, they adapt to maintain the normal circadian variation in blood pressure (see below). They also maintain elevated arterial blood pressure in systemic hypertension. Sensory input to the reflex is reduced in disorders of the autonomic nervous system, and in the prolonged weightlessness of space flight.

Blood volume

The circulating blood volume is relatively small, and a large proportion is contained in the veins (Fig. 16.1.3.6) so that any change in blood volume will affect venous return and, therefore, cardiac output and blood pressure. When blood volume is large and the veins full, there is little reduction in venous return on standing and cardiac output is maintained. However, when effective blood volume is reduced and the veins are relatively empty, on standing there is pooling of blood in the veins of the legs and a reduction in venous return and cardiac output so that arterial blood pressure falls. Baroreceptor responses become evident within a couple of beats, the heart rate increases, and cardiac output and blood pressure are restored. Circulating blood volume is kept relatively constant by a combination of mechanisms which involve the actions of natriuretic peptides, the renin–angiotensin–aldosterone system, vasopressin, and osmolality.

Natriuretic peptides

The discovery of secretory granules in the atria of the heart, and the demonstration in 1981 that they produce a natriuretic factor that inhibits the reabsorption of sodium in the distal tubule of the kidney, enhanced understanding of the regulation of blood volume and cardiac performance. Three natriuretic peptides have subsequently been identified.

◆ Atrial natriuretic peptide is present in the circulation, and concentrations increase during volume expansion. The right atrium contains about 2 to 4 times as much activity as the left, and release of the hormone is mediated largely by atrial distension. The effect is to produce a diuresis and to reduce cardiac and circulating blood volume. Atrial natriuretic peptide also has a vasodilator action and opposes the vasoconstricting effects of noradrenaline and angiotension II.

◆ The second natriuretic peptide was identified in brain tissue and is referred to as brain natriuretic peptide. Large amounts were later found in the ventricles of the heart, and circulating levels are increased in ventricular hypertrophy and cardiac failure. Brain and atrial natriuretic peptides have similar actions.

◆ The third natriuretic peptide to be identified was C-type natriuretic peptide. It is distributed widely in tissues, circulating concentrations are low, and it appears to have actions similar to the other two peptides, but with a greater vasodilator effect on veins.

These three peptides contribute to the regulation of cardiac and circulating blood volume and of blood pressure. Both B-type natriuretic peptide and N-terminal pro-brain natriuretic peptide are useful adjuncts to the clinical evaluation of dyspnoeic patients in that levels are elevated when the dyspnoea is due to cardiac failure.

Renin–angiotensin system

This system, which is both local and systemic, is of major importance in the regulation of circulating blood volume and the maintenance of normal blood pressure. Enhanced activity of systemic renin and angiotensin increases the production of aldosterone, which promotes reabsorption of sodium by the kidney and expansion of circulating blood volume. All components of the renin–angiotensin system are distributed widely throughout tissues—including the brain and the heart—and increased activation of the system increases the risk of cardiovascular events. Angiotensin II is a potent vasoconstrictor that also enhances the proliferation of smooth muscle cells. The angiotensin-converting enzyme (ACE) inhibitors in clinical use diminish angiotension II production locally and in the circulating blood. Both local and general effects appear important in mediating the benefits that accrue from the use of these drugs in the management of hypertension and congestive cardiac failure, and in the reduction in rates of recurrence of coronary events in ischaemic heart disease. The mechanisms mediating the latter include antioxidant effects and a reduction in the production of potentially damaging free radicals, anti-inflammatory effects, and augmentation of the profibrinolytic effects of bradykinin. The more recently developed angiotensin II receptor blocking drugs have now been shown to produce similar outcomes.

Regulation of nitric oxide production

A recently recognized contribution to endothelial function, which affects the afterload, is related to nitric oxide production, and its inhibition by asymmetric dimethylarginine (ADMA). Asymmetric dimethylarginine is produced by the physiological degradation of methylated proteins. ADMA inhibits the production of nitric oxide, which is derived directly from L-arginine, present in all cells. ADMA levels are regulated by the balance between its production and its metabolism. The balance may be disrupted in clinical situations, for example in renal impairment. Reduced renal function increases the level of ADMA and this reduces endothelial dilatation.

Ventricular volume and afterload

Ventricular volume also has a major effect on afterload, as pressure is equal to force per unit area. The force acting radially on the inner surface of the whole ventricle at any time during systole is the product of the intraventricular pressure and ventricular surface area at that time. If the left ventricle is assumed to be a sphere (surface area = πd^2), the force opposing ejection at any time during contraction is the product of the intracavity pressure and πd^2 at that time. Thus, a doubling in left ventricular diameter from a normal value of 5 cm to 10 cm would result in a fourfold increase in the force opposing ejection for the same intracavity systolic pressure; the ventricle would need to develop greatly increased wall tension to overcome that force. Because wall tension developed during systole is the major determinant of myocardial oxygen consumption, the contraction will clearly be much less efficient in the larger heart for the same stroke volume and ejection pressure (stroke work).

During a normal heartbeat, the afterload is greatest at the beginning of ejection (rapid rise in pressure and maximum volume; Fig. 16.1.3.3), but decreases thereafter as the pressure reaches a plateau and then declines as the ventricle becomes smaller. There is, therefore, a matching of the afterload to the declining intensity of the contraction as it proceeds to completion, and fibres shorten at a relatively constant rate. This is less obvious in a large heart where the volume change during ejection is a smaller proportion of the total ventricular volume.

The end-diastolic volume is influenced by preload, afterload, circulating blood volume, the inotropic state of the ventricle, heart rate, and neurohumoral influences. It is smaller in the erect than in the horizontal position because of reduced venous return, and it decreases with a moderate increase in heart rate because of an associated positive inotropic effect. The proportion of end-diastolic volume ejected during systole, the ejection fraction

(normal 50–70%), is a useful index of overall left ventricular function and is easily measured noninvasively by gated blood-pool scanning and two-dimensional echocardiographic techniques. The ejection fraction increases with exercise and with positive inotropic interventions. Values for right ventricular ejection fraction are of the same order as those for the left side of the heart.

Myocardial contractility and inotropic state

Myocardial function is greatly altered by changes in inotropic state or contractility. Positive inotropic effects are thought to be mediated by activation of excitation–contraction coupling mechanisms and are associated with an increased influx of calcium ions into myocardial cells and a more powerful contraction. Changes in the intensity of excitation–contraction coupling are independent of the Frank–Starling mechanism. Increases in the intensity shift the curve upwards and to the left, and decreases shift it downwards and to the right (Fig. 16.1.3.5). With a positive inotropic effect, the force of contraction, however measured, is increased for a given end-diastolic fibre length and, if the afterload is the same, the initial velocity of fibre shortening is also increased (Fig. 16.1.3.4); in the intact heart, there is more complete emptying during systole. Increased sympathetic stimulation, some drugs, and an increase in heart rate itself (the staircase or Bowditch phenomenon; postectopic potentiation, see below) have positive inotropic effects. Myocardial depressants, such as hypoxia and most anaesthetic drugs, have negative inotropic effects. Increased parasympathetic stimulation produces acetylcholine-mediated negative inotropic effects that are confined almost entirely to the atria because of the anatomical distribution of vagal endings in the myocardium.

It is difficult to measure inotropic changes accurately in the human heart because changes in the intensity of excitation–contraction coupling and changes in the Frank–Starling relationship, though separate, are nevertheless closely linked. The peak rate of change of intraventricular pressure (peak dp/dt) is a useful index of

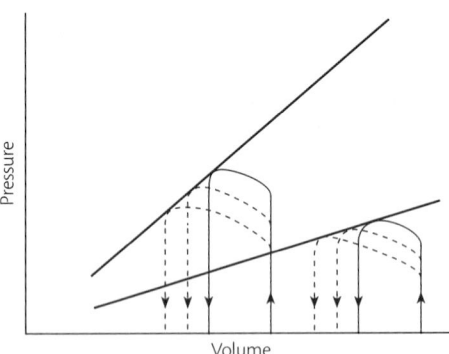

Fig. 16.1.3.7 Diagrammatic representation of intraventricular pressure and volume relationships during the cardiac cycle at two levels of myocardial contractility; three separate beats with the same end-diastolic volume are shown for each. The loops on the left of the diagram were obtained when contractility is increased and those on the right when it is reduced. There is a linear end-systolic pressure–volume relationship with different afterloads (pressures) for each level of contractility. The slope of the end-systolic pressure–volume relationship for any inotropic state is relatively insensitive (see text) to changes within physiological ranges in afterload and preload, although changes in preload are not shown in this diagram. The volume change seen on the horizontal axis for each beat is the stroke volume. This increases with reduction in pressure (afterload).

change in contractility, provided that preload, afterload, and heart rate remain constant.

An approach that appears relatively insensitive to changes in both preload and afterload is that of Suga and Sagawa, using the ventricular pressure–volume-loop diagram. There is an approximately linear relationship between end-systolic pressure (or wall stress) and end-systolic volume when measured over a narrow physiological range in the human left ventricle. Increased contractility shifts the relationship upwards and to the left, as illustrated in Fig. 16.1.3.7, allowing the separation of enhanced from reduced contractility in the same heart, and poorly contracting from normally contracting ventricles. Stroke volume is shown on the abscissa as the difference between end-diastolic and end-systolic volumes. The efficacy of reduction in afterload in assisting reduced ventricular function is also easily explained from the diagram. With a reduced afterload, the aortic valve opens at a lower pressure and a greater stroke volume is ejected; a new end-systolic pressure–volume point is reached, which is shifted downwards on the same linear relationship. There has been no change in contractile state.

Heart rate

Frequency of contraction is the fourth essential determinant of cardiac performance. Heart rate during rest and exertion may vary from 45 to 200 beats/min in the healthy young adult. As changes can occur within seconds, an increase in heart rate is the usual and most effective way of producing a rapid increase in cardiac output. It plays the major role in the response to exercise, during which stroke volume does increase (more so in athletes and when in the erect, rather than the supine, position) but the changes are less marked than those of rate. In addition, an increase in contraction frequency itself produces a positive inotropic effect, whereby the force of contraction increases and reaches a new steady state within a few beats. This is termed the 'positive staircase', Treppe, or Bowditch effect. It may be a consequence of an augmented movement of calcium ions into myocardial cells with increased frequency of action potentials, combined with diminished time for outward movement of calcium between beats. More forceful contractions also follow premature beats—the phenomenon of postextrasystolic potentiation—and the mechanism is probably the same. The extrasystole occurring prematurely is a weak contraction because of decreased filling time and an uncoordinated activation of the ventricle when the ectopic focus is within the ventricle. The next beat is delayed because of the refractory period of the extrasystolic beat, but is a more powerful contraction because of increased filling time and ventricular volume, and increased contractility. Calcium-dependent changes similar to those of the Bowditch effect are probably responsible for the latter.

Coronary blood flow

Coronary blood flow accounts for about 4% of the cardiac output. The heart extracts most (70%) of the oxygen carried in the coronary circulation; the arteriovenous difference for oxygen across the heart being about 110 ml/litre, while that for the whole body is only about 40 ml/litre under resting conditions. Therefore, large increases in myocardial oxygen requirements must be met largely by increases in coronary blood flow, and this may increase five- or sixfold during strenuous exercise. The greater part of this flow is to the left ventricle, of which at least two-thirds occurs during diastole because

of the throttling effect systole has on myocardial perfusion. The main coronary arteries are on the superficial surface of the heart, and because of this, and the hindrance to coronary flow during systole, the subendocardial region of the left ventricle is more vulnerable to perfusion deficits in relation to oxygen need than the outer two-thirds of the muscle wall. Despite these mechanical problems, flow is normally evenly distributed throughout the myocardium so that when regional coronary blood flow is measured using injected radioactive microspheres (in dogs), the ratio of endocardial to epicardial flow is approximately unity. In fact, the inner layers of the heart probably receive slightly more blood (up to 10%) than the outer layers. This is consistent with the subendocardium developing more tension than the subepicardium, and is evidence for a greater rate of myocardial oxygen consumption in the inner layers.

Myocardial oxygen requirements and coronary blood flow are finely adjusted: for information on how such adjustments are made, see Chapter 16.1.1.

The nervous system and the heart

The heart is richly supplied with adrenergic nerves, whose terminals reach atrial and ventricular muscle fibres and impinge upon all pacemaker tissue, including the sinoatrial and atrioventricular nodes and Purkinje fibres. Sympathetic stimulation leads to an increase in myocardial contractility and heart rate, and in the rate of spread of the activation wave through the atrioventricular node and the Purkinje system. This is mediated by local noradrenaline release, which interacts with β-adrenergic receptors. The key elements in these regulatory mechanisms are calcium ions and cAMP. The activated β-receptor increases adenylcyclase activity and the conversion of ATP to cAMP. Peptide cotransmitters, released with noradrenaline and acetylcholine, have recently been isolated and also influence autonomic function. Neuropeptide Y is a peptide of 36 amino acids that is colocated with noradrenaline in most sympathetic nerves and is released with sympathetic stimulation. It is a powerful pressor agent with direct arteriolar vasoconstrictor action and also potentiates the pressor action of noradrenaline.

The distribution of parasympathetic fibres is much more limited, being confined to the sinoatrial and atrioventricular nodes and the atria, with few, if any, fibres reaching the ventricles in humans, except perhaps in relation to coronary arteries and Purkinje tissue. The effects of parasympathetic nerve stimulation are mediated by local acetylcholine release, which slows the heart rate and speed of conduction through the atrioventricular node and Purkinje tissue, and depresses atrial contractility. The negative inotropic effects are associated with a lowering of the concentration of intracellular cAMP.

The effect of the nervous system on the heart at any one time is the sum of the activities of these two opposing control systems. They usually vary reciprocally. Under resting conditions, vagal inhibitory effects predominate, maintaining a slow heart rate, there being virtually no sympathetic outflow. With exercise, there is withdrawal of vagal activity and an increase in sympathetic outflow. Afferents from stretch receptors in the carotid sinus and aortic arch—the baroreceptors—also have a considerable effect on cardiac performance, this effect being mediated via the adrenergic nervous system and vagal withdrawal. A fall in blood pressure reduces stretching in the carotid sinus and inhibitory afferent traffic so that the sympathetic outflow increases. As a consequence of this combined vagal and adrenergic effect, there is a quickening of the heart rate within one or two beats, a positive inotropic effect, and also a constriction of veins and arterioles that increases preload and afterload. Elevation of pressure in the carotid sinus has the reverse effects. In cardiac failure, there is a reduced variability in heart rate due to these autonomic mechanisms as there is then a predominance of adrenergic activity.

There are also mechanoreceptors in all four chambers of the heart (identified in dogs) and in the coronary vessels, which give rise to depressor reflexes. Their clinical relevance is uncertain, but they may contribute, e.g. to the bradycardia and hypotension occurring in some patients with acute myocardial infarction and to the syncope that patients with critical aortic stenosis may experience with the onset of exercise when there is sudden left ventricular distension. Vagal afferents from reflexogenic areas in the infarcting left ventricle may be responsible for the bradycardia, gastric distension, nausea, and vomiting which frequently occur with the onset of inferior or posterior myocardial infarction, but not usually of anterior infarction, which is generally associated with a marked increase in sympathetic activity. The cardiac receptors connected to afferent fibres running in cardiac sympathetic nerves, however, are very important because they are responsible for the perception of cardiac pain. Receptors have also been identified (in animals) at the junction of pulmonary veins with the atrial wall. These respond to mechanical distension with increased sympathetic outflow to the sinus node and inhibition of secretion of antidiuretic hormone from the posterior lobe of the pituitary gland. The result is a quickening of the heart rate and diuresis.

Autonomic efferent activity

The autonomic outflow to the heart is controlled by multiple integrative sites within the central nervous system, with complex interactions between afferent and central inputs. Autonomic responses are mediated through the suprapontine and bulbospinal pathways—both those arising 'reflexively' and those arising from various types of volitional or central 'command'. Nevertheless, intrinsic mechanisms are sufficient for adequate cardiac function in the absence of autonomic control, as prolonged survival after cardiac transplantation has shown. But in the denervated heart, there is blunting of the normally rapid physiological adjustments mediated by the autonomic nervous system.

Diurnal variation in autonomic function

Variations in vascular tone and control of blood pressure and of hormone secretion and platelet function occur in a predictable way throughout the 24-h cycle. In normal subjects, there is a circadian rhythm of blood pressure changes that is not seen in patients, after cardiac transplantation, who have denervated hearts. There is a decline in both blood pressure and heart rate at night, and increases in both soon after wakening. This is due to a normal adrenergic surge in the early morning, which results in increased vascular tone and blood pressure. Increased forearm vascular resistance in the morning, with a reduction in the afternoon and evening, can be clearly identified in humans by assessing responses to α-adrenergic blockade. It is presumed that this occurs in coronary vessels as well. Measurable early morning increases in circulating catecholamines and in the propensity for platelets to aggregate can also be documented.

The circadian rhythm of autonomic function is correlated with a significant tendency for myocardial infarction and sudden cardiac death to occur more frequently in the morning, soon after wakening. There is also an increase in the occurrence of angina pectoris in the early morning, independent of the level of physical activity.

Exercise and the heart: cardiac reserve

The heart responds to exercise with an increase in cardiac output, and values of 30 litres/min may be achieved in a trained athlete. Exercising muscles extract more oxygen from the blood, but the response of the cardiac output is the ultimate determinant of delivery of oxygen to tissues and is the limiting factor for aerobic exercise.

The cardiac response to exercise involves all the mechanisms already discussed. Interaction within the central nervous system between higher and autonomic centres augments sympathetic discharge, and there is a withdrawal of parasympathetic outflow. The heart rate increases immediately, and redistribution of peripheral flow increases venous return and preload. There is venoconstriction, particularly in the large-volume splanchnic circulation, and vasoconstriction and increased oxygen extraction in inactive parts. In active parts, there is vasodilation. This is most evident in the vascular beds of the exercising skeletal muscles and of the heart. The overall effect is a marked lowering of total peripheral vascular resistance, which reduces afterload and encourages greater systolic emptying of the left ventricle. Stroke volume increases during exercise in the upright position. During light to moderate exercise (running or cycling), up to about 80% of maximum exercise capacity there is an almost linear relationship between work intensity and heart rate response, cardiac output, and oxygen uptake. With further exercise, the heart rate and cardiac output responses level off while additional increases in oxygen consumption (c.500 ml) occur by increased oxygen extraction and a greater widening of the arteriovenous difference for oxygen.

The venous return increases in relation to the elevated cardiac output. Vasodilation in the working muscles that receive the bulk of the redirected blood permits high flow rates into the capacitance vessels. Because of adrenergically mediated venoconstriction, the capacity of this system is reduced, so that blood moves rapidly into the right atrium. Venous return is also enhanced by the pumping action of the rhythmically contracting working muscles, by a decrease in intrathoracic pressure with forced inspiration, and by an increase in intra-abdominal pressure. The augmented pulmonary blood flow results in only slight increases in pulmonary artery pressure because of the distensibility of the large pulmonary arteries, an increased area of the pulmonary capillary bed due to the recruitment of more capillaries, and the low resistance offered by the normal pulmonary circulation (see Table 16.1.3.1).

The elevated cardiac output and larger stroke volume result in increased systolic blood pressure and pulse pressure, even though the afterload itself is reduced. Enhanced neurohumoral activity from adrenergic stimulation of the heart and the suprarenal glands (increased circulating adrenaline and noradrenaline) effect positive inotropic changes, to which tachycardia also contributes because of the Bowditch effect. There is a shift in the Frank–Starling relationship to the left, increased speed and force of cardiac contraction, and elevated ejection fraction and stroke volume. Peak dp/dt is increased, and there is a rapid rise in coronary blood flow to meet myocardial oxygen requirements that increase linearly with the product of systolic blood pressure and heart rate. During moderate exercise, these changes together result in a decreased or unaltered end-diastolic volume and decreased end-systolic volume. With severe exercise, end-diastolic dimensions and end-diastolic fibre length are slightly increased and the Frank–Starling mechanism then operates and further augments the force of contraction.

The haemodynamic and ventilatory responses evoked by an increase to a new steady workload take about 2 to 3 min to equilibrate and adjust oxygen supply to the greater demand. Protocols for exercise testing are therefore usually based on work increments at 3-min intervals to allow time for a new 'steady state' to occur, e.g. in the standard Bruce Exercise Protocol. A steady state becomes progressively more difficult to maintain as maximal exercise capacity is approached. Glycogen is used by the working skeletal muscles as a source of stored energy, and the anaerobic metabolism which ensues produces lactic acidosis and thereby further increases ventilation. As all cardiopulmonary transport mechanisms reach maximum levels, shortness of breath, fatigue, and muscle pain become limiting symptoms; motivation is then the final determinant of the duration of exercise. Ageing reduces the efficacy of cardiopulmonary transport mechanisms and, of course, exercise capacity. The heart rate response at peak exercise reflects this. In healthy individuals aged 20 years it is about 200 beats/min, and at 65 years about 170 beats/min.

When exercise stops, the cardiopulmonary and metabolic changes return rapidly to resting levels, the rate following an exponential pattern in the first few minutes; the excretion and metabolism of lactate and other substances, and the dissipation of heat generated take longer (time constant of about 15 min or more). Reduced circulatory function slows the recovery rate.

Training effects

Regular exercise to about 60% of maximal heart rate for 20 to 30 min three times a week is the minimum requirement for improved effort tolerance due to a training effect. The resting heart rate becomes slower, while the cardiac output is maintained by an increased end-diastolic volume and ejection fraction, and therefore stroke volume. In a 'trained' exercising individual, there is a reduced heart rate response to a standard submaximal workload, and systemic blood flow is more effectively distributed away from visceral and skin circulations to working muscles. Changes in

muscle mitochondria permit increased oxygen consumption. There is suggestive animal evidence that prolonged endurance training increases the calibre of coronary arteries and enlarges capillary surface area relative to cardiac muscle mass. Myocardial protein synthesis increases. Adrenergic mechanisms appear to be involved in mediating this response. Rhythmic exercise (e.g. running) and isometric exercise (e.g. weightlifting) have different physiological effects. The blood pressure rises disproportionately during the latter. The mechanisms are partly reflex and partly mechanical from the contracting muscles. Isometric exercise training is not recommended for cardiac patients because of the increased afterload it imposes.

Regular exercise has other effects: it increases feelings of well-being and lowers blood pressure in normotensive and mildly hypertensive subjects. There are also diverse exercise-related hormonal changes, including the reduction of glucose-stimulated insulin secretion—of particular relevance to patients with type 2 diabetes. Regular exercise also improves the availability of nitric oxide, with its important vascular effects. These are considered elsewhere.

To summarize, changes in the four essential determinants of cardiac function—preload, afterload, heart rate, and contractility—combine to augment cardiac output and oxygen delivery during exercise. Measurement of the cardiovascular response to exercise is essential for the objective assessment of cardiac function.

Further reading

Ganong WF (2005). *Review of medical physiology*, 22nd edition. McGraw Hill, New York.

Jones NL, Killian KJ (2000). Exercise limitation in health and disease. *N Engl J Med*, **243**, 632–41.

Katz, Arnold M (2006). *Physiology of the Normal Heart*, 4th edition, Lippincott Williams and Wilkins, Philadelphia.

Libby P, *et al.* (eds) (2008). *Braunwald's Heart Disease; a textbook of cardiovascular medicine*, 8th edition, Saunders Elsevier, Philadelphia.

Young ME (2006). The circadian clock within the heart: potential influence on myocardial gene expression, metabolism, and function. *Am J Physiol Heart Circ Physiol*, **290**, 1–16.[†] It is with regret that we report the death of Professor Poole-Wilson during the preparation of this edition of the textbook.

Clinical presentation of heart disease

Contents

16.2.1 Chest pain, breathlessness, and fatigue

J. Dwight

Essentials

Chest pain, breathlessness, and fatigue are common diagnostic challenges. They have a broad differential diagnosis that includes a number of life-threatening pathologies.

Chest pain

The most reliable discriminating feature for angina, as opposed to other causes of chest pain, is a fixed and predictable relationship to exertion that is relieved, within a few minutes, by rest or glyceryl trinitrate.

The ECG is used to triage patients with chest pain on admission to the Emergency Department, with treatment by thrombolysis or angioplasty after a brief confirmatory history in patients with significant ST elevation. However, these represent only a small fraction of those presenting with chest pain, and patients without ST elevation present the greater diagnostic challenge. A detailed history is needed to establish whether the pain is cardiac, and to inform the risk-stratification process that determines the nature and time course of subsequent therapy and investigation.

The character of pain in acute coronary syndromes is similar to exertional angina, but usually more severe. It usually reaches maximal intensity over the course of a few minutes: pain reaching its maximum intensity instantaneously suggests an alternative cause.

Aortic dissection is a rare but important cause of chest pain: its pain is very sudden in onset, usually described as tearing or ripping, and the patient may report that it migrates from the front to the back of the chest. Pain with this description, loss of peripheral pulses, blood pressure difference between the two arms (>20 mmHg), and mediastinal widening on the chest radiograph are the most helpful diagnostic indicators.

Pericarditis occurs most commonly following myocardial infarction or viral infection. The pain is usually sharp and precordial, its onset is often sudden, and it is characteristically worse on inspiration, but is relieved by sitting up and leaning forward. A pericardial friction rub heard over the sternum may be positional and can appear and disappear within hours.

Breathlessness and fatigue

Most patients find it impossible to distinguish between cardiac and pulmonary causes of dyspnoea. The New York Heart Association classification is used to classify the extent of disability.

In the diagnosis of left ventricular failure, the most helpful features in the history are exertional breathlessness, orthopnoea, paroxysmal nocturnal dyspnoea, or a history of myocardial infarction. Tachycardia, cyanosis, and an elevated jugular venous pressure are features of heart failure, but they are also features of the major differential diagnoses. A displaced apex on palpation is helpful and relatively specific. A third heart sound has a high specificity (90–97%) but low sensitivity (31–51%) for detecting left ventricular dysfunction. Basal inspiratory crackles are suggestive of pulmonary oedema but have a sensitivity and specificity as low as 13 and 35%, respectively.

Other considerations

The cardiovascular history routinely includes assessment of risk factors and those aspects of the patient's past medical history that make cardiovascular disease more likely. The presence of numerous risk factors may, on occasion, prompt the physician to proceed to further investigation even in the face of a relatively unconvincing history.

Most diagnoses are made on the basis of the history, and the physician is always compelled to return to the initial history and examination to put the findings of any investigations into context and to plan therapy appropriate for the individual patient.

Introduction

The symptoms of chest pain, breathlessness, and fatigue present a frequent diagnostic challenge in the outpatient and acute medical departments as well as the Emergency Department. They have a broad differential diagnosis that includes a number of life-threatening pathologies.

As with all clinical presentations, the initial presenting symptom will prompt a differential diagnosis that the physician must narrow down, using a thorough history, to one or two possibilities. The onset, nature, and precipitating causes of symptoms need to be accurately defined, with carefully directed questions used to assess their relevance. The process involves a partnership between the patient and their doctor, and is enhanced by explaining the reasoning behind the questions asked and their relevance to making a diagnosis. In this way history-taking is a useful opportunity to assist the patient to a better understanding of their symptoms and to improve their compliance with any management plan.

The cardiovascular history routinely includes assessment of risk factors such as age, occupation, diabetes, hypertension, smoking, hypercholesterolaemia, drugs (both therapeutic and recreational), and a family history. It should also record those aspects of the patient's past medical history that make cardiovascular disease more likely, e.g. stroke, transient ischaemic attack, claudication, vascular surgery, renal disease, or connective tissue disease. The presence of numerous risk factors may, on occasion, prompt the physician to proceed to further investigation even in the face of a relatively unconvincing history.

Armed with a differential diagnosis obtained from the history, the physical examination is directed to identifying further supporting evidence. In isolation, however, there are surprisingly few examination findings that will provide a definitive diagnosis.

The cardiologist has a large armamentarium of diagnostic tools available to assist in making a diagnosis—ECG, echocardiography, coronary angiography, MRI, etc. These may appear to threaten to displace history-taking with the allure of high-definition images and impressive software. However, most diagnoses are made on the basis of the history, and the physician is always compelled to return to the initial history and examination to put the findings of any investigations into context and to plan therapy appropriate for the individual patient.

Chest pain

Chest pain accounts for up to 20% of all medical consultations and is one of the commonest presentations to the Emergency Department. In the community setting musculoskeletal or gastrointestinal causes are most common, whereas cardiac causes are more frequent in the Emergency Department (Table 16.2.1.1).

The circumstances of chest pain

Chest pain on exertion: angina pectoris

> They who are afflicted with it are seized while they are walking (more especially if it be uphill and soon after eating) with a painful and most disagreeable sensation of the breast, which seems as if it would extinguish life, if it were to increase or continue, but the moment they stand still, all this uneasiness vanishes. (Heberden 1768)

Unfortunately for the physician, the descriptors used by patients with angina are highly variable and include burning, heaviness,

Table 16.2.1.1 Cardiovascular causes of chest pain and differential diagnoses

Frequency as cause of chest pain	Cardiovascular	Noncardiovascular
Common	Angina	Oesophageal reflux
	Acute coronary syndromes	Pleurisy
	Pericarditis	Spinal root compression
	Pulmonary embolism	Costochondritis
	Syndrome X	Muscular/ arthropathies
	Tachyarrhythmias	
Uncommon	Valvular heart disease	Pneumothorax
	Pulmonary hypertension	Herpes zoster
	Aortic dissection	Peptic ulcer disease
	Myocarditis	Pulmonary or mediastinal tumours
		Mediastinitis

tightness, pressure, squeezing, aching, and strangling. Patients may not describe pain and it is preferable to ask for symptoms of discomfort in the chest. Most patients with angina recognize the pain as being worrying or serious. The location of the discomfort is usually retrosternal and may radiate to the arms, neck, and jaw (Fig. 16.2.1.1). Less commonly the pain may be felt in the back and upper abdomen.

The most reliable discriminating feature for angina as opposed to other causes of chest pain is a fixed and predictable relationship to exertion that is relieved within a few minutes by rest or glyceryl trinitrate. The discomfort characteristically occurs when walking on an incline and compels the patient to stop. In some cases the characteristic symptoms occur at the start of exertion and then ease, which is termed 'walk-through angina'. Surprisingly, patients may still be able to perform substantial anaerobic exercise without limitation. Angina is often worse in cold weather, in a cold wind, or after eating. Occasionally the pain is only present at the start of the day, when the patient is shaving or brushing their teeth. Symptoms of chest discomfort occurring after rather than during exertion, or which are present continuously throughout the day, are not due to angina.

Taking a careful history of the time course of relief with rest and glyceryl trinitrate is important. Many patients mistakenly report a response to glyceryl trinitrate when their pain has taken more than 15 min to resolve, but a response to glyceryl trinitrate is only helpful diagnostically when it occurs within a few minutes. Oesophageal spasm also responds to glyceryl trinitrate and may produce similar discomfort, but the pain is not related to exertion and is nearly always associated with symptoms of reflux.

Chest pain at rest

Chest pain due to ischaemia that occurs at rest has a broader differential diagnosis. Arrhythmias, e.g. paroxysmal atrial fibrillation, may precipitate angina at rest and a history of palpitations should be sought in those with unpredictable symptoms. Emotional stress may also precipitate an attack. Nocturnal angina may be precipitated by nightmares or the onset of pulmonary oedema, but a history of

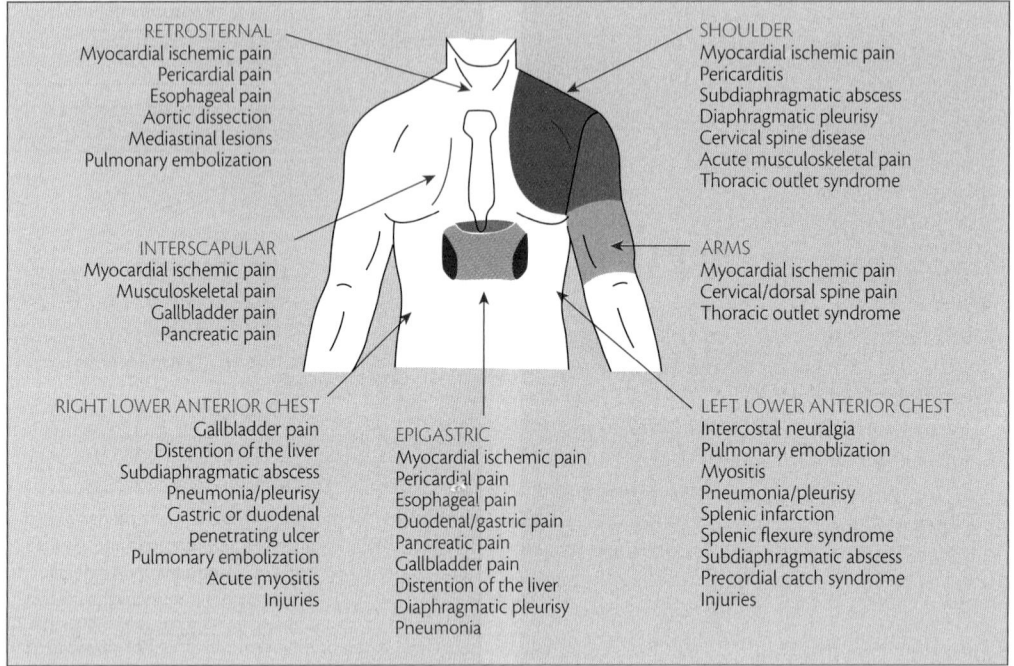

Fig. 16.2.1.1 Differential diagnosis of chest pain according to location and radiation. Serious intrathoracic or sub diaphragmatic diseases are usually associated with pains that begin in the left anterior chest, left shoulder, or upper arm, the interscapular region, or the epigastrium. The scheme is not all inclusive (e.g. intercostal neuralgia occurs in locations other than the left, lower anterior chest area).
From Miller AJ: Diagnosis of Chest Pain. New York, Raven Press (LWW), 1988, p 175.

exertional angina is nearly always present. Where nocturnal chest pain is present in the absence of exertional symptoms a history of acid reflux (relief on sitting up or with antacids, and discomfort on drinking hot fluids) should be sought. Reflux symptoms are common and may coexist with angina, and the patient may find it impossible to differentiate between the two.

Once alternative causes have been excluded, newly presenting ischaemic-sounding chest pain at rest, or which is rapidly progressive (indicated by a sudden reduction in the patient's exercise tolerance over days or weeks), usually points to a diagnosis of an acute coronary syndrome.

Particular causes of chest pain

Acute coronary syndromes

The term 'acute coronary syndrome' encompasses myocardial infarction and unstable angina, conditions which are usually caused by a common pathology, the rupture or erosion of an atheromatous plaque. Because of the need for rapid assessment and treatment, the ECG is often used to triage patients with chest pain on admission to the Emergency Department. Where there are classic features of ST elevation infarction, treatment is commenced with thrombolysis or angioplasty after a brief confirmatory history (see Chapter 16.13.5). However, patients with ST elevation represent only a small fraction of those presenting with chest pain, and those without ST elevation present the greater diagnostic challenge. Some will simply have dyspepsia or musculolskeletal pain, whereas those at the other end of the spectrum will be at imminent risk of myocardial infarction. The history has two important roles: first to establish whether the pain is cardiac, and secondly to contribute to the risk-stratification process that determines the nature and time course subsequent therapy and investigation.

The character of pain in acute coronary syndromes is similar to exertional angina, but usually more severe. It usually reaches maximal intensity over the course of a few minutes. Pain reaching its maximum intensity instantaneously suggests an alternative cause. The patient should be asked to describe exactly what they were doing at the onset of the pain: sudden onset during a specific movement will suggest a musculoskeletal origin.

The classical description of the pain of myocardial infarction is of a heavy, crushing or constricting pain. In comparison to angina the duration of pain in myocardial infarction is longer (>15 min), and with increasing duration myocardial infarction is more likely, but the pain rarely lasts more than a few hours. Infarction is more likely to be associated with systemic symptoms (breathlessness, sweating, nausea and vomiting) and does not respond to glyceryl trinitrate. About one-half of patients will have a history suggestive of worsening exertional angina, or short-lived episodes of chest pain at rest before presentation. The pain of an acute coronary syndrome usually discourages the patient from attempting any exertion and does not improve with exercise. Although the history alone cannot definitively rule out myocardial infarction, it can be used to assess the probability of this condition (Box 16.2.1.1).

During the examination the patient should be asked to map out the distribution of the pain. Highly localized pain of less than a few centimetres in distribution is unlikely to ischaemic in origin. Tenderness on palpation of the chest wall or pain exacerbated by rotation of the thorax or passive movements of the arms or neck suggest musculoskeletal pain.

Components of the history, the ECG, and markers of myocardial damage are used in non-ST elevation acute coronary syndromes to determine the risk of subsequent events in the TIMI (Thrombolysis in Myocardial Infarction) risk score (Table 16.2.1.2). Great emphasis

Low risk

- Pain that is pleuritic, positional, or reproducible with palpation, or is described as stabbing

Probably low risk

- Pain not related to exertion or that occurs in a small inframammary area of the chest

Probably high risk

- Pain described as pressure, is similar to that of a prior myocardial infarction or worse than prior anginal pain, or is accompanied by nausea, vomiting, or diaphoresis

High risk

- Pain that radiates to one or both shoulders or arms or is related to exertion

has been placed on the use of troponin estimation in determining the risk of subsequent events in these patients and this is undoubtedly a useful tool. However, in the absence of definitive ECG changes or troponin rise, the patient may still score 5 on the history alone, giving a risk of 25% of major cardiovascular adverse events in the next 14 days. For further discussion see Chapter 16.13.5.

There are no specific findings on cardiovascular examination in acute coronary syndromes. In the context of severe coronary disease the patient may present with the clinical features of left ventricular failure (see below) or cardiogenic shock. Features of increased sympathetic tone, pallor, tachycardia, and sweating are often present in infarction, but are also features of all causes of severe chest pain and of fear. A pansystolic murmur may indicate the development of a ventricular septal defect or papillary muscle rupture and severe mitral regurgitation, complications which are usually associated with haemodynamic compromise and left ventricular failure.

The presence or peripheral vascular disease increases the probability of coexistent coronary disease and the patient should be examined for carotid, femoral, and renal bruits and an abdominal aortic aneurysm. The foot pulses should also be assessed.

Table 16.2.1.2 TIMI risk score for non-ST elevation acute coronary syndromes

Clinical feature	Points
Age ≥65 years	1
At least three risk factors for coronary disease[a]	1
Prior demonstration of significant coronary artery stenosis	1
ST deviation on ECG	1
Severe anginal symptoms (e.g. ≥2 anginal events in the last 24 h)	1
Use of aspirin in previous 7 days	1
Elevated cardiac markers (e.g. troponin)	1

[a] Family history, hypertension, hypercholesterolaemia, diabetes, current smoking.
From Antman et al JAMA 2000; 284:835–842.

The presence of neck and/or chest-wall tenderness will point to alternative diagnoses such as cervical spondylopathy, costochondritis, or nerve entrapment. Hypochondrial tenderness suggests a gastrointestinal cause, e.g. peptic ulcer disease, pancreatitis, or gallstones.

Coronary spasm, Prinzmetal's angina, syndrome X, atypical angina

Patients with unpredictable angina due to the occurrence of coronary spasm, either in the context of coronary disease or with normal coronary arteries, have been described. The diagnosis should only be considered in the patient with a classical description of ischaemic chest pain that usually responds rapidly to glyceryl trinitrate, preferably in the context of ECG changes (ST elevation in the case of Prinzmetal's angina). Cocaine abuse is now a frequent cause of this presentation to the Emergency Department.

Syndrome X, as its name suggests, is poorly understood. This label (whether it can properly be called a diagnosis is debatable) is often attached to patients with cardiac-sounding chest pain and a normal angiogram. This finding is more common in women. The pain often has features atypical of angina. It is often of submammary location or radiation, and precipitating factors are highly variable. This diagnosis should only be considered after other causes of chest pain have been carefully excluded, since it may expose the patient to a lifetime of inappropriate treatment and anxiety.

The term 'atypical chest pain' is meaningless (especially for the patient) and is best avoided. There are, however, many patients for whom a confident diagnosis cannot be made. Serious pathology can be excluded and the patient can be reassured that they have an excellent prognosis. It is better to leave the diagnosis at 'chest pain,? cause' than to inappropriately label the patient as having 'atypical angina' or syndrome X.

Aortic dissection

Aortic dissection is a rare but important cause of chest pain: up to half of all patients with an untreated proximal aortic dissection die within 48 h. The pain of aortic dissection is very sudden in onset, is usually described as tearing or ripping, and the patient may report that it migrates from the front to the back of the chest. There should be a particularly high index of suspicion when chest pain is associated with neurological features such as hemiplegia or paraplegia due to involvement of the carotid vessels and spinal arteries, but these are present in less than 20% of cases. Risk factors in the history include hypertension, Marfan's syndrome, a bicuspid aortic valve, previous aortic valve replacement, cocaine usage, and the third trimester of pregnancy. Of the clinical features (see Box 16.2.1.2) aortic pain (as described above), loss of peripheral pulses, blood pressure difference between the two arms (>20 mmHg), and mediastinal widening on the chest radiograph are the most helpful. In the absence of these features the incidence of aortic dissection is less than 5%. The absolute level of blood pressure in unhelpful in discriminating aortic dissection from other causes of chest pain.

Pericarditis

Pericarditis occurs most commonly following a myocardial infarction or viral infection. The patient may describe a preceding viral illness with fever and cough. The pain is usually sharp and precordial. The onset is often sudden. It is characteristically worse on

Box 16.2.1.2 Clinical features associated with aortic dissection

- Sudden onset tearing, ripping chest pain that migrates to the back
- Loss of peripheral pulses
- Blood pressure difference >20 mmHg between arms
- Hemiparesis
- Paraparesis
- Diastolic murmur
- Pleural effusion (usually left sided)
- Hoarseness
- Horner's syndrome
- Bilateral testicular tenderness
- Pulsatile stenoclavicular joint
- Superior vena cava obstruction
- Pulsus paradoxus (with pericardial tamponade)

inspiration and relieved by sitting up and leaning forward, and it can be accompanied by classic pleuritic pain. A less typical description occurs when a pericardial effusion has developed and the pain arises from pericardial distension, when the pain may be a dull restrosternal ache or pressure. Radiation of pericarditic pain occurs to all those areas associated with myocardial infarction, but radiation to the trapezius ridges is pathognomic of the diagnosis.

The patient is usually well and not compromised haemodynamically (except where there is pericardial tamponade). Clinical examination may initially be normal. A pericardial friction rub heard over the sternum may be positional and appear and disappear within hours. Repeated examination may be helpful, including auscultation of the patient lying flat in expiration. The ECG finding of concave ST elevation in multiple lead is helpful, but ECG findings are equivocal or normal in 40 to 50% of cases.

Breathlessness and fatigue

Breathlessness (or dyspnoea, derived from Greek words meaning painful or difficult breathing) is the endpoint of a variety of pathologies and is mediated by a series of neural pathways, the sensory inputs of which originate in the lungs, chest wall, and peripheral and sensory chemoreceptors (see Fig. 16.2.1.2). Patients may describe the sensation of breathlessness as tightness, wheeze, 'inability to get enough air', sighing, choking, or suffocating. Heart failure, asthma, and chronic obstructive airways disease account for about three-quarters of hospital admissions with breathlessness in industrialized nations. Symptom clusters have been described for these pathologies, but most patients find it impossible to distinguish between cardiac and pulmonary causes of dyspnoea.

The time course of the illness is an important aid to the diagnosis in patients with dyspnoea but must be interpreted in the context of the patient's day-to-day activities. Even when the disease progresses gradually the patient may report a recent onset of symptoms because they have (often subconsciously) adapted their lifestyle over the course of many months. This is particularly true of patients with chronic heart failure.

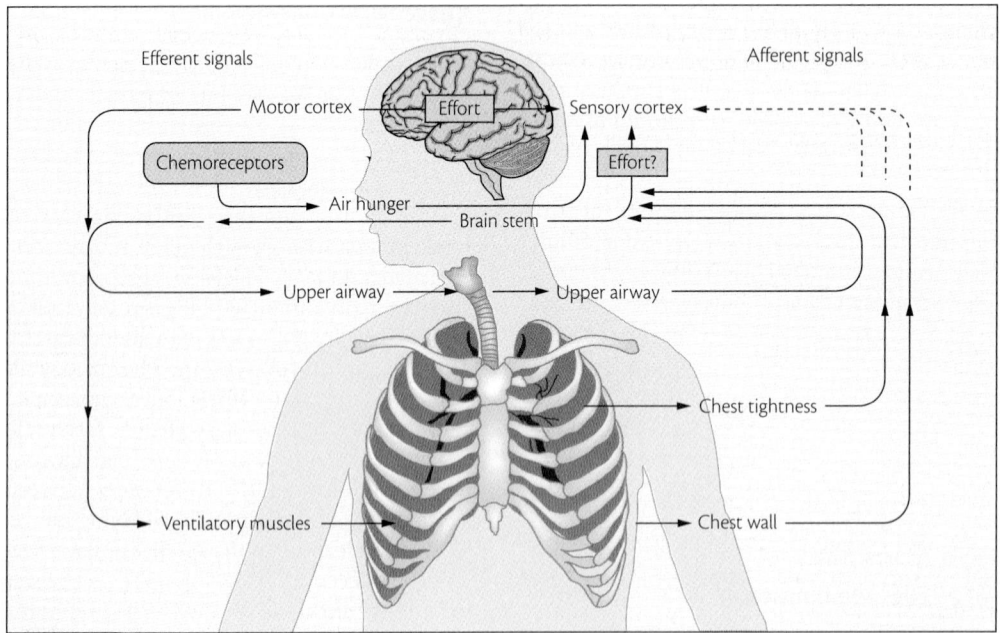

Fig. 16.2.1.2 Efferent and afferent signals that contribute to the sensation of dyspnea. The sense of respiratory effort is believed to arise from a signal transmitted from the motor cortex to the sensory cortex coincidently with the outgoing motor command to the ventilatory muscles. The arrow from the brainstem to the sensory cortex indicates that the motor output of the brainstem may also contribute to the sense of effort The sense of air hunger is believed to arise, in part, from Increased respiratory activity within the brainstem, and the sensation of chest tightness probably results from stimulation of vagal-irritant receptors. Although afferent Information from airway, lung, and chest-wall receptors most likely passes through the brainstem before reaching the sensory cortex, the dashed lines indicate uncertainty about whether some afferents bypass the brainstem and project directly to the sensory cortex.
From Manning.H.L Schwartzstein RM New England Journal of Medicine. 333. 1547–1553. http://content.nejm.org/cgi/content/extract/333/23/1547.

Table 16.2.1.3 New York Heart Association classification of breathlessness according to severity

Class I	No limitation—ordinary physical activity does not cause undue fatigue, dyspnoea, or palpitation
Class II	Slight limitation of physical activity—comfortable at rest, but ordinary physical activity results in fatigue, dyspnoea, or palpitation
Class III	Marked limitation of physical activity—comfortable at rest, but less than normal activity produces symptoms
Class IV	Inability to carry out any physical activity without discomfort

Until relatively recently, symptoms of fatigue and breathlessness in heart failure have been assumed to be due purely to a combination of poor cardiac output and pulmonary congestion. However, in patients with heart failure the correlation between symptoms and left ventricular ejection fraction is very poor. Changes in skeletal and respiratory muscle function appear to contribute significantly to symptoms, a hypothesis that is supported by the response observed to exercise training programmes in patients with chronic heart failure, and which may account for part of the considerable variability in disability in patients with similar haemodynamic and echocardiographic findings. Because of the contribution of fatigue it is more helpful to ask about a change in exercise tolerance in patients with suspected heart failure, since this may correlate more closely with the underlying pathology. The New York Heart Association classification is used to classify the extent of disability (Table 16.2.1.3).

The time course of onset of breathlessness can be particularly useful in determining the underlying pathology (Table 16.2.1.4).

Breathlessness of dramatic onset (over minutes) is suggestive of pulmonary embolism, pulmonary oedema, upper airway obstruction, or a pneumothorax. Chronic dyspnoea presents in the context of worsening breathlessness over a period of months or years and is typical of chronic obstructive airways disease, interstitial lung disease, or anaemia, but may be a feature of heart failure. Acute on chronic dyspnoea indicates an exacerbation of breathlessness in a patient with established disease.

Chronic obstructive airways disease, asthma, and heart failure are common in the population of industrialized countries and most elderly patients presenting to the Emergency Department with breathing difficulties will have a prior history of pulmonary or cardiac disease. However, it is important not to automatically attribute any deterioration in symptoms as being due to progression of their underlying disease process. Alternative causes should be considered, and this situation is often a major diagnostic challenge. A common example is a sudden deterioration in the patient with long-standing well-controlled heart failure, which should prompt consideration of further pathology such as a silent myocardial infarction, pulmonary embolism, or arrhythmia.

Breathlessness at rest occurs in pulmonary embolism or pulmonary oedema, and with a pneumothorax. Exertional dyspnoea occurs in left ventricular failure and chronic obstructive airways disease. Psychogenic breathlessness is frequently present at rest and is associated with sighing, features of hyperventilation such as perioral or peripheral paraesthesiae, and chest tightness. The presence of breathlessness at rest but not on exertion strongly suggests a functional origin.

Particular causes of breathlessness

Left ventricular failure

The incidence of left ventricular failure in the community is 1 to 2%. It is important to attempt to identify the cause during the initial assessment. A history of ischaemic or valvular heart disease, alcohol abuse, smoking, diabetes, hypertension, and a family history are important.

Patients with left ventricular failure commonly present to the outpatient clinic, but may present for the first time to the

Table 16.2.1.4 Conditions causing breathlessness classified by the rate of onset

Acute	Acute on chronic	Chronic
Asthma	Infective exacerbation of COPD	COPD
Myocardial infarction	Decompensated chronic heart failure	Cardiac failure
Pulmonary embolism	Pulmonary embolism complicating congestive cardiac failure or COPD	Anaemia
Cardiogenic pulmonary oedema (secondary to ischaemia, valvular disease, arrhythmias)	Pneumothorax complicating COPD or asthma	Pulmonary vascular disease (pulmonary embolism, pulmonary hypertension)
Pneumonia	Atrial fibrillation/flutter complicating COPD or cardiac failure	Parenchymal lung disease, e.g. UIP, sarcoid
Noncardiogenic pulmonary oedema	Chordal rupture in chronic nonrheumatic mitral regurgitation	Pleural disease, e.g. effusion, asbestosis
Pulmonary haemorrhage		Chest wall disease e.g. kyphosis, ankylosing spondylitis.
Spontaneous pneumothorax		Neuromuscular disorders, e.g. muscular dystrophy, polio, myasthenia gravis
Chest trauma		Malignancy
Upper airway obstruction		Obesity/deconditioning
Hyperventilation syndrome		Sleep apnoea
		Silent myocardial ischaemia

Emergency Department. An acute presentation is more likely when there has been a rapid rise in the left atrial pressure generating pulmonary oedema. In severe cases this is associated with haemoptysis in the form of frothy pink sputum. This type of presentation occurs with myocardial infarction, mitral valve papillary muscle or chordal rupture, malignant hypertension, tachyarrhythmias, and endocarditis with major valve destruction. Where a rise in left atrial pressure occurs over a longer time course, sustained elevated left atrial pressures are compensated for by increased lymphatic drainage and structural changes in the pulmonary capillary and alveolar basement membrane (see Chapter 16.15.3) and patients more commonly present with fatigue, exertional breathlessness, and orthopnoea. Prolonged increases in left atrial pressure are associated with pulmonary hypertension and the associated clinical features of right ventricular enlargement, tricuspid regurgitation, and a loud pulmonary second sound. This type of presentation is more frequently a feature of patients with an idiopathic, ischaemic, hypertensive, or alcoholic cardiomyopathy.

Clinical findings that help in assessing impaired left ventricular function or elevated left atrial filling pressures are shown in Table 16.2.1.5.

The most helpful features in the history are exertional breathlessness, orthopnoea, paroxysmal nocturnal dyspnoea, or a history of myocardial infarction. Breathlessness that is worse on lying flat and relieved promptly on sitting up is characteristic for orthopnoea. Patients with chronic obstructive airways disease may also describe orthopnoea, but this is usually present only in the setting of severe disease and chronic breathlessness at rest. Paroxysmal nocturnal dyspnoea is due to the development of interstitial oedema and typically occurs 2 to 4h after the onset of sleep. The patient usually stands up or sits on the side of the bed and symptoms resolve over the course of 10 to 15min. This is usually a frightening and memorable experience for the patient, and to avoid these symptoms they will sleep propped up on pillows or, in severe cases, in a chair. However, a history of paroxysmal nocturnal dyspnoea or orthopnoea is only present in 20% of patients and its absence does not exclude the diagnosis of heart failure. Ankle oedema is supportive of a diagnosis of heart failure, but dependent oedema is often present in older people and in patients with chronic obstructive airways disease, and the astute physician should avoid the common mistake of assuming that 'ankle oedema means cardiac failure means diuretic prescription'.

The clinical examination findings are used to support a suspected diagnosis of heart failure, but they are not always helpful. Tachycardia, cyanosis, and an elevated jugular venous pressure are features of heart failure, but they are also features of the major differential diagnoses, pulmonary embolism, and chronic obstructive airways disease. Although jugular venous pressure correlates with left atrial pressure it may be misleading in the presence of isolated right ventricular dysfunction, tricuspid regurgitation, and pulmonary hypertension. A displaced apex on palpation is helpful and relatively specific. Basal inspiratory crackles (rales) are suggestive of pulmonary oedema but can be present in fibrotic lung disease infection and chronic airways disease and have a sensitivity and specificity as low as 13% and 35% respectively. The third sound—a low-pitched sound heard in mid diastolic, best with the bell of the stethoscope placed lightly over the apex—can be confused with a split second sound, but is later in diastole and has a much longer duration. It has a high specificity (90–97%) but low sensitivity (31–51%) for detecting left ventricular dysfunction.

Fever and purulent sputum usually point to a diagnosis of an infective exacerbation of chronic bronchitis or chest infection. In older people, however, a chest infection may precipitate decompensation of heart failure.

Left ventricular failure is highly unlikely in the presence of a genuinely normal ECG, whilst the presence of Q waves in the anterior chest leads is highly predictive of left ventricular dysfunction.

The most useful finding on chest radiography is cardiomegaly, but heart size may be normal, particularly in diastolic heart failure. Changes of pulmonary venous distension, pulmonary oedema, and pleural effusion are more common in acute presentations, but are frequently absent in patients presenting with chronic breathlessness.

Following clinical assessment, including ECG and chest radiography, there may still be considerable uncertainty about the diagnosis of the cause of breathlessness, particularly in patients presenting to the Emergency Department. Measurement of blood brain natriuretic peptide (BNP) may assist in a more rapid and accurate diagnosis in this circumstance, a level below 100 pg/ml (>300 pg/ml for NT-proBNP) making the diagnosis of left ventricular failure highly unlikely, such that alternative diagnoses should be considered. High levels (>500 pg/ml) are strongly suggestive of heart failure, but intermediate levels are more difficult to interpret as there are a number of confounding factors for BNP measurement (Table 16.2.1.6)

As with troponin (see Chapter 16.13.5), BNP levels must be interpreted in the context of the history, clinical findings and other investigations. A scoring system has been devised for using BNP and other clinical and investigation findings in acute dyspnoea (Fig. 16.2.1.3).

Table 16.2.1.5 Helpful clinical findings for predicting heart failure in patients presenting with dyspnoea

	Increased filling pressure	Ejection fraction <40%
Very helpful findings (significant in all studies)	Jugular venous distension	Abnormal apical impulse
	Radiographic redistribution	Anterior Q waves
		Left bundle branch block
		Radiographic cardiomegaly or redistribution
Somewhat helpful findings (significant in most studies)	Orthopnoea	Any previous myocardial infarction
	Tachycardia	Pulse >90/min
	Low systolic blood pressure	Systolic blood pressure <90 mmHg
	Proportional blood pressure[a] <25%	Proportional pulse pressure[a] <33%
	Abnormal abdominojugular reflux	Third heart sound
	Crepitations	Crepitations
	Radiographic cardiomegaly	Raised CK (troponin)
Findings only helpful when present (highly specific)	Leg oedema	Jugular venous distension
		Oedema

[a] Pulse pressure/systolic pressure.
Adapted from Badgett R.G., Lucey C.R., Mulrow.C.D., Can the clinical examination diagnose left-sided heart failure in adults? JAMA 1997;277:1712–1719.

Table 16.2.1.6 Confounding factors in the interpretation of BNP measurements

Increased BNP	Decreased BNP
Increasing age	Obesity
Female sex	Cardioactive drugs
Pulmonary disease	ACE inhibitors
Systemic hypertension	Spironolactone
Hyperthryoidism	β-Blockers (long term)
Cushing's syndrome	Diuretics
Glucocorticoid usage	
Conn's syndrome	
Hepatic cirrhosis with ascites	
Renal failure	
Paraneoplastic syndrome	
Subarachnoid haemorrhage	

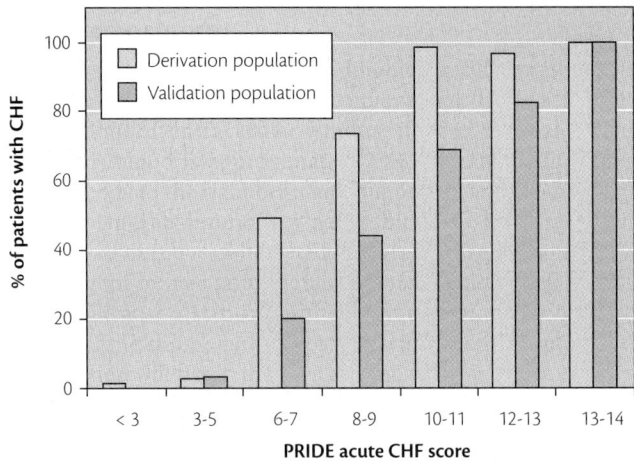

Fig. 16.2.1.3 Scoring system to predict whether a patient presenting to the Emergency Department has congestive heart failure (CHF). The patient's total score (maximum 14) is obtained by adding the points that they score for each clinical or investigation feature:

Clinical and investigation findings	Points
Elevated NT-proBNP	4
Interstitial oedema on chest radiograph	2
Orthopnoea	2
Absence of fever	2
Current loop diuretics	1
Age >75	1
Crepitations (rales) on lung examination	1
Absence of cough	1

Reprinted from *Am J Heart*, Vol 151 (1), Baggish A.L et al, A validated clinical and biochemical score for the diagnosis of acute heart failure: the Pro-BNP Investigation of Dyspnoea in the Emergency Department (PRIDE) acute heart failure score, pp48–54. Copyright (2006), with permission from Elsevier.

Given the relatively poor predictive value of the clinical history and physical signs in the diagnosis left ventricular failure, open access to echocardiography may appear superior to clinical assessment. However, there are important arguments for careful clinical assessment. Firstly, echocardiography is not always available in the emergency setting. Secondly, cardiac and noncardiac causes of dyspnoea (particularly chronic obstructive pulmonary disease (COPD) often coexist, and where there is dual pathology, deciding which treatment to escalate is more dependent on the appropriate interpretation of the symptoms, clinical signs, and chest radiographic findings than echocardiographic parameters. Thirdly, heart failure may be present in the presence of apparently preserved systolic function on echocardiography.

Airways disease

The clinical features of heart failure and airways disease are often difficult to distinguish. Patients with lung disease tend to use the terms 'chest tightness' or 'restriction', whereas the patient with heart failure is more inclined to describe the sensation of 'not being able to get enough air'. Patients are more likely to have COPD if they have a self-reported history of COPD, wheezing on examination (although this can be a feature of heart failure), and a forced expiratory time ≥9 s and laryngeal descent. Clearly COPD is very unlikely in the absence of a smoking history and in patients under 45 years of age. Patients with COPD and left ventricular failure may suffer from a chronic cough, although in the case of heart failure this is usually a dry cough and more prominent at night.

Fluid retention giving rise to an elevated jugular venous pressure and ankle oedema can occur in association with hypoxia, but only if saturations are persistently less than 94%. Ankle oedema may also be a feature of chronic CO_2 retention. Although often cited as a cause of the clinical features of right heart failure in COPD, true right ventricular failure is relatively uncommon and the mechanism of fluid retention is complex. COPD and heart failure often coexist.

The chest radiograph may be unhelpful and patients with emphysema and left ventricular failure may not have any radiological features of pulmonary congestion or oedema. In these situations systolic heart failure can only be ruled out by echocardiography.

Pulmonary embolism

Pulmonary embolism is a common differential diagnosis in patients with breathlessness and should be considered in any presenting with breathlessness without clinical signs of left ventricular failure. The acute presenting symptoms are of breathlessness (usually of sudden onset), chest pain (classically pleuritic, but central with large pulmonary emboli), and less commonly haemoptysis, cough, and syncope. The differential diagnosis depends on the predominant presenting feature, i.e. pleuritic pain (chest infection with pleurisy, pericarditis), central chest pain (myocardial infarction), dyspnoea (COPD or heart failure). Chronic pulmonary embolic disease and pulmonary hypertension present with exertional breathlessness, and patients may complain of central chest pain that is due to right ventricular subendocardial ischaemia. The diagnosis of pulmonary embolism cannot easily be excluded without investigation and the exclusion of an alternative, more likely, cause of breathlessness is crucial to the initial assessment.

Most patients with acute pulmonary embolism are breathless or tachypnoeic (respiratory rate >20/min) and in the absence of these findings haemoptysis and pleuritic chest pain are usually due to another cause. See Chapter 16.16.1 for further discussion of examination findings and diagnostic strategy in patients with suspected pulmonary embolism.

Dyspnoea with preserved left ventricular function

Where breathlessness is present in the context of preserved left ventricular function, diastolic heart failure should be considered. This diagnosis can only be made in the context of an appropriate history and examination findings. Echocardiographic parameters of diastolic dysfunction (see Chapter 16.3.2) are common in the community setting, but more than 50% of individuals with such an echocardiographic diagnosis are asymptomatic and the presence of diastolic dysfunction in a patient with breathlessness should not automatically lead to a diagnosis of the clinical syndrome of diastolic heart failure. COPD, ischaemic heart disease, and obesity are common in individuals with diastolic dysfunction, and diastolic heart failure can be overdiagnosed. Hypertension, coronary disease, and left ventricular hypertrophy are important causes of diastolic dysfunction and in their absence diastolic heart failure is rare. Alternative causes for dyspnoea should be always be excluded, in particular, chronic thromboembolic disease, airways disease, sleep apnoea, and silent ischaemia.

Further reading

Badgett RG, Lucey CR, Mulrow CD (1997). Can the clinical examination diagnose left-sided heart failure in adults? *JAMA*, **277**, 1712–19.

Bugiardini R, Merz CNB (2005). Angina with normal coronary arteries. A changing philosophy. *JAMA*, **293**, 477–84.

Cayley WE (2005). Diagnosing the cause of chest pain. *Am Fam Physician*, **72**, 2012–21.

Chunilal SD, *et al.* (2003). Does this patient have pulmonary embolism? *JAMA*, **290**, 2849–58.

Davie AP, *et al.* (1997). Assessing diagnosis in heart failure: which features are any use? *Q J Med*, **90**, 335–9.

Gehlbach BK, Geppert E (2004). The pulmonary manifestations of left heart failure. *Chest*, **125**, 669–82.

Hurst JW, Morris DC (2001). *Chest pain*. Futura, Armonk, NY.

Klompas, M (2002). Does this patient have acute thoracic aortic dissection? *JAMA*, **287**, 2262–2272.

Mahler, DA (1990). *Dyspnoea*. Futura, Armonk, NY.

Manning HL, Schwartzstein RM (1995). Pathophysiology of dyspnea. *N Engl J Med*, **333**, 1547–53.

Marcus GM, *et al.* (2005). Association between phonocardiographic third and fourth heart sounds and objective measures of left ventricular function. *JAMA*, **293**, 2238–44.

Miller AJ (1988). *Diagnosis of chest pain*. Raven Press, New York.

Scano G, Stenardi L, Grazzini M (2005). Understanding dyspnoea by its language. *Eur Resp J*, **25**, 380–5.

Straus SE, *et al.* (2000). The accuracy of patient history, wheezing, and laryngeal measurements in diagnosing obstructive airway disease. CARE-COAD1 Group. Clinical assessment of the reliability of the examination-chronic obstructive airways disease. *JAMA*, **283**, 1853–7.

Swap CJ, Nagurney JT (2005). Value and limitations of chest pain history in the evaluation of patients with suspected acute coronary syndromes. *JAMA*, **294**, 2623–9.

Wang CS, *et al.* (2005). Does this dyspneic patient in the emergency department have congestive heart failure? *JAMA*, **294**, 1944–56.

16.2.2 **Syncope and palpitations**

A.C. Rankin, A.D. McGavigan, and S.M. Cobbe

Essentials

Syncope is a transient episode of loss of consciousness due to cerebral hypoperfusion. Its causes can be subdivided based on pathophysiology, including (1) neurally mediated—or reflex—syncope; (2) orthostatic hypotension; (3) cardiac causes; and (4) cerebrovascular or psychogenic causes.

Neurocardiogenic syncope, or simple faint, is the commonest cause and is benign, but it is always important to exclude or establish the diagnosis of cardiac syncope, because this has an adverse prognosis that may be improved with appropriate treatment. Cardiac arrhythmia should be considered in all patients who have syncope associated with any of the following: (1) exertion, chest pain, or palpitations; (2) a past medical history of heart disease; (3) abnormal cardiovascular findings on examination; and (4) an abnormal ECG.

Initial assessment of the patient with syncope by clinical history, examination, and 12-lead ECG will indicate a probable diagnosis in most patients and guide further investigation (if required). Documentation of cardiac rhythm during syncope is extremely useful, especially if it is associated with palpitations, but this is usually difficult to obtain because of the intermittent and typically infrequent nature of the symptom. External or implanted loop-recorders, which can store the rhythm before, during, and after an episode, are increasingly used when the diagnosis remains unclear. In patients with structural heart disease in whom arrhythmia is suspected, programmed electrical stimulation of the ventricles may induce sustained monomorphic ventricular tachycardia: this is a relatively specific response, shows that the patient is at risk of recurrent ventricular arrhythmia, and makes an arrhythmic origin of syncope likely, but the diagnostic yield of electrophysiological testing is low in patients with a structurally normal heart.

Palpitation is the awareness of one's heart beating—it may be due to an awareness of an abnormal cardiac rhythm, or an abnormal awareness of normal rhythm. It is most commonly due to premature beats and is benign. Correlation between symptoms and cardiac rhythm is the initial aim of investigations in patients presenting with palpitations.

Syncope

Definition

Syncope is defined as a transient loss of consciousness, with loss of postural tone, usually resulting in falling. It is often of sudden onset, with prompt spontaneous recovery. The underlying mechanism is reduced cerebral perfusion, which may be due to a variety of cardiovascular—or less commonly cerebrovascular—causes. It is a common presentation, producing 1 to 3% of Emergency Department visits and up to 6% of hospital admissions. The cause is often initially uncertain and assessment must first differentiate syncope from other causes of loss of consciousness, such as epileptic seizures.

Box 16.2.2.1 Features associated with cardiac syncope

History of syncopal episode

- Occurs during exertion
- Associated palpitations
- Associated chest pain

Past medical history

- Known structural heart disease
- Previous myocardial infarction
- History of heart failure
- Valvular heart disease

Family history

- Family history of sudden death

Examination

- Presence of murmur
- Signs of heart failure
- Carotid bruit

12-lead ECG

- Evidence of atrioventricular block
- Bundle branch block
- Evidence of previous infarction
- Left ventricular hypertrophy
- Long QTc interval
- Features of Brugada syndrome

Prognosis

The prognosis depends on the aetiology, with most patients having a benign condition, although recurrent syncope can produce anxiety and reduction in quality of life regardless of the underlying cause. The exceptions are cardiac causes of syncope, which have been reported to have 1-year mortality rates as high as 18 to 33%. An important aim in the evaluation of syncope is to identify this subgroup of patients: clues may come from the history, examination, and the 12-lead ECG (Box 16.2.2.1).

Differential diagnosis

The initial evaluation of the patient with possible transient loss of consciousness should include history, examination, supine and upright blood pressure, and 12-lead ECG (Fig. 16.2.2.1). It is important to establish that loss of consciousness (syncope) occurred to enable differentiation from nonsyncopal causes such as falls, drop attacks, and transient ischaemic attacks. In the absence of features of cardiac syncope (Box 16.2.2.1) and with a normal 12-lead ECG, a single episode of syncope requires no further investigation or treatment, other than reassurance. In patients with recurrent syncope, or a single episode in a high-risk individual, further investigation and treatment will depend on the suspected diagnosis.

The causes of syncope can be subdivided on the basis of pathophysiology, namely (1) neurally-mediated—or reflex—syncope, (2) orthostatic hypotension, (3) cardiac causes, and (4) cerebrovascular or psychogenic causes (Table 16.2.2.1). The history is most important. For example, it may strongly suggest a vasovagal origin, or an epileptic seizure. However, the diagnosis may be complicated by an overlap in features, such as convulsive movements during a vasovagal episode due to anoxic convulsive seizures. It is increasingly recognized that many patients who attend clinics for epilepsy have been misdiagnosed and are suffering from recurrent syncope: some of these patients have potentially lethal ventricular arrhythmias for which they should be receiving treatment.

Neurally mediated syncope

There are many disorders of autonomic control that can cause syncope. The most common is neurocardiogenic syncope, or simple faint, which is due to an increased sensitivity of normal reflex responses. By contrast, autonomic dysfunction may produce abnormal neurovascular control that results in orthostatic hypotension.

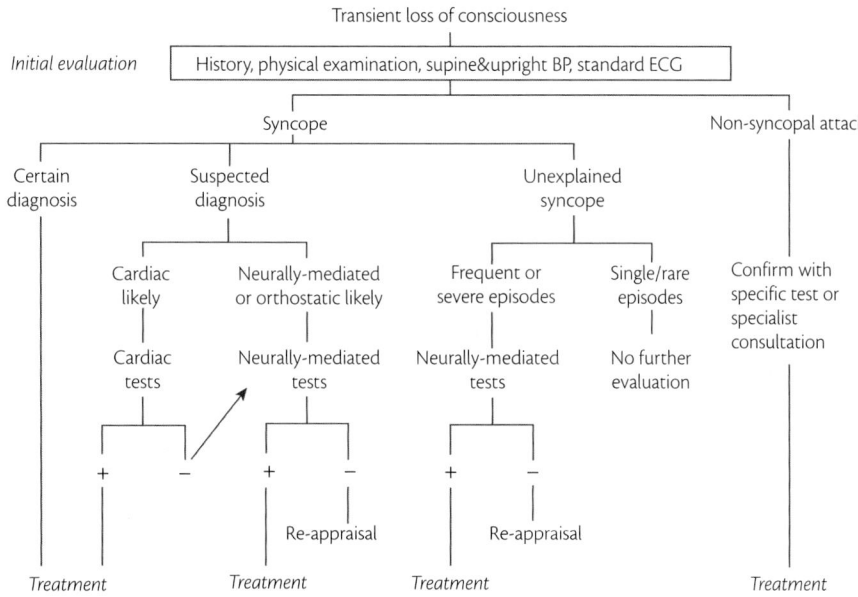

Fig. 16.2.2.1 A flow-diagram showing the evaluation of loss of consciousness, proposed by the Task Force on Syncope of the European Society of Cardiology. The most useful cardiac tests are echocardiography, prolonged ECG monitoring, stress test, electrophysiological study and implantable loop recorder. Neurally mediated tests include tilt test, carotid sinus massage and implantable loop recorder. BP, blood pressure; ECG electrocardiogram.
Reproduced with permission from Brignole M, et al (2004) *Guidelines on management (diagnosis and treatment) of syncope--update 2004. Europace* 6, 467–537.

Table 16.2.2.1 Causes of syncope

Neurally mediated	Vasovagal or neurocardiogenic syncope
	Carotid sinus hypersensitivity
	Situational (micturition, defecation, cough, swallow)
Orthostatic hypotension	Primary autonomic failure
	Pure autonomic failure
	Multiple system atrophy (parkinsonian, cerebellar)
	Secondary autonomic failure (diabetic, amyloid neuropathy)
	Postural orthostatic tachycardia syndrome
	Drugs and alcohol
	Volume depletion (haemorrhage, diarrhoea)
Cardiac syncope	
Bradycardia	Atrioventricular block
	Sinoatrial disease
Tachycardia	Ventricular arrhythmia
	Structural heart disease
	Previous myocardial infarction
	Cardiomyopathy
	Structurally normal heart
	Long-QT or Brugada syndrome
	Supraventricular arrhythmia
Structural cardiovascular disease	Aortic stenosis
	Hypertrophic cardiomyopathy
	Atrial myxoma or thrombus
	Pulmonary embolism
Cerebrovascular or psychogenic	
Neurological	Migraine
	Subclavian steal
	Vertebrobasilar disease
Psychogenic	Anxiety, depression, and hyperventilation

Vasovagal syncope

Vasovagal or neurocardiogenic syncope is the most common cause of syncope. It can affect all age groups and varies from infrequent episodes associated with obvious triggering factors to frequent unprovoked collapses, which may be debilitating. The pathophysiology most commonly involves venous pooling of blood and reduced venous return to the heart in response to upright posture. Reduced cardiac output and blood pressure stimulate arterial baroreceptors with resultant increased sympathetic activity and catecholamine levels. The vigorous contraction of relatively empty ventricles results in the activation of mechanoreceptors that would normally respond to stretch in the left ventricular wall. Afferent nerve fibres conduct to the cerebral medulla and activate the reflex

withdrawal of peripheral sympathetic tone and activation of vagal parasympathetic activity. The resultant vasodilatation and bradycardia cause reduced cerebral perfusion and loss of consciousness. However, there is debate about these mechanisms and other factors may be involved in the aetiology of syncope, as illustrated by the documentation of neurocardiogenic syncope—despite cardiac denervation—in orthotopic heart transplant recipients. Certainly, it is well recognized that vasovagal syncope can result from other stimuli, such as pain, emotional shock, or the sight of blood: in these instances the reflex activation is central in origin.

The development of tilt testing has allowed the study of the pathophysiology of neurocardiogenic syncope. The patient is strapped to a tilt table and is tilted, head upright, usually at 70° for up to 45 min. Protocols that use additional provocation with isoprenaline or nitrates are commonly used. Blood pressure and cardiac rhythm are monitored throughout the tilt test. In neurocardiogenic syncope, the patient classically maintains normal blood pressure initially, until the sudden onset of syncope is associated with severe hypotension and bradycardia, often preceded by tachycardia. These features resolve with return to the supine posture. Some patients have a mainly vasodepressor response, with hypotension and little change in heart rate, while others have a marked cardioinhibitory response, with severe bradycardia or asystole of several seconds duration (Fig. 16.2.2.2). Most have a mixed response of hypotension and bradycardia.

Carotid sinus hypersensitivity

An abnormal sensitivity of a normal reflex is responsible for syncope. Activation of the carotid sinus baroreceptors (e.g. by physical pressure, such as carotid sinus massage) results in sympathetic withdrawal and parasympathetic activation. Bradycardia is usually a prominent feature.

Situational reflex-mediated syncope

In susceptible individuals, similar abnormal reflex sensitivity can result in syncope in response to afferent activity from other mechanoreceptor activation. Syncopal responses to cough, micturition, defecation, or swallowing have been reported.

Orthostatic hypotension

Hypotension may occur in patients in whom there are abnormalities in the autonomic control of cardiovascular function.

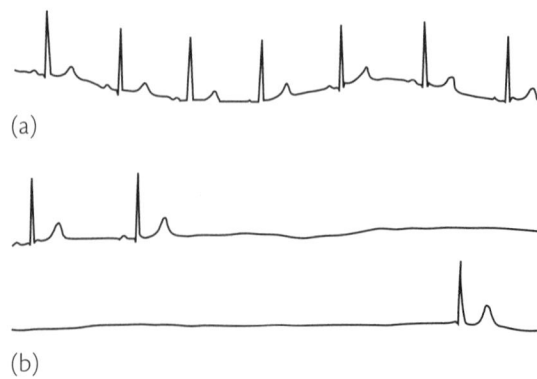

(a)

(b)

Fig. 16.2.2.2 Cardioinhibitory response to tilt testing. (a) After 6 min of head-up tilting at 70° the patient complained of presyncope. Heart rate was 60/min but blood pressure was 70 mmHg. (b) By 7 min the patient had lost consciousness, associated with an asystolic pause of 10 s duration and an unrecordable blood pressure. Recovery was rapid following the patient's return to the supine position.

Box 16.2.2.2 Drugs that may cause postural hypotension

- Diuretics
- α-Adrenergic receptor blockers
- β-Adrenergic receptor blockers
- ACE inhibitors
- Angiotensin II receptor antagonists
- Calcium-channel blockers
- Nitrates
- Opiates
- Ethanol
- Tricyclic antidepressants
- Bromocriptine
- Phenothiazines
- Levodopa

Abnormalities of afferent or efferent pathways, or of peripheral vascular control, can result in low blood pressure in the upright posture, i.e. orthostatic hypotension. This may be diagnosed by a fall in systolic pressure of more than 20 mmHg, or to less than 90 mmHg, within 3 min of standing. During tilt testing there may be an immediate drop in blood pressure with head-upright tilting, or a progressive fall may be observed in some patients, in contrast to those with reflex-mediated syncope in whom blood pressure is maintained until the sudden onset of symptoms.

Orthostatic hypotension is more common in elderly patients, where it may be multifactorial, often exacerbated by drugs (Box 16.2.2.2). Nocturnal symptoms may occur, with a fall in blood pressure exacerbated by sudden rising from a warm bed.

Autonomic failure is an uncommon cause of syncope and patients may present with other features, including disturbances of bowel, bladder, or sexual function. Pure autonomic failure can be acute or chronic, primary (of unknown origin) or secondary to systemic disease. Multiple system atrophy is characterized by autonomic dysfunction, parkinsonism, and ataxia. Orthostatic hypotension may be a marked feature (the Shy–Drager syndrome), with additional parkinsonian features or cerebellar symptoms. Secondary autonomic failure can result from the central or peripheral involvement of certain diseases, including multiple sclerosis, cerebral tumour, diabetes and amyloidosis. A milder form of autonomic dysfunction, the postural orthostatic tachycardia syndrome (POTS), causes symptoms because of inappropriate tachycardia on standing, and occasionally syncope secondary to hypotension.

Cardiac syncope

Loss of consciousness of cardiac origin may result from some substantial disturbance of cardiovascular function or from abnormalities of heart rhythm, with resultant reduced cerebral perfusion. The importance in establishing the diagnosis of cardiac syncope is the associated adverse prognosis, which may be improved with appropriate treatment. The probability of cardiac syncope is increased in the presence of structural cardiovascular disease identified from the history, clinical examination, or the ECG (Box 16.2.2.1).

Tachycardia

Syncope may be caused by tachycardia, most commonly ventricular, but supraventricular tachycardia can also be associated with loss of consciousness if it is very fast or in patients with structural heart disease. Syncope, rather than cardiac arrest, may result from self-terminating ventricular tachycardia or from sustained tachycardia with hypotension at the onset, but with a subsequent recovery of blood pressure. Whether or not a tachycardia causes syncope is related to its rate, underlying left ventricular function, and the patient's baroreceptor sensitivity.

Cardiac arrhythmia should be considered in all patients with structural heart disease presenting with syncope. Ventricular tachycardia most commonly occurs in patients with structural heart disease, e.g. prior myocardial infarction, but may also occur in patients with structurally normal hearts. For example, torsades de pointes in a patient with the long-QT syndrome is an important diagnosis to consider in young people with a history of loss of consciousness and possible epilepsy, in whom the episodes of collapse may be due to syncope caused by ventricular arrhythmia.

Bradycardia

A sudden decrease in heart rate, onset of ventricular standstill, or asystole may be a cause of syncope. When due to sinoatrial dysfunction (sick-sinus syndrome) this is not associated with a poor prognosis, but syncope due to intermittent complete atrioventricular block is. Syncope in a patient with a permanent pacemaker may indicate pacemaker malfunction.

Structural cardiovascular disease

Aortic stenosis may be associated with syncope, particularly during sudden exertion when the demand for increased cardiac output cannot be met because of the mechanical obstruction. Hypertrophic cardiomyopathy may also be associated with syncope, either because of outflow obstruction or ventricular arrhythmia. Obstruction of blood flow through the mitral valve by an atrial myxoma or thrombus is an uncommon cause of syncope. A number of other cardiac diseases may be associated with loss of consciousness by a variety of mechanisms (arrhythmia, reflex-mediated, or haemodynamic), including myocardial infarction, pulmonary embolism, congenital heart disease, or cardiac tamponade. Vascular diseases may also be involved, such as aortic dissection and extracranial vascular disease.

Cerebrovascular or psychogenic causes of syncope

When epilepsy is excluded, neurological conditions are rare causes of loss of consciousness, but possible diagnoses include migraine, transient ischaemic attacks, vertebrobasilar vascular disease, and subclavian steal syndrome. However, in most cases these will not result in true syncope.

A psychogenic origin of loss of consciousness implies the absence of neurally mediated, neurological, or cardiac abnormalities, and may occur in association with anxiety, depression, and conversion disorders. For instance, apparent syncope may occur during tilt testing but with normal pulse and blood pressure. Hyperventilation may be an associated mechanistic factor in psychogenic syncope.

Assessment of the patient with syncope

Careful assessment of the patient's history, a full physical examination and the 12-lead ECG will indicate a likely diagnosis in over

50% of patients with a history of syncope. Further investigations will be prompted by the initial evaluation (Fig. 16.2.2.1).

History

The importance of the clinical history in assessing a patient with syncope cannot be overemphasized. If possible, an eyewitness description of the patient during the syncopal event should be obtained. Features associated with increased risk of cardiac syncope should be sought (Box 16.2.2.1).

Provocative factors

Vasovagal syncope is classically associated with upright posture, often with aggravating circumstances such as prolonged standing, a hot environment, or hunger. However, episodes may also occur when seated, including while driving. Specific stimuli may be responsible for neurocardiogenic syncope in susceptible individuals. Ventricular arrhythmia, in particular torsades de pointes in the Long-QT syndrome, may be provoked by sudden stimuli such as a noise, e.g. an alarm clock, or exercise, in particular swimming. Exertional syncope is a feature of aortic stenosis or hypertrophic cardiomyopathy.

Preceding symptoms

Sweating and feeling hot or nauseated may precede vasovagal syncope. Cardiac arrhythmia may be associated with palpitation, chest pain, or breathlessness. Bradycardia, such as intermittent complete heart block, may produce no preceding symptoms and may cause loss of consciousness without warning. Sinoatrial dysfunction is a cause of symptoms of dizziness and light-headedness in addition to syncope. A psychogenic origin may be suggested by multiple associated symptoms including hyperventilation, paraesthesiae in fingers and lips, palpitation, and chest pain, which may precede syncope. Epilepsy may be preceded by a characteristic aura, which would strongly point away from syncope as the diagnosis.

The syncopal episode

In syncope the duration of loss of consciousness is usually short, with recovery after a few minutes. A longer duration of loss of consciousness would suggest an alternative diagnosis. An exception to this is when the patient has remained upright during the attack, possibly aided by well-meaning but misguided helpers. Incontinence is a feature of epileptic seizure but may also occur (uncommonly) with syncope. Description of the patient during the episode is of great value. The classic description of an episode of syncope due to cardiac arrhythmia—in particular sudden-onset severe bradycardia—is of a sudden loss of colour, becoming deathly pale, with flushing on recovery (Stokes–Adams attack). Cyanosis may be a feature of an arrhythmic origin of syncope. Convulsive movements during the episode would raise the possibility of epilepsy, but they also occur with syncope. Although any cause of syncope can be associated with injury, its absence may point to a nonsyncopal or psychogenic origin.

The recovery period

By contrast to the postictal phase following epilepsy, there is commonly a rapid recovery of cerebral function following syncope. Vasovagal syncope may be followed by persisting nausea or vomiting.

Family history

There are a few specific causes of syncope in which a family history of syncope or sudden death may have prognostic significance. Long-QT syndrome is hereditary and may be associated with sudden death. A family history of syncope is of adverse prognostic significance in hypertrophic cardiomyopathy.

Investigation

The investigation of cardiac disease and arrhythmia are dealt with in the appropriate chapters, but the approach to the patient with syncope will be described briefly. Dependent on the history, further investigations may not be necessary with the exception of a 12-lead ECG. For example, the diagnosis of vasovagal syncope is a clinical one and other investigations are likely to have a low diagnostic yield. By contrast, if the history or examination points to a clear cause of syncope, investigations appropriate to the underlying cause should be performed.

Electrocardiogram

An ECG should be performed on all patients with syncope. This may provide evidence of aetiology of syncope, such as the long-QT syndrome, or of structural heart disease, such as prior myocardial infarction or left ventricular hypertrophy. An arrhythmia may be documented if it is sustained, and there may be evidence of sinoatrial disease or conduction system disease, such as trifasicular block, bundle-branch block, or first- or second-degree block. After first ensuring the absence of carotid bruits, carotid sinus massage with digital pressure to the carotid artery for up to 5 s may cause marked bradycardia in carotid sinus hypersensitivity, with pauses of more than 3 s duration.

Ambulatory monitoring

Documentation of cardiac rhythm during syncope is extremely useful, especially if it was associated with palpitations, but is difficult to obtain because of the intermittent and usually infrequent nature of the symptom. Holter monitoring is unlikely to record the rhythm during an episode but may provide evidence of lesser degrees of abnormality, which may support a diagnosis such as sinoatrial dysfunction. Real-time event-recorders are also of limited value in the investigation of syncope because they require a conscious patient to make the recording. Patient-activated loop-recorders, which can store the rhythm before, during, and after an episode, may be of more value. Implantable loop-recorders are being increasingly used when the diagnosis remains unclear.

Tilt-testing

When the history is suggestive of vasovagal syncope, the tilt test may be of value in confirming the diagnosis, but a negative test does not exclude the diagnosis. Adjuvant provocation (isoprenaline or nitrate) may increase the sensitivity, but the incidence of false positive tests with tilt testing has been reported as 5 to 20%. As such, its use is probably best limited to investigation of recurrent symptoms with an atypical history in patients in whom there are no features to suggest cardiac syncope.

Electrophysiological testing

Abnormal sinus node function or evidence of atrioventricular conduction disease may be elicited by electrophysiological testing, but demonstrating bradycardia during ambulatory monitoring more reliably makes both these diagnoses. In patients with structural heart disease in whom arrhythmia is suspected, programmed electrical stimulation of the ventricles can induce sustained monomorphic ventricular tachycardia. This is a relatively specific response, shows that the patient is at risk of recurrent ventricular arrhythmia, and makes an arrhythmic origin of syncope likely. The diagnostic yield of electrophysiological testing is low in patients with a structurally normal heart.

Other investigations

Assessment for structural heart disease is important. Physical examination will detect most significant valve disease, but other diagnoses, e.g. hypertrophic cardiomyopathy or atrial myxoma, may produce little in the way of clinical signs. An echocardiogram is therefore worthwhile in cases where the diagnosis remains unclear. A strong suspicion of diagnoses other than syncope should lead to other investigations, including EEG and brain imaging, but these have a low diagnostic yield in patients with syncope and should not be routine.

Treatment

Neurocardiogenic syncope may require no treatment other than reassurance and avoidance of provocative factors. Management of vasovagal syncope, bradycardia, and cardiac arrhythmia are discussed in Chapters 24.5.4 and 16.4. In up to one-third of patients the aetiology of syncope may not be found: these patients have a good outcome unless they have underlying heart disease.

Palpitation

The symptom of palpitation is defined as an awareness of one's heart beating. This may be due to an awareness of an abnormal heart rhythm but it may also be due to an abnormal awareness of normal rhythm. A careful and detailed history can provide a likely diagnosis. The most important aim in investigation is to correlate symptoms with cardiac rhythm.

History

A description of the symptom should include an estimate of heart rate, duration of symptom, regularity of rhythm, suddenness of onset and offset. It may be helpful to ask the patient to tap with their finger to describe their palpitation. Trigger factors, including exercise, and aggravating factors such as alcohol and caffeine should be detailed. The length of history may be of interest.

Sinus tachycardia

An awareness of a rapid heart rate of gradual onset and offset is often associated with feelings of alarm and panic in patients with anxiety.

Premature beats

Atrial and ventricular beats commonly occur in normal individuals and may be associated with symptoms. The patient may describe 'missed beats' or forceful beats. These symptoms relate to the pause that follows a premature beat. The premature beat produces a short diastolic filling interval and the low ventricular volume results in reduced ventricular contraction with a small stroke volume. However, the subsequent pause provides a long diastolic filling period and the resultant stretching of the ventricular walls is associated with an increased and forceful systolic contraction. The combination of the diminished premature beat and the enhanced postextrasystolic beat is responsible for the symptoms.

Atrial fibrillation

This common arrhythmia may produce a variety of symptoms depending on ventricular rate, irregularity, and persistence. Paroxysmal atrial fibrillation is characterized by self-terminating

episodes of atrial fibrillation, when there may be a rapid and irregular ventricular response. The patient is aware of an increased heart rate and often describes the irregular nature of the symptom. The variations in diastolic interval produce symptoms by similar mechanisms to that described above for premature beats, with 'missed' and 'forceful' beats. Patients with sinoatrial dysfunction may be most symptomatic on termination of the atrial fibrillation, which can be followed by sinus bradycardia or prolonged sinus pauses. Atrial fibrillation may be persistent or permanent, and the severity of symptoms will be related to the ventricular rate and irregularity.

Paroxysmal supraventricular tachycardia

A history of sudden onset, rapid, regular palpitation in a healthy patient with no underlying structural heart disease is suggestive of paroxysmal supraventricular tachycardia. It may stop spontaneously or with vagotonic manoeuvres, or the patient may have had to attend hospital for intravenous therapy. In addition to palpitation, patients commonly report fatigue, malaise, light-headedness, or dyspnoea, but because they have normal hearts such episodes of tachycardia are usually well tolerated. Polyuria is a common associated symptom, which results from the release of atrial natriuretic peptide secondary to atrial stretch.

Ventricular tachycardia

Ventricular arrhythmias can present with the symptom of palpitation, but more severe symptoms such as syncope or cardiac arrest also occur. Characteristically the symptom of palpitation would be of sudden onset and offset of a rapid regular heart rhythm. A history of structural heart disease should be sought.

Investigation

Electrocardiogram

The first aim is to document cardiac rhythm during symptoms. This may be possible with a standard ECG if the arrhythmia is sustained or persistent. Atrial or ventricular premature beats, or evidence of structural heart disease, e.g. myocardial infarction, may be documented. The presence of pre-excitation indicates the diagnosis of Wolff–Parkinson–White syndrome and suggests symptoms due to episodes of atrioventricular reentry tachycardia.

Ambulatory monitoring

The success of ambulatory monitoring in documenting the rhythm during symptoms will be dependent on the frequency of symptoms. If they occur daily then a 24- or 48-h Holter recording should suffice. However, palpitation is often infrequent and other patient-activated devices can be of more value. These include hand-held, patient-activated event recorders that allow the telephonic transmission of recordings. These devices do not allow retrospective recording and require symptoms of sufficient duration to allow their use. Shorter episodes may be captured using loop-recorders.

Electrophysiological studies

Invasive studies are of most value in determining the mechanism of a previously documented tachyarrhythmia, particularly with a view to treatments such as radiofrequency catheter ablation.

Management

Documentation of the cardiac rhythm during palpitation allows appropriate management, with reassurance as the only treatment in those with sinus tachycardia or premature beats. The treatment of other cardiac arrhythmias is discussed in Chapter 16.4.

Further reading

Benditt DG, Sutton R (2005). Tilt-table testing in the evaluation of syncope. *J Cardiovasc Electrophysiol*, **16**, 356–8.

Brignole M, *et al.* (2004). Guidelines on management (diagnosis and treatment) of syncope–update 2004. *Europace*, **6**, 467–537.

Brignole M. (2007). Diagnosis and treatment of syncope. *Heart*, **93**, 130–6.

Grubb BP (2005). Neurocardiogenic syncope and related disorders of orthostatic intolerance. *Circulation*, **111**, 2997–3006.

Moya A, Sutton R, Ammirati F, *et al.* (2009). Guidelines for the diagnosis and management of syncope (version 2009): the Task Force for the Diagnosis and Management of Syncope of the European Society of Cardiology (ESC). *Eur Heart J*, **30**, 631–71.

Strickberger SA, *et al.* (2006). AHA/ACCF Scientific Statement on the evaluation of syncope: from the American Heart Association Councils on Clinical Cardiology, Cardiovascular Nursing, Cardiovascular Disease in the Young, and Stroke, and the Quality of Care and Outcomes Research Interdisciplinary Working Group; and the American College of Cardiology Foundation: in collaboration with the Heart Rhythm Society: endorsed by the American Autonomic Society. *Circulation*, **113**, 316–27.

Clinical investigation of cardiac disorders

Contents

16.3.1 **Electrocardiography**

Andrew R. Houghton and David Gray

Essentials

The resting 12-lead ECG

The ECG has been recognized as a valuable diagnostic tool since the end of the 19th century. The normal ECG waveform consists of P, QRS, and T waves (and sometimes U waves)—P waves result from atrial depolarization, QRS complexes from ventricular depolarization, and T waves from ventricular repolarization. The standard 12-lead ECG utilizes 4 limb electrodes and 6 precordial electrodes to generate 12 leads or 'views' of the heart's electrical activity. There are six limb leads (termed I, II, III, aVR, aVL, and aVF) and six precordial leads (termed V1, V2, V3, V4, V5, and V6). Supplementary 'views' can be obtained by using additional leads, such as V7, V8, and V9 to assess the posterior aspect of the heart and right-sided chest leads to look for a right ventricular myocardial infarction.

Assessment of the 12-lead ECG—this should be done in a methodical manner, working through each aspect in turn. Conventionally, the heart rate, rhythm and axis are assessed before inspection of each component of the waveform in turn—the P wave, PR interval, QRS complex, ST segment, T wave, QT interval, and U wave, with each component having its own range of normal attributes.

Myocardial hypertrophy—the ECG can be a specific but generally insensitive tool for detecting myocardial hypertrophy: (1) left ventricular hypertrophy can be assessed using a number of diagnostic criteria, including the Cornell criteria and the Romhilt–Estes scoring system; (2) right ventricular hypertrophy is indicated by a dominant R wave in lead V1 with right axis deviation; (3) left atrial hypertrophy is indicated by broad, bifid P waves; and (4) right atrial hypertrophy by tall P waves.

Conduction blocks—(1) left anterior hemiblock results from a block of conduction in the anterosuperior fascicle and is a cause of left-axis deviation; (2) left posterior hemiblock results from a block of conduction in the posteroinferior fascicle and is a cause of right-axis deviation; (3) left and right bundle branch blocks both cause broadening of the QRS complexes by prolonging ventricular depolarization, and both exhibit characteristic diagnostic features.

Ventricular pre-excitation—causes shortening of the PR interval and can result from Wolff–Parkinson–White-type pre-excitation, short PR-type pre-excitation, or Mahaim-type pre-excitation (for discussion of the 12-lead ECG in arrhythmia, see Chapter 16.4).

Acute coronary syndromes

The ECG is the most useful bedside triage tool in acute coronary syndromes, with utility in diagnosis, in location of the site of ischaemia/infarction, and as a prognostic indicator.

ST elevation myocardial infarction (STEMI)—the first indication of infarction on the ECG is usually ST segment elevation, which occurs within a few hours. The J point (the origin of the ST segment at its junction with the QRS complex) is elevated by 1 mm or more in two or more limb leads, or by 2 mm in two or more precordial leads. The ST segment returns to the baseline over the next 48 to 72 h, during which Q waves and symmetrically inverted T waves appear. Some patients develop left bundle branch block, either transiently or permanently. The ECG of a completed infarct shows new Q waves greater than 2 mm, R waves reduced in size or absent, and inverted T waves.

Non-ST-elevation myocardial infarction (NSTEMI)—ECG changes are more variable than in STEMI. The ECG may be normal on first presentation and remain unchanged throughout the acute admission; there may be transient ST segment depression indicative of myocardial ischaemia; in 20 to 30% the only change will be T-wave inversion.

Difficulties in interpretation of the ECG in acute coronary syndromes—the ECG diagnosis of acute myocardial infarction can pose challenges in the setting of right ventricular infarction, atrial infarction, coronary artery spasm, reciprocal changes, 'stuttering' infarction, noninfarct ST segment elevation, late presentation, left bundle branch block, prior infarction, pre-excitation, and T-wave inversion.

Clinical decision-making—incorrect interpretation of an ECG can lead to inappropriate patient triage, either missing the opportunity to provide appropriate reperfusion therapy, or leading to inappropriate thrombolysis with attendant risk. Up to 12% of those with a high-risk ECG are missed on admission to the Emergency Department, yet pressure to provide treatment promptly to fulfil audit 'targets', e.g. door-to-needle time for thrombolysis, should not replace accuracy in diagnosis. It is sometimes better to wait a short while, control symptoms, give aspirin, and repeat the ECG than to make an incorrect diagnosis. It is easy to place too much reliance on minor changes on the ECG; it is gross changes of ST elevation or depression within the parameters above that should determine treatment.

Exercise ECG testing

Exercise ECG testing is better as an indicator of prognosis than as a diagnostic tool. The sensitivity of exercise ECG testing, the proportion with coronary disease correctly identified by the test, is 68% (range 23–100) and specificity, the proportion free of disease correctly identified by the test, is 77% (range 17–100). In multivessel disease, these figures are 81% (range 40–100) and 66% (range 17–100), respectively. This means that exercise testing frequently yields both false-positive results—incorrectly diagnosing disease when coronary arteries are normal or minimally diseased—and false-negative results—missing coronary disease when a flow-limiting, even critical left main stem, coronary stenosis is present.

Appearance of symptoms or ECG changes early in an exercise test is generally associated with more severe and extensive coronary disease and a poor prognosis. Changes within the first 3 min usually indicate severe coronary disease affecting the left main stem or the proximal segments of at least one major coronary artery. Multivessel coronary disease is more likely with ST segment down-sloping, delayed ST normalization after exercise, increased number of leads affected, and lower workload at which ECG changes appear.

The resting 12-lead ECG

History

The first electrocardiogram (ECG), of an exposed frog's heart, was performed by Marey in 1876 using the mercury capillary electrometer that had recently been invented by Gabriel Lippmann. Two years later the British physiologists John Burdon Sanderson and Fredrick Page demonstrated that recordings of the frog heart's electrical activity consisted of two phases (which were subsequently to become known as the QRS complex and T wave). The first human ECG was published in 1887 by Augustus D Waller, who had worked under Sanderson in the Department of Physiology at the University College of London. While working at St Mary's Hospital, London, Waller used a capillary electrometer to record the ECG of a laboratory technician, Thomas Goswell.

Electrocardiography was developed further by the Dutch physiologist Willem Einthoven, who witnessed a demonstration by Waller at the First International Congress of Physiology in Basle, Switzerland, in 1889. Although Einthoven made considerable improvements to the technique of recording ECGs with the capillary electrometer, it was only with his invention of the string galvanometer at the turn of the century that high-quality ECG recording became possible. Within a decade of Einthoven's publication of the first string galvanometer ECG recordings in 1902, a commercial ECG machine became available. Manufactured by the Cambridge Scientific Instrument Company, the first machine was delivered to Sir Thomas Lewis, who would play a major role in developing the clinical application of elecrocardiography. Einthoven's invention led to him being awarded the Nobel Prize in 1924.

Einthoven was also the first to use the PQRST notation to describe the ECG waveforms. In the early ECG recordings, the waveforms were named ABCD (four deflections were recognized). Mathematical correction, using differential equations, was used to correct and improve ECG recordings, and it was traditional that mathematical notation used letters from the latter half of the alphabet. The letters N and O were already used elsewhere, so it was decided to begin the notation at P.

Over the following years further refinements were undertaken, most notably in the 1930s when the use of the chest leads was first described. At around the same time Frank Wilson invented the 'indifferent electrode' (also known as the 'Wilson central terminal'). This led to the development of the 'unipolar' limb leads VR, VL, and VF ('V' stands for 'voltage'). In 1942 the American cardiologist Emanual Goldberger increased the voltage of these leads by 50%, leading to the term 'augmented' leads (aVR, aVL, and aVF), and the 12-lead ECG which remains familiar today finally took shape.

Although the format of the 12-lead ECG has remained essentially unchanged since that time, there have nevertheless been other significant developments in electrocardiography over more recent years. Ambulatory ECG recorders have gained a central role in the investigation of patients with suspected arrhythmias, and the use of intracardiac ECG recording has enable the rapid development and widespread use of electrophysiological studies.

Normal ECG appearances

The ECG waveform

The three fundamental deflections on the normal ECG are termed the P wave, the QRS complex, and the T wave (Fig. 16.3.1.1). The origins of each deflection are as follows.

P wave

The P wave results from depolarization of the atrial myocardium. Depolarization of the sinoatrial node itself, which triggers normal atrial depolarization, cannot be seen on the surface ECG (although it can be identified in intracardiac recordings). However, the presence of a P wave with normal morphology and orientation is generally taken to infer normal sinoatrial node depolarization.

Repolarization of the atrial myocardium is represented on the ECG by the Ta wave (the atrial equivalent of the ventricular T wave). The Ta wave is seen as a small asymmetrical deflection after

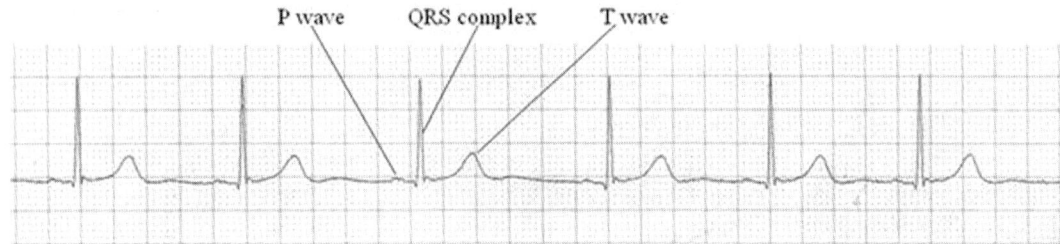

Fig. 16.3.1.1 Basic ECG waveform.

the P wave, with an opposite polarity to the preceding P wave. The Ta wave is often hidden within the QRS complex and is therefore not easily seen—in fact, it is unusual to be able to appreciate the Ta wave at all. However, it can extend right through to the following ST segment, where it can be mistaken for the ST segment depression of myocardial ischaemia (particularly because the Ta wave is most likely to be seen extending into the ST segment during exercise-induced sinus tachycardia). There is one case report of a positive Ta wave (after an inverted P wave) giving the erroneous impression of an acute ST segment elevation myocardial infarction.

QRS complex

The QRS complex represents depolarization of the ventricular myocardium. Of all the deflections, the QRS complex can exhibit the greatest variability in appearance. As a result, the individual components of the QRS complex can be labelled in upper case (Q, R, or S) or lower case (q, r, or s) to represent the relative size of the component. For example, QRS complexes with a small Q wave deflection can be termed qRS complexes, and those QRS complexes with no Q wave component and a small R wave component can be termed rS complexes.

T wave

The T wave (together with the preceding ST segment) represents repolarization of the ventricular myocardium.

The 12 conventional ECG leads

Lead nomenclature

It is important to emphasize that the term 'lead' does not refer to the electrode connecting the ECG machine to the patient. For a standard 12-lead ECG recording, 10 electrodes are used to generate the 12 conventional ECG leads. The 12 leads can be categorized as limb (or frontal plane) leads (I, II, III, aVR, aVL, aVF) and chest (or precordial) leads (V1, V2, V3, V4, V5, V6). The 12 leads can also be categorized as bipolar (I, II, III) or unipolar (aVR, aVL, aVF, V1, V2, V3, V4, V5, V6). The leads aVR, aVL, and aVF can be further described as 'augmented' leads, as they are modified versions of the original VR, VL, and VF leads, having a voltage amplification of 50%.

The bipolar leads are generated by measuring the potential (voltage) between two electrodes. One electrode acts as a positive terminal and the other as a negative terminal. For instance, lead I measures the potential between the left arm electrode (positive) and right arm electrode (negative). Lead I is obtained by subtracting the right arm vector from the left arm vector. Similarly, lead II measures the potential between the left leg electrode and the right arm electrode, and lead III measures the potential between the left leg electrode and the left arm electrode.

The augmented unipolar leads measure the voltage between a single positive electrode and a 'central' point of reference generated from the other limb electrodes. Thus aVR uses the right arm electrode as the positive terminal, aVL uses the left arm electrode, and aVF uses the left leg electrode. The three bipolar leads and the three augmented unipolar leads together comprise the six limb leads that view the heart in the frontal plane.

The unipolar chest leads measure the voltage between six electrodes placed across the surface of the chest and a central point of reference, providing a view of the heart that is perpendicular to the frontal plane leads. For all 12 ECG leads, it is conventional that a wave of depolarization moving towards a lead generates a positive (upward) deflection on the ECG recording and vice versa.

The six limb leads (frontal plane leads)

Because the limbs act as linear conductors, it does not matter whereabouts the limb electrodes are attached on each limb. The six limb leads provide general spatial information (being less localized than the six chest leads). Figure 16.3.1.2 shows the orientation of

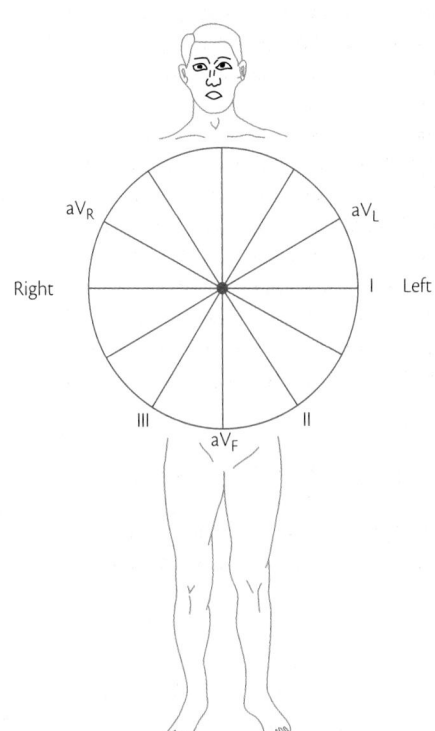

Fig. 16.3.1.2 The six limb leads and their 'view' of the heart. Note that leads II, III, and aVF are inferior to the heart, I and aVL are anterolateral to the heart, and aVR looks into the cavity of the heart.

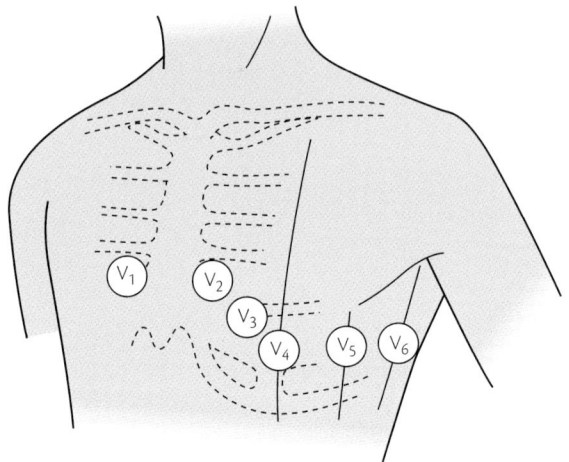

Fig. 16.3.1.3 Surface positions of the chest electrodes.

the six limb leads in relation to the heart. In simple terms one can visualize lead aVR as 'looking' at the heart from the right shoulder, lead aVL from the left shoulder and lead aVF from the feet. Lead I 'looks' at the heart from the left horizontal position. Similarly, the 'views' of leads II and III are shown in Fig. 16.3.1.2.

The six chest leads (precordial leads)

For the chest (precordial) leads, each of the six electrodes is attached to a particular site on the chest wall. The chest electrodes act as positive terminals, and the indifferent terminal is formed from a combination of leads R, L and F. The location of each electrode is important, in contrast to the limb leads. The surface positions of the chest electrodes is shown in Fig. 16.3.1.3, and the relation between the chest leads and the heart in Fig. 16.3.1.4. The electrodes are placed as follows:

- The V_1 electrode is placed at the upper right sternal edge in the fourth intercostal space
- The V_2 electrode is placed at the upper left sternal edge in the fourth intercostal space
- The V_3 electrode is placed midway between the V_2 and V_4 electrodes

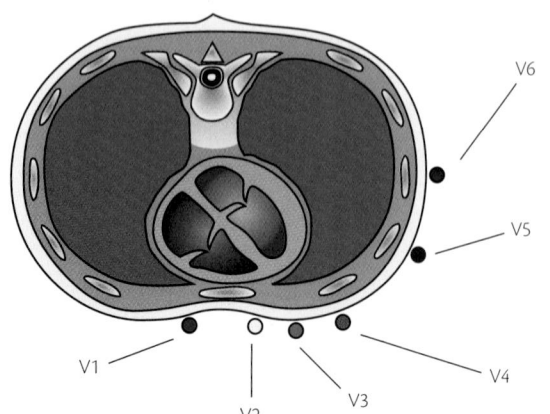

Fig. 16.3.1.4 The chest leads and their anatomical relationship to the heart.

- The V_4 electrode is placed at the left midclavicular line in the fifth intercostal space
- The V_5 electrode is placed at the left anterior axillary line in a horizontal line with V_4
- The V_6 electrode is placed at the left midaxillary line in a horizontal line with V_4 and V_5

Reading a normal 12-lead ECG

Figure 16.3.1.5 shows a normal 12-lead ECG. As is conventional, this shows the leads arranged in four columns, each column containing three leads. In addition, a rhythm strip runs along the bottom of the ECG across its whole width. This is conventionally lead II, but any one of the 12 leads can be used for the rhythm strip as required. The ECG is recorded at a paper speed of 25 mm/s, and at a sensitivity of 10 mm/mV. The speed and sensitivity settings can also be adjusted on most ECG machines, if required, and so it is important that the actual recording speed and sensitivity are always noted on the ECG for future reference.

In the following paragraphs we will describe the appearances of the normal ECG, looking at each wave, interval and segment in turn. We will assume that the patient is in normal sinus rhythm, and that a standard paper speed (25 mm/s) and calibration (10 mm/mV) have been used—this should always be checked before reading any ECG.

Identification details

Before reading the ECG, check the patient's details (the patient's name and at least one other form of identification, such as date of birth or identification number, should be recorded on the ECG) and the date and time on which the ECG was recorded. It is good practice to note on the ECG any relevant clinical features. For instance, a record that the patient was experiencing chest pain or palpitations at the time the ECG was recorded can prove invaluable later on. Indeed, ECG interpretation should always take into account the appropriate clinical context. For instance, the ECG shown in Fig. 16.3.1.5 can be interpreted as showing normal sinus rhythm in a patient who is well. However, in a patient who is unconscious and pulseless, the same ECG would be interpreted as showing pulseless electrical activity, a cardiac arrest rhythm. Before interpreting any ECG it is therefore appropriate (and important) to ask, 'How is the patient?'

Rate

A normal heart rate is between 60 and 100 beats/min. A rate below 60 beats/min is termed bradycardia; a rate greater than 100 beats/min is termed tachycardia. Heart rate normally applies to the ventricular rate, as shown on the ECG by the rate of QRS complexes. However, the atria have their own rate, as shown by the P wave rate. The atrial and ventricular rates are usually the same, and there is a 1:1 ratio between P waves and QRS complexes. However, the rates can differ; for instance, in complete heart block, the atrial rate is usually greater than the ventricular rate, and both rates should therefore be quoted.

Ventricular rate can be calculated in two different ways. One method necessitates counting the number of large (5 mm) squares between two adjacent QRS complexes. This figure is then divided into 300 to give the ventricular rate per minute. For instance, if there are 5 large squares between QRS complexes, the ventricular rate is 300/5 = 60 beats/min. The same method can be used

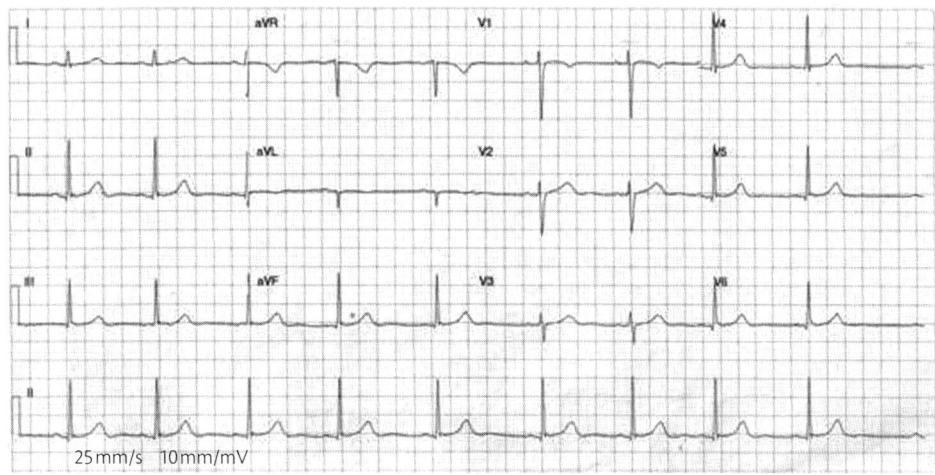

Fig. 16.3.1.5 A normal 12-lead ECG.

to calculate atrial rate, counting the large squares between two consecutive P waves.

If the heart rhythm is irregular, the square-counting method is not so useful. An alternative method is to count the number of QRS complexes in a certain time period, and then multiply the number up to obtain a rate per minute. Traditionally one counts the number of QRS complexes in a period of 30 large squares, which equates to 6 s of recording (a paper speed of 25 mm/s covers 5 large squares per second, or 300 large squares per minute). One then multiplies the result by 10 to obtain the rate per minute. Thus if there are 8 QRS complexes within 30 large squares, then the ventricular rate is 8 × 10 = 80 beats/min. Once again, the same method can be used to calculate atrial rate.

Rhythm

A detailed description of arrhythmias can be found in Chapter 16.4. In general terms, the assessment of rhythm on the ECG requires careful attention to the following:

- Whether there is ventricular activity (QRS complexes) and what is the ventricular rate

- Whether there is atrial activity (P waves) and what is the atrial rate

- Whether the heart rhythm is regular or irregular

- Whether the QRS complexes are normal or broad (broad complexes indicating either a ventricular origin to the rhythm or aberrant conduction of a supraventricular rhythm)

- Whether there is a relationship between P waves and QRS complexes

Assessing the ECG along these lines will provide a basis upon which to describe the rhythm and begin to identify the nature of the arrhythmia.

Axis

The concept of axis is often regarded as one of the hardest principles to grasp when learning ECG interpretation. The concept is, nonetheless, straightforward: axis refers to the overall direction in which the wave of depolarization travels. There is a QRS (ventricular) axis, which is what most people refer to when discussing

cardiac axis, but the P wave has its own axis too, representing the overall direction of depolarization in the atria. The T wave also has an axis, in this case referring to the overall direction of the wave of repolarization. In this section the discussion is confined to the QRS (ventricular) axis, but the same principles apply to P wave and T wave axes too.

As the ventricles depolarize, the wave of depolarization travels through the atrioventricular node, into the bundle of His, and then to the ventricular myocardium via the Purkinje fibres. The overall direction of this depolarization wavefront is usually towards the apex of the heart. If, by convention, we regard the 'view' that lead I has of the heart (a horizontal line to the left of the heart) as 0°, and any angle clockwise from that line is positive (and any angle anticlockwise from that line is negative), then the normal ventricular depolarisation wavefront travels through the ventricles at an angle of approximately +60° (Fig. 16.3.1.6).

As Fig. 16.3.1.6 illustrates, the six limb leads 'view' the heart from different angles. Lead I is taken as the horizontal reference point, 0°. Moving in a clockwise (positive) direction, lead II views the

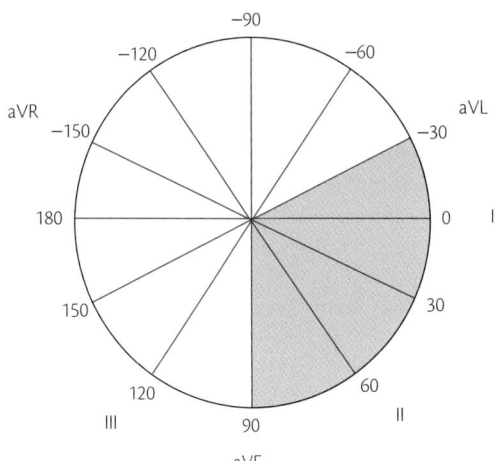

Fig. 16.3.1.6 The standard convention for describing the orientation of cardiac axis, and the corresponding 'views' of each of the six limb leads. The shaded area represents the normal range for the QRS axis.

heart from an angle of +60°, lead aVF from an angle of +90°, and lead III from an angle of +120°. Moving anticlockwise from lead I, lead aVL views the heart from an angle of −30°, and lead aVR from an angle of −150°. This system of looking at axis, using the six limb leads, is known as the hexaxial reference system.

The shaded area in Fig. 16.3.1.6 shows the normal range for the QRS axis, which lies between −30° and +90°. This does vary with body morphology—tall, slim individuals tend to have axes towards the rightward (+90°) end of the normal range; short, overweight individuals have axes towards the leftward (−30°) end of the normal range. An axis more negative (anticlockwise) than −30° is abnormal and termed left axis deviation. Similarly, an axis more positive (clockwise) than +90° is abnormal and termed right axis deviation. Left axis deviation is seen in left anterior hemiblock (see below), inferior myocardial infarction and also in ostium primum atrial septal defect. Right axis deviation is seen in left posterior hemiblock, right ventricular hypertrophy, lateral myocardial infarction, ostium secundum atrial septal defect, and Wolff–Parkinson–White (WPW) syndrome.

There are a number of ways to calculate the QRS axis. One method is to look for which of the six limb leads has a QRS complex in which the R wave and S wave are closest to being equal (i.e. in which the positive and negative deflections cancel each other out). The QRS axis will be at right angles to this 'equipolar' lead, but could be pointing in either direction. For instance, if the equipolar lead is lead III (which looks at the heart from +120°), then the QRS axis will be at right angles to this, namely either +30° or −150° (refer back to Fig. 16.3.1.6). Next, find which lead is at right angles to the equipolar lead—in this example, the answer would be lead aVR. Now, if the QRS axis is −150°, then you would expect a positive QRS complex in lead aVR (because the wave of depolarization would be travelling directly towards it). If, however, the QRS complex in lead aVR is negative, the depolarization must be moving away from it and the QRS axis must be therefore be +30°. This method works whichever limb lead is equipolar, as every limb lead has another lead at right angles to it.

An alternative and quick method of checking whether the QRS axis is within the normal range is simply to look at leads I and II. If the QRS complex in lead I is positive (or at least equipolar), then the QRS axis must lie somewhere in the range of −90° to +90°. Similarly, if the QRS complex in lead II is positive, then the QRS axis must lie somewhere in the range -30° to +150°. Therefore we can say that if the QRS complexes in leads I and II are both positive then the QRS axis must lie somewhere in the range −30° to +90°. Thus a positive QRS complex in leads I and II means the QRS axis is within the normal range; a positive QRS complex in lead I and a negative QRS complex in lead II indicate left axis deviation; a negative QRS complex in lead I and a positive QRS complex in lead II indicate right axis deviation.

More precise calculations of the QRS axis can be made by measuring the individual R and S waves in each of the limb leads and using vector analysis to plot out the overall direction of depolarization, but this degree of precision is usually unnecessary.

P wave

The P wave represents atrial depolarization. P waves are usually upright except in leads aVR and V1 (and sometimes V2), where they can be inverted (or biphasic). P waves are seen most clearly in lead II and this is usually the lead of choice for the rhythm strip so that atrial activity can be assessed clearly.

P waves can be inverted in other leads, indicating that atrial depolarization has been initiated somewhere other than the sinoatrial node. For instance, an ectopic focus of depolarization near the atrioventricular node will give rise to inverted P waves in the inferior leads (II, III, and aVF) as the wave of atrial depolarization will spread upwards rather than downwards.

P waves are normally no broader than 3 small squares (0.12 s) and no taller than 2.5 mm. The features of atrial hypertrophy are discussed later.

PR interval

The PR interval is measured from the beginning of the P wave to the beginning of the QRS complex. A normal PR interval is between 0.12 s and 0.20 s in adults.

A long fixed PR interval is termed first-degree atrioventricular block and results from a delay in conduction between the atria and ventricles (Fig. 16.3.1.7). In second-degree atrioventricular block the PR interval may gradually increase with each beat before a P wave is not conducted (Mobitz type I or Wenckebach phenomenon), or may be fixed and long (or normal) with intermittent nonconduction of P waves (Mobitz type II). In third-degree atrioventricular block and also in atrioventricular dissociation the PR interval will vary because of the absence of any association between atrial and ventricular activity. See Chapter 16.4 for further discussion.

A short PR interval is seen in ventricular pre-excitation (see below) or when the focus of atrial depolarization arises not from the sinoatrial node but from the vicinity of the atrioventricular node.

QRS complex

The QRS complex represents ventricular depolarization. The first negative deflection of the complex is termed the Q wave and the first positive deflection the R wave (whether or not it follows a Q wave). A negative deflection after an R wave is termed an S wave. If the deflections are small, lower-case letters (q, r, and s) are used. Thus it is possible to have QRS complexes, qRS complexes, rS complexes, and so on.

Normal 'physiological' q waves are usually narrow (no more than 0.04 s in duration) and small (less than 25% the amplitude of the following R wave) and result from the left to right depolarization of the interventricular septum ('septal q waves'). Larger Q waves may be pathological, although can be normal in leads III and aVR, and may also been seen in lead aVL if the QRS axis is greater than +60°.

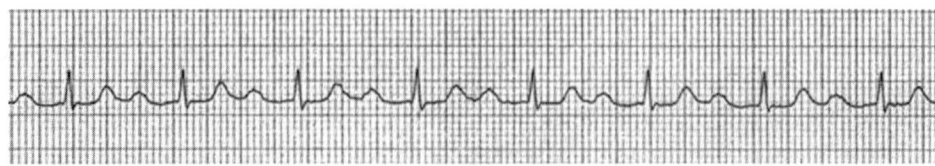

Fig. 16.3.1.7 First-degree atrioventricular block (long PR interval).

The normal QRS complex duration is less than 0.12 s. The amplitude of the QRS complex varies normally from lead to lead and, in the precordial leads, normally increases progressively from lead V1 to V6. At least one R wave in the precordial leads must be at least 8 mm in height, and the tallest R wave should be no more than 27 mm (and the deepest S wave no more than 30 mm), and the sum of the tallest R wave and the deepest S wave should be no more than 40 mm. In the limb leads, the R wave height should be no more than 13 mm in lead aVL and 20 mm in lead aVF.

ST segment

The ST segment should be horizontal and should not normally deviate by more than 1 mm above or below the isoelectric line (which is the line between end of the T wave and the start of the subsequent P wave).

T wave

T waves in the limb leads are normally concordant—if the QRS complex is positive, the subsequent T wave is upright, and vice versa. The T wave is normally inverted in lead aVR and upright in leads I and II.

With regard to the precordial leads, normal T waves are always upright in leads V4 to V6. A flat or inverted T wave is found in lead V1 in 20% of adults, and in lead V2 in 5% of adults (in which case, the T wave should be inverted in lead V1 as well). An inverted T wave in lead V3 can, rarely, be found in normal young adults. T waves should not change their orientation—an inverted T wave is not normal if previous ECGs show that it was previously upright.

There are no strict criteria for normal T wave size, so 'tall' and 'small' T waves are not well defined and deciding on their presence tends to be a subjective judgement. 'Tall' T waves can occur in early acute myocardial infarction ('hyperacute' T waves) and in hyperkalaemia ('tented' T waves). Small T waves can be seen in hypokalaemia.

QT interval

The QT interval is measured between the start of the QRS complex and the end of the T wave. The normal range for the QT interval varies according to heart rate. It is therefore convenient to correct the measured QT interval to what it would be if the heart rate were 60 beats/min. This is done using Bazett's formula, in which the measured QT interval (in seconds) is divided by the square root of the RR interval (in seconds), to give the corrected QT interval (QTc). The normal range for the QT interval at a heart rate of 60 beats/min, and thus for the QTc, is between 0.35 s and 0.44 s (men) or 0.45 s (women).

U wave

The T wave is occasionally followed by a U wave, most clearly seen in the right precordial leads, which has the same orientation as the T wave and is usually no more than one-third of its size. The physiological origin of the U wave is still debated, but is often said to relate to afterdepolarizations in the ventricles.

Myocardial hypertrophy

Left ventricular hypertrophy

Evidence of left ventricular hypertrophy on the ECG is a significant risk factor for cardiovascular morbidity and mortality. A number of diagnostic ECG criteria for left ventricular hypertrophy have

---

> **Box 16.3.1.1** Diagnostic criteria for left ventricular hypertrophy
>
> **Limb leads**
> - R wave >11 mm in lead aVL
> - R wave >20 mm in lead aVF
> - S wave >14 mm in lead aVR
> - Sum of R wave in lead I and S wave in lead III >25 mm
>
> **Precordial leads**
> - R wave of ≥25 mm in the left precordial leads
> - S wave of ≥25 mm in the right precordial leads
> - Sum of S wave in lead V1 and R wave in lead V5 or V6 >35 mm (Sokolow–Lyon criteria)
> - Sum of tallest R wave and deepest S wave in the precordial leads >45 mm

been developed which, in general, are relatively specific (>90%) but not very sensitive (20–60%). The diagnostic criteria shown in Box 16.3.1.1 are commonly used.

The Cornell criteria involve measuring the S wave in lead V3 and the R wave in lead aVL. Left ventricular hypertrophy is indicated by a sum of more than 28 mm in men and more than 20 mm in women.

The Romhilt–Estes scoring system allocates points for the presence of certain criteria, with a score of 5 indicating left ventricular hypertrophy and a score of 4 indicating probable left ventricular hypertrophy. Points are allocated as follows:

- 3 points for (a) R or S wave in limb leads of 20 mm or more, (b) S wave in right precordial leads of 25 mm or more, or (c) R wave in left precordial leads of 25 mm or more
- 3 points for ST segment and T wave changes ('typical strain') in a patient not taking digitalis (1 point with digitalis)
- 3 points for P-terminal force in V1 greater than 1 mm deep with a duration greater than 0.04 s
- 2 points for left axis deviation (beyond –15°)
- 1 point for QRS complex duration greater than 0.09 s
- 1 point for intrinsoid deflection (the interval from the start of the QRS complex to the peak of the R wave) in V5 or V6 greater than 0.05 s

A left ventricular 'strain' pattern (ST-T wave abnormalities) is associated with around double the risk of myocardial infarction and stroke as left ventricular hypertrophy in the absence of strain.

Left ventricular hypertrophy cannot be assessed reliably using the ECG in patients with bundle branch block, previous myocardial infarction or WPW syndrome; visualization via echocardiography or cardiac MRI is required.

An example of left ventricular hypertrophy is shown in Fig. 16.3.1.8.

Right ventricular hypertrophy

As with left ventricular hypertrophy, the ECG criteria for right ventricular hypertrophy tend to be relatively specific but not very sensitive. Right ventricular hypertrophy shifts the QRS complex

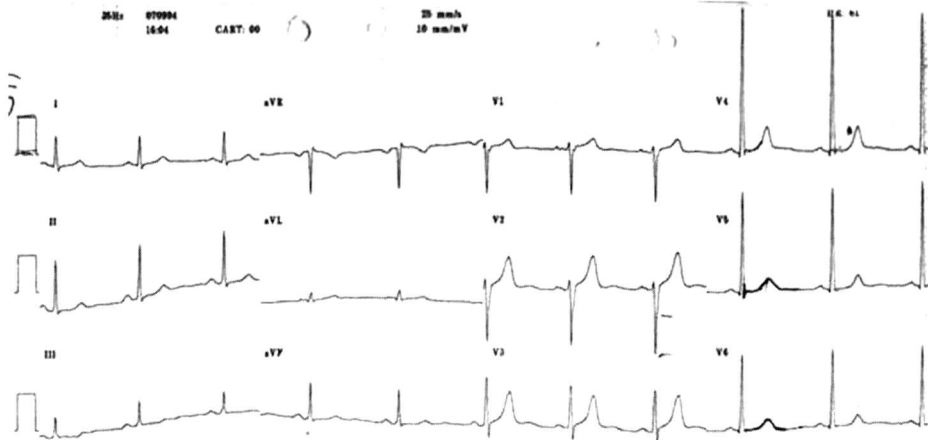

Fig. 16.3.1.8 Left ventricular hypertrophy.

axis rightwards as well as producing higher-voltage QRS complexes in the right precordial leads. ECG criteria include:

- a dominant R wave (R wave ≥ S wave) in lead V1, in the presence of a normal QRS duration
- a QRS complex axis of greater than +90°

These criteria are supported by:

- ST segment depression and T wave inversion in the right precordial leads
- deep S waves in the lateral precordial and limb leads

It is not essential for all these criteria to be present, but the greater the number of features present, the greater the likelihood of right ventricular hypertrophy. It is prudent to remember that a dominant R wave in lead V1 can also be seen in right bundle branch block, WPW syndrome, and a posterior wall myocardial infarction.

Atrial hypertrophy

Left atrial hypertropy

Left atrial depolarization is responsible for the terminal portion of the normal P wave. Left atrial hypertrophy increases the voltage and duration of this depolarization, and thus usually evidences itself by abnormalities of the terminal portion of the P wave. The P wave duration is prolonged, and it becomes bifid in lead II and biphasic, with a predominant negative component, in lead V1. So-called 'P mitrale' can be seen in the left atrial enlargement that results from mitral valve stenosis (hence the term) and also in association with conditions that cause left ventricular hypertrophy, such as hypertension (most commonly) and aortic stenosis (Fig. 16.3.1.9).

Right atrial hypertrophy

Right atrial hypertrophy increases the voltage, but not the duration, of the P wave, and this is usually best seen in the inferior and right precordial leads. A P wave height greater than 2.5 mm is regarded as abnormal. So called 'P pulmonale' can result from right ventricular hypertrophy or from tricuspid valve stenosis (Fig. 16.3.1.10).

The hemiblocks

The left bundle branch divides into anterosuperior and posteroinferior fascicles. A block of either fascicle (hemiblock) causes a deviation of the QRS axis.

Left anterior hemiblock

Block of the anterosuperior fascicle leads to left anterior hemiblock. This causes a leftward shift in the QRS axis, as the right/inferior region of the left ventricle depolarizes first (via the posteroinferior fascicle) and then the wave of depolarization spreads to the left/superior region. Although this hemiblock introduces a minor delay in ventricular depolarization, the QRS duration remains within the normal range (up to 120 ms). The QRS axis shifts to the left (beyond −30°). As a similar axis shift can result from an inferior myocardial infarction, the diagnosis of left anterior hemiblock requires the presence of left axis deviation in the absence of an abnormal q wave in lead aVF.

Left posterior hemiblock

Block of the posteroinferior fascicle leads to left posterior hemiblock. This causes a rightward shift in the QRS axis, as the left/superior region of the left ventricle depolarizes first (via the anterosuperior fascicle) and then the wave of depolarization spreads to the right/inferior region. As with left anterior hemiblock, the QRS duration remains within the normal range (up to 120 ms). The QRS axis shifts to the right (beyond +90°). However, right axis deviation can occur in several conditions (most commonly right ventricular hypertrophy, but also in lateral myocardial infarction and WPW syndrome). It is therefore not possible to diagnose left posterior hemiblock with certainty from the 12-lead ECG alone.

Bundle-branch block

Left bundle branch block

Left bundle branch block (LBBB) leads to a delay in left ventricular depolarization, as the left ventricle is depolarized via the right-sided

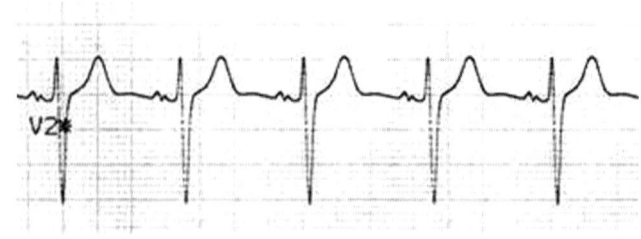

Fig. 16.3.1.9 Left atrial hypertrophy ('P mitrale').

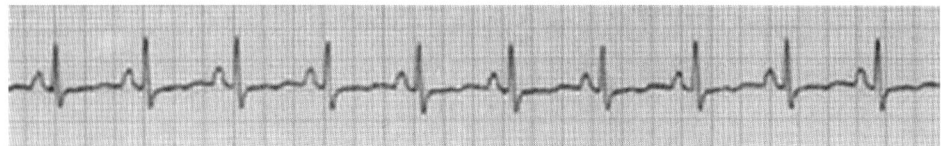

Fig. 16.3.1.10 Right atrial hypertrophy ('P pulmonale').

Purkinje system. In addition, the interventricular septum depolarizes from right to left instead of the usual left to right. Thus, in LBBB:

◆ The QRS duration is prolonged (≥120 ms)

◆ The normal 'septal' q waves usually seen in the lateral leads are absent

◆ A secondary r wave is not seen in lead V1 (this distinguishes LBBB from RBBB with clockwise cardiac rotation)

These findings may be accompanied by ST segment depression and T wave inversion in the lateral precordial and limb leads, broad QS waves in the right precordial leads and broad R waves in the lateral leads, and R wave notching ('M-shaped' QRS complexes).

An example of LBBB is shown in Fig. 16.3.1.11. The extensive nature of the ECG changes means that further interpretation of the QRS complexes, ST segments or T waves cannot be made. The difficulties of diagnosing myocardial infarction in the setting of LBBB are discussed later.

Right bundle branch block

Right bundle branch block (RBBB) leads to a delay in right ventricular depolarization, as the right ventricle is depolarized via the left-sided Purkinje system. However, the normal left to right activation of the interventricular septum is preserved. The ECG changes seen in RBBB are therefore not as extensive as in LBBB. The QRS duration is prolonged (≥120 ms) and the right ventricular leads contain a second positive wave (and, conversely, the left ventricular leads contain a second negative wave). Thus, in RBBB:

◆ the QRS duration is prolonged (≥120 ms)

◆ lead V1 contains a second positive wave (rsR′)

◆ lead V6 contains a second negative wave (qRs)

These findings may be accompanied by deep slurred S waves in the lateral precordial and limb leads, and abnormal ST-T wave changes in the right precordial leads.

An example of RBBB is shown in Fig. 16.3.1.12.

Ventricular pre-excitation

The normal progression of a wave of depolarization is from the sinoatrial node through the atria to the atrioventricular node, and then through the bundle of His and the Purkinje fibres to the ventricular myocardium. However approximately 1 in 1000 of the population has an accessory pathway—an alternative pathway from atria to ventricles that bypasses part of this normal route. Such a pathway initiates depolarization of the ventricles at a slightly earlier stage in the cardiac cycle than would otherwise be the case, hence the term 'ventricular pre-excitation'. This is because the accessory pathway lacks the inherent delay to conduction that is normally found in the atrioventricular node, thus allowing faster conduction of the wave of depolarization from atria to ventricles.

There are several types of pathway that can give rise to ventricular pre-excitation.

WPW-type pre-excitation

WPW-type pre-excitation is exemplified by WPW syndrome. In WPW syndrome an accessory pathway, the bundle of Kent,

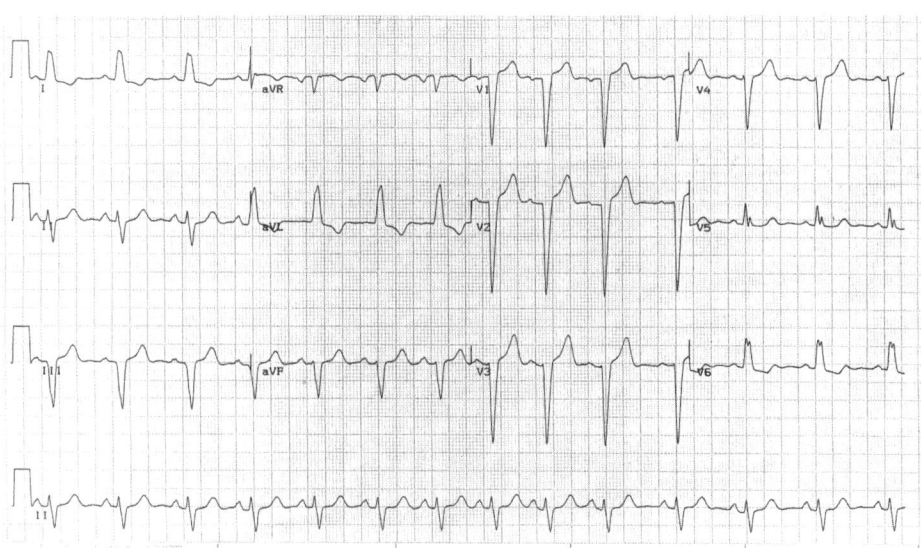

Fig. 16.3.1.11 Left bundle branch block.

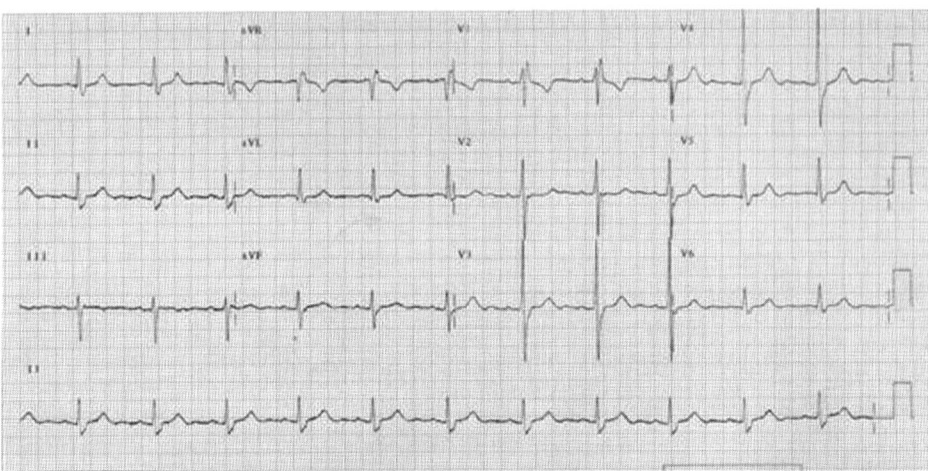

Fig. 16.3.1.12 Right bundle branch block.

connects the atria to the ventricles and bypasses the atrioventricular node altogether. This shortens the time between the onset of atrial depolarization and the onset of ventricular depolarization, and hence one of the ECG features of WPW syndrome is a short PR interval (<0.12 s). Because the accessory pathway leads directly to the ventricular myocardium, and not into the His–Purkinje system, the subsequent initial ventricular depolarization progresses slowly, as conduction of the wave of depolarization cannot take advantage of the rapidly-conducting Purkinje fibres. This gives rise to a delta wave—a slurred initial upstroke of the QRS complex. These features can be seen in the ECG from a patient with WPW syndrome in Fig. 16.3.1.13.

Conduction between atria and ventricles can be via the accessory pathway, or via the atrioventricular node, or via both routes, or can vary from one to another. If conduction does not occur via the accessory pathway, the ECG will appear normal and the pathway is said to be 'concealed'.

The appearances of the delta wave can vary from patient to patient. Indeed, the ECG appearances of the QRS complex can be used, to a limited extent, to predict the likely location of the accessory pathway. However, the exact location can only be found with electrophysiological studies. The QRS complex morphology

in WPW syndrome can mimic LBBB, RBBB, or acute myocardial infarction. WPW syndrome can also lead to repolarization (and therefore T wave) abnormalities. Great care must be thus taken in diagnosing these conditions in the presence of WPW syndrome.

The existence of two atrioventricular pathways (the normal atrioventricular node and the abnormal bundle of Kent) provides a substrate for atrioventricular re-entry tachycardia, which is discussed in more detail in Chapter 16.4.

Short PR-type pre-excitation

A short PR interval in the absence of a delta wave/abnormal QRS complex is often referred to as Lown–Ganong–Levine syndrome, in which an atrio-His accessory pathway bypasses the slow-conducting part of the atrioventricular node. Identical appearances can also seen with a fast-conducting atrioventricular node. The presence of an atrio-His accessory pathway is a substrate for atrioventricular nodal re-entry tachycardia. For further discussion see Chapter 16.4.

Mahaim-type pre-excitation

Mahaim fibres, first described in the 1930s, are atriofascicular or atrioventricular accessory pathways that connect the atrioventricular

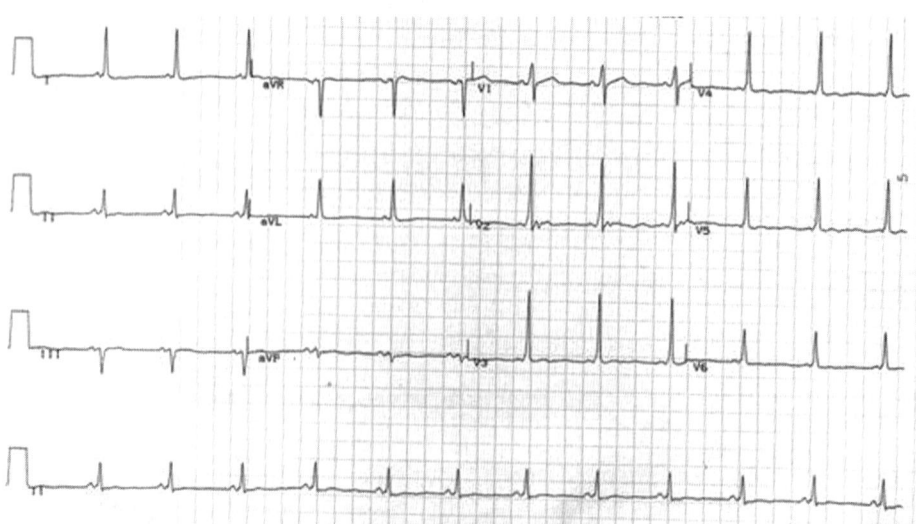

Fig. 16.3.1.13 WPW syndrome, showing the short PR interval and delta wave.

node to the right bundle or the right ventricle. Patients with Mahaim-type pre-excitation have a normal PR interval with a LBBB QRS complex morphology and are prone to re-entry tachycardia. For further discussion see Chapter 16.4.

Acute coronary syndromes

Sudden disruption of existing coronary plaque may partially or totally occlude a coronary artery, causing myocyte necrosis. Symptoms of severe, centrally located chest pain develop suddenly, usually accompanied by breathlessness due to left ventricular dysfunction and tachycardia, pallor, sweating, nausea and extreme anxiety due to sympathetic drive. The American College of Cardiology and the European Society of Cardiology classification of myocardial ischaemia and infarction recognizes that acute changes in coronary atheroma produce a spectrum of disease, the acute coronary syndromes (ACS):

- Unstable angina, where coronary plaque has ruptured but stabilizes without major change in the lumen of the coronary artery: the ECG may be normal, or indicate a previous myocardial infarction, or dynamic ST depression and/or T wave inversion may appear. Serum troponin level, a marker of myocyte necrosis, is within normal limits.

- Non-ST elevation myocardial infarction (NSTEMI), where plaque is ruptured with partial occlusion of a major coronary artery: ECG signs are variable—the ECG may be normal, or indicate a previous myocardial infarction, or ST depression may appear transiently or symmetrically inverted T waves may appear. Troponin levels are elevated.

- ST elevation myocardial infarction (STEMI) where thrombosis from a ruptured plaque completely occludes a coronary artery: the ECG shows ST segment elevation initially, then resolves within a day or two, with new Q waves and inverted T waves appearing in the leads subtending the infarcted area. Troponin levels are elevated.

For discussion of the clinical features and management of acute coronary syndromes, see Chapters 16.2.1, 16.13.5, and 16.13.6.

Role of the ECG in acute coronary syndromes

The ECG remains the most useful bedside triage tool in the emergency setting, whether in the community, en route to hospital, or in the Emergency Department. Accurate interpretation is essential—misinterpretation of the ECG can be as high as 12% and lead to inappropriate management. The ECG is used to diagnose acute coronary syndromes, to locate the site of ischaemia and infarction (see Table 16.3.1.1) and to identify areas of impaired perfusion (see 'Reciprocal changes').

Of those who suffer a STEMI, the initial ECG is diagnostic in 50%, abnormal but not diagnostic in 40%, and normal in the remainder. Repeat ECGs may be necessary to confidently diagnose or exclude an acute coronary syndrome, as diagnostic changes may not appear for several hours. Serial recordings increase the sensitivity to 95%.

The presenting ECG and prognosis in acute coronary syndrome

About 22% of all patients with acute chest pain will present with T wave inversion, 28% with ST segment elevation, 35% with ST segment depression, and 15% with a combination of ST segment

Table 16.3.1.1 Location of infarction and affected coronary artery

ECG leads affected	Site of infarction	Most likely artery occluded (positive predictive value)
V3 and V4 I, aVL and V1 to V6 (in extensive infarction)	Anterior	Left anterior descending (96%)
V1 and V2	Septal	
V1 to V4	Anteroseptal	
I, aVL and V3 to V6	Anterolateral	
II, III and aVF	Inferior	Right coronary (80%) Right or circumflex (94%)
I, aVL and V6 I and aVL (high lateral)	Lateral	Circumflex (75%)
ST depression in V1 and V2 followed by development of prominent R waves in lead V1 or V2	Posterior	Circumflex (75%)
	Lateral or posterior	Right or circumflex (94%)
II, III and aVF with aVL, V5 and V6	Inferolateral	Right coronary (93%)

elevation and depression. T wave inversion is most likely to be associated with angiographically normal coronary arteries. Those with ST segment depression are more likely to have three-vessel disease. Mortality at 1 month is 1.7% in those with T wave changes, 5.1% with ST segment elevation or depression, and 6.6% with both depression and elevation. Severe ST segment depression (>2 mm in two contiguous leads) is associated with an increased risk of death at 1 year.

The presenting ECG and probability of acute coronary syndrome

New, or presumed new, ST segment deviation greater than 0.05 mV, however transiently, or T wave inversion greater than 0.2 mV, is highly indicative of ACS. Q waves, ST segment displacement or T waves have an intermediate probability of ACS. T wave flattening inverted or normal ECG has a low probability of ACS. The likelihood of NSTEMI is increased threefold in chest pain with ST segment depression in three leads or >0.2 mV.

The presenting ECG and triage

The presenting ECG can be used to triage patients with acute cardiac-sounding chest pain:

- ST elevation present: immediate reperfusion should be considered, either by primary percutaneous coronary intervention (PCI) or by intravenous thrombolysis

- ST elevation not evident: immediate treatment with anti-platelet drugs and infusion of an intravenous glycoprotein IIb/IIIa inhibitor, with consideration of coronary angiography in those with a Troponin above the normal range

- ST elevation present transiently: thrombolysis is not appropriate but monitor on a coronary care unit; repeat ECG in 1 h or if pain recurs or increases; if ST elevation is present, consider PCI or intravenous thrombolysis

ST segment elevation myocardial infarction

The ECG changes of myocardial infarction, first described in 1920, reflect myocardial ischemia, injury, and myocyte necrosis. Within an hour or so of occlusion of a coronary artery, the T wave becomes more prominent, exceeding one-half the height of the preceding R wave in the ECG leads subtending the infarcted area (see Fig. 16.3.1.14). Many patients present later than this, so these changes may pass unnoticed. In up to 50%, the presenting ECG is normal. The first documented indication of infarction is usually ST segment elevation which occurs within a few hours. The J point (the origin of the ST segment at its junction with the QRS complex) is elevated by 1 mm or more in two or more limb leads, or by 2 mm in two or more precordial leads.

The ST segment returns to the baseline over the next 48 to 72 h, during which Q waves and symmetrically inverted T waves appear. Some patients develop LBBB, either transiently or permanently. The ECG of a completed infarct shows new Q waves greater than 2 mm, R waves reduced in size or absent, and inverted T waves. This classical evolution of STEMI is seen in about 50 to 66% of patients.

Reperfusion therapy, whether by PCI or thrombolysis, may alter this natural sequence of changes in the ECG, as both have the potential to unblock the occluded coronary artery. If treatment is given with thrombolysis, then an ECG performed 90 min after initiation should show that ST elevation has been reduced by at least 50% from pretreatment levels (Fig. 16.3.1.15). If chest pain persists and the ST segments remain elevated, coronary angiography and rescue PCI should be considered. Where available, primary PCI may be offered in preference to thrombolysis.

Resolution of ST segment elevation predicts 30-day mortality. With greater than 70% ST segment resolution, mortality is 2.1%; with 30–70% ST segment resolution 5.2%; with no ST segment resolution 5.5%; and with worsening ST segment elevation 8.1%.

Non-ST elevation myocardial infarction

ECG changes in NSTEMI are more variable than in STEMI. The ECG may be normal on first presentation and remain unchanged throughout the acute admission. There may be transient ST segment depression indicative of myocardial ischaemia. In 20 to 30%, the only change will be T wave inversion. Risk-scoring systems have been developed, e.g. by the Trials In Myocardial Infarction group (www.timi.org), for use in patients with acute coronary syndromes. These are described in Chapter 16.13.5: with regard to non-ST-elevation myocardial infarction, ST segment deviation greater than 0.5 mm is one of the recorded parameters.

The extent of ST depression identifies those who are most likely to benefit from early revascularization (FRISC II trial). Mortality with early invasive therapy is 4% with ST segment depression, 2% with no ECG changes, and 0.2% with T wave inversion.

Difficult diagnoses in acute myocardial infarction

Right ventricular infarction

The ECG provides prognostic as well as diagnostic information. An inferior infarction generally carries a good prognosis unless it is associated with a right ventricular infarction, when there is a sixfold increased risk of a major in-hospital complication, including ventricular fibrillation, reinfarction, and death. The right ventricle is involved in about 50% of those with an inferior infarction, occurring with occlusion of the right coronary artery, causing a transmural infarct of the inferoposterior wall and the posterior septum.

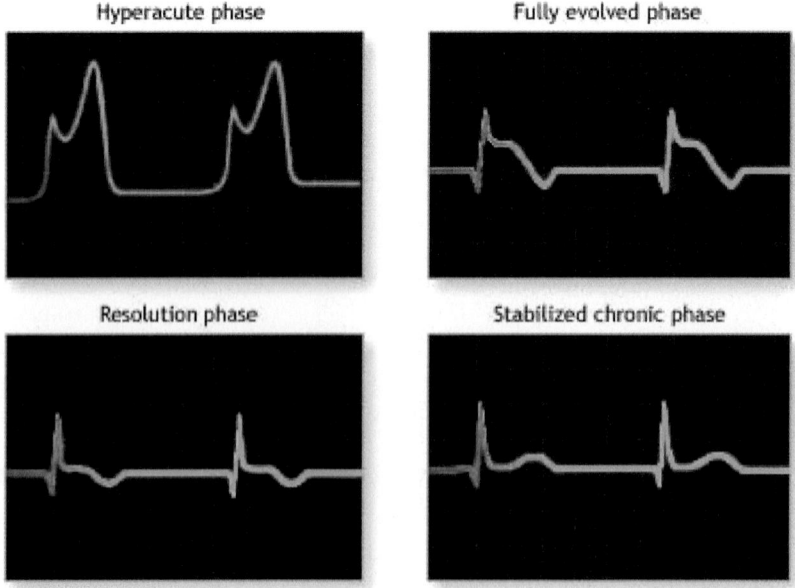

Fig. 16.3.1.14 Evolution of STEMI over several days.

The evolving infarction: ST elevation, followed by development of new Q waves and inverted T waves

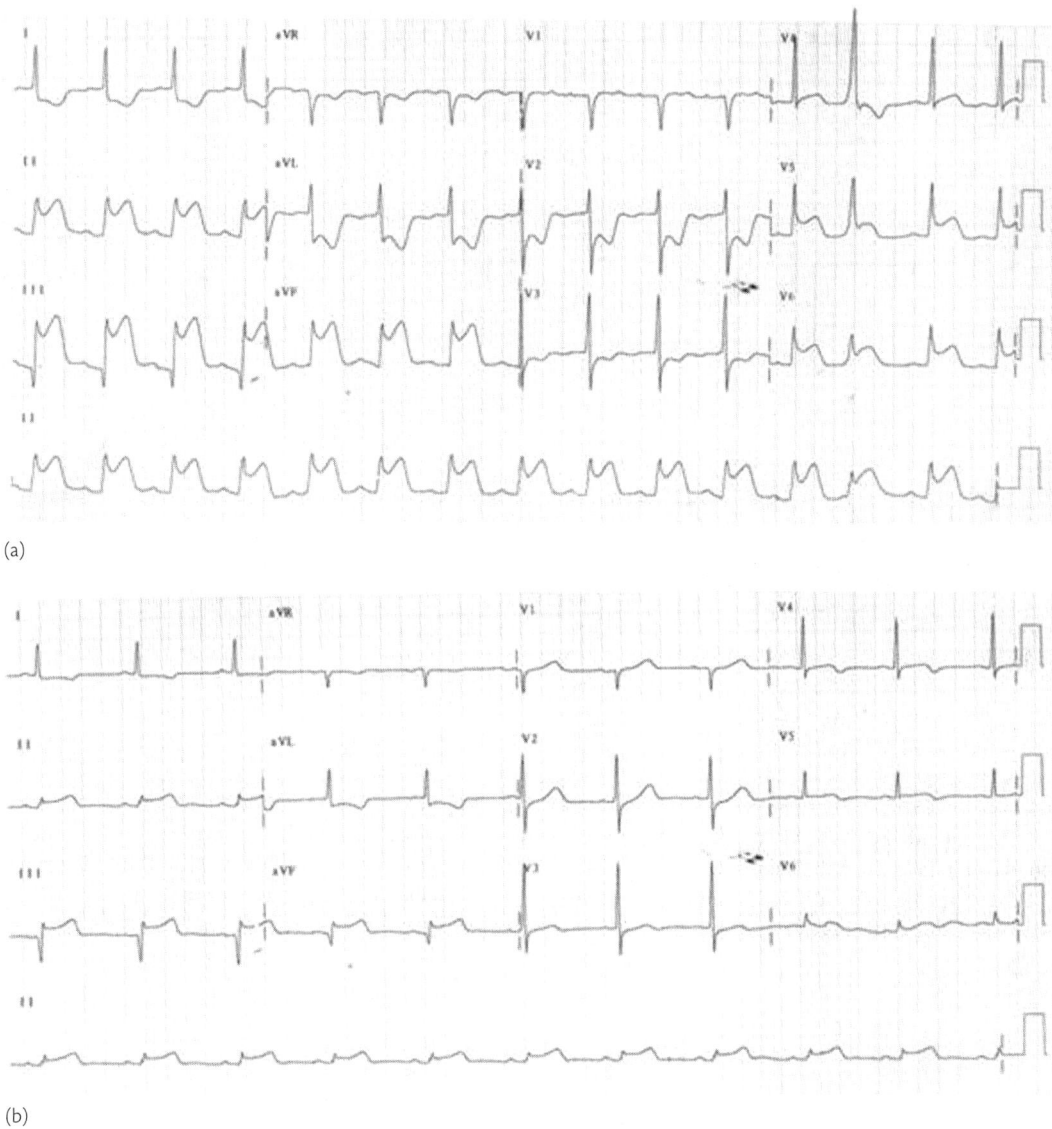

(a)

(b)

Fig. 16.3.1.15 (a) Acute inferolateral ST segment elevation myocardial infarction. (b) Substantial (but not complete) resolution of ST segment elevation 90 min after the initiation of thrombolysis.

To determine whether the right ventricle is involved in an inferior infarction, an ECG should be recorded with the anterior chest leads placed on the right side of the chest, in equivalent (but mirrored) positions to a standard 12-lead ECG. The right ventricle is involved if there is greater than 1 mm ST segment elevation in chest lead 'right V4' (RV4); this has a sensitivity of 100%, specificity of 87%, and positive predictive value of 92% for occlusion of the right coronary artery proximal to the right ventricular branch. If these changes are absent, the right ventricle has been spared (Fig. 16.3.1.16).

Atrial infarction

This occurs in up to 10% of myocardial infarcts in conjunction with ventricular infarction. A clue to its presence is PR segment displacement but there may also be an abnormal P wave. It can cause rupture of the atrial wall and is frequently associated with atrial arrhythmias including atrial fibrillation, atrial flutter, and atrioventricular nodal rhythm.

Coronary artery spasm

The pain of Prinzmetal's or variant angina is not usually triggered by exercise, emotion, cold, or a meal but tends to occur at rest, accompanied by transient, marked ST segment elevation. This rapidly reverts to normal when the pain resolves spontaneously or with glyceryl trinitrate. Atrioventricular block or ventricular arrhythmia may accompany spasm-induced myocardial ischaemia. Spasm sufficient to cause myocardial ischaemia, myocardial infarction, and sudden death can follow cocaine use.

Reciprocal changes—septal ischaemia or posterior infarction?

ST or 'reciprocal' depression may be seen in leads remote from the site of a STEMI. For example, ST depression may be seen in leads V1 to V4 in an inferior STEMI. There are two explanations. First, in a right-dominant system (70% of the population), the right

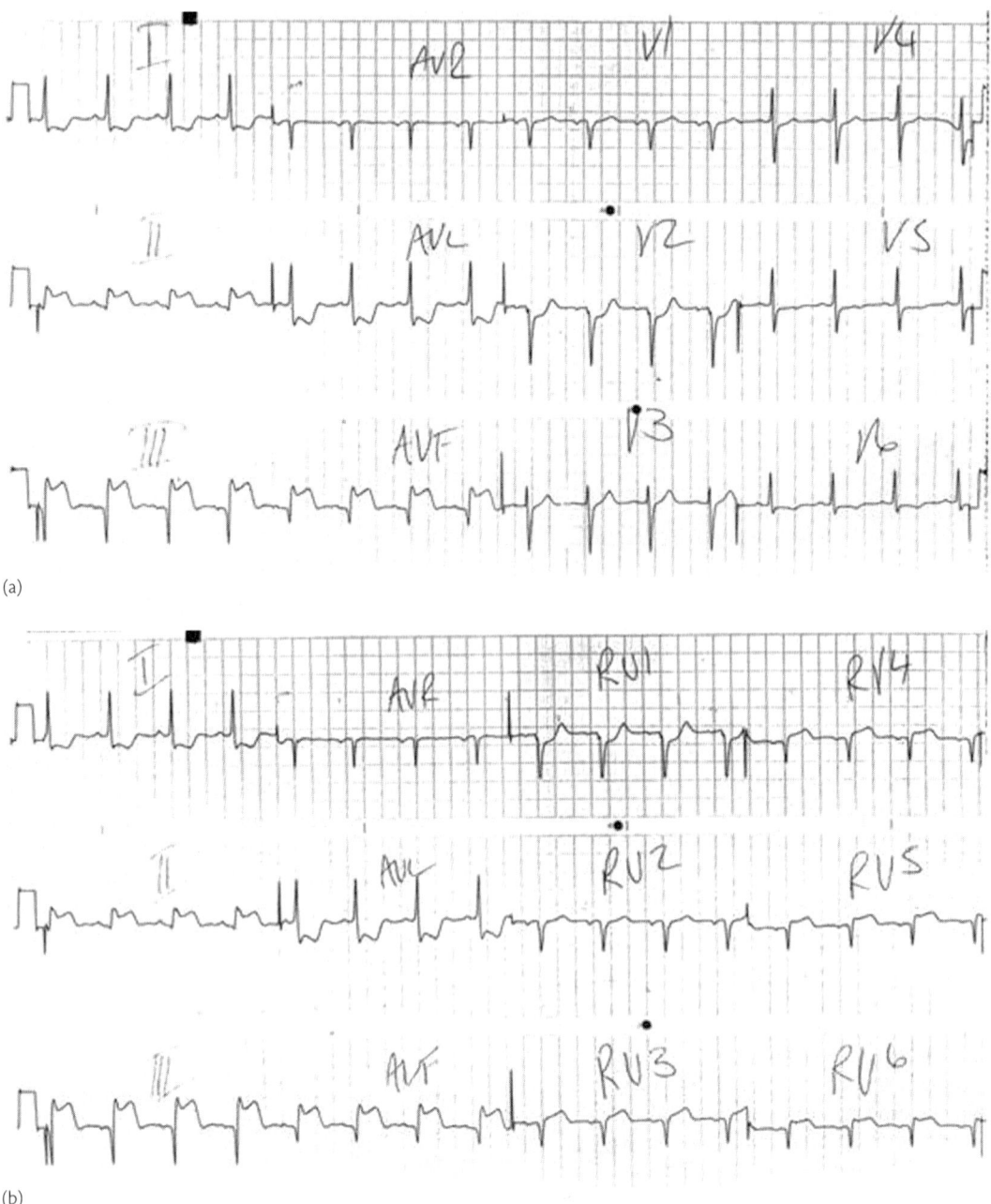

Fig. 16.3.1.16 (a) Inferior ST segment elevation myocardial infarction. (b) Inferior ST segment elevation myocardial infarction with right ventricular involvement (note the right ventricular chest leads, with ST segment elevation in lead RV4).

coronary artery supplies the posterior interventricular septum, which becomes ischaemic with an inferior STEMI; the ischaemia resolves within a few days as septal perforating arteries from the left anterior descending artery dilate in response to ischaemic stress. Second, in a left-dominant system, the circumflex supplies the posterior interventricular septum; if this occludes, a 'true posterior infarction' follows.

Difficulties in diagnosing STEMI

'Stuttering' infarction

Symptoms of myocardial infarction are usually severe and of sudden onset. Occasionally, the onset of symptoms is not so clear cut and chest pain may resolve but recur at intervals over several hours. The time of arterial occlusion is at best a guess but for practical purposes is taken as the time that symptoms increase or are at their worst.

Noninfarct causes of ST segment elevation

Pericarditis may mimic the pain of myocardial infarction but is usually relieved by sitting forward and is accompanied by a pericardial rub. The ST segments are elevated diffusely, do not fit the usual lead pattern for an inferior or anterior infarction, and, unlike the convexity of STEMI, are concave upwards. Prinzmetal's angina, caused by coronary artery spasm, can also mimic myocardial infarction. This usually occurs at rest, with marked ST elevation during pain and a brisk response to glyceryl trinitrate. The ST segment can be elevated chronically in left ventricular aneurysm, left ventricular hypertrophy, LBBB, hypertrophic cardiomyopathy, acute cor pulmonale, hypothermia, and cocaine abuse. A normal variant is so-called 'high take-off' where serial ECGs show consistent ST elevation across most ECG leads; patients should be given a copy of the ECG to show to medical personnel to avoid unnecessary investigations and treatment.

Late presentation

Patients who present to hospital outside the 12-h time limit for thrombolysis are sometimes diagnosed as 'missed infarction'. The ECG may show signs characteristically seen later in the infarction process, with ST segments only slightly elevated, with established Q waves and inverted T waves. Over the next few days, the ST segment fully returns to baseline and Q waves and T waves deepen.

LBBB

A septal Q wave is absent in LBBB, because the septum is initially activated from right to left. A Q wave will not be detected when a myocardial infarction occurs in a patient with pre-existing LBBB. On first presentation, it may not be known whether LBBB is 'old' or 'new'. Although there may be subtle clues on the ECG that may help diagnose an acute infarction, patients with LBBB have a better outcome with thrombolysis.

ECG changes of 'old' infarction

Q waves, once formed, usually persist indefinitely and so are a reliable indicator of a previous myocardial infarction (Fig. 16.3.1.17). However there are several other causes of a Q wave that may cause confusion, the most common being hypertrophic cardiomyopathy and idiopathic cardiomyopathy. Rarer causes include myocarditis, cardiac amyloid, neuromuscular disorders (e.g. muscular dystrophy, myotonic dystrophy, Friedreich's ataxia), scleroderma, sarcoidosis and an anomalous coronary artery.

Pre-excitation

WPW syndrome makes interpretation of the ECG more complicated. It may mask a myocardial infarction if conduction via the bypass tract is towards the left ventricle, as a Q wave will not be apparent. WPW may also simulate an infarction due to a negative delta wave in the inferior leads producing Q waves. Serial or previous ECGs will reveal the true diagnosis. Patients with WPW syndrome should be given a copy of their ECG to avoid confusion and unnecessary future investigations.

T wave inversion

Atypical ECG features are seen in up to half of all infarctions in the early stages. Alone, these changes are not diagnostic. They can occur in ventricular aneurysm, electrolyte abnormalities, myocarditis, and subarachnoid haemorrhage, and with some drugs. Serial ECGs are necessary to establish a firm diagnosis.

Deep, symmetrical 'arrowhead' T waves developing during an infarction are most often due to proximal occlusion of the left anterior descending coronary artery (Fig. 16.3.1.18).

Where errors occur

Incorrect interpretation of an ECG leads to inappropriate patient triage and misses the opportunity to provide reperfusion therapy, whether by angioplasty or thrombolysis. In the worst case scenario, inappropriate thrombolysis might lead to a haemorrhagic stroke or ruptured aneurysm. Up to 12% of those with a high-risk ECG, i.e. ST segment elevation of at least 0.1 mV, ST segment depression of at least 0.05 mV, or T wave inversion of at least 0.2 mV in 2 or more contiguous leads, are missed on admission to the Emergency Department.

The ECG provides a 'snapshot' of electrical events within the heart, when the clinician really needs a 'movie' to monitor the dynamic changes of an acute coronary syndrome. If a diagnosis cannot be made on the presenting ECG but the history suggests an acute coronary syndrome, the patient should be admitted to a monitored area, a review by a specialist should be arranged, and the ECG should be repeated if symptoms get worse or if ST segment changes are seen are seen on the monitor. This will ensure prompt and appropriate treatment.

While it may be important to provide treatment promptly to fulfil audit targets, e.g. door-to-needle time for thrombolysis, speed should not replace accuracy in diagnosis. It is sometimes better to wait a short while, control symptoms, give aspirin, and repeat the ECG than to make an incorrect diagnosis. It is easy to place too much reliance on minor changes on the ECG; it is gross changes of ST elevation or depression within the parameters above, that should determine treatment.

Exercise ECG testing

ECG changes on exercise were first reported in patients with chronic stable angina in the early 1900s. Exercise testing was adopted into routine clinical practice soon after a standardized exercise protocol was developed.

Cardiovascular responses to exercise in normal subjects and in coronary disease

Normally on treadmill exercise, heart rate increases as a result of diminished vagal and increased sympathetic outflow. Heart rate increases on commencing exercise and reaches a plateau during

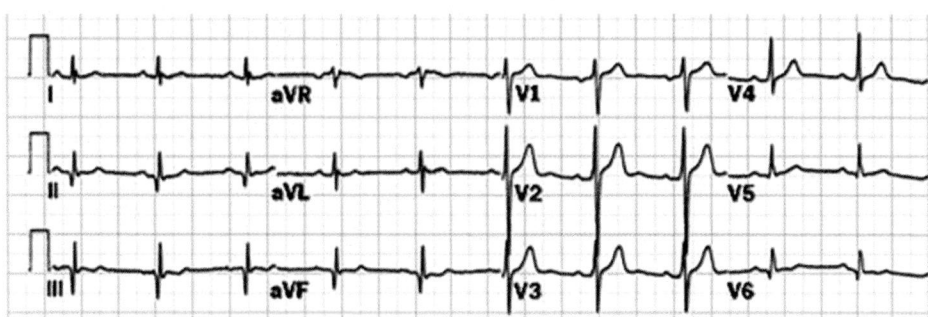

Fig. 16.3.1.17 'Old' inferior myocardial infarction: pathological Q waves in leads II, III, and aVF.

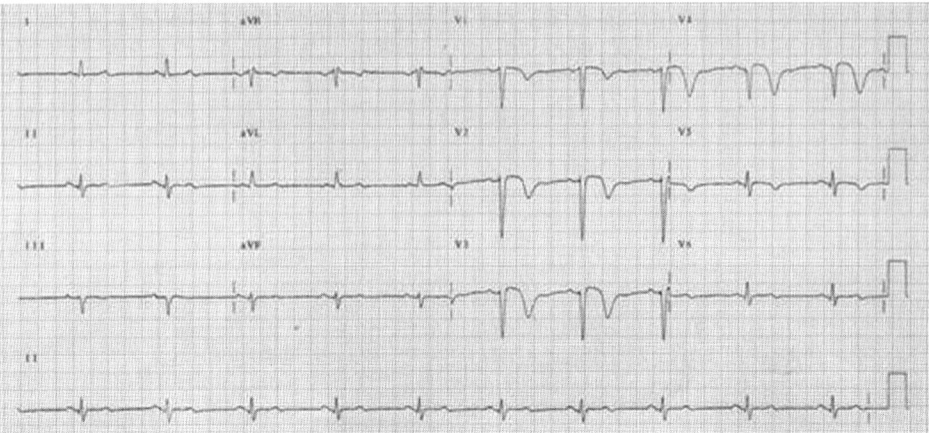

Fig. 16.3.1.18 Recent anterior ST segment elevation myocardial infarction with 'arrowhead' T wave inversion.

each stage of the exercise test. A rapid increase may be due to lack of fitness, prolonged bed rest, anaemia, or dehydration. Systolic blood pressure increases in line with increased cardiac output, while diastolic pressure is near constant or falls slightly due to vasodilatation. On stopping the test, heart rate slows within a few minutes to pretest levels and both systolic and diastolic blood pressure falls, often to below pretest levels, as a result of vasodilatation.

With cardiac disease, the maximum cardiac rate may be attenuated (even in the absence of a β-blocker) due to sinus node disease, coronary heart disease, or postinfarction (with or without β-blockade). Failure to achieve the maximum predicted heart rate, calculated as 220 minus age, is suggestive of cardiac disease. Brady- and tachyarrhythmias including atrial fibrillation may occur. Exercise-induced hypotension, even a transient fall in blood pressure at (near-)maximum heart rate, is indicative of severe heart disease and increases the risk of ventricular fibrillation. On stopping exercise, systolic pressure falls to resting levels (or lower) within minutes, where it may remain for several hours. In some, venous pooling may cause a precipitous drop in systolic pressure.

ECG changes with exercise in normal subjects and in coronary disease

In normal subjects, exercise-induced tachycardia causes shortened PR, QRS, and QT intervals, increased P wave amplitude, and down-sloping of the PR segment. R waves and T waves may diminish and S waves increase at maximum exercise. The J point (the isoelectric point where the S wave reaches the baseline) may become depressed in all leads and the ST segment may become up-sloping.

The most helpful ECG marker of exercise-induced myocardial ischaemia is the ST segment which becomes depressed with increasing heart rate. This is due to shortening of the action potential due to ischaemia, setting up electrical gradients between endocardium and epicardium. Horizontal or down-sloping ST depression, measured 60 to 80 ms after the J point, of 1 mm (0.10 mV) or more for 80 ms in at least three complexes is considered significant (Fig. 16.3.1.19), but the leads in which ST depression appear do not reliably localize the site of myocardial ischaemia.

Other indicators of myocardial ischaemia include:

♦ ST segment elevation—this indicates severe ischaemia due to proximal disease or coronary spasm, or an aneurysmal or dyskinetic left ventricle. Unlike exercise-induced ST segment depression, the ECG site of ST segment elevation is relatively specific for the coronary artery involved

♦ T wave inversion—this may occur with exercise-induced hyperventilation

♦ Normalization of an inverted T wave—this alone is not indicative of coronary disease

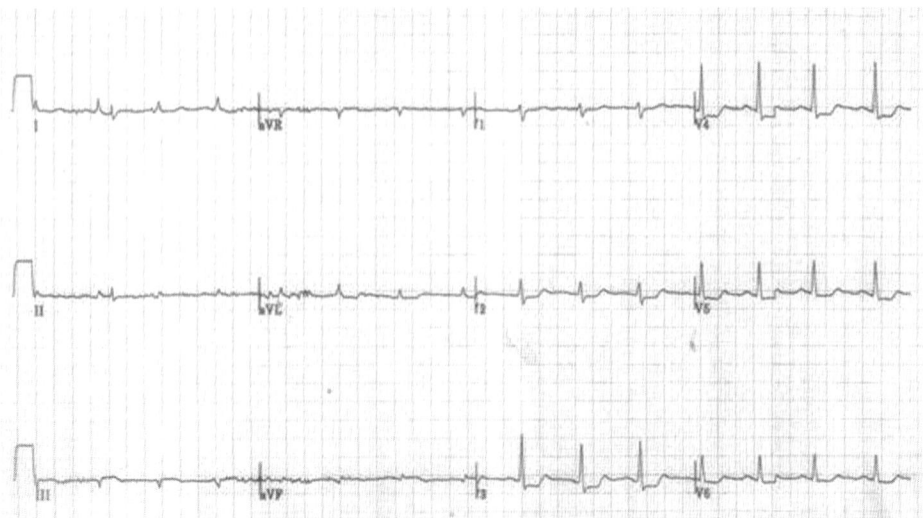

Fig. 16.3.1.19 ECG recorded during an exercise treadmill test, showing anterolateral ST segment depression after 3 min of exercise using the Bruce protocol.

◆ U wave inversion—this is relatively specific for coronary artery disease but is relatively insensitive; in precordial leads, it usually indicates left anterior descending coronary artery disease

Exercise protocols

Various protocols have been developed but the most widely used are the following.

Bruce protocol

This is a multistage test with 3-min walking periods during which a steady state is reached before the workload is increased by increasing the speed and slope of the treadmill. It is clearly only suitable for those whose walking is not limited by other considerations, e.g. musculoskeletal or neurological. For older patients or those with limited exercise capacity, the test can be modified to include two stages with lower workload demands.

Bicycle ergometry

This is often combined with radionuclide imaging (see Chapter 16.3.3), which increases the sensitivity and specificity of the test. Cycling avoids motion artefact, and so ECG recordings are clearer. The patient pedals at a comfortable speed of between 60 and 80 revolutions/min; the test is terminated if speed cannot be maintained above 40 revolutions/min. Exercise workload begins at 25 W and resistance is increased every 2 min in 25-W increments by applying either an electronic or mechanical brake.

The workload achieved during exercise is measured in metabolic equivalents or METs. This allows comparison of different protocols. A MET is 3.5 ml/min per kg, the resting V_{O_2} for a 40-year-old 70-kg male. METs equivalent to normal daily activities have been estimated (Table 16.3.1.2).

Conducting the exercise test

Who should have an exercise test?

Deciding who should and who should not undergo an exercise test requires clinical judgement and the test should not be organized as a routine. Exercise testing is used to:

◆ assess functional capacity and estimate prognosis in the evaluation of chest pain

◆ assess patients considered at intermediate or high risk of coronary disease, based on gender, age and symptomatology

◆ establish prognosis after myocardial infarction either predischarge (submaximal test) or 4–6 weeks postdischarge (symptom-limited)

◆ assess the effectiveness of coronary revascularization

◆ assess patients with symptoms of exercise-induced cardiac arrhythmia

◆ risk-stratify before noncardiac surgery in patients with or at high risk of coronary disease

◆ determine the efficacy of rate-responsive pacemakers

Exercise testing may also be indicated in selected asymptomatic individuals:

◆ in specific occupations for licensing purposes (e.g. airline pilots, bus or heavy good vehicle drivers; see Chapter 16.13.8)

◆ with more than two cardiovascular risk factors for risk stratification

◆ wishing to commence a strenuous exercise programme

◆ to assess cardiovascular risk due to prior to major surgery

Who should not have an exercise test?

Some conditions are considered to be absolute contraindications to exercise testing but even in these patients a submaximal test may be informative.

Exercise testing is inappropriate:

◆ in healthy individuals with a low risk factor profile—the false positive rate is increased (see below)

◆ with unstable medical conditions such as unstable angina; severe congestive cardiac failure; uncontrolled ventricular or supraventricular arrhythmia; myocarditis; severe pulmonary hypertension; drug toxicity; haemodynamic instability; symptomatic aortic stenosis; active thromboembolic disease; hypertension with systolic blood pressure >200 or diastolic blood pressure >110 mmHg

◆ in extreme obesity

◆ when taking specific medication—digoxin depresses the ST segment; type 1 antiarrhythmics and tricyclic antidepressants may be proarrhythmic

◆ in vasoregulatory disorders—pulse and blood pressure changes are unpredictable

Patients with aortic stenosis may fail to report symptoms of angina, breathlessness, and syncope. Although aortic stenosis is considered an absolute contraindication to exercise testing, a medically supervised symptom-limited test may identify those who warrant cardiac catheterization and valve replacement.

Who should supervise an exercise test—cardiac technician, specialist nurse or physician?

Patients with new- or recent-onset chest pain thought to be angina are often referred to a rapid-access chest pain clinic for assessment, where a specialist nurse carries out an initial assessment and then an exercise test. Experience shows that this approach is safe, provided a physician is available for consultation and advice. There are some high-risk situations where the test, if it must be carried out, should be supervised by a physician. These include patients whose symptoms are unstable, aortic stenosis, known severe coronary disease, severe or moderate systemic or pulmonary hypertension,

Table 16.3.1.2 Table of MET equivalents

Occupation	METs	Activity	METs
Receptionist	1–2	Carrying a suitcase	7
Professional (active)	1.5–2.5	Cleaning floor	4
Housewife	1.5–4	Washing clothes	5
Farm worker	3.5–7.5	Cooking	3
Construction worker	4–8.5	Gardening	4
Miner	4–9	Push mower	5
Postman	2.5–5	Sex	5
		Bed-making	5–6

severe left ventricular dysfunction, congestive or hypertrophic cardiomyopathy, or a history of ventricular tachycardia or second or third-degree atrioventricular block.

Risks of exercise testing

Exercise testing is generally considered a safe procedure but full resuscitation facilities, including defibrillator, emergency drug kit, airways management equipment, and oxygen are essential. Serious complications are rare. The risk of myocardial infarction and sudden death is less than 1 in 1000, more when testing patients after myocardial infarction or with malignant ventricular arrhythmia.

When to stop an exercise test

Reasons for stopping a test include:

- achieving 90% of the maximum predicted heart rate

- symptoms—establish if these are typical symptoms of chest pain or breathlessness; exercise may continue provided that symptoms are not distressing or severe

- systolic blood pressure—if systolic blood pressure falls below baseline levels or if systolic increases to greater 250 mmHg or diastolic to greater than 115 mmHg

- change in ECG—if more than 2 mm ST segment depression or more than 1 mm ST segment elevation; or if left bundle branch block (this may look remarkably like ventricular tachycardia at fast heart rate) or arrhythmia develops

- clinical signs—if signs of poor peripheral perfusion such as cyanosis appear

- symptoms of central nervous system dysfunction—dizziness, near syncope or ataxia

- serious arrhythmia—ventricular tachycardia, multifocal ectopics, ventricular triplets or couplets

- technical difficulties—failure of blood pressure recording or poor ECG trace

- patient request—distressing symptoms of fatigue, breathlessness, wheeze or claudication; maximal patient effort; or inability to maintain speed of treadmill

Recovery period

It is important to observe the patient into the recovery period until the pretest heart rate and blood pressure have been restored. Minor ECG abnormalities early in recovery are common but late changes usually indicate myocardial ischaemia.

Interpreting the results of an exercise test

Like all medical tests, the exercise test is not a perfect indicator of the presence or absence of disease. Nevertheless, a test is often described as:

- positive—chest pain develops with or without ST displacement; blood pressure falls; arrhythmia occurs; the patient fails to complete the first two stages of the Bruce protocol or reach 90% of predicted maximum heart rate

- negative—the patient completes uneventfully three stages of the Bruce protocol or reaches 90% of predicted maximum heart rate

- indeterminate—90% predicted heart rate is not reached; symptoms occur which are not typical of cardiac pain with a normal ECG throughout

A positive test does not necessarily mean that the patient has coronary disease, nor does a negative test mean the patient has some other, noncardiac, cause for chest pain. The exercise test has limited use as a diagnostic test for coronary disease.

Limitations and strengths of the exercise test

The exercise test as a diagnostic tool

The sensitivity of the exercise test, the proportion with coronary disease correctly identified by the test, is 68% (range 23–100) and specificity, the proportion free of disease correctly identified by the test, is 77% (range 17–100). In multivessel disease, these figures are 81% (range 40–100) and 66% (range 17–100) respectively.

This means that exercise testing frequently yields false-positive results, incorrectly diagnosing disease when coronary arteries are normal or minimally diseased; and false-negative results, missing coronary disease when a flow-limiting, even critical left main stem, coronary stenosis is present.

Selection of patients for exercise testing is important as a false positive result is more likely when an individual has few predisposing risk factors for coronary disease or the prevalence of coronary disease prevalence in the population is low.

Example 1

A positive test in a middle aged man with multiple coronary risk factors (smoking, dyslipidaemia, hypertension, diabetes mellitus, and family history) and typical chest pain on exertion (who is highly likely to have coronary disease) is most likely to be correct.

Example 2

A positive test in a young woman with atypical chest pain and few or no cardiovascular risk factors is likely to be incorrect and may lead to other, more invasive tests including coronary angiography. The prevalence of coronary disease is lower in women than men and the specificity of exercise testing is lower in women, which means that the test is more likely to be positive in the absence of coronary disease, possibly due to increased catecholamine secretion during exercise contributing to coronary vasoconstriction.

The exercise test as an indicator of prognosis

Although the exercise test is of limited value as an aid to diagnosis, it is more reliable as a marker of prognosis.

Generally, appearance of symptoms or ECG changes early in the test is associated with more severe and extensive coronary disease and a poor prognosis (Table 16.3.1.3). Changes within the first 3 min usually indicate severe coronary disease affecting the left main stem or the proximal segments of at least one major coronary artery.

Multivessel coronary disease is more likely with ST segment down-sloping, delayed ST normalization after exercise, increased number of leads affected, and lower workload at which ECG changes appear.

Difficulties with exercise testing

Baseline ECGs that make interpretation of the exercise test difficult

ECG patterns that may make exercise-induced changes hard to recognize include:

- ST depression or elevation at rest

- ventricular strain patterns—left and right ventricular hypertrophy

Table 16.3.1.3 Prognostic indicators on treadmill testing

	Indicators of a good prognosis	Indicators of a poor prognosis
ST segment	No displacement or up-sloping	2 mm or more depression in stage 1 Bruce- within 3 minutes Down-sloping or horizontal
Duration of exercise	9 minutes (>9 METs)	Unable to complete stage 2 Bruce or equivalent (<6.5 METs)
Heart rate at onset of limiting symptoms	Reaches maximum predicted heart rate (220 – age)	Unable to attain >120/min off β-blocker
Systolic BP response	Maintained or increased	Sustained decrease >10 mmHg or failure to rise with exercise
Changes on exercise	No changes	Ventricular tachycardia U wave inversion T wave normalization
Recovery	Recovers normal heart rate <10 min	Delayed recovery >10 min
Symptoms	None or atypical	Test terminated due to increasing angina on exercise

◆ T wave changes—inversion secondary to previous infarction or 'strain'

◆ conduction abnormalities—left bundle branch block affects ST segment and T wave; right bundle branch block affects ST segment and T wave changes in V1, V2, and V3

◆ prolonged QT interval

Alternative tests that do not rely on the ECG to identify myocardial ischaemia are dobutamine stress echocardiography, radionuclide thallium or MIBI stress test, or cardiac MRI (see Chapters 16.3.2 and 16.3.3).

Medication and exercise testing

β-Blockers and rate-modifying calcium antagonists may mask myocardial ischaemia by limiting exercise-induced tachycardia and so delay the appearance of ST depression. Blood pressure lowering medication may blunt the normal exercise-induced rise in pressure. Digoxin may induce or accentuate ST depression on the resting ECG.

Medication may be continued if the indication for exercise testing is to assess the efficacy of treatment but should be temporarily stopped in all other circumstances. Specific rules apply if assessing for driving licensing purposes—always check local rules, but generally, antianginal drugs must be stopped at least 48 h prior to the assessment; blood pressure lowering drugs can be continued.

ST segment depression in the absence of symptoms

Asymptomatic, exercise-induced ST segment depression, or 'silent ischaemia', is seen in 60% of patients with coronary disease but does not increase the risk of cardiac death compared with those who report angina.

Technical issues

Current ECG machines filter out motion and muscle artefact to facilitate measurement of the ST segment. Because leads placed on the limbs produce motion artefact, moving these to the torso exaggerates the degree of change and increases the amplitude of the R wave, potentiating exercise-induced ST segment changes. It can be difficult to identify ST segment depression during exercise. If there is any doubt about the extent of ST segment depression on the running ECG, most automated machines will provide a filtered 12-lead ECG for comparison with baseline.

Exercise testing in special groups
Peri- and postmyocardial infarction

Exercise testing after myocardial infarction may be performed for risk stratification and selection for revascularization. A submaximal predischarge test to identify residual ischaemia appears to be safe, with 0.05% morbidity and 0.02% mortality. An abnormal blood pressure response or low exercise capacity predicts a poor outcome and is an indication for urgent revascularization.

More commonly, an exercise test is recommended 6 weeks or so after discharge from hospital. Evidence of myocardial ischaemia, especially at low workload, is an indication for referral for coronary angiography.

Elderly patients

Advanced age alone is not a contraindication to exercise testing, provided that the individual can walk at a reasonable speed. If mobility is limited, dobutamine stress echocardiography, radionuclide thallium or MIBI stress test, or cardiac MRI are alternative means of identifying ischaemia (see Chapters 16.3.2 and 16.3.3).

Asymptomatic individuals

Testing may be undertaken in asymptomatic individuals, generally a low-risk population, as part of health screening, for insurance purposes, or for risk stratification. Up to 12% of middle-aged men and up to 30% of women will have an abnormal exercise test in the absence of symptoms; the risk of a cardiac event is low unless the test result indicates a poor prognosis. The presence of cardiovascular risk factors increases the likelihood of coronary disease.

Cardiac arrhythmia

Exercise testing can be useful in evaluating cardiac arrhythmia, supplementary to ambulatory monitoring and electrophysiological studies. In about 10%, it may provoke an arrhythmia.

Further reading

Bruce, RA, Fisher LD (1987). Exercise-enhanced assessment of risk factors for coronary heart disease in healthy men. *J Electrocardiol*, **20** (Suppl. October), 162.

Cura FA, *et al.* (2004). ST segment resolution 60 minutes after combination treatment of abciximab with reteplase or reteplase alone for acute myocardial infarction (30-day mortality results from the resolution of ST segment after reperfusion therapy substudy). *Am J Cardiol*, **94**, 859–863.

Einthoven W (1912). The different forms of the human electrocardiogram and their signification. *Lancet*, **1**, 853–861.

Gianrossi R, *et al.* (1989). Exercise-induced ST segment depression in the diagnosis of coronary artery disease: a meta-analysis. *Circulation*, **80**, 87–98.

Houghton AR, Gray D (2008). *Making sense of the ECG*, 3rd edition. Hodder Arnold, London.

Joint European Society of Cardiology/American College of Cardiology Committee (2000). Myocardial infarction redefined—a consensus document of the joint European Society of Cardiology/American College of Cardiology Committee for the Redefinition of Myocardial Infarction. *Eur Heart J*, **21**, 1502–13.

Knaapen P, van Loon RB, Visser FC (2005). A rare cause of ST segment elevation. *Heart*, **91**, 188.

Levy D, *et al.* (1990). Determinants of sensitivity and specificity of electrocardiographic criteria for left ventricular hypertrophy. *Circulation*, **81**, 815–20.

Lloyd Jones DM, *et al.* (1998). Electrocardiographic and clinical predictors of acute myocardial infarction in patients with unstable angina pectoris. *Am J Cardiol*, **81**, 1182–6.

Marey EJ (1876). Des variations électriques des muscles et du coeur en particulier étudiés au moyen de l'électromètre de M Lippman. *C R Acad Sci (Paris)*, **82**, 975–7.

Mueller C, *et al.* (2004). Prognostic value of the admission electrocardiograph in patients with unstable angina/ST segment elevation myocardial infarction treated with very early revascularisation. *Am J Med*, **117**, 145–50.

Savonitto S, *et al.* (1999). Prognostic value of the admission electrocardiogram in acute coronary syndromes. *JAMA*, **281**, 707–13.

Waller AD (1887). A demonstration on man of electromotive changes accompanying the heart's beat. *J Physiol (Lond)*, **8**, 229–34.

16.3.2 Echocardiography

Adrian P. Banning and Andrew R.J. Mitchell

Essentials

Ease of use, rapid data provision, portability, and safety mean that echocardiography has become the principal investigation for a variety of cardiac conditions. A modern, transthoracic echocardiography examination combines real-time two-dimensional imaging of the myocardium and valves with information about velocity and direction of blood flow obtained by Doppler and colour flow mapping. A complete examination can be performed in most patients in less than 30 min.

Valvular heart disease—echocardiography has revolutionized the diagnosis and follow-up of patients with these conditions. Serial cardiac catheterization to assess severity and progress of valvular stenosis has been almost completely superseded by Doppler echocardiography, and the role of invasive investigation is increasingly limited to the assessment of the coronary arteries prior to revascularization.

Transoesophageal echocardiography—this is now a routine investigation in many centres. Under sedation, an ultrasound probe is passed into the oesophagus to a position behind the heart, producing excellent resolution of cardiac structures. It is used diagnostically in many emergency situations, including aortic dissection and suspected prosthetic mechanical valve dysfunction, and as an additional method of monitoring cardiac performance during cardiac and noncardiac surgery.

Other technological developments—these include (1) stress echocardiography—used to detect occult coronary disease and predict cardiac risk; (2) use of contrast agents—these improve visualization of the endocardium in patients with poor acoustic windows and allow some estimation of myocardial perfusion; and (3) real-time three-dimensional imaging—this is available on most new machines and allows detailed assessment of myocardial and valvular function.

History of echocardiography

In 1842, Christian Doppler noted that the pitch of a sound wave varied if the source of sound was moving. His mathematical formulae are still in use today, and his discovery coined the name of the eponymous technique. Ultrasound was developed in 1880 by applying an electric charge to a crystal. In 1912, the British engineer Richardson identified that sound waves could be used to detect underwater objects, leading to the development of sonar. In 1929, the Soviet scientist Sergei Sokolov developed a technique using ultrasound to identify flaws in metal components of ships and tanks. This technology then remained of military interest until after the Second World War, when medical applications of ultrasound were discovered.

Carl Herz and Inge Edler from Sweden are credited with the origins of clinical echocardiography. Their development of the cardiac 'supersonic reflectoscope', in 1954, allowed the movements of the posterior heart wall to be seen for the first time. The A-mode and M-mode techniques were subsequently refined and used to detect mitral stenosis, pericardial effusions, left atrial tumours, and aortic stenosis. Meanwhile, a Japanese group started to use Doppler techniques to examine the functioning of the heart.

In the 1960s, multielement scanners allowed the development of two-dimensional (2D) echocardiography, and when it was realized in the 1970s that Doppler could be used to determine pressure gradients across valves, echocardiography took off as an important clinical investigation. Transoesophageal echocardiography and stress echocardiography were subsequently developed in the late 1970s.

Further refinement of these echocardiography techniques has occurred over the last 30 years. Miniaturization of the transducers now permits intracardiac and intracoronary ultrasound. Transpulmonary contrast agents are allowing myocardial perfusion to be examined. Tissue Doppler imaging, tissue tracking, and spectral Doppler are providing more detailed analysis of myocardial function. Real-time three-dimensional (3D) echocardiography is now becoming a standard feature on modern equipment, and echocardiography is now able to determine pressures in all cardiac chambers, precisely measure cardiac function, and accurately assess valvular disease, making the days of invasive assessment obsolete.

Principles of echocardiography

The transducer used for most echocardiographic examinations contains piezoelectric crystals that emit ultrasound frequencies of 2.5 to 5 MHz. Most of the sound energy is scattered or absorbed, but reflection occurs at interfaces between tissues of different acoustic impedance (e.g. between blood and muscle). The transducer collects these reflections and the time delay between emission and reception is calculated. This allows the depth of the reflection to be derived and its position to be displayed on a screen as a dot (pixel). The brightness of the dot is related to the magnitude of the reflected signal. In general, higher-frequency transducers allow better discrimination between structures, but the increased attenuation leads to reduced penetration.

There are three main echocardiographic techniques: 2D (cross-sectional), M-mode, and Doppler.

2D echocardiography (cross-sectional)

Cross-sectional images are constructed as the ultrasound beam sweeps across the heart in a sector (Fig. 16.3.2.1). Between 50 and

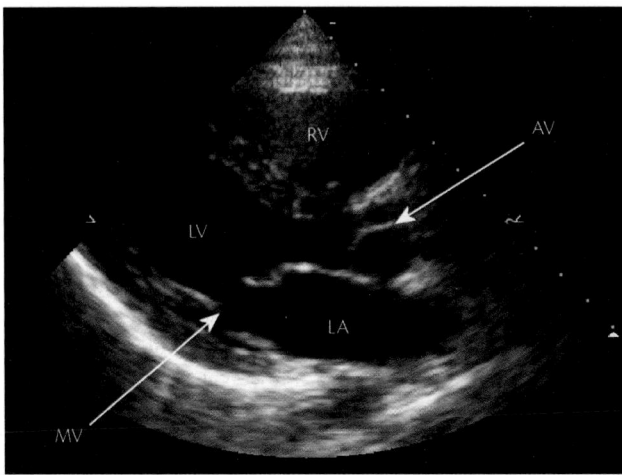

Fig. 16.3.2.1 Parasternal long-axis view of the heart using 2D echocardiography. The sector images through the right ventricle (RV) to the left ventricle (LV). In this view, 2D echocardiography provides useful data on the structure and function of the aortic valve (AV) and mitral valve (MV).

100 cross-sections are presented each second, giving the impression of a moving picture. These images are readily interpretable by an observer with knowledge of cardiac anatomy, and this technique is the cornerstone of modern echocardiography.

M-mode echocardiography

M-mode echocardiography preceded modern 2D imaging. Unlike 2D imaging, which uses a series of sweeps across the heart, M-mode uses a single static beam of very frequent ultrasound pulses. The narrow beam is analogous to a vertical mineshaft passing through various layers of rock. Displayed in real time, this results in reflections from cardiac structures being displayed as horizontal lines, with superficial structures at the top of the screen and the deeper structures at the bottom (Fig. 16.3.2.2). These data are

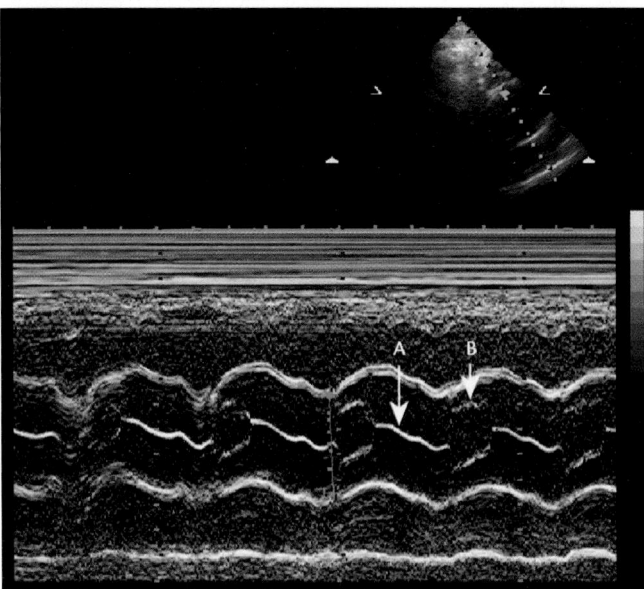

Fig. 16.3.2.2 M-Mode view of the aortic valve imaging the closure (point A) and opening (point B) of the valve. The high imaging frequency of M-mode allows accurate measurements of structures to be made, in this case the aortic root.

interpretable when one knows which structure each line represents. The technique has excellent spatial resolution; hence, with the advent of 2D echocardiography and Doppler, M-mode is now principally used for measurement of cardiac chamber dimensions and observation of the relative movement of cardiac structures to each other, e.g. the relationship of the anterior leaflet of the mitral valve to the septum in hypertrophic cardiomyopathy.

Doppler echocardiography

The Doppler principle allows the velocity and direction of movement of an object (or moving blood in the case of cardiac ultrasonography) to be calculated from the shift in the frequency of a reflected waveform relative to the observer. Cardiac imaging employs pulsed-wave, continuous-wave, and colour-Doppler techniques. Pulsed-wave Doppler allows information about flow to be obtained from a particular point within the heart. The range of detectable velocities is limited, and the technique is used for sampling normal and low velocities, e.g. mitral valve flow. Continuous-wave Doppler identifies the peak velocity encountered along the ultrasound beam and is particularly valuable for measuring high-velocity jets, e.g. as seen in aortic valve disease (Fig. 16.3.2.3). It is important to remember that failure to align the transducer exactly parallel to flow results in measurement of artefactually low velocities and potentially an underestimation of valvular stenosis.

Colour Doppler allows a dynamic representation of the direction and velocity of flow to be superimposed onto a 2D image of the heart. Velocities towards the transducer are usually coded in red and velocities away in blue (Fig. 16.3.2.4). Turbulent and high-velocity flow produces variable velocities and results in a mosaic pattern that is ideal for characterization of regurgitant lesions. This technique is now so sensitive that it can detect trivial regurgitation during the closure of many normal heart valves.

Transthoracic echocardiography

Imaging is usually performed with dedicated echocardiography equipment with the patient lying on their left hip in the left lateral position and with their left arm behind their head. Ultrasound cannot travel through bone and thus cardiac imaging is performed via intercostal spaces to the left of the sternum and at the apex of the heart in the axillary line. These 'echo windows' provide standard views described as the parasternal short and long axis and apical two-, four-, and five-chamber views. Useful additional views can also be obtained from the subcostal and suprasternal approach in some patients. A standard echocardiography examination involves 2D imaging from the parasternal, apical, and subcostal approaches supported by M-mode measurements, continuous, pulsed, and colour Doppler.

Valvular heart disease

Transthoracic echocardiography is the investigation of choice for patients with suspected valvular heart disease. All four cardiac valves can be visualized and interrogated by Doppler and 2D echocardiography. Concomitant abnormalities in ventricular performance can be assessed simultaneously.

Aortic stenosis

2D echocardiography can usually image the aortic valve cusps; if they are thin and freely mobile, it is unlikely that there is significant aortic stenosis. However, if the valve cusps are thickened and

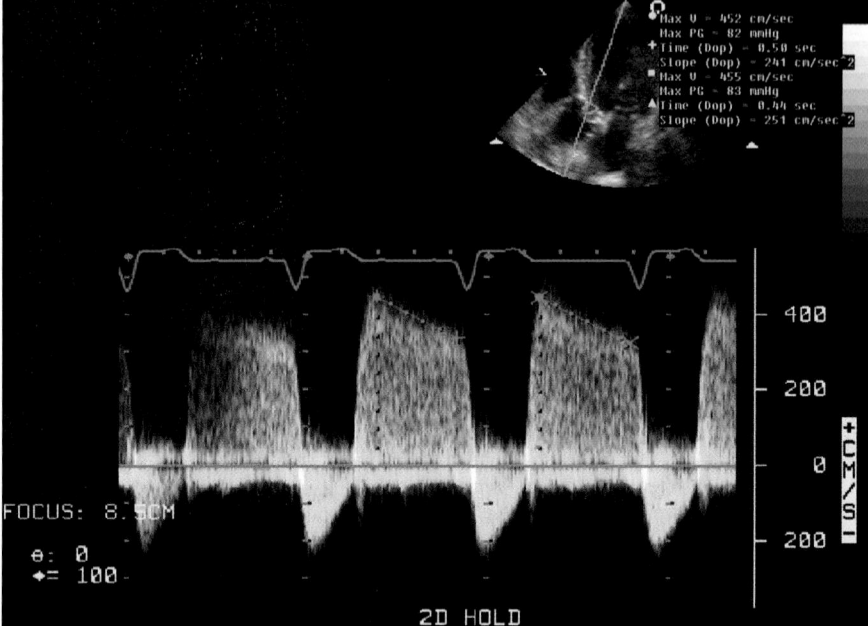

Fig. 16.3.2.3 Continuous wave Doppler of the aortic valve showing aortic regurgitation (flow towards the probe above the line). Calculations can be performed using on-machine software to instantly provide useful haemodynamic data.

calcified, interrogation by continuous-wave Doppler is mandatory. The severity of aortic stenosis is usually expressed as the peak pressure difference (or gradient) across the valve, and is calculated from the maximum flow velocity (V) using the modified Bernoulli equation (pressure gradient = $4V^2$). In patients with normal left ventricular systolic function, a peak gradient measured by Doppler of over 65 mmHg or a mean gradient of over 40 mmHg suggests significant aortic stenosis (Fig. 16.3.2.5).

When chronic critical outflow obstruction results in declining left ventricular function and reduced cardiac output, the gradient produced by any degree of valve obstruction also falls. Doubt about the severity of the stenosis can usually be resolved by calculating the valve area using the continuity equation, which uses data from Doppler and 2D echocardiography. In experienced hands this provides valuable additional information, but accurate measurement of the left ventricular outflow-tract diameter can be difficult and if the findings are not consistent with other data, the investigation should be either be repeated or the patient should be referred for

cardiac catheterization. A valve area of less than 1 cm^2 usually represents severe aortic stenosis.

Aortic regurgitation

Assessment of the mechanism and severity of aortic regurgitation requires a combination of all three echocardiography modalities. M-mode may demonstrate fluttering of the anterior leaflet of the mitral valve and, in the setting of acute, severe aortic regurgitation, may reveal premature closure of the mitral valve. 2D echocardiography will occasionally demonstrate prolapse of one more of the aortic cusps, but even severe aortic regurgitation can occur through an aortic valve that appears to be structurally normal.

The severity of aortic regurgitation can be estimated using continuous-wave and colour Doppler (see Chapter 16.14.1, Figs. 16.14.1.3 and 16.14.1.4), although assessment can be difficult as it is influenced by left ventricular function. Doppler-derived pressure half-time and measurement of regurgitant fraction and/or flow convergence zone are valuable when there is uncertainty over

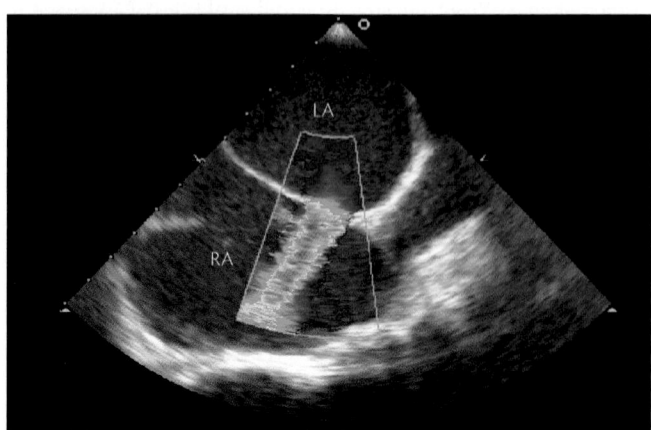

Fig. 16.3.2.4 Colour flow mapping of an atrial septal defect. There is high velocity flow from the left atrium (LA) to the right atrium (RA).

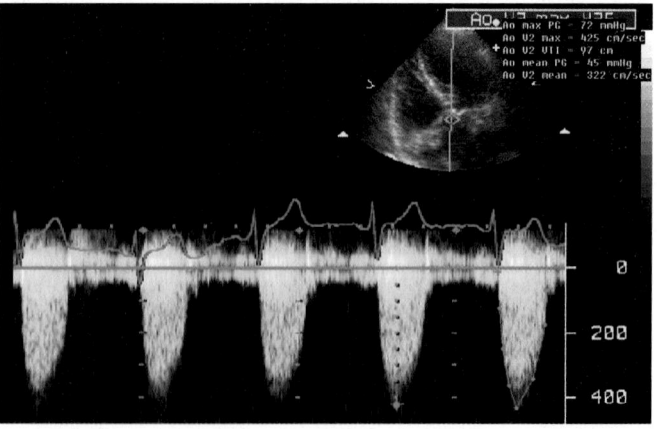

Fig. 16.3.2.5 Continuous wave Doppler through the aortic valve. The peak velocity is 425 cm/s. This equates to a peak pressure gradient (A_0 max PG) of 72 mmHg and a mean of 45 mmHg.

lesion severity. M-mode and colour Doppler can be combined and, when the regurgitant jet fills more than 50% of the left ventricular outflow tract, the regurgitation is classified as severe.

In patients with severe asymptomatic aortic regurgitation, a serial increase in left ventricular dimensions or a progressive fall in ejection fraction are indications for surgery. However, any increase in ventricular dimension should be at least 0.5 cm before it is regarded as significant, given the limited reproducibility of echocardiographic parameters.

Mitral stenosis

Mitral valve stenosis is well visualized using either M-mode or cross-sectional echocardiography. Its severity can be determined by estimating the area of the valve orifice either by direct planimetry of the 2D short-axis image or from the Doppler pressure half-time (mitral valve area = 220/pressure half-time). A valve area of less than 1.0 cm^2 usually indicates severe mitral stenosis (Fig. 16.3.2.6). Transthoracic echocardiography is also used to assess the suitability of the mitral valve for balloon dilation, although transoesophageal imaging is necessary to exclude left atrial thrombus.

Mitral regurgitation

Transthoracic echocardiography will usually demonstrate the mechanism and severity of mitral regurgitation. 2D imaging identifies abnormalities of the valve leaflets and colour flow shows jet direction and area (Fig. 16.3.2.7). Severe mitral regurgitation is suggested by increased left ventricular end-diastolic dimension and hyperdynamic wall motion due to volume overload. Precise quantification of the amount of regurgitation is demanding as it is influenced by left ventricular function, the direction of the jet, and left atrial size. Various algorithms have been devised to improve quantification of mitral regurgitation, including measurement of the flow convergence zone and the proximal isovelocity surface area (PISA) method, but most centres simply classify the extent of regurgitation as mild, moderate, or severe (Table 16.3.2.1).

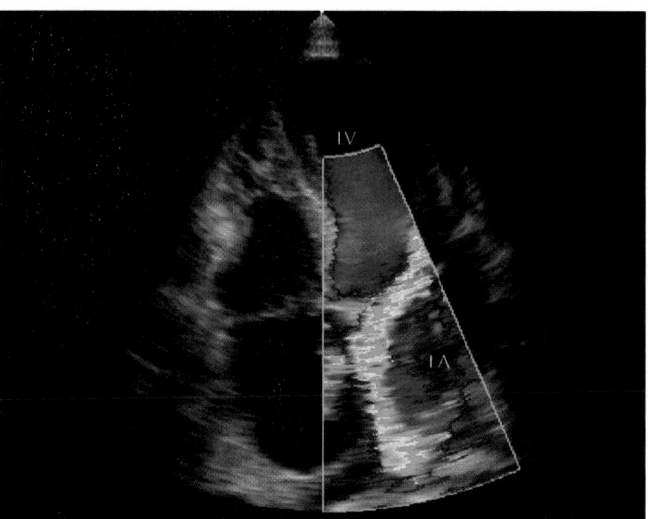

Fig. 16.3.2.7 Apical four-chamber view with colour flow demonstrating an eccentric jet of mitral regurgitation from the left ventricle (LV) to the left atrium (LA). In this case the leak is due to prolapse of the posterior mitral valve leaflet.

Pulmonary and tricuspid valve disease

In adults, 2D imaging of the pulmonary valve may be difficult, particularly if there is lung disease. Despite this, accurate Doppler information is usually obtainable. Tricuspid stenosis is very uncommon, but some degree of tricuspid regurgitation is detectable even in healthy individuals. Measurement of the peak velocity of tricuspid regurgitation (V) is valuable as, in the absence of

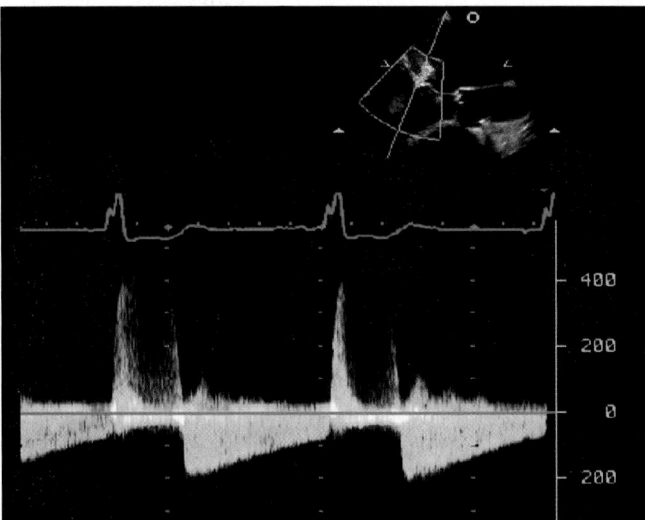

Fig. 16.3.2.6 Continuous wave Doppler through the mitral valve in a patient with mitral valve disease. The pressure tracing below the line (flow through the mitral valve) takes a long time to decay (a long pressure half-time). This is highly suggestive of severe mitral stenosis.

Table 16.3.2.1 Classification of mitral regurgitation

	Mild	Severe
Specific signs of severity		
Vena contracta	<0.3 cm	>0.7 cm
Jet size	<4 cm^2 or <20% left atrium	>40% left atrium
	Small and central	Large and central or wall-impinging and swirling
PISA radius	None/minimal (<0.4 cm)	Large (>1 cm)
Pulmonary vein flow		Systolic reversal
Valve structure		Flail or rupture
Supportive signs of severity		
Pulmonary vein flow	Systolic dominant	
Mitral inflow	A-wave dominant	E-wave dominant (>1.2 m/s)
CW trace	Soft and parabolic	Dense and triangular
LV and LA	Normal size LV if chronic MR	Enlarged LV and LA if no other cause

CW, continuous wave; LA, left atrium; LV, left ventricle; PISA, proximal isovelocity surface area.

pulmonary valve disease, it can be used to estimate pulmonary artery (PA) systolic pressure:

$$\text{PA systolic pressure (mmHg)} = 4V^2 + \text{right atrial pressure}$$
$$\text{(usually 5–10 mmHg)}$$

Prosthetic valves

Transthoracic echocardiography is commonly performed as part of the routine follow-up of prosthetic valves. It is usually able to assess biological valves accurately, but for mechanical mitral valve prostheses in particular, attenuation artefact produced by the metal may be problematic. Transoesophageal imaging is recommended when transthoracic imaging is suboptimal or if improved resolution is required, for example, in patients with suspected prosthetic valve endocarditis.

Abnormal left ventricular function

In most patients, a full transthoracic echocardiography study will confirm or refute a clinical suspicion of left ventricular dysfunction and identify the likely aetiology of any abnormality. Systolic and diastolic left ventricular function can be assessed and a variety of methods can be used to derive an estimate of left ventricular ejection fraction. In patients with ischaemic heart disease, assessment of regional wall motion is valuable and may occasionally demonstrate evidence of aneurysm formation. Left ventricular hypertrophy is detected by echocardiography and a measurement of left ventricular mass can also be derived. Echocardiography is recommended in suspected heart failure as patients can have a combination of impaired systolic and diastolic dysfunction. Transthoracic echocardiography may also detect intracardiac thrombus, particularly in patients with impaired systolic ventricular function (Fig. 16.3.2.8).

Left ventricular hypertrophy

Minor concentric left ventricular hypertrophy is common in patients with hypertension. In hypertrophic cardiomyopathy, 2D imaging may demonstrate asymmetrical septal hypertrophy with disproportionate thickening of the interventricular septum compared with the left ventricular free wall, or dramatic concentric hypertrophy with left ventricular cavity obliteration. Other characteristic features of hypertrophic cardiomyopathy include systolic anterior motion of the mitral valve and partial midsystolic closure of the aortic valve, which usually correlates with the presence of outflow tract obstruction. In the absence of conditions that may induce ventricular hypertrophy, for example, aortic stenosis, these findings are diagnostic of hypertrophic cardiomyopathy. Colour Doppler can demonstrate turbulence in the outflow tract and continuous-wave Doppler may detect characteristic 'dynamic' gradients that increase in severity as systole progresses. Other associated echocardiographic abnormalities in hypertrophic cardiomyopathy include mitral regurgitation and severe diastolic dysfunction.

Atrial fibrillation

Most patients with atrial fibrillation should undergo echocardiography as it excludes a structural cause for atrial fibrillation (e.g. mitral stenosis) and facilitates thromboembolic risk stratification. It also allows measurement of left atrial dimensions, which is valuable as cardioversion is less likely to be successful when this is large. Identification of left ventricular hypertrophy can guide the choice of antiarrhythmic drug therapy. Transoesophageal echocardiography can be useful to facilitate cardioversion in patients with atrial fibrillation of unknown duration by excluding intracardiac thrombus, particularly in the left atrial appendage (Fig. 16.3.2.9).

Following an embolic event or stroke

Echocardiography is the investigation of choice when a cardiac source of an embolus is suspected. It should be considered in all patients presenting with embolic occlusion of a peripheral artery, or thromboembolic episodes in more than one vascular territory. Echocardiography should not, however, be performed in circumstances when the result is unlikely to influence patient management. In patients with ischaemic stroke and a low likelihood of atheromatous arterial disease, an echocardiogram can be considered as, occasionally, it will detect occult abnormalities such as a cardiac thrombus or atrial myxoma (Fig. 16.3.2.10). Contrast studies with Valsalva manoeuvre should be considered to exclude paradoxical embolism through a cardiac shunt from the right heart.

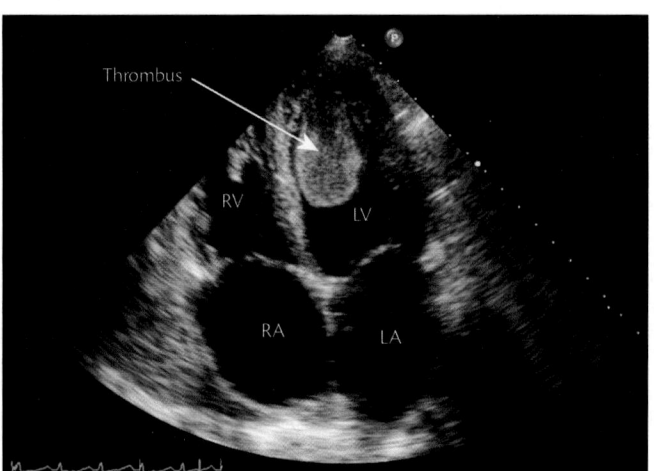

Fig. 16.3.2.8 Apical four-chamber view showing the left ventricle (LV), left atrium (LA), right ventricle (RV), and right atrium (RA). There is a large thrombus attached to the left ventricular apical septum.

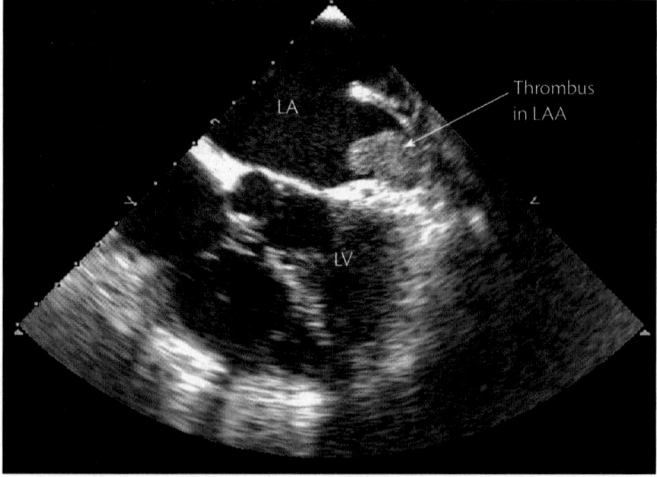

Fig. 16.3.2.9 Transoesophageal echocardiography of a patient with atrial fibrillation. There is a large thrombus filling (and extending from) the left atrial appendage (LAA). LA, left atrium; LV, left ventricle.

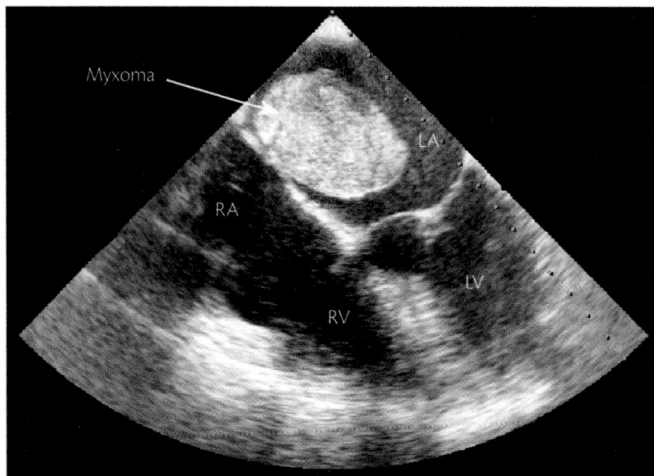

Fig. 16.3.2.10 Transoesophageal echocardiography revealing a large atrial myxoma attached to the interatrial septum. LA, left atrium; LV, left ventricle; RA, right atrium; RV = right ventricle,.

In patients with a high clinical suspicion of a cardiac source of embolus, in whom transthoracic echocardiography is normal, transoesophageal echocardiography is recommended.

Pericardial disease

Echocardiography is not routinely indicated in patients with uncomplicated pericarditis. It can, however, diagnose the presence of pericardial fluid and is useful when a pericardial effusion is suspected and percutaneous drainage is being considered. Echocardiographic signs of pericardial tamponade include exaggerated respiratory variation in the mitral valve Doppler, presystolic closure of the aortic valve, and (particularly) right atrial and right ventricular diastolic collapse (Fig. 16.3.2.11). Constrictive pericarditis is a difficult diagnosis to make using standard echocardiographic techniques. Patients may complain of episodic breathlessness and fluid retention, have characteristic abnormalities of the venous pressure, and have subtle abnormalities on mitral and tricuspid valve inflow Doppler patterns.

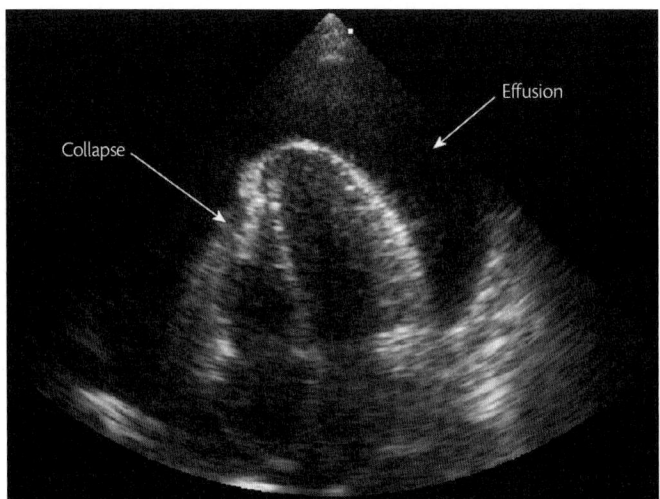

Fig. 16.3.2.11 Apical four-chamber view demonstrating a large pericardial effusion. There is collapse of the right ventricle (arrowed) suggesting cardiac tamponade.

Pulmonary embolism

Echocardiography can be useful in patients with pulmonary embolism as it can demonstrate right ventricular dilation and/or impaired right ventricular systolic function. Tricuspid regurgitant velocity can be used to estimate pulmonary artery systolic pressure, although it is unusual for this to be more than 70 mmHg acutely. Exceptionally, 2D imaging may show a thrombus within the right heart or the proximal pulmonary arteries. Although echocardiography is diagnostically useful when it demonstrates features consistent with pulmonary embolism, it cannot exclude the diagnosis.

Infective endocarditis

Echocardiography cannot be used to exclude endocarditis but is valuable when endocarditis is suspected clinically while there is insufficient data to make a formal diagnosis. Under these circumstances, a typical vegetation detected by an experienced observer is regarded as a major criterion in the Duke diagnostic classification, and this may facilitate appropriate management. Transoesophageal echocardiography should be performed when there is a suspicion of aortic root abscess, if prosthetic endocarditis is suspected, or occasionally, in cases where there is persistent diagnostic doubt and the additional sensitivity and spatial resolution of echocardiography might be valuable.

Congenital heart disease

Echocardiography is the diagnostic modality of choice for patients with suspected congenital heart disease. Detailed transthoracic cardiac imaging is possible in cooperative infants and children, but occasionally sedation or a short anaesthetic may be required. Rates of cardiac catheterization have been reduced by miniaturization of transoesophageal probes that facilitate diagnosis and follow-up of complex congenital heart disease. Fetal echocardiography is performed when surveillance obstetric ultrasound is abnormal or in cases where previous history suggests a possible cardiac problem.

Transoesophageal echocardiography

Transoesophageal echocardiography is now available in many centres (Fig. 16.3.2.12). The ultrasound probe is similar to the endoscope used for upper gastrointestinal investigation, except

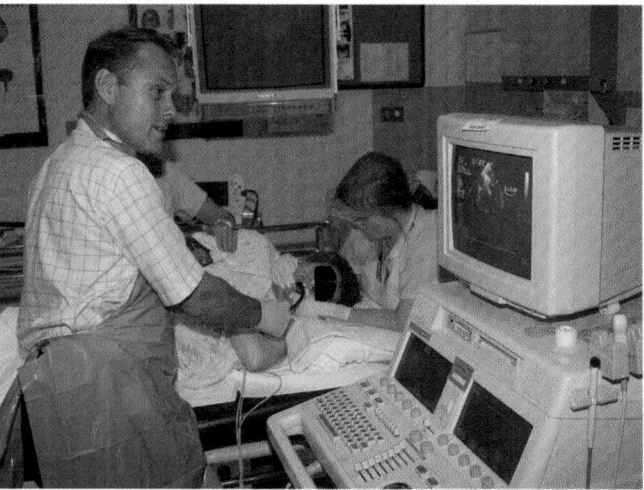

Fig. 16.3.2.12 Transoesophageal echocardiography.

that there are no optical fibres. Transoesophageal echocardiography is an invasive procedure for which the patient's written consent is (usually) required. After fasting for a minimum of 4 h, a local anaesthetic spray (10% lidocaine) is applied to the upper pharynx and the patient is usually sedated, typically with a short-acting intravenous benzodiazepine (e.g. midazolam 2 mg). The probe is manipulated into the oesophagus where its position behind the heart produces excellent resolution, particularly of posterior cardiac structures. Blood pressure and oxygen saturation are monitored throughout, and both resuscitation equipment and the benzodiazepine antagonist flumazenil should be readily available.

Even though transoesophageal echocardiography is commonly performed in high-risk, haemodynamically unstable patients, the rate of serious complications (aspiration and oesophageal rupture/tears) is less than 1%. Absolute contraindications to transoesophageal echocardiography include oesophageal tumours, strictures, diverticulae, and varices.

Who should have a transoesophageal echocardiogram?

The principal indications for transoesophageal echocardiography are listed in Box 16.3.2.1. The principal advantages over transthoracic imaging are improved spatial resolution and the ability to image posterior structures such as the left atrium and descending aorta. It is valuable in a number of emergency situations, including suspected aortic dissection, prosthetic mechanical valve failure, and possible endocarditis. Transoesophageal echocardiography may be used to image the heart in patients in whom data from transthoracic imaging is unsatisfactory due to obesity, lung disease, or chest deformity. Other indications include screening for left atrial thrombus before cardioversion of atrial fibrillation, and monitoring cardiac performance during cardiac and some noncardiac surgery.

Valve disease

Patients with mitral stenosis are at particular risk of thromboembolism, and transthoracic echocardiography has limited sensitivity for the detection of left atrial thrombus. Transoesophageal echocardiography is recommended in those patients with mitral stenosis if embolic events occur despite therapeutic anticoagulation, and may demonstrate spontaneous echocardiography contrast (smoke-like echoes produced by the interaction of erythrocytes and plasma proteins under conditions of stasis). This is an independent predictor of left atrial thrombus and cardiac thromboembolic events. Transoesophageal echocardiography is also used to assess anatomy and exclude left atrial thrombus before balloon valvuloplasty in patients with mitral stenosis and to assess anatomy, severity, and suitability for surgical repair in patients with mitral regurgitation. In patients with mitral prostheses, reverberation artefact overlying the left atrium limits the ability of transthoracic imaging to detect paraprosthetic regurgitation. Transoesophageal imaging provides excellent visualization of the left atrium and is particularly recommended under these circumstances.

Endocarditis

Characteristic vegetations or evidence of abscess formation identified by echocardiography are increasingly used as diagnostic criteria in patients with possible endocarditis. The excellent spatial resolution (<1 mm) of transoesophageal echocardiography makes it superior to transthoracic imaging for the detection of vegetations and

---

> **Box 16.3.2.1** Principal indications for transoesophageal echocardiography
>
> **Valve disease**
> - Mitral stenosis—to assess suitability for percutaneous balloon commisurotomy and exclude left atrial thrombus
> - Mitral regurgitation—to assess anatomy, severity and suitability for surgical repair
> - Prosthetic valves—particularly to assess prosthetic mitral regurgitation
>
> **Infective endocarditis**
> - Possible aortic root abscess
> - Failure to respond to antibiotics, or recurrent fever in a patient with endocarditis
> - High clinical suspicion of endocarditis with no diagnostic abnormality on transthoracic imaging
> - Possible prosthetic valve endocarditis
>
> **Aortic disease**
> - Possible acute aortic dissection
> - Follow-up of patients with known aortic pathology
> - Imaging aortic atheroma before surgery or patients with possible cholesterol embolization
>
> **Potential cardiac source of embolism**
> - Before elective cardioversion of atrial fibrillation
> - Patients with valvular heart disease and a definite embolic episode despite anticoagulation
> - Patients with a definite embolic episode and a 'normal heart' on transthoracic imaging
>
> **Incomplete or impractical transthoracic imaging**
> - Chest deformity or pulmonary disease
> - Patients undergoing mechanical ventilation
> - Congenital heart disease
> - Perioperative imaging of cardiac function and surgical procedures

---

its sensitivity may exceed 90% (Fig. 16.3.2.13). Transoesophageal echocardiography should be considered when there is a high clinical suspicion of endocarditis but blood cultures are sterile and transthoracic imaging is not diagnostic, or under circumstances when the sensitivity of transthoracic imaging is particularly poor, for example prosthetic valves or calcific valvular disease. Transoesophageal echocardiography is also recommended if there is a possibility of aortic root abscess formation as this complication is not easily identified using transthoracic imaging and surgery may be required.

Aortic disease

Transthoracic imaging of the aorta is limited to the proximal aortic root and the arch in most patients. Using transoesophageal imaging, most of the ascending and the entire descending thoracic

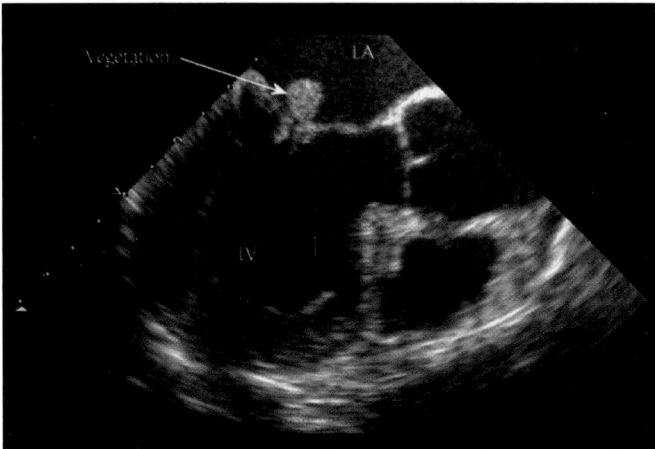

Fig. 16.3.2.13 Transoesophageal echocardiography demonstrating a large vegetation attached to the mitral valve. LA, left atrium; LV, left ventricle.

aorta can be visualized and image quality is improved. This is particularly useful in patients with suspected acute aortic dissection and, in many cases, it is the only imaging necessary before emergency surgery (see Chapter 16.14.1, Figs. 16.14.1.8 and 16.14.1.9). Large, mobile, or pedunculated aortic atheromas in the descending aorta which can be associated with ischaemic stroke may be detected by transoesophageal echocardiography (Fig. 16.3.2.14). Transoesophageal imaging of the aorta has also been recommended in suspected cases of cholesterol embolization and to assess thromboembolic risk prior to cardiac intervention or surgery.

Thromboembolism

In patients with thromboembolism, there has been extensive debate over the value of imaging with transoesophageal echocardiography. Clinical examination, electrocardiography, and transthoracic echocardiography provide sufficient information to determine optimal management in the majority. However, transoesophageal echocardiography is indicated when embolic events occur in anticoagulated patients with native or prosthetic valvular heart disease, especially if endocarditis is suspected, or when transthoracic images are inconclusive. In patients with unexplained or cryptogenic

ischaemic stroke, wider use of transoesophageal echo has been advocated. Transthoracic echocardiography and exclusion of alternative pathologies such as thrombophilia and carotid stenoses should precede the transoesophageal examination, but under these circumstances minor cardiac structural abnormalities are more likely to be clinically relevant.

Transoesophageal echocardiography is superior to the transthoracic approach for imaging the interatrial septum for atrial septal aneurysm (a redundant bulge in the area of the fossa ovale, with respiratory movement >10 mm) and assessing patency of the foramen ovale (Fig. 16.3.2.15). However, the clinical relevance of such atrial septal abnormalities can be questionable as the relationship to the thromboembolic event is commonly speculative. Currently, anticoagulation is the usual management following an otherwise unexplained, single, embolic event, but occasionally a percutaneous or surgical correction of the defect is recommended.

Stress echocardiography

Diagnosis of reversible ischaemic myocardial dysfunction is now possible using echocardiography. Imaging can be performed either during or immediately after exercise, but more commonly an intravenous infusion of dobutamine is used to mimic the cardiac response to exercise. Development of reversible systolic regional wall-motion abnormalities suggests coronary artery disease. Stress echocardiography also has an increasing role in risk stratification before general surgical procedures and in assessing myocardial viability before revascularization. The use of transpulmonary contrast agents reduces the number of inconclusive scans, allows more accurate assessment of left ventricular function, and allows some measure of myocardial perfusion to be made (Fig. 16.3.2.16).

Intracardiac echocardiography

Miniaturization of echocardiography probes has led to the development of echocardiography from within the heart. Small, flexible catheters with ultrasound transducers can be manoeuvred within the heart to provide very-high-resolution images of intracardiac structures. This has been particularly useful during percutaneous

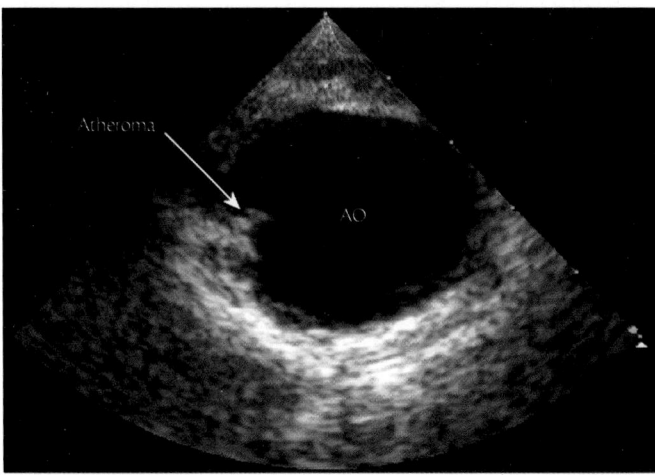

Fig. 16.3.2.14 Transoesophageal echocardiography of the descending aorta (AO). There is a prominent, eccentric atherosclerotic plaque.

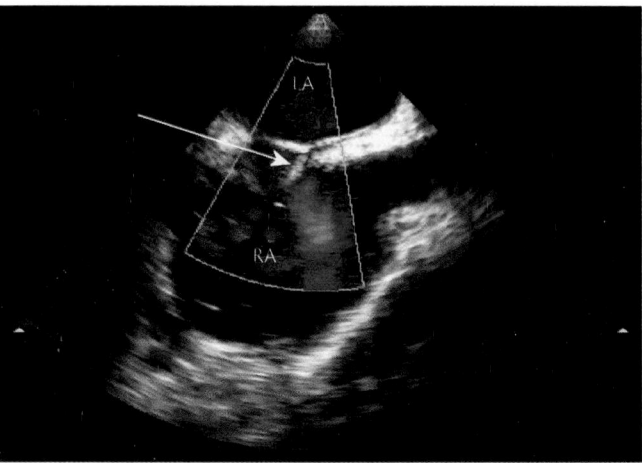

Fig. 16.3.2.15 Transoesophageal echocardiography of the interatrial septum. The flap of the patent foramen ovale can be seen where the septum primum is overlapped by the septum secundum. There is colour flow through it (arrowed) from the left atrium (LA) to the right atrium (RA).

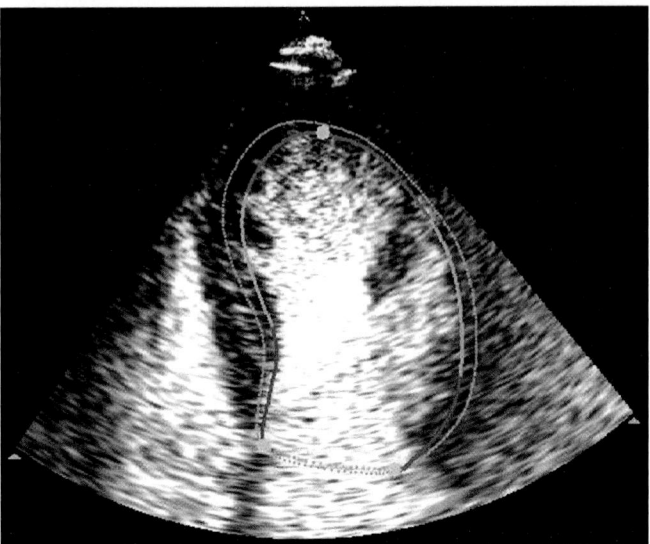

Fig. 16.3.2.16 Stress echocardiography in the apical four-chamber view. A transpulmonary contrast agent has been used to improve border definition and automatic border tracking software is being used to measure systolic function.

closure of atrial septal defects and during radiofrequency ablation procedures (Fig. 16.3.2.17).

3D echocardiography

Real-time, 3D image acquisitions are now available on most high-end echocardiography machines. Some systems acquire a series of gated images to reconstruct the entire heart during a cardiac cycle. This image can then be manoeuvred and slices cut away to visualize the area of interest (Fig. 16.3.2.18). Regional wall tracking can also allow a 3D model of left ventricular function to be acquired and provides an accurate assessment of left ventricular function as well as identifying areas of left ventricular dysynchrony.

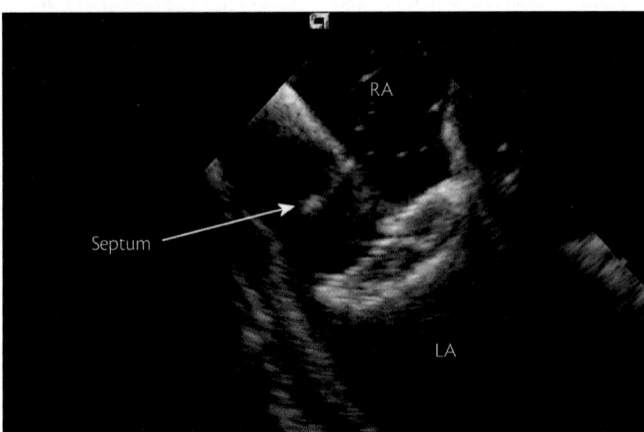

Fig. 16.3.2.17 Intracardiac echocardiography from the right atrium (RA). An atrial septal defect is being closed using a percutaneous approach. The disk in the left atrium (LA) has been deployed and is about to be pulled tight to the interatrial septum.

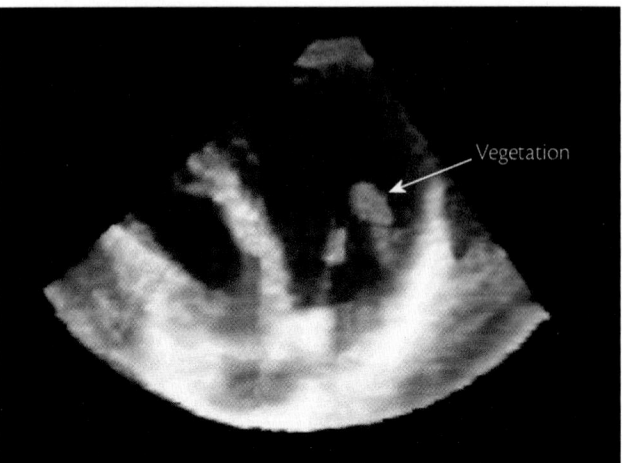

Fig. 16.3.2.18 3D echocardiography of the mitral valve. The images show a vegetation at the tip of the mitral valve leaflet.

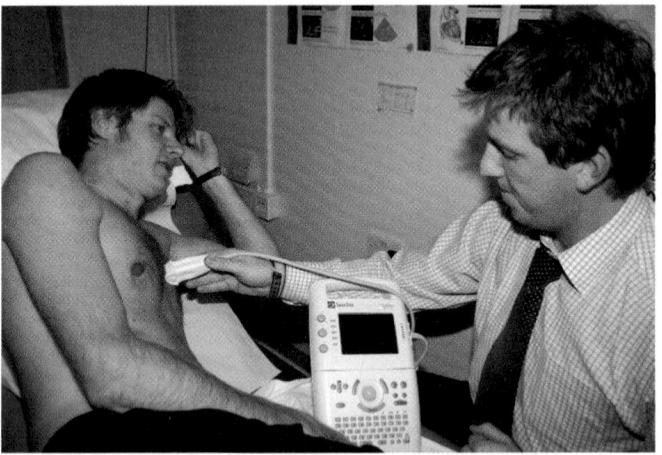

Fig. 16.3.2.19 Hand-held echocardiography allows rapid assessment of cardiac function and can exclude a pericardial effusion.

Portable echocardiography

Echocardiography equipment increases in sophistication but also continues to miniaturize, and now there are several small portable machines available (Fig. 16.3.2.19). These are increasingly available in emergency and intensive care departments. A hand-held 'screening echocardiogram' can be performed in a matter of seconds to exclude pericardial effusion, recognize left ventricular dysfunction, and diagnose most valvular abnormalities. This is proving extremely useful in the management of the critically ill. A more detailed echocardiogram examination can be performed if the screening scan is abnormal or inconclusive.

Further reading

Cheitlin MD, *et al.* (2003). ACC/AHA/ASE guideline update for the clinical application of echocardiography: summary article. *Circulation*, **108**, 1146.

Feigenbaum H (2004). *Feigenbaum's echocardiography*. Lea & Febiger, Philadephia.

Flachskampf FA, *et al.* (2001). Recommendations for performing transesophageal echocardiography. *Euro J Echocardiol*, **2**, 8.

Leeson P, Becher H, Mitchell ARJ (2007). *Echocardiography (Oxford specialist handbooks in cardiology)*. Oxford University Press, Oxford.

Rimington H, Chambers J (1998). *Echocardiography: a practical guide for reporting*. Parthenon, London.

16.3.3 Cardiac investigation— nuclear and other imaging techniques

Nikant Sabharwal and Harald Becher

Essentials

Myocardial perfusion scintigraphy

Three radioisotopic tracers are routinely used in single photon emission computed tomography (SPECT) imaging: thallium-201 and technetium-99 m (bound to either sestamibi or tetrofosmin). Imaging can be performed at rest or with stress (exercise or pharmacological), comparison allowing determination of whether regional perfusion is normal, or there is ischaemia, or there is infarction/scar.

Myocardial perfusion imaging is minimally invasive, and—in contrast to other methods of investigation—is not limited by exercise capacity, airways disease, abnormalities of the resting ECG, pacemakers, or acoustic windows.

In the investigation of the patient with possible coronary artery disease, a normal SPECT study is very reassuring, predicting a very low chance of a major cardiac endpoint event in the following few years (<1% per year). High-risk markers on SPECT provide additional prognostic value to clinical and electrocardiographic variables, and decisions about revascularization can be usefully informed by SPECT imaging.

ECG-gated SPECT allows images to be taken throughout the cardiac cycle, when comparison of end-systolic and end-diastolic images then allows volumetric analysis and calculation of left ventricular ejection fraction.

Positron emission tomography (PET)

Perfusion can be assessed with nitrogen-13 ammonia or rubidium-82, and metabolism with fluorine-18 fluorodeoxyglucose (FDG). Cardiac PET studies tend to be confined to research institutions, with the metabolic tracer FDG considered to be the 'gold standard' for assessment of myocardial viability.

Cardiac MRI

Cardiac MRI can reveal images of spectacular similarity to anatomical cross-sections and is the best method available for quantifying ventricular volumes, ejection fraction, myocardial mass, and differentiating viable (preserved myocytes) from nonviable (fibrotic) myocardium (although echocardiography—which is cheaper and more readily available—remains the first choice in routine clinical practice for many of these indications).

Cardiac MRI provides the highest quality images of patients with congenital heart disease and is particularly indicated for those with complex conditions or in whom it is difficult to obtain good echocardiographic pictures.

Cardiac CT

Multislice spiral computed tomography (MSCT) is indicated to assess pericardial thickening/calcification and is a fast and noninvasive method for the visualization of the coronary arteries. It can also be used to quantify the amount of coronary and aortic valve calcium.

Cardiac CT does not yet match invasive coronary angiography, but many studies have shown a very high negative predictive value, hence cardiac CT appears to be a reasonable test to rule out coronary stenoses in patients with low-to-intermediate likelihood of disease. However, with further developments it is likely that coronary CT will replace invasive coronary angiography for diagnostic purposes.

Nuclear imaging

Within cardiovascular medicine nuclear imaging is an important technique with the following capacity:

- Identification of ischaemic heart disease, with ability to make a prognostic assessment
- Identification of the quantity of viable myocardium in a patient with heart failure
- Assessment of regional and global myocardial function
- Provision of insights into molecular processes via targeted imaging

The procedure is versatile and minimally invasive, and is not limited by exercise capacity, airways disease, abnormalities of the resting ECG, pacemakers, or acoustic windows. Indeed, it is very difficult to identify any patient who is not suitable for nuclear perfusion imaging, and as a result the technique has matured into an almost comprehensive procedure for assessment of coronary artery disease. Over 5 million nuclear cardiology procedures were undertaken in the USA in 2001.

Myocardial perfusion scintigraphy

Basic principles

An intravenous injection of a radiopharmaceutical tracer is administered, which is taken up by intact myocardial cells, the cellular uptake being dependent on the myocardial blood flow at the time of the injection. Rest and peak stress images are required to assess for reversible ischaemia, and comparison of these images determines whether regional perfusion is normal (no hypoperfusion), or due to infarction/scar (hypoperfusion at rest and stress) or ischaemia (hypoperfusion at stress only) (Fig. 16.3.3.1).

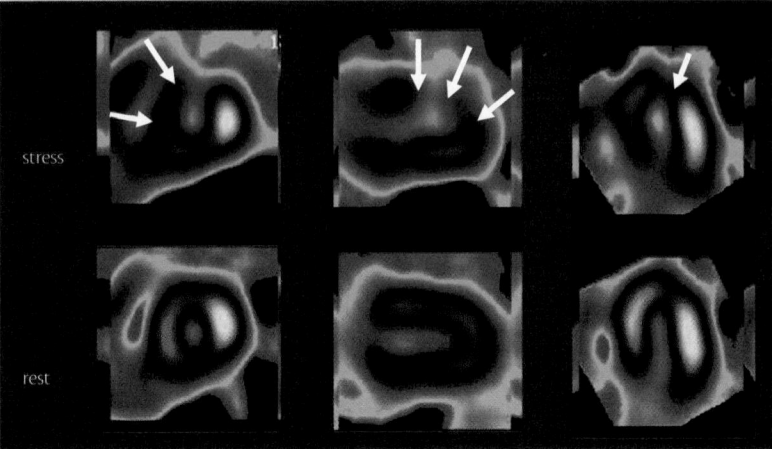

Fig. 16.3.3.1 Myocardial perfusion imaging—an example of inducible ischaemia in the anteroseptal myocardium. Panels from left to right show short axis (SA), horizontal long axis (HLA), and vertical long axis (VLA) projections, with normal uptake of the tracer at rest and perfusion defect (arrows) at peak stress.

There are currently three radioisotopic tracers used in single photon emission computed tomography (SPECT) imaging. The oldest is thallium-201, which is an analogue of the potassium ion; it has a half-life of 73 h and emits photons of varying energies (predominantly 68–80 keV). Uptake is dependent upon an intact Na^+,K^+-ATPase membrane pump. A dose of 80 Mbq is injected at peak stress (exercise or vasodilator), with imaging after 5 to 10 min. Myocardial perfusion defects fill with tracer (by redistribution) 3 to 4 h after initial injection, although areas subtended by severely stenotic coronary arteries may not redistribute for many hours and delayed imaging up to 24 h later may be required. Reinjection of thallium-201 at rest is sometimes added to protocols after redistribution imaging to improve the overall accuracy.

The other two tracers contain technetium-99m, which emits γ-rays at 140 keV and has a half-life of 6 h, bound to either sestamibi or tetrofosmin before intravenous injection. Both tracers enter viable myocardial cells and are fixed—there is no/minimal redistribution—hence separate injections (250–1000 MBq) are required for rest and peak stress imaging. Imaging can then occur at a more convenient time after stress, e.g. 45 to 90 min, reducing motion artefact from overbreathing.

Photons emitted from the patient are identified by a gamma camera and reconstructed to form an image on a computer workstation. The gamma camera rotates around the patient in a 180° arc from right anterior oblique (RAO) to left posterior oblique (LPO). Acquisition usually takes less than 15 min, newer solid state cameras promise two minute acquisition times. The images are ECG gated to allow functional as well as perfusion analysis and are reconstructed and displayed in the following three planes to allow analysis of each region in more than one view—short axis (SA), horizontal long axis (HLA), and vertical long axis (VLA).

Principles of stress testing

The varied stress modalities available to nuclear cardiology are one of its major advantages. Exercise (or physiological) stress can be achieved with a treadmill or bicycle following a specified protocol, e.g., Bruce protocol. The preferred method, which mimics 'real world' stress and also provides valuable ECG data, is for the isotope to be injected at peak stress and the patient asked to maintain exercise for a further minute to allow circulation of the radiotracer.

Patients unable to exercise can undergo pharmacological stress instead. Vasodilators such as adenosine or dipyridamole can be injected intravenously to induce hyperaemia and provide flow heterogeneity between coronary vascular beds. These vasodilators are contraindicated in patients with significant airways disease, significant atrioventricular node disease, hypotension, methylxanthine exposure in last 48 h, and acute myocardial infarction (<2 days). Selective adenosine A_{2A} receptor agonists have fewer serious side effects. If a patient cannot undergo vasodilator stress, then inotropic stress with escalating doses of dobutamine (± atropine) can be used. GTN-enhanced rest technetium-99m studies have also been shown to demonstrate viable myocardium. It is very unlikely that any patient cannot undergo some form of stress imaging with nuclear cardiology techniques.

Some practical considerations

The overall radiation exposure of a patient undergoing a stress-rest technetium study is approximately 10 mSv, which is greater than a diagnostic coronary angiogram but without the invasive and vascular complications.

Cost-effectiveness analyses have been performed with SPECT. Studies in Europe and the United States of America have confirmed that utilizing a strategy involving these techniques is associated with cost savings as well as fewer invasive tests. This has helped to drive a significant increase in the number of SPECT procedures performed worldwide.

Clinical uses of nuclear imaging

Investigation of coronary artery disease

In a large meta-analysis of 33 studies the sensitivity and specificity of myocardial perfusion imaging were 87% and 73% respectively. The normalcy rate, which removes the referral bias of false-positive patients being referred on for coronary angiography, was 91%. Similar results are available for vasodilator and dobutamine stress. More importantly, there is a wealth of prognostic data available. The value of a normal SPECT study is beyond doubt, with a meta-analysis including just under 21 000 patients followed up for 2.3 years demonstrating a major cardiac endpoint event rate of 0.7% per year. Follow-up studies extending up to 7 years have demonstrated similar low event rates.

High-risk markers on SPECT have incremental prognostic value over electrocardiographic and clinical variables. These include multivessel disease patterns, large burdens of ischaemia (>10% of myocardium), transient ischaemic left ventricular dilatation, left ventricular ejection fraction (LVEF) <0.4 (see below) and lung uptake (only with thallium-201). SPECT is also able to further risk stratify when risk scores such as the Duke treadmill score are applied to exercise ECG variables (Fig. 16.3.3.2), and can provides additional prognostic value in specific populations such as patients after myocardial infarction or with diabetes mellitus, women and patients with an abnormal ECG. e.g. left bundle branch block.

Nuclear techniques are well suited to the identification of myocardial viability and predict functional recovery (identified by echocardiography) in approximately 80% of segments after revascularization. This means that decisions about revascularization can be usefully informed by SPECT: studies have clearly demonstrated that patients with low ischaemic burdens on SPECT have the same cardiac event rate if treated with either medical therapy or revascularization, and that those with significantly abnormal scans have lower event rates with revascularization compared to medical therapy. Comparative studies with low dose dobutamine echocardiography (see Chapter 16.3.2), positron emission tomography (PET), and cardiovascular magnetic resonance (CMR) have been performed. Each test is broadly similar in its ability to predict functional recovery. SPECT has also been used to assess success of revascularization procedures.

In the acute setting, resting SPECT injections have been performed in patients attending Emergency Departments with chest pain and a nondiagnostic initial ECG. A normal perfusion scan was associated with a lower risk of future events, lower likelihood of requiring cardiac catheterization, and lower costs owing to the shorter hospital stay and fewer subsequent investigations.

Assessment of left ventricular volume and function

ECG-gated SPECT allows images to be taken throughout the cardiac cycle, when comparison of end-systolic and end-diastolic images then allows volumetric analysis and calculation of LVEF. There are three methods for calculation of volumes, regional function, and ejection fraction with nuclear techniques—first pass radionuclide ventriculography, equilibrium radionuclide ventriculography, and gated SPECT.

First pass radionuclide ventriculography This relies on an intravenous injection of technetium-99 m DTPA or pertechnate while the patient is already lying under the gamma camera. The circulation of

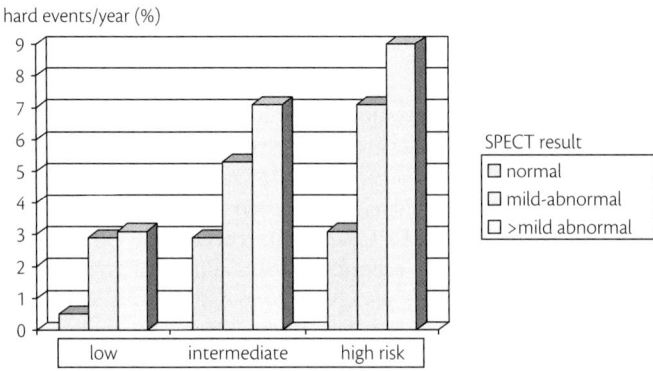

hard events/year (%)

Result of exercise ECG (Duke treadmill score)

SPECT result
□ normal
□ mild-abnormal
□ >mild abnormal

Fig. 16.3.3.2 Incremental value of myocardial perfusion imaging over exercise ECG: Hard event rates per year as a function of exercise SPECT in patients initially stratified by low, intermediate and high Duke treadmill scores.

isotope is studied in the right- and then left-sided cardiac chambers. The radioactivity is proportional to the volume of blood in the chamber. The technetium is not bound to sestamibi or tetrofosmin and therefore no myocardial uptake occurs. Right-to-left shunts can be detected by this method.

Equilibrium radionuclide ventriculography This technique, also known as multigated acquisition (MUGA), relies on technetium-99 m pertechnate radiolabelled erythrocytes, which are prepared in vivo to accept the technetium with a preceding injection of stannous pyrophosphate. The radiolabelled erythrocytes are allowed to circulate within the circulating volume with acquisition after 10 min. All four cardiac chambers are identified at the same time and so accurate camera positioning is required to reduce overlap. Images are gated to the R wave and many hundreds of cycles are acquired to produce an average. Regional motion can be identified on end systolic and diastolic frames. Left ventricular and right ventricular ejection fractions are also calculated. Acquisition time for both techniques is short (typically 10–15 min).

ECG-gated SPECT This relies on endomyocardial border definition from techneiutm-99 m sestamibi or tetrofosmin to produce end-systolic and diastolic frames (Fig. 16.3.3.3). Regional analysis, volumes, and LVEF are calculated.

The first two techniques are well established and validated and until recently were considered the 'gold standard' for volumetric analysis. Gated SPECT provides accurate assessment without requiring a blood pool injection. Alternatives such as echocardiography and X-ray ventriculography are not as reproducible, although cardiac MRI is now considered the gold standard for volumetric analysis.

The addition of volumes and LVEF to SPECT increases the prognostic value of myocardial perfusion imaging. Changes in post-stress LVEF are likely to represent sub-endocardial ischaemia, which may help to assess patients with 'balanced' multivessel ischaemia who may not have obvious regional perfusion defects.

Positron emission tomography (PET)

Basic principles

PET relies on coincidence detection of 512-keV photons. Perfusion can be assessed with nitrogen-13 ammonia or rubidium-82. Metabolism is assessed with fluorine-18 fluorodeoxyglucose (FDG). Nitrogen-13 ammonia and FDG have a short half-life and need to be produced in a cyclotron, which restricts their use. Nevertheless these tracers allow quantitation of myocardial flow, and the metabolic tracer (FDG) is considered to be the gold standard for assessment of myocardial viability. Cardiac PET studies tend to be confined to research institutions, but the increase in oncological studies requiring combined PET/CT machines may increase the availability of this technique for cardiac studies.

Comparison with other techniques

For myocardial perfusion the alternatives to PET include exercise electrocardiography, stress (exercise or dobutamine) echocardiography, and CMR (pharmacological stress). The exercise electrocardiogram is inferior mainly due to its dependence on exercise ability and a normal resting ECG. Stress echocardiography is a rapidly improving technique with a slightly lower sensitivity but a superior specificity in comparative studies: it is physician intensive

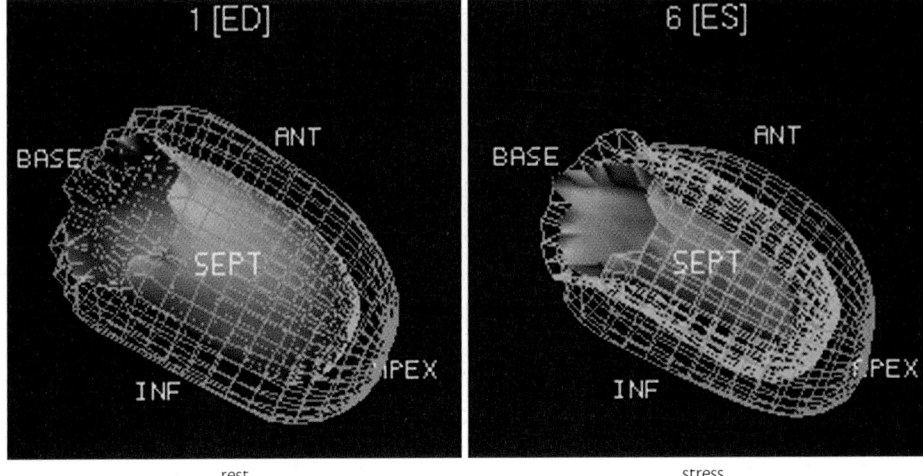

Fig. 16.3.3.3 Gated SPECT to assess global and regional left ventricular wall motion. Ant, anterior; ED, end diastole; ES, end systole; Inf, inferior; Sept, septum.

and operator dependent, but harmonic imaging and microbubble contrast agents have made an enormous difference to the technique so that it is comparable to PET in expert hands. CMR is an evolving technique that is showing great promise with regard to perfusion using gadolinium as a contrast agent (although recent experience suggests that gadolinium is not entirely benign, see below). Multislice CT (MSCT) may provide ischaemia/infarct imaging, but this is still at an experimental phase. As mentioned earlier, CMR is the gold standard for volumetric and functional analysis, although echocardiography is more versatile and accessible.

Cardiac MRI

For cardiac investigations standard MRI scanners have to be upgraded with a cardiac program (ECG gating, etc.) to allow for the movement of the heart, but can then reveal images of spectacular similarity to anatomical cross-sections. MRI also has the advantage over other techniques described in this chapter of not exposing the patient to radiation, although recently nephrogenic systemic fibrosis has been reported after application of the MRI contrast agent gadolinium. Those with impaired renal function are most susceptible to this complication, hence a patient's serum creatinine, allowing derivation of estimated glomerular filtration rate (eGFR), should be obtained before an MRI scan. In patients with an eGFR below 30ml/min exposure to gadolinium MRI contrast agents should be avoided if possible, but imaging with gadolinium may be performed if no other imaging modalities are available to make the diagnosis and the diagnostic information is vital.

Traditional concerns about MRI of patients with implantable cardiac devices include possible movement of the device, programming changes, and induced lead currents that might cause heating and cardiac stimulation. The presence of a permanent pacemaker or implantable cardioverter defibrillator (ICD) is therefore currently considered a relative contraindication to MRI. However, if the information provided by cardiac MRI cannot be obtained using other imaging modalities, it may be necessary to take the small risk of MRI imaging. Clinical studies have shown that—as long as the patient is not dependent on antibradycardic pacing—noncardiac and cardiac MRI can be performed safely in patients with selected implantable pacemaker and defibrillator systems.

Clinical uses of cardiac MRI

Assessment of ventricular function and mass

For this indication no contrast agent is needed and the technique has become the gold standard for quantifying ventricular volumes, ejection fraction, and myocardial mass. The image quality of native MRI recordings is usually excellent, with substantial differences in contrast between blood and myocardial tissue (Fig.13.3.3.4), which allows for accurate contour finding that is the prerequisite for reliable measurements of volumes and mass, particularly when the ventricular shape deviates from the assumed geometric model, as in patients with aneurysms or other major wall motion abnormalities.

With the availability of cardiac MRI, MUGA scanning—although also very accurate—has become less important for assessment of left ventricular volumes and function because of the radiation exposure that it requires. Cardiovascular MRI yields more accurate values for left ventricular parameters than planar imaging methods such as two-dimensional echocardiography or angiography. Newer echocardiographic techniques such as three-dimensional echocardiography and contrast echocardiography come close to cardiac MRI for assessment of left ventricular volumes and left ventricular function, but for accurate measurement of left ventricular mass MRI still appears to be superior to echocardiography. Therefore, in routine clinical practice the cheaper echocardiography remains first choice, but cardiac MRI is indicated when echocardiographic image quality is suboptimal.

Display of acute and chronic myocardial damage and assessment of myocardial viability

By using the MRI-specific contrast agent gadolinium it is possible to display small areas of damaged myocytes or loss of myocytes and replacement by scar tissue. Gadolinium chelates are extracellular tracers that cannot cross cell membranes. In normal myocardium the myocytes are densely packed and the extracellular space and vascular volume represents less than 15% of the myocardial volume, hence after injection of gadolinium there are only few gadolinium molecules in a myocardial sample volume. By contrast, when the membranes of myocytes rupture, gadolinium molecules can penetrate into the myocytes and stay there, even late after gadolinium injection, such that in scar tissue the interstitial space

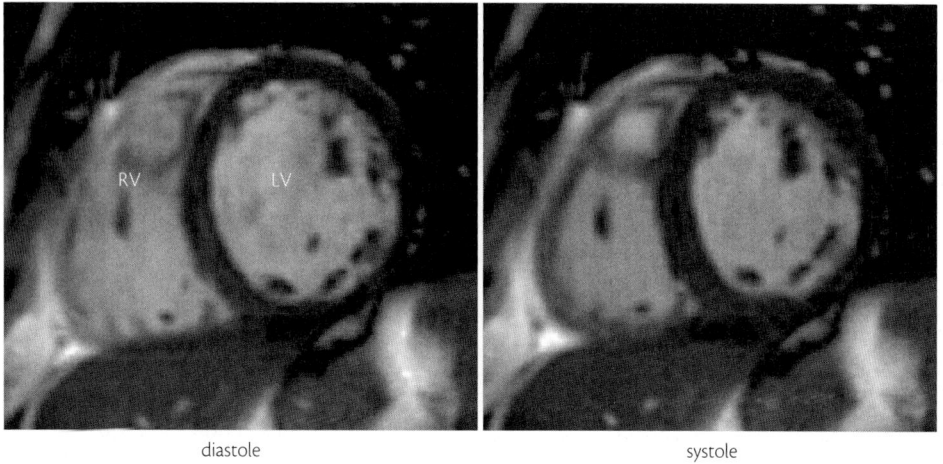

diastole   systole

Fig. 16.3.3.4 End-diastolic and end-systolic images of left ventricle (LV) and right ventricle (RV): note the good delineation of the myocardium from the blood and the surrounding tissue.
Courtesy of Dr Saul Myerson, Oxford Centre for Clinical Magnetic Resonance Research.

is expanded and increased gadolinium concentration is found (Fig. 16.3.3.5).

Late gadolinium enhancement (LGE)

LGE in coronary artery disease

Late after injection of gadolinium the intravascular contrast molecules are washed out and only the few gadolinium molecules in the interstitial space persist in normal myocardium. More gadolinium molecules remain in acutely damaged myocardium and scar tissue. The display of acute myocardial damage and scar tissue is independent from the underlying disease, hence LGE cannot distinguish between acute and chronic infarcts, but the pattern may differ in different ischaemic and inflammatory heart diseases (Fig. 16.3.3.6).

The need for cardiac MRI in acute myocardial infarction is limited, but LGE reflects irreversibly injured myocardium and MRI is an excellent method for displaying the extent of myocardial infarction. For larger infarcts this is not clinically relevant because SPECT and

echocardiography can do the same, but due to its higher spatial resolution LGE appears to be the best method for detection of small subendocardial infarctions—even the small infarcts that may occur during percutaneous coronary interventions.

LGE imaging is of more clinical relevance in chronic ischaemic disease and in many centres it has become the method of choice for assessing myocardial viability in chronic coronary artery disease. Alternative methods are SPECT and PET, which expose the patient to radiation, or echocardiography, which needs to be performed with dobutamine stress.

In patients with coronary artery disease impaired myocardial contraction can be due to necrosis of myocytes and subsequent fibrosis, or hibernating or stunned myocardium. Cardiac MRI appears to be the best imaging modality to differentiate viable (preserved myocytes) from nonviable (fibrotic) myocardium. Such assessment of viability is an important step in the consideration of patients with ischaemic cardiomyopathy, because percutaneous coronary interventions or bypass grafting are only indicated in vessels that supply viable myocardium. Myocardial tissue showing LGE is not likely to recover after revascularization of the supplying coronary artery and the transmural extent of LGE correlates negatively with the outcome after revascularization, but the threshold is

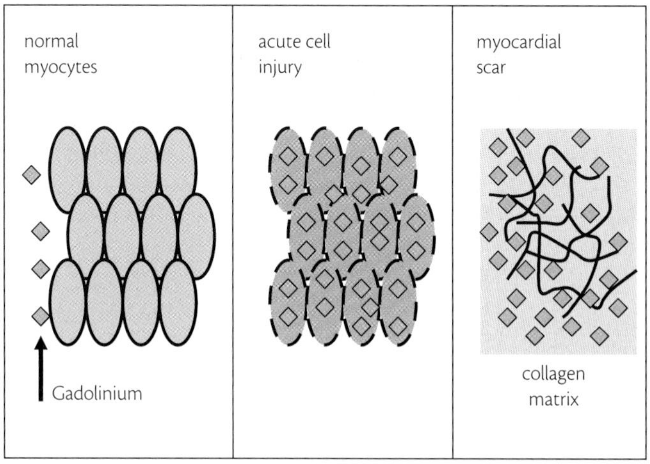

Fig. 16.3.3.5 Mechanism for late gadolinium enhancement (LGE) in acute and chronic myocardial damage: (a) Densely packed myocytes with intact cell membrane—gadolinium chelates only in the vessels and extracellular space. (b) Acute myocardial damage with ruptured cell membranes of myocytes—intracellular accumulation of gadolinium chelates. (c) Chronic myocardial damage with loss of myocytes and replacement by scar tissue—mostly collagen fibres that are filled with gadolinium chelates.

normal myocytes

Gadolinium

acute cell injury

myocardial scar

collagen matrix

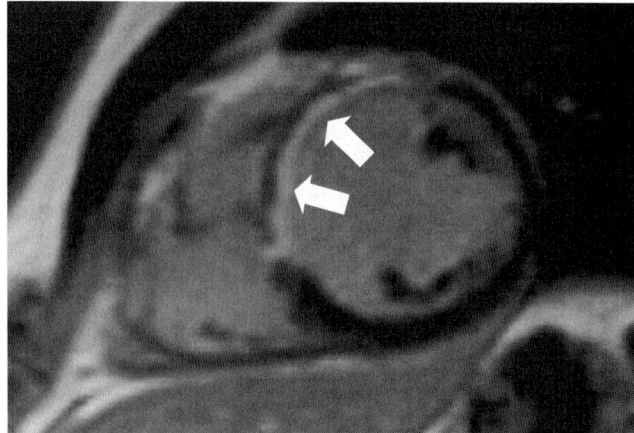

Fig. 16.3.3.6 Late gadolinium enhancement (LGE) showing as a white rim (arrowed) in a patient with transmural myocardial infarction.
Courtesy of Dr Saul Myerson, Oxford Centre for Clinical Magnetic Resonance Research.

not clear. To improve the sensitivity and specificity for prediction of functional recovery additional assessment of contractile reserve using low dose dobutamine may be considered, with imaging by echocardiography or MRI.

LGE in dilated cardiomyopathy

Subendocardial or transmural LGE related to the territories supplied by coronary arteries is typical for ischemic cardiomyopathy, but can also found in patients with diffuse reduction in contractility and only minor plaques seen by coronary angiography. This is probably caused by transient obstruction or spasm of the corresponding coronary arteries. By contrast, in dilated cardiomyopathy there may be no LGE, or a patchy or streaky pattern in the mid wall of the left ventricle.

LGE—often multifocal and patchy—is a frequent finding in patients with hypertrophic cardiomyopathy, but the clinical implication is not yet understood.

LGE in inflammatory and infiltrative heart disease

The diagnosis of acute myocarditis is often difficult using laboratory findings, ECG, and echocardiography. Cardiac MRI can confirm a clinical suspicion, typically revealing LGE in the myocardium in a patchy epicardial distribution, or band-like in the inferolateral wall. Cardiac involvement in sarcoidosis, which is otherwise difficult to diagnose, can also show a patchy LGE pattern.

Amyloidosis is another indication for cardiac MRI, with the gadolinium contrast agent diffusing into the amyloid that is deposited in the interstitium: hyperenhancement is diffuse, but more pronounced in the endocardial layers. In Fabry's disease enhancement is diffuse or focal in the inferolateral midwall.

Congenital heart disease

In many patients echocardiography is sufficient for clinical purposes, but all the information obtained in an echocardiographic examination is provided by MRI, and MRI images are more comprehensive because the window to the heart is not limited, and the images are often of better quality than the corresponding echocardiographic recordings.

Sedation is required in small children and monitoring is demanding in critically ill infants, hence CMR is usually performed following, and as an adjunct to, transthoracic echocardiography in neonates and infants. When readily available, it becomes a first-line technique in older children, adolescents, or adults, in patients with more complex anatomy, and at any age after surgery because body habitus and interposition of scar tissue and lungs become an increasing problem for transthoracic echocardiography. As discussed previously, cardiac MRI provides precise and reproducible quantification of ventricular volumes, mass, and function, and this is especially the case for the right ventricle, which is usually the chamber implicated in and stressed by repair of congenital heart disease. Cardiac MRI is also very effective for the evaluation of anomalies of the thoracic aorta and conduits.

Assessment of coronary arteries and myocardial perfusion

MRI is indicated to define congenital or inflammatory changes of the coronary arteries. The spatial resolution and image quality of MRI are inferior to multislice CT, but for disease and anomalies affecting the proximal coronary arteries cardiac MRI appears to be the first choice as it does not entail exposure to radiation.

Cardiac MRI offers two methods for diagnosis of inducible myocardial ischaemia: firstly, assessment of left ventricular wall motion and thickening using dobutamine stress to provoke wall motion abnormalities in a territory supplied by a stenosed coronary artery; secondly, direct display of myocardial perfusion using gadolinium combined with adenosine stress, similar to nuclear imaging. Both methods compete with stress echocardiography and nuclear imaging, and CMR has similar sensitivity and specificity for detection of coronary disease. The choice of perfusion imaging technique depends in practice on local availabilities, with stress echocardiography and nuclear imaging usually less expensive than MRI techniques and more widely available.

Cardiac CT

Multislice spiral computed tomography (MSCT) has become a valuable diagnostic procedure for a variety of diseases. It is indicated to assess pericardial thickening/calcification and is a fast and noninvasive method for the visualization of the coronary arteries, with the entire coronary circulation revealed in a single breath-hold with modern techniques. MSCT provides a unique opportunity to exclude significant coronary stenosis and to quantify the amount of coronary and aortic valve calcium.

For cardiac indications a volume data set is acquired, covering the distance from the carina to the diaphragmatic side of the heart. Native scanning is sufficient for assessment of coronary calcium. For display of the coronary lumen the investigation is longer and exposes the patient to more radiation, equivalent to the amount required for conventional coronary angiography, and intravenous infusion of a large amount of contrast agent (currently 100 ml) is needed. Other limitations of the technique are shown in Box 16.3.3.1.

The high spatial resolution and contrast between the myocardium/valves and the blood pool means that an excellent display of various cardiac structures can be achieved. For many indications cardiac MRI and echocardiography are preferable because they do not require radiation or contrast agents, but there are two areas where cardiac CT can play a major role—the display of coronary calcification and arteriosclerotic lesions, and luminal obstructions of the coronary arteries.

Clinical uses of cardiac CT

Coronary calcification

The accuracy of CT techniques to detect and quantify calcified structures is unbeaten by other imaging techniques. The presence of calcifications is assumed if contiguous pixels with a density of more than 130 Hounsfield units (HU) are found within the coronary

---

Box 16.3.3.1 Limitations of MSCT

- Radiation exposure
- Calcium scoring 1.5–2 mSv
- Coronary angiography 4–12 mSv
- Needs iodinated contrast agents
- Needs low heart rate to avoid motion artefacts[a]
- Calcium/stents can impair the judgement of the lumen

[a] For visualization of coronary artery lumen only.

artery system. The Agatston score is used to quantify the amount of coronary calcium, which takes into account the area and the CT density of calcified coronary lesions.

Coronary calcium is a surrogate marker for coronary arteriosclerosis, only patients with renal failure have coronary calcifications without arteriosclerotic plaques. However, not every coronary plaque is calcified, and coronary calcium does not indicate or exclude instability of the plaque. The amount of coronary calcium correlates moderately closely with the amount of coronary arteriosclerosis, but there is only a weak correlation with the angiographic severity of obstructive coronary lesions. Significant obstruction of the coronary arteries is very unlikely, but not impossible, if no calcium is found in the coronary artery tree. Measurement of the coronary calcium score can be used for risk stratification of asymptomatic patients or patients with atypical angina (Figs. 16.3.3.7 and 16.3.3.8).

Visualization of the coronary artery lumen

Selective coronary angiography via the direct arterial approach has been the method of choice for accurate assessment of coronary obstructions (see Chapter 16.3.4). Cardiac CT (termed coronary CT angiography for this purpose) provides a less invasive approach to display the coronary arteries, and numerous studies have been undertaken to compare the accuracy of detection of coronary stenoses by the two techniques. Cardiac CT does not yet match invasive coronary angiography, but many studies have shown a very high negative predictive value, ranging from 92 to 100%, hence cardiac CT appears to be a reasonable test to rule out coronary stenoses in patients with low to intermediate likelihood of disease (Fig. 16.3.3.9).

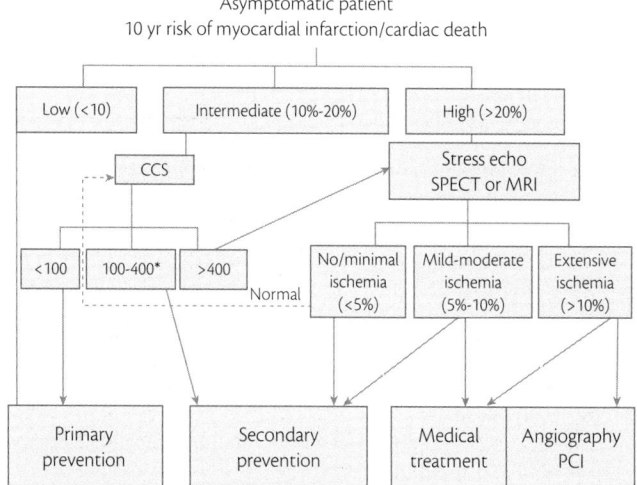

Fig. 16.3.3.8 Approach to use of coronary calcium scanning and nuclear testing in screening for coronary artery disease in asymptomatic patients. CCS, coronary calcium score; PCI, percutaneous coronary intervention; revasc, revascularization; Sx, symptoms. *Consider SPECT/PET in higher-risk subsets.
(Modified from Berman DS, *et al.* (2006). Roles of nuclear cardiology, cardiac computed tomography, and cardiac magnetic resonance: noninvasive risk stratification and a conceptual framework for the selection of noninvasive imaging tests in patients with known or suspected coronary artery disease. *J Nuclear Med*, **47**, 1107–18.)

Coronary CT angiography is an extremely reliable tool for investigation of patients with known or suspected congenital coronary anomalies. The only alternative technique is cardiac MRI, but this can be more challenging to perform and interpret. With further developments it is likely that coronary CT will replace invasive coronary angiography for diagnostic purposes.

The display of a coronary lesion is very helpful to establish the diagnosis of coronary artery disease. However, the management of the patient also depends on the results of functional imaging—in particular on the amount of myocardial ischaemia and viability—hence

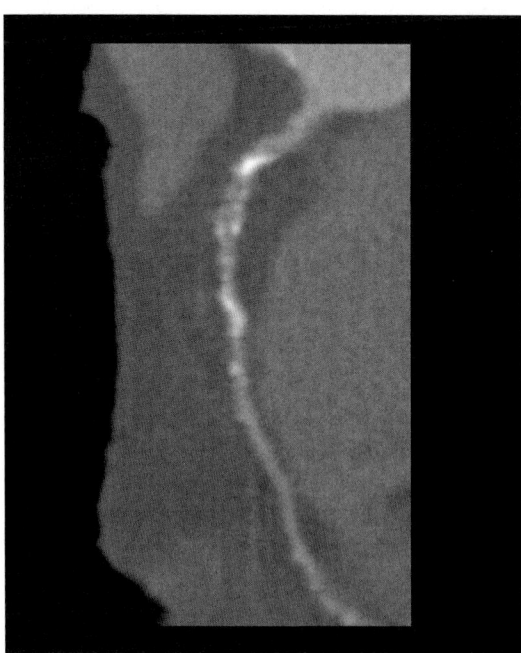

Fig. 16.3.3.7 Multislice spiral computed tomography (MSCT) showing a calcified middle segment of the right coronary artery. The calcium is displayed as bright areas superimposed on the coronary artery. Note that it is not possible to display the lumen and possible vessel obstructions in calcified segments.
Image courtesy of Dr E Nicol, National Heart and Lung Institute, London.

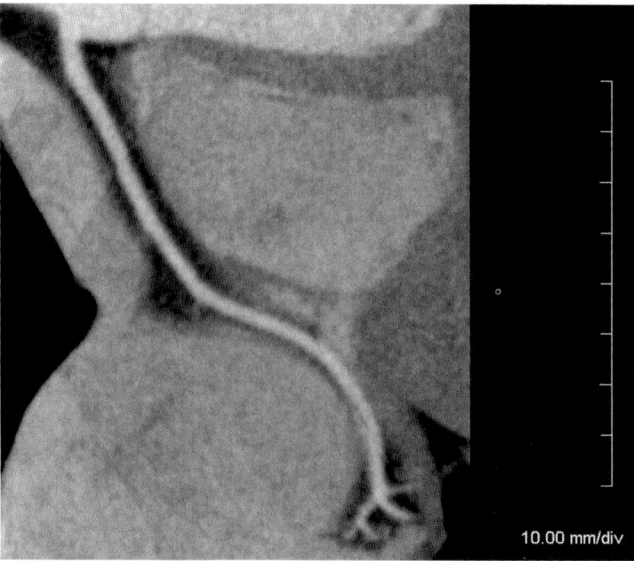

Fig. 16.3.3.9 CT coronary angiography showing a normal right coronary artery.
Image courtesy of Dr E Nicol, National Heart and Lung Institute, London.

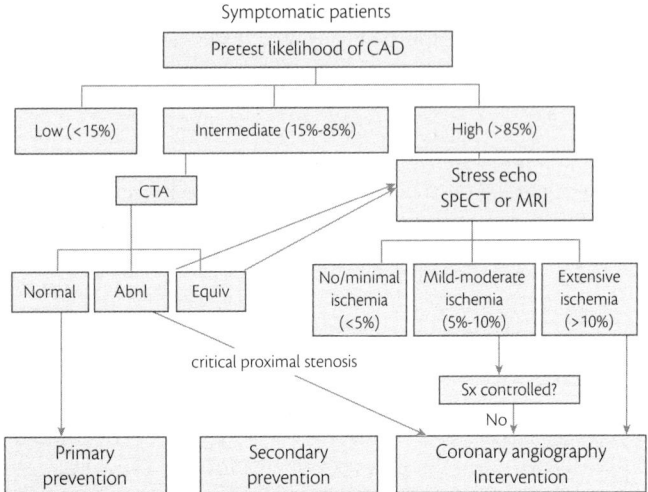

Fig. 16.3.3.10 Approach to diagnosis and management of coronary artery disease in symptomatic patients using coronary CT angiography (CTA) and stress SPECT or stress echocardiography. Abnl, abnormal; CAD, coronary artery disease; Equiv, equivocal; revasc, revascularization; Sx, symptoms.
(Modified from Berman DS, et al. (2006). Roles of nuclear cardiology, cardiac computed tomography, and cardiac magnetic resonance: noninvasive risk stratification and a conceptual framework for the selection of noninvasive imaging tests in patients with known or suspected coronary artery disease. J Nuclear Med, **47**, 1107–18.)

the anatomical information provided by coronary angiography cannot be interpreted without the results of functional imaging performed with nuclear, echocardiographic, or MRI methods. Often these methods will provide enough information for patient management such that direct visualization of the coronary tree is not needed (Fig. 16.3.3.10).

Further reading

Achenbach S, Daniel WG (2007). Current role of cardiac computed tomography. *Herz*, **32**, 97–107.

Berman DS, et al. (2006). Roles of nuclear cardiology, cardiac computed tomography, and cardiac magnetic resonance: noninvasive risk stratification and a conceptual framework for the selection of noninvasive imaging tests in patients with known or suspected coronary artery disease. *J Nuclear Med*, **47**, 1107–18.

Dilsizian V, Narula J (2009). *Atlas of nuclear cardiology*, 3rd edition. Springer, New York.

Hendel RC, et al. (2006). ACCF/ACR/SCCT/SCMR/ASNC/NASCI/ SCAI/SIR 2006 appropriateness criteria for cardiac computed tomography and cardiac magnetic resonance imaging: a report of the American College of Cardiology Foundation Quality Strategic Directions Committee Appropriateness Criteria Working Group, American College of Radiology, Society of Cardiovascular Computed Tomography, Society of Cardiovascular Magnetic Resonance Imaging, American Society of Nuclear Cardiology, North American Society of Cardiac Imaging, Society of Cardiovascular Angiography and Interventions and Society of Interventional Radiology. *J Am Coll Cardiol*, **48**, 1475–97.

Sabharwal NK, Loong C, Kelion A (2008). *Oxford handbook of nuclear cardiology*. Oxford University Press. Oxford.

Marcu CB, Beek AM, van Rossum AC (2006). Clinical applications of cardiovascular magnetic resonance imaging. *CMAJ*, **175**, 911–17.

Nazarian S, et al. (2006). Clinical utility and safety of a protocol for noncardiac and cardiac magnetic resonance imaging of patients with permanent pacemakers and implantable-cardioverter defibrillators at 1.5 Tesla. *Circulation*, **114**, 1277–84.

Pennell DJ, et al. (2004). Clinical indications for cardiovascular magnetic resonance (CMR): Consensus Panel report. *Eur Heart J*, **25**, 1940–65.

Vohringer M, et al. (2007). Significance of late gadolinium enhancement in cardiovascular magnetic resonance imaging. *Herz*, **32**, 129–37.

Zaret B, Beller GA (2005). *Clinical nuclear cardiology: state of the art and future directions*, 3rd edition. Mosby, London.

16.3.4 **Cardiac catheterization and angiography**

Edward D. Folland

Essentials

Cardiac catheterization/angiography is indicated for evaluation of patients with coronary, valvular, and congenital heart disease in whom diagnostic or therapeutic decisions cannot be made on the basis of noninvasive tests. Most patients presenting for cardiac catheterization have coronary artery disease: no other imaging modality can, as yet, provide the detailed anatomy of the entire coronary circulation that is needed for planning revascularization procedures.

Technique and diagnostic utility—vascular access is usually obtained percutaneously from the femoral or radial artery (for the left heart), or the femoral or brachial/antecubital vein (for the right heart). Key information that can be obtained by cardiac catheterization/angiography include (1) pressures within cardiac chambers; (2) cardiac output; (3) quantitative estimation of left ventricular function; (4) diagnosis and quantitation of intracardiac shunts; (5) calculation of systemic and pulmonary vascular resistances; (6) assessment of cardiac valves; and (7) details of coronary arterial anatomy and function.

Therapeutic utility—cardiac catheterization/angiography permits interventions, particularly coronary angioplasty/stenting (see Chapters 16.13.5 and 16.13.6), that are of great and increasing therapeutic importance.

Introduction

Invasive cardiac diagnosis by means of catheterization and angiography developed hand in hand with cardiac surgery throughout the 20th century. It answered the need for precise information about cardiac physiology and anatomy, which arose in the 1940s when surgical techniques for the treatment of congenital and rheumatic heart disease first became available. A few years earlier, in 1929, Werner Forsman of Germany successfully and safely passed a filiform urinary catheter from a median basilic vein into the right atrium of his own heart and documented it on X-ray film.

Although this feat cost him his own job, it enabled Andre Cournand and Dickenson Richards a decade later to use catheters for sampling blood, measuring pressure and flow, and injecting radio-opaque contrast medium (angiography) into the intact, beating human heart, ushering in the era of invasive cardiac diagnosis. Cournand and Richards later won the Nobel Prize for their important work. This chapter will review the diagnostic applications of cardiac catheterization and angiography.

Indications for cardiac catheterization and angiography

Catheterization entails some degree of risk and discomfort, and is expensive, hence patients should be carefully selected. In broadest terms, it is indicated for detailed evaluation of those with coronary, valvular, and congenital heart disease, once they have been identified as candidates for surgery or other forms of intervention. It may also be indicated for patients whose diagnosis is uncertain from noninvasive evaluation.

Coronary artery disease

Most patients presenting for cardiac catheterization have coronary artery disease. Angiography of the coronary arteries performed during cardiac catheterization is essential for patients in whom revascularization is indicated. In spite of the limitations discussed later in this chapter, no other imaging modality, including MRI and CT (see Chapter 16.3.3), can as yet provide the detailed anatomy of the entire coronary circulation that is needed for planning revascularization procedures such as coronary artery bypass surgery and percutaneous intervention.

Coronary angiography is indicated for patients with chronic stable angina that persists in spite of reasonable efforts at pharmacological therapy. It is also indicated for patients whose survival would be improved by revascularization, regardless of symptoms. Such patients are those with severe stenosis of the main left coronary artery and those with severe two- and three-vessel coronary artery disease in combination with impaired left ventricular function. These patients may be identified by the following features of stress testing: ischaemia at low workload (especially in stage 1 of the Bruce protocol), marked depression of the electrocardiographic ST segment (>2 mm), failure to augment systolic blood pressure during exercise, and large exercise-induced defects or increased lung uptake during radionuclide perfusion imaging (see Chapters 16.3.1 and 16.3.3). In addition, patients with high-risk clinical presentations such as acute myocardial infarction, unstable angina, and post-myocardial infarction ischaemia are candidates for angiography. Patients having acute myocardial infarction are best served by immediate percutaneous coronary intervention if this is available in a timely manner (see Chapters 16.13.5 and 16.13.6). Finally, catheterization is sometimes indicated to obtain a definitive diagnosis when noninvasive testing has yielded equivocal or inconsistent results.

Valvular disease

Catheterization was once considered essential prior to the surgical treatment of valvular heart disease. This is no longer the case because of advances in noninvasive testing using ultrasound and Doppler techniques. Nevertheless, catheterization is frequently helpful for gathering the information needed to properly select patients for surgical therapy, and to guide the surgeon in providing optimum treatment, the most common issue being to assess the need for coronary artery revascularization, particularly among those with aortic stenosis, who commonly have coronary artery disease. Haemodynamic studies may also be necessary in cases where noninvasive diagnostic data are limited or equivocal. By contrast, it is often possible to avoid catheterization in young patients in whom noninvasive studies yield unequivocal conclusions and there is no evidence of coronary artery disease.

Congenital disease

Most patients with congenital heart defects can be definitively diagnosed by transthoracic or transoesophageal ultrasound, CT, or MRI (see Chapters 16.3.2 and 16.3.3). As in valvular disease, catheterization is most useful in cases where the abnormality is unusually complex, the noninvasive data are incomplete, or the patient is suspected of having coronary artery disease. Catheterization is particularly useful in quantifying shunt flow and pulmonary vascular resistance, both of which are important considerations in the treatment of intracardiac defects. The physical passage of a systemic venous catheter across the atrial septum into a pulmonary vein or the left ventricle is diagnostic of an atrial septal defect.

Pericardial disease

Pericardial tamponade and constriction lend themselves particularly well to diagnosis by catheterization. Although ultrasonography has superseded catheterization as a rapidly available method of confirming the clinical diagnosis of tamponade, it is usually inconclusive for patients with pericardial constriction. At catheterization, patients with both conditions usually demonstrate equalization of all intracardiac diastolic pressures, with unique pressure waveforms exhibited in the right atrium and right ventricle usually distinguishing the two diagnoses (Fig. 16.3.4.1).

Congestive heart failure

The aetiology and pathophysiology of congestive heart failure are readily elucidated by catheterization. States of pressure and volume

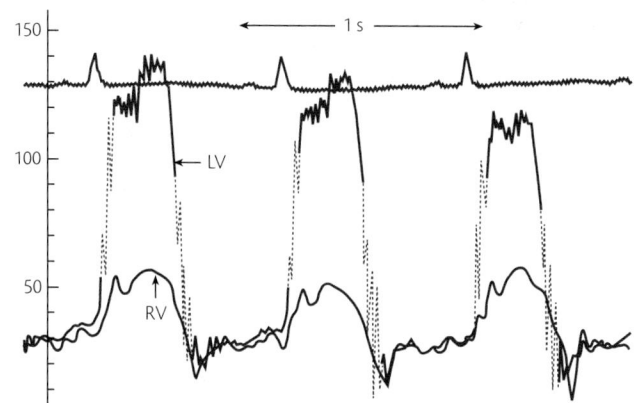

Fig. 16.3.4.1 Pericardial constriction. This is a tracing of simultaneous left ventricular (LV) and right ventricular (RV) pressure in a patient with pericardial constriction. Generally, the diastolic pressure of the left ventricle is higher than that of the right ventricle. For patients with a constriction, the pericardium determines the diastolic compliance of both chambers, causing the diastolic pressures to be equal. Note also the typical 'dip–plateau' pattern or 'square-root sign' of both chambers in diastole. Although diastolic ventricular pressures are also equal for patients having tamponade, the dip–plateau pattern is usually absent.

overload as well as systolic and diastolic dysfunction of the ventricles can be easily identified, as explained in detail later in this chapter. Furthermore, catheterization is uniquely suited for identifying transient or reversible causes of left ventricular dysfunction caused by ischaemia or myocardial hibernation due to underlying coronary artery disease. Sometimes exercise or other interventions are performed during a catheter study to elicit transient abnormal haemodynamic function. Myocardial biopsy performed during catheterization can sometimes identify the aetiology of primary myocardial dysfunction.

Pulmonary vascular disease

Patients with primary pulmonary hypertension (see Chapter 16.15.2) should undergo catheterization to measure pulmonary vascular pressure and resistance. Certain vasodilating drugs may or may not benefit the patient, depending upon their effect on pressure and resistance during acute administration. Pulmonary angiography performed during right heart catheterization is still regarded as the most definitive test for pulmonary embolism, although in most cases the diagnosis can be secured by radioisotope lung scanning and spiral CT.

Practicalities of cardiac catheterization

Preparing the patient

Precatheterization evaluation should consist of a careful history and examination, particularly aimed at eliciting details of prior cardiac procedures, reactions to contrast medium, renal function, peripheral vascular status, and haemostatic function. The patient should be carefully advised of the indications, alternatives, risks, discomforts, and expected benefits of the procedure. The skilled clinician does this while building the patient's confidence and avoids creating undue alarm. Following an uncomplicated diagnostic catheterization the patient should usually expect to go home the same day and to resume customary physical activities within a day or two.

Vascular access

The traditional approach to vascular access is via a cut-down near the antecubital fossa, with isolation and mobilization of the brachial or antecubital vein and the brachial artery for right and left heart catheterization thereby allowing arterial and venous access. After the procedure the arterial entry site is repaired by suture and the vein is usually tied off. However, although this approach has the advantage of enabling early postprocedure ambulation and the security of direct arterial closure in anticoagulated patients, it has the disadvantage of being time-consuming for most physicians and less cosmetic for the patient, hence the cut-down approach is now seldom used, with percutaneous arterial catheterization becoming increasingly popular.

Percutaneous vascular access is achieved by direct puncture with a needle through which a flexible spring guide wire is passed into the vessel. Catheters may then be passed into the vessel over the guide wire. Following the procedure haemostasis is achieved by applying pressure over the puncture site until bleeding stops. Percutaneous access is frequently employed at the femoral site, although it may also be used at brachial, axillary, internal jugular, and radial locations. It has the advantage of speed, simplicity, and—when performed from the femoral vessels—frees the upper body

and arms during angiographic filming. However, it has the disadvantage of sometimes requiring several hours' immobilization of the catheterization site following the procedure. Nevertheless, the femoral approach has become the preferred choice in most cases, with use of smaller catheters (4 and 5 French) and closure devices for the arterial puncture site enabling earlier ambulation, but the percutaneous radial approach has become increasingly popular for outpatients.

Right heart catheterization

Right heart catheterization can be performed from any of the approaches described above. Although traditionally performed with a stiff, woven Dacron, end-hole catheter, it is often done with a flexible, balloon-tip, flow-directed catheter (Swan–Ganz) because this is safer and enables the measurement of cardiac output by thermodilution.

Catheterization of the right heart is indicated by itself for the study of pulmonary vascular disease and haemodynamic response to exercise or drug administration. It is indicated in combination with left heart catheterization for patients requiring haemodynamic study of valvular, congenital, or myocardial disease, and for patients being studied primarily for coronary artery disease who also have heart failure, valvular, or pulmonary disease.

Left atrial pressure can be measured indirectly via right heart catheterization by wedging the tip of the catheter in a pulmonary arteriole, or by occluding a pulmonary artery branch with the inflated balloon at the tip of a Swan–Ganz catheter. In either case, this creates a static column of blood from the tip of the catheter, through the pulmonary capillary bed, to the left atrium. This static column of blood has the effect of extending the tip of the catheter to the left atrium for pressure-measuring purposes. The resulting pressure is identical to the directly measured left atrial pressure, except that it is delayed temporally by approximately 80 ms. This pressure, commonly known as the pulmonary (artery) capillary wedge (PCW) pressure, is very useful in the management of left heart failure and shock, and for estimating the diastolic gradient across the mitral valve in patients with mitral stenosis.

Left heart catheterization

Left heart catheterization is generally performed in conjunction with coronary angiography, but is specifically required for the assessment of left ventricular function and assessment of stenosis or regurgitation of the left-sided valves (mitral and aortic). It is most often accomplished by femoral or brachial arterial access, and by retrograde crossing of the aortic valve to enter the left ventricle. Left heart catheterization may also be achieved by controlled puncture of the interatrial septum with a catheter originating from the right femoral vein (trans-septal left heart catheterization): this can then be used to measure left atrial pressure directly, and be passed antegradely through the mitral valve to measure pressure and perform angiography of the left ventricle. Retrograde access of the left atrium from the left ventricle is technically difficult and seldom done.

The left ventricle may also be entered via transthoracic needle puncture. This approach, known as direct left ventricular puncture, is occasionally necessary for studying patients who have both mitral and aortic mechanical prosthetic valves. The passage of the needle into the left ventricle from the cardiac apex is facilitated by echocardiographic guidance.

Information obtained from cardiac catheterization and angiography

Intracardiac pressures

Methodology

Pressure at the tip of the catheter is transmitted through the fluid inside the catheter (usually saline) to a transducer, which converts the pressure signal to an electrical signal that can then be amplified and displayed on a screen or on a strip-chart paper recording. Once calibrated, the pressure at the tip of the catheter can be read graphically from the recording screen or paper. The fidelity of recording depends upon the physical characteristics of the fluid-filled catheter, stopcocks, connecting tubing, and the pressure transducer itself. A fluid-filled system is usually capable of responding to transient pressure changes up to 20 or occasionally 30 Hz, which is of sufficient fidelity to reproduce diagnostically useful pressure waveforms from the heart. However, it is not responsive enough to accurately reproduce the rate of rise of left ventricular pressure during the isovolumic phase of systole (dP/dt). This requires responsiveness to transient pressure changes of at least 60 Hz, of which fluid-filled catheter systems are not capable. For such applications catheter-tip manometers are available (Millar catheters) in which the transducer is placed at the catheter tip, eliminating the need for an intervening column of fluid. These devices are expensive and are used only when such fidelity is required, usually in research applications.

Normal intracardiac pressures

The upper limits of all normal intracardiac pressures measurable from a right heart catheter are approximate multiples of six, hence they are easily remembered by the 'rule of sixes' (Table 16.3.4.1). For example, the mean right atrial pressure is 6 mmH g or less, mean left atrial pressure is 12 mmHg or less. A further aid to remembering normal pressures is the 'corollary of continuity', which means that contiguous chambers have a common pressure when the intervening valve is open. For example, the right ventricle and right atrium are essentially a common chamber when the tricuspid valve is open in diastole, therefore the upper limit of right ventricular end-diastolic pressure is the same as the upper limit of the normal right atrial pressure, or 6 mmHg. This assumes there is no significant stenosis or regurgitation across the tricuspid valve, and that the right ventricle has normal compliance. The same condition applies to the mitral valve in diastole and the pulmonic and aortic valves in systole. Another practical rule is that the pulmonary artery diastolic and pulmonary artery capillary pressures approximate each other in the absence of severe pulmonary vascular disease. Once this has been established for any given patient, the pulmonary artery diastolic pressure can be followed as a surrogate for pulmonary capillary wedge pressure in situations where a pulmonary artery catheter is used for intensive-care monitoring.

All intracardiac pressures rise and fall phasically with breathing due to transmission of shifting intrapleural pressure during respiratory effort. Usually this variation is no more than a few mmHg from inspiration to expiration, but it can be quite marked in patients with obstructive lung disease. Standards of normal pressure are based upon measurements taken during resting respiration, averaging several respiratory cycles. Pressures in the catheterization laboratory should be similarly measured: asking a patient to hold their breath may generate misleading data.

Table 16.3.4.1 Normal intracardiac pressures[a]

Location	Phasic pressure (mmHg)	Mean pressure (mmHg)
Right atrium		3 ± 2
Right ventricle	24 ± 4	
Systole	5 ± 3	
Diastole		
Pulmonary artery	24 ± 6	13 ± 5
Systole	13 ± 5	
Diastole		
Pulmonary capillary		9 ± 3
Wedge		
Left atrium		9 ± 3
Left ventricle		
Systole	120 ± 18	
Diastole	10 ± 5	

[a] These values are derived from 100 consecutive catheterization studies of patients proven to have no evidence of heart disease at the West Roxbury Veterans Administration Hospital from 1955 to 1980. An easy way to remember the upper limits of normal values (≤2 standard deviations above mean) is that they are generally multiples of the number 6.

Waveforms

The shape of intracardiac pressure waveforms carries useful diagnostic information. Atria and ventricles have characteristic waveforms, the left-sided chambers normally demonstrating similar patterns at relatively higher pressures than right-sided chambers. The state of volume loading and the relative compliance or 'stiffness' of the respective ventricles during diastolic filling determines pressures in the right and left atria. The left ventricle is generally thicker, stiffer, and less compliant to the stretch of increasing volume than the right ventricle; hence the left atrial and left ventricular diastolic pressures are higher than the respective pressures in the right heart. Conditions such as pericardial constriction and tamponade alter this normal relationship (see Fig. 16.3.4.1).

Cardiac flow and output

Measurement of cardiac output was one of the earliest applications of catheterization. Most methods entail application of the indicator dilution theory (the Fick principle), summarized graphically in Fig. 16.3.4.2, which can be stated simply as follows: the rate of flow can be measured if an indicator substance is added to the moving vehicle (e.g. blood) at a known rate, and the concentration of the indicator is also known proximal and distal to the point where the indicator is added. The indicator can be any readily measured substance such as oxygen, indocyanine green dye, or saline, the temperature of which is known and different from that of the bloodstream.

Cardiac output by oximetry

In this method, commonly called the Fick method, the indicator is oxygen that is carried physiologically by the blood. The method requires that the subject be in a metabolic steady state where the use of oxygen is constant. Such a steady state exists at rest and also

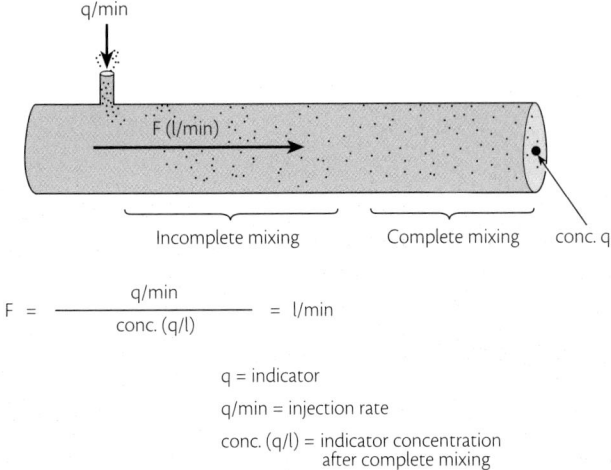

$$F = \frac{q/min}{conc.\ (q/l)} = l/min$$

q = indicator

q/min = injection rate

conc. (q/l) = indicator concentration
after complete mixing

Fig. 16.3.4.2 The Fick principle. The flow rate (F) through a vessel (cardiac output, in this case) can be measured if an indicator is added to the flowing liquid at a known rate (q/min) and the concentration (q/L) of the indicator is measured after complete mixing has occurred.

during exercise, provided that the workload is constant for at least 3 min. As seen in Fig. 16.3.4.3, the pulmonary blood flow can be calculated when the oxygen consumption rate is known and the oxygen contents of blood in systemic and pulmonary arteries are known. In the absence of intracardiac shunts the pulmonary blood flow equals the systemic blood flow, or cardiac output.

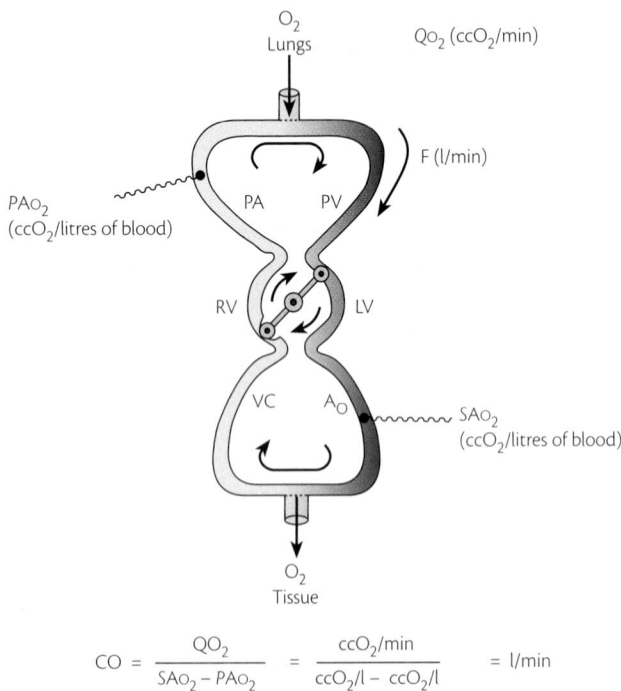

$$CO = \frac{QO_2}{SAO_2 - PAO_2} = \frac{ccO_2/min}{ccO_2/l - ccO_2/l} = l/min$$

Fig. 16.3.4.3 Cardiac output measured by oximetry. This is an application of the Fick principle in which oxygen is the indicator carried by flowing blood. The patient's metabolism must be at steady state, a condition where oxygen consumption and utilization are matched. It requires three measurements: oxygen consumption rate (QO_2), systemic arterial oxygen content (SAO_2), and pulmonary arterial oxygen content (PAO_2). Ao, aorta; cc, volume in ml; CO, cardiac output; LV, left ventricle; PV, pulmonary vein; RV, right ventricle; VC, vena cava.

Dye dilution

This method entails the rapid injection of a known quantity of indocyanine dye into the pulmonary artery. Blood is then sampled by withdrawal at a constant rate from a systemic artery. The sampled blood passes through a spectrophotometer, which is calibrated to measure the concentration of dye. A concentration curve is inscribed when the injected bolus of dye passes the sampling point (Fig. 16.3.4.4). Dividing the quantity of dye injected by the area of the time–concentration curve (corrected for recirculation) yields the cardiac output.

Thermodilution

Measurement of cardiac output by thermodilution uses the same principle as dye dilution, with the indicator being 'negative calories' (the difference between the caloric content of the injected bolus of cool saline and the caloric content of the same quantity of the subject's blood). The downstream 'concentration' of injected negative calories is measured as a transient drop in temperature by a thermistor at the tip of the injection catheter several centimetres from the point of injection. Dividing the negative calories injected by the area of the distal time–temperature curve yields cardiac output. The advantages of speed, automaticity, and repeatability of this method make it particularly suitable for serial measurements during different haemodynamic states.

Angiographic output

This is the only commonly used method that does not employ the indicator dilution or Fick principle. The left ventricular stroke volume calculated from quantitative angiography is multiplied by the heart rate to yield the left ventricular output. In the absence of valvular regurgitation this is the same as cardiac output. As explained in greater detail later in the chapter, this method is particularly useful in assessing mitral and aortic valvular regurgitation.

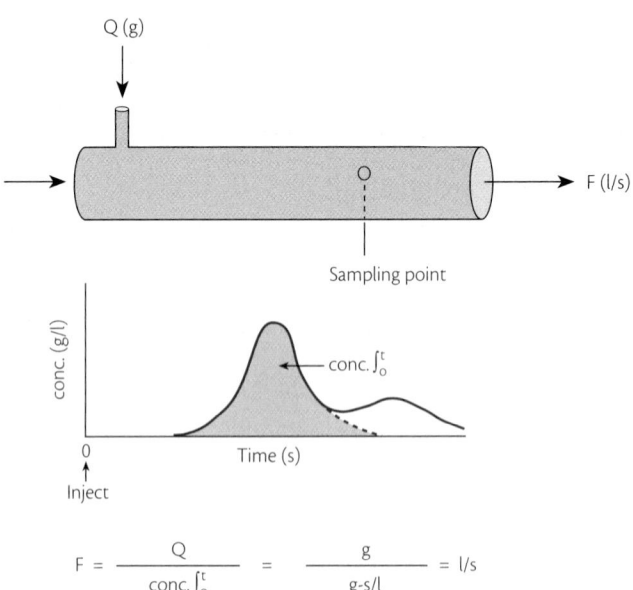

$$F = \frac{Q}{conc.\ \int_0^t} = \frac{g}{g\text{-}s/l} = l/s$$

Fig. 16.3.4.4 Cardiac output measured by dye curve. The concentration curve of indocyanine green dye generated by sampling distal to an injection point can be analysed to yield cardiac output. See text for more details. Thermodilution cardiac output employs the same principle, except that temperature is the measured indicator. F, flow or cardiac output; Q, quantity of indicator injected.

Quantitative angiography

Quantitative left ventricular angiography enables the measurement of left ventricular volume at instants throughout the cardiac cycle. Radiographic contrast medium is injected rapidly into the left ventricle and the shadow image of the opacified ventricle captured on film or electronically at a particular frame rate in any chosen projection. The most common projection is 30° right anterior oblique at a filming rate of 30 frames/s. In this view the image of the left ventricle is parallel to its long axis, resembling an ellipse. Arvidsson and Greene first suggested that the volume of the left ventricle could be calculated from the volume formula for an ellipsoid, the three-dimensional structure created by rotating an ellipse on its long axis. Dodge and Sandler improved upon this concept by deriving the minor hemi-axes from an idealized ellipse of the same length and area as the projected image of the ventricle. This method is still commonly used and is often referred to as the area–length method. Images captured at end diastole and end systole are analysed and corrected for magnification to yield end-diastolic and end-systolic volumes, the difference between these volumes being the stroke volume and the product of the stroke volume and heart rate, the angiographic left ventricular output. These indices are useful in the assessment of left ventricular function and valvular regurgitation as discussed later in this chapter.

Intracardiac shunts

The same methods of oximetry and indicator dilution utilized in measuring cardiac output can be employed for the detection and quantitation of intracardiac shunts. Under normal resting conditions, blood is approximately 75% saturated as it returns from the body to the right heart and pulmonary artery. As it leaves the lungs in the pulmonary veins blood is 99% saturated. Intracardiac shunts can be detected, localized and quantified by measuring the oxygen saturation in various locations. Left-to-right shunts will cause a step-up in the saturation of the blood at the location of the shunt; e.g. in a patient with an atrial septal defect the saturation will rise in the right atrium, whereas with a ventricular septal defect the saturation will rise in the right ventricle. A patient with Eisenmenger's syndrome (pulmonary hypertension and right-to-left shunting) will exhibit a drop in saturation at the location of the shunt, namely at the left atrium or ventricle in the case of atrial and ventricular septal defects, respectively. The degree of the change in saturation is proportional to the size of the shunt, and enables calculation of the shunt flow in either direction in litres/min. Figure 16.3.4.5 presents a scheme and formulae for calculating shunt volume.

Vascular resistance

Blood flow through the pulmonary and systemic circulations can be compared to the flow of an electric current through a circuit. Pressure is the driving force analogous to voltage, flow rate is analogous to current, and the impediment to flow through the vascular bed is resistance. Pressure, flow, and resistance relate to each other in a fashion analogous to Ohm's law:

$$\text{resistance} = \text{pressure/flow}$$

In the above formula 'pressure' is the difference in mean pressure across the systemic vascular bed (systemic arterial pressure – right atrial pressure) or the pulmonary vascular bed (pulmonary artery pressure – left atrial pressure). In the absence of intracardiac

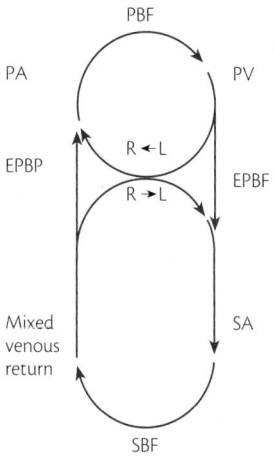

$$SBF\ (l/min) = \frac{O_2\ \text{consumption (ml/min)}}{(SAO_2 - \text{mixed }VO_2) \times 10}$$

$$PBF\ (l/min) = \frac{O_2\ \text{consumption (ml/min)}}{(PVO_2 - PAO_2) \times 10}$$

$$EPBF\ (l/min) = \frac{O_2\ \text{consumption (ml/min)}}{(PVO_2 - \text{mixed }VO_2) \times 10}$$

Shunt flow (l/min):
$$L \to R = PBF - EPBF$$
$$R \to L = SBF - EPBF$$

Fig. 16.3.4.5 Quantitation of intracardiac shunts. Shunts between the left and right sides of the heart due to septal defects can be quantified by oximetry using this scheme. EPBF, effective pulmonary blood flow, i.e. that part of the systemic venous return that actually passes through the lungs and is oxygenated; PBF, pulmonary blood flow; mixed VO_2, mixed systemic venous oxygen content; PAO_2, pulmonary artery oxygen content; PVO_2, pulmonary vein oxygen content; SAO_2, systemic artery oxygen content; SBF, systemic blood flow.

shunts 'flow' is the same for both circulations and is measured as cardiac output by methods already described. In cases of intracardiac shunting the systemic and pulmonary flows will differ according to the degree of shunting, and can be calculated as described under the section on cardiac shunts. Normal values for pulmonary vascular and systemic vascular resistance are expressed either in dyne s cm^{-5} or Wood units and are shown in Table 16.3.4.2. Total pulmonary resistance is a useful concept for expressing the total resistance against which the right ventricle must work, and includes not only the pulmonary vascular resistance but also the resistance engendered by the static pressure in the left atrium. Hence, pulmonary vascular disease, left heart failure, or both, can increase the total pulmonary resistance.

Measurement of resistance is useful for assessing the state of the pulmonary circulation in congenital heart disease with intracardiac shunting: high pulmonary vascular resistance may preclude the safe correction of an intracardiac shunt, particularly if the shunt is from right to left. It is also useful in diagnosing the relative contribution of left heart failure and pulmonary vascular disease in patients with pulmonary hypertension, and is the best indicator of the effectiveness of vasodilating drugs for patients with pulmonary hypertension.

Table 16.3.4.2 Normal vascular resistance[a]

Location	Resistance (dynes s cm^{-5})[b]
Total systemic resistance	1276 ± 371
Total pulmonary resistance	185 ± 57
Pulmonary vascular resistance	55 ± 18

[a] The values are derived from 100 consecutive catheterization studies of patients proven
  to have no evidence of cardiac disease at the West Roxbury Veterans Administration
  Hospital during the years 1955–1980.
[b] Divide these values by 10 to obtain values in MPa s/m^3.

Valvular stenosis

Valvular stenosis is assessed by measuring the transvalvular pressure gradient and by calculating the valvular orifice area using a formula introduced in the late 1940s by cardiologist Richard Gorlin and his father, an engineer. The Gorlin formula for valve area was initially developed for patients with rheumatic mitral stenosis. It is based upon a study which utilized data from right heart catheterization alone, validated by relatively crude intraoperative estimates of valve area using the index finger of surgeon Dwight Harken during closed mitral commissurotomy operations at the Peter Bent Brigham Hospital in Boston, Massachusetts. Although its validation was relatively crude, the formula has stood the test of time and remains the standard for the haemodynamic assessment of valvular stenosis. In its generalized form it is expressed as follows:
where K is a constant unique to mitral or aortic valve analysis (38

$$\text{valve area} = \text{TFR}/K \sqrt{m}$$

and 44.5, respectively) and TFR is the transvalvular flow rate, and m is the mean pressure gradient in mmHg during the time when the valve is open.

In aortic valve applications TFR (i.e. cardiac output normalized for the time that the valve is actually open) is the cardiac output divided by the product of heart rate and systolic ejection period. In mitral valve applications it is the cardiac output divided by the product of heart rate and diastolic filling period. Cardiac output is the effective systemic blood flow as determined by Fick, thermodilution, or dye dilution methods, unless there is associated valvular regurgitation, in which case it is the total left ventricular output as determined by quantitative left ventricular angiography.

Figure 16.3.4.6 shows tracings that demonstrate typical gradients from patients with aortic and mitral stenosis. The ranges of calculated valve area associated with various levels of stenosis for both aortic and mitral valves are displayed in Table 16.3.4.3. In general, procedures performed for the relief of anatomical stenosis are expected to be beneficial in symptomatic patients with severe valvular obstruction. However, many factors enter into such a decision and individual clinical judgement is required. Although patients with large transvalvular gradients generally experience the best result from intervention, the gradient by itself can be misleading due to its exponential relationship to cardiac output.

Valvular regurgitation

Qualitative assessment

Regurgitation of all four cardiac valves can be qualitatively assessed by angiography. The downstream side of the valve in question is opacified by a rapid injection of radiographic contrast medium. Regurgitation is visualized as upstream leakage of contrast across

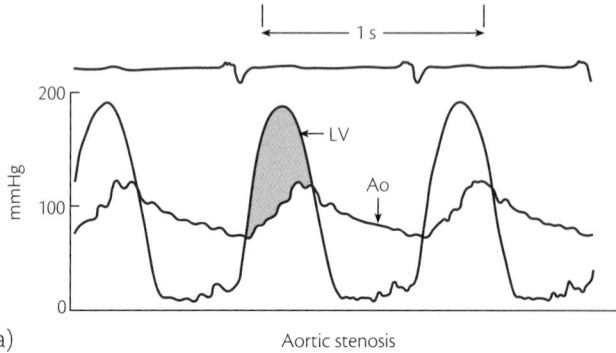

(a)   Aortic stenosis

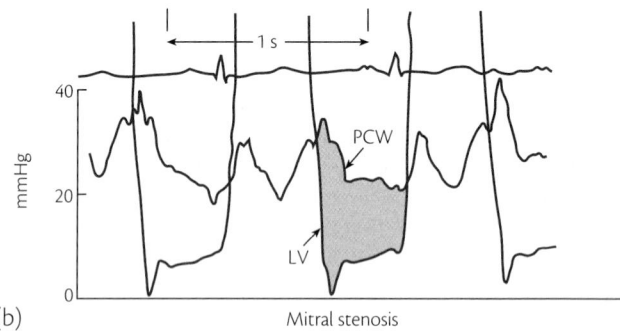

(b)   Mitral stenosis

Fig. 16.3.4.6 Pressure gradients associated with valvular stenosis. The upper panel shows simultaneous tracings of left ventricular (LV) and ascending aortic (Ao) pressure in a patient with severe aortic stenosis. The mean systolic gradient across the aortic valve is 60 mmHg. The lower panel shows simultaneous tracings of left ventricular (LV) and pulmonary capillary wedge (PCW) pressure in a patient with severe mitral stenosis. The mean diastolic pressure gradient across the valve is 16 mmHg. The respective valvular gradients are cross-hatched.

the closed valve. In the case of mitral regurgitation systolic opacification of the left atrium occurs during injection of the left ventricle. In aortic regurgitation diastolic opacification of the left ventricle occurs during supravalvular injection of the aorta. The degree of regurgitation is graded on an arbitrary scale from mild (1+) to severe (4+).

Quantitative assessment

Aortic and mitral regurgitation can be quantified in terms of regurgitant flow in litres/min or regurgitant fraction as a percentage of left ventricular output. Regurgitant flow is the difference obtained by subtracting the effective forward flow (Fick method described earlier) from the total left ventricular output (angiographically derived). It is the best method for measuring the severity of regurgitation, provided that the left ventricular angiogram, which itself changes cardiac output, is performed soon after the Fick measurement.

Table 16.3.4.3 Calculated valve areas associated with various degrees of mitral and aortic stenosis

Severity	Valve area (cm^2)	
	Aortic	**Mitral**
Mild	>1.2	>2.0
Moderate	0.8–1.2	1.1–2.0
Severe[a]	< 0.8	≤1.0

[a] 'Severe' stenosis is generally considered to be sufficient to warrant surgical correction.

Furthermore, both measurements must be made with considerable care to ensure accuracy. Regurgitation is considered clinically severe when 50% or more of the total left ventricular output is simply shuttling or regurgitating across the defective valve. The ability to quantify regurgitation across either valve is lost when both mitral and aortic valves are leaky.

Left ventricular function

Global function

Global function of the left ventricle is broadly described by its ability to generate pressure and flow under particular conditions of preload and afterload. Plotting the pressure and volume of the left ventricle at instants in time for a single cardiac cycle generates a pressure–volume loop displayed in Fig. 16.3.4.7. Most of the commonly used indices of left ventricular function can be derived from such a loop, including end-diastolic volume, end-systolic volume, stroke volume, ejection fraction, end-diastolic pressure, and dP/dt. Of these, the ejection fraction is most useful because it correlates with prognosis in a variety of cardiac diseases.

Grading angiographic wall motion in various segments of the left ventricle as normal, hypokinetic, akinetic, or dyskinetic assesses the regional function of the left ventricle. Regions of abnormal function generally correspond to locations of infarcted or ischaemic myocardium.

Contractility

This parameter is difficult to assess in the intact heart because all pressure and volume indices are dependent upon preload and afterload. Although ejection fraction is clinically useful it can be misleading in situations of high afterload (e.g. severe aortic stenosis) and low afterload (e.g. severe mitral regurgitation). The concept of 'elastance' has gained favour as a useful index of intrinsic contractility because it is relatively independent of loading conditions. Elastance is the slope of the line generated by plotting the end-systolic left ventricular pressure from a series of pressure–volume loops generated at differing afterloads created by the infusion of pressor or vasodilator drugs. The method is laborious and generally reserved for research applications.

Diastolic function

Diastolic function of the left ventricle is best appreciated from the slope of the pressure–volume loop during the period from mitral valve opening to its closure at the onset of systole. The curve becomes steeper as the left ventricle becomes less compliant due to the effects of hypertrophy, ischaemia, or infiltrative disease. In general, left ventricular end-diastolic pressure (LVEDP) rises as diastolic compliance falls, accounting for the high left atrial pressure and heart failure seen in diastolic left ventricular dysfunction.

Assessment of coronary arterial anatomy and function

Disease of the coronary arteries can be characterized at catheterization by both anatomical and functional assessment. Coronary angiography images the lumen of the vessel, which has been rendered radio-opaque by injection of radiographic contrast medium. It is a shadowing technique that displays the impact of the lesion on the arterial lumen but does not image the plaque *per se*. Intracoronary ultrasonography provides a tomographic image of the vessel wall and is capable of demonstrating the thickness and sonic density of the vessel wall and any associated plaque, hence angiography and intravascular ultrasonography are complementary methods of assessing vascular anatomy. To learn the haemodynamic importance of a coronary lesion it may be necessary to analyse its effect on function by measuring pressure and flow in the affected vessel. All these anatomical and functional modalities may be accomplished by catheterization.

Coronary arteriography or angiography

Coronary arteriography or angiography is presently the single most essential application of cardiac catheterization. The anatomy of coronary arteries in living, conscious humans was first demonstrated by nonselective injection of the aortic root. In the early 1960s David Littmann developed a loop catheter that enabled the injection of contrast medium preferentially in the outer circumference of the aortic root, opacifying the left and right coronary arteries simultaneously. At the time it was commonly believed that selective injection of contrast material into a coronary artery would have fatal consequences. This changed when Mason Sones accidentally performed the first selective coronary angiogram without harm. He was intending to inject the left ventricle, but the catheter recoiled across the aortic valve and into the right coronary artery. Sones, a cardiologist by training, went on to develop a safe method of selective coronary angiography from the brachial artery cut-down approach using the flexible-tip catheter bearing his name. At the same time Melvin Judkins, a radiologist by training, was perfecting his own method of selective coronary angiography, using preshaped catheters, from a percutaneous femoral artery approach. Both methods have continued to be practised, although the percutaneous femoral, or Judkins' approach, has become most popular because of its speed and simplicity. However—as stated previously—in recent years there has been a return to the arm approach using percutaneous catheterization of the radial artery, which enables more rapid patient ambulation, and the radial artery

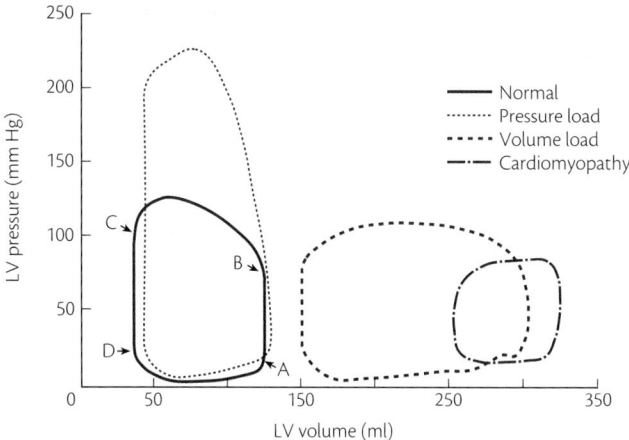

Fig. 16.3.4.7 Pressure–volume loops. Simultaneously plotting the instantaneous pressure and volume of the left ventricle throughout a single cardiac cycle produces these loops. The loop is a synthesis of most information relevant to left ventricular function. In this figure a loop from a normal patient is contrasted with those from patients with pressure load (hypertension or aortic stenosis), volume load (aortic or mitral regurgitation), and cardiomyopathy. Point A represents mitral valve closure; segment A–B, isovolumic contraction; point B, aortic valve opening; segment B–C, systolic ejection; point C, aortic valve closure; segment C–D, isovolumic relaxation; point D, mitral valve opening; and segment D–A, diastolic filling.

approach is also associated with fewer serious access site complications.

Normal coronary anatomy is demonstrated in Fig. 16.3.4.8. A patient's anatomy is considered to be right (80%)- or left (20%)-dominant, depending upon whether the posterior descending artery arises from the right or left coronary artery, respectively.

Atherosclerotic disease is manifest by lesions that encroach upon the opacified lumen of the coronary artery (Fig. 16.3.4.9). Various approaches are used to grade the severity of these lesions. Most commonly a visual estimate of the percentage of the stenotic reduction in luminal diameter is given to each lesion, with severity quantified by comparing the minimal lumen diameter within a lesion to the diameter of the nearest normal segment of artery. This can be done manually using calipers or automatically using computer-based systems for edge detection and contrast densitometry. Quantitative coronary angiography is a complex subject because it requires attention to many variables, such as selection of view and frame, and choice made from among several analytical techniques.

Early work by Lance Gould determined that a lesion must impair coronary blood flow to be clinically important. Although flow at rest is not usually reduced until stenosis reduces vessel diameter by 90%, flow under stress may be impaired when the diameter is reduced by 70%. The clinical impact of a stenosis of any given severity is also dependent upon the degree of collateral flow into the vascular bed distal to the stenosis.

Flow and pressure may be directly measured in the coronary artery by means of special guide wires that have pressure transducers or Doppler flow transducers mounted near their tips. As mentioned above, the flow at rest may be normal across a particular coronary artery stenosis. Coronary flow normally increases after maximal vasodilatation induced by local vasodilators. The quotient of the vasodilated flow divided by the resting flow is called the coronary flow reserve, which is normally greater than 2. If not, the lesion in question is considered to be haemodynamically important. Pressure can be measured in the coronary artery at a location distal to a lesion using a guide wire with a transducer at its tip. The quotient of pressure distal to a lesion compared to the proximal pressure during maximal vasodilatation is called the fractional flow reserve. A quotient less than 0.75 is considered to be clinically important.

Intravascular ultrasonography (IVUS)

IVUS is accomplished by advancing a catheter over a guide wire previously placed into a coronary artery. The catheter has a miniature ultrasound transducer near its tip, which enables rotational Doppler imaging of the vessel wall in a plane perpendicular to

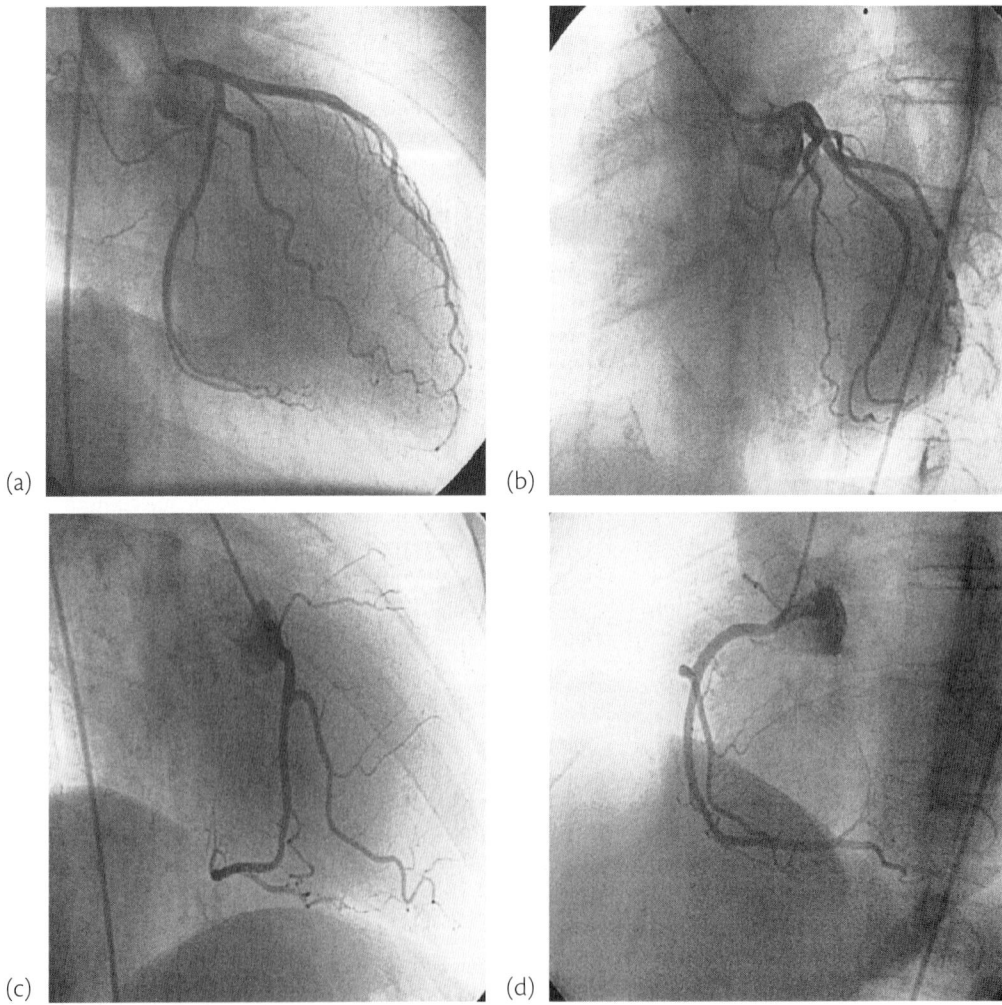

Fig. 16.3.4.8 Normal coronary anatomy. Left coronary angiogram showing main stem, left anterior descending, and left circumflex arteries from right anterior oblique view (a) and left anterior oblique view (b). Right coronary angiogram showing right coronary and posterior descending arteries from right anterior oblique view (c) and left anterior oblique view (d).

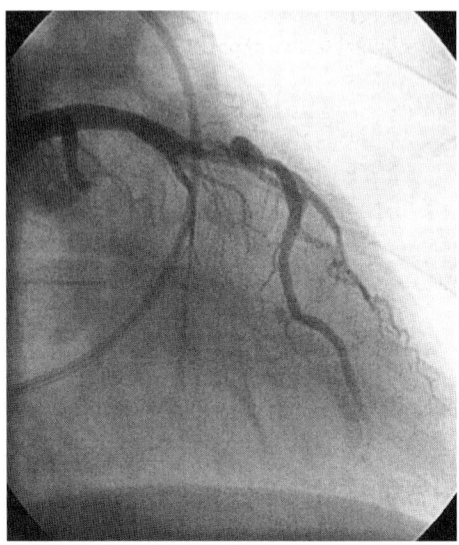

Fig. 16.3.4.9 Atherosclerotic coronary artery disease. The constrictions and blunt terminations seen in this patient's coronary angiogram represent atherosclerotic lesions.

Table 16.3.4.4 Complications of cardiac catheterization from a prospective study of 1559 procedures performed on 1483 United States veterans having valvular heart disease during the years 1977–1982[a]

Type of complication	Frequency (%)
Death within 24 h	0.1
Death between 24 h and 30 days	0.1
Stroke	0.3
Transient cerebral ischaemia	0.1
Myocardial infarction	0.2
Peripheral arterial embolism	0.1
Access site complications	1.7
Cardiac tamponade	0.3
Ventricular fibrillation	0.5
Arrhythmia other than ventricular fibrillation	1.5
Primary hypotension	0.5
Reaction to contrast medium (allergic and renal)	1.8
Arterial perforation or dissection	0.3
Miscellaneous complications	1.4
Patients having one or more of the above complications	6.9

[a] Although this is a high-risk group of patients undergoing extensive study, the rates are very comparable to what should be expected today. In fact, some complications, especially bleeding, are now more frequent because of aggressive anticoagulation and antiplatelet treatments given to many patients before and during catheterization.

its axis. IVUS is particularly useful for assessing the nature of angiographically questionable lesions, determining the true size of the vessel prior to stent deployment, and assessing the completeness of stent deployment. It is also probably the best method for serial studies of coronary anatomy during drug treatment trials, because it is able to image the plaque itself and is therefore a more sensitive method than angiography.

Complications of cardiac catheterization

Although cardiac catheterization is a relatively safe procedure, it is nevertheless important for both the patient and the referring physician to recognize the nature and likelihood of potential complications. Table 16.3.4.4 lists the complications of bilateral heart catheterization, including coronary, left ventricular, and aortic angiography, in a prospective study of valvular heart disease from the United States Veterans Administration. Even though these data were collected over 20 years ago from a particularly high-risk group of patients, the frequency of complication is a realistic estimate of what should currently be expected. The rate of each particular complication will vary with the age and general health of the patient. For example, the risk of vascular complication is considerably increased by the presence of vascular disease, and the risk of renal failure due to contrast medium is particularly high in diabetic patients with pre-existing renal dysfunction. Access site complications (bleeding, haematoma, arteriovenous fistula, pseudoaneurysm,

and occlusion) have received particular attention in recent years because of the use of aggressive anticoagulation and antiplatelet treatments during percutaneous coronary intervention. Use of smaller gauge catheters and careful location of arterial puncture site is important. Vascular closure devices enable earlier ambulation of patients having femoral procedures.

In counselling the patient regarding the likelihood of untoward events it is important to give individualized advice based upon the patient's particular circumstances. The decision to recommend catheterization must be based upon the anticipation that its benefits justify its risk and cost.

Further reading

Baim DS, Grossman W (eds) (2005). *Cardiac catheterization, angiography, and intervention*, 7th edition. Lippincott/Williams and Wilkins, Baltimore, MD.
Kern MJ (2003). *The cardiac catheterization handbook*, 4th edition. Mosby-Year Book, St Louis, MO.

16.4

Cardiac arrhythmias

S.M. Cobbe, A.D. McGavigan, and A.C. Rankin

Essentials

The term cardiac arrhythmia (or dysrhythmia) is used to describe an abnormality of cardiac rhythm of any type. The spectrum of cardiac arrhythmias ranges from innocent extrasystoles to immediately life-threatening conditions such as asystole or ventricular fibrillation.

The key to the successful diagnosis of cardiac arrhythmias is the systematic analysis of an ECG (see Chapter 16.3.1) of optimal quality obtained during the arrhythmia.

Continuous monitoring is necessary for identification when arrhythmias are intermittent. Ambulatory electrocardiographic recordings are of most value when they provide correlation between the patient's symptoms and the cardiac rhythm at that moment. Alternative strategies for the detection of infrequent arrhythmias include the use of a patient-activated recorder, which is applied and activated during symptoms, or an external or implanted loop recorder.

More detailed investigation of cardiac arrhythmias is undertaken by invasive cardiac electrophysiological testing. Multipolar electrodes are inserted transvenously to record electrograms from the atrium, ventricle, His bundle, and commonly from the coronary sinus. Electrophysiological mapping is an essential part of radiofrequency ablation.

Bradycardias

Bradycardia is defined as a ventricular rate of less than 60 beats/min. The principal indications for active intervention in bradycardia are symptomatic (disturbances of consciousness, fatigue, lethargy, dyspnoea, or bradycardia-induced tachyarrhythmias) or prognostic (prevention of sudden cardiac death).

In the presence of haemodynamic compromise, immediate attempts to increase heart rate should be employed, using atropine, isoproterenol (isoprenaline), and/or temporary cardiac pacing (transvenous or transcutaneous). Following stabilization, factors causing or contributing to the presentation should be sought and corrected—especially, acute ischaemia and infarction, concomitant drug therapy, or electrolyte disorders.

Specific disorders causing bradycardia include (1) sinoatrial disease ('sick sinus syndrome'); (2) neurocardiogenic syncope (e.g. carotid

sinus hypersensitivity); and (3) atrioventricular (AV) conduction disorders ('heart block').

AV block—the commonest cause of AV block is idiopathic fibrosis of the His–Purkinje system, and the severity (degree) of block can be classified as (1) first-degree—defined as a PR interval greater than 0.2 s, which produces no symptoms and does not require treatment; (2) second-degree—when there is intermittent failure of conduction from atrium to ventricle, either with (Mobitz type I, Wenckebach) or without (Mobitz type II) a characteristic pattern of increasing PR-interval duration preceding the nonconducted P wave; pacemaker implantation is not necessary for type I in most cases, but is required for type II; (3) third-degree (complete) AV block—when there is complete dissociation between atrial and ventricular activity, which is an indication for permanent pacemaker implantation, except in the context of an acutely reversible condition.

Tachycardias

The principal mechanisms responsible for tachyarrhythmias are (1) abnormal automaticity; (2) triggered activity; or (3) re-entry. Most clinically important sustained tachycardias appear to arise on the basis of re-entry, which requires the presence of a potential circuit comprising two limbs with different refractoriness and conduction properties.

The first and most important step in the diagnosis and management of tachycardias is to determine whether the arrhythmia arises within the atria and/or AV junction, or from the ventricles, which can often be achieved by careful analysis of a 12-lead ECG.

Diagnosis—it is safe to assume that virtually all narrow-complex tachycardias have a supraventricular origin, but wide-complex tachycardias (QRS duration ≥0.12 s) may arise either from the ventricle or from supraventricular mechanisms, and few areas in cardiology cause more difficulty—or result in more mismanagement—than the diagnosis of wide-complex tachycardias. Careful scrutiny of the 12-lead ECG may reveal diagnostic features, but the commonest reason for error is that the clinical context is not considered, or erroneous conclusions are drawn from it: key issues to recognize are

(1) elderly patients or those with a history of ischaemic heart disease are most likely to have ventricular arrhythmia; (2) the patient's haemodynamic status is a poor predictor of the type of tachycardia; (3) ventricular tachycardia can present with a history of paroxysmal self-terminating episodes.

Treatment—R-wave synchronized, direct-current (DC) cardioversion under general anaesthesia or deep sedation is the most effective and immediate means of terminating sustained tachycardias, and should be employed when tachycardia is associated with haemodynamic compromise. In patients with tachycardia who are haemodynamically stable, manoeuvres that produce transient vagal stimulation, such as the Valsalva manoeuvre or carotid sinus massage, may be employed. The response to intravenous adenosine, which will often terminate arrhythmias dependent on the AV node, may be of therapeutic or diagnostic value, and should be considered in all patients with tolerated regular tachycardia. In the long term, tachycardias can be treated with antiarrhythmic drugs (usefully categorized by the Vaughan Williams classification), implantable cardioverter–defibrillators (ICDs), radiofrequency ablation, or arrhythmia surgery.

Atrial fibrillation

Cardioversion—if it is clinically appropriate to attempt cardioversion, the drugs of choice are the class Ic agents (e.g. flecainide) for patients without significant underlying heart disease; class III drugs are somewhat less effective but are safer in the presence of left ventricular dysfunction or ischaemic heart disease (e.g. sotalol or amiodarone). Normally, only one drug should be tried in any individual patient: if drug therapy fails, DC cardioversion is commonly effective.

Risk of thromboembolism—because atrial fibrillation is a risk factor for the development of intracardiac thrombus formation, cardioversion—by chemical or electrical means—should not be attempted if arrhythmia has been present for longer than 48 h. Anticoagulation plus rate control with a β-blocker, calcium-channel blocker, or digoxin should be considered in these circumstances. Prophylaxis against thromboembolism should be considered in all patients with atrial fibrillation.

Paroxysmal atrial fibrillation—drug therapy may not be necessary for patients with infrequent paroxysms, or a 'pill-in-the-pocket' approach can be used in those without structural heart disease, whereby they take a dose of an antiarrhythmic drug after the onset of arrhythmia. No drug is entirely satisfactory for recurrent paroxysmal atrial fibrillation: a β-blocker is often prescribed as first-line therapy.

Persistent atrial fibrillation—usually requires electrical cardioversion to achieve sinus rhythm and has a high recurrence rate even after successful cardioversion. The key decision is whether to employ a rhythm or rate-control strategy. In general, a rate-control strategy (AV nodal blocking drug, e.g. β-blocker, calcium channel blocker, or digoxin) should be employed in patients with few or minor symptoms, elderly patients, and those with contraindications to antiarrhythmic therapy or cardioversion. A rhythm-control strategy (elective cardioversion) may be best in more severely symptomatic or younger patients, or in those with atrial fibrillation due to a treated precipitant.

Atrial flutter

It is important to attempt to terminate atrial flutter since the ventricular rate is often poorly controlled by AV nodal blocking drugs: this may be achieved by chemical or electrical cardioversion. Prophylaxis against thromboembolism should be given as for atrial fibrillation.

Supraventricular tachycardias

The term supraventricular tachycardia (also called junctional re-entry tachycardia) is commonly reserved for those in which the AV node is an obligate part of a re-entry circuit—AV nodal re-entrant tachycardia (AVNRT) or AV re-entry tachycardia (AVRT).

Termination of an attack of AV nodal re-entrant tachyxardia is achieved by producing transient AV nodal block by vagotonic manoeuvres, adenosine or by verapamil. Drug prophylaxis is undertaken with β-blockers, a combined β-blocker/class III agent such as sotalol, or AV nodal blocking drugs such as verapamil or digoxin. Curative treatment is by radiofrequency ablation.

Attacks of AV re-entry tachycardia are treated in the same way as is AV nodal re-entrant tachycardia. Antiarrhythmic prophylaxis may be effective, but radiofrequency ablation offers high success rates with low incidence of complications and should be considered early.

Pre-excitation syndromes

The term 'pre-excitation' refers to the premature activation of the ventricle via one or more accessory pathways that bypass the normal AV node and His–Purkinje system. The commonest type is Wolff–Parkinson–White (WPW) syndrome, where a δ-wave is characteristically seen on the ECG, and the main prognostic concern is pre-excited atrial fibrillation, which can be very rapid and degenerate into ventricular fibrillation. Patients with symptomatic WPW syndrome should be offered radiofrequency ablation as first-line therapy.

Ventricular tachycardia

Ventricular tachycardia normally occurs in individuals with overt heart disease, but is also seen in young and apparently healthy subjects, when occult cardiac disease or cardiac genetic syndromes should be considered.

Sustained ventricular tachycardia is a medical emergency. Immediate DC cardioversion is necessary if the patient is hypotensive; haemodynamically tolerated VT may be terminated pharmacologically, with intravenous lidocaine (lignocaine) or sotalol being the usual first-choice options. Unless there is a clear precipitating factor, the risk of sudden death is high and patients should be considered for an implantable cardioverter-defibrillator.

Polymorphic ventricular tachycardia, of which torsades de pointes is a well-recognized type associated with acquired or congenital prolongation of the QT interval, is an unstable rhythm with varying QRS morphology that undergoes spontaneous termination or degenerates into ventricular fibrillation. In patients with this condition, it is essential to discontinue predisposing drugs or other agents and to avoid empirical antiarrhythmic drug therapy. Intravenous magnesium sulphate is a safe and effective emergency measure.

Ventricular fibrillation

The management of cardiac arrest due to ventricular fibrillation is discussed in Chapter 17.1. Patients who survive an episode should be assessed carefully to determine the risk of recurrence and may require an implantable cardioverter-defibrillator or antiarrhythmic therapy as for patients with ventricular tachycardia.

Genetic syndromes

The congenital long-QT syndromes are inherited conditions due to mutations in genes encoding ion-channel proteins: their prognosis, if untreated, is poor. β-Blockers are highly effective in the commonest form of the condition.

The Brugada syndrome is an autosomal dominant condition where there is an unusual pattern of variable ST-segment elevation and partial right bundle branch block in the right precordial leads, associated with a risk of polymorphic ventricular tachycardia and sudden death. Patients with congenital long QT or Brugada syndrome considered at high risk of sudden death should be considered for an implantable cardioverter-defibrillator.

General principles

Definition

The term cardiac arrhythmia (or dysrhythmia) is used to describe an abnormality of cardiac rhythm of any type. Normal cardiac electrophysiology is discussed in Chapter 16.3.1. The spectrum of cardiac arrhythmias ranges from innocent extrasystoles to immediately life-threatening conditions such as asystole or ventricular fibrillation. Arrhythmias may occur in the absence of cardiac disease, but are more commonly associated with structural heart disease or external provocative factors.

Symptoms of cardiac arrhythmias

The symptoms produced by bradyarrhythmias depend on the extent of cardiac slowing. They may include sudden death, syncope (Stokes–Adams attacks), or dizziness (presyncope). Continuous bradycardia without asystolic pauses may produce symptoms of fatigue, lethargy, dyspnoea, or mental impairment.

The symptoms caused by tachyarrhythmias depend on a variety of factors including the heart rate, the difference between the rate during the arrhythmia and the preceding heart rate, the degree of irregularity of the rhythm, and the presence or absence of underlying cardiac disease. Symptoms of tachycardia include a feeling of rapid palpitation, angina or dyspnoea, syncope or sudden death. The differential diagnosis of palpitation and syncope is discussed in Chapter 16.2.2.

Investigation of arrhythmias

History taking must include a detailed description of the symptoms associated with the arrhythmia. Evidence should be sought for factors that may precipitate the arrhythmia (e.g. exercise, alcohol) and for the presence of underlying cardiac disease, in particular valvular heart disease, myocardial ischaemia/infarction, or congestive heart failure. Examination of the pulse may be unremarkable if the arrhythmia is intermittent. Physical examination for evidence of structural heart disease is essential. Further investigations to establish the presence of structural heart disease and to determine ventricular function may include 12-lead ECG, chest radiography, echocardiography, exercise stress testing, coronary arteriography, or MRI.

Electrocardiography

The key to the successful diagnosis of cardiac arrhythmias is the systematic analysis of ECG (see Chapter 16.3.1)of optimal quality obtained during the arrhythmia (Table 16.4.1). Ideally, this should comprise all 12 leads recorded on a multichannel recorder, which can allow the identification of P-waves in one lead while they may be absent or equivocal in another.

Ambulatory electrocardiography

Continuous monitoring is necessary for identification when arrhythmias are intermittent. Ambulatory (Holter) electrocardiography is normally performed for periods of 24 to 48h using a portable recorder. High-speed or automatic replay facilities enable the identification of intermittent arrhythmias, as well as the quantification of extrasystoles and assessment of parameters of heart rate variability. Interpretation of recordings requires knowledge of possible artefacts, such as those caused by movement, or variations in tape speed in recorders that use magnetic tape. It is important to allow for physiological variability in the sinus rate, also appreciating that minor abnormalities such as extrasystoles or brief (3–4 beat) runs of supraventricular arrhythmias are usually of no significance. Ambulatory electrocardiographic recordings are of most value when they provide correlation between the patient's symptoms and the cardiac rhythm at that moment. Patients should be issued with a diary card and asked to note any symptoms suggestive of arrhythmia during the recording.

Alternative strategies for the detection of infrequent arrhythmias include the use of a patient-activated recorder, which is applied and activated during symptoms, or an external or implanted

Table 16.4.1 Principles of ECG diagnosis of arrhythmias

Obtain 12-lead or multichannel recordings if possible	
Atrial activity	P-waves visible?
	Normal P-wave morphology and axis?
	Flutter/fibrillation waves?
	Atrial rate?
Ventricular activity	Ventricular rate?
	Regular or irregular?
	Normal QRS morphology and duration?
	Bundle-branch block or bizarre QRS morphology?
	Variation in QRS morphology/axis?
Atrioventricular relationship	PR interval—fixed or varied?
	Retrograde P-waves?
	Atrial versus ventricular rate?

loop recorder. Loop recorders continually record the electrocardiographic signal, but only have sufficient memory to retain a few minutes of data. In the event of symptoms, the patient activates the device, thus 'fixing' the previous few minutes of recording for subsequent analysis. External loop recorders are usually used for up to 7 days, while an implanted event recorder can last for up to 18 months.

Cardiac electrophysiological study

More detailed investigation of cardiac arrhythmias is undertaken by invasive cardiac electrophysiological testing. Multipolar electrodes are inserted transvenously to record electrograms from the atrium, ventricle, His bundle, and commonly from the coronary sinus (Fig. 16.4.1). The site of conduction delays within the heart may be identified, or accessory pathways localized. Sustained arrhythmias may be initiated and terminated by extrastimuli (Fig. 16.4.2), and their pattern of activation in the heart studied in detail. Electrophysiological mapping is an essential part of radiofrequency ablation (see below), and modern three-dimensional mapping systems have facilitated ablation of complex arrhythmias.

Bradycardias

Aetiology and mechanisms

Bradycardia is defined as a ventricular rate of less than 60/min, and results from a reduction in the rate of normal sinus pacemaker activity, or from disturbances of atrioventricular (AV) conduction. Sinus bradycardia may be physiological, e.g. during sleep in young people, and in athletes. Pathological bradyarrhythmias can result from intrinsic degenerative disease of the sinus or AV node, or the conducting system. Bradycardia may also be due to extraneous factors such as sympathetic withdrawal, vagal stimulation, drug effects, myocardial ischaemia/infarction, infiltration, or surgical trauma and also miscellaneous conditions such as hypothyroidism, hypothermia, jaundice, or raised intracranial pressure.

General principles of management

The principal indications for active intervention in bradycardia are symptomatic (disturbances of consciousness, fatigue, lethargy, dyspnoea, or bradycardia-induced tachyarrhythmias) or prognostic (prevention of sudden cardiac death). Particular attention should be given to the history and ECG documentation of the

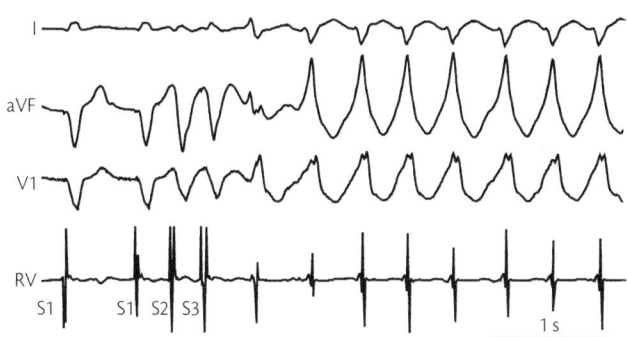

Fig. 16.4.2 Induction of ventricular tachycardia by programmed stimulation. Ventricular pacing stimuli (S1) at 100 beats/min are followed by two extra-stimuli (S2 and S3). Sustained monomorphic ventricular tachycardia is induced. Surface leads I, aVF, V₁, and the intracardiac electrogram from right ventricular apex (RV) are shown.

rhythm disturbance. Drugs interfering with sinoatrial or AV nodal function should be withdrawn if possible, although under certain circumstances (e.g. tachycardia–bradycardia syndrome) it may be necessary to combine pacemaker implantation with continued drug therapy.

Acute management of bradycardia

General principles can be applied to patients presenting with overt bradycardia, regardless of aetiology (Table 16.4.2). In the presence of haemodynamic compromise, immediate attempts to increase heart rate should be employed. Transient increases in sinus rate or the ventricular escape rate in complete AV block may be achieved with atropine or isoproterenol (isoprenaline). However, drug treatment is only of temporary value, and temporary cardiac pacing is indicated for persistent bradycardia (see 'Pacemaker therapy', below). Temporary pacing is also indicated where frequent Stokes–Adams attacks are occurring. Pacing can be performed transcutaneously

Table 16.4.2 General principles of acute management of the patient with bradycardia

Assess the patient	Respiratory status
	Blood pressure
	Symptoms
Examine the ECG	Sinus rate
	Ventricular rate
	AV relationship
	QRS morphology and duration
If haemodynamic compromise	Atropine
	Isoproterenol
	Temporary pacing
Look for precipitants	Ischaemia/infarction
	Vasovagal episode
	Thyroid status
	Electrolyte imbalance
	Hypothermia
	Drug therapy

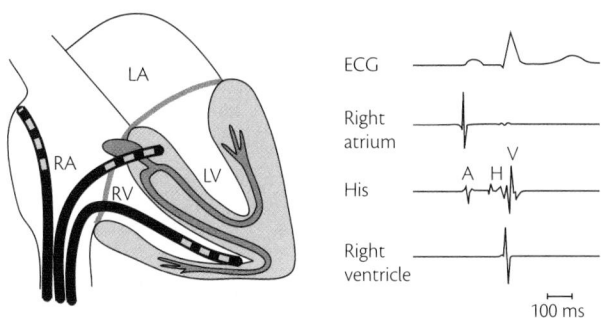

Fig. 16.4.1 Electrophysiological study. Illustration of lead placement (left). Quadripolar leads have been inserted from the femoral vein and the tips are shown positioned to allow recording and pacing from the high right atrium, His bundle, and the right ventricular apex. Intracardiac electrograms (right) show recordings from atrium (A), His bundle (H), and right ventricle (V).

Fig. 16.4.3 Sinus bradycardia. The heart rate is less than 40 beats/min, and the sinus rate is so slow that an escape junctional beat is seen (open circle), preceding the P wave.

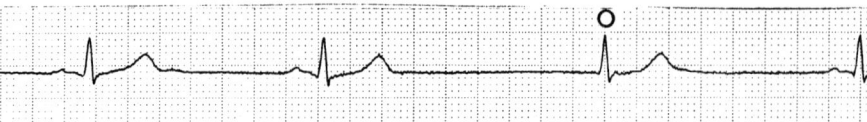

using an external pacing system in the emergency situation if facilities for transvenous pacing are not immediately available.

Following stabilization, factors causing or contributing to the presentation should be sought and corrected, especially acute ischaemia and infarction, concomitant drug therapy, or electrolyte disorders. Analysis of the ECG will allow identification of the conduction disorder and plans for long-term management can be instituted.

Specific causes of brachycardia

Sinoatrial disease

Sinoatrial disease, often referred to as 'sick sinus syndrome', results in inappropriate sinus bradycardia, sinus pauses, or junctional rhythm (Fig. 16.4.3) in the absence of extrinsic factors. The condition is most commonly caused by idiopathic degeneration of the sinus nodal cells, particularly in older people, and is associated in about 20% of cases with idiopathic bundle branch fibrosis (see below). Occasionally, sinoatrial disease is caused by ischaemia due to obstruction of the right coronary artery. Conduction block may occur between the sinus node and the atrium (sinoatrial block), resulting in 'dropped' P-waves (Fig. 16.4.4). More prolonged suppression of sinus node activity results in periods of sinus arrest, which are terminated by an escape beat from the sinus node, AV junction, or ventricle (Fig. 16.5.5a). Where the sinus rate is permanently slower than the junctional rate, continuous AV junctional rhythm will be present. Patients with sinoatrial disease have an increased predisposition to atrial tachyarrhythmias (tachycardia–bradycardia syndrome), and prolonged pauses may follow termination of tachycardia (Fig. 16.4.5b).

Sinoatrial disease can cause symptomatic bradycardia, dizziness, or syncope, but may be asymptomatic. The diagnosis is normally made from 12-lead or ambulatory ECG recording. Investigation should focus on excluding extrinsic causes of bradycardia, and on demonstrating the correlation between bradycardia or pauses and symptoms. Pacemaker implantation is indicated for the relief of symptoms (see below). Prognosis is not improved by pacemaker implantation in sinus nodal disease and thus pacemaker implantation in asymptomatic patients is not indicated.

Neurocardiogenic syncope

Conditions where patients suffer reflex-induced attacks of bradycardia or hypotension are described in Chapter 16.2.2.

Patients with carotid sinus hypersensitivity and symptoms of presyncope or syncope should undergo permanent pacemaker implantation (see below). In patients with recurrent vasovagal syncope, the optimal treatment is uncertain. Medical therapy with agents as diverse as α-agonists, β-blockers, vagolytic agents (disopyramide, hyoscine), ephedrine, or antidepressants is often tried, but the evidence base for the efficacy of drug therapy is weak. Spontaneous resolution of symptoms occurs in many patients. Nonpharmacological treatments, such as isometric manoeuvres (e.g. leg crossing or arm tensing) at the onset of symptoms may reduce the severity of episodes and prevent syncope. There is little evidence to support pacemaker implantation even in those with predominant bradycardia as the response to tilt testing, but it may be considered in selected individuals with intractable symptoms.

Atrioventricular conduction disorders

Impairment of AV conduction may occur either within the AV node (intranodal) or within the His–Purkinje system (infranodal). Intranodal block is not associated with QRS abnormalities, while distal (infranodal) block is commonly associated with bundle branch block.

Aetiology of atrioventricular block

The causes of AV block are shown in Box 16.4.1. The commonest is idiopathic fibrosis of the His–Purkinje system, which occurs with increasing frequency from the seventh decade of life onwards, is associated with sinoatrial disease in up to 25% of cases, and results in progressive impairment of AV conduction.

Atrioventricular block may occur acutely in myocardial infarction (Fig. 16.4.6). Inferior myocardial infarction predominantly affects AV nodal conduction by vagal overactivity, and possibly adenosine release from ischaemic myocardium. First-degree, second-degree type I (Wenckebach), or third-degree AV block may occur, but are commonly transient. Spontaneous recovery of normal conduction generally occurs within 7 to 10 days. By contrast, AV block secondary to anterior myocardial infarction is normally due to extensive infarction of the interventricular septum involving both the left and right bundle branches. This may result in type II second-degree block or complete AV block, with a lower probability of recovery of normal conduction.

Any drug slowing AV conduction may potentially produce AV block. The risk is greater when such drugs are used in combination. Intravenous verapamil in patients already receiving β-adrenoceptor blockers is particularly hazardous. Vagally mediated conduction disturbances occur as a physiological finding in highly trained athletes, and in young people during sleep,

Fig. 16.4.4 Sinoatrial block. A pause occurred because of the absence of a P wave (open arrow). The timing of the sinus beats, however, is not interrupted, indicating that the sinus node discharged but the impulse failed to excite the atria.

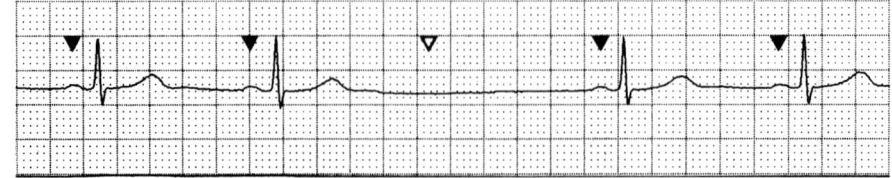

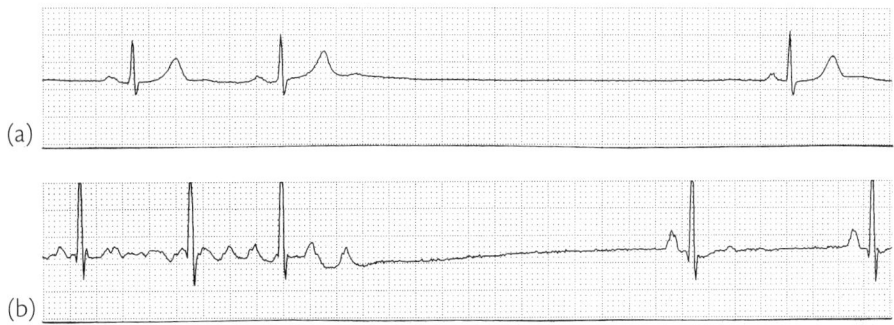

(a)

(b)

Fig. 16.4.5 Sinus arrest. (a Pause of 4 s results from failure of the sinus node to discharge. (b) Termination of atrial fibrillation is followed by a sinus pause of 2.5 s due to sinus arrest in a patient with bradycardia/tachycardia syndrome.

or in neurocardiogenic syncope. Atrioventricular conduction disturbances arise in structural congenital heart disease such as endocardial cushion defects, but also as an isolated congenital abnormality, commonly in association with maternal systemic lupus erythematosus.

First-degree atrioventricular block

First-degree AV block is defined as a PR interval greater than 0.20 s (Fig. 16.4.7). This produces no symptoms and does not require treatment, although the risk of progression to higher-degree AV block should be considered.

Second-degree atrioventricular block

In second-degree AV block, there is intermittent failure of conduction from atrium to ventricle. In type I (Wenckebach) second-degree block, a characteristic pattern of increasing PR interval duration followed by a non-conducted P-wave is seen (Fig. 16.4.8). The QRS morphology is commonly normal. Type I (Wenckebach) second-degree AV block usually indicates block in the AV node, and is normally associated with a reliable subsidiary pacemaker and a low risk of progression to complete heart block. In most instances pacemaker implantation is not necessary unless recurrent presyncope or syncope suggest the occurrence of an intermittent higher-degree block. By contrast, in type II second-degree AV block (commonly called Mobitz type II AV block) there is a sudden failure of conduction, without a preceding increase in the PR interval (Fig. 16.4.9). Regular non-conducted P-waves may result in

high-degree block, with 2:1 or 3:1 conduction. Type II second-degree AV block is generally indicative of extensive infranodal conduction abnormality, with a high risk of progression to complete AV block. Guidelines therefore recommend permanent pacemaker implantation even in the absence of symptoms.

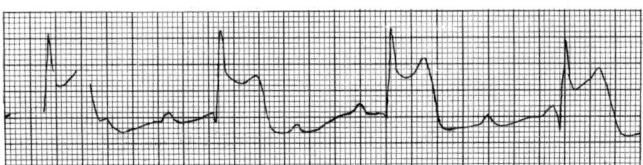

Fig. 16.4.6 Complete heart block in a patient with acute myocardial infarction. There is a narrow QRS complex escape rhythm with ST-segment elevation, ventricular rate 45 beats/min.

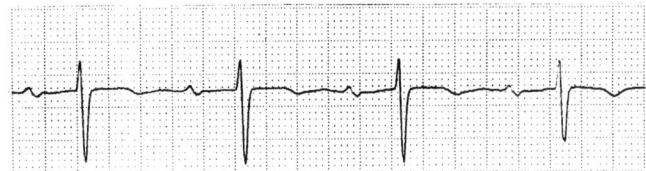

Fig. 16.4.7 First-degree heart block. The PR interval is prolonged (0.32 s).

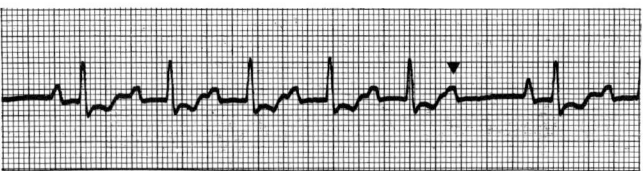

Fig. 16.4.8 Second-degree heart block, type I (Wenckebach). The PR interval progressively prolongs until there is a failure of conduction following a P wave (arrow).

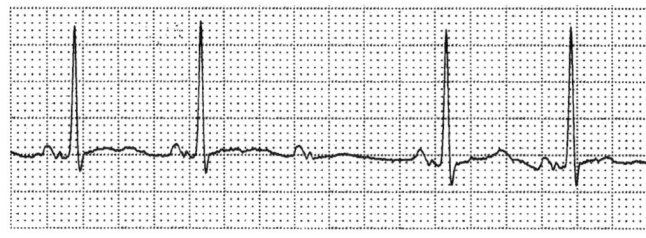

Fig. 16.4.9 Second-degree heart block, type II. A non-conducted P wave occurs without preceding prolongation of the PR interval.

Box 16.4.1 Causes of atrioventricular block

- Idiopathic conducting system fibrosis
- Acute myocardial ischaemia/infarction
- Infiltration—calcific aortic stenosis, sarcoidosis, scleroderma, syphilis, tumour
- Infection—diphtheria, rheumatic fever, endocarditis, Lyme disease
- Drugs—digoxin, verapamil or diltiazem, β-blockers, antiarrhythmic drugs
- Surgical trauma, radiofrequency ablation
- Congenital heart block, congenital heart disease
- Vagal—athletic heart, carotid sinus, and vasovagal syndrome
- Myotonic dystrophy

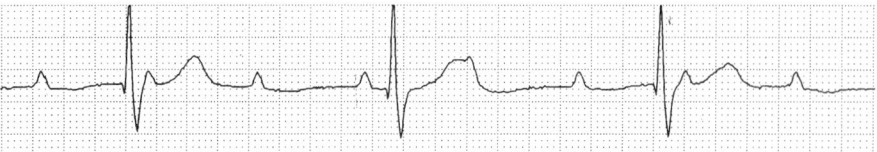

Fig. 16.4.10 Third-degree (complete) heart block. Atrial activity does not conduct to the ventricles, and there is a regular escape rhythm of 35 beats/min.

Third-degree atrioventricular block

The characteristic feature of third-degree (complete) AV block is dissociation between atrial and ventricular activity (Figs. 16.4.6 and 16.4.10). The ventricular rate is regular and slower than the atrial rate. An escape rhythm arising above the bifurcation of the bundle of His will produce a narrow QRS morphology, commonly with a relatively stable escape rhythm (50–60/min). A more distal escape rhythm results in widened, bundle branch block morphology complexes with a slower escape rate (20–30/min). When complete AV block coexists with atrial fibrillation, it is recognized by the presence of a slow, regular ventricular response. High-degree AV block can be intermittent, and the resting ECG may be normal or only show evidence of mild conducting system disturbance such as first-degree AV block or bundle branch block. If there is clinical suspicion, ambulatory ECG recording is required, for prolonged periods if necessary.

The presence of complete AV block, except in the context of an acutely reversible condition, should be regarded as an indication for permanent pacemaker implantation. This is urgent in patients who are having Stokes–Adams attacks; their prognosis is poor without pacemaker implantation, and markedly improved by permanent pacing, after which outcome will depend on the presence and extent of any underlying cardiac disease. Permanent pacing also improves prognosis in asymptomatic patients with complete AV block. One exception to this general rule is congenital complete heart block, where the escape rhythm is often relatively fast (50–60/min) with a narrow QRS morphology. Many patients remain asymptomatic well into adult life, although there is a small risk of syncope or sudden death. Pacemaker implantation should be considered if there are symptoms, if there are abrupt pauses, if the average heart rate is below 50/min, or in patients over 40 years of age.

Asystole

The term asystole is used when the electrocardiogram shows a complete cessation of both atrial and ventricular activity. This appearance may be mimicked by disconnected ECG cables or other artefacts, but since asystole causes cardiac arrest the distinction is virtually always obvious. The management of asystole is discussed in Chapter 17.1.

Pacemaker therapy

Basic principles

The basis of pacemaker therapy is the local depolarization of the myocardium by an electric current passed through an electrode in contact with the heart (atrium or ventricle). Activation of the remainder of the atria or ventricles occurs by direct cell-to-cell conduction. The minimum current necessary to stimulate the heart during diastole is known as the pacing threshold. Pacemaker systems comprise one or more intracardiac catheter electrodes, introduced into the heart via the venous system, and a pulse generator, which contains the circuitry for generating and timing the pacing stimulus, as well as for sensing spontaneous cardiac depolarizations.

The pacing stimulus is delivered between the active pole at the tip of the electrode catheter and an indifferent electrode sited either on the same catheter 1–2 cm proximal to the tip (bipolar pacing), or utilizing the can of an implanted pulse generator (unipolar pacing). Satisfactory pacing requires stable electrode contact with the myocardium. The standard sites for endocardial atrial and ventricular pacing are the right atrial appendage and the right ventricular apex respectively (Fig. 16.4.11), although screw-in active fixation leads allow placement at other atrial and ventricular sites.

An external pulse generator is used for temporary pacing. For permanent pacing, it is usually implanted deep to the subcutaneous fat layer in the prepectoral region (Fig. 16.4.11). The generator contains a timer set to deliver pacing stimuli at a preset pulse interval (e.g. 1000 ms). Pacemakers normally operate in the demand mode, whereby if spontaneous activation of the cardiac chamber is sensed via the electrode, the delivery of a pacing stimulus is inhibited and the timer circuit of the generator is reset. Pacing in the fixed rate mode results in the delivery of stimuli regardless of the spontaneous activity of the chamber being paced.

Temporary ventricular pacing

Temporary pacing is indicated in patients with bradycardia causing haemodynamic compromise, or as a prelude to permanent pacemaker implantation in those with significant recurring

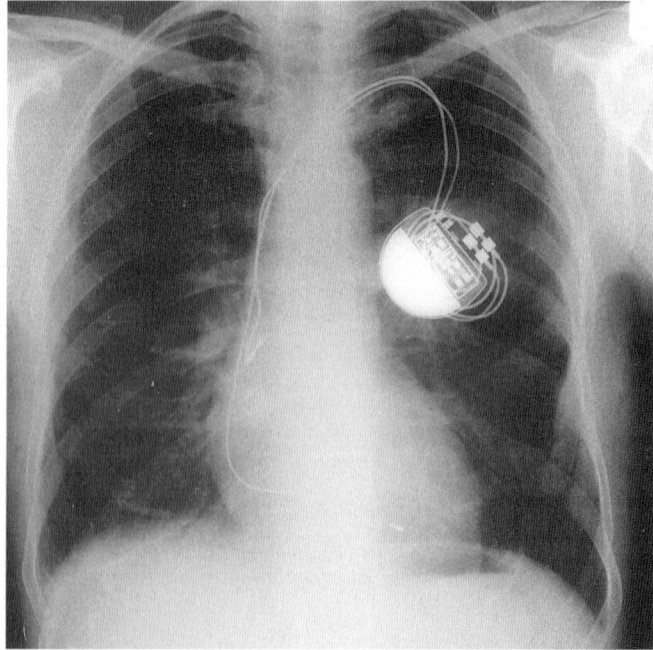

Fig. 16.4.11 Dual-chamber permanent pacemaker. Chest radiograph showing the pacemaker generator (in a subcutaneous pocket in the pectoral region), which is connected to electrodes that pass via the left subclavian vein and superior vena cava to the heart. The tips of the electrodes are in the right atrial appendage and the right ventricular apex.

symptoms, or high-risk AV block. Facilities for radiographic screening, continuous electrocardiographic monitoring, and defibrillation are required. The pacing electrode is introduced under aseptic conditions via an intravascular sheath into the subclavian, internal jugular, or femoral vein and the tip advanced under radiographic guidance to the right ventricular apex. Nonsustained ventricular tachycardia, or occasionally ventricular fibrillation, may occur during catheter manipulation. Once the electrode is at an acceptable site, pacing is initiated, and the minimum output necessary to achieve stable ventricular capture is determined. The pacing threshold should normally be less than 1 V, at a pulse width of between 0.5 and 2 ms. If the pacing threshold is unsatisfactory, the electrode is repositioned until an acceptable site is found. Care should be taken to determine that the electrode is stable by asking the patient to take deep breaths or to cough while pacing at threshold. The electrode is then secured at the site of insertion and the pulse generator set to an output of at least 3 V above the pacing threshold.

Permanent pacemaker implantation

Permanent pacing electrodes are normally inserted via the left or right subclavian or cephalic vein. Once the electrode is in a satisfactory position, it is secured and connected to the implanted pulse generator. Most pulse generators are powered by lithium batteries and have a life of approximately 6 to 8 years, after which the generator is replaced. The rate, output voltage, pulse width, and other pacemaker functions can be modified noninvasively by means of telemetry via a transmitter/receiver placed on the skin over the pulse generator. The amplitude and pulse width of the pacing stimulus are usually set at nominal values (e.g. 5 V, 1 ms), but are adjustable and can be reduced to prolong the life of the battery, providing there is a sufficient safety margin between the pulse generator output and the pacing threshold.

Pacing mode selection

The nomenclature used to describe pacing mode is given in Table 16.4.3, and electrocardiographic examples of the principal pacing modes are shown in Fig. 16.4.12. Atrial demand (AAI) pacing is used for sinoatrial disease in the absence of AV block. Ventricular pacing (VVI) is the simplest and technically easiest mode of pacing, and is required for AV conduction disturbances. However, VVI pacing does not permit AV synchrony or an increase in pacing rate in response to an increase in sinus (atrial) rate. Dual-chamber (DDD) pacemakers have electrodes in both the right atrium and ventricle. If the sinus cycle length is greater than the pulse interval, atrial demand pacing occurs. Following the atrial stimulus, a programmable AV delay commences. If no spontaneous ventricular depolarization is sensed before the end of this

Table 16.4.3 Pacemaker mode nomenclature

Chamber-paced		Chamber-sensed		Mode		Additional features	
A	Atrium	A	Atrium	I	Inhibited	R	Rate responsive
V	Ventricle	V	Ventricle	T	Triggered		
D	Dual (A and V)	D	Dual (A and V)	D	Dual (I and T)		
		O	Neither	O	Fixed rate		

See text for examples.

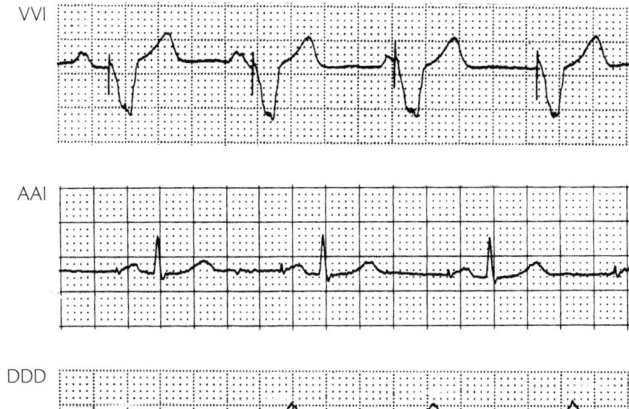

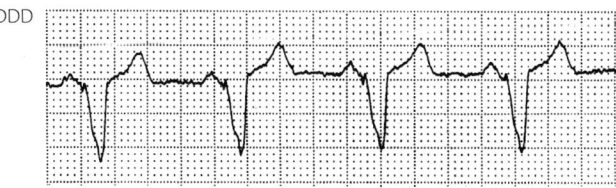

Fig. 16.4.12 Permanent pacemaker modes. Ventricular demand pacing, VVI (upper) with broad-complex ventricular complexes following the stimulus. Dissociated atrial activity can be seen. Atrial demand pacing, AAI (middle) with low amplitude bipolar pacing spike preceding the P-waves. Dual-chamber pacemaker, DDD (lower) with paced ventricular complexes following each P-wave (atrial tracking).

interval, a pacing stimulus is delivered via the ventricular electrode. If the sinus cycle length is shorter than the pulse interval, no atrial stimulus is given, but the AV delay is triggered by the sensed atrial activity, followed by a paced ventricular beat, if a conducted ventricular activation does not occur. By this means, the ventricular rate tracks the atrial rate up to a programmable maximum, allowing the heart to increase its rate in a physiological manner in response to metabolic demand. An alternative, and simpler, approach to achieve a rate response is the use of an activity sensor such as an accelerometer in the pulse generator. Such devices detect bodily movement and increase the pacing rate according to a programmable algorithm. Rate response can be utilized in either single- or dual-chamber pacemakers, and is designated by the suffix 'R' (e.g. AAIR, VVIR, DDDR).

The advantage of DDD pacing over VVI pacing lies in the maintenance of AV synchrony and rate responsiveness, but this is achieved at the expense of increased complexity, complications, and cost. DDD pacing reduces the risk of atrial fibrillation by virtue of pacing the atrium and avoiding retrograde atrial activation via the AV node and has a lower incidence of the pacemaker syndrome (see below). However, large-scale randomized trials comparing DDD with VVI(R) pacing have failed to substantiate survival benefits from DDD pacing, at least during follow-up periods of up to 3 years.

Complications of pacemaker insertion

Complications of temporary or permanent pacemaker implantation include those of central venous cannulation (e.g. pneumothorax), perforation of the heart by the electrode tip leading to pericardial effusion and cardiac tamponade, and macroscopic or microscopic displacement of the electrode resulting in an increase in the pacing threshold or failure to capture. A chest radiograph should always be taken after pacemaker insertion to exclude pneumothorax and to confirm that the electrode position is satisfactory.

Permanent pacing may be complicated by the development of infection around the pulse generator, or by mechanical erosion of the generator through the skin. Once infection is established, or the skin is breached, it is almost never possible to eradicate infection with antibiotics: removal and replacement of the pacing system is required. The development of oedema and inflammation around the implanted electrode tip may result in a steady rise in the pacing threshold over the first few weeks, which can lead to an increase of the pacing threshold such that capture is lost (Fig. 16.4.13a), although the process is normally mild and self-limiting.

Demand pacemakers require an adequate intracardiac signal to recognize activation of the chamber in question, to inhibit output. The pacing stimulus will not be suppressed ('undersensing') if the intracardiac signal is of insufficient amplitude, resulting in inappropriate pacemaker firing (Fig. 16.4.13b). This phenomenon is commoner in atrial pacing, owing to the lower amplitude of atrial compared with ventricular electrograms. Conversely, detection of extraneous electrical activity (e.g. skeletal muscle activity) via the pacing electrode can result in inappropriate inhibition of the pacemaker output (oversensing) (Fig. 16.14.13c). Oversensing is commoner with unipolar than bipolar pacing modes because of the inclusion of the pulse generator can in the electrical circuit, and its proximity to the pectoral muscles. For the same reason, unipolar pacemaker systems are more prone to the problem of local skeletal muscle stimulation. Damage to the conductor or insulation of the pacing electrode may occur due to trauma at the site of ligation or to compression between the clavicle and first rib. This may result in oversensing, skeletal muscle stimulation, or short-circuiting leading to premature battery depletion.

Patients receiving AAI pacemakers may subsequently develop AV block, resulting in a recurrence of syncope and requiring upgrade of the pacing system to a DDD unit. Some patients with VVI pacemakers, particularly those with sinoatrial rather than AV disease, will manifest retrograde ventriculoatrial conduction during ventricular pacing. This sometimes causes symptoms of fatigue, dizziness, or hypotension ('pacemaker syndrome'), which are associated with the presence of atrial cannon waves occurring as a result of simultaneous atrial and ventricular contraction. Upgrade of the system to a dual-chamber unit is necessary if symptoms are troublesome. Newer pacing systems allow DDD pacemakers to act as single-chamber atrial pacemakers, automatically switching to dual-chamber pacing should AV conduction fail, providing the benefits of atrial pacing with less risk of pacemaker syndrome.

Follow-up

Many patients with long-standing heart block treated by permanent pacing have no underlying cardiac rhythm, hence failure of the pacing system for whatever reason may be fatal and patients require follow-up in a pacemaker clinic. As well as detection of the complications described above, the function of such a clinic is to assess the status of the pulse generator battery, and to maximize its life by programming the pulse generator output to the minimum consistent with a satisfactory safety margin. The design of pulse generators and the battery characteristics normally allow prediction of the expected replacement date several months if not years ahead. However, premature battery depletion or pacemaker failure does occur, and patients should therefore be assessed at least annually by the clinic.

Tachycardias

Mechanisms of arrhythmogenesis

The principal mechanisms responsible for tachyarrhythmias are those of abnormal automaticity, triggered activity, or re-entry (Fig. 16.4.14). There is a complex interaction between the underlying substrate, such as previous myocardial infarction, a triggering event such as an extrasystole, and modulating influences, of which sympathetic stimulation and myocardial ischaemia are the most important.

Automaticity

Abnormal automaticity is defined as an inappropriate increase in the rate of discharge of a tissue that has physiological pacemaker

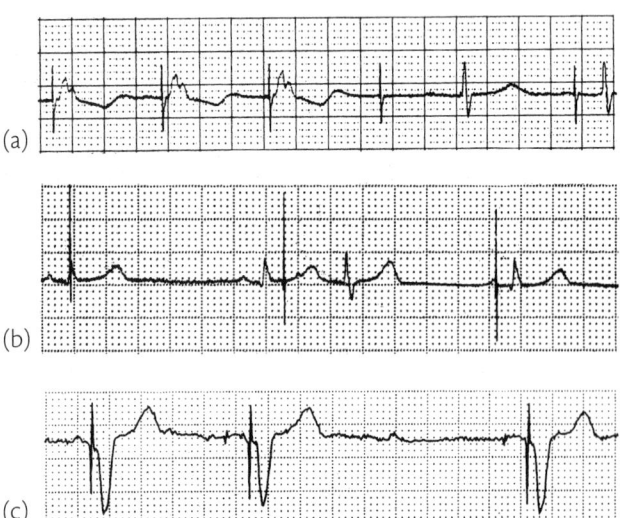

Fig. 16.4.13 Pacemaker malfunction. (a) Failure to capture. The fourth stimulus fails to capture the ventricle. (b) Undersensing. The atrial pacemaker has failed to sense the preceding atrial activity and therefore delivered the second stimulus. This has captured the atrium, with the P-wave in the ST segment, and subsequent conduction to the ventricle. (c) Oversensing. This dual-chamber pacemaker has sensed an electrical artefact through the ventricular lead and as a result has suppressed ventricular pacing, with the absence of ventricular activation following the third P-wave.

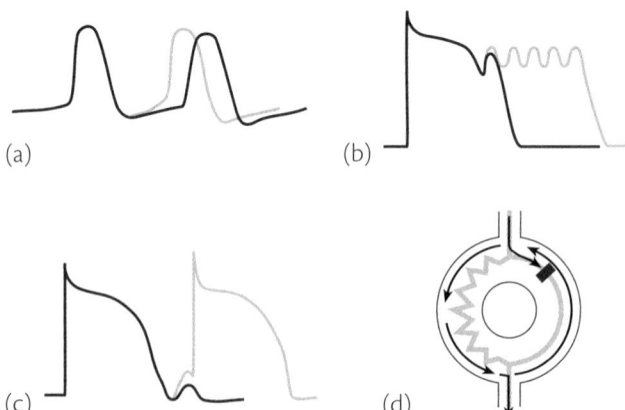

Fig. 16.4.14 Mechanisms of arrhythmia. (a) Increased automaticity. (b) Triggered activity due to early after-depolarizations. (c) Triggered activity due to delayed after-depolarizations. (d) Re-entry circuit. See text for details.

properties (sinus node, AV node, or Purkinje fibres) or the pathological development of automaticity in atrial or ventricular myocytes (Fig. 16.4.14a). Such abnormalities are most commonly seen in the presence of ischaemia, sympathetic stimulation, or drug toxicity, especially digoxin. Automatic tachycardias are characterized by an absence of initiation by extrasystoles, either spontaneously or during electrophysiological testing.

Triggered activity

The term 'triggered activity' is used to define an impulse initiation associated with a preceding action potential, and can be induced *in vitro* in tissues that do not demonstrate physiological automaticity. Two characteristic forms of depolarization may cause triggered activity.

Early after-depolarizations

These occur during the plateau phase of the action potential, prior to repolarization (Fig. 16.4.14b), and are more evident at slow heart rates, particularly in the presence of hypokalaemia and hypomagnesaemia. Mutations in cardiac Na+ or K+ channels, or drugs that prolong myocardial repolarization by inhibiting one or more components of the outward potassium current, I_K, (including class IA and class III antiarrhythmics, tricyclic antidepressants, antihistamines, organophosphorous insecticides, and many others) predispose to the appearance of early after-depolarizations *in vitro*. These changes are associated with the congenital and acquired long QT syndromes and the arrhythmia torsades de pointes (see below).

Delayed after-depolarizations

These are subthreshold depolarizations occurring after full repolarization of the action potential (Fig. 16.4.14c). Their amplitude is increased by tachycardia or intracellular calcium overload, and may reach a threshold at which an action potential is generated, potentially initiating a sustained tachycardia. Delayed after-depolarizations can be induced experimentally by digitalis overload, and are the likely mechanism of digitoxic arrhythmias.

Re-entry

Most clinically important sustained tachycardias, whether of atrial, junctional, or ventricular origin, appear to arise on the basis of re-entry. The establishment of a re-entry tachycardia requires the presence of a potential circuit comprising two limbs with different refractoriness and conduction properties (Fig. 16.4.14d). A premature beat can be conducted in one limb of the circuit, but the other limb may still be refractory, resulting in unidirectional conduction block. If conduction is sufficiently slow, the tissue distal to the site of block in the refractory limb will have regained excitability before the arrival of the depolarizing wavefront, and conducts the activity retrogradely. This results in reactivation of the initial conducting pathway and thus a circus movement tachycardia is established. Macro re-entry is defined as the occurrence of a re-entry circuit over a large area of the heart, such as in the presence of an accessory pathway (Fig. 16.4.15a). Micro re-entry occurs in a relatively small area of the heart, for example at the border zone of an old myocardial infarction, where conduction velocity is markedly slowed (Fig. 16.4.15b). The characteristic feature of a re-entrant tachycardia is that an appropriately timed extrastimulus can induce unidirectional block and initiate the arrhythmia. The tachycardia may be terminated by extrastimuli that depolarize the tissue ahead of the circulating wave front and thus interrupt the circus movement.

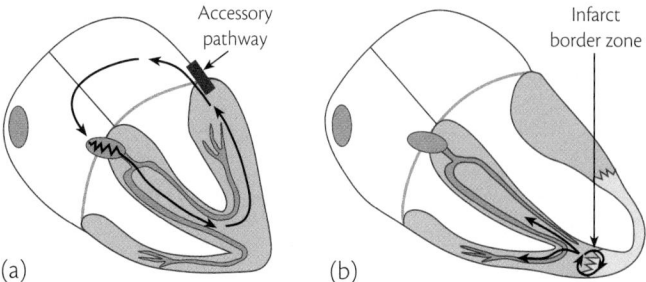

Fig. 16.4.15 Examples of re-entry tachycardias. (a) Macro re-entry circuit involving an accessory pathway, which results in atrioventricular re-entry tachycardia. (b) Micro re-entry circuit at the border zone of a myocardial infarction.

Differential diagnosis of tachycardias

General principles

The first and most important step in the diagnosis and management of tachycardias is to determine whether the arrhythmia arises within the atria and/or AV junction, or from the ventricles. An essential element in the differential diagnosis is to distinguish between tachycardias with normal QRS-complex morphology and duration ('narrow-complex tachycardias'), and those where the QRS complexes are abnormal in morphology and increased in duration ('wide-complex tachycardias'). A guide to the differential diagnosis of tachyarrhythmias is provided in Fig. 16.4.16.

Narrow-complex tachycardias

Narrow-complex tachycardias arise through mechanisms that result in ventricular activation via the AV node and His–Purkinje system and therefore show normal QRS morphology and duration (≤0.12 s) during tachycardia. Careful study of all leads of the electrocardiogram is necessary to assess regularity of QRS complexes and to identify the presence of atrial activity (P-waves) (Fig. 16.4.16). The relationship of the PR to the RP interval is helpful in determining mechanism of narrow-complex tachycardias. In supraventricular tachycardias (see below), P waves may not be visible, or may occur immediately following the QRS complex. A long RP interval is found in atrial tachycardia, atypical AV nodal re-entry tachycardia and AV re-entry involving a slowly conducting accessory pathway as the retrograde limb. Atrial flutter waves are most commonly evident in the inferior limb leads or in lead V1.

Wide-complex tachycardias

Few areas in cardiology cause more difficulty, or result in more mismanagement, than the diagnosis of wide-complex tachycardias. Whereas it is safe to assume that virtually all narrow-complex tachycardias have a supraventricular origin, wide-complex tachycardias (QRS duration ≥0.12 s) may arise either from the ventricle or from supraventricular mechanisms, the latter occurring if there is bundle branch block, either pre-existing or functional (aberration) as a result of the high rate (Fig. 16.4.16). An additional cause of aberrant conduction is activation of the ventricles via an accessory pathway.

If the wide QRS morphology during tachycardia is identical to that in sinus rhythm, then a supraventricular origin is likely, with fixed bundle branch block. However, no ECG in sinus rhythm may be available, and difficulties in diagnosis and management arise when ventricular tachycardia is not recognized and is

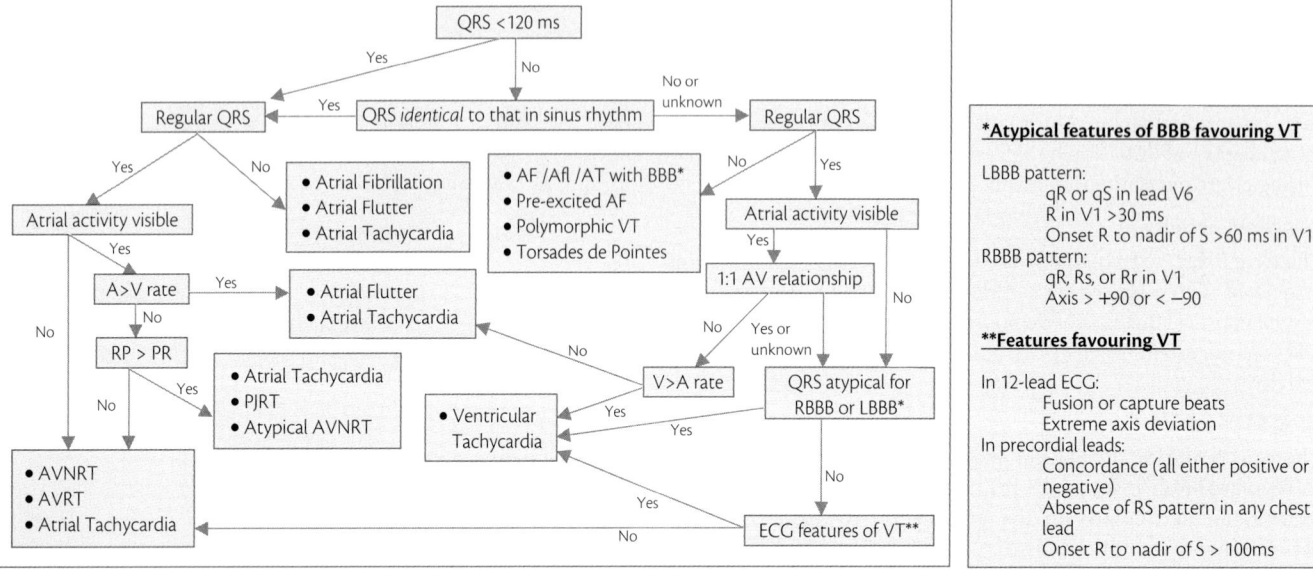

Fig. 16.4.16 Algorithm for diagnosis of tachycardia from 12-lead ECG. A, atrial rate; AF, atrial fibrillation; Afl, atrial flutter; AT, atrial tachycardia; AVNRT, atrioventricular nodal reentrant tachycardia; AVRT, atrioventricular reentrant tachycardia; BBB, bundle branch block; LBBB, left bundle branch block; PJRT, permanent junctional reciprocating tachycardia; PR, PR interval; RBBB, right bundle branch block; RP, RP interval; V, ventricular rate; VT, ventricular tachycardia. See text for details.

misdiagnosed as 'SVT with aberration'. This usually happens as a result of a number of failings and misconceptions, the commonest being that the clinical context is not considered:

♦ The age of the patient—middle-aged or elderly individuals presenting with a recent history of wide-complex tachycardia, and who give a history of myocardial infarction or congestive heart failure, are more likely to have ventricular than supraventricular tachycardia. However, ventricular tachycardia can also arise in young patients.

♦ The haemodynamic status of the patient—it is often assumed that ventricular tachycardia should cause haemodynamic collapse, whereas patients may in fact be haemodynamically stable if the rate is not excessively fast or if underlying cardiac function is good. Conversely, supraventricular tachycardias may cause syncope, hypotension, or shock if sufficiently rapid, or if there is underlying heart disease.

♦ The nature of the episodes of palpitation—it is often not appreciated that ventricular tachycardia can present with a typical history of paroxysmal self-terminating episodes, just as in the case of supraventricular tachycardia.

The importance of making a correct diagnosis in wide-complex tachycardia is twofold. First, inappropriate acute therapy of the tachyarrhythmia can be avoided. In particular, the use of verapamil in ventricular tachycardia misdiagnosed as supraventricular tachycardia is associated with a high risk of haemodynamic collapse as a result of its negative inotropic effect, coupled with its lack of efficacy in terminating ventricular tachycardia. Secondly, if the original arrhythmia has been misdiagnosed, then the adverse prognostic significance of ventricular tachycardia will be overlooked. Appropriate investigation and long-term management may not be instituted. It is therefore important that a diagnosis of SVT with aberration is made only if the ECG displays typical left or right bundle branch block with none of the features suggestive of VT

listed in Fig. 16.4.16. In addition to attention to the history and 12-lead ECG, the response to transient AV nodal blockade with adenosine will assist diagnosis in many patients (Table 16.4.4).

General principles of management

Many cardiac arrhythmias are benign and require no intervention. The main indications for treatment are to relieve symptoms, or to prevent complications such as myocardial ischaemia, cardiac failure, embolism, or arrhythmic sudden death. Precipitating factors such as myocardial ischaemia/infarction, infection, thyrotoxicosis, alcohol, electrolyte disorders, or drug toxicity must be sought and treated if possible. The therapy indicated will commonly be influenced by the presence of underlying structural heart disease such as myocardial ischaemia/infarction or left ventricular dysfunction and can include drug therapy, device implantation, or radiofrequency ablation.

Acute management of tachycardia

An algorithm for the treatment of tachyarrhythmias is shown in Fig. 16.4.17. Assessment of the patient's cardiorespiratory status

Table 16.4.4 Diagnostic use of intravenous adenosine

Arrhythmia	Response
Atrial tachycardia Atrial flutter Atrial fibrillation	Transient AV block reveals atrial arrhythmia Rarely terminated
AVNRT AVRT	Terminates tachycardia by anterograde (AV) block
Ventricular tachycardia	Not terminated 1:1 VA conduction may be blocked, revealing AV dissociation

For abbreviations, see Fig. 16.4.16.

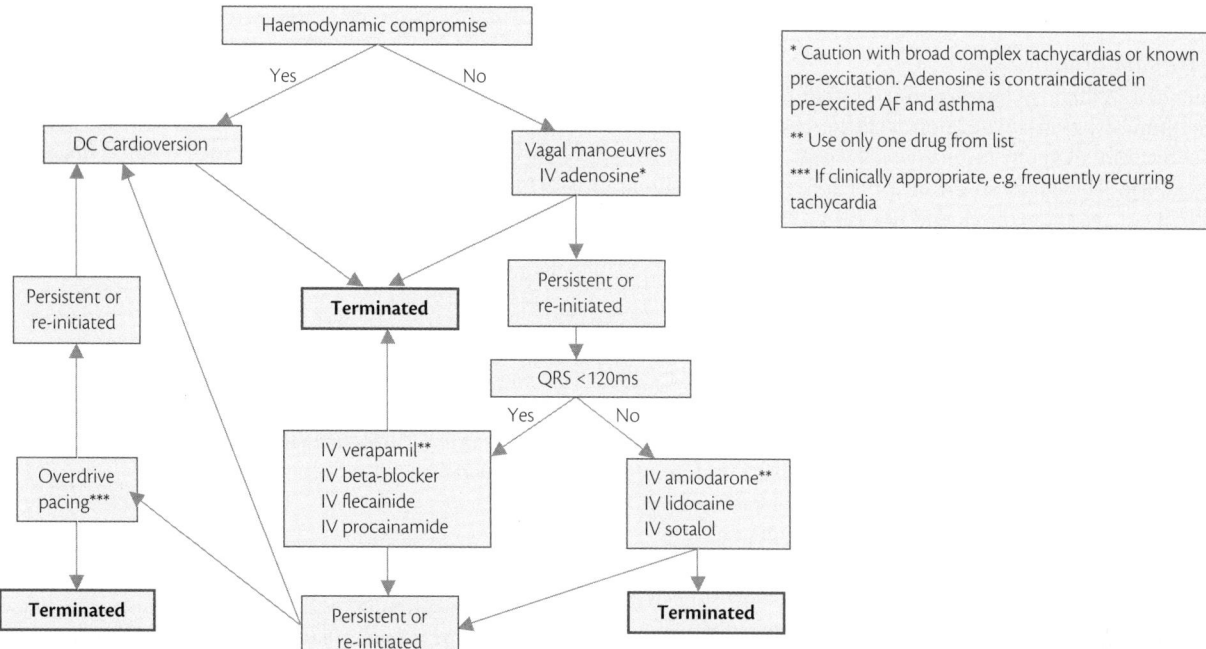

Fig. 16.4.17 Algorithm for the acute management of tachyarrhythmias.

takes precedence. R-wave synchronized, direct current (DC) cardioversion under general anaesthesia or deep sedation is the most effective and immediate means of terminating sustained tachycardias, and should be employed when the tachycardia is associated with haemodynamic compromise (Fig. 16.4.18). Although atrial flutter may respond to low-energy cardioversion (50–100 J), other arrhythmias normally require energies of 100 to 360 J for termination (100–150 J for biphasic shocks). The use of nonsynchronized DC shock in the termination of ventricular fibrillation is discussed in Chapter 16.3.

In patients with haemodynamically stable tachycardias, manoeuvres that produce transient vagal stimulation such as the Valsalva manoeuvre or carotid sinus massage may be employed. Similarly, adenosine (see below) is used pharmacologically to produce transient slowing or block of the sinus node or AV node. Vagal manoeuvres or adenosine will often terminate arrhythmias dependent on the AV node, and are also useful diagnostic tools, since transient interruption of AV nodal conduction may reveal the tachycardia mechanism (Table 16.4.4). Atrial tachyarrhythmias

will not normally be terminated by vagal stimulation or adenosine, but an increase in AV block reveals the underlying atrial rhythm.

Re-entry tachycardias may be terminated by the delivery of appropriately timed extrastimuli that depolarize part of the re-entry circuit prior to the arrival of the wave front and interrupt the arrhythmia. Simple overdrive pacing can be effective in the termination of atrial flutter, AV nodal re-entry, AV (orthodromic) re-entry tachycardia, or sustained ventricular tachycardia (Fig. 16.4.19). The cardiac chamber in question is paced for brief periods, e.g. 6 to 12 beats, at a rate just above that of the tachycardia, with repeated attempts sometimes necessary at gradually increasing rates. Overdrive atrial or ventricular pacing may result in degeneration into atrial and ventricular fibrillation respectively, hence facilities for immediate defibrillation must be available. Implantable antitachycardia pacing facilities are incorporated into implantable cardioverter-defibrillators (see below).

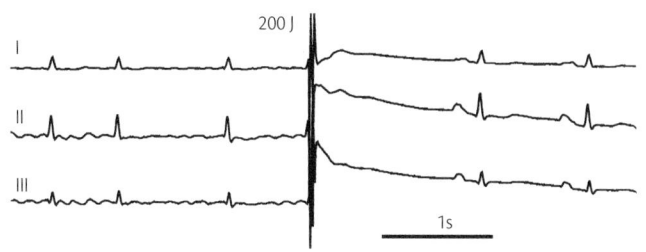

Fig. 16.4.18 Synchronized DC cardioversion of atrial fibrillation. A DC shock, 200 J, is delivered during atrial fibrillation to coincide with the R wave of the QRS complex. This shock terminates the arrhythmia with restoration of normal sinus rhythm.

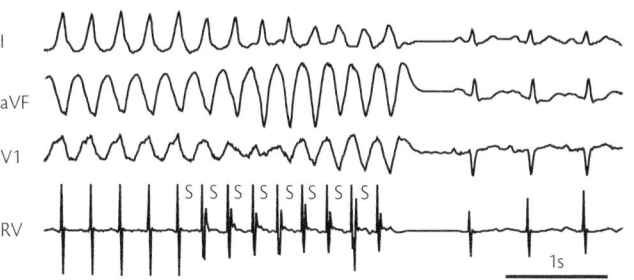

Fig. 16.4.19 Termination of ventricular tachycardia by overdrive ventricular pacing. During ventricular tachycardia a burst of eight stimuli (S) results in termination of the tachycardia and resumption of normal sinus rhythm. Surface leads I, aVF, V1, and intracardiac electrograms from the right ventricular apex (RV) are shown.

Treatments for tachycardias
Antiarrhythmic drug therapy
The Vaughan Williams classification is based on the effects of antiarrhythmic drugs in isolated normal tissue, and although many drugs act by more than one mechanism, the classification is still in widespread use. The effects of the major classes of antiarrhythmic drug activity at the tissue level, and the associated electrocardiographic changes, are listed in Table 16.4.5. Individual drugs are described in Table 16.4.6.

Class I activity
Class I antiarrhythmic drugs act by inhibiting the rapid inward sodium current. Class Ia agents (e.g. quinidine, procainamide, and disopyramide) increase the cardiac action potential duration and have intermediate effects on the onset and recovery kinetics of the sodium channel and hence on intracardiac conduction. Class Ib agents (e.g. lidocaine and mexiletine) shorten the cardiac action potential duration and have very rapid offset kinetics that result in minimal slowing of normal intracardiac conduction. Class Ic drugs (e.g. flecainide and propafenone) have no major effect on action potential duration, but produce the most long-lasting effect on cardiac sodium channel kinetics and the most marked slowing of intracardiac conduction.

Class II activity
Class II activity is defined as antagonism of the arrhythmogenic effects of catecholamines. The commonest agents in this class are the competitive β-adrenoceptor blockers. Other agents such as propafenone have a weak β-receptor blocking activity, and amiodarone (see below) exhibits a noncompetitive sympatholytic effect.

Class III activity
The class III mode of antiarrhythmic activity comprises lengthening of the cardiac action potential duration and hence of the effective refractory period. Drugs in this class possess a broad spectrum of activity against atrial, supraventricular, and ventricular arrhythmias. Currently available class III agents act by inhibiting the rapid component of the outward potassium current I_{Kr}. Dofetilide and ibutilide are examples of drugs with 'pure' class III antiarrhythmic actions. Sotalol is a non-selective β-adrenoceptor antagonist

that also possesses class III activity. Amiodarone possesses antiarrhythmic activity in all four Vaughan Williams classes.

Class IV activity
Class IV drugs (e.g. verapamil and diltiazem) reduce the inward calcium current I_{Ca} in sinoatrial and AV nodal tissues. They are used to prevent or interrupt re-entry arrhythmias involving the AV node (e.g. AV nodal re-entry tachycardia), or to slow the ventricular response in atrial fibrillation or flutter. The dihydropyridine calcium antagonists, such as amlodipine and nifedipine, have no antiarrhythmic action.

Digoxin
The antiarrhythmic activity of digoxin is not explained within the Vaughan Williams classification and appears to be mediated predominantly through vagal stimulation. It is used to slow ventricular rate in atrial fibrillation.

Adenosine
Adenosine, a naturally occurring purine nucleoside, is used pharmacologically to produce transient slowing or block of the sinus node or atrioventricular node. It is of particular value in view of its extremely short plasma half-life (c.2 s), which confers safety. It must be administered by rapid intravenous bolus injection, using incremental doses from 3 to 12 mg, to achieve the desired therapeutic effect. Adenosine is contraindicated in pre-excited atrial fibrillation or in severe asthma and cautioned in patients with known pre-excitation syndrome (see below).

Nonpharmacological therapy
Cardioversion External electrical cardioversion, as described above, can be used electively to restore normal rhythm in patients with persistent arrhythmia. Failure of external cardioversion of atrial fibrillation occurs in some patients as a result of various factors, including increased transthoracic impedance due to obesity, prolonged atrial fibrillation, left ventricular dysfunction, and left atrial dilatation. Internal cardioversion can be successful in many of these patients. The procedure involves the introduction of specialized electrode catheters that permit DC-shock delivery between electrodes in the right atrium and the pulmonary artery or coronary sinus, providing a current field that achieves depolarization of both atria.

Table 16.4.5 Classification of antiarrhythmic drug activity

Class		ECG effect				Tissue effect			
		HR	PR	QRS	QT	SA node	Atrium	AV node	Ventricle
Class	Ia	0	0/−	+	++	0	++	−	++/−
	Ib	0	0	0	0/−	0	0	0	++/−
	Ic	0	+	++	+	0	++	0/+	++/−
Class	II	−	+	0	0	++	++	++	+/0
Class	III	0/−	0/+	0	++	0/+	++	0/+	++/−
Class	IV	0/−	+	0	0	0/+	+/−	++	0
Digoxin		0/−	+	0	0	0/+	0/−	++	0/−
Adenosine		−	+	0	0	++	0/−	++	0

ECG effect: +, increases; −, decreases; 0, no effect; HR, heart rate.
Tissue effect: +, antiarrhythmic activity; −, potential adverse or proarrhythmic effect; 0 no effect

Table 16.4.6 Commonly used antiarrhythmic drugs

	Principal indication	Dose		Adverse effects
		IV	Oral	
Class Ia				
Quinidine	AF cardioversion	–	1–2 g/day	Hypersensitivity, GI symptoms, QT prolongation, hypotension
Disopyramide	AF prophylaxis VT termination	2 mg/kg	300–600 mg/day	Negative inotropy, QT prolongation, parasympathetic blockade (accelerated AV conduction, urinary retention, dry mouth, blurred vision)
Procainamide	AF cardioversion VT termination	100 mg/5 min up to 1000 mg1–6 mg/min	2–6 g/day	Hypotension, QT prolongation, GI upset, lupus syndrome
Class Ib				
Lidocaine (lignocaine)	VT termination VT/VF prophylaxis	100 mg bolus 1–4 mg/min	Ineffective	CNS—confusion, dysarthria, fits
Class Ic				
Flecainide	AF cardioversion AF prophylaxis WPW prophylaxis	2 mg/kg	100–300 mg/day	Proarrhythmia, negative inotropy, CNS disturbance
Propafenone	AF cardioversion AF prophylaxis WPW prophylaxis	–	450–900 mg/day	Proarrhythmia, negative inotropy, CNS disturbance, bronchoconstriction
Class II				
Various, e.g. atenolol	AF prophylaxis AF rate control SVT prophylaxis Sudden death prophylaxis	–	50–100 mg/day	Bradycardia, -ve inotropy, cold extremities, bronchoconstriction, lethargy
Class III				
Sotalol	AF termination AF prophylaxis WPW prophylaxis VT prophylaxis	2 mg/kg	160–480 mg/day	Bradycardia, negative inotropy, cold extremities, bronchoconstriction, lethargy, QT prolongation
Amiodarone	AF termination AF prophylaxis WPW prophylaxis VT prophylaxis	300 mg in30 min, then 1200 mg/24 h	0.6–1.2 g/day loading first 2 weeks, then100–400 mg/day	Bradycardia, photosensitivity, skin pigmentation, hypo- or hyperthyroidism, alveolitis, hepatitis, peripheral neuropathy, epidydimitis
Class IV				
Verapamil	SVT termination SVT prophylaxis AF rate control	5–10 mg	240–480 mg/day	Negative inotropy, AV block, flushing, constipation
Other				
Digoxin	AF rate control		0.125–0.5 mg/day ineffective	Anorexia, nausea, vomiting, AV block, atrial and ventricular arrhythmias
Adenosine	SVT termination	3–12 mg by incremental bolus		Flushing, chest pain, bronchospasm, transient AV block

AF, atrial fibrillation; SVT, supraventricular tachycardia (atrioventricular nodal and atrioventricular re-entrant tachycardia); VT, ventricular tachycardia; WPW, Wolff–Parkinson–White syndrome.

Implantable cardioverter-defibrillators Patients identified as being at high risk of sudden cardiac death, e.g. a history of spontaneous or inducible sustained ventricular arrhythmias or out-of-hospital cardiac arrest, may be treated with an implantable cardioverter–defibrillator (ICD). A transvenous rate-sensing/shocking electrode is introduced via the subclavian vein to the right ventricular apex, with the generator implanted in the pectoral region (Fig. 16.4.20). If a heart rate above the limit programmed by the device is recognized, a shock is delivered between the intracardiac shocking electrode and the generator casing. Some devices also include a right atrial electrode to sense atrial activation. This improves the distinction between sinus or atrial tachyarrhythmias

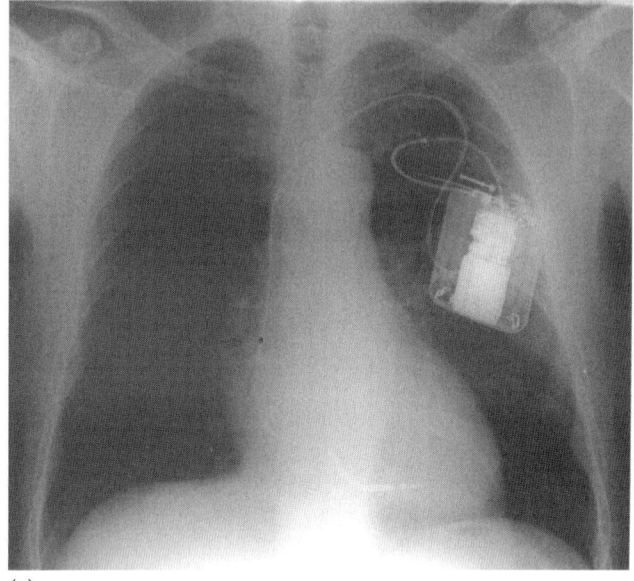

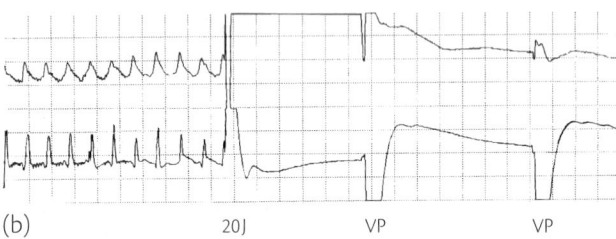

Fig. 16.4.20 Implantable cardioverter–defibrillator (ICD). (a) Chest radiograph showing the ICD generator in the left pectoral region, connected to a lead which passes via the left subclavian vein and superior vena cava to the heart. The tip of the lead is in the right ventricular apex. Cardiac rhythm is sensed from the electrodes at the tip of the lead, and shocks can be delivered between the metal casing of the generator and the right ventricular coil (thickened portion of lead). (b) Discharge from an ICD. A rapid polymorphic ventricular tachycardia is terminated by a 20-J shock from the device. Electrograms shown are retrieved from the memory of the device, upper tracings from the shocking circuit (generator can to ventricular coil) and lower tracings from the sensing circuit (bipolar electrodes at the tip of the catheter in the right ventricle. The shock is followed by ventricular pacing (VP).

and ventricular tachycardia, and reduces the risk of an inappropriate shock being delivered. A third lead lying in a tributary of the coronary sinus can be implanted to pace the left ventricle and help restore electromechanical synchrony in those with heart failure, reduced ejection fraction and evidence of dyssynchrony (cardiac resynchronization therapy). An ICD can be programmed to deliver initial antitachycardia ventricular pacing for tolerated tachycardias, with shock delivery available for faster rates or if pace-termination fails. ICDs are expensive, complex, and require regular specialist follow-up.

Radiofrequency ablation Selective ablation of part of a re-entry circuit, an arrhythmic focus, or of the AV node is used increasingly in the management of arrhythmias, and offers the opportunity of curative treatment. Radiofrequency energy is delivered between the tip of an intracardiac electrode positioned at the appropriate site and an indifferent surface electrode placed over the scapula. The energy produces a localized necrotic lesion 2 to 3 mm in diameter,

Table 16.4.7 Indications for radiofrequency ablation

Diagnosis	Ablation target	Success	Comments
AVRT	Accessory pathway	+++	
Pre-excited AF	Accessory pathway	+++	
AVNRT	Slow pathway	+++	0.5–1% risk of CHB
Atrial flutter	TVA–IVC isthmus	+++	
Focal atrial tachycardia	Tachycardia focus	++	
Paroxysmal AF	Pulmonary vein isolation	++	High recurrence rate
Persistent AF	Extensive LA ablation	+	Often requires >1 procedure
Permanent AF	AV node	+++	Requires permanent pacing
Scar-related ventricular tachycardia	Re-entry circuit	+	High recurrence rate
Focal ventricular tachycardia	Site of origin	++	Especially RVOT focus

AVRT, atrioventricular (orthodromic) re-entry tachycardia; AF, atrial fibrillation; AVNRT, atrioventricular nodal re-entry tachycardia; LA, left atrial; CHB, complete heart block; TVA, tricuspid valve annulus; IVC, inferior vena cava; RVOT, right ventricular outflow tract.

which results in local conduction block. Current indications for radiofrequency ablation are listed in Table 16.4.7, and specific issues are discussed below in relation to individual arrhythmias.

Arrhythmia surgery The 'maze' procedure for atrial fibrillation involves creating a series of lines of conduction block in the left and right atria, either by incisions or by ablation. This prevents the development of atrial re-entry circuits while permitting AV conduction. Surgical management of recurrent ventricular tachycardia by mapping and resection of the re-entry circuit is occasionally performed, but has been largely superseded by ablation or ICD therapy.

Specific causes of arrhythmias

Extrasystoles

The term extrasystole is used to describe a premature beat arising from a focus other than the sinus node. Extrasystoles are also described as premature beats, premature contractions, premature depolarizations, or ectopic beats.

Atrial extrasystoles

Atrial extrasystoles are recognized by a premature P-wave of different morphology from the sinus P-wave (Fig. 16.4.21a), which can be hidden within the ST segment or T wave of the preceding sinus beat. Premature atrial extrasystoles that occur before full recovery of the AV node will be followed by prolongation of the PR interval, or, if sufficiently premature, complete failure of conduction (Fig. 16.4.21b). Nonconducted atrial extrasystoles must be distinguished from sinus arrest or second-degree AV block.

An atrial extrasytole will commonly reset the sinoatrial node, such that the next sinus beat occurs earlier than expected with

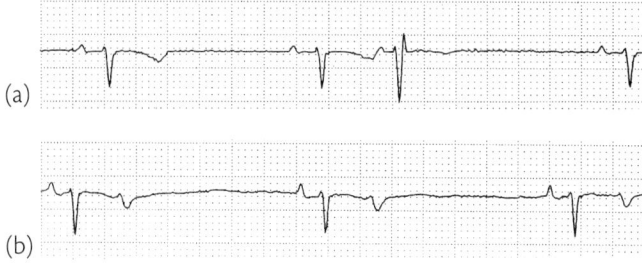

Fig. 16.4.21 Atrial extrasystoles. (a) An atrial extrasystole, with an abnormal P wave at the end of the preceding T wave, occurs following a sinus beat. (b) Blocked atrial extrasystoles. In the same patient, atrial extrasystoles occur following each sinus beat. They are earlier than those in (a), and the AV node is refractory because of the proximity of the atrial extrasystoles to the preceding beat, and conduction is blocked.

respect to the preceding sinus beat, and the pause is less than compensatory.

Atrial extrasystoles are a common finding in healthy people, particularly with increasing age, but are more frequent in the presence of increased atrial pressure or stretch such as in cardiac failure or chronic mitral valve disease. Patients should be reassured that the arrhythmia is benign and that drug treatment is rarely necessary. If treatment is required on symptomatic grounds, β-adrenergic blockers may be used, but class I antiarrhythmic drugs should be avoided in view of their proarrhythmic risk.

Junctional extrasystoles

Junctional extrasystoles are identified by the appearance of a premature, normal QRS complex in the absence of a preceding atrial extrasystole. The atria as well as the ventricles may be activated, resulting in an inverted P-wave simultaneous with the QRS complex, or inscribed within the ST segment. The significance and management of junctional extrasystoles are similar to those of atrial extrasystoles.

Ventricular extrasystoles

Ventricular extrasystoles are identified by the appearance of a bizarre, wide QRS complex not preceded by a P-wave (Fig. 16.4.22). There is commonly ST segment depression and T wave inversion. Ventricular extrasystoles may be intermittent, or occur with a fixed relationship to the preceding normal beats, i.e. 1:2, 1:3 (bigeminy or trigeminy). Ventricular extrasystoles occur in otherwise normal hearts, but are found particularly in the presence of structural heart disease. They occur commonly in the acute phase of myocardial infarction, but are also seen in the postinfarction phase, and in the presence of severe left ventricular hypertrophy or dysfunction of whatever cause. Extrasystoles may produce symptoms that require treatment in a minority of cases. The safest option is β-blockade.

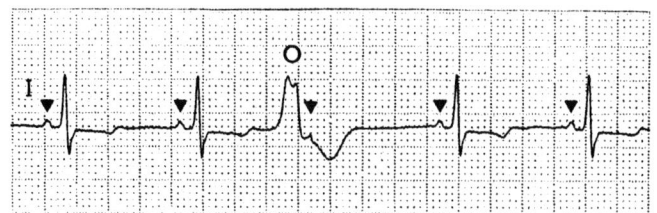

Fig. 16.4.22 Ventricular extrasystole (open circle). No retrograde atrial activation occurs, and the P wave sequence is undisturbed (arrowed).

Atrial arrhythmias

Atrial fibrillation

Mechanisms

Studies of patients with paroxysmal atrial fibrillation suggest that the arrhythmia may be triggered by one or more rapidly discharging foci, which are commonly situated in the pulmonary veins.

The underlying mechanism for maintenance of fibrillation is thought to be re-entry, with multiple wavelets (probably a minimum of six) circulating through the atria. Rapid atrial activation induces a process of electrical remodelling, which renders cardioversion and maintenance of sinus rhythm more difficult ('atrial fibrillation begets atrial fibrillation'). The initial mechanism of remodelling is thought to be intracellular calcium overload resulting in shortening of the atrial refractory period, although more prolonged atrial tachyarrhythmias result in downregulation of calcium entry and dedifferentiation of atrial myocytes towards a fetal phenotype. Structural changes, including interstitial fibrosis, also occur and further perpetuate the arrhythmia.

Clinical features

The prevalence of atrial fibrillation increases with advancing age and may be as high as 5 to 10% in very elderly individuals. There are numerous causes of the arrhythmia (Box 16.4.2), but in many instances no obvious aetiological factor can be identified, and the patient is described as having 'lone' atrial fibrillation. Atrial fibrillation carries adverse prognostic significance, in part through its association with organic heart disease but also as an important risk factor for the development of stroke and systemic embolism as a result of stasis and thrombus formation in the left atrium. The risk of stroke is particularly high in patients with mitral stenosis or mitral valve replacement and chronic atrial fibrillation.

Atrial fibrillation results in loss of the atrial contribution to left ventricular filling, which can result in a worsening of heart failure. More commonly, symptoms and impairment of left ventricular function ('tachycardiomyopathy') arise as a result of a rapid uncontrolled ventricular rate. In addition, uncontrolled atrial fibrillation

---

Box 16.4.2 Aetiology of atrial fibrillation

- Increased atrial pressure—mitral valve disease, congestive heart failure,
- left ventricular hypertrophy, restrictive cardiomyopathy, pulmonary embolism
- Atrial volume overload—atrial septal defect
- Myocardial ischaemia/infarction
- Thyrotoxicosis
- Alcohol
- Sinoatrial disease
- Infiltration—constrictive pericarditis, tumour
- Infection— systemic, e.g. pneumonia
- Infection— cardiac: myo/pericarditis
- Retrograde activation—WPW syndrome, ventricular pacing
- Cardiac or thoracic surgery
- Idiopathic—'lone' atrial fibrillation

can cause further impairment of ventricular filling in mitral stenosis and conditions associated with left ventricular diastolic dysfunction, or the development of angina in patients with coexisting coronary artery disease.

Diagnosis

The characteristic ECG findings in atrial fibrillation of recent onset are of rapid, irregular 'f' waves at a rate of 350 to 600/min. These are associated with an irregular ventricular response because of variable conduction through the AV node (Fig. 16.4.23). With increasing duration of chronic atrial fibrillation, the amplitude of the 'f' waves diminishes until they are no longer visible. Under these circumstances, atrial fibrillation is diagnosed by the absence of P-waves and the irregular ventricular response (Fig. 16.4.23b).

Atrial fibrillation is classified into three patterns: paroxysmal, persistent, or permanent. In paroxysmal atrial fibrillation, spontaneously terminating attacks of palpitation last anything from a few seconds to a few days. The ventricular rate is often rapid and the patient may be severely symptomatic. The term 'persistent atrial fibrillation' is used to describe instances where the arrhythmia is not self-terminating, but where sinus rhythm can be restored by electrical or pharmacological cardioversion. Permanent atrial fibrillation describes the situation where restoration of sinus rhythm is no longer possible. At this stage, the ventricular rate is often slower and the patient may be unaware of the irregular pulse or of palpitations.

Acute management

Appropriate management of atrial fibrillation depends on the presence or absence of symptoms, haemodynamic status, duration of arrhythmia and the presence of factors affecting the successful maintenance of sinus rhythm. Atrial fibrillation of recent onset may terminate spontaneously, particularly if associated with an acute febrile illness. However, outside of the context of an acute febrile illness, an attempt to restore sinus rhythm should be made unless the arrhythmia is obviously long-standing (>48 h) or is associated with advanced organic heart disease. Underlying precipitating factors such as thyrotoxicosis should be corrected before attempting cardioversion.

Chemical cardioversion may be achieved with class Ia, Ic, or III agents. Class Ia agents accelerate the ventricular rate by virtue of their anticholinergic action on the AV node and must be used in combination with AV nodal blocking agent (e.g. digoxin, beta-blocker, or calcium channel blocker). For patients without significant underlying heart disease, the current drugs of choice are the class

Ic agents (e.g. flecainide 2 mg/kg intravenously over 30 min). Class III drugs are somewhat less effective but are safer in the presence of left ventricular dysfunction or ischaemic heart disease. Options include sotalol (1.5 mg/kg intravenously over 30 min) or amiodarone (300 mg intravenously over 30 min followed by 1200 mg/24 h until cardioversion). The pure class III agent ibutilide is approved for this indication in the United States of America. Normally, only one drug should be tried in any individual patient. If drug therapy fails, direct current (DC) cardioversion is commonly effective.

Given that atrial fibrillation is a risk factor for the development of intracardiac thrombus formation, cardioversion, by chemical or electrical means, should not be attempted if arrhythmia has been present for longer than 48 h. Anticoagulation plus rate control with a β-blocker, calcium channel blocker, or digoxin should be considered in these circumstances. However, in the presence of haemodynamic compromise, the benefit of achieving sinus rhythm may outweigh the potential risk of embolism and attempt to restore sinus should be made. Transoesophageal echocardiography is useful in this situation to exclude left atrial thrombus.

Prevention of thromboembolism

Prophylaxis against thromboembolism should be considered in all patients with atrial fibrillation, as stroke risk exists with paroxysmal, persistent, or permanent atrial fibrillation. Chronic anticoagulation with warfarin is indicated in patients in atrial fibrillation with rheumatic mitral valve disease. Meta-analysis of trials of patients with nonrheumatic atrial fibrillation shows that warfarin anticoagulation with a target range for the international normalized ratio (INR) of between 2.0 and 3.0 reduces the risk of thromboembolic events by about 60%. Aspirin is a significantly less effective alternative, achieving a risk reduction of around 20%. As such, the choice of antithrombotic prophylaxis depends on balancing the risk of thromboembolism against the risk of haemorrhagic complications, as well as the local facilities for anticoagulant control. The presence of high risk features such as previous stroke, history of heart failure, age over 75 years, hypertension, and diabetes favours warfarin, although the balance of risk vs benefit has to be assessed on an individual basis (Box 16.4.3). See Chapter 16.16.1 for further discussion.

Paroxysmal atrial fibrillation

Paroxysmal atrial fibrillation is a self-terminating, recurrent arrhythmia, often associated with marked symptoms of palpitations. The goal of treatment is the maintenance of sinus rhythm and the amelioration of symptoms. In patients with infrequent paroxysms, drug therapy may not be necessary, or a 'pill in the pocket' approach can be used with selected patients without structural heart disease. For this, the patient takes a dose of an antiarrhythmic drug after the onset of arrhythmia, e.g. flecainide 200 to 300 mg, if this has previously been shown to be safe and effective under hospital supervision.

In those with recurrent paroxysmal atrial fibrillation, prophylactic therapy should be considered. No drug is entirely satisfactory and a β-blocker is often prescribed as first-line therapy. If this is ineffective, other antiarrhythmic therapy should be started. Class Ic agents (flecainide or propafenone) are effective and reasonably safe in the absence of underlying ischaemia or left ventricular dysfunction. Sotalol (80–160 mg twice daily) is also effective and well tolerated. Amiodarone is effective but can be associated with significant adverse effects and should be reserved for when the

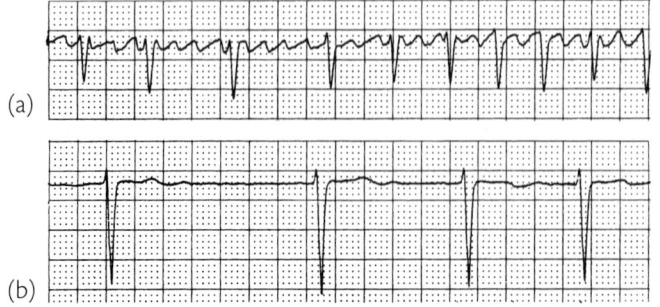

Fig. 16.4.23 Atrial fibrillation. (a) Coarse atrial fibrillation of recent onset. (b) Fine atrial fibrillation in a patient with long-standing valvular disease. Surface V1 leads are shown.

above measures fail. In the tachycardia–bradycardia syndrome, implantation of a permanent pacemaker may be required to control bradycardia and to allow antiarrhythmic therapy for the treatment of tachycardia. Finally, radiofrequency ablation should be considered for those in whom pharmacological therapy has failed. Foci arising from the pulmonary vein are targeted by placing lesions at the pulmonary vein antrum to achieve electrical isolation, with clinical success rates of 70 to 80%.

Persistent atrial fibrillation

Persistent atrial fibrillation is not self-terminating, usually requires electrical cardioversion to achieve sinus rhythm, and has a high recurrence rate even after successful cardioversion. The key decision is whether to employ a rhythm or rate control strategy. The AFFIRM trial showed no overall benefit of a rhythm control strategy. In general, a rate control strategy should be employed in asymptomatic or mildly symptomatic individuals, in older people, and in those with contraindications to antiarrhythmic therapy or cardioversion. This group should be treated as having permanent atrial fibrillation. In more severely symptomatic or younger patients, or in those with atrial fibrillation due to a treated precipitant, a rhythm control strategy may be more appropriate. However, treatment choice has to be tailored to the individual and both options should be discussed with the patient. Prophylaxis of thromboembolism should be considered in both groups.

If a rhythm control strategy is adopted, elective cardioversion should be scheduled. Given that cardioversion may be associated with embolism, patients undergoing this procedure should ideally be treated with warfarin for at least 4 weeks beforehand and warfarin should be continued for a minimum of 4 weeks afterwards since atrial mechanical function recovers slowly. There is a high risk of recurrent atrial fibrillation (up to 50% at 1 year) and antiarrhythmic prophylaxis should be considered. First-line therapy is often a simple β-blocker followed by a class Ic agent if there is no structural heart disease. Amiodarone may also be considered, and treatment prior to cardioversion increases the likelihood of its success. Finally, radiofrequency ablation may be employed but this requires more extensive left atrial ablation compared to paroxysmal atrial fibrillation (Fig. 16.4.24), with a lower success rate, and often requires more than one procedure.

Permanent atrial fibrillation

In permanent atrial fibrillation, restoration of sinus rhythm is not feasible or is unsuccessful and chronic management involves control of ventricular rate. Traditionally, the mainstay of treatment has been digoxin, at a dose titrated to achieve adequate slowing in the ventricular rate at rest, with therapeutic plasma concentrations. However, despite adequate rate control at rest, patients commonly have an uncontrolled heart rate on exercise. Control of rate response with other AV nodal blocking drugs such as β-blockers or verapamil is associated with improved rate control which is especially important if the duration of diastole is critical, as in mitral stenosis or ischaemic heart disease. Often a combination of AV

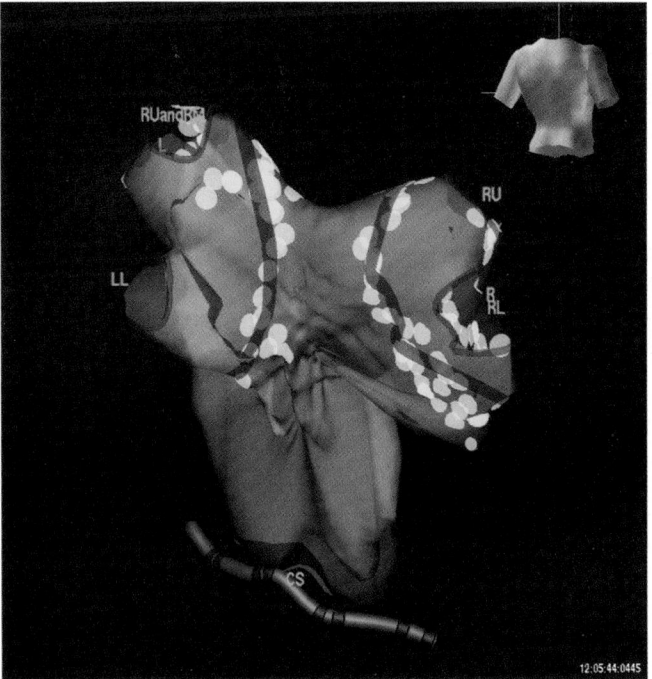

Fig. 16.4.24 Virtual geometry of the left atrium using the Ensite NavX systems (St Jude Medical, Minnesota). The view is a posterior view (as illustrated by the torso, upper right). The ostia of the pulmonary veins are shown (red lines) and the veins are labelled (RU, right upper; RL, right lower; RM, right middle; LL, left lower). A multipolar catheter in the coronary sinus (CS) is shown. Lesions produced by sequential application of radiofrequency energy are shown by the yellow dots, encircling the pulmonary veins to produce electrical isolation.

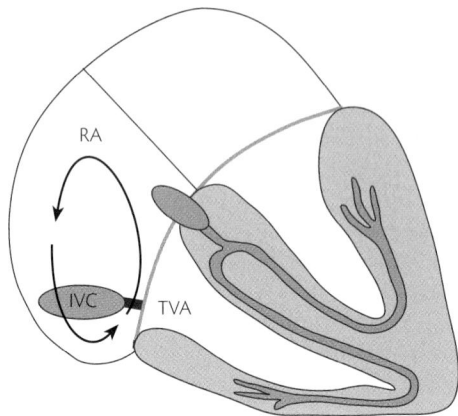

Fig. 16.4.25 Mechanism of atrial flutter. Typical atrial flutter results from a counter-clockwise re-entry circuit in the right atrium. The isthmus between the tricuspid valve annulus (TVA) and inferior vena cava (IVC) forms a critical part of this circuit, and linear ablation to create block can prevent recurrent atrial flutter.

nodal blocking drugs is required. In cases where adequate rate control cannot be achieved despite combination therapy, radiofrequency ablation of the AV node and implantation of a permanent pacemaker is an option, although this commits the patient to lifelong pacemaker therapy.

Atrial flutter

Atrial flutter is caused by a macro re-entrant circuit in the right atrium (Fig. 16.4.25), which produces a typical electrocardiographic 'sawtooth' pattern of atrial activity with a rate close to 300/min (Fig. 16.4.26). In the common form of the arrhythmia, flutter waves are negative in leads II, III, and aVF and positive in lead V1. Atrial flutter may be associated with either a regular or irregular ventricular response. Flutter with 2:1 AV conduction produces a regular tachycardia of 150/min and should always be considered in the differential diagnosis of a regular, narrow-QRS tachycardia of this rate. Occasionally, flutter occurs with 1:1 AV conduction producing a ventricular rate approaching 300/min. Class I antiarrhythmic

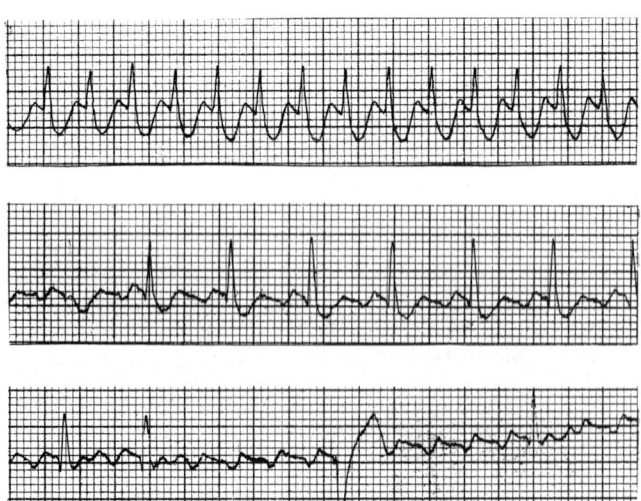

Fig. 16.4.26 Atrial flutter with 1:1 AV conduction (above), 2:1 conduction (middle), and following adenosine administration (below) (6 mg intravenous injection 10 s previously).

drugs may predispose to this by causing a relative slowing of the atrial rate and allowing 1:1 conduction through the AV node. The flutter waves may not be seen easily with faster ventricular rates, and transient slowing of AV conduction may be necessary to make the diagnosis (Fig. 16.4.26).

The underlying causes of atrial flutter are the same as those of atrial fibrillation (Box 16.4.2). Although atrial flutter may last for many months or occasionally years, it usually degenerates into chronic atrial fibrillation unless cardioversion is undertaken. Atrial flutter also carries a risk of thromboembolism, and anticoagulation is indicated before and after cardioversion as for atrial fibrillation. It is important to attempt to terminate atrial flutter since the ventricular rate is often poorly controlled by AV nodal blocking drugs. Termination may be achieved by chemical or electrical cardioversion as described above for atrial fibrillation. Bursts of atrial overdrive pacing at a rate approximately 10% above the atrial flutter rate are also used: this may restore sinus rhythm or precipitate atrial fibrillation. Prophylaxis against atrial flutter is undertaken using the same agents as in paroxysmal atrial fibrillation; indeed the conditions often coexist and patients may manifest either flutter or fibrillation at different times. Treatment of atrial flutter by radiofrequency ablation creates a line of conduction block between the tricuspid valve annulus and the inferior vena cava, interrupting the isthmus through which the re-entry circuit must pass (Fig. 16.4.25). This achieves cure in 90% of cases and is increasingly used as a first-line therapy.

Atrial tachycardia

Atrial tachycardia usually results in an atrial rate between 120 and 250/min. There may be a degree of AV block, although 1:1 AV conduction can occur. The ECG shows regular P-waves which do not show the same 'sawtooth' appearance as in atrial flutter (Fig. 16.4.27). Atrial tachycardia may occur as a result of sinus node re-entry, with sudden paroxysms of tachycardia with a normal P-wave morphology. Automatic atrial tachycardia manifests an abnormal P-wave morphology, commonly with a prolonged PR interval. The rate characteristically accelerates or 'warms up' before reaching a rate of 125 to 200/min. Atrial tachycardia with AV conduction block is a manifestation of digitalis toxicity. Multifocal atrial tachycardia, in which rapid, irregular P-waves of three or four different morphologies are seen, may occur in severely ill elderly patients or in association with acute exacerbation of pulmonary disease.

Management includes drug treatment or cardioversion, as for atrial fibrillation. Focal atrial tachycardia may be amenable to treatment with radiofrequency ablation with success rates approaching 75%, although recurrence rate is high.

Supraventricular tachycardia

Although all atrial arrhythmias are by definition supraventricular in origin, the term supraventricular tachycardia is commonly reserved for those in which the AV node is an obligate part of a re-entry circuit—AV nodal re-entrant tachycardia (AVNRT) or

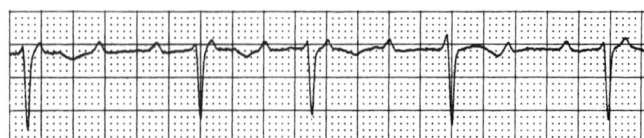

Fig. 16.4.27 Atrial tachycardia, with variable AV conduction. Lead V1.

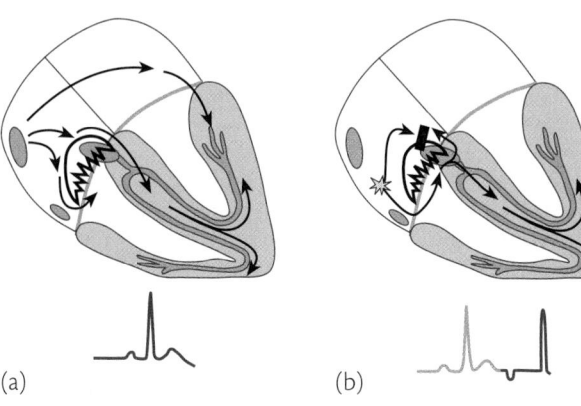
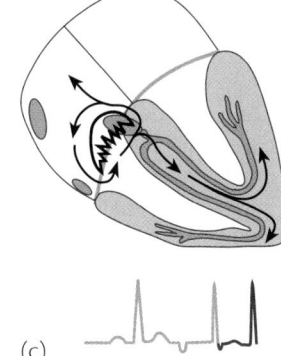

(a)   (b)   (c)

Fig. 16.4.28 Atrioventricular nodal re-entry tachycardia. Mechanism of initiation by atrial extrasystole. See text for details.

AV re-entry tachycardia (AVRT)—also known as junctional re-entry tachycardias. Correct recognition of these arrhythmias has achieved additional importance with the development of effective curative measures.

Atrioventricular nodal re-entry tachycardia

Mechanism
This is the commonest cause of paroxysmal re-entry tachycardia manifesting regular, normal QRS complexes. The basis of the arrhythmia is the presence of two functionally distinct pathways in the region of the AV node (Fig. 16.4.28). The 'fast' pathway conducts more rapidly, but has a longer refractory period. The 'slow' pathway has slower conduction properties but a shorter refractory period. During sinus rhythm, AV nodal conduction occurs via the fast pathway with a normal PR interval (Fig. 16.4.28a). If a sufficiently premature atrial extrasystole arises, conduction in the fast pathway is blocked, but slow pathway conduction may continue, resulting in an abrupt increase in the AH interval as recorded in the His bundle electrogram. This corresponds to an increased PR interval on the surface ECG. If conduction down the slow pathway is sufficiently delayed to allow the fast pathway to recover excitability before activation reaches the distal end of the pathways, retrograde activation occurs via the fast pathway (Fig. 16.4.28b). The stage is then set for a re-entry circuit with anterograde conduction via the slow pathway and retrograde conduction via the fast pathway ('slow/fast AV nodal re-entry') (Fig. 16.4.28c). Characteristically, anterograde activation of the ventricles and retrograde activation of the atria occur virtually simultaneously, resulting in the P-wave being 'buried' within the QRS complex, or producing a very small distortion of the terminal QRS, recognition of which requires careful comparison with the ECG during sinus rhythm (Fig. 16.4.29).

A less common variant of AV nodal re-entry tachycardia may arise where anterograde conduction during tachycardia is via the fast pathway with retrograde conduction via the slow pathway ('fast/slow AV nodal re-entry'). Under these circumstances, the atrium is activated well after the QRS complex, characteristically producing an inverted P′ wave, with the RP′ interval greater than the P′ interval during tachycardia (Fig. 16.4.30).

Clinical features
Atrioventricular nodal re-entry tachycardia commonly presents for the first time in childhood or adolescence, although it may appear at any age. The natural history is of episodic paroxysmal tachycardia. Attacks occur at random intervals, although clustering of attacks may occur interposed with periods of relative freedom from symptoms. Atrioventricular nodal re-entry tachycardia has no specific association with other organic heart disease. Palpitations are normally well tolerated unless the tachycardia is particularly rapid, prolonged, or if the patient has other heart disease.

Management
Termination of an attack of AV nodal re-entry tachycardia is achieved by producing transient AV nodal block. This may be achieved by vagotonic manoeuvres, by intravenous adenosine (3–12 mg) (Fig. 16.4.29), or by intravenous verapamil (5–10 mg). Drug prophylaxis of AV nodal re-entry tachycardia is undertaken with β-blockers, a combined β-blocker/class III agent such as sotalol, or AV nodal blocking drugs such as verapamil or digoxin. Curative treatment of AV nodal re-entry tachycardia by radiofrequency ablation is increasingly used as a first-line therapy, and is indicated if patients are refractory to drugs, intolerant of side effects, or unwilling to take long-term medication. Radiofrequency energy is delivered to the 'slow' pathway, which lies between the compact AV node and the tricuspid annulus. Ablation at this site is normally curative in over 90% of cases, but carries a small risk (0.5–1%) of inducing complete heart block.

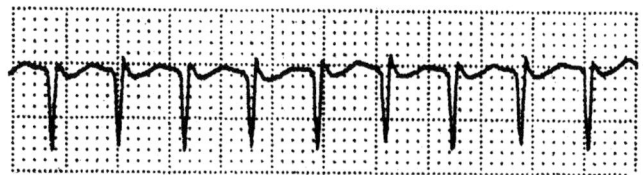

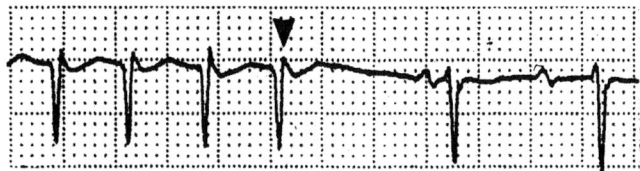

Fig. 16.4.29 Atrioventricular nodal re-entrant tachycardia. Rapid narrow-complex tachycardia with no apparent P waves (upper) responding to 6 mg adenosine with restoration of sinus rhythm (lower). Close inspection reveals a positive deflection of the terminal QRS during tachycardia (arrow) which is absent during sinus rhythm. This is due to retrograde atrial activity coincident with ventricular activation. Lead V1.

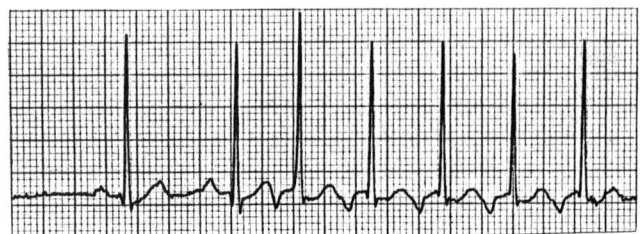

Fig. 16.4.30 Atypical atrioventricular nodal re-entry tachycardia ('long RP'). Inverted P waves precede the QRS complex during tachycardia (compare with preceding sinus beats)

Atrioventricular re-entry tachycardia

Mechanism

In contrast to AV nodal re-entry tachycardia, the substrate for AV re-entry is the presence of a second atrioventricular connection, separate from the AV node. This accessory pathway can lie anywhere along the mitral or tricuspid annuli. Anterograde pathway conduction produces ventricular pre-excitation and is discussed in the 'Pre-excitation syndromes' section below. However, most pathways conduct only in the retrograde (ventriculoatrial) direction and are termed 'concealed', since there is no clue to their presence on the resting ECG. The anterograde limb of the re-entrant circuit is the AV node, with retrograde atrial activation occurring over the accessory pathway (see Fig. 16.4.31). This is termed orthodromic tachycardia and normally produces a narrow complex QRS morphology. Retrograde atrial activation can be identified by the presence of a characteristic inverted P′ wave early in the ST segment, an important diagnostic feature of AV re-entry tachycardia (Fig. 16.4.32). Rarely, an accessory pathway with slow retrograde conduction may allow a stable, incessant re-entrant circuit with a long RP interval, referred to as permanent junctional reciprocating tachycardia.

Clinical features

Features are similar to AV nodal re-entry tachycardia, although accessory pathways are the more common tachycardia substrate in children. Patients have a similar relapsing course of symptoms interspersed with periods of relative quiescence. Multiple pathways can be present within the same patient and are more common if there is coexisting Ebstein's anomaly (see Chapter 16.12).

Management

As with AV nodal re-entry tachycardia, the AV node is an obligate part of the circuit and attacks may be aborted by vagotonic manoeuvres or with intravenous adenosine or verapamil. Antiarrhythmic therapy may be effective, but radiofrequency ablation offers high success rates with low incidence of complications and should be considered early in a patient's treatment.

Pre-excitation syndromes (Wolff–Parkinson–White syndrome)

The term 'pre-excitation' refers to the premature activation of the ventricle via one or more accessory pathways that bypass the normal AV node and His–Purkinje system. The commonest of the pre-excitation syndromes is the Wolff–Parkinson–White syndrome, in which accessory pathways with electrophysiological properties of normal myocardium may lie at any point in the AV ring, the commonest sites being in the left free wall or the posteroseptal region (Fig. 16.4.31). The characteristic electrocardiographic appearance is of early activation of the ventricular myocardium adjacent to the insertion of the accessory pathway. There is no AV delay via the pathway, hence the PR interval is shortened, but slow intraventricular conduction results in slurred initiation of the QRS complex (the delta wave) (Fig. 16.4.33), before the remainder of the ventricle is excited via the normal His–Purkinje system. The ECG appearances of a delta wave occur in approximately 1.5 per 1000 of the population, but many individuals never experience paroxysmal tachycardias. The degree of pre-excitation during sinus rhythm is variable: it may be intermittent if the refractory period of the accessory pathway is close to the sinus cycle length (Fig. 16.4.33), or inapparent if the delta wave is obscured due to rapid AV nodal conduction. In such instances, transient slowing of AV nodal conduction (e.g. by adenosine) will enhance the proportion of the ventricle excited by the accessory pathway and reveal pre-excitation.

Mechanisms of orthodromic and antidromic tachycardia

The mechanism for orthodromic AV re-entry tachycardia is illustrated in Fig. 16.4.31. A premature atrial extrasystole may find the pathway refractory but be conducted through the AV node to the ventricles (Fig. 16.4.31b). If sufficient delay has occurred by the time the ventricular insertion of the accessory pathway is depolarized, the pathway may have recovered excitability and allow retrograde activation from the ventricle to atrium, with the establishment

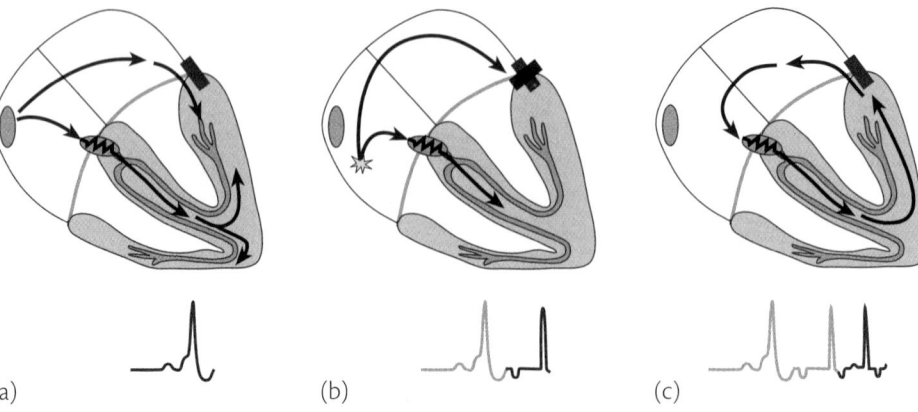

Fig. 16.4.31 Atrioventricular re-entry tachycardia. Mechanism of initiation by atrial extrasystole. See text for details: if the accessory pathway were concealed the ECG in sinus rhythm would not show the characteristic delta wave.

(a)   (b)   (c)

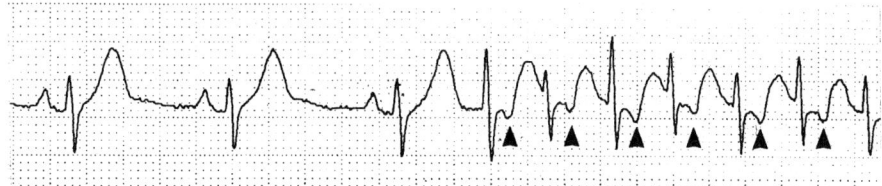

Fig. 16.4.32 Initiation of atrioventricular re-entry tachycardia. The third sinus beat is followed by the onset of narrow-complex tachycardia, initiated by an atrial extrasystole (obscured by T-wave). Retrograde atrial activation, with inverted P waves in the ST segment (arrows), are seen during tachycardia.

of a re-entry circuit (Fig. 16.4.32c). Since the circuit involves activation of the ventricles via the His–Purkinje system, the QRS morphology during re-entry tachycardia is normal, unless a rate-related bundle branch block develops.

A rare form of AV re-entry tachycardia has anterograde conduction via the accessory pathway and retrograde conduction via the AV node (antidromic tachycardia). The QRS morphology of this tachycardia is grossly abnormal with appearances dependent upon the site of insertion of the accessory pathway.

Pre-excited atrial fibrillation

The major prognostic concern in Wolff–Parkinson–White syndrome is pre-excited atrial fibrillation. Conduction via an accessory pathway with a short refractory period, bypassing the normal AV nodal slowing, may result in very rapid ventricular conduction (Fig. 16.4.34) that can degenerate into ventricular fibrillation. The degree of pre-excitation during atrial fibrillation varies, giving a characteristic pattern of an irregular ventricular response with QRS morphology ranging from normal to fully pre-excited. The risk of sudden death is increased if the shortest R–R interval is <250 ms during pre-excited atrial fibrillation, and is an indication for urgent cardioversion and early radiofrequency ablation.

Management of the symptomatic patient with ventricular pre-excitation

The AV node is a part of the re-entry circuit in both ortho- and antidromic tachycardia, and adenosine and other AV nodal blocking drugs may be effective. However, adenosine may precipitate pre-excited atrial fibrillation and should be used with caution. In patients with known Wolff–Parkinson–White syndrome presenting with AV re-entrant tachycardia, drugs which also act on the accessory pathway such as flecainide or sotalol may be preferred. In pre-excited atrial fibrillation, AV nodal blocking drugs such as digoxin or verapamil should be avoided, because of the risk of ventricular fibrillation; treatment should be with antiarrhythmic therapy such as flecainide or by DC cardioversion. Patients with symptomatic Wolff–Parkinson–White syndrome should be offered radiofrequency

ablation as first-line therapy. This abolishes the risk of pre-excited atrial fibrillation as well as preventing further attacks of AV re-entry tachycardia. Careful mapping of the AV annulus using an electrode catheter is necessary to identify the site of the accessory pathway, at which the interval between the atrial and ventricular electrograms is at a minimum. Passage of the radiofrequency current causes heating of the catheter tip and results in the disappearance of accessory pathway conduction within a few seconds (Fig. 16.4.35). The success rate of ablation varies according to the location of the pathway, but is usually over 90% in experienced hands.

Approach to the asymptomatic patient with ventricular pre-excitation

Patients with Wolff–Parkinson–White syndrome should be evaluated carefully for the risk of pre-excited atrial fibrillation, even in the absence of symptoms. The risk of sudden death due to rapid pre-excited atrial fibrillation is very low among those who have not had any symptomatic tachycardias, but is higher in symptomatic patients. If pre-excitation is intermittent, this indicates a long refractory period of the pathway and a low risk of life-threatening tachycardias. Abrupt disappearance of the delta wave in response to exercise testing, or during Holter monitoring, or with the administration of a class Ia or Ic antiarrhythmic drug, also suggests a low risk. Some centres advocate diagnostic electrophysiological studies to identify a high-risk group with short pathway refractory periods and inducible tachycardia or pre-excited atrial fibrillation. The general tendency is for accessory pathway conduction to become slower with increasing age, and spontaneous disappearance of conduction is well documented.

Other pre-excitation syndromes

Other forms of pre-excitation include the Mahaim pathway, a direct AV or atriofasicular connection with slow conduction properties similar to AV nodal tissue. Evidence for direct atrionodal pathways associated with a short PR interval but no delta wave (Lown–Ganong–Levine syndrome) remains controversial and has not been established histologically.

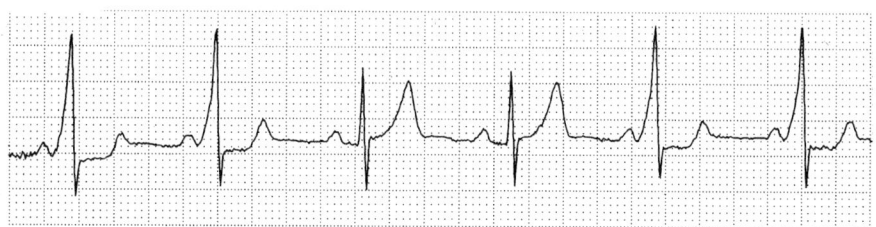

Fig. 16.4.33 Intermittent pre-excitation in Wolff–Parkinson–White syndrome. The first two beats show the characteristic short PR interval and delta wave. The middle two beats, however, show that the pre-excitation was intermittent. The pathway has become refractory, with normal PR interval and QRS morphology. Pathway conduction returns to cause pre-excitation in the final two beats.

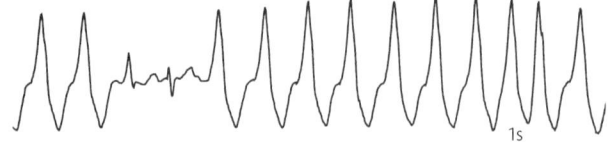

Fig. 16.4.34 Pre-excited atrial fibrillation. Conduction via an accessory pathway results in an irregular wide-complex tachycardia. The third and fourth beats show less pre-excitation, with activation mainly through the normal conducting system, with more normal QRS-complex morphology. Lead V1.

Ventricular tachycardia

Definitions

Ventricular tachycardia is defined as the presence of three or more consecutive ventricular beats at a rate of 120/min or greater. It is considered to be sustained if an individual salvo lasts for 30 s or more, and nonsustained if the duration is between 3 beats and 30 s. Monomorphic ventricular tachycardia demonstrates a consistent QRS morphology during each paroxysm,. Polymorphic ventricular tachycardia demonstrates a constantly changing QRS morphology, often without discrete QRS complexes. Polymorphic ventricular tachycardia may degenerate into ventricular fibrillation and the electrocardiographic distinction between the two is difficult. Torsades de pointes is a polymorphic VT in association with QT interval prolongation and is discussed in more detail later in the chapter.

ECG characteristics

The presence of AV dissociation is a particularly important feature to seek in a wide-complex tachycardia as it makes the diagnosis of ventricular tachycardia virtually certain (Fig. 16.4.36a). A careful search for P-waves perturbing the QRS complex or T-waves is necessary, ideally using multilead recordings. Occasionally, a fortuitously timed P-wave allows the development of a capture beat of normal QRS morphology without interrupting the tachycardia.

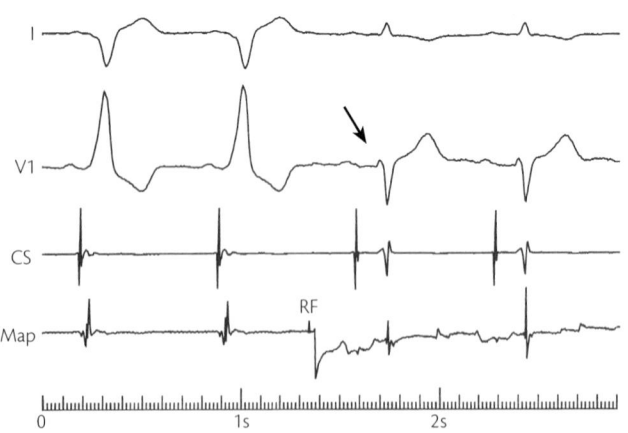

Fig. 16.4.35 Radiofrequency ablation of an accessory pathway. The patient had Wolff–Parkinson–White syndrome with evidence of ventricular pre-excitation on the surface electrogram during sinus rhythm (short PR interval, delta wave). One beat after switching on the radiofrequency (RF) current the QRS becomes normal, indicating successful ablation of the accessory pathway. This was a left-sided accessory pathway, as shown by the short interval between left atrial and left ventricular activation recorded from the coronary sinus (CS). This interval is prolonged following ablation of the pathway. Surface leads I, V1, and intracardiac electrograms from CS and mapping catheter (Map) are shown.

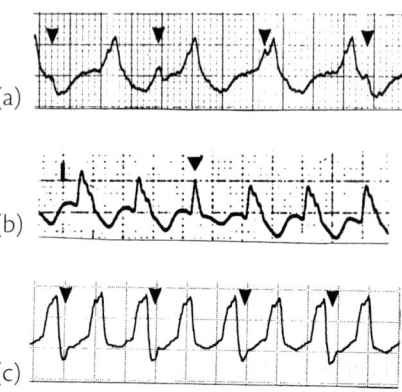

Fig. 16.4.36 Sustained monomorphic ventricular tachycardia. (a) Ventricular tachycardia with atrioventricular dissociation. P-waves (arrowed) are seen to have no relationship to the ventricular activation. Lead V1. (b) Ventricular tachycardia with fusion beat (arrow). Lead V1. (c) Ventricular tachycardia with 2:1 ventriculoatrial conduction. Lead III. Inverted P-waves (arrows) follow every second ventricular complex.

A fusion beat occurs when activation of the ventricle is partly via the normal His–Purkinje system and partly from the tachycardia focus (Fig. 16.4.36b). Fusion and capture beats are diagnostic of ventricular tachycardia, but are commonly present only if the ventricular rate is relatively slow. Where dissociated P-wave activity cannot be recognized with certainty on the surface ECG, direct recording of atrial activity by an oesophageal or right atrial electrogram may aid the diagnosis. Although AV dissociation is diagnostic of ventricular tachycardia, it is not invariable. Retrograde ventriculoatrial conduction may occur, giving either 1:1 conduction or higher degrees of block (Fig. 16.4.36c).

The QRS duration in ventricular tachycardia is commonly greater than 0.12 s, and values greater than 0.14 s are particularly suggestive of ventricular tachycardia. Although the QRS morphology may superficially resemble left or right bundle branch block, the morphology is commonly atypical (see Fig. 16.4.16). Ventricular tachycardia arising from the right ventricular free wall has a left bundle branch block-like pattern, whereas left ventricular free wall tachycardias show right bundle branch block morphology. The presence of concordant positive or negative QRS complexes across the chest leads is suggestive of ventricular tachycardia, as is the existence of extreme axis deviation. Electrocardiographic features consistent with VT are listed in Fig. 16.4.16.

Aetiology

Sustained monomorphic ventricular tachycardia commonly occurs in the presence of structural heart disease, but also arises in structurally normal hearts. It rarely occurs in the acute phase of myocardial infarction, but may be seen in the subacute phase (>48 h), or may arise many years later, particularly in association with left ventricular dilatation and aneurysm formation. The arrhythmia also occurs in other conditions associated with ventricular dilatation or fibrosis such as dilated cardiomyopathy, hypertrophic cardiomyopathy, or previous ventriculotomy (e.g. following repair of Fallot's tetralogy). Ventricular tachycardia may degenerate into ventricular fibrillation (see below). Sustained monomorphic tachycardia can occur as a proarrhythmic response to antiarrhythmic drugs, particularly class I agents.

Although ventricular tachycardia normally occurs in individuals with overt heart disease, it is also seen in young and apparently healthy subjects. In these, occult cardiac disease or cardiac genetic syndromes should be considered (see below). There remain a few patients with documented ventricular tachycardia in whom no structural heart disease is evident on clinical, ECG, or echocardiographic examination. The tachycardia may arise from the outflow tract of the right or (rarely) left ventricle, or from one of the fascicles of the left bundle branch, and is amenable to radiofrequency ablation.

Acute management of ventricular tachycardia

Rapid ventricular tachycardia may present with cardiac arrest, syncope, shock, anginal chest pain, or left ventricular failure, but slower tachycardias in patients with preserved cardiac function may be well tolerated. Sustained ventricular tachycardia is a medical emergency. If the patient is pulseless or unconscious, immediate DC cardioversion is necessary. If the patient is conscious but hypotensive, urgent DC cardioversion under general anaesthesia or deep sedation is used. Haemodynamically tolerated tachycardias may be terminated by drug therapy (see Fig. 16.4.17). Adenosine may be administered if there is diagnostic uncertainty, but is likely to be ineffective (see Table 16.4.5). Intravenous lidocaine (lignocaine) 100 mg, repeated if necessary after 5 min, may restore sinus rhythm in about 30% of patients, and is usually well tolerated. Sotalol 1.5 mg/kg intravenously is more effective, but its use is restricted by its negative inotropic action. Second-line drugs for the termination of ventricular tachycardia include procainamide, disopyramide, and amiodarone. Amiodarone has a relatively slow onset of action but may be effective if the tachycardia is well tolerated. Flecainide is contraindicated in view of the risk of developing incessant tachycardia. Verapamil should be avoided as it may cause clinical deterioration. The only exception to this is in the rare instance of patients with structurally normal hearts who have ventricular tachycardia that is known to respond to verapamil, e.g. left ventricular fascicular tachycardia. All antiarrhythmic drugs have significant negative inotropic actions that may further impair the haemodynamic status of the patient if sinus rhythm is not restored. For this reason, no more than one antiarrhythmic drug should normally be given before recourse to alternative therapy, usually DC cardioversion. Overdrive termination of ventricular tachycardia following insertion of a temporary pacing lead may be effective, particularly if the tachycardia is relatively slow. Facilities for cardioversion must be available in view of the risk of acceleration or degeneration into ventricular fibrillation.

Secondary prevention

Ventricular tachycardia is a potentially life-threatening condition. Unless the acute episode was clearly precipitated by some transient or reversible factor, there is a high probability of recurrent attacks, which may result in sudden death. Prognosis is worse if the arrhythmia was poorly tolerated, or if there is severe left ventricular dysfunction. The 3-year cardiac survival rate varies from 80% in patients in whom arrhythmia induction is suppressed by antiarrhythmic drug therapy to 40% in those in whom no effect of suppression is achieved and/or empirical therapy is used.

Clinical evaluation of the patient after restoration of sinus rhythm should be supported by electrocardiography, echocardiography, and/or radionuclide ventriculography. In those with ischaemic heart disease, exercise testing should be undertaken to identify the presence of reversible ischaemia, which may act as a trigger to ventricular tachycardia, and coronary arteriography to determine the extent of arterial disease. Unless there is a clear precipitating factor such as drug toxicity, electrolyte abnormality, or acute ischaemia, the risk of sudden death is high and patients should be considered for an ICD (see Fig. 16.4.20). A meta-analysis of three secondary prevention trials of patients resuscitated from ventricular fibrillation or ventricular tachycardia causing haemodynamic compromise showed defibrillators to be better than antiarrhythmic drug therapy in preventing death from any cause (Fig. 16.4.37a).

Primary prevention

Patients with left ventricular dysfunction of any cause are at risk of sudden death from ventricular tachycardia or fibrillation and implantable defibrillators are appropriate for a subgroup of these patients as part of a primary prevention strategy. Those with nonsustained ventricular tachycardia, in whom sustained tachycardia can be induced at electrophysiological testing, have a better survival with defibrillator implantation compared with drug therapy. The Sudden Cardiac Death in Heart Failure Trial (SCD-HeFT) expanded the indications to include patients with class II/III heart failure and an ejection fraction <30%, even in the absence of known arrhythmia (Fig. 16.4.37b). Patients with a QRS duration greater than 120 ms appear to derive the largest benefit.

Antiarrhythmic therapy

Implantable defibrillator therapy is not affordable in all countries, and not appropriate for patients with other conditions causing a severely limited prognosis. Medical therapy is necessary for many patients, but is limited by a relative lack of evidence from randomized controlled trials. β-Adrenoceptor blockers are comparable to conventional antiarrhythmic agents in the prevention of recurrent ventricular tachyarrhythmias. Since they have been shown to reduce the risk of sudden death in unselected survivors of myocardial infarction and in patients with chronic heart failure, they should be used routinely in the prophylaxis of ventricular tachycardia if tolerated. Of the conventional antiarrhythmic agents, there is evidence that the class III drugs sotalol and amiodarone are superior to class I antiarrhythmic agents, which should not be used for this indication. However, sotalol and amiodarone have not been tested against placebo or conventional β-adrenoceptor blockers in randomized trials, although observational studies suggest they are of benefit in the prevention of arrhythmic death.

Other therapies

Radiofrequency ablation is used in the management of ventricular tachycardia, particularly in those with no structural heart disease. Right ventricular outflow tract and fascicular tachycardia are particularly amenable to ablation. Location and ablation of critical areas of slow conduction in ventricular tachycardias of an ischaemic origin is feasible but technically difficult. Success rates are lower than for other types of ablation and this approach is often reserved for the treatment of frequently recurrent tachycardia in patients with implantable defibrillators.

Direct surgical management of recurrent ventricular tachycardia involves aneurysmectomy, endocardial mapping, and resection of the subendocardial area containing the micro re-entry circuit. The indications for surgery have been reduced considerably since the advent of the ICD, since the surgical mortality is up to 10 to 15%, compared with 0.5% for defibrillator implantation. Where medically intractable ventricular tachyarrhythmias are associated with very poor left ventricular function, the only possible therapeutic option is cardiac transplantation.

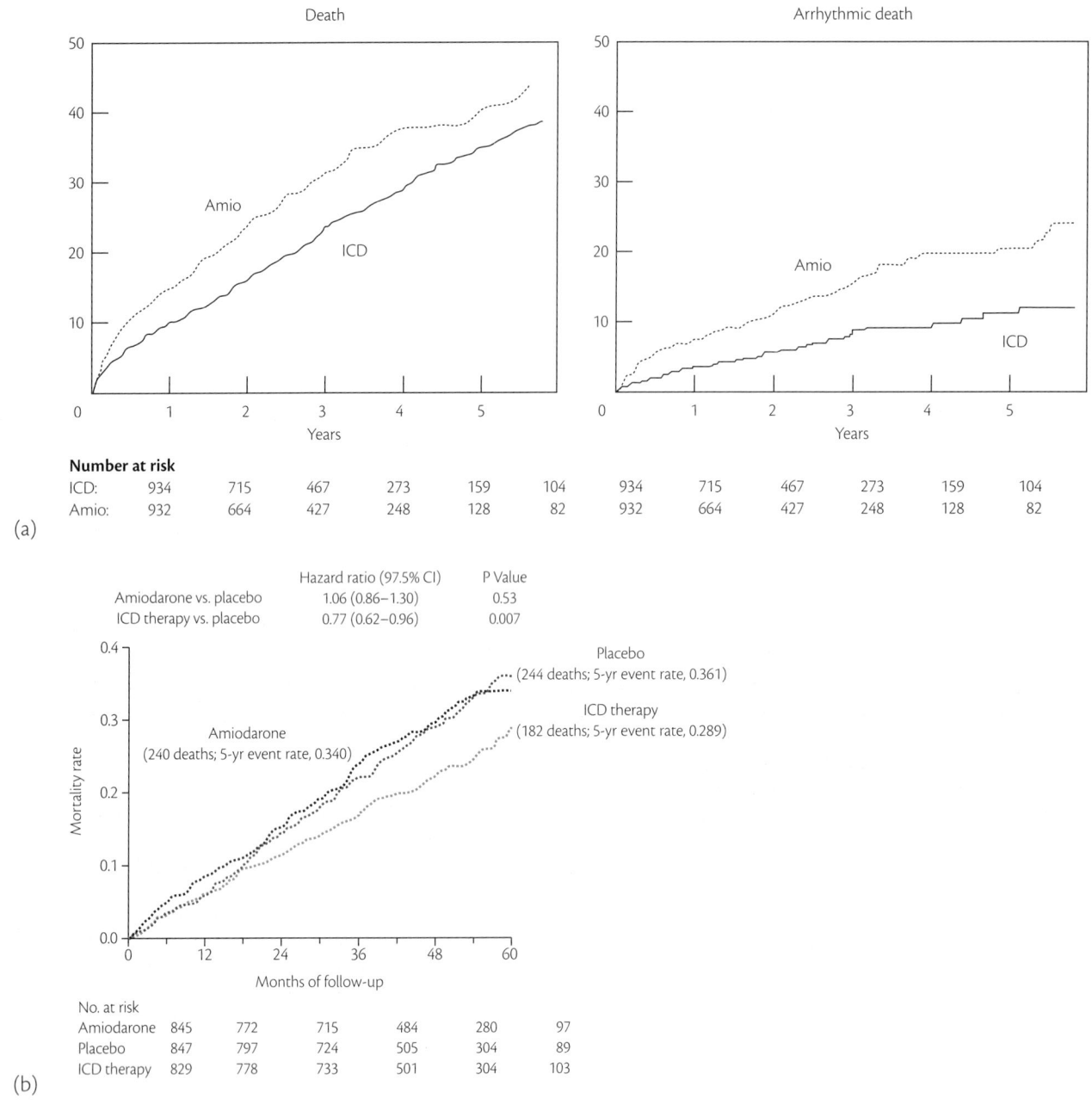

Fig. 16.4.37 Improved survival with the implantable cardioverter defibrillator (ICD). (a) Cumulative risk of fatal events for ICD or amiodarone (amio) from a meta-analysis of trials of secondary prevention, showing reduced death with ICD (left panel), due to reduced arrhythmic death (right panel). (b) Improved survival with ICD compared to amiodarone or placebo in a study of primary prevention in patients with heart failure.

a) Reproduced with permission from Connolly SJ et al, *European Heart Journal* (2007) 28, 1598–1660.

b) Bardy GH, et al (2005), New England Journal of Medicine 352, 230. Copyright ©2005 Massachusetts Medical Society. All rights reserved.

Nonsustained ventricular tachycardia

The mechanism and causes of nonsustained ventricular tachycardia (Fig. 16.4.38) are similar to those of sustained ventricular tachycardia. There is often slight variation in the RR interval, particularly if the salvo involves only a few beats. Short salvos of nonsustained ventricular tachycardia are often asymptomatic. Apart from the instances where nonsustained ventricular tachycardia produces troublesome symptoms, the major clinical significance of the arrhythmia is as a risk marker for sustained ventricular tachycardia or sudden cardiac death in patients with left ventricular dysfunction or hypertrophy. Patients with structural heart disease, in particular those with severe left ventricular dysfunction, with QRS duration >120 ms or inducible ventricular arrhythmias, should be considered for an implantable defibrillator as primary prevention of sudden cardiac death. If no significant organic heart disease is present, and the patient is asymptomatic, no treatment is indicated as long-term follow-up of such patients indicates a good prognosis with no excess risk of sudden death.

Polymorphic ventricular tachycardia

Polymorphic ventricular tachycardia is an unstable rhythm with varying QRS morphology. It is most commonly seen in the acute

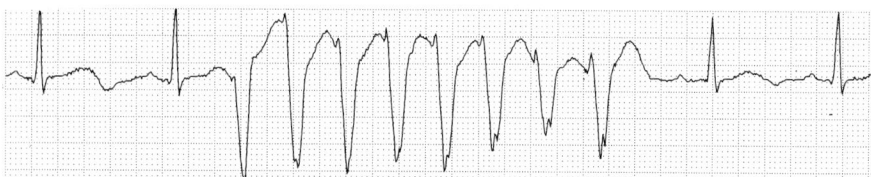

Fig. 16.4.38 Nonsustained ventricular tachycardia.

phase of myocardial infarction and is due to unstable re-entry circuits. As such, it either undergoes spontaneous termination or degenerates into ventricular fibrillation. If episodes of polymorphic ventricular tachycardia are frequent in the early hours of myocardial infarction, they can be suppressed by intravenous lidocaine (lignocaine), although there is no evidence that this improves survival. Short, infrequent episodes are commonly left untreated.

Torsades de pointes and the long-QT syndromes

Torsades de pointes is a characteristic type of polymorphic ventricular tachycardia with a typical undulating variation in QRS morphology as a result of variation in axis. It occurs in association with a prolonged QT interval during sinus rhythm. Long-QT syndromes may be acquired or congenital. The latter are discussed later in the chapter.

Aetiology

Although class Ia and III antiarrhythmic drugs are the best-known causes of acquired long QT syndrome, a very large number of noncardiac drugs inhibit the outward potassium current I_{Kr}, and may cause significant lengthening of the QT interval singly or in combination (Table 16.4.8). Episodes of torsades de pointes are often multifactorial in origin, with prolongation of the QT interval by an I_{kr} inhibitor in association with predisposing factors such as bradycardia or pauses, hypokalaemia, or hypomagnesaemia. All of these predispose to early after-depolarizations *in vitro* and this mechanism appears to be the likely cause of torsades de pointes in the acquired syndromes. The prognosis of the acquired long QT syndromes is excellent, provided the underlying predisposing

factors are identified and corrected. However, it is increasingly recognized that there is a genetic predisposition to the development of acquired long QT syndrome in the face of predisposing factors, leading to the concept that patients developing acquired long QT syndrome have reduced 'repolarization reserve' as a result of a *forme fruste* of the congenital syndrome.

ECG characteristics

Torsades de pointes is an atypical ventricular tachycardia characterized by a continuously varying QRS axis ('twisting of points') (Fig. 16.4.39). Episodes of torsades are commonly repetitive and normally self-terminating, although they may degenerate into ventricular fibrillation. Paroxysms of torsades de pointes are associated in the preceding beats with evidence of marked QT prolongation, and frequently with morphological abnormalities of the T-wave such as T–U fusion, gross increases in T-wave amplitude, or T-wave alternans. In the acquired long-QT syndromes a slowing of the heart rate, and in particular a postextrasystolic pause, is often associated with initiation of the arrhythmia. This produces a characteristic 'short–long–short' sequence of initiation (Fig. 16.4.39).

Acute management

The common clinical presentation is of recurrent dizziness or syncope, and the condition may easily be misdiagnosed as self-terminating polymorphic ventricular tachycardia or ventricular fibrillation unless the characteristic morphology of torsades de pointes and the associated QT interval prolongation is recognized. It is essential to discontinue predisposing drugs or other agents and to avoid empirical antiarrhythmic drug therapy, which may worsen the arrhythmia. Individual paroxysms of torsades de pointes are normally self-limiting, but if they are persistent, cardiac arrest will occur and emergency defibrillation is necessary. Intravenous magnesium sulphate (8 mmol over 10–15 min, repeated if necessary) is

Table 16.4.8 Causes or contributory factors in acquired long-QT syndromes

Drug induced	Antiarrhythmic drugs —classes ia, iii
	Macrolide antibiotics —erythromycin
	Antifungals —ketoconazole
	Vasodilators —prenylamine, ketanserin, lidoflazine
	Psychotropics —tricyclic/tetracyclic antidepressants, antipsychotics
	Antihistamines —terfenadine, astemizole
	Cholinergic antagonists —cisapride
	Synthetic opioid —methadone
Electrolyte disturbances	Hypokalaemia, hypomagnesaemia, hypocalcaemia
Metabolic	Hypothyroidism, starvation, anorexia nervosa, liquid protein diet
Bradycardia	Sinoatrial disease, AV block
Toxins	Organophosphorous insecticides, heavy metal poisoning

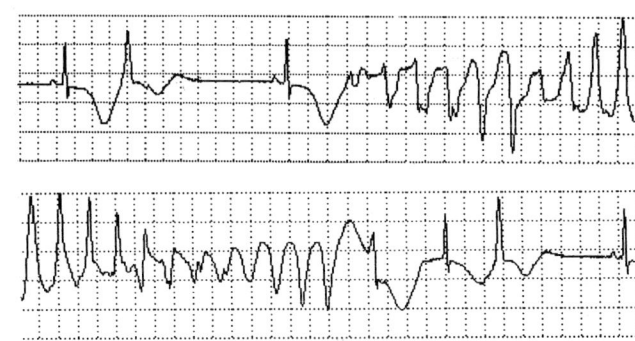

Fig. 16.4.39 *Torsades de pointes.* Note the marked QT interval prolongation in the sinus beats, and the "short-long" pattern of RR intervals immediately prior to initiation of the arrhythmia. Ambulatory monitoring recording is shown (continuous tracing).

a safe and effective emergency measure for the prevention of recurrent paroxysms of tachycardia. If torsades de pointes is associated with bradycardia and pauses, the heart rate should be increased to between 90 and 100/min by atrial or ventricular pacing or isoproterenol (isoprenaline) infusion. Hypokalaemia should be sought and corrected if necessary.

Accelerated idioventricular rhythm

The term 'accelerated idioventricular rhythm' is used to describe a continuous ventricular rhythm with a rate less than 120/min. Idioventricular rhythm commonly occurs in the setting of acute myocardial infarction and appears to be a marker of successful reperfusion therapy. No active treatment is necessary.

Ventricular fibrillation

Ventricular fibrillation is defined as a chaotic, disorganized arrhythmia with no identifiable QRS complexes (Fig. 16.4.40). The mechanism is of multiple, unstable re-entry circuits. The electrocardiographic pattern depends on the duration of fibrillation: recent-onset fibrillation is described as 'coarse', with a peak-to-peak amplitude of around 1 mV (1 cm). With increasing duration of cardiac arrest, the amplitude of ventricular fibrillation diminishes and such 'fine' ventricular fibrillation is less likely to be amenable to successful electrical defibrillation.

Ventricular fibrillation may occur during acute myocardial ischaemia often initiated by an R on T extrasystole, and is the principal cause of death in the first 2 h following acute myocardial infarction (Fig. 16.4.40). Ventricular fibrillation during myocardial infarction is subdivided into primary, occurring without warning in an otherwise stable patient, and secondary, where fibrillation occurs in the context of left ventricular failure or cardiogenic shock. Ventricular fibrillation occurring in chronic heart disease is most commonly a result of degeneration of rapid ventricular tachycardia, whose causes have been described above. Rarer causes of fibrillation are listed in Box 14.4.4.

Ventricular fibrillation is rarely self-terminating, and normally causes cardiac arrest with the rapid onset of pulselessness, unconsciousness, and apnoea. The management of cardiac arrest due to ventricular fibrillation is discussed in Chapter 17.1.

Patients who survive an episode of ventricular fibrillation should be assessed carefully to determine the risk of recurrence. If ventricular fibrillation has occurred in the first few hours of a typical ST-elevation myocardial infarction, the risk of recurrent cardiac arrest is low, and no specific prophylactic therapy other than assessment and treatment of residual ischaemia and conventional postinfarction β-blockade is indicated. However, in many instances ventricular fibrillation arises as a result of acute ischaemia in patients with known, extensive heart disease who have not sustained an acute infarction. These patients remain at high risk of

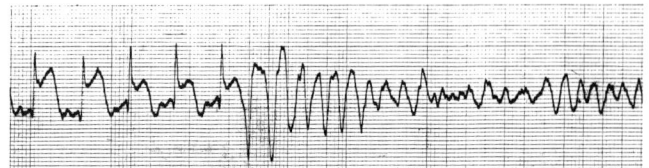

Fig. 16.4.40 Ventricular fibrillation complicating acute myocardial infarction. The arrhythmia is initiated by an 'R on T' ventricular extrasystole.

Box 16.4.4 Causes of ventricular fibrillation

- Acute myocardial ischaemia
- Acute myocardial infarction—primary or secondary
- Advanced organic heart disease with poor LV or RV function
- Severe LV hypertrophy
- Ventricular tachycardia/torsades de pointes
- Electrical—electrocution, lightning, unsynchronized DC shock, competitive ventricular pacing
- Pre-excited atrial fibrillation
- Profound bradycardia
- Hypoxia, acidosis
- Genetic syndromes (e.g. long QT-syndrome, Brugada syndrome)

---

recurrent ventricular fibrillation, and should be evaluated fully by exercise testing and coronary arteriography with a view to revascularization, and managed with an ICD or antiarrhythmic therapy as discussed in the section on ventricular tachycardia.

Genetic syndromes

Congenital long-QT syndromes

The congenital long-QT syndromes are inherited conditions due to mutations in genes encoding ion channel proteins. They are mainly autosomal dominant and are subclassified according to the underlying gene defect (Table 16.4.9). Most cases are either LQT1 or LQT2, due to mutations affecting either the slow (I_{Ks}) or rapid (I_{Kr}) components of the outward potassium current. In the less common LQT3, the inward sodium current (I_{Na}) is affected. Lengthening of ventricular repolarisation, and hence of the QT interval, occur as a result either of reduced outward current flow via I_{Kr} or I_{Ks} or increased duration of current flow via I_{Na}. The arrhythmia, torsades de pointes, has characteristics consistent with triggered activity.

Attacks of torsades de pointes in the congenital syndromes are commonly associated with sympathetic stimulation such as exercise, waking, or fright, and are associated with increases in sinus rate. Cardiac events are particularly associated with exercise in LQT1, with auditory stimulation in LQT2, and can occur during sleep in LQT3.

Table 16.4.9 Congenital long-QT syndromes

Subtype	Chromosome	Gene	Protein	Ion current affected	Frequency
LQT1	11	KCNQ1	KvLQT1	$\downarrow I_{Ks}$	c.50%
LQT2	7	KCNH2	HERG	$\downarrow I_{Kr}$	30–40%
LQT3	3	SCN5A	Nav 1.5	$\uparrow I_{Na}$	5–10%
LQT4	4	ANK2	Ankyrin-B	$\downarrow$ Multiple	Rare
LQT5	21	KCNE1	minK	$\downarrow I_{Ks}$	Rare
LQT6	21	KCNE2	MiRP1	$\downarrow I_{Kr}$	Rare
LQT7	17	KCNJ2	Kir2.1	$\downarrow I_{K1}$	Rare
LQT8	12	CACNA1C	Cav1.2	$\uparrow I_{CaL}$	Rare

Paroxysms may produce syncope, which if prolonged may be complicated by convulsion, leading to misdiagnosis as epilepsy. A family history of recurrent syncope or sudden death may be obtained. Sinus bradycardia is commonly seen in these syndromes.

The prognosis of untreated congenital long-QT syndrome is poor, with a high incidence of sudden death in childhood. Increased risk of syncope or sudden death is associated with a corrected QT interval (QTc) of more than 500 ms. Males with LQT3 are at increased risk regardless of the degree of QT interval prolongation. LQT1 has a better prognosis than other subtypes. Episodes of torsades de pointes and T wave alternans on Holter monitoring also confer a higher risk.

β-Blockers are highly effective in LQT1 but are less protective in LQT2 and LQT3. Selective high left stellate ganglionectomy has been employed successfully in cases with recurrent events despite β-blockers. Permanent pacing at rates of 70 to 80/min, in combination with β-blockers, may also be effective in reducing symptoms but defibrillator implantation is necessary for resistant cases, and is commonly used as first-line therapy if episodes of torsades de pointes have resulted in cardiac arrest or in those thought to be at high risk of sudden death.

Short-QT syndrome

This is a recently described entity with autosomal dominant inheritance characterized by a gain of function mutation in the outward potassium currents (I_{Kr} and I_{Ks}). It produces a markedly shortened QTc, often less than 280 ms, and predisposes to atrial and ventricular fibrillation.

Brugada syndrome

The Brugada syndrome is an autosomal dominant condition which has a risk of sudden cardiac death associated with characteristic ECG abnormalities and a structurally normal heart. There is an unusual pattern of variable ST-segment elevation and partial right bundle branch block in the right precordial leads, associated with a risk of polymorphic ventricular tachycardia and sudden death. Mutations of genes encoding the rapid sodium channel (SCN5a), causing partial inactivation, have been identified in about 20% of patients. Patients with a history of syncope or a family history of sudden death should be considered for defibrillator therapy.

Catecholaminergic polymorphic ventricular tachycardia

This is a rare arrhythmia characterized by polymorphic or bidirectional ventricular tachycardia occurring in situations of strenuous exercise, psychological stress or emotion, often presenting in childhood. It is associated with mutations of genes involved in controlling intracellular calcium handling. Mutations of the cardiac ryanodine receptor have autosomal dominant transmission, whereas mutations of the gene encoding for calsequestrin have autosomal recessive transmission. The resting ECG has no diagnostic features and the heart is structurally normal. β-Blockers may prevent syncope but an ICD may be indicated for recurrent symptoms or high risk of cardiac arrest.

Hypertrophic cardiomyopathy

Hypertrophic cardiomyopathy has a prevalence of 0.2% in the population, and is associated with a wide range of mutations encoding structural or regulatory proteins of the cardiac myofibrillar apparatus. The mode of inheritance is autosomal dominant in 70% of cases, with variable penetrance. Although symptoms are often related to impaired haemodynamics, left ventricular hypertrophy and myofibrillar disarray increase the risk of re-entrant arrhythmias and sudden death. Patients with sustained ventricular tachycardia or fibrillation should be considered for defibrillator therapy. Risk assessment should be performed in all patients with hypertrophic cardiomyopathy. Unexplained syncope, nonsustained ventricular tachycardia, ventricular septal thickness greater than 3 cm, a family history of sudden cardiac death, and a hypotensive response to exercise are all associated with increased risk. An ICD may be considered if two or more high-risk features are present. See Chapter 16.7.2 for further discussion.

Arrhythmogenic right ventricular cardiomyopathy

Arrhythmogenic right ventricular cardiomyopathy (dysplasia) is an autosomal dominant condition associated with replacement of the right ventricular free wall with fat and fibrous tissue. These patients may have no symptoms or signs of cardiac disease, but typical ECG changes (epsilon wave in V1, or T wave inversion in the right precordial leads) are associated with variable degrees of dilatation of the right ventricle demonstratable by echocardiography or MRI. This creates a substrate for ventricular tachycardia and fibrillation and many patients will ultimately require defibrillator therapy.

Further reading

Diagnosis and treatment

Echt DS, *et al.* (1991). Mortality and morbidity in patients receiving encainide, flecainide, or placebo. *N Engl J Med*, **324**, 781–8.

Eckardt L, *et al.* (2006). Approach to wide complex tachycardias in patients without structural heart disease. *Heart*, **92**, 704–11.

Hall MC, Todd DM. (2006) Modern management of arrhythmias. *Postgrad Med J*, **82**, 117–25.

Morady F. (1999). Radio-frequency ablation as treatment for cardiac arrhythmia. *N Engl J Med*, **340**, 534–44.

Roden DM. (2000). Antiarrhythmic drugs: from mechanisms to clinical practice. *Heart*, **84**, 339–46.

Bradycardia

Fitzpatrick A, Sutton R. (1992). A guide to temporary pacing. *BMJ*, **304**, 365–9.

Gammage MD. (2000). Temporary cardiac pacing. *Heart*, **83**, 715–20.

Gregoratos G, *et al.* (2002) ACC/AHA/NASPE 2002 guideline update for implantation of cardiac pacemakers and antiarrhythmia devices: a report of the American College of Cardiology/American Heart Association Task Force on Practice Guidelines (ACC/AHA/NASPE Committee on Pacemaker Implantation). *Circulation*, **106**, 2145–61.

Healey JS, *et al.* (2006) Cardiovascular outcomes with atrial-based pacing compared with ventricular pacing: meta-analysis of randomized trials, using individual patient data. *Circulation*, **114**, 11–17.

Morley-Davies A, Cobbe SM (1997). Cardiac pacing. *Lancet*, **349**, 41–6.

Atrial arrhythmias

Calkins H, *et al.* (2007) HRS/EHRA/ECAS Expert Consensus Statement on Catheter and Surgical Ablation of Atrial Fibrillation: Recommendations for Personnel, Policy, Procedures and Follow-Up: A report of the Heart Rhythm Society (HRS) Task Force on Catheter and Surgical Ablation of Atrial Fibrillation developed in partnership with the European Heart Rhythm Association (EHRA) and the European Cardiac Arrhythmia Society (ECAS). *Europace*, **9**, 335–79.

Camm AJ, Savelieva I (2007). Some patients with paroxysmal atrial fibrillation should carry flecainide or propafenone to self treat. *BMJ*, **334**, 637.

Earley MJ, Schilling RJ. (2006) Catheter and surgical ablation of atrial fibrillation. *Heart*, **92**, 266–74.

Fuster V, *et al.* (2006) ACC/AHA/ESC 2006 Guidelines for the Management of Patients with Atrial Fibrillation: a report of the American College of Cardiology/American Heart Association Task Force on Practice Guidelines and the European Society of Cardiology Committee for Practice Guidelines. *Circulation*, **114**, e257–354.

Haïssaguerre M, *et al.* (1998). Spontaneous initiation of atrial fibrillation by ectopic beats originating in the pulmonary veins. *N Engl J Med*, **339**, 659–66.

Hart RG, Pearce LA, Aguilar M. (2007) Meta-analysis: antithrombotic therapy to prevent stroke in patients who have nonvalvular atrial fibrillation. *Ann Intern Med*, **146**, 857–67.

Lip GY, Boos CJ. (2006) Antithrombotic treatment in atrial fibrillation. *Heart*, **92**, 155–61.

Wijffels MCEF, *et al.* (1995). Atrial fibrillation begets atrial fibrillation: a study in awake chronically instrumented goats. *Circulation*, **92**, 1954–68.

Wyse DG, *et al.* (2002). A comparison of rate control and rhythm control in patients with atrial fibrillation. *N Engl J Med*, **347**, 1825–33.

Supraventricular tachycardias

Blomstrom-Lundquist C, *et al.* (2003). ACC/AHA/ESC guidelines for the management of patients with supraventricular arrhythmias—executive summary: a report of the American College of Cardiology/American Heart Association Task Force on Practice Guidelines and the European Society of Cardiology Committee for Practice Guidelines. *Circulation*, **108**, 1871–909.

Calkins H. (2001) Radiofrequency catheter ablation of supraventricular arrhythmias. *Heart*, **85**, 594–600. [Review of the role of catheter ablation in the management of patients with supraventricular tachycardia.]

Holdgate A, Foo A. (2006) Adenosine versus intravenous calcium channel antagonists for the treatment of supraventricular tachycardia in adults. *Cochrane Database Syst Rev*, **4**, CD005154.

Ventricular arrhythmias

Bardy GH, *et al.* (2005). Amiodarone or an implantable cardioverter-defibrillator for congestive heart failure. *N Engl J Med*, **352**, 225–37.

Connolly SJ, *et al.* (2000) Meta-analysis of the implantable cardioverter defibrillator secondary prevention trials. AVID, CASH and CIDS studies. Antiarrhythmics vs Implantable Defibrillator study. Cardiac Arrest Study Hamburg. Canadian Implantable Defibrillator Study. *Eur Heart J*, **21**, 2071–8.

Gupta A, *et al.* (2007) Current concepts in the mechanisms and management of drug-induced QT prolongation and torsade de pointes. *Am Heart J*, **153**, 891–9.

Zipes DP, *et al.* (2006) ACC/AHA/ESC 2006 Guidelines for Management of Patients With Ventricular Arrhythmias and the Prevention of Sudden Cardiac Death: a report of the American College of Cardiology/American Heart Association Task Force and the European Society of Cardiology Committee for Practice Guidelines. *Circulation*, **114**, e385–484.

Genetic syndromes

Brugada J, Brugada R, Brugada P. (1998). Right bundle branch block and ST-segment elevation in leads V1 through V3: a marker for sudden death in patients without demonstrable structural heart disease. *Circulation*, **97**, 457–60.

Kies P, *et al.* (2006) Arrhythmogenic right ventricular dysplasia/cardiomyopathy: screening, diagnosis, and treatment. *Heart Rhythm*, **3**, 225–34.

Maron BJ, *et al.* (2003). American College of Cardiology/European Society of Cardiology clinical expert consensus document on hypertrophic cardiomyopathy. A report of the American College of Cardiology Foundation Task Force on Clinical Expert Consensus Documents and the European Society of Cardiology Committee for Practice Guidelines. *J Am Coll Cardiol*, **42**, 1687–713.

McKenna WJ, Behr ER. (2002). Hypertrophic cardiomyopathy: management, risk stratification, and prevention of sudden death. *Heart*, **87**, 169–76.

Priori SG, *et al.* (2003). Risk stratification in the long-QT syndrome. *N Engl J Med*, **348**, 1866–74.

Shah M, Akar FG, Tomaselli GF (2005). Molecular basis of arrhythmias. *Circulation*, **112**, 2517–29.

Wilde AA, Bezzina CR (2003). Genetics of cardiac arrhythmias. *Heart*, **91**, 1352–8.

Wilde AA, *et al.* (2002). Proposed diagnostic criteria for the Brugada syndrome: consensus report. *Circulation*, **106**, 2514–19.

16.5

Cardiac failure

Contents

16.5.1 Clinical features and medical treatments

Martin R. Cowie and Badrinath Chandrasekaran

Essentials

Heart failure is a clinical syndrome that results from any structural or functional cardiac disorder that reduces the ability of the heart to function as a pump. It affects 1 to 2% of the population, and mortality may be as high as 30% in the year after diagnosis, falling to between 5 and 10% annually thereafter with best treatment. The most common underlying pathophysiological abnormality is systolic dysfunction of the left ventricle (LV), but a few patients—particularly elderly people—have no obvious valvular or systolic impairment of the heart and are assumed to have diastolic abnormalities.

Clinical features and diagnosis—heart failure is usually associated with dyspnoea, fatigue, and fluid retention, but these are nonspecific, hence diagnosis depends on careful clinical examination supplemented by tests, in particular echocardiography. Measurement of the plasma concentration of B-type natriuretic peptide (BNP) is the best test for ruling out heart failure in a particular patient.

Management

Treatment usually involves lifestyle measures and drug therapy. Implantable devices, such as pacemakers and cardioverter-defibrillators, are being used increasingly, but surgical interventions only apply to a few patients.

Lifestyle measures—few recommendations are supported by a large evidence base, but those that are widely advised include salt restriction (with a maximum daily intake of 6 g), smoking cessation, and supervised exercise training.

Drug therapy—most of the evidence base for the management of heart failure relates to heart failure due to LV systolic dysfunction—'systolic heart failure'; the best management for heart failure due to valvular disease or diastolic heart failure is less clear. Relating to particular drugs (1) diuretics—these are the most effective means of removing retained fluid, and their introduction often produces rapid symptomatic relief; (2) angiotensin-converting enzyme (ACE) inhibitors—in chronic heart failure these reduce the relative risk of death by 23% and of worsening heart failure by 35%; (3) angiotensin receptor blockers (ARBs)—proven in randomized trials to reduce the risk of mortality and heart failure deterioration, and now generally used in patients who cannot tolerate an ACE inhibitor due to cough; (4) β-blockers—reduce the relative risk of death by about 25% and reduce the risk of death from heart failure by 35%; (5) spironolactone—reduces the risk of death by 30% in patients with moderate to severe heart failure despite treatment with diuretic and ACE inhibitor; eplerenone is a more selective aldosterone antagonist that is often prescribed in place of spironolactone if gynaecomastia develops while on that drug. However, it is important to recognize that the treatment of patients with heart failure with diuretics and/or ACE inhibitors or ARBs and/or β-blockers and/or spironolactone (or eplerenone) is often difficult, with problems arising from hypotension, bradycardia, hyperkalaemia, and deterioration of renal function. Close monitoring and careful clinical judgement are required.

Cardiac resynchronization—up to 20% of patients with heart failure have mechanical dyssynchrony due to native left bundle branch block, which means that the interventricular septum and lateral free wall of the LV do not contract at the same time, reducing the efficiency of pumping. An atriobiventricular pacing system, where conventional right atrial and right ventricular pacing wires are supplemented by a third lead placed in a lateral coronary vein via the coronary sinus to allow pacing of the LV system, can reduce the dyssynchrony (cardiac resynchronization therapy, CRT). Large clinical trials have demonstrated that this can produce a substantial reduction in mortality (up to 40%) in patients with left bundle branch block and moderate to severe symptoms of heart failure despite optimal drug therapy. The risk of sudden cardiac death can be further reduced by combining CRT with an implantable cardioverter defibrillator (ICD).

End of life—palliative care skills are an important component of good management of heart failure.

Introduction

Heart failure is a clinical syndrome that results from any structural or functional cardiac disorder that reduces the ability of the heart to function as a pump. Any condition that damages the heart can lead to heart failure.

Heart failure is not in itself a complete diagnosis, which requires consideration of the underlying abnormality of the heart, the severity of the syndrome, the aetiology, the precipitating and exacerbating factors, the identification of concomitant disease relevant to management, and an estimation of prognosis. The diagnosis has serious implications both for the patient and the health care system. Mortality may be as high as 30% in the year after diagnosis, but with optimal drug and device therapy drops to between 5 and 10% annually thereafter. In addition, heart failure impacts on quality of life more than almost any other chronic medical condition. Comorbidity—such as renal dysfunction, cognitive impairment, and chronic airways disease—is common and may complicate management.

Heart failure is common, affecting 1 to 2% of the population, with the average age at diagnosis being 75 years. The management of heart failure accounts for 1 to 2% of the health care budget of most developed countries, largely due to the cost of the often lengthy hospitalizations required to restabilize the syndrome after deterioration.

Diagnosis is increasingly straightforward as a result of improvements in cardiac imaging and biochemical assays. Treatment has changed markedly in the past two decades through better understanding of the underlying pathophysiology and many large clinical trials of drug and devices. In a rapidly changing field, communication between health care professionals, education of patients and carers, and better chronic disease management remain key to improving patient outcomes.

Diagnosis

Heart failure is usually associated with dyspnoea, fatigue, and fluid retention. Other symptoms may include nocturia, anorexia, abdominal bloating and discomfort, constipation, and cerebral symptoms such as confusion, dizziness, and memory impairment. None of these symptoms is specific for heart failure, and several other conditions can present in the same way (Box 16.5.1). Symptoms alone cannot therefore be relied upon to make the diagnosis: good clinical skills with history taking and a careful physical examination need to be supplemented by further tests.

Useful tests in patients with suspected heart failure

A patient with suspected heart failure should have the following investigations:

- 12-lead electrocardiogram (ECG)

> **Box 16.5.1** Other conditions that may present with symptoms similar to heart failure
>
> - Obesity
> - Chest disease—including lung, pleura, diaphragm, or chest wall disease
> - Venous insufficiency in lower limbs
> - Drug-induced ankle swelling (e.g. amlodipine, nifedipine, felodipine)
> - Drug-induced fluid retention (e.g. steroids, NSAIDs)
> - Hypoalbuminaemia
> - Intrinsic renal or hepatic disease
> - Pulmonary embolic disease
> - Depression and/or anxiety
> - Severe anaemia
> - Severe thyroid disease
> - Bilateral renal artery stenosis

- Chest radiograph—principally to exclude other conditions such as lung cancer or pneumonia, but it may help confirm the diagnosis if it shows cardiomegaly and pulmonary congestion
- Blood biochemistry (including urea, creatinine, glucose, electrolytes), haemoglobin, thyroid and liver function tests, and blood lipids
- Urinalysis to detect proteinuria or glycosuria
- Cardiac imaging—usually a transthoracic echocardiogram, which can rapidly provide detailed information about the structure and function of the cardiac chambers, valves, and pericardium

The algorithm for the diagnosis of heart failure currently recommended by the National Institute for Health and Clinical Excellence (NICE) in the United Kingdom is shown in Fig. 16.5.1. Echocardiography is the key imaging test that is generally available.

These tests will not only help confirm the clinical diagnosis, but will also help exclude other pathologies that may masquerade as heart failure, such as renal failure or severe anaemia. They may also identify comorbidities that can influence management. In most cases the investigations described will rapidly confirm the clinical diagnosis of heart failure, but some cases may be more difficult and the input of a specialist may be required.

If the resting ECG is completely normal then heart failure due to left ventricular (LV) systolic dysfunction is unlikely. A better 'rule out' test is measurement of the plasma concentration of B-type natriuretic peptide (BNP) or N-terminal pro-BNP (NT-proBNP). For patients with new symptoms, heart failure (whatever the cause) is unlikely if the BNP level is low (<100 pg/ml), and other conditions should be considered first. If either (or both) the ECG and BNP are abnormal, then further cardiac investigation is likely to prove worthwhile, with imaging of the heart being the key test to confirm cardiac dysfunction.

The ECG is useful for reasons other than helping to exclude heart failure. It can confirm a clinical diagnosis of atrial fibrillation, and may give clues as to the aetiology of heart failure (e.g. Q waves from previous myocardial infarction; voltage criteria for LV hypertrophy

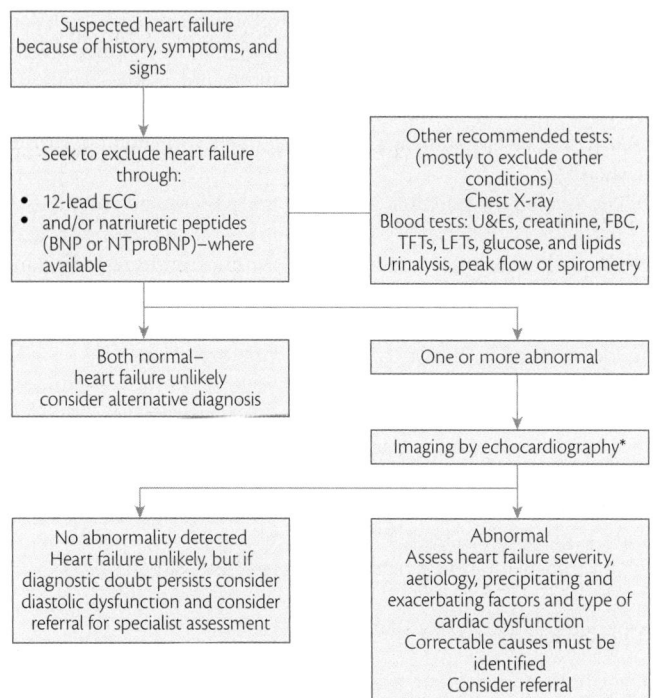

* Alternative methods of imaging the heart should be considered when a poor image is produced by transthoracic. Doppler 2D echocardiography – alternatives include transcesophageal Doppler 2D echocardiography, radionuclde imaging or cardiac magnetic resonance imaging

Key:	
BNP	B-type natriuretic peptide
ECG	Electrocardiogram
FBC	Full blood count
LFTs	Liver function tests
NTproBNP	N-terminal pro-B-type natriuretic peptide
TFTs	Thyroid function tests
U&Es	Urea and electrolytes

Fig. 16.5.1 Algorithm for diagnosis of heart failure, as recommended by NICE (2003).
NICE CHF guideline.

in hypertension, aortic stenosis or hypertrophic cardiomyopathy). It may also indicate where a pacemaker may be required—such as in complete heart block—or where cardiac resynchronization therapy may be useful (left bundle branch block).

The most common underlying pathophysiological abnormality of the heart in patients with heart failure is systolic dysfunction of the LV. The ventricle contracts poorly in systole and is usually dilated. The term 'systolic heart failure' is often applied to this condition, which is easily detected by echocardiography (or cardiac MRI). A few individuals with heart failure, particularly elderly patients, have no obvious valvular or systolic impairment of the heart and are assumed to have diastolic abnormalities. This is more likely if there is a history of hypertension. A definitive diagnosis can only be made at cardiac catheterization, but the echocardiogram may give some pointers towards this diagnosis.

Doppler echocardiography

Doppler echocardiography (see Chapter 16.3.2) provides useful information on overall LV systolic function, regional wall motion abnormalities (suggesting previous myocardial infarction), LV wall thickness, indirect assessment of diastolic function through Doppler measurement of flow through the mitral valve in diastole

or by measurement of movement of ventricular walls during diastole (M-mode measurements or Tissue Doppler), assessment of structure and function of the cardiac valves, indirect estimation of pulmonary artery pressure, and assessment of right ventricular function. It is important that the echocardiogram is performed by a trained operator on high resolution equipment, with interpretation of results depending on the clinical situation.

In some patients, often those who are obese or who have chronic airways disease, echocardiography does not provide useful images. Cardiac MRI is particularly useful in such cases. Radionuclide blood pool multiple gated acquisition (MUGA) scanning can also provide an accurate estimation of the systolic function of the left ventricle, but does not detect valve dysfunction and exposes the patient to radiation. See Chapter 16.3.3 for further information about these techniques.

Determining the aetiology of heart failure

Determining the underlying cause of heart failure is important in that treatment for primary valve disease differs from treatment for LV systolic impairment, and several causes of heart failure have a strong genetic component with implications for family screening and counselling regarding reproduction (e.g. hypertrophic cardiomyopathy). Echocardiography is very useful, in addition to good history taking and clinical examination, in determining the most likely aetiology, with the most common causes listed in Table 16.5.1.

There is still debate as to how important it is to determine whether the underlying cause of LV systolic impairment is coronary artery disease or not. Drug treatment may differ for this group of patients from those with dilated cardiomyopathy, e.g. statins and aspirin generally recommended for patients with coronary artery disease, and several trials are examining whether revascularization of patients with heart failure due to coronary artery disease is beneficial. Most centres now recommend noninvasive assessment of the likelihood of coronary artery disease, with stress echocardiography or myocardial perfusion imaging as a preliminary step before coronary angiography is considered.

Acute heart failure

There is no universally agreed definition of acute heart failure, but it is generally considered to represent the relatively abrupt onset of symptoms severe enough to merit hospitalization. It can occur as the first manifestation of a failing heart (acute *de novo* heart failure), or can occur on the background of chronic heart failure, where the term 'acute decompensation' is often applied.

The clinical presentation of acute heart failure varies: perhaps 70% present with peripheral fluid retention, 15% acute pulmonary oedema, 10% hypertensive heart failure, and 5% cardiogenic shock with hypotension and poor organ perfusion. Patients with acute *de novo* heart failure are more than twice as likely to present with pulmonary oedema or cardiogenic shock than patients with decompensation of chronic heart failure.

Prognosis

Heart failure has a substantial impact on life expectancy. The syndrome is progressive, despite the many therapeutic advances in the past two decades. Mortality remains around 20 to 30% in the first year after diagnosis, reducing to around 10% annually thereafter. Survival is affected by age, the extent of comorbidity, and the

Table 16.5.1 Aetiology of heart failure (NB: more than one factor may be aetiologically important in an individual)

Anatomical category	Aetiology	Examples	Approximate UK prevalence (%)
Pericardial		Constrictive pericarditis	<1
Myocardial	Coronary artery disease (CAD)	Myocardial infarction	50–60
	Dilated (no CAD)	Viral, bacterial	10–20
	Idiopathic*	Thyroid disease	
	Infective	Alcohol	
	Metabolic	Thiamine	
	Toxin	Mitochondial myopathy	
	Deficiency		
	Genetic		
	Peripartum		
	Hypertrophic		5–10 (NB Hypertension rare as sole aetiology, but history of this in 60% of patients)
	Hypertension		
	Genetic defect		
	Restrictive	Amyloidosis Haemochromatosis	<1
Endocardial	Valvular heart disease	Aortic stenosis	10
Arrhythmia		Atrial fibrillation	Found in 30–40% of heart failure patients, but rarely sole abnormality
High-output states		Paget's disease Ateriovenous fistula	5
Congenital heart disease		Ventricular septal defect	<1

* In the absence of known causes.

severity of the syndrome. The severity of the syndrome is graded by the degree of exertion that causes breathlessness—typically by using the New York Heart Association (NYHA) grading scheme (Table 16.5.2).

Table 16.5.2 New York Heart Association classification of symptomatic severity of heart failure

NYHA class	Description	Category
I	No limitation: ordinary physical activity does not cause fatigue, breathlessness or palpitations	Asymptomatic
II	Slight limitation in physical activity: comfortable at rest but ordinary activity results in fatigue, breathlessness or palpitations	Mild
III	Marked limitation of physical activity: comfortable at rest but less than ordinary activity results in fatigue, breathlessness or palpitations	Moderate
IV	Unable to carry out any physical activity without discomfort: symptoms of cardiac failure at rest with increased discomfort with any physical activity	Severe

The mode of death is more likely to be from progressive heart failure in the more severe grades of heart failure (often after several decompensations requiring hospitalization), but sudden death can occur at any time. Predicting likely life expectancy is more difficult than in terminal malignancies, making management decisions more difficult.

The overall in-hospital mortality for patients admitted with heart failure is between 4 and 8%, but for those presenting with cardiogenic shock (low cardiac output with organ hypoperfusion) it is around 40%. Within 12 weeks of initial discharge, 1 in 4 acute heart failure patients are readmitted to hospital and around 15% are dead, rising to 30% at 12 months from discharge.

There are several prognostic scoring systems. The most commonly used is the Heart Failure Survival Score, which takes into account seven variables: aetiology (ischaemic or not), resting heart rate, QRS duration on the ECG, serum sodium concentration, peak oxygen consumption on cardiopulmonary exercise testing, pulse pressure, and LV ejection fraction. This is generally used only in patients in whom transplantation is being considered (see Chapter 16.5.1).

Treatment

The aims of treatment are to improve life expectancy and to improve quality of life. The relative importance of these aims may differ between patients and may change with time, and the patient's preferences should be taken into account.

The treatment of heart failure usually involves lifestyle measures and drug therapy. Electrical devices, such as pacemakers and implantable cardioverter defibrillators (ICDs), are being used in an increasing proportion of patients. Surgical intervention—such as valve repair or replacement, LV assist devices, or transplantation—apply only to a minority of patients.

Lifestyle measures

Lifestyle changes can have an important impact on the control of the heart failure syndrome, although few recommendations are supported by a large evidence base.

Salt and fluid restriction

Fluid restriction is rarely necessary for patients with mild and stable symptoms, but can be useful for those with resistant fluid retention or hyponatraemia. Such patients can be advised to suck ice cubes or suck boiled sweets to assuage thirst, rather than to drink. Salt restriction is generally recommended for anyone with heart failure, with a maximum daily intake of 6 g, but this can be difficult to achieve, particularly if convenience (processed) foods are eaten. Patients with heart failure should avoid 'low salt' substitutes as they contain substantial amounts of potassium, which may affect serum levels and the propensity to arrhythmia (unless they are known to be hypokalaemic, perhaps as a consequence of diuretic therapy, and serum potassium concentration is monitored).

Alcohol

Chronic consumption of alcohol, probably at a level of more than 10 units each day for at least 5 years, may lead to heart failure. Abstinence from alcohol in such patients can lead to substantial improvement in LV function and should be recommended. Those affected are likely to require substantial support to achieve this. For those patients in whom alcohol is not thought to be aetiologically important, drinking within currently recommended levels is probably safe, although the fluid load may be important for some patients. Variable alcohol consumption can have a marked affect on anticoagulation control.

Cigarette smoking

Those who continue to smoke are likely to have a worse outcome than those who abstain, although the evidence is not robust. However, smoking has other harmful effects on health and smoking cessation is strongly recommended in all heart failure guidelines. Patients should be provided with the necessary support to achieve this, which is likely to include counselling and nicotine replacement therapy.

Physical activity

Inactivity can lead to physical deconditioning and worsening of exercise intolerance and fatigue. Training can improve exercise performance through adaptation of peripheral muscles, without adversely affecting cardiac function. Both aerobic exercise and resistive exercise are likely to improve symptoms, exercise performance, and quality of life, although compliance with a programme may be difficult and the long-term effects are not known. Many heart failure programmes now offer supervised exercise training along with other elements of rehabilitation therapy. One caveat to a recommendation for regular physical exercise is that swimming may produce rather marked and potentially harmful changes in central haemodynamics: alternative forms of exercise should be encouraged.

Bed rest is still recommended for patients with marked and acute deterioration in the heart failure syndrome (NYHA Class IV), but early mobilization once the syndrome is improving is sensible.

Sexual activity

There are no published studies of the effects of sexual activity in patients with heart failure. Breathlessness on exertion and inability to lie flat may clearly interfere with sexual activity, and anxiety about the potential harmful effects may impair enjoyment for both the patient and the partner. Sexual activity increases energy expenditure by a factor of 3 to 5 in healthy men, but with a wide interindividual variation. As a simple guide, if a patient can perform moderate exercise without difficulty, then sexual activity is unlikely to cause a problem. Such issues should be discussed with the patient and their partner. Sildenafil has been used by men with heart failure and erectile problems, but must not be taken with nitrates as this can lead to prolonged hypotension.

Nutritional supplements

There is no convincing evidence of benefit from nutritional supplements in heart failure. For patients with advanced heart failure and cachexia, protein and calorie supplements are frequently prescribed, but the evidence for benefit is scant. Various fruit juices may interact with medication: cranberry juice increases the potency of warfarin, and grapefruit juice interferes with the metabolism of simvastatin. St John's wort (bought over the counter to treat low mood/depression) may interact with a number of drugs frequently prescribed to heart failure patients, e.g. warfarin, digoxin, eplerenone, and selective serotonin reuptake inhibitors, and the effect of different preparations of St John's wort can vary markedly.

Complementary therapies

There are few robust studies of the impact of aromatherapy, reflexology, or relaxation therapy in patients with heart failure. They may improve some aspects of quality of life and may also provide benefit in terms of increased social interaction. There is no evidence of harm.

Psychological therapies

The provision of psychological therapy by a trained professional—whether education, counselling, stress management, or cognitive behavioural therapy—has not been robustly assessed in heart failure. Anxiety and depression are common and at times may be difficult to distinguish from the heart failure syndrome itself. It is unlikely that psychological therapies would cause harm and they may be a useful starting point before considering drug therapy for psychological or psychiatric disorder. Most guidelines recommend that if drug therapy is to be considered for depression in patients with heart failure, then newer-generation serotonin reuptake inhibitors should be used rather than tricyclic antidepressants.

Air travel

There are no pathophysiological reasons why most patients with stable heart failure and well-controlled symptoms should not be able to travel by air. Patients with decompensated heart failure, including pulmonary oedema, may become more hypoxic during air travel, as may those who are symptomatic at rest or on minimal exertion. Obviously, if oxygen is needed at rest on the ground, then hypoxia will be worse during air travel. However, for many patients with heart failure the most difficult part of air travel is the long walk within the airport, or the need to stand still and queue for long periods. Assistance may be required to enable easier check-in and transfer to the departure gate.

Vaccination

Patients with chronic cardiac conditions—including heart failure—should receive annual vaccination against influenza. Pneumococcal vaccination is also recommended, and may have to be repeated every 5 years to maintain protection.

Drug therapy

Most of the evidence base for the management of heart failure relates to heart failure due to LV systolic dysfunction—'systolic heart failure'. The best management for heart failure due to valve disease or heart failure with preserved ejection fraction (HFPEF) is less clear.

Diuretics

Diuretics are the most effective means of removing retained fluid, and their introduction often produces rapid symptomatic relief in patients with heart failure, whatever the underlying cause of the cardiac dysfunction. Most patients with heart failure require at least a small dose of regular diuretic. It is common practice to start diuretic therapy at a low dose, and to increase the dose as required to control fluid retention provided renal function does not deteriorate substantially. The dose can often be reduced once an angiotensin converting enzyme (ACE) inhibitor or angiotensin receptor blocker (ARB) has been introduced.

Most patients who require diuretic therapy are treated with a loop diuretic (e.g. furosemide, bumetanide, or torasemide) because these are more powerful than thiazide diuretics. Table 16.5.3 lists the diuretics that are generally used in heart failure. The combination of a loop diuretic with a potassium-sparing diuretic (e.g. amiloride) can increase diuresis and also guard against hypokalaemia. The risk

Table 16.5.3 Diuretics used in the treatment of heart failure (based on recommendations from NICE)

Drug	Initial dose (mg)	Maximum recommended daily dose (mg)
Loop diuretics		
Bumetanide	0.5–1.0	5–10
Furosemide	20–40	250–500
Torasemide	5–10	100–200
Thiazides		
Bendroflumethiazide	2.5	5
Metolazone	2.5	10
Potassium-diuretic		
Amiloride	2.5–5[a]	20–40[a]*
Triamterene	25–50[a]	100–200[a]

[a] Lower range appropriate for patient on ACE inhibitor or ARB.
NICE CHF guideline.

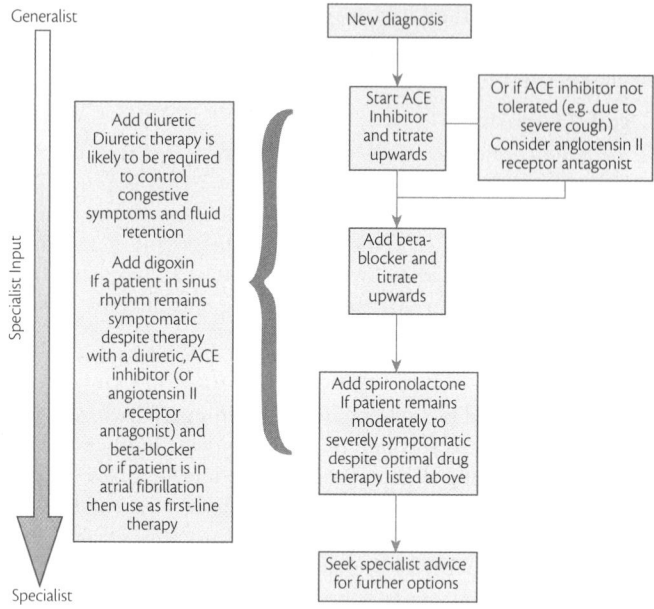

Fig. 16.5.2 Algorithm for the treatment of heart failure due to LV systolic dysfunction, based on the recommendations from NICE (2003).
NICE CHF guideline.

of hypokalaemia is less if the patient is taking an ACE inhibitor, ARB, or aldosterone antagonist. In the case of resistant fluid retention in severe heart failure, the combination of a loop and thiazide diuretic can be useful. High dose furosemide infusion may also produce a more powerful diuresis than bolus dosing.

The minimum dose of diuretic required to control fluid retention should be used: this will vary from one patient to another, and also may vary in an individual patient over time, particularly if there is change in other medication, intercurrent illness, or nonadherence to dietary restriction of salt intake. However, on its own diuretic therapy exacerbates neurohormonal activation and the modern therapy of heart failure due to LV systolic dysfunction demands the use of drugs to antagonize this. A simplified algorithm for treatment is shown in Fig. 16.5.2, modified from the NICE recommendations.

The main drug classes used are ACE inhibitors, ARBs, β-blockers, and aldosterone blockers such as spironolactone and eplerenone.

ACE inhibitors

ACE inhibitors improve both mortality and morbidity in a wide range of clinical settings, including patients with heart failure due to LV systolic dysfunction, asymptomatic LV systolic dysfunction, and also heart failure or asymptomatic LV systolic dysfunction after myocardial infarction. They should be considered in all such patients. The benefit in chronic heart failure is a reduction in the relative risk of death of 23% and of worsening heart failure of 35%.

Important side effects include cough (perhaps 10% of patients), hypotension, worsening renal dysfunction, and hyperkalaemia. Angio-oedema occurs rarely but requires the immediate withdrawal of the ACE inhibitor. Patients with bilateral renal artery stenosis may suffer a marked and rapid decline in renal function when challenged with an ACE inhibitor (or ARB) and if this occurs the drug should be withdrawn and imaging of the renal arteries considered.

The ACE inhibitor should be started at a low dose and the dose doubled at two weekly intervals with monitoring of blood pressure, renal function and electrolytes, until the target dose is achieved, or failing that the highest tolerated dose below that (Table 16.5.4). Caution is needed if the patient has significant hyperkalaemia (K+ >5 mmol/litre), renal dysfunction (serum creatinine >220 μmol/

litre), symptomatic hypotension or severe asymptomatic hypotension (systolic blood pressure <90 mmHg).

The typical cough induced by an ACE inhibitor is unproductive. Other causes should be excluded, in particular lung disease or pulmonary oedema due to worsening heart failure. Many patients can tolerate the cough if it is mild, but if it is bothersome an ARB can be used instead of the ACE inhibitor. If hypotension is a problem, other drugs that lower blood pressure should be discontinued if possible (e.g. nitrates, calcium channel antagonists), and the dose of diuretic can be reduced if there are no symptoms or signs of congestion. If these measures do not help, then the dose of ACE inhibitor may have to be reduced.

Table 16.5.4 Drugs used in the treatment of heart failure (as recommended by the Scottish Intercollegiate Guidelines Network)

	Starting dose	Target dose
ACE inhibitors		
Captopril	6.25 mg three times daily	50 mg three times daily
Enalapril	2.5 mg twice daily	10–20 mg twice daily
Lisinopril	2.5–5 mg once daily	20 mg once daily
Ramipril	2.5 mg once daily	5 mg twice daily or 10 mg once daily
Trandolapril	0.5 mg once daily	4 mg once daily
ARBs		
Candesartan	4 or 8 mg once daily	32 mg once daily
Valsartan	40 mg twice daily	160 mg twice daily
β-Blockers		
Bisoprolol	1.25 mg once daily	10 mg once daily
Carvedilol	3.125 mg twice daily	25–50 mg twice daily
Nebivolol	1.25 mg once daily	10 mg once daily

Adapted with permission from SIGN Guideline 95 - *Management of Chronic Heart Failure*

Some rise in urea, creatinine, and potassium is usual in patients taking an ACE inhibitor. An increase in K^+ to <5.5 mmol/litre is acceptable, but will require continued close monitoring. Potassium-retaining drugs such as spironolactone, eplerenone, amiloride, and triamterene may have to be stopped. Most physicians will accept a rise in creatinine of up to 50 μmol/litre, or to a level of 250 μmol/litre, whichever is the smaller. Nephrotoxic drugs such as nonsteroidal anti-inflammatory drugs (NSAIDs) should be discontinued. The dose of diuretic can be reduced, provided there are no symptoms or signs of congestion.

Serial monitoring of blood biochemistry and blood pressure is essential when introducing and up-titrating an ACE inhibitor (or ARB or β-blocker) in patients with heart failure. Intercurrent illness, particularly if it causes fever or changes in fluid balance, e.g. vomiting or diarrhoea, may have a profound effect on blood pressure and renal function in patients with severe heart failure. This may require cessation of or temporary reduction in the dose of ACE inhibitor, but this should be titrated upwards again once the patient has stabilized.

ARBs

ARBs block the action of angiotensin at one of its receptor subtypes and thus mimic the effect of ACE inhibitors without producing a rise in bradykinin, hence they do not have the side effect of cough. In other respects their side-effect profile and the actions to take if there are changes in blood pressure or renal function are identical to those for ACE inhibitors.

ARBs proven in randomized trials to reduce the risk of mortality and heart failure deterioration (valsartan and candesartan) are now generally used in patients who cannot tolerate an ACE inhibitor because of cough. This applies to chronic heart failure due to LV systolic dysfunction (candesartan) or heart failure, LV systolic dysfunction, or both after myocardial infarction (valsartan). Candesartan may also be added to therapy with an ACE inhibitor and β-blocker in chronic heart failure, with evidence that this reduces the risk of cardiovascular death or hospitalization for chronic heart failure.

β-Blockers

Many randomized clinical trials have shown the benefit of β-blockers in patients with heart failure, with an approximate 25% reduction in the relative risk of death and a 35% reduction in the risk of death from heart failure. This benefit has been seen with a wide range of β-blockers, including bisoprolol, metoprolol, nebivolol (all cardioselective), and carvedilol (non-cardioselective). One caveat to this is that the evidence for metoprolol is strongest for long-acting metoprolol succinate (which is not available in the United Kingdom), rather than the shorter-acting tartrate.

Although providing substantial benefit for patients with heart failure, the introduction of a β-blocker can lead to deterioration in the control of the syndrome. It is therefore important that the β-blocker is introduced at a low dose and titrated up slowly, with close monitoring of blood pressure, heart rate, renal function, and side effects. A β-blocker should not be used in patients with definite asthma, second- or third-degree heart block, or symptomatic hypotension. The cardioselective β-blockers can be used in chronic irreversible airways disease. The starting dose and target dose for the β-blockers proven to be of benefit in heart failure are shown in Table 16.5.4.

If heart failure worsens on the introduction of a β-blocker— manifest by increasing breathlessness, fatigue, oedema, or weight gain—then the dose of diuretic can be increased, but if this fails to improve the situation the dose of β-blocker should be reduced, but it is rarely necessary to stop the β-blocker completely.

An ECG should be done to exclude heart block if marked bradycardia develops. In the absence of heart block, if symptoms are worsening and the resting heart rate is below 50/min, then the dose of β-blocker can be halved, but again it is rarely necessary to withdraw it. Other rate-slowing medication should be reduced or stopped in preference to reducing the β-blocker dose, e.g. digoxin, amiodarone.

Symptomatic hypotension should trigger the stopping of other blood pressure lowering medications such as nitrates or calcium channel blockers. If there are no symptoms or signs of congestion, the dose of diuretic can be reduced. If these measures are not successful then the dose of β-blocker should be reduced, or in exceptional circumstances it should be stopped. If there is a problem with symptomatic hypotension, most physicians will prefer to have a patient on a medium dose of both an ACE inhibitor (or ARB) and β-blocker, rather than a high dose of only one of these agents.

Aldosterone antagonists

Two drugs that block the action of aldosterone on its receptor have been shown to be of benefit in heart failure. Spironolactone reduces the risk of death by 30% in patients with moderate to severe heart failure despite treatment with diuretic and ACE inhibitor. This drug, used at a dose of 25–50 mg once a day, can produce gynaecomastia (particularly when digoxin is also prescribed), hyperkalaemia, and renal dysfunction, hence monitoring of renal function and electrolytes is essential, particularly with initiation of therapy or dose adjustment. Changes in fluid balance status can have a marked effect on renal function and serum potassium levels such that frequent monitoring is essential during inter-current illness. Spironolactone should not be used in those with a baseline K^+ above 5 mmol/litre or in those with a serum creatinine above 220 μmol/litre, and there is no evidence to support its use in patients with mild heart failure or in the immediate period after myocardial infarction.

Eplerenone is a more selective aldosterone antagonist than spironolactone and therefore much less likely to cause gynaecomastia. It is often prescribed in place of spironolactone if gynaecomastia develops on that drug. The evidence for its use is in patients with a low ejection fraction (≤ 40%) and either diabetes or heart failure up to 2 weeks after acute myocardial infarction. It reduces the risk of sudden death by 20%, and the risk of death or hospitalization from cardiovascular causes by 13%. The dose of eplerenone is 25 mg once daily to start, aiming for 50 mg once daily provided renal function and serum potassium concentration are satisfactory. As with spironolactone, it should not generally be prescribed to patients with a baseline K^+ of more than 5 mmol/litre or serum creatinine above 220 μmol/litre.

Monitoring of renal function and electrolytes should be done frequently after initiation of an aldosterone antagonist (e.g. at 1, 4, 8, 12 weeks) and then every 3 to 6 months thereafter. Changes in the dose of spironolactone or eplerenone (or other heart failure drugs) should trigger a check on renal function and electrolytes, as should any intercurrent illness. NSAIDs should be avoided if at all possible. 'Low salt' substitutes, which contain significant potassium, should not be used in cooking. Drugs that increase serum potassium such as amiloride, triamterene, ACE inhibitors, and ARBs should be watched carefully. The combination of ACE inhibitor, ARB, and spironolactone (or eplerenone) is particularly likely to lead to hyperkalaemia and should only be used under specialist supervision. If serum K$^+$ rises above 5.5 mmol/litre (or creatinine to above 220 µmol/litre), then the dose of the aldosterone antagonist should be reduced. If the K$^+$ rises above 6 mmol/litre (or creatinine above 310 µmol/litre) it should be stopped completely. Diarrhoea or vomiting should trigger the temporary stopping of the aldosterone antagonist, which can be reintroduced with appropriate monitoring of renal function and electrolytes once the patient is stable.

Digoxin

There is little evidence that digoxin improves the overall outcome for patients with heart failure in sinus rhythm. It may reduce the risk of worsening heart failure and the need for hospitalization, but it is generally reserved for patients with systolic heart failure who have failed to respond to conventional treatment with diuretic, ACE inhibitor or ARB, β-blocker, and spironolactone.

Digoxin is used to help control ventricular rate in patients with heart failure and fast atrial fibrillation. In this setting a β-blocker is also indicated and likely to have additional benefit. If the combination of a β-blocker and digoxin causes bradycardia, the digoxin should be stopped in preference to the β-blocker.

The usual daily dose of digoxin is 125 to 250 µg if the serum creatinine is normal: in older people and in those with renal dysfunction the dose should be reduced. A number of drugs can alter its pharmacokinetics, the most common problems occurring with antiarrhythmic drugs affecting renal clearance or volume of distribution (verapamil, amiodarone, propafenone, and quinidine), drugs increasing its absorption (erythromycin, omeprazole, tetracycline), and drugs decreasing its absorption (colestipol, cholestyramine). A more complete list can be found in the British National Formulary (http://bnf.org).

Digoxin has a narrow therapeutic window, with arrhythmia and gastrointestinal side effects being the most common clinical reasons for withdrawal. There is little relationship between the serum level of digoxin and its therapeutic effect, but measurement of the serum level may be useful to confirm compliance or the clinical suspicion of toxicity. It is important to realize that toxicity can occur even with 'normal' serum levels, and is likely to be worse when serum potassium concentration is deranged.

Amiodarone

Amiodarone is effective against most ventricular arrhythmia but does not improve the overall mortality in patients with heart failure at risk of sudden death (see Chapter 16.4). It can be used to try and cardiovert atrial fibrillation back to sinus rhythm, and to reduce the need for DC shocks in patients with recurrent ventricular arrhythmia and an ICD.

Amiodarone has numerous side effects, including photosensitivity, thyroid dysfunction, pulmonary fibrosis, liver dysfunction, and neuropathy. Corneal microdeposits are common but rarely necessitate stopping the drug. The need to continue its prescription should be reviewed regularly, with regular monitoring of thyroid and liver function, and a careful watch for signs of pulmonary toxicity.

Nitrate and hydralazine combination

This combination was shown to reduce mortality in heart failure in the pre-ACE inhibitor era, but is less effective than ACE inhibitors. In African-American patients the combination appears to reduce the risk of death or hospitalization from heart failure in patients with moderate to severe symptoms and on top of treatment with diuretic, ACE inhibitor or ARB, and β-blocker. In white patients the combination of nitrates and hydralazine is reserved those intolerant of an ACE inhibitor or ARB because of renal dysfunction or hyperkalaemia. When used at the correct dosage, vasodilator side effects are common, and rarely hydralazine can induce a lupus-like syndrome.

Statins and PUFA

In randomized trials, statins have had a neutral effect on outcome in patients with heart failure, whether ischaemic or non-ischaemic in aetiology. n-3 polyunsaturated fatty acid supplementation of 1g/day reduced mortality by 9% in one randomized trial.

Anticoagulants and antiplatelet agents

Warfarin should be prescribed for patients with heart failure and atrial fibrillation (whether paroxysmal or persistent) as it reduces the risk of thromboembolism including stroke. In those in whom the risk of warfarin is considered too high, aspirin at the dose of 300 mg daily can be considered, but is likely to be less effective than warfarin at preventing thromboembolism. See Chapter 16.16.1 for further discussion.

In sinus rhythm the balance of risk and benefit is more difficult, but warfarin should be considered for those with intracardiac thrombus, LV aneurysm, or a history of thromboembolism.

Many patients with heart failure have coexisting atherosclerotic disease and are likely to be on long-term aspirin therapy. There is some debate as to the potential harmful effects of this agent in chronic heart failure, with some evidence that it may increase the risk of decompensation. Most physicians use aspirin at a dose of 75 mg once daily for patients with coexisting symptomatic atherosclerosis (e.g. previous myocardial infarction, angina, stroke, or transient ischaemic attack).

Calcium channel blockers

Calcium channel blockers do not improve the outcome in patients with heart failure. Amlodipine and felodipine (long-acting dihydropyridines) are not harmful and may be useful in patients with concomitant angina, although β-blockers should be considered first. Verapamil, diltiazem, and short-acting dihydropyridines (e.g. nifedipine) can cause clinical deterioration and should not be used.

Drugs used in acute decompensation, including inotropes

Most patients hospitalized with heart failure have had a previous diagnosis of the condition and are already on disease-modifying therapy e.g. with ACE inhibitors, ARBs, and/or β-blockers. The treatment of acute decompensation of chronic heart failure depends on the clinical status of the patient. Table 16.5.5 shows a practical approach, classifying patients depending on their fluid status ('wet' or 'dry') and organ perfusion ('warm' or 'cold'). If the patient is warm but wet, then intravenous diuretic therapy and vasodilators such as intravenous nitroglycerine can be used. If the patient is cold and dry, then careful intravenous fluid replacement should be tried, under close monitoring. If this fails to increase

Table 16.5.5 Simple clinical classification and approach to treatment of the patient with acute heart failure

Congestion / Perfusion	Not present: patient is 'dry'	Present: patient is 'wet'
Good: patient is 'warm'	Well compensated—alteration in management is probably not required (good prognosis)	Diuretics ± vasodilators
Poor: patient is 'cold'	May be over-diuresed: careful fluid replacement ± inotropes	Inotropes ± diuretics (poorest prognosis)

organ perfusion then inotropic agents can be used, which are also first line for the cold and wet patient. Inotropic agents increase cardiac output and organ perfusion and may dramatically improve the clinical condition of the patient, reducing pulmonary wedge pressure, clearing pulmonary oedema, and allowing a diuresis as renal perfusion improves.

The inotropic agent most often used is dobutamine, although the evidence base is weak. It acts on β-adrenoreceptors and may therefore be less effective in patients on β-blockers, in which case the phosphodiesterase inhibitors (such as milrinone or enoximone) may be more effective. Dobutamine may induce sinus tachycardia and more serious cardiac arrhythmia, may exacerbate myocardial ischaemia due to increased myocardial oxygen consumption, and may lose effect with prolonged treatment ('tachyphylaxis'). The phosphodiesterase inhibitors cause vasodilatation in addition to increasing myocardial contractility, which may be useful, but they also increase myocardial oxygen consumption and can induce arrhythmia. Excessive peripheral vasodilatation may exacerbate hypotension.

Levosimendan is a newer inotropic agent with vasodilator properties, not yet available in the United Kingdom, but may be better tolerated and slightly more effective than dobutamine. Nesiritide (synthetic human B-type natriuretic peptide) is used in North America as a powerful vasodilator with some natriuretic effect, although there is some concern about a possible harmful effect on renal function in some patients.

Chronic therapy with oral inotropes (such as the phosphodiesterase inhibitors) is not used because it increases mortality.

Drugs in development

There are a large number of drugs in development, including adenosine antagonists and arginine vasopressin antagonists. Other therapies have been tried but found to be unhelpful or harmful (antitumour necrosis factor, endothelin antagonists, minoxidil).

Drugs to avoid or use with caution

Patients with heart failure may have significant renal (and hepatic) impairment. Drugs cleared predominantly by the kidney (and liver) can therefore accumulate in these patients, causing toxicity, and this can include drugs used to treat heart failure itself such as ACE inhibitors and digoxin.

NSAIDs may exacerbate fluid retention and renal dysfunction in patients with heart failure and should be used with caution. This applies to both nonselective agents and the newer COX-2 selective agents. Oral and intravenous steroids may also exacerbate fluid retention.

Drugs with a negative inotropic effect should also be avoided, including verapamil, dilitazem and Class I antiarrhythmic agents. Other drugs to be avoided include glitazones (fluid retention),

metformin (lacticacidosis in severe heart failure), tricyclic antidepressants (arrhythmia and reduced contractility), carbenoxolone (fluid retention), macrodlide antibiotics, and some antifungal agents (QT prolongation and increased risk of arrhythmia). Fuller details can be found in the British National Formulary (http://bnf.org).

Nonprescription drugs (such as herbal remedies) can have important interactions with prescription drugs taken by patients with heart failure. St John's wort can affect serum levels of digoxin and warfarin. Liquorice and dandelion can lead to fluid retention. Ginko, garlic, aescin and dong quai can increase the risk of bleeding. More details can be found on the website http://herbmed.org.

Comorbidity and its impact on drug therapy

The average age of a new patient with heart failure in the UK is 75 years, hence comorbidity is common. This may complicate management and increase the risk of adverse events with 'standard' therapy.

Renal dysfunction

Most patients with heart failure will have at least mild derangement of renal function, which can be worsened by excessive diuresis, hypotension, or the use of ACE inhibitors/ARBs and aldosterone antagonists. The serum creatinine can appear relatively normal, despite marked impairment of renal function, because of old age and low muscle bulk, and estimated glomerular filtration rate (eGFR) should always be considered.

Asthma and chronic airways disease

β-Blockers are absolutely contraindicated in asthma, but in chronic airways disease where there may be little reversibility a cardioselective β-blocker (such as bisoprolol or nebivolol) should be tried under careful supervision.

Angina

β-Blockers are the drugs of choice for concomitant angina. Nitrates (both sublingual and oral) are safe to use in heart failure, provided blood pressure is satisfactory. Only long-acting dihydropyridine calcium antagonists (such as amlodipine) can be safely used in heart failure: nifedipine, diltiazem, and verapamil should not be used. Revascularization may have to be considered if patients remain symptomatic from angina.

Atrial fibrillation

Paroxysmal or persistent atrial fibrillation affects 30 to 40% of patients with heart failure and the best management for this is unclear, excepting that they require anticoagulation with a target INR of 2.5. Most physicians will attempt to restore sinus rhythm at least once unless the ventricular function is so poor or the atrial size so large that the chances of success are deemed too low. The usual approach is to attempt chemical cardioversion with oral amiodarone, and if this fails after 4–6 weeks to perform a DC cardioversion. The amiodarone is continued for some months but can usually be stopped if sinus rhythm is maintained for 6 months or more. If the chance of cardioversion is deemed low, or cardioversion has failed before, then the aim is to control the ventricular rate, usually with a combination of β-blocker and digoxin. In some patients this is difficult and atrioventricular nodal ablation with permanent pacing (perhaps with a biventricular rather than right ventricular system) is necessary to control a high resting ventricular rate. The role of atrial ablation in patients with heart failure is unclear: success in routine practice in the typical patient with much structural heart damage is likely to be low, but trials are under way.

Anaemia

Many patients with heart failure are anaemic, some due to iron deficiency from blood loss from the gastrointestinal tract or poor dietary intake, but many due to concomitant renal dysfunction or the heart failure syndrome itself. Those with anaemia have a worse prognosis than those without, but there is no convincing evidence that treatment with a combination of erythropoietin and intravenous iron improves mortality. Most physicians will treat anaemia with these drugs in patients with heart failure and moderate to severe renal dysfunction while the results of large randomized controlled trials are awaited, and it seems sensible practice to correct severe anaemia with blood transfusion (slowly, with diuretic cover and close clinical supervision) in patients admitted to hospital with exacerbation of heart failure.

Gout

Gout is not uncommon in patients with heart failure, particularly those who require high dose diuretics to control fluid retention. NSAIDs should be avoided because they worsen renal function and the tendency to fluid retention. Most physicians treat acute attacks with colchicine, adding in allopurinol when the attack has settled in an attempt to reduce the risk of a subsequent attack. Occasionally a short course of oral steroid is needed to abort the attack, but this can lead to fluid retention.

Treatment of heart failure with preserved ejection fraction

Most of the evidence base relating to the drug treatment of heart failure has come from trials with patients with obvious impairment of LV systolic function. Many patients, particularly elderly people with a history of hypertension and/or diabetes, do not have systolic dysfunction but a presumed abnormality of diastole—termed 'diastolic' or heart failure with preserved ejection fraction. This is most usually a diagnosis of exclusion and the physician should check that there is not another (noncardiac) explanation for symptoms. An elevated plasma BNP concentration, in the absence of marked renal dysfunction, helps confirm the diagnosis.

If the diagnosis of nonsystolic heart failure is secure, then the patient requires treatment. This will include a diuretic, at as low a dose as possible to control fluid retention because high doses are tolerated poorly, with the stiff ventricle requiring adequate filling pressure to maintain its output. Concomitant atrial fibrillation needs treatment in its own right because patients with stiff ventricles tend to tolerate this arrhythmia particularly poorly.

There is little direct evidence for the use of ACE inhibitors in this condition, although theoretically they should be helpful. There is some, not very robust, evidence that the ARB candesartan can reduce the risk of cardiovascular mortality or heart failure hospitalization in patients with non-systolic heart failure, but a large randomized trial of irbesartan found no such effect. β-Blockers and rate-limiting calcium antagonists (such as diltiazem or verapamil) are used to increase the filling time of the ventricular cycle, but there is little hard evidence to prove that this is clinically useful.

Comorbidites such as obesity, hypertension, and diabetes should be treated on their own merits.

Devices used to treat heart failure

Implantable pacemakers

Permanent pacing has been used to treat symptomatic bradycardia in patients with heart failure for many years. It may alleviate heart failure when this is associated with complete heart block.

Dual chamber (atrio-right ventricular) pacing for the treatment of heart failure in the absence of symptomatic bradycardia or heart block produces no haemodynamic benefit and may have a detrimental effect on LV function. This is probably due to the fact that right ventricular apical pacing results in a left bundle branch block pattern of ventricular activation that induces 'mechanical dyssynchrony', with regions of early and late contraction: the interventricular septum contracts early relative to the delayed contraction of the LV lateral free wall. In its most severe form such dyssynchrony can result in contraction of the septum whilst the lateral wall is still relaxing and vice versa. With failure of opposing ventricular walls to contract together, a significant amount of blood is simply shifted within the ventricular cavity instead of being ejected into the circulation, thereby reducing cardiac output. The proportion of the cardiac cycle available for LV filling and ejection is also reduced by dyssynchronous contraction, leading to a further decrease in the pumping ability of the heart.

Patients with mechanical dyssynchrony due to native left bundle branch block (perhaps up to 20% of all heart failure patients) are increasingly likely to be considered for sophisticated pacing using an atriobiventricular system to reduce the dyssynchrony (cardiac resynchronization therapy, CRT). With this therapy the conventional right atrial and right ventricular pacing wires are supplemented by a third lead placed in a lateral coronary vein via the coronary sinus, thus allowing pacing of the left ventricle transvenously (Fig. 16.5.3). This can lead to an improvement in LV systolic function, reduction in ventricular dimensions, increase in LV filling time, reduction in pulmonary capillary wedge pressure, and increase in cardiac output and systemic blood pressure. Large clinical trials have demonstrated a substantial reduction in mortality (up to 40%) in patients with left bundle branch block

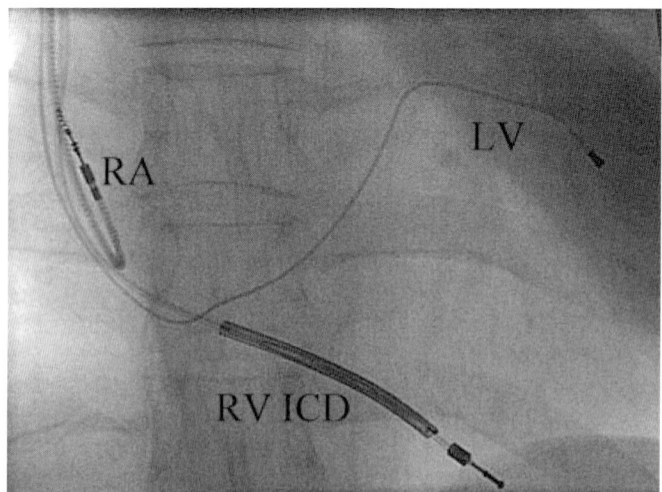

Fig. 16.5.3 Chest radiograph from a patient with heart failure with cardiac resynchronization therapy and ICD. LV, left ventricular lead (place in a lateral coronary vein via the coronary sinus); RA, right atrial lead; RV ICD, right ventricular ICD lead.

and moderate to severe symptoms of heart failure despite optimal drug therapy. Symptoms, the risk of rehospitalization, and quality of life also improve. A few patients, however, do not respond to this therapy: work is ongoing to determine the best way of identifying these. It is still not clear if patients with atrial fibrillation benefit as much as those in sinus rhythm. Recent trials suggest there may also be a role for CRT in patients with milder symptoms.

Implantable cardioverter defibrillator (ICD) therapy

ICD therapy reduces mortality in patients with coronary artery disease, impaired LV systolic function, and failed sudden death or evidence of ventricular arrhythmias, when compared to optimal medical therapy alone. Patients with coronary artery disease, very poor LV systolic function (ejection fraction <30%), and a broad QRS complex (>120 ms) are also identified as a group at high risk of sudden death, and ICD implantation is recommended, even in the absence of documented ventricular arrhythmia—but not within 4 weeks of an acute myocardial infarction. Patients with severely symptomatic heart failure (NYHA Class IV) are generally not considered suitable for such therapy: the risk of death is substantially greater from progressive heart failure, and a sudden death in these circumstances may not be the worst outcome.

The evidence for the use of ICDs in patients with heart failure not due to coronary artery disease is less robust, but at least one large trial suggests that an ICD benefits these patients as much as those with coronary artery disease. Amiodarone appeared to be no better than placebo in terms of reduction in mortality in heart failure patients, although it suppresses ventricular arrhythmia and may reduce the frequency of (appropriate) shocks in patients with ICDs.

Combined therapy with CRT and ICD (CRT-D)

It is possible to combine CRT with an ICD in one device. Such an approach is likely to maximize the impact on reducing mortality in patients with heart failure. Opinion differs as to which patients should be considered for combined therapy, but increasingly if a CRT device is being fitted, the physician will opt for the more expensive CRT-D system to provide greater protection against sudden death.

LV assist devices

The worldwide experience of using implantable ventricular assist devices is steadily increasing, with a small number of patients continuing on such mechanical support for more than 2 years. Although accepted as an appropriate 'bridge to transplant' for patients deteriorating while on a cardiac transplantation waiting list, the role of these devices as 'destination therapy' is unclear. There is evidence that in some patients the heart may recover whilst being supported by such devices, but how best to identify such patients and how to stimulate the heart to recover is as yet unclear. The use of such devices outside the context of a heart transplantation programme is not recommended. See Chapter 16.5.2 for further discussion.

Other interventions for heart failure

Valve replacement/repair

Heart failure due to primary valve disease is potentially curable. It is thus vital that this is detected. Good clinical examination supplemented by a high-quality Doppler echocardiogram is essential. The timing of valve replacement can be difficult and is based on the cardiac anatomy, severity of the disease, comorbidities, ventricular function, haemodynamics, and rate of progression of the valve disease. Rapid deterioration suggests the possibility of a change in cardiac rhythm (e.g. onset of atrial fibrillation) or infection (endocarditis) and requires specialist input.

Severe aortic stenosis may present in elderly people with heart failure. The risk of valve replacement is often considered too high, but recent developments in percutaneous valve replacement may offer a new therapeutic avenue. An expandable stented valve is placed percutaneously through the orifice of the native aortic valve, and is then expanded under considerable pressure. The 'new' valve then operates as a better conduit for blood from the left ventricle, with a reduction in afterload. The procedure is being performed in more specialist cardiac centres, but is still in development.

A similar procedure can be used for percutaneous pulmonary valve replacement in patients with congenital heart disease. Percutanous mitral valve repair for patients with moderate to severe functional mitral regurgitation is at an earlier stage of development, and relies upon percutaneous access to the coronary sinus.

See Chapter 16.6 for further discussion of valvular disease.

Revascularization

Although ischaemic heart disease is the most common cause of heart failure in the United Kingdom and other developed countries, the benefits of revascularization in chronic heart failure are not well established. The risk of coronary artery bypass surgery in patients with poor LV systolic function can be high, and many surgeons are reluctant to take on such candidates despite evidence from some studies that they have the most to gain from surgery.

There is considerable heterogeneity in the effect of coronary artery disease on the LV myocardium in such patients, with regional variation in the extent of scar, viable but noncontractile ('hibernating') tissue, and viable and contracting ('normal') tissue. A variety of imaging techniques can be used to try to determine the extent of such hibernation, including stress echocardiography, nuclear imaging, and cardiac MRI, as discussed in Chapters 16.3.2 and 16.3.3. Several randomized trials are examining whether revascularizing those with significant hibernating myocardium is beneficial.

For those with symptoms of angina or breathlessness due to inducible ischaemia, revascularization for symptom improvement is generally considered reasonable after optimization of medical treatment if the coronary anatomy is suitable.

Transplantation

The number of heart transplantations performed worldwide has been falling for the past decade. This relates to both a reduction in the supply of organs and better drug therapies for patients with heart failure. There are no randomized studies of transplantation, but case series suggest benefit in those with severe heart failure, no significant comorbidity, and an expected survival of less than 70% at 5 years. See Chapter 16.5.2 for further discussion.

Other surgical procedures

Patients with severe LV dilatation often have severe 'functional' mitral regurgitation sue to stretching of the valve ring.

Surgical correction of the regurgitation is possible, but more data are needed before those most likely to benefit can be clearly identified.

Ventricular reduction surgery—particularly where an area of scar tissue can be removed—may be of benefit in selected patients with heart failure. Use of this in patients with globally dilated left ventricles and little regional variation in the extent of scar is not currently recommended.

Cardiomyoplasty, a procedure where skeletal muscle is wrapped around the ventricle and 'trained' to contract more like cardiac muscle, has been examined, but remains an experimental technique with considerable technical challenge.

Ultrafiltration

Ultrafiltration can be used to treat hospitalized patients with resistant fluid retention or pulmonary oedema. Smaller bedside devices that can be managed on a coronary care unit have been developed, but experience to date is limited.

Noninvasive ventilation

Sleep-disordered breathing is found in 50% of patients with heart failure, with central sleep apnoea predominating in more severe heart failure. Cheyne–Stokes respiration is a particular type of central sleep apnoea. Obstructive sleep apnoea can, and should be, treated with continuous positive airways pressure (CPAP), which can now be safely and easily organized in a patient's home. There is as yet no evidence that treating central sleep apnoea with CPAP or servoassisted ventilation improves outcome, but a large randomized trial is under way.

Patients presenting with acute pulmonary oedema may benefit from CPAP therapy or other forms of assisted ventilation, particularly if the work of breathing is consuming a large proportion of the limited cardiac output. This should be considered in consultation with the intensive care unit staff.

Disease monitoring and communication with patient and carer

Traditionally patients with heart failure have been assessed periodically in primary or secondary care by clinical examination (noting the extent of fluid retention, jugular venous pressure, and lung auscultatory findings) supplemented by checking of blood biochemistry. Recent randomized studies have suggested that serial monitoring of plasma BNP and adjustment of therapy to reach a target level of BNP may improve the clinical outcome compared with standard care, but this is not as yet routine.

Box 16.5.2 lists some of the subjects to discuss with a heart failure patient and their family. Clearly, not all of these topics can be covered in one consultation, and written or visual material can be very helpful in reinforcing key information and self-management. Experienced heart failure physician and nurse teams reliably reduce hospitalization rates in patients with heart failure, the key element probably being close contact between the nurse and the patient/carer, enabling early identification of clinical deterioration. Patients can monitor their weight and be educated to adjust their diuretic dose at an early stage of decompensation.

Telemonitoring (generation of clinically relevant data that are transmitted remotely to a health care professional) has been

---

> **Box 16.5.2** Subjects to discuss with a patient with heart failure and their family and carers
>
> **General advice**
> - What is heart failure?
> - Why do symptoms occur?
> - How to recognize symptoms?
> - What to do if symptoms worsen
> - Self-weighing
> - Rationale for treatments
> - Importance of adherence to lifestyle and drug therapy
> - Smoking cessation
> - Anxiety and depression
> - Prognosis
>
> **Lifestyle measures**
> - Dietary restrictions, including salt, fluid, and alcohol
> - Rest and exercise
> - Sexual activity
> - Travel
>
> **Drug counselling**
> - Drug effects
> - Dose and timing
> - Adverse effects
> - Self-management (particularly diuretic dose)
> - Vaccination

---

examined in a number of randomized trials. Although the details differ markedly from one telemonitoring system to another, the evidence suggests that such an approach is safe and acceptable to patients and their families, and although not necessarily reducing hospitalizations it does reduce mortality. This is presumably due to better compliance with drug therapy and earlier identification of decompensation.

Modern generations of CRT and ICDs can also provide information useful for chronic disease monitoring in heart failure, e.g. frequency and duration of episodes of atrial fibrillation, heart rate variability (reflecting sympathetic tone in the autonomic nervous system), patient activity, and even intrathoracic impedance or indirectly estimated pulmonary artery pressure. It is likely that such data could be used by health care professionals to better manage patients with these devices, although this area is in its infancy.

'Heart failure' has strongly negative connotations for lay people, who equate it with 'cardiac arrest'. Feedback from patient and carer focus groups suggests that an early and frank discussion of the diagnosis and treatment options is greatly appreciated. Such discussion will also improve the patient's understanding of the disease and empower them (and their carer) to take more of an active role in management. Health care professionals should be sensitive to the information needs of their patients and tailor the method and content of their communications appropriately. The detection of anxiety and depression is important, particularly as these are common in patients with heart failure: counselling, cognitive behavioural therapy, and (if necessary) drug therapy are likely to improve quality of life.

End of life issues

Palliative care skills are an important component of good management of heart failure, particularly in the terminal stages of the condition (see Chapter 31.1). Good communication between the health care professionals (in primary and secondary care) and the patient and family is particularly crucial at this point. General palliative care can be given by the heart failure team, working with the primary care services. More specialist input may be necessary at times. Local arrangements vary markedly. Key issues are symptom management, decision making, withdrawal of unnecessary or inappropriate therapies (including drugs and defibrillation), emotional support, and coordination of care. Patient preferences may change over time.

Further reading

Authors/Task Force Members, Dickstein K, Cohen-Solal A, *et al.* (2008). ESC Guidelines for the diagnosis and treatment of acute and chronic heart failure 2008: The Task Force for the Diagnosis and Treatment of Acute and Chronic Heart Failure 2008 of the European Society of Cardiology. Developed in collaboration with the Heart Failure Association of the ESC (HFA) and endorsed by the European Society of Intensive Care Medicine (ESICM). *Eur Heart J.* **29**, 2388–442.
Jessup M, Abraham WT, Casey DE, *et al.* (2009). Focused Update: ACCF/AHA Guidelines for the Diagnosis and Management of Heart Failure in Adults: A Report of the American College of Cardiology Foundation/American Heart Association Task Force on Practice Guidelines: Developed in Collaboration With the International Society for Heart and Lung Transplantation. *Circulation.* **119**, 1977–2016.
National Collaborating Centre for Chronic Conditions (Royal College of Physicians of London) (2003). *NICE Guidance No. 5. Chronic heart failure: national clinical guideline for diagnosis and management in primary and secondary care.* (http://guidance.nice.org.uk/CG5/Guidance/pdf/English).
Scottish Intercollegiate Guidelines Network (2007). *Management of chronic heart failure: a national clinical guideline (No. 95)* (http://www.sign.ac.uk/pdf/sign95.pdf).

Information for patients, families, and carers

British Heart Foundation. http://www.bhf.org.uk [A useful website for patient information and basic questions about heart failure and other cardiovascular conditions.]
Heart Failure Association of the European Society of Cardiology. http://www.heartfailurematters.org [Useful patient website.]
National Institute for Health and Clinical Excellence (NICE). http://guidance.nice.org.uk/CG5 [Guidance for patients with heart failure.]
National Heart Lung and Blood Institute. http://www.nhlbi.nih.gov/ [A large website with useful information about heart failure, and good links to other sites.]

16.5.2 Cardiac transplantation and mechanical circulatory support

Jayan Parameshwar

Essentials
Cardiac transplantation

Cardiac transplantation is the treatment of choice for selected patients with advanced heart failure: median survival exceeds 10 years and recipients enjoy an excellent quality of life, but availability is severely limited by shortage of donor organs. The need for life-long immunosuppression is associated with side effects, including an increased incidence of malignancy. Newer immunosuppressive agents offer promise in reducing nephrotoxicity of conventional regimens and in delaying the onset of (currently inevitable) cardiac allograft vasculopathy.

Mechanical circulatory support

Ventricular assist devices (VADs) are mechanical blood pumps that work in parallel or series with the native ventricle: there are two main types—pulsatile, also referred to as volume displacement, and rotary. Significant complications arise from bleeding, thromboembolism, and infection.

Short-term use—several devices are available for use in patients who need support for days to periods of up to 4 to 6 weeks: these are invaluable in postcardiotomy cardiogenic shock and in patients who present *in extremis* with multiorgan failure.

Longer-term use—implantation of a device in patients with chronic heart failure must be viewed either as a bridge to heart transplantation or as permanent support. The REMATCH study (Randomized Evaluation of Mechanical Assistance for the Treatment of Congestive Heart Failure) randomized patients with endstage heart failure to best medical therapy or the implantation of the HeartMate I assist device: survival was improved in the device group (52% vs 25% at 1 year; 23% vs 8% at 2 years).

Heart transplantation

In 1964 James Hardy transplanted a chimpanzee heart into a 68-year old man with ischaemic heart failure, but the patient did not survive surgery. The first human-to-human heart transplant was performed in Cape Town on 3 December 1967 by Christiaan Barnard; the patient died 18 days afterwards of infective complications. By the end of 1968, 102 patients had received heart transplants in 50 hospitals in 17 countries: mean survival was only 29 days and there was widespread disenchantment with the procedure. Few institutions continued clinical cardiac transplantation in the 1970s, the team at Stanford University under the leadership of Norman Shumway being pre-eminent among them. By the late 1970s 1-year survival at Stanford had increased to 65%, establishing the place of heart transplantation. The introduction of new immunosuppressive drugs in the 1980s led to further improvement in outcome and an explosion of activity around the world. Over the last decade there has been a decline in the number of heart transplants performed owing to a lack of donor organs.

Before transplantation

Recipient selection

Heart transplantation is the treatment of choice for selected patients with endstage heart failure. However, the number of available donor organs is only a small fraction of the number of potential recipients. Careful selection of patients is therefore crucial to use scarce donor organs to best effect. Patients with NYHA Class IIIB and Class IV heart failure are best discussed with the local heart failure/transplant centre to optimize medical management and to consider high-risk nontransplant surgery where appropriate (see Chapter 16.5). Patients with chronic heart failure should be referred before they develop significant renal and hepatic dysfunction and irreversible pulmonary hypertension. Box 16.5.2.1 summarizes criteria used to select patients for transplantation, with the use of cardiopulmonary exercise testing to objectively quantify functional capacity and to estimate prognosis is an important part of the assessment process. Box 16.5.2.2 outlines the important contraindications.

Matching of donor and recipient

Donor and recipient blood groups need to be compatible. Appropriate size matching is also generally thought to be necessary to minimize donor organ failure. HLA matching is not routinely carried out, but there is some evidence that HLA-DR matching results in fewer episodes of acute rejection.

After transplantation

Most patients spend 2 to 3 weeks in hospital after a heart transplant and are fit to return to work after 4 to 6 months. In the first year they need to return to the transplant centre frequently to monitor immunosuppression, and to have endomyocardial biopsies to diagnose acute rejection.

Immunosuppression

Immunosuppression is commenced at surgery and continued for life. The intensity of immunosuppression is greatest early post-transplant, with a gradual decrease in the dosage of drugs over the first year. Box 16.5.2.3 lists the agents commonly used for maintenance immunosuppression: some patients receive additional antibody therapy for the first few days after the transplant. At least 50%

Box 16.5.2.1 Indications for heart transplantation

- Ongoing symptoms of heart failure at rest or minimal exertion despite optimal medical therapy. Functional capacity measured by peak oxygen uptake on exercise <14 ml/kg per min (or 50% predicted). For patients receiving β-blockers a value of 12 ml/kg per min has been recommended

- History of recurrent admissions to hospital with worsening heart failure

- Refractory ischaemia not amenable to revascularization associated with severe impairment of left ventricular function

- Recurrent symptomatic ventricular arrhythmia associated with severe impairment of ventricular function

---

Box 16.5.2.2 Contraindications to heart transplantation

- Active infection (including chronic viral infections, e.g. HIV, hepatitis B)

- Symptomatic peripheral or cerebrovascular disease

- Diabetes mellitus with end-organ damage (nephropathy, neuropathy, proliferative retinopathy)

- Coexistent or recent neoplasm

- Severe lung disease (FEV_1 and FVC <50% predicted)

- Renal dysfunction with creatinine clearance less than 40 ml/min

- Recent pulmonary thromboembolism

- Pulmonary hypertension (pulmonary artery systolic pressure >60 mm Hg, transpulmonary gradient ≥15 mmHg and/or pulmonary vascular resistance >5 Wood units)

- Psychosocial factors including history of noncompliance with medication, inadequate support, drug or alcohol abuse

- Obesity (body mass index >30 or weight >140% of ideal body weight

- Age (usually >65 years)

---

of patients can be safely weaned off prednisolone in the first 2 years after surgery. Episodes of acute rejection (usually confirmed by endomyocardial biopsy) are treated with intravenous methylprednisolone and are almost always reversible.

Outcome

Figure 16.5.2.1 shows the survival of patients after heart transplantation. Median survival now exceeds 10 years in most large centres. Annual mortality after the first year is approximately 3.5% per year. Most patients enjoy an excellent quality of life after a heart transplant, with minimal or no functional limitation. Successful pregnancy is possible after heart transplantation: management requires close collaboration between transplant and obstetric teams. Maternal morbidity is higher than in the general population and there is a higher incidence of small for date babies. Teratogenicity does not seem to be a significant problem with the immunosuppressive regimens used in the 1980s and most of the 1990s (steroids, azathioprine, calcineurin inhibitors), but the same cannot be said of many of the newer agents.

Complications

General complications related to immunosuppression include an increase in opportunistic infection and malignancy, in particular squamous cell carcinoma of the skin and non-Hodgkin's B-cell lymphoma (which affects 2% of heart transplant recipients).

Box 16.5.2.3 Immunosuppressive drugs

- Calcineurin inhibitor: ciclosporin or tacrolimus

- Antimetabolites: mycophenolate mofetil or azathioprine

- Corticosteroid: usually prednisolone

- Target of rapamycin (TOR) inhibitor: sirolimus or everolimus

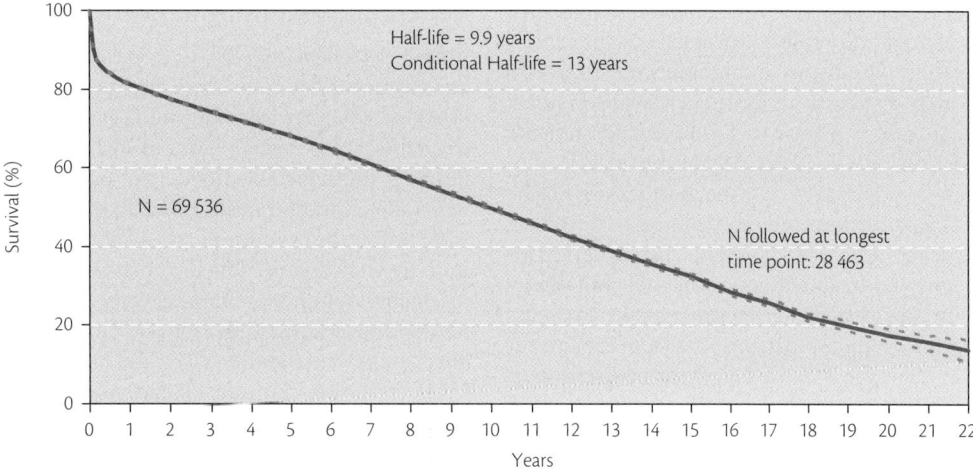

Fig. 16.5.2.1 Survival after heart transplantation. Survival was calculated using the Kaplan–Meier method, incorporating information from all transplants for whom any follow-up has been provided between January 1982 and June 2004. The half-life is the estimated time point at which 50% of all recipients have died; the conditional half-life is the estimated time point at which 50% of the recipients who survive to at least 1 year have died.
From Taylor DO, et al. (2006). Registry of the International Society for Heart and Lung Transplantation: *Twenty-third Official Adult Heart Transplantation Report* 2006, J Heart Lung Transplant, 25, 8697–9.

Calcineurin inhibitors can cause headaches, tremor, hypertension, nephropathy, and peripheral neuropathy, and exacerbate myalgia/myositis associated with statin use. Corticosteroids are associated with osteoporosis and diabetes. Ciclosporin can cause hirsutism and gum hypertrophy. These are discussed in detail in Chapter 21.7.3. Issues particular to cardiac transplantation are described below.

Hyperlipidaemia

Abnormalities in lipid levels have been reported in up to 80% of patients on standard immunosuppressive drug regimes. Pretransplant abnormalities are common in patients transplanted for heart failure secondary to coronary artery disease. Use of statins early post-transplant has been shown to delay the onset of cardiac allograft vasculopathy and reduce mortality after heart transplantation and is now standard practice in most units.

Renal dysfunction

The most serious specific side effect of calcineurin inhibitors is renal dysfunction. Data from the International Society for Heart and Lung Transplantation indicate that about 20% of patients have some degree of renal dysfunction at 1 year after transplantation. Afferent renal arterial vasoconstriction is believed to be the cause of early renal dysfunction and is reversible. Late renal dysfunction is related to tubular damage and tends to be progressive, even when the offending drug is discontinued. At least 5 to 6% of heart transplant patients progress to require renal replacement therapy in the first 10 years post-transplant, and their prognosis on dialysis is poor. The recent introduction of calcineurin inhibitor-free regimes will, it is hoped, decrease the incidence of renal failure. Selected patients with good cardiac function can be considered for renal transplantation.

Cardiac allograft vasculopathy

This term is used to describe concentric narrowing of the coronary arteries (and sometimes veins) of the transplanted heart. It is believed to be an immune mediated disease and is also referred to as 'chronic rejection', although nonimmune mechanisms probably contribute to pathogenesis. It is the commonest cause of late death

after heart transplantation but occasionally presents as a fulminant process that causes death within the first year. Conventional risk factors like smoking and hyperlipidaemia are associated with earlier disease, but cardiac allograft vasculopathy occurs in children and in the absence of other risk factors.

The basic pathological lesion is a diffuse and progressive thickening of the intima that occurs in epicardial and intramyocardial arteries. The disease tends to affect the arterial tree diffusely, although there is heterogeneous involvement of different parts of the arteries. The degree of intimal thickening that occurs in the first year (measured by intravascular ultrasonography) is a predictor of the development of angiographic disease and death or retransplantation for cardiac allograft vasculopathy, risk factors for which are shown in Box 16.5.2.4.

Box 16.5.2.4 Risk factors for cardiac allograft vasculopathy

Immunological

- Number of episodes of acute rejection
- HLA DR mismatch between donor and recipient
- Anti-HLA antibodies in the recipient (associated with the deposition of antibody and complement in the vasculature of the allograft)

Nonimmunological

- Donor age
- Recipient age and gender
- Coronary artery disease as the cause for transplantation in the recipient
- Cytomegalovirus infection
- Smoking
- Obesity
- Hyperlipidaemia

Most patients with cardiac allograft vasculopathy present with signs and symptoms of heart failure, although angina can be experienced despite denervation. The disease is commonly first seen during surveillance coronary angiography. Revascularization is rarely feasible because the disease is diffuse, but occasionally patients have focal proximal lesions that are amenable to angioplasty.

Intravascular ultrasonography (IVUS) is the most sensitive technique for diagnosis of early disease and most clinical trials of new immunosuppressive drugs include IVUS-derived parameters as an endpoint. The only definitive treatment for cardiac allograft vasculopathy is retransplantation, which—given the shortage of donor organs—is an option for only a few patients. Target of rapamycin (TOR) inhibitors may delay the onset and slow the progression of cardiac allograft vasculopathy.

Mechanical circulatory support

The concept of arterial counterpulsation to unload the heart in systole was introduced in the early 1960s. This led to the development of the intra-aortic balloon pump, which was first applied clinically by Kantrowitz in 1967. In 1966 DeBakey reported the first successful clinical application of a true ventricular assist device in a 37-year old woman who could not be weaned from cardiopulmonary bypass following aortic and mitral valve replacement. In 1984 Stanford University reported the first successful heart transplant following bridging with a left ventricular assist device (LVAD).

Ventricular assist devices (VADs) are mechanical blood pumps that work in parallel or series with the native ventricle. A LVAD draws blood from the left atrium or ventricle and returns it to the aorta; a right ventricular assist device (RVAD) draws blood from the right atrium or ventricle and returns it to the pulmonary artery (Fig. 16.5.2.2).

The contexts for using mechanical circulatory support

Bridge to transplantation

Successful cardiac transplantation provided the stimulus for the development of devices that could be used to support patients until a suitable donor organ became available. The availability of donor hearts is unpredictable, hence the patient with acute haemodynamic deterioration needs other methods of circulatory support when intravenous inotropic therapy does not maintain adequate flow to vital organs. Renal and hepatic function improves on mechanical support, pulmonary vascular resistance falls, and nutrition and muscle strength recover. This reduces the risk of subsequent transplantation. Box 16.5.2.5 outlines guidance for use of a LVAD as a bridge to transplantation and factors affecting risk of perioperative complications.

Permanent support

Depending on definition, the prevalence of severe heart failure between the ages of 65 and 75 years is 0.5 to 1.2%. Most of these patients will not be candidates for heart transplantation by virtue of age and comorbidity. VADs were originally developed as a long-term treatment for heart failure and patients who are not transplant candidates can be considered for this form of therapy.

The REMATCH study (Randomized Evaluation of Mechanical Assistance for the Treatment of Congestive Heart Failure) randomized patients with endstage heart failure to best medical therapy or the implantation of the HeartMate I assist device. Survival at 1 year was 52% in the device group and 25% in the medical group; at 2 years it was 23% and 8% respectively. Quality of life was significantly improved at 1 year in the device group, but with a higher frequency of serious adverse events. Survival in the centres with the best outcomes has improved significantly since the REMATCH study, with 60% of patients surviving 2 years.

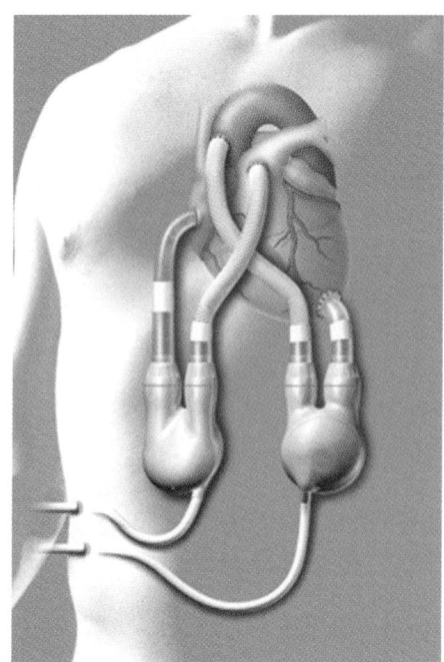

Fig. 16.5.2.2 Stylized picture of a patient with left and right ventricular assist devices.
Courtesy of Thoratec.

Box 16.5.2.5 Guidelines for the use of LVAD as a bridge to transplantation

Inclusion criteria

- The patient is a candidate for transplantation, or is likely to become one with mechanical support
- Haemodynamics (usually on intravenous inotropic therapy; cardiac index <2.0 litres/min per m²; systolic blood pressure <80 mmHg; pulmonary capillary wedge pressure >20 mmHg)

Exclusion criteria

- Technical—aortic regurgitation, right-to-left shunt, abdominal aortic aneurysm, prosthetic valves, left ventricular thrombus
- Severe right ventricular failure (would need BIVAD)

Factors increasing the risk of perioperative complications

- Right atrial pressure >16 mmHg
- Prothrombin time >16 s
- Reoperation
- White blood cell count >15 × 10⁹/litre; pyrexia
- Urine output <30 ml/h
- Mechanical ventilation

The United States Food and Drug Administration approved the HeartMate I device for permanent support in 2002, and several devices have been used in Europe for permanent support. LVAD insertion is not approved for permanent support in the United Kingdom, although there is central funding for bridging to transplantation. Clinical parameters required by the funding agencies in the United States of America include: NYHA IV heart failure that has failed to respond to optimal medical management for at least 60 of the last 90 days; left ventricular ejection fraction less than 25%; functional limitation with peak oxygen consumption less than 12 ml/kg per min, or need for continuous intravenous inotropic therapy.

Several other devices, including continuous flow devices, are undergoing clinical trials as long-term treatment for heart failure. A trail randomizing patients to either Heartmate I or HeartMate II device is due to report in late 2009 and it is expected that the latter device will receive FDA approval for long-term support.

Bridge to recovery

Patients dying from fulminant myocarditis can be supported with mechanical circulatory support and it is not uncommon to see recovery of myocardial function to the point where the device can be removed. Recovery has also been reported in patients with idiopathic dilated cardiomyopathy. LVADs unload the ventricle to a degree that cannot be achieved by drug therapy, and there is a considerable body of evidence to show that the myocardium recovers at the cellular and molecular level with mechanical circulatory support. Structural improvement detectable by echocardiography occurs much less frequently, and clinical recovery to the point where the device can be removed safely is rarer still (<10% of patients in most series, although there are intriguing reports of higher rates of clinical recovery from a few centres). Studies are ongoing, but at present implantation of a device in patients with chronic heart failure must be viewed as a bridge to heart transplantation or as permanent support.

Short-term support

Several devices are available for use in patients who need support for days to periods of up to 4 to 6 weeks. These are invaluable in postcardiotomy cardiogenic shock and in patients who present *in extremis* with multiorgan failure. In the latter group a short-term device may be a bridge to a longer-term device or to heart transplantation, but occasionally patients may improve to the point where the device can be removed and they can be stabilized on medical therapy.

Types of VADs

There are many devices available for clinical use. Box 16.5.2.6 shows a classification of devices and examples of each type: a brief description of selected devices in each category follows.

Pulsatile devices

Pulsatile devices, also referred to as volume displacement VADs, have been used for over 20 years in several thousand patients. An inflow cannula carries blood from the apex of the left ventricle to the device, while the outflow cannula connects to the ascending aorta. Porcine or mechanical valves direct blood flow in the cannulae.

Thoratec PVAD and IVAD

This device (Fig. 16.5.2.3) was originally used as a paracorporeal pump (PVAD), but is now also available in an implantable version (IVAD). It is the only pulsatile VAD that can be used to support

---

Box 16.5.2.6 Classification of VADs

Short-term devices
- Abiomed BVS 5000
- Impella
- Levitronix Centrimag

Long-term devices
Pulsatile (volume displacement)
- Thoratec (PVAD and IVAD)
- HeartMate I
- Novacor

Continuous flow
- Berlin Incor
- HeartMate II
- Jarvik 2000
- Micromed DeBakey
- Ventracor VentrAssist
- Heartware

---

either or both ventricles. It has a 65-ml stroke volume pumping chamber and produces flows of up to 7 litres/min. The implantable version has a percutaneous lead, which connects to the driver. Patients can be discharged home with the device while awaiting a transplant. Anticoagulation is required with a coumarin derivative (maintaining an INR of 2.5–3.5) and antiplatelet therapy may also be needed.

HeartMate XVE

This is a vented electric implantable device (Figs. 16.5.2.4 and 16.5.2.5) that has been used in several thousand patients. The HeartMate is unique in that it has a textured inner surface that promotes a nonthrombogenic pseudoendothelium such that it is the only device for which a coumarin derivative is not required; antiplatelet therapy with aspirin is used. However, the same layer

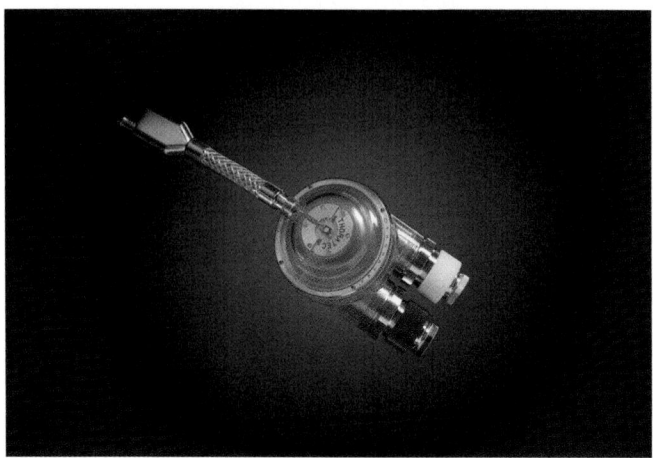

Fig. 16.5.2.3 A Thoratec ventricular assist device.
Courtesy of Thoratec.

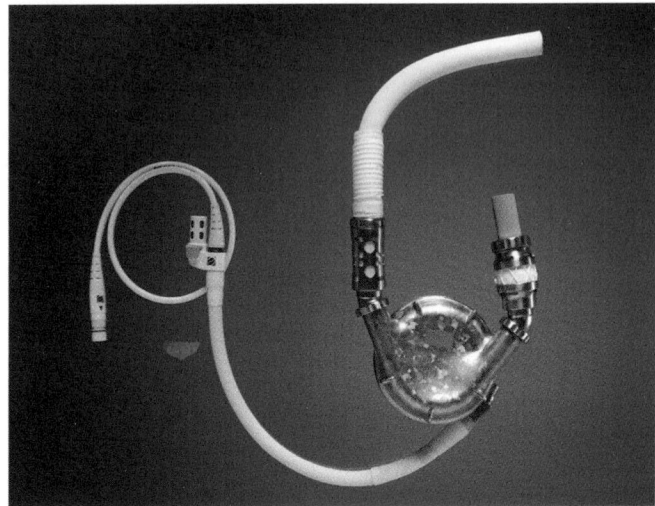

Fig. 16.5.2.4 A Heartmate XVE.
Courtesy of Thoratec.

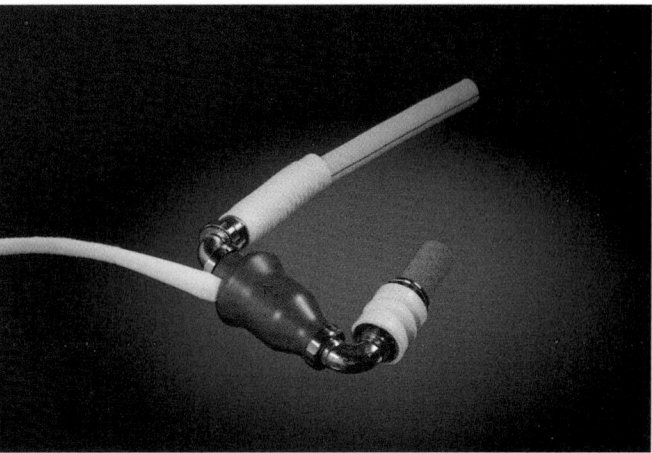

Fig. 16.5.2.6 A Heartmate II.
Courtesy of Thoratec.

may be immunologically active and give rise to antibodies in the patient that complicate subsequent transplantation. Power is supplied by two batteries (worn on a belt) and an external controller. The two batteries supply power for 4 to 7 h. The maximum stroke volume of the pump is 83 ml and flow of between 4 and 10 litres/min can be produced.

Rotary VADs

The pulsatile devices are large and often not suitable for small adults and children. Rotary devices are smaller, have a limited blood contact surface, and lack valves, vents, or compliance chambers: newer pumps also lack bearings and it is hoped will be more

durable. Implantation is generally easier and infections are less common because of a small pump pocket and smaller drive line.

As their name suggests, rotary pumps have a rotating component that has one or more impellers (a disk, cylinder, or blades that propel blood) supported within the pump. They provide continuous flow and are therefore not 'physiological'; patients usually do not have a palpable pulse and blood pressure measurement requires Doppler devices. Pulsatile devices are preload responsive and relatively afterload insensitive: rotary pumps are preload and afterload sensitive such that they require complex feedback algorithms to ensure adequate flow while avoiding ventricular suction. The absence of prosthetic valves makes them simpler and results in less haemotrauma, but in the event of pump stoppage free regurgitation back into the ventricle may occur. Depending on native left ventricular function, some pulsatility may be seen as the aortic valve opens allowing ventricular ejection. Pump thrombosis has been a problem with some of these devices and all rotary pumps currently require anticoagulation with warfarin and antiplatelet agents.

Several continuous flow devices have been in use for the last decade: none has been universally accepted as superior to others and clinical trials with newer devices are ongoing. In the bridge to transplant setting, patient survival has been similar to that with pulsatile devices, although quality of life may be better.

One rotary device is the Heartmate II (Fig. 16.5.2.6). This consists of an internal blood pump with a percutaneous lead that connects the pump to an external computer controller and power source. The blood pump is a 12mm diameter straight tube made of titanium alloy. It connects via cannulae to the left ventricular apex and ascending aorta. The controller and batteries are wearable, the latter providing two to four hours of power. The pump weighs about 350 g, is about 7 cm in length, and is capable of generating flow of up to 10 litres/min. The VentrAssist (Fig. 16.5.2.7) and HeartWare devices are examples of "third generation" continuous flow devices that have completed pivotal trials and been awarded the CE mark in Europe. The HeartWare pump weighs 145 g, has a volume of 45 ml and sits within the pericardial space. The wide-bladed impeller is the pump's only moving part and is held in place by a combination of magnetic and hydrodynamic forces. The lack of bearings in these devices will, it is hoped, result in fewer mechanical problems during long-term support.

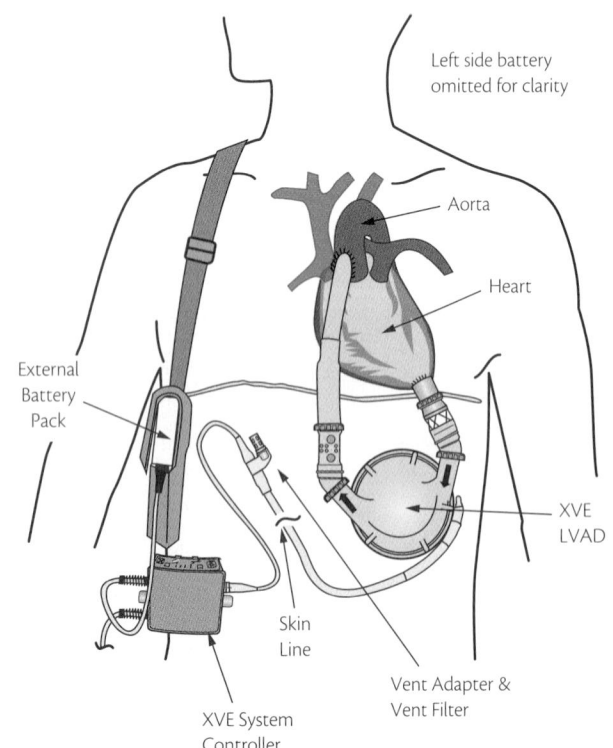

Fig. 16.5.2.5 Stylized picture of a patient with a Heartmate XVE LVAD.
Courtesy of Thoratec.

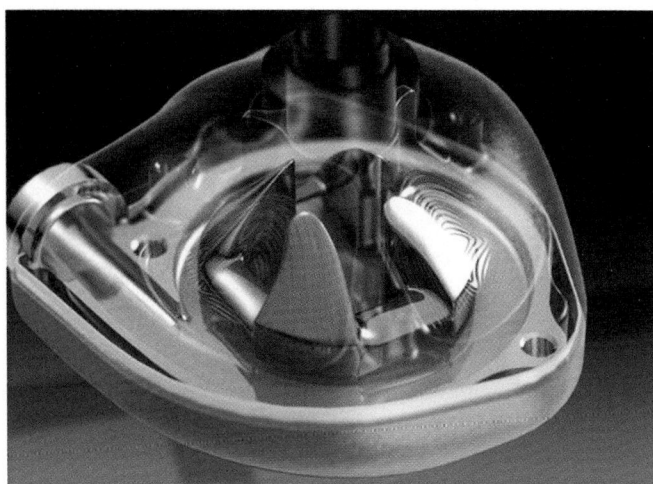

Fig. 16.5.2.7 A VentrAssist.
Courtesy of Ventracor.

Complications of ventricular assist devices

There are three main complications in the peri-implant period: bleeding related to a coagulopathic state in the patient, and surgical bleeding; acute right ventricular failure; neurological events from particulate matter from within the pump or air.

The major complications in the postimplant period include infection, of either pump pocket or drive line site (in up to 25% of patients); thromboembolism, related to device or patient (in up to 20% of patients); haemolysis, which may be less of a problem with rotary pumps; and device malfunction (usually a late complication).

Further reading

Barnard CN (1967). A human cardiac transplant: an interim report of a successful procedure performed at Groote Schuur Hospital, Capetown. *S Afr Med J*, **41**, 12717–4.

Billingham ME (1992). Histopathology of graft coronary disease. *J Heart Lung Transplant*, **11**, 5384–4.

Birks EJ, *et al.* (2006). Left ventricular assist device and drug therapy for the reversal of heart failure. *N Eng J Med*, **355**, 18738–4.

Hill DJ, *et al.* (2006). Positive displacement ventricular assist devices. In Frazier OH, Kirklin JK (eds) *Mechanical circulatory support*, pp. 537–6. Elsevier, Philadelphia.

Kapadia SR, *et al.* (1998). Development of transplantation vasculopathy and progression of donor-transmitted atherosclerosis. *Circulation*, **98**, 26727–8.

Mancini DM, *et al.* (1991). Value of peak oxygen consumption for optimal timing of cardiac transplantation in ambulatory patients with heart failure. *Circulation*, **83**, 7788–6.

Mehra MR, *et al.* (2006). Listing criteria for heart transplantation: International Society for Heart and Lung Transplantation Guidelines for the Care of Cardiac Transplant Candidates-2006. *J Heart Lung Transplant*, **25**, 10244–2.

Rose EA, *et al.* (2001). Long-term use of a left ventricular assist device for end-stage heart failure. *N Engl J Med*, **345**, 14354–3.

Taylor DO, *et al.* (2006). Registry of the International Society for Heart and Lung Transplantation: Twenty-third Official Adult Heart Transplantation Report 2006. *J Heart Lung Transplant*, **25**, 8697–9.

16.6

Heart valve disease

Michael Henein

Essentials

Rheumatic valve disease remains prevalent in developing countries, but over the last 50 years there has been a decline in the incidence of rheumatic valve disease and an increase in the prevalence of degenerative valve pathology in northern Europe and North America. In all forms of valve disease, the most appropriate initial diagnostic investigation is almost always the echocardiogram.

Mitral stenosis

The most common cause is rheumatic valve disease. Other causes include mitral annular calcification, congenital mitral stenosis, infective endocarditis (very rarely), and systemic lupus erythematosus (SLE) (Liebman–Sachs endocarditis).

The important consequences of mitral stenosis are its effect on left atrial pressure, size, and the pulmonary vasculature; it commonly causes atrial fibrillation. Presenting symptoms are typically exertional fatigue and breathlessness; systemic embolism can occur. Characteristic physical signs are irregular pulse, tapping apex beat, loud first heart sound, opening snap, and an apical low-pitched rumbling mid-diastolic murmur.

Management—the only medical treatments in mitral stenosis are (1) prophylactic measures against rheumatic fever and endocarditis; (2) anticoagulation to prevent systemic embolism; and (3) diuretics for raised left atrial pressure. Patients who are symptomatic need intervention by either surgical valvotomy or catheter–balloon valvuloplasty, whether or not they have pulmonary hypertension. Early intervention—before the development of atrial fibrillation and an enlarged left atrium—is recommended, provided a conservative operation is possible. Mitral valve replacement is reserved for cases where the mitral valve cannot be repaired.

Mitral regurgitation

The most common causes are ischaemic myocardial dysfunction, mitral valve prolapse, and dilated cardiomyopathy. Other causes include congenital valve disease, infective endocarditis, endomyocardial fibrosis, and connective tissue diseases (including Marfan's syndrome).

Mitral regurgitation is an isolated volume overload on the left ventricle, providing the physiological equivalent of afterload reduction so that a normal forward cardiac output is maintained by the combination of increased ejection fraction and higher preload. Patients with mild regurgitation may not have any symptoms: those with severe regurgitation are likely to present with dyspnoea. Characteristic physical signs are an apex beat that may be prominent and displaced, an apical pansystolic murmur, and a third heart sound. The loudness of the murmur generally correlates with severity of regurgitation. The cardinal signs of mitral prolapse are a mid-systolic click followed by a murmur.

Management—prophylaxis against endocarditis is recommended. Patients in atrial fibrillation should be given anticoagulants. The development of symptoms suggests the need for surgical correction to avoid development of irreversible left ventricular dysfunction. Assessment during routine follow-up should identify those likely to need surgical intervention even in the absence of symptoms, with an effective regurgitant orifice of over $40\,mm^2$ being one proposed indication. It is generally considered that a left ventricular end-systolic dimension more than 50 mm indicates a poor prognosis and that surgical intervention is unlikely to be of benefit. If technically possible, mitral valve repair results in a much better clinical outcome than does valve replacement, but mitral replacement by a mechanical valve or bioprosthesis is the only option for irreparable valves.

Aortic stenosis

Aortic stenosis may be at subvalvar, valvar, or supravalvar level, the commonest being valvar stenosis. Age-related degenerative calcific disease is the commonest cause in western Europe and the United States of America. Other causes include congenital bicuspid aortic valve and rheumatic disease (always associated with aortic regurgitation, 'mixed aortic valve disease', and usually with rheumatic mitral disease).

With the increase in outflow-tract resistance in aortic stenosis, left ventricular wall stress increases and hypertrophy develops, preserving overall ventricular systolic function, but potentially at the expense of subendocardial ischaemia. Patients with mild disease may be asymptomatic, and even severe stenosis may be silent, but breathlessness, angina, and syncope are typical. Characteristic physical signs are a slowly rising, low-amplitude pulse, a narrow pulse pressure, a sustained apex beat, and a long and harsh ejection systolic murmur that is loudest at the base (second right intercostal space, also known as the aortic area) of the heart, and in most cases radiates to the carotids (where a thrill may be palpable).

Management—patients with moderate or severe disease should be advised to avoid strenuous exercise. Prophylaxis against endocarditis is required. Asymptomatic patients with mild or moderate aortic stenosis require follow-up; those with severe disease (pressure gradient >70 mmHg) need aortic valve replacement.

Aortic regurgitation

Aortic regurgitation is caused by leaflet disease or aortic root dilatation, the commonest causes being isolated medionecrosis, rheumatic disease, infective endocarditis, and Marfan's syndrome.

The left ventricular stroke volume is significantly increased, which is accommodated by an increase in left ventricular cavity size. As disease progresses, end-systolic volume increases out of proportion to stroke volume, and eventually these changes lead to irreversible damage. The onset of symptoms, particularly breathlessness, coincides with the onset of left ventricular disease. Characteristic physical signs of chronic severe aortic regurgitation are a large amplitude 'collapsing' pulse (which when severe can induce pulsations in many parts of the body), a low diastolic blood pressure (<50 mmHg) and/or a high pulse pressure (>80 mmHg), an apex beat that is sustained and/or displaced, and an early diastolic, decrescendo murmur, loudest at the left sternal border. Acute aortic regurgitation causes the patient to be cold and shut down, with tachycardia, hypotension, and a short early diastolic murmur that is easily missed.

Management—medical treatment of chronic aortic regurgitation includes angiotensin converting enzyme (ACE) inhibitors and/or calcium channel blockers to reduce afterload. Patients with a dilated aortic root should be given β-blockade with ACE inhibition/angiotensin receptor blockers. Prophylaxis against endocarditis is required. Although patients with severe chronic aortic regurgitation may remain asymptomatic, valve replacement should be offered when there is progressive increase in left ventricular end

systolic dimension, which should not be allowed to reach more than 40 mm.

Right heart valve disease

Many of the conditions that cause right-sided valve diseases are congenital, and are excluded from further discussion here (see Chapter 16.12).

Tricuspid stenosis—this is rare, but most often caused by rheumatic disease that almost invariably simultaneously affects the mitral valve. Symptoms include fatigue, dyspnoea, and fluid retention. On auscultation at the left or right sternal edge, a mid-diastolic murmur is heard and a tricuspid opening snap may be present. Diuretics can help to minimize fluid retention. Severe tricuspid stenosis needs surgical repair, or replacement if additional regurgitation is present.

Tricuspid regurgitation —significant disease is most commonly secondary to pulmonary hypertension and/or right heart dilatation; the commonest noncongenital primary cause is infective endocarditis. Symptoms include fluid retention and hepatic congestion. A raised venous pressure with prominent V-wave is expected. Other signs include a pansystolic murmur at the left or right sternal edge (in one-third of cases), expansile pulsation of the liver (in most), and peripheral oedema/ascites. Diuretics and ACE inhibitors may reduce systemic venous pressure and right ventricular size, even restoring valve competence in some cases. Valve repair or replacement may be advised in some cases.

Pulmonary stenosis—a rare condition usually caused by rheumatic disease or carcinoid syndrome. Fatigue and dyspnoea are the main symptoms. Characteristic physical signs are a prominent venous 'a' wave in the neck and an ejection systolic murmur loudest at the upper left sternal edge. Balloon valvuloplasty is the procedure of choice if intervention is warranted.

Pulmonary regurgitation—significant disease is rare, but usually caused by rheumatic disease, carcinoid, and endocarditis. The characteristic physical sign is a soft early diastolic murmur in the left upper parasternal region. Arrhythmia or progressive right ventricular dilatation are indications for surgery, using homograft or conduit and valve.

Introduction

Over the last 50 years there has been a significant shift in the causes of heart valve disease in Northern Europe and North America, with a decline in the incidence of rheumatic valve disease and an increase in the prevalence of degenerative valve pathology. Rheumatic valve disease remains prevalent in the developing countries, particularly in areas with limited clinical services. The commonest valve involved with rheumatic pathology is the mitral valve, but the aortic and tricuspid valves can also be involved. The apparent increase in the diagnosis of valve disease could be due either to ageing of the population or to the extensive use of echocardiography in cardiology clinics. Age affects the valves, making leaflets thicker with fibrous strands and adipose tissue deposition at the closure lines of

the leaflets. Isolated myxomatous changes may also occur in the valve fibrosa. In patients with a suspected diagnosis of endocarditis these changes can add to diagnostic difficulty since they may look like small vegetations, and they also need to be distinguished from papillary muscle fibroelastoma.

Medical treatment of valve disease is limited, focusing mostly on prophylaxis against endocarditis and ventricular dysfunction as well as optimizing haemodynamics. Although surgical repair is the main conventional treatment of severe valve disease, the need for this is 5 to 10 times less than that for coronary artery disease.

Valve-related mortality is more common in aortic valve disease than mitral valve disease, largely due to the frequent development of left ventricular dysfunction that causes congestive heart failure.

Other causes of death in valve disease are additional pathologies such as coronary artery disease, endocarditis, or arrhythmia.

The mitral valve

Normal mitral valve anatomy and function

Optimum function of the mitral valve depends on the intact function of all its components—leaflets, chordae, annulus, and papillary muscles, in addition to the left atrium and the left ventricle. A normal mitral valve does not close passively. In addition to the pressure difference between the ventricle and atrium in systole, the annular contraction and papillary muscle contraction play an important role in the competence of the mitral valve. The anterior mitral valve leaflet represents a continuation of the posterior aortic root wall. The annular fibrous ring is located mainly posteriorly; it is usually D-shaped but there is significant variability in different individuals. The normal diameter of the mitral annulus is around 3 cm with a circumference of 8 to 9 cm: it is not a passive structure, so in addition to its normal movement towards the apex in systole, the contraction of the posterior myocardial muscle shortens its diameter by 25%, with such movement being a very important component in the mechanism of mitral valve competence.

Change in the size and shape of the left atrial cavity is a cause for incompetence of the mitral valve by enlarging the annular diameter. Loss of atrial mechanical function may contribute significantly to the development of mitral regurgitation in patients with atrial fibrillation. Likewise, atrial fibrillation itself has been shown to contribute to the enlargement of the left atrium and consequently the development of mitral regurgitation.

The two leaflets of the mitral valve meet at the medial and lateral commissures. The area of the U-shaped anterior leaflet is larger than that of the posterior leaflet, which is wider and shorter than the anterior leaflet. The posterior leaflet is made up of a number of scallops, commonly three. The two leaflets coapt at the zone of apposition, leaving an overlapping segment 5 mm long.

The chordal anatomy of the mitral valve is complicated, with around 12 primary chordae rising from each papillary muscle. These divide into secondaries and numerous tertiary branches that attach themselves to the margins of the two leaflets. In addition, a number of basal chordae also attach themselves to the ventricular surface of the leaflets and to the commissures. The location of the chordae follows that of the papillary muscles anterolaterally and posteromedially. Any rupture or redundancy of the chordae or extra tissue in the leaflets results in mitral regurgitation.

Mitral stenosis

Causes

The most common cause of mitral stenosis, which affects women more than men (2:1), is rheumatic valve disease. The rheumatic process involves not only the leaflets but may also affect the chordae and the annulus, causing fibrosis and superimposed calcification. The rheumatic leaflets become thickened and fibrosed, and the commissures fuse. The end result of this pathology is a reduction in mitral valve area, the rigid movement of the leaflets and the commissural fusion together contributing to the limited flow across the mitral valve orifice and hence stenosis. It is not uncommon for the fibrotic process to involve the subvalvar region in an aggressive way, thus causing flow to be limited at the level of the subvalvar apparatus. In such cases the chordae become short and the inflow tract of the left ventricle become tunnel-like.

Mitral annular calcification is another cause of raised filling velocities: this is seen in older people with the calcification limited to the annulus and the proximal segments of the leaflets, but the leaflets themselves are normal. A very uncommon cause of mitral stenosis is congenital mitral stenosis, which may be associated with other cardiac abnormalities. Infective endocarditis with bulky vegetations may rarely cause restriction of mitral flow, and patients with systemic lupus erythematosus (SLE) can develop fibrosis of the mitral cusps with commissural fusion following Liebman–Sachs endocarditis.

Pathophysiology and complications

The important consequence of mitral stenosis is its effect on left atrial pressure and size and on the pulmonary vasculature. As the valve area falls progressively, left atrial pressure rises, its size increases, and the pulmonary venous pressure also increases. In most patients with rheumatic mitral valve disease the left ventricle is normal in size and systolic function unless the valve stenosis is severe and making the ventricle under filled.

With a mild degree of mitral stenosis, reduced orifice area is compensated by increased flow during atrial systole. As the valve stenosis becomes more severe, the left atrial pressure increases, the pressure difference between the atrium and the ventricle increases, and the filling occurs throughout diastole. In severe mitral stenosis the pressure difference may be as high as 25 to 30 mmHg. Long-standing disease may result in irreversible pulmonary hypertension secondary to the raised left atrial pressure. Atrial fibrillation also develops, with loss of mechanical atrial function.

A normal mitral valve area is of the order of 5 cm^2, compared to a valve area in a patient with severe mitral stenosis of less than 1 cm^2. Effective mitral valve area changes very little with increase in heart rate compared to aortic valve area (which increases), the reason probably being the smaller number of commissures that assist opening of the mitral valve compared to the aortic valve. During exercise, particularly in atrial fibrillation, diastolic time falls and the fixed valve area causes raised left atrial pressure and pulmonary venous pressure.

Left atrial dilatation

Progressive reduction in mitral valve orifice area causes progressive increase in left atrial pressure and size and pulmonary venous pressure. Left atrial dilatation is associated with reduction in its mechanical function that slows down intra-atrial blood circulation (swirling). With progressive disease and development of atrial fibrillation, the circulation in the atrium becomes very sluggish and echocardiography may demonstrate spontaneous echo-contrast, particularly on transoesophageal images. Such patients are given anticoagulants in order to avoid clot formation and hence the risk of transient ischaemic attacks (TIA). Almost one-fifth of the patients undergoing surgery for mitral stenosis have left atrial thrombus, and in one-third of them the thrombus is restricted to the atrial appendage.

Atrial fibrillation

This is the most common complication of mitral stenosis and its prevalence increases with age, being found in 70% of patients in their thirties and in 80% of those in their fifties. The presence of pulmonary hypertension raises the prevalence of atrial fibrillation.

The Framingham study estimated a 20-fold increase in risk of stroke in patients with atrial fibrillation and mitral stenosis compared to only 5-fold increase in those without mitral valve disease. Left atrial thrombus may also form in patients with a dilated left atrium with spontaneous echo-contrast who are in sinus rhythm. The loss of left atrial appendage mechanical function has been proposed as a possible mechanism behind blood stagnation and thrombus formation.

Left ventricular dysfunction

Although in most cases of mitral stenosis the left ventricle is normal in size and systolic function, in some diastolic function may be impaired and end-diastolic pressure raised. This could be related to additional pathology, e.g. systemic hypertension and diabetes. The left ventricle is dilated only in the presence of additional coronary artery disease. Primary rheumatic myocardial disease was proposed years ago, but no convincing evidence has ever come to light.

Pulmonary hypertension

With the increase in left atrial pressure, the pulmonary venous pressure increases and hence pulmonary arterial pressure also rises. Although pulmonary artery pressure corresponds to the degree of increase in left atrial pressure, a discrepancy between the two may reflect a raised pulmonary vascular resistance. A normal pressure drop across the pulmonary bed is of the order of 10–15 mmHg. The pulmonary hypertension is not always reversible after valve surgery. For any degree of mitral stenosis patients can display a wide range of pulmonary pressures, but it is very rare for secondary pulmonary hypertension to develop with left atrial pressure <20 mmHg in the setting of isolated mitral stenosis.

Right heart disease

With the development of pulmonary hypertension the right ventricle becomes hypertrophied and its cavity dilates. This is also reflected in right atrial size. Patients with rheumatic mitral valve disease may have additional tricuspid valve involvement in particular, the annulus dilating and causing significant tricuspid regurgitation. Patients with severe tricuspid regurgitation may complain of fluid retention that needs careful management in order to maintain the left-sided cardiac output and obtain tissue perfusion. Long-standing significant tricuspid regurgitation and raised right atrial pressure may cause further deterioration of right ventricular function and congestive heart failure. By that stage the damage is usually irreversible despite any successful mitral valve surgery.

Clinical presentation

Symptoms

Patients may remain asymptomatic with mild mitral stenosis. As the disease progresses, early symptoms are exertional fatigue and breathlessness. With severe mitral stenosis shortness of breath is accompanied by orthopnoea and paroxysmal nocturnal dyspnoea. With the development of pulmonary hypertension, right ventricular dysfunction and tricuspid regurgitation patients may present with fluid retention as well as recurrent chest infection. Atrial fibrillation may be an early symptom in patients with mitral stenosis, particularly palpitations on exercise. Major systemic embolus can also be a presenting symptom, and the condition may be detected for the first time during pregnancy as patients complain of disproportionate dyspnoea.

Physical examination

Long-standing mitral stenosis characteristically causes weight loss and a malar flush. The pulse character is normal, but pulse volume may be reduced and atrial fibrillation is likely. The jugular venous pressure is usually normal unless there is tricuspid regurgitation and/or pulmonary hypertension (see below). The apex is not displaced, but the first heart sound is sometimes palpable ('tapping apex'), and less frequently the opening snap is also.

The characteristic auscultatory features of rheumatic mitral stenosis are an opening snap in early diastole, a mid-diastolic murmur, and a loud first heart sound. The opening snap is caused by the abrupt tension that develops in the fibrosed leaflets at the termination of the opening movement. It is best heard at the lower left sternal edge or apex, becoming closer to the second heart sound as left atrial pressure rises, and it is absent with leaflet calcification. The diastolic murmur is low pitched and maximal at the apex. It is caused by increased blood flow velocity between the left atrium and left ventricle and is accentuated in late diastole by atrial contraction in patients in sinus rhythm. The longer the mid-diastolic murmur, the more likely that the mitral stenosis is severe. The loud first heart sound is associated with fibrosis of the anterior leaflet and is lost with leaflet calcification. Many patients with mitral stenosis have some degree of mitral regurgitation, which is not significant in the presence of severe stenosis.

In the presence of pulmonary hypertension the jugular venous pressure is raised, there may be a palpable right ventricular heave, and the second heart sound is usually loud. In patients with significant tricuspid regurgitation, whether secondary to pulmonary hypertension or due to rheumatic tricuspid valve, there is a clear V-wave and deep Y descent in the jugular venous pulse, and expansile pulsation of the liver. The murmur of tricuspid regurgitation is not usually prominent.

Investigations

Chest radiograph and electrocardiogram

Early in the disease a chest radiograph may show a completely normal cardiac silhouette. Later, as the disease progresses, left atrial enlargement appears and a prominent left atrial appendage contour becomes very evident (Fig. 16.6.1). Left atrial double-density and elevation of left main bronchus may also be evident. In patients with raised left atrial pressure, pulmonary vascular redistribution manifest as 'dilated upper lobe veins' and interstitial pulmonary oedema 'Kerley B lines' may be seen. The central pulmonary arteries become prominent as pulmonary hypertension develops, and upper lobe deviation is also seen. Finally, right-sided dilatation may also be seen as tricuspid regurgitation develops.

The electrocardiogram can show a broad and notched P-wave due to left atrial hypertrophy ('P mitrale') as a classical finding in mitral stenosis, but will more often reveal atrial fibrillation.

Echocardiography

Echocardiography is the investigation of choice in mitral valve disease. A typical picture of rheumatic valve disease is a short, fibrosed, and stiff posterior leaflet; a fibrosed anterior leaflet that bows down towards the ventricle in diastole; and narrow valve area (Fig. 16.6.2). Short axis images clearly demonstrate the fused commissures and two-dimensional images show the extent of chordal fibrosis. Planimetry of the mitral valve area in diastole gives an estimate of the degree of stenosis. Continuous wave Doppler assesses the blood flow velocity across the valve. In mild stenosis,

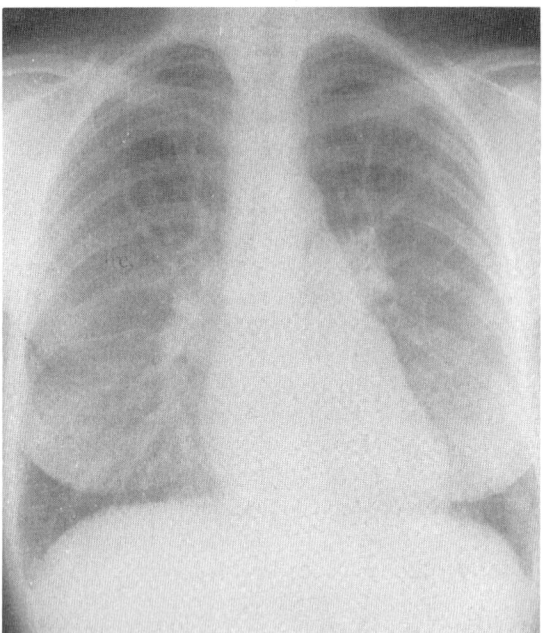

Fig. 16.6.1 Chest radiograph from a patient with pure mitral stenosis. The heart size is normal, but the left atrial appendage is enlarged. The upper lobe vessels are dilated and there are Kerley lines at both bases.

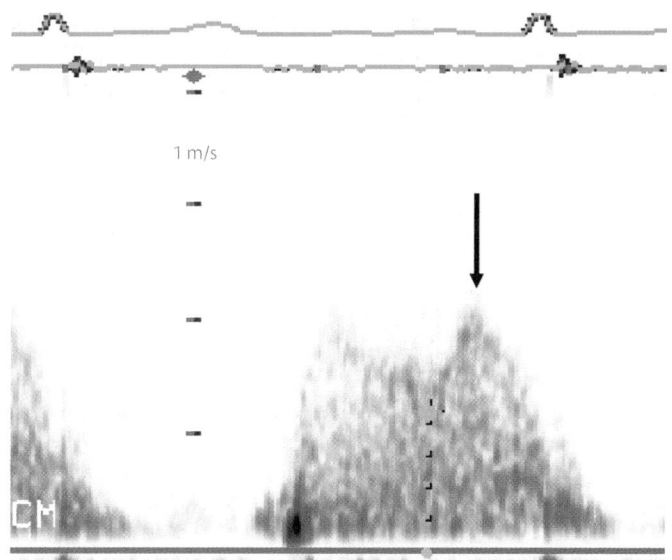

Fig. 16.6.3 Continuous wave Doppler of left ventricular filling from a patient with mitral stenosis, showing raised velocities (>2 m/s, arrowed) across the mitral valve as the ventricle fills in diastole. A mean velocity of more than 1.3 m/s at the mitral valve leaflet tips is abnormal.

transmitral Doppler demonstrates a peak velocity in late diastole compared to in early diastole in severe stenosis. With atrial fibrillation there is a single early diastolic filling component to the left ventricle. A transmitral mean pressure gradient of more than 4 mmHg suggests a moderate degree of stenosis (Fig. 16.6.3), and a mean pressure gradient of more than 8 mmHg suggests severe stenosis. Colour flow Doppler can provide a quantitative approach for assessing mitral stenosis severity using the proximal isovelocity surface area (PISA) method or the vena contracta method (the vena contracta being the narrowest region of the stenotic jet, just downstream of the valve orifice and reflecting the size of that orifice). Although the latter is easy to use it has its limitations since it varies more with deformation of the mitral orifice area and shape.

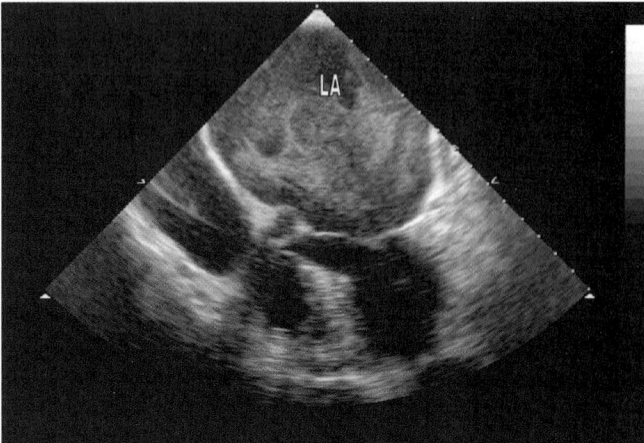

Fig. 16.6.2 Transoesophageal echocardiogram from a patient with severe rheumatic mitral stenosis showing a dilated left atrium (LA) with spontaneous echo contrast.

Colour flow Doppler will also show any mitral regurgitation jet and give some indication of its severity.

Echocardiography also assesses any involvement of the aortic valve or the tricuspid valve by the same or other pathologies. It is now common practice that most patients with mitral valve disease are studied by transoesophageal echo because this provides more detailed assessment of the mitral valve, the subvalvar apparatus, and the presence of left atrial spontaneous contrast and appendage clots.

Cardiac catheterization

Echocardiography has replaced cardiac catheterization in making the diagnosis of mitral stenosis. Catheterization may provide additional information on pulmonary vascular resistance and coronary artery disease before surgery.

Differential diagnosis

The diagnosis of mitral stenosis is usually straightforward on the basis of clinical findings supported by echocardiography, which should distinguish the presence of an Austin–Flint murmur caused by aortic regurgitation (see below) and the rare conditions of left atrial myxoma (see Chapter 16.10) and cor triatriatum (see Chapter 16.12).

Management

There is a significant time lag between the acute event of rheumatic fever and the presentation of mitral stenosis with mild symptoms, which could be up to 15 years. Patients may need another 10 years to develop signs and symptoms of severe stenosis. The likely reason behind this delay is the time needed for rheumatic leaflet fibrosis and calcification to develop and cause raised left atrial pressure. This time lag between acute rheumatic fever and clinical presentation varies significantly between developed and developing countries. In Europe and North America patients need valve surgery for mitral stenosis in their fifties, whereas those in developing countries need it in their thirties. The clinical outcome of patients with unoperated rheumatic mitral stenosis has changed significantly over time, with 20-year follow-up mortality dropping from historically 85% to recently 44% in those who refuse surgery.

Medical

The only medical treatments in mitral stenosis are the prophylactic measures against rheumatic fever (penicillin prophylaxis, see Chapter 16.9.1) and endocarditis (see Chapter 16.9.2), anticoagulation to prevent systemic embolism, and diuretics for raised left atrial pressure. There is no medication that has a direct effect on slowing disease progress.

Patients with mitral stenosis should be followed up clinically using noninvasive investigations, particularly Doppler echocardiography. The frequency of follow-up should be tailored according to individual patient's clinical condition and the severity of disease. Whilst this could be every 2 years in a patient with mild stenosis and regurgitation, closer attention is required for the patient with severe stenosis and evidence of pulmonary hypertension. Particularly close follow-up is advised for pregnant women who have mitral stenosis.

In patients who develop atrial fibrillation, attempts to restore sinus rhythm are usually unsuccessful unless associated with surgery. To maintain sinus rhythm the organic mitral lesion should be dealt with either interventionally or surgically. In addition to heart rate control, digoxin may keep a patient with a modestly dilated left atrium in sinus rhythm. However, once atrial fibrillation is established, attention should be diverted to rate control with digoxin, β-blockers, or calcium channel blockers. With persistent atrial fibrillation anticoagulation is essential and INR level should be monitored and maintained at 2.5 to 3.5. Patients recommended for percutaneous mitral valvuloplasty should receive stable anticoagulation therapy for at least 3 months before the procedure and transoesophageal echo should exclude left atrial clot. Those who need surgical intervention may receive a maze procedure as a means for restoring the sinus rhythm, which involves surgically creating a single electrical pathway from the sinus node to the atriventricular node, while isolating the abnormal electrical activity of the left and right atrial tissue. Recently, electrophysiological mapping with isolation of pulmonary veins has offered an alternative procedure. The success of the maze procedure varies considerably, ranging between 25% and 80% even after an initially successful procedure. See Chapter 16.4 for further discussion.

Patients who are symptomatic need intervention by either surgical valvotomy or catheter balloon valvuloplasty, whether or not they have pulmonary hypertension. Early intervention is highly recommended, before the development of atrial fibrillation and an enlarged left atrium, provided a conservative operation is possible. The percutaneous mitral valvuloplasty procedure involves inserting an Inoue balloon into the mitral valve orifice and inflating it until an increase in mitral valve area is achieved (Fig. 16.6.4). Contraindications to this procedure are left atrial appendage thrombus, calcified subvalvar apparatus, and/or mitral regurgitation. Early results of this technique are satisfactory, particularly if patients are well selected, e.g. those with relatively mobile, noncalcified leaflets that are not greatly thickened, and without subvavlular thickening. Mitral stenosis may recur following this procedure after the healing period of the split of the fused commissures.

Surgical

Closed mitral valvotomy has been replaced by percutaneous mitral valvuloplasty, but its results are not optimal. There is thus still

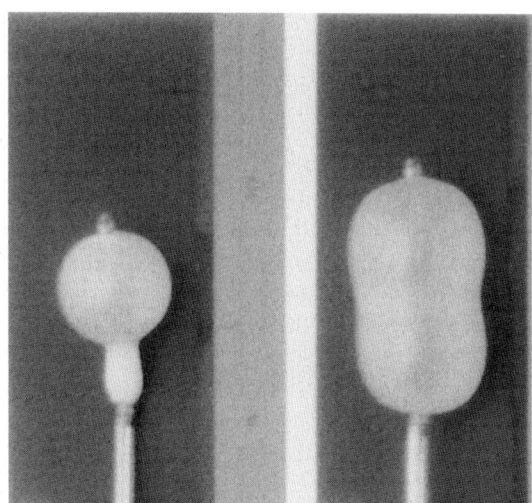

Fig. 16.6.4 Inoue balloon catheter, as used for mitral valvuloplasty, partially (left) and completely (right) inflated.

room for surgical repair of the mitral valve. This is better suited to patients with minimal calcification and those with short chordae. The technique offers the advantage of avoiding replacing the mitral valve, which has effects on left ventricular function. However, in a patient with an irreparable mitral valve the only remaining option is mitral valve replacement.

Closed mitral commissurotomy

This historic procedure aimed at opening the mitral valve by applying a dilator through the ventricular apex, with the *surgeon using their finger* to feel the valve leaflets and orifice to judge when the desired valve area was achieved. The first successful operations were carried out in 1948. It has been intensively used in the United Kingdom and other countries, with an average mortality of 3 to 4%.

Open mitral valvotomy

This operation requires the use of an extracorporeal circulation and aims at direct visualization of the mitral valve through a medial sternotomy with careful dissection of the fused commissures under direct vision. In contrast to the closed operation, the surgeon is able to deal with the subvalvar apparatus and the fused chordae, and correct chordal shortening if required. The left atrial appendage can also be visualized, and if there is thrombus present it can be removed. With appropriate patient selection and preoperative evaluation open commissurotomy is feasible in most patients, with an operative mortality of approximately 1%.

Mitral valve replacement:

Mitral valve replacement involves either a mechanical or a tissue valve substitute. Surgical mortality varies according to other comorbidities: it is of the order of 3% in patients with isolated mitral valve stenosis but can be as high as 12% in patients with additional pulmonary hypertension. The life of biological mitral valve substitutes, particularly porcine xenografts, is limited to less than 10 years in most adults, hence their use tends to be restricted to very elderly patients. Cryopreserved mitral homografts have been proposed recently as a better option, as has the use of a pulmonary autograft in a Dacron tube, but experience is limited.

Mitral regurgitation

Causes

The most common causes of mitral regurgitation are ischaemic myocardial dysfunction, mitral valve prolapse, and dilated cardiomyopathy. Other causes are given in Table 16.6.1.

Ischaemic mitral regurgitation

The posteromedial papillary muscle is predisposed to ischaemic dysfunction and infarction because it is supplied by a single branch of the posterior descending artery and tends to have only a few collaterals. The anterolateral papillary muscle receives blood from branches of both the left anterior descending artery and the circumflex artery, so it is less susceptible to ischaemia. Ischaemic disturbances of left ventricular function contribute to the development of mitral regurgitation through a number of mechanisms: (1) regional wall motion abnormalities with adverse ventricular remodelling and systolic tenting of the valve leaflets, (2) left ventricular dilatation and shape change that alters normal alignment of the papillary muscles and results in leaflet tethering and inadequate closure, and (3) annular dilatation leading to inadequate annular contraction. These mechanisms may contribute to further enlargement of the left ventricle and deterioration of its function, which itself would add to the severity of mitral regurgitation. Four clinical presentations are seen in ischaemic mitral regurgitation: acute myocardial infarction, papillary muscle rupture, reversible ischaemic myocardial dysfunction in the presence of preserved left ventricular systolic function, and endstage ischaemic cardiomyopathy with reduced function.

Table 16.6.1 Common causes of mitral regurgitation

Structure primarily affected	Anatomical defect	Cause
Valve cusps	Congenital cleft	Primary atrial septal defect Isolated
	Redundant cusp	Mitral valve prolapse Marfan's syndrome
	Perforation	Infective endocarditis
	Scarring	Rheumatic fever Ergot-derived dopamine receptor agonists
Chordae	Redundant	Mitral valve prolapse Marfan's syndrome Other connective tissue disease
	Rupture	Acute myocardial infarction Mitral valve prolapse Marfan's syndrome Other connective tissue disease Infective endocarditis Rheumatic fever
	Shortening	Rheumatic fever Endomyocardial fibrosis
Papillary muscle	Dysfunction	Ischaemia
Valve annulus	Dilatation	Severe left ventricular disease of any cause—'dilated cardiomyopathy'

Acute myocardial infarction

Significant mitral regurgitation complicates 3 to 16% of acute myocardial infarctions. Most present within the obvious context of acute myocardial infarction, but some with pulmonary oedema from the acute development of mitral regurgitation. Most patients presenting with myocardial infarction complicated by mitral regurgitation have right and circumflex coronary artery disease that causes inferior wall dysfunction. Mitral regurgitation does not therefore seem to be related to infarct size, but to the extent of ischaemic dysfunction and involvement of the posteromedial papillary muscle. The resulting poor support to the posterior leaflet, referred to as tethering, causes lack of leaflet coaption and valve incompetence. When severe mitral regurgitation develops it carries a poor prognosis, with mortality rising to 25% at 30 days and over 50% at 1 year. The effect of reperfusion on mitral regurgitation remains controversial.

Papillary muscle rupture

Complete papillary muscle rupture causes severe mitral regurgitation and cardiogenic shock that is usually fatal—70% within 24 h without emergency surgery. Surgical repair of the papillary muscle is not feasible in most cases because tissues are necrotic: valve replacement is necessary, with risk influenced by other factors including the severe left ventricular disease that is usually present.

Ischaemic mitral regurgitation in a normal left ventricle

Patients with long-standing ischaemic myocardial dysfunction usually have exertional reversible ischaemia. If this affects the posterior wall of the left ventricle it leads to further deterioration of posterior wall function and consequently the posterior leaflet function with the development of mitral regurgitation. Exertional breathlessness in these patients does not always have to be due to raised end-diastolic pressure and may be caused by a sudden increase in left atrial pressure through the development of mitral regurgitation with exercise, particularly in those with a dilated left atrium. Stress echocardiography is ideal for demonstrating the stress induced ischaemic ventricular dysfunction and the development of mitral regurgitation and raised left atrial pressure, when antianginal therapy and afterload reduction may be beneficial. Patients who develop significant mitral regurgitation with stress and who are accepted for coronary artery bypass surgery should receive mitral valve repair and a ring insertion at the time of surgical revascularisation.

Ischaemic mitral regurgitation in ventricular dysfunction

Mitral regurgitation is very common in patients with longstanding ischaemic left ventricular dysfunction and/or endstage ventricular disease. Since the valve leaflets appear morphologically normal, the mitral regurgitation is described as 'functional'. However, three-dimensional echocardiographic assessment of the mitral valve proves that it is not entirely normal, with long-standing progressive changes in the interleaflet relations and subvalvar apparatus. Reducing ventricular pressures may improve left ventricular geometry, and lowering blood pressure may reduce mitral regurgitation severity.

Mitral valve prolapse

Mitral valve prolapse is a genetic connective tissue disorder that affects the mitral leaflets, chordae, and annulus, with an autosomal dominant pattern of inheritance and variable penetrance. Histologically the leaflets show thickening of the spongiosa and disruption of the fibrosa with fragmentation. Collagen is also abnormal with high rate of synthesis, deficiency in type III collagen, and splitting of collagen with fibre disarray. The cause has not yet been identified: defects in a collagen gene or in a gene encoding a component of microfibrils, similar to that involved in Marfan's syndrome, have obviously been considered. The condition is common: 1.5 to 6% of adults have mitral prolapse, depending on definition, and screening of first-degree family members demonstrates prolapse in approximately 30% of cases.

Mitral prolapse can be classified into two types: a benign condition that is seen in young people, commonly women, that does not always progress; and the 'myxomatous mitral valve disease' seen in older people, often causing significant mitral regurgitation that needs surgical repair. Overall survival in patients with mitral prolapse is 97% at 6 years and 88% at 8 years, but those with myxomatous mitral valve disease and a flail leaflet have a 10-year survival much less. With posterior leaflet myxomatous prolapse, progressive chronic mitral regurgitation is associated with progressive dilatation of the left atrium and left ventricle.

The commonest site for posterior mitral prolapse is the middle scallop (P_2). Significant mitral regurgitation occurs in less than 10% of patients with posterior prolapse compared to 25% of those with anterior leaflet prolapse. In contrast, the incidence of atrial fibrillation and heart failure is significantly higher in posterior leaflet prolapse than in anterior leaflet prolapse. In general severe mitral regurgitation is associated with redundant leaflets, a longer posterior leaflet, and a larger annulus. Chordal distribution may also be abnormal, and there may be a relative scarcity of chordae to the central scallop of the posterior leaflet, increased chordal division or a higher incidence of chordal rupture.

There is a clear relationship between mitral valve prolapse, arrhythmia and sudden death. The annual rate of sudden death in mitral prolapse is approximately 2%, which significantly falls after surgical repair. The risk of endocarditis is estimated at three to eight times that of the general population, the substrate being that leaflet prolapse causes significant turbulence of the blood flow across the valve orifice, disrupting platelet and fibrin deposition on the valve surface and subsequently resulting in vulnerability to infection. There is controversy regarding the relationship between mitral prolapse and embolic events.

Dilated cardiomyopathy

Mitral regurgitation is common in dilated nonischaemic cardiomyopathy. Dilatation of the left ventricle disturbs the normal closure of the mitral valve, the leaflets fail to coapt and hence mitral regurgitation occurs.

Pathophysiology and complications
Regurgitant orifice and jet

The regurgitant volume of mitral regurgitation is calculated as the regurgitant flow over the regurgitant area. The flow velocity through the orifice is related to the ventricular–atrial systolic pressure difference. A high left ventricular systolic pressure, e.g. systemic hypertension, increases mitral regurgitation volume, and low left ventricular pressure reduces it. Left atrial pressure in acute mitral regurgitation is raised, with a V-wave in late systole due to the increased volume and the velocity of blood entering it (although the absence of such a wave on the left atrial or pulmonary wedge pressure trace does not exclude the diagnosis of severe mitral regurgitation).

Mitral regurgitation is often a dynamic lesion, with the size of the regurgitant orifice and regurgitant volume varying with the pressure gradient across the valve and with changes in left ventricular volume and geometry. The use of medical therapy to reduce left ventricular volume and improve its systolic function may therefore assist in reducing the severity of mitral regurgitation.

Left atrium

Left atrial volume increases in patients with mitral regurgitation in response to the increase in its pressure, to the transmission of the mitral regurgitation kinetic energy to the left atrial wall, and also to the development (in some cases) of atrial fibrillation. These effects balance those of the mitral regurgitation jet on left atrial pressure, which is normal in compensated patients. In contrast to mitral stenosis, the fast regurgitant jet in the left atrium reduces the risk of thrombus formation.

Afterload

Mitral regurgitation is an isolated volume overload on the left ventricle, providing the physiological equivalent of afterload reduction so that a normal forward cardiac output is maintained by the combination of increased ejection fraction and higher preload. Therefore, unlike the situation with pressure overload, the coronary blood flow is normal and the increase in myocardial oxygen consumption in mitral regurgitation is only mild. Left ventricular dysfunction, manifest by increased end-systolic diameter, is one of the most important determinants of outcome.

Right heart

The risk of right heart disease and dysfunction in mitral regurgitation is very similar to that in mitral stenosis. The raised left atrial pressure and pulmonary venous pressure are directly reflected in right ventricular systolic pressure. Right ventricular dysfunction as a complication of pulmonary hypertension is an important determinant of outcome.

Clinical presentation
Symptoms

Patients with mild mitral regurgitation may not have any symptoms: those with severe regurgitation are likely to present with dyspnoea. It is sometimes reported that mitral valve prolapse may be associated with nonspecific symptoms such as chest pain and fatigue, but this is debatable.

Physical examination

The patient with nonrheumatic mitral regurgitation is usually in sinus rhythm, but with severe mitral regurgitation of any cause patients may present in atrial fibrillation. The pulse is likely to be of normal character, but is sometimes reported as 'jerky', meaning of normal amplitude but rapid upstroke. The venous pressure is normal unless there is significant pulmonary hypertension or associated tricuspid disease.

The apex beat may be prominent and displaced, may be double due to a palpable third heart sound, and there may be a palpable systolic thrill in severe cases. A palpable left parasternal heave may be due to systolic expansion of the left atrium and/or right ventricular hypertrophy.

The first heart sound is normal or soft, the most prominent findings on auscultation being an apical pansystolic murmur and a third heart sound. The loudness of the murmur generally correlates with severity of regurgitation, a murmur of less than grade 2/6 (meaning that it can be heard only with special effort) indicating mild disease, with the notable exception that no murmur may be audible with acute mitral regurgitation (when the mitral valve may effectively be absent). The cardinal signs of mitral prolapse are the mid-systolic click, due to the backward movement of the mitral leaflet into the left atrium, and the late systolic mitral regurgitation that occurs after the click. The murmur extends throughout systole as mitral regurgitation becomes severe.

The radiation of a mitral regurgitant murmur depends on the direction of the regurgitant jet. A posterolateral jet—seen in ischaemic mitral regurgitation, anterior leaflet disease and dilated cardiomyopathy—radiates from the apex to the axilla, and even to the back. An anterosuperior jet due to posterior leaflet prolapse is heard better at the lower left sternal edge or cardiac base (second right intercostal space, also known as the aortic area), and even on the carotids.

Other physical signs depend on the severity of mitral regurgitation and possible complications, e.g. pulmonary hypertension.

Investigations

Chest radiograph and electrocardiogram

The chest radiograph reflects the haemodynamic disturbance (Fig. 16.6.5). The overall heart size is often normal or only moderately enlarged, with selective enlargement of the left atrium, although not to the same extent as with mitral stenosis (see Fig. 16.6.1). However, considerable cardiac enlargement develops due to secondary left ventricular disease if mitral regurgitation is severe and long standing.

The ECG usually shows sinus rhythm. There may also be evidence of left atrial hypertrophy, left ventricular hypertrophy and frequent ventricular ectopic beats.

Echocardiography

Two-dimensional echocardiography provides a thorough assessment of the anatomy and function of the mitral valve apparatus, including the leaflets and annular diameter, as well as left ventricular size and function, left atrial size, and pulmonary artery pressure. The echocardiographic criterion for mitral prolapse is the presence of at least 2 mm of late systolic posterior displacement of the leaflets across the mitral annular plane (Fig. 16.6.6). Severe myxomatous degeneration is associated with thickening of the leaflets and the appearance of extensive folding or redundancy of the leaflets in diastole, chordal elongation, and systolic anterior motion of the leaflets. Secondary mitral prolapse can easily be distinguished from primary prolapse in patients such as those with Marfan's syndrome, where the leaflets (particularly the anterior) are thin and long, and also in hypertrophic cardiomyopathy, with long leaflets and anterior motion of the mitral valve. Transthoracic echocardiography is perfectly adequate, but transoesophageal echocardiography is recommended if images are limited in quality.

Because it is noninvasive, echocardiography is an ideal tool for the follow up of patients to allow early identification of worsening of regurgitation or deterioration in ventricular function. Many echocardiographic methods for determining the severity of regurgitation have been described (Fig. 16.6.7), three-dimensional reconstruction of the mitral regurgitation jet being a very promising tool for obtaining accurate regurgitant volume assessment since it avoids the conventional cross-sectional limitations. The extent of left ventricular cavity activity directly reflects the severity of volume overload, thus limiting the accuracy of using ejection fraction as a measure of ventricular function in such patients, hence changes in left ventricular end-systolic volume or dimensions should be taken as marker of ventricular dysfunction. Patients recommended for surgical repair need detailed transthoracic and transoesophageal echocardiographic assessment of the anatomy of the valve and subvalvular apparatus to assist surgeons in planning.

Findings that support pulmonary hypertension, in particular enlargement of the right side of the heart and increase in the retrograde pressure drop across the tricuspid valve, are easily obtained

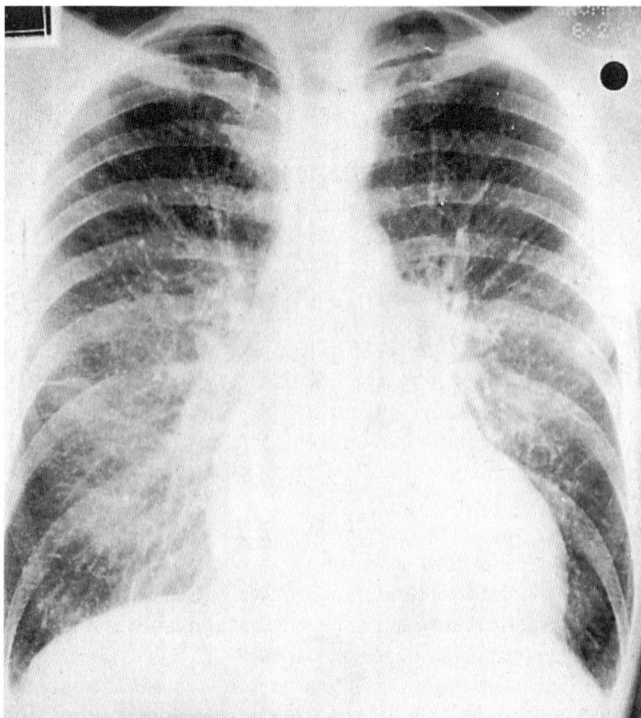

Fig. 16.6.5 Chest radiograph showing acute pulmonary oedema due to acute mitral regurgitation resulting from ruptured chordae tendinae.

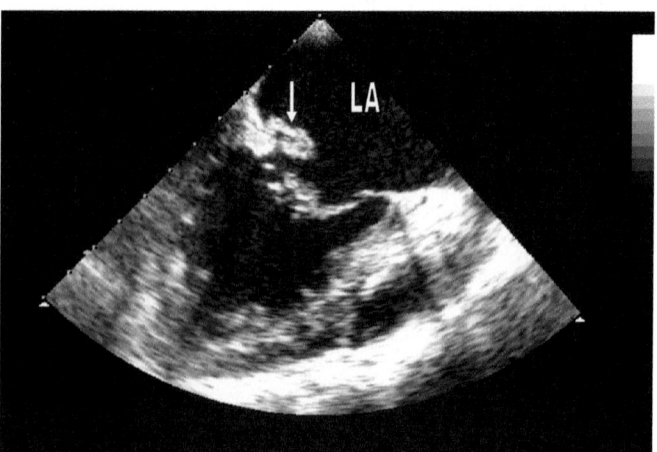

Fig. 16.6.6 Transoesophageal echocardiogram from a patient with posterior mitral leaflet prolapse (arrow). LA, left atrium.

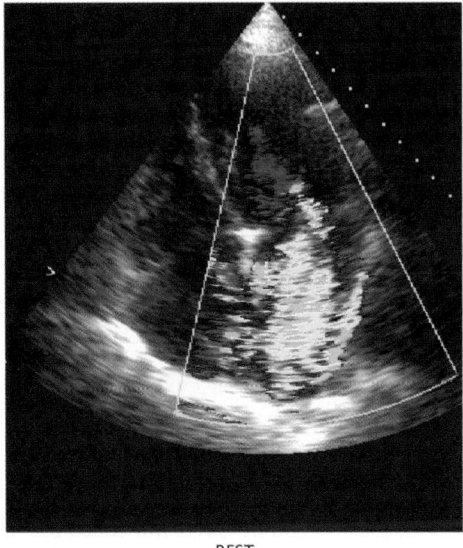 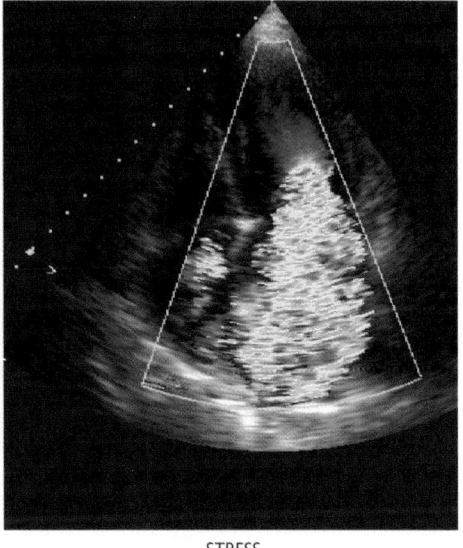

REST   STRESS

Fig. 16.6.7 Apical four-chamber views from a patient with coronary artery disease and ischaemic mitral regurgitation at rest (left) and stress (right). Note the significant increase in mitral regurgitation severity with stress as the ventricle became ischaemic.

from a conventional Doppler echocardiographic study. Tricuspid leaflet prolapse is seen in 20% of patients with mitral valve prolapse, but aortic involvement is much less frequent.

Cardiac catheterization

This is not indicated for diagnostic purposes but may be required for preoperative assessment of the coronary arteries.

Differential diagnosis

Mitral regurgitation needs to be distinguished from ventricular septal defect (VSD), aortic valve disease, and tricuspid regurgitation.

Congenital VSDs are discussed in Chapter 16.12, but the commonest scenario in adult practice where distinction between mitral regurgitation and VSD needs to be made is the patient who deteriorates shortly after a myocardial infarction and is found to have a pansystolic murmur. It is impossible to distinguish reliably between the two by physical examination, although if the murmur is heard over the back VSD is most likely. Echocardiography and/or right heart catheterization with measurement of oxygen tension in the various cardiac chambers are required (see Chapter 16.13.5).

The systolic murmur of aortic valve disease can radiate to the apex, and sometimes be louder there than at the base (aortic area). The latter can lead to misdiagnosis of mitral valve disease, and the former can lead to confusion as to whether both aortic and mitral valves are diseased. Aside from looking for other evidence of aortic valve disease (see later in this chapter), the key thing is to establish the precise timing of the murmur. Mitral valve disease should only be diagnosed if the murmur is pansystolic, extending right up to and even obliterating the second heart sound (or right up to the onset of the early diastolic murmur of aortic regurgitation).

The murmur of tricuspid regurgitation is typically loudest at the lower left sternal border, is loudest during inspiration, and is associated with elevation of the venous pressure with systolic waves.

Management

Patients with chronic mitral regurgitation may survive for a long time with no limiting symptoms. Once symptoms develop they suggest the need for surgical correction of valve regurgitation to avoid development of irreversible left ventricular dysfunction.

Assessment during routine follow up identifies those likely to need surgical intervention even in the absence of symptoms, with an effective regurgitant orifice of over 40 mm^2 being the cut-off recommended value. Although patients with acute regurgitation secondary to papillary muscle rupture need emergency surgery, this does not necessarily apply to those with ruptured chordae or chronic ischaemic regurgitation. Such patients need to be stabilized and other risk factors and comorbidities identified and optimally managed.

Medical

There is no medical therapy that cures mitral regurgitation or mitral valve prolapse. Endocarditis prophylaxis is strongly recommended for those with regurgitation, although isolated mitral prolapse in the absence of regurgitation might not be counted as a definite indication. Symptomatic supraventricular arrhythmia needs optimum therapy, usually with β-blockers, and patients with ventricular tachycardia and syncope should be evaluated for implantable defibrillator (see Chapter 16.4). Those in atrial fibrillation should be given anticoagulants and INR adjusted at 2.5 to 3.5.

Appropriate pacing for dilated cardiomyopathy has been reported as reducing the severity of mitral regurgitation. Vasodilators improve prognosis and also reduce preload and the venous return, which improves leaflet coaption and reduces mitral regurgitation. Their effect on the afterload improves the forward flow and also reduces the retrograde flow across the mitral valve. Carvedilol has been shown to reduce long axis length over diameter ratio ('cardiac index') and reduce mitral regurgitation severity. Similar findings have been documented in patients receiving ACE inhibitors or angiotensin receptor antagonists.

Surgical

A number of factors predict surgical outcome after correction of mitral regurgitation. As might be expected, the more complex the surgical procedure the higher the surgical risk. Age-related operative mortality is of the order of 12% in patients over 75 years of age and 1% in younger patients. Symptoms related to mitral regurgitation are important predictors: patients in New York Heart Association (NYHA) classes I and II carry a mortality of 0.5%, but for those in classes III and IV it is 10% or more. The aetiology of mitral regurgitation is another determinant, with 1 to 3% mortality in rheumatic mitral valve disease, compared to 9% in ischaemic mitral regurgitation.

Ventricular dysfunction adds to the surgical risk, in particular having an end-systolic dimension greater than 45 to 50 mm. However, recent data suggest that even significant left ventricular dysfunction should not be used as an exclusion criterion for correction of mitral regurgitation, although the general belief remains that a systolic dimension of more than 50 mm indicates a poor prognosis and that surgical intervention is unlikely to be of benefit. Pulmonary hypertension is another important predictor of outcome that carries a poor prognosis: correction of mitral regurgitation does not always guarantee normalization of pulmonary artery pressure, particularly if long-standing, which indicates that surgical intervention should be considered before development of this complication.

Mitral valve prolapse accounts for approximately 25% of mitral valve surgical procedures. The benefit of surgical intervention and ring insertion into patients with dilated cardiomyopathy remains controversial.

Mitral valve repair

The intention of mitral valve repair is to preserve the integrity of the valve, which—if successful—results in a much better clinical outcome for patients with mitral regurgitation than does valve replacement. Preservation of the chordal attachment is crucial, keeping the continuity between the mitral leaflets and the papillary muscles which control the long axis function of the left ventricle. This itself also affects the sphericity of the left ventricle and hence overall performance of the cavity.

Mitral valve repair avoids the use of anticoagulants that are needed for life in patients with mechanical prostheses, and even those who develop atrial fibrillation from mitral valve repair might not need the higher dose of anticoagulants necessary for those who receive a mechanical valve. The risk of endocarditis is much lower from mitral valve repair compared to replacement.

As for any operation, patient selection for mitral valve repair is important. Although historical results of mitral valve repair for rheumatic regurgitation showed a success rate of 50%, better results have been reported recently, with a reoperation in approximately 20% of patients at 10 years. Surgical repair for rheumatic mitral valve disease is also affected by rheumatic aortic and tricuspid valve disease.

The most common procedure is the quadrilateral resection of the posterior leaflet, removing excess valve tissue, reapproximating the scallops, and reducing the annulus, with or without mitral annuloplasty. The success rate of this technique is of the order of 90%. Although historically anterior leaflet repair was not so easy as that of the posterior leaflet, recent advances have made it as successful. An alternative approach (not widely accepted in the surgical community) is the Alfieri repair, which involves suturing the posterior and anterior leaflets together in the central section and creating a double-orifice mitral valve.

Recently, nonsurgical mitral valve repair procedures have developed 'clip-procedure' with fast growing experience.

It is now routine practice to use intraoperative transoesophageal echocardiography to provide detailed assessment and detect signs of valve dysfunction immediately on completion of surgery on the valve: residual regurgitation can be dealt with before closure of the chest.

In addition to mitral repair, patients with atrial fibrillation may be considered for arrhythmia ablation—surgically or by radiofrequency—to restore sinus rhythm. Results of the combined procedure have been satisfactory, even with chronic atrial fibrillation before surgery.

Mitral valve replacement

Mitral valve replacement has a higher operative mortality than aortic valve replacement for aortic stenosis or regurgitation, or conservative operation for mitral stenosis. Although survival from mitral valve replacement surgery has improved significantly over the years, probably because of the better selection, improved myocardial preservation, and surgical techniques, it remains of concern, particularly in patients with ischaemic mitral regurgitation, where 5-year survival is 75%.

The ideal valve would be a homograft in the mitral position, but this can only be achieved by use of a composite including the mitral valve and related structures and placing it attached to the annulus, which avoids cutting the papillary muscle heads and the chordae and preserves the continuity between the mitral valve apparatus and the left ventricle. However, such attempts have proved uniformly unsuccessful. Pulmonary autograft has been used in the mitral position with satisfactory results, but in only a small group of patients in one or two centres.

Mitral replacement by a mechanical valve or bioprosthesis is the only option for irreparable valves. It has a very satisfactory success rate, particularly when papillary muscles and chordae are preserved. Bileaflet or tilting disc are currently the most commonly used mechanical valves.

Mixed mitral valve disease

Mixed mitral disease is nearly always due to rheumatic valve disease. In general, it occurs in older patients than pure mitral stenosis, and the valve is more likely to be calcified with limited cusp mobility and scarred subvalve apparatus. The mitral regurgitation is not usually severe, but the increased stroke volume increases the diastolic pressure drop across the valve.

Symptoms are the same as for mitral stenosis or regurgitation. On examination the first heart sound is not palpable or loud, the pansystolic murmur is usually loudest towards the axilla, and there is a mid-diastolic murmur.

The chest radiograph (Fig. 16.6.8) may show more advanced changes than in pure mitral stenosis (see Fig. 16.6.1): the left atrium can be extremely large. Echocardiography is likely to show thickened cusps with reduced motion in addition to mitral regurgitation. When symptoms merit, valve replacement is usually required.

Aortic valve disease

Aortic stenosis

Causes

Aortic stenosis is caused by congenital, rheumatic or senile disease. It may be at subvalvar, valvar, or supravalvar level, the commonest being valvar stenosis.

Age-related degenerative calcific disease is now the commonest cause of aortic stenosis in western Europe and the United States of America. The commonest congenital valvar aortic disease is the bicuspid aortic valve, which may remain completely silent for years,

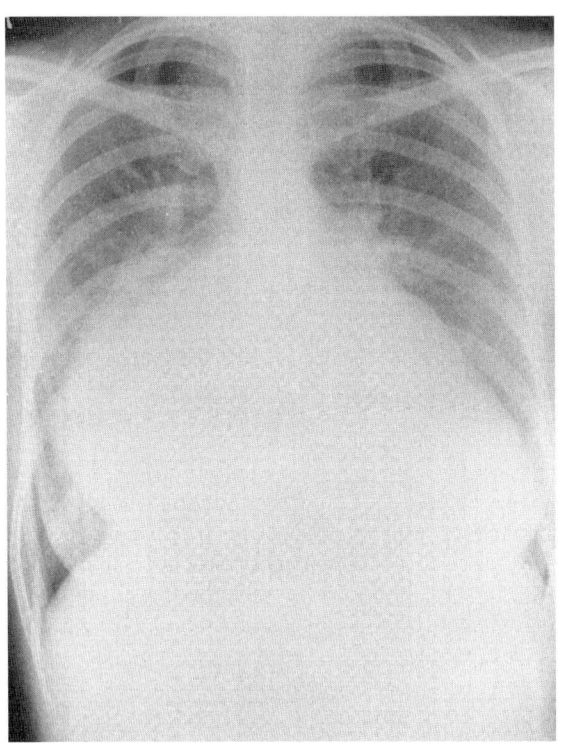

Fig. 16.6.8 Chest radiograph of a patient with mixed mitral valve disease, showing gross cardiac enlargement, mainly due to dilatation of the left atrium.

but as age advances the leaflets become thickened and calcified resulting in significant reduction in valve area, raised transvalvar velocities and pressure drop (gradient) across the valve. Rheumatic aortic stenosis is nearly always associated with aortic regurgitation (mixed aortic valve disease, see below) and with rheumatic mitral disease. Symptomatic valvar aortic stenosis is more prevalent in men.

Subvalvar aortic stenosis is caused by a membrane (shelf) or a hypertrophied upper septal segment bulging into the outflow tract. Subaortic membrane is a congenital anomaly that commonly progresses with age. Hypertrophy of the upper septum is an acquired syndrome that affects the elderly, particularly those with long standing hypertension. Supravalvar aortic stenosis is rare: when found it is commonly part of Williams' syndrome (OMIN 194050; 'elfin' facies with low nasal bridge, unusual behaviours and mental retardation, transient hypercalcaemia; supravalvar aortic stenosis).

Pathophysiology and complications

In addition to the anatomical narrowing of the aortic valve, left ventricular function plays an important role in determining the transvalvar velocities. Patients with severe aortic stenosis and poor left ventricular function may have underestimated velocities and pressure drop. By contrast, those with mild valve narrowing but a hyperactive ventricle (e.g. hyperdynamic circulation) may present with overestimated velocities across the valve; in particular, significant aortic regurgitation can lead to overestimation of the degree of valve stenosis because of increased stroke volume. Despite various attempts to determine the most sensitive marker of aortic stenosis, valve gradient (pressure drop) remains the most appropriate measure in clinical practice.

Left ventricular response

With the increase in outflow tract resistance in aortic stenosis, left ventricular wall stress increases and hypertrophy develops. This compensatory mechanism preserves overall ventricular systolic function. Most patients develop concentric left ventricular hypertrophy and increased mass, which regresses after removal of the stenosis. Patients with untreated aortic stenosis may present very late with left ventricular cavity dilatation, reduced ejection fraction and dyssynchrony. Left ventricular subendocardial ischaemia may result from long-standing ventricular hypertrophy and outflow tract obstruction, and diastolic left ventricular function also become impaired, resulting in increased end-diastolic pressure and left atrial pressure. Most patients with aortic stenosis who are allowed to reach this degree of ventricular dysfunction complain of progressive breathlessness and finally pulmonary oedema.

Coronary circulation

Even in the absence of significant coronary artery disease (atherosclerosis), the coronary circulation plays an important role in the pathophysiology and clinical presentation of aortic stenosis. Proximal coronary artery size is often increased, probably as a compensatory mechanism for the increased myocardial oxygen demand because of left ventricular hypertrophy, but coronary flow reserve remains suboptimal. This limited coronary flow reserve is manifested in the subendocardium, which may become irreversibly damaged, and the more severe the aortic stenosis, the greater the impairment of subendocardial function. Furthermore, left ventricular relaxation is usually prolonged in left ventricular hypertrophy, which further reduces coronary flow. The combination of hypertrophy-related altered coronary flow and increased myocardial work probably contributes to the angina-like symptoms, even in the absence of epicardial coronary disease. Regression of left ventricular hypertrophy after aortic valve replacement improves coronary flow reserve.

Clinical presentation
Symptoms

Mild aortic stenosis does not give any symptoms, and even severe stenosis may be silent. Breathlessness or exercise intolerance is the most common symptom. Progressive deterioration of left ventricular function and increased end-diastolic pressure leads to acute pulmonary oedema and florid heart failure. Angina is the second most frequent symptom, but less common than breathlessness. When it happens it represents a significant mismatch between myocardial oxygen supply and demand, and it may be exercise limiting even in the absence of epicardial coronary artery disease. The third symptom is syncope, which in some patients is clearly related to exertion. This can be caused by reduced cardiac output due to outflow tract obstruction, or by arrhythmia (transient atrioventricular block, ventricular arrhythmia, and carotid sinus hypersensitivity have all been described), with exercise-induced peripheral vasodilatation in the face of a fixed cardiac output the likely explanation for those who collapse when exercising.

Physical examination

The physical signs of significant aortic stenosis are very characteristic. Proper examination of the character of the pulse is crucial: a slowly rising, low-amplitude carotid (or brachial) pulse has high specificity for diagnosing severe aortic stenosis, and there may be a carotid thrill. Arterial pulse pressure is narrow.

The venous pressure is usually normal until late in the disease, but a small 'a' wave is often present. This is known as a Bernheim 'a' wave and appears to be related in some little-understood way to the presence of left ventricular hypertrophy: it should not be taken in isolation as evidence of pulmonary hypertension.

The apex beat is often sustained and may be double, due to an additional left atrial impulse. On palpation of the praecordium there may be a systolic thrill over the aortic area in severe cases.

On auscultation the first heart sound is normal or soft, and may be preceded by a fourth heart sound. The characteristic long and harsh ejection systolic murmur is loudest at the base (second right intercostal space, also known as the aortic area) of the heart, and in most cases it radiates to the carotids. The murmur is often heard at the lower left sternal border, and in a minority the ejection systolic murmur may also be referred to the apex. A systolic ejection click may be heard, typically in patients with an uncalcified bicuspid valve. The second heart sound in aortic stenosis is typically single because of the limited cusp movement in a heavily calcified valve, but in young patients with severe aortic stenosis and mobile leaflets the splitting of the second sound is reversed. A normal split second heart sound is a reliable sign for mild aortic stenosis. A third heart sound may be heard when left ventricular cavity dilatation and raised left atrial pressure have developed. A soft early diastolic murmur is often present, which does not necessarily imply haemodynamically significant aortic regurgitation.

It is important to note these physical signs are modified as ventricular disease progresses and stroke volume falls. Pulse volume drops and the pulse loses its slow rising quality, the systolic murmur becomes shorter and softer and may even disappear, and a functional mitral regurgitant murmur can appear along with a third heart sound. Such 'silent' but critical aortic stenosis cannot be diagnosed reliably on the basis of physical signs: a high index of suspicion and a good quality echocardiogram are required to prevent misdiagnosis of 'congestive cardiomyopathy, cause unknown'.

Investigations

Chest radiograph and electrocardiogram

The chest radiograph may be completely normal in patients with uncomplicated aortic stenosis. Post stenotic dilatation of the ascending aorta may be seen. Associated left ventricular disease leads to pulmonary venous congestion.

In most patients the ECG shows evidence of left ventricular hypertrophy based on voltage criteria, but in some cases it can be completely normal. Advanced hypertrophy may be associated with nonspecific T-wave changes. With progressive left ventricular dysfunction QRS duration broadens and left bundle branch block may develop. Inverted U wave may be seen in patients with severe left ventricular disease.

Echocardiography

Echocardiography is the investigation of choice for patients with aortic stenosis, providing comprehensive information on valve anatomy and function and left ventricular size and function, as well as other associated cardiac abnormalities that may contribute to patient's symptoms, e.g. mitral valve regurgitation. Transthoracic echocardiography is mandatory in all patients with suspected aortic stenosis. Transoesophageal echocardiography may assist in examining the aortic root and the proximal ascending aorta.

The most clinically valuable measure of severity of aortic stenosis is transvalvular velocity using continuous wave Doppler. The blood flow sounds under two-dimensional echocardiographic guidance assist in deciding on the optimum positioning of the probe for velocity recordings, with the beam as parallel as possible to the jet direction. Peak velocities across the aortic valve are converted into a pressure drop (pressure gradient) using the modified Bernoulli equation, $P = 4V^2$.

Timing of peak velocity across the valve is a good indicator of the degree of aortic stenosis: in mild stenosis velocities peak in early systole, but in severe stenosis velocities peak in mid systole, in parallel with the rise in aortic pressure.

Aortic stenosis can be quantified as valve area, which can be calculated from Doppler velocity data using the continuity equation based on the fact that the flow rate across the stenotic valve and the normal subvalvar area are equal. Valve area is therefore calculated based on the relative increase in blood velocity across the aortic valve with respect to the subvalvar region, in conjunction with an estimate of the subvalvar cross-sectional area. Thus, an increase in peak velocity across the aortic valve by five times that of subvalvar velocity, with a pressure gradient of at least 35 mmHg, is consistent with a fivefold drop in aortic valve area and suggests severe aortic stenosis (Fig. 16.6.9).

An important application of this principle is seen in patients who have a moderate aortic pressure drop and in whom it is not clear whether this is simply because stenosis is not severe, or because stroke volume is low due to impaired left ventricular function. Stress echocardiography is a useful investigation in these circumstances (Fig. 16.6.10). With increase in heart rate the increased blood flow across the valve differentiates between severe valve narrowing and severe left ventricular disease. A significant increase in transvalvular velocities and pressure gradient reflects fixed valve area and hence the diagnosis of severe aortic stenosis. By contrast, failure of aortic velocities to increase significantly with stress suggests impaired left ventricular function as the cause of the low cardiac output and symptoms rather than aortic stenosis.

Colour flow Doppler will reveal the presence of mild aortic regurgitation in most patients with aortic stenosis, and in those with impaired left ventricular function and raised end-diastolic pressure Doppler recordings of aortic regurgitation should be assessed carefully to avoid overestimating the degree of regurgitation because of raised left ventricular end-diastolic pressure.

Echocardiography can provide accurate measurements of left ventricular dimensions and systolic function, as well as left ventricular hypertrophy and mass, from which mass index can be calculated. Left ventricular filling pattern guides towards assessment of left atrial pressure. Most patients with aortic stenosis and left ventricular hypertrophy have a small early diastolic filling component and dominant late diastolic one. With progressive left ventricular disease and increase in end-diastolic pressure, the left atrial pressure increases and ventricular filling becomes of the restrictive pattern, with a dominant early diastolic filling component with short deceleration time and a very small late diastolic filling component with flow reversal in the pulmonary veins. Most patients presenting with this pattern of physiology have a dilated left atrium and some may even present with atrial arrhythmia. The extent of the commonly found mitral regurgitation can also be assessed, and other parameters enable estimation of the presence and degree of pulmonary hypertension. Mitral annular calcification is a very common finding in patients with severe aortic stenosis but rarely contributes to any increase in atrial pressure or results in mitral stenosis.

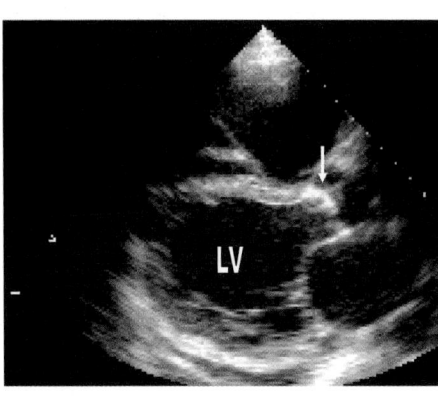

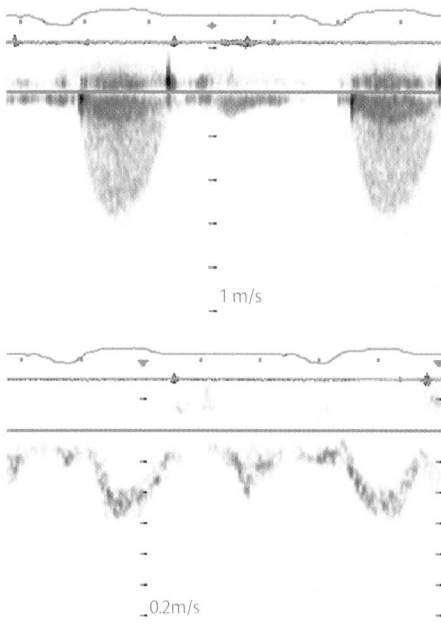

Fig. 16.6.9 Parasternal long axis views from a patient with severe calcific aortic stenosis (arrow) and poor left ventricular function showing a dilated cavity with increased end-systolic dimension (LV). Transvalvar peak velocity of 3.0 m/s (upper right panel) and subvalvar velocity of 0.6 m/s (lower right panel).

Cardiac catheterization

High-standard echocardiographic estimation of the severity of aortic stenosis is clinically very reliable and does not need to be reconfirmed by catheterization. The traditionally measured aortic pressure gradient during cardiac catheterization, using a pull-back technique to record the difference between peak left ventricular and aortic pressure, is a less satisfactory measure than that possible echocardiographically because the two peaks do not occur simultaneously. A further problem with estimation of aortic gradient by cardiac catheterization occurs because left ventricular pressure may not be uniform, hence the measured pressure difference depends on the location of catheter tip in the ventricle, particularly in the presence of significant hypertrophy as in most cases of aortic stenosis. The difficulty increases since aortic pressure also depends on its distance from the valve leaflets and the aortic wall, as well as the pressure recovery process in the aortic root. Such estimates should thus be regarded as semiquantitative.

Cardiac catheterization is needed only to assess possible coronary artery disease, which frequently accompanies aortic stenosis. CT coronary angiography can now provide similar information.

Differential diagnosis

The commonest differential diagnosis that needs to be considered is aortic sclerosis, when examination of an elderly patient reveals an ejection systolic murmur at the base or left sternal edge. Other features of aortic stenosis—slow rising pulse, narrow pulse pressure, radiation of the murmur to the carotids, presence of a thrill—are not present.

Most often in a younger patient the possibility of hypertrophic cardiomyopathy needs to be considered, but here the carotid pulse is normal or jerky rather than slow rising (see Chapter 16.7.2). Fixed subaortic stenosis also needs to be considered in children and young adults (see Chapter 16.12).

All of these differential diagnoses can be distinguished from aortic stenosis by echocardiography.

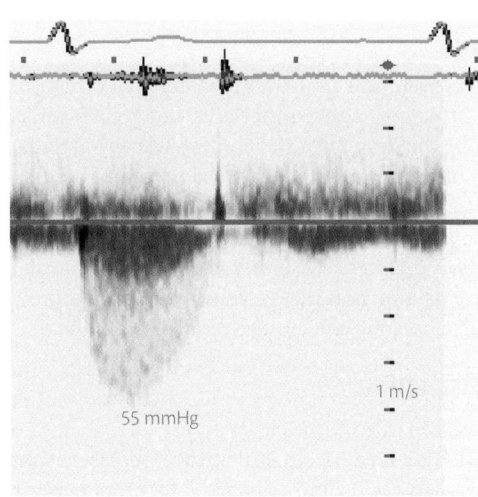

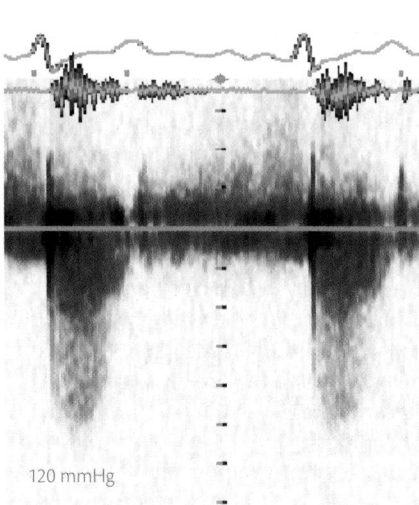

Fig. 16.6.10 Continuous wave Doppler of transaortic valve velocities at rest (left panel) and peak stress (right panel) showing significant increase in velocities and consequently gradient from 55 to 120 mmHg.

Management

Progression of aortic stenosis is generally slow. Symptoms are variable but overall reflect left ventricular disease. Patients with a congenital bicuspid aortic valve tend to develop symptoms at an average age of 50 years, whereas those with senile valve disease do so at the age of 70 to 80 years. Patients with significant congenital aortic valve stenosis may develop symptoms earlier in life. Some 50% of patients with severe aortic stenosis die suddenly.

Raised aortic velocities and gradient, and the rate of increase in velocities over time, are the most accurate predictors of outcome, the rate of deterioration being faster in senile disease than rheumatic aortic stenosis. Once symptoms develop the outcome is poor without surgical intervention, with 5-year survival less than 50%. Autopsy series showed that the average time from symptom development to death is 2 years in patients with exertional syncope, 3 years in those with dyspnoea, and 5 years in those with angina. It should be highlighted that prognosis is much better in patients with a high valve gradient rather than those with low gradient due to severe left ventricular disease. Recent data suggests that patients presenting with an ejection fraction below 20% fail to thrive even after successful aortic valve replacement surgery.

Approximately 50% of adults with aortic stenosis who need surgery have additional coronary artery disease. Patients with angina-like symptoms who have only mild aortic stenosis are likely to have significant epicardial coronary disease, but a new onset of angina in patients with severe aortic stenosis may reflect a further deterioration of the degree of aortic stenosis and subendocardial ischaemia. A particularly difficult group of patients to manage are those with moderate aortic stenosis and angina-like symptoms.

Medical

There is no medical treatment for aortic stenosis that will stop disease progression. Asymptomatic patients with mild or moderate aortic stenosis require follow-up; those with severe aortic stenosis need aortic valve replacement. It is prudent to advise those with moderate or severe disease to avoid strenuous exercise. A pressure gradient of more than 70mmHg across the aortic valve is a good indication for surgery, particularly in those who are symptomatic. Patients with severe aortic stenosis and left ventricular disease who present with heart failure should be stabilized before referral for surgery: diuretics are important, as well as β-blockers for controlling the heart rate; vasodilators, including ACE inhibitors, are contraindicated. Once a patient develops raised left atrial pressure and pulmonary hypertension the outcome is less than satisfactory, even with surgery.

Instructions on endocarditis prophylaxis and the use of antibiotics before dental and surgical procedures should be given. Patients with other comorbidities and risks, in particular hyperlipidaemia, should have these addressed. The effect of statins on the rate of progression of aortic stenosis seems to be negligible.

Surgical

Recent advances in aortic valve surgery—earlier intervention, changes in the procedures used, improved methods of myocardial preservation—have resulted in a significant fall in surgical mortality to 2.7 to 8.3% in adults under 70 years of age. Concurrent coronary artery disease, ventricular dysfunction, and pulmonary hypertension are important surgical risks. Older patients with aortic stenosis, particularly those over the age of 80 years, tend to have a higher mortality, but age is not a contraindication to surgery.

Surgical intervention in octogenarians has been shown to provide improvement in quality of life, with a 5-year postoperative survival compared to only 1 year for the unoperated.

Aortic valve repair

In young people aortic valvotomy is an acceptable procedure, but the option of valve repair in adults remains uncertain. It may provide a medium-term solution for a clinical problem, but further surgical intervention will definitely be required in the long term.

Tissue valves

Tissue valves do not need anticoagulants in the absence of atrial fibrillation. Although their durability is significantly lower than that of mechanical valves, indications for their use are clear: older people, young pregnant women, and patients with limited access to anticoagulant therapy. Over the years the durability of tissue valves has significantly improved: for patients over the age of 60, modern, third-generation, glutaraldehyde-preserved valves provide 90% survival at 15 years. Stentless tissue valves have better durability and are associated with faster recovery of ventricular function, but they are more difficult to implant.

The best option to replace a native valve is a human valve (homograft), but availability is limited. An aortic valve homograft replacement is particularly indicated in patients with endocarditis that involves the aortic root and is associated with abscess formation, because a mechanical valve replacement in this scenario compromises eradication of the infection. Aortic homograft implantation techniques have evolved from a two-layer subcoronary implantation to conduit implantation, which involves replacing the valve and sinus of Valsalva by a full root and valve. This still is considered more challenging than mechanical or tissue valve implantation. Under the age of 30 years aortic homografts tend to fail within 10 years: in older patients the mean survival of the valve is 15 to 18 years.

An alternative procedure is the pulmonary autograft or 'Ross procedure'. This goes back to 1967 when Donald Ross transferred a patient's own living pulmonary valve to the aortic position and inserted a homograft in the pulmonary position. In children these autograft valves, unlike any other valve substitute, are capable of growth. A pulmonary homograft is placed in the right ventricular outflow tract, where because of the lower pressures on the right side of the circulation the mean survival of the valve is 20 years. More recently, percutaneous replacement of the aortic (TAVI procedure) valve has become a possibility.

Mechanical valves

Over the years technical improvement in valve design has been remarkable, providing larger orifice area and greater resistance to thrombosis. In the long term the commonest problem, affecting less than 5% of patients with mechanical prostheses, is paravalvular dehiscence. While this may not always be haemodynamically significant, it may be responsible for haemolytic anaemia due to shear stress on red blood cells, and it is a focus for infective endocarditis. Valve dysfunction due to subvalvar tissue ingrowth that influences valve opening and closure remains a problem.

Aortic regurgitation

Causes

Aortic regurgitation is caused by either leaflet disease or aortic root dilatation (Table 16.6.2), the commonest causes being isolated

Table 16.6.2 Causes of aortic regurgitation

Structure primarily affected	Anatomical defect	Cause
Cusp	Distortion	Rheumatic Rheumatoid Ergot-derived dopamine receptor agonists—pergolide, cabergoline (treatments for Parkinson's disease) Fenfluramine, phentermine (appetite suppressants)
	Perforation	Infective endocarditis
Root disease	Dilatation	Isolated medionecrosis Marfan's syndrome Syphilis Ankylosing spondylitis or other connective tissue disease
Loss of support		Dissecting aneurysm of aortic root Subaortic ventricular septal defect

medionecrosis, rheumatic disease, infective endocarditis, and Marfan's syndrome.

Pathophysiology and complications

The left ventricular stroke volume, which equals the forward stroke volume plus the regurgitant volume, is significantly increased in aortic regurgitation. This is accommodated by an increase in left ventricular cavity size, a process that is progressive in a similar fashion to that of mitral regurgitation, although the degree of ventricular dilatation is greater. Another difference between the two conditions is the peripheral vascular resistance, which is significantly raised only in patients with aortic regurgitation. This combination of volume overload and raised peripheral resistance results in a progressive increase in left ventricular wall thickness and mass. In uncomplicated aortic regurgitation, the left ventricular ejection fraction is maintained, but as the disease progresses end-systolic volume increases out of proportion to stroke volume, and eventually these changes lead to irreversible damage which persists even after surgical correction of the aortic regurgitation.

Whether or not aortic regurgitation is accompanied by some degree of aortic stenosis due to intrinsic valve leaflet disease, the increase in stroke volume causes high systolic velocities across the aortic valve. Pressure relations between the aorta and the left ventricle in diastole are of great importance, in particular the end-diastolic pressure difference that depends not only on aortic but also on left ventricular end-diastolic pressure: the higher the left ventricular end-diastolic pressure the lower the pressure difference across the valve. In mild aortic regurgitation the pressure drop between the aorta and the left ventricle is maintained throughout diastole. By contrast, with acute aortic regurgitation the pressure difference between the aorta and the left ventricle falls to 15 mmHg or even less before end of diastole, either because of the very low resistance at the valve level or because the left ventricle is stiff, hence a relatively small regurgitant volume causes a disproportionate left ventricular diastolic pressure rise. This disturbed physiology has major implications because the aortic–left ventricular diastolic pressure gradient is the pressure head supporting the coronary flow. Coronary autoregulation stops at a

perfusion pressure difference between the aorta and the left ventricle of 40 mmHg, and with acute aortic regurgitation—or even severe chronic aortic regurgitation—the gradient is less than this, resulting in significant myocardial ischaemia and progressive ventricular dysfunction. This disturbed physiology may be tolerated in chronic severe aortic regurgitation, but in acute severe aortic regurgitation it may contribute to rapid clinical deterioration. The limitation of coronary flow by a raised ventricular end-diastolic pressure is further exacerbated by the increased oxygen demand of the myocardium as a result of the hyperdynamic ventricular state, as well as (in chronic regurgitation) the hypertrophy resulting from the volume overload. This results in subendocardial ischaemia, particularly with stress.

Clinical presentation
Symptoms

Patients with aortic regurgitation may remain asymptomatic for a long time. The onset of symptoms, particularly breathlessness, coincides with the onset of left ventricular disease, a significant rise in end-diastolic pressure, and development of pulmonary venous hypertension. Angina is an uncommon symptom in chronic aortic regurgitation, but when it occurs it should suggest significant subendocardial ischaemia as a result of the mismatch between the coronary artery flow and myocardial mass. It is more common in those with acute aortic regurgitation. Any sudden worsening of symptoms may reflect acute deterioration of the degree of aortic regurgitation or impairment of left ventricular function.

Physical examination

The physical signs of significant chronic aortic regurgitation are characteristic. The pulse has large amplitude and is 'collapsing' in nature ('water hammer', Corrigan's pulse) due to the increased stroke volume and rapid fall-off in aortic pressure during diastole. When severe, this can induce pulsations in many parts of the body, generating many eponyms that describe what is effectively a single physical finding. Amongst the better known of these are Quincke's capillary pulsations (best demonstrated by blanching a portion of a fingernail by applying gentle pressure and observing the pulsating border between the white and the red segments), de Musset's sign (bobbing of the head in time with the arterial pulse, named after the French poet who had the condition), and pulsations of various organs or their parts (uvula—Muller's sign, retinal arteries—Becker's sign).

The same pathophysiology underlies two peripheral arterial signs. Pistol shot sounds are short, loud sounds that can be heard over large peripheral arteries if the stethoscope is lightly applied: they occur because of sudden expansion and tensing of the walls during systole. Duroziez's sign is a double to-and-fro (systolic and diastolic) murmur heard over the brachial or femoral artery if the stethoscope is firmly applied: the diastolic component results from reversal of flow in the artery during diastole.

A diastolic blood pressure of less than 50 mmHg and/or a pulse pressure of 80 mmHg or more suggest moderate or severe regurgitation in patients who have a characteristic murmur (but are of no significance with regard to the aortic valve if no murmur is present). The venous pressure is normal until late in the course of disease, although a dominant Bernheim 'a' wave may be seen. The apex beat is sustained and/or displaced because of the left ventricular hypertrophy and/or dilatation.

On auscultation the classical murmur of aortic regurgitation is diastolic, starting immediately after the second heart sound, decrescendo in nature, and loudest at the left sternal border. It may be short, or extend throughout diastole. It may radiate to the right sternal border if it is caused by aortic root dilatation, and rarely it is loudest at the apex or even in the left axilla. The louder the murmur, the more severe is the regurgitation. The heart sounds may not demonstrate any specific change in aortic regurgitation, or—as with aortic stenosis—the aortic component of the second heart sound may be absent. An ejection systolic murmur due to increased stroke volume is nearly always present. At the apex a low-pitched mid-diastolic murmur (Austin–Flint murmur) mimicking that of mitral stenosis may be heard: it is usually assumed that this is due to the aortic regurgitant jet striking the anterior leaflet of the mitral valve, but other hypotheses have been advanced.

In acute aortic regurgitation—usually caused by infective endocarditis, thoracic aortic dissection, or disintegration of a tissue valve replacement—the physical signs are quite different, based on the fact that the stroke volume in acute regurgitation does not increase by the same magnitude as in chronic regurgitation. The patient is cold and shut down due to a low cardiac output, with tachycardia, a low systolic blood pressure and low pulse pressure, and a short early diastolic murmur that is easily missed. The apex is not displaced and peripheral signs are absent. There may be a loud third heart sound.

Investigations

Chest radiograph and electrocardiogram

The chest radiograph may show increased cardiothoracic ratio and dilatation of the aortic root (Fig. 16.6.11). In isolation these appearances cannot be taken as diagnostic, but they are very useful for follow-up of a known case.

The 12-lead ECG may demonstrate increased voltage and a 'strain' pattern that correlates with increase in left ventricular cavity dimensions, hypertrophy, and wall stress. The voltage pattern may fall significantly after correction of the aortic regurgitation and regression of left ventricular mass. Nonspecific T-wave changes may occur with exercise, reflecting either the development of subendocardial ischaemia or increase in systolic left ventricular volume. Increased QRS duration is a marker of left ventricular disease. A long PR interval may indicate aortic root abscess, particularly in those with other clinical suspicion of endocarditis.

Echocardiography

Doppler echocardiography is an invaluable investigation in the assessment of patients with aortic regurgitation (Fig. 16.6.12). Two-dimensional images can identify the exact cause of regurgitation, revealing the valve anatomy, leaflet number, calcification, or evidence of infection. The diameter of the aortic root and proximal ascending aorta can also be measured. Transoesophageal examination is always recommended if this is not achievable on transthoracic images, particularly in patients with Marfan's syndrome or those presenting with suspected dissection. Left ventricular size, dimensions, wall thickness and ejection fraction can easily be measured, and muscle mass calculated using simple formulae. Colour Doppler detects the presence of aortic regurgitation and gives some idea of its severity: the finding of large vena contracta, a large regurgitant orifice area, penetration of the regurgitant jet into the left ventricle, and jet diameter more than 50% of the aortic root diameter are all consistent with significant regurgitation. Continuous wave Doppler is ideal for assessing regurgitation severity as well as pressure differences between the aorta and the left ventricle (Fig. 16.6.13): in general, the faster the pressure decline on the aortic regurgitation trace, the more severe is the regurgitation likely to be, although this does not apply in patients with raised end-diastolic pressure. Doppler can also confirm severity of aortic regurgitation by demonstrating flow reversal in the descending aorta or femoral arteries. In patients with symptoms disproportionate to the degree of aortic regurgitation, a diagnosis of left ventricular disease should be considered, e.g. hypertension or coronary heart disease.

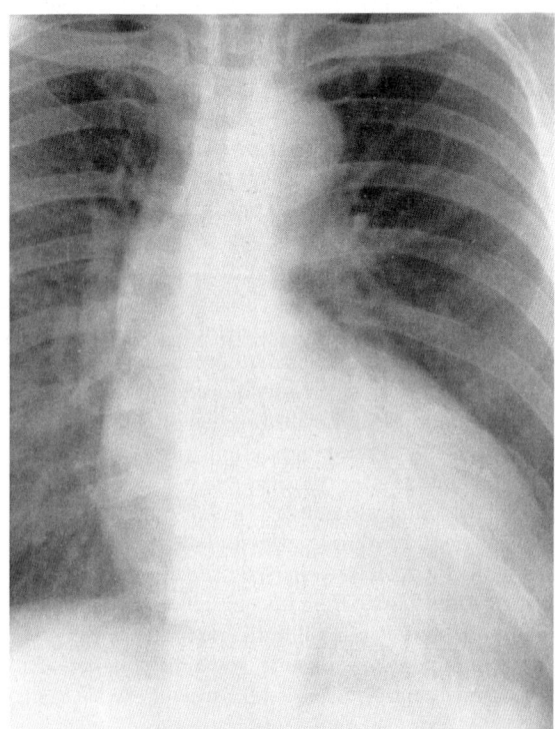

Fig. 16.6.11 Chest radiograph of a patient with chronic aortic regurgitation showing cardiac enlargement and dilatation of the ascending aorta.

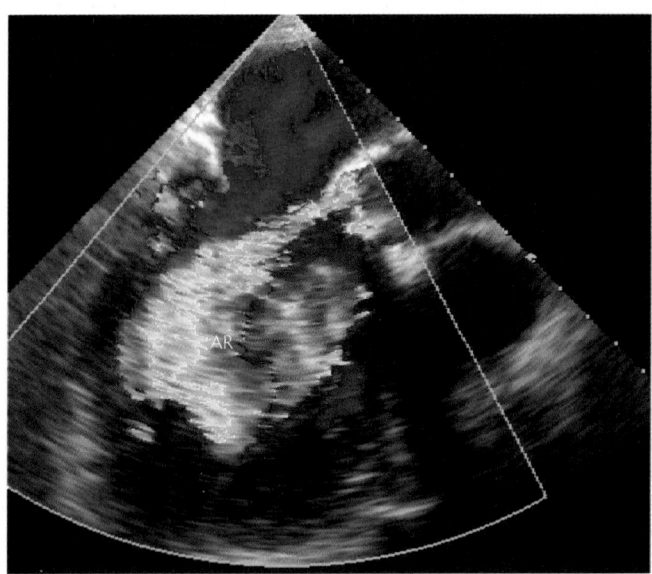

Fig. 16.6.12 Transoesophageal echocardiogram from a patient with aortic regurgitation on colour flow Doppler.

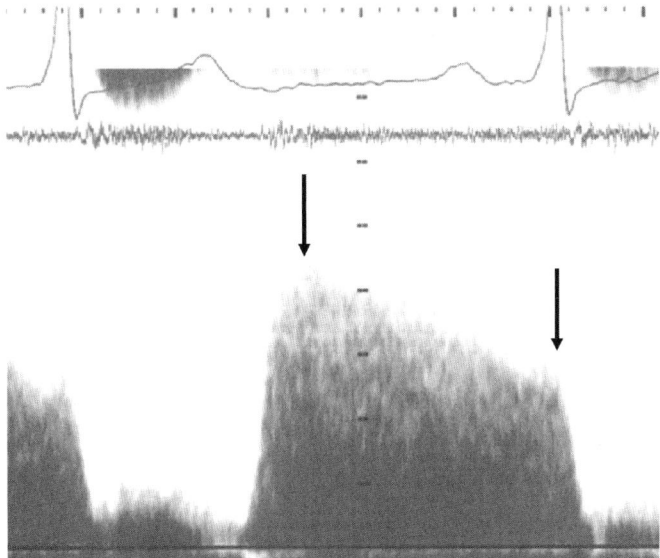

Fig. 16.6.13 Continuous wave Doppler from the same patient as shown in Fig. 16.6.12 showing significant regurgitation based on the rate of transvalvar pressure decline in diastole (between the arrows).

In acute aortic regurgitation echocardiography demonstrates clearly the cause of the disease; endocarditis with its complications or disintegrating homograft or bioprosthesis. M-mode echocardiography shows premature mitral valve closure which, together with the left ventricular activity, support the diagnosis of acute aortic regurgitation.

Cardiac catheterization

Cardiac catheterization is not needed to assess the severity of aortic regurgitation: it is only needed to confirm the presence of additional coronary artery disease, particularly before surgical intervention.

Differential diagnosis

It can sometimes be difficult to distinguish the early diastolic murmur of aortic regurgitation from that caused by pulmonary regurgitation (Graham–Steell murmur). In this circumstance no other features of aortic regurgitation are expected, and pulmonary regurgitation is usually associated with other signs indicating the presence of significant pulmonary hypertension (including a large pulmonary artery on the chest radiograph).

Other causes of aortic run-off, including persistent ductus arteriosus, ruptured sinus of Valsalva aneurysm, and coronary arteriovenous fistula, can also produce auscultatory findings that can be confused with aortic incompetence. However, they all cause a continuous murmur, rather than one confined to diastole.

Management

It is uncommon for mild aortic regurgitation to progress rapidly to severe regurgitation, hence the importance of Doppler echocardiography in the follow-up of patients. Identification of the cause of aortic regurgitation helps in determining how often patients should be reviewed: those with mild aortic regurgitation due to aortic root or ascending aorta disease should be followed up more closely than those with stable valve disease. Patients with moderate or severe aortic regurgitation may have no symptoms for years. As symptoms always reflect ventricular dysfunction, a progressive increase in end-systolic dimension/volume should be taken as an indication for serious consideration of surgery, even in the absence of symptoms. Ejection fraction cannot be taken as a marker of ventricular function in aortic regurgitation because of the volume overload and overestimation of the ejection performance: an end-systolic dimension up to 40 mm carries a good prognosis, whereas a dimension more than 50 mm is associated with 20% possibility of developing ventricular dysfunction, symptoms, or even death over a course of 5 years.

In the same way that patients with aortic regurgitation secondary to aortic valve disease are managed, those with aortic regurgitation associated with or causing aortic root dilatation should be followed up to assess the aortic root dimensions, with the aim of preventing progressive dilatation and the potential risk thereof. Some patients with a bicuspid aortic valve develop progressive dilatation of the aortic root because of the eccentric jet, as well as the accompanying aortopathy. Another group of patients who need regular follow-up and careful aortic root assessment are those with Marfan's syndrome, in whom aortic root aneurysmal dilatation and dissection are the major causes of morbidity and mortality. In addition to using conventional Doppler echocardiography, CT scanning and MRI can play a useful role in the follow-up of patients with aortic root or ascending aorta disease, and three-dimensional echocardiography for assessment of left ventricular size and function (see Chapters 16.3.2 and 16.3.3 for further discussion).

Medical

Medical management in aortic regurgitation aims at slowing down its progression, supporting the left ventricle, and determining the optimal time of surgical intervention. The increased afterload in patients with aortic regurgitation should be managed medically to reduce the wall stress and the diastolic driving pressure across the valve. Doing so decreases the pressure and the volume overload on the left ventricle and prevents progressive left ventricular dilatation and systolic dysfunction, and can delay the need for surgery. This effect has been demonstrated using ACE inhibitors and calcium channel blockers, the choice of the pharmacological agent for left ventricular afterload reduction depending on the other comorbidities, e.g. coronary artery disease, as well as patient tolerance.

Patients with aortic root dilatation should not be treated with vasodilators alone. In this instance β-blockers are recommended because they decrease aortic wall stress, blood pressure, and the rate of pressure increase in systole. Although patients with Marfan's may remain completely asymptomatic, the rate of aortic root dilatation is the most important risk factor. It may be that the combination of β-blockade with ACE inhibition/angiotensin receptor blockers (possibly acting through inhibition of TGF-β signalling) may prove effective in retarding or even preventing dilatation. However, when dilatation does occur previous guidelines have suggested that aortic root dimension larger than 55 mm is a good indication for surgical intervention, although recent recommendations have advocated an earlier surgical approach, particularly in the presence of family history of dissection. See Chapter 16.11 for further discussion.

As is the case with all valve disease, oral hygiene should be encouraged in patients with aortic regurgitation and prophylactic antibiotics prescribed to cover dental, proctological, urological, and gynaecological surgeries.

Surgical

Although patients with severe chronic aortic regurgitation may remain asymptomatic, surgical intervention should be offered when there is progressive increase in systolic dimension. A left ventricular end-systolic dimension of 40 mm is a cut-off value for preserved left ventricular systolic function, particularly for an active ventricle. Predictors of outcome after valve surgery are severe aortic regurgitation, age, severe symptoms, exercise intolerance, and evidence for left ventricular hypertrophy on echocardiography. Raised left ventricular end-diastolic pressure and the ratio of wall thickness to chamber dimension have also been identified as potential predictors of outcome. An additional risk is the presence of coronary artery disease. These patients should be carefully evaluated by preoperative cardiac catheterization and receive myocardial revascularization surgery and coronary grafting at the same setting with aortic valve replacement surgery. There is evidence to suggest that patients with aortic regurgitation and ventricular dysfunction develop faster reverse remodelling and fall of left ventricular mass index following successful valve replacement if they receive a stentless rather than a stented valve. Details of surgical procedures for aortic regurgitation are as described in the preceding section on aortic stenosis.

Acute aortic regurgitation, irrespective of its aetiology, should be managed as an emergency with surgical intervention. While diagnostic evaluation is in progress the patient should be treated with afterload reduction. Aortic balloon counter pulsation is contraindicated because it increases afterload. Cases caused by infective endocarditis should receive optimal antibiotic therapy following blood culture and emergency valve replacement, which could be life saving.

Mixed aortic disease

Mild to moderate aortic regurgitation often accompanies aortic stenosis but does little to alter the overall clinical picture. The combination can result from a bicuspid aortic valve or chronic rheumatic heart disease, or be the result of endocarditis or conservative surgery on a stenosed valve. The main haemodynamic disturbance is increased resistance to ejection, but the superimposition of even a moderately increased stroke volume due to regurgitation on the small, stiff left ventricle of pure aortic stenosis can lead to high filling pressures, left atrial enlargement, and even pulmonary hypertension. Breathlessness and chest pain are the most prominent symptoms. The arterial pulse is bisferiens, and typical ejection systolic and early diastolic murmurs are expected. Patients with symptoms are likely to require valve replacement.

Right heart valve disease

Many of the conditions that affect right sided valves are congenital: these are discussed in detail in Chapter 16.12. Particular pulmonary and tricuspid valve diseases that develop later in life are discussed here, after general discussion of effects of abnormal right-sided haemodynamics on right heart function and diagnostic techniques.

Pathophysiology and complications
Right ventricular response to valve disease
The right ventricle responds to chronic pressure overload, e.g. caused by pulmonary stenosis or pulmonary hypertension, by hypertrophy and early dilatation. With increased afterload and right ventricular dilatation the ventricle adapts by making the intraventricular septum function as part of the right heart.

This can be identified by studying septal movement during various phases of the cardiac cycle using M-mode echocardiography, revealing that it becomes reversed in systole and in diastole. Right ventricle dilatation includes the tricuspid annulus and results in tricuspid regurgitation. Eventually right ventricular systolic function deteriorates, which may become irreversible even after correcting the volume or pressure overload. With right ventricular volume overload the ventricle is very active, readily apparent on recording its free wall movement at the level of the tricuspid ring. However, assessing right ventricular ejection fraction and overall systolic function is difficult because of its complex anatomy, being made of an inlet portion and an outlet portion that are at a significant angle to each other, and a trabecular portion at the apex.

Assessment of right ventricular size and function
A three-dimensional approach to the assessment of right ventricular systolic function is the ideal method, but other cross-sectional echocardiographic and MRI techniques have developed over the years and proved sensitive in assessing right ventricular ejection fraction. Right ventricular inlet diameter can be used as a marker of cavity dilatation. Free wall long axis movement studied by M-mode and tissue Doppler imaging from the lateral angle of the tricuspid annulus is an easy measure of systolic function and correlates closely with right ventricular ejection fraction. Likewise, right ventricular outflow tract diameter has been shown a sensitive measure of systolic function. In patients with reversed septal movement it is crucial to exclude any shunt as a cause for volume overload in the right ventricle.

Estimation of pulmonary artery pressure is an essential component in the evaluation of patients with right-sided valve disease. The retrograde flow velocity across the tricuspid valve gives an indication of systolic right ventricular pressure by use of the simplified Bernoulli equation. In all patients systolic pulmonary artery pressure equals the retrograde peak pressure drop across the tricuspid valve added to the estimated right atrial pressure, according to the collapsibility of the inferior vena cava. These measurements are clinically useful in patients without pulmonary stenosis.

Investigation of valve stenosis and regurgitation
The methods used in clinical practice for investigating possible tricuspid and pulmonary valve stenosis and regurgitation are the same as those used in assessment of conditions affecting the left side of the heart. Colour Doppler detects the level at which there are increased velocities as a sign of valve narrowing, which can be confirmed by continuous wave Doppler. In patients with valve regurgitation colour Doppler assesses the jet diameter, direction, and area which, with respect to the right atrial area in cases of tricuspid regurgitation, gives some indication of the severity of tricuspid regurgitation. Transoesophageal echo images, particularly in tricuspid valve disease, provide detailed assessment of valve pathology.

Transthoracic images of the pulmonary valve can be somewhat limited technically, but in most cases Doppler studies can exclude significant valve disease based on forward and backward velocities and pressure drop. Transoesophageal echo provides a clearer image of the pulmonary valve and so is best suited for determining the level of valve stenosis. The degree of pulmonary stenosis and regurgitation severity is assessed by continuous wave Doppler, with timing of reversal of regurgitant pulmonary flow another confirmation of its severity. Mild pulmonary regurgitation occupies the whole of diastole, while in severe regurgitation there is early pressure equalization between the two chambers. A jet diameter of 7 mm or more also supports the diagnosis of severe pulmonary regurgitation.

MRI is another good noninvasive technique for assessment of right-sided chamber size and valve function, in particular the pulmonary valve. The level of narrowing can easily be determined, the degree of stenosis by velocity mapping, and severity of regurgitation by estimating the regurgitant volume.

Tricuspid stenosis

Tricuspid stenosis is a rare condition, most often caused by rheumatic disease, which almost invariably simultaneously affects the mitral valve. Other (even rarer) causes are carcinoid disease, infective endocarditis, and Whipple's disease. A right atrial myxoma or extension of hypernephroma into the inferior vena cava and right atrium can in very rare instances present with signs and symptoms of right ventricular inflow tract obstruction, similar to tricuspid stenosis.

Symptoms include fatigue, dyspnoea, and fluid retention. In patients with chronic rheumatic heart disease the problem is to recognize that the tricuspid valve has been affected in addition to the mitral (and perhaps the aortic valve as well). If the patient is in sinus rhythm there may be an 'a' wave in the venous pulse, which would be unusual in the presence of pulmonary hypertension and mitral stenosis alone (when the patient is very likely to be in atrial fibrillation). On auscultation at the left or right sternal edge a mid-diastolic murmur (usually higher in pitch than the murmur of mitral stenosis) is heard, and a tricuspid opening snap may be present (later in the cardiac cycle than a mitral opening snap, and varying in timing in relation to P_2 with respiration), although it is not possible to differentiate this reliably from the mitral opening snap that is likely to coexist.

The chest radiograph shows a large right atrium with normal pulmonary artery size and clear lung fields. Echocardiography shows a dilated right atrium and demonstrates clearly the valve anatomy and function, as well as other intracardiac pathologies. The echocardiographic signs of rheumatic tricuspid disease are similar to those of the mitral valve, including commissural fusion, fibrosed leaflets that dome in diastole, short and fibrosed chordae, and raised transtricuspid forward flow velocities.

Tricuspid valve disease progresses very slowly and needs careful follow-up. Medical treatments are not satisfactory: diuretics can help to minimize fluid retention, but at the expense of reduced cardiac output if pushed too hard. Mild and moderate tricuspid stenosis is generally tolerated; severe tricuspid stenosis needs surgical repair, or replacement if additional regurgitation is present.

Tricuspid regurgitation

Mild tricuspid regurgitation is found in 50% of normal individuals. Causes of significant tricuspid regurgitation are shown in Table 16.6.3, the commonest being secondary to either pulmonary hypertension or right heart dilatation.

Endocarditis is commonly caused by intravenous access, either in those who abuse drugs intravenously, or in patients who required prolonged right-heart catheters for medical therapy. Endomyocardial fibrosis, which is prevalent in tropical Africa, causes fibrosis of the papillary muscle tips and thickening and

Table 16.6.3 Causes of tricuspid regurgitation

Cause	Type of condition	Disease
Primary	Congenital	Ebstein's anomaly
		Atrioventricular defect
		Prolapsing cusp
	Acquired	Rheumatic fever
		Infective endocarditis
		Permanent pacemaker wires
		Endomyocardial fibrosis
		Blunt trauma to the chest
		Carcinoid syndrome
		Ergot-derived dopamine receptor agonists
		Following radiotherapy to the chest
Secondary	'Functional'	Pulmonary hypertension or right heart dilatation
		Ischaemic right ventricular disease

shortening of tricuspid valve leaflets and chordae. Permanent pacemaker wires across the tricuspid valve may rarely cause leaflet adhesions and dysfunction. Blunt trauma to the chest may be complicated by tricuspid regurgitation through the papillary muscle or chordal lacerations. Metastatic carcinoid tricuspid valve disease is rare, but echocardiographic findings of carcinoid involvement of the tricuspid valve are very characteristic, showing short, fibrosed, and thickened leaflets resulting in larger areas of incomplete coaption and severe tricuspid regurgitation. Tricuspid valve prolapse is occasionally seen in patients with mitral valve prolapse.

The symptoms of tricuspid regurgitation are usually nonspecific. When it develops in a patient with mitral stenosis it is often associated with increased fatigue rather than breathlessness. Some patients will present with increasing peripheral oedema, and hepatic congestion may cause nausea or upper abdominal pain exacerbated by exercise. Diarrhoea caused by a protein-losing enteropathy (thought to be secondary to venous congestion of the gut) has been reported.

The main physical sign is a raised venous pressure with prominent V-wave, without which the diagnosis of significant tricuspid regurgitation is very difficult to sustain. In about one-third of cases a pansystolic tricuspid regurgitation murmur can be heard at the left or right sternal edge: this tends to increase in intensity with inspiration as the venous return increases, and it can radiate into the epigastrium. Expansile pulsation of the liver is present in most cases, but hepatic fibrosis (and jaundice) can occur if regurgitation is long-standing and this physical sign then disappears. Most patients with severe regurgitation have peripheral oedema, ascites, or both.

The findings on a chest radiograph depend mainly on whether or not the patient has any other cardiac disease, but there may be enlargement of the heart shadow towards the right. The ECG may show right atrial hypertrophy. Echocardiography is the best way to make the diagnosis (Fig. 16.6.14). Cardiac catheterization is not required for assessment of tricuspid regurgitation but may be indicated for diagnosis or assessment of other concurrent heart disease.

Many patients tolerate tricuspid regurgitation for a long time, but some present with symptoms that significantly limit their exercise capacity and lifestyle. Medical treatment with diuretics and ACE inhibitors may reduce systemic venous pressure and right ventricular size, even restoring competence to the tricuspid valve in some cases. Attempts should be made to treat pulmonary

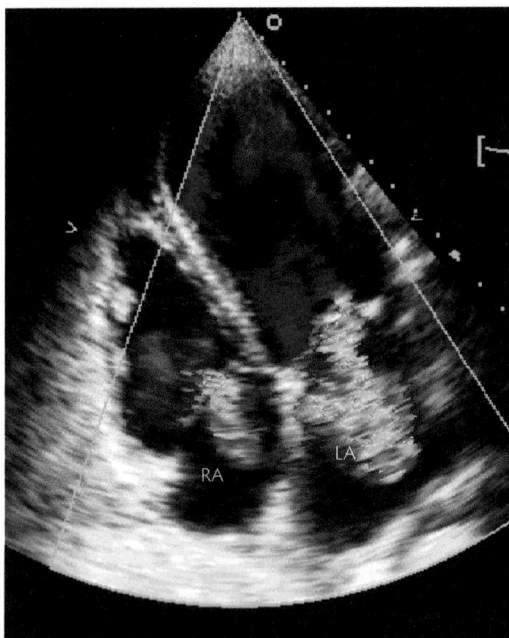

Fig. 16.6.14 Apical four-chamber view from a patient with tricuspid regurgitation secondary to left-sided dilated cardiomyopathy and mitral regurgitation: regurgitation into both left atrium (LA) and right atrium (RA) can be seen.

hypertension if this is the primary cause of right ventricular dilatation and tricuspid regurgitation. If fluid retention is severe and refractory to medical treatment, careful consideration should be given to surgical correction of tricuspid regurgitation before the patient develops irreversible right ventricular damage. Repair and replacement of the tricuspid valve are problematic operations, with the former sometimes failing to prevent regurgitation and the latter leading to a significant diastolic pressure drop between the right atrium and ventricle, creating a problem of iatrogenic tricuspid stenosis, but in specialist centres the current approach is less conservative than it used to be.

Tricuspid valvuloplasty is often performed at the time of mitral valve surgery for rheumatic disease. Annuloplasty involves a full ring, incomplete ring, or suture plication of the annulus. A semicircular ring has the advantage of maintaining annular flexibility and avoiding conduction disturbances, but residual tricuspid regurgitation occurs less often with a circular angioplasty ring than with a semicircular one. Tricuspid valve replacement by a mechanical prosthesis has a potential risk for endocarditis, particularly in drug abusers. Bioprostheses have a much lower thrombogenicity and resistance to flow in the tricuspid position and are therefore the preferred choice.

The surgical mortality of tricuspid valve surgery depends particularly on the degree of preoperative hepatic congestion. Survival following tricuspid valve replacement is not purely related to the surgical procedure itself or to valve function, but is significantly affected by right ventricular dysfunction that is almost always masked by the volume overload before surgery.

Pulmonary stenosis

Pulmonary stenosis is congenital in 95% of cases (see Chapter 16.12): rarely it is caused by rheumatic valve disease or carcinoid syndrome. Patients can tolerate moderate pulmonary stenosis (gradient <50 mmHg) for years, fatigue and dyspnoea due to reduced cardiac output being the main symptoms in those with severe disease. Physical examination reveals a prominent venous 'a' wave in the neck and an ejection systolic murmur at the upper left sternal edge that radiates to the suprasternal notch and left side of the neck. With severe pulmonary stenosis the pulmonary component of the second sound may be delayed, but it is often inaudible. An ejection click may be heard at the upper left sternal edge. Echocardiography and MRI show the level of stenosis. Doming leaflets are consistent with congenital valve disease. MRI imaging is particularly good for demonstrating supravalvar stenosis. Event-free survival is related to the pressure gradient across the pulmonary valve.

Balloon valvuloplasty is the procedure of choice for children and adults with significant pulmonary stenosis. On average transpulmonary gradient drops by two-thirds of the baseline value without development of significant pulmonary regurgitation. Additional subvalvar stenosis may underestimate the success of the procedure. Surgical valvotomy may be considered if balloon valvuloplasty fails, and valve replacement may be needed for those with iatrogenic significant pulmonary regurgitation, especially after repair of tetralogy of Fallot. Homograft replacements might be advantageous to avoid anticoagulation and thrombogenicity.

Pulmonary regurgitation

A small amount of pulmonary regurgitation is common. Significant pulmonary regurgitation is very rare and most commonly preceded by intervention to the pulmonary valve during childhood. Although the outcome of repair of tetralogy of Fallot is excellent in most cases, many of its complications are related to pulmonary regurgitation. Rare causes of pulmonary regurgitation are rheumatic disease, carcinoid, and endocarditis. Many patients with pulmonary hypertension and dilatation of the right ventricular outflow tract will demonstrate some degree of pulmonary regurgitation.

The typical murmur of pulmonary regurgitation is a soft early diastolic murmur that is best heard in the left upper parasternal region. It begins after the pulmonary component of the second sound and may be accompanied by an ejection systolic murmur caused by increased stroke volume. Most patients have enlarged neck veins and other evidence of pulmonary hypertension.

Most patients with mild pulmonary regurgitation remain completely asymptomatic for years. Although those with severe regurgitation may remain asymptomatic, correction of valve incompetence may save them irreversible damage of the right ventricle. Arrhythmia or progressive right ventricular dilatation are indications for surgery, using homograft or conduit and valve. Normalization of right ventricular size and function following pulmonary homograft insertion occurs in some but not all patients, probably depending on preoperative ventricular dysfunction that could be masked by volume overload.

Further reading

Henein MY, et al. (2004). *Clinical Echocardiography*. Springer.
Henein MY (2009). *Valvular Heart Disease in Clinical Practice*. Springer.

Mitral valve disease

Alpert JS (1999). Mitral stenosis. In: Alpert JS, Dalen JE, Rahimtoola SH (eds) *Valvular heart disease*. Lippincott Williams & Wilkins, Philadelphia.

Bonow RO, *et al.* (2006). ACC/AHA 2006 guidelines for the management of patients with valvular heart disease: a report of the American College of Cardiology/American Heart Association Task Force on Practice Guidelines (writing Committee to Revise the 1998 guidelines for the management of patients with valvular heart disease) developed in collaboration with the Society of Cardiovascular Anesthesiologists endorsed by the Society for Cardiovascular Angiography and Interventions and the Society of Thoracic Surgeons. *J Am Coll Cardiol*, **48**, e1–148.

Bonow RO, *et al.*(2008). American College of Cardiology/American Heart Association Task Force on Practice Guidelines. *J Am Coll Cardiol*, **52**, e1–142. [2008 focused update incorporated into the ACC/AHA 2006 guidelines for the management of patients with valvular heart disease: a report of the American College of Cardiology/American Heart Association Task Force on Practice Guidelines (Writing Committee to revise the 1998 guidelines for the management of patients with valvular heart disease). Endorsed by the Society of Cardiovascular Anesthesiologists, Society for Cardiovascular Angiography and Interventions, and Society of Thoracic Surgeons.]

Breithardt OA, *et al.* (2003). Acute effects of cardiac resynchronization therapy on functional mitral regurgitation in advanced systolic heart failure. *J Am Coll Cardiol*, **41**, 765–70.

Devereux RB (1995). Recent developments in the diagnosis and management of mitral valve prolapse. *Curr Opin Cardiol*, **10**, 107–16.

Devereux RB, Kramer-Fox R, Kligfield P (1989). Mitral valve prolapse: causes, clinical manifestations, and management. *Ann Intern Med*, **111**, 305–17.

Duren DR, Becker AE, Dunning AJ (1988). Long-term follow-up of idiopathic mitral valve prolapse in 300 patients: a prospective study. *J Am Coll Cardiol*, **11**, 42–7.

Enriquez-Sarano M, *et al.* (2005). Quantitative determinants of outcome in asymptomatic mitral regurgitation. *N Engl J Med*, **352**, 875–83.

Horstkotte D, Niehues R, Strauer BE (1991). Pathomorphological aspects, aetiology and natural history of acquired mitral valve stenosis. *Eur Heart J*, **12** Suppl, 60.

Sharma SK, *et al.* (1992). Clinical, angiographic and anatomic findings in acute severe ischemic mitral regurgitation. *Am J Cardiol*, **70**, 77–280.

Waller BF (1988). Etiology of mitral stenosis and pure mitral regurgitation. In: Waller BF (ed.) *Pathology of the heart and great vessels*, pp. 101–48. Churchill Livingstone, New York.

Rothlisberger C, *et al.* (1993). Results of percutaneous balloon mitral valvotomy in young adults. *Am J Cardiol*, **72**, 73–7.

Aortic valve disease

Borer JS, *et al.* (1998). Prediction of indications for valve replacement among asymptomatic or minimally symptomatic patients with chronic aortic regurgitation and normal left ventricular performance. *Circulation*, **97**, 525–34.

Cohn LH, Narayanasamy N (2007). Aortic valve replacement in elderly patients: what are the limits?. *Curr Opin Cardiol*, **22**, 92–5.

Enriquez-Sarano M, Tajik AJ (2004). Clinical practice. Aortic regurgitation. *N Engl J Med*, **351**, 1539–46.

Frank S, Johnson A, Ross J, Jr (1973). Natural history of valvular aortic stenosis. *Br Heart J*, **35**, 41–6.

Kvidal P, *et al.* (2000). Observed and relative survival after aortic valve replacement. *J Am Coll Cardiol*, **35**, 747–56.

Lombard JT, Selzer A (1987). Valvular aortic stenosis. A clinical and hemodynamic profile of patients. *Ann Intern Med*, **106**, 292–8.

Malouf JF, *et al.* (2002). Severe pulmonary hypertension in patients with severe aortic valve stenosis: clinical profile and prognostic implications. *J Am Coll Cardiol*, **40**, 789–95.

Marsalese DL, *et al.* (1989). Marfan's syndrome: natural history and long-term follow-up of cardiovascular involvement. *J Am Coll Cardiol*, **14**, 422–8.

O'Brien MF, *et al.* (2001). The homograft aortic valve: a 29-year, 99.3% follow up of 1,022 valve replacements. *J Heart Valve Dis*, **10**, 334–44.

Otto CM, *et al.* (1997). Prospective study of asymptomatic valvular aortic stenosis. Clinical, echocardiographic, and exercise predictors of outcome. *Circulation*, **95**, 2262–70.

Pohle K, *et al.* (2001). Progression of aortic valve calcification: association with coronary atherosclerosis and cardiovascular risk factors. *Circulation*, **104**, 1927–32.

Richards AM, *et al.* (1984). Syncope in aortic valvular stenosis. *Lancet*, **ii**, 1113–1116.

Rosenhek R, *et al.* (2000). Predictors of outcome in severe, asymptomatic aortic stenosis. *N Engl J Med*, **343**, 611–17.

Ross DN (1967). Replacement of aortic and mitral valves with a pulmonary autograft. *Lancet*, **ii**, 956–958.

Vahanian A, *et al.*(2008). *Eur J Cardiothorac Surg*, **34**, 1–8.[Transcatheter valve implantation for patients with aortic stenosis: a position statement from the European Association of Cardio-Thoracic Surgery (EACTS) and the European Society of Cardiology (ESC), in collaboration with the European Association of Percutaneous Cardiovascular Interventions (EAPCI).]

Tricuspid and pulmonary valve disease

Hansing CE, Rowe GG (1972). Tricuspid insufficiency. A study of hemodynamics and pathogenesis. *Circulation*, **45**, 793–799.

Lindqvist P, Calcutteea A, Henein M.(2008). Echocardiography in the assessment of right heart function. *Eur J Echocardiogr*, **9**, 225–34.

Pellikka PA, *et al.* (1993). Carcinoid heart disease. Clinical and echocardiographic spectrum in 74 patients. *Circulation*, **87**, 1188–96.

Weinreich DJ, *et al.* (1985). Isolated prolapse of the tricuspid valve. *J Am Coll Cardiol*, **6**, 475–81.

Diseases of heart muscle

Contents

16.7.1 Myocarditis

Jay W. Mason

Essentials

Myocarditis has many infectious and noninfectious aetiologies; in most regions, viral infections are the main cause, with notable exceptions such as Chagas' myocarditis in South America. The condition often results in congestive heart failure and is a common cause of chronic dilated cardiomyopathy, and it can also present with chest pain and/or ventricular arrythmias.

Patients with lymphocytic myocarditis are usually young (average age in the forties) and often report an antecedent viral illness. The disease can be diagnosed specifically by demonstration of lymphocyte infiltration and adjacent myocyte damage on endomyocardial biopsy. Detection of viral genomic material and tissue markers of immune activation in biopsy specimens, MRI and other imaging techniques, and presence of circulating biomarkers are also helpful in establishing the diagnosis. Adverse immune activation is the primary cause of myocardial damage in most cases.

Appropriately timed immunosuppressive therapy, most commonly with a steroid (prednisolone), may improve outcome in some cases, but efficacy is limited to special cases. Other immunomodulatory therapies and antiviral therapies have also been used, usually in patients who are deteriorating, but without proof of benefit. Specific forms of myocarditis include peripartum myocarditis, Lyme carditis, cardiac sarcoidosis, giant cell myocarditis, and Chagas' carditis, each of which requires specific diagnostic and therapeutic measures.

Introduction

Myocarditis has captured the interest of clinicians and scientists because of its varied aetiology, its diagnostic and therapeutic challenges, and the possibility that myocarditis may be the primary cause of dilated cardiomyopathy. Scientific study of myocarditis is facilitated by the availability of numerous easily manipulated animal models of the disease and by new molecular probes.

Clinical features

Myocarditis affects young people: the average age of patients in the United States Myocarditis Treatment Trial was 42 years. There was a slight male predominance (62%) in that trial, but other series have not demonstrated a sex predilection. The true incidence of myocarditis is unknown: autopsy studies have reported figures of up to 3%, but varying histological criteria were used, and myocarditis may occur as an incidental complication of other fatal illnesses. About 10% of patients with influenzal infections have electrocardiographic abnormalities, but it is not known if these are the result of myocarditis. The incidence of fatal myocarditis was estimated in a retrospective review of United States Air Force recruits undergoing boot camp training: there were 8 such deaths over 1 606 167 person days, which yields an estimate of 4/100 000 per year in people aged 17 to 28 years. This incidence is probably greater than would be expected in the general population in the United States of America, who would not be exposed to similar levels of intense exercise or high probability of transmission of viral illnesses.

In Europe and North America most cases of myocarditis present with congestive heart failure of unknown cause. In many cases there is a history of recent upper respiratory tract infection or of a 'flu-like' illness. This is followed by symptoms of cardiac decompensation, usually fatigue, breathlessness, and cough. Chest pain occurs in a substantial minority of patients. A few present with ventricular tachyarrhythmias and minimal or no cardiac dilatation. Typically, the duration of symptoms due to infection is brief, less than 1 month in approximately 50% of patients and nearly always less than 1 year. Myocarditis should always be suspected when a patient presents with unexplained congestive heart failure with a rapid onset, especially if there is a viral prodrome.

Clinical examination typically reveals signs of cardiac failure. The ECG may show conduction abnormalities and ST/T-wave changes, or arrhythmias (atrial or ventricular). The chest radiograph shows cardiomegaly and pulmonary oedema. The echocardiogram reveals four-chamber dilatation and reduced contractility, and is notable for the fact that valvular disease is absent or minimal. Cardiac scintigraphy with indium-111 antimyosin antibodies and single photon emission computed tomography (SPECT) can be used to detect myocarditis. Contrast-enhanced MRI allows assessment of the regional extent of myocardial involvement. Should coronary angiography be performed, the vessels are normal or show only minor abnormalities. The role of myocardial biopsy will be discussed later. Creatine phosphokinase (CPK-MB) elevation is common.

Although viruses are thought to be the most common cause of myocarditis, viral titres are rarely useful in diagnosis and treatment. Although the cardiotrophic enteroviruses, including echoviruses and coxsackieviruses, are the predominant aetiological agents, dozens of viruses have been implicated and many more undoubtedly, cause myocarditis in humans. Thus, it is impractical to exclude them all. In addition, patients usually present a substantial length of time after the viral infection has cleared, making it difficult or impossible to document an acute rise in titre. Knowledge of a specific virus, or any virus, as the cause in a given case of myocarditis has little, if any, therapeutic relevance. Even if viricidal therapy (which is not yet a proven treatment; see below) is being considered, negative titres for the common viral agents do not exclude a viral aetiology.

A small number of patients, perhaps about 10%, present with a secondary form of myocarditis: these special presentations are discussed below.

Aetiology and pathogenesis (Table 16.7.1.1)

The most common form of myocarditis in Europe and North America is known as lymphocytic myocarditis or nonspecific lymphocytic myocarditis. Other frequently applied terms are viral or postviral myocarditis, because an antecedent viral infection is common. Indeed, some experts believe that nearly all lymphocytic myocarditides are the result of viral infections, presumed to be subclinical in those patients with no awareness of a viral prodrome.

In animal models enteroviruses, such as coxsackie B3, can cause two phases of myocarditis. The first is the result of direct injury of myocytes by replicating virus and the resulting acute immune response. A delayed immune response brings about the second phase, and it is this that is thought to be the more common cause of overt congestive heart failure. The underlying mechanisms are complex and incompletely understood, but most hypotheses suggest that autoimmune phenomena play a major role. In some instances molecular mimicry may be involved, in which the similarity of a viral antigen to a myocardial protein triggers an autoimmune reaction. In others an autoimmune response to cellular proteins released during the viral replication phase may occur, and myosin has been implicated in this regard. Cytokines arising from immune

Table 16.7.1.1 Aetiologies of myocarditis

INFECTION
Viruses
Adenovirus
Arbovirus
Arenavirus
Coronavirus
Coxsackievirus (A, B)
Cytomegalovirus
Echovirus
Encephalomyocarditis
Epstein–Barr
Hepatitis B
Hepatitis C
Herpes simplex
Human immunodeficiency
Influenza (A, B)
Junin
Parvovirus (B19)
Mumps
Polio
Rabies
Respiratory syncytial
Rubella (German measles)
Rubeola (measles)
Vaccinia
Varicella-zoster virus
Variola
Bacteria, spirochaetes, and Bacteria-like organisms
β-Haemolytic streptococci
Borrelia burgdorferi (Lyme disease)
Brucella spp.
Campylobacter jejuni
Chlamydia psittaci (psittacosis)
Chlamydia trachomatis (trachoma)
Clostridia spp.
Corynebacterium diphtheriae
Francisella tularensis (tularaemia)
Gonococcus
Haemophilus influenzae
Legionella pneumophila
Leptospira spp.
Listeria monocytogenes
Mycobacterium spp.
Mycoplasma pneumoniae

(Continued)

Table 16.7.1.1 *(Cont'd)* Aetiologies of myocarditis

Neisseria gonorrhoeae
Neisseria meningitidis
Salmonella typhi
Streptococcus pneumoniae
Staphylococcus spp.
Treponema pallidum (syphilis)
Tropheryma whippleii
Rickettsia
Coxiella burnetii (Q fever)
Orientia tsutsugamushi (scrub typhus)
Rickettsia rickettsii (Rocky Mountain spotted fever)
Rickettsia prowazekii (typhus)
Protozoa
Entamoeba histolytica
Leishmania spp.
Toxoplasma gondii
Trypanosoma cruzi (Chagas' disease)
Helminths
Cysticerus
Echinococcus spp.
Schistosoma spp.
Toxocara spp.
Trichinella spp.
Fungal
Actinomyces spp.
Aspergillus spp.
Blastomyces dermatitides
Candida spp.
Coccidioides immitis
Cryptococcus neoformans
Fusarium
Oxysporum
Histoplasma capsulatum
Mucor
Nocardia spp.
Sporothrix schenckii
DRUGS AND CHEMICALS
Toxicity
2-Interferon
Amphetamines
Animal & insect toxins
Anthracyclines
Arsenic
Catecholamines

Table 16.7.1.1 *(Cont'd)* Aetiologies of myocarditis

Chloroquine
Cocaine
5-Fluorouracil
Interleukin 2
Lithium
Paracetamol
Hypersensitivity
Aminophylline
Ampicillin
Benzodiazepines
Digoxin
Ephedrine
Frusemide
Hydrochlorthiazide
Methyldopa
Penicillin
Phenytoin
Tetracycline
Tricyclic antidepressants
AUTOIMMUNITY
Antigenic mimicry
Autoimmune disease associated
Cardiac myosin
Cytokines
Dressler's syndrome
Post-cardiotomy syndrome
Postinfectious
Post-radiation

activation and cellular necrosis probably play a role in some cases, bringing about further cellular damage, such as through activation of matrix metalloproteinases. Viral persistence appears to induce a chronic adverse immune response and, as a result, to correlate with a poor prognosis. Although all of these mechanisms have been well delineated in murine models, they have not been proven to cause myocarditis in humans.

Myocarditis may result from a hypersensitivity reaction to a drug or other agent (see Table 16.7.1.1). In these cases eosinophils accompany the inflammatory lymphocytic infiltrate. A number of other specific causes of myocarditis, each with differing pathogeneses and presentations, are discussed below.

Relationship to idiopathic dilated cardiomyopathy

Classic lymphocytic myocarditis usually resolves, with resultant improvement in cardiac function over weeks or months. In the United States Myocarditis Treatment Trial, the mean left ventricular ejection fraction (LVEF) improved during the year after initial presentation by more than 10 EF units (from 24 to 36%; normal >55%). However, residual cardiac dilatation and dysfunction were common, and mortality was high, reaching 55% at 5 years. In those patients who do not recover fully, the ensuing clinical picture cannot be distinguished from that of idiopathic dilated cardiomyopathy. The possibility that myocarditis may occur without an obvious viral prodrome therefore raises the interesting possibility that viral myocarditis may be a common covert cause of idiopathic dilated cardiomyopathy. In the United States trial, only 10% of patients with suspected myocarditis had positive biopsies. Hence, the fact that endomyocardial biopsy does not reveal myocarditis in patients with idiopathic dilated cardiomyopathy may be the result of timing of the biopsy after resolution of the lymphocytic infiltrate, sampling error, or absence of a lymphocytic response in some patients. The presence of viral genomic material in some of these negative biopsies lends support to the viral aetiology hypothesis. Absence of viral genome in the rest of them does not eliminate postviral autoimmune processes, proceeding despite complete viral clearing, as a possible aetiology. The fact that immunomodulatory therapy may improve cardiac function in patients with dilated cardiomyopathy but without lymphocytic myocardial infiltrates adds indirect evidence that idiopathic dilated cardiomyopathy has an inflammatory origin in some cases.

Treatment of postviral and nonspecific lymphocytic myocarditis

As stated above, nonspecific lymphocytic myocarditis is believed by most to have a viral aetiology, even in the absence of a clinically apparent viral prodrome. In the acute phase of viral myocarditis, the direct cytolytic effect of viral myocyte infection may lead to congestive heart failure, although this is uncommon. In this early phase, the immune response is likely, on balance, to be beneficial. Thus, antiviral therapy might be expected to be helpful, but on theoretical grounds immunosuppressive therapy would not. However, though antiviral therapies have shown promise, none have been adequately tested in humans.

In the second stage of myocarditis, thought to result from an adverse immune response to previous infection, immunosuppressive therapy has appeared to be beneficial in uncontrolled trials. However, no benefit was demonstrated in the United States Myocarditis Treatment Trial, the only prospective, randomized trial performed in patients with myocarditis defined histologically. In that trial the 'Dallas' criteria defined myocarditis histologically as a lymphocytic infiltrate with associated myocyte necrosis (Fig. 16.7.1.1). Treatment with prednisone combined with either ciclosporin or with azathioprine did not improve outcome, as defined by change in left ventricular ejection fraction. However, it is appropriate to consider other diagnostic criteria, such as presence of viral genomic material and HLA up-regulation on biopsy, circulating antiheart antibodies and imaging in the diagnosis and treatment of myocarditis.

An algorithm for the diagnosis and treatment of suspected myocarditis is shown in Fig. 16.7.1.2. Spontaneous improvement in left ventricular function can be anticipated in many patients. In most cases it is reasonable to use standard therapy for congestive heart failure, without performing a biopsy or administering steroids, and to observe the patient, using echocardiography to monitor left

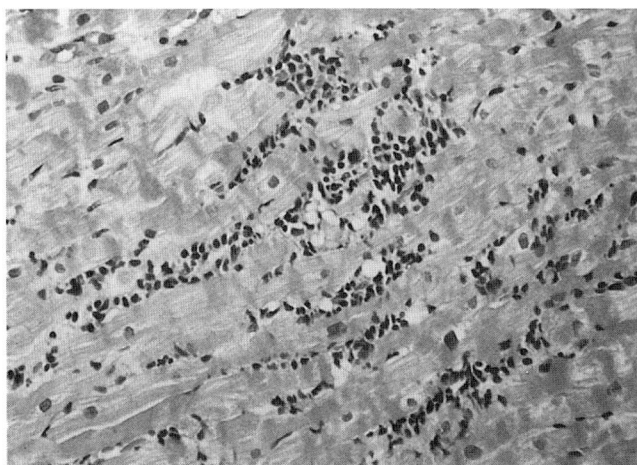

Fig. 16.7.1.1 An example of acute myocarditis, with lymphocytic infiltration adjacent to frayed myocytes.

ventricular function. However, in patients who deteriorate, or who present in cardiogenic shock, an endomyocardial biopsy should be performed. Many experts would also base a diagnosis of myocarditis on proven imaging techniques, such as contrast-enhanced MRI, in combination with a circulating biomarker such as cardiac-specific antibodies. If myocarditis is present, immunosuppressive therapy should be administered, typically beginning with prednisone at 1.25 mg/kg per day, tapering to 0.15 mg/kg per day over 1 month. It must be admitted, however, that the efficacy of such treatment has not been proved. If the patient worsens despite this therapy, antiviral or immunomodulatory therapy can be offered in an investigative setting. Direct antiviral treatments that have been tested or proposed include aciclovir, ganciclovir, foscarnet, and amantadine. Immunomodulatory treatments include immunoadsorptive apheresis, interferons, immune globulins, pentoxifylline, and cytokines such as interleukin-6.

Management of ventricular tachyarrhythmias in patients with myocarditis

Lymphocytic myocarditis, with or without a viral prodrome, may present with ventricular tachyarrhythmias and little or no cardiac dilatation and dysfunction. An endomyocardial biopsy should be considered in all cases of ventricular tachycardia of recent onset if no aetiology is apparent, because the presence of myocarditis can substantially change treatment strategy. Since myocarditis is often a self-limiting disorder, the patient's risk of recurrent ventricular tachyarrhythmias may resolve, and it may be unnecessary to subject the patient to electrophysiological study and/or cardioverter–defibrillator implantation. If arrhythmia does not improve spontaneously, a trial of immunosuppressive therapy should be considered. In such cases it is difficult to know how long to continue with antiarrhythmic drugs. The risks of ventricular arrhythmia should not be underestimated, but nor should those of long-term treatment with agents such as amiodarone. If 24-h ECG monitoring at 6 months shows no sinister abnormalities, then many would withdraw antiarrhythmic treatment at that point, but others advocate repeat endomyocardial biopsy to document complete resolution of myocarditis before taking this step.

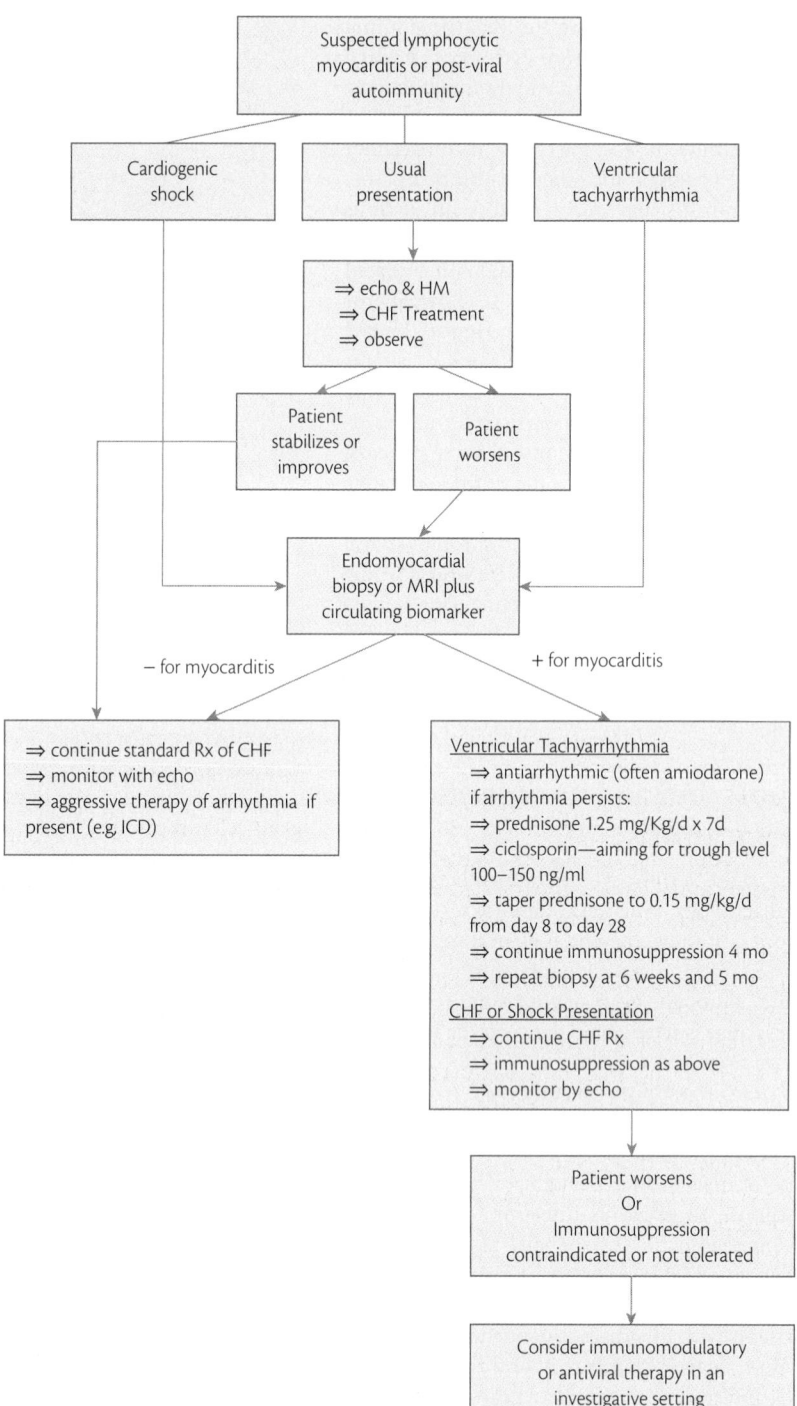

Fig. 16.7.1.2 Algorithm for diagnosis and treatment of suspected myocarditis. ACE, angiotensin converting enzyme; CHF, congestive heart failure; echo, echocardiogram; HM, Holter monitor; ICD, implantable cardioverter–defibrillator.

Specific forms of myocarditis

Specific forms of myocarditis are shown in Fig. 16.7.1.3.

Peripartum myocarditis

Dilated cardiomyopathy developing during the last trimester of pregnancy or within 6 months of delivery is known as peripartum or postpartum cardiomyopathy (see Chapter 14.6). In some series the dominant cause is myocarditis. When heart failure develops rapidly in the first few weeks after delivery, myocarditis is more likely to be found on endomyocardial biopsy than when the onset is insidious and delayed, and those with early, rapid onset are more likely to recover quickly and completely. While steroid therapy has been used and is recommended by some, its efficacy has not been proved, and spontaneous resolution of peripartum cardiomyopathy is well documented. The usual prohibition against future pregnancy has been debated; it is very clear that some women risk recurrent heart failure, while others do not. In those women in whom severe heart failure persists, cardiac transplantation is an appropriate therapy. After transplantation, successful pregnancies have occurred without recurrence of cardiomyopathy.

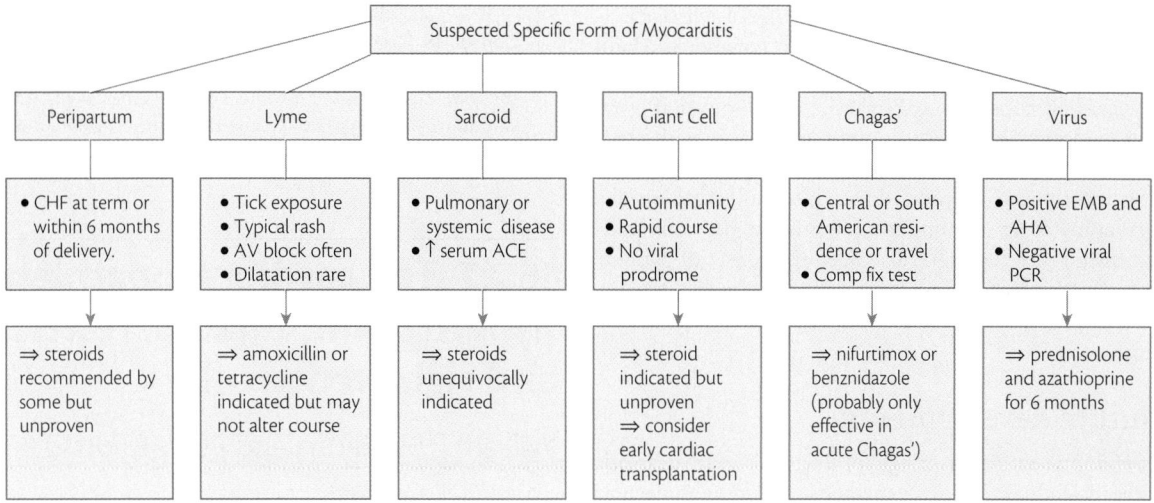

Fig. 16.7.1.3 Suspected specific forms of myocarditis. ACE, angiotensin converting enzyme; CHF, congestive heart failure; Comp fix, complement fixation; EMB, endomyocardial biopsy;AHA, anti-heart antibody;PCR, polymerase chain reaction.

Lyme carditis (see Chapter 7.6.32)

Borrelia burgdorferi, a spirochaete, infects humans following *Ixodes* tick bites. Lyme disease, which results from this infection, has been reported in 48 of the 50 United States as well as in Europe and Asia. It is characterized by an erythema migrans rash and flu-like symptoms, followed by arthritis, carditis, and neurological disorders in some patients. Carditis is detected in approximately 8% of cases. Both lymphocytic infiltration and the bacterium itself can be demonstrated by endomyocardial biopsy. The usual cardiac manifestation is varying degrees of atrioventricular block. Infrequently, cardiac dilatation occurs. Atrioventricular block is usually transient, though permanent complete heart block has been reported. The site of block appears to be the atrioventricular node in most cases, but block within the His bundle has been documented by electrophysiological study, and the common occurrence of intraventricular conduction delays suggests that bundle branch block may also occur. Temporary pacing is usually sufficient, though recovery of antegrade conduction may take a week or longer. Lyme carditis should be considered in any case of heart block of unknown cause, especially in young individuals.

Antibiotic therapy is recommended in Lyme carditis, but it is not known if this alters the course of carditis and atrioventricular block.

Cardiac sarcoidosis

Less than 10% of patients with pulmonary or systemic sarcoidosis have clinically manifest cardiac involvement, ranging from conduction disturbances and arrhythmias to cardiac dilatation. Endomyocardial biopsy reveals typical sarcoid granulomas. The most serious complications of cardiac sarcoidosis are complete heart block, ventricular tachyarrhythmias, and dilated cardiomyopathy. The relatively high incidence of sudden death in patients with sarcoidosis is thought to result from sudden complete heart block or ventricular fibrillation. Patients with sarcoidosis who develop significant conduction disease, arrhythmias, or congestive heart failure should receive steroids. Occasionally, cardiac involvement will occur without detectable systemic manifestations of sarcoidosis. Thus, cardiac sarcoidosis is in the differential diagnosis of any undiagnosed ventricular arrhythmia, dilated cardiomyopathy, or atrioventricular block. See Chapter 16.7.3 for further discussion.

Giant cell myocarditis

Early recognition of this rapidly progressive form of myocarditis is required, as it has a prognosis considerably worse than that of nonspecific lymphocytic myocarditis. The endomyocardial biopsy is distinguished by the presence of multinucleated giant cells and scattered lymphocytic infiltrates with eosinophils. The aetiology of giant cell myocarditis is unknown, but thought to be autoimmune, given its association with myasthenia gravis, thymoma, Crohn's disease, and other immune disorders. It should be suspected in patients—particularly those with a history of an autoimmune condition—who present with disease which progresses unusually rapidly, without viral prodrome, and who do not respond to standard therapy of congestive heart failure. Endomyocardial biopsy should be performed if giant cell myocarditis is suspected, because immunosuppressive therapy appears to be helpful, though not yet proved. Patients with giant cell myocarditis should be considered for early cardiac transplantation if they do not respond to therapy.

Chagas' disease (see Chapter 7.8.11)

Chagas' disease, caused by *Trypanosoma cruzi*, is the leading cause of myocarditis and dilated cardiomyopathy in some Central and South American countries, but uncommon in the United States of America. Overt acute myocarditis with congestive heart failure, arrhythmias, and conduction disease may develop, but cardiac involvement in early Chagas' disease is usually subclinical. Years later, chronic Chagas' disease may develop and may involve the heart. In the chronic phase, right bundle branch block and biventricular failure are present, and right heart failure predominates. Myocarditis occurs in both the acute and chronic phases, when immune mediation of myocyte injury is well documented. Antiprotozoal treatment with nifurtimox or benznidazole is beneficial in the acute phase. These agents are also indicated in the chronic phase, but—while they do reduce or eliminate serological immune markers of disease—it is not known if they improve outcome.

Virus-negative myocarditis

An entity known as virus-negative myocarditis is defined as chronic systolic heart failure with histological and immunochemical evidence of lymphocytic inflammation, but without evidence of a viral aetiology, as determined by negative comprehensive polymerase chain reaction detection of RNA or DNA of known cardiotropic viruses on endomyocardial biopsy tissue. Frustaci and colleagues showed recently in a randomized trial that immunosuppression with prednisolone and azathioprine improved left ventricular size and performance in virus-negative myocarditis. This result supports the hypothesis that inefficacy of immunosuppression in previous studies resulted from exacerbation of disease in the subset of patients with on-going viral infection, and it provides a rationale for rigorously excluding presence of inflammation in patients with chronic heart failure.

Likely future developments

The use of endomyocardial histology for diagnosis of myocarditis will be replaced gradually by other methods, including molecular assessments of biopsy tissue and noninvasive methods. In addition to diagnosis, new techniques will identify subsets of patients likely to respond to specific therapies more accurately. The most important advances will lead to prevention of the causative infections through vaccination and other prophylactic measures. These developments could profoundly reduce the incidence of dilated cardiomyopathy throughout the world.

Further reading

Aretz HT, *et al.* (1987). Myocarditis. A histopathologic definition and classification. *Cardiovasc Pathol*, **1**, 3–14.

Cooper LT, Berry GJ, Shabetai R (1997). Idiopathic giant-cell myocarditis—natural history and treatment. *N Engl J Med*, **336**, 1860–6.

Baughman KL (2006). Diagnosis of myocarditis: death of Dallas criteria. *Circulation*, **113**, 593–5.

Felker GM, *et al.* (2000). Myocarditis and long-term survival in peripartum cardiomyopathy. *Am Heart J*, **140**, 785–91.

Frustaci A, *et al.* (2003). Immunosuppressive therapy for active lymphocytic myocarditis: virological and immunologic profile of responders versus nonresponders. *Circulation*, **107**, 857–63.

Frustaci A, et al. (2009). Randomized study on the efficacy of immunosuppressive therapy in patients with virus-negative inflammatory cardiomyopathy: The TIMIC study. *Euro Heart J*, **30**, 1995–2002.

Gauntt CJ, *et al.* (1995). Molecular mimicry, antcoxsackievirus B3 neutralizing monoclonal antibodies, and myocarditis. *J Immunol*, **154**, 2983–95.

McManus BM, *et al.* (1993). Direct myocardial injury by enterovirus: a central role in the evolution of murine myocarditis. *Clin Immunol Immunopathol*, **68**, 159–69.

McNamara DM, *et al.* (2001). A controlled trial of intravenous immune globulin in recent-onset dilated cardiomyopathy. *Circulation*, **103**, 2254–9.

Mahrholdt H, *et al.* (2004). Cardiovascular magnetic resonance assessment of human myocarditis: a comparison to histology and molecular pathology. *Circulation*, **109**, 1250–8.

Mason JW, *et al.* (1995). A clinical trial of immunosuppressive therapy for myocarditis. *N Engl J Med*, **333**, 269–75.

Matsumori A, Sasayama S (2001). The role of inflammatory mediators in the failing heart: immunomodulation of cytokines in experimental models of heart failure. *Heart Failur Rev*, **6**, 129–36.

Muller JG, *et al.* (2000). Immunoglobulin adsorption in patients with idiopathic dilated cardiomyopathy. *Circulation*, **101**, 385–91.

Rose NR, Hill SL (1996). The pathogenesis of postinfectious myocarditis. *Clin Immun Immunopath*, **80**, S92–S99.

Skouri HN, *et al.* (2006). Noninvasive imaging in myocarditis. *J Am Coll Cardiol*, **48**, 2085–93.

Wojinicz R, *et al.* (2001). Randomized, placebo-controlled study for immunosuppressive treatment of inflammatory dilated cardiomyopathy: two-year follow-up results. *Circulation*, **104**, 39–45.

16.7.2 The cardiomyopathies: hypertrophic, dilated, restrictive, and right ventricular

William J. McKenna and Perry Elliott

Essentials

The term cardiomyopathy is used to describe heart muscle disease unexplained by abnormal loading conditions (hypertension, valve disease, etc.), congenital cardiac abnormalities, and ischaemic heart disease. Cardiomyopathies associated with systemic diseases are described in Chapter 16.7.3. This chapter describes the various forms of 'idiopathic' disease, although the discovery of more and more disease-causing mutations makes the term idiopathic increasingly redundant.

Hypertrophic cardiomyopathy

The diagnosis of hypertrophic cardiomyopathy is based upon the demonstration of unexplained myocardial hypertrophy, defined as a wall-thickness measurement exceeding two standard deviations above normal for gender and age. In practice, in an adult of normal size, the presence of a left ventricular myocardial segment of 1.5 cm or greater in thickness is diagnostic. Less stringent criteria should be applied to first-degree relatives of an unequivocally affected individual. Ninety per cent of patients have familial disease, usually with autosomal dominant inheritance. Mutations in genes encoding proteins of the cardiac sarcomere are most common (60% of cases).

Symptomatic presentation may be at any age, with breathlessness on exertion, chest pain, palpitation, syncope, or sudden death. In children and adolescents, the diagnosis is most often made during screening of siblings and offspring of affected family members. In most patients the physical examination is unremarkable, but characteristic features include a rapid upstroke arterial pulse, a forceful left ventricular cardiac impulse with palpable atrial beat, an ejection systolic murmur, and a fourth heart sound.

Investigation and diagnosis—the 12-lead ECG is the most sensitive diagnostic test, with ST-segment depression and T-wave changes being the most common abnormalities, usually associated with voltage changes of left ventricular hypertrophy and/or deep S waves in the anterior chest leads V1 to V3. Echocardiography reveals left ventricular hypertrophy that may be symmetric or asymmetric and localized to the septum or the free wall, but most commonly to both the septum and free wall with relative sparing of the posterior wall.

Management—β-adrenoceptor blockers and calcium antagonists, especially verapamil, are the mainstay of symptomatic pharmacological therapy. Surgery is considered for patients with obstruction (typically resting left ventricular outflow-tract gradient of more than 50 mmHg) and/or mitral valve abnormalities, with the commonest operation being removal of a segment of the upper anterior septum (myotomy/myectomy) via a transaortic approach. Injection of alcohol into the septal artery that supplies the 'obstructing' septal muscle has been developed as a percutaneous, nonpharmacological approach to gradient reduction.

Prognosis—annual mortality is 1 to 2%, but the risk of death and other disease-related complications varies between individuals. Prevention of sudden death relies on risk factor stratification to identify a high-risk cohort.

Dilated cardiomyopathy

Dilated cardiomyopathy is defined by dilatation and impaired systolic function of the left ventricle or both ventricles in the absence of coronary artery disease, valvular abnormalities, or pericardial disease. At least 25% of cases are familial, with a large number of disease-causing gene mutations described.

Initial presentation is usually with symptoms of cardiac failure, but other presentations include arrhythmia, systemic embolism, or the incidental finding of an electrocardiographic or radiographic abnormality. Physical examination may reveal cardiac enlargement and signs of congestive heart failure.

Investigation and diagnosis—on echocardiography, the presence of ventricular end-diastolic dimensions greater than two standard deviations above the mean and fractional shortening less than 25% are generally sufficient to make the diagnosis.

Management—symptomatic therapy involves the treatment of heart failure with diuretics, angiotensin converting enzyme (ACE) inhibitors, and β-blockers. Anticoagulation with warfarin is advised in patients in whom an intracardiac thrombus is identified echocardiographically, or those with a history of thromboembolism. Internal cardioverter defibrillators are warranted if sustained or symptomatic arrhythmias are documented during 24-h ECG monitoring or exercise testing. Biventricular or left ventricular pacing can improve symptoms and prognosis in selected patients, and cardiac transplantation may be appropriate for those with progressive deterioration.

Restrictive cardiomyopathy

Restrictive cardiomyopathies are defined by restrictive ventricular physiology in the presence of normal or reduced diastolic volumes of one or both ventricles, normal or reduced systolic volumes, and normal ventricular wall thickness. In the Western world, amyloidosis is the commonest cause; in the tropics, endomyocardial fibrosis.

Presentation is usually insidious: left-sided disease may present with symptoms of pulmonary congestion and/or mitral regurgitation; right-sided disease with raised jugular venous pressure, hepatomegaly, ascites, and tricuspid regurgitation. Echocardiography confirms the diagnosis, typically showing that ventricular dimensions and wall thickness are normal, but the atria are grossly enlarged.

Congestive symptoms from raised right atrial pressure can be improved with diuretics, though too great a reduction in ventricular filling pressure will lead to a reduction in cardiac output. Prognosis of advanced disease is poor.

Arrhythmogenic right ventricular cardiomyopathy

Arrhythmogenic right ventricular cardiomyopathy is a heart muscle disease characterized by progressive fibrofatty replacement of right ventricular myocardium, associated with ventricular arrhythmia, heart failure, and sudden cardiac death. It is inherited in at least 50% of cases.

Symptomatic presentation is usually with palpitation and/or syncope from sustained ventricular arrhythmia, but the first presentation of the disease may be with sudden cardiac death. There is no single diagnostic test, and the diagnosis is based on the presence of major and minor criteria encompassing structural, histological, electrocardiographic, arrhythmic, and genetic factors. The most common electrocardiographic abnormality is T-wave inversion in leads V1 to V3 in the absence of right bundle branch block. Typical echocardiographic findings include right ventricular dilatation, regional hypokinesia or dyskinesia, and other abnormalities.

Management—patients with symptomatic, non-life-threatening ventricular arrhythmias are treated empirically with β-blockers, amiodarone, or sotalol. Those with a history of sustained, haemodynamically compromising ventricular arrhythmia should be offered an implantable cardioverter–defibrillator.

Introduction

Heart muscle disease has traditionally been divided into idiopathic (cardiomyopathies) and secondary types (specific heart muscle diseases); the cardiomyopathies are classified further according to specific morphological and physiological characteristics into hypertrophic, dilated, right ventricular, and restrictive forms. This descriptive classification is useful when describing natural history, treatment, and prognosis, but the discovery of disease-causing mutations in all forms of cardiomyopathy means that the term 'idiopathic heart muscle disease' is increasingly redundant. For the purposes of this chapter, the term cardiomyopathy will be used to describe heart muscle disease unexplained by abnormal loading conditions (hypertension, valve disease, etc.), congenital cardiac abnormalities, and ischaemic heart disease. Heart muscle disease associated with systemic or extracardiac diseases are described in more detail in Chapter 16.7.3.

Hypertrophic cardiomyopathy

Definition

Hypertrophic cardiomyopathy (HCM) is defined clinically by the presence of increased myocardial thickness in the absence of loading conditions (hypertension, valve disease, etc.) sufficient to cause the observed degree of hypertrophy. Historically, ventricular thickening caused by systemic diseases such as amyloidosis and glycogen-storage disease has been excluded from the definition in order to separate conditions in which there is myocyte hypertrophy from those in which left ventricular mass and wall thickness are increased by interstitial infiltration or intracellular accumulation of metabolic substrates. In everyday clinical practice, however, it is frequently impossible to differentiate these two entities using noninvasive imaging, and hence metabolic and infiltrative disease should be considered in the differential diagnosis of hypertrophic cardiomyopathy.

Causes

Pedigree analysis reveals familial disease in 40 to 50% of patients, but when cardiovascular evaluation of first-degree relatives using electrocardiography and echocardiography is performed, 90% of patients have familial disease. In most cases, the inheritance is autosomal dominant.

Approximately 60% of patients with familial hypertrophic cardiomyopathy have mutations in genes encoding proteins of the cardiac sarcomere: specifically cardiac β-myosin heavy chain, cardiac myosin-binding protein C, essential and regulatory myosin light chain, α-tropomyosin, cardiac troponin T and I, cardiac actin, titin, and α-myosin. Most mutations involve a single base-pair change in exons encoding highly conserved regions that result in amino acid substitutions. *De novo* mutations occur, but appear to account for less than 10% of cases.

Variable expression and incomplete penetrance is common, even within families bearing the same gene defect, but some phenotypes do seem to associate with particular mutations. β-Myosin heavy chain mutations that are fully penetrant are associated with worse prognosis (such as Arg403Glu or Arg453Cys), while disease complications are uncommon in patients with mutations that cause mild or no clinical expression (such as Leu908Val). This contrasts with troponin T disease, which although associated with mild hypertrophy and few symptoms can still cause premature sudden death. Mutations in myosin-binding protein C cause 20 to 30% of disease; most are major deletions rather than single base-pair changes. Disease expression can occur later in life, sometimes associated with mild hypertension. Once disease expression occurs (abnormal ECG and/or echocardiogram), patients are at the same risk from symptoms and disease-related complications as patients with disease onset in early life. The expression of disease in patients with troponin I mutations is variable; such mutations may cause restrictive physiology in the absence of severe hypertrophy and may mimic restrictive cardiomyopathy.

Clinical presentation with left ventricular hypertrophy under the age of 3 years is usually caused by metabolic or mitochondrial disorders (Table 16.7.2.1) and is uncommon in autosomal dominant hypertrophic cardiomyopathy.

Pathology

Hypertrophic cardiomyopathy may involve the left or both ventricles (Fig. 16.7.2.1). Hypertrophy in the left ventricle is usually asymmetric, involving the anterior and posterior septum and the free wall to a greater extent than the posterior wall. Right ventricular hypertrophy, which is usually symmetric, is seen in up to 30% of patients; isolated right ventricular hypertrophy (in the absence of pulmonary hypertension or right ventricular outflow obstruction) has not been reported. Many patients have structural abnormalities of the mitral valve, including increased leaflet area and length, and malposition or anomalous insertion of the papillary muscles. A common macroscopic finding is a patch of endocardial

Table 16.7.2.1 Causes of left ventricular hypertrophy at age 3 years or less

Metabolic*	Pompe's disease (GSD II)
	Forbes' disease (GSD III)
	Total lipodystrophy
	Hurler's syndrome
	Infant of a diabetic mother
Hypertrophic cardiomyopathy with associated syndromes	Noonan's syndrome
	LEOPARD syndrome
	Friedreich's ataxia
	Beckwith–Wiedemann syndrome
	Mitochondrial myopathy
	MELAS
	MERFF
	NADH–coenzyme Q reductase deficiency
	Cytochrome *b* deficiency
Miscellaneous causes	Hypertension
	In utero ritodrine HCl exposure
	Swyer's syndrome (46, XY pure gonadal dysgenesis)

* The main metabolic causes of left ventricular hypertrophy.
GSD, glycogen storage disorder; MELAS, myopathy, encephalopathy, lactic acidosis, stroke-like episodes; MERFF, myoclonic epilepsy and ragged red fibres.

thickening just below the aortic valve, which results from contact of the septum with the anterior mitral leaflet in patients with dynamic left ventricular outflow-tract obstruction.

The histological findings in hypertrophic cardiomyopathy are distinctive and provide the basis for the pathological diagnosis. Affected myocardium shows interstitial fibrosis with gross disorganization of the muscle bundles resulting in a characteristic whorled pattern. The cell-to-cell orientation of muscle cells is lost (disarray) and there is disorganization of the myofibrillar architecture within cells. Myocardial cells are broad, short, and often bizarre in shape. Foci of disorganized cells are often interspersed among areas of hypertrophied muscle cells that are otherwise normal in appearance. Such changes are not completely specific: small amounts of myofibre disarray may be seen in congenitally abnormal hearts and in secondary left ventricular hypertrophy; disarray is also present at the junction of the septum with the anterior and posterior walls of the left ventricle in normal subjects. However, the extent of myocyte disarray in normal subjects rarely exceeds 5%, while in hypertrophic cardiomyopathy up to 40% of the myocardium may be involved. As well as contributing to diastolic and systolic dysfunction, the disorganized myocardial architecture provides a substrate for electrical instability.

Pathophysiology

Diastolic dysfunction

Diastolic abnormalities caused by myocardial hypertrophy, myocardial ischaemia, myocyte disarray, and fibrosis are common but variable in severity. Typically, left ventricular end-diastolic pressure and atrial pressures are elevated as a consequence of abnormal left ventricular diastolic filling and reduced compliance. The isovolumic

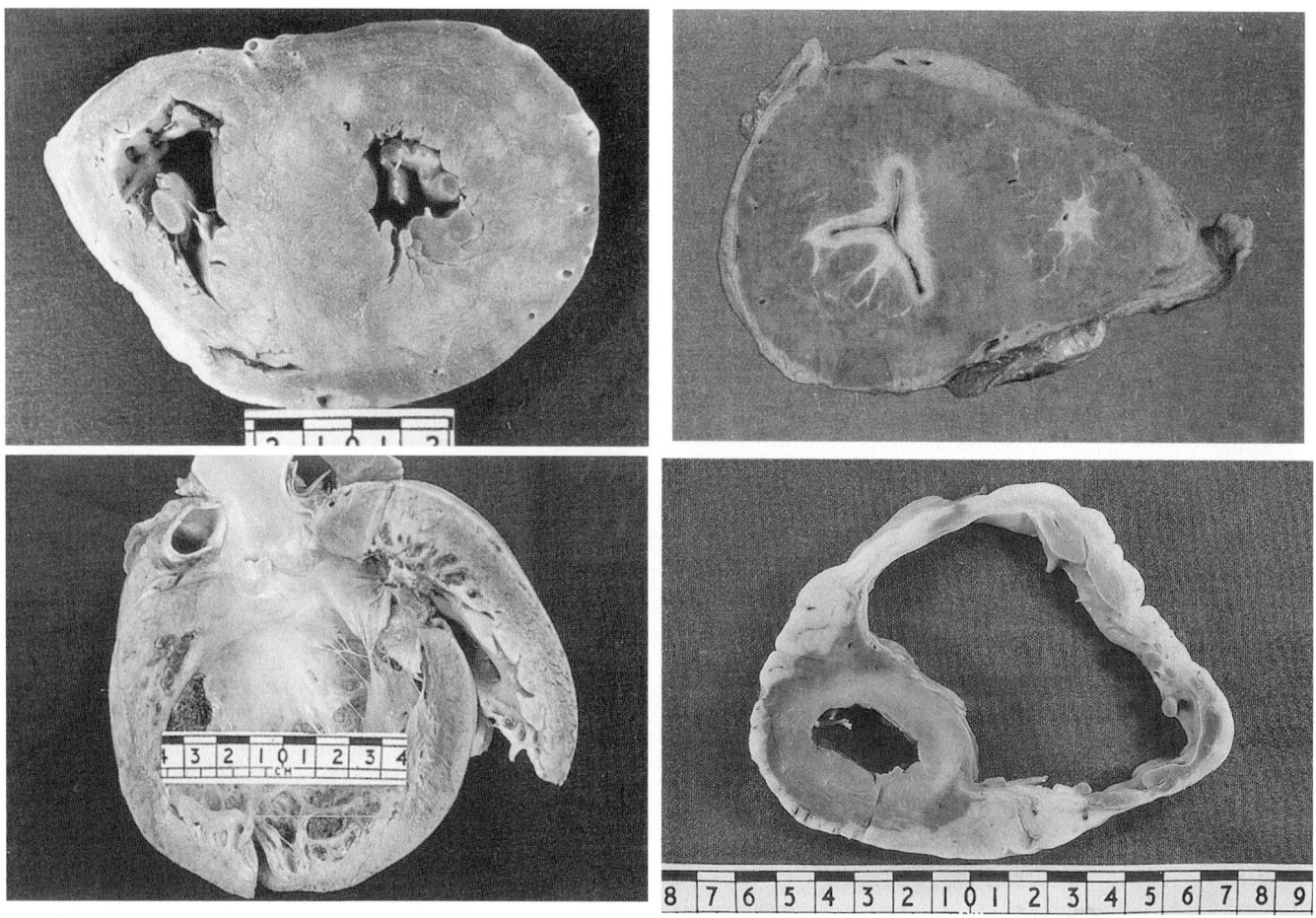

Fig. 16.7.2.1 Transverse short-axis section through the ventricles from patients with cardiomyopathy. Upper left shows symmetrical left ventricular hypertrophy in hypertrophic cardiomyopathy. Upper right shows dense white fibrous tissue obliterating the apex of both ventricles in endomyocardial fibrosis. Lower left shows a globular, dilated left ventricle in a child with dilated cardiomyopathy. Lower right shows a grossly dilated right ventricle with adipose infiltration of the right ventricular free wall in arrhythmogenic right ventricular dysplasia.
Davies MJ, 1986, Colour atlas of cardiovascular pathology, Oxford University Press.

relaxation time is prolonged, left ventricular filling is slow, and the proportion of filling volume that results from atrial systolic contraction (while still preserved) may be increased. Occasionally, there is rapid early filling with restrictive physiology similar to that seen in constrictive pericarditis or endocardial fibrosis (see Chapter 16.8).

Systolic function and dynamic outflow-tract obstruction

Most patients with hypertrophic cardiomyopathy have rapid and near-complete ventricular emptying resulting in an increase in measured ejection fraction. 'Endstage' hypertrophic cardiomyopathy—characterized by severe impairment of contractile performance, restrictive left ventricular physiology, and heart-failure symptoms—can develop at any age including childhood and adolescence, but, in most, the time from onset of symptoms to diagnosis of severe systolic impairment is long (a mean of 14 years).

Approximately 30% of patients have a gradient between the body and outflow tract of the left ventricle at rest; an additional 20 to 25% develop such a gradient following manoeuvres that increase myocardial contractility or that reduce ventricular afterload or venous return. The presence and magnitude of a gradient is determined by left ventricular outflow-tract size and geometry, which are in turn a function of the severity of septal hypertrophy, mitral leaflet morphology, and papillary muscle size and position.

The conventionally accepted mechanism of the gradient is that Venturi forces from increased ejection velocity in the narrowed outflow tract draw the anterior and/or posterior mitral leaflets towards the septum. More recent data suggest that the abnormally positioned mitral valve leaflets are 'driven' into the septum.

Myocardial ischaemia

Patients with hypertrophic cardiomyopathy have reduced coronary flow reserve and evidence for myocardial ischaemia during rapid atrial pacing and pharmacological stress. Myocardial ischaemia is almost certainly a major cause of exertional symptoms and may be a trigger for ventricular arrhythmia. However, detection of ischaemia in everyday clinical practice is challenging because conventional markers of ischaemia such as ST-segment change and reversible perfusion abnormalities on single photon emission computed tomography (SPECT) imaging correlate poorly with more objective biochemical markers of ischaemia.

Diagnosis

Left ventricular hypertrophy in the absence of moderate to severe hypertension and valve disease occurs in about 1 in 500 adults. The population frequency of unexplained left ventricular hypertrophy in children is unknown, but the annual incidence of left ventricular hypertrophy ranges between 0·3 and 0·5 per 100 000. The diagnosis of hypertrophic cardiomyopathy is based upon the demonstration of unexplained myocardial hypertrophy, defined as a wall-thickness measurement exceeding two standard deviations for gender and age. In practice, in an adult of normal size the presence of a left ventricular myocardial segment of 1.5 cm or greater in thickness is diagnostic. Less stringent criteria should be applied to first-degree relatives of an unequivocally affected individual, where the probability of carrying the disease gene is 1 in 2 (Table 16.7.2.2).

Problems in diagnosis often arise in patients with moderate to severe hypertension. The determinants of the hypertrophic response in a patient with hypertension are unknown, but are partly influenced by racial origin, with a greater increase in left ventricular mass in African-Caribbean individuals. In general, however, hypertrophic cardiomyopathy should be suspected in any individual with hypertension and a wall thickness in excess of 1.5 cm, particularly if the ECG shows widespread repolarization abnormalities and there is evidence of good blood pressure control.

The physiological changes of athletic training can rarely mimic hypertrophic cardiomyopathy. Athletes who participate in events that combine both isometric and isotonic activities (e.g. rowing and cycling) have the greatest increases in left ventricular wall thickness. Pure strength training is associated with an increase in left ventricular mass and wall thickness relative to the left ventricular cavity size, but is rarely associated with an increase in absolute wall thickness (unless the athlete also uses anabolic steroids). A diagnosis of hypertrophic cardiomyopathy in an elite athlete is likely when left ventricular wall thickness exceeds 1.6 cm in males and 1.4 cm in females and when they are symptomatic or have a family history of hypertrophic cardiomyopathy and premature sudden death. In athletes, the ECG frequently displays voltage criteria for left ventricular hypertrophy, sinus bradycardia, and sinus arrhythmia. Marked repolarization abnormalities are rare in elite athletes and should always raise suspicion of myocardial disease. Echocardiographic features favouring hypertrophic cardiomyopathy include small left ventricular cavity dimensions, left atrial enlargement, left ventricular outflow gradients, and diastolic impairment.

Clinical features

History

Symptomatic presentation may be at any age with breathlessness on exertion, chest pain, palpitation, syncope, or sudden death. Hypertrophic cardiomyopathy is occasionally found at autopsy in a stillborn baby or presents during infancy with cardiac failure, which is usually fatal. In children and adolescents, the diagnosis is most often made during screening of siblings and offspring of affected family members. Paroxysmal symptoms or mild impairment of exercise tolerance are often present, but in the absence of a murmur may not prompt cardiac evaluation.

About 50% of adults present with symptoms; in the remainder the diagnosis is made during family screening or following the detection of an unsuspected abnormality on physical, electrocardiographic, or echocardiographic examination. Dyspnoea is common (>50%) as a consequence of elevated left atrial and pulmonary capillary wedge pressures resulting from impaired left ventricular relaxation and filling, and about 50% complain of chest pain, which is exertional, atypical, or both in similar proportions of patients. Atypical pain may have no obvious precipitant; more commonly it follows exercise- or anxiety-related tachycardia, when it persists for up to several hours after the stress has been removed without enzymatic evidence of myocardial damage. Syncopal episodes occur in 15 to 25%, but in only a few are there findings suggestive of an arrhythmia or evidence of overt conduction disease: in most patients, the mechanism cannot be determined. Patients rarely present with paroxysmal nocturnal dyspnoea, ascites, or peripheral oedema.

Physical examination

In most patients with hypertrophic cardiomyopathy the physical examination is unremarkable. There may be a rapid upstroke arterial pulse reflecting dynamic left ventricular emptying. In about one-third, the jugular venous pulse may demonstrate a prominent 'a' wave, reflecting diminished right ventricular compliance secondary to right ventricular hypertrophy. Many patients have a forceful left ventricular cardiac impulse, best appreciated on full-held expiration in the left lateral position, when there may be a palpable atrial beat reflecting forceful atrial systolic contraction that may or may not be associated with significant forward flow of blood.

The first and second heart sounds are usually normal, and—unless the patient is in atrial fibrillation—there is likely to be a loud

Table 16.7.2.2 Major and minor criteria for the diagnosis of hypertrophic cardiomyopathy in adult members of affected families. Criteria are fulfilled if (1) one major echocardiographic, or (2) two minor echocardiographic, or (3) one minor echocardiographic plus two minor electrocardiographic abnormalities are seen

Major criteria	Minor criteria
Echocardiography	
Left ventricular wall thickness ≥13 mm in the anterior septum or posterior wall or ≥15 mm in the posterior septum or free wall	Left ventricular wall thickness of 12 mm in the anterior septum or posterior wall or of 14 mm in the posterior septum or free wall
Severe SAM (septal–leaflet contact)	Moderate SAM (no septal–leaflet contact)
	Redundant mitral valve leaflets
Electrocardiography	
Left ventricular hypertrophy + repolarization changes (Romhilt and Estes)	Complete bundle branch block or (minor) interventricular conduction defect (in LV leads)
T-wave inversion in leads I and aVL (≥3 mm) (with QRS–T-wave axis difference ≥30°), V3–V6 (≥3 mm) or II and III and aVF (≥5 mm)	Minor repolarization changes in LV leads
Abnormal Q (>40 ms or >25% R wave) in at least two leads from II, III, aVF (in absence of left anterior hemiblock), V1–V4; or I, aVL, V5–V6.	Deep S in V2 (>25 mm)
Clinical	
There are no clinical major criteria	Unexplained chest pain, dyspnoea, or syncope

LV, left ventricular; SAM, systolic anterior motion of the mitral valve.
Reproduced from *Heart*, McKenna WJ et al, 77:130–2. Copyright 1997, with permission from BMJ Publishing Group Ltd.

fourth heart sound, reflecting increased atrial systolic flow into a non-compliant ventricle. However, in those patients (20–30%) who have a resting left ventricular outflow-tract gradient, the most obvious physical sign is an ejection systolic murmur. This murmur starts well after the first heart sound and ends well before the second. It is best heard at the left sternal border, radiating towards the aortic and mitral areas, but not into the neck or the axilla. The intensity varies with changes in ventricular volume; it can be increased by physiological and pharmacological manoeuvres that decrease afterload or venous return (amyl nitrate, standing, Valsalva, etc.), and decreased by manoeuvres that increase afterload and venous return (squatting, phenylephrine, etc.). Occasionally there is an ejection sound at the onset of the systolic murmur.

Most patients with a left ventricular gradient also have mitral regurgitation, which may be difficult to distinguish by auscultation. Doppler examination reveals that mitral regurgitation usually begins just before (30–40 ms) the onset of the gradient and continues for the duration of systole. Radiation of the systolic murmur to the axilla is often the best auscultatory clue to the presence of coexistent mitral regurgitation, which may be moderate to severe, either alone or in association with a left ventricular outflow-tract gradient. A mid-diastolic rumble may sometimes result from increased transmitral flow in patients with severe mitral regurgitation.

Early diastolic murmurs of aortic incompetence may develop following surgical myotomy/myectomy or infective endocarditis involving the aortic valve. Although such murmurs are rare in the absence of such complications, they appear to occur more commonly than would be expected by chance and may reflect traction on the non-coronary cusp of the aortic valve by the septum. An ejection systolic murmur in the pulmonary area, reflecting right ventricular outflow-tract obstruction, is also rare; when present, it is usually associated with severe biventricular hypertrophy in the young or in those with coexistent Noonan's syndrome and a dysplastic pulmonary valve (see Chapter 16.12).

Prognosis

Patients with hypertrophic cardiomyopathy experience slow progression of symptoms and gradual deterioration of left ventricular function, and are at risk of sudden cardiac death throughout life. Annual mortality rates are in the range of 1 to 2%, but the risk of death and other disease-related complications varies between individuals and within individuals during the course of the disease.

Severe heart failure symptoms may develop in association with progressive myocardial wall thinning caused by myocardial fibrosis and severe reduction in left ventricular systolic performance and/or diastolic filling. Patients who experience such deterioration occasionally present with a clinical picture resembling restrictive cardiomyopathy, with grossly enlarged atria, signs of right heart failure, and relative preservation of left ventricular systolic performance. The development of systolic failure is associated with a poor prognosis, with rapid progression from onset to death or transplantation, and an overall mortality rate of up to 11% per year.

Atrial dilatation and the development of atrial fibrillation/flutter are important features in the clinical course, leading to a risk of embolic stroke as well as of acute or chronic cardiac deterioration. Early onset of atrial fibrillation was considered to be an ominous development, but is part of the evolution of patients with diastolic

dysfunction, and with appropriate management need not represent a major cause of morbidity or mortality.

Left ventricular hypertrophy develops during childhood and adolescence, but is not progressive in adults. The trigger and other determinants of disease expression in late-onset disease are uncertain.

Investigations

Cardiological evaluation of patients with hypertrophic cardiomyopathy is performed to confirm the diagnosis, to guide symptomatic therapy, and to assess the risk of complications, particularly that of sudden death.

Electrocardiography

The 12-lead ECG is the most sensitive diagnostic test, although occasionally normal (*c*.5%), particularly in the young. Five to ten per cent of patients are in atrial fibrillation at the time of diagnosis. Many have an intraventricular conduction delay and 20% have left-axis deviation, but complete right bundle or left bundle branch block is uncommon (c.5%). The latter may develop following surgery and is occasionally seen in elderly patients. ST-segment depression and T-wave changes are the most common abnormalities and are usually associated with voltage changes of left ventricular hypertrophy and/or deep S waves in the anterior chest leads V1 to V3. Isolated repolarization changes or giant negative T waves are occasionally seen. Voltage criteria for left ventricular hypertrophy are rare in the absence of repolarization changes. About 20% of patients have abnormal Q waves, either inferiorly (II, III, and aVF), or less commonly in leads V1 to V3. P-wave abnormalities of left and/or right atrial overload are common. The distribution of the PR interval is similar to that in the normal population, but occasionally a short PR interval may be associated with a slurred upstroke to the QRS complex, similar to that seen in the Wolff–Parkinson–White syndrome. At electrophysiological study, such changes are not usually associated with evidence of pre-excitation, although patients with hypertrophic cardiomyopathy and accessory pathways have been described. Despite the many electrocardiographic abnormalities, there is no ECG that is typical of hypertrophic cardiomyopathy; a useful rule is to consider the diagnosis whenever the ECG is bizarre, particularly in younger patients.

The incidence of arrhythmias during 48-h ambulatory electrocardiographic monitoring increases with age. Non-sustained ventricular tachycardia is detected in 20 to 25% of adults and, although usually asymptomatic, is associated with an increased risk of sudden death. Supraventricular arrhythmias are also common in adults: these are poorly tolerated if sustained (>30 s)—unless the ventricular response is controlled—and they carry an increased risk of thromboembolism. By contrast, most children and adolescents are in sinus rhythm, and arrhythmias during ambulatory electrocardiographic monitoring are uncommon. The increased incidence of supraventricular arrhythmias with age is not surprising: their development is related to increased left atrial dimensions and increased left ventricular diastolic pressure, both of which increase with age. The aetiology of ventricular arrhythmias is not known, but may relate to myocyte loss and myocardial fibrosis. Documented sustained ventricular tachycardia is uncommon, but is a recognized complication in patients with an apical out-pouching or aneurysm, which may develop as a consequence of midventricular obstruction.

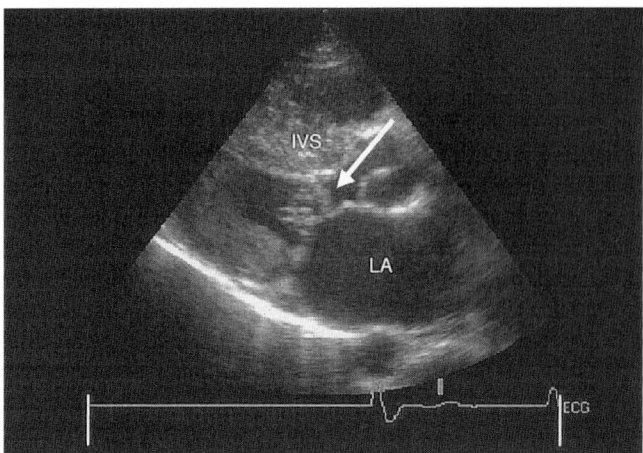

Fig. 16.7.2.2 An echocardiogram (parasternal long-axis view) of a patient with hypertrophic obstructive cardiomyopathy demonstrating hypertrophy of the interventricular septum (IVS), enlargement of the left atrium (LA), and systolic anterior motion of the mitral valve, bringing it into contact with the septum (arrow).

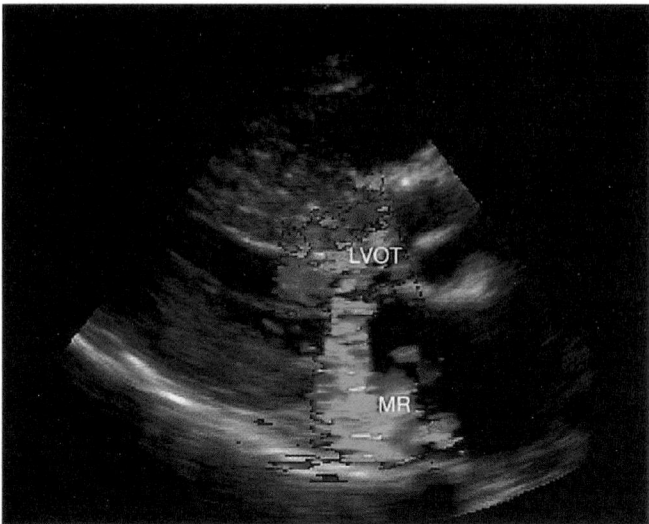

Fig. 16.7.2.3 Colour flow Doppler image (parasternal long-axis view) of the same patient as shown in Fig. 16.7.2.2, demonstrating left ventricular outflow tract (LVOT) turbulence and mitral regurgitation (MR) with a posteriorly directed jet.

Chest radiography

The chest radiograph may be normal or show evidence of left and/ or right atrial or left ventricular enlargement; if left atrial pressure has been chronically elevated, there may be evidence of redistribution of blood flow to upper lung zones. Mitral valve annular calcification is seen, particularly in elderly patients.

Echocardiography

Left ventricular hypertrophy may be symmetric or asymmetric and localized to the septum or the free wall, but most commonly to both the septum and free wall with relative sparing of the posterior wall (Fig. 16.7.2.2). Isolated apical hypertrophic cardiomyopathy appears to be common in Japan, but is rare in the West, although about 10% of patients have left ventricular hypertrophy that is maximal in the distal ventricle from the level of the papillary muscles down to the apex. Approximately one-third of patients also have hypertrophy of the right ventricular free wall, the presence and severity of which is strongly related to the severity of left ventricular hypertrophy. Typically, left ventricular end-systolic and end-diastolic dimensions are reduced, and the left atrial dimension is increased. Indices of systolic function such as ejection fraction may be increased, but systolic function is often impaired, which may be best appreciated by measurement of long-axis rather than short-axis function.

Colour Doppler provides a sensitive method of detecting left ventricular outflow-tract turbulence (Fig. 16.7.2.3), and when combined with continuous-wave Doppler the peak velocity (V_{max}) of left ventricular blood flow can be measured and left ventricular outflow-tract gradients calculated. Doppler gradients (pressure gradient (mmHg) = $4V_{max}^2$) are seen in 20 to 30% of patients and correlate well with those measured invasively. Systolic anterior motion of the mitral valve is usually present when the calculated outflow tract gradient is more than 30 mmHg, and early closure or fluttering of the aortic valve leaflets is often seen in association with such motion. A posteriorly directed mitral regurgitant jet is seen in association with and related to the magnitude of the outflow-tract gradient (Fig. 16.7.2.3). An anterior regurgitant jet or mitral regurgitation in the absence of obstruction suggests the coexistence of structural mitral valve abnormalities.

Other imaging techniques

Good-quality echocardiography suffices for diagnostic and therapeutic purposes in most patients with hypertrophic cardiomyopathy, but MRI is useful in selected cases to assess right ventricular, apical, and lateral left ventricular involvement. Gadolinium-enhanced cardiac MRI permits detection of myocardial fibrosis, the extent of which may predict evolution to the burnt-out phase and risk of sudden death.

Cardiac catheterization

Two-dimensional echo/Doppler evaluation has replaced invasive haemodynamic measurements and angiography as the method of assessing left ventricular structure and function in hypertrophic cardiomyopathy. Cardiac catheterization is not necessary for diagnosis and is rarely indicated unless symptoms are refractory and direct measurement of cardiac pressures is potentially informative, particularly in assessing the severity of mitral regurgitation. Coronary arteriography may be necessary to exclude coexistent coronary artery disease in older patients who have significant angina or ST-segment changes during exercise. The left coronary arteries are usually large in calibre. The left anterior descending and septal perforator arteries may demonstrate narrowing during systole in the absence of fixed obstructive lesions, but such changes do not appear to relate to symptoms. Left ventricular angiography is rarely indicated, but recognition of the abnormally shaped ventricle, which typically ejects at least 75% of its contents in association with mild mitral regurgitation, may provide a valuable diagnostic clue when hypertrophic cardiomyopathy was not suspected before catheterization.

Exercise testing

Maximal exercise testing in association with respiratory gas analysis provides useful functional and prognostic information, which can be monitored serially. Oxygen consumption at peak exercise (peak V_{O_2}) is usually moderately reduced, even in patients who claim their exercise tolerance is not limited. Continuous measurement of the blood pressure during upright treadmill or bicycle exercise reveals that about one-third of younger patients (<40 years) have an abnormal blood pressure response, with either a drop of more than 10 mmHg from peak recordings or a failure to rise by 20 mmHg or more despite an appropriate increase in cardiac output. Such changes are usually asymptomatic but are associated with an increased risk of sudden death. The mechanism of the hypotensive response during exercise in hypertrophic cardiomyopathy is uncertain, but may relate to myocardial mechanoreceptor activation and altered baroreflex control causing inappropriate drops in systemic vasculature resistance and to a poor cardiac output response. ST-segment depression of 2 mm from baseline is documented in 25% of patients, but appears not to be of prognostic significance.

Electrophysiological studies

Electrophysiological studies may occasionally be necessary in patients with sustained, rapid palpitation to identify associated accessory pathways or aid management of sustained monomorphic ventricular tachycardia. Conventional, programmed ventricular stimulation does not aid the identification of high-risk patients (see below).

Tests for specific causes of hypertrophic cardiomyopathy

A number of clinical features that suggest particular causes of hypertrophic cardiomyopathy are listed in Table 16.7.2.3; the presence of such clues should trigger appropriate biochemical and genetic testing.

Management

Screening and follow-up of asymptomatic patients

It is now possible to offer relatively rapid genetic testing to individuals with unequivocal disease. If a disease-causing mutation is identified, relatives can be offered predictive testing, but this should only be performed after appropriate genetic counselling.

Table 16.7.2.3 Clinical features suggesting the aetiology of HCM

Clinical feature	Examples
Symptoms	Acroparaesthesiae, tinnitus, deafness (Anderson–Fabry disease). Skeletal muscle weakness (desminopathy, mitochondrial cytopathy, etc.)
Physical examination	Retinitis pigmentosa (mitochondrial, Danon disease, etc.) Postural hypotension (amyloid) Angiokeratoma (Anderson–Fabry disease) Lentigines (LEOPARD syndrome) Facial morphology (Noonan, Anderson–Fabry disease, etc.)
Electrocardiogram	Pre-excitation/premature conduction disease (AMP kinase) Low-voltage/infarct pattern (amyloid)
Echocardiography	Concentric/biventricular hypertrophy (infiltrative, metabolic disease, etc.) Valve thickening (Anderson–Fabry disease, amyloid, etc.)
Family history	X-linked inheritance (Anderson–Fabry disease, Danon, etc.) Diabetes, epilepsy, and deafness (mitochondrial)
Biochemistry	Creatine kinase (Glycogen storage disease, mitochondrial, etc.) Lactate (mitochondrial) Renal dysfunction (Anderson–Fabry disease, mitochondrial, etc.) Paraproteinaemia (amyloid)
Exercise testing	Severe premature acidosis (mitochondrial)

In children and adolescents with a sarcomeric protein-gene mutation, ECG and echocardiographic manifestations of myocardial hypertrophy often develop during or following growth spurts. For this reason, young people should be assessed annually during adolescence. In adults, *de novo* development of unexplained left ventricular hypertrophy is less common, but does occur, particularly in patients with myosin-binding protein C gene mutations. Asymptomatic normal adults with a family history of hypertrophic cardiomyopathy but no identifiable mutation should be offered rescreening every 5 years, or sooner should they develop symptoms.

Pharmacological

The goal of therapy is to improve symptoms and prevent complications, in particular sudden death. β-Adrenoceptor blockers, particularly propanolol, and calcium antagonists, especially verapamil, are the mainstay of symptomatic pharmacological therapy. Both drugs have several potentially beneficial actions, including a decrease in myocardial oxygen consumption and blunting of the heart rate response during exercise, thereby increasing time for filling. Both agents exert a negative inotropic effect, thereby reducing hyperdynamic systolic function and left ventricular gradients, and they may improve diastolic function, verapamil by improving relaxation and β-blockers by increasing compliance. The side effects of propranolol are rarely serious, but the suppressant effect of verapamil on atrioventricular nodal conduction may cause problems in patients with unsuspected pre-existing conduction disease, and its vasodilatory and negative inotropic effects can result in acute pulmonary oedema and death in very symptomatic patients with severe obstruction and pulmonary hypertension.

Endocarditis is a rare complication of hypertrophic cardiomyopathy, occurring predominantly in patients with left ventricular outflow tract turbulence and/or mitral regurgitation. Antibiotic prophylaxis should be recommended in any patient with an outflow tract gradient or intrinsic valve disease.

Surgical

Surgery is a therapeutic option in patients with obstruction and/or mitral valve abnormalities. The conventional indication for surgery has been a resting left ventricular outflow tract gradient of more than 50 mmHg in patients refractory to medical therapy, and the commonest operation has been to remove a segment of the upper anterior septum (myotomy/myectomy) via a transaortic approach. Transventricular approaches have been used, but these are associated with a higher incidence of late complications, particularly of cardiac failure. Mitral valve repair and papillary muscle remodelling may be required, and mitral valve replacement has also been advocated; excellent results have been achieved, particularly in elderly patients with severe mitral regurgitation. Specialist hypertrophic cardiomyopathy centres report perioperative mortality of 1% or less, with 90% success in abolishing gradients and improving symptoms.

Alcohol septal ablation

Injection of alcohol into the septal artery that supplies the 'obstructing' septal muscle has been developed as a percutaneous, nonpharmacological approach to gradient reduction. Most experienced centres have reported symptomatic improvement in 70% of patients. As for surgery and dual-chamber (DDD) pacing (see below), patient selection—in particular, regarding the mechanism of the gradient—and technical considerations are important determinants of outcome. The major complication has been the need for a pacemaker in up to 30%, and concerns remain about long-term left ventricular function and arrhythmia risk. At present, alcohol septal ablation offers a therapeutic option in older patients with suitable anatomy who are refractory to drugs.

Pacing

Alteration of the ventricular activation sequence by pacing the right ventricular apex may result in reduction of gradients and filling pressures and improved symptoms in selected patients. The role of atrioventricular synchronous pacing (DDD pacing) in symptomatic management of obstruction has been evaluated in two randomized multicentre trials, demonstrating symptomatic improvement and gradient reduction (50%), but no change in exercise capacity. However, the placebo effect of the procedure was considerable: 40% reported significant symptomatic improvement with the pacemaker programmed to a standby mode. Nevertheless, pacing offers a therapeutic option in patients with obstruction that is refractory to drug treatment, and in whom surgery is either not acceptable or inappropriate. It appears that elderly patients with localized septal hypertrophy and without significant free wall involvement or mitral regurgitation may do particularly well.

Clinical approach to individual symptoms

Dyspnoea

Dyspnoea most often occurs in patients who also experience chest pain or discomfort. Treatment depends on the predominant mechanism. In patients with dyspnoea who have slow filling that continues throughout diastole, β-blockers and verapamil are appropriate. Conversely, those with rapid, early filling may benefit from a relative tachycardia and do better without negative chronotrophic agents. When dyspnoea is associated with significant obstruction—meaning at least 50% of stroke volume remaining in the left ventricle at the onset of the gradient—β-blockers, disopyramide, and (failing these) myotomy/myectomy or the other nonpharmacological options may be beneficial. Disopyramide should be used in the maximum tolerated dose (anticholinergic side effects may limit higher doses) in conjunction with a conventional β-blocker. Occasionally, dyspnoea is associated with severe mitral regurgitation and responds well to mitral valve replacement.

Chest pain

Exertional chest pain usually responds to therapy with propranolol or verapamil, and when refractory can respond to very high doses of these agents (propranolol at 480 mg daily, verapamil at 720 mg daily). Short-acting nitrates, diuretics, and high-dose verapamil may be useful in selected patients, perhaps by reducing filling pressures and improving coronary flow to subendocardial layers. Atypical chest pain may persist long after the initial stimulus has been removed.

Arrhythmia

Arrhythmias are a common complication of hypertrophic cardiomyopathy. Treatment with anticoagulants and verapamil or β-blockers is appropriate once atrial fibrillation is established, the aims being to control the ventricular response and prevent emboli. Most patients who develop atrial fibrillation during electrocardiographic monitoring are unaware of changes from sinus rhythm to atrial fibrillation as long as the ventricular response is well controlled. However, in a few cases the loss of atrial systolic contribution to

filling volume is important, when electrical cardioversion can be facilitated by prior therapy (4–6 weeks) with amiodarone (300 mg daily) if pharmacological cardioversion does not occur first.

Sustained (>30 s) episodes of paroxysmal atrial fibrillation or supraventricular tachycardia can cause haemodynamic collapse and systemic emboli. Low-dose amiodarone (1000–1400 mg weekly) is effective in suppressing such episodes and also provides control of the ventricular response should breakthrough occur. If episodes persist, the threshold for anticoagulation should be low as embolic complications are common, even when atrial dimensions are only moderately increased.

Nonsustained episodes of supraventricular arrhythmia are common, and although often asymptomatic they are a marker (albeit of low positive predictive accuracy) for the subsequent development of established atrial fibrillation. The threshold to introduce amiodarone, with or without anticoagulation, should be low if they occur in the presence of atrial enlargement. Episodes of nonsustained ventricular tachycardia are common but are rarely symptomatic: therapy is warranted only if it can be shown to improve prognosis (see below).

Prevention of sudden death

Sudden death is a consequence of multiple interacting mechanisms. The histological abnormalities—particularly myocyte disarray, small vessel disease, and replacement scarring—contribute to the underlying substrate. Events may be triggered by haemodynamic alterations, myocardial ischaemia, and arrhythmias, including ventricular tachycardia, atrial fibrillation, atrioventricular block, and rapid conduction of a supraventricular arrhythmia via an accessory pathway. Intense physical exertion may also contribute to the above triggers. The interaction of triggers and substrate may be modified by inappropriate peripheral vascular responses and the development of myocardial ischaemia.

Risk stratification

Prevention of sudden death relies on risk factor stratification to identify a high-risk cohort. Several adverse features that can be elicited from the clinical history and noninvasive evaluation have been identified (Box 16.7.2.1). Their relative importance varies with age; for example, the finding of nonsustained ventricular tachycardia on 24-h electrocardiographic monitoring in children and adolescents is uncommon (<5%), but is associated with an eightfold increased risk of sudden death, whereas in adults this

---

Box 16.7.2.1 Risk factors for sudden death

- Family history of sudden death (≥2 premature (<40 years) sudden deaths)
- Unexplained syncope within previous year
- Abnormal exercise blood pressure
- Nonsustained ventricular tachycardia (≥3 beats at ≥120 beats/min)
- Severe left ventricular hypertrophy (>3 cm)
- Severe left ventricular outflow tract obstruction (>90 mmHg)
- Cardiac arrest (or sustained ventricular tachycardia)

arrhythmia is common (20–25%), but in isolation confers only a twofold increased risk.

In young people (<25 years) the finding of nonsustained ventricular tachycardia, severe and extensive left ventricular hypertrophy, unexplained syncope (particularly if recurrent or exertional), or a family history where a high proportion of affected individuals experienced premature (<40 years) sudden death warrants prophylactic treatment. Such patients usually also exhibit abnormal blood pressure responses to exercise; indeed, the finding of a normal exercise blood pressure response appears to identify the low-risk younger (<40 years) patient (negative predictive accuracy 97%), allowing appropriate reassurance that is also clinically important. In adults aged 25 to 60 years, the positive predictive accuracy for each of the risk factors is much lower (15–20%): in general, prophylactic treatment is reserved for those with two or more risk factors who will have a predicted risk of sudden death of at least 3% per year.

It is important to consider risk in all patients, even those who are asymptomatic or who have mild echocardiographic features of hypertrophic cardiomyopathy. Although children and adolescents with severe congestive symptoms may be at greater risk, the data reveals that the severity of chest pain, dyspnoea, and exercise limitation are not reliable predictors of the risk of sudden death in adults. In addition, it is recognized that most patients who die suddenly have mild (1.5–2.0 cm) or moderate (2.0–2.5 cm) left ventricular hypertrophy, while some genetic defects (e.g. cardiac troponin T) may cause sudden death in the absence of symptoms or hypertrophy.

The presence of a left ventricular outflow tract gradient is also associated with sudden death. The management of symptomatic patients should be focused on gradient reduction; in asymptomatic patients, severe left ventricular outflow tract obstruction should be considered in the overall risk profile of the patient. Diastolic impairment with abnormal Doppler filling patterns and atrial enlargement is associated with symptomatic limitation and poor prognosis, but not with premature sudden death.

Some investigators have suggested that the induction of sustained ventricular arrhythmias during programmed electrophysiological stimulation is associated with a higher risk of sudden death. However, the predictive accuracy is low, and as most high-risk patients can be identified using noninvasive clinical markers, the inherent risks and inconvenience associated with programmed stimulation dictate that it should not be used routinely to assess risk in hypertrophic cardiomyopathy.

Dilated cardiomyopathy

Definition

Dilated cardiomyopathy is a heart muscle disorder defined by dilatation and impaired systolic function of the left ventricle or both ventricles in the absence of coronary artery disease, valvular abnormalities, or pericardial disease. A number of different cardiac and systemic diseases are associated with left ventricular dilatation and impaired contractility (see Chapter 16.7.3). When no identifiable cause is found, the condition is referred to as idiopathic dilated cardiomyopathy.

Dilated cardiomyopathy has been described in Western, African, and Asian populations, affecting both genders and all ages. In North America and Europe, symptomatic dilated cardiomyopathy has an incidence and prevalence of 20 and 38 per 100 000, respectively, and is the commonest indication for cardiac transplantation.

Causes

Pedigree analysis reveals familial disease in at least 25% of cases; a further 10 to 20% of relatives have mild abnormalities of left ventricular performance that evolve into dilated cardiomyopathy in about one-third. Inheritance is usually autosomal dominant with incomplete penetrance, with a smaller number of families having X-linked transmission. Penetrance is age dependent and has been estimated to be 10% in those aged less than 20 years, 34% in young adults aged 20 to 30 years, 60% in adults aged 30 to 40 years, and 90% in those over 40 years. Guidelines for the diagnosis of familial disease based on the identification of major and minor criteria are shown in Box 16.7.2.2. The diagnosis of familial dilated cardiomyopathy is fulfilled in a first-degree relative of a proband in the presence of one major criterion, or left ventricular dilatation plus one minor criterion, or three minor criteria.

Disease-causing mutations are reported in numerous genes including dystrophin, taffazin (Barth's syndrome), metavinculin, cardiac actin (autosomal dominant), lamin A/C (associated with premature conduction disease), desmin, myosin-binding protein C, troponin T and C, β-myosin heavy chain, and Z-line associated protein (ZASP). Lamin A/C mutations also cause Emery–Dreifuss and limb-girdle muscular dystrophy and familial partial lipodystrophy; desmin may cause conduction disease with restrictive cardiomyopathy; dystrophin mutations cause childhood (Duchenne) and adult (Becker) forms of muscular dystrophy.

Different patterns of disease expression are recognized. Disease progression appears to be slow (over decades) in most cases, and conduction disturbance is a late complication related to disease severity. However, in some families (<20%), particularly those with mutations in the lamin A/C gene, the early stages are characterized by progressive conduction disease, and left ventricular

---

Box 16.7.2.2 Major and minor criteria for the diagnosis of familial dilated cardiomyopathy in adult members of affected families (see text for details)

Major criteria

- A reduced ejection fraction of the left ventricle (<45%) and/or fractional shortening (<25%) as assessed by echocardiography, radionuclide scanning, or angiography

- An increased left ventricular end-diastolic diameter corresponding to >117% of the predicted value corrected for age and body surface area

Minor criteria

- Unexplained supraventricular or ventricular arrhythmia

- Ventricular dilatation (>112% of the predicted value)

- An intermediate impairment of left ventricular dysfunction

- Conduction defects

- Segmental wall motion abnormalities in the absence of intraventricular conduction defect or ischaemic heart disease

- Unexplained sudden death of a first-degree relative or stroke before 50 years of age

dilatation and impairment are later manifestations, in the 4th to 6th decade. Families are also recognized in whom dilated cardiomyopathy develops in later decades in individuals who have had sensorineural hearing loss since childhood, or in association with skeletal myopathy (dystrophin gene mutations).

Pathology and pathophysiology

Macroscopic examination of hearts with dilated cardiomyopathy reveals dilated cardiac chambers (see Fig. 16.7.2.1), mural thrombi, and platelet aggregates with normal extra- and intramural coronary arteries. Myocardial mass is increased, but ventricular wall thickness is normal or reduced. Histology is nonspecific with patchy perimyocyte and interstitial fibrosis, various stages of myocyte death, as well as myocyte hypertrophy and often extensive myofibrillary loss, resulting in a vacuolated appearance of the myocytes. An interstitial T-lymphocyte infiltrate and focal accumulations of macrophages associated with individual myocyte death are common.

The identification of disease-causing mutations in genes encoding various components of the cardiac myocyte cystoskeletal and sarcomeric contractile apparatus shows that the pathogenesis of dilated cardiomyopathy is heterogeneous. Two models have been proposed to explain ventricular remodelling in dilated cardiomyopathy. In the 'final common pathway' hypothesis, dilated cardiomyopathy reflects a nonspecific degenerative state, which may result from a variety of stimuli, including genetic mutations, viral infections, toxins, and volume overload. The alternative hypothesis suggests that a number of distinct, independent, pathways can remodel the heart and cause dilated cardiomyopathy—in other words, the different causes of dilated cardiomyopathy share a common histopathology, but their molecular biology is distinct. The final common pathways resulting in dilated cardiomyopathy remain speculative, but may include altered myocyte energetics and calcium handling.

Clinical features

History

Initial presentation is usually with symptoms of cardiac failure (fatigue, breathlessness, decreased exercise tolerance, etc.), but arrhythmia (atrial fibrillation, ventricular tachycardia, atrioventricular block, etc.), systemic embolism, or the incidental finding of an electrocardiographic or radiographic abnormality during routine screening may prompt earlier diagnosis.

Physical examination

Physical examination may be entirely normal or may reveal evidence of myocardial dysfunction with cardiac enlargement and signs of congestive heart failure. Systolic blood pressure is usually low, with a narrow pulse pressure and a low-volume arterial pulse. Pulsus alternans may be present in patients with severe left ventricular failure, and the jugular veins may be distended, with a prominent V wave reflecting tricuspid regurgitation. In such patients, the liver is often engorged and pulsatile, and there is usually peripheral oedema and ascites. The precordium often reveals a diffuse and dyskinetic left (and occasionally right) ventricular impulse. The apex is usually displaced laterally, reflecting ventricular dilatation. The second heart sound is usually normally split, but paradoxical splitting may be present when there is left bundle branch block, which occurs is about 15% of patients. With severe disease and the development of pulmonary hypertension, the

pulmonary component of the second heart sound may be accentuated. Characteristically, a presystolic gallop or fourth heart sound is present before the development of overt cardiac failure. However, once cardiac decompensation has occurred, ventricular gallop or third heart sound is often present. When there is significant ventricular dilatation, systolic murmurs are common, reflecting mitral and (less commonly) tricuspid regurgitation.

The development of unexplained cardiac failure within the last month of pregnancy or 5 months postpartum is termed peripartum cardiomyopathy. There is usually uncertainty whether the cardiac failure is acute (e.g. potentially myocarditic) or chronic and exacerbated by the haemodynamic stress of pregnancy and labour (e.g. dilated cardiomyopathy). When the heart failure is acute and there is persistence of left ventricular chamber dilatation or impaired systolic performance, the diagnosis of peripartum cardiomyopathy can legitimately be made. The mechanism and true natural history is uncertain, though it is probable that the adverse prognostic effect of subsequent pregnancies is less important than the literature would suggest, particularly in those with only mild residual abnormalities of left ventricular structure and function. For further discussion of cardiac disease in pregnancy, see Chapter 14.6.

Prognosis

The prognosis of dilated cardiomyopathy is uncertain because the diagnosis is usually not made until clinical features, which are late manifestations of the disease, become obvious. Follow-up of asymptomatic first-degree relatives suggests that disease progression is insidious over decades. An upper respiratory tract infection or a salt or fluid load often precipitates clinical presentation. Symptoms develop when filling pressures rise or when stroke volume diminishes sufficiently to cause salt and water retention and oedema. Once clinical symptoms of impaired ventricular performance are apparent, prognosis is poor and related to the degree of left ventricular dilatation and impaired contractile performance. Data in adults and children in the 1970s and 1980s demonstrated 50% mortality from progressive heart failure or its complications in the 2 years following referral diagnosis. Survival has been substantially improved since then by early recognition of mild disease, and by modern management with angiotensin converting enzyme (ACE) inhibitors, β-blockade, aggressive treatment of arrhythmias, and cardiac transplantation. Estimated annual mortality is now 4%, predominantly from sudden death, even in those who improve or stabilize.

Arrhythmia

Atrial arrhythmias, particularly atrial fibrillation, are common and associated with the severity of symptoms, left ventricular dysfunction, and poor prognosis, but atrial fibrillation is not an independent predictor of disease progression or sudden death. Occasionally, however, persistent atrial tachycardia or atrial fibrillation may cause gradual deterioration in left ventricular function, resembling dilated cardiomyopathy ('tachycardiomyopathy'): systolic function usually returns to normal with control of the arrhythmia.

Ventricular arrhythmias are also common and like supraventricular arrhythmias are markers of disease severity. Nonsustained ventricular tachycardia during ECG monitoring is seen in about 20% of asymptomatic or mildly symptomatic patients and in up to 70% of those who are severely symptomatic. The prognostic significance of this arrhythmia is controversial: its presence early in the course of disease, when left ventricular function is relatively preserved, is probably an independent marker of sudden death risk, whereas in general markers of haemodynamic severity (such as ejection fraction, left ventricular end-diastolic dimension, or filling pressures) are more predictive of disease-related mortality and sudden death. Sudden-death risk in patients with severe disease (New York Heart Association, NYHA class III or IV) increases approximately threefold when syncope is present.

Investigation

Electrocardiography

The electrocardiographic features of dilated cardiomyopathy are nonspecific and highly variable. Sinus tachycardia is common (particularly in children and infants); nonspecific ST-segment and T-wave changes may be seen, most commonly in the inferior and lateral leads; and pathological Q waves may be present in the septal leads in patients with extensive left ventricular fibrosis. Atrial enlargement is common, and in advanced disease may be associated with bundle branch block. All degrees of atrioventricular block may also be seen and should raise the possibility of mutations in the lamin A/C gene if associated with relatively mild impairment of left ventricular function, or when present in a young patient.

Chest radiography

The chest radiograph is usually abnormal in patients with dilated cardiomyopathy, except in a rare subset of patients with acute viral myocarditis associated with left ventricular systolic impairment and preserved cavity dimensions. An increased cardiothoracic ratio (>0.5) is typically seen, reflecting left ventricular and left atrial dilatation. Increased pulmonary vascular markings and pleural effusions may be present in patients with elevated left ventricular filling pressures.

Echocardiography

Echocardiography is used to identify the presence of left ventricular cavity dilatation and systolic impairment, which are the typical features of the condition. In general, the presence of ventricular end-diastolic dimensions more than two standard deviations above body surface area-corrected mean values and fractional shortening less than 25% are sufficient to make the diagnosis (Fig. 16.7.2.4). Two-dimensional echocardiography is also used to determine whether intracavitary thrombus is present in the ventricles.

Colour flow Doppler may be used to determine the presence and quantify the severity of functional mitral (and/or tricuspid) regurgitation (Fig. 16.7.2.5). Pulsed wave and continuous wave Doppler can be used to estimate pulmonary artery pressures. Patients with dilated cardiomyopathy usually have abnormalities of diastolic left ventricular function in addition to systolic impairment: these can be assessed using mitral inflow, pulmonary vein, and tissue Doppler parameters.

Cardiac biomarkers

The serum creatine kinase should be measured in all patients with dilated cardiomyopathy because this simple test may provide an important clue to the aetiology of the condition (e.g. muscular dystrophy, lamin A/C defect, etc.). Other cardiac biomarkers, e.g. troponin I and troponin T, may also be elevated in dilated cardiomyopathy, particularly in association with an inflammatory cause. Plasma natriuretic peptide levels are elevated in chronic heart failure and predict mortality.

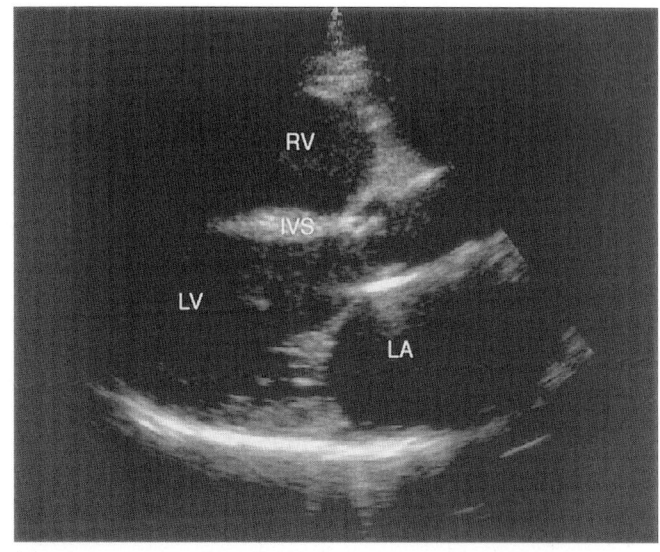

(a)

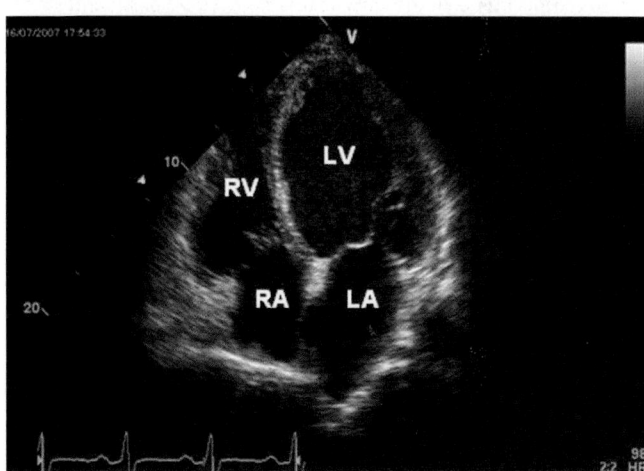

(b)

Fig. 16.7.2.4 Echocardiographic appearances of two patients with familial dilated cardiomyopathy. Panel A: parasternal long-axis view showing significant left atrial (LA) and biventricular dilatation with a thin intraventricular septum (IVS). Panel B: apical four-chamber view demonstrating a globular dilated left ventricle. LA, left atrium; LV, left ventricle; RA, right atrium; RV, right ventricle.

Many of the systemic diseases that are associated with heart muscle disorders have typical clinical, immunological, and biochemical features (see Chapter 16.7.3), and in the absence of clinical clues to suggest a systemic disease an exhaustive 'routine screen' is probably not cost effective. There are, however, several potential reversible secondary causes of heart muscle disorder that may simulate dilated cardiomyopathy, and basic screening tests should include serum phosphorus (hypophosphataemia), serum calcium (hypocalcaemia), serum creatinine and urea (uraemia), thyroid function tests (hypothyroidism), and serum iron/ferritin (haemochromatosis).

Exercise testing

Symptom-limited exercise testing (treadmill or bicycle) combined with respiratory gas analysis is a useful technique to assess functional limitation in patients with dilated cardiomyopathy and provides a means of objectively evaluating disease progression. The detection of respiratory markers of severe lacticacidaemia during metabolic

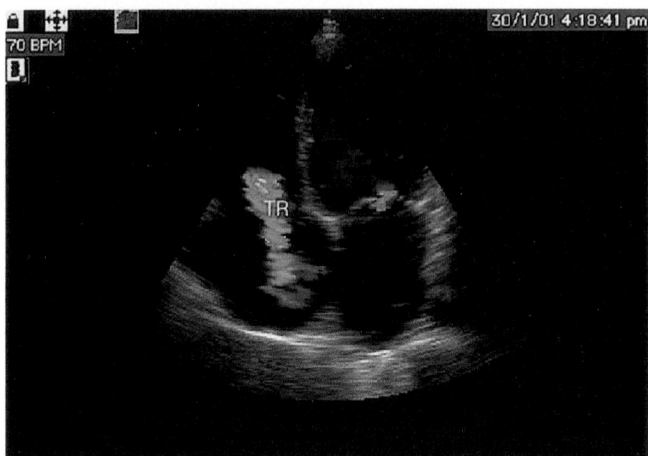

Fig. 16.7.2.5 Colour flow Doppler image of the same patient as shown in Fig. 16.7.2.4A demonstrating a regurgitant tricuspid jet (TR).

exercise testing may suggest a mitochondrial or other metabolic cause for dilated cardiomyopathy. Assessment of exercise capacity is essential in the assessment of patients prior to cardiac transplantation.

Cardiac catheterization

Cardiac catheterization is performed to exclude coronary artery disease as a cause of impaired systolic function. Haemodynamic assessment of left ventricular end-diastolic and pulmonary artery pressures is performed as part of cardiac-transplant work-up. Endomyocardial biopsy may be diagnostic for myocarditis and for some metabolic or mitochondrial disorders, but the diagnostic yield is low.

Cardiac MRI

Cardiac MRI may be a useful alternative imaging technique in patients with poor echocardiographic windows. In addition, the detection of fibrosis with gadolinium contrast enhancement may provide additional prognostic and diagnostic information.

Electrophysiological testing

Programmed electrical stimulation is of limited clinical value in the identification of high-risk patients. Polymorphic ventricular tachycardia is inducible in up to 30% of cases, but this is a nonspecific finding. Approximately 10% of patients have inducible sustained monomorphic ventricular tachycardia; about one-third of these die suddenly, but most (75%) who die in this way do not have inducible ventricular tachycardia during programmed stimulation. In some patients (as many as 40% in one series), ventricular tachycardia arises as the consequence of bundle branch re-entry. This tachycardia is typically rapid (mean cycle length 280 ms) and uses a macro re-entrant circuit that involves the His–Purkinje system, usually with right bundle branch anterograde conduction and left bundle branch retrograde conduction. Differentiation from myocardial ventricular tachycardia is confirmed by the presence of a His or right bundle branch potential preceding each QRS: diagnosis is important since catheter ablation of either the left or right bundle branch usually is curative.

Management

Management in dilated cardiomyopathy aims to improve symptoms, to attenuate disease progression, and prevent arrhythmia, stroke, and sudden death.

Pharmacological treatment

Symptomatic therapy is the treatment of heart failure with reliance on diuretics, ACE inhibitors, and β-blockers (see Chapter 16.5).

Diuretics

Loop and/or thiazide diuretics should be used in all patients with fluid retention to achieve a euvolaemic state, but they should never be used as monotherapy as they exacerbate neurohormonal activation, thereby worsening disease progression. The aldosterone antagonist, spironolactone, reduces the overall risk of death by 30% in adults with severe heart failure (NYHA class IV and ejection fraction <35%): side effects include hyperkalaemia (infrequent in the presence of normal renal function) and painful gynaecomastia.

ACE inhibitors and angiotensin receptor blockers

Activation of the renin–angiotensin–aldosterone system is central to the pathophysiology of heart failure, regardless of the underlying aetiology, and ACE inhibitors should be considered in all patients with dilated cardiomyopathy. Many clinical trials have shown that ACE inhibitors improve symptoms, reduce hospitalizations, and reduce cardiovascular mortality in adults with symptomatic heart failure, and reduce the rate of disease progression in asymptomatic patients. ACE inhibitors are usually well tolerated, the most common side effects being cough and symptomatic hypotension.

The angiotensin receptor blockers (ARBs) have similar haemodynamic effects to ACE inhibitors. Clinical trials in adults with heart failure have shown similar haemodynamic effects, efficacy, and safety to ACE inhibitors, such that ARBs are currently recommended in adults who are intolerant of ACE inhibitors. Combination treatment with ACE inhibitors and ARBs may be more beneficial at preventing ventricular remodelling than either drug alone, but with little additional benefit on overall survival.

β-Blockers

Excess sympathetic activity contributes to heart failure and numerous multicentre placebo-controlled trials—using carvedilol, metoprolol, and bisoprolol—have shown substantial reductions in mortality (both sudden death and death from progressive heart failure) in adults with NYHA class II and III heart-failure symptoms. β-Blockers are usually well tolerated, but side effects include bradycardia, hypotension, and fluid retention, and they are generally contraindicated in asthma. β-Blockers should be started at low doses and slowly up-titrated; they should not be started in patients with decompensated heart failure.

Digoxin

Digoxin improves symptoms in patients with heart failure, but no survival benefit has been demonstrated in large study cohorts. High serum digoxin levels may be associated with increased mortality in some patients. Digoxin should be used only in patients who remain symptomatic in spite of treatment with diuretics, ACE inhibitors, and β-blockers, or to control heart rate in patients with permanent atrial fibrillation.

Anticoagulation

The prevalence of intramural thrombi and systemic thromboembolism ranges between 3 and 50%, with an incidence between 1.5 and 3.5% per year. Anticoagulation with warfarin is, therefore, advised in patients in whom an intracardiac thrombus is identified echocardiographically, or those with a history of thromboembolism. There are no trial data to guide prophylactic anticoagulation in dilated cardiomyopathy, but patients with severe ventricular dilatation and moderate to severe systolic impairment may also benefit from warfarin therapy.

Treatment of arrhythmia in dilated cardiomyopathy

If sustained or symptomatic arrhythmias are documented during 24-h ECG monitoring or exercise testing, conventional treatment is warranted (see Chapter 16.4). Many commonly prescribed antiarrhythmic agents should be avoided or used with caution because of their negative inotropic and proarrhythmic effects. Data on amiodarone are contradictory, but the recent Sudden Cardiac Death in Heart Failure Trial (SCD-HeFT) showed that amiodarone had no beneficial effect on survival when compared with implantable cardioverter–defibrillators. It can, however, be used safely to prevent or treat atrial arrhythmias.

Nonpharmacological treatment

Permanent pacing can correct two important intracardiac conduction abnormalities. First, a small subset of patients who have marked PR interval prolongation (>220 ms), usually secondary to atrioventricular nodal disease, experience deleterious effects on left ventricular haemodynamics with reduction in diastolic ventricular filling time and the development of end-diastolic tricuspid and mitral regurgitation. Correction of PR interval prolongation with short atrioventricular delay dual-chamber pacing may increase stroke volume and blood pressure, thus decreasing mitral regurgitation with dramatic clinical improvement. Second, patients with marked intraventricular conduction delay (left bundle branch block >150 ms) have dyssynchronous contraction of the left ventricular free wall and interventricular septum (which may decrease ejection fraction) and late activation of the anterolateral papillary muscle (which may increase functional mitral regurgitation). Biventricular or left ventricular pacing with specialized leads via the coronary sinus can correct both problems and has been shown to improve symptoms and prognosis in randomized trials. In addition, the resultant increase in blood pressure and pacemaker maintenance of the desired minimum heart rate permits use of higher doses of β-blockade and ACE inhibition with potential secondary benefit.

Surgical removal of nonviable (Dor procedure) and/or viable myocardium (Batista procedure) to improve haemodynamics by reducing left ventricular volume has been advocated, but these and other surgical volume-reduction procedures (partial left ventriculotomy) probably have no role in dilated cardiomyopathy. Mitral valve repair may occasionally be helpful.

Cardiac transplantation may be appropriate in patients with progressive deterioration. In addition, improvements in left ventricular assist devices and artificial heart technology provide alternatives that are now reasonably seen as viable future treatment options. These issues are discussed in Chapter 16.5.2.

Restrictive cardiomyopathy

Definition

Restrictive left ventricular physiology is characterized by a pattern of ventricular filling in which increased stiffness of the myocardium causes ventricular pressure to rise precipitously with only small increases in volume. The definition of restrictive cardiomyopathy has been confusing because this pattern can occur with a wide range of different pathologies. For the purposes of this chapter, restrictive cardiomyopathies are defined by restrictive ventricular physiology in the presence of normal or reduced diastolic volumes of one or both ventricles, normal or reduced systolic volumes, and normal ventricular wall thickness. Historically, systolic function was said to be preserved in restrictive cardiomyopathy, but it is rare for contractility to be truly normal.

Causes

Restrictive cardiomyopathy is the least common of the cardiomyopathies. Many causes have been identified, including infiltrative and storage disorders, and endomyocardial disease. In the Western world, amyloidosis is the commonest cause in adults, with some familial cases caused by mutations in the transthyretin gene. In the tropics, endomyocardial fibrosis is the commonest cause in adults, and probably also in children.

Rare reports of familial restrictive cardiomyopathy associated with autosomal dominant skeletal myopathy, autosomal recessive musculoskeletal abnormalities, and Noonan's syndrome have been described in children. Mutations in the gene encoding desmin (an intermediate filament protein) cause restrictive cardiomyopathy associated with skeletal myopathy and, in some cases, abnormalities of the cardiac conduction system. Mutations in the gene encoding cardiac troponin I (a cardiac sarcomeric contractile protein) are reported in 50% of apparently idiopathic restrictive cardiomyopathy in adults. In infants, mutations in other sarcomeric protein genes (troponin I and actin) are reported.

Pathology

Restrictive cardiomyopathy is best regarded as a heterogeneous group of conditions with different aetiologies rather than single disease entity. Macroscopically, restrictive cardiomyopathy is characterized by marked biatrial dilatation in the presence of normal heart weight, a small ventricular cavity, and no left ventricular hypertrophy. The histological features of idiopathic restrictive cardiomyopathy are usually nonspecific, with patchy interstitial fibrosis that may range in extent from very mild to severe. There may also be fibrosis of the sinoatrial and atrioventricular nodes. Myocyte disarray is not uncommon in patients with pure restrictive cardiomyopathy, even in the absence of macroscopic ventricular hypertrophy.

In endomyocardial fibrosis the cardiac pathology is distinctive, with endocardial fibrosis and overlying thrombosis involving the inflow tracts and the apices, but sparing the outflow tracts of one or both ventricles. Necrotic, thrombotic, and fibrotic stages have been defined in patients with endomyocardial fibrosis and hypereosinophilia. In the necrotic stage, there is an acute inflammatory reaction characterized by eosinophilic abscesses in the myocardium, with associated necrosis and arteritis. The endocardium is often thickened and mural thrombi may develop. The thrombotic stage is characterized by endocardial thrombus formation that may be severe, with massive intracavitary thrombosis causing restriction to ventricular filling and a low-output state with high filling pressures. There is a risk of systemic emboli. During the necrotic and thrombotic stages the disease may mimic a hyperacute rheumatic carditis (see Chapter 16.9.1). If the patient survives, healing by fibrosis with hyaline fibrous tissue occurs. There is no further evidence of inflammation and the impact of the disease is caused by the effect of the dense fibrous tissue on ventricular filling volume and atrioventricular valve function.

Clinical features and investigation

Disease onset is usually insidious. Left-sided disease may present with symptoms of pulmonary congestion and/or mitral regurgitation; right-sided disease with raised jugular venous pressure, hepatomegaly, ascites, and tricuspid regurgitation. Radiographic and electrocardiographic appearances are nonspecific, showing evidence of raised left and/or right atrial pressure and cardiomegaly with left ventricular hypertrophy. Pulmonary infiltrates, nonspecific repolarization changes, and fascicular blocks may be seen.

Two-dimensional echocardiography confirms the diagnosis, allowing visualization of the structural abnormalities involving the endocardium and atrioventricular valves as well as demonstration of the abnormal physiology with restriction to filling (Fig. 16.7.2.6). There may be intracavitary thrombus with apical cavity obliteration, or bright echoes from the endocardium of the right or left ventricle with tethering of the chordae and reduced excursion of the posterior mitral valve leaflet. Typically, ventricular dimensions and wall thickness are normal, whereas the atria are grossly enlarged. Left ventricular filling terminates early and is followed by a plateau phase coincident with the third heart sound.

The principal haemodynamic consequence of endomyocardial scarring is a restriction to normal filling. Early diastolic pressures are normal, but there is a rapid mid-diastolic rise (square root sign), which plateaus and is not associated with impairment of systolic performance. A similar functional haemodynamic abnormality is seen in pericardial constriction (see Chapter 16.8), but in the latter condition end-diastolic pressures are usually closely similar within the two ventricles, whereas in endomyocardial fibrosis there is usually inequality of the end-diastolic pressures. Mitral and tricuspid regurgitation may be severe and both ventricles appear abnormal in shape on angiography due to obliteration of the apices. This may be particularly marked in the right ventricle in which the infundibulum is hypertrophied and hypocontractile. In addition, the fibrotic process results in smoothing of the internal architecture of the ventricle with loss of the normal trabeculae. The presence of intracavitary thrombi in the left ventricle may give rise to the erroneous diagnosis of a cardiac tumour.

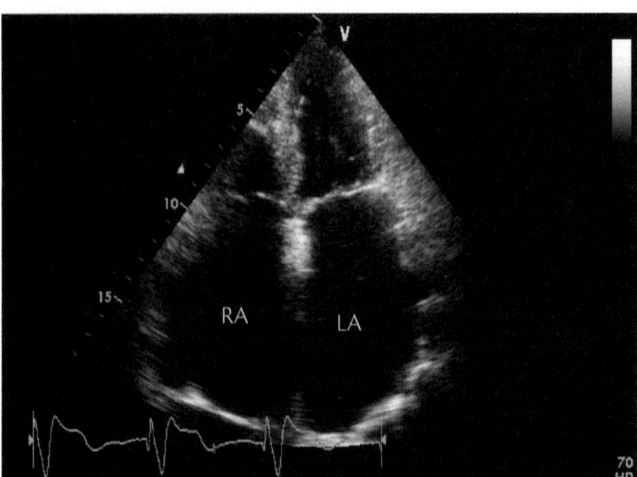

Fig. 16.7.2.6 Two-dimensional echocardiogram (apical four-chamber view) showing normal-sized ventricles with massive dilatation of left (LA) and right (RA) atria.

The structural and physiological abnormalities that can be demonstrated with two-dimensional echocardiography or during cardiac catheterization result from the thrombotic and fibrotic stages of the disease. Diagnosis may be difficult during the early acute phase, when the appearances of the left and right ventricle are far less abnormal, and may require confirmation by endomyocardial biopsy. In later stages, however, the diagnosis should be readily apparent and the risk of biopsy is excessive.

Management

There is no good medical treatment for advanced disease and the prognosis is poor, with 35 to 50% 2-year mortality. Congestive symptoms from raised right atrial pressure can be improved with diuretics, though too great a reduction in ventricular filling pressure will lead to a reduction in cardiac output. Arrhythmias are common, but their prognostic significance is uncertain and they should not be treated unless they are sustained or associated with symptoms. Antiarrhythmic drugs that significantly slow the heart rate may be deleterious because of the small stroke volume. Digoxin may be helpful to control the ventricular response in atrial fibrillation, but cannot be expected to improve congestive symptoms as systolic function is usually well preserved. Anticoagulants may help to prevent venous thrombosis and systemic emboli; both warfarin and antiplatelet drugs are advised.

Surgery with either mitral and/or tricuspid valve replacement, with or without decortication of the endocardium, has been carried out in some patients with endomyocardial fibrosis. Good long-term results have been obtained, but there is significant perioperative mortality (15–20%).

Arrhythmogenic right ventricular cardiomyopathy

Definition

Arrhythmogenic right ventricular cardiomyopathy (ARVC, which replaces the term 'arrhythmogenic right ventricular dysplasia' initially used to describe the condition) is a heart muscle disease characterized by progressive fibro-fatty replacement of right ventricular myocardium, initially with regional and later with global right and left ventricular involvement, associated with ventricular arrhythmia, heart failure, and sudden cardiac death, with as many as 20% of such deaths in young individuals and athletes attributable to the condition. Arrhythmogenic right ventricular cardiomyopathy occurs worldwide, in all ethnic groups. The prevalence is unknown, but is conservatively estimated to be between 1 in 1000 and 1 in 5000.

Causes

Systematic family studies have shown that arrhythmogenic right ventricular cardiomyopathy is inherited in at least 50% of cases. The mode of transmission is usually autosomal dominant with variable penetrance, but rare autosomal recessive forms have provided the first insights into the genetic basis of the condition. Two autosomal recessive syndromes characterized by arrhythmogenic right ventricular cardiomyopathy, woolly hair, and palmoplantar keratoderma (Naxos disease (OMIM 601214) and Carvajal–Huerta syndrome (OMIM 605676)) are caused by mutations in the genes encoding plakoglobin and desmoplakin, respectively. These proteins are important components of the desmosome, with key roles in cell-to-cell adhesion and transduction of mechanical stress. Analysis of these and similar proteins in families with the more common autosomal dominant form of disease have revealed mutations in desmoplakin, plakophilin, desmoglein, and desmocollin. Nondesmosomal gene mutations reported in some families with arrhythmogenic right ventricular cardiomyopathy include the ryanodine-2 receptor (more typically associated with catecholaminergic polymorphic ventricular tachycardia) and transforming growth factor β.

Pathology and pathophysiology

Segmental disease is usual in arrhythmogenic right ventricular cardiomyopathy, with involvement of the diaphragmatic, apical, and infundibular regions of the right ventricular free wall (the 'triangle of dysplasia'). Evolution to more diffuse right ventricular involvement and left ventricular abnormalities with heart failure are more common than the earlier literature suggested. Macroscopic examination of the heart may show diffuse thinning of the right ventricular wall, with aneurysms present in up to 50% of cases. The fibro-fatty replacement of the myocardium may be focal or widespread, usually involves the subepicardial layer of the right ventricular free wall and, when severe, may appear transmural. Histologically, arrhythmogenic right ventricular cardiomyopathy is characterized by replacement myocardial fibrosis with thinning and discrete bulges of the right ventricular free wall, often in association with lymphocytic infiltrates surrounding degenerating or necrotic myocytes. Animal and in vitro studies support the hypothesis that mutations in plakoglobin or analogous genes involved in cell adhesion may cause myocytes under mechanical stress to detach and die, with subsequent fibro-fatty replacement. Other aetiopathogenic factors have been postulated, including enteroviral and adenoviral infection.

Suggested arrhythmic mechanisms include re-entry circuits arising from fibro-fatty myocardial replacement and heterogeneous conduction resulting from destabilization of cell-adhesion complexes and gap junctions.

Clinical features

Symptomatic presentation is usually with palpitation and/or syncope from sustained ventricular arrhythmia, but the first presentation of the disease—especially in young people—may be with sudden cardiac death in an individual who was previously entirely asymptomatic. Occasionally, the victim will have experienced syncope in the months preceding their death (particularly during exercise). Other symptoms are presyncope and chest pain, and features of right and later biventricular failure may be present, including dyspnoea on exertion, as the disease progresses. 'Hot phases' are recognized, during which previously stable patients may suffer repeated episodes of ventricular arrhythmia and be prone to sudden death.

Investigation

There is no single diagnostic test for arrhythmogenic right ventricular cardiomyopathy, and the diagnosis is based on the presence of major and minor criteria encompassing structural, histological, electrocardiographic, arrhythmic, and genetic factors, proposed by the Study Group on Arrhythmogenic Right Ventricular Dysplasia/Cardiomyopathy of the Working Group Myocardial and Pericardial Disease of the European Society of Cardiology and of the Scientific

Council on Cardiomyopathies of the International Society and Federation of Cardiology (Table 16.7.2.4). The diagnosis of arrhythmogenic right ventricular cardiomyopathy is fulfilled in the presence of two major criteria, or one major plus two minor criteria, or four minor criteria from different categories. However, these criteria are currently being revised in the light of new family data showing that at least 30% of patients have left ventricular involvement in the form of regional or global left ventricular dysfunction, and many have subclinical left ventricular fibrosis (evident on magnetic resonance) affecting particularly the posterolateral segments.

Family studies have shown that first-degree relatives of affected individuals may have minor cardiac abnormalities, which—although not fulfilling the above diagnostic criteria—are likely to represent disease expression in the context of an autosomal dominant disease. Modified diagnostic criteria for the diagnosis of arrhythmogenic right ventricular cardiomyopathy in family members of affected individuals have been proposed.

Electrocardiography

The most common electrocardiographic abnormality is T-wave inversion in leads V1 to V3 in the absence of right bundle branch block (but note that this is a normal finding in children and therefore cannot be used as a diagnostic criterion) (Fig. 16.7.2.7). Other electrocardiographic features include QRS dispersion (localized prolongation of the QRS complex in the right ventricular leads, with a difference in QRS duration of at least 40 ms between right and left precordial leads), right intraventricular conduction delay (progressing to right bundle branch block in some patients) and the presence of an epsilon wave (a terminal notch in the QRS complex), typically seen in lead V1. Ventricular tachycardia is of left bundle branch block morphology suggesting a right ventricular origin.

The signal-averaged ECG is used to detect late potentials and predicts susceptibility to ventricular arrhythmia in different cardiac diseases. Up to 80% of patients with arrhythmogenic right ventricular cardiomyopathy have late potentials on the signal-averaged electrocardiogram, which may correlate with the risk of ventricular arrhythmia and disease progression.

Exercise testing

The role of exercise testing in arrhythmogenic right ventricular cardiomyopathy is primarily to detect ventricular arrhythmias induced by physical activity. Ventricular ectopy and nonsustained ventricular tachycardia of right ventricular origin have been described in young patients. Cardiopulmonary exercise testing may be useful as an objective measure of functional capacity in patients with advanced disease.

Echocardiography

Echocardiography is used to confirm the diagnosis and to exclude congenital heart disease, which may present as a differential diagnosis for arrhythmogenic right ventricular cardiomyopathy. Typical echocardiographic findings include right ventricular dilatation, regional hypokinesia or dyskinesia, free wall aneurysms, increased echogenicity of the moderator band, and right ventricular apical hypertrabeculation. Left ventricular involvement with posterior wall hypokinesia or ventricular dilatation may be seen in up to 30% of cases. In patients in whom the right ventricle is difficult to visualize adequately using standard two-dimensional echocardiography, injection of echocardiographic contrast may provide improved definition

Table 16.7.2.4 Criteria for the diagnosis of arrhythmogenic right ventricular cardiomyopathy (ARVC). Criteria are fulfilled if two major criteria, or one major plus two minor criteria, or four minor criteria are seen

Major	Minor
Family history	
Familial disease confirmed at autopsy or surgery	Family history of premature sudden death (<35 years) caused by ARVC Family history (clinical diagnosis based on present criteria)
ECG depolarization/conduction abnormalities	
Epsilon waves or localized prolongation (>110 ms) of the QRS complex in the right precordial leads (V1–V3)	Late potentials seen on signal- averaged ECG
Repolarization abnormalities	
	Inverted T waves in right precordial leads (V2 and V3) in individuals aged >12 years and in the absence of right bundle branch block
Tissue characterization of walls	
Fibrofatty replacement of myocardium on endomyocardial biopsy	
Global and/or regional dysfunction and structural alterations[a]	
Severe dilatation and reduction of right ventricular ejection fraction with no (or only mild) left ventricular impairment	Mild global right ventricular dilatation and/or ejection fraction reduction with normal left ventricle
Localized right ventricular areas with aneurysms (akinetic or dyskinetic diastolic bulging)	Mild segmental dilatation of the right ventricle
Severe segmental dilatation of the right ventricle	Regional right ventricular hypokinesia
Arrhythmias	Left bundle branch block type or ventricular tachycardia (sustained or nonsustained) documented on ECG, Holter monitoring, or during exercise testing
	Frequent ventricular extrasystoles(>1000/24 h) on Holter monitoring

[a] Detected by echocardiography, angiography, MRI, or radionuclide scintigraphy.
Reproduced from *Br Heart J*, McKenna WJ *et al*, 71:215–18. Copyright 1994, with permission from BMJ Publishing Group Ltd.

of the right ventricular endocardial border and allow the identification of subtle wall-motion abnormalities or diastolic bulging.

Cardiac magnetic resonance imaging

Assessment of the right ventricle using echocardiography is challenging, even in experienced hands. Cardiovascular MRI has the advantage that it is a three-dimensional technique with no limitations imposed by acoustic windows (Fig. 16.7.2.8). When performed with a dedicated protocol by experienced operators, in both children and adults, the technique has a high sensitivity for detecting right ventricular abnormalities in individuals who fulfil conventional diagnostic criteria, and may help to confirm individuals with early disease who fulfil the modified familial criteria. Reproducibility and accuracy are still, however, strongly operator dependent. Late enhancement with gadolinium has been shown to correlate with fibro-fatty changes in arrhythmogenic right ventricular cardiomyopathy.

Endomyocardial biopsy

Although a histological diagnosis of arrhythmogenic right ventricular cardiomyopathy may be definitive, the sensitivity of endomyocardial biopsies is low because of (1) the segmental nature of the disease, (2) the amount of tissue usually obtained is insufficient to differentiate fibro-fatty replacement from islands of adipose tissue that are not infrequently seen between myocytes in the right ventricle of normal subjects, and (3) the fact that samples are usually taken from the septum, a region that is less frequently involved. The complication rate—which includes cardiac perforation and tamponade

because of thinning of the right ventricular wall—is also relatively high, hence endomyocardial biopsies are no longer considered part of the routine diagnostic work-up for the condition.

Management

Treatment in arrhythmogenic right ventricular cardiomyopathy is individualized according to the presence of symptoms, arrhythmia, and perceived risk of sudden death. Patients with symptomatic, non-life-threatening ventricular arrhythmias are treated empirically with β-adrenoreceptor blockers, amiodarone, or sotalol.

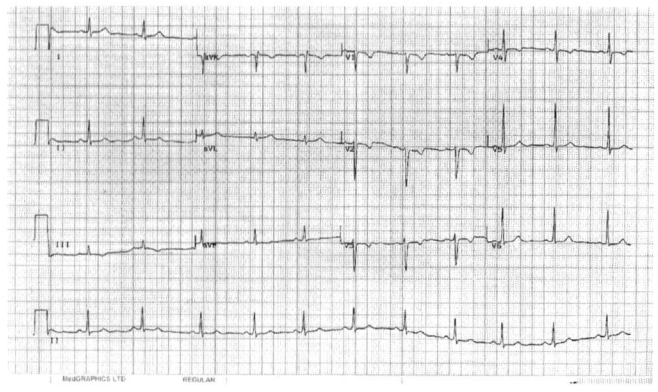

Fig. 16.7.2.7 A 12-lead ECG from a young woman showing the most common electrocardiographic abnormality found in arrhythmogenic right ventricular cardiomyopathy, T-wave inversion in the precordial leads V1–V4.

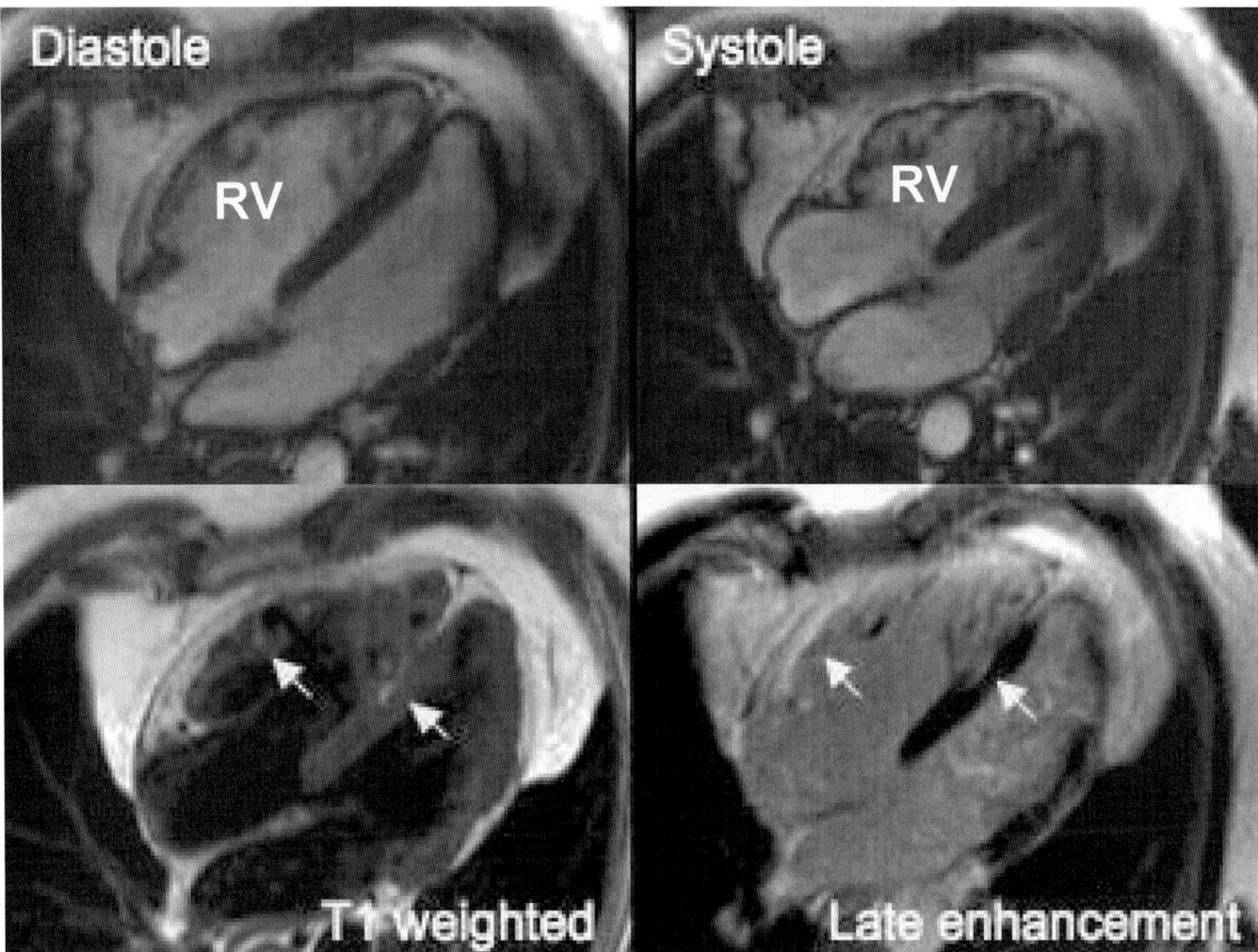

Fig. 16.7.2.8 Arrhythmogenic right ventricular cardiomyopathy. On the cine images (top) the right ventricle (RV) is globally dilated with multiple RV wall-motion abnormalities. There are two areas of LV involvement with wall thinning (free wall, apex). On T_1-weighted imaging, fat can be seen in the septum and RV trabeculae (arrows). After contrast, late enhancement representing fibrosis is also seen (arrows).

β-Blockers are particularly effective at treating symptoms related to exercise-induced arrhythmia, and sotalol suppresses ventricular arrhythmia in most patients. Those with a history of sustained, haemodynamically compromising ventricular arrhythmia should be offered an implantable cardioverter–defibrillator (ICD). Studies in such patients have shown a high rate of appropriate device discharges, ranging from 15 to 22% per year. More problematic is the prevention of sudden death in patients without such a history. A number of markers of increased risk have been proposed, including unexplained syncope, symptomatic ventricular tachycardia, family history of sudden death, young age, left ventricular involvement, and diffuse right ventricular dilatation. However, population-based survival studies are needed to evaluate the significance of these and other factors (such as asymptomatic nonsustained ventricular tachycardia).

Patients with severe right ventricular or biventricular involvement should be treated according to current heart-failure treatment guidelines, including the use of diuretics, ACE inhibitors, and anticoagulation. Patients with advanced disease are candidates for cardiac transplantation (see Chapters 16.5.1 and 16.5.2).

Further reading

Hypertrophic cardiomyopathy

Davies MJ, McKenna WJ (1995). Hypertrophic cardiomyopathy: pathology and pathogenesis. *Histopathology*, **26**, 493–500.

Elliott P, McKenna WJ (2004). Hypertrophic cardiomyopathy. *Lancet*, **363**, 1881–91.

Maron BJ (2002). Hypertrophic cardiomyopathy. A systematic review. *JAMA*, **287**, 1308–20.

Maron BJ, *et al.* (2003). American College of Cardiology Foundation Task Force on Clinical Expert Consensus Documents; European Society of Cardiology Committee for Practice Guidelines. American College of Cardiology/European Society of Cardiology Clinical Expert Consensus Document on Hypertrophic Cardiomyopathy. A report of the American College of Cardiology Foundation Task Force on Clinical Expert Consensus Documents and the European Society of Cardiology Committee for Practice Guidelines. *Eur Heart J*, **24**, 1965–91.

Richard P, *et al.* (2003). Hypertrophic cardiomyopathy: distribution of disease genes, spectrum of mutations, and implications for a molecular diagnosis strategy. *Circulation*, **107**, 2227–32.

Seidman JG, Seidman C (2001). The genetic basis for cardiomyopathy: from mutation identification to mechanistic paradigms. *Cell*, **104**, 557–67.

Watkins H (2003). Genetic clues to disease pathways in hypertrophic and dilated cardiomyopathies. *Circulation*, **107**, 1344–46.

Wigle ED, *et al.* (1985). Hypertrophic cardiomyopathy. The importance of the site and the extent of hypertrophy. A review. *Progr Cardiovasc Dis*, **28**, 1–83.

Dilated cardiomyopathy

Burkett EL, Hershberger RE (2005). Clinical and genetic issues in familial dilated cardiomyopathy. *J Am Coll Cardiol*, **45**, 969–81.

Dec GM, Fuster V (1994). Idiopathic dilated cardiomyopathy. *N Engl J Med*, **331**, 1564–75.

Mestroni L, *et al.* (1999). Guidelines for the study of familial dilated cardiomyopathies. Collaborative Research Group of the European Human and Capital Mobility Project on Familial Dilated Cardiomyopathy. *Eur Heart J*, **20**, 93–102.

Shaw T, Elliott P, McKenna WJ (2002). Dilated cardiomyopathy: a genetically heterogeneous disease. *Lancet*, **360**, 654–5.

Restrictive cardiomyopathy

See Chapter 16.7.2.

Arrhythmogenic right ventricular dysplasia

Corrado D, Thiene G (2006). Arrhythmogenic right ventricular cardiomyopathy/dysplasia: clinical impact of molecular genetic studies. *Circulation*, **113**, 1634–7.

Hulot JS, *et al.* (2004). Natural history and risk stratification of arrhythmogenic right ventricular dysplasia/cardiomyopathy. *Circulation*, **110**, 1879–84.

McKenna WJ, *et al.* (1994). Diagnosis of arrhythmogenic right ventricular dysplasia/cardiomyopathy. *Br Heart J*, **71**, 215–18.

Sen-Chowdhry S, *et al.* (2004). Arrhythmogenic right ventricular cardiomyopathy: clinical presentation, diagnosis, and management. *Am J Med*, **117**, 685–95.

16.7.3 **Specific heart muscle disorders**

William J. McKenna and Perry Elliott

Essentials

Autoimmune rheumatic disorders and the vasculitides

Cardiovascular involvement is very common, although it may be occult and often goes undetected. Any anatomical structure in the heart may be involved, hence patients may present with pericarditis, myocarditis, endocarditis, or coronary vasculitis. There is usually no correlation between the extent of systemic disease and cardiac involvement.

Systemic lupus erythematosus (SLE)—more than 50% have cardiovascular involvement at some time; 30% have clinical pericarditis; myocarditis can occasionally present with heart failure or arrhythmias; marantic endocarditis can be identified in at least 30% at autopsy, but is rarely clinically significant; neonates born to mothers with SLE

who have anti-Ro/anti-La antibodies frequently develop complete heart block; atherosclerosis is the leading cause of late death in SLE.

Systemic sclerosis—symptomatic cardiac involvement is uncommon (10%), but is frequently detected at autopsy (60%), when the most common features are chronic pericarditis and myocardial fibrosis; pulmonary hypertension is common, usually secondary to lung involvement, and has a very poor prognosis.

Rheumatoid arthritis—10 to 15% have clinical cardiac involvement, 60% on echocardiography: pericarditis is most frequent, with up to 40% having an effusion on echocardiography; myocarditis is frequent at autopsy but rarely causes symptoms; vasculitis affecting epicardial arteries, nonspecific valvitis, and conduction disturbances are reported.

Seronegative arthropathies—associated with pancarditis, proximal aortitis, aortic incompetence, and varying degrees of conduction abnormalities.

Takayasu's arteritis—proximal coronary arteries are involved in 15 to 20%; dilatation of the aortic root may cause aortic regurgitation; pulmonary artery aneurysms and stenoses are common; involvement of the renal arteries can cause malignant hypertension; aortic, coronary, pulmonary, and bronchial arterial fistulae are reported.

Kawasaki disease—myocarditis is frequent (35%) in the acute stage, often in association with a pericardial effusion; coronary artery involvement occurs in 20%, resulting in aneurysm formation and thrombotic occlusion, such that—in the longer term—patients can present with myocardial ischaemia.

Other conditions

Amyloid—in systemic AL (primary) amyloidosis up to 50% have cardiac involvement; systemic AA (secondary) amyloidosis is almost never associated with clinical cardiac amyloidosis; the heart is frequently involved in familial amyloid polyneuropathy. The clinical picture most frequently mimics hypertrophic cardiomyopathy with restrictive physiology. The ECG may show diminished voltages, loss of R waves in precordial leads, and Q waves in the inferior leads. Echocardiography may show a characteristic 'sparkling' appearance to the myocardium. Symptomatic heart disease typically occurs late in the course of amyloidosis and is an ominous feature.

Sarcoidosis—cardiac involvement is clinically apparent in less than 10% of cases, but sudden (presumed arrhythmic) death is not infrequent amongst these.

Endocrine disorders—diabetes is associated with an increased risk of developing heart failure; hyperthyroidism can cause a low output state with symptoms of heart failure and echocardiographic demonstration of dilated cardiomyopathy and systolic dysfunction; hypothyroidism frequently causes pericardial effusion, but heart failure generally represents exacerbation of pre-existing cardiac disease by thyroid deficiency.

Neuromuscular disorders—myocardial dysfunction is common in the muscular dystrophies.

Inherited metabolic disorders—hereditary haemochromatosis causes thickening of the ventricular walls, dilatation of the ventricular chambers, and heart failure; cardiac disease is particularly important in lysosomal storage diseases, including hypertrophic and dilated cardiomyopathy, coronary artery disease, and valvular disease.

Cardiac disease in autoimmune rheumatic disorders

The autoimmune rheumatic disorders (connective tissue diseases) are a heterogeneous group of conditions with multisystem involvement. Cardiovascular involvement is very common, although it may be occult and often goes undetected. As any anatomical structure in the heart may be involved, patients may present with one or more features consistent with pericarditis, myocarditis, endocarditis, and vasculitis. There is usually no correlation between the extent of systemic disease and cardiac involvement. For details of the cardiac manifestations of autoimmune rheumatic diseases and the vasculitides, see Tables 16.7.3.1 and 16.7.3.2.

Systemic lupus erythematosus (SLE)

SLE is a multisystem immune disorder characterized by the formation of autoantibodies to various cell antigens. The prevalence of cardiovascular involvement at some time in the illness is more than

Table 16.7.3.1 Cardiac manifestations of autoimmune rheumatic diseases and the vasculitides

Disease	Cardiac manifestation
Systemic lupus erythematosus	Accelerated atherosclerosis
	Noninfective endocarditis (Libman–Sacks)
	Myocarditis
	Pericarditis
Rheumatoid arthritis	Coronary arteritis
	Aortic and mitral regurgitation
Seronegative arthropathies—ankylosing spondylitis, Reiter's syndrome, psoriatic arthritis, ulcerative colitis, Crohn's disease	Pancarditis
	Proximal aortitis
	Conduction disease
Systemic sclerosis	Myocarditis
	Pericarditis
	Arrhythmias
Wegener's granulomatosis	Constrictive pericarditis
	Atrioventricular block
Churg–Strauss syndrome	Congestive cardiac failure
	Pericarditis
	Coronary arteritis/myocardial infarction
	Arrhythmias
Polyarteritis nodosa	Hypertension
	Congestive heart failure
	Partial or complete coronary artery occlusion
	Pericarditis
	Arrhythmias
Takayasu's syndrome	Pericarditis
	Aortic arch vasculitis
	Heart failure

50%. The pericardium is most commonly affected, with as many as 30% of patients having clinical pericarditis at some stage, and up to 80% affected at autopsy. Progression to constrictive pericarditis or tamponade is extremely rare.

Clinically evident myocardial involvement occurs less frequently, but is reported in 40 to 50% of patients at autopsy: signs and symptoms are uncommon, but patients may occasionally present with heart failure or arrhythmias. Other factors that may contribute to ventricular dysfunction in SLE include atherosclerosis, hypertension, and drugs (e.g. chloroquine).

As many as one-third of patients with SLE have systolic murmurs, which are usually caused by hyperdynamic flow. The classic verrucous vegetations adherent to the endocardium described by Libman and Sacks in 1924 (marantic endocarditis) can be identified in 30% or more at autopsy. These lesions most commonly affect the mitral valve but are rarely clinically significant.

Neonates born to mothers with SLE who have anti-Ro/anti-La antibodies frequently develop complete heart block (see Chapter 14.14). Various degrees of heart block and bundle branch block can be seen in adults, but complete heart block is rare. Arrhythmias such as atrial fibrillation and flutter may also occur, particularly in association with pericarditis.

Myocardial infarction is very uncommon in patients with systemic lupus erythematosus, but accelerated or premature atherosclerosis is the leading cause of late death in SLE. Its cause is unknown, but suggested contributory factors include chronic inflammation, immune complex deposition, antiphospholipid antibodies, hypertension, dyslipidaemia, and hyperglycaemia (caused by chronic steroid administration).

Death from the cardiac complications of lupus is rare. Mild pericardial disease may respond to nonsteroidal anti-inflammatory drugs, heart failure is treated conventionally, and conduction defects may require pacing. Coronary vasculitis and/or lupus myocarditis are usually treated with steroids and other immunosuppressants, but there are no trials to guide therapeutic decision making in these rare conditions.

Antiphospholipid syndrome

The antiphospholipid syndrome is recognized both in patients without (primary) and with SLE. It is a thrombophilic disorder characterized by arterial and venous occlusions, recurrent fetal loss, thrombocytopenia, increased maternal complications of pregnancy, and associated with persistently raised titres of anticardiolipin antibodies. Involvement of the mitral and aortic valves is particularly common. Dramatic response to prednisolone has been described (see Chapter 15.14 for further information).

Systemic sclerosis

Systemic sclerosis is characterized by abnormal collagen deposition in various organ systems. Symptomatic cardiac involvement is uncommon (10%), but is frequently detected at autopsy (60%), when the most common features are chronic pericarditis (70%) and myocardial fibrosis (37%). Clinically these cause heart failure, ventricular arrhythmia, and conduction disease. Rare cases of tamponade are reported. Valve involvement is less common, except for tricuspid regurgitation, which occurs in 40% of patients and is usually associated with pulmonary hypertension. Pulmonary hypertension is present in 47% of patients, usually secondary to

Table 16.7.3.2 Cardiac involvement in the more common autoimmune rheumatic disorders

	Pericardial involvement	Myocardial involvement	Valvular involvement	Coronary/arteritis	Conduction system involvement
Rheumatoid arthritis	16–40% at autopsy 10–15% clinical pericarditis	4–20% at autopsy Symptomatic in <5%	> 50% valvulitis at autopsy Symptoms rare	11–20% involvement of coronary vessels at autopsy Vasculitis affecting the aorta rare	Any part of conduction system involved Varying degrees of heart block in 0.1%
Systemic lupus erythematosus	45–66% at autopsy 20–30% clinical pericarditis	30% at autopsy Symptomatic in <10%	Libman–Sacks lesions in 30% at autopsy	Coronary vessels involved in <10% Vasculitis affecting the aorta rare	Any part of conduction system involved Varying degrees of heart block in <1%
Systemic sclerosis and variants	70% at autopsy 7–15% clinical pericarditis	Up to 60% at autopsy Symptoms rare	Rare, AR and MVP described Symptoms in <10%	Reversible perfusion defects in up to 40% Vasculitis demonstrated rarely	Any part of conduction system involved; Abnormal ECG in 50%
Polymyositis/ dermatomyositis	Clinical involvement rare (usually in children with dermatomyositis)	Up to 25% at autopsy Symptoms in 13–26%	MVP common Other lesions rare		Any part of conduction system involved Symptoms extremely rare
Seronegative spondyloarthro pathies	< 1% incidence of pericarditis in AS and Reiter's	Myocardial involvement/ dysfunction common on ECHO in AS Symptoms rare	Aortic incompetence most common: 1–10% in AS, 1–15% in Reiter's MR very rare	Aortitis: 1–10% in AS, 1–15% in Reiter's	Heart block: 8% in AS, 8% in Reiter's, rare in other forms of spondyloarthropathy

AR, aortic regurgitation; AS, ankylosing spondylitis; MR, mitral regurgitation; MVP, mitral valve prolapse; SLE, systemic lupus erythematosus.

lung involvement, and is associated with a 1-year survival of only 50%. Involvement of the large epicardial blood vessels is not a feature of systemic sclerosis, but microvascular dysfunction is common and may contribute to myocardial ischaemia and patchy myocardial fibrosis. In the limited form of systemic sclerosis (formerly known as CREST syndrome) the overall prognosis is more favorable: pulmonary hypertension without severe lung disease occurs in 10–15%, and subclinical left ventricular dysfunction is reported.

Rheumatoid arthritis

Cardiac involvement is found in up to 60% of patients on echocardiography, but only in 10 to 15% clinically. The presence of cardiac disease correlates with the severity of joint disease and the presence of rheumatoid nodules, male gender, age, high titres of rheumatoid factor, and other systemic markers of disease activity. Histological changes consist of a nonspecific inflammatory infiltrate, myocyte necrosis, and fibrosis affecting any part of the heart. Rheumatoid nodules may accompany this, and the heart may be affected rarely 5% by secondary amyloidosis. Myocarditis is reported in up to 40% at autopsy, but symptoms are uncommon. Pericarditis occurs more frequently, and up to 40% of patients have an effusion on echocardiography, but progression to constrictive pericarditis or tamponade is rare. Acute vasculitis involving the larger epicardial arteries has been reported but is uncommon. Nonspecific valvitis may affect the mitral and particularly the aortic valve: this may eventually lead to scarred, hyalinized, and even incompetent valves. Rheumatoid nodules may occasionally deform the mitral valve and lead to valvular incompetence. Conduction disturbances may be secondary to infiltration by rheumatoid nodules: the commonest ECG abnormality is first-degree heart block, but left bundle branch block and complete heart block are also described. Although pericarditis is usually responsive to steroids, it is unclear whether steroids or disease-modifying drugs alter the other cardiac manifestations.

Seronegative arthropathies

This group of disorders is characterized by the absence of rheumatoid factor and includes ankylosing spondylitis, Reiter's syndrome, and psoriatic and gastrointestinal arthropathies. These may all be associated with cardiac involvement, in particular pancarditis, proximal aortitis, aortic incompetence, and varying degrees of conduction abnormalities. They may also result in amyloid deposition. On occasion cardiac disease may present before joint disease. Treatment is empirical and based on symptomatology.

Polymyositis and dermatomyositis

Cardiac symptoms in polymyositis or dermatomyositis are rare, but post-mortem and clinical studies suggest that left ventricular diastolic dysfunction and conduction disturbances are present in 40 to 50% of cases. When cardiac symptoms are present they are associated with a poor prognosis. Rare cases of cardiac tamponade are reported. Interstitial lung disease, found in 5 to 30% of cases, may lead to right heart failure. Treatment is symptomatic.

Cardiac disease in the vasculitides

Takayasu's arteritis

Takayasu's arteritis is a rare inflammatory arteritis that predominantly affects the thoracic aorta and the proximal portions of its major branches, the pulmonary arteries and the coronary vessels. Asians are affected more than other ethnic groups, with a 10:1 female to male ratio. The disease typically evolves from an early inflammatory stage to a fibrotic obliterative phase with arterial aneurysms, stenoses, and occlusions. The proximal coronary arteries are involved in 15 to 20% of cases. Dilatation of the aortic root may cause aortic regurgitation. Pulmonary artery aneurysms and stenoses are common and can cause pulmonary hypertension, right heart failure, and pulmonary haemorrhage. Involvement of the renal arteries can cause malignant hypertension. Aortic, coronary, pulmonary and bronchial arterial fistulae are reported. Subclinical myocardial involvement, in the absence of coronary lesions, is reported in up to 50% of patients. Pericarditis is rare.

Polyarteritis nodosa

Classic polyarteritis nodosa (PAN) is a rare, nongranulomatous, necrotizing arteritis of small and medium-sized vessels without microscopic angiitis or glomerulonephritis. The most typical cardiovascular complication is malignant hypertension caused by renal artery vasculitis. Coronary vasculitis causing aneurysms, myocardial infarction, and cardiomyopathy are reported, but they are probably rare. Pericarditis and clinically important conduction system involvement is uncommon. Valve disease appears not be a feature.

Giant cell (temporal) arteritis

Giant cell arteritis is a granulomatous arteritis of the aorta and its major branches, in particular the carotid artery. It usually affects people older than 50 years of age. Five to ten per cent of patients have cardiac involvement, the most common lesions being thoracic aortic aneurysms and aortic regurgitation. Coronary involvement is rare.

Kawasaki's disease

Kawasaki's disease (or mucocutaenous lymph node syndrome) is an acute vasculitis of small and medium-sized vessels that typically presents in children aged less than 5 years, with a peak at 1 year and a small male predominance (1.5:1). In the acute stage, myocarditis is frequent (35%), often in association with pericardial effusions, treatment being with aspirin and high dose gammaglobulin. Coronary artery involvement occurs in 20%, resulting in aneurysm formation and thrombotic occlusion, such that in the longer term patients can present with acute coronary syndromes and myocardial ischaemia, which are managed conventionally. See Chapter 19.11.8 for further discussion.

Microscopic polyangiitis

Microscopic polyangiitis is a disorder of capillaries, venules, and arterioles with occasional involvement of medium-sized vessels. In one series, 50% of patients had cardiac involvement in the form of pericarditis, heart failure, and myocardial infarction.

Wegener's granulomatosis

Wegener's granulomatosis is a necrotizing vasculitis of medium and small vessels associated with granulomatous lesions in the upper and lower respiratory tract. Pericarditis and valvulitis are the most frequently reported abnormalities, but their frequency varies substantially between series. Coronary arteritis is relatively common at post-mortem, but rarely causes myocardial infarction. Myocarditis and complete heart block are rare (2%).

Behçet's disease

Behçet's disease is a relapsing inflammatory disorder characterized by oral and genital ulceration, uveitis, and arterial and venous thrombosis. The disease is common in the eastern Mediterranean and eastern Asia. Cardiac disease, including myocarditis, atrioventricular block, pericarditis, and valve disease, is present in less than 5% of patients. Coronary artery disease is very rare (<1%) but poses challenges for revascularization because of tissue fragility and pseudoaneurysm formation. Aneurysms may also be seen in the pulmonary (Hugues–Stovin syndrome), coronary, and other arteries.

Amyloid

Amyloidosis describes a group of diverse protein-deposition diseases (see Chapter 12.12.3). As many as 50% of patients with systemic AL (primary) amyloidosis have cardiac involvement, which will manifest clinically in up to one-half of these. Systemic AA (secondary) amyloidosis is almost never associated with clinical cardiac amyloidosis. The heart is frequently involved in familial amyloid polyneuropathy, which is the most common type of hereditary amyloidosis that can be caused by one of more than 70 mutations in the transthyretin gene. Senile amyloidosis is extremely common; indeed, almost all individuals over the age of 80 years will have scattered deposits of amyloid, particularly affecting the aorta: clinical involvement is variable, depending on the extent of deposition, but tends to be unimportant.

The extracellular deposition of amyloid results in a firm, thickened, noncompliant myocardium. Deposition occurs throughout the atrial and ventricular muscle. Conducting as well as nodal tissue may be affected: fibrosis of these structures may occur. Valvular function is rarely affected, although deposition in and thickening of cardiac valves is common. Intramural coronary arteries and veins frequently contain deposits, which can occasionally compromise the lumina of these vessels.

Amyloid heart disease most frequently mimics hypertrophic cardiomyopathy with restrictive physiology. The reduced compliance of the myocardium produces the characteristic diastolic dip and plateau (square root sign) in the ventricular pressure waveform that may simulate constrictive pericarditis. An impaired rate of early diastolic filling is characteristic and systolic dysfunction may also occur, leading to congestive heart failure.

Progressive infiltration of the autonomic nervous system results in orthostatic hypotension in 10% of cases. Arrhythmias are common, in particular ventricular premature beats and atrial fibrillation. Complex ventricular arrhythmias may be harbingers of sudden death.

The chest radiograph may show cardiomegaly in patients with systolic dysfunction but is often normal in those with restrictive cardiomyopathy, although pulmonary congestion may be prominent. The ECG shows diminished voltages in about 50% of patients, and loss of R waves in precordial leads; the presence of Q waves in the inferior leads may simulate myocardial infarction. Echocardiography reveals an increased thickness of the ventricular walls with small ventricular chambers, dilated atria, intra-atrial septal thickening, left ventricular dysfunction, and a characteristic 'sparkling' appearance to the myocardium. Asymmetrical septal hypertrophy has also been recognized. Scintigraphy with technetium-99 pyrophosphate may be strongly positive. CT and MRI may also be helpful, as may endomyocardial biopsy.

Symptomatic heart disease typically presents late in the course of amyloidosis and the presence of clinical signs is an ominous feature, with mortality approaching 100% at 2 years. Treatment is supportive in combination with measures to suppress the underlying amyloidogenic condition. This ranges from myeloma-type chemotherapy in AL amyloidosis to liver transplantation in familial amyloid polyneuropathy. Digoxin and calcium channel antagonists should be used with caution as they selectively bind to amyloidal fibrils, enhancing their effect. Patients with symptomatic conduction system disease require a pacemaker. Diuretics and vasodilators should be used cautiously as they may aggravate hypotension. Transplantation is feasible in selected cases, but is a palliative procedure without treatment of the underlying process.

Sarcoid

Sarcoid is a multisysytem granulomatous disorder of unknown aetiology. Myocardial involvement is seen in 20 to 30% of patients at autopsy, but is clinically apparent in less than 10% of cases. Primary cardiac involvement is extremely rare.

Noncaseating granulomas may involve any region of the heart, although the left ventricular free wall and interventricular septum are the most commonly affected sites. The granulomas can be localized or widespread, and healing may result in the formation of scars. The ventricular muscle eventually becomes increasingly noncompliant, leading to defects in contractile function as well as wall motion. Replacement of large portions of the ventricle by sarcoid tissue may lead to aneurysm formation. Granulomas and fibrosis may also extend to involve nodal or conducting tissue. Isolated pericardial involvement is rare, although pericardial effusions are commonly seen on echo. Valvular dysfunction occurs in less than 5% of patients and may be the result of infiltration of papillary muscles or direct valvular involvement, which is less common.

Clinical manifestations of myocardial sarcoidosis are shown in Table 16.7.3.3. Chest pain has been described in up to 28% of patients, and since about half of these will have abnormal thallium perfusion scans despite arteriographically normal coronary arteries, this is thought to be secondary to microvascular dysfunction.

Sudden death is one of the most common and feared manifestations of myocardial sarcoidosis, occurring in about 65% of affected patients. It is thought to be predominantly secondary to arrhythmias, including ventricular tachycardia and fibrillation. The presence of a ventricular aneurysm may be associated with resistant

Table 16.7.3.3 Clinical manifestations in myocardial sarcoidosis

Abnormality	Reported percentage of patients affected
Atrioventricular block	41–52
Ventricular ectopics	31–47
Congestive heart failure	12–19
Sudden death	21–38
Bundle branch block	26–34
Supraventricular tachycardia	11–25
Ventricular tachycardia	12–23
Simulating myocardial infarction on ECG	14–18
Pericarditis/pulmonary embolism	4–8

ventricular arrhythmias and necessitate its resection. Conduction disturbances such as complete heart block are a frequent occurrence and may also predict sudden death. The electrocardiogram is frequently abnormal, with T wave abnormalities and varying degrees of intraventricular or atrioventricular block. Pathological Q waves may simulate myocardial infarction when myocardial involvement becomes extensive. Echocardiography most commonly shows features of restrictive or occasionally dilated cardiomyopathy. Systolic and/or diastolic dysfunction as well as regional wall motion abnormalities may also be seen. Gallium or technetium pyrophosphate scanning and MRI have all been used to detect affected areas of myocardium. Endomyocardial biopsy can be diagnostic, but is rarely done due to the patchy nature of the disease.

Steroids have been shown to improve symptoms as well as electrocardiographic and echocardiographic features and myocardial perfusion defects, although there is a theoretical risk of increased aneurysm formation. Amiodarone may be of benefit in resistant arrhythmia, and the insertion of an implantable defibrillator may protect against sudden death in susceptible patients. Transplantation may improve prognosis and quality of life in patients who remain symptomatic despite these measures, although recurrence has been documented. The average survival from the onset of symptomatic cardiac involvement has been reported as 1 to 2 years.

Cardiac disease in endocrine disorders
Diabetes

A man with diabetes has a relative risk of developing heart failure that is 2.4 times higher than that of a man without diabetes, and the equivalent relative risk for a woman is 5:1. The risk has been shown to be independent of age, systolic blood pressure, serum cholesterol, and weight. People with diabetes have elevated end-diastolic pressures, reduced ejection fractions, left ventricular dilatation, and hypertrophy, even in the absence of coronary artery disease. Diastolic dysfunction as well as a diffuse hypokinesis of the myocardium has also been demonstrated. Implicated mechanisms include small-vessel disease and autonomic neuropathy.

The most prominent histopathological finding is myocardial fibrosis. Occasionally a picture resembling restrictive heart disease is seen, with a small left ventricular chamber and reduced compliance of the left ventricle.

The treatment of heart failure is the same as in patients without diabetes, although β-blockers with intrinsic sympathomimetic activity are preferred. Preload and afterload reducing agents should be used cautiously because of autonomic dysfunction. It is unclear whether tight glucose control affects the progression of diabetic 'cardiomyopathy', but it is clearly prudent for other reasons to optimize control as well as to reduce obesity and control hypertension.

Hyperthyroidism

In general, excess thyroid hormone results in a high output state with tachycardia, increased cardiac contractility, and peripheral vasodilatation. In the long term this can result in ventricular hypertrophy and an increase in ejection fraction. However, some patients may develop a low output state with symptoms of heart failure and echocardiographic demonstration of dilated cardiomyopathy and systolic dysfunction. These changes may be a result of long-standing tachycardia and increased cardiac work, but thyroxine itself may directly alter the expression of cardiac proteins involved in cardiac function, and there is also some evidence that direct autoimmune attack on the myocardium may occur in Graves' disease.

Typical cardiac symptoms of hyperthyroidism include angina-like chest pain, fatigue, palpitations, and exertional dyspnoea. Cardiac findings include sinus tachycardia and atrial flutter or fibrillation in 17 to 20%. These may be complicated by thromboembolism in up to 40%; also by congestive heart failure. Mitral valve prolapse has been reported in patients with Graves' disease.

Control of the ventricular rate in atrial fibrillation may be obtained with digoxin, β-blockers, or calcium channel antagonists. The increased metabolic clearance of digoxin may necessitate a higher maintenance dose. Attempts at cardioversion should generally be deferred until the patient is euthyroid, at which time they may have spontaneously reverted to sinus rhythm. The presence of an already dilated vascular bed means that diuretics should be used with caution and vasodilators are generally contraindicated.

Hypothyroidism

Patients suffering from hypothyroidism, whether in its mild form or full-blown myxoedema, present a wide variety of symptoms. Complaints of fatigue, lethargy, mental slowness, and cold intolerance usually dominate. Less frequently, symptoms suggestive of cardiac dysfunction such as dyspnoea on exertion, syncope, or angina-like chest pain may be prominent. The most common cardiac abnormality is pericardial effusion, which is usually asymptomatic but reported in at least 30% of untreated patients. Heart failure generally represents exacerbation of pre-existing cardiac disease by the superimposed haemodynamic consequences of thyroid deficiency—bradycardia, diminished myocardial contractility, and increased peripheral vascular resistance. Rarely, hypothyroidism alone can closely resemble cardiomyopathy and be severe enough to cause heart failure. Echocardiographic evidence of asymmetric thickening of the interventricular septum as well as reduced dimensions of the left ventricular outflow tract has been reported. The characteristic ECG findings are sinus bradycardia, prolongation of the QT interval, and a reduction in voltages if there is an associated pericardial effusion.

The management of heart failure involves the identification of any primary cardiac disease that may coexist; both ischaemic heart disease and aortic stenosis may be exacerbated by thyroid replacement. Thyroxine (T_4) significantly enhances myocardial performance within 1 week. It is generally used as first-line treatment of hypothyroidism, but in those with known or suspected coronary artery disease it should be initiated at a lower dose than usual, typically 25 μg/day, and increased slowly at 4- to 6-week intervals until the thyroid-stimulating hormone is within the normal range. Tri-iodothyronine (T_3) may be preferable in severe cases as clinical improvement occurs sooner. β-Blockade can be used prophylactically or added if treatment with thyroxine exacerbates ischaemic heart disease.

Cardiac disease in neuromuscular disorders

Cardiac involvement is very common in the whole spectrum of neuromuscular disorders. Myocardial dysfunction is particularly common in the muscular dystrophies, a group of disorders characterized by progressive skeletal and cardiac muscle involvement (Table 16.7.3.4). Dystrophic effects on skeletal muscle result in fibre necrosis, followed by fibrosis and fatty replacement. These structural and functional changes, which occur in the ventricles, can lead to the development of cardiomyopathy, in particular dilated cardiomyopathy and heart failure. The effect on the specialized conducting tissue may lead to bradyarrhythmias, conduction defects, malignant arrhythmias, and sudden death.

Duchenne and Becker muscular dystrophy are progressive disorders arising from abnormalities (deletion, duplication, or point mutation) in the genes involved in the manufacture of the extrasarcomeric cytoskeletal protein dystrophin. In addition to defects in dystrophin, other defects that might be responsible for muscular dystrophy and dilated cardiomyopathy include those affecting the genes for the intracellular proteins, emerin (a transmembrane protein that is embedded in the inner nuclear cell membrane), and lamin A–C (filament-like proteins that form a proteinaceous mesh underlying and attached to the inner nuclear membrane). The mechanism by which alterations in these proteins may lead to cardiomyopathy remains unclear.

In general, treatment of the cardiomyopathy of neuromuscular disorders is empirical and based on symptomatology and evidence of arrhythmia or conduction block. Should advances in the treatment of neuromuscular disorders by gene therapy or other means result in prolonged survival, then cardiac failure may become the limiting factor.

Cardiac disease in inherited metabolic disorders

Haemochromatosis

Hereditary haemochromatosis is the most common single-gene disorder in people of northern European origin, where approximately 3 to 5 persons per 1000 are homozygous for the condition. It results in excessive and inappropriate mucosal absorption of iron, which is then deposited predominantly in the heart, liver, gonads, and pancreas. Deposition in the heart results in thickening of the ventricular walls together with dilatation of the ventricular chambers and heart failure. Histopathologically, myocardial degeneration and fibrosis occur over time and may extend to involve the conducting system of the heart.

The ECG most commonly reveals changes in ST and T waves. Supraventricular arrhythmias are characteristic, with atrioventricular conduction defects and ventricular arrhythmias being less common. Echocardiography typically shows a mixed dilated and restrictive cardiomyopathy with thickened ventricular walls, ventricular chamber enlargement, systolic and/or diastolic dysfunction. Endomyocardial biopsy may be useful to confirm the diagnosis but cannot rule it out. Treatment involves repeated phlebotomy and/or desferrioxamine.

The type of the inherited mutation may determine the development of cardiomyopathy, with some possibly causing cardiomyopathy by a mechanism(s) unrelated to excessive iron.

Lysosomal diseases

Cardiac disease is particularly important in lysosomal glycogen storage diseases (Pompe's and Danon's diseases), mucopolysaccharidoses and in glycosphingolipidoses (Anderson–Fabry

Table 16.7.3.4 Cardiovascular abnormalities in neuromuscular disorders

Condition	Inheritance	Cardiac disease	Noncardiac manifestations	Genetic defects
Duchenne	X-linked 1:3500 male births HCM and DCM reported Symptoms uncommon	Begins in first decade, 62% have ECG changes by age 10 years: short PQ, prolonged QT, tall R in V1 Conduction system anomalies/dependency by age 12 Death in adolescence	Severe muscle weakness, proximal-girdle distribution at 2–5 years in males Calf pseudohypertrophy, mild cognitive impairment, high CPK Wheelchair	Xp21; dystrophin gene mutations
Becker	X-linked 1:15 000 male births	High incidence of clinical cardiac involvement, heart failure is the most common cause of death DCM seen ECG usually abnormal: reduced R wave or prominent Q in1, AVL and V6 Arrhythmias and heart block in <10%	Mild to moderate muscle weakness, proximal girdle distribution from childhood, and ambulation preserved at least until late teens Calf pseudohypertrophy, high CPK Lifespan usually dependent on severity of cardiac involvement	Xp21; dystrophin gene mutations
X-linked dilated cardiomyopathy	X-linked (rare)	Second or third decade onset CM and heart failure, rapid cardiac progression Milder variants possible Heart block not reported, arrhythmias in <10%	No muscular weakness. Muscle cramps, myalgias CPK usually elevated	Xp21; altered or selective loss of cardiac dystrophin
Limb girdle	AD	Variable degrees of AV block, AF, with high degree block, bradycardia, palpitations, and syncope	Mild to moderate muscle weakness, proximal limb girdle distribution. CPK elevated	Lamin A–C gene, 1q11–21.
1B		DCM in 5%		Allelic to AD-EDMD and isolated cardiomyopathy with conduction system disease mapped to 1q
2A	AR	Cardiac involvement rare	Muscle weakness, proximal-girdle distribution CPK elevated	15q15 Calpain-3 (calcium activated neutral protease)
with sarcoglycan deficiency	AR	DCM reported Arrhythmias uncommon	Proximal-girdle distribution of muscle weakness Calf pseudohypertrophy. CPK elevated Severity varies from Duchenne to Becker -like	α-Sarcoglycan, 17q12 β-Sarcoglycan, 4q12 γ-Sarcoglycan, 13q12 δ-Sarcoglycan, 5q3
Myotonic (1:8000)	AD	Conduction defects and arrhythmias common yet most remain asymptomatic ECG changes in 23–80%: prolonged PR and QRS intervals Left and right bundle branch block, AF, a flutter and bradycardias MVP common DCM and HCM detected rarely	Muscle weakness, may be associated with frontal balding, cataracts, hypogonadism, and myotonia	19q13.3 Myotonin-protein kinase gene mutations (unstable CTG trinucleotide repeats)
Emery–Dreifuss	X-linked	AV block is the most common feature, high incidence of sudden death (pacemaker advised) Sinus node disease as well as tachyarrhythmias are common DCM is rare	Childhood onset of contractures, mild muscle weakness in humeroperoneal distribution Lower extremities affected first CPK elevated moderately No calf pseudohypertrophy	Xq28 defect of nuclear transmembane protein emerin
	AD (actually more common than X-linked)	DCM associated with conduction system disease commonly seen Ventricular fibrillation reported despite pacing	Same as X-linked form May be little evidence of skeletal myopathy	1.q11–21 Laminin A–C mutation (allelic to LGMD1B)

AD, autosomal dominant; AR, autosomal recessive; AF, atrial fibrillation; AV, atrioventricular; CPK, creatinine phosphokinase; DCM, dilated cardiomyopathy; EDMD, Emery–Dreifuss muscular dystrophy; HCM, hypertrophic cardiomyopathy; MVP, mitral valve prolapse.
Table adapted from Cox *et al.* (1997). Dystrophies and heart disease. Current Opinion in Cardiology 12, 329–42.

disease). Various disease manifestations may be observed, including hypertrophic and dilated cardiomyopathy, coronary artery disease, and valvular disease.

Anderson–Fabry disease (angiokeratoma corporis diffusum universale)

Anderson–Fabry disease is an X-linked condition caused by mutations in the gene encoding the lysosomal enzyme α-galactosidase A, which leads to intralysosomal accumulation of neutral glycosphingolipids, mainly globotriaosylceramide (Gb_3), in various organ systems. The disease is characterized by progressive clinical manifestations and premature death from renal disease, stroke and cardiac disease. The electrocardiogram often shows left ventricular hypertrophy, a short PR interval, conduction defects, and arrhythmias. Echocardiography usually demonstrates increased thickness of the left ventricle, which may simulate hypertrophic cardiomyopathy. Differentiation from other hypertrophic or restrictive processes may require MRI or endomyocardial biopsy. A low leucocyte α-galactosidase activity is diagnostic in males.

Gaucher's disease

Gaucher's disease is the most common sphingolipidosis, caused by a deficiency in β-glucocerebrosidase that leads to lysosomal accumulation of glucocerebroside within macrophages. Lipid-laden macrophages (Gaucher cells) accumulate within the reticuloendothelial system resulting in hepatosplenomegaly, bone marrow-replacement, anaemia and thrombocytopenia. Valvular and aortic calcification, heart failure, and pericarditis are reported, but the heart is not involved in most patients. Pulmonary hypertension occurs in up to 30% of untreated patients, with enzyme replacement treatment reducing the prevalence to 7.4%.

Further reading

Benson MD (1997). Aging, amyloid, cardiomyopathy. *N Engl J Med*, **336**, 502–4.

Braunwald E (ed.) (1998). *Heart disease: a textbook of cardiovascular medicine*, 5th edition, pp. 1427–35. W B Saunders, Philadelphia.

Cox GF, Kunkel LM (1997). Dystrophies and heart disease. *Curr Opin Cardiol*, **12**, 329–42.

Guertl B, Noehammer C, Hoefler G (2000). Metabolic cardiomyopathies. *Int J Exp Pathol*, **81**, 349–72.

Landerson PW (1990). Recognition and management of cardiovascular disease related to thyroid dysfunction. *Am J Med*, **88**, 638–41.

Shabina H, Isenberg DA (1999). Autoimmune rheumatic diseases and the heart. *Hospl Med*, **60**, 95–9.

Shammas RL (1993). Sarcoidosis of the heart. *Clin Cardiol*, **16**, 462–72.

Pericardial disease

Michael Henein

Essentials

The most common clinical presentations of pericardial disease are pericarditis, effusion, tamponade, and constriction.

Acute pericarditis

The most common proven causes are viral infection or as a complication of myocardial infarction, but a wide range of other conditions including autoimmune rheumatic disorders and tuberculosis need to be considered. No firm cause is established in many cases, which are regarded as 'idiopathic' (presumed viral).

The main clinical features are chest pain, the presence of a pericardial rub, and widespread ST segment elevation on the ECG. Idiopathic disease is self limiting: treatment is with analgesics and/ or nonsteroidal anti-inflammatory agents.

Pericardial effusion

Acute rapid collection is usually caused by traumatic injury, iatrogenic ventricular puncture, or aortic dissection. Presentation is with pericardial tamponade (see below).

Chronic fluid accumulation is most commonly caused by viral infection, uraemia, autoimmune rheumatic disease, myocardial infarction, myxoedema, or malignancy. Patients may remain asymptomatic despite the presence of a large volume of fluid in the pericardium due to corresponding increase in the capacity of the pericardial cavity. Examination may reveal distant heart sounds and increase in the area of cardiac dullness to percussion. The chest radiograph typically shows a large globular heart and clear lung fields. Echocardiography is the investigation of choice for confirming the presence of effusion and for assessing its volume.

Pericardial tamponade

Pericardial tamponade is a condition of haemodynamic instability caused by chamber compression because increased intrapericardial pressure is greater than the filling pressure of the right and left ventricles.

Presentation is typically with shortness of breath or circulatory collapse. The key physical findings are tachycardia, pulsus paradoxus (an exaggeration of the normal fall in systolic blood pressure on inspiration) of greater than 10 mmHg, and elevation of the venous pressure. Echocardiography is the most important investigation, providing clear evidence of fluid collection around the heart and presence of diastolic right ventricular or right atrial collapse. Immediate management is by pericardial aspiration.

Pericardial constriction

A stiff pericardium loses its stretching ability to accommodate normal changes in intracardiac pressures. Most patients present with leg or abdominal swelling and dyspnoea. The key physical findings are elevated venous pressure (with a characteristic 'M' or 'W' waveform), a pericardial knock, hepatomegaly, ascites, and oedema.

Investigation and diagnosis—Doppler echocardiography is the best noninvasive investigation. Cardiac catheterization demonstrates a difference of less than 5 mmHg between end-diastolic pressures in the two ventricles, persisting with respiration and fluid loading; a peak right ventricular pressure of less than 50 mmHg; and a ratio of end-diastolic to peak right ventricular pressure of more than 0.33.

Management—fluid retention in early pericardial constriction can be managed by diuretics, with pericardiectomy recommended for patients who are resistant.

Anatomy and physiology

The pericardium consists of two layers, a visceral layer lined by mesothelial cells and a parietal or fibrous layer also lined by mesothelial cells, but with attached fat and fibrous tissue. The mesothelial layer secretes about 50 ml of clear pericardial fluid that allows both surfaces to slide together during the cardiac cycle. The innermost layer of the visceral pericardium is adherent to the outer myocardial layer, the epicardium. The fibrous layer is usually 1 mm in thickness, and the visceral layer is a transparent membrane on the surface of the heart. The fibrous pericardium attaches the heart to the diaphragm below and the great vessels above.

Intrapericardial pressure normally ranges between −2 and +2 mmHg, thus it is less than that of the right heart. It falls with the intrapleural pressure during inspiration, resulting in a fall in right-sided cardiac pressures. This causes a modest increase in right heart filling velocities with inspiration. These effects are often exaggerated in patients with clinically significant pericardial disease.

The most common clinical presentations of pericardial disease are pericarditis, effusion, tamponade, and constriction.

Pericarditis

Causes

Infection

The most common causes of acute viral pericarditis are coxsackie B, flu, mumps, hepatitis B, rubella, echovirus 8, and HIV. The typical presentation is with 'flu-like' upper respiratory tract infection along with chest pain that is related to breathing. Sending blood tests for viral titres is not usually conclusive in routine clinical practice. The condition is usually self-limiting.

Bacterial infection (other than tuberculous) is a very rare cause of pericarditis, usually caused by staphylococci, pneumococci, or streptococci spreading directly from the lungs or pleura, particularly in patients with impaired immunity.

Tuberculous infection is an important cause of bacterial pericardial disease, particularly in developing countries. It may take the form of acute pericarditis, pericardial effusion, or constriction. The primary response is an acute pericarditis due to allergic reaction. Chronic pericardial effusion and constriction both reflect granulomatous disease complicated by fibrosis and calcification. Both parietal and visceral layers of the pericardium may be involved, including the epicardial layer of the myocardium. In sub-Saharan Africa most patients (>80%) with tuberculous pericarditis will be HIV positive. This needs to be established before treatment: antituberculous chemotherapy is the first line of management for all, but if there is pericardial effusion or constriction steroids are used for the first few weeks to limit the development of adhesions; hence the need for pericardiectomy in those who are HIV-negative.

Actinomycosis, coccidioidomycosis, histoplasmosis, and hydatid disease can rarely cause pericarditis in endemic areas.

Myocardial infarction

This may be complicated by acute pericarditis in 15% of cases, particularly in patients with transmural infarction, when the ECG demonstrates ST and T wave changes that are more generalized than the segmental distribution of the infarct. A friction rub may be heard and a small effusion may be seen on transthoracic echocardiographic examination. A delayed response 3 to 4 weeks after an acute infarct may present as Dressler's syndrome, with fever and pericardial rub. Although this condition is self limiting it may respond to nonsteroidal anti-inflammatory medications (NSAIDs) and (if needed) steroids.

Autoimmune diseases

Pericardial involvement can be a serious manifestation of rheumatoid disease, systemic lupus erythematosus, systemic sclerosis, and Churg–Strauss syndrome. Presentation can be with pericardial pain, effusion, or even constriction. A small pericardial effusion is seen in most cases of rheumatic fever, but this hardly ever develops into a significant problem. If adhesions develop they may later mature in the form of constriction, a pathology which can be confirmed at the time of valve surgery.

Other medical conditions

Inadequately treated chronic renal failure may be complicated by pericarditis and pericardial effusion. Pericardial tamponade may develop if the effusion remains untreated. Hypothyroidism may be complicated by pericarditis, usually accompanied by a small fluid collection that is unlikely to require drainage.

Irradiation

Irradiation can cause pericarditis soon after treatment, with typical ECG presentation, fluid collection or even constriction. Late presentation can be seen years after irradiation, when the pericardium is thickened and fibrosed.

Clinical features

There are three main features of the clinical syndrome of acute pericarditis—chest pain, pericardial rub, and electrocardiographic changes.

The chest pain occurs at rest and varies with posture and respiration. It is typically sudden in onset (although often preceded by the nonspecific symptoms of a viral illness), retrosternal, continuous, sharp or 'raw' in character, worse on inspiration, radiating to the trapezius ridge, and relieved by sitting up. It needs to be distinguished from ischaemic cardiac pain (particularly in the context of recent myocardial infarction), oesophageal pain, and musculoskeletal pain.

On examination the main feature is the presence of a pericardial rub. This scratching or creaking sound, variably described as being like 'walking on fresh snow' or the 'creaking of new leather', is usually loudest at the left sternal border, but may be heard anywhere in the chest. It often changes with posture, may be louder with inspiration, and can be fleeting, coming and going over a matter of hours. Other elements of the cardiovascular examination are normal unless pericarditis is associated with the presence of sufficient pericardial fluid to cause tamponade, or with pericardial constriction.

The typical ECG change is generalized ST elevation, usually concave upwards, by 1 mm or more. Nonspecific T-wave changes may follow later, after the acute episode has resolved. These changes usually resolve, but they may persist for years afterwards in some cases.

The chest radiograph is not usually helpful in diagnosis: it may show cardiac enlargement, but may be completely normal. Echocardiography is the best technique to show any fluid collection around the heart and to assess its physiological significance.

Although the underlying cause of pericarditis should always be sought, the final diagnosis is often 'idiopathic' or 'presumed viral'. Idiopathic pericarditis is self-limiting and needs only analgesics. Small effusions due to other causes rarely need drainage, but with symptoms the patient may benefit from NSAIDs.

Pericardial effusion

The diagnosis of pericardial effusion is only made when the volume of the fluid in the pericardial space is more than the physiological amount of 50 ml. Two-dimensional echocardiography can detect 100 ml fluid in the pericardial space.

Pericardial effusion can be secondary to cardiac or noncardiac causes. Acute rapid collection is usually caused by traumatic injury, iatrogenic ventricular puncture, or aortic dissection. The common causes of chronic fluid accumulation are viral infection, uraemia, autoimmune rheumatic disease, myocardial infarction, myxoedema, and malignancy. Conditions associated with generalized salt and water retention such as congestive cardiac failure, renal failure, and hepatic cirrhosis may also be complicated by pericardial effusion.

A small, rapidly accumulated effusion may result in raised pericardial pressure and development of symptoms (see 'Pericardial tamponade', below), whereas with a slowly accumulating effusion patients may remain asymptomatic despite the presence of a large volume of fluid because of the corresponding increase in the capacity of the pericardial cavity. Symptoms in uncomplicated pericardial effusion are nonspecific—reduced exercise tolerance or dull aching chest pain—but patients may develop symptoms of mediastinal syndrome: cough caused by bronchial compression, dyspnoea due to lung compression, or hoarseness of voice caused by recurrent laryngeal nerve compression.

On examination distant heart sounds and increase in the area of cardiac dullness to percussion may be the only physical signs until tamponade develops.

The chest radiograph does not always confirm the presence of pericardial effusion if it is less than 250 ml, but when the effusion is large there is an increased cardiothoracic ratio and the cardiac shadow is globally enlarged (Fig. 16.8.1). The ECG may show low voltage QRS complexes, and electrical alternans may be present if the effusion is large, with the heart swinging two and fro within it (Fig. 16.8.2).

Echocardiography is the investigation of choice for confirming the presence of pericardial effusion and for assessing its volume (Fig. 16.8.3). An echo-free space in the pericardium, on both M-mode and two-dimensional images, should be distinguished from anterior pericardial fat pad. Quantitation of pericardial effusion is quite reliable from two-dimensional echocardiographic images: a 1-cm global collection around the heart suggests an approximate amount of 200 ml. With localized effusion, a comparative assessment of the effusion size with that of the left ventricle gives a rough estimation of the collection volume. The haemodynamic effects of pericardial effusion depend on the pressure–volume relation of the pericardium, the speed of fluid collection and the volume of the effusion. Ventricular compliance may also add to the haemodynamic effects of pericardial effusion in patients with ventricular disease.

Pericardial tamponade

Pericardial tamponade is a condition of haemodynamic instability caused by chamber compression because increased intrapericardial pressure is greater than the filling pressure of the right and left ventricles.

Pathophysiology

Provided the pericardium can stretch slowly, more than 2000 ml of fluid can be accumulated without a significant increase in pressure, but rapid accumulation of as little as 200 ml increases pericardial pressure. Inability of the pericardium to distend acutely causes its pressure to rise above right atrial pressure, followed by right ventricular pressure, and eventually results in right ventricular collapse. Intrapericardial and intrapleural pressures normally fall equally during inspiration, but with tamponade intrapericardial pressure does not fall as much, resulting in a reduced pressure gradient between intrathoracic pressure/pulmonary veins and left atrium/left ventricle. This results in reduced left-sided filling velocities during inspiration and hence stroke volume. On the right side of the heart the normal increase in right ventricular dimensions during inspiration enhances right-sided filling and ejection. Progressive increase in pericardial pressure and right ventricular pressure may affect the left heart further, adding to the compromise of its filling during inspiration and exacerbating reduction in stroke volume. The combined effect of these two mechanisms eventually compromises cardiac output.

Pericardial pressure greater than 10 mmHg results in right ventricular collapse and raised diastolic pressures of both ventricles as well as increased capillary wedge pressure. This leads to inspiratory fall of aortic pressure and hence hypotension with pulsus paradoxus (see below). Left ventricular and left atrial collapse are much less commonly seen with tamponade.

Causes

The most common cause of tamponade is malignant effusion or acute fluid collection after cardiac surgery. Intrapericardial clot formation after cardiac surgery or as a complication of an interventional procedure, e.g. trans-septal puncture, may result in signs of tamponade due to the rapid increase in intrapericardial pressure, even in the absence of a significantly large fluid volume. Left ventricular invagination caused by localized collection around the free wall has been reported after open heart surgery. Significant localized posterior effusion is usually caused by anterior adhesions between the right ventricle, the right atrium, and pericardium.

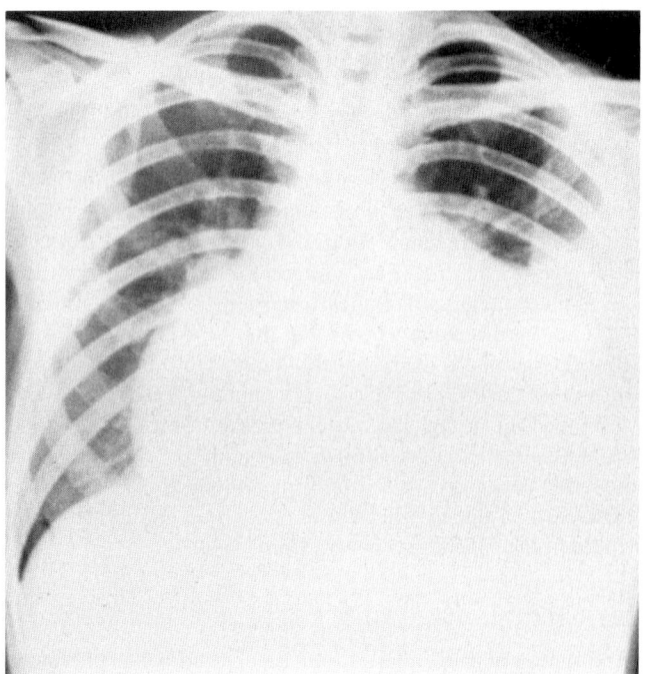

Fig. 16.8.1 Posteroanterior chest radiograph of a patient with a large pericardial effusion. The heart shadow is greatly enlarged and globular in shape. Those parts of the lung fields that can be seen are normal.

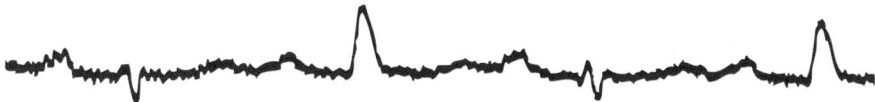

Fig. 16.8.2 ECG from a patient with a massive malignant pericardial effusion. All QRS complexes are sinus beats with a constant PR interval, but the QRS axis alternates, hence the term 'electrical alternans'.

Clinical features

Patients with cardiac tamponade present with shortness of breath or circulatory collapse. The key physical findings to make the diagnosis are tachycardia, pulsus paradoxus of more than 10 mmHg, and elevation of the venous pressure.

Tachycardia (>100/min) is almost invariable, but clearly not specific for tamponade. Pulsus paradoxus describes an exaggeration of the normal fall in systolic blood pressure (up to 10–12 mmHg) on inspiration. With the patient breathing normally, the best way to detect this sign is to stop deflation of the blood pressure cuff as soon as the first Karotkoff sound is heard, in which case in the presence of pulsus paradoxus the sound will disappear on every inhalation and reappear on every exhalation. After noting the systolic pressure reading, the cuff is then gradually deflated until the Karotkoff sound is heard throughout the respiratory cycle, at which point the pressure is again noted—the difference between the two readings is the measurement of the amount of paradox. A pulsus paradoxus of over 10 mmHg is found in 98% of patients with tamponade, over 20 mmHg in 78%, over 30 mmHg in 49%, over 40 mmHg in 38% and total (pulse not palpable on inspiration) in 23%. The most common reason for pulsus paradoxus to be absent in tamponade is profound hypotension. However, although pulsus paradoxus is a sensitive sign of tamponade, it must be noted that it is not specific: it can be seen not infrequently in severe asthma, also (uncommonly) in constrictive pericarditis, right ventricular infarction, and pulmonary embolism.

The venous pressure is always high in cardiac tamponade: if it is not, then the diagnosis is wrong. Usually it is very high, which can make it difficult to see the top. The venous pressure normally falls on inspiration because right heart pressures drop as intrathoracic pressure decreases. Kussmaul's sign is an increase in venous pressure during inspiration, which can be observed (infrequently if at all in most series) in tamponade because of the inability of the right atrium and ventricle to accommodate greater influx of blood.

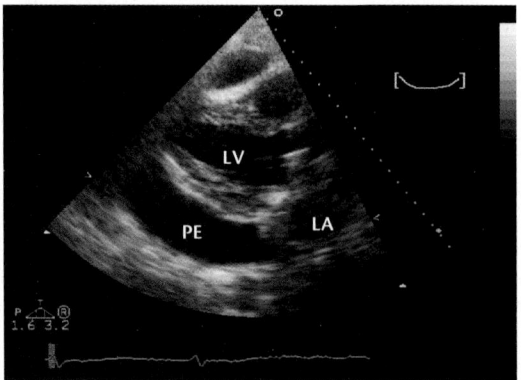

Fig. 16.8.3 Parasternal long axis echocardiographic view from a patient with a large pericardial effusion (Pe), located mostly posteriorly to the left ventricle (Lv). La, left atrium.

Abnormalities of the venous wave form are not helpful in making the diagnosis of tamponade.

In addition to tachycardia, pulsus paradoxus, and elevated venous pressure, patients with tamponade will usually have tachypnoea and cool peripheries, and they may have a pericardial rub.

Differential diagnosis

The main requirement is for the doctor to consider the diagnosis, even if only briefly, when confronted with any patient in unexplained circulatory shock. Tamponade must be distinguished from the common causes of such a presentation, namely hypovolaemia, overwhelming sepsis, severe ventricular disease (e.g. acute myocardial infarction), and pulmonary embolism.

If the patient is shocked with a high venous pressure, then particular consideration needs to be given to pulmonary embolism, right ventricular infarction, and (less commonly) pericardial constriction.

Investigations

The chest radiograph typically shows a large globular heart, which unlike congestive heart failure is not associated with pulmonary venous congestion (Fig. 16.8.1): if pulmonary oedema is present it suggests additional myocardial disease. The ECG shows tachycardia, often with low-voltage QRS complexes, and may reveal electrical alternans (Fig. 16.8.2).

Echocardiography is the most important investigation. It provides clear evidence for fluid collection around the heart, which is usually large with tamponade (Fig. 16.8.3), and is likely to show evidence for diastolic right ventricular or right atrial collapse. Right ventricular collapse is a sensitive (92%) and highly specific (100%) diagnostic sign for tamponade, reflecting transient negative transmural early diastolic pressure as pericardial pressure exceeds right ventricular pressure. Right atrial collapse is less sensitive (82%) but equally specific (100%). In the absence of a haemodynamically significant pericardial effusion, right ventricular diastolic collapse may be caused by bilateral large pleural effusions (Fig. 16.8.4). Right ventricular collapse may be delayed by myocardial hypertrophy, pulmonary hypertension, or free wall adhesions, commonly associated with malignant effusions. Swinging of the heart inside the pericardial fluid may be seen. Doppler recordings of right and left cardiac filling and ejection show inspiratory dominance in the right with reciprocal changes in the left (Fig. 16.8.5). Finally, echocardiography can exclude the presence of large pleural effusion as a potential cause of the clinical and physiological disturbances: it is essential for the echocardiographer to identify the high-intensity echo of the fibrous pericardium posterior to the left ventricle on the left parasternal image—a pericardial effusion is inside this layer and a pleural effusion outside it.

Management

Pericardial tamponade is a medical emergency, particularly when there is clear evidence for arterial paradox, or if the effusion is collecting rapidly. Pericardial aspiration should be performed in an

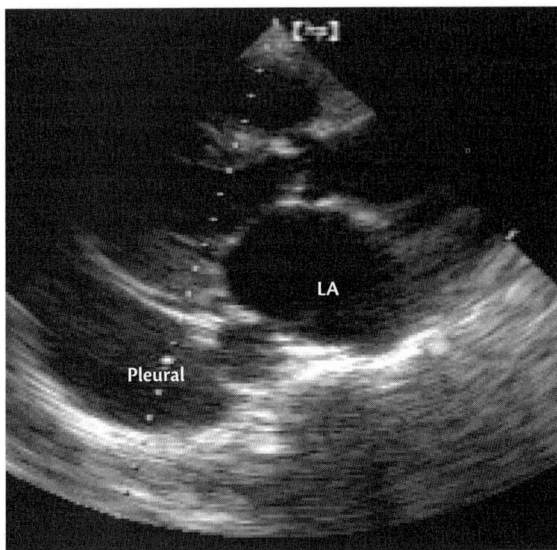

Fig. 16.8.4 Parasternal long axis view showing pleural effusion posterior to the LV.

area where resuscitation facilities are available. Echocardiography is used to determine where to insert the needle and to estimate the depth and direction of advancement. The subcostal route is the most popular because it avoids possible injury to the coronary artery (left anterior descending). After a local anaesthetic is given a larger needle or polythene cannula is introduced into the effusion, followed by a pigtail catheter inserted over a guide wire. A maximum of 500 ml of fluid is removed initially to relieve haemodynamic instability: rapid withdrawal of a larger volume can provoke cardiovascular collapse. Continuous drainage is then commenced and the rest of the effusion drained over the next few hours.

Many pericardial effusions are heavily bloodstained, particularly those that are malignant. The aspirated fluid can be distinguished from blood (usually to the great relief of the doctor performing the procedure) by its colour (dark because very desaturated) and failure to clot (because defibrinated). Fluid should be sent for culture and cytological analysis, and biochemical analysis (glucose and protein) can sometimes be useful.

Surgical creation of a pericardial window is recommended for recurrent or rapidly accumulating effusions, which permits therapeutic pressure relief, fluid drainage, and pericardial biopsy (for culture and histological examination).

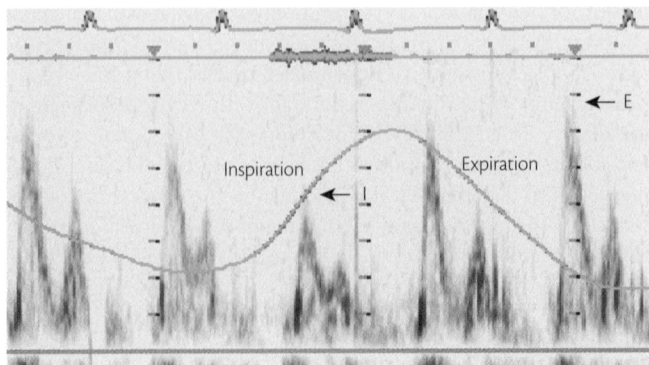

Fig. 16.8.5 Transmitral pulsed Doppler velocities from a patient with large pericardial effusion and tamponade demonstrating significant fall in left ventricular filling velocities with inspiration (arrow, I) compared to expiration (arrow, E).

Constrictive pericarditis

Pericardial constriction is a pathological condition characterized by pericardial thickening and fibrosis that results in adhesion of its two layers. Chronic constrictive pericarditis frequently proves to be 'idiopathic'; a (presumed) viral aetiology frequently invoked when no other cause is found. Tuberculosis is currently an uncommon cause, particularly in developed countries. Other causes include radiation, autoimmune rheumatic disease, chronic renal failure, neoplastic disease, and previous cardiac surgery.

Pathophysiology

The stiff pericardium loses its stretching ability to accommodate normal changes in intracardiac pressures. This is demonstrated by equalization of a raised end-diastolic pressures in the right and left ventricles, with the 'dip and plateau pattern' a cardinal sign for diagnosing pericardial constriction (see Fig. 16.3.4.1).

Pericardial constriction also leads to characteristic abnormalities in the venous pressure waveform, with prominent X and Y descents. The X descent, which occurs after atrial contraction (A wave), is caused by two processes: (1) right atrial relaxation (followed by a positive C wave that is not visible on inspection) and (2) the atrioventricular tricuspid valve ring moving downwards during systole, increasing the volume of the right atrium. A fibrosed and unstretchable pericardium, being adherent to the epicardial layer of the myocardium, can limit its normal movement during the cardiac cycle along the ventricular transverse axis, particularly in systole. It cannot, however, affect shortening and lengthening of the longitudinal myocardial fibres that are located in the subendocardium, hence the downward displacement of the tricuspid ring and valve in systole is preserved, allowing a column of blood to enter the atrium rapidly, thereby producing a characteristic exaggerated X descent (Fig. 16.8.6). Following the X descent the V wave represents right atrial filling, with the Y descent beginning the moment that the tricuspid valve opens at the beginning of diastole and allows blood to enter the ventricle. In pericardial constriction the Y descent is prominent because, from a high venous pressure, diastolic filling is not impaired at the beginning of diastole, only when the relaxing ventricle meets the rigid pericardium. Similar features can be seen in the left-heart physiology.

It should be noted that simply the presence of a thickened pericardium on imaging technique is not a sufficient diagnostic criterion for constrictive physiology. Furthermore, in rare cases of rapidly increasing ventricular volumes, as in dilated cardiomyopathy, the pericardium may be completely normal and yet demonstrate an external constricting effect, thus adding to the deterioration of the clinical condition.

Clinical features

Most patients with constrictive pericarditis present with leg or abdominal swelling and dyspnoea. Rarely the patient can present with jaundice, or with features of nephrotic syndrome or protein-losing enteropathy. The key physical findings are elevated venous pressure, a pericardial 'knock', hepatomegaly, ascites, and oedema.

As with pericardial tamponade, the venous pressure is always high; if it is not, then the diagnosis is almost certainly wrong. However, unlike with pericardial tamponade, the form of the venous waveform is characteristic, with exaggerated X and Y descents (for reasons explained above) that create two conspicuous

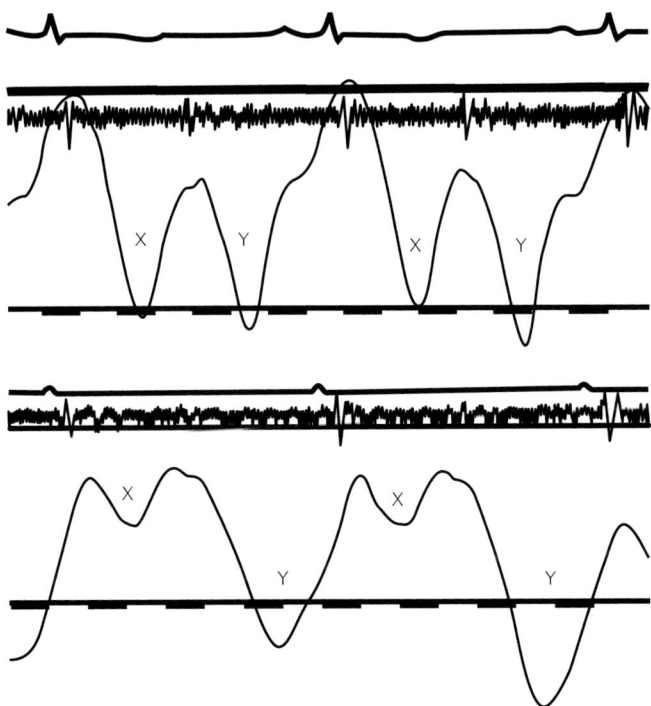

Fig. 16.8.6 Systemic venous pulse from a patient with constrictive pericarditis before (top) and after (bottom) pericardiectomy. Note the 'M' or 'W' pattern, with deep X descent that disappears after pericardiectomy.

dips per cardiac cycle, making the waveform appear to follow an 'M' or 'W' pattern with each arterial pulse (Fig. 16.8.5). Kussmaul's sign (an increase in venous pressure during inspiration) is seen in 50% of cases. Sometimes the changes in venous pressure are transmitted to the liver, which then pulses twice with each cardiac cycle.

A pericardial knock is a loud, high-frequency sound, typically best heard between the left lower sternal border and the apex. It is caused by sudden cessation of ventricular filling as it meets the constriction, and is reported in about 50% of cases in most series.

Other common findings are atrial fibrillation, a mild degree of pulsus paradoxus (≤20 mmHg), and systolic retraction of the apical impulse. A pericardial rub can be heard in some cases.

Differential diagnosis

The main differential diagnosis of constrictive pericarditis is restrictive myocardial disease (see Chapters 16.7.2 and 16.7.3). Distinction between these can be difficult. In restriction ventricular filling becomes limited to early diastole, with high acceleration and deceleration frequently associated with right-sided third heart sound. Respiratory variation of ventricular filling and ejection velocities may be present in constriction but is absent in restrictive right ventricular disease. Imaging (see below) can help to determine if the main abnormality is likely to be pericardial or myocardial.

Pericardial constriction also needs to be distinguished from other causes of raised venous pressure, including obstruction of the superior vena cava, tricuspid stenosis, or tricuspid regurgitation.

Investigations

The chest radiograph is usually normal but may show pericardial calcification, either as multiple plaques or as a rim covering the diaphragmatic and anterior surfaces of the heart. The ECG is not diagnostic, but can show low-voltage QRS complexes and nonspecific T-wave changes. On CT scanning or MRI the pericardium may appear thickened, but this is an insensitive marker for constriction.

Doppler echocardiography is the best noninvasive investigation to demonstrate the systolic descent in the jugular venous pressure and systolic filling of the right atrium from the superior and inferior vena cavae during ventricular systole. Ventricular filling is nonspecific, depending on additional myocardial disease. In constrictive pericarditis there is less intracardiac than extracardiac respiratory variation, particularly on the right side, when compared to that seen with pericardial tamponade. A raised right atrial pressure during inspiration (Kussmaul's sign) and dilated inferior vena cava are nonspecific signs of constriction. Spontaneous contrast in the inferior vena cava, resulting from the limited venous return, may also be an additional finding in favour of constrictive pericarditis.

Cardiac catheterization demonstrates the following diagnostic features for constriction:

♦ A difference of less than 5 mmHg between end-diastolic pressures in the two ventricles, persisting with respiration and fluid loading

♦ A peak right ventricular pressure of less than 50 mmHg

♦ A ratio of end-diastolic to peak right ventricular pressure of more than 0.33

Management

Fluid retention in early pericardial constriction can be managed by diuretics, with pericardiectomy recommended for patients who are resistant. After surgical removal of the pericardium, which is often very difficult, the venous pressure drops and the X descent disappears from the jugular venous pressure (Fig. 16.8.6). This is not always instantaneous and may take up to few days or even weeks to settle.

Pericardial complications after open heart surgery

Apart from the commonly seen pericardial collection, other significant complications may occur that have a major impact on clinical management.

Pericardial clot

A collection of clot in the pericardial space, with or without pericardial effusion, is often associated with delayed postoperative clinical recovery. It may have an important physiological effect on overall cardiac function, irrespective of the amount present. The clinical presentation is typically with cooling of the peripheries, hypotension, and fall in urine output over minutes to hours, and the condition should be suspected particularly in any patient who has bled rather heavily at operation, especially if the blood flow from the chest drains suddenly falls. There are no specific abnormalities on the chest radiograph or ECG; transthoracic echocardiography rarely gives good images immediately postoperatively; transoesophageal echocardiography may show clot alongside the heart. Reopening the chest to remove the clot surgically is the best management, with early detection and removal securing complete recovery.

'Tight' pericardium

In the absence of postoperative pericardial effusion, intrapericardial pressure may be raised to the extent that it affects right-sided physiology so that superior vena caval flow occurs only during inspiration. This condition mimics left ventricular disease and may lead to inappropriate administration of inotropic agents. The jugular venous pressure is raised and right sided filling and ejection is predominantly inspiratory. On two-dimensional echocardiographic images there is no evidence for right atrial or ventricular collapse. Although these signs usually resolve with time, delayed sternal closure has proved beneficial when the clinical manifestations are severe. The condition tends to settle within days or weeks after surgery, with complete normalization of venous pressure.

Restrictive pericarditis

This is a rare clinical presentation that has been documented after open heart surgery, presenting with resistant fluid retention and raised venous pressure. Two-dimensional echocardiographic images may not show any specific abnormality, although MRI may demonstrate a thickened pericardium. The underlying pathology seems to be chronic combined pericardial and epicardial inflammation that results in massive fibrosis and adhesions between the two layers, with myocardial involvement. Patients with this condition are usually resistant to medical therapy, demonstrating signs of restrictive physiology on both sides of the heart with a dominant early diastolic filling component and short deceleration time. Cases resistant to medical therapy may respond to surgical decortication of the pericardium.

Pericardial tumours

The commonest tumours of the pericardium are secondaries from elsewhere, most frequently carcinoma of the breast and lung, malignant melanoma, lymphoma, and leukaemia. They invade the pericardium either directly, or via lymphatics, or by haematogenous dissemination. Primary tumours are rare but include malignant mesothelioma and sarcomas. Whereas carcinomas metastasize in the pericardium in the form of localized masses, lymphomas and leukaemia present in the form of uniform pericardial infiltration and thickening, which may cause tumour incarceration of the heart and hence the clinical syndrome of 'constrictive physiology'. A mild degree of pericardial thickening can easily be missed on echocardiography, but the pattern of ventricular wall motion is characteristic. MRI or CT scanning may be better at showing pericardial thickening. See Chapter 18.19.4 for further discussion.

Recurrent pericardial effusion of unknown aetiology should always suggest malignancy until otherwise proved, as should pericardial effusion in the presence of an intracardiac mass.

Congenital pericardial disease

Congenital anomalies of the pericardium are rare. Pleuropericardial defect, either complete or partial (80% of cases), is the most common form. The left side is most commonly involved in the partial form, allowing the left atrial appendage or part of the left ventricle (if the defect is large) to herniate through the defects. The chest radiograph is characteristic, demonstrating a shift of the heart to the left and prominent main pulmonary artery. Defects in the diaphragmatic portion of the pericardium are extremely rare. In most instances pericardial defects are asymptomatic, but about one-third of cases are associated with congenital abnormalities of the heart and lungs.

Pericardial cysts are very rare, difficult to diagnose, and if present do not cause any clinical problem. Their presence can only be confirmed when found surgically and removed. See Chapter 18.19.4 for further discussion.

Pericardial constriction due to fibrosis of unknown cause may contribute to the clinical picture of Mulibrey (muscle, liver, brain, eye) nanism, which is an autosomal recessive condition characterized by growth failure, a triangular face (often with a hydrocephalus), hypotonia, a peculiar voice, large liver, and yellowish dots and pigment dispersion in the optic fundi.

Further reading

Bertog SC, et al. (2004). Constrictive pericarditis: etiology and cause-specific survival after pericardiectomy. *J Am Coll Cardiol*, **43**, 1445–52.

Callahan JA, et al. (1985). Two-dimensional echocardiographically guided pericardiocentesis: experience in 117 consecutive patients. *Am J Cardiol*, **55**, 476–479.

Cameron J, et al. (1987). The etiologic spectrum of constrictive pericarditis. *Am Heart J*, **113**, 354–360.

Clare GC, Troughton RW (2007). Management of constrictive pericarditis in the 21st century. *Curr Treat Options Cardiovasc Med*, **9**, 436–42.

Clinical Echocardiography by Michael Y. Henein, Mary Sheppard, John R. Pepper, and Michael Rigby. Springer (2004).

Guberman BA, et al. (1981). Cardiac tamponade in medical patients. *Circulation*, **64**, 633–40.

Hatle LK, Appleton CP, Popp RL (1989). Differentiation of constrictive pericarditis and restrictive cardiomyopathy by Doppler echocardiography. *Circulation*, **79**, 357–70.

Henein MY, et al. (1999). Restrictive pericarditis. *Heart*, **82**, 389–92.

Henein MY, et al. (2004). *Clinical Echocardiography*. Springer.

Kochar GS, Jacobs LE, Kotler MN (1990). Right atrial compression in postoperative cardiac patients: detection by transesophageal echocardiography. *J Am Coll Cardiol*, **16**, 511–16.

McGee SR (2001). *Evidence-based physical diagnosis*. W B Saunders, Philadelphia.

Price S, et al. (2004). Tamponade following cardiac surgery: terminology and echocardiography may both mislead. *Eur J Cardiothorac Surg*, **26**, 1156–60.

Reddy PS, et al. (1978). Cardiac tamponade: hemodynamic observations in man. *Circulation*, **58**, 265–272.

Sagrista-Sauleda J, et al. (2004). Effusive-constrictive pericarditis. *N Engl J Med*, **350**, 469–75.

Shabetai R, et al. (1965). Pulsus paradoxus. *J Clin Invest*, **44**, 1882–98.

Shabetai R, Fowler NO, Guntheroth WG (1970). The hemodynamics of cardiac tamponade and constrictive pericarditis. *Am J Cardiol*, **26**, 480–9.

Singh S, et al. (1984). Right ventricular and right atrial collapse in patients with cardiac tamponade—a combined echocardiographic and hemodynamic study. *Circulation*, **70**, 966–71.

Troughton RW, Asher CR, Klein AL (2004). Pericarditis. *Lancet*, **363**, 717–27.

Cardiac involvement in infectious disease

Contents

16.9.1 Acute rheumatic fever

Jonathan R. Carapetis

Essentials

Acute rheumatic fever is an immunologically mediated multisystem disease induced by recent infection with group A streptococcus. About 5% of people have the potential to develop acute rheumatic fever after infection by a strain of streptococcus with propensity to cause the condition. Most cases (97%) occur in developing countries, particularly in sub-Saharan Africa, Pacific nations, Australasia, and the Indian subcontinent. Children aged 5 to 15 years are most commonly affected, and rheumatic heart disease remains the most common acquired heart disease of childhood in the world.

Presentation—after a latent period (1–5 weeks in most cases, but up to 6 months for presentation with chorea) the disease presents with one or more of the following major criteria: (1) carditis—most typically manifest as an apical pansystolic murmur of mitral regurgitation; (2) polyarthritis—severe, large-joint, and migratory; (3) chorea; (4) subcutaneous nodules; (5) erythema marginatum. Other minor criteria that can support the diagnosis include fever, polyarthralgia, elevated acute phase reactants or neutrophil count, prolongation of the PR interval on the ECG.

Diagnosis—in addition to the criteria described above, evidence of preceding group A streptococcal infection is required: (1) positive throat culture, or (2) elevated or rising anti-Streptolysin O or other streptococcal antibody, or (3) rapid antigen test for group A streptococcus, or (4) recent scarlet fever (contentious).

Prognosis and management—untreated acute rheumatic fever lasts for about 3 months. All patients with acute disease should be given penicillin to eradicate the group A streptococcus that precipitated the attack. Children with arthritis or severe arthralgia should be treated with nonsteroidal anti-inflammatory medication (usually salicylates). For severe carditis, many clinicians use oral prednisone or prednisolone at a dose of 40 to 60 mg/day (1–2 mg/kg per day in children), tapering after 2 or 3 weeks, but benefit is not proven. Important prognostic factors are the severity of the acute carditis and the number of recurrences: 30 to 50% of patients with a first episode of acute rheumatic fever will develop chronic rheumatic heart disease, but more than 70% of those with severe carditis at the first episode, or with recurrent episodes.

Secondary prophylaxis—every patient with acute rheumatic fever should immediately commence intramuscular benzathine penicillin G every 3 or 4 weeks, or twice daily oral penicillin V. In patients without carditis, this should continue for 5 years or until age 18, whichever comes later; with mild or healed carditis, for 10 years or until age 25, whichever is longer; those with more severe valvular disease or after valve surgery should have secondary prophylaxis for life.

Primary prophylaxis—a full course of penicillin treatment commencing within 9 days of the onset of symptomatic group A streptococcal pharyngitis will prevent the subsequent development of acute rheumatic fever in most cases, but this is not widely practised in most developing countries and would not prevent those cases of acute rheumatic fever which do not follow a sore throat.

Introduction

Acute rheumatic fever is an immunologically mediated multisystem disease induced by recent infection with group A streptococcus. Most medical practitioners in industrialized countries will rarely, if ever, see a case. However, the dramatic decline in incidence of acute rheumatic fever in industrialized countries during the second half of the 20th century was not replicated in many developing countries, or among some indigenous and other populations living in poverty in industrialized countries. Moreover, acute rheumatic fever has recently returned as an important public health problem in some middle-class regions of the United States of America. Rheumatic heart disease remains the most common acquired heart disease of childhood in the world.

Epidemiology

It was recently estimated that between 15 and 19 million people are affected by rheumatic heart disease, with approximately 280 000 new cases and 230 000 deaths occurring each year as a result. Ninety-seven per cent of acute rheumatic fever cases and deaths occur in developing countries. Although acute rheumatic fever and rheumatic heart disease are relatively common in all developing countries, they occur at particularly high rates in sub-Saharan Africa, Pacific nations, Australasia, and the Indian subcontinent (Fig. 16.9.1.1).

There have been dramatic declines in incidence in recent decades in many Latin American and Asian countries with improving economic and living conditions. In most populations with high incidence, the predisposing conditions are those that promote endemicity and high levels of transmission of group A streptococci: these include overcrowded housing, poor personal and community hygiene, poor access to medical services, and, in some circumstances, widespread skin infection and scabies infestation.

Outbreaks of acute rheumatic fever occurred in middle-class areas of the United States during the 1980s and 1990s. These outbreaks arose because of the emergence of virulent strains of group A streptococci, particularly belonging to M serotypes 1, 3, and 18. By contrast, outbreaks of acute rheumatic fever have rarely, if ever, been described from developing countries; most cases appear to arise from the ongoing circulation of pathogenic group A streptococcal strains in the population.

Recurrent episodes are almost as common as primary episodes in many populations with high incidence rates of acute rheumatic fever. These may lead to accumulated cardiac valvular damage and are therefore responsible for many cases of rheumatic heart disease, yet they are almost entirely preventable using secondary prophylaxis (see later).

In many developing countries, females are affected more than males, although this gender association is stronger for rheumatic heart disease (especially mitral stenosis) than for acute rheumatic fever; this may reflect a greater tendency to recurrences among females. Any female preponderance may relate to inherited characteristics, to greater exposure to group A streptococci because of the increased involvement of girls and young women in child-rearing in most cultures, or to reduced access by females to primary and secondary prophylaxis.

The maximum incidence of acute rheumatic fever is between the ages of 5 and 15 years in all populations. Approximately 5% of cases occur in children younger than 5 years, but very rarely are children younger than 3 years affected. This age distribution parallels that of group A streptococcal pharyngitis, and supports the hypothesis that all cases of acute rheumatic fever follow this condition. However, it may be that cases do not occur in infants or very young children because of the need for maturity of the immune system (particularly of cellular immunity), or sensitization of the immune response by prior streptococcal infections. New cases occur occasionally up to age 30, but rarely beyond. Hypotheses to explain the

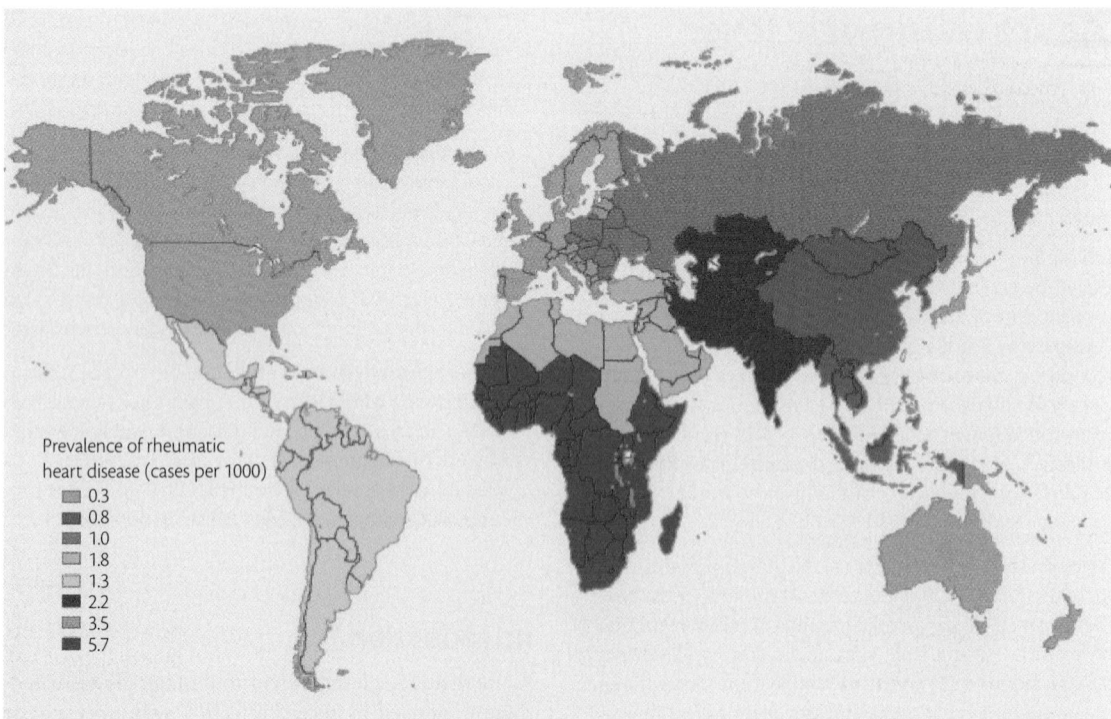

Fig. 16.9.1.1 Prevalence of rheumatic heart disease in children aged 5–14 years. Circles within Australia and New Zealand represent indigenous populations, and also Pacific Islanders in New Zealand.
Reprinted from *The Lancet Infectious Diseases*, Vol. 5, Carapetis JR et al, *The global burden of group A streptococcal diseases*, pp685–94. Copyright (2005), with permission from Elsevier.

reduced incidence in adulthood include development of non-type-specific immunity to primary group A streptococcal infections, further maturation of immune responses, or reduced sensitization by recurrent streptococcal infections.

Pathogenesis

Despite a century of research, the pathogenesis of acute rheumatic fever remains incompletely understood. The presumed pathogenetic pathway is summarized in Fig. 16.9.1.2.

Host factors

Epidemiological evidence suggests that less than 5 to 6% of people have the potential to develop acute rheumatic fever after relevant streptococcal exposure, and that this proportion does not vary substantially between populations. Attack rates of acute rheumatic fever after untreated group A streptococcal pharyngitis vary from less than 1 to 3%. Genetic susceptibility to acute rheumatic fever was first suggested by its familial aggregation and by a greater concordance in monozygotic than in dizygotic twins. The mode of inheritance is uncertain; autosomal recessive or autosomal dominant with partial penetrance have been suggested.

The basis for genetic susceptibility is not known. Recent work suggests an association of rheumatic heart disease with certain HLA class II alleles. A B-cell alloantigen (D8/17) is expressed in a high percentage of B cells from patients with acute rheumatic fever and their family members in many populations. However, D8/17 may not predict susceptibility in all populations; studies in India suggest that different B-cell alloantigens may identify patients with acute rheumatic fever there. However, it is not yet clear whether these putative markers are involved in the pathogenesis of acute rheumatic fever.

Organism factors

The observation that outbreaks of pharyngitis due to certain sero-types of group A streptococcus resulted in high attack rates of acute rheumatic fever, whereas no cases occurred after infection with other serotypes, led to the concept of 'rheumatogenicity'—that only some strains of group A streptococcus have the potential to cause acute rheumatic fever. M serotypes 1, 3, 5, 6, 14, 18, 19, 24, 27, and 29 were most frequently implicated in studies predominantly from the United States of America. However, recent studies from regions with high endemicity of group A streptococcal infections have not found consistent M serotype, or emm genotype, associations with acute rheumatic fever. There may be substantial genetic diversity among strains belonging to a particular M serotype, and not all strains of 'rheumatogenic serotypes' appear to cause acute rheumatic fever. Therefore, rheumatogenicity may be strain specific rather than serotype specific; i.e. any group A streptococcus may acquire the potential to cause acute rheumatic fever.

The pathogenic factor(s) are not known. Parts of the organism have immunological cross-reactivity with human tissue; there is close homology between regions of the M protein and human myosin, tropomyosin, keratin, actin, laminin, vimentin, and N-acetylglucosamine. Other components of group A streptococci, including the hyaluronic acid capsule, the cell-wall associated group-specific carbohydrate, and the cell membrane, cross-react with a variety of human tissues damaged in acute rheumatic fever, including components of heart muscle and valves, joints, and brain. Acute rheumatic fever-associated strains of group A streptococcus also tend to be heavily encapsulated with hyaluronic acid, and not to express opacity factor. Group A streptococci possess components which act as superantigens, selectively stimulating subsets

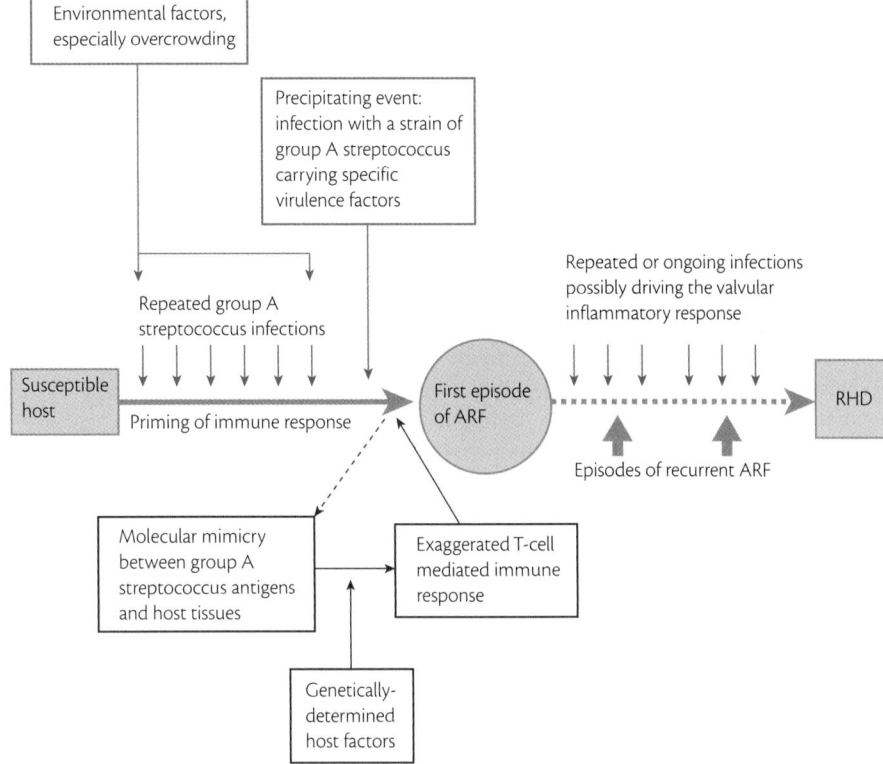

Fig. 16.9.1.2 Pathogenetic pathway for acute rheumatic fever and rheumatic heart disease. Simplified approach to understanding the pathogenesis of acute rheumatic fever. ARF, acute rheumatic fever; RHD, rheumatic heart disease.
Reprinted from The Lancet, Vol. 366, Carapetis JR, McDonald M, Wilson NJ, *Acute rheumatic fever*, pp155–68. Copyright (2005), with permission from Elsevier.

of T cells without the need for antigen presentation. Their role in acute rheumatic fever pathogenesis is not yet clear.

Site of infection

Although it is widely accepted that acute rheumatic fever may result from group A streptococcal infection of the upper respiratory tract, but not of the skin, there is some evidence that this may not always be the case. Upper respiratory tract infection certainly accounts for most, if not all, episodes of acute rheumatic fever in countries with a temperate climate. However, in tropical countries where streptococcal impetigo is highly endemic but group A streptococcal pharyngitis less common, it may be that skin infection accounts for many cases of acute rheumatic fever, either *de novo* or after subsequent throat infection. Determining whether group A streptococcal skin infection may have a role in pathogenesis of acute rheumatic fever would have enormous public health implications, as it may redirect present approaches to primary prevention (see later).

The immune response

Molecular mimicry between group A streptococcal epitopes and human tissue is the basis for the autoimmune response that leads to rheumatic fever. It is thought that epitopes in cardiac myosin, normally sequestered from the immune response, are exposed by normal cardiac cell turnover. This leads to sensitization of T cells, which may then be recalled following subsequent exposure to group A streptococci. However, myosin cross-reactivity with M protein does not explain the valvular damage that is the hallmark of rheumatic carditis. The link may be laminin, another α-helical coiled-coil protein like myosin and M protein, which is found in cardiac endothelium and is recognized by anti-myosin, anti-M protein T cells. Moreover, antibodies to cardiac valve tissue cross-react with the *N*-acetylglucosamine of group A streptococcal carbohydrate, and there is some evidence that these antibodies may be responsible for valvular damage. Overall, it is not entirely clear if the initial damage in rheumatic fever is primarily due to cellular or humoral immunity, but it does appear that ongoing damage is mainly due to T cell and macrophage infiltration.

Clinical manifestations

There is always a latent period between group A streptococcal infection and the development of acute rheumatic fever. This varies from 1 to 5 weeks in most cases (usually *c*.3 weeks), but may be shorter in recurrences. Chorea may occur up to 6 months after the precipitating streptococcal infection. The preceding infection is asymptomatic in about two-thirds of cases.

The tissues most commonly affected are the heart, joints, and brain. Although the symptoms due to each can be disabling in the short term, only cardiac damage may be permanent and progressive. Therefore, the focus in controlling or treating acute rheumatic fever is always to prevent the development of rheumatic heart disease.

The frequency with which the various clinical manifestations have occurred in recent descriptions of acute rheumatic fever is listed in Table 16.9.1.1.

Carditis

Although inflammation in acute rheumatic fever may affect the pericardium (causing pericardial rubs and occasionally pleuritic

Table 16.9.1.1 Frequency of clinical manifestations in acute rheumatic fever

Manifestation	Proportion of patients with manifestation (%)	
	Chorea[a] absent	Chorea[a] present
Carditis	40–60	20–30
Polyarthritis	50–75	<10
Erythema marginatum	1–10	0–1
Subcutaneous nodules	1–10	0–1
Fever >37.5 °C	>90	10–25
Arthralgia	<10–20	<5
Elevated acute phase reactants	>90	10–25
Prolonged PR interval	30–50	5–10

[a] Chorea is present in <10% to >30% of patients with acute rheumatic fever, depending on the population.

chest pain) or the myocardium (sometimes causing cardiac failure, and evident on biopsy with pathognomonic Aschoff bodies), endocardial inflammation is the most important cause of cardiac damage. If either acute cardiac failure or chronic cardiac disease occurs, it is almost always due to damage to the cardiac valves.

A murmur is the most common evidence of acute valvular disease, usually the apical pansystolic murmur of mitral regurgitation, with or without a low-pitched mid-diastolic (Carey–Coombs) murmur. Occasionally an aortic regurgitant murmur may be heard, mainly in older adolescents or young adults. Murmurs of tricuspid or pulmonary regurgitation are rare and are usually secondary to increased pulmonary venous pressures resulting from mitral regurgitation or stenosis. Sinus tachycardia or gallop rhythms may also be present in acute carditis.

Valves affected by rheumatic carditis may have a characteristic appearance or pattern of regurgitation on Doppler echocardiography (when interpreted by experienced technicians), which may be found even in the absence of a cardiac murmur. This may be useful for diagnosis when other clinical manifestations are not definitive. However, echocardiographic criteria have not yet been standardized, and it is difficult to distinguish acute carditis from previous rheumatic valve damage.

Mitral or aortic stenosis may develop as later complications of severe and/or recurrent acute carditis due to scarring and contraction following the acute inflammatory process. Rarely, mitral stenosis may occur in young children with acute rheumatic fever—so-called 'juvenile mitral stenosis'—the reasons for the development of this condition are not clear.

Damage to the electrical conduction pathways may result in prolongation of the PR interval on electrocardiography. Although a subset of healthy people may have this finding, the presence of a prolonged PR interval that resolves over the ensuing few days to weeks may be a useful diagnostic feature in cases where the clinical manifestations are not clear. Occasionally, in the acute phase, second- or third-degree heart block or a nodal rhythm may be present (Fig. 16.9.1.3).

Arthritis

The characteristic joint manifestation of acute rheumatic fever is severe, large-joint, migratory polyarthritis. The knees, ankles, wrists, and elbows are most commonly involved; only rarely, and

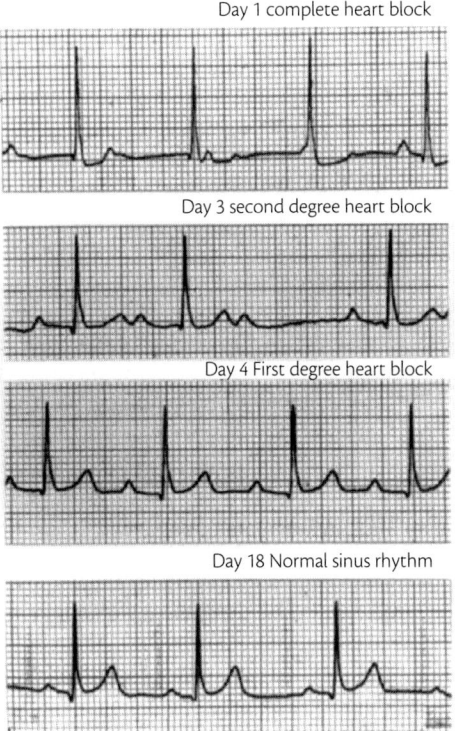

Fig. 16.9.1.3 Electrocardiographic changes in a young adult with acute rheumatic fever, showing evolution over 18 days from complete heart block, to second-degree (Wenckebach) block, to first-degree block, and then to normal sinus rhythm.
From Bishop W et al. (1996). A subtle presentation of acute rheumatic fever in remote northern Australia. Australian and New Zealand Journal of Medicine 26, 241–2. http://www3.interscience.wiley.com/journal/119957992/abstract.

usually only when the patient is untreated for several days, are the hips or small joints of the hands or feet inflamed. One joint characteristically becomes exquisitely painful and inflamed as another is waning. Most patients have only one or two joints affected at any one time, and each joint may be involved for just a few hours or up to 1 or 2 days. The arthritis is so responsive to nonsteroidal anti-inflammatory medication (NSAIDs) that its persistence more than 1 or 2 days after commencing high-dose aspirin should lead one to consider alternative diagnoses.

Arthritis of a single large joint is increasingly described in acute rheumatic fever from regions with high rates of disease. This is sometimes, but not always, due to early administration of anti-inflammatory medication, before the typical migratory pattern has emerged. Other causes of mono-arthritis, including septic arthritis, should first be excluded before a diagnosis of acute rheumatic fever is entertained. Arthralgia (joint pain without objective evidence of inflammation) is usually migratory and affects large joints, and like the arthritis of acute rheumatic fever is very responsive to NSAIDs.

Sydenham's chorea

In 1686 the English physician Thomas Sydenham described rheumatic chorea, initially naming it 'St Vitus' dance'. It is the most intriguing manifestation of acute rheumatic fever, particularly as it commonly occurs in the absence of other manifestations, usually follows a prolonged latent period (up to 6 months) after the precipitating group A streptococcal infection, and occurs most commonly

in females (and almost never in postpubertal males). The rapid, jerky, involuntary movements affect predominantly the upper limbs and face, may be asymmetrical, and may be sufficiently severe to render the patient unable to eat, drink, walk, or perform other activities of daily living. Mild chorea can sometimes be detected by having the patient join palms above the head to reveal occasional twitches of the arms or the head. Typical signs include the 'milkmaid's grip' (rhythmic squeezing when the patient grasps the examiner's fingers), spooning of extended hands (caused by flexion of the wrists and extension of the fingers), darting of the protruded tongue, and the 'pronator sign' (the arms and palms turn outwards when held above the head). As with other forms of chorea, the disorder usually becomes more evident with anxiety or purposeful movements (such as drinking or writing). Movements may appear semi-purposeful, and symptoms subside during sleep. Sydenham's chorea is often associated with excessive emotional lability or personality changes, which may precede the abnormal movements.

Most patients can be reassured that Sydenham's chorea will resolve completely and leave no long-lasting effects, usually within 6 weeks and almost always within 6 months, but rarely lasting up to 3 years.

Subcutaneous nodules and erythema marginatum

Both of these manifestations are found in less than 2% of patients with acute rheumatic fever, although they were described in up to 10 to 20% of patients in earlier studies from the United States of America and the United Kingdom. Subcutaneous nodules are firm, painless lumps, usually between 0.5 and 2 cm in diameter, commonly found in crops of three or more, and usually appear 2 to 3 weeks after the onset of acute rheumatic fever. They occur mainly over extensor surfaces or bony protuberances, particularly the hands, feet, occiput, and back. The nodules are similar, though often smaller, to those found in rheumatoid arthritis, and are most likely to be associated with severe carditis. Nodules usually last from a few days to 2 or 3 weeks.

The characteristic rash, erythema marginatum, appears as a light pink macule that spreads outwards with a serpiginous, well-demarcated edge, while the central portion clears. It appears, disappears, or moves before the observer's eyes. Multiple areas are often involved, usually over the trunk, occasionally over the proximal portions of the limbs, but rarely, if ever, the face. It usually appears together with the other initial symptoms of acute rheumatic fever, but may recur intermittently for weeks or even months. This does not indicate ongoing rheumatic inflammation, and patients can be reassured that the rash will eventually disappear without complications.

Fever

With the exception of those with pure chorea, 90% of patients will have a temperature at presentation higher than 37.5 °C. Although it has been reported that the temperature usually exceeds 39 °C, others have found only 25% of confirmed cases with fever to that level. Any temperature above 37.5 °C should be considered a minor manifestation. As with arthritis, fever is very sensitive to NSAIDs, usually resolving completely within 1 or 2 days of commencing high-dose salicylates.

Elevated acute phase reactants

Almost all patients, except those with pure chorea, have a dramatically elevated erythrocyte sedimentation rate or serum C-reactive protein. There appears little difference between these measurements in their diagnostic usefulness. The C-reactive protein may return to normal more rapidly than the sedimentation rate when rheumatic activity subsides. Mild to moderate peripheral leucocytosis is common, although this is a less sensitive marker of rheumatic inflammation.

Other features

Severe central abdominal pain is found at presentation in a small proportion of patients. It may be associated with other features of acute rheumatic fever; if not, these features usually appear within 1 or 2 days. The pain responds quickly to NSAIDs. Epistaxis was reported frequently in historical accounts of acute rheumatic fever, but does not feature prominently in recent descriptions. Pulmonary infiltrates may be found in patients with acute carditis; this has been labelled 'rheumatic pneumonia' although it is not clear whether the infiltrates represent rheumatic inflammation or another process. There may be microscopic haematuria, pyuria, or proteinuria; also mild elevations of liver transaminases: these are nonspecific and not usually severe.

Associated poststreptococcal syndromes

Poststreptococcal reactive arthritis has been differentiated from rheumatic fever by some authors because it has a shorter incubation period after streptococcal infection, sometimes follows non-group A β-haemolytic streptococcal infection, may have a different pattern of arthritis (including small joint involvement), and is less responsive to NSAIDs. Because of the lack of cardiac involvement, these patients are said not to require secondary prophylaxis. However, descriptions of patients who have subsequently developed carditis have led other authors to question the distinction between poststreptococcal reactive arthritis and rheumatic fever. If poststreptococcal reactive arthritis is diagnosed, secondary prophylaxis should be prescribed for at least 1 year and discontinued if there is no evidence of carditis. In populations with high incidence rates of acute rheumatic fever, it may be prudent to treat all cases of possible poststreptococcal reactive arthritis as acute rheumatic fever.

The frequent finding of emotional lability, motor hyperactivity, and occasional obsessive–compulsive symptoms in patients with Sydenham's chorea led to the observation that group A streptococcal infections may precipitate or exacerbate other disorders of the basal ganglia. These include tic disorders, Tourette's syndrome, and obsessive–compulsive disorder, and the term PANDAS (paediatric autoimmune neuropsychiatric disorders associated with streptococcal infections) has been coined. The existence of PANDAS is not universally accepted. Patients with PANDAS are said not to be at risk of developing carditis. There is evidence that these patients, and some children with autism, have high proportions of circulating B cells expressing D8/17 antigen, which is a proposed marker of rheumatic fever susceptibility. It is not yet clear whether these syndromes are linked with acute rheumatic fever.

Diagnosis

Because of the diversity of symptoms and signs, and the nonspecific nature of most of them, Dr T Duckett Jones developed a set of criteria to aid in the diagnosis of acute rheumatic fever in 1944. The Jones criteria have subsequently been revised and updated a number of times to improve their positive and negative predictive values, most recently in 1992. These 1992 criteria are to be used only for the diagnosis of the initial episode of acute rheumatic fever. In response to uncertainty about how to use the Jones criteria for the diagnosis of recurrent episodes, a World Health Organization (WHO) expert committee published the 2002–2003 WHO Criteria, which are now the standard for acute rheumatic fever diagnosis (Table 16.9.1.2).

The manifestations are divided into major, those which are most predictive of acute rheumatic fever, and minor, those which are commonly found in acute rheumatic fever but are less specific. The diagnosis of an initial episode requires the presence of either two major, or one major and two minor criteria, plus the demonstration of a current or recent group A streptococcal infection. Evidence of group A streptococcal infection is not required for chorea, where the onset may be delayed up to 6 months after streptococcal infection, and late-onset carditis, when low-grade inflammation may persist for prolonged periods after the precipitating infection. Recurrences can be diagnosed with less stringent criteria.

Proof of a recent group A streptococcal infection can include demonstrating the organism in the upper respiratory tract, either by culture or rapid antigen techniques. However, most children with acute rheumatic fever no longer have a group A streptococcus detectable by these methods, and up to 15 to 25% of normal children in temperate climate countries may carry the organism in their throats. Serological techniques are therefore most commonly used, particularly the antistreptolysin O, anti-DNase B, or antihyaluronidase titres. One of any two of these tests will be positive in well over 90% of recent streptococcal infections. Their usefulness is increased by performing more than one serological test, or by demonstrating rising titres in paired sera. Serology is of limited value in regions with high prevalence rates of streptococcal impetigo, where children may have positive antistreptococcal titres most of the time. There is therefore a need for a better diagnostic test of recent streptococcal infection, or an objective diagnostic test for acute rheumatic fever itself.

The most common clinical presentation, that of a child with fever and polyarthritis, raises multiple differential diagnoses that will vary by region. Table 16.9.1.3 lists some alternative diagnostic possibilities for the three most common major manifestations.

Treatment

If untreated, acute rheumatic fever lasts on average for 3 months. Except in the case of life-threatening acute carditis, there is no evidence that presently available treatments alter the outcome. Most treatments are designed to provide symptomatic relief or are based on theoretical (but unproven) approaches to attenuating the long-term damage.

If practical, all patients with acute rheumatic fever should be admitted to hospital to confirm the diagnosis, perform baseline investigations to ascertain the status of the heart, provide adequate treatment for the acute phase, commence secondary prophylaxis, allow communication of details to personnel responsible for long-term follow-up of the patient, and begin education of the patient and family. The mainstays of treatment are bed rest, penicillin, and salicylates.

Bed rest

Previous recommendations that children with acute rheumatic fever be rested in bed until all signs of active inflammation abated

Table 16.9.1.2 2002–03 World Health Organization criteria for the diagnosis of rheumatic fever and rheumatic heart disease (based on the 1992 revised Jones criteria)

Diagnostic categories	Criteria
Primary episode of rheumatic fever[a]	Two major or one major and two minor manifestations plus evidence of preceding group A streptococcal infection
Recurrent attack of rheumatic fever in a patient without established rheumatic heart disease	Two major or one major and two minor manifestations plus evidence of preceding group A streptococcal infection
Recurrent attack of rheumatic fever in a patient with established rheumatic heart disease[b]	Two minor manifestations plus evidence of preceding group A streptococcal infection[c]
Rheumatic chorea Insidious onset rheumatic carditis[b]	Other major manifestations or evidence of group A streptococcal infection not required
Chronic valve lesions of rheumatic heart disease (patients presenting for the first time with pure mitral stenosis or mixed mitral valve disease and/or aortic valve disease)[d]	Do not require any other criteria to be diagnosed as having rheumatic heart disease
Major manifestations	Carditis
	Polyarthritis
	Chorea
	Erythema marginatum
	Subcutaneous nodules
Minor manifestations	Clinical: fever, polyarthralgia
	Laboratory: elevated ESR or leucocyte count[e]
	Electrocardiogram: prolonged PR interval
Supporting evidence of a preceding streptococcal infection within the last 45 days	Elevated or rising anti-Streptolysin O or other streptococcal antibody, or A positive throat culture, or Rapid antigen test for group A streptococcus, or Recent scarlet fever[e]

[a] Patients may present with polyarthritis (or with only polyarthralgia or monoarthritis) and with several (three or more) other minor manifestations, together with evidence of recent group A streptococcal infection. Some of these cases may later turn out to be rheumatic fever. It is prudent to consider them as cases of 'probable rheumatic fever' (once other diagnoses are excluded) and advise regular secondary prophylaxis. Such patients require close follow up and regular examination of the heart. This cautious approach is particularly suitable for patients in vulnerable age groups in high incidence settings.

[b] Infective endocarditis should be excluded.

[c] Some patients with recurrent attacks may not fulfil these criteria.

[d] Congenital heart disease should be excluded

[e] 1992 Revised Jones criteria do not include elevated leucocyte count as a laboratory minor manifestation (but do include elevated C-reactive protein), and do not include recent scarlet fever as supporting evidence of a recent streptococcal infection.

WHO Expert Consultation on *Rheumatic Fever and Rheumatic Heart Disease, Rheumatic fever and rheumatic heart disease: report of a WHO Expert Consultation* (WHO Technical Report Series, 923), p23. Copyright (2004) Geneva; World Health Organization. Reproduced with permission.

Table 16.9.1.3 Differential diagnoses of common major presentations of acute rheumatic fever

	Presentation		
	Polyarthritis and fever	Carditis	Chorea
Differential diagnoses	Septic arthritis (including gonococcal)	Innocent murmur	SLE
	Connective tissue and other autoimmune disease[a]	Mitral valve prolapse	Drug intoxication
	Viral arthropathy[b]	Congenital heart disease	Wilson's disease
	Reactive arthropathy[b]	Infective endocarditis	Tic disorder[c]
	Lyme disease	Hypertrophic cardiomyopathy	Choreoathetoid cerebral palsy
	Sickle cell anaemia	Myocarditis—viral or idiopathic	Encephalitis
	Infective endocarditis	Pericarditis—viral or idiopathic	Familial chorea (including Huntington's)
	Leukaemia or lymphoma		Intracranial tumour
	Gout and pseudogout		Lyme disease
			Hormonal[d]

SLE, systemic lupus erythematosus.

[a] Includes rheumatoid arthritis, juvenile chronic arthritis, inflammatory bowel disease, systemic lupus erythematosus, systemic vasculitis, sarcoidosis, among others.

[b] Mycoplasma, cytomegalovirus, Epstein–Barr virus, parvovirus, hepatitis, rubella vaccination, and yersinia and other gastrointestinal pathogens.

[c] Possibly including PANDAS (pediatric autoimmune neuropsychiatric disorder associated with streptococcal infection).

[d] Includes oral contraceptives, pregnancy (chorea gravidarum), hyperthyroidism, hypoparathyroidism.

Reprinted from *The Lancet*, Vol. 366, Carapetis JR, McDonald M, Wilson NJ, *Acute rheumatic fever*, pp155–68. Copyright (2005), with permission from Elsevier.

were probably more extreme than is necessary. Once symptoms of arthritis have subsided and any cardiac failure is controlled, the child may begin gentle mobilization, which may be increased as tolerated. There is no evidence that bed rest beyond the period where mobilization leads to exacerbation of pain or cardiac failure has any long-term benefit.

Penicillin

All patients with acute rheumatic fever should be given penicillin to eradicate the group A streptococcus that precipitated the attack. This is based on an early finding that, in some cases, prolonged group A streptococcal infection led to more severe acute rheumatic fever. Although in most cases the precipitating organism cannot be cultured, a treatment course of penicillin is prudent in case the strain remains present in low numbers, and to prevent its transmission to other contacts. As the aim is eradication of group A streptococcal infection, penicillin may be administered either as a single intramuscular injection of benzathine penicillin G at a dose of 1.2 million units (600 000 U for patients <30 kg) into the gluteal or quadriceps muscles, or as a 10-day course of oral phenoxymethyl penicillin (V) at a dose of 500 mg (adolescents and adults) or

250 mg (children) given either two or three times daily. In the case of penicillin allergy, the present recommendation is to use oral erythromycin at 20 to 40 mg/kg per day given two to four times daily for 10 days, although in some regions levels of erythromycin resistance among group A streptococci are increasing.

Salicylates

Children with arthritis or severe arthralgia should be treated with NSAIDs; salicylates have been most widely used. Aspirin at a dose of 80 to 100 mg/kg per day (4–8 g/day in adults) usually results in defervescence and resolution of arthritis and arthralgia within 1 to 2 days. Sometimes these doses lead to nausea or vomiting, which can be minimized by increasing from lower starting doses. After a few days or up to 2 weeks, when the initial symptoms are abating, the dose can be reduced to 60 to 70 mg/kg per day for the remaining 2 to 4 weeks. Arthritis or arthralgia may return up to 2 to 3 weeks after discontinuation of therapy; this is usually a brief and mild recrudescence, often associated with increased erythrocyte sedimentation rate or C-reactive protein, and can be managed either with rest and reassurance or a short course of lower-dose NSAIDs.

When the diagnosis is uncertain, salicylates should be withheld for a day or two to look for the development of characteristic migratory polyarthritis. In such cases, paracetamol or codeine can be used to control pain until the diagnosis is confirmed. There is no evidence that salicylates reduce the severity of acute carditis or the risk of chronic cardiac valve damage.

Corticosteroids

For many years, corticosteroids have been used in acute rheumatic fever, particularly for patients with severe carditis. Two meta-analyses have found no evidence that they reduce the risk of long-term valve damage. However, the studies included in these meta-analyses were all conducted more than 40 years ago and used corticosteroid medications not in common usage today. Many clinicians continue to use oral prednisone or prednisolone at a dose of 40 to 60 mg/day (1–2 mg/kg per day in children), tapering after 2 or 3 weeks, in the belief that this might reduce the severity of acute carditis.

Treatment of cardiac failure

There is no doubting the need to treat cardiac failure. Diuretics, angiotensin-converting enzyme (ACE) inhibitors (especially in aortic regurgitation), and fluid restriction are most commonly employed. Digoxin is usually restricted to cases where atrial fibrillation coexists with cardiac failure, often found in older patients with established mitral stenosis.

If medical therapy fails, cardiac surgery should be considered, even during the acute phase. In populations where fulminant acute carditis is relatively common (e.g. South Africa), mitral valve repair or replacement can be life saving and surgeons have developed techniques for undertaking these procedures despite friable, acutely inflamed valvular and perivalvular tissues. In recent years, there has been a greater tendency to undertake valve repair rather than replacement, or to use homografts or xenografts rather than mechanical prostheses. This is to avoid high rates of thromboembolic complications associated with mechanical prostheses, particularly in populations where compliance with anticoagulation chemotherapy is suboptimal and there are difficulties in monitoring coagulation indices.

Treatment of chorea

Sydenham's chorea always resolves, and in most cases there is no need for medical treatment. However, medications may reduce abnormal movements in moderate or severe chorea. Carbamazepine or sodium valproate are recommended as first-line treatment, haloperidol less commonly because of its side-effect profile. Other medications sometimes employed include pimozide, chlorpromazine, or benzodiazepines. All of these medications should be used sparingly and only for limited periods, and the tendency to try multiple medications should be avoided.

Salicylates and steroids have no role in treatment of chorea. Psychotherapeutic interventions have little role in the short to medium term, and may increase the stigma of this self-limited organic disease. However, behavioural therapy should be considered if longer-term behavioural abnormalities persist (e.g. emotional lability, obsessive–compulsive traits).

Newer therapies

Because of the autoimmune nature of acute rheumatic fever, immunomodulatory therapies have been tried. Intravenous immune globulin (IVIG) has been given in some small trials. One study showed no apparent benefit on rate of improvement of clinical, laboratory, or echocardiographic parameters of acute carditis, but another suggested that it may accelerate recovery from chorea. Other therapies have yet to be formally assessed.

Prognosis and follow-up

The most important prognostic factors are the severity of the acute carditis and the number of recurrences. Overall, approximately 30 to 50% of patients with a first episode of acute rheumatic fever will develop chronic rheumatic heart disease. This increases to more than 70% in patients with severe carditis at the first episode, or in those who have had at least one recurrence.

Any patient with acute rheumatic fever requires long-term follow-up. Follow-up assessments should focus on cardiac status, adherence to secondary prophylaxis, early treatment of group A streptococcal pharyngitis, and prevention of streptococcal pyoderma (including hygiene and treatment or prevention of scabies infestation). Patients with evidence of cardiac valve damage should be assessed regularly by specialist physicians and considered for cardiac surgery before substantial left ventricular dysfunction occurs. Vasoactive drugs, particularly ACE inhibitors, may delay the need for operation in asymptomatic patients with chronic aortic regurgitation. Regular echocardiography may be useful to follow the progress of rheumatic heart disease, especially in populations where follow-up may be irregular or in whom communication or cultural differences make clinical assessment difficult.

Recurrences

About 75% of all recurrences occur within 2 years of an episode of acute rheumatic fever. The reasons for this are not known, but are thought to relate to a time-dependent sensitization of the immune response. The clinical features of recurrences tend to mimic those present at the initial episode, particularly in the case of chorea. However, this rule is not absolute, and the risk of developing other manifestations, particularly carditis, increases with each recurrence. The practical implication of this is that the absence of carditis at the first episode does not help to identify patients who may not need secondary prophylaxis.

Prevention of acute rheumatic fever

Secondary prophylaxis

Every patient with acute rheumatic fever should immediately commence secondary prophylaxis: long-term, regular antibiotics to prevent primary group A streptococcal infections. This strategy is proven to reduce the incidence of recurrences and the risk of developing chronic rheumatic heart disease.

The optimal regimen is 1.2 million units of intramuscular benzathine penicillin G every 3 or 4 weeks, and this is commonly given in populations with high incidences of acute rheumatic fever and programmes in place to support the regimen. Higher doses (1.8 or 2.4 million U) given every 4 weeks may have similar effect, but further evidence is needed before such regimens can be recommended routinely. An alternative strategy is to use oral penicillin V at a dose of 250 mg twice daily; this is almost as effective as using benzathine penicillin G, but adherence is usually less reliable.

For patients proven to be allergic to penicillin, the present recommendation is to use oral erythromycin at a dose of 250 mg twice daily. Recent trials have shown newer oral cephalosporins to be effective at eliminating upper respiratory tract carriage of group A streptococci. However, none of these antibiotics have been evaluated for their ability to prevent acute rheumatic fever.

The duration of secondary prophylaxis is dictated by the reducing risk of recurrence with increasing age, with time since the last episode, and the possible consequences of recurrences. In patients without carditis, secondary prophylaxis should continue for 5 years following the most recent episode or until age 18 years, whichever comes last. In patients with mild or healed carditis, prophylaxis should be continued for 10 years following the most recent episode or until age 25 years, whichever is longer. Patients with more severe valvular disease or those who have undergone valve surgery should have secondary prophylaxis for life.

Primary prophylaxis

A full course of penicillin treatment commencing within 9 days of the onset of symptomatic group A streptococcal pharyngitis will prevent the subsequent development of acute rheumatic fever in most cases. After the diagnosis has been confirmed by a throat culture or rapid antigen diagnostic test, the treatment of choice is penicillin, administered either as a single intramuscular injection of benzathine penicillin G (600 000 U for children who weigh <30 kg, or 1.2 million U for larger children and adults) or as a full 10 days of oral (phenoxymethyl) penicillin V (250 mg for children or 500 mg for adults given two to three times daily). The importance of completion of the 10-day course, even if symptoms abate quickly, should be stressed to patients and parents. Shorter courses of oral penicillin treatment are associated with higher risks of acute rheumatic fever. There has never been a clinical isolate of group A streptococcus that is resistant to penicillin; therefore, the use of other antibiotics for primary prophylaxis should be restricted to patients who are allergic to penicillin.

In the case of penicillin allergy, a 10-day course of an oral macrolide such as erythromycin is recommended. First-generation oral cephalosporins may also be considered. However, these agents have not been evaluated in populations with high incidences of acute rheumatic fever. Shorter courses (e.g. 5 days) of some later-generation oral cephalosporins and azolides appear to be effective in eradicating carriage, but because of their expense and broader spectrum of antimicrobial activity they should be considered as second-line agents.

It is not possible to predict which episodes of group A streptococcal pharyngitis will precipitate acute rheumatic fever, so this treatment must be offered in all cases to be effective. Unlike prevention of recurrent episodes, which is virtually complete using secondary prophylaxis, penicillin treatment of streptococcal pharyngitis will at best prevent only the one-third or so of cases of acute rheumatic fever that follow a sore throat. However, this important intervention may arrest the spread of pathogenic group A streptococci in the community. Penicillin treatment of group A streptococcal pharyngitis should begin as early as possible in patients with a history of acute rheumatic fever, should they not be taking secondary prophylaxis, but even then may not prevent a recurrence, hence the need for secondary prophylaxis.

In recent years the use of primary prophylaxis has been questioned in some industrialized countries where acute rheumatic fever is now rare. It is argued that the strategy prevents few cases of acute rheumatic fever but contributes to overuse of antibiotics. Similar arguments were raised in the United States of America during the 1970s, but faded somewhat with the resurgence of acute rheumatic fever in that country during the 1980s. Any country considering abandoning primary prophylaxis should first have in place effective surveillance to detect changes in the epidemiology of primary group A streptococcal infections and the appearance of cases of acute rheumatic fever.

Primary prophylaxis is unsuccessful in many developing countries. It requires trained health workers, microbiology laboratories, transportation and communication infrastructure, the availability of penicillin, and a population likely to seek and adhere to treatment for sore throats. In some high-risk populations, all patients with sore throats receive intramuscular benzathine penicillin G without further attempts at diagnosis; the cost-effectiveness of this strategy has not been fully determined. Clinical algorithms to identify patients with group A streptococcal pharyngitis without resorting to laboratory tests have not been validated sufficiently for them to be recommended universally. Even if primary prophylaxis were to be instituted effectively in developing countries, acute rheumatic fever would not disappear, as most cases do not follow a sore throat.

Other methods of primary prevention are clearly needed in developing countries. Improved living standards and access to primary health care seem to be years or decades away in many places. Although streptococcal skin infections may be linked to acute rheumatic fever pathogenesis, there are no trials of impetigo control programmes to prevent acute rheumatic fever. There is a current focus on attempts to develop a group A streptococcal vaccine. Clinical trials of one prospective vaccine are under way, and others are imminent, but the process will take many years, and recent experience suggests that new vaccines are often beyond the financial reach of most developing countries. For the foreseeable future at least, acute rheumatic fever prevention in many developing countries will depend on improving adherence to secondary prophylaxis and developing new strategies for primary prophylaxis.

Further reading

Anonymous (1995). Strategy for controlling rheumatic fever/rheumatic heart disease, with emphasis on primary prevention: memorandum from a joint WHO/ISFC meeting. *Bull World Health Organ*, **73**, 583–7.

Bach JF, *et al.* (1996). 10-year educational programme aimed at rheumatic fever in two French Caribbean islands. *Lancet*, **347**, 644–8.

Batzloff MR, *et al.* (2003). Protection against group A streptococcus by immunization with J8-diptheria toxoid: contribution of J8-and diptheria toxoid-specific antibodies to protection. *J Infect Dis*, **187**, 1598–1608.

Bisno AL (1991). Group A streptococcal infections and acute rheumatic fever. *N Engl J Med*, **325**, 783–93.

Bisno AL, *et al.* (2005). Prospects for a group A streptococcal vaccine: rationale, feasibility, and obstacles—report of a National Institute of Allergy and Infectious Diseases workshop. *Clin Infect Dis*, **41**, 1150–6.

Carapetis JR, McDonald M, Wilson NJ (2005). Acute rheumatic fever. *Lancet*, **366**, 155–68.

Carapetis JR, *et al.* (2005). The global burden of group A streptococcal diseases. *Lancet Infect Dis*, **5**, 685–94.

Cilliers AM (2006). Rheumatic fever and its management. *BMJ*, **333**, 1153–6.

Cilliers AM, Manyemba J, Saloojee H (2003). Anti-inflammatory treatment for carditis in acute rheumatic fever. *Cochrane Database Syst Rev*, CD003176.

Cunningham MW (2000). Pathogenesis of group A streptococcal infections. *Clin Microbiol Rev*, **13**, 470–511.

Cunningham MW (2004). T cell mimicry in inflammatory heart disease. *Mol Immunol*, **40**, 1121–7.

Hu MC, *et al.* (2002). Immunogenicity of a 26-valent group A streptococcal vaccine. *Infect Immun*, **70**, 2171–7.

Kaplan EL (1993). T. Duckett Jones Memorial Lecture. Global assessment of rheumatic fever and rheumatic heart disease at the close of the century. Influences and dynamics of populations and pathogens: a failure to realize prevention? *Circulation*, **88**, 1964–72.

Lennon D (2000). Rheumatic fever: a preventable disease? The New Zealand experience. In: Martin DR, Tagg JR (eds) *Streptococci and streptococcal diseases: entering the new millennium*, pp. 503–512. Securacopy, Auckland.

Lennon D (2004). Acute rheumatic fever in children: recognition and treatment. *Paediatr Drugs*, **6**, 363–73.

Martin DR, *et al.* (1994). Acute rheumatic fever in Auckland, New Zealand: spectrum of associated group A streptococci different from expected. *Pediatr Infect Dis J*, **13**, 264–9.

McDonald M, Currie BJ, Carapetis JR (2004). Acute rheumatic fever: a chink in the chain that links the heart to the throat? *Lancet Infect Dis*, **4**, 240–5.

McDonald M, *et al.* (2005). Preventing recurrent rheumatic fever: the role of register-based programs. *Heart*, **91**, 1131–3.

National Heart Foundation of Australia (RF/RHD guideline development working group) and the Cardiac Society of Australia and New Zealand (2006). *Diagnosis and management of acute rheumatic fever and rheumatic heart disease in Australia—an evidence-based review*. National Heart Foundation of Australia, Melbourne.

Quinn RW (1989). Comprehensive review of morbidity and mortality trends for rheumatic fever, streptococcal disease, and scarlet fever: the decline of rheumatic fever. *Rev Infect Dis*, **11**, 928–53.

Robertson KA, Volmink JA, Mayosi BM (2005). Antibiotics for the primary prevention of rheumatic fever: a meta-analysis. *BMC Cardiovasc Disord*, **5**, 11.

Special Writing Group of the Committee on Rheumatic Fever Endocarditis and Kawasaki Disease of the Council on Cardiovascular Disease in the Young of the American Heart Association (1992). Guidelines for the diagnosis of rheumatic fever. Jones Criteria, 1992 update. *JAMA*, **268**, 2069–73.

Steer AC, *et al.* (2002). Systematic review of rheumatic heart disease prevalence in children in developing countries: the role of environmental factors. *J Paediatr Child Health*, **38**, 229–34.

Stollerman GH (2001). Rheumatic fever in the 21st century. *Clin Infect Dis*, **33**, 806–14.

Tubridy-Clark M, Carapetis JR (2007). Subclinical carditis in rheumatic fever: A systematic review. *Int J Cardiol*, **119**, 54–8.

Veasy LG, Tani LY, Hill HR (1994). Persistence of acute rheumatic fever in the intermountain area of the United States. *J Pediatr*, **124**, 9–16.

Wannamaker LW (1973). The chain that links the heart to the throat. *Circulation*, **48**, 9–18.

WHO Expert Consultation on Rheumatic Fever and Rheumatic Heart Disease (2004). *Rheumatic fever and rheumatic heart disease: report of a WHO Expert Consultation, Geneva, 29 October–1 November 2001*. WHO Technical Report Series 923, World Health Organization, Geneva.

16.9.2 Infective endocarditis

William A. Littler

Essentials

Endocarditis predominantly affects the valves of the left side of the heart: a large autopsy series revealed mitral involvement in 86%, aortic 55%, tricuspid 20%, and pulmonary 1%. In the developing world rheumatic heart disease is the commonest predisposing factor, but in developed countries over 50% of patients have no known pre-existing cardiac lesion.

Clinical features

Presenting symptoms and signs include those of a bacteraemic illness, tissue destruction (heart valve(s) and adjacent structures), systemic or pulmonary embolism, and phenomena thought to be related to circulating immune complexes, e.g. splinter and conjunctival haemorrhages, Osler's nodes, Janeway lesions, vasculitic rash, Roth spots, and nephritis. Right-sided infective endocarditis accounts for only 5% of cases overall, is usually associated with intravenous drug abuse or indwelling intravascular devices, and often causes septic pulmonary emboli that can lead to cavitating pulmonary infarcts.

Investigation and diagnosis—blood culture is the most important laboratory investigation in the diagnosis of endocarditis, with prolonged incubation requested in circumstances where endocarditis is strongly suspected. Serological tests can aid in the identification of organisms that are difficult to isolate. Echocardiography should be performed as soon as possible when endocarditis is suspected: its principal role is to detect vegetations, but it is not sufficiently sensitive to allow the clinician to exclude the diagnosis confidently on the basis of a negative result. Diagnosis is based on pathological criteria (demonstration of microorganisms by culture or histological examination, or histological evidence of active endocarditis) or—more usually—a combination of major and minor clinical criteria, with the major clinical criteria relating to (1) positive blood cultures of 'typical' or 'consistent' organisms, and (2) evidence of endocardial involvement detected on physical examination (new murmur) or by echocardiography.

Causes and management

The causes of endocarditis are viridans streptococci (up to 58%), *Staphylococcus aureus* (30% of community acquired and 46% of hospital acquired), *Streptococcus bovis* (up to 12%), enterococcus species (up to 10%), fungal (up to 10%), coagulase-negative staphylococci (5% of native valve endocarditis), the HACEK group of organisms (3%), and others.

Best management is provided by a multidisciplinary team involving cardiologists, microbiologists, infectious disease specialists, and cardiac surgeons. Bactericidal antibiotics are the mainstay of treatment. Recommended empirical therapy for the patient with suspected endocarditis presenting acutely is flucloxacillin (8–12 g/day IV in four to six divided doses) plus gentamicin (1 mg/kg body weight IV 8-hourly, modified according to renal function), and for the patient presenting with a more indolent course is penicillin (7.2 g/day IV in six divided doses) or ampicillin/amoxicillin (2 g IV 6-hourly) plus gentamicin (as above). This should be modified to a definitive antibiotic treatment regimen when the pathogen is known (see text for details). Surgery is required in about 30% of cases during the acute phase and in 20 to 40% of cases thereafter, with the main indications being haemodynamic instability, persistent infection, and annular or aortic abscesses.

Prevention

Until recently, antibiotic prophylaxis in 'at risk' patients—meaning any with a wide variety of cardiac lesions undergoing a wide variety of medical/surgical procedures—were accepted as reasonable, but there is no good evidence to support this practice. Recommendations from relevant UK, European and American professional bodies are now much more restrictive. UK (National Institute for Health and Clinical Excellence) guidelines state that antibiotic prophylaxis should only be given to patients at risk if they are undergoing a gastrointestinal or genitourinary procedure at a site where there is suspected infection. Most cardiologists feel that this is too restrictive and prefer European and American guidelines which recommend prophylaxis before dental and non-dental procedures for patients at high risk, including those with prosthetic cardiac valves or other prosthetic material within their hearts, previous infective endocarditis, and some forms of congenital heart disease.

When prophylaxis is recommended for dental and other procedures, regimen typically include amoxicillin (or clindamycin if penicillin-allergic), with the addition of gentamicin if risks are thought to be high, and substitution of vancomycin (or teicoplanin) for amoxicillin if the patient is penicillin-allergic (or has taken more than a single dose of penicillin in the previous month).

Historical background

Lazerous Riverius recorded the first case of what is now known as infective endocarditis in 1723. He described a French magistrate with an irregular pulse, oedema, and congestion, who at autopsy had fleshy masses 'the size of hazelnuts' obstructing the aortic ostia. Some 50 years later, Morgani (1769) made the link between infection (fulminating gonorrhoea) and 'whitish polypus concretions on the upper part of the aortic valve near its borders'.

The clinical picture of endocarditis was first described by Jean Baptiste Bouillard, in 1835: 'fever, an irregular pulse, cardiomegaly (by percussion) and a bellows murmur in the heart'. He gave the disease the name 'endocarditis', or an inflammation of the inner membrane of the heart and fibrous tissues of the valve, and was the first to use the term 'vegetations' for the valvular lesions.

Winge used the term 'mycoses endocardi' for the groups of microorganisms that he saw when he examined vegetations under the microscope in 1870. In 1886, Wyssecokowitch cultured *Staphylococcus aureus* from an endocardial vegetation. Lenthartz, in 1901, was the first to use blood cultures in the diagnosis of endocarditis. 'Infective endocarditis' was the term used by Thomas Horder, in 1901, to describe the syndrome consisting of (1) the presence of valvular disease, (2) the occurrence of systemic embolism, and (3) the discovery of microorganisms in the bloodstream.

Epidemiology

Infective endocarditis was universally fatal before the advent of antibiotic therapy. About 200 deaths are recorded each year in the United Kingdom, but this is almost certainly an underestimate. A recent review of papers published between 1993 and 2003 found the mean age of patients varied between 36 and 69 years, the median incidence being 3.6 per 100 000 population per year (range 0.3–22.4), increasing from 5 or less in individuals aged younger than 50 years to 15 or more in those older than 65 years. The median in-hospital mortality rate was 16% (range 11–26%). The incidence is greater in men, in those over 65 years of age and in those with prosthetic heart valves. In intravenous drug users, the incidence of infective endocarditis is estimated as 150 to 200 per 100 000 person years.

Pathogenesis

Normal vascular endothelium is resistant to microbial infection and very few patients potentially at risk actually develop infective endocarditis. Bacteraemia may occur spontaneously during chewing, tooth brushing, and other normal activities. Since low-grade bacteraemia occurs frequently in everyone, a defence mechanism must exist that can eradicate microbes adherent to vegetations. Platelets play a pivotal role in the antimicrobial host-defence mechanism and human platelets have been found to contain at least 10 different bactericidal proteins or 'thrombocidins'.

Damage to the endothelial surface of the heart or blood vessels induces platelet and fibrin deposition producing a sterile thrombotic vegetation; infective endocarditis is initiated by the binding of microbes, discharged into the general circulation from a peripheral site, to these vegetations. These microbes become rapidly encased in further depositions of platelets and fibrin, and multiply.

The pathogenesis of infective endocarditis involves complex interactions between microbes and the host-defence mechanisms, both circulating and at the site of endothelial damage. An essential step is the activation of the clotting system and the formation of a fibrin clot on the endothelial surface. Experimental evidence suggests that the main pathogens in infective endocarditis (streptococci and staphylococci) can bind to endothelial cells and induce functional changes within these cells causing monocyte adhesion. The endothelial cells respond to local inflammation by expressing β1-integrins which promote the adhesion of pathogens that carry fibronectin-binding proteins on their surface. The combination of damaged endothelial cells, bacteria, and endothelial bound monocytes results in the induction of tissue-factor-dependent procoagulant activity which initiates clot formation. Polymorphonuclear leucocytes which are recruited to the infected endothelial site may be subsequently involved in the disease progression, with the contents of lysosomes released by the activated leucocytes probably causing softening and separation of valve tissue, leading to its destruction.

In endocarditis, the vegetations are found predominately on the left side of the heart (85%). In a large autopsy series of more than 1000 cases reported over 50 years ago, the mitral valve was involved in 86%, the aortic in 55%, the tricuspid in 20%, and the pulmonary valve in only 1%. The predominance of left-sided lesions has led to the belief that the higher pressures and velocities encountered in the left side of the heart and the proximal aorta must impose a greater mechanical stress on the valves and endocardium, which in turn leads to local damage.

Endocarditis is classically associated with 'jet lesions', where blood flowing from a high-pressure area through an orifice to an area of lower pressure produces a high-velocity jet. Vegetations are usually found in the lower-pressure area, e.g. on the atrial surface of the mitral valve in mitral regurgitation, or the ventricular surface of the aortic valve in aortic regurgitation. This particular deposition of vegetations has been explained on the basis of the Venturi effect.

Once a vegetation is established, it determines the subsequent clinical picture by four basic processes: bacteraemia, local tissue destruction, embolization, and the formation of circulating immune complexes.

Clinical features

Early reports of infective endocarditis described a low-grade, febrile illness caused by viridans streptococci from the mouth in a patient with chronic rheumatic heart disease. Night sweats, anorexia, and weight loss were followed by the development of splinter haemorrhages and Osler nodes, finger clubbing, and splenomegaly. The infection progressed relentlessly with increasing cachexia, and the patient died from cardiac failure or a major embolic episode. The term 'subacute bacterial endocarditis' was used to describe this illness. 'Acute or malignant endocarditis' described an aggressive form of the disease, usually caused by *Staph. aureus* or other virulent bacteria.

During the past 50 years, there has been a striking change in the pattern of endocarditis. The proportion of patients in developed countries with endocarditis who have no known pre-existing cardiac lesion has risen to over 50%. This change is related both to the decline in rheumatic heart disease and to the increase in extracardiac predisposing factors, including intravenous drug abuse, haemodialysis, and the use of intravascular devices. Prosthetic heart valves are an important predisposing factor and cardiac surgery for complex congenital lesions has increased the lifespan of patients who would previously have died prematurely. Antibiotic-resistant organisms have emerged. The longevity of the populations of developed countries has resulted in an increasing age of patients with infective endocarditis, with mean age rising from under 40 years, before 1940, to 60 to 70 years today.

Features of a bacteraemic illness

Discharge of the infecting agent into the circulation produces constant bacteraemia which may present as pyrexia, rigors, malaise, anorexia, headache, confusion, arthralgia, and anaemia. Some cases of endocarditis may present without fever, particularly in older people.

Features of tissue destruction

Endocarditis initially affects valve cusps, leaflets, or chordae tendineae. Tissue destruction results in valvular incompetence, cusp perforation, or rupture of the chordae, producing an appropriate cardiac murmur that may change in character during the course of the illness: 80% of patients present with a murmur, and 15 to 20% develop one during their hospital stay. Large vegetations rarely obstruct a native valve, but mechanical obstruction of prosthetic valves is more common and clinically more difficult to detect.

As the infective process progresses, it may extend beyond the valve into the paravalvular structures. Aortic root abscess is a serious complication: extension through the aortic wall into other tissues or cavities can create a fistula or pseudoaneurysm. Particular problems can include sinus of Valsalva aneurysm and involvement of the coronary ostia, and septal abscesses can lead to progressive conduction defects evidenced by prolongation of the PR interval on the ECG and eventually complete heart block.

Paravalvular abscess is more common in native aortic valve endocarditis than in mitral valve infection. Infection of a mechanical valve involves the sewing ring and may lead to valve dehiscence. In the case of a mechanical aortic valve, where infection is often localized to the junction between the sewing ring and the aortic annulus, a large false aneurysm may develop in this area. Free wall myocardial abscesses may rupture and cause sudden death.

Features of systemic or pulmonary emboli

Fragments of an infected vegetation may be dislodged into the systemic or pulmonary circulation, producing emboli in 20 to 40% of cases (up to 50% reported in autopsy series). These may lodge in any part of the circulation and present as a cerebrovascular accident, arterial occlusion of a limb, myocardial infarction, sudden unilateral blindness, or infarction of the spleen or a kidney. Septic embolism from the left side of the heart may result in the formation of a cerebral abscess. In right heart endocarditis, recurrent septic pulmonary emboli may be misinterpreted as 'pneumonia'.

Mycotic aneurysms arise from embolism of the vasa vasorum that weakens the arterial wall: these have been reported in almost 3% of clinical cases but are found in up to 15% at autopsy. In the cerebral circulation, such aneurysm may produce subarachnoid haemorrhage or intracerebral haemorrhage. The popliteal artery is a common site for mycotic aneurysms.

Emboli are characteristic of *Staph. aureus* infections and large emboli are a feature in HACEK (see below) and fungal endocarditis. They usually occur before or within the first few days after starting antimicrobial therapy. Anterior mitral valve-leaflet vegetations are more likely to embolize than aortic valve vegetations, especially if they are highly mobile. Vegetation size does not predict systemic embolization, but large vegetations (>10 mm) are associated with a poor outcome overall.

After an embolic complication, recurrent episodes are likely to follow, especially if vegetations persist on echocardiography. In more than 50% of cases, such recurrence occurs within 30 days of the first episode. This is not reduced by treatment with anticoagulants such as warfarin or antiplatelet therapy such as aspirin: both may increase the risk of bleeding and should be avoided unless they are essential.

Features of circulating immune complexes

The infected vegetation acts as an antigen that triggers an immune response. Chronic antigenaemia stimulates generalized

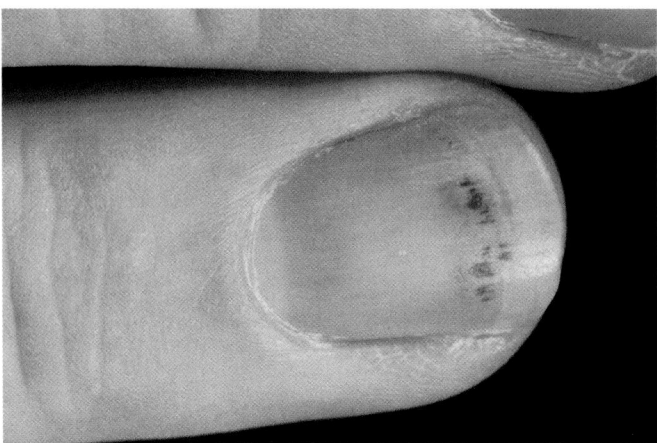

Fig. 16.9.2.1 Splinter haemorrhages in a case of infective endocarditis.

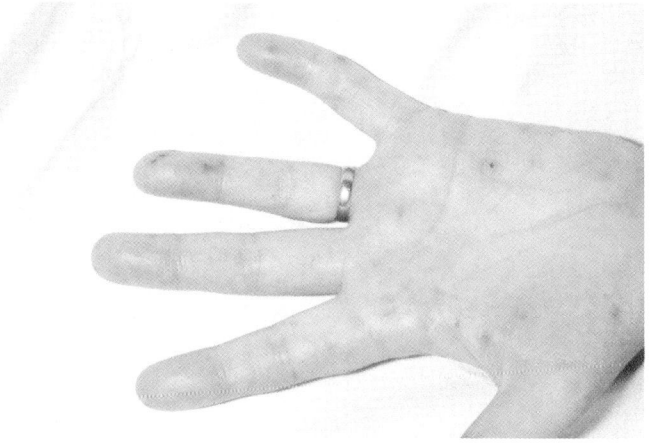

Fig. 16.9.2.3 Osler's nodes involving the fingers and the thenar and hypothenar eminences.

hypergammaglobinaemia such that after several weeks of infection a variety of autoantibodies can be detected. Immune complex deposition probably causes many of the extracardiac manifestations of infective endocarditis, but these classical signs are relatively uncommon and are often absent in individual patients.

♦ Splinter haemorrhages—these are found in the nail bed of the fingers and less commonly the toes, and are linear in form (Fig. 16.9.2.1). They occur in 5 to 15% of cases

♦ Conjunctival haemorrhages (Fig. 16.9.2.2)

♦ Osler's nodes—these transient painful erythematous nodules are found at the ends of fingers and toes and the thenar and hypothenar eminences (Fig. 16.9.2.3). They occur in 5 to 10% of cases, and may be due to minute infected emboli rather than immune complex deposition

♦ Janeway lesions—irregular painless erythematous macules found in roughly the same distribution as Osler's nodes (Fig. 16.9.2.4); they tend to blanch with pressure

♦ Vasculitic rash—immunoglobulin and complement deposits are found in the walls of skin capillaries (Fig. 16.9.2.5). Vasculitis may account for some of the neurological findings in infective endocarditis

♦ Roth spots—boat-shaped haemorrhages in the retina are often called Roth spots, but true Roth spots are white retinal exudates

that may be surrounded by haemorrhage. They consist of perivascular collections of lymphocytes and occur in 5 to 10% of cases.

♦ Splenomegaly—clinical splenomegaly is less common than was reported in earlier literature. CT scanning of the abdomen shows the spleen to be enlarged in at least 50% of cases and often demonstrates splenic infarcts (Fig. 16.9.2.6). Splenic abscesses sometimes occur and splenic rupture can be fatal

♦ Nephritis—immune complexes can cause glomerulonephritis, manifest as proteinuria, haematuria, and decline in renal function, with immunoglobulin and complement deposition within glomeruli on renal biopsy (see Chapters 21.8.5, 21.8.6, and 21.1.9). Key investigations are simply dipstick testing of the urine (with microscopy if more than 1+ positive for blood and/or protein) and measurement of serum creatinine

♦ Arthralgia—the joint manifestations of infective endocarditis may result from immune complex deposition in the synovial membrane

Other features

Up to 30% of patients with endocarditis present with neurological symptoms: these are most common in staphylococcal infection, in which one-third present with the clinical features of meningitis.

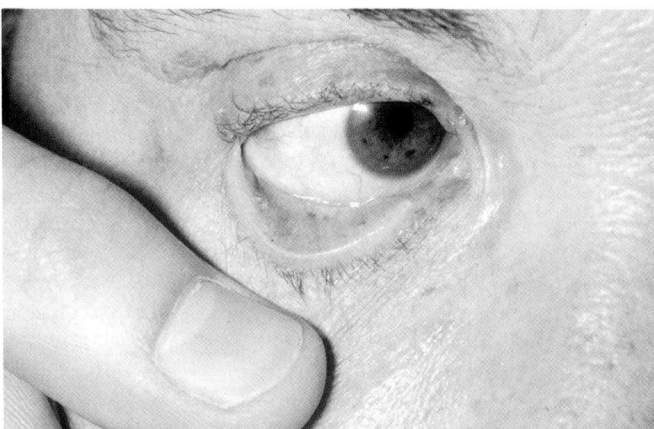

Fig. 16.9.2.2 Subconjuctival haemorrhages in a case of endocarditis.

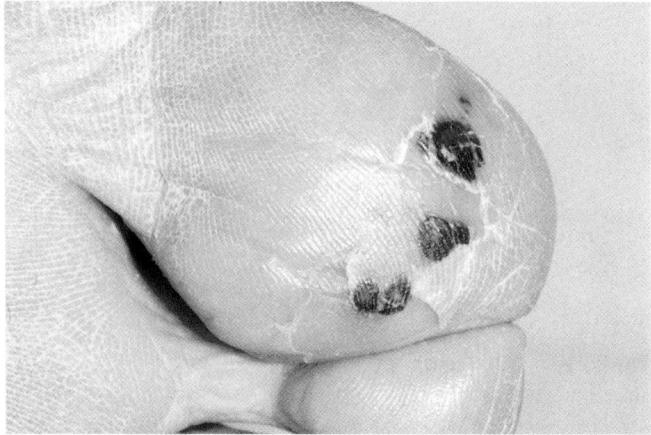

Fig. 16.9.2.4 Janeway lesions on the under surface of the left big toe in a case of endocarditis.

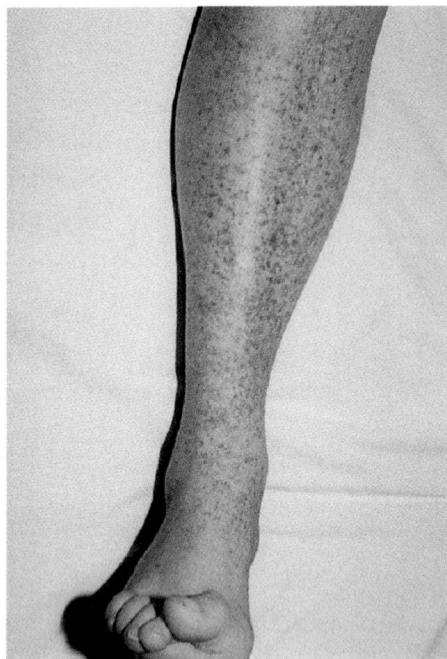

Fig. 16.9.2.5 Vasculitic rash on lower limb of a patient with infective endocarditis.

Headaches, confusion, and toxic psychosis can be present as well as encephalomyelitis. It is not certain whether some of these neurological manifestations result from repeated small emboli or from a vasculitic process within the cerebral circulation as a consequence of immune complex deposition. The cerebrospinal fluid can show an increase in white cells, but is usually sterile on culture, although very occasionally it may be positive for staphylococcal infection.

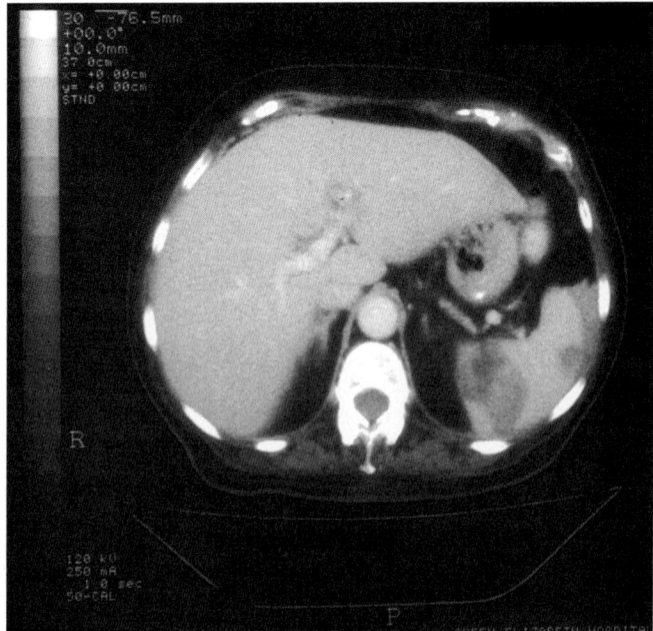

Fig. 16.9.2.6 CT scan in a case of endocarditis showing multiple splenic infarcts in an enlarged spleen.

Although immune-mediated glomerulonephritis has been regarded as the typical renal lesion of infective endocarditis, this assumption was based on small series predating modern treatment regimens. More recent work indicates that the commonest renal histological finding is infarction, usually septic. Circulatory compromise can rarely cause severe renal impairment as a result of renal cortical necrosis.

Finger clubbing is one of the classical features of infective endocarditis, usually seen after 1 or 2 months of the illness. It is seldom seen now, but when present is still a useful sign because it rarely occurs in conditions with which infective endocarditis can be confused.

Specific types or circumstances of endocarditis

Prosthetic valve endocarditis

Patients with prosthetic heart valves have a small, but constant, risk of infective endocarditis, estimated at 0.2 to 1.4 events per 100 patient years. The incidence of prosthetic valve endocarditis is about 3% in the first postoperative year, with the highest risk during the first 3 months. Prosthetic valve endocarditis is five times more common in the aortic area than the mitral area and may involve mechanical, xenograft, and homograft valves.

Prosthetic valve endocarditis has been classified as early or late according to its temporal relationship to surgery. Early prosthetic valve endocarditis usually occurs within 60 days of open heart surgery and accounts for 30% of cases. It is caused either by contamination of the prosthetic valve at implantation or by perioperative bacteraemia from intravenous catheters, arterial lines, urethral catheters, or endotracheal tubes. The commonest organisms are coagulase-negative staphylococci.

Late prosthetic valve endocarditis accounts for 70% of cases and usually occurs 60 days or more after surgery. The pathogens are those seen in native valve endocarditis, with a preponderance of viridans streptococci and staphylococci, but with a higher incidence of other organisms. Some patients with late prosthetic valve endocarditis will have acquired the infection at the time of surgery, but a bacteraemia is usually the principal cause.

Bacteraemia in a patient with a prosthetic valve must always be taken seriously, but it may not always be the result of endocarditis. The clinical picture of prosthetic valve endocarditis is typically fever, malaise, and weakness, with the more classical signs usually absent. The condition is often insidious and difficult to diagnose clinically. A new murmur may appear, and heart failure and embolic phenomena cause high mortality (20–50%). Infection in a mechanical valve is located in the sewing ring, from which the infection can spread into the host tissues producing annular/myocardial abscesses, paravalvular leak, and prosthetic dehiscence as described above. Infection of a tissue valve usually involves the valve leaflets, resulting in destruction or perforation and valvular incompetence. Vegetations may cause obstruction with all forms of prosthetic valve.

The diagnosis of prosthetic valve endocarditis requires a high index of clinical suspicion, blood cultures, and transoesophageal echocardiography, which is far superior to the transthoracic approach for finding vegetations and identifying periprosthetic spread of infection. Vegetations are more difficult to identify in patients with mechanical valves than those with bioprostheses.

Right-sided endocarditis

Right-sided infective endocarditis accounts for only 5% of cases overall, but centres that treat large numbers of intravenous drug users will have a higher incidence. The clinical picture differs significantly from left-sided disease. It is usually associated with intravenous drug addiction or indwelling intravascular devices, including pacemakers, central venous lines of all types, and septal occluder devices. *Staph. aureus* is the commonest pathogen and the tricuspid valve is more commonly affected (80%) than the pulmonary. Fever is almost always present and a cardiac murmur is found in 80% of cases. There may be septic pulmonary emboli (Fig. 16.9.2.7) and the resultant pulmonary infarcts may cavitate. Symptoms include cough, haemoptysis, and pleuritic chest pain; a chest radiograph shows pulmonary infiltrates often misdiagnosed as 'patches of pneumonia'. Renal involvement has been described in over one-half of cases, most commonly abscess formation or diffuse pyelonephritis. Myocarditis is more common in right-sided involvement than left. Peripheral stigmata, splenomegaly, and central nervous system involvement are rare (no more than 5% of cases). Death is most commonly due to sepsis, rarely to heart failure.

Endocarditis in intravenous drug users

Endocarditis is a serious complication of intravenous drug abuse. The right side of the heart is affected most commonly, but the left may also be involved in a substantial number of patients (37%), and both right and left side in a few (7%). On the left side, mitral and aortic valves are equally infected. A history of previous heart disease is only found in some 25% of cases.

Staph. aureus is responsible for 40% of all cases. Gram-negative bacilli are next most frequent, *Pseudomonas aeruginosa* and *Serratia marcescens* accounting for most of these. Candida can cause endocarditis in intravenous drug users, and polymicrobial endocarditis accounts for 5% of cases.

The skin is the commonest site from which pathogens enter the bloodstream via needles. Gram-negative bacilli are rarely recovered

from needles or the drug itself, and it has been suggested that these organisms come from tap water, sinks, or lavatory pans.

The clinical picture of intravenous drug use-associated endocarditis depends on which side of the heart is affected. Right-sided disease is described above; left-sided disease behaves like that seen in nondrug cases, with a high incidence of heart failure, arterial embolism, central nervous system involvement, and peripheral stigmata.

The overall mortality depends on when the patient presents: it is high if they present late, reflecting among other things the difficulty in dealing with addicts because of their poor compliance and reluctance to discontinue their drug habit. The principles of management are similar to those in patients who are not drug abusers. The duration of intravenous antibiotics should be at least 4 weeks, but this is frequently impossible to do in practice, and in right-sided endocarditis simple removal of the valve without replacement appears to be the best strategy.

Endocarditis in children

Endocarditis does occur in children but is rare, especially in the first decade of life. In the older literature, tetralogy of Fallot was the commonest cardiac problem associated with infective endocarditis. Complex cyanotic disease, congenital heart disease corrected with prosthetic material, and small ventricular septal defects make up the bulk of cases now.

Diagnosis of infective endocarditis

Laboratory methods

Blood culture

This is the most important laboratory investigation in the diagnosis of endocarditis (Table 16.9.2.1). Isolation of the pathogen enables an effective antibiotic treatment regimen to be devised. Optimal technique is necessary to avoid false-positive cases due to contaminating organisms from the skin. Each set of blood cultures should be taken from a separate venepuncture and at least 10 ml of blood be injected into each culture bottle. Blood cultures should be taken before antibiotics are given; if they have already been given, cultures should still be done and, if possible, the giving of further antibiotics delayed for a few days. However, previous antibiotics may render the blood sterile for some time, and the chances of recovering the pathogen, particularly when it is a viridans streptococcus, are very low. Much mystique has been attached to the number and timing of blood cultures in cases of suspected endocarditis. What is known is that the bacteraemia is usually constant, and that whenever the blood is obtained for culture, and however many sets are taken, then in most cases all bottles will grow the pathogen. There are, of course, rare exceptions when only a few bottles taken are positive, and this is one reason why it is conventional to take two or three sets. Another reason for several cultures is to assess the relevance of the common skin contaminants, particularly the coagulase-negative staphylococci but also corynebacterium, that can cause endocarditis.

In most laboratories, blood culture systems are automated, with continuous monitoring that flags up growth for further investigation. Most cultures become positive within 48 h and after this the chances of isolating the pathogen recede, with the exception of fastidious organisms of the HACEK group that may take much longer to recover from the blood. In most laboratories,

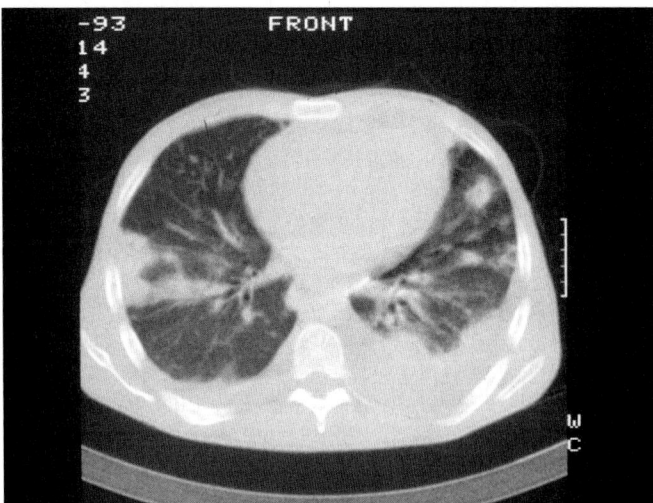

Fig. 16.9.2.7 CT scan of the chest showing multiple pulmonary infarcts in a case of right sided endocarditis of the tricuspid valve in an intravenous drug abuser.

Table 16.9.2.1 Microbiological diagnosis of infective endocarditis

Organism	Estimated incidence	Relevant clinical history	Blood cultures	Serology
Staphylococcus aureus	30% of community community-acquired 46% of hospital acquired	IVDA/IV access devices	Usually positive	Under development (lipid S)
Coagulase-negative staphylococci	5% of native valve IE	Vasectomy/angiography/ haemodialysis IVDA	Usually positive	In progress
Viridans streptococci	Up to 58%	Dental abscess/poor oral hygiene	Positive, if no previous antibiotics	In progress
Streptococcus bovis	up to 12%	Gastrointestinal malignancy/ presumed normal heart valves/ older patient population	Positive, if no previous antibiotics	None
HACEK	3%	Dental treatment/URTI/IVDU	Most positive in 6 days with high CO_2 concentrations	None
Fungal	Up to 10%	Prosthetic valves/IVDU/ immunosuppression/long-term intravenous lines	Filamentous fungi rarely positive. Candida commonly positive	Fungal serology not validated for IE
		Should be performed if multiple risk factors for fungal IE		
Enterococcus spp.	Up to 10%	Urinary catheter insertion/ gastrointestinal malignancy	Positive, if no previous antibiotics	In progress
Brucella spp.	1–4%	Endemic area/contaminated milk consumption	Positive in 80%. %. May need prolonged incubation	Reference assay = tube agglutination
Coxiella burnetii (Q fever)	3–5%	Farming background/exposure to domestic ruminants/raw milk consumption/previous valvulopathy/endemic area	Rarely positive. Tissue cell culture reported as optimal method	Major criteria for modified Duke criteria: Anti phase 1 IgG >800 and IgA antibody >100 is highly sensitive Reference assay = microimmunofluorescence
Bartonella	Up to 3%	Homelessness/alcoholism/ exposure to cats	Rarely positive	Reference assay = microimmunofluorescence
Legionella	<1%	Usually an outbreak/institution Role unclear for prosthetic valves/pneumonia	Rarely positive IE. Urinary antigen. Bronchial washings/ sputum	High antibody levels Reference assay = microimmunofluorescence
Chlamydia	Unknown due to cross-reactivity with bartonella	Pneumonia Significance is controversial	Rarely positive. Needs tissue cell culture	Cross-reaction with *Bartonella* spp.
				Reference assay = microimmunofluorescence

IE, infective endocarditis; IV, intravenous; IVDU, intravenous drug abuse; URT, upper respiratory tract infection.
Reprinted from Journal of Infection, Vol 47, Watkin *et al*, *The microbial diagnosis of infective endocarditis*, pp1–11. Copyright (2003), with permission from Elsevier and the British Infection Society.

blood cultures are incubated for 5 to 7 days, but this may not be long enough for the rare fastidious slow grower. The onus is on the clinical microbiologist or clinician to request prolonged incubation for blood cultures from patients in whom endocarditis is strongly suspected, who have not had previous antibiotics, and whose blood cultures are sterile after a week's incubation.

Other routine blood tests
In infective endocarditis, an elevated ESR and C-reactive protein are almost invariable, and these inflammatory markers are used most commonly to monitor the activity of the disease. A normochromic normocytic anaemia is often present and a polymorphonuclear leuco-cytosis is found in most cases. Hypergammaglobulinaemia and a low serum complement may be present, together with a false-positive rheumatoid factor. Circulating immune complexes may be detected.

Serological tests aid in the identification of organisms that are difficult to isolate, including bartonella, coxiella (Q fever), chlamydia, mycoplasma, legionella, brucella, and fungi. Candida antibodies are of no diagnostic value.

Echocardiography
In suspected cases of endocarditis, echocardiography should be performed as soon as possible and interpreted by an experienced cardiologist. Its principal role is to detect vegetations (Fig. 16.9.2.8), but it is not sufficiently sensitive to allow the clinician to exclude the diagnosis confidently on the basis of a negative result. The sensitivity depends on the size of the vegetations and the time course of the disease: it can resolve vegetations as small as 1 to 2 mm, but it is more difficult with prosthetic than native valves and more difficult with mechanical than biological prostheses.

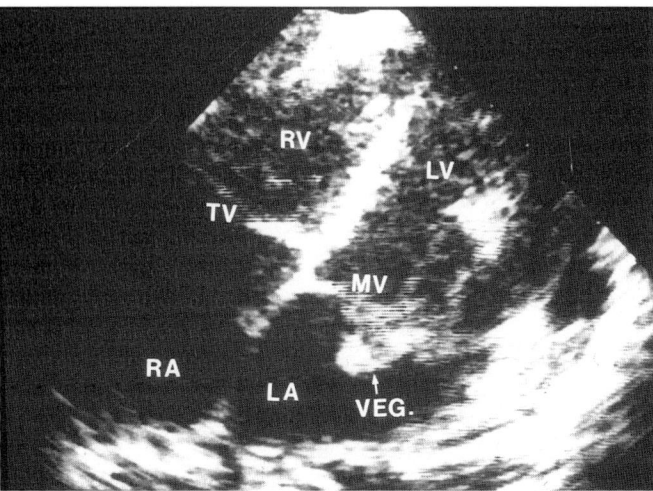

Fig. 16.9.2.8 A transthoracic echocardiogram in a case of endocarditis showing a large vegetation involving the posterior leaflet of the mitral valve and prolapsing into the left ventricle. LA, left atrium; LV, left ventricle; MV, mitral valve; RA, right atrium; RV, right ventricle; TV, tricuspid valve; VEG, vegetation.

Vegetations appear as thick, ragged, nonuniform echoes oscillating on or around a cardiac valve or in the path of a regurgitant jet. They do not usually restrict leaflet mobility and they exhibit valve-dependent motion. On native valves, vegetations are usually attached to the ventricular side of the aortic valve and the atrial side of the mitral and tricuspid valves (Fig. 16.9.2.9).

Two-dimensional echocardiography should be employed initially in all cases of suspected endocarditis. Transoesophageal echocardiography has improved the rate of diagnosis of infective endocarditis over that of transthoracic echocardiography, particularly in the presence of a prosthetic valve. It has also made it easier to recognize many complications of prosthetic valve endocarditis, such as abscesses, fistulas, and paravalvular leak. In addition to vegetations, echocardiography may demonstrate indirect signs of valvular integrity, such as excessive systolic expansion of the left atrium in mitral incompetence or fluttering of the anterior leaflet of the mitral valve in aortic incompetence. Ventricular size and contractility are both easily assessed.

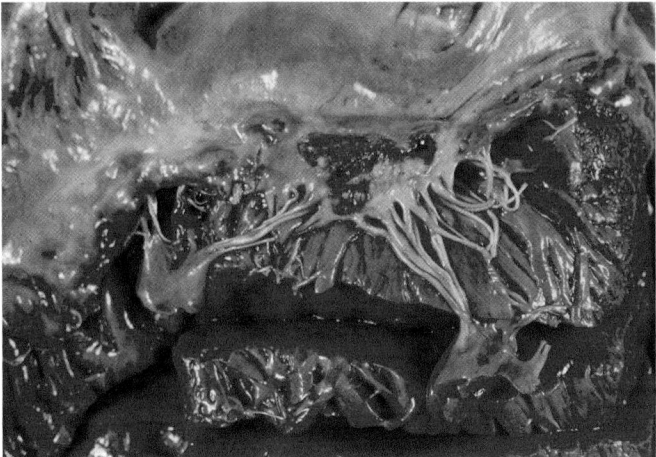

Fig. 16.9.2.9 Bacterial vegetations on the mitral valve in a case of infective endocarditis—the patient had died as a result of a large cerebral embolus.

The diagnosis of right-sided endocarditis has been greatly facilitated by echocardiography, particularly transoesophageal echocardiography. Vegetations tend to be larger on the right side and can be demonstrated in 80 to 100% of cases.

Vegetations need to be differentiated from other conditions which produce echo-density on cardiac valves, including calcification, myxomatous degeneration, and atrial myxoma.

Examination of the heart valve and other tissues

Histology

Histology remains the gold standard for explanted valves. When valve replacement is undertaken, valvular tissue (including vegetation) should be examined histologically and cultured for the presence of microorganisms, which may allow postoperative antibiotics to be tailored accordingly. However, the isolation of microorganisms by valvular culture in infective endocarditis is infrequent: only 15% in one large series, with staphylococci being most common. Fastidious and rare microorganisms have been demonstrated on heart valves by various staining techniques.

Nucleic acid-based techniques

There are now several papers in the literature describing the application of polymerase chain reaction techniques to samples obtained from heart valves, vegetations, and embolic tissue in patients with suspected endocarditis. The intention is to allow identification of the infecting microorganism when blood cultures are negative due to prior antibiotic therapy, or the causative organism is fastidious or cannot be cultured. This is not yet routine practice because of the following issues. Firstly, bacterial DNA is present within heart valves for many months and possibly years following successful treatment. Secondly, contamination of samples with any bacterial DNA leads to false-positive results. Thirdly, false-negative results can occur due to polymerase chain reaction inhibitory factors present within blood and other bodily fluid.

Criteria for the diagnosis of infective endocarditis

In 1994, Durack and his colleagues introduced criteria for the diagnosis of infective endocarditis that have been accepted as the 'Duke criteria', which categorize patients into definite, possible, and rejected groups. Although these criteria have been shown to be superior to previous diagnostic tools, they have limitations: in particular, there is a possibility of misclassification when blood cultures remain negative or echocardiography is inconclusive. Negative blood cultures occur in 5 to 31% of cases of infective endocarditis, commonly due to prior antibiotic therapy, also because of fastidious and atypical microorganisms. Transthoracic echocardiography visualizes vegetations in only about 50% of cases: transoesophageal echocardiography has a higher sensitivity for detecting signs of endocarditis on both native and prosthetic valves, but will only be diagnostic in 50 to 94% of cases. These issues mean that the number of patients who may be incorrectly diagnosed as having possible infective endocarditis, as opposed to definite, could be as high as 24%.

Modification of the Duke criteria to increase their sensitivity has been suggested by several authors (Table 16.9.2.2). Positive serology for typical microorganisms and the use of polymerase chain reaction techniques have been suggested as major criteria, and the following additional minor criteria have been proposed—the

Table 16.9.2.2 Duke Criteria for the diagnosis of infective endocarditis (IE) and proposed modifications

Duke criteria	Suggested modifications
Pathological criteria	
Microorganisms demonstrated by culture or histological examination.	
Active endocarditis demonstrated by histological examination	
Major criteria	
Positive blood cultures	To be added:
Typical microorganisms consistent with endocarditis from two separate blood cultures.	Positive serology for *Coxiella burnetii*.
Microorganisms consistent with endocarditis from persistently positive blood cultures	Bacteraemia due to *Staphylococcus aureus*.
	Positive molecular assay for specific gene targets and universal loci for bacteria and fungi.
	Positive serology for *Chlamydia psittaci*.
	Positive serology for *Bartonella* species.
Evidence of endocardial involvement	
Echocardiography - oscillating structures, abscess formation, new partial dehiscence of prosthetic valve.	
Clinical - new valvar regurgitation	
Minor criteria	
Predisposing heart disease	To be omitted:
Fever> 38° C	Suspect echocardiography (no major criterion)
Vascular phenomenaImmunological phenomena	To be added:
Microbiological evidence (no major criterion)	Elevated CRP, elevated ESR, splenomegaly,
Suspect echocardiography (no major criterion)	haematuria, clubbing, splinter haemorrhages, petechiae, purpura.
	Identified IE organism from metastatic lesions.
Categories	
Definite:	
Pathological criteria positive	
or 2 major criteria positive	
or 1 major and 2 minor criteria positive	1 major and 1 minor criterion positive
or 5 minor criteria positive	3 minor criteria positive
Possible:	
All cases which cannot be classified as definite or rejected.	
Rejected:	
Alternative diagnosis.	
Resolution of the infection with antibiotic treatment for< 4 days.	
No histological evidence.	

CRP, C reactive protein; ESR erythrocyte sedimentation rate.
Reproduced from Heart, Prendergast B. D, Vol 92, pp. 879–885. Copyright (2006) with permission from BMJ Publishing Group Ltd.

presence of newly diagnosed clubbing, splenomegaly, splinter haemorrhages and petechiae, microscopic haematuria, a high erythrocyte sedimentation rate or a high CRP, also the presence of central nonfeeding lines and peripheral lines.

Microbiology

Although almost any microorganism can cause infective endocarditis, particularly when this involves a prosthetic valve, certain species do so much more commonly than others. The predominant species involved in the infection have not changed significantly in their incidence in the past three decades. Overall, viridans streptococci and staphylococci account for about two-thirds of cases. However, endocarditis cannot be considered as a microbiologically homogeneous entity as the incidence of any specific organism depends (1) on the patient, whether an intravenous drug user or not; (2) on the valve, whether native or prosthetic—and if native, whether previously abnormal or not, and if prosthetic whether mechanical or a bioprosthesis, and whether the infection was acquired early or late; and (3) where (and how) the infection was acquired, whether in the community or (as increasingly these days) in hospital, usually via an infected intravascular device.

The more common species encountered will be considered individually.

Streptococci

The genus *Streptococcus* includes species of differing virulence and pathogenicity as well as differing normal habitat in humans. The genus has undergone numerous taxonomic revisions over the past decade or more, and the previous dependence on haemolytic activity on blood agar and serological reactions has been superseded, in many cases, by molecular and chemotaxonomic approaches. Examples of such taxonomic change include the assignment of the faecal streptococci to the genus *Enterococcus*, and of *Streptococcus morbillorum* to *Gemella morbillorum*, and of the nutritionally dependent streptococci previously known as *Streptococcus adjacens* and *Streptococcus defectivus* to the genus *Abiotrophia*. There are many other examples, but taxonomic change is of limited interest to clinicians and has no bearing on the management of infection.

Viridans streptococci

For many years, it has been conventional to refer to a group of streptococci that produce greening (α-haemolysis) on blood agar as viridans streptococci; indeed, many still refer (inaccurately) to a microbe 'Streptococcus viridans'. Although most of these streptococci are virtually specific to the normal oropharyngeal flora and are rarely encountered at other sites, some are not found in the oropharynx at all, e.g. *Strep. bovis*, and others are found at many sites including the oropharynx, e.g. the milleri group of streptococci. The viridans streptococci are the commonest cause of community-acquired native valve endocarditis and community-acquired late-onset prosthetic endocarditis. The commonest species of the viridans streptococci specific to the oropharynx are *Strep. sanguis*, *Strep. oralis*, and *Strep. mutans*, but there are others. Dextran formation may be a virulence factor in these streptococci. Contrary to popular belief, they do not require a dental extraction to enter the bloodstream and cause frequent bacteraemias after chewing, tooth brushing, etc. They are organisms of low virulence and thus usually only infect previously abnormal heart valves. Whereas *Strep. oralis* and *Strep. sanguis* are occasionally isolated from blood cultures of patients who do not have endocarditis, the isolation of *Strep. mutans* from the blood is virtually synonymous with endocarditis.

Streptococcus bovis

This streptococcus, which may appear 'viridans' on blood agar, is part of the normal intestinal flora, but may initially be mistaken for an oral streptococcus. In common with the enterococci, it bears the Lancefield group D antigen and thus can also be mistaken for *Enterococcus faecalis*, though it is sensitive to penicillin whereas the latter is resistant. There is a significant association between *Strep. bovis* bacteraemia (and hence endocarditis) and colonic pathology, and any patient with *Strep. bovis* endocarditis thus warrants appropriate investigation. *Strep. bovis* endocarditis is much less common than that caused by oral streptococci.

Pyogenic streptococci

These organisms, often referred to as β-haemolytic streptococci, cause endocarditis less frequently than the viridans streptococci, but are more aggressive microbes and likely to affect (and often rapidly destroy) a previously normal valve. The commonest pyogenic streptococcus to cause endocarditis is the Lancefield group B β-haemolytic streptococcus (GBS), sometimes referred to as *Strep. agalactiae*. This organism is found as normal flora in the genital and gastrointestinal tracts. As with *Staph. aureus*, any patient with community acquired group B β-haemolytic streptococcus bacteraemia should be assumed to have infection in bone, joint, or on a heart valve until proved otherwise. Groups C and G β-haemolytic streptococci occasionally cause endocarditis, and group A even more rarely.

The milleri group of streptococci are best regarded as pyogenic streptococci: they form part of the normal flora of all mucous membranes and occasionally cause endocarditis, though much more often cause abscesses at many different sites. The milleri group consists of three species, *Strep. constellatus*, *Strep. intermedius*, and *Strep. anginosus*. Interestingly, these streptococci can bear the Lancefield antigens A, C, G, or F (or none); all group F streptococci are milleri, but not all milleri are group F.

Streptococcus pneumoniae (pneumococcus)

Pneumococcal endocarditis accounted for about 10% of cases of endocarditis in the preantibiotic era, but is now rarely seen, although it is sometimes diagnosed at autopsy of patients with fatal pneumococcal infection. The pneumococcus is a virulent pathogen and attacks normal heart valves. Patients with endocarditis generally have pneumonia and sometimes meningitis.

Enterococci

Enterococci form part of the normal gastrointestinal flora. They are more virulent than viridans streptococci and more resistant to antibiotics. The past decade has seen an increase in enterococcal endocarditis, particularly in older people, but this infection is still much less common than that caused by viridans streptococci. Whilst there are many species of enterococci, those causing endocarditis are usually *E. faecalis* and occasionally *E. faecium*. Most cases are community acquired, but the infection can sometimes be acquired in hospital as a result of urological instrumentation. Any patient admitted from the community with *E. faecalis* in the blood should be investigated for endocarditis.

Staphylococci

Staphylococci now account for about one-third of cases of community-acquired endocarditis and are the commonest cause of hospital-acquired endocarditis. Most of these staphylococci are *Staph. aureus*, but an increasing proportion are now coagulase-negative staphylococci. All staphylococci are skin organisms and patients become infected from their own skin flora, or in the case of methicillin-resistant *Staph. aureus* (MRSA) from that of others by cross-infection.

Staphylococcus aureus

Staph. aureus is an important and aggressive pathogen in community-acquired native valve endocarditis. Sometimes a trivial skin lesion can be identified as the source of the organism, but there is often no obvious lesion. *Staph. aureus*, and increasingly now MRSA, is the commonest cause of hospital-acquired endocarditis. Prosthetic valves can become infected with *Staph. aureus*, both early as result of sternal wound sepsis and late as with native valves. *Staph. aureus* is the commonest pathogen causing endocarditis in intravenous drug users.

Coagulase-negative staphylococci

Although still regarded by many as pathogens of prosthetic rather than native valves, coagulase-negative staphylococci also cause native valve infection. This has become more common, or certainly more commonly recognized, in the last two decades. The infecting species is most often *Staph. epidermidis*, but in many reports the designation '*Staph. epidermidis*' tends to be used for any unspeciated coagulase-negative staphylococcus. Many other species have been reported in native valve endocarditis, including *Staph. lugdunensis*, *Staph. simulans*, *Staph. warneri*, *Staph. capitis*, *Staph. caprae*, and *Staph. sciuri*. As in community-acquired *Staph. aureus* endocarditis, there is sometimes a presumptive predisposing skin lesion. Most patients have a pre-existing cardiac abnormality. Many of these staphylococci can be as virulent as *Staph. aureus* and share some of the same virulence factors.

Other organisms

A wide variety of organisms account for the few cases of endocarditis that are not caused by streptococci, staphylococci, or enterococci: only a few warrant a specific mention here.

HACEK group

These are fastidious, slow-growing species that are oropharyngeal commensals and have a predilection for heart valves such that their presence in blood cultures is virtually synonymous with this infection. The group consists of *Haemophilus aphrophilus/paraphrophilus*, *Actinobacillus actinomycetemcomitans*, *Cardiobacterium hominis*, *Eikenella corrodens*, and *Kingella kingae*. *A. actinomycetmecomitans*, in particular, seems more likely to infect prosthetic than native valves. The large vegetations thought to be characteristic of HACEK organisms in native valve infection may be the result of diagnostic delay and prolonged illness rather than any inherent property of the microbes.

Organisms that cannot be cultured by routine techniques

Endocarditis is a rare (and late) sequel of acute *Coxiella burnetii* (Q fever) infection, mostly in middle-aged men with pre-existing valve disease. The reservoir of the organism is usually sheep or cattle, but the source and mode of transmission in many cases is unknown. The diagnosis is usually made serologically, although *C. burnetii* can be recovered from the blood and excised valves by special techniques. The disease is almost certainly underdiagnosed, with some cases labelled 'culture negative' endocarditis.

Bartonella quintana endocarditis was first recognized in 1995 in homeless, alcoholic patients; *B. henselae* infection may be associated with cat or cat-flea contact, and other species of bartonella have also been described as causing endocarditis. Bartonella infection is usually diagnosed by serology, although these bacteria can be recovered from the blood and excised valves by special culture techniques and their presence detected by polymerase chain reaction. False-positive serology for chlamydia has been reported with bartonella infections, but chlamydia species, particularly *Chlamydia psittaci*, can also cause endocarditis (very rarely). It is possible that some cases attributed to chlamydia in the past on the basis of serology may have been caused by bartonella.

Fungi

Fungal endocarditis is very rare and more likely to occur on prosthetic than native valves, except in intravenous drug users. Most infections are acquired in hospital, with infection at intravascular access sites and broad-spectrum antibiotics predisposing to candida infections. Candida species, usually *Candida albicans*, are the commonest fungi, but *Aspergillus* spp. and more exotic genera have also been reported. Blood cultures are only likely to be positive with candida, and often only intermittently; for other fungi, the diagnosis must be made by serology and culture of the fungus from the excised valve or detection on valve histology.

Blood culture negative endocarditis

The possibility that an illness is not due to endocarditis should always be entertained when blood cultures are repeated negative. However, in 5 to 31% of definite cases of endocarditis the blood cultures will be negative. The commonest explanation for this is previous administration of antibiotics. In a few cases the pathogen will be recovered from another site, including the excised valve, excised emboli, or—specifically in right-sided endocarditis—respiratory specimens. Other causes of negative blood cultures are infection with organisms that cannot be grown by conventional blood culture methods, and infections that are diagnosed by serology such as *C. burnetii*, bartonella, and chlamydia.

Treatment

Initial therapy

The treatment of infective endocarditis ideally should be undertaken by a multidisciplinary team involving cardiologists, microbiologists, infectious disease specialists, and cardiac surgeons. Where possible, patients should be treated in cardiac centres that undertake cardiac surgery. Bactericidal antibiotics are the mainstay of treatment. The choice and duration of treatment depend upon the type of microorganism and its susceptibility profile, whether infection involves a native or prosthetic valve, and whether the patient is allergic to any antimicrobials.

In those patients who have been ill for many weeks, antibiotic treatment can be deferred until the blood cultures are positive and the pathogen known. Antibiotic treatment should be started immediately after taking blood cultures in patients who are acutely ill, using a broad-spectrum combination that can be adjusted when the pathogen is known. However, endocarditis is often not suspected initially in many patients who are acutely ill with native valve infection: there may be no obvious signs of this and antibiotics are started for 'septicaemia'. When methicillin-resistant staphylococci (whether *Staph. aureus* or coagulase-negative staphylococci) are likely pathogens, vancomycin or teicoplanin are an essential component of any combination. If empirical therapy is indicated the choice of antimicrobial agent should be dictated by the type of presentation, whether or not there is an intracardiac prosthesis in place, and on the expected causative organism as indicated from the clinical picture (Table 16.9.2.3).

Definitive therapy

There are various national guidelines for the treatment of specific organisms. It is important to realize that these are consensus based because there are no randomized controlled trials to show the efficacy of any particular regimen. It is conventional to estimate the minimum inhibitory concentration (MIC) of the antibiotic for the pathogen, but in practice routine disc sensitivity tests are quite satisfactory in many cases. Although it is widely believed that prosthetic endocarditis requires a longer duration of antibiotic treatment than native valve infection, there are few data to support this.

Table 16.9.2.3 Recommendations for empirical therapy of suspected endocarditis

Acute presentation	Flucloxacillin (8–12 g/d IV in 4 -6 divided doses) plus gentamicin (1 mg/kg/body weight IV 8 hourly *)
Indolent presentation	Penicillin (7.2 g IV daily in 6 divided doses) or ampicillin/amoxicillin (2 g IV 6 hourly) plus gentamicin (1 mg/kg/body weight IV 8 hourly *)
Penicillin allergy Intracardiac prosthesis Suspected MRSA	Vancomycin (1 g 12 hourly IV *) plus rifampicin (300 – 600 mg 2 hourly by mouth) plus gentamicin (1 mg/kg/body weight IV 8 hourly *)

* modified according to renal function and with monitoring of blood levels
Elliott et al, J. Antimicrobial Chemotherapy (2004), Guidelines for the antibiotic treatment of endocarditis in adults: report of the Working Party of the British Society for Antimicrobial Chemotherapy, 54:971–981. Reproduced with permission from the British Society for Antimicrobial Chemotherapy.

Recommendations for the treatment of the commonest causative organisms are taken from guidelines published by the British Society for Antimicrobial Chemotherapy (Tables 16.9.2.4–16.9.2.6).

HACEK endocarditis

If amoxicillin-sensitive, 2 g amoxicillin/ampicillin should be administered intravenously 4 to 6-hourly, plus gentamicin 1 mg/kg body weight according to renal function (for the first 2 weeks only) and with regular monitoring of drug levels. If amoxicillin-resistant, ceftriaxone 1 to 2 g (maximum 4 g) should be administered intravenously once daily, plus gentamicin as above.

Other uncommon causes of endocarditis

Treatments for uncommon culture-negative causes of endocarditis are shown in Table 16.9.2.7.

Fungal endocarditis

For candida, amphotericin B 1 mg/kg per day and flucytosine 100 mg/kg should be administered in four divided doses according to renal function (first choice), or fluconazole 400 mg 12-hourly orally (second choice), or caspofungin 70 mg as a loading dose, followed by 50 mg once daily (70 mg per day if weight >80 kg) (first choice if intolerance or resistance precludes other options).

Table 16.9.2.4 Summary of treatment options for streptococcal endocarditis

Penicillin MIC (mg/litre)	Penicillin and gentamicin 2 weeks	Penicillin 4 weeks	Ceftriaxone 4 weeks	Vancomycin 4 weeks	Ampicillin or amoxicillin by continuous infusion	Vancomycin or penicillin 4–6 weeks and gentamicin 2 weeks	Penicillin 4–6 weeks and gentamicin 4–6 weeks	Vancomycin 4–6 weeks and gentamicin 4–6 weeks
Viridans streptococci and S. bovis								
≤0.1	√	√	√	√				
≥0.1–>0.5		√		√		√		
0.5–>16					√		√	√
≥16								√
Group A streptococcus	√	√	√					
Group B, C, G streptococcus								
<0.5						√		
≥0.5							√	√
S. pneumoniae								
<0.1		√	√	√				
≥0.1			√	√				
Nutritionally variant streptococci							√	√
Prosthetic valve endocarditis								
≤0.1						√		
>0.1							√	√

Streptomycin is an alternative to gentamicin for streptomycin-sensitive, gentamicin-resistant isolates. (see sections on susceptibility testing, drug toxicity, and monitoring levels).
Penicillin and gentamicin for 2 weeks should not be used if there is an intracardiac abscess or extracardiac focus of infection.
If gentamicin or streptomycin is contraindicated (unacceptable risk of toxicity or a resistant bacterium).
Use only for isolates that are susceptible to ceftriaxone (MIC<0.5 mg/litre).
6 weeks treatment
Dosage (NB all need to be adjusted in renal impairment):penicillin, 1.2 – 2.4 4 g, 4-hourly or by continuous infusion: gentamicin, 1 mg/kg (ideal body weight) 8–12-hourly; ampicillin or amoxicillin, 12 g over 24 h;vancomycin, 1 g, 12-hourly; streptomycin, 7. mg/kg body weight, 12-hourly.
Elliott et al, J. Antimicrobial Chemotherapy (2004), Guidelines for the antibiotic treatment of endocarditis in adults: report of the Working Party of the British Society for Antimicrobial Chemotherapy, 54:971–981. Reproduced with permission from the British Society for Antimicrobial Chemotherapy.

Table 16.9.2.5 Summary of treatment recommendations for staphylococcal endocarditis

Methicillin sensitive	Flucloxacillin (2 g 4–6-hourly IV)
Methicillin resistant/ penicillin allergy	Vancomycin (1 g IV 12-hourly [a])
	plus
	Rifampicin (300–600 mg 12-hourly by mouth)[b]
	or
	Gentamicin (1 mg/kg body weight 8-hourly[a])
	or
	Sodium fusidate (500 mg 8-hourly by mouth)[b]
Endocarditis in presence of intracardiac prosthesis	Flucloxicillin (2 g 4–6-hourly IV)
	or
	Vancomycin (1 g IV 12-hourly [a])
	plus
	Rifampicin (300–600 mg 12-hourly by mouth)[b]
	and/or
	Gentamicin (1 mg/kg bodyweight 8-hourly[a])
	and/or
	Sodium fusidate (500 mg 8-hourly by mouth)[b]

[a] Modified according to renal function and with monitoring of drug levels.
[b] According to sensitivity.
Elliott et al, J. Antimicrobial Chemotherapy (2004), Guidelines for the antibiotic treatment of endocarditis in adults: report of the Working Party of the British Society for Antimicrobial Chemotherapy, 54:971–981. Reproduced with permission from the British Society for Antimicrobial Chemotherapy.

Table 16.9.2.6A Recommended regimens for treatment of enterococcal endocarditis caused by ampicillin-susceptible (MIC ≤8 mg/litre) isolates

Antimicrobial regimen	Dose and route	Duration (weeks)	Comment
1. Ampicillin (or penicillin)	2 g 4-hourly IV (2.4 g 4-hourly)	≥4	
plus gentamicin	1 mg/kg 8–12-hourly IV	≥4	
2. Vancomycin	1 g 12-hourly IV[b]	≥4	Alternative for patient with penicillin allergy provided vancomycin-susceptible (MIC ≤4 mg/litre)
plus gentamicin[a]	1 mg/kg 8–12-hourly IV[b]	≥4	
3. Teicoplanin	10 mg/kg 24-hourly IV[b]	≥4	Alternative for patient with penicillin allergy provided teicoplanin-susceptible (MIC ≤4 mg/litre)
plus gentamicin	1 mg/kg 8–12-hourly IV[b]	≥4	

[a] Provided isolate is high-level gentamicin-susceptible (MIC ≤128 mg/litre).
[b] Modified according to renal function and with monitoring of drug levels.
Elliott et al, J. Antimicrobial Chemotherapy (2004), Guidelines for the antibiotic treatment of endocarditis in adults: report of the Working Party of the British Society for Antimicrobial Chemotherapy, 54:971–981. Reproduced with permission from the British Society for Antimicrobial Chemotherapy.

Table 16.9.2.6B Regimens for treatment of enterococcal endocarditis caused by ampicillin-resistant isolates (MIC >8 mg/litre)

Antimicrobial regimen	Dose	Duration (weeks)
1. Vancomycin	1 g 12-hourly IV[b]	≥4
plus gentamicin[a]	1 mg/kg 8–12-hourly IV[b]	≥4
2. Teicoplanin	10 mg/kg 24-hourly IV[b]	≥4
plus gentamicin[a]	1 mg/kg 8–12-hourly IV[b]	≥4

[a] If high-level gentamicin-susceptible (MIC ≤128 mg/litre) isolate
[b] Modified according to renal function and with monitoring of drug levels.
Elliott et al, J. Antimicrobial Chemotherapy (2004), Guidelines for the antibiotic treatment of endocarditis in adults: report of the Working Party of the British Society for Antimicrobial Chemotherapy, 54:971–981. Reproduced with permission from the British Society for Antimicrobial Chemotherapy.

For aspergillus, voriconazole 6 mg/kg 12-hourly for two doses (loading) should be administered, then 4 mg/kg 12-hourly intravenously, or 400 mg 12-hourly for 24 h followed by 200 mg 12-hourly orally, or amphotericin B 1 mg/kg per day according to renal function.

Monitoring of treatment

Serum bactericidal titres against the infecting organism are no longer recommended. There was always great variation in the monitoring methods used for these tests and in the interpretation of their results. At best, they could only predict bacteriological not clinical cure, and bacteriological failure is very rare. The most useful

Table 16.9.2.6C Regimens for treatment of enterococcal endocarditis caused by high-level gentamicin-resistant (MIC >128 mg/litre) isolates

Antimicrobial regimen	Dose and route	Duration (weeks)	Comment
1. Ampicillin or (penicillin)	2 g 4-hourly IV (2.4 g IV 4-hourly)	≥4	Ampicillin-susceptible isolate (MIC ≤8 mg/litre)
plus streptomycin*	7.5 mg/kg 12-hourly IM	≥4	
2. Vancomycin	1 g 12-hourly IV**	≥4	Alternative for patient with penicillin allergy or ampicillin-resistant isolate (MIC >8 mg/litre)
plus streptomycin*	7.5 mg/kg 12-hourly IM	≥4	
3. Teicoplanin	10 mg/kg 24-hourly IV**	≥4	Alternative for patient with penicillin allergy or ampicillin-resistant isolate (MIC >8 mg/litre)
plus streptomycin*	7.5 mg/kg 12-hourly IM	≥4	

[a] Streptomycin can be added if the isolate is not high-level resistant. If streptomycin is considered appropriate or the isolate is streptomycin resistant, the cell-wall-acting agent should be continued for a minimum of 8 weeks.
[b] Modified according to renal function and with monitoring of drug levels.
Elliott et al, J. Antimicrobial Chemotherapy (2004), Guidelines for the antibiotic treatment of endocarditis in adults: report of the Working Party of the British Society for Antimicrobial Chemotherapy, 54:971–981. Reproduced with permission from the British Society for Antimicrobial Chemotherapy.

Table 16.9.2.7 Management of known causes of culture-negative endocarditis

Pathogen	Proposed treatment
Brucella	Doxycycline plus rifampicin or cotrimoxazole (>3 months' treatment)
Coxiella burnetti	Doxycycline plus hydroxychloroquine or doxycycline plus quinolone(>18 months' treatment)
Bartonella	β-Lactams or doxycycline plus aminoglycoside (>6 weeks' treatment)
Chlamydia	Doxycycline or new fluoroquinolones (long-term treatment, optimum duration unknown)
Mycoplasma	Doxycycline or new fluoroquinolones (>12 weeks treatment)
Legionella	Macrolides plus rifampicin or new fluoroquinolones (>6 months treatment)
Tropheryma whipplei	Cotrimoxazole or β-lactam plus aminoglycoside (long-term treatment; optimum duration unknown)

Reproduced from *Heart*, Prendergast B. D, 92:879–885. Copyright (2006) with permission from BMJ Publishing Group Ltd.

Table 16.9.2.8 Cardiac conditions at risk for infective endocarditis—international consensus

Cardiac diseases with the highest risk	Prosthetic valves—5–10 times higher risk than native valves
	Congenital heart disease causing cyanosis
	Previous infective endocarditis
	Surgically constructed conduits
Other cardiac diseases at risk	Valvular heart disease—AR, MR, AS, MS (including MVP with MR, and bicuspid aortic valve)
	Congenital heart disease which does not cause cyanosis, except IAC
	Hypertrophic obstructive cardiomyopathy
Cardiac disease not at risk for infective endocarditis	IAC
	MVP without MR, functional MI, mitral ring calcifications
	Coronary artery-bypass grafting
	Cardiac pacemakers
	Implantable defibrillators
	Corrected left-to-right shunts

AR, aortic regurgitation; AS, aortic stenosis; IAC, interatrial communication; MI, mitral insufficiency; MR, mitral regurgitation; MVP, mitral valve prolapse.

Catherine Leport and the Endocarditis Working Group of International Society of Chemotherapy (2008). Antibiotic prophylaxis for infective endocarditis. Clin Microbial Infect 4, 3S56–3S61 (table 5 p3s59). With permission from Wiley-Blackwell.

laboratory test for monitoring the response to treatment (which is usually obvious clinically) is serial estimation of C-reactive protein; this is of much more use than the ESR, which is much slower to fall.

Relapse of endocarditis usually occurs within 2 months of cessation of treatment. The relapse rate is lowest for patients with native valve endocarditis caused by penicillin-sensitive viridans streptococci. Relapse rate in prosthetic valve endocarditis is between 10 and 15%.

Prevention and prophylaxis

Antibiotic prophylaxis in 'at risk' patients is generally accepted as reasonable. This is largely based on indirect data from *in vitro* studies, experimental animal models, and studies of clinical bacteraemia, but there are many uncertainties about its value, and data confirming its clinical effectiveness are lacking. However, many authorities continue to recommend antibiotic prophylaxis to cover certain procedures associated with predictable and significant bacteraemia in patients known to be at high risk, but accept that this might fail, even with the recommended regimens, and that significant adverse reactions to antibiotics are important, even if relatively uncommon.

The most controversial area for the use of prophylactic antibiotics concerns dental treatment. A working party of the British Society of Antimicrobial Chemotherapy first recommended that the practice of giving all patients with cardiac abnormalities antibiotics before dental treatment should be stopped, except for those who have a history of healed infective endocarditis, prosthetic heart valves, or surgically constructed conduits. Many other groups vigorously opposed this recommendation, not least because some cases of endocarditis that involve dental procedures have resulted in litigation, and in most of these legal cases, endocarditis was judged to be caused by dental manipulations on the basis of the dental procedure, cardiac pathology, infecting microorganism, and the temporal link between the onset of endocardial infection and the dental manipulation.

In 2007 the American Heart Association revised its guidelines limiting the use of antibiotic prophylaxis to the highest risk patients who were undergoing the highest risk procedures (Tables 16.9.2.8–16.9.2.9); in the case of dental treatment these were manipulation of gingival tissue, the periapical region of teeth or perforation of the oral mucosa.

The National Institute for Health and Clinical Excellence (NICE) has developed guidelines for adoption by the National Health Service in England, Wales and Northern Ireland. Based on its findings that (1) there is no consistent association between having an interventional procedure and infective endocarditis, (2) that the clinical effectiveness of antibiotic prophylaxis is not proven, (3) that the risk of antibiotic associated adverse effects exceeds the benefits, and (4) that prophylaxis is not cost effective, NICE concluded that antibiotic prophylaxis should not be given to any at risk patients undergoing an interventional procedure. NICE made one exception; namely in patients undergoing a gastrointestinal or genitourinary procedure where there is suspected pre-existing infection, who should receive an antibiotic that covers endocarditis causative organisms.

Most recently the ACC/AHA Task Force on Practice Guidelines has downgraded from Class 1 (mandatory) to Class 2 (reasonable practice) the recommendation for antibiotic prophylaxis for high risk patients.

Not surprisingly these departures from established practice have met with mixed reactions; the dental profession in the UK has welcomed the NICE proposals, but many British cardiologists and cardiovascular surgeons have opposed them. A sensible approach

Table 16.9.2.9 Procedures at risk for infective endocarditis—international consensus

Dental	All procedures
Upper respiratory tract	Tonsillectomy, adenoidectomy
Gastrointestinal	Oesophageal dilatation or surgery
	Endoesophageal laser procedures
	Sclerosing procedures of oesophageal varices
	Abdominal surgery
	ERCP
Urological	Instrumental procedures involving the ureter or the kidney
	Biopsy or surgery of prostate or urinary tract
Procedures for which the risk of infective endocarditis is controversial	
Upper respiratory tract	Fibreoptic bronchoscopy
	Endotrachial tube insertion
Gastrointestinal	Colonoscopy with or without biopsy
Genital	Vaginal hysterectomy, vaginal delivery[a]

[a] However, antibiotic treatment is required in cases of concomitant infection.
Catherine Leport and the Endocarditis Working Group of International Society of Chemotherapy (2008). Antibiotic prophylaxis for infective endocarditis. Clin Microbial Infect 4, 3S56–3S61 (table 6 p3s59). With permission from Wiley-Blackwell.

would appear to be to allow individual doctors to do what they feel is best for their patients and to be encouraged to discuss their reasons for taking a particular stance on antibiotic prophylaxis with those patients. Patients themselves should be taught the importance of good oral hygiene and to recognize symptoms that might indicate infective endocarditis and when to seek expert help. Suitable prophylactic antibiotic regimens are described in Table 16.9.2.10

Surgical treatment of infective endocarditis

Surgery will be required in about 30% of cases during the acute phase (first 4 months) of endocarditis, and in 20 to 40% of cases thereafter. Since surgery may be required at any time during an episode of endocarditis, it is essential to involve a cardiac surgeon in the overall management from the outset, which in practice means transferring the patient to a centre with cardiac surgery whenever possible. Surgery for endocarditis carries a risk of 10 to 25% mortality, with up to 25% of patients developing a paravalvular leak requiring a further operation. The main predictive factors for mortality associated with surgery are prosthetic valve endocarditis, infections due to staphylococci or candida, perioperative shock, or late referral.

The timing of surgery is all-important and demands experience and clinical judgement. The main indications are haemodynamic instability, persistent infection, and annular or aortic abscesses. In such cases surgery should never be delayed, even if only hours or days of antibiotic treatment have been given. The primary goals of the surgeon are to remove all infected material and to reconstruct the heart and/or restore valvular function at the lowest operative risk. An understanding of the surgical anatomy of infective endocarditis is a precondition for surgical success, which means the involvement of an experienced surgical team. Wherever possible, surgeons now strive to preserve the native valve, either by removal of the vegetation(s) or by valve repair. In prosthetic valve endocarditis, removal of all foreign material is mandatory. Actuarial survival figures indicate a 75% survival at 5 years and a 61% survival at 10 years after cardiac surgery for infective endocarditis.

Table 16.9.2.10 Prevention of endocarditis in patients with known cardiac risk[a]

Procedure	Dose/route	Comment
Dental procedures[b] (under local or no anaesthesia)		
Patients who have not received more than a single dose of a penicillin in the previous month, including those with a prosthetic valve (but not those who have had endocarditis)	Oral amoxicillin 3 g 1 h before the procedure; children <5 years to receive one-quarter of adult dose, aged 5–10 years, then half the adult dose.	
Patients who are penicillin-allergic	Oral clindamycin 600 mg 1 h before procedure; children <5 years to receive one-quarter the adult dose, aged 5–10 years, half the adult dose.	
Patients who have had previous endocarditis	Amoxicillin + gentamicin	As under general anaesthesia
Dental procedures[b] (under general anaesthetic)		
No special risk		
(including patients who have not received more than a single dose of penicillin in the previous month)	*Either* IV amoxicillin 1 g at induction, then oral amoxicillin 500 mg 6 h later; children <5 years to receive one-quarter of adult dose, aged 5–10 years, half the adult dose.	
	Or oral amoxicillin 3 g 4 h before induction, then oral amoxicillin 3 g as soon as possible after the procedure; children <5 years to receive one-quarter of adult dose, aged 5–10 years half the adult dose.	
	Or oral amoxicillin 3 g + oral probenecid 1 g 4 h before procedure.	

Table 16.9.2.10 (*cont'd*) Prevention of endocarditis in patients with known cardiac risk[a]

Procedure	Dose/route	Comment
Special risk		
Patients with a prosthetic valve or who have had endocarditis	IV amoxicillin 1 g + IV gentamicin 1.5 mg/kg at induction, then oral amoxicillin 500 mg 6 h later; children <5 years to receive amoxicillin at one-quarter of adult dose + gentamicin 2 mg/kg; aged 5–10 years amoxicillin half the adult dose + gentamicin 2 mg/kg.	
Patients who are penicillin-allergic or who have received more than a single dose of penicillin in the previous month	*Either* IV vancomycin 1 g over at least 100 min, then IV gentamicin 120 mg at induction or 15 min before procedure; children <10 years to receive vancomycin 20 mg/kg + gentamicin 2 mg/kg.	
	Or IV teicoplanin 400 mg + gentamicin 120 mg at induction or 15 min before procedure; children <14 years to receive teicoplanin 6 mg/kg + gentamicin 2 mg/kg.	
	Or IV clindamycin 300 mg over at least 10 min at induction or 15 min before procedure, then oral or IV clindamycin 150 mg 6 h later; children <5 years to receive one-quarter of adult dose, aged 5–10 years, half the adult dose.	
Other procedures		
For genitourinary, gastrointestinal, respiratory, or obstetric/gynaecological procedures in patients at risk of endocarditis		
Ampicillin/amoxicillin	IV amoxicillin 1 g (<5 years of age 250 mg; 5–10 years of age 500 mg)	A single dose given just before the procedure or at induction of anaesthesia
+ gentamicin	1.5 mg/kg IV	
If allergic to penicillin		
Teicoplanin	400 mg IV (children <14 years 6 mg/kg)	Given just before the procedure or at induction of anaesthesia
+gentamicin	1.5 mg/kg IV	
Multistage procedures		
Amoxicillin + clindamycin	Amoxicillin 3 g + clindamycin 600 mg	Alternating oral doses 1 h before procedure are recommended

[a] Advice on the prevention of endocarditis reflects the recommendations of a Working Party of the British Society for Antimicrobial Chemotherapy, *Lancet* 1982, **2**, 1323–6; *idem*, 1986, **1**, 1267; *idem*, 1990, **335**, 8–9; *idem*, 1922, **339**, 292–3; *idem*, 1997, **350**, 1100; *J Antimicrob Chemother*, 1993; **31**, 437–8. *J Antimicrob Chemother*, 2006; **57**, 1035–42.

[b] Antibiotic prophylaxis for dental procedures may be supplemented by with chlorhexidine gluconate gel 1% or chlorhexidine gluconate mouthwash 0.2% used 5 min before procedure, but there is no proof that this is beneficial.

Reproduced from *J. Antimicrobial Chemotherapy* (2006) 57:1035–1042. With permission from Oxford University Press.

There are several unresolved issues with regards to the surgical treatment of endocarditis. First, the use of surgery when embolization has taken place remains controversial. Recurrent emboli, persistent vegetation, after a major systemic embolus, and vegetation size (>10 mm), have all been put forward as indications, but there are no controlled trials to support a firm recommendation. Secondly, the optimal timing of surgery in patients who have had a cerebrovascular accident, either as a result of an embolic stroke or from haemorrhage due to a ruptured mycotic aneurysm: as a general rule, delay of at least 1 week is suggested if haemorrhage is detected by CT scanning, but surgery can be undertaken within 72 h if there is no haemorrhage present. Thirdly, the duration of antibiotic treatment postoperatively: if the excised valve is sterile, it is doubtful whether further antibiotics are of any benefit, but if the pathogen is isolated from the excised valve a continuance of 2 weeks of antibiotics seems reasonable, although if debridement is incomplete whatever antibiotics are given may fail.

Further reading

Baine RJI, *et al.* (1988). Impact of a policy of collaborative management on mortality and morbidity from infective endocarditis. *Int J Cardiol*, **19**, 47–54.

Brooks, N (2009). Prophylactic antibiotic treatment to prevent infective endocarditis: new guidance from the National Institute for Health and Clinical Excellence. *Heart*, **95**, 774–80.

Cohen PS, Maguire JH, Weinstein L (1980). Infective endocarditis caused by gram negative bacteria: a review of the literature 1945–1977. *Prog Cardiovasc Dis*, **22**, 205–241.

Elliott TSJ, *et al.* (2004). Guidelines for the antibiotic treatment of endocarditis in adults. Report of the Working Party of the British Society for Antimicrobial Therapy. *J Antimicrob Chemother*, **54**, 971–81.

Habib G, *et al.* (2009). Guidelines on the prevention diagnosis and treatment of infective endocarditis. *European Heart Journal*, **30**, 2369–413.

Hoen B, *et al.* (1995). Infective endocarditis in patients with negative blood cultures: analysis of 88 cases from a one year nationwide survey in France. *Clin Infect Dis*, **20**, 501–6.

Moreillon P, Que Y-A (2004). Infective endocarditis. *Lancet*, **363**, 139–49.

Mylonakis E, Calderwood SB (2001). Infective endocarditis in adults. *N Engl J Med*, **345**, 1318–29.

NICE clinical guideline 64 (2008). Prophylaxis against infective endocarditis: antimicrobial prophylaxis against infective endocarditis in adults and children undergoing interventional procedures. www.nice.org.uk

Prendergast BD (2006). The changing face of endocarditis. *Heart*, **92**, 879–85.

Rick A, *et al.* (2008). ACC/AHA 2008 guideline update on valvular heart disease: focused update on infective endocarditis. *Circulation*, **118**, 887–96.

Watkin R, *et al.* (2003). The microbiological diagnosis of infective endocarditis. *J Infect*, **47**, 1–11.

16.9.3 Cardiac disease in HIV infection

Peter F. Currie

Essentials

Symptomatic heart disease can affect up to 10% of HIV-positive patients and cause death in around 2%. Echocardiographic screening is recommended.

In resource-poor countries where access to antiretroviral drugs is limited the typical manifestations are (1) HIV heart-muscle disease—this occurs in the late stages of HIV infection, with dilated cardiomyopathy having a dismal prognosis, the median survival after diagnosis being about 100 days; angiotensin converting enzyme (ACE) inhibitors and β-blockers may produce unacceptable side effects; (2) pericardial effusion—a common finding, but most are symptomless; significant effusions are often due to mycobacterial infection or malignant infiltration, particularly with non-Hodgkin's lymphoma; and (3) isolated pulmonary hypertension—this is rare and has a grave prognosis (50% survival at 1 year), but highly active antiretroviral therapy (HAART) may be beneficial.

In the developed world premature coronary artery disease is more common in patients with HIV than in controls. There is a two- to threefold increase in the incidence of acute coronary events in HAART-treated HIV patients, which is thought to be related to HIV lipodystrophy, an ill-defined syndrome that resembles the non-HIV metabolic syndrome and is found in up to 35% of patients after 12 months of protease inhibitor therapy.

Sudden death due to cardiac-rhythm abnormalities is well recognized in HIV infection and may account for 20% of cardiac-related deaths.

Introduction

Cardiovascular manifestations of HIV infection are well recognized and have been reported in up to 40% of autopsies and about 25% of echocardiographic studies performed on patients with AIDS. Although most of these lesions are minor, symptomatic heart disease can affect up to 10% of HIV-positive patients and cause death in around 2%.

Heart muscle disease was previously the dominant cardiac complication of HIV infection in the developed world. However, the development of highly active anti-retroviral therapy (HAART) has significantly altered the course of HIV infection and has most likely reduced the incidence of many forms of heart disease in AIDS. However, HAART-induced dyslipidaemia may be an important factor for the development of premature coronary artery disease, which is becoming increasingly common. HIV heart-muscle disease, pericardial effusion, and pulmonary hypertension continue to predominate in resource poor countries where access to antiretroviral drugs is limited.

The common cardiovascular manifestations of HIV infection are listed in Table 16.9.3.1.

HIV/AIDS and the pericardium

Pericardial effusion was found frequently in early autopsy studies, often in association with generalized fluid retention and advanced HIV infection. Small effusions remain common, but most are symptomless. Cardiac tamponade is rare, but the finding of unexplained breathlessness, raised jugular venous pressure, or

Table 16.9.3.1 Cardiac manifestations of HIV/AIDS

Pericardial effusion	Idiopathic
	Infectious (viral, bacterial—especially tuberculous, and fungal)
	Neoplastic (Kaposi's sarcoma and non-Hodgkin's lymphoma)
Heart muscle disease	Myocarditis (idiopathic/lymphocytic, specific infections, toxins)
	Dilated cardiomyopathy
Left ventricular dysfunction	
Isolated right ventricular dysfunction	
Endocarditis	Marantic (nonbacterial thrombotic endocarditis)
	Infective
Pulmonary hypertension	Primary
	Secondary (recurrent bronchopulmonary infections, thromboembolism)
Premature atherosclerosis and coronary artery disease	
Adverse drug effects	Hyperlipidaemia
	Induction of arrhythmia
Vascular disease	Coronary artery disease
Autonomic dysfunction	Sudden death

radiographic cardiomegaly should prompt early echocardiographic assessment (see Chapter 16.8).

In Africa up to 72% of patients with serosanguinous effusions have been found to be HIV positive, and *Mycobacterium tuberculosis* or *M. avium-intracellulare* pericarditis is common. Appropriate antituberculous and antiviral therapies may be helpful, but it is not clear if corticosteroids are beneficial in this situation and they are generally avoided. Herpes simplex virus, cytomegalovirus, and other unusual organisms may clinically be implicated, but significant pericardial effusions are often due to malignant infiltration, particularly with non-Hodgkin's lymphoma.

Pericardiocentesis and pericardiectomy can be used to treat tamponade in HIV infection, but surgical intervention may not be appropriate in patients with very advanced disease. Clearly, however, culture of pericardial biopsy or fluid from symptomatic effusions may be useful in identifying treatable opportunistic infections or malignancy.

Cardiac tumours in HIV/AIDS

In AIDS patients, Kaposi's sarcoma (KS) is a disseminated visceral disease with cardiac involvement in up to 25% of cases. Isolated cardiac Kaposi's sarcoma is rare. The tumour often invades the subpericardial fat around coronary arteries and may infiltrate the pericardium or myocardium. However, despite this, Kaposi's sarcoma is not usually associated with cardiac symptoms and significant effusion is rare. The prevalence of cardiac Kaposi's sarcoma in HIV/AIDS appears to be falling.

Primary cardiac lymphoma is extremely rare in HIV-negative individuals, although disseminated lymphoma may involve the myocardium more frequently. Both patterns of malignant cardiac involvement occur in AIDS patients, and non-Hodgkin's lymphoma in particular may involve the pericardium or myocardium. In contrast to Kaposi's sarcoma, cardiac lymphoma is commonly associated with tamponade, symptomatic heart failure and conduction abnormalities. This diagnosis should therefore be considered in AIDS patients with rapidly progressive cardiovascular symptoms, unexpected arrhythmias or heart block.

Endocardial disease in HIV/AIDS

Marantic or nonbacterial thrombotic endocarditis was a frequent finding in early AIDS port-mortem series. Noninfectious, systemic thromboembolism was a common sequel and hence the condition is associated with significant morbidity and mortality. It is now rarely described as a complication of AIDS.

Although AIDS patients are susceptible to bacterial infections, infective endocarditis rarely occurs in HIV infection outwith the setting of injection drug use (see Chapter 16.9.2). Asymptomatic HIV infection *per se* appears to have little effect on the susceptibility to, or the mortality from, the condition, although bacterial endocarditis runs a more fulminant course in the late stages of AIDS. As with infective endocarditis in patients who are HIV negative, in intravenous drug users the tricuspid valve is most commonly involved and *Staphylococcus aureus* or *Streptococcus viridans* are the most frequently isolated organisms. *Aspergillus fumigatus*, *Pseudallescheria boydii*, and other forms of bacterial and fungal endocarditis occur in end stage AIDS.

Just as for patients without AIDS, adequate bacteriological investigations are required when endocarditis is suspected in HIV-positive individuals, but initial 'best guess' antimicrobial treatment (see Chapter 16.9.2) may have to be widened, particularly if fungal endocarditis is suspected. Valvular heart surgery has been described in HIV positive intravenous drug users with endocarditis, but continued drug use often results in a poor prognosis.

Heart muscle disease

HIV heart muscle disease occurs in the late stages of HIV infection and is associated with low CD4 counts. Before HAART, symptomatic, congestive cardiac failure was found in around 5% of HIV patients. However, the signs and symptoms of heart failure were frequently mistakenly attributed to anaemia or bronchopulmonary infection, and left ventricular systolic dysfunction—either isolated or in the form of a dilated cardiomyopathy—could be found echocardiographically in 10 to 15% of patients with AIDS.

The cause or causes of HIV heart muscle disease remain unknown, but are almost certainly complex. It is likely that an autoimmune lymphocytic myocarditis plays a key pathogenic role, in line with current thinking on the pathogenesis of idiopathic dilated cardiomyopathy in HIV-negative patients. Some form of myocarditis can be found by biopsy or at autopsy in up to 40% of patients with AIDS, and rarely specific organisms may be identified, e.g. *Toxoplasma gondii* or cytomegalovirus, usually in the setting of disseminated infection. Some *in situ* hybridization studies have suggested that HIV-1 may be present in the myocardium of patients with HIV heart muscle disease, although clear evidence for a primary HIV myocarditis is still lacking. It is possible that the myocarditis is secondary to an autoimmune reaction mediated through cytokines or circulating cardiac autantibodies, but other potential co-factors include specific micronutrient deficiencies (especially selenium) or the cardiotoxic side effects of antiretroviral agents.

HIV-related dilated cardiomyopathy has a dismal prognosis, with median survival after diagnosis being about 100 days (Fig. 16.9.3.1). Conventional anti-heart failure treatment is used, but vasodilating agents such as ACE inhibitors are often poorly tolerated and β-blockers may produce unacceptable side effects. Diuretics, digoxin, and aldosterone antagonists may be more useful. The incidence of myocarditis, heart muscle disease, and symptomatic heart failure appears to have decreased in the HAART era.

Right ventricular dysfunction and pulmonary hypertension in HIV/AIDS

Right ventricular dysfunction may occur as part of HIV heart muscle disease but can occur in isolation, without pulmonary hypertension, and is of unknown significance (Fig. 16.9.3.1). Bronchopulmonary infections should be treated aggressively and intravenous drug use, which may result in microvascular emboli, should be discouraged.

Isolated pulmonary hypertension (Fig. 16.9.3.2) is a rare complication of HIV infection and has a grave prognosis, with a 50% survival at 1 year. The condition has little correlation with CD4 counts and may be related to the action of viral proteins or cytokines on the endothelial cell. Characteristic pathological lesions including intimal fibrosis and plexiform lesions confirm its similarity to non-HIV primary pulmonary hypertension. Right heart catheterization may be worthwhile to determine if pulmonary hypertension is reversible. Oxygen, calcium channel antagonists, vasodilators, phosphodiesterase V inhibitors, and nitric oxide therapy may be

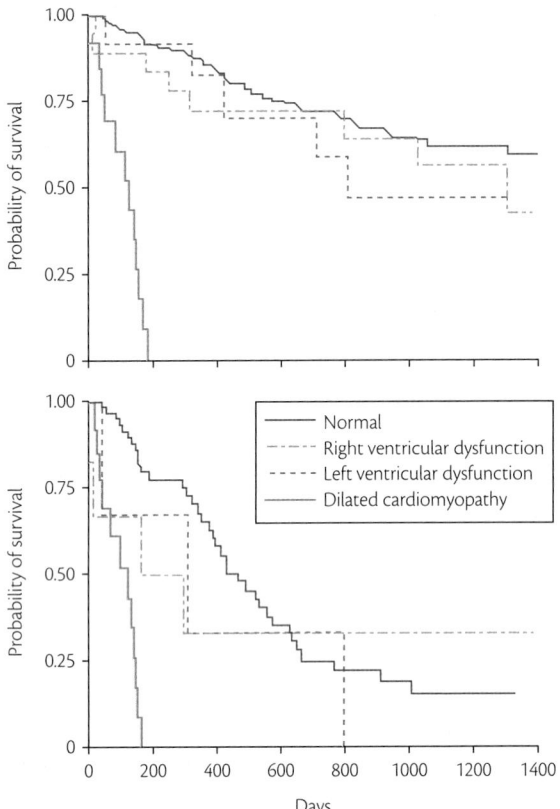

Fig. 16.9.3.1 Top: Survival curves for 296 patients who were HIV positive with structurally normal hearts or cardiac dysfunction. Bottom: Survival time to death related to AIDS in 81 subjects with CD4 cell count <20 × 10⁶/litre.
Reproduced from *BMJ*, Currie *et al*, 309:1605–1607. Copyright (1994) with permission from BMJ Publishing Group Ltd.

considered, but are unproven therapies in this circumstance and do not necessarily improve prognosis, but HAART itself may prove beneficial in terms of outcome.

Coronary artery disease in HIV infection

HIV lipodystrophy is an ill-defined syndrome that resembles the non-HIV metabolic syndrome and includes dyslipidaemia and insulin resistance. It is dependent on the type and duration of antiretroviral therapy, but can be found in up to 35% of patients after 12 months of protease inhibitor therapy.

The significant changes in lipid metabolism noted in the recipients of protease inhibitors have led to fears of an epidemic of premature atherosclerotic disease in this population. The first cases of acute myocardial infarction in treated HIV patients emerged in the late 1990s. Acute myocardial infarction appears to be the commonest presentation of coronary heart disease in HIV populations and it is plausible that—because acute coronary syndromes involve low-volume, lipid-rich plaques—HAART may promote development of vulnerable lesions or influence plaque rupture. Similarly, most HIV patients with coronary symptoms will have been diagnosed with AIDS, which raises the possibility that opportunistic infections may also be involved in this process. A case of coronary arteritis due to HIV has been described, but acute coronary events are not clearly related to HIV replication as one-third of patients have undetectable plasma HIV RNA at the time of symptoms.

Coronary angiography can be carried out safely in patients with HIV and frequently reveals proximal vessel involvement and single vessel disease. Percutaneous coronary intervention is a reasonable therapy, with use of drug eluting stents advocated by some because of concerns over the possibility of aggressive restenosis. Fibrinolysis and coronary artery bypass have also been used with acceptable survival rates, hence it is reasonable that the clinical situation should determine the use of coronary treatments in the same manner as for the non-HIV population.

It may be necessary to consider drug treatment for hyperlipidaemia, particularly if antiretroviral treatment cannot be changed or interrupted. Like protease inhibitors, most HMG CoA reductase inhibitors (statins) are metabolized through the cytochrome P450 system. Coprescription of these drugs may therefore result in competitive inhibition, significantly increased plasma statin levels, and increased risk of myopathy and rhabdomyolysis. Pravastatin is metabolized by a different pathway and for this reason it is recommended that hypercholesterolaemia in HIV patients receiving protease inhibitors is initially treated with pravastatin 20 mg daily, with careful monitoring of virological parameters and creatine kinase levels. Rosuvastatin, a more power statin, metabolized in a similar manner, may be used with care in some cases. Bile acid sequestrants, although attractive from the point of view of drug interactions, may have adverse effects on serum triglyceride levels or impair absorption of antiretrovirals.

Sudden death

Sudden death due to cardiac rhythm abnormalities is well recognized in HIV infection and may account for 20% of cardiac-related deaths

Fig. 16.9.3.2 (a) Long-axis and (b) short-axis parasternal view of a two-dimensional echocardiogram from an HIV-positive intravenous drug user with idiopathic pulmonary hypertension illustrating dilatation of the right ventricle and flattening of the interventricular septum. LV, left ventricle; RV, right ventricle.

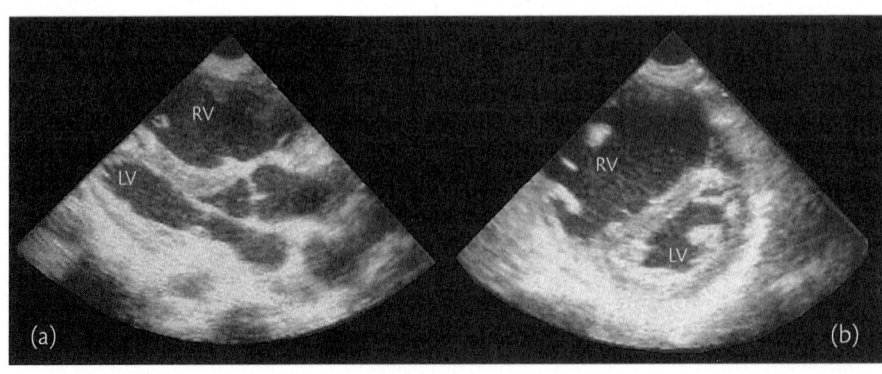

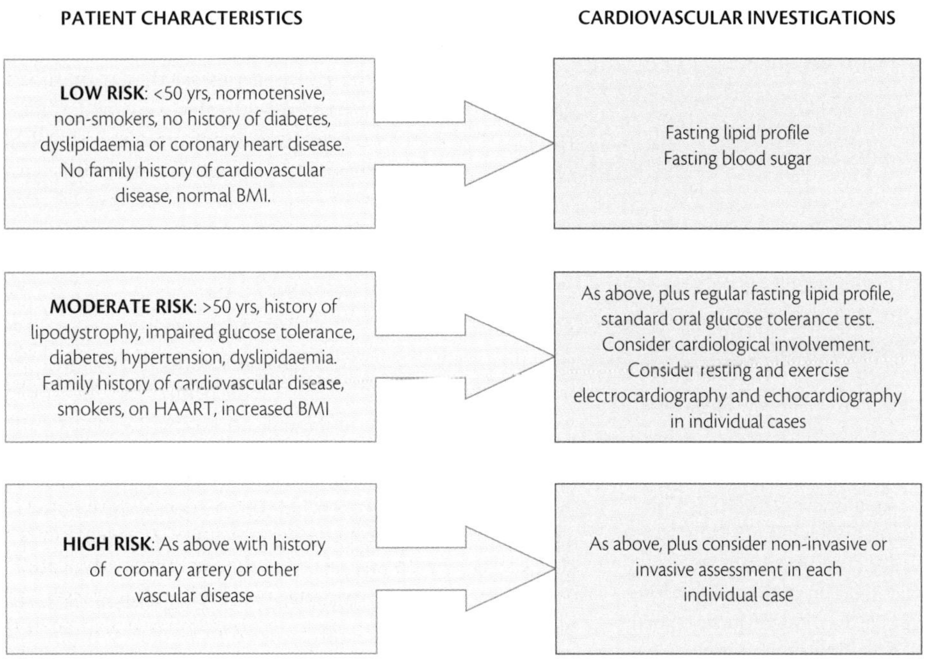

PATIENT CHARACTERISTICS   CARDIOVASCULAR INVESTIGATIONS

> **LOW RISK**: <50 yrs, normotensive, non-smokers, no history of diabetes, dyslipidaemia or coronary heart disease. No family history of cardiovascular disease, normal BMI.

> Fasting lipid profile
> Fasting blood sugar

> **MODERATE RISK**: >50 yrs, history of lipodystrophy, impaired glucose tolerance, diabetes, hypertension, dyslipidaemia. Family history of cardiovascular disease, smokers, on HAART, increased BMI

> As above, plus regular fasting lipid profile, standard oral glucose tolerance test. Consider cardiological involvement. Consider resting and exercise electrocardiography and echocardiography in individual cases

> **HIGH RISK**: As above with history of coronary artery or other vascular disease

> As above, plus consider non-invasive or invasive assessment in each individual case

Fig. 16.9.3.3 An approach to cardiovascular assessment in patients with HIV.

in this population. Arrhythmia may be secondary to other cardiac pathology or be a consequence of some forms of treatment. Pentamidine and ganciclovir in particular may be arrhythmogenic, especially in the setting of electrolyte disturbance. Autonomic dysfunction, with excessive sympathetic tone, small vessel vasculitis, and neural tissue fibrosis may also predispose to syncopal events or death.

Cardiovascular assessment of the patient with HIV/AIDS

Echocardiography

The usefulness of echocardiographic assessment of patients with HIV has been demonstrated in many studies. It can easily identify many cardiac conditions common in HIV-positive patients that are associated with a poor outcome, including useful information on the appearance of the right ventricle, an indirect assessment of pulmonary pressures, and regional wall motion abnormalities suggestive of coronary artery disease. Any HIV-positive patient at high risk of developing cardiovascular disease, or with any potential clinical manifestation of it, should therefore have an echocardiogram performed, with repeated imaging every 1 to 2 years. It may be justifiable to perform a baseline study at the time of diagnosis of HIV in any patient, with 1- to 2-yearly examination of asymptomatic patients and closer monitoring on discovery of cardiovascular abnormalities or in those with significant viral infection or unexplained pulmonary symptoms.

Assessment of cardiovascular risk

Traditional cardiovascular risk profiling has become more important in the care of HIV-positive patients. The prevalence of heavy cigarette smoking in HIV-infected patients is as high as 40%.

Diabetes mellitus requiring treatment is common, and HIV patients appear to be at higher risk of developing hypertension at a younger age than the general population such that blood pressure screening is recommended. A careful history should also identify a family history of premature vascular disease, recreational drug use, poor diet, and lack of physical exercise. A risk score may be calculated to help guide investigation and treatment (Fig. 16.9.3.3).

Further reading

Chen Y, *et al.* (1999). Human immunodeficiency virus – associated pericardial effusion: report of 40 cases and review of the literature. *Am Heart J*, **137**, 516–21.

Currie PF, *et al.* (1994). Heart muscle disease related to HIV infection: prognostic implications. *BMJ*, **309**, 1605–7.

Hsue PY, Waters DD (2005). What a cardiologist needs to know about patients with human immunodeficiency virus infection. *Circulation*, **112**, 3947–57.

Huang L, *et al.* (2006). Intensive care of patients with HIV infection. *New Engl J Med*, **355**, 173–81.

Nahass RG, *et al.* (1990). Infective endocarditis in intravenous drug users: a comparison of human immunodeficiency virus type 1—negative and positive patients. *J Infect Dis*, **162**, 967–70.

Pugliese A, *et al.* (2000). Impact of highly active antiretroviral therapy in HIV-positive patients with cardiac involvement. *J Infect*, **40**, 282–4.

Saidi A, Bricker JT (1998). Pulmonary hypertension in patients infected with HIV. In: Lipshultz SE (ed.) *Cardiology in AIDS*, pp. 187–94. Chapman & Hall, New York.

Vittecoq D, *et al.* (2003). Coronary heart disease in HIV-infected patients in the highly active antiretroviral treatment era. *AIDS*, **17**, Suppl 1, S70–6.

Volberding PA, *et al.* (2003). The Pavia consensus statement. *AIDS*, **17**, Suppl 1, S170–9.

16.9.4 Cardiovascular syphilis

Krishna Somers

Essentials

Clinicians need to be aware of cardiovascular syphilis in patients at risk of infection, with the time taken from initial infection to clinical manifestation ranging from 10 to 25 years, although this is accelerated in patients with HIV infection. Inadequate or interrupted antibiotic therapy may confound the development of cardiovascular syphilis and make diagnosis difficult.

Presentation may be with (1) asymptomatic aortitis; (2) aortic regurgitation—the commonest manifestation resulting from annular dilatation of the aortic ring and eventually affecting 70% of patients with untreated syphilis; (3) coronary ostial stenosis; (4) aneurysm of the aorta; or (5) a combination of these. Syphilitic aortitis must be included in the differential diagnosis of aortic regurgitation in older people and those with predisposing factors.

Diagnosis—serological testing is the mainstay: latent or inadequately treated syphilis should be suspected with the finding of a positive nonspecific treponemal serological test (e.g. rapid plasma reagin, RPR) and a positive specific treponemal antibody test (e.g. *Treponema pallidum* haemagglutination, TPHA), but negative serology does not absolutely exclude infection with *T. pallidum*, particularly in an immunocompromised host.

Management—parenteral penicillin remains the treatment of choice for cardiovascular syphilis: the World Health Organization and European and United States guidelines recommend benzathine penicillin 2.4×10^6 units administered once weekly for 3 weeks by the intramuscular route. Modern imaging technology with MRI and three-dimensional CT enables innovative surgical approaches in the repair of syphilitic aortitis.

Introduction

At the beginning of the 20th century cardiovascular syphilis accounted for 5 to 10% of deaths due to cardiovascular disease. The institution of public health measures—early recognition of syphilis and treatment with penicillin since the 1940s—produced a sharp decline in its incidence and hence in the tertiary manifestations and mortality from cardiovascular and neurosyphilis.

The rarity of syphilitic aortitis in recent times has led to publication of case reports describing challenges in diagnosis and management. With the re-emergence of syphilis in both developed and developing countries, particularly in South East Asia and sub-Saharan Africa, delayed cardiovascular complications of syphilis are likely to be seen with increasing frequency.

An increased rate of infection with the causative organism, *Treponema pallidum*, prevails in sexually promiscuous individuals, intravenous drug abusers, men who have unsafe sex with men, sex workers trafficked from 'east to west', clients of sex workers, and so-called 'bridging populations', such as men who have both male and female sexual partners. Increase in syphilis infection rates amongst homosexual men is well documented in several cities in the United States of America and also in Europe, Canada, and Australia.

Clinicians need to be aware of cardiovascular syphilis in groups considered to have been at risk of infection. Inadequate or interrupted antibiotic therapy may confound the development of cardiovascular syphilis and make diagnosis difficult.

Pathogenesis and pathology of cardiovascular syphilis

Syphilis is spread through body fluids and is usually acquired by sexual contact with an infected person. In the preantibiotic era, 50 to 75% of partners of persons with primary or secondary syphilis were liable to become infected. Spontaneous healing of the early lesions of primary and secondary syphilis is followed by a long latent period, the time taken from initial infection to clinical manifestation of cardiovascular syphilis, ranging from 10 to 25 years. The 2-year mortality rate after diagnosis of untreated syphilitic aneurysm is about 80%.

T. pallidum has a predilection for small vessels, especially in the aorta and also the nervous system. In tertiary syphilis, obliterative endarteritis of the vasa vasorum of the media and the adventitia of the aorta is characterized by the presence of an inflammatory cuff composed of lymphocytes and plasma cells around the affected vessels, causing ischaemic necrosis of collagen and elastic tissue in the aortic media. Syphilis classically involves the proximal ascending aorta, presumably because the vasa vasorum are more plentiful in that region.

The pathological hallmark of syphilitic aortitis is 'tree-barking', a description of longitudinal wrinkling of the aortic intima resulting from contraction of fibrous scars in the aortic media. Fibrosis of the media in the proximal ascending aorta results in dilatation of the aortic root and aneurysm formation, leading to aortic regurgitation, the most common complication of syphilitic aortitis afflicting 20 to 30% of patients. A rarer form of cardiovascular syphilis is 'gummatous' myocarditis, which is usually diagnosed post-mortem.

Clinical presentation

Cardiovascular syphilis may present in one of four forms, but the features may be mixed.

- Asymptomatic aortitis—the most prevalent form, and usually diagnosed at necropsy with the unexpected finding of characteristic 'tree-barking' of the aortic intima

- Aortic regurgitation—the commonest manifestation of cardiovascular syphilis that results from annular dilatation of the aortic valve ring in syphilitic aortitis affecting the ascending aorta (the valve cusps remain normal); 70 to 80% of patients with untreated syphilis eventually develop aortic regurgitation

- Coronary ostial stenosis—occurs in up to 30% of cases of cardiovascular syphilis, and frequently coexists with aortic regurgitation as a complication of aortitis affecting the proximal ascending aorta

- Syphilitic aneurysm of the aorta—the least common manifestation of cardiovascular syphilis, occurring in 10 to 15% of patients with untreated syphilis; usually saccular but may be fusiform, and can occur as solitary aneurysm anywhere along the aorta, with characteristic radiographic appearance of dilatation

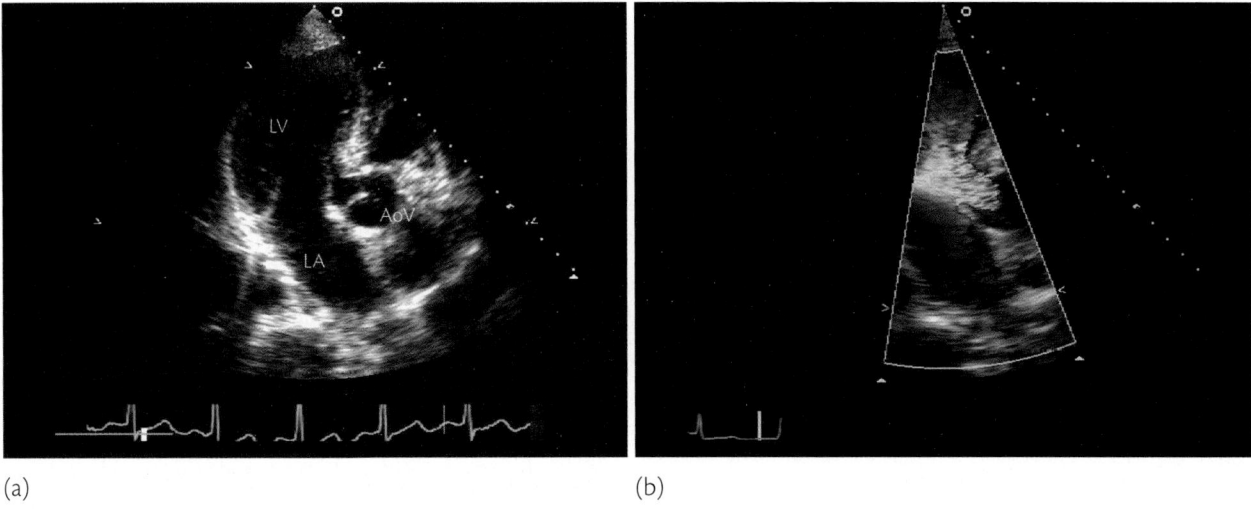

(a)   (b)

Fig. 16.9.4.1 Transthoracic echocardiography of a 61-year-old woman with syphilitic aortitis. A. Apical long-axis view of the left ventricle in mid-diastole. The aortic valve leaflets are closed. The diameter of the ascending aorta is 4.8 cm (normal <3 cm) with the dilatation extending to the arch. AoV, aortic valve; LA, left atrium LV, left ventricle. B. Apical long-axis colour Doppler study in mid-diastole showing severe aortic regurgitation.

Aortic regurgitation

With typical location of syphilitic disease in the ascending aorta, the murmur of syphilitic aortic regurgitation may be more prominent along the right sternal edge, in contrast to the left side in rheumatic aortic regurgitation. Transthoracic echocardiography will demonstrate that the aortic regurgitation is a result of dilatation of the aortic root (Fig. 16.9.4.1). Patients with syphilitic aortitis of the ascending aorta die of heart failure resulting from aortic valve regurgitation.

Coronary ostial stenosis

Angina or acute myocardial infarction may be the first presentation of syphilitic heart disease (Fig. 16.9.4.2) and may also result from associated coronary atherosclerosis. In the South African literature in the 1980s there were several reports of acute myocardial infarction and death due to syphilitic ostial stenosis (see 'Syphilis and HIV infection' below), hence patients found, at coronary angiography, to have bilateral coronary ostial stenosis but no distal coronary disease should be screened for syphilis, especially if they have known risk factors.

Syphilitic aneurysm

Nearly half the cases of syphilitic aneurysm occur in the ascending aorta, 30 to 40% in the aortic arch, and the remainder in the descending aorta. Mural thrombus, often with calcification, may obliterate the lumen of an aneurysm. Aneurysm of the aortic arch may compress and erode contiguous structures, such as a bronchus, resulting in pulmonary atelectasis; great veins, with presentation of superior mediastinal obstruction; the left recurrent laryngeal nerve, causing cough and hoarseness; and the vertebral bodies or sternum, causing pain. Aneurysm of the aortic arch may also produce tracheal tug, stridor, and dysphagia. Sternal erosion may be an early manifestation of syphilitic aortitis, as the junction between the ascending aorta and the aortic arch is near to the sternum, and massive aortic aneurysm may present as a pulsatile swelling in the right anterior thoracic cage. Rupture of an aortic aneurysm (70% of cases) into a bronchus—resulting in massive and fatal haemoptysis—or into the pleural space or pericardium may be the first clinical manifestation of syphilitic aneurysm.

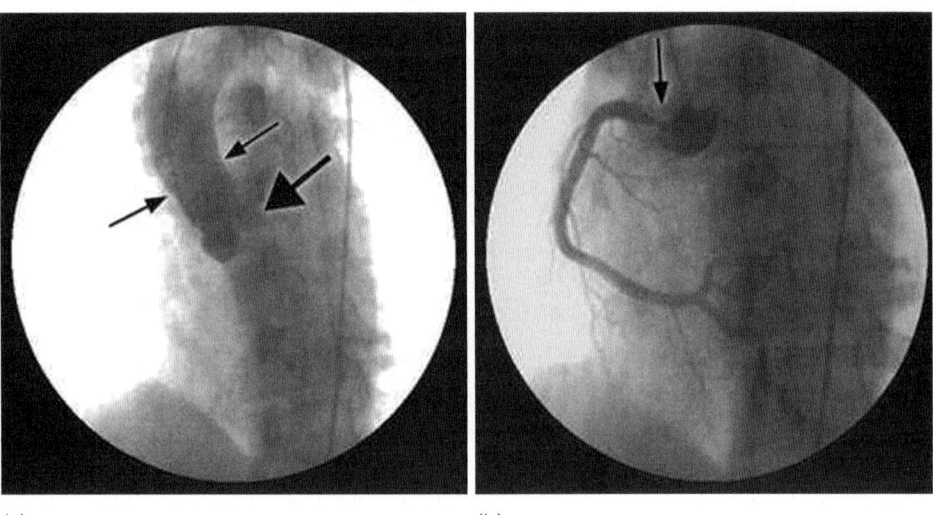

(a)   (b)

Fig. 16.9.4.2 Coronary angiogram of a 40-year-old Indonesian man who presented with severe, central chest pain. Note tapering of the aortic root (panel A, thin arrows), left main coronary artery stump (panel A, arrowhead), and 90% ostial lesion of the right coronary artery (panel B, arrow). Emergency coronary artery grafting was performed. Serology obtained afterwards proved positive for syphilis.
Tong SYC *et al* (2006). MJA, 184; 241-3.
© Copyright 2006. The Medical Journal of Australia.

Although extremely rare, tertiary syphilis should be considered in the differential diagnosis of thoracic aneurysms, even in the setting of atherosclerotic disease in older subjects. Patients with syphilitic aneurysm of the thoracic aorta, if untreated, have a mean life expectancy of 6 to 9 months from the onset of symptoms.

Aneurysm of the abdominal aorta due to syphilitic aetiology is rare and (if asymptomatic) of unknown prognosis, but it may present with lumbar or abdominal pain and—extremely rarely—as spontaneous aortocaval fistula.

Diagnosis

A high index of suspicion is required to make the diagnosis in a patient found to have aortic regurgitation or aortic aneurysm, but syphilitic disease should be considered, especially if the patient belongs to a group at high risk of syphilitic infection or is elderly with a suggestive background risk factor, such as birth in a country where diagnosis and treatment of syphilis are likely to have been inadequate. With appropriate questioning a history of syphilis and its treatment may be obtained, but patients will often not volunteer such information. The diagnosis of syphilitic aortitis is often overlooked because atherosclerosis has greatly surpassed it as a cause of aortic aneurysm (Fig. 16.9.4.3).

Laboratory investigation

Serological testing is the mainstay of diagnosis. Rapid plasma reagin (RPR) is currently the most widely available non-specific

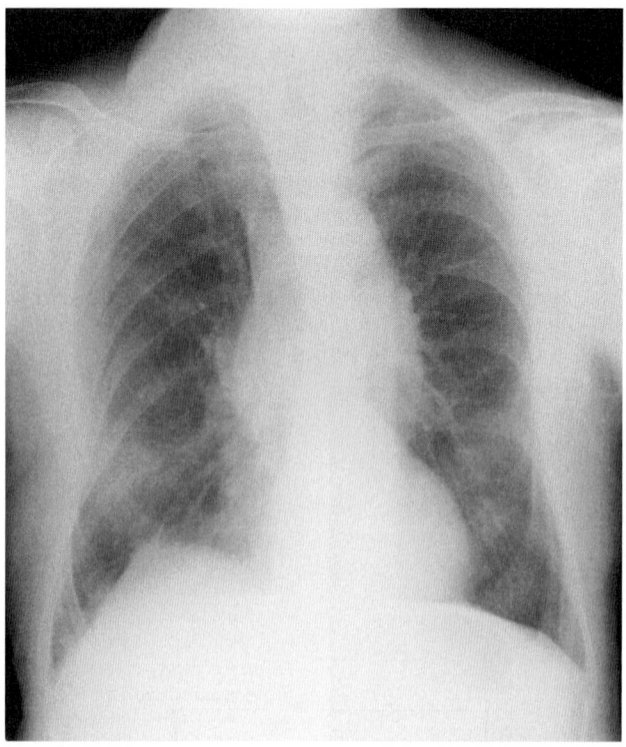

Fig. 16.9.4.3 Chest radiograph showing aneurysm of the ascending aorta in an elderly man with cardiovascular syphilis. Note the typical linear calcification in the wall of the dilated ascending aorta. Atherosclerotic aneurysm of the ascending aorta in diffuse atherosclerotic disease may present a similar picture, although calcification—when present—is usually limited to the aortic knuckle and descending aorta.

treponemal test: if positive in high titre, it may indicate latent or inadequately treated disease and be used to gauge response to treatment, but false positives are not uncommon—it is always positive in patients with nonvenereal treponematosis, and it may be negative in cardiovascular syphilis. Specific treponemal antibody tests such as *T pallidum* haemagglutination (TPHA) detect antibodies to *T. pallidum*-specific antigen and are almost always positive in cardiovascular syphilis, indicating prior infection with this organism. However, negative serology does not absolutely exclude infection with *T. pallidum*, particularly in an immunocompromised host. Latent syphilis, defined by the presence of positive serological tests in the absence of clinical evidence of syphilis, may progress to cardiovascular and gummatous manifestations of tertiary syphilis. Even when confirmatory tests are not readily available, treatment should be initiated on suspicion of diagnosis.

The diagnostic gold standard remains direct identification of *T. pallidum* in clinical specimens obtained at surgery. Polymerase chain reaction (PCR) assay can provide definite diagnosis of spirochaetal infection when biopsy material is available.

Between 10 and 20% of patients with cardiovascular syphilis have coexisting neurosyphilis, hence cerebrospinal fluid examination is recommended.

Syphilis and HIV infection

Syphilis promotes the transmission of HIV infection. and both infections can interact with each other. Cardiovascular syphilis develops more quickly in patients who are HIV seropositive (40 months from the time of primary infection) compared to those who are HIV seronegative (102 months), suggesting that coinfection with HIV hastens progression to late syphilis, perhaps due to immunosuppression. Even though new cases of cardiovascular syphilis remain rare, it has been suggested that the decline of tertiary syphilis in males in the 1990s could be attributed to mortality from AIDS.

As a general principle, consideration of one sexually transmissible infection should lead to consideration of another. After appropriate consent, any person with syphilis should be studied for antibodies to HIV and hepatitis B virus, and vice versa, and contacts traced for evidence of infection.

Medical treatment

In spite of discrepancies in dosage regimens, international consensus supports the use of parenteral penicillin as first-line treatment for all stages of syphilitic infection. *T. pallidum* has remained sensitive to penicillin despite over 60 years of its use in the treatment of syphilis. A standard course cures most patients, although some authorities have recorded serological failure rates as high as 25%.

It is thought that tertiary syphilis requires a longer course of treatment than early syphilis, since the treponemes may be dividing very slowly in the later stage of infection. The World Health Organization and European and United States guidelines recommend treatment of cardiovascular syphilis with benzathine penicillin 2.4×10^6 units administered once weekly for 3 weeks by the intramuscular route. United Kingdom guidelines propose 750 mg procaine benzyl penicillin once daily for 17 days by the intramuscular route. The Australian recommendation for the treatment of all forms of tertiary syphilis is benzyl penicillin 1.8 g intravenously 4-hourly for 15 days. Doxycycline, 100 mg by mouth twice daily

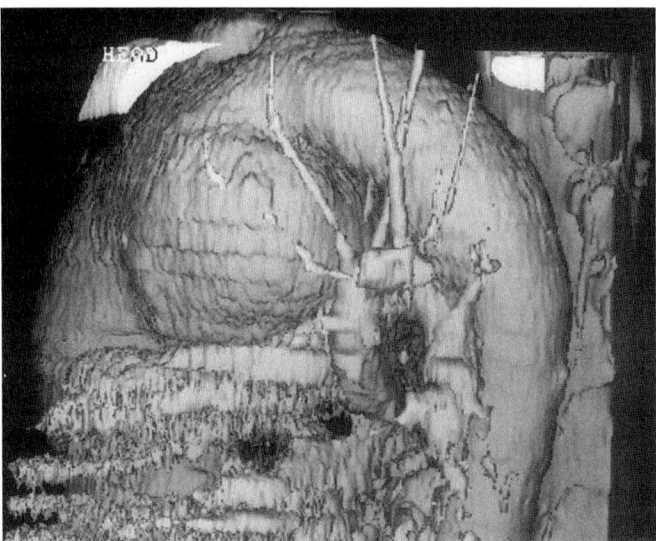

Fig. 16.9.4.4 Three-dimensional left-profile reconstruction of the thoracic aorta and adjacent structures in a 51-year-old man with the finding, on routine chest radiography, of an aortic aneurysm that proved to be syphilitic.
de Cannière D et al. 1999. 21st Century Imaging for a 19th-Century Disease, Circulation: 100; 884 – 885 (http://circ.ahajournals.org/cgi/content/extract/100/8/884).

for 28 days, is recommended by the United States Centers for Disease Control in those with penicillin allergy; United Kingdom guidelines suggest that doxycycline 200 mg twice daily for 28 days is preferable.

An unusual feature in the antibiotic treatment of syphilis is the Jarisch–Herxheimer reaction. The mechanism of the reaction, which comprises malaise and fever within 24 h of penicillin treatment, is uncertain and may be due to release of endotoxins from the massive death of treponema. In patients with cardiovascular syphilis, the Jarisch–Herxheimer reaction can be avoided by prednisolone 10 to 20 mg three times daily for 3 days, starting 24 h before commencement of penicillin therapy. Established aortic aneurysm and aortic regurgitation cannot be reversed or halted by medical treatment.

All patients with cardiovascular syphilis require clinical and serological follow-up 6 and 12 months after treatment. Syphilis serology is often difficult to interpret after treatment, as post-treatment treponemal tests usually remain positive even after completion of successful treatment. Treatment failure could be indicated by failure of nonspecific treponema antibody titres to decline fourfold within 6 months of treatment. There is a higher rate of syphilis treatment failure in HIV-positive patients.

Surgical treatment

Digital subtraction aortography, MRI, or three-dimensional CT scanning enables visualisation of the anatomy of syphilitic aortitis and can inform surgical strategy (Fig. 16.9.4.4). The aortic valve, if it is involved, may be replaced by the insertion of a prosthetic valve if there is normal aortic tissue upstream. Alternatively, a Bentall procedure, which involves replacement of the ascending aortic arch, may be the surgical treatment of choice. Coronary ostial lesions have been conventionally treated, with favourable results, using internal mammary grafts or combination with saphenous vein grafting.

Isolated aortic aneurysm may be treated with endovascular stent-graft repair, especially in patients with comorbidities who may be at high risk for open surgery, provided the lesion is considered anatomically suitable with adequate proximal and distal vessels. Conventional surgery, combined with endovascular repair, may be tried in the patients with syphilitic aortic aneurysm involving the aortic arch and the descending thoracic aorta, with the 30-day mortality of such intervention ranging from 5 to 10%.

Further reading

Bodhey NK, et al. (2003). Early sternal erosion and luetic aneurysms of thoracic aorta. *Eur J Cardiothorac Surg*, **28**, 499–501.

Cheng TO (2001). Syphilitic aortitis is dying but not yet dead. *Catheter Cardiovasc Interv*, **52**, 240–1.

Goh BT (2005). Syphilis in adults. *Sex Transm Infect*, **81**, 448–52.

Golden MR, Marra CM, Holmes KK (2003). Update on syphilis: resurgence of an old problem. *JAMA*, **290**, 1510–14.

Goldstein B, Carroccio A, Ellozy SH (2003). Combined open and endovascular repair of a syphilitic aortic aneurysm. *J Vasc Surg*, **38**, 1422–5.

Jackman JD, Radolf JD (1989). Cardiovascular syphilis. *Am J Med*, **87**, 425–33.

Kennedy JLW, Barnard JJ, Prahlow JA (2006). Syphilitic coronary ostial stenosis resulting in acute myocardial infarction and death. *Cardiology*, **105**, 25–9.

Maharajan M, Sampath Kumaar G (2005). Cardiovascular syphilis in HIV infection: a case-controlled study at the Institute of Sexually Transmitted Diseases, Chennai, India. *Sex Transm Infect*, **81**, 361.

Parkes R, et al. (2004). Review of current evidence and comparison of guidelines for effective syphilis treatment in Europe. *Int J STD AIDS*, **15**, 73–88.

Tong SYC, Haqqani H, Street AC (2006). A pox on the heart: five cases of cardiovascular syphilis. *MJA*, **184**, 241–3.

16.10

Tumours of the heart

Thomas A. Traill

Essentials

Cardiac myxoma

Cardiac myxomas are rare benign tumours that grow in the lumen of the atria, usually the left. Most are sporadic, but they can be associated with the Carney complex, where unusual freckling is typically the most obvious clinical clue.

Symptoms and signs most commonly mimic those of mitral stenosis. Systemic emboli occur in about 40% of cases. Constitutional effects predominate in a few patients who present with what seems to be an obscure multisystem disorder. In many patients, specific cardiovascular signs are inconspicuous or absent: an audible 'tumour plop' in early diastole, analogous to a mitral opening snap, is often reported only after the diagnosis is established.

The diagnosis is almost always made by echocardiography. Treatment is by urgent surgical removal. Recurrence is uncommon, provided excision has been complete, except in Carney complex.

Other tumours of the heart

The most common tumour seen in adult patients is the benign papillary fibroelastoma, which should be surgically removed only if it has been discovered in the search for a source of otherwise unexplained embolism.

Primary cardiac sarcomas are found more often in the right heart than in the left. Surgical resection is often attempted for obstructive symptoms, but recurrence and metastasis are common, and long-term outcome is very poor.

Microscopic secondary deposits within the myocardium can often be found in patients who die of metastatic cancer, but these are rarely of clinical importance. Intraluminal spread of cancer to the heart by direct extension up the inferior vena cava is a particular feature of renal cell carcinoma.

Cardiac myxoma

Cardiac myxomas are benign, typically golfball-sized, tumours that grow in the lumen of the atria, usually the left, attached by a stalk to the atrial septum. They are not common, but are important because they can present in a number of ways to general physicians, and because most can straightforwardly and permanently be removed by heart surgery. They are easily demonstrated by conventional transthoracic echocardiography, and it is usually the echocardiographer who makes the diagnosis; seldom has the patient been referred with this possibility in mind. Estimates of the prevalence of such a rare condition are necessarily approximate and range from 1 to 5 per 10 000 in autopsy series, or 2 per 100 000 in the general population, with a sex ratio of 2:1 in favour of women. As a cause of left atrial obstruction, myxomas are 200 to 400 times less common than mitral stenosis. Most patients are between 30 and 60 years, but there are reports of tumours occurring in infants and in older people.

Most myxomas are sporadic, unassociated with other diseases, but there is at least one mendelian syndrome involving myxoma, best named the Carney complex. This is caused by mutation in the protein kinase A regulatory subunit-1-alpha gene (Carney complex type 1) or mutations in other genes and characterized by lentiginosis, multiple myxomas (most of them cardiac), skin fibromas, and various kinds of endocrine overactivity, which has included Cushing's syndrome caused by pigmented adrenocortical hyperplasia, acromegaly, and Sertoli cell tumour. Unlike the usual kind of atrial myxoma, myxomas in Carney's syndrome may arise anywhere in the heart, are commonly multiple, and frequently recur. Inheritance of this rare disease is autosomal dominant, with centrofacial freckling as the most obvious outward marker of the phenotype. This freckling often involves unusual areas, for instance the lips, conjunctiva, and vulva.

Pathology

Cardiac myxomas are benign. Local invasion is unknown and metastatic growth is exceptional, despite the lesions' situation in the bloodstream. They take the form of polypoid masses arising from a stalk, ranging in size from 3 cm to as much as 10 cm or more, with a smooth or lobulated surface and gelatinous consistency. They are frequently covered with more or less adherent thrombus. More than 75% occur within the left atrium, with the base of the pedicle arising from the fossa ovalis or its rim. Occasionally, they arise from the base of the mitral valve leaflets, from the posterior part of the left atrium, or from within the right atrium. Sometimes they grow in both atria, in the form of a dumbbell. Ventricular myxomas are exceptional and seen almost exclusively as part of Carney's syndrome. Left atrial myxomas are not generally as large as those in the right atrium at the time they are first detected. The latter may almost fill the right atrium before they begin to obstruct systemic venous return.

The histology is that of a loosely woven, sparsely cellular, connective tissue tumour with very infrequent mitotic figures. Several cell types are identifiable, including undifferentiated stellate and polygonal cells, as well as smaller numbers of fibroblasts, smooth muscle cells, and endothelial cells. Among these are found macrophages and plasma cells, and rarely other mesodermal tissues, including bone. Cytogenetic studies fit with the general presumption that these indolent masses are indeed neoplastic, but immunohistochemical studies of differentiation markers do not clearly define the cell type of origin. It is suggested that the source is a primitive multipotential mesenchymal cell and that the predilection of these tumours for the atrial septum reflects the abundance of such cells in this region.

Clinical features

Left atrial obstruction

The most common symptoms and signs mimic those of mitral stenosis, with left ventricular inflow obstruction as the chief pathophysiological change. The presenting symptoms are progressive breathlessness, orthopnoea, paroxysmal nocturnal dyspnoea, fluid retention, and atrial arrhythmias. Examination suggests rheumatic heart disease, and before the routine use of ultrasonography a few such patients were referred for mitral valve surgery and the lesion was first diagnosed at operation. Some patients may develop pulmonary hypertension before the diagnosis becomes apparent.

Systemic embolism

Systemic emboli occur in about 40% of patients and are frequently the first manifestation of disease. By contrast to mitral stenosis, such emboli often occur while patients are in sinus rhythm. Emboli may be sizeable, large enough even to occlude the aortic bifurcation, and, besides thrombus, they frequently contain tumour material, hence histological examination may be diagnostic. When systemic emboli are removed from patients, they should always be sent for histological analysis. Typically, patients with systemic embolism are referred for echocardiography, and the diagnosis is then easily made.

Constitutional effects

Constitutional effects of the neoplasm predominate in a few patients who present with what seems to be an obscure multisystem disorder. Symptoms and signs include fever, weight loss (which is more conspicuous than in mitral stenosis and often occurs without severe left atrial obstruction), Raynaud's phenomenon (rare), finger clubbing (rare), a raised erythrocyte sedimentation rate (present in about 60% of patients), and abnormal serum proteins with elevated immunoglobulin levels. These changes are usually attributed to abnormal proteins secreted by the tumour, although the nature of these has not been determined. Other haematological abnormalities include anaemia, which may be due to mechanical haemolysis, polycythaemia, associated particularly with right atrial tumours,

leucocytosis, and thrombocytopenia. Such constitutional changes may prompt an initial diagnosis of infective endocarditis in patients who have heart murmurs, or lead to the suspicion of autoimmune rheumatic or vasculitic disease, or of occult cancer.

Physical signs

In many patients, specific cardiovascular signs of myxoma are inconspicuous or absent. In others, they vary from a prominent first heart sound to obvious changes similar to those of mitral valve disease. These include apical systolic murmurs, somewhat more common than diastolic rumbles, and—in some patients—signs of pulmonary hypertension, with accentuated pulmonary closure and tricuspid regurgitation. Some may have an audible 'tumour plop' in early diastole, analogous to a mitral opening snap, but this is often reported only after echocardiographic diagnosis. On combined echocardiographic and phonocardiographic recordings, the plop is seen to coincide with the end of the tumour's downward movement into the ventricle, usually a short time after mitral valve opening. A rare but specific feature of the condition is variation of the auscultatory findings with change in posture; this may be particularly obvious in right atrial tumours.

Investigations

Chest radiography and electrocardiography do not help to distinguish myxoma from mitral valve disease. Left atrial enlargement is common but seldom marked, and signs of pulmonary venous hypertension are infrequent. Calcification within the tumour is rarely demonstrable.

Echocardiography

While the first account of left atrial myxoma diagnosed during life was not until 1951, it is now exceptional for the diagnosis to be made first at autopsy. This is chiefly attributable to the wide availability of echocardiography, which has proved itself both reliable and specific for recognizing these tumours. It is no accident that the echocardiographic appearance of these lesions was among the first clinical reports by ultrasonographers in 1959. Figure 16.10.1 illustrates a typical two-dimensional echocardiogram from a

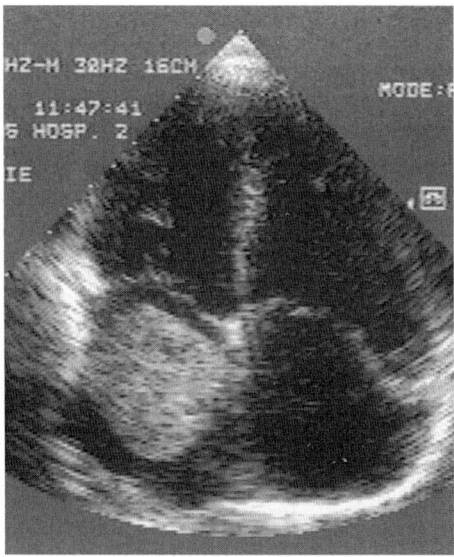

Fig. 16.10.1 Echocardiogram in the four-chamber view showing a myxoma occupying much of the left atrium.

patient with left atrial myxoma. A video recording would demonstrate the mobility of the mass as it flops to and fro within the atrium, restrained only by its peduncle.

Transoesophageal echocardiography affords the opportunity to examine the tumour and its attachment with great precision; generally this extra clarity is unnecessary, but on occasion the transoesophageal technique is helpful if there is difficulty in differentiating tumour from an atrial thrombus.

The differential diagnosis of left atrial myxoma is seldom difficult. Large masses may occasionally be difficult to distinguish from left atrial ball thrombus—a lesion that is even rarer than myxoma. Smaller left atrial masses may be papillary fibroelastomas or infective vegetations caused by endocarditis. These can usually be distinguished by their clinical context. Masses in the right atrium may also be due to thrombus, sometimes propagated from the inferior vena cava, or occasionally venous extension of abdominal cancers, particularly renal cell cancer. In a few patients, abundant strands of the Chiari network of right atrial trabeculation may give rise to similar echocardiographic appearances.

Cardiac catheterization

The echocardiographic appearance is so characteristic that angiography no longer has a role in diagnosis of myxoma, although it may be required as a prelude to surgery in the older patient in whom there is, or might be, coronary artery disease.

Treatment and prognosis

Atrial myxoma is treated by urgent surgical removal. The risk is low, comparable with that of surgery for mitral valve disease. It is important to ensure complete removal of the base by excising a full-thickness button of the atrial septum, the resulting defect being repaired with a small patch.

Functional results of surgery are good. Some patients are left with mitral regurgitation, but this is seldom severe. Recurrence is uncommon, provided excision has been complete, except in Carney's syndrome. In these patients, regular echocardiographic follow-up is required, at intervals of 6 months. The rare occurrence, after excision, of the usual kind of myxoma generally occurs within the first 2 years; thereafter, follow-up can safely be infrequent.

Other tumours of the heart

While each individually is rare, taken together the other tumours of the heart have an incidence that roughly equals that of myxoma. They include benign lesions, seen especially in children, sarcomas, and secondary involvement by metastasis or direct tumour extension. They are generally first recognized or suspected during echocardiography. MRI, or occasionally echo-directed transvenous biopsy, usually yields the diagnosis.

Benign cardiac tumours

Papillary fibroelastoma

The most common tumour seen in adult patients is the papillary fibroelastoma, a small pedunculated mass that hangs off one of the left-sided valve leaflets, usually the mitral valve. Its echocardiographic appearance is very characteristic. The size of the mass and presence of a peduncle distinguish this small tumour from the usual kind of Lambl's excrescence, but histologically they are identical and, like Lambl's excrescences, papillary fibroelastomas probably arise through organization of fibrinous material that collects at the trailing edges of the valve leaflets. Their importance lies in the fact that they have been labelled as a potential source of systemic embolism, and that some authors have recommended that they should be removed as a matter of routine. The evidence to support this view is thin, and the author's recommendation is to remove them only if they have been discovered in the search for a source of otherwise unexplained embolism. If they are an incidental echocardiographic finding, then it is safe to leave them alone; aspirin treatment may be recommended.

Fibroma, rhabdomyoma, hamartoma, and haemangioma

These are tumours of childhood, rhabdomyoma being the characteristic cardiac tumour in patients with tuberous sclerosis. In contrast to myxomas and fibroelastomas, they grow within the myocardium, not into the lumen of the heart. Rhabdomyomas are usually asymptomatic, and when they are they should be left alone, since most regress spontaneously. Fibromas and hamartomas are both very rare, presenting with arrhythmias (particularly ventricular hamartomas or Purkinje cell tumours) or with haemodynamic abnormalities caused by their mass effect. They require surgical excision, and when this is feasible the long-term results of treatment are very good. Haemangiomas, also very rare, tend to grow and to develop multiple feeding vessels, so that surgical excision is usually recommended.

Cardiac sarcoma

Primary cardiac sarcomas are found more often in the right heart than in the left, and can have one of several cell types. Haemangiosarcoma is the most common, typically developing in the right atrium. Rhabdomyosarcoma may develop in the ventricular septum or in the right ventricular outflow tract, as may the still rarer osteosarcoma, or tumours that are undifferentiated. Since these tumours often present with mechanical effects, typically obstruction at the atrial or outflow tract level, surgical resection is often attempted. However, recurrence and metastasis are common, and long-term outcome is very poor.

Cardiac involvement by other malignancies

Microscopic secondary deposits within the myocardium can often be found in patients who die of metastatic cancer, but intramyocardial secondaries of a size large enough to be of clinical importance are very rare. By contrast, pericardial involvement by lymphoma, or by cancers of the lung, breast, pancreas, and other tumours is not uncommon, and may sometimes be the first presentation of the tumour (see Chapter 16.8). Treatment is analogous to that of malignant pleural effusions, with drainage, creation of a window, or intrapericardial chemotherapy, depending on the rest of the clinical situation.

Intraluminal spread of cancer, by direct extension up the inferior vena cava, is a particular feature of renal cell carcinoma. Diagnosis by echocardiography is generally obvious as the tumour has a very characteristic appearance as it waves, like seaweed, in the right atrium and even dangles through the rest of the right heart. It may prove possible to resect the cava, along with the kidney and the tumour mass, under circulatory arrest.

Further reading

Cardiac myxoma

Casey M *et al.* (2000). Mutations in the protein kinase A R1alpha regulatory subunit cause familial cardiac myxomas and Carney complex. *J Clin Invest*, **106**, R31–8.

Greenwood WF (1968). Profile of atrial myxoma. *Am J Cardiol*, **21**, 367–75.

Pucci A, Gagliardotto P, Zanini C *et al.* (2000). Histopathologic and clinical characterization of cardiac myxoma: review of 53 cases from a single institution. *Am Heart J*, **140**, 134–8.

Schaff HV, Mullany CJ (2000). Surgery for cardiac myxomas. *Semin Thorac Cardiovasc Surg*, **12**, 77–88.

Wilkes D, McDermott DA, Basson CT (2005). Clinical phenotypes and molecular genetic mechanisms of Carney complex. *Lancet Oncol*, **6**, 501–8.

Other tumours of the heart

Burke A, Jeudy J Jr, Virmani R (2008). Cardiac tumours: an update. *Heart*, **94**, 117–23.

Cardiac involvement in genetic disease

Thomas A. Traill

Essentials

Many clinicians find themselves faced, from time to time, with a patient who has a family history of a known disorder, such as Marfan's syndrome, or who has noncardiac features that suggest a syndrome.

Syndromic congenital heart disease

Down's syndrome—25 to 50% have congenital heart disease, most characteristically atrioventricular canal defect.

Turner's syndrome—causes two principal abnormalities of the aorta: coarctation and congenital abnormalities of the aortic valve (usually bicuspid).

Noonan's syndrome—the most common heritable syndrome that characteristically causes congenital heart disease. Mutations in an intracellular signalling molecule protein tyrosine phosphatase SHP-2 account for 40% of cases. Characteristics include short stature, with a facies that is variously described as elfin or triangular, ocular hypertelorism, ears that are set low and rotated forwards, and webbing of the neck (the most obvious of the features that may lead to confusion with Turner's syndrome). The most typical cardiac lesion is pulmonary stenosis.

Williams' syndrome—caused by macrodeletions of chromosome 7 that include the elastin gene; includes the cardiovascular features of familial supravalvar aortic stenosis along with a characteristic facial appearance, with round, blue eyes, a distinctive stellate pattern of the irises, depression of the nasal bridge, outwards tilting of the nostrils, abnormal dentition, and big lips.

Other conditions—many other genetic syndromes have significant cardiac and vascular manifestations.

Connective tissue disorders

Marfan's syndrome—caused by mutations of the fibrillin-1 gene (*FBN1*); characteristic cardiovascular findings are aneurysmal dilatation of the aorta, and occasionally other large arteries, and floppy mitral valve. Diagnosis is based on the presence of particular major or minor criteria, the major criteria being (1) aortic aneurysm, (2) lens subluxation, (3) characteristic skeletal abnormalities, and (4) dural ectasia. Aortic dissection and rupture are the commonest causes of death in untreated cases. β-Blockers are commonly given to slow the progression to aneurysm, but the benefit is probably modest and recent work suggests that angiotensin-II receptor blockers may be much more effective. Surgical replacement of the aortic root is generally recommended when the maximum measurement across the aorta reaches 5 cm.

Other conditions—the Ehlers–Danlos syndromes and many other genetic disorders have significant cardiac and vascular manifestations.

Introduction

Singling out a few of the more prominent mendelian disorders seen by cardiologists may seem a somewhat arbitrary basis for a chapter, especially in an age when we are exploring the molecular genetic basis for so many more of the common heart diseases, but this works in practice. Many clinicians find themselves faced, from time to time, with a patient who has a family history of a known disorder, such as Marfan's syndrome, or who has noncardiac features that suggest a syndrome, perhaps Noonan's. They may wonder how to make the diagnosis, what else to look for, and how to screen family members.

Inherited diseases of the contractile machinery of the heart, which lead to familial hypertrophic and dilated cardiomyopathy, are covered in Chapters 16.7.2 and 16.7.3 and ion-channel mutations that underlie long-QT syndromes and other inherited causes of paroxysmal ventricular tachycardia are covered in Chapter 16.4.

The first part of this chapter deals with developmental syndromes that include congenital cardiac defects, with coverage restricted to a few relatively common disorders that are seen in adult patients. The second part describes the two common connective tissue disorders—Marfan's and Ehlers–Danlos syndromes—and the recently described Loeys–Dietz syndrome that shares some pathogenetic mechanisms with Marfan's. A number of other heritable diseases that affect the heart are listed in a table, without discussion in the text. Haemochromatosis (Chapter 12.7.1) and Friedreich's ataxia (Chapter 24.7.5) are discussed elsewhere in this textbook; the others, though important to other organ systems, offer little opportunity to the cardiologist for diagnosis or management.

Syndromic congenital heart disease

Aneuploidy disorders

The two commonest chromosomal disorders in adult patients are Down's and Turner's syndromes, and each includes characteristic cardiac abnormalities. A third, Klinefelter's syndrome, does not.

Some 25 to 50% of patients with Down's syndrome have congenital heart disease. The characteristic lesion, present in about half of the affected hearts, is atrioventricular canal defect. This ranges from the relatively simple primum atrial septal defect to the complete type, in which the defect involves both the atrial and ventricular septa, between which there lies a single atrioventricular valve ring. In other patients, ventricular septal defect, tetralogy of Fallot, and persistent ductus arteriosus are seen in roughly equal numbers. Patients with Down's syndrome undergo heart surgery most easily when they are infants, and the tendency has shifted from the nihilistic approach of past years to correcting serious cardiac malformations early in life.

Turner's syndrome causes abnormalities of the aorta, the two principal lesions being coarctation and congenital abnormalities of the aortic valve, usually a bicuspid valve. Most patients with coarctation have a bicuspid aortic valve as well, and patients with either lesion frequently have some degree of annuloaortic ectasia. In some patients with Turner's syndrome, the whole aorta is abnormal—either hypoplastic or weakened by the presence of cystic medial necrosis. Aortic dissection may occur, and aortic surgery, e.g. to repair coarctation, can sometimes be very difficult, owing to the fragile nature of the aortic wall. Other congenital heart abnormalities are not common in Turner's syndrome, except for anomalies of pulmonary venous return.

Mendelian syndromes that include congenital heart disease

Noonan's syndrome

Noonan's syndrome (OMIM 163950) is the most common heritable syndrome that characteristically causes congenital heart disease. The syndrome shares some features with the Turner phenotype, and the two were confused between 1930 and Noonan's studies in the 1960s, which coincided with the advent of cytogenetics. In 1963, Noonan described a small series of patients with pulmonary stenosis who shared a characteristic facial appearance. Since then, the phenotype has been well described and shown to be associated with a normal karyotype and autosomal dominant inheritance. Cardiac involvement has been recognized to include not only pulmonary stenosis, but also a wide variety of other lesions, much wider than in Turner's syndrome. Mutations in an intracellular signalling molecule protein tyrosine phosphatase SHP-2 (the gene is called *PTPN11*) account for 40% of cases, but the disease is genetically heterogeneous. The pathogenetics are further complicated by both clinical and genetic overlap. Another syndrome—LEOPARD syndrome (OMIM 151100)—is also caused by *PTPN11* mutations, and the Noonan phenotype is closely related to disorders caused by mutations affecting other members of the RAS-ERK intracellular signalling cascade.

Patients with Noonan's syndrome are of short stature, with a facies that is variously described as elfin or triangular (Fig. 16.11.1). There is ocular hypertelorism, and the palpebral fissure may slope downwards (the antimongoloid slant), which may be emphasized by ptosis or an epicanthal fold. The ears are set low and rotated forwards so that the lobes are prominent, and there is characteristic webbing of the neck—the most obvious of the features that may lead to confusion with Turner's syndrome. Pectus deformities are common, as are other miscellaneous skeletal abnormalities, including cubitus valgus. Patients with Noonan's syndrome are prone to develop keloid scars. Cryptochidism is common, as is delayed sexual maturation, but not infantilism as in Turner's syndrome. Unlike Turner's syndrome, many patients with

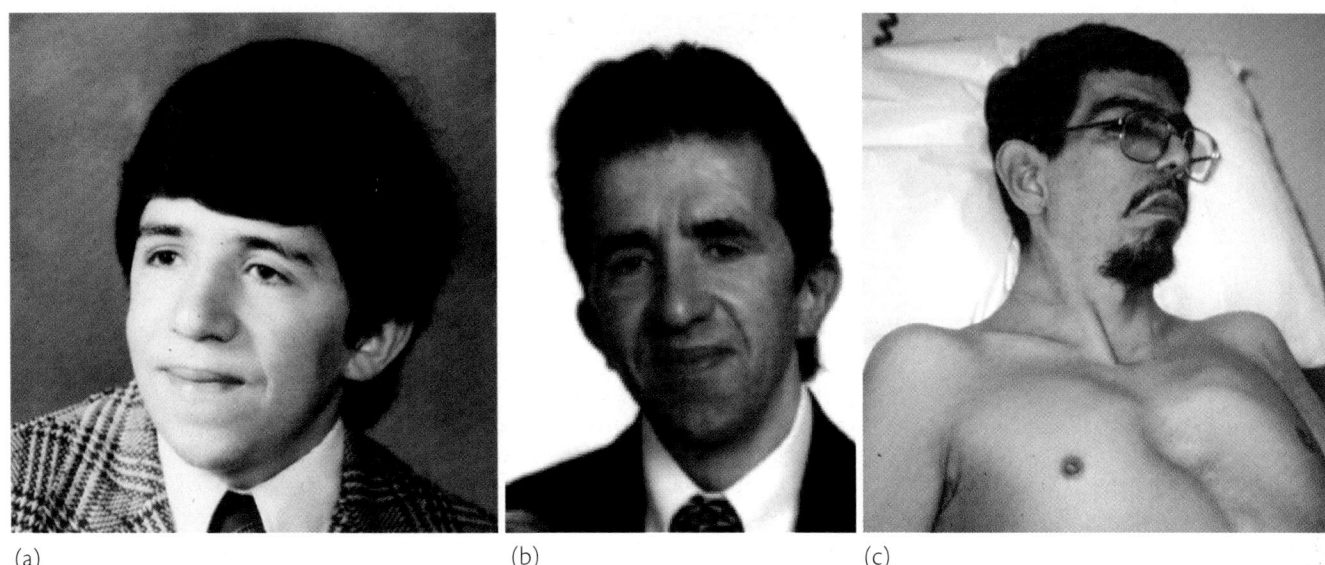

(a)   (b)   (c)

Fig. 16.11.1 Two patients with Noonan's syndrome. A and B: Patient 1 aged 18 and 40. C: Patient 2—note scars at site of plastic surgery for pterygium colli.

Noonan's syndrome have a degree of mental retardation, but this is quite variable. Among this author's patients with Noonan's syndrome are a physician, an architect, a certified accountant, and a high-school mathematics teacher.

The frequency of cardiac involvement in Noonan's syndrome is unknown because the diagnosis is so easily missed in the absence of congenital heart disease. The most characteristic lesion is pulmonary stenosis, but in contrast to the almost stereotypical cardiovascular findings in Turner's syndrome, the range in Noonan's syndrome is broad. In many patients, the stenotic pulmonary valve leaflets are not simply fused, as in nonsyndromic pulmonary stenosis, but may be dysplastic, thickened, and immobile—unsuitable for simple balloon or surgical valvotomy. Other congenital lesions found in Noonan's syndrome are ventricular and atrial septal defects, tricuspid atresia, single ventricle, and abnormalities of the left ventricle, including congenital mitral stenosis, subaortic stenosis, and a combination of these two lesions. The electrocardiogram often shows a superior axis (left-axis deviation), even when there is pulmonary stenosis and right ventricular hypertrophy.

The most ominous complication of Noonan's syndrome is cardiomyopathy, taking the form of myocardial hypertrophy complicated by progressive fibrosis. This leads, over the course of 5 to 15 years, to low cardiac output with very high ventricular diastolic pressures—the pathophysiology of restrictive cardiomyopathy.

Since the valvular abnormalities are for the most part correctable, this hypertrophic restrictive cardiomyopathy is the main factor limiting life expectancy.

Familial supravalvar aortic stenosis and Williams' syndrome

Familial supravalvar aortic stenosis is caused by loss-of-function mutation or deletion affecting the gene for elastin located on chromosome 7. Affected patients develop a tight, fleshy constriction of the aorta, or sometimes the pulmonary artery at the level of the sinotubular junction above the semilunar valve (Fig. 16.11.2). In some patients, both great arteries are affected. Supravalvar aortic stenosis can lead to severe left ventricular outflow obstruction, with left ventricular failure or even sudden death. This is not a setting for balloon dilation or stenting, but the results of surgery are good, for either lesion or for both.

Williams' syndrome (OMIM 194050) is one of the best-documented examples of a contiguous gene phenomenon seen in adult medicine. It is caused by macrodeletions of chromosome 7 that include the elastin gene. Hence, Williams' syndrome includes the cardiovascular features of familial supravalvar aortic stenosis described in the previous paragraph. In addition, more far-reaching effects caused by deletion of contiguous genes accompany these vascular abnormalities. The full syndrome comprises a characteristic facial appearance, with round, blue eyes,

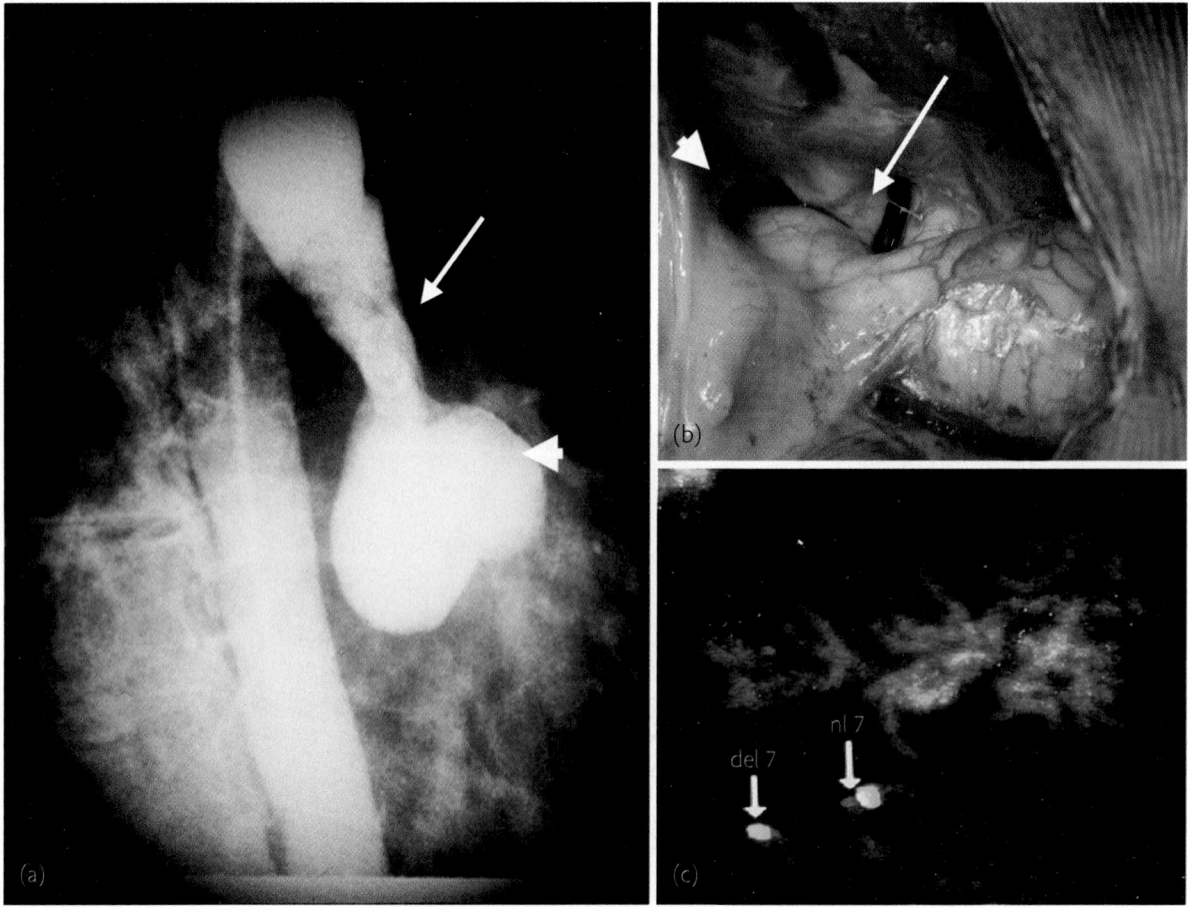

Fig. 16.11.2 Supravalvar aortic stenosis. A. Contrast angiogram of the thoracic aorta showing normal sinuses of Valsalva (broad arrow) with constriction at the sino–tubular junction (narrow arrow). B. Operative photograph. The patient's head is to the right. Arrows as in panel A. C. Fluorescence *in situ* hybridization (FISH) showing two markers for chromosome 7 (bright fluorescence), but only one for the elastin gene (orange fluorescence).

a distinctive stellate pattern of the irises, depression of the nasal bridge, outwards tilting of the nostrils, abnormal dentition, and big lips, together with small stature, mental retardation, and a history of infantile hypercalcaemia. Mental retardation in Williams' syndrome takes on very individual forms, the patients often being articulate and socially adept: several purported idiot savants have had Williams'syndrome. As in the purely cardiac syndrome, surgery may be required to relieve severe left (or right) ventricular outflow obstruction.

DiGeorge and velocardiofacial syndromes (chromosome 22 deletion syndrome)

DiGeorge syndrome (OMIM 188400), described in 1965, comprises abnormalities of the parathyroid glands, absence or hypoplasia of the thymus, and conotruncal abnormalities of the heart such as pulmonary atresia and severe forms of tetralogy of Fallot. A number of affected patients have learning disabilities or schizophrenia. It was recognized soon after the original description that the syndrome is generally caused by deletions in a region of chromosome 22.

Velocardiofacial syndrome (OMIM 192430), or Shprintzen's syndrome, described in 1981, comprises similar cardiac abnormalities along with cleft palate, a characteristic facies, and learning difficulty. It has since proved to be caused by deletions in the same region of chromosome 22, now often referred to as the DiGeorge critical region (DGCR). A third syndrome, known as 'conotruncal anomalies face', is also linked to this site.

With a broad spectrum of phenotypic variation, and deletions that are often quite large, it was suspected for some time that these syndromes are related manifestations of a contiguous gene phenomenon, just as in Williams' syndrome. However, it has emerged that the size of the deletion does not predict the extent of the phenotype, and that within a family the same (presumably stable) deletion can be the cause of a wide range of phenotypes. Two candidate genes lie within the DGCR—*TBX1* and *UFDIL*; it remains to be seen whether either can be implicated as the cause of the entire group of phenotypes.

Heart–hand syndromes

The two commonly recognized heart–hand syndromes are Holt–Oram syndrome and Ellis–van Creveld syndrome.

Holt–Oram syndrome (OMIM 142900)

Holt–Oram syndrome, inherited as an autosomal dominant trait, was described in 1960. It includes a secundum atrial septal defect and skeletal abnormalities, principally affecting the upper limbs and shoulder girdle, never the legs, and usually more pronounced in the left arm (Fig. 16.11.3). Within a family, affected individuals may have skeletal abnormalities, congenital heart disease, or both. The limb abnormalities cover a wide spectrum from just a triphalangeal thumb to phocomelia. Abnormalities of the hand and forearm always involve the radial side and thumb (in contrast to Ellis–van Creveld syndrome). The characteristic cardiac abnormality is fossa ovalis (secundum) atrial septal defect, but affected patients may have other relatively simple lesions, e.g. ventricular septal defect or pulmonary stenosis.

Holt–Oram syndrome is caused by mutation in a transcription factor, TBX5, a close homologue of a transcription factor seen as phylogenetically far away as the fruit fly, where mutations produce abnormalities of the wing.

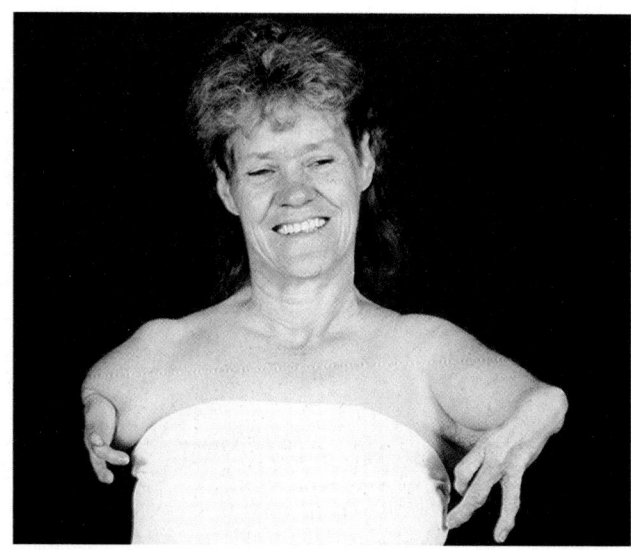

Fig. 16.11.3 Holt–Oram syndrome.

Ellis–van Creveld syndrome (OMIM 225500)

Ellis–van Creveld syndrome is inherited as a recessive trait, hence the more complete clinical descriptions have come from studies in genetically circumscribed communities, notably the Old Order Amish of Pennsylvania where, thanks to a founder effect, the gene is common and homozygotes abound. The syndrome, described in 1940, includes dwarfism, caused mainly by shortening of the forearms and lower legs, and symmetrical polydactyly affecting the ulnar side with accessory sixth and even seventh digits attached to or beyond the little finger. Cardiac involvement is very common, present probably in three-quarters of homozygotes. The characteristic lesion is common atrium—a lesion that has the appearance, on echocardiography and to the surgeon, of a very large primum atrial septal defect. A few patients have more complete forms of atrioventricular canal defect, and—at least among the Amish—there is a high perinatal mortality rate among affected infants, suggesting the possibility of still more extensive cardiac involvement. The gene has been mapped to chromosome 4 and sequenced, but the protein's function is unknown.

Connective tissue disorders

Marfan's syndrome

Thanks principally to the work of McKusick and his collaborators, beginning in 1955, Marfan's syndrome (OMIM 154700) has become the paradigm for the clinical, genetic, and molecular investigation of the heritable disorders of connective tissue. The importance of the syndrome is heightened by the fact that its recognition and treatment have had a dramatic impact on survival among those affected. Untreated, patients had a median survival into the fourth decade before death from aortic dissection and rupture (Fig. 16.11.4). Today, affected patients have a near-normal lifespan, and there are reasons to hope that recent advances in understanding the molecular pathogenesis may yet make this genetic disease, in a sense, 'curable'.

In 1896, Marfan described a weak, generally hypotonic child, with what he termed arachnodactyly. In the century since, it has been appreciated that the syndrome is mendelian and pleiotropic,

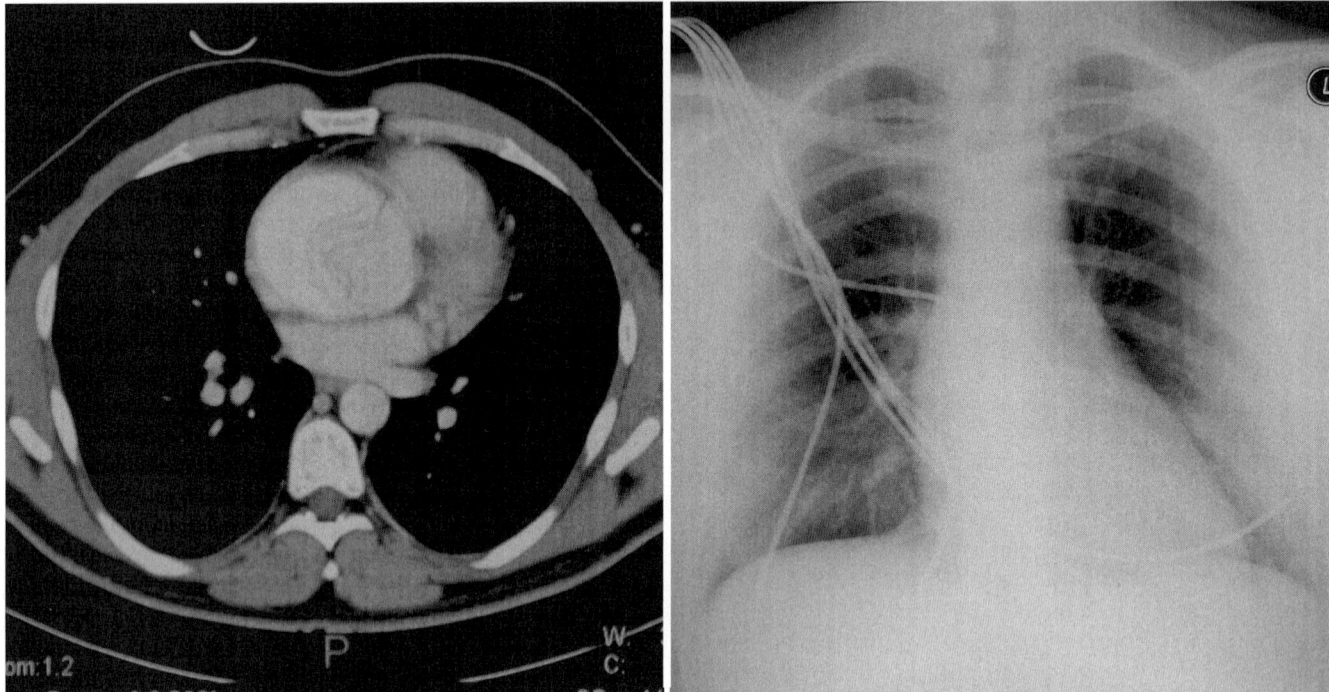

Fig. 16.11.4 Aortic ectasia and dissection in a patient with Marfan's syndrome. Note that the aortic root enlargement, to 7 cm, is not apparent from the chest radiograph.

involving several apparently unrelated organs whose common feature proves to be the importance of elastic tissue to their structural integrity. Ocular involvement, with the lens subluxed because of failure of its suspensory ligament, was recognized early in the 20th century. Cardiovascular involvement was noted incidentally in the 1940s, and studied systematically from the 1950s onwards. Skeletal involvement includes—besides long limbs and arachnodactyly—scoliosis and other abnormalities of the thoracic cage. The sternum may be pushed outwards or inwards by the abnormally long ribs, hence pectus carinatum and/or excavatum, often asymmetrical. Skin involvement is identified by light-coloured striae, which should be looked for over the deltopectoral groove and the flanks. Less common findings are dural ectasia, which can sometimes be so marked as to cause radicular symptoms, and pulmonary involvement leading to spontaneous pneumothorax or apical blebs. In severely affected children, like the one Marfan described, there may be generalized weakness and hypotonia.

The characteristic cardiovascular findings in Marfan's syndrome are aneurysmal dilatation of the aorta, and occasionally other large arteries, and floppy mitral valve. The former was recognized in the 1920s, but not really addressed until McKusick showed that it was the principal cause of early death in the disease. Shortly afterwards, echocardiography became available to identify and follow these abnormalities, and surgical techniques were developed by Bentall and Gott to repair the aneurysms. Until then, median life expectancy for men with Marfan's syndrome had been 45 years, for women a year or two longer.

Fibrillin-1 mutations

The syndrome (OMIM 134797) is caused by mutations of the fibrillin-1 gene (*FBN1*) on chromosome 15. It has recently emerged that besides a purely structural role, one that could hardly be replaced by any form of treatment, fibrillin-1 acts to modulate cell-to-cell

signalling during development and, at least in a mouse model, after birth. The dominant negative hypothesis, in which the mutated fibrillin protein was believed to have its effect by interfering with polymerization of the product of the nonmutated allele, thus proves to have been an oversimplification. Rather, the pleiotropic effects of *FBN1* mutations prove to be mediated through paradoxical up-regulation of the signalling pathway transforming growth factor β1 (TGFβ1), which is modulated by fibrillin-1. Such findings have led to the likelihood of pharmacological treatment for the disease. Losartan, an angiotensin-II receptor blocker, which like the other members of its class also blocks TGFβ1 signalling, has been shown dramatically to prevent aortic dilation in a mouse model, also in a small clinical cohort study.

The fibrillin molecule is large, and most of the disease-causing mutations have yet to be described, hence genetic diagnosis by screening for known mutations is often not possible and diagnosis usually depends on applying clinical criteria. There are many polymorphisms within the gene, so in some kindreds it is possible, by tracking particular haplotypes, to determine which is associated with the disease and therefore contains the pathogenetic mutation. This has allowed diagnosis of the syndrome in individual family members in whom the clinical findings were uncertain, and has been used for prenatal diagnosis. Furthermore, the technique makes it possible to infer the existence of a fibrillin-1 mutation in kindreds where the phenotype has not met clinical criteria for Marfan's syndrome; if aortic ectasia segregates with a particular fibrillin-1 haplotype, then the chances are high that a fibrillin mutation somewhere in that copy is the pathogenetic mechanism.

Diagnostic criteria

The clinical diagnosis of Marfan's syndrome rests on major and minor criteria. In an index case, involvement of three organ systems is required, with major criteria in two. Major criteria can be aortic aneurysm, lens subluxation, characteristic skeletal abnormalities, or dural ectasia. Minor criteria can be striae, mitral valve prolapse, joint laxity, the facies, or moderate pectus excavatum. Characteristic skeletal abnormalities can be arachnodactyly (encircling the wrist with the thumb and little finger, the 'wrist sign', and making a fist with a protruding thumb, the 'thumb sign'), marked pectus deformity, increased wingspan to 5% more than the height, and scoliosis. In the relative of an index case, the positive family history becomes another major criterion.

In clinical practice, determining whether a patient satisfies these criteria may be fairly subjective and requires experience with the syndrome. Often, it is enough to know whether or not there is cardiovascular involvement, and there are numerous families with aortic aneurysms or ectasia who do not satisfy clinical criteria for Marfan's syndrome, yet whose long-term management is identical. Indeed, in a busy cardiac surgery practice with expertise in aortic root replacement, such 'nonsyndromic' familial aortopathy represents a significant proportion of patients treated, and some of these families have yielded other loci as sites for the cause of their disease. On the other hand, a lanky patient who has a normal aorta needs only infrequent follow-up, even though there may be a suspicion that he has a mild case of the syndrome.

Clinical management

Patients with Marfan's syndrome should be followed up with annual or 6-monthly echocardiograms to examine the aortic root. If there is reason to suspect that the aorta may be dilated above the echo plane, then CT scanning or MRI is required at least once to validate the echo measurement. When the maximum measurement across the aorta reaches 5 cm, we generally recommend surgical replacement of the aortic root, to prevent aortic dissection (see Chapter 16.14.1), which becomes a real risk once the dimension reaches 6 cm. The traditional and very successful approach is with the composite graft, whereby a mechanical aortic valve prosthesis—to which is indissolubly attached a tubular vascular prosthesis—is used to replace the entire aortic root and annulus. The coronary artery ostia are excised from the native aorta and reattached to the prosthetic root. Recently, to avoid anticoagulation in certain patients, there has been interest in a valve-sparing technique of root replacement in which a vascular prosthesis is fitted snugly over the aortic valve commissures, with the native leaflets suspended in their normal anatomical arrangement. Long-term success with this approach will depend on the degree to which the valve leaflets themselves degenerate because of the connective tissue abnormality. The Ross (pulmonary autograft) procedure is not appropriate in Marfan's syndrome. After surgery, and especially in patients whose surgery was done as an emergency for dissection, follow-up is with periodic imaging by CT or MRI to keep the remaining aorta under surveillance. Management of mitral prolapse and regurgitation in Marfan's syndrome is the same as in other patients. Surgery is required for severe or symptomatic regurgitation; mitral valve repair has proved surprisingly successful.

It is usual to treat patients who have aortic involvement with β-adrenergic blockers to slow the progression to aneurysm, but the benefit is probably modest. In mice with fibrillin-1 mutations in which the Marfan phenotype is well reproduced, β-adrenergic blockade had only slight effect on aortic ectasia. This was in contrast to the dramatic effect of losartan, alluded to in a previous paragraph, and many clinicians now recommend use of this drug.

We generally advise against excessively demanding sports, particularly competitive basketball, but in all affected children it is important to balance the risks of aortic disease against the importance of normal psychological development. Pregnancy is not contraindicated in all women with Marfan's syndrome, but genetic counselling should be offered, and it is advised that women not become pregnant if the aorta is enlarged to over 4 cm. Indeed, aortic dissection has been reported in a very few affected patients during pregnancy, even when they did not previously have aortic enlargement. In this autosomal dominant condition with high penetrance, the risk for the offspring of affected mothers or fathers is 50%. This can be mitigated, when the disease-causing mutation has been identified, by preimplantation genetic diagnosis or even by screening the fetus by chorionic villus sampling.

Loeys–Dietz syndrome

If the pathogenesis of Marfan's syndrome lies with abnormal TGFβ signalling, then it should not come as a surprise that mutations in the TGFβ receptors also cause abnormalities of vascular and other tissues. Recently, this was confirmed in the description of Loeys–Dietz syndrome (OMIM 609192, 610380, 610168, 608967), a disease that shares some aspects of the Marfan's phenotype and is associated with mutations of either of the two TGFβ receptors. Patients with Loeys–Dietz syndrome have more diffuse vascular involvement than those with Marfan's, and may have dissection even in vessels that are only mildly dilated. In this, they resemble patients affected by the vascular form of Ehlers–Danlos syndrome, and the phenotypes may be very difficult to distinguish. Prominent nonvascular features include ocular hypertelorism with malar hypoplasia, bifid or broad uvula (Fig. 16.11.5), cleft palate,

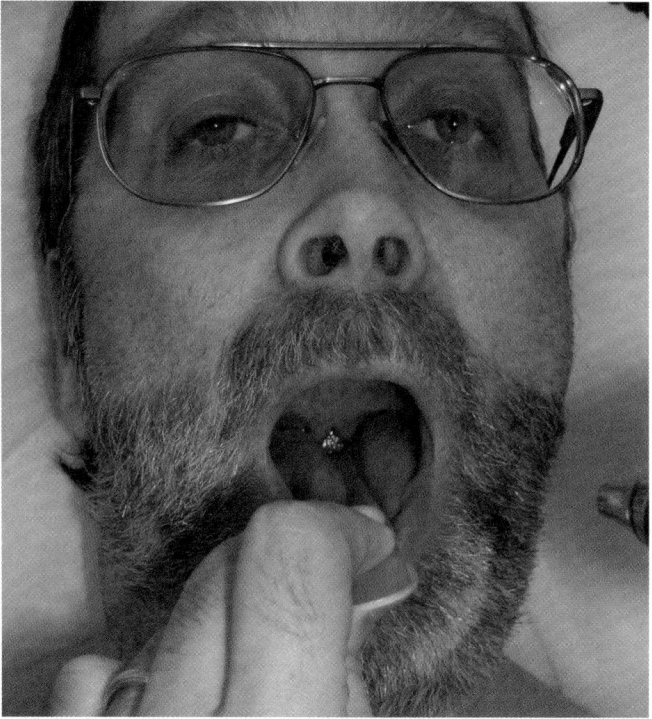

Fig. 16.11.5 Loeys–Dietz syndrome, illustrating the characteristic bifid uvula.

arachnodactyly, scoliosis, and pectus excavatum, yet excessive height is uncommon.

Ehlers–Danlos syndromes

In the early part of the 20th century, Ehlers and Danlos independently described an association between hyperextensibility of the skin, atrophic scarring, and hypermobility of the large joints. In the following 75 years, numerous accounts were published of what we now recognize to be a group of related conditions, so that by 1988 a new classification of the Ehlers–Danlos syndrome included ten separate phenotypes in an unwieldy classification. For practical purposes, clinicians distinguish 'classical' Ehlers–Danlos, formerly types I and II, from the potentially fatal 'vascular' form, previously type IV.

Classical Ehlers–Danlos (OMIM 130000, 130010)

This is characterized by skin elasticity, abnormal scars, and joint hypermobility, and is inherited as a dominant trait. Skin hyperextensibility is obvious, e.g. on tugging at the side of the neck or face. Joint laxity is much more marked than in Marfan's syndrome, and allows for tricks like placing the feet behind the head or other contortionist performances, besides permitting a remarkable span on the piano or violin. It also leads eventually to severe degenerative arthritis, often with considerable deformity of the hands. Ability to touch the nose with the tip of the tongue may also provide a clue to the diagnosis. The third aspect of the phenotype, atrophic scarring, if not immediately apparent, may be sought by inspecting the knees for the results of minor childhood injuries: there one may find

Table 16.11.1 Rare mendelian disorders affecting the cardiovascular system

	Biochemical abnormality	Noncardiac features	Cardiovascular features
Osteogenesis imperfecta (OMIM 166200, and others)	Heterogeneous, abnormalities of type 1 procollagen	Bony fractures and deformity, blue scleras (four types described)	Mitral valve prolapse and regurgitation Aortic root enlargement and aortic regurgitation.
Pseudoxanthoma elasticum (OMIM 264800)		Areas of thickened skin and pseudoxanthomas Vascular fragility and haemorrhage Fundus: angioid streaks	Extensive vascular narrowing and calcification with angina, claudication, and limb ischaemia
Hunter's syndrome (MPS II) (OMIM 309900)	Iduronate sulphate sulphatase	X-linked usually severe with dwarfing, mental retardation, gargoylism	Cardiomyopathy, coronary narrowing, valve lesions
Scheie's syndrome (MPS IS) (OMIM 607016)	α-Iduronidase (as in the much more severe, allelic, Hurler's syndrome, MPS IH)	Arthropathy, hepatosplenomegaly, corneal clouding	Aortic regurgitation Abnormal valve leaflets
Morquio's syndrome (MPS IV) (OMIM 253000 and others)	Galactosamine-6-sulphate sulphatase or α-galactosidase	Dwarfism, deafness, spinal cord compression and injury	Aortic regurgitation and stenosis
Homocystinuria (OMIM 236200)	Cystathionine-α-synthase	Osteoporosis, sternal deformity, lens subluxation, mental retardation	Vascular thrombosis, precocious coronary atherosclerosis
Fabry's disease (OMIM 301500)	α-Galactosidase A	Painful neuropathy, CNS disease, renal failure, corneal opacity	Coronary artery disease, myocardial infarction, mitral valve dysfunction
Friedreich's ataxia (OMIM 229300)	Frataxin	Spinocerebellar degeneration	Cardiomyopathy with increased wall thickness and restrictive physiology Ventricular arrhythmias
Duchenne's muscular dystrophy (OMIM 310200)	Dystrophin	X-linked muscular dystrophy with rapid progression during childhood and adolescence	Dilated cardiomyopathy, characteristic ECG
Becker's muscular dystrophy (OMIM 300376)	Dystrophin	X-linked muscular dystrophy, less severe than Duchenne's	Dilated cardiomyopathy, variable severity
Dystrophia myotonica (OMIM 160900)	Myotonin protein kinase	Weakness and myotonia, ptosis, cataracts, frontal balding, intellectual slowing	Bundle branch block, bradyarrhythmias, less frequently VT
Haemochromatosis (OMIM 235200 and others)	HFE protein	Diabetes, liver disease, pigmentation, arthritis, pituitary dysfunction	Dilated or restrictive cardiomyopathy
Arrhythmogenic right ventricular dysplasia (OMIM 107970 and others)	Transforming growth factor-beta-3 (and others)	None	Palpitations, syncope, sudden death

CNS, central nervous system; MPS, mucopolysaccharidosis; VT, ventricular tachycardia.

characteristic wide, atrophic ('cigarette paper') scars still obvious from bygone years.

Cardiovascular findings in classical Ehlers–Danlos are for the most part benign. Affected patients frequently have mitral valve prolapse, as do many people with joint laxity who do not have diagnosable Ehlers–Danlos syndrome. Relatively few progress to develop severe mitral reflux or to the point of requiring surgery. Enlargement of the aortic sinuses of Valsalva may occur, but only rarely is this severe or progressive. Surgical replacement of the aortic root, as is performed in Marfan's syndrome, is unusual in Ehlers–Danlos syndrome.

Vascular Ehlers–Danlos (OMIM 130050)

This, by contrast to classical Ehlers–Danlos, is a potentially fatal condition, with a natural history worse than Marfan's syndrome. It is genetically and biochemically well characterized: patients have mutations in the COL3A1 gene which encodes for type III procollagen, with inheritance as a dominant trait. The collagen defect leads to excessive fragility of blood vessels, the bowel, and the uterus, and the natural history of the condition is to present with spontaneous rupture of one of these three (in the case of the uterus, during pregnancy). Because of the intrinsic weakness of the affected tissues, surgical repair is challenging and these complications frequently prove fatal. Furthermore, in patients who have once undergone vascular or bowel rupture, the likelihood of a second event is high.

The joint and skin features of the vascular phenotype are less obvious than those of the classical form. Joint hypermobility is not seen, nor the resulting arthropathy. However, the skin feels soft and thin, and is abnormally translucent such that the veins are easily seen through it as one examines the shoulders and upper chest. The face is often thin and bony and the nose pinched.

Vascular complications are hard to anticipate. Aortic ectasia and aneurysm occur only in a few patients. Moreover, arterial rupture—as common as dissection—may occur in medium-sized vessels of the brain, thorax, or abdomen just as often as the aorta. In these regards, the vascular complications of this disease are comparable to those of the Loeys–Dietz syndrome. In affected patients and their families, detailed genetic evaluation is important and should include screening of COL3A1 and biochemical analysis of type III collagen obtained from skin biopsy and cultured fibroblasts. If these prove negative, then screening the TGF-β receptor genes would be appropriate.

Other heart-related connective tissue and metabolic disorders

Osteogenesis imperfecta causes aortic and mitral regurgitation, as do several of the mucopolysaccharidoses (Table 16.11.1). It is striking, particularly in the case of osteogenesis imperfecta, how healing is almost nonexistent where there is foreign material. If the opportunity arises, even years later, to inspect the operative result in a patient who has undergone valve replacement, the sutures look as though they had only just been placed, with minimal endothelial reaction and scar-tissue formation.

Further reading

Brooke BS, et al. (2008). Angiotensin II blockade and aortic-root dilation in Marfan's syndrome. *N Engl J Med*, **358**, 2787–95.

Gelb BD, Tartaglia M. (2006). Noonan syndrome and related disorders: dysregulated RAS-mitogen activated protein kinase signal transduction. *Hum Mol Genet*, **15** (Review Issue 2), R220–6.

Habashi JP, et al. (2006). Losartan, an AT1 antagonist, prevents aortic aneurysm in a mouse model of Marfan syndrome. *Science*, **312**, 117–21.

Judge DP, Dietz HC (2005). Marfan's syndrome. *Lancet*, **366**, 1965–76.

Lowery MC, et al. (1995). Strong correlation of elastin deletions, detected by FISH, with Williams syndrome: evaluation of 235 patients. *Amer J Hum Genet*, **57**, 49–53.

McKusick VA (2000). Ellis–van Creveld syndrome and the Amish. *Nat Genet*, **24**, 203–4.

Oderich GS et al. (2005). The spectrum, management and clinical outcome of Ehlers–Danlos syndrome type IV: a 30-year experience. *J Vasc Surg*, **42**, 98–106.

Pyeritz RE (1983). Cardiovascular manifestations of heritable disorders of connective tissue. *Progr Med Genet*, **5**, 191–302.

Radonic T, et al. (2010). Losartan therapy in adults with Marfan syndrome: study protocol of the multi-center randomized controlled COMPARE trial. *Trials*, **11**, 3 [Epub ahead of print].

Sund KL, et al. (2009). Analysis of Ellis van Creveld syndrome gene products: implications for cardiovascular development and disease. *Hum Mol Genet*, **18**, 1813–24.

Yamagishi H et al. (1999). A molecular pathway revealing a genetic basis for human cardiac and craniofacial defects. *Science*, **283**, 1158–61.

16.12

Congenital heart disease in the adult

S.A. Thorne

Essentials

Adults with congenital heart disease are a growing population, and now outnumber children with congenital heart disease in the UK. Many adult survivors have complex, surgically-altered hearts and circulations that reflect the surgical and interventional practices of the preceding two decades. For some, their long term outlook is unknown and they remain at lifelong risk of complications that may require further intervention. The organization of services to provide specialist care is key to their long term survival.

Classification of congenital heart disease

The classification and description of complex congenital heart disease can appear intimidating, but should be easily understood by using a simple physiological approach that takes into account whether a condition is cyanotic or acyanotic, whether there is a shunt, and the implications of the morphology for pulmonary blood flow.

The description of the congenitally malformed heart is aided by a sequential segmental analysis of the relationship of the three cardiac segments, which makes it possible to understand and describe how a complex heart is connected. The three segments to be considered are: (1) The atria; (2) The ventricles; (3) The great vessels. The next step is to describe each segment and its relation to the next segment:

(1) Atria:

♦ Situs solitus is the usual arrangement of the atria (and other asymmetrical structures)

♦ Atrial situs inversus is the mirror-image arrangement of the atria

♦ Isomerism describes abnormal symmetry of paired structures that usually show laterality – eg bilateral morphological left atria in left atrial isomerism.

(2) How the atria connect to the ventricles, ie the atrioventricular connections, and the morphology of the atrioventricular valves:

♦ Atrioventricular concordance, which is the normal arrangement, with the right atrium connecting to the right ventricle via a

tricuspid valve, and the left atrium connecting to the left ventricle via a mitral valve

♦ Atrioventricular discordance, which is abnormal: the right atrium connects to the left ventricle via a mitral valve, and the left atrium connects to the right ventricle via a tricuspid valve.

(3) How the ventricles connect to the great vessels, ie the ventriculo-arterial connections, and the morphology of the great arteries:

♦ Ventriculo-arterial concordance, which is the normal arrangement, with the right ventricle connecting to the pulmonary artery via a pulmonary valve, and the left ventricle connecting to the aorta via an aortic valve

♦ Ventriculo-arterial discordance, which is abnormal: the right ventricle connects to the aorta via an aortic valve, and the left ventricle connects to the pulmonary artery via a pulmonary valve.

Important general aspects

Cyanosis

Cyanosis occurs as a result of a right to left shunt, with its natural history determined by the pulmonary blood flow. If pulmonary blood flow is limited (e.g. by pulmonary stenosis in the presence of a large VSD), then pulmonary blood flow and arterial oxygen will be low, as will pulmonary artery pressure. Cyanotic patients with low or normal pulmonary artery pressure are usually amenable to surgical repair that abolishes the cyanosis. By contrast, if the pulmonary circulation is unprotected (e.g. if the defect includes a large ventricular septal defect and no pulmonary stenosis), then pulmonary blood flow will be high and at high pressure, pulmonary vascular remodelling will occur, and - without intervention - pulmonary vascular disease will eventually develop (pulmonary arterial hypertension; the Eisenmenger syndrome). Once pulmonary vascular disease is established, it is not possible to repair the defect and abolish the right to left shunt.

The right ventricle

The right ventricle is a key factor in the long term outcome of many congenital cardiac conditions. It may fail as a result of either

Acknowledgement: Dr P J Oldershaw wrote with Dr S Thorne on this subject in the fourth edition of the *Oxford Textbook of Medicine*. Some of that material has been retained in this edition, and we acknowledge Dr Oldershaw's contribution.

longstanding pressure or volume overload. (1) Pressure loading – this occurs in patients in whom the right ventricle supports the systemic circulation, such as those with congenitally corrected transposition of the great arteries, and in those who underwent interatrial repair (Mustard or Senning operation) of simple transposition of the great arteries. The right ventricle is hypertrophied, and ultimately fails, with tricuspid regurgitation secondary to annular dilatation hastening the decline. (2) Volume loading – this commonly occurs as a result of pulmonary regurgitation secondary to pulmonary valvotomy or repair of tetralogy of Fallot in early life. There may be no audible murmur because there are often only remnants of pulmonary valve tissue, such that the regurgitant flow is laminar. Partly because of the lack of physical signs, and partly because pulmonary regurgitation is usually tolerated for many years before the right ventricle begins to fail, patients may present very late with a very dilated and impaired ventricle. Longstanding large atrial septal defects produce similar right ventricular volume loading effects. The right ventricle may be inherently abnormal, as in Ebstein anomaly where a combination of a functionally small ventricle and volume loading from tricuspid regurgitation may cause the right ventricle to fail.

The Fontan circulation

Hearts which have only one functional ventricle present a particularly difficult challenge. Patients are cyanosed, and only a few will reach adulthood if left unoperated. The ultimate aim for patients with only one functional ventricle is a Fontan circulation: a palliative approach that reduces ventricular volume loading and abolishes cyanosis. It is critically dependent on a low pulmonary vascular resistance, hence early control of pulmonary blood flow is paramount. If pulmonary blood flow is too high, it is controlled by placing a pulmonary artery band: i.e. by the creation of iatrogenic, protective pulmonary stenosis. If pulmonary blood flow is too low, the infant will not thrive, and pulmonary blood supply is augmented by means of a systemic to pulmonary artery shunt. There are many variations of the Fontan operation, but all involve the separation of pulmonary and systemic circulations by using the single ventricle to support the systemic circulation and by connecting the systemic veins directly (or via the right atrium) to the pulmonary artery. There is thus no 'pump' in the pulmonary circulation, so although cyanosis is abolished, the Fontan circulation is one of

a chronic low output state. Thus, although the Fontan approach enables most patients with a single ventricle to reach adulthood, they have a fragile circulation and will develop a range of complications. They are particularly at risk if they have a tachyarrhythmia or acute non-cardiac illness, since they tolerate such insults poorly and are dependent on their medical teams' understanding of their circulation to ensure good hydration, avoidance of vasodilatation and rapid restoration of sinus rhythm.

Tachyarrhythmia

Tachyarrhythmias are a major cause of sudden death in patients with congenital heart disease, with scar related atrial tachyarrythmias being common in those who have had previous cardiac surgery, and probably a commoner cause of death than ventricular arrhythmias. Atrial tachyarrhymias are the reason that patients who underwent interatrial repair (Mustard or Senning operations) of transposition of the great arteries are the congenital cardiac group with the highest incidence of sudden death. Their surgically created atrial 'baffles' mean that atrial function is abnormal, and ventricular filling is impaired, particularly at high heart rates. Atrial flutter is common post Mustard or Senning, and patients are usually able to conduct 1:1 at a rate of 300bpm, resulting in cardiovascular collapse. Correct management is rapid restoration of sinus rhythm, followed by flutter ablation. Patients with a Fontan circulation are similarly vulnerable to interatrial re-entry tachyarrythmias. Ventricular and atrial tachycardias may both occur in most survivors of complex congenital heart disease, particularly post repair of tetralogy of Fallot. If ablation is not successful, consideration should be given to an internal cardiovertor defibrillator.

Pregnancy and contraception

Most women with congenital heart disease wish to consider pregnancy. For most this can be undertaken with only a small increased risk, but for some pregnancy carries a significant risk of complication, long term morbidity and death. Outcomes can be optimised by pre-conception counseling and specialist joint cardiac and obstetric care. Access to safe and effective contraception is important to allow patients to avoid potentially high risk pregnancies. Estrogen containing preparations are not suitable for those at risk of intracardiac thrombus or who have a right to left shunt; long acting progestogen-only methods offer safe and effective alternatives.

Introduction

The growing number of adult survivors of congenital heart disease will encounter medical staff from all areas of medicine and surgery. It is therefore important that all doctors have an understanding of the principles of congenital heart disease and enough knowledge to know when to refer such patients to a specialist centre.

As a result of advances in paediatric cardiac surgery and intervention, the outlook for the approximately 8 per 1000 babies born with congenital heart disease has changed dramatically in the last half century. Fifty years ago, 70% of children born with congenital heart disease died before their 10th birthday; now more than 80% survive to adulthood and there are more adults than children living in the United Kingdom with congenital heart disease.

Despite such advances, only those with the simplest conditions, e.g. isolated secundum atrial septal defect or anomalous pulmonary

venous drainage successfully repaired in childhood, may be considered cured of their heart disease. Most patients need continued specialist follow-up since they have residual lesions that may progress over many years and require timely intervention.

Surgical techniques continually evolve, creating new populations with different, surgically modified conditions and long-term outcomes. Careful follow-up is therefore crucial, not only to provide high standards of clinical care, but also to provide feedback about late results in order to inform initial management in infancy. As a result of such long-term follow-up information, the operation of choice for transposition of the great arteries is now the arterial switch, because of the late problems encountered in patients who had undergone interatrial repair with the Senning or Mustard operations.

Surgical advances mean that patients with new surgically modified conditions are reaching adulthood. Their outlook and the complications they may face are not known, so lifelong specialist

Table 16.12.1 Classification of congenital heart disease

Acyanotic				Cyanotic Obligatory right-to-left shunt					
No shunt		Left-to-right shunt		Eisenmenger syndrome		High pulmonary blood flow		Normal or low pulmonary blood flow	
Level of lesion	Example of specific lesion	Level of shunt	Example of specific lesion	Level of shunt	Example of specific lesion	Level of shunt	Example of specific lesion	Level of shunt	Example of specific lesion
R inflow	Ebstein's anomaly	Atrial	PAPVD ASD AVSD	Atrial	Large ASD (uncommon cause)	Atrial	Large ASD	Atrial, with obstruction to pulmonary blood flow	Severe pulmonary stenosis with ASD Left SVC to LA connection
L inflow	Congenital mitral stenosis Cor triatatrium	Ventricular	VSD	Ventricular	Large VSD	Ventricular	Large VSD	Ventricular, with obstruction to pulmonary blood flow	Tetralogy of Fallot, Pulmonary atresia VSD, Univentricular heart with pulmonary stenosis
R outflow	Infundibular stenosis Pulmonary stenosis	Arterial	PDA Aortopulmonary window	Arterial	Large PDA Aortopulmonery window	Arterial	Large PDA Aortopulmonery window	Extra cardiac	Pulmonary AVM
L outflow	Subaortic stenosis Bicuspid aortic valve	Multiple	AVSD	Multiple	Large AVSD	Multiple	Large AVSD		
Arterial	Supravalvar stenosis Coarctation of the aorta								

ASD, atrial septal defect; AVSD, atriventricular septal defect; LA, left atrium; PAPVD, partial anomalous pulmonary venous drainage; SVC, superior vena cava; VSD, ventricular septal defect.

surveillance is important. Survivors of the hypoplastic left heart syndrome will be the largest such new group reaching the adult clinics in the next decade.

Classification and nomenclature

The classification and description of complex congenital heart disease can appear intimidating. Nonetheless, a grasp of the basic principles is important to understand the anatomy and pathophysiology of congenital cardiac conditions. A simple physiological approach to classifying congenital heart disease takes into account whether a condition is cyanotic or acyanotic, whether there is a shunt, and the implications of the morphology for pulmonary blood flow (Table 16.12.1).

Sequential segmental analysis

The description of the congenitally malformed heart is aided by a segmental approach, which makes it possible to understand and describe how a complex heart is connected. Any heart can be described by considering it as three segments (the atrial chambers, the ventricular mass, and the great arteries) and describing in a sequential manner how each segment is arranged and connected to the next segment (Box 16.12.1).

Atrial arrangement

Situs solitus is the usual arrangement of asymmetrical structures, i.e. morphological left atrium on the left and right atrium on the right; morphological left main bronchus on the left and right main bronchus on the right; stomach on the left, liver on the right. Situs inversus is the mirror image arrangement of these structures.

Isomerism describes abnormal symmetry of paired structures that usually show laterality, as shown in Table 16.12.2. The presence

of isomerism of the atrial appendages should alert the physician to the coexistence of complex associated lesions, including a variety of abnormalities of venous connections that may cause technical difficulties at cardiac catheterization and permanent pacemaker insertion. Right isomerism is commoner in males and left isomerism in females. Survival to adulthood with right isomerism is uncommon because of associated asplenia and severe cyanotic heart disease,

---

Box 16.12.1 Segmental analysis

◆ The arrangement of the atria (situs) is described first—see text below for discussion of abnormal situs/isomerism

◆ The atrioventricular (AV) connections and the morphology of the AV valves are described:

 • AV concordance—normal; the RA connects to the RV via a tricuspid valve; the LA connects to the LV via a mitral valve

 • AV discordance—abnormal; the RA connects to the LV via a mitral valve; the LA connects to the RV via a tricuspid valve

◆ The ventriculoarterial (VA) connections and the morphology of the great arteries are described:

 • VA concordance—normal; the RV connects to the PA via a pulmonary valve, the LV connects to the aorta via an aortic valve

 • VA discordance—abnormal; the RV connects to the aorta via an aortic valve, the LV connects to the PA via a pulmonary valve

◆ Associated malformations are then described

Table 16.12.2 Diagnosis of atrial arrangement

	Atrial situs solitus (normal)	Atrial situs inversus	Right isomerism	Left isomerism
Atrial morphology	Normal: R-sided morphological RA L-sided morphological LA	Mirror image: R-sided morphological LA L-sided morphological RA	Bilateral morphological RA, extensive pectinate muscles	Bilateral morphological LA, pectinate muscles confined to appendages
Atrial appendages[a]	Normal: Broad based RA appendage, long narrow LA appendage	Mirror image	Bilateral broad based RA appendages	Bilateral long narrow LA appendages
Sinus node	Single, R-sided	Single, L-sided	Bilateral	Absent
Pulmonary morphology	R lung trilobed L lung bilobed	R lung bilobed L lung trilobed	Bilateral trilobed lungs	Bilateral Bilobed lungs
Bronchial morphology[b]	R-sided main bronchus: short, L- sided main bronchus: long,	Mirror image	Bilateral short morphological R bronchi	Bilateral long morphological L bronchi
Abdominal arrangement[c] Aorta IVC Stomach Liver Spleen	To L of spine To R of spine L-sided R-sided R-sided	Normal or mirror image	Aorta and IVC on same side. IVC anterior to aorta. Usually L sided. Midline Usually absent	Aorta and azygos on same side. Azygos posterior to aorta. Usually R sided. Midline Often polysplenia.

IVC, inferior vena cava; L, left; LA, left atrium; R right; RA, right atrium; SVC, superior vena cava.

[a] Readily identified on transoesophageal echocardiography.

[b] Since bronchopulmonary situs nearly always follows atrial situs, atrial situs can be inferred from the chest radiograph.

[c] Echocardiography shows the intra-abdominal relations of the great vessels. In left isomerism, there is usually interruption of the IVC, and the abdominal venous return connects to the heart via a (right-sided) azygos or (left-sided) hemiazygos vein. The hepatic veins can be identified draining separately into the atria.

including obstructed anomalous pulmonary venous drainage (the pulmonary venous confluence is a left atrial structure). The lesions associated with left isomerism tend to produce left-to-right shunts and little if any cyanosis.

Cyanosis: a multisystem disorder

Cyanosis occurs as a result of a right-to-left shunt. Cyanotic heart disease is a multisystem disorder; its manifestations are listed in Table 16.12.3.

Secondary erythrocytosis

Chronic hypoxia is the stimulus to the increased red blood cell mass and high haematocrit found in cyanotic heart disease. This physiological response increases the oxygen-carrying capacity of the blood and may improve tissue oxygenation sufficiently to reach a new equilibrium at a higher haematocrit. However, adaptive failure occurs if the increase in blood viscosity brought about by the high haematocrit impairs oxygen delivery and negates the beneficial effects of erythrocytosis.

The secondary erythrocytosis of cyanotic heart disease is a physiological response, often associated with thrombocytopenia. It is fundamentally different from the generaliszed increase in all haemopoietic stem cell lines found in the malignant disease, polycythaemia rubra vera. Failure to differentiate between these two phenomena has contributed to the persistent mismanagement of erythrocytosis in cyanotic heart disease. Three misconceptions lead to inappropriate venesection in cyanotic heart disease:

♦ 'Volume replacement is not necessary'—if venesection is performed without simultaneous volume replacement, the sudden fall in systemic blood flow, oxygen delivery and cerebral perfusion may result in cardiovascular collapse. Simultaneous infusion of an equal volume of 0.9% saline or colloid should be given.

♦ 'Venesection is performed to reduce the risk of stroke'—the risk of stroke in adults with cyanotic heart disease does not relate to the haematocrit, but rather to microcytosis and iron deficiency brought on by injudicious venesection.

Table 16.12.3 Complications of cyanotic congenital heart disease

Haematological	Secondary erythrocytosis Iron deficiency (overvenesection, menorrhagia) Thrombocytopenia Haemorrhage Coagulopathy	→Hyperviscosity →Hyperviscosity ↑ Risk of CVA
Neurological	CVA Cerebral abscess	2° to paradoxical embolism
Hyperuricaemia	Impaired renal clearance of uric acid Increased uric acid production?	→Gout
Renal abnormalities	↓ Uric acid clearance Glomerular proteinuria Mesangial matrix thickening Capillary and hilar arteriole dilatation	→High risk of iatrogenic renal failure
Bilirubin kinetics	↑ Haem breakdown	→Pigment gallstones
Digits and long bones	Clubbing Hypertrophic osteoarthropathy	
Dental	Gingival hypertrophy	→↑ Risk of endocarditis
Infection	Endocarditis Cerebral abscess	
Skin	Acne	

CVA, cardiovascular accident.

Box 16.12.2 Symptoms of hyperviscosity

- Headache
- Faint, dizzy, light-headed
- Depressed mentation, sense of distance
- Blurred vision, amaurosis fugax
- Paraesthesiae
- Tinnitus
- Fatigue, lethargy
- Myalgia, muscle weakness
- Chest and abdominal pain
- Restless legs

- 'Venesection should be done routinely to keep the haematocrit below 65%'—the only indication for venesection is for the temporary relief of symptoms of hyperviscosity in hydrated, iron-replete individuals with haematocrit greater than 60 to 65% (Box 16.12.2 and Tables 16.12.4).

Any dehydration should be corrected before assessing the need for venesection, and if the patient does not gain symptomatic improvement then further venesection is unlikely to be beneficial. Some patients reach a stable equilibrium with a haematocrit above 70%; venesection is not indicated if there are no symptoms of hyperviscosity, the only exception being the preoperative patient with thrombocytopenia and a high haematocrit, when venesection may cause a temporary rise in platelet count and a reduction in perioperative bleeding.

Microcytic, hypochromic iron-deficient erythrocytes require a higher haematocrit and therefore higher blood viscosity to achieve the same oxygen-carrying capacity as iron-replete cells. Iron deficiency also causes muscle weakness and myalgia, independent of its effect on blood viscosity. If standard doses of iron supplements are given, uncontrolled erythropoiesis occurs and the haematocrit rises rapidly, resulting in a cycle of excessive venesection and iron deficiency leaving the patient symptomatic from both haematocrit-

Table 16.12.4 Guidelines for venesection in adults with cyanotic heart disease

Symptoms of hyperviscosity	Haematocrit and serum iron	Action
No	Any	Venesection not indicated
Yes	Hct >60% Iron replete No dehydration	Isovolumic venesection (400–500 ml)
Yes	Hct <65%, iron deficient	Treat underlying cause of iron deficiency No venesection Consider low dose iron therapy, closely monitoring Hct
Yes	>65% iron deficient	Seek underlying cause of iron deficiency Avoid venesection if possible Consider cautious low dose iron ± hydroxyurea

HCT, haematocrit.

induced and iron-deficiency-induced hyperviscosity. Low dose iron replacement (ferrous sulphate 200 mg/day) combined with close monitoring of the blood count so that iron therapy is withdrawn as soon as the haematocrit rises (often within a week) should allow the gradual recovery of iron stores and the avoidance of counter-productive venesection and further iron deficiency. Hydroxyurea is an antitumour agent that may have a role in suppressing the erythrocytotic response to iron therapy in patients with a high haematocrit, but it also causes thrombocytopenia and neutropenia and so should be used with caution.

Menorrhagia is common in women with cyanotic heart disease and may be sufficient to cause iron-deficiency anaemia. It may be difficult to manage, the combined oral contraceptive pill being contraindicated because of the prothrombotic effects of the oestrogen it contains, and tranexamic acid may similarly be associated with thrombosis. Norethisterone may provide short-term relief. Progestogen-only contraceptives have unpredictable effects on menstruation: a subdermal implant (e.g. Implanon) is safe and causes oligoamenorrhoea in some women. Mirena IUS is a progestogen-eluting intrauterine device that causes oligoamenorrhoea in most women, but it is not generally recommended in those with cyanotic heart disease or who have not undergone previous vaginal delivery because insertion may a vasovagal response and cardiovascular collapse. If menorrhagia is due to uterine fibroids, catheter embolization of the feeding uterine artery is safe and may be successful.

Disorders of coagulation and blood vessels

It is poorly understood why patients with cyanotic disease are at increased risk of haemorrhage and thrombosis. There is often a mild thrombocytopenia that may be due partly to shortened platelet survival time, and the large multimeric forms of von Willebrand factor and other clotting factors may be depleted. Coagulation testing may yield spurious results in patients with haematocrit over 55% unless the amount of citrate anticoagulant is reduced.

Bleeding may be minor and mucocutaneous, but major haemorrhage may occur during surgery, or from the lungs. Pulmonary artery thrombosis is discussed below (see 'Eisenmenger syndrome: defects with secondary pulmonary vascular disease', below). Interestingly, systemic arterial atherosclerosis is exceedingly rare in the cyanotic population, perhaps because of a combination of thrombocytopenia, upregulated nitric oxide, hyperbilirubinaemia, and hypocholesterolaemia.

Other complications of cyanotic heart disease

The risk of is increased in cyanotic heart disease, with independent risk factors being intravenous lines, arterial hypertension, atrial fibrillation, and the strongest risk factor, red cell microcytosis.

Right-to-left shunting creates a risk of paradoxical embolism causing stroke and cerebral abscess, as well as air emboli from venous lines not fitted with filters. Patients who require transvenous pacing should be anticoagulated with warfarin to prevent paradoxical thromboembolism from pacing leads.

Despite the high incidence of hyperuricaemia, attacks of acute gout are uncommon and asymptomatic hyperuricaemia does not require treatment. Acute attacks should be treated with colchicine, avoiding nonsteroidal anti-inflammatory agents (NSAIDs) because of their detrimental effects on haemostasis and renal function. As in primary hyperuricaemia, allopurinol is useful in preventing recurrence.

The renal abnormalities outlined in Table 16.12.3 are frequently not associated with abnormal baseline renal function. However, renal failure may be precipitated by hypotension and dehydration, especially in combination with radiographic contrast media, NSAIDs or aminoglycoside antibiotics. Acne is a common complaint in adolescents and adults with cyanotic disease and may be widespread and psychologically debilitating. When severe it may also increase the risk of bacteraemia and endocarditis.

Digital clubbing is almost universal in cyanotic heart disease, and some degree of hypertrophic osteoarthropathy of the long bones may occur in up to one-third of patients. Symptoms include aching and tenderness of the long bones of the forearms and legs. There is oedema and cellular infiltration, causing lifting of the periosteum that is visible radiographically, with new bone formation and resorption. Localized activation of endothelial cells by an abnormal platelet population, with the ensuing release of fibroblast growth factors, may play a central role in the pathogenesis of both phenomena.

Cyanotic patients become more hypoxic during air travel as the partial pressure of oxygen in a pressurized aircraft is lower than that at sea level. However, such travel seems to be well tolerated and supplemental oxygen should not normally be necessary. Travellers should be warned to avoid dehydration and to plan their journeys to avoid having to carry baggage for long distances within large airports.

Eisenmenger syndrome: defects with secondary pulmonary vascular disease

Eisenmenger syndrome is a condition where there is pulmonary hypertension at systemic level. It occurs when a communication between the systemic and pulmonary circulations results in high pulmonary blood flow and the development of high pulmonary vascular resistance, which in turn results in a reversed or bidirectional shunt. The communication may be at atrial, ventricular or arterial levels.

Surgery in infancy should usually prevent the development of this irreversible syndrome, but when patients do present their management is dependent on a good understanding of their condition.

Clinical findings

Symptoms of breathlessness relate to the degree of hypoxia; many patients feel worse in hot weather or after a hot bath because the resulting systemic vasodilatation is not accompanied by a reduction in pulmonary vascular resistance, so the right-to-left shunt is enhanced and they become more hypoxic. Exercise-induced syncope may occur, and is exacerbated by hot weather and dehydration. Haemoptysis is common and may be fatal.

Whatever the underlying defect, some examination findings are shared. Patients are cyanosed and clubbed and may be plethoric. There is a right ventricular heave and the pulmonary component of the second heart sound is palpable and loud. A pulmonary ejection click and pulmonary regurgitation may be audible. A soft systolic flow murmur may be heard from the dilated pulmonary artery. No systolic murmur can be heard from the lesion responsible for the pulmonary vascular disease since the chambers on both sides of the lesion are at equal pressure.

It is frequently possible to distinguish between the common lesions associated with the Eisenmenger syndrome on clinical grounds. The patient with an Eisenmenger duct has differential cyanosis and clubbing since fully saturated blood from the left ventricle supplies the aortic arch and its branches before mixing occurs with desaturated pulmonary arterial blood via the patent duct. The right hand may therefore be pink with no clubbing, the left may be slightly more cyanosed because of the origin of the left subclavian artery opposite the duct, and the toes are more deeply cyanosed and clubbed. The second heart sound may be closely or normally split. In contrast, cyanosis and clubbing is uniform when the right-to-left shunt occurs at atrial, ventricular or ascending aortic (as in truncus arteriosus or aortopulmonary window) levels. The second sound is single in ventricular septal defect (VSD), AV septal defect (AVSD), and truncus, but may be split in an atrial septal defect (ASD).

Investigations

The chest radiograph shows a dilated pulmonary trunk because of high pulmonary blood flow in earlier life, but reduced blood flow as pulmonary vascular resistance rose means that the lung fields are oligaemic (Fig. 16.12.1). Unless cardiac failure intervenes, the heart size is usually normal, the effects of volume overload having regressed as pulmonary vascular resistance increased and the left-to-right shunt diminished and disappeared.

The ECG shows P pulmonale and biventricular hypertrophy. The echocardiogram should establish the site of the shunt and allow an estimation of pulmonary arterial pressure and ventricular function.

Cardiopulmonary exercise testing may be used with caution: patients with Eisenmenger syndrome are among the most limited of those with congenital heart disease and maximal exercise testing may induce potentially fatal syncope. The less strenuous but still objective 6-min walk test is the preferable measure of exercise capacity in these patients.

Multislice CT scanning demonstrates the hypertensive pulmonary vasculature and any collateral vessels. It is also the investigation of choice to show in situ pulmonary thrombus and pulmonary artery aneurysms, and to demonstrate the site of any pulmonary haemorrhage. Care should be taken to avoid contrast-induced nephropathy by ensuring adequate hydration.

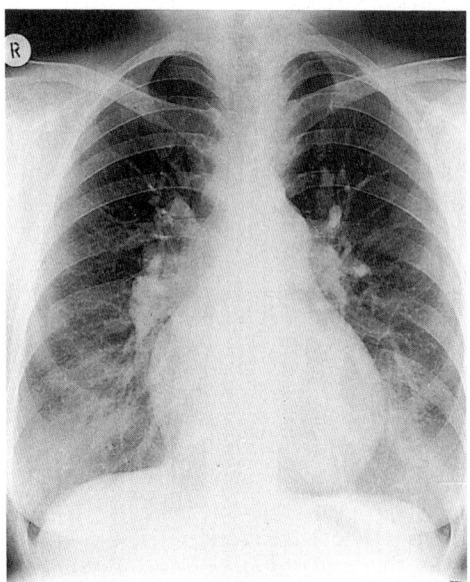

Fig. 16.12.1 Chest radiograph of a 35-year-old woman with Eisenmenger secundum atrial septal defect. The aortic knuckle is small and the central pulmonary arteries enlarged, indicating pulmonary arterial hypertension; the lung fields are clear. The cardiac silhouette is not enlarged.

Cardiac catheterization is unnecessary and potentially dangerous for patients with established pulmonary vascular disease. The only indication is for those patients whose pulmonary vascular disease is suspected to be reversible and who would be considered for surgical repair if reversibility can be confirmed. This situation is rarely encountered in the adult population.

Histologically, pulmonary vascular disease progresses from medial hypertrophy through intimal proliferation with migration of smooth muscle cells, to progressive fibrosis and obliteration, dilatation, the development of angiomata and finally fibrinoid necrosis. Those who have developed fibrotic and obliterative changes are likely to have irreversible pulmonary vascular disease. Routine lung biopsy is not recommended; it carries a high risk in the pulmonary hypertensive adult and is unlikely to show reversible pathology. In addition, thoracotomy scars from open lung biopsy are a relative contraindication to heart–lung transplantation.

Outcome and complications

Survival into adulthood with Eisenmenger syndrome is common. Life expectancy may be around 20 years less than for the general population, but this is markedly better than for those with idiopathic pulmonary arterial hypertension. Markers of poorer prognosis include complex anatomy and physiology, decline in functional class, and the development of heart failure and clinical arrhythmia. Serum uric acid increases with disease progression and may also be used as a long term predictor of mortality.

The patient with Eisenmenger syndrome is prone to all the complications of cyanotic heart disease discussed above.

Haemoptysis is usually due to rupture of small hypertensive intrapulmonary vessels, or more rarely to thrombosis *in situ* and pulmonary infarction. All patients should be admitted to hospital and the systemic pressure kept low by bed rest and β-blockade; the pulmonary artery pressure being the same as that measured in the brachial artery. NSAIDs should be stopped and vasodilators should not be given. If the haemoptysis is massive, diamorphine should be administered, fresh frozen plasma or cryoprecipitate may be given, and consideration should be given to selectively intubating the nonbleeding lung. Bronchoscopy has no role and may worsen the haemorrhage.

In situ thrombosis in the dilated pulmonary arteries of adults with Eisenmenger syndrome is common (prevalence of 20–30%) and relates to the degree of cyanosis. It is best detected and quantified using multislice CT scanning. Anticoagulation of any sort has not been shown to resolve such thrombus, and patients are at risk of pulmonary embolic episodes. Warfarin may increase the risk of bleeding while failing to reduce the thrombus, and aspirin should be avoided as it may exacerbate haemorrhage associated with thrombocytopenia.

Right ventricular failure may be precipitated by atrial arrhythmia and usually occurs after the age of 30 years. Decline may be heralded by the onset of right ventricular failure, supraventricular arrhythmia and haemoptysis. Death may be sudden and due to arrhythmia or massive haemoptysis. In some patients death follows progressive hypoxia terminating in bradycardia and asystole from which they cannot be resuscitated.

Intercurrent illness and noncardiac surgery may pose major risks. The latter is particularly dangerous when carried out without the benefit of expert cardiology, anaesthetic and perioperative care. A sound understanding of the pathophysiology is vital (Box 16.12.3).

> **Box 16.12.3** Checklist for patients at high risk[a] of iatrogenic complications during the perioperative period or during intercurrent illness
>
> - Maintain hydration—intravenous fluids (via air filter if cyanotic to avoid the risk of paradoxical embolism) when nil by mouth
> - Maintain haemoglobin commensurate with degree of cyanosis to optimise oxygen carrying capacity
> - Avoid vasodilator agents—especially at induction of anaesthesia
> - Protect the kidneys—maintain hydration, avoid nephrotoxic agents (NSAIDs, aminoglycosides), use minimal volumes of contrast agents.
>
> [a] Patients at high risk include those who are cyanotic and those with Eisenmenger syndrome or Fontan circulation.

Treatment options

Until recently, treatment has been palliative and symptom led, directed at avoiding iatrogenic and natural complications. Although this approach is still the mainstay of treatment, selective pulmonary vasodilators including phosphodiesterase inhibitors (eg sildenafil) and endothelin receptor antagonists may improve outcome. They have been shown to improve outcome in other forms of pulmonary hypertension, and data from initial short-term randomized controlled studies of bosentan suggests that it may be beneficial in Eisenmenger syndrome.

Pregnancy and contraception

Pregnancy carries a particularly high risk, 25–40% maternal mortality. Pregnancy and contraception in congenital heart disease are discussed below, and in heart disease in general in Chapter 14.6. All women with pulmonary hypertension of any cause should be counselled of the risks and given access to safe, effective contraception. If a woman with Eisenmenger syndrome does become pregnant and chooses not to have a termination, she should be referred to a specialist centre.

Valve and outflow tract lesions

Isolated pulmonary valve stenosis

Isolated pulmonary stenosis is common, occurring in up to 10% of patients with congenital heart disease. There is usually fusion of the valve cusps leading to a doming appearance. Syndromic associations are not unusual and include Noonan's, Williams's and Alagille's syndromes.

Significant pulmonary stenosis results in right ventricular hypertrophy and high right-sided pressures; right-to-left shunting causing cyanosis may occur if there is a coexistent ASD or patent foramen ovale.

Pulmonary stenosis is a better-tolerated lesion than aortic stenosis, with an excellent survival. Severe pulmonary stenosis usually presents in childhood, either as an asymptomatic murmur, or with failure to thrive, chest pain, dyspnoea, or cyanosis.

Physical signs

Patients are acyanotic unless there is an interatrial communication, in which case cyanosis is severe. The venous pressure is raised only if the right ventricle has begun to fail and there is tricuspid regurgitation. There may be a right ventricular heave. The pulmonary component of the second heart sound is soft and there is a pulmonary ejection systolic murmur. An early diastolic murmur may also be present if there is coexistent pulmonary regurgitation.

Investigations
The ECG may demonstrate right ventricular hypertrophy. This regresses after relief of the stenosis. The chest radiograph reveals poststenotic dilation of the proximal pulmonary artery, and the lung fields may be oligaemic if the pulmonary stenosis is severe.

Transthoracic echocardiography confirms the diagnosis and allows functional assessment of the severity of pulmonary stenosis and regurgitation as well as right ventricular hypertrophy, dilatation, and function.

Management
Adults with trivial (<20 mmHg) pulmonary stenosis do not require regular follow-up, since progression is unlikely. Approximately 20% of adults with mild stenosis (<50 mmHg) may progress and ultimately require intervention, and most of those with a peak pulmonary valve gradient greater than 50mmHg require intervention.

Balloon pulmonary valvotomy is the treatment of choice, unless associated anomalies require a surgical approach. Valvotomy is usually successful and it is uncommon for stenosis to recur, however, the procedure invariably results in a degree of pulmonary regurgitation and so long-term follow-up is required.

Lone infundibular stenosis and double-chambered right ventricle
Abnormally placed muscle bands cause either infundibular obstruction or—if placed more inferiorly—subinfundibular obstruction and a double-chambered right ventricle. The degree of obstruction may be mild in childhood, but progresses in adult life and causes symptoms as the right ventricle hypertrophies. A perimembranous VSD usually coexists and may close spontaneously. Treatment is by surgical resection of the obstructing muscle bands.

Ebstein's anomaly
This rare, complex defect of the tricuspid valve occurs in 1 in 20 000 live births and affects both sexes equally. The risk may be increased by maternal exposure to lithium during the first trimester. Ebstein's anomaly is characterized by a spectrum of features:

* Adherence of the tricuspid valve leaflets to the underlying myocardium due to failure of delamination in fetal life, resulting in apical displacement of the functional tricuspid valve tethering, redundancy, and fenestrations of the valve leaflets

* Apical displacement of the tricuspid valve annulus:
  * As a result of the failure of delamination the septal and posterior (mural) leaflets insert further into the body of the right ventricle than in the normal heart (in which the mitral and tricuspid valves are offset so that the tricuspid valve is displaced up to 1.5 cm towards the right ventricular apex).
  * the 'atrialized' portion of the right ventricle is often thinner walled than the functional right ventricle due to congenital partial absence of the myocardium

* as a result the functional size of the right ventricle is reduced and of the right atrium increased
* Dilation of the functional right atrium
* Dilatation of the true tricuspid valve annulus at the AV junction

This combination of features usually results in tricuspid regurgitation (or very rarely stenosis) and right heart dilation, providing a substrate for atrial and ventricular arrhythmias.

Associated abnormalities
A patent foramen ovale or ASD is present in most cases, and allows cyanosis to develop as the disease progresses and of right-to-left shunting occurs. Left heart abnormalities occur as a consequence of alterations in left ventricular geometry due to leftwards displacement of the interventricular septum; e.g. mitral valve prolapse may occur as result of relatively long chordae in a left ventricle of reduced cavity size. Coexistent Wolfe–Parkinson–White syndrome, usually with single or multiple right-sided pathways, occurs in 20% of patients.

Ebstein's anomaly may also form part of other complex congenital lesions, including pulmonary stenosis and atresia and tetralogy of Fallot. When it coexists with congenitally corrected transposition of the great arteries, the tricuspid valve is the systemic AV valve.

Clinical presentation and course
There is a broad spectrum of severity, ranging from intrauterine or neonatal death to presentation in late adulthood. Mortality, both with and without surgery, is influenced by age at presentation, the condition of the tricuspid valve, the cardiac rhythm, and the functional capacity of the right ventricle, including the severity of right ventricular outflow tract obstruction and the size of the right atrium in relation to the other cardiac chambers.

Arrhythmia is the commonest mode of initial presentation in adult life; presentation earlier in life is usually associated with severe disease and additional cardiac lesions.

Cyanosis may develop in adulthood if there is an associated ASD or patent foramen ovale; as the right ventricular filling pressure increases there is a parallel rise in right atrial pressure, and a right-to-left interatrial shunt is established. These patients are at risk of paradoxical embolism, but the risk of endocarditis is low because the tricuspid regurgitant jet is of low velocity.

Heart failure may intervene as a result of the combination of severe tricuspid regurgitation and the onset of atrial fibrillation or flutter. These atrial arrhythmias may be particularly troublesome if a coexistent accessory pathway allows a rapid ventricular response rate. The onset of atrial fibrillation is a predictor of death within 5 years, and may account for the increased death rate in the fifth decade.

Physical signs
The patient may be acyanotic or cyanosed and clubbed. Even when tricuspid regurgitation is severe the jugular venous pressure may not be particularly high or the v wave prominent because of the capacity of the right atrium and thin-walled atrialized right ventricle to accommodate the low pressure regurgitant volume. Once right ventricular failure develops the jugular venous pressure rises further and the a and v waves become more prominent. In the uncommon situation of tricuspid stenosis, the a wave is increased and may be giant. The first heart sound is widely split with a delayed tricuspid component, due to the extra distance that the large anterior leaflet has to

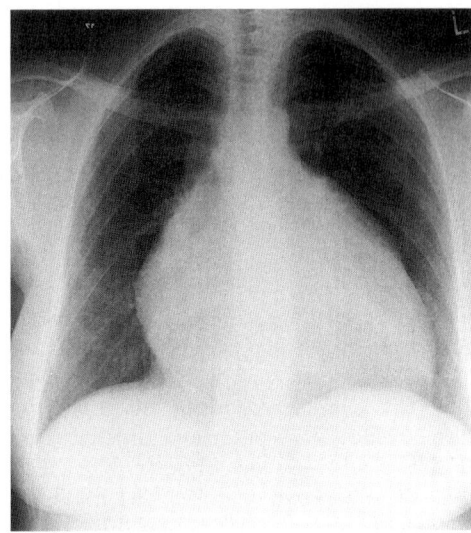

Fig. 16.12.2 Chest radiograph of a 43-year-old woman with classic cardiac silhouette of Ebstein's anomaly due to right atrial enlargement. The aortic knuckle and pulmonary arteries are inconspicuous and the lung fields oligaemic.

travel to reach the limit of its systolic excursion. The second heart sound may be single because low pressure in the right ventricular outflow tract renders the pulmonary component inaudible, or it may be widely split reflecting right bundle branch block. Third or fourth ventricular filling sounds may be present. The systolic murmur of tricuspid regurgitation varies from inaudible to loud enough to generate a thrill, but is classically decrescendo and scratchy. Once the right ventricle begins to fail and the venous pressure rises, hepatomegaly, ascites and peripheral oedema are common.

Investigations

The chest radiograph is characteristic (Fig. 16.12.2). The ECG typically shows a superior axis and right atrial enlargement, with or without right bundle branch block. The p wave may be peaked and the PR interval prolonged, reflecting the prolonged conduction in the large right atrium, or there may be evidence of pre-excitation. Right bundle branch block may occur due to abnormal activation and conduction in the atrialized right ventricle.

Echocardiography establishes the diagnosis, severity, and associated abnormalities of Ebstein anomaly. The atrialized and functional portions of the right ventricle can be identified, as can the precise attachments and degree of tethering of the anterior leaflet of the tricuspid valve. Echocardiography is the investigation of choice in planning surgical intervention, tethering and restricted motion of the anterior leaflet and a small right ventricle being strong predictors of the need for tricuspid valve replacement rather than repair. Cardiac catheterization is only necessary if specific haemodynamic questions remain after noninvasive assessment.

Cardiopulmonary exercise testing is invaluable in assessing functional capacity when planning timing of surgery.

Treatment

Patients should be anticoagulated when atrial arrhythmias develop, particularly if there is an ASD. If re-entry tachycardias cannot be controlled with antiarrhythmic drugs, radiofrequency ablation of accessory pathways may be performed. However, ablation may be made difficult by the size and abnormal shape of the right atrium and abnormal position of the accessory pathway or pathways.

Symptomatic patients should be assessed for surgery. In addition, the asymptomatic patient with severe tricuspid regurgitation and normal cardiopulmonary exercise tolerance should be considered for repair if right ventricular function has begun to deteriorate. The timing of surgery may be difficult to decide in the adult patient, even in the few centres with reasonable experience. Once the patient has developed overt right heart failure with a raised venous pressure, hepatomegaly, ascites, and atrial fibrillation, ventricular function may have deteriorated such that repair of the valve is no longer possible and transplantation may need to be considered.

Successful repair of the ebsteinoid valve is difficult, as evidenced by the many techniques described. The aim is to achieve a competent native valve with its insertion at the true annulus and a reduction in right atrial size. Where possible, valve replacement should be avoided, since long term outcomes are better with repair. A maze procedure should also be considered to reduce the long-term risk of atrial flutter and fibrillation.

For high-risk patients in whom the right ventricle is thought to be unable to support the pulmonary circulation with a competent tricuspid valve, techniques to reduce its workload may be considered. The '1½' ventricle repair combines tricuspid valve repair with a cavopulmonary anastomosis so that upper body systemic venous return is directly to the pulmonary arteries, thus offloading the right ventricle. A single ventricle repair may also be used, resulting in a Fontan circulation (see below).

Other right ventricular anomalies

Uhl's anomaly and arrhythmogenic right ventricular cardiomyopathy (see also Chapter 16.7.2) are rare sporadic or familial conditions affecting the right ventricle. Table 16.12.5 list the key distinguishing features.

Early diagnosis and the screening of family members of affected individuals is challenging and requires experience. MRI and multislice CT are useful tools, but early abnormalities are subtle and may be over interpreted.

Cor triatatrium and congenital mitral valve anomalies

Cor triatatrium

This is a very rare defect in which one of the atria (nearly always the left) is partitioned by a fibromuscular membrane into an upper chamber that receives the pulmonary veins, and a lower chamber connecting with the atrial appendage and mitral valve. This is

Table 16.12.5 Right ventricular cardiomyopathy and Uhl's anomaly

	Arrhythmogenic right ventricular cardiomyopathy	Uhl's anomaly 'Parchment heart'
Morphology	Patchy, localized fibro-fatty replacement of parietal myocardium mostly affecting outflow tract. Other parts of right and occasionally left ventricle may be involved	Congenital absence of parietal ventricular myocardium with direct apposition of endocardium and epicardium. Normal interventricular septum and left ventricle
Sex ratio	2:1 male:female	Equal
Typical presentation	As young adult Exercise-induced ventricular tachycardia: palpitation, syncope, sudden death	In infancy Congestive cardiac failure

thought to occur due to a failure of the common pulmonary venous chamber to incorporate into the body of the left atrium early in fetal life. As a result, a persistent membrane inserts into the atrial septum at the fossa ovalis and into the posterolateral wall just above the mouth of the left atrial appendage. An ASD coexists in about 50% of cases, allowing communication between the right and left atria. The membrane may be intact, or pierced by one or more holes that are usually restrictive, causing supramitral stenosis.

If the membrane obstructs pulmonary venous inflow, presentation is early in life, and adult survivors will have undergone surgical resection. First presentation in adulthood is unusual unless the membrane is nonrestrictive or coexists with a large ASD. Patients may have signs of an ASD or mitral stenosis. New symptoms in adulthood may be due to fibrosis or calcification of the membrane so that it becomes restrictive, or from progressive mitral regurgitation.

The diagnosis is made by echocardiography. The chest radiograph may also be characteristic, showing signs of pulmonary venous congestion, but not the left atrial appendage enlargement that accompanies valvar mitral stenosis, since the appendage lies in the low pressure atrial chamber. The lateral chest radiograph may show enlargement of the pulmonary venous compartment of the left atrium.

Treatment is unnecessary if the membrane is unobstructive and there are no significant associated lesions. The results of surgical resection of obstructive membranes and the postoperative prognosis are good.

Congenital mitral valve anomalies

These are rare and frequently coexist with other lesions. A supramitral ring often coexists with congenital mitral stenosis. It differs from cor triatriatum in that the ring is sited inferiorly to the os of the appendage and lies immediately above the mitral valve.

Shone's syndrome consists of four levels of left heart obstruction: supramitral ring, parachute mitral valve, subaortic stenosis, and coarctation of the aorta. Parachute mitral valve occurs when the two papillary muscles are fused or there is hypoplasia or absence of one papillary muscle; the valve and its apparatus are often additionally dysplastic. Obstruction occurs at the level of the abnormal papillary muscles. The parachute mitral valve may also be regurgitant if the chordae are elongated and not significantly fused.

Isolated cleft mitral valve differs from the 'cleft' seen in an AVSD in being in the anterior (aortic) leaflet, directed towards the aortic outflow tract, rather than being in the space between the bridging leaflets and pointing towards the septum. The isolated cleft can be readily repaired to resemble a competent normal mitral valve.

Left ventricular outflow tract obstruction
Bicuspid aortic valve

This is the commonest congenital cardiac anomaly, occurring in 1 to 2% of the population. Bicuspid aortic valve is four times more common in males than females. In 20% of cases it is associated with other lesions such as patent arterial duct and coarctation. There is also an association with aortic root dilatation and dissection. Symptoms occur late in young people with aortic valve disease, hence regular follow-up is particularly important. Exercise testing is useful in planning the timing of surgery in those with asymptomatic aortic stenosis and left ventricular hypertrophy: ST segment changes and a failure of blood pressure to rise appropriately in response to stress indicate that intervention should be considered. Aortic stenosis and regurgitation are discussed in Chapter 16.6.

Supravalvar aortic stenosis

In this least common form of left ventricular outflow tract obstruction there is a localized narrowing of the aorta immediately above the aortic sinuses. Fibromuscular thickening of the aortic wall at the site of obstruction may encroach into the coronary ostia or onto the aortic valve leaflets and adversely influence prognosis. Unlike other forms of left ventricular outflow obstruction, the coronary arteries lie proximal to the obstruction and so are exposed to high left ventricular pressures, resulting in premature atherosclerosis. The condition may be associated with Williams' syndrome when the prognosis may be worse since there is diffuse arterial involvement that may also involve the pulmonary and renal arteries (see Chapter 16.11).

Subaortic stenosis

Subaortic stenosis may be due to a discrete fibromuscular ridge or ring, or a long muscular tunnel. It may exist in isolation or as part of another lesion such as AVSD, where the aorta is 'unwedged'; the left ventricular outflow tract elongated, and abnormal insertion of the left AV valve may all cause obstruction. Whether discrete or tunnel-like, subaortic stenosis tends to progress and may recur following surgical resection. It may result in functional disruption of the aortic valve and secondary aortic regurgitation, which can progress even after resection of subaortic stenosis.

Atrial septal defects

Interatrial communications are common both in congenital heart disease and in the general population. The different types of ASD are illustrated in Fig. 16.12.3. ASDs account for around 10% of congenital heart disease.

Patent foramen ovale

Patent foramen ovale (PFO) is a normal variant that occurs in 20 to 30% of the population. There is no deficiency of atrial septal tissue, but after birth—when left atrial (LA) pressure exceeds right atrial (RA) pressure and closes the PFO—the valve of the foramen ovale fails to fuse with the septum.

Interest has risen in PFO in recent years because of its potential to be a route for paradoxical embolism or for thrombosis *in situ*, especially if associated with an aneurysmal interatrial septum. PFO is associated with cryptogenic embolic stroke in young adults, with neurological decompression sickness in divers, and with migraine

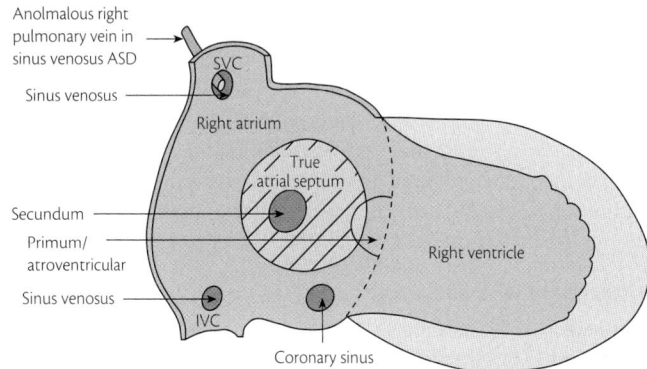

Fig. 16.12.3 Sites of atrial septal defects. The shaded area delineates the true atrial septum. Sinus venosus and coronary sinus defects are therefore not strictly atrial septal defects although they permit shunting at atrial level.

with aura. Device closure of a PFO appears to protect against recurrent stroke and decompression sickness. Whether closure of PFO will be beneficial for some sufferers of migraine is the subject of current research.

Careful consideration should be given to all risk factors in assessing a patient with an embolic stroke and a PFO for suitability for device closure of the PFO. If there are multiple risk factors for arterial disease, such as advanced age, smoking history, diabetes, hyperlipidaemia, hypertension, or proven existing atherosclerotic disease, then device closure of a PFO is unlikely to reduce the risk of a further embolic event. The same is true for patients with risk factors for left-sided intracardiac thrombosis, such as atrial fibrillation, mitral valve disease with a dilated left atrium, or left ventricular aneurysm. In contrast, patients with a PFO and previous embolic stroke who have risk factors for venous thrombosis, such as a thrombophilia or previous venous thomboembolism, may well be protected against further events by device closure.

Ostium secundum atrial septal defect

Secundum ASD accounts for 40% of left-to-right shunts in adults aged over 40 years. It is commoner in females, with a sex ratio of 2:1, and may be familial. It may occur as an isolated abnormality with autosomal dominant inheritance, be associated with Holt–Oram syndrome (autosomal dominant skeletal abnormalities and AV conduction defects due to *TBX5* mutation), and is a common association with Down's syndrome.

ASD may be an incidental finding in an elderly patient at autopsy, and diagnosis in life may be delayed well into adulthood because of the absence of symptoms and subtlety of clinical signs. However, the natural history of this lesion is not benign: historically only 50% with unoperated nonrestrictive (large) ASD survived to the age of 40 years, and 10% beyond 60 years of age.

Presentation in adulthood may be with symptoms of exertional dyspnoea or palpitation, or as a result of incidental clinical or radiographic findings. However, 20% may have developed atrial fibrillation by 40 years, with the figure rising to around 60% by the age of 60 years. Similarly, the volume-loaded right ventricle is well tolerated for many years, but may ultimately fail, usually after the fifth decade.

Contributing factors to progression of symptoms with age may be increased left-to-right shunting due to an age-related reduction in left ventricular compliance causing an increase in left ventricular end diastolic pressure and therefore left atrial pressure, and development of mitral regurgitation causing an increase in left atrial pressure. In addition, modest pulmonary arterial hypertension increases with age so the right ventricle is exposed to pressure as well as volume overload, precipitating right ventricular failure.

A left-to-right shunt at atrial level predisposes to paradoxical embolus since simple manoeuvres such as the Valsalva are sufficient to increase right atrial pressure and reverse the shunt. Patients with unoperated ASD are therefore at risk of embolic stroke, and should not dive because of the risk of paradoxical gas embolism.

Interactions with coexisting heart disease

Acquired disease may coexist and interact with congenital heart disease, especially in the ageing patient. Left ventricular dysfunction due to coronary artery disease and systemic hypertension may increase the left-to-right interatrial shunt, resulting in a more rapid clinical deterioration. Similarly, mitral regurgitation increases the effective interatrial shunt and mitral valve abnormalities may be acquired secondary to the effects of a secundum ASD. There may be distortion of the anterior mitral valve leaflet with fibrotic shortened chordae due to the abnormal position of the interventricular septum as a result of chronic right ventricular overload. Lutembacher's syndrome is the association of mitral stenosis with secundum ASD.

Mitral valve disease is underestimated in the presence of an ASD because the LA is able to decompress through the ASD. If significant mitral stenosis or regurgitation is overlooked at the time of ASD repair, left atrial pressure will rise and the patient may decompensate dramatically. It is therefore vital to ensure thorough assessment of the mitral valve in any patient in whom ASD closure is planned. Since LV dysfunction may also be masked by an ASD, the defect serving to allow the LV to offload, ventricular function must also be assessed carefully prior to ASD closure, particularly in elderly patients.

Coexisting pulmonary stenosis may be overestimated in the presence of an ASD, since Doppler velocities are increased in the presence of a left-to-right shunt.

Pulmonary vascular disease and atrial septal defect

Mild pulmonary hypertension with ASD is a common finding with advancing age, but pulmonary vascular resistance is rarely >6 Wood units and advanced pulmonary hypertension is rare. Few ASDs develop a right-to-left shunt secondary to pulmonary vascular disease, and a causal relationship between ASD and the Eisenmenger reaction remains controversial. In ASD, unlike other lesions which may cause the Eisenmenger reaction such as large VSD, the pulmonary vasculature is not exposed to increased flow at systemic pressure.

ASD with a right-to-left shunt due to pulmonary vascular disease and pulmonary hypertension occurs most commonly in young women, and in some cases may be due to idiopathic pulmonary arterial hypertension with an incidental ASD. In this combination, the prognosis may be better than for idiopathic pulmonary arterial hypertension with intact atrial septum, the septal defect protecting the right heart from pressure overload by allowing right-to-left shunting. Persistence of the fetal pulmonary vascular pattern may be implicated in the development of pulmonary hypertension in some young patients with ASD. Patients living or born at high altitude have a higher incidence of pulmonary vascular disease.

Clinical signs

If the defect is nonrestrictive the a and v waves of the jugular venous pulse tend to be equal. In older patients with reduced left ventricular compliance, the left and therefore right atrial pressure is raised, reflected by an elevated jugular venous pressure. A right ventricular heave may be felt at the left sternal border, and the dilated pulmonary artery may be palpable in the left second intercostal space. The first sound is loud because of increased diastolic flow across the tricuspid valve. If the left-to-right shunt is greater than approximately 2:1, the second heart sound is widely split and fixed, and there is loss of normal sinus arrhythmia. There may be a pulmonary flow murmur at the upper left sternal edge. Only if the ASD has a high gradient across it will it generate a murmur itself, usually a soft continuous murmur. This is the case if the defect is small and restrictive and the left atrial pressure high, e.g. if there is associated mitral stenosis. If the patient has pulmonary vascular disease, the signs will be the same as for pulmonary hypertension with right-to-left shunt (see above).

Investigations

The ECG may show sinus node dysfunction, prolongation of the PR interval, right axis deviation, and QRS prolongation with rSr′ in lead V1—which does not represent incomplete right bundle branch block, but occurs since the last part of the myocardium to depolarize is the right ventricular outflow tract that is enlarged and thickened due to volume overload. Postoperatively the ECG may show sinus node dysfunction due to damage when the superior vena cava (SVC) is cannulated, and the PR interval returning to normal as right atrial size decreases. Macro re-entry circuits at the site of atrial surgery may result in postoperative ectopic atrial tachycardias.

The typical chest radiograph shows dilated proximal pulmonary arteries with a small aortic knuckle, plethoric lung fields, and cardiomegaly secondary to dilatation of the right atrium and ventricle.

Transthoracic echocardiography demonstrates the volume-overloaded right atrium and ventricle. The size of the shunt can be estimated and colour flow Doppler facilitates the detection of the site of the shunt. If transcatheter device closure is considered, a transoesophageal approach is necessary to define the site and size of the ASD precisely and to identify the pulmonary veins.

Cardiac catheterization is indicated only to calculate pulmonary vascular resistance if there is a suspicion of pulmonary hypertension, or to exclude coexisting congenital or acquired cardiac pathology such as coronary artery disease.

Indications for closure of atrial septal defect

Closure of an ASD is indicated if there is right heart volume overload, left-to-right shunt is 1.5:1 or more, and the ASD is at least 10 mm in diameter. Prevention of recurrent paradoxical embolism is an additional indication for closure. Contraindications to closure are significant pulmonary hypertension (which may be suggested by a right-to-left shunt on exercise or at rest) and severe left ventricular dysfunction. In addition, merely closing the ASD in the presence of significant mitral valve disease is contraindicated.

Irrespective of age, the benefits of device closure should be improved functional class, exercise capacity, and breathlessness. Repair of a large isolated secundum ASD by the third decade results in a normal life expectancy. Between the ages of 25 and 41 years it results in a good but shorter than normal life expectancy, but beyond the age of 41 years morbidity and mortality remain significantly higher than normal. Nonetheless, functional status and longevity are improved following repair over the age of 40 years, 5- and 10-year survival being estimated as 98% and 95% respectively for patients who underwent repair, and 93% and 84% for those treated medically. Repair in older patients does not reduce the risk of late atrial arrhythmia, particularly if there is right ventricular dysfunction, elevated pulmonary artery pressure or pre-existing atrial arrhythmia. Whether the incorporation of a modified maze procedure or cryoablation into the surgical repair of ASD will reduce the long-term incidence of existing or *de novo* atrial arrhythmia remains to be determined.

Secundum ASDs up to 4 cm stretched diameter may be closed by transcatheter devices so long as the surrounding rim of atrial septal tissue is sufficient. Criteria for device closure of secundum ASD are size less than 4 cm; a situation away from the AV valves, pulmonary, and caval veins; and normal pulmonary venous drainage. The risk of major complication during device closure is 1 to 2%.

Following closure, antiplatelet or anticoagulant therapy is recommended for 3 to 6 months. Surgical repair carries also carries a low mortality and morbidity, but perioperative atrial fibrillation is common and recovery time is longer.

Other forms of atrial septal defect

Sinus venosus atrial septal defect

Sinus venosus defects account for 2 to 3% of ASDs and have an equal sex incidence. They are not truly defects of the atrial septum, but since they allow shunting at atrial level, they are included in the classification of ASDs. The inferior border of the more common SVC type of sinus venosus defect is made by the superior limbus of the fossa ovalis, and the upper border comprises the junction of the SVC with the atrial mass. The superior caval vein overrides the atrial septum, connecting to both atria, and the right upper pulmonary vein drains anomalously into the SVC. There may be an ectopic atrial pacemaker because the defect is located in the area of the sinoatrial node. This may be reflected by a leftwards p wave axis and an inverted p wave in lead III.

The sinus venosus defect may not be visualized with transthoracic echocardiography, and a transoesophageal approach is usually necessary to define the defect and is associated anomalous pulmonary venous drainage.

They are unsuitable for transcatheter device closure, both because there is no superior rim and because of anomalous drainage of one or more of the right pulmonary veins. The proximity of the sinus node to the SVC type of defect makes it vulnerable to damage during surgical repair; postoperative atrial pacing may be required.

Coronary sinus defect

The rarest form of ASD, this defect is at the site of entry of the coronary sinus to the right atrium. The unroofed coronary sinus is a variation of coronary sinus defect in which the partition between the coronary sinus and the left atrium is absent as the coronary sinus runs posteriorly along the floor of the left atrium. In this condition, a left SVC commonly connects directly to the left atrium, producing a right-to-left shunt and cyanosis.

Ostium primum atrial septal defect

This is a defect in the true atrial septum that exists as part of an AV septal defect and is discussed below.

Ventricular septal defects

With the exceptions of bicuspid aortic valve and mitral valve prolapse, ventricular septal defect (VSD) is the commonest congenital cardiac malformation, occurring in around 3 per 1000 live births. It occurs equally in both sexes. Defects may exist in isolation, in association with other lesions such as coarctation of the aorta, or as an integral part of lesions such as tetralogy of Fallot. This section deals with isolated VSDs.

Morphology and classification

An understanding of the basic anatomy of the ventricular septum is necessary to appreciate the various types of VSD. A VSD arises when there is failure of one of the components of the ventricular septum to develop correctly. The septum comprises four parts and is described as viewed from the right ventricle (Fig. 16.12. 4):

- Inlet septum—separates the mitral and tricuspid valves

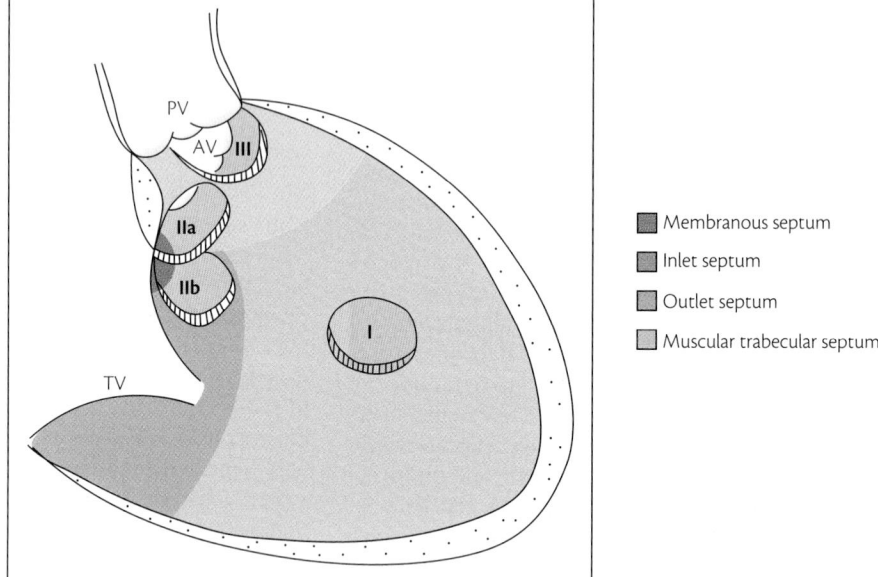

Fig. 16.12.4 Schematic representation to show the sites of different types of VSDs. The heart is in cross-section, viewed from the right ventricular aspect. I, muscular VSD; IIa, perimembranous outlet VSD; IIb perimembranous inlet VSD; III doubly committed subarterial VSD. AV Aortic valve, seen through VSD; PV Pulmonary valve; TV Tricuspid valve.

- ◆ Muscular trabeculated septum—extends from the tricuspid valve leaflet attachments to the muscle separating the tricuspid and pulmonary valves (the crista supraventricularis)
- ◆ Outlet septum—extends from the crista to the pulmonary valve
- ◆ Perimembranous septum—small fibrous area bordered by the aortic and tricuspid valves

VSDs are classified by their location within the septum and by their borders, again viewed from the right ventricle. There are three types: muscular, perimembranous and doubly committed subarterial (Figs. 16.12.4 and 16.12.5). The position of muscular and perimembranous VSDs may be inlet, trabecular or outlet, depending on which part of the right ventricle they open into. Perimembranous VSD is the commonest type of defect; only 5 to 7% of VSDs in Europe and North America are doubly committed subarterial defects, whereas they account for up to 30% of defects in Asian patients.

Clinical presentation and complications of unoperated VSD

The presentation of an isolated VSD depends on its size and haemodynamic effects (Table 16.12.6). Perimembranous and doubly committed subarterial VSDs may be associated with the development of aortic valve leaflet prolapse and aortic regurgitation, and the conduction tissue in these types of defects is vulnerable to damage at operation.

Adults with isolated unoperated restrictive VSDs are usually asymptomatic and acyanotic, with normal arterial and jugular venous pulses. There may be a thrill at the left sternal border, the left ventricular apex may be thrusting if the defect is large enough to cause volume overload, and a dilated pulmonary artery may be palpable. The second heart sound is usually normally split. There is a loud harsh pansystolic murmur at the left sternal edge, which is softer and shorter (early systolic) in very small defects.

Late complications of unoperated small VSDs include significant risk of endocarditis due to the high-velocity jet from left to right ventricle, particularly if the jet is directed onto tricuspid valve tissue; aortic regurgitation if the aortic valve forms part of the border of the VSD; atrial arrhythmia if there is left heart volume overload; and small increased risk of sudden death and ventricular arrhythmia.

Larger VSDs rarely present for repair in adulthood since the large left-to-right shunt is unlikely to allow unoperated survival unless pulmonary vascular disease has developed. Nonrestrictive defects are not associated with the classical VSD murmur since left and right ventricular pressures are equal.

Investigations

Investigation should determine the type and number of VSDs, the size of the defect (restrictive or nonrestrictive), an estimation of the size of the shunt (Qp:Qs), pulmonary artery pressure and resistance, and assessment of left and right ventricular function and volume and pressure overload. Associated lesions that may alter management should be identified, especially aortic regurgitation, subaortic stenosis, and right ventricular outflow tract obstruction.

The chest radiograph is normal if the defect has been small from birth. If the VSD is (or has been) larger, the left ventricle, left atrium, and pulmonary trunk may be dilated and there may be increased

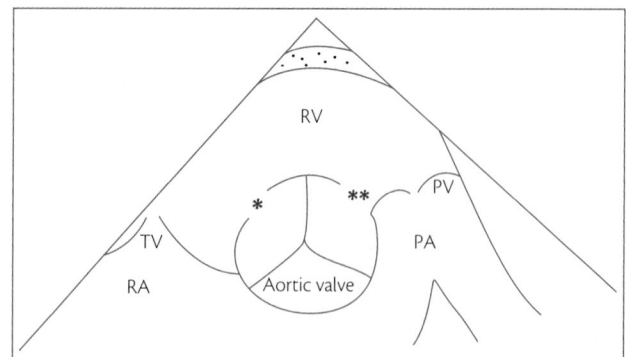

Fig. 16.12.5 Schematic representation of the transthoracic echocardiographic parasternal short axis view, to demonstrate sites of VSDs. **, site of doubly committed subarterial VSD—the aortic and pulmonary valves are in continuity and form the roof of the VSD. *, site of subaortic perimembranous VSD. PA, pulmonary artery; PV, pulmonary valve; RA, right atrium; RV, right ventricle; TV, tricuspid valve; VSD, ventricular septal defect.

Table 16.12.6 Grading of ventricular septal defects by size

	Small	Moderate	Large	Eisenmenger syndrome
Pulmonary artery pressure: systemic pressure ratio	<0.3	0.3–0.6	RV=LV pressure	RV≥LV pressure
Qp:Qs	<1.4: 1	1.4–2.2: 1	>2.2:1	<1.5: 1
Clinical grading	Negligible haemodynamic changes, normal LV	LA and LV enlargement and reversible pulmonary hypertension	Pulmonary vascular disease (Eisenmenger syndrome) will develop unless there is RVOTO	
	Restrictive (RV pressure < LV pressure in absence of RVOTO)		Non-restrictive (equal RV and LV pressures in absence of RVOTO)	

Qp, pulmonary blood flow; Qs, systemic blood flow; RVOTO, right ventricular outflow tract obstruction.

pulmonary vascularity. The ECG shows a normal QRS axis unless there are multiple defects, when there may be left axis deviation. In the presence of a large left-to-right shunt the p wave may be broad and there may be evidence of left ventricular hypertrophy. Two-dimensional echocardiography identifies the number and site of defects as well as describing the morphology and associated defects. Doppler is used to estimate the size and direction of the shunt, and right ventricle to left ventricle pressure difference, but this may not be accurate if there is an obliquely lying muscular VSD. Cardiac catheterization is important to measure the size of shunt and pulmonary vascular resistance, with reversibility studies if baseline resistance is high.

Indications for repair and postoperative sequelae

Repair of a VSD is indicated in the presence of symptoms, if Qp:Qs is greater than 2:1, or if there is ventricular dysfunction with right ventricular pressure overload or left ventricular volume overload. Repair should also be undertaken if there are coexisting lesions such as significant right ventricular outflow tract obstruction, or more than mild aortic regurgitation or aortic valve prolapse in the presence of an outlet VSD. An episode of endocarditis may also be considered as an indication for VSD closure. If the pulmonary artery pressure is more than two-thirds systemic pressure, repair should only be considered if Qp:Qs exceeds 1.5:1 or if there is evidence of reversibility in response to pulmonary vasodilators such as oxygen and nitric oxide.

The surgical approach aims at avoiding damage to important structures such as the conducting tissues, which are especially vulnerable in perimembranous defects. Transatrial repair reduces the risk of postoperative ventricular arrhythmias by avoiding a right ventriculotomy. Transient postoperative complete heart block is associated with an increased risk of late high degree block, and permanent pacemaker implantation is indicated in the 1 to 2% of patients in whom complete heart block persists, even if they are asymptomatic, because there is a significant risk of late sudden death.

The prognosis after VSD repair in the early years of life is good, but if repair is delayed into late childhood left ventricular dilatation may persist and systolic function be impaired. Long-term postoperative survival depends on the presence of pulmonary hypertension, left ventricular dysfunction, and complications such as aortic regurgitation and endocarditis.

Transcatheter device closure of VSDs is possible providing that valvar apparatus can be avoided. Both muscular and selected perimembranous VSDs may be device closed, the latter requiring experienced hands to avoid damage to the aortic valve and heart block.

This approach is particularly useful for defects that are difficult to access or close surgically, and a hybrid surgical/interventional technique may be used.

Atrioventricular septal defect

The key feature of an atrioventricular septal defect (AVSD) (previously termed endocardial cushion defect or AV canal) is a common atrioventricular (AV) junction and AV valve ring (Fig. 16.12.6). The AV septum is absent and the AV valves share a common junction and fibrous ring, with a five-leaflet AV valve. Since they share common leaflets, the valves are not correctly called mitral and tricuspid valves, but left and right AV valves. As a consequence the normal offsetting of the right AV valve towards the right ventricular apex is absent. In addition, the aorta is 'unwedged' from its normal position between the left and right AV valves. The left ventricular outflow tract is therefore elongated ('gooseneck') and has the propensity to develop obstruction. 'Cleft mitral valve' refers to the commissure between the anterior and posterior bridging leaflets that renders the left AV valve potentially regurgitant. The left ventricular papillary muscles are abnormally placed anteriorly and posteriorly instead of in the normal anterolateral and posteromedial positions. Ostium primum defect describes the atrial component of an AVSD.

There are two types of AVSD, partial and complete. Both have a common AV junction, but in a partial AVSD the right and left AV valves have separate orifices and the VSD is usually small or absent, and in a complete AVSD there is a common AV valve and valve orifice, and the VSD is usually large.

AVSD occurs with equal sex incidence. The complete form of the defect is most commonly associated with Down's syndrome. A single gene defect may be responsible for AVSD with normal chromosomes, when the recurrence risk is about 10% if the mother has an AVSD, less if the father is affected.

The physiological consequences of an AVSD are the same as for other conditions with left-to-right shunting at atrial or ventricular level, but may be complicated by left AV valve regurgitation or left ventricular outflow tract obstruction. Pulmonary vascular disease may develop if the VSD is large and nonrestrictive. Patients with Down's syndrome are at particular risk of this complication, and coexisting upper airway obstruction and sleep apnoea, and abnormal pulmonary parenchyma may be contributory factors.

Investigations

The ECG is distinctive, with a left and superior QRS axis and notching of S waves in the inferior leads. The chest radiograph

☐ Superior bridging leaflet

☐ Inferior bridging leaflet

☐ Left mural leaflet

☐ Right inferior leaflet

☐ Right anterosuperior leaflet

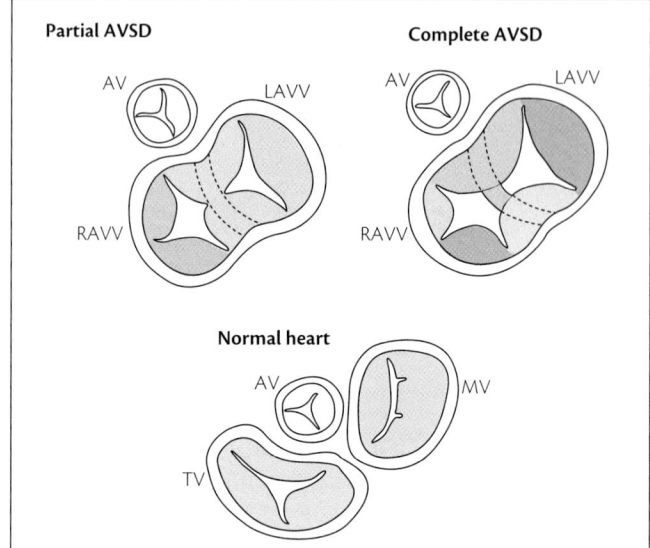

Fig. 16.12.6 Schematic representation of the atrioventricular junction in AVSD. Short axis view, seen from the atrial aspect. In both forms of AVSD, there is a common atrioventricular valve ring guarded by five valve leaflets. In the partial defect, the superior and inferior bridging leaflets fuse to create two separate valve orifices. This fusion does not occur in complete AVSD, so there is a common valve orifice. AV, aortic valve; LAVV, left atrioventricular valve; RAVV, right atrioventricular valve.

appearances depend on the degree of interatrial shunting and left AV valve regurgitation, the former producing cardiomegaly due to left heart dilatation and the latter left atrial enlargement. There may be increased pulmonary vascularity, particularly in young patients with complete AVSD and high pulmonary blood flow.

Transthoracic echocardiography reveals the detailed anatomy of the defect and establishes the site and degree of shunting, the presence and nature of left ventricular outflow tract obstruction, and the function and anatomy of the AV valves.

The indications for cardiac catheterization are the same as for secundum ASD, namely to exclude inoperable pulmonary vascular disease. In addition useful information may be obtained regarding the severity of left AV valve regurgitation and left ventricular outflow tract obstruction.

Clinical course

First presentation may occur in adulthood if the left-to-right shunt is small and the left AV valve is competent. Physical signs are the same as in other ASDs, and there may also be an apical pansystolic murmur. Paradoxical embolism is less common than in secundum ASD because the position of the primum defect low in the interatrial septum avoids the streaming of blood from the inferior vena cava that is most likely to carry emboli and is directed towards the midportion of the septum.

Most adult patients have undergone surgery to repair the defect and left AV valve: others have survived unoperated and may have developed pulmonary vascular disease.

Late complications after repair of AVSD include recurrent AV valve regurgitation, the severity of which may increase with age in response to changes in the left ventricle due to ageing, ischaemia, or systemic hypertension; residual ASD or VSD; residual or recurrent left ventricular outflow tract obstruction, which may be difficult to relieve surgically if it involves left AV valve tissue; complete heart block, related to the abnormally positioned AV node that is particularly vulnerable to intraoperative damage; atrial arrhythmia—it is vital to read the original operation note when planning ablation, since the mouth of the coronary sinus is often left opening into the left atrium making it inaccessible to the electrophysiologist; and endocarditis—relating largely to the left AV valve.

Arterial disorders

Coarctation of the aorta

Aortic coarctation is a narrowing of the aorta, usually sited near the ligamentum arteriosum. It is one of the commonest congenital cardiac lesions, occurring in 1 in 12 000 live births, with a male to female ratio of 3:1. There is considerable variation in anatomy and severity, ranging from a mild obstruction to interruption of the aorta, and from a discrete fibromuscular shelf to hypoplasia of the arch. Coarctation is most strongly associated with bicuspid aortic valve, which coexists in up to 80% of cases. Other associations are VSD, patent ductus arteriosus, subaortic ridge, and mitral valve abnormalities. It is a frequent finding in Turner's syndrome and is also associated with congenital aneurysm of the circle of Willis.

Presentation

Most patients present in infancy, but some survive into adulthood before being diagnosed at routine examination or during investigation for hypertension, leg claudication, angina, heart failure, or cerebral haemorrhage. More than 75% with unoperated coarctation die by age 50 years, from premature coronary disease, stroke, or aortic dissection.

Clinical findings include upper body hypertension: the leg blood pressure is lower, as is that in the left arm if the subclavian artery is involved in the coarctation. If there is a good collateral supply, femoral arteries may be easily palpable, but they are usually reduced, with radiofemoral delay. Intercostal collaterals may be both visible and palpable over the patient's back. There is an ejection systolic murmur from the site of coarctation, and systolic collateral murmurs may be heard. Fundoscopy shows a typical corkscrew appearance of the retinal vessels and there may be evidence of hypertensive retinopathy.

Investigations

There may be electrocardiographic evidence of left ventricular hypertrophy. The chest radiograph (Fig. 16.12.7) has a typical appearance.

Transthoracic echocardiography may show left ventricular hypertrophy, with the coarctation site visualized on two-dimensional

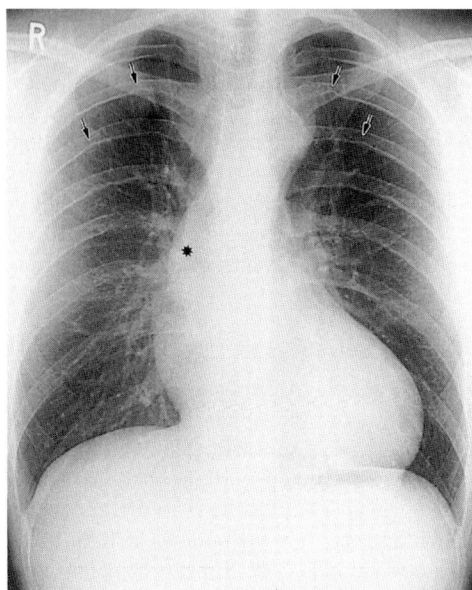

Fig. 16.12.7 Chest radiograph of an 18-year-old man with unoperated coarctation of the aorta and bicuspid aortic valve. There is bilateral rib notching (arrows) and a prominent deformed aortic knuckle. The ascending aorta is dilated (*).

imaging and its severity assessed using Doppler mode from the suprasternal notch. A peak gradient of over 20 mmHg is significant, especially if accompanied by a diastolic tail.

MRI provides definitive non-invasive haemodynamic data and two- and three-dimensional images of the coarctation site, collaterals and related vessels (Fig. 16.12.8). It may obviate the need for angiography unless coronary disease is suspected. In the adult, diagnostic angiography is usually reserved for assessing coronary disease.

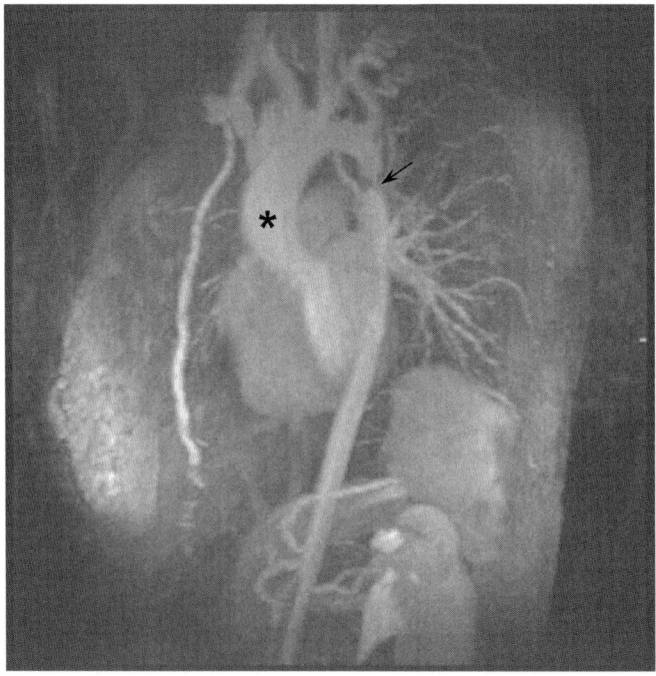

Fig. 16.12.8 MRI of a 20-year-old woman who presented with hypertension. There is a severe discrete coarctation (↓), multiple tortuous collaterals and a dilated ascending aorta (*) associated with a bicuspid aortic valve.

Repair of native coarctation

Surgical repair is the conventional approach in neonates and children, with a risk of less than 1% for those with simple coarctation. Extensive collateral vessels and nonelastic diseased aortic tissue make surgical repair of adult coarctation challenging, and this is associated with significant morbidity. The incidence of perioperative spinal cord ischaemia and paraplegia is up to 0.4%, those patients without an abundant collateral circulation probably being most at risk. Those with well-developed collaterals are at risk of significant intraoperative haemorrhage. Early postoperative hypertension is common and may be difficult to control, and postoperative intestinal ileus may persist for several days.

Transcatheter balloon dilatation and primary stenting of native coarctation in adults are alternatives to surgery. The use of primary stents, particularly covered stents, is likely to support the aorta following dilatation and to reduce the risk of aortic dissection or late aneurysm formation. However, this interventional approach is controversial and should only be performed in specialist centres; careful follow-up is required.

Follow-up after coarctation repair

Follow-up after repair of coarctation should be lifelong, since late complications are frequent: residual or recoarctation, aneurysm formation, persistent hypertension despite adequate repair, premature atherosclerotic disease, and progression of associated lesions such as bicuspid aortic valve. Older age at repair is the main risk factor influencing longevity. Late survival is 92% for patients repaired in infancy, 25-year survival is 75% for those repaired between ages and 40 years, but 15-year survival is only 50% for those repaired at age more than 40 years.

Recoarctation may be diagnosed when the resting arm–leg systolic blood pressure gradient is 20 mmHg at rest and 50 mmHg after exercise. This occurs most commonly following neonatal repair by end-to-end anastomosis, and the diagnosis should be sought when there is new or persisting hypertension. Blood pressure should be recorded in the both arms of all such patients; spuriously low readings may be obtained if one of the subclavian arteries (usually the left) is involved in the repair or recoarctation.

MRI is the investigation of choice for both recoarctation and aneurysm formation after coarctation repair. Multislice CT is used following stent repair of coarctation (Fig. 16.12.9), since the artefact produced by the stent renders MRI unhelpful. Balloon angioplasty with or without stent insertion is used to relieve most recoarctations, but reoperation is required for some patients with complex anatomy.

The 14-year incidence of aneurysm formation at the site of repair is up to 27%; it occurs most commonly in adults and in those with Dacron patch repair. An aneurysm may rupture into the bronchial tree, hence any patient with a history of coarctation who presents with haemoptysis should undergo emergency noninvasive diagnostic imaging (MRI or CT) and surgical repair. Bronchoscopy and conventional angiography are contraindicated since they may cause further damage to the ruptured area.

Hypertension is a major risk factor for atherosclerotic disease and may persist despite an apparently good result from surgical repair. Continuing hypertension relates in part to older age at time of surgery. Nonetheless, even if repaired in adulthood, systolic hypertension becomes easier to control.

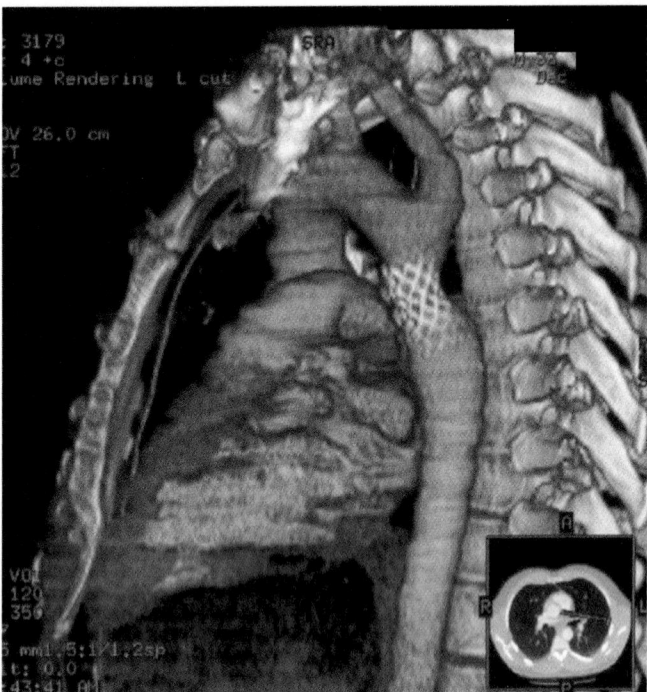

Fig. 16.12.9 Multislice CT scan demonstrating stent deployed at native coarctation site.

Patent arterial duct

The pathophysiological consequences of a patent arterial duct in adulthood depend on the size of the shunt. Small ducts are of no haemodynamic significance and are associated with a low risk of infective endarteritis. Moderate-sized ducts may cause left heart volume overload and late atrial fibrillation and ventricular dysfunction. A large nonrestrictive duct may cause pulmonary vascular disease (see 'Eisenmenger syndrome', above).

Duct closure is usually recommended if a duct is clinically detectable, i.e. there is a machinery murmur in the left subclavicular area, to avoid long-term haemodynamic complications. Ducts up to 14 mm in diameter are usually suitable for transcatheter device closure. Pulmonary vascular disease should be excluded before repair of large ducts is undertaken.

Aortopulmonary window

In this rare condition there is a direct communication between adjacent portions of the proximal ascending aorta and pulmonary artery. The communication is usually large and the physiological consequences are the same as for a patent arterial duct. Rare patients surviving unoperated into adulthood are likely to have developed the Eisenmenger reaction. If pulmonary vascular resistance is low at the time of childhood repair, long-term postoperative survival is good.

Truncus arteriosus/common arterial trunk

This condition accounts for 1 to 4% of all congenital heart disease. It may coexist with interrupted aortic arch, coarctation, coronary anomalies and DiGeorge syndrome. A single great artery arises from the heart and gives rise to the coronary arteries, aorta and pulmonary arteries. There is a single semilunar 'truncal' valve that has three or more leaflets, and a subtruncal VSD.

Most patients present in infancy with heart failure. If left unoperated, pulmonary vascular resistance rises, cyanosis becomes more marked, and the Eisenmenger reaction becomes established. Repair before pulmonary vascular disease develops involves closure of the VSD, detachment of the pulmonary arteries from the common arterial trunk, and placement of a valved right ventricular to pulmonary artery conduit. The truncal valve then functions as the aortic valve. Late complications following repair include truncal regurgitation, truncal (aortic root) dilation, ventricular dysfunction, and the need to replace stenotic conduits.

Sinus of Valsalva aneurysm

There is dilation of one of the aortic valve sinuses between the aortic valve annulus and sinotubular junction, and the aneurysm progressively dilates and ruptures. The right and noncoronary cusps are most often affected; rupture of the noncoronary sinus aneurysm is nearly always into the right atrium and of the right coronary sinus into the right ventricle or atrium. Involvement of the left coronary sinus is rare. Rupture usually occurs in early adulthood and may be precipitated by endocarditis. If sudden it is accompanied by tearing chest pain, breathlessness, and congestive cardiac failure with a loud continuous murmur. Small perforations may remain asymptomatic for many years. The diagnosis and site of the rupture is confirmed echocardiographically and/or angiographically before surgical or transcatheter repair.

Coronary artery anomalies

The importance of congenital coronary anomalies lies in their potential to impair myocardial blood flow and cause ischaemia and sudden death. Evidence of ischaemia is the main indication for repair.

Anomalous origin of the coronary arteries from an inappropriate aortic sinus

Ischaemia is particularly associated with an anomalous proximal coronary course between the aorta and pulmonary trunk, an intramural proximal segment of the coronary artery inside the aortic wall, and acute angulation between the origin of an anomalous coronary artery and the aortic wall.

Anomalous origin of the left coronary artery from the pulmonary artery

This rare condition usually presents in infancy with myocardial ischaemia and left ventricular failure when pulmonary vascular resistance decreases. However, 10 to 15% survive into adulthood because an adequate intercoronary collateral circulation is established. Adults may be asymptomatic or present with myocardial ischaemia or mitral regurgitation due to papillary muscle dysfunction. Survival following surgical repair depends on the amount of ischaemic myocardial damage and degree of mitral regurgitation.

Congenital coronary arteriovenous fistulae

The coronary arteries arise normally from their aortic sinuses, but a fistulous branch communicates directly with the right ventricle in 40% of cases, the right atrium in 25%, pulmonary artery in 15%, or rarely the SVC or pulmonary vein. Survival to adulthood is usual, but lifespan may be reduced, depending on the size of the fistulous connection and the presence of myocardial ischaemia resulting from any coronary steal phenomenon. Symptoms increase with age and there is a risk of endocarditis, heart failure, arrhythmia,

Box 16.12.4 Major types of coronary anomaly

- Anomalous origin from inappropriate aortic sinus or coronary vessel
  - LAD from right aortic sinus or RCA
  - Absent LMS (separate origins of LAD and Cx)
  - Cx from right aortic sinus or RCA or absent cx
  - RCA from left aortic sinus, posterior sinus or LAD
  - Single coronary artery from right or left aortic sinus
- Anomalous origin from other systemic artery (rare)
  - Innominate, subclavian, internal mammary, carotid, bronchial arteries, or descending aorta
- Anomalous origin from pulmonary artery
- Coronary arteriovenous fistulae

Cx, circumflex; LAD, left anterior descending; LMS, left main stem; RCA, right coronary artery.

myocardial ischaemia and infarction, and sudden death. Surgical repair is recommended unless there is a trivial isolated shunt. Some smaller fistulae are suitable for transcatheter device occlusion.

Systemic venous anomalies

These anomalies frequently form part a more complex lesion, particularly atrial isomerism. Normal systemic venous drainage is illustrated in Fig. 16.12.10.

Superior caval vein anomalies

A persistent left-sided SVC occurs in 0.3% of the general population, approximately 3% of patients with congenital heart disease, and 15% with tetralogy of Fallot. The left SVC may be visible on the chest radiograph. It usually drains to the right atrium via the coronary sinus, which is seen to be dilated on two-dimensional echocardiography (Fig. 16.12.11). A right-sided SVC is usually also present, but the two caval veins do not usually communicate via the brachiocephalic vein. This common anomaly should be sought routinely at cardiac catheterization; although it does not have any haemodynamic significance, it may cause technical difficulties during transvenous pacemaker insertion and cardiac surgery (Fig. 16.11.12).

Other SVC anomalies are rare. An absent right SVC is associated with arrhythmias including AV block, sinus node dysfunction, and atrial fibrillation. The left, or rarely the right, SVC may connect directly to the left atrium, causing an obligatory right-to-left shunt and cyanosis. This may be associated with isomerism of the atrial appendages.

Inferior caval vein anomalies

Azygos continuation of the inferior vena cava (IVC) occurs in 0.6% of patients with congenital heart disease. The infrahepatic portion of the IVC is absent and continues to the SVC via an azygos vein; the hepatic veins drain directly into the right atrium. This is often associated with complex lesions, particularly left atrial isomerism. The chest radiograph reveals an absence of the IVC at the junction of the diaphragm with the right heart border and a dilated azygos vein (Fig. 16.12.13). Direct connection of the IVC to the LA is rare: the patient is cyanosed, as in the SVC–LA connection.

Pulmonary venous anomalies

Total anomalous pulmonary venous drainage

Total anomalous pulmonary venous drainage occurs in 1 in 17 000 live births. All four pulmonary veins drain into the right atrium, either directly or via a common vein into a systemic vein. The anomalous veins may follow (1) a supracardiac course draining to the SVC, azygos, or brachiocephalic veins; (2) a cardiac course, draining to the right atrium directly or to the coronary sinus directly or via a persistent left SVC connection; or (3) an infradiaphragmatic course, draining to the portal vein or IVC.

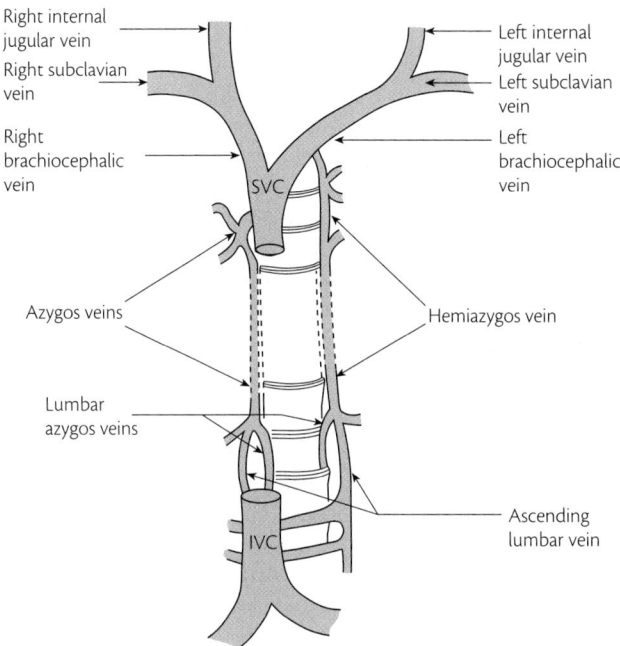

Fig. 16.12.10 Schematic diagram of normal systemic venous drainage.

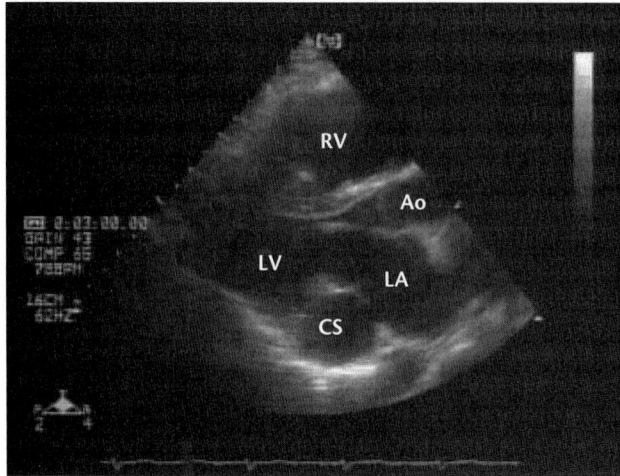

Fig. 16.12.11 Persistent left superior vena cava. Transthoracic two-dimensional echocardiogram, parasternal long axis view. The coronary sinus, receiving the persistent left superior vena cava, is dilated. Ao, aorta; CS, coronary sinus; LA, left atrium; LV, left ventricle; RV, right ventricle.

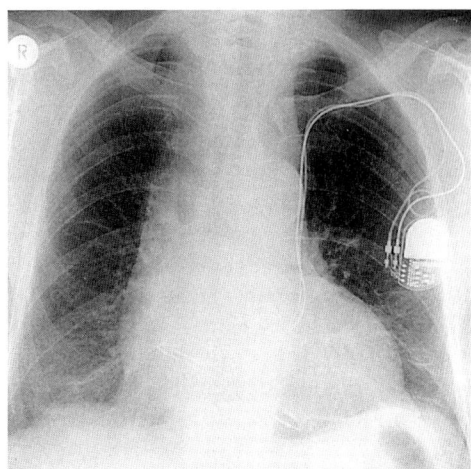

Fig. 16.12.12 Chest radiograph of a 56-year-old man with bicuspid aortic valve, aortic regurgitation, and coarctation. A left superior vena cava draining via the coronary sinus to the right atrium is marked by the path taken by the transvenous pacing leads, inserted for complete heart block.

The presence of pulmonary venous obstruction is the most important predictor of a poor outcome. Associated anomalies include an obligatory right-to-left shunt, nearly always at atrial level.

The condition presents in infancy, hence 98% of patients reaching the adolescent or adult clinic will have survived corrective surgery in early life. Unless there is residual pulmonary hypertension most such adults should be asymptomatic, have a normal cardiovascular examination, and an excellent prognosis. Patients who are still growing may develop obstruction of the redirected pulmonary venous pathway and present with dyspnoea, signs of pulmonary oedema, evidence of pulmonary venous congestion on the chest radiograph, and an obstructive echo Doppler flow signal at the site of the stenosis.

The rare patient who reaches adulthood unoperated is likely to have survived because of a large ASD and unobstructed pulmonary

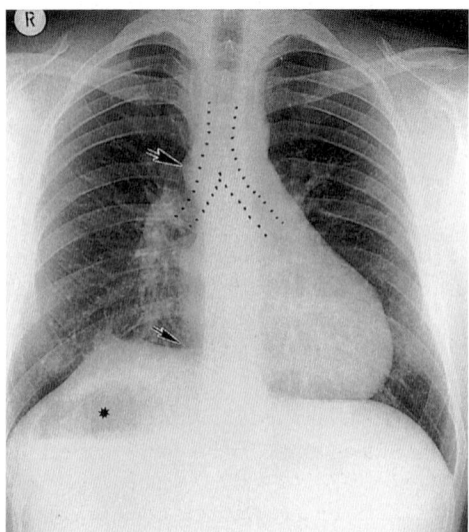

Fig. 16.12.13 Chest radiograph of a 50-year-old man with abdominal situs inversus (*) and laevocardia. Left atrial isomerism is inferred from the symmetrical long bronchi. The inferior vena cava is absent at the level of the diaphragm (small arrow), and the azygos vein receiving inferior caval venous blood is prominent (large arrow).

venous drainage. They will be cyanosed, have developed pulmonary vascular disease, and be at risk of atrial tachyarrhythmias and right heart failure. The chest radiograph has the appearance of a large ASD with a small aortic knuckle, cardiomegaly, and a dilated main pulmonary artery. In addition, the anomalous veins may cause an abnormal vascular shadow.

Partial anomalous pulmonary venous drainage

There is anomalous drainage of some of the pulmonary veins to the right atrium. In 90% of cases the anomalous pulmonary venous connection is between the right upper or middle pulmonary vein to the SVC or right atrium, usually in association with an ASD, 10 to 15% of all ASDs and 80 to 90% of SVC-type sinus venosus ASDs being associated with partial anomalous pulmonary venous connection.

Partial anomalous pulmonary venous drainage may present in adult life with signs of a left-to-right shunt at atrial level; the pathophysiological consequences are the same as for an ASD with an equivalent shunt.

The chest radiograph may reveal the abnormally draining pulmonary vein. Transthoracic echocardiography may be indicative of a shunt at atrial level, but in adults it may not be possible to image the pulmonary veins and a transoesophageal approach is likely to be necessary. The identification of all the pulmonary veins is crucial in assessing the suitability of a secundum ASD for transcatheter device closure, this technique being contraindicated in the presence of anomalous pulmonary veins (see 'Atrial septal defects', above).

The indications for surgical repair are the same as those for repair of an ASD. In the most common variant of right pulmonary venous connection to the SVC in association with a sinus venosus defect, the patch closing the ASD is placed to direct the anomalous vein into the left atrium.

Scimitar syndrome

Partial anomalous pulmonary venous drainage also occurs as part of the rare familial 'scimitar syndrome' in which part or all of the right pulmonary venous drainage is to the IVC below the diaphragm. The affected lung lobes are usually hypoplastic (Fig. 16.12.14) and are supplied with arterial blood from the descending aorta. Recurrent infection and bronchiectasis may develop in the hypoplastic lobes or lung. MRI demonstrates the abnormal arterial supply and venous drainage of the affected lung segment, and may obviate the need for diagnostic cardiac catheterization. Surgical repair may be complicated by difficulty in maintaining perfusion to the affected lung, and lobectomy may be required. In view of this it should be remembered that patients presenting with scimitar syndrome for the first time in adult life have a good unoperated prognosis, similar to that of a small ASD.

Transposition complexes

The nomenclature of the transposition complexes may cause confusion. There are two types:

• Complete transposition of the great arteries (TGA)—this condition is described as AV concordance, VA discordance (Fig. 16.12.15), previously known as D-TGA. Without intervention this is not compatible with life once the arterial duct and foramen ovale have closed, because there is complete separation of the

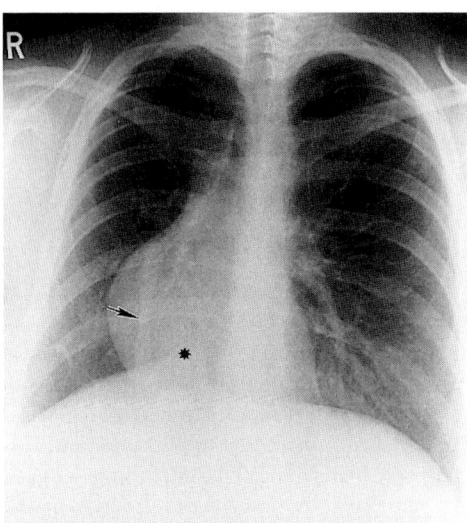

Fig. 16.12.14 Chest radiograph of a 25-year-old woman with scimitar syndrome. The heart is shifted into the right hemithorax because the right lung is small. The 'scimitar' shadow (arrow) is produced by the anomalous descending venous channel which drains into the dilated inferior vena cava(*).

systemic and pulmonary circulations such that deoxygenated blood from the systemic veins recirculates to the aorta, and oxygenated blood from the pulmonary veins recirculates to the pulmonary artery.

◆ Congenitally corrected TGA (cTGA)—this condition is described as AV and VA discordance (Fig. 16.12.16), previously known as L-TGA. cTGA is congenitally physiologically 'corrected': deoxygenated systemic venous blood reaches the pulmonary

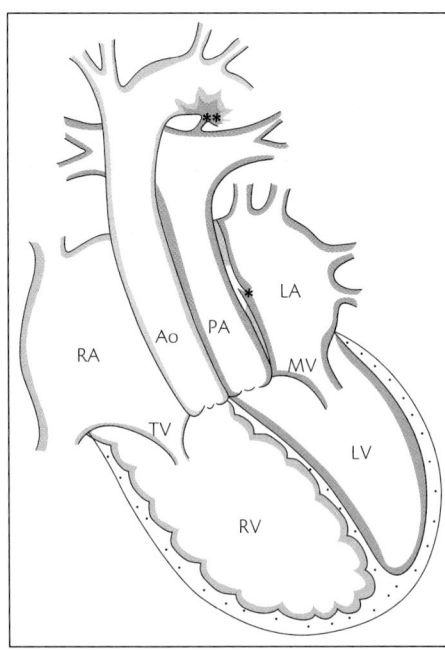

Fig. 16.12.15 Schematic representation of complete transposition of the great arteries (ventriculoarterial discordance). The pulmonary and systemic circulations are completely separate once the arterial duct and foramen ovale close. Without intervention, the condition is not compatible with life. Ao, aorta; LA, left atrium; LV, left ventricle; MV, mitral valve; PA, pulmonary artery; RA right atrium; RV right ventricle; TV tricuspid valve; *, patent arterial duct; **, patent foramen ovale.

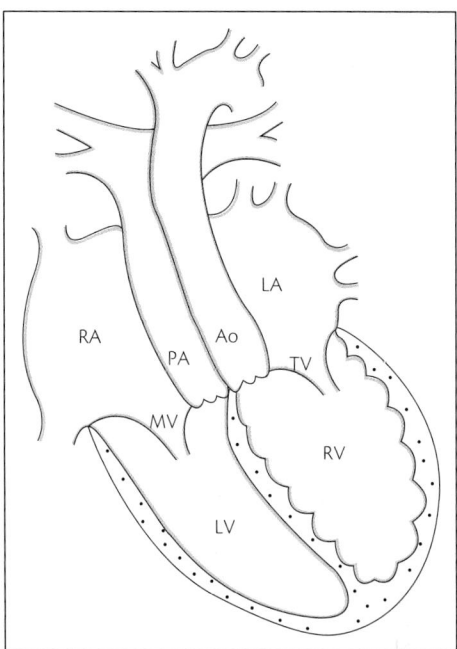

Fig. 16.12.16 Schematic representation of congenitally corrected transposition of the great arteries (atrioventricular and ventriculoarterial discordance). The circulation is congenitally physiologically 'corrected' in that systemic venous blood reaches the pulmonary artery (via the LV) and pulmonary venous blood reaches the aorta (via the RV). Ao, aorta; LA, left atrium; LV, left ventricle; MV, mitral valve; PA, pulmonary artery; RA, right atrium; RV, right ventricle; TV, tricuspid valve.

artery, albeit via the morphological left ventricle; oxygenated pulmonary venous blood reaches the aorta, but via the morphological right ventricle.

Complete transposition of the great arteries (TGA) (AV concordance, VA discordance)

This accounts for about 5% of congenital cardiac malformations and is four times more common in males than females. Associated anomalies such as VSD and pulmonary stenosis occur in approximately one-third of patients. As described above, unoperated survival after closure of the foramen ovale and arterial duct have closed is dependent upon the presence of other associated lesions, such as a VSD, which allow mixing of the two circulations. Without intervention, 30% die within the first week and only 10% survive their first year.

Immediate management in the neonatal period requires a prostaglandin infusion to maintain patency of the arterial duct until a balloon atrial septostomy is performed. The neonate remains cyanosed, but there is usually adequate mixing to allow it to thrive until definitive surgery. There are survivors of four operative approaches in adult clinics.

Interatrial repair: Mustard or Senning operations

This approach was first described in 1957 and can be used for those with TGA or TGA with VSD. Interatrial repair involves excision of the atrial septum and placement of a saddle-shaped patch ('baffle') to direct pulmonary venous blood into the right atrium and right ventricle and thence to the aorta (Fig. 16.12.17). Systemic venous blood is directed into the left atrium, left ventricle, and pulmonary artery. The right ventricle and tricuspid valve therefore support the systemic circulation.

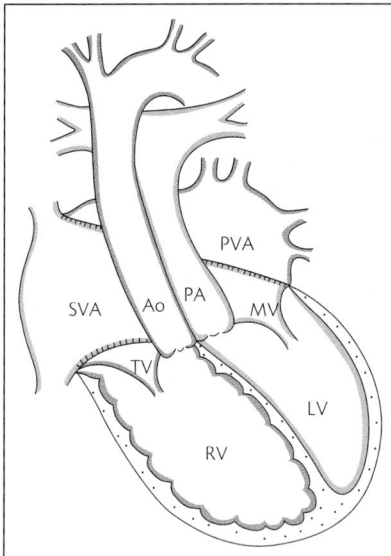

Fig. 16.12.17 Schematic representation of intra-atrial repair for complete TGA (Senning or Mustard operation). Ao, aorta; LV, left ventricle; MV, mitral valve; PA, pulmonary artery; PVA, pulmonary venous atrium; RV, right ventricle; SVA, systemic venous atrium; TV, tricuspid valve.

Clinical signs and complications after interatrial repair

The systemic right ventricle causes a parasternal heave. The aortic component of the second heart sound may be palpable and loud, and the second sound single, due to the anterior-lying aorta. The presence of cyanosis suggests a baffle leak allowing right-to-left shunting between the systemic and pulmonary venous atria. Systemic venous pathway obstruction may be associated with elevation of the jugular venous pressure and hepatomegaly.

Complications after interatrial repair include:

- Progressive bradycardias and sinus node disease, due to damage to the sinus node during repair

- Atrial flutter and interatrial re entry tachycardias, due to extensive atrial surgical scarring—these are often poorly tolerated, are associated with sudden death, and should be treated with urgent DC cardioversion rather than antiarrhythmic drugs, since the latter can precipitate cardiovascular collapse if there is underlying impaired ventricular function. After an episode of flutter, ablation should be performed.

- Systemic venous pathway obstruction, which usually only causes symptoms if both the IVC and SVC pathways are narrowed—if only one pathway is narrowed, the systemic venous blood flows along the azygos vein and drains to the heart via the unobstructed pathway; obstruction can usually be relieved by balloon dilation or stenting

- Pulmonary venous pathway obstruction such that flow into the atrium and systemic ventricle is obstructed—the patient will be breathless, but clinical signs are few; it is demonstrated by echocardiography or MRI; surgical repair is usually necessary; transcatheter intervention is usually unsatisfactory

- Baffle leak—holes along the baffle suture lines allow shunting which may be left to right, or right to left, causing cyanosis; an interventional approach sometimes allows successful closure of these interatrial communications

- Systemic AV valve regurgitation—the tricuspid valve is poorly designed to support systemic pressures and commonly becomes regurgitant; if right ventricular function is adequate, valve replacement should be performed because valve repair is rarely successful

- Systemic ventricular failure—the right ventricle may fail because it is inherently unsuitable to support the systemic circulation in the long term, because of long-standing tricuspid regurgitation, and because of poor ventricular filling from the surgically constructed atrial pathways

There has been much interest in whether placement of a pulmonary artery band to 'retrain' the left ventricle to enable it to support the systemic circulation will allow takedown of the Mustard operation and performance of an arterial switch operation. This approach only appears possible in young children, or in older patients with a degree of left ventricular outflow tract obstruction in whom the left ventricle has always retained near systemic pressures.

Arterial switch operation

As a result of the late complications of interatrial repair, a different surgical approach was developed that restored the left ventricle to the systemic circulation and avoided extensive atrial surgery: the arterial switch.

Since the 1980s anatomical correction by the arterial switch operation has superseded interatrial repair as the operation of choice for most patients with TGA. Blood is redirected at arterial level by switching the aorta and pulmonary arteries so that the left ventricle becomes the subaortic ventricle supporting the systemic circulation. The coronary arteries are reimplanted into the neo-aortic root.

Late follow-up appears good for these patients, but vigilance is required to detect late problems including myocardial ischaemia due to coronary anastomotic stenosis; neo-aortic or pulmonary valve regurgitation; neo-aortic root dilation; and pulmonary arterial stenosis.

Rastelli operation

This operation is performed for patients with TGA, VSD, and pulmonary stenosis (Fig. 16.12.18). The VSD is closed so that the left ventricle carrying oxygenated blood empties into the aorta. The stenotic pulmonary artery is ligated and a conduit is placed between the right ventricle and pulmonary artery. The main advantage of this operation is that the left ventricle supports the systemic circulation, but it commits the patient to several further conduit replacement operations.

'Palliative' Mustard/Senning or arterial switch operations

These procedures are performed for patients with TGA, VSD, and pulmonary vascular disease to improve mixing of blood and oxygenation. The VSD is left open. These patients should be treated in the same way as other patients with Eisenmenger syndrome.

Congenitally corrected transposition of the great arteries (cTGA) (AV, VA discordance)

This rare condition accounts for less than 1% of all congenital heart disease. Both atrial and arterial connections to the ventricles are discordant, so pulmonary venous blood passes through the left atrium, through the right ventricle and into an anteriorly lying aorta (Fig. 16.12.16). Similarly, systemic venous blood reaches the

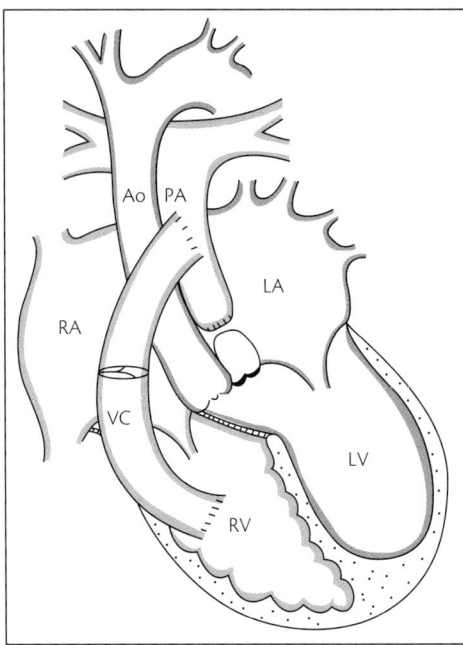

Fig. 16.12.18 Schematic representation of Rastelli operation for TGA with ventricular septal defect and pulmonary stenosis. Ao, aorta; LA, left atrium; LV, left ventricle; PA; pulmonary artery; RA, right atrium, RV, right ventricle, VC, valved conduit.

pulmonary trunk via the left ventricle. The circulation is therefore physiologically 'corrected', but the morphological right ventricle and tricuspid valve support the systemic circulation.

More than 95% of cases have associated anomalies, most commonly VSD and pulmonary stenosis, but also Ebstein anomaly of the systemic (tricuspid) AV valve, aortic stenosis, AVSD, abnormalities of situs, and coarctation. Congenital complete heart block occurs in around 5% of patients and may develop at any stage of life, particularly following surgery to the AV valve.

Presentation depends on associated lesions. Patients with isolated cTGA may remain asymptomatic and undiagnosed into old age, but failure of the systemic ventricle, systemic AV valve regurgitation, or the onset of complete heart block and atrial arrhythmias usually result in presentation with symptoms from the fourth decade onwards. Those with VSD and pulmonary stenosis may be cyanosed, and those with VSD alone may present with pulmonary hypertension.

A parasternal heave is usually palpable from the pressure-loaded anteriorly lying systemic right ventricle; this may be especially prominent if it is also volume-loaded by systemic (tricuspid) AV valve regurgitation. There may be a prominent aortic pulsation in the suprasternal notch and the aortic component of the second heart sound may be palpable and loud. The pulmonary component is soft or inaudible due to the posterior position of the pulmonary artery.

The ECG may show varying degrees of AV block or evidence of pre-excitation due to accessory pathways (associated with Ebstein-like anomalies of the systemic AV valve). There may be left axis deviation. The right and left bundles are inverted, so the initial septal activation is right-to-left, resulting in Q waves in V1–2 and an absent Q in V5–6; this pattern may be wrongly interpreted as a previous anterior myocardial infarction. The chest radiograph has a

typical appearance (Fig. 16.12.19). Echocardiography confirms the discordant relations and assesses ventricular and systemic (tricuspid) AV valve function as well as other associated lesions. Ebstein anomaly may be diagnosed if the tricuspid valve is apically displaced by more than $8\,mm/m^2$. Cardiac catheterization is indicated to assess the haemodynamic importance of associated lesions.

Angiotensin converting enzyme (ACE) inhibitors may be useful when there is systemic ventricular dysfunction or AV valve regurgitation, but there are no trial data to support their use. Transvenous AV sequential pacing is indicated for complete heart block; active fixation ventricular leads are required because of the absence of coarse apical trabeculations in the morphologically left subpulmonary ventricle. If there are associated intracardiac shunts, patients should be formally anticoagulated to reduce the risk of paradoxical embolism, or epicardial pacing should be considered.

The conventional surgical approach to systemic AV valve regurgitation is tricuspid valve replacement (repair is rarely successful), but if systemic ventricular function is poor (ejection fraction <40%) transplantation may be the only option. Where there is coexistent VSD and pulmonary stenosis, classical repair involved closure of the VSD and insertion of a valved conduit between the left ventricle and pulmonary artery, with the right ventricle continuing to support the systemic circulation.

Anatomical repair, so that the morphological left ventricle supports the systemic ventricle, has had success in children with systemic AV valve regurgitation and systemic ventricular dysfunction. For patients with an associated non-restrictive VSD the left ventricle is at systemic pressure and therefore 'pretrained' to support the systemic circulation. If there is no pulmonary stenosis, a 'double switch' may be performed, combining an interatrial repair (usually a Senning operation) with an arterial switch operation. If there is also pulmonary stenosis, the Senning operation is combined with a Rastelli-type repair. The regurgitant tricuspid valve and right ventricle are therefore placed in the pulmonary circulation. For children with corrected transposition whose left ventricle is at low

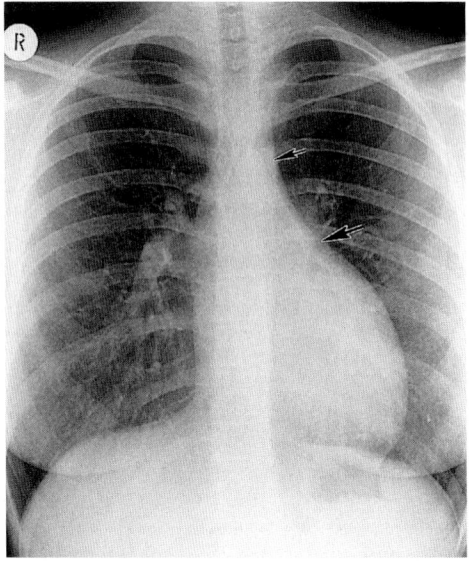

Fig. 16.12.19 Chest radiograph of a 23-year-old woman with congenitally corrected transposition of the great vessels. There is a narrow pedicle due to the abnormally related great arteries (small arrow) and the left heart border is straight (large arrow) due to the abnormal position of the left-lying anterior ascending aorta.

pressure, a period of left ventricular 'training' is required before a double switch operation can be performed, which is achieved by placing a pulmonary artery band to increase left ventricular pressure and induce hypertrophy. Pulmonary artery banding *per se* may improve symptoms, since the increased left ventricular pressure causes the interventricular septum to move towards the systemic ventricle, reducing systemic AV regurgitation.

The long-term outcome of these anatomical approaches to corrected transposition is not yet known; complications relating to the dysfunction of the retrained left ventricular, conduit replacement, neo-aortic valve regurgitation, and arrhythmia may become significant. There are reports of adults with VSD and pulmonary stenosis having successfully undergone Mustard–Rastelli repair, but it is probably not possible to adequately 'train' an adult left ventricle that has been at low pressure for many years.

Tetralogy of Fallot

Tetralogy of Fallot is the commonest cyanotic defect, occurring in 1 in 3600 live births; it affects males and females equally. Most patients reaching the adult clinics have undergone radical repair, but some natural and palliated survivors may present.

The fundamental abnormality in tetralogy of Fallot is anterocephalad deviation of the outlet septum which creates the four key features: subvalvar pulmonary stenosis, VSD, an aortic valve that overrides the VSD, and right ventricular hypertrophy (Fig. 16.12.20). There is great anatomical variation, ranging from minimal aortic override to double outlet right ventricle (DORV), and from minimal pulmonary stenosis to pulmonary atresia. The VSD is perimembranous and there is usually additional pulmonary valvar stenosis.

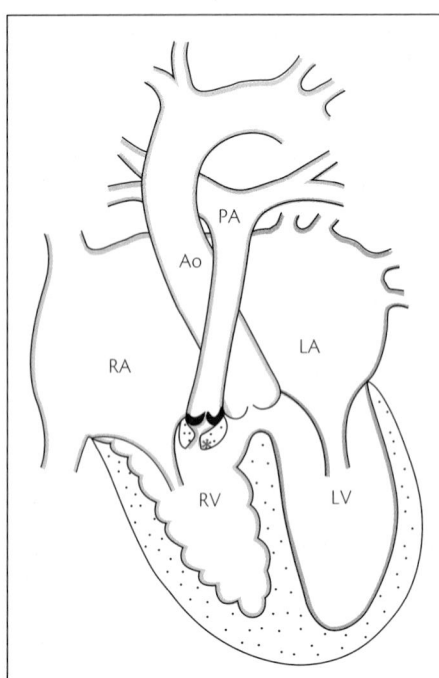

Fig. 16.12.20 Schematic representation of tetralogy of Fallot. *Anterocephalad deviation of outlet septum creates ventricular septal defect, subpulmonary stenosis, aorta overriding crest of interventricular septum, and secondary right ventricular hypertrophy. Ao, aorta, LA, left atrium, LV, left ventricle, PA, pulmonary artery, RA, right atrium, RV, right ventricle.

Associations

Microdeletions of chromosome 22q11 may occur in association with tetralogy of Fallot, especially in its most severe form with pulmonary atresia and associated with a broad spectrum of phenotypic abnormalities in the velocardiofacial syndrome (which includes DiGeorge syndrome) with (1) other cardiac defects—Fallot with right aortic arch, truncus arteriosus, pulmonary atresia with VSD, interrupted aortic arch; (2) facial abnormalities—cleft palate, hare lip, hypertelorism, narrow eye fissures, puffy eyelids, a small mouth, deformed earlobes; (3) psychiatric disorders and learning difficulties; and (4) neonatal immune deficiency (thymic hypoplasia) and hypocalcaemia (parathyroid hypoplasia).

Cardiac defects associated with tetralogy of Fallot include a right-sided aortic arch in 16%, a left SVC in around 15%, additional VSDs in 5%, and a secundum ASD ('pentalogy' of Fallot) in 8%. The most important associated coronary anomaly is the crossing of the right ventricular outflow tract by a left anterior descending coronary artery arising anomalously from the right coronary sinus: this is vulnerable to damage during surgical repair.

Clinical course and management

Without surgical intervention, only 2% of patients survive to their fortieth year. Those that do survive may be a selected group in whom subpulmonary stenosis was not severe in early life, but progressed with advancing age. Unoperated patients are at risk of the complications of cyanosis, endocarditis, atrial and ventricular arrhythmias, progressive ascending aortic dilatation (without the high risk of dissection found in Marfan's syndrome), aortic regurgitation—causing volume overload of both ventricles and subsequent biventricular failure, and systemic hypertension—adding additional pressure overload to the work of both ventricles and further contributing to the onset of biventricular failure.

There is cyanosis and clubbing, a right ventricular heave, and sometimes a thrill over the right ventricular outflow tract. A right-sided aorta may be palpable to the right of the sternum. The second heart sound is usually single, and there is a loud pulmonary ejection murmur. There may be aortic regurgitation.

The ECG shows right axis deviation and right ventricular hypertrophy, and the QRS duration may be prolonged in older patients. The classical cardiac silhouette is a 'coeur en sabot', i.e. a clog-shaped heart, but this is more likely to be seen in tetralogy with pulmonary atresia (see below). The heart size is usually normal and pulmonary vascularity reduced. There may be a right-sided aortic arch indenting the right of the trachea, and there may be a prominent dilated ascending aorta.

Two-dimensional echocardiography reveals infundibular stenosis with or without pulmonary valve stenosis, right ventricular hypertrophy, the typical VSD, and varying degrees of aortic override. There may be evidence of left ventricular volume overload, aortic root dilatation and aortic regurgitation.

Cardiac catheterization should be performed prior to radical repair in adults. The anatomy of the right ventricular outflow tract obstruction and pulmonary arteries is defined, and pulmonary vascular resistance assessed. Selective coronary angiography demonstrates any anomalous origin and course as well as acquired coronary disease. Aortography shows aortic root dilatation and any aortopulmonary collaterals. MRI may be performed instead of conventional cardiac catheterization, except that it does not provide pulmonary vascular resistance data.

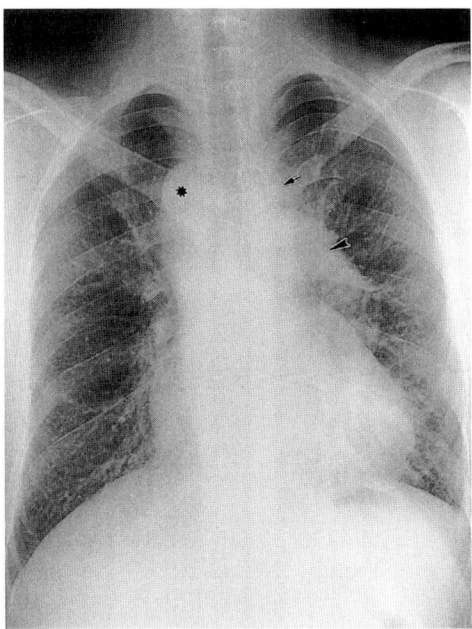

Fig. 16.12.21 Chest radiograph of a 36-year-old man with tetralogy of Fallot palliated by a classic left Blalock–Taussig shunt (small arrow). There is secondary dilatation of the left pulmonary artery (large arrow) and a right aortic arch (*).

Palliated history

Helen Taussig first suggested palliative surgery in 1943, and the first Blalock–Taussig shunt was performed in 1945 (Fig. 16.12.21 and Table 16.12.7). Nowadays, palliative shunts are usually performed as a staging procedure in small infants; however, occasional patients reach the adult clinic having had palliation without subsequent radical repair. They are cyanosed and clubbed and have a continuous murmur under the clavicle and over the scapula on the side of the shunt. In a classical Blalock–Taussig shunt the ipsilateral radial pulse is diminished or absent and the hand often small. Late complications of systemic to pulmonary artery shunts include infective endarteritis, acquired pulmonary atresia, aortic regurgitation, and biventricular failure, with increasing cyanosis and bronchopulmonary collateral development if the shunt blocks or is outgrown, and pulmonary vascular disease if the shunt is too big.

Table 16.12.7 Systemic to pulmonary arterial shunts

Classical Blalock–Taussig shunt	Subclavian artery divided distally. Proximal subclavian artery anastomosed end-to-side to pulmonary artery
Modified Blalock–Taussig shunt	Prosthetic graft between subclavian and pulmonary arteries
Central shunts:	
Waterston shunt[a]	Side-to-side anastomosis between ascending aorta and (right) pulmonary artery
Potts shunt*	Side-to-side anastomosis between descending aorta and (left) pulmonary artery
Other	Prosthetic graft between aorta and pulmonary artery

[a] Now obsolete because not possible to adequately control the size of the shunt.

Radical repair

Radical repair involves patch closure of the VSD with infundibular resection with or without pulmonary valvotomy or replacement: 86% of patients who undergo such surgery survive to 32 years of age, these being the majority of tetralogy patients seen in the adult clinic. However, they remain at risk of late complications including pulmonary regurgitation and stenosis, aortic regurgitation, ventricular dysfunction, endocarditis, arrhythmia, and sudden death. Those repaired in early childhood and by a transannular approach have a better long-term prognosis than those repaired later or by a transventricular approach.

In many patients repair involves placing a patch across the annulus of the pulmonary valve in order to create an unobstructed right ventricular outflow. As a result, most of these patients have free pulmonary regurgitation, which although well tolerated for many years may result in progressive right ventricular dilation and dysfunction, impaired exercise tolerance, and increased risk of atrial and ventricular arrhythmias. A widening of the QRS complex beyond 180 ms may be a marker for right ventricular dilation and dysfunction, these being risk factors for developing worsening functional class, sustained ventricular tachycardia and sudden death. Pulmonary valve replacement is indicated if there is impaired exercise tolerance, sustained arrhythmia, progressive right ventricular dilation or any evidence of right ventricular dysfunction.

Pulmonary regurgitation is worsened in the presence of pulmonary arterial stenosis that may occur at the site of a previous shunt. Right ventricular outflow tract obstruction may recur, especially if a valved right ventricular to pulmonary artery conduit was placed, this being due to excessive formation of neointima (peel) in the conduit or to calcification of the valve.

Most patients have right bundle branch block after repair (Fig. 16.12.22) due to surgical damage to the right bundle as it runs in the floor of the VSD. Bifasicular block and transient postoperative complete heart block carry a risk of developing late complete heart block. Atrial arrhythmias occur in 30% of long-term survivors and are a major cause of morbidity. Those with left-sided volume overload and left atrial dilatation secondary to residual VSD or previous shunts are at particular risk of atrial flutter and fibrillation. Rapidly conducted atrial flutter is particularly poorly tolerated and is likely to be responsible for a proportion of sudden deaths. Ventricular arrhythmias occur in up to 45% of patients. However, the incidence of late sudden death is only 1 to 5%, so nonsustained ventricular arrhythmias are not an independent risk factor. Sustained monomorphic ventricular tachycardia is likely to be a significant risk factor for sudden death, as are atrial arrhythmias and heart block.

Adverse right ventricular risk factors include dilatation and dysfunction, outflow tract obstruction, hypertrophy, aneurysm, impaired myocardial blood flow and pulmonary regurgitation. Surgical risk factor for late sudden death include transventricular versus transatrial repair, large ventriculotomy scar, residual VSD, previous complex or multiple operations, impaired left ventricular function, older age at operation, and length of follow-up.

Tetralogy of Fallot with absent pulmonary valve syndrome

This variation accounts for approximately 3% of cases of tetralogy. There is a ring-like, usually stenotic malformation, with failure of

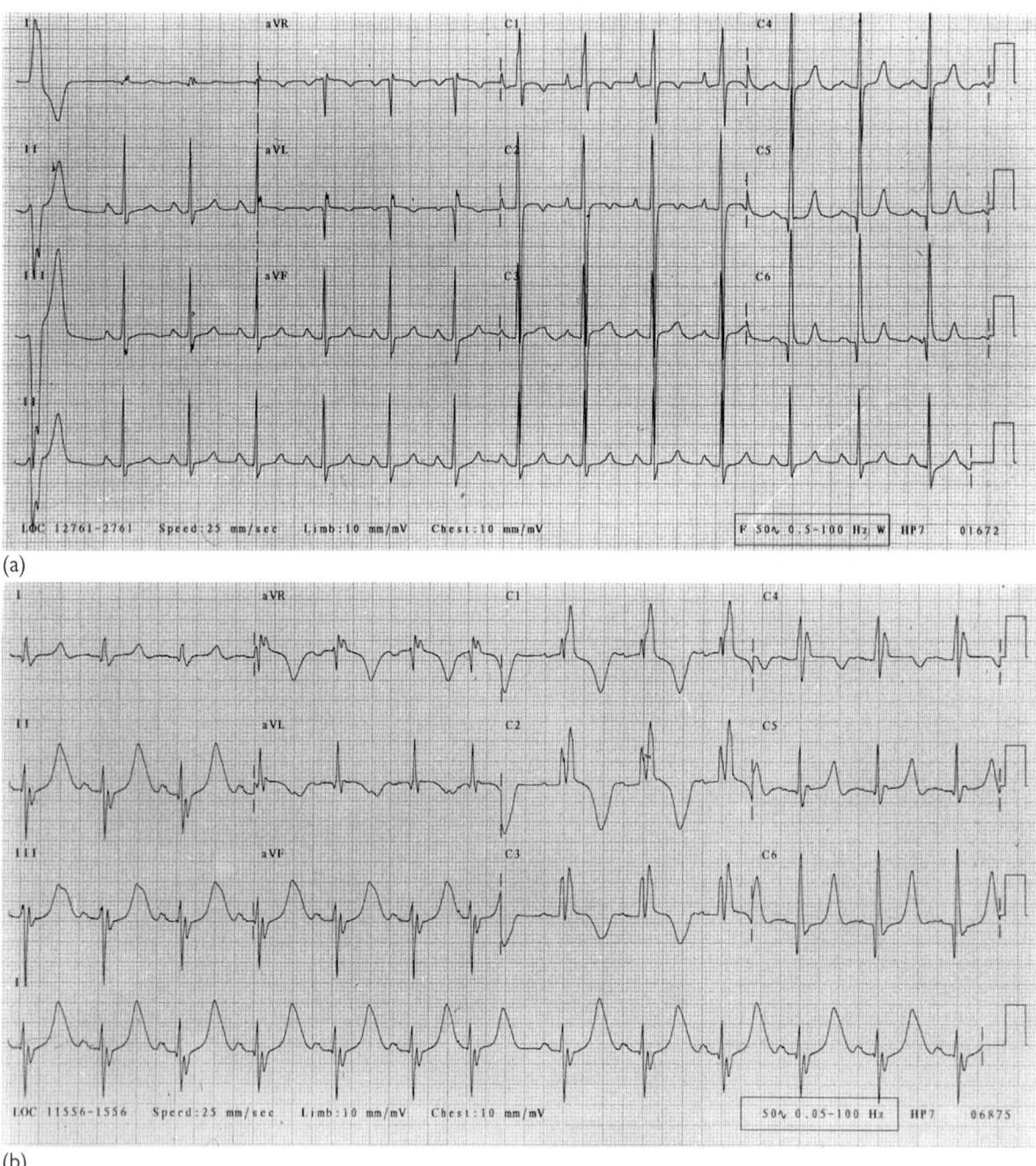

(a)

(b)

Fig. 16.12.22 Electrocardiograms of a 35-year-old woman who underwent radical repair of tetralogy of Fallot. Preoperatively (a) there is right ventricular hypertrophy, postoperatively (b) there is right bundle branch block, due to damage to the right bundle as it runs in the floor of the ventricular septal defect.

development of the pulmonary valve cusps. The central pulmonary arteries are usually hugely dilated or aneurysmal.

Double outlet right ventricle

In double outlet right ventricle (DORV) more than half the circumference of both great vessels arises from the morphological right ventricle. A complete or partial muscular infundibulum usually lies beneath each arterial valve. The anatomy and physiology are enormously varied, as are the surgical approaches to repair. The degree of pulmonary stenosis and the relation of the VSD to the great vessels determine the haemodynamics.

Most (80%) subaortic defects have pulmonary stenosis and Fallot-like physiology. The Taussig–Bing anomaly accounts for less than 10% of DORV and describes a subpulmonary defect without pulmonary stenosis. There is transposition-like physiology with cyanosis and high pulmonary blood flow. As the pulmonary vascular resistance rises, pulmonary blood flow falls and cyanosis increases. Unoperated survival to adulthood is uncommon, but occurs occasionally if the pulmonary vascular resistance establishes adequate but not excessive pulmonary blood flow. If such a survivor also has a patent arterial duct, there will be reversed differential cyanosis. Deoxygenated blood selectively enters the aorta to supply the arch vessels, whereas oxygenated blood enters the pulmonary artery and supplies the descending aorta via the duct; thus the fingers are more cyanosed and clubbed than the toes.

If the VSD is remote from the great vessels, a biventricular repair may not be possible and a single ventricle repair (Fontan) may be necessary.

Pulmonary atresia with ventricular septal defect

This is a complex and heterogeneous cyanotic condition. The intracardiac anatomy is the same as tetralogy of Fallot, but the right ventricular outflow tract is blind-ended (atretic). The pulmonary blood supply is derived entirely from three different types of systemic vessels: (1) a large muscular duct that resembles a collateral; (2) a diffuse plexus of small 'bronchial' arteries arising from mediastinal and intercostal arteries; and (3) large tortuous systemic arterial collaterals known as MAPCAs (major aortopulmonary collateral arteries), which arise directly from the descending aorta, from its major branches (usually the subclavian artery), or from bronchial arteries, and may connect with central pulmonary arteries or supply whole segments or lobes of lung independently, leading this variation to have been termed 'complex pulmonary atresia'.

Prognosis and management depends largely on the pulmonary vasculature, in which there is considerable anatomical variation. Confluent pulmonary arteries with pulmonary vessels having a near normal arborization pattern to all segments of the lungs are associated with the best prognosis. Here radical repair, with recruitment of MAPCAs to the native pulmonary arteries, an RV to PA conduit, and closure of the VSD is likely to be possible, and the pulmonary vascular resistance is likely to be low. The 20-year survival after radical repair is about 75%. The outlook is worse if there are no native pulmonary arteries and multiple tortuous MAPCAs with poor arborization. Radical repair may be extremely challenging or impossible, and pulmonary vascular resistance likely to be high. Such patients may be suitable for no or only palliative surgery and will remain cyanosed. Following surgical palliation, 20-year survival is around 60%; unoperated survival is very poor, only about 8% reaching 10 years of age, and those that do reach adulthood have a mean age of death of 33 years.

Clinical findings

Examination findings in the unoperated or palliated patient are similar to those of the unoperated Fallot without pulmonary atresia, except that there are continuous collateral murmurs and often a collapsing pulse.

The chest radiograph shows a right aortic arch in 25% of cases and has a typical appearance (Fig. 16.12.23). The pulmonary collateral vessels may follow a bizarre pattern. Colour flow Doppler may identify collateral vessels, but conventional angiography is required to precisely delineate their origin, degree of ostial stenosis, and intrapulmonary course (Fig. 16.12.24). Multislice CT and MRI are useful tools in imaging complex pulmonary vasculature.

Late complications in unoperated or palliated survivors include increasing cyanosis due either to the development of pulmonary vascular disease in lung segments perfused at systemic pressure through nonstenosed collaterals, or to the progressive stenosis of collateral vessels. In the latter, good symptomatic relief may be obtained from stenting. The aortic root may become markedly dilated and aortic regurgitation may develop, resulting in

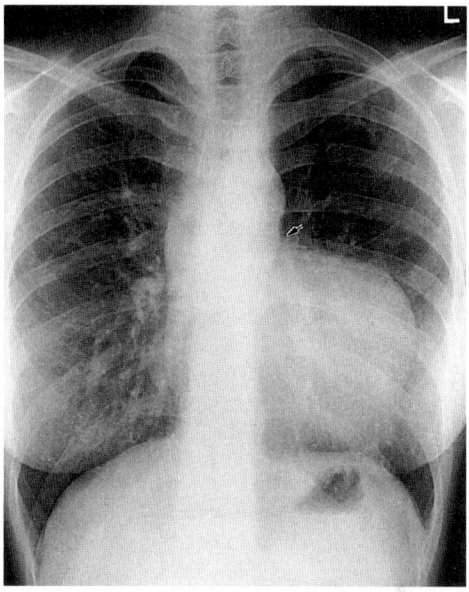

Fig. 16.12.23 Chest radiograph of a 21-year-old woman with tetralogy of Fallot and pulmonary atresia, no central pulmonary arteries, and multiple aortopulmonary collaterals which create an abnormal pulmonary vascular pattern. The typical 'coeur en sabot' silhouette is due to right ventricular hypertrophy and the pulmonary bay where the pulmonary artery should be (arrow).

biventricular volume overload and failure. Aortic valve endocarditis is a particular risk.

Late complications after radical repair include those that follow repair of tetralogy of Fallot. In addition, patients face inevitable repeated conduit replacements, and right ventricular failure secondary to high pulmonary vascular resistance.

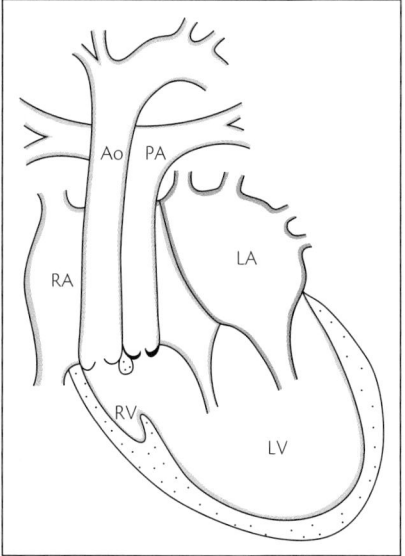

Fig. 16.12.24 Schematic representation of double inlet left ventricle with VA discordance. Both atria connect to the LV via the tricuspid and mitral valves, so that systemic and pulmonary venous blood mix in the LV and the patient is cyanosed. The LV supports both the systemic and pulmonary circulations. The aorta arises from the rudimentary RV via the VSD. If the VSD is restrictive, it creates obstruction to systemic blood flow. Ao, aorta; LA, left atrium; LV, left ventricle; PA, pulmonary artery; RA, right atrium; RV, right ventricle; VA, ventriculoarterial; VSD, ventricular septal defect.

Hearts with univentricular AV connection

Also known as univentricular or single-ventricle hearts, these hearts are defined by the connection of both atria to one ventricle, or by the absence of one of the AV connections. There is one dominant ventricle, with a second rudimentary and incomplete ventricle. When the rudimentary ventricle is of right morphology, it nearly always lies anteriorly. Less commonly, there is a posteriorly lying morphologically left rudimentary ventricle, and rarely, there is solitary ventricle of indeterminate morphology.

The two most common variants are double inlet left ventricle (DILV) and tricuspid atresia (Figs. 16.12.24 and 16.12.25) which together account for around 4 to 5% of congenital heart disease. This section will consider these two conditions, a discussion of more complex variants being beyond the scope of this text.

Clinical course

Presentation depends largely on pulmonary blood flow, which in turn is dependent on the degree of pulmonary stenosis. Those with severe obstruction to pulmonary blood flow present as neonates with severe cyanosis. Neonates without pulmonary stenosis have excessively high pulmonary blood flow and present in congestive cardiac failure with breathlessness and only mild cyanosis. The presence of subaortic stenosis or other obstruction to systemic blood flow such as coarctation exacerbates heart failure and results in early presentation.

The outcome is most favourable for patients with left ventricular morphology, moderate pulmonary stenosis, and no subaortic stenosis, and for those with 'balanced' pulmonary and systemic blood flow, i.e. moderately severe pulmonary stenosis and no obstruction to systemic blood flow. Unoperated survival into adulthood is uncommon: 50% of patients with DILV die before 14 years, 50% with double inlet right ventricle die by 4 years of age.

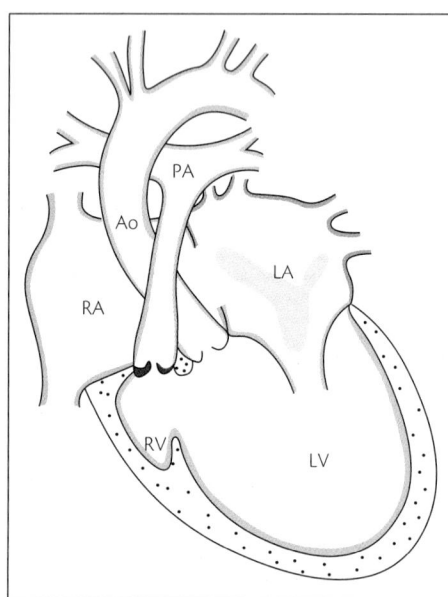

Fig. 16.12.25 Schematic representation of tricuspid atresia. Systemic venous blood leaves the RA via an atrial septal defect and mixes with pulmonary venous blood in the LA. The LV thus supports both the systemic and pulmonary circulations and the patient is cyanosed. The rudimentary RV does not play a functional role. Ao, aorta; LA, left atrium; LV, left ventricle; PA, pulmonary artery; RA, right atrium; RV, right ventricle.

Nonetheless, rare patients with balanced circulation reach their sixth decade without surgical intervention.

There is cyanosis and clubbing. A giant a wave may be present in the jugular venous pulse in tricuspid atresia. An absent right ventricular impulse and prominent left ventricular impulse are characteristic of DILV and tricuspid atresia. There may be a precordial thrill from pulmonary stenosis, particularly if the pulmonary artery lies anteriorly. If there are discordant ventriculoarterial connections the aortic pulsation of the anteriorly lying aorta may be prominent in the suprasternal notch. The second heart sound is usually single.

If pulmonary vascular disease has developed there will be additional signs of pulmonary hypertension. Signs of congestive heart failure may be present in the ageing patient, particularly with the onset of atrial arrhythmia, such that the venous pressure is raised, with hepatomegaly and peripheral oedema.

The chest radiograph shows cardiomegaly due to chronic ventricular volume overload. If ventriculoarterial connections are discordant, there is a narrow pedicle and the ascending aorta forms a straight edge along the left heart border. Pulmonary vascularity reflects the pulmonary blood flow, the main pulmonary arteries being small where there is significant pulmonary stenosis, with large main pulmonary arteries indicating high pulmonary blood flow, either past or present.

In tricuspid atresia the ECG usually shows right atrial hypertrophy, normal PR interval, small or absent right ventricular forces, and left axis deviation. There are left axis deviation and large left ventricular forces in DILV. If the rudimentary chamber lies to the right the PR interval is usually normal, but if it lies to the left the PR interval may be prolonged or there may be complete heart block.

Two-dimensional echocardiography and colour flow Doppler allow detailed assessment of the anatomy and physiology, including ventricular morphology and pulmonary and sub-aortic stenosis. Cardiac catheterization is required to assess pulmonary artery anatomy and resistance.

Surgical management of univentricular hearts: the Fontan operation

Management requires a staged approach, the ultimate aim of which is to achieve a pink patient in whom the functionally single ventricle supports only the systemic circulation: the Fontan operation.

The first stage is to obtain control of pulmonary blood flow. In those with excessive flow a pulmonary artery band is placed to create supravalvar pulmonary artery stenosis and limit pulmonary flow. In neonates with severe pulmonary stenosis a systemic artery to pulmonary artery shunt is placed to augment pulmonary blood flow.

As the child grows and becomes more cyanosed the central shunt is replaced with a superior vena cava to pulmonary artery anastomosis (Glenn, or cavopulmonary anastomosis), as illustrated in Fig. 16.12.26. This reduces cyanosis, perfuses the pulmonary arteries at low pressure, and reduces the volume load on the single ventricle. However, as the child grows, the relative contribution of the SVC to the circulation diminishes, resulting in progressive cyanosis.

Completion of the Fontan operation is usually performed by age 4 to 6 years. The principle of this approach is to separate the systemic and pulmonary circulations. This is achieved by using the single functional ventricle to support the systemic circulation and leaving the pulmonary circulation without a ventricle, i.e. with

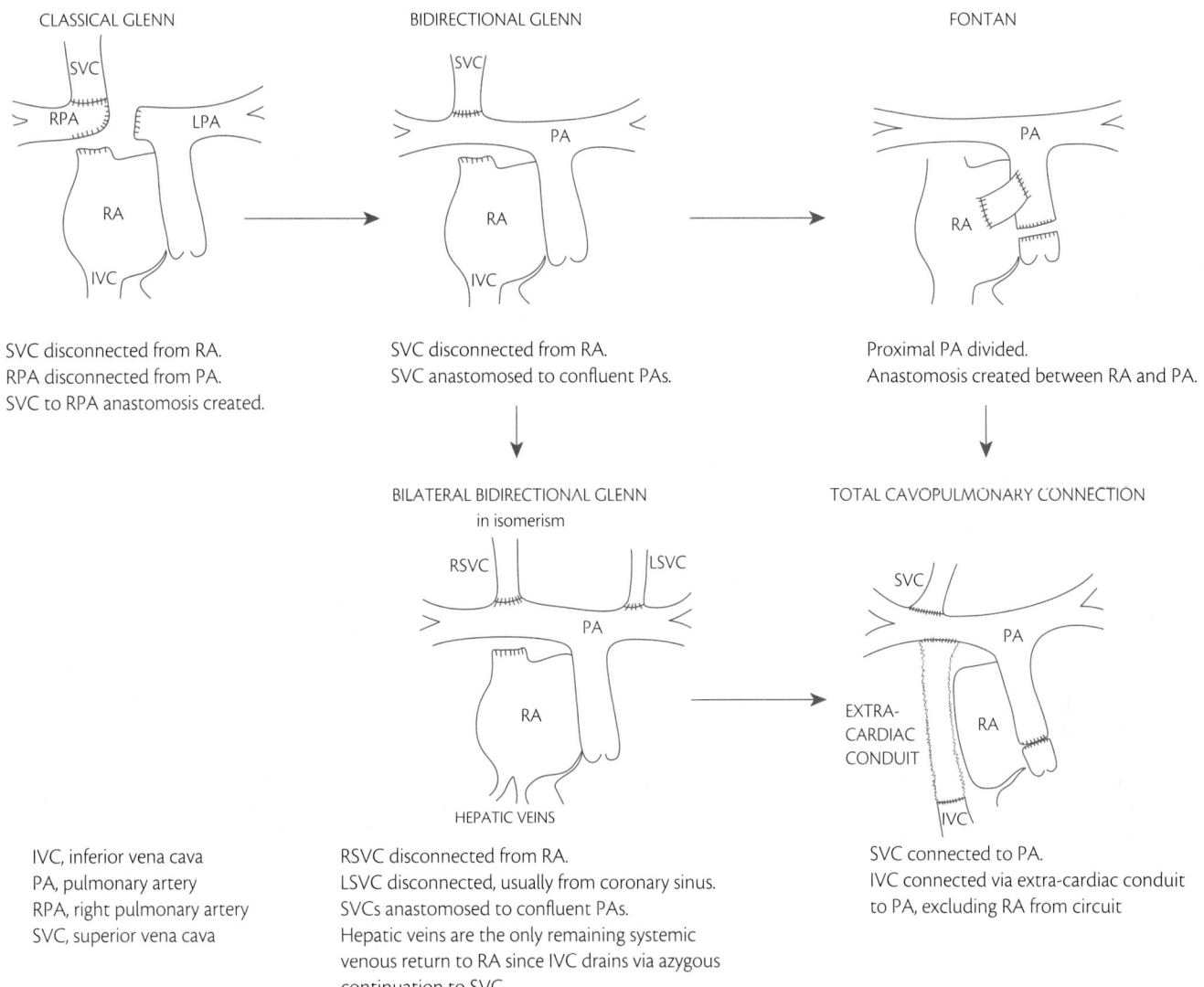

Fig. 16.12.26 Evolution of Fontan and total cavopulmonary connection. IVC, inferior vena cava; PA, pulmonary artery; RPA, right pulmonary artery; SVC, superior vena cava.

phasic rather than pulsatile flow. Since its first description in 1972 the atriopulmonary Fontan operation has evolved, so that now several variations exist. The favoured approach nowadays is the total cavopulmonary connection (TCPC), which avoids some of the late complications of the original approach. Nonetheless, all the variations result in the same basic physiology, the 'Fontan circulation'.

The Fontan circulation is one of a chronic low cardiac output state, critically dependent upon adequate systemic venous filling pressure to drive forward flow across the pulmonary vascular bed. It is a fragile circulation in which small changes in haemodynamics can result in a serious, sometimes catastrophic, fall in cardiac output. Problems that can cause trouble include dehydration, stenosis at the site of connection of the right atrium or systemic veins to the pulmonary artery, pulmonary embolism from *in situ* right atrial thrombus, a rise in pulmonary vascular resistance, atrial flutter, mitral regurgitation, a rise in left ventricular end-diastolic pressure, aortic or subaortic stenosis, drug-induced vasodilatation (e.g. anaesthetic induction agents, nitrates), and positive pressure ventilation that reduces systemic venous return.

Clinical features after the Fontan operation

Most patients are acyanotic: new or worsening cyanosis is cause for concern. The jugular venous pulse is usually slightly raised and the second heart sound single. No murmur arises from the Fontan connection. There may be a murmur of mitral regurgitation. It patients with VA discordance, a loud systolic murmur raises suspicion of subaortic stenosis (which may be at the level of the VSD). The liver edge is often palpable, but new or increasing hepatomegaly is a worrisome finding. Ascites often precedes peripheral oedema in young patients with complications post Fontan.

A combination of echocardiography and MRI provide anatomical and physiological data. Cardiac catheterization is needed to assess pulmonary vascular resistance. Cardiopulmonary exercise testing is a useful indicator early signs of decompensation.

Complications after the Fontan operation

Patient selection is important in ensuring a good outcome of Fontan surgery. Survival post Fontan ranges from 81% at 10 years for 'perfect candidates' to 60 to 70% for all patients. Preoperative risk factors for a poor outcome are pulmonary vascular resistance

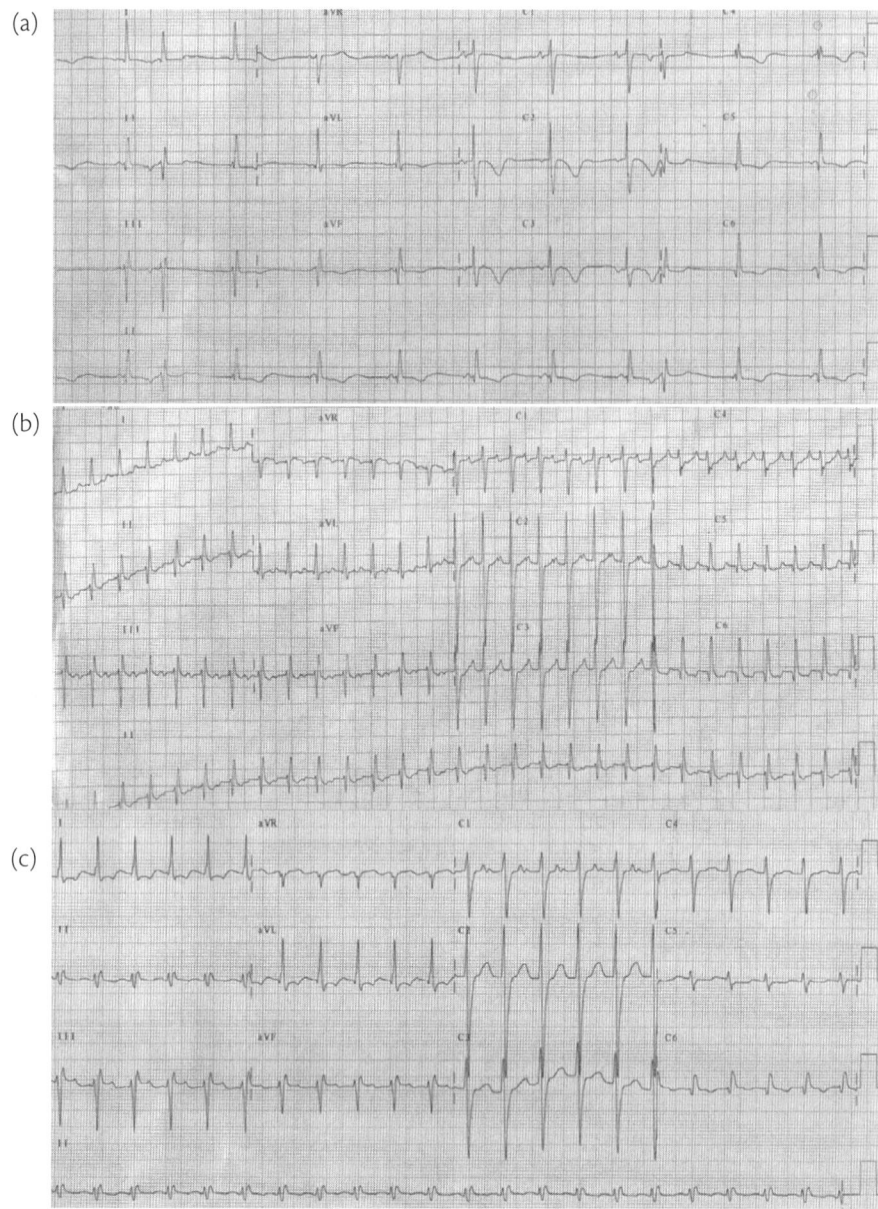

Fig. 16.12.27 ECGs from a 24-year-old woman with tricuspid atresia and previous Fontan surgery. a shows sinus rhythm. b and c show interatrial re-entry tachycardias which were poorly tolerated and required urgent DC cardioversion.

greater than 4 Wood units, mean pulmonary artery pressure more than 15 mmHg, ventricular hypertrophy, impaired systolic ventricular function, severe AV valve regurgitation, aortic outflow obstruction, and small or distorted pulmonary arteries. However, even patients with none of these risk factors are at risk of a great range of late complications which include intra-atrial reentry tachycardia (IART)/atrial flutter, sinus node dysfunction, progressive ventricular dysfunction, AV valve regurgitation, development of subaortic stenosis, pathway obstruction, right lower pulmonary vein compression by dilated right atrium, thromboembolism (all adult patients should be anticoagulated), recurrent effusions, ascites, peripheral oedema, cyanosis (due to development of venous collaterals to the left atrium or pulmonary arteriovenous fistulas), protein-losing enteropathy, and hepatic dysfunction.

A detailed discussion of these many complications is beyond the scope of this book, but atrial flutter/IART merits further discussion because it may be an acutely life-threatening complication (Fig. 16.12.27). Flutter is common post Fontan, and, as discussed above, is

poorly tolerated. Time may be wasted once medical attention is sought because the ECG appearances are often atypical and may be misinterpreted as sinus tachycardia. If in doubt, intravenous adenosine will reveal flutter waves and confirm the diagnosis, but will not terminate the arrhythmia. Other intravenous antiarrhythmics should be avoided since they may precipitate cardiovascular collapse. The safest approach is DC cardioversion. Intravenous fluids should be given while the patient is nil by mouth to maintain systemic venous filling pressure. Care must be taken to avoid excessive systemic vasodilation at induction of anaesthesia, and allowance must be made for the fall in cardiac output that accompanies ventilation.

Hypoplastic left heart syndrome (HLHS)

Until very recently this condition was not discussed in adult texts, since there were no survivors to adulthood. With the introduction of the three-staged Norwood operation, resulting in a complex

Table 16.12.8 Risk of maternal mortality in different cardiac conditions

Low risk (<1%)	Significant risk (1–10%)	High risk, pregnancy contraindicated (>10%)
Unoperated, small or mild: Pulmonary stenosis Septal defects Patent arterial duct	Mechanical valve	Pulmonary hypertension
Most repaired septal defects	Systemic right ventricle	Impaired systemic ventricular function
Successfully repaired coarctation	Cyanosis without pulmonary hypertension	Aortic aneurysm
Repaired tetralogy of Fallot	Fontan circulation	Severe left-sided obstruction, e.g. mitral and aortic stenosis
Most regurgitant valvar lesions		

Table 16.12.9 Risks of infective endocarditis or endarteritis in congenital heart disease

Unoperated	Operated
Low risk: lesions with no or low velocity turbulence and no prosthetic material	
Anomalous pulmonary venous drainage	Anomalous pulmonary venous drainage
Secundum ASD	Secundum ASD
Ebstein's anomaly	Ebstein's anomaly with repaired native valve
Mild pulmonary stenosis	VSD/tetralogy of Fallot without residual lesions
Isolated corrected transposition	Patent ductus arteriosus
Eisenmenger syndrome without valvar regurgitation	Fontan type procedures
	Arterial switch for transposition without residual lesions
Moderate risk	
Systemic AV valve regurgitation	Residual regurgitation of repaired native aortic or systemic AV valve
Subaortic stenosis	Nonvalved conduits
Moderate—severe pulmonary stenosis	
Tetralogy of Fallot	
Double outlet right ventricle	
Univentricular heart with pulmonary stenosis	
Truncus arteriosus	
Coarctation	
Restrictive patent ductus arteriosus	
High risk	
Bicuspid aortic valve	Prosthetic valves
Aortic regurgitation secondary to VSD or subaortic stenosis	Aortopulmonary shunts e.g. Gore-Tex, modified Blalock–Taussig
Restrictive VSD	Valved conduits

ASD, atrial septal defect; AV, atrioventricular; VSD, ventricular septal defect.

Fontan-type circulation, survivors are on the cusp of reaching the adult clinic.

HLHS is a heterogeneous syndrome in which the left side of the heart is unable to support the systemic circulation because of hypoplasia, stenosis, or atresia at different levels of the left side of the circulation. In early series only about 50% survived the three operations, but survival now approaches 70%. Those who reach the adult clinic will face the complications of any Fontan circulation, and in addition they are at risk of complications from ascending aorta and coarctation repair sites, coronary arteries arising from the hypoplastic remnant of ascending aorta, left pulmonary artery stenosis at site of arch repair, and failure of the right ventricle and tricuspid valve as they support the systemic circulation.

Pregnancy and contraception in congenital heart disease

Cardiac disease is the leading cause of pregnancy-related death in the United Kingdom. All patients with congenital heart disease should be counselled from adolescence on their risk of pregnancy and their contraceptive options. Pregnancy and contraception in heart disease is discussed in detail in Chapter 14.6, but the risk of pregnancy in congenital heart disease ranges from being the same as that of the general population to a 50% risk of maternal death in pulmonary hypertension. Each patient requires specialist individual assessment before embarking on pregnancy. An outline of the risks associated with different conditions is shown in Table 16.12.8: it should be remembered that risks are additive, so a repaired septal defect with poor ventricular function moves from a low-risk to high-risk category.

Two principles should be remembered when considering contraceptive options: efficacy of the method, and cardiovascular safety of the method. The risk of oestrogen-containing preparations (which include the combined oral contraceptive pill) relates to their thrombogenicity. Patients at risk of intracardiac or pulmonary thrombosis and those with right-to-left shunts should not use these preparations. Progestogen-only preparations are safe in cardiac disease, but the mode of delivery may carry risk. For example—as stated earlier in this chapter—insertion of a progestogen-eluting intrauterine device (Mirena) carries a risk of vasovagal syncope in nulliparous women, a reaction that can provoke cardiovascular collapse in cyanotic or

post-Fontan patients. In addition, although the progestogen-only 'minipill' is safe, its efficacy is poor. The newer progestogen-only pill Cerazette combines cardiovascular safety with an efficacy equal to that of the combined pill. Other safe and effective methods useful for most women with cardiac disease are the subdermal implant Implanon and the injectable DepoProvera.

Bacterial endocarditis

Endocarditis is discussed in Chapter 16.9.2; the risks for specific congenital lesions are outlined in Table 16.12.9.

Further reading

Anderson RH, Becker AE (1997). *Controversies in the description of congenitally malformed hearts.* Imperial College Press, London.
Campbell M (1970). Natural history of coarctation of the aorta. *Br Heart J,* **32**, 633–640.

Campbell M (1970). Natural history of atrial septal defect. *Br Heart J*, **32**, 820–6.

Cherian G, *et al.* (1983). Pulmonary hypertension in isolated atrial septal defect. *Am Heart J*, **105**, 952–7.

Clapp S, *et al.* (1990). Down's syndrome, complete AV canal and pulmonary vascular obstructive disease. *J Thorac Cardiovasc Surg*, **100**, 115–21.

Del Sette M, *et al.* (1998). Migraine with aura and right-to-left shunt on trancranial Doppler: a case-control study. *Cerebrovasc Dis*, **8**, 327–30.

Diller GP, *et al.* (2006). Presentation, survival prospects and predictors of death in Eisenmenger syndrome: a combined retrospective and case-control study. *Eur Heart J*, **27**, 1737–42.

Driscoll DJ, *et al.* (1992). Five to fifteen year follow-up after Fontan operation. *Circulation*, **85**, 469–96.

Dupuis C, *et al.* (1992). The 'adult' form of the scimitar syndrome. *Am J Cardiol*, **70**, 502–7.

Fyfe A, *et al.* (2005). Cyanotic congenital heart disease and coronary artery atherogenesis. *Am J Cardiol*, **96**, 283–90.

Hagen PT, Scholz DG, Edwards WD. (1984). Incidence and size of patent foramen ovale during the first 10 decades of life: an autopsy study of 965 normal hearts. *Mayo Clin Proc*, **59**, 17–20.

Harinck E, *et al.* (1996). Air travel and adults with cyanotic congenital heart disease. *Circulation*, **93**, 272–6.

Ho SY, *et al.* (1995). *Colour atlas of congenital heart disease. Morphological and clinical correlations.* Mosby-Wolfe, London.

Khairy P, O'Donnell CP, Landzberg MJ. (2003). Transcatheter closure versus medical therapy of patent foramen ovale and presumed paradoxical thromboemboli: a systematic review. *Ann Intern Med*, **139**, 753–**0**.

Kirklin JW, Barratt-Boyes BG (1993). *Cardiac surgery*, 2nd edition. Churchill Livingstone, New York.

Koller M, Rothlin M, Senning Å (1987). Coarctation of the aorta: review of 362 operated patients. Long term follow up and assessment of prognostic variables. *Eur Heart J*, **8**, 670–9.

Konstanides S, *et al.* (1995). A comparison of surgical and medical therapy for atrial septal defects in adults. *New Engl J Med*, **333**, 469–73.

MacMahon B, McKeown T, Record RG (1953). The incidence and life expectation of children with congenital heart disease. *Br Heart J*, **15**, 121–9.

Moodie DS, Ritter DJ, Tajik AJ, O'Fallon WM (1984). Long term follow up in the unoperated univentricular heart. *Am J Cardiol*, **53**, 1124–8.

Moon RE, Camporesi EM, Kissolo JA (1989). Patent foramen ovale and decompression sickness in divers. *Lancet*, **i**, 513–14.

Murphy JG, *et al.* (1993). Long-term outcome in patients undergoing surgical repair of tetralogy of Fallot. *New Engl J Med*, **329**, 593–9.

Overell JR, Bone I, Kees KR (2000). Interatrial septal abnormalities and stroke: a meta-analysis of case-control studies. *Neurology*, **55**, 1172–9.

Perloff JK (1994). *The clinical recognition of congenital heart disease*, pp. 293–380. W B Saunders, Philadelphia.

Perloff JK, Child JS (1998). *Congenital heart disease in adults*. B Saunders, Philadelphia.

Redington AN, *et al.* (1998). *The right heart in congenital heart disease.* Greenwich Medical Media, London.

Roberts WC (1986). Major anomalies of coronary arterial origin seen in adulthood. *Am Heart J*, **111**, 941–62.

Sarris GE, *et al.* (2006). European Congenital Heart Surgeons Association. Results of surgery for Ebstein anomaly: a multicentre study from the European Congenital Heart Surgeons Association. *J Thorac Cardiovasc Surg*, **32**, 50–7.

Schamroth CL, *et al.* (1987). Pulmonary arterial thrombosis in secundum atrial septal defect. *Am J Cardiol*, **60**, 1152–6.

Stark J, de Leval MR (eds) (1994). *Surgery for congenital heart defects*. W B Saunders, London.

Thorne SA (1998). Management of polycythaemia in adults with cyanotic congenital heart disease. *Heart*, **79**, 315–16.

Thorne S, MacGregor A, Nelson-Piercy C (2006). Risks of contraception and pregnancy in heart disease. *Heart*, **92**, 1520–5.

Warnes CA (2006). Transposition of the great arteries. *Circulation*, **114**, 2699–2709.

Wood P (1958). Eisenmenger syndrome: or pulmonary hypertension with reversed central shunt. *Br Med J*, **ii**, 701–709, 755–762.

16.13

Coronary heart disease

Contents

16.13.1 Biology and pathology of atherosclerosis

Clare Dollery and Peter Libby

Essentials

Atherosclerosis is a systemic inflammatory disease. The initial steps of atherogenesis involve cholesterol accumulation in the intima that is thought to mediate recruitment of inflammatory leucocytes, followed by development of a fibro-fatty plaque comprising a lipid core and macrophages that ultimately evolve into lipid-rich foam cells.

Initiation of atheroma

Lipoprotein particles accumulate in the arterial intima soon after initiation of hypercholesterolaemia and undergo oxidative and other chemical modifications that can confer proinflammatory properties such as induction of adhesion molecules that mediate leucocyte adherence.

During the initial phases of atherogenesis, endothelial cells express molecules such as vascular cell-adhesion molecule-1 (VCAM-1) in a patchy distribution that reflects the ultimate location of arterial plaques.

Oxidized low-density lipoprotein (LDL) in the arterial intima can mediate other proinflammatory effects, such as (1) stimulating endothelial and smooth muscle cells to produce potent chemokines, which can encourage adherent leucocytes to migrate through the endothelium into the arterial intima to initiate plaque formation; (2) activating leucocytes after their recruitment into the plaque, leading to the production of further inflammatory molecules, such as cytokines, and small molecules, such as biologically active eicosanoids.

Antiatherogenic processes oppose this potent cocktail of proatherogenic events, including reverse cholesterol transport—whereby high-density lipoproteins (HDL) unload cholesterol from lipid-laden plaque macrophages and carry it away from the arterial wall for breakdown and disposal.

Evolution of atheroma

Inflammatory monocytes and T cells enter the arterial wall along a chemokine gradient, forming the earliest microscopic lesion of atheroma. The recruited monocytes mature into macrophages, promoting expression of the scavenger receptors that permit the unregulated uptake of cholesterol-laden, modified, lipoprotein particles and leading them to become foam cells, which form a small fatty streak that progresses gradually to become an atheromatous plaque.

As the fatty streak matures, the smooth muscle cells produce extracellular matrix and the fibrous components that produce the characteristic structure of a subendothelial fibrous cap overlying a lipid-rich core and deeper islands of smooth muscle cells and macrophages. Events within the atheromatous plaque are complex: endothelial cells form internal, immature, leaky haemorrhage-prone microvessels that provide a new site for entry into the lesion of inflammatory monocytes that perpetuate the atherosclerotic process; they also present a potential site for the intraplaque bleeding associated with plaque progression. Some plaques show deposition of calcium over time in a process similar to bone mineralization.

Atheromatous plaques are unpredictable—atheroma progresses through very gradual cellular accumulation, as described above, punctuated by crises that promote lesion development. These crises may occur when a plaque erodes or ruptures, exposing its thrombogenic core and causing sudden, partial luminal thrombosis.

Acute coronary syndromes

Acute coronary syndromes follow sudden thrombotic events related to the exposure of circulating platelets to thrombogenic components of the plaque via either superficial erosions or rupture of the plaque's fibrous cap. Careful anatomopathological study has given rise to the concept of the 'vulnerable' plaque—an intact plaque similar to those present beneath the site of a fatal coronary thrombosis that is characterized by a thin fibrous cap, a relative paucity of smooth muscle cells, and an abundance of inflammatory cells, particularly macrophages. Plaques that rupture are not necessarily those that cause high-grade stenoses: intravascular ultrasound studies and autopsy data show that many individuals have multiple high-risk or vulnerable plaques as well as ruptured plaques, causing symptomatic or fatal acute coronary syndromes.

Introduction

Cardiovascular disease—already the leading cause of death in Europe (4.35 million/year) and the United States of America (2600/day)—will probably become the leading cause of death worldwide. Atherosclerosis causes about one-half of these deaths from coronary heart disease and one-third from stroke. In the face of this growing threat to the world's health, researchers are working to develop a greater understanding of the mechanisms of atheromatous vascular disease.

According to the traditional view, atherosclerosis resulted from storage of excessive cholesterol in the arterial intima, forming atheromatous lesions that would eventually lead to stenosis, causing symptoms of angina, or ultimately occlusion, causing myocardial infarction. This concept disregarded the common clinical scenario of myocardial infarction or sudden cardiac death as a first manifestation of coronary atherosclerosis without premonitory ischaemic signs or symptoms. Moreover, evidence accumulated from autopsy and clinical studies showed that only 25 to 33% of lethal coronary thrombi occurred at sites of the most stenotic segments in the infarct-related artery. The discrepancy between the substantial benefits of cholesterol-lowering therapies in altering cardiovascular event rates in the face of minimal changes in severity of coronary stenoses fuelled further doubts about this concept of atherogenesis (Fig. 16.13.1. 1).

Today we appreciate a more complex interaction between critical cells of the artery wall and the blood, which helps us better understand the molecular messages they exchange. Our current knowledge supports the theory of inflammation as the driving force behind initiation, progression, and catastrophic thrombotic complications of atherosclerosis. These three phases may occur simultaneously in the arterial tree of an individual, illustrating the nonlinear nature of atherogenesis. Recent studies reveal that patients with acute coronary syndromes may have more than one potentially unstable lesion in addition to the culprit responsible for the acute presentation. These changes in our view of atherogenesis favour the concept of atherosclerosis as a systemic inflammatory disease in which acute revascularization may accomplish important relief of ischaemia due to fixed stenoses and limit damage during ST-segmented elevation myocardial infarction, but does not address the underlying processes governing the condition. Here we review the evolving concepts of pathophysiology of atheroma that help us understand the disease and approach patient diagnosis and management more rationally than in the past.

The normal vessel wall

Diet and lifestyle in the Western world have rendered the normal artery relatively rare outside childhood. Arteries comprise three concentric layers—the tunica intima, tunica media, and adventitia (Fig. 16.13.1.2).

The intima

The innermost layer—the intima—consists of a thin layer of endothelial cells that form the critical interface with the circulating blood. In healthy vessels, endothelial cells produce nitric oxide (NO) to maintain the arterial bed in a continuous state of relaxation, resist thrombosis and limit inflammation: 'atheroprotective' functions often lost in arteries subjected to risk factors for atherosclerosis or disturbed local flow. Endothelial cells also powerfully resist blood clot formation by expressing heparan sulphate proteoglycans on their surface and producing endogenous fibrinolytic agents such as tissue and urokinase plasminogen activators. The endothelium rests on a basement membrane of nonfibrillar collagens such as laminin and type IV collagen, but with age the intima may thicken and incorporate more complex fibrillar collagens (I and III) elaborated by smooth muscle cells.

The tunica media

The media comprises a layer of smooth muscle cells and extracellular matrix, which differs in large and small arteries. The larger vessels have multiple elastin-rich laminae interspersed with smooth muscle cells, while smaller vessels lack these elastic layers, enmeshing the cells directly in the matrix. In both types of arteries, endothelial and smooth muscle cells proliferate very slowly if at all, and, importantly, a balance prevails between extracellular matrix synthesis and breakdown, which preserves the vessel's structural integrity. The external elastic lamina borders the media and demarcates the outer layer of the artery, the adventitia.

The adventitia

This last layer of the arterial wall contains a loose mesh of collagen fibrils encompassing the vaso vasorum, the nerve supply to the vessel wall, and cells such as fibroblasts and mast cells. Long neglected in comparison to the other layers of the vessel wall, the adventitia has become the focus of more studies, particularly in light of the recognition of the importance of neovascularization in plaque stability.

For fuller discussion of the biology of blood vessels and the endothelium, see Chapter 16.1.1.

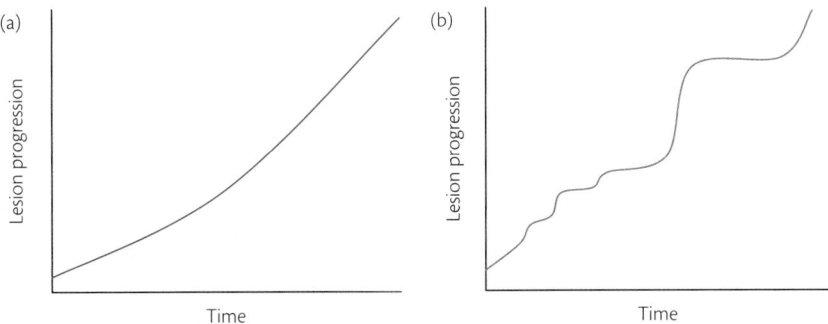

Fig. 16.13.1.1 Atherogenesis is not a linear process. Panel A shows the historical view of the time scale of atherogenesis in which a continuous accumulation of cholesterol ultimately leads to arterial occlusion sufficient to cause symptoms of angina or myocardial infarction. Our current concept of atheroma is shown in panel B, where periods of little or no progression are interspersed with crises such as plaque rupture in which thrombosis leads to sudden increases in plaque burden. Increases in plaque size do not necessarily lead to changes in degree of stenosis due to positive remodelling.

Initiation of atheroma

Atherogenesis and risk factors for coronary disease

The initial steps to atherogenesis involve cholesterol accumulation in the intima that is thought to mediate recruitment of inflammatory leucocytes followed by development of a fibro-fatty plaque comprising a lipid core and macrophages that will ultimately evolve into lipid-rich foam cells (Fig. 16.13.1.3). Pivotal observational studies in the United Kingdom, Europe, and the United States of America have improved our understanding of risk factors for coronary heart disease such as hypercholesterolaemia, cigarette smoking, hypertension, and diabetes, but the biological links between these risk factors and the pathobiology of atheroma remain incompletely understood.

Hyperlipidaemia links consistently with human and experimental atheroma. Many atherogenesis studies use mice with genetic modification that causes profound dyslipidaemia to stimulate rapid atherogenesis. Studies of such atherosclerosis-prone animals show that lipoprotein particles accumulate in the arterial intima soon after initiation of hypercholesterolemia. The lipids bind to proteoglycans, prolonging their residence in the intima, a site sequestered from certain plasma antioxidants. There, the retained lipoprotein particles can undergo oxidative and other chemical modifications that can confer proinflammatory properties such as induction of adhesion molecules that mediate leukocyte adherence. Endothelial cells express leucocyte adhesion molecules such as vascular cell adhesion molecule-1 (VCAM-1) during the initial phases of atherogenesis in a patchy distribution, principally at branch points and sites of disturbed flow where there is low shear stress. This nonrandom and discontinuous distribution of VCAM-1 induction reflects the ultimate location of arterial plaques in both animals and humans.

Oxidized low-density lipoprotein (LDL) in the arterial intima can mediate other proinflammatory effects such as stimulating endothelial and smooth muscle cells to produce potent chemokines such as monocyte chemoattractant protein-1 (MCP-1), which can encourage adherent leucocytes to migrate through the endothelium into the arterial intima to initiate plaque formation. Oxidized LDL activates these leucocytes after their recruitment into the plaque and the cells produce further inflammatory molecules such as cytokines and small molecules such as biologically active eicosanoids.

Hypertension may exert some of its deleterious effects on the vasculature via angiotensin II, which can promote production of reactive oxygen species and mediate expression of adhesion molecules on endothelial cells, encouraging leucocyte recruitment. In addition, angiotensin II can advance plaque formation by making smooth muscle cells express chemoattractants such as MCP-1 and proinflammatory cytokines such as interleukin-6 (IL-6).

Diabetes confers substantial cardiovascular risk, and individuals may often have additional risk factors such as hypertension and hyperlipidaemia. Oxidative stress, hyperglycemia, and development of advanced glycation products may enhance inflammation in diabetic vasculopathy. Products of advanced glycation, for example, can promote the release of proinflammatory atherogenic soluble CD40L from megakaryocytes *in vitro*. Whether good glycaemic control can reduce inflammation and/or reduce

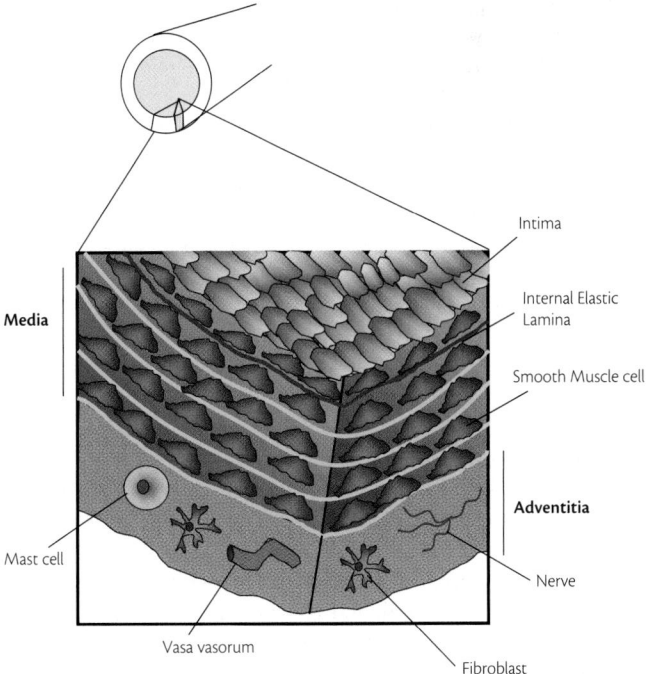

Fig. 16.13.1.2 Structure of the normal artery—a normal elastic artery is shown with the typical cellular constituents of the intima, media, and adventitia.

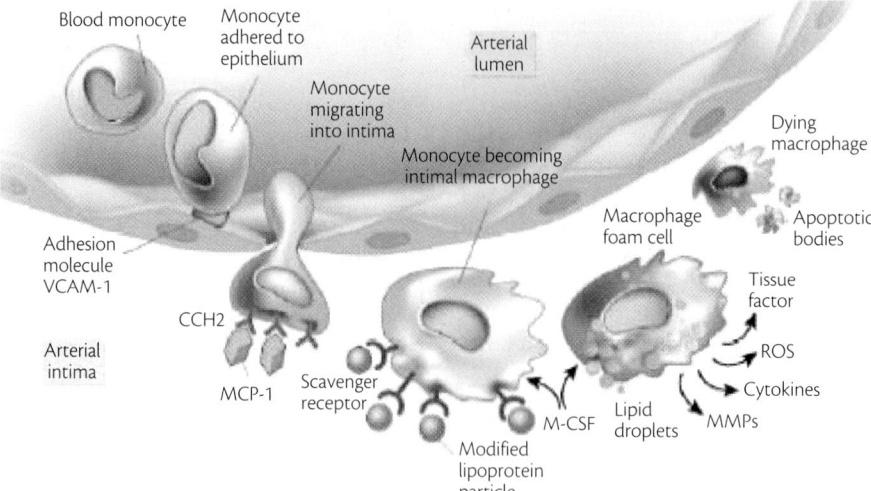

Fig. 16.13.1.3 Mononuclear phagocytes in atherogenesis. This figure schematizes steps in the recruitment of mononuclear phagocytes to the nascent atherosclerotic plaque and some of the functions of these cells in the mature atheroma. The steps are depicted in an approximate time sequence proceeding from left to right. The normal arterial endothelium resists prolonged contact with leukocytes including the blood monocyte. When endothelial cells undergo inflammatory activation, they increase their expression of various leucocyte adhesion molecules. In the context of monocyte recruitment to the atheroma, vascular cell adhesion molecule-1 (VCAM-1) seems to have a major role. Once adherent to the activated endothelial layer, the monocyte diapedeses between intact endothelial cells to penetrate into the tunica intima, or the innermost layer of the arterial wall. This directed migration requires a chemoattractant gradient. Various chemokines seem to participate in this process, particularly interaction of monocyte chemoattractant protein-1 (MCP-1) with its receptor CCR2. Once resident in the intima, the monocyte acquires characteristics of the tissue macrophage. In the atheroma in particular, the macrophage expresses scavenger receptors that bind internalized lipoprotein particles, modified e.g. by oxidation or glycation. These processes give rise to the arterial foam cell, a hallmark of the arterial lesion, so named because of its foamy appearance under the microscope, which is the result of accumulation of lipid droplets within the cytoplasm. Within the arterial intima, the macrophage serves many functions related to atherosclerosis and its complications. Notably, the foam cell secretes pro-inflammatory cytokines that amplify the local inflammatory response in the lesion, as well as reactive oxygen species. The activated mononuclear phagocyte has a key role in the thrombotic complications of atherosclerosis by producing matrix metalloproteinases (MMPs) that can degrade extracellular matrix that lends strength to the plaque's fibrous cap. When the plaque ruptures as a consequence, it permits the blood to contact another macrophage product, the potent procoagulant protein tissue factor. Eventually the macrophages congregate in a central core in the typical atherosclerotic plaque. Macrophages can die in this location, some by apoptosis, hence producing the so-called 'necrotic core' of the atherosclerotic lesion. M-CSF, macrophage colony stimulating factor; ROS, reactive oxygen species; VCAM, vascular cell adhesion molecule.
Reprinted by permission from Macmillan Publishers Ltd: *Nature* 40(6917):868–74, copyright (2002).

vascular events in diabetes remains controversial. Agonists of the peroxisome proliferator-activated receptor (PPAR)-α and PPAR-γ nuclear receptors have attracted interest as regulators of key metabolic pathways that may regulate inflammation in diabetes. Human trials have not yet demonstrated that drugs targeting these nuclear receptors reduce cardiovascular disease.

Coronary artery disease affecting transplanted hearts represents an extreme case of atherogenesis accelerated by adaptive immune responses. Recent reviews have highlighted the features of this disease compared to the more common native atherosclerosis.

Leucocyte recruitment

Recruitment of leucocytes into the developing atherosclerotic plaque provides the building blocks for intense local inflammation. Expression of adhesion molecules such as VCAM-1 on the vascular endothelial cells provides the anchor for leucocytes to attach to the vessel wall via their surface very late antigen 4 (VLA4). Mice deficient in important adhesion molecules such as selectins or expressing dysfunctional truncated VCAM-1 exhibit reduced severity of atheroma. After adhesion, locally produced chemokines such as MCP-1 can attract the leucocyte into the vessel wall. Monocytes participate fundamentally in atherogenesis as they evolve into macrophages that accumulate lipids via their scavenger receptors and become lipid-rich foam cells. These foam cells can produce abundant proinflammatory cytokines and proteases, which potentially

promote changes in plaque biology that can precipitate clinical events.

Monocytes accumulate continuously in both early and late plaques in hypercholesterolemic mice, suggesting that leucocyte recruitment reflects an ongoing dynamic process rather than an early trigger of atheroma. Specific monocyte subsets have particular propensity to enter plaques, and certain chemokine receptors (CCR2 and CX3C-chemokine receptor 1) participate in this trafficking. These receptors may form important therapeutic targets, particularly CX3C chemokine receptor 1, which appears more specific to atheroma than general inflammation. The recruitment of monocytes into established plaques in both early and advanced atheroma suggests that modifying the process would require long-term interventions. T cells and mast cells also appear in atherosclerotic plaques, originating not only from the luminal endothelium of the vessel but also from the vasa vasorum that penetrate in to the plaque, probably primarily from the adventitia. Most T cells in the plaque predominantly produce Th1-type cytokines such as interferon-γ (IFN-γ), tumour necrosis factor α (TNFα) and interleukins (IL) 12, 15, and 18. These proatherosclerotic factors promote macrophage activation, production of further Th1 differentiated T cells, protease production and activation, and diminished collagen synthesis and smooth muscle cell proliferation. Long recognized as denizens of the adventitia, and as a small portion of the leucocyte population in plaques, mast cells may also promote atherogenesis, not only by elaborating small-molecule mediators (e.g. histamine), but also proinflammatory cytokines and proteinases.

Cellular senescence

Advanced senescence of white cells of patients with coronary artery disease correlates with adverse outcomes. Telomere (nucleotide repeats on the ends of chromosomes) length reflects cellular senescence, which in youth may be 10 000 to 20 000 base pairs long but which gradually reduces with cell division and age. Endothelial cells from patients with coronary disease have shorter telomeres. In one nested case-control trial of the West of Scotland Primary Prevention Study, shorter mean telomere length not only predicted future coronary events but also indicated who would benefit most from statin treatment. Telomere length may relate to events associated with inflammation in addition to an inherited component (chromosome 12). Senescent arterial endothelial cells express more ICAM-1 and less NO, while oxidative stress accelerates telomere attrition.

Molecular biology of atheroprotection

Antiatherogenic processes oppose this potent cocktail of proatherogenic events. One of the foremost is reverse cholesterol transport—the ability of high-density lipoproteins (HDL) to unload cholesterol from lipid-laden plaque macrophages and carry it away from the arterial wall for breakdown and disposal. The ABCA1 and ABCG1 lipid transporters mediate this process. HDL particles also oppose atherogenesis by reducing cytokine-induced expression of adhesion molecules in endothelial cells and by providing a source of antioxidants such as paroxonase-1 to oppose the proinflammatory effects of phospholipids. HDL also interacts with NO, increasing production and activation of the enzyme nitric oxide synthase. In turn, NO dilates arteries, opposes leucocyte recruitment into the vessel wall, and combats platelet aggregation. As NO production and stability increase at sites of laminar shear stress, the atheroprotective properties of this gas may in part explain the predilection of regions of disturbed flow to atheroma formation.

The immune system can also defend against atherosclerosis. While adaptive immunity mediated by T cells secreting Th1 type cytokines (e.g. interferon-γ) can aggravate atherosclerosis, Th2 cells (in addition to platelets, macrophages, endothelial cells, and smooth muscle cells) produce antiatherogenic cytokines such as IL-10 and TGFβ. Gain of function or loss of function experiments in atherosclerotic mice have shown a clear atheroprotective role for IL10. In studies of mice with T cells expressing dominant negative TGFβ receptors, two models exhibited marked inflammation and poor matrix formation after prevention of this cytokine's T-cell-related functions, thus supporting a role for TGFβ in T-cell-mediated suppression of inflammation. TGFβ stimulates collagen production, and these studies also demonstrate its role in enhancing features of plaques linked to resistance to rupture. Humoral immunity can also mitigate atherosclerosis: for example, administration of antibodies raised against oxidized LDL can reduce atherosclerosis, and interference with B cell function can promote lesion formation.

Evolution of atheroma

In the earliest stage of atheroma, LDL particles accumulate in the arterial intima and undergo oxidation as described above. Products of LDL oxidation in turn stimulate endothelial cells to express vital adhesion molecules such as ICAM and VCAM. Inflammatory monocytes and T cells begin to roll along the arterial wall and adhere to the now 'sticky' endothelium. These white cells then enter the arterial wall along a chemokine gradient, forming the earliest microscopic lesion of atheroma. Factors such as macrophage colony-stimulating factor (M-CSF) cause recruited monocytes to mature into macrophages and promote subsequent expression of the scavenger receptors that permit the unregulated uptake of cholesterol-laden modified lipoprotein particles and become foam cells (so called due to the microscopic foamy appearance of the pool of intracellular lipid). This process repeats itself, amplifying the atherogenic events within the arterial wall. Foam cells form a small fatty streak that progresses gradually to become an atheromatous plaque (Fig. 16.13.1.4).

Smooth muscle cells

The dysfunctional endothelial cell crucially instigates atherogenesis because it recruits cells that mediate inflammation within the wall and has hampered NO production. As the fatty streak matures, the smooth muscle cells and macrophages within the plaque steer much of its subsequent development. While some smooth muscle cells may populate the intima of normal human arteries, intimal inflammation encourages smooth muscle cells from the media to migrate into the intima. The macrophages and foam cells within the plaque secrete chemoattractants such as platelet-derived growth factor (PDGF), which promote smooth muscle cell migration. In contrast to the early response to arterial injury following balloon angioplasty or stenting, proliferation of smooth muscle cells occurs quite slowly in atherosclerosis. Mitoses occur in fewer than 1% of cells in advanced plaques. The combination of smooth muscle cell migration and proliferation during the lengthy development time of atherosclerosis allows smooth muscle cells to contribute to lesion expansion.

Extracellular matrix

The smooth muscle cell produces much of the arterial extracellular matrix, which supplies the fibrous components that add volume to the developing fibro-fatty plaque. The major extracellular matrix macromolecules in plaque include interstitial collagens (types I and III) and proteoglycans such as versican, biglycan, aggrecan, and decorin. Elastin fibres may also accumulate in atherosclerotic plaques and may display more active turnover than previously thought. The matrix components function beyond furnishing a scaffold for the plaque. Some constituents (notably proteoglycans) bind lipoproteins, prolong their residence in the intima, and render them more susceptible to oxidative modification and glycation. The resultant oxidized phospholipids and advanced glycation end-products promote the inflammatory response within the vessel wall, advancing atherogenesis. The matrix can also serve as a storage site for growth factors, and cleaving certain components such as laminin releases sequestered mediators that promote cellular migration. The vascular smooth muscle cell produces these matrix molecules in both diseased and normal arteries. Cytokines such as TGFβ and PDGF derived from T cells, platelets, macrophages, and monocytes stimulate smooth muscle cells to produce excess extracellular matrix. This process not only increases plaque size but also allows the formation of its characteristic structure, with a subendothelial fibrous cap overlying the lipid-rich core and deeper islands of smooth muscle cell macrophages (Fig. 16.13.1.5).

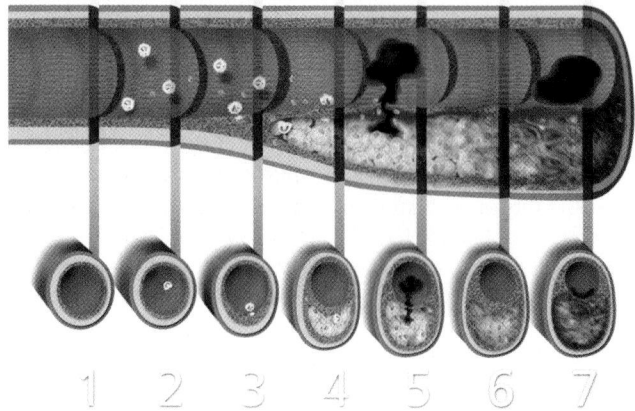

Fig. 16.13.1.4 Initiation, progression, and complication of human coronary atherosclerotic plaque. Top: longitudinal section of artery depicting 'timeline' of human atherogenesis from normal artery (1) to atheroma causing clinical manifestations by thrombosis or stenosis (5, 6, 7). Bottom: cross-sections of artery during various stages of atheroma evolution. 1. Normal artery. Note that in human arteries, the intimal layer is much better developed than in most other species; the intima of human arteries contains resident smooth muscle cells often as early as first year of life. 2. Lesion initiation occurs when endothelial cells, activated by risk factors such as hyperlipoproteinemia, express adhesion and chemoattractant molecules that recruit inflammatory leucocytes such as monocytes and T lymphocytes. Extracellular lipid begins to accumulate in the intima at this stage. 3. Evolution to fibro-fatty stage. Monocytes recruited to the artery wall become macrophages and express scavenger receptors that bind modified lipoproteins. Macrophages become lipid-laden foam cells by engulfing modified lipoproteins. Leucocytes and resident vascular wall cells can secrete inflammatory cytokines and growth factors that amplify leucocyte recruitment and cause smooth muscle cell migration and proliferation. 4. As the lesion progresses, inflammatory mediators cause expression of tissue factor, a potent procoagulant, and of matrix-degrading proteinases that weaken fibrous cap of plaque. 5. If the fibrous cap ruptures at the point of weakening, coagulation factors in blood can gain access to the lipid core which contains thrombogenic tissue factor, causing thrombosis on nonocclusive atherosclerotic plaque. If the balance between prothrombotic and fibrinolytic mechanisms prevailing at that particular region and at that particular time is unfavourable, occlusive thrombus causing acute coronary syndromes may result. 6. When thrombus resorbs, products associated with thrombosis such as thrombin and mediators are released from degranulating platelets, including platelet-derived growth factor and transforming growth factor β, can cause healing response, leading to increased collagen accumulation and smooth muscle cell growth. In this manner, the fibro-fatty lesion can evolve into advanced fibrous and often calcified plaque, one that may cause significant stenosis, and produce symptoms of stable angina pectoris. 7. In some cases, occlusive thrombi arise not from fracture of the fibrous cap but from superficial erosion of the endothelial layer. Resulting mural thrombus, again dependent on local prothrombotic and fibrinolytic balance, can cause acute myocardial infarction. Superficial erosions often complicate advanced and stenotic lesions, as shown here. However, superficial erosions do not necessarily occur after fibrous cap rupture, as depicted in this idealized diagram.
Libby P, *Current Concepts of the Pathogenesis of the Acute Coronary Syndromes, Circulation*, 104 (3):365–372.

Matrix breakdown also participates in plaque progression. Catabolism of extracellular matrix macromolecules at the leading edge of inflammatory monocytes, macrophages, and smooth muscle cells probably facilitates their migration into the intima. In the arterial wall there is a delicate balance between matrix breakdown and synthesis. Four groups of proteases within the vasculature break down the extracellular matrix: metalloproteinases (MMPs), cysteine proteases, serine proteases, and the newest group, distintegrin metalloproteases (or ADAMs). Tight regulation of proteases happens not only at transcriptional level but also through activation, in the case of the metalloproteinases, and endogenous inhibitors. For example, the tissue inhibitors of the metalloproteinases oppose the actions of the MMPs while cystatin C hinders the cysteine proteases such as the cathepsins.

Cell death in the plaque

The importance of programmed cell death within the plaque is increasingly recognized. In more advanced atheromatous plaques, fragmentation of smooth muscle cell DNA occurs, suggesting apoptotic cell death. Proinflammatory T cells may mediate these events because they prompt expression of Fas, which can bind Fas ligand on the smooth muscle cell surface, promoting cell death. The death of lipid-laden macrophages can lead to extracellular deposition of tissue factor (TF), some in particulate form. The extracellular lipid that accumulates in the intima can coalesce and form the classic lipid-rich 'necrotic' core of the atherosclerotic plaque.

Neovascularization

As plaques develop, smooth muscle cells and macrophages are not the only cell types to proliferate. Oxidized phospholipids within the plaque can stimulate the production of important angiogenic factors such as vascular endothelial growth factor (VEGF) isoforms in both monocytes and endothelial cells. Endothelial cells then form immature, leaky, haemorrhage-prone microvessels within the plaque. These neovessels provide a new site for entry into the lesion of inflammatory monocytes that perpetuate the atherosclerotic process. The microvessels also present a potential site for the intraplaque bleeding associated with plaque progression. Haem-derived iron deposited extracellularly due to haemorrhage in plaques from disrupted microvessels can catalyse reactions that form reactive oxygen species that promote oxidative stress in plaques.

Plaque calcification

Some plaques show deposition of calcium over time in a process similar to bone mineralization. Some smooth muscle cells elaborate bone morphogenic proteins related to TGFβ. Plaque calcification, even when microscopic, can produce biomechanical changes in plaques that prompt clinical complications. Quantitation of plaque calcification by radiographic techniques may provide a noninvasive

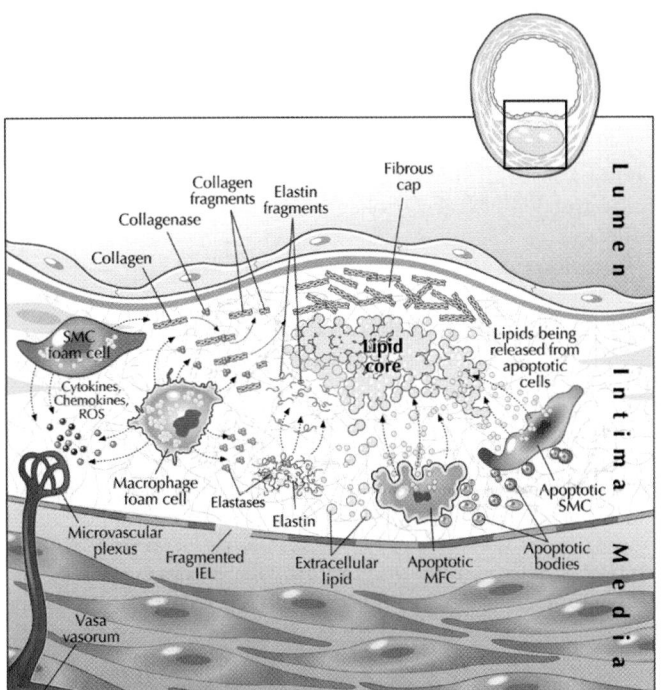

Fig. 16.13.1.5 Maturation of the atherosclerotic plaque. More mature lesions develop a fibrous cap composed of a dense extracellular matrix containing collagen and elastin. Underneath the fibrous cap, a lipid core forms that contains many macrophages, dead or dying macrophages, cellular debris including apoptotic bodies, and extracellular lipid accumulations. Proinflammatory mediators released from activated white cells and endothelial cells and smooth muscle cells (SMC) can potentiate cell death by apoptosis in the advancing lesion. As SMCs die within lesions, fewer remain to renew the extracellular matrix in the plaque's fibrous cap. Activated cells in the lesion, notably the macrophages, secrete proteinases that can degrade the macromolecules of the extracellular matrix, thus weakening the fibrous cap. Elastases can break down elastin required for migration of cells within the lesion, and arterial remodelling occurs during compensatory enlargement, and in the extreme, aneurysm formation. During this phase of atherogenesis neovessels form in the intima, often arising as extensions of vasa vasorum that originate in the adventitial layer. IEL, internal elastic lamina; MFC, macrophage foam cell; ROS, reactive oxygen species.
Reprinted from JACC, 48 (9), Libby P and Ridker PM, *Inflammation and Atherothrombosis: From Population Biology and Bench Research to Clinical Practice*, ppA33–46. Copyright (2006), with permission from the American College of Cardiology.

assessment of plaque burden. Whether calcium scores provide important prognostic information beyond risk prediction algorithms that do not require imaging remains a matter of debate.

Arterial calcification accelerates in patients with hypercalcaemia related to renal disease in which coronary calcification can affect up to 88% of 20- to 30-year-olds on dialysis, compared to 5% in an age-matched control group. Coronary calcification in renal failure correlates with adverse prognosis. Atherosclerosis of renal failure has features distinct from coronary disease in the general population but still represents the same disease.

Disease progression and positive remodelling

Some of the pathological events associated with atheroma described above suggest a gradual inevitability in progressive arterial stenosis. This model does not fit the pattern seen in experimental or clinical settings. Rather, atheroma progresses through very gradual cellular accumulation punctuated by crises that promote lesion development. These crises may occur when a plaque erodes or ruptures, exposing its

thrombogenic core and causing sudden partial luminal thrombosis. These ruptures probably occur frequently and very often remain subclinical. The healing phase that follows may involve further smooth muscle cell proliferation and matrix deposition, which may stabilize but also enlarge the plaque and promote stenosis by constrictive remodelling. In this respect, a plaque is like the cinder cone of an active volcano, which expands with each small eruption but whose size alone does not help predict a catastrophic eruption.

The lack of correlation between pre-existing plaque size and future coronary events also relates to positive remodelling within the arterial wall. Interventional angiographically based therapies for coronary artery disease (see Chapter 16.13.6) depend only on the luminal size when assessing lesion severity. This approach allows relevant therapy to treat the often relatively fibrous occlusive lesions that cause stable angina. However, intravascular ultrasound studies have shown that larger areas of plaque burden may exist in regions of the arteries with little or no luminal stenosis. Compensatory outward expansion of the artery's external elastic lamina can accommodate plaques with large lipid cores that do not appear on angiogram but may nonetheless rupture suddenly, causing thrombus formation and acute coronary syndromes.

Acute coronary syndromes

Acute coronary syndromes form an increasingly large part of the clinical manifestation of coronary artery disease and comprise unstable angina (angina of increasing frequency and severity), non-ST elevation myocardial infarction, and ST elevation myocardial infarction. These definitions have evolved as our ability to detect myocardial necrosis through biomarkers such as troponin I and T has become more sensitive and moves beyond definitions based on the ECG. Acute coronary syndromes follow sudden thrombotic events related to exposure of circulating platelets to thrombogenic components of the plaque via either superficial erosions or rupture of the plaque's fibrous cap (Fig. 16.13.1.6).

Plaque erosion

Understanding of the mechanisms of plaque erosion has lagged behind that of plaque rupture. Plaque erosion comprises an acute thrombus in direct contact with the intima in an area absent of endothelium. The crucial event appears to be endothelial loss, which follows either apoptosis of endothelial cells or shedding of cells from the basement membrane via the action of proteases such as gelatinases on type IV collagen or other components of the basement membrane upon which endothelial cells rest. Coronary vasospasm may explain the observed lack of endothelium and intact, relatively thick media at erosion sites compared to sites of plaque rupture. Sites of plaque erosion may not exhibit prominent macrophage and lymphocyte accumulation. The underlying plaque in erosions consists of a thickened intima or fibrous cap atheroma, and lesions may be eccentric or calcified. Plaque erosion is found in 20% of all sudden deaths and in 40% of coronary thrombi in patients dying suddenly with coronary artery atherosclerosis. Fatal thrombosis due to plaque erosion associates with smoking, especially in women. Compared to fibrous cap rupture, death due to plaque erosion occurs more often in younger individuals and may affect less severely narrowed arteries at the site of fatal thrombosis. Plaque erosion accounts for more than 80% of thrombi occurring in women less than 50 years of age.

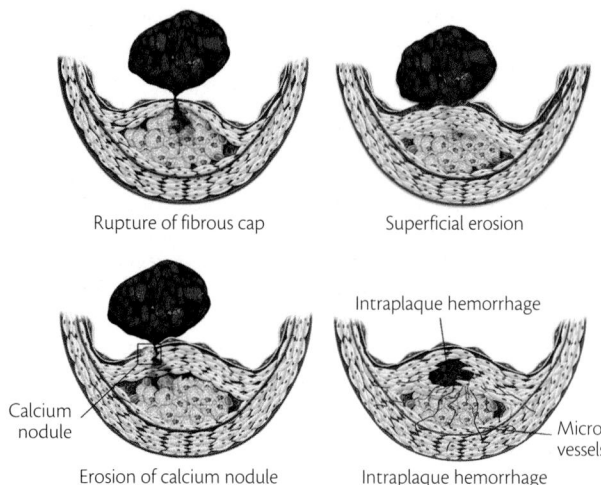

Fig. 16.13.1.6 Microanatomy of coronary arterial thrombosis and acute occlusion. Rupture of fibrous cap (upper left) causes some two-thirds to three-quarters of fatal coronary thromboses. Superficial erosion (upper right) occurs in one-fifth to one-quarter of all cases of fatal coronary thromboses. Certain populations such as diabetic individuals and women appear more susceptible to superficial erosion as mechanism of plaque disruption and thrombosis. Erosion of a calcium nodule may also cause plaque disruption and thrombosis (lower left). In addition, friable microvessels in the base of atherosclerotic plaque may rupture and cause intraplaque haemorrhage. Consequent local generation of thrombin may stimulate SMC proliferation, migration, and collagen synthesis, promoting fibrosis and plaque expansion on subacute basis. Severe intraplaque haemorrhage can cause sudden lesion expansion by mass effect acutely as well.
Libby P, Theroux P, *Pathophysiology of Coronary Artery Disease, Circulation*, 11 (25):3481–3488.

Plaque rupture

Careful anatomopathological study has given rise to the concept of the 'vulnerable' plaque—an intact plaque similar to those present beneath the site of a fatal coronary thrombosis. A thin fibrous cap, a relative paucity of smooth muscle cells, and an abundance of inflammatory cells, particularly macrophages, characterize plaques that have provoked fatal coronary thrombosis. The plaques have a lipid core of variable size formed of foam cells and debris from dead or dying phagocytes that deposited their cholesterol into the plaque. Deposition of cholesterol-rich red cell membranes due to intraplaque haemorrhages from fragile neovessels may also contribute to formation of the plaque's lipid core. These atheromatous, lipid-rich plaques, distinct from more fibrous and often highly calcified plaques, have shoulder regions where macrophages and T cells accumulate relatively close to the fibrous cap and lumen of the vessel.

The small number of smooth muscle cells likely contributes to the lack of extracellular matrix and the more meager fibrous cap. The interstitial collagens (types I and II) would normally confer mechanical stability on the plaque, but IFN-γ derived from T cells and macrophages reduces production of these structural plaque components in areas of inflammation. IFN-γ also inhibits smooth muscle cell proliferation, contributing further to the lack of smooth muscle cells and matrix in these plaques.

Matrix breakdown within the fibrous cap that reveals the thrombogenic core may trigger rupture, and interstitial collagenase MMP-1, as well as MMP-2, MMP-3, MMP-9, and tissue inhibitors of MMPs (TIMP-1 and TIMP-2), localize in plaques. Shoulder regions of carotid plaques have abundant foam cells, show evidence

of collagenolysis in situ, and express MMPs -9, -3, and -1. MMPs colocalize with intraplaque haemorrhages, areas of increased wall stress in human atheroma, and occur in plaques with histological features associated with vulnerability. The interstitial collagenases (MMP-1, -8 and -13) share the unusual ability to initiate collagenolysis by cleaving intact triple helical collagen. MMP collagenases colocalize with cleaved collagen fragments *in situ* in human lesions.

Breakdown of elastin, a structural component of the arterial wall, may be important in expansive and occlusive remodelling. Human atheromata contain smooth muscle-derived cathepsins S, K, and L, potent elastases that localize at sites of breaks in the elastic laminae. Interestingly, normal vessels contain little or no cathepsins, while fatty streaks—thought to be an early stage of atheroma—have widely distributed cathepsins S and K. More advanced atheroma macrophages express these proteinases in addition to cathepsins B, D, and F, which degrade elastin and collagen. Macrophages in the shoulders of human carotid plaques express the serine proteinase known as neutrophil elastase, and CD40L regulates this enzyme. Serine proteases urokinase-type plasminogen activator (uPA) and tissue plasminogen activator (tPA) occur in intimal smooth muscle cells and macrophage-derived foam cells. Macrophages localized on the necrotic core margin express particularly high levels of uPA while both tPA and uPA abound in the neomicrovessels of plaques, suggesting a role in plaque angiogenesis.

CD40L is an important inflammatory mediator that localizes in plaques and promotes proteolysis. Pathological studies of human atheroma and in mice implicate CD40L in atherogenesis and disease progression. Endothelial cells, smooth muscle cells and macrophages all express the CD40 receptor, and its ligation activates these cell types to produce key molecules in atherogenesis such as cytokines IL-1, IL-6, and IL-8 and adhesion molecules ICAM-1, VCAM-1, and E-selectin. CD40L can prompt production of each MMP listed above. It also enhances thrombogenicity by inducing tissue factor expression within the plaque.

A number of processes foster rapid thrombosis following plaque rupture. Exposure of blood to collagen fibres within the disrupted plaque leads to platelet aggregation. Tissue factor produced by smooth muscle cells and macrophages also potently activates the coagulation cascade. This process promotes thrombin generation, which further activates platelets, endothelial cells, smooth muscle cells, and macrophages. These processes within the plaque interact with the blood. Patients with obesity or diabetes exhibit higher circulating levels of plasminogen activator inhibitor-1 (PAI-1), which disrupts fibrinolytic processes. In addition, disrupted plaques or dying endothelial cells may release tissue factor and microparticles bearing this procoagulant into the blood, causing an additional circulating threat. Accordingly, changes in the fluid phase of blood as well as the solid state of the plaque may enhance susceptibility to acute cardiac events.

Vulnerable plaque and the vulnerable patient

The concept of the vulnerable plaque enhances our understanding of atherogenesis and its crises—the acute coronary syndromes. It may, however, have led to an erroneous expectation regarding the potential to identify threatening plaques and deliver local stabilizing agents—perhaps via interventional techniques—that would alter prognosis. Recent clinical trial data confirm that coronary intervention in stable angina does not reduce death, myocardial

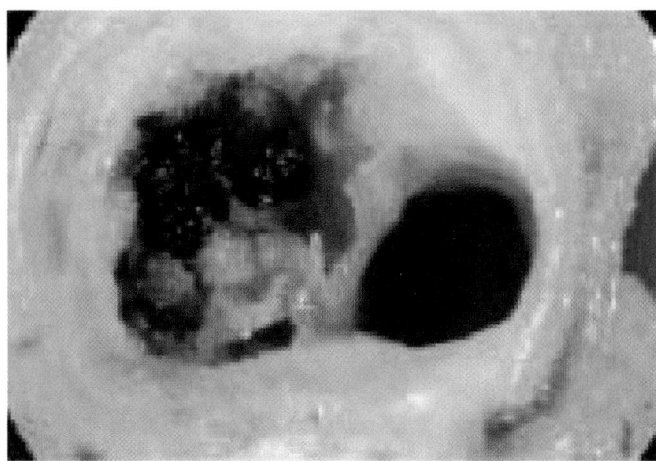

Fig. 16.13.1.7 A plaque 5 days after thrombolysis. There is a cavity containing some residual thrombus which communicates with the arterial lumen via a hole in the plaque cap. The lipid in the core has been washed out *in vivo* to create the cavity.
Reproduced from Davies MJ. Atlas of coronary artery disease, publishers Lippincott-Raven.

infarction, or cardiovascular events compared with optimal medical therapy. These clinical trial results make sense, as plaques that rupture do not necessarily cause the high-grade stenoses that comprise the most appropriate target for revascularization. Both intravascular ultrasound studies and autopsy data also show that many individuals have multiple high-risk or vulnerable plaques as well as ruptured plaques, causing symptomatic or fatal acute coronary syndrome (Fig. 16.13.1.7). Attention now focuses on systemic therapies such as statins, which in animal studies alter the character of plaques to a more fibrous, less inflamed type. Quantitative coronary angiographic studies such as the FATs study show that lovastatin and colestipol versus usual therapy correlates with only a –0.3% change in luminal calibre of the fixed stenoses, but a profound 73% reduction in death, myocardial infarction, or repeat intervention for ischaemia.

Interest now focuses on identifying biomarkers that may predict the vulnerable patient who has a modifiable cardiovascular risk. An increased risk of primary or recurrent vascular events is associated with fibrinogen, IL-1, IL-6, IL-8, myeloperoxidase, MMP-9, sCD40L, lipoprotein-associated phospholipase A$_2$, soluble ICAM-1, VCAM-1, P-selectin, leptin, and adiponectin, in addition to the connection with reduced telomere length previously discussed. C-reactive protein, measured with a high-sensitivity assay, currently constitutes the most clinically practical marker of inflammation. Numerous trials of both primary and secondary prevention of cardiovascular risk have found an association between CRP and cardiovascular risk, although CRP probably does not have a direct pathological role. The current most effective treatments for preventing cardiovascular events—the statins—address not only lipid lowering but also other atherogenic processes implicated in reducing systemic inflammation, and appear to stabilize plaques. Thus, these systemic therapies may protect both the vulnerable plaque and the vulnerable patient.

Further reading

American Heart Association (2005). *Heart disease and stroke statistics 2005—Update.*
Berliner JA, Watson AD (2005). A role for oxidized phospholipids in atherosclerosis. *N Engl J Med*, **353**, 9–11.
Boden WE, *et al.* (2007). Optimal medical therapy with or without PCI for stable coronary disease. *N Engl J Med*, **356**, 1503–16.
Brouilette SW, *et al.* (2007). Telomere length, risk of coronary heart disease, and statin treatment in the West of Scotland Primary Prevention Study: a nested case-control study. *Lancet*, **369**, 107–14.
Brown BG, *et al.* (1993). Lipid lowering and plaque regression. New insights into prevention of plaque disruption and clinical events in coronary disease. *Circulation*, **87**, 1781–91.
Chen CH, Walterscheid JP (2006). Plaque angiogenesis versus compensatory arteriogenesis in atherosclerosis. *Circ Res*, **99**, 787–9.
Dollery CM, Libby P (2006). Atherosclerosis and proteinase activation. *Cardiovasc Res*, **69**, 625–35.
Hackett D, Davies G, Maseri A (1988). Pre-existing coronary stenoses in patients with first myocardial infarction are not necessarily severe. *Eur Heart J*, **9**, 1317–23.
Libby P, Plutzky J (2007). Inflammation in diabetes mellitus: role of peroxisome proliferator-activated receptor-alpha and peroxisome proliferator-activated receptor-gamma agonists. *Am J Cardiol*, **99**, 27B–40B.
Libby P, Theroux P (2005). Pathophysiology of coronary artery disease. *Circulation*, **111**, 3481–8.
Petersen SPV, *et al.* (2005). *European cardiovascular disease statistics 2005.* British Heart Foundation, London.
Rahmani M, *et al.* (2006). Allograft vasculopathy versus atherosclerosis. *Circ Res*, **99**, 801–15.
Virmani R, *et al.* (2006). Pathology of vulnerable plaque. *J Am coll cardiol*, **47**, C13–8.

16.13.2 Coronary heart disease: epidemiology and prevention

Harry Hemingway and Michael Marmot

Essentials

Unlike many medical conditions that are common, disable, and kill, cardiovascular disease (CVD)—already the most common cause of death in the world, and expected to account for a growing proportion of all deaths—is almost entirely preventable.

Socioeconomic factors and habits of society, including (1) a diet high in saturated fat, (2) sedentary living, and (3) smoking, are important underlying determinants of the population rate of coronary disease. Myocardial infarction (MI) mortality rates vary widely between countries (e.g. more than 10-fold higher in Russia than Japan) and change rapidly over time within countries (e.g. 50% decline in 20 years in western Europe; increases in Russia in the 1990s). Coronary heart disease (CHD) is the most common cause of death in women, and while there is a male excess in MI incidence, women are less protected from angina pectoris.

There are strong, unconfounded relationships between several risk factors and CHD mortality and nonfatal myocardial infarction.

Those with the strongest effect are (1) age, (2) country, and (3) presence of symptomatic or preclinical disease. Based on recent individual patient data meta-analysis, systolic blood pressure and cholesterol have a log-linear relation with CHD mortality, with no evidence of lower threshold at every age up to the ninth decade of life. A lower blood pressure is associated with a lower risk, whatever the starting level. The implications of this are profound: shifting the distribution of such a risk factor in the whole population by an apparently small amount has a major effect on population rates of disease, e.g. a 5-mmHg reduction in the population mean systolic blood pressure (e.g. achieved through reductions in dietary salt) is predicted to decrease event rates by 20%.

Observations in cohort studies that specific dietary components—including antioxidant vitamins (A, C, and E), B vitamins, folate, and ω – 3 fats (from fish)—may reduce the rate of coronary events have not been supported by the available randomized trial evidence. Likewise, hormone replacement therapy appeared protective in observational studies, but the Women's Health Initiative and other trials showed that it was not.

Nine simple risk factors together may account for 90% of the population attributable risk of myocardial infarction across 52 countries in the Interheart study. Yet, despite this apparent triumph of explanation, meta-analyses of peripheral blood markers of inflammatory, haemostatic, and other processes support medium to strong associations for a number of novel factors, independent of established risk factors. The causal significance, or the contribution to prediction, of these 'biomarkers' awaits clarification.

Genetic factors—meta-analyses support a small effect of more than 10 common polymorphisms in the aetiology of CHD, although how they interrelate with other genes, or with the environmental factors is not known. Even an apparently 'simple' (one gene, dominant inheritance, and complete penetrance) disorder, familial hypercholesterolaemia, probably has complex interactions with the environment in determining the distal phenotype of premature coronary death.

While simple risk factors combine to predict CHD events in individuals, most events occur among people who are not at high risk. For this reason, treatment of high-risk individuals is a palliative action in public health terms.

A major challenge for CHD epidemiology in the future is to understand the macroeconomic and societal forces which influence population rates in the context of the molecular and genetic mechanisms through which they operate.

Introduction

Diseases desperate grown
By desperate remedy are relieved
Or not at all

Hamlet, Shakespeare

Coronary heart disease (CHD) has, in several senses, grown desperate: from a global perspective, more people are dying from it than ever before, with the largest numbers in India, China, and Russia. For decades we have known the major determinants of the population rate in coronary disease, but for complex reasons this knowledge has not averted exporting the Western epidemic of coronary disease around the world. From the perspective of high-income

countries, more people are living with coronary disease than previously, despite the declines in mortality rate observed in western Europe, North America, and Australia since the late 1960s. From a life-course perspective, coronary disease is a paediatric condition, with atherosclerotic changes established in the first and second decades of life. How desperate that primordial prevention has failed to such an extent that, not only in the United States of America and Europe, but also in China and India, there is an epidemic of obesity.

What then is the epidemiological evidence for remedial strategies aimed at preventing CHD? This chapter has three objectives. First, to understand the implications, societally profound, for 'remedy' which are provided by recent studies of the large variations in population rate of coronary disease between countries, over time, and in different demographic groups. Second, to consider new large-scale evidence for causes, ranging from distal socioeconomic factors through behavioural and psychosocial factors to more proximal causes 'under the skin', including new insights offered by '-omic' disciplines and imaging. Third, to draw implications for national and international public health policy and practice.

Two remedial strategies are required to avert, or mitigate, the onset of coronary disease: population-wide measures which seek to shift the mean distribution of risk factors in the whole population and lower the population rate; and high-risk approaches which seek to identify and modify the behaviour of a minority of individuals (the traditional health care approach).

Historical perspective

Many of the causes put forward for angina pectoris in the century after its first description in 1768 were explored, confirmed, or refuted—at least for myocardial infarction (MI) and coronary death—during the second half of the 20th century, largely through the complementary approaches of observational epidemiological studies and randomized trials (Table 16.13.2.1). For example, Heberden noted patients 'inclining to be fat', while Black in 1819 noted the paradox of the low rates of coronary disease in France, despite their rich diet. This illustrates an important phenomenon (apart from the observation that there are few new ideas!); the natural history of a risk factor hypothesis is long. It is about 100 years since the first blood pressure–mortality relationships were described in large populations. After the Second World War, cohort studies, such as Framingham and Seven Countries, were established as highly successful study designs and reported associations between, literally, hundreds of putative 'risk factors' and coronary events. This is remarkable: the apparent luxury of associations is not found for cancer and other chronic diseases, but poses a challenge—which ones are real and important?

In the 1980s Geoffrey Rose argued that public health importance relates to the mean distribution of risk factors in populations as a whole. By the 1990s it was realized that the now scores of cardiovascular cohort studies were individually small (e.g. reporting only hundreds of events), and might usefully be combined using meta-analytic techniques. In the early 21st century, the exponential proliferation of new information available in large population collections, principally from high-throughput blood-based measures, including single nucleotide polymorphisms (SNPs) and other biomarkers, and imaging capabilities (ultrasound, CT), poses the challenge of how to reconcile the molecular and the macroeconomic influences on coronary disease in populations.

Table 16.13.2.1 Field synopsis of CHD epidemiology: factors associated with CHD aetiology according to their frequency, size of summarized evidence, and relative risk

Size of effect[a]	Risk factor[b]	Definition of high-risk vs low-risk groups[c]	Prevalence of risk group (%)[d]	No. of CHD cases	Relative risk (age adjusted)[e]	Meta-analysis (or large dataset) reference
Very large (RR ≥3.0)	Age	Top vs bottom thirds	33	5070	23	Illustration from male population of Finland aged 40–84 years; approximately one-third of the population is aged 49 years and under, and one-third 59 years and older
	Country	Russia vs Japan	–	10^5	14	Illustration from WHO Mortality database 2002, comparing male rates aged 65–74 years
	Symptomatic disease	Second-year MI survivor vs no MI	5	1237	5	Illustration of 60-year-old British man (Law et al. 2002)
	Preclinical disease					
	Exercise ECG	ST depression vs none	3–16	10^2	2–21	US preventive task force(Fowler-Brown et al. 2004)
	Coronary artery calcium	Agatston score >400 vs 0	20	143	10	Pletcher et al. 2004
Large (RR 1.75–2.99)	Social position	Low vs high education	77–92	263000	1.7	Illustration of women aged 60–74 years (Huisman et al. 2005)
	Sex (MI or CHD death)	Men vs women	50	12292	2.2	Illustration from WHO mortality database, UK age 65–74
	Smoking	Current vs never	20–30	12461	2.9	Interheart (Teo et al. 2006)
	Diabetes	Diabetic vs not	5	7570	2.1	Effect is stronger in women (Huxley et al. 2006)
	Depression	Depressed vs not	15	6362	1.8	Nicholson et al. 2006
	Systolic blood pressure	Top vs bottom third	33	34000	1.9[f]	Prospective studies collaboration (Lewington et al. 2002)
	Cholesterol	Top vs bottom third	33	34000	1.9[f]	Prospective studies collaboration
	ApoB/ApoAI ratio	Top vs bottom third	33	15152	2.5	Interheart (Yusuf et al. 2004)
	Waist-to-hip ratio	Top vs bottom third	33	12461	2.0	Interheart (Yusuf et al. 2005) 1.37 after full adjustment)
	Lipoprotein (a)	Top vs bottom third	33	5436	1.7	Danesh et al. 2000
	Fibrinogen	Top vs bottom third	33	7118	2.3[f]	Danesh et al. 2005
	Creatinine	15–60 ml/min/1.73 m^2 vs >60	8	3262[g]	1.8[f]	In blacks (Weiner et al. 2005)
	Ankle brachial pressure index	<0.9 vs ≥0.9	10	388	2.3	Doobay et al. 2005
Medium (1.30–1.74)	Family history	CVD in first-degree relative vs none	20	15152	1.6	Interheart (Yusuf et al. 2004)
	Ethnicity	South Asian vs white in England	2	15619	1.5	Wild et al. 1997
	Exercise	Sedentary vs vigorous	45	1646	1.6	Oguma et al. 2004
	Von Willebrand factor	Top vs bottom third	33	1524	1.5	Whincup et al. 2002
	C-reactive protein	Top vs bottom third	33	2459	1.5	Danesh et al. 2005
	Genotype					
	APOE E2, E3, E4	4 4 vs 3 3	23	15492	1.4	Song et al. 2004
	eNOS Glu298Asp	Asp298++ vs Glu298++	11	13876	1.4	Casas et al. 2006
Small (<1.30)	Sex (angina)	Men vs women	50	119000	1.1	Hemingway et al. 2006
	Alcohol	Never vs light/moderate	20	66118	1.2	Corrao et al. 2000

(Continued)

Table 16.13.2.1 *(Cont'd)* Field synopsis of CHD epidemiology: factors associated with CHD aetiology according to their frequency, size of summarized evidence, and relative risk

Size of effect[a]	Risk factor[b]	Definition of high-risk vs low-risk groups[c]	Prevalence of risk group (%)[d]	No. of CHD cases	Relative risk (age adjusted)[e]	Meta-analysis (or large dataset) reference
Small (<1.30) (cont'd)	Nondiabetic fasting glycaemia	Glucose 4.7–6.1 mmol/litre; per 1.1 mol/litre		2 033[g]	1.2	Levitan *et al.* 2004
	Homocysteine	25% higher usual homocysteine		5 073	1.2	Homocysteine Study Collaboration 2002
	Gene (polymorphism)					
	APOB signal peptide ins/del	D+	52	6 007	1.2	Chiodini 2003
	CETP TaqIB	B1+ vs B22	68	7 681	1.2[f]	Boekholdt *et al.* 2005
	Paroxonase-1 Q192R	R192+ vs QQ	21	5 723	1.2	Wheeler *et al.* 2003
	ACE insertion/ deletion	DD vs I+	28	14 292	1.2	Morgan *et al.* 2003
None, inconsistent, or confounded	Vitamin E	Low vs high		1 491[g]	1.6	Hooper *et al.* 2001
	Fish oils	Low vs high	20	1 929[g]	1.1	Hooper *et al.* 2006
	Hormone replacement therapy	Current vs never	25		1.0	Adjusted for social status (Nelson *et al.* 2002)

[a] Size of effect: the cut points separating small, medium, large and very large effects are somewhat arbitrary. Different subgroups (e.g. women vs men), adjustments, may change the size of effect of some risk factors, particularly between medium and large categories.

[b] Eligible risk factors defined by the availability of large-scale studies or systematic reviews with more than 1000 CHD cases from cohort or case control studies; scores of polymorphisms and biomarkers have been the subject of literature based meta-analysis, and only a selection are shown here; eligible preclinical measures of disease were defined by the availability of any systematic review, irrespective of size.

[c] Definition of risk groups: for continuous variables top vs bottom tertiles (thirds) have been used where available. For categorical variables country and sex, the effects vary, and illustrative examples are given.

[d] Overall prevalence of risk factor is given, but in all cases will vary within populations (e.g. by age, sex, social position and ethnicity), between populations, or both.

[e] Relative risks are age adjusted (except the effect for age) and are shown as risks, rather than as protective effects (e.g. alcohol, exercise).

[f] Individual participant data meta-analysis.

[g] Outcome included noncoronary events, such as stroke, and all-cause death.

Rates: disease burden: geographical, temporal, and demographic variations

What is 'CHD'?

A clinician distinguishes between stable and unstable angina, between ST elevation and non-ST elevation MI (STEMI and non-STEMI), and between ventricular arrhythmias which cause sudden cardiac death, because the underlying vascular, myocardial, and electrophysiological pathology; the prognosis; and the treatment differ. Not so the epidemiologist. By contrast with the clinician 'splitters', epidemiologists have been 'lumpers.' Overwhelmingly, coronary disease in epidemiological studies refers to fatal coronary disease, or nonfatal MI, defined largely without troponins or electrocardiographic subtyping. Such aggregate markers of 'CHD,' or even more broadly cardiovascular disease (which includes atherothrombotic disease of the cerebral and peripheral circulations) have served public health well; improving risk factor burden in individuals and populations lowers CHD mortality. However, increasingly there is evidence that the causes of sudden as compared to nonsudden cardiac death, or acute as compared with chronic coronary syndromes, may differ.

Morbidity

People who die from coronary disease commonly suffer beforehand. Death may be sudden (presumed cardiac) in that there are no premonitory symptoms within 24 h, but in many cases this is a consequence of earlier, clinically manifest, coronary disease. The conglomerate of codes for coronary death in the International Classification of Disease has been widely used in epidemiological studies, but is a measure that conflates aetiology (first onset) and prognosis (case fatality). Age-specific incidence rates of nonfatal MI are declining in the West. However, the term 'incident MI' usually refers to the first MI, which may have been preceded by stable angina, in Framingham and other studies a common initial presentation of coronary disease. There is a lack of age-specific incidence data for stable angina and unstable angina, but first admission with chest pain, and unstable angina show an increasing trend from 1990 to 2000 among people aged under and over 75 years (Fig. 16.13.2.1). The prevalence of stable angina pectoris, using standardized questionnaires, has shown little evidence of decline over the last two decades. The age specific burden of heart failure is also projected to increase over the next 20 years, due improved survival among patients with coronary disease.

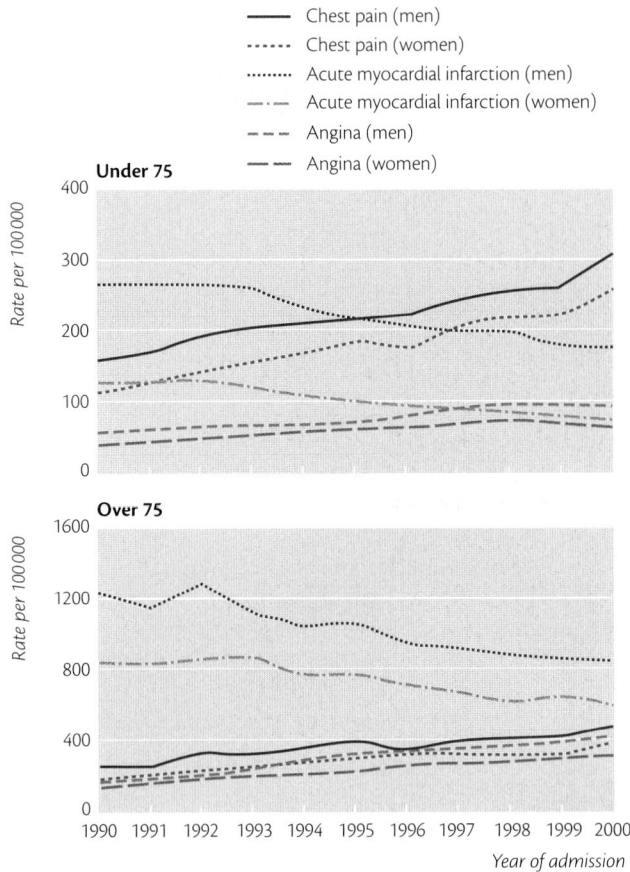

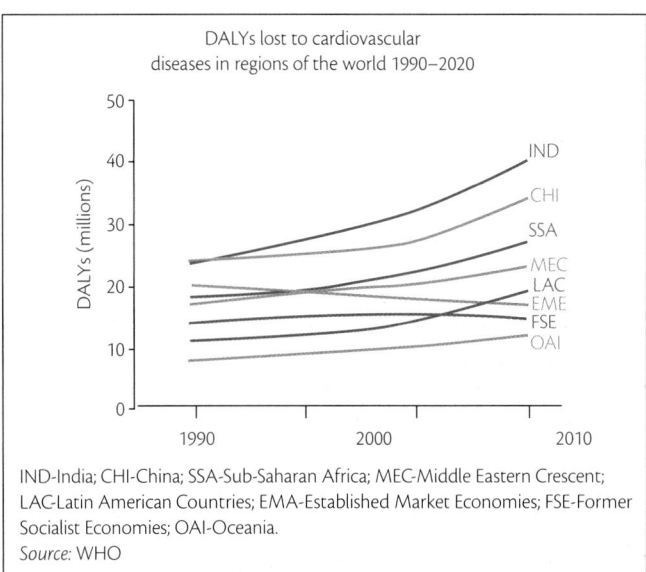

IND-India; CHI-China; SSA-Sub-Saharan Africa; MEC-Middle Eastern Crescent; LAC-Latin American Countries; EMA-Established Market Economies; FSE-Former Socialist Economies; OAI-Oceania.
Source: WHO

Fig. 16.13.2.2 Disability-adjusted life years lost to CVDs in regions of the world 1990–2020.
Reproduced from *Cardiovascular Health* with kind permission of the International Bank for Reconstruction and Development, The World Bank.

Fig. 16.13.2.1 Trends in hospitalization for first admissions with chest pain, myocardial infarction, and unstable angina in Scotland 1990–2000.
Reproduced from BMJ, Murphy *et al*, 328:1413–1414. Copyright (2004) with permission from BMJ Publishing Group Ltd.

Global increases and regional declines in mortality: epidemiological transitions

Of all the estimated 57 million deaths in the world in 2002, CVD was the largest single cause—resulting in 17 million deaths. CVD, particularly if atherothrombotic, is an indicator of a society's economic development. The widespread urbanization accompanying economic development is associated with the uptake of high-fat diets, tobacco use, and sedentary habits. Disability adjusted life-years (DALYs) lost to CVD are increasing globally (Fig. 16.13.2.2). Developed countries experienced marked declines in communicable disease before their epidemic in CVDs; the epidemiological transition currently being experienced in developing countries is different, with a double burden of the emerging noncommunicable diseases coexisting with communicable disease. There are very large variations in rates of coronary mortality and MI incidence between countries, with approximate fourfold differences in European women illustrated in Fig. 16.13.2.3. Among Russian men aged 65–74 years, rates of CHD mortality in 2002 were about 14 times higher than those in Japan (Table 16.13.2.1). In the West, CHD mortality rates have declined by around 60% since the mortality peak in the late 1960s, though it remains the leading cause of death in women and men.

Social class gradient in economically developed countries

Societies with medium or high income *per capita* demonstrate an inverse relation between social position and coronary disease incidence and mortality. Coronary disease rates are higher with each step down the social strata, whether indexed by occupation, education or income. Figure 16.13.2.4 shows that the inverse gradient according to social class was modest at the start of the decline in CHD mortality in 1971, but by 1981 the gradient had become considerably steeper in relative and absolute terms, and by 1991 the rate was more than double in unskilled manual workers (social class V) (230/100 000 men) compared to social class I (80/100 000 men). In 1991 the CHD mortality rate among unskilled manual workers was little different from 1971. In contrast, the CHD rate among professional workers was 60% lower than at the height of the epidemic. Using a different marker of social position, educational level, there are large differences across Europe; at all ages from 45 to aged 75 years and older, absolute mortality rate differences between those with high and low education were highest for coronary disease.

Psychosocial factors

The causal mechanisms are beginning to be understood by which occupational status, education, or income influence coronary disease. Habits of living such as smoking are undoubtedly important, but independent of behavioural factors there is evidence that a range of psychosocial factors may be involved. Depression has been the most extensively investigated psychosocial factor in cohort studies and is associated with an effect of about 1.8 (Fig. 16.13.2.5) in a meta-analysis illustrating a potential bias whereby studies which reported effects adjusted for established risk factors had a higher unadjusted effect than studies which did not (1.9 vs 1.5). Randomized trials of cognitive-behavioural and other interventions which have reduced depression scores have not been associated with lower coronary event rates.

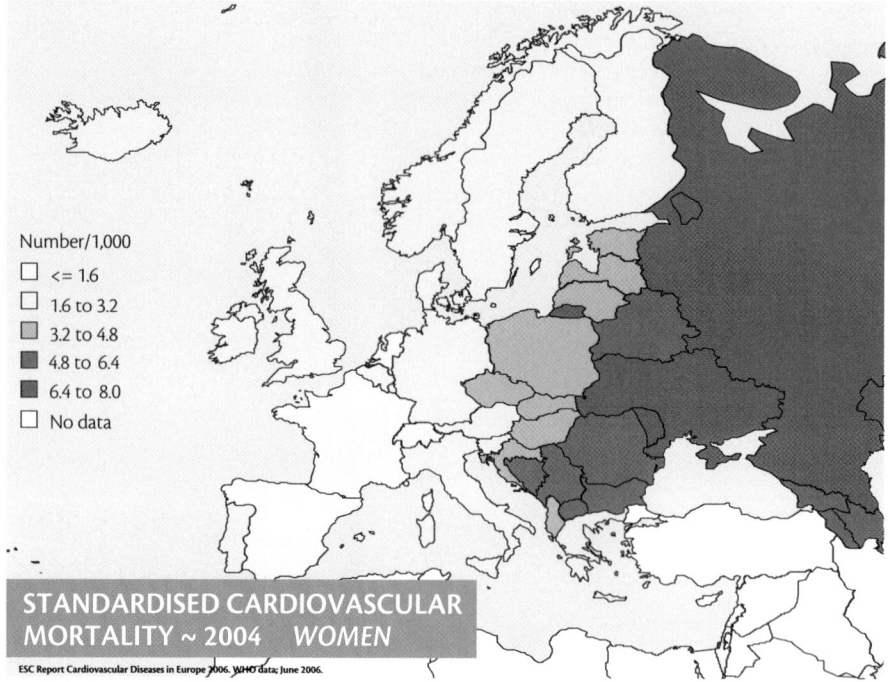

Fig. 16.13.2.3 Geographical variations in cardiovascular mortality in Europe 2004 among women. ESC report, cardiovascular diseases in Europe 2006. WHO data June 2006. P15. Report online at http://www.escardio.org/guidelines-surveys/ehs/Documents/EHS-CVD-report-2006.pdf

Prospective studies show that working conditions are associated with risk of incident CHD; low control, high demands, and low support at work, effort–reward imbalance, job insecurity, and organizational injustice have each been associated with cardiovascular risk. The Interheart study, a 52-country case control study of MI, found that stress at home and at work, financial stress, stressful life events, low locus of control, and depression were associated with CHD risk, accounting for 33% of the population attributable risk of MI.

Basic science describes a number of plausible physiological mechanisms that may translate chronic stress into increased coronary risk. Altered functioning of stress-related autonomic and endocrine axes has been identified among men with increased CHD

risk and low self-reported control at work. Prospectively, chronic work stress increases the risks of metabolic syndrome and obesity in a dose–response manner after adjustment for smoking, diet, and physical activity levels.

Ageing societies

Age is the strongest risk factor for all forms of coronary disease, with approximate doubling of mortality every 5 years, and doubling of incidence for each 10 years of age. The effect of age dwarfs that of other risk factors and, along with country of origin, has been proposed as the only robust measure of screening for individual risk in asymptomatic individuals. The effect of age, like that of sex, is not fixed and inevitable; it varies in different societies, e.g. with some rural populations showing little evidence of increasing blood pressure with age, within a high-rate country.

Age at presentation is increasing; the upper age limit of MI in the MONICA study of 65 years is now about the mean age of MI in many countries. The percentage of the population over the age of 65 is increasing in low, middle, and high income countries. Aided by improved survival following MI, the absolute numbers living with CVD is increasing. From the age of 50 it has been estimated that 20% of remaining life expectancy is spent living with CVD. Much of the gains in life expectancy in developed countries in recent years have come from the reduction in CVD mortality.

Women, MI, and angina pectoris

CHD is the most common cause of death in women in most developed countries. The rate of decline in the death rate due to CVD has been less in women than in men. The incidence of nonfatal and fatal MI shows a male excess (albeit of varying magnitude) across countries with widely differing absolute rates of MI mortality. When CHD rates are plotted on a log scale, there is no evidence of a threshold increase in women around the age of the menopause; the male excess in CHD mortality diminishes continuously with age.

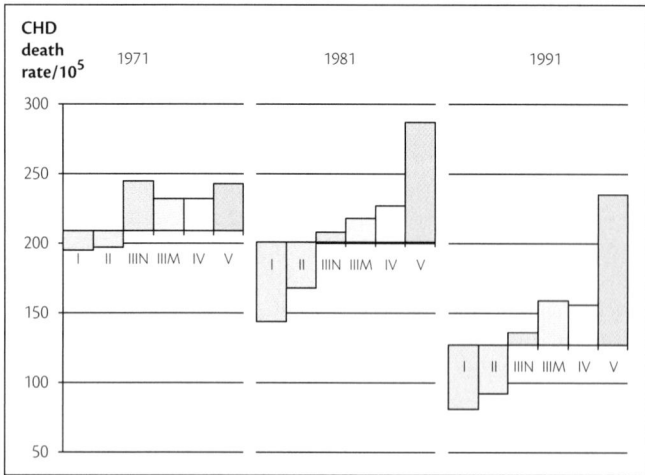

Fig. 16.13.2.4 Death rates from CHD by social class in Great Britain 1971–91 in men. Rates are age standardized by the direct method for comparison across the three national censuses.

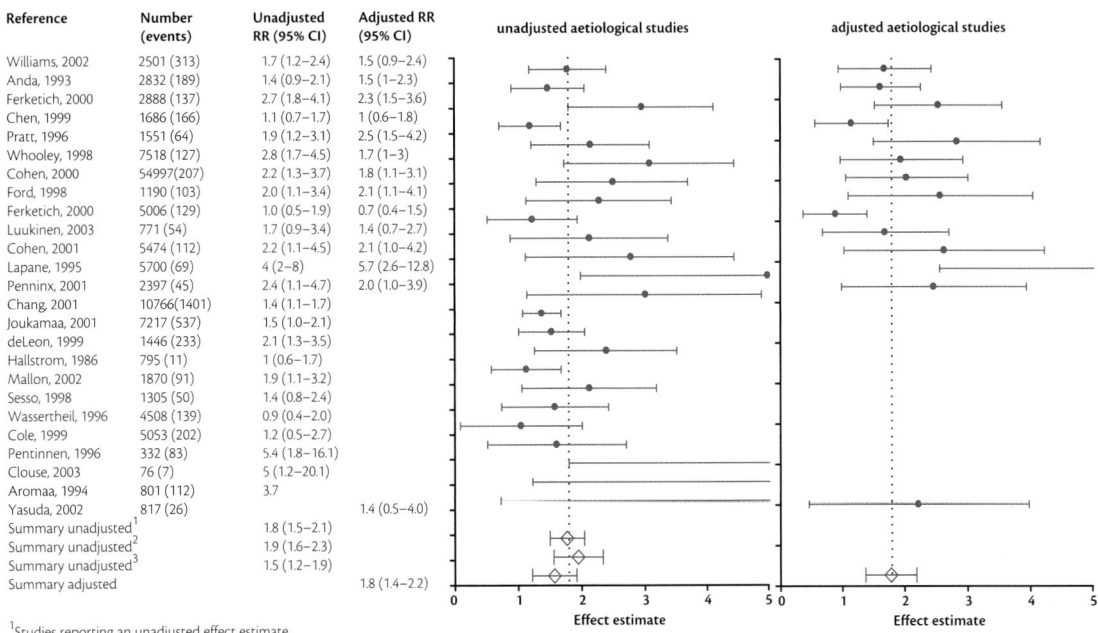

Reference	Number (events)	Unadjusted RR (95% CI)	Adjusted RR (95% CI)
Williams, 2002	2501 (313)	1.7 (1.2–2.4)	1.5 (0.9–2.4)
Anda, 1993	2832 (189)	1.4 (0.9–2.1)	1.5 (1–2.3)
Ferketich, 2000	2888 (137)	2.7 (1.8–4.1)	2.3 (1.5–3.6)
Chen, 1999	1686 (166)	1.1 (0.7–1.7)	1 (0.6–1.8)
Pratt, 1996	1551 (64)	1.9 (1.2–3.1)	2.5 (1.5–4.2)
Whooley, 1998	7518 (127)	2.8 (1.7–4.5)	1.7 (1–3)
Cohen, 2000	54997 (207)	2.2 (1.3–3.7)	1.8 (1.1–3.1)
Ford, 1998	1190 (103)	2.0 (1.1–3.4)	2.1 (1.1–4.1)
Ferketich, 2000	5006 (129)	1.0 (0.5–1.9)	0.7 (0.4–1.5)
Luukinen, 2003	771 (54)	1.7 (0.9–3.4)	1.4 (0.7–2.7)
Cohen, 2001	5474 (112)	2.2 (1.1–4.5)	2.1 (1.0–4.2)
Lapane, 1995	5700 (69)	4 (2–8)	5.7 (2.6–12.8)
Penninx, 2001	2397 (45)	2.4 (1.1–4.7)	2.0 (1.0–3.9)
Chang, 2001	10766 (1401)	1.4 (1.1–1.7)	
Joukamaa, 2001	7217 (537)	1.5 (1.0–2.1)	
deLeon, 1999	1446 (233)	2.1 (1.3–3.5)	
Hallstrom, 1986	795 (11)	1 (0.6–1.7)	
Mallon, 2002	1870 (91)	1.9 (1.1–3.2)	
Sesso, 1998	1305 (50)	1.4 (0.8–2.4)	
Wassertheil, 1996	4508 (139)	0.9 (0.4–2.0)	
Cole, 1999	5053 (202)	1.2 (0.5–2.7)	
Pentinnen, 1996	332 (83)	5.4 (1.8–16.1)	
Clouse, 2003	76 (7)	5 (1.2–20.1)	
Aromaa, 1994	801 (112)	3.7	
Yasuda, 2002	817 (26)		1.4 (0.5–4.0)
Summary unadjusted[1]		1.8 (1.5–2.1)	
Summary unadjusted[2]		1.9 (1.6–2.3)	
Summary unadjusted[3]		1.5 (1.2–1.9)	
Summary adjusted			1.8 (1.4–2.2)

[1]Studies reporting an unadjusted effect estimate
[2]Studies reporting an unadjusted effect estimate that also report an adjusted effect estimate
[3]Studies reporting an unadjusted effect estimate that do not report an adjusted effect estimate

Fig. 16.13.2.5 Association of depression and CHD aetiology: literature based meta-analysis comparing adjusted and unadjusted studies.
Reproduced with permission from Nicholson, A., Kuper, H., & Hemingway, H., *Depression as an aetiologic and prognostic factor in coronary heart disease: a meta-analysis of 6362 events among 146 538 participants in 54 observational studies, Eur.Heart J.*, (2006) vol. 27, no. 23, pp. 2763–2774.

By contrast, the male excess is not so clear for angina pectoris. Male sex is not associated with physician-defined angina occurrence in either a small (146 cases in women) healthy population study (Framingham) or in a large (67 832 cases in women) study of primary care patients in Finland as shown in Fig. 16.13.2.6. In the Finnish study angina was defined by new, filled prescriptions for nitrates (reasonably specific for the diagnosis of angina, upper panel) and, separately, among patients with ischaemic abnormalities on coronary angiography or exercise electrocardiography (lower panel). While both case definitions were associated with increased coronary mortality rates in women and men, the nitrate cases showed a slight female excess, and the test-positive cases a male excess. Evidence that the latter may be biased by access to investigation for women comes from a meta-analysis, based on almost 25 000 angina cases in women and men from 31 countries, using a standardized questionnaire for assessing angina symptoms in the general population, independent of diagnostic or treatment decisions. This found that women had a slightly higher prevalence of stable angina pectoris compared to men, with a pooled sex ratio of 1.20, consistent across countries with widely differing MI mortality rates. These findings suggest that, globally, symptoms of heart disease represent an important burden in women as well as men.

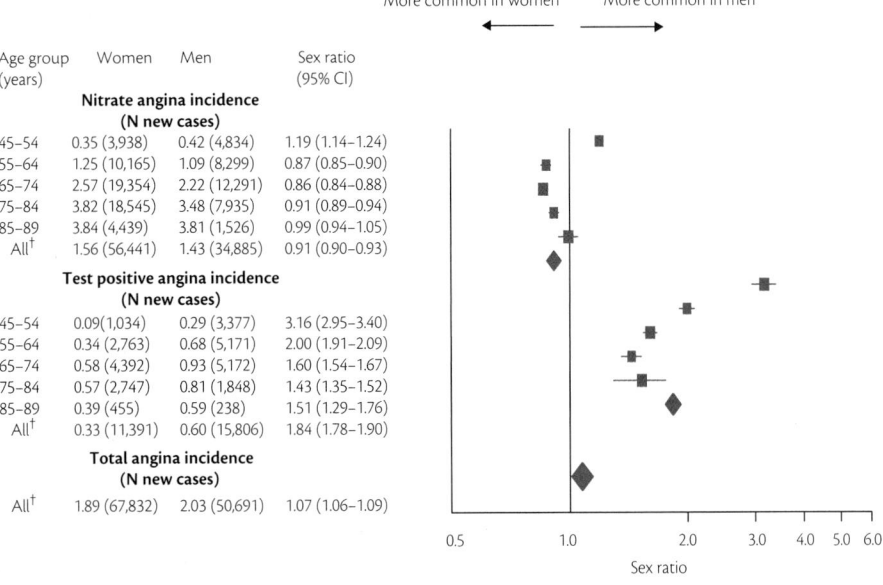

Age group (years)	Women	Men	Sex ratio (95% CI)
	Nitrate angina incidence (N new cases)		
45–54	0.35 (3,938)	0.42 (4,834)	1.19 (1.14–1.24)
55–64	1.25 (10,165)	1.09 (8,299)	0.87 (0.85–0.90)
65–74	2.57 (19,354)	2.22 (12,291)	0.86 (0.84–0.88)
75–84	3.82 (18,545)	3.48 (7,935)	0.91 (0.89–0.94)
85–89	3.84 (4,439)	3.81 (1,526)	0.99 (0.94–1.05)
All[†]	1.56 (56,441)	1.43 (34,885)	0.91 (0.90–0.93)
	Test positive angina incidence (N new cases)		
45–54	0.09 (1,034)	0.29 (3,377)	3.16 (2.95–3.40)
55–64	0.34 (2,763)	0.68 (5,171)	2.00 (1.91–2.09)
65–74	0.58 (4,392)	0.93 (5,172)	1.60 (1.54–1.67)
75–84	0.57 (2,747)	0.81 (1,848)	1.43 (1.35–1.52)
85–89	0.39 (455)	0.59 (238)	1.51 (1.29–1.76)
All[†]	0.33 (11,391)	0.60 (15,806)	1.84 (1.78–1.90)
	Total angina incidence (N new cases)		
All[†]	1.89 (67,832)	2.03 (50,691)	1.07 (1.06–1.09)

Fig. 16.13.2.6 Incidence of stable angina pectoris as first manifestation of CHD by gender and age.

Standard risk factors poorly explain the male excess in CHD mortality. While meta-analyses of observational studies suggested that current hormone replacement therapy (HRT) might be protective for women, this effect was not seen among studies controlling for socioeconomic status. The Women's Health Initiative trial found increased CHD events (HR 1.29) among women randomized to HRT. Since there is little sex difference in aortic calcium, or in intimal thickening in intracoronary ultrasound studies among heart transplant patients, factors related to plaque development and rupture may be important. The explanation for the high burden of anginal symptoms in women, despite their lower burden of obstructive disease in the epicardial coronary arteries, may relate to microvascular disease. Indeed, a direct measure of microvascular disease in the general population, the ratio of retinal arteriole:venule diameters was strongly related to coronary events in women, but not in men, in the ARIC study.

Ethnicity

South Asians

With continuing economic development, market economy countries attract migrants from poorer nations. For some migrant groups, coronary disease rates increase to approximate those of the host country (Japanese migrants to the United States of America), but this is not the case for two broad ethnic groups in the United Kingdom. Globally, migrants from South Asia have higher rates of CHD mortality than the indigenous population. South Asians living in England and Wales have about 50% higher coronary mortality than whites, and the rate of decline between 1971 and 1991 in coronary mortality was slower in South Asians. The 1999 Health Survey for England found that the prevalence of angina was higher, particularly among Bangladeshi men compared to whites. Despite similar blood pressures and lower total cholesterol levels than whites, South Asians have a higher prevalence of diabetes, higher fasting and postglucose serum insulin concentrations, higher plasma triglyceride, and lower high-density lipoprotein (HDL) cholesterol concentrations. However, these risk factors did not explain the excess risk among South Asians in one of the few prospective studies. Some South Asian communities are socioeconomically deprived, but the ways in which material or psychosocial factors, or access to preventive health care, might influence coronary incidence in South Asians are unclear.

Afro-Caribbeans

By contrast, British people born in the Caribbean or West Africa have lower coronary mortality rates than whites. Afro-Caribbeans have higher mean blood pressure, left ventricular mass, and body mass index, and a higher prevalence of diabetes compared to whites. African Americans have a similar profile of risk factors and similar HDL and LDL cholesterol values to those in whites, and intriguingly the Multi Ethnic Study of Atherosclerosis showed that blacks in the general population have a lower prevalence of any coronary artery calcium and a lower mean distribution of calcium scores, after adjustment for risk factors (Fig. 16.13.2.7). The prognostic validity of coronary artery calcium in different ethnic groups awaits demonstration, but this may shed light on different stages in the disease process. Incidence of nonfatal MI among people aged 60–74 years is lower in African Americans than whites in the ARIC study, yet mortality from CHD (which incorporates case fatality) shows a small excess among African Americans.

Risk factors and reversal: aetiological and prognostic factors

The current causal model for CHD in populations is that a modest number of risk factors (around 10) answers, with varying degrees of success, two fundamentally different questions: Why is the rate of CHD high in a given population? Why does a particular individual have CHD? In this section the risk factors which have been most extensively investigated for a causal role in CHD are discussed in relation to the strength of observational and, where available, randomized trial evidence.

Smoking

Observational evidence

All forms of tobacco consumption increase the risk of MI, with a relative risk approaching 3 between current and never smokers. This risk increases by about 6% for every additional cigarette smoked. Second-hand smoke (passive smoking) also has an effect of about 1.15. The population attributable risks of active smoking are particularly high in young men (58%) compared with older women (6%). Smoking continues to exert an effect among those who have stopped smoking more than 20 years earlier.

Interventions

At the population level, the WHO Framework Convention on Tobacco Control, introduced in 2005, sets international standards on tobacco price, advertising, packaging, education, public awareness cessation measures, illicit trade, sales to minors, and support for economically viable alternatives. In England, bans on advertising (2003) and smoking in public places and workplaces (2007) are expected to further reduce the prevalence of smoking. Among the poorest people in the United Kingdom as much as 20% of total household expenditure is spent on tobacco. Effective interventions aimed at individual smokers, include telephone counselling, busproprion, and nicotine patches.

Blood pressure

Observational evidence

Unlike the categorical association of smoking and coronary disease—where the goal is abolition of smoke exposure—for some other coronary risk factors the relationship is continuous. In terms of global causal impact this is best understood for blood pressure and cholesterol. There is a continuous association between blood pressure values (down to 115 mmHg systolic) and the risks of CHD. At every age there is a straight line relationship between CHD risk (log scale) and blood pressure. There is no threshold, so a lower blood pressure is associated with lower risk, irrespective of the starting level. Risk approximately doubles between the 25th and 75th centile. Most events occur at those with 'normal' blood pressures (Fig. 16.13.2.8).

Interventions

The rise of blood pressure with age is related to four dietary related factors: salt (NaCl) intake, low potassium intake, obesity, and excessive alcohol consumption; these are the targets for intervention aimed at shifting the mean blood pressure in the whole population (see Fig. 16.13.2.9). Some 26% of the world's population (972 million people) are estimated to have elevated blood pressure, of whom 639 million are in developing countries. At an individual

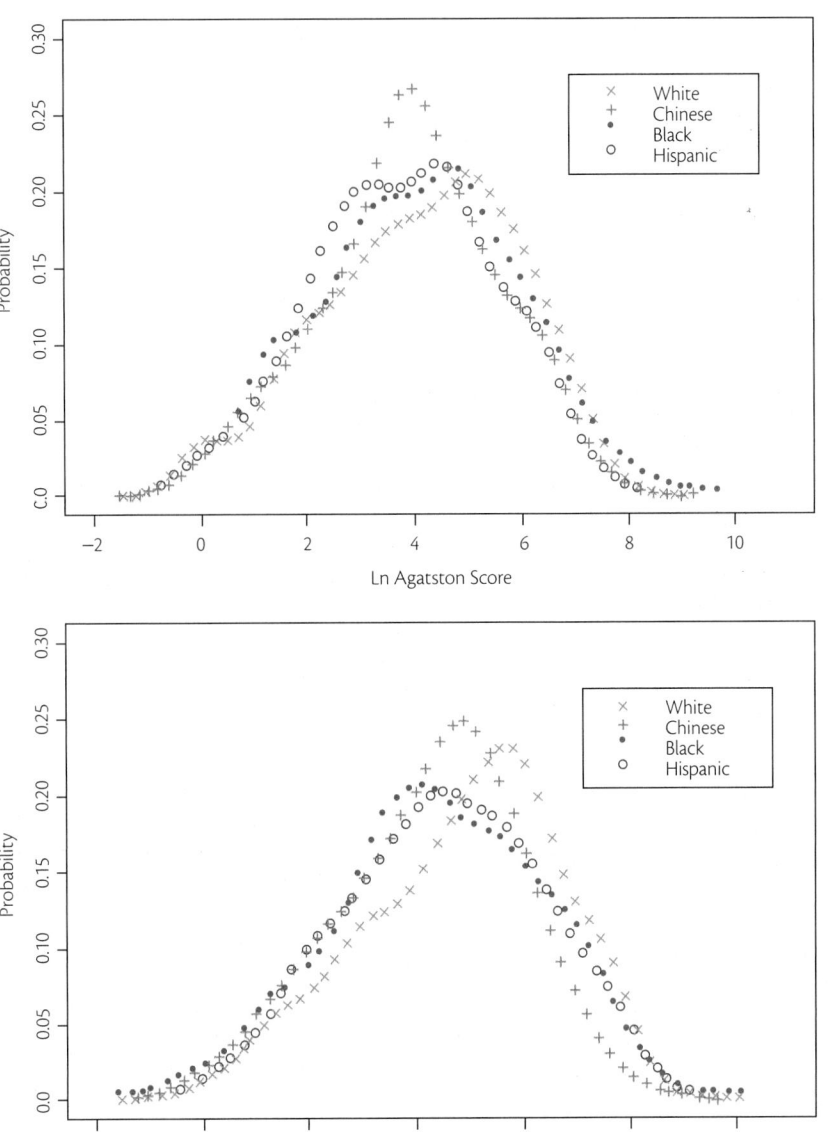

Fig. 16.13.2.7 Coronary artery calcium score among those with any calcium by gender and ethnicity. Women (upper panel): 45% of whites and 37% of blacks had some coronary artery calcium Men (lower panel): 70% of whites and 52% of blacks had some coronary artery calcium.
Bild, D. E., Detrano, R., Peterson, D., Guerci, A., Liu, K., Shahar, E., Ouyang, P., Jackson, S., & Saad, M. F. 2005a, "Ethnic differences in coronary calcification: the Multi-Ethnic Study of Atherosclerosis (MESA)", Circulation, vol. 111, no. 10, pp. 1313–1320. (http://circ.ahajournals.org/cgi/content/abstract/111/10/1313)0.)

level, dietary change, reduced alcohol, and reduced weight can all lower blood pressure. Pharmacological blood pressure lowering among people with blood pressure >140/90 clearly reduces cardiovascular events, and probably coronary events.

Diet and lipids

Dietary habits cause coronary disease; the evidence is strong for saturated fat (via effects on serum cholesterol), good for the multiple dietary influences which affect blood pressure, but lacking—or controversial—for antioxidant vitamins (β-carotene, vitamin C and vitamin E), B vitamins and folate, and fish oils.

Saturated fat, cholesterol, and other lipid subfractions
Total cholesterol, LDL cholesterol
Observational evidence Saturated fat consumption is associated with serum cholesterol levels. Attempts to define 'normal' for serum cholesterol levels are misleading: there is a strong and continuous

between-country correlation between average serum cholesterol and coronary mortality, ranging from 6 mmol/litre in Britain to 3–3.5 in rural China. LDL cholesterol, about 2 mmol/litre lower than total cholesterol, is responsible for much of the atherogenic effect of lipids, and the effects in observational studies and trials for LDL and total cholesterol tend to match closely. Within populations the relationship between total cholesterol and CHD mortality is log linear, which links the proportional change in the cholesterol to an absolute change in CHD mortality. There is no threshold; even in China, where the overall mean was low, there is a dose–response relation with CHD mortality.

Interventions Population reduction of saturated fat consumption by about 7% of total calories would lead to about a 0.6 mmol/litre reduction in serum cholesterol. This has occurred in the United States of America and in Finland. For example, the North Karelia project in Finland reduced the intake of saturated fat from liquid

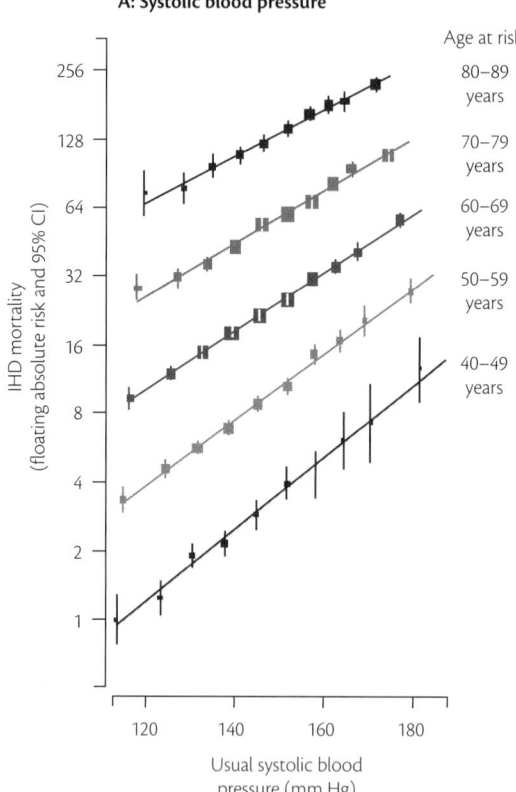

A: Systolic blood pressure

Age at risk:

80–89 years

70–79 years

60–69 years

50–59 years

40–49 years

Fig. 16.13.2.8 CHD mortality in each decade of age vs usual blood pressure at the start of that decade.
Reprinted from *The Lancet, Vol. 360, Lewington et al, Age-specific relevance of usual blood pressure to vascular mortality: a meta-analysis of individual data for one million adults in 61 prospective studies*, pp. 1903–1913. Copyright (2002), with permission from Elsevier.

dairy products and spreadable fat by two-thirds between 1972 and 1992, with reductions in mean cholesterol levels. Denmark has banned industrially produced *trans*-fatty acids on the grounds that they adversely affect LDL levels and can be removed without effect on the taste, price, or availability of foods. At the international policy level it has been claimed that the European Union has maintained subsidies to producers of full-fat milk and beef while keeping the cost of fruits and vegetables high. Individual dietary change can achieve relatively modest (e.g. 5%) reductions in serum cholesterol. Statins reduce coronary event rates, among people with established CVD (Heart Protection Study) and among individuals without established CHD.

HDL cholesterol, apolipoproteins B and A1

High density lipoprotein (HDL) is protective for coronary disease; in cohort studies an absolute increase of 0.12 mmol/litre is associated with a 15% decrease in CHD and treatment with recombinant apolipoprotein A1 is associated with regression of coronary atherosclerosis. Statins increase HDL by only about 5%, so this effect on CHD events is small. HDL cholesterol is highly correlated with apoliporotein A1, and LDL cholesterol with apolipoprotein B; the apolipoproteins have the advantage of not requiring a fasting sample for measurement. The ratio of apoB/apoA is strongly related to MI with relative risk of about 2.5 for top vs bottom third (see Table 16.13.2.1).

Genes, lipids, and the environment

Environmental factors influence an individual's cholesterol level via pathways under genetic control, although for the most part the genes responsible are not known. Familial hypercholesterolaemia (prevalence 1 in 500) is an exception; caused by mutations in a single gene (for the LDL receptor), familial hypercholesterolaemia is inherited as a simple mendelian dominant trait, and has such large effects on cholesterol levels it might be considered as a linear, deterministic factor in causing CVD (see Chapter 12.6). Recent evidence suggests that this may not be the case. Based on a large pedigree of 250 individuals, with probands selected during screening (and not on the basis of having suffered CVD), mortality was not increased in carriers of the mutation during the 19th and early 20th century; it rose after 1915 and reached its maximum between 1935 and 1964 (standardized mortality ratio 1.78, 95% confidence interval 1.13–2.76), and fell thereafter (Fig. 16.13.2.10). Furthermore, mortality differed significantly between two branches of the pedigree. This large variability over time and between branches of the pedigree points to a strong interaction with environmental factors, such as changing dietary patterns and medical care. In contrast with familial hypercholesterolaemia, CHD and stroke are complex diseases that are known to aggregate in families but not to segregate in a mendelian fashion. Under the common disease/common variant hypothesis a number of genes, each with modest effects, are thought to operate. People with the *E4* allele of the apololipoprotein E (*APOE*) gene have higher serum cholesterol concentrations than those without the allele and this accounts for an appreciable proportion (about 7%) of the variability in cholesterol levels in the general population. *E4* allele frequency differs widely between populations, with a lower prevalence in Japan (7%) compared to Finland (19%), and a gradient of decreasing prevalence from north to south Europe. The *APOE* gene *E4* allele has been shown in a recent meta-analysis of 48 studies with over 15 000 cases to be associated with coronary artery disease with a relative risk of 1.42.

B vitamins, folate, homocysteine

Plasma homocysteine is associated with CHD, with meta-analyses suggesting a relative risk of 1.13 for a 2.6 µmol/litre higher homocysteine. In global public health terms this observation is of particular interest because there is a simple intervention—increasing folate consumption substantially decreases homocysteine levels. However, there is major scope for confounding (homocysteine levels are associated with smoking and low social position) and reverse causality (CVD may lead to elevated homocysteine levels). Recently common genetic variants have been used to help understand whether specific environmental exposures are causal. A common genetic variant in the *MTHFR* gene (677C to T substitution) is associated with homocysteine levels, such that those with the TT genotype have about 2.6 µmol/litre higher homocysteine levels than those with the CC genotype. Since, under Mendel's second law, assortment of alleles at the time of gamete formation is random, confounders are likely to be evenly distributed by genotype, a situation analogous to a randomized controlled trial. Under the Mendelian randomization design, the association between genotype and coronary disease predicts that TT individuals have a risk of 1.16, which is very close to that observed, lending some support to causal inference. The complementary randomized trials of folate supplementation in a primary prevention (aetiological) setting are awaited, although trials in a secondary prevention (prognostic) setting have been negative.

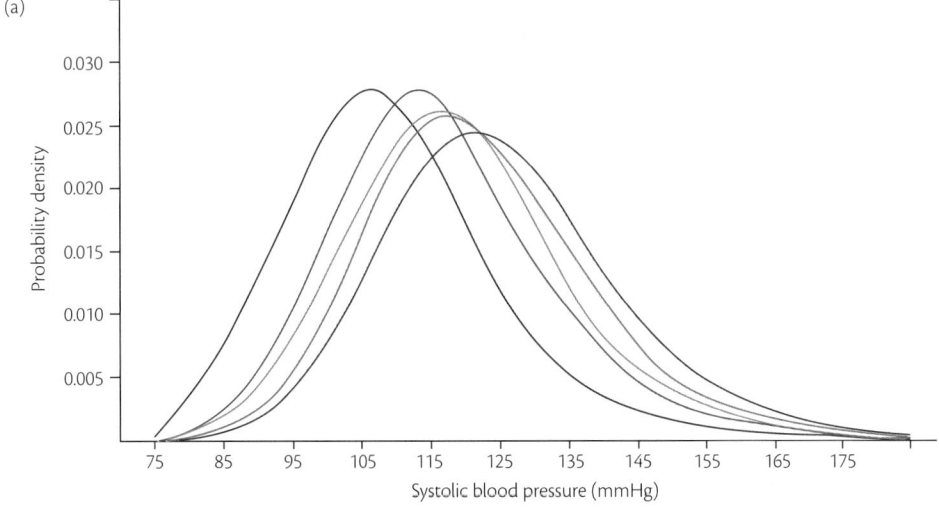

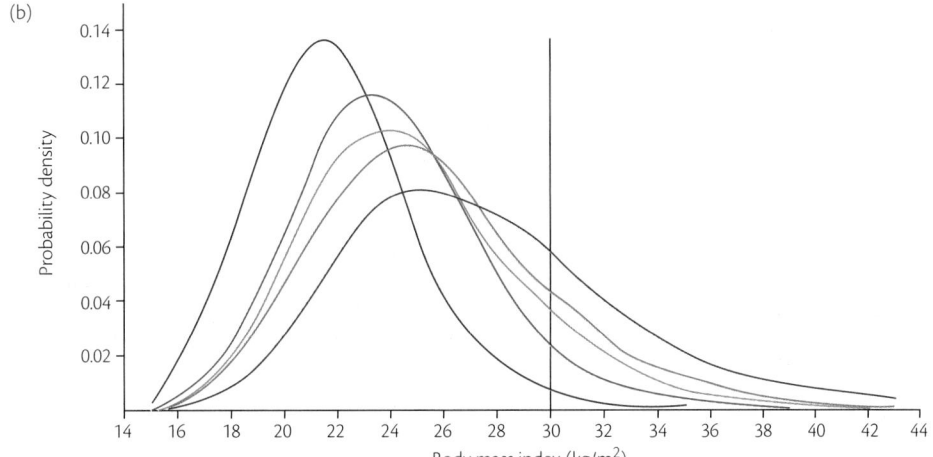

Fig. 16.13.2.9 Distribution of systolic blood pressure (upper panel) and body mass index (lower panel) of five population groups. It is estimated that changing the population mean in SBP by 5 mmHg will result in a 21% lower CV event rate, which has been observed in randomized trials. Similarly, decreasing the population mean of BMI by 1 unit is predicted to decrease the incidence of CV events by 10%.
Reproduced from Rose, G. 1992, *The Strategy of Preventive Medicine*. With permission of Oxford University Press.

Other dietary components

The search for other causal moieties in diet has seen a pattern of apparently promising associations in observational studies not being confirmed in randomized trials. The antioxidant vitamins β-carotene, vitamin C, and vitamin E have each fallen at the hurdle of intervention, and ω – 3 polyunsaturated fatty acids do not show clear and consistent associations in observational studies or trials. However, available evidence does not exclude an important effect of ω – 3 fats on coronary events; less biased trials reporting more events are required. Whole dietary patterns may be additionally important.

Alcohol

There is a J-shaped relationship between alcohol consumption and CHD, with risks elevated slightly in never drinkers, and those who drink excessively. However bi-directional confounding may be important in this relationship. People who report light alcohol consumption have a lower prevalence of 27/30 risk factors and behaviours compared to nondrinkers. By contrast, in heavy drinkers, confounding will obscure rather than exaggerate any coronary protection because of their heart-unhealthy behaviours. Thus the evidence for a coronary-protective effect is probably stronger for moderate to heavy drinking than for light to moderate drinking. In public health terms a more important question is not whether any given level of alcohol consumption is protective for coronary disease, but its overall relation with harms. Light to moderate drinking might have a small, unconfounded protective association with CHD; but any increase in the mean population *per capita* alcohol consumption will increase the prevalence of heavy drinking with its known (noncoronary) harms.

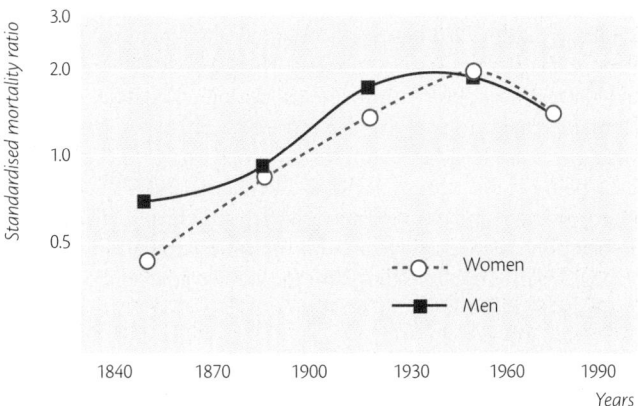

Fig. 16.13.2.10 Mortality in familial hypercholesterolaemia, according to sex and time in 250 individuals in a pedigree with 0.5 probability of carrying V408M. Reproduced from BMJ, Sijbrands, E. J. *et al*, 322:1019–1023. Copyright (2001) with permission from BMJ Publishing Group Ltd.

Exercise

Physical activity, through pleiotropic effects on blood pressure, lipids, glucose and fat utilization, obesity, and cardiorespiratory fitness, is causally associated with the incidence of coronary disease. While the optimal type, intensity, duration, and frequency of exercise are continued grounds for debate, there is a dose–response relationship, with CHD risk decreasing with increasing amounts of physical exercise. Even walking for 1 h/week is associated with reduced risk of CVD outcomes. Higher resting heart rate, strongly associated with sedentary habits, is a consistent predictor of coronary events, particularly sudden cardiac death. Low heart rate rise with exercise, and fall after exercise, may also predict sudden death.

Obesity and diabetes

Obesity

The combination of gluttony and sloth, more socially patterned than individually chosen, is causing an epidemic of obesity from childhood onwards in developed, and developing, countries throughout the world. The general thesis that obesity causes coronary disease is not contested, but there is much debate about how best to measure obesity and the mechanisms of causality. Based on 74 analytic cohorts with 60 374 deaths during follow-up, the associations between body mass index (BMI) and CHD mortality were modest with relative risk 1.51 in men for obesity (BMI >30) as compared to individuals with BMI 18.5 to <25. There was little evidence that overweight (BMI 25 to <30) was associated with mortality. In Interheart BMI showed a modest and graded association with myocardial infarction that was substantially reduced after adjustment for waist-to-hip ratio (1.12), and nonsignificant after adjustment for other risk factors. Among people with established disease a meta-analysis of 40 studies found lower cardiovascular mortality among the overweight and mildly obese groups. Waist-to-hip ratio is a simple surrogate measure of visceral obesity, a key determinant of metabolic abnormalities. Waist-to-hip ratio was associated with risk of MI (odd ratios for top vs bottom third 2.0), even after adjustment for other risk factors.

Diabetes and impaired glucose tolerance

The number of diabetics in the world is estimated to rise to 221 million by the year 2010 (from 124 million in 1997), with Asia and Africa experiencing the greatest increases. Diabetes is a strong risk factor for CHD, stronger in women than in men. There is some evidence that the 2-h blood glucose is a better predictor of deaths from CVD than is fasting glucose. Nondiabetic hyperglycaemia may have a weak (risk ratio 1.19) association with CHD. The environments that cause obesity also cause type 2 diabetes. Interactions with genes are likely to be important, with one promising candidate being transcription factor 7-like 2 gene (*TCF7L2*). Unlike many previous polymorphisms reported for chronic diseases, the association has been replicated in multiple populations, appears strong, (relative risk exceeding 2 for the homozygote) and population attributable risk is high (21%).

Interventions for obesity and diabetes

Obesity may represent 'normal physiology within a pathological environment' encompassing sedentary lifestyles and overly rich nutrition. Strategies that specifically reduce abdominal obesity have not been developed, but overall weight loss probably reduces abdominal obesity. Exercise is associated with improved CVD risk factors even if no weight is lost. Diabetes is potentially preventable by implementation of dietary changes at the prediabetic stage of impaired glucose tolerance.

Clusters of risk factors: the metabolic syndrome

Although it is clear that risk factors cluster within individuals, it remains unclear that the whole of the (variously) defined metabolic syndrome predicts risk of CHD events beyond the individual component variables. A recent meta-analysis of eight studies examining CHD incidence reported an effect for the metabolic syndrome of 1.5. In nine European population-based cohorts the prevalence of the metabolic syndrome differed widely according to definitions: WHO (27% in men, 20% in women), the National Cholesterol Education Program (26%, 23%), NCEP revised (32%, 29%) and the International Diabetes Federation (36%, 34%). With CVD mortality as the outcome, the respective hazard ratios were 2.1, 1.7, 1.7, and 1.5 in men, and consistently lower in women—1.6, 1.4, 1.1, and 1.5. With a few exceptions, the hazard ratios for full definitions of the syndrome were not significantly different from those for their single components. Serum triglycerides, which are strongly related to LDL and HDL cholesterol, may be associated with CHD risk, but the independence of this association remains contentious.

Combining risk factors to predict risk in individuals

Combinations of risk factors may be used to predict the risk of coronary events in individuals and the use of scores is increasing in clinical practice. Figure 16.13.2.11 shows how the absolute risk of coronary events at a given level of one risk factor is determined by the levels of other risk factors. The premise of risk prediction is that those at higher absolute risk have the greatest individual benefits from risk factor reduction, and people who perceive themselves at risk may be more motivated to change their health related behaviours. A further advantage is one of explicit prioritization; patients at a given level of risk may be targeted, irrespective of how that risk was reached.

However, the identification of individuals at risk is not straightforward. Existing scores, based on combinations of risk factors, do not reliably identify a minority of high-risk patients who will experience the majority of CHD events. Most events occur in people who are not at high risk. Nor can risk factor screening in the population identify a group of individuals who will not benefit from reductions in risk factors. The technology of calculating risk in individuals has not been tested in randomized trials. Two simple pieces of information—older age and living in a country with a high rate of CVD—are the most robust identifiers of risk (see Table 16.13.2.1). To date the hope that novel biomarkers might substantially improve risk prediction has not been substantiated. If causal risk factors for disease have—thus far—been poor screening tools, then measuring the consequences of early, preclinical stages of disease may be more helpful.

Inflammatory, haemostatic, and other circulating biomarkers

The hypothesis that markers of inflammation may be causally associated with coronary events has had some empirical support, although the effects of C-reactive protein (CRP) appears modest, and Mendelian randomization studies suggest that the effect might be confounded by its strong associations with established risk factors. Fibrinogen is the only biomarker which has been the subject of

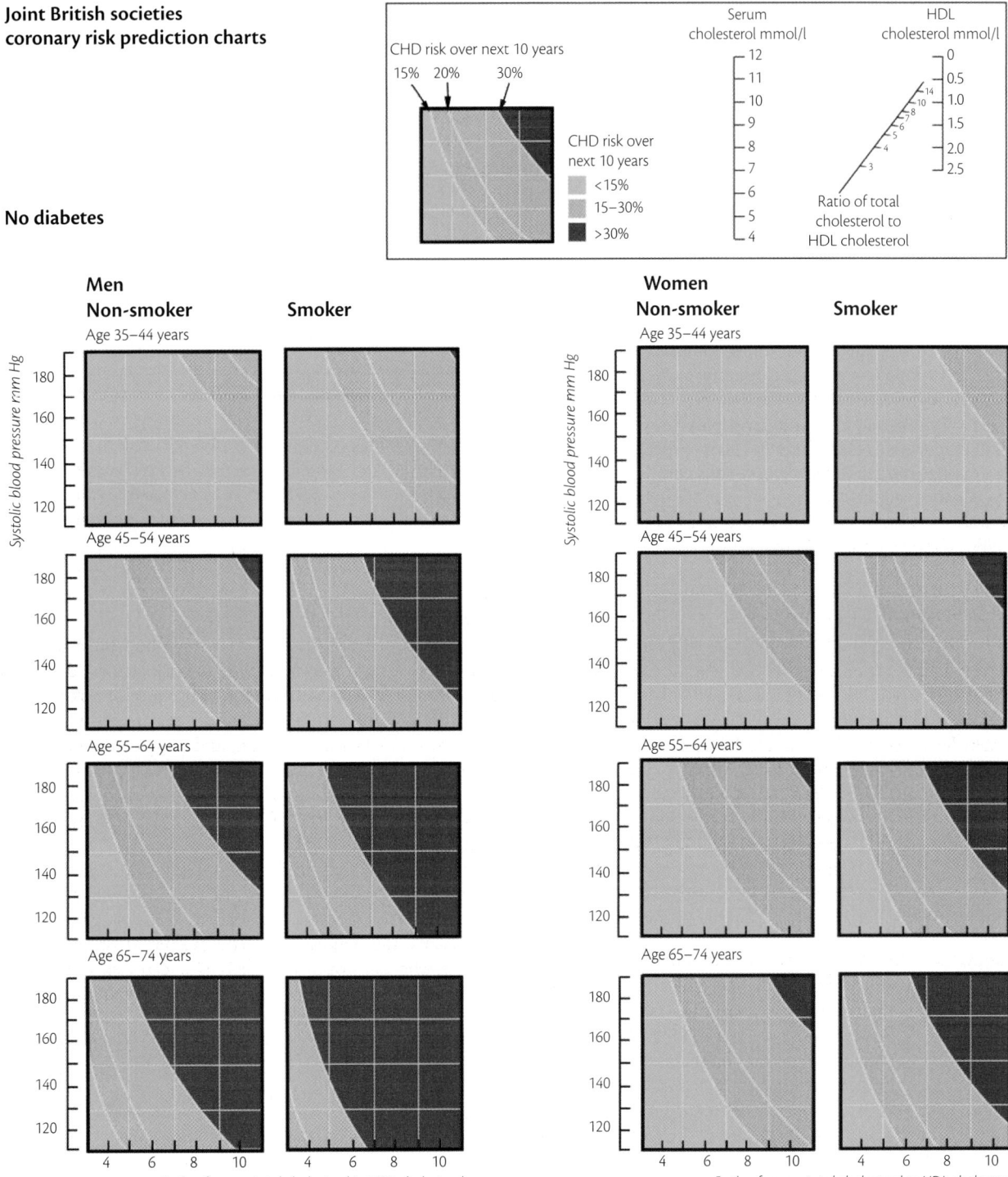

Fig. 16.13.2.11 Absolute risk prediction of 10 year rates of CHD death and nonfatal MI in individuals using risk factors: a model from Framingham.

large individual patient data meta-analysis. While fibrinogen is associated more strongly (2.3) with CHD events, similar genetic evidence suggests these effects might be confounded. A further challenge in assessing the causal contribution of these factors comes from the absence of specific therapeutic agents which alter CRP or fibrinogen activity. A potentially promising line of enquiry involves relating the risk of inflammatory disorders, e.g. psoriasis

or rheumatoid arthritis, to risk of subsequent disease. Although issues of confounding still pertain, the reported risks are of intrinsic clinical interest.

Lipoprotein (a) (Lp(a)) is a putative biomarker subject to less confounding by environmental factors because of its high heritability (0.93–0.98). With a homology to plasminogen and therefore a potential role in haemostasis, Lp(a) is associated with coronary events with a relative risk of about 1.7. Serum creatinine level, a ubiquitously performed test in which there is little direct commercial interest, may offer clues to aetiology of importance to clinical practice. In an individual patient data meta-analysis, a glomerular filtration rate between 15 and 60 ml/min per 1.73 m^2 was associated with CVD events in black individuals more strongly than in whites. This may reflect more frequent or severe subclinical vascular disease secondary to hypertension or diabetes in black individuals.

Over 100 circulating biomarkers have been associated with coronary disease aetiology or prognosis, and more than 10 of these biomarkers have been subjected to meta-analytic scrutiny; emerging findings suggest that individual biomarker effects tend to be modest, confounded, or subject to biased reporting. Even if a biomarker were found with a very large effect (odds ratio of 3 or more), this may add little to risk prediction. Combining sets of biomarkers in panels, and taking a systems biology approach may offer more promise, although there has been little empirical support to date. A recent study found that measuring multiple acute phase reactants, proinflammatory molecules and markers of endothelial activation in the post-MI setting added little beyond established risk factors to risk prediction (Fig. 16.13.2.12).

Genetic influences

Parental history of CHD confers an approximate doubling of risk of CHD among the offspring and, in the Framingham study, those with a sibling with CVD were also at increased risk beyond that conferred by parental CVD and established risk factors. The possibility that the sibling effect may be stronger than the parental effect suggests that early life environment, as well as shared genes, may be important. Many quantitative traits including measures of disease phenotype—proximal coronary artery stenosis, coronary artery calcification—and intermediate phenotypes (including blood pressure, BMI, cholesterol) show modest to high heritability coefficients (0.2–0.8). Genome-wide association studies investigating tens of thousands of SNPs have identified a small number of genes significantly associated with MI. Candidate gene approaches, summarized in literature based meta-analysis, have identified SNPs in more than 10 genes that are associated with MI. The risk alleles are common, but the reported effects are small, commonly less than 1.3. How these genes inter-relate with other genes or with environmental factors is not known. Within a generation, heritable changes in function and expression of genes not involving DNA sequence (epigenetics) are emerging as important mechanisms by which the environment might influence disease.

Life-course influences

Trajectories of change in blood pressure, cholesterol, and markers of carbohydrate metabolism have their origins in early life; values track within individuals over time and measurements made in the second and third decade of life predict manifest coronary disease in mid and later life. Correlations between ischaemic heart disease mortality with both neonatal and postneonatal mortality stimulated the hypothesis that impaired fetal growth may influence adult coronary disease. Identifying which aspects of growth and development are most important is ongoing, although recent meta-analyses suggest that birthweight is not causally associated with either systolic blood pressure or cholesterol in adult life. See Chapter 16.13.3 for further discussion.

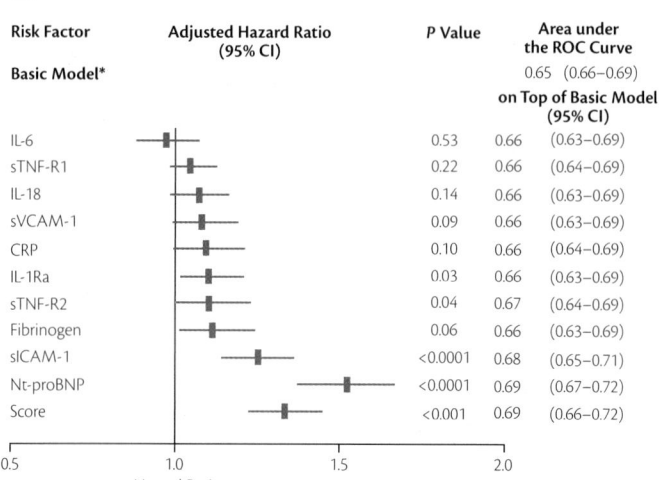

(a)

Risk Factor	Adjusted Hazard Ratio (95% CI)	P Value	Area under the ROC Curve
Basic Model*			0.65 (0.66–0.69)
			on Top of Basic Model (95% CI)
IL-6		0.53	0.66 (0.63–0.69)
sTNF-R1		0.22	0.66 (0.64–0.69)
IL-18		0.14	0.66 (0.63–0.69)
sVCAM-1		0.09	0.66 (0.63–0.69)
CRP		0.10	0.66 (0.64–0.69)
IL-1Ra		0.03	0.66 (0.63–0.69)
sTNF-R2		0.04	0.67 (0.64–0.69)
Fibrinogen		0.06	0.66 (0.63–0.69)
sICAM-1		<0.0001	0.68 (0.65–0.71)
Nt-proBNP		<0.0001	0.69 (0.67–0.72)
Score		<0.001	0.69 (0.66–0.72)

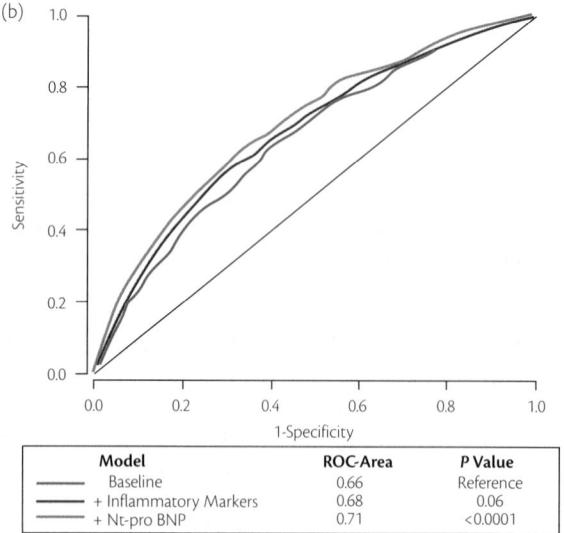

(b)

Model	ROC-Area	P Value
Baseline	0.66	Reference
+ Inflammatory Markers	0.68	0.06
+ Nt-pro BNP	0.71	<0.0001

Fig. 16.13.2.12 Independent and incremental prognostic value of novel biomarkers beyond conventional risk factors, for the prediction of cardiovascular events among patients with established CVD. (a) Independent effects. After adjustment for conventional risk factors, novel risk factors, with the exception of N-terminal pro-BNP, had small effects. (b) Incremental effects. Compared to the predictive discrimination provided by simple risk factors (baseline), the inflammatory markers added little prognostic information.
Blankenberg, McQueen, Smieja, Pogue, Balion, Lonn, Rupprecht, Bickel, Tiret, Cambien, Gerstein, Munzel, & Yusuf 2006. "Comparative impact of multiple biomarkers and N-Terminal pro-brain natriuretic peptide in the context of conventional risk factors for the prediction of recurrent cardiovascular events in the Heart Outcomes Prevention Evaluation (HOPE) Study", Circulation, vol. 114, no. 3, pp. 201–208. (http://circ.ahajournals.org/cgi/content/abstract/114/3/201).

Imaging and screening for preclinical coronary disease

Measuring arterial, myocardial, or electrophysiological disease processes before the first symptomatic manifestation of disease is important, both to understand disease mechanisms and potentially as screening tools to improve the identification of high risk individuals. The absolute risk of coronary events according to the presence and absence of abnormalities on preclinical disease measures is illustrated in Fig. 16.13.2.13. Although individual studies were small and take variable account of established risk factors, Fig. 16.13.2.13

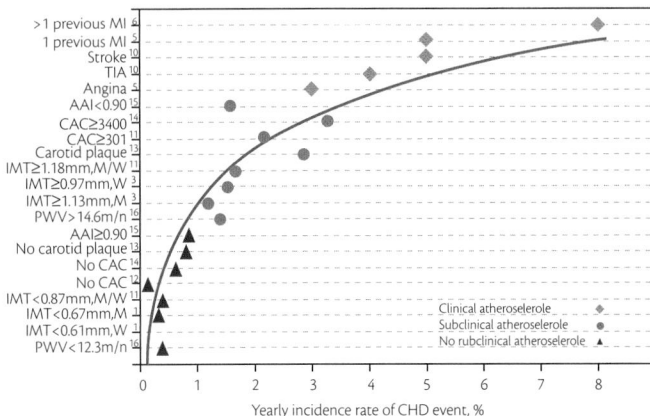

Relation of yearly CHD incidence with absence and presence of subclinical atherosclerosis and presence of clinical arterial disease. M, men; W, women; CAC, coronary artery calcium; AAI, ankle arm index; TIA, transient ischemic attack. Superscript number on the y axis legends indicates bibliographic reference.

Fig. 16.13.2.13 One-year absolute risk of CHD among people with and without markers of sub-clinical atherosclerosis and clinically manifest disease.
Simon, Chironi, & Levenson 2006. "Performance of subclinical arterial disease detection as a screening test for coronary heart disease", Hypertension, vol. 48, no. 3, pp. 392–396. (http://hyper.ahajournals.org/cgi/content/abstract/48/3/392).

illustrates the principle of a continuum of risk; coronary event rates are lowest among those without subclinical disease, intermediate among those with subclinical disease, and substantially higher among those with manifest disease. A growing number of measures are available, although optimal combinations or sequential testing strategies await clarification.

Electrocardiography

The resting ECG is the most widely assessed measure of subclinical disease, although robust estimates of the predictive value of its many parameters have not been subjected to systematic review. At least one (categorical) ischaemic abnormality on the resting electrocardiogram is found in about 25% of the 'healthy' population, and even changes that have been termed 'minor' are associated with subsequent coronary event rates. Left ventricular hypertrophy, a less common abnormality, is associated with an approximate threefold increase in events. Continuous measures, such as QRS/T angle and high QRS nondipolar voltage, may further add predictive information. For exercise ECG, population-based studies of asymptomatic, healthy middle-aged people show that ST depression is a strong predictor of CHD events, with relative risk of 2.8 to 10 (based on 9 studies).

Coronary artery imaging for calcium

Currently the only direct population-based measure of the presence and extent of coronary artery disease comes from calcium scores, using electron beam CT. Although atherosclerosis may be present in the absence of calcium, the presence of calcium in the coronary arteries is highly specific for atherosclerosis. Among asymptomatic middle-aged individuals about 70% of white men and 45% of white women have some coronary artery calcium. Early evidence suggests a strong dose response relationship between increasing score and increasing coronary event rates. Compared to individuals with no coronary artery calcium, the odds ratios (coronary artery calcium scores) in a recent small meta-analysis were 2.1 (1 to 100), 5.4 (101–400), and 10 (>400).

Structure and function of peripheral arteries

Population studies increasingly incorporate measures of large and small artery structure and function outside the coronary circulation.

The ratio of the systolic blood pressure assessed in the brachial and ankle arteries is associated with cardiovascular mortality, independent of other risk factors, with a relative risk of about 2. The ankle brachial index is a simple, low-cost measure, with high reliability. Common carotid intima media thickness, assessed with B mode ultrasound, is associated with risk factors and predicts future coronary events. For example, using the cut point of 1 mm, the relative risk in the ARIC study was 5.07 in women and 1.85 in men. Systemic arterial stiffness and pulse wave velocity have also been related to coronary events. Small-artery compliance or stiffness is a marker for endothelial dysfunction that induces a functional change in the microcirculation and is a predictor of adverse cardiovascular events.

Synthesis and strategy: implications for policy

High-risk approach to prevention

Geoffrey Rose presented two complementary strategies for prevention. The 'high-risk' strategy, the traditional medical approach to prevention, identifies individuals at high risk of subsequent CVD events who are then offered behavioural or pharmacological interventions. However, there are limitations to the high-risk approach to preventing coronary disease, the first being that current risk prediction tools have modest discriminatory performance.

The second limitation is that while there are effective methods to modify dietary and smoking behaviour, their influence on blood pressure, cholesterol or BMI has tended to be disappointing. Unfortunately, there are no satisfactory clinical trials that evaluate the effect of a 30% fat or a 20% low-fat diet on clinical CHD. Pharmacological modification of risk factors such as lipid levels (with statins) and blood pressure has been demonstrated to have an effect in randomized trials. Controversially, it has been proposed that individuals aged 55 and over should be offered a combination pill ('polypill') containing low doses of hydrochlorothiazide, atenolol, enalapril, simavastatin, aspirin, and folic acid. Although randomized trials have yet to be carried out, such an approach is predicted to lead to a reduction in ischaemic heart disease events by 88%.

A third issue is that even when quality of care can be defined, international surveys repeatedly show that it is suboptimal. For example, in a survey in 15 European countries of patients with coronary disease, behavioural modification and pharmacological control of cardiovascular risk factors was poor.

A fourth matter is that uptake of screening or interventions may favour higher socioeconomic groups, and this may contribute to the slower declines e.g. in smoking prevalence in more deprived groups.

It is also the case that compliance with treatment regimens in chronic asymptomatic diseases remains difficult to achieve, and most fundamental of all, the high-risk approach is palliative and temporary in that it does not seek to alter the underlying causes of the disease but to identify individuals who are particularly susceptible to those causes.

Population-based strategies for prevention

A more radical approach to prevention, the 'population strategy', seeks to control the determinants of incidence in the population as a whole. The risk associated with many clinical variables—blood pressure, cholesterol—is continuous with no evidence of threshold (see Fig. 16.13.2.8). Such variables are strong, consistent predictors of CVD in groups, but are poor predictors of susceptibility in individuals. Figure 16.13.2.9 shows the distributions of blood pressure (top panel) in five populations taken from the Intersalt study; with increasing median values their normal distributions shift rightward, towards higher risk. Interventions on the whole population will shift the distribution of a risk factor in a favourable direct (to the left in this case); a 5 mmHg lowering of the population mean blood pressure would correspond to about a 20% reduction in the coronary event rates.

Globalization and risk factors

An important mechanism for bringing about improvements of the cardiovascular health of whole populations lies in national and international fiscal, regulatory, and legislative change—so-called 'health protection'—in which individual members of the population need have no knowledge or understanding of the changes, nor how they may be linked to health. The changing ways in which people now interact across physical, temporal, and cognitive boundaries, most commonly referred to as globalization, is increasing interdependence, integration, and interaction between people and companies in disparate locations and influencing cardiovascular health in disparate ways. Public health policies need to take into account the role that agriculture, trade, education, the physical environment, town planning, and transport have on CVD aetiology.

Explaining temporal and geographical variations with risk factors

The Interheart study concluded that nine risk factors—smoking, apoB/apoA, high blood pressure, diabetes, abdominal obesity, psychosocial factors, fresh fruit and vegetables, alcohol, and physical activity accounted for 90% of the population attributable risk for myocardial infarction. The WHO Multinational Monitoring of Trends and Determinants in Cardiovascular Disease (MONICA) Project found that trends in risk factors, measured since the 1980s in 38 populations from 21 countries, explained much of the variation in population trends in MI before age 65 years. However, several countries continue to offer paradoxes. The rapid increase, and then decrease, of CHD mortality in Russia during the 1990s occurred without major changes in smoking, blood pressure, and cholesterol; it may have reflected social and economic stressors, in combination with high alcohol consumption. Japan has had a substantially lower coronary mortality rate than other developed countries despite a prevalence of cigarette smoking among the highest in developed countries, cholesterol levels comparable to those of the United States of America, and increasing prevalence of obesity and diabetes.

Likely future developments

If globally the CVD epidemic is growing more desperate, future remedies must be commensurate; policy approaches to the prevention of CHD will increasingly take an international or global perspective. The WHO Commission on Social Determinants of Health, which reports in 2008, is expected to demonstrate the preeminent role of social and economic factors in defining the risk behaviours, and their psychosocial context within countries, and to make recommendations for achievable ways in which societies

across the development spectrum, should change. WHO is shortly to announce its guidelines for the prevention of CVD.

A key tension for the future is the reconciliation of two perspectives: the cultural and the cellular, the macroeconomic and the molecular. Such wide variations in the rate of CHD across the globe and, particularly, such rapid changes in CHD rate over time among migrants and indigenous populations have, traditionally, been interpreted as leaving little scope for the play of genetic factors in global cardiovascular health. In the next decade this position is likely to be nuanced, if not recast. Epigenetics might prove a core discipline in this regard, with early reports suggesting strong associations e.g. between smoking and CpG island methylation, and animal models suggesting that environmental interventions (diet) can lead to epigenetic changes, which in turn lead to altered gene expression. Already population geneticists are reporting large genetic differences across current political borders over which there has been large and recent two-way migration. Black and white populations show large differences in frequency of common polymorphisms affecting the metabolism of an increasingly prevalent set of environmental exposures—therapeutic medication. Improvements in individualized risk prediction for CHD are likely, although the process of sifting the huge amount of information into knowledge is likely to be slow and complex. Using a panel of information derived from large numbers of '-omic' variables might generate signatures that supplant and surpass current efforts to identify high risk individuals; expression studies are already claiming this for the prognosis of cancer.

However, without refining the measures of disease outcome—separating plaque development, plaque rupture, thrombotic and necrotic processes—efforts to dissect out the molecular causes may be blunted. Epidemiological studies will increasingly complement the study of the presence or absence of coronary disease (usually undifferentiated MI) with measures of how much coronary artery disease and which manifestation. Higher endpoint resolution of known phenotypes and 'class discovery' of new phenotypes are both important. As radiation dose decreases for CT techniques, it may be possible to image the coronary arteries in the general population for plaque burden and (with molecular imaging) composition.

Over the next decade epidemiology as applied to CHD is likely to become more complex. There has been much success with the epidemiological paradigm, likened to a game of billiards, where one exposure of interest (the cue ball) is linearly associated with one outcome, independent of confounders (a third ball getting in the way). It remains to be seen how this (simple) paradigm evolves in relation to new insights from a widening range of disciplines: from social science, through to systems biology and bioinformatics. From a public health perspective epidemiology is predicted to remain, as William Petty wrote in 1690, political arithmetic.

Further reading

Barrett-Connor E (1997). Sex differences in coronary heart disease. Why are women so superior? The 1995 Ancel Keys Lecture. *Circulation*, **95**, 252–64.

Bild DE, *et al.* (2005). Ethnic differences in coronary calcification: the Multi-Ethnic Study of Atherosclerosis (MESA). *Circulation*, **111**, 1313–20.

Blankenberg S, *et al.* (2006). 'Comparative impact of multiple biomarkers and N-terminal pro-brain natriuretic peptide in the context of conventional risk factors for the prediction of recurrent cardiovascular events in the Heart Outcomes Prevention Evaluation (HOPE) Study. *Circulation*, **114**, 201–8.

British Heart Foundation (2006). http://www.heartstats.org/temp/Chaptersp1%281%29hs1hs.pdf.

Chandola T, Brunner E, Marmot M (2006). Chronic stress at work and the metabolic syndrome: prospective study. *BMJ*, **332**, 521–5.

Clouse ME (2006). How useful is computed tomography for screening for coronary artery disease? Noninvasive screening for coronary artery disease with computed tomography is useful. *Circulation*, **113**, 125–46.

Corrao G, *et al.* (2000). Alcohol and coronary heart disease: a meta-analysis. *Addiction*, **95**, 1505–23.

Dahlof B, *et al.* (2005). Prevention of cardiovascular events with an antihypertensive regimen of amlodipine adding perindopril as required versus atenolol adding bendroflumethiazide as required, in the Anglo-Scandinavian Cardiac Outcomes Trial-Blood Pressure Lowering Arm (ASCOT-BPLA): a multicentre randomised controlled trial. *Lancet*, **366**, 895–906.

Danesh J, Collins R, Peto R (2000). Lipoprotein(a) and coronary heart disease. Meta-analysis of prospective studies. *Circulation*, **102**, 1082–5.

Daviglus ML *et al.* (1999). Association of nonspecific minor ST-T abnormalities with cardiovascular mortality: the Chicago Western Electric Study [see comments]. *JAMA*, **281**, 530–536.

Doobay AV, Anand SS (2005). Sensitivity and specificity of the ankle-brachial index to predict future cardiovascular outcomes: a systematic review. *Arterioscler Thromb Vasc Biol*, **25**, 1463–9.

Ezzati M, *et al.* (2005). Rethinking the 'diseases of affluence' paradigm: global patterns of nutritional risks in relation to economic development. *PLoS Med*, **2**, e133.

Forouhi NG, *et al.* (2006). Do known risk factors explain the higher coronary heart disease mortality in South Asian compared with European men? Prospective follow-up of the Southall and Brent studies, UK. *Diabetologia*, **49**, 2580–8.

Fowler-Brown A, *et al.* (2004). Exercise tolerance testing to screen for coronary heart disease: a systematic review for the technical support for the U.S. Preventive Services Task Force. *Ann Intern Med*, **140**, W9–24.

Fraga MF, *et al.* (2005). Epigenetic differences arise during the lifetime of monozygotic twins. *Proc Natl Acad Sci. U S A*, **102**, 10604–9.

Galassi A, Reynolds K, He J (2006). Metabolic syndrome and risk of CVD: a meta-analysis. *Am J Med*, **119**, 812–19.

Grant SF, *et al.* (2006). Variant of transcription factor 7-like 2 (*TCF7L2*) gene confers risk of type 2 diabetes. *Nat Genet*, **38**, 320–3.

Hemingway H, *et al.* (2005). Does autonomic function link social position to coronary risk? The Whitehall II Study. *Circulation*, **111**, 3071–7.

Hemingway H, *et al.* (2006). Incidence and prognostic implications of stable angina pectoris among women and men. *JAMA*, **295**, 1404–11.

Homocysteine Studies Collaboration (2002). Homocysteine and risk of ischemic heart disease and stroke: a meta-analysis. *JAMA*, **288**, 2015–22.

Hooper L, *et al.* (2006). Risks and benefits of omega 3 fats for mortality, CVD, and cancer: systematic review. *BMJ*, **332**, 752–60.

Huisman M, *et al.* (2005). Educational inequalities in cause-specific mortality in middle-aged and older men and women in eight western European populations. *Lancet*, **365**, 493–500.

Huxley R, Barzi F, Woodward M (2006). Excess risk of fatal coronary heart disease associated with diabetes in men and women: meta-analysis of 37 prospective cohort studies. *BMJ*, **332**, 73–8.

Huxley R, Neil A, Collins R (2002). Unravelling the fetal origins hypothesis: is there really an inverse association between birthweight and subsequent blood pressure? *Lancet*, **360**, 659–65.

Huxley R, *et al.* (2004). Birthweight and subsequent cholesterol levels: exploration of the 'fetal origins' hypothesis. *JAMA*, **292**, 2755–64.

Kayser M, *et al.* (2005). Significant genetic differentiation between Poland and Germany follows present-day political borders, as revealed by Y-chromosome analysis. *Hum Genet*, **117**, 428–43.

Kearney PM, *et al.* (2005). Global burden of hypertension: analysis of worldwide data. *Lancet*, **365**, 217–223.

Klerk M, *et al.* (2002). MTHFR 677C T polymorphism and risk of coronary heart disease: a meta-analysis. *JAMA*, **288**, 2023–31.

Kuh D, Ben Shlomo Y (2004). *A life course approach to chronic disease epidemiology*, 2nd edition. Oxford University Press, New York.

Kuulasmaa K, *et al.* (2000). Estimation of contribution of changes in classic risk factors to trends in coronary-event rates across the WHO MONICA Project populations [see comments]. *Lancet*, **355**, 675–87.

Lampe FC, *et al.* (2005). Trends in rates of different forms of diagnosed coronary heart disease, 1978 to 2000: prospective, population based study of British men. *BMJ*, **330**, 1046.

Law MR, Wald NJ, Thompson SG (1994). By how much and how quickly does reduction in serum cholesterol concentration lower risk of ischaemic heart disease? *BMJ*, **308**, 367–72.

Lewington S, *et al.* (2002). Age-specific relevance of usual blood pressure to vascular mortality: a meta-analysis of individual data for one million adults in 61 prospective studies. *Lancet*, **360**, 1903–13.

Malyutina S, *et al.* (2002). Relation between heavy and binge drinking and all-cause and cardiovascular mortality in Novosibirsk, Russia: a prospective cohort study. *Lancet*, **360**, 1448–54.

Marmot MG (1998). 'Improvement of social environment to improve health', *Lancet*, vol. 351, no. 9095, pp. 57–60.

Marmot M (2005). Social determinants of health inequalities. *Lancet*, **365**, 1099–1104.

McGee DL (2005). Body mass index and mortality: a meta-analysis based on person-level data from twenty-six observational studies. *Ann Epidemiol*, **15**, 87–97.

Murphy NF, *et al.* (2004). Hospital discharge rates for suspected acute coronary syndromes between 1990 and 2000: population based analysis. *BMJ*, **328**, 1413–14.

Murray CL (1994). *Global comparative assessments in the health sector*. World Health Organization, Geneva.

Nelson HD (2002). Assessing benefits and harms of hormone replacement therapy: clinical applications. *JAMA*, **288**, 882–4.

Nicholson A, Kuper H, Hemingway H (2006). Depression as an aetiologic and prognostic factor in coronary heart disease: a meta-analysis of 6362 events among 146 538 participants in 54 observational studies. *Eur Heart J*, **27**, 2763–74.

Oguma Y, Shinoda-Tagawa T (2004). Physical activity decreases CVD risk in women: review and meta-analysis. *Am J Prev Med*, **26**, 407–18.

Pletcher MJ, *et al.* (2004). Using the coronary artery calcium score to predict coronary heart disease events: a systematic review and meta-analysis. *Arch Intern Med*, **164**, 1285–92.

Qiao Q (2006). Comparison of different definitions of the metabolic syndrome in relation to cardiovascular mortality in European men and women. *Diabetologia*, **49**, 2837–46.

Romero-Corral A, *et al.* (2006). Association of bodyweight with total mortality and with cardiovascular events in coronary artery disease: a systematic review of cohort studies. *Lancet*, **368**, 666–78.

Rose G (1992). *The strategy of preventive medicine*. Oxford University Press, New York.

Sijbrands EJ, *et al.* (2001). Mortality over two centuries in large pedigree with familial hypercholesterolaemia: family tree mortality study. *BMJ*, **322**, 1019–23.

Simon A, Chironi G, Levenson J (2006). Performance of subclinical arterial disease detection as a screening test for coronary heart disease. *Hypertension*, **48**, 392–6.

Song Y, Stampfer MJ, Liu S (2004). Meta-analysis: apolipoprotein E genotypes and risk for coronary heart disease. *Ann Intern Med*, **141**, 137–47.

Teo KK, *et al.* (2006). 'Tobacco use and risk of myocardial infarction in 52 countries in the INTERHEART study: a case-control study', *Lancet*, vol. **368**, no. 9536, pp. 647–658.

Tuomilehto J, *et al.* (2001). Prevention of type 2 diabetes mellitus by changes in lifestyle among subjects with impaired glucose tolerance. *N Engl J Med*, **344**, 1343–1350.

Turnbull F (2003). Effects of different blood-pressure-lowering regimens on major cardiovascular events: results of prospectively-designed overviews of randomised trials'. *Lancet*, **362**, 1527–35.

Verschuren WM, *et al.* (1995). Serum total cholesterol and long-term coronary heart disease mortality in different cultures. Twenty-five-year follow-up of the seven countries study. *JAMA*, **274**, 131–6.

Wald NJ, Law MR (2003). A strategy to reduce CVD by more than 80%. *BMJ*, **326**, 1419.

Weiner DE, *et al.* (2004). Chronic kidney disease as a risk factor for CVD and all-cause mortality: a pooled analysis of community-based studies. *J Am Soc Nephrol*, **15**, 1307–15.

WHO (2003). *World health report 2003—shaping the future.* World Health Organization, Geneva.

Wild S, Mckeigue, P (1997). Cross sectional analysis of mortality by country of birth in England and Wales, 1970–92. *BMJ*, **314**, 705.

Wong TY, *et al.* (2002). Retinal arteriolar narrowing and risk of coronary heart disease in men and women. The Atherosclerosis Risk in Communities Study. *JAMA*, **287**, 1153–9.

Yusuf S, *et al.* (2004). Effect of potentially modifiable risk factors associated with myocardial infarction in 52 countries (the INTERHEART study): case-control study. *Lancet*, **364**, 937–52.

16.13.3 Influences acting *in utero* and in early childhood

D.J.P. Barker

Essentials

The search for the environmental causes of ischaemic heart disease is generally guided by a 'destructive' model, where the causes to be identified are thought to act in adult life and accelerate destructive processes such as the formation of atheroma, rise in blood pressure, and loss of glucose tolerance. By contrast, a 'developmental' model for the disease focuses on causes acting on the baby and argues that in responding to undernutrition and other adverse influences, the baby ensures its continued survival and growth at the cost of premature death from ischaemic heart disease.

Low birthweight is associated with increased rates of ischaemic heart disease and the related disorders—stroke, hypertension, and type 2 diabetes. These associations, which have been extensively replicated in studies in different countries, extend across the normal range of birthweight, and depend on lower birthweights in relation to the duration of gestation rather than the effects of premature birth. They are thought to be consequences of developmental plasticity—the phenomenon by which one genotype can give rise to a range of different physiological or morphological states in response to different environmental conditions during development.

Impaired growth in infancy and rapid childhood weight gain exacerbate the effects of impaired prenatal growth. The placenta is likely to play a key role in programming the baby.

The fetal origins hypothesis

Over the past 15 years epidemiological studies have shown that people who had low birthweight, or who were thin or short at birth, are at increased risk of developing ischaemic heart disease and the related disorders stroke, hypertension, and type 2 diabetes. Associations between small size at birth and later disease, first recorded in the United Kingdom, have now been extensively replicated in studies in Europe and the United States of America. The associations extend across the whole range of birthweight and depend on lower birthweights in relation to the duration of gestation rather than the effects of premature birth. They are not the result of confounding variables acting in later life, such as low socioeconomic status and smoking.

These observations gave rise to the 'fetal origins hypothesis', which proposes that cardiovascular disease originates through adaptations that are made by a fetus when it is undernourished. Unlike adaptations made in adult life, those made during early development tend to have permanent effects on the body's structure and function—a phenomenon sometimes referred to as 'programming'.

Fetal nutrition

In common with other living creatures, human beings are 'plastic' in their early life, and their organs and systems are shaped by their environment at that time. The development of the sweat glands provides a simple example of this. All humans have similar numbers of sweat glands at birth, but none of them function. In the first 3 years after birth a proportion of the glands become functional, depending on the temperature to which the child is exposed. The hotter the conditions, the greater the number of sweat glands that are programmed to function. After 3 years the process is complete and the number of sweat glands is fixed. Thereafter the child who has experienced hot conditions will be better equipped to adapt to similar conditions in later life, because people with more functioning sweat glands cool down faster.

This brief description encapsulates the essence of developmental plasticity: a critical period when a system is plastic and sensitive to the environment, followed by loss of plasticity and a fixed functional capacity. For most organs and systems the critical period occurs *in utero*. There are good reasons why it may be advantageous in evolutionary terms for the body to remain plastic during development. It enables the production of phenotypes that are better matched to their environment than would be possible if the same phenotype was produced in all environments. Developmental plasticity is formally defined as the phenomenon whereby one genotype can give rise to a range of different physiological or morphological states in response to different environmental conditions during development.

The fetus responds to undernutrition in a number of ways. It can redistribute its cardiac output to protect key organs, the brain in particular; it can alter its metabolism, e.g. by switching from glucose to amino acid oxidation; and it can change the production of, or tissue sensitivity to, hormones regulating growth, importantly insulin. Slowing of growth is adaptive because it reduces the requirement for substrate. Experiments show that even minor modifications to the diets of pregnant animals may be followed by lifelong changes in the offspring in ways that can be related to human disease, for example raised blood pressure and altered glucose–insulin metabolism.

Effects of fetal and postnatal growth on adult diseases

Ischaemic heart disease

An important clue suggesting that ischaemic heart disease originates during fetal development came from studies of death rates among babies in the United Kingdom during the early 1900s. The usual certified cause of death in newborn babies at that time was low birthweight. Death rates in the newborn differed considerably between one part of the country and another, being highest in the northern industrial towns and the poorer rural areas in the north and west. This geographical pattern in death rates was shown to closely resemble today's large variations in death rates from ischaemic heart disease, variations that form one aspect of the continuing inequalities in health in the United Kingdom. This led to the hypothesis that low rates of growth before birth are linked to the development of ischaemic heart disease in adult life.

The subsequent studies that confirmed this association were based on the simple strategy of examining men and women in middle and late life whose body size at birth was recorded. In the first study of this kind 16 000 men and women born in Hertfordshire (southern England) during 1911 to 1930 were traced from birth. Death rates from ischaemic heart disease fell twofold between those at the lower and upper ends of the birthweight distribution (Fig. 16.13.3.1). Later studies showed that it was people who were small at birth because they failed to grow, rather than because they were born early, who were at increased risk of the disease. The graded nature of the association between birthweight and ischaemic heart disease, shown in Fig. 16.13.3.1, implies that normal variations in the food supply from normal healthy mothers to their babies have profound long-term effects.

The association between low birthweight and ischaemic heart disease has since been confirmed in studies in Finland, Sweden, the United Kingdom, and the United States of America. Among 80 000 women in the American Nurses Study there was a twofold fall in the relative risk of nonfatal ischaemic heart disease across the range of birthweight. An association between low birthweight and prevalent ischaemic heart disease has also been shown in a small study in South India.

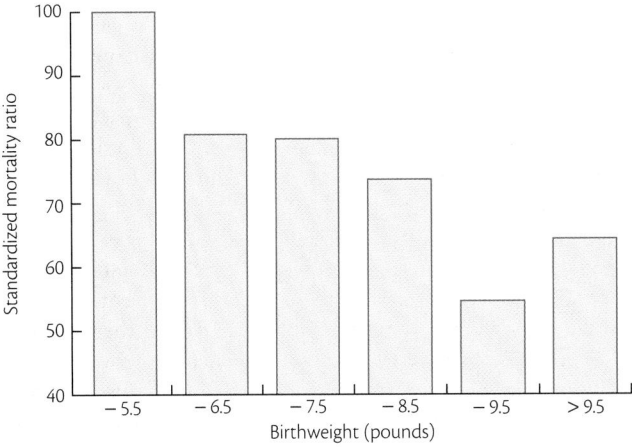

Fig. 16.13.3.1 Death rates from ischaemic heart disease in 15 726 men and women born in Hertfordshire according to their birthweights.
Reprinted from *The Lancet*, Vol. 334, Barker DJP *et al*, *Weight in Infancy and Death from Ischaemic Heart Disease* pp. 577–80. Copyright (1989), with permission from Elsevier.

Stroke

The pattern of body proportions at birth which predicts stroke is different to that which predicts ischaemic heart disease. Studies in Sheffield (northern England) and Helsinki (Finland) found increased rates among people who had a low ratio of birthweight to head circumference. One interpretation of this is that normal head growth was sustained at the cost of interrupted growth of the body in late gestation. 'Brain-sparing' patterns of growth can result from diversion of cardiac output to the brain at the expense of the abdominal viscera, importantly the liver. Preliminary evidence suggests that this has lasting effects on liver function, including altered regulation of low density lipoprotein (LDL) cholesterol.

Type 2 diabetes

Studies of the mechanisms linking low birthweight with cardiovascular disease have shown that the progressive fall in disease rates across the range of birthweight (Fig. 16.13.3.1) is paralleled by progressive falls in type 2 diabetes, a major risk factor for the disease. The original observation made among men in Hertfordshire (Table 16.13.3.1) has now been extensively replicated in men and women. Both insulin resistance and deficiency in insulin production are thought to be important in the pathogenesis of type 2 diabetes, and there is evidence that both may originate during fetal life. There is now a substantial literature showing that low birthweight is associated with insulin resistance. Men and women who had low birthweight also have a high prevalence of the 'metabolic syndrome' in which impaired glucose tolerance, hypertension, and raised serum triglyceride concentrations occur in the same patient: they are insulin resistant and hyperinsulinaemic.

A number of studies have shown that people who had low birthweight are already insulin resistant in childhood. A study of men and women who were *in utero* during the wartime famine in the Netherlands provides direct evidence that maternal undernutrition can programme insulin resistance and type 2 diabetes in the offspring. The 'Dutch famine' began abruptly in November 1944 and ended with the liberation of the Netherlands in 1945. The official rations varied between 400 and 800 calories per day. Men and women exposed to the famine *in utero* had higher 2-h plasma glucose concentrations after a standard oral glucose challenge than those born before or conceived after it. They also had higher fasting plasma proinsulin and 2-h plasma insulin concentrations, indicating insulin resistance.

Table 16.13.3.1 Percentage of men in Hertfordshire with type 2 diabetes or impaired glucose tolerance (2-h plasma glucose concentration 7.8 mmol/litre or more) according to birthweight

Weight (pounds)	% of men	Odds ratio (95% CI)[a]
≤5.5	40	6.6 (1.5–28)
–6.5	34	4.8 (1.3–17)
–7.5	31	4.6 (1.4–16)
–8.5	22	2.6 (0.8–8.9)
–9.5	13	1.4 (0.3–5.6)
>9.5	14	1.0
p for trend	<0.001	

[a] Adjusted for current BMI.

Table 16.13.3.2 Hazard ratios (95% confidence intervals) for ischaemic heart disease according to birthweight and BMI at 2 years of age: boys and girls combined

Birthweight (kg)	BMI at age 2 (kg/m²)		
	<16	16–17	>17
<3.0	1.9 (1.3–2.8)	1.9 (1.2–3.0)	1.3 (0.7–2.2)
3.0–3.5	1.5 (1.0–2.1)	1.6 (1.1–2.2)	1.2 (0.8–1.8)
>3.5	1.7 (1.2–2.5)	1.5 (1.1–2.2)	1.0

Cardiovascular disease and postnatal growth

Postnatal growth modifies the increased risk of ischaemic heart disease associated with small body size at birth. One important source of information on this is the Helsinki birth cohort comprising 13 000 people born in Helsinki during 1934–44. The height and weight of each infant was measured on an average of eight occasions between birth and 2 years of age, and on a further eight occasions between 2 and 11 years. This made it possible to examine, for the first time, the paths of childhood growth that precede the development of cardiovascular disease and type 2 diabetes in adult life. The mean body size of the boys and girls who later had ischaemic heart disease, stroke, or type 2 diabetes was below the average at birth. Between birth and 2 years of age their body size fell further in relation to that of other children, so that at 2 years they were thin or short. After that age those who developed ischaemic heart disease or type 2 diabetes put on weight rapidly, reaching the average weight and body mass index before 10 years of age. Those who developed type 2 diabetes gained weight most rapidly. Tables 16.13.3.2 and 16.13.3.3 show the combined effects of low birthweight, low body mass index (BMI) at 2 years, and high BMI at 11 years on the later risk of ischaemic heart disease in men and women.

In contrast to the findings for ischaemic heart disease, children who later developed stroke grew slowly in height after 2 years and remained short and thin. This observation may be relevant to the wider ecology of cardiovascular disease. Ischaemic heart disease is a disorder of Westernization, one feature of which is improved childhood nutrition and more rapid gain in body mass index. Stroke is common in the developing countries and among poorer communities in the Western world, where failure to thrive before and after birth may not be followed by compensatory weight gain in later childhood.

Hypertension

A clinical study of people aged 60 years in the Helsinki birth cohort showed that two different paths of growth preceded the development of two different groups of patient with hypertension.

Table 16.13.3.3 Hazard ratios (95% confidence intervals) for ischaemic heart disease according to children's BMI at 2 and 11 years of age.

BMI at age 2 (kg/m²)	BMI at age 11 (kg/m²)		
	<16	16–17.5	>17.5
<16	1.6 (0.8–3.3)	2.4 (1.2–4.9)	3.0 (1.4–6.3)
16–17	1.4 (0.7–3.1)	1.6 (0.8–3.3)	1.9 (0.9–3.9)
>17	1.0	1.3 (0.6–2.7)	1.1 (0.5–2.3)

Table 16.13.3.4 Percentage prevalence of hypertension according to birthweight and current weight among men and women in Helsinki

Birthweight (kg)	Fifths of current weight (kg)					All
Men	–74.8	–81.5	–88.0	–96.5	>96.5	
Women	–62.6	–68.7	–75.2	–83.9	>83.9	
–3.0	28	36	33	50	63	40(396)
–3.5	18	22	25	40	56	32(792)
–4.0	19	25	18	34	52	30(612)
>4.0	4	19	22	21	35	24(202)
All	20(401)	26(400)	24(401)	38(400)	52(400)	32(2002)

Figures in parentheses are numbers of subjects.

One group was obese and insulin resistant, two features of the metabolic syndrome, and were already being treated for hypertension. They had small body size at birth and low weight gain from birth to 2 years, but grew rapidly after that. Table 16.13.3.4 shows the combined effects of birthweight and current adult weight on the prevalence of hypertension in this group. The prevalence ranges from 4% among people with birthweight above 4 kg but current weights in the lowest fifth, to 63% among those with birthweight of 3 kg or less but current weights in the highest fifth. A second group of patients had atherogenic lipid profiles and had not been previously diagnosed as having hypertension, but their blood pressures were classified as hypertensive under current definitions. They were short at birth, had low weight gain from birth to 2 years, and remained small after 2 years of age. The first of these two different paths of growth is the one associated with ischaemic heart disease, whilst the second is the one associated with stroke. The two paths are shown in Fig. 16.13.3.2. They may lead to hypertension and cardiovascular disease through different biological mechanisms, and may therefore respond differently to medication.

Associations between low birthweight and raised systolic and diastolic pressure in childhood and adult life have been extensively

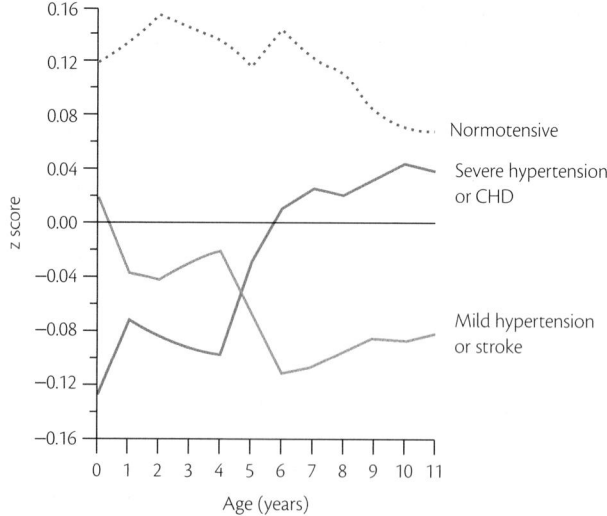

Fig. 16.13.3.2 Mean standard deviation scores (Z scores) for weight in the first 11 years after birth among children who developed hypertension as adults. CHD, coronary heart disease.

Eriksson JG et al. *Childhood Growth and Hypertension in Later Life, Hypertension.* 49:1415–1421.

documented around the world, but the associations tend to be small. A 1 kg difference in birthweight is associated with around 3 mmHg difference in systolic pressure. The contrast between this small effect and the large effect on hypertension (Table 16.13.3.4) suggests that lesions that accompany poor fetal growth and tend to elevate blood pressure have a small influence on blood pressure within the normal range because counter-regulatory mechanisms can maintain normal blood pressure levels for many years. Studies in humans and animals show that slow fetal growth is accompanied by a reduced number of nephrons at birth, which is a lifelong allocation as there is little capacity to develop new nephrons after birth. One hypothesis seeks to link this to the subsequent development of hypertension by arguing that a reduced nephron number results in hyperfiltration of each nephron. Hyperfiltration leads to glomerular hypertension and sclerosis and—ultimately—to nephron death, when counter-regulatory mechanisms are no longer able to maintain homeostasis and there begins a cycle of rising blood pressure, resulting in further nephron death, leading to a further rise in blood pressure. Rapid increase in body size after birth may exacerbate glomerular injury because greater body size leads to increased excretory loads and enhanced glomerular hyperfiltration. Indirect evidence in support of this has come from a study of the kidneys of people killed in road accidents: those being treated for hypertension had fewer, but larger, glomeruli.

The processes that link slow growth during infancy with later hypertension and stroke are not known. One possibility is that it is accompanied by impaired development of the cerebral vasculature at a critical period of early postnatal life. There is also evidence that it is accompanied by impaired development of the liver and altered set points for the regulation of cholesterol.

Other considerations

Role of the placenta

The placental weight of a baby at birth is associated with its risk of developing hypertension and ischaemic heart disease in later life. Associations with low placental weight have been found in some studies, while associations with high placental weight have been found in others. These two different associations may reflect different placental responses to undernutrition. Observations in animals show that in response to undernutrition in pregnancy the placenta may reduce its growth or, if the mother was well nourished at the time of conception, the placenta may enlarge. There is preliminary evidence of a similar phenomenon in humans. Placental enlargement may be an adaptive response to undernutrition that allows the fetus to extract more nutrients from the mother. The placenta is highly responsive to nutrition, oxygen, and its hormonal environment, its biology suggesting that it must play a central role in the genesis of cardiovascular disease, though one about which remarkably little is known.

Maternal nutrition

The nutrition of the fetus depends on the nutrition of the mother. In recent years 'maternal nutrition' has been equated with the diets of pregnant women. This is too limited a definition. The availability of nutrients to the fetus is influenced by the mother's nutrient stores and metabolism, as well as by her diet during pregnancy. In developing countries many babies are undernourished because their mothers are chronically malnourished. Despite current levels of nutrition in Western countries, the nutrition of many fetuses and infants remains

suboptimal because the nutrients available are unbalanced or because their delivery is constrained by maternal metabolism. Mellanby wrote in 1933 that "it is certain that the significance of correct nutrition in child-bearing does not begin in pregnancy itself or even in the adult female before pregnancy. It looms large as soon as a female child is born and indeed in its intrauterine life". Maternal nutrition defined in this way encompasses the nutritional experience of the mother through fetal life and childhood, and into adolescence and adult life. The mother's early nutritional experience establishes her metabolism and hormonal profile, and during pregnancy these shape the baby's development. The ecology of cardiovascular disease—stroke in particular—may depend more on the mother's early nutritional experience than on events during pregnancy.

The mother's body composition before and during pregnancy is an important influence in programming the fetus. The children of overweight mothers are at increased risk of ischaemic heart disease and type 2 diabetes. The raised plasma glucose concentrations in overweight women, which necessarily lead to higher glucose intakes by the fetus, may be one adverse influence. There is now a strong body of evidence suggesting that mothers who are thin also afford an unfavourable environment to their fetuses, leading to insulin resistance and raised blood pressure in the offspring. In the Dutch famine, for example, it was people born to mothers with the lowest weights in pregnancy who had the highest 2-h plasma glucose concentrations. Maternal thinness may have different consequences for the fetus depending on whether it reflects low body muscularity, low body fat, or low weight gain in pregnancy. Mothers' diet in pregnancy has been directly related to cardiovascular risk factors in the offspring during adult life in studies in Scotland. The blood pressures of men and women were related to the balance of animal protein and carbohydrate in their mothers' diets in late pregnancy, while high intakes of fat and protein were associated with insulin deficiency.

Conclusion

Figure 16.13.3.3 gives a framework of possible mechanisms through which fetal undernutrition could lead to ischaemic heart disease. We are beginning to understand the biological processes that may underlie these mechanisms. Changes occur at different levels and include allocation of stem cells and alteration of gene expression in the embryo; changes in heart, renal and liver growth; and alteration in metabolic and hormonal setpoints. These changes can make systems more vulnerable to disruptive influences in postnatal life, which include rapid weight gain, oxidative stresses (including smoking), environmental stress, and an inappropriate diet.

Studies of programming in fetal life and infancy are now established in the agenda for medical research. They have refocused attention on maternal nutrition and fetal growth. The search for the environmental causes of ischaemic heart disease has hitherto been guided by a 'destructive' model, where causes to be identified act in adult life and accelerate destructive processes: the formation of atheroma, rise in blood pressure, and loss of glucose tolerance. There is now a 'developmental' model for the disease, where the causes to be identified act on the baby, in responding to which the baby ensures its continued survival and growth at the expense of premature death from ischaemic heart disease.

The effects of low birthweight on later disease have been shown to be conditioned by the presence of genetic polymorphisms. Interactions between the effects of genes and nutrition during

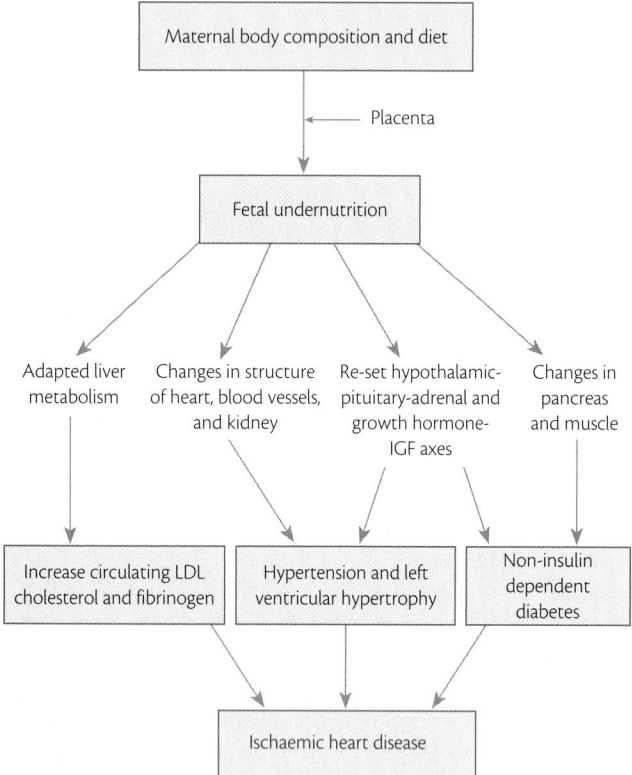

Fig. 16.13.3.3 Framework of possible mechanisms linking fetal undernutrition and ischaemic heart disease.

development would be expected as a manifestation of phenotypic plasticity. The effects of birthweight on later disease are also modified by the postnatal environment, by living conditions during childhood, by adult lifestyles and by the path of postnatal growth. It seems that the pathogenesis of cardiovascular disease and type 2 diabetes cannot be understood within a model in which risks associated with adverse influences at different stages of life add to each other. Rather, disease is the product of branching paths of development, with the environment triggering the branching. The path of development that follows each branch determines the individual's vulnerability to the next adverse influence that lies ahead.

Further reading

Barker DJP, *et al.* (1990). Fetal and placental size and risk of hypertension in adult life. *BMJ*, **301**, 259–62.

Barker DJP (1998). *Mothers, babies and health in later life*, 2nd edition. Churchill Livingstone, Edinburgh.

Barker DJP (ed.) (2000). *Fetal origins of cardiovascular and lung diseases.* NIH Monograph Series, Marcel Decker, New York.

Gluckman P, Hanson M (eds) (2006). *Developmental origins of health and disease.* Cambridge University Press, Cambridge.

Harding JE (2001). The nutritional basis of the fetal origins of adult disease. *Int J Epidemiol*, **30**, 15–23.

McCance RA. (1962). Food, growth and time. *Lancet*, **ii**, 621–6.

Mellanby E. (1933). Nutrition and child-bearing. *Lancet*, **ii**, 1131–7.

Phillips DIW (1996). Insulin resistance as a programmed response to fetal undernutrition. *Diabetologia*, **39**, 1119–22.

Stearns S (ed.) (1998). *Evolution in health and disease.* Oxford University Press, Oxford.

16.13.4 **Management of stable angina**

Adam D. Timmis

Essentials

Angina—the pain provoked by myocardial ischaemia—is usually caused by obstructive coronary artery disease that is sufficiently severe to restrict oxygen delivery to the cardiac myocytes. Quality of life is impaired in direct proportion to the severity of symptoms.

Clinical history remains the most useful basis for diagnosis and referral decisions to specialist services, the commonest indications being (1) new-onset angina, (2) exclusion of angina in high-risk individuals with atypical symptoms, (3) worsening angina in a patient with previously stable symptoms, (4) new or recurrent angina in a patient with history of myocardial infarction or coronary revascularization, (5) assessment of occupational fitness (e.g. airline pilots).

Investigation—noninvasive testing is used primarily for diagnosis, but whatever test is employed—exercise ECG, myocardial perfusion imaging, stress echocardiography, or multidetector CT—the incremental diagnostic value is greatest for patients with an intermediate pretest probability of coronary artery disease in whom uncertainty is greatest. Such tests also have a role in risk assessment to inform decisions about the urgency and aggressiveness of treatment in individual cases.

Medical treatment of angina involves (1) dealing with exacerbating comorbidities, (2) secondary prevention by lifestyle modification (smoking cessation, exercise training, Mediterranean-style diet, etc.) and drugs (aspirin, statins, angiotensin-converting enzyme (ACE)-inhibitors, etc.), (3) antianginal drugs (most commonly β-blockers, short acting nitrates, and calcium channel blockers).

Patients with continuing moderate or severe stable angina despite optimal medical treatment should undergo coronary angiography, as should those identified as being at high risk on noninvasive testing. In symptomatic patients, revascularization is generally indicated if one or more of the major coronary arteries—or their large branches—have flow-limiting stenoses (>70% luminal narrowing) or occlusions. Percutaneous coronary intervention (PCI) and coronary artery bypass grafting (CABG) produce comparable symptomatic benefit. With regard to life expectancy, PCI does not produce survival benefit in patients with stable angina. By contrast, studies more than 20 years ago showed that CABG produced small gains in life expectancy in some patients.

With current management strategies, patients with angina are living longer, but a few remain symptomatic with poor quality of life despite optimal medical treatment and having exhausted revascularization options. Psychological support is important to treat anxiety and depression and improve confidence, and neuromodulatory techniques are sometimes employed.

Introduction

Angina—the pain provoked by myocardial ischaemia—is usually caused by obstructive coronary artery disease that is sufficiently severe to restrict oxygen delivery to the cardiac myocytes (Box 16.13.4.1). It is the most common initial manifestation of coronary artery disease, the only manifestation that occurs almost as commonly in women as in men, and the only manifestation that is not declining in incidence. When angina occurs in patients without coronary artery disease it may be attributable to other ischaemic mechanisms such as severe anaemia resulting in inadequate oxygen delivery to the cardiac myocytes, or left ventricular hypertrophy secondary to hypertension or aortic stenosis resulting in increased oxygen demand. The appropriately called syndrome X is a diagnosis of exclusion in patients with angina and unobstructed coronary arteries for which there is no clear cause despite full cardiac investigation: abnormal microvascular function is one proposed mechanism, but although symptoms are often resistant to treatment, prognosis is usually good in terms of life expectancy.

In most patients with angina caused by coronary artery disease, quality of life is impaired in direct proportion to the severity of symptoms (Fig. 16.13.4.1). Prognosis is often good, particularly in patients with chronic stable symptoms receiving contemporary secondary prevention therapy, but in those with recently diagnosed angina risk is greater, with a 2 to 3% incidence of death or nonfatal myocardial infarction in the first year. Recognition of the need for early investigation has led to the widespread implementation of chest pain clinics both in the United Kingdom and elsewhere to provide patients with suspected angina prompt treatment to relieve symptoms and reduce risk.

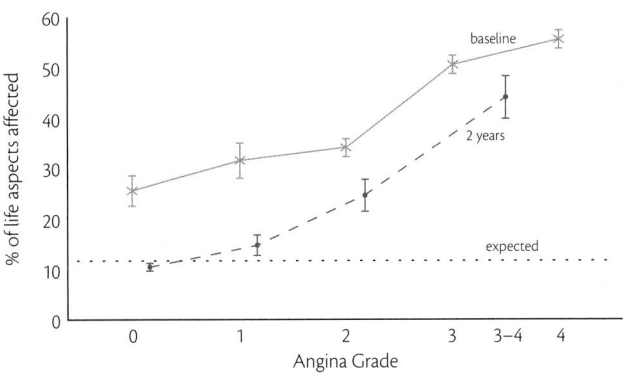

Fig. 16.13.4.1 Effect of angina on quality of life. Data are at baseline and 2 years after randomization in the RITA trial, showing impact of angina on life aspects encoded in part 2 of the Nottingham Health Profile. Note how quality of life deteriorates rapidly with worsening angina.
Pocock SJ, Henderson RA, Seed P, Treasure T, Hampton JR. Quality of life, employment status, and anginal symptoms after coronary angioplasty or bypass surgery. 3-year follow-up in the Randomized Intervention Treatment of Angina (RITA) Trial. Circulation 1996;94:135–42.

Referral for specialist assessment

Referral for specialist assessment (Box 16.13.4.2) is indicated in all patients with known coronary artery disease—particularly those with previous myocardial infarction or coronary revascularization—who experience abrupt worsening of symptoms, often indicating plaque rupture and risk of impending infarction.

However, referral decisions may be more difficult in patients presenting for the first time with chest pain. A noncardiac diagnosis accounts for most cases, but it is the task of the primary care or general physician to ensure that all those with suspected angina receive specialist assessment for confirmation of the diagnosis and risk stratification to identify those at greatest risk who need more intensive treatment. As in any screening process, false-negative diagnoses in which patients receive inappropriate reassurance must be avoided. By contrast, a proportion of false-positive diagnoses and referrals is acceptable, and among patients referred from primary care to chest pain clinics 75% have a noncardiac diagnosis.

In primary care, screening is based largely on the character of the symptoms and the age and gender of the patient, other risk factors further helping to identify those with a high probability of coronary artery disease (see below). Access to noninvasive diagnostic tests can be helpful in primary care or the nonspecialist clinic, but there is often insufficient recognition of their limitations,

---

Box 16.13.4.1 Causes of angina

Reduced myocardial oxygen supply

- Coronary artery disease
  - Atherosclerosis
  - Spasm
  - Vasculitic disorders
  - Post radiation therapy
- Severe anaemia

Increased myocardial oxygen demand

- Left ventricular hypertrophy
  - Hypertension
  - Aortic stenosis
  - Aortic regurgitation
  - Hypertrophic cardiomyopathy
- Right ventricular hypertrophy
  - Pulmonary hypertension
  - Pulmonary stenosis
- Rapid tachyarrhythmias

Indeterminate mechanism

- Syndrome X

Box 16.13.4.2 Angina—indications for specialist cardiological referral

- New-onset angina
- Exclusion of angina in high-risk individuals with atypical symptoms
- Worsening angina in a patient with previously stable symptoms
- New or recurrent angina in a patient with history of:
  - Myocardial infarction
  - Coronary revascularization
- Assessment of occupational fitness (e.g. airline pilots)

the exercise ECG (for example) having a diagnostic sensitivity of only about 50%, which means that up to one-half of all cases with coronary disease are missed. For this reason, the clinical history remains the most useful basis for diagnosis and referral decisions. Thresholds for referral should be lowered in high-risk patients, including those with previous myocardial infarction and diabetes, and also in airline pilots and public service drivers whose occupations might put others at risk in the event of myocardial infarction or sudden death.

The recommendation that all patients with suspected angina be referred for specialist assessment leaves little room for prevarication. Yet studies repeatedly show inequitable management of patients with chest pain, those with the greatest need often being the very patients who receive the least intensive treatment. Thus elderly patients with chest pain and those of south Asian origin are both high-risk groups, but are less likely than their younger and white counterparts to receive referral to chest pain clinics. Women are also disadvantaged and are less likely than men to be referred, even though it is increasingly recognized that angina in women is almost as common as in men and prognosis little better (Fig. 16.13.4.2). The reasons for this inequity are complex and poorly understood, but the consequences for health care are important.

Diagnosis of angina

Angina varies considerably in its clinical presentation and its overlap with other entities can make the differential diagnosis of chest pain difficult. A detailed description of the symptom complex is the most important step in the diagnostic process and in the context of other factors, particularly age and gender, allows the clinician to estimate the probability of coronary artery disease. The extent of work-up required to exclude a noncardiac cause needs to be individually determined. The diagnosis is informed by the clinician's intuition, experience, and interviewing skills, supported by investigations such as resting ECG, stress testing, and coronary angiography.

Clinical evaluation

A careful history of the character, location, radiation, provocation, and duration of the chest pain provides the most useful diagnostic information. Typically angina is experienced as a constricting, centrally located chest discomfort, radiating to the arms, throat, or jaw, provoked by exertion, less commonly by stress, and relieved by rest usually within 5–10 min. Symptoms are often worse in the morning, shortly after getting up, probably because catecholamine levels and blood pressure peak at this time of day. For similar reasons angina tends to be worse in cold weather and also after a heavy meal. In addition to age and gender, diagnostic probability is also influenced by a family history of premature coronary artery disease and also by other risk factors—particularly diabetes, smoking, hypertension, and dyslipidaemia. Thus, in the patient with chest pain, the probability of coronary disease is very low in men and women under 30, almost regardless of the typicality of the symptoms, while in men and women over 60 with multiple risk factors the probability of coronary disease is high even when the history has atypical features. The experienced clinician makes these probability judgements intuitively in the consulting room and they provide the main basis for the diagnosis of angina. For further discussion see Chapter 16.2.1.

Despite the reliance on clinical history in making a diagnosis of angina, it can be misleading, with atypical features, such as exertional dyspnoea in the absence of chest pain. Atypical presentations are said to be more common in patients with diabetes but, contrary to popular belief, there is little evidence that this also applies in women and South Asian people.

The physical examination is often normal in the patient with angina but may contribute to diagnosis if signs of major risk factors are identified, particularly hypertension, cutaneous manifestations of dyslipidaemia, and complications of diabetes such as retinopathy and neuropathy. Patients with signs of peripheral vascular disease (e.g. absent pulses, arterial bruits) have associated coronary involvement in most cases.

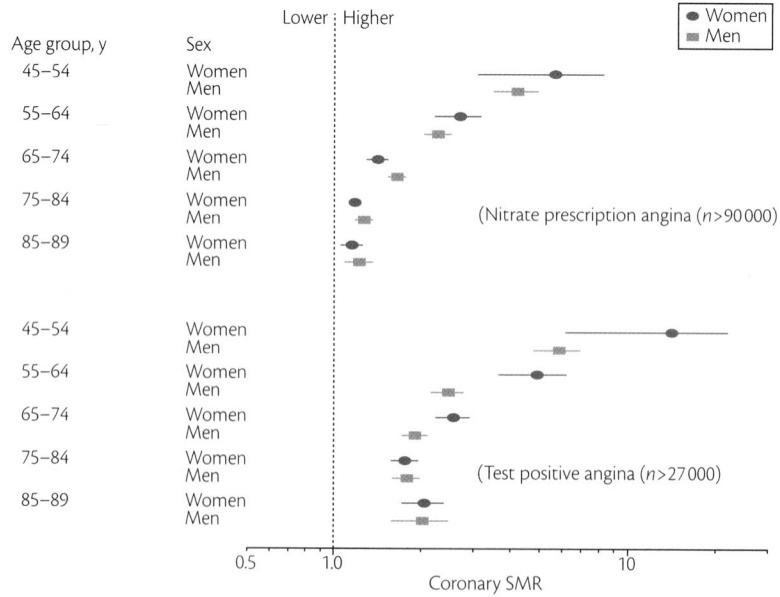

Fig. 16.13.4.2 Prognosis of angina in women and men. Primary care electronic records for Finland linked with mortality data have permitted estimation of the prognosis of angina for men and women, presented here as standardized mortality ratios. Two mutually exclusive case definitions of angina were used based on nitrate prescription and test positivity, yielding >90 000 and >27 000 cases, respectively. The data show that the contemporary prognosis of angina is not always good and at all ages is similar for men and for women. SMR, standardized mortality ratio. Hemingway H, McCallum A, Shipley M, Manderbacks K, Martikainen P, Keskimaki I. Incidence and prognostic implications of stable angina pectoris among women and men. JAMA 2006;295:1404–11.

CI indicates confidence interval.

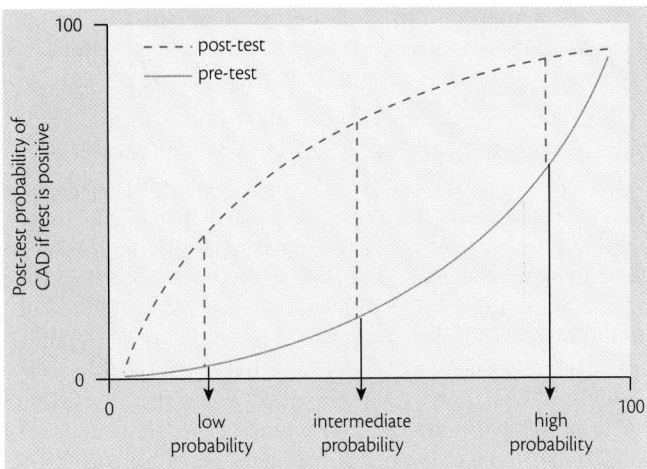

Fig. 16.13.4.3 Diagnosis of coronary artery disease—probability analysis. If the pretest probability of coronary artery disease (CAD) is very low (e.g. a young patient with very atypical chest pain) or very high (e.g. an elderly patient with typical angina), stress testing is generally unhelpful for diagnostic purposes because a positive test does not increase the probability of CAD very much. By contrast, in patients with an intermediate probability of disease, where there is real uncertainty about the diagnosis, a positive test produces a much larger increase in the probability of disease.

Simple laboratory investigations may also contribute to diagnosis by identifying groups at heightened risk of coronary disease due to renal dysfunction, dyslipidaemia or diabetes. Anaemia is also important to document because it may cause or—more commonly—exacerbate myocardial ischaemia.

Noninvasive investigation

Noninvasive testing is used primarily for diagnosis of coronary artery disease, but also has a role in risk assessment (see below). By tradition, nearly all patients presenting with chest pain have an ECG, although it is of limited diagnostic value. Many patients with angina have a normal recording and, although regional ST segment or T wave changes are commonly associated with coronary disease,

only pathological Q waves, reflecting previous myocardial infarction, are diagnostic. Other features of the ECG of potential relevance include tachycardia—particularly in patients with atrial fibrillation—and evidence of left ventricular hypertrophy, either of which may cause or exacerbate myocardial ischaemia.

Diagnostic indications for noninvasive testing depend largely on the level of uncertainty following the clinical assessment. Thus, a 60-year-old man with multiple risk factors who experiences constricting chest pain relieved by rest when he walks up stairs does not need noninvasive testing for diagnostic purposes—he clearly has angina and a negative test would do nothing to change that diagnosis. Similarly, a 25-year-old with transient stabbing pains in the left side of the chest unrelated to exertion does not have angina and a positive test would not modify that diagnostic judgement. These bayesian considerations apply to all noninvasive tests that commonly provide false-positive or false-negative results with little incremental value when the probability of coronary disease based on clinical assessment is respectively very low or very high. Incremental diagnostic value is greatest for patients with an intermediate pretest probability of coronary artery disease in whom uncertainty is greatest (Fig. 16.13.4.3). In these patients the results of noninvasive testing, positive or negative, can help resolve the uncertainty and contribute to the appropriate further management (Fig. 16.13.4.4). Noninvasive testing also provides an important means of risk assessment in patients with chest pain (see below).

Exercise ECG

This is the most widely used noninvasive test for diagnosis of coronary artery disease, with a sensitivity and specificity of 50% and 90%, respectively, after correcting for referral bias. Details are described in Chapter 16.3.1. The diagnostic value of the exercise ECG tends to be lower in women than in men. The regional development of planar or down-sloping ST segment depression, with gradual recovery when exercise stops, is usually diagnostic, particularly when associated with typical chest pain (Fig. 16.13.4.5a). The exercise ECG also provides important prognostic information: low exercise tolerance, ST depression early during exercise, an exertional fall in blood pressure, or exercise-induced ventricular arrhythmias all point to an increased risk of myocardial infarction

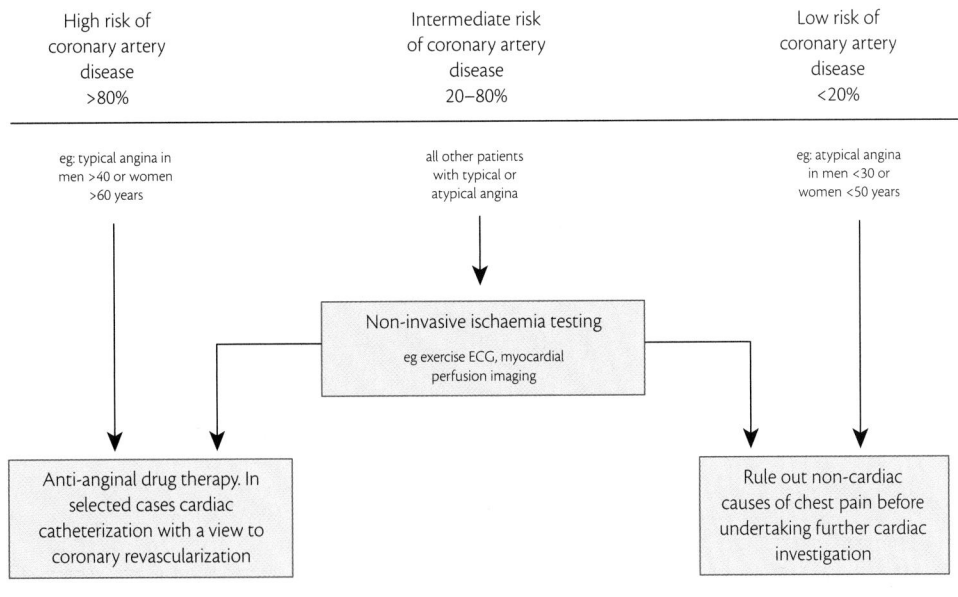

Fig. 16.13.4.4 Risk-based management strategy in chronic stable angina.
(Timmis AD, Nathan AW, Sullivan ID. Essentials of Cardiology (3rd Edition). Oxford. Blackwell Scientific Publications 1997.)

or sudden death. The Duke treadmill score, which takes into account duration of exercise, degree of ST segment deviation, and angina provides a quantitative prognostic assessment and a useful basis for determining the urgency of coronary arteriography.

Myocardial perfusion imaging

This is also widely used for diagnostic purposes and, although more costly and time-consuming than the exercise ECG, has enhanced diagnostic accuracy with a sensitivity and specificity of about 90% for detection of coronary artery disease. Details are described in Chapter 16.3.3. Fixed defects, present at rest and during stress, indicate areas of myocardial infarction (Fig. 16.13.4.5b). Perfusion imaging also provides useful prognostic information, the extent and severity of perfusion defects (fixed or reversible), the degree of lung uptake of radio-isotope (reflecting level of pulmonary capillary pressure), and the calculated ventricular volume and ejection fraction all predicting risk of future events.

Stress echocardiography

This is used increasingly for diagnostic purposes, but is more dependent than other noninvasive tests on the technical and interpretive skills of the operator. Details are described in Chapter 16.3.2. In expert hands it has similar sensitivity to exercise electrocardiography but higher specificity for diagnosing coronary artery disease in patients with suspected angina. Left ventricular imaging during

dobutamine infusion permits assessment of regional wall motion in response to adrenergic stress, with decreasing systolic wall motion or wall thickening indicating ischaemia and the likelihood of coronary artery disease.

Multidetector CT (MDCT)

Multidetector (or multislice) CT scanners with up to 64 detectors have sufficient image acquisition speed and spatial resolution to provide noninvasive coronary arteriograms that are becoming comparable to those obtained in the catheter laboratory, as reflected by sensitivity and specificity values of greater than 90% for detection of high-grade coronary stenoses (Fig. 16.13.4.6). Details are described in Chapter 16.3.3. Unlike conventional coronary arteriography information is also provided about the arterial wall, particularly the severity and distribution of coronary calcification which relates to the severity of coronary atherosclerosis. MDCT provides real promise for delivery of noninvasive coronary arteriography which, if fulfilled, will revolutionize the outpatient assessment of patients with chest pain.

Risk assessment of angina

Recent clinical trials of patients with chronic angina show that aggressive treatment under cardiological supervision reduces risk considerably such that long-term prognosis is good, with all-cause

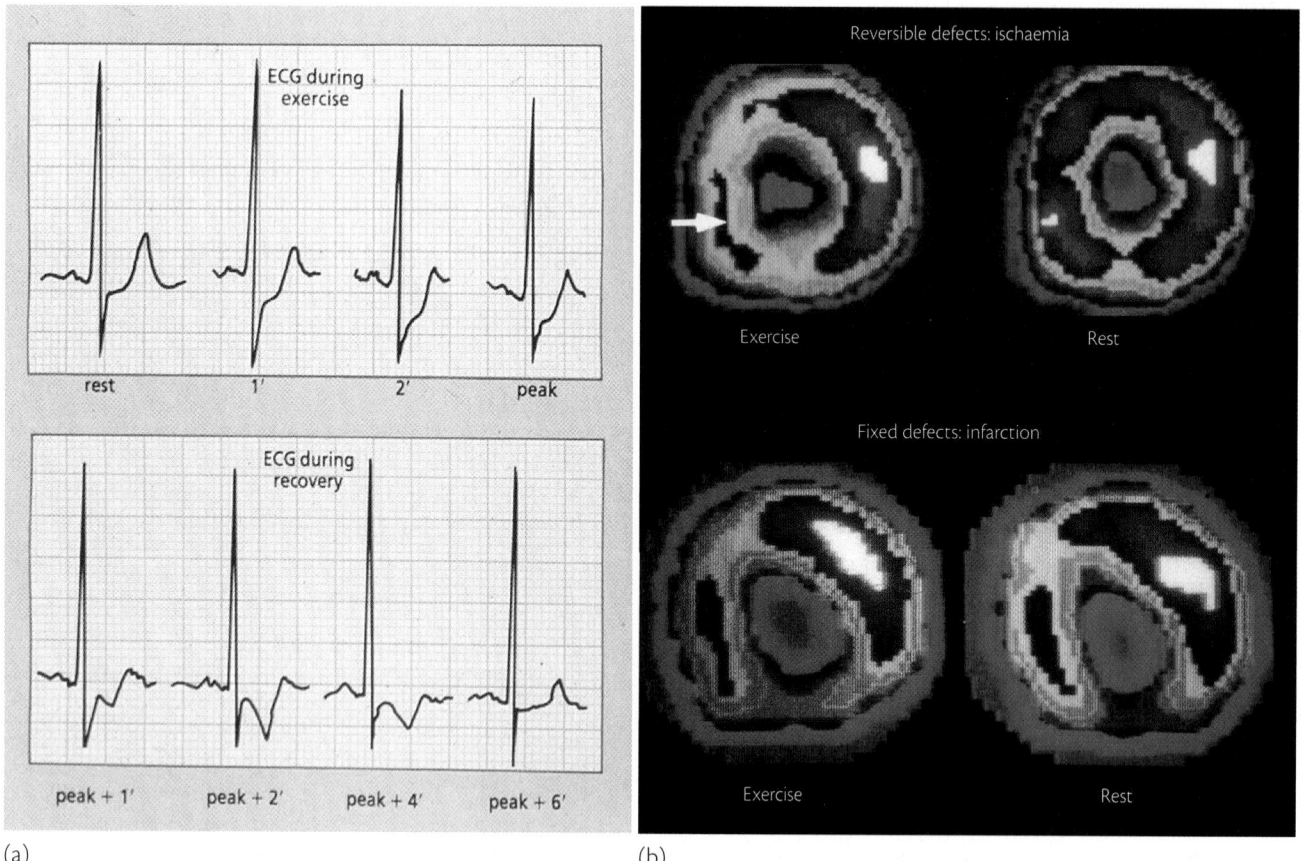

(a)   (b)

Fig. 16.13.4.5 Noninvasive testing for diagnosis of myocardial ischaemia. (a) Exercise ECG: lead V2 of the ECG is shown. Exercise produces progressive ST segment depression with gradual resolution during the recovery period. (b) Isotope perfusion imaging. These are colour-coded perfusion images obtained during exercise stress. The upper panels shows reversible ischaemia with an exertional perfusion defect (arrowed) affecting the lateral LV wall with resolution at rest. The lower panels show fixed perfusion defects denoting prior infarction.

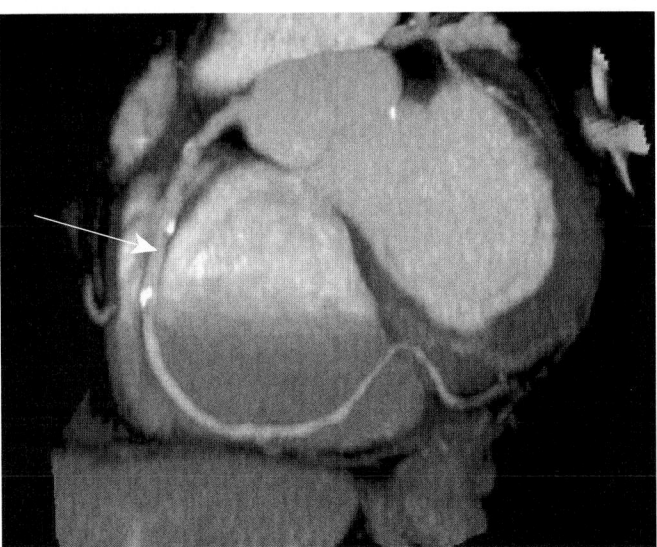

Fig. 16.13.4.6 Non-invasive coronary angiography by MDCT. The right coronary artery (arrowed) is patent but has localized areas of dense calcification in its proximal and mid segments denoting atherosclerosis.

mortality rates of about 1.5% per year. However, prognosis is worse in cohorts attending chest pain clinics in the early weeks or months after symptom onset, with mortality rates in excess of 3% in the first year. Identification of high-risk patients is therefore an important part of the initial assessment to inform decisions about the urgency and aggressiveness of treatment in individual cases.

Clinical indicators of risk

As with diagnosis, it is the clinical assessment that provides the most useful prognostic information in angina. Risk is greatest in patients who are old, those with typical symptoms and—contrary to conventional wisdom—those with more severe symptoms. Women and south Asians, with angina do not appear to be at greater risk. Risk increases with the number of 'reversible' risk factors, particularly diabetes, smoking, hypertension, and dyslipidaemia, all of which are important targets for treatment. Risk is also increased in patients with a history of myocardial infarction or stroke. Tachycardia is associated with increased risk, although treatment to slow the heart rate is directed primarily at preventing exertional ischaemia. Heart failure increases risk substantially. The most useful laboratory markers of risk are blood concentrations of lipids (particularly LDL cholesterol and apolipoproteins) and glucose. In patients with renal dysfunction, risk rises in proportion to reduction in creatinine clearance.

Noninvasive testing for risk assessment

Abnormalities of the resting ECG, particularly pathological Q waves and left bundle branch block, are associated with heightened risk in the patient with angina. Other noninvasive tests, including the exercise ECG and isotope perfusion imaging, are also used for risk assessment (see above). Generally speaking, negative test results indicate a good prognosis and a low level of urgency for further invasive investigation. However, when test results suggest severe and extensive ischaemia, risk is often high with important implications for future management.

Risk scores

Many scores have been developed for determining cardiovascular risk in healthy populations and in patients with acute myocardial infarction. Scores are also available for risk assessment in chronic stable angina based on many of the clinical and laboratory variables described above, plus echocardiographic measurement of left ventricular function. As yet, angina risk scores have not found major application in clinical practice.

Invasive testing for risk assessment

In patients with angina, risk of myocardial infarction and cardiovascular death is related to the extent and severity of angiographic coronary artery disease. Risk is particularly high when disease (luminal stenosis >50%) affects all three of the major coronary arteries. In patients with left main coronary artery disease urgent revascularization is necessary to prevent certain death in the event of left main occlusion.

Novel biomarkers

A range of inflammatory markers, including C-reactive protein, have been assessed in stable patients with coronary artery disease, but their incremental predictive value for future coronary events is very low once conventional risk factors have been taken into account. Brain natriuretic peptide may be more useful in this group of patients, although currently its main clinical application is in the diagnosis of heart failure (see Chapter 16.2.1).

Treatment of angina

The purpose of treatment is to correct symptoms and reduce risk, thereby improving both the quality of life and its duration (Fig. 16.13.4.7).

General measures

Comorbidities that exacerbate angina include anaemia, obesity, and thyrotoxicosis, all of which need treating. Most important, however, is hypertension, which increases myocardial oxygen demand in proportion to its severity. Simple lowering of blood pressure will often correct angina without the need for additional symptomatic treatment. Atrial fibrillation is also important because it is common, particularly in elderly patients, and increases myocardial oxygen demand due to tachycardia. Symptom relief can often be achieved by heart rate control or cardioversion. Aortic stenosis is another cause of angina that can be corrected by valve replacement.

Secondary prevention

The risk of myocardial infarction, stroke, and cardiovascular death can be reduced by lifestyle modification and specific drug therapy. Logic also requires that major atherogenic risk factors—particularly diabetes, smoking, hypertension, and dyslipidaemia—are treated vigorously in patients with angina, evidence for risk reduction being best for blood pressure control, smoking cessation, and LDL cholesterol reduction. Strict glycaemic control in type 2 diabetes, on the other hand, provides little demonstrable protection against cardiovascular endpoints although microvascular complications (renal failure and retinopathy) are effectively diminished. There is some evidence that drugs that increase insulin sensitivity, particularly metformin, may reduce cardiovascular risk in obese people with diabetes, but this requires confirmation in randomized trials.

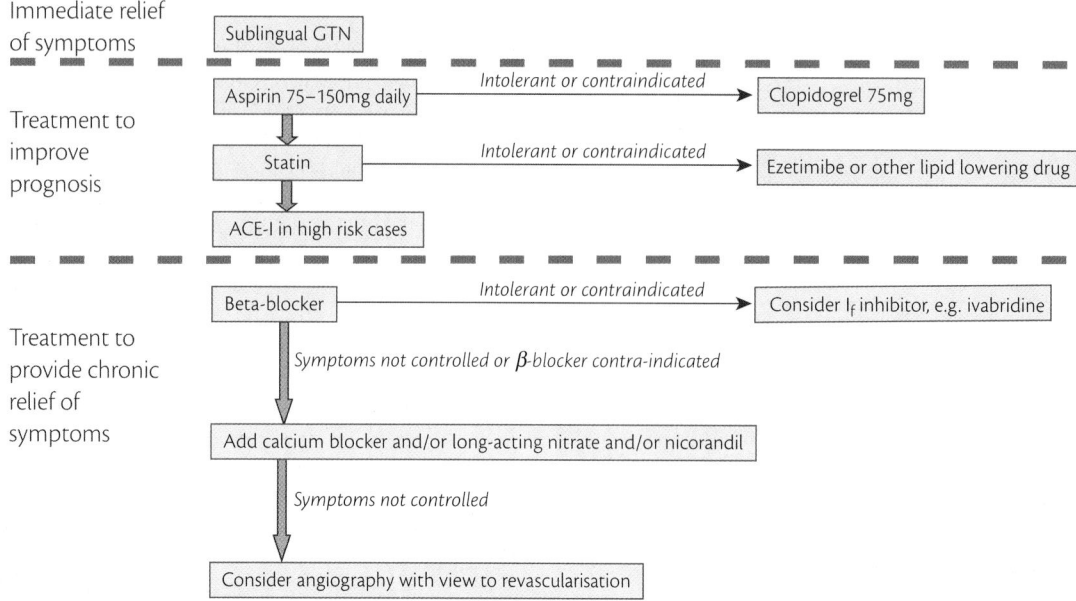

Fig. 16.13.4.7 Medical management of stable angina.
European Society of Cardiology guidelines (Eur Heart J 2006;27:1341–81).

Lifestyle modification

Evidence-based recommendations are for smoking cessation, exercise training and a Mediterranean-style diet characterized by low intake of total and saturated fats and increased intake of marine or plant ω – 3 fatty acids, fresh fruits and vegetables, and cereals rich in fibre, antioxidants, minerals, vegetable proteins and B group vitamins. Weight reduction in obese patients is also recommended, particularly those with hypertension, dyslipidaemia, or diabetes.

Secondary prevention drugs

All patients with angina should receive aspirin 75–150 mg daily, its antiplatelet activity reducing the thrombotic response to plaque rupture and protecting against myocardial infarction and stroke. Patients intolerant of aspirin despite proton pump inhibition should be treated with clopidogrel, which offers equivalent protection.

Patients with angina should also receive statin therapy to lower LDL cholesterol, thereby reducing lipid accumulation in the arterial wall and stabilizing the atherosclerotic plaque against rupture. Risk reduction is independent of baseline LDL cholesterol concentration, but the more it is lowered the greater the protection against cardiovascular events. At present, therefore, recommendations are to treat to a target of 4 mmol/litre for total cholesterol and 2 mmol/litre for LDL cholesterol. If this cannot be achieved with simvastatin 40 mg (the conventional first line statin in the United Kingdom), the dose needs increasing or a more potent statin such as atorvastatin or rosuvastatin needs to be substituted. In patients who cannot be treated to target or who are unable to tolerate statins, ezetimibe is usually added (or substituted) to reduce cholesterol absorption from the bowel, although there is no current evidence of prognostic benefit. The cardiovascular risk attributable to low HDL is well established, but it is not yet known if treatment to increase HDL with nicotinic acid derivatives is beneficial in patients with coronary artery disease.

Angiotensin converting enzyme (ACE) inhibition provides additional protection against cardiovascular endpoints in patients with angina, evidence being best for high-risk subgroups such as elderly patients, those with diabetes, and those with previous myocardial infarction. However, given the extended indications for these drugs in hypertension, diabetes, and left ventricular dysfunction, most patients with angina are suitable candidates for treatment. The mechanism of benefit with ACE inhibition may extend beyond blood pressure reduction, there being evidence for anti-inflammatory and antiproliferative effects which inhibit the atherogenic process and stabilize coronary plaques.

β-Blockers, though widely used for symptomatic treatment, have no clear evidence-based indication for secondary prevention in patients with angina unless there is associated left ventricular dysfunction, when prognostic benefit is well established. Antioxidant vitamins C and E have failed the test of clinical trials for secondary prevention in coronary artery disease. Similarly, there is no role for hormone replacement therapy for protecting against coronary events in postmenopausal women.

Antianginal drugs

Drugs used to treat angina reduce ischaemia by improving the balance between myocardial oxygen supply and demand (Fig. 16.13.4.8). Guideline recommendations are that medical therapy with antianginal drugs should be tried before angioplasty or surgery is considered, except in the few patients with stable angina who have a demonstrated survival advantage with revascularization (e.g. left main stem coronary disease, or two- to three-vessel coronary disease with proximal left anterior descending coronary artery involvement).

The three most widely used groups of antianginal drugs are β-blockers, nitrates, and calcium channel blockers. A meta-analysis of randomized trials concluded that β-blockers should be considered the first line treatment, but in clinical practice the three groups of drugs are used with approximately equal frequency, often in combination when benefits are additive.

β-Blockers

These drugs reduce myocardial oxygen demand, principally by slowing the heart rate, although reductions in left ventricular wall

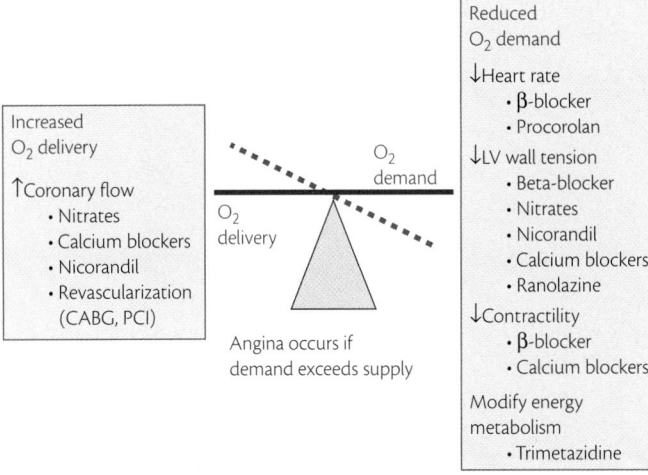

Fig. 16.13.4.8 Symptom relief with drugs.

tension (blood pressure) and contractility also contribute. Choice of β-blocker is largely determined by patient acceptability, with preference given to once-daily cardioselective agents such as atenolol or bisoprolol. Effective relief of exertional angina can often be obtained without recourse to other drugs if the heart rate response to exercise can be reduced sufficiently. There is a clear indication for β-blockers when angina occurs in patients with heart failure or asymptomatic left ventricular dysfunction. They are usually well tolerated, but noncardiac side effects, particularly fatigue and erectile dysfunction, may be troublesome even with cardioselective agents. β-Blockers are contraindicated in patients with bronchial asthma.

Nitrates

These drugs improve myocardial oxygen delivery and reduce demand by direct coronary and peripheral vascular dilatation. Sublingual glyceryl trinitrate by tablet or spray should be given to all patients with angina, rapid absorption through the buccal mucosa providing symptomatic relief within 3 min. It can also be used prophylactically to prevent angina during exertion. Long-acting isosorbide mononitrate for regular oral administration is widely used, although variable tolerance to its therapeutic action may occur. Side effects are rarely troublesome apart from headache during the first few days of treatment.

Calcium blockers

Like nitrates, these are vasodilators and improve myocardial oxygen balance by their effect on coronary flow and peripheral resistance. Angina complicated by hypertension provides a clear indication for drugs of this class when amlodipine is usually the preferred agent. Diltiazem and verapamil are also useful because, in addition to vasodilator activity, they often produce minor reductions in heart rate, although combination therapy with β-blockers is best avoided. Nifedipine, which tends to increase heart rate, is not recommended for treatment of angina. Side effects of calcium blockers are related to vasodilatation and include facial flushing, postural dizziness, and mild ankle oedema.

Potassium channel openers

Nicorandil is the only drug in this group licensed to treat angina. It is a vasodilator with effects comparable to those of long-acting nitrates. The principal side effect is headache.

Trimetazidine

This interesting compound is licensed for treatment of angina in a number of European countries (not the United Kingdom). Its pharmacological effects are metabolic, not haemodynamic, with coupling between glycolysis and carbohydrate oxygenation restored by shifting cardiac energy metabolism from oxygenation of fatty acids (the preferred myocardial substrate) to glucose, thus preserving intracellular ATP levels. Antianginal effects are comparable to other agents and are additive to those of β-blockers and calcium blockers. Side effects, including gastrointestinal disturbance, are rarely troublesome.

Ivabridine

This recently licensed compound inhibits the I_f channel in the sinus node, reducing the slope of diastolic depolarization and slowing the heart rate. The effect of ivabridine on heart rate is comparable to that of β-blockers, but because I_f channels are largely restricted to the heart and the retina blood pressure is unaffected and many of the noncardiac effects of β-blockers, particularly fatigue and erectile dysfunction, do not occur. Mild visual side effects tend to resolve during treatment. Antianginal efficacy appears to be comparable to β-blockers and calcium blockers and the drug is now licensed for treatment of angina in patients with normal sinus rhythm (rate reduction does not occur in atrial fibrillation) who have a contraindication to or intolerance of β-blockers.

Ranolazine

This newly developed agent now has a licence for use in chronic angina where other antianginals have been inadequate. Its mechanism of action has not been fully characterized but appears to involve inhibition of the late inward sodium channel which indirectly prevents calcium overload of ischaemic myocytes and reduces diastolic wall tension and oxygen demand. Heart rate or blood pressure are unaffected. Antianginal effects are additive to those of β-blockers and calcium blockers. Side effects including constipation and dizziness are rarely troublesome.

Revascularization

In the patient with angina, revascularization provides a nonpharmacological means of improving myocardial oxygen delivery by restoring coronary flow to the ischaemic myocardium. More than 60% of all revascularization procedures in stable angina are now by percutaneous intervention (PCI) using balloon angioplasty and stenting (Fig. 16.13.4.9). The remainder are by coronary artery bypass surgery (CABG), the choice depending largely on the extent and severity of coronary artery disease. At present, this can only be determined by coronary angiography which is an essential prerequisite of revascularization in the management of angina. See Chapters 16.13.6 and 16.13.7 for further discussion.

Which patients with stable angina should undergo coronary angiography?

This question has received little attention from clinical trialists, but guideline recommendations are for angiography in patients with continuing moderate or severe angina despite optimal medical treatment. Other groups for whom angiography is recommended include those identified as being at high risk on noninvasive testing (see above), those who have been successfully resuscitated from sudden cardiac death or who have life-threatening ventricular

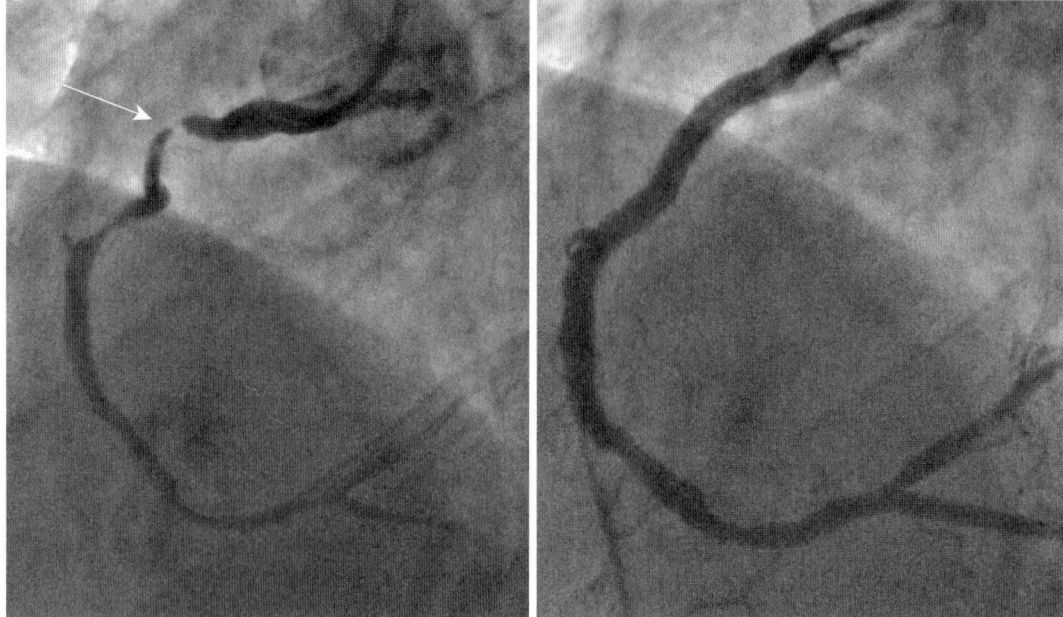

Fig. 16.13.4.9 Coronary stenting. Right coronary arteriogram (a) before stenting and (b) after deployment of a drug-eluting stent across the diseased segment (arrowed) in the proximal part of the vessel. The patient had stable angina and experienced complete relief of symptoms after the procedure.

arrhythmias. Occasionally angiography is indicated in asymptomatic patients with suspected or known coronary artery disease whose jobs (e.g. piloting aircraft, driving public service vehicles) are dependent on a normal or fully revascularized coronary circulation. It may also be indicated in patients unwilling or unable to take antianginal drugs, or those in whom there is important diagnostic uncertainty despite noninvasive investigation.

Choice of revascularization procedure—CABG vs PCI

In symptomatic patients who have undergone cardiac catheterization, revascularization is generally indicated if one or more of the major coronary arteries—or their large branches—have flow-limiting stenoses (>70% luminal narrowing) or occlusions. The choice of revascularization procedure is dependent on a range of factors:

- Coronary anatomy—historically, PCI has been preferred for single-vessel and two-vessel coronary artery disease and CABG for more extensive disease. This preference has been based largely on evidence of prognostic benefit for CABG in patients with three-vessel or left main stem disease (see below), but also on technical factors, particularly the relative inefficacy of PCI in total coronary occlusions and in densely calcified lesions when coronary dissection or failure of adequate dilatation have been commonplace. However, technological developments, including drills and stents, and improvements in operator technique, now allow successful procedures in many cases that until recently were considered exclusively surgical. Choice of procedure is therefore now less dependent on anatomical considerations, and more on operator experience and patient preference.

- Patient preference—PCI is often preferred because it avoids surgery, requires no more than 48 hours hospitalization (day case PCI is now feasible) and permits early return to normal activities within a few days of the procedure.

- Procedural risk—mortality is lower for PCI than CABG (0.9% vs 2.2%). Stroke risk is also lower but rates of nonfatal myocardial infarction are comparable.

- Symptomatic benefit—this is comparable for PCI and CABG, but recurrence of symptoms and need for repeat revascularization is higher for PCI because of coronary restenosis in the months following a successful procedure. Indeed restenosis has been the Achilles heel of PCI, and until the introduction of coronary stents affected 30% or more of all patients. Since then stenting has become widespread, producing more effective coronary patency although reductions in rates of restenosis to less than 10% had to await the introduction of drug-eluting stents that deliver antiproliferative drugs (e.g. sirolimus, paclitaxel) locally within the coronary artery. The prospect of providing long-term relief of symptoms without the need for repeat procedures has considerably enhanced the clinical value of PCI.

- Prognostic benefit—to date there have been no studies showing survival benefit for PCI in patients with stable angina. For CABG, small gains in life expectancy have been reported in patients with left main stem coronary disease, three-vessel disease and two-vessel disease with severely stenosed proximal left anterior descending artery. These reports, however, are from studies more than 20 years ago and their contemporary relevance may have changed with advances both in surgical techniques and in medical therapy. Indeed it is generally accepted that improvements in the prognosis of coronary artery disease in the last 25 years have little to do with revascularization, but much to do with lifestyle changes and advances in secondary prevention therapy.

Management of refractory angina

With current management strategies patients with angina are living longer, but a proportion, perhaps 5 to 10%, remain symptomatic on optimal medical treatment, having exhausted revascularization options. These patients commonly have extensively collateralized coronary circulations and well-preserved left ventricular function such that prognosis is not worse than other patients with angina, but the quality of life is poor because of refractory symptoms. Psychological support is important to treat anxiety and depression and improve confidence. Options for further antianginal therapy, however, are limited.

Neuromodulation

Stellate ganglion block has a time-honoured role in the treatment of refractory angina, local anaesthetic injection interrupting sensory traffic from the myocardium with variable relief of symptoms. Repeated treatments are available for responders.

Transcutaneous electrical nerve stimulation (TENS) finds application in a variety of acute and chronic pain syndromes. Its use is not based on any well-substantiated therapeutic mechanism, but some patients find it helpful.

Spinal cord stimulation (SCS) also finds application in a variety of pain syndromes without a well substantiated therapeutic mechanism. Clinical trials confirm that SCS reduces myocardial ischaemia with amelioration of symptoms in patients with refractory angina, but because effective blinding is impossible placebo effects may contribute significantly to clinical benefit.

Other techniques

Enhanced external counterpulsation (EECP) works on the same principle as the intra-aortic balloon pump. Pressure cuffs applied to the lower limbs are inflated sequentially during diastole, resulting in augmented diastolic central aortic pressure and increased coronary perfusion pressure. Compression of the vascular bed of the legs also increases venous return and cardiac output. Rapid and simultaneous decompression of the cuffs at the onset of systole permits systolic unloading and decreased cardiac workload. Clinical benefit has been reported, but again the contribution of placebo response is hard to quantify.

A single study of autologous bone marrow cells injected via the coronary sinus produced variable benefit in patients with refractory angina. More studies are needed to determine whether this treatment will have a useful clinical role.

Further reading

Blankenberg S, et al. (2006). Comparative impact of multiple biomarkers and N-terminal pro-brain natriuretic peptide in the context of conventional risk factors for the prediction of recurrent cardiovascular events in the Heart Outcomes Prevention Evaluation (HOPE) Study. Circulation, 114, 201–8.

Braunwald E, et al. (2004). Angiotensin-converting-enzyme inhibition in stable coronary artery disease. N Engl J Med, 351, 2058–68.

Clayton TC, et al. (2005). Risk score for predicting death, myocardial infarction, and stroke in patients with stable angina, based on a large randomised trial cohort of patients. BMJ, 331, 869–73.

Collins R, et al. (2004). Effects of cholesterol-lowering with simvastatin on stroke and other major vascular events in 20536 people with cerebrovascular disease or other high-risk conditions. Lancet, 363, 757–67.

Fox KM, et al. (2003). Efficacy of perindopril in reduction of cardiovascular events among patients with stable coronary artery disease: randomised, double-blind, placebo-controlled, multicentre trial (the EUROPA study). Lancet, 362, 782–8.

Heidenreich PA, et al. (1999). Meta-analysis of trials comparing beta-blockers, calcium antagonists, and nitrates for stable angina. JAMA, 281, 1927–36.

Hemingway H, et al. (2006). Incidence and prognostic implications of stable angina pectoris among women and men. JAMA, 295, 1404–11.

Hulley S, et al. (1998). Randomized trial of estrogen plus progestin for secondary prevention of coronary heart disease in postmenopausal women. Heart and Estrogen/progestin Replacement Study (HERS) Research Group. JAMA, 280, 605–13.

LaRosa JC, et al. (2005). Intensive lipid lowering with atorvastatin in patients with stable coronary disease. N Engl J Med, 352, 1425–35.

Messerli FH, et al. (2006). Guidelines on the management of stable angina pectoris: executive summary: The Task Force on the Management of Stable Angina Pectoris of the European Society of Cardiology. Eur Heart J, 27, 2902–3.

Morice MC, et al. (2002). Randomized study with the sirolimus-coated Bx velocity balloon-expandable stent in the treatment of patients with de novo native coronary artery lesions. A randomized comparison of a sirolimus-eluting stent with a standard stent for coronary revascularization. N Engl J Med, 346, 1773–80.

Pocock SJ, et al. (1996). Quality of life, employment status,and anginal symptoms after coronary angioplasty or bypass surgery. 3-year follow-up in the Randomized Intervention Treatment of Angina (RITA) Trial. Circulation, 94, 135–42.

Poole-Wilson PA, et al. (2004). Effect of long-acting nifedipine on mortality and cardiovascular morbidity in patients with stable angina requiring treatment (ACTION trial): randomised controlled trial. Lancet, 364, 849–57.

Sekhri N, et al. (2007). How effective are rapid access chest pain clinics? Prognosis of incident angina and non-cardiac chest pain in 8762 consecutive patients. Heart, 93, 458–63.

Serruys PW, et al. (2001). Comparison of coronary-artery bypass surgery and stenting for the treatment of multivessel disease. N Engl J Med, 344, 1117–24.

Timmis AD (1985). Probability analysis in the diagnosis of coronary artery disease. Br Med J, 291, 1443–4.

UK Prospective Diabetes Study (UKPDS) Group (1998). Intensive blood-glucose control with sulphonylureas or insulin compared with conventional treatment and risk of complications in patients with type 2 diabetes (UKPDS 33). Lancet, 352, 837–53.

16.13.5 Management of acute coronary syndrome

Keith A.A. Fox

Essentials

The acute coronary syndrome (ACS) is precipitated by an abrupt change in an atheromatous plaque, resulting in increased obstruction to perfusion and ischaemia or infarction in the territory supplied by the affected vessel. The clinical consequences of plaque rupture can range from an entirely silent episode, through to unstable symptoms of ischaemia without infarction, to profound ischaemia complicated by progressive infarction, heart failure, and risk of sudden death.

The choice and timing of management strategy is critically dependent on the extent and severity of myocardial ischaemia, with the spectrum of ACS broken down into three elements: (1) Unstable angina: typical ischaemic symptoms without ST elevation on ECG and without elevated biomarkers of necrosis. (2) Non-ST-elevation myocardial infarction (MI): typical ischaemic symptoms without ST elevation on ECG but with biomarkers of necrosis above the diagnostic threshold. (3) ST-elevation MI: typical ischaemic symptoms with ST elevation on ECG and with biomarkers of necrosis above the diagnostic threshold.

An acute reperfusion strategy (primary percutaneous coronary intervention (PCI) or thrombolysis) is of proven benefit only in ST segment elevation infarction (or MI with new bundle branch block).

Prompt relief of pain is important, not only for humanitarian reasons, but also because pain is associated with sympathetic activation, vasoconstriction, and increased myocardial work. Effective analgesia is best achieved by the titration of intravenous opioids, with concurrent administration of an antiemetic. High-flow oxygen should be given, especially to those who are breathless or those with any features of heart failure or shock.

The management of prehospital cardiac arrest requires special attention: at least as many lives can be saved by prompt resuscitation and defibrillation as by reperfusion. Patients may also require management of arrhythmic and haemodynamic complications, including heart failure.

Acute coronary syndromes without ST elevation (unstable angina/non-ST elevation MI)

Patients without ST elevation or left bundle branch block can be triaged into low, intermediate, and high-risk categories. (1) High-risk—patients with typical clinical features of ischaemia and ST-segment depression or transient ST-segment elevation, or with troponin elevation and a high-risk score (Risk calculator downloadable from http://www.outcomes.org/grace or http://www.timi.org/files/riskscore/ua_calculator.htm). Patients are also at high risk when ischaemia provokes arrhythmias or haemodynamic compromise. (2) Intermediate or low risk—patients with clinical features of acute coronary syndrome and nonspecific ECG changes (T wave inversion, T wave flattening, minor conduction abnormalities, etc.). (3) Low risk or an alternative diagnosis—patients with a normal ECG, normal biomarkers, normal cardiac examination, and normal echo.

Patients at high risk—(1) High-risk patients with acute ischaemia at initial presentation, or those who develop such features after hospital admission, and especially those with haemodynamic compromise, require emergency assessment for revascularization and potentially benefit from glycoprotein IIb/IIIa inhibition. (2) Those proceeding to emergency revascularization should receive (a) aspirin; (b) thienopyridine, e.g. clopidogrel; (c) glycoprotein IIb/IIIa inhibition, e.g. abciximab, eptifibatide, and tirofiban; and (d) unfractionated or low molecular weight heparin (LMWH), or a direct thrombin inhibitor, e.g. bivalirudin. (3) Some patients should receive anti-ischaemic therapy (e.g. nitrates, β-blockers, calcium entry blockers, potassium channel activators, etc.), and some will require antiarrhythmic management or haemodymamic support (e.g. intra-aortic balloon pump to reduce ischaemia and stabilize the patient for revascularization).

Patients developing ST elevation require emergency reperfusion by primary percutaneous coronary intervention (PCI), or—if PCI is not available—by thrombolysis (see below).

Patients at intermediate or low risk—patients with non-ST-elevation ACS and an intermediate risk score require dual antiplatelet therapy (aspirin plus thienopyridine, e.g. clopidogrel) plus anticoagulation (e.g. heparin, LMWH, fondaparinux, or bivalirudin). They are candidates for an early elective revascularization strategy (within c.72 h).

Clinically stable patients with minor or nonspecific ECG abnormalities and a low risk score (including negative repeat troponin) are at very low risk for in-hospital, major cardiac events. Such patients may, nevertheless, have significant underlying coronary artery disease. They require stress testing or perfusion scanning, ideally prior to discharge.

Specific interventions—anti-ischaemic therapies—(1) nitrates—effective in reducing ischaemia in the in-hospital management of non-ST elevation ACS, but there is no evidence that they improve mortality; (2) β-blockers—patients with suspected acute coronary syndromes should be initiated on β-blocker therapy unless contraindicated; (3) dihydropyridine calcium entry blockers—should be employed with β-blockers in acute coronary syndromes to avoid reflex tachycardia. In patients unable to tolerate β-blockers, a heart-rate-slowing calcium antagonist, e.g. diltiazem or verapamil, may be appropriate. Short-acting dihydropyridines should not be used in isolation in ACS.

Antiplatelet therapies—(1) aspirin 75–325 mg daily—indicated in all patients with acute coronary syndromes unless there is good evidence of aspirin allergy or evidence of active bleeding; (2) thienopyridine—patients with non-ST-elevation ACS should be given clopidogrel as an initial 300-mg loading dose, followed by continued treatment at a dose of 75 mg daily, in combination with aspirin. Clopidogrel should be given alone to patients with contraindications to aspirin (same regimen). Clopidogrel should be maintained for 12 months, unless the risks of bleeding exceed potential benefits. In patients undergoing PCI, a loading dose of 600 mg of clopidogrel may be used to achieve more rapid inhibition of platelet function. Following PCI, the duration of clopidogrel administration should take account of the type of stent implanted (bare metal or drug-eluting) and the risks of bleeding/thrombosis; Prasugrel is a more potent thienopyridine than clopidogrel (TRITON Study) and has improved outcomes (mainly reduced MI), especially in diabetics. It results in fewer stent thromboses. However there is more bleeding, and it should be avoided in patients with previous intracerebral bleeding or transient ischaemic attack. (3) GPIIb/IIIa inhibitors—e.g. abciximab, eptifibatide, tirofiban—result in improved outcome in patients requiring urgent percutaneous intervention for non-ST-segment-elevation ACS and in those at intermediate to high risk. Should be administered with oral antiplatelet agents (aspirin and thienopyridines) and anticoagulants (heparin or LMWH). Ticagrelor, a non thienopyridine P2Y12 platelet antagonist also has improved outcomes compared with clopidogrel (fewer infarctions and fewer deaths and fewer stent thromboses) (PLATO study). Overall rates of bleeding were not increased but non-CABG bleeding was increased. It is not yet approved in ACS.

Anticoagulation—this is required in addition to antiplatelet therapy. LMWH is better than unfractionated heparin and is most commonly used. In the absence of an urgent/early invasive strategy, fondaparinux (a synthetic pentasaccharide that selectively binds antithrombin and causes inhibition of factor Xa) has the most favourable efficacy/safety profile.

ST-segment-elevation myocardial infarction

Patients with clear-cut evidence of ST-elevation infarction (STEMI) require immediate triage to reperfusion therapy. 'Fast-track' systems have been developed to minimize in-hospital delay to reperfusion: these aim to achieve clinical assessment and electrocardiography within 15 min of arrival and rapid transfer for percutaneous coronary intervention or the institution of thrombolytic therapy within 30 min. Audit programmes and continuous training are necessary for centres to achieve this 30-min median 'door-to-needle' time.

PCI—Randomized clinical trials of primary PCI vs thrombolysis have shown consistent findings: primary PCI is better, providing more effective restoration of vessel patency, achieving better ventricular function, and improving important clinical outcomes with lower rates of death, re-infarction, stroke, major bleeding, and recurrent ischaemia. Particular gains are seen in haemodynamically compromised patients. In consequence, primary PCI is the preferred therapeutic option in national and international guidelines.

Thrombolysis—prehospital thrombolysis is the next best option if a primary PCI programme is not available, or if transfer times are sufficiently prolonged that reperfusion may not be achieved within 90 min of patient call.

The current reference standard for the comparison of fibrinolytic agents is the accelerated infusion regimen of alteplase (tPA), or—for simplicity—the single-bolus administration of tenecteplase (TNK), which does not require an infusion pump or refrigeration and hence is particularly suited for pre-hospital administration. Internationally, streptokinase remains the most widely used fibrinolytic agent, principally because it is relatively inexpensive.

Antiplatelet agents and anticoagulants—(1) Aspirin 75–325 mg daily—indicated in all patients with acute coronary syndromes unless there is good evidence of aspirin allergy or evidence of active bleeding. (2) Thienopyridine—clopidogrel (regimen as described above) should be given to all patients, continuing for at least 1 month in patients managed with fibrinolysis (or as determined by the type of stents implanted). (3) GP IIb/IIIa inhibitors—e.g. abciximab, eptifibatide, tirofiban—are indicated in patients managed with primary PCI, but not in those managed with fibrinolysis. (4) Anticoagulants—patients treated with fibrinolytic therapy should receive LMWH or fondaparinux (a factor Xa inhibitor).

Secondary prevention measures in patients with ACS

Patients require advice and help regarding cessation of smoking (including the avoidance of passive smoking), dietary modification, exercise, rehabilitation, and management of obesity.

The following therapies have been shown to reduce the risk of subsequent cardiovascular events: (1) antiplatelet therapy—aspirin in a dose of 75 mg/day, clopidogrel 75 mg/day; (2) β-blockers in those without contraindications; (3) lipid lowering with 3-hydroxy-3-methylglutaryl coenzyme A (HMG CoA) reductase inhibitors (statins); (4) angiotensin converting enzyme (ACE) inhibitors/angiotensin receptor blockers (ARB), especially in those with left ventricular dysfunction and heart failure, and benefit is also possible in other patients with vascular disease.

Introduction

The term 'acute coronary syndrome' (ACS) describes the clinical manifestations of a heterogeneous spectrum of conditions that share key pathophysiological features: disruption or erosion of coronary atheromatous plaque, changes in vascular tone, and a variable extent of thrombotic occlusion. The clinical presentations are determined by the extent of coronary obstruction, the volume of ischaemic myocardium, and temporal pattern of the atherothrombotic disease process. Acute coronary syndrome occurs in patients with underlying, symptomatic or occult coronary artery disease and flow-limiting or non-flow-limiting atheromatous plaques in the coronary arterial wall (Fig. 16.13.5.1).

The ACS is precipitated by an abrupt change in an atheromatous plaque, resulting in increased obstruction to perfusion and ischaemia or infarction in the territory supplied by the affected vessel. For discussion of the mechanisms involved, see Chapter 16.13.1. The pattern and severity of clinical manifestations are dependent not only upon the degree of obstruction to perfusion, but also on the presence or absence of collateral perfusion, the extent and distribution of fragmented microthrombi, and myocardial oxygen demand in the perfused territory. Thus, the clinical consequences of plaque rupture can range from an entirely silent episode, through to unstable symptoms of ischaemia without infarction, to profound ischaemia complicated by progressive infarction, heart failure, and risk of sudden death.

The goals of early management of ACS are to relieve ischaemia (by reducing myocardial oxygen demand, inhibiting thrombotic occlusion, and reducing coronary obstruction), to prevent further thrombotic occlusion, and to prevent or manage complications. The choice and timing of management strategy, including pharmacological treatment and percutaneous or surgical revascularization, is critically dependent on the extent and severity of myocardial ischaemia. Despite sharing key pathophysiological mechanisms across the spectrum of ACS, ST-segment-elevation acute myocardial infarction (STEMI) and non-ST-elevation ACS (unstable angina and non-STEMI) need to be considered separately because an acute reperfusion strategy (primary percutaneous coronary intervention (PCI) or thrombolysis) is of proven benefit in STEMI (or MI with new bundle branch block), but not in the remainder of the syndrome. Thus, although the management of STEMI differs, the remainder of the ACS should be managed as a continuous spectrum, but influenced by risk stratification.

Clinical presentation and definition of ACS

The ACS may present *de novo* (as new-onset angina), with typical ischaemic discomfort at rest (rest angina) or on minimal exertion. Alternatively, a previously stable pattern of angina may change, resulting in episodes of typical rest angina or angina provoked by minor exertion (crescendo angina). New-onset exertional angina has not previously been recognized as part of 'acute coronary syndrome', but the outcomes are similar (*c*.7% develop nonfatal MI and 4% die, and a further 19% require revascularization within 15 months) and such patients may fulfill the clinical and ECG/biomarker characteristics of the syndrome (Euroheart survey, GRACE, and CRUSADE registries).

There are three components to the clinical diagnosis of ACS: the symptom description, the ECG, and biomarker evidence of myocyte necrosis. The symptoms must be distinguished from noncardiac

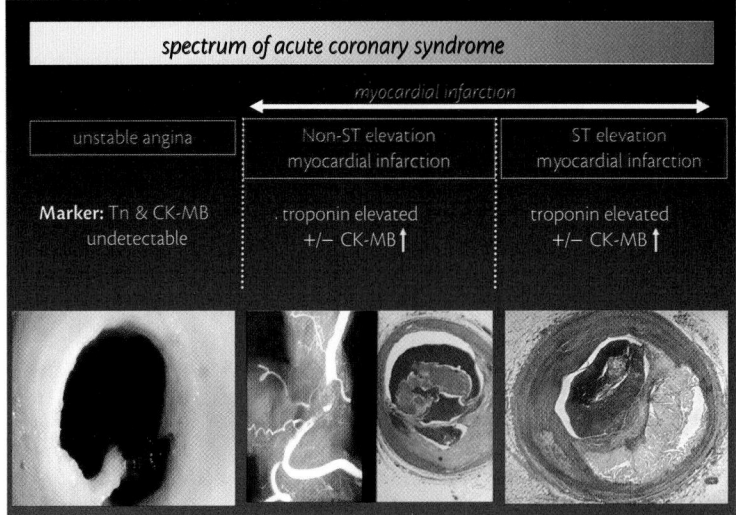

Fig. 16.13.5.1 The spectrum of acute coronary syndromes.

pain, and from stable angina. To improve the specificity of diagnosis, clinical trials use a more restricted definition, requiring at least 15 to 20 min of typical ischaemic discomfort or two 5-min episodes at rest. The specificity is further improved when the definition requires objective evidence of ischaemia or evidence of underlying coronary artery disease. ST segment depression on the ECG, especially in association with typical pain, is highly predictive, whereas the less specific ECG abnormalities, including T wave inversion, are less strong predictors. Markers of myocardial damage (troponins or cardiac enzymes) are powerfully predictive, in the presence of a typical clinical syndrome. ST elevation or depression on the ECG and elevated biomarkers of necrosis are markers of higher risk and adverse outcome (Table 16.13.5.1). In the absence of such markers, documented evidence of underlying coronary artery disease (prior infarction or angiographically demonstrated coronary disease) helps to confirm the diagnosis.

In brief, the three components of ACS comprise:

- unstable angina—typical ischaemic symptoms without ST elevation on ECG and without elevated biomarkers of necrosis

- non-STEMI—typical ischaemic symptoms without ST elevation on ECG but with biomarkers of necrosis above the diagnostic threshold

- STEMI—typical ischaemic symptoms with ST elevation on ECG and with biomarkers of necrosis above the diagnostic threshold

Table 16.13.5.1 Prognostic value of admission ECG for early risk stratification in 12 142 patients with an acute coronary syndrome

	ST elevation + ST depression (%)	ST elevation (%)	ST depression (%)	T wave inversion (%)	p
Patients	15	28	35	23	
Acute infarction on admission	87	81	47	31	<0.0001
Death	6.8	5.0	5.0	1.8	<0.001
(Re)infarction	6.9	5.1	6.7	4.3	<0.001

Death and reinfarction at 30 days follow-up.
Data from the GUSTO IIb trial.

The definition of MI has recently been revised by a 'Global Task Force' of the European Society of Cardiology, the American College of Cardiology, the American Heart association, and others and has identified five subtypes of MI (Box 16.13.5.1).

Outcome of ACS

Trial data and large-scale observational registry studies

Overall, based upon large-scale registries with consistent disease definitions, there are approximately two patients with non-STEMI ACS for each patient with STEMI. Previously, inclusion of patients with chest pain—but without diagnostic features of acute ischaemia—under the term 'unstable angina' may have masked the true hazards of the syndrome. Comparisons between studies may be confounded by different disease definitions and varying use of more sensitive markers of myocyte necrosis (troponins), but on the basis of data from randomized trials and prospective registry studies there is no doubt that patients with ACS (with or without persistent ST elevation) are at substantial risk of subsequent cardiac events despite current therapy. About 9 to 11% suffer death or

---

Box 16.13.5.1   The subtypes of MI

- Type 1—spontaneous MI related to ischaemia due to a primary coronary event such as plaque fissuring, erosion or rupture, or dissection

- Type 2—myocardial infarction secondary to ischaemia due either to increased oxygen demand or to decreased supply (e.g. coronary spasm or embolism, anaemia, arrhythmias, hypertension, or hypotension)

- Type 3—sudden unexpected cardiac death, including cardiac arrest, with symptoms suggestive of myocardial ischemia, accompanied by new ST elevation, or new left bundle branch block, or definite new thrombus by coronary angiography (death before blood samples obtained) or in the lag phase of cardiac biomarkers

- Type 4—MI associated with PCI

- Type 5—MI associated with CABG

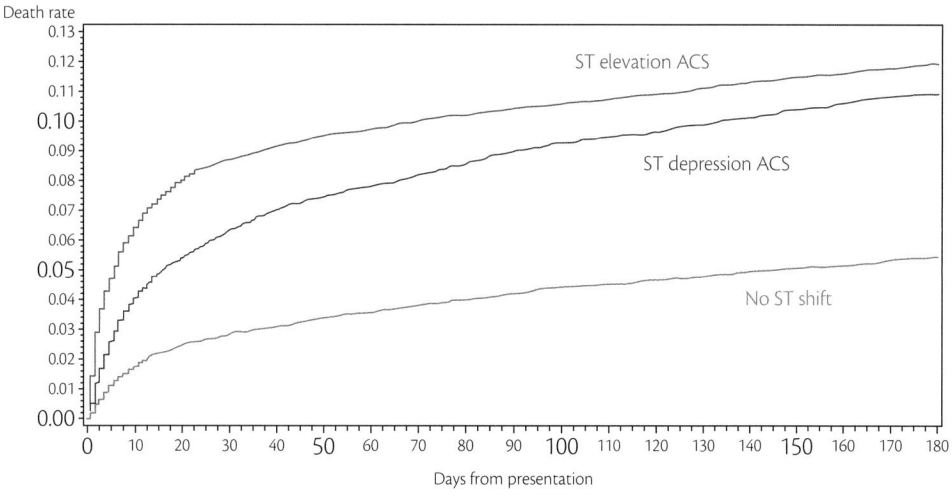

Fig. 16.13.5.2 Mortality over the first 180 days following presentation with ACS: patients stratified according to ST shift on presentation to hospital. Reproduced with permission from Bassand J-P et al, *Guidelines for the Diagnosis and Treatment of Non-ST-Segment Elevation Acute Coronary Syndromes. European Heart Journal* (2007) 28, 1598–1660.

MI in the first 6 months following presentation, and almost half of this risk is within the first 7 days (GUSTO IIb, OASIS Registry, and GRACE Registry). Whereas patients with STEMI are most at risk of death, especially in the first hours of symptom onset, those with non-STEMI ACS are at higher risk after discharge (Fig. 16.13.5.2 and Table 16.13.5.2).

The clinical syndrome and outcome

The Braunwald classification categorizes unstable angina according to the mode of onset and time course (Table 16.13.5.3). It was empirically based, but has been validated by prospective studies. Patients with unstable ischaemic pain at rest and those with ST depression have the highest risk of an adverse cardiac event. Similarly, those with unstable angina following acute MI are at an increased risk. Although the classification is useful, many of the patients that present with ACS are in Braunwald class 3B and additional methods of risk characterization are required to optimize management.

A diagnostic triage system can be developed for patients with suspected ACS (see below). This is based on ECG changes,

Table 16.13.5.2 Mortality in hospital and at 6 months in low-, intermediate-, and high-risk categories in registry populations according to the GRACE (Global Registry of Acute Coronary Events) risk score, which assigns risk on the basis of the following patient characteristics on admission: age, heart rate, systolic blood pressure, serum creatinine, evidence of congestive heart failure, also the presence/absence of cardiac arrest, ST-segment deviation and elevated cardiac enzymes/markers. For calculations, see http://www.outcomes.org/grace

Risk category (tertiles)	GRACE risk score	In-hospital deaths (%)
Low	≤108	<1
Intermediate	109–140	1–3
High	>140	>3
Risk category (tertiles)	GRACE risk score	Post-discharge to 6 months deaths (%)
Low	≤88	<3
Intermediate	89–118	3–8
High	>118	>8

From Fox KA, et al. (2006). Prediction of risk of death and myocardial infarction in the six months after presentation with acute coronary syndrome:prospective multinational observational study (GRACE). *BMJ*, **333**, 1091–4.

biomarker release, and stress or perfusion testing. Patients with evolving STEMI are identified, and those with higher risk separated from those with lower risk. The respective categories of patients require different management strategies.

The ECG and outcome

The 12-lead ECG (performed on admission) provides direct prognostic information (Table 16.13.5.1). The greatest risk of death and subsequent MI is seen in patients with simultaneous ST elevation and depression; the next highest risk is seen in those with transient ST segment elevation or ST segment depression; isolated T wave inversion carries a lower risk. The number of leads demonstrating ST deviation also yields prognostic information: among those with ST deviation in the anterior leads a rate of death or MI of 12.4% was seen at 1 year—higher than seen with similar changes in other locations (TIMI III trial). Patients with a left main and three-vessel coronary artery disease may show a combination of ST-segment elevation and depression.

Ambulatory ST segment recording can identify patients with unstable angina and either silent or symptomatic myocardial ischaemia with an increased risk for major subsequent cardiac events. However, conventional ambulatory monitoring usually requires offline analysis and is not suitable for the prediction of imminent events. Computer-assisted, continuous, multilead, ECG monitoring techniques has become available for real-time ECG and ST segment monitoring. The occurrence and extent of ischaemic territory identified by such continuous recordings can provide additional

Table 16.13.5.3 Classification of unstable angina (Braunwald)

Class		A Secondary unstable angina	B Primary unstable angina	C Postinfarction (<2 weeks) unstable angina
I	New-onset, severe or accelerated angina	IA	IB	IC
II	Subacute rest angina (<48 h ago)	IIA	IIB	IIC
III	Acute rest angina (within 48 h)	IIIA	IIIB	IIIC

From Braunwald E. Circulation 1989, 80, 410–14 (http://circ.ahajournals.org/cgi/reprint/80/2/410).

prognostic information over and above the admission ECG. The information can be combined with biomarkers and, together, they provide additional prognostic information (FRISC study).

Biochemical markers and outcome

Enzymes and biomarkers of necrosis are gradually released into the systemic circulation following complete or transient occlusion of the coronary artery, or fragmentation of a thrombus and embolization. Following total occlusion of the vessel, troponins and creatine kinase (or more specifically CK-MB) are released and are detectable at clearly abnormal levels about 6 to 8 h after the event unless there is extensive collateral perfusion.

The cardiac isoforms of troponin I and troponin T are exclusively expressed in cardiac myocytes and provide specific evidence of myocardial damage. Following infarction, troponins are released from the cytosolic pool and first appear in the circulation in detectable concentrations between 3 and 4 h after the ischaemic event, and reach diagnostic concentrations at 6 to 8 h. Troponin release is evidence of myocardial injury and carries prognostic significance: the greater the troponin release, the greater the risk of subsequent MI and death. However, it is important to recognize that other causes of myocyte necrosis (including myocarditis, pulmonary embolism, and severe heart failure) can give rise to detectable troponin concentrations in the circulation; so the diagnosis of ACS requires the presence of an appropriate clinical syndrome.

When should the cardiac enzymes be measured? The time course of the release of troponins (or enzymes) from myocardium is such that diagnostic concentrations may not be achieved until between 6 and 8 h after an ischaemic event. Thus, a normal value for a patient on arrival does not exclude infarction or unstable angina, but an elevated value is highly predictive of subsequent infarction. Troponins should be measured on arrival and at approximately 8 to 12 h: these provide the highest predictive accuracy.

Among those with persistently negative troponins and without significant ECG changes, there is a very low risk of subsequent infarction and death (provided that severe underlying coronary artery disease is excluded). Such patients should undergo pre-discharge stress testing, the best tests being myocardial perfusion scanning or stress echocardiography, but treadmill ECGs on exercise are more widely available (see Chapter 16.3.1).

Markers of inflammation

Inflammatory changes in the vessel wall promote plaque fissuring or erosion, and inflammatory changes also follow episodes of minor myocardial damage. In ACS there is evidence that inflammatory markers (C-reactive protein (CRP), interleukin (IL)-6, and IL-1) are independent predictors of adverse outcome. After the acute phase, continuing inflammation—e.g. with elevated C-reactive protein—occurs in one-half of those whose levels are acutely elevated and identifies a category of patients at increased risk. However, although inflammatory mechanisms are implicated in plaque growth and plaque destabilization, specific anti-inflammatory therapies have not yet been demonstrated to improve outcome, and measurement of CRP or other inflammatory markers is not part of routine clinical practice.

Risk characterization in ACS

The timing and the nature of key management decisions in ACS are dependent upon risk estimation. For example, the choice of reperfusion therapy in ST elevation may be influenced by the presence of comorbidity, bleeding risk, and time delay from symptom onset. Similarly, in non-STEMI ACS, ongoing ischaemia with ST depression or the presence of hypotension or a high risk score may initiate very early re-vascularization. Specific pharmacological (e.g. glycoprotein IIb/IIIa inhibitors) or interventional therapies (PCI) have demonstrated benefit in high- or moderate-risk patients but not in low-risk patients (5-year outcome: RITA 3, FRISC II).

In patients with ACSs, risk can be separated into two components: 'prior risk' and 'acute ischaemic risk'. Prior risk is determined by patient characteristics (age and gender), prior ischaemic heart disease (MI, heart failure, prior angina, etc.), and systemic factors that influence risk (hypertension, diabetes, renal dysfunction, and other life-threatening systemic disorders). These can be considered as the background level of risk that the patients bring with them to the point of presentation. Although several of the individual risk components may not be modifiable, the combined impact of prior risk influences the balance between benefit and risk for each of the therapeutic strategies in ACS. Thus, prior risk 'sets the baseline' for risk–benefit decisions.

By contrast, 'acute ischaemic risk' is potentially modifiable and determined by the severity of coronary obstruction and the extent of the territory affected. Collateral perfusion, embolization, myocardial oxygen demand, and cytoprotection mechanisms all influence the extent of ischaemia. Patients with similar clinical features may have experienced transient complete occlusion, or severe subtotal occlusion complicated by distal embolization of fragments of a platelet-rich thrombus, and altered vascular tone in the distal territory. Clinical markers of acute ischaemic risk include ECG changes, release of biomarkers of necrosis into the systemic circulation, and mechanical and arrhythmic complications of the ischaemic episode.

Simplistically, prior risk can be regarded as the 'baggage' that the patient carries with them, and acute ischaemic risk as an 'acquired hazard' arising from the new ischaemic event. The distinction is important because management strategies for prior risk aim to treat heart failure, underlying coronary and systemic disease, and risk factors. The management of acute ischaemic risk aims to reverse the impact of acute coronary obstruction and thrombosis and is the first priority in the management of patients with ACS. Assessment of the extent and impact of underlying coronary artery disease (e.g. with stress testing) and assessment of left ventricular function can take place later in the management of these patients (Box 16.13.5.2).

Box 16.13.5.2 Practical steps to assess risk (in addition to clinical symptoms)

- 12-lead ECG—obtained directly after first medical contact, repeated after recurrent symptoms
- Troponin estimation (cTnT or cTnI)—repeated after 6–12 h, if the initial test is negative
- Apply a risk score (such as GRACE, TIMI—see Fig. 16.13.5.2)
- An echocardiogram may be required to rule in/out alternative diagnoses
- In patients with no recurrence of pain, normal ECG and no troponin elevation, a noninvasive stress test may be required.

Management of ACS without ST elevation (unstable angina/non-STEMI)

Anti-ischaemic therapy

Anti-ischaemic therapy can decrease myocardial oxygen consumption by reducing heart rate, lowering blood pressure, or depressing left ventricular contractility, and may also act by inducing vasodilatation. In consequence, anti-ischaemic therapy can limit the progression of occlusion and improve perfusion and improve the supply–demand imbalance. Mechanical revascularization (PCI and coronary bypass surgery) also aims to relieve obstruction and reduce a patient's susceptibility to ischaemia—these interventions will be considered separately (see below and Chapter 16.13.6).

Nitrates

Nitrates act by venodilatation and—in higher dose—by arteriolar dilatation, and hence reduce preload and afterload, thereby decreasing oxygen demand. In addition, nitrates can also induce coronary vasodilatation. They are effective in relieving symptoms of ischaemia. In the acute phase of the syndrome, where dose titration is required, they are most conveniently administered intravenously. Once dose titration is no longer required, oral administration is feasible.

Continuous nitrate administration can induce tolerance; so when symptoms are controlled, oral nitrates should be prescribed with appropriate nitrate-free intervals. An alternative is to use drugs with nitrate-like properties but without the same problems of tolerance, such as a potassium channel activator (see below).

Large outcome trials have been conducted with nitrates in acute MI but not in other ACS. However, patients without ST-segment elevation or bundle branch block were randomized within the ISIS-4 trial: their mortality was 5.3% for nitrate treatment and 5.5% for placebo treatment, a nonsignificant difference.

Nitrates are effective in reducing ischaemia in the in-hospital management of non-ST elevation ACS, but there is no evidence that they improve mortality.

β-Blockers

β-Adrenoceptor antagonists reduce heart rate and blood pressure and myocardial contractility and hence decrease myocardial oxygen consumption. They are primarily employed to reduce ischaemia in ACS. Large-scale trials have not been conducted in patients with non-ST elevation ACS. However, in the context of acute MI, β-blockers reduce mortality by approximately 10 to 15%. They may act be reducing ventricular arrhythmias, reinfarction, and myocardial rupture. A meta-analysis of five trials involving 4700 patients with threatened MI (treated with intravenous β-blockers followed by oral therapy for c.1 week) resulted in a 13% reduction in the risk of MI. Patients with significantly impaired atrioventricular conduction or asthma or acute left ventricular dysfunction should not receive β-blockers. Although β-blockers may exacerbate acute heart failure, extensive trials have produced strong evidence of a benefit for the gradual introduction of β-blockers in ambulant patients with heart failure (see Chapter 16.5).

Patients with suspected ACS should be initiated on β-blocker therapy unless contraindicated.

Calcium entry blockers

These agents inhibit the slow inward current induced by the entry of extracellular calcium through the cell membrane, especially in cardiac and arteriolar smooth muscle. They act by lowering myocardial oxygen demand, reducing arterial pressure, and reducing contractility. Calcium channel blockers can provide symptom relief in patients already receiving nitrates and β-blockers, and may be useful in patients with contraindications to β-blockade. Some agents induce a reflex tachycardia (e.g. nifedipine, nicardipine, amlodipine) and are best administered in combination with a β-adrenoceptor antagonist. By contrast, diltiazem and verapamil are suitable for patients who cannot tolerate a β-blocker because they inhibit conduction through the atrioventricular (AV) node and tend to cause bradycardia. All calcium antagonists reduce myocardial contractility and may aggravate heart failure. Calcium entry blockers have been demonstrated to reduce the frequency of angina in patients with variant angina.

A meta-analysis of calcium entry blockers in ACS indicates a nonsignificant trend towards a higher mortality in treated vs control patients (5.9% vs 5.2%, in 7551 patients). In individual trials, diltiazem has been compared with propranolol, and both agents produced a similar reduction in anginal episodes.

Dihydropyridine calcium-entry blockers should be employed with β-blockers in ACS to avoid reflex tachycardia. In patients unable to tolerate β-blockers, a heart-rate-slowing calcium antagonist may be appropriate. Short-acting dihydropyridines should not be used in isolation in ACSs.

Potassium channel activators

These agents (e.g. nicorandil) have arterial and venous dilating properties, but do not exhibit the tolerance seen with nitrates. They have been shown to be better than placebo in relieving the symptoms of angina. A randomized trial of nicorandil (a combined nitrate-like and potassium channel activator) suggested benefit on a composite clinical endpoint (IONA study), and this drug may be considered as an alternative to nitrate administration.

The following recommendations for anti-ischaemic therapy are based on current clinical and trial evidence:

♦ Anti-ischaemic therapy should be administered in conjunction with antithrombotic and interventional therapy (see below), with the overall strategy guided by risk evaluation of the patient (see risk stratification).

♦ Patients with suspected ACS should be initiated on nitrate and β-blocker therapy, unless there are contraindications to the use of β-blockers

♦ In patients with contraindications to β-blockers, heart rate-slowing calcium antagonists should be employed

♦ The combination of a calcium antagonist and β-blocker is superior to either agent alone

♦ Angiography and revascularization should be considered in patients with recurrent or persistent ischaemia, or patients with troponin elevation (including non-STEMI). The timing of angiography should be guided by the risk status of the patient.

Antiplatelet therapy

Aspirin

Exposure of the contents of atheromatous plaque to circulating blood triggers platelet activation by several different pathways. Aspirin is a potent and irreversible inhibitor of platelet cyclo-oxygenase, blocking the formation of thromboxane A_2 and inhibiting platelet aggregation. Although the effects of aspirin can be overcome in the presence of potent thrombogenic stimuli, nevertheless the benefits of aspirin treatment in unstable angina are clearly defined and substantial. The Antiplatelet Trialists Collaboration demonstrated a reduction of 36% in death or MI with antiplatelet treatment (predominantly aspirin) vs placebo in unstable angina trials. Aspirin treatment significantly reduces subsequent MI, stroke, and vascular death, with the largest reductions seen amongst patients at highest risk. In patients with unstable angina, four key studies have demonstrated that aspirin significantly reduces the risk of cardiac death or nonfatal MI by approximately 50%.

The efficacy of lower-dose aspirin (75 mg/day) therapy has been demonstrated in several studies, including those of Wallentin and colleagues where long-term effects were evaluated in men under 70 years of age with unstable coronary artery disease. After 6 and 12 months of aspirin treatment, the risk of MI or death was reduced by 54% and 48%, respectively (risk ratio 0.52 with 95% confidence intervals 0.37–0.72). The strength of evidence and magnitude of benefit demonstrated with aspirin treatment in non-ST-segment-elevation ACS is such that aspirin is indicated in all patients with ACS, unless there is a clear contraindication. Nevertheless, patients with ACS remain at significant risk despite aspirin therapy. In prospective registry studies of unstable angina/non-STEMI, and in spite of aspirin treatment in more than 80% of patients, the risk of death or MI is approximately 10% at 6 months and the risk of death/MI or refractory angina is approximately 22 to 33% over the same period (OASIS Registry, PRAIS Registry).

Aspirin treatment (75–325 mg daily) is indicated in all patients with ACS unless there is good evidence of aspirin allergy or evidence of active bleeding.

ADP antagonists (thienopyridines)

Ticlopidine and clopidogrel are adenosine diphosphate receptor antagonists, and they block the ADP-induced pathway of platelet activation by inhibiting of the P2Y12 ADP receptor.

Clopidogrel has replaced ticlopidine on account of a superior safety profile and has been tested in a large-scale trial of patients with unstable angina/non-STEMI (n = 12 562, CURE trial). The agent was used on top of existing therapy, and in addition to aspirin. It reduced death, nonfatal MI, and stroke from 11.4 to 9.3% (95% confidence interval 0.72–0.90, p < 0.001). For every 1000 patients treated, there were 28 fewer major cardiovascular complications but six more transfusions. Importantly, benefits were seen across risk groups (diabetics, hypertensives, biomarker elevation or not, revascularization or not). In a substudy (PCI-CURE), clopidogrel also reduced death and MI in those undergoing percutaneous re-vascularization (2.9% clopidogrel vs 4.4% for placebo). Thus, with the combination of clopidogrel and aspirin, there is evidence of early and sustained reductions in the risks of death and MI in patients that present with ACS.

A number of smaller studies have used higher loading doses of clopidogrel (usually 600 mg), and these show more rapid inhibition of platelet aggregation than that achieved with 300 mg. Thus, higher loading doses of clopidogrel are feasible and may have advantages in the context of early percutaneous coronary intervention. A large-scale outcome and safety study testing higher loading and maintenance doses of clopidogrel is underway (CURRENT OASIS-7).

Triple antiplatelet therapy (aspirin, clopidogrel, and IIB/IIa inhibitor) has been shown to be superior in preventing ischaemic events (compared to no IIb/IIIa inhibitor) in combined analysis of percutaneous coronary intervention trials and in the ISAR-REACT-2 trial. Hence, dual antiplatelet therapy (with aspirin and clopidogrel) is not sufficient in high-risk patients undergoing percutaneous coronary intervention.

Long-term clopidogrel administration was tested in the CHARISMA study of 15 603 patients with documented vascular disease or risk factors for vascular disease. Overall, there was no difference in the primary endpoint of cardiovascular death, MI, or stroke. However, in the subgroup of patients with documented cardiovascular disease, the same endpoint was significantly reduced with dual antiplatelet therapy, when compared with aspirin (6.9 vs 7.9%, relative risk 0.88, 95% confidence interval 0.77–0.99). Thus, longer-term treatment with dual antiplatelet therapy should only be considered in those in whom the risk of ischaemic events exceeds the risk of bleeding complications.

Newer P2Y12 inhibitors with more potent receptor affinity and more rapid onset of action are currently under evaluation (e.g. prasugrel, cangrelor, AZD6140).

Recommendations for thienopyridines are:

◆ Patients with non-ST-elevation ACS should be given clopidogrel as an initial 300-mg loading dose, followed by continued treatment at a dose of 75 mg daily in combination with aspirin at a dose of 75–325 mg daily. Clopidogrel should be given alone to patients with contraindications to aspirin (same regimen).

◆ Clopidogrel should be maintained for 12 months unless the risks of bleeding exceed potential benefits.

◆ In patients undergoing percutaneous coronary intervention, a loading dose of 600 mg of clopidogrel may be used to achieve more rapid inhibition of platelet function. Following percutaneous coronary intervention, the duration of clopidogrel administration should take account of the type of stent implanted (bare metal or drug eluting) and the risks of bleeding/thrombosis.

Glycoprotein IIb/IIIa inhibitors

Platelet adhesion is the initial step in haemostasis after disruption of an atheromatous plaque. It is triggered by damage to the vessel wall and exposure of the subendothelium, and is followed by platelet activation and aggregation. Regardless of the agonist, the final common pathway leading to the formation of a platelet aggregate is mediated by the glycoprotein (GP) IIb/IIIa receptor. GPIIb/IIIa receptor antagonists inhibit platelet aggregation irrespective of the agonist, and they prevent binding of fibrinogen to its receptor on the platelet surface.

Three GPIIb/IIIa receptor antagonists have been approved for clinical use: abciximab, eptifibatide, and tirofiban. Abciximab is a chimeric human–murine monoclonal antibody that binds with high affinity to the receptor: it has a long biological half-life of 6 to 12 h, and low levels of receptor occupancy are detected even 2 weeks after treatment. Eptifibatide is a synthetic cyclic heptapeptide with high affinity for the arginine–glycine–aspartic acid ligand-adhesion site of the IIb/IIIa receptor. It inhibits platelet aggregation in a dose-dependent manner and is readily reversible due to competitive binding and a short half-life of approximately 2.5 h. Tirofiban is a nonpeptide tyrosine derivative which also binds to the arginine–glycine–aspartic acid site with high specificity. It inhibits platelet aggregation in a dose- and concentration-dependent manner and is rapidly reversible, with platelet function approaching normal levels in 90% of patients within 4 to 8 h.

Although it is convenient to group glycoprotein IIb/IIIa receptor antagonists together, and undoubtedly there is evidence of a class effect, there are biological and pharmacological differences between the agents.

Trials of GPIIb/IIIa inhibitors

More than 32 000 patients have been randomized in clinical trials involving GPIIb/IIIa inhibitors (16 trials). A highly significant ($p < 0.001$) benefit is observed for the combined endpoint of death or MI at 48 to 96 h, 30 days, and 6 months. At 30 days the odds ratio is 0.76, or 20 fewer events per 1000 patients treated, and a highly significant benefit is observed for the combined endpoint of death/MI or revascularization at all time points. By contrast, mortality benefits are seen only at 48 to 96 h, with no significant benefit at 30 days or 6 months. Figure 16.13.5.3 shows summary data from a subset of these trials. A pooled analysis of abciximab trials has revealed a net mortality benefit, but there is no evidence of benefit for abciximab in medically treated patients (GUSTO-4-ACS).

The impact of GPIIb/IIIa inhibitors is influenced by the risk status of the patient and whether administered in the context of percutaneous coronary intervention. In a meta-analysis of 29 570 patients, there was a 9% reduction in relative risk overall, but with no significant benefit in those who were medically managed (death and MI at 30 days of 9.3% for IIb/IIIa vs 9.7% placebo, OR 0.95, 95% confidence interval 0.86–1.04). Significant benefit was observed when GP IIb/IIIa inhibitors were maintained during percutaneous coronary intervention (10.5 vs 13.6%, OR 0.74, 95% confidence interval 0.57–0.96). Similarly, there is no convincing evidence of benefit in low-risk patients, irrespective of interventional strategy.

Indications for treatment with GPIIb/IIIa inhibitors are:

- Treatment with glycoprotein IIb/IIIa inhibitors results in improved outcome in patients at intermediate to high risk—e.g. those with elevated troponins, ST depression, or diabetes.
- GPIIb/IIIa inhibitors should be administered with oral antiplatelet agents (aspirin and thienopyridines) and anticoagulants (heparin or low-molecular-weight heparin (LMWH)).

- Glycoprotein IIb/IIIa inhibitors result in improved outcome in patients requiring urgent percutaneous intervention for non-ST-segment elevation ACS.
- Bivalirudin may be used as an alternative to GP IIb/IIIa inhibitors plus UFH/LMWH (see below).

Anticoagulants

Unfractionated heparin

Unfractionated heparin is widely used for the treatment of non-ST-elevation ACS, but the evidence on which this is based is less robust than for other widely adopted treatment strategies. In practice, unfractionated heparin is difficult to control because of its unpredictable levels of binding to plasma proteins, and this may be amplified by the acute-phase response. In addition, heparin has reduced effectiveness against platelet-rich and clot-bound thrombin.

Oler and colleagues conducted a meta-analysis of the influence of adding heparin to aspirin in the treatment of patients with unstable angina. Only six randomized trials were available, with 1353 patients included: there were 55 deaths or MIs in the aspirin plus heparin arm and 68 in the aspirin-alone arm, giving a risk reduction of 0.67 and a 95% confidence interval of 0.44 to 1.02. These results do not produce conclusive evidence of benefit from adding heparin to aspirin, but it must be stressed that appropriately powered, larger-scale trials have not been conducted. Nevertheless, clinical practice has adopted unfractionated heparin treatment with aspirin as a pragmatic extrapolation of the available evidence.

LMWH

Trials vs placebo

The FRISC trial tested dalteparin against placebo in aspirin-treated patients with unstable angina/non-STEMI. Some 1506 patients were randomized to receive dalteparin (twice daily for the first 6 days and then once daily at a lower dose for approximately 6 weeks), and the trial showed a highly significant reduction in the frequency of death or new MI at 6 days (1.8% vs 4.8%, with a risk ratio of 0.37).

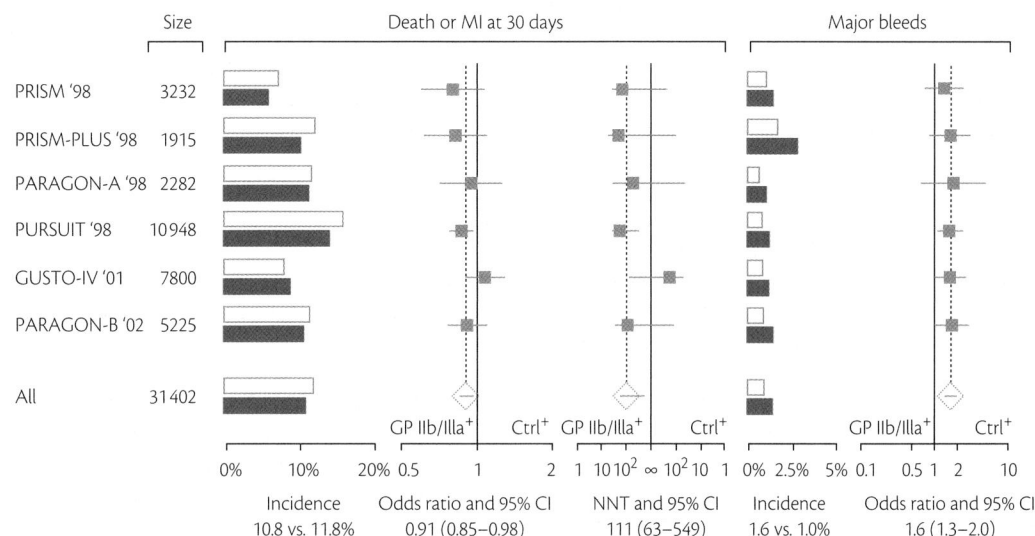

Fig. 16.13.5.3 Death, MI, and major bleeds at 30 days in randomized trials of glycoprotein IIb/IIIa inhibitors (filled bars) vs control (open bars) in a conservative strategy. NNT, number of patients who needed to be treated to avoid one event.
(From the European Society of Cardiology Guidelines (2007). *Eur Heart J*, **28**, 230–68.)

The effects were sustained to 42 days, but were attenuated at 6 months, the differences no longer maintaining significance. Nevertheless, this trial clearly showed the benefit of LMWH over placebo in the presence of aspirin.

Trials vs unfractionated heparin

LMWH possesses enhanced anti-Xa activity in relation to anti-IIa (antithrombin) activity, compared with unfractionated heparin. It also exhibits decreased sensitivity to platelet factor 4 (PF4), has more predictable anticoagulant effect, and lower rates of thrombocytopenia. In view of its enhanced bioavailability, it offers the substantial practical advantage of subcutaneous administration based on a dose per kilogram of body weight and without the need for laboratory monitoring.

Acute-phase treatment (c.2–8 days)

In the FRIC trial, dalteparin was tested against unfractionated heparin in 1400 patients with unstable angina: it had limited power to show a difference, and no significant difference was seen between unfractionated heparin and dalteparin.

The ESSENCE trial was double-blinded and placebo-controlled and tested enoxaparin against unfractionated heparin. The treatments were given for 2 to 8 days (median 2.6 days) and the primary endpoints were death, MI, or recurrent angina. Enoxaparin reduced the primary endpoint from 19.6% to 16.6% at 14 days (odds ratio 0.80 and confidence intervals 0.67–0.98) (see Fig. 16.13.5.4). A similar and significant odds ratio was maintained at 30 days and 1 year. At 1 year, there were 3.7 fewer events/100 patients ($p = 0.022$). The study was not powered for death/MI alone, but demonstrated corresponding trends for these endpoints.

The TIMI 11b trial was also double-blinded and tested enoxaparin vs unfractionated heparin, but additionally it examined 72 h of treatment vs 43 days of treatment. The results up to 14 days mirrored those seen in the ESSENCE trial: at 14 days the primary outcome occurred was 16.6% (heparin) vs 14.2% (enoxaparin), risk ratio 0.85 ($p = 0.03$). A combined analysis of ESSENCE and TIMI 11b indicated an absolute reduction of 3.1 per 100 for death/MI/refractory angina, and showed a similar risk ratio of 0.79

(confidence interval 0.65–0.96) for death and MI. Taken together, these findings indicate that short-term treatment with enoxaparin results in about 3 per 100 fewer major cardiac endpoints compared to unfractionated heparin treatment, and this is achieved without additional major bleeding.

Prolonged outpatient treatment

The FRAXIS trial tested fraxaparin, for 6 or 14 days, against unfractionated heparin in 3468 patients; no difference was seen in efficacy, but there was a significant excess of major bleeds with longer-term outpatient treatment. In TIMI 11b, the curves remained separated over the succeeding treatment interval: at 43 days there were 19.6% events (heparin) vs 17.3% (enoxaparin) ($p = 0.049$), with no evidence of a further separation of the curves. There was 1.4% absolute excess in major bleeds over the chronic phase.

Conclusions from the LMWH studies

There is convincing evidence in aspirin-treated patients (heparin or LMWH is not indicated in the absence of antiplatelet therapy) that LMWH is better than placebo (FRISC trial). The two trials using enoxaparin have provided consistent data in favour of LMWH over unfractionated heparin when administered as an acute regimen. The other trials have produced a similar outcome for the acute phase of treatment and it can be concluded that acute treatment is at least as effective as unfractionated heparin (Fig. 16.13.5.4). There is no convincing evidence to support longer-term treatment with LMWH.

Evidence supports the following conclusions regarding the use of heparin:

♦ LMWH is superior to placebo in aspirin-treated patients

♦ LMWH is at least as effective as unfractionated heparin

♦ LMWH can be used in place of unfractionated heparin and has practical advantages over unfractionated heparin

Direct thrombin inhibitors

Direct thrombin inhibitors (e.g. hirudin, bivalirudin) bind directly to thrombin (factor IIa) and inhibit thrombin-induced conversion

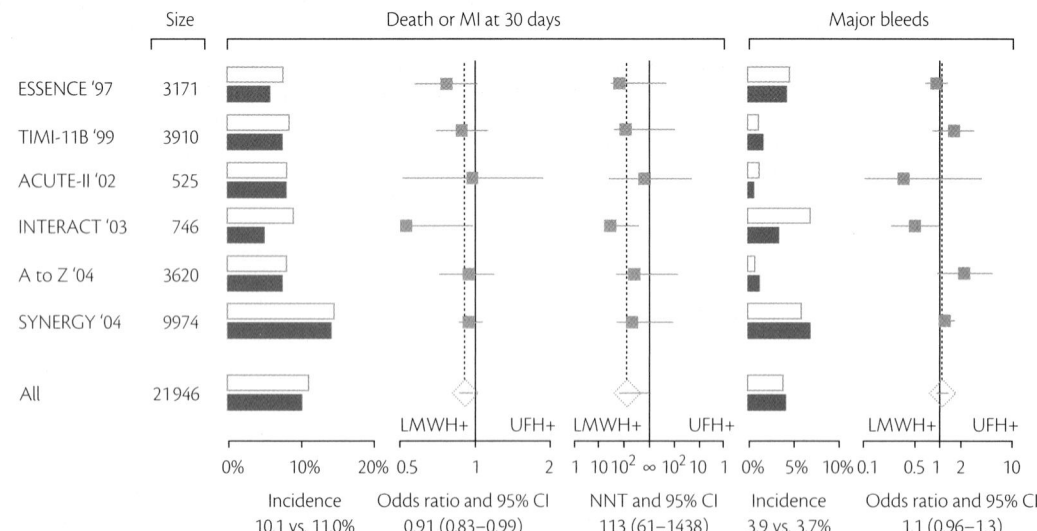

Fig. 16.13.5.4 Death, MI, and major bleeds at 30 days in randomized trials of enoxaparin (filled bars) vs unfractionated heparin (open bars). NNT, number of patients who needed to be treated to avoid one event.

Reproduced with permission from Bassand J-P et al, *Guidelines for the Diagnosis and Treatment of Non-ST-Segment Elevation Acute Coronary Syndromes. European Heart Journal* (2007) 28, 1598–1660.

of fibrinogen to fibrin. They inactivate fibrin-bound thrombin as well as thrombin in the circulation. They do not bind to plasma proteins nor interact with PF4, and hence their anticoagulant effect is predictable.

Hirudin has been tested in large-scale trials (e.g. OASIS-1, OASIS-2, TIMI 9b, GUSTO IIb) against heparin and a combined analysis suggests a 22% relative-risk reduction in cardiovascular death or MI at 72 h, 17% at 7 days, and 10% at 35 days. This combined analysis is significant at 72 h and 7 days but not beyond. Hirudin is licensed for heparin-induced thrombocytopenia but not for ACS.

Bivalirudin was tested in the open-label randomized ACUITY trial in 13 819 patients with moderate- to high-risk non-ST-elevation ACS with a planned invasive strategy. The composite endpoints included death, MI, or unplanned revascularization for ischaemia, major bleeding (noncoronary artery bypass graft (CABG)-related), and net clinical outcome (composite ischaemia or major bleeding). Bivalirudin plus GPIIb/IIIa had similar outcomes (noninferior) to heparin/LMWH plus GPIIb/IIIa and similar rates of bleeding. Bivalirudin alone had similar outcome (noninferior composite) to heparin/low-molecular-weight heparin plus GPIIb/IIIa, but had superior safety (less bleeding). An interaction with the effects of clopidogrel was evident; benefits were seen with clopidogrel but not without.

Anti-Xa inhibitors

Fondaparinux is a synthetic pentasaccharide that selectively binds antithrombin and causes inhibition of factor Xa. In the OASIS-5 study, 20 078 patients with non-ST-elevation ACS were randomized (double-blind design) to receive 2.5 mg subcutaneous fondaparinux once daily vs subcutaneous enoxaparin 1 mg/kg twice daily for up to 8 days. Fondaparinux was noninferior at 9 days (the primary endpoint), but subsequently those randomized to fondaparinux had reduced mortality and approximately half the rate of major bleeding. In those undergoing PCI, there was an excess of catheter-related thrombi, and administration of this agent requires additional antithrombin therapy (the excess thrombi were not seen when combined with unfractionated heparin and there was no evidence of excess bleeding with this combination).

Anticoagulation for non-ST-elevation ACS:

◆ Anticoagulation is required in addition to antiplatelet therapy

◆ Anticoagulant options include unfractionated heparin (UFH), LMWH, fondaparinux, and bivalirudin, with choice dependent on the initial strategy (early invasive, or not) and the bleeding risk

◆ With an urgent invasive strategy, unfractionated heparin, enoxaparin, or bivalirudin are treatment options

◆ In the absence of an urgent/early invasive strategy, fondaparinux has the most favourable efficacy/safety profile

Revascularization

The aim of revascularization in non-ST-elevation ACS is to relieve angina, to alleviate myocardial ischaemia, and to prevent progression to MI or death. The indications for myocardial revascularization are dependent on the risk status of the patients and the presence or absence of evidence of ongoing myocardial ischaemia and/or evidence that the ischaemia has resulted in mechanical or electrical complications. Following angiography, the choice of PCI

or coronary artery bypass grafting is dependent on the extent and severity of angiographic stenoses and the comorbidity of the patient. Angiographic analyses from the TIMI-3B and FRISC-2 studies demonstrates that about 30 to 38% of patients with non-ST-elevation ACS have single-vessel disease and 44 to 60% have multivessel disease (>50% diameter stenosis).

Observational studies

Large-scale observational studies have demonstrated wide variations between countries in the use of cardiac catheterization and revascularization for patients with acute ischaemic syndromes and a paradox whereby lower-risk patients are less likely to receive aggressive antithrombotic and interventional treatment than moderate- or higher-risk patients. Similar findings have been observed in the United States of America in the CRUSADE registry. Nevertheless, there is clear evidence over time of increasing use of guideline-indicated therapies (especially class 1 indicated treatments) in non-ST-elevation ACS, including angiography and interventional procedures. Overall, the changing pharmacological and interventional therapies have been associated with striking improvements in outcome, including a halving of new heart failure and a reduced risk of death. Higher rates of revascularization have been associated with an increased frequency of procedural complications, including stroke and major bleeding. Definitive assessment of the impact of revascularization on outcomes requires randomized trials and longer-term follow-up.

Randomized trial data

Several smaller and older trials (including TIMI 3B and VANQWISH) tested the impact of an interventional strategy in ACS. These largely predated modern antithrombotic therapy and modern interventional technology (including PCI and stents). For the sake of completeness, all the randomized trials are included in the overall meta-analysis (see below), but the larger and more recent trials require further description.

The FRISC-II trial compared an invasive strategy with a conservative strategy in patients who were initially stabilized with approximately 6 days of treatment with LMWH. Coronary angiography was performed within the first 7 days and revascularization performed in 71% of those in the invasive arm and 9% of those in the noninvasive arm within 10 days. This was, therefore, the first trial to achieve substantial separations in strategy and to include an appropriately powered population. After 6 months, death or MI occurred in 9.4% of the invasive group compared with 12.1% of the noninvasive group (a risk ratio of 0.78, $p = 0.031$) and the results remained significant at 1 year, but the mortality and the death or MI outcomes were no longer significant at 5 years. However, the results at 5 years clearly demonstrate that most benefit was seen in higher-risk patients, with no evidence of benefit in low-risk patients. A similar relationship between patient risk status and long-term outcome had been demonstrated in the RITA 3 trial.

The FRISC-II and the RITA 3 trials demonstrated that invasive therapy was associated with an excess early (within 30 days) rate of death or MI due to periprocedure complications. Overall, there was a consistency of benefit (for the efficacy endpoints) across the FRISC-II, TACTICS and RITA-3 trials. RITA 3 demonstrated that most benefit in the first year was in preventing refractory angina, but over 5 years there was a significant benefit in death or MI, and in preventing cardiovascular death, in those randomized to intervention. The more recent ICTUS trial was smaller and had

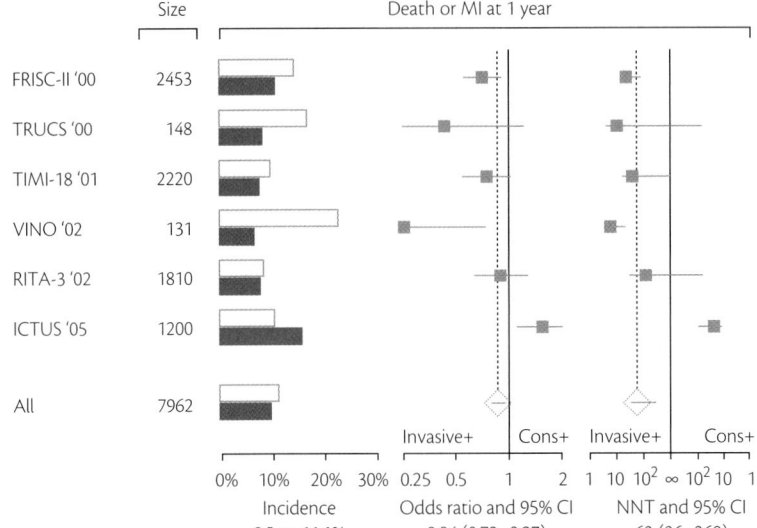

Fig. 16.13.5.5 Death or MI in six contemporary randomized trials comparing early invasive (filled bars) vs conservative strategy (open bars). NNT, number of patients who needed to be treated to avoid one event. Reproduced with permission from Bassand J-P et al, *Guidelines for the Diagnosis and Treatment of Non-ST-Segment Elevation Acute Coronary Syndromes. European Heart Journal* (2007) 28, 1598–1660.

a high rate of intervention in the 'selective invasive' arm of the trial, about as high as the intervention arm in RITA 3 and only modestly lower than in the intervention arm of FRISC-II. ICTUS employed a high rate of adjunctive therapies (including GPIIb/IIIa inhibitors), and the trial did not show an overall benefit for intervention. Differences in trial design, in the risk status of the trial populations, and in the definitions of MI in the respective trials must be taken into consideration. Nevertheless, a pooled analysis of all the trials is likely to represent the most reliable interpretation of all of the randomized trial data.

In a meta-analysis of all the trials, published in the European Society of Cardiology Guidelines (*Eur Heart J*, 2007), there was clear evidence for overall benefit on the outcomes of death or MI at 1 year (9.5% death/MI with intervention, 11.1% conservative strategy; odds ratio 0.84; 95% confidence interval 0.73–0.97) (Fig. 16.13.5.5). The number needed to treat to prevent one death or MI was 63. However, on the basis of the findings that most benefit was seen in moderate-to higher-risk patients and little or no benefit in lower-risk patients, the European Society of Cardiology Guidelines strongly recommend risk stratification of the patients as the basis for deciding who requires emergency or urgent revascularization, and who does not.

Risk stratification of patients with non-ST-elevation ACS

Risk stratification is required to guide management and therapeutic decisions in patients with non-ST-elevation ACS. Some patients are clearly at high risk at the time of initial presentation, e.g. those with typical ongoing ischaemic pain and ST depression on the ECG. However, for the remainder it may not be possible to identify higher-risk patients on the basis of the clinical features and ECG findings alone. Several studies have demonstrated that simple risk scores can accurately predict short- and longer-term outcome, not only in those with defined characteristics of ACS, but also in patients with suspected cardiac chest pain (GRACE and TIMI risk scores). Using a handheld device, a computer, or a scorecard, risk status can be calculated in less that a minute (risk calculator downloadable from http://www.outcomes.org/grace or http://www.timi.org/files/riskscore/ua_calculator.htm, Fig. 16.13.5.2). International comparisons have demonstrated superior predictive accuracy for

the GRACE score and the European Society of Cardiology 2007 Guidelines for non-ST-elevation ACS recommend this score. The European Society of Cardiology Guidelines also recommend that risk status be re-evaluated, especially if clinical or biochemical features change.

Troponin (cTnT or cTnI) measurement should be performed at presentation (on the basis that those with elevated markers of necrosis on arrival are at increased risk) and repeated after 6 to 12 h if the initial test is negative. Echocardiography may be required to demonstrate the presence or absence of contractile dysfunction or to rule out alternative diagnoses.

Markers of long-term risk include the following:

◆ Increased age, heart rate, blood pressure, or Killip class

◆ Previously documented coronary disease, MI, or diabetes

◆ ST-segment depression, elevated troponin, or renal dysfunction

◆ Impaired left ventricular function, three-vessel or left main disease

◆ High risk score

An integrated approach to the patient with non-ST-elevation ACS

Patients with ACS may present to primary care physicians or directly to emergency hospital services. In addition, 15 to 20% of those presenting directly to chest pain clinics have ACS. Among patients presenting with an ACS, approximately 40% have evidence of prior coronary artery disease (e.g. MI, angiographically demonstrated disease, documented angina with a positive stress test).

The evaluation of patients with suspected ACS needs to be considered in a stepwise approach, proceeding from initial assessment and formulation of a working diagnosis (on the basis of clinical evaluation and the results of immediately available diagnostic tests) to confirmation of the diagnosis and stratification of the patients for emergency, urgent, and elective management.

Emergency Department–triage and establishing a working diagnosis

For the patient with chest pain, two issues must be resolved urgently. First, is the chest pain/discomfort thought to be of cardiac origin? This is a clinical judgement and requires prompt and skilled assessment. Secondly, in those with suspected cardiac pain, is there evidence of evolving infarction?

Patients with evolving infarction (ST-segment elevation or bundle branch block and clinical features of infarction) require emergency reperfusion with primary angioplasty, or if unavailable, thrombolysis (see below).

Patients without ST elevation or left bundle branch block can be triaged into low, intermediate, and high-risk categories (Fig. 16.13.5.6):

+ High-risk ACS—patients with typical clinical features of ischaemia and ST segment depression or transient ST segment elevation, or with troponin elevation and a high risk score. Patients are also at high risk when ischaemia provokes arrhythmias or haemodynamic compromise.

+ Intermediate or low-risk ACS—patients with clinical features of ACS and nonspecific ECG changes (e.g. T wave inversion, T wave flattening, minor conduction abnormalities).

+ Patients with a normal ECG, normal biomarkers, normal cardiac examination, and normal echo are potentially low-risk ACS or may have an alternative diagnosis.

Management of patients with non-ST-elevation and high-risk status

High-risk patients with acute ischaemia at initial presentation, and especially those with haemodynamic compromise, require

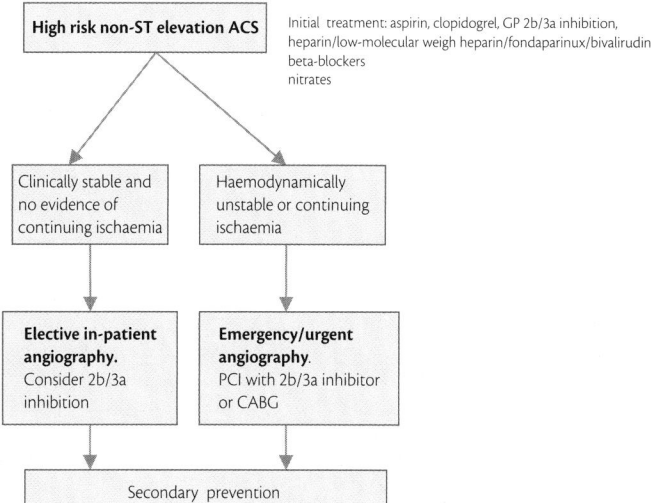

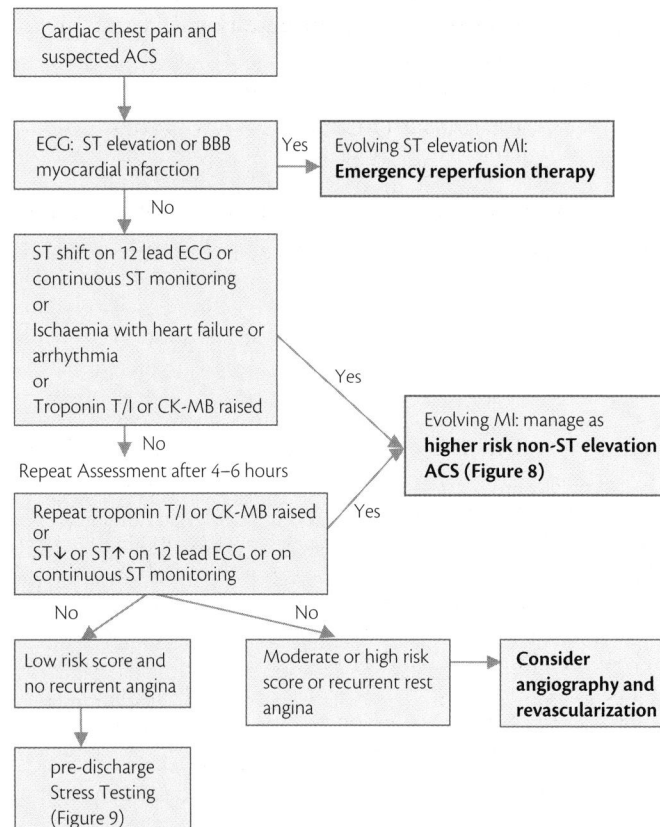

Fig. 16.13.5.6 Diagnostic triage for suspected acute coronary syndromes. Flow chart to illustrate the key diagnostic features for evolving MI, for higher-risk unstable angina and for low-risk patients.

Fig. 16.13.5.7 Flowchart to illustrate the key management steps for patients with non-ST-elevation acute coronary syndrome and high-risk status.

emergency assessment for revascularization (Fig. 16.13.5.7). Such patients potentially benefit from glycoprotein IIb/IIIa inhibition (Fig. 16.13.5.3). Trial evidence also supports an improved outcome with glycoprotein IIb/IIIa inhibition amongst the remainder of patients with troponin positivity or ST-segment depression. Those proceeding to emergency revascularization should receive (1) aspirin, (2) thienopyridine, e.g. clopidogrel, (3) glycoprotein IIb/IIIa inhibition, and (4) unfractionated heparin or LMWH, or bivalirudin. In addition, patients should receive anti-ischaemic therapy (see above) and some patients require antiarrhythmic management or haemodymamic support (e.g. intra-aortic balloon pump to reduce ischaemia and stabilize the patient for revascularization).

Management of patients with non-ST-elevation ACS at intermediate or low risk

Patients without high-risk features on initial presentation require further assessment to guide management (Fig. 16.13.5.8). Application of a risk score will reveal that a significant proportion have unsuspected higher risk (approximately one-third based on registry studies). Such patients require monitoring and repeat ECGs (ideally ST segment continuous analysis) and evaluation in a dedicated chest pain, cardiac, or combined assessment unit (while awaiting the results of biomarker and other investigations).

+ Patients who develop high-risk features after initial presentation should be considered for urgent angiography and re-vascularization (within 24–72 h). Such patients also fulfill guideline criteria for GPIIb/IIIa inhibitors (initiated prior to angiography) and anticoagulant and antiplatelet therapy (as above) and a revascularization strategy. Those developing ST elevation require emergency reperfusion (by primary percutaneous coronary intervention or—if PCI not available—by thrombolysis).

+ Patients with non-ST-elevation ACS and an intermediate risk score require dual antiplatelet therapy (aspirin plus thienopyridine, see above) plus anticoagulation (heparin, LMWH, fondaparinux or bivalirudin, see above). They are candidates for an early elective revascularization strategy (within approx 72 h).

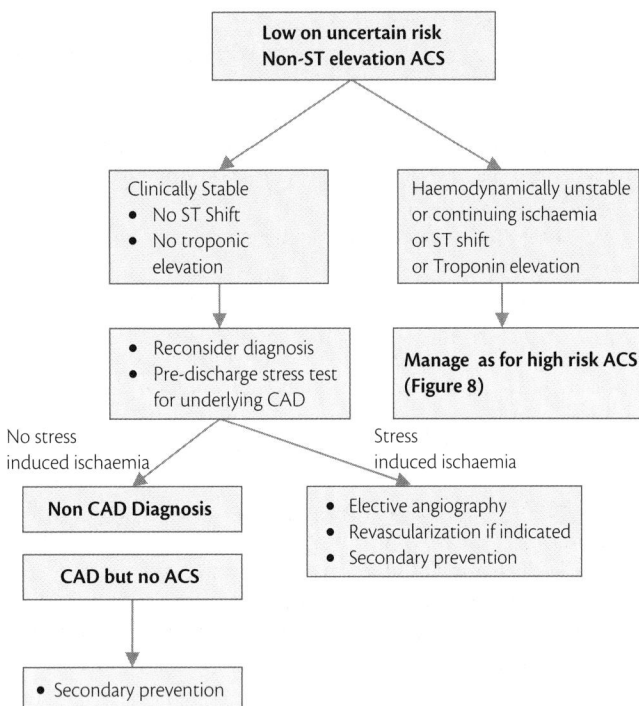

Fig. 16.13.5.8 Flowchart to illustrate the key management steps for patients with non-ST-elevation acute coronary syndrome and low or uncertain risk status.

◆ Clinically stable patients with minor or nonspecific ECG abnormalities and a low risk score (including negative repeat troponin) are at very low risk for in-hospital major cardiac events. Such patients may, nevertheless, have significant underlying coronary artery disease. They require stress testing or perfusion scanning, ideally prior to discharge.

Other considerations

Coronary artery bypass surgery

As demonstrated by the FRISC II study, those with three-vessel or left main coronary artery disease and an ACS can be stabilized in the acute phase with antiplatelet and anticoagulant therapy and can proceed to coronary artery bypass surgery with a low perioperative and postoperative morbidity and mortality in experienced centres (c.2%, 30-day mortality). Based on the findings of the CURE study, bleeding risk is minimized if the thienopyridine (clopidogrel) is stopped for 5 or more days prior to surgery. Patients at high risk for thrombotic events in the presurgery phase may require an intravenous small molecule GP IIb/IIIa inhibitor (to provide more potent but reversible platelet inhibition up until the time of surgery). See Chapter 13.7 for further discussion.

Secondary prevention

All patients with ACS require cardiovascular secondary prevention measures including lifestyle modification (smoking cessation, diet, exercise), oral pharmacological therapy (antiplatelet, cholesterol-lowering, ACE inhibitor/ARB) and the management of established and newly detected comorbidities (e.g. diabetes, hypertension, renal dysfunction, heart failure). These are the same in patients with non-ST-elevation ACS as they are for those with STEMI (see below for details).

ST segment elevation MI (STEMI)

Outcome in STEMI is critically determined by the extent and severity of myocardial ischaemia. In addition, the eventual extent of irreversibly injured myocardium is influenced by residual myocardial perfusion (via collaterals or subtotal coronary occlusion), the duration of myocardial ischaemia, and cytoprotective mechanisms including preconditioning. As a result, the clinical consequences of abrupt coronary occlusion can range from an entirely silent episode, to profound ischaemia with major cardiac rhythm disturbances (ventricular fibrillation or asystole), to acute mechanical decompensation with heart failure or cardiogenic shock. The outcome is influenced by the extent to which ischaemia is modified by prompt and effective reperfusion and the presence or absence of significant complications, especially arrhythmias (ventricular tachycardia, ventricular fibrillation, and asystole) and acute heart failure. Prompt and successful reperfusion, e.g. within the first hour of symptom onset, may 'abort' or greatly attenuate the eventual extent of MI. Importantly, prompt and effective resuscitation for early ventricular arrhythmias (especially ventricular fibrillation) may have a big impact on survival and freedom from cardiac complications.

The priorities in the management of STEMI are to manage acute life-threatening complications (resuscitation), relieve acute distress, limit the extent of infarction, and treat complications. Beyond the acute phase, attention focuses on secondary prevention and rehabilitation.

Outcome in STEMI

Historically, community-based studies in various populations demonstrated that the case fatality from acute MI, prior to the advent of resuscitation and reperfusion and other modern therapies, was approximately 50% by 1 month after the onset (MONICA studies). About one-half of those deaths were within the first 2 h of symptom onset. However, the risk of death, prior to hospitalization, varies with age: 80% of those above 85 years die before reaching hospital but only 40% of those below 55 years. Before the introduction of cardiac care units in the 1960s, in-patient mortality was in the range of 25 to 30%, and in the 1980s—before the introduction of reperfusion—inpatient mortality averaged about 18%. More recently, the MONICA study from five cities has indicated that the 28-day mortality for patients admitted to hospital with a MI ranged from 13 to 27%, and other studies have provided figures of 10 to 20%.

There is a marked discrepancy between mortality figures from randomized clinical trials and those from observational studies. Publications reporting the outcome for individuals ineligible for inclusion in trials have demonstrated substantially higher death rates than seen in those entered into contemporaneous trials in the same centres. Clinical trials can provide accurate information on what is possible in defined populations (often excluding patients with important comorbidity), and carefully conducted registries can provide an accurate reflection of 'real-world' clinical practice. Both approaches are required.

The multinational GRACE registry has demonstrated a decline in in-hospital mortality from 8.4 to 4.6% and new heart failure from 19.5 to 11.0% between 1999 and 2006. The more widespread application of evidence-based pharmacological and reperfusion therapy is closely linked with the improved outcome (with no change in the risk status of patients at presentation), highlighting the importance of 'closing the gap' between evidence from guidelines and clinical trials and application in clinical practice. International organizations including the American College of Cardiology and the European Society of Cardiology have stressed this. Special attention needs to be drawn to the more comprehensive provision of acute resuscitation and defibrillation in the community and to the provision of early effective reperfusion.

Prehospital care

The priorities in prehospital care are to establish a prompt diagnosis of suspected acute infarction, to provide effective resuscitation (especially for ventricular fibrillation), and to initiate prehospital thrombolysis if primary PCI is not available. In addition, patients require effective analgesia and the management of acute complications. Where available, telemetry of the ECG can confirm the diagnosis, expedite emergency transfer for primary PCI, and prepare the cardiac team for receiving the patient in the cardiac catheter laboratory. The aim is to provide reperfusion within 90 min of symptom onset. Although this has been demonstrated to be feasible in many centres and various countries, there are major logistic challenges. 'Door-to-balloon' times exclude the prehospital phase and, in many instances, 'door-to-balloon' times are longer than 90 min, just for this phase of treatment. In rural and other communities with prolonged transfer times to a hospital with PCI facilities, appropriate equipment and training needs to be established to allow prehospital thrombolysis to be administered safely and effectively.

Making a diagnosis of suspected infarction and initiating treatment

A working diagnosis of suspected infarction is based upon typical severe chest discomfort of more than 15 min duration which is unresponsive to glyceryl trinitrate. Characteristically, the pain may radiate to the neck, lower jaw, and arms, and is often accompanied by autonomic features including sweating and pallor. Unless complications are present, physical examination may reveal no significant abnormalities, other than those associated with autonomic disturbance, but signs can include tachycardia or bradycardia, the presence of a third or fourth heart sound, and features of heart failure (see Chapter 16.2.1).

The initial ECG is seldom normal, but may not show the classical features of ST segment elevation or evidence of Q waves (unless prior MI had occurred). Hyperacute T wave changes can be present within minutes of the onset of ischaemia due to coronary occlusion, and this may be followed by the evolution of characteristic ST segment elevation. However, minor or nonspecific ECG abnormalities in conjunction with a characteristic history may signal the early stages of infarction. The working diagnosis relies heavily on the clinical history, and when this suggests MI, repeat ECG within 30 to 60 min (or continuous ST analysis) will frequently reveal the evolution of recognizable ECG changes. It is critically important that infarction that evolves after initial presentation should be detected promptly.

In the prehospital setting, a paramedic or primary care physician may have to rely on the clinical findings to establish the working diagnosis and to initiate immediate treatment. Prompt relief of pain is important, not only for humanitarian reasons, but because pain is associated with sympathetic activation, vasoconstriction, and increased myocardial work. Effective analgesia is best achieved by the titration of intravenous opioids, although some paramedic

crews only have access to nonopioid analgesia. Side effects of analgesia include nausea and vomiting, hypotension, and respiratory depression. Antiemetics can be administered concurrently; hypotension and bradycardia will usually respond to atropine and respiratory depression to naloxone. Oxygen should be administered, especially to those who are breathless or those with any features of heart failure or shock (see Chapter 17.1 for information on basic and advanced life support in the management of cardiac arrest or ventricular fibrillation).

The logistics of providing acute care for patients with MI depend upon the locally available facilities. Guidelines recommend an integrated service involving prehospital emergency care (ambulance and paramedic personnel, primary care physicians, etc.) and hospital-based specialists, including cardiologists and emergency care physicians. Within an urban setting, with relatively short transfer times, the shortest delays and the most prompt initiation of reperfusion occurs when the patient seeks an emergency medical ambulance and achieves direct transfer to a hospital with available primary PCI facilities. Studies have shown that once the diagnosis is confirmed (e.g. by telemetry of the ECG) substantial time can be saved by direct transfer of the patient to the catheterization laboratory for PCI rather than transfer via an Emergency Department.

Prehospital thrombolysis

If a primary PCI programme is not available, or if transfer times are sufficiently prolonged that reperfusion may not be achieved within 90 min of patient call, then prehospital thrombolysis is the next best option. The combined analysis of primary PCI vs thrombolysis trials clearly shows superior outcome (deaths, recurrent MI, stroke, etc.) and less bleeding complications (especially intracerebral bleeds) for primary PCI. However, whether primary PCI—with the inherent transfer delays—is superior to very early thrombolysis (administered within the first hour of symptom onset) remains untested in trials of sufficient power.

To date, eight trials have been conducted comparing prehospital with in-hospital administration of thrombolytic therapy. Depending upon the clinical setting, between 30 and 130 min are saved by prehospital thrombolysis (fibrinolytic drug plus aspirin). Overall, for the complete study population of 6607 patients, the 30-day mortality was 10.7% for those receiving in-hospital administration of thrombolysis, and 9.1% for those where it was administered prior to hospital admission. This amounts to a 17% relative reduction in early mortality with a p value of 0.02 (1.6% absolute reduction). Complication rates were similar for community-treated and hospital-initiated thrombolysis, although ventricular fibrillation occurred more frequently with community administration and necessitated well-trained staff and the availability of defibrillators. The greatest benefit is seen when prehospital treatment is applied in remote settings where transport delays are more than 1 h. Several studies have indicated that about 20 patients with chest pain require evaluation for each patient found to be eligible for thrombolytic therapy in the community. Nevertheless, with appropriate training and facilities, prehospital care can provide a gain of approximately 20 lives per 1000 treated amongst eligible patients.

Prehospital cardiac arrest

The management of prehospital cardiac arrest requires special attention. At least as many lives can be saved by prompt resuscitation and defibrillation as by reperfusion. For these reasons, emergency assessment of the patient with suspected infarction necessitates that the clinician or paramedic has access to a defibrillator and the skills to manage cardiac arrest promptly and effectively. The provision of basic or advanced life-support training to paramedic ambulance crews, together with semiautomatic defibrillators, has resulted in a substantial increase in the number of patients surviving out-of-hospital cardiac arrest. Before the institution of such programmes, successful resuscitations were opportunistic and often relied on the availability of a bystander with medical or nursing training. Nationwide figures indicate that resuscitation now achieves survival in 7 to 10% of those patients found with cardiac arrest and in whom the initial rhythm is thought to be ventricular fibrillation. With effective integrated programmes, higher success rates have been achieved: for instance, in the south-eastern region of Scotland, about 14% survive to reach hospital alive, and in Seattle, with a well-established community training and resuscitation programme, the figure exceeds 20%. About one-half of those reaching hospital alive survive to be discharged home.

Emergency Department triage and management

Ideally, in those with typical clinical features and ST elevation on the ECG, a working diagnosis has been made in the prehospital setting (by paramedics with ECG telemetry or by a primary care physician) and early management initiated prior to hospital arrival. Where facilities are available, the patient should be transferred directly to the catheterization laboratory (with the team alerted while the patient is in transit), or if the decision is made for thrombolysis, then this is administered before arrival in hospital.

In-hospital evaluation is required in the remainder, where the symptoms are unclear, the ECG not diagnostic, or where significant comorbidity is present (e.g. bleeding risks). The priority immediately after arrival at the hospital is to identify those patients with ST elevation infarction for prompt reperfusion therapy (Fig. 16.13.5.9). Triage is usually performed in the Emergency Department, or, in some institutions, patients with a high probability of infarction gain direct access to a cardiac care assessment area. An integrated strategy involving the paramedic or ambulance system, the emergency physicians, and the cardiologists is required. 'Fast track' systems have been developed to minimize in-hospital

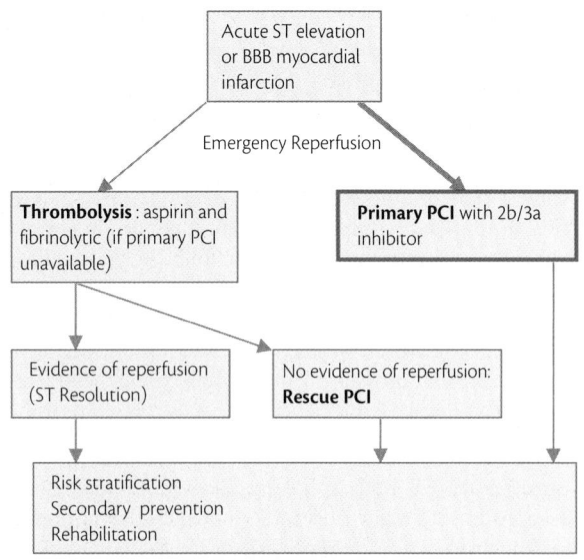

Fig. 16.13.5.9 Management of acute MI.

delay to reperfusion: these are facilitated by specifically trained medical and nursing staff, with the aim of ensuring clinical assessment and ECG within 15 min of arrival and rapid transfer for PCI or the institution of thrombolytic therapy within 30 min. Audit programmes and continuous training are necessary for centres to achieve this 30-min median 'door-to-needle' time.

Definite vs suspected infarction

Rapid triage systems allow the identification of patients with clearly defined clinical and ECG features of infarction, i.e. characteristic symptoms of infarction which persist at rest and are not relieved by glyceryl trinitrate, in the presence of at least 1-mm ST segment elevation in two or more contiguous leads, or the development of bundle branch block. Clinical trials have employed ECG criteria of a 1-mm ST elevation for limb leads and 2 mm for chest leads, a definition that improves specificity, but is associated with reduced sensitivity.

Amongst those without diagnostic ECG changes, a working diagnosis of suspected MI or non-ST-elevation ACS can be established. Such patients require repeat clinical and ECG assessments or continuous ST analysis to detect those with evolving infarction and separate them from those with unstable angina or non-ST-elevation infarction.

The rationale for minimizing delays to reperfusion

Experimental and clinical data demonstrate that the duration of ischaemia prior to reperfusion is a critical determinant of the eventual extent of myocardial damage. These data are supported by the improved outcome seen with prehospital vs in-hospital thrombolysis, also observational data from large clinical trials in which survival gain diminishes with each additional hour of ischaemia. The Fibrinolytic Trials Overview suggests about 1.6 additional deaths per hour of delay per 1000 treated, and a more recent meta-analysis suggests that early time delay is especially important.

The relationship between the duration of ischaemia and the extent of infarction is nonlinear: the greatest potential for salvage occurs when reperfusion is initiated within 60 min of the onset of infarction. Under such circumstances, a proportion of patients (5–7%) will have the infarction aborted and will not develop Q waves or significant enzyme elevation despite characteristic ST elevation on the initial ECG. Minimizing the time delay is, therefore, critical in salvaging myocardium. Based on data from individual trials, and from the Fibrinolytic Trials Overview, most benefit occurs within the first 3 h of the onset of infarction, and highly significant benefits still occur at up to 6 h. Statistically significant gains are still present at 12 h, but beyond 12 h the benefits are marginal. However, some patients present with a stuttering pattern and in the presence of persistent or intermittent ST segment elevation and continuing symptoms of ischaemia, reperfusion beyond 12 h may salvage significant ischaemic myocardium.

Differential diagnosis

Critically, thrombolytic therapy or angiography for anticipated primary angioplasty will be of no benefit to those who do not have MI and may convey significant hazards. Such patients suffer the dual hazards of thrombolysis or angiography in the acute phase of their illness and the delay in initiating appropriate treatment. Furthermore, those treated inappropriately with thrombolysis will experience the bleeding hazards of the drug (a net increase in intracerebral haemorrhage of c.0.5%) and the disrupted coagulation system will render other emergency surgery (e.g. for perforated peptic ulceration) more hazardous. Alternative cardiac diagnoses include non-ST-segment-elevation ACS, myocarditis, pericarditis, and aortic dissection. Noncardiac diagnoses include gastrointestinal pain of oesophageal, peptic, or biliary origin; pancreatitis; pulmonary embolism; and respiratory and musculoskeletal disorders.

Aortic dissection presents a particular problem when it extends proximally to the origin of the right coronary artery and produces inferior infarction. CT, MRI, or transoesophageal echocardiography may be required to establish the diagnosis (see Chapter 16.14.1).

Transthoracic echocardiography can be valuable when infarction is suspected, but characteristic ECG features are absent: normal left ventricular function excludes significant infarction, and conversely a regional contraction abnormality helps to confirm the diagnosis of ischaemia or possible infarction. However, in those with prior myocardial damage, the differentiation of new from old mechanical dysfunction is complex and requires specialist assistance.

Cardiac enzymes are helpful when abnormal, but most patients present within 3 h of the onset of symptoms and insufficient time has elapsed to produce a diagnostic release of biomarkers of necrosis (troponins, creatine kinase (CK), or CK-MB). Patients with suspected infarction but normal ECGs require further clinical ECG and biomarker estimations 4 to 6 h after the suspected event.

Among elderly and very elderly patients (>90 years of age), the presentation of infarction is often atypical. They may not experience a typical pattern of symptoms and concomitant multisystem disorders may obscure the diagnosis. MI must be considered in the differential diagnosis of abrupt collapse, haemodynamic disturbance of sudden onset, or severe nonspecific symptoms in elderly patients.

Continuing management in the Cardiac Department

Administration of analgesia, management of rhythm and haemodynamic compromise, and initiation of antithrombotic therapy (heparin, LMWH, aspirin, clopidogrel, GPIIb/IIIa inhibitors, etc.) should have been initiated shortly after the diagnosis of ST-elevation MI is made (in the Emergency Department or Cardiac Assessment Area or prehospital). The first priority is for emergency reperfusion (primary PCI, or if unavailable thrombolysis). Patients may require management of heart failure and arrhythmias and pain relief while in transit to reperfusion therapy, but every effort should be made to avoid delays to reperfusion.

Percutaneous coronary intervention
Primary PCI

Primary angioplasty is defined as PCI without concomitant fibrinolytic therapy. It requires prompt availability of a highly skilled interventional cardiology team with substantial experience of the procedure.

Randomized clinical trials of primary PCI vs thrombolysis have shown consistent findings: primary PCI has superior outcomes. In experienced centres it is more effective in restoring patency, achieves better ventricular function, and improves important clinical outcomes, with lower rates of death, reinfarction, stroke, major bleeding, and recurrent ischaemia (Table 16.13.5.4). Particular gains are seen in haemodynamically compromised patients and those with cardiogenic shock. In consequence, primary PCI is the preferred therapeutic option in national and international guidelines (SIGN, European Society of Cardiology PCI Guidelines, American College of Cardiology, and American Heart Association).

Table 16.13.5.4 Advantages of primary percutaneous coronary intervention over thrombolysis

Clinical indices	Event rate (%)		Absolute risk (%)	Relative risk (%)	NNT
	Thrombolysis	PCI			
Short-term mortality (4–6 weeks)	8	5	3	36	33
Long-term mortality (6–18 months)	8	5	3	38	33
Stroke	2	<1	2	64	50
Re-infarction	8	3	5	59	20
Recurrent ischaemia	18	7	11	59	9
Death or nonfatal reinfarction	12	7	5	44	20
Need for CABG	13	8	5	36	20

Data from Hartwell D et al. Clinical Effectiveness and Cost-Effectiveness of Immediate Angioplasty for Acute Myocardial Infarction: Systematic Review and Economic Evaluation. Health Technology Assess 2005; 9(17).

Patients are transferred as an emergency to the cardiac catheterization laboratory and angiography undertaken (radial artery or femoral artery access) to establish coronary anatomy and the nature of the vessel occlusion. A flexible guide wire is then passed across the occluded lesion and balloon angioplasty (usually accompanied by stent implantation) performed ('primary PCI'), thereby restoring patency to the previously occluded coronary artery.

Adjunctive GPIIb/IIIa inhibitors are indicated for primary PCI. Meta-analysis of 11 trials and 27 115 patients has demonstrated reduced short-term (30 day) and long-term (6–12 months) mortality (absolute relative risk, 1 and 1.8% respectively; relative relative risk 29%), as well as a reduction in 30-day reinfarction (absolute relative risk 0.9%) with the use of abciximab in primary PCI.

- Primary percutaneous coronary angioplasty (PCI) is the treatment of choice in patients with STEMI.

- Primary PCI requires a highly experienced interventional team with 24-h availability and an integrated approach to management to achieve reperfusion with the minimum of delay—ideally within 90 min of symptom onset.

- GP IIb/IIIa inhibitors are indicated for patients receiving primary PCI.

- Where primary PCI is unavailable, the patient should undergo prompt thrombolytic therapy, provided no contraindications are present.

- The limit in treating all potentially eligible patients with reperfusion therapy has not been reached. Internationally, at least one-third of all MIs (without a major bleeding risk) receive neither thrombolysis nor primary PCI.

Rescue PCI

Thrombolytic therapy may fail to achieve effective reperfusion in 30% or more of those in whom it is administered for STEMI. Patients experience continuing symptoms of ischaemia and failure of resolution of ST elevation on the ECG (<50% resolution of the ST elevation within 1 h of administration). Rescue PCI is more effective than repeat thrombolysis or conservative treatment in improving outcome (REACT trial). Thus, in centres where primary PCI is not available, logistics need to be established for prompt transfer for rescue percutaneous coronary intervention of patients in whom thrombolysis does not result in signs of reperfusion.

Facilitated PCI

The combination of full-dose or reduced-dose fibrinolysis followed by emergency PCI has been tested in large-scale trials and shown worse outcomes and greater bleeding risks (ASSENT 4 Trial). Hence, planned emergency PCI after thrombolysis is not recommended. although later PCI—after the impact of thrombolysis has resolved—may be of benefit (GRACIA 2 Study). The latter approach should be considered as part of the strategy to deal with residual stenoses after PCI (prior to hospital discharge), rather than as 'facilitated' PCI.

Thrombolytic treatment

Thrombolytic treatment refers to the combination of antiplatelet therapy (aspirin and clopidogrel) with fibrinolytic treatment. The fibrinolytic agent, directly or indirectly, converts plasminogen to plasmin and plasmin lyses fibrin in the clot. Cross-linked fibrin is more resistant to fibrinolytic drugs than a newly formed fibrin clot.

The combination of aspirin and a fibrinolytic agent has undergone extensive clinical testing in trials involving more than 100 000 patients. Additional trials have been conducted comparing one fibrinolytic agent with another. For patients presenting within 6 h of symptom onset, and with ST elevation or bundle branch block, approximately 30 deaths are prevented per 1000 patients treated. For those presenting between 7 and 12 h, approximately 20 deaths are prevented per 1000 patients treated, and beyond 12 h the benefits are inconclusive. Thrombolysis is a very cost-effective treatment for acute MI. A sustained benefit on survival has been demonstrated 14 years after thrombolysis.

The ISIS-2 trial demonstrated that the benefits of aspirin treatment were additional to those of fibrinolytic treatment, each achieving about 25 lives saved per 1000 patients treated (for the whole of the study population). Thus, in combination, about 50 lives are saved per 1000 patients treated, but the benefits are larger than this among those presenting within 3 h of infarction with ST segment elevation or bundle branch block.

Overall, the largest absolute benefit is seen in patients at highest risk, although the proportional benefit may be similar for all. High-risk patients include those over 65 years of age, those with a systolic blood pressure below 100 mmHg, and those with anterior infarction or more extensive ischaemia (see primary angioplasty below). The absolute benefit in lives saved per 1000 treated is 11 ± 3 for those under 55 years of age; 18 ± 4 for those between 55 and 64; 27 ± 5 for those 65 to 74; and 10 ± 13 for those over 75. However, for ST depression there is a net hazard of 14 lives lost per 1000 treated, and for those with a normal ECG 7 lives lost per 1000 treated (Fibrinolytic Trials Overview). Thus, evidence supports thrombolysis treatment only for those patients with ST elevation or bundle branch block.

Hazards of thrombolysis

Thrombolytic therapy is associated with a significant excess of haemorrhagic complications, including cerebral haemorrhage. Overall, about 2 nonfatal strokes occur per 1000 patients treated, and of these half are moderately or severely disabling. An additional 2 strokes per 1000 patients are fatal, and the net impact on mortality includes such patients. The risk of stroke increases with age, especially for those over 75 years of age, and for those with systolic hypertension. There is also an excess of noncerebral bleeds of about 7 per 1000 treated. Bleeding occurs at arterial and venous puncture sites, hence blood sampling or cannulation of vessels should be limited to sites where external compression can achieve haemostasis.

Streptokinase and other streptokinase-containing agents can produce hypotension and, rarely, allergic reactions. Routine administration of hydrocortisone is not indicated. When hypotension occurs, it can be managed by interrupting the streptokinase infusion, lying the patient flat or head down, and by the administration of atropine or intravascular volume expansion.

Comparison of thrombolytic agents

The most widely used thrombolytic agents are streptokinase, alteplase (tissue plasminogen activator, tPA), tenecteplase (TNK), and reteplase (rPA). The GISSI International Trial and ISIS-3 international trial both failed to find a difference in outcome between streptokinase and tPA. However, the GUSTO trial (Global Utilization of Streptokinase and Tissue plasminogen active for Occluded coronary arteries) employed an accelerated administration of alteplase over 90 min and intravenous heparin adjusted using the activated partial thromboplastin time, finding 10 fewer deaths per 1000 patients treated with alteplase compared with the streptokinase group. Meta-analysis confirms the superiority of clot-specific agents (e.g. alteplase, tenecteplase) over streptokinase.

The current reference standard for the comparison of fibrinolytic agents is the accelerated infusion regimen of alteplase (tPA), or for simplicity the single-bolus administration of tenecteplase (TNK). Tenecteplase does not require an infusion pump nor refrigeration and hence is particularly suited for prehospital administration, but internationally streptokinase remains the most widely used fibrinolytic agent, principally because it is relatively inexpensive.

Which combinations of treatments are effective?
Combination of fibrinolytic therapy or primary PCI with glycoprotein IIb/IIIa inhibitors

Despite the benefits in STEMI of antiplatelet therapy with aspirin, and with aspirin plus clopidogrel, large-scale randomized trials (ASSENT-3 and GUSTO V) have not shown significant overall benefit from use of GPIIb/IIIa inhibitors in combination with fibrinolysis in this condition. By contrast, there is evidence to support the use of GPIIb/IIIa inhibitors with primary PCI.

Combination of fibrinolytic therapy or primary PCI with clopidogrel

Clopidogrel is indicated for primary and elective PCI after MI in order to reduce thrombotic risks. Guidelines suggest that higher loading doses of clopidogrel can be used to minimize delays to effective antiplatelet therapy (e.g. 600-mg loading dose). This approach does not appear to increase bleeding risks, but large-scale trials of higher loading (600 mg vs 300 mg clopidogrel) and higher initial maintenance doses (150 mg vs 75 mg) are being tested (CURRENT trial). Whether newer thienopyridines (e.g. prasugrel) will have advantages over clopidogrel in PCI is uncertain: at the time of writing, this is being tested in ACS patients undergoing PCI (TRITON trial).

In patients treated with thrombolysis, there is clear evidence that the addition of clopidogrel provides further benefit, although with significant increases in bleeding risk. This has been tested in a trial of coronary patency (CLARITY) and in a very large-outcome trial (COMMIT). Thus, there is clear evidence—at least for about 1 month of treatment—for improved outcomes by adding clopidogrel to fibrinolytic therapy plus aspirin.

Combination of fibrinolytic therapy with unfractionated or LMWH or fondaparinux

The combination of LMWH with fibrinolytic therapy for STEMI was tested in a very large double-blind randomized trial ($n = 20\,506$ patients) of enoxaparin vs unfractionated heparin. Death or recurrent MI occurred in 12% of patients with unfractionated heparin and 9.9% with enoxaparin, with the major benefit being reduced reinfarction. There was an increase in major bleeding (2.1% vs 1.4%), but not in intracranial bleeding. Hence enoxaparin has clear advantages, including subcutaneous administration without laboratory monitoring, over unfractionated heparin in ST-elevation myocardial intervention.

Fondaparinux (a factor Xa inhibitor) has been tested against placebo in patients with STEMI in whom the investigator had not planned to give a form of heparin (e.g. streptokinase administration or no fibrinolysis). There was clear advantage for the fondaparinux (OASIS 6 trial), with no increase in bleeding but improved survival and improved reinfarction. Thus, in these groups of patients fondaparinux has clear benefits and no disadvantages. In a second stratum of the same study, fondaparinux was tested against heparin/LMWH (in these patients, the investigator had planned to give a form of heparin). Similar efficacy and lower bleeding was seen with fondaparinux. The only limitations were in patients proceeding to primary or other PCI, where fondaparinux was associated with an increase in the rate of catheter-related thrombotic events. However, it appears that these events may be avoided by supplementary unfractionated heparin (exact amount to be defined). Thus fondaparinux may offer an attractive anticoagulant option, especially in patients without a planned PCI.

Coronary artery bypass surgery (CABG)

In the acute phase of MI, the role of CABG is limited to those patients with acute mechanical complications, such as ventricular septal defect or mitral regurgitation due to papillary muscle rupture. Unless such mechanical complications are present, the hazards of acute bypass surgery are significantly increased compared to delayed revascularization in a stabilized patient. The Danish DANAMI study investigated the role of revascularization in those with ischaemia during the recovery phase of MI. It suggested that, following infarction, individuals with symptomatic or electrocardiographic ischaemia on stress testing experience significant long-term benefit from surgical revascularization.

Further in-hospital management

The period of hospitalization for reperfused and uncomplicated patients following STEMI has progressively shortened, and is now in the range of 3 to 5 days. Thus there are time pressures to initiate lifestyle modifications, drug therapy for secondary prevention, and rehabilitation measures. It is essential to initiate these management steps before hospital discharge to minimize the risk that they are not carried out afterwards.

The main aims of further in-hospital management are the identification and treatment of acute complications of infarction, identification of patients at increased risk for subsequent cardiac events, and initiation of secondary prevention and rehabilitation.

Major complications may be apparent at the time of presentation and haemodynamic, arrhythmic, or ischaemic complications may be evident shortly thereafter. Nevertheless, in the period beyond the first 12 to 24 h, it is appropriate to focus attention on the points listed above.

Identification and treatment of complications of infarction
Failure of reperfusion

Electrocardiographic markers of failed thrombolysis reperfusion are the persistence of ST segment elevation together with clinical and haemodynamic features of continuing ischaemia. Continuous computed ST analysis allows the most accurate definition of ECG changes, but an approximation can be obtained with repeated 12-lead ECGs and measurement of ST segment elevation. In those with successful reperfusion, ST segments decrease to less than 50% of peak elevation within 60 min.

In addition, some patients exhibit reperfusion arrhythmias (ventricular tachycardia, idioventricular rhythm, and—rarely—ventricular fibrillation). Such arrhythmias are more common in the presence of marked ischaemia and prompt reperfusion within 60 to 90 min of occlusion.

Rescue angioplasty is the appropriate management for failed reperfusion, and consists of mechanical recanalization of the occluded vessel with percutaneous intervention, including stent implantation. This strategy achieves an 'open artery', and randomized trial data (REACT Trial) shows superior outcome compared with repeat thrombolysis or conservative management.

Cardiogenic shock

In cardiogenic shock, mechanical contractile abnormalities of the left ventricle or acute haemodynamic complications (papillary muscle rupture or ventricular septal defect) lead to reduced blood pressure and impaired tissue perfusion. Clinically, the condition is recognized by a systolic blood pressure of less 90 mmHg together with impaired tissue flow, as reflected by oliguria, impaired cerebral function, and peripheral vasoconstriction. Between 5 and 20% of those patients admitted to hospital with acute MI demonstrate cardiogenic shock, although the frequency has been reduced by thrombolytic therapy and primary PCI. The mortality rate when cardiogenic shock complicates an acute coronary event is in excess of 70%, if acute revascularization is not possible.

Time delay is critically important in the management of cardiogenic shock: mortality rises progressively if more than 2 h have elapsed since its onset. Treatment aims to improve the recovery of acutely ischaemic myocardium (mechanical and surgical revascularization) and to support the circulation with a combination of inotropes, vasodilators, and loop diuretics. Evidence suggests that the most important treatment may be to reopen the infarct-related artery. In addition, the SHOCK trial has demonstrated that aggressive treatment with intra-aortic balloon pumping (IABP) followed by surgical revascularization may also significantly reduce mortality.

In addition to achieving reperfusion, management of the patient with cardiogenic shock after MI may require inotropic support in addition to intra-aortic baloon pumping. Dopamine is commonly used, initially at a low 'renal dose' (1–5 µg/kg per min) that activates dopaminergic receptors (but also has an effect on the circulation), but if necessary at higher doses of 5 to 20 µg/kg per min that have positive inotropic and chronotropic effects. In doses above 20 µg/kg per min, these activate α-adrenoceptors with undesirable peripheral vasoconstriction and a decline in renal perfusion.

Dobutamine acts mainly as a β_1-adrenoceptor agonist and is used in the range of 2 to 40 µg/kg per min. Phosphodiesterase inhibitors have both inotropic and vasodilator effects and, although they have produced favourable haemodynamic responses, the studies conducted have not shown an improvement in outcome.

The management of pulmonary oedema consists of opiates (to relieve distress and to reduce vascular resistance), oxygen, vasodilators, and diuretics. If it is severe, patients may require positive end-expiratory ventilation or even full mechanical ventilation. Vasodilators (including nitrates, salbutamol, and sodium nitroprusside) reduce venous and pulmonary arterial pressure, but tachycardia may be a limiting feature and their use is limited in those who are profoundly hypotensive. Loop diuretics are employed in bolus intravenous doses or by infusion.

In all instances, decisions to proceed to mechanical external support of the circulation or mechanical ventilation need to take account of the extent to which the cardiac dysfunction may be reversible, the presence of comorbidity, and the wishes of the patient and their family.

Left ventricular dysfunction and heart failure
Large-scale trials of angiotensin-converting enzyme (ACE) inhibitors and angiotensin receptor blockers (ARB) have been conducted in patients with left ventricular dysfunction and those with clinical and radiological features of heart failure (see Chapter 16.5). Clear evidence demonstrates improved short- and long-term outcome with ACE inhibitors/ARBs in patients with heart failure and those with asymptomatic left ventricular dysfunction.

Caution must be exercised with the introduction of ACE inhibitors in patients with intravascular volume depletion, when they can cause hypotension, and in patients with low arterial pressure or renal impairment. ACE inhibition should commence with a very small dose (e.g. 6.25 mg of captopril), with dosages increased progressively in conjunction with clinical monitoring. They can provoke deterioration in renal function in patients with renal artery stenosis and in those with significant pre-existing renal impairment, hence it is important to check serum electrolytes and creatinine during early treatment and follow-up.

Arrhythmias
A wide variety of arrhythmias can be seen in the context of acute MI and its treatment. The most serious, including ventricular fibrillation, ventricular tachycardia, and heart block, can lead to cardiac arrest. However, routine administration of antiarrhythmic agents is not indicated. They are almost invariably negatively inotropic, and they may also be pro-arrhythmic in the context of acute coronary ischaemia. An overview of randomized trials into the use of prophylactic lignocaine (lidocaine) showed that it increased mortality. Ventricular fibrillation should be treated with direct current (DC) cardioversion, and recurrent ventricular arrhythmias require antiarrhythmics (e.g. amiodarone). Importantly, attention should be paid to electrolyte imbalance and the correction of reversible ischaemia or other factors provoking arrhythmias. (see Chapter 16.4 for details of the diagnosis and treatment of arrhythmias).

Heart block of any degree can occur after acute MI. It is more common with inferior than anterior infarction because the right coronary artery supplies the atrioventricular node, and also because vagal reflexes are more likely from this area. It is often transient, and does not necessarily imply a large infarct, except when it occurs with anterior infarction, in which case the prognosis is grave.

Temporary transvenous pacing is justified when bradycardia compromises the circulation, but is not advocated 'prophylactically'.

Ventricular septal defect, papillary muscle rupture, and myocardial rupture
Rupture of the interventricular septum occurs in up to 3% of acute infarctions and is responsible for about 5% of deaths due to MI. Rupture in the apical area may complicate anterior infarction and in the basal inferior area may complicate inferior infarction. Clinically, the condition is associated with the development of a new pansystolic murmur and clinical features of a left-to-right shunt with increased pulmonary congestion. The findings are confirmed on echocardiography or cardiac catheterization. Surgery should be undertaken as soon as possible: the outlook for those who are not operated upon is very bleak, with few surviving. However, some patients with small shunts survive the acute phase, in which case they may suffer the later consequences of the shunt.

Papillary muscle rupture occurs as a result of acute ischaemic damage due to obstruction of either the left anterior descending or circumflex coronary arteries. It causes the abrupt onset of severe mitral regurgitation and accounts for 5% of deaths after acute MI. The complication generally occurs within the first week after infarction, and may be recognized as the abrupt onset of acute pulmonary oedema. It is often accompanied by a new systolic murmur, but when the left atrial pressure rises acutely the murmur may be insignificant. The findings are confirmed with echocardiography. The management is acute surgical repair with or without revascularization.

In the patient who deteriorates haemodynamically after MI—with hypotension, pulmonary oedema, or both—it is important to consider the possibility of a ventricular septal defect or acute mitral regurgitation. However, it can be impossible to distinguish between the two on clinical grounds. Both classically produce a new pansystolic murmur, and although differences between the murmurs have been described, these are not robust enough to discriminate with certainty in the individual case. Acute mitral regurgitation is best diagnosed by echocardiography, but transthoracic echocardiography may be unable to detect a ventricular septal defect in a reliable manner. Transoesophageal echocardiography is better, as is the use of a contrast-enhanced technique. If this is unavailable, an alternative approach is to pass a flow-directed pulmonary catheter and take blood samples from the pulmonary artery, right ventricle, and right atrium. A step-up in oxygen tension between the right atrium and the pulmonary artery indicates the presence of a left-to-right shunt and confirms the diagnosis of a ventricular septal defect.

Myocardial rupture may follow acute infarction, usually involving the free wall of the left ventricle. It is responsible for approximately 10% of all deaths in acute MI. Half of the ruptures occur within the first week, and 90% within 2 weeks. The location of rupture is usually within the infarcted area, but may be at the junction with adjacent normal myocardium. In most cases, death is immediate and due to electromechanical dissociation. The patient is unresponsive to resuscitation measures but, rarely—with subacute rupture—patients can be supported until surgical repair is performed. The diagnosis is made on clinical and echocardiographic criteria with assessment for possible cardiac tamponade (see Chapter 16.8). In some patients, partial rupture of the free wall can result in the late development of a false aneurysm.

Left ventricular thrombus

A left ventricular thrombus can be detected using echocardiography in up to 40% of patients with acute anterior MI. The thrombus is usually located at the apex in association with a dyskinetic or aneurysmal section of myocardium with impaired contractile function. The thrombus may be large, and is associated with risks of embolization (in 15–20% of cases). Anticoagulation with heparin followed by warfarin is advised in patients with extensive infarction and those in whom apical aneurysms or mural thrombi are detected. Both, thrombolysis and surgical repair, have been successfully conducted. However, there is no clear evidence that either strategy is superior (provided there is no evidence of embolization).

Pericarditis

Pericarditis may complicate an extensive MI, and may be manifest clinically as a pericardial friction rub accompanied by pleuritic chest pain. A small pericardial effusion may be detected using echocardiography. Dressler's syndrome is a rare late complication and is associated with pericarditis between 2 weeks and 3 months after acute infarction. It has an autoimmune basis, often accompanied by pleural and pericardial effusions. It is managed with salicylates or nonsteroidal anti-inflammatory agents. The frequency of both pericarditis and Dressler's syndrome is reduced with acute reperfusion.

An integrated approach to the management of STEMI

Pre-hospital management

In a patient with suspected acute infarction, the priorities are to establish whether typical clinical features and ST elevation (or left bundle branch block) are present, and if so to initiate reperfusion with the absolute minimum of delay. Where possible, the diagnosis is confirmed and the transfer of the patient arranged by telemetry of the ECG. The phrase 'time is muscle' has been coined for acute STEMI. Acute resuscitation may be required for cardiac arrest or major arrhythmic complications, especially ventricular fibrillation. Additional priorities are to provide analgesia and oxygen. Prehospital thrombolysis may be given by appropriately trained paramedic crews, when transfer times to a PCI hospital are such that more than 90 min will lapse from diagnosis to PCI.

In-hospital management

Initial triage and management

Initial assessment involves the identification of those with clear-cut evidence of STEMI (based on clinical and diagnostic ECG criteria). Such patients require immediate triage to reperfusion therapy (primary PCI, or if unavailable thrombolysis with a fibrinolytic agent plus an antiplatelet agents). In transit to primary PCI or while preparing pharmacological reperfusion, patients may require further analgesia and management of arrhythmic and haemodynamic complications, including heart failure.

Patients in whom the diagnosis of MI is suspected, but the ECG criteria are not diagnostic, should be managed in an intensive care setting (in the Emergency Department or Cardiac Care Unit with repeat ECG evaluation at 30-min intervals (or ST segment analysis). Cardiac biomarkers (troponins) may be elevated at presentation, if sufficient time has lapsed from onset of ischaemia (4–6 h), or they may become elevated following arrival (repeat measurement at 8–12 h). Such patients may be divided into those with evidence of non-STEMI (ECG and troponin elevation) and those with unstable angina (T wave inversion, ST segment depression, or transient ST segment elevation, without elevated cardiac troponins). Among those with minor or nonspecific ECG changes and no enzyme elevation, re-evaluation should take place for alternative diagnoses, and stress testing performed subsequently to detect underlying coronary artery disease (Fig. 16.13.5.9). A key component of initial evaluation of those without ST elevation or left bundle branch block involves risk stratification (see above). Echocardiography may be valuable to detect signs of ischaemia/infarction or to demonstrate normal contractile function in those with an alternative diagnosis.

Later in-hospital management

During this phase the management of complications, initiation of secondary prevention, and early cardiac rehabilitation should take place. In high-risk patients (those with recurrent acute ischaemia or those with failure of ST segment resolution and continuing pain), emergency PCI or surgical revascularization can be performed in appropriately equipped centres (Fig. 16.13.5.9).

Regular clinical and electrocardiographic assessments are required during the recovery phase to detect acute mechanical and arrhythmic complications, and to identify impaired contractile function in patients who will benefit from ACE inhibitor/ARB treatment. This treatment is indicated in those with overt heart failure in the acute phase and also indicated for secondary prevention in patients with established vascular disease (HOPE trial). Thus, ACE inhibitors or ARBs are indicated for those with vascular disease, irrespective of whether there is evidence of overt heart failure or impaired left ventricular function in acute phase. Patients also require lipid-lowering therapy: robust evidence demonstrates that all patients with MI or non-ST-elevation ACS will benefit (MRC/BHF Heart Protection Study). There is evidence to support management of diabetes with glucose and insulin during the in-hospital and early posthospital phase.

All patients will benefit from smoking cessation, the management of hypertension (systolic pressure to less than 140 mmHg), and dietary and lifestyle modification (including exercise) (SIGN Guideline 2007). After STEMI, patients benefit from participation in a rehabilitation programme, with improved quality of life, symptom relief, and return to an active lifestyle or occupation.

Secondary prevention measures in those with STEMI or non-STEMI ACS

Following an ACS, patients require dietary and lifestyle advice including the support necessary to discontinue smoking (including nicotine replacement therapy) (SIGN Guideline 2007). Lipids should be measured within the first 24 h of admission, with evidence supporting the use of lipid-lowering therapy. Individuals with documented coronary artery disease, and especially those with left ventricular contractile dysfunction or heart failure, have reduced long-term risks of death and MI if maintained on an ACE inhibitor or ARB. In addition, patients may require antianginal therapy if revascriztion is incomplete and all should receive long-term, low-dose aspirin. Clopidogrel should be given for at least 1 month in STEMI (the limits of the evidence) and a year for non-ST-elevation ACS (or as determined by the type of stents implanted).

Nonpharmacological interventions

Evidence supports the following nonpharmacological interventions in secondary prevention: cessation of smoking (including the avoidance of passive smoking); dietary modification; exercise; rehabilitation; and management of obesity.

Pharmacological interventions

Trial evidence supports therapeutic interventions to modify the following conditions: hyperlipidaemia; left ventricular dysfunction and heart failure; diabetes mellitus; and hypertension.

Reduction of cardiovascular risk

Evidence (summarized in Tables 16.13.5.5 and 16.13.5.6) supports the following therapies to reduce the risk of subsequent cardiovascular events: antiplatelet therapy (aspirin in a dose of 75 mg/day, clopidogrel 75 mg day); β-blockers in those without contraindications; lipid-lowering with 3-hydroxy-3-methylglutaryl coenzyme A (HMG CoA) reductase inhibitors (statins); ACE inhibitor or ARB

Table 16.13.5.5 Estimated benefits of long-term secondary prophylactic treatment/intervention after MI

Treatment/intervention		Problems prevented per 1000 patient-years of treatment
All post-MI patients (unless specific contraindications exist)		
Aspirin (meta-analysis)	7	vascular deaths
	9	nonfatal reinfarctions
	3	nonfatal strokes
Oral β-blocker	21	deaths
	21	re-infarctions
Statin (hyperlipidaemia, post-MI)	7	deaths
	11	re-vascularizations
	12	nonfatal MIs
	3	strokes
	4	congestive heart failure
	13	angina
Statin (average cholesterol, post-MI, CARE)	2	deaths
	9	re-vascularizations
	4	nonfatal MIs
	2	strokes
	4	unstable angina
Smoking cessation	15	deaths
(observational studies)	46	re-infarctions
Post-MI patients with LVD or heart failure (additional treatment unless specific contraindications exist)		
ACE inhibitor	12	deaths
(left ventricular ejection fraction ≤ 40%)	9	MIs
	10	congestive heart failure (requiring hospital admission)
ACE inhibitor (heart failure)	45	deaths
	26	congestive heart failure (severe)

LVD, left ventricular dysfunction.
Sivers F Evidence-based strategies for secondary prevention of coronary heart disease, 2nd edn. A&M Publishing, Guildford, Surrey. - now owned by Wiley.

Table 16.13.5.6 Comparison of the treatment benefits from interventions to prevent cardiovascular events

Problems/therapy	Events prevented	NNT*
Severe hypertension (DBP 115–129 mmHg)	Death or stroke or MI	3
Coronary artery bypass surgery for left main stem stenosis	Death	6
Aspirin for transient ischaemic attack	Death or stroke	6
Statin for hyperlipidaemia, post-MI/angina (4S)	Death or nonfatal MI or CABG/PTCA or cerebrovascular event	6
Warfarin for atrial fibrillation	Stroke	7
ACE inhibitor for LV dysfunction post-MI	CV death or hospitalization for CHF	10
Statin for average cholesterol post-MI (CARE trial) or stroke	Death or nonfatal MI or CABG/PTCA	11
Aspirin post-MI	CV death or stroke or MI	12
Statin for average/elevated cholesterol, post-MI/unstable angina (LIPID trial)	Death or nonfatal MI or CABG/PTCA or stroke	15
Beta-blocker post-MI	Death	20
ACE inhibitor for LV dysfunction	CV death or hospitalization for CHF	21
ACE inhibitor for vascular disease (HOPE)	Deaths	50
	MI	42
	Stroke	67
Statin for hypercholesterolaemia in primary prevention	Death or nonfatal MI or CABG/PTCA or stroke	26
Mild hypertension (DBP 90–109 mmHg)	Death or stroke or MI	141

ACE, angiotensin converting enzyme; CABG, coronary artery bypass grafting; CARE, Cholesterol and Recurrent Events Trial; CHF, congestive heart failure; CV, cardiovascular; DBP, diastolic blood pressure; HOPE, Heart Outcomes Prevention Evaluation Trial; LIPID, Long-term Intervention with Pravastatin in Ischaemic Disease Trial; LV, left ventricle; MI, myocardial infarction; NNT, estimated number of patients that need to be treated for 5 years to prevent one event; PTCA, percutaneous transluminal coronary angioplasty.
Sivers F Evidence-based strategies for secondary prevention of coronary heart disease, 2nd edn. A&M Publishing, Guildford, Surrey.

especially in those with left ventricular dysfunction and heart failure, and benefit is also possible in other patients with vascular disease (Table 16.13.5.6).

Anticoagulants

These are indicated in those with high risks of embolism due to left ventricular or atrial thrombus. There is evidence to support the use of anticoagulants in post-MI patients but no definitive evidence that such treatment is superior to aspirin therapy. Current trials are evaluating the role or oral antithrombins and oral anti-Xa inhibitors following ACS.

Hormone replacement therapy (HRT)

HRT is not indicated for risk reduction after ACS. When used to relieve menopausal symptoms, HRT is associated with a small, but increased, risk of thrombotic events.

Calcium channel blockers

An overview of data from 19 000 patients, based on all randomized trials of acute infarction and unstable angina, suggests that the available calcium channel blockers are unlikely to reduce the rate of subsequent infarct development, infarct size, or subsequent infarction. They may, however, have indications for the relief of angina (especially heart-rate-lowering calcium antagonists).

Antiarrhythmic agents

A review of the effects of antiarrhythmic agents (with the exception of β-blockers) does not demonstrate a beneficial impact on mortality. Many have significant proarrhythmic complications and negative inotropic effects.

Further reading

Antithrombotic Trialists Collaboration (2002). Collaborative meta-analysis of randomised trials of antiplatelet therapy for prevention of death, myocardial infarction, and stroke in high risk patients. *BMJ*, **324**, 71–86.

Antman EM, et al. (1996). Cardiac-specific troponin I levels to predict the risk of mortality in patients with acute coronary syndromes. *N Engl J Med*, **335**, 1342–9.

Antman EM, et al. (1999). Abciximab facilitates the rate and extent of thrombolysis: results of the thrombolysis in mycocardial infarction (TIMI) 14 trial. *Circulation*, **99**, 2720–32.

Antman EM, et al. (1999). Assessment of the treatment effect of enoxaparin for unstable angina/non-Q-wave myocardial infarction. TIMI IIB–ESSENCE meta-analysis. *Circulation*, **100**, 1602–8.

Antman EM, et al. (2006). Enoxaparin versus unfractionated heparin with fibrinolysis for ST elevation mycocardial infarction. *N Engl J Med*, **354**, 1477–88.

Armstrong PW, et al. (1998). Acute coronary syndromes in the GUSTO-IIb trial: prognostic insights and impact of recurrent ischemia. *Circulation*, **98**, 1860–8.

ASSENT-2 Investigators (1999). Single-bolus tenecteplase compared with front-loaded alteplase in acute myocardial infarction: the ASSENT-2 double-blind randomised trial. *Lancet*, **354**, 716–22.

ASSENT-3 Investigators (2001). Efficacy and safety of tenecteplase in combination with enoxaparin, abciximab, or unfractionated heparin: the ASSENT-3 randomised trial in acute mycocardial infarction. *Lancet*, **358**, 605–13.

Bassand J-P, et al. (2007). Guidelines for the diagnosis and treatment of non-ST-segment elevation acute coronary syndromes. *Eur Heart J*, **28**, 1598–660.

Bhatt DL, et al. (2004). Utilization of early invasive management strategies for high-risk patients with non-ST-segment elevation acute coronary syndromes: results from the CRUSADE Quality Improvement Initiative. *JAMA*, **292**, 2096–104.

Bhatt DL, et al. (2006). Clopidogrel and aspirin versus aspirin alone for the prevention of atherothrombotic events. *N Engl J Med*, **354**, 1706–17.

Bode C, et al. (1999). Randomised comparison of coronary thrombolysis achieved with double-bolus reteplase (recombinant plasminogen activator) and front-loaded, accelerated alteplase (recombinant tissue plasminogen activator) in patients with acute myocardial infarction. *Circulation*, **94**, 891–8.

Boden WE, et al. (1998). Outcomes in patients with acute non-Q-wave myocardial infarction randomly assigned to an invasive as compared with a conservative management strategy. Veterans Affairs Non-Q-Wave Infarction Strategies in Hospital (VANQWISH) Trial Investigators. *N Engl J Med*, **38**, 1785–92.

Boersma E, et al. (2002). Platelet glycoprotein IIb/IIIa inhibitors in acute coronary syndromes: a meta-analysis of all major randomized clinical trials. *Lancet*, **359**, 189–98.

Boersma E (2006). Does time matter? A pooled analysis of randomized clinical trials comparing primary percutaneous coronary intervention and inhospital fibrinolysis in acute mycocardial infarction patients. *Eur Heart J*, **27**, 779–88.

Bradley EH, et al. (2006). Strategies for reducing the door-to-balloon time in acute myocardial infarction. *N Engl J Med*, **355**, 2308–20.

Braunwald E (1989). Unstable angina: a classification. *Circulation*, **80**, 410–14.

Braunwald E, et al. (1994). Effects of tissue plasminogen activator and a comparison of early invasive and conservative strategies in unstable angina and non-Q-wave myocardial infarction, results of the TIMI III trial. *Circulation*, **89**, 1545–56.

Briel M, et al. (2006). Effects of early treatment with statins on short-term clinical outcomes in acute coronary syndromes: a meta-analysis of randomized controlled trials. *JAMA*, **295**, 2046–56.

Cannon CP, et al. (1995). Prospective validation of the Braunwald classification of unstable angina: results from the Thrombolysis in Myocardial Ischemia (TIMI) III Registry. *Circulation*, **92**, 1–19.

Cannon CP, et al. (2001). Comparison of early invasive and conservative strategies in patients with unstable coronary syndromes treated with the glycoprotein IIb/IIIa inhibitor tirofiban. *N Engl J Med*, **344**, 1879–87.

CAPTURE Investigators (1997). Randomised placebo-controlled trial of abciximab before and during coronary intervention in refractory unstable angina: the CAPTURE study. *Lancet*, **349**, 1429–35.

Chen ZM, et al. (2005). Addition of clopidogrel to aspirin in 45,852 patients with acute myocardial infarction: randomised placebo-controlled trial. *Lancet*, **366**, 1607–21.

Cohen MD, et al. (1997). A comparison of low-molecular-weight heparin with unfractionated heparin for unstable coronary artery disease. *N Engl J Med*, **337**, 447–52.

Collinson J, et al. (2000). Clinical outcomes, risk stratification and practice patterns of unstable angina and myocardial infarction without ST elevation: Prospective Registry of Acute Ischaemic Syndromes in the UK (PRAIS-UK). *Eur Heart J*, **21**, 1450–7.

Cox J, Naylor CD (1992). The Canadian Cardiovascular Society grading scale for angina pectoris: is it time for refinements? *Ann Int Med*, **117**, 677–83.

de Araujo Goncalves P, et al. (2005). TIMI, PURSUIT, and GRACE risk scores: sustained prognostic value and interaction with revascularization in NSTE-ACS. *Eur Heart J*, **26**, 865–872.

de Lemos JA, Braunwald E (2001). ST segment resolution as a tool for assessing the efficacy of reperfusion therapy. *J Am Coll Cardiol*, **38**, 1283–94.

De Luca G, et al. Abciximab as adjunctive therapy to reperfusion in acute ST-segment elevation myocardial infarction: a meta-analysis of randomized trials. *JAMA*, **293**, 1759–65.

de Winter RJ, et al. (2005). Early invasive versus selectively invasive management for acute coronary syndromes. *N Engl J Med*, **353**, 1095–104.

Eikelboom JW, et al. (2000). Unfractionated heparin and low-molecular-weight heparin in acute coronary syndrome without ST elevation: a meta-analysis. *Lancet*, **355**, 1936–42.

Eikelboom JW, et al. (2006). Adverse impact of bleeding on prognosis in patients with acute coronary syndromes. *Circulation*, **114**, 774–82.

Fibrinolytic Therapy Trialists' (FTT) Collaborative group (1994). Indications for fibrinolytic therapy in suspected acute myocardial infarction: collaborative overview of early mortality and major morbidity results from all randomised trials of more than 1000 patients. *Lancet*, **343**, 311–22.

Fox KA, et al. (2004). Benefits and risks of the combination of clopidogrel and aspirin in patients undergoing surgical revascularization for non-ST-elevation acute coronary syndrome: the Clopidogrel in Unstable angina to prevent Recurrent ischemic Events (CURE) Trial. *Circulation*, **110**, 1202–8.

Fox KA, *et al.* (2005). 5-year outcome of an interventional strategy in non-ST-elevation acute coronary syndrome: the British Heart Foundation RITA 3 randomised trial. *Lancet*, **366**, 914–20.

Fox KA, *et al.* (2006). Prediction of risk of death and mycocardial infarction in the six months after presentation with acute coronary syndrome: prospective multinational observational study (GRACE). *BMJ*, **333**, 1091–4.

Fox KA, *et al.* (2007). Intervention in acute coronary syndromes: do patients undergo intervention on the basis of their risk characteristics? The global registry of acute coronary events (GRACE). *Heart*, **93**, 177–82.

Fox KA, *et al.* (2007). Decline in rates of death and heart failure in acute coronary syndromes, 1999–2006. *JAMA*, **297**, 1892–900.

FRAX.I.S. Study Group (1999). Comparison of two treatment durations (6 days and 14 days) of a low molecular weight heparin with a 6-day treatment of unfractionated heparin in the initial management of unstable angina or non-Q wave myocardial infarction: FRAX.I.S. (FRAxiparine in Ischaemic Syndrome). *Eur Heart J*, **20**, 1553–62.

FRISC II Investigators (1999). Invasive compared with non-invasive treatment in unstable coronary artery disease: FRISC II prospective randomised multicentre study. *Lancet*, **354**, 708–15.

Gandhi MM, Lampe FC, Wood DA (1995). Incidence, clinical characteristics, and short-term prognosis of angina pectoris. *Br Heart J*, **73**, 193–8.

Gershlick AH, *et al.* (2005). Rescue angioplasty after failed thrombolytic therapy for acute myocardial infarction (REACT Trial). *N Engl J Med*, **353**, 2758–68.

GISSI (Gruppo Italiano per lo Studio Della Streptochinasi Nell'Infart Miocardico) (1988). Effectiveness of intravenous thrombolytic treatment in acute myocardial infarction. *Lancet*, **i**, 397–402.

Fox KA, *et al.* (2002). Management of acute coronary syndromes. Variations in practice and outcomes: findings of the Global Registry of Acute Coronary Events (GRACE). *Eur Heart J*, **23**, 1177–89.

Grines CL, *et al.* (2007). Prevention of premature discontinuation of dual antiplatelet therapy in patients with coronary artery stents. A Science Advisory from the American Heart Association, American College of Cardiology, Society for Cardiovascular Angiography and Interventions, American College of Surgeons, and American Dental Association, with Representation from the American College of Physicians. *Circulation*, **115**, 813–8.

GUSTO Investigators (1993). An international randomised trial comparing four thrombolytic strategies for acute myocardial infarction. *N Engl J Med*, **329**, 673–82.

GUSTO-V Investigators (2001). Reperfusion therapy for acute myocardial infarction with fibrinolytic therapy or combination reduced fibrinolytic therapy and platelet IIb/IIIa inhibition: the GUSTO V trial. *Lancet*, **357**, 1905–14.

Hamm CW, *et al.* (1992). The prognostic value of serum troponin T in unstable angina. *N Engl J Med*, **327**, 146–50.

Hamm CW, *et al.* (1997). Emergency room triage of patients with acute chest pain by means of rapid testing for cardiac troponin T or troponin I. *N Engl J Med*, **337**, 1648–53.

Hartwell D, *et al.* (2005). Clinical effectiveness and cost-effectiveness of immediate angioplasty for acute myocardial infarction: systematic review and economic evaluation. *Health Technol Assess*, **9**(17). http://www.hta.ac.uk/fullmono/mon917.pdf

Hasdai D, *et al.* (2002). A prospective survey of the characteristics, treatments and outcomes of patients with acute coronary syndromes in Europe and the Mediterranean basin. The Euro Heart Survey of Acute Coronary Syndromes. *Eur Heart J*, **23**, 1190–201.

Held PH, Yusuf S, Furberg CD (1989). Calcium channel blockers in acute myocardial infarction and unstable angina: an overview of randomized trials. *BMJ*, **299**, 1187–92.

Herrington DM (1999). *Erratum*, Comparison of the Heart and Estrogen/Progestin Replacement Study (HERS) cohort with women with coronary disease from the National Health and Nutrition Examination Survey III (NHANES). *Am Heart J*, **138**, 800. [First published in *Am Heart J* 1998, **136**, 115–24].

HOPE Study Investigators (The Heart Outcomes Prevention Evaluation) (2000). Effects of an angiotensin-converting-enzyme inhibitor, ramipril, on death from cardiovascular causes, myocardial infarction, and stroke in high-risk patients. *N Engl J Med*, **342**, 145–53.

IONA Study Group (2002). Effect of nicorandil on coronary events in patients with stable angina: the Impact Of Nicorandil in Angina (IONA) randomized trial. *Lancet*, **359**, 1269–75.

ISIS-2 (Second International Study of Infarct Survival) Collaborative Group (1988). Randomised trial of intravenous streptokinase, oral aspirin, both, or neither among 17,187 cases of suspected acute myocardial infarction. *Lancet*, **ii**, 349–60.

ISIS-3 (Third International Study of Infarct Survival) Collaborative Group (1992). A randomised comparison of streptokinase *vs* tissue plasminogen activator *vs* anistreplase and of aspirin plus heparin *vs* aspirin alone among 41 299 cases of suspected acute myocardial infarction. *Lancet*, **339**, 153–70.

ISIS-4 (Fourth International Study of Infarct Survival Collaborative Group) (1995). A randomised factorial trial assessing early oral captopril, oral mononitrate, and intravenous magnesium sulphate in 58,050 patients with suspected acute myocardial infarction. *Lancet*, **345**, 669–85.

Kastrati A, *et al.* (2006). Abciximab in patients with acute coronary syndromes undergoing percutaneous coronary intervention after clopidogrel pretreatment: the ISAR-REACT 2 randomized trial. *JAMA*, **295**, 1531–8.

Keeley EC, Boura JA, Grines CL (2003). Primary angioplasty versus intravenous thrombolytic therapy for acute myocardial infarction: a quantitative review of 23 randomized trials. *Lancet*, **361**, 13–20.

Kong DF, *et al.* (1998). Clinical outcomes of therapeutic agents that block the platelet glycoprotein IIb/IIIa integrin in ischemic heart disease. *Circulation*, **98**, 2829–35.

Lagerqvist B, *et al.* (2002). A long-term perspective on the protective effects of an early invasive strategy in unstable coronary artery disease: two-year follow-up of the FRISC-II invasive study. *J Am Coll Cardiol*, **40**, 1902–14.

Lewis WR, Amsterdam EA (1994). Utility and safety of immediate exercise testing of low-risk patients admitted to the hospital for suspected acute myocardial infarction. *Amer J Card*, **74**, 987–90.

Lindhal B, Venge P, Wallentin L (1996). Relation between troponin T and the risk of subsequent cardiac events in unstable coronary artery disease. *Circulation*, **93**, 1651–7.

Luescher MS, *et al.* (1997). Applicability of cardiac troponin T and I for early risk stratification in unstable coronary disease. *Circulation*, **96**, 2578–85.

Maas ACP, *et al.* (1999). Sustained benefit at 10–14 years follow-up after thrombolytic therapy in myocardial infarction. *Eur Heart J*, **20**, 819–26.

Madsen JK, *et al.* (1997). Danish multicentre randomised study of invasive versus conservative treatment in patients with inducible ischaemia after thrombolysis in acute myocardial infarction (DANAMI). *Circulation*, **96**, 748–55.

Mehta SR, *et al.* (2001). Effects of pretreatment with clopidogrel and aspirin followed by long-term therapy in patients undergoing percutaneous coronary intervention: the PCI-CURE study. *Lancet*, **358**, 528–33.

Mehta SR, *et al.* (2005). Routine vs selective invasive strategies in patients with acute coronary syndromes: a collaborative meta-analysis of randomized trials. *JAMA*, **293**, 2908–17.

Mehta RH, *et al.* (2006). Recent trends in the care of patients with non-ST-segment elevation acute coronary syndromes: insights from the CRUSADE initiative. *Arch Intern Med*, **166**, 2027–34.

Montalescot G, *et al.* (2006). Enoxaparin versus unfractionated heparin in elective percutaneous coronary intervention. *N Engl J Med*, **355**, 1006–17.

MRC/BHF Heart Protection Study (HPS Study) of cholesterol lowering with simvastatin in 20,536 high-risk individuals: a randomised placebocontrolled trial. *Lancet*, **360**, 7–22.

Nunn CM, *et al.* (1999). Long-term outcome after primary angioplasty. Report from the primary angioplasty in mycocardial infarction (PAMI-I) trial. *J Am Coll Cardiol*, **33**, 640–6.

Oler A, *et al.* (1996). Adding heparin to aspirin reduces the incidence of mycocardial infarction and death in patients with unstable angina. A meta-analysis. *JAMA*, **276**, 811–15.

Petersen JL, *et al.* (2004). Efficacy and bleeding complications among patients randomized to enoxaparin or unfractionated heparin for antithrombin therapy in non-ST-segment elevation acute coronary syndromes: a systematic overview. *JAMA*, **292**, 89–96.

Pitt B, *et al.* (1999). Effects of losartan versus captopril on mortality in patients with symptomatic heart failure: rationale, design, and baseline characteristics of patients in the Losartan Heart Failure Survival Study—ELITE II. *J Cardiac Fail*, **5**, 146–54.

Pocock SJ, *et al.* (1995). Meta-analysis of randomised trials comparing coronary angioplasty with bypass surgery. *Lancet*, **346**, 1184–9.

PRISM. The Platelet Receptor Inhibition in Ischemic Syndrome Study Investigators (1998). A comparison of aspirin plus tirofiban with aspirin plus heparin for unstable angina. *N Engl J Med*, **338**, 1498–505.

PRISM-PLUS. The Platelet Receptor Inhibition in Ischemic Syndrome Management in Patients Limited by Unstable Signs and Symptoms Study Investigators (1998). Inhibition of the platelet glycoprotein IIb/IIIa receptor with tirofiban in unstable angina and non-Q-wave mycocardial infarction. *N Engl J Med*, **338**, 1488–97.

Ravkilde J, *et al.* (1995). Independent prognostic value of serum creatine kinase isoenzyme MB mass, cardiac troponin T and myosin light chain levels in suspected acute mycocardial infarction. Analysis of 28 months of follow-up in 196 patients. *J Am Coll Cardiol*, **25**, 574–81.

Rawles J, *et al.* (1994). Halving of mortality at 1 year by domiciliary thrombolysis in the Grampian Region Early Anistreplase Trial (GREAT). *J Am Coll Cardiol*, **23**, 1–5.

Ryan TJ (1999). Early revascularisation in cardiogenic shock—a positive view of a negative trial. *N Engl J Med*, **341**, 687–8.

Sabatine MS, *et al.* (2005). Addition of clopidogrel to aspirin and fibrinolytic therapy for mycocardial infarction with ST-segment elevation. *N Engl J Med*, **352**, 1179–89.

Savonitto S, *et al.* (1997). Prognostic value of the admission electrocardiogram in acute coronary syndromes. Results from the GUSTO-IIb trial. *Eur Heart J*, **18** (Suppl), **335**, 5–82.

SIGN (SIGN) (2007). *Risk estimation and the prevention of cardiovascular disease.* SIGN Publication no. 97, Scottish Intercollegiate Guidelines Network, Edinburgh. http://www.sign.ac.uk.

Sivers F (1999). *Evidence-based strategies for secondary prevention of coronary heart disease*, 2nd edition. A&M Publishing, Guildford.

Stone GW, *et al.* (2006). for the ACUITY Investigators. Bivalirudin for patients with acute coronary syndromes. *N Engl J Med*, **355**, 2203–16.

Tunstall-Pedoe H, *et al.* (1996). Sex differences in myocardial infarction and coronary deaths in the Scottish MONICA population of Glasgow 1985–1991. *Circulation*, **93**, 1981–92.

Van de Werf F, *et al.* (2005). Access to catheterization facilities in patients admitted with acute coronary syndrome: multinational registry study. *BMJ*, **330**, 441.

Yusuf S, *et al.* (1985). B-blockade during and after mycocardial infarction: an overview of the randomized trials. *Progr Cardiovasc Dis*, **27**, 335–71.

Yusuf S, *et al.* (1998). Variations between countries in invasive cardiac procedures and outcomes in patients with suspected unstable angina or myocardial infarction without initial ST elevation. *Lancet*, **352**, 507–14.

Yusuf S, *et al.* (2001). Effects of clopidogrel in addition to aspirin in patients with acute coronary syndromes without ST-segment elevation. *N Engl J Med*, **345**, 494–502.

Yusuf S, *et al.* (2004). Effect of potentially modifiable risk factors associated with myocardial infarction in 52 countries (the INTERHEART study): case–control study. *Lancet*, **364**, 937–52.

Yusuf S, *et al.* (2006). Effects of Fondaparinux, a factor Xa inhibitor, on mortality and reinfarction in patients with acute myocardial infarction presenting with ST-segment elevation. Organization to Assess Strategies for Ischemic Syndromes (OASIS)-6 Investigators. *JAMA*, **295**, 1519–30.

Yusuf S, *et al.* (2006). Efficacy and safety of fondaparinux compared to enoxaparin in 20,078 patients with acute coronary syndromes without ST segment elevation. The OASIS (Organization to Assess Strategies in Acute Ischemic Syndromes)-5 Investigators. *N Engl J Med*, **354**, 1464–76.

16.13.6 Percutaneous interventional cardiac procedures

Edward D. Folland

Essentials

Percutaneous coronary intervention (PCI) is the term applied to a variety of percutaneous, catheter-based procedures that accomplish revascularization either by angioplasty (enlargement of a vessel lumen by modification of plaque structure), stenting (deployment of an internal armature or stent), atherectomy (removal or ablation of plaque), or thrombectomy (removal of thrombus).

The most common single indication for PCI is acute coronary syndrome. Randomized trials have shown that direct intervention for ST-elevation myocardial infarction (STEMI) is superior to initial thrombolytic therapy when performed in appropriate centres, and it can be used as a salvage procedure after failed thrombolytic therapy.

Balloon angioplasty is the traditional, basic technique of coronary intervention, but it is now uncommonly employed as a stand-alone treatment and finds its chief application in deployment of balloon-expandable stents, which have become the intervention of choice in about 90% of cases undergoing PCI. A variety of percutaneous techniques can be used to remove atheroma or thrombus from coronary arteries as a prelude to angioplasty/stenting.

There are two main types of coronary stent—'bare metal' and 'drug eluting'. The latter contain a drug (e.g. sirolimus, paclitaxol, etc.) that inhibits smooth muscle proliferation and thereby considerably reduces the risk of restenosis, which is the most common complication of stenting. Restenosis typically presents as exertional angina at 1 to 6 months following intervention: if it is not present at 6 months, it is unlikely to occur.

Percutaneous techniques can also be used to treat valvular stenosis and close cardiac defects in (highly) selected cases.

Introduction

The birth of interventional vascular medicine is generally credited to Charles Dotter, a radiologist from Portland, Oregon, who in 1964 first dared to relieve atherosclerotic stenosis of a patient's femoral artery by passage of a percutaneously introduced dilator. Although Dr Dotter had a few notable successes, which were widely publicized in the lay press, the scientific community scorned him.

His radical concept lay dormant until a decade later when Andreas Gruentzig, a young German radiologist studying in Zurich, revived it. Dr Gruentzig was convinced that percutaneous dilatation of atherosclerotic stenosis was a sound concept and proposed that Dotter's solid dilator be replaced by a catheter with an inflatable cylindrical balloon at its tip. Using catheters he created in his own kitchen, he proceeded carefully and logically in applying his technique first to animal models, then to human peripheral vessels, and finally in 1977 to his ultimate goal, the human coronary artery. News of Gruentzig's percutaneous transluminal coronary angioplasty (PTCA) was quickly embraced by the medical community, and the era of percutaneous coronary intervention (PCI) was born. This chapter deals with percutaneous approaches to treating coronary, valvular, and congenital heart disease.

Percutaneous coronary intervention

Percutaneous coronary intervention (PCI) is the current general term applied to a variety of percutaneous, catheter-based procedures that accomplish revascularization either by angioplasty (enlargement of a vessel lumen by modification of plaque structure), stenting (deployment of an internal armature or stent), atherectomy (removal or ablation of plaque), or thrombectomy (removal of thrombus). Several different devices have been developed to perform these procedures. The interventional cardiologist chooses among these approaches to best suit the particular requirements of each individual patient.

Indications

The indications for percutaneous revascularization have expanded dramatically during the past 30 years. In the early days of PTCA it was indicated for subtotal, proximal occlusions of single vessels in patients with chronic, stable angina pectoris who had failed medical therapy. As experience grew and equipment improved, patients with unstable angina, total occlusions, bypass grafts, multivessel disease, and acute myocardial infarction were added to the list. Currently, the most common single indication for PCI is acute coronary syndrome (see Chapter 16.13.5).

PCI has traditionally been performed only in hospitals having cardiac surgical backup. However, as the procedure has become safer and the need for emergency bypass surgery less common (currently <1% of all cases), it has become more common, particularly in Europe, for these procedures to be performed in facilities where surgical backup is not on-site. Likewise, all patients undergoing PCI were once required to be potential candidates for bypass surgery in case of failure of the percutaneous procedure. Now some patients who are poor surgical candidates may undergo salvage intervention as their best or only avenue for revascularization. The choice of initial treatment (pharmacological, interventional, or surgical) for patients with each of the above coronary syndromes has been guided by evidence from a number of randomized clinical trials and will be treated in more detail in the later section headed 'Outcomes'.

Devices and techniques

Balloon angioplasty

Balloon angioplasty is the traditional, basic technique of coronary intervention, although it is now uncommonly employed as a stand-alone treatment. Nevertheless, it is fundamental to the deployment

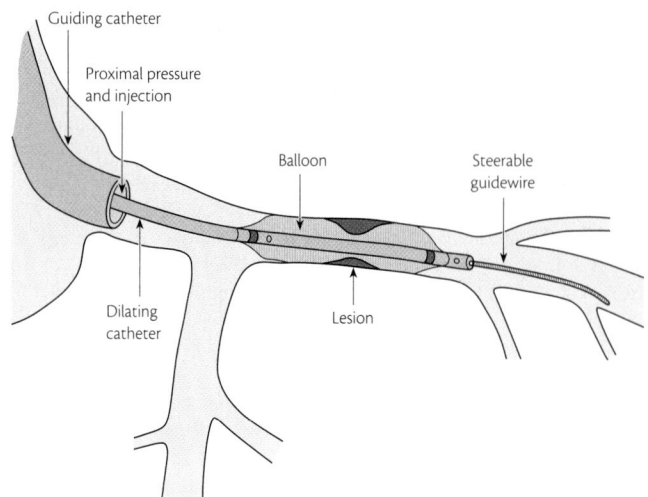

Fig. 16.13.6.1 Balloon angioplasty. The guiding catheter gives access to the coronary artery and provides a platform against which the dilating apparatus can be advanced. The steerable guide wire is passed down the vessel being treated and provides a rail over which the balloon catheter can be advanced. Once centred on the atherosclerotic lesion, the balloon is inflated under pressure to dilate the narrowed segment of artery.

of coronary stents, which are currently the most widely utilized of the interventional devices. The equipment for angioplasty is shown in Fig. 16.13.6.1 and consists of a coaxial array of guiding catheter, balloon catheter, and steerable guide wire. The procedure is accomplished by first engaging the left or right coronary orifice with the tip of the guiding catheter to access the vessel containing the target lesion and to provide backup support during advancement of the guide wire and balloon across the lesion (Fig. 16.13.6.2a). Next, the guide wire is advanced through the guide catheter into the appropriate vessel and across the lesion to be treated. Typical guide wires are 0.0014 of an inch in diameter (c.0.36 mm) and have a flexible spiral coil tip that can be directed by rotating their proximal end outside the body. The balloon catheter is then advanced over the guide wire until the deflated balloon lies across the target lesion. Finally, the balloon is inflated with a solution of dilute contrast medium to a pressure sufficient to expand the cylindrical balloon to its nominal manufactured diameter (Fig. 16.13.6.2b). The balloon size is selected to match the estimated diameter of the nearest segment of normal vessel and the length of the target lesion. Sometimes intravascular ultrasound is used to assist in this choice. The balloon is then withdrawn and the result assessed by angiography and, occasionally, by ultrasound (Fig. 16.13.6.2c).

Traditional angioplasty now finds its chief application in deployment of balloon-expandable stents. However, angioplasty may serve as a stand-alone interventional technique for the treatment of lesions of small vessels (<2.5 mm in diameter) and lesions located far distally or beyond tortuous segments where more rigid devices such as stents cannot reach. In experienced hands, with appropriate case selection, the initial success rate of balloon angioplasty should exceed 95%. Abrupt closure of the vessel might be expected in about 3% of cases (usually due to dissection), but most of these can be corrected by deployment of a stent, resulting in a need for emergency bypass surgery in less than 1% of cases. The clinical consequence of vessel closure is often insufficient to justify surgery in vessels too small or distal for grafting.

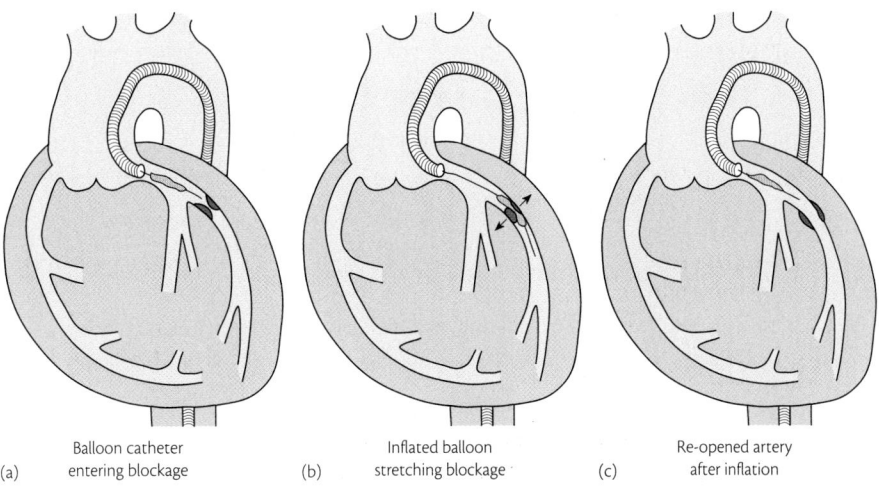

(a) Balloon catheter entering blockage   (b) Inflated balloon stretching blockage   (c) Re-opened artery after inflation

Fig. 16.13.6.2 A typical lesion (a) before, (b) during, and (c) after balloon angioplasty.

The technology of guide, balloon, and guide wire systems has advanced to the point where few locations in the coronary anatomy are inaccessible. Totally occluded vessels can usually be successfully crossed with appropriate manipulation of the right guide wire, enabling successful angioplasty. The success rate for angioplasty of totally occluded vessels depends upon the age, length, and composition (thrombus vs plaque) of the occlusion; it is well over 90% in cases of acute thrombotic occlusion, and over 50% in cases of chronic occlusion (>3 months). The chief disadvantage of balloon angioplasty is the phenomenon of restenosis, which will be discussed in more detail later in this chapter, and which spurred the development of newer devices in the hope of preventing restenosis.

Stenting

Bare metal stents

Stenting has become the intervention of choice in about 90% of cases undergoing PCI. A modern-day vascular stent is actually an armature, or internal skeleton, for restoring and maintaining the cylindrical structure of the diseased vessel. Most stents are made from a thin-walled stainless steel or cobalt–chromium steel tube in which slots have been carved. The slotted tube is then mounted securely on a deflated angioplasty balloon and deployed at the target lesion of the coronary artery by inflating the balloon at high pressure with dilute contrast medium. When the balloon is deflated the stent remains expanded against the vessel wall, its slots stretched into diamond-shaped apertures (Fig. 16.13.6.3). Approximately 20% of the vessel wall is covered by metal, the remainder being an intrastrut aperture. This accounts for the surprisingly high patency of side branches following stent deployment, and the ability to access these side branches when necessary for further intervention.

A variation of the slotted-tube stent is a balloon-deployed coiled wire (Wallstent and others). A coiled wire made from nitinol, or another alloy with shape-retaining characteristics, is compressed into a tubular delivery sheath, which is advanced over a guide wire across the target lesion. Once in its proper position the sheath is drawn back, allowing the stent to expand to its original size and shape (Fig. 16.13.6.4). As with slotted-tube stents, pre- or post-deployment dilation with a balloon may be necessary, depending upon the nature of the lesion treated and the device used. Although one of the original stent designs, the self-expanding stent is now used less commonly for coronary artery applications, but it still finds use in many peripheral vascular cases. Most current stent designs are hybrids, which incorporate desirable properties of both the slotted-tube and coiled-wire designs.

Stents have gained remarkable popularity, mainly for three reasons. First, immediate complications are reduced because abrupt closure of the vessel due to dissection is less likely, emphasized by the fact that a stent is the best treatment for a balloon-induced dissection. Second, the immediate result is better in terms of the diameter and smoothness of the lumen, which turns out to be of more than cosmetic value because the early gain in lumen size relates directly to the late outcome. Thirdly, stents have been demonstrated in randomized clinical trials to be effective in reducing the likelihood of late restenosis. However, stents do have some disadvantages, which include the fact that they cannot be deployed under some circumstances, their propensity to subacute thrombosis, and the persistence of some degree of restenosis (depending upon the size of the vessel and length of the lesion). Subacute thrombosis, a complication unique to stents, usually occurs within a few weeks after stent deployment. By contrast to restenosis, which is a gradual phenomenon, stent thrombosis is usually sudden, presenting as acute myocardial infarction and requiring emergency revascularization, usually by balloon angioplasty. The likelihood of subacute thrombosis has been reduced to less than 1% by antiplatelet therapy with a combination of aspirin along with clopidogrel, ticlopidine or prasugrel.

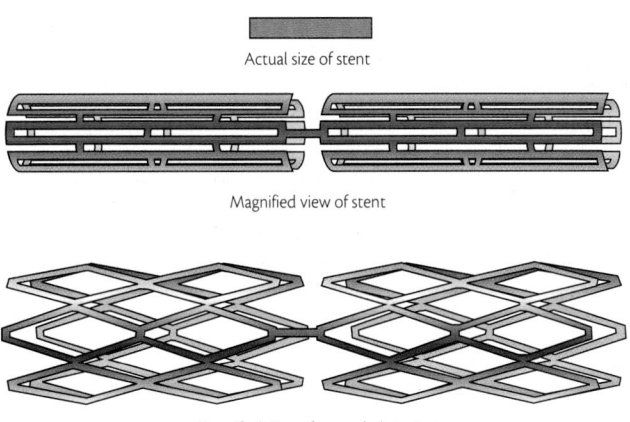

Actual size of stent

Magnified view of stent

Magnified view of expanded stent

Fig. 16.13.6.3 A balloon-deployed coronary artery stent (a) before and (b) after deployment.

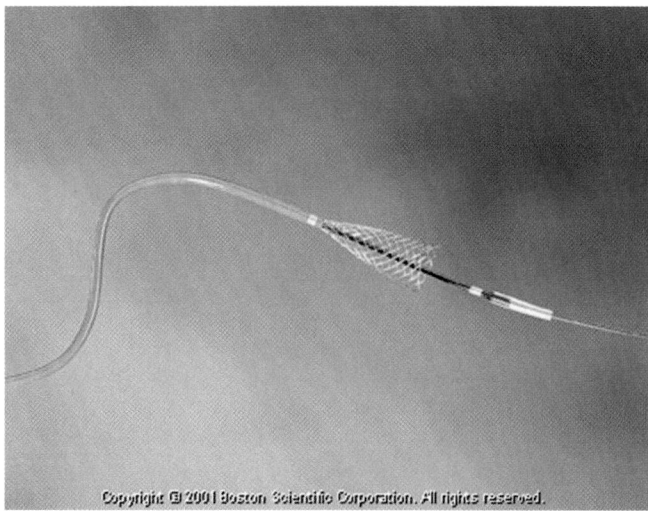

Fig. 16.13.6.4　A self-deploying coil stent. The stent unfurls as its delivery (containment) sheath is pulled back.
Copyright 2001. Boston Scientific Corporation.

Drug-eluting stents

The development of stents that gradually elute a drug into the surrounding vessel wall has reduced the need for repeat intervention due to restenosis from approximately 15% for bare metal stents to less than 5%. This technology is largely responsible for the rapid and sustained growth in popularity of stent procedures such that most patients requiring coronary revascularization are now treated by percutaneous rather than surgical techniques. The design of the drug-eluting stent incorporates a polymer matrix coating that contains a drug which inhibits the proliferation of smooth muscle cells in the surrounding vessel wall. The active drug slowly elutes from this coating into the underlying tissue while the vascular response to injury caused by vessel dilation is most active. Drug elution is usually complete by two months following stent deployment, but by modulating the proliferation of smooth muscle cells the growth of neo-intima covering the stent struts is limited, reducing the likelihood of restenosis of the treated vessel. The first two types of drug-eluting stents to be commercially available use sirolimus and paclitaxol as the active drug. These drugs inhibit cell proliferation through different mechanisms, but have proven to be equally effective. Other drugs are currently under investigation. Although excessive neo-intimal growth is undesirable, some is needed in order to cover the stent struts and prevent thrombosis. Dual antiplatelet drug therapy is necessary to minimize this risk as long as the struts are exposed. Bare metal stents are usually fully covered by 2 months, but drug-eluting stents may remain uncovered for 6 months or longer. For this reason, most cardiologists recommend that clopidigrel ticlopidine, or prasugrel be continued along with aspirin for at least 1 year following deployment of drug-eluting stents.

Cutting balloon

The cutting balloon has several tiny longitudinally mounted blades that become erect when the balloon is inflated and create linear cuts along the vessel wall. This was conceived as a method to dilate a vessel less traumatically and thereby reduce the likelihood of restenosis. This goal was never realized for *de novo* lesions, but the device has been advantageous for treatment of recurrent stenosis within previously deployed stents (in-stent restenosis) and for

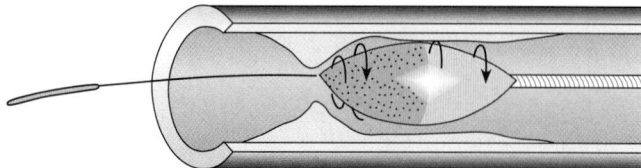

Fig. 16.13.6.5　Rotational atherectomy. The rotating burr pulverizes plaque as it is advanced over the guide wire into the lesion.

dilating lesions located at the ostium of a vessel, which are otherwise often subject to elastic recoil when dilated.

Atherectomy

Rotational ablation

Rotational ablation (Rotablator) is a method of pulverizing plaque into particles smaller than the size of a capillary, which wash away with the circulating blood. This process is accomplished by means of a diamond-studded burr, which rotates at approximately 150 000 rev/min (Fig. 16.13.6.5) and is advanced along a guide wire into the plaque. The diamond studs on the forward face of the olive-shaped burr selectively cut into hard substances such as plaque and calcium, sparing the soft surface of normal tissue. During rotational atherectomy a vasodilating solution is infused into the artery proximal to the burr to prevent spasm and to maintain maximal coronary flow, which carries away particulate debris. Burrs are manufactured in sizes ranging from 1.5 mm to 2.5 mm in diameter. Atherectomy often requires the use of two or three burrs of progressively larger size until an adequate lumen size is achieved. Although occasionally used as a stand-alone procedure, rotational ablation is usually employed to 'debulk' lesions prior to final dilatation with a balloon or stent.

Rotational ablation was originally conceived as a potential solution to the problem of postintervention restenosis. Unfortunately, it has failed to outperform balloon angioplasty in this regard and has assumed the role of a 'niche' device for special situations. It is most commonly used in the treatment of heavily calcified lesions that do not respond well to balloons and stents. It is also useful in treating diffuse, osteal, and bifurcating lesions. The frequency with which rotational ablation is employed varies by operator, but averages less than 5% of most centres' cases. It has the disadvantages of being an expensive addition to other interventional modalities, is unable to adequately increase the lumen of large vessels, and is contraindicated in lesions containing thrombus. Due to its tendency to transiently decrease contractility during the ablation process, it is also relatively contraindicated in patients whose left ventricular function is severely impaired.

Directional coronary atherectomy

Directional coronary atherectomy (DCA) is achieved with a device illustrated in Fig. 16.13.6.6 that utilizes a rotating cylindrical blade which is advanced across an open aperture near the tip of a cone-shaped catheter directed by a guide wire. Opposite the aperture is an eccentric balloon, which when inflated compresses plaque of the opposite vessel wall into the aperture, where it is cut away by the rotating blade and pushed into the nose cone. The direction of the aperture can be rotated so that slices of plaque are removed in a radial fashion by multiple cuts taken at different locations around the circumference of the vessel. The catheter can then be withdrawn and the excised plaque removed from the

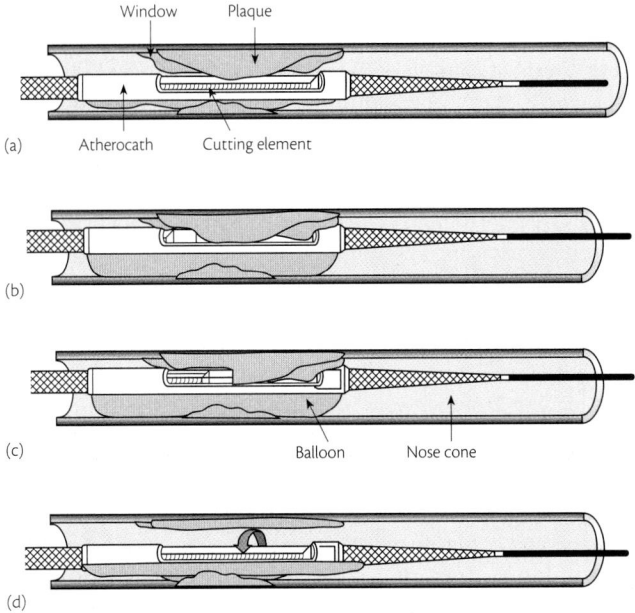

Fig. 16.13.6.6 Directional coronary atherectomy. (a) The catheter is inserted such that the blade housing is adjacent to the plaque to be removed; (b) the balloon on the opposite side of the blade housing is inflated, pushing the aperture over the plaque; (c) the rotating cylindrical blade is advanced across the window of the housing and cuts away plaque, packing it into the nose cone; (d) the catheter can be rotated to remove plaque elsewhere on the circumference of the vessel.

nose cone. The catheter may be reintroduced, if necessary, for more atherectomy.

Although DCA was originally devised with the hope of reducing the incidence of restenosis, it has failed to outperform balloon angioplasty in most circumstances. It has therefore assumed the role of a 'niche' technology, which is useful in particular situations such as very eccentric proximal lesions, and lesions involving the ostia of major side branches. Removal of plaque at branch points seems to reduce the likelihood of plaque shifting from one branch to another as the respective lesions are dilated with balloons or stents. However, DCA has the disadvantage of requiring a rather large, stiff device, limiting its application to proximal lesions of large vessels. Furthermore, the removal of plaque seems to have surprisingly little effect on restenosis. DCA is currently employed in less than 5% of interventional cases.

Other devices

The transcutaneous excision catheter (TEC) device was developed at about the same time as directional coronary atherectomy. It employs a rotating conical blade that cuts away plaque and clot as it is advanced over a guidewire. The resulting debris is sucked back through the catheter into a reservoir outside the body. Although originally developed as an atherectomy device, it has found its chief application in treating clot-laden lesions, but it has not gained wide usage.

Excimer laser coronary atherectomy (ELCA) employs a fibreoptic catheter directed by a guide wire to deliver bursts of excimer laser energy to the plaque. Disintegrated plaque washes away in the circulation. However, ELCA has also failed to solve the restenosis problem, is used uncommonly in most centres, but remains the sole surviving member of a number of laser applications that have been tried and failed over the past 30 years. It finds its most frequent application in treatment of osteal lesions, stent restenosis, and diffuse calcified disease. Because of the limitations of fibre size it is usually followed by balloon or stent treatment.

Thrombectomy

Thrombectomy is an adjunct to angioplasty and stent procedures in patients with acute myocardial infarction and thrombus-laden lesions. Its purpose is to prevent distal embolization by removing the thrombus prior to balloon dilation and stent deployment. The devices for achieving this have become simpler over time. The simplest and least expensive is called a Pronto, which is a catheter delivered over a guide wire that has a relatively large inner lumen that is attached to a suction syringe. As blood is withdrawn through the catheter, its tip is moved back and forth through the thrombus, picking it up and removing it. A more complex device called AngioJet uses the Venturi effect from a high-velocity jet of water, which draws thrombus into a window near the tip of a catheter directed by a guide wire and propels it into a reservoir. Another device called the Excisor employs a helical screw at the end of a catheter, which breaks up the clot so that it can be withdrawn through the catheter. Both these devices currently find their chief application in the treatment of degenerated and clot-laden vein-graft lesions.

Distal protection

Distal protection devices are methods of capturing and collecting thrombus and other debris that may embolize distally from the target lesion during the use of many of the interventional tools mentioned above. They may be particularly beneficial during the treatment of old, degenerated vein grafts in which distal embolization is especially common. Two general approaches are employed. The simplest is a guide wire with a filter on its end (Filterwire, Fig. 16.13.6.7). The filter looks like a windsock and catches debris released proximal to it. The other approach (PercuSurge) is to use a guide wire with a balloon near its tip which is progressively inflated until it occludes the distal portion of the vessel being treated. Intervention is then performed over the guide wire proximal to the occlusion balloon. Once the intervention is complete an export catheter is advanced over the guide wire and any debris removed by suction. Finally, the distal balloon is deflated, restoring flow and the guide wire removed.

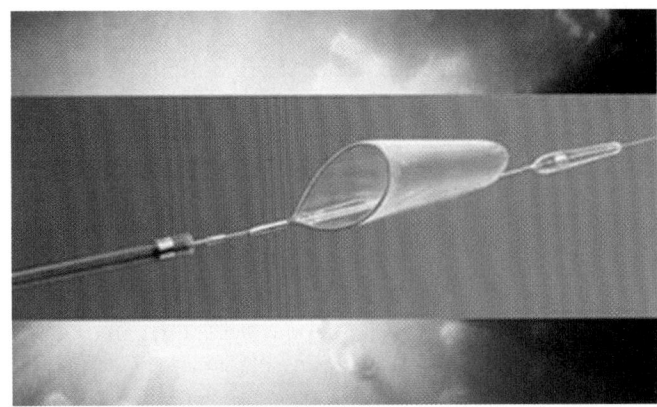

Fig. 16.13.6.7 Distal protection device: FilterWire
Copyright 2001. Boston Scientific Corporation.

Brachytherapy

The local, catheter-based delivery of β or γ radiation has been demonstrated to reduce the incidence of recurrent stent restenosis. Radiation is delivered with the assistance of a radiation therapist after initial treatment of stent restenosis with a cutting balloon, Rotablator, or conventional balloon. The benefit of brachytherapy appears to be limited to treatment of stent restenosis and it is not recommended following initial deployment of a stent. Brachytherapy also prolongs the period of risk for subacute thrombosis, making it necessary to treat patients with both aspirin and clopidogrel for at least 6 months following treatment. However, the need for brachytherapy has been virtually eliminated by drug-eluting stents. Not only is restenosis less likely after initial deployment of a drug eluting stent, but restenosis—when it does occur—is most effectively treated by concentric deployment of a second drug-eluting stent.

Complications

PCI exposes the patient to all the potential complications of cardiac catheterization presented in Chapter 16.3.4. In addition, it carries the risk of other complications unique to interventional procedures. Most of these stem from four general processes that cause adverse outcomes in coronary artery intervention: abrupt closure, distal embolization, stent thrombosis, and restenosis. Patient characteristics such as age, acute coronary syndrome, previous bypass surgery, and renal insufficiency are major determinants of risk. When considering PCI for a patient, it is important to weigh the likelihood of these adverse outcomes against the expected chance of adverse events without intervention. The approximate frequencies of various specific complications from percutaneous coronary intervention are listed in Table 16.13.6.1. As in diagnostic catheterization, the likelihood of these complications also depends upon operator skill.

Abrupt closure and distal embolization

Abrupt closure and distal embolization account for most of the immediate complications of PCI, especially acute myocardial infarction and emergency coronary artery bypass surgery. Dissection, spasm, and thrombosis are the leading causes of abrupt closure. The availability of stents has reduced the need for emergency bypass surgery to less than 1% because these are an effective treatment for acute dissection in most cases. Nevertheless, dissection

Table 16.13.6.1 Complications of percutaneous coronary intervention

Complication	Frequency (%)[a]
Death	0.5–2
Acute myocardial infarction	2–5
Emergency bypass surgery	0.5–3
Abrupt closure	1–2
Subacute stent thrombosis	1–3
Peripheral arterial complications	5
Restenosis (clinical)	10–30

[a] These rates are approximate and vary widely with the clinical setting and patient characteristics. These are in addition to the usual complications of cardiac catheterization presented in Chapter 16.3.4.

sometimes extends with the addition of each stent, and occasionally the stent itself can be the cause of dissection at one of its edges. Acute thrombosis may occur in spite of routine prophylactic treatment with heparin and aspirin: glycoprotein IIb/IIIa inhibitors may stop this process and are often given prophylactically, especially in high-risk cases. Incomplete stent deployment seems to be a leading cause of thrombotic occlusion. Distal embolization is surprisingly uncommon, except when patients have acute coronary syndromes or visible thrombus. It is especially troublesome for patients with degenerated or thrombus-laden vein grafts. Embolization may result in discrete occlusion of branch vessels or the phenomenon called 'no reflow', which is manifest by reduced flow without identifiable occlusion and thought to be due to capillary plugging from showers of microemboli. Distal protection devices (Fig. 16.13.6.7) may help prevent these problems. Both abrupt closure and no reflow usually cause some degree of myocardial infarction, the likelihood of infarction being a matter of how it is defined: non-ST elevation infarction indicated only by a rise of troponin or creatine kinase enzymes is more common than ST elevation (Q wave) infarction.

Stent thrombosis

Thrombosis is a serious complication of particular concern for stents. It rarely occurs after the first 24 h following isolated balloon angioplasty or atherectomy. However, when a stent is deployed it may occur at a later time and is manifest by acute myocardial infarction. It is a medical emergency that must be managed in a fashion similar to spontaneous acute infarction. Emergency reperfusion by balloon angioplasty is usually preferred, unless a catheterization laboratory is unavailable, in which case thrombolytic therapy is recommended. In the early days of stenting this complication occurred in over 3% of cases in spite of vigorous anticoagulation including intravenous heparin and warfarin, a treatment that required several days of hospital stay for the initiation of warfarin therapy and delayed the widespread acceptance of stenting. However, once the current treatment of oral antiplatelet agents was proven to be superior, the length of hospital stay and local bleeding complications were reduced, and the use of stents grew rapidly. Stent thrombosis now occurs in less than 1% of cases. Thrombosis is defined as subacute when it occurs between 1 day and 1 month following stent deployment. Subacute thrombosis is equally likely for bare metal and drug-eluting stents. Thrombosis occurring more than 1 month after stent deployment is called late stent thrombosis and is particularly associated with drug-eluting stents. To minimize the risk of late stent thrombosis, dual antiplatelet therapy with aspirin and clopidigrel should be continued without interruption for at least 1 year following implantation of drug-eluting stents.

Restenosis

Restenosis was once the Achilles heel of coronary intervention. In patients undergoing isolated balloon angioplasty the likelihood of restenosis at 6 months following intervention lies between 30 and 50% if defined by angiographic criteria, and approximately 25% if defined by the clinical recurrence of symptoms. The use of bare metal stents reduced the angiographic rate of restenosis to about 25% and the clinical rate to as little as 10%. Drug-eluting stents have further reduced the rate to 5% or less, depending upon clinical and anatomic circumstances. The risk of restenosis varies according to individual factors such as vessel diameter and lesion length. Restenosis typically presents clinically as exertional angina at 1 to 6 months following intervention: if it is not present at 6 months, it is unlikely to occur. As described above, it is caused by the proliferation and migration of smooth muscle cells into the lumen of the treated vessel, a process that can be significantly modulated by use of drug-eluting stents.

Outcomes

Chronic stable angina

Randomized clinical trials have shown that patients with single- and double-vessel disease experience a more rapid and complete resolution of symptoms, and a greater improvement in treadmill exercise performance, when treated by balloon angioplasty rather than by pharmacological therapy for chronic stable angina pectoris. However, this comes at the price of a greater likelihood of repeat intervention or bypass surgery at 6 months, largely due to the need to treat restenosis. Nevertheless, the rate of bypass surgery becomes equal in both groups by 3 years. When compared to coronary bypass surgery, angioplasty provides similar relief of symptoms and similar rates of mortality and myocardial infarction at 5-year follow-up, with the exception of diabetic patients who have somewhat better 5-year survival rates when treated surgically. Otherwise, the main difference between patient groups randomly assigned to surgery or angioplasty is that repeat catheterization or revascularization is less frequent for those having surgery. Again, this difference is largely due to the effect of restenosis in the angioplasty group. Few of the interventionally treated patients in these trials received stents, so the likelihood of repeat procedures might be expected to be less using current devices. See Chapter 16.13.4 for further discussion.

Unstable angina

The choice between initial aggressive treatment (catheterization and revascularization) and initial conservative treatment (medical therapy with catheterization and revascularization only for those who have continued evidence of ischaemia) for patients with unstable angina has been controversial. However, recent studies favour an aggressive approach to these patients. See Chapter 16.13.5 for further discussion.

Acute myocardial infarction

Percutaneous intervention has been shown to be an effective treatment for acute myocardial infarction with ST segment elevation (STEMI), both as a salvage procedure after failed thrombolytic therapy and as a direct initial approach to reperfusion. Randomized trials have shown that direct intervention for STEMI is superior to initial thrombolytic therapy when performed in centres with expert interventionists and catheterization facilities that are available around the clock. Direct PCI is also an option for patients presenting outside these centres provided that they can be transferred and effectively treated in less than 90 min. In any case, direct PCI is the treatment of choice for patients in whom thrombolytic therapy is contraindicated and for patients who are haemodynamically unstable. See Chapter 16.13.5 for further discussion.

Economic considerations

The cost of equipment and supplies for percutaneous coronary procedures may become a limiting factor, particularly in developing countries and in health care systems with stringent budgets.

Most catheters, guide wires, and other supplies are intended for one-time use. Expendable supplies alone cost approximately £750 ($US 1200) for a simple balloon angioplasty procedure. That cost may be multiplied several-fold when drug-eluting stents are used—these are two to three times more costly than bare metal stents, although the added cost is offset somewhat by the reduced likelihood of repeat procedures necessitated by restenosis. The coverage of this additional cost varies considerably throughout the world depending upon insurance and government policies. Nevertheless, the cost of a single percutaneous revascularization procedure usually remains less than that of a comparable coronary bypass operation. However, when the added cost of repeat percutaneous revascularizations necessitated by restenosis is considered, the price difference between the two therapeutic approaches narrows.

Percutaneous treatment of valvular disease

Allain Cribier of France developed the treatment of valvular stenosis by means of balloon catheters in the 1980s. The clinical utility of the procedure depends upon the valve treated and the age of the patient. Percutaneous aortic valve replacement and treatment for mitral regurgitation are emerging technologies.

Mitral stenosis

Balloon valvuloplasty of the mitral valve has become the treatment of choice for selected patients with rheumatic mitral stenosis. The concept is similar to the aortic valvuloplasty illustrated in Fig. 16.13.6.8. The most common approach to the mitral valve is via trans-septal puncture of the left atrium from percutaneous access of the right femoral vein. After passing a stiff guide wire with a curved soft tip across the mitral valve, an appropriately sized balloon is centred on the valve and inflated with dilute contrast medium, tearing open the fused commissures and allowing the valve to open more normally. A dumbbell-shaped balloon, named after Dr Inoue, is often utilized, preventing the balloon from slipping off the valve during inflation. Clinical improvement, complications, and durability of the outcome from balloon mitral valvuloplasty have been shown to be comparable to surgical commissurotomy in appropriately

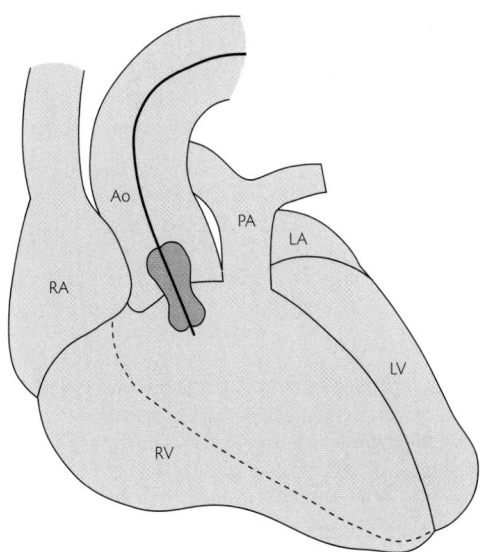

Fig. 16.13.6.8 Percutaneous balloon aortic valvuloplasty. The balloon is centred on the stenotic valve and inflated to tear open the fused commissures.

selected patients. To be a candidate for balloon mitral valvuloplasty a patient must have no evidence of thrombus in the left atrium. Other features which auger poorly include immobility of the valve leaflets, severe calcification, thickening of the chordae tendineae, and more than mild regurgitation.

Mitral regurgitation

Percutaneous treatment of mitral regurgitation is being approached by two different strategies. The first involves applying a clip to the mitral valve commissures, effectively creating a dual orifice valve. The second approach is to pass a ring into the coronary sinus which constricts the mitral valve annulus, enabling better coaptation of the valve leaflets. Both of these procedures are emerging technologies that are largely investigational at the time of writing this chapter.

Aortic stenosis

Experience with balloon valvuloplasty for patients with aortic stenosis has been disappointing, largely due to an almost universal tendency for the stenosis to recur within 1 year. Consequently, the procedure is now performed only under unusual circumstances. It is occasionally used as a bridge to later surgery for patients who are initially too ill to safely undergo valve replacement. It is also sometimes performed for the temporary palliation of patients who are not candidates for valve replacement. It also has a role for children with congenital aortic stenosis, where temporary treatment by valvuloplasty may allow the child to complete growth before requiring surgical valve replacement. Percutaneous implantation of a bioprosthetic valve has been performed in hundreds of patients worldwide: it is presently an investigational procedure, but holds promise for future development.

Pulmonary stenosis

Balloon valvuloplasty is the treatment of choice for patients with pulmonary stenosis. Most are children whose valves respond well to this treatment, the advantage of avoiding surgery outweighing the moderate tendency for restenosis of these valves.

Percutaneous closure of cardiac defects

Atrial septal defects and patent ductus arteriosus can be closed percutaneously with catheter-delivered devices. One such device, called a clamshell, has been used for this purpose for a number of years. It is now available throughout the world and is useful for closing smaller defects, although larger defects still require surgical closure.

Closure of patent foramen ovale can be accomplished by devices similar to the clamshell used for atrial septal defect. This is indicated as an alternative to surgery in patients who have had embolic stroke due to paradoxical embolism through the defect.

Further reading

Boden WE, Eagle K, Granger CB (2007). Reperfusion strategies in acute ST-segment elevation myocardial infarction: a comprehensive review of contemporary management options. *J Am Coll Cardiol*, **50**, 917–29.

Bravata DM, *et al.* (2007). Systematic review: the comparative effectiveness of percutaneous coronary interventions and coronary artery bypass graft surgery. *Ann Intern Med*, **147**, 703–16.

Daemen J, Serruys PW. (2006). Optimal revascularization strategies for multivessel coronary artery disease. *Curr Opin Cardiol*, **21**, 595–601.

Sharma SK, Chen V. (2006). Coronary interventional devices: balloon, atherectomy, thrombectomy and distal protection devices. *Cardiol Clin*, **24**, 201–15.

Spaulding C, *et al.* (2007). A pooled analysis of data comparing sirolimus-eluting stents with bare-metal stents. *N Engl J Med*, **356**, 989–97.

Stettler C, *et al.* (2007). Outcomes associated with drug-eluting and bare-metal stents: a collaborative network meta-analysis. *Lancet*, **370**, 937–48.

Topol EJ (ed.) (2002). *Textbook of interventional cardiology*, 4th edition. W B Saunders, Philadelphia.

Vahanian A, Acar C (2005). Percutaneous valve procedures: what is the future? *Curr Opin Cardiol*, **20**, 100–6.

16.13.7 Coronary artery bypass surgery

Graham Cooper

Essentials

Patients with left main-stem stenosis and three-vessel disease merit surgery for prognosis, regardless of symptom severity, especially if ventricular function is impaired. Coronary artery bypass is also an effective therapy for angina pectoris that is not controlled with medical treatment.

Despite a worsening risk profile in the population undergoing coronary artery bypass, operative mortality remains low. Ten years after operation, about 80% of patients are still alive and two-thirds are free of angina. Contemporary results are likely to be better than this due to increasing use of arteries instead of veins as bypass grafts, and improvements in secondary prevention.

The evidence shows that coronary artery bypass gives patients with coronary artery disease longer survival than percutaneous intervention, even with the use of drug-eluting stents.

Introduction

The coronary artery bypass operation is arguably the most studied operation in the history of surgery. It is also one of the most successful.

Historical perspectives

The development of coronary angiography and cardiopulmonary bypass in the 1960s allowed a direct surgical approach to coronary artery disease. Before this various attempts to improve myocardial blood supply had been ineffective and the coronary artery bypass operation rapidly gained favour. Between 1972 and 1984, three prospective randomized trials established its superiority to medical treatment. Between 1977 and 2003 the number of operations performed in the United Kingdom increased 10-fold to 25 000 per year.

Indications

Coronary artery bypass is principally indicated for relief of angina pectoris or to improve the prognosis of a patient with coronary artery disease (Table 16.13.7.1). In some cases both indications apply. For any patient the decision to proceed requires an assessment that the benefits outweigh the risk, although those at highest operative risk often have the most to gain.

Meta-analysis of the three major and four smaller prospective randomized trials conducted in the late 1970s and early 1980s shows a survival advantage for coronary artery bypass surgery compared to medical treatment alone (Fig. 16.13.7.1). This improvement in survival is greatest in those at highest risk, risk being defined by the extent of coronary artery disease. Mortality reduction with surgery is 68% at 5 years in left main stem stenosis and 42% with three-vessel disease. Subsequent registry data has enabled benefit to be defined according to ventricular function, extent of ischaemic myocardium, and severity of angina as well as coronary anatomy.

Angina pectoris

In asymptomatic patients or those with nonlimiting angina, operation is advised for those in whom it will improve prognosis. This encompasses patients with left main stem stenosis (flow-limiting stenosis of the left coronary artery before division into left anterior descending and circumflex arteries) or equivalent (flow-limiting stenosis of proximal left anterior descending and proximal circumflex arteries) and three-vessel disease (stenosis of all three coronary arteries).

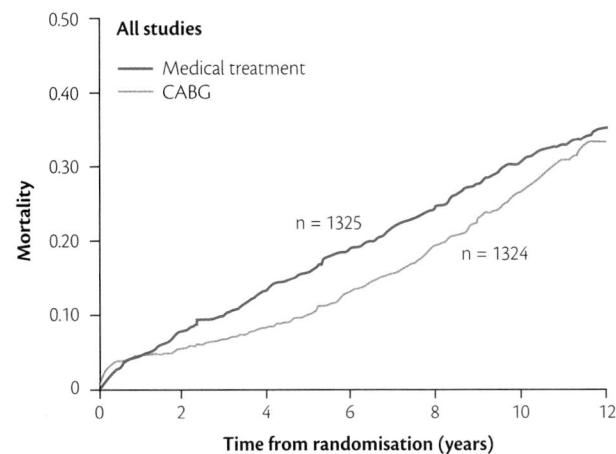

Fig. 16.13.7.1 Survival after coronary artery bypass surgery (CABG) compared to medical treatment.

In the presence of limiting angina despite adequate medical treatment, coronary artery bypass is indicated provided the coronary arteries are suitable for grafting and the operative risk is not prohibitive.

Non-ST-elevation myocardial infarction (non-STEMI)

After non-STEMI the indications for coronary bypass are as indicated in Table 16.13.7.1. The timing of surgery is critical: operative risk is increased two- to three fold in the first week and gradually declines over the next month, but delaying operation to ameliorate this risk has to be balanced against the risk of an adverse event during the period of waiting.

ST-elevation myocardial infarction (STEMI)

In contemporary practice coronary artery bypass has little place in the management of acute STEMI. After the acute phase the caveats associated with non-STEMI apply.

The coronary artery bypass operation

Access to the heart is provided by a median sternotomy incision. The left internal mammary artery is mobilized and divided distally. Proximally it is left connected to the left subclavian artery. If the right internal mammary artery is used, this may be left attached to the right subclavian artery or detached and used as a free graft. Enough long saphenous vein is mobilized from the leg. The radial artery is mobilized from the nondominant arm if required.

Cannulae are inserted to allow cardiopulmonary bypass and the bypass machine is started. The ascending aorta is clamped and the heart arrested in diastole by infusing cardioplegia solution with a high potassium concentration into the aorta on the cardiac side of the cross clamp. It may also be administered retrogradely through the coronary sinus.

Longitudinal incisions (2–3 mm) are made in the coronary arteries distal to the stenosis and the bypass grafts are sutured to them. The left anterior descending coronary artery is grafted with the left internal mammary artery. If a free right internal mammary artery graft or radial artery graft is used, the proximal anastomosis is made either to the aorta or to the side of the left internal mammary artery. The proximal ends of vein grafts are attached to the ascending aorta. Removal of the cross clamp reperfuses the heart, washing

Table 16.13.7.1 Indications for coronary artery bypass surgery

Coronary anatomy	Reduced left ventricular function	Extensive myocardial ischaemia on noninvasive testing	Limiting angina	Class of evidence	Level of evidence
Left main-stem stenosis				I	A
Left main-stem equivalent				I	A
Three-vessel disease	Yes			I	C
Three-vessel disease		Yes		I	C
Three-vessel disease			Yes	I	A
Proximal left-anterior descending stenosis	Yes			I	B
Proximal left anterior descending stenosis		Yes		I	B
One- or two-vessel disease			Yes	I	B

out the cardioplegia solution, and cardiac contraction restarts spontaneously. When adequate cardiac contraction is achieved the patient is separated from cardiopulmonary bypass.

The operation may also be performed without the use of cardiopulmonary bypass. A special retractor is used to stabilize the heart and provide a still operative field. At present there are no conclusive data showing the superiority for the coronary artery bypass operation performed with or without cardiopulmonary bypass.

Complications

Operative mortality

With time, the risk profile for patients undergoing coronary artery bypass has steadily increased. This has been contributed to by an ageing population, extension of the indications for the operation, and increasing treatment of low risk patients with percutaneous coronary intervention (PCI). However, despite a worsening risk profile the operative mortality for isolated coronary artery bypass has steadily declined and was 1.5% in the United Kingdom in 2008. Patients less than 60 years of age without significant comorbidity have an operative mortality of 0.4%. Operative mortality is adversely influenced by advancing age, reduced left ventricular function, urgency of the operation, female sex, and more extensive coronary artery disease. Repeat operation trebles operative risk.

Neurological injury

Permanent neurological injury occurs in around 3% of patients. Increasing age, previous stroke, carotid artery disease, and ascending aortic atheroma are risk factors for the development of this complication. Up to 30% of postoperative strokes are associated with carotid artery disease. Preoperative carotid endarterectomy may be indicated in patients with severe carotid artery disease, especially if symptomatic.

Local and cardiac complications

Sternal wound infection

Dehiscence of the sternal wound with mediastinitis occurs in around 1% of patients and is predisposed to by diabetes mellitus and obesity. For this reason use of both internal mammary arteries is avoided in obese diabetics. Treatment generally requires surgical revision of the wound and may require the use of muscle flaps.

Pleural effusion

With use of the internal mammary artery grafts pleural effusions are common, but these are generally small and self-limiting. If large enough to cause shortness of breath they should be aspirated.

Pericardial effusion

Between 25% and 50% of patients develop a pericardial effusion following operation, but in only a few per cent is this large enough to cause cardiac tamponade. Percutaneous drainage may be possible with echocardiographic control: if not surgical drainage is required. Pericardial effusions generally develop within a few days of surgery but may present some weeks later.

Postcardiotomy syndrome

Postcardiotomy syndrome is characterized by fever and anterior chest pain. A pericardial friction rub, lymphocytosis, and persistent pericardial and pleural effusions are often associated.

Nonsteroidal anti-inflammatory drugs are generally effective. Steroids are second line treatment.

Atrial fibrillation

Around 30% of patients suffer postoperative atrial fibrillation, which can be reduced by peri- and postoperative β-blockade. If it is persistent, patients should be anticoagulated. Amiodarone usually restores sinus rhythm and should be continued for 6 weeks. Electrical cardioversion is required if amiodarone is unsuccessful.

Outcomes

Long-term survival

In a heterogeneous group of patients 10-year survival is around 80%. Half of late deaths are from cardiac causes. The use of a pedicled left internal mammary artery to the left anterior descending coronary artery, in place of a saphenous vein graft, gives a 10% survival advantage at 10 years which persists for at least another 5 years. Using both left and right internal mammary arteries further improves outcome (Fig. 16.13.7.2).

Recurrent angina

Two-thirds of patients are free from angina 10 years after operation, although contemporary results are expected to be better due to increased use of arterial grafts and improved secondary prevention. Relief of angina after coronary artery bypass largely depends upon continued bypass graft patency, although progression of native coronary artery disease and incomplete revascularization play a part.

The presence of a left internal mammary artery to the left anterior descending coronary artery reduces late myocardial infarction and reoperation, but its impact on recurrent angina is less certain. Use of both internal mammary arteries extends the benefits of a single mammary artery; angina-free survival is improved and reoperation reduced.

A strategy of total arterial revascularization has not been shown to be superior to two mammary arteries and supplementary vein grafts. It may be useful for selected younger patients and those in whom there is no venous conduit. The radial artery is widely used

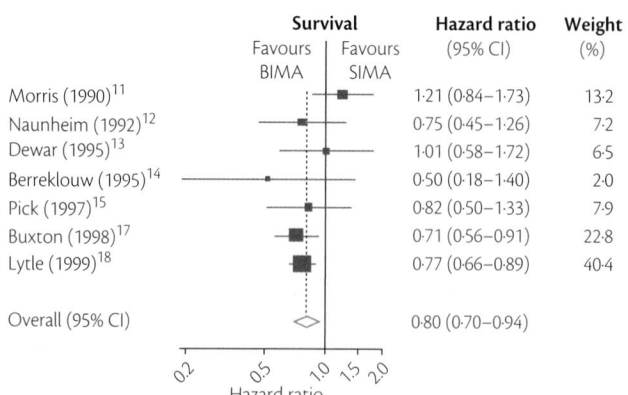

Effects of bilateral IMA compared with single IMA
Random-effects meta-analysis of data from seven studies. Horizontal lines indicate 95% CI.

Fig. 16.13.7.2 Effects of bilateral internal mammary artery (IMA) compared with single IMA.

as an arterial conduit and there is increasing data to suggest that it has improved patency compared to saphenous vein.

Secondary prevention

General measures such as smoking cessation and weight loss are beneficial. All patients should be offered cardiac rehabilitation, which improves postoperative exercise tolerance. Specific attention should be paid to antiplatelet therapy and cholesterol reduction, which improve graft patency as well as their known role in secondary prevention for cardiovascular disease.

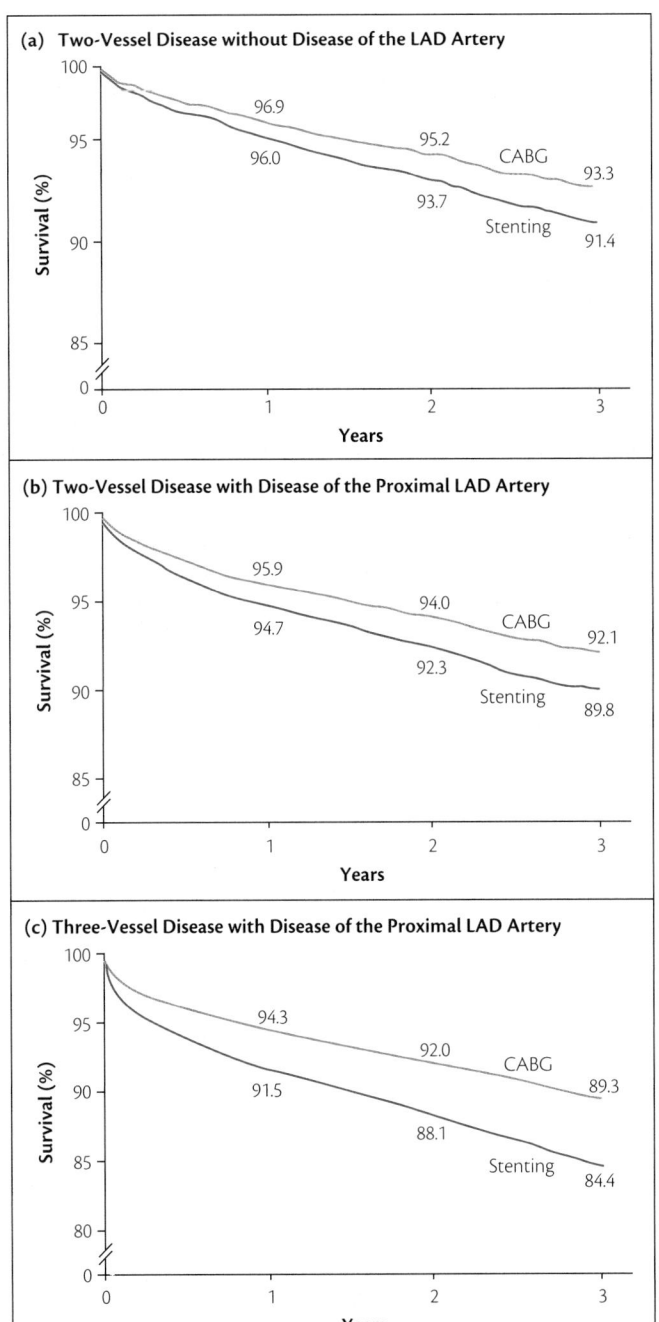

Fig. 16.13.7.3 Long-term survival after coronary artery bypass and percutaneous intervention with bare metal stents according to extent of coronary artery disease.

Antiplatelet therapy

Aspirin reduces vein graft thrombosis from 23% to 13% in the first postoperative year. Doses of between 75 and 300 mg per day are effective, with the first given early after operation and certainly within 48 h. Clopidogrel should be used if aspirin is not tolerated. The superiority of a combination of aspirin and clopidogrel is not established. Warfarin is not indicated to improve graft patency.

Cholesterol reduction

Aggressive reduction of LDL cholesterol to less than 2.5 mmol/litre with a statin reduces saphenous vein graft disease progression and the need for further revascularisation by 30%.

Coronary artery bypass and percutaneous intervention

Randomized studies comparing coronary artery bypass with balloon angioplasty typically show reintervention rates of 50% in the angioplasty group compared to 10% in the surgical arms. The use of bare metal stents halves reintervention after angioplasty. Procedural mortality is similar in both groups, but for patients with diabetes survival at 7 years is 76% with surgery and 56% with PCI. Patients with extensive coronary artery disease have a survival advantage with coronary artery bypass (Fig. 16.13.7.3). Although drug-eluting stents have a reduced restenosis rate in clinical trials, registry data suggest that this may not be as prominent in routine practice. Even with the use of drug-eluting stents, coronary artery bypass remains the gold standard treatment for patients with left main stem stenosis and three-vessel disease.

Further reading

BARI Investigators (2000). Seven year outcome in the bypass angioplasty revascularisation investigation (BARI) by treatment and diabetic status. *J Am Coll Cardiol*, **35**, 1122–9.

Eagle KA, *et al.* (2004). *ACC/AHA guideline update for coronary artery bypass graft surgery.* http://www.acc.org/clinical/guidelines/cabg/cabg.pdf.

Fitzgibbon GM, *et al.* (1991). Coronary bypass graft fate: long term angiographic study. *J Am Coll Cardiol*, **17**, 1075–80.

Goldman S, *et al.* (1989). Saphenous vein graft patency 1 year after coronary artery bypass surgery and effects of antiplatelet therapy. Results of a Veterans Administration Cooperative Study. *Circulation*, **80**, 1190–7.

Hannan EL, *et al.* (2005). Long-term outcomes of coronary-artery bypass grafting versus stent implantation. *N Engl J Med*, **352**, 2174–83.

Hannan EL, *et al.* (2008). Drug-eluting stents vs coronary-artery bypass grafting in multi-vessel coronary disease. *N Engl J Med*, **358**, 331–41.

Loop FD, *et al.* (1986). Influence of the internal mammary artery graft on 10 year survival and other cardiac events. *N Engl J Med*, **314**, 1–6.

Roques F, *et al.* (1999). Risk factors and outcome in European Cardiac surgery: Analysis of the EuroSCORE multinational database of 19030 patients. *Eur J Cardiothorac Surg*, **15**, 816–22.

Serruys PW *et al.* (2009). Percutaneous coronary intervention versus coronary-artery bypass grafting for sever coronary artery disease. *N Engl J Med*, **360**, 961–72.

Society for Cardiothoracic Surgeons (2009). *Sixth national adult cardiac surgical database report 2008.* Dendrite Clinical Systems, Henley-on-Thames.

Taggart DP, D'Amico R, Altman DG (2001). Effect of arterial revascularisation on survival: a systematic review of studies comparing bilateral and single internal mammary arteries. *Lancet*, **358**, 870–75.

Yusuf S, *et al.* (1994). Effect of coronary artery bypass graft surgery on survival: overview of ten-year results from randomized trials by the Coronary Artery Bypass Graft Surgery Trialist Collaboration. *Lancet*, **344**, 563–70.

16.13.8 The impact of coronary heart disease on life and work

Michael C. Petch

Essentials

Coronary heart disease is common and lethal: these facts are well known and have a profound influence on attitudes of victims and others—their families, friends, and employers.

The presence of heart failure and/or significant areas of cardiac ischaemia is the principal determinant of prognosis, and can be determined by history, examination, and noninvasive testing, with common sense and experience being the best tools for assessing an individual's fitness to resume life and work following the development of coronary heart disease.

Following a cardiac event such as myocardial infarction or coronary artery bypass grafting, patients with an acceptable exercise response are often enrolled into a rehabilitation programme. Following myocardial infarction or unstable angina, those with no complications and good exercise tolerance may return to work in about 4 weeks.

The risk of sudden disability and death through ventricular fibrillation is the major factor affecting work capacity amongst victims of coronary heart disease. Workers whose sudden incapacity would place themselves and others at risk are described as being in 'safety-critical' jobs. The best approach to determine whether someone should be able to return to work is to define what level of risk is acceptable, and then decide whether their medical condition places them within the predetermined limits of acceptability. The Civil Aviation Authority was the first to adopt this approach with what is now known as the '1% rule', based on assumptions and calculations indicating that a pilot with a 1% annual risk of a cardiac event has the same risk of 'failing' when flying as other elements of the aircraft.

Ordinary driving may be resumed 1 month after a cardiac event, provided that the driver does not suffer from angina that may be provoked at the wheel. Vocational driving may be permitted at 6 weeks, subject to a satisfactory outcome from noninvasive testing.

Despite modern treatments, some patients will experience multiple coronary events that eventually lead to extensive ventricular damage: they—with their partners, if appropriate—should be given the opportunity of a frank discussion about their prognosis, but some would rather not know and that attitude should be respected.

Introduction

Coronary heart disease is common and lethal (Tables 16.13.8.1 and 16.13.8.2). In developed countries, heart attacks account for about one-quarter of all deaths. Death is often sudden. These facts are well known and have a profound influence on attitudes towards the victims of heart disease. Employers are reluctant to take back people who have lost time off work as a result of a heart problem. Spouses become overprotective. The survivors are acutely aware that they have received an intimation of their mortality; some fail to cope. The first manifestation of coronary heart disease, which is usually chest pain, prompts re-evaluation of the remainder of life and work. The spectre of cardiac pain and death hangs over many a middle-aged man, including employers, politicians, public health physicians, journalists, and others in positions of influence. In most developed countries there is therefore public pressure to prevent the development of coronary disease (primary prevention), to prevent a recurrence (secondary prevention), and to put in place measures that will reduce the risk of harm to the individual and others in the event of sudden incapacity/death of a worker in a 'safety-critical' job.

Women are not immune, but for them coronary heart disease tends to strike later, often after usual retirement age. Nevertheless, the impact of coronary heart disease can be as devastating: older women are often the most important carers in a family. Although there are minor differences between the sexes in the presentation and management of coronary heart disease, the comments in this chapter should be taken to apply to both sexes.

Life before coronary heart disease

Most people do not think about their health until it goes wrong. With advancing years people become aware that their contemporaries are suffering from mortal diseases and belatedly begin to look at their own lifestyle. Many believe the results of the latest research quoted in the press and attempt to adapt their habits by increasing their intake of vitamin E, or fish oil, or red wine, or by reducing the amount of coffee and animal fat that they consume, or by undergoing stress counselling, or by purchasing an exercise machine that they never use. Then along comes a new report and another fashion is spawned.

There are a few public health issues on which the medical profession can speak with authority. Cigarette smoking is the prime example. Doctors, nurses, and other health care professionals have a duty to discourage this habit by example and by persuasion. No other habit enjoys such powerful evidence that mandates a lifestyle change. Regular exercise is to be commended. A prudent diet is capable of different interpretations, but the old adage 'a little of what you fancy does you good' dates back many generations to a time when coronary heart disease was much less common. Food can be one of life's great pleasures. The current political ambition to change national lifestyles is not heeded by those most at risk and has never been clearly shown to have lasting benefit.

A sensible compromise for most societies is to prevent smoking, encourage exercise, promote the sale of fruit and vegetables, and reduce the availability of junk foods in shops and workplace canteens, but not to go to such lengths that people feel guilty when faced with a delicious steak. The fact that most doctors share this epicurean attitude makes it all the more persuasive. The use of drugs such as aspirin and statins to reduce the risk of a coronary event can

Table 16.13.8.1 Deaths by cause, sex, and age, 2006, United Kingdom

		All ages	Under 35	35–44	45–54	55–64	65–74	75+
All causes	Men	273 488	9 015	7 439	14 300	31 856	56 175	154 703
	Women	297 546	4 823	4 416	9 421	20 775	40 175	217 936
	Total	571 034	13 838	11 855	23 721	52 631	96 350	372 639
All diseases of the circulatory system (I10–I99)								
	Men	94 987	548	1 521	4 254	10 068	19 276	59 320
	Women	102 780	315	634	1 537	3 892	11 279	85 123
	Total	197 767	863	2 155	5 791	13 960	30 555	144 443
Coronary heart disease (I20–I25)								
	Men	52 585	114	834	2 809	6 802	11 885	30 141
	Women	41 796	34	185	588	1 883	5 494	33 612
	Total	94 381	148	1 019	3 397	8 685	17 379	63 753
Stroke (I60–I69)								
	Men	21 267	113	220	578	1 284	3 295	15 777
	Women	33 831	77	193	490	927	2 821	29 323
	Total	55 098	190	413	1 068	2 211	6 116	45 100

Notes: ICD codes in parentheses.
Source: England and Wales, Office for National Statistics (2008) personal communication.
Scotland, General Register Office (2008) personal communication.
Northern Ireland, General Register Office Statistics and Research Agency (2008) personal communication.

likewise only be justified in those individuals whose risk is especially high, as judged by their family history and other risk factors.

Health screening is another controversial topic. In (over)-developed societies screening services have become very popular and assessment of cardiovascular risk in businessmen is a useful source of income for some clinics. Certainly the measurement of blood pressure can be supported and, in some circumstances, the estimation of serum lipids. Beyond that the advice that may be offered boils down to common sense—don't smoke, take more exercise, and eat less.

Table 16.13.8.2 Inpatient cases by main diagnosis and sex, National Health Service hospitals, 2006/07, England and Scotland

	England		Scotland	
	Men	**Women**	**Men**	**Women**
All diagnoses	6 483 429	6 940 203	603 757	676 463
All diseases of the circulatory system (I00–I99)	705 822	549 768	75 155	62 882
Coronary heart disease (I20–I25)	276 900	151 013	30 223	18 351
Angina pectoris (I20)	71 343	52 446	6 600	5 026
Acute myocardial infarction (I21)	70 404	42 757	9 654	6 412
Other coronary heart disease (I25)	135 153	55 810	13 969	6 913
Heart failure (I50)	51 541	8 941	5 392	5 196
Stroke (I60–I69)	84 271	92 181	9 483	10 648

Notes: Finished consultant episodes; ordinary admissions and day cases combined.
Pregnancy cases are not included. ICD codes (10th version) in parentheses.
Source: Department of Health (2008) Hospital Episode statistics 2006/07.
www.hesonline.nhs.uk
Information services Division Scotland (2008) Main diagnosis discharges from hospital 2006/07. www.isdscotland.org

Health screening nowadays commonly includes exercise testing with ECG monitoring. False-positive results suggesting silent coronary disease occur in up to 15% of middle-aged people, depending upon the criteria used. The psychological effect can be devastating. This investigation can only be justified when the individual is aware of the possible outcomes of screening and/or is in a safety-critical job. The ability of multislice CT to detect coronary calcification has further complicated this area of medical practice: it is readily available to those who are prepared to pay, and the subsequent management of those individuals is uncertain because long-term follow-up of those with abnormal findings is not available. The radiation exposure means that the investigation should not be undertaken without due consideration. The finding of minimal calcification is particularly difficult to interpret and has prompted the aphorism 'the normal person is merely the one who has not been adequately investigated'.

Life and work with coronary heart disease

The risk of sudden disability and death through ventricular fibrillation is the major factor affecting work capacity amongst victims of coronary heart disease. The risk is greatest in the early days following the development of symptoms and in those with most extensive coronary disease and/or with most myocardial damage.

Common sense and experience (i.e. clinical judgement) remain the best tools for assessing an individual's fitness to resume life and work following the development of coronary heart disease. The onset of cardiac pain, or change in the nature of pain in someone with known ischaemic heart disease, should prompt rapid evaluation. Stable angina pectoris, preferably confirmed by exercise testing, usually requires no change in lifestyle: modern drug therapy is very effective and often comprises just aspirin, glyceryl trinitrate, and a statin. Unstable angina or myocardial infarction is a different matter and necessitates hospital admission, with further investigation. Even then clinical judgement remains the basis for advice about lifestyle changes, supplemented by noninvasive tests.

The presence of heart failure and/or significant areas of ischaemia are the principal determinants of prognosis. The former may be identified by history, clinical examination, chest radiography and echocardiography; the latter by the development of angina and electrocardiographic ST segment shift on exercise testing. An exercise test may also reveal cardiovascular incapacity in other ways, e.g. exhaustion, inappropriate heart rate and blood pressure responses, and arrhythmia.

Following myocardial infarction or unstable angina, assessment of prognosis along the lines outlined above is recommended: those with no complications and good exercise tolerance may return to work in about 4 weeks. This applies particularly to younger individuals whose employers need have little hesitation in taking them back to their former job, perhaps part-time initially. A few will take longer to recover, and some will need a change of job.

Limitation of working capacity and the risk of sudden incapacity can both be well judged in populations by specialist opinion, aided by the results of noninvasive tests. However, the progression of coronary disease can be unpredictable, and individuals judged to be at low risk from further cardiovascular events can suffer recurrences. This difference between the individual and the population is not well understood by employers and employees and can be a source of misunderstanding and confusion. Nevertheless, individual exceptions do not invalidate the principles on which recommendations are made.

Percutaneous coronary intervention (PCI)

Patients with persistent angina, or those with a very abnormal exercise response, should undergo coronary arteriography with a view to myocardial revascularization. PCI invariably nowadays involves the insertion of a stent and is a straightforward, safe procedure that can be very effective in relieving angina. Resumption of normal activities, including work, is normally possible a few days afterwards. Recurrent angina is much less common with the more widespread use of drug-eluting stents, which have reduced the risk of restenosis almost to zero. There is a small risk of late stent thrombosis, but the absolute risk is so small that there should be no significant impact on lifestyle and ability to work. Recovery is rapid and most people are back at work within a few days.

Acute myocardial infarction with ST segment elevation is now best managed by immediate coronary angiography and stenting, which is preferable to thrombolytic treatment provided that the intervention can be performed within two hours. Acute coronary syndromes should similarly prompt early angiography and intervention when appropriate. With increasing experience of the success of acute PCI, guidelines concerned with the resumption of normal activities following a coronary event, e.g. work and travel, are likely to recommend even shorter periods of convalescence. This is both because recovery times are shorter than with previous therapy and because the state of the coronary arteries and left ventricle are known, hence further risk assessment is superfluous.

Coronary artery bypass grafting

Coronary artery bypass grafting is also remarkably safe, with most centres reporting mortality rates of less than 1% for elective operations. Recovery is rapid and most patients resume work within 2 to 3 months of surgery. Almost all are relieved of their angina. Patients who were able to work before surgery should generally be able to do so afterwards, and restrictions that may have been appropriate previously should no longer be relevant. However, since surgery is a dramatic event, it may prompt overprotective attitudes amongst family members, friends, employers, or even medical advisers. Many individuals who could and should return to work fail to do so for this reason, rather than because of continuing incapacity. No special restrictions are usually necessary after return to work. Coronary graft stenosis and occlusion leads to recurrence of angina at a rate of about 4% per year. This is generally less severe than previously but will affect long-term occupational planning. The short recovery times, safety, and efficacy of PCI has meant that this procedure is the preferred method of myocardial revascularization, with approximately three times as many procedures being performed in most developed countries; 73 000 PCI procedures as compared with 25 000 bypass operations in the United Kingdom in 2005.

Rehabilitation programmes

Rehabilitation programmes are now well established in many hospitals and communities. These enable patients to make a full physical and psychological recovery following a cardiac event such as myocardial infarction or coronary artery bypass grafting. An acceptable exercise response is a prerequisite for enrolment into a rehabilitation programme. The participants are thus the fittest survivors, selected for physical retraining on the strength of their satisfactory performance on the treadmill. Definite measures of benefit, such as reduction in recurrent myocardial infarction or death, are lacking.

The popularity of cardiac rehabilitation owes much to the enthusiasm of the participants—patients and staff alike—but may also be a reflection of modern cardiological practice with its mechanistic approach, haste, and failure to recognize the psychological and lifestyle implications of a diagnosis of heart disease. Sex, for example, is rarely discussed except in rehabilitation classes, yet for many patients it is a burning issue. The mechanistic view is that the physical effort required is equivalent to two flights of stairs or stage 3 of the Bruce protocol; the psychological aspects are less easy to quantitate.

Risk evaluation

The 1% rule

Workers whose sudden incapacity would place themselves and others at risk are described as being in 'safety-critical' jobs. The traditional approach to this dilemma was to exclude anyone with heart disease from working in such an environment. This may still be appropriate in occupations where any increased risk of incapacity is unacceptable: drivers of mainline passenger trains and captains of ocean-going vessels are two current examples. However, this blanket exclusion is patently unfair to some, and may waste the skills and experience of a valued employee. Also, no individual is totally free of risk of an incapacitating event, and a few accidents as a result of sudden illness in apparently normal people are inevitable.

A better approach is to define what level of risk is acceptable, and then decide whether the medical condition places an individual within the predetermined limits of acceptability. This has the great merit of objectivity, and is a well-tried engineering practice.

The Civil Aviation Authority was the first to adopt this approach with what is now known as the '1% rule'. Aircraft engineers have always recognized that a disaster may occur as a result of component failure, and have recommended design and safety features so that the risk of failure is 'extremely improbable' ($1/10^9$ flying hours). If a number of assumptions are made this approximates to a risk of an incapacitating event in a pilot of 1% per year, which happens to be the average annual risk of a heart attack in men aged 45 to 64 years. A pilot with a medical condition may therefore be regarded as a component of aircraft safety and hold a licence if his risk of a cardiovascular event is comparable, i.e. his risk is no greater than his peers or other parts of the aircraft.

There are a number of difficulties in applying the approach described above to other situations and other industries. First, who decides an acceptable level? Second, the epidemiological data generally describe events such as death or heart attack, which may not be the relevant parameter. A heart attack, for example, is a rare cause of road traffic accident; more commonly the driver is found in his vehicle on the verge, 'slumped over the wheel with the engine still running'. Death may have been sudden in epidemiological terms, but it was not instantaneous; the victim had sufficient warning to pull over to the side of the road. Third, some incapacitating events, neurocardiogenic syncope for example, are clearly relevant to many safety-critical jobs, and yet there are scant data on which to base an objective decision. Fourth, cardiovascular event rates have fallen since the 1% rule was formulated. Nevertheless, the approach is to be commended, and objectivity may be further improved by the use of quantifiable investigations such as exercise testing and echocardiography.

Exercise testing

The data on exercise testing in coronary heart disease are the best established for evaluating the risk of incapacity in employees in safety-critical jobs, e.g. vocational driving. The guidelines relating to vocational drivers were developed in the United Kingdom and adapted by a Task Force of the European Society of Cardiology. They are now being applied more widely to other groups of workers whose occupation may involve an element of risk to themselves or others should that individual suffer cardiovascular collapse.

The protocol for which most information is available is that described by Bruce. He and Fisher examined strategies for risk evaluation of sudden cardiac incapacitation in men in occupations affecting public safety: 2373 men with clinically manifest coronary artery disease who had undergone exercise evaluation were followed up for a mean of 61 months; 300 sudden cardiac incapacitations (cardiac arrest or sudden cardiac death) occurred. Exercise testing in all age groups defined low- and high-risk populations with annual incapacitation rates of 1 and 3%, respectively. The former were those who could reach stage 3 of the Bruce protocol with no chest pain, attain 85% of age-predicted maximal heart rate, and manifest less than 1 mm of ischaemic ST segment depression. A similar message came from the study of 4083 medically treated patients in the Coronary Artery Surgical Study registry. The 32% of patients who could exercise into stage 3 of the Bruce protocol with less than 1 mm ST segment depression on ECG (10 METS) had an annual mortality of 1% or less. By contrast, the annual mortality rate of the 730 patients with 2 mm or greater ST depression was 3.6%, ranging from 5.6% for those patients achieving stage 1 or less of exercise to 2.0% for those patients achieving stage 3. The study also confirmed the overriding prognostic importance of left ventricular function and the poor survival of patients with heart failure. An ability to exceed stage 3 of the Bruce protocol with less than 2 mm of ST segment depression is the best criterion for identifying a population with an annual risk of death of less than 2%.

Driving

Since decisions concerning fitness to drive should be objective and evidence-based whenever possible, a similar approach to that described for pilots is being adopted. An attempt is also being made to be consistent, so that all forms of illness that might cause sudden incapacity should be considered in comparable manner. One condition for which good data are available is epilepsy. Currently the agreed annual acceptable risk of a seizure in the United Kingdom is 2% for vocational drivers and 20% for ordinary drivers, and a driver's licence entitlement can be determined by reference to well-validated tables of risk, e.g. following a head injury.

The risk of incapacity in drivers with cardiovascular disorders is less easy to quantify; incapacitating syncope occurs in elderly drivers with no structural cardiovascular disorder, whilst others who are apparently at high risk of a cardiac arrest remain asymptomatic for years. However, some drivers with heart disease can be identified as being at an increased risk of an incapacitating event, and attempts are being made in the transport industry and elsewhere to provide objective criteria, which will be applicable across a range of disease processes. Detailed advice is available from http://www.dvla.gov.uk in the section entitled 'Medical rules, at a glance guide'.

The 2% rule may prove to be the correct criterion for vocational drivers and other workers in similar occupations who suffer from cardiovascular disorders. Society already accepts drivers with vocational licences up to the age of 80 years, by which time their annual risk of a cardiovascular event is 4%. If the assumption is made that half of the events are incapacitating then the acceptable risk accords with the epilepsy criteria, so those drivers whose annual risk of a cardiovascular event is 4% (or death 2%) or greater should not be entitled to hold a vocational licence.

For ordinary drivers a 20% annual risk also seems reasonable for cardiovascular disorders; such a level of risk is in accord with existing guidelines, e.g. shortly after a heart attack. Ordinary driving may be resumed 1 month after a cardiac event provided that the driver does not suffer from angina that may be provoked at the wheel. Vocational driving may be permitted at 6 weeks, subject to a satisfactory outcome from noninvasive testing. In the United Kingdom, ordinary driving licence holders do not need to notify the Driver and Vehicle Licensing Agency (DVLA) if they have made a good recovery and have no continuing disability, but vocational drivers must notify the DVLA. Insurance companies vary in their requirements, but most policies are temporarily invalidated by illness.

Special circumstances

Stress

In the 1950s Friedman and his colleagues developed the idea that chronic psychological stress had a role in the aetiology of coronary heart disease. They described the 'type A personality' who had hectic work patterns marked by long hours and organizational chaos, competitiveness, time urgency, and aggression; such individuals seemed particularly prone to heart attacks and sudden cardiac death. Subsequent studies in Europe had difficulty in identifying the type A personality, but better definition of personality traits, such as concealed hostility and failure to cope have been incorporated into questionnaires that have permitted the conclusion that chronic psychological stress is a risk factor for the development of coronary heart disease. Scientific respectability for the role of chronic stress as a risk factor for the development of myocardial infarction came with the publication of the INTERHEART study, which assessed psychological stress from four simple questions about stress at work and at home, financial stress, and major life events in the preceding year, with additional questions assessing the perceived ability to control life circumstances and the presence of depression.

The idea that an acutely stressful incident may trigger a heart attack is also well embedded in Western culture. This has always enjoyed biological plausibility and has more recently acquired scientific credibility. John Hunter was the first to observe that stress could cause angina when he said that he "was at the mercy of any man that would provoke him". Some increase in the incidence of myocardial infarction or sudden cardiac death has long been recognized after environmental disturbances such as a major earthquake or military assault. However, to argue that such events are triggers is more difficult because the background level of myocardial infarction or sudden cardiac death in any developed community is very high. There are approximately 12 deaths an hour from coronary heart disease in the United Kingdom. Acute physical and psychological distress is likewise very common. Patients and their relatives can almost invariably point to a stressful incident prior to a heart attack and may forget that life is a series of stressful incidents, that heart attacks are extremely common, and coincidences are inevitable, but studies using the epidemiological case crossover control method have identified some events as occurring so much more frequently before a heart attack or sudden cardiac death that they can be recognized as a trigger. The best evidence relates to sudden unaccustomed vigorous effort shortly before (within 2 h of) the attack, especially in emotionally distressed individuals. Anger or acute psychological distress by itself may be a trigger, but this is more difficult to substantiate because of the problem of quantifying psychological stress. The preceding event obviously needs to be sufficiently disturbing to promote the release of catecholamines and provoke the 'fight or flight' reaction with an acceleration of heart rate, surge in systolic blood pressure, and increase in ventricular irritability.

The relationship between stress and coronary heart disease has assumed importance for two reasons. First, there may be therapeutic implications: counselling to reduce stress levels before or after a heart attack is commercially available, but there are no outcome data. Second, there has been a huge tide of litigation, generally initiated by bereaved relatives who have been encouraged by solicitors to pursue a claim on the grounds that an action triggered a heart attack. Hitherto a Court of Law has required very persuasive evidence of a causal relationship for a case to succeed: 'shopkeeper dies chasing thieves' would be such an example; chronic stress has not yet been accepted as a reason for a settlement.

Travel

Following a cardiac event such as myocardial infarction, individuals should convalesce at home and not travel far for 4 to 6 weeks. Those with no evidence of continuing myocardial ischaemia or heart failure can then travel freely within their own country for pleasure, e.g. a holiday. Business and overseas travel is more problematic because the physical and psychological demands are greater. Additional difficulties for the overseas traveller include the uncertain provision of coronary care facilities in some countries and the justifiable reluctance of insurance companies to provide health cover. Such travel is best deferred until 3 months have elapsed and any necessary further investigations and treatment have been carried out to ensure cardiovascular fitness.

Overseas travel for those with continuing cardiovascular unfitness need not be ruled out. Utilizing the airport services for disabled travellers can ease a passenger through the irritations of customs and passport control at major airports. Modern aircraft can be very comfortable. The cabins are kept at a pressure equivalent to 2000 m so that those with angina are not likely to experience an attack. Businessmen with continuing cardiac disorders may therefore fly to Europe, North America, and other countries with good coronary care services with very little risk. But flights in unpressurized aircraft, work in undeveloped countries or in remote areas of the world, and work in a hostile environment (both climatic and political) are best avoided.

Aircrew are subject to guidelines drawn up by the Joint Aviation Authorities. In the United Kingdom the regulatory agency is the Civil Aviation Authority, whose advice should always be sought.

Cardiac deaths are uncommon in trekkers or workers at high altitude (2440–4570 m). The increase in cardiac output at altitude will exacerbate symptoms in those who already experience symptoms at sea level, but asymptomatic individuals with coronary heart disease are unlikely to be at special risk.

Particular occupations

Exposure to toxic substances

Work involving exposure to certain hazardous substances may aggravate pre-existing coronary heart disease and careful consideration should be given to patients who are returning to jobs involving exposure to chemical vapours and fumes. Methylene chloride, a main ingredient of many commonly used paint removers, is rapidly metabolized to carbon monoxide in the body, and in poorly ventilated work areas blood levels of carboxyhaemoglobin can become elevated enough to precipitate angina or even myocardial infarction. A blood carboxyhaemoglobin level of 2 to 4% has been shown to be associated with impairment of cardiovascular function in patients with angina pectoris. The World Health Organization recommends a maximum carboxyhaemoglobin level of 5% for healthy industrial workers and a maximum of 2.5% for susceptible persons in the general population exposed to ambient air pollution: this level may also be applied to workers whose jobs entail specific exposure to carbon monoxide, such as car park attendants and furnace workers. To ensure that the 2.5% carboxyhaemoglobin level is not exceeded, the ambient carbon monoxide concentration should not be higher than 10 ppm over an 8-h working day: equivalent to exposure to the current occupational exposure standard (50 ppm) for no more than 30 min. Occupational exposure to carbon disulphide in the viscose rayon manufacturing industry is a recognized causal factor of coronary heart disease, but the mechanism remains unclear.

Reports of sudden death from angina are well recognized in dynamite workers, particularly after a period of 36 to 72 h away from work and following re-exposure, an effect almost certainly related to direct action of nitroglycerine on the blood vessels of the heart or peripheral circulation. Individuals with clinical evidence of coronary heart disease should avoid occupational exposure to these substances.

Solvents such as trichloroethylene or 1,1,1-trichloroethane may cause sudden death in workers receiving heavy exposure in poorly ventilated workplaces. The chlorofluorocarbon CFC-113 has been implicated in sudden cardiac deaths and CFC-22 has been reported to cause arrhythmias. Some industrial workers will need proper assessment of their workplace by an occupational physician and occupational hygienist so that they can be advised on their suitability for work handling chlorinated hydrocarbon solvents or involving exposure to gases.

There are no formal medical requirements for workers who have to enter confined spaces where there may be hazards of oxygen deficiency or a build up of toxic gases. Those with heart disease or severe hypertension may need to be excluded. Certain occupations may require the use of special breathing apparatus either routinely (e.g. asbestos-removal workers), or in emergencies (e.g. water workers handling chlorine cylinders). The additional cardiorespiratory effort required while wearing a respirator, combined with the general physical exertion that may be required, usually means that people with a previous history of coronary heart disease are excluded from such work.

Seafarers

The Merchant Shipping (Medical Examination) Regulations in the United Kingdom have recently been revised along the lines of DVLA to take into account the nature of the job, and the likelihood of a further coronary event. The previously draconian regulation that any manifestation of ischaemic heart disease rendered the seafarer unfit to return to sea has been rescinded. The current regulations apply to vessels registered in the United Kingdom above a certain size (a small coaster upwards). They do not necessarily apply to vessels registered in other countries. For more detail see http://www.mcga.gov.uk.

Working in hot conditions

Working in hot conditions may prove hazardous for some patients with heart disease. High ambient temperatures or significant heat radiation from hot surfaces or liquid metal, added to the physical strain of heavy work, will produce vasodilatation of muscle and skin vessels. Compensatory vascular and cardiac reactions to maintain central blood pressure may be inadequate and lead to reduced cerebral or coronary artery blood flow. The possibility of syncope will be enhanced by the use of drugs with vasodilating and negative inotropic actions; some reduction in dosage may be necessary.

Working in cold conditions

Cold exacerbates myocardial ischaemia. Individuals with coronary heart disease should therefore exercise caution. Impaired circulation to the limbs will result in an increased likelihood of claudication, risk of damage to skin (frostbite), and poor recovery from accidental injury to skin and deeper structures.

Implanted devices

Cardiac pacemakers are generally implanted into older patients who have idiopathic degeneration of their conduction system.

However, both heart block and sinoatrial disorder are well-recognized complications of coronary heart disease. Single- and dual-chamber (invariably VVI or DDD) pacemakers are rarely vulnerable to electromagnetic interference and no modification of lifestyle is necessary, although patients should know that their device can trigger alarms at airports and elsewhere.

The implantable cardioverter–defibrillator (ICD) has the capacity to detect and treat ventricular tachycardia and fibrillation, either by antitachycardia pacing or by a shock, in patients in whom a further cardiac arrest is anticipated. Both the shock and the arrhythmia are potentially incapacitating. In North America and Europe, patients with ICDs have restrictions placed upon them, e.g. with regard to driving. They commonly have severe underlying heart disease and may well not be able to work, but if they can do so, then this should be in an environment that is free from electromagnetic interference. There has been one report of ICD malfunction in the vicinity of an electronic antitheft surveillance system.

There has been considerable interest in the possibility that mobile telephones might interfere with pacemakers and ICDs. Studies have shown that this is a theoretical possibility and that reprogramming of a pacemaker can be achieved under exceptional circumstances if the telephone is held close (<20 cm) to the pacemaker. In practice no clinically significant interference has yet been reported, but individuals are advised to use the hand and ear furthest from the pacemaker and not to 'dial' with the telephone near to the pacemaker.

Retirement and end of life

Despite modern treatments some patients will experience multiple coronary events that eventually lead to extensive ventricular damage and persisting symptoms of fatigue and dyspnoea, with signs of heart failure. Such individuals should be warned of their limited prognosis. Some should be advised to retire, which is never an easy decision.

There is commonly a discrepancy between an individual's symptoms and the objective cardiac data. For some patients a heart attack proves devastating: the man who has always enjoyed robust good health may appear to be very symptomatic despite good ventricular function and no evidence of continuing myocardial ischaemia. One explanation for this is the profound psychological disturbance that sometimes follows the development of cardiovascular disease. At the other extreme some patients seem well and active despite appalling ventricular function, although puzzlingly for the lay observer they are prone to experience sudden cardiac death despite apparently being 'so well'. As always, common sense has to override the results of investigations, and individuals can defy the predictions made on the basis of good epidemiological outcome data.

Patients (with their partners if appropriate) should be given the opportunity of a frank discussion about their prognosis, but some would rather not know and that attitude should be respected. However, most need to put their affairs in order, and what to say exactly is one of the most difficult problems in cardiology. The victim's quality of life may be excellent. There is no point in advising a restricted lifestyle or retirement. The only definite lifestyle trigger of a heart attack, namely sudden unexpected vigorous exercise, should be avoided. Otherwise, normal activities should continue, with the knowledge that the chance of successful resuscitation following a coronary event are greater in developed countries, in fact better in most of Europe and North America than in the United Kingdom.

Early retirement on grounds of ill health following a coronary event is sometimes seen as an attractive option. However, most permanent sickness policies contain a clause which states that benefit will only be payable if the subscriber is 'totally unable to follow his former occupation', which is often not the case after a heart attack or coronary artery bypass grafting. Advice about retirement should only be given after due consideration and a review of the job terms and conditions.

Further reading

Joy MD (ed.) (1999). Second European Workshop in Aviation Cardiology. *Eur Heart J*, Suppl D.

Petch MC (1998). Task Force Report: driving and heart disease. *Eur Heart J*, **19**, 1165–77.

Price A, Petch MC (2007). Cardiovascular disorders. In: Palmer K, Cox RAF, Brown I (eds) *Fitness for work*, 4th edition. Oxford University Press, Oxford.

Rosengren A, *et al.* (2005). Association of psychological risk factors with risk of acute myocardial infarction in 11 119 cases and 13 648 controls from 52 countries (the INTERHEART study): case-control study. *Lancet*, **364**, 953–62.

Stansfield SA, Marmot MG (2002). *Stress and the heart*. BMJ Books, London.

16.14

Diseases of the arteries

Contents

16.14.1 Thoracic aortic dissection

Andrew R.J. Mitchell and Adrian P. Banning

Essentials

Acute dissection of the thoracic aorta is uncommon, but if left unrecognized and untreated it carries a mortality rate of up to 2% per hour and 50% within the first few weeks.

Clinical presentation—the pain of acute dissection is typically of instantaneous onset, cataclysmic in severity, pulsatile and tearing in quality, located either in the anterior thorax or back, and migrating as it follows the course of the dissection through the thorax. Patients usually appear shocked, but blood pressure may be normal or raised and heart rate relatively slow. Physical signs typically reflect the region of the aorta involved in the dissection and effects of pressure on adjacent structures: evidence of new aortic regurgitation or development of pulse deficits should be actively sought.

Diagnosis—abnormalities on the chest radiograph and ECG are common, but neither investigation is diagnostic and further imaging is always necessary by MRI, contrast-enhanced CT, or transoesophageal echocardiography, depending on local availability and the clinical condition of the patient.

Management—every patient with a clinical suspicion of dissection should receive effective pain relief and antihypertensive medication (intravenous labetalol or esmolol), aiming to maintain systolic blood pressure <120 mmHg. For confirmed dissection of the ascending aorta (type A), emergency surgery is indicated. When the ascending aorta is spared (type B), aggressive control of blood pressure is the usual initial management, with surgery being considered if there is evidence of further progression of dissection or ischaemic complications. In the long term, strenuous efforts to control blood pressure are indicated for all patients who have survived aortic dissection, with repeat imaging at least once a year.

Other related aortic conditions—modern imaging techniques have demonstrated variants of acute aortic dissection, including spontaneous intramural haematoma, with 50% of patients subsequently developing dissection or aortic rupture, and penetrating atherosclerotic ulcer, which has a high risk of rupture.

Introduction

Aortic dissection is one of the acute thoracic aortic syndromes, encompassing aortic dissection, intramural haematoma, and penetrating aortic ulcer. It should be considered, even if only briefly, in the differential diagnosis of most patients complaining of acute chest pain. The history and presenting signs often clinch the diagnosis, which is confirmed by appropriate noninvasive investigations. The consequences of missing aortic dissection can be disastrous.

Pathogenesis

The aortic wall is composed of three layers: a thin intimal lining, a thicker medial layer (largely composed of elastin fibres that provide strength), and a thinner adventitial outer layer from which small blood vessels (the vasa vasorum) arise to nourish the outer layers of the media. Dissection occurs when a breach in the integrity of the intima allows blood at high pressure to penetrate the media. Through this tear, pulsatile blood flow can then propagate distally, parallel to the lumen, often spiralling and splitting the arterial wall into an inner (intima–medial) and outer layer (media–adventitia). This process of tearing within the wall results in the

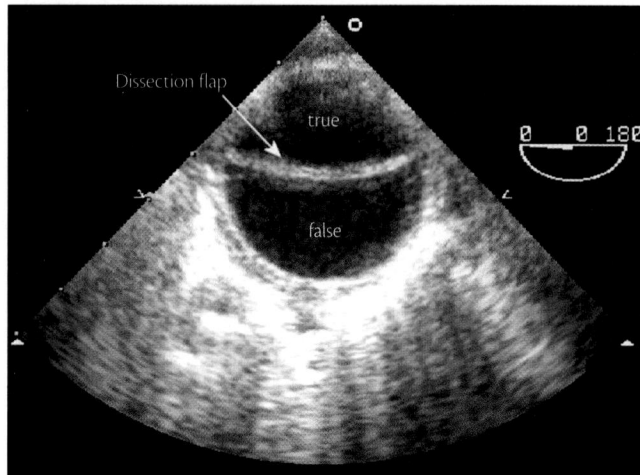

Fig. 16.14.1.1 Transoesophageal echocardiography of the descending aorta showing a dissection flap separating the true and false lumens.

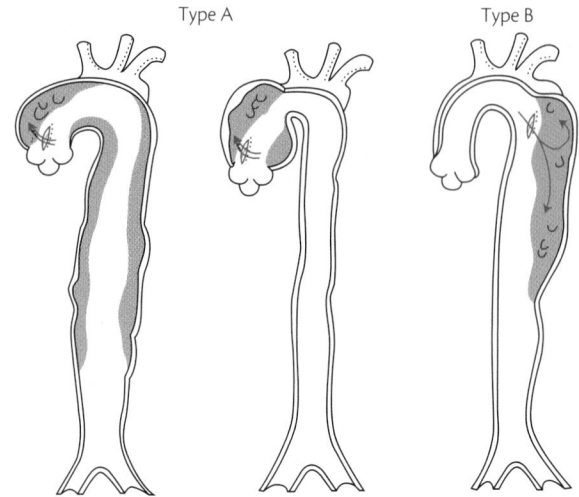

Fig. 16.14.1.2 The Stanford classification of aortic dissection. Type A dissection involves the ascending aorta, irrespective of the distal extent of dissection.

formation of a false lumen, parallel to the original true lumen, and commonly of a similar or larger size (Fig. 16.14.1.1).

Further communication between the lumens (or re-entry tears) can occur and may reduce the pressure within the false lumen, thus limiting propagation of the dissection. However, the process often extends along the entire length of the aorta to the common iliac arteries, threatening the origins of branch vessels that may be avulsed or narrowed by the mass effect of the false lumen, and leading to ischaemia in the dependent vascular territories. When dissection extends retrogradely towards the heart it can cause occlusion of a coronary artery and distortion of the aortic valve, resulting in acute aortic regurgitation. Dissection may also rupture into the pericardial space, causing cardiac tamponade. The weakened aortic wall can rupture at any point along its length, which is usually fatal.

Classification

The commonest sites for thoracic aortic dissection to originate are in the ascending aorta, just above the sinuses of the aortic valve, and in the upper descending aorta just beyond the origin of the left subclavian artery. The Stanford group proposed a classification that is directly linked to patient management (Fig. 16.14.1.2). Aortic dissection that involves the ascending thoracic aorta is classified as type A and demands consideration of immediate surgery, whereas dissection that spares the ascending aorta is classified as type B and initial management is usually medical.

Aetiology

The most common predisposing risk factor (70% of patients) for aortic dissection is hypertension. Although the processes involved in the initiation of dissection remain incompletely understood, medial haemorrhage from rupture of vasa vasorum appears to be important. When this process is self-limiting and there is no expansion of the resultant haematoma by recurrent bleeding, healing may occur with reabsorption of the haemorrhage. Alternatively, and particularly when the bleeding is extensive or recurrent, a large intramural haematoma may form around the circumference

of the aorta. This alters the distribution of tensile stresses within the aorta, with much of the redistributed stress affecting the intima/endothelium overlying the mass. An intimal tear may then result in splitting and separation of the media, propagation of a false lumen, and dissection.

Patients with Marfan's syndrome (see Chapter 16.11) may present with aortic dissection or aortic root dilatation and aortic regurgitation (Fig. 16.14.1.3). Abnormal fibrillin within the aortic media results in intimal instability, particularly when aortic dilation leads to increased wall stress. Although the absolute risk of dissection rises with increasing size of the ascending aorta, it is important to remember that all patients with Marfan's syndrome are at risk, particularly when there is a family history of aortic

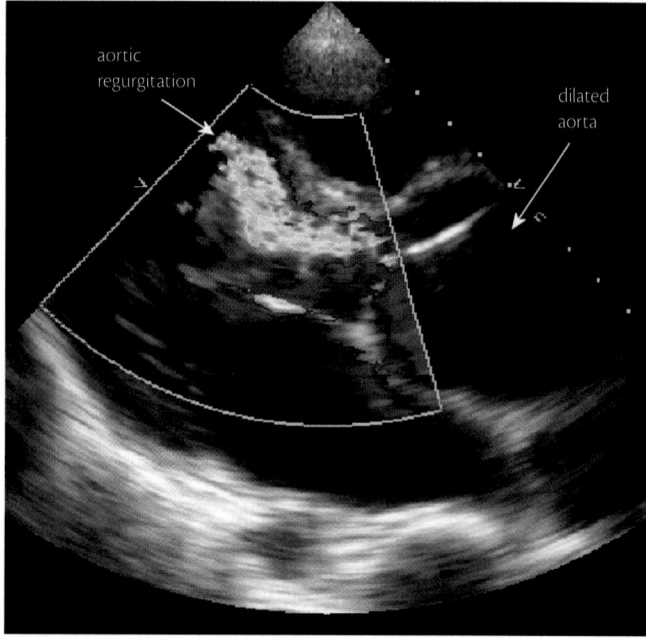

Fig. 16.14.1.3 Transthoracic echocardiography in a patient with Marfan syndrome. The aortic root is significantly dilated with a central jet of aortic regurgitation.

dissection. Patients with Ehlers–Danlos syndrome are also at risk of spontaneous dissection, not only of the aorta but of its principal branches, including the coronary arteries.

Patients with coarctation of the aorta and those with bicuspid aortic valves also appear to be at increased risk of dissection, possibly related to defects in aortic wall composition. Dissection may also occur in patients with Turner's syndrome, Noonan's syndrome, and in the later stages of pregnancy, particularly in patients with Marfan's syndrome. In high-risk patients with Marfan's syndrome with dilated aortas or a family history of dissection, deferring pregnancy until after elective aortic root replacement may be advisable.

Clinical features

Most patients present with characteristic symptoms and clinical findings, in which case the diagnosis of dissection can be made with reasonable assurance. However, a few present atypically and it is worth considering the possibility of aortic dissection in any patient who is haemodynamically unstable without satisfactory explanation.

The pain of acute dissection of the aorta can be described in terms of its (1) instantaneous onset, (2) cataclysmic severity, (3) pulsatile and tearing quality, (4) location either in the anterior thorax or back, and (5) migration as it follows the course of the dissection through the thorax. Careful interrogation about the presence of these five features will usually allow differentiation from other causes of chest pain. The instant onset, tearing/pulsatile quality, and migratory pattern contrast with the pain of cardiac ischaemia, which is usually gradual in onset (over minutes), tight or crushing, and more unchanging in its distribution in the anterior chest. Syncope shortly after the onset of typical pain is not common, but is another characteristic presentation of dissection, often caused by rupture of the false lumen into the pericardial cavity. Other uncommon modes of presentation include stroke and limb ischaemia, with or without pain, and very occasionally congestive heart failure resulting from severe aortic regurgitation.

Although patients with dissection usually appear shocked, their blood pressure may be normal or raised and their heart rate relatively slow. The distribution of the abnormalities detected by physical examination usually reflect the region of the aorta involved in the dissection and pressure on adjacent structures. Signs of aortic regurgitation or tamponade are likely to be found in a patient with dissection involving the ascending aorta, whereas absent upper limb pulses and cerebral abnormalities suggest involvement of the aortic arch. Expansion of the arch may compress venous return and cause engorgement of one or both jugular veins. Similarly, hoarseness and Horner's syndrome can follow pressure on the left recurrent laryngeal nerve and superior cervical ganglion, respectively. Tenderness over a carotid artery may be due to dissection extending up the artery from the arch. Involvement of the descending aorta can result in visceral and lower limb ischaemia.

Although traditional teaching emphasizes the relevance of blood pressure discrepancy between the arms, this is not a particularly sensitive sign, particularly when dissection spares the ascending aorta and arch. However, evidence of new aortic regurgitation or development of pulse deficits are specific signs of dissection and should be actively sought by the examining physician.

Clinical investigation

Abnormalities of the chest radiograph and electrocardiogram are common in patients with dissection, but neither investigation is diagnostic and further imaging is always necessary.

Chest radiograph

Potential abnormalities on the chest radiograph include a widened aortic contour, aortic kinking, tracheal deviation, left pleural effusion and a widened mediastinum (Fig. 16.14.1.4). The 'calcium sign' is medial displacement of the calcium in the aortic knuckle by more than 6 mm and occurs in 20% of cases. The chest radiograph is normal in 10% of patients with acute aortic dissection.

ECG

Nonspecific ST segment and T wave changes on the ECG are often found, as are changes of left ventricular hypertrophy related to previous hypertension. The ECG is normal in one-third of patients. Actual involvement of a coronary artery is relatively uncommon, but the right coronary artery is most likely to be affected. An atypical distribution of ST elevation changes (i.e. generalized acute changes, affecting the anterior and inferior leads) is well recognized and should always alert the physician to the possibility of a diagnosis other than acute myocardial infarction and thereby reduce the possibility of inadvertent administration of thrombolytic treatment.

Blood tests

The diagnosis of aortic dissection should not be delayed while the results of blood tests are awaited. Nevertheless, immunoassays of monoclonal antibodies to smooth muscle myosin heavy chains have a high sensitivity and specificity for the diagnosis of aortic dissection. Cardiac enzymes are usually normal, but an elevated cardiac troponin on admission is a marker for a worse in-hospital outcome. If there is haemolysis of blood in the false lumen, lactate

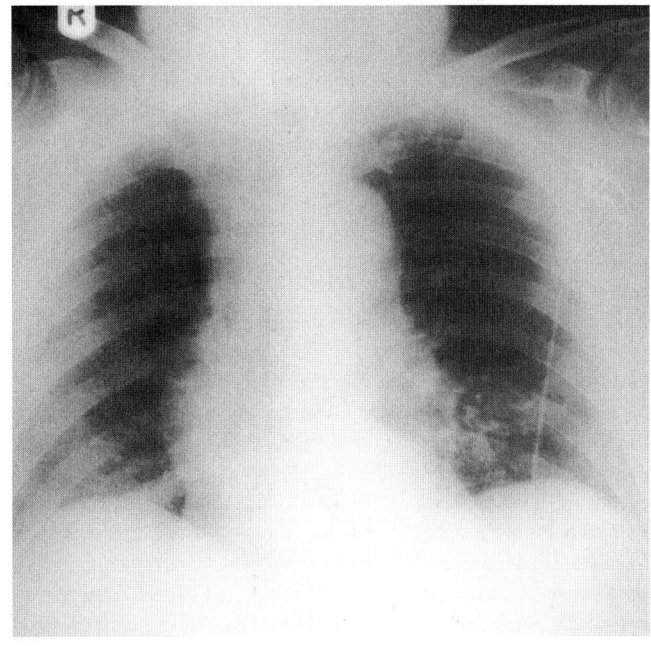

Fig. 16.14.1.4 Chest radiograph in aortic dissection showing mediastinal enlargement.

Table 16.14.1.1 Sensitivity and specificity of investigations for the diagnosis of aortic dissection

Investigation	Sensitivity (%)	Specificity (%)
Magnetic resonance imaging	99–100	99–100
Computed tomography	96–100	96–100
Transoesophageal echocardiography	98	95
Transthoracic echocardiography	59–85	63–96
Aortography	77–88	94

dehydrogenase may be elevated. Haemoglobin may be reduced if there has been significant leakage of blood from the aorta. A mildly raised leucocyte count is common.

Key imaging studies

The priorities when imaging a patient with suspected dissection are to confirm the diagnosis and to decide if the ascending aorta is involved (Stanford type A), as this will determine whether or not surgery is required. The surgeon wants to know the entry site of the dissection, if the aortic valve is competent, if there is a pericardial effusion or tamponade, and if there is involvement of the coronary arteries. Several diagnostic techniques are available (Table 16.14.1.1).

Historically, aortography was the investigation of choice, but it has several disadvantages. These include delay during the assembly of the catheter laboratory team, the risk of aortic rupture during catheter manipulation, and the nephrotoxicity of radiological contrast media when renal function may already be compromised by hypotension or renal artery involvement. CT, MRI, and echocardiography all have proven advantages over aortography.

Contrast-enhanced CT is noninvasive, but requires the use of radiological contrast medium. Its sensitivity and specificity is at least equivalent to aortography, but its accuracy is inferior to MRI, although this has been improved by the use of newer multislice CT scanners. MRI is noninvasive and provides excellent images of the whole aorta. Its sensitivity and specificity for dissection are up to 100% in some series, and the addition of cardiac gated and ciné techniques can give information on luminal blood flow and valvular regurgitation (Fig. 16.14.1.5). MRI is therefore the investigation of choice for most diseases affecting the aorta, but it has several limitations in patients with suspected acute dissection of the aorta. These include the requirement for patient transfer to the scanner, with attendant delays, restricted access to the patient during scanning, and the high degree of patient cooperation required to obtain artefact-free images.

The limited sensitivity and specificity of transthoracic echocardiography mean that it cannot be used to exclude aortic dissection. However, in some patients dissection of the ascending aorta can be confidently diagnosed using parasternal and suprasternal imaging, mandating urgent transfer to a surgical centre where additional information can be obtained by transoesophageal echocardiography in the anaesthetic room. Transoesophageal echocardiography provides detailed anatomical information about the morphology of a dissection and can also demonstrate the consequences of proximal extension, including the presence of aortic regurgitation, pericardial effusion, and involvement of the coronary artery ostia, thus making complementary investigations such as angiography unnecessary (Fig. 16.14.1.6).

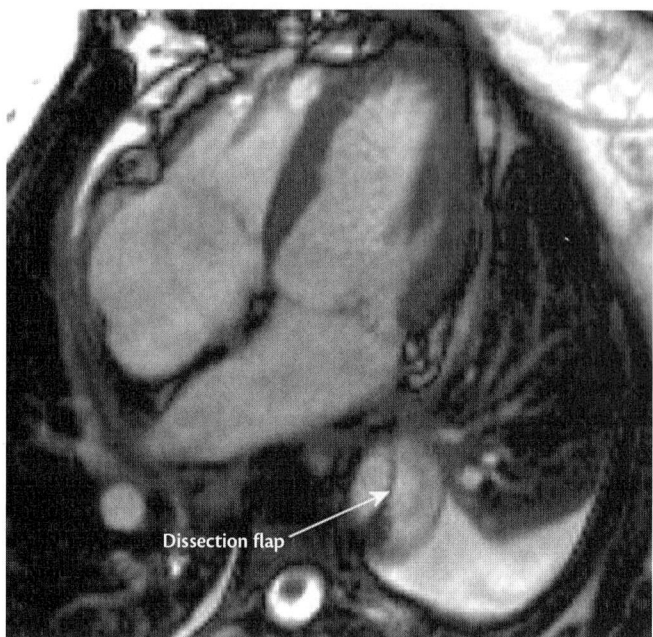

Fig. 16.14.1.5 MRI of the chest. A dissection flap in the descending aorta and a left-sided pleural effusion are visible.

Management

Emergency management

Lowering systolic blood pressure and limiting shear stress reduces the likelihood of progression of dissection. Every patient with a clinical suspicion of dissection should therefore receive effective pain relief (intravenous morphine is usually required) and antihypertensive medication pending a definitive diagnosis by imaging. Patients should be cared for in a high-dependency area with continuous monitoring of the electrocardiogram and regular blood pressure and urine output measurement. Ideally, systolic blood pressure should be maintained below 120 mmHg, using intravenous labetalol (initial dose 50 mg bolus followed by 1–2 mg/min) or intravenous esmolol. Both of these agents produce a rapid and titratable reduction in blood pressure, with β-blockade particularly appropriate in this context because it reduces the force of cardiac contraction and the rate of rise of the arterial pressure (dP/dt). If blood pressure control remains suboptimal, an additional infusion of sodium nitroprusside may be used (0.5–8 µg/kg per min). Intravenous nitrates and oral calcium antagonist are alternatives in patients who are intolerant of β-blockers.

The optimal management of patients with aortic dissection requires close liaison between those who admit patients as medical emergencies and cardiac surgical centres, using local guidelines for investigation that should reflect the available expertise and surgical opinion. Patients with a low clinical index of suspicion of dissection who are in a stable cardiovascular state should undergo prompt investigation in their local hospital, using a nominated noninvasive technique—usually CT scanning. Unless noninvasive imaging is available immediately, unstable patients with a high clinical index of suspicion should receive medical treatment and be transferred immediately to a surgical centre for both diagnostic imaging and management. This approach minimizes delay, a critical aspect of the management of acute aortic dissection.

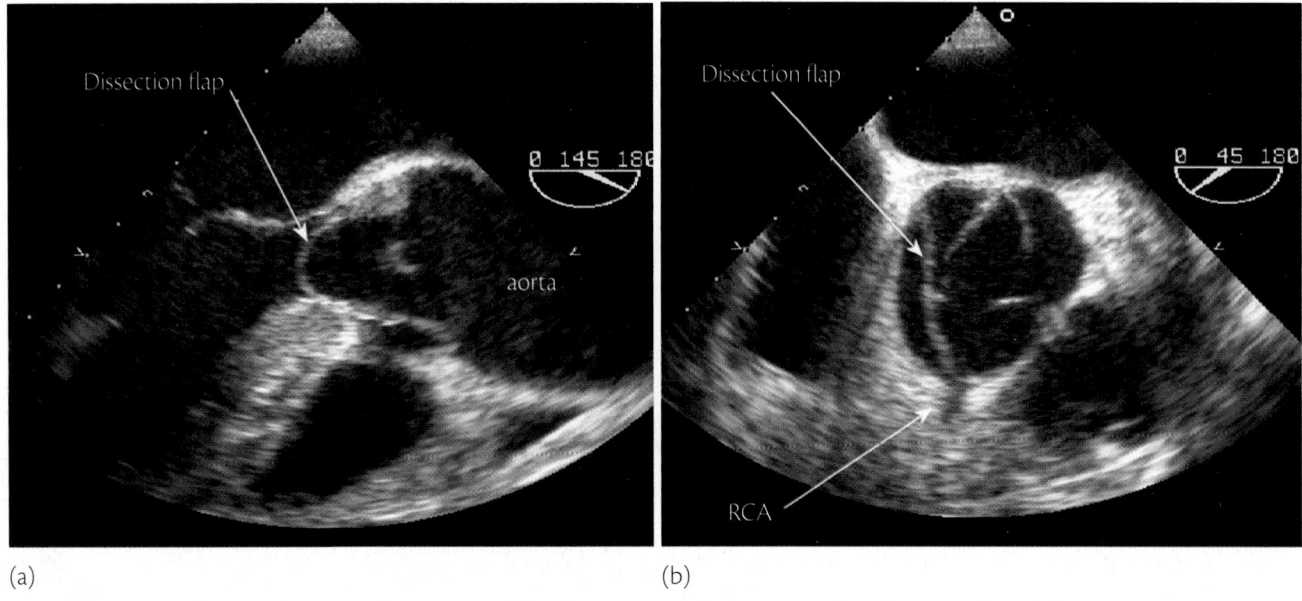

(a)   (b)

Fig. 16.14.1.6 Transoesophageal echocardiography at the level of the aortic valve. Panel (a) shows a view along the aorta and Panel (b) a cross-sectional view. There is a large dissection flap in the ascending aorta (type A) that nearly involves the ostium of the right coronary artery (RCA).

Surgery

When the dissection involves the ascending aorta (type A), immediate surgery is required as there is a high risk of proximal extension causing dissection of the coronary arteries, incompetence of the aortic valve, and rupture into the pericardium. Surgery usually involves excision of the intimal tear in the ascending aorta and interposition of a Dacron graft. This procedure protects the lower ascending aorta and valve from progressive dissection and prevents distal extension by reducing pressure within the false lumen. The false lumen may subsequently thrombose, or—in cases with multiple intimal tears—may remain patent but decompressed.

Replacement of the aortic valve is usually performed only when resuspension of the valve is not possible. However, in patients with Marfan's syndrome the ascending aorta and valve are usually replaced with a composite graft to prevent subsequent annular dilatation. In cases where dissection extends into the aortic arch, some surgeons advocate that the arch and great vessels should be included in the initial repair as arch involvement is a strong predictor of a requirement for repeat surgery. However, extended surgery can increase the duration of the operation and the risk of central nervous system damage, hence inclusion of the arch in dissection repair is generally restricted to centres with particular expertise.

Further management of descending aortic dissection

Proximal extension towards the heart is less likely when the dissection begins distal to the left subclavian artery (type B). These patients tend to be older than those with ascending aortic involvement and are more likely to have comorbidity. Diligent blood pressure management is the usual initial treatment as surgery upon the descending thoracic aorta carries significant mortality and morbidity, including impaired blood supply to the spinal cord and paraplegia. However, some centres recommend elective surgery (after several weeks) in selected patients with Marfan's syndrome, in younger patients with dissection associated with large aneurysms, and if thrombosis of the false lumen fails to occur.

Surgery for type B dissection should be considered if there is evidence of proximal extension of the dissection, progressive aortic enlargement threatening external rupture, or ischaemic complications from involvement of major arteries, e.g. the prognosis is extremely poor when ischaemia occurs in the territory of a major abdominal artery, in which case emergency surgical fenestration of the intimal flap can be life-saving.

Encouraging results have recently been achieved using endovascular stenting for patients with complicated dissection starting distal to the left subclavian artery. Using vascular access from a groin incision, a covered stent can be delivered to cover the intimal tear. In suitable cases this obliterates flow into the false lumen, relieving branch ischaemia and preventing further aneurysmal dilatation.

Follow-up and prognosis

Strenuous efforts to control blood pressure are indicated for all patients who have survived aortic dissection. β-Blocking drugs are the agents of choice for most, with other agents added as required. Most patients will require a combination of antihypertensive agents to achieve satisfactory blood pressure control (systolic <120–130 mmHg). Imaging at least once a year is recommended, using the modality with which there is most local expertise. Increased frequency of imaging is recommended following any acute event, for example severe chest pain, and for some patients with Marfan's syndrome.

The long-term survival of patients with type A aortic dissection who have surgery and survive to discharge is encouraging: 90% are still alive at 3 years. Although patients who are treated medically have extremely high in-hospital mortality (50%), two-thirds of patients who survive to hospital discharge are alive 3 years later. The mortality is often not related to dissection but from other cardiovascular conditions. Patients with a history of atherosclerosis or prior cardiac surgery are at increased risk of death. In hospital mortality for patients treated medically with type B dissection is 10%, and 3-year survival is approximately 70%.

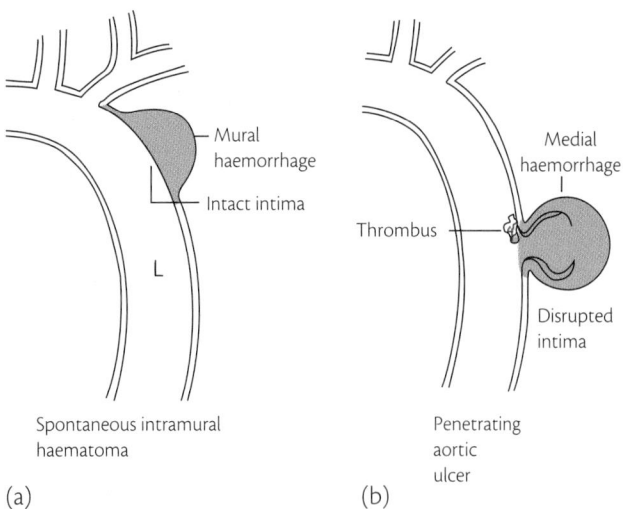

Fig. 16.14.1.7 Mechanism of acute thoracic aortic syndromes. Panel (a), spontaneous intramural haematoma; Panel (b), penetrating atherosclerotic ulcer.

Other causes of thoracic aortic syndrome

Modern imaging techniques have shown that variants of acute aortic dissection occur. They include spontaneous intramural haematoma and penetrating atherosclerotic ulcer, which present in much the same way as classic dissection and may be considered part of the acute aortic syndromes (Fig. 16.14.1.7).

Spontaneous intramural haematoma

Spontaneous intramural haematoma was described by pathologists in 1920. It occurs when the small arterioles that run in the outer media of the aorta (the vasa vasorum) rupture and bleed. It is a medial/adventitial event, with the intima remaining intact, and there is no false lumen. The clinical presentation may mimic that of dissection

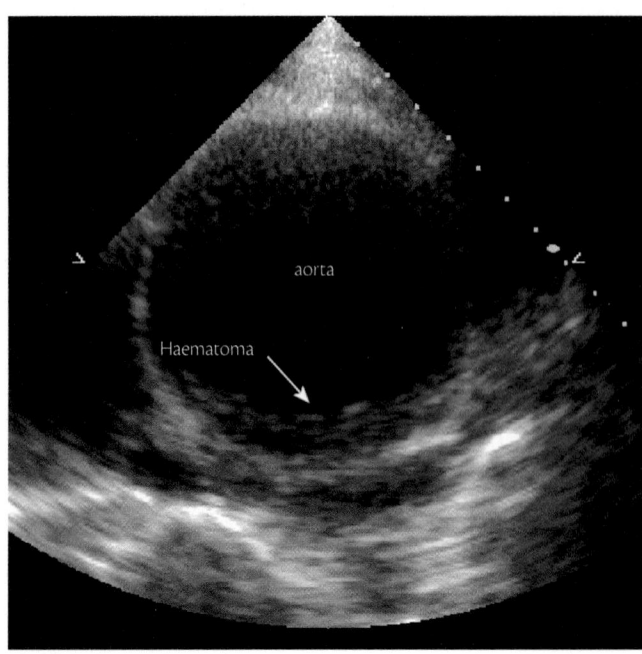

Fig. 16.14.1.8 Transthoracic echocardiography of the ascending aorta. The aorta is dilated and there is a posterior intramural haematoma.

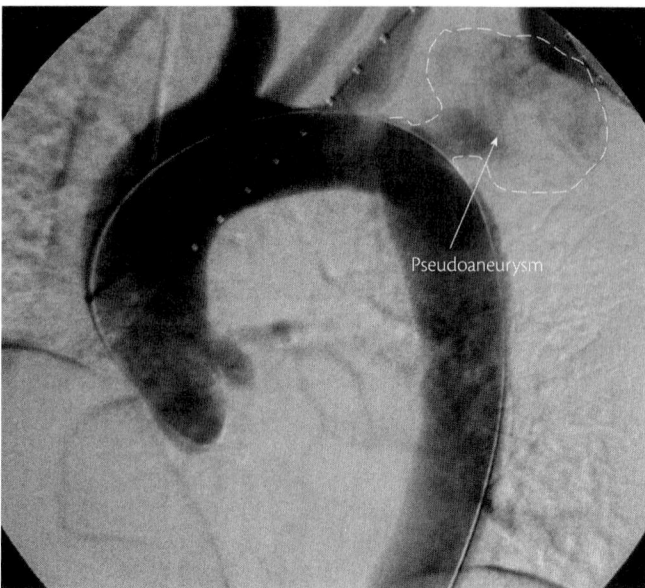

Fig. 16.14.1.9 Emergency aortography during endovascular closure of a pseudoaneurysm occurring due to a penetrating atherosclerotic ulcer.

and the diagnosis can only be made by exclusion of an intimal tear or a penetrating atherosclerotic ulcer. The intramural haematoma is not readily identifiable by aortography, but using noninvasive imaging, a circular or crescentic thickening of the aortic wall of more than 7 mm in depth associated with central displacement of any intimal calcification supports the diagnosis (Fig. 16.14.1.8).

As outlined earlier, there is increasing evidence that spontaneous intramural haematoma may be a precursor of aortic dissection. Clinical studies have supported this assertion: despite aggressive blood pressure control, up to 50% of patients with an intramural haematoma develop dissection or aortic rupture. Surgery is generally indicated when the ascending aorta is involved.

Penetrating atherosclerotic ulcer

Penetrating atherosclerotic ulcer presents with similar symptoms to aortic dissection, usually in elderly patients with disseminated atheroma. Intimal disruption caused by atheroma results in perforation and secondary haemorrhage into the media. Imaging demonstrates an out-pouching from the lumen into the aortic wall with localized haemorrhage and evidence of diffuse atheroma. Rarely, this can cause a localized dissection, but the main threat is the high incidence of rupture. Pseudoaneurysm formation can occur (Fig. 16.14.1.9). Treatment is usually with endovascular stenting to cover the ulcer, or with high risk surgery.

Further reading

Dake MD, *et al.* (1999). Endovascular stent graft placement for the treatment of acute aortic dissection. *N Engl J Med*, **340**, 1546–52.

Estrera AL, *et al.* (2006). Outcomes of medical management of acute type B aortic dissection. *Circulation*, **114**, 384–9.

Evangelista A, *et al.* (2005). Acute intramural hematoma of the aorta. A mystery in evolution. *Circulation*, **111**, 1063–70.

Kodolitsch Y, *et al.* (2004). Chest radiography for the diagnosis of acute aortic syndrome. *Am J Med*, **116**, 73–7.

Macura KJ, *et al.* (2003). Pathogenesis in acute aortic syndromes: aortic dissection, intramural hematoma, and penetrating atherosclerotic aortic ulcer. *Am J Roentgenol*, **181**, 309–16.

Nienaber CA, *et al.* (1993). The diagnosis of thoracic aortic dissection by non-invasive imaging procedures. *N Engl J Med*, **328**, 1–9.

Nienaber CA, Eagle KA (2003). Aortic dissection: new frontiers in diagnosis and management. Part I: from etiology to diagnostic strategies. *Circulation* **108**, 628–35; Part II: Therapeutic management and follow-up. *Circulation* **108**, 772–8.

Trimarchi S, *et al.* (2006). Role and results of surgery in acute type B aortic dissection: insights from the international registry of acute aortic dissection (IRAD). *Circulation*, **114**, 357–64.

Tsai TT (2005). Acute aortic syndromes. *Circulation*, **112**, 3802–13.

Tsai TT, *et al.* (2006). Long-term survival in patients presenting with type A acute aortic dissection: insights from the international registry of acute aortic dissection (IRAD). *Circulation*, **114**, 350–356.

Vilacosta I, *et al.* (1998). Penetrating atherosclerotic ulcer: documentation by transoesophageal echocardiography. *J Am Coll Cardiol*, **32**, 83–9.

16.14.2 Peripheral arterial disease

Janet Powell and Alun Davies

Essentials

The most common presentations of peripheral arterial disease are intermittent claudication and abdominal aortic aneurysm. In patients under 50 years of age the cause of disease is most likely to be genetic, congenital, immunological, infectious, or traumatic; over 50 years the principal risk factor is smoking.

Diagnosis—the main diagnostic method used to confirm the diagnosis of peripheral arterial disease is Doppler ultrasonography, in particular to estimate the ratio of systolic blood pressure at the ankle and in the arm, the ankle–brachial pressure index (ABPI; normal value 1.0–1.4, <0.9 abnormal). Ultrasonography is the standard technique for demonstrating abdominal aortic aneurysms, usually defined as being when the maximum aortic diameter exceeds 3 cm.

Critical leg ischaemia is defined as gangrenous change, ulceration, tissue loss, or rest pain lasting for 2 weeks, with an absolute ankle pressure of less than 50 mmHg.

Acute leg ischaemia

Presents as a painful, pale and pulseless limb, and is usually caused by thrombosis at the site of an atherosclerotic stenosis. Requires administration of analgesia and, if appropriate, rapid surgical intervention: (1) for irreversible ischaemia the options are amputation or palliative care; (2) for severe but potentially reversible ischaemia (white leg), surgery is usually the treatment of choice; and (3) for moderate limb ischaemia (no paralysis and only mild sensory loss), arteriography with consideration of thrombolysis, endovascular angioplasty/stenting, or surgical embolectomy/endarterectomy/bypass.

Chronic leg ischaemia

Most commonly presents with claudication affecting the calf and thigh. This is associated with high cardiovascular risk, but only 5% will go on to lose a limb, and surgical or endovascular intervention is not usually required. Key elements in management are smoking cessation, aspirin, and statins.

Abdominal aortic aneurysm

Ruptured abdominal aortic aneurysm typically causes collapse and severe back or abdominal pain: less than 20% reach hospital alive, and almost half of those undergoing emergency surgical die within 30 days.

By standard definition, more than 5% of men older than 55 years have an abdominal aortic aneurysm, but most of these are small (3–5.5 cm). These should be managed by ultrasound surveillance, with attention to modification of cardiovascular risk factors.

Repair is generally recommended for asymptomatic aneurysms greater than 5.5 cm (perhaps >5 cm in women), or symptomatic aneurysms of any size. Minimally invasive endovascular aneurysm repair has an operative mortality of about 2%, which is only one-third of that associated with traditional open repair, but within 2 years the mortality advantage of endovascular repair has been lost and long-term outlook is unknown.

Introduction

Peripheral arterial disease, defined for the purpose of this chapter as diseases of the abdominal aorta and its branches, has risk factors and features that overlap with, but can be distinguished from, those of coronary artery disease. The two conditions often coexist, but patients with coronary disease are almost always referred directly to physicians, whereas those with peripheral arterial disease are referred directly to vascular surgeons, particularly in regions where angiology is a poorly developed specialty, since medical therapies are limited. Vascular surgeons also manage patients with arterial disease in the carotid vessels and upper limbs. These aspects will receive only passing mention in this chapter: for discussion regarding the clinical features and management of carotid artery disease, see Chapter 24.10.1.

The most common presentations of peripheral arterial disease are intermittent claudication and abdominal aortic aneurysm. Most peripheral arterial disease remains asymptomatic. It is not a new disease that results from a modern Westernized lifestyle. Atherosclerotic disease, partially occluding the peripheral arteries, has been described in the mummies of ancient Egypt. Life as a cavalry officer was associated with an increased risk of popliteal aneurysm, a condition treated by ligation by John Hunter, the pioneering 18th-century surgeon. Albert Einstein died of a ruptured abdominal aortic aneurysm.

Techniques for repairing abdominal aortic aneurysms were not developed until the middle of the 20th century. This was the golden era for the development of vascular surgery as a specialty, with the increasing use of bypass surgery that reduced the need for amputation. Today newer, less-invasive approaches are being employed—angioplasty and endovascular stenting—but few specific medical therapies are on the horizon.

Aetiology and epidemiology

Peripheral arterial disease may occur in the young, but the prevalence increases sharply with age. Both young and old may suffer from occlusive (stenosing) disease of the peripheral arteries or dilating (aneurysmal) disease, while vasospastic disease is uncommon. However, the underlying causes of peripheral arterial disease in those below and above 50 years of age tend to be very different.

Peripheral arterial disease in patients less than 50 years old

In younger patients, the cause of disease is most likely to be genetic, congenital, immunological, infectious, or traumatic. Patients with familial hypercholesterolaemia and related inherited disorders of lipid metabolism may present with peripheral limb ischaemia. There are also congenital causes of early onset leg ischaemia. These include aortic hypoplasia, which occurs during the embryonic fusion of the distal aortas, and popliteal entrapment, where the popliteal artery takes an unusual course through the head of the gastrocnemius muscle, with exercise involving knee flexion causing intermittent occlusion of the artery and calf pain that resembles intermittent claudication. A fierce immunological inflammatory response to smoking causes Buerger's syndrome, which involves the artery, vein, and associated nerves in both the legs and the arms. This disease, seen principally in men, is particularly prevalent in the Indian subcontinent, and may resolve if the patient stops smoking. Sudden thrombotic occlusion of the iliac and distal arteries may occur in those below 50 years of age, suggesting the presence of an inherited thrombotic disorder. Embolic occlusion from a proximal source is also possible.

Marfan's syndrome may sometimes be confirmed only after a patient has presented with a ruptured abdominal aortic aneurysm. In some variants of Ehlers–Danlos syndrome, patients with mutations in type III collagen present with visceral artery aneurysms. In South Africa (and elsewhere), aneurysms of the abdominal, femoral, or popliteal arteries in those under 50 years have been attributed to infectious causes, from HIV to tuberculosis. Syphilitic aneurysms, which used to affect principally the thoracic aorta, are now rare.

Peripheral arterial disease in patients over 50 years old

For patients over 50 years of age, the principal risk factor for peripheral arterial disease—stenosing, aneurysmal, or vasospastic—is smoking. The pathology is atherosclerotic change with superimposed thrombosis. Of patients who present with peripheral arterial disease, less than 5% have never smoked. For this reason, more men than women presented with peripheral arterial disease in the past, but recently more women are affected, perhaps a reflection of the increasing number who smoke. Nevertheless, unlike Buerger's disease, cessation of smoking is not associated with an immediate dramatic improvement in symptoms and it may take several years without smoking to improve prognosis.

Diabetes is another important risk factor for stenosing peripheral arterial disease. Other risk factors include hypertension, raised levels of plasma fibrinogen, and hyperlipidaemia, with elevated plasma triglycerides being a common finding. The risk factors for dilating arterial disease are similar, with the exception of diabetes, which is rare.

For aortic aneurysms, although strong familial clustering has been observed, no specific common genetic mutations associated with aneurysmal disease have been identified yet and atherosclerotic change is commonplace. White and northern European populations appear to be at higher risk of aneurysmal disease than black populations. Stenosing and aneurysmal disease are associated with degenerative changes of the artery wall, the prevalence of both diseases increasing sharply with age (Table 16.14.2.1).

Table 16.14.2.1 The increasing prevalence of peripheral arterial disease with age in the populations of northern Europe

Population	Age (years)	Asymptomatic peripheral arterial disease (ABPI < 0.9) (%)	Intermittent claudication (%)	Abdominal aortic aneurysm (>3 cm) (%)
Men	55–64	8	1.2	5
Women	55–64	7	0.8	0.7
Men	65–74	16	2.5	7.5
Women	65–74	11	1.2	1.3
Men	75+	>30	4.0	9
Women	75+	>30	1.5	1.5

Most peripheral arterial disease, both stenosing and dilating, is asymptomatic. The data have been derived from several studies and geographical variation may occur. ABPI, ankle–brachial pressure index.

Epidemiological studies also indicate a difference between stenosing and aneurysmal disease, with death from aneurysmal disease (aortic aneurysm) being more common amongst those of higher social classes and in affluent geographical areas.

Clinical features of leg ischaemia

The terms acute and chronic relate purely to the length of time that symptoms have been present and must not be confused with terms related to severity, such as critical limb ischaemia.

Critical leg ischaemia

Critical leg ischaemia is defined as gangrenous change, ulceration, tissue loss, or rest pain lasting for 2 weeks, with an absolute ankle pressure of less than 50 mmHg, although patients with diabetes are difficult to include in this classification.

Acute leg ischaemia

The incidence of acute leg ischaemia, which presents as a painful, pale, and pulseless limb, is 1 in 12 000 patients per year. It can be due either to an embolic event or thrombosis of an atherosclerotic stenosis. The commonest cause of a peripheral embolus used to be rheumatic heart disease in a patient with atrial fibrillation, but this is now uncommon, and other sources of emboli, such as an aortic aneurysm, must be considered. The development of a thrombosis at the site of an atherosclerotic stenosis, either in the superficial femoral artery or popliteal artery, is undoubtedly now the commonest cause of acute leg ischaemia. However, it should be stressed that, whatever the cause, there is no difference on clinical examination of the acutely ischaemic limb.

Arterial trauma due to road traffic accidents and knife or gunshot wounds is becoming commoner, as is iatrogenic trauma following the insertion of intra-arterial catheters for diagnosis or therapy. A rare but dramatic cause of acute leg ischaemia is phlegmasia cerulea dolens, in which massive thrombosis of all the major veins of the limb occurs with gross swelling that obstructs the arterial supply.

Patients with a thrombosis of a popliteal aneurysm may present with classic symptoms of pain, paralysis, loss of power, paraesthesia, pallor, lack of pulse, and perishing cold. If the blood supply is not restored, fixed blue staining of the skin is a further sign of irreversible ischaemia, as is a tense calf with plantar flexion. However, most patients presenting with acute ischaemia have symptoms that are less severe.

Chronic leg ischaemia

Chronic leg ischaemia is much more common than acute ischaemia (Table 16.14.2.1), and its main cause is atherosclerosis. In the young patient, one should also consider cystic adventitial disease, entrapment of the popliteal artery, and occasionally fibromuscular hyperplasia of the iliac arteries, particularly in women.

Symptoms are pain on walking, claudication affecting the calf and thigh, rest pain, ulceration, and gangrenous change. Less commonly, patients may present with buttock claudication and impotence (Leriche's syndrome). Although the differential diagnoses of the acutely ischaemic limb are few, in the chronically ischaemic limb pain may be due to spinal stenosis or nerve-root compression (spinal claudication) or arthritis of the hip or knee. Classically the patient with claudication will complain of cramp-like pain in the calf, appearing after walking a particular distance, relieved by a few minute's rest, and recurring again at the same distance if the patient resumes walking. Failure of the pain to disappear on resting, or its reappearance after a shorter distance after each rest, suggest a possible musculoskeletal cause, particularly if distal pulses are present on examination. However, it should also be remembered that distal pulses may be felt at rest in the limbs of patients with claudication due to peripheral vascular disease, but disappear on exercise to the point of pain.

Investigation of the patient with an ischaemic leg

The main diagnostic method used to confirm the diagnosis of peripheral arterial disease is Doppler ultrasonography (duplex scanning), an example of which is shown in Fig. 16.14.2.1. The ratio of systolic blood pressure at the ankle and in the arm, the ankle–brachial pressure index (ABPI), provides a physiological measure of blood flow at the level of the ankle. At rest, in a normal leg, the ankle–brachial pressure index lies between 1.0 and 1.4. As the blood flow in the leg is compromised, the ABPI falls sharply and values below 0.9 are considered abnormal and likely to confirm the diagnosis of peripheral vascular disease. To emphasize the important overlap between this condition and coronary artery disease, a reduction in ABPI nearly always signals the presence of coronary artery disease, which is the cause of death in most patients with peripheral arterial disease.

Exercise testing provides an objective method of assessing walking distance and helps with the identification of disease processes, such as angina, that may be limiting. It only needs to be used in those people who have a history of claudication but have normal resting ABPI, and can be used as a way of eliminating or suggesting other diagnoses.

In addition to establishing the diagnosis of peripheral arterial disease, duplex ultrasonography is able to determine the site of disease and indicate the degree of stenosis or length of an occlusion and hence aid in the planning of interventional treatment. Other imaging modalities such as CT scanning and magnetic resonance (MR) angiography can provide three-dimensional reconstructions of the diseased vessels and may be used for planning surgical treatment.

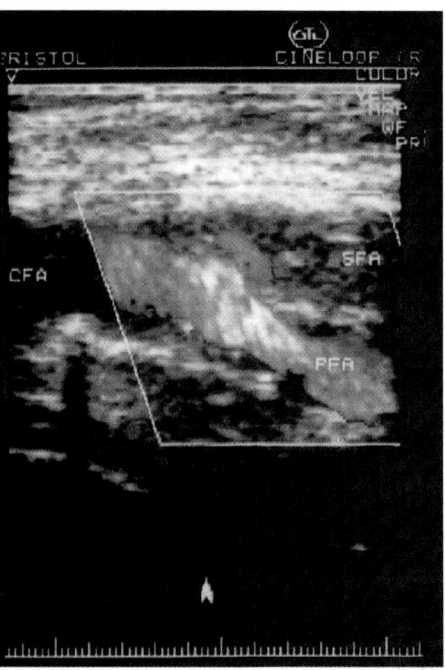

Fig. 16.14.2.1 Occlusion of the superficial femoral artery demonstrated by colour-coded duplex ultrasonography. On the left, the common femoral artery (CFA) lies outside the colour box. In the colour box antegrade flow through the profunda femoris artery (PFA) is shown in blue. The red flash represents rebound flow against the occluded origin of the superficial femoral artery (SFA).

Angiography is only required as an adjuvant to endovascular treatment, for surgical planning in some circumstances, or in the management of the acutely ischaemic limb.

Attention to risk factors, in particular smoking, blood pressure, and exercise, are important issues.

Management of critical and acute limb ischaemia

Critical limb ischaemia requires administration of analgesia and rapid surgical intervention. The severity of ischaemia will determine the treatment options considered. However, all patients with a severely ischaemic limb should be given adequate analgesia and 5000 units of heparin intravenously. Many will be old and frail, with significant medical comorbidities. These issues must be considered in deciding whether or not surgical intervention is appropriate for any individual case, with action taken to improve those aspects of the patient's medical condition that can be improved before surgery, or as part of continuing medical management.

For a patient with irreversible ischaemia (fixed skin staining and tense muscles), the main decision is whether a primary amputation or palliative care should be offered. If severe but potentially reversible ischaemia is present (white leg), surgery is usually the treatment of choice. Delay while thrombolytic therapy is tried is not advisable in this group. For patients with moderate limb ischaemia, where there is no paralysis and only mild sensory loss, arteriography with consideration of the potential use of thrombolysis should be performed. However, it should be remembered that thrombolysis is associated with numerous potential complications, most notably gastrointestinal haemorrhage and stroke. If the limb is salvageable, it may be possible to offer the patient an endovascular procedure, such as an angioplasty (with or without stenting). Surgical treatment can involve simple embolectomy, but may require a bypass procedure or endarterectomy, and in the severely ischaemic limb fasciotomies may be needed to treat or prevent a compartment syndrome. For at least 10% of patients, it will not be possible to offer revascularization: a few of these may benefit from the use of a prostacyclin analogue (iloprost), which might diminish amputation rates and alleviate pain. Any benefits of gene therapy, with vascular endothelial growth factor (VEGF) or other molecular mediators, on avoidance of amputation are far from established. Limb-salvage rates for patients presenting with critical limb ischaemia are variable, probably 50 to 60% at 2 years, dependent on the severity of disease.

In a patient presenting with acute leg ischaemia the outlook is poor, with only about 60% leaving hospital with an intact limb. The 30-day mortality for this group of patients can be as high as 30%, the main cause of death being cardiac disease. The strategy for management is described in Fig. 16.14.2.2. Controversial areas in the treatment of acute leg ischaemia include the role of arteriography, and which technique of thrombolysis is the safest and most cost effective.

In the patient who has had an embolic event, long-term anticoagulation should not be forgotten, and nor should a search for the source of embolus. If the patient is not in atrial fibrillation, has normal cardiac enzymes and 12-lead ECG, then they should have an echocardiogram to exclude any valvular lesion, a 24-h ECG to look for arrhythmia, an ultrasound to exclude abdominal aortic aneurysm, and a screen for thrombophilia.

Management of the chronically ischaemic leg

In chronic limb ischaemia, management depends upon the severity of the disease. Most patients present with claudication, which is relatively benign: only about 5% will go on to lose a limb, but claudication identifies patients with a threefold increased risk of death from either heart disease or cerebrovascular disease compared with age- and sex-matched controls. It is important when planning treatment that all the potential risk factors are covered. In the past surgical intervention was usually considered unnecessary: at least one-third will have improvement of symptoms with simple medical treatment and exercise. However recent trials have suggested

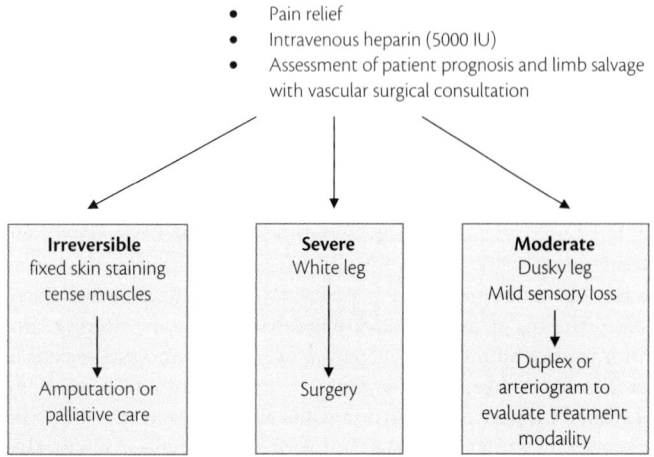

Fig. 16.14.2.2 Management of the patient with an acutely ischaemic leg.

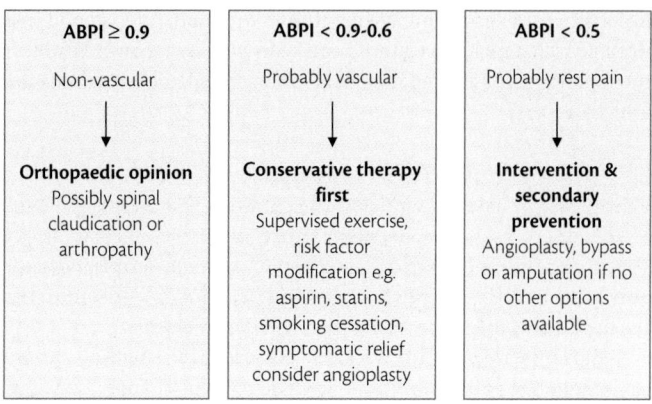

Fig. 16.14.2.3 Management of the patient with chronic lower leg pain, but no tissue loss, stratified by ankle brachial pressure index (ABPI).

that either angioplasty with adjunct and stents or coated balloons or angioplasty combined with exercise therapy may offer early benefits (to 2 years) and longer term results are awaited eagerly. The current treatment of patients with chronic lower leg pain is shown in Fig. 16.14.2.3.

General management

Careful attention must be paid to the cleanliness of ischaemic feet to avoid infection, and particular care should be given to the cutting of toenails. In many patients this is best done by a careful younger relative or chiropodist, since apparently minor lacerations can lead to ulcers, infection, and gangrene. Patients are recommended to exercise. Walking to the point of claudication is not harmful, and may improve collateral circulation with beneficial results. Supervised exercise therapy appears to be more effective than merely providing advice to exercise more.

Smoking is by far the most significant risk factor for occlusive arterial disease and every effort should be made to encourage smokers to stop. If patients undergo surgical treatment, then the long-term patency rate following arterial reconstruction is four times greater in smokers who stop than in those who persist.

Pharmacological treatment

Since coronary artery disease is the main cause of death in those with peripheral arterial disease, patients with the latter condition should receive similar cardiovascular risk reduction therapy to patients with coronary heart disease. Low-dose aspirin therapy (75–325 mg/day) should be recommended for all. If aspirin cannot be tolerated, ADP-receptor antagonists, such as clopidogrel, are equally effective in reducing the risk of cardiovascular events (stroke, myocardial infarction, and vascular deaths).

Secondary prevention trials have demonstrated the benefits of statin therapy in reducing cardiovascular morbidity and mortality in those with stenosing atherosclerotic disease of the peripheral arteries. Statins also may improve operative cardiovascular morbidity and mortality, but neither fibrates nor chelation therapy offer benefits.

The options for facilitating smoking cessation are increasing and nicotine replacement therapy can be used with either buproprion or varenicline if necessary, although many will not stop smoking until surgery threatens.

There is good evidence that cilostazol (a selective cAMP phosphodiesterase inhibitor) improves walking distance in those with intermittent claudication, although the mechanism of action is not clear, side effects are frequent, and the drug is contraindicated in patients with congestive heart failure.

Surgical treatment

In general, surgeons are conservative with respect to interventional treatment for patients with claudication, despite a possible early benefit for those having an endovascular procedure. However, in the patient who has severe claudication, with symptoms that significantly affect their quality of life, it is certainly possible and appropriate to offer interventional treatment.

Both endovascular techniques (angioplasty with or without stent) and bypass surgery are effective treatments, with little to choose between the two. For infrainguinal bypass, good-quality autologous vein is the conduit of choice. However, reasonable results can be obtained with synthetic grafts, particularly where the distal anastomosis is above the knee. Below the knee, an adjuvant vein interposition in the form of either a Miller cuff or Taylor patch is used. Stenting is used widely, but its use is contentious, and, at least in the iliac arteries, it may not be of value. The role of exercise therapy compared with angioplasty in the treatment of mild to moderate claudication continues to be debated, but it might be prudent to consider the conjoint treatment of angioplasty with exercise therapy.

Ischaemia of the arm

Ischaemia of the arm is usually a result of embolism from the heart. Occasionally the subclavian artery is diseased or has suffered traumatic injury or radiation damage following radiotherapy. The basic principles of investigation and management are the same as for the leg. However, it should be noted that the upper limb has multiple interconnection of collateral vessels, hence occlusion of the major arterial supply may still leave a viable limb. The other disease process that needs to be considered in differential diagnosis is the thoracic outlet syndrome, which gives rise to symptoms in the arm as a result of arterial, venous, or neurological compression caused by an additional cervical rib or by scalene bands. Management may require surgical intervention, either cervical rib excision or thoracic outlet decompression with the removal of the first rib.

Mesenteric ischaemia

Mesenteric ischaemia is uncommon. Over one-third of cases of acute mesenteric ischaemia are due to arterial embolism, with emboli lodging at the ostium of the superior mesenteric artery in many cases. Patients with acute mesenteric artery thrombosis have often had symptoms of mesenteric ischaemia prior to the acute episode. Chronic mesenteric ischaemia typically presents with weight loss and abdominal pain on ingestion of food, the classic story being that the patient is constantly hungry, but frightened to eat. Other causes of acute mesenteric ischaemia include venous thrombosis and nonocclusive ischaemia secondary to hypoperfusion.

Patients with acute mesenteric ischaemia will usually present with abdominal pain, but the abdominal physical signs may be much less dramatic than would be anticipated from the subsequent clinical course. Suspicion of the diagnosis should be heightened in the presence of atrial fibrillation or widespread atheromatous vascular disease. Patients may deteriorate suddenly and present in shock.

The diagnosis of acute mesenteric ischaemia is difficult to make. In the acute situation, clues to look for include leucocytosis, hyperamylasaemia, and unexplained acidosis. Liver function tests are usually normal. Radiological imaging is rarely able to make a positive diagnosis, although it can be very useful in excluding other possibilities. Angiography is not always accurate. CT scanning can be helpful in the diagnosis of mesenteric venous thrombosis.

Intensive resuscitation to replace fluids is essential. Surgery is usually necessary for the patient to survive, and the possibility of acute mesenteric ischaemia remains one of the dwindling number of reasons for requiring an emergency diagnostic laparotomy. Depending on the findings, resection of small bowel may suffice, but formal arterial surgery may be necessary, and in some unfortunate instances the extent of irreversible ischaemia can preclude any attempt at resection or revascularization. In cases where the surgeon is unsure of the viability of bowel remaining after resection, a second laparotomy may be planned to assess the situation a few days later. Repeat laparotomy may also be required to examine, and if necessary resect, more bowel in the patient who is not 'doing well' postoperatively. The prognosis for patients who present with acute mesenteric ischaemia is poor.

For patients who present with chronic mesenteric ischaemia, the aim of treatment is to improve blood flow and to act as a prophylactic procedure to prevent the catastrophic disaster of arterial occlusion. The potential options, having identified the site of the disease process by duplex scanning and angiography, include angioplasty, endarterectomy, reimplantation, or a surgical bypass procedure.

Abdominal aortic aneurysm

Definition

There is no fixed definition of an abdominal aortic aneurysm beyond agreement that it is a localized dilatation of the abdominal aorta, usually fusiform, with dilation starting distal to the renal arteries. Some would apply the term when the maximum aortic diameter is more than 1.5 times the diameter of the undilated proximal aorta.

Manual palpation to detect abdominal aortic aneurysms is unreliable, unless undertaken by a specialist on a nonobese patient. The most convenient method of screening for the presence of these aneurysms is ultrasonography, measuring the anterior–posterior diameter. Since the reproducibility of ultrasound measurements of the suprarenal aorta is poor, a convenient working definition of an abdominal aortic aneurysm is when the maximum diameter exceeds 3 cm, which in most people is more than 1.5 times the diameter of the undilated proximal aorta. In practice, it is only aneurysms of 4 cm or greater in diameter that have been of clinical concern.

Epidemiology

Population screening studies in northern Europe have shown that the disease is usually without symptoms, much more common in men than in women (Table 16.14.2.1), and is strongly associated with smoking. The associations with hypertension and hyperlipidaemia are inconsistent. The prevalence of large aneurysms (>5 cm in diameter) detected by screening is only about 1% in men and the large majority of screen-detected aneurysms are 3 to 5 cm in diameter. The natural history of abdominal aortic aneurysms is progressive enlargement (with the diameter increasing by 2–5 mm each year) without symptoms, until the aortic wall is so weakened that it ruptures, which is a catastrophic event.

The infrarenal aorta is by far the most common site of aneurysmal dilatation, and usually the abdominal aorta is the only site of dilatation. When patients present with aneurysms of the iliac, femoral, or popliteal arteries, abdominal aortic aneurysm is often present and screening for this is mandatory. This emphasizes the tendency of some patients to have a more generalized form of dilating arterial disease.

Most patients (60%) with abdominal aortic aneurysm die from cardiovascular causes, and up to 25% of other male family members may develop occult aneurysms.

Ruptured aneurysms

The symptoms of a ruptured abdominal aortic aneurysm are collapse (shock) and severe back or abdominal pain. Rarely a ruptured aneurysm will present with gastrointestinal bleeding from an aortoduodenal fistula or high-output cardiac failure from an aortocaval fistula.

Less than 20% of patients with a ruptured abdominal aortic aneurysm reach hospital alive, and even among those that undergo emergency surgical repair almost one-half will die within 30 days. With this bleak prognosis and the very significant costs associated with emergency repair following rupture, evidence has accumulated that screening of men over 65 years to detect those with the largest aneurysms, at highest risk of rupture, is cost effective. Accordingly, there are plans for national screening programmes for abdominal aortic aneurysm in the United Kingdom and other countries.

Management of ruptured aneurysms requires:

- Access lines, cross-matched blood, and resuscitation—maintaining moderate hypotension at ~70 mmHg may be beneficial
- Confirmation of diagnosis—ultrasound (to show aneurysm); CT scan or experienced vascular surgeon (to confirm diagnosis of rupture)
- Rapid assessment of whether patient would benefit from emergency repair
- If yes, immediate surgical or endovascular repair

Aneurysms detected before rupture

Abdominal aortic aneurysms are commonly symptomless, but rupture—as explained above—is catastrophic. However, elective repair of an abdominal aortic aneurysm, a major surgical procedure, is not without risk. Traditionally, larger aneurysms have been repaired by cross-clamping of the aorta and insertion of a Dacron inlay graft at open surgery. This is a durable procedure and effectively 'cures' the patient. However, although some specialized surgical centres report an operative mortality of less than 2% associated with this elective procedure, on a population basis the mortality is more likely to be 5 to 8%, which is an important reason for avoiding surgery in those with small aneurysms.

Minimally invasive endovascular aneurysm repair, via femoral access vessels, has developed rapidly. Only about one-half of patients have an aneurysm that is anatomically suitable for this mode of repair, but randomized trials have shown that the operative mortality associated with endovascular repair is less than 2%, which is only one-third of the mortality associated with traditional open repair. However, within 2 years the mortality advantage of endovascular repair has been lost and a significant proportion of patients with endovascular repair require further interventions to ensure continued exclusion of the aneurysm. Hence patients with endovascular repair are likely to require lifelong surveillance. The cost-effectiveness, long-term durability, or patient preference for this new technique has not been established. In the UK endovascular repair now is considered cost-effective for elective procedures (www.nice.org.uk/TA167). The majority of patients would prefer endovascular repair although some still prefer open repair principally because there is no requirement for long-term follow up. The long-term durability of endovascular repair remains to be established and late rupture may be a greater problem than for open repair. Although the endovascular approach initially was developed for patients not considered fit for open surgery because of numerous comorbidities, the operative mortality rises to 9% in this cohort and there is no evidence that endovascular aneurysm repair prolongs patient survival.

Two randomized trials have shown that for aneurysms of 4.0 to 5.5 cm in diameter a policy of early elective surgery confers no long-term survival benefit, and hence early surgery should not be recommended. For such patients surveillance, with measurement of ultrasound diameter every 6 months, is a safe policy that engenders little patient anxiety, and the risk of aneurysm rupture is very low—1% per year. By contrast, for patients with aneurysms greater than 6 cm in diameter the risk of rupture may be as high as 25% per year, and in most such cases elective repair is recommended. Over 90% of the patients enrolled in the trials were men, and it is possible that the diameter threshold for considering surgery should be 5 cm in women.

Repair is also recommended when symptoms are attributed to the aneurysm, whatever its size, the commonest being back or abdominal pain, or tenderness to palpation. It is assumed that such aneurysms are at high risk of rupture and need early repair. As the aneurysm dilates, onion skin layers of laminated thrombus deposit in the lumen, to leave a blood-flow channel of approximately normal aortic diameter. These layers of thrombus are very stable and only in rare circumstances are the sources of emboli to the legs. The aneurysms which most often provoke symptoms have very thick, inflamed, fibrotic walls, which entrap nerves and may become adherent to other tissues. These are known as inflammatory aneurysms and the thickened wall can often be detected by CT or MRI. They are technically demanding to repair. There is no convincing evidence that a course of preoperative corticosteroids is beneficial. In the Japanese population, inflammatory aneurysms have been associated with active cytomegalovirus infection.

A strategy for the management of abdominal aortic aneurysms detected before rupture is shown in Fig. 16.14.2.4. Patients with

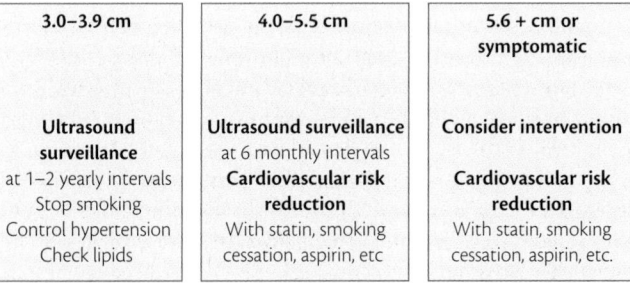

3.0–3.9 cm	4.0–5.5 cm	5.6 + cm or symptomatic
Ultrasound surveillance at 1–2 yearly intervals Stop smoking Control hypertension Check lipids	**Ultrasound surveillance** at 6 monthly intervals **Cardiovascular risk reduction** With statin, smoking cessation, aspirin, etc	**Consider intervention** **Cardiovascular risk reduction** With statin, smoking cessation, aspirin, etc.

Fig. 16.14.2.4 Management of men with asymptomatic, unruptured abdominal aortic aneurysm stratified by aneurysm diameter.

small aneurysms should stop smoking and have their blood pressure controlled. Since screening detects mainly small aneurysms, it would clearly be beneficial if a treatment to limit aneurysm growth were available. Although β-blockers have proved effective in limiting the dilation of the proximal aorta in patients with Marfan's syndrome, there is no evidence that they are effective for abdominal aortic aneurysms. Furthermore, many patients with abdominal aortic aneurysm have impaired lung function, perhaps through smoking, and β-blockers often are poorly tolerated. However, effective control of blood pressure and cessation of smoking are both likely to minimize the rate of aneurysm growth and the risk of rupture, and statins may also be helpful. Intervention to exclude the aneurysm remains the only available treatment for aneurysms larger than 5.5 cm in diameter.

Medical management

Just as for patients with limb ischaemia, patients with abdominal aortic aneurysm are at high risk of cardiovascular events. All patients with abdominal aortic aneurysm should be offered statin therapy to reduce the risk of morbidity and mortality from other forms of coexistent cardiovascular disease. Antiplatelet therapy should be considered, and there is some evidence that, for hypertensive patients, angiotensin converting enzyme (ACE) inhibitors minimize the chance of aneurysm rupture.

Conventional surgical management

Preoperative evaluation requires CT or MRI to define the anatomy and extent of the aneurysm. Cardiac, pulmonary, and renal function should always be assessed and optimal treatment instituted before surgery: poor renal and lung function are associated with an increased risk of postoperative morbidity and mortality.

The most common surgical approach to an abdominal aortic aneurysm is through a transperitoneal incision under general anaesthesia. The retroperitoneal approach, which avoids bowel manipulation and permits a more rapid return to oral diet, has similar cross-clamp, operating, and recovery times. The transperitoneal approach offers the advantage of exploring the abdominal cavity for other pathology. In this approach, after the bowel has been removed from the operative field, the aorta is exposed anteriorly from the left renal vein to the bifurcation. The infrarenal neck of the aneurysm is exposed anteriorly and laterally so that an occluding clamp may be applied. Both common iliac arteries are exposed for the placement of the distal occluding clamps. The aneurysm is opened longitudinally on the anterior surface and the remainder of the procedure performed from inside the aneurysm cavity. Usually following a small dose of intravenous heparin, arterial clamps are applied. Clot and debris are evacuated and any back-bleeding lumbar or mesenteric arteries ligated. A Dacron prosthesis is then sutured, end-to-end, to the normal-diameter aorta above the aneurysm. This anastomosis is tested for leaks before the graft is trimmed to appropriate length and sutured in place above the aortic bifurcation. The aneurysmal sac is closed over the prosthesis, before replacement of abdominal contents. Such tube grafts are the most common type, but when the iliac arteries are dilated or diseased a bifurcated prosthesis is used. The cross-clamp time should be less than 1 h and the whole procedure completed within 2 to 4 h. The longest procedures involve inflammatory aneurysms and cases where the proximal aneurysm neck lies above the renal arteries. The patient should be ready to leave hospital 7 to 12 days after the operation, with a durable repair.

Endovascular aneurysm repair

The technique of endovascular repair was introduced in the early 1990s and the technology has now stabilized. The procedure may be performed under general, regional, or even local anaesthesia. This flexibility allows endovascular repair in patients where general anaesthesia is risky, and the avoidance of aortic cross-clamping is an additional benefit for those with limited cardiac reserve.

Preoperative investigation to evaluate the extent and size of the aneurysm (spiral CT or MRI) is of critical importance. The length of the aneurysm neck below the renal arteries, angulation of the aorta, and tortuosity of the iliac arteries must be evaluated precisely so that the correct size of graft can be placed via the femoral artery. The insertion of the graft is performed under fluoroscopic control. This requires the use of significant amounts of contrast material, which may underlie the unfavourable results reported in patients with pre-existing renal impairment. The proximal end of the graft is held in place either by hooks and barbs, balloon, or self-expandable stents.

The length of the procedure is similar to that for open repair but the transfusion requirements are similar to those for open repair but the transfusion requirements are less and the patient recovers more rapidly and is ready to leave hospital within 2 to 5 days. The long-term success of the procedure depends on the successful exclusion of the aneurysmal sac and the security of the proximal attachment to prevent graft migration. Endoleaks may develop when the aneurysm is not completely excluded, the graft migrates or fatigues, or there is back-bleeding from lumbar vessels or the inferior mesenteric artery into the aneurysm sac. These are associated with an important risk of continued aneurysm expansion and rupture. For these reasons, continued vigilance and repeated evaluation of the aneurysm with duplex or CT scanning is necessary at annual intervals.

The endovascular revolution has affected the management of all categories of peripheral arterial disease, although in many instances the advantages and indications for the use of the (often more expensive) endovascular approach are not based on evidence from randomized trials.

Further reading

ACC/AHA (2006). 2005 guidelines for the management of peripheral arterial disease. *J Am Coll Cardiol*, **47**, 123–312.
BASIL Trial Participants (2005). Bypass versus angioplasty in severe ischaemia of the leg (BASIL): multicentre, randomized controlled trial. *Lancet*, **366**, 1925–34.
Bhatt DL, et al. (2006). Clopidogrel and aspirin versus aspirin alone for the prevention of atherothrombotic events. *N Engl J Med*, **354**, 1706–17.
Brady AR, Powell JT (2004). Detection, management and prospects for the medical treatment of small abdominal aortic aneurysms. *Arterioscler Thromb Vasc Biol*, **24**, 241–5.
EVAR Trial Participants. Endovascular aneurysm repair versus open repair in patients with abdominal aortic aneurysm (EVAR trial 1): randomised controlled trial. *Lancet*, **365**, 2179–86.
Fowkes FGR (1988). The epidemiology of atherosclerotic arterial disease in the lower limbs. *Euro J Vasc Surg*, **2**, 283–91.
Hankey GJ, Norman PE, Eikelboom JW (2006). Medical treatment of peripheral arterial disease. *JAMA*, **295**, 547–53.
Powell JT, et al. (2007). Final 12-year follow-up of surgery versus surveillance. 94, 702–8.
Tetteroo E et al. (1998). Randomised comparison of primary stent placement versus primary angioplasty followed by selective stent

placement in patients with iliac artery occlusive disease. *Dutch Iliac Stent Trial Group. Lancet*, **351**, 1153–9.

Thompson PD, *et al.* (2002). Meta-analysis of results from eight randomized, placebo-controlled trials on the effect of cilostazol on patients with intermittent claudication. *Am J Cardiol*, **90**, 1314–9.

16.14.3 Cholesterol embolism

Christopher Dudley

Essentials

Cholesterol embolism occurring after vascular surgery or intra-arterial angiographic procedures is not uncommon, but is often unrecognized. The clinical features mimic a number of conditions, including contrast nephropathy and systemic vasculitis, and—if mis-diagnosed—can result in the inappropriate use of powerful immuno-suppressive drugs. A high index of suspicion is required when an elderly patient with widespread vascular disease develops a nonspe-cific systemic illness with progressive renal impairment, particularly after vascular surgery or arteriography. Biopsy of affected tissue, especially skin or kidney, is diagnostic—showing biconvex, needle-shaped cholesterol clefts within the lumen of arteries or arterioles. Treatment is supportive and the prognosis is often poor.

Introduction

When atheromatous plaques ulcerate and become denuded of their endothelial covering, the underlying cholesterol-rich extracellular matrix can become detached and embolize. If the dislodged plaque and superimposed thrombi is sufficiently large, occlusion of a major systemic artery results in infarction of the organ or ischaemia of the limb supplied. This has been termed 'thromboembolism'. By contrast, 'atheroembolism' or cholesterol-crystal embolism occurs when much smaller and more numerous particles, composed prin-cipally of cholesterol crystals, lodge in a number of small arteries simultaneously. The presence of a collateral circulation usually prevents infarction, and the event frequently passes unrecognized by the patient or their physician. However, tissue damage in a number of organs can result from multiple showers of emboli. Because severe ulcerative atherosclerosis is most frequently present in the abdominal aorta, cholesterol embolism commonly affects the legs, gastrointestinal tract, and kidneys. The condition usually presents as a complication of vascular surgery or angiographic pro-cedures, when mechanical dislodgement of crystals from ulcerated plaques occurs. Anticoagulant and thrombolytic use has also been implicated as a predisposing factor. The clinical features are those of a systemic disorder with renal failure that can mimic vasculitis, although more indolent cases with stable renal failure have been observed.

Epidemiology

The incidence of cholesterol-crystal embolism found at post-mortem is high: 77% after aortic surgery, 30% after aortography,

and 25.5% after cardiac catheterization. By contrast, the clinical syndrome of cholesterol-crystal embolism is rare, complicating less than 2% of cardiac catheterizations.

Since the condition occurs in patients with severe atheromatous disease, it is most often seen in older male patients with obvious risk factors (hypertension, diabetes mellitus, smoking, etc.) and overt vas-cular disease (ischaemic heart disease, abdominal aortic aneurysm, cerebrovascular disease, etc.). Although spontaneous cholesterol embolism can occur, it is much more common after vascular sur-gery or invasive radiology including aortography, angiography, and angioplasty. Under these circumstances, direct trauma to the vessel may result in detachment of atheromatous material from a ruptured plaque, or denude the endothelial lining of the vessel exposing the underlying atheroma for subsequent embolization. Anticoagulant use has been associated with cholesterol embolism, and it has been proposed that by preventing thrombosis of ulcerating atheromatous plaques, anticoagulants favour the dissemination of atheromatous material. However, a causal relationship is unproven and many patients with widespread atherosclerosis coincidentally receive anti-coagulants for a variety of reasons. Cholesterol embolism following the use of thrombolytic agents has been rarely reported.

Prevention

Prevention is important, particularly with the increasing number of older patients submitted to invasive angiography. Noninvasive methods of arterial imaging such as CT or magnetic resonance (MR) angiography are to be preferred in patients with diffuse atherosclerosis. When invasive angiography is unavoidable, careful attention must be paid to the angiographic technique, including the arterial approach (brachial, or radial instead of femoral, for cardiac catheterization), use of softer, more flexible catheters, and reduced catheter manipulation.

Clinical features

Symptoms are often nonspecific with fever, weight loss, and myalgia. The clinical features are, otherwise, determined by the pattern of organ involvement and are usually referable to the gastrointestinal tract, kidneys, and legs. Bilateral skin changes over the lower extremities are the commonest physical finding and include livedo reticularis, a purpuric rash, 'trash feet', blue toes (acral cyanosis), and focal digital necrosis (Figs. 16.14.3.1 and 16.14.3.2). Ulceration, nodules, and petechiae have also been described. Despite these skin changes and the presence of calf claudication (or frank myositis), pedal pulses may be felt easily, emphasizing that small vessels are occluded in this disorder. Carotid and femoral bruits are frequently heard, reflecting widespread and generalized atherosclerosis.

Abdominal pain, gastrointestinal bleeding, and pancreatitis may occur, and embolism to the stomach, small bowel, colon, gall-bladder, and spleen have all been reported. The most frequently involved of these sites is the colon.

Because of their large blood supply and proximity to the abdom-inal aorta, the kidneys are commonly affected. This usually mani-fests as a subacute stepwise deterioration in renal function over 2 to 6 weeks, invariably accompanied by a worsening of pre-existing hypertension that can be labile and difficult to control. Cardiac failure with pulmonary oedema is a common accompaniment. Acute renal failure with necrotizing glomerulonephritis and cres-cent formation on renal biopsy has been described, but is rare.

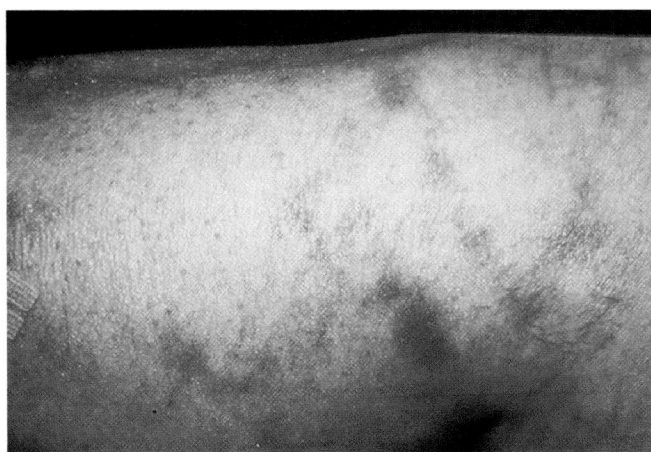

Fig. 16.14.3.1 Livedo reticularis and vasculitic-like erythematous nodules on the leg of a patient in whom cholesterol-crystal embolization occurred after coronary angiography.

Thus, a typical case is an elderly man presenting after angiography with progressive renal failure accompanied by a low-grade fever, abdominal pain, livedo reticularis of the lower body, and purpura over the feet with focal digital ischaemia of the toes.

Transient ischaemic attacks, amaurosis fugax, and strokes can occur when embolism is from the carotid arteries or aortic arch. Retinal cholesterol-crystal emboli may be observed on ophthalmoscopy as bright refractile plaques within the retinal arterioles, especially at their bifurcation. Spinal cord infarction has also been reported.

Differential diagnosis

The diagnosis is frequently missed during life, or confused with that of acute renal failure induced by radiocontrast media (contrast nephropathy) when renal failure occurs after arteriography. A high index of clinical suspicion is therefore required, particularly in elderly patients with evidence of atherosclerotic disease who develop renal failure after arteriography or following aortic or cardiac surgery; cholesterol embolism should also be considered in the differential diagnosis of a multisystem disease in elderly patients. Spontaneous cholesterol-crystal embolism associated with renal failure, fever, rash, and eosinophilia may, not surprisingly,

be misdiagnosed as a vasculitic illness such as Wegener's granulomatosis, microscopic polyangiitis, Churg–Strauss syndrome, polyarteritis nodosa, or bacterial endocarditis (see Chapter 21.10.2). A false-positive antineutrophil cytoplasmic antibody (ANCA) test (not uncommonly by immunofluorescence, rarely to specific antigen) may further compound the diagnostic difficulty. Under these circumstances, renal biopsy is mandatory to make the correct diagnosis.

Clinical investigation

Laboratory findings are non-specific, but frequently include a raised erythrocyte sedimentation rate (ESR), plasma viscosity, and C-reactive protein (CRP). Leucocytosis and a transient eosinophilia are common and may be pronounced. Depending on the tissue involvement, an elevation in creatine phosphokinase, amylase, lactate dehydrogenase (LDH), serum aspartate aminotransferase (AST), and alkaline phosphatase may all be seen. Hypocomplementaemia is rare and usually mild. As stated above, ANCA have been reported, and their presence may further confuse the diagnosis with a multisystem vasculitic process. Mild proteinuria is generally present, and nephrotic-range proteinuria has been reported. Urine microscopy may be bland or reveal red cells, white cells (particularly eosinophils), and hyaline and granular casts. Renal failure is frequently nonoliguric.

Histology

The definitive histological diagnosis of cholesterol-crystal embolism can usually be made from biopsies of kidney, skin, or muscle (including clinically uninvolved areas), although sampling error may miss the lesion due to its patchy distribution. Ante-mortem histological diagnoses have also been made from other tissues, including a gastric biopsy, prostatic currettings, and a bone marrow biopsy. The diagnostic feature is of biconvex, needle-shaped cholesterol clefts within the lumen of arteries or arterioles that remain after the crystals have dissolved during routine histological preparation (Fig. 16.14.3.3). In fresh samples, the crystals can be identified by birefringence under polarized light or by specific histochemical staining of cholesterol. In the kidneys, the typical finding is occlusion of small arteries and arterioles of between 150 and 200 μm in diameter,

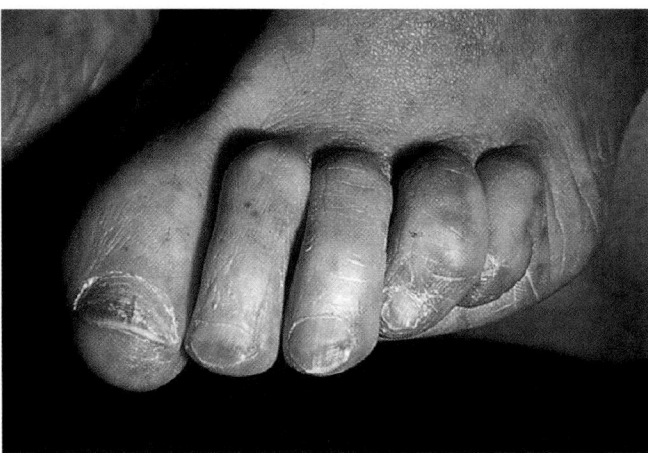

Fig. 16.14.3.2 Purpuric spots and acral cyanosis of the toes from cholesterol embolism after aortic aneurysm repair.

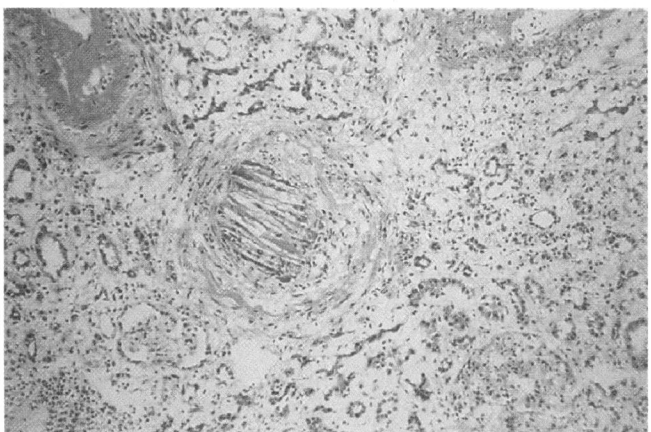

Fig. 16.14.3.3 Renal biopsy demonstrating the characteristic needle-shaped cholesterol clefts occluding a medium-sized renal arteriole with surrounding inflammatory cell infiltration, intimal proliferation, thickening, and concentric fibrosis. There is extensive autolysis (post-mortem sample).

such as the arcuate and interlobular arteries, resulting in patchy areas of ischaemia and small areas of infarction. Crystals can also be seen within the glomeruli. In chronic cases, ischaemia produces a wedge-shaped lesion involving all components of the renal cortex radiating towards the capsule. The glomeruli appear ischaemic and sclerosed and the tubules become atrophic and separated by interstitial fibrosis. Grossly, the kidneys may be reduced in size with a rough granular surface and wedge-shaped scars.

Based on animal studies involving the injection of atheromatous material, the presence of cholesterol crystals in the vascular lumen is thought to trigger a localized inflammatory and endothelial vascular reaction. Inflammatory cells (mainly macrophages and eosinophils) infiltrate, and multinucleated giant cells engulf the cholesterol crystals, but these are resistant to the scavenger effects of macrophages and may persist for many months. The inflammatory phase is followed by marked intimal thickening with concentric fibrosis and occlusion of the vessel. Depending on the extent of organ involvement, these pathological changes result in ischaemia, infarction, or—rarely—necrosis of the distal tissue.

Management

There is no effective therapy. Steroids, aspirin, dipyridamole, and low-molecular weight dextran have all been tried, but without any clear effect. There are anecdotal reports of a response to hydroxyl methyl glutaryl coenzyme A (HMG CoA)-reductase inhibitors (statins, theoretically inducing plaque stabilization), but recovery may have been spontaneous. Anticoagulants are of no proven benefit and should be avoided given their potential role in the pathogenesis of the disorder. Encouraging results with iloprost and low density lipoprotein (LDL) apheresis have been reported, but these observations require replication.

CT scanning of the aorta has been used to identify the precise source (e.g. aortic aneurysm, localized aortic plaque) of cholesterol emboli, and surgical replacement of the diseased vessel with a graft has been advocated. However, major surgery in elderly patients with widespread vascular disease and renal impairment carries significant risks and is generally avoided.

Supportive therapy is directed at stopping anticoagulation unless essential, avoiding further angiographic or vascular surgical procedures, controlling hypertension, and appropriate management of renal failure. Use of angiotensin converting enzyme (ACE) inhibitors or angiotensin receptor blockers (ARB) has been advocated, but careful monitoring of renal function is required.

Prognosis

Mortality is high, due to the coexistence of cardiac and vascular disease with renal failure in elderly patients. Renal impairment may remain stable, but frequently progresses such that dialysis is required, although partial recovery has been reported, even after several months of dialysis. The mechanism of this recovery is uncertain.

Further reading

Belenfant X, Meyrier A, Jacquot C (1999). Supportive treatment improves survival in multivisceral cholesterol crystal embolism. *Am J Kidney Dis*, **33**, 840–50.

Elinav E, Chajek-Shaul T, Stern M (2002). Improvement in cholesterol emboli syndrome after iloprost therapy. *BMJ*, **324**, 268–9.

Fine MJ, Kapoor W, Falanga V (1987). Cholesterol crystal embolization: a review of 221 cases in the English literature. *Angiology*, **38**, 769–84.

Hasegawa M, Sugiyama S (2003). Apheresis in the treatment of cholesterol embolic disease. *Ther Apher Dial*, **7**, 435–8.

Hyman BT, *et al.* (1987). Warfarin-related purple toes syndrome and cholesterol microembolization. *Am J Med*, **82**, 1233–7.

Keen RR, *et al.* (1995). Surgical management of atheroembolization. *J Vasc Surg*, **21**, 773–81.

Mannesse CK (1991). Renal failure and cholesterol crystal embolization: a report of 4 surviving cases and a review of the literature. *Clin Nephrol*, **36**, 240–5.

Meyrier A (2006). Cholesterol crystal embolism: diagnosis and treatment. *Kidney Int*, **69**, 1308–12.

Scolari F, *et al.* (2000). Cholesterol crystal embolism: a recognizable cause of renal disease. *Am J Kidney Dis*, **36**, 1089–90.

Scolari *et al.* (2007). The challenge of diagnosing atheroembolic renal disease: clinical features and prognostic factors. *Circulation*, **116**(3), 298–304.

16.14.4 Takayasu's arteritis

Yasushi Kobayashi

Essentials

Takayasu's arteritis is a chronic granulomatous vasculitis of unknown cause characterized by stenosis, occlusion, and aneurysm of large elastic arteries, mainly the aorta and its branches. It mainly affects young women, predominantly in Asian, Middle Eastern, and South American countries.

Clinical presentation—symptoms in the acute stage are nonspecific, such as general fatigue and fever, which can persist for months to years. Symptoms in the chronic stage depend on the anatomical location of the vascular lesions, with typical complaints relating to ischaemia of the brain, eyes, or arms. The commonest finding on physical examination is a weak or absent pulse in one or both brachial, radial, and/or ulnar arteries. Bruits can often be heard over affected arteries. Hypertension and aortic insufficiency are strongly associated with poor prognosis.

Diagnosis—comprehensive angiographic imaging is required for diagnosis, evaluation of the extent of disease, and to guide therapy. American College of Rheumatology diagnostic criteria require the presence of three out of the following six to diagnose Takayasu's arteritis: (1) age of onset less than 40 years; (2) claudication of a limb; (3) decreased brachial artery pulse; (4) systolic pressure difference between two limbs greater than 10 mmHg; (5) bruit over aorta or subclavian arteries; and (6) angiographic narrowing/occlusion of aorta, its primary branches, or large arteries in proximal arms or legs.

Treatment—is with prednisolone and antiplatelet agents, with other immunosuppressants added if necessary. Surgical bypass graft procedures are often required.

Introduction

Takayasu's arteritis is a chronic granulomatous vasculitis characterized by stenosis, occlusion, and aneurysm of large elastic arteries, mainly the aorta and its branches, including the coronary arteries (Fig. 16.14.4.1). The pulmonary arteries can also be affected. Pathologically the condition is defined as vasa vasoritis of the aorta, which generally affects young women during their reproductive period.

Acute severe inflammation sometimes causes dilatation of vessel walls and/or aneurysm formation. Chronic inflammation causes arterial stenosis and occlusion due to thrombus. In the early stages patients often have nonspecific inflammatory symptoms such as intermittent fever, fatigue, and malaise,which may exist for months to years prior to the onset of full-blown vasculitis, when clinical manifestations then depend on the arteries involved.

Historical perspective

Takayasu's arteritis was described by Mikito Takayasu at the 12th Annual Meeting of the Japanese Ophthalmology Society in 1908. He reported a case of a 21-year-old woman who had a peculiar wreath-like arteriovenous anastomosis, termed a 'coronary anastomosis', around the optic papilla (Fig. 16.14.4.2). As is often the case for eponymous diseases, the condition had almost certainly been observed before. In 1761 Morgagni reported a 40-year-old woman in Italy whose radial pulses were impalpable for many years. In 1856 Savoy described a young woman in whom the main arteries of both arms and of the left side of the neck were completely obliterated.

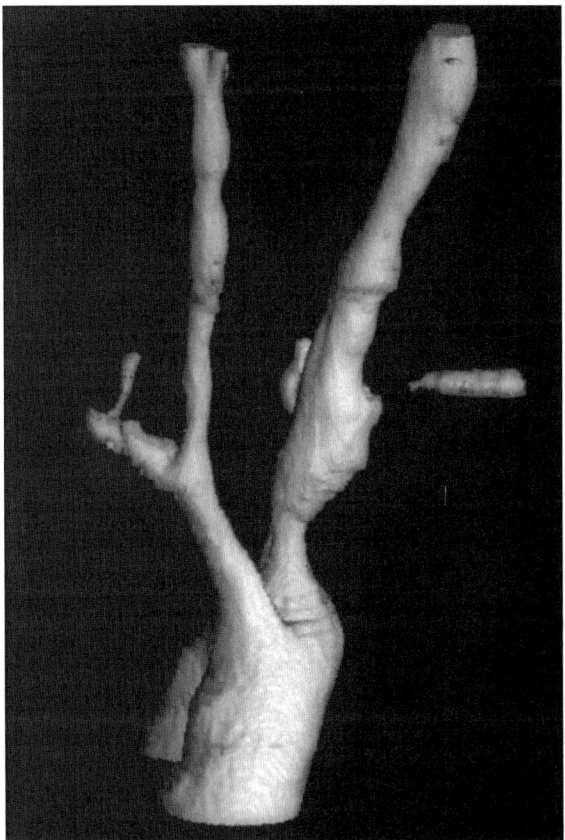

Fig. 16.14.4.1 Three-dimensional CT image showing narrowing and aneurysmal dilatation in the aorta and vessels arising from the aorta in Takayasu's arteritis.

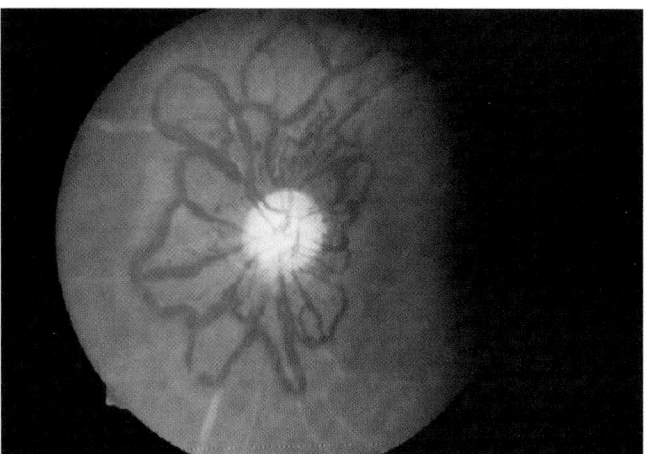

Fig. 16.14.4.2 Typical coronary anastomosis of retinal vessels in Takayasu's arteritis.

Takayasu's arteritis has also been called pulseless disease, aortitis syndrome, aortic arch syndrome, long-segment atypical coarctation of the aorta, Martorell's syndrome, and occlusive thrombo-aortopathy.

Aetiology and pathology

The aetiology of Takayasu's arteritis remains unknown. For a long time tuberculosis was suspected to be the cause in India and Mexico, but the incidence of proven tuberculosis in patients with Takayasu's arteritis was not higher than that in the general population and it is not now considered to be a causative agent. Takayasu's arteritis after hepatitis B vaccination has also been reported, but so far no clear bacterial or viral organism has been incriminated as the cause, although it may be that aberrant host response to infection is a trigger.

The observations that there is a strong predilection for women, higher incidence in Asian, Middle Eastern, and South American populations, and that cases have been described in monozygotic twins, are all consistent with a role for genetic factors in causing Takayasu's arteritis. But balanced against this must be the fact that only 1% of Japanese patients with Takayasu's arteritis have affected relatives.

HLA studies in Japan revealed positive associations of Takayasu's arteritis with the class II alleles HLA DRB1*1502 and DPB1* 0901, and with the class I alleles B*5201 and B*3902, with the two class II alleles mentioned in strong linkage disequilibrium with HLA B*5201 in Japanese population. An association of HLA with Takayasu's arteritis has also been reported in Mexico and Colombia. Such HLA associations suggest that specific antigen may be related to the cause of inflammation in Takayasu's arteritis.

Pathologically Takayasu's arteritis is defined as an inflammatory vasculopathy that involves mainly large and mid-sized vessels. The aorta is thick and often rigid secondary to fibrosis of all three arterial layers, particularly the adventitia and intima. It is characteristic that narrowings of the aortic lumen may alternate with aneurysmal dilatations of the aortic wall ('skipped lesions'). The gross appearance of the intima may be of cobblestones, with smooth, round, white, gelatinous, well-circumscribed plaques of variable size alternating with intervening normal intima. When thickened the intima may reveal longitudinal wrinkling and ridges that give the gross appearance of tree bark. In endstage Takayasu's arteritis the aorta may have a 'lead pipe' appearance.

Takayasu's arteritis may be divided into an acute florid inflammatory phase and a chronic healed fibrotic phase, with both types sometimes seen simultaneously suggesting recurrent inflammation. In the acute phase the inflammatory lesions originate in the vasa vasorum and are characterized by perivascular cuffing, mainly composed of γδT lymphocytes, cytotoxic T cells, and helper T cells. Luminal stenosis of small adventitial arteries due to intimal thickening is relatively common, and an increase in the adventitial thickness due to fibrosis is a histopathological feature found in the chronic phase. Inflammatory infiltrates in the arterial wall are typically arranged in granulomas that are dependent on T cells regulating the activity and integrity of macrophages. The media has neovascularization often accompanied by infiltrates of lymphocytes, plasma cells and occasional Langerhans type giant cells. Patches of medial coagulation necrosis surrounded by a fence-like arrangement of epithelioid cells are occasionally seen at the periphery. In the chronic stage of Takayasu's arteritis, intimal fibrosis is often accompanied by well-formed fibrous atherosclerotic plaques and calcification. Extension of the adventitial fibrosis and round cell infiltration to adjacent structures may result in retroperitoneal fibrosis.

Epidemiology

Although Takayasu's arteritis has been reported from all over the world, there is a wide variation in its prevalence in different geographical regions. It is predominantly found in Asian, Middle Eastern, and South American countries, although recently patients with the condition have been increasingly recognized in Africa, Europe, and North America. The incidence rate of Takayasu's arteritis in Japan in 2005 was 4.2 persons per 100 000 population; by contrast, in Sweden and the United States of America the prevalence was reported to be between 0.26 and 0.64 persons per 100 000 population.

Takayasu's arteritis affects healthy young women, the average age of onset in Japanese and Indian patients being 15–35 years old.

Clinical features

Some patients are asymptomatic and diagnosed as having Takayasu's arteritis incidentally when they are found to lack pulses, have a significant difference in blood pressure between their arms, or to have raised inflammatory markers on blood testing. When they occur, clinical symptoms may be divided into those of acute and chronic stages.

In the acute stage the symptoms of Takayasu's arteritis are usually nonspecific and generalized, including fever, easy fatigability, general malaise, neck pain, weight loss, and arthralgia. Faintness and/or dizziness are sometimes reported, perhaps due to hypersensitivity of the baroreceptors in the aortic arch leading to hypotension. The vague and nonspecific nature of these symptoms means that the diagnosis is often missed for a long time. Stroke and sudden blindness may be caused by thrombosis of cerebral arteries.

In the chronic stage most patients with Takayasu's arteritis present with features related to specific vascular lesions, although they may also have the constitutional symptoms described above. In east Asian countries the condition affects the aortic arch most frequently, hence typical complaints relate to ischaemia of the brain, eyes, or arms, namely dizziness, syncope, visual disturbance, and easy fatigability of the arms, with pain due to intermittent claudication. By contrast, in south Asian countries Takayasu's arteritis tends to affect the abdominal arteries such that hypertension may be the first clue. This may be caused by atypical coarctation of the aorta, loss of vascular compliance of the aorta, aortic insufficiency, or renal artery stenosis.

The commonest finding on physical examination is a weak or absent pulse in one or both brachial, radial, and/or ulnar arteries (usually on the left side), which is noted in about 80% of Japanese patients. Reduced blood pressure in one or both arms is often observed. Bruits can often be heard over affected arteries. A 'bird face' due to atrophy of facial muscles (Fig. 16.14.4.3), intermittent claudication of the jaw muscles and perforation of the nasal septum – all due to ischaemia – are helpful diagnostic clues.

Cardiac manifestations of Takayasu's arteritis are associated with poor prognosis and are the commonest cause of death in Japanese patients. Aortic insufficiency is present in almost one-third in Japanese series, typically caused by annulo-aortic ectasia, and left ventricular hypertrophy is often observed, presumed related to hypertension. The combination of aortic insufficiency and left ventricular hypertrophy may eventually result in heart failure. The inflammation of Takayasu's arteritis may involve the ostia of the coronary arteries and thus lead to exertional angina or acute myocardial infarction.

Pulmonary lesions are frequently found with imaging techniques, but clinical symptoms such as haemoptysis and dyspnoea are uncommon. Isolated pulmonary arteritis has rarely been reported.

Renal artery involvement in Takayasu's arteritis causes hypertension and renal dysfunction. In India almost one-half of all patients with Takayasu's arteritis exhibit ostial and/or proximal renal arterial involvement. Hypertension, nephritic/nephrotic syndrome and renal failure are reported consequences or associations.

Acute gastrointestinal bleeding may be the first symptom in Takayasu's arteritis, and Crohn's disease, ulcerative colitis, and nonspecific inflammatory colitis are rarely associated with the condition.

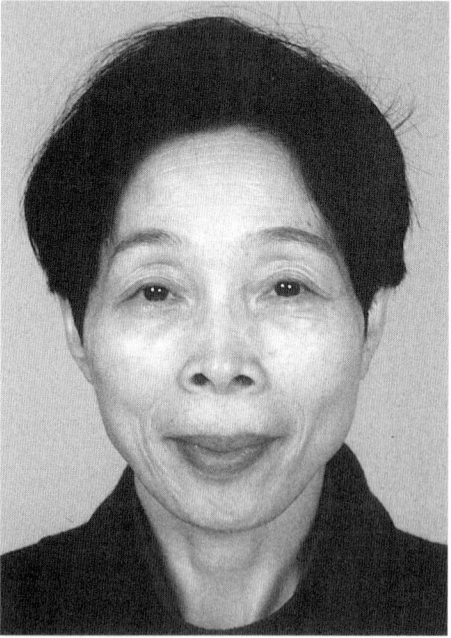

Fig. 16.14.4.3 The 'bird face' of Takayasu's arteritis: note the hollow cheeks and eye sockets.

The ocular complications of Takayasu's arteritis are decreasing due to advances in early diagnosis and therapy. Emboli may cause sudden blindness in the acute stage. Hypertensive retinopathy is commonly reported, with other ocular complications including cataracts, optic atrophy, loss of eye reflexes, iris atrophy, and rubeosis iris.

Erythema nodosum is the most common skin lesion associated with Takayasu's arteritis in white populations, and ulcerative subacute nodular lesions have been described in Mexico and Japan.

Differential diagnosis

The nonspecific symptoms of the acute stage of Takayasu's arteritis are most commonly misdiagnosed as being due to viral infection, tuberculosis, rheumatoid arthritis, or other causes of a 'fever of unknown origin'. The differential diagnosis of the chronic stage includes atherosclerosis, inflammatory abdominal aortic aneurysm, Behçet's disease, syphilitic aortitis, temporal arteritis, and congenital vascular abnormality.

Investigation

The most frequent laboratory abnormalities are elevation of erythrocyte sedimentation rate (70–90% of cases) and C-reactive protein (50–70%), which are good indices of acute disease activity. The white blood cell count (40%) and gammaglobulin level are often elevated, and mild anaemia (50%) and elevation of complement factors are also observed. Coagulopathies and platelet activation are seen in the acute stage. HLA typing may help with prognosis of Takayasu's arteritis in some countries.

On the chest radiograph, segmental, fine dystrophic calcification with abrupt termination is very suggestive of Takayasu's arteritis in a young patient (Fig. 16.14.4.4). Rib notching due to aortic aneurysm or dilatation of ascending aorta may also be found.

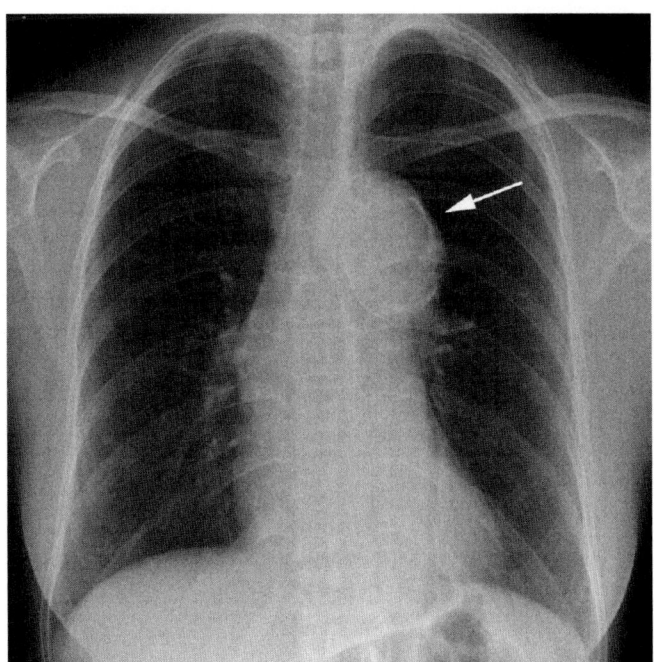

Fig. 16.14.4.4 Chest radiograph showing calcification along the aorta (arrow) in Takayasu's arteritis.

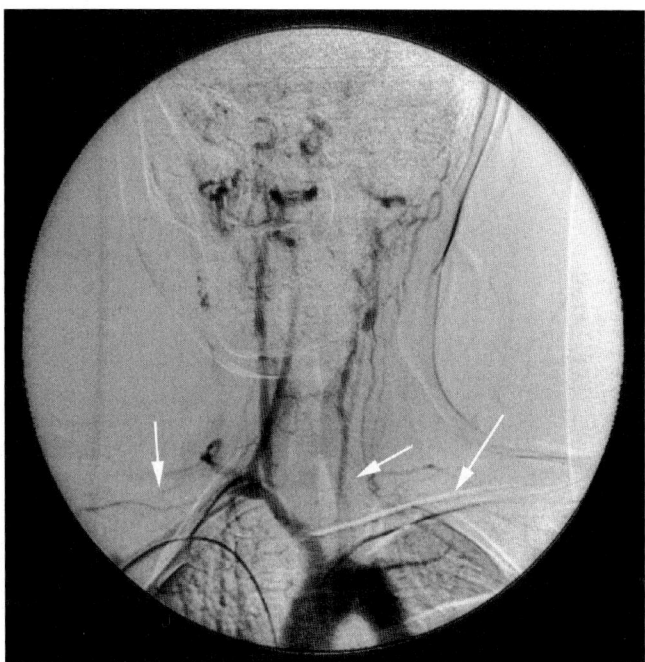

Fig. 16.14.4.5 Angiogram showed marked narrowing of the left common carotid artery and both subclavian arteries (arrows) in Takayasu's arteritis.

A comprehensive angiogram is performed to diagnose Takayasu's arteritis and evaluate the extent of disease and guide therapy (Fig. 16.14.4.5). Digital subtraction angiography (DSA), CT, and magnetic resonance angiography (MRA) may also provide valuable information. Localized narrowing or irregularities of the aortic wall are early changes on arteriography. Obliterative vascular lesions range from narrowing and stenosis to complete occlusion. The vessel may be dilated or aneurismal, and there may be a combination of obstruction and aneurismal dilatation. The classification proposed by the international cooperative study on Takayasu's arteritis is used to standardize description of disease based on location of vascular lesion (Table 16.14.4.1); involvement of coronary or pulmonary arteries is designated as C(+) or P(+), along with any of the types.

Aortic insufficiency and cardiac function should be assessed by echocardiography. Doppler ultrasonography can demonstrate lesions of the carotid artery and estimate intimal thickness, which may reflect disease activity, as can the use of MRI to detect vessel wall oedema. ^{18}F-fluorodeoxyglucose positron emission tomography (^{18}F-FDG PET) can show inflammatory activity and—in conjunction with CT or MRI—define its anatomical location, potentially enabling early diagnosis of Takayasu's arteritis with estimation of the inflammatory burden (Fig. 16.14.4.6). However, ^{18}F-FDG can

Table 16.14.4.1 Classification of Takayasu's arteritis

Type	Site of involvement
I	Branches of aortic arch
II	Ascending aorta, aortic arch, and its branches
III	Ascending aorta, aortic arch, and its branches, and thoracic descending aorta
IV	Abdominal aorta and/or renal arteries
V	Combination of types IIb and IV

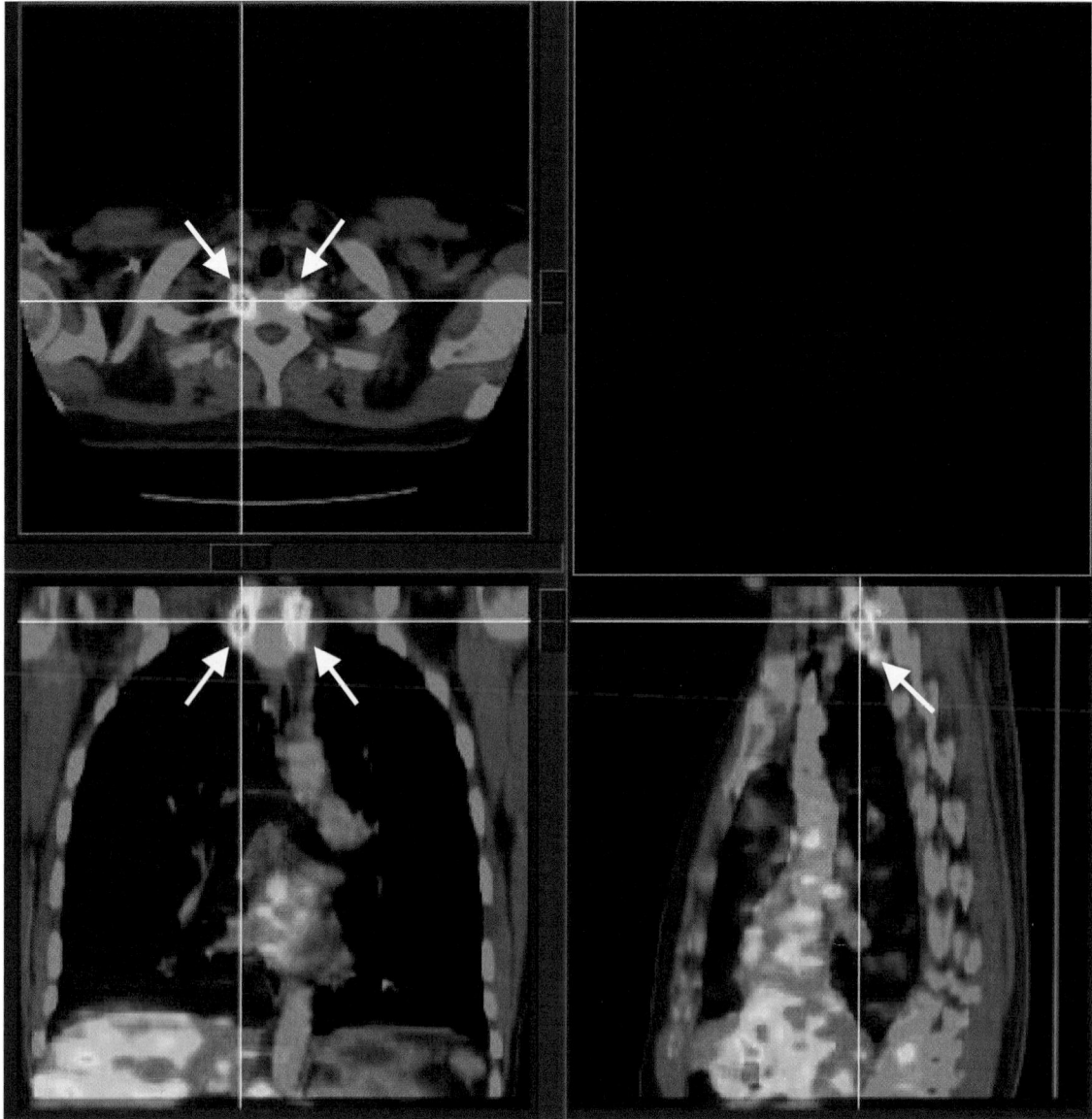

Fig. 16.14.4.6 ^{18}F-FDG PET showing inflammation in both vertebral arteries (arrows) in Takayasu's arteritis.

also be accumulated in atherosclerotic lesions and other vascular diseases, hence FDG-PET data must be interpreted carefully in conjunction with other clinical and laboratory findings.

Criteria for diagnosis

The diagnosis of Takayasu's arteritis is based on the finding of vascular lesions in large and middle size vessels by angiogram, CT, or MRI. Age of onset should also be considered in making the diagnosis. The American College of Rheumatology has proposed following diagnostic criteria, which are generally accepted, with presence of three out of the six required for diagnosis:

1 Age of onset <40 years old

2 Claudication of an extremity

3 Decreased brachial artery pulse

4 Difference of more than 10 mm Hg systolic pressure between two limbs

5 Bruit over subclavian arteries or the aorta

6 Angiographic evidence of narrowing or occlusion of the aorta, its primary branches, or large arteries in the proximal upper or lower extremities

Treatment

Medical management of Takayasu's arteritis in the acute stage is with corticosteroids as a first line therapy. The use of low dose aspirin or other antiplatelet drugs in addition reduces the likelihood of ischaemic complication. A typical initial regimen would be oral prednisolone at a dose of 0.5–1 mg/kg per day, depending upon the clinical symptoms and general inflammatory markers. About 60 to 80% of patients will go into remission, but relapse during corticosteroid taper occurs in more than 50%. If patients cannot then be tapered to an alternate-day regimen without disease exacerbation, a cytotoxic agent such as ciclosporin, cyclophosphamide, azathioprine, or methotrexate can be used, ciclosporin typically being administered as a daily oral dose of 1 to 3 mg/kg per day in conjunction with prednisolone 10 to 20 mg daily.

Established vascular lesions are usually not reversible with medical treatment alone, hence surgical intervention may be needed if severe ischaemic organ dysfunction is present. This is commonly required in patients with severe complications of Takayasu's arteritis, particularly for cerebrovascular disease due to cervicocranial vessel stenosis, coronary artery disease, severe to moderate aortic regurgitation, severe coarctation of the aorta, renovascular hypertension, limb claudication and progressive aneurysm enlargement. Bypass graft procedures are often performed, with good long-term outcomes reported.

Takayasu's arteritis is a disease that affects women of childbearing age, but it does not alter fertility, hence it sometimes presents during pregnancy and around the time of delivery, and recurrences may also occur at these times. Inflammation during pregnancy may be managed with prednisolone, with dose based on the activity of inflammation. Management of labour and/or the decision to proceed to caesarean section are based on standard assessment of maternal and fetal risk factors.

Prognosis

Earlier diagnosis of Takayasu's arteritis, attributable to increased clinical awareness of the condition and advances in imaging techniques, mean that the reported prognosis of the condition has improved. In recent series most patients are well controlled, with no or minimal symptoms, and many are on no treatment. However, 25 to 30% have a poor prognosis, the major factors contributing to this being cardiovascular complications, particularly aortic insufficiency and hypertension causing congestive heart failure.

Cerebrovascular events, myocardial infarction, and pulmonary infarction may be fatal.

Further reading

Arend WP, et al. (1990). The American College of Rhematology: Criteria for the determination of Takayasu arteritis. *Arthritis Rheum*, **33**, 1129–34.

Andrews J, Mason JC (2006). Takayasu's arteritis—recent advances in imaging offer promise. *Rheumatology*, **46**, 6–15.

Gravanis MB (2000). Giant cell arteritis and Takayasu aortitis: morphologic, pathogenetic and etiologic factors. *Int J Cardiol*, **75** Suppl 1, S21–33.

Hashimoto Y, et al. (1992). Aortic regurgitation in patients with Takayasu arteritis: assessment by color Doppler echocardiography. *Heart Vessels*, **7** Suppl, 111–5.

Hata A, et al. (1996). Angiographic findings of Takayasu arteritis: new classification. *Int J Cardiol*, **54** Suppl, S155–63.

Hoffman GS, et al. (1994). Treatment of glucocorticoid-resistant or relapsing Takayasu arteritis with methotrexate. *Arthritis Rheum*, **37**, 578–82.

Jennette JC, et al. (1994). Nomenclature of systemic vasculitides. Proposal of an international consensus conference. *Arthritis Rheum*, **37**, 187–92.

Kerr GS, et al. (1994). Takayasu arteritis. *Ann Intern Med*, **120**, 919–29.

Kimura A, et al. (2000). Mapping of the HLA-linked genes controlling the susceptibility to Takayasu's arteritis. *Int J Cardiol*, **75** Suppl 1, S105–10.

Kobayashi Y, et al. (2005). Aortic wall inflammation due to Takayasu arteritis imaged with ^{18}F-FDG PET coregistered with enhanced CT. *J Nuclear Med*, **46**, 917–22.

Miyata T, et al. (2003). Long-term survival after surgical treatment of patients with Takayasu's arteritis. *Circulation*, **108**, 1474–80.

Numano F (2000). Vasa vasoritis, vasculitis and atherosclerosis. *Int J Cardiology*, **75** Suppl, 1–8.

Numano F, et al. (2000). Takayasu's arteritis. *Lancet*, **356**, 1023–5.

The pulmonary circulation

Contents

Many neural and humoral mediators can influence pulmonary vascular tone, including nitric oxide and prostacyclin. Alveolar hypoxia causes constriction of the small pulmonary arteries, whereas systemic arteries dilate when hypoxic: this hypoxic pulmonary vasoconstriction can reduce venous admixture and improve arterial oxygenation in the presence of bronchial obstruction. Despite large regional differences in the matching of ventilation and perfusion within the normal lung, the overall lung ventilation–perfusion ratio is maintained remarkably steady at around 0.85.

16.15.1 Structure and function

Nicholas W. Morrell

Essentials

The normal pulmonary circulation distributes deoxygenated blood at low pressure and high flow to the pulmonary capillaries for the purposes of gas exchange. The structure of pulmonary blood vessels varies with their function—from large elastic conductance arteries, to small muscular arteries, to thin-walled vessels involved in gas exchange.

Pulmonary vascular resistance (PVR) is about one-tenth of systemic vascular resistance, with the small muscular and partially muscular arteries of 50 to 150 μm diameter being the site of the greatest contribution to resistance. The gas-exchanging capillary surface area (*c.* 125 m^2) contains a blood volume of about 150 ml at any one time, with the blood–gas barrier being only 0.2 to 0.3 μm thick at its thinnest part. In the normal pulmonary circulation, a large increase in cardiac output causes only a small rise in mean pulmonary arterial pressure because PVR falls on exercise: this is accomplished by a combination of vascular distensibility and recruitment. Pulmonary blood flow is heterogeneous: gravity causes increased blood flow in the more dependent parts of the lung; within a horizontal region—or within an acinus—blood-flow heterogeneity is imposed by the branching pattern of the vessels.

Introduction

The main function of the pulmonary circulation is respiratory gas exchange, a vital function that the lungs take over from the placenta at birth. The structure of the pulmonary circulation is highly adapted to fulfil this role. It receives the entire cardiac output from the right ventricle during each cardiac cycle, and this mixed venous blood is delivered at high flow but low pressure to the delicate alveolar structures where gas exchange occurs. Blood flow is matched closely to the regional ventilation within the lung to optimize and maintain systemic arterial oxygenation. This chapter discusses the anatomy and physiology of the pulmonary circulation.

Structure of the pulmonary circulation

The pulmonary arteries and bronchi, together with lymphatics, run in a single connective tissue sheath in the centre of pulmonary segments and lobules, the so-called bronchovascular bundle. The 'conventional' pulmonary arteries branch dichotomously and symmetrically, along with the airways, and they also give off extra branches between the conventional branching points, called 'supernumerary' or short branches. The intrapulmonary veins pursue a different course along the edges of lobules and segments, in the interlobular septa. The branching pattern of veins is similar to that of the pulmonary arteries.

The branching pattern of the pulmonary arteries can be described by a 'divergent' approach, where the main pulmonary artery is called generation 1, with each division giving rise to generation 2, 3, etc. An alternative is the 'convergent' approach where the most peripheral branch is numbered 'order 1', and the orders increase until the main pulmonary artery (order 17) is reached.

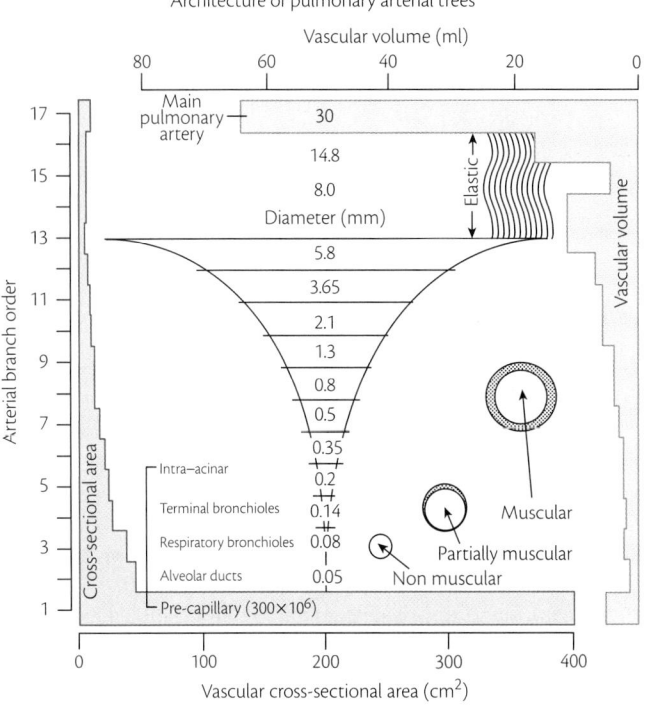

Fig. 16.15.1.1 Map of the pulmonary arterial tree showing how vascular volumes, cross-sectional areas, diameters, and wall structure vary with branch order number.

Fig. 16.15.1.1 shows this arrangement going from the pre-capillary arteriole of order 1, whose diameter is about 13 µm, to the main pulmonary artery (order 17) with a diameter of 30 000 µm. Note the ninefold expansion in cross-sectional area of the pulmonary vascular bed from order 2 to order 1: it is these precapillary vessels that are often involved in disease processes that affect the pulmonary circulation. In the normal lung, the site of the greatest pulmonary vascular resistance (PVR) is in the small partially muscular and muscular pulmonary arteries (orders 4 to 6; 50–150 µm diameter).

The wall structure of the pulmonary arteries changes along their length depending on the function of the vessel (Fig. 16.15.1.2).

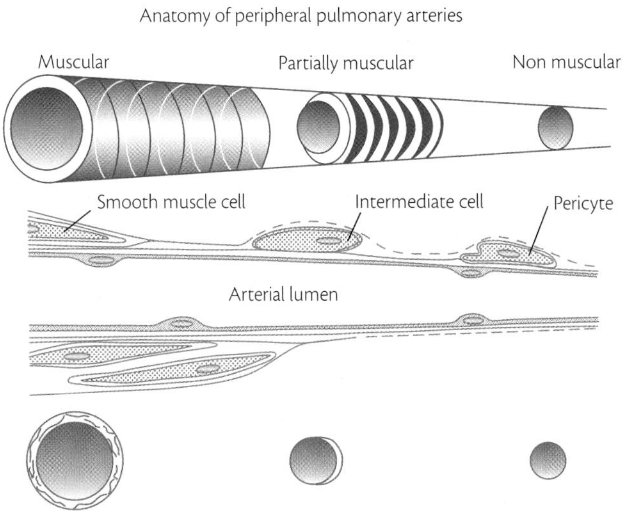

Anatomy of peripheral pulmonary arteries

Muscular   Partially muscular   Non muscular

Smooth muscle cell   Intermediate cell   Pericyte

Arterial lumen

Fig. 16.15.1.2 The changing structure of pulmonary arteries.

All pre-acinar arteries have a complete muscular coat, but the muscle layer may be incomplete or absent in smaller intra-acinar vessels.

◆ Elastic arteries (orders 17–13): these larger arteries have adventitial, muscular, and intimal layers. The media, or muscular layer, is bounded by internal and external elastic laminae, with three or more elastic laminae within the muscle coat. Medial thickness is about 1 to 2% of external diameter.

◆ Muscular arteries (orders 13–3): these small arteries have a thicker muscle layer in relation to their external diameter (2–5%), and they possess only internal and external elastic laminae; in the smallest arteries, the internal elastic lamina disappears.

◆ Partially muscular arteries (orders 5–3): the smooth muscle fibres investing the smallest pulmonary arteries taper off in a spiral, leading to an incomplete muscular coat (Fig. 16.15.1.2). Most arteries of 50 to 100 µm external diameter are partially muscular.

◆ Nonmuscular arteries (orders 5–1): these arteries have no elastic laminae. The smooth muscle cell is replaced by pericytes whose basement membrane fuses with that of the endothelial cell lining the vascular lumen.

◆ Supernumerary arteries: these are small, relatively thin-walled arteries that branch sharply from the parent vessel between bifurcations of the conventional branching system, starting from orders 11 to 12. They provide a short cut for blood supplying the alveoli adjacent to the conduit arteries and bronchi, which would otherwise require a long and circuitous supply by the axial route.

◆ Pulmonary veins: the branching pattern and organization of the pulmonary veins is similar to that of the arteries, but with only 15 orders, because the 4 pulmonary veins converge on the left atrium without joining up to form an additional 2 orders. Veins do not have an internal elastic lamina. Their walls contain more elastic tissue and less muscle than arteries of the same size. There are supernumerary veins like the supernumerary arteries.

◆ Capillary network: the 300 million precapillary vessels lead into a network of alveolar septal capillaries with a blood volume (150 ml) equal to that in the pulmonary arterial or venous systems. The capillary surface area is about 125 m² (c.86% of the alveolar surface area). Individual capillaries are not much wider than a single erythrocyte, hence the microvascular bed at normal vascular pressures is essentially a sheet of blood one red cell thick, exposed to alveolar gas on both sides. Alveolar capillaries have a thick side and a thin side. The thin side consists of the cytoplasmic extensions of the luminal endothelial cell and the alveolar epithelial cell with their fused basement membrane (0.2–0.3 µm across). The thick side, up to 2 µm across, contains collagen, elastin, and fibroblast processes to give structural support to the alveolus.

Pulmonary vascular resistance

The pulmonary circulation is a high-flow, low-pressure system whose vascular resistance is one-tenth of systemic vascular resistance. PVR is the ratio of the mean pulmonary arterial–venous pressure difference (Ppa – Ppv) to mean pulmonary blood flow (Qp):

$$(P\text{pa} - P\text{pv})/Q\text{p} = \text{PVR (mmHg/litre per min)}$$

The normal PVR is less than 2 mmHg/litre per min at rest.

The main determinants of PVR are captured in the equation for Poiseuille flow (steady flow of a Newtonian fluid through long, straight, unbranched tubes):

$$PVR \sim 8\mu L/\pi D^4$$

where L is vascular path length, μ is the viscosity of blood, and D is vessel diameter. L/D^4 is known as the geometric factor, the importance of which can be seen by considering that a 16% decrease in D leads to a twofold increase in PVR. In reality, the situation is more complicated because blood flow in the lungs is not of uniform velocity, but is, of course, pulsatile.

PVR normally falls on exercise despite the increase in cardiac output, hence Ppa rises only modestly, perhaps from 15 mmHg at rest to 23 mmHg. The fall in PVR during exercise is accomplished by a combination of vascular 'distensibility' (vascular compliance) and 'recruitment' (number of parallel pathways with flow). Vascular recruitment means that a vessel goes from a state of zero flow to one of finite flow. An increase in pulmonary arterial pressure during exercise can distend pulmonary arteries. The total compliance of the pulmonary circulation is about 20 ml/mmHg, hence on heavy exercise, if all vascular pressures rose by 10 mmHg, pulmonary vascular volume would increase by 200 ml, provided vessels had not reached their limiting size.

The distribution of PVR can be partitioned into a three-segment model, which can be described as having (1) arterial, (2) 'middle', and (3) venous segments. In isolated lungs, about 20% of the total PVR lies in the distensible 'middle' segment (capillaries and small arteries and veins), with 40% each in the arterial and venous segments. This distribution can be altered by factors, e.g. hypoxia, that increase resistance predominantly in the 'middle' segment. Blood viscosity is a further factor that affects PVR, e.g. when polycythaemia increases PVR.

Distribution of pulmonary blood flow

Blood flow within the lung is heterogenous in distribution. For example, between lung regions of secondary lobule size ($c.10\,cm^3$) there is a modest amount of gravity-dependent heterogeneity, with flow increasing with vertical distance (more to the lower zones than the upper zones). Within these lung regions and within the respiratory acinus there is a greater degree of heterogeneity, which is independent of gravity.

Gravity-dependent flow

The effects of gravity are best illustrated by considering that, in the erect posture at rest in man, mean pulmonary artery pressure (Ppa) at the level of the hilum is about 18 cmH$_2$O, whereas the apex of the lung is 20 cmH$_2$O above the hilum. Consequently, the apex of the lung will only be perfused during the systolic pressure peak. In the supine position, the apical blood flow increases, with the result that the distribution from apex to base becomes more uniform. During exercise, with the increase in cardiac output, both upper and lower zone blood flow increases, but the upper increases more than the lower, so that flow becomes more even. The role of gravity in determining pulmonary blood flow was extended by West and encompassed in the three-zone model of pulmonary circulation (Fig. 16.15.1.3). This model relies on the assumption that the site of major flow resistance is in the small vessels whose extravascular pressure is the alveolar pressure ($Palv$). There is no flow in zone I

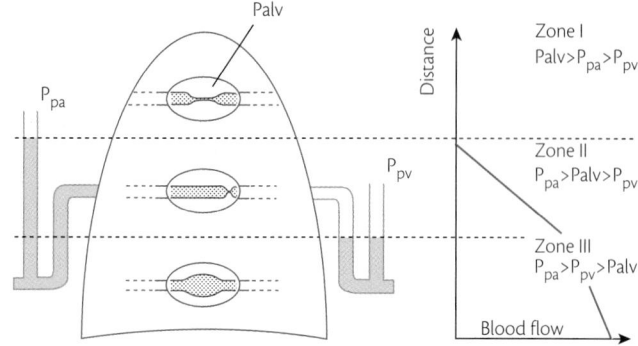

Three zone model of pulmonary blood flow distribution

Fig. 16.15.1.3 The three-zone model of pulmonary blood flow distribution.

because $Palv$ is greater than Ppa. Flow increases down zone II because the driving pressure increases by 1 cm of H$_2$O for each 1 cm distance down the lung. Flow increases with distance down zone III, although ΔP ($Ppa - Ppv$) remains constant, because local PVR decreases due to capillary distension and recruitment. The driving pressure for blood flow is determined by the relationship between $Palv$, Ppa, and pulmonary venous pressure (Ppv) down the upright lung. A further zone (zone IV) is found at the lung base: in this zone, blood flow is observed to decrease with distance down the lung due to increased perivascular pressure in extra-alveolar vessels.

Gravity-independent flow

The branching pattern of pulmonary arteries imposes changes in perfusion that are independent of gravity. Within any given horizontal level of the upright lung, there is a decrease in blood flow in peripheral lung regions compared to central hilar regions. This is thought to be due to the reduction in Ppa in small acinar arteries with increasing distance from the hilum. This pattern is also seen at the level of the secondary lobule (the group of acini supplied by one terminal bronchiole), with a decreasing gradient of blood flow from the centre to the periphery.

Regulation of pulmonary vasomotor tone

The pulmonary circulation differs from the systemic in that it is under minimal resting tone and is almost fully dilated under normal conditions. Circulating and local production of vasodilators and vasoconstrictors contribute to the resting tone, with the balance tipped in favour of vasodilators. Nitric oxide, produced locally by endothelial cells, and the arachidonic acid metabolite prostacyclin, are important vasodilators that contribute to this low pulmonary vascular tone.

The autonomic nervous system interacts with humoral mediators and haemodynamic forces in the control of pulmonary vascular tone, autonomic innervation of the lung being via parasympathetic (cholinergic: predominantly vasodilator) and sympathetic (adrenergic: predominantly vasoconstrictor) nerves in the periarterial plexus.

Hypoxic pulmonary vasoconstriction

The pulmonary circulation responds to a reduction in the partial pressure of alveolar oxygen by vasoconstriction. This is opposite to the response to hypoxia in the systemic circulation, where tissue hypoxia leads to vasodilatation, hence improving tissue oxygen delivery. Hypoxic pulmonary vasoconstriction (HPV) probably

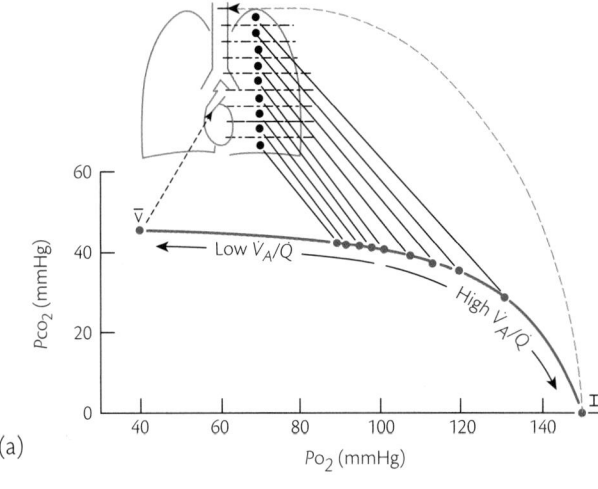

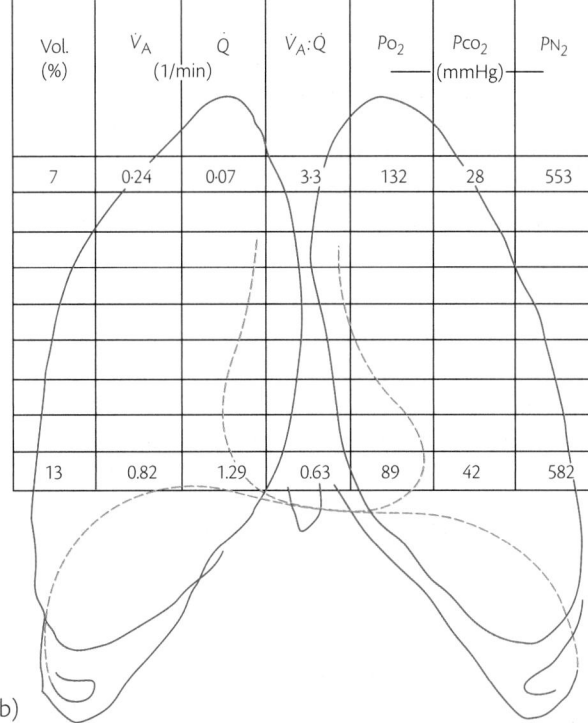

Vol. (%)	$\dot{V}_A$ (1/min)	$\dot{Q}$ (1/min)	$\dot{V}_A:\dot{Q}$	P_{O_2} (mmHg)	P_{CO_2} (mmHg)	P_{N_2}
7	0.24	0.07	3.3	132	28	553
13	0.82	1.29	0.63	89	42	582

Fig. 16.15.1.4 Panel A: O_2–CO_2 diagram showing how the change in ventilation–perfusion ratio up the lung determines the regional composition of alveolar gas. Dashed lines show the composition of mixed venous (pulmonary arterial) blood and inspired (tracheal) gas. Panel B: Effects of change in ventilation–perfusion ratio up the lung on the regional composition of alveolar gas, with volumes of lung slices, ventilations, and blood flows also shown.

plays little role in the normal distribution of pulmonary blood flow or regulation of ventilation–perfusion relationships in humans. However, in diseases characterized by airway obstruction, such as acute asthma or chronic obstructive lung disease, HPV can divert blood flow away from poorly ventilated lung regions, reducing venous admixture (shunt through poorly ventilated lung regions) and preserving arterial oxygenation. The magnitude of the response varies widely between individuals and is, at best, 50% efficient. It is noteworthy that populations indigenous to high-altitude regions, e.g. Tibetans, lack HPV with no obviously detrimental effect.

At high altitude, with low atmospheric partial pressures of oxygen, HPV would lead to generalized vasoconstriction and pulmonary hypertension, which is presumably more detrimental than the lack of HPV.

Ventilation–perfusion relationships

In the normal lung, it is remarkable that pulmonary blood flow and ventilation are, in general, well matched given the heterogeneity of blood flow described above. Of course, regional ventilation is also under similar constraints and forces as the blood flow. For further discussion of the structure and function of the airways and alveoli see Chapter 18.1.2, but, in brief, the airways run with the arteries in the bronchovascular bundle and the branching patterns are similar. Regional ventilation is under the influence of gravity: the lung sits in the thorax under its own weight, which leads to a gradient of intrapleural pressure, with more negative pressures at the top of the lung than at the bottom in the upright position. This means that the lung is more expanded at the apex than at the base at the end of a normal breath (functional residual capacity). Thus, the upper and lower parts of the lung are operating on different portions of their pressure–volume curves. The result is that, during normal breathing, greater ventilation is delivered to the bottom than to the top of the lung. This gradient of regional ventilation down the lung is reminiscent of the gradient of blood flow described above. In fact, with increasing distance up the lung, the rate of change of ventilation per unit of alveolar volume is somewhat less than the rate of change of perfusion (about one-third). This leads to large regional differences in the ventilation–perfusion ratio up the lung (Fig. 16.15.1.4): alveoli at the bottom of the lung are relatively overperfused, leading to a low ventilation–perfusion ratio (c.0.6); by contrast, alveoli at the apex of the lung are relatively under-perfused, leading to ventilation–perfusion ratios over 3.0. Nevertheless, the overall ventilation–perfusion ratio for the whole lung is approximately 0.85. The regional ventilation–perfusion ratio will determine the partial pressures of oxygen and CO_2 found in the alveoli at a given level of the lung, and this will be reflected in the gas tensions found in pulmonary venous blood draining those alveoli. The result is that the P_{O_2} is higher, and the P_{CO_2} lower, in blood draining from the top of the lung, compared with the bottom. The matching of ventilation and perfusion in the normal lung ensures that the overall ventilation–perfusion ratio remains fairly constant with changes in posture or exercise.

Further reading

De Mello DE, Reid LM (1997). Arteries and veins. In: Crystal RG, *et al.* (eds.) *The lung: scientific foundations*, 2nd edition, pp. 1117–27. Lippincott-Raven, Philadelphia.

Hughes JMB (1997). Distribution of pulmonary blood flow. In: Crystal RG, *et al.* (eds.) *The lung: scientific foundations*, 2nd edition, pp. 1523–36. Lippincott-Raven, Philadelphia.

Hughes JMB, Morrell NW (2001). *Pulmonary circulation: from basic mechanisms to clinical practice.* Imperial College Press, London.

Singhal S, *et al.* (1973). Morphometry of the human pulmonary arterial tree. *Circ Res*, **33**, 190–7.

West JB, Dollery CT, Naimark A. (1964). Distribution of blood flow in isolated lung: relation to vascular and alveolar pressures. *J Appl Physiol*, **19**, 713–24.

West JB (1985). *Ventilation/blood flow and gas exchange*, 4th edition. Blackwell Scientific Publications, Oxford.

16.15.2 Pulmonary hypertension

Nicholas W. Morrell

Essentials

Symptoms of unexplained exertional breathlessness or symptoms out of proportion to coexistent heart or lung disease should alert the clinician to the possibility of pulmonary hypertension, and the condition should be actively sought in patients with known associated conditions, such as scleroderma, hypoxic lung disease, liver disease, or congenital heart disease. Heterozygous germ-line mutations in the gene encoding the bone morphogenetic protein type II receptor (*BMPR2*) are found in over 70% of families with pulmonary arterial hypertension (PAH).

Pulmonary hypertension is defined as a mean pulmonary arterial pressure greater than 25 mmHg at rest, or 30 mmHg on exercise, and may be due to increased pulmonary vascular resistance (e.g. PAH), increased transpulmonary blood flow (e.g. congenital heart disease), or increased pulmonary venous pressures (e.g. mitral stenosis). Exercise tolerance and survival in pulmonary hypertension is ultimately related to indices of right heart function, such as cardiac output.

Investigation—echocardiography is a good screening tool for the presence of pulmonary hypertension, but right heart catheterization is needed to confirm the diagnosis and guide treatment. CT pulmonary angiography and high-resolution CT are important to exclude underlying parenchymal lung disease and chronic thromboembolic pulmonary hypertension. In idiopathic PAH a vasodilator study should be undertaken at the time of right heart catheterization to detect the few (5–10%) patients who will have good long-term survival on calcium channel blockers.

Management—new treatments for PAH include prostanoids, endothelin receptor antagonists, and phosphodiesterase inhibitors, which improve symptoms of breathlessness, exercise tolerance, quality of life, and probably survival. Chronic thromboembolic pulmonary hypertension (CTEPH) is an important diagnosis to make because selected patients with predominantly proximal disease can be cured by pulmonary endarterectomy.

Introduction

The normal pulmonary circulation, as described in Chapter 16.15.1, is a low-pressure, high-flow system that delivers the output of the right ventricle to the alveolar capillary network during each cardiac cycle for the purposes of gas exchange. Pulmonary hypertension is defined as a sustained elevation of mean pulmonary arterial pressure to greater than 25 mmHg at rest, or 30 mmHg on exercise.

Many diseases can lead to an elevation of pulmonary arterial pressure. Therefore, the term 'pulmonary hypertension' is not a final diagnosis, but a starting point for further investigation. In general terms, the main causes of pulmonary hypertension are (1) a narrowing or obstruction of the precapillary pulmonary arteries, (2) an increase in pulmonary venous pressure, or (3) a persistent elevation of pulmonary blood flow. This simplified approach is worth keeping in mind during the assessment of patients found to have pulmonary hypertension, because it has major consequences for prognosis and management.

Classification of pulmonary hypertension

Table 16.15.2.1 shows the World Health Organization (2003) classification of pulmonary hypertension as determined by an international panel of experts. The grouping of causes in this classification takes into account similarities in aetiology, pathology, and haemodynamic assessment at right heart catheterization. The classification helps to understand the underlying cause of pulmonary hypertension in a given patient and to plan management, hence it is a useful framework to consider the various causes of pulmonary hypertension, described in more detail below.

Pulmonary arterial hypertension

The term pulmonary 'arterial' hypertension (PAH) refers to conditions characterized predominantly by a precapillary obstruction to blood flow through the pulmonary vascular bed. This elevation of pulmonary vascular resistance increases the driving pressure required to maintain blood flow through the lungs: pulmonary arterial pressure rises to maintain adequate left ventricular filling. The normal mean pulmonary arterial pressure (*c*.17 mmHg) is about one-fifth of the systemic mean blood pressure. In PAH, mean pulmonary arterial pressure may approach systemic levels. The normally thin-walled right ventricle struggles to cope with the increasing pressure. At first it undergoes a degree of hypertrophy, which increases its ability to generate higher pressures, but ultimately it begins to fail and cardiac output declines. It is the reduction in cardiac output that generates most of the clinical symptoms in patients, with dyspnoea and fatigue being the most common (Fig. 16.15.2.1). The function of the right heart is the main determinant of prognosis in patients with PAH.

Epidemiology and aetiology

PAH is broadly divided into idiopathic PAH (previously known as primary pulmonary hypertension), and PAH found with other known associated conditions or triggers. Idiopathic PAH is further divided into familial or sporadic disease, with about 10% of patients with idiopathic PAH having an affected relative. Idiopathic PAH is a rare disorder with an estimated incidence of 1 to 2 per million per year. It is more common in women (female:male sex ratio = 2.3:1), can occur at any age, but most commonly occurs between the ages of 20 and 45 years.

PAH that is pathologically indistinguishable from the idiopathic form can occur in a range of associated conditions (Table 16.15.2.1). Of the autoimmune rheumatic diseases, the most common association is with systemic sclerosis, where PAH can complicate the clinical course in 15 to 20% of patients in the absence of interstitial lung disease. Other associated conditions include mixed connective tissue disease and systemic lupus erythematosus, and more rarely rheumatoid arthritis, dermatopolymyositis, and primary Sjögrens' syndrome.

There is a well-recognized association of PAH with congenital heart disease leading to left-to-right shunts. Overall, the prevalence of PAH is 15 to 30%, but varies depending on the nature of the underlying cardiac defect. Portal hypertension, usually associated with cirrhosis, is associated with PAH in less than 5% of patients.

Table 16.15.2.1 Clinical Classification of Pulmonary Hypertension (Venice 2003)

1. Pulmonary arterial hypertension (PAH)

  1.1. Idiopathic (IPAH)
  1.2. Familial (FPAH)
  1.3. Associated with (APAH):

    1.3.1. Collagen vascular disease
    1.3.2. Congenital systemic-to-pulmonary shunts**
    1.3.3. Portal hypertension
    1.3.4. HIV infection
    1.3.5. Drugs and toxins
    1.3.6. Other (thyroid disorders, glycogen storage disease, Gaucher disease, hereditary hemorrhagic telangiectasia, hemoglobinopathies, myeloproliferative disorders, splenectomy)

  1.4. Associated with significant venous or capillary involvement

    1.4.1. Pulmonary veno-occlusive disease (PVOD)
    1.4.2. Pulmonary capillary hemangiomatosis (PCH)

  1.5. Persistent pulmonary hypertension of the newborn

2. Pulmonary hypertension with left heart disease

  2.1. Left-sided atrial or ventricular heart disease
  2.2. Left-sided valvular heart disease

3. Pulmonary hypertension associated with lung diseases and/or hypoxemia

  3.1. Chronic obstructive pulmonary disease
  3.2. Interstitial lung disease
  3.3. Sleep-disordered breathing
  3.4. Alveolar hypoventilation disorders
  3.5. Chronic exposure to high altitude
  3.6. Developmental abnormalities

4. Pulmonary hypertension due to chronic thrombotic and/or embolic disease

  4.1. Thromboembolic obstruction of proximal pulmonary arteries
  4.2. Thromboembolic obstruction of distal pulmonary arteries
  4.3. Non-thrombotic pulmonary embolism (tumor, parasites, foreign material)

5. Miscellaneous

Sarcoidosis, histiocytosis X, lymphangiomatosis, compression of pulmonary vessels (adenopathy, tumor, fibrosing mediastinitis)

**Guidelines for classification of congenital systemic-to-pulmonary shunts

1. Type

Simple
Atrial septal defect (ASD)
Ventricular septal defect (VSD)
Patent ductus arterious
Total or partial unobstructed anomalous pulmonary venous return
Combined
Describe combination and define prevalent defect if any
Complex
Truncus arteriosus
Single ventricle with unobstructed pulmonary blood flow
Atrioventricular septal defects

2. Dimensions

Small (ASD≤2.0 cm and VSD≤1.0 cm)
Large (ASD>2.0 cm and VSD>1.0 cm)

3. Associated extracardiac abnormalities

4. Correction status

Noncorrected
Partially corrected (age)
Corrected: spontaneously or surgically (age)

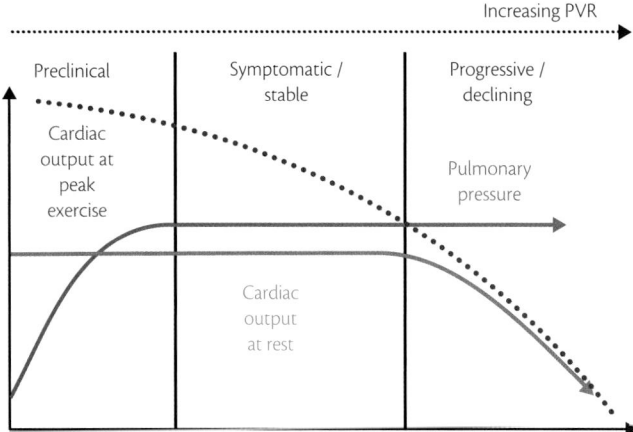

Fig. 16.15.2.1 Relationship between pulmonary hypertension, right ventricular function, and symptoms in pulmonary hypertension. PAH is characterized by progressively increasing pulmonary vascular resistance. In the early stages, the disease is asymptomatic and only manifests during exercise or during unusually demanding activities, but over time there is a progressive reduction in cardiac output and increasing PVR, eventually progressing to cardiac failure and death. PVR, pulmonary vascular resistance.

There is an unusually high prevalence of PAH (c.0.5%) in patients with HIV infection. Epidemiological studies have confirmed the association of PAH with amphetamine-like diet pills. In the 1970s, increased numbers of patients with PAH were found to have been exposed to Aminorex. In the 1990s, further studies confirmed an association of PAH with appetite-suppressant drugs of the fenfluramine and dexenfluramine group. An epidemic of PAH also occurred in Spain in the 1980s, following the ingestion of contaminated rape seed oil. Other more rarely associated conditions are listed in Table 16.15.2.1.

The classification of PAH includes two other rare pulmonary vascular diseases—pulmonary veno-occlusive disease and pulmonary capillary haemangiomatosis. Both are rarer than idiopathic PAH, but their true prevalence is unknown. Persistent pulmonary hypertension of the newborn is a disorder characterized by a failure of vascular transition from fetal to a neonatal circulation and estimated to affect 0.2% of live-born term infants.

Genetics

Familial PAH is a rare autosomal dominant condition, with reduced penetrance. It is indistinguishable on clinical or pathological grounds from idiopathic PAH. Linkage studies localized the gene to the long arm of chromosome 2 (2q33). In 2000, heterozygous germ-line mutations were identified in the *BMPR2* gene encoding the bone morphogenetic protein type II receptor, which is a constitutively active serine-threonine kinase that acts as a receptor for bone morphogenetic proteins (BMPs), these being members of the transforming growth factor β(TGFβ) superfamily. Mutations in BMPR-II have now been identified in over 70% of cases of familial PAH, and similar mutations are also found in 15 to 26% of patients thought to have sporadic or idiopathic disease. Many of these are unexpected examples of familial disease with low penetrance, although *de novo* mutations have also been reported. BMPR-II mutations have been identified in most of the 13 exons of the *BMPR2* gene, most (c.70%) being nonsense or frameshift mutations predicted to cause haploinsufficiency due to nonsense-mediated mRNA decay of the mutant transcript: only the wild-type

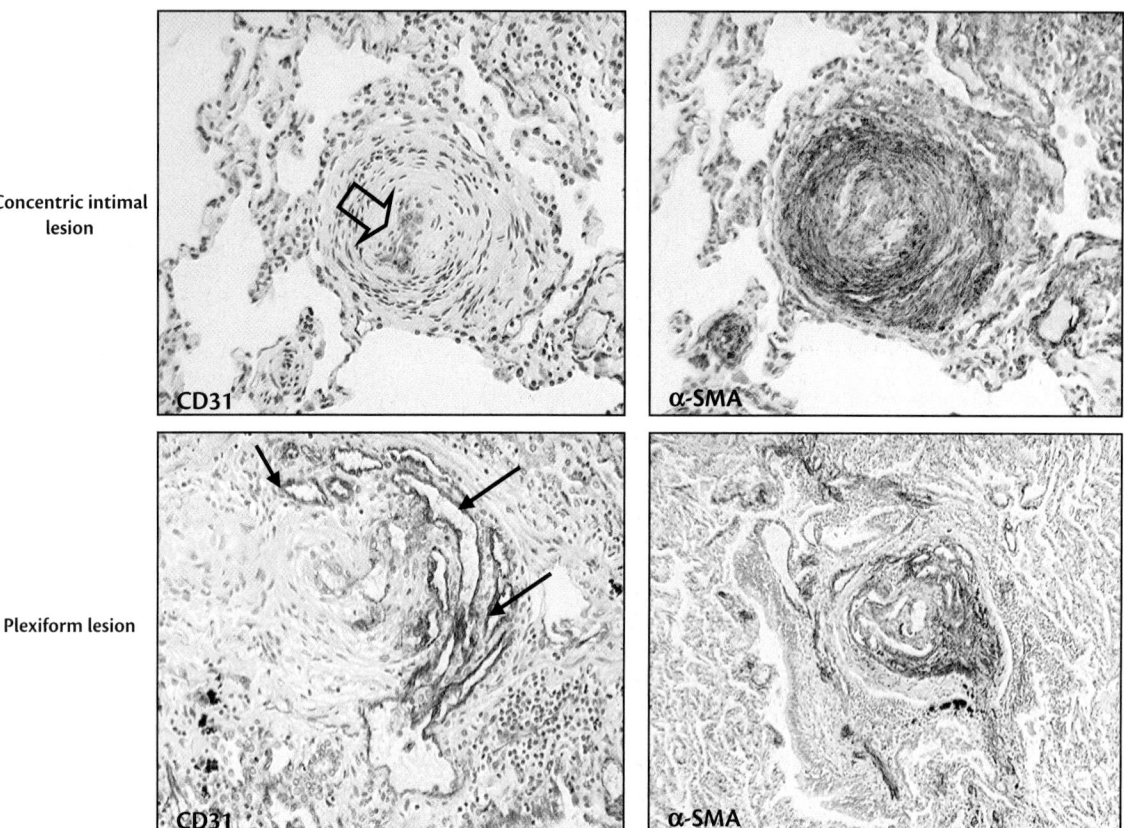

Fig. 16.15.2.2 Representative images of vascular lesions in idiopathic PAH immunostained for the endothelial marker CD31, or the smooth muscle cell marker α-smooth muscle specific actin (α-SMA). In concentric intimal lesions, a single layer of cells adjacent to the vascular lumen stains for CD31 (upper left panel, open arrow), with concentric layers of cells comprising the vascular wall staining for α-SMA (upper right panel). In plexiform lesions, CD31 stains a single layer of cells lining endothelial channels (lower left panel, arrows), with the supporting stroma staining for α-SMA (lower right panel).
Atkinson, C et al. *Primary Pulmonary Hypertension Is Associated With Reduced Pulmonary Vascular Expression of Type II Bone Morphogenetic Protein Receptor*, *Circulation*. 105:1672–1678.

allele is expressed in these cases, reducing the amount of BMPR-II protein to about 50% of normal. About 30% of the mutations are mis-sense mutations, which cause retention of mutant protein within the endoplasmic reticulum or affect important functional domains of the receptor, such as the ligand-binding domain or the kinase domain. Mutations in BMPR-II have also been found in a small proportion (c.10%) of patients with PAH associated with appetite suppressants, and in children with complicated PAH associated with congenital heart disease.

Mutations in another TGFβ receptor, ALK-1, have also been reported is association with PAH. These are usually found in families with hereditary haemorrhagic telangiectasia, but occasionally some family members develop severe PAH. These findings have highlighted the central role of the TGFβ signalling pathway in the pathogenesis of PAH.

Pathology

Typical morphological appearances include increased muscularization of small (<200 μm diameter) arteries and thickening or fibrosis of the intima, referred to as concentric intimal fibrosis (Fig. 16.15.2.2). In severe cases, dilatation of small pulmonary arterioles is seen and, sometimes, fibrinoid necrosis. In the larger elastic arteries, aneurysmal dilatation and atherosclerotic change may occur, the latter being otherwise extremely unusual in the normotensive pulmonary artery. The term plexogenic arteriopathy is used to describe the presence of plexiform lesions (200–400 μm), which are

tangles of capillary-like channels adjacent to small pulmonary arteries. Plexiform changes are found in some 50% of cases of idiopathic PAH, but also in other causes of severe pulmonary hypertension, such as that due to congenital heart disease.

In some cases of idiopathic PAH, there are pathological changes in the pulmonary venous circulation as well as in the arterial. If the venous changes dominate the pathology, the diagnosis is pulmonary veno-occlusive disease (PVOD), which has some distinct clinical features (see below). The pathological hallmark of pulmonary veno-occlusive disease is the extensive and diffuse occlusion of pulmonary veins by intimal fibrous tissue, which may be loose and oedematous or dense and sclerotic. The intimal thickening is confined usually to the smaller veins. Accompanying arterial changes, particularly muscular hypertrophy, often coexist. Pulmonary and pleural lymphatics are dilated, and longstanding venous hypertension may lead to oedema and fibrosis.

A further distinct pathological entity is pulmonary capillary haemangiomatosis (PCH), characterized by the presence of numerous foci of proliferating, congested, thin-walled capillaries, which invade alveolar tissue, as well as the pleural, bronchial, and vascular tissue.

Pathogenesis

The process of pulmonary vascular remodelling described above involves proliferation of smooth muscle cells, fibroblasts, and endothelial cells in the vessel wall (Fig. 16.15.2.3). Endothelial dysfunction contributes to the pathogenesis of PAH, manifesting as an

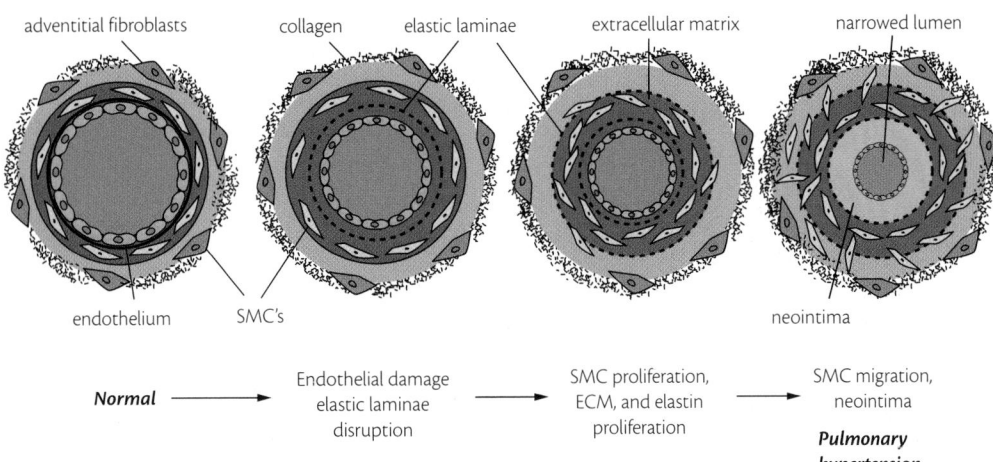

Fig. 16.15.2.3 Cellular mechanisms of pulmonary vascular remodelling. ECM, extracellular matrix; SMC, smooth muscle cell. By Doig Simmonds. From *Pulmonary Circulation: Basic Mechanisms to Clinical Practice* (2001). With permission of Imperial College Press.

increase in the release of vasoconstrictors and a deficiency of endogenous vasodilators. Initially, there is an increased tendency towards endothelial cell apoptosis, though clonal survival of endothelial cells may lead to the plexiform lesions seen in severe PAH. The increase in medial and adventitial thickness and cell number may result from increased proliferation, but also from migration of precursor cells from within the vessel wall, the surrounding interstitium, and from circulating progenitor cells. At least in some forms of PAH, increased vasoreactivity may precede the structural changes in the vessels.

A number of mediators and growth factors have been shown to be involved in driving the cellular changes (Fig. 16.15.2.4). Increased circulating and local pulmonary vascular expression of endothelin-1 is observed in patients with PAH. As well as being a potent vasoconstrictor, endothelin stimulates smooth muscle and fibroblast proliferation via the endothelin A (ET_A) and/or endothelin B (ET_B) receptors, the expression of which is increased in small hypertensive pulmonary arteries—ET_B receptors on the endothelium-mediating endothelin-1 clearance as well as release of nitric oxide and prostacyclin. Circulating levels of serotonin (5HT) are also elevated in PAH and the known association of severe PAH with appetite-suppressant drugs of the fenfluramine/dexfenfluramine group is thought, partly, to be due to increased serotonergic signalling by metabolites of these drugs. Serotonin stimulates mitogenesis of vascular cells via serotonin receptors, including the $5HT_{2A}$, $5HT_{2B}$, and $5HT_{1B}$ receptors. In human pulmonary artery smooth muscle cells, a major proliferative pathway involves activation of mitogen-activated protein kinases via the serotonin transporter, increased expression of which is found in hypertensive arteries.

A relative deficiency of vasodilator pathways is observed in severe PAH, leading to an imbalance that enhances the activity of mitogenic and vasoconstrictor pathways. Patients with PAH produce less endothelial-derived prostacyclin. They also exhibit reduced expression of nitric oxide synthase in their small pulmonary arteries, and consequently less nitric oxide release. More recent studies have also shown a deficiency of the neuropeptide vasodilator vasoactive intestinal polypeptide (VIP) in the lungs of patients with PAH. Many of these important vasodilator pathways also exert antiproliferative effects on smooth muscle cells and fibroblasts via production of the cyclic nucleotides cAMP and cGMP. Deficiency of these key vasodilator pathways has provided the rationale for many of the new therapies that have emerged over the past decade (see below).

Another important pathway involved in the process of pulmonary vascular remodelling includes loss of potassium channel (Kv1.5 and Kv2.1) expression and function, promoting smooth muscle cell contraction and survival. Activation of vascular elastases within the vessel media and disruption of the elastic laminae is also a key step in disease pathogenesis. Inflammatory cells may also contribute, especially in PAH associated with autoimmune conditions, accompanied by increased expression of inflammatory cytokines and chemokines in small pulmonary arteries.

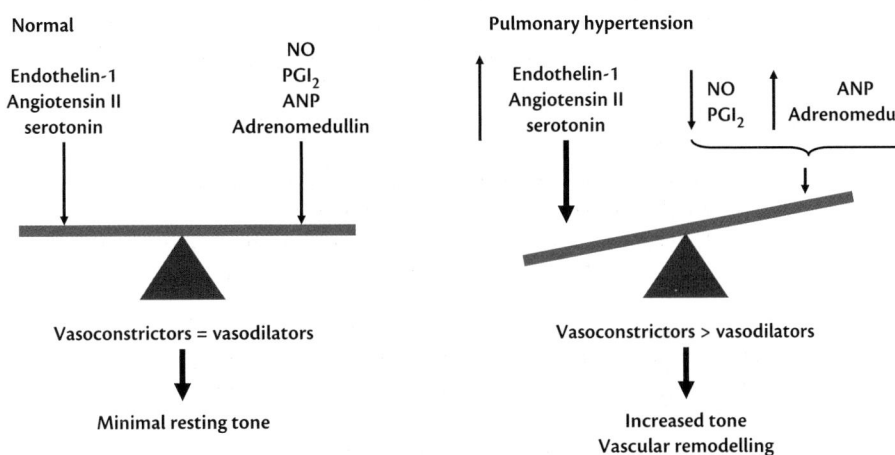

Fig. 16.15.2.4 An imbalance of pulmonary vascular vasodilators and vasoconstrictors contributes to the vascular constriction and remodelling in pulmonary hypertensio ANP, atrial natriuretic pep NO, nitric oxide; PGI$_2$, pros

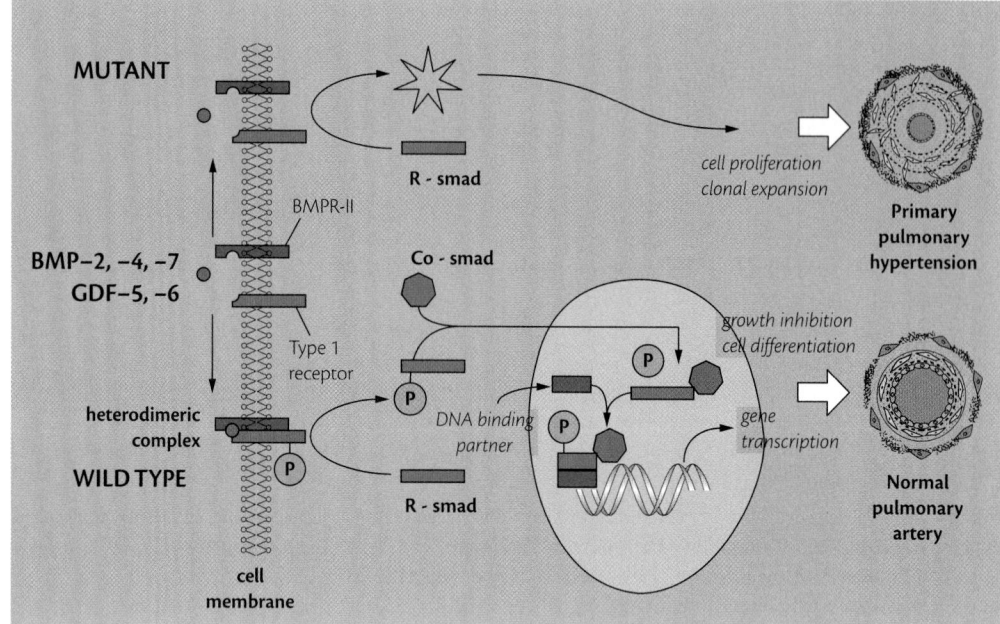

Fig. 16.15.2.5 The potential role of mutations in the bone morphogenetic protein type II receptor (BMPR-II) in familial PAH. The wild-type receptor signals in response to ligands by activating receptor-regulated Smad proteins (R-Smads), which dimerize with common partner Smads (Co-Smads) to regulate gene expression in the vascular cell. Mutation in BMPR-II disrupts Smad signalling and leads to abnormal vascular cell proliferation. BMP, bone morphogenetic protein; GDF, growth differentiation factors.
By Doig Simmonds. From *Pulmonary Circulation: Basic Mechanisms to Clinical Practice* (2001). With permission of Imperial College Press.

Pathological studies have identified the presence of thrombosis in small pulmonary arteries of patients with PAH. It is not clear whether this represents *in situ* thrombosis as a consequence of the reduced blood flow, or embolic phenomena. Platelet dysfunction has also been recognized in PAH, and an increased frequency of antiphospholipid antibodies associated with an increased thrombotic risk.

The identification of mutations in the BMPR-II receptor has highlighted the important role of the TGFβ superfamily in the pathogenesis of familial PAH. Most mutations lead to a reduction in a critical signalling pathway, the Smad pathway, downstream of BMP receptors. This, in turn, leads to the failure of BMPs, particularly BMP2 and BMP4, to activate transcription of important target genes. In smooth muscle cells, BMPR-II mutation leads to a failure of the normal growth suppressive and pro-apoptotic effects of bone morphogenetic proteins, favouring excessive pulmonary artery smooth muscle cell proliferation and survival (Fig. 16.15.2.5). In endothelial cells, by contrast, BMPR-II mutation promotes endothelial dysfunction and endothelial cell apoptosis. The combination of endothelial cell dysfunction and smooth muscle cell proliferation within the pulmonary circulation favour the development of vascular obliterative lesions and pulmonary hypertension. Clonal expansion of apoptosis-resistant endothelial cells may contribute to the formation of plexiform lesions. However, this simple model does not explain all of the features of familial PAH. In particular, it does not explain why disease is confined to the lung circulation, while BMPR-II is widely expressed in many tissues. In addition, it does not explain why the presence of the mutation is not sufficient on its own to cause disease, with gene penetrance as low as 20% in some families. These observations indicate that additional environmental and/or genetic factors are necessary for disease manifestation. This putative 'second hit' may further impact on BMP signalling pathways, leading to a critical reduction in bone morphogenetic signalling via Smad proteins and initiation of the process of pulmonary vascular remodelling.

Although mutations in BMPR-II are not generally found in most secondary forms of PAH, it is now becoming clear that dysfunction of the BMPR-II pathway is involved in their pathogenesis. Further research is likely to reveal further clues to the involvement of this important pathway in vascular disease.

Clinical features

Symptoms

The three main presenting symptoms are dyspnoea, chest pain, and syncope. The severity of symptoms is related to prognosis. A modified New York Heart Association score is a useful way to assess symptom severity and follow response to treatment (Box 16.15.2.1).

Unexplained breathlessness on exertion should always raise the possibility of PAH, particularly in the setting of conditions known to be associated with pulmonary hypertension (Table 16.15.2.1).

Box 16.15.2.1 Modified New York Heart Association functional classification of pulmonary hypertension

◆ Class I—pulmonary hypertension without resultant limitation of physical activity. Ordinary physical activity does not cause undue dyspnoea or fatigue, chest pain, or near syncope

◆ Class II—pulmonary hypertension resulting in slight limitation of physical activity. The patient is comfortable at rest. Ordinary physical activity causes undue dyspnoea or fatigue, chest pain, or near syncope

◆ Class III—pulmonary hypertension resulting in marked limitation of physical activity. The patient is comfortable at rest. Less than ordinary activity causes undue dyspnoea or fatigue, chest pain, or near syncope

◆ Class IV—Pulmonary hypertension with inability to carry out any physical activity without symptoms. These patients manifest signs of right heart failure. Dyspnoea and/or fatigue may be present at rest. Discomfort is increased by any physical activity

The condition may have an insidious onset: frequently, there is a delay of up to 3 years between the onset of first symptoms and diagnosis. Syncope is an ominous sign, usually reflecting severe right ventricular dysfunction. Other symptoms include lassitude, abdominal swelling from ascites, and ankle swelling. Small haemoptysis may occur at later stages.

Clinical signs

Tachypnoea may be present, even at rest. Peripheral cyanosis is common due to a low cardiac output. Central cyanosis occurs later as pulmonary gas exchange deteriorates or right-to-left shunting occurs through a patent foramen ovale. The jugular venous pulse may be elevated with a prominent 'a' wave, reflecting the increased force of atrial contraction, or—if tricuspid regurgitation is present—there may be a large 'V' wave. There may be a right ventricular heave and a pulsatile liver. On auscultation, forceful closure of the pulmonary valve leads to an accentuated pulmonary arterial component of the second heart sound. There are often a third and fourth right heart sound. The murmurs of tricuspid regurgitation (systolic) or pulmonary regurgitation (diastolic) may be heard. Jaundice, ascites, and peripheral oedema may be present at advanced stages of the disease.

Differential diagnosis

If the symptoms and clinical signs suggest pulmonary hypertension, the differential diagnosis should be considered with reference to the classification in Table 16.15.2.1. Most importantly, the presence of left heart disease, parenchymal lung disease, or congenital heart disease should be excluded. Pulmonary hypertension due to chronic thromboembolic disease is important to detect because specific surgical treatment is available. Idiopathic PAH remains a diagnosis of exclusion.

Clinical investigation

The investigation of a patient with suspected pulmonary hypertension involves (1) the exclusion of other underlying causes and (2) an assessment of severity of pulmonary hypertension and right heart failure for prognosis and treatment. The investigations that are useful in identifying the aetiology of newly diagnosed, unexplained pulmonary hypertension are listed in Table 16.15.2.2.

Blood tests

A thrombophilia screen, including antithrombin III, protein C and S, factor V Leiden, anticardiolipin antibodies, and lupus anticoagulant should be performed, and may reveal clotting abnormalities predisposing to chronic thromboembolic pulmonary hypertension (CTEPH). Thyroid function should be checked since both hypo- and especially hyperthyroidism are commonly reported associations. An autoantibody screen should be performed to exclude underlying autoimmune rheumatic or vasculitic disease: positive antinuclear antibodies can be found in 30 to 40% of patients with idiopathic PAH, but a positive test for antineutrophil cytoplasmic antibodies (ANCA) would be uncommon. Since there is an increased incidence of unexplained pulmonary hypertension in HIV-positive patients, this diagnosis should always be considered.

Imaging

The plain chest radiograph shows enlargement of the proximal pulmonary arteries, which may be dramatic, with peripheral pruning of the pulmonary vascular pattern, giving rise to increased peripheral

Table 16.15.2.2 Investigation of the patient with suspected IPH

Blood tests
Full blood count/film/differential
Hb electrophoresis
Urea and electrolytes
Liver function including gamma GT
Thyroid function
Thrombophilia screen
Antithrombin III
Protein C
Protein S
Factor V Leiden
Anti-cardiolipin antibody
Lupus anticoagulant
CMV deaff
Autoantibodies
RhF
ANA
ENAs
anti-dsDNA
anti-cardiolipin IgG and IgM
anti-SM/anti-SCL/anti-SS
complement C3,C4,CH50
ANCA
Serum angiotensin converting enzyme
Hepatitis screen
HIV test
Imaging
Chest X-ray
Ventilation-perfusion lung scan
High resolution and spiral CT
Pulmonary artery angiography
Lung function
Pulmonary function tests
Exercise tests with saturation monitoring
Arterial blood gases on air
Cardiac function
ECG
Echocardiogram
Diagnostic cardiac catheterization
Miscellaneous
Urine microscopy
Abdominal ultrasound? cirrhosis

radiolucency. If heart failure is present the heart may be enlarged, with particular enlargement of the right atrium (Fig. 16.15.2.6). The chest radiograph may also give clues to underlying diagnoses such as interstitial lung disease.

Spiral contrast-enhanced CT will detect proximal pulmonary arterial obstruction suggestive of acute or chronic thromboembolic disease (Fig. 16.15.2.7). A pattern of mosaic perfusion of the lung

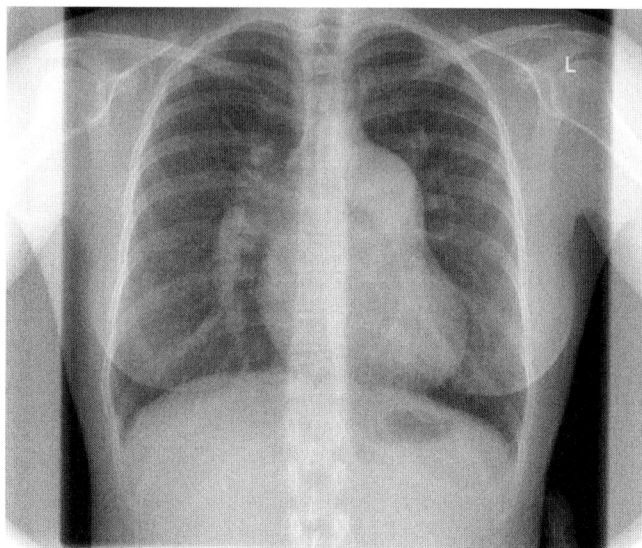

Fig. 16.15.2.6 Chest radiograph demonstrating cardiomegaly with dilated right heart chambers and dilatation of the proximal pulmonary arteries in a patient with PAH secondary to an atrial septal defect.
Courtesy of Dr Nick Screaton, Addenbrooke's Hospital.

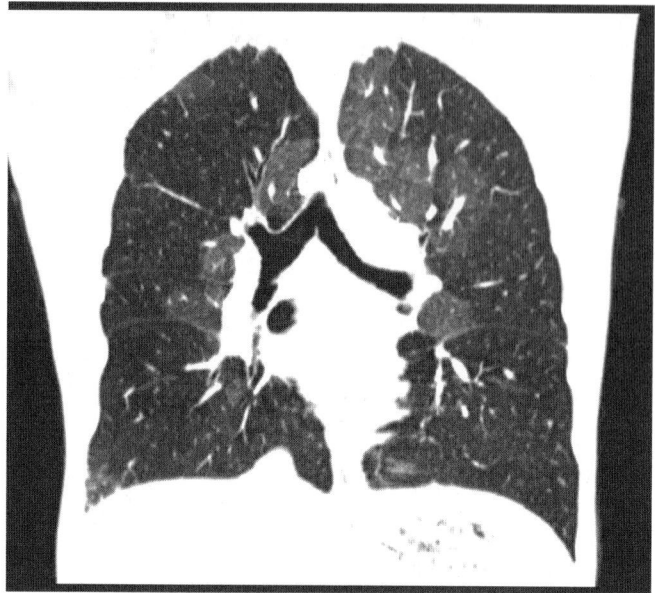

Fig. 16.15.2.8 Coronal multiplanar reconstruction demonstrating extensive mosaic perfusion in both lungs in a patient with CTEPH.
Courtesy of Dr Nick Screaton, Addenbrooke's Hospital.

parenchyma is also a feature of CTEPH, and may be the only sign in predominantly distal disease (Fig. 16.15.2.8). A high-resolution CT scan will pick up unsuspected parenchymal abnormalities, such as fibrosis. CT scanning is also useful to indicate more uncommon forms of PAH, such as pulmonary veno-occlusive disease, when there may be a degree of mediastinal lymphadenopathy and septal lines in the lung periphery, presumably indicating lymphatic and venous obstruction (Fig. 16.15.2.9).

On ventilation–perfusion lung scanning, the pattern of ventilation is usually normal in idiopathic PAH, and uneven ventilation should suggest underlying lung disease. The pattern of perfusion is also virtually normal, although small patchy perfusion defects may be present. This is in contrast to the appearance in CTEPH when segmental or larger perfusion defects persist, often indistinguishable from the pattern of acute pulmonary embolism (Fig. 16.15.2.10).

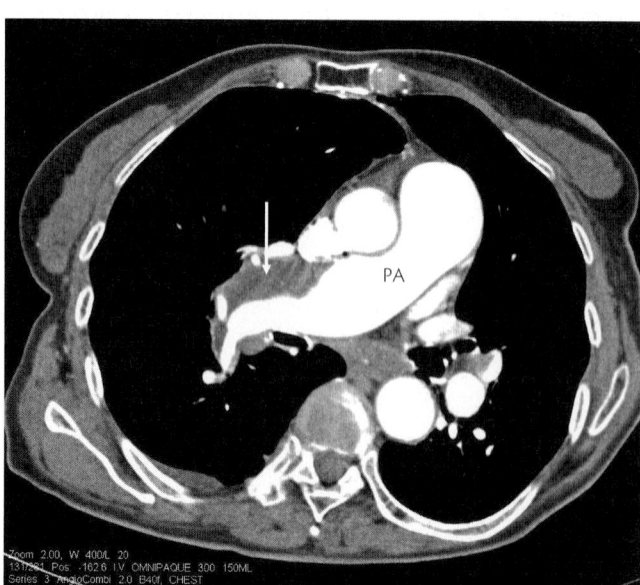

Fig. 16.15.2.7 Image from a CT pulmonary angiogram at the level of the right main pulmonary artery demonstrating dilatation of the main pulmonary artery (PA) with laminated thrombus in the distal right pulmonary artery (arrow) in keeping with proximal CTEPH.
Courtesy of Dr Nick Screaton, Addenbrooke's Hospital.

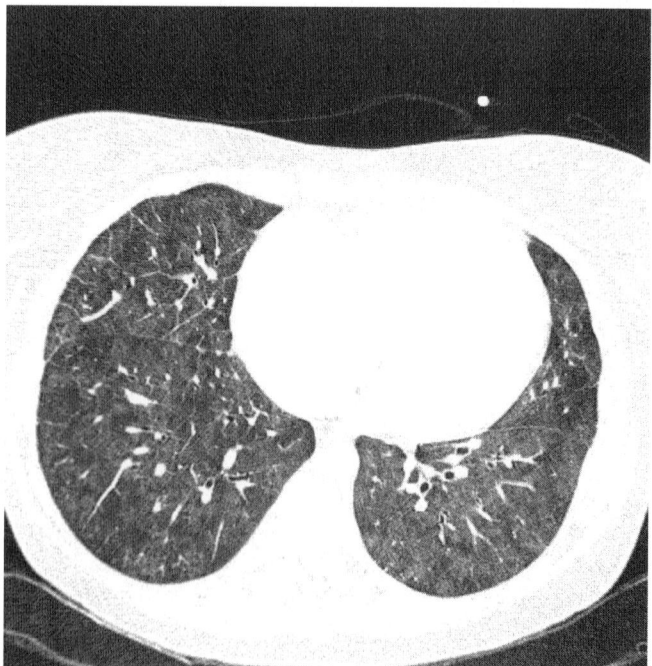

Fig. 16.15.2.9 Transverse CT image through the lower zones demonstrating heterogeneous attenuation of the lung parenchyma, centrilobular ground-glass opacities, and smooth thickening of the interlobular septa in a patient with pathologically proven veno-occlusive disease.
Courtesy of Dr Nick Screaton, Addenbrooke's Hospital.

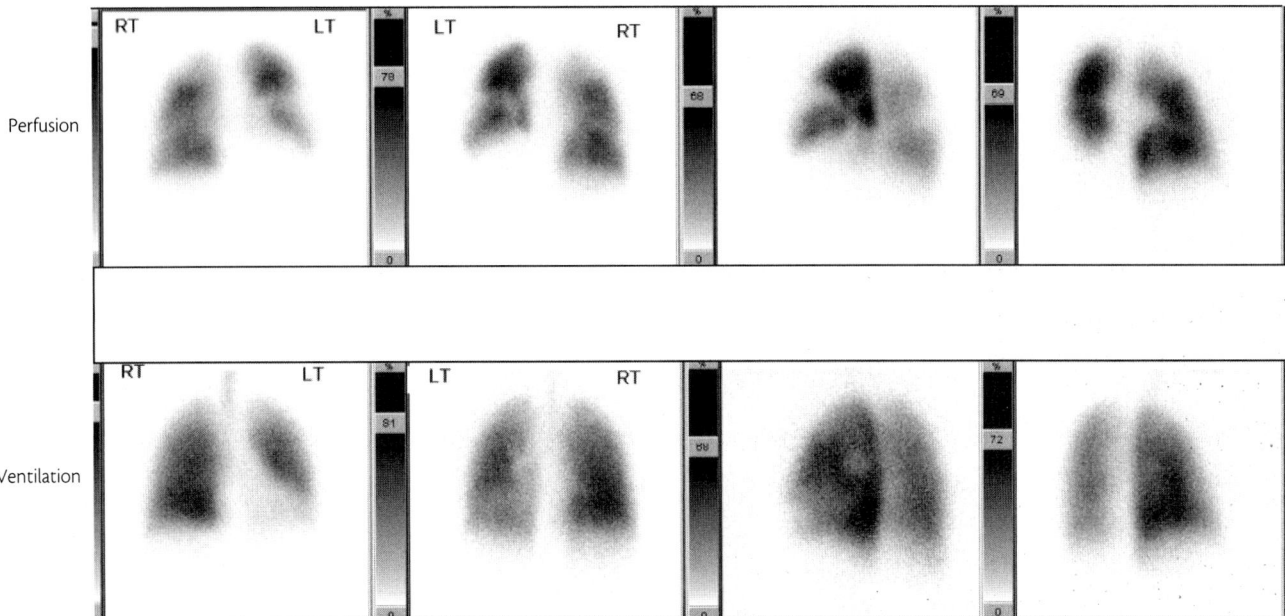

Fig. 16.15.2.10 Perfusion scintigram demonstrates multiple perfusion defects in a patient with CTEPH.
Courtesy of Dr Nick Screaton, Addenbrooke's Hospital.

Pulmonary artery angiography is really only required if the diagnosis is likely to be CTEPH, in which situation angiography will provide precise anatomical information regarding the location of vascular obstruction, indicated by abrupt cut-off of vessels or intravascular webs, that may be of great use if surgical endarterectomy is being contemplated.

The main contribution of MRI is in the assessment of patients with suspected intracardiac shunts or with anomalous vascular anatomy, e.g. if a shunt is suspected on the basis of right heart catheterization but cannot be demonstrated by echocardiography. MRI can also provide further pulmonary angiographic images.

Pulmonary function tests

The typical pattern for standard pulmonary function test for disease confined to the pulmonary circulation is to find normal lung volumes; normal forced expiratory volume in 1 s (FEV_1)/vital capacity (VC) ratio (>0.75), indicating no airflow obstruction; and low transfer factor (diffusing capacity, TLco), and low transfer coefficient (Kco).

The low diffusing capacity probably results from a combination of a reduced cardiac output and disease affecting the small arterioles, thereby reducing local perfusion. Additional findings in the pulmonary function tests—such as marked airflow obstruction (e.g. severe chronic obstructive pulmonary disease) or a restrictive defect (e.g. pulmonary fibrosis)—would indicate the presence of an underlying cause for the pulmonary hypertension. However, subtle changes in lung volumes and mild airflow obstruction have been reported in a few patients with PAH. In some groups of patients at high risk of developing PAH, e.g. in scleroderma, the low transfer coefficient can be monitored at intervals, with breathlessness accompanied by a fall in the low transfer coefficient sometimes being the first sign of this complication.

Exercise testing

Significant PAH is always associated with a reduced exercise capacity, one of the most useful tests of this being the 6-min walk test, with monitoring of heart rate and oxygen saturation. This can readily be repeated to assess patients over time and as a measure of response to treatment. A normal distance is more than 500 m, with a low 6-min walk predictive of a poor survival.

Full cardiopulmonary exercise testing is technically more demanding to perform and is only recommended if the diagnosis is in doubt, e.g. if there was a need to document cardiovascular limitation on exercise. Peak oxygen uptake on exercise is low and the anaerobic threshold is reduced to about 40% of normal. There is excessive ventilation for a given degree of oxygen consumption or CO_2 output, even at rest. There is no ventilatory impairment when underlying lung disease is absent. There is often a pronounced tachycardia at submaximal exercise, and usually arterial oxygen desaturation.

ECG

In symptomatic PAH, the ECG is abnormal in 80 to 90% of cases, but it has inadequate sensitivity (55%) and specificity (70%) as a screening tool for detecting pulmonary hypertension. The typical appearances are right-axis deviation (more than + 120°) in the limb leads, and a dominant R wave and T wave inversion in the right precordial leads, accompanied by a dominant S wave in the left precordial leads, suggesting right ventricular hypertrophy (Fig. 16.15.2.11). Tall, peaked P waves in the right precordial and inferior leads denote right atrial enlargement. Right bundle branch block is common.

Echocardiography

Echocardiography remains the best screening test for significant pulmonary hypertension. It detects the presence, and direction, of intracardiac shunts. Usually, this is possible using conventional transthoracic techniques, but if visualization is poor or a small shunt is still suspected, then transoesophageal echocardiography may be necessary. In addition, the left ventricle can be assessed to determine whether there is a contribution from left ventricular systolic or diastolic dysfunction to elevated pulmonary arterial pressure. The function of the right side of the heart can also be

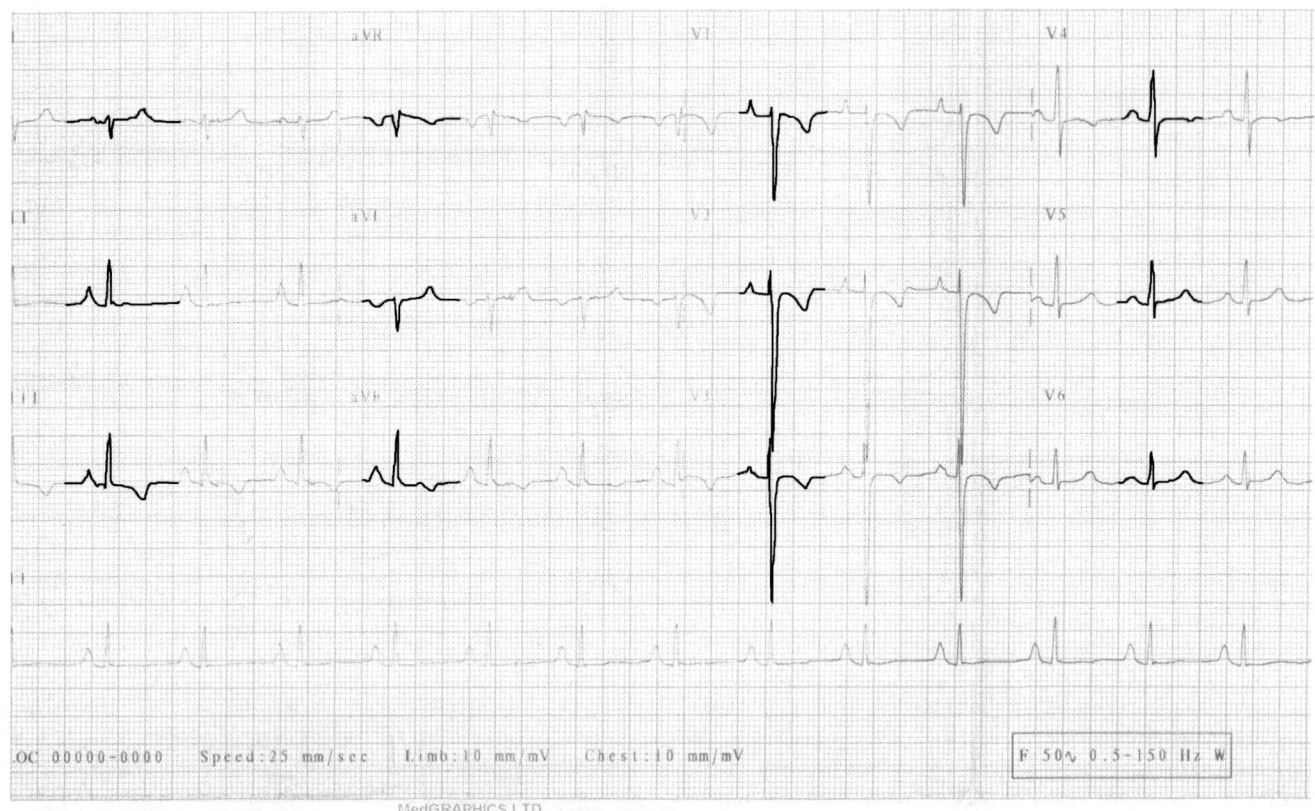

Fig. 16.15.2.11 12-lead ECG from a patient with idiopathic PAH showing a rightward axis, p pulmonale, poor R wave progression and ST segment changes indicative of right ventricular strain in the anterior chest leads.

assessed qualitatively and quantitatively. Atrial and ventricular dimensions and wall thickness can be measured, and paradoxical bowing of the intraventricular septum into the left ventricular cavity may be seen during systole as a consequence of greatly elevated right-sided pressures. Continuous-wave Doppler echocardiography is used to measure high-flow velocities across cardiac valves, one of the most commonly derived indices in the right heart being the pulmonary artery systolic pressure estimated by Doppler echocardiography from measurement of the velocity of the tricuspid regurgitant jet (c.80% of patients with PAH and 60% of normal subjects, have measurable tricuspid regurgitation). The maximum flow velocity (v) of the regurgitant jet is measured and inserted into the modified Bernoulli equation for convective acceleration pressure change, giving an estimate of right ventricular systolic pressure (RVSP):

$$RVSP = 4v^2 + RAP$$

where RAP is right atrial pressure, which can be estimated clinically from the height of the jugular venous pressure. In the absence of pulmonary valve stenosis, the right ventricular systolic pressure is equal to the pulmonary artery systolic pressure (PASP). There is a reasonable correlation between Doppler estimates of pulmonary artery systolic pressure and catheter measurements. Newer echocardiographic techniques such as three-dimensional echo and tissue Doppler are being evaluated.

Right heart catheterization

Right heart catheterization remains the best technique for confirming the diagnosis of pulmonary hypertension and for providing important prognostic information. An elevated mean pulmonary arterial pressure of greater than 25 mmHg at rest, or 30 mmHg on exercise, is the accepted definition. In patients with idiopathic PAH the mean pulmonary arterial pressure may exceed 60 mmHg. The pulmonary capillary wedge pressure (PCWP) can also be determined at catheterization, which is an approximation of left atrial pressure. An elevated PCWP (>15 mmHg) generally indicates left heart disease, but can also be elevated in pulmonary veno-occlusive disease. Measurement of PCWP is often unreliable in the presence of CTEPH. Sampling of venous blood oxygen saturation as the catheter passes down from the right atrium to right ventricle may detect a sudden 'step-up' in oxygenation, which would indicate the presence of a left-to-right shunt. Cardiac output can be determined by thermodilution or the Fick method.

Indicators of right heart failure, and hence poorer prognosis, include (1) an elevated right atrial pressure (>10 mmHg), (2) an elevated right ventricular end-diastolic pressure (>10 mmHg), (3) a reduced mixed venous oxygen saturation (Svo_2 <63%), and (4) reduced cardiac output (<2.5 litre/min).

Vasoreactivity studies

A subgroup (10–15%) of patients with idiopathic and anorexigen-associated PAH demonstrate a marked reduction in pulmonary vascular resistance following the administration of a vasodilator. These patients are the only group that respond favourably to long-term treatment with vasodilator therapy in the form of calcium channel blockers (see below), and are thus an important group to identify. Vasodilator studies are undertaken at the time of right heart catheterization, the preferred agent being inhaled nitric oxide, or an intravenous infusion of prostacyclin or adenosine. A positive response is defined as a fall in mean pulmonary arterial pressure of at least 10 mmHg to below 40 mmHg, accompanied by an increase or no change in cardiac output.

Conventional treatments

All patients with suspected severe PAH are best referred to a specialist centre for initial assessment and treatment. A multidisciplinary team approach to planning treatment is preferred, with input from respiratory physicians and cardiologists, transplant physicians and cardiothoracic surgeons, radiologists, specialist nurses, and palliative care specialists. Assisting patients to adapt to the uncertainty associated with chronic, life-shortening disease is essential if they are to successfully adjust to the demands of their illness and its treatment. The overall aims are to improve symptoms and quality of life, increase exercise capacity, and improve prognosis.

Supportive medical therapy

Patients with right heart failure and fluid retention may require diuretics. Decreasing cardiac preload with diuretics is often enough to alleviate episodes of right heart failure. However, caution should be exercised because faced with a reduction in vascular filling pressures, patients with severe PAH will not be able to increase cardiac output effectively, which may result in systemic hypotension and syncope.

Antiarrhythmics may be required for sustained or paroxysmal atrial fibrillation. Patients with severe PAH are prone to this complication because of stretching of the overloaded right atrium, and atrial fibrillation can significantly compromise the already reduced cardiac output in patients with PAH, hence it should be treated aggressively. Rate control with digoxin is possible, but if not contraindicated, pharmacological cardioversion with amiodarone is preferable. Electrophysiological mapping of arrhythmias and ablation of arrhythmogenic pathways may be indicated in selected patients.

Anticoagulation

Warfarin therapy to maintain the international normalized ratio (INR) between 2 and 3 is recommended in all patients with idiopathic and familial PAH. Two retrospective, and one small prospective, studies have demonstrated a survival benefit of anticoagulation, almost doubling survival rate in idiopathic PAH over a 3-year period. The consensus is that patients with PAH associated with autoimmune rheumatic tissue disease should also receive warfarin, unless contraindicated. The risk–benefit ratio of anticoagulation in other forms of PAH is undetermined.

Oxygen therapy

Oxygen therapy is indicated for symptomatic relief of breathlessness. There are no published trials of the benefit of long-term oxygen therapy in hypoxaemic patients with PAH. Nocturnal oxygen has been shown to be of no benefit in Eisenmenger's syndrome. Ambulatory oxygen may be beneficial if there is evidence of correctable desaturation between 4% and 90% during a 6-min walk test. Consideration should be given to in-flight supplemental oxygen for air travel.

Disease-targeted therapies

Calcium channel blockers

Patients with idiopathic PAH and a documented acute vasodilator response at cardiac catheterization, as defined above, should be offered long-term treatment with a calcium channel blocker. This is associated with very significant improvement in symptoms and prognosis in this subset of patients, although only 50% of those who respond in the cardiac catheterization laboratory will maintain a long-term response. Calcium channel blockers should be avoided in any patient with significant signs of right ventricular failure, or until this is controlled, because of their negative inotropic effects. For this reason, and the risk of systemic hypotension, calcium channel blockers should not be prescribed without confirmation of a vasodilator response at cardiac catheterization: indiscriminate prescribing will lead to increased mortality in the PAH population. Treatment should be started in hospital, using diltiazem, amlodipine, or nifedipine, and carefully titrated against systemic blood pressure. The aim is to increase the dose to the maximum tolerated.

Newer agents

Over the last 10 years, remarkable advances have been made in the availability of therapeutic agents for PAH. In the early 1980s, carefully timed heart–lung transplantation was the only option known to improve prognosis. We now have a range of pharmacological agents available and licensed for treatment in this condition, based on data from clinical trials that have almost exclusively recruited patients with idiopathic and anorexigen-associated PAH, although often including a subset of patients with PAH associated with systemic sclerosis. The drugs are used to reduce pulmonary vascular resistance and improve cardiac output: they all improve exercise performance and some prolong life. Fig. 16.15.2.12 presents an algorithm summarizing the pharmacological approach to treating PAH, based on current recommendations. Disease-targeted therapy is usually only licensed for treatment of patients in New York Heart Association (NYHA) class III and IV.

Prostanoids

Prostacyclin was the first treatment to be developed for the treatment of PAH during the 1980s. This has minimal oral bioavailability, has a half-life in the circulation of less than 2 min, and thus must be given by continuous intravenous infusion. It produces acute haemodynamic effects in some patients; most experience a fall in pulmonary vascular resistance with long-term use even in the absence of acute improvements. These observations support the view that long-term administration of these agents may reverse some of the vascular remodelling, as well as having a vasodilator effect. Prostacyclin has been shown to improve haemodynamics, exercise tolerance, quality of life, and survival in patients in NYHA class III and IV. The dose may have to be increased on a regular basis because of tachyphylaxis, and side effects are usually experienced when starting prostacyclin or when escalating the dose, including jaw pain, cutaneous flushing, nausea, and diarrhoea, as well as myalgias. Acute withdrawal of prostacyclin, e.g. if the infusion pump fails, can causes severe rebound pulmonary hypertension that can be fatal. Recurrent sepsis due to line infection can also be problematic.

Although prostacyclin remains a proven therapy in PAH, the complexity of its administration and the availability of newer oral agents mean that its use tends to be reserved for patients with severe haemodynamic compromise. Stable analogues of prostacyclin have been developed with longer half lives and improved bioavailability: iloprost can be given by the intravenous or inhalation route; treprostinil can be given subcutaneously or intravenously and is approved for use in patients in NYHA class II, III, and IV; and

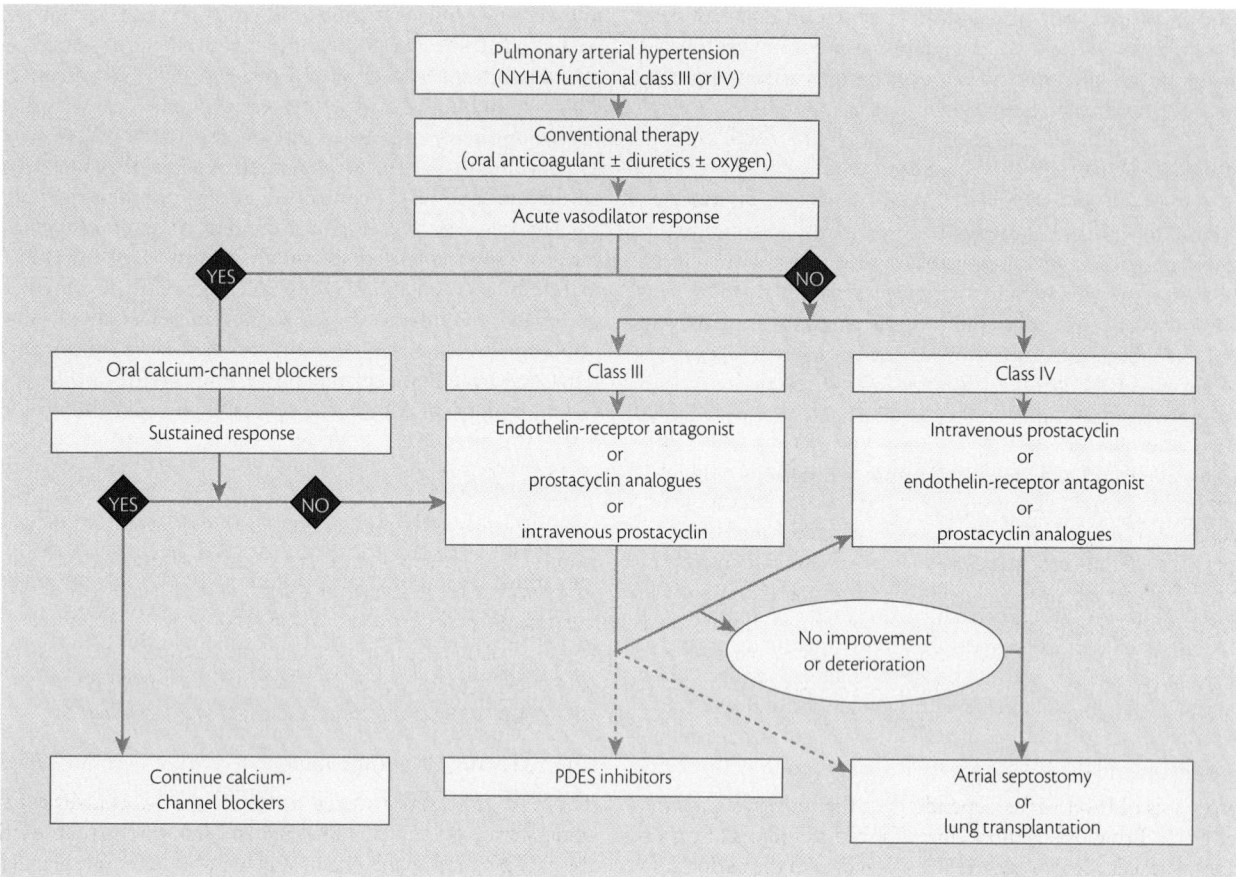

Fig. 16.15.2.12 Algorithm showing the approach to treatment in patients with severe PAH. PDE5, phosphodiesterase type V.
Reproduced from Humbert M, Sitbon O, Simonneau G. Treatment of Pulmonary Arterial Hypertension. N Engl J Med, Vol. 351, No. 14, September 30, 2001 Copyright © 2004 Massachusetts Medical Society. All rights reserved.

beraprost is an orally available prostacyclin analogue, although the dose may be limited by gastrointestinal side effects and it is presently only available in Japan.

Endothelin receptor antagonists
Bosentan, an orally active dual-selective ET_A/ET_B receptor antagonist, has been shown to improve exercise capacity, functional class, haemodynamics, echocardiographic, and Doppler variables, and time to clinical worsening in idiopathic PAH. Its most significant side effect is elevation of the hepatic transaminases, which is usually reversible on stopping the drug. Sitaxsentan and ambrisentan are newer ET_A selective agents with similar efficacy to bosentan in short-term studies, and favourable safety profiles. All patients on these agents require monthly monitoring of liver function tests.

Phosphodiesterase inhibitors
Sildenafil is an orally active selective inhibitor of cGMP-phosphodiesterase type 5. It acts by inhibiting the breakdown of cGMP, with vasorelaxant and antiproliferative effects in pulmonary vascular smooth muscle. Sildenafil improves exercise tolerance and pulmonary haemodynamics in short-term studies in PAH. Longer-acting phosphodiesterase (PDE5) inhibitors such as tadalafil also show promise.

Combination therapy
There is considerable theoretical and experimental evidence to support the use of combinations of the above disease-targeted therapies in PAH, which is a progressive disease. Most patients eventually deteriorate on monotherapy, and the addition of further agents has been shown to provide clinical benefit, although the evidence for precise recommendations is lacking at present.

Other strategies
Atrial septostomy
Atrial septostomy involves creating a right-to-left shunt between the atria, the preferred technique being percutaneous graded balloon dilatation. The rationale for this procedure is that patients with PAH and a patent foramen ovale have improved survival. Creating the shunt reduces right ventricular preload, which relieves the failing right ventricle and can increase cardiac output and improve exercise capacity. The increase in cardiac output is at the expense of a reduction in systemic arterial oxygen saturation, but systemic oxygen delivery is usually improved. The procedure is usually reserved for patients who are failing on maximal medical therapy or as a bridge to transplantation for PAH patients in NYHA class IV. Patient selection is vital. A high right atrial pressure (>20 mmHg) and low arterial oxygen saturation (<80% on air) prior to septostomy are associated with a high mortality related to the procedure, although impact on survival has not been formally assessed.

Transplantation
Transplantation of the lungs or heart and lungs developed as a treatment for endstage PAH during the 1980s. The advent of modern, targeted therapies has reduced the number of patients referred

for transplantation, but the long-term outcome of patients who remain in NYHA functional class III or IV remains poor. Lung or heart–lung transplantation therefore remains an important mode of treatment for patients failing medical therapy. Patients with pulmonary veno-occlusive disease and pulmonary capillary haemangiomatosis have a particularly poor outlook; they respond poorly to available medical therapies and should be referred early for transplantation assessment.

In general, patients presenting with NHYA class IV symptoms should be referred for transplantation assessment at the time of presentation, because their prognosis is poor. Additional indicators of poor prognosis include (1) a 6-min walking distance less than 332 m, (2) peak oxygen consumption less than 10.4 ml/min per kg, (3) cardiac index less than 2 litre/min per m², (4) right atrial pressure greater than 20 mmHg, (5) mean pulmonary arterial pressure greater than 55 mmHg, (6) mixed venous oxygen saturation of less than 63%. Those with significant improvement after 3 months of medical therapy can be removed or suspended from listing for transplant. The choice of procedure varies between centres, but single lung, bilateral lung, and heart–lung transplantation are used in patients with PAH. International registry figures show that the 1-year mortality post-transplantation is highest in patients with idiopathic PAH, compared with any other indication, with median survival post-transplantation between 4 and 5 years.

Prognosis

The prognosis of PAH varies depending on the underlying association or cause. Prognosis is most closely linked to indices of cardiac function, especially cardiac index. Historical data in the period prior to the availability of modern, targeted therapies suggest an expected median survival for idiopathic pulmonary arterial hyper tension between 2.5 and 4 years, and a 3-year survival of about 60%. The prognosis is worse for patients with underlying systemic sclerosis, autoimmune rheumatic disease, HIV disease, and anorexigen-associated PAH, and that for patients surviving to adulthood with PAH associated with a congenital intracardiac defect is substantially better than patients with idiopathic disease. At least in patients with idiopathic PAH, targeted therapies seem to improve survival to some extent, though definitive studies are awaited. Women with severe PAH should be advised that pregnancy carries a very high mortality because of the associated increased burden on the right heart.

Miscellaneous conditions associated with pulmonary hypertension

Pulmonary hypertension is detectable in some 5% of patients with sarcoidosis. This may develop in the context of endstage pulmonary fibrosis, but may also present as an isolated sarcoid vasculopathy in patients with relatively little parenchymal lung involvement. A falling diffusion coefficient for carbon monoxide in the face of preserved lung volumes may be the first clue to this in a sarcoid patient with worsening dyspnoea. In patients with vasculopathy, there may be a marked response to immunosuppression with prednisolone, which is worth trying before embarking on targeted PAH therapy.

It is often stated that the commonest worldwide cause of pulmonary hypertension is schistosomiasis. When one considers how many patients are infected with schistosomiasis, this may be true, but true prevalence figures are hard to come by. The clinical picture in schistosomiasis is usually dominated by the effect on the urinary tract (*Schistosoma haematobium*) or liver (*S. mansoni* and *S. japonica*). Pulmonary hypertension is thought to be due to granulomata in or adjacent to pulmonary arterioles caused by the reaction to the presence of schistosome eggs.

One of the commonest causes of pulmonary hypertension is that occurring as a complication of chronic obstructive pulmonary disease (COPD), which is due to a combination of hypoxic pulmonary vasoconstriction, hypoxia-driven pulmonary vascular remodelling, and a reduction in capillary cross-sectional area in emphysema. Lung hyperinflation and polycythaemia may also contribute. The prevalence of pulmonary hypertension in patients with severe chronic obstructive pulmonary disease may be as high as 50%, but the average mean pulmonary arterial pressure is of the order of 25 mmHg and progresses slowly (less than 1 mmHg/year). It is likely that ventilatory impairment due to obstructed airways contributes most to the exercise limitation in these patients. Nevertheless, there are relatively unusual cases of chronic obstructive pulmonary disease in which the pulmonary hypertension dominates. These patients are often profoundly hypoxic, have emphysema on CT scanning, and demonstrate a low diffusion coefficient for carbon monoxide. The level of pulmonary hypertension is similar to that seen in idiopathic PAH and these patients warrant targeted therapy for PAH in addition to optimization of their chronic obstructive pulmonary disease medication.

Likely future developments

The next few years will see further important advances in our understanding of the pathobiology of PAH. Intensive research into the TGFβ/BMP signalling pathway in pulmonary vascular cells and tissues should elucidate the mechanisms by which mutation in the *BMPR2* gene leads to PAH. This knowledge will allow the development of new therapies aimed at prevention, arrest, or reversal of the process of pulmonary vascular remodelling in PAH. Already trials are under way to explore the impact of growth factor inhibition in PAH, and the next few years is likely to see more of these experimental studies using drugs initially developed for use in oncology. Cell-based therapy using circulating progenitor cells is also being evaluated. New pathways are being targeted which impact on ion channels, cell survival, and endothelial function, including drugs such as statins and activators of the peroxisome proliferator-activated receptors. Novel biomarkers of disease activity and progression are being identified. Imaging modalities using the latest advances in echocardiography, CT scanning, and MRI are being developed to maximize the information derived from these techniques, which may then replace invasive right heart catheterization.

Chronic thromboembolic pulmonary hypertension (CTEPH)

Pathogenesis

CTEPH occurs when a clot fails to resolve completely after an acute pulmonary embolic event. The rate of resolution of clots after acute pulmonary embolism varies and is longer in patients with pre-existing cardiopulmonary disease, but normal perfusion should be restored by 4 to 6 weeks after an acute event. To some extent, the rate of resolution depends on the initial clot burden or the size of the acute pulmonary embolism. If the clot fails to resolve, it becomes organized before it can be completely fibrinolysed, and this organized thrombus is incorporated into the wall of the pulmonary artery, becomes covered by endothelial cells, and forms a false intima. The organized material occludes the vascular lumen, which increases pulmonary vascular resistance and leads to pulmonary hypertension.

The true prevalence of CTEPH is hard to ascertain, because it is not usually sought in patients who are recovering from acute pulmonary embolism (PE), but it is almost certainly underdiagnosed. One well-designed study found that 4% of patients with a history of acute pulmonary embolism had a persistent elevation of pulmonary arterial pressure after 2 years. Those with a higher initial clot burden (massive PE) are more likely to develop CTEPH than those with minor pulmonary embolism. The more widespread use of thrombolysis for acute pulmonary embolism is often assumed to reduce the prevalence of CTEPH, but no data at present support this view.

It is of note that some of the classic risk factors for acute deep vein thrombosis (DVT)/PE are not found with increased frequency in the population that develops CTEPH. For example, the factor V Leiden polymorphism, which leads to activated protein C resistance and is found with high prevalence in the population of patients with acute DVT, is not overrepresented in patients with CTEPH. By contrast, the prevalence of protein C and S deficiency is increased in patients with CTEPH, but these conditions account for only a small minority of patients. In addition, some 10% of patients with CTEPH may have circulating antiphospholipid antibodies. Recent research points to a deficiency in the ability to fibrinolyse established clots as a predisposing factor. Other important predisposing factors include previous splenectomy and inflammatory bowel disease.

Clinical presentation

Patients often present with persistent symptoms of dyspnoea after an acute embolic event despite the recommended period of anticoagulation, up to 60% having a prior documented episode of previous venous thromboembolism, although some patients may present with gradually worsening dyspnoea in the absence of acute events. On physical examination, there may be pulmonary flow murmurs resulting from turbulent flow across partially obstructed large pulmonary arteries: these are audible on chest auscultation in up to 30% of patients with CTEPH. Otherwise, the clinical presentation is similar to that described above for PAH.

Investigation

The work-up of patients referred with a suspected diagnosis of CTEPH requires a multidisciplinary approach involving surgeons, physicians, and radiologists. Imaging plays a key role in determining whether a patient is suitable for the surgical procedure of choice, pulmonary endarterectomy. CT pulmonary angiography with modern multislice scanners is a rapid and noninvasive technique that can provide several important pieces of information in the assessment of patients with suspected CTEPH, both assessing the presence of any associated lung disease or tumours, and most importantly giving an accurate assessment of the extent of proximal organized clots (Fig. 16.15.2.7). Although occlusion of very small arteries cannot be visualized directly in the case of predominantly distal disease, the characteristic appearance of 'mosaic perfusion' suggests the presence of peripheral disease (Fig. 16.15.2.8), and ventilation–perfusion lung scans also usually show multiple segmental perfusion defects not matched by defects in ventilation in this circumstance (Fig. 16.15.2.10). CT can also reveal the extent of right ventricular hypertrophy and dilatation, although this is probably best seen by MRI. Three-dimensional reconstruction of the two-dimensional CT and MR images can help decide whether the distribution of disease is suitable for pulmonary endarterectomy. The use of a combination of these techniques means that the more invasive traditional pulmonary angiogram can be avoided in most patients.

Treatment

About 60% of cases of CTEPH is potentially suitable for surgery. Of the patients who are not suitable for surgical management, many may be suitable for targeted therapy with the new pharmacological agents described previously for PAH.

Pulmonary endarterectomy involves removal of organized thrombi from the proximal pulmonary arteries. The procedure is a major operation that usually requires the patient to undergo

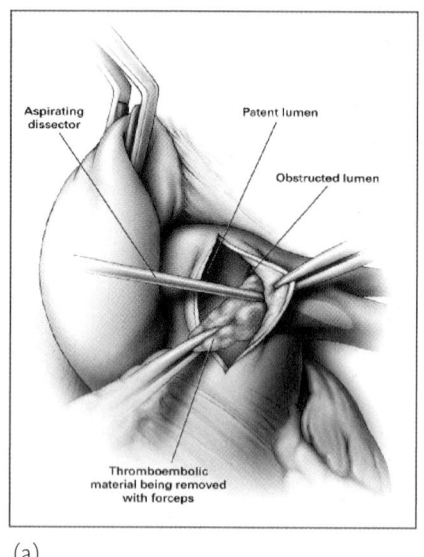

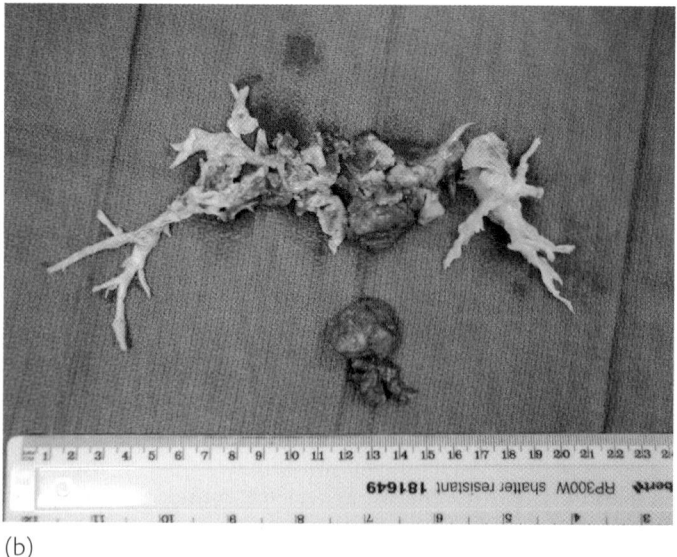

(a)   (b)

Fig. 16.15.2.13 The surgical technique of pulmonary endarterectomy (a) and the surgical specimen obtained from a patient undergoing surgery for CTEPH (b).
Reproduced from from N Engl J Med, Vol. 345, No. 20, November 15, 2001 Copyright © 2001 Massachusetts Medical Society. All rights reserved.

repeated cycles of cardiopulmonary bypass with cerebral cooling, which ensures a bloodless field of view for the surgeon, who can then enter the left and right main pulmonary arteries via an arteriotomy. The aim is to identify a dissection plane along the base of the false intima and to dissect distally as far as possible, when it is often possible to remove organized material down to the level of segmental pulmonary arteries (Fig. 16.15.2.13). With successful clearance of proximal clots the pulmonary vascular resistance can fall dramatically postoperatively, and near normalization of resistance can be achieved in the long term.

There are two main aspects to patient selection for this procedure. Comorbidities are important predictors of perioperative mortality and require careful assessment. A further important consideration is the distribution of the disease, as organized clots need to be anatomically accessible to the surgeon. If the organized material is predominantly of a distal distribution within the pulmonary arteries, i.e. involves subsegmental vessels, there is a high risk that pulmonary vascular resistance will not decrease after the procedure and that the patient will be left with significant pulmonary hypertension.

Despite careful patient selection, the operation is high risk, with perioperative mortality varying between 7 and 20% depending on the experience of the centre. However, in those who survive surgery, the long-term outlook is often excellent after a successful procedure, with marked improvements in exercise capacity, NYHA functional status, and quality of life. To prevent further thromboembolism, patients have an inferior vena cava filter sited prior to the operation and are maintained on lifelong warfarin.

Likely future developments

Much remains unknown about the natural history of CTEPH and the risk factors for failure of resolution of an acute embolic event. Large studies designed to prospectively follow up patients with acute embolism over many years will be necessary to get a clearer picture of the underlying causes. Whether chronic thromboembolic pulmonary embolism always results from embolic phenomena or whether *in situ* thrombosis also contributes remains uncertain. The distinction between CTEPH leading to occlusion of small peripheral pulmonary arteries and idiopathic PAH can be difficult in some cases, and indeed they may be part of the same spectrum of disease.

Selection of patients likely to respond favourably to surgery can be difficult, and improved imaging or physiological assessments are needed. These, along with advances in anaesthetic technology and surgery, are likely to improve further the already impressive results of surgery. The response of inoperable CTEPH to targeted pharmacological therapy requires further evaluation, and we are also likely to see medical interventions aimed at reducing the incidence of CTEPH after acute pulmonary embolism.

Further reading

Abenhaim L, et al. (1996). Appetite-suppressant drugs and the risk of primary pulmonary hypertension. N Engl J Med, 335, 609–16.

Archibald CJ, et al. (1999). Long-term outcome after pulmonary thromboendarterectomy. Am J Respir Crit Care Med, 160, 523–8.

Barst RJ, et al. (1994). Survival in primary pulmonary hypertension with long-term continuous intravenous prostacyclin. Ann Intern Med, 121, 409–15.

Barst RJ, et al. (1996). A comparison of continuous intravenous epoprostenol (prostacyclin) with conventional therapy for primary pulmonary hypertension. N Engl J Med, 334, 296–301.

Bonderman D, et al. (2007). Predictors of outcome in chronic thromboembolic pulmonary hypertension. Circulation, 115, 2153–8.

Deng Z, et al. (2000). Familial primary pulmonary hypertension (gene PPH1) is caused by mutations in the bone morphogenetic protein receptor-II gene. Am J Hum Genet, 67, 737–44.

Fedullo PF, et al. (2001). Chronic thromboembolic pulmonary hypertension. N Engl J Med, 345, 1465–72.

Fuster V, et al. (1984). Primary pulmonary hypertension: natural history and the importance of thrombosis. Circulation, 70, 580–7.

Galie N, et al. (2005). Sildenafil citrate therapy for pulmonary arterial hypertension. N Engl J Med, 353, 2148–57.

Heath D, Segel N, Bishop J (1966). Pulmonary veno-occlusive disease. Circulation, 34, 242–8.

Heath D (1996). Pulmonary vascular disease. In: Hasleton PS (ed.) Spencer's pathology of the lung, pp. 649–93. McGraw-Hill, London.

Higenbottam T, et al. (1984). Long-term treatment of primary pulmonary hypertension with continuous intravenous epoprostenol (prostacyclin). Lancet, i, 1046–7.

Hoeper MM, et al. (2002). New treatments for pulmonary arterial hypertension. Am J Respir Crit Care Med, 165, 1209–16.

Humbert M, et al. (2004). Cellular and molecular pathobiology of pulmonary arterial hypertension. J Am Coll Cardiol, 43(12, Suppl 1), S13–24.

Humbert M, Sitbon O, Simonneau G (2004). Treatment of pulmonary arterial hypertension. N Engl J Med, 351, 1425–36.

Kay JM, Smith P, Heath D (1971). Aminorex and the pulmonary circulation. Thorax, 26, 262–70.

Loyd JE, Primm RK, Newman JH (1984). Familial primary pulmonary hypertension: clinical patterns. Am Rev Respir Dis, 129, 194–7.

Moser KM, et al. (1983). Chronic thrombotic obstruction of major pulmonary arteries. Results of thromboendarterectomy in 15 patients. Ann Intern Med, 99, 299–304.

Newman JH, et al. (2004). Genetic basis of pulmonary arterial hypertension: current understanding and future directions. J Am Coll Cardiol, 43(12, Suppl 1), S33–39.

Olschewski H, et al. (2002). Inhaled iloprost for severe pulmonary hypertension. N Engl J Med, 347, 322–9.

Palevsky HI, et al. (1989). Primary pulmonary hypertension: vascular structure, morphometry, and responsiveness to vasodilator agents. Circulation, 80, 1207–21.

Pengo V, et al. (2004). Incidence of chronic thromboembolic pulmonary hypertension after pulmonary embolism. N Engl J Med, 350, 2257–64.

Pepke-Zaba J, et al. (1991). Inhaled nitric oxide as a cause of selective pulmonary vasodilatation in pulmonary hypertension. Lancet, 338, 1173–4.

Rich S, Kaufmann E, Levy PS (1992). The effect of high doses of calcium-channel blockers on survival in primary pulmonary hypertension. N Engl J Med, 327, 76–81.

Rich S, et al. (1987). Primary pulmonary hypertension. A national prospective study. Ann Intern Med, 107, 216–23.

Rubin LJ, et al. (2002). Bosentan therapy for pulmonary arterial hypertension. N Engl J Med, 346, 896–903.

Rudarakanchana N, et al. (2002). Functional analysis of bone morphogenetic protein type II receptor mutations underlying primary pulmonary hypertension. Hum Mol Genet, 11, 1517–25.

International PPH Consortium et al. (2000). Heterozygous germ-line mutations in BMPR2, encoding a TGF-b receptor, cause familial primary pulmonary hypertension. Nat Genetics, 26, 81–4.

Wagenvoort C, Wagenvoort N (1970). Primary pulmonary hypertension: a pathological study of vessels in 156 clinically diagnosed cases. Circulation, 42, 1163–84.

16.15.3 Pulmonary oedema

Nicholas W. Morrell and John D. Firth

Essentials

The formation of pulmonary oedema depends on the balance between capillary hydrostatic pressure, interstitial tissue pressure, plasma colloid osmotic pressure, endothelial permeability, and lymphatic function. The efficiency of lymphatic drainage of interstitial fluid (which can increase >10-fold) is critical in determining the onset and extent of hydrostatic oedema.

Pulmonary capillary pressures in the range 25 to 35 mmHg increase the filtration of water and small solutes; interstitial oedema and pleural effusions result. Pulmonary capillary pressures greater than 35 mmHg cause blood and gas barrier disruption (stress failure); protein-rich fluid and red cells fill the air spaces. Endothelial disruption leads to oedema fluid with a high protein content and activation of coagulation, predisposing towards interstitial fibrosis. The dangerous combination of hydrostatic and high-permeability pulmonary oedema (which is slower to resolve) occurs in neurogenic and high-altitude pulmonary oedema.

Clinical features—the characteristic symptom of pulmonary oedema is breathlessness, which comes on more or less acutely in the first instance. Orthopnoea and paroxysmal nocturnal dyspnoea develop later because of postural hydrostatic factors. Typical physical signs are of diminished breath sounds and fine lung crepitations at the bases, but in the most dramatic cases the patient produces pink, frothy fluid from their mouth and looks as though they are about to die (which they will without immediate effective treatment).

Investigation—in early hydrostatic pulmonary oedema, the chest radiograph initially shows distended lymphatics (Kerley septal lines), followed by signs of interstitial oedema such as 'cuffing' of airways and arteries. As alveolar oedema becomes established, there is a loss of lucency around the hila in a 'butterfly' pattern.

Management—should be aimed at the underlying physiological abnormality where possible, e.g. correction of plasma oncotic pressure or reduction in capillary hydrostatic pressure. General supportive measures involve putting the patient in the 'trunk up, legs down' position to help pool blood in the dependent parts and reduce central venous pressure, and giving high-flow oxygen, diuretics, intravenous nitrates, and morphine. If these are ineffective and oxygen administration at normal airway pressure cannot maintain the arterial partial pressure of oxygen and/or hypercapnia develops, then application of a continuous positive airway pressure (CPAP) mask, noninvasive ventilation, or tracheal intubation and intermittent positive pressure ventilation need to be considered.

Acknowledgement: Much of the chapter written for the third edition of this textbook by the late J S Prichard has been retained here.

Introduction

Acute fulminant pulmonary oedema is a terrifying event in which patients literally drown in their own body fluids. Much more commonly, the clinician is called to treat pulmonary oedema in its less acute form, for breathlessness disturbs the patient long before serious alveolar flooding has begun.

Because pulmonary oedema is very commonly seen as a manifestation of left-sided heart disease—where its relief by diuretics is so effective—there is a temptation to forget the very wide range of other causes. Indeed, it is prudent to make the diagnosis of hydrostatic pulmonary oedema of cardiac origin only when other manifestations of heart disease are present, and to consider wider possibilities in all other circumstances. Pulmonary oedema has many possible causes, which occur in combination more often than is usually recognized (Box 16.15.3.1). Only by careful and clear analysis of clinical and pathophysiological data can the contributing factors be identified and the clinical situation fully understood.

Pathogenesis

Fluid balance between the capillaries and the interstitial space

The continuous movement of water from the lung capillaries into the interstitium is regulated by the permeability of the endothelium to water and protein and by the imbalance of hydrostatic and osmotic forces across the membrane. The Starling hypothesis suggests that perturbation of any one of several factors could lead to oedema (Figs. 16.15.3.1 and 16.15.3.2). These include capillary hydrostatic pressure (P_{cap}), interstitial tissue pressure (P_{int}), plasma colloid osmotic (oncotic) pressure (π_{cap}), endothelial permeability (expressed by k and s), and lymphatic function. Abnormalities in the first four will cause oedema by increasing water entry to the interstitial space, while impaired function of the last will diminish drainage. Interstitial colloid osmotic pressure (P_{int}) has not been included as an independent variable as it is determined by the plasma protein concentration and endothelial permeability.

Experimentally, the development of pulmonary oedema may be characterized by the relationship between tissue water and microvascular hydrostatic pressure (Fig. 16.15.3.3). In the normal lung, the water content rises only slowly until the capillary pressure reaches 25 to 30 mmHg: thereafter, the rise is rapid. The curve is shifted leftwards by decreased interstitial pressure, increased endothelial permeability, decreased plasma oncotic pressure, or impaired lymphatic drainage. Fig. 16.15.3.3 illustrates the interactions between these factors: at low and normal hydrostatic pressures, changes in oncotic pressure, permeability, and lymphatic drainage do not readily cause oedema, but at higher hydrostatic pressures their effect is much more dramatic. The fact that pulmonary capillary pressure may be raised to 25 to 30 mmHg before there is any significant accumulation of water in a normal lung is a considerable 'safety factor', due principally to the behaviour of the lymphatic system. In response to faster transcapillary water flux from whatever cause (see below), the lymphatic system can increase its activity so much that flow accelerates to between 3 and 10 times the basal level before the drainage becomes overwhelmed. The situation in which the lung water content has increased only a little while the transcapillary and lymph fluxes have increased considerably emphasizes that pulmonary oedema is a dynamic

Box 16.15.3.1 Causes of pulmonary oedema

Hydrostatic pulmonary oedema

- Pulmonary venous hypertension—cardiogenic. Left ventricular failure; mitral stenosis and regurgitation; left atrial thrombosis; left atrial myxoma; cor triatriatum; loculated pericarditis

- Pulmonary venous hypertension—noncardiogenic. Veno-occlusive disease; congenital pulmonary venous stenosis; mediastinal granulomas, fibrosis, masses; neurogenic

- Pulmonary arterial hypertension. Hyperkinetic states (extreme exercise, left-to-right shunts, hypoxia, anaemia, thyrotoxicosis); pulmonary emboli; high altitude

Permeability oedema

- Drugs and circulating toxic substances—hydrochlorthiazide, phenylbutazone, aspirin, methylsalicylate, nitrofurantoin, hydralazine, bleomycin, heroin, morphine, methadone, dextropropoxyphene, paraquat, alloxan, α-naphthylthiourea, coral snake venom, silver nitrate, ammonium chloride, ammonium sulphate, chelating agents, oleic acid (fat embolus), diltiazem, iodine-containing contrast media, interleukin-2

- Immunological—Goodpasture's syndrome, antilung serum, Stevens–Johnson syndrome

- Radiation

- Viral infection

- Aspirated toxic substances—fresh water, salt water, stomach contents

- Inhaled toxic substances—smoke, nitrogen oxides, ozone, chlorine, cadmium oxide, oxides of sulphur, carbonyl chloride, phosgene, lewisite, oxygen

- Metabolic—hepatic failure, renal failure

- Mechanical endothelial disruption—?neurogenic pulmonary oedema

- Mechanical epithelial disruption—?pulmonary hyperinflation

- Other causes of permeability oedema—adult respiratory distress syndrome. Particularly: shock lung, septicaemia, pancreatitis, burns, fat embolism, cardiopulmonary bypass, banked unfiltered blood, amniotic fluid embolism

Reduced alveolar septal tissue interstitial pressure

- Upper airway obstruction—acute. Laryngospasm, epiglottitis, laryngotracheobronchitis, spasmodic croup, foreign body, tumour, upper airway trauma, strangulation, peritonsillar abscess, Ludwig's angina, angio-oedema; near-drowning, ?asthma

- Upper airway obstruction—chronic. Obstructive sleep apnoea; adenoidal, tonsillar, or nasopharyngeal mass; thyroid goitre; acromegaly

Reduced plasma-colloid osmotic pressure

- Rare as sole cause. Contributes to oedema caused by adult respiratory distress syndrome, hepatic and renal failure, fluid overload, myocardial infarction. Important when hypoproteinaemia occurs with other conditions predisposing to oedema.

Failure of lymphatic clearance

- Lymphangitis carcinomatosa; mediastinal obstruction; lung transplant; contributes to oedema in adult respiratory distress syndrome, malaria, silicosis

phenomenon, in which tissue swelling is but the endstage reached when lymphatic drainage capacity is exceeded. Only then does fluid accumulation begin—slowly at first in the interstitial space, but then rapidly as alveolar flooding begins.

Mechanisms of pulmonary oedema

Hydrostatic

Any increase in capillary hydrostatic pressure, whether from cardiac failure, fluid overload, or pulmonary venous occlusion, speeds the rate of water flow into the interstitium. Provided the increase in pressure is not too great, this process will be self-limiting. Thus, molecular sieving, by allowing water to enter the interstitial space more readily than macromolecular solutes, will reduce π_{int}. Increased interstitial water increases the interstitial hydrostatic pressure P_{int} and decreases the macromolecular exclusion volume—again increasing P_{int}. So, as long as lymphatic pumping can keep pace, tissue water will expand only slightly. However, once the capacity of the lymphatic drainage is exceeded, accumulation of an oedema fluid with low protein content begins. This starts in the lower parts of the lung (because it is here that hydrostatic pressures are greatest) and is associated with a characteristic redistribution of blood flow away from the lung bases.

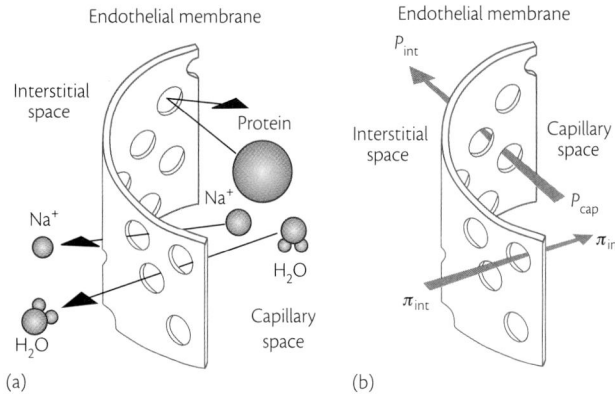

Fig. 16.15.3.1 (a) The lung endothelial membrane is permeable to water and electrolytes but less permeable to macromolecules. (b) The Starling equation: $Q_1 = K(P_{cap} - P_{int}) - Ks(\pi_{cap} - \pi_{int})$, where Q_1 is the net fluid filtration rate, K is the filtration coefficient, s is the reflection coefficient, $(P_{cap} - P_{int})$ is the hydrostatic pressure gradient from the capillary lumen to interstitial space, and $(\pi_{cap} - \pi_{int})$ is the oncotic pressure difference across the capillary membrane.

The activity of lung lymphatics is critical in determining the onset and extent of hydrostatic oedema, and therefore it is not surprising to find that, in conditions where pulmonary venous pressures are chronically elevated, the lymphatics undergo hypertrophy as a protective mechanism. Consequently, acute elevations of pulmonary vascular pressure will produce acute life-threatening oedema at levels that, when reached chronically, cause little distress and are registered clinically only by the characteristic radiological changes of lymphatic hypertrophy.

High permeability

Endothelial damage speeds water flux into the interstitial space, but—unlike hydrostatic oedema—there is also an increase in protein flux so that the oedema fluid has a high protein content. This has four consequences:

1 The oncotic pressure of the interstitial fluid increases and one of the major mechanisms for limiting the progress of oedema becomes unavailable.

2 Much of the protein reaching the tissue and alveoli is fibrinogen, which coagulates. Initially, the damage from interstitial coagulation is limited by fibrinolysis by plasminogen, but this defence is soon exhausted and mobilization of the coagulum ceases.

3 The residual coagulum impairs lymphatic drainage.

4 The residual coagulum promotes the development of lung fibrosis.

By far, the most common cause of high permeability pulmonary oedema is the acute respiratory distress syndrome, which is discussed in Chapter 17.5. Less common causes include toxic gases and fumes (Chapter 18.14.11) and drugs (Chapter 18.14.13).

Reduced plasma oncotic pressure

A reduction in plasma oncotic pressure increases fluid transudation into the lung and leads to pulmonary oedema at lower hydrostatic pressures than would otherwise be expected. Although this is readily demonstrable experimentally, it is frequently overlooked in clinical practice, where it may be of importance following myocardial infarction, after transfusion of crystalloids, and in adult respiratory distress syndrome. A useful clinical guide to the danger is the difference between pulmonary wedge pressure (measured by a Swann–Ganz catheter) and colloid osmotic pressure (the COP–PAW gradient). The normal lower limit of this index is about $-12\,mmHg$, but at levels below $-9\,mmHg$ the risk of oedema is considerably enhanced. A practical problem in applying this method has been the difficulty in standardizing and maintaining protein oncometers: the alternative of using serum protein measurements is valuable but slower.

Lymphatic oedema and the role of the lung lymphatics

The lymphatic system provides the lung with its major 'safety factor'. It is capable of increasing the tissue clearance rate at least 10-fold before becoming overwhelmed. In chronic venous and capillary hypertension, as in mitral stenosis, even larger lymph flows occur because of lymphatic hypertrophy.

Oedema soon develops when lymphatic drainage is occluded experimentally. This has clinical relevance for patients with lung transplants, whose lung lymphatic pathways are severed and in whom initial alveolar flooding is common. Lymphatic oedema also

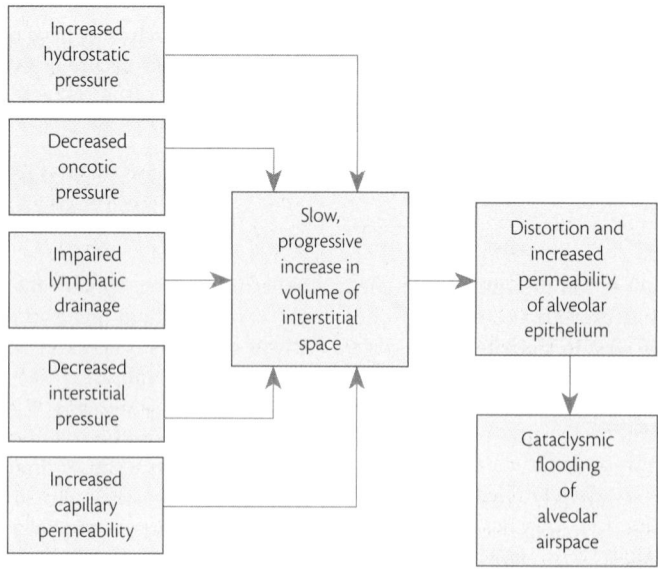

Fig. 16.15.3.2 The initiation of pulmonary oedema and the sequence of development.

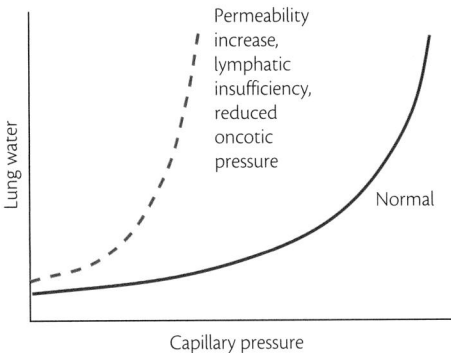

Fig. 16.15.3.3 Lung water content and capillary pressure. In the normal lung tissue, the water content does not begin to increase until the capillary pressure is approximately 30 mmHg. Where colloid osmotic pressure (e.g. plasma protein concentration) is reduced, endothelial permeability is increased or the lymphatic pump is impaired, the whole curve is shifted to the left.
Reproduced from Prichard JS (1982). Edema of the lung. Charles C. Thomas, Springfield, Illinois.

plays a part in pulmonary oedema from lymphangitis carcinomatosa and in facilitating oedema in patients with silicosis and malaria.

Reduced interstitial pressure

Tissue pressure within the interstitial space is one of the determinants of transendothelial fluid movement. It can be altered independently of intravascular events by changes in the intrapleural pressure. Thus, when extreme negative intrapleural pressures occur, the interstitial perialveolar tissue pressure can fall considerably below its normal subatmospheric level and accelerate the rate of fluid movement into the interstitium. Oedema will appear if the rate of fluid entry exceeds the rate at which it can move through the interstitium and be removed by the lymphatics.

The sequence of oedema accumulation

When oedema fluid begins to accumulate in lung tissue—irrespective of the underlying cause—it does so first around fissures, blood vessels, and airways because these tissues are 'loose' and swell easily without great change in tissue pressure. When this 'sump' has become near maximally dilated, swelling and thickening of alveolar walls begins. This is the interstitial phase of pulmonary oedema (up to 400 ml capacity). Pulmonary gas exchange is not affected at this stage, because the fluid is confined to the thick side of the alveolar septum. Excess filtrate is also accommodated in the pleural space, which in terms of fluid balance can be regarded as an extension of the interstitium of the lungs. Finally, after a phase of progressive alveolar wall thickening, fluid begins to accumulate in the alveoli themselves. This occurs mainly in the dependent zones of the lung where, because of gravity, capillary pressures are greatest. In addition, stress failure of the blood and gas barrier is most likely to occur in these regions, promoting alveolar filling with a protein-rich fluid. This final phase begins at a point where total lung water has increased by about 30% (Fig. 16.15.3.4).

At first, the fluid in the alveoli is confined to the alveolar angles. Subsequently, complete flooding of individual alveoli occurs. A striking feature of the microscopic appearance at this stage is the way in which alveoli are either completely filled with fluid or else have only minimal accumulation in the angles. There are no half-filled alveoli: flooding is a 'quantal' event, with flooded alveoli scattered at random throughout the affected area. Atelectasis is

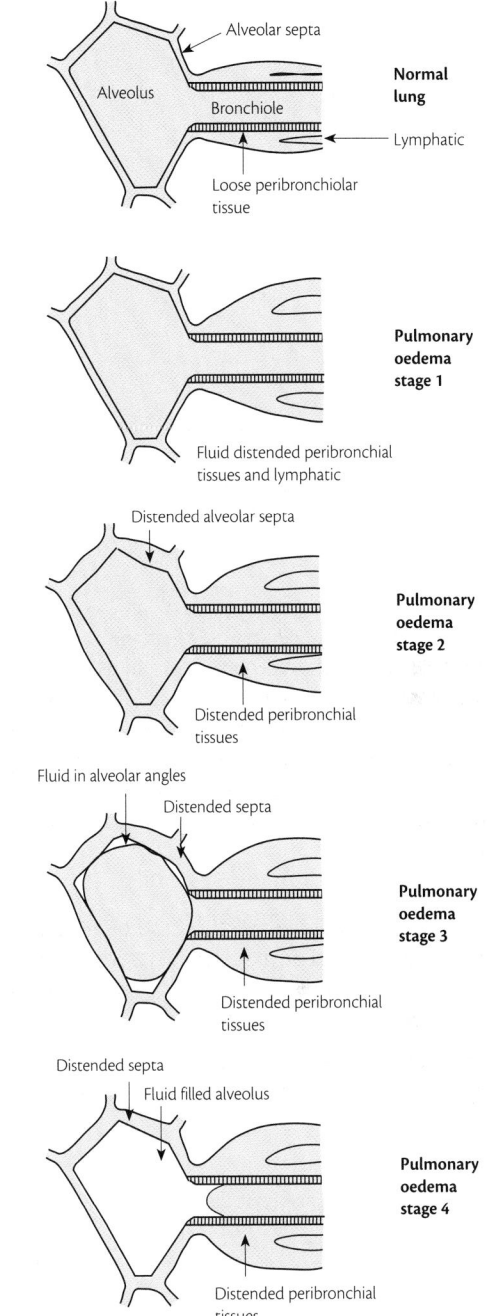

Fig. 16.15.3.4 Stages in the development of pulmonary oedema.
Stage 1: peribronchial swelling; stage 2: distended alveolar septa; stage 3: limited accumulation of fluid in alveolar angles; stage 4: alveolar flooding.
Reproduced from Prichard JS (1982). Edema of the lung. Charles C. Thomas, Springfield, Illinois.
http://www.ccthomas.com/css_permission.cfm.

uncommon and air is rarely trapped, although the volume of each alveolus is smaller when fluid-filled than when air-filled.

The quantal nature of alveolar flooding arises from the interaction of surface and tissue forces (Fig. 16.15.3.5). The immediate precipitating factor is probably an increase in alveolar epithelial permeability caused by the distortion and swelling of the alveolar wall, which allows water to flood from the interstitium into the air space. An alternative, less likely, hypothesis is that fluid entry occurs via pores in the epithelium of the terminal airways. Irrespective

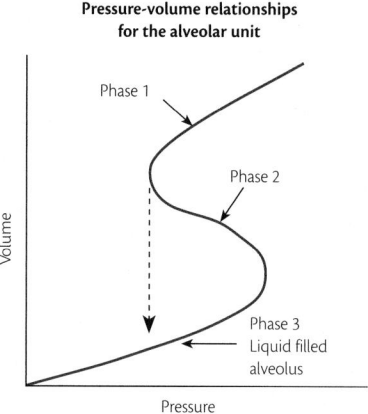

Pressure-volume relationships for the alveolar unit

Phase 1

Phase 2

Phase 3
Liquid filled
alveolus

Volume

Pressure

Fig. 16.15.3.5 Pressure–volume relationships in the alveolus. Phase 1 represents the normal alveolus lined by surfactant. Tissue elasticity, osmotic balance, and the presence of surfactant combine to produce a direct, mechanically stable relationship between pressure and volume. Phase 2 represents the situation in which alveolar permeability has increased. Any influx of fluid into the alveolus decreases the overall surface area. At these lower dimensions, surfactant is inoperative and surface tension is independent of area. The relationship between volume and pressure is that of an air bubble in liquid ($P = 2T/R$) and is unstable, a situation only resolved when the alveolus has flooded. The air volume, therefore, shrinks as air is expelled until phase 3 is reached. Here the remaining air is a 'bleb' at the bronchiolar orifice.

of the route, the ease of fluid entry now makes the relationship between pressure and volume inverse and unstable, as explained in the legend to Fig. 16.13.3.5.

The resolution of pulmonary oedema

The extent and rapidity of resolution of pulmonary oedema depend upon its cause. Hydrostatic oedema and that due to low oncotic pressure can resolve completely and rapidly, but this is rarely the case with permeability oedema, where slow disappearance and permanent lung damage may result.

Resolution of hydrostatic oedema occurs in two phases: return of the capillary pressure towards normal, and then lymphatic and osmotic resorption of tissue and alveolar fluid. Once hydrostatic pressure has been reduced, fluid is removed from the interstitial space by lymphatic drainage, which can be increased (three to fourfold) for as long as 24 h after an acute episode in experimental models. Oncotic resorption into the circulation can also play a significant part. However, the mechanism of alveolar clearance is not well understood. Much fluid is removed by coughing and ciliary drainage, and final resorption seems to occur as a result of active sodium ion transport, although it is uncertain whether this takes place in the alveolar or terminal airway epithelium.

The clearance mechanisms in high-permeability oedema are considerably less efficient than in hydrostatic oedema because fibrin has coagulated in the interstitium, lymphatics, and alveoli, and because the tissues have often been damaged. Regeneration of epithelium and endothelium is frequently necessary.

Clinical aspects

Causes of pulmonary oedema

Box 16.13.3.1 lists the main causes of pulmonary oedema classified according to the predominant pathophysiological mechanism. However, the clinician should never forget that more than one cause may be operating (Table 16.15.3.1), and must not neglect one remediable factor at the expense of another, or allow therapy itself to intensify the problem. For example, overvigorous fluid replacement following pulmonary endothelial damage may be the very factor that accelerates water and protein flow into the interstitium and provokes oedema.

Descriptions of the clinical manifestations and management of the more common diseases listed in Box 16.15.3.1 are provided elsewhere, but particular aspects are noted here.

Pulmonary oedema in heart failure

Heart failure, discussed in detail in Chapter 16.5, is the cause of the commonest form of pulmonary oedema, but two features deserve comment. The first is the symptom of orthopnoea in which the oedema either first appears or, if already present, intensifies after

Table 16.15.3.1 The multifactorial nature of pulmonary oedema

	Hydrostatic pressure increase	Oncotic pressure decrease	Endothelial permeability increase	Lymphatic drainage impairment	Reduced interstitial pressure	Reduced alveolar surfactant
Shock lung	From therapy	Yes	Yes	Yes		(Yes)
Hepatic failure		Yes	Yes			
Renal failure	Yes	(Yes)	Yes			
Neurogenic oedema	Yes		Yes			
Fluid overload	Yes	(Yes)				
Pulmonary emboli	Yes		Yes			
MI	Yes	(Yes)				
Carcinomatosis		Yes		Yes		
High altitude	Yes		Yes			
Re-expansion		(Yes)			Yes	(Yes)
Airway obstruction	(Yes)				Yes	

Parentheses indicate minor contributions.
MI, myocardial infarction.

a period of lying down. The cause is a shift of blood from the systemic to the pulmonary circulation, which occurs because of the change in posture. This leads to an increase in intracapillary hydrostatic pressure, which in turn triggers oedema. The symptom is at its most dramatic in paroxysmal nocturnal dyspnoea. The second feature—and one that frequently causes confusion because it is contrary to expectation—is the tendency of the blood pressure to rise as the patient progresses into left heart failure. The cause is probably increasing sympathetic activity and circulating catecholamines, which lead to intense systemic arterial and venous vasoconstriction, thereby increasing afterload and central venous pressure inappropriately and so intensifying the development of oedema.

Loculated constrictive pericarditis

Loculated constrictive pericarditis, predominantly involving the left ventricle, can occur in patients with chronic renal failure who are undergoing dialysis. Echocardiography is helpful in diagnosis, which may be difficult because the characteristic signs of pericardial tamponade may be missing. When located posteriorly, the fluid is difficult to aspirate percutaneously, but open drainage is rarely necessary because strict attention to fluid regulation during and between dialyses usually leads to resolution.

Pulmonary venous thrombosis

This is a rare condition that is difficult to diagnose. It may be idiopathic or may be a manifestation of conditions such as polyarteritis nodosa, other vasculitic disorders, and occult neoplastic disease. The idiopathic condition is most common in middle-aged women. Presenting symptoms are of increasing lassitude and breathlessness, sometimes with a low-grade fever. Gross-effort dyspnoea and pulmonary oedema, usually with pleural effusions, develop later. Signs of pulmonary hypertension are present. Difficulty in obtaining a clear pulmonary arterial wedge pressure tracing and normal left atrial pressure (measured directly by the trans-septal route) should alert suspicion. Pulmonary artery angiography demonstrates poor segmental drainage in the regions affected by thrombosis. Open lung biopsy will confirm the diagnosis, but this is dangerous and should be undertaken only when there is real fear of missing an alternative cause of the oedema.

Left atrial myxoma, ball thrombus of the left atrium, and cor triatriatum

These are rare, but must not be missed as they are remediable by surgery. Their clinical presentation may be very similar to that of pulmonary venous thrombosis. All three conditions also enter into the differential diagnosis of tight mitral stenosis. Echocardiography is the key investigation.

High-altitude oedema

Some apparently normal people experience acute pulmonary oedema on ascending rapidly to high altitude (see Chapter 9.4). The condition tends to occur in those individuals who have an exaggerated acute pulmonary arterial pressor response to hypoxia. These develop pulmonary hypertension at high altitude, with oedema probably resulting from inhomogeneity of vasoconstriction and consequent extreme hyperperfusion of those areas not vasoconstricted. A further contribution may arise from hypoxic inhibition of sodium transport and inflammation.

Neurogenic pulmonary oedema

A large variety of intracranial lesions leading to raised intracranial pressure may occasionally be associated with acute pulmonary oedema. It is probable that damage to the nucleus of the tractus solitarus and the hypothalamus lead to severe systemic vasoconstriction ('sympathetic storm'), which shifts blood to the pulmonary circulation, causing an extreme paroxysm of pulmonary hypertension. In addition, there is evidence to suggest that pulmonary venoconstriction also occurs, thus causing a rise in pulmonary capillary pressure even in excess of that predicted from pulmonary arterial pressure measurements. The extreme high blood pressure in the capillaries first induces hydrostatic oedema and if sufficiently severe also damages the endothelium, leading to a less easily resolved permeability oedema.

Pulmonary thromboembolism

This may occasionally lead to florid pulmonary oedema, for which two hypotheses have been proposed: local overperfusion caused by diversion of blood flow away from the occluded site and humoral alteration of permeability. It is possible that both mechanisms may play a part, and also that the causes may be different in micro- and macroemboli. Evidence for the over-perfusion mechanism originates from experiments in which balloon occlusion of the major pulmonary vessels leads to oedema and increased flow of low-protein lymph from other areas.

Expansion pulmonary oedema

Pulmonary oedema after expansion of a collapsed lung is rare, but more likely when the lung (or lobe) has been collapsed for some time. The likelihood may be reduced by ensuring that negative pressure in the pleural space during re-expansion does not exceed $10 \, cmH_2O$, that the procedure is terminated if cough develops, and that not more than 1500 ml of fluid is aspirated at any one time when collapse is related to an effusion. The mechanism is uncertain. Permeability change is likely as high protein oedema has been found in both clinical and experimental situations. The mechanism of damage may be from toxic, oxygen free radicals, as in cardiac reperfusion injury. Additional contributing factors could be loss of surfactant during the period of collapse and increased negativity of interstitial pressure during re-expansion.

Postobstructive pulmonary oedema

The initiating event is a markedly negative intrapleural pressure generated by forceful inspiratory effort against an obstructed upper airway, which is then transmitted to the pulmonary interstitial space. During normal breathing, intrapleural pressures rarely fall below $-5 \, cmH_2O$, but in upper airway obstruction the value may be as low as $-50 \, cmH_2O$. Postobstructive oedema should, therefore, be suspected wherever there is the rapid onset of dyspnoea, cyanosis, frothy pink sputum production, and radiological pulmonary infiltrates after the rapid relief of upper airway obstruction. The onset is usually immediate but occasionally delays of up to 2 h have been reported. The chronic form occurs in patients with obstructive sleep apnoea, in whom negative intrapleural pressures as low as $-100 \, cmH_2O$ have been recorded.

Lymphatic oedema and lymphatic obstruction

Surprisingly little is known of pulmonary lymphatic failure in clinical practice. Lymphatic occlusion underlies the oedema and dyspnoea of lymphangitis carcinomatosa. In cases where cardiac failure and pneumoconioses coexist, it has been found that oedema develops at lower capillary pressures than would be expected, and this has been attributed to lymphatic blockage. Mechanical lymphatic disruption is probably a contributing factor to the ease with which lungs develop oedema immediately after transplantation.

Disorders of capillary permeability

Many of the conditions associated with adult respiratory distress syndrome (see Chapter 17.5) can also be associated with less dramatic degrees of oedema. It is a good rule always to consider the possibility that a permeability abnormality might exist as an associated cause in all cases of pulmonary oedema. The history can be particularly helpful, particularly with regards to possible infections, use of drugs, and occupational chemicals. The possibility of oxygen toxicity should be borne in mind in all patients in intensive care.

Unilateral oedema

This frequently causes diagnostic confusion. Unilateral oedema on the same side as pre-existing lung abnormalities (ipsilateral oedema) may arise from posture (lying on one side during oedema development), increased perfusion of one lung secondary to a systemic to pulmonary shunt, unilateral venous occlusion (either from unilateral veno-occlusive disease or from extrinsic compression), or unilateral lymphatic pathology such as lymphangitis carcinomatosa. Contralateral oedema is seen where the pre-existing pathology protects that lung. Instances include congenital unilateral pulmonary artery, Swyer–James–McLeod syndrome, unilateral thromboembolism, and unilateral fibrosis causing unilateral hypoxia and vasoconstriction.

The diagnosis of pulmonary oedema

The diagnosis of pulmonary oedema is by clinical observation and chest radiography.

Clinical features

The characteristic symptom of pulmonary oedema is breathlessness, probably generated by an awareness of inappropriate respiratory effort and by firing of J (juxta-alveolar) receptors. This dyspnoea comes on more or less acutely in the first instance, often following exercise. Later, paroxysmal nocturnal dyspnoea develops because of postural hydrostatic factors. Only then are signs of diminished breath sounds at the bases and fine, lung crepitations found. The crepitations (crackles) characteristic of pulmonary oedema are intermittent, explosive sounds that each last for less than 20 ms. They are probably caused by the sudden opening of a succession of small airways, the acoustic wave being produced either by equalization of downstream and upstream pressures or by sudden alterations in the tension of the airway walls. They thus relate to the 'all-or-none' features of alveolar flooding observed physiologically. The rhonchi or wheezes that are sometimes heard, and which may cause considerable diagnostic confusion in the dyspnoeic patient, can arise either from bronchiolar wall oedema or from vagally mediated reflex bronchospasm.

In dramatic cases the patient is sitting up, terrified, gasping for breath, barely able to speak, cyanosed, cold and clammy, and pink, frothy oedema fluid may be coming from their mouth *in extremis*. Auscultation of the chest reveals crackles all over. See Chapter 17.3 for

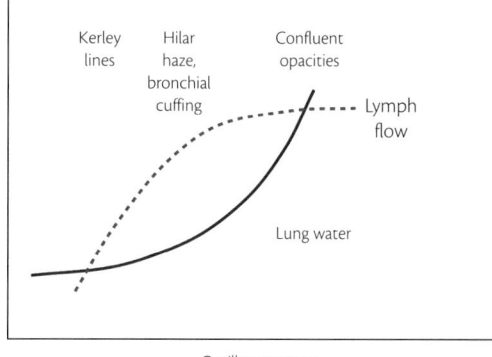

Fig. 16.15.3.6 Radiological signs and pulmonary pathophysiology. Kerley lines are a particularly useful radiological sign, as they occur at a stage where lymph flow and transinterstitial water flow have both increased but where appreciable tissue swelling has not yet appeared.
Reproduced from Prichard JS (1982). Edema of the lung. Charles C. Thomas, Springfield, Illinois.

discussion of how to proceed in this circumstance (put out a cardiac arrest call/get help from intensive care unit (ICU) immediately).

Chest radiography

The chest radiograph is a sensitive and easily available tool for spotting early pulmonary oedema (Figs. 16.15.3.6 and 16.15.3.7). Most radiographical studies have been made during cardiogenic oedema where changes of oedema are necessarily superimposed on other circulatory alterations. Three successive and overlapping phases can be identified.

Pre-oedema

This reflects cardiac and circulatory changes and the increased flow of fluid that occurs through the lymphatics before swelling of the tissue takes place. The cardiothoracic ratio on a posteroanterior film is usually more than 0.5 (>0.57 for an anteroposterior film is standard when geometry is preserved). Distension and engorgement of blood vessels occur, particularly in the upper zone, with inverse changes at the bases leading to reversal of the usual pattern. Distended lymphatics subsequently become identifiable as septal lines, perilobular lines, and rosettes. Septal lines were originally identified by Kerley: type A lines are ragged, unbranched, and run centripetally towards the hilum; type C lines are fine, interlacing, and seen most easily in the central and perihilar regions; type B lines are the best known and most commonly seen. They are short,

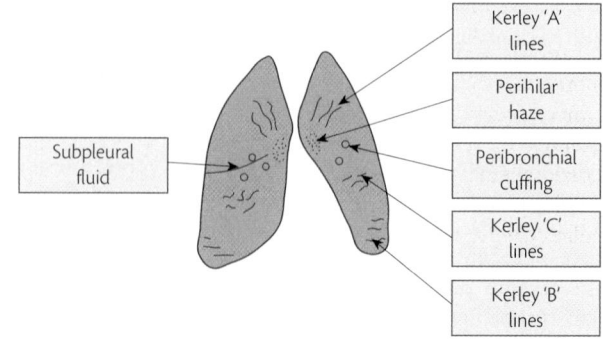

Fig. 16.15.3.7 Characteristic radiological appearances in interstitial oedema (see text).
Reproduced from Prichard JS (1982). Edema of the lung. Charles C. Thomas, Springfield, Illinois.

sharp, horizontal, and found in the costophrenic angles. They occur most often in pulmonary oedema due to chronic pulmonary venous hypertension. Indeed, there is excellent correlation between the density of Kerley B lines and left atrial pressure in mitral stenosis. The lines are rarely seen below a mean left atrial pressure of 13.5 mmHg, are commonly found in the region of 22 mmHg, and are invariably present when the left atrial pressure exceeds 30 mmHg. Perilobular lines and rosettes are found on close inspection in about 3% of radiographs and probably represent the lymphatics running around the respiratory acini.

Interstitial oedema

This first appears in areas of 'loose' connective tissue when wedge pressure begins to rise above 15 mmHg (see sequence of oedema accumulation, above). Visible interlobar and accessory lung fissures are the first manifestations. These are followed by perivascular and peribronchial cuffs, which contribute (respectively) to the homogeneous circular shadows formed by the already distended vessels and to the 'ring' shadows around bronchi seen close to the hilum. Micronoduli consist of small, round densities (<3 mm) arising from the accumulation of fluid around the smaller blood vessels. Blurring and hazing of the hilar regions represent the beginning of true alveolar septal interstitial oedema and, in hydrostatic oedema, begin at wedge pressures of around 20 mmHg. A diffuse increase in lung density (clouding) represents the final phase.

Alveolar oedema

This starts when wedge pressure reaches 25 to 28 mmHg. It is seen as a 'fluffy' loss of lucency, either around the hila in a butterfly or bat's wing pattern, or predominantly in the lower zones, usually reflecting a 'gravitational' distribution. Associated changes are the development of effusions and a loss of lung volume caused by a fall in lung compliance.

Radiologically, the permeability oedemas follow the pattern of the hydrostatic except that (1) the distribution of alveolar oedema tends to be patchy; and (2) the characteristic vascular and cardiac changes are not present.

The presence of pre-existing lung disease—particularly chronic obstructive pulmonary disease—may modify the radiological appearance of pulmonary oedema considerably. Hyperinflation may render the silhouette of a large heart unremarkable; with the onset of interstitial oedema, a hyperinflated lung may shrink to normal size; the distribution of oedema shadowing may be patchy and only evident where parenchyma is sufficiently preserved; Kerley lines may be difficult or impossible to identify.

Other investigations

CT scanning is not necessary for the diagnosis of pulmonary oedema, but the appearances are characteristic, with thickening and increased visualization of interlobular septa and associated thickening of subpleural and peribronchial interstitial spaces. Alveolar oedema leads to varying degrees of alveolar consolidation. As in the plain radiograph, there may be associated heart and vascular changes and pleural effusions.

Pulmonary function in oedema of the lung

The oedematous lung shows a mixture of restrictive and obstructive defects, although the former dominate. The restrictive component arises from decreased compliance, which is a result of vascular congestion (in cardiogenic and fluid overload oedema), interstitial oedema, and surfactant washout. Of these, the interstitial oedema contributes surprisingly little so that restrictive changes are indicative of an engorged vascular system to start with and later of alveolar flooding.

Sometimes, airflow resistance may cause easily audible wheeze and rhonchi (so-called 'cardiac asthma') and a reduction in forced expiratory volume in 1 s/forced vital capacity (FEV_1/FVC), but—more usually—it is difficult to detect by simple methods because it occurs predominantly in the small airways of 1 to 2 mm diameter, which contribute relatively little to overall resistance. There could be a number of causes for such airflow obstruction. In the pre-oedematous phase of heart failure the smallest airways may be compressed by the distension of adjacent vessels in the bronchovascular bundle. In frank interstitial oedema, it has been suggested that perivascular cuffing could do the same, but this has not been substantiated. However, submucosal oedema and vagally mediated reflex bronchoconstriction are proven and probably responsible for most of the effect. Restriction and obstruction may combine to reduce vital capacity, and serial measurements of this can be a good index of severity of and recovery from pulmonary oedema.

Tachypnoea is a prominent feature of all forms of pulmonary oedema. This is associated with a low tidal volume, but total ventilation (V_E)—both at rest and during exercise—is high relative to the prevailing level of arterial carbon dioxide tension. Most of this increase is accounted for by deadspace ventilation; hence, unless the patient is progressing into severe alveolar oedema (see below), he or she remains normocapnic. The mechanism underlying this tachypnoea is uncertain. Hypoxic effects upon the central carbon dioxide chemostat do not appear to be an explanation, and evidence using perialveolar local anaesthetic suggests that the J (juxta-alveolar) receptor—an unmyelinated nerve ending in the vicinity of the alveoli, which responds to interstitial swelling and distension—is only involved at more severe levels of oedema. Respiratory muscle fatigue is a possibility.

In acute, severe oedema the usual blood gas abnormalities are hypocapnia and hypoxia. The hypoxia is a result of ventilation/perfusion mismatching. The hypocapnia is accounted for by the reflex tachypnoea leading to increased alveolar ventilation, which more than compensates for the increased pulmonary deadspace (volume of deadspace/volume of tidal air ratios, V_D/V_T ratio). However, in about 20% of severe cases, hypercapnia (with respiratory acidosis) is seen, even when no chronic airflow disease coexists. A number of mechanisms have been proposed, including uncontrolled oxygen administration accompanied by low central CO_2 sensitivity, respiratory muscle fatigue, and severe ventilation/perfusion imbalance. In acute oedema, blood gas abnormalities are usually accompanied by a mild metabolic acidosis, but occasionally the base excess may exceed −15 mmol/litre. This frank metabolic acidosis is most likely in patients with severe oedema who already have carbon dioxide retention.

In the more chronic permeability oedemas—as in adult respiratory distress syndrome—the overwhelming problem is continuing severe hypoxaemia. Three mechanisms have been proposed: (1) diffusion impairment; (2) low ventilation/perfusion (V_A/Q) values; and (3) shunt (V_A/Q <0.005). Using both, the arterial oxygen response to changing fractional inspired oxygen concentration (Fio_2) and the inert-gas technique, it has been shown that diffusion impairment plays little part: shunt and ventilation/perfusion mismatch are more important, but their contribution varies greatly from patient to patient.

Treatment of pulmonary oedema

As described previously, pulmonary oedema may result from increased microvascular hydrostatic pressure, decreased tissue interstitial pressure, decreased plasma colloid oncotic pressure, increased microvascular permeability, or impaired lymphatic drainage. Treatment of each form should include measures designed to reverse the specific cause. However, with the exception of a reduction of elevated hydrostatic pressure and relief of upper airway obstruction, these are rarely available and the clinician has to rely upon general supportive measures combined with meticulous attention to fluid balance and monitoring of plasma oncotic pressure. (See Chapters 17.3 and 17.5 for discussion of the clinical approach to the severely ill and breathless patient.)

Acute cardiogenic and fluid overload pulmonary oedema

By far the most common causes are acute and chronic left-sided heart disease, although the overenthusiastic use of intravenous fluid regimens containing normal saline is frequently an additional factor. The patient is most comfortable in the 'trunk up, legs down' position to help pool blood in the dependent parts and reduce central venous pressure. Oxygen, diuretics, intravenous nitrates, and morphine are the fundamentals of treatment. Thigh cuffs inflated to occlude venous return can help as a form of a bloodless phlebotomy and venesection, and removal of 200 to 500 ml of blood is an effective treatment when other measures are not available.

Hypoxia is relieved with a standard face mask, nasal prongs, or reservoir bag, delivering oxygen at high flow rates—up to 10 litres/min—providing an inspired concentration of up to 60%. The fractional inspired oxygen concentration given should be as high as is necessary to keep the arterial partial pressure of oxygen near to the normal level—and no more—because, in permeability oedema: (1) high oxygen levels may lead to absorption atelectasis in areas of low ventilation/perfusion; (2) oxygen toxicity may become a problem where prolonged administration is necessary. If oxygen administration at normal airway pressure cannot maintain the arterial partial pressure of oxygen and/or hypercapnia develops, then application of a continuous positive airway pressure (CPAP) mask, non-invasive ventilation, or tracheal intubation and intermittent positive pressure ventilation will need to be considered (see Chapter 17.5).

A bolus dose of furosemide (frusemide) (or other loop diuretic), administered intravenously, is usually given. This acts both as a venous dilator and as a diuretic. Diuretics are at their most valuable where pulmonary oedema is a component of congestive cardiac failure and where the volume of extracellular fluid is generally increased. By contrast, when left ventricular failure has come on acutely, significant fluid retention has not occurred and pulmonary oedema is a result of fluid shift from the systemic circulation, then overvigorous use of diuretics runs the risk of causing hypovolaemia. It is wise to catheterize the bladder if the patient is *in extremis* or heavily sedated, for—as a result of the diuresis—bladder distension may induce intense reflex systemic vasoconstriction leading, on occasion, to disastrous cardiac overload.

Intravenous nitrates, in particular isosorbide dinitrate at a dose between 2 and 20 mg/h, can effectively reduce venous pressure and alleviate pulmonary oedema. Arterial hypotension is the effect that usually limits dosage, the combination of heart failure with low blood pressure and pulmonary oedema being difficult to treat and of grave prognosis.

Morphine acts centrally to relieve the distress of dyspnoea and also dilates the systemic venous system. This reduces venous filling pressure to the heart and shifts blood from the pulmonary to the systemic circulation. It is best administered by slow intravenous injection in a total dose of 2 to 10 mg at a rate of 2 mg/min, together with an appropriate antiemetic.

Aminophylline has diuretic, bronchodilator, cardiac inotropic, and respiratory muscle inotropic effects. Its use would seem logical, but it is now scarcely ever given because of its capacity to induce arrhythmias and the availability of other effective treatments. If it is to be administered, a dose of 250 to 500 mg should be given intravenously in not less than 20 min.

Other types of pulmonary oedema

A reduction in oncotic pressure may contribute to pulmonary oedema, as in crystalloid fluid overload, hepatic failure, or nephrotic syndrome. In fluid overload, the most appropriate therapy is the use of diuretics, for these not only reduce the extracellular and blood volumes but also return oncotic pressure towards normal. It is more difficult to be certain about therapy in true hypo-oncotic states: even where there is no evidence of endothelial damage, the effects of salt-free albumin and plasma concentrate are disappointing.

In high-permeability pulmonary oedema, the best form of management would be to block the inappropriate activation and progress of the cascades that are responsible for the condition (see Chapter 17.5). Unfortunately, there is no therapy that allows this at present and management, aside from aiming to treat any precipitating disorder, is supportive.

Further reading

Artigas A, et al. (1992). *The adult respiratory distress syndrome*. Churchill Livingstone, Edinburgh.

Flick MR, Matthay MA (2000). Pulmonary edema and acute lung injury. In: Murray JF et al. (eds) *Textbook of respiratory medicine*, 3rd edition, pp.1575–1630. W B Saunders, Philadelphia.

Gammage M. (1998). Commentary. Treatment of acute pulmonary oedema: diuresis or vasodilatation? *Lancet*, **351**, 382–3.

Guyton AO, Lindsey AW (1959). Effect of elevated left atrial pressure and decreased plasma protein concentration upon the development of pulmonary oedema. *Circ Res*, **7**, 649.

Kreiger BP, de la Hoz RE (1999). Altitude related pulmonary disorders. *Crit Care Clin*, **15**, 265–80.

Miserrochi G, Ngrini D (1997). Pleural space: pressures and fluid dynamics. In: Crystal RG et al. (eds) *The lung: scientific foundations*, 2nd edition, pp. 1217–25. Lippincott-Raven, Philadelphia.

Morgan PW, Goodman LR (1991). Imaging of diffuse lung diseases: pulmonary oedema and adult respiratory distress syndrome. *Radiol Clin N Amer*, **29**, 943–63.

Pang D, et al. (1998). The effects of positive pressure airway support on mortality and the need for intubation in cardiogenic pulmonary oedema: a systematic review. *Chest*, **114**, 1185–92.

Prichard JS (1982). *Edema of the lung*. Charles C. Thomas, Springfield, IL.

Sacchetti AD, Harris RH (1998). Acute cardiogenic pulmonary edema. What's the latest in emergency treatment? *Postgrad Med*, **103**, 145–7, 153–4, 160–2.

Schuster DP (1998). Pulmonary oedema. In: Fishman AP *et al.* (eds) *Fishman's pulmonary diseases and disorders*, 3rd edition, pp. 1331–56. McGraw-Hill, New York.

Simon RD (1993). Neurogenic pulmonary edema. *Neurol Clin*, **11**, 309–23.

Szidon PS (1989). Pathophysiology of the congested lung. *Cardiol Clin*, **7**, 39–48.

Taylor AE, *et al.* (1997). Fluid balance. In: Crystal RG *et al.* (eds) *The lung: scientific foundations*, 2nd edition, pp. 1549–66. Lippincott-Raven, Philadelphia.

Trimby J, *et al.* (1990). Mechanical causes of pulmonary oedema. *Chest*, **98**, 973–9.

West JB, Mathieu-Costello O (1995). Vulnerability of pulmonary capillaries in heart disease. *Circulation*, **95**, 622–31.

Wiedemann HP, Matthay MA (eds) (2000). Adult respiratory distress syndrome. *Clin Chest Med*, **21**, 401–620.

Venous thromboembolism

Contents

16.16.1 Deep venous thrombosis and pulmonary embolism

Paul D. Stein and John D. Firth

Essentials

Deep venous thrombosis

Deep venous thrombosis (DVT) is diagnosed in 1 to 2% of hospitalized patients, but is often silent and is found much more frequently at autopsy. Patients typically complain of pain and/or swelling of the leg, but often the diagnosis will be considered only when the physician detects unilateral leg swelling.

Investigation—given the sinister nature of untreated DVT, it is important to confirm or refute the diagnosis with appropriate investigations whenever clinical suspicion is aroused, unless the general condition of the patient makes this inappropriate. Management algorithms have been developed to guide strategy for investigation. These typically use scoring systems to stratify the clinical probability that the particular patient has a DVT (or pulmonary embolism). Those with a low clinical probability proceed to D-dimer testing, with further investigation not pursued if this is negative. Patients with either a high clinical probability, or a low clinical probability but elevated D-dimer, proceed to tests for the presence of thrombus in the leg veins, typically by ultrasonography.

Management—a first episode of symptomatic isolated calf venous thrombosis, diagnosed by noninvasive testing, should be treated with anticoagulation for 3 months. Longer duration of treatment may be recommended for those whose thrombosis occurred in the absence of a reversible risk factor or in those with a thrombophilic condition. Indefinite treatment is recommended for those with two or more episodes of thromboembolism. Treatment is initiated with heparin (low molecular weight or unfractionated) for ≥ 5 days and warfarin (or other vitamin K antagonist), with the heparin stopped when the international normalized ratio (INR) is greater than 2.0 or ≥ 24 h.

DVT carries extensive morbidity irrespective of pulmonary embolism: severe postphlebitic syndrome occurs in 9% of patients by 5 years.

Pulmonary embolism

Acute pulmonary embolism (PE) is the third most common cardiovascular problem after coronary heart disease and stroke. It is a complication of DVT, with emboli originating in the legs in 80% or more of cases. Immobilization, irrespective of the cause, is the most frequent predisposing factor.

Common symptoms are dyspnoea (c.75%), pleuritic chest pain (c.50%), cough (c.35%), and calf or thigh pain or swelling (c.40%). Circulatory collapse (systolic blood pressure <80 mmHg or loss of consciousness) is an uncommon (8–15%) mode of presentation in patients entered into clinical trials, but likely to be more frequent in routine clinical practice. Tachypnoea (respiratory rate ≥20 cycles/min or greater) is the most common physical sign (50–70%), and abnormalities may be found on respiratory (30–50%) or cardiac (20–30%) examination.

Investigation—algorithms similar to those used to guide management of patients with suspected DVT are used when PE is suspected or needs to be excluded. Patients with a low clinical probability and negative D-dimer are not investigated further. Patients with a moderate or high clinical probability, and patients with an elevated D-dimer, proceed to tests for the presence of pulmonary emboli, typically by contrast-enhanced spiral CT in combination (in many centres) with CT venous-phase imaging.

Management—treatment with anticoagulants while awaiting the outcome of diagnostic tests may be appropriate, particularly if the tests cannot be obtained immediately. All patients who are hypoxic should be given supplementary oxygen at high concentration.

Anticoagulation is as described for DVT. Thrombolytic therapy is not indicated for routine treatment, but is advised for those that are hypotensive or have continuing hypoxemia whilst receiving high-flow oxygen.

Inferior vena cava filter—this is recommended for patients with proximal DVT or PE if anticoagulants are contraindicated, PE has recurred whilst on adequate anticoagulant therapy, or PE is severe and any recurrent PE may be fatal.

A very few survivors of acute PE (0.1–0.2%) develop chronic pulmonary thromboembolic hypertension.

Introduction

Deep venous thombosis (DVT) and pulmonary embolism (PE) are sometimes described together using the term 'thromboembolism'. PE is a complication of DVT, with thrombi in 80% or more of cases originating in the legs. Management strategies have been developed that are based on the diagnosis of either PE or DVT, provided the patient has good respiratory reserve. Treatment with anticoagulants is the same for both, although some physicians believe that patients can be managed better if it is known whether acute PE is present, even if a diagnosis of DVT is already established.

Prognosis of untreated disease

The frequency of fatal PE in patients with untreated DVT has diminished as diagnostic tests have made it possible to diagnose DVT before it becomes extensive. In 1955, prior to the use of sensitive noninvasive tests for the early detection of DVT, the risk of fatal PE in untreated patients with clinically apparent DVT was 37%. Based on a diagnosis by radioactive fibrinogen scintiscans, the risk of fatal PE in patients with untreated DVT, most of which were subclinical, was about 5%.

Early diagnosis has also reduced the risk of death from PE. In the early 1960s the mortality in untreated patients with acute PE, diagnosed on the basis of clinical features, was 26 to 37%, and an additional 36% died of recurrent PE. In 1998, the estimated case fatality rate from acute PE was 7.7%. In recent years, among patients with mild PE who inadvertently escaped treatment, the mortality was 5%.

Deep venous thrombosis

Incidence and pathology

In 1999 DVT was diagnosed in 1.3% of hospitalized patients in the United States of America. The condition is often silent: among patients with DVT detected by screening with ^{125}I-fibrinogen scans, clinical evidence was present in 49%. Proximal DVT was found at autopsy in 22% of patients who died of various causes in a tertiary care hospital.

Thrombosis of the leg veins usually occurs without inflammation. Inflammation of the walls of the veins, when it occurs, is usually secondary to the thrombosis. No clear evidence indicates that inflammation of the veins prevents embolization, or that embolization is more frequent in those patients with thrombi not associated with venous inflammation. The valve pockets are a frequent site of origin of thrombi.

Clinical features

Patients may complain of pain or swelling of the leg, but physical examination remains the means by which attention is usually drawn to the potential diagnosis of DVT. DVT sometimes, but not always, leads to swelling of the leg. If restricted to the popliteal and calf veins, swelling is confined to below the knee, but if thrombosis involves the femoral and pelvic veins (or inferior vena cava), then swelling of the thigh is also expected. A difference of circumference of the calves of 1.0 cm or more, measured 10 cm below the tibial tuberosity, is abnormal. It is important to repeat the measurement of circumference of the calves and thighs at frequent intervals: proximal extension of a thrombus is likely to cause increased swelling, and to allow repeated measurements to be made from a fixed point it is good practice for the position of the first measurement to be marked indelibly on the patient's skin.

Homans' sign is positive when active and/or passive dorsiflexion of the foot associated with any of the following: (1) pain, (2) incomplete dorsiflexion (with equal pressure applied) to prevent pain, or (3) flexion of the knee to release tension in the posterior muscles with dorsiflexion. This sign was present in 44% of patients with DVT of the lower leg, and in 60% of patients with femoral venous thrombosis.

The elicitation of pain with inflation of a blood pressure cuff around the calf to 60 to 150 mm Hg has been recommended as a test for DVT. However, this test has not been shown to be more helpful than the assessment of direct tenderness or leg circumference.

In one study, the sensitivity of oedema, erythema, calf tenderness, palpable cord, or Homans' sign alone, or 1 cm or more calf asymmetry alone was 55 to 80%, but the specificity was only 49%. The combination of one of these signs plus 1 cm or more ipsilateral calf asymmetry increased the specificity to 87%, but decreased the sensitivity to 15 to 33%. The specificity increased to 91% with one of these signs in combination with 2 cm or more calf asymmetry. Only 3 to 10% of patients had one or more qualitative signs plus 3 cm or more ipsilateral calf asymmetry: in these the specificity for DVT was 96%.

Other clinical features of DVT, whose sensitivity and specificity have not been tested, include increased temperature on the affected side, cyanotic discoloration of the limb, and persistent engorgement of superficial veins. Superficial varicose veins almost always empty when the patient lies down: if they remain engorged, this suggests problems with drainage through the deep veins. In very rare cases, tense venous oedema can cause arterial compression and venous gangrene.

Differential diagnosis

The clinical diagnosis of DVT is not always straightforward. Many of the findings described above can also be found in those with muscular strains and bruising, ruptured Baker's cyst or plantaris tendon, superficial thrombophlebitis, cellulitis, and other traumatic conditions. The presence of bruising near either malleolus suggests ruptured Baker's cyst or other cause of calf haematoma.

Given the sinister nature of untreated DVT it is important to confirm or refute (so far as is possible) the diagnosis with appropriate investigations whenever clinical suspicion is aroused, unless the general condition of the patient makes this inappropriate.

Investigation

Detection of evidence of thrombus within the circulation: D-dimer

D-dimer is a specific degradation product released into the circulation by endogenous fibrinolysis of a cross-linked fibrin clot. A D-dimer measured by enzyme-linked immunosorbent assay (ELISA) below a cut-off of 300 to 540 ng/ml (the values differ slightly from one study to another) make the diagnosis of DVT (or PE) unlikely. However, a concentration of D-dimer above the cut-off level is not useful for making a positive diagnosis because of the large number of false positive tests.

Conventional ELISA assays are cumbersome and not suited for emergency use, which limited the practical utility of D-dimer measurements until the development of rapid ELISA assays. These provide the best balance of sensitivity and specificity among the various assays for the safe diagnostic handling of patients with suspected DVT and PE.

Detection of the physical presence of thrombus in leg veins

The 'gold standard' is contrast venography, but this can be unpleasant for patients, time consuming for radiology departments, and expensive. This has driven the search for acceptable noninvasive methods of diagnosis and contrast venography is now rarely performed, except as part of research protocols.

In most centres contrast venography has been replaced by B-mode ultrasonography as the preferred first line diagnostic technique. Among patients with DVT proven by contrast venography, B-mode ultrasonography using compression showed a 95% sensitivity in symptomatic patients. In asymptomatic patients who were evaluated because of a high risk of DVT, venous compression ultrasound showed a sensitivity of only 67%. Regarding veins of the calves, venous compression ultrasound was 93% sensitive in symptomatic patients, but only 26% sensitive in asymptomatic high-risk patients with DVT. In all instances, specificity was 97 to 99%.

Venous-phase contrast-enhanced spiral CT is useful for imaging the veins of the pelvis and thighs, particularly in combination with spiral CT pulmonary angiograms. This offers a comprehensive study for thromboembolism.

Gadolinium-enhanced magnetic resonance venography following an intravenous injection, was sensitive for DVT in the veins of the thighs and pelvis but often technically inadequate. Specificity in all regions was 95 to 100%. Usage is restricted by cost, availability and risk of nephrogenic systemic fibrosis/nephrogenic fibrosing dermopathy in patients with poor renal function.

Fibrinogen uptake radionuclide scanning was used extensively in the 1960s. It is more sensitive for DVT in the calves than in the thighs, meaning that its value is limited because of the greater risk of PE with the former rather than with the latter.

Strategy for diagnosis

Management algorithms have been developed to identify patients at low risk of DVT or PE who can be spared extensive testing. These algorithms typically use scoring systems to stratify the clinical probability that the particular patient has a DVT (or PE) and then proceed to D-dimer testing of those with low probability. Patients with a low clinical probability and a negative D-dimer test are not investigated further. Patients with either a high clinical probability, or a low clinical probability but elevated D-dimer, proceed to tests for the presence of thrombus in the leg veins, typically by ultrasonography. An example of a pretest scoring system and management algorithm is shown in Table 16.16.1.1.

Prevention

The prevention of DVT is critical in the prevention of PE. Risk factors for DVT are almost certainly the same as those for PE (see later section in this chapter). Recommendations for the prevention of DVT are shown in Tables 16.16.1.2–16.16.1.7.

Treatment

Proximal DVT leads to PE more frequently than DVT confined to the calf. Even so, symptomatic isolated calf venous thrombosis, diagnosed by noninvasive testing, should be treated with anticoagulation for 3 months. If anticoagulation cannot be given, serial noninvasive studies of the leg veins should be performed over the next 7 to 14 days to assess for proximal extension of the thrombus. Recommendations for treatment are shown in Table 16.16.1.8, with further details discussed in Chapter 16.16.2.

Complications

DVT itself carries extensive morbidity irrespective of PE. Severe postphlebitic syndrome (venous ulcer or combinations of pain, cramps, heaviness, pruritus, paresthesia, pretibial oedema, induration, hyperpigmentation, venous ectasia, redness or pain with calf compression) occurs in 9% of patients by 5 years after a 3-month course of treatment with anticoagulants. Randomized controlled trials have shown that elastic compression stockings applied directly after an episode of DVT can reduce the chances of the patient developing postphlebitic syndrome by about 70%, but there is no clear evidence on which to recommend how long such stockings should be worn after an acute episode.

Acute pulmonary embolism

Incidence

Acute PE is the third most common cardiovascular problem after coronary heart disease and stroke.

The population-based rate of PE in the United States of America in 1999 was 51/100 000. In hospitalized patients in the United States, from 1979 through 1999, 0.4% of adults had acute PE, with age-adjusted rates that were similar in men and women. Silent PE has been reported in 38 to 51% of patients with DVT. The incidence of acute PE increases exponentially with age and is much more frequent in adults than in children, but it is not rare in children.

In autopsy studies encompassing university as well as nonuniversity hospitals, when the pathologist judged that PE contributed to death or caused death, the diagnosis was unsuspected ante-mortem in over one-half of cases. Some of these were in patients who died of malignancy, in whom a diagnosis of PE may (appropriately) not have been actively pursued. However, the time-honoured point remains as valid today as ever: a high index of suspicion is necessary to reduce the number of patients with unsuspected PE.

Predisposing factors

Immobilization, irrespective of the cause, is the most frequent predisposing factor (Table 16.16.1.9). Immobilization of even 1 or 2 days may predispose to PE and most patients with PE are immobilized less than 2 weeks. Obesity is also a risk factor.

Table 16.16.1.1 Pre-test clinical probability scoring system and care pathway for the patient with suspected deep venous thrombosis

(a) Pre-test probability score

Criteria	Score
Active cancer	+1
Paralysis, plaster cast	+1
Bed rest >3 days, surgery within 4 weeks	+1
Tenderness along veins	+1
Entire leg swollen	+1
Calf swollen >3 cm	+1
Pitting oedema	+1
Collateral veins	+1
Alternative diagnosis likely	−2

(b) Pre-test probability

Low	0
Moderate	1 or 2
High	3 or more

(c) Management algorithm

Pre-test probability score	Action	Result	Further action
0 or 1	Perform D-dimer	Negative	No further investigation
		Positive	Perform ultrasonography
2 or more	Do not perform D-dimer		
	Perform ultrasonography	Negative	Withhold treatment and repeat ultrasonography in 10–14 days. If serial ultrasonography is negative, pulmonary embolism rarely occurs.
		Positive	Diagnosis of venous thrombosis established

Notes
1. Pre-test probability score from Wells *et al.* (1997).
2. This management algorithm is typical of many used, but further prospective evaluation is warranted.
3. If the physician's judgement is that deep venous thrombosis is very likely in a particular case, then they should proceed to investigations directed at detecting thrombus in leg veins whatever the scoring algorithm would suggest. If the result of ultrasonography is negative, and repeat ultrasonography in 10–14 days is also negative, pulmonary embolism rarely occurs.
4. All patients who are discharged with 'deep venous thrombosis excluded' should be given written information describing how they can be reassessed if symptoms worsen or fail to settle over the next few days.

Thromboembolic events have been linked to oestrogen-containing oral contraceptives, but the absolute risk is low and their frequency has been reduced with the use of preparations that contain less than 50 μg of oestrogen. Oral contraceptives may increase the risk of venous thromboembolism after surgery even if their oestrogen content is low.

Pregnancy-associated DVT has increased in recent years, the rate being over twice that in nonpregnant women. The rate of DVT following caesarean section is twice the rate following vaginal delivery. By contrast, higher rates of PE have not been shown in pregnancy, but this may be because of reluctance to perform imaging studies in pregnant women.

There has been much interest in the subject of genetic predisposition to thromboembolism. Heterozygosity for the factor V Leiden mutation increases susceptibility three- to eight-fold in a variety of circumstances. Other genetic and acquired thrombophilic factors include protein C deficiency, protein S deficiency, antithrombin deficiency, prothrombin 20 201A, high concentration of factor VIII, hyperhomocystinaemia, heparin cofactor II deficiency, dysfibrinogenaemia, decreased levels of plasminogen, decreased levels of plasminogen activators, antiphoslipid antibodies, heparin-induced thrombocytopenia, and myeloproliferative disorders. For full discussion of these and related issues, see Chapter 22.6.4.

Clinical features

The clinical characteristics of acute PE have been derived from prospectively acquired data of patients recruited in trials of diagnostic investigations or therapies such as the Prospective Investigation of PE Diagnosis (PIOPED) studies. Such trials clearly only include those in whom there was sufficient clinical suspicion to lead physicians to obtain diagnostic tests: whether subtle PE was overlooked is undetermined. The specificity of signs, symptoms, and ordinary clinical tests was low among patients with suspected PE in whom the diagnosis was eventually excluded.

Symptoms

In patients in whom the diagnosis is not confused by pre-existing cardiac or pulmonary disease, dyspnea is the most common

Table 16.16.1.2 Recommendations for prevention of deep venous thrombosis in patients undergoing general, vascular, gynecological, urological and laparoscopic surgery

Indication	Recommendation
General surgery	
Low risk patients (minor procedure, age <40 years, no additional risk factors)	Early and persistent mobilization
Moderate-risk (age 40–60 years with no additional risk factors, or major surgery and age <40 years with no additional risk factors).	Unfractionated heparin 5000 U twice daily or LMWH ≤3400 U once daily or fondaparinux
Higher-risk general surgery (nonmajor surgery and age >60 years or have additional risk factors, or major surgery and age >40 years or have additional risk factors)	Unfractionated heparin 5000 U three times daily or LMWH >3400 U daily or fondaparinux
High-risk general surgery (multiple risk factors).	Unfractionated heparin 5000 U three times daily or LMWH > 3400 U daily or fondaparinux combined with graduated compression stockings and/or intermittent pneumatic compression
High risk of bleeding	Properly fitted compression stockings or intermittent pneumatic compression
Selected high-risk general surgery patients, including major cancer surgery	Post-hospital discharge prophylaxis with LMWH uto 28 days
Vascular surgery	
If no additional risk factors	Early and persistent mobilization
If additional risk factors	Low dose unfractionated heparin or LMWH or fondaparinux
Gynecological surgery	
Brief procedures of ≤30 min for benign disease	Early and persistent mobilization
Laparoscopic procedures, additional risk factors present	Unfractionated heparin 5000 U twice daily or LMWH, or intermittent pneumatic compression, or graduated compression stockings or combinations
Major gynecological surgery for benign disease, without additional risk factors	Unfractionated heparin 5000 U twice daily or LMWH ≤3400 U daily until hospital discharge, or intermittent pneumatic compression started just before surgery and used continuously whilst the patient is not ambulating
Extensive surgery for malignancy, or patients with additional risk factors	Unfractionated heparin 5000 U three times daily or LMWH >3400 U/day or fondaparinux + graduated compression stockings or intermittent pneumatic compression. All continued until discharge from hospital. Alternatively intermittent pneumatic compression alone, continued until hospital discharge
Particularly high risk, including cancer surgery and age > 60 years or previous PE or DVT	Continue prophylaxis upto 28 days after hospital discharge
Urological surgery	
Transurethral or other low risk	Early and persistent mobilization
Major open procedures	Unfractionated heparin 5000 U twice or three times daily. Alternatives include intermittent pneumatic compression and/or graduated compression stockings LMWH fondaparinux or combination
Actively bleeding or very high risk for bleeding	Graduated compression stockings and/or intermittent pneumatic compression Start pharmacological prophylaxis when risk of bleeding decreases
Laparoscopic surgery	
No additional risk factors	Aggressive mobilization
Additional risk factors	Low dose unfractionated heparin or fondaparinux or LMWH, or intermittent pneumatic compression, or graduated compression stockings or combination

LMWH, low molecular weight heparin.
Adapted from Geerts, W.H. *et al.* (2004). Prevention of venous thromboembolism: the Seventh ACCP Conference on Antithrombotic and Thrombolytic Therapy. Chest 126(Suppl) 338S–400S. (http://chestjournal.chestpubs.org/content/126/3_suppl/338S.abstract).

symptom, occurring in 73% of cases both in PIOPED and PIOPED II (Table 16.16.1.10), with dyspnoea only on exertion in 16%. Dyspnoea (at rest or during exertion) and orthopnoea were more frequent in patients with PE in main or lobar pulmonary arteries than in patients in whom the largest vessel with PE was a segmental pulmonary artery. The onset of dyspnoea occurred within seconds or minutes in 72% of cases, and within seconds, minutes, or hours in 83%. In some, however, the onset of dyspnoea occurred over days.

Pleuritic chest pain (66% of patients with PE and no pre-existing cardiopulmonary disease in PIOPED and 44% in PIOPED II)

Table 16.16.1.3 Recommendations for prevention of DVT in patients undergoing orthopaedic surgery

Surgical procedure	Recommendation
Elective total hip replacement	LMWH (at a usual high-risk dose, started 12 h before surgery or 12–24 h after surgery, or 4–6 h after surgery at half the usual high-risk dose and then increasing to the usual high-risk dose the following day) for 10–35 days
	or Fondaparinux, (2.5 mg started 6–24 h after surgery) for 10–35 days
	or Vitamin K antagonist started preoperatively or on the evening after surgery (INR 2.0–3.0) for 10–35 days
Elective total knee arthroplasty	As with total hip replacement, although intermittent pneumatic compression is an alternative
Hip fracture surgery	Fondaparinux *or* LMWH at usual high-risk dose *or* vitamin K antagonist (INR 2.0–3.0) *or* low dose unfractionated heparin for 10–35 days
	If surgery is delayed—low dose unfractionated heparin or LMWH while waiting
	Mechanical prophylaxis if high risk of bleeding

INR, international normalized ratio; LMWH, low molecular weight heparin.
Adapted from Geerts, W.H. *et al.* (2004). Prevention of venous thromboembolism: the Seventh ACCP Conference on Antithrombotic and Thrombolytic Therapy. Chest 126(Suppl) 338S–400S. (http://chestjournal.chestpubs.org/content/126/3_suppl/338S. abstract).

Table 16.16.1.5 Recommendations for prevention of DVT in patients following trauma, acute spinal cord injury and burns

Indication	Recommendation
Trauma	LMWH. Continue after hospital discharge with LMWH or a vitamin K antagonist (INR 2.0 to 3.0) if major impaired mobility Intermittent pneumatic compression ±, graduated compression stockings if bleeding or a high risk for bleeding
Acute spinal cord injury	Intermittent pneumatic compression with low dose unfractionated heparin or LWMH Intermittent pneumatic compression and/or graduated compression stockings is recommended if anticoagulant prophylaxis is contraindicated During rehabilitation phase continue LMWH or convert to oral vitamin K antagonist (INR 2.0–3.0).
Burns if advanced age, morbid obesity, extensive or lower extremity burns, concomitant lower extremity trauma, use of a femoral venous catheter, and/or prolonged immobility	Low dose unfractionated heparin or LMWH Intermittent pneumatic compression ±, graduated compression stockings if high risk for bleeding

INR, international normalized ratio; LMWH, low molecular weight heparin.
Adapted from Geerts, W.H. *et al.* (2004). Prevention of venous thromboembolism: the Seventh ACCP Conference on Antithrombotic and Thrombolytic Therapy. Chest 126(Suppl) 338S–400S.

Table 16.16.1.4 Recommendations for prevention of DVT in patients undergoing neurosurgery

Surgical procedure	Recommendation
Elective spine surgery	
No additional risk factors Additional risk factors (advanced age, malignancy, neurological deficit, previous VTE, or an anterior surgical approach)	Early and persistent mobilization Low dose unfractionated heparin *or* LMWH *or* perioperative intermittent pneumatic compression *or* perioperative graduated compression stockings *or* perioperative intermittent pneumatic with compression stockings
Neurosurgery	
No additional risk factors	Intermittent pneumatic compression ± graduated compression Alternatively, low dose unfractionated heparin *or* postoperative LMWH
High risk	Graduated compression stockings *and/or* intermittent pneumatic compression) and low dose unfractionated heparin or LMWH

LMWH, low molecular weight heparin.
Adapted from Geerts, W.H. *et al.* (2004). Prevention of venous thromboembolism: the Seventh ACCP Conference on Antithrombotic and Thrombolytic Therapy. Chest 126(Suppl) 338S–400S. (http://chestjournal.chestpubs.org/content/126/3_suppl/338S.abstract).

Table 16.16.1.6 Recommendations for prevention of DVT in patients hospitalized with medical conditions and in critical units

Medical conditions in hospital	Recommendation
Heart failure or severe respiratory disease	Low dose unfractionated heparin, LMWH or fondaparinux
Patients confined to bed and have cancer, previous VTE, sepsis, acute neurological disease, or inflammatory bowel disease	Compression stockings *or* intermittent pneumatic compression if high risk of bleeding
Critical care	
Moderate risk (medically ill or postoperative)	Low dose unfractionated heparin or LMWH
Higher risk (major trauma or orthopaedic surgery)	LMWH
High risk of bleeding	Compression stockings and/or intermittent pneumatic compression

LMWH, low molecular weight heparin.
Adapted from Geerts, W.H. *et al.* (2004). Prevention of venous thromboembolism: the Seventh ACCP Conference on Antithrombotic and Thrombolytic Therapy. Chest 126(Suppl) 338S–400S. (http://chestjournal.chestpubs.org/content/126/3_suppl/338S.abstract).

Table 16.16.1.7 Recommendations for prevention of DVT during long-distance air travel

Long distance travel (flights of >8 h duration)	Avoid constrictive clothing around the lower extremities or waist; avoid dehydration; frequent calf muscle contraction
Additional risk factors	Below-knee graduated compression stockings providing 15–30 mmHg of pressure at ankle, or single dose of LMWH prior to departure

LMWH, low molecular weight heparin.
Adapted from Geerts, W.H. *et al.* (2004). Prevention of venous thromboembolism: the Seventh ACCP Conference on Antithrombotic and Thrombolytic Therapy. Chest 126(Suppl) 338S–400S. (http://chestjournal.chestpubs.org/content/126/3_suppl/338S.abstract).

occurred much more often than haemoptysis (13% in PIOPED and 5% in PIOPED II).

Cough was common (37% and 34% in PIOPED and PIOPED II) among patients with PE and no pre-existing cardiopulmonary disease. This was nonproductive or productive of bloody (typically blood-streaked, but it can be pure blood or blood-tinged) or purulent (5% of cases) sputum.

Signs

Tachypnoea (respiratory rate 20/min or greater) was the most common sign of acute PE among patients with no prior cardiac or pulmonary disease (70% of patients in PIOPED and 54% in PIOPED II) (Table 16.16.1.11). Tachycardia (heart rate greater than 100/min) occurred in 30% and 24% of patients with PE in PIOPED and PIOPED II, and the pulmonary component of the second sound was accentuated in 23% and 15% of cases. DVT was clinically apparent in 11% of patients with PE in PIOPED, but more frequently in PIOPED II (47%). A right ventricular lift, third heart sound, or pleural friction rub were uncommon, each occurring in 4% or less of patients with PE.

Most patients with PE who had rales (crepitations) had pulmonary parenchymal abnormalities, atelectasis, or a pleural effusion on the chest radiograph.

Among patients with PE and no other source of fever, temperature below 39.9°C was present in 12% and fever of 39.9°C or higher occurred in 2%. Fever in patients with pulmonary haemorrhage/infarction was not more frequent than among those with no pulmonary haemorrhage/infarction. Clinical evidence of DVT was often present in patients with PE and otherwise unexplained fever.

Table 16.16.1.8 Recommendations for treatment of DVT and/or pulmonary thromboembolism

Condition	Treatment
High clinical suspicion of DVT or PE	Give anticoagulants while awaiting outcome of diagnostic tests
Confirmed DVT or PE	LMWH or intravenous heparin (or subcutaneous unfractionated heparin with DVT or nonmassive PE) or fondaparinux for ≥5 days
	Intravenous unfractionated heparin–aPTT prolongation corresponding to plasma heparin levels 0.3–0.7 IU/ml anti-Xa activity by the amidolytic assay. If large doses fail to achieve therapeutic aPTT, measure anti-Xa level for dose guidance
	Subcutaneous unfractionated heparin–an initial dose of 17500 U twice daily SC, with subsequent dosing to maintain the aPTT in the therapeutic range
	LMWH - subcutaneously once or twice daily as an outpatient if possible for DVT. If severe renal failure, intravenous unfractionated heparin is preferred.
	Start vitamin K antagonists with LMWH or unfractionated heparin on first treatment day and discontinue heparin when INR is stable and >2.0 for 24 h
	Ambulate as tolerated
Nonmassive PE	LMWH preferred over unfractionated heparin
Massive PE, hemodynamically unstable	Systemic thrombolytic therapy, short infusion time preferred
Massive PE, highly compromised patients unable to receive thrombolytic therapy or whose critical status does not allow sufficient time to infuse thrombolytic therapy	Catheter extraction or fragmentation or pulmonary embolectomy
Extensive DVT	Catheter-directed thrombolysis: followed by balloon angioplasty and stents or systemic thrombolytic therapy. Thrombus fragmentation and/or aspiration if expertise and resources are available.
PE or DVT and contraindication to anticoagulants or recurrent thromboembolism despite adequate anticoagulation	Inferior vena cava filter
Condition	**Duration of treatment**
First episode DVT or PE, reversible risk factor	Vitamin K antagonist for 3 months
First episode, idiopathic DVT or PE	Vitamin K antagonist for 3 months; then consider indefinite treatment (INR 2.0–3.0)
DVT or PE and cancer	LMWH for 3-6 months followed by indefinite duration of anticoagulation or until cancer is resolved.
Two or more episodes DVT or PE	Indefinite treatment

aPTT =activated partial thromboplastin, LMWH, low molecular weight heparin.
Adapted from Geerts, W.H. *et al.* (2004). Prevention of venous thromboembolism: the Seventh ACCP Conference on Antithrombotic and Thrombolytic Therapy. Chest 126(Suppl) 338S–400S. (http://chestjournal.chestpubs.org/content/126/3_suppl/338S.abstract).

Table 16.16.1.9 Predisposing factors for PE in all patients irrespective of previous cardiac or pulmonary disease (n = 383)

Predisposing factor	Cases (%)
Immobilization	54
Surgery	42
Lung disease	27
Malignancy	18
Coronary heart disease	20
Thrombophlebitis—ever	19
Myocardial infarction	13
Trauma—lower extremities	12
Heart failure	12
Chronic obstructive pulmonary disease	10
Stroke	10
Asthma	7
Pneumonia—acute	7
Prior pulmonary embolism	6
Oestrogen	6
Collagen vascular disease	4
Postpartum—3 months or less	2
Interstitial lung disease	2

Unpublished data from PIOPED in Stein PD (In press). Pulmonary Embolism. Blackwell publishing, Oxford, UK.

Table 16.16.1.10 Symptoms of PE in patients without pre-existing cardiac or pulmonary disease

Symptoms	PE (%)	
	PIOPED I (n=117)	PIOPED II (n=127–133)
Dyspnea		
Dyspnea (rest or exertion)	73	73
Dyspnea (at rest)		55
Dyspnea (exertion only)		16
Orthopnea (≥2 pillow)		28
Pleuritic pain	66	44
Chest pain (not pleuritic)	4	19
Cough	37	34
Haemoptysis	13	5[a]
Purulent		5
Clear		5
Nonproductive		20
Wheezing	9	21
Palpitations	10	
Calf or thigh swelling		41
Calf swelling only	28	33
Calf and thigh swelling		7
Thigh swelling only		1
Calf or thigh pain		44
Calf pain only	26[b]	23
Calf and thigh pain		17
Thigh pain only		3

[a] Haemoptysis, patients with PE: 2, slightly pinkish; 4, blood-streaked; 1, all blood (<1 teaspoonful).
[b] 'Leg pain'.
Data from Stein PD, *et al.* (1991). Clinical, laboratory, roentgenographic and electrocardiographic findings in patients with acute pulmonary embolism and no pre-existing cardiac or pulmonary disease. *Chest*, **100**, 598–603 and Stein PD, *et al.* (2007). Clinical characteristics of patient with acute pulmonary embolism: data from PIOPED II. *Am J Med*, **120**, 871–9.

Circulatory collapse (systolic blood pressure <80 mmHg or loss of consciousness) was an uncommon mode of presentation: 15% in PIOPED and in 8% in PIOPED II. However, patients with circulatory collapse may not be candidates for recruitment into trials of diagnostic investigations or therapies, and patients with circulatory collapse often die within the first few hours, hence it may be that the incidence of circulatory collapse as determined from published series is falsely low. Patients with pulmonary infarction have less severe PE than patients with isolated dyspnoea, and those with circulatory collapse probably have the most severe of all.

Combinations of symptoms and signs

Dyspnoea or tachypnoea (respiratory rate 20/min or greater) was present in 90% and 84% of patients with acute PE and no pre-existing cardiac or pulmonary disease in PIOPED and PIOPED II. Dyspnoea or tachypnoea or pleuritic pain was present in 97% and 92% respectively. Dyspnea or tachypnea or pleuritic pain or radiographic evidence of atelectasis or a parenchymal abnormality was present in 98%. The remaining patients usually had either DVT or an unexplained low Pao_2. PE was rarely diagnosed in the absence of dyspnoea or tachypnoea or pleuritic pain.

Dyspnea or tachypnea occurred in 92% of all patients with PE (irrespective of pre-existing cardiopulmonary disease) in whom the pulmonary emboli were in main or lobar pulmonary arteries, but in only 65% of patients in whom the largest PE was in segmental pulmonary arteries. Dyspnoea or tachypnoea or pleuritic pain occurred in 97% of patients with proximal PE and 77% of patients with pulmonary emboli in only segmental pulmonary arteries.

Accuracy of clinical assessment

To emphasize the point that the diagnosis of PE is difficult to make, senior staff physicians and postgraduate fellows taking part in the PIOPED study were uncertain of the diagnosis in most patients. Using individual judgement without any specific predetermined criteria, senior staff were correct in the diagnosis in 88% of cases when their clinical assessment indicated a high probability of PE. When their clinical assessment indicated a low probability of PE, senior staff correctly excluded PE in 86%. Postgraduate fellows, on the basis of clinical assessment, were more accurate in excluding PE than they were in making the diagnosis. Objective scoring systems for the probability of acute PE give probability assessments similar to those of experienced physicians and do not require experience or clinical judgement. An example of an objective scoring system is shown in Table 16.16.1.12.

Table 16.16.1.11 Signs of PE in patients without pre-existing cardiac or pulmonary disease

Signs	PE (%)	
	PIOPED I **(n=117)**	**PIOPED II** **(n=127–133)**
General		
Tachypnea (≥20/min)	70	54
Tachycardia (>100/min)	30	24
Diaphoresis	11	2
Cyanosis	1	0
Temperature >38.5°C (>101.3°F)	7	1
Cardiac examination (any)		21
Increased P2	23	15
Third heart sound	3	
Fourth heart sound	24	
Right ventricular lift	4	4
Jugular venous distension		14
Lung examination (any abnormality)		29
Rales (crackles)	51	18
Wheezes	5	2
Rhonchi		2
Decreased breath sounds		17
Pleural friction rub	3	0
DVT		
Calf or thigh	11	47[a]
Calf only		32
Calf and thigh		14
Thigh only		2
Homans' sign	4	

P2, pulmonary component of second sound.

[a] Number of patients with PE who had one or more signs of DVT: oedema, 55; erythema, 5; tenderness, 32; palpable cord, 2.

Data from Stein PD *et al*, (1991). Clinical, laboratory, roentgenographic and electrocardiographic findings in patients with acute pulmonary embolism and no pre-existing cardiac or pulmonary disease. *Chest* **100**, 598–603 and Stein PD, *et al.* (2007). Clinical characteristics of patient with acute pulmonary embolism: data from PIOPED II. *Am J Med*, **120**, 871–9.

Differential diagnosis

The commonest presentation of acute PE is with dyspnoea and/or pleuritic chest pain. There are several other possible causes of these symptoms, the commonest being musculoskeletal pain and pneumonia. Musculoskeletal chest pain can be very similar to that caused by pleurisy, and splinting of the chest can lead to a perception of breathlessness that may be exacerbated by anxiety. If there is an obvious history of local trauma to the chest, then the patient will rarely present to the physician, but it is worthwhile to ask specifically whether there has been any trauma or unaccustomed physical activity, whether the pain can be brought on by particular movements, and to examine carefully for local tenderness of the ribs, muscles, or costal margins. Tenderness can sometimes be

Table 16.16.1.12 A model to determine the clinical probability of PE according to Wells and associates

Clinical feature	Score (points)
Clinical signs and symptoms of DVT (objectively measured leg swelling and pain with palpation in the deep vein system)	3.0
Heart rate > 100/min.	1.5
Immobilization ≥3 consecutive days (bed rest except to access bathroom) or surgery in previous 4 weeks	1.5
Previous objectively diagnosed PE or DVT	1.5
Haemoptysis	1.0
Malignancy (cancer patients receiving treatment within 6 months or receiving palliative treatment)	1.0
PE as likely or more likely than alternative diagnosis (based on history, physical examination, chest radiograph, ECG, and blood tests)	3.0

Score: <2.0, low probability; 2.0–6.0, moderate probability; >6.0, high probability.
Data from Wells PS, *et al.* (2001). Excluding PE at the bedside without diagnostic imaging: management of patients with suspected PE presenting to the emergency department by using a simple clinical model and D-dimer. *Ann Intern Med*, **135**, 98–107.

found in cases of pleurisy, but with appropriate history clearly supports a diagnosis of musculoskeletal pain.

Pneumonia complicated by pleurisy can cause dyspnoea and chest pain. Important features to look for in the history include preceding systemic upset ('flu-like' symptoms), high fever, and rigors, and on examination, high fever, 'toxic appearance', and chest signs of pneumonic consolidation. If a positive diagnosis of another cause of dyspnoea and/or pleuritic chest pain cannot be made, then the default position should be to assume that the patient has PE until proven otherwise.

Investigation

Detection of evidence of thrombus within the circulation: D-dimer

As when considering the diagnosis of DVT, a 'negative' D-dimer test is useful for excluding PE in patients who are clinically thought to be at low risk, but a 'positive' result does not establish the diagnosis. Hence, when used in the appropriate clinical context, D-dimer testing is useful in defining a group of patients with suspected PE who do not require further investigation.

In ranking the D-dimer assays according to their sensitivity values and likelihood of increasing certainty for ruling out PE, the enzyme-linked immunosorbent assay (ELISA) and quantitative rapid ELISA assays are significantly superior to the semiquantitative latex and whole blood agglutination assays. The quantitative rapid ELISA assay is more convenient than the conventional ELISA and provides a high level of certainty for a negative diagnosis of PE as well as DVT.

Detection of the physical presence of thrombus in the pulmonary circulation

Ventilation–perfusion lung scans

By 2001 in the United States of America the use of CT pulmonary angiography surpassed the use of ventilation–perfusion lung scans for the diagnosis of acute PE. Even so, radiation exposure from ventilation–perfusion lung scans is much lower than with CT

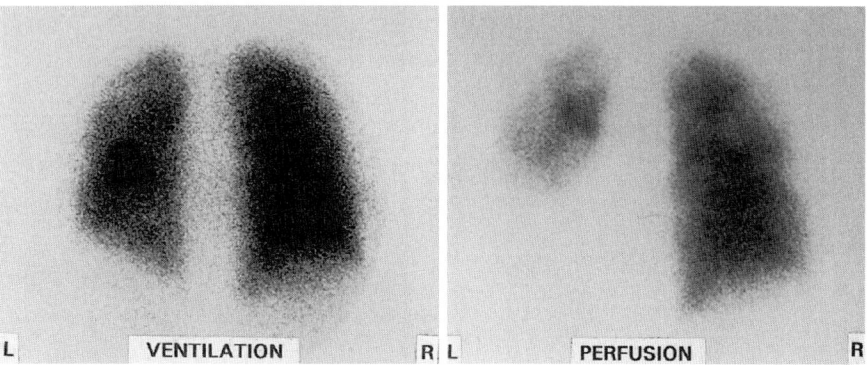

Fig. 16.16.1.1 Ventilation lung scan (left panel) and perfusion lung scan (right panel): posterior views with left (L) and right (R) indicated. The ventilation scan, equilibrium phase, shows nearly normal ventilation. The perfusion scan shows absent perfusion in the left lower lobe and mismatched perfusion defects in the left upper lobe. Perfusion defects (grey areas) are also shown in the right lung. This ventilation–perfusion lung scan was interpreted as showing high probability for PE.

pulmonary angiography, and some suggest that a ventilation–perfusion lung scan is the imaging test of choice in pregnant women and women of reproductive age.

A high probability lung ventilation–perfusion scan (Fig. 16.16.1.1) indicates PE in 87% of patients (Table 16.16.1.13) and a normal scan excludes PE. In the absence of any other information an intermediate probability scan indicates a 30% chance of PE and a low probability scan 14%. A low probability ventilation–perfusion scan by the criteria used in PIOPED does not therefore exclude PE. Intermediate and low probability interpretations may be grouped as 'nondiagnostic', which was frequently the case in PIOPED. However, since PIOPED, some have shown that in patients with suspected acute PE and a normal chest radiograph the perfusion lung scan was diagnostic (high probability, normal or very low probability) in 79% of patients. Also, since PIOPED, criteria for the interpretation of very low probability lung scans (positive predictive value <10%) have been developed and tested.

Prior clinical assessment in combination with interpretation of the ventilation–perfusion scan improves diagnostic validity (Table 16.16.1.13). If the ventilation–perfusion scan is interpreted as high probability for PE, and if the clinical impression is concordantly high, then the positive predictive value for PE is 96%. If the ventilation–perfusion scan is low probability and the clinical suspicion is concordantly low, then PE is excluded in 96% of patients.

The probability of PE can be determined based on the number of mismatched defects. A further refinement of probability can be made if the ventilation–perfusion scan is interpreted after being stratified according to prior cardiopulmonary disease. Fewer mismatched perfusion defects are required to diagnose PE among patients with no prior cardiopulmonary disease. Adding clinical assessment to the stratification results in a more accurate evaluation.

Although not routine practice in most centres, it can be useful to obtain a posttherapy baseline ventilation–perfusion lung scan for use in the event of suspected recurrent PE. This will assist in determining if abnormalities subsequently discovered on a ventilation–perfusion scan are new or residual. A residual abnormality of perfusion 1 year after PE is more frequent among patients with prior cardiopulmonary disease than among patients with none.

Pulmonary angiography
Pulmonary angiography is useful and remains the diagnostic gold standard for PE (Fig. 16.16.1.2). However, it is associated with serious complications in about 1% of patients and has been generally replaced by contrast-enhanced CT.

Contrast-enhanced spiral computed tomography
The sensitivity of single-slice CT angiography for the diagnosis of acute PE, based on pooled data, was 73%. Those with 3 mm collimation showed a sensitivity of 78% and specificity was 90%. Data with single-slice CT using 5 mm collimation showed a sensitivity of 68% and specificity of 83%.

The sensitivity of multidetector CT angiography alone and in combination with CT venous-phase venography were investigated in PIOPED II. The CT angiogram among 824 patients was of insufficient quality for a conclusive interpretation in 6.2%. Among 773

Table 16.16.1.13 The probability of PE using clinical assessment in combination with ventilation–perfusion lung scans

Clinical science probability (%)	80–100		20–79		0–19		All probabilities	
Scan category	PE+/No of patients[a]	%	PE+/No of patients	%	PE+/No of patients	%	PE+/No of patients	%
High probability	28/29	96	70/80	88	5/9	56	103/118	87
Intermediate probability	27/41	66	66/236	28	11/68	16	104/345	30
Low probability	6/15	40	30/191	16	4/90	4	40/296	14
Near normal/normal	0/5	0	4/62	6	1/61	2	5/128	4
Total	61/90	68	170/569	30	21/228	9	252/887	28

[a] PE+ indicates angiogram reading that shows PE or determination of PE by the outcome classification committee on review. PE status is based on angiogram interpretation for 713 patients, on angiogram interpretation and outcome classification committee reassignment for 4 patients, and on clinical information alone (without definitive angiography) for 170 patients.

Reproduced from A National Investigation by the PIOPED Investigators (1990). Value of the ventilation/perfusion scan in acute pulmonary embolism - results of the prospective investigation of pulmonary embolism diagnosis (PIOPED). Copyright 1990 American Medical Association.

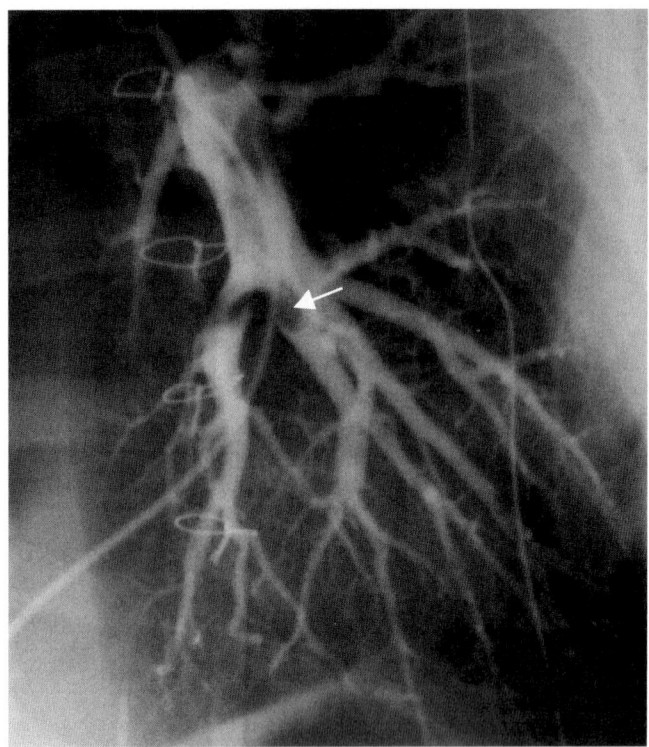

Fig. 16.16.1.2 Selective digital subtraction pulmonary angiogram of the left pulmonary artery showing multiple intraluminal filling defects indicative of pulmonary thromboemboli. One of these has been identified with an arrow.

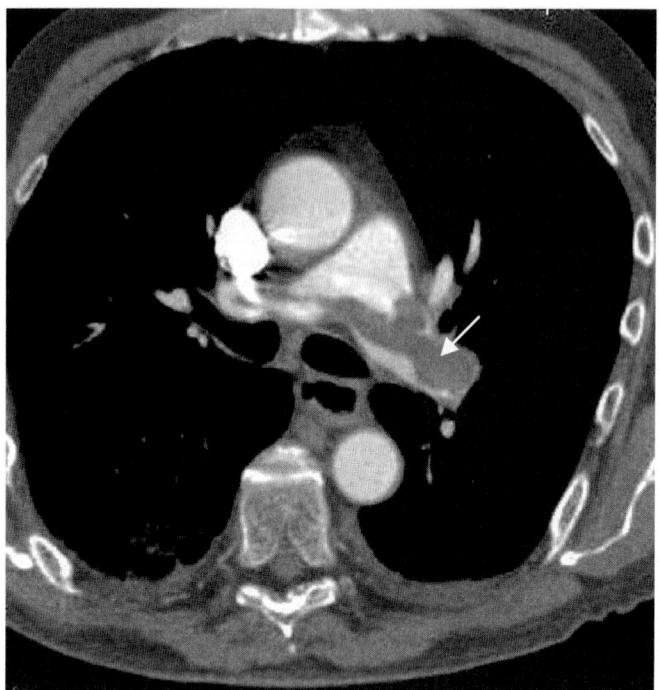

Fig. 16.16.1.3 Contrast-enhanced spiral CT showing a large intraluminal filling defect (arrow).

patients with an adequate CT angiogram, the sensitivity of CT angiography was 83% and specificity was 96% (Fig. 16.16.1.3): positive predictive value was 86% and negative predictive value was 95%. Positive predictive values were 97% for PE in a main or lobar artery, 68% in those in whom the largest vessel with PE was a segmental pulmonary artery, and 25% among only a few patients in whom the largest PE was in a subsegmental branch.

The combination CT angiogram with venous-phase imaging of the pelvic and thigh veins (CT venogram) among 824 patients was of insufficient quality for a conclusive interpretation in 11%. Among the 737 patients with an adequate CT angiogram/CT venogram combination, the sensitivity was 90% and specificity was 95%, with positive predictive value 85% and negative predictive value 97%.

As with ventilation–perfusion scans, better prediction can be made if imaging results are interpreted in the light of clinical information (Table 16.16.1.14). Among patients with a high or intermediate probability prior clinical assessment based on the Wells score, a positive CT angiogram had a positive predictive value for PE of 96% and 92% respectively. In patients with a low or intermediate probability prior clinical assessment and a negative CT angiogram, the negative predictive values for exclusion of PE were 96% and 89% respectively. Positive and negative predictive values were considerably reduced when scan results were discordant with clinical probabilities.

MRI

Preliminary observations suggest that gadolinium-enhanced magnetic resonance (MR) angiography during a single breath hold shows promise as a useful imaging technique (Fig. 16.16.1.4). Among the potential advantages are that it does not involve the use

of iodinated contrast agents, it is minimally invasive, and patients are not exposed to ionizing radiation. In small studies it shows a sensitivity for PE in proximal or segmental branches that ranges from 77% to 100% and specificity that ranges from 95 to 98%. Gadolinium-enhanced venous-phase imaging of the veins of the pelvis and thighs in combination with imaging of the pulmonary arteries would permit a comprehensive study for thromboembolism comparable to the combination of contrast-enhanced spiral CT of the pulmonary arteries in combination with venous-phase CT

Table 16.16.1.14 Positive and negative predictive values of CT pulmonary angiography in relation to prior clinical assessment

	High clinical probability (Wells score >6) n/N (%)	Intermediate clinical Probability (Wells score 2–6) n/N (%)	Low clinical probability[a] (Wells score <2) n/N (%)
CTA positive (positive predictive value)	22/23 (96)	93/101 (92)	22/38 (58)
CTA or CTV positive (positive predictive value)	27/28 (96)	100/111 (90)	24/42 (57)
CTA negative (negative predictive value)	9/15 (60)	121/136 (89)	158/164 (96)[a]
CTA and CTV negative (Negative Predictive Value)	9/11 (82)	114/124 (92)	146/151 (97)[a]

[a] To avoid bias for calculation of the negative predictive value in patients with a low probability prior clinical assessment, only patients with a reference test diagnosis by V/Q scan or conventional pulmonary digital subtraction angiography were included.
CTA, computed tomographic pulmonary angiography; CTV = computed tomographic venous-phase imaging.
Modified from Stein PD *et al.* (2006). PK for the PIOPED II Investigators. Multidetector computed tomography for acute pulmonary embolism. N Eng J Med 354:2317–2327. With permission.

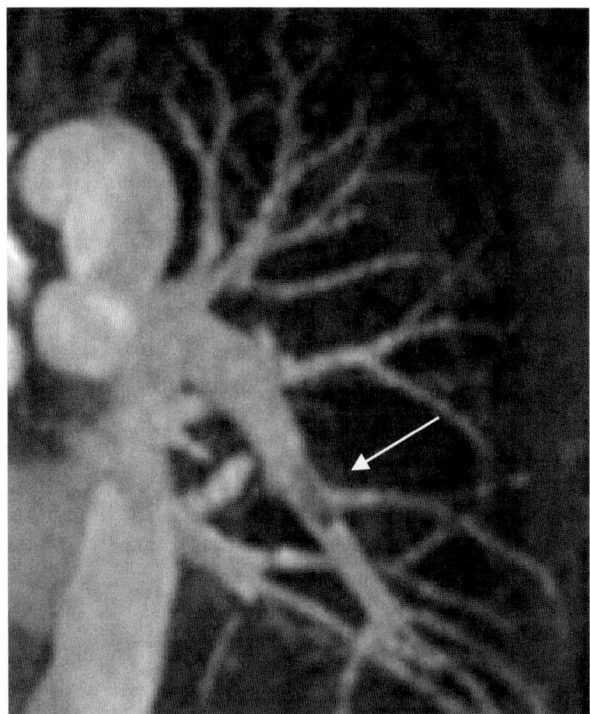

Fig. 16.16.1.4 Contrast-enhanced MRA using a single bolus of an iron-based contrast agent (Clariscan) showing PE (arrow).
Courtesy of Pamela K. Woodard, MD, Department of Radiology, Mallinckrodt Institute of Radiology, Washington University, St. Louis, Missouri. Reproduced from Stein PD (In press). Pulmonary Embolism. Blackwell publishing, Oxford, UK.

Table 16.16.1.15 Electrocardiographic manifestations of pulmonary embolisms in patients without prior cardiac or pulmonary disease (n=89)

Patients with electrocardiographic findings[a]	(%)
Rhythm disturbances	
Atrial flutter	1
Atrial fibrillation	4
Atrial premature contractions	4
Ventricular premature contractions	4
P wave	
P pulmonale	2
QRS abnormalities	
Right axis deviation	2
Left axis deviation	13
Incomplete right bundle branch block	4
Complete right bundle branch block	6
Right ventricular hypertrophy	2
Pseudoinfarction	3
Low voltage (frontal plane)	3
ST segment and T wave	
Nonspecific ST segment or T wave abnormalities	49

[a] Some patients had more than one abnormality.
Data from Stein PD, *et al.* (1991). Clinical, laboratory, roentgenographic and electrocardiographic findings in patients with acute pulmonary embolism and no pre-existing cardiac or pulmonary disease. *Chest*, **100**, 598–603.

of the veins of the lower extremities. There are difficulties, however, in obtaining technically adequate images, both in pulmonary arteries and veins of the thighs.

Nephrogenic systemic fibrosis (also known as nephrogenic fibrosing dermopathy) has been reported in patients with moderate or severe renal failure and in patients on dialysis following MR angiography with gadolinium-containing contrast agents. Other diagnostic approaches are recommended in such patients.

Other tests

Electrocardiography

Electrocardiographic abnormalities are common in acute PE (Table 16.16.1.15), with a normal electrocardiogram found in only 30% of patients. Acute ventricular dilatation is speculated to be the most likely cause of the electrocardiographic changes. Abnormalities of the ST segment and T wave are by far the most frequent observation, with nonspecific ST segment or T wave changes seen in about 50% of patients in whom the severity of PE ranged from mild to severe. Atrial flutter or atrial fibrillation in patients with acute PE is nearly always limited to individuals with prior heart disease.

Electrocardiographic manifestations of acute cor pulmonale ($S_1Q_3T_3$, complete right bundle branch block, P pulmonale, or right axis deviation) are less common than ST segment or T wave changes. One or more of these abnormalities occurred in 26% of patients with submassive or massive acute PE not associated with cardiac or pulmonary disease (32% of patients with massive PE). Left axis deviation occurs more frequently than right axis deviation.

The electrocardiogram may simulate an inferior infarction with Q waves and T wave inversion in leads II, III, and aVF, or anteroseptal infarction characterized by QS or QR waves in V1 and T-wave inversion in the right precordial leads. The development of Q waves and extensive T wave inversion in the anterior and lateral leads has also been observed. However, a pseudoinfarction pattern is seen in only 3% of patients.

Inversion of the T waves is the most persistent electrocardiographic abnormality, disappearing in only 22% of patients 5 or 6 days after the PE was diagnosed, although resolving in 49% by 2 weeks. Depression of the ST segment tends to resolve somewhat faster, and abnormalities of depolarization resolve more quickly than abnormalities of repolarization. Well over half of the electrocardiograms that showed pseudoinfarction, S1S2S3, S1Q3T3, right ventricular hypertrophy or right bundle branch block no longer show these abnormalities 5 or 6 days after the diagnosis is made.

Patients with ST segment abnormalities, T wave inversion, pseudoinfarction patterns, S1Q3T3 patterns, incomplete right bundle branch block, right axis deviation, right ventricular hypertrophy, or ventricular premature beats have larger perfusion defects on the lung scan or larger defects on the pulmonary arteriogram than those with normal electrocardiograms. Such patients have higher pulmonary arterial pressures and in general have a low partial pressure of oxygen in arterial blood.

Chest radiography

The findings on the plain chest radiograph—when used together with the history, physical examination, electrocardiogram and simple laboratory tests—assist in identifying PE. The chest radiograph, when normal in a patient who is dyspneic, hints that PE is a diagnostic possibility. Among patients with no prior cardiopulmonary disease a normal chest radiograph is found in 16% (Table 16.16.1.16). Atelectasis or a pulmonary parenchymal abnormality are the most frequent abnormalities present (68%). Pleural effusions are found in about half of cases and are usually small, with most limited to blunting of the costophrenic angle. In some studies, an elevated hemidiaphragm is the most frequent abnormality. Westermark's sign (a prominent central pulmonary artery and decreased pulmonary vascularity) is identified by radiologists in only 7% of patients with PE.

In cases of PE, those with a normal plain chest radiograph have the lowest pulmonary artery mean pressures. The highest pulmonary artery mean pressures are in patients with a prominent central pulmonary artery or cardiomegaly.

Echocardiography

Echocardiography may show right ventricular dilatation and evidence of pulmonary hypertension, which—in the proper clinical setting—may strengthen the clinical impression that PE has occurred. Transesophageal echocardiography sometimes may show proximal pulmonary emboli, but it has limited value in this regard.

Arterial blood gases and alveolar–arterial oxygen difference

A low partial pressure of oxygen in arterial blood (Pao_2) is typical of acute PE and supports the diagnosis, but patients with acute PE can have a normal Pao_2. Among patients with acute PE and no prior cardiopulmonary disease who have measurements of the Pao_2 while breathing room air, 24% have a Pao_2 of 80 mmHg (10.5 kPa) or higher, and even among patients with submassive or massive acute PE, 12% have a Pao_2 of this level or higher. A normal alveolar–arterial oxygen difference (alveolar–arterial oxygen gradient) does not exclude acute PE. No value of the alveolar–arterial oxygen difference is diagnostic of PE, and no value can exclude the diagnosis.

Other routine blood tests

Among patients in whom a possible or definite cause for leucocytosis is eliminated, 80% of patients with PE have a normal white blood cell count, 6% a count of 10.1–11.9 × 10⁹/litre, and 13% a count of higher than this. A white blood cell count of 20 x 10⁹/litre or greater is rarely if ever seen. Leucocytosis is not more frequent in patients with the pulmonary haemorrhage/infarction syndrome than in other patients with acute PE.

Table 16.16.1.16 Chest radiograph findings in pulmonary embolism in patients with no previous cardiac or pulmonary disease (n =117)

Patients with radiographic finding	(%)
Atelectasis or pulmonary parenchymal abnormality	68
Pleural effusion	48
Pleural based opacity	3
Elevated diaphragm hemidiaphragm	24
Decreased pulmonary vascularity	21
Prominent central pulmonary artery	15
Cardiomegaly	12
Westermark's sign[a]	7

[a] Prominent central pulmonary artery and decreased pulmonary vascularity.
Data are modified from Stein PD *et al*, (1991). Clinical, laboratory, roentgenographic and electrocardiographic findings in patients with acute pulmonary embolism and no pre-existing cardiac or pulmonary disease. Chest 100, 598–603. with permission.

Strategy for diagnosis

With increasing severity of PE, from pulmonary infarction to isolated dyspnoea to circulatory collapse, trends suggest that the prevalence of signs and symptoms increases, but generally recognized symptoms may be absent, even in patients with large pulmonary emboli. Clues that can assist the physician in assessing the possibility of PE, and avoiding inadvertent exclusion of the diagnosis are as follows:

- Dyspnoea—onset is usually, but not always, within minutes or hours, and may be present only on exertion. Frequent in patients with large pulmonary emboli, but often absent in those with small pulmonary emboli

- Orthopnea—often present in dyspnoeic patients with PE

- Circulatory collapse—may occur with PE in patients who do not have dyspnoea or tachypnoea or pleuritic pain

- Tachypnoea—frequent in patients with large pulmonary emboli, but often absent in those with small pulmonary emboli

- Crepitations (rales)—common among patients with pulmonary infarction, but less so in those with isolated dyspnoea or circulatory collapse; they occur in those with radiographic evidence of a parenchymal abnormality

- Electrocardiogram—a normal ECG is frequent in patients with the pulmonary infarction syndrome, but uncommon in those with isolated dyspnoea; nonspecific ST segment and T wave changes are the most frequent abnormality

- Chest radiograph—abnormalities are more common among patients with pulmonary infarction but are often observed in those with isolated dyspnoea; patients with circulatory collapse may have a normal chest radiograph

- Ventilation–perfusion scan—a high probability interpretation occurs in a minority of patients with the pulmonary infarction syndrome but in the majority of those with the isolated dyspnea syndrome; a low probability scan may occur in patients with PE and circulatory collapse

- Oxygenation—a Pao_2 higher than 80 mmHg (10.5 kPa) is not uncommon in patients with the pulmonary infarction syndrome, but such levels are uncommon in those with the isolated dyspnoea syndrome

Subjecting all patients who might have a pulmonary embolus to complex, expensive and/or invasive tests is best avoided. Management algorithms have been developed to identify those at very low risk, who can then be spared imaging tests. These algorithms typically use scoring systems to stratify the clinical probability that the particular patient has a pulmonary embolus, proceeding to D-dimer testing of those with low or intermediate probability. Patients with a low clinical probability and negative D-dimer (or low or intermediate clinical probability and negative D-dimer by rapid ELISA) are not investigated further. Patients with a high clinical probability and patients with an elevated D-dimer proceed to tests for the presence of pulmonary emboli, typically by contrast-enhanced spiral CT in combination with CT venous-phase imaging. Recommendations for the approach to the diagnosis of acute PE based on use of a pretest scoring system (Table 16.16.1.12) and D-dimer followed by imaging are as follows.

Patients with low probability clinical assessment

A D-dimer test should be performed, with no further testing if the D-dimer is normal. If the D-dimer is elevated, CT angiography in combination with CT venography (restricted to the femoral and popliteal veins to reduce radiation exposure) is recommended for most patients. If CT angiography or CT angiography in combination with CT venography is negative, then treatment is unnecessary. With main or lobar pulmonary emboli on CT angiography, treatment is indicated; with segmental or subsegmental pulmonary emboli the certainty of the CT diagnosis should be reassessed, and CT angiography or CT angiography/CT venography should be repeated if image quality is poor.

In patients with segmental or subsegmental pulmonary emboli, pulmonary scintigraphy, a single venous ultrasound examination in those evaluated by CT angiography only, serial venous ultrasound examinations, or pulmonary digital subtraction angiography are optional.

Patients with a moderate probability clinical assessment

A D-dimer test using the rapid ELISA method should be performed: no further testing is necessary if this is negative, but a venous ultrasound examination or MR venography is optional. If the D-dimer is positive, or if the rapid ELISA test is not available, then CT angiography in combination with CT venography is recommended for most patients.

Treatment with anticoagulants while awaiting the outcome of diagnostic tests may be appropriate, particularly if the tests cannot be obtained immediately.

No treatment is necessary if CT angiography or the combination of CT angiography with CT venography is negative, but venous ultrasonography is recommended for those with a negative CT angiogram alone. Treatment is clearly to be recommended if CT angiography in main or lobar pulmonary arteries or CT venography are positive. With segmental or subsegmental pulmonary emboli the certainty of the CT diagnosis should be reassessed and options followed according to recommendations for patients with a low probability clinical assessment.

Patients with a high probability clinical assessment

D-dimer testing should not be done because a negative D-dimer in a patient with a high probability clinical assessment does not exclude PE. The patient should be treated with anticoagulants while awaiting the outcome of diagnostic tests. CT angiography in combination with CT venography is recommended for most patients. If CT angiography is negative and CT angiography in combination with CT venography was not done or was technically inadequate, then a venous ultrasound examination is recommended. If CT angiography or CT angiography with CT venography is negative, other options include serial venous ultrasound examinations, pulmonary digital subtraction angiography, and pulmonary scintigraphy. Treatment is clearly to be recommended if CT angiography or CT venography are positive.

Other considerations

A venous ultrasound examination prior to imaging with CT angiography or CT angiography in combination with CT venography or prior to imaging with a ventilation–perfusion lung scan is optional and may guide treatment if positive. However, about 50% of patients with PE have negative noninvasive leg tests for DVT, even though DVT is the source of the PE.

Allergy to iodinated contrast material

D-dimer testing in conjunction with clinical assessment is recommended to exclude PE. Patients with mild iodine allergies may be treated with steroids prior to CT imaging, with venous ultrasonography and pulmonary scintigraphy recommended as alternative diagnostic tests in patients with severe iodine allergy. Serial venous ultrasonography is an option.

Patients with impaired renal function

Patients with mildly impaired renal function (eGFR 30–60 ml/min, CKD stage 3) can usually be managed with standard protocols described above. For patients with more severe renal impairment there is concern that the contrast load required for CT angiography/venography can be deleterious to renal function, and gadolinium-enhanced MRI carries the risk of nephrogenic sclerosing fibrosis. As with any investigation a cost–benefit analysis needs to be made by the physician responsible for the individual patient. In the usual manner D-dimer testing in conjunction with clinical assessment is recommended to exclude PE, followed—if CT with contrast is to be avoided—by venous ultrasonography. Treatment is indicated if this is positive, and pulmonary scintigraphy is recommended if it is negative. Serial venous ultrasonography is an option if scintigraphy is nondiagnostic.

Women of reproductive age

If D-dimer is elevated, venous ultrasonography as the next diagnostic test is optional, with pulmonary scintigraphy recommended by some as the next imaging test. A CT angiogram with venous ultrasound is an acceptable alternative. It is advisable to start at the acetabulum to reduce gonadal irradiation if a CT venogram is deemed necessary.

Pregnant women

As usual, D-dimer testing in conjunction with clinical assessment is required. Venous ultrasonography is recommended before imaging tests with ionizing radiation if the D-dimer is positive. Some recommend pulmonary scintigraphy and some a CT angiogram if further imaging is necessary.

Patients in extremis

Echocardiography and leg ultrasonography are recommended as rapidly obtainable bedside tests. In an appropriate clinical setting right ventricular enlargement or poor right ventricular function, or a positive venous ultrasound, can be interpreted as indicating PE. A portable perfusion scan is recommended by some, and immediate transfer to an interventional catheterization laboratory is recommended by others, but such tests are not always readily available. A combination of a negative bedside echocardiogram and venous ultrasonography indicates the need for CT angiography if this is feasible.

An alternative strategy

An alternative strategy for the diagnosis of PE that avoids CT scanning is based on ventilation–perfusion scanning and ultrasonography to detect and treat DVT. Such a strategy can apply only to patients with adequate cardiorespiratory reserve (no pulmonary oedema, no loss of consciousness within 1 week, systolic blood pressure 90 mmHg or higher, no leg oedema, heart rate less than 120/min in association with atrial fibrillation or atrial flutter, Pao_2 above 50 mmHg or $Paco_2$ less than 45 mmHg while breathing room air) because even a small recurrent pulmonary embolus might be dangerous if cardiorespiratory reserve is poor. If the patient has a high probability or a normal ventilation–perfusion scan, then treatment can be given or withheld accordingly. If the ventilation–perfusion scan is nondiagnostic (intermediate or low probability), serial ultrasonography of the legs can be obtained over a period of 2 weeks, with the patient treated if DVT is shown. The risk of PE is low if serial leg tests show no DVT.

Treatment—general measures

All patients who are hypoxic should be given supplementary oxygen at high concentration (enough to restore normal Pao_2). In the early stages continuous monitoring of arterial oxygen tension by pulse oximetry is advised, with particularly careful clinical and arterial blood gas monitoring of those with coincident chronic chest disease in case CO_2 retention is problematic.

Resuscitation

Patients with massive PE and circulatory collapse may look as though they are about to die, with cool peripheries, cyanosis, profound hypotension, and marked elevation of the jugular venous pulse. Features typical of long-standing pulmonary hypertension (palpable right ventricular heave, right ventricular gallop, loud P2, hepatomegaly, ascites, peripheral oedema) are unlikely to be present. This dramatic haemodynamic picture may not be simply due to the direct anatomical effects of occlusion of main pulmonary vessels (the same picture is not seen after pneumonectomy, when one pulmonary artery is tied off completely), but also secondary to pulmonary neurogenic reflexes and local release of vasoactive substances, including 5-hydroxytryptamine and thromboxane from activated platelets.

Every effort should be made to support the circulation until measures designed to deal with the embolus (usually thrombolysis—see below) can be applied and take effect.

Treatment—antithrombotic

It is common and sensible to begin anticoagulant treatment as soon as the diagnosis of PE is suspected unless there are serious concerns about the potential side effects of anticoagulation or imaging is immediately available. The antithrombotic regimen is the same as for DVT: see Table 16.16.1.8 and Chapter 16.16.2.

Thrombolytic therapy

Thrombolytic therapy is not indicated for the routine treatment of PE. Hypotension and continuing hypoxemia whilst receiving high fractions of inspired oxygen (Fio_2) are indications for intervention. Right ventricular dysfunction on the echocardiogram may indicate impending hemodynamic instability.

A more rapid lysis of pulmonary thromboemboli occurs with thrombolytic agents than occurs spontaneously in patients treated only with anticoagulants, but pulmonary reperfusion as demonstrated on perfusion lung scans is similar after 2 weeks in patients treated with thrombolytic agents and patients treated with anticoagulants.

In 1973 the Urokinase Pulmonary Embolism Trial showed no improvement of mortality and no difference of the rate of recurrence of PE among stable patients treated with thrombolytic therapy and patients treated with anticoagulants. There have been no subsequent prospective randomized trials to contradict these results, although a trend suggesting a lower rate of recurrent PE

has been shown among patients with right ventricular dysfunction who were treated with tissue plasminogen activator.

Thrombolysis has risks. Based on pooled data the frequency of major bleeding from tissue plasminogen activator among patients with PE in randomized trials was 14.7%. This occurred despite the fact that all studies excluded patients at a high risk of bleeding, such those with recent surgery, recent biopsy, peptic ulcer disease, blood dyscrasia, or severe hepatic or renal disease. The risk of intracranial haemorrhage with tissue plasminogen activator (2%) was higher among patients with PE than among patients who received tissue plasminogen activator for myocardial infarction.

Regimens of thrombolytic therapy

Regimens approved by the United States Food and Drug Administration for treatment of acute PE are:

◆ streptokinase 250 000 IU over 30 min followed by 100 000 IU/h for 24 h

◆ urokinase 4400 IU/kg over 10 min followed by 4400 IU/kg per h for 12 to 24 h

◆ tissue plasminogen activator 100 mg (50 million IU)/2 h

Potentially advantageous regimens of thrombolytic therapy that have not been fully evaluated for treatment of PE are:

◆ urokinase 3 000 000 U/2 h

◆ streptokinase 1 500 000 U/1–2 h

◆ reteplase 10 U, repeat 10 U in 30 min

◆ saruplase 80 mg/30 min

◆ staphylokinase 20 mg/30 min

◆ tenecteplase single bolus in 5 s, 30–50 mg depending on weight

◆ anistreplase 5 or 10 mg × 3 doses

It is recommended that heparin be discontinued during thrombolytic therapy and reinstituted upon discontinuation of thrombolytic therapy. None of the regimens approved by the United States Food and Drug Administration utilize concomitant heparin.

Inferior vena cava occlusion

An inferior vena cava filter is recommended in a patient with proximal DVT or PE if anticoagulants are contraindicated, PE has recurred while on adequate anticoagulant therapy, or PE is severe (hypotension, right ventricular failure on physical examination) and any recurrent PE may be fatal. Insertion of an inferior vena cava filter is also strongly recommended in patients following pulmonary embolectomy.

Routine insertion of an inferior vena cava filter is not indicated only on the basis of a continuing predisposition for DVT, although in special circumstances this may be the best approach, e.g. in high-risk patients with DVT, severe pulmonary hypertension, and minimal cardiopulmonary reserve.

Several vena cava filters have been designed for percutaneous insertion and many are retrievable. They differ in outer diameter of the delivery system, maximal caval diameter into which they can be inserted, hook design, retrievability, biocompatibility, and filtering efficiency. They may be effective alone in preventing PE, but anticoagulant therapy after insertion of a filter is recommended.

Complications of permanent vena cava filters include improper anatomic placement, filter deformation, filter fracture, insufficient opening of the filter, and filter migration; also perforation, thrombosis, and stenosis of the cava wall. Symptomatic occlusion of the inferior vena cava is the most frequent complication, occurring in about 9% of patients. Complications at the site of insertion of the catheter do not differ from complications observed locally with other catheter techniques. DVT at the puncture site generally has been reported in 8% to 25%. Retrievable vena cava filters typically are successfully removed after 1 to 3 months, but some have been successfully removed after 1 year.

PE after insertion of an inferior vena cava filter is uncommon (1%), and fatal embolism is rare. Possible mechanisms that can explain PE after filter insertion are (1) ineffective filtration, especially with tilting of the filter, (2) growth of trapped thrombi through the filter, (3) thrombosis on the proximal side of the filter, (4) filter migration, (5) filter retraction from the caval wall, (6) embolization through collaterals, (7) embolization from sites other than the inferior vena cava, and (8) incorrect position of the filter.

Catheter interventions

Catheter-tip devices for the extraction or the fragmentation of PE have the potential of producing immediate relief from massive PE. Such interventions may be particularly useful in patients in whom there is a contraindication to thrombolytic therapy. A suction-tip device for extraction of PE has been used in some patients, and thrombus fragmentation with a guide wire, angiographic catheter, balloon catheter, or specially designed devices has been reported in small case series or case reports. The release of fragmented thromboemboli into the distal pulmonary arterial branches is not a problem. A registry of management strategies used by hospitals throughout Germany showed use of thrombus fragmentation in 1.3% to 6.8% of patients with PE, depending on severity.

Although originally it was thought that catheter embolectomy or fragmentation could substitute for thrombolytic therapy, it now appears to be an adjunct to thrombolysis, allowing a larger surface area of the fragmented emboli to be exposed to thrombolytic agent. Among patients who undergo fragmentation with standard angiographic catheters, the rate of successful clinical outcome with a local infusion of thrombolytic agents in combination with fragmentation is higher than with a systemic infusion.

Pulmonary embolectomy

Medical therapy is likely to give better results than embolectomy, although the latter may have life-saving potential in some instances. The average operative mortality among 253 patients operated from 1985 to 2006 was 20%, and higher in those who experienced a preoperative cardiac arrest. A candidate for pulmonary embolectomy should meet the following criteria: (1) massive PE, angiographically documented if possible, (2) haemodynamic instability (shock) despite heparin therapy and resuscitative efforts, and (3) failure of thrombolytic therapy or a contraindication to its use.

Chronic pulmonary thromboembolic hypertension

Pulmonary emboli resolve because of natural thrombolytic processes. Among patients with no prior cardiopulmonary disease who were treated with anticoagulants, resolution of 90% or more on perfusion lung scans was shown at 1 year in 91% of patients, compared with only 72% of those with prior cardiopulmonary disease. The residual emboli undergo fibrovascular organization, causing chronic obstruction to pulmonary arterial blood flow. In a very few patients—0.1 to 0.2% of survivors of acute PE—this process results in chronic pulmonary thromboembolic hypertension. See Chapter 16.15.2 for further discussion.

Further reading

Buller, HR *et al.* (2004). Antithrombotic therapy for venous thromboembolic disease: the Seventh ACCP Conference on Antithrombotic and Thrombolytic Therapy. *Chest*, **126** Suppl, 401–28S.

Collaborative Study by the PIOPED Investigators (1990). Value of the ventilation/perfusion scan in acute pulmonary embolism—results of the Prospective Investigation of Pulmonary Embolism Diagnosis (PIOPED). *JAMA*, **263**, 2753–59.

Doyle RL, *et al.* (2004). Surgical treatments/interventions for pulmonary arterial hypertension: ACCP evidence-based clinical practice guidelines: the Seventh ACCP Conference on Antithrombotic and Thrombolytic Therapy. *Chest*, **126** Suppl, 63–71S.

Geerts WH, *et al.* (2004). Prevention of venous thromboembolism. American College of Chest Physicians evidence-based clinical guidelines (8th edition), *Chest*, **133**, 381S–453S.

Geerts WH, *et al.* (2004). Prevention of venous thromboembolism: the Seventh ACCP Conference on Antithrombotic and Thrombolytic Therapy. *Chest*, **126** Suppl, 338–400S.

Kearon CJS, *et al.* (2001). Management of suspected deep venous thrombosis in outpatients by using clinical assessment and D-dimer testing. *Ann Intern Med*, **135**, 108–11.

Kearon C, *et al.* (2008). Antithrombotic therapy for venous thromboembolic disease. American College of Chest Physicians evidence-based clinical guidelines (8th edition), *Chest*, **133**, 454S–545S.

National Cooperative Study (1973). The Urokinase Pulmonary Embolism Trial. *Circulation*, **47** Suppl II, II-1–108.

Stein PD (2007). *Pulmonary embolism*, 2nd edition. Blackwell, Oxford.

Stein PD, *et al.* (1991). Clinical, laboratory, roentgenographic and electrocardiographic findings in patients with acute pulmonary embolism and no pre-existing cardiac or pulmonary disease. *Chest*, **100**, 598–603.

Stein PD, *et al.* (2004). D-dimer for the exclusion of deep venous thrombosis and acute pulmonary embolism: a systematic review. *Ann Intern Med*, **140**, 589–602.

Stein PD, *et al.* (2004). Venous thromboembolism in pregnancy: 21 year trends. *Am J Med*, **117**, 121–5.

Stein PD, *et al.* (2006). Diagnostic pathways in acute pulmonary embolism: Recommendations of the PIOPED II investigators. *Am J Med*, **119**, 1048–55.

Stein PD, *et al.* (2006). Multidetector computed tomography for acute pulmonary embolism. *N Engl J Med*, **354**, 2317–27.

Stein PD, *et al.* (2007). Clinical characteristics of patient with acute pulmonary embolism: data from PIOPED II. *Am J Med*, **120**, 871–9.

Tapson VF (2008). Acute pulmonary embolism. *N Engl J Med*, **358**, 1037–52.

Wells PS, *et al.* (1997). Value of assessment of pretest probability of deep-vein thrombosis in clinical management. *Lancet*, **350**, 1795–8.

Wells PS, *et al.* (2001). Excluding PE at the bedside without diagnostic imaging: management of patients with suspected PE presenting to the emergency department by using a simple clinical model and D-dimer. *Ann Intern Med*, **135**, 98–107.

16.16.2 Therapeutic anticoagulation

David Keeling

Essentials

Heparin is needed in the initial treatment of venous thromboembolism. Warfarin can be commenced on the day of diagnosis and heparin must be continued for 5 days or until the international normalized ratio (INR) is greater than 2.0 for 2 consecutive days, whichever is the longer.

Low molecular weight heparins (LMWH) have largely replaced unfractionated heparin. Their much more predictable anticoagulant response combined with high bioavailability after subcutaneous injection means that the dose can be calculated by body weight and given subcutaneously without any monitoring or dose adjustment. Their widespread use has enabled most patients with deep vein thrombosis to be managed as outpatients, and this is also increasingly the case for uncomplicated pulmonary embolism.

Particular issues—(1) in patients with cancer, giving LMWH for the first 6 months of long-term anticoagulant therapy has been shown to be superior to switching to a vitamin K antagonist; (2) high-dose loading regimens of warfarin are unnecessary and may increase the risk of overanticoagulation and bleeding; (3) warfarin for venous thromboembolism and atrial fibrillation should be given with a target INR of 2.5 (range 2.0–3.0); for patients with prosthetic heart valves the target INR is usually greater; (4) indefinite anticoagulation is required for patients with atrial fibrillation or a mechanical heart valve; for venous thromboembolism a careful clinical decision is required regarding duration of treatment; (5) for patients with atrial fibrillation and other risk factors for stroke, the superior efficacy of warfarin as compared to aspirin makes it the treatment of choice; (6) if warfarin needs to be stopped for surgery, full-dose heparin does not have to be given perioperatively unless the risk of thromboembolism is high, and warfarin can be continued in patients having dental extractions; (7) new oral anticoagulants specifically targeting thrombin or factor Xa have been developed and may replace warfarin for many indications over the next decade.

Introduction

The main indications for therapeutic anticoagulation are venous thromboembolism (deep vein thrombosis and pulmonary embolism, see Chapter 16.16) and the prevention of stroke in patients with atrial fibrillation or mechanical heart valves. Oral vitamin K antagonists (in the United Kingdom, mostly warfarin) are the mainstay of treatment. However, initial anticoagulation with heparin is required in acute venous thromboembolism because warfarin takes time to become effective. The new oral direct thrombin inhibitors and Xa inhibitors are reporting their clinical trials and are likely to replace warfarin for many indications.

Therapeutic anticoagulation for venous thromboembolism

Deep vein thrombosis and pulmonary embolism are aspects of the same disease—venous thromboembolism. Forty per cent of patients with deep vein thrombosis without clinical evidence of pulmonary embolism have evidence of emboli on lung scanning. The principles of therapeutic anticoagulation are the same for both. In proximal deep vein thrombosis (DVT) and pulmonary embolism (PE), this involves immediate anticoagulation with heparin followed by a period of anticoagulation with warfarin (or other oral vitamin K antagonist). Distal DVT can be managed in the same way, but an alternative strategy is to use serial noninvasive testing (e.g. ultrasonography), which only reliably detects proximal thrombosis, to ensure that suspected distal thrombosis does not extend above the knee, withholding treatment if it does not.

There is clear evidence that heparin is needed in the initial phase and that anticoagulation with oral vitamin K antagonists alone is inadequate. Warfarin can be commenced on the first day and heparin is continued for 5 days or until the international normalized ratio (INR) is greater than 2.0 for 2 consecutive days, whichever is the longer. Extending the period of heparinization from 5 to 10 days is not more effective and increases the risk of heparin-induced thrombocytopenia. However, for massive PE or severe iliofemoral thrombosis, a longer period of heparin therapy may be considered.

Heparin

Heparin, a glycosaminoglycan, is composed of alternating uronic acid and glucosamine saccharides that are sulphated to a varying degree. Its mode of action is to potentiate the activity of the serine protease inhibitor (serpin) antithrombin, whose main mode of action is to inhibit thrombin, but which also inhibits several other coagulant proteases such as factor Xa. A specific pentasaccharide sequence determined by the sulphation pattern along the heparin chain binds to antithrombin and causes a conformational change, giving it full activation against factor Xa but only partial activation against thrombin. Heparins of 18 saccharides (molecular weight (MW) 5 400) or more can extend across the intermolecular gap and also bind to thrombin giving full antithrombin activity, which is lost if the chains are shorter. Unfractionated or standard heparins are a mixture of chains of different lengths (MW 5 000–35 000, mean 13 000) and low-molecular-weight heparins (LMWH, MW 2 000–8 000, mean 5 000) are derived from them by enzymatic or physicochemical cleavage. LMWH have, with good reason, largely replaced unfractionated heparin for the treatment of venous thromboembolism, but the use of the latter will be discussed first.

Anticoagulation with unfractionated heparin

Unfractionated heparin has most often been given by continuous intravenous infusion, the rate of which has to be adjusted, usually by measuring the activated partial thromboplastin time (APTT). An inadequate APTT response in the first 24 h may increase the risk of recurrence of thromboembolism, although this does not seem to be critical if the starting infusion rate is at least 1 250 IU/h. A validated regimen is to give a bolus dose of 80 IU/kg and to start the infusion at 18 IU/kg/h, performing the first APTT estimate after 6 h. The dose is then usually adjusted to maintain the APTT between 1.5 to 2.5 times the average laboratory control value. With older

APTT reagents, this corresponded to a therapeutic heparin level of 0.2 to 0.4 IU/ml by protamine titration or 0.3 to 0.7 IU/ml by anti-Xa assay. However, many current APTT reagents show an increased sensitivity to unfractionated heparin and, with these, higher ratios should be aimed for. The local laboratory should advise on the appropriate therapeutic range with its reagent. When the dose is therapeutic, the APTT should be checked daily.

An alternative is to give unfractionated heparin subcutaneously once every 12 h, and a meta-analysis suggested that this might be more effective and at least as safe as continuous intravenous infusion. A reasonable starting dose is 250 IU/kg, adjusting the dose according to the mid-interval APTT.

Anticoagulation with LMWH

Although much is made of the greater anti-Xa/antithrombin ratio of the LMWH, their key clinical property is that they produce a much more predictable anticoagulant response than unfractionated heparin. This, combined with the fact that they have very high bioavailability after subcutaneous injection, means that the dose can be calculated by body weight and be given subcutaneously without any monitoring or dose adjustment. The actual dosage used differs slightly with the different LMWH and the manufacturers' recommendations should be followed, but a typical dose is 200 IU/kg once a day. They are at least as effective and at least as safe as unfractionated heparin, even when given once a day. Their widespread use has enabled most patients with DVT to be managed as outpatients, and this is also increasingly the case for uncomplicated PE. LMWH is renally excreted and so should be used with caution in patients with renal failure: it is possible to adjust the dose based on anti-Xa levels, but renal impairment is one of the few situations where unfractionated heparin, monitored by the APTT, may be preferred by some physicians.

In patients with cancer, giving LMWH for the first 6 months of long-term anticoagulant therapy has been shown to be superior to switching to vitamin K antagonist.

Complications of heparin treatment

If a patient on intravenous unfractionated heparin is excessively anticoagulated, it is usually sufficient simply to stop the infusion, the half-life being 1 to 2 h. If bleeding is severe, the heparin can be neutralized with protamine sulphate, giving 1 mg for every 100 IU that has been infused over the previous hour. The reversal of LMWH is more problematic. Although protamine sulphate may not neutralize the smaller chains, it is often clinically effective, though estimating an appropriate dose is more difficult (the maximum dose is 50 mg, so this is often given if the subcutaneous injection was recent).

Heparin-induced thrombocytopenia is a feared complication, but much less common now that short courses of LMWH are used. It is due to the development of an antibody to the heparin–platelet factor 4 complex and can be associated with serious venous and arterial thrombosis. Patients on heparin for 5 or more days should have their platelet count checked. Heparin must be stopped if heparin-induced thrombocytopenia is likely and an alternative substituted in full dosage (e.g. danaparoid or lepirudin).

Warfarin

The oral vitamin K antagonists remain the mainstay of long-term anticoagulant therapy. Warfarin is the commonest vitamin K antagonist given; acenocoumarol (which has a shorter half-life)

and phenindione (which has a higher incidence of skin rashes) are seldom used in the United Kingdom. The procoagulant factors II, VII, IX, and X (and the anticoagulants protein C and protein S) need vitamin K for the γ-carboxylation of the glutamic acid residues that form their gla domains. Without this post-translational modification they cannot bind calcium, and as a consequence cannot bind to anionic phospholipid surfaces such that assembly of the key coagulation complexes is disrupted.

Warfarin takes a number of days to become effective, during which period heparin is given. When warfarin is started, the vitamin K-dependent factors fall according to their half-lives. Factor VII and protein C have the shortest half-lives, so that despite a prolongation of the INR due to factor VII deficiency, warfarin may initially be procoagulant. This is the mechanism for the rare problem of warfarin-induced skin necrosis, most often described in those with protein C deficiency.

Initiation and monitoring of anticoagulation with warfarin

Monitoring of warfarin treatment is by the INR. This is a manipulation of the prothrombin time (PT) to allow for the different sensitivities of various laboratory reagents to the warfarin-induced coagulopathy. The INR equals $(PT/MNPT)^{ISI}$ where MNPT is the (mean normal) control PT and ISI is the international sensitivity index of the thromboplastin used in the assay. For the treatment of DVT and PE, the target INR should be 2.5 (target range 2.0–3.0). If a recurrence occurs despite an INR of 2.0 to 3.0, then the target is usually increased to 3.5 (target range 3.0–4.0).

If the initial coagulation tests are not prolonged, it has been customary to give 10 mg of warfarin on the first evening and check the INR the following morning, adjusting the dose according to the daily INR results until the patient is stable. With these regimens, most patients received 10 mg of warfarin on the first 2 days. Recent studies have shown that regimens that start with 5-mg doses, or a single 10-mg dose followed by 5-mg doses, may be preferable to regimens that start with repeated 10-mg doses. This is certainly the case in patients with an increased risk of bleeding, e.g. elderly people (>60 years old), and those with liver disease or cardiac failure. The dosing algorithm used in Oxford is shown in Table 16.16.2.1.

When patients are stable, they may go for up to 8 weeks between INR checks. If the INR is unstable, patients are seen more frequently, but it should be noted that with warfarin it takes approximately 1 week (5 times the half-life of 36 h) to reach a new steady state after dose adjustment, hence more frequent dosage alteration is inadvisable.

Duration of anticoagulation after venous thromboembolism

It is a difficult clinical decision to decide how long to continue warfarin—a matter of balancing the risks of recurrence against the risks of warfarin. The latter are well known: 1 to 2% of people on warfarin have a major bleed each year and 0.5% suffer an intracranial bleed, of which 50% die, giving a fatality rate of 0.25% per year. However, warfarin is highly (90–95%) effective at preventing recurrence. The risk of a recurrent venous thromboembolism after a first DVT is approximately 5% per year, when a case-fatality rate of 5% would also give a fatality rate of 0.25% per year. Other factors that may either increase the risk of bleeding or increase the risk of recurrence need to be taken into account. The risk of recurrence is higher for the first 3 months, it is higher for proximal DVT and PE than for distal DVT, and it is lower if a transient risk factor was present (e.g. recent surgery, use of the contraceptive pill).

Table 16.16.2.1 A warfarin induction regimen

Days 1 and 2	Day 3		Day 4	
	INR	Dose (mg)	INR	Dose (mg)
Give 5 mg each evening if baseline INR < 1.4	<1.5	10	<1.6	10
	1.5–2.0	5	1.6–1.7	7
	2.1–2.5	3	1.8–1.9	6
	2.6–3.0	1	2.0–2.3	5
	>3.0	0	2.4–2.7	4
			2.8–3.0	3
			3.1–3.5	2
			3.6–4.0	1
			>4.0	0
	and seek advice on further management			

Six months of anticoagulation has been shown to be more effective than six weeks of anticoagulation and three months has been shown to be equivalent to six months. For patients with a first episode of distal DVT (whether provoked or unprovoked), or a first episode of proximal DVT or PE secondary to a transient (reversible) risk factor, treatment is recommended for 3 months. For patients with a first episode of idiopathic proximal DVT or PE, treatment is recommended for at least 3 months and consideration should be given to long-term treatment where there are no risk factors for bleeding and where anticoagulant control is good. Raised D-dimers after discontinuing anticoagulation and antiphospholipid antibodies increase the risk of recurrence. Deficiencies of antithrombin, protein C or protein S may increase the risk of recurrence. Factor V Leiden and the prothrombin mutation do not do so to a clinically significant degree and therefore should not influence duration of treatment. For patients with two or more episodes of objectively documented venous thromboembolism or those with a first event and an on-going risk factor (such as cancer), indefinite treatment should be considered. Taking all this into account, a reasonable approach is indicated in Table 16.16.2.2.

Complications of warfarin treatment

The only major complication of warfarin treatment is bleeding. Risk factors for bleeding are increasing age, a history of stroke, a history of gastrointestinal bleeding, anaemia, renal impairment, diabetes, and recent myocardial infarction. A major problem in control is the starting and stopping of other medication. Many drugs interact with warfarin (see Table 16.16.2.3 for those with the most evidence) such that patient (and doctor) education and

Table 16.16.2.2 Duration of warfarin treatment

1st calf DVT 1st proximal DVT with TRFª	1st unprovoked proximal DVT	1st proximal DVT with on-going risk factor Recurrent VTE
3 months	3 months or long term	long-term

ªTRF = transient risk factor, e.g. surgery, combined pill, pregnancy, plaster cast

Table 16.16.2.3 Many drugs interact with warfarin; the evidence is strongest for those listed

Potentiation	Inhibition
Amiodarone	Barbiturates
Cimetidine	Carbamazepine
Clofibrate	Chlordiazepoxide
Cotrimoxazole	Cholestyramine
Erythromycin	Griseofulvin
Fluconazole	Rifampicin
Isoniazid	Sucralfate
Metronidazole	
Miconazole	
Omeprazole	
Paracetamol	
Phenylbutazone	
Piroxicam	
Propafenone	
Propanolol	
Statins	
Sulphinpyrazone	

constant vigilance are essential. Close monitoring of the INR is advised when concomitant medication is altered.

The approach taken to reverse overanticoagulation with warfarin depends on the circumstances (see Box 16.16.2.1). Prothrombin complex concentrates, unlike fresh frozen plasma, reliably and rapidly correct the defect and should be used in life-threatening situations such as intracranial bleeding. Small doses of phytomenadione (vitamin K_1) can lower a high INR without making subsequent anticoagulation difficult, as is the case if high doses are given.

Fibrinolysis for venous thromboembolism

Thrombolytic agents dissolve thrombi by directly or indirectly activating the zymogen plasminogen to plasmin. Plasmin then degrades fibrin to soluble peptides, but cannot distinguish fibrin in pathological thrombi from fibrin in haemostatic plugs.

The use of thrombolytic agents for venous thromboembolism requires careful individual assessment. It is rarely given in DVT, though its use can be considered in massive iliofemoral thrombosis. Although thrombolytic therapy for PE achieves more rapid resolution than heparin alone, there is no clear evidence of lasting benefit. Patients with PE who survive long enough to have the diagnosis made and treatment with heparin begun have an excellent prognosis, unless they have associated severe medical disease. Thrombolytic therapy—which carries a much greater risk of bleeding—is, therefore, reserved for those cases of massive PE with haemodynamic instability threatening the patient's life (see Chapter 16.16).

Streptokinase (which forms a complex with plasminogen that then activates free plasminogen), urokinase, and tissue plasminogen

Box 16.16.2.1 Management of overanticoagulation with warfarin

Major bleeding

◆ Stop warfarin

◆ Give PCC (30 IU/kg) or FFP (15 ml/kg) if PCC not available

◆ Give phytomenadione 5 mg intravenously

No bleeding/minor bleeding

◆ Stop warfarin until INR < 5

◆ If INR < 8: no other action is required

◆ If INR 8–12: give phytomenadione, 0.5 mg intravenously or 2.5 mg orally

◆ If INR > 12: give phytomenadione, 1 mg intravenously or 5 mg orally

FFP, fresh frozen plasma; PCC, prothrombin complex concentrates. PCC should be used for life-threatening bleeding.

activator (tPA) have all been used. For PE, streptokinase is recommended as a 250 000-IU loading dose followed by an infusion for 24 h at 100 000 IU/h. Urokinase is given as a 4400 IU/kg loading dose followed by 2200 IU/kg for 12 h. Following the success of rapid fibrinolytic regimens in myocardial infarction, tPA given as 100 mg over 2 h has been used for PE, and the use of more rapid regimens with the other two agents has also been suggested (see Chapter 16.16 for further discussion).

Anticoagulation in particular clinical circumstances

Treatment of venous thromboembolism in pregnancy

Heparin does not cross the placenta and can be used in pregnancy. As pregnant women are excluded from clinical trials, evidence for with LMWH is limited. However, experience seems to indicate that LMWH, with all its logistical advantages, can be used effectively and safely in pregnancy. Indeed osteopenia, sometimes seen with prolonged use of unfractionated heparin, seems to be less of a problem with LMWH. Warfarin, which crosses the placenta, can cause an embryopathy if given between 6 and 12 weeks of gestation. At any time, it can cause fetal bleeding and has been associated with central nervous system abnormalities.

The usual treatment recommended for venous thromboembolism in pregnancy is to continue with full-dose subcutaneous heparin until term. Warfarin can be used for the 6 weeks of the puerperium: women taking warfarin can breastfeed.

Therapeutic anticoagulation for atrial fibrillation

Atrial fibrillation affects 2 to 5% of people over the age of 60, and is associated with a stroke rate of 5% a year. In patients with atrial fibrillation, warfarin given to a target INR of 2.5 (target range 2.0–3.0) prevents two-thirds of fatal or disabling stokes, though it becomes less effective when the INR is less than 2.0. Aspirin reduces stroke in atrial fibrillation by approximately 20%.

In patients with atrial fibrillation, the following increase the risk of stroke: congestive heart failure, hypertension, age greater than

75 years, diabetes, previous ischaemic stroke, or transient ischaemic attack. One scheme used to assess patients (CHADS$_2$) gives a point for each of these (with the exception of 2 points for previous ischaemic stroke or transient ischaemic attack). Aspirin alone is sufficient in patients with atrial fibrillation and no risk factors (a CHADS$_2$ score of 0), whereas in patients with a score of 3 or more, warfarin is the treatment of choice. For those with a score of 1 or 2 (risk of stroke 3–4% per year), the decision between warfarin and aspirin is more balanced.

For outpatients who do not require rapid anticoagulation, a slow-loading regimen (such as starting patients on 3 mg of warfarin daily for 1 week and determining subsequent doses by weekly INR measurement) is safe and achieves therapeutic anticoagulation in most patients within 3 to 4 weeks. This appears to avoid overanticoagulation and bleeding associated with rapid loading.

A target INR of 2.5 is recommended for 3 weeks before and 4 weeks after cardioversion. In order to minimize cardioversion cancellations due to low INRs on the day of the procedure, a higher target INR, e.g. 3.0, can be used prior to the procedure.

Therapeutic anticoagulation in patients with prosthetic heart valves

Vitamin K antagonists are recommended for all patients with mechanical prosthetic heart valves, the overall risk of embolic stroke if not anticoagulated being 8% per year. Emboli are more common from mitral prosthetic valves than aortic prosthetic valves, and caged-ball valves are more thrombogenic than bi-leaflet or tilting-disk valves.

Various national and international recommendations are made regarding the target INR in patients with prosthetic valves, with 3.5 traditionally being advised. This is still treasonable for caged-ball valves, but for tilting-disks and bi-leaflet valves the target INR can possibly be lower, e.g. 2.5 (range 2.0–3.0) for aortic valves and 3.0 (range 2.5–3.5) for mitral valves. When a new valve is inserted, it is recommended that unfractionated heparin or LMWH be given until the INR is stable and at a therapeutic level for 2 consecutive days.

Perioperative management of therapeutic anticoagulation

Warfarin does not need to be stopped for dentistry, nor for some minor surgery. For many operations, however, warfarin will need to be temporarily discontinued. It can generally be stopped 5 days before surgery and the INR be checked on the day of surgery (checking the day before obviates the risk of cancellation as a small dose of oral vitamin K can be given if necessary). The main clinical decision is whether to give bridging therapy with treatment-dose heparin perioperatively when the INR is less than 2.0. This depends on balancing the risk of bleeding with the risk of thromboembolism. For those at high risk of thromboembolism, such as patients with a prosthetic mitral valve, treatment-dose heparin is usually given (Table 16.16.2.4). For those at low risk, such as patients with uncomplicated atrial fibrillation, full dose heparin probably carries more risk than withholding anticoagulation. For other patients, such as those with aortic prosthetic valves, an individual decision is needed. It is worth noting that if an aortic valve carries a risk of embolism of 4% per annum off anticoagulation, then stopping anticoagulation for 4 to 5 days carries a risk of 1 in 2000.

Table 16.16.2.4 Management of anticoagulation perioperatively

	Preoperatively	Postoperatively until INR > 2
High risk e.g. VTE within 1 month; prosthetic mitral valve; AF and history of stroke	Treatment-dose heparin (either IV UFH or SC LMWH)*	Treatment-dose heparin (either IV UFH or SC LMWH)
Low risk e.g. AF without previous stroke	Nil or prophylactic LMWH	Prophylactic LMWH

AF, atrial fibrillation; IV, intravenous; LMWH; low molecular weight heparin; SC, subcutaneous; UFH, unfractionated heparin; VTE, venous thromboembolism.

a Stop full dose IV UFH 6 h before surgery and check APTT before operation begins, omit full dose SC LMWH on day of surgery. Therapeutic dose heparin must not be given for at least 48 hours after high bleeding risk surgery.

New anticoagulants

The ideal anticoagulant would be orally active, have a wide therapeutic index, predictable pharmacokinetics and dynamics, with minimal interactions with other drugs and food (negating the need for monitoring), a rapid onset of action, an antidote, and minimal nonanticoagulant side effects. Heparin needs to be given parenterally. Warfarin has a slow onset of action, a narrow therapeutic index, and unpredictable pharmacokinetics and dynamics, plus significant drug and dietary interactions that make regular monitoring essential. New anticoagulants are, therefore, much needed, and various parts of the coagulation cascade have been targeted by potential new drugs (Fig. 16.16.2.1), some of which are discussed below.

Indirect Xa inhibitors

Fondaparinux is the pentasaccharide of heparin, chemically synthesized and modified. Like heparin, it binds to antithrombin and enhances its inhibition of factor Xa (unlike heparin it does not enhance inhibition of thrombin). Given once a day, subcutaneously, it is as effective as heparin for the initial treatment of venous thromboembolism. It does not appear to cause heparin-induced thrombocytopenia. A hypermethylated derivative, idraparinux, with half-life of 80 h is under investigation as a possible once-a-week treatment.

Oral direct Xa inhibitors

The development of fondaparinux showed that inhibition of Xa can be an effective anticoagulant strategy. Pharmaceutical companies are now developing oral direct Xa inhibitors such as rivaroxaban, which is in phase III clinical trials.

Direct thrombin (IIa) inhibitors

Lepirudin directly inhibits thrombin, meaning that it does not require antithrombin for its action. However, it does require parenteral administration, but the development of oral direct thrombin inhibitors has raised much optimism. The first of these, ximelagatran, was shown to be effective for the treatment of acute DVT and as effective as warfarin for preventing stroke in atrial fibrillation. Unfortunately, it caused abnormal liver function tests

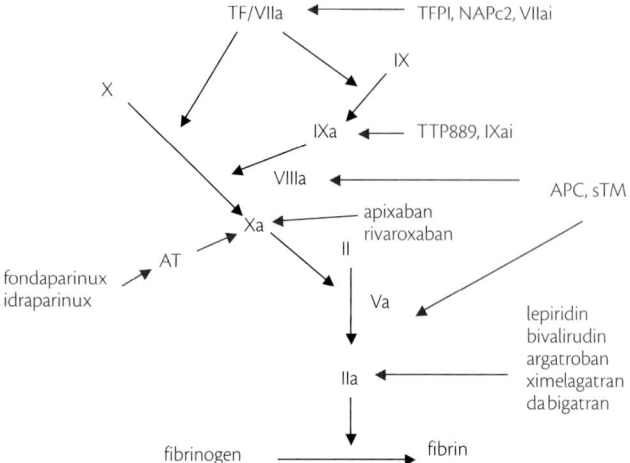

Fig. 16.16.2.1 New anticoagulants. Roman numerals represent the coagulation factors (a - indicates the activated forms), TF – tissue factor, AT – antithrombin, TFPI – tissue factor pathway inhibitor, NAPc2 – nematode anticoagulant peptide, VIIai and IXai – active site inhibited VIIa and IXa, TTP899 - IXa inhibitor in development, APC – activated protein C, sTM – soluble thrombomodulin

in 8% of patients, and has been withdrawn from development. Other oral direct thrombin inhibitors are in development, and dabigatran etexilate is in phase III clinical trials.

Introducing new anticoagulants into clinical practice

Oral direct thrombin inhibitors and oral direct Xa inhibitors are entering clinical practice, possibility to be followed by drugs targeting other coagulation factors. They will be expensive but, unlike warfarin, will not require monitoring. Unless they are suitable for all patients and all indications (and there seems to be a reluctance to test them in patients with prosthetic heart valves), we will have to keep the infrastructure in place to monitor warfarin.

Further reading

Anonymous (1998). Guidelines on oral anticoagulation: 3rd edition. *Br J Haematol*, **101**, 374–87.

Baglin T, *et al.* (2006). Guidelines on the use and monitoring of heparin. *Br J Haematol*, **133**, 19–34.

Baglin TP, Keeling DM, Watson HG (2006). Guidelines on oral anticoagulation (warfarin): 3rd edition—2005 update. *Br J Haematol*, **132**, 277–85.

Buller HR, *et al.* (2004). Antithrombotic therapy for venous thromboembolic disease: the Seventh ACCP Conference on Antithrombotic and Thrombolytic Therapy. *Chest*, **126**, 401–28S.

Dunn AS, Turpie AG (2003). Perioperative management of patients receiving oral anticoagulants: a systematic review. *Arch Intern Med*, **163**, 901–8.

Lee AY, *et al.* (2003). Low-molecular-weight heparin versus a coumarin for the prevention of recurrent venous thromboembolism in patients with cancer. *N Engl J Med*, **349**, 146–53.

Salem DN, *et al.* (2004). Antithrombotic therapy in valvular heart disease—native and prosthetic: the Seventh ACCP Conference on Antithrombotic and Thrombolytic Therapy. *Chest*, **126**, 457S–482S.

Weitz JI, Bates SM (2005). New anticoagulants. *J Thromb Haemost*, **3**, 1843–53.

16.17

Hypertension

Contents

16.17.1 Essential hypertension—definition, epidemiology, and pathophysiology

Bryan Williams

Essentials

'Essential hypertension' is high blood pressure for which there is no clearly defined aetiology. From a practical perspective, it is best defined as that level of blood pressure at which treatment to lower blood pressure results in significant clinical benefit—a level which will vary from patient to patient depending on their absolute cardiovascular risk.

Most guidelines define 'hypertension' as an office blood pressure greater than or equal to 140/90 mmHg. When using 24-h ambulatory blood pressure or home blood pressure averages to define hypertension, the diagnostic thresholds are lower than those used with office measurement.

Isolated diastolic hypertension (systolic blood pressure (SBP) < 140 mmHg, dialstolic blood pressure (DBP) > 90 mmHg) is more common in younger people, and isolated systolic hypertension (SBP > 140 mmHg, DBP < 90 mmHg) is the most common form of hypertension in older people.

Recent American guidelines have recently included a new category of 'prehypertension' (SBP 120–139 mmHg and/or diastolic blood pressure, DBP 80–89 mmHg), the reason for this being that blood pressure in this range is associated with both adverse cardiovascular outcome and a high rate of progression to hypertension.

Epidemiology

In 2000, it was estimated 25% of the world's adult population were hypertensive, and predicted that this would rise to 29% by 2025. By the age of 60, more than one-half of adults in most regions of the world will be hypertensive.

There is a continuous relationship between blood pressure and cardiovascular risk from blood pressure values as low as 115/75 mmHg. The relationship is steeper for stroke than it is for coronary heart disease, and is magnified by age. There is a doubling in risk of stroke and ischaemic heart disease mortality for every 20/10 mmHg increase in blood pressure.

Most people with hypertension are over the age of 50 years, and in these systolic blood pressure is by far the most important contributor to the burden of cardiovascular disease attributable to hypertension.

Pathogenesis and pathophysiology

The pathogenesis of essential hypertension is a complex interplay between (1) genetic predisposition, (2) lifestyle and environmental influences, and (3) disturbances in vascular structure and neurohumoral control mechanisms.

Genetic predisposition—blood pressure runs in families, with a remarkably consistent level of correlation of around 0.2 between first-degree relatives found in many studies. This means that if the blood pressure of one member of the family deviates from the norm by + 10 mmHg, the first-degree relative will deviate by + 2 mmHg on average. Variants in a large number of genes, involving virtually all of the main physiological systems affecting blood pressure, have shown association with blood pressure in one or more studies, but the effect of any individual variant is likely to be modest.

Lifestyle and environmental influences—the exploding prevalence of hypertension in economically developing regions reflects lifestyle changes, so-called 'Westernization', more than anything else, with the most important influences on blood pressure being sodium intake, obesity, and alcohol intake.

Pathophysiology—a characteristic finding in essential hypertension is an inappropriate increase in peripheral vascular resistance relative to the cardiac output. This is due to remodelling of small arteries (arterioles), which is characterized by an increase in their media/ lumen ratio, but it is not clear whether these changes are a consequence or a cause of raised blood pressure. The functional integrity of large conduit arteries, i.e. the aorta, which becomes stiffer, also influences the development of hypertension—especially systolic hypertension. Endothelial dysfunction and decreased nitric oxide production are found in hypertension, but are more likely a consequence than a cause of elevated blood pressure. The specific role of the renin–angiotensin–aldosterone system in the development of essential hypertension remains unclear, but therapeutic agents that inhibit this system have proved to be very effective treatments. The sympathetic nervous system is involved in the acute and chronic regulation of blood pressure, but whether disturbances in it play a major role in the initiation and maintenance of chronic essential hypertension remains unknown.

The hypertensive phenotype and target-organ damage

Although blood pressure measurement is used to define hypertension, hypertension is more than just blood pressure. Essential hypertension is commonly associated with metabolic disturbances (the 'insulin-resistance phenotype') and multisystem structural damage that conspire to enhance cardiovascular risk beyond that which can be attributed to blood pressure alone.

Left ventricular hypertrophy is a classic feature of untreated or inadequately treated long-standing hypertension, and is a very potent predictor of premature cardiovascular disease and death. Inhibition of the renin–angiotensin–aldosterone system is particularly effective at regressing left ventricular hypertrophy, which is associated with dramatically improved prognosis for people with hypertension.

Hypertension is the single most important risk factor for stroke, and is increasingly recognized as a major factor contributing to the rate of cognitive decline in later life. Patients with renal disease often have hypertension, people with hypertension can develop renal disease, and the age-related decline in GFR is more rapid in people with essential hypertension, but renal function is usually well preserved throughout life in patients with mild to moderate essential hypertension. Retinal changes caused by hypertension are discussed in Chapter 16.17.2.

Implications of the evolution of hypertensive injury

The process of hypertensive injury to target organs evolves silently over many years. Current treatment guidelines have been developed from an evidence base relating to changes in hard clinical endpoints derived from studies in very elderly patients at the end of the hypertensive disease process. Future treatment strategies must surely focus on preventing the evolution of the silent disease process, rather than simply battling with its consequences.

Definitions of hypertension

The commonest form of hypertension has been termed 'essential hypertension', i.e. hypertension for which there is no clearly defined aetiology. Blood pressure is normally distributed within populations and thus the definition of 'hypertension' is a moving target. From a practical perspective it is best defined as that level of blood pressure at which treatment to lower blood pressure results in significant clinical benefit, which will change as new evidence from clinical trials emerges. This statement also highlights the conundrum in definition of 'hypertension' because the risk associated with blood pressure is a continuum and the level of pressure at which treatment results in 'significant clinical benefit' for any individual will depend on their absolute cardiovascular risk.

There is substantial evidence that treating systolic pressure (SBP) above 160 mmHg and/or a diastolic pressure (DBP) above 100 mmHg is beneficial; there is also evidence that treating pressures above 140/90 mmHg is worthwhile, especially in higher-risk patients. Most guidelines therefore define 'hypertension' as an office blood pressure ≥140/90 mmHg. Various grades of hypertension are also specified (Table 16.17.1.1). The hypertension guidelines in the United States of America have recently included a new category of 'prehypertension' (SBP 120–139 mmHg and/or DBP 80–89 mmHg), which is discussed later in this chapter.

It is important to note that the diagnostic thresholds for hypertension vary according to the method of measurement. The aforementioned blood pressure thresholds for diagnosis have been defined according to seated blood pressure measurements, so-called 'office blood pressures'. When using 24-h ambulatory blood pressure or home blood pressure averages to define hypertension, the diagnostic thresholds are lower than these office blood pressures.

Subtypes of hypertension

Various categories of blood pressure can be identified in populations, with isolated diastolic hypertension (IDH) (SBP <140 mmHg, DBP >90 mmHg) being more common in younger people and isolated systolic hypertension (ISH) (SBP >140 mmHg, DBP <90 mmHg) being the most common form of hypertension in older people, with systolic/diastolic hypertension (SDH) (SBP>140 mmHg and DBP >90 mmHg) bridging the two extremes of age (Fig. 16.17.1.1).

Table 16.17.1.1 Classification of hypertension. Grades 1–3 replace the old terminology of 'mild', 'moderate', and 'severe'. The 'high normal' blood pressure range corresponds to 'prehypertension' in the United States guideline

Category	Systolic		Diastolic
Optimal	<120	and	<80
Normal	120–129	and/or	80–84
High normal	130–139	and/or	85–89
Grade 1 hypertension	140–159	and/or	90–99
Grade 2 hypertension	160–179	and/or	100–109
Grade 3 hypertension	>180	and/or	>110
Isolated systolic hypertension	>140	and	<90

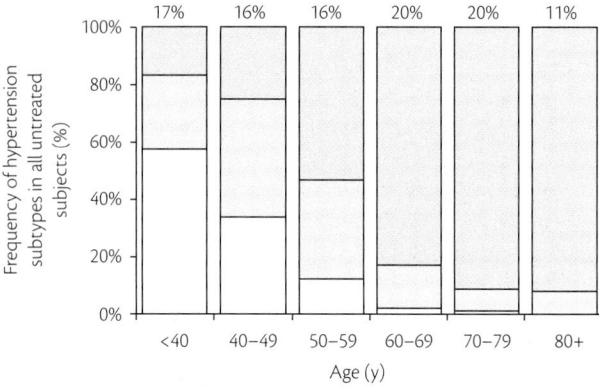

Isolated systolic hypertension (SBP >140 mm Hg and DBP <90 mm Hg)

Systolic/diastolic hypertension (SBP >140 mm Hg and DBP >90 mm Hg)

Isolated diastolic hypertension (SBP <140 mm Hg and >DBP 90 mm Hg)

Fig. 16.17.1.1 Blood pressure subtypes in the United States of America according to age. The percentage values at the top of each column indicate the prevalence of hypertension in that age band.
Reproduced from Franklin SS et al, Predominance of Isolated Systolic Hypertension Among Middle-Aged and Elderly US Hypertensives , Hypertension 2001;37:869–874 with permission of Wolters Kluwer Health.

Although traditionally DBP was considered to carry the greatest prognostic significance, it is now clear that this is no longer the case. Most people with hypertension are over the age of 50 years, and in them SBP is by far the most important contributor to the burden of cardiovascular disease attributable to hypertension. The different patterns of blood pressure and the relative importance of DBP and SBP with regard to prognosis reflect progression of the underlying pathology. The pathogenesis of hypertension in younger people is characterized by an increased peripheral vascular resistance. This results in an increased diastolic pressure, with any associated rise in systolic pressure 'cushioned' by a compliant aorta, hence the commonly observed IDH. With ageing there is progressive stiffening of the aorta, a consequent reduction in large-artery compliance, and a reduced capacity to sustain diastolic pressure and to cushion systolic pressure. The result is an age-related widening of pulse pressure as diastolic pressure falls alongside a progressive rise in SBP, hence the emergence of ISH (Fig. 16.17.1.2).

Epidemiology

Global prevalence

The global prevalence of hypertension when defined either as a blood pressure of ≥140/90 mmHg, or the use of antihypertensive medication, was estimated to be 972 million in the year 2000, representing about 25% of the world's adult population. The global prevalence of hypertension is expected to rise dramatically by about 60% by 2025, representing 29% of the world's adult population and affecting 1.6 billion people (Fig. 16.17.1.3). Most of this increase in the worldwide burden of hypertension is expected to result from an increase in the number of people with hypertension in economically developing regions, hence almost 75% of the world's hypertensive populations will be in economically developing regions by 2025.

The prevalence of hypertension in almost all regions of the world increases with age and more steeply in women. By the age of 60, more than one-half of adults in most regions of the world will be hypertensive. India and Asia have and will most likely continue have the lowest rates of hypertension, whereas the highest rates are likely to remain in Latin America, the Caribbean, former Socialist Republics, and sub-Saharan Africa. Consequently, hypertension is set to remain the single most important preventable cause of premature death worldwide over the next two decades, with the World Health Organization estimating that about 7.1 million deaths per year may be attributable to hypertension, and that suboptimal blood pressure (SBP ≥115 mmHg by their definition) is responsible for 62% of cerebrovascular disease and 49% of ischaemic heart disease worldwide, with little variation by sex.

Lifetime risk

The prevalence of hypertension increases with age, affecting over one-half of those aged 60 to 69 years and over three-quarters of those aged over 70 years in the United States of America and most developed countries. As indicated above, almost all of the age-related rise in the prevalence of hypertension is due to a progressive rise in SBP. The lifetime probability of developing hypertension is about 90% for men and women who were not hypertensive at 55 or 65 years old and survived to age 80 to 85 (Fig. 16.17.1.4).

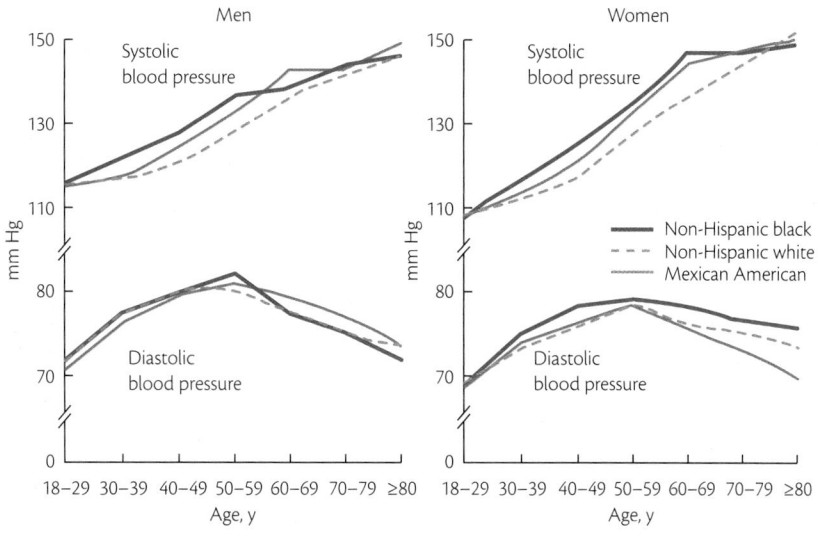

Fig. 16.17.1.2 Data from the United States of America NHANES III population survey (1988–91) showing the progressive rise in SBP with age and the rise in DBP up until age c.50 years, after which DBP falls and pulse pressure widens. This pattern is typical of Westernized countries and explains the high prevalence of isolated systolic hypertension in older people in these countries.
Reproduced from Burt VL et al, Prevalence of Hypertension in the US Adult Population, Hypertension, 1995;23:305–313 with permission of Wolters Kluwer Health.

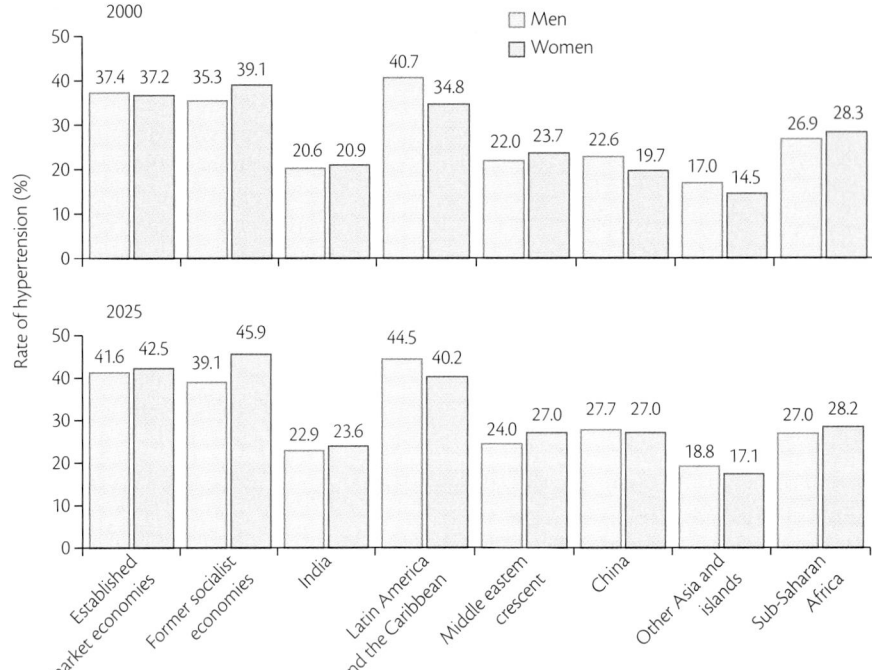

Fig. 16.17.1.3 Frequency of hypertension in people aged 20 years and older by world region and gender in 2000 (upper panel) and projected to 2025 (lower panel).
Reprinted from *The Lancet*, Vol. 365, Kearney PM, *et al*, *Global burden of hypertension: analysis of world-wide data*, pp217–23. Copyright (2005), with permission from Elsevier.

Cardiovascular morbidity and mortality associated with hypertension

Elevated blood pressure increases the risk of cardiovascular morbidity and mortality. Data from observational studies of over 1 million people has indicated a continuous relationship between blood pressure and cardiovascular risk from blood pressure values as low as 115/75 mmHg (Fig. 16.17.1.5). The relationship is steeper for stroke than it is for coronary heart disease and is magnified by age. For every 20/10 mmHg increase in blood pressure, there is a doubling in risk of stroke and ischaemic heart disease mortality. Hypertension also increases the risk of congestive cardiac failure, endstage renal disease, and dementia. Moreover, data from the Framingham Heart Study also indicates that there is a doubling of risk of cardiovascular complications in patients with blood pressure levels above normal but not yet classified as having overt hypertension (Fig. 16.17.1.6). This was the basis for the American guidelines

introducing the term 'prehypertension' (SBP 120–139 mmHg and/or DBP 80–89 mmHg) to emphasize that this level of blood pressure (1) is not benign, (2) is associated with an elevated cardiovascular disease risk, and (3) predicts with a high degree of certainty that blood pressure is on an upward trajectory and that affected people are almost certain to develop more severe hypertension, unless there is intervention with effective in lifestyle changes and/or drug therapy.

Systolic blood pressure as the main risk factor

For many years DBP was considered the main denominator for defining the threshold and treatment targets for hypertension. This is no longer the case. As indicated above, there is a progressive rise in DBP up to about the age of 50 years and thereafter it usually falls. By contrast, SBP begins to rise relentlessly from the age of around 40 years (Figs. 16.17.1.1 and 16.17.1.2). Thus, at the age of peak prevalence of hypertension, i.e. older than 60 years, SBP is the

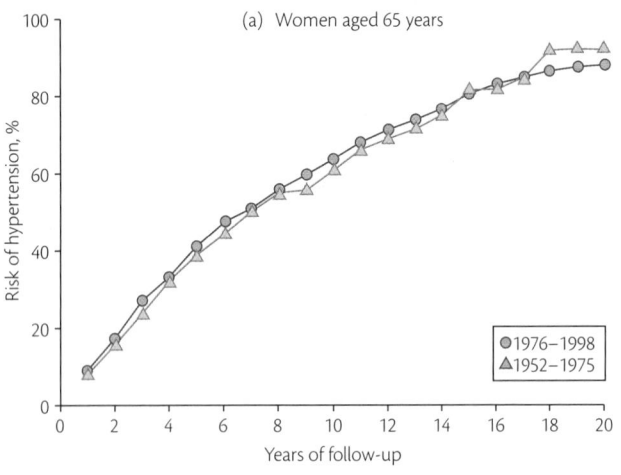

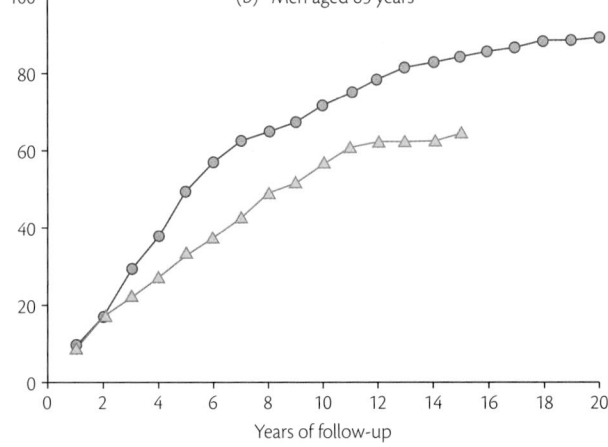

Fig. 16.17.1.4 Lifetime risk of hypertension in women and men aged 65 years.
JAMA 2002; 287:1003–1010.

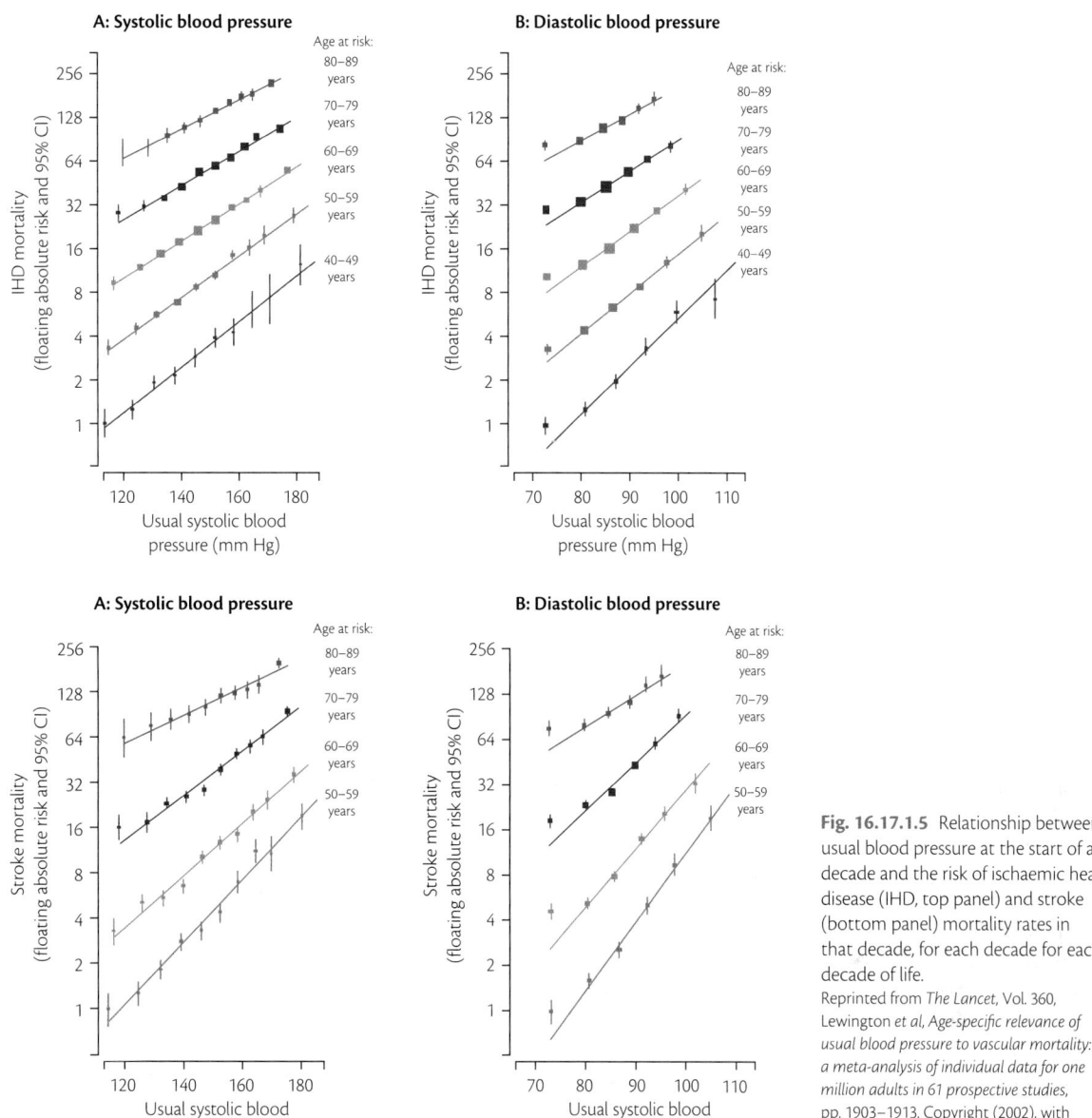

Fig. 16.17.1.5 Relationship between usual blood pressure at the start of a decade and the risk of ischaemic heart disease (IHD, top panel) and stroke (bottom panel) mortality rates in that decade, for each decade for each decade of life.
Reprinted from *The Lancet*, Vol. 360, Lewington *et al*, *Age-specific relevance of usual blood pressure to vascular mortality: a meta-analysis of individual data for one million adults in 61 prospective studies*, pp. 1903–1913. Copyright (2002), with permission from Elsevier.

major contributor to the diagnosis of the condition and its associated risk. Below the age of 50 years, DBP is also important. Fig. 16.17.1.7 illustrates the shift in the major risk burden attributable to hypertension, from DBP to SBP, at about the age of 50 years. However, because most hypertension, i.e. >75%, occurs over the age of 50 years, SBP rather than DBP is by far the most important contributor to the huge global cardiovascular risk burden attributable to hypertension. SBP is also the most difficult to treat, which has led some to argue that for patients over the age of 50 years the attention of doctors should be focused solely on the SBP.

Pathogenesis and pathophysiology of hypertension

The pathogenesis of essential hypertension has remained something of an enigma, in part reflecting the fact that the basis for the diagnosis, i.e. an elevated blood pressure, has so many potential causes. From a physiological perspective, the pressure in the circulation is

the product of the cardiac output (CO) and impedance to flow, i.e. peripheral resistance (PR):

$$\text{blood pressure} = \text{CO} \times \text{PR}$$

Both CO and PR can be influenced by a number of control mechanisms, including activity of the renin–angiotensin–aldosterone system, activity of the sympathetic nervous system, and other factors influencing salt and water homeostasis. In addition, vascular structural changes associated with hypertension play a role in accentuating its severity and conferring resistance to treatment. These structural changes include small-artery remodelling that results in a reduced media/lumen ratio (which increases peripheral resistance) and large-artery stiffening (which changes pulse wave characteristics and reduces the compliance of the circulation). Recent reports suggest that a reduced diameter of the proximal aorta may also be a factor contributing to the development of hypertension. Whether structural changes precede and predispose to the onset of hypertension, or follow it, or both, remains a subject of considerable debate.

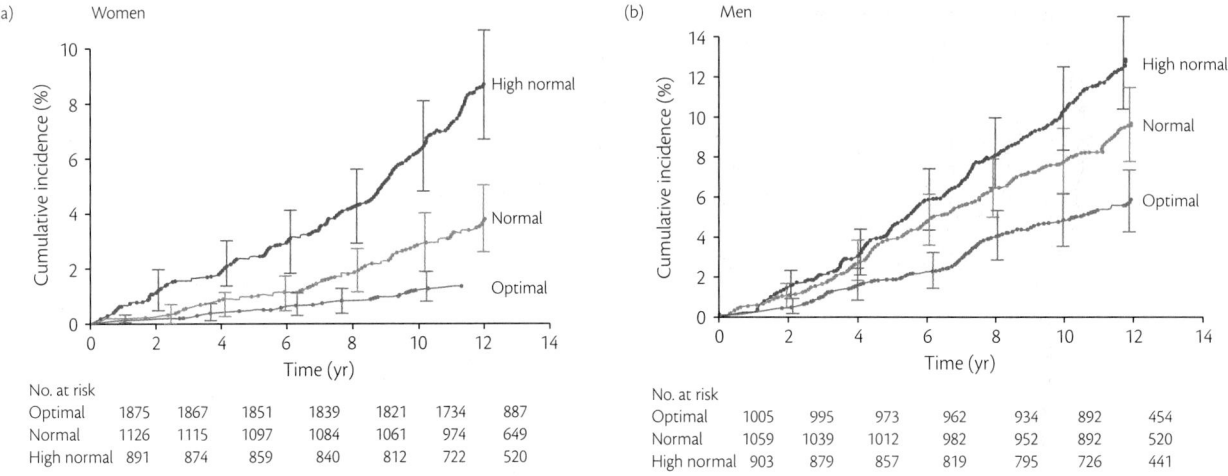

Fig. 16.17.1.6 High normal blood pressure and the risk of cardiovascular disease. Cumulative incidence of cardiovascular events in women (a) and men (b) without hypertension, according to blood-pressure category at the baseline examination. For this analysis, optimal blood pressure was defined as SBP <120 mmHg and DBP <80 mmHg, normal blood pressure as SBP 120–129 mmHg and/or DBP 80–84 mmHg, and high-normal BP as SBP 130–139 mmHg and/or DBP 85–89 mm Hg. 95% confidence intervals are shown.
N Engl J Med 2001; 345:1291–1297.

In some cases (probably <10%) a discrete cause for hypertension will be identified (see Chapter 16.17.3). In most other circumstances the pathogenesis of essential hypertension, i.e. hypertension that is not due to a recognized secondary cause, is a complex interplay between (1) genetic predisposition (2) lifestyle and environmental influences, and (3) disturbances in structure and the aforementioned control mechanisms. These are in turn compounded by the effects of ageing on the cardiovascular and renal systems.

Genetic factors (this section written by Prof. Nilesh Samani)

Historical perspective

The history of the genetics of hypertension is marked by a celebrated debate in the 1950s and 1960s between Platt and Pickering, two doyens of British medicine. On the basis of a finding of a bimodal distribution of blood pressures in some families of patients with hypertension, and evidence of hypertension transmitted over three generations in a few pedigrees, Platt argued that hypertension was a distinct genetic disorder with a likely autosomal dominant mode of

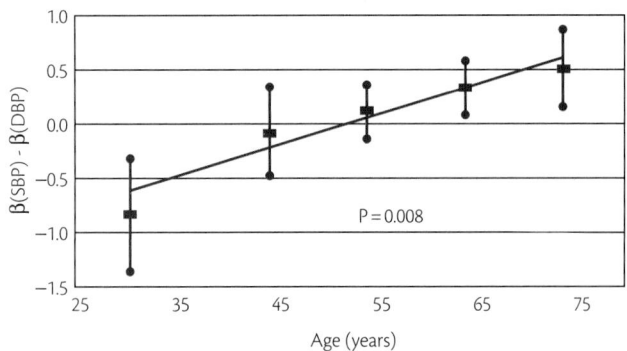

Fig. 16.17.1.7 The impact of DBP and SBP on the risk of coronary heart disease as a function of Age: A β-coefficient level less than 0.0 indicates a stronger effect of DBP on CHD risk, a β-coefficient level greater than 0.0 indicates a greater importance of SBP. The 'switch' from DBP to SBP occurs at around age 50 years.
Franklin SS, *et al.* Circulation 2001; 103:1245. (http://circ.ahajournals.org/cgi/content/abstract/103/9/1245).

inheritance. By contrast, Pickering and colleagues showed that in the general population there was no obvious discontinuity of blood pressure distribution and that the familial resemblance of blood pressure spanned the whole range of blood pressures, and was not different for those with hypertension. Thus, Pickering argued that blood pressure, like height and weight, was a quantitative trait, and that although there was a significant genetic contribution, this was polygenic and that hypertension represented one extreme of the trait but was not a distinct disorder, except perhaps for rare monogenetic forms embedded in the blood pressure distribution curve. Today, the overwhelming mass of evidence supports the Pickering concept, although several mendelian disorders that predispose to hypertension have been described (see Chapter 16.17.4).

Genetic epidemiology of blood pressure and hypertension

The extent of familial aggregation of blood pressure has been studied in diverse ethnic groups living in distinct places, ranging from Polynesians to Middle Americans. A remarkably consistent level of correlation of around 0.2 between first-degree relatives has been found, meaning that if the blood pressure of one member of the family deviates from the norm by +10 mmHg, the first degree relative will deviate by +2 mmHg on average. Studies in children and infants suggest that the familial resemblance in blood pressure starts very early and is maintained throughout life.

Attempts to partition the familial resemblance of blood pressure between shared genes and shared environment have been made through studies of adoptees and twins. In the Montreal Adoption Study, correlations between natural siblings compared with adoptive siblings, and between parents and natural children compared with parents and adopted children, were at least twice as great. Similarly, several studies have documented much higher correlations in blood pressure between monozygotic twins (0.55 to 0.85) compared with dizygotic twins (0.25 to 0.50), although the results from twin studies have to be viewed with caution as there is substantial evidence of excess sharing of sociocultural environments by twin pairs, especially monozygotic.

However, taken altogether the epidemiological data suggest that genetic factors account for about 40 to 45% of the population variability of blood pressure, common household environment for about 10 to 15%, and nonfamilial factors for the remaining 40 to 45%.

Although determination of familial correlations of blood pressure provides an overall view of the impact of heredity in determining blood pressure, a more relevant measure of the importance of genetic factors in determining susceptibility to hypertension is relative risk. This is the ratio of the risk of an individual developing the condition given its presence in a first-degree relative compared with the overall population risk. For relatively rare monogenetic conditions such as cystic fibrosis, relative risk is as high as 500. For common and complex polygenic disorders, relative risk tends to be much lower. For hypertension, relative risk estimates vary between 2 and 5 depending on the criteria used to define family history. Values are highest when both parents have hypertension before the age of 55 years.

Genes involved in 'essential hypertension'

Given the importance of hypertension as a risk factor for several cardiovascular diseases, a huge effort has been made in the last 20 years to identify genes where variants affect blood pressure and increase risk of hypertension or hypertension-related end-organ damage. Most of the studies have involved association analyses of so-called candidate genes whose products are known, or suspected to, be involved in regulation of blood pressure. A smaller number have used linkage analyses in collections of affected sib pairs to identify genetic loci in a systematic manner. Variants in a large number of genes, involving virtually all the main physiological systems affecting blood pressure such as the renin–angiotensin–aldosterone system (Table 16.17.1.2) and the sympathetic system have shown association with blood pressure in one or more studies. The findings to date suggest that the effect of any individual variant is likely to be modest. For example, a meta-analysis of 32 case–control studies (corresponding to 13 760 patients) of the methionine to threonine (M235T) polymorphism in the angiotensinogen gene, one of the most studied variants, found that the *TT* genotype conferred a 31% increased risk of hypertension compared with the *MM* genotype. There is evidence that variants may act in an additive or epistatic fashion. For example, one prospective study of 678 initially normotensive subjects found that combined carriage of the angiotensin-converting enzyme *DD* genotype (at the insertion (I)/deletion (D) polymorphism in the gene), the tryptophane (Trp) allele at codon 460 in the α-adducin gene, and the *CC* genotype at the −344C/T promoter polymorphism in aldosterone synthase *CC* genotype, increased the risk of developing hypertension by

Table 16.17.1.2 Some genes with evidence for common variants influencing blood pressure or risk of hypertension

Gene	Role
Angiotensinogen	Substrate for renin
Angiotensin converting enzyme	Converts angiotensin 1 to angiotensin I
Angiotensin receptor (type 1)	Main vascular receptor for angiotensin II
Aldosterone synthase	Promotes synthesis of aldosterone
α-Adducin	Cytoskeletal protein involved in sodium homeostasis
G protein β3 subunit	Involved in G-protein signalling

From Cusi D et al. (1997). Polymorphisms of α-adducin and salt sensitivity in patients with essential hypertension. *Lancet*, **349**, 1353–7.

252% over a median follow-up of 9.1 years compared with other genotypes.

The Trp allele of α-adducin, part of a ubiquitous α/β heterodimeric cytoskeletal protein which affects sodium absorption in the kidney, has also been associated with greater blood-pressure-lowering response to thiazide diuretics, and in one study of hypertensive subjects diuretic therapy was associated with a lower risk of combined myocardial infarction or stroke than other antihypertensive therapies in carriers of this adducin variant. Such findings raise the prospect of better prediction and individually tailored treatment for hypertension. However, inconsistent findings between studies reflecting, at least in part, poorly understood gene–gene and gene–environment interactions have hampered progress and significant clinical application so far.

While genetic dissection of essential hypertension has proved challenging, the genetic basis of several monogenic forms of hypertension has been elucidated during the same period. The findings have provided novel and illuminating insights into the molecular regulation of blood pressure and particularly the role of the kidney and sodium homeostasis. See Chapter 16.17.4 for further discussion.

Environmental and lifestyle influences on the development of hypertension

The prevalence of hypertension can be powerfully influenced by local lifestyles and customs. There are a number of lines of evidence that support this conclusion, including studies of migrant populations, comparisons between different communities, prospective population studies, and randomized trials of lifestyle interventions. There is little doubt that the exploding prevalence of hypertension in economically developing regions reflects lifestyle changes, so-called 'Westernistation', more than anything else.

Migrant studies

Migration studies have provided powerful evidence to illustrate the importance of the local environment and lifestyle on the level of blood pressure and the prevalence of hypertension. Studies of migration from rural to urban areas of Africa and Australia typically report marked increases in migrant blood pressure, body weight, and sodium intake, coincident with the adoption of more sedentary lifestyles, usually within months of migration. This latter point is important because it helps discriminate between powerful lifestyle factors and genetics—i.e. the changes in blood pressure are more nurture than nature.

Population studies

Studies of specific populations are often very informative. Populations in specific regions of the world, e.g. primitive rural populations such as the Yanamamo Indians of Brazil, do not show much evidence of an age-related rise in blood pressure, suggesting that the progressive rise in systolic blood pressure seen in urban populations is not inevitable. This could reflect genetic differences in vascular structure in discrete populations, but most likely reflects influence of the local environment, and customs. Evidence in support of this conclusion comes from a classic study which compared Italian nuns with a control group of women from the same town. In the control group, blood pressure typically rose with age, whereas the nuns, from a similar genetic background, showed no such rise in blood pressure over 20 years of follow-up. Thus, essential hypertension is undoubtedly a 'disease of urbanization', reflecting the impact of a number of specific lifestyle factors.

Specific lifestyle influences on blood pressure

The most important lifestyle/environmental influences on blood pressure are sodium intake, obesity, and alcohol intake. Early nutritional deficiency may be important, and recent evidence suggests that psychosocial factors are likely to play some role in the development of essential hypertension. A small socioeconomic gradient of blood pressure has also been observed. Interestingly, this gradient is negative for developed countries and positive for developing countries, which probably reflects the higher prevalence of obesity and higher intakes of alcohol and salt among those of higher socioeconomic status in developing countries, compared to the reverse in more economically developed regions of the world. With regard to dietary influences on blood pressure, recent evidence (discussed later) suggests that diets rich in fruit and vegetables with low total and saturated fats may protect against hypertension. Low calcium intake, although associated with hypertension in population studies, is now considered to play no part in pathogenesis.

Dietary salt intake

There has been vigorous debate about the role of dietary salt in the genesis of hypertension. It is clear that sodium balance is a key factor determining the blood pressure of an individual. Moreover, it is intriguing that the various monogenic forms of hypertension that have been characterized by genetic studies all involve disturbances to renal sodium handling (see Chapter 16.17.4). Review of the evidence from population-based studies and studies of dietary intervention support the hypothesis that dietary sodium intake has an important impact on blood pressure, and recent studies have also highlighted the importance of salt intake in the genesis of hypertension in children and the effectiveness of sodium restriction at reducing blood pressure. That said, there will clearly be some patients whose blood pressure will be more sensitive to dietary sodium intake than others. As indicated in Chapter 16.17.2, dietary sodium restriction forms part of the lifestyle interventions recommended by all guidelines as part of the treatment strategy for hypertension, and to delay the development of hypertension in people with prehypertension.

A related but different question is whether dietary sodium restriction could influence not only blood pressure, but also cardiovascular disease outcomes. Recent studies suggest that this is likely to be the case. People allocated to a sodium restricted diet experienced a 30% lower incidence of cardiovascular events in the next 10–15 years, irrespective of sex, ethnic origin, age, body mass, and blood pressure. As the people randomized into these studies were not hypertensive (blood pressure c.125/85 mmHg) it is conceivable that the benefits, impressive as they are, might have been even greater in a hypertensive population. These findings support current guideline recommendations and underscore the importance of education and national health policies to reduce dietary sodium intake.

Obesity and blood pressure

Fat people generally have higher blood pressures than lean people. Fat arms can lead to overestimation of blood pressure when small cuffs are used, but the relation between body weight and blood pressure persists after correcting for arm circumference. Although body mass index (BMI) is often used to define obesity, visceral adiposity seems to be more important in defining the relationship between blood pressure and obesity. Visceral obesity also increases the likelihood of coexisting 'metabolic syndrome' (see below) in people

with hypertension. In untreated hypertensive people, fat tends to preferentially accumulate intra-abdominally and intrathoracically, and the magnitude of the visceral adiposity is quantitatively related to the blood pressure. Importantly, the adiposity–blood pressure link is observable from early childhood and a key predictor of the likelihood of developing overt hypertension.

Recent analysis of longitudinal data from the Bogalusa Heart Study tracked the association between obesity in childhood and the risk of developing hypertension. Excess adiposity was present in one-fifth of those with normal blood pressure, one-third of those with prehypertension and more than one-half of those with hypertension. Moreover, these associations were evident in people as young as 4 to 11 years, suggesting that the avoidance of obesity could markedly reduce the prevalence of hypertension in middle-aged adults. In support of the strength of the association between BMI and the risk of developing hypertension, in a study of 36 424 Israel Defense Forces employees (mean age c.35 years), BMI was the strongest predictor of prehypertension, with a 10 to 15% increase in risk for every 1 kg/m² increase in BMI. The strong cause and effect relationship between obesity and hypertension has been confirmed by intervention studies showing that weight reduction results in a fall in blood pressure.

Alcohol intake and blood pressure

Epidemiological data have consistently shown an association between alcohol intake and blood pressure, and intervention trials confirm that blood pressure falls when alcohol is withdrawn from heavy drinkers. Analysis of data from the National Health and Nutrition Examination Survey (NHANES) (1999–2000) showed that an alcohol intake of up to two drinks per day had no effect on blood pressure, which is consistent with previous reports that moderate drinking (2–3 units daily) does not appear to exert a pressor effect. Heavier alcohol intakes, patterns of alcohol consumption, and the types of alcohol consumed can also influence blood pressure. Binge drinking can exert a pressor effect, but the mechanism accounting for the pressor effects of alcohol remain undefined. However, whatever the mechanism, data from the WHO Global Burden of Disease survey in 2000 attributed 16% of all hypertensive disease to alcohol.

There has been controversy about whether moderate alcohol consumption might actually reduce cardiovascular disease risk. For example, in a prospective study of almost half a million men and women in the United States of America, the relative risk of death from cardiovascular disease in moderate drinkers compared with nondrinkers was 0.7 for men and 0.6 for women. However, it is important to emphasize that these kind of analyses run the risk of confounding by an unmeasured disease effect modifier that tracks with different patterns of alcohol consumption.

Sleep and blood pressure

Blood pressure characteristically falls during sleep. A recent longitudinal analysis of the first NHANES ($n = 4810$) examined the impact of sleep duration on the risk of developing hypertension. This risk was increased by about twofold in adults in middle age who sleep for less than 5 h each night. Even after adjusting for obesity and diabetes (the risk of which also increase with sleep deprivation), the risk remained around 1.6-fold. There are a number of mechanisms that might account for this relationship: it may simply reflect a longer duration of sympathetic nervous system activation as a consequence of less time asleep and hence a higher 24-h average blood pressure load, giving rise to a higher risk of longer-term cardiovascular structural damage and hence to sustained hypertension.

There is also a clear association between obstructive sleep apnoea and hypertension. An apnoea–hypopnoea index of ≥15 (i.e. breathing decreases or stops ≥15 times per hour of sleep) is associated with a threefold increase in the risk of developing hypertension. Moreover, in such patients continuous positive airway pressure can be effective in lowering both night-time and, to a lesser extent, daytime blood pressure. Doctors should therefore consider sleep deprivation and obstructive sleep apnoea in their assessment of people developing hypertension.

Psychosocial stress and blood pressure

Blood pressure elevation is a well-recognized acute stress response, and the act of taking the blood pressure can increase the systolic by up to 75 mmHg in some patients. However, the role of chronic stress in the pathogenesis of hypertension has been difficult to assess, (1) because of individual variability in the response to stress, (2) because it is difficult to objectively measure chronic stress, and (3) because stress can induce behavioural and lifestyle choices that could influence blood pressure independently of stress *per se*.

One measure of stress that does appear to be robust in predicting blood pressure is an individual's perception of control in their employment. Using ambulatory blood pressure monitoring it has been shown that in men—but not in women—job strain is associated with an elevated blood pressure, both at work and also while at home and during sleep. Job strain in this context was defined as having a highly demanding job, but with the individual having little control over it. By contrast, people employed in equally demanding jobs, but where they have an element of control over their work, have less stress and less elevation of blood pressure. This effect of job strain on blood pressure is independent of other environmental and lifestyle influences, and is as strong as the impact of obesity.

Early origins of hypertension—impact of fetal and infant growth

An associated between low birth weight and risk of developing hypertension and premature cardiovascular disease has been recognized in many epidemiological studies. A large family-based study recently explored the mechanisms underlying the associations of birth weight and gestational age with systolic blood pressure measured at 17 to 19 years of age. This suggested that the inverse associations of birth weight and gestational age with systolic blood pressure are not explained by confounding resulting from a family's socioeconomic status, or other factors that are shared by siblings. Variations in maternal metabolic or vascular health during pregnancy or placental implantation and function may explain these associations. Other studies have suggested that this relationship may relate to fetal programming of increased risk for hypertension via a reduction in nephron number, thereby increasing salt sensitivity. For further discussion of the impact of fetal growth on cardiovascular disease, see Chapter 16.13.3.

Another hypothesis has suggested that increased nutritional support to promote 'catch-up growth' in the immediate postnatal period for babies who are small for gestational age could ameliorate the risk for developing hypertension. This hypothesis was tested in a cohort of small for gestational age babies who had been fed with either a standard or nutrient-enriched (28% more protein than standard) formula after birth. The enriched feed promoted faster postnatal weight gain and was associated with higher (not lower) blood pressure in later childhood, which does not support the promotion of faster weight gain in infants born small for gestational age.

Prehypertension predicts hypertension

The presence of mild elevation in blood pressure for age predicts the likelihood of developing hypertension. In a study of patients with prehypertension (SBP 120–139 mmHg and/or DBP 80–89 mmHg) the annual rate of progression to hypertension (≥140/90 mmHg) was greater than 15% per year despite lifestyle advice. In addition to an elevated blood pressure, people with prehypertension often also have the characteristic metabolic phenotype associated with hypertension (see below) and evidence of endothelial dysfunction and cardiovascular structural damage. This may explain why an analysis of data from the Women's Health Study in the United States of America, involving over 60,000 women followed for 7 years, showed that the presence of prehypertension was associated with an almost doubling in risk of any cardiovascular event—including death, myocardial infarction, stroke, or hospitalization for heart failure—when compared to those with normal blood pressure. Prehypertension was also more common in people with diabetes, when it was associated with an almost fourfold increase in risk of cardiovascular disease when compared to people without diabetes and normal blood pressure.

Kidney, vascular structure, and neurohumoral control systems and the development of hypertension

The maintenance of an adequate mean arterial pressure is fundamental to life, hence there are many homeostatic mechanisms designed to achieve this despite fluctuations in posture, volume status, exercise and other metabolic demands. There is considerable redundancy within these control systems, such that inhibition of one system is compensated for by increased activity of another, which is important when considering the design of effective strategies to lower blood pressure.

Kidney

The kidney is important for blood pressure regulation via two key mechanisms (1) the regulation of sodium and volume homeostasis, and (2) the regulation of the activity of the renin–angiotensin–aldosterone system. The transplantation of a kidney from a genetically hypertensive rat into a normotensive control rat results in the development of hypertension in the recipient, and the converse is also true. In humans, significant renal impairment is invariably associated with hypertension, which in large part relates to disturbances in sodium handling, and as stated previously almost all of the single gene defects resulting in the development of hypertension involve disturbances in the renal tubular handling of sodium (see Chapter 16.17.4).

The kidney is also intimately involved with sensing and setting of blood pressure via the activity of the renin–angiotensin–aldosterone system. Reduced renal perfusion pressure (e.g. in renal artery stenosis) results in activation of the renin–angiotensin–aldosterone system, which in turn elevates blood pressure to try and restore renal perfusion pressure via a number of mechanisms (see below).

Structure of small arteries

A characteristic finding in essential hypertension is an inappropriate increase in peripheral vascular resistance relative to the cardiac output. The main site of this resistance is small arteries (arterioles), which undergo inward eutrophic remodelling that is characterized by an increase in their media/lumen ratio. These changes result from vascular remodelling, i.e. rearrangement of existing material in the vascular media around a smaller lumen, and there is often also evidence of some hypertrophy and/or hyperplasia of the resident myocytes.

There has been much debate about whether these changes in small artery structure antedate and thus contribute to the development of hypertension, and/or whether they are the consequence of an elevated blood pressure and the trophic effects of neurohumoral activation (i.e. sympathetic nervous system and the renin–angiotensin–aldosterone system) in people with hypertension. Whatever the mechanism, recent studies of small arteries isolated from biopsies in humans, or retinal vascular structural changes (especially narrowing), suggest that the magnitude of structural changes of the small arteries is strongly predictive of future cardiovascular events. It is also predictive of the likelihood and magnitude of structural changes elsewhere, i.e. left ventricular hypertrophy.

Structure of large arteries

The functional integrity of large conduit arteries, i.e. the aorta, also influences the development of hypertension, especially systolic hypertension. The pulsatile nature of blood flow exerts chronic cyclical stress on the walls of these arteries, and over time this results in deterioration in their elastic properties as a consequence of thinning, splitting, and fragmentation of the elastin fibres within the media. This process is accelerated in people with hypertension, resulting in progressive dilatation in aortic root diameter and arterial stiffening. In turn, this reduction in arterial compliance increases pulse wave velocity, increases systolic pressure and central aortic pulse pressure, and reduces diastolic pressure. This explains the very high prevalence of systolic hypertension with advancing age (see Fig. 16.17.1.2) and the progressive age-related disappearance of diastolic hypertension.

The process of age-related stiffening of the aorta is accelerated by post-translational modification of vascular wall proteins such as collagen by the formation of advanced glycation end products (AGEs). AGE formation is accelerated in people with diabetes, thereby explaining the earlier onset of isolated systolic hypertension in patients with this condition. It is conceivable that if aortic function and especially its elasticity were genetically determined, then accelerated degeneration of aortic elastic function could also be a factor in the development of systolic hypertension in younger people. Aside from aortic function, there is current debate about whether the diameter of the aortic root is causally related to the likelihood of developing hypertension. This has been prompted by recent observations that central aortic pulse pressure appears to be inversely related to aortic root diameter, prompting speculation that a smaller effective root diameter might also contribute to the development of hypertension.

Endothelium

The endothelium plays a key role in the regulation of vascular tone. Endothelial cells form nitric oxide (NO) from L-arginine via the activity of nitric oxide synthase (eNOS), which is tonically activated by shear stress and relaxes vascular tone. NO also inhibits platelet aggregation and inhibits vascular smooth muscle cell proliferation. Hypertension, even in its earliest stages, has been associated with 'endothelial dysfunction', usually by demonstrating a reduction in forearm blood flow in response to agents that promote NO release such as acetyl choline or its mimetics. NO production has also been shown to be decreased in people with hypertension.

It is not clear whether endothelial dysfunction and decreased NO production are a cause or consequence of an elevated blood pressure, but the latter seems most likely. Whatever the mechanism, a reduction in NO production would be expected to increase vascular tone and may also contribute to vascular proliferation and remodelling (see above). NO-donors such as glyceryl trinitrate (GTN) are very effective at lowering blood pressure in the acute setting, and are especially effective at reducing central aortic pressure. However, the use of NO-donors to lower blood pressure outside of the acute setting has been bedevilled by their short duration of action and the fact that tolerance to them develops rapidly. The actions of some commonly used antihypertensive drugs, i.e. ACE inhibitors and angiotensin receptor blockers (ARBs), have in part been attributed to their local potentiation of NO.

The endothelium also produces a powerful vasoconstrictor, endothelin. This seems less important in the chronic regulation of blood pressure, even though inhibitors of endothelin have been shown to lower it. The biology and actions of NO and endothelin are discussed in greater detail elsewhere (Chapter 16.1.1).

Oxidative stress

Numerous studies in experimental animals and humans have indicated that hypertension is associated with markers of increased systemic oxidative stress, i.e. the increased production of oxygen free radicals such as superoxide and hydrogen peroxide. These are short-lived reactive species that have the potential to cause cellular damage via oxidation of proteins, lipids and DNA. They also react with and inactivate NO, thereby providing a mechanism for reduced NO levels and increased vascular tone. The mechanism for increased oxidative stress in hypertension is not known, but studies have suggested that this may in part relate to activation of NADH/NADPH oxidase within vascular cells. Of interest, this vascular oxidase is activated by angiotensin II, which provides a link between the renin–angiotensin–aldosterone system and endothelial dysfunction and may contribute to the pressor effect of angiotensin II.

Renin–angiotensin–aldosterone system

The renin–angiotensin–aldosterone system, whose main effector molecules are angiotensin II and aldosterone, plays an important role in the regulation of blood pressure via a number of mechanisms. Angiotensin II is produced by an enzymatic cascade (Fig. 16.17.1.8). Renin—the rate-limiting step for the production of angiotensin II—may be synthesized in a number of tissues apart from the kidney, including the adrenal, heart, the blood vessel wall, and brain. In the kidney it is produced by the juxtaglomerular apparatus in response to falls in renal perfusion pressure, sodium depletion, and increased sympathetic nerve activity. However, the renin–angiotensin–aldosterone system is active both in the circulation and locally within tissues.

The two principle angiotensin receptors are AT1 and AT2. The major actions of angiotensin II are via the AT1 receptor, which is the target for the ARB class of blood-pressure-lowering agents. The AT2 receptor is less ubiquitously expressed than the AT1 receptor, is markedly up-regulated during tissue repair, and its activation produces effects that appear to oppose those of AT1 activation, suggesting that the two receptors may operate a Yin–Yang relationship.

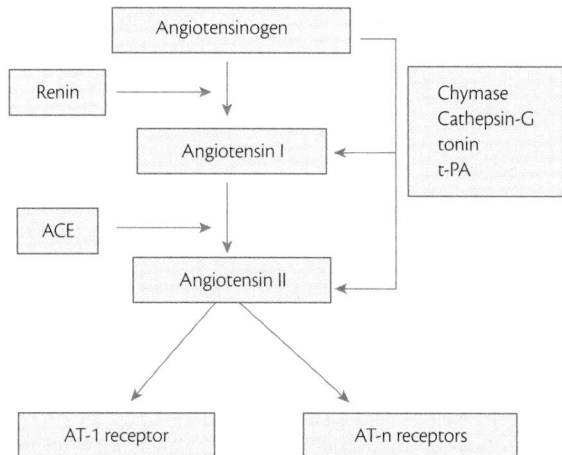

Fig. 16.17.1.8 The renin–angiotensin system. The enzyme renin cleaves its substrate angiotensinogen to generate the decapeptide angiotensin I, which is then cleaved by angiotensin converting enzyme (ACE) to generate angiotensin II, which binds to a family of specific angiotensin receptors. Its main effect on blood pressure regulation is via the AT-1 receptor, the functions of other angiotensin receptors (AT-n) being poorly defined. Angiotensin II can also be generated by other proteolytic enzyme systems such as chymases and tissue plasminogen activators (t-PA). These pathways may be important for local angiotensin II generation in disease.

Angiotensin II elevates blood pressure by a number of different mechanisms: (1) it is a direct pressor agent promoting vasoconstriction, and it also increases superoxide production by the endothelium, which reduces NO availability (see above); (2) it increases sodium reabsorption by the kidney via direct tubular effects and via simulation of aldosterone release from the adrenal cortex; (3) it can have trophic effects on vascular cell growth and has been implicated in the small artery remodelling process that results in increased peripheral vascular resistance; (4) it acts centrally on AT1 receptors in the nucleus tractus solitaris to desensitize the afferent component of the baroreceptor reflex.

In addition to these pressor actions, angiotensin II has also been implicated in the development of end-organ damage through (1) trophic effects on the myocardium, resulting in left ventricular hypertrophy; (2) the development of glomerular hypertension, albuminuria and interstitial fibrosis, leading to chronic renal disease; (3) pro-oxidant effects, contributing to the development of atherosclerosis. Consequently, the renin–angiotensin–aldosterone system has become a popular target for drug therapy to lower blood pressure and limit its cardiovascular consequences.

Aldosterone is the other effector molecule of the renin–angiotensin–aldosterone system. It is produced by the adrenal cortex in response to many stimuli, including sodium and volume depletion, angiotensin II, excess potassium intake, trauma and stress. It acts on the distal tubule of the kidney to promote sodium absorption in exchange for potassium. An inappropriate increase in production of aldosterone can lead to the development of hypertension (e.g. Conn's syndrome and adrenal hyperplasia), as discussed in Chapter 16.17.3.

The specific role of the renin–angiotensin–aldosterone system in the development of essential hypertension remains unclear, although therapeutic agents that inhibit this system have proved to be very effective treatments. Plasma renin levels vary widely in essential hypertension, from low (30%), to normal (50%), to high (20%): they are inversely related to sodium loading and tend to decline with ageing. Thus patients with low renin levels are generally older and have volume-dependent hypertension. Hypertensive patients with higher renin levels are generally younger, and their increased renin may reflect increased levels of sympathetic nervous system activity (see below). Blacks at any age have a high prevalence of low renin hypertension, suggesting a primary role for sodium retention in the pathogenesis of their hypertension. Although the baseline renin level is rarely measured in routine clinical practice, age has been used as a surrogate in the recent hypertension guidelines in the United Kingdom for predicting the most effective initial therapy in people with essential hypertension. If plasma renin levels are measured, it is important to recognize that they can be affected by concomitant blood-pressure-lowering therapy, with almost all commonly used classes of antihypertensive drugs increasing plasma renin, the main exception being β-blockers which suppress plasma renin.

Sympathetic nervous system

The sympathetic nervous system is involved in the acute and chronic regulation of blood pressure. It is known to be involved in the regulation of arteriolar resistance, cardiac output and volume regulation, renin release by the kidney, and catecholamine and mineralocorticoid release by the adrenal gland. It is by necessity a complex system that involves (1) vasomotor control centres within the brain; (2) the peripheral nervous system providing efferent and afferent signals, and (3) the adrenal medulla. Several nuclei within the central nervous system are involved in the regulation of blood pressure, with control integrated in the rostral ventrolateral nucleus of the medulla oblongata—the vasomotor centre—that is particularly influenced by the nucleus tractus solitarius (NTS) which receives its input from peripheral afferents such as baroreceptor activation in the aortic arch, carotid sinus, and cardiac ventricles and atria. The NTS also receives excitatory and inhibitory inputs from other regions of the brain, i.e. the brain stem and cortex, and its outputs to the vasomotor centre tend to inhibit sympathetic outflow and thus buffer acute rises in blood pressure—the baroreceptor reflex arc. Another important influence on the rostral ventrolateral nucleus–NTS complex is the action of angiotensin II. The area postrema in the floor of the IV ventricle does not have a blood–brain barrier, which allows circulating angiotensin II to blunt the inhibitory effect of the NTS on the rostral ventrolateral nucleus, thereby increasing central sympathetic outflow. The various inputs and outputs are summarized in Fig. 16.17.1.9.

Environmental and behavioural impacts on blood pressure are primarily coordinated via the hypothalamus. The posterolateral hypothalamus is responsible for the classical 'flight or flight' response, and lesions in this area reduce blood pressure. By contrast, lesions in the anterior hypothalamus can substantially increase blood pressure.

The peripheral vascular α-adrenergic system (α_1 receptors) is also important in maintaining enhanced vascular resistance in hypertension, with some studies suggesting that peripheral α-adrenergic responsiveness might be especially enhanced in blacks with hypertension.

The importance of the sympathetic nervous system in the regulation of blood pressure is beyond question, but a key unanswered question is whether disturbances to the regulation of the sympathetic nervous system play a major role in the initiation

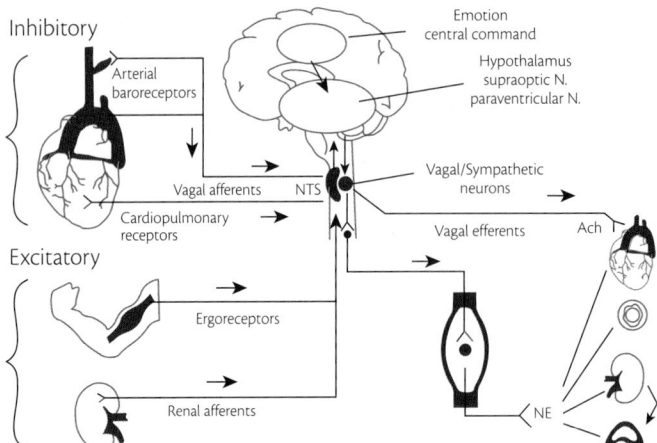

Fig. 16.17.1.9 Organization of the nervous system control of blood pressure. Peripheral inhibitory and excitatory inputs are integrated in the nucleus tractus solitarius (NTS), whose central inputs are integrated via the hypothalamus. The NTS regulates sympathetic outflow via the rostral centrolateral nuclei of the medulla oblongata. The balance of sympathetic and vagal outflow influences cardiac output, heart rate, vasoconstrictor tone, renin release, and renal blood flow, also catecholamine and mineralocorticoid release via the (From Abboud FM (1982).

Adapted from Abboud F.M. The sympathetic system in hypertension. State-of-the-art review. Hypertension, 1982; 4 (Suppl II); 208-225. (http://hyper.ahajournals.org/cgi/content/abstract/4/3/208).

and maintenance of chronic essential hypertension. Most surveys of younger people with prehypertension or stage 1 hypertension indicate the presence of an elevated heart rate, indicative of sympathetic nervous system activation. Other studies have reported elevated circulating catecholamine levels in young patients with prehypertension, and that such elevations predict the risk of developing hypertension. Further studies have used radiolabelled norepinephrine to demonstrate enhanced 'spillover' indicative of enhanced sympathetic nervous system activity, or microneurography to demonstrate increased sympathetic nervous system activity in young hypertensives. It must be emphasized, however, that simple demonstration of enhanced activity of a particular system at a single snap shot in time cannot be taken as evidence of a direct causal role—the critical question is whether the level of activity is appropriate or inappropriate in the context of the overall integrated physiological regulation of blood pressure. In this regard, a full understanding of the role of the sympathetic nervous system in the genesis of essential hypertension in humans has been hindered by the complexity of the system under study and the rather crude instruments used to evaluate the system *in vivo*. Some remain to be convinced of the importance of the sympathetic nervous system in the genesis of essential hypertension, while others argue that given the importance of the sympathetic nervous system in regulating blood pressure, then—even if essential hypertension has an unrelated aetiology—abnormal activity of the sympathetic nervous system must be permissive in maintaining blood pressure elevation.

Sympathetic nervous system, obesity, and the metabolic syndrome

Obesity is associated with increased muscle sympathetic nerve activity, and increased sympathetic nervous system activity has been implicated in the pathogenesis of obesity-related hypertension. Hypertension is often associated with features of a metabolic syndrome (see below) characterized by insulin resistance, dyslipidaemia, and impaired glucose tolerance. Increased sympathetic nervous system activity has also been implicated in the development of this syndrome, and drugs therapies that reduce central sympathetic outflow or block α_1 adrenergic receptors improve insulin sensitivity and features of the metabolic syndrome.

Natriuretic peptides

The natriuretic peptide system—including atrial natriuretic peptide (ANP), brain natriuretic peptide (BNP), and C-type natriuretic peptide (CNP)—is an endocrine system that is involved in the regulation of salt and water homeostasis. ANP is secreted primarily by the right atrium in response to atrial wall stretch. BNP was initially identified in the brain (hence the name), but is predominantly produced in the ventricles in response to stretch. CNP is produced by vascular endothelial cells and in the kidney. These natriuretic peptides bind to specific cell membrane receptors on target tissues and induce natriuresis and diuresis; they also decrease renin secretion and aldosterone, and induce vasodilatation and a modest fall in blood pressure. These physiological actions suggested a potential role for reduced natriuretic peptide levels or action in the pathogenesis of hypertension, hence these have been measured in patients with essential hypertension. The results have been conflicting, with no clear pattern emerging. This in part reflects the fact that levels of natriuretic peptides, especially BNP, will be elevated in people with early or established left ventricular dysfunction and other hypertension related complications, but it does not preclude a future role for drugs that augment the activity of natriuretic peptides in the clinical management of hypertension.

The hypertensive phenotype and target organ damage in hypertension

Although blood pressure measurement is used to define hypertension, hypertension is more than just blood pressure. Essential hypertension is commonly associated with metabolic disturbances and multisystem structural damage that conspire to enhance cardiovascular risk beyond that which can be attributed to blood pressure alone.

Hypertension and the metabolic syndrome

Few people with essential hypertension simply have an elevated blood pressure: many also have associated disturbances in metabolism which are typical of the 'insulin resistance phenotype', notably predisposition to impaired glucose tolerance, elevated triglyceride levels, reduced HDL-cholesterol values, and hyperuricaemia. These metabolic disturbances appear to precede and may even predict the likelihood of developing hypertension: in large prospective population studies in the United States of America and Europe the development of hypertension could be predicted by a person's initial metabolic profile. Even in those with optimal initial blood pressure levels (<120/80 mmHg), increasing obesity and the aforementioned abnormal lipid profile were major predictors of the development of hypertension.

With regard to obesity, the accumulation of visceral fat (i.e. abdominal obesity) is most strongly associated with hypertension and attendant metabolic disturbances. Indeed, the link between visceral fat content and indices of insulin resistance and metabolic syndrome is demonstrable even in lean patients when MRI is used to quantify visceral fat. Moreover, the link between visceral adiposity and blood pressure is present from early childhood and explains the approximately two-fold increase in risk of developing type 2 diabetes in patients with essential hypertension.

The frequent coexistence of obesity with other features of metabolic syndrome in patients with hypertension underscores the need to view hypertension as more than just blood pressure in the context of cardiovascular disease risk management, and it points to the importance of early lifestyle interventions as the foundation for prevention and treatment.

Vascular structural changes and atherosclerosis

Aorta and large arteries

The arterial system is designed to convert the pulsatile flow generated by cardiac contraction into steady flow in the capillary bed. Thus the aorta is both a conduit and an elastic reservoir designed to buffer pulsatile blood flow. Over time, recurrent pulsatile stress produces uncoiling, disruption and calcification of elastic fibres within the aortic wall. At the same time, relatively inelastic collagen is increased and made more rigid by post translational modification by the accumulation of advanced glcyation end products (AGEs). Such age-related processes cause loss of the normal elastic reservoir function of the aorta and other large arteries. These changes are accelerated by the presence of high blood pressure and hence occur at an earlier age in hypertensive patients.

In addition to these structural changes, elevation in pressure itself contributes to a loss of large artery compliance and buffering because, as pressure increases, the elastic fibres become fully stretched, thereby transferring load-bearing function to the relatively inelastic collagen fibres. As a result of these changes, the pressure wave generated by left ventricular contraction is no longer buffered by the aorta and proximal large arteries, but instead is transmitted into the arterial tree with greater amplitude. This is manifested clinically as increased brachial pulse pressure, with higher systolic and lower diastolic pressures. More importantly, the resulting increase in pulse wave velocity and changes in arterial haemodynamics contribute to an elevation in central aortic systolic and pulse pressures and an increase in ventricular loading conditions—changes that cannot always be appreciated by measurement of the brachial blood pressure alone.

Increased large artery stiffening and reduced compliance also reduces the sensitivity of the carotid and aortic baroceptors to stretch, which blunts the normal rapid buffering of changes in blood pressure. As a result, blood pressure becomes more labile and the circulatory adaptation to acute changes, i.e. postural, may become impaired, producing symptoms of postural dizziness in older people.

Resistance vessels

The characteristic structural change in the smaller arteries and arterioles of hypertensive patients is an increase in wall/lumen ratio, the characteristics and pathogenesis of which have been discussed above. These changes have important functional consequences. The vessels can still dilate in response to stimuli such as warmth or drugs, but maximal vasodilatation is reduced. The converse is also true; responsiveness to pressor agents or stimuli becomes enhanced. These structural changes in resistance vessels also contribute to the characteristic increase in vascular resistance in hypertension, and they render vital organs more susceptible to ischaemic damage at the small vessel level, e.g. small vessel ischaemic brain damage.

Atheroma in hypertension

Hypertension is associated with an increased risk of generalized atherosclerotic disease. This is likely to result from an interplay of many factors, including pressure and haemodynamic stress, metabolic disturbances, inflammatory and oxidative stresses, endothelial disturbances, neurohumoral activation, and many other factors.

The overwhelming importance of haemodynamic factors and pressure is illustrated by (1) the predilection for atheroma to develop at sites of increased haemodynamic stress within the circulation, i.e. arterial bifurcations; and (2) the fact that atheroma is rarely observed in a low pressure circulation, i.e. the pulmonary circulation or venous system (unless pulmonary hypertension develops, or veins are grafted into the arterial circulation). Two recent studies have been important in establishing a direct link between pressure and the development and/or regression of atherosclerosis. Using a mouse genetically prone to develop atheroma, the placement of a suprarenal clip was used to generate aortic constriction (a high renin state) and hypertension. Atheromatous plaque area was greatly increased by the presence of hypertension and was not obviously ameliorated by administration of angiotensin receptor blockade. This study therefore suggested that pressure and not activation of the renin–angiotensin–aldosterone system was the main cause of accelerated atheroma in this model. Further data from a human study that used intravascular ultrasonography to quantify changes in coronary atheroma suggested that the patients' in-trial blood pressure determined whether there was progression, stabilization or regression of atheromatous plaque over a 2-year period. Thus, a large body of evidence supports the hypothesis that blood pressure plays a key role in the initiation and progression of atheroma in humans. It is also likely that haemodynamic stress plays an important role in the process of plaque rupture, as well as the plaque burden.

The heart in hypertension

Left ventricular hypertrophy is a classic feature of untreated, or inadequately treated, long-standing hypertension. In this regard it can be considered the hypertensive equivalent of the glycated Hb_{Alc} for patients with diabetes: it is an index of the prevailing blood pressure load. Left ventricular hypertrophy is demonstrable in about 50% of untreated hypertensive patients using echocardiography, but only 5 to 10% when using conventional ECG criteria (Sokolov–Lyon or Cornell duration product). Pressure load on the left ventricle is unquestionably the most important pathogenic factor, with ambulatory monitoring blood pressure measurements much better correlated with left ventricular hypertrophy than clinic measurements of pressure. Pressure load is compounded by stiffening of the aorta with ageing, but neurohumoral factors, including the activity of the sympathetic nervous system and renin–angiotensin–aldosterone system, also appear to be important.

Left ventricular hypertrophy is a very potent predictor of premature cardiovascular disease and death. Its presence on the ECG, especially when associated with a characteristic 'strain pattern' (see Chapter 16.3.1), is associated with a two- to threefold increase in risk of cardiovascular disease morbidity and mortality, including a marked increased risk of stroke and heart failure. Using echocardiography to characterize left ventricular hypertrophy, recent studies suggest that concentric hypertrophy carries a worse prognosis that eccentric hypertrophy (Fig. 16.17.1.10).

Pathological features

There are two pathological features of the cardiac changes in hypertension that culminate in the development of left ventricular hypertrophy: an increase in size of cardiomyocytes, which increases the muscular mass of the left ventricle, and an increase in extracellular matrix deposition within the ventricle, which contributes to an increase in wall stiffness. The increase in left ventricular mass and stiffness manifests initially as impaired relaxation during diastole, which is often detectable on echocardiography in hypertensive patients at diagnosis, even before the left ventricular mass is sufficiently increased to be classified as indicating hypertrophy. Over time, in untreated or poorly treated patients, cardiac changes will progress to impaired systolic function and ultimately overt heart failure.

Myocardial ischaemia

In addition to impaired cardiac diastolic and systolic function, the hypertensive heart is also predisposed to myocardial ischaemia

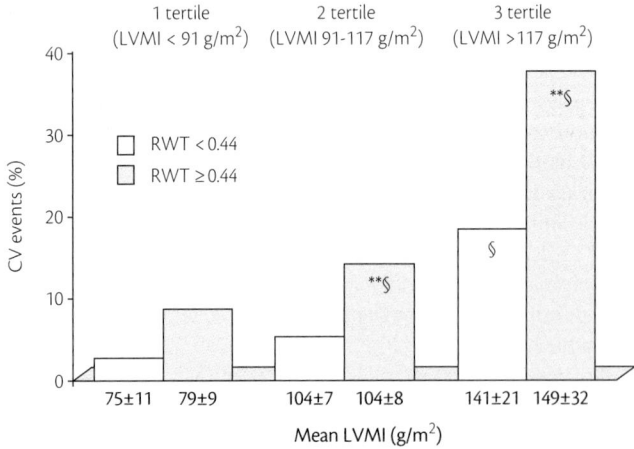

Fig. 16.17.1.10 Concentric vs eccentric left ventricular hypertrophy and cardiovascular risk in hypertensive patients. All patients had echocardiographic evidence of left ventricular hypertrophy (LVH), concentric LVH being defined according to the relative wall thickness (RWT), i.e. LVH + RWT greater than or equal to 0.44 was defined as concentric LVH. Cardiovascular events increased progressively per LVH tertile at follow-up, and were greater in each tertile of LVH in those with concentric LVH. CV, cardiovascular; LVMI, left ventricular mass index.
Data from Lorenza M, et al, Hypertension 2004.

because of (1) increased myocardial oxygen consumption due to increased cardiac afterload, (2) impaired endocardial blood flow due to the structural and functional changes in small arteries described above, (3) an increase in the systolic time interval and reduced diastolic filling time and pressures due to large artery stiffening and impaired ventricular–vascular coupling, and (4) increased risk of coronary atheroma in people with hypertension.

Cardiac arrhythmias

The aforementioned structural and ischaemic changes also predispose to an increased prevalence of simple and complex ventricular arrhythmias in people with hypertensive left ventricular hypertrophy. In addition, it has recently become recognized that atrial fibrillation is much commoner in older people with hypertension. Moreover, in hypertensive patients with left ventricular hypertrophy the risk of developing atrial fibrillation is at least twofold greater, and increases further as a function of advancing age, increased systolic pressure, increased left ventricular mass, and increased left atrial diameter. The combination of these latter two cardiac features is a particularly potent predictor of the risk of developing atrial fibrillation in hypertensive patients.

Regression of left ventricular hypertrophy

Recent clinical studies suggest that inhibition of the renin–angiotensin–aldosterone system is particularly effective at regressing left ventricular hypertrophy. This is important, because there is now clear evidence that regression of the ECG manifestations of left ventricular hypertrophy is associated with dramatically improved prognosis for people with hypertension (50% reduction in risk of cardiovascular death over 5 years). Moreover, blockade of the renin–angiotensin–aldosterone system may be particularly effective at reducing the risk of developing atrial fibrillation in people with hypertensive left ventricular hypertrophy. Consensus in guidelines is that blood pressure lowering is of paramount importance for patients with left ventricular hypertrophy, but that effective renin–angiotensin–aldosterone system blockade should also be part of the treatment strategy.

The brain and hypertension

Hypertension is the single most important risk factor for stroke and is increasingly recognized as a major factor contributing to the rate of cognitive decline in later life. All categories of stroke—ischaemic (large and small vessel), haemorrhagic, and embolic—are increased in hypertensive patients.

Cerebral (atherothrombotic) infarction

Infarction accounts for about 80% of the strokes suffered by patients with hypertension. It is usually attributable to atheroma of one of the larger cerebral arteries (usually the middle cerebral artery), or to small vessel (lacunar) infarction. Although poorly characterized, it is likely that embolic stroke is also more common in people with hypertension, especially those with left ventricular hypertrophy, because of the increased likelihood of paroxysmal or sustained atrial fibrillation on a background of increased left atrial size.

Intracerebral haemorrhage

This accounts for 10 to 15% of strokes in patients with hypertension and is usually the result of rupture of a small intracerebral degenerative microaneurysm (Charcot–Bouchard aneurysm).

These lesions develop in the small ($<200\,\mu m$ diameter) perforating arteries in the region of the basal ganglia, thalamus, and internal capsule. Hyaline degeneration (lipohyalinosis) occurs in the aneurysmal wall, with a defect in the media at the neck of the aneurysm. The incidence of Charcot–Bouchard aneurysms is closely correlated with age and blood pressure, the two factors acting additively so that lesions are rarely if ever seen in younger normotensive people. The relationship between blood pressure and haemorrhagic stroke appears to be steeper in people of Chinese Asian origin.

The remaining strokes in hypertensive patients are due to subarachnoid haemorrhage. Transient ischaemic attacks due to disease of extracranial vessels are also more frequent in hypertensive subjects.

Hypertension and cognitive function

Hypertension is increasingly recognized as an important cause of dementia, with increased blood pressure in mid life associated with an increased risk of dementia in later life. Cognitive decline is related to diffuse small vessel cerebrovascular disease in untreated hypertension and in older patients. Functional imaging studies have shown relative reductions in blood flow in parietal and forebrain areas in hypertensive patients during memory tasks and areas of cortical and subcortical hypometabolism. More advanced vascular disease gives rise to multiple, punctate, hyperintense white matter lesions on MRI scanning. These are due to focal ischaemia, either as a result of lipohyalinosis or microatheromatous disease, tortuosity, and narrowing of the perforating arteries. All degrees of impairment of cognitive performance may occur as a result of these lesions, ranging from effects only detectable with sensitive psychometric testing, to lacunar strokes and Binswanger's disease.

Hypertensive encephalopathy

The brain is protected from wide fluctuations in blood pressure by blood flow autoregulation, i.e. the intrinsic capacity of the cerebral vessels to constrict in the face of increased pressure and dilate in the face of decreased pressure to maintain a constant flow. Resistance vessel remodelling and hypertrophy may enhance protection against higher perfusion pressures, thereby extending the upper limits of the autoregulatory range in long-standing hypertension. However, such remodelling may also impair the autoregulation of blood flow when faced with decreased pressure because of impaired capacity of hypertrophied resistance vessels to dilate, thereby predisposing to small vessel ischaemia. In severe hypertension focal areas of vasodilatation can develop if blood pressure rises above the autoregulatory range, resulting in localized perivascular oedema and fibrinoid necrosis. Focal haemorrhages, ischaemia, and infarction may result, giving rise to the clinical picture of encephalopathy (see Chapter 16.17.5).

The kidney in hypertension

Patients with renal disease often have hypertension, and people with hypertension can develop renal disease. The age-related decline in GFR is more rapid in people with essential hypertension. However, GFR is usually well preserved throughout life in patients with mild to moderate essential hypertension, hence the development of endstage renal disease in such patients is unusual in the absence of any other renal lesions. The decline in GFR, when it does occur, is due to progressive glomerulosclerosis, most likely driven by raised intraglomerular capillary pressures, which also explain the increased urinary albumin excretion rates in these patients.

Increased urinary albumin excretion rate has in turn been linked to increased likelihood of more widespread endothelial/vascular dysfunction and an increased risk of premature cardiovascular disease and death, hence the kidney—and urinary albumin excretion rate in particular—has been proposed as the earliest clinical indicator of significant pressure mediated vascular injury.

Significant hypertension-induced glomerulosclerosis is much more likely in two settings (1) severe and accelerated hypertension, resulting in so-called hypertensive nephropathy; and (2) in the presence of intrinsic renal disease, i.e. due to diabetes or glomerulonephritis. Effective control of blood pressure is of substantial importance in retarding the progression of renal impairment in these settings.

Another important association between hypertension and renal disease is atheromatous renal vascular disease. In these patients, hypertension is usually moderate to severe, and the condition is characteristically associated with a progressive ischaemic nephropathy due either to proximal renal artery (often ostial) disease and/or smaller branch artery disease. It may be associated with small vessel cholesterol embolization, the affected patients usually being older, with evidence of widespread atheromatous disease.

The eye in hypertension

The findings in the retina of patients with hypertension range from mild generalized retinal–arteriolar narrowing, through to the development of more significant changes of flame-shaped or blot-shaped haemorrhages, cottonwool spots, hard exudates, microaneurysms, or a combination of all of these factors. Swelling of the optic disc can also be seen. The classification of these changes and their pathophysiology and significance are discussed in Chapter 16.17.2.

The evolution of hypertensive injury—from physiology to philosophy

The process of hypertensive injury to target organs evolves silently over many years, the magnitude and rate of progression determined largely by the level of blood pressure, but also by individual susceptibility (Fig. 16.17.1.11). In the prehypertensive phase, patients may already have disturbances in blood pressure regulation, i.e. responses to pressor stimuli, visceral obesity, and subtle features of the metabolic syndrome. The injurious process and metabolic disturbances then progress though a silent phase, often lasting many years, during which there is subtle damage to many target organs as cited above, i.e. vascular wall, myocardium, brain, kidney, and eye. This subtle early damage is potentially preventable and/or reversible, but progresses if untreated to more sinister markers of more advanced damage—the so-called intermediate or surrogate disease markers that can be detected in many cases by simple tests such as the ECG, or urinalysis for albumin or protein. Untreated or poorly treated, this progressive hypertension-mediated damage culminates in overt cardiovascular, renal, and cerebrovascular disease and clinical events—the so-called 'hard clinical endpoints' that form the evidence base for treatment guidelines. Alongside, the metabolic syndrome is evolving, increasing the risk of developing diabetes and magnifying the cardiovascular risk burden associated with the blood pressure elevation. Along the way, the conduit arteries are stiffening with damage and age, and the systolic pressure is rising and becoming more difficult to treat.

Current treatment guidelines have been developed from an evidence base relating to changes in hard clinical endpoints derived

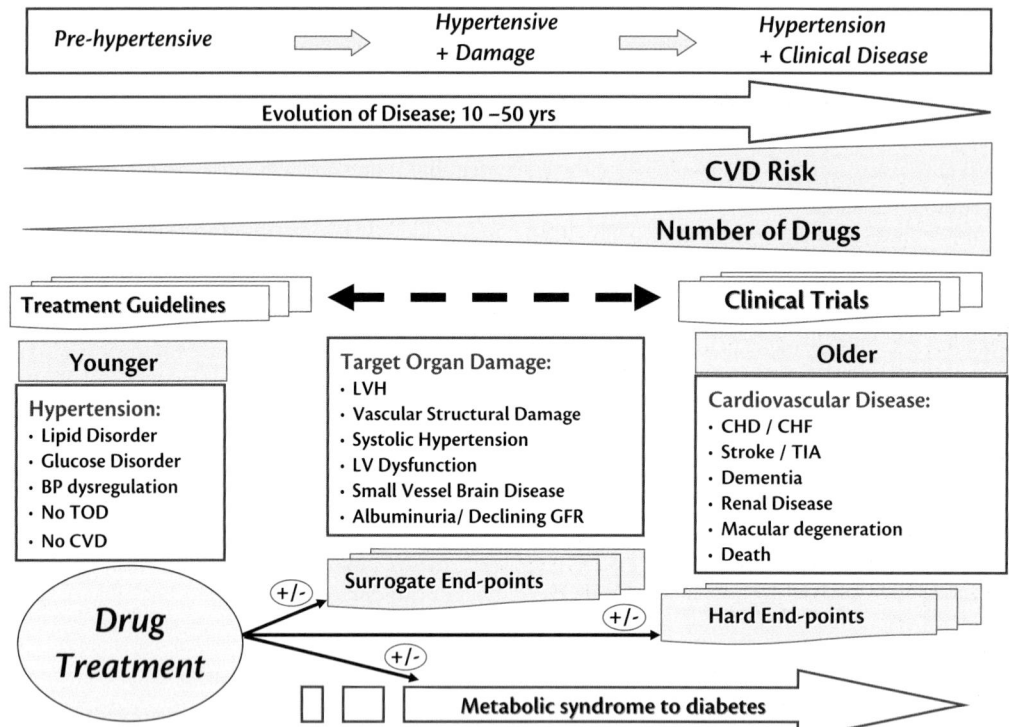

Fig. 16.17.1.11 The clinical progression of hypertension. BP, blood pressure; CHD, coronary heart disease; CHF, congestive heart failure; CVD, cardiovascular disease; GFR, glomerular filtration rate; LV, left ventricular; TIA, transient ischaemic attack; TOD, target organ damage.

from studies in very elderly patients at the end of the hypertensive disease process. Somehow, we have to try to translate that evidence into strategies for treating younger patients at the start of the disease process when their risk of clinical events is low. Future treatment strategies must surely focus on preventing the evolution of the silent disease process, rather than simply battling with its consequences. To meet that challenge, we need more and better studies of younger patients with hypertension to better characterize the impact of treatments on the evolution of hypertensive disease, and to determine the robustness of the associated intermediate or surrogate disease markers at predicting treatment benefit.

Further reading

Epidemiology

Asia Pacific Cohort Studies Collaboration (APCSC) (2005). Joint effects of systolic blood pressure and serum cholesterol on cardiovascular disease in the Asia Pacific region. *Circulation*, **112**, 3384–90.

Chobanian AV (2007). Isolated systolic hypertension in the elderly. *N Engl J Med*, **357**, 789–96.

Ezzati M, *et al.* (2002). Selected major risk factors and global and regional burden of disease. *Lancet*, **360**, 1347–60.

Franklin SS, *et al.* (1997). Hemodynamic patterns of age-related changes in blood pressure: the Framingham Heart Study. *Circulation*, **96**, 308–15.

Lawes CMM, *et al.* (2006). Blood pressure and the global burden of disease 2000. Part I: estimates of blood pressure levels. *J Hypertens*, **24**, 413–22.

Lawes CMM, Vander Horn S, Rodgers A (2008). Global burden of blood pressure related disease, 2001. *Lancet*, **371**, 1513–18.

Lewington S, *et al.* (2002). Age-specific relevance of usual blood pressure to vascular mortality: a meta-analysis of individual data for one million adults in 61 prospective studies. *Lancet*, **360**, 1903–13.

MacMahonS, Meal B, Rodgers A (2005). Hypertension—time to move on. *Lancet*, **365**, 1108–9.

Staessen JA, *et al.* (2003). Cardiovascular prevention and blood pressure reduction: a quantitative overview updated until 1st March 2003. *J Hypertens*, **21**, 1055–76.

Vasan RS, *et al.* (2001). Impact of high-normal blood pressure on the risk of cardiovascular disease. *New Engl J Med*, **345**, 1291–7.

Wang Y, Wang QJ (2004). The prevalence of prehypertension and hypertension among US adults according to the new joint national committee guidelines: new challenges of the old problem. *Arch Intern Med*, **164**, 2126–34.

William B, Lindholm LH, Sever PS (2008). Systolic pressure is all that matters. *Lancet*, **371**, 2219–21.

Yusuf S, *et al.* (2004). Effect of potentially modifiable risk factors associated with myocardial infarction in 52 countries (the INTERHEART study): case-control study. *Lancet*, **364**, 937–52.

Pathophysiology

Aksnesa TA, *et al.* (2007). Prevention of new-onset atrial fibrillation and its predictors with angiotensin II-receptor blockers in the treatment of hypertension and heart failure. *J Hypertens*, **25**, 15–23.

Cusi D, *et al.* (1997). Polymorphisms of α-adducin and salt sensitivity in patients with essential hypertension. *Lancet*, **349**, 1353–57.

Devereux RB, *et al.* (2004). Prognostic significance of left ventricular mass change during treatment of hypertension. *JAMA*, **292**, 2386–8.

Drukteinis J, *et al.* (2007). Cardiac and systemic hemodynamic characteristics of hypertension and prehypertension in adolescents and young adults. the Strong Heart Study. *Circulation*, **115**, 221–7.

Elliott WJ, Meyer PM (2007). Incident diabetes in clinical trials of antihypertensive drugs: a network meta-analysis. *Lancet*, **369**, 201–207.

Lip GYH, Blann AD (2000). Does hypertension confer a prothrombotic state? Virchow's triad revisited. *Circulation*, **101**, 218–20.

Mancia G, *et al.* (2007). The sympathetic nervous system and the metabolic syndrome. *J Hypertension*, **25**, 909–20.

Mancini JGB, Dahlof B, Diez J (2004). Surrogate markers for cardiovascular disease. *Circulation*, **109** Suppl, IV22–30.

Mason JM, *et al.* (2005). The diabetogenic potential of thiazide-type diuretic and beta-blocker combinations in patients with hypertension. *J Hypertens*, **23**, 1777–81.

Okin PM, *et al.* (2004). Electrocardiographic strain pattern and prediction of cardiovascular morbidity and mortality in hypertensive patients. *Hypertension*, **44**, 48–54.

Okin PM, *et al.* (2006). Electrocardiographic strain pattern and prediction of new-onset congestive heart failure in hypertensive patients: the Losartan Intervention for Endpoint Reduction in Hypertension (LIFE) study. *Circulation*, **113**, 67–73.

Pepine CJ, Cooper-DeHoff RM (2004). Cardiovascular therapies and risk of the development of diabetes. *J Am Coll Cardiol*, **44**, 609–12.

Psaty BM, *et al.* (2002). Diuretic therapy, the alpha-adducin gene variant, and the risk of myocardial infarction or stroke in persons with treated hypertension. *JAMA*, **287**, 1680–9.

Sironi AM, *et al.* (2004). Visceral fat in hypertension. *Hypertension*, **44**, 127–33.

Srinivasan SR, Myers L, Berenson GS (2006). Changes in metabolic syndrome variables since childhood in prehypertensive and hypertensive subjects: the Bogalusa Heart Study. *Hypertension*, **48**, 33–9.

Staessen JA, *et al.* (2001). Effects of three candidate genes on prevalence and incidence of hypertension in a Caucasian population. *J Hypertens*, **19**, 1349–58.

Stevens LA, *et al.* (2006). Assessing kidney function—measured and estimated glomerular filtration rate. *N Engl J Med*, **354**, 2473–83.

Swales JD (1985). *Platt versus Pickering: an episode in recent medical history.* Keynes Press, London.

Taddei S, *et al.* (2000). Endothelial dysfunction in hypertension. *J Nephrol*, **13**, 205–10.

Wang JG, *et al.* (2006). Carotid intima-media thickness and antihypertensive treatment: a meta-analysis of randomized controlled trials. *Stroke*, **37**, 1933–40.

Ward R (1990). Familial aggregation and genetic epidemiology of blood pressure. In: Laragh JH, Brenner BM (eds) *Hypertension: pathophysiology, diagnosis and management*, pp. 81–100. Raven Press, New York.

Williams B (1994). Insulin resistance: the shape of things to come. *Lancet*, **344**, 521–4.

Wong T, Mitchell P (2007). The eye in hypertension. *Lancet*, **369**, 425–35.

16.17.2 Diagnosis, assessment, and treatment of essential hypertension

Bryan Williams

Essentials

Essential hypertension is almost invariably symptomless, and usually detected by routine screening or opportunistic measurement of blood pressure. Key questions to answer in the assessment of a person presenting with an elevated blood pressure are: (1) Do they have hypertension, i.e. is the blood pressure persistently elevated? (2) Are there any associated clinical features that might warrant further evaluation to exclude secondary causes of hypertension? (3) Are there factors that might be contributing to an elevated blood pressure, including lifestyle or dietary factors or concomitant medication? (4) Is there any associated target organ damage or comorbidity that influences the overall cardiovascular disease risk and subsequent treatment of the patient?

Diagnosis

It is normal to find large variations in blood pressure measured in a single individual, hence it should be measured as accurately as possible using the British Hypertension Society protocol. All adults should have their blood pressure measured routinely at least every 5 years. Ambulatory blood pressure measurement (ABPM) recordings provide much more information than standard office blood pressure measurements with regard to diagnosis and efficacy of treatment of hypertension.

The appropriate thresholds for diagnosis of hypertension depending on the method of blood pressure measurement are (1) office or clinic—systolic blood pressure (SBP) 140 mmHg, diastolic blood pressure (DBP) 90 mmHg; (2) APPM 24 h—SBP 125 to 130 mmHg, DBP 80 mmHg; daytime—SBP 130 to 135 mmHg, DBP 85 mmHg; night-time—SBP 120 mmHg, DBP 70 mmHg; and (3) home measurements—SBP 130–135 mmHg, DBP 85 mmHg. The European Society of Hypertension classification of hypertension is described in Chapter 16.17.1.

Isolated office hypertension ('white coat' hypertension) should be diagnosed whenever office blood pressure is greater than or equal to 140/90 mmHg on at least three occasions, while 24-h mean and daytime blood pressures are within their normal range.

Clinical examination and investigation

Fundoscopy is the most convenient method of directly visualizing vascular pathology and provides important prognostic information: three grades are recognized: (1) mild—generalized and focal arteriolar narrowing, arteriolar wall opacification, and arteriovenous nipping; (2) moderate—as (1) plus flame-shaped blot haemorrhages and/or cotton wool spots and/or hard exudates and/or microaneurysms; and (3) severe—as (2) plus swelling of the optic disc.

Aside from measurement of blood pressure and fundal examination as detailed above, particular features to look for on examination are evidence of secondary effects of sustained hypertension on the heart, and features that might suggest the presence of a secondary cause of hypertension (coarctation—absent/delayed femoral pulses, cardiac murmur; and renovascular disease—renal bruit).

Patients with essential hypertension need only a limited number of routine investigations, which must include (1) urine strip test for protein and blood; (2) serum creatinine and electrolytes; (3) blood glucose—ideally fasted; (4) lipid profile—ideally fasted; and (5) electrocardiogram (ECG).

Management

The treatment of hypertension is directed towards reducing risk rather than treating symptoms. There is international consensus that, for office blood pressure, an optimal treatment target should be less than 140/90 mmHg, with a lower target of less than 130/80 mmHg proposed for higher-risk patients, i.e. those with established cardiovascular or renal disease or diabetes. Although early studies focused primarily on diastolic blood pressure as the treatment target, systolic blood pressure is invariably more difficult to control and should be the main focus of treatment.

The most effective lifestyle interventions for reducing blood pressure are (1) modifications to diet to induce weight loss, (2) regular aerobic exercise, and (3) restrictions in alcohol and sodium intake. Many patients will require more than one drug to control blood pressure: monotherapy is rarely sufficient. The blood pressure response to an individual class of blood pressure-lowering medication is heterogeneous, hence there is no 'perfect drug' for every patient, but some trials have indicated that certain comorbidities or target organ damage provide compelling indications for inclusion of specific classes of drug therapy in the treatment regimen.

There is wide variation in the international guidelines with regard to the preferred initial therapy for essential hypertension: (1) the (American) Joint National Committee (JNC) VII guideline recommends low-dose thiazide-type diuretic therapy as initial therapy for all patients (unless contraindicated); (2) the recent European guideline suggests that all five main classes of blood pressure-lowering drugs (angiotensin converting enzyme (ACE) inhibitors, angiotensin receptor blockers, β-blockers, calcium channel blockers, and diuretics) are all suitable as initial therapy; (3) the British Hypertension Society/NICE guideline suggests that a calcium channel blocker (C) or alternatively a diuretic (D) are most likely to deliver the most effective initial blood pressure lowering in older people (i.e. ≥55 years), whereas an ACE inhibitor or an angiotensin receptor blocker (A) are preferred initial therapy for younger patients (<55 years), with the caveat that C or D would be the preferred therapy for people of black African origin at any age.

All guidelines recognize that combinations of blood pressure lowering drugs are often required to achieve recommended blood pressure goals, especially in those with high cardiovascular disease risk or comorbidities who are targeted to lower pressures. Only the British guideline provides explicit guidance on preferred combinations of treatment at step 2, i.e. A + C or A + D, and step 3, i.e. A + C + D.

Patients with hypertension and deemed to be at high cardiovascular risk (>20% over 10 years) should receive advice to adjust their lifestyles and be considered for treatment with statin therapy and low-dose aspirin to optimize their risk reduction.

Indications for specialist referral include uncertainty about the decision to treat, investigations to exclude secondary hypertension, severe and complicated hypertension, and resistant hypertension.

Clinical presentation

Symptoms

Essential hypertension is invariably symptomless and usually detected by routine screening or opportunistic measurement of blood pressure. However, once a patient has been labelled as 'hypertensive' it is not uncommon for them to associate preceding symptoms to their elevated blood pressure. Some patients will claim that they can recognize when their blood pressure is elevated, usually on the basis of symptoms such as plethoric features, palpitations, dizziness, or a feeling of tension. Screening surveys have demonstrated that these symptoms occur no more commonly in untreated hypertensive patients than they do in the normotensive population. However, there are two important caveats to the symptomless nature of essential hypertension: (1) symptoms may develop as a consequence of target organ damage, (2) headache may be a feature of severe hypertension.

Headache

Most headaches in hypertensive patients are tension headaches, not related to blood pressure at all, although they become more common when patients become aware of the diagnosis. The classic hypertensive headache is present on waking in the morning, situated in the occipital region, radiating to the frontal area, throbbing in quality, and wears off during the course of the day. It is more commonly associated with more severe hypertension. Effective treatment of hypertension reduces the incidence of such headaches. Morning headaches in obese hypertensive patients may be related to sleep apnoea.

Epistaxis

Epistaxis is not associated with mild hypertension but is more common in moderate to severe hypertension. However, the associated anxiety can elevate blood pressure when patients present with bleeding, hence it is particularly important that patients are not automatically labelled as hypertensive, with care taken to dissociate hypertension as a cause of epistaxis from a pressor response to the epistaxis itself.

Male impotence

Patients rarely volunteer information about impotence, but there is an increased prevalence of erectile dysfunction in untreated hypertensive men. This is related to two factors: remodelling of small arteries and increased risk of atheroma, both of which vascular changes can reduce penile blood flow despite the elevation in blood pressure. Furthermore, erectile dysfunction can develop or worsen as a consequence of treatment, for the most part related to the reduction in blood pressure before any concomitant change in vascular structure.

Nocturia

This is common in people with untreated hypertension as a consequence of a reduction in urine-concentrating capacity. The symptoms usually improve with treatment.

Symptoms associated with target organ damage

If patients develop cardiac, vascular, cerebrovascular, and/or renal complications as a consequence of long-standing untreated or poorly treated hypertension, then symptoms related to these complications may be present. Target organ damage and associated symptoms are discussed in the Chapter 16.7.1.

Aims of assessment

There are several important issues that must be considered in the assessment of people presenting with an elevated blood pressure:

- Does the patient have hypertension, i.e. is the blood pressure persistently elevated?

- Are there any associated clinical features that might warrant further evaluation to exclude secondary causes of hypertension? (see below and Chapter 16.7.3)

- Are there factors that might be contributing to an elevated blood pressure, including lifestyle or dietary factors or concomitant medication?

- Is there any associated target organ damage or comorbidity that influences the overall cardiovascular disease risk and subsequent treatment of the patient?

These factors, along with the age and ethnicity of the patient, will inform the decision to treat, the urgency of the need to treat, the need for further investigation, and the choice of treatment.

Physical examination

Blood pressure measurement

Large variations in blood pressure measured in a single individual are normal, hence it should be measured as accurately as possible using the British Hypertension Society (BHS) protocol (Box 16.17.2.1). Blood pressure should initially be measured in both arms because there can be large inter-arm difference in blood pressure. The finding of a difference of greater than 10 mmHg may indicate the presence of underlying vascular disease, especially subclavian stenosis. When there is a significant inter-arm difference in blood pressure reading, the arm with the higher pressure should be used for all subsequent measurements.

All adults should have their blood pressure measured routinely at least every 5 years. Those with high-normal blood pressure (systolic blood pressure (SBP) 130–139 mmHg or diastolic blood pressure (DBP) 85–89 mmHg) and those who have had high blood pressure readings at any time previously should have their blood pressure re-measured annually. These measurements can be made in the clinic, in the home setting, or using ambulatory blood pressure monitoring (ABPM) (see below).

Seated blood pressure recordings are generally sufficient, with the patient seated and rested for a few minutes beforehand. At least two measurements should be taken, and if the first is >10 mmHg higher than the subsequent measurement, then it should be discarded and further reading taken. Standing blood pressure (after at least 2 min standing) should be measured in elderly or diabetic patients to exclude significant orthostatic hypotension.

The timing of blood pressure measurement should take account of the timing of medication. Treatment decisions should not be based on single blood pressure readings: the average of two readings at each of at least three visits (depending on severity) should be used to guide the decision to treat. The time between visits will vary according to the severity of the hypertension, ranging from days, weeks to months. In patients with severe hypertension, especially when there is unequivocal evidence of target organ damage, the decision to treat may be made at the time of first presentation.

When measuring blood pressure, the upper arm should be supported at heart level during recordings, and it is important that an appropriate cuff size is used, with the bladder encircling at least 80% of the upper arm. Using too large a cuff results in an underestimation of blood pressure and too small a cuff will lead to overestimation. If the auscultatory method is used to measure blood pressure, then Korotkoff phase I (first appearance of sound) and phase V sounds (disappearance of sound) should be taken for systolic and diastolic pressures, respectively. If phase V goes to zero, then phase IV (muffling of sound) should be recorded.

The beat-to-beat variability associated with atrial fibrillation can make blood pressure measurement difficult and semiautomatic or automated devices can be very inaccurate in such circumstances, in which case multiple readings of auscultatory measurements are recommended.

Blood pressure monitors

The sphygmomanometer has been the mainstay of blood pressure measurement for over 100 years, but its use is likely to decline as a consequence of the decommissioning of mercury-based devices and the emergence of automated and semiautomated devices for routine blood pressure measurement in the office and home and for ABPM.

It is important to note that there are different diagnostic thresholds for the diagnosis of hypertension dependent on the method of measurement, i.e. when using multiple home or ambulatory blood pressure values to measure an average blood pressure, then the average value used to define hypertension is lower than the equivalent office blood pressure threshold of 140/90 mmHg (Table 16.17.2.1) and it should be noted—as stated above—that automated devices are inaccurate in patients with atrial fibrillation. Detailed guidance on blood pressure measurement and a wide range of validated monitors is available from http://www.bhsoc.org.

Ambulatory blood pressure measurements (ABPM)

ABPM recordings provide much more information than standard office blood pressure measurements with regard to diagnosis and efficacy of treatment of hypertension. When compared to office blood pressure, there is a much steeper relationship between ABPM averages and target organ damage indices and cardiovascular events, no doubt reflecting that fact that more measurements are

---

Box 16.7.2.1 British Hypertension Society protocol for blood pressure measurement

- Use a properly maintained, calibrated, and validated device
- Measure sitting blood pressure routinely: standing blood pressure should be recorded at the initial estimation in elderly and diabetic patients
- Remove light clothing, support arm at heart level, ensure hand relaxed and avoid talking during the measurement procedure
- Use cuff of appropriate size
- Lower mercury column slowly (2 mm/s)
- Read blood pressure to the nearest 2 mmHg
- Measure diastolic as disappearance of sounds (phase V)
- Take the mean of at least two readings. more recordings are needed if marked differences between initial measurements are found
- Do not treat on the basis of an isolated reading

Reprinted by permission from Macmillan Publishers Ltd: *Journal of Human Hypertension* 18, 139–185 (2004).

Table 16.7.2.1 Diagnostic thresholds for hypertension according to different methods of measurement

	SBP (mmHg)	DBP (mmHg)
Office or clinic	140	90
24-hour	125–130	80
Day	130–135	85
Night	120	70
Home	130–135	85

DBP, diastolic blood pressure; SBP, systolic blood pressure.

obtained and the 'white coat effect (see below) is eliminated. Generally, ABPM devices are programmed to record blood pressure at 20 min intervals during the day and 30 min intervals at night. A diary is provided to record activity and sleep patterns. In addition to the 24-h blood pressure average, ABPM also provides information on blood pressure profiles, e.g. daytime and night time averages, the 'dipper status', i.e. the relationship between night time and day time blood pressure averages, blood pressure variability throughout the day, the morning surge in blood pressure, and—more recently indices—of aortic function via the ambulatory stiffness index. Each of these parameters adds value over and above the assessment of office blood pressure, hence such techniques are increasingly used for the assessment of people with hypertension. Clinical indications for the use of ABPM are shown in Box 16.17.2.2.

Home blood pressure measurements

The concept of patients measuring their own blood pressure at home is becoming increasingly popular and may improve adherence to treatment. Validated devices should be used, with an average of duplicate morning and evening home blood pressure measurements recorded daily for 7 days. The measurements should be recorded seated after 5 min rest, with those taken on the first day discarded, leaving at least 24 measurements to be averaged to obtain the home blood pressure average.

'White coat' or isolated office hypertension

In some patients office blood pressure is persistently elevated although their 24-h blood pressure or home blood pressure averages are within the normal range. This has been termed 'white coat' hypertension or isolated office hypertension. It is important to note that blood pressure will generally fall with repeated readings in all patients, hence it is the chronicity of the office blood pressure elevation that is important to establish the diagnosis.

White coat or isolated office hypertension should be diagnosed whenever office blood pressure is 140/90 mmHg or more on at least three occasions, while 24-h mean and daytime blood pressures are within their normal range. The diagnosis can also be based on home blood pressure values, i.e. average home readings below 135/85 mmHg and office values 140/90 mmHg or more.

Surveys suggest that white coat or isolated office hypertension may be present in as many as 15% of the general population and approximately one-third of all hypertensives. There is considerable debate about its prognostic significance: some studies report

Box 16.17.2.2 Possible indications for ambulatory blood pressure monitoring

- Unusual blood pressure variability
- Possible 'white coat' hypertension
- Informing equivocal treatment decisions
- Evaluation of nocturnal hypertension
- Evaluation of drug-resistant hypertension
- Determining the efficacy of drug treatment over 24 h
- Diagnoses and treatment of hypertension in pregnancy
- Evaluation of symptomatic hypotension

association with evidence of hypertensive target organ damage, but others do not. However, overall it appears that white coat hypertension is not benign, with the associated risk probably sitting between those with hypertension confirmed by office readings and ABPM, and those with definitively normal pressures by all methods of measurement. When white coat hypertension is diagnosed, the best advice is to monitor blood pressure and target organ damage via ABPM or home blood pressure averages and not treat unless these pressures are persistently elevated.

Masked hypertension

Less attention has been paid to masked hypertension, i.e. patients with a normal office blood pressure but elevated ABPM or home blood pressure averages, than to those with white coat hypertension. Estimates of prevalence range from 10 to 30% of the population, hence a normal office blood pressure does not exclude hypertension. Moreover, as home blood pressure measurement becomes more popular, the detection of masked hypertension will increase. These patients are more likely to have target organ damage and are at increased cardiovascular risk, perhaps more so than those with white coat hypertension. Masked hypertension should be considered in patients who have clinical evidence of hypertensive target organ damage, but in whom office blood pressure appears normal. Treatment should be offered to such patients, aimed at controlling the home blood pressure average.

Fundal examination

Fundoscopy is the most convenient method of directly visualizing vascular pathology and provides important prognostic information. Signs of hypertensive retinopathy are frequently seen in adults 40 years and older, and are predictive of incident stroke, congestive heart failure, and cardiovascular mortality—independently of traditional risk factors.

The Keith Wagener classification of fundal appearances has been used for many years, but has serious shortcomings. This classification identified four grades of hypertensive retinopathy. Grade I and II changes, which result from arteriolar thickening, are often difficult to differentiate from each other, and the prognostic significance of the grade I and II subclassification is unclear. A more practical three-grade classification (i.e. mild, moderate, and severe) has been proposed (Table 16.17.2.2). The mild changes of generalized retinal–arteriolar narrowing and arteriovenous nipping are related to both the blood pressure at diagnosis and chronic exposure to an elevated blood pressure, hence they appear to be an index of the chronicity of blood pressure elevation (Fig. 16.17.2.1a). The changes of moderate hypertensive retinopathy are the changes of mild retinopathy plus flame-shaped or blot-shaped haemorrhages, cotton

Table 16.7.2.2 Modern classification of hypertensive retinopathy

Mild hypertensive retinopathy	Retinal arteriolar signs, such as generalized and focal arteriolar narrowing, arteriolar wall opacification, and arteriovenous nipping
Moderate hypertensive retinopathy	The signs above plus flame-shaped or blot-shaped haemorrhages, cotton-wool spots, hard exudates, microaneurysms, or a combination of all of these factors.
Severe hypertensive retinopathy	The signs above plus swelling of the optic disc

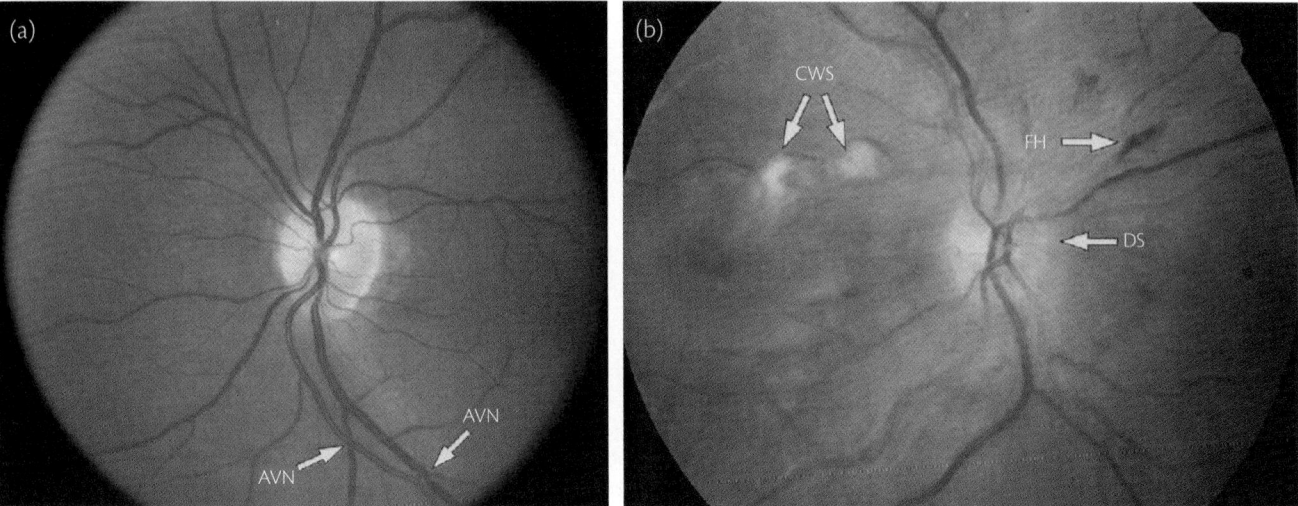

Fig. 16.17.2.1 (a) Signs of mild hypertensive retinopathy. (b) Signs of severe hypertensive retinopathy. AVN, arteriovenous nipping; CWS, cotton wool spots; DS, swelling of the optic disc; FH, flame-shaped retinal haemorrhage.
Reprinted from *The Lancet*, Vol. 369, Wong T, Mitchell P, *The eye in hypertension* pp. 425–35. Copyright (2007), with permission from Elsevier.

wool spots, hard exudates, microaneurysms, or a combination of all of these factors. Severe retinopathy (malignant or accelerated hypertension) is characterized by all of the aforementioned changes plus swelling of the optic disc (Fig. 16.17.2.1b). These moderate and severe fundal changes are more closely related to more recent elevation of blood pressure, suggesting they are the consequence of more transient and severe blood pressure elevation.

The flame-shaped haemorrhages are superficial and shaped due to constraints imposed by nerve fibres. Dot and blot haemorrhages are deeper than the nerve fibres and thus are not so constrained. Haemorrhages usually disappear after a few weeks of effective blood pressure control. There are two types of exudates: hard or waxy exudates represent the end result of fluid leakage into the fibre layers of the retina from damaged vessels, with fluid reabsorption leaving a protein–lipid residue that is slowly removed by macrophages; soft exudates or cotton wool patches are usually larger than hard exudates and have a woolly, ill-defined edge, but they are not true exudates, rather nerve fibre infarcts caused by hypertensive vascular occlusion. Unlike hard exudates, these lesions disappear within a few weeks of establishing adequate antihypertensive therapy.

Severe fundal changes are characterized by disc swelling (i.e. papilloedema) resulting from raised pressure in the disc head secondary to severe vascular damage and increased permeability. Venous distension is followed by increased vascularity of the optic disc, which has a pink appearance with blurring of the disc margins and loss of the optic cup. Raising of the optic disc with anterior displacement of the vessels occurs later. The surrounding retina often shows oedema, small radial haemorrhages, and cotton wool exudates. Moderate or severe fundal changes represent malignant or accelerated hypertension and carry the same adverse prognosis and should be treated as a medical emergency (see Chapter 16.17.5).

Other fundal changes associated with hypertension

Hypertension also predisposes to the development of a number of sight-threatening complications that can be detected by fundoscopy.

Retinal vein occlusion

This is characterized by dilated and tortuous retinal veins and the presence of retinal haemorrhages, cotton wool spots, and oedema of the macula and optic disc. In the case of central retinal vein occlusion, all four fundal quadrants are involved (Fig. 16.17.2.2a); only one fundal quadrant is involved if there is a branch vein occlusion (Fig. 16.17.2.2b). Central retinal vein occlusion can either be ischaemic or nonischaemic, patients with an ischaemic central retinal vein occlusion typically having poor visual acuity and a relative afferent pupillary defect. Ophthalmic follow-up is needed to diagnose and prevent the two main complications of retinal vein occlusion, namely neovascularization and macular oedema.

Retinal arteriolar embolization

Due to cholesterol crystals, platelet/fibrin clot, or calcium, this is twice as common in people with hypertension compared to those who are normotensive, with the risk further accentuated in cigarette smokers and those with diabetes.

Retinal artery occlusion

Also more common in people with hypertension, central retinal artery occlusion typically presents with a sudden, painless, unilateral loss of vision, associated with a cherry red spot (Fig. 16.17.2.3a). Branch retinal artery occlusion (Fig. 16.17.2.3b) will present with a sudden, painless, visual field defect, and there may be only minimal impairment of central vision.

Retinal arterial macroaneurysms

These can be either fusiform or saccular. They are uncommon, but are usually only seen in patients with hypertension. When they occur, about 20% are bilateral and 10% are multiple. They are usually discovered by routine fundoscopy in asymptomatic hypertensive patients, but can present acutely, with visual loss secondary to haemorrhage or exudation.

Nonarteritic ischaemic optic neuropathy

This is also more common in people with hypertension, occurring (in one series) with a yearly incidence of 1 in 10 000. It presents with sudden unilateral visual loss and optic disc oedema. There is no effective treatment and prospects for visual recovery are poor.

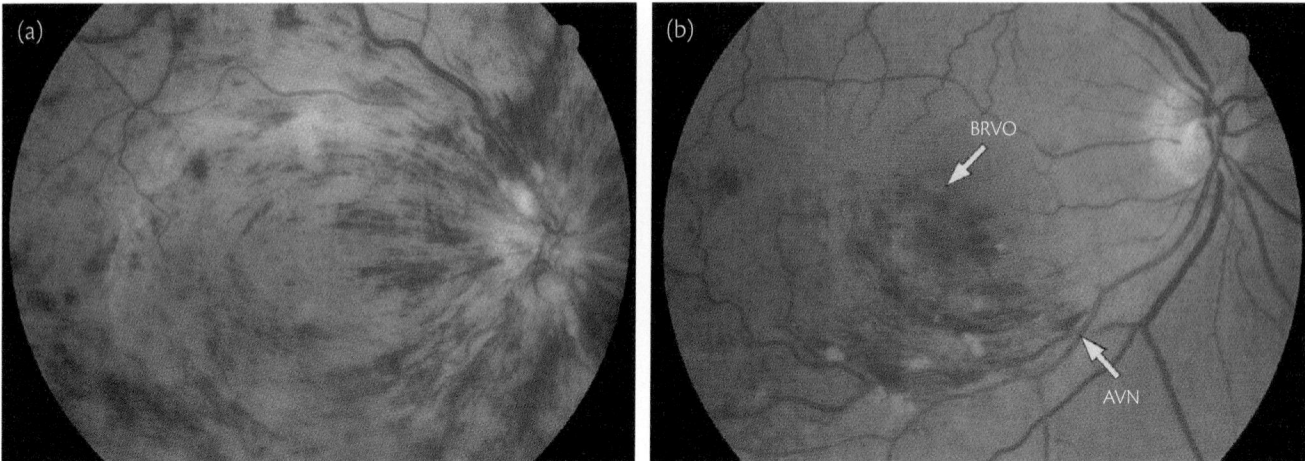

Fig. 16.17.2.2 (a) Central retinal vein occlusion involving all four fundal quadrants. (b) Branch retinal vein occlusion (BRVO) involving a single fundal quadrant, also showing a good example of arteriovenous nipping (AVN).
Reprinted from *The Lancet*, Vol. 369, Wong T, Mitchell P, *The eye in hypertension* pp. 425–35. Copyright (2007), with permission from Elsevier.

Other systems

All patients with hypertension should have a thorough physical examination (Box 16.17.2.3). Aside from measurement of blood pressure and fundal examination as detailed above, particular features to look for are evidence of secondary effects of sustained hypertension on the heart, features that might suggest the presence of a secondary cause of hypertension, and evidence of other vascular pathology (absent pulses, arterial bruits).

Cardiac examination may reveal a sustained apex beat, or features of cardiac failure that might be secondary to hypertension. It is sometimes said that the second component of the aortic sound is loud in moderate or severe hypertension, but this is not a reliable finding.

In coarctation of the aorta the femoral pulses will be absent or diminished and delayed, and there may be various murmurs (usually as systolic murmur at the sternal border and a continuous murmur at the back of the chest), also visible or palpable collateral arteries on the back of the chest or in the axillae. Blood pressure measured in the legs will be lower than that in the arms.

Abdominal bruits are reported in 4 to 20% of normal people, most commonly in those aged less than 40 years, when it is typically systolic and audible only between the xiphisternum and the umbilicus. In patients with severe hypertension that is difficult to control, the finding of an abdominal bruit in both systole and diastole strongly supports the diagnosis of renovascular hypertension, but a bruit confined to systole is much less likely to be of significance.

Routine investigation

Patients with essential hypertension need only a limited number of routine investigations, which must include:

♦ urine strip test for protein and blood

♦ serum creatinine and electrolytes

♦ blood glucose—ideally fasted

♦ lipid profile—ideally fasted

♦ ECG

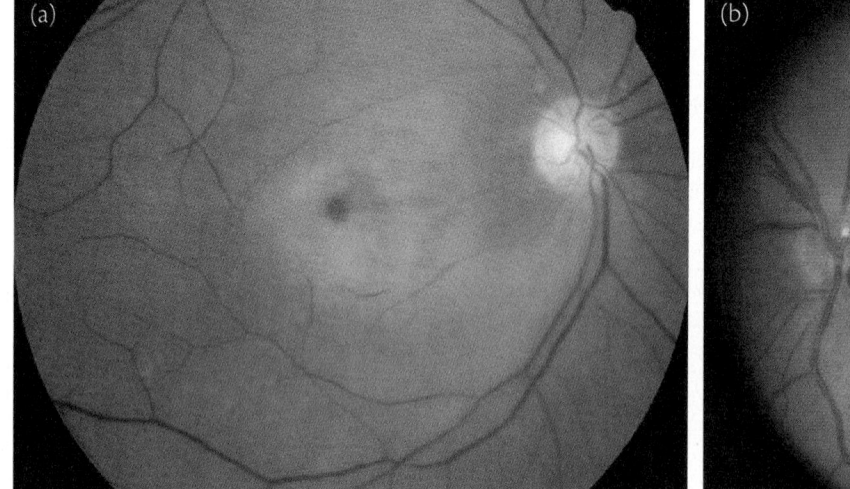
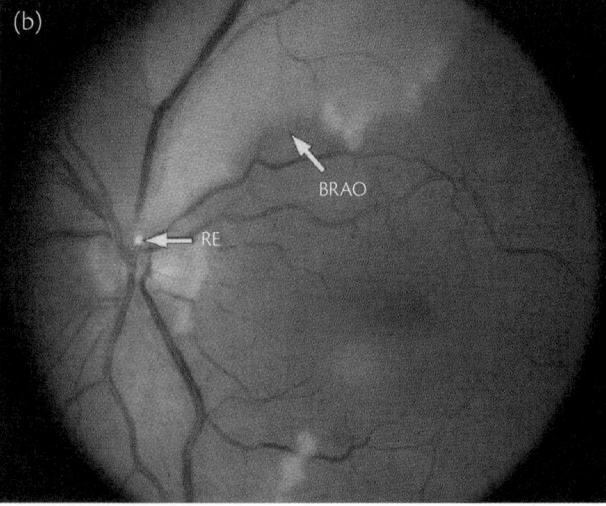

Fig. 16.17.2.3 (a) Central retinal artery occlusion with a characteristic cherry red spot. (b) Retinal–arteriolar emboli (RE) and retina branch artery occlusion (BRAO).
Reprinted from *The Lancet*, Vol. 369, Wong T, Mitchell P, *The eye in hypertension* pp. 425–35. Copyright (2007), with permission from Elsevier.

Box 16.17.2.3 Initial assessment of the patient with hypertension

- ◆ Causes of hypertension
  - · Drugs (NSAIDs, oral contraceptive, steroids, liquorice, sympathomimetics, i.e. some cold cures)
  - · Renal disease (present, past or family history, proteinuria and/or haematuria: palpable kidney(s)—polycystic, hydronephrosis, or neoplasm)
  - · Renovascular disease (abdominal or loin bruit)
  - · Phaeochromocytoma (paroxysmal symptoms)
  - · Conn's syndrome (tetany, muscle weakness, polyuria, hypokalemia)
  - · Coarctation (radiofemoral delay or weak femoral pulses)
  - · Cushings (general appearance)
- ◆ Contributory factors
  - · Overweight
  - · Excess alcohol (>3 units/day)
  - · Excess salt intake
  - · Lack of exercise
  - · Environmental stress
- ◆ Complications of hypertension/target organ damage
  - · Stroke, TIA, dementia, carotid bruits
  - · LVH and/or LV strain on ECG, heart failure
  - · Myocardial infarction, angina, CABG or angioplasty
  - · Peripheral vascular disease
  - · Fundal hemorrhages or exudates, papilledema
  - · Proteinuria
  - · Renal impairment (raised serum creatinine)
- ◆ Cardiovascular disease risk factors
  - · Smoking
  - · Diabetes
  - · Total cholesterol:high-density lipoprotein-cholesterol ratio
  - · Family history
  - · Age
  - · Sex
- ◆ Drug contraindications

CABG, coronary artery bypass graft; LVH, left ventricular hypertrophy; NSAIDs, nonsteroidal anti-inflammatory drugs; TIA, transient ischaemic attack.

These routine investigations help inform the assessment of target organ damage and cardiovascular disease risk. With regard to renal function, many laboratories now report an 'estimated' GFR (eGFR) calculated using an algorithm based on the serum creatinine measurement (see Chapters 21.4 and 21.6). If urinary stick testing for protein is positive, this should be followed by quantification on a spot urine sample of the urinary albumin/creatinine ratio (ACR). More sophisticated assessment tools are available, but the list above is sufficient for routine clinical practice. Note that only two of these routine investigations contribute to the detection of underlying causes of hypertension, namely urinalysis (renal causes) and serum creatinine and electrolytes (renal causes and mineralocorticoid excess), although the ECG may rarely show U waves as a clue to one of the hypokalaemic syndromes. Indications for further investigation for causes of secondary hypertension are given in Chapter 16.7.3.

A chest radiograph and urine microscopy are not routinely required. Echocardiography is more sensitive at detecting left ventricular hypertrophy than an ECG, but is not required routinely, although it is valuable to confirm or refute the presence of left ventricular hypertrophy when the ECG shows voltage criteria suggestive of this.

Assessment of cardiovascular disease risk

The cardiovascular risk associated with hypertension is not eliminated by the treatment of blood pressure alone. This is because many patients have established cardiovascular damage which may not necessarily reverse with treatment of blood pressure, also lifestyle habits such as smoking and dietary factors that may not have changed since therapy was initiated. Other factors are also important: patients with high blood pressure often have associated disturbances in their metabolic profile (especially lipids and glucose tolerance) that also contributes to their risk, which has led many international guidelines to recommend that cardiovascular risk should be formally assessed in all patients with hypertension to determine whether they are at low, medium, or high risk.

Risk calculations based on the Framingham cohort have been used in the United States of America and the United Kingdom, and European guidelines have used a risk score based on mortality data from European countries. Pragmatism in risk assessment is important, with the risk factors cited in the guidelines being conventional markers that can easily be documented in a basic clinical setting, i.e. systolic blood pressure, age, gender, low-density lipoprotein (LDL) cholesterol, presence of diabetes, smoking history, and the presence or absence of structural damage, e.g. ECG evidence of left ventricular hypertrophy. Recent surveys suggest that >90% of population attributable risk for cardiovascular disease can be explained by these risk factors. The use of more sophisticated risk assessment by adding any of the recently advocated biomarkers, such as C-reactive protein, adds little to the conventional methods of cardiovascular risk estimation.

Cardiovascular disease risk thresholds for intervention currently define 'high risk patients' as having a 10-year Framingham-derived cardiovascular disease risk of 20% or more. The typical hypertensive male aged 55 years or more has this level of cardiovascular disease risk, and it is likely that even lower thresholds would be cost-effective for intervention. Formal cardiovascular disease risk estimation is not necessary for patients with hypertension and established cardiovascular disease, diabetes, or overt end organ damage: they are already at sufficient cardiovascular disease risk to benefit from multifactorial risk factor intervention.

Patients with hypertension and deemed to be at high risk should receive strong advice to adjust their lifestyles and be considered for treatment with statin therapy and low dose aspirin to optimize their risk reduction (see below).

Clinical management

Initial considerations

Blood pressure is elevated sporadically in everybody. Key objectives in the assessment of essential hypertension are to establish whether blood pressure is persistently elevated; the level to which blood pressure is elevated, i.e. the severity of hypertension; and the presence or absence of hypertension-mediated target organ damage. The initial assessment is usually followed by a period of observation, the duration of which will be dependent on the severity of the hypertension and the associated cardiovascular disease risk and damage. Lifestyle advice should be provided during this observation period, with drug therapy initiated depending on the level of blood pressure and overall cardiovascular disease risk at the end of the observation period.

Establishing the diagnosis

Patients with essential hypertension usually present in one of three ways:

◆ As an asymptomatic individual whose blood pressure has been measured at routine examination for employment, insurance, or as a result of screening or preoperatively—the most common presentation

◆ As a patient whose blood pressure has been measured opportunistically when presenting with an unrelated disorder; or

◆ As a result of symptoms produced by hypertension, or by the acute or chronic complications of hypertension—the least common presentation

Repeated blood pressure measurements over a period of observation are usually necessary to establish the diagnosis. Exceptions to this are patients presenting with severe hypertension in whom fundal examination or other assessment of target organ damage (e.g. left ventricular hypertrophy or renal impairment) clearly reveals the presence of hypertension-mediated damage, indicative of the fact that the blood pressure needs treatment.

The period of observation required before initiating drug therapy is dependent on the severity of the hypertension and the presence or absence of cardiovascular disease, diabetes and/or target organ damage. Those with more severe hypertension and disease require emergency or urgent intervention with drug therapy to lower their blood pressure, whereas those with less severe hypertension and/or the absence of damage or disease can be monitored over a longer period—up to many months—before initiating drug therapy. This period of observation is important because it is used to repeat blood pressure measurements, confirm the presence of sustained hypertension, and get a more accurate appreciation of the associated risk, also to implement lifestyle interventions that may reduce blood pressure.

Diagnostic thresholds for therapeutic intervention and the observation period

The diagnostic thresholds for the levels of hypertension severity are shown in Fig. 16.17.2.4 and Table 16.17.1.1, and the recommended period of observation for different grades of hypertension are shown in Table 16.17.2.3. Although there is general consensus about the management of grade II (i.e ≥160/100 mmHg) or more severe hypertension, the British guidelines have traditionally been more cautious than other guidelines with regard to drug therapy for uncomplicated grade I hypertension (140–159/90–99 mmHg) (Table 16.17.2.3). Most other guidelines recommend treating all patients with a blood pressure sustained above 140/90 mmHg, whereas the British guidelines have recommended drug therapy for those with grade I hypertension only when there is associated cardiovascular disease or target organ damage, or a calculated risk of cardiovascular disease at least 20% over 10 years. There is genuine uncertainty about the cost-effectiveness of treating otherwise low risk people with grade I hypertension, but this must be balanced by recognition that the greatest burden of blood pressure attributable

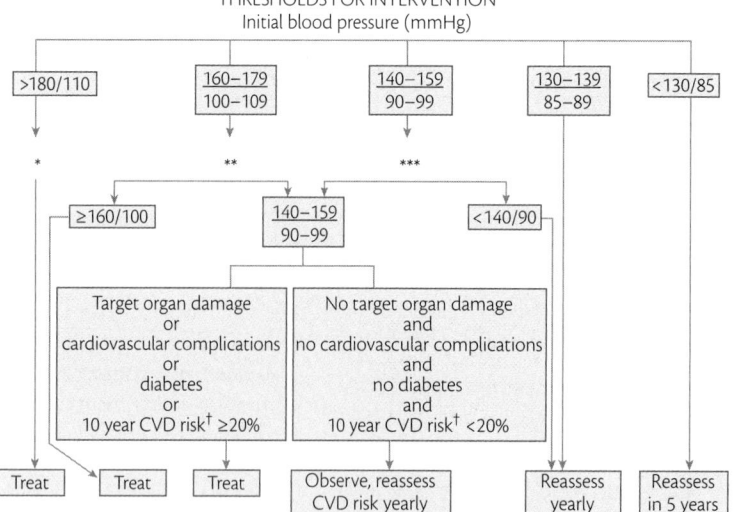

Fig. 16.17.2.4 Thresholds for blood pressure intervention.
From Williams B (2004). *et al. BMJ*, **328**, 634–40.

* Unless malignant phase of hypertensive emergency confirm over 1–2 weeks then treat
** If cardiovascular complications, target organ damage or diabetes is present, confirm over 3–4 weeks then treat, if absent re-measure weekly and treat if blood pressure persists at these levels over 4–12 weeks
*** If cardiovascular complications, target organ damage, or diabetes is present, confirm over 12 weeks then treat if absent re-measure monthly and treat if these levels are maintained and if estimated 10 year CVD resk is ≥20%
† Assessed with CVD risk chart

Table 16.17.2.3 Typical observation periods for different grades of hypertension and associated cardiovascular disease, diabetes, and/or target organ damage

Grade of hypertension	Typical observation period
Accelerated (malignant) hypertension (papilloedema and/or fundal haemorrhages and exudates or with acute cardiovascular complications e.g. aortic dissection)	Immediate treatment—usually requiring acute hospital admission (see Chapter 16.17.5)
BP ≥220/120 mmHg	Treat immediately—hospital admission not usually required
Grade III hypertension BP >180–219/110–119 mmHg	Confirm by repeated measurements over 1–2 weeks, then treat
Grade II hypertension BP 160–179/100–109 mmHg	In the presence of cardiovascular disease, diabetes, or target-organ damage: confirm over 3–4 weeks, then treat No cardiovascular disease, diabetes, or target-organ damage: lifestyle measures, re-measure weekly initially, and treat if BP persists at these levels over 4–12 weeks
Grade I hypertension: BP 140–159/90–99 mmHg	Cardiovascular disease, diabetes, or target-organ damage: confirm within weeks, then treat No clinical cardiovascular disease, diabetes or target-organ damage: lifestyle advice and re-measure BP at monthly intervals for 3–6 months. If mild hypertension persists, estimate 10-year cardiovascular diseases risk and treat if this is ≥20% (if <20%, keep under annual review).

From Williams. B et al. (2004). BMJ, **328**, 364–40.

disease in populations is in those with grade I hypertension because it is so common. Moreover, blood pressure will invariably continue to rise in patients with grade I hypertension, and there is concern that the subtle vascular damage that is occurring while these patients remain untreated may not be reversible when treatment is eventually initiated at higher levels of pressure. Thus, while a prolonged period of observation and lifestyle intervention for uncomplicated, low risk, grade I hypertension is considered acceptable, it is inevitable that most of these patients will eventually (if not immediately) require drug treatment.

Initial advice

The treatment of hypertension is directed towards reducing risk rather than treating symptoms. It is imperative, therefore, to explain the significance of high blood pressure at the earliest opportunity. Many patients find difficulty in grasping the concept of blood pressure variability and are often alarmed by the inevitable occasional high reading. Discussion of the rationale for evaluation and treatment, together with an explanation of the nature of high blood pressure and its very high prevalence, reassures patients and may improve adherence to treatment. Further comprehensive advice for patients may be obtained from http://www.bpassoc.org.uk.

Treatment targets

The evidence base identifying the optimal blood pressure treatment targets for hypertension is less substantial than it should be. There is international consensus that for office blood pressure an

optimal treatment target should be <140/90 mmHg, and a lower target of <130/80 mmHg has been recommended for higher risk patients, i.e. those with established cardiovascular or renal disease or diabetes. Whether such targets are appropriate for very elderly individuals (i.e. >80 years) has been debated, with a recent study suggesting that at target blood pressure of <150/90 mmHg is appropriate for this age group. It is important to note that as people age, diastolic blood pressure generally falls and systolic blood pressure rises, hence the systolic blood pressure assumes the greatest importance with regard to the treatment target, although it is generally more difficult to control.

Lifestyle advice

Blood pressure is strongly influenced by lifestyle factors such as diet and exercise and their consequences such as weight. Effective lifestyle modification for patients with grade I hypertension may lower blood pressure as much as a single blood pressure lowering drug, and combinations of two or more lifestyle modifications may be even more effective. Lifestyle interventions may reduce the need for drug therapy for people with mild hypertension, can enhance the antihypertensive effects of blood pressure lowering medication, and can favourably influence overall cardiovascular disease risk.

The most effective lifestyle interventions for reducing blood pressure in clinical trials are modifications to diet to induce weight loss, regular aerobic exercise, and restrictions in alcohol and sodium intake. The expected reduction in blood pressure with these lifestyle manoeuvres are shown in Table 16.17.2.4, and recommended lifestyle interventions to reduce blood pressure and/or cardiovascular disease risk are shown in Box 16.17.2.4.

Patients are often enthusiastic to try lifestyle changes rather than take drug therapy. This is a reasonable initial option in patients with grade I hypertension who do not have associated target organ damage or high cardiovascular disease risk. In patients with more severe hypertension or those at high risk, lifestyle measures should be recommended alongside drug therapy. This is important because these measures may improve the effectiveness of drug therapy and also contribute to a reduction in overall cardiovascular risk.

Table 16.17.2.4 Blood pressure reductions associated with lifestyle interventions for patients with hypertension

Intervention	Recommendation	Expected SBP reduction (range)
Weight reduction	Maintain ideal BMI 20–25 kg/m²)	5–10 mmHg per 10 kg weight loss
DASH eating plan	Consume diet rich in fruit, vegetables, low fat dairy products with reduced content of saturated and total fat	8–14 mmHg
Dietary sodium restriction	Reduce dietary sodium intake to <100 mmol/day (<2.4 g sodium or <6 g sodium chloride)	2–8 mmHg
Physical activity	Engage in regular aerobic physical activity, e.g. brisk walking lor at least 30 min most days	4–9 mmHg
Alcohol moderation	Men ≤21 units/week	2–4 mmHg
	Women ≤14 units/week	

BMI, body mass index; SBP, systolic blood pressure.

> **Box 16.17.2.4** Lifestyle measures that lower blood pressure and reduce cardiovascular disease risk
>
> **Lifestyle measures that lower blood pressure**
> - Weight reduction
> - Reduced salt intake
> - Limitation of alcohol consumption
> - Increased physical activity
> - Increased fruit and vegetable consumption
> - Reduced total fat and saturated fat intake
>
> **Measures to reduce cardiovascular disease risk**
> - Cessation of smoking
> - Reduced total fat and saturated fat intake
> - Replacement of saturated fats with monounsaturated fats
> - Increased oily fish consumption

Note, however, that effective implementation of lifestyle measures requires enthusiasm, knowledge, patience, and considerable time spent with patients and other family members. It is best undertaken by well-trained health professionals, e.g. practice or clinic nurses, and should be supported by clear written information.

Weight reduction

Many patients with hypertension are overweight and weight reduction by calorie restriction is an appropriate recommendation. The blood pressure lowering effect of weight reduction may be enhanced by increased regular aerobic physical exercise, by alcohol moderation in heavy drinkers, and by a reduction in sodium intake. On average, blood pressure may fall by as much as 1 mmHg per kg weight loss, although results vary in studies and the maximum overall effect of combined lifestyle interventions is an average of 10 mmHg fall in systolic blood pressure. Body mass index is frequently used as a measure of overweight, but other measures of obesity—particularly central obesity—are better markers of adverse cardiovascular outcomes in people with hypertension. In this regard, weight reduction also has beneficial effects on associated risk factors such as insulin resistance, risk of developing diabetes, and dyslipidaemia.

Dietary salt reduction

Sodium intake influences blood pressure and all international guidelines recommend dietary sodium restriction. Dietary salt reduction from an average of 10 to 5 g/day (5 g = 1 teaspoon) lowers blood pressure by about 5/2 mmHg, with larger blood pressure falls in elderly people, blacks, and in those with higher initial blood pressure levels. About one-third of people will achieve a reduction of 5/5 mmHg or more. These effects are additive to the blood pressure lowering effect of a healthy diet, e.g. the Dietary Approaches to Stop Hypertension (DASH) diet http://www.nhlbi.nih.gov/health/public/heart/hbp/dash/ (see below).

Many patients will already be aware of the relationship between salt and blood pressure will have discontinued adding salt at the table and even when cooking, but few are aware of the large amount of salt in processed foods, such as bread (one slice contains 0.5 g salt), some breakfast cereals, ready prepared meals, and flavour enhancers such as stock cubes or manufactured sauces. Patients, and those who cook for patients, should be provided with specific written advice, such as that from http://www.bpassoc.org.uk.

Increased fruit and vegetable consumption

Using the DASH diet, which increased vegetable consumption from two to seven portions per day, blood pressure was lowered by around 7/3 mmHg in hypertensive patients. Hypertensive patients should therefore be given clear advice to increase fruit and vegetable intake to at least five portions per day. When this is combined with an increased use of low-fat dairy products and reduction of total and saturated fat, then blood pressure falls averaging 11/6 mmHg are seen. The mechanism whereby fruit and vegetable consumption are thought to lower blood pressure is uncertain, but it may be due to an associated increase in potassium intake, which is compatible with some supplementation studies.

Physical activity

Regular physical activity, especially when combined with dietary measures, can be particularly effective at reducing blood pressure (Table 16.17.2.4). The activity should be regular, aerobic (e.g. brisk walking), and tailored to the individual. For example, three vigorous training sessions per week may be appropriate for fit younger patients, or brisk walking for 20 min/day in older patients. This activity will be expected to reduce systolic blood pressure and diastolic blood pressure by about 2–3 mmHg, with the combination of exercise and diet reducing both by 5–6 mmHg. Heavy physical exercise should be discouraged in people with severe hypertension or those in whom hypertension is poorly controlled. Exercise can be recommended once drug therapy has been started and blood pressure is better controlled.

In addition to its effects on blood pressure, physical exercise appears to exert a strong protective effect against cardiovascular mortality and is associated with a lower risk of coronary heart disease in men and women. Protection is lost when exercise is discontinued. Any activity appears to be of benefit, but those that are more active appear to gain more protection. A reasonable strategy is regular aerobic exercise (e.g. brisk walking) for at least 30 min, ideally on most days, but at least three days per week.

Alcohol intake

An alcohol intake of above 21 units per week is associated with blood pressure elevation, and binge drinking is associated with an increased risk of stroke. Hypertensive patients should be advised to limit their alcohol intake to 21 units per week (men) and 14 units per week (women). On average, structured interventions to reduce alcohol consumption have a small effect on blood pressure, reducing systolic blood pressure (and possibly diastolic blood pressure) by about 2–3 mmHg. Consumption of smaller amounts of alcohol, up to the recommended limit, may protect against cardiovascular disease and should not be discouraged.

Sleep and blood pressure

Blood pressure characteristically falls during sleep, and sleep duration impacts on the risk of developing hypertension. The risk of developing hypertension in one survey was increased by about twofold in adults in middle age who sleep 5 h or less each night. This may simply reflect a higher 24-h average blood pressure load and longer duration of sympathetic nervous system activation as a consequence of less time asleep, which in turn would give rise to a higher risk of longer term cardiovascular structural damage, leading to sustained hypertension. Whatever the mechanism, sleep deprivation should be considered in the assessment of people developing hypertension. Consistent with the association between sleep deprivation and hypertension, high blood pressure is more common in patients with obstructive sleep apnoea. Although this could be explained by the fact that both conditions are commoner in males and in obese individuals, a few studies indicate that continuous positive airways pressure can reduce blood pressure, particularly nocturnal pressures, implying a causal relationship.

Lifestyle strategies to reduce cardiovascular risk in hypertensive patients

Cigarette smoking

Patients with hypertension should be encouraged and given support to stop smoking. Nicotine replacement therapy and other strategies are safe and effective in people with hypertension and double the chance of quitting smoking. Those who fail on their first attempt to quit should be encouraged to continue trying: the chance of success increases with the number of quit attempts. Although smoking is not a major contributor to an elevated blood pressure, it does significantly amplify the cardiovascular risk associated with hypertension. Smoking is a major factor related to the persistent increase in coronary and stroke mortality in men with treated hypertension. Those who stop smoking experience a rapid decline in risk, by as much as 50% after 1 year, but up to 10 years may be needed to reach the risk level of those who have never smoked.

Reduced dietary saturated fat intake

Reducing dietary fat intake can reduce serum cholesterol values, which can reduce the risk of cardiovascular disease. All patients should be advised to keep total dietary intake of fat to less than one-third of their total energy intake, to keep the intake of saturated fats to less than one-third of their total fat intake, and to replace saturated fats by an increased intake of monounsaturated fats. These dietary changes can be very effective, but reduce serum cholesterol by only about 6% on average, in part because of difficulty in sustaining such dietary discipline. A regular intake of fish and other sources of $\omega - 3$ fatty acids (at least two servings of fish per week) will further improve lipid profiles and has been shown to reduce blood pressure.

Lifestyle modifications that are ineffective at lowering blood pressure

Dietary supplements The best available evidence does not support the use of calcium, magnesium, or potassium supplementation (i.e. tablets), individually or in combination, to achieve a worthwhile reduction in blood pressure. Inadequate information is available from randomized controlled trials to support the recommendation for garlic, herbal, or other complementary medicines.

Psychological stress reduction Structured interventions to reduce stress e.g. stress management programmes, meditation, yoga, cognitive therapies, breathing exercises, biofeedback, and acupuncture have been shown to modestly reduce blood pressure in some but not all studies. However, many of these interventions are time consuming and have been short term, and it is difficult to know whether they would be an effective intervention for adequate blood pressure control over the longer term.

Clinical management

Pharmacological treatments

The treatment of hypertension has been subjected to many large randomized controlled trials that have compared active treatments with placebo, and different treatment strategies with each other. Hypertension has the most impressive evidence base in medicine to guide treatment decisions, and analysis of this has provided important guiding principles with regard to treatment strategies:

- Effective blood pressure lowering is overwhelmingly important in reducing the risk of major cardiovascular events in people with hypertension, thus the first priority in treatment is to control blood pressure.

- Many patients will require more than one drug to control blood pressure; monotherapy is rarely sufficient.

- Although early studies focused primarily on diastolic blood pressure as the treatment target, systolic blood pressure is invariably more difficult to control and should now be the main focus of treatment.

- The blood pressure response to an individual class of blood pressure lowering medication is heterogeneous, hence there is no 'perfect drug' for every patient.

- Some trials have indicated that certain comorbidities or target organ damage provide compelling indications for inclusion of specific classes of drug therapy in the treatment regimen.

- There is inadequate clinical outcome data for treatment studies of younger patients as most of the studies, especially the more recent ones, have been conducted in patients over the age of 55 years, and typically with a mean age over 65 years.

Blood pressure lowering therapy is effective at reducing the risk of stroke, myocardial infarction, heart failure, chronic renal disease, peripheral vascular disease, and death. It may also be effective at reducing the risk of vascular dementia. On average, lowering blood pressure by 20/10 mmHg will reduce the risk of major cardiovascular events by one-half, with the reduction in stroke risk appearing to follow the predicted reduction in risk based on the epidemiological association between stroke and blood pressure. There appears to be a shortfall in the reduction in risk of ischaemic heart disease with blood pressure lowering when compared to epidemiological predictions, which is best addressed by attention to concomitant risk factors. Importantly, the risk reduction associated with blood pressure lowering appears to be continuous across a wide range of blood pressures, thus the absolute benefit from treatment is greatest in those with the highest absolute cardiovascular disease risk. This provides the rational for advocating the use of complementary strategies to reduce cardiovascular disease risk, e.g. statins and antiplatelet therapy, in those with established vascular disease, target organ damage, or at high calculated cardiovascular disease risk, i.e. a calculated cardiovascular disease risk of 20% or more over 10 years.

The main classes of blood pressure lowering therapies are summarized below. The over-riding treatment priority is to control blood pressure, but there is general consensus amongst international guidelines about indications and contraindications for the use of specific classes of blood pressure lowering therapy in specific clinical situations, and these are detailed in Tables 16.17.2.5 and 16.17.2.6.

Table 16.17.2.5 Indications favouring the use of specific classes of blood pressure lowering drugs

Thiazide diuretics	Isolated systolic hypertension (elderly)
	Heart failure
	Hypertension in blacks
ACE inhibitors	Heart failure
	LV dysfunction
	Postmyocardial infarction
	Diabetic nephropathy
	Nondiabetic nephropathy
	LVhypertrophy
	Carotidatherosclerosis
	Proteinuria/microalbuminuria
	Atrial fibrillation
	Metabolic syndrome
Angiotensin receptor blockers	Heart failure
	Post-myocardial infarction
	Diabetic nephropathy
	Proteinuria/microalbuminuria
	LV hypertrophy
	Atrial fibrillation
	Metabolic syndrome
	ACB-induced cough
β-Blockers	Angina pectoris
	Post-myocardial infarction
	Heart failure
	Tachyarrhythmias
	Glaucoma
	Pregnancy
Calcium antagonists (dihydropyridines)	Isolated systolic hypertension (elderly)
	Angina pectoris
	LV hypertrophy
	Carotid/Coronary Atherosclerosis
	Pregnancy
	Hypertension in blacks
Diuretics (antialdosterone)	Heart failure
	Postmyocardial infarction
Calcium antagonist (verapamil/diltiazem	Angina pectoris
	Carotid atherosclerosis
	Supraventricular tachycardia
Loop diuretics	Endstage renal disease
	Heart failure

It is important to note that these lists are not comprehensive and are subject to change as new evidence emerges, and the reader is directed towards the information sheets for each specific drug for more detailed prescribing information.

Diuretics

Thiazides

Thiazide-type diuretics were the first major class of drug used to treat hypertension on a large scale and they remain one of the main therapeutic options for the treatment of essential hypertension. Commonly used examples include chlorthalidone, hydrochlorthiazide, and bendroflumethiazide. Thiazide-type diuretics lower blood pressure by a complex series of mechanisms. Urinary loss of sodium resulting from a blockade of renal tubular reabsorption of sodium is integral to the antihypertensive effect. The early changes in salt and water balance are often accompanied by

Table 16.17.2.6 Compelling and possible contraindications to specific classes of blood pressure lowering therapies

	Compelling	Possible
Thiazide diuretics	Gout	Metabolic syndrome
		Glucose intolerance
		Pregnancy
β-Blockers	Asthma	Peripheral artery disease
	AV block (grade 2 or 3)	Metabolic syndrome
		Glucose intolerance
		Athletes and physically active patients
		Chronic obstructive pulmonary disease
Calcium antagonists (dihydropiridines)		Tachyarrhythmias
		Heart failure
Calcium antagonists (verapamil, diltiazem)	AV block (grade 2 or 3)	
	Heart failure	
ACE inhibitors	Pregnancy	
	Angioneurotic oedema	
	Hyperkalemia	
	Bilateral renal artery stenosis	
Angiotensin receptor antagonists	Pregnancy	
	Hyperkalemia	
	Bilateral renal artery stenosis	
Diuretics (antialdosterone)	Renal failure	
	Hyperkalaemia	

ACE, angiotensin converting enzyme; AV, atrioventricular.
Data from Williams *et al.* BHS Guidelines 2004. *Guidelines for management of hypertension: report of the fourth working party of the British Hypertension Society*, 2004—BHS IV.

counter-activation of several vasoconstrictor mechanisms including the renin–angiotensin–aldosterone system, which may transiently raise peripheral vascular resistance and attenuate blood pressure lowering. There is subsequently a gradual reduction in peripheral vascular resistance and a new steady state of reduced total body sodium and blood pressure.

The sustained actions of thiazide/thiazide-like diuretics on the kidney make them preferable to loop diuretics for the control of blood pressure. This is because loop diuretics are shorter acting, and the short-term sodium and water loss is usually compensated for by sodium retention during the latter part of the dosing interval and reduced blood pressure lowering efficacy. There is really no place for loop diuretics in the routine management of essential hypertension, but thiazide-type diuretics become ineffective in patients with a glomerular filtration rate below 30 ml/min and in such patients loop diuretics are often required for effective blood pressure lowering, especially when there is clinical evidence of sodium and water retention.

The main adverse effects of thiazide-type diuretics are hypokalaemia, hyponatraemia (less commonly), impaired glucose tolerance, and small increments in blood levels of LDL cholesterol and triglycerides. Thiazide-type diuretics also elevate serum uric acid levels and should be avoided in patients predisposed to gout, also avoided in those receiving lithium because of a high risk of lithium toxicity. An incidental advantage of thiazides may be reduction in osteoporosis as a result of calcium retention.

To minimize the adverse effects of thiazide-type diuretics, low doses of these drugs have been recommended by guidelines for the treatment of essential hypertension, and these are well tolerated. On the basis of some small studies it has been assumed that the dose response to thiazide-type diuretics is generally flat (unlike the adverse affect profile), and this has been used to further justify the low dose strategy for thiazide-type diuretics, but it should be emphasized that some patients do respond to and tolerate higher doses. Moreover, when thiazides are combined with drugs that block the renin–angiotensin system, e.g. ACE inhibition, then the dose response is steeper and higher doses may be used in patients with more resistant hypertension (see below).

Potassium-retaining diuretics

Potassium-retaining diuretics, e.g. spironolactone or amiloride, are effective blood pressure lowering agents that are much less commonly used for the routine treatment of hypertension. They can be very effective in combination with thiazide-type diuretics, and are increasingly used as part of a multidrug strategy for the treatment of resistant hypertension (see below). They are used and effective in large doses in the treatment of primary aldosteronism. They have the advantage over thiazide-type diuretics in not causing hypokalemia or hyperuricaemia and do not impair glucose tolerance, but spironolactone causes nipple tenderness and gynaecomastia in some patients, which is dose dependent and can limit its use. Moreover, if potassium-sparing diuretics are used in combination with drugs that block the activity of the renin–angiotensin system or in patients with renal impairment, then monitoring of serum potassium is required because of the increased risk of hyperkalaemia.

β-Adrenoceptor blocking drugs (β-blockers)

β-Blockers reduce blood pressure and cardiovascular events in patients with hypertension. Most β-blockers, with the exception of those with strong intrinsic sympathomimetic activity, reduce cardiac output due to their negative chronotropic and inotropic effects. As with diuretics, short-term haemodynamic responses can be offset by counter-activation of vasoconstrictor mechanisms, which may limit initial blood pressure lowering. Longer term reduction in arterial pressure, which occurs over days, is due to restoration of vascular resistance to pretreatment levels. Partial blockade of renin release from the kidney may contribute to the later haemodynamic response.

β-Blockers differ in their duration of action, their selectivity for β_1 receptors, lipophilicity, and partial agonist activity. Side effects include lethargy, aches in the limbs on exercise, impaired concentration and memory, erectile dysfunction, vivid dreams, and exacerbation of symptoms of peripheral vascular disease and Raynaud's syndrome. They are contraindicated in asthma and can cause adverse metabolic effects, including impaired glucose tolerance and worsening of dyslipidaemia—notably reduced HDL-cholesterol and raised triglycerides. There is accumulating evidence that β-blockers increase the likelihood of new-onset diabetes, particularly when combined with thiazide-type diuretics. Moreover, recent meta-analyses suggest that there is a shortfall in cardiovascular protection with β-blocker-based treatment for hypertension (especially in stroke reduction) when compared to treatment with other main drug classes. As a consequence, recent British guidelines suggest that β-blockers are no longer preferred as an initial therapy for routine hypertension and should only be used when there is a compelling indication other than blood pressure control, e.g. in patients with hypertension and angina or chronic heart failure. One caveat is in younger women of childbearing potential, in whom β-blockers are often very effective at lowering blood pressure, perhaps due to higher renin levels of younger people, and are safer than ACE inhibition or angiotensin receptor blockers in those anticipating pregnancy.

Calcium channel blockers

This class of drug has been extensively used in treating hypertension since the 1970s: they are very effective at reducing blood pressure and have an extensive evidence base supporting their use. In addition to their blood pressure-lowering properties, they are also effective antianginal agents.

There are two main groups of calcium channel blocker (CCB), the dihydropyridines (e.g. amlodidpine, nifedipine) and the nondihydropyridines (e.g. diltiazem, verapamil). The dihydropyridine CCBs act mainly by inducing relaxation of arterial smooth muscle by blocking L-type calcium channels, thereby inducing peripheral vascular relaxation with a fall in vascular resistance and arterial pressure. Nondihydropyridine CCBs also block calcium channels in cardiac muscle and reduce cardiac output. Verapamil has an additional antiarrhythmic action through its effects on the atrioventricular node.

The earlier formulations of some dihydropyridines, such as capsular nifedipine, had a rapid onset of action, unpredictable effects on blood pressure, and were accompanied by reflex sympathetic stimulation and tachycardia. With the availability of longer-acting formulations of dihydropyridine CCBs, these shorter-acting CCBs have no place in the management of hypertension, even (and especially) in the emergency setting (see Chapter 16.17.5).

Side effects of dihydropyridine CCBs include dose-dependent peripheral oedema, which is not due to fluid retention but results from transudation of fluid from the vascular compartments into the dependent tissues due to precapillary arteriolar dilatation. This oedema does not respond to diuretic therapy but is alleviated by limb elevation, and there is emerging evidence that it may be also reduced by coadministration of an ACE inhibitor or angiotensin receptor blocker because of their effects on venous capacitance. Gum hypertrophy can occur with dihydropyridine CCBs, but is rarely seen with nondihydropyridine CCBs. Nondihydropyridine CCBs cause less peripheral oedema but are negatively inotropic and negatively chronotropic and should therefore be avoided in patients with compromised left ventricular function, and used with caution in combination with β-blockers. Verapamil use is commonly accompanied by constipation.

Blockade of the renin–angiotensin system

The renin–angiotensin system (RAS) has become a very popular target for drug development to treat hypertension. Inhibition of the renin–angiotensin system is predictably effective at lowering blood pressure by inhibiting the various central and peripheral pressor effects of angiotensin II, and blockade may also lower blood pressure by other mechanisms involving improvements in endothelial function, vagal tone and baroreceptor function, and via inhibition of the renal tubular reabsorption of sodium. In addition, inhibition of the renin–angiotensin system has been promoted by clinical trial evidence showing reduced morbidity and mortality with these treatments in patients with heart failure, delay the progression of renal disease, and reduction in cardiovascular events in patients at high cardiovascular risk.

ACE inhibitors

The ACE inhibitors, which block the conversion of angiotensin I to angiotensin II, were the first effective strategy to inhibit the renin–angiotensin system and have been used to treat hypertension since the late 1970s. The resulting reduction in levels of angiotensin II leads to vasodilatation and a fall in blood pressure. Angiotensin II has many additional actions that are potentially harmful to the cardiovascular system and have been implicated in the pathogenesis of structural changes in the heart, blood vessels, and kidneys in hypertension.

Sharp falls in blood pressure following the introduction of ACE inhibitors may occur when the renin–angiotensin system is activated, e.g. in patients who are dehydrated, in heart failure, or have accelerated hypertension. This is rarely a problem when therapy is initiated in uncomplicated hypertensive patients. Side effects of ACE inhibitors include the development of a persistent dry cough in about 20% of users. This is more common in women and in people from Asia, and only disappears after discontinuation of the drug. Another rare but important complication is angio-oedema, which occurs in around 1% but is much more common in the black population (c.4%). ACE inhibitors should be avoided in women of childbearing potential because of the danger of fetal renal malformation. They should not be used in patients with bilateral renal artery disease because they may precipitate deterioration in renal function and renal failure. Careful monitoring of renal function and serum potassium is also required in patients with more advanced renal impairment of any cause because of the risk of hyperkalaemia.

Angiotensin receptor blockers

In the 1990s, the angiotensin receptor blockers (ARBs), which are highly selective inhibitors of the angiotensin II type 1 receptor (AT-1), emerged as an alternative to ACE inhibition. In general they are as effective as ACE inhibitors at reducing blood pressure, but appear to have a longer duration of action, and in common with ACE inhibitors they inhibit the actions of angiotensin II on the cardiovascular system and kidney. They are very well tolerated by patients, with a placebo-like adverse effect profile. Cough and angio-oedema are much less likely to occur than with ACE inhibitors and most guidelines recommend switching patients to an ARB when an ACE-induced cough occurs. Cautions and contraindications are similar to those outlined for ACE inhibitors.

Direct renin inhibition

A third strategy to inhibit the renin–angiotensin system for the treatment of hypertension is direct renin inhibition, the first non-peptide, orally active, direct renin inhibitor being aliskiren. This has high specificity for renin and is a potent renin inhibitor with a long half life (c.24 h). It inhibits the rate-limiting step in angiotensin production, notably the renin-dependent conversion of angiotensinogen to angiotensin I, and appears to have similar blood pressure lowering efficacy to other means of inhibiting the renin system, i.e. ACE inhibition or ARBs, but with less side effects than ACE inhibition. The contraindications to use of direct renin inhibitors are similar to those for ACE inhibition or ARBs. The results

of ongoing clinical trials will ultimately define their role in the hierarchy of treatment.

α-Adrenergic blocking drugs

The original members of this class (e.g. prazosin) were short acting drugs that blocked the activation of α_1 adrenoceptors in the vasculature, leading to vasodilatation. The dosages that were initially recommended were too high, and postural hypotension and syncope proved serious problems that retarded the acceptance of this class of drugs, although the use of lower doses and the development of longer-acting agents (e.g. doxazosin) has largely overcome this problem. Blockade of sphincteric receptors improves symptoms in patients with benign prostatic hypertrophy, and occasionally these same sphincteric effects can worsen symptoms of stress incontinence in women. Uniquely amongst antihypertensive drugs, the α_1-antagonists produce modest favourable changes in plasma lipids, with a reduction in total and LDL cholesterol and triglycerides, and an increase in high-density lipoprotein (HDL) cholesterol.

Centrally acting sympatholytic drugs

Some of the earliest drugs developed to treat hypertension targeted the activation of the sympathetic nervous system at various levels, including the cardiovascular regulatory nuclei in the brainstem, the peripheral autonomic ganglia, and the post ganglionic sympathetic neuron. With one or two exceptions, few of these agents have any residual role to play in the modern treatment of hypertension because side effects are common, often unpleasant, and potentially harmful.

Methyldopa

Methyldopa reduces sympathetic outflow from the brainstem. It was originally developed in the late 1950s and for many years it was one of the mainstays of antihypertensive therapy. However, it frequently causes sedation, impaired psychomotor performance, dry mouth, and erectile dysfunction. This unfavourable impact upon quality of life led to it being replaced by more effective drugs, although it is still used extensively in the management of hypertension of pregnancy, which is now its main indication.

Clonidine

Clonidine is now rarely used because of its short duration of action and risk of a withdrawal syndrome after discontinuing the drug; sudden discontinuation results in a rebound rise in catecholamines with features that may resemble phaeochromocytoma, such as severe hypertension, tachycardia, and sweating. This is exacerbated when patients are also receiving nonselective β-blockers such as propranolol. The syndrome is treated by readministering the drug and then gradually discontinuing it, or the intravenous infusion of labetalol in an emergency.

Moxonidine

Moxonidine is a newer centrally acting agent that is an imidazoline receptor agonist, acting to reduce sympathetic outflow and blood pressure. It has a lower incidence of side effects and is better tolerated than other centrally acting agents.

Direct vasodilators

Hydralazine

Hydralazine was previously extensively used as part of a stepped care regimen. However, its main disadvantages were sympathetic activation and the development of a lupus-like syndrome, particularly in patients with the slow acetylator genotype, which together with the need for multiple daily dosage have resulted in its replacement by other agents, except for occasional use in severe hypertension and hypertension associated with pregnancy. No endpoint trials have been carried out.

Minoxidil

Minoxidil is a very potent vasodilator. Its used is confined to specialist centres for the treatment of severe and resistant hypertension because of its side effects, which include stimulation of body hair growth, tachycardia, and severe fluid retention. For this reason, combination with a potent loop diuretic and a β-blocker is almost always necessary.

Pharmacological treatment strategies

Initial drug therapy

After a suitable period of observation and after assessment of concomitant risk factors, comorbid disease and overall cardiovascular disease risk, a decision may be reached to treat the patient with drug therapy. However, even when this is contemplated it is important to continue to emphasize the importance of lifestyle changes to reduce cardiovascular risk and enhance the efficiency of blood pressure lowering medications, and it is also important to view the patient's blood pressure in the context of their overall cardiovascular risk burden and decide whether other therapies such as statins and antiplatelet therapy might also be appropriate.

Once a decision has been made to initiate drug therapy, it is usual to commence treatment with a single drug. Monotherapy will on average reduce systolic pressure by 7 to 13 mmHg and diastolic pressure by 4 to 8 mmHg. This will give some indication as to whether monotherapy is likely to be effective at achieving the recommended blood pressure goal, but there is marked heterogeneity in response among individuals to particular drugs. Treatment should normally commence with a low dose of the drug selected. If an adequate response is not obtained, the dose of the initial drug can be increased. However, if there has not been much response to the starting dose and the patient's blood pressure remains well short of the target blood pressure, then a more appropriate action would be to add a second drug, either separately or as a combination tablet, mindful of the fact that most people with hypertension require two or more drugs to adequately control their blood pressure. Alternatively, if the initial drug produced a weak response, or none at all, and the patient could conceivably get to their blood pressure

goal on monotherapy, then the first drug could be discontinued and replaced with another class of antihypertensive agent.

Initial therapy with a two drug combination

The heterogeneity of blood pressure responses to different classes of BP-lowering drugs and the likelihood that most people will be uncontrolled by monotherapy, has led to the suggestion that more people should be initiated on treatment with low-dose combination therapy. Low-dose two-drug combination therapy has been recommended in European and American hypertension guidelines for the treatment of patients whose blood pressure is greater than 20/10 mmHg above their goal blood pressure and therefore unlikely to achieve their goal blood pressure with monotherapy (Fig. 16.17.2.5). The United States guideline has been explicit in stating that this combination would usually involve a diuretic. The concept of initial therapy with a two-drug combination has in part been driven by concern that the up-titration of treatment in people at high risk may be too slow and leave them at risk for too long.

Choice of initial therapy

There is wide variation in the international guidelines with regard to the preferred initial therapy for essential hypertension. In the United States of America, the Joint National Committee (JNC) VII guideline recommended low dose thiazide-type diuretic therapy as initial therapy for all patients (unless contraindicated), reflecting a view that the most important driver of benefit was blood pressure control and that the low dose diuretic was the most cost-effective way to deliver that.

The recent European guideline suggested that all five main classes of blood pressure lowering drugs (ACE inhibitors, angiotensin receptor blockers, β-blockers, calcium channel blockers, and diuretics) were all suitable as initial therapy and that choice would in part reflect physician preference and the concomitant conditions and specific indications and contraindications for different drug classes in an individual patient (Table 16.17.2.6).

The British Hypertension Society/NICE guideline adopted a different approach. Their analysis of the data suggested that a calcium channel blocker (C) or alternatively a diuretic (D) would be most likely to deliver the most effective initial blood pressure lowering in older people (i.e. ≥55 years), whereas an ACE inhibitor or an angiotensin receptor blocker (A) would be the preferred initial therapy for younger patients (<55 years), with the caveat that C or D would be the preferred therapy for people of black African

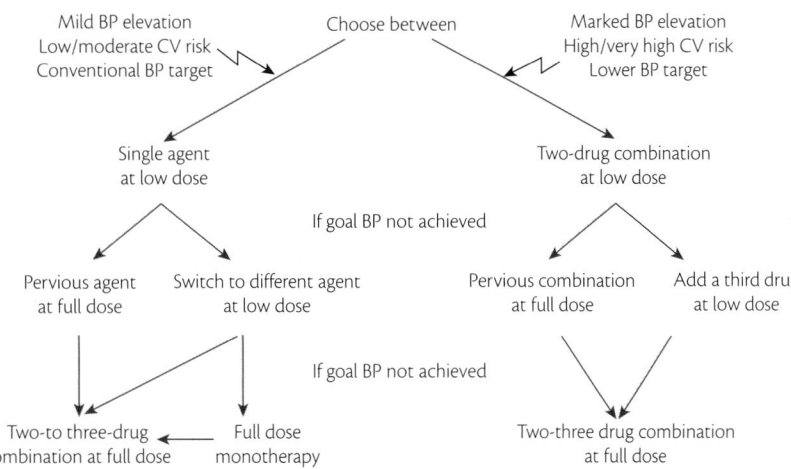

Fig. 16.17.2.5 European Society of Hypertension/European Society of Cardiology 2007 guideline recommendation for treatment strategies for hypertension.
European Society of Hypertension Guideline, 2007. From Journal of hypertension, 2007 ESH-ESC Practice Guidelines for the Management of Arterial Hypertension: ESH-ESC Task Force on the Management of Arterial Hypertension, 2007, 25:1751–1762. (http://journals.lww.com/jhypertension/Citation/2007/09000/2007_ESH_ESC_Practice_Guidelines_for_the.1.aspx) - fig 4.

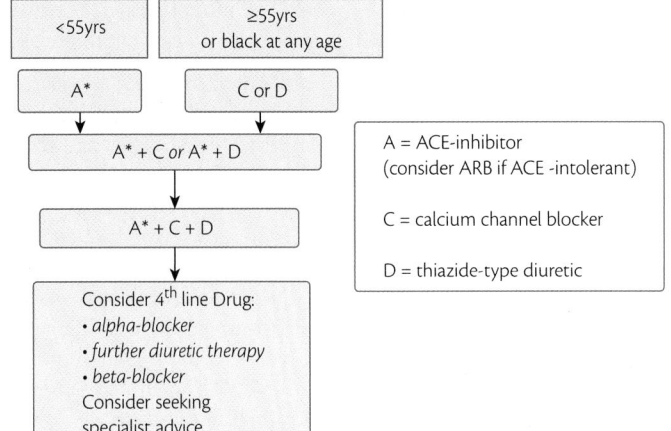

Fig. 16.17.2.6 British Hypertension Society/NICE treatment algorithm for the treatment of essential hypertension.
National Institute for Health and Clinical Excellence (2006) CG 34 Hypertension: management of hypertension in adults in primary care. London: NICE. Available from www.nice.org.uk/CG34 Reproduced with permission.

origin at any age (Fig. 16.17.2.6). The rationale for this recommendation was founded on the observation that plasma renin levels fall as people age and are lower in blacks at any age. Therefore drugs that target the renin system are more likely to be more effective initial therapy in higher renin younger patients, whereas the converse in true with ageing. These guidelines also recommended against the use of β-blockers as a preferred initial therapy (especially for older patients), unless there were compelling indications, because (1) they appear less effective at reducing the risk of stroke than the alternatives, (2) they are associated with an increased risk of developing diabetes, and (3) they are the least cost-effective treatment option for essential hypertension.

Combination therapy for controlling blood pressure

All guidelines recognize that combinations of blood pressure lowering drugs are often required to achieve recommended blood pressure goals, especially in those with high cardiovascular disease risk or comorbidities who are targeted to lower pressures. The European guidelines provide a diagram to illustrate suitable combinations of treatment (Fig. 16.17.2.7). The American JNC VII guidelines suggest that whatever combination is used, it should usually include a diuretic, consistent with the fact that they have recommended that initial therapy would usually be with a diuretic. Only the British guideline provides explicit guidance on preferred combinations of treatment at step 2, i.e. A + C or A + D, and step 3, i.e. A + C + D (Fig. 16.17.2.6). The recent ACCOMPLISH study suggested that A+C may be more effective than A+D at preventing cardiovascular events, despite similarities in BP control.

Resistant hypertension

Drug-resistant hypertension can be defined as blood pressure that is not controlled despite treatment with an appropriate combination of three drug therapies (e.g. A + C + D—see Fig. 16.17.2.6) prescribed at their maximum recommended and tolerated doses. In the absence of evidence of target organ damage, white coat hypertension should be excluded by 24-h ambulatory monitoring. Other causes for resistant hypertension include (1) secondary hypertension (e.g. renovascular or endocrine); (2) ingestion of drugs that may raise blood pressure (e.g. nonsteroidal anti-inflammatory agents); (3) heavy alcohol intake; (4) sodium and fluid retention as a result of inadequate diuretic therapy; and (5) poor patient adherence to treatment.

Most patients with drug-resistant hypertension are likely to be retaining sodium and will respond to further diuretic therapy.

A suppressed plasma renin despite treatment with A + C + D would be indicative of sodium retention because these treatments would be expected to elevate plasma renin, hence the preferred initial approach to treatment in this situation is further diuretic therapy, either with increased dosage of the thiazide diuretic, or using low dose spironolactone (e.g. 25 mg/day), or amiloride (10–20 mg/day), with careful monitoring of electrolytes. For some patients with very severe drug resistant hypertension it may be necessary use a combination of monoxidil, loop diuretic, and β-blocker to improve blood pressure control.

Poor adherence to therapy is often difficult to detect in hypertensive patients and can lead to expensive investigations for secondary causes. One way of detecting effectiveness of treatment is to use ABPM to monitor blood pressure after directly observed consumption of medication. Although this may not resolve the problem of adherence with treatment, it will identify whether the treatment is effective if adhered to, thus avoiding the need for further investigations.

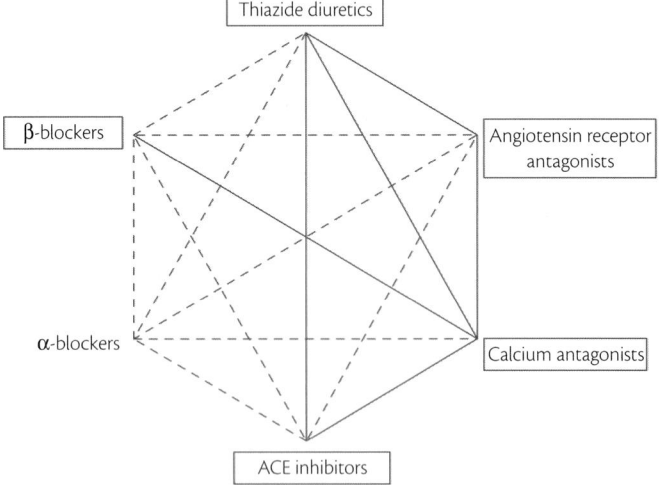

Fig. 16.17.2.7 European Society of Hypertension/European Society of Cardiology 2007 guideline recommendations for combining drugs to lower blood pressure. The preferred combinations in the general hypertensive population are represented as thick lines. The frames indicate classes of agents proven to be beneficial in controlled intervention trials.
European Society of Hypertension Guideline, 2007. From Journal of hypertension, 2007 ESH-ESC Practice Guidelines for the Management of Arterial Hypertension: ESH-ESC Task Force on the Management of Arterial Hypertension, 2007, 25:1751–1762. (http://journals.lww.com/jhypertension/Citation/2007/09000/2007_ESH_ESC_Practice_Guidelines_for_the.1.aspx) - fig 4

Where adherence is obviously poor, a number of manoeuvres can help to improve it. The treatment should be made as simple as possible, using once-daily drugs and combination tablets, and a carer needs to be involved in administering medication to those who are confused. Whenever possible, effective communication with full information and involvement of the patient in his or her treatment is essential. Nurses, pharmacists, and other health professionals can play a vital role in this process.

Follow-up

It is essential that patients are monitored regularly and it is important that this message is conveyed to the patient. In the early stages of treatment the frequency of monitoring will be determined by the response to therapy, comorbidities, and the complexity of the treatment regimen required to control the blood pressure. Once blood pressure is controlled, patients should be reviewed at least annually, and most will be reviewed every 6 months. Patients are increasingly monitoring their own blood pressure in the intervening period.

Withdrawal of therapy

The vast majority of patients with hypertension require lifelong therapy. Some with grade 1 hypertension who make substantial adjustments to their lifestyle may obtain sufficient fall in their blood pressure to warrant withdrawal of monotherapy. However, patients with target organ damage or those at high cardiovascular disease risk should not usually have their therapy withdrawn, unless there is a compelling clinical reason to do so. It is also important to note that in patients with previously severe hypertension that has subsequently been well controlled, treatment withdrawal may not always result in an immediate increase in blood pressure. This can sometimes convey the false impression that treatment may no longer be required because blood pressure can sometimes take many months to progressively rise back to dangerously high pretreatment values. Thus, any patient who discontinues therapy must remain under review with regular monitoring of their blood pressure, and all but a very few will require treatment again.

Other issues

Indications for specialist referral

There are circumstances when referral to a specialist centre is indicated for the management of hypertension. These include uncertainty about the decision to treat, investigations to exclude secondary hypertension, severe and complicated hypertension, and resistant hypertension, among others as detailed in Box 16.17.2.5.

Medication to reduce cardiovascular risk

Blood pressure should not be treated in isolation and should be considered as part of a comprehensive strategy to reduce cardiovascular disease risk. In this regard, patients at high risk, i.e. those with established cardiovascular disease, target organ damage, and/or diabetes, or those with a calculated cardiovascular disease risk which is elevated (e.g. ≥20% over 10 years), should be considered for additional interventions to reduce risk. These include reinforcement of lifestyle advice, especially smoking cessation, and treatment with statin therapy to further reduce their risk of stroke and coronary disease. In recent studies the routine use of statins to reduce total cholesterol values by 1 mmol/litre has been associated with a reduction in the risk of ischaemic heart disease events by about one-third and stroke by about one-fifth, over and above the benefit already accrued from blood pressure lowering.

Box 16.17.2.5 Recommended and possible indications for specialist referral for patients with hypertension

Urgent treatment needed

- Accelerated hypertension (severe hypertension with grade III—IV retinopathy)
- Particularly severe hypertension (>220/120 mmHg)
- Impending complications (e.g. transient ischaemic attack, left ventricular failure)

Possible underlying cause

- Any clue in history or examination of a secondary cause, e.g. hypokalemia with increased or high normal plasma sodium (Conn's syndrome)
- Elevated serum creatinine
- Proteinuria or haematuria
- Sudden-onset or worsening of hypertension
- Resistance to multidrug regimen, i.e. ≥3 drugs
- Young age (any hypertension <20 years; needing treatment <30 years)

Therapeutic problems

- Multiple drug intolerance
- Multiple drug contraindications
- Persistent nonadherence or noncompliance

Special situations

- Unusual blood pressure variability
- Possible white coat hypertension
- Hypertension in pregnancy

Moreover, the relative risk reduction associated with statin therapy in higher risk hypertensive patients was not dependent on a high baseline cholesterol value.

Once blood pressure has been controlled, higher risk hypertensive patients should also be considered for treatment with low dose aspirin (75 mg/day). This has been shown to reduce the incidence of myocardial infarction in higher-risk patients over 50 years old and should be offered routinely to patients who fall in this category and who do not have contraindications. In view of the increased incidence of haemorrhage, it is not indicated in lower-risk hypertensive patients.

Hypertension in specific groups of patients

People of black African origin

Hypertension is more prevalent in blacks, is associated with more target organ damage and consequently carries a worse prognosis, with a particularly high risk of stroke. Black patients as a group tend to respond better to diuretics, calcium channel blockers, and dietary salt restriction than white patients. ACE inhibitors, angiotensin receptor blockers, and β-blockers are generally less effective as initial therapy, but become more effective when combined with diuretics and/or calcium channel blockers.

Older people

Most people with hypertension are elderly. If a blood pressure of 140/90 mmHg or more is used to define hypertension, then over 70% of people over the age of 60 years will be hypertensive, with most of these having isolated systolic hypertension. Surveys suggest that doctors consistently underestimate the risks and undertreat hypertension in older people, which is somewhat paradoxical in that elderly people have much higher absolute risk than younger people with hypertension and therefore much to gain from blood pressure lowering. There are, however, some important considerations when treating older people:

- The arterial wall stiffening that gives rise to systolic hypertension and increased pulse pressure (isolated systolic hypertension) is also associated with impaired baroreflex sensitivity, with increased risk of orthostatic hypotension, hence it is important to record lying and standing blood pressure in elderly patients.

- eGFR declines with age and renal conservation of sodium and fluid in the face of depletion is impaired, thus elderly patients are more prone to dehydration as a result of diuretic therapy.

- Clearance of drugs and their active metabolites is decreased as a result of declining hepatic and renal function.

- Cardiac function and reserve are often reduced, such that patients are much more likely to develop cardiac failure. This explains why endpoint trials of hypertension treatment have consistently shown reductions in morbidity and mortality from cardiac failure.

- Comorbidity is much more common.

- Communication and adherence with therapy may be more difficult with decline in cognitive function. Some evidence from clinical trials suggests that this decline may be retarded by antihypertensive treatment.

Despite these considerations, elderly people tolerate blood pressure lowering medications well, and the benefits of blood pressure reduction are impressive with regard to reductions in morbidity and mortality due to stroke, ischaemic heart disease, and heart failure. As a general rule, drug regimens should be as simple as possible and dosages increased more gradually, the greatest danger resulting from lowering pressure too much and too rapidly. Until recently there was uncertainty about the risks and benefits of treating hypertension in very elderly people, i.e. those over the age of 80 years, but a recent study in this age group confirmed that treatment was well tolerated and associated with impressive reductions in the risk of stroke, heart failure, and mortality. Thus, there is no reason to manage very elderly patients any differently from those who are not as old. Biological rather than chronological age should be the deciding factor in initiating antihypertensive treatment, but there is never any substitute for clinical common sense—the elderly man with mild cognitive impairment, prone to falls, and with occasional dizziness on standing up, is not likely to be well served by the doctor who advocates medication to reduce marginally elevated blood pressure.

Children

Although secondary hypertension is more common in children than in adults, no specific cause is found for hypertension in most adolescents. The criteria for drug treatment, however, have to be modified because of the lower normal blood pressure range. The JNC guidelines recommend that blood pressures above the 95th percentile—taking into account age, height, and sex—should be considered elevated. In principle, treatment regimens are the same as those recommended for adults, with appropriate dose adjustment.

Further reading

Blood pressure measurement

Agabiti-Rosei E, *et al.* (2007). Central blood pressure measurements and antihypertensive therapy: A consensus document. *Hypertension*, **50**, 1–7.

European Society of Hypertension (2008). Guidelines for blood pressure monitoring at home: a summary report of the Second International Consensus Conference on Home Blood Pressure Monitoring. *J Hypertens*, **26**, 1505–26.

Kikuya M, *et al.* (2007). Diagnostic thresholds for ambulatory blood pressure monitoring based on 10-year cardiovascular risk. *Circulation*, **115**, 2145–52.

O'Brien E, *et al.* (2003). European Society of Hypertension recommendations for conventional, ambulatory and home blood pressure measurement. *J Hypertens*, **21**, 821–48.

Pickering TG, *et al.* (2008). Call to action on use and reimbursement for home blood pressure monitoring: a joint scientific statement from the American Heart Association, American Society of Hypertension, and Preventive Cardiovascular Nurses Association. *Hypertension*, **52**, 10–29.

Verdecchia P, *et al.* (2002). Properly defining white coat hypertension. *Eur Heart J*, **23**, 106–9.

Lifestyle interventions

Appel LJ, *et al.* (1997). A clinical trial of the effects of dietary patterns on blood pressure. *N Engl J Med*, **336**, 1117–24.

Beilin LJ, Puddey IB (2006). Alcohol and hypertension—an update. *Hypertension*, **47**, 1035–8.

Cook NR, *et al.* (2007). Long term effects of dietary sodium reduction on cardiovascular disease outcomes: observational follow-up of trials of hypertension prevention. *BMJ*, **334**, 885–92.

Dickinson HO, *et al.* (2006). Lifestyle interventions to reduce raised blood pressure: a systematic review of randomized controlled trials. *J Hypertens*, **24**, 215–33.

Gangwisch JE, *et al.* (2006). Short sleep duration as a risk factor for hypertension: analyses of the First National Health and Nutrition Examination Survey. *Hypertension*, **47**, 833–9.

He FJ, MacGregor GA (2006). Importance of salt in determining blood pressure in children meta-analysis of controlled trials. *Hypertension*, **48**, 861–9.

Clinical trials and pharmacological treatment

Blood Pressure Lowering Treatment Trialists' Collaboration (2003). Effects of different blood-pressure-lowering regimens on major cardiovascular events: results of prospectively-designed overviews of randomised trials. *Lancet*, **362**, 1527–45.

Hanon O, *et al.* (2003). Effect of antihypertensive treatment on cognitive functions. *J Hypertens*, **24**, 2101–7.

Jamerson K, Weber MA, Bakris GL, *et al.* (2008). Benazepril plus amlodipine or hydrochlorothiazide for hypertension in high-risk patients. *N Engl J Med*, **359**, 2417–28.

Julius S, *et al.* (2006). for the Trial of Preventing Hypertension (TROPHY) Study Investigators. Feasibility of treating prehypertension with an angiotensin-receptor blocker. *N Engl J Med*, **354**, 1685–97.

Lawes CM, *et al.* (2004). Blood pressure and stroke: An overview of published trials. *Stroke*, **35**, 776–85.

Lindholm LH, Carlberg B, Samuelsson O (2005). Should β blockers remain first choice in the treatment of primary hypertension? A meta-analysis. *Lancet*, **366**, 1545–53.

Mancia G, Grassi G (2002). Systolic and diastolic blood pressure control in antihypertensive drug trials. *J Hypertens*, **20**, 1461–4.

Staessen JA, et al. (2003). Cardiovascular prevention and blood pressure reduction: a quantitative overview updated until 1st March 2003. *J Hypertens*, **21**, 1055–76.

Williams B (2004). Protection against stroke and dementia: an update on the latest clinical trial evidence. *Curr Hypertens Rep*, **6**, 307–13.

Williams B (2005). Recent hypertension trials: implications and controversies. *J Am Coll Cardiol*, **45**, 813–27.

Williams B (2007). Beta-blockers and the treatment of hypertension. *J Hypertens*, **25**, 1351–3.

Williams B (2007). Hypertension in the young—preventing the evolution of disease versus prevention of clinical events. *J Am Coll Cardiol*, **50**, 840–2.

Zhang H, Thijs L, Staessen JA (2006). Blood pressure lowering for primary and secondary prevention of stroke. *Hypertension*, **48**, 187–95.

Other therapies to reduce cardiovascular risk in hypertensive patients

Emberson J, et al. (2004). Evaluating the impact of population and high-risk strategies for the primary prevention of CVD. *Eur Heart J*, **25**, 484–91.

Gaziano TA, Opie LH, Weinstein MC (2006). Cardiovascular disease prevention with a multidrug regimen in the developing world: a cost-effectiveness analysis. *Lancet*, **368**, 679–86.

Heart Protection Study Collaborative Group (2002). MRC/BHF Heart Protection Study of antioxidant vitamin supplementation in 20 536 high-risk individuals: a randomised placebo-controlled trial. *Lancet*, **360**, 23–33.

Patrono C, et al. (2005). Low-dose aspirin for the prevention of atherothrombosis. *N Engl J Med*, **353**, 2373–83.

Sever PS, et al. (2003). Prevention of coronary and stroke events with atorvastatin in hypertensive patients who have average or lower-then-average cholesterol concentrations, in the Anglo Scandinavian Cardiac Outcomes Trial-Lipid Lowering Arm (ASCOT-LLA): A multicentre randomised controlled trial. *Lancet*, **361**, 1149–58.

Wald NJ, Law MR (2003). A strategy to reduce cardiovascular disease by more than 80%. *BMJ*, **326**, 1419–23.

Treatment guidelines

Adams, Jr, HP, et al. (2007). Guidelines for the early management of adults with ischemic stroke. *Circulation*, **115**, e478–534.

Broderick J, et al. (2007). Guidelines for the management of spontaneous intracerebral hemorrhage in adults: update. *Stroke*, **38**, 2001–2023.

Chobanian AV, et al. (2003). The seventh report of the Joint National Committee on Prevention, Detection, Evaluation and Treatment of High Blood Pressure: the JNC VII Report. *JAMA*, **289**, 2560–72.

Colhoun DA, et al. (2008). Resistant hypertension: Diagnosis evaluation and treatment. A scientific statement from the American heart association professional education committee of the council for high blood pressure research. *Hypertension*, **117**, e510–26.

Conroy RM, et al. (2003). Estimation of ten-year risk of fatal cardiovascular disease in Europe: the SCORE project. *Eur Heart J*, **24**, 987–1003.

Douglas JG, et al. (2003). The Hypertension in African Americans Working Group. Management of high blood pressure in African Americans. *Arch Intern Med*, **163**, 525–41.

Higgens B, et al. (2007). Pharmacological management of hypertension. *Clin Med*, **7**, 612–16. [Key features of the UK BHS/NICE hypertension guideline update in 2006, with link to the full guideline resource: http://www.nice.org.uk/CG034guidance.]

Mendis S, et al. (2007). World Health Organization (WHO) and International Society of Hypertension (ISH) risk prediction charts: assessment of cardiovascular risk for prevention and control of cardiovascular disease in low and middle-income countries. *J Hypertens*, **25**, 1578–82.

Task Force for the Management of Arterial Hypertension of the European Society of Hypertension (ESH) and of the European Society of Cardiology (ESC). (2007). Guidelines for the management of arterial hypertension. *J Hypertens*, **25**, 1105–87.

Williams B, et al. (2004). Guidelines for management of hypertension: report of the fourth working party of the British Hypertension Society, 2004-BHS IV. *J Hum Hypertens*, **18**, 139–85.

Williams B (2006). Evolution of hypertensive disease: a revolution in guidelines. *Lancet*, **368**, 6–8.

Williams B. (2009). Resistant hypertension. *Lancet*, **374**, 1396–1398.

Recent reviews

Messerli FH, Williams B, Ritz E (2007). Essential hypertension. *Lancet*, **370**, 591–603.

Williams B (2006). The year in hypertension. *J Am Coll Cardiol*, **48**, 1698–711.

Williams B (2008). The year in hypertension. *J Am Coll Cardiol*, **51**, 1803–17.

16.17.3 Secondary hypertension

Morris J. Brown

Essentials

The term 'secondary hypertension' is used to describe patients whose blood pressure is elevated by a single, identifiable cause, with an important subdivision being into reversible and irreversible causes: clinically, it is important to exclude the former, but not necessarily to find the latter.

In the first two decades of life, the prevalence of secondary hypertension is greater than that of essential hypertension; thereafter, a patient is much more likely to have essential hypertension, but investigations for secondary hypertension should still be assiduous in the twenties and thirties because the alternative entails so many years of tablet-taking.

All patients with hypertension should have a minimum set of investigations (see Chapter 16.7.2). Common indications for further investigations are (1) any evidence of an underlying cause on history or examination; (2) proteinuria, haematuria, or elevated serum creatinine (eGFR<30; CKD 4/5); (3) hypokalaemia, even if caused by diuretics; (4) accelerated (malignant) hypertension; (5) documented recent onset or recent worsening of hypertension; (6) resistant hypertension (not controlled with three antihypertensive drugs); (7) young age—any hypertension at less than 20 years; any hypertension needing treatment at less than 35 years.

The minimum screen in younger patients should include plasma bicarbonate, plasma renin, and a 24-h urine test to exclude phaeochromocytoma; 24-h electrolyte excretion should be measured either in all patients, or in those with abnormal renin levels.

Renovascular hypertension

This is most commonly due to intrinsic disease of the intima (acquired, atherosclerosis, etc.) or media (congenital, fibromuscular dysplasia (FMD), etc.). FMD accounts for only 10–20% of all cases, but is the commonest cause under the age of 40.

Most cases of renovascular hypertension are probably not diagnosed because of the absence of sensitive clinical or biochemical markers. The main clinical clue is the finding in 50% of cases of a bruit anteriorly or posteriorly over a renal area, but it is important to remember that such a bruit is never diagnostic. The diagnosis is made radiologically, most commonly by CT or MR angiography.

In FMD, angioplasty is usually curative, with about three-quarters of patients able to discontinue antihypertensive treatment. In atheromatous disease, angioplasty is much less likely to be successful: complete cure of hypertension is rare, and often the purpose of intervention is to protect declining renal function.

Coarctation of the aorta

Coarctation causes less than 1% of all cases of hypertension. The classical clinical finding is radio–femoral pulse delay. Diagnosis is confirmed by two-dimensional echocardiography, or by CT or MR angiography. Treatment is by surgery, balloon dilatation, or stenting.

Primary hyperaldosteronism (Conn's syndrome)

Primary hyperaldosteronism causes increased sodium retention through the epithelial sodium channel (ENaC) in the distal tubule and cortical collecting duct, which leads to hypertension. It can be caused by (1) Conn's adenoma—a small (0.5–3.5 cm) benign tumour of the adrenal gland; (2) bilateral adrenal hyperplasia—where there are macro- or micronodules in the adrenal cortex; (3) the very rare condition of glucocorticoid-remediable aldosteronism (see Chapter 16.7.4).

Diagnosis—the classic clinical picture is hypertension with plasma electrolytes showing low K^+, elevated bicarbonate, and Na^+ typically at the upper end of the normal range, together with suppressed plasma renin and elevated aldosterone—but these findings are not invariable and diagnosis can be difficult. The adrenals are usually easily imaged by either CT or MRI, but functional lateralization can be difficult, although essential for predicting that removal of one adrenal will have a substantial benefit, as well as indicating which adrenal to remove. The most reliable technique is adrenal vein sampling: all samples need to be assayed for aldosterone and cortisol, with the ratio compared between the two sides.

Management—medical treatment is preferred for bilateral adrenal hyperplasia, before surgery for adenoma, in older patients with adenoma who are well controlled, or where there is any doubt about diagnosis or lateralization. High doses of spironolactone or amiloride are most commonly used. Elective surgery is indicated for younger patients with macroadenoma, and older patients intolerant of—or uncontrolled by—medical treatment.

Phaeochromocytoma

Phaeochromocytomas are rare tumours of chromaffin tissue that account for 0.1 to 1% of cases of hypertension: 90% are benign and 90% are located in the adrenal gland. Most are sporadic, but some are associated with genetic syndromes, including von Hippel–Lindau and multiple endocrine neoplasia type 2.

Hypertension, usually in association with one or more symptoms of headache, sweating, and palpitations, is the most common presentation. Other rarer presentations include unexplained heart failure or paroxysmal arrhythmia. Four per cent of adrenal incidentalomas are phaeochromocytomas.

Diagnosis—this is usually not difficult once the possibility of phaeochromocytoma has been entertained; more difficult is excluding the diagnosis in patients who have clinical and/or biochemical features of physiological catecholamine excess. Investigation must first determine whether the patient has a phaeochromocytoma, and then where the tumour is. The best screening test is to measure plasma or 24 h urine normetanephrine (normetadrenaline) and metanephrine (metadrenaline): their assay in a reliable laboratory is more sensitive and specific than measurement of catecholamines or vanillylmandelic acid (VMA). Detection of elevated metadrenaline is a useful clue to the usual adrenal location of the phaeochromocytoma. A pharmacological suppression test can be performed where doubt about the diagnosis remains: physiological elevations of noradrenaline release are temporarily suppressed by administration of the ganglion-blocking drug pentolinium, or the centrally acting α_2-agonist clonidine, but these drugs do not suppress autonomous secretion by tumour. CT or MRI scanning usually provides excellent imaging of the adrenal. Radioisotope scanning with the iodinated analogue of noradrenaline, m-iodobenzylguanidine (mIBG), can be helpful in localizing extra-adrenal tumours. Selective venous sampling is occasionally required.

Management—the task for the physician is to make surgery—the definitive treatment that cures hypertension in most patients—safe. This should be done by α-blockade with phenoxybenzamine, with a low dose of a β_1-selective blocker used to prevent tachycardia.

Introduction

The term 'secondary hypertension' is used to describe patients whose blood pressure is elevated by a single, identifiable cause. Until recently, there has been an optimistic view that description of new causes of hypertension would mean that those regarded as having 'essential hypertension' would be an ever-diminishing group. However, as discussed in Chapter 16.17.1, genome-wide investigation into the genetic bases of hypertension have shown that there are no common inherited susceptibility alleles that can explain more than 1 to 2mmHg of a person's blood pressure. Hence it is now almost certain that essential hypertension differs from secondary hypertension not only in being unexplained, but in being, within each patient, due to a multiplicity of inherited and acquired characteristics.

An important subdivision of secondary hypertension is into reversible and irreversible causes: clinically it is important to exclude the former, but not necessarily to find the latter. Their elucidation may lead to improved medical therapy, e.g. by predicting the best diuretic in the monogenic causes of low-renin hypertension, or help assess prognosis, as in the patient with proteinuria. However, the resource implications of finding causes, which can be considerable, need to be balanced against achievable gains. These in turn are influenced by the patient's age, usually meaning that a search for secondary causes is easier to justify in young patients in whom small benefits are multiplied over many years.

Age-related prevalence of secondary hypertension

Whereas essential hypertension is clearly an age-related phenomenon, the same is less true of secondary hypertension, although different causes predominate at different ages. The net likelihood of a given patient with hypertension having a secondary cause is higher at a young age (Fig. 16.17.3.1). In the first two decades, essential

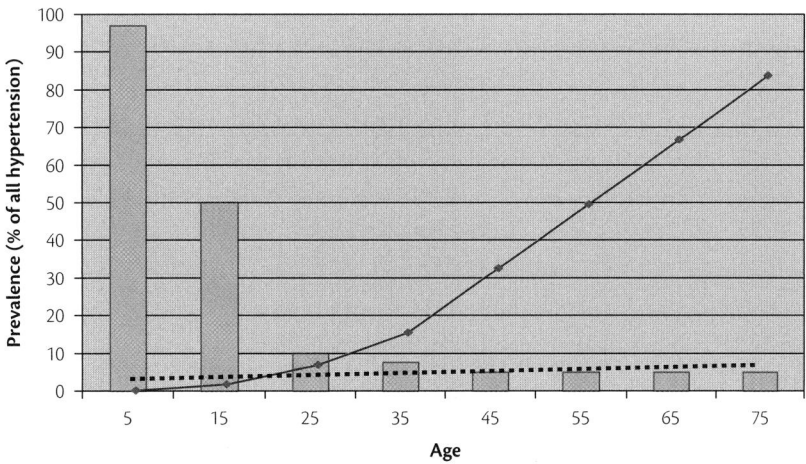

Fig. 16.17.3.1 The age-related prevalence of secondary hypertension. The red line shows the prevalence of essential hypertension by age (years), the dotted line the prevalence of secondary hypertension by age, and the bars show the percentage of all hypertensives with a secondary cause.

hypertension is so uncommon that even the absolute prevalence of secondary hypertension is greater than that of essential hypertension. Thereafter, a patient is much more likely to have essential hypertension, but investigations for secondary hypertension should still be aggressive in patients in their twenties and thirties because the alternative entails so many years of tablet-taking.

In the first decade of life the main causes of secondary hypertension are the monogenic syndromes causing low-renin (Na⁺-dependent) hypertension and congenital causes (e.g. coarctation). However, the rarity of blood pressure measurement or of complications in the first decade means diagnosis is often later, hence these are also the main causes of hypertension diagnosed in the second decade. Additional causes by this time are some acquired renal diseases, and the familial phaeochromocytoma syndromes. Conn's syndrome becomes the commonest cause for the next two to three decades. From the fifth decade onwards, atheromatous renal artery stenosis is the main secondary cause of hypertension.

The clinical approach to secondary hypertension

All patients with hypertension should have a minimum set of investigations, as described in Chapter 16.7.2. Common indications for further investigations are shown in Box 16.17.3.1.

Box 16.17.3.1 Indications for investigation for secondary causes of hypertension

- Any evidence of an underlying cause in the history or examination (Table 16.17.3.1)
- Proteinuria, haematuria, or elevated serum creatinine (eGFR<30; CKD 4/5)
- Hypokalaemia even if caused by diuretics
- Accelerated (malignant) hypertension
- Documented recent onset or recent worsening of hypertension
- Resistant hypertension (not controlled with three antihypertensive drugs)
- Young age—any hypertension <20 years; any hypertension needing treatment <35 years

---

If possible, patients with blood pressure requiring treatment in their twenties or thirties should be investigated before initiation of treatment because this is rarely pressing at a young age, and some of the tests are easier to interpret off treatment.

The minimum screen in younger patients should include plasma bicarbonate, plasma renin, and a 24-h urine test to exclude phaeochromocytoma; 24-h electrolyte excretion should be measured either in all patients, or in those with abnormal renin levels, with the trend to using metanephrine excretion for phaeochromocytoma screening allowing a single collection (without preservative) to be used for both purposes. Sodium intake is most readily estimated at steady state (i.e. no recent change in diet or drugs) by measuring sodium excretion: intakes between 100 and 200 mmol (*c.*6–12 g)/day have little effect upon plasma renin, whereas outside this range there is a steep inverse relationship.

Further investigations pursuing specific diagnoses that might be considered in particular cases (Table 16.17.3.1) are described in the following sections.

Renal hypertension

The principal curable cause is renovascular hypertension. This is usually due to a stenosis in one or both renal arteries, but can be due to a suprarenal aortic stenosis. Other curable causes include renal tumours (hypernephroma and, the rarest of all secondary causes, a juxtaglomerular renin-secreting tumour); a unilateral, poorly functioning scarred or hydronephrotic kidney which hypersecretes renin, and can be removed without unacceptable loss of renal function; and various causes of acute/subacute glomerulonephritis, some associated with systemic disorders whose treatment by immunosuppression cures the hypertension and underlying disorder.

Renovascular hypertension

This is most commonly due to intrinsic disease of the intima (acquired, atherosclerosis) or media (congenital, fibromuscular dysplasia). Extrinsic narrowing can be caused by ligamentous bands, or by tumours, e.g. neurofibromas.

Fibromuscular dysplasia (FMD) accounts for only 10 to 20% of all patients with renovascular hypertension, but is the commonest cause under the age of 40. It is a nonatherosclerotic and noninflammatory disease of small and medium arteries, usually affecting

Table 16.17.3.1 Evidence in history, examination, or routine investigations suggesting a secondary cause for hypertension

Clinical	Evidence	Condition to consider
History	Paroxysmal features—palpitation, sweating, pallor, panic, pain in head or chest	Phaeochromocytoma
	Personal or family history of renal disease	Renal hypertension
	Drug history—oestrogen-containing oral contraceptives; non-steroidal anti-inflammatory drugs; sympathomimetics (cold cures, nasal decongestants); corticosteroids; ciclosporin; carbenoxalone; sodium bicarbonate; ergotamine; mono-amine oxidase inhibitors (with tyramine-containing foods); erythropoietin	Drug-induced hypertension
	Tetany, muscle weakness	Conn's syndrome
Examination	General appearance	Cushing's syndrome, Acromegaly
	Palpable kidney(s)	Adult polycystic kidney disease, Tuberous sclerosis
	Abdominal or loin bruits	Renovascular disease
	Delayed or weak femoral pulses	Coarctation of the aorta
Investigations	Proteinuria, haematuria, or elevated serum creatinine (eGFR<30; CKD 4/5)	Renal or renovascular disease
	Hypokalaemia	Conn's syndrome

the media, less commonly the adventitia (<25%), and rarely the intima. The classical 'string of beads' appearance seen at arteriography results from proliferation of the extracellular matrix and disruption of the internal elastic lamina, causing multiple stenoses and poststenotic saccular aneurysms. The condition affects women more often than men, and there is usually no family history of hypertension. FMD involves extrarenal arteries in about one-quarter of patients, with cerebral infarction recorded due to relative hypotension and hypoperfusion of FMD-affected carotid arteries following successful renal angioplasty.

The typical medial form of FMD does not affect the proximal part of the renal arteries and is bilateral in about one-third of cases. Other vascular beds, e.g. the cerebral arteries, can be affected. Complications (other than renal ischaemia) are rare, whereas dissection or thrombosis can ensue in the rarer intimal or adventitial form of FMD. Rupture of renal artery aneurysms is rare.

Atheromatous renal artery stenosis has the same risk factors as atheromatous disease of other arteries, which often coexists. It is thus commoner in older men, and whereas FMD rarely causes renal impairment, atheromatous disease often presents with impaired renal function rather than hypertension, with intervention undertaken to protect renal function as much as to lower blood pressure. Apart from the obvious difference in biology of FMD and atheromatous renovascular hypertension, there is a difference in location of the stenosis, which is more likely to be proximal in atheromatous disease (Fig. 16.17.3.2).

Mechanism of hypertension

Unilateral renal artery stenosis gives rise to an endocrine disorder, because reduced pressure in the afferent arteriole causes juxtaglomerular hyperplasia and increased renin secretion. The consequent increase in angiotensin II formation causes hypertension, partly by vasoconstriction and partly through increased aldosterone secretion. Although secondary hyperaldosteronism is not usually a marked feature of renal artery stenosis, the combination of hypokalaemia and hyponatraemia should raise suspicion of the diagnosis, the latter being dilutional and due to the inhibition by angiotensin II of free water clearance. The effect on renin secretion is less predictable when renal artery stenosis affects both renal arteries: sometimes it is high, but sometimes bilateral reduction in GFR leads to sufficient sodium retention that renin is suppressed.

Diagnosis

Most cases of renovascular hypertension are probably not diagnosed because of the absence of sensitive clinical or biochemical markers. Lack of a family history of hypertension in younger patients, or recent onset (or exacerbation) of hypertension in older patients is more likely than in essential hypertension. Acute shortness of breath, due to flash pulmonary oedema, can be the presenting feature of bilateral renal artery stenosis. However, the main clinical clue is the finding, in about one-half of the patients, of a bruit anteriorly or posteriorly over a renal area. But it is important to remember that such a bruit is never diagnostic: normal abdominal arteries can give rise to innocent flow murmurs in younger patients, and in older patients a bruit could arise from any of a number of arteries within the abdomen. The response to antihypertensive drugs can also give clues, in particular poor response to β-blockade in younger patients, or rapid worsening of renal function in older patients.

The diagnosis of renal artery stenosis is made radiologically. The cheapest investigation is a nuclear medicine scan using technetium-labelled MAG3, both the uptake and elimination of this being delayed on the ischaemic side, with the difference in excretion rate between sides greatly increased following a single dose of captopril (25 mg) because of dilatation of the efferent arterioles in glomeruli and consequent reduction in filtration fraction. For this reason the scan is best performed initially with captopril; if abnormal, it is repeated on a subsequent visit without captopril, with partial or complete normalization being evidence that the previous abnormality was due to vascular rather than renal parenchymal disease. However, the MAG3 scan is not always positive, with chronic use of ACE inhibitors being a cause of some false negatives, and it may also miss bilateral renal artery stenoses that do not cause significant asymmetry between the kidneys.

Partly for these reasons, nuclear imaging is not performed for suspected renal artery stenosis in many centres, with investigation proceeding to direct imaging of the renal arteries by CT or MR angiography (Fig. 16.17.3.2). In patients under 20 years of age, some form of angiography should always be undertaken, except in those with low-renin syndromes, because of the high likelihood of a secondary cause being present, and that this will be a vascular abnormality. As well as providing an accurate estimate in most patients of the severity of any stenosis, angiography will also detect

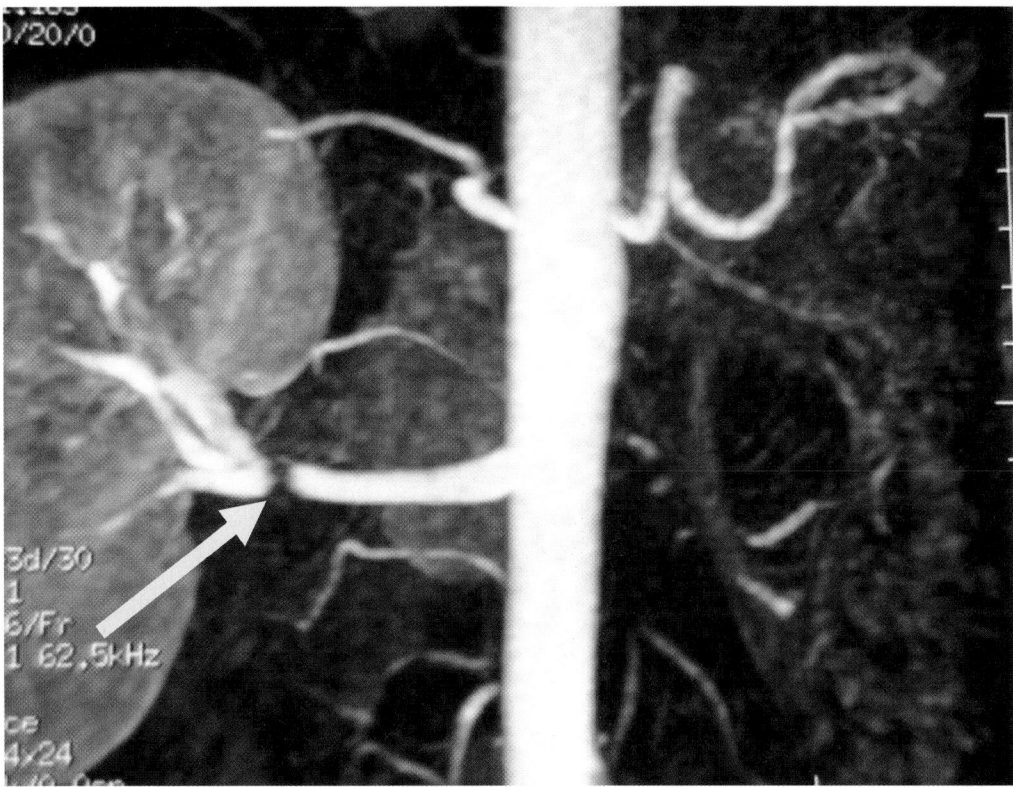

Fig. 16.17.3.2 MR angiogram demonstrating fibromuscular dysplasia of the right renal artery causing stenosis (arrow).

suprarenal aortic stenoses. False-positive and false-negative diagnoses still occur; e.g. the poststenotic dilatations of FMD can—if they expand proximally around the artery—be a cause of stenosis being missed. However, the risk of diagnostic error can be reduced by careful review of images taken in more than one projection, and it is useful to remember that stenoses are not usually isolated lesions in both FMD and atheromatous disease.

Some centres use Doppler flow measurements for diagnosis, but these are more user-dependent than angiography, which is still required subsequently for anatomical diagnosis. On the other hand, there are some patients in whom an anatomical diagnosis is made first, but the severity is in question. Here it can be useful to perform Doppler or MAG3 scan as the second investigation before proceeding to treatment. Another investigation that is sometimes helpful at this stage is renal vein sampling for renin determination, the main use for which is before removing a kidney thought responsible for causing hypertension through elevated renin secretion. The contralateral—anatomically normal—kidney has often sustained microvascular damage as a consequence of prolonged hypertension and renin excess, and is found to secrete as much renin as (or more than) the diseased kidney. Nephrectomy should not normally be contemplated where significant renal function remains, but in any circumstance there would rarely be an indication for removing a kidney showing less than 25% excess renin secretion compared to the contralateral side.

Treatment

There are several options, one of which is simply to continue optimal drug treatment if for any reason the risks of other intervention appear excessive. Among interventions, the options are as for any other arterial stenosis, namely angioplasty, stenting or surgery.

For FMD, angioplasty is usually curative, and about three-quarters can discontinue antihypertensive treatment. In atheromatous disease, angioplasty is much less likely to be successful, especially for lesions at the origin of the artery, and restenosis can occur. It is reasonable to recommend stenting as a backup procedure when angioplasty has failed. Complete cure of hypertension is very much less likely than in FMD. In the past, the purpose of intervention was often to protect or improve renal function. The ASTRAL trial has largely rebutted this objective, although some argue that patients were excluded from this trial where clinicians were certain of benefit from intervention.

Sometimes angioplasty is unsuccessful because balloon inflation fails to dent the stenosis. Surgery is required in this situation, or when failure can be predicted because stenosis is due to external compression or there is complete occlusion. As renovascular surgery is not common today outside the transplant arena, a favoured surgical procedure is autotransplantation to the pelvis.

Coarctation of the aorta

Coarctation of the aorta, a congenital cause of hypertension, was described pathologically in the 1700s and recognized clinically in the early 1900s. The term describes a constriction of the aorta at the point where the fetal ductus arteriosus originates, and the condition should ideally be diagnosed in early childhood, with most cases treated before hypertension develops. Coarctation represents 5– to 8% of all causes of congenital heart disease, but less than 1% of all cases of hypertension. However, sometimes diagnosis is delayed until the patient presents in adulthood with hypertension, and high blood pressure can sometimes develop even after surgical cure of the coarctation. The mechanism of hypertension is

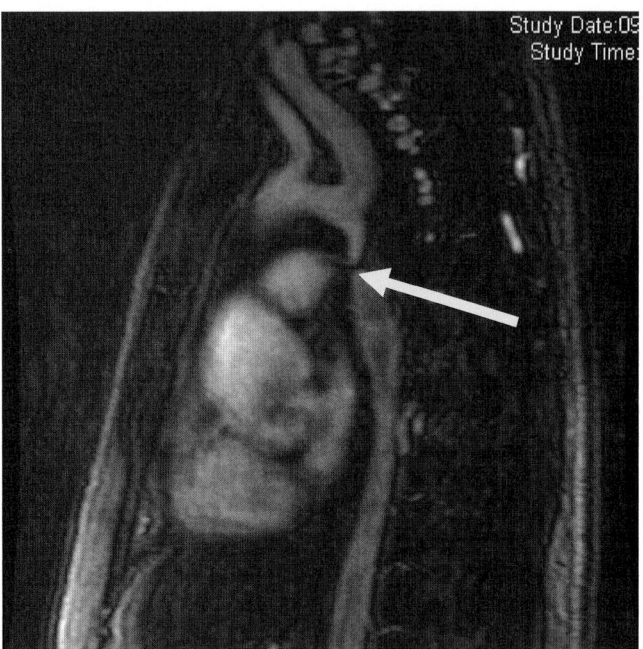

Study Date:09
Study Time:

Fig. 16.17.3.3 MR angiogram showing coarctation of the aorta (arrow).

predominantly the relative renal ischaemia consequent on low perfusion pressure in the aorta beyond the coarctation.

The classical clinical finding in coarctation is radiofemoral pulse delay, confirmed by measurement of reduced blood pressure in the legs. Of greater sensitivity and specificity in the clinic is a bruit—systolic or continuous—over the front and back of the praecordium, which arises in the intercostal collaterals.

The diagnosis should be confirmed by two-dimensional echocardiography (suprasternal view) or by CT or MR angiography (Fig. 16.17.3.3). Treatment is by surgery, balloon dilatation or stenting. Surgery or balloon dilation are the preferred approaches in childhood, balloon dilation and stent implantation in adolescents and adults. Although upper limb hypertension is usually cured, recurrence has been attributed to a variety of unproven factors, including a systemic vasculopathy.

Primary hyperaldosteronism (Conn's syndrome)

History

With the words 'to our surprise and delight, a cortical adenoma was observed to be arising from the right adrenal gland', Jerome Conn reported the first observation of the benign aldosterone-secreting tumour that now bears his name. The patient had presented with severe hypertension and hypokalaemia, shortly after discovery of aldosterone ('electrocortin') in London by the Taits. On detecting a high level of aldosterone in the patient's urine, Conn decided to remove both adrenals. There is an historical irony in this entirely right decision: not so much because the patient retained her left adrenal, but because the finding of unilateral disease in this patient has largely pre-empted the same decision being made in patients with truly bilateral disease.

Conn's report led to a flurry of similar diagnoses and optimism that as much as 20% of hypertension might be due to his tumour. However, it soon became apparent that no adenoma could be found in perhaps 50% of patients with the clinical and biochemical features of primary hyperaldosteronism, some being diagnosed instead as having bilateral nodular hyperplasia. With waning enthusiasm for finding a curable cause of hypertension, estimated prevalence fell to less than 1% of hypertension, but the picture again reversed with the recognition that not all patients with primary hyperaldosteronism have an elevated plasma aldosterone concentration. However, the popularization of the aldosterone/renin ratio as a single diagnostic test led to some blurring of the definition of primary hyperaldosteronism, confusing primary hyperaldosteronism with the low-renin end of the spectrum of essential hypertension: this chapter will concentrate on the potentially curable end of that spectrum.

Aetiology and pathology

Conn's adenoma is a small (0.5–3.5 cm) benign tumour. Although aldosterone is normally secreted selectively by the (outer) zona glomerulosa of the adrenal, most of the tumours arise from the cortisol-secreting zona fasciculata, and secrete more cortisol than aldosterone, which in larger tumours may be sufficient to cause suppression of the contralateral adrenal.

Bilateral adrenal hyperplasia is a distinct condition in which either radiologically or histologically there are macro- or micronodules in the adrenal cortex where the monolayered arcades of the normal zona glomerulosa are replaced by bi- or multicellular layered arcades. In the one type of primary hyperaldosteronism of known cause—glucocorticoid remediable aldosteronism (see Chapter 16.17.4)—there is no anatomical lesion in the adrenals other than expansion of the zona glomerulosa.

It remains unknown whether some patients develop single adenomas on the background of nodular hyperplasia, with suppression of all but the dominant nodule, or whether unilateral adenomas are usually a different condition from hyperplasia. In favour of the latter are a number of biochemical and pharmacological differences, and the fact that patients with glucocorticoid remediable hyperaldosteronism never develop a superadded adenoma. Patients with Conn's adenomas show an exaggerated diurnal rhythm in aldosterone, consistent with an enhanced ACTH-dependent cAMP pathway. By contrast, patients with hyperplasia show exaggerated aldosterone response to stimulation by angiotensin II and therefore have higher erect than supine aldosterone levels.

Primary hyperaldosteronism causes increased sodium retention through the epithelial sodium channel (ENaC) in the distal tubule and cortical collecting duct. The chronic sodium retention leads to hypertension, which is an essential feature of Conn's syndrome. Electroneutrality in the tubular cell is retained by secreting K^+ and/or H^+ ions in exchange for the Na^+, with consequent hypokalaemic alkalosis.

Epidemiology

Adenomas are slightly commoner in women, bilateral hyperplasia commoner in men. Conn's syndrome is not a cause of childhood hypertension, except for the rare monogenic syndrome of glucocorticoid remediable hyperaldosteronism. Hyperplasia is said to be commoner among older patients with hypertension, but in this context it also becomes more difficult clinically to distinguish true hyperplasia from common-or-garden low-renin hypertension, and furthermore there is commonly confusion between functioning and nonfunctioning adrenal adenomas ('incidentalomas'), which are present in at least 4% of people over 50, but uncommon in those who are younger.

Overall prevalence remains a very contentious issue. In younger patients, where nonfunctioning adenomas and low-renin hypertension are both uncommon, and response to surgery is more clear cut, the prevalence is 1 to 2% of those with hypertension. The proportion of older patients with hypertension benefiting from surgery is probably no higher, but a larger number merit investigations because of the prevalence of the differential diagnoses—low-renin hypertension, and adrenal incidentalomas. Recent estimates that 10 to 15% of patients with hypertension have primary hyperaldosteronism are incorrect if the term is used to denote a curable, secondary cause of hypertension. It remains likely, however, that excess aldosterone secretion is a common factor in the low-renin hypertension of older patients.

Clinical features

Patients with primary hyperaldosteronism 'escape' from the effects of aldosterone before sufficient Na^+ is retained to cause overt oedema, hence the clues and confirmation of the diagnosis are largely biochemical. The classic picture in Conn's syndrome is hypertension in which the plasma electrolytes show a low K^+, elevated bicarbonate, and a Na^+ typically at the upper end of the normal range, but sometimes above this. The hypertension is often resistant to treatment with conventional treatment for the patient's age group—e.g. ACE inhibition in a younger patient, or to multiple drugs including a thiazide diuretic in the older age groups. It is important to mention, however, that the classical hallmark—hypokalaemia—is not always present, and yet the consequences of K^+ depletion—weakness, tiredness, U wave on ECG—might still be manifest. The severity of hypokalaemia varies steeply with the Na^+ load presented to ENaC, this depending partly on dietary Na^+ intake and partly on drugs—principally thiazide diuretics—which affect the proportion of the filtered Na^+ load reaching the distal tubule. The commonest reason for the biochemical features of Conn's to be masked is concurrent treatment with a calcium channel blocker, hence when considering the possibility of Conn's in a patient with hypertension apparently resistant to conventional treatment, it is important to look not just at the current plasma electrolytes but at an historical set of results for any finding of hypokalaemia or alkalosis, also to reflect that hypokalaemia on a low-dose of thiazide is a reason for pursuing (rather than dismissing) the diagnosis of primary hyperaldosteronism.

Differential diagnosis

The hypokalaemic hypertensive is an interesting diagnostic challenge that can usually be solved by a series of logical moves. The finding of a Conn's adenoma is the most satisfying outcome because most likely to lead to long-term cure. The other curable cause is liquorice which, taken in excess, inhibits the enzyme 11β-hydroxysteroid dehydrogenase (11HSD) and permits cortisol access to the mineralocorticoid excess (see 'Apparent mineralocorticoid excess' in Chapter 16.17.4). Excess production of cortisol in Cushing's syndrome can also mimic Conn's. This is most likely to happen when there is ectopic ACTH production, resulting in gross excess of cortisol, and consequent saturation of the 11HSD enzyme.

Clinical investigation

Electrolytes

The critical tests in the investigation of hypokalaemic hypertension are plasma and urine electrolytes, and plasma renin and aldosterone. If the recommendations described above for screening tests in young patients with hypertension have been observed, all but the plasma aldosterone should already have been performed. The urine K^+ (which can be performed on a spot sample) should be >20 mmol/litre if hypokalaemia is due to increased urinary loss, but this test is valuable only when performed when plasma K^+ is low. Because transient hypokalaemia is common, and hypokalaemia commonly transient even in Conn's syndrome, it is important not to postpone urine K^+ estimation and risk missing a one-off opportunity for sparing a patient the further investigations required for renal K^+ loss.

Renin

Of the triad of hypokalaemia, suppressed plasma renin and elevated aldosterone, the renin is of most importance in the diagnosis of Conn's—although still not invariable, even in untreated patients. The diagnosis should be entertained even in the absence of an elevated aldosterone in patients with resistant hypertension and a suppressed renin despite multiple drugs which normally elevate rennin: the detection and removal of an adrenal microadenoma (<5 mm) can have dramatic benefit in such cases.

The main confounders in interpretation of the plasma renin level are drugs. A low renin in the presence of β-blockade is of no significance, and a β-blocker (which is unlikely to help with blood pressure control in Conn's) should be discontinued or substituted by an ACE inhibitor 2 weeks before renin measurement. Conversely, spironolactone or amiloride will at some dose cause desuppression of renin in most patients, and this should be borne in mind if the patient was already receiving one of these drugs prior to investigation.

Renin itself is very stable in blood, providing this is not chilled (which cryoactivates the renin precursor, prorenin). Although changes in posture and activity cause two- to threefold changes in renin, the range of renin between high- and low-renin patients is some 1000-fold, hence it is simple to interpret results taken in routine outpatients or surgeries, providing the blood sample (taken into an EDTA tube) reaches the laboratory for plasma separation on the same day as the blood is taken.

Aldosterone

Plasma aldosterone is often elevated above the normal range (100–400 pmol/litre), and is generally higher in patients with macroadenomas (>1 cm) than in those with microadenomas or hyperplasia. In patients with adenomas there is an exaggerated influence of ACTH leading to pronounced diurnal variation in aldosterone levels, which are more likely to be normal when sampled in the afternoon. By contrast, patients with hyperplasia have and exaggerated response to angiotensin II, so that levels may actually rise during the day in response to activity and be normalized by drugs blocking the renin system, particularly angiotensin receptor blockade. However, the most profound influences are serum K^+ and the use of calcium channel blocker treatment, which as already stated are probably now the commonest reason for the diagnosis of Conn's syndrome to be missed.

Aldosterone/renin ratio

The recognition that aldosterone is often normal—even, sometimes, after correction of hypokalaemia and withdrawal of calcium channel blocker—led to the concept of the aldosterone/renin ratio.

However, in practice, because renin is log-normally distributed and aldosterone distribution is normal, the aldosterone/renin ratio is always high in low-renin patients (except in the rare low-renin, low-aldosterone differential diagnoses considered above for hypokalaemic hypertension) and the vast majority of those with an elevated aldosterone/renin ratio do not have primary hyperaldosteronism, hence the key question is how to avoid unnecessary investigations in these cases. The empirical answer is that in the absence of other clues—hypokalaemia, high/high-normal plasma Na^+, alkalosis—investigation be undertaken only in patients with resistant hypertension. In younger patients with completely suppressed plasma renin, a useful strategy is to treat for one month with bendroflumethiazide 5 mg (or hydrochlorothiazide 50 mg), which will unmask hypokalaemia in most patients with a macroadenoma.

Fludrocortisone suppression

A possible dynamic test before proceeding to radiological investigations is the fludrocortisone suppression test, which in principle is equivalent to the outpatient dexamethasone test for Cushing's syndrome (see Chapter 13.7.1). In practice the classical test prescribes sodium and potassium loading during the 3 days of suppression by fludrocortisone 400 μg daily, and the consequent risk of severe hypertension necessitates close observation. Simplified protocols using either fludrocortisone or saline suppression alone are now entering practice, but with insufficient experience so far to recommend as a routine.

Genetic testing

This is rarely required, but if there is a family history of early-onset hypertension, and particularly of strokes at a young age, the patient should be screened for glucocorticoid remediable aldosteronism (see Chapter 16.17.4), of which there are only a few known families in the United Kingdom.

Scanning

The adrenals are easily imaged by either CT or MR, except when there is a dearth of intra-abdominal fat (Fig. 16.17.3.4). There is no proven advantage of one modality over the other, but it is valuable to check that the radiologist and department can provide coronal images, which may the only view to convincingly demonstrate an adenoma. Visualization of the right adrenal vein is also helpful if the patient proceeds to the next stage of adrenal venous sampling. Neither MRI nor CT can differentiate functional from incidental adenomas, but the latter are rare in younger patients (<35 years) although problematic in those who are older, with 5% of people over 55 years having one. In younger patients whose biochemistry is equivocal, or in whom it is difficult to alter their drugs to clarify the result, it is reasonable to proceed at an early stage to CT/MRI. In older patients the bar for proceeding to imaging should be set somewhat higher in the expectation that many scans will not resolve the diagnosis, and the next stage of investigation will therefore be required.

Functional lateralization

This is the key and, unfortunately, most difficult stage of diagnosis. Lateralization is essential in predicting that removal of one adrenal will have a substantial benefit, as well as indicating which adrenal to remove, although it might occasionally be omitted in younger patients with macroadenomas, or where the tumour is more than 3.5 cm in diameter and needs to be removed to exclude a mixed adrenal carcinoma. However, even such 'clear cut' cases still render occasional surprises, and are valuable positive controls for the centre's experience of lateralization. Whatever technique is used, it is vital that lateralization is not masked by desuppression of renin. Since it is not always possible to withdraw treatment altogether, it is adequate to check that renin is in the lower third of the normal range, and if necessary reduce spironolactone dosage to achieve this.

The most reliable form of lateralization at present is adrenal vein sampling, which is technically demanding and should be undertaken only by experienced radiologists (Fig. 16.17.3.5). On the left side, the adrenal vein is the only vein to enter the renal vein superiorly, and cannulation is relatively straightforward. On the right, however, the adrenal vein is one of several small veins (<1 mm diameter) entering the inferior vena cava posteriorly. A fish-hooked 'Cobra' catheter

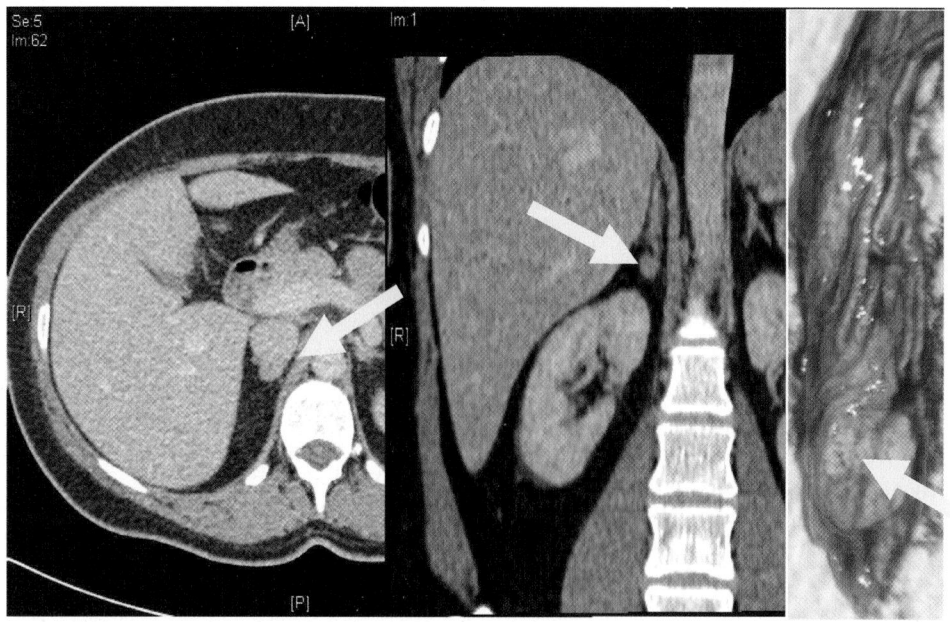

Fig. 16.17.3.4 Conn's adenoma (arrow): CT transverse view (left), coronal view (middle), surgical specimen (right).

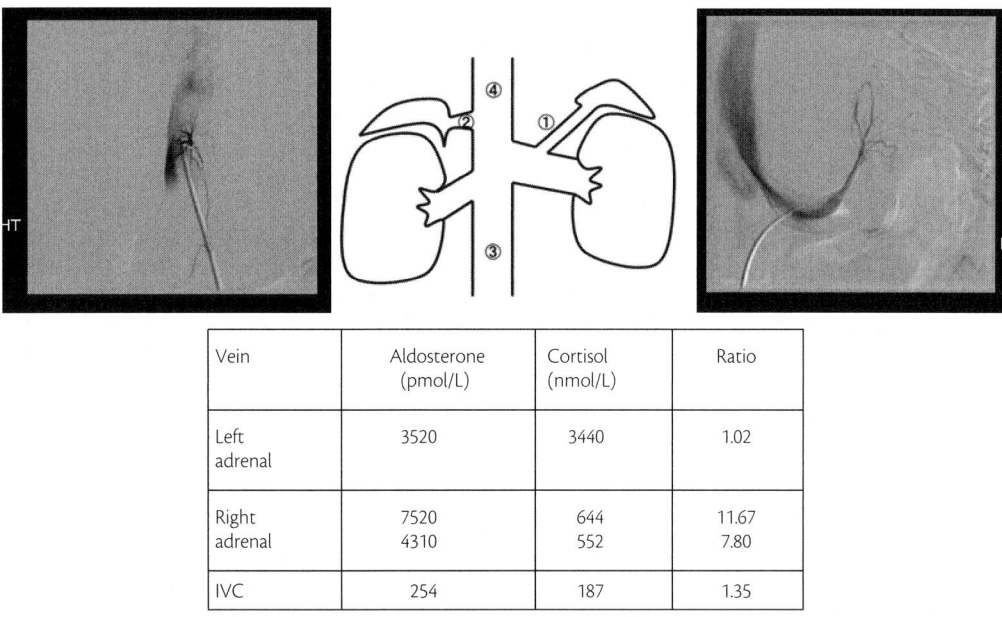

Vein	Aldosterone (pmol/L)	Cortisol (nmol/L)	Ratio
Left adrenal	3520	3440	1.02
Right adrenal	7520 4310	644 552	11.67 7.80
IVC	254	187	1.35

Fig. 16.17.3.5 Adrenal vein sampling for a right adrenal adenoma.

with side-holes maximizes the chances of success at 90 to 95%, providing several veins are sampled, with reference samples also taken in the inferior vena cava above and below the adrenal veins.

All samples need to be assayed for aldosterone and cortisol, with the ratio compared between the two sides: a ratio above 4 is usually diagnostic, and above 10 is definitive. Ratios of two- to fourfold can be compatible with lateralization, but are best confirmed on repeat sampling. In such cases reproducibility is probably more useful than trying to enhance the ratio by ACTH stimulation, but opinions about this vary. When the right adrenal vein cannot be cannulated—revealed by a cortisol concentration less than 20% above that in the inferior vena cava—it is very risky to draw conclusions from the left sample alone: concentrations of aldosterone can be very high, even in a normal vein, because adrenal vein blood flow is so low.

Isotope scans can also be used for lateralization. ^{131}I-cholesterol can be generated for scanning in any nuclear medicine department, but ^{11}C-metomidate (Fig.16.17.3.6) only in centres with a cyclotron and positron emission tomographic (PET) scanner. The former relies on cholesterol's role as precursor of steroid synthesis, and the scan is performed 1 week after isotope administration to permit cholesterol turnover and elimination from nonadrenal sites. However, the technique has a generally unreliable record, possibly because the dexamethasone taken during the week of investigation has variable influence on zona glomerurlosa as well as zona fasciculata uptake. Metomidate binds to synthetic enzymes in both the aldosterone and cortisol pathway, increased uptake by functional adenomas may be due to upregulated 2-pore K+channels.

Treatment

Medical

Medical treatment is preferred for bilateral adrenal hyperplasia, before surgery for adenoma, in older patients with adenoma who are well controlled, or where there is any doubt about diagnosis or lateralization.

Chronic medical treatment is by K+-sparing diuretic, preferably spironolactone or amiloride. Spironolactone is a competitive

antagonist of aldosterone, hence patients with very high aldosterone levels may require higher doses than used in resistant hypertension. While this is possible for preoperative use, long-term administration causes gynaecomastia. High-dose amiloride (20–40 mg daily) is better tolerated but a little less effective. Eplerenone also avoids the gynaecomastia of spironolactone, but again is less effective. A possible strategy is to combine eplerenone or a low dose of spironolactone (≤25 mg daily) with amiloride, but vigilant monitoring of plasma electrolytes is required.

It may not be possible to control blood pressure entirely by diuresis, especially in older patients with microadenomas, when calcium channel blockers or α-blockers can usefully be added. In patients who are difficult to control the maximum useful dose of diuretic can be found by titrating dose against plasma renin: once this is desuppressed it becomes logical to add ACE inhibition or angiotensin receptor blockade, which, as already remarked, may be effective in patients with bilateral hyperplasia, even when renin is suppressed.

Surgical

Elective surgery is indicated for younger patients with macroadenoma, and older patients intolerant of medical treatment, or uncontrolled

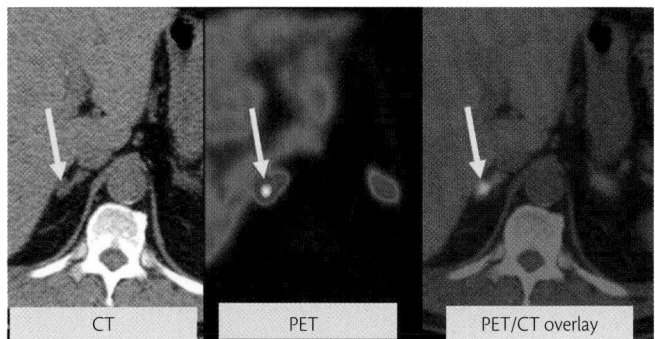

Fig. 16.17.3.6 11C-metomidate PET/CT scan of a right adrenal aldosteronoma. Uptake correctly differentiated hot and cold nodules, as confirmed by presence and absence of aldosterone secretion from the nodules when cultured post-operatively.

by it. A good blood pressure response to spironolactone augurs well for cure by surgery, but the opposite is not necessarily true (a poor response does not exclude benefit from surgery). It is best not to promise any patient complete cure, but rather a substantial reduction in number of medicines required to control blood pressure. A bonus in many patients is alleviation of chronic fatigue, presumably attributable to total body K^+ depletion.

Surgery should be undertaken by a surgeon experienced in laparoscopic adrenalectomy, but patients warned that anatomical anomalies—or peroperative eventualities such as tear of the inferior vena cava—may necessitate conversion to open adrenalectomy in about 1/20 procedures. No special preoperative care is required. Diuretics should be withdrawn from the time of surgery, but any additional antihypertensive treatment continued until the course of blood pressure improvement becomes clear over the following weeks.

Prognosis

Most (70–80%) younger patients with adenomas are cured of hypertension and hypokalaemia. Older patients are less likely to come off all antihypertensive treatment, but hypokalaemia is rarely persistent if they have been well selected for surgery, and the average number of medicines is more than halved, with improved blood pressure control in the remainder. The lesser success of surgery in older patients is due to a mixture of longer duration of hypertension, associated essential hypertension, and lingering suspicion that microadenomas are part of the bilateral hyperplasia spectrum, with residual disease in the contralateral adrenal. Residual hypertension can be exquisitely sensitive to low doses of an angiotensin receptor blocker, and there may be a role for routine prophylactic treatment of older patients to prevent hyperplasia of the remaining adrenal.

Phaeochromocytoma

Aetiology and pathology

Catecholamine biochemistry

Catecholamine biochemistry is summarized in Fig. 16.17.3.7. The final step in the biosynthetic pathway is the *N*-methylation of noradrenaline (norepinephrine) to adrenaline (epinephrine), which outside the brain occurs only in the adrenal medulla because the enzyme phenylethanolamine *N*-methyltransferase in the adrenal is dependent for induction on glucocorticoids, secreted at high concentration into the adrenal portocapillary circulation. The clinical importance of this is that extra-adrenal phaeochromocytomas rarely produce adrenaline.

The metabolism of catecholamines is different from normal in phaeochromocytoma in that adrenaline and noradrenaline are liberated directly into the bloodstream, rather than mainly into the synaptic gap around sympathetic nerve endings. Noradrenaline released from these is largely recaptured by neuronal and extraneuronal uptake, and metabolized before any free amine escapes into the bloodstream. Consequently, the proportion of parent amine (noradrenaline) to metabolite (adrenaline) is usually higher in blood and urine in the presence of a phaeochromocytoma than in any other cause of elevated catecholamine production.

Pathology

Phaeochromocytomas arise in chromaffin tissue and their anatomical distribution closely parallels the sites where this tissue is present

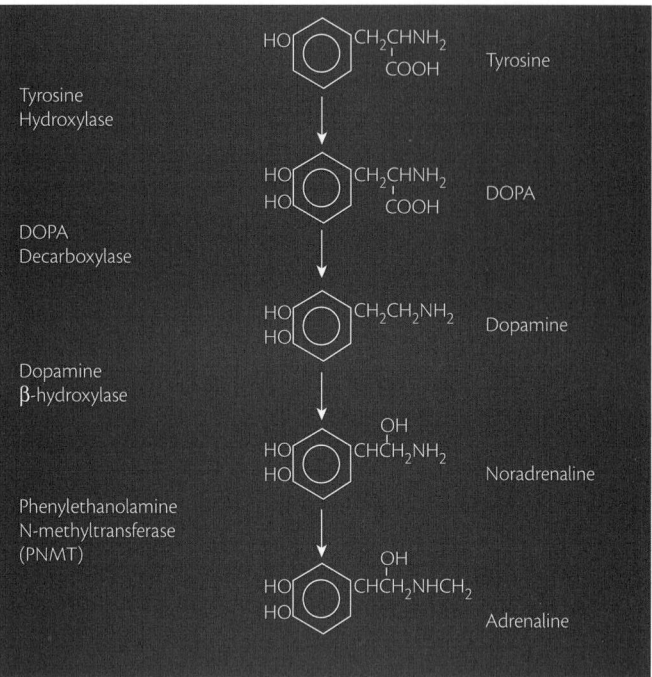

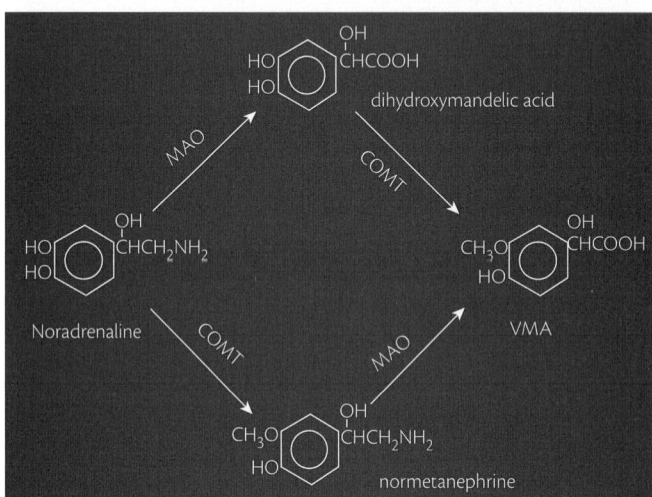

Fig. 16.17.3.7 The biosynthetic pathway for epinephrine and norepinephrine (upper panel), and for metabolism of norepinephrine (lower panel). COMT, catechol-*O*-methyltransferase; DOPA, dihydroxyphenylalanine; MAO, monoamine oxidase; VMA, vanillylmandelic acid.

at the time of birth. The term phaeochromocytoma reflects the dusky colour of the cut surface of the tumour, whereas the term chromaffin refers to the brownish colour caused by contact with dichromate salts, which oxidize the catecholamines.

Most phaeochromocytomas are benign, but the pathologist can rarely provide a clear distinction between those that are benign and those that are malignant: benign tumours can appear to be invading the capsule of the tumour, which is often ill-defined, while malignant tumours may show no mitoses because of their slow rate of division.

Genetics

Several mutations cause syndromes that include phaeochromocytoma (Table 16.17.3.2), the clinical and biochemical features of which are variable. Only tumours associated with mutations of

Table 16.17.3.2 Genes associated with familial forms of phaeochromocytoma

Gene	Chromosome	Exons	Protein	Frequency of germ-line mutations in apparent sporadic phaeochromocytoma (%)	Frequency of malignant disease (%)
VHL	3p25–26	3	pVHL19 and pVHL30	2–1	5
RET	10qll.2	21	Tyrosine-kinase receptor	<5	3
NF1	17qll.2	59	Neurofibromin	Unknown	11
SDHB	1P36.13	8	Catalytic iron-sulphur protein	3–10	50
SDHD	Hq23	4	CybS (membrane-spanning subunit)	4–7	<3

VHL, von Hippel–Lindau syndrome; RET, a proto-oncogene encoding a receptor tyrosine kinase; NF1, neurofibromatosis type 1; SDHB, succinate dehydrogenase B; SDHD, succinate dehydrogenase D.

succinate dehydrogenase (SDH, subunits B or D) commonly occur outside the adrenal, where they are sometimes referred to as paragangliomas rather than extra-adrenal phaeochromocytomas, and parangangliomas in the head or neck are restricted to SDHD (or rarely SDHC) mutations. VHL and RET mutations may cause multiple tumour types, the site of these being determined by the site of mutation in the gene: e.g. VHL type 2c missense mutations cause only phaeochromocytoma, while the gene deletions of type 1 cause renal cell carcinoma but not phaeochromocytoma. The main value of genotyping has become prediction of multiple (but usually benign) extra-adrenal phaeochromocytomas in patients with SDHD mutations, while patients with SDHB mutations have a high incidence of malignancy.

Some of the mutations in VHL or SDH also occur in sporadic tumours. This observation, together with the biochemical connection between VHL and SDH, has suggested that one underlying cause of phaeochromocytoma is failure to suppress hypoxia-induced cell proliferation. Oxygen detection by prolyl hydroxylases normally leads to degradation of hypoxia inducible factors in a process that requires the VHL protein: if VHL is defective, or prolyl hydroxylases are inhibited by accumulation of succinate, then the degradation of hypoxia inducible factors is altered and cell proliferation is stimulated.

Epidemiology

Phaeochromocytoma is a rare tumour, responsible for probably 0.1 to 1% of hypertensives, although it is possible that some its non-blood-pressure presentations are overlooked and that we selectively detect patients in whom pressure natriuresis no longer compensates the effect of vasoconstriction upon blood pressure. However, despite its rarity, phaeochromocytoma justifies the disproportionate interest that it commands among physicians, combining the potential for being lethal if not diagnosed and treated, and for cure in most patients if diagnosed. The need for maintaining a high awareness of the condition is emphasized by the small number of deaths each year due to undiagnosed phaeochromocytoma in both anaesthetic and obstetric practice.

Clinical features

Hypertension is the most common presentation of phaeochromocytoma in clinical practice, but other rare presentations include unexplained heart failure or paroxysmal arrhythmia. Patients with large tumours occasionally remain asymptomatic, and this is the norm for small phaeochromocytomas detected through regular screening of patients with a genetic diagnosis.

In hypertensive patients a spontaneous history or direct enquiry will usually reveal at least one of a group of characteristic symptoms. The classical triad is comprised of headache, sweating, and palpitations; less frequent are episodes of pallor, a feeling of 'impending doom', and paraesthesiae. Spontaneous haemorrhage and infarction in the tumour can be associated with local pain and (on occasion) systemic features of tissue necrosis, and rarely the patient can present with the features of full-blown retroperitoneal haemorrhage, coupled to a pathognomonic swinging blood pressure.

Most of the symptoms of phaeochromocytoma can be readily ascribed to the expected effects of catecholamine excess, and disappear rapidly on initiation of appropriate treatment. Because large tumours principally secrete noradrenaline, even when arising within the adrenal gland, tachycardia is usually only modest, and can be replaced altogether by reflex bradycardia when episodes of hypertension are triggered by release of noradrenaline alone. The bradycardia can be severe enough—if the hypertension is high enough—to be misdiagnosed as asystolic cardiac arrest, and the correct treatment is not atropine but phentolamine to reduce the blood pressure. Severe bradycardia is also recorded in response to the paradoxical rise in blood pressure when patients with phaeochromocytoma are inadvertently given a nonselective β-blocker such as propranolol. Often, however, the clinical features are less impressive than might be expected, possibly because the adrenoceptors have been down-regulated by years of exposure before the diagnosis is first entertained.

Examination may reveal a bruit over the tumour. A Raynaud's type of discolouration over the extremities and the larger joints in the limbs can be caused by ischaemia.

Clinical investigation

The diagnosis of phaeochromocytoma is usually not difficult once the possibility has been entertained; often more difficult is excluding the diagnosis in patients who have clinical and/or biochemical features of physiological catecholamine excess. There are two distinct questions to ask in order. 'Does the patient have a phaeochromocytoma?', and 'Where is it?'. It is unwise to use radiological tests to answer the first question because of the risk of false positives and false negatives.

Biochemical analyses of catecholamines and their metabolites

24-h urine samples measure integrated catecholamine release and provide the best screening test, with catecholamine metabolites less temperamental to assay than the more unstable catecholamines themselves. Vanillylmandelic acid (VMA) measured by HPLC is least prone to interference, L-DOPA and paracetamol being the main concerns, and although now regarded as less sensitive than some alternatives it is still the exception for VMA to be entirely normal in a patient with hypertension due to a phaeochromocytoma. Metanephrines (sometimes called metadrenalines) measured by radioimmunoassay or gas chromatography–mass spectrometry (GCMS) are more sensitive and more specific than VMA, with the assay of 'fractionated metanephrines' permitting separate evaluation of noradrenaline and adrenaline secretion, also the use of 24-h collections without addition of acid preservatives. The ability to differentiate physiological release of noradrenaline from sympathetic nerve endings from pathological secretion from a phaeochromocytoma arises because of the presence of two different enzymes in the two locations: monoamine oxidase (MAO) in sympathetic nerves, and catechol-O-methyltransferase (COMT) in the adrenal medulla and phaeochromocytoma (see Fig. 16.17.3.7).

The measurement of free catecholamines in plasma (which have a very short half-life) by high-performance liquid chromatography (HPLC) with electrochemical detection allows short bursts of secretion during a possible phaeochromocytoma crisis to be detected. However, the technique is susceptible to interference, especially in the adrenaline peak, and the finding of an adrenaline concentration that is higher than that of noradrenaline should be regarded as suspect. Dopamine levels are usually undetectable in plasma, whereas it is the major catecholamine in urine as a product of renal decarboxylation of plasma dihydroxyphenylalanine. Only several-fold increases in urinary dopamine are of diagnostic value, and are more likely to indicate neuroblastoma (in a child) or melanoma (which secretes dopamine as a by-product of melanin synthesis) than phaeochromocytoma.

Most adrenal phaeochromocytomas secrete adrenaline (and therefore metadrenaline), the exceptions being patients with very large tumours, which completely disrupt the portocapillary supply of cortisol required to induce phenylethanolamine N-methyltransferase, and patients with VHL, who often have normal adrenaline levels even when their tumour is small. By contrast, in patients with multiple endocrine neoplasia an elevated plasma adrenaline concentration is the first biochemical abnormality. Usually the normal adrenal predominance of adrenaline over noradrenaline is reversed as the tumour enlarges. Occasionally even large tumours secrete mainly adrenaline if *either* the tumour's centre is infarcted leaving a rim still exposed to cortical cortisol supply or the tumour itself is secreting ACTH or CRF. This secretion may be triggered by alpha-blocker therapy, and typical Cushing's features are then absent (as with any ectopic ACTH tumour).

Phaeochromocytomas often secrete one or more neuropeptides: somatostatin may exaggerate the episodic nature of catecholamine discharge by inhibiting catecholamine release as soon as a discharge starts, and it may also contribute to a reversible form of diabetes in phaeochromocytoma.

Suppresssion tests

The use of plasma or urine metanephrine measurements, in a reliable laboratory, has reduced the number of patients with ambiguous results. In deciding which of the 'grey zone' patients need further investigations, it is also helpful to remember that modest increases in noradrenaline secretion are usually insufficient to cause severe hypertension. This is partly because of receptor (and postreceptor) desensitization, and partly volume depletion consequent on pressure natriuresis. Where doubt about the diagnosis remains, a pharmacological suppression test can be performed prior to imaging. Whereas physiological elevations of noradrenaline release are temporarily suppressed by administration of the ganglion-blocking drug pentolinium, or the centrally acting α_2-agonist clonidine, these drugs do not suppress autonomous secretion by tumour.

Pentolinium should not be used in patients with an eGFR less than 60 ml/min. After resting supine for 30 min, plasma catecholamines are measured in two baseline samples taken 5 min apart from an intravenous cannula, and in two further samples taken 10 and 20 min after an intravenous bolus of pentolinium 2.5 mg. Patients should remain supine for a further 60 min, and their erect arterial pressure checked before they are allowed to leave the clinic. A normal response to pentolinium is a fall of both plasma noradrenaline and adrenaline concentrations into the normal range, or by 50% from baseline. However, there may be little fall in plasma catecholamine values when the basal levels are already within the normal range.

In the clonidine test, blood is taken hourly for 3 h before and after oral administration of clonidine 300 μg. Plasma noradrenaline or normetanephrine should fall by 50%, but adrenaline is little affected. Clonidine is more useful than pentolinium for patients with normal basal levels of noradrenaline or normetanephrine.

Localization of phaeochromocytomas

A substantial clue to localization is provided by measurement of plasma adrenaline (or metadrenaline) or fractionated urinary metanephrines (as stated previously, extra-adrenal tumours rarely produce adrenaline), and CT or MRI scanning provide excellent imaging of the adrenal, where 90% of phaeochromocytomas are found (Fig. 16.17.3.8). They are usually much larger than Conn's tumours, and may appear nonhomogeneous.

It is best to withhold CT/MRI scanning for extra-adrenal phaeochromocytomas until the radiologist can be given some clue as to where to concentrate. This can be achieved by radioisotope scanning with the iodinated analogue of noradrenaline, m-iodobenzylguanidine (mIBG), in about 85% of patients. This may carry either an [123I] or [131I] label, the former being more sensitive but also more expensive, and may be misinterpreted if users are unaware that normal adrenal glands also accumulate mIBG. There is a case for undertaking mIBG scanning in addition to CT, even for patients found to have an adrenal phaeochromocytoma, to identify extra-adrenal secondary deposits when tumours are malignant, and because there may be coexisting adrenal and extra-adrenal phaeochromocytomas. PET scans have been used and may be positive when mIBG is unhelpful, that using the tracer ^{18}F-DOPA appearing to be the most promising of these, with no reports of false-negative scans.

Selective venous sampling remains useful when diagnostic problems persist. About 25 samples of blood are collected under fluoroscopic guidance from various sites, with an arterial sample invaluable for interpreting the results because it enables sites with a positive veno-arterial difference to be readily detected. Because of the short half-life of catecholamines in the circulation (c. 1 min), the concentration at the tumour site is usually several-fold greater than elsewhere. This procedure should not usually be used for adrenal phaeochromocytomas, an exception being patients with von Hippel–Lindau syndrome with small adrenal masses, in whom all other biochemical tests may be normal, and the diagnosis of phaeochromocytoma is suggested by a reversal of the normal excess of adrenaline to noradrenaline in the adrenal vein.

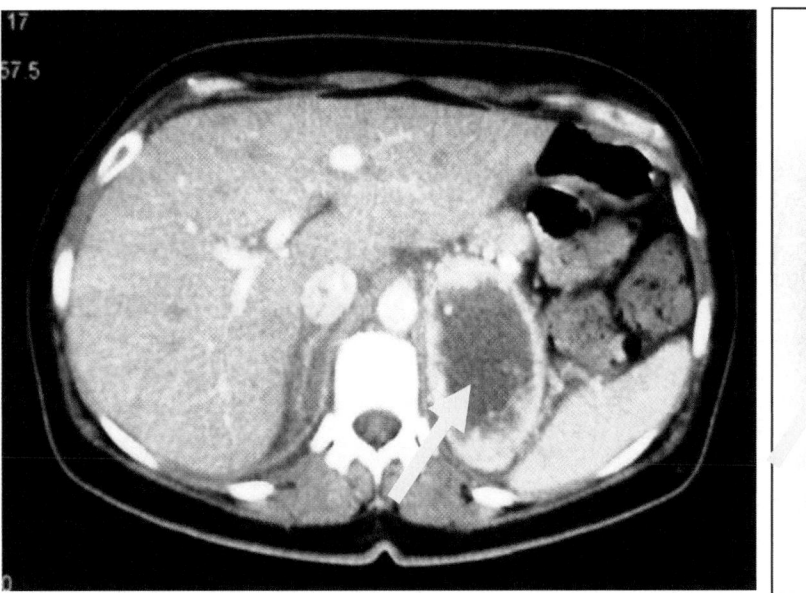
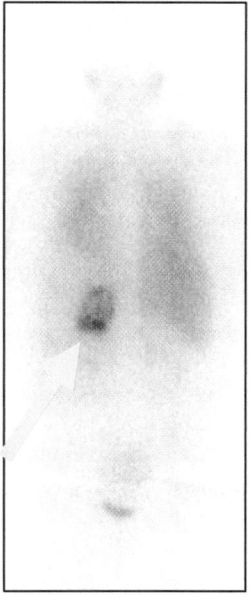

Fig. 16.17.3.8 CT (left) and *m*-iodobenzylguanidine (mIBG) scan (right) of a patient with a left adrenal phaeochromocytoma. Both scans illustrate typical nonhomogeneous appearance due to large area of haemorrhage/infarction at the centre of the tumour.

Because phaeochromocytomas are vascular tumours, they provide a good tumour blush, and occasionally angiography is required to resolve equivocal scans. Patients must be fully α-blocked and preferably also β-blocked prior to angiography.

Other investigations

It is important to check blood glucose in every patient as there may be α-mediated inhibition of insulin release prior to effective treatment, and all patients should be screened for an associated medullary carcinoma of the thyroid (see Chapter 13.5). Routine slit lamp examination of the fundi has resulted in more frequent diagnosis of von Hippel–Lindau syndrome, sometimes as a *de novo* occurrence.

Treatment

Medical management before surgery

The definitive treatment for phaeochromocytoma is surgical, with laparoscopic surgery possible for most adrenal tumours. Even the small number of phaeochromocytomas that are recognized to be malignant preoperatively (e.g. by the presence of bone or liver metastases) may still benefit from resection of the primary tumour. The task for the physician is to make surgery safe, for which the mainstay of medical treatment is α-blockade, but not all patients—especially those without elevated plasma adrenaline levels—require β-blockade. The objective of treatment is not solely control of blood pressure, but also the expansion of blood volume, which is always reduced. Indeed, phaeochromocytoma represents the pure vasoconstriction end of the vasoconstriction-volume spectrum, and the hypertensive patient is best seen as the exception where pressure natriuresis has failed to compensate adequately for vasoconstriction. Normotension is an indication, not contraindication, for the use of α -blockade to restore volume pre-operatively.

The α-blocker of choice is phenoxybenzamine, which is an irreversible blocker that actually destroys the α-receptor by alkylation. More modern α-blockers, such as doxazosin, and the mixed α- and β-blocker labetalol, cause competitive blockade, which can be overcome by a surge of noradrenaline release from the tumour.

An additional advantage of phenoxybenzamine is that it will block both α_1- and α_2-receptors, with blockade of the latter possibly advantageous because extrasynaptic α_2-receptors mediate some of the direct vasoconstriction caused by circulating (non-neuronal) catecholamines. The diabetogenic effect of catecholamines is also an α_2-mediated response. The starting dose of phenoxybenzamine is 10 mg once or twice daily, with increases titrated against blood pressure up to a maximum of 90 mg daily. The effect of irreversible antagonists is cumulative, with the effect of the drug—and each subsequent dose increment—taking several days to reach maximum.

There is rarely any urgency for surgery, which should not normally be considered in less than 1 month after initiation of treatment in patients with symptomatic phaeochromocytomas. Indeed, the more severe the initial clinical picture, the greater the need for prolonged α-blockade to expand intravascular volume. In most patients there is a low filling pressure at presentation, evident clinically as a jugular venous pressure visible only when the patient lies flat, and any postural hypotension should be assumed to reflect continuing hypovolaemia, not excessive α-blockade, until the venous pressure is normalized. Usually volume expansion will occur spontaneously with phenoxybenzamine treatment, but expansion should be achieved with intravenous saline if there is persistent hypovolaemia when patients are admitted a few days before surgery, and during the preoperative admission the dose of phenoxybenzamine should be increased until there is at least a 10 mmHg postural fall in blood pressure.

The need for β-blockade is indicated by tachycardia, which may become apparent only after treatment with phenoxybenzamine, and the dose of β-blocking drug necessary is generally lower than that used in the treatment of hypertension. It is usually better to use a β_1-selective agent so that the peripheral vasodilatation mediated by β_2-receptors is not affected. Occasionally, pronounced β_2-receptor mediated effects, including tachycardia or tremor, can oblige use of a non-selective β-blocker, although blood pressure control may then be more difficult and require addition of a calcium blocker. The reason for using as low a dose of β-blocker as possible is that there may be a period of hypotension immediately upon removal of the phaeochromocytoma, despite the preoperative preparation that has been outlined. This hypotension should normally be offset by the ability to mount a tachycardia. The correct treatment is by volume replacement, supplemented if necessary by β-agonists, most vasoconstrictor drugs being ineffective because of the slow washout of phenoxybenzamine.

Malignant phaeochromocytomas

The treatment of malignant phaeochromocytomas remains uncertain and unsatisfactory. The rate of growth is usually slow, but the prognosis for affected individuals can vary between the extremes of local recurrence at intervals of many years, and rapid demise sometimes precipitated by surgery. The tumours are not particularly sensitive either to chemotherapy or to radiotherapy, although the variability of response may still make them worth trying. There has been interest in the use of therapeutic doses of mIBG as a means of targeting high doses of radioactivity to the tumour: some patients show considerable regression after such treatment, but long-term results are less certain.

It is rare for the pharmacological effects of the tumour to be the principal problem if the primary tumour has been removed or debulked. High doses of phenoxybenzamine are preferable to α-methyltyrosine, used as an inhibitor of noradrenaline synthesis. There is anecdotal evidence that therapy with high doses of an angiotensin receptor blocker might slow progression through reflex activation of renin and hence AT_2-receptor mediated apoptosis.

Prognosis and genetic screening

Most (90%) phaeochromocytomas are benign, and the proportion is probably even higher for adrenal tumours, whereas those that are extra-adrenal have a greater than 10% likelihood of proving malignant. The latter should be screened for mutations in the SDHB gene, which carry greater than 50% risk of malignancy. Other genetic screening will be influenced by a mixture of clinical features and cost considerations. A history (or family history) of other relevant tumours will lead to a search for VHL or Multiple Endocrine Neoplasia type 2. There is some consensus that all patients presenting under the age of 45 should have structured genetic counselling and screening, and this is particularly important in much younger patients. All patients should be followed indefinitely with at least an annual measurement of arterial pressure and analysis of one of the indices of catecholamine secretion. The removal of a phaeochromocytoma cures hypertension in most patients, especially those that are young.

Other endocrine causes of hypertension

Conn's syndrome and phaeochromocytoma have been singled out for attention in this chapter as the two endocrine conditions most likely to present as hypertension. However, hypertension is a feature of several other endocrinopathies: Cushing's syndrome (Chapter 13.7.1), acromegaly (Chapter 13.2), hyperparathyroidism (Chapter 13.6), and is a common complication of type 2 diabetes. The hypertension of Cushing's syndrome is usually modest, except

in ectopic ACTH where there is saturation by high cortisol levels of 11β-hydroxysteroid dehydrogenase 2 (which normally converts cortisol to the inactive cortisone). The cause of the hypertension in other syndromes is unclear and often not corrected by surgical cure of the primary problem.

Further reading

Renovascular hypertension and coarctation

Caliezi C, Reber P (2006). Images in clinical medicine. Fibromuscular dysplasia of the renal artery. *N Engl J Med*, **355**, 2131.

Rosenthal E (2005). Coarctation of the aorta from fetus to adult: curable condition or life long disease process? *Heart*, **91**, 1495–1502.

Safian RD, Textor SC (2001). Renal-artery stenosis. *N Engl J Med*, **344**, 431–42.

White CJ (2006). Catheter-based therapy for atherosclerotic renal artery stenosis. *Circulation*, **113**, 1464–73.

Primary hyperaldosteronism

Brown MJ, Hopper RV (1999). Calcium-channel blockade can mask the diagnosis of Conn's syndrome. *Postgrad Med J*, **75**, 235–6.

Dluhy RG, Lifton RP (1999). Glucocorticoid-remediable aldosteronism. *J Clin Endocrinol Metab*, **84**, 4341–4.

Ganguly A (1998). Primary aldosteronism. *N Engl J Med*, **339**, 1828–34.

Gordon RD, *et al.* (1994). High incidence of primary aldosteronism in 199 patients referred with hypertension. *Clin Exp Pharmacol Physiol*, **21**, 315–318.

Hood SJ, *et al.* (2007). The Spironolactone, Amiloride, Losartan, and Thiazide (SALT) double-blind crossover trial in patients with low-renin hypertension and elevated aldosterone-renin ratio. *Circulation*, **116**, 268–75.

Kaplan NM (2004). The current epidemic of primary aldosteronism: causes and consequences. *J Hypertens*, **22**, 863–9.

Mulatero P, *et al.* (2006). Comparison of confirmatory tests for the diagnosis of primary aldosteronism. *J Clin Endocrinol Metab*, **91**, 2618–23.

Stewart PM (1999). Mineralocorticoid hypertension. *Lancet*, **353**, 1341–7.

Stowasser M, *et al.* (2003). High rate of detection of primary aldosteronism, including surgically treatable forms, after 'non-selective' screening of hypertensive patients. *J Hypertens*, **21**, 2149–57.

Young WF Jr (2007). The incidentally discovered adrenal mass. *N Engl J Med*, **356**, 601–610.

Phaeochromocytoma

Allison DJ, *et al.* (1983). Role of venous sampling in locating a phaeochromocytoma. *BMJ*, **286**, 1122–4.

Brown MJ, *et al.* (1981). Increased sensitivity and accuracy of phaeochromocytoma diagnosis achieved by use of plasma epinephrine estimations and a pentolinium suppression test. *Lancet*, **i**, 174–7.

Brown MJ *et al.* (2009). Pheochromocytoma. *Horm Metab Res*, **41**, 655–7.

Col V, *et al.* (1999). Laparoscopic adrenalectomy for phaeochromocytoma: endocrinological and surgical aspects of a new therapeutic approach. *Clin Endocrinol (Oxf)*, **50**, 121–5.

Manger WM (1997). *Pheochromocytoma*. Springer Verlag, Berlin.

Richards FM, *et al.* (1998). Molecular genetic analysis of von Hippel-Lindau disease. *J Intern Med*, **243**, 527–33.

Sisson JC, Shulkin BL (1999). Nuclear medicine imaging of pheochromocytoma and neuroblastoma. *Q J Nucl Med*, **43**, 217–23.

16.17.4 Mendelian disorders causing hypertension

Nilesh J. Samani

Essentials

Several mendelian disorders with hypertension as the predominant manifestation have been characterized at the molecular level. Features that may suggest one of these very rare conditions include a young age of onset, moderate to severe hypertension, strong family history, consanguinity (for the autosomal recessive disorders), and electrolyte abnormalities, particularly of potassium (although this is not invariable).

Glucocorticoid remediable aldosteronism—an autosomal dominant condition caused by a chimeric gene where the regulatory elements of the 11β-hydroxylase gene become attached to the coding region of aldosterone synthase. Hypertension responds to a low daily dose of exogenous glucocorticoid.

Apparent mineralocorticoid excess—an autosomal recessive disorder caused by mutations causing loss of function in the type 2 11β-hydroxysteroid dehydrogenase gene that normally inactivates cortisol in the kidney and prevents it binding to the mineralocorticoid receptor. The hypertension responds to spironolactone or amiloride.

Liddle's syndrome—an autosomal dominant condition caused by activating mutations in genes encoding the β- or γ-subunits of the trimeric epithelial sodium channel. Hypertension responds to direct inhibitors triamterene or amiloride.

Pseudohypoaldosteronism type 2 (PHA2, Gordon's syndrome)—an autosomal dominant condition, some cases of which are caused by mutations in serine-threonine kinases (WNK1 and WNK4) that regulate salt reabsorption by the Na-Cl cotransporter (SLC12A3) and the linked process of potassium secretion by the renal outer medullary potassium channel (ROMK). The hypertension and physiological abnormalities are corrected by thiazide diuretics.

Introduction

Several rare mendelian disorders where hypertension is the predominant manifestation have been characterized at the molecular level (Box 16.17.4.1). These include glucocorticoid remediable aldosteronism, the syndrome of apparent mineralocorticoid excess, Liddle's syndrome and Gordon's syndrome. Hypertension and hypokalaemia are features of 11β-hydroxylase and 17β-hydroxylase deficiency—two rare recessive gene disorders of adrenal steroid-synthesizing enzymes that, among others, cause congenital adrenal hyperplasia. 11β-Hydroxylase deficiency usually presents in infancy or early childhood with virilization of both sexes, while presentation of 17β-hydroxylase deficiency may be delayed until adolesecence or adulthood. Hypertension due to a phaeochromocytoma may be a feature of multiple endocrine neoplasia type 2 (MEN2, Sipple's syndrome), which when familial is inherited in an autosomal dominant pattern, or rarely to be a feature of neurofibromatosis (von Recklinghausen's disease).

Glucocorticoid-remediable aldosteronism

Glucocorticoid-remediable aldosteronism (GRA) is a form of mineralocorticoid hypertension that is inherited in an autosomal dominant fashion. The hypertension is accompanied by hypokalaemia (not invariably), a tendency to metabolic alkalosis, an elevated plasma aldosterone level and a suppressed renin level, and it often responds to thiazides or spironolactone. Patients are usually suspected of having primary aldosteronism (Conn's syndrome, see Chapter 16.17.4), although the age of onset, usually in the first two decades of life, is younger than typical of primary aldosteronism. Intracranial aneurysms are common and the first manifestation may be a presentation with intracranial haemorrhage.

The two hallmarks features of GRA are the presence of large amounts of two abnormal steroids—18-hydroxycortisol and 18-oxocortisol—in the urine, and the paradoxical response of the hypertension, with return of plasma aldosterone to a normal level and disappearance of the abnormal steroids, following treatment over a few days with a low daily dose of exogenous glucocorticoid, e.g. 0.5 to 1.0 mg of dexamethasone (hence the name).

Patients with GRA have a chimeric gene due to an unequal crossing-over event at meiosis between two adjacent and highly homologous genes involved in adrenocorticosteroid synthesis—aldosterone synthase (CYP11B2) (normally expressed only in the zona glomerulosa, involved in aldosterone synthesis and regulated by angiotensin II) and 11β-hydroxylase (CYP11B1) (expressed in the zona fasciculata, involved in glucocorticoid synthesis and regulated by ACTH). In the chimeric gene, the regulatory elements of CYP11B1 have become attached to the aldosterone synthase coding region of CYP11B2 (Fig. 16.17.4.1a). This leads to ACTH-driven production of aldosterone (and the other abnormal hormones) in the zona fasciculata, hence the clinical syndrome and its suppression by glucocorticoids.

Box 16.17.4.1 Mendelian forms of blood pressure variation

Hypertension

- Glucocoticoid-remediable aldosteronism (GRA)
- Syndrome of apparent mineralocorticoid excess (AME)
- Liddle's syndrome
- Gordon's syndrome (pseudohypoaldosteronism type II, PHA-II)
- Hypertension exacerbated by pregnancy
- Hypertension with brachydactyly
- 11β-Hydroxylase deficiency
- 17β-Hydroxylase deficiency
- Multiple endocrine neoplasia type 2 (Sipple's syndrome) with phaeochromocytoma

Hypotension

- Pseudohypoaldosteronism type 1
- Gittleman's syndrome
- Bartter syndrome
- 11β-hydroxylase deficiency
- Aldosterone synthase deficiency

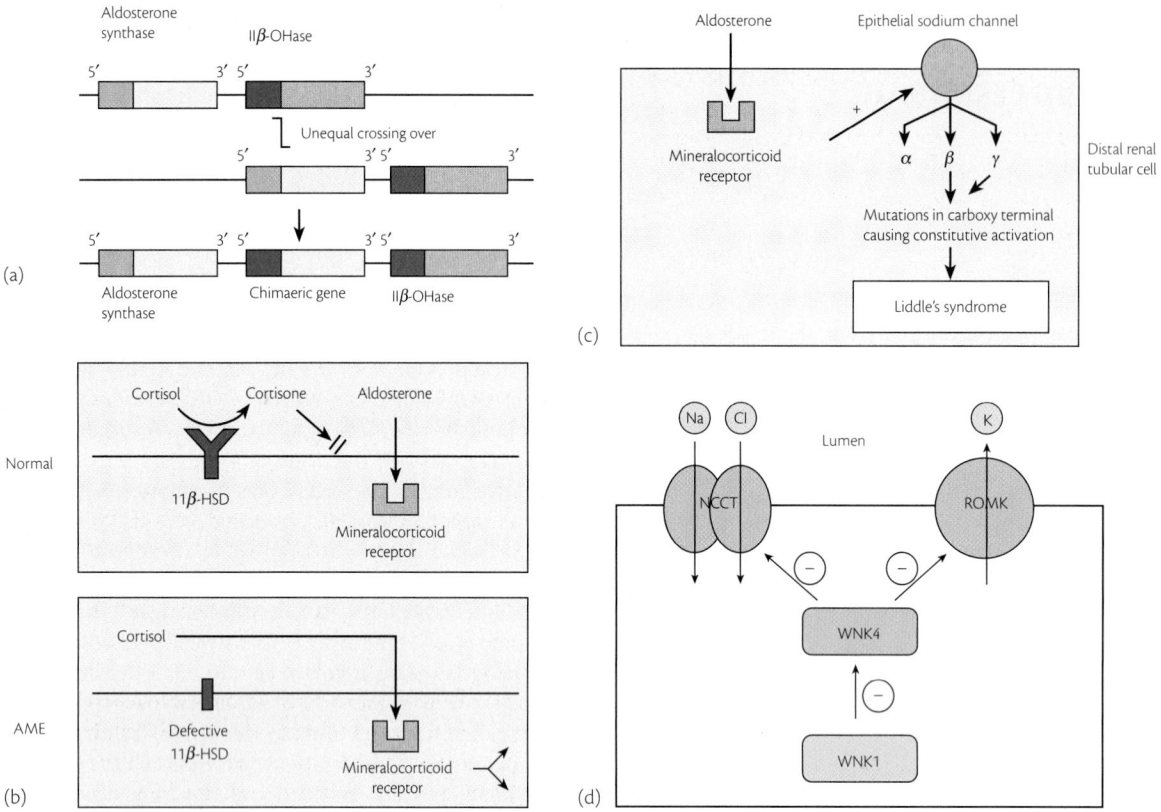

Fig. 16.17.4.1 Mechanisms underlying four forms of monogenetic hypertension. (a) Glucocorticoid remediable aldosteronism (GRA). In GRA an unequal crossing event leads to a chimeric gene where the coding region of aldosterone synthase (light pink bar) becomes attached to the regulatory region for 11β-hydroxylase (magenta bar). The chimeric gene produces excess amounts of aldosterone under the regulation of ACTH. (b) Syndrome of apparent mineralocorticoid excess (AME). The mineralocorticoid receptor in the distal renal tubule is normally protected from stimulation by cortisol by the activity of the 11β-hydroxysteroid dehydrogenase enzyme. In AME, mutations in the enzyme allow cortisol to gain access to the receptor. (c) Liddle's syndrome. The trimeric epithelial sodium channel mediates sodium reuptake in the distal renal tubule under regulation by the mineralocorticoid receptor. In Liddle's syndrome, mutations in the β and γ subunits of the channel render the channel constitutively active. (d) Gordon's syndrome. WNK4 is a negative regulator of the thiazide-sensitive sodium-chloride co-transporter (NCCT) in the distal nephron and also a negative regulator of potassium secretion via ROMK. Mutations in WNK4 relieve its inhibition of NCCT but maintain or increase its inhibition of ROMK, resulting in hypertension and hyperkalaemia. WNK1 mutations cause Gordon's syndrome by affecting WNK4.

The mainstay of treatment for GRA is glucocorticoids, with physiological doses (or only slightly higher, e.g. 0.125 mg of dexamethasone or 2.5 mg of prednisolone daily) sufficing. Response can be monitored by measuring the suppression of aldosterone production. Selective mineralocorticoid receptor blockers, such as spironolactone, can provide useful adjunctive treatment.

Syndrome of apparent mineralocorticoid excess

The syndrome of apparent mineralocorticoid excess (AME) is an autosomal recessive disorder that usually presents in childhood with hypertension, hypokalaemia, and low renin activity. Despite the clinical features of mineralocorticoid excess, levels of all known mineralocorticoid hormones are low, yet the hypertension responds to spironolactone or amiloride. Patients with the disorder cannot metabolize cortisol to its inactive metabolite cortisone normally, resulting in a prolonged half-life of cortisol and a characteristic increase in urinary cortisol (compound F) compared with cortisone (compound E) ratio.

Elucidating the defect causing AME first required the solution of another paradox—why cortisol, which circulates at a level several-fold greater than aldosterone, does not overwhelmingly activate the renal mineralocorticoid receptor *in vivo* despite the two having equal affinity *in vitro*. The reason relates to the enzyme 11β-hydroxysteroid dehydrogenase (11β-HSD), which has two isoforms. Type 1 11β-HSD is located in the liver, adipose tissue and gonad and converts cortisone to cortisol. Type 2 11β-HSD is expressed in the mineralocorticoid target tissues—kidney, colon, and salivary gland—and inactivates cortisol to cortisone. In the kidney the enzyme plays the crucial role of protecting the mineralocorticoid receptor on the distal tubule from activation by cortisol. In subjects with AME a variety of loss-of-function mutations in the type 2 11β-HSD gene cause a deficiency of the enzyme, allowing cortisol access to the mineralocorticoid receptor (Fig. 16.17.4.1b).

The severe form of AME, due to disabling mutations in type 2 11β-HSD, usually presents in childhood. Recently a milder form, termed AME type II, has been described, which is characterized by a later age of presentation (>30 years), a more variable degree of hypertension, and less impact on biochemical parameters. These patients have alterations in 11β-HSD2 that produce a partial rather than absolute decrease in enzymatic activity. The mainstay of treatment of either form of AME is spironolactone. A low-salt diet is also important.

AME resembles the syndrome observed in subjects ingesting large amounts of liquorice or taking the now redundant antiulcer drug carbenoxolone, both of which contain glycyrrhetinic acid, an inhibitor of type 2 11β-HSD, thus explaining the hypertension and hypokalaemia observed with these compounds. Spillover access of cortisol to the mineralocorticoid receptor may also, at least partly, explain the hypertension accompanying some forms of Cushing's syndrome and glucocorticoid resistance.

Liddle's syndrome

Liddle described a family in which the siblings were affected by early-onset hypertension and hypokalaemia, but with low renin and aldosterone levels. The clue to the nature of the molecular defect underlying this autosomal dominant disorder came from the observation that the hypertension does not respond to spironolactone, the mineralocorticoid receptor antagonist, but does respond to direct inhibitors (such as triamterene or amiloride) of the epithelial sodium channel, which mediates the effects of activation of the mineralocorticoid receptor. This indicated that the defect lay downstream of the mineralocorticoid receptor, with subsequent work revealing activating mutations in genes (SCNN1B, SCNN1G) encoding the β- or γ-subunits of the trimeric epithelial sodium channel (Fig. 16.17.4.1c), which is located in the distal nephron and represents the final effector molecule of the renin–angiotensin–aldosterone system in the kidney. All mutations so far identified cause an alteration or deletion of a proline-rich (PY) motif in the C-terminal cytoplasmic tails of the subunits that is necessary for regulatory proteins such as Nedd4 to bind and internalize the channel. When this is impaired the channel remains constitutively active at the cell surface, leading to over-reabsorption of sodium and water.

Pseudohypoaldosteronism type 2 (Gordon's syndrome)

Pseudohypoaldosteronism type 2 (PHA2), also known as Gordon's syndrome, is an autosomal dominant disorder that causes elevated blood pressure accompanied by hyperkalaemia, despite normal renal glomerular filtration. Mild hyperchloraemia, metabolic acidosis, and suppressed plasma renin activity are variable associated findings. Hypercalciuria can also be a feature, leading to osteopenia, osteoporosis, and kidney stone disease. The hypertension and physiological abnormalities are corrected by thiazide diuretics.

Recent studies have established that at least some cases of PHA2 are due to mutations in two members, WNK1 and WNK4, of the WNK (With No K, K = lysine) family of serine-threonine kinases. Both proteins localize to the distal nephron, where they contribute to regulation of the salt reabsorption by the Na-Cl cotransporter (SLC12A3) and the linked process of potassium secretion by the renal outer medullary potassium channel (ROMK). WNK4 is a negative regulator of both channels (Fig. 16.17.4.1d). PHA2-causing mutations in WNK4 result in loss of its inhibition of the Na-Cl cotransporter but at the same maintain or increase its ability to inhibit potassium secretion via ROMK, providing an explanation for why the hypertension caused by WNK4 mutations is accompanied by hyperkalaemia. Current evidence suggests that WNK1 acts as a negative regulator of WNK4: PHA2-causing mutations in WNK1 are associated with increased expression of the protein and hence are expected to relieve WNK4- mediated suppression of the Na-Cl cotransporter. The Na-Cl transporter is the target for thiazide diuretics, which explains the specific clinical response of PHA2 to this class of drugs.

Defects in the Na-Cl cotransporter lead to the salt-losing Gitelman's syndrome, which as described below is the mirror image of PHA2.

Other monogenetic forms of hypertension

A missense mutation in the ligand-binding domain of the mineralocorticoid receptor has been found to cause an autosomal dominant form of hypertension that is markedly accelerated in pregnancy. The mutation, MR S810L, causes partial, aldosterone-independent activation of the receptor, causing carriers to develop hypertension before age 20. Compounds such as progesterone that normally bind to but do not activate the mineralocorticoid receptor are all potent agonists of the mutant receptor, hence MR S810L carriers have dramatic acceleration of hypertension during pregnancy stimulated by the 100-fold rise in progesterone. Although the MR S810L mutation is extremely rare, the finding does raise the question of whether related mechanisms may underlie other forms of hypertension in pregnancy.

A gene causing autosomal dominant hypertension in conjunction with type E brachydactyly in a large Turkish kindred has been mapped to chromosome 12p. The hypertension in this syndrome, unlike most of the disorders described above, closely resembles essential hypertension with no evidence of volume expansion or electrolyte imbalance. The genetic defect is unknown.

Genetic defects causing hypotension

A number of mendelian syndromes where hypotension is a feature have recently been characterized at the molecular level (Table 16.17.4.1). Many are mirror images of the genetic abnormalities causing the mendelian forms of hypertension described above.

Pseudohypoaldosteronism type 1 (PHA1) occurs in two forms, autosomal recessive and autosomal dominant. Both are characterized by life-threatening dehydration in the neonatal period, hypotension, salt wasting, hyperkalaemia, metabolic acidosis, and marked elevation of renin and aldosterone. The autosomal recessive form is due to inactivating mutations (compare with Liddle's syndrome) in one of the genes SCNN1A, SCCN1B or SCNN1G, encoding (respectively) the α, β, and γ subunits of the

Table 16.17.4.1 Biochemical and therapeutic characteristics of Glucocorticoid remediable aldosteronism (GRA), syndrome of apparent mineralocorticoid excess (AME), Liddle's syndrome, and Gordon's syndrome

	GRA	AME	Liddle's	Gordon's
Plasma electrolytes	↑Na ↓K	↑Na ↓K	↑Na ↓K	↑Na ↑K
Plasma aldosterone	↑	↓	↓	↑↓
Plasma renin	↓	↓	↓	↓
Specific treatment	Dexamethasone	Spironolactone	Amiloride	Thiazide

Note that while the biochemical changes are characteristic, they are not invariably present.

epithelial sodium channel, while the autosomal dominant form is due to loss-of-function mutations in the gene (*NR3C2*) encoding the mineralocorticoid receptor.

Gitelman's syndrome is an autosomal recessive disorder characterized by hypotension, neuromuscular abnormalities, hypokalaemia, hypomagnesaemia, hypocalciuria, metabolic alkalosis, and an activated renin–angiotensin system. It arises due to inactivating mutations in the gene encoding the renal thiazide-sensitive Na-Cl cotransporter (*SLC12A3*), and typically presents in adolescence or early adulthood with neuromuscular signs and symptoms.

Bartter's syndrome is caused by mutations in one of the genes that encode regulators of chloride transport within the thick ascending limb of nephron. Defects in genes encoding bumetanide-sensitive sodium-(potassium)-chloride co-transporter 2 (*SLC12A1*), ATP-regulated potassium channel ROM-K (*KCNJ1*), chloride channel Kb (*CLCNKB*), and barttin (*BSDN*) are responsible for four types of Bartter's syndrome. The manifestation of these autosomal recessive disorders is heterogeneous, but the most typical clinical presentations include early onset (infancy or childhood), hypovolaemia and polyuria, low or normal blood pressure, elevated prostaglandin levels and nephrocalcinosis. The recently identified Bartter-like syndrome occurring in subjects with mutations in the *CASR* gene (that encodes extracellular basolateral calcium sensing receptor) manifests as hypocalcemic hypercalciuria. For further discussion of Gitelman's and Bartter's syndrome, see Chapter 21.2.2.

Does my patient have a recognized form of monogenetic hypertension?

Identification that a patient has GRA, AME, Liddle's syndrome, or Gordon's syndrome has important consequences for treatment (Table 16.17.4.1) and family screening. Phenotypic expression is highly variable, but all of the syndromes are extremely rare and suspicion will usually go unrewarded. Features that may suggest a diagnosis of mendelian hypertension include a young age of onset, moderate to severe hypertension, strong family history, consanguinity (for the autosomal recessive disorders), and electrolyte abnormalities, particularly of potassium (although this is not invariable). A good starting point, as described in Chapter 16.17.4, is the measurement of plasma renin activity and plasma aldosterone. If the aldosterone is significantly elevated then the differential diagnosis lies between the various forms of Conn's syndrome and GRA. Diagnosis of GRA would be supported by the finding of elevated 18-hydroxycortisol and 18-oxocortisol in the urine, and a positive dexamethasone suppression test, suppression of plasma aldosterone levels to less than 4 ng/dl with 0.75 to 2.0 mg/day for at least 2 days being reported to have a greater than 90% specificity and sensitivity for the diagnosis, and GRA can now also be relatively easily confirmed by finding a chimeric gene fragment with DNA testing.

If the aldosterone level is suppressed, then finding an increased ratio of cortisol/cortisone metabolites in the urine would support a diagnosis of AME. The presence of hyperkalaemia, hyperchloraemia and metabolic acidosis would suggest a diagnosis of Gordon's syndrome. No biochemical abnormalities specifically support a diagnosis of Liddle's syndrome. Ultimately, diagnosis of AME, Liddle's syndrome, and Gordon's syndrome also requires DNA confirmation, but this is not as straightforward as it is with GRA since several different mutations can give rise to each syndrome.

Further reading

Geller DS, *et al.* (2000). Activating mineralocorticoid receptor mutation in hypertension exacerbated by pregnancy. *Science*, **289**, 119–23.

Lifton RP, *et al.* (1992). A chimaeric 11 ß-hydroxylase/aldosterone synthase gene causes glucocorticoid-remediable aldosteronism and human hypertension. *Nature*, **355**, 262–65.

Lifton RP, *et al.* (2001). Molecular mechanisms of human hypertension. *Cell*, **104**, 545–56.

Mune T, *et al.* (1995). Human hypertension caused by mutations in the kidney isozyme of 11 -hydroxysteroid dehydrogenase. *Nat Genet*, **10**, 394–9.

Shimkets RA, *et al.* (1994). Liddle's syndrome: Heritable human hypertension caused by mutations in the β subunit of the epithelial sodium channel. *Cell*, **79**, 407–14.

Wilson FH, *et al.* (2001). Human hypertension caused by mutations in WNK kinases. *Science*, **293**, 1107–12.

16.17.5 Hypertensive urgencies and emergencies

Gregory Y.H. Lip and D. Gareth Beevers

Essentials

Hypertensive urgencies and emergencies occur most commonly in patients with previous hypertension, especially if inadequately managed. About 40% of cases have an underlying cause, most commonly renovascular disease, primary renal diseases, phaeochromocytoma, and connective tissue disorders. Hypertensive emergencies occur when severely elevated or sudden marked increase in blood pressure is associated with acute end-organ damage.

The key pathophysiological process is intense peripheral vasoconstriction, resulting in a rapid rise in blood pressure and a vicious circle of events, including ischaemia of the brain and peripheral organs.

Hypertensive urgencies

Malignant-phase hypertension is a rare condition (1–3 per 100 000 per year, more common in blacks) characterized by very high blood pressure, with bilateral retinal haemorrhages and/or exudates or cotton wool spots, with or without papilloedema.

Presentation is typically with visual disturbance, with or without headaches. Urinalysis may demonstrate proteinuria and haematuria, even in the absence of primary renal disease. Some patients with mild renal impairment at first presentation may improve, or even regain normal renal function, but this is unlikely to occur in those with more severe renal impairment at presentation.

Patients with severe hypertension who are asymptomatic require controlled reduction in blood pressure with oral antihypertensive agents. Over-rapid blood pressure reduction may be hazardous, leading on occasion to ischaemic complications such as stroke, myocardial infarction, or blindness. The maximum initial fall in blood pressure should not exceed 25% of the presenting value, with the initial aim of treatment being to lower the diastolic pressure to about 100 to 105 mmHg over a period of 2 to 3 days. The first-line oral antihypertensive agent is either a short-acting calcium antagonist (such as nifedipine, 10–20 mg of the tablet formulation: sublingual or capsular preparations should never be used) or a β-blocker (such as atenolol, 25 mg initial dose).

Hypertensive emergencies

Patients who are symptomatic with acute life-threatening complications of severe hypertension, such as hypertensive encephalopathy, hypertensive left ventricular failure, or aortic dissection, require parenteral antihypertensive therapy to promptly reduce the blood pressure in a carefully controlled manner. Blood pressure should be reduced by 25% over several hours, depending on the clinical situation, usually with a target diastolic blood pressure of less than 100 to 110 mmHg. The first-line treatment for most hypertensive emergencies is either intravenous sodium nitroprusside or intravenous labetolol, with β-blockade essential in patients with aortic dissection.

Hypertensive emergencies and urgencies carry a poor short- and long-term prognosis unless adequately managed. Initial over-rapid reduction of blood pressure to a normal value is dangerous, but—in the long term—blood pressure should eventually be reduced to accepted blood pressure targets.

Introduction

Hypertensive emergencies occur when severe hypertension is associated with acute end-organ damage. These can take a variety of forms and can occur at any age. They may be acute life-threatening medical conditions, and are associated with either severe hypertension or sudden marked increases in blood pressure (Box 16.17.5.1). Symptomatic patients with complications such as aortic dissection and hypertensive encephalopathy require parenteral antihypertensive therapy to reduce the blood pressure promptly, but in a controlled manner and with careful monitoring because over-rapid treatment may in itself be hazardous, leading, on occasions, to ischaemic complications such as stroke, myocardial infarction, or blindness. Thus, in patients who have severe hypertension but are asymptomatic, slower controlled reduction in blood pressure should be achieved with oral antihypertensive agents, making such situations hypertensive 'urgencies' rather than 'emergencies'.

In general, there has been a decline in the incidence of hypertensive emergencies over the past 20 years in the Western world, which may possibly be the result of the more effective detection, diagnosis, and treatment of mild to moderate hypertension.

If patients with hypertensive emergencies are not recognized or treated appropriately, the mortality and morbidity can be very high, with the 1-year mortality being 70 to 90%, and the 5-year mortality 100%. With adequate blood pressure control, the 1-year and 5-year mortality rates decrease to 25 and 50%, respectively.

Hypertensive emergencies occur most commonly in patients with previous hypertension, especially if inadequately managed. Nevertheless, some patients can present with hypertensive emergencies *de novo*, without any previous history of hypertension.

Very severe and malignant hypertension are more likely to be associated with underlying causes such as renovascular disease, primary renal diseases, phaeochromocytoma, and connective tissue disorders, but malignant hypertension complicating primary hyperaldosteronism (Conn's syndrome) is very rare. About 40% of patients with malignant hypertension have an underlying cause.

Pathophysiology

The common denominator in hypertensive emergencies is intense peripheral vasoconstriction, resulting in a rapid rise in blood pressure and a vicious circle of events, including ischaemia of the brain and peripheral organs. This ischaemia stimulates neurohormone and cytokine release, exacerbating vasoconstriction and ischaemia, further increasing blood pressure, and resulting in target organ damage. In addition, myointimal proliferation in the vasculature may exacerbate the situation, as can disseminated intravascular coagulation. Also, renal ischaemia leads to activation of the renin–angiotensin system, causing further rise in blood pressure and microvascular damage.

With mild to moderate elevation of blood pressure, the initial response of the vasculature is arterial and arteriolar vasoconstriction—such autoregulation maintaining tissue perfusion at a relatively constant level and preventing the raised blood pressure from damaging smaller, more distal blood vessels. Later, arteriolar hypertrophy also minimizes the transmission of pressure to the capillary circulation. In normotensive subjects, the upper limit of autoregulation can be a mean arterial pressure of 120 mmHg (equivalent to 160/100 mmHg), but in chronic hypertension, where the vessels are hypertrophied by long-standing hypertension, the lower limit of autoregulation of cerebral blood flow is shifted towards higher blood pressures (Fig. 16.17.5.1), with impairment of the tolerance to acute hypotension. However, the process of autoregulation fails with rapid and severe rises in blood pressure, leading to a rise in

---

Box 16.17.5.1 Hypertensive emergencies and urgencies

Hypertensive emergencies

◆ Hypertensive encephalopathy

◆ Hypertensive left ventricular failure

◆ Hypertension with myocardial infarction or unstable angina

◆ Hypertension with aortic dissection

◆ Severe hypertension with subarachnoid haemorrhage or stroke

◆ Phaeochromocytoma crisis

◆ Recreational drugs (amphetamines, LSD, cocaine, MDMA (ecstasy), etc.)

◆ Perioperative hypertension

◆ Severe pre-eclampsia or eclampsia

Hypertensive urgencies

◆ Malignant hypertension

◆ Chronic renal failure

◆ Pre-eclampsia

◆ Severe nonmalignant hypertension

LSD, lysergic acid diethylamide; MDMA, 3,4-methylenedioxymethamphetamine.

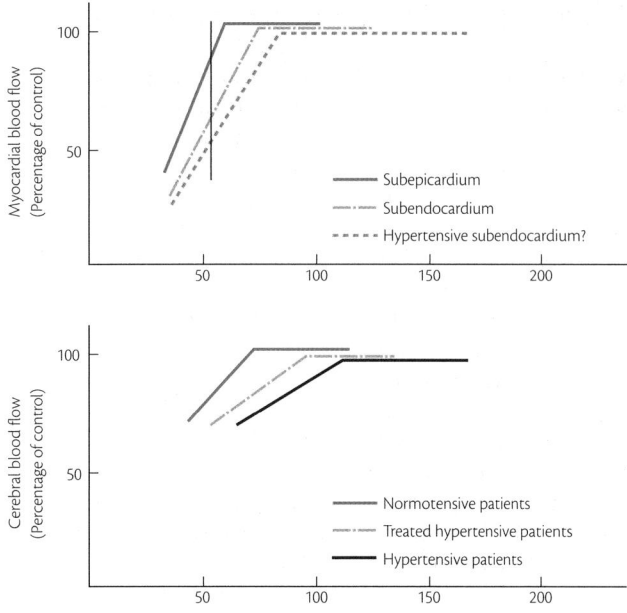

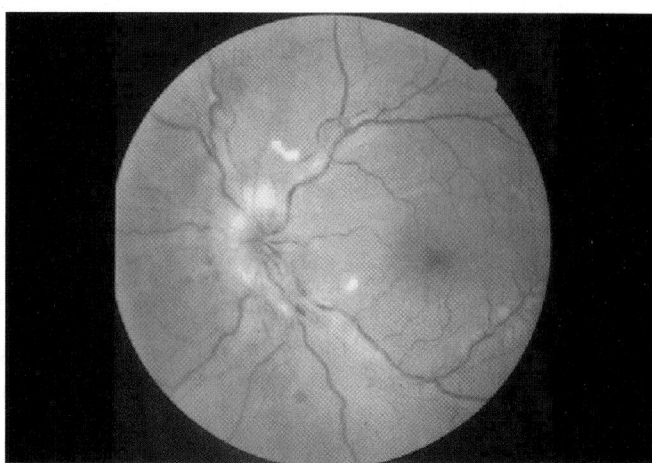

Fig. 16.17.5.2 Ocular fundus in hypertension, showing papilloedema, exudates, and a few haemorrhages.

Fig. 16.17.5.1 Autoregulation of myocardial and cerebral blood flow in normotensive and hypertensive patients.
Reprinted from *The Lancet*, Vol. 330, Strandgaard S and Haunsø S, *Why does antihypertensive treatment prevent stroke but not myocardial infarction?*, pp658-60. Copyright (1987), with permission from Elsevier.

pressure in the arterioles and capillaries, causing vascular damage. Disruption of the endothelium allows plasma constituents (including fibrinoid material) to enter the vessel wall, narrowing or obliterating the lumen in many tissue beds, the level at which fibrinoid necrosis occurs depending upon the baseline blood pressure. In the cerebral circulation, this can lead to the development of cerebral oedema and the clinical picture of hypertensive encephalopathy.

In addition to protecting the tissues against the effects of hypertension, autoregulation maintains perfusion during the treatment of hypertension via arterial and arteriolar vasodilatation. However, falls in blood pressure below the autoregulatory range can lead to organ ischaemia, and the arteriolar hypertrophy induced by chronic hypertension means that target organ ischaemia will occur at a higher pressure than in previously normotensive subjects.

Malignant hypertension, a hypertensive 'urgency'

The malignant phase of hypertension is a rare condition characterized by very high blood pressure, with bilateral retinal haemorrhages and/or exudates or cotton wool spots, with or without papilloedema (Fig. 16.17.5.2). Its pathophysiological definition is based on the histological hallmark of fibrinoid necrosis of arterioles in many tissues, particularly the kidney—changes which are broadly similar to those seen in the haemolytic–uraemic syndrome or scleroderma. Mucoid intimal proliferation in renal interlobular arteries and ischaemic collapse of the glomerular tufts may also be seen. Myointimal hyperplasia is a common finding in black patients, with the consequent intrarenal vascular disease leading to ischaemia of the juxtaglomerular apparatus and activation of the renin–angiotensin system with further vasoconstriction and wall damage, as well as exacerbation of hypertension.

Epidemiology

Malignant hypertension may be becoming rarer in some countries, particularly amongst white populations, but it still remains a common problem in developing countries and in other populations with health and social deprivation, where it is an important cause of endstage renal failure. In west Birmingham in the United Kingdom, the incidence of malignant hypertension is around 1 to 2 per 100 000 population per year, with no clear reduction between 1970 and 2006 in the number of new cases seen, the mean duration of known hypertension before presentation, presenting blood pressures, or the number of antihypertensive drugs that were being used. These data are reinforced by an analysis, from Amsterdam, of 122 patients with malignant hypertension in a multiethnic population, where the incidence rate was approximately 2.6 per 100 000 per year, and was higher among blacks.

Although essential hypertension is usually the most common underlying cause of malignant hypertension in adults, secondary causes (especially renal disease) are more prevalent among younger patients, being identified in up to 40% of white and 10% of black subjects. In children (aged <16 years) with malignant hypertension, parenchymal renal disease is the commonest cause (63%), with 33% having renovascular hypertension (aortoarteritis and fibromuscular dysplasia), and only 5% with essential hypertension.

There is an association between cigarette smoking and malignant hypertension that remains unexplained. Very rarely, the oral contraceptive pill may be implicated, consistent with the well-recognized increase in blood pressure in some women taking the combined oestrogen/progesterone oral contraceptive pill. It is uncertain whether oral contraceptives cause hypertension directly, or whether they simply exaggerate a tendency in women who already have a propensity to raised blood pressure.

Malignant hypertension can occur in older people, and is more common in Afro-Caribbean than in white and Indo-Asian populations. Possible reasons for this include the relative resistance of black patients to some antihypertensive therapies and, perhaps, poorer drug compliance. In many series, black individuals had higher systolic blood pressures and more renal dysfunction than whites.

One reason for the failure of malignant hypertension to decline in some centres may be inadequate medical screening facilities among poorly educated people with a limited understanding of the nature of the disease and the need to comply with antihypertensive therapy. Any reduction in the incidence of malignant hypertension may be because increasing use of drug therapy in milder grades of hypertension prevents progression to the malignant phase. Nevertheless, it is possible that there has been no real decline in malignant hypertension, but merely a failure to recognize this life-threatening condition.

Clinical features

The predominant presenting symptom is visual disturbance with or without headaches, but some patients with malignant hypertension remain asymptomatic, and others present at a late stage of their disease, this proportion ranging from 10 to 75% in one series from Nigeria.

In the west Birmingham series, the presenting mean systolic and diastolic blood pressures have remained surprisingly similar over the 30 years surveyed (average blood pressure 229/142 mmHg), despite improvements in antihypertensive therapy. Heart failure, angina, or myocardial infarction are complicating features in approximately 20% of patients, and the ECG shows that many patients to have cardiomegaly and left ventricular hypertrophy. Nevertheless, some patients do have normal chest radiographs, ECGs, or echocardiograms despite very high blood pressure, suggesting that hypertension may have been of recent onset.

Investigation

All patients with malignant hypertension need a detailed clinical history and examination, and investigation with blood tests (full blood count, serum biochemistry—including electrolytes and renal function), 12-lead ECG, chest radiography, and urinalysis. Fundoscopy and retinal photography are mandatory. Urinalysis may demonstrate proteinuria and haematuria, even in the absence of primary renal disease, but the presence of proteinuria is a poor prognostic sign. The kidneys should be imaged by abdominal ultrasonography to assess renal size and appearance, with a low threshold for proceeding to renal angiography to look for renal artery stenosis if the kidneys are asymmetric. A 24-h urinary collection is necessary for catecholamines (see Chapter 16.17.3) and so is protein excretion assessment in all patients (or the latter can be estimated by albumin/creatinine ratio, ACR). These initial screening tests serve to identify patients in whom additional investigations may be appropriate to detect an underlying cause of hypertension.

The full blood count and film may reveal the anaemia of chronic renal failure or occasionally a microangiopathic haemolytic anaemia—with red cell fragmentation and intravascular haemolysis—possibly related to the degree of arteriolar fibrinoid necrosis. Serum urea and creatinine should initially be measured daily: renal impairment may have significant prognostic implications. Mild hypokalaemia due to secondary hyperaldosteronism may be present, which usually resolves after control of the hypertension. Only very rarely does hypokalaemia indicate primary hyperaldosteronism (Conn's syndrome), but if it is extreme or persists despite good blood pressure control, then the characteristic findings of low renin levels, but high aldosterone concentrations, may be present. More commonly, both plasma renin and aldosterone levels are high in malignant hypertension, usually attributed to juxtaglomerular ischaemia. Inflammatory markers (erythrocyte sedimentation rate (ESR) and C-reactive protein (CRP)) are often modestly elevated in malignant hypertension, but measurement of autoantibodies (antinuclear antibodies and antineutrophil cytoplasmic antibodies) can be used to discern uncommon cases due to vasculitis. Renal biopsy is required to make a specific diagnosis in some instances, but should not be performed until blood pressure is controlled.

The chest radiograph may show cardiomegaly and the presence of pulmonary oedema. In a recent series of patients with malignant hypertension undergoing echocardiography, cardiac hypertrophy was common and associated with systolic dysfunction and a dilated left atrium, irrespective of the duration of known hypertension. These structural/functional abnormalities may predispose patients to cardiovascular complications including heart failure and cardiac arrhythmias, such as atrial fibrillation.

Complications

Retinopathy

As described above and in Chapter 16.17.2, the most widely used classification of hypertensive changes in the fundus is that of Keith, Wagener, and Barker—the strength of this being the correlation in the original description between clinical findings and prognosis (Table 16.17.5.1). However, this classification has now been made obsolete by advances in the understanding of the pathophysiology of arterial hypertension and the availability of effective antihypertensive therapy. Ophthalmoscopic grading of the retinal changes in hypertension has been simplified into mild, moderate, and severe levels (see Chapter 16.17.2), and can be further reduced into two

Table 16.17.5.1 The Keith, Wagener, and Barker classification of hypertensive retinopathy

	Grade 1	Grade 2	Grade 3	Grade 4
Retinal findings	Mild narrowing or sclerosis of the retinal arterioles	Moderate to marked sclerosis of the retinal arterioles	Retinal oedema, cotton wool spots and haemorrhages	All the above and optic disc oedema
		Exaggerated arterial light reflex	Sclerosis and spastic lesions of retinal arterioles	
		Venous compression at arterio-venous crossings ('nipping')	Macular star	
Percentage surviving in original series				
1 year	90	88	65	21
3 years	70	62	22	6
5 years	70	54	20	1

Grades 1 and 2 are broadly similar and are related to age and general cardiovascular status as well as blood pressure. Grades 3 and 4 are much more alike and both are now considered to be 'malignant'. See Chapter 16.17.2 for further discussion.

groups: grade A (nonmalignant)—arteriolar narrowing and focal constriction, which also correlate with age and general cardiovascular status as well as blood pressure; and grade B (malignant)—linear flame-shaped haemorrhages, and/or exudates, and/or cotton wool spots, with or without disc swelling. Papilloedema is an unreliable physical sign, and its presence or absence in the context of other grade-B changes does not indicate a worse prognosis.

Similar retinal appearances with haemorrhages and papilloedema can occur in severe anaemia, connective tissue disease, and infective endocarditis. Idiopathic intracranial hypertension with bilateral papilloedema is itself associated with hypertension and obesity but this is not indicative of hypertension entering its malignant phase. Nevertheless, severe hypertension and lone bilateral papilloedema may be a variant of malignant hypertension, with similar clinical features and prognosis. The retinal features of malignant hypertension regress over a period of 2 to 3 months, if good blood pressure control is achieved.

Renal involvement

Renal involvement in malignant hypertension has been referred to as malignant nephrosclerosis, manifest as haematuria, proteinuria, and (sometimes) acute renal failure. Renal failure is the commonest cause of death, with presenting urea and creatinine levels independent predictors of survival.

When antihypertensive therapy is initiated and blood pressure control achieved, the effect on renal function is variable. In the short term, renal function stabilizes in 10% of cases, deteriorates progressively in 30%, and deteriorates transiently before improving over a matter of weeks in the remainder. Renal failure is more frequent (two- to threefold) in black, than in white, individuals (Fig. 16.17.5.3), but mainly because of higher serum creatinine levels at presentation.

Isles and co-workers have suggested that the renal outcome of patients with malignant hypertension can be considered in three groups, each with a different renal prognosis: (1) patients whose serum creatinine is less than 300 μmol/litre at presentation, who do well with effective antihypertensive therapy; (2) patients with chronic renal failure (serum creatinine >300 μmol/litre) who do not require renal dialysis immediately, but are unlikely to maintain or recover renal function, except possibly in the short term, and commonly progress to endstage renal failure; and (3) a small group with acute renal failure. It is possible that some of these patients may have poststreptococcal acute nephritic syndrome, characterized by retinopathy, fluid retention, and usually complete renal recovery.

In the west Birmingham series, Lip *et al.* did not find such a clear distinction based on serum creatinine and found that renal function continued to deteriorate among many patients with malignant hypertension, despite good blood pressure control at follow-up. About half of the patients with severe renal impairment at presentation demonstrated either static or improved renal function, and there was no evidence that those cases where renal function remained static were those with less renal impairment at presentation. The severity of malignant hypertension at presentation did not predict outcome, but the quality of control of systolic blood pressure at follow-up and the height of the serum creatinine at presentation did, suggesting that careful monitoring of renal function and aggressive treatment of blood pressure is mandatory in patients with this condition.

High serum urate levels are associated with greater renal impairment at baseline, as well as higher diastolic blood pressures, but are not predictive of deterioration in renal function or overall survival in patients with malignant hypertension.

There are varying reports of the frequency of renovascular disease in malignant hypertension, which may be due to the frequency with which renal angiography is performed. In older patients, renal artery stenosis is likely to be due to atheromatous disease, which itself may be a consequence of chronic hypertension and chronic hyperlipidaemia, as well as cigarette smoking. In younger patients, and particularly in women, renal artery stenosis may be due to fibromuscular dysplasia of the renal arteries, with the characteristic 'string of beads' appearance on renal angiography. The value of surgical or angioplastic correction of atheromatous disease is debatable, possibly producing no better results than effective blood pressure control with antihypertensive drugs. In patients with fibromuscular dysplasia, however, renal angioplasty with stenting is worthwhile and will often lead to a normal blood pressure level.

Management

All patients with malignant hypertension require assessment, investigation, and commencement of therapy under supervision, preferably as an in-patient. Blood pressure should be measured 4-hourly, with the initial aim of treatment being to lower the diastolic pressure near about 100 to 105 mmHg over a period of 2 to 3 days, with oral therapy and dose escalation at daily intervals, if necessary. The maximum initial fall in blood pressure should not exceed 25% of the presenting value, gradual reduction allowing adaptation of disordered tissue autoregulation and avoidance of target organ ischaemia. More aggressive antihypertensive therapy is both unnecessary and dangerous, as it may reduce the blood pressure to below the autoregulatory range, leading to ischaemic events such as strokes, heart attack, or renal failure.

The first line oral antihypertensive agent is either a short-acting calcium antagonist (such as nifedipine) or a β-blocker (such as atenolol). An appropriate dose of nifedipine is 10 to 20 mg of the

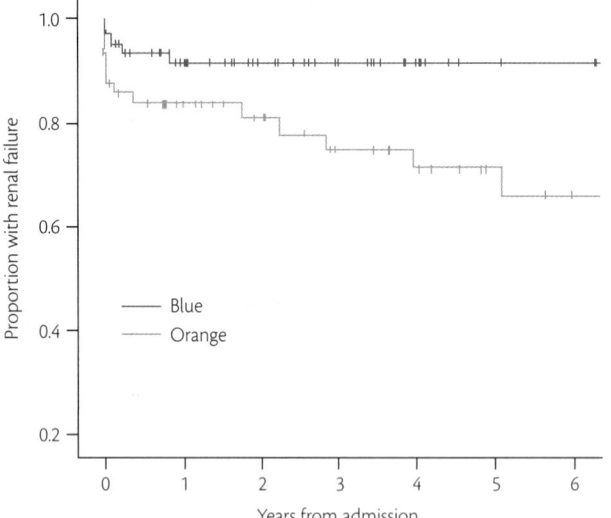

Fig. 16.17.5.3 Proportion with renal failure after presentation with malignant hypertension, stratified for ethnicity.
From van den Born *et al* 2006 - Van den Born BJ et al (2006). Ethnic disparities in the incidence, presentation and complications of malignant hypertension. J Hypertens 24, 2299-304 (http://journals.lww.com/jhypertension/Abstract/2006/11000/Ethnic_disparities_in_the_incidence,_presentation.27.aspx).

tablet formulation, which can be repeated or increased, as necessary, to bring about gradual reduction in blood pressure. Nifedipine is not absorbed from the oral mucosa, and there have been reports of complications including visual loss, cerebral infarction, and myocardial infarction with nifedipine therapy using the short-acting sublingual capsules, which produce unpredictable falls in blood pressure and should never be used. β-Blockers are useful alternatives, but should be avoided in patients with asthma or where there is a high suspicion of an underlying phaeochromocytoma. It is sensible to start with small doses, such as 25 mg of atenolol, increasing dose as necessary. The combination of oral atenolol and nifedipine is often a well-tolerated and effective regime.

Diuretics should be restricted to those with evidence of fluid overload. Some patients are volume depleted, presumably secondary to a pressure-related diuresis and activation of the renin–angiotensin system. Captopril and the other angiotensin converting enzyme (ACE) inhibitors can produce rapid and dangerous falls in blood pressure, particularly in patients with hypokalaemic secondary hyperaldosteronism and hyponatraemia secondary to juxtaglomerular ischaemia or renovascular disease, which may be unrecognized in the acute situation.

Over a period of about 1 to 2 weeks, further antihypertensive drugs should be added in to achieve a gradual reduction of blood pressure to less than 140/85 mmHg. Triple or quadruple drug regimens are invariably necessary in the long term.

Drugs for the treatment of hypertensive emergencies and urgencies anre summarized in Tables 16.17.5.2 and 16.17.5.3.

Prognosis

If malignant hypertension is left untreated, around 80% of patients die within 2 years, hence the name. In west Birmingham, between 1965 and 2006, after a median follow-up of 103 months (range 1–539 months), 40% were alive and not requiring renal replacement therapy, 3.2% were on long-term haemodialysis, and 40%

Table 16.17.5.2 Oral drugs for hypertensive emergencies and urgencies

Category	Example	Comment
β-Blockers	Atenolol (25–50 mg)	Safe unless contraindicated
Calcium channel blockers	Nifedipine capsules	Dangerous
	Nifedipine tablets (10–20 mg)	Safe
	Amlodipine	Onset of action is slow (c.5 days)
	Verapamil	Useful if tachycardia or associated supraventricular arrhythmia
	Nicardipine	Not better than nifedipine by mouth
α-Blockers	Prazosin	Little experience
	Doxazosin	Little experience
	Phenoxybenzamine	Phaeochromocytoma
Diuretics	Thiazides	Slow onset
	Loop diuretics	Only if heart failure
ACE inhibitors	Captopril (6.25–50 mg, 3 times a day)	If patient on diuretic, or if renal artery stenosis is undiagnosed, may cause rapid falls in blood pressure and acute renal failure

were dead, with the remainder lost to follow-up. The commonest causes of death were renal failure (39.7%), stroke (23.8%), myocardial infarction (11.1%), and heart failure (10.3%).

The advent of effective and tolerable antihypertensive drug therapy has improved prognosis. For example, in the west Birmingham series, 5-year survival rates improved from 31.4% prior to 1967 to 91.9% for the years 1997 to 2006. (Fig. 16.17.5.4). The series by Scarpelli and coworkers reported a 12-year survival rate of about 69%, although patients with malignant hypertension diagnosed after 1980 had a 100% survival rate. More contemporaneous data from the Amsterdam series, describing patients incident between 1993 and 2005, showed that 10% had died and 19% needed renal replacement therapy after a mean follow-up of 4 years. Hence, whatever the cause of malignant hypertension, progressive renal impairment is still a common complicating factor, with many patients needing dialysis in the long term.

The importance of early diagnosis is emphasized as patients tend to develop clinical symptoms only at a late stage of their disease. Black men with malignant hypertension have a poor prognosis when compared with other ethnic groups or women; they also present with more severe hypertension and greater renal damage, which are independent predictors of outcome and explain the poorer prognosis.

Hypertensive emergencies

Hypertensive left ventricular failure

Hypertension causes heart failure by a number of mechanisms: these include pressure overload on the heart due to the raised peripheral vascular resistance, reduced left ventricular compliance (e.g. in left ventricular hypertrophy), an increased risk for coronary artery disease and the precipitation of cardiac arrhythmias (such as atrial fibrillation). Severe hypertension results in a significant increase in afterload and may result in decompensation of the failing heart.

In very severe hypertension with marked pulmonary oedema, intravenous sodium nitroprusside may be necessary to reduce preload and afterload in addition to conventional management with opioids and loop diuretics. However, metabolism of nitroprusside to cyanide, possibly leading to the development of cyanide or (rarely) thiocyanate toxicity, may be a limitation. This manifests with altered mental status and lactic acidosis, and can be fatal. The risk of toxicity is increased in children, also with prolonged treatment (>24–48 h), underlying renal insufficiency, and requirement for high doses (>2 µg/kg per min). An infusion of sodium thiosulphate can be used in affected patients to provide a sulphur donor to detoxify cyanide into thiocyanate.

Nitrates may also be used to treat hypertensive left ventricular failure, but they are less potent than sodium nitroprusside. ACE inhibitors should be considered only after the patient's condition is stabilized, when they are well established to be life-saving in those with left ventricular systolic impairment, lead to long-term regression of left ventricular hypertrophy, and may also improve heart failure secondary to diastolic dysfunction.

Hypertensive encephalopathy

Hypertensive encephalopathy refers to the presence of signs of cerebral oedema caused by breakthrough hyperperfusion following severe and sudden rises in blood pressure. There is failure of autoregulatory vasoconstriction with focal or generalized dilatation of small arteries and arterioles. This leads to high cerebral

Table 16.17.5.3 Parenteral drugs for the treatment of hypertensive emergencies

	Action	Administration	Use and adverse effects	Comment
Sodium nitroprusside	Dilates both arterioles and veins via generation of cGMP which then activates calcium-sensitive potassium channels in the cell membrane	IV infusion; rapid onset and offset of action, minimizing the risk of hypotension Recommended starting dose is 0.25–0.5 µg/kg per min, increased as necessary to a maximum dose of 8–10 µg/kg per min, for up to 10 min Nitroprusside should not be given to pregnant women	Can cause intrapulmonary shunting and coronary 'steal' Thiocynate and cyanide toxicity manifest by clinical deterioration, muscle twitching, altered mental status, and lactic acidosis, and can be fatal	The most effective parenteral drug for most hypertensive emergencies Easy to control on a minute-to-minute basis
Nitroglycerine (glyceryl trinitrate)	Similar action to nitroprusside, but greater venodilatation	IV infusion, 5–100 µg/min Onset of action is 2–5 min, duration of action 5–10 min	Headache (due to direct vasodilatation) and tachycardia (reflex sympathetic activation) Vomiting Methaemoglobinaemia	Most useful in patients with symptomatic coronary disease and in those with hypertension following surgery
Labetalol	Combined β- and α-blocker	Rapid onset of action (5 min or less) Bolus of 20 mg initially, followed by 20–80 mg every 10 min to a total dose of 300 mg The infusion rate is 0.5–2 mg/min	Avoid in patients with contraindications to β-blockers	Safe in patients with active coronary disease since it does not increase the heart rate Also useful in the perioperative care of patients with severe hypertension
Esmolol	β-Blocker	Rapid onset and offset of action IV infusion, titrated to heart rate and blood pressure response	Reduces myocardial ischaemia Avoid in patients with contraindications to β-blockers	Useful in tachycardias, hyperdynamic heart, arrhythmias (e.g. atrial fibrillation), perioperative hypertension, aortic dissection
Nicardipine	Dihydropyridine calcium channel blocker	IV infusion at 5–15 mg/h	Headache and flushing Tachycardia	Becoming more popular Useful for most hypertensive emergencies, except acute heart failure
Diazoxide	Arteriolar vasodilator that has little effect on the venous circulation	IV bolus 50–150 mg or infusion 2–10 mg/h Peak effect seen within 15 min, lasts for 4–24 h	Do not use in patients with angina pectoris, myocardial infarction, pulmonary oedema, or a dissecting aortic aneurysm Can cause marked fluid retention and a diuretic may be needed	Give β-blocker to block reflex activation of the sympathetic nervous system Rarely used nowadays as may cause excessive blood pressure reduction which is difficult to reverse
Hydralazine	Direct arteriolar vasodilator	IV bolus Initial dose is 10–20 mg Fall in blood pressure begins within 10–30 min and lasts 2–4 h	Tachycardia, flushing, headache, vomiting Aggravation of angina Hypotensive response to hydralazine is less predictable	Used in pregnant women
Phentolamine	α-Adrenergic blocker	IV bolus, 5–10 mg every 5–15 min as necessary	Severe hypertension due to phaeochromocytoma and other syndromes of increased catecholamine activity, such as drug abuse, MAO-induced hypertension, etc.	Tachyphylaxis means that doses need to be escalated

IV, intravenous; MAO, monoamine oxidase.

blood flow, dysfunction of the blood–brain barrier, and the formation of brain oedema, which is thought to cause the clinical symptoms. The condition is now very rare, and it is essential to perform a CT or an MRI scan to ensure that this hypertensive emergency is distinguished from other neurological syndromes associated with high blood pressure, including intracerebral or subarachnoid haemorrhage, ischaemic stroke, or lacunar infarction.

Hypertensive encephalopathy is usually associated with a history of hypertension that has been inadequately treated, or where previous treatment has been discontinued. It is characterized by the insidious onset of headache, nausea, and vomiting, followed by visual disturbances and fluctuating, nonlocalizing neurological symptoms such as restlessness, confusion, and—if the hypertension is not treated—seizures and coma. Severe retinopathy is frequently, but not always, present.

CT or MRI may demonstrate white matter oedema, and one of these tests is mandatory to exclude cerebral haemorrhage or infarction. Indeed, the increased use of CT scanning has demonstrated that almost all patients who appear to have hypertensive encephalopathy have cerebral infarction or haemorrhage with surrounding oedema and space-occupying cerebral symptoms. Lumbar puncture is not indicated in the management of patients with malignant hypertension; but if obtained (perhaps in ignorance of the diagnosis) the cerebrospinal fluid is usually normal, although at an

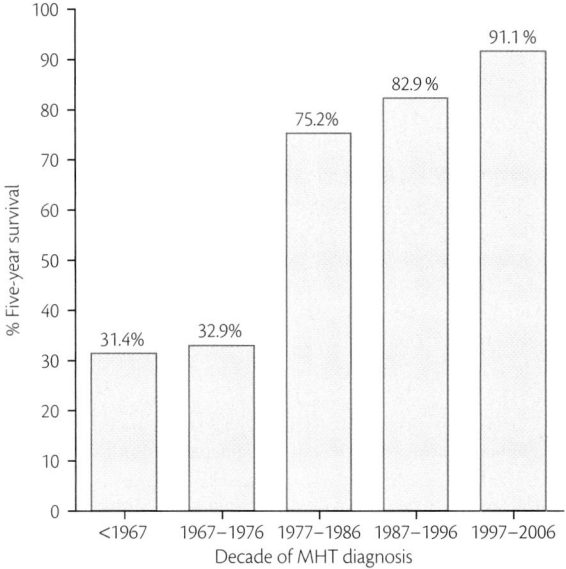

Fig. 16.17.5.4 Five-year survival by decade of diagnosis. MHT, malignant phase hypertension.
Reprinted by permission from Macmillan Publishers Ltd: American Journal of Hypertension, Lane DA, Lip GYH, Beevers DG, Improving survival of malignant hypertension patients over 40 years. 22: 1199–204, copyright (2009).

increased pressure. The ECG may show variable transient, focal, or bilateral abnormalities.

Sodium nitroprusside is the drug of choice for genuine hypertensive encephalopathy, but is not usually given if there is a cerebral infarct or haemorrhage. Parenteral labetalol and nitrates have also been used successfully. Rarely, diazoxide and hydralazine have been given, but they can cause precipitate and life-threatening acute falls in blood pressure, and they require concurrent β-blocker administration to minimize reflex sympathetic stimulation. Sublingual nifedipine capsules should never be used (see above). Phentolamine is used only in patients with severe hypertension due to increased catecholamine activity, such as that seen in phaeochromocytoma, or after tyramine ingestion in a patient being treated with a monoamine oxidase inhibitor. ACE inhibitors are best avoided in the early stage as they may, even in a very low dose, cause precipitate falls in blood pressure and life-threatening reduction in cerebral perfusion, particularly when patients are fluid depleted due to diuretic therapy or in the presence of renal artery stenosis.

Severe pre-eclampsia and eclampsia are discussed in detail elsewhere (see Chapter 14.4). They may present with clinical features similar to hypertensive encephalopathy, and treatment is broadly similar, with labetolol infusions, magnesium sulphate, and early delivery of the fetus.

Hypertension with unstable angina or acute myocardial infarction

In a patient presenting with an acute coronary syndrome (unstable angina or acute myocardial infarction) and severe hypertension, a 'true' hypertensive emergency, such as aortic dissection, must first be ruled out. The risk of bleeding and stroke is significantly increased if anticoagulation with heparin, antiplatelet therapies (such as glycoprotein IIb/IIIa inhibitors), or thrombolytic therapy is administered.

The appropriate initial treatment of patients with severe hypertension (>180/110 mmHg) and an acute coronary syndrome should include the initiation of intravenous nitrates, with intravenous labetalol, sodium nitroprusside, or nicardipine as alternatives. The reduction of blood pressure should not be too abrupt: as, with malignant hypertension, a gradual reduction is recommended in an endeavour to avoid further myocardial or brain ischaemia. As stated previously, sublingual nifedipine—once considered as a first line drug—should not be used in view of its negligible oral absorption and the unpredictable hypotensive effects from later gastric absorption. Anticoagulation or thrombolytic therapy can be administered when the blood pressure is adequately controlled (<180/110 mmHg), or revascularization with primary percutaneous coronary angioplasty can be considered as an alternative for acute ST segment elevation myocardial infarction (STEMI).

Hypertension with acute stroke and after a stroke

It is common to find modestly elevated blood pressure in patients admitted to hospital following an acute stroke. Cerebral autoregulation is commonly impaired in this context, with flow becoming pressure dependent. Thus, excessive antihypertensive treatment may serve to worsen the cerebral damage resulting from intracerebral infarction or haemorrhage, and stroke physicians are very wary about lowering the blood pressure. There are few randomized controlled trials to inform the management of this common problem. Current consensus only recommends acute blood pressure lowering where there is associated acute end-organ damage—e.g. cardiac (acute myocardial infarction, severe left ventricular failure) or vascular urgencies (aortic dissection), hypertensive encephalopathy, acute renal failure, concurrent coagulant therapy (thrombolysis, intravenous heparin, etc.), or persistent blood pressure elevation with a threshold of greater than 200/120 mmHg for ischaemic stroke and greater than 180/105 mmHg for haemorrhagic stroke. In these cases, oral therapy with small doses of nifedipine or atenolol may be required. Parenteral treatment or sublingual nifedipine is always contraindicated. The calcium antagonist nimodipine has beneficial effects on cerebral vasospasm following subarachnoid haemorrhage, but these effects are not related to the small fall in blood pressure with this drug.

Severe hypertension after a stroke is a risk factor for further stokes, and long-term treatment is worthwhile. It is unclear whether the immediate treatment of mild hypertension is of benefit. The role of antihypertensive medication before, during, and after a stroke can, therefore, be summarized as follows:

1 Before a stroke, it is of benefit to have blood pressure reduced to below 140/85 mmHg, as stroke prevention can be achieved.

2 During a stroke, it is detrimental to have hypertension treated aggressively, in view of the disordered cerebral autoregulation.

3 After a stroke, the epidemiological associations of hypertension with recurrent stroke have not been entirely consistent, with some studies showing no association or a J-shaped relationship.

In the last decade, many studies have reported on the effects of antihypertensive drugs—predominantly ACE inhibitors or angiotensin receptor blockers—in the poststroke setting. The Heart Outcomes Prevention Evaluation (HOPE) study reported a subset of 1013 subjects with a previous history of stroke or transient ischaemic attack (TIA), where there was a nonsignificant 15% reduction in total stroke recurrence with ramipril. In the PROGRESS trial, 6105 normotensive and hypertensive patients with a history of ischaemic or haemorrhagic stroke or TIA were randomized to perindopril (± indapamide), which reduced recurrent stroke by 28% and major vascular events by 26% during 4 years of follow-up. The Morbidity and Mortality after Stroke Eprosartan Study (MOSES) compared eprosartan (an angiotensin receptor blocker) to nitrendipine (a dihydropyridine calcium channel blocker) in hypertensive-stroke survivors and found a 21% risk reduction in the primary endpoint of all cardiovascular and cerebrovascular events and a 25% reduction in recurrent cerebrovascular events in the eprosartan-treated patients.

Management of blood pressure in a patient with aortic dissection

The detailed presentation, diagnosis, and treatment of aortic dissection is discussed in Chapter 16.14.1. On suspicion of the diagnosis, whether or not surgery is indicated, all patients should be treated pharmacologically to reduce the systolic blood pressure to around 110 mmHg and the heart rate to 60 to 70 beats/min, thus reducing the force of systolic ejection to reduce aortic shear stress and limit the size of the dissection. Labetalol is an effective agent, or alternatively, sodium nitroprusside in conjunction with a β-blocker may be used. Patients should ideally have haemodynamic monitoring with an arterial line in position. Diagnostic tests are then performed on an urgent basis to confirm the dissection, identifying whether the ascending aorta is involved, and defining any vascular abnormalities resulting from the dissection.

Further reading

Bloxham CA, Beevers DG, Walker JM (1979). Malignant hypertension and cigarette smoking. *Br Med J*, **i**, 581–3.

Gudbrandsson T, *et al.* (1979). Malignant hypertension. Improving prognosis in a rare disease. *Acta Med Scand*, **206**, 495–9.

Harvey JM, *et al.* (1992). Renal biopsy findings in hypertensive patients with proteinuria. *Lancet*, **340**, 1435–6.

Isles CG, McLay A, Boulton Jones JM (1984). Recovery in malignant hypertension presenting as acute renal failure. *Q J Med*, **212**, 439–52.

Jhetam D, *et al.* (1982). The malignant phase of essential hypertension in Johannesburg blacks. *S Afr Med J*, **61**, 899–902.

Kadiri S, Olutade BO (1991). The clinical presentation of malignant hypertension in Nigerians. *J Hum Hyper*, **5**, 339–43.

Keith NM, Wagener HP, Barker NW (1939). Some different types of essential hypertension: their course and prognosis. *Am J Med Sci*, **196**, 332–43.

Kumar P, *et al.* (1996). Malignant hypertension in children in India. *Neph Dial Trans*, **11**, 1261–6.

Lane DA, Lip GYH, Beevas DG (2009). Improving survival of malignant hypertension patients over 40 years, *Am J hypertns*, **22**, 1199–204.

Leishman AWD (1959). Hypertension—treated and untreated: a study of 400 cases. *Br Med J*, **i**, 1361–3.

Lim KG, *et al.* (1987). Malignant hypertension in women of childbearing age and its relation to the contraceptive pill. *BMJ*, **294**, 1057–9.

Lip GYH *et al.* (1995). Severe hypertension and lone bilateral papilloedema: a variant of malignant phase hypertension. *Blood Press*, **4**, 339–42.

Lip GYH, *et al.* (1995). Malignant hypertension in the elderly. *Q J Med*, **88**, 641–7.

Lip GYH, Beevers M, Beevers DG (1997). Does renal function improve following diagnosis of malignant phase hypertension? *J Hypertens*, **15**, 1309–15.

Lip GYH, Beevers M, Beevers DG (2000). Serum urate is associated with baseline renal dysfunction but not survival or deterioration in renal function in malignant phase hypertension. *J Hypertens*, **18**, 97–101.

Mamdani BH, *et al.* (1974). Recovery from prolonged renal failure in patients with accelerated hypertension. *N Engl J Med*, **291**, 1343–4.

Pitcock JA, *et al.* (1976). Malignant hypertension in blacks. Malignant intrarenal arterial disease as observed by light and electron microscopy. *Hum Pathol*, **7**, 333–46.

Scarpelli PT, *et al.* (1997). Accelerated (malignant) hypertension: a study of 121 cases between 1974 and 1996. *Nephrology*, **10**, 207–15.

Schrader J, *et al.* (2005). Morbidity and mortality after stroke, eprosartan compared with nitrendipine for secondary prevention: principal results of a prospective randomized controlled study (MOSES). *Stroke*, **36**, 1218–26.

Strandgaard S, Paulson OB (1996). Antihypertensive drugs and cerebral circulation. *Eur J Clin Invest*, **26**, 625–30.

Van den Born BJ, *et al.* (2006). Ethnic disparities in the incidence, presentation and complications of malignant hypertension. *J Hypertens*, **24**, 2299–304.

Veriava Y, *et al.* (1990). Hypertension as a cause of end-stage renal failure in South Africa. *J Hum Hypertens*, **4**, 379–83.

Webster J, *et al.* (1993). Accelerated hypertension—patterns of mortality and clinical factors affecting outcome in treated patients. *Q J Med*, **86**, 485–93.

Zampaglione P, *et al.* (1996). Hypertensive urgencies and emergencies. Prevalence and clinical presentation. *Hypertension*, **27**, 144–7.

Chronic peripheral oedema and lymphoedema

Peter S. Mortimer

Essentials

Lymph transport, not venous capillary reabsorption, is the main process responsible for interstitial fluid drainage. Oedema develops when the microvascular filtration rate exceeds lymph drainage for a sufficient period, either because the filtration rate is high or because lymph flow is low, or a combination of the two. In the United Kingdom the prevalence of lymphoedema is just over 0.1%, rising to 0.5% in those over 65 years of age.

Causes of lymphoedema

Lymph drainage may fail either because of a defect intrinsic to the lymph conducting pathways (primary lymphoedema), or because of irreversible damage from some factor(s) originating from outside the lymphatic system (secondary lymphoedema).

Primary lymphoedema—can be caused by mutations in the vascular endothelial growth factor receptor-3 gene (Milroy's disease) or in the forkhead transcription factor gene *FOXC2* (lymphoedema—distichiasis), but for most forms the genetic cause is unknown. Congenital lymphoedema may occur in isolation or as part of a syndrome.

Secondary lymphoedema—filariasis is by far the most common cause of lymphoedema worldwide. In the United Kingdom 25% of cases are due to malignancy.

Clinical features and management

Lymphoedema causes persistent swelling that does not resolve with overnight elevation and is associated with cellulitis. Response to diuretics is poor. The oedema does pit, but prolonged pressure is required to do so, and the skin is thickened and warty. The investigation of choice for confirming that oedema is primarily of lymphatic origin is lymphoscintigraphy (isotope lymphography).

No drug or surgical therapy is known to improve lymph drainage. Treatment relies on improving lymph drainage through the application of simple physiological principles known to stimulate lymph flow, while at the same time restoring any excessive capillary filtration to as near normal as possible. Patients with leg lymphoedema often notice that walking reduces swelling, and the addition of a bandage or stocking can enhance the effect of movement by creating an outer collar to the leg that resists expansion of the calf muscle during contraction. This generates a high interstitial pressure during muscle contractions to drive lymph filling and drainage, but allows low pressures during skeletal muscle relaxation and hence permits lymphatic vessel refilling before further muscle contraction repeats the cycle. Compression without movement (active or passive exercises) does not improve lymph drainage. Manual lymphatic drainage therapy, a specific form of lymphatic massage, operates on the same principle of stimulating alternating rises and falls in interstitial pressure and is used to decongest more proximal regions of the body.

Prevention and prompt treatment of cellulitis is crucial to the control of lymphoedema, because this contributes to further decline in lymph drainage, which in turn encourages more infection.

Introduction

Oedema is an excess of interstitial fluid and is an important sign of ill health in clinical medicine. In medical practice peripheral oedema tends to be pigeon holed according to possible systemic or peripheral causes, e.g. heart failure, nephrotic syndrome, venous obstruction, or lymphoedema. This view point fails to appreciate the many dynamic physiological forces contributing to oedema development and in particular the central role of the lymphatic drainage system in tissue fluid (and consequently plasma volume) homeostasis.

Hence the clinician's approach to peripheral oedema is often misguided and the necessary medical intervention inappropriate, e.g. empirical use of diuretics. Management of peripheral oedema is better based on physiological principles that can then guide treatment.

Pathophysiology

Lymph transport, not venous capillary reabsorption, is the main process responsible for interstitial fluid drainage. Oedema develops

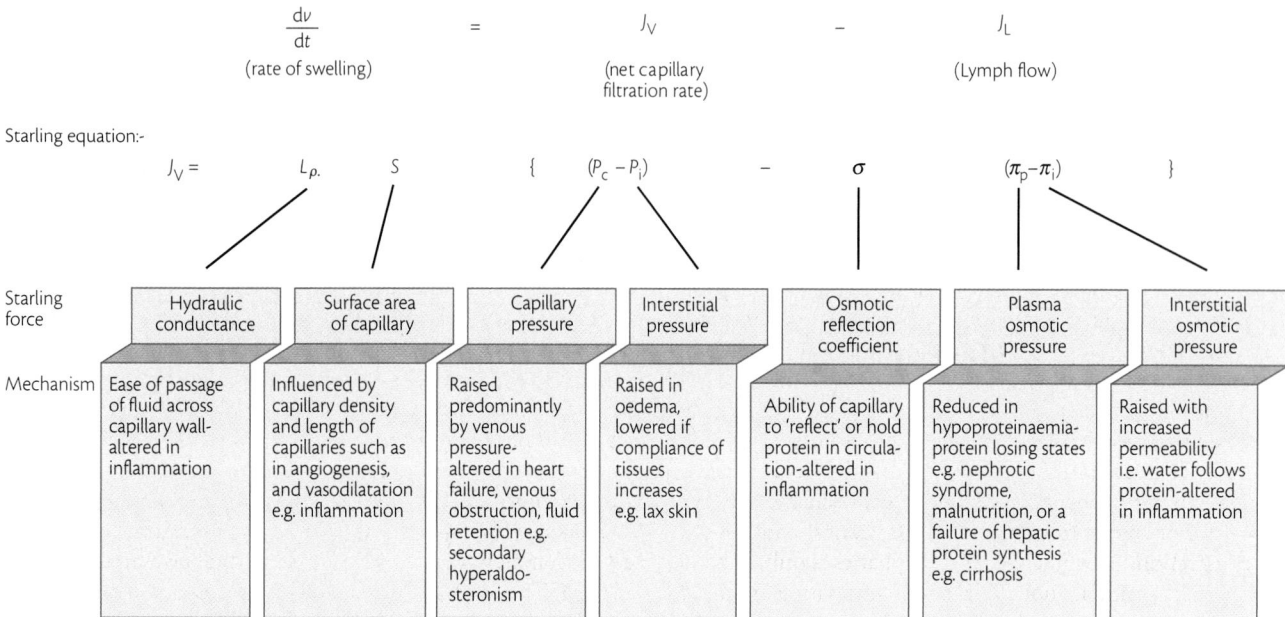

Fig. 16.18.1 Physiology of oedema.

when the microvascular (from capillaries and venules) filtration rate exceeds lymph drainage for a sufficient period, either because the filtration rate is high or because lymph flow is low, or a combination of the two. Filtration rate is governed by the Starling principle of fluid exchange, which is described succinctly and quantitatively by the Starling equation for flow across a semipermeable membrane (Fig. 16.18.1).

In simple terms, filtration of fluid from capillary into interstitium is driven by the hydraulic (water) pressure gradient across the wall $(P_c - P_i)$ and is opposed by the osmotic pressure gradient $(\pi_p - \pi_i)$, which is the 'suction' force keeping fluid in the circulation.

The Starling equation provides a logical approach for classifying oedema that is due to increased filtration:

1 Raised capillary pressure. Capillary pressure is more susceptible to changes in venous pressure than systemic (arterial) blood pressure because postcapillary resistance is much lower than precapillary resistance. Peripheral venous pressure is raised in:

- right ventricular failure
- salt and water overload (e.g. overtransfusion)
- venous obstruction
- venous reflux (chronic venous disease) e.g. following deep vein thrombosis, primary varicose veins
- dependency (the effect of gravity)

2 Reduced plasma osmotic pressure (COP). This essentially means hypoalbuminaemia, which can arise from:

- malnutrition
- intestinal disease (malabsorption or protein loss)
- nephrotic syndrome
- hepatic failure to synthesize albumin—due to liver disease or chronic inflammatory states

3 Increased capillary permeability

Inflammation can cause a breakdown in the endothelial barrier, facilitating the passage of both plasma proteins and water across the capillary wall. In addition, vasodilatation causes a rise in capillary pressure (and blood flow).

Traditionally it has been taught that the arterial end of capillaries filter fluid while the venous end reabsorbs the bulk of fluid filtered. This view is not supported by modern evidence, which demonstrates that in most vascular beds there is a net but dwindling filtration along the entire length of well-perfused capillaries. The sum of all Starling forces is not an absorptive force in venous capillaries but a slight filtration force, except e.g. following haemorrhage, when capillary pressure drops sufficiently for transient absorption to occur. Even under such circumstances Starling forces soon re-equilibrate and slight filtration is restored. Sustained reabsorption of fluid is a normal feature of some microcirculatory beds, namely intestinal mucosa, renal peritubular, and lymph node capillaries, but not peripheral tissues. Since the old concept of sustained fluid absorption by venous capillaries is no longertenable, the major responsibility for drainage of interstitial fluid is through the lymphatic system.

Restraining factors against oedema include (1) elevation of interstitial fluid pressure, (2) fall in interstitial COP, and (3) increased lymph flow. Stiffness in tissues resists swelling. A small increase in interstitial fluid in a stiff tissue (low compliance) will cause a relatively large increase in interstitial pressure (P_i), which then opposes filtration, e.g. subfascial muscle compartment. Placing a bandage or rigid stocking around a leg will reduce compliance and resist stretch. Consequently P_i will increase more steeply for a given interstitial volume increase and the increased P_i will oppose filtration. Relating to interstitial COP, an increase in filtration rate will dilute the interstitial protein concentration and consequently reduce the osmotic pressure (π immediately outside the semipermeable membrane). The resulting increase in the osmotic pressure gradient will raise the suction force keeping fluid within the blood compartment.

Increases in interstitial fluid pressure and volume stimulate lymph flow. Lymph drainage is a complex process involving absorption of protein and fluid (as well as other macromolecules, microorganisms, immune cells, and cancer cells) from the interstitium into initial lymphatic vessels (also known as lymphatics) and then downstream through vessels of ever-enlarging diameter until reaching the main collecting lymphatics that pump lymph to the sentinel lymph nodes. Valves ensure unidirectional flow. Transport of interstitial fluid into and along initial lymphatics is largely a passive process dependent upon changes in tissue (interstitial) pressure from movement (active and passive exercise), massage, and local arterial pulsation and—in more central tissues—breathing. The larger collecting lymphatics contract and are mainly responsible for pumping lymph against gravity. Successive segments of collecting lymphatics behave like 'mini hearts' in series, and their contractile cycle bears striking similarities to the cardiac cycle. Sympathetic input influences the pumping rate, while the diastolic filling (preload or supply from upstream lymphatics) controls the force of contraction. Flow in collecting lymphatics is only as good as the supply from initial (noncontractile) lymphatics. Influx of calcium ions is important for smooth muscle contraction in the walls of the collecting lymphatics, hence calcium channel blocking agents are likely to work at least in part on the lymphatic system in causing peripheral oedema.

The lymph vessels return the capillary filtrate back to the bloodstream via the lymph nodes and eventually the thoracic duct. This completes the extravascular circulation of fluid and protein and maintains tissue volume homeostasis. Lymph flow should respond to increases in capillary filtration and so prevent oedema. By failing to compensate for increased capillary filtration and so permitting swelling, the lymphatic is to some extent failing in its duty in all types of oedema. This could help explain differences in the degree of leg oedema seen in patients with right-sided heart failure. True lymphoedema is strictly oedema arising from reduced lymph transport that is unable to cope with normal levels of capillary filtration. Most oedema arises from increased capillary filtration overwhelming lymph transport capacity for a sustained period of time. Once high lymph flow cannot be sustained and transport capacity fails, 'true' lymphoedema ensues. This pathophysiology is comparable with that occurring in high-output cardiac failure.

Aetiology

Lymph drainage may fail either because of a defect intrinsic to the lymph conducting pathways (primary lymphoedema, Fig. 16.18.2a) or because of irreversible damage from some factor(s) originating from outside the lymphatic system (secondary lymphoedema, Fig. 16.18.2b).

Physiologically there are only a limited number of ways that lymphatics can fail. They may be reduced in number (aplasia/hypoplasia), obliterated or damaged without repair (failed lymphangiogenesis), obstructed, lose contractility (pump failure), or become incompetent (valvular reflux). A lack of sensitive methods for investigation makes it difficult to distinguish between these mechanisms.

Primary lymphoedema

A defining moment in lymphatic research came with the discovery of the receptor vascular endothelial growth factor receptor-3 (VEGFR-3) and its ligands VEGF-C and VEGF-D as the main signalling mechanism for lymphangiogenesis. Lymph sacs appear in humans at 6 to 7 weeks of gestation, with lymphatic endothelial cells arising from embryonic veins with the *PROX1* gene committing to a lymphatic lineage and *VEGFC* driving lymphatic capillary sprouting and migration. In mice, deletion of *Flt4* (= VEGFR-3) leads to defects in blood as well as lymphatic vessels and embryonic death, indicating an early role in both cardio- and lymphovascular function for this gene. Heterozygous missense point mutations leading to tyrosine-kinase inactivation have been found in *FLT4* in patients with congenital familial lymphoedema (Milroy's disease, OMIM 153100). The phenotype manifests with lymphoedema at or soon after birth, with swelling confined to one or both feet and ankles due to a reduction in functioning initial lymphatics.

The forkhead transcription factor FOXC2 is involved in the specification of the lymphatic capillary vs collecting lymphatic vessel phenotype. It is also important for the development and maintenance of lymphatic (and venous) valves. Heterozygous loss-of-function mutations in FOXC2 cause lymphoedema–distichiasis (LD, OMIM 153400), a dominantly inherited late-onset (postpubertal) lymphoedema associated with a double row of (ingrowing) eyelashes (distichiasis). Unlike Milroy's disease the lymphatic vasculature is well formed or even hyperplastic, but a defect in lymphatic valves results in lymph reflux. Swelling may not manifest until the fifth decade, indicating how genetic abnormalities can cause late-onset lymphoedema. The phenotype may possess congenital heart disease, emphasizing the close relationship between cardiovascular and lymphatic development.

Congenital lymphoedema may be sporadic and involve several limbs, genitalia, or even the face. A failure in lymphatic development may also manifest with internal lymphatic abnormalities such as pleural effusion, pulmonary or intestinal lymphangiectasia. Obstruction to intestinal lymph drainage may result in chylous reflux, with chyle re-routing to various parts of the body, e.g. chylous effusion or ascites. The fat as well as protein content of such fluids should be measured for diagnosis. Congenital lymphoedema may occur in isolation or as part of a syndrome, e.g. Turner's, Noonan's or Proteus. It is not unusual for lymphoedema to associate with hypertrophy of other tissues giving rise to increased limb girth or length.

For most forms of primary lymphoedema the genetic cause remains unknown. Swelling usually presents at or after puberty, particularly in females, and affects the distal leg. Familial forms in which lymphangiograms demonstrate a reduction in size and number of superficial lymphatic collecting vessels are called Meige's disease (OMIM 153200). Lymphoedema of the proximal obstructive type with unilateral whole-limb swelling is sporadic in type. Lymphangiograms of this form of lymphoedema demonstrate obstruction at the inguinal nodes, but no cause can be found. In such cases it is of the utmost importance to exclude tumour or iliac vein thrombosis.

Those cases of unilateral limb swelling associated with vascular abnormalities such as port wine stain and/or varicose veins are likely to be a form of Klippel–Trenaunay syndrome. The yellow nail syndrome, although given an OMIM number (153300), rarely has a family history and is of unknown cause.

Secondary lymphoedema

Filariasis is by far the most common cause of lymphoedema worldwide (filarial elephantiasis). It is endemic in eastern Asia, the Indian

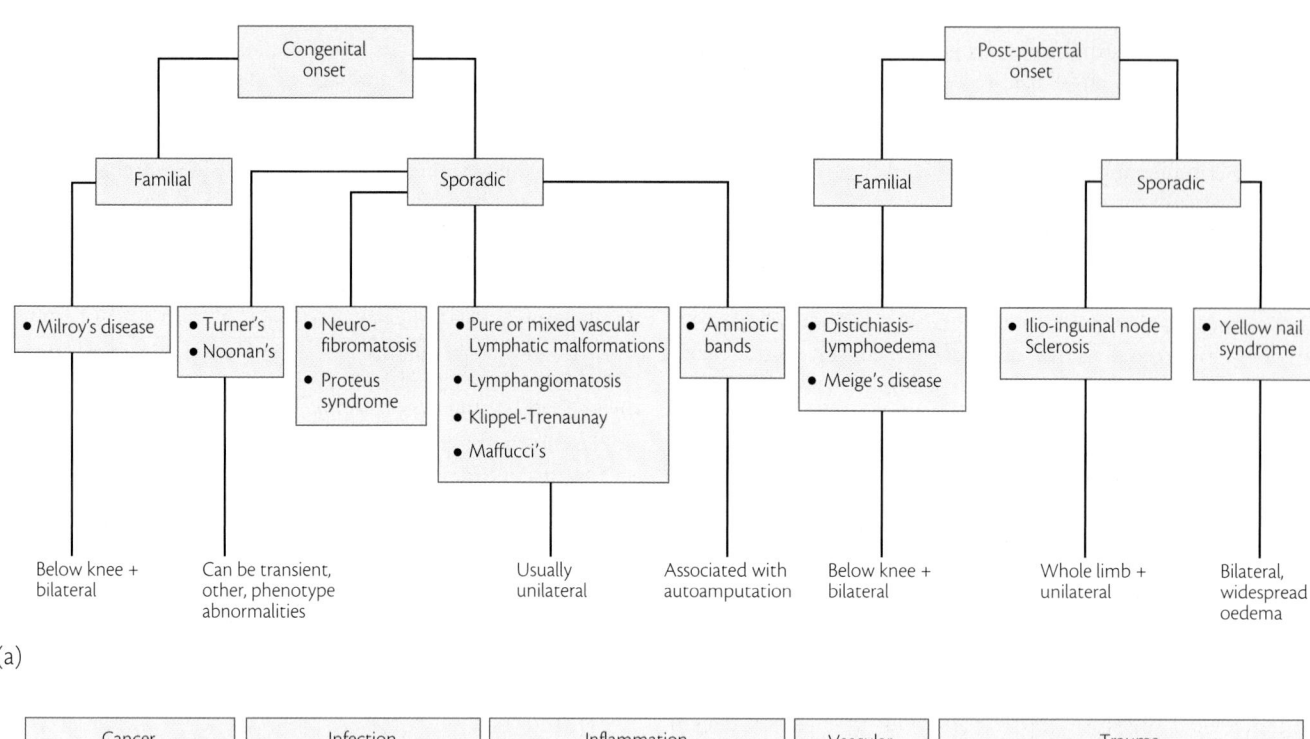

(a)

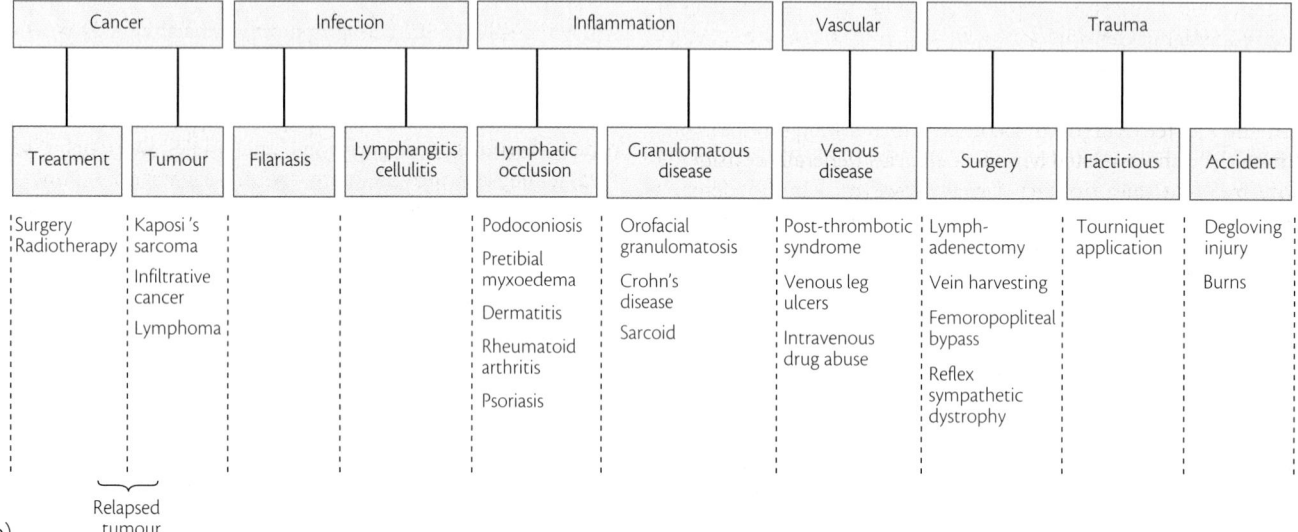

(b)

Fig. 16.18.2 (a) Causes of primary lymphoedema. (b) Causes of secondary lymphoedema.

subcontinent, west and east Africa, Brazil, and the Caribbean. Microfilaria introduced into the skin by mosquitoes migrate towards and enter initial lymphatics. Adult worms develop within the main collector vessels close to the nodes, resulting in lymphatic dilatation and lymphadenitis.

In developed countries surgical removal or irradiation (or both) of lymph nodes for cancer treatment results in lymphoedema. In breast-cancer-related lymphoedema the exact mechanisms for development are unclear, but a simple 'stopcock' obstruction in the axilla from scarring seems unlikely. Lymphoedema can develop in some patients after one (sentinel) node removal, but not in others who have had a complete auxiliary clearance. Nevertheless, in general the more extensive the damage to lymph-conducting pathways from elective surgery or accidental trauma, the more likely is permanent swelling to occur. It is probably the failure

of lymphatics to regrow or reconstitute functional channels (lymphangiogenesis) that represents the fundamental cause.

Cancer rarely presents with lymphoedema, except in advanced disease, but relapsed tumour frequently results in lymphoedema due to obstruction or infiltration of collateral lymphatic routes that have hitherto permitted escape of lymph. Kaposi's sarcoma is a neoplasm characterized by vascular plaques in skin such that lymphoedema can result. The condition is associated with infection by human herpesvirus 8. The transcriptional profile of Kaposi's sarcoma cells is closely related to normal lymphatic endothelial cells.

Lymphangitis or cellulitis probably only cause lymphoedema when the lymphatics are perilously vulnerable. Any patient suffering recurrent lymphangitis/cellulitis in the same region is likely to have impaired lymphatic function. Recurrent attacks of cellulitis frequently head to a stepwise deterioration in swelling.

Podoconiosis (endemic elephantiasis) is a form of endemic non-filarial lymphoedema caused by microparticles of silica that penetrate the feet during barefoot walking in soil containing silica and aliminosilicates in tropical west and east Africa, certain volcanic islands, and Central America (see Chapter 9.5.8).

Functional lymphoedema may develop as a result of immobility and dependency due to infirmity following stroke, severe arthritis, or respiratory disease, with long periods spent in a chair. It is probably the lack of exercise as much as increased weight that causes lymphoedema to develop with obesity and sleep apnoea syndrome.

Lymphoedema is a common consequence of post-thrombotic syndrome (following deep vein thrombosis) and severe long-standing venous reflux due to varicose veins. High filtration rates from the ambulatory venous hypertension slowly exhaust lymph drainage in a manner equivalent to high output cardiac failure. Irreversibly impaired lymph drainage eventually results. Lymphoedema can also result from long-term inflammatory states such as rheumatoid arthritis and chronic hand or foot dermatitis (with or without infection).

Epidemiology

An estimated 15 million people suffer from leg lymphoedema in filariasis-endemic areas of the world. Other lymphatic manifestations such as genital lymphoedema and hydrocoele are equally common.

In the United Kingdom secondary forms of lymphoedema, particularly cancer-related lymphoedema, are generally considered more frequent than primary forms. However, lymphoedema is more common than is usually recognized, and noncancer forms are commoner than those related to malignancy. A study investigating lymphoedema in south-west London ascertained a prevalence of 1.33 per 1000 population, rising to 1 in 200 over 65 years of age, and with three noncancer patients for every cancer patient identified. 29% of the cases had experienced cellulitis in the preceding year, with one-quarter of them requiring admission. Time off work was attributed to the lymphoedema in 80% of cases, with employment status affected in 9%. Quality of life suffered. with clear deficits in many domains of the well-validated SF-36 questionnaire.

In cancer practice the prevalence of lymphoedema following breast cancer treatment is approximately 25% lifetime risk, reducing to approximately 7% with sentinel node techniques. Other cancers such as gynaecological, prostate, head and neck, melanoma, testicular, and sarcoma have smaller numbers presenting with lymphoedema as a result of treatment or through progressive disease. One study of lower limb lymphoedema in gynaecological cancer identified an overall prevalence of 18%, but 47% following treatment for vulval cancer.

Prevention

Identification of patients at risk of lymphoedema relies on awareness of its causes. Nevertheless, as cancer-related lymphoedema epidemiology demonstrates, it is difficult to predict who will develop lymphoedema, particularly as there may be several years delay between causative event and onset of swelling. Known risk factors are genetic predisposition, infection (e.g. cellulitis), advanced venous disease, immobility, and obesity.

Clinical features

Lymphoedema is rarely considered at presentation and consequently diagnosis is usually delayed while other possible causes of swelling are investigated and excluded. Any chronic oedema, irrespective of cause, will mean some degree of lymphatic failure.

Lymphoedema most commonly affects the extremities, particularly the leg, although midline swelling affecting head and neck or genitalia can be an isolated finding. Truncal oedema is often observed in the adjoining quadrant of the trunk to an affected limb because of the shared lymph drainage route. Oedema that is symmetrical (equal between right and left legs) is more likely to have systemic origins, e.g. right-sided heart failure or hypoproteinaemia. Oedema that is asymmetrical (more in one leg than the other) implies a local cause, e.g. impaired venous or lymph drainage, but both systemic and local causes can coexist. In a patient with advanced cancer leg oedema may result from a combination of hypoproteinaemia (liver metastases), impaired lymph drainage (original lymphadenectomy and/or lymphatic infiltration by tumour), venous obstruction (deep vein thrombosis or vein compression by tumour), immobility, and dependency.

History

Swelling frequently develops rapidly—within a day—but may be mild and intermittent at first. Pain may feature initially, prompting diagnoses such as deep vein thrombosis, soft tissue injury, or infection (although cellulitis often triggers lymphoedema). With time, oedema becomes more permanent and painless, although discomfort, aching and heaviness are common symptoms. Functional impairment is slight until swelling becomes more severe (Fig. 16.18.3).

Lymphoedema does not respond to elevation or diuretics, except in the early stages or when it is compounded by increased capillary filtration. Chronic oedema that does not reduce significantly overnight is likely to be lymphatic in origin.

Clinical signs

It is often said that lymphoedema does not pit, but this is not true until the advanced stages of fibrosis (elephantiasis). To demonstrate pitting in lymphoedema sustained pressure for some 20 s may be necessary, owing to the firmer (and thicker) nature of the skin and subcutaneous tissues. The skin may double in thickness in lymphoedema, particularly at the base of the second toe, where it may be impossible to pinch up a fold of skin, which is called the (Kaposi–) Stemmer sign (Fig. 16.18.4, Table 16.18.1). Skin creases become enhanced and a warty texture (hyperkeratosis) develops.

Accumulation of lymph under pressure in dermal lymphatics can result in lymph blisters that bulge on the surface (lymphangiectasia) and weep lymph. When associated with dermal fibrosis the surface bulges are firmer and resemble cobblestones (papillomatosis). The resemblance of the skin texture to elephant hide explains the term elephantiasis. Intestinal lymph that is rerouted or refluxes into more dependent regions of the body will appear milky (chyle) due to its high fat content. Chyle may reflux into the lower limbs, genitalia, peritoneal cavity, urinary and genital tracts, pleural cavity, and other cavities such as synovial joints and pericardium. Chyle will only appear if the lymphatic incompetence extends up to the preaortic lymphatics and cisterna chyli.

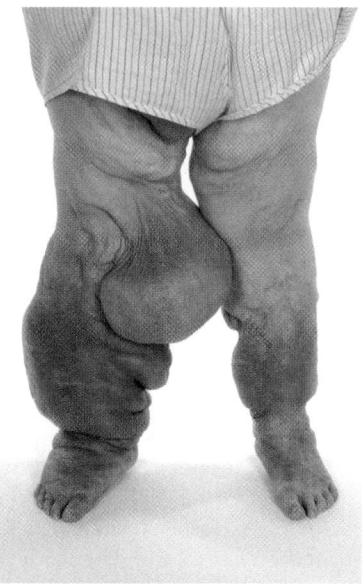

Fig. 16.18.3 Lymphoedema exhibiting characteristic skin changes (thickened skin with warty surface change and in more advanced cases 'cobblestone' papillomatosis) together with loss of shape and folds developing around the ankles.

Cellulitis

In addition to swelling, impaired lymph drainage also predisposes to infection because of the role the lymphatic system plays in immunosurveillance. Acute inflammatory episodes identical to cellulitis can often be recurrent and frequent. In filarial lymphoedema secondary bacterial infections appear to be important for the progression of the condition. 'Acute attacks' manifest with increased oedema, pain, fever, or flu-like symptoms and can be largely prevented with long-term penicillin and improvements in skin hygiene. In primary and cancer-related lymphoedema recurrent cellulitis can be an equally common and difficult problem to that seen in filariasis, suggesting that altered immunity associated with lymphoedema is the fundamental cause.

Differential diagnosis of the swollen limb

Both excessive capillary filtration and compromised lymph drainage frequently coexist (Fig. 16.18.5).

'Venous' oedema

Most cases of chronic venous disease giving rise to venous hypertension do not manifest with oedema because of increased lymph flow in response to increased capillary filtration. This suggests that the development of oedema in post-thrombotic syndrome and venous ulceration is as much a failure of lymph drainage to compensate as it is due solely to overwhelming filtration. Chronic 'congestion' in the lower leg resulting from both increased capillary filtration and impaired lymph drainage will often result in lipodermatosclerosis, usually seen just above the medial malleolus or anterior gaiter region (Fig. 16.18.6). The expansion of the venous pool in the leg due to dilatation of the veins will also contribute to an increase in limb girth.

'Armchair' legs (dependency syndrome)

This syndrome refers to those patients who sit in a chair day and night with their legs dependent. Immobility results in minimal

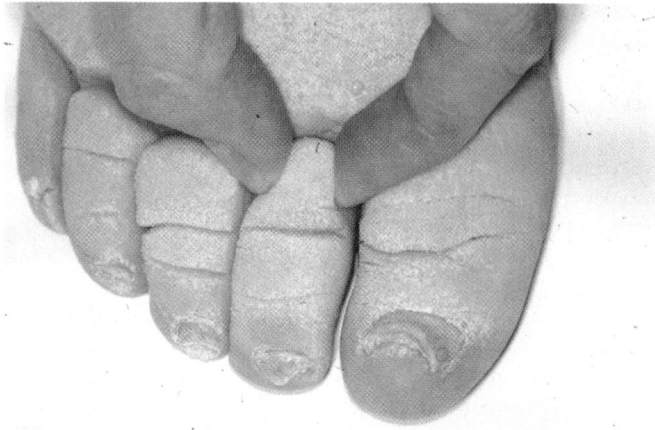

Fig. 16.18.4 Kaposi–Stemmer sign: the inability to pinch and pick up a fold of skin at the base of the second toe (due to thickened skin).

lymph drainage and 'functional lymphoedema' ensues, i.e. there is no stimulation of lymph drainage from movement, compounded by increased capillary filtration from gravitational forces. Predisposed are those suffering cardiac or respiratory failure who cannot lie flat, those paralysed from stroke or spinal damage including spina bifida, and those with crippling arthritis, particularly rheumatoid. An increasing problem is excessively obese individuals with or without obstructive sleep apnoea.

Lipoedema (lipodystrophy, lipohypertrophy, lipidosis)

Frequently misdiagnosed as lymphoedema, lipoedema is almost exclusive to females with onset at or after puberty. Lipoedema (lip = fat, oedema = swelling) results in excessive fat deposition below the waist (and sometimes upper arms), but not affecting the feet. A disproportionate large pear-shaped lower half with thick, heavy, chunky legs results (Fig. 16.18.7). The skin is soft, tender, and bruises easily. Pain may be a striking feature, Lipoedema is not influenced by dieting and is distinct from morbid obesity.

Clinical investigation

The investigation of choice for confirming that oedema is primarily of lymphatic origin is lymphoscintigraphy (isotope lymphography).

Table 16.18.1 Criteria for diagnosis of lymphoedema

Symptoms	Persistent swelling (can be intermittent at first)
	Oedema does not resolve with overnight elevation
	Poor response to diuretics
	Associated with cellulitis
Signs	Pitting oedema (but difficult to pit)
	Thickened, warty skin
	Kaposi–Stemmer sign
Investigation	Abnormal lymph drainage routes or impaired transport on lymphoscintigraphy

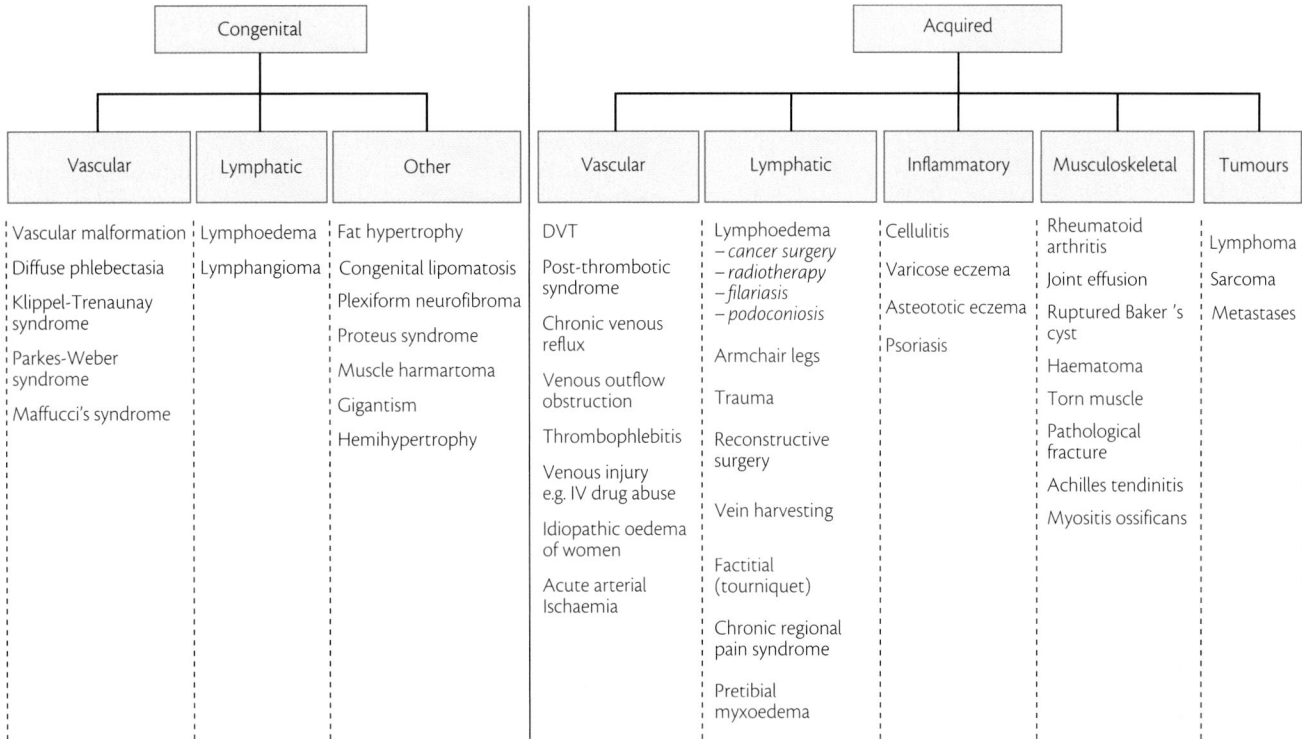

Fig. 16.18.5 Causes of a swollen limb.

Traditional direct-contrast radiographic lymphography is now rarely undertaken to investigate lymphoedema. MRI or CT is of value in identifying a cause for lymphatic obstruction, e.g. cancer.

Lymphoscintigraphy

A radiolabelled protein or colloid is administered via a subcutaneous or intradermal injection and its absorption and transport through lymphatic vessels to lymph nodes is imaged by gamma camera. Theoretically lymphoscintigraphy permits examination of lymph drainage from any site to which radiolabelled tracer can be administered, as has happened with sentinel node mapping for melanoma,

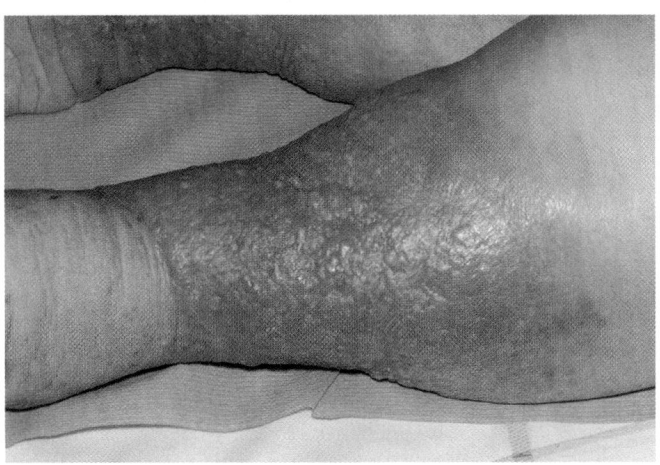

Fig. 16.18.6 Lipodermatosclerosis, a consequence of chronic congestion, manifests with fixed plum-red discolouration of skin, subcutaneous induration, and oedema—and is often mistaken for cellulitis.

breast, and genital cancer management. For the investigation of a swollen limb tracer is administered bilaterally into feet or hands. Lymph drainage routes can be crudely imaged and abnormalities identified (Fig. 16.18.8). Offline calculation of time–activity curves over regions of interest permit quantitative analysis of lymph drainage. Lymphoscintigraphy is very specific, i.e. there are few false positives, but only 90% sensitive and may miss lymphoedema.

MRI

MRI (or CT) demonstrates a thicker skin and a 'honeycomb' pattern in the swollen subcutaneous compartment of lymphoedema. Following deep vein thrombosis of the leg the subfascial muscle compartment is enlarged, but not so in lymphoedema. MRI and CT are more sensitive than ultrasonography for identifying enlarged lymph nodes or pathology responsible for lymphatic obstruction such as pelvic tumour, and to differentiate lipoedema (fat) from lymphoedema (fluid).

Colour Doppler duplex ultrasound

Venous disease (primary varicose veins or post-thrombotic syndrome) may cause or contribute to lower limb swelling. Venous duplex ultrasonography is helpful for identifying venous reflux. Iliac vein thrombosis or compression can be a cause of whole-leg swelling.

Gene testing

Gene testing for Milroy's disease (FLT4 mutations) and lymphoedema–distichiasis (FOXC2 mutations) is now available if the phenotype is appropriate.

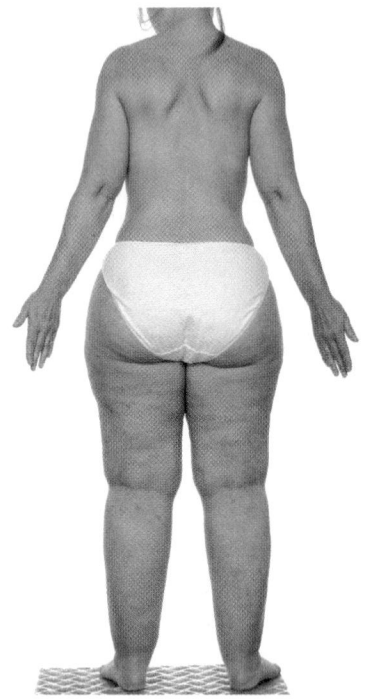

Fig. 16.18.7 Lipoedema—a condition almost exclusive to women resulting in excess subcutaneous fat on hips, buttocks, thighs, or legs giving rise to disproportionately large lower limbs and often mistaken for lymphoedema.

Treatment

Physical therapy

No drug or surgical therapy is known to improve lymph drainage. The treatment of lymphoedema relies on improving lymph drainage through the application of simple physiological principles known to stimulate lymph flow, while at the same time restoring any excessive capillary filtration to as near normal as possible. The principles of treatment are generic, but obviously vary according to individual circumstances dependent on site, e.g. facial vs leg lymphoedema, and cause, e.g. genetic lymphoedema in a child vs lymphoedema in advanced cancer.

Unlike blood flow, which is predominantly driven by the heart, lymph flow falls to low levels unless stimulated by movement and in particular exercise. Alternating changes in interstitial fluid pressure (by active or passive exercise or massage) increase initial lymphatic filling and flow within initial lymphatics. Increases in lymph load to collecting lymphatics will stimulate greater contractility within these main pumping vessels. Patients with leg lymphoedema often notice that walking reduces swelling. The addition of a bandage or stocking will enhance the effect of movement. The idea of compression is not to squeeze fluid out of the limb with force like squeezing toothpaste out of a tube, but to create an outer collar to the leg that resists expansion of the calf muscle during contraction. This generates a high interstitial pressure during muscle contractions to drive lymph filling and drainage, but allows low pressures during skeletal muscle relaxation and hence permits lymphatic vessel refilling before further muscle contraction repeats the cycle. Compression without movement (active or passive exercises) does not improve lymph drainage. Such treatment as provided by compression will be particularly helpful in circumstances where lymphatic collector contractility is impaired. It has the added benefit of lowering venous pressure in the leg, so reducing filtration.

Manual lymphatic drainage therapy (MLD), a specific form of lymphatic massage, operates on the same principle of stimulating alternating rises and falls in interstitial pressure and is used to decongest more proximal regions of the body, e.g. the adjoining quadrant of the trunk to a swollen limb, through which lymph from the limb needs to pass before being directed to a normally functioning lymphatic basin. In right-arm lymphoedema MLD would serve to direct collateral lymph drainage to normally draining lymph routes in the contralateral left axilla and so complement the effect of any compression and exercise to the right arm.

Fig. 16.18.8 Lymphoscintigraphy is the investigation of choice for determining if limb swelling is due to lymphoedema. Following a web space injection (hand or foot) of a radiolabelled colloid (^{99m}Tc–antimony sulphide colloid) the transport of radioactivity is imaged by gamma camera. Image abnormalities or a quantitative reduction in radioactivity in a region of interest within draining lymph nodes indicates lymphoedema. (a) Normal lymphoscintigraphy. (b) A patient with Milroy's disease and identified mutation in the *FLT4* gene giving rise to dysfunctional initial (absorbing) lymphatics in the feet. (c) A patient with lymphoedema–distichiasis due to mutation in the *FOXC2* gene that results in lymph reflux due to lymphatic valve failure.

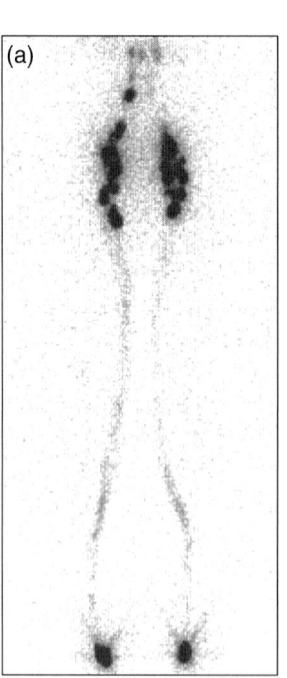

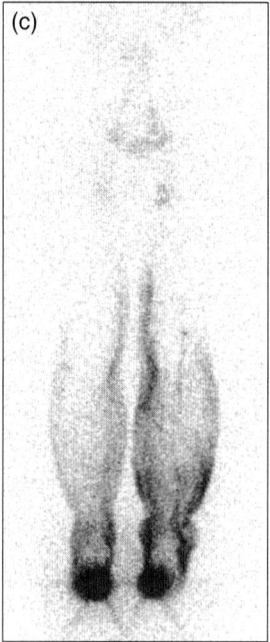

In moderate to severe lymphoedema treatment with an intensive course of MLD, multilayer lymphoedema bandaging and exercise can reverse more or less all the comorbidity from swelling, including 'elephantiasis' skin changes. Once swelling has been reduced and limb shape improved, control is maintained through exercise while wearing appropriately fitted compression hosiery. In elderly and infirm individuals the application and removal of hosiery can be problematic, but technique can be helped and aids to application provided.

Elevation of the legs is often wrongly chosen over exercise as treatment. Elevation helps oedema by lowering venous pressure and consequently reducing capillary pressure, not by improving lymph drainage. While exercise is preferred to elevation as treatment, elevation is recommended during periods of rest.

Pneumatic compression pumps probably displace fluid as much as improve lymph flow. Nevertheless, they may prove helpful for patients spending considerable time in chairs and in cases of oedema associated with high filtration.

Drug therapy

Too often diuretics are prescribed for oedema on an empirical basis without due thought for the underlying pathophysiology. Diuretics have very little effect in established lymphoedema because their main action is to reduce capillary filtration. They should only be prescribed in circumstances of salt and water retention, whereupon spironolactone may be preferred. Rutoside (a glycoside) has been advocated, but clinical effect is minimal.

Calcium channel blockers should be avoided in lymphoedema because they encourage oedema. The mechanism is unclear, but lymphatic pumping is paralysed in animal studies.

Prevention of infection

Prevention of cellulitis is crucial to the control of lymphoedema because it contributes to further decline in lymph drainage, which in turn encourages more infection. Care of the skin, good hygiene, treatment of any dermatitis or fungal infection, and antisepsis following minor wounds are important. Consensus recommendations for the treatment of cellulitis with lymphoedema are given in Table 16.18.2.

Surgery

Surgery can involve removal of excess tissue (reducing/debulking operations or liposuction) or bypassing of local lymphatic defects. Availability of centres offering microsurgical lymphovenous, lymphatic–lymphatic anastomoses remains limited. Surgery rarely if ever obviates the need for long-term compression hosiery.

Genital lymphoedema

Genital lymphoedema may arise from a genetic fault in lymphatic development, in which case internal lymph problems, e.g. intestinal lymphangiectasia, may coexist. Acquired forms may result from cancer treatment, infection (cellulitis), Crohn's disease, and hidradenitis suppurativa. Control of any inflammation is essential for control of oedema.

Facial lymphoedema

Impaired lymph drainage within skin and subcutaneous local lymphatics is likely to be a factor in cases of facial swelling, particularly periorbital oedema associated with rosacea, dermatomyositis, and thyroid disease.

Table 16.18.2 Treatment of cellulitis in lymphoedema[a]

Situation	First-line antibiotics	If allergic to penicillin	Second-line antibiotics	Comments
Acute infectious episode + septicaemia (inpatient admission)	Amoxicillin IV 2 g every 8 h or benzylpenicillin 1.2–2.4 g every 6 h + flucloxacillin 500 mg every 6 h	Clindamycin IV 600 mg q6 h	Clindamycin IV 600 mg every 6 h (if poor or no response by 48 h)	Switch to amoxicillin 500 mg every 8 h or clindamycin 300 mg every 6 h when: Temperature down for 48 h; Inflammation much resolved; Falling CRP; Then continue as below
Acute infectious episode (home care)	Amoxicillin 500 mg every 8 h[b]	Clarithromycin 500 mg every 12 h	If fails to resolve, convert to IV regimen as in row 1, column 2	Give for a minimum of 2 weeks; Continue antibiotics until the acute inflammation has completely resolved; this may take 1–2 months
Prophylaxis if 2+ acute infectious episodes per year	Phenoxymethylpenicillin 500 mg o.d. (1 g if weight >75 kg)	Erythromycin 250 mg o.d. or clarithromycin 250 mg o.d	Clindamycin 150 mg o.d. or clarithromycin 250 mg o.d.	After 1 year, halve the dose of phenoxymethylpenicillin; if an acute infectious episode develops after discontinuation, treat the acute episode and then commence lifelong prophylaxis
Emergency supply of antibiotics 'in case of need' (when away from home)	Amoxicillin 500 mg every 8 h	Clindamycin 300 mg every 6 h	If fails to resolve, or constitutional symptoms develop, convert to IV regimen as in row 1, column 2 above	

IV, intravenous; o.d., once daily.
[a] By mouth unless stated otherwise.
[b] If *Staphylococcus aureus* infection suspected (pus formation, crusted dermatitis), add flucloxacillin 500 mg every 6 h.
Adapted from Twycross RG, et al. (2007). *Palliative care formulary*, 3rd edition. palliativedrugs.com, Nottingham.

Further reading

Badger C, *et al.* (2004). Physical therapies for reducing and controlling lymphoedema of the limbs. *Cochrane Database Syst Rev*, **4**, CD 003141.

Badger C, *et al.* (2004). Antibiotics/anti inflammatory for reducing acute inflammatory episodes in lymphoedema of the limbs. *Cochrane Database Syst Rev*, **2**, CD 003143.

British Lymphology Society (2005). *Consensus document on the management of cellulitis in lymphoedema.* http://www.thebls.com/concensus.php

Brorson H (2000). Liposuction gives complete reduction of chronic large arm lymphoedema after breast cancer. *Acta Oncol*, **39**, 407–20.

Browse NL, Burnand KG, Mortimer PS (2003). *Diseases of the lymphatics.* Arnold, London.

Burnand KG, *et al.* (2002). Value of isotope lymphography in the diagnosis of lymphoedema of the leg. *Br J Surg*, **89**, 74–8.

Foldi M, Foldi E, Kubik S (2003). *Textbook of lymphology for physicians and lymphoedema therapists.* Urban & Fischer, San Francisco.

International Society of Lymphology (2003). Consensus document on the diagnosis and treatment of peripheral lymphoedema. *Lymphology*, **36**, 84–91.

Lymphoedema Framework Project (2006). *Best practice for the management of lymphoedema, international consensus.* Medical Educsation Partnership, London.

Moffatt C, *et al.* (2003). Lymphoedema: an underestimated health problem. *Q J Med*, **96**, 731–8. Available at: www.library.nhs.uk/Best practice for the management of lymphoedema: International consensus.

Mortimer PS, Levick JR (2004). Chronic peripheral oedema: the critical role of the lymphatic system. *Clin Med*, **4**, 4448–53.

Nutman TB (ed.) (2000). *Lymphatic filariasis.* Imperial College Press, London.

Tammela T, Alitalo K (2010). Lymphangiogenesis: Molecular mechanisms and future promise. *Cell*, **19**(140), 460–76.

Twycross RG, *et al.* (2007). *Palliative care formulary*, 3rd edition. palliativedrugs.com, Nottingham.

Zuther JE (2005). *Lymphedema management.* Thieme, New York.

Idiopathic oedema of women

John D. Firth

Essentials

Idiopathic oedema is an unsatisfactory label that is applied to women who complain of swelling, typically variable, with diagnosis requiring exclusion of known causes of oedema and (most authors would agree) demonstration of weight gain, from morning to evening, of more than 1.4 kg.

The cause of idiopathic oedema is (by definition) unknown, but the blood vessels of affected women are more permeable to albumin than normal. There is no clear relationship to the menstrual cycle.

Use and abuse of diuretics can complicate and exacerbate the problem.

Management is difficult, but patients can be helped by a sympathetic approach from the physician and (1) encouragement to lose weight if they are obese, (2) avoidance of excess dietary salt, (3) weaning from consumption of high doses of diuretics that can cause or exacerbate the tiredness, lethargy, weakness, and dizziness that are suffered by many.

Definition and diagnosis

In some women fluid retention occurs in the absence of any clear explanation and is termed idiopathic oedema. Since the condition typically fluctuates in severity from one time to another it is sometimes called cyclical or periodic oedema, but these terms mislead; first, because there is rarely any recognizable periodicity, and second, because the condition is not related to menstrual periods. Most women retain fluid just before the menses and lose this fluid immediately afterwards. Idiopathic oedema occurs most commonly in women aged 20 to 40 years, but has no clear relationship with the menstrual cycle and can persist after the menopause or oophorectomy.

The diagnosis of idiopathic oedema depends on the exclusion of other causes of oedema, including cardiac, hepatic, renal, allergic, or hypoproteinaemic disease, venous or lymphatic obstruction, and use of some medications. The role of diuretics, causally or in treatment, is contentious, as discussed below. However, it is always unsatisfactory when a diagnosis is made by exclusion of other conditions rather than on the basis of 'positive' criteria. Such criteria for the diagnosis of idiopathic oedema have not been universally agreed, although both Thorn and McKendry (see Kay *et al.* for discussion) have made proposals that (1) require evidence of substantial weight gain during the course of the day from morning to evening, with a figure of more than 1.4 kg often quoted, although this does not provide a clear-cut separation from normal, and (2) demand the presence of (loosely specified) emotional or psychological factors. Many authors comment on the aggravation of swelling by prolonged sitting or standing, but this does not feature in the diagnostic criteria mentioned.

Clinical features

The patient's complaint is of swelling, which usually waxes and wanes but can be constant. In the morning the face and eyelids feel swollen and heavy. By the end of the day the areas worst affected are the hands, breasts, trunk, abdomen, thighs, ankles, and feet. Rings no longer fit the swollen fingers, and undergarments and clothes can feel uncomfortably tight such that they have to be removed or replaced with something larger. The feet and ankles may be relatively spared, hence the disposition of oedema tends to be different from that in most other oedematous states, where it begins distally in the feet and ankles and progresses proximally.

Episodes or exacerbations of fluid retention often occur unpredictably, but obesity, emotional stress, and consumption of high-carbohydrate food are thought to be triggers in some. Sufferers are often mentally and physically lethargic during periods of fluid retention, frequently expressing the view that they feel bloated and ugly, even though this may not be apparent to the observer. Many appear to be emotionally labile or anxious and some are depressed, invariably (and perhaps correctly) claiming that this is secondary to the fluid retention. Other common symptoms include carpal tunnel syndrome, nonarticular rheumatism, palpitations, nonulcer dyspepsia, and headaches.

Aside from oedema, which may or may not be present at the time of medical assessment, examination is unremarkable, as are routine investigations for the cause of oedema. Those patients that have used diuretics may have a hypokalaemic hypochloraemic metabolic alkalosis.

Pathophysiology

The cause of idiopathic oedema is not known (by definition). Diurnal weight fluctuation of more than 1.4 kg is required for diagnosis, but weight may fluctuate from day to day by up to 4 or 5 kg. During periods of weight gain the patient may be oliguric, passing low volumes of urine in which there is little sodium (<20 mmol/litre).

The blood vessels of women with idiopathic oedema are more permeable to albumin, the fractional catabolic rate of albumin is increased, both intravascular and total body albumin pools are smaller, and the plasma volume decreases by more on standing than in normal controls. Activation of the sympathetic nervous system, renin–angiotensin–aldosterone system, and high levels of antidiuretic hormone (ADH) in the plasma that are consistent with intravascular volume depletion have all been reported, as has reduction in dopaminergic activity. These changes provide a plausible explanation for why the kidney retains salt and water in idiopathic oedema, but the prime mover remains uncertain. They also form the background to postural water-loading or sodium-loading tests that have been advocated as diagnostic tools, although these are not used routinely in clinical practice. After similar loading on two separate occasions, patients with idiopathic oedema who remain upright throughout the test excrete less water or sodium than they do if they remain supine.

Many patients seen in hospital practice will already be taking diuretics or have taken them in the past, and some will be consuming large doses of loop agents every day. One influential study reported 10 such patients who started to take diuretics because of concern about swelling or their body weight and who continued to take them because cessation provoked rapid weight gain, facial bloating, and abdominal distension. When prevailed upon to stop diuretics they each gained weight (up to 5 kg), reaching a maximum in 4 to 10 days, but by 20 days 7 of the 10 had fallen to below their previous weight, and 9 of the 10 remained free of oedema over a long period of follow-up without taking diuretics. This led the authors to suggest that diuretic abuse might be the cause of all cases of idiopathic oedema. This view is not held by most with experience in the field, but rebound oedema on diuretic withdrawal can undoubtedly be an exacerbating feature, and it is appropriate to look for evidence of diuretic abuse if the patient denies taking such drugs and yet routine biochemical testing of blood and urine suggests the possibility (see Chapter 21.2.2 for further discussion).

Management

Women with idiopathic oedema frequently complain that doctors have not taken their condition seriously, and there is no doubt that it is a frustrating disorder for both patients and their physicians. Sympathetic explanation of the nature of the problem helps management.

A patient who is obese should be given advice as to how to lose weight, and—independent of any effect on weight—some find that reducing dietary carbohydrate helps. They should be advised to avoid long periods of standing or sitting and to wear loose-fitting clothing, although most will have discovered these things for themselves. Avoidance of an excessive dietary intake of sodium is a sensible recommendation. On theoretical grounds the use of elastic stockings would also seem appropriate, since these might reduce the postural reduction in plasma volume seen in idiopathic oedema. However, few find that their benefits outweigh their disadvantages and it is difficult to get most patients to persist with them for long enough to see whether or not they really would be of help.

Diuretics are a real problem. It seems intuitively obvious to most patients and to many doctors that someone who is retaining fluid would benefit from a diuretic, hence many patients with idiopathic oedema end up on very large doses of loop agents, often combined with amiloride or spironolactone. Rather than helping, these may worsen symptoms of tiredness, lethargy, weakness, and dizziness by exacerbating intravascular volume depletion, and attempts to stop typically lead to rebound oedema. Explanation is the key here, in that if patients recognize rebound oedema for what it is and relieve oedema with supine rest rather than renewed consumption of high doses of diuretics, then there is a reasonable chance that they can be weaned off diuretics with benefit.

A range of agents including levodopa, carbidopa, bromocriptine, and captopril have been tried in idiopathic oedema. None is of proven benefit. There is a single report that aminaphtone (aminophenazone) produced improvement in 70% of cases in a small series, but this drug (formerly used as an antipyretic and analgesic, but which can cause leucocytopenia) is not widely available.

Further reading

Kay A, Davis CL (1999). Idiopathic edema. *Am J Kidney Dis*, **34**, 405–23.

MacGregor GA, et al. (1979). Is 'idiopathic' oedema idiopathic? *Lancet*, **i**, 397–400.

Marks AD (1983). Intermittent fluid retention in women. Is it idiopathic edema? *Postgrad Med*, **73**, 75–83.

Pereira de Godoy JM (2008). Aminaphtone in idiopathic cyclic oedema syndrome. *Phlebology*, **23**, 118–19.

Sabatini S (2001). Hormonal insights into the pathogenesis of cyclic idiopathic edema. *Semin Nephrol*, **21**, 244–50.

Streeten DH (1995). Idiopathic edema. Pathogenesis, clinical features, and treatment. *Endocrinol Metabol Clin North Am*, **24**, 531–47.

SECTION 17

Critical care medicine

17.1

Cardiac arrest

Jasmeet Soar, Jerry P. Nolan, and David A. Gabbott

Essentials

Cardiovascular disease is the most common cause of sudden cardiac arrest, which causes over 60% of adult coronary heart disease deaths. In Europe, the annual incidence of out-of-hospital cardiopulmonary arrests treated by emergency medical systems is 38 per 100 000.

Survival from cardiac arrest depends on a sequence of interventions—the Chain of Survival—comprising (1) early recognition and call for help, (2) early cardiopulmonary resuscitation (CPR), (3) early defibrillation, and (4) postresuscitation care. The division between basic life support and advanced life support (ALS) is arbitrary—the resuscitation process is a continuum.

Starting CPR

1 Check the patient for a response—and if they do not respond.

2 Turn the patient on their back, open the airway, and check for breathing and circulation—and if the patient has no signs of life, no pulse, or if there is any doubt.

3 Start CPR immediately.

Initial resuscitation

1 The compression to ventilation ratio is 30:2, with a chest compression rate of 100/min and depth for compression of 4 to 5 cm.

2 Use whatever equipment is available immediately for airway and ventilation.

3 Do continuous chest compressions with no pause for ventilations once the trachea is intubated—good quality chest compressions with minimal interruption for other procedures improves outcome.

4 When the defibrillator arrives, apply the electrodes to the patient and analyse the rhythm.

Advanced life support

Continue CPR and proceed to:

1 Treat shockable cardiac arrest rhythms (ventricular fibrillation/pulseless ventricular tachycardia—VF/VT) with attempted defibrillation.

2 Treat nonshockable rhythms (asystole and pulseless electrical activity, PEA) by treating the underlying cause.

3 Identify and treat reversible causes—hypoxia, hypovolaemia, electrolyte (hyperkalaemia, hypokalaemia, hypocalcaemia) or metabolic disorders (acidaemia), hypothermia, tension pneumothorax, tamponade, toxic substances, thromboembolism (pulmonary embolism or coronary thrombosis).

4 Minimizing interruptions to chest compressions will improve patient survival.

Postresuscitation care

The quality of postresuscitation care determines the patient's final outcome if resuscitation is successful. Consider therapeutic hypothermia and early percutaneous coronary intervention (PCI) in comatose survivors of cardiac arrest to improve neurological outcome and survival.

Do not attempt resuscitation (DNAR)

Do not attempt (cardiopulmonary) resuscitation decisions should be used to prevent CPR in patients who will not benefit from it or do not wish to have it. The most senior doctor available should enter a DNAR decision and the reasons for it in the medical records, the decision should be communicated effectively to all members of the team involved in the patient's care, and it should be reviewed regularly in the light of changes in the patient's condition.

Introduction

Survival from cardiac arrest depends on a sequence of interventions—the 'chain of survival' (Fig. 17.1.1)—all four links in the chain must be strong:

◆ Early recognition and call for help

◆ Early cardiopulmonary resuscitation (CPR)

◆ Early defibrillation

◆ Postresuscitation care

Historical perspective

Current CPR techniques were first described relatively recently: the first report of external defibrillation was in 1956, mouth-to-mouth ventilation in 1958, and chest compressions in 1960.

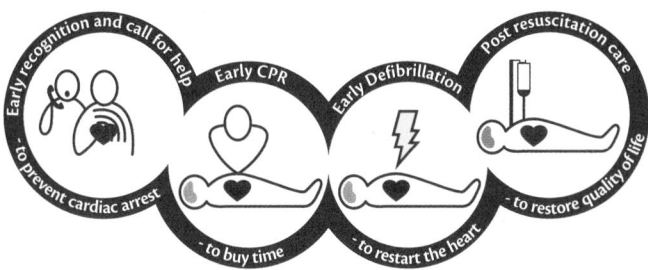

Fig. 17.1.1 The chain of survival.

Epidemiology

Sudden cardiac arrest causes over 60% of adult coronary heart disease deaths. In Europe, the annual incidence of out-of-hospital cardiopulmonary arrests treated by emergency medical services is 38 per 100 000, with the annual incidence of VF/VT arrest being 17 per 100 000. Survival to hospital discharge is 10.7% for all-rhythm and 21.2% for VF cardiac arrest.

One-third of those developing a myocardial infarction die before reaching hospital. Usually the presenting rhythm is VF/VT in 25% of cases. The initial treatment for VF/VT is attempted defibrillation—with each minute's delay without CPR the chances of a successful outcome decrease by 7 to 10%.

Factors influencing the incidence of in-hospital cardiac arrest include the criteria for hospital admission and use of do not attempt (cardiopulmonary) resuscitation (DNAR) orders. The incidence of primary cardiac arrest in hospital is 1.5 to 3.0/1000 admissions, with 15 to 20% survival to hospital discharge. In two-thirds of in-hospital cardiac arrests the first monitored rhythm is asystole or pulseless electrical activity (PEA).

Prevention

Out-of-hospital, recognition of the importance of chest pain enables victims or bystanders to call the emergency medical service who can initiate treatment that can prevent cardiac arrest. In-hospital cardiac arrests are usually not sudden or unpredictable: in about 80% there is deterioration in clinical signs during the preceding few hours. Hypoxia and hypotension are often unnoticed, or are recognized but not acted upon or treated poorly. The cardiac arrest rhythm is usually PEA or asystole and prognosis is poor. Earlier recognition and treatment can prevent some cardiac arrests, deaths, and unanticipated intensive care unit (ICU) admissions. Earlier recognition also enables decision making about DNAR orders.

Cardiopulmonary resuscitation

The division between basic life support and advanced life support (ALS) is arbitrary—the resuscitation process is a continuum. The keys steps are:

- Cardiorespiratory arrest is recognized immediately.
- Help is summoned.
- CPR (chest compressions and ventilations) is started immediately and, if indicated, defibrillation attempted as soon as possible (ideally, within 3 min of collapse).

The sequence of actions and outcome depends on:

- Location—out-of-hospital/in-hospital? Witnessed/unwitnessed? Monitored/unmonitored?
- Skills of the responders—in some public places (e.g. airports, railway stations) staff may be trained in CPR and defibrillation. Automated external defibrillator (AED) programmes with rapid response times in airports, on aircrafts, or in casinos, and studies using police officers have achieved survival rates as high as 49 to 74%. General practitioners and dental practitioners should have an AED on their premises.
- Number of responders—single responders must ensure that help is coming. If others are nearby, several actions can be undertaken simultaneously.
- Equipment available—AEDs are available in some public places. Staff working in hospitals usually have immediate access to resuscitation equipment and drugs.
- Response system to cardiac arrest and medical emergencies—outside hospital the emergency medical service should be summoned. In hospital, the resuscitation team can be a traditional cardiac arrest team (called when cardiac arrest is recognized). Alternatively, hospitals can have strategies to recognize patients at risk of cardiac arrest and summon a team (e.g. medical emergency team, rapid response team, or critical care outreach team) before cardiac arrest occurs.

Risks to the rescuer

There are few reports of harm to rescuers from doing CPR. Gloves should be worn: eye protection, aprons, and face masks may be necessary. A pocket mask with filter, or a barrier device with one-way valve, should be used to minimize risk during rescue breathing. However, the risk of infection is lower than perceived: there are reports of transmission of tuberculosis and severe acute respiratory syndrome (SARS), but HIV transmission has never been reported. It is sensible to wear full personal protective equipment when the victim has a serious infection (e.g. tuberculosis or SARS). Mouth-to-mouth ventilation should be avoided in hydrogen cyanide or hydrogen sulphide poisoning, as should contact with corrosive chemicals (e.g. strong acids, alkalis, paraquat) or substances (e.g. organophosphates) that are absorbed through the skin or respiratory tract.

Starting CPR

CPR should be started as shown in Box 17.1.1.

Cardiopulmonary resuscitation—mechanism of action

Chest compressions create blood flow by increasing intrathoracic pressure and compressing the heart directly. However, perfusion of the brain and myocardium is (at best) 25% of normal. The coronary perfusion pressure achieved during CPR correlates with return of spontaneous circulation (ROSC). In the presence of VF, chest compressions increase the likelihood that attempted defibrillation will be successful, and pauses in chest compressions of just 5 s before shock delivery almost halves the chances of successful defibrillation. Frequent interruptions in chest compressions reduce survival from cardiac arrest. Each time chest compressions are stopped the coronary perfusion pressure decreases rapidly, and on

Box 17.1.1 Starting CPR

1 Check the patient for a response

- If you see a patient collapse or apparently unconscious:
  - shout for help
  - assess responsiveness (shake their shoulders) and seek a verbal response

2 If the patient does not respond

- Agonal breathing (occasional gasps, slow, laboured, or noisy breathing) is common immediately after cardiac arrest—do not mistake this for a sign of life.
- Turn patient on to their back and open the airway.

3 Open airway, check breathing, and check for circulation

- Open the airway using a head tilt chin lift.
- Look in the mouth and remove any visible foreign body or debris.
- A patent airway takes priority over concerns about a potential cervical spine injury, but minimize neck movement if cervical spine injury is suspected.
- Keeping the airway open, look, listen, and feel (for up to 10 s) to determine if the patient is breathing normally (an occasional gasp, slow, laboured, or noisy breathing is not normal) and simultaneously feel for a carotid pulse.

4 If the patient has no signs of life, no pulse, or if there is any doubt, start CPR immediately

- Ensure help is coming.
- If alone, leave the patient to get help.
- Give 30 chest compressions (depth 4–5 cm, rate 100 compressions/min) followed by two ventilations (compression–ventilation ratio=30:2).

- The hand position for chest compression is the middle of the lower half of the sternum.
- Allow the chest to recoil completely after each compression.
- Take the same amount of time for compression and relaxation.
- Use whatever equipment is available immediately for airway and ventilation. Use a pocket mask (which can be supplemented with an oral airway), a laryngeal mask airway (LMA) and self-inflating bag, or bag mask. Attempt tracheal intubation only if trained and competent to do so.
- Use an inspiratory time of 1 s and enough volume to produce a normal chest rise. Add supplemental oxygen as soon as possible.
- Avoid rapid or forceful breaths to prevent gastric distension.
- Once the patient's trachea has been intubated, continue chest compressions uninterrupted at a rate of 100/min, and ventilate the lungs at approximately 10 breaths/min.
- If airway and ventilation equipment are unavailable, give mouth-to-mouth ventilation. If there are clinical reasons to avoid mouth-to-mouth contact, or you are unwilling or unable to do this, do chest compressions until help or airway equipment arrives.
- When the defibrillator arrives, apply the electrodes to the patient and analyse the rhythm. See ALS for further steps.
- Providing CPR is tiring—change the individual undertaking compressions every 2 min.

5 If the patient is not breathing and has a pulse (respiratory arrest)

- Ventilate the patient's lungs (as described above) and check for a circulation every 10 breaths (about every minute).
- If there are any doubts about the presence of a pulse, start chest compressions.

resuming chest compressions it takes time to build up to the coronary perfusion pressure present just before compressions were interrupted (Fig. 17.1.2).

Advanced life support (ALS)

The ALS algorithm enables a standardized approach to cardiac arrest management (Fig. 17.1.3). Once CPR has started, assess the patient's rhythm as soon as possible. Heart rhythms associated with cardiac arrest comprise:

- Shockable rhythms—VF/VT. In adults, the most common rhythm at the time of cardiac arrest is VF, which may be preceded by a period of VT, by a bradyarrhythmia, or less commonly by supraventricular tachycardia (SVT).
- Nonshockable rhythms—asystole and pulseless electrical activity (PEA). PEA is cardiac electrical activity in the absence of any palpable pulses.

Treatment of shockable rhythms (VF/VT)

Shockable rhythms should be treated as shown in Box 17.1.2.

During CPR

Resume chest compressions immediately after a shock. Even if a defibrillation attempt is successful in restoring a perfusing rhythm, it is rare for a pulse to be palpable immediately after defibrillation, and delay in trying to palpate a pulse will further compromise the myocardium if a perfusing rhythm has not been restored. If a perfusing rhythm has been restored, giving chest compressions does not increase the chance of VF recurring.

The vasopressor adrenaline is given to increase coronary perfusion pressure during CPR. A recent meta-analysis showed no statistically significant difference between vasopressin and adrenaline for ROSC, death within 24 h, or death before hospital discharge.

There is no evidence that giving any antiarrhythmic drug routinely during human cardiac arrest increases survival to hospital discharge. In the prehospital setting, the use of amiodarone (300 mg intravenously) in VF refractory to shock (three failed defibrillation attempts) improves the short-term outcome of survival to hospital admission in comparison with placebo and lidocaine.

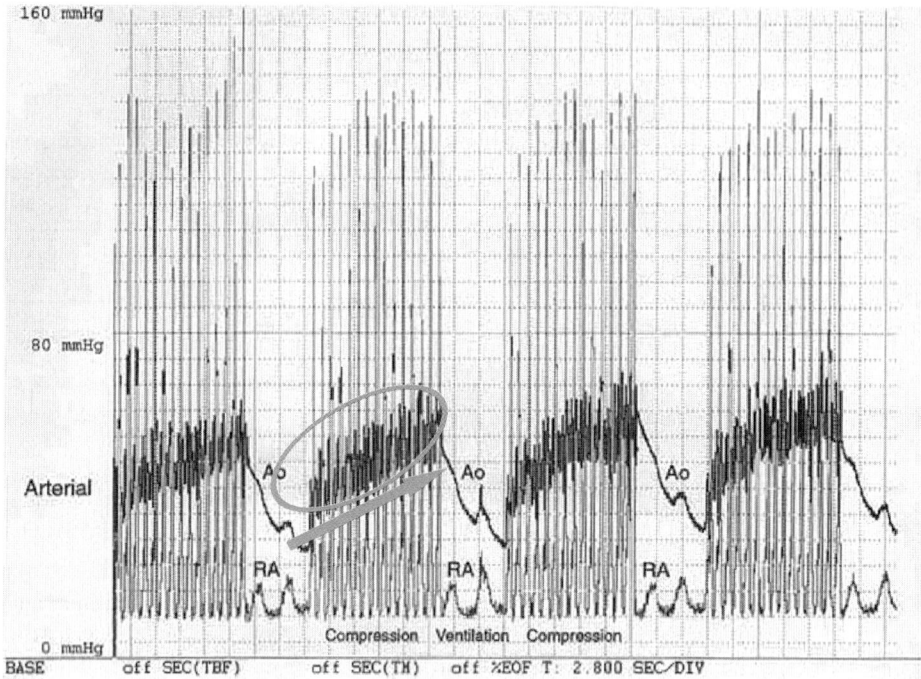

Fig. 17.1.2 Effect of chest compressions on coronary perfusion pressure. Coronary perfusion pressure (CPP) is determined by the difference between aortic diastolic pressure and right atrial pressure. The lower border of the dark band (marked by the orange ellipse) depicts the aortic diastolic pressure and thus CPP. This increases progressively as chest compressions are continued but decreases to base levels each time compressions are stopped. Note also that CPP continues to increase and does not plateau after 15 compressions. Uninterrupted chest compressions will generate a higher CPP.
Reproduced from Resuscitation, 39;3;10, Efficacy of chest compression-only BLS CPR in the presence of an occluded airway, Kern, Hilwig, Berg & Ewy, © 1998 with permission from BMJ Publishing Group Ltd.

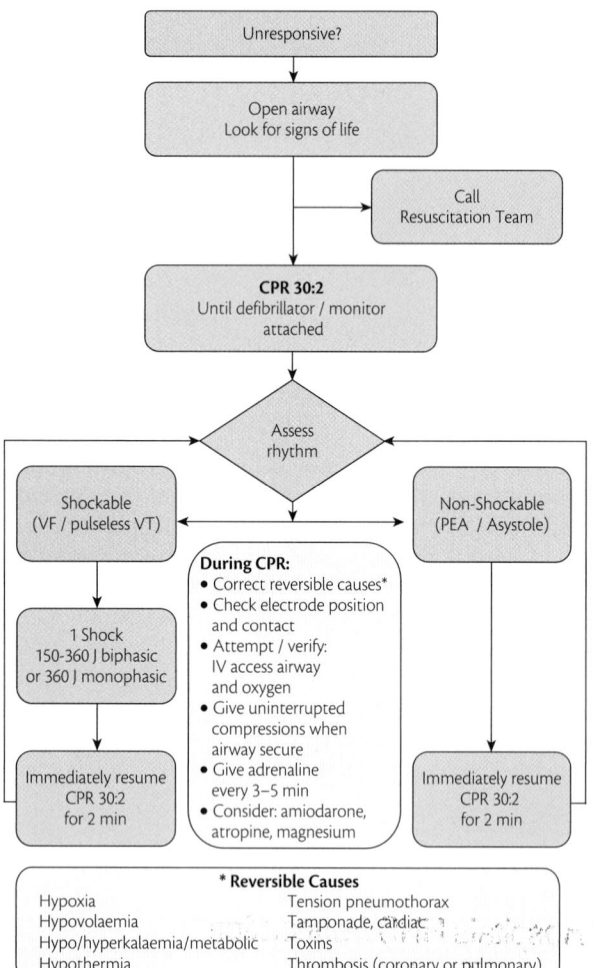

Fig. 17.1.3 The advanced life support algorithm.
Reproduced with permission of the Resuscitation Council (UK)

Monitored and witnessed cardiac arrest

If a patient has a monitored and witnessed cardiac arrest: confirm cardiac arrest and shout for help; consider a precordial thump if the rhythm is VF/VT and a defibrillator is not available for immediate delivery of a shock; if the initial rhythm is VF/VT and a defibrillator is available for immediate shock delivery, then give a shock, starting CPR immediately after the shock is delivered.

The precordial thump

The mechanical energy of a precordial thump is converted to electrical energy, which may be sufficient to achieve cardioversion. The electrical threshold of successful defibrillation increases rapidly after the onset of arrhythmia, and the amount of electrical energy generated falls below this threshold within seconds. A precordial thump is most likely to be successful in converting VT to sinus rhythm. Successful treatment of VF by precordial thump is much less likely unless the precordial thump is given within the first 10 s of VF (Fig. 17.1.4). Recent evidence suggests that the precordial thump rarely works.

Nonshockable rhythms (PEA and asystole)

Nonshockable rhythms should be treated as shown in Boxes 17.1.3 and 17.1.4, with care taken to identify and treat reversible causes of PEA and asystole during CPR, as described below.

Airway and ventilation

Tracheal intubation provides the most reliable airway during CPR, but should be attempted only by trained rescuers. Acceptable alternatives include the Combitube, laryngeal mask airway (LMA), ProSeal LMA, or Laryngeal Tube, which are supraglottic devices that can be inserted without the need for laryngoscopy. Compared with bag mask ventilation, early ventilation with a supraglottic device reduces the incidence of gastric distension and subsequent regurgitation, and enables more effective ventilation of the lungs of an unconscious patient. Continuous chest compressions should be performed without stopping for ventilations if such an alternative

Box 17.1.2 Treatment of shockable rhythms (VF/VT)

- Start CPR and assess rhythm to diagnose VF/VT: if using an old monophasic defibrillator, consider resuming chest compressions while charging the defibrillator (older equipment is slow to charge).

- Give one shock of 150 to 200 J biphasic (360 J monophasic).

- Immediately resume chest compressions (30:2) without reassessing the rhythm or feeling for a pulse.

- Continue CPR for 2 min, then pause briefly to check the monitor.

- If VF/VT persists:
  - Give a further (2nd) shock of 150 to 360 J biphasic (360 J monophasic).
  - Resume CPR immediately and continue for 2 min.
  - Pause briefly to check the monitor.

- If VF/VT persists:
  - Give adrenaline 1 mg intravenously followed immediately by a (3rd) shock of 150 to 360 J biphasic (360 J monophasic). Do not delay a shock to wait for adrenaline—if the adrenaline is not ready, give it after delivery of the shock.
  - Resume CPR immediately and continue for 2 min.
  - Pause briefly to check the monitor.

- If VF/VT persists:
  - Give amiodarone 300 mg intravenously followed immediately by a (4th) shock of 150 to 360 J biphasic (360 J monophasic).
  - Resume CPR immediately and continue for 2 min.
  - Give adrenaline 1 mg intravenously immediately before alternate shocks (i.e. approximately every 3–5 min).
  - Give further shocks after each 2 min period of CPR and after confirming that VF/VT persists.

- If organized electrical activity compatible with a cardiac output is seen, check for a pulse.

- If a pulse is present, start postresuscitation care.

- If no pulse is present, continue CPR and switch to the non-shockable algorithm (Boxes 17.1.3 and 17.1.4).
  - If asystole is seen, continue CPR and switch to the non-shockable algorithm (Boxes 17.1.3 and 17.1.4).

airway has been inserted, but if excessive gas leakage results in inadequate ventilation of the patient's lungs, then chest compressions should be interrupted to enable ventilation.

Drug delivery

Peak drug concentrations are higher and circulation times are shorter when drugs are injected into a central vein compared with a peripheral vein. However, insertion of a central venous catheter requires interruption of CPR and is associated with several potential complications: peripheral venous cannulation is quicker, easier, and safer. Flush drugs injected peripherally with at least 20 ml of fluid and elevate the extremity for 10 to 20 s to facilitate drug delivery to the central circulation. Consider the intraosseous or tracheal routes in adults when the intravenous route is impossible, the intraosseous route being more effective than the tracheal route.

Reversible causes

Reversible causes should be identified and treated during CPR in all cardiac arrests. These can be divided into two groups of four, based upon their initial letter—either H or T:

- Hypoxia
- Hypovolaemia
- Hyperkalaemia, hypokalaemia, hypocalcaemia (acidaemia and other metabolic disorders)
- Hypothermia
- Tension pneumothorax
- Tamponade
- Toxic substances
- Thromboembolism (pulmonary embolism or coronary thrombosis)

Defibrillation

Defibrillation is the passage of sufficient current across the myocardium to depolarize a critical mass of the cardiac muscle simultaneously, which enables the natural pacemaker tissue to resume control. Success is defined as termination of fibrillation or—more precisely—the absence of VF/VT at 5 s after shock delivery, although the ultimate goal is ROSC.

Factors affecting defibrillation success

Transthoracic impedance

In adults, impedance is normally 70 to 80 Ω, but in the presence of poor technique it may rise to 150 Ω, halving the current delivered and thereby reducing the chance of successful defibrillation. The factors influencing transthoracic impedance are listed in Table 17.1.1.

Electrode position

During defibrillation, transmyocardial current is likely to be maximal when electrodes are placed so that the part of the heart

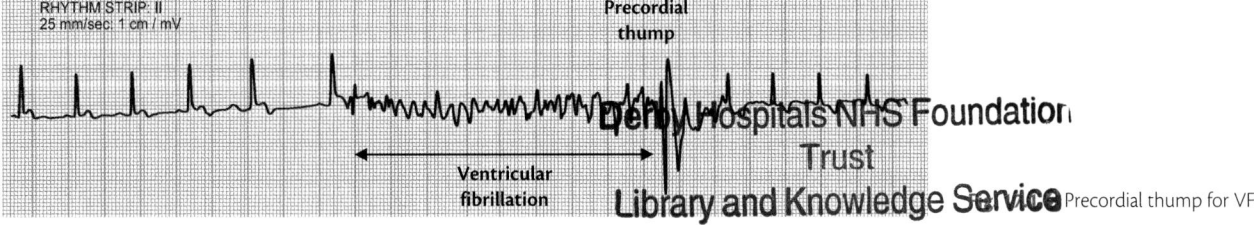

Precordial thump for VF.

Box 17.1.3 Treatment for PEA

- Start CPR 30:2.
- Give adrenaline 1 mg intravenously as soon as intravascular access is achieved.
- Continue CPR 30:2 until the airway is secured—then continue chest compressions without pausing during ventilation.
- Recheck the rhythm after 2 min:
  - If organized electrical activity is seen, check for a pulse and/or signs of life.
- If pulse and/or signs of life are present, start postresuscitation care.
- If no pulse and/or signs of life are present (PEA):
- Continue CPR.
- Recheck the rhythm after 2 min and proceed accordingly.
- Give further adrenaline 1 mg intravenously every 3 to 5 min (alternate loops).
  - If VF/VT at rhythm check, change to the shockable side of algorithm (Box 17.1.2).
  - If asystole or an agonal rhythm seen at rhythm check:
- Continue CPR.
- Recheck the rhythm after 2 min and proceed accordingly.
- Give further adrenaline 1 mg intravenously every 3 to 5 min (alternate loops).

---

that is fibrillating lies directly between them (i.e. ventricles in VF/VT, atria in AF). This means that the optimal electrode position may not be the same for ventricular and atrial arrhythmias.

Pads versus paddles

Self-adhesive defibrillation pads are safe, effective, and preferable to defibrillation paddles. When used for initial monitoring of a rhythm

---

Box 17.1.4 Treatment for asystole and slow PEA (rate <60/min)

- Start CPR 30:2.
- Check that the leads are attached correctly without stopping CPR.
- Give adrenaline 1 mg intravenously as soon as intravascular access is achieved.
- Give atropine 3 mg intravenously (once only)—this dose will provide maximum vagal blockade and blocks any excessive vagal discharge.
- Continue CPR 30:2 until the airway is secured, then continue chest compressions without pausing during ventilation.
- Recheck the rhythm after 2 min and proceed accordingly.
- If VF/VT occurs, change to the shockable rhythm algorithm (Box 17.1.2).
- Give adrenaline 1 mg intravenously every 3 to 5 min (alternate loops).

Table 17.1.1 Factors influencing transthoracic impedance

Chest hair	Hair increases impedance and can cause burns to the patient's chest
Electrode size	The total electrode area should be a minimum of 150 cm². Larger electrodes have lower impedance, but excessively large electrodes may result in less transmyocardial current flow
Coupling agents	If using manual paddles, gel pads are preferable to electrode pastes and gels because the latter can spread between the two paddles, creating the potential for a spark
Paddle force	Apply paddles firmly to the chest wall to reduce transthoracic impedance by improving electrical contact at the electrode–skin interface and reducing thoracic volume. The optimal force of application is 8 kg in an adult

and shock delivery, both pads and paddles enable quicker delivery of the first shock compared with attaching standard ECG electrodes. Pads make it easier to minimize interruption to chest compressions.

Shock energy and waveforms

There are currently two main types of waveforms used for defibrillation (Fig. 17.1.5): monophasic and biphasic (e.g. truncated exponential, rectilinear). The optimal defibrillation energy dose should achieve defibrillation and ROSC and minimize myocardial injury, and also reduce the need for repetitive shocks (which also limits myocardial injury). Although energy levels are selected for defibrillation, it is the transmyocardial current flow that actually achieves defibrillation, the optimal current for defibrillation using a monophasic waveform being in the range of 30 to 40 A, with indirect evidence suggesting 15 to 20 A using biphasic waveforms. Because they require less energy, biphasic devices have smaller capacitors and need less battery power, hence they are smaller, lighter, and more easily portable.

First-shock efficacy for long duration VF/VT is greater with biphasic (86–98%) than monophasic waveforms (54–91%), although a survival advantage has yet to be demonstrated. Some defibrillator manufacturers recommend escalating energy doses with successive shocks, while others favour fixed-energy dose shocks. There is currently no evidence supporting one strategy over the other.

Defibrillator safety

The operator must ensure that everyone is clear of the patient before delivering a shock, also that no oxygen is flowing across the chest. Oxygen masks should be moved to a distance greater than 1 m away, with tracheal tubes or supraglottic devices left connected to a breathing circuit or bag device. Safety checks should be rapid to ensure that the preshock pause is not prolonged.

Postresuscitation care

The quality of postresuscitation care significantly influences the patient's ultimate outcome. The airway, breathing, circulation, disability, and exposure (ABCDE) system approach should be applied.

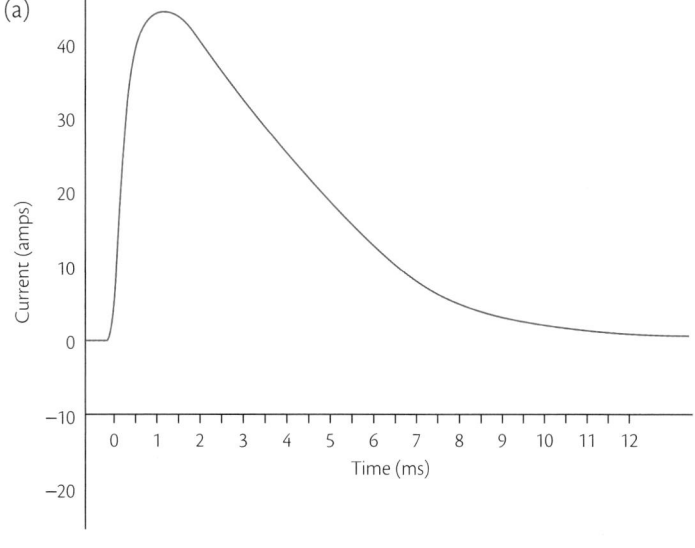

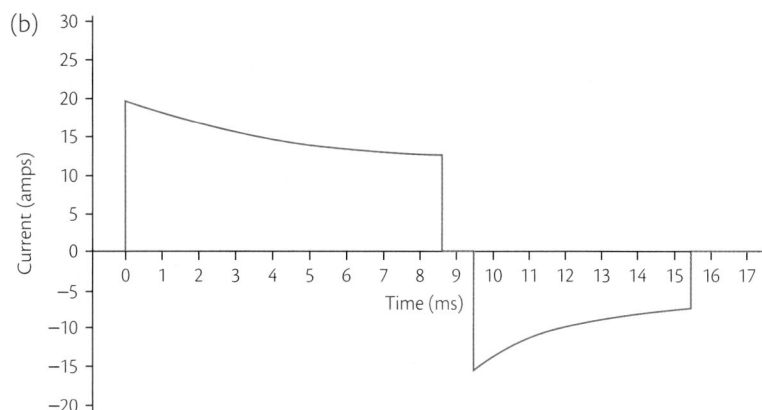

Fig. 17.1.5 Defibrillation waveforms: (a) monophasic waveform and (b) biphasic truncated exponential waveform.

Airway and breathing

Consider tracheal intubation, sedation and controlled ventilation in patients with obtunded cerebral function after ROSC. Hypocapnia induced by hyperventilation causes cerebral ischaemia after cardiac arrest. There are no data to support the targeting of a specific P_aCO_2 after resuscitation in this situation, but it is reasonable to adjust ventilation to achieve normocapnia and the inspired oxygen concentration to achieve adequate arterial oxygen saturation.

Circulation

Haemodynamic instability is common after cardiac arrest and manifests as hypotension, low cardiac output, and arrhythmia. This is partly caused by reperfusion injury and is usually transient, often reversing within 24 to 48 h. The postresuscitation period is associated with marked elevation in plasma cytokine concentrations and with a sepsis-like syndrome and multiple organ dysfunction.

A 12-lead ECG should be recorded as soon as possible. Acute S-T segment elevation or new left bundle branch block in a patient with a typical history of acute myocardial infarction is an indication for reperfusion therapy by thrombolysis or emergency percutaneous coronary intervention.

Disability and exposure

Cerebral perfusion

Immediately after ROSC there is a period of cerebral hyperaemia, but global cerebral blood flow decreases after 15 to 30 min of reperfusion and there is generalized hypoperfusion. Normal cerebral autoregulation is lost, leaving cerebral perfusion dependent on mean arterial pressure. Under these circumstances, hypotension will compromise cerebral blood flow severely and will compound any neurological injury, hence after ROSC the aim should be to maintain mean arterial pressure at the patient's usual level.

Control of seizures

Seizures and/or myoclonus occur in 5 to 15% of patients who achieve ROSC and in about 40% of those who remain comatose. Per se, they are not related significantly to outcome, but status epilepticus—and in particular status myoclonus—is a poor prognostic sign. Prolonged seizures can cause cerebral injury and should be controlled with benzodiazepines, phenytoin, propofol, or a barbiturate.

Temperature control
Treatment of hyperthermia

Hyperthermia is common in the first 48 h after cardiac arrest, and the risk of a poor neurological outcome increases for each degree of body temperature over 37°C. Any hyperthermia occurring in the first 72 h after cardiac arrest should be treated with antipyretics or active cooling.

Therapeutic hypothermia

Mild hypothermia suppresses many of the chemical reactions associated with reperfusion injury, including free radical production, excitatory amino acid release, and calcium shifts, which can in turn lead to mitochondrial damage and apoptosis (programmed cell death).

Unconscious adult patients with spontaneous circulation after out-of-hospital VF cardiac arrest should be cooled to a temperature of 32 to 34°C as soon as possible and maintained at this level for at least 12 to 24 h. Induced hypothermia might also benefit unconscious adult patients with spontaneous circulation after out-of-hospital cardiac arrest from a nonshockable rhythm, or cardiac arrest in hospital. The patient should be rewarmed slowly (0.25°C/h), with avoidance of hyperthermia, but the optimum target temperature, rate of cooling, duration of hypothermia, and rate of rewarming have yet to be determined.

Prediction of prognosis after cardiac arrest

Of 24 132 patients admitted to ICUs in the United Kingdom after cardiac arrest, 42.9% survived to leave intensive care and 28.6% survived to hospital discharge. Of those discharged from hospital, 80% return immediately to their normal residence.

Two-thirds of those dying after admission to ICU following out-of-hospital cardiac arrest do so from neurological injury, as do a quarter of those admitted following in-hospital cardiac arrest. A means of predicting neurological outcome that can be applied to individual patients immediately after ROSC would be extremely useful, but none is available.

Clinical tests

There are no neurological signs that can predict outcome in the first few hours after ROSC. By 3 days after the onset of coma relating to cardiac arrest, 50% of patients with no chance of ultimate recovery have died. The absence of pupillary light reflexes or an absent motor response to pain on day 3 are independently predictive of a poor outcome (death or vegetative state) with very high specificity. The use of therapeutic hypothermia influences the reliability of these clinical predictors and may mean that prognostication has to be delayed until 3 days after the return to normothermia.

Electrophysiological tests

Median nerve somatosensory evoked potentials in normothermic patients, comatose for at least 72 h after cardiac arrest, predict poor outcome with 100% specificity. Bilateral absence of the N20 component of the evoked potentials in comatose patients with coma of hypoxic-anoxic origin is uniformly fatal. A normal or a grossly abnormal EEG both predict outcome reliably, but an EEG between these extremes does not.

Other issues

Cardiac electrophysiological assessment

The possible requirement for an implantable cardioverter defibrillator (ICD) should be considered in any patient who has been resuscitated from cardiac arrest in a shockable rhythm outside the context of proven acute ST segment elevation myocardial infarction. All such patients should be referred before discharge from hospital for assessment by a cardiologist with expertise in heart rhythm disorders.

Audit and research

All CPR attempts should be audited to ensure that practice complies with published standards. Lack of uniformity in cardiac arrest reporting makes it difficult to evaluate the impact on survival of individual factors, such as new drugs or techniques. New interventions that improve survival rate only slightly are highly significant because cardiac arrest is common and kills thousands of people every year. However, individual hospitals or health care systems are unlikely to have sufficient patients to identify subtle effects or eliminate confounders, but by adopting uniform definitions and collecting standardized data on the process and outcome of CPR in many patients and systems it may be possible to identify relatively small but important changes in outcome. Changes in the resuscitation process could then be introduced and evaluated more widely.

The Utstein style template was established by consensus among a group of resuscitation experts and this standardized format should be followed when collecting data for audit or research.

Many countries are now establishing national cardiac arrest registries that collate data from individual hospitals, e.g. National CPR registry in the USA and National Cardiac Arrest Audit in the UK.

Decisions relating to cardiopulmonary resuscitation

It is essential to identify patients for whom cardiopulmonary arrest represents an anticipated terminal event and in whom CPR is inappropriate. All institutions should ensure that there is a clear and explicit resuscitation plan for all patients, and for some patients this will involve a DNAR decision. In the United Kingdom, national guidelines from the British Medical Association, Resuscitation Council (United Kingdom), and the Royal College of Nursing provide a framework for formulating local policy, and a written policy about resuscitation decisions should be available in all hospitals.

If a resuscitation plan has not been made and the wishes of the patient are unknown, resuscitation should be attempted when cardiac arrest occurs. Withholding of resuscitation should be considered in the following conditions:

- The patient's condition indicates that effective CPR is unlikely to be successful.
- CPR is not in accord with the recorded, sustained wishes of the patient who is mentally competent.
- CPR is not in accord with an applicable advance decision ('living will').
- Successful CPR is likely to be followed by a length and quality of life that is not in the best interests of the patient.

The most senior doctor available should enter a DNAR decision and the reasons for it in the medical records, the decision should be communicated effectively to all members of the team involved in the patient's care, and it should be reviewed regularly in the light of changes in the patient's condition.

Likely developments over the next few years

International CPR guidelines are updated every 5 years. Defibrillator technology is evolving rapidly, and many have several other functions as well as defibrillation. New defibrillators already have the ability to provide real-time feedback on depth and rate of chest compression, and on ventilation rate and volumes. In the near future, AEDs will be able to analyse the rhythm without interruption of chest compressions, which will enable continuous CPR with just a short pause for shock delivery. Analysis of VF waveforms will indicate when a shock is likely to achieve ROSC and will reduce the incidence of postshock asystole or PEA, thus minimizing the number of ineffective and potentially harmful shocks given to the patient.

Several mechanical chest compressing devices are available, but as yet none have been shown to improve long-term survival after cardiac arrest. It is likely that the efficiency of these devices will be improved.

The use of transthoracic echocardiography in the peri-arrest period to identify reversible causes of cardiac arrest will become more popular. This will require increased training in echocardiography and wider availability of echocardiography machines.

Hypothermia provides significant protection from ischaemia and hypoxia. The possibility of cooling patients rapidly just before cardiac arrest, e.g. during exsanguinating haemorrhage in the military setting, may enable the patient to be transported for definitive surgery in a state of 'suspended animation'. This technology has been applied successfully in animal models.

Further reading

Abella BS, et al. (2005). Quality of cardiopulmonary resuscitation during in-hospital cardiac arrest. *JAMA*, **293**, 305–310.

Atwood C, et al. (2005). Incidence of EMS-treated out-of hospital cardiac arrest in Europe. *Resuscitation*, **67**, 75–80.

Bernard SA, et al. (2002). Treatment of comatose survivors of out-of-hospital cardiac arrest with induced hypothermia. *N Engl J Med*, **346**, 557–563.

Cretikos M, et al. (2006). Guidelines for the uniform reporting of data for Medical Emergency Teams. *Resuscitation*, **68**, 11–25.

Cullinane M, et al. (2005). *An acute problem? National Confidential Enquiry into Patient Outcome and Death 2005 report.* http://www.ncepod.org.uk/2005report/.

Deakin CD, Nolan JP, European Resuscitation Council (2005). European Resuscitation Council Guidelines for Resuscitation 2005. Section 3: Electrical therapies: automated external defibrillators, defibrillation, cardioversion and pacing. *Resuscitation*, **67** Suppl 1, S25–37.

Decisions relating to cardiopulmonary resuscitation. Joint statement from the BMA, the Resuscitation Council (UK) and RCN (October 2007) www.resus.org.uk.

Edelson DP, et al. (2006). Effects of compression depth and pre-shock pauses predict defibrillation failure during cardiac arrest. *Resuscitation*, **71**(2), 137–45.

Gabbott D, et al. (2005). Cardiopulmonary resuscitation standards for clinical practice and training in the UK. *Resuscitation*, **64**, 13–19.

Hypothermia after Cardiac Arrest Study Group (2002). Mild therapeutic hypothermia to improve the neurological outcome after cardiac arrest. *N Engl J Med*, **346**, 549–56.

International Liaison Committee on Resuscitation (2005). Proceedings of the 2005 International Consensus on Cardiopulmonary Resuscitation and Emergency Cardiovascular Care Science with Treatment Recommendations. *Resuscitation*, **67**, 157–341.

Koster RW (2009). Precordial thump: Friend or enemy? *Resuscitation*, **80**(1), 2–3.

Langhelle A, et al. (2005). Recommended guidelines for reviewing, reporting, and conducting research on post-resuscitation care: the Utstein style. *Resuscitation*, **66**, 271–83.

Lloyd MS, et al. (2008). Hands-on defibrillation: an analysis of electrical current flow through rescuers in direct contact with patients during biphasic external defibrillation. *Circulation*, **117**, 2510–2514.

Nolan J, et al. (eds) (2006). *Advanced life support*, 5th edition. Resuscitation Council UK, London.

Nolan JP, et al. (2005). European Resuscitation Council guidelines for resuscitation 2005. Section 4. Adult advanced life support. *Resuscitation*, **67** Suppl 1, S39–86.

Nolan JP, et al. (2008). Post-cardiac arrest syndrome: epidemiology, pathophysiology, treatment, and prognostication. A Scientific Statement from the International Liaison Committee on Resuscitation; the American Heart Association Emergency Cardiovascular Care Committee; the Council on Cardiovascular Surgery and Anesthesia; the Council on Cardiopulmonary, Perioperative, and Critical Care; the Council on Clinical Cardiology; the Council on Stroke. *Resuscitation*, **79**(3), 350–79.

Nolan JP. Soar J (2008). Airway and ventilation techniques. *Curr Opin Crit Care*, **14**, 279–86.

Nolan JP. Soar J (2009). Defibrillation in clinical practice. *Curr Opin Crit Care*, **15**, 209–15.

Sandroni C, et al. (2007). In-hospital cardiac arrest: incidence, prognosis and possible measures to improve survival. *Intensive Care Med*, **33**, 237–245.

Soar J, et al. (2005). European Resuscitation Council guidelines for resuscitation 2005. Section 7. Cardiac arrest in special circumstances. *Resuscitation*, **67** Suppl 1, S135–170.

Soar J, Nolan JP (2008). Cardiopulmonary resuscitation for out of hospital cardiac arrest, Editorial. *BMJ*, **336**, 782–3.

Zandbergen EG, de Haan RJ, Hijdra A (2001). Systematic review of prediction of poor outcome in anoxic-ischaemic coma with biochemical markers of brain damage. *Intensive Care Med*, **27**, 1661–67.

17.2

Anaphylaxis

Anthony F.T. Brown

Essentials

The term anaphylaxis describes both IgE immune-mediated reactions and nonallergic, nonimmunologically triggered events. Comorbidities such as asthma or infection, exercise, alcohol, or stress and concurrent medications such as β-blockers and aspirin increase the risk known as 'summation anaphylaxis'.

Aetiology and pathogenesis—activated mast cells and basophils release preformed, granule-associated mediators and newly formed lipid mediators, and generate cytokines and chemokines. These cause vasodilatation, increased capillary permeability, and smooth muscle contraction, as well as attract new cells to the area. Positive feedback mechanisms amplify the reaction in a 'mast cell—leucocyte cytokine cascade', although conversely reactions can be self-limiting. Parenteral penicillins, hymenopteran stings, and food are the most common causes of IgE immune-mediated fatalities, with radiocontrast media, aspirin, and other nonsteroidal anti-inflammatory drugs most commonly responsible for nonallergic fatalities.

Diagnosis—anaphylaxis is a clinical diagnosis and is highly likely when any one of the following three criteria is fulfilled: (1) acute onset (minutes to hours) of an illness with involvement of the skin, mucosal tissues, or both, together with (a) respiratory compromise, or (b) hypotension/syncope/collapse; (2) two or more of the following that occur rapidly after exposure to a likely allergen for that patient: (a) involvement of the skin, mucosal tissues, or both, (b) respiratory compromise, (c) hypotension/syncope/collapse, or (d) persistent abdominal symptoms; (3) reduced blood pressure after exposure (minutes to hours) to a known allergen for that patient.

Clinical features—80 to 95% of patients with anaphylaxis have cutaneous manifestations, which assist prompt early diagnosis, but cutaneous or mucosal features alone do not constitute anaphylaxis. Deaths occur by hypoxia from upper airway asphyxia or severe bronchospasm or by profound shock from vasodilatation and extravascular fluid shift.

Management—if anaphylaxis is suspected, any potential causative agent, e.g. intravenous drug/infusion, should be stopped immediately. First-line treatment is with (1) oxygen—high flow; (2) adrenaline—0.01 mg/kg to a maximum of 0.5 mg (0.5 ml of 1:1000 adrenaline) given intramuscularly into the lateral thigh which acts to reverse all the features of anaphylaxis, as well as inhibiting further mediator release; (3) intravenous fluid—crystalloids (0.9% saline) at 10 to 20 ml/kg are essential in shock.

Other issues relating to immediate management—(1) Intravenous adrenaline is only ever needed if there is rapidly progressive vascular collapse with shock, imminent airway obstruction, or critical bronchospasm: it should be given as a dilute solution (0.5 mg diluted to 50 ml with 0.9% saline), slowly (0.5–1.5 ml/min), and titrated against clinical response. Nebulized adrenaline (5 mg, i.e. 5 ml of undiluted 1:1000 adrenaline) can be given while parenteral adrenaline is being prepared, particularly for upper airway oedema and bronchospasm. (2) The roles of H1 and H2 antihistamines, steroids, glucagon, and aminophylline are unclear: they should only be considered once cardiovascular stability has been achieved with first-line agents. (3) Patients must be observed for 4 to 6 h after full recovery before discharge from immediate medical care, when a clear plan for further management is essential.

Further management—(1) Referral to an immunologist is needed for all those who have had significant, recurrent, unavoidable, or unknown reactions. (2) Patient education is important for successful long-term care. (3) Self-injectable adrenaline should be given to patients with anaphylaxis after known allergen exposure outside of a medical setting, patients with food allergy (particularly to nuts or peanuts), and those in whom the reaction was severe and/or the cause unknown, including idiopathic anaphylaxis. Whoever takes responsibility for prescribing must explain and demonstrate exactly how to use the device provided, educating both the patient and another caregiver, particularly in children with anaphylaxis.

Introduction

The term anaphylaxis, literally meaning 'against protection', was introduced by Richet and Portier in 1902 (Fig. 17.2.1). It represents the most catastrophic of the immediate-type, generalized hypersensitivity reactions and remains the quintessential medical emergency. Anaphylaxis following exposure to a trigger can range from mild to severe, gradual in onset to fulminant, and may involve

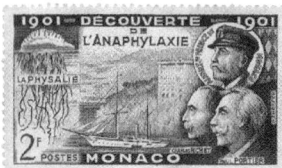

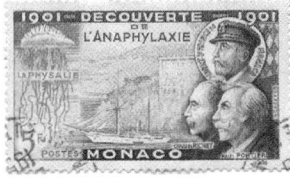 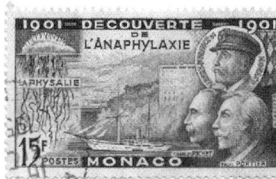

Fig. 17.2.1 The discovery of anaphylaxis in 1901. Stamps showing Charles Richet, Paul Portier, and Prince Albert of Monaco.

multiple organ systems or cause isolated shock or wheeze. It presents unheralded in otherwise healthy people, and mandates prompt clinical diagnosis based on pattern recognition and probability in the absence of any immediate confirmatory test. All clinicians and other health care workers must be familiar with the condition: urgent treatment can prevent death from hypoxia or hypotension.

Definition

There is still no agreement on the classification, diagnosis, or severity grading of anaphylaxis. The European Academy of Allergology and Clinical Immunology Nomenclature Review Committee proposed a broad definition in 2003 that 'Anaphylaxis is a severe, life-threatening, generalized or systemic hypersensitivity reaction' (Working Group of the Resuscitation Council (UK), 2008). Meanwhile, the National Institute of Allergy and Infectious Disease (NIAID) and the Food Allergy and Anaphylaxis Network (FAAN) in the United States of America convened international meetings in 2004 and 2005 that recommended a brief, broad definition as 'Anaphylaxis is a serious allergic reaction that is rapid in onset and may cause death', with the full definition agreeing on aims to capture more than 95% of clinical cases with three diagnostic criteria (see Box 17.2.1). Criterion 1 should identify at least 80% of anaphylaxis cases, even if the allergic status of the patient and potential cause of the reaction may be unknown, as most anaphylactic reactions include skin symptoms. Criterion 2 is anaphylaxis in the absence of cutaneous features such as in children with food allergy, or insect sting allergy, but requires a known allergic history and possible exposure: gastrointestinal symptoms are included. Criterion 3 captures the rare patient with an acute hypotensive episode after exposure to a known allergen. This inclusive definition for anaphylaxis should be used by researchers, unless refined by future prospective data.

Severity grading

There is no prospectively validated grading system linking the clinical features of anaphylaxis with its severity, urgency, treatment, or outcome. One system based on retrospective multivariate analysis of over 1000 clinically diagnosed generalized hypersensitivity reactions defined three grades (Table 17.2.1). Mild cases were generalized

---

Box 17.2.1 Definition of anaphylaxis: clinical criteria for diagnosis

Anaphylaxis is highly likely when any one of the following three criteria is fulfilled:

1. Acute onset of an illness (minutes to several hours) with involvement of the skin, mucosal tissue, or both (e.g. generalized hives, pruritus or flushing, swollen lips–tongue–uvula), and at least one of the following:
   - Respiratory compromise (e.g. dyspnoea, wheeze-bronchospasm, stridor, reduced PEF, hypoxaemia)
   - Reduced BP or associated symptoms of end organ dysfunction (e.g. hypotonia (collapse), syncope, incontinence)

2. Two or more of the following that occur rapidly (minutes to several hours) after exposure to a likely allergen for that patient:
   - Involvement of the skin–mucosal tissue (e.g. generalized hives, itch-flush, swollen lips–tongue–uvula)
   - Respiratory compromise (e.g. dyspnoea, wheeze-bronchospasm, stridor, reduced PEF, hypoxaemia)
   - Reduced BP or associated symptoms (e.g. hypotonia (collapse), syncope, incontinence)
   - Persistent gastrointestinal symptoms (e.g. crampy abdominal pain, vomiting)

3. Reduced BP after exposure (minutes to several hours) to known allergen for that patient:
   - Infants and children: low systolic BP (age specific) or >30% decrease in systolic BP[a]
   - Adults: systolic BP of <90 mmHg or >30% decrease from that person's baseline

BP, blood pressure; PEF, peak expiratory flow.
[a]Low systolic blood pressure for children is defined as <70 mmHg from 1 month to 1 year; <70 mmHg + (2 × age) from 1 to 10 years; and <90 mmHg from 11 to 17 years.
Reproduced from Journal of Allergy and Clinical Immunology, 117, Hugh A. Sampson et al, Second Symposium on the definition and management of anaphylaxis: Summary report - Second National Institute of Allergy and Infectious Disease/Food Allergy and Anaphylaxis Network symposium, 391–397, 2006 with permission from Elsevier.

---

allergic reactions confined to the skin and subcutaneous tissues, but moderate and severe grades with multisystem involvement correlated with the need for adrenaline and represent true anaphylaxis according to the NIAID/FAAN criteria. This grading system should again be used as a starting point by researchers for descriptive purposes, until future prospective data refine the criteria.

Aetiology

IgE-dependent activation of mast cells and basophils is the key trigger for most cases of antigen-induced, immune-mediated allergic anaphylaxis. An identical clinical syndrome known as nonallergic anaphylaxis (a term now preferred to anaphylactoid) follows non-immunological mechanisms, with the release of identical inflammatory mediators. Nonallergic anaphylaxis may occur on first exposure to an agent and does not require a period of sensitization.

Table 17.2.1 Severity grading system for generalized hypersensitivity reactions

Grade	Defined by
1. Mild[a] (skin and subcutaneous tissues only)	Generalized erythema, urticaria, periorbital oedema, or angioedema
2. Moderate[b] (features suggesting respiratory, cardiovascular, or gastrointestinal involvement)	Dyspnoea, stridor, wheeze, nausea, vomiting, dizziness (presyncope), diaphoresis, chest or throat tightness, or abdominal pain
3. Severe[b] (hypoxia, hypotension, or neurological compromise)	Cyanosis or SpO_2 ≤92% at any stage, hypotension (systolic blood pressure <90 mmHg in adults), confusion, collapse, loss of consciousness, or incontinence

[a] Mild reactions can be further subclassified into those with and without angioedema.
[b] Grades 2 and 3 constitute true anaphylaxis.
Reproduced from Journal of Allergy and Clinical Immunology, 114, Simon G. A. Brown, Clinical features and severity grading of anaphylaxis, 371–376. 2004, with permission from Elsevier.

Important clinical categories of anaphylaxis include anaphylaxis related to medications, biologicals, and vaccines, as well as insect stings, food, anaesthesia, latex exposure, exercise, and idiopathic anaphylaxis (see Table 17.2.2).

Table 17.2.2 Causes of anaphylaxis

IgE-dependent mechanisms	*Drugs, chemicals, and biological agents:* Penicillins, cephalosporins, sulphonamides, muscle relaxants, vaccines, insulin, thiamine, protamine, gamma globulin, antivenoms, formaldehyde, ethylene oxide, chlorhexidine, semen *Foods:* Peanuts, tree nuts, shellfish, finfish, milk, eggs, fruits, vegetables, flour *Hymenopteran sting venom, insect saliva, other venoms:* Bees, wasps, ants, hornets, ticks, triatomid bugs, snakes, scorpions, jellyfish *Latex* *Environmental:* Pollen, horse dander, hydatid cyst rupture
Non-IgE-dependent mechanisms	*Physical factors:* Exercise, cold, heat *Medications and biological agents:* Opiates, aspirin and NSAIDs, ACEI, vancomycin, radiocontrast media, N-acetylcysteine, fluorescein *Food additives:* Metabisulphite, tartrazine
Idiopathic/unknown	

ACEI, angiotensin converting-enzyme inhibitors; NSAIDs, nonsteroidal, anti-inflammatory drugs.
Note: Cross-reactivity occurs, and both IgE-dependent and non-IgE-dependent reactions may happen with the same agent. Several mechanisms may coexist such as exercise-induced following food.
Non-IgE-dependent mechanisms include complement activation, kinin production or potentiation, and direct mediator release.

Drug-induced anaphylaxis

Penicillin is the most common cause of drug-induced anaphylaxis, with around 1:500 patient courses having an apparent allergic reaction, mostly urticaria alone. True allergic cross-reactivity to cephalosporins occurs in under 4% of cases and is largely with the first-generation cephalosporins. Aspirin and nonsteroidal anti-inflammatory drugs (NSAID) are the next most common cause of drug-induced anaphylaxis. Reactions appear to be medication specific as there is no clinical cross-reactivity with structurally unrelated NSAIDs.

There are no valid tests for IgE-mediated reactions for most drugs or biological agents, with the exception of penicillins.

Insect sting anaphylaxis

Reactions to stings from bees, wasps, and ants of the order Hymenoptera are second only to drug-induced anaphylaxis and occur in up to 3% of the population. Reactions are often rapid and may be fatal within 30 min, mandating the early use of adrenaline, including by self-administration. Nonanaphylactic toxic, large local, or late serum sickness-like reactions also occur following a sting (see Chapter 9.2).

Food-induced anaphylaxis

This cause of anaphylaxis is most common in the young, particularly following the ingestion of peanuts, tree nuts such as walnuts and pecans, fish, shellfish, milk, and eggs. Cross-reactivity with other foods is unpredictable, or reactions may occur to additives such as carmine, metabisulphite, and tartrazine. Mislabelling and contamination during manufacturing or at home can lead to inadvertent exposure, and associated factors, such as exercise after food, must be recognized (see later).

Although fatalities are rare and usually associated with pre-existing asthma, biphasic reactions are seen as symptoms subside then recur several hours later. Patient and carer education is paramount, and schools in particular need to be prepared to respond with adrenaline in an emergency.

Anaesthesia-related anaphylaxis

The incidence of anaesthesia-related anaphylaxis ranges from 1:10 000 to 1:20 000 cases, with 4–10% of reported reactions being fatal. Neuromuscular blocking drugs (muscle relaxants), latex, antibiotics, and induction agents cause most cases of anaphylaxis, but opioids, colloids, blood products, radiocontrast dye, isosulphan or methylene blue, methyl methacrylate, chlorhexidine, and protamine may be responsible. Muscle relaxants cause 60% of reactions, with suxamethonium and rocuronium most commonly responsible. Reactions to suxamethonium and other relaxants occur in the absence of prior use: this suggests cross-reactivity and renders large-scale preoperative testing untenable.

Latex-induced anaphylaxis

The highest risk group for latex allergy includes health care workers, children with spina bifida and genitourinary abnormalities, and occupational exposure. Reactions follow direct contact, parenteral contamination, or aerosol transmission. Patients at known risk must be treated in a latex-free environment with glass syringes and nonlatex containing gloves, stethoscopes, breathing systems, blood pressure cuffs, intravenous tubing, and administration ports.

Exercise-induced anaphylaxis

Anaphylaxis can occur with a variety of physical activities. Up to 50% of cases are associated with the prior ingestion of a food, or follow aspirin or NSAID use. Prophylactic medication is not useful, unlike with exercise-induced asthma.

Idiopathic anaphylaxis

This is defined as anaphylaxis in which no discernible causative allergen or inciting physical factor can be identified: most cases occur in adults, but it is seen in children; diagnosis is by exclusion.

'Summation anaphylaxis'

Various comorbidities and concurrent medications increase the risk of anaphylaxis, giving rise to the concept of 'summation anaphylaxis'. These include asthma, intercurrent infection, psychological stress, exercise, alcohol, and drugs such as β-blockers, angiotensin-converting enzyme inhibitors, NSAIDs, and, to a lesser extent, angiotensin II blockers and α-blockers. Summation anaphylaxis may also explain an individual's unpredictable response to recurrent antigen exposure.

Pathophysiology

Mast cells and basophils release inflammatory mediators following binding of multivalent allergen that cross-links surface, high-affinity IgE Fc receptors (FcεRI), or from cell membrane perturbation. This is coupled with mobilization of calcium in the endoplasmic reticulum and leads to the release of preformed, granule-associated mediators by exocytosis, or the *de novo* synthesis of lipid mediators based on arachidonic acid metabolism, and the activation of genes for various cytokines and chemokines.

Mast cell and basophil inflammatory mediators

The preformed mediators released by mast cells and basophils include histamine, proteases such as tryptase, chymase, and carboxypeptidase A, and proteoglycans such as heparin and chondroitin sulphate E. Newly synthesized lipid mediators include prostaglandin D_2 and thromboxane A2 via the cyclo-oxygenase pathway, and the leukotrienes LTC4, LTD4, and LTE4 via the lipoxygenase pathway. The cytokines released include TNF-α, various interleukins such as IL-3, IL-4, IL-5, IL-6, IL-8, IL-13, and IL-16, and granulocyte-macrophage colony-stimulating factor (GM-CSF). The chemokines include platelet activating factor, neutrophil chemotactic factor, and eosinophil chemotactic factor, plus macrophage inflammatory protein-1α.

Mediator actions

Mediators act to induce vasodilatation, increase capillary permeability and glandular secretion, cause smooth muscle spasm—particularly bronchoconstriction—and to attract new cells such as eosinophils, leucocytes, and platelets to the area. Positive feedback mechanisms amplify and perpetuate reactions to recruit further effector cells to release increasing amounts of mediators in a 'mast cell–leucocyte cytokine cascade' effect. By contrast, other anaphylactic reactions self-limit, with spontaneous recovery related to endogenous compensatory mechanisms including increased secretion of adrenaline, angiotensin II and endothelin I.

Epidemiology

The true incidence of anaphylaxis is unknown. Data—which are unreliable with lack of a standard definition—are almost exclusively in the form of diverse, retrospective case collections from the emergency department, anaesthetic department, or the allergist/immunologist's office. Under-reporting is common due to missed diagnoses, or following spontaneous recovery, prehospital treatment, or fatality. However, all the data from western countries show the incidence of anaphylaxis is increasing.

Emergency department anaphylaxis

Between 1:439 and 1:1100 presentations of adults to the emergency department are with anaphylaxis, representing up to one adult presentation per 3400 population per year. Anaphylaxis is the cause of about 1:1000 of paediatric emergency department presentations, although generalized allergic reactions in children (without multisystem involvement) are almost 10 times more common than this.

A causative agent is found in 75% of cases of anaphylaxis presenting to the emergency department, recognized from a prior reaction or by close temporal association with the onset of symptoms. The most frequent in childhood are food-induced or drug-related, whereas in adults drug-related and hymenopteran stings predominate. Respiratory features appear more common in paediatric anaphylaxis and cardiovascular features in adults.

Fatal anaphylaxis

Fatalities are rare: less than one per million population per year. When they do happen, fatal reactions are rapid, with a median time to cardiorespiratory arrest of just 5 min if iatrogenic, 15 min for venom, and 30 min following foods. Adrenaline is given in only 14% cases prior to arrest, and not at all in 38% of fatalities.

Deaths follow hypoxia in upper airway swelling with asphyxia, bronchospasm, and mucus plugging, and/or shock related to vasodilatation, extravascular fluid shift, and direct myocardial depression. Tachycardia is usual in shock, but bradycardia related to a neurocardiogenic, vagally mediated mechanism (Bezold–Jarisch reflex) has occasionally been observed.

Clinical features

Anaphylaxis characteristically affects fit people and is rarely seen or described in critically ill or shocked patients, other than asthmatics. The speed of onset relates to the mechanism of exposure and the severity of the reaction. Parenteral antigen exposure may cause life-threatening anaphylaxis within minutes, whereas symptoms can be delayed for some hours following oral or topical exposure.

Between 80 and 95% of patients with anaphylaxis have cutaneous features, which assist prompt early diagnosis. However, alerting cutaneous features may be absent because of prehospital treatment or their spontaneous resolution, be subtle clinically and missed, or the onset of other life-threatening complications such as laryngeal oedema or shock may precede them. Cutaneous or mucosal changes alone do not constitute anaphylaxis, the hallmark of anaphylaxis being the precipitate onset of respiratory, cardiovascular, gastrointestinal, and/or neurological dysfunction (see Table 17.2.3).

Table 17.2.3 Clinical features of anaphylaxis

Cutaneous	Tingling or warmth, erythema (flushing), urticaria, pruritus (itch), angioedema
	Rhinorrhoea, conjunctival injection, lacrimation
Respiratory	Throat tightness, cough, dyspnoea, hoarseness, stridor, aphonia
	Tachypnoea, wheeze, SaO$_2$ ≤92%[a], cyanosis[a]
Cardiovascular and neurological	Tachycardia (rarely bradycardia), hypotension[a], arrhythmias, cardiac arrest[a]
	Light-headedness, sweating, incontinence[a], syncope[a], confusion[a], coma[a]
Gastrointestinal	Odynophagia (difficult or painful swallowing), abdominal cramps, nausea, vomiting, diarrhoea
Nonspecific	Premonitory aura, anxiety, feeling of impending doom
	Pelvic cramps

SaO$_2$, oxygen saturation (on pulse oximetry).
[a] Indicates severe reaction. (See Table 17.2.1).

Cutaneous and general reactions

A premonitory aura, tingling or warm sensation, anxiety, and feeling of impending doom precede generalized erythema, urticaria with pruritus, and angioedema of the neck, face, lips, and tongue (Fig. 17.2.2). Rhinorrhoea, conjunctival injection, and tearing are seen.

Respiratory manifestations

Throat tightness and cough precede mild to critical respiratory distress due to oropharyngeal or laryngeal oedema with dyspnoea, hoarseness, stridor, and even aphonia; or related to bronchospasm

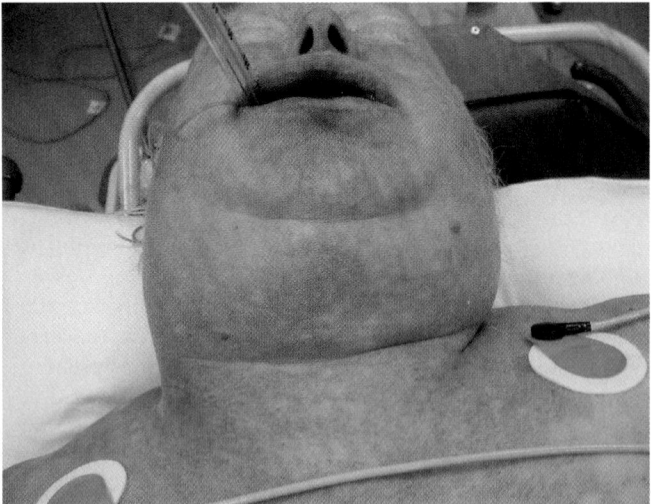

Fig. 17.2.2 Massive facial and body oedema with cardiovascular collapse in rapid sequence induction-related anaphylaxis, within 2 min of intravenous drug bolus. Picture reproduced with permission.

with tachypnoea and wheeze. Hypoxia with oxygen saturation less than 92% on pulse oximetry and central cyanosis indicate severe anaphylaxis and the need for immediate treatment (see severity grading in Table 17.2.1).

Cardiovascular and neurological manifestations

Light-headedness, sweating, syncope, incontinence, or coma may precede or accompany cardiovascular collapse with tachycardia, hypotension, and cardiac arrhythmias. These may appear to be benign supraventricular rhythms, particularly in children, but with an impalpable pulse.

Gastrointestinal manifestations

Difficult or painful swallowing, nausea, vomiting, diarrhoea with soiling, and abdominal cramps may be associated with a severe reaction, but are usually overshadowed by more immediately life-threatening features.

Differential diagnosis

The protean manifestations of anaphylaxis have a potentially vast differential diagnosis, although the rapidity of onset, accompanying cutaneous features, and relationship to a likely or known potential trigger suggest the diagnosis in most cases, but the following may need to be considered.

Wheeze and difficulty breathing—bronchial asthma, cardiogenic pulmonary oedema, foreign body inhalation, irritant chemical exposure, and tension pneumothorax are distinguished by the history, comorbidity, and associated presenting features.

Light-headedness and syncope—an anxiety or vasovagal reaction need to be considered when there is a history of fearing an actual reaction, or in the context of a painful procedure such as an injection or local anaesthetic infiltration. Bradycardia, sweating and pallor without urticaria, erythema or itch, associated with a brief prodrome and rapid response to the recumbent position favour the diagnosis of a vasovagal reaction.

Facial swelling or angioedema—bacterial or viral infections usually cause fever and/or pain, and traumatic or anticoagulant-related bleeding causes recognizable bruising. Angioedema in the absence of urticaria or pruritus can be caused by actual or functional C1 esterase inhibitor deficiency, which may be hereditary (autosomal dominant, associated with prominent abdominal symptoms and recurrent attacks related to minor stress) or acquired (lymphoproliferative and some connective tissue disorders). Measurement of serum C4 is a rapid and inexpensive screening test, followed by the more specific C1 esterase inhibitor assay to confirm the diagnosis if the C4 is low. Management is with C1 esterase inhibitor concentrate (or fresh frozen plasma if this is not available) in a serious attack.

Flushing—scombroid poisoning following ingestion of spoiled fish, carcinoid syndrome, and alcohol-induced and systemic mastocytosis all produce flushing and require differentiation by a careful history and investigation.

Other forms of shock—hypovolaemic, septic, and cardiogenic shock, tension pneumothorax, and other forms of shock should all be apparent from the history and examination. These are commonly associated with tachypnoea, but not with the other cutaneous and respiratory features of anaphylaxis.

Clinical investigation

The diagnosis of anaphylaxis is clinical: no immediate laboratory or radiological test confirms the process, and these must never delay immediate management.

Disease progress may be monitored by pulse oximetry, haematocrit level (may rise with fluid extravasation), and arterial blood gases (looking for respiratory or metabolic acidosis). Measurement of electrolytes and renal function, blood glucose, chest radiography, and ECG are indicated if there is a slow response to treatment, or when there is doubt about the diagnosis.

Mast cell tryptase and histamine

Despite initial promise, mast cell tryptase in blood taken from 1 to 6 h after a suspected episode cannot be totally relied upon to diagnose anaphylaxis. It is not elevated consistently, particularly following food allergy, and it may be elevated post-mortem in non-anaphylactic deaths. However, measuring serial levels, or specific allelic subtypes such as mature β tryptase, may improve diagnostic value. When possible, three samples should be taken: one immediately following resuscitation; the next 1 to 2 h after symptoms onset; the last at 24 h or during convalescence to establish the patient's baseline tryptase level.

Histamine levels are impractical to measure as they are unstable and evanescent, only remaining elevated for 30 to 60 min maximum.

IgE skin testing, *in vitro* testing, and challenge testing

Skin or blood tests for specific IgE antibodies must be done by those trained in their performance and interpretation. Skin prick testing is the more sensitive: standardized extracts should be used with correct technique, supervised by an experienced physician in case of the occasional severe reaction. *In vitro* testing

for allergen-specific IgE is less sensitive and depends on clinical correlation and the availability of specific assays. Over 500 different allergens are available for testing with the ImmunoCAP system, or clinicians may use a radioallergosorbent (RAST) test.

Challenge testing may be particularly useful in the diagnosis of nonallergic anaphylaxis: false positive and false negative reactions do occur, but are much less likely than with skin prick or *in vitro* testing; supervision by an experienced physician is essential.

Immediate treatment

A patient with anaphylaxis may present directly to his or her family doctor, or the emergency department, or the reaction may happen in hospital on a ward, in the operating theatre, the radiology department, and even in outpatients. Make certain that an ambulance is called at an early stage for all out-of-hospital anaphylactic reactions.

Stop any potential causative agent such as an intravenous drug or infusion immediately. Manage the patient in a monitored resuscitation area, or bring equipment including at least a pulse oximeter, a noninvasive blood pressure device, and an ECG monitor to them.

Obtain a brief history of possible allergen exposure and perform a rapid assessment of the extent and severity of the reaction. Look particularly for signs of upper airway swelling, bronchospasm, or circulatory shock.

The first priority is to achieve cardiorespiratory stability by giving oxygen, adrenaline, and fluids with the patient supine. Antihistamines and steroids play no role until this has been achieved, and even then their value is debatable (see Box 17.2.2).

Oxygen and airway patency

Give oxygen by face mask to all patients, aiming for an oxygen saturation above 92%. Place the patient supine, preferably with the legs elevated to optimize venous return in shock. Elevate the head and torso if respiratory distress is prominent or worsened. Call urgently for experienced anaesthetic assistance if there are signs of impending airway obstruction such as worsening stridor or hoarseness, or rapidly progressive respiratory failure with tachypnoea and wheeze.

Cyanosis and exhaustion indicate imminent respiratory arrest, but sedative or muscle relaxant drugs should never be given unless the physician is trained in the management of the difficult airway. Endotracheal intubation and mechanical ventilation are extremely challenging. Create a surgical airway via the cricothyroid membrane as a last resort, but before hypoxic cardiac arrest occurs.

Adrenaline

Adrenaline is the drug of choice for acute anaphylaxis, whether allergic IgE-mediated or nonallergic. This should be given in all but the most trivial cases, certainly if there is progressive airway swelling, bronchospasm, or hypotension. It has beneficial α-, β$_1$- and β$_2$-adrenergic effects that counteract the profound vasodilatation, mucosal oedema, and bronchospasm. Equally important is that adrenaline, via β$_2$-adrenergic receptors, triggers a rise in intracellular cAMP and thereby inhibits further mast cell and basophil mediator release, thus attenuating the severity of the reaction when given early.

Box 17.2.2 Initial treatment of anaphylaxis

- Stop delivery of any potential causative agent
- Call for help
- Give adrenaline 0.01 mg/kg intramuscularly into lateral thigh, to maximum 0.5 mg (0.5 ml of 1:1000 adrenaline)
  - May be repeated every 5–15 minutes
  - Alternatively, use the patient's EpiPen if readily available—may be given through clothing
- Lay supine (or elevate legs) for shock
- Give high flow oxygen
- Insert large-bore intravenous cannula (14 G or 16 G) and give crystalloid fluid bolus of 10–20 ml/kg

The patient who is failing to respond or deteriorating rapidly:

- Start adrenaline infusion 1 ml (1 mg) of 1:1000 adrenaline in 100 ml normal saline at 30–90 ml/h (5–15 µg/min) titrated to response
  - Patient must be on ECG monitor
  - Give adrenaline faster in cardiopulmonary collapse/arrest
- Consider assisted ventilation and endotracheal intubation by skilled doctor, which may be extremely difficult

Intramuscular adrenaline

Intramuscular adrenaline is recommended when anaphylaxis is treated early, is progressing slowly, if venous access is difficult or delayed, or in the unmonitored patient. The dose is 0.01 mg/kg up to a maximum of 0.5 mg (1:1000 aqueous adrenaline up to a maximum of 0.5 ml), repeated every 5 to 15 min as necessary. This should be given into the upper outer thigh and may be injected through clothing in an emergency, including when self-administered prehospital using an EpiPen. Intramuscular adrenaline is superior to subcutaneous, and the vastus lateralis muscle in the thigh is preferred to the arm deltoid muscle.

Safe and practical intramuscular adrenaline doses in children are 0.3 mg (0.3 ml of 1:1000 aqueous adrenaline) for children aged 6 to 12 years and 0.15 mg (0.15 ml of 1:1000 aqueous adrenaline) for children aged less than 6 years (Working Group Resuscitation Council UK, 2008).

Intravenous adrenaline

Intravenous adrenaline is only ever needed if there is rapidly progressive vascular collapse with shock, imminent airway obstruction, or critical bronchospasm. It should only be given by practitioners experienced in its regular use, with the patient on an ECG monitor. It must be given with extreme care, suitably diluted, slowly, and titrated to response to avoid potentially lethal complications such as cardiac arrhythmias, myocardial ischaemia, and cerebrovascular accident. The initial intravenous dose is 0.75 to 1.5 μg/kg (i.e. 50–100 μg) given slowly over up to 5 minutes depending on the rapidity and severity of the patient's decline, with the dose repeated according to response. Although 1:10 000 adrenaline containing 100 μg/ml is readily available, e.g. as the Minijet preparation, it is difficult to give slowly enough (10 μg/min) for intravenous use. An infusion of adrenaline containing 1 mg in 100 ml 0.9% saline (10 μg/ml) can be given at 30 to 90 ml/h (5–15 μg/min) and titrated to response, continuing for up to 60 min after the resolution of all symptoms and signs of anaphylaxis, then weaning over the next 30 min and stopping while watching closely for any recurrence.

Nebulized adrenaline (5 mg, which is 5 ml of undiluted 1:1000 adrenaline) can be given while parenteral adrenaline is being prepared as described above, particularly for upper airway oedema and bronchospasm.

Fluid replacement

A large-bore intravenous cannula should be inserted as soon as possible in patients showing signs of shock to give an initial fluid bolus of 10 to 20 ml/kg 0.9% saline, with up to 50 ml/kg needed in total to counter the massive intravascular fluid shifts and peripheral vasodilatation that occurs in minutes with anaphylactic shock. There are no outcome data favouring colloids over crystalloids.

Second-line treatments

Once oxygen, adrenaline, and fluids have been given to optimize the cardiorespiratory status and tissue oxygenation, the following drugs may be administered in a support role.

Vasopressors

Vasopressors such as noradrenaline, metaraminol, phenylephrine, and vasopressin have anecdotally been reported as treatments for hypotension resistant to initial adrenaline and fluid therapy.

As with intravenous adrenaline, these agents should only be given by those experienced in their use.

H1 and H2 antihistamines

There is only weak evidence to support the use of antihistamines, which should be reserved for the symptomatic relief of skin symptoms such as urticaria, mild angioedema, and pruritus, although the Resuscitation Council (UK) recommends chlorphenamine 10 to 20 mg intramuscularly or (given slowly) intravenously to counter histamine mediated vasodilation and bronchoconstriction. They must never be relied upon as sole therapy in significant anaphylaxis. Side effects of sedation, confusion, and vasodilatation can be troublesome, particularly if given parenterally.

The combination of an H2 antihistamine with an H1 antihistamine is better at attenuating the cutaneous manifestations of a generalized allergic reaction than an H1 antagonist alone. However, there are no data in severe anaphylaxis and their combined use remains controversial.

Corticosteroids

As with the antihistamines, there are no placebo-controlled trials to confirm the effectiveness of steroids in anaphylaxis, despite their many theoretical benefits on mediator release and tissue responsiveness. Most clinicians give prednisone 1 mg/kg (up to 50 mg) orally or hydrocortisone 1.5 to 3 mg/kg intravenously, particularly in patients with airway involvement and bronchospasm, based purely on their important role in asthma. It is also thought that steroids prevent a biphasic reaction with recrudescence of symptoms following recovery, but again supporting data are unconvincing, although they are essential in the management of recurrent idiopathic anaphylaxis.

Glucagon, atropine, and salbutamol

Patients taking β-blockers are prone to very severe or treatment-refractory anaphylaxis. Glucagon should be given if adrenaline has been ineffective, 1 to 5 mg intravenously, followed by an infusion at 5 to 15 μg/min titrated to response. This raises cAMP by a nonadrenergic mechanism, but may cause nausea and vomiting.

Some patients with anaphylactic shock develop bradycardia resistant to adrenaline, possibly mediated by a neurocardiogenic vagal reflex. Atropine 0.6 mg intravenously up to 0.02 mg/kg has been successful in this situation.

Nebulized salbutamol can be given in addition to adrenaline for resistant bronchospasm, which has the advantage of familiarity.

Observation

Most anaphylactic reactions are uniphasic and respond rapidly and completely to treatment. However, some patients develop protracted reactions with an incomplete response to adrenaline, or deteriorate on attempted weaning from adrenaline. Such patients with unstable vital signs should be monitored and admitted to an intensive care facility.

Biphasic anaphylaxis

Patients who relapse after apparent complete resolution of all their initial symptoms and signs are described as having biphasic anaphylaxis, which is reported in 1 to 20% of all cases. It is unknown if this is predisposed to or caused by more severe presenting features, delayed or inadequate doses of adrenaline, or the failure to give steroids. However, the risk of a biphasic response means that patients with systemic anaphylactic reactions, including all those who have received adrenaline, must be observed for at least 4 to 6 h after apparent full recovery. Those with reactive airways disease should be kept under close watch a little longer because most deaths from anaphylaxis occur in this group. Observation is safely performed in the emergency department if a suitable holding area exists: ECG monitoring is not essential.

Continuing treatment

All patients should be given a letter to take home detailing the nature and circumstances of the anaphylactic reaction, the treatment given, and the suspected causative agent(s). Before discharge, the need for take-home medication, self-injectable adrenaline, and allergist/immunologist referral must be considered.

Oral medication

Although there are no good data to support or refute their use, it is common practice to prescribe a 2- or 3-day discharge supply of combined H1 and H2 antihistamines plus oral steroids to prevent early relapse. Consider cetirizine 10 mg once daily, ranitidine 150 mg every 12 h, and prednisolone 50 mg once daily in adults with predominant cutaneous features such as urticaria following a generalized allergic reaction, or in those with bronchospasm.

Self-injectable adrenaline

The quandary of who to prescribe self-injectable adrenaline to, and what to write in an action plan, is well described. As a guide, this should be given to patients with anaphylaxis after known allergen exposure outside of a medical setting, patients with food allergy (particularly to nuts or peanuts), and those in whom the reaction was severe and/or the cause unknown, including idiopathic anaphylaxis.

The EpiPen or Anapen with 0.3 mg (300 μg) of adrenaline, and the EpiPen Jr or Anapen Junior containing 0.15 mg (150 μg) are approved for self-administered intramuscular use. However, there is no general agreement on who should receive self-injectable adrenaline, and the availability, cost, and licensing regulations differ from country to country. Attitudes vary as to whether the emergency physician or general practitioner should initiate its use, rather than waiting for specialist allergist/immunologist review. However, whoever takes responsibility must explain and demonstrate exactly how to use these devices, and educate both the patient and another caregiver, particularly in children with anaphylaxis. Both need to be able to recognize the symptoms and signs of anaphylaxis and actually use the device, particularly if distant from a health care facility. Recipients must be reminded that self-injectable adrenaline has a relatively short shelf life, and must be shown how to look after it.

Allergist/immunologist referral

Disappointingly, few patients who suffer an episode of anaphylaxis are referred for specialist allergist/immunologist follow-up. This should be mandatory for anyone prescribed a self-injectable adrenaline device and for patients following a wasp or bee sting suitable for immunotherapy, suspected food-induced, drug-induced, or exercise-induced anaphylaxis, and those with severe reactions without an obvious trigger. To assist the allergist/immunologist it is useful to ask the patient to write a brief diary of events in the 6 to 12 h preceding the reaction, particularly when the cause is unclear. This should include all foods ingested, drugs taken (including non-proprietary), cosmetics used, and activities performed outside as well as indoors. Later recall of events will be flawed unless documented contemporaneously.

Prevention

Education

A written anaphylaxis action plan suitable for the patient, carer, or school (in children) is essential, particularly for anyone given self-injectable adrenaline. Patients must understand the nature and cause of the reaction, how to recognize anaphylaxis, and the importance of carrying an EpiPen at all times. Individualized antigen elimination measures such as hymenopteran avoidance must be explained, with information on hidden or unexpected sources of antigen such as salicylate in over-the-counter preparations, trace food elements such as nuts, and possible cross-reactions to unrelated substances.

It is sensible to recommend that the patient wears an alert bracelet such as the MedicAlert following a severe reaction that may recur with sufficient severity to prevent them from giving a history, particularly highlighting drug or vaccine allergy to avoid inadvertent iatrogenic exposure.

A variety of web-based resource material is now available, including from the British Society for Allergy and Clinical Immunology (http://www.bsaci.org.uk), The Anaphylaxis Campaign (http://www.allergyinschools.org.uk), the American Academy of Allergy, Asthma & Immunology (http://www.aaaai.org), the American College of Allergy, Asthma & Immunology (http://www.acaai.org) and from the Australasian Society of Clinical Immunology and Allergy (http://www.allergy.org.au).

Pretreatment

There is no convincing justification for pretreatment. In particular, the practice of giving prophylactic corticosteroids and/or antihistamines to reduce the risk of serious iodinated contrast media reactions during radiological procedures is neither reliable, nor supported by the literature, and should be abandoned.

Skin testing and short-term desensitization

Skin testing should be considered in certain clinical circumstances, such as when penicillin is considered essential but there is a history of possible penicillin allergy. If positive, it should be followed by short-term desensitization over several hours, with increasing doses at 15 min intervals under strict medical control in a monitored area. There are well-tried desensitization regimes for other β-lactams and sulphonamides, and some that are empirically derived for a variety of other antimicrobials.

Long-term desensitization (immunotherapy)

Hyposensitization immunotherapy is reserved for hymenoptera venom in wasp and bee allergy because these reactions may become life-threatening and yet are preventable in over 90% of cases. Patients with asthma or on β-blockers or ACE inhibitors require careful risk–benefit evaluation. Therapy needs to be continued for at least 3 to 5 years.

Drug and allergen avoidance

Wherever possible give drugs orally or, if intravenously, administer slowly. Avoid drugs known to predispose to reactions in allergic patients, particularly aspirin, NSAIDs, and ACE inhibitors, as well as β-blockers. Patients at risk of recurrent anaphylaxis with hypertension or ischaemic heart disease should ideally be taken off β-blockers, with care taken not to substitute an ACE inhibitor. This may need discussion with the patient's other specialists to be certain that the overall risk–benefit favours medication change.

Patients should be advised to reduce the chance of allergen exposure risk by destroying nearby wasp nests and removing allergenic foods from the house, also to avoid insect sting with appropriate clothing and certain foods by always checking the manufacturer's label.

Areas of uncertainty and future developments

Progress in anaphylaxis research is hampered by the lack of a universally accepted definition, or an agreed grading system for severity. Prospective data collection, preferably in multiple sites, is essential to improve the evidence base and allow validation of assessment, treatment, and follow-up protocols. Particular areas that need elucidating include which symptoms or signs most reliably predict the risk of severe anaphylaxis; which laboratory test(s) should be employed to confirm and ideally quantify the severity of an anaphylactic reaction; what predicts a biphasic reaction; and finally whether novel treatments such as anti-IgE therapy in peanut allergy, sublingual immunotherapy for food allergy, or even sublingual adrenaline for self-medication will prove effective and acceptable.

Further reading

Association of Anaesthetists of Great Britain and Ireland (2009). Suspected anaphylactic reactions associated with anaesthesia. *Anaesthesia*, **64**, 199–211.

Axon AD, Hunter JM (2004). Editorial III: Anaphylaxis and anaesthesia—all clear now? *Br J Anaesth*, **93**, 501–504.

Braganza SC, et al. (2006). Paediatric emergency department anaphylaxis: different patterns from adults. *Arch Dis Child*, **91**, 159–63.

Brown AFT (2004). Anaphylaxis gets the adrenaline going. *Emerg Med J*, **21**, 128–9.

Brown AFT, McKinnon D, Chu K (2001). Emergency department anaphylaxis: A review of 142 patients in a single year. *J Allergy Clin Immunol*, **108**, 861–6.

Brown SG (2006). Anaphylaxis: clinical concepts and research priorities. *Emerg Med Australas*, **18**, 155–69.

Brown SG (2004). Clinical features and severity grading of anaphylaxis. *J Allergy Clin Immunol*, **114**, 371–6.

Brown SG, Mullins RJ, Gold MS (2006). Anaphylaxis: diagnosis and management. *Med J Aust*, **185**, 283–89.

Brown SG, et al. (2004). Insect sting anaphylaxis: Prospective evaluation and treatment with intravenous adrenaline and volume resuscitation. *Emerg Med J*, **21**, 149–54.

Caughey GH (2006). Tryptase genetics and anaphylaxis. *J Allergy Clin Immunol*, **117**, 1411–14.

Chang TW, Shiung YY (2006). Anti-IgE as a mast cell-stabilizing therapeutic agent. *J Allergy Clin Immunol*, **117**, 1203–12.

Douglass JA, O'Hehir RE (2006). Diagnosis, treatment and prevention of allergic disease: the basics. *Med J Aust*, **185**, 228–33.

Galli SJ (2005). Pathogenesis and management of anaphylaxis: current status and future challenges. *J Allergy Clin Immunol*, **115**, 571–4.

Johansson SGO, et al. (2004). Revised nomenclature for allergy for global use: Report of the Nomenclature Review Committee of the World Allergy Organization, October 2003. *J Allergy Clin Immunol*, **113**, 832–6.

Lenchner K, Grammer LC (2003). A current review of idiopathic anaphylaxis. *Curr Opin Allergy Clin Immunol*, **3**, 305–11.

Leung D, Schatz M (2006). Consultation and referral guidelines citing the evidence: How the allergist-immunologist can help. *J Allergy Clin Immunol*, **117**, S495–S523.

Lieberman P (2005). Biphasic anaphylactic reactions. *Ann Allergy Asthma Immunol*, **95**, 217–26.

Lieberman P, et al. (2005). The diagnosis and management of anaphylaxis: An updated practice parameter. *J Allergy Clin Immunol*, **115**, S483–S523.

Prussin C, Metcalfe DD (2006). IgE, mast cells, basophils, and eosinophils. *J Allergy Clin Immunol*, **117**, S450–6.

Pumphrey RS (2000). Lessons for management of anaphylaxis from a study of fatal reactions. *Clin Exp Allergy*, **30**, 1144–50.

Ring J, Darsow U (2002). Idiopathic anaphylaxis. *Curr Allergy Asthma Rep*, **2**, 40–45.

Sampson HA (2006). Anaphylaxis: Persistent enigma. *Emerg Med Australas*, **18**, 101–2.

Sampson HA, et al. (2006). Second symposium on the definition and management of anaphylaxis: summary report—Second National Institute of Allergy and Infectious Disease/Food Allergy and Anaphylaxis Network symposium. *J Allergy Clin Immunol*, **117**, 391–7.

Sampson HA, et al. (2005). Symposium on the definition and management of anaphylaxis: summary report. *J Allergy Clin Immunol*, **115**, 584–91.

Sheikh A, et al. (2007). H1-antihistamines for the treatment of anaphylaxis: Cochrane systematic review. *Allergy*, **62**, 830–7.

Sicherer SH, Leung DY (2005). Advances in allergic skin disease, anaphylaxis, and hypersensitivity reactions to food, drugs, and insects. *J Allergy Clin Immunol*, **116**, 153–63.

Sicherer SH, Simons FE (2005). Quandaries in prescribing an emergency action plan and self-injectable epinephrine for first-aid management of anaphylaxis in the community. *J Allergy Clin Immunol*, **115**, 575–83.

Simons FE (2006). Anaphylaxis, killer allergy: long-term management in the community. *J Allergy Clin Immunol*, **117**, 367–77.

Simons FE (2009). Anaphylaxis: Recent advances in assessment and treatment. *J Allergy Clin Immunol*, **124**, 625–36.

Tramèr MR, et al. (2006). Pharmacological prevention of serious anaphylactic reactions due to iodinated contrast media: systematic review. *BMJ*, **333**, 675–8.

Working Group of the Resuscitation Council (UK) (2008). Emergency treatment of anaphylactic reactions—guidelines for healthcare providers. *Resuscitation*, **77**, 157–169.

The clinical approach to the patient who is very ill

John D. Firth

Essentials

When dealing with emergency admissions (and sometimes in other contexts), always ask yourself the question 'is this patient well, ill, very ill, or nearly dead?' Airway, breathing, and circulation (ABC) must be assessed immediately in the patient who is very ill or worse, a key further question being 'do you think that this patient can keep breathing like this for the next 10 min?' If not, summon help from someone with advanced airway skills immediately.

Key things to remember and/or do when dealing with a patient who is very ill include:

(1) Hypoxia kills, hypercarbia merely intoxicates—give oxygen in as high a concentration as possible by face mask—and remember that elective intubation and ventilation are preferable to cardiorespiratory arrest.

(2) Always consider tension pneumothorax and decompress the chest immediately if this is present.

(3) Obtain venous access safely: if veins in the forearm or antecubital fossa cannot be cannulated in the patient who is hypovolaemic, then cannulate the femoral vein, which lies medial to the femoral artery (nerve, artery, vein, Y-fronts—NAVY). An attempt to insert a central venous cannula into the internal jugular or subclavian vein of a patient who is *in extremis* can kill.

(4) If the patient is clearly volume depleted, give 500 ml of blood, plasma expander, or 0.9% saline/balanced salt solution (as appropriate and as available) as fast as possible, then recheck the signs (peripheral perfusion, pulse rate, blood pressure). Repeat cycles of rapid infusion until there is clear evidence of improvement. Consider vasopressors, inotropes, or vasodilators when this is not sufficient (see Chapter 17.4).

(5) As soon as resuscitation is underway, attention must turn towards making a diagnosis. A pragmatic approach uses a 'surgical sieve' technique to look for features on history, examination, and investigation to diagnose conditions that can kill. In many cases treatment must be started 'on suspicion', in particular if the diagnoses of pulmonary embolism or sepsis are possible.

(6) Do not forget to speak to the patient's relatives.

Introduction—recognizing the problem

The first priority in the management of patients who are very ill is to recognize that this is the situation. It is a sensible discipline when dealing with emergency admissions (and sometimes in other contexts) to ask yourself the question: 'Is this patient well, ill, very ill, or nearly dead?' Some physicians will recognize this intuitively; those who do not can learn to do so; and all can be improved by training and experience. In most circumstances, the physician's approach to the patient begins with the history, followed by the examination, and sometimes the ordering and appraisal of the results of investigations, before a diagnosis is reached and treatment commences. This approach can be fatal in those who are very ill or nearly dead at the start.

Key features—summarized as airway, breathing, and circulation (ABC)—to assess immediately in the patient who is very ill or worse are shown in Table 17.3.1. If in any doubt, the most important of the questions to answer is: 'Do you think that this patient can keep breathing like this for the next 10 min?' If the answer is no, then you need to get help immediately: this will usually involve summoning someone with advanced airway skills, often directly from the intensive care unit, or putting out a 'cardiac arrest' call. It is better to do this 10 min before the heart stops than 2 min afterwards, a strategy emphasized by increasing use of Medical Early Warning Scoring (MEWS) systems to trigger nursing and medical staff to call medical emergency or critical care outreach teams if a patient's vital signs are poor. This seems intuitively reasonable, although review of randomized trials does not prove better outcome, but there is no doubt that one nurse or one doctor is not enough to deal optimally with a patient who is *in extremis*, and it seems to be common sense to call for help sooner rather than later.

Table 17.3.1 Key questions to ask when assessing someone with cardiorespiratory collapse

Airway and breathing

- Is the airway patent?
- Is the patient making a respiratory effort, and is the chest expanding with it?
- Is the chest expanding symmetrically? Could there be a tension pneumothorax? (trachea deviated, mediastinum shifted, absent breath sounds on hyperinflated side of the chest)
- Does the patient look as though they could keep this breathing up for the next 10 min?

Circulation

- Do the peripheries feel cold or hot?
- Can you feel the pulse, and what is the rate and rhythm?
- What is the blood pressure?
- Is there a postural drop if the patient is moved from lying to being propped up?
- What is the jugular venous pressure? If you can't see it: is it too high or too low?

Immediate management of airway and breathing

The immediate treatment priorities for the patient with cardiorespiratory collapse are shown in Table 17.3.2.

Airway and oxygen

If a patient is having problems breathing, then is there a difficulty in maintaining the upper airway? If a head tilt/chin lift manoeuvre is beneficial, then a gentle attempt to insert an oropharyngeal airway should be made. This should not be done against resistance—a fight is much more likely to do harm than good—and if the patient spits the airway out it means that it is not necessary.

All patients who are extremely ill should be given oxygen in as high a concentration as possible by face mask. A fraction of inspired oxygen (Fio_2) of around 60% can be obtained using a standard face mask with a reservoir bag and an oxygen flow rate of 10 litre/min. An obvious concern is that this may induce carbon dioxide retention in some patients, most typically those with chronic obstructive pulmonary disease, but denying oxygen can be fatal: hypoxia kills, hypercarbia merely intoxicates. Arterial blood gas analysis should be performed within a few minutes of commencing high flow oxygen, and if this shows that the patient

Table 17.3.2 Immediate treatment priorities for the patient with cardiorespiratory collapse

Airway and breathing

- Give high-flow oxygen (10 l/min) via face mask with reservoir bag
- Consider oropharyngeal airway
- Give intravenous naloxone if any suspicion that patient has received opioids
- Consider elective intubation and ventilation
- If tension pneumothorax, decompress immediately

Circulation

- Obtain intravenous access using a safe technique (see text)
- See Table 17.3.5 for further information.

is retaining carbon dioxide, the Fio_2 can gradually be reduced if oxygenation allows, or elective ventilation can be arranged (if appropriate).

If a patient with respiratory difficulty has received opioids within the past 48 h, or could have done so (have they got small pupils?), then give intravenous naloxone (0.2–0.4 mg in those who have received opioids; 0.8–2.0 mg repeated to a maximum of 10 mg in case of overdosage). This sometimes produces a dramatic response.

Elective ventilation

The patient should be electively intubated and ventilated if breathing seems to be failing despite the measures indicated above, although in some circumstances noninvasive ventilation may be an appropriate alternative. There is no substitute for wise clinical judgement in deciding when this should be done, and it is easy for the inexperienced to be led astray. Too soon is better than too late. A 'normal' respiratory rate of, say, 12 breaths/min may indicate normality, but is also compatible with near death in the patient with a severe respiratory problem who is becoming exhausted. A blood gas level that 'does not seem too bad', meaning perhaps a Po_2 of 9 kPa and Pco_2 of 5.5 kPa, which may not be a cause for any concern at all in a patient who is comfortable and breathing room air, is not at all reassuring if the patient is breathing 60% oxygen and looks very tired.

The work of breathing accounts for up to one-third of the body's oxygen consumption, hence taking this burden from patients by sedating, paralysing, and ventilating them can have a dramatically beneficial effect, whatever the reason for their predicament. However, one note of caution: while being ventilated can be very helpful, the minute or two when the patient is being sedated, paralysed, and intubated is a time of very high risk, since the pharmacological agents used can, to varying degrees, induce profound hypotension culminating in a 'crash'. The chances of this happening can be reduced by giving the patient a bolus of fluid (a rapid infusion of 500 ml of 0.9% saline or colloid) immediately before induction, with dilute adrenaline (1:10 000; not 1:1000) given as 1 ml intravenous pushes (up to one push/min) in the event of a dramatic fall in blood pressure. While the anaesthetist is attending to the airway, the experienced physician will not skulk off into a corner but stand by a site of intravenous access with such a syringe in their hand and keep a careful watch.

Tension pneumothorax

If the patient has a tension pneumothorax, then this should be decompressed immediately by inserting a large-bore venous cannula into the chest and then withdrawing the stylet. This can either be done in the second intercostal space in the midclavicular line, or in the midaxillary line above the level of the nipple, the latter being easier, particularly in muscular men. The response is dramatic and satisfying. A chest drain with underwater seal can then be inserted at (relative) leisure.

The prospect of performing chest decompression is daunting for many junior physicians, and even more so for most of their senior colleagues. Remember that the physical signs are not subtle, the patient with '? minor shift of the trachea' as the only relevant sign does not have a tension pneumothorax. If the patient is blue and cannot breathe, one side of the chest looks blown up and there are no breath sounds over it, then—after attending to the

Table 17.3.3 Clinical evaluation of volume status

Clinical signs of intravascular volume depletion[a]

♦ Low jugular venous pressure[b]
♦ Hypotension, particularly postural hypotension with a drop in systolic pressure of more than 20 mmHg (lying and sitting if lying and standing not possible)
♦ Postural pulse increment >30/min or severe postural dizziness
♦ Cool peripheries (nose, fingers, toes) and collapsed peripheral veins

Clinical signs of volume overload

♦ High jugular venous pressure[b]
♦ Gallop rhythm
♦ Hypertension, basal crepitations, liver congestion, peripheral oedema

[a]Reduced skin turgor, dry mouth and tongue, and sunken eyes are not reliable indicators of intravascular volume depletion. All may be present in patients who are dehydrated, meaning deficient in body water, which is not the same as having intravascular volume depletion. Many elderly patients have low skin turgor; nasal blockage and tachypnoea causes a dry mouth and tongue; and to wait until the eyes sink is to leave things much too late.
[b]Absolute values are deliberately not given. The normal right atrial pressure is in the range +4 to +8mmHg (measured from the mid-axillary line), that is, the jugular venous pressure can range from not being visible when the patient is lying with their torso at 45° to elevated a few centimetres above the angle of Louis. In some circumstances the optimal jugular venous pressure may be considerably outside this normal range, for example much higher if there is pulmonary hypertension.

airway and oxygen and calling the cardiac arrest team—stick in the cannula. There is much to be gained from doing so, and little to be lost if it does not lead to improvement.

Immediate management of the circulation

In a patient who is very ill, if the pulse rate is less than about 60 to 70/min, or above 120/min other than with a sinus tachycardia, then manoeuvres to speed it up (atropine, isoprenaline, pacing) or slow it down (DC cardioversion or antiarrhythmics, but avoiding any of the latter that are negatively inotropic excepting in rare circumstances) are likely to improve the circulation (see Chapter 16.4 for further information).

Most patients who are very ill will have a sinus tachycardia, when there is no advantage in attempting to alter pulse rate and rhythm, indeed there is much to be lost from ill-advised attempts to do so. The key question then becomes: Is the filling pressure optimal?

Does the patient need to be given fluid, or is there too much fluid on board? Those who do not see many very ill patients might think that it should be easy to tell the difference, but the answer is not always obvious, and yet the physician must decide rapidly, often without anything other than clinical judgement to guide them. Although they may yearn for a measurement of central venous or pulmonary artery occlusion ('wedge') pressure, or for a chest radiograph to see whether or not there is pulmonary oedema, to delay management might be fatal. The clinical features to look for are listed in Table 17.3.3, and the appropriate responses discussed in Table 17.3.4.

The patient who is volume depleted

Obtaining venous access

The need is to insert a cannula into a decent-sized vein quickly, and with as low a risk of complication as possible. Try initially for a peripheral vein in the forearm or antecubital fossa, but if these are constricted and cannot be cannulated and the patient is *in extremis*, then go for the femoral vein, which lies medial to the artery in the groin (nerve, artery, vein, Y-fronts, NAVY). The procedure is easiest if the patient can lie flat, but can be performed with the patient propped up if respiratory difficulty means that lying down is impossible. Feel for the femoral pulse just below the crease of the groin and, after giving local anaesthetic, insert the needle (with the bevel pointing forwards) one finger breadth medial to the point of maximum pulsation at an angle of about 60° to the skin and parallel to the long axis of the leg. The only significant complication of this procedure is inadvertent arterial puncture (Table 17.3.5), the consequences of which are much less likely to be severe in the groin than in the neck or below the clavicle.

An attempt to insert a central venous cannula into the internal jugular or subclavian vein of a patient who is *in extremis* has led to more deaths than such catheters have prevented. If the patient's intravascular volume is depleted, then the veins are constricted and small, cannulation is very difficult, and the procedure tends to degenerate into what is known in the trade as the 'sewing machine technique', where multiple stabs culminate in something being hit, often not the vein that was being (increasingly loosely) targeted. If patients are volume overloaded and in respiratory difficulty, then

Table 17.3.4 Immediate clinical response to determination of volume status

Main problem	Key clinical signs	Immediate management
Hypotension	Peripheries cool and shut down Postural hypotension Low jugular venous pressure	Intravenous fluid given rapidly until clear evidence that physical signs are being restored to normal, then slower infusion
Breathing difficulty	High jugular venous pressure Gallop rhythm Basal crepitations	Do not give fluid Sit up Consider intravenous loop diuretic and/or venodilator Consider need for ventilation
Hypotension and breathing difficulty	Peripheries cool and shut down Jugular venous pressure likely to be high May be gallop rhythm Likely to be basal crepitations	Likely to need urgent ventilation, preferably before suffering cardiorespiratory arrest (see text for details of medical management of this process) Trial of fluid infusion may be appropriate: give 200 ml of plasma expander, keeping patient under continuous observation and terminating infusion immediately in the event of clinical deterioration

All patients should be given high-flow oxygen.
Vigorous attempts should be made to diagnose and treat the underlying condition concurrent with efforts to resuscitate.
If the patient remains hypotensive despite 'optimization' of intravascular volume, then consideration can be given to the use of inotropes and vasoactive agents: see Chapter 17.4 for further discussion.

Table 17.3.5 Complications during insertion of 5465 central venous catheters

Approach	Number of procedures	Complication					
		Pneumothorax (%)	Arterial puncture (%)	Repeated puncture, meaning two or more consecutive attempts to puncture a vein using the same approach (%)	Necessity to shift to another approach (%)	Failure to cannulate central vein, even after shifting to another approach (%)	Malposition of catheter (%)
Femoral vein	1014	Not relevant	9	5	4	0.1	0.1
High approach to internal jugular	460	0	7.7	9	22	0.5	4.5
Low lateral approach to internal jugular	1767	0	1.2	3.3	12	0.1	0.8
Axial approach to internal jugular	104	1	7	12	20	1	2
Infraclavicular approach to subclavian vein	1273	2.5	2.8	6.5	8.6	0.4	2.6
Supraclavicular approach to subclavian vein	847	1.1	3.6	4	8	0.2	1.4

Data from Journal of Vascular Access 1, 100-7, M. Pittiruti et al., Which is the easiest and safest technique for central venous access? A retrospective survey of more than 5,400 cases, 2000

they will not tolerate being laid flat for the cannulation attempt: if you try to make them do so, they won't lie still for long, and if they do become still it might be because they have died.

When the patient who is volume depleted has had intravascular volume restored, or when the situation of the patient who is volume overloaded and breathless has been rendered safe (perhaps by intubation and ventilation), then the insertion of a central venous catheter can be helpful in diagnosis (e.g. to allow passage of a right heart catheter for measurement of the pulmonary artery occlusion pressure), monitoring (e.g. of a fall in the central venous pressure indicating further gastrointestinal haemorrhage), and treatment (e.g. infusion of vasopressors, inotropes, other drugs, or parenteral nutrition).

The approaches for internal jugular and subclavian vein cannulation using 'landmark methods' are shown in Figs. 17.3.1 and 17.3.2. Details of safety and reliability in one large study are shown in Table 17.3.5. While there is no doubt that experienced operators can achieve high rates of successful cannulation with few complications, failure rates of up to one in three have been reported in the literature, and it is clear that complications can lead to substantial morbidity and (on occasion) mortality. Guidance has been issued in the United Kingdom that two-dimensional imaging ultrasonography guidance should be considered in most clinical circumstances where central venous catheter insertion is necessary, but it must be emphasized that this is not a panacea: the inadequately trained operator with an ultrasonography machine will perform less well and put their patients at greater risk than the experienced operator using a landmark approach that they are familiar with.

What fluid should you give, and how much?

A great deal of heat, but little light, has been generated in the literature on the subject of when to replace fluid, what to give, and how much. For patients with penetrating trauma to the torso it has been shown that delayed resuscitation, where venous access is

established but fluid is not given until the patient is in the operating theatre, is preferable to immediate resuscitation, but there is no obvious analogy between this situation and that of the vast majority of patients with circulatory collapse and the rule, in general, remains that resuscitation should start as soon as possible.

It is logical that the fluid given to the patient whose intravascular volume is depleted should be one that remains substantially within the intravascular compartment. Solutions based on dextrose (with zero or low concentration of sodium) are most certainly not appropriate, since they partition throughout the body water and relatively little remains in the intravascular compartment, but beyond this it is not possible to make any firm recommendation. If the patient has lost blood, then it would seem sensible to give blood, and most physicians would recommend this. Whether isotonic crystalloid (usually 0.9% saline), hypertonic crystalloid (usually saline), or various types of colloid are best in other situations is not clear. Cochrane reviews have failed to find significant differences between the use in critically ill patients of crystalloid or colloid, between isotonic or hypertonic fluids, or between different types of colloid solution.

Although some advocate the use of algorithms, at the outset it is not possible to judge precisely how much fluid will be needed to resuscitate a patient. The only way to determine this is by frequent clinical examination as fluid is given. In the patient who is very unwell and clearly volume depleted, standard practice is to give 500 ml of blood, plasma expander, or 0.9% saline (as appropriate and as available) as fast as the giving set and venous cannula will allow (applying pressure to the bag by manual or mechanical compression if the patient is *in extremis*). A second 500 ml infusion is commenced while checking peripheral perfusion, pulse rate, blood pressure, and the jugular venous pressure. Rapid infusion is continued until there is clear evidence that the situation is beginning to improve, as manifest by warming of the peripheries, slowing of

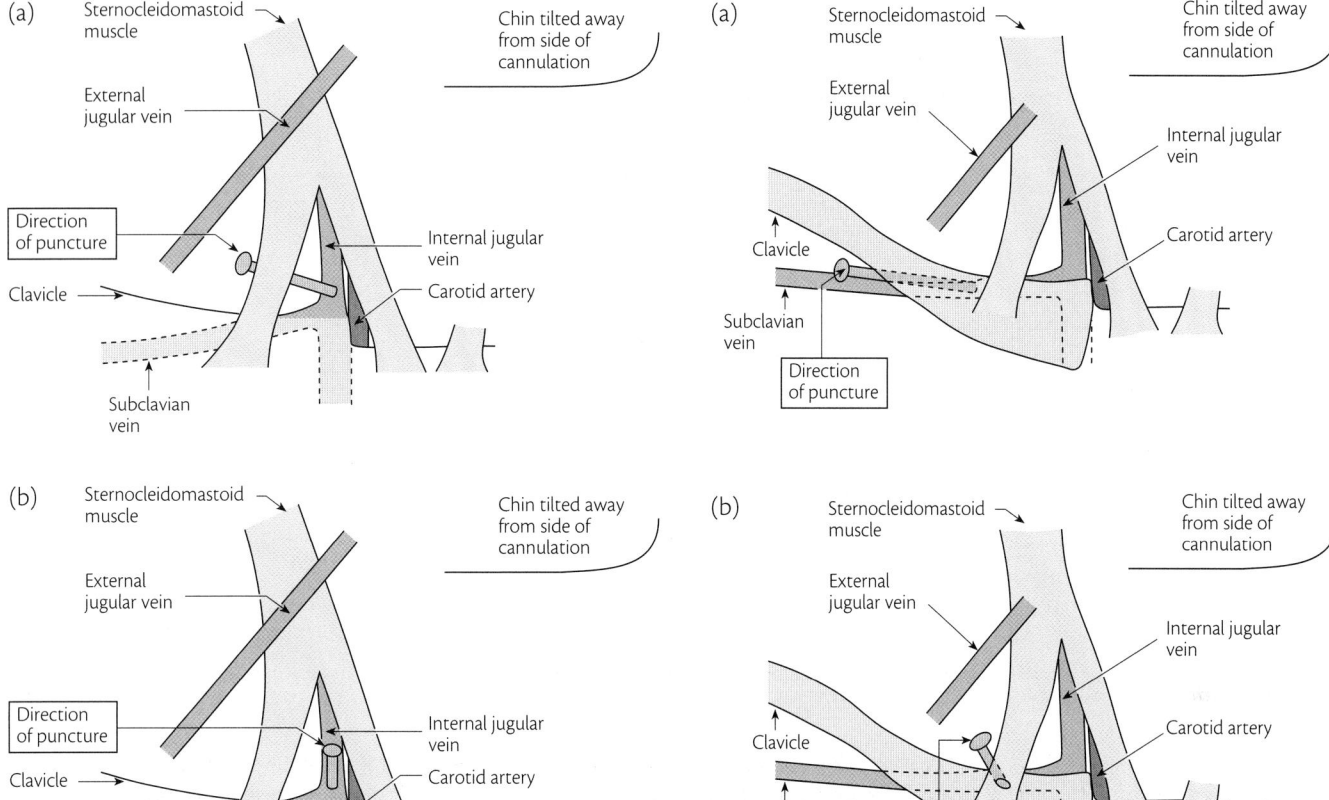

Fig. 17.3.1 The low lateral (a) and axial (b) approaches to the internal jugular vein. In (a) the patient is supine with the head turned away from the side of the puncture. A towel may be placed under both shoulders to extend the neck. After preparation of the skin and drapes, and insertion of local anaesthetic, the bed is tilted to a 25° head down position. The needle is inserted just lateral to the posterior border of the clavicular head of the sternocleidomastoid muscle, about one finger breadth above the clavicle. It is then advanced parallel to the line of the clavicle and just behind the sternocleidomastoid muscle. The internal jugular vein, which lies superficially at this point, is cannulated close to its junction with the subclavian vein. As soon as the vein is entered, the needle is angulated caudally to ease cannulation, the guidewire passing directly into the innominate vein. The risk of complications was lower with this technique than for any other method of central venous cannulation used in one large series (see Table 17.3.5). (b) The patient is positioned as described for the low lateral approach to the internal jugular vein. The needle is inserted just above the mid point of the triangle formed by the two heads of the sternocleidomastoid muscle and the clavicle and advanced caudally at about 45° to the skin. See Table 17.3.5 for details of complications using this approach.

Fig. 17.3.2 The infraclavicular (a) and supraclavicular (b) approaches to the subclavian vein. (a) The patient is positioned as described for the low lateral approach to the internal jugular vein (Fig. 17.3.1a), except that instead of a towel being placed under both shoulders it should be positioned under the spine, allowing the shoulders to retract to reduce the risk of pneumothorax. The needle enters the skin below the midpoint of the lower border of the clavicle and is advanced under the clavicle towards the upper edge of the junction of the clavicle with the manubrium. See Table 17.3.5 for details of complications using this approach. (b) The patient is positioned as described for the infraclavicular approach to the subclavian vein. The needle is inserted into the angle between the superior border of the clavicle and the posterior border of the clavicular head of the sternocleidomastoid and advanced caudally, medially, and ventrally. See Table 17.3.5 for details of complications using this approach.

the pulse rate, and rise in blood pressure. Interpretation of change in the height of the jugular venous pressure requires some care. It rises as fluid starts to be given, but may then fall for two reasons: first, if there is further fluid loss, most typically haemorrhage; and second, as venoconstrictor tone diminishes in the patient who is 'warming up' with adequate resuscitation. Their different effects on peripheral perfusion, pulse rate, and blood pressure easily distinguish these two eventualities.

As soon as it is clear that the patient's circulation is beginning to improve, the rate of fluid infusion should be slowed so as not to risk precipitating pulmonary oedema by forcing very high

hydrostatic pressures in a circulation that is still 'tight' due to the effect of endogenous vasoconstrictors. Hence, the patient who has lost, say, 2 litres of blood, may be optimally treated by receiving the first litre as quickly as possible, followed by the second litre over the next 2 h or so as the circulation 'relaxes'.

When resuscitation is complete—meaning that peripheral perfusion, pulse rate, blood pressure, and jugular venous pressure have all returned to acceptable levels—fluid input should then be given with regard to fluid output. At this stage it is good practice to insert a urinary catheter into any patient who has presented with severe cardiorespiratory disturbance. Urinary flow rate reflects renal perfusion, which is a marker of the overall state of the circulation, and accurate measurement of urinary output is essential

Table 17.3.6 Examination and investigation of the patient with cardiorespiratory collapse

Diagnosis		Key finding on examination	Key initial investigation	Definitive investigations
Cardiovascular	Myocardial infarction	No specific findings likely	ECG	ECG, cardiac enzymes
	Arrhythmia	Pulse rate and rhythm	ECG	ECG
	Aortic dissection	Absence or reduction in one or more peripheral pulses, especially left radial. Blood pressure lower in left arm than right	Chest radiograph showing widened mediastinum	Imaging of aorta, usually by CT scan or trans-oesophageal echocardiography
	Cardiac tamponade	Raised jugular venous pressure. Pulsus paradoxus (pulse becomes impalpable on inspiration in extreme cases)	Chest radiograph may show globular heart. ECG may show low-voltage complexes or electrical alternans	Echocardiography
Cardiorespiratory	Pulmonary embolus	Raised jugular venous pressure. Right ventricular heave. Loud P2. Right ventricular gallop rhythm. Signs of deep vein thrombosis in leg	ECG may show features of acute right heart strain	Ventilation/perfusion scan. Imaging of pulmonary vessels by CT scan or pulmonary angiography
	Pulmonary oedema	Gallop rhythm. Crackles (see text)	Chest radiograph	Usually cardiac—ECG, echocardiography
Respiratory	Tension pneumothorax	Tracheal deviation. Hyperexpansion of one side of chest. Mediastinal shift. Absent breath sounds on one side of chest	Chest radiograph—but should be treated on basis of clinical diagnosis (see text)	Chest radiograph— but should be treated on basis of clinical diagnosis (see text)
	Pneumonia	May have high fever. Signs of consolidation or pleurisy	Chest radiograph	Chest radiograph. Blood culture. Serological tests
	Asthma	Wheezes, but beware of silent chest	Response to treatment (β-agonist), but chest radiograph excludes other respiratory diagnoses	Peak flow measurements before and after β-agonist
	Exacerbation of chronic obstructive pulmonary disease	Features of chronic obstructive pulmonary disease	A clinical diagnosis, but chest radiograph excludes other respiratory diagnoses	See Chapter 18.8
Abdominal	Gastrointestinal haemorrhage	Usually obvious, but don't forget rectal examination for blood/melaena in the patient with unexplained hypotension	A clinical diagnosis	Endoscopy
	Perforated viscus	Peritonism	Erect abdominal radiograph to look for free air	CT scan or laparotomy, depending on clinical situation
	Pancreatitis	Peritonism. Bruising in flanks	Serum amylase	Imaging of pancreas, usually by CT scan
	Ruptured abdominal aortic aneurysm	Peritonism. Palpable aneurysm. Bruising in flanks	A clinical diagnosis	CT scan or laparotomy, depending on clinical situation
Sepsis		May have high fever. May have warm peripheries and bounding pulse, but could be cold and shut down. No specific findings likely, but look for rash or localized infection, such as abscess	A clinical diagnosis	Blood culture
Metabolic	Many possible causes, such as renal failure, hepatic failure, profound acidosis, but collectively these are rare causes of presentation with cardiorespiratory collapse	May have evidence of organ failure, or of drug overdose. May have no specific findings	Electrolytes, renal and liver function tests. Blood gases	As indicated following initial tests
Anaphylaxis		Facial, tongue, and throat swelling. Stridor. Wheeze. Urticarial rash. Skin erythema or extreme pallor	A clinical diagnosis	Serum mast cell tryptase. Specific IgE for suspect allergens. See Chapter 17.2 for further information

Primarily neurological disorders may compromise the airway or ventilation, but rarely cause cardiovascular collapse. If a patient with cardiovascular collapse has a severely depressed conscious level (Glasgow coma scale less than 8) or focal neurological signs, then the assumption—until proven otherwise—should be that the neurological impairment is secondary to the cardiovascular collapse and not the cause of it.

to judge continuing fluid requirement. If patients have developed acute tubular necrosis with oliguria as a result of hypotension, they will not be well served by continued prescription of (say) 3 litres of fluid per day to follow on from that given to resuscitate. This will inevitably lead to pulmonary oedema if continued in the face of diminished urinary output. A daily input equal to the last 24-h output (from all sources), plus 500 to 1000 ml for insensible losses, is appropriate in these circumstances, with the patient examined at least twice a day for signs of volume depletion or overload to allow adjustment of fluid infusion rate as required.

The patient who is volume overloaded

Acute volume overload manifests as pulmonary oedema, which can be a most terrifying condition. When severe, patients cannot get their breath and, with good reason, think they are going to die. As for patients in extreme respiratory difficulty, they sit up and use their accessory muscles. They are sweaty, cool peripherally, tachycardic, hypertensive (usually), centrally cyanosed, the jugular venous pressure is raised, and there is a gallop rhythm, although this may be hard to appreciate amidst the widespread crackles and wheezes in the chest. In extreme forms, frothy pink oedema fluid may come from the mouth. For further information see Chapter 16.15.3. The main features of treatment are shown in Table 17.3.4.

Other manoeuvres to support the circulation

In many patients the circulation will be restored to normal simply by correction of fluid deficit. When this alone is not sufficient, benefit may be obtained by use of vasopressors, inotropes, or vasodilators: see Chapter 17.4 for further details.

The underlying condition

The initial management of patients who are desperately ill does not depend on making a precise diagnosis of the cause of their predicament. However, as soon as resuscitation is underway, attention must turn towards making a diagnosis. Although the naive might think that the more severe the illness, the more obvious the cause should be, the opposite is often the case. When dead, all patients look identical, and the same is true just before they die. Patients who are *in extremis*, whether due to profound hypoxia or with next to no blood pressure, are not lucid historians, and it may be that the only question that they can usefully answer is: 'Do you have any pain?' If they indicate their chest or their abdomen, this might be a helpful clue.

The pragmatic approach to making a diagnosis in the patient with cardiorespiratory collapse is to use a 'surgical sieve' technique, looking systematically for features on examination and investigation to diagnose conditions that can kill (Table 17.3.6). Details of the management of the many specific disorders listed in Table 17.3.6 can be found in the relevant sections of this book, but one general point is extremely important: if initial investigations do not give any clear diagnostic lead, then treatment must be started 'on suspicion', especially for disorders that cannot reliably be diagnosed or excluded by clinical examination or by tests that

are rapidly available. In particular, pulmonary embolism and sepsis should always be considered. If the clinical context makes pulmonary embolism likely, for instance the patient has collapsed after an operation a week or so ago, then—in the absence of other explanation for the problem—it is sensible to start therapeutic anticoagulation with intravenous heparin (which can be reversed if necessary) immediately, pending definitive imaging, but it would be unwise to give thrombolytic agents until the diagnosis was established. If a patient who looks unwell is hypotensive for no obvious reason, then give broad-spectrum parenteral antibiotics as soon as blood cultures have been taken. And with regard to sepsis, ask the patient where they have travelled recently and consider malaria, which still kills in temperate parts of the world, sometimes because 'the doctor didn't think of the diagnosis'.

Communication

Once resuscitation and diagnostic endeavours are underway, and certainly when you have a clear idea what the diagnosis is, do not forget to speak to the patient's relatives. Always give them an honest account of the situation, including any uncertainties about diagnosis, an outline of the management plan, and a realistic assessment of the likely outcome, and record in the medical notes what you have told them. Part of the business of looking after very ill patients is looking after their relatives, and one of the most common causes of the complaints that are made with increasing frequency if a patient dies is that 'the doctors didn't tell us what was going on … they never told us how ill he was'. It is well worth spending 5 min talking to the relatives and 2 min writing an account of this in the notes.

Further reading

Alderson P, *et al.* (2004). Human albumin solution for resuscitation and volume expansion in critically ill patients. *Cochrane Database Syst Rev* 2004, **4**, CD001208.

Bickell WH, *et al.* (1994). Immediate versus delayed fluid resuscitation for hypotensive patients with penetrating torso injuries. *N Engl J Med*, **331**, 1105–9.

Bunn F, Trivedi D, Ashraf S (2008). Colloid solutions for fluid resuscitation. *Cochrane Database Syst Rev*, **1**, CD001319.

National Institute for Clinical Excellence. *Technology Guidance—No.49 (2002). Guidance on the use of ultrasound locating devices for placing central venous catheters.* http://www.nice.org.uk/nicemedia/pdf/ Ultrasound_49_GUIDANCE.pdf

Perel P, Roberts I (2007). Colloids versus crystalloids for fluid resuscitation in critically ill patients. *Cochrane Database Syst Rev*, **4**, CD000567.

Pittiruti M, *et al.* (2000). Which is the easiest and safest technique for central venous access? A retrospective survey of more than 5400 cases. *J Vasc Access*, **1**, 100–7.

McGaughey J, *et al.* (2007). Outreach and Early Warning Systems (EWS) for the prevention of Intensive Care admission and death of critically ill adult patients on general hospital wards. *Cochrane Database Syst Rev*, **3**, CD005529.

McGee S (2007). *Evidence-based physical diagnosis*, 2nd edition. W B Saunders.

17.4

Circulation and circulatory support in the critically ill

Michael R. Pinsky

Essentials

Cardiovascular dysfunction is common in the critically ill patient and is the primary cause of death in a vast array of illnesses. The prompt identification and diagnosis of its probable cause, coupled to appropriate resuscitation and (when possible) specific treatments, are cornerstones of intensive care medicine.

Cardiovascular monitoring and diagnosis—cardiovascular performance can be assessed clinically at the bedside and through haemodynamic monitoring, and with therapeutic or other proactive interventions. Diagnostic approaches or therapies based on data derived from invasive haemodynamic monitoring in the critically ill patient assume that specific patterns of derangement reflect specific disease processes, which will respond to appropriate intervention.

Interpretation of haemodynamic variables—the various adaptive cardiovascular controls and varying metabolic demands make rules about specific haemodynamic variables of limited clinical utility. It is simply not possible to say that, when looking after a critically ill patient, the central venous pressure, or any other single measurable variable, must be kept at x or y. Key points in this context are: (1) tachycardia is never a good thing; (2) hypotension is always pathological; (3) there is no such thing as a normal cardiac output; (4) central venous pressure is only elevated in disease; and (5) peripheral oedema is of cosmetic concern.

Oxygen delivery—while there is no level of cardiac output which is 'normal', there are oxygen delivery thresholds below which normal metabolism can no longer occur. One cardinal sign of increased circulatory stress is an increased O_2 extraction ratio, which manifests itself as a decreasing mixed venous O_2 saturation (Svo_2): a value of less than 70% connotes circulatory stress, less than 60% identifies significant metabolic limitation, and less than 50% frank tissue ischaemia.

Pathophysiology of shock

Circulatory shock can be defined as a decreased effectiveness of circulatory blood flow to meet the metabolic demands of the body. Four basic functional aetiologies are recognized.

(1) Hypovolaemic shock (e.g. haemorrhage, dehydration)—effective circulating blood volume is inadequate to sustain a level of cardiac output necessary for normal function without supplemental sympathetic tone or postural changes to ensure adequate amounts of venous return.

(2) Cardiogenic shock (e.g. myocardial infarction)—pump dysfunction can be due to either left ventricular (LV) or right ventricular (RV) failure, or both. LV failure is usually manifest by an increased LV end-diastolic pressure, left atrial pressure and (by extension) pulmonary artery occlusion ('wedge') pressure, which must exist to sustain an adequate LV stroke volume.

(3) Obstructive shock—mechanical obstruction of blood flow (e.g. pulmonary embolism) or of ventricular filling (cardiac tamponade). In the acute setting, neither pulmonary vascular resistance nor mean pulmonary artery pressure need be grossly elevated for RV failure to occur. In cardiac tamponade, the cardinal sign is diastolic equalization of all pressures, central venous pressure, pulmonary arterial diastolic pressure, and pulmonary artery occlusion ('wedge') pressure.

(4) Distributive shock—loss of blood flow regulation occurs as the endstage of all forms of circulatory shock, but as the initial presenting process it is common in sepsis, neurogenic shock, and adrenal insufficiency. The haemodynamic profile of sepsis is one of increased cardiac index, normal pulmonary artery occlusion ('wedge') pressure, elevated Svo_2, and a low to normal arterial pressure, consistent with loss of peripheral vasomotor tone.

Circulatory support of the haemodynamically unstable patient

If the cause of hypotension is intravascular volume loss, either absolute or relative, then cerebral and coronary perfusion pressures must be maintained while fluid resuscitation is begun, otherwise cardiac pump failure may develop and limit the effectiveness of fluid resuscitation.

Pharmacotherapies for cardiovascular insufficiency—these are directed at the pathophysiological processes that either induce or compound the problem. They can be loosely grouped into one of three types: (1) vasopressor therapy—agents that increase vascular smooth muscle tone include noradrenaline (norepinephrine), adrenaline (epinephrine), dopamine, and phenylephrine; (2) inotropic support—agents that

Acknowledgement: The author's work was supported in part by NIH grants HL67181 and HL07820.

that increase cardiac contractility include dobutamine, dopexamine, and phosphodiesterase inhibitors; (3) vasodilator therapy—agents that decrease smooth muscle tone include sodium nitroprusside and glyceryl trinitrate (nitroglycerine). It is important to recognize that most inotropes and vasopressors in clinical use are sympathomimetics that have direct effects on the adrenoreceptor system, and there is a quantitatively unpredictable variation in adrenoreceptor density and function in many pathophysiological states, hence agents acting upon them need to be titrated to effect rather than being given at a defined infusion rate.

Resuscitation strategies—the only prospective clinical trials documenting benefit from particular interventions were applied early in the course of sepsis or in high-risk surgical patients. However, it makes physiological sense to prevent organ ischaemia by maintaining blood flow, hence the following strategies seem warranted.

(1) Loss of vasomotor tone requires both fluid resuscitation to achieve the increased vascular volume needed to restore an effective pressure gradient for venous return, and increased α-adrenergic tone via sympathomimetic agents to restore arterial and venous vasomotor tone. Targets for resuscitation are an SvO_2 less than 70% with a MAP greater than 60 mmHg.

(2) Impaired contractility requires afterload reduction, as tolerated, up to a decrease in MAP to approximately 70 mmHg, targeting pulmonary artery occlusion ('wedge') pressure less than 18 mmHg and SvO_2 greater than 70%. In sepsis, SvO_2 is usually elevated following fluid resuscitation, hence resuscitation targets usually focus on reaching elevated levels of oxygen delivery (e.g. >450 ml/min per m²).

(3) In RV failure, maintaining a MAP greater than pulmonary arterial pressure is essential to minimize RV myocardial ischaemia.

Introduction

Cardiovascular dysfunction is common in the critically ill patient and is the primary cause of death in a vast array of illnesses including sepsis, pulmonary embolism, and acute respiratory failure, as well as in those with cardiac disease. The prompt identification of cardiovascular dysfunction, the diagnosis of its probable cause, and appropriate specific treatments (when possible) coupled to appropriate resuscitation and restorative management are cornerstones of intensive care medicine.

Cardiovascular performance can be assessed at the bedside and through haemodynamic monitoring and therapeutic or other proactive interventions. Diagnostic approaches or therapies based on data derived from invasive haemodynamic monitoring in the critically ill patient assume that specific patterns of derangement reflect specific disease processes, which will respond to appropriate intervention. Why such constellations of measured abnormalities occur is due to the underlying cardiovascular interactions that define normal and pathological states, hence it is essential that the practising clinician be well versed in the underlying principles of cardiovascular physiology and pathophysiology in order to appropriately diagnose and then treat the critically ill.

Principles of cardiovascular homeostasis

Physicians often consider disease states as involving only one organ, such as the heart, during acute coronary ischaemia or the circulation during haemorrhage. However, no organ system operates in the body without numerous and redundant feedback processes which both amplify and inhibit the specific response of the organ and the rest of the body to stress, disease, and treatment. These interactions form the basis of haemodynamic profile pattern recognition. Specific combinations of changing cardiovascular and metabolic variables better reflect specific disease processes than do individual values for specific variables. Furthermore, the change in these variables in response to time and treatment define the progression or resolution of disease, its severity, and subsequent responsiveness to therapy.

Although specific combinations of haemodynamic variables often reflect certain disease states, there may be considerable overlap of haemodynamic data sets among markedly different pathological states, which may require different therapies. These vagaries reflect individual patient differences, complex cardiovascular interactions not considered in the original logic, and also inaccuracies in the measures themselves and incorrect assumptions as to what the primary force is, and what is its response. This confusion can be minimized, however, by performing an experiment at the bedside to force the cardiovascular system into doing one thing or another. This is the essence of a 'clinical trial' of positive pressure breathing, passive leg raising, fluid therapy, diuresis, or increased inotropy. Thus, by examining the specific haemodynamic response of the individual to a specific therapy, the clinician at the bedside can gain essential insight into the process that is dysfunctional and also tailor therapy to the individual. Let us first consider normal cardiovascular physiology, then pathophysiology, and finally how to diagnose and treat.

Ventricular pump function

Frank–Starling relationship

Our understanding of cardiac pump function has evolved greatly since the initial studies of Frank and Starling in the 1890s. Frank, a German physiologist, noted that when cardiac muscle strips were stretched they (unlike skeletal muscle strips) increased their force of contraction. Starling used these data to reason that since the left ventricular (LV) cavity approximated a sphere, increases in LV end-diastolic volume (EDV) should proportionally increase LV myocardial fibre stretch. Thus, he explained the observation that the force of LV contraction was related to left ventricular end-diastolic volume (LVEDV). Based on this construct, increasing LVEDV when LV function is normal will increase LV stroke volume and—for a constant heart rate—cardiac output as well. However, if LV pump function is impaired, then for the same increase in LVEDV stroke volume will not increase as much, if at all. Most studies of ventricular function revolve around LV function, assuming that the right ventricle follows suit.

The Frank–Starling relationship is central to most diagnostic and therapeutic protocols used to assess cardiac function. In fact, clinically, the immediate treatment of acute cardiovascular insufficiency and arterial hypotension is to increase intravascular volume. If arterial pressure increases, then the subject is said to be 'preload responsive' and the presumptive diagnosis of hypovolaemia is made.

However, this common therapeutic response of fluid resuscitation will only increase cardiac output in half the patients who are haemodynamically unstable, hence understanding better the determinants of cardiovascular insufficiency and how to assess them are important goals in the training of critical care physicians.

When modelling LV pump function, one assesses both stroke volume and pressure work, or stroke work, needed to cause that flow. LV stroke volume varies inversely with outflow pressure (arterial pressure) for a constant LVEDV and LV contractility, whereas stroke work will remain constant. Thus, LV stroke work, rather than stroke volume, is often used to assess LV functional status because it is relatively pressure (afterload) independent. If stroke work is less for the same LVEDV, then LV contractility is also said to be less under this condition (Fig. 17.4.1).

The measure of LV function best used to assess cardiovascular status is highly dependent on the question being asked. If the question is the adequacy of LV output to meet the metabolic demands of the body, then stroke volume and cardiac output are the relevant measures. However, if the question is 'what is the functional status of the heart, and can it be counted on to sustain blood flow as ejection pressures rise?', which in essence is asking 'what is the level of myocardial contractile reserve, independent of the level of blood flow?', then the change in LV stroke work relative to the change in LVEDV is a better index.

LV pressure–volume loop

LV pump behaviour is best described using the LV pressure–volume relation, wherein a single cardiac cycle is described as a loop with LV volume on the x-axis and pressure on the y-axis (Fig. 17.4.2). In this construct no time units are used. Filling occurs during diastole when LV chamber pressure decreases to less than left atrial pressure. The slope of the passive LV distention is diastolic compliance. At end-diastole, defined by the electromechanical coupling of contraction, the pressure/volume ratio is at its minimum. This point is often used to assess diastolic compliance, but is influenced by external forces independent of the LV, such as the pericardium, lungs, and right ventricle. LVEDV is synonymous with LV preload as applied to the Frank–Starling relationship.

With mechanical contraction, the LV intracavitary pressure rises, forcing mitral valve closure and changing the shape of the LV

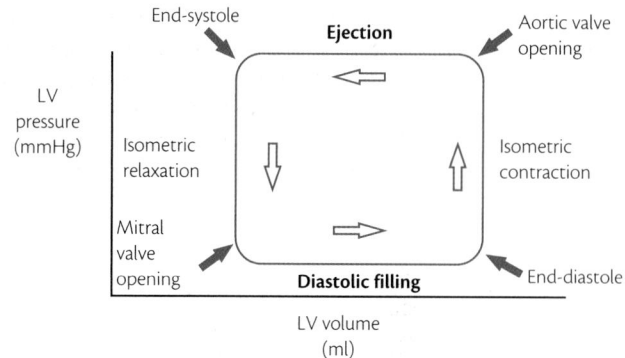

Fig. 17.4.2 The LV pressure–volume relationship describing all aspects of the cardiac cycle.

from an elongated ellipsoid into more of a sphere. As contraction progresses, intracavitary pressure rises as the end-diastolic blood volume is trapped in the LV. Once intracavitary pressure exceeds aortic pressure the aortic valve passively opens and ejection begins. In a subject with a normal heart, the point where ejection occurs represents the maximal LV wall stress, itself the product of radius of curvature and developed pressure. Thus, diastolic arterial pressure is a major determinant of LV wall stress, and this LV wall stress is the LV afterload. Any therapy which selectively decreases diastolic arterial pressure will then reduce LV afterload more than therapies which selectively decrease systolic arterial pressure. Similarly, if an inovasodilator, such as dopexamine, were given that decreased LVEDV but increased LV stroke volume and ejection pressure, one may erroneously conclude that LV afterload increased, when in fact it decreased.

Ejection occurs as LV volume decreases and both LV pressure and aortic pressure rise. Due to the filling characteristics of the aorta, aortic pressure increases most towards the end of ejection as the distensible volume of the aorta is finally reached. Thus, most of the increase in arterial pressure occurs when the LV volume is already small. As a result, the maximal LV wall stress usually occurs at the start of ejection and the LV unloads itself during ejection. That the left ventricle unloads itself during ejection has important clinical implications. First, systolic hypertension is better tolerated without much increase in myocardial oxygen demand (MVo_2) than is diastolic hypertension. However, if LVEDV is increased such that LV volumes do not decrease much during ejection, as is the case in congestive heart failure, then systolic pressure will be a major contributor to both LV wall stress and MVO_2. Accordingly, in dilated heart failure states the LV performance is sensitive to changes in systolic arterial pressure, and end-systolic volume (ESV) then is a function of both afterload and contractility. As such, increases in afterload will increase ESV whereas increases in contractility will decrease ESV.

LV relaxation occurs once ejection has finished. Diastolic relaxation or lusitropy is an energy-dependent process, causes LV intracavitary pressure to decrease faster than would be predicted by passive relaxation alone, and is impaired by myocardial ischaemia. Impaired active diastolic relaxation is the earliest manifestation of myocardial ischaemia and can be readily identified by echocardiography and as an S3 gallop on cardiac auscultation. Since coronary artery blood flow occurs primarily in diastole, when LV wall stress is low

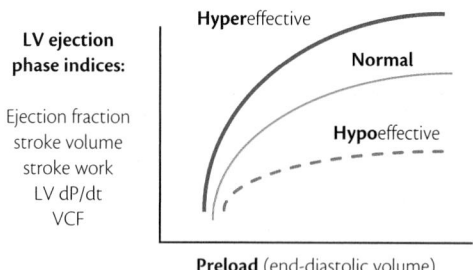

Fig. 17.4.1 Relationship between LV end-diastolic volume (preload) and LV ejection phase indices, including ejection fraction, stroke volume, stroke work, rate of change of LV pressure (dP/dt), and velocity of circumferential fibre shortening (VCF). Shown in the example are three curves of varying performance referred to as hypereffective, normal, and hypoeffective performance. Each ejection phase index is affected to a greater or lesser extent by changes in afterload and contractility.

and perfusion pressure is high, any process which impairs diastolic relaxation will decrease coronary blood flow.

Time-varying elastance

The entire LV contractile process can be understood better from the perspective, not of a single pressure–volume loop, but of the pressure–volume domain of contraction. In this context, as time progresses from the start of contraction to end ejection, the left ventricle becomes progressively more stiff (e.g. more elastic), such that the pressure may increase and the volume may decrease independent of preload and afterload characteristics, but where on the pressure–volume domain this point lies is a function of the stiffness or elastance of the ventricle. Time-varying elastance (E(t)) describes the progressive stiffening through systole and then its relaxation in diastole in the pressure–volume domain. It can be calculated as a plot of the slopes of the isochronic (similar point in time) pressure–volume relations during ejection as end-diastolic volume is rapidly varied (Fig. 17.4.3) by either rapid volume loading or occlusion of venous drainage. The slopes of these sequential pressure–volume lines reflect the obligatory LV pressure–volume domain that must be followed during systole.

The end-systolic elastance (Ees) is usually calculated from the regression line of the end-systolic pressure–volume data pairs of repetitive LV pressure–volume loops as either preload or afterload are rapidly varied. Ees is also referred to as the LV end-systolic pressure–volume relationship (ESPVR). Maximal elastance (Emax) is the maximal LV pressure–volume ratio and usually occurs just after end-systole due to the inertial and impedance hydrodynamic characteristics of the arterial tree. Increased contractility results in both a more rapid rise of (E(t)) to Ees and a higher Ees value. Using this construct, it becomes clear that the Frank–Starling relationship is the unidimensional description of the mechanical quality of ventricular ejection as described by time-varying elastance.

Applied cardiac physiology at the bedside

The preload-dependent nature of LV performance is central to the understanding of applied cardiac physiology. In fact, documenting that LVEDV is above some minimal value, despite cardiac output and stroke work both being depressed, is essential for the diagnosis of cardiac pump dysfunction. Similarly, demonstrating that LVEDV is reduced in the setting of haemodynamic instability presumes the diagnosis of inadequate circulating blood volume as

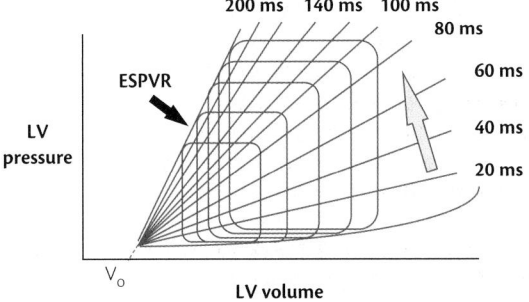

Fig. 17.4.3 Multiple LV pressure–volume relations over time with isochronic pressure–volume domains (time-varying elastance) drawn for all ventricles ending at the end-systolic pressure–volume relationship (ESPVR). Isochronic lines at 20-ms intervals. Note that LV time-varying elastance increases progressively from end diastole to end systole.

the most likely cause of the haemodynamic instability, even though other aetiologies, such as tamponade, cor pulmonale, and restrictive cardiomyopathies can coexist and require different treatments.

However, knowing LVEDV does not predict if LV stroke volume will increase in response to volume loading. Since a fundamental aspect of haemodynamic monitoring is to predict which patients will be preload-responsive, meaning that their cardiac output will increase in response to a fluid challenge, this lack of concordance between right atrial pressure, pulmonary artery occlusion pressure ('wedge' pressure), and even ventricular volumes, and subsequent changes in cardiac output in response to volume challenge can be disquieting. Still, it is a reality. However, there are three techniques of proven utility in defining preload responsiveness: the classic volume challenge, noting the magnitude of (1) the arterial pulse pressure or (2) left ventricular stroke volume variation during fixed tidal volume positive pressure ventilation, and (3) noting the change in mean cardiac output in response to a passive leg raising manoeuvre. For either pulse pressure variation (PPV, the ratio of maximal minus minimal pulse pressure to mean pulse pressure over five or more breaths) or stroke volume variation (SVV, the ratio of maximal minus minimal stroke volume to mean stroke volume over five or more breaths) to reflect preload responsiveness, the tidal volume must be fixed during unassisted positive pressure breathing and the sequential R-R intervals must be constant (i.e. no arrhythmias). In patients who are breathing spontaneously, and those with arrhythmias, the mean increase in flow 20 s after a passive leg raising to 30° gives a similar predictive value. In all cases, having a PPV greater than 13% or a SVV or mean increase in flow of more than 10% accurately predicts preload responsiveness as validated by many independent studies. PPV can be measured from the arterial pressure waveform and SVV calculated using numerous devices that assess beat-to-beat stroke volume using the arterial pressure waveform.

Arterial pressure and the vascular circuit

Organ perfusion is dependent on organ perfusion pressure and local vasomotor tone. Local vasomotor tone varies inversely with local tissue metabolic demand. For most organs, except the kidneys and heart, independent changes in arterial pressure above some minimal value are associated with increased vasomotor tone to maintain organ perfusion constant, hence this is essentially independent of cardiac function and cardiac output. In this circumstance, cardiac output is only important to allow parallel circuits to maintain flow without inducing hypotension, and cardiac function is only important in sustaining cardiac output and a given output pressure without causing too high a back pressure in the venous circuits.

Operationally, mean arterial pressure (MAP) is the input pressure to all organs other than the heart. Diastolic aortic pressure is the input pressure for coronary blood flow. Usually, MAP is equal to the diastolic pressure plus one-third the pressure pulse between diastole and systole. If, in a previously nonhypertensive subject, MAP decreases below 65 mmHg, then tissue perfusion will decrease independent of metabolic demand. Hypotension directly reduces organ blood flow and is synonymous with cardiovascular instability and is the essence of circulatory shock.

However, the assumption is often false that because MAP is the major central determinant of organ perfusion pressure, then organ perfusion must be adequate if MAP exceeds some minimal value. Intraorgan vascular resistance and venous outflow pressure are the two other determinants of organ blood flow. Furthermore, in severe stress situations, such as shock states, normal homeostatic mechanisms functioning through carotid body baroreceptors vary arterial vascular tone to maintain MAP relatively constant despite varying cardiac output, this vasoconstriction being done to maintain cerebral and coronary blood flow at the expense of the remainder of the body. In subjects with normal renal function, immediate oliguria is the manifestation of this adaptive response, reflecting marked reduction in renal blood flow and solute clearance by the kidneys despite persisting normal arterial blood pressure, hence normotension does not insure haemodynamic sufficiency. Indirect measures of sympathetic tone, such as heart rate, respiratory rate, and peripheral capillary filling and peripheral cyanosis are better estimates of cardiovascular status than is MAP.

Despite the lack of sensitivity of MAP to reflect haemodynamic sufficiency, measures of MAP are essential in the assessment and management of haemodynamically unstable subjects for several reasons. Measures that increase MAP will also increase organ-perfusion pressure. Hypotension causes coronary hypoperfusion, impairing cardiac function and cardiac output. Vasoconstrictor therapies will increase vasomotor tone in nonvital peripheral organs, but will maintain flow to the cerebral and coronary beds. It is also important to remember that the normal mechanism allowing autoregulation of blood flow distribution is local changes in organ inflow resistance, such that organs with increased metabolic demand vasodilate to increase their blood flow. If there is hypotension, then local vasodilation will not result in increased blood flow because the pressure gradient for that flow will also be reduced. Thus, hypotension impairs autoregulation of blood flow distribution. Vasopressor therapy can reverse systemic hypotension, but at a price: the only way that it can increase MAP is by reducing blood flow through vasoconstriction. Importantly, cerebral and coronary vascular circuits have minimal α-adrenergic receptors so their beds will not constrict. Regrettably, in hypovolaemic states vasopressor support may improve transiently both global blood flow and MAP, but at the expense of worsening local nonvital blood flow and hastening tissue ischaemia. Initial resuscitative efforts should therefore always include an initial volume expansion component and fluid challenge or other diagnostic approaches that identify preload-responsive shock states, before relying on vasopressors alone to support the unstable patient.

Cardiac output, oxygen delivery, and oxygen consumption

To support cellular metabolism, the circulation must deliver adequate amounts of oxygen (Do_2) and blood flow (cardiac output) to support oxidative phosphorylation. Do_2 is the product of cardiac output and arterial O_2 content. Within this construct, cardiac output and Do_2 are often used interchangeably, primarily because the greatest gain in Do_2 comes from varying cardiac output, not arterial O_2 content. However, like all simplification constructs, this one is also limited. Nonmetabolic blood flow, such as renal and splanchnic and skin blood flow, are essential to normal homeostasis. All of these processes need to be maintained under normal conditions and cannot be excluded for long in stress states without inducing marked end organ dysfunction.

Haemodynamic homeostasis

Since the primary goal of the cardiorespiratory system is to continuously maintain adequate Do_2 to meet the metabolic demands of the tissues, how can one assess its adequacy? As described above, neither LV preload nor MAP are sensitive or specific measures of adequacy of cardiovascular function. Although the best measure of circulatory sufficiency is the maintenance of normal bodily functions, this analysis is often difficult to assess accurately at the bedside during states of stress. Furthermore, since metabolic demand can vary widely, there is no value of cardiac output or Do_2 that ensures circulatory sufficiency. Under normal conditions, Do_2 and metabolic demand vary in parallel. However, as metabolic demands start to exceed Do_2 limits, either because of increased metabolic demand (e.g. seizures, fever, fighting the ventilator) or decreased delivery (e.g. circulatory shock and respiratory failure), the ability of the cardiovascular system to sustain O_2 consumption is stressed.

One cardinal sign of increased circulatory stress is an increased O_2 extraction ratio, which manifests itself as a decreasing mixed venous O_2 saturation (Svo_2). However, even this concept is useful only in limited conditions. Muscular activity effectively extracts O_2 from the blood because of the set-up of the microcirculatory flow patterns and the large concentration of mitochondria in these tissues. Thus, normal vigorous muscular activity can be associated with a marked decrease in Svo_2 despite a normal circulatory system. Muscular activities, such as moving in bed or being turned, 'fighting the ventilator', and breathing spontaneously increase O_2 consumption. In the patient with an intact and functioning cardiopulmonary apparatus, this will translate into an increase in both Do_2 and O_2 consumption and a decrease in Svo_2. However, in the sedated and ventilated patient, Svo_2 is a very sensitive marker of circulatory stress. There is no level of cardiac output which is 'normal', but there are Do_2 thresholds below which normal metabolism can no longer occur. Using Svo_2 as a sensitive but nonspecific marker of circulatory stress, values less than 70% connote circulatory stress, less than 60% identify significant metabolic limitation, and values less than 50% frank tissue ischaemia.

The various adaptive cardiovascular controls and varying metabolic demands make rules about specific haemodynamic variables of limited clinical utility. It is simply not possible to say that, when looking after a critically ill patient, the central venous pressure, or any other single measurable variable, must be kept at x or y. Table 17.4.1 lists some haemodynamic monitoring key points relevant to the critically ill patient.

Pathophysiology of shock

The heart, vascular integrity, vasomotor tone, and autonomic control all interact to sustain circulatory sufficiency. Circulatory shock reflects a failure of this system and results in an inadequate perfusion of the tissues to meet their metabolic demand, which can lead to cellular dysfunction and death. Numerous disease processes can result in circulatory shock, displaying surprisingly similar gross phenotypic expressions despite being caused by divergent processes whose treatments are equally different.

Weil and Shubin defined circulatory shock in 1968 as a decreased effectiveness of circulatory blood flow to meet the metabolic demands of the body. Four basic functional aetiologies of circulatory shock can be defined: (1) hypovolaemic, due to inadequate venous return (haemorrhage, dehydration), (2) cardiogenic, due

Table 17.4.1 The critically ill patient: haemodynamic monitoring key points

Key point	Explanation
Tachycardia is never a good thing	Tachycardia defines stress or an adaptation to stress. It may be necessary to sustain adequate blood flow, as in heart failure, but it still reflects heart failure.
Hypotension is always pathological	Hypotension impairs blood flow distribution and thus any patient with a MAP <65 mmHg is impaired. They may have hepatic cirrhosis with adequate tissue blood flow at rest, but they have a markedly limited ability to adapt to increased metabolic demand.
There is no such thing as a normal cardiac output	Since blood flow is regulated to meet the metabolic demand of the body, and that metabolic demand can vary widely and rapidly, there is no value of total cardiac output that guarantees adequate tissue perfusion. Blood flow is either adequate or inadequate, no matter what the absolute value is.
Central venous pressure is only elevated in disease	Under most conditions, the central venous pressure is very close to zero as the heart pumps all venous return immediately back to the body. The CVP will rise if either right or left sided heart failure develops, or fluid overload (due to renal failure and/or iatrogenic). The presence of an elevated CVP before medical intervention connotes disease of some sort.
Peripheral oedema is of cosmetic concern	Tissue perfusion is independent of interstitial fluid accumulation. Since the primary concern is maintenance of organ perfusion, which requires an adequate venous return and MAP, restricting fluid resuscitation in an unstable patient because of peripheral oedema is illogical and should be avoided.

CVP, central venous pressure; MAP, mean arterial pressure.

to inadequate ventricular pump function (myocardial infarction), (3) obstructive, due to vascular obliteration (pulmonary embolism or tamponade), and (4) distributive, due to loss of vasoregulatory control (sepsis).

Tissue hypoperfusion is common in all forms of shock, with the possible exception of hyperdynamic septic shock. This results in tissue hypoxia and a switch from aerobic to anaerobic metabolism, inducing hyperlactacidaemia and metabolic acidosis. However, hyperlactacidaemia, per se, is not a marker of ongoing tissue hypoperfusion because lactate clearance is often delayed or impaired in shock states, and processes such as exercise (seizure activity) can induce hyperlactacidaemia without cardiovascular insufficiency. Sustained circulatory shock results in cellular damage, not from anaerobic metabolism alone, but also from an inability to sustain intermediary metabolism and enzyme production necessary to drive normal mitochondrial performance. Metabolic failure due to sustained tissue hypoxia may explain why preoptimization and early goal-directed therapy improve outcome, whereas aggressive resuscitation after injury is not effective at reducing mortality from a variety of insults.

As stated above, measures of cardiac output, MAP and their changes in response to both shock and its treatment poorly reflect both regional blood flow and microcirculatory blood flow. Since most forms of haemodynamic monitoring measure global parameters like arterial pressure, heart rate, other vascular pressures, and cardiac output, it is clear that assessment of severity of shock and its initial response to therapy is often limited if monitoring is limited to these variables alone. Potentially, measuring Svo_2 or the difference between tissue Pco_2 and arterial Pco_2, referred to as the Pco_2 gap, would allow one to assess effective tissue blood flow since decreases in capillary blood flow initially causes CO_2 from aerobic metabolism to accumulate. Gastric tonometry describing Pco_2 gaps identifies gastric ischaemia and may be useful in guiding resuscitation in critically ill patients: sublingual Pco_2 gaps are much easier to measure and offer a readily simple bedside monitoring approach. However, gastric tonometry is confounded by CO_2 production from nonoxidative phosphorylation, and sublingual Pco_2 is not yet validated as a routine measure. Thus, at the present time, we are forced to use global measures of circulatory function, and determine which of the four shock categories is the most likely cause of organ dysfunction by noting their characteristic groupings of abnormalities, referred to as haemodynamic profile analysis.

Hypovolaemic shock

Hypovolaemia is the cardiovascular state in which the effective circulating blood volume is inadequate to sustain a level of cardiac output necessary for normal function without supplemental sympathetic tone or postural changes to ensure adequate amounts of venous return. It is a relative process and can occur through absolute blood loss, as with haemorrhage and trauma, or fluid and electrolyte loss, as with massive diuresis, diarrhoea, vomiting, or evaporation from large burn surfaces. The normal reflex response to hypovolaemia is increased sympathetic tone, vasoconstriction, and tachycardia. Cardiac output is often sustained by these mechanisms such that heart rate is increased and stroke volume decreased, whereas blood flow distribution is diverted away from the skin, resting muscles, and gut. With tissue hypoperfusion, lactic acidosis develops as a marker of tissue anaerobic metabolism. Thus, hypovolaemia initiates as tachycardia, reduced arterial pulse pressure, and (often) hypertension with a near normal resting cardiac output, followed by signs of organ hypoperfusion (oliguria, confusion) as cardiac output decreases. Systemic hypotension is the final presentation of hypovolaemic shock and—if the clinician waits for this before acting—ischaemic tissue injury is almost always present.

Cardiogenic shock

Cardiac pump dysfunction can be due to either LV or RV failure, or both. LV failure, as described above, is usually manifest by an increased LV end-diastolic pressure, left atrial pressure, and (by extension) pulmonary artery occlusion ('wedge') pressure, which must exist to sustain an adequate LV stroke volume. Tachycardia is universal in the patient who is not β-blocked.

The most common cause of isolated LV failure in the critically ill patient is acute myocardial infarction. Usually, LV stroke work is reduced and heart rate increased. In chronic heart failure both cardiac output and systemic vasomotor tone may be normal, whereas in acute LV failure states both may be reduced. These combined haemodynamic interactions lead Forrester and colleagues to use a pulmonary artery occlusion ('wedge') pressure of 18 mmHg and a cardiac index of 2.2 as the cut-off to define heart failure states following acute myocardial infarction. However, neither cardiac output nor systemic vascular resistance is a sensitive marker of LV failure until cardiogenic shock develops. Since pulmonary artery occlusion ('wedge') pressure is the back pressure to pulmonary blood flow, increases associated with LV failure may lead to pulmonary oedema and hypoxaemia, and secondary pulmonary hypertension may subsequently impair RV ejection, inducing biventricular failure, peripheral venous hypertension, and peripheral oedema formation, the so-called 'backward failure'.

The normal adaptive response of the host to impaired LV contractile function is to increase sympathetic tone, induce tachycardia, activate the renin-angiotensin system, retain sodium by the kidneys, and thus increase the circulating blood volume. Fluid retention takes time, whereas acute impairments of LV contractility can occur over seconds in response to myocardial ischaemia. Thus, the haemodynamic profile of acute and chronic LV failure can be different. Acute LV failure is manifest by increased sympathetic tone (tachycardia, hypertension), impaired LV function (increased filling pressure and reduced stroke volume), with minimal RV effects (normal central venous pressure), and increased O_2 extraction manifest by a low Svo_2. Cardiac output need not be reduced and may in fact be elevated, owing to the release of catecholamines as part of the acute stress response; vascular resistance is increased. By contrast, in chronic heart failure, although sympathetic tone is elevated, the heart rate is rarely over 105/min, and filling pressures are elevated in both ventricles consistent with combined LV failure and fluid retention. Again, cardiac output is not reduced except in severe heart failure states, but a cardinal finding is the inability of the heart to increase output in response to a volume load or metabolic stress (exercise). Furthermore, owing to the increased sympathetic tone, splanchnic and renal blood flows are reduced and can lead to splanchnic or renal ischaemia.

Obstructive shock

Obstruction in this context means mechanical obstruction of blood flow or ventricular filling. The most common cause of obstructive shock is pulmonary embolism leading to acute RV failure, but isolated RV dysfunction can occur in the setting of an acute inferior wall myocardial infarction, also as a consequence of pulmonary vascular disease (chronic obstructive pulmonary disease, primary pulmonary hypertension). When RV dysfunction predominates and is induced by pulmonary parenchymal disease, it is referred to as cor pulmonale, which is associated with signs of backward failure, elevated RV volume and pressures, systemic venous hypertension, low cardiac output, as well as reduced renal and hepatic blood flow. LV diastolic compliance decreases as the right ventricle dilates due to ventricular interdependence, either from intraventricular septal shift or absolute limitation of biventricular volume due to pericardial restraint. Thus, pulmonary artery occlusion ('wedge') pressure is often elevated for a specific LV stroke work, giving the erroneous appearance of impaired LV contractility, but if LVEDV were measured it is possible that no change in LV function would be seen if this were plotted against LV stroke work.

Neither pulmonary vascular resistance nor mean pulmonary artery pressure need be grossly elevated for RV failure to be present. Indeed, and importantly, if pulmonary arterial pressures are greater than 30 to 35 mmHg, then pulmonary hypertension is probably chronic in nature because acute elevations of pulmonary arterial

pressures above this level are not consistent with life. Elevations in central venous pressure of more than 12 mmHg also reflect fluid retention, suggesting further that there is a state of compensated RV failure.

Cardiac tamponade can occur from either (1) ventricular dilation limiting biventricular filling due to pericardial volume limitation, (2) acute pericardial effusion due to either fluid (inflammation) or blood (haemorrhage), which needs not be great in quantity, and (3) hyperinflation, which can act like pericardial tamponade to limit biventricular filling. The first two aetiologies are rarely seen, whereas the third commonly occurs. The cardinal sign of tamponade is diastolic equalization of all pressures, central venous pressure, pulmonary arterial diastolic pressure, and pulmonary artery occlusion ('wedge') pressure. Since RV compliance is greater than LV compliance, early on in tamponade there may be selective reduction in RV filling.

Distributive shock

Loss of blood flow regulation occurs as the endstage of all forms of circulatory shock, but as the initial presenting process it is common in sepsis, neurogenic shock, and adrenal insufficiency. Sepsis is a systemic process characterized by activation of the intravascular inflammatory mediators and generalized endothelial injury, but it is not clear that tissue ischaemia is an early aspect of this process. Acute septicaemia is associated with increased sympathetic activity (tachycardia, diaphoresis) and increased capillary leak with loss of intravascular volume. Before fluid resuscitation this combination of processes resembles simple hypovolaemia, with decreased cardiac output, normal to increased peripheral vasomotor tone, and very low Svo_2, reflecting systemic hypoperfusion. LV function is often depressed, but only in parallel with depression of other organs, and this effect of sepsis is usually masked by the associated hypotension that maintains low LV afterload. However, most patients with such a clinical presentation receive initial volume expansion therapy such that the clinical picture of sepsis reflects a hyperdynamic state rather than hypovolaemia, which has been referred to as 'warm shock' in contrast to all other forms of shock. The haemodynamic profile of sepsis is one of increased cardiac index, normal pulmonary artery occlusion ('wedge') pressure, elevated Svo_2, and a low to normal arterial pressure, consistent with loss of peripheral vasomotor tone.

Acute spinal injury, spinal anaesthesia, general anaesthesia, and central nervous system catastrophe all induce a loss of sympathetic tone. The resulting hypotension is often not associated with compensatory tachycardia, hence systemic hypotension can be profound and precipitate cerebral vascular insufficiency and myocardial ischaemia. Since neurogenic shock reduces sympathetic tone, biventricular filling pressures, arterial pressure, and cardiac output all decrease. Treatment consists of reversing the primary process and supporting the circulation with infusion of an α-adrenergic agonist, such as phenylephrine, dopamine, or noradrenaline.

Acute adrenal insufficiency can present with hyperpyrexia and circulatory collapse. This is more common than might be guessed, based on the epidemiology of adrenal cortical disease, because many patients are receiving chronic corticocosteroid therapy for the management of systemic and localized inflammatory states, such as asthma or rheumatoid arthritis, and in such cases the added stress of trauma, surgery, or infection can precipitate secondary adrenal insufficiency, as can the (unwise) discontinuation of long-term steroid treatment. Presentation is with nausea and vomiting, diarrhoea, confusion, hypotension, and tachycardia. Cardiovascular collapse is similar to that seen in neurogenic shock, except that the vasculature is not as responsive to sympathomimetic support. Accordingly, failure to respond to vasoactive pharmacological support in a patient who is hypotensive should suggest the diagnosis of adrenal insufficiency, when giving stress doses of corticosteroids usually reverses the unresponsive nature of the shock process.

Circulatory support of the haemodynamically unstable patient

If the cause of hypotension is intravascular volume loss, either absolute, as would occur with haemorrhage or massive diarrhoea, or relative, as would occur with loss of vasomotor tone or increased capillary endothelial permeability, then cerebral and coronary perfusion pressures must be maintained while fluid resuscitation is begun, otherwise cardiac pump failure may develop and limit the effectiveness of fluid resuscitation. Infusions of vasoactive agents will increase both cardiac output and MAP at the expense of the remaining vascular beds, hence fluid resuscitation to achieve an adequate intravascular blood volume is essential for sustaining isolated vasopressor therapy in the setting of systemic hypotension. Many pathological states and acute stress conditions are associated with either adrenergic exhaustion or blunted responsiveness to otherwise adequate circulating levels of catecholamines, e.g. diabetes, adrenal insufficiency, hypothermia, hypoglycaemia, and hypothyroidism. Furthermore, acute sepsis and systemic inflammation are associated with reduced adrenergic responsiveness. Thus, even if the host makes an otherwise adequate sympathetic response, the vasomotor and inotropic response may be inadequate, requiring transient use of potent sympathomimetic agents to sustain cardiovascular homeostasis.

Pharmacotherapy for cardiovascular insufficiency is directed at the pathophysiological processes that either induce or compound it. These therapies can be loosely grouped into one of three processes: (1) those that increase vascular smooth muscle tone (vasopressor therapy), (2) those that increase cardiac contractility (inotropic support), and (3) those that decrease smooth muscle tone (vasodilator therapy). Infusion of vasopressor agents are indicated to sustain a MAP greater than 60 mmHg to prevent coronary or cerebral ischaemia, while other resuscitative measures, like volume resuscitation, and specific treatment of the underlying condition are ongoing. This level of MAP is clearly arbitrary since some patients maintain adequate coronary and cerebral blood flow at lower MAP levels, whereas others—notably those with either pre-existent systemic hypertension or atherosclerotic cerebrovascular disease—may not tolerate MAP decreasing more than 30 mmHg from their baseline values. Once an adequate MAP has been achieved and intravascular volume losses corrected, care shifts toward maintaining adequate blood flow to metabolically active tissues to sustain organ performance.

Adrenergic receptor physiology

Most inotropes and vasopressors in clinical use are sympathomimetics that have direct effects on the adrenoreceptor system. Adrenoreceptors are complex membrane glycoproteins whose intracellular signal transduction is commonly, although not exclusively, mediated through G proteins and adenylate cyclase in an amplification type system. Adrenoreceptors are classically subtyped into six functional classes: myocardial β_1 and smooth muscular β_2, postsynaptic α_1 and dopamine$_1$ (DA_1), and presynaptic α_2 and DA_2. Despite several recent reports indicating that there are more classes of adrenoreceptors, conceptually the six subtypes serve clinicians well, with most functional issues relating only to α and β adrenergic receptor modulation. Importantly, there is a quantitatively unpredictable variation in adrenoreceptor density and function in many pathophysiological states, hence agents acting upon them need to be titrated to effect rather than being given at a defined infusion rate.

Vasopressor agents

Phenylephrine

The only noncatecholamine sympathomimetic used, phenylephrine differs chemically from other sympathomimetics by the absence of a hydroxyl group on position 4 of the benzene ring. This deletion reduces its potency relative to other sympathomimetics. It acts as a moderately potent α_1-agonist and is used in those patients in whom hypotension is due to decreased arterial elastance (it only activates β-adrenoreceptors at high doses). A modest direct coronary vasoconstrictor effect appears to be offset by autoregulatory mechanisms in the absence of flow-limiting coronary disease. It is not metabolized by catecholamine O-methyltransferase (COMT), which metabolizes catecholamines, and therefore its absolute half-life is considerably longer than catecholamine sympathomimetics.

Noradrenaline (norepinephrine)

Noradrenaline has significant activity at α and β_1-adrenoreceptors, resulting in a positive vasoconstrictor and inotropic effect. Its β_1 activity makes it the α_1-agonist of choice in the patient with hypotension and known LV dysfunction. Its positive vasopressor effect may enhance renal perfusion and indices of renal function in haemodynamically stable patients, and this effect may also be seen at higher doses when noradrenaline is used as a vasopressor in those with sepsis. Both observations are likely related to elevation of MAP, the input pressure for organ perfusion. However, concerns regarding renovascular vasoconstriction have led some practitioners to supplement high-dose noradrenaline infusions with a low-dose dopamine infusion to blunt potential ischaemic nephrotoxicity, with support for this practice coming from an animal investigation.

Adrenaline (epinephrine)

Adrenaline is a very potent catecholamine sympathomimetic that has markedly increased β_2-adrenoreceptor activity compared with its molecular substrate, noradrenaline. Adrenaline has potent chronotropic, inotropic, β_2-vasodilatory, and α_1-vasoconstrictor properties. Its net vasopressor effect is the end result of the balance between adrenaline-mediated β_2 and α_1 adrenoreceptor stimulation. At low doses this balance may result in no net pressor effect, with a fall in the diastolic blood pressure. Adrenaline, like noradrenaline, is known to have potent renovascular and splanchnic vasoconstrictor properties. Clearance rates are variable and mediated by both the COMT and monoamine oxidase systems.

Dopamine

Dopamine is the most controversial of the clinically utilized catecholamine sympathomimetics. This stems largely from claims for selective, dose-dependent, splanchnic and renovascular vasodilatory properties. Its dopaminergic properties do not reduce the incidence of renal failure in patients with shock when compared to noradrenaline. Dopamine stimulates the release of noradrenaline from sympathetic nerve terminals in a dose-dependent manner, with this indirect noradrenaline effect accounting for up to half of dopamine's clinically observed physiological activity. Cardiomyocyte noradrenaline stores are finite, accounting for tachyphylaxis to the positive inotropic effects of dopamine observed after approximately 24 h in patients with acute myocardial infarction.

Inotropic agents

Dobutamine

Dobutamine is a synthetic analogue of dopamine. It is utilized by continuous infusion as a positive inotrope, with the improvement in cardiac output noted to potentially increase renal blood flow, creatinine clearance, and urine output. As a β_1-agonist it will increase myocardial oxygen consumption, although autoregulatory increases in coronary blood flow usually fully compensate in the absence of flow-limiting coronary artery disease. A noted problem with dobutamine is the development of tachyphylaxis with prolonged (as little as 72 h) infusions, suggested to be due to the down-regulation of β_1-adrenoreceptors.

Dopexamine

Dopexamine is a synthetic dopamine analogue with significant β_2-adrenoreceptor agonist activity. Its splanchnic blood flow effects and positive inotropic activity have lead to enthusiasm for potential utility outside its primary indication, acute heart failure syndromes with hypertension and oliguria. Randomized controlled clinical investigations have demonstrated improvement in morbidity and mortality outcomes when dopexamine was utilized as the pharmaceutical of choice in achieving goal-oriented oxygen delivery values in perioperative critically ill patients.

Phosphodiesterase inhibitors

These agents are not widely used in the management of circulatory shock, but the two most commonly employed agents in this class are amrinone and milrinone. Both are bipyridines, and the class of drugs is otherwise known as 'inodilators' with reference to the two predominant dose-dependent modes of action identified. Conventional wisdom is that these agents are much more potent vasodilators than inotropes, with the difference in potency approaching 10 to 100-fold. Milrinone has a shorter half-life and is a more potent (10–15-fold) inotropic agent than amrinone, but from all other aspects they are similar agents. Both are eliminated by conjugation, with amrinone's biological half-life known to be extended in the presence of congestive heart failure. Their mechanism of action is not precisely known, but at least part of their activity is related to inhibition of phosphodiesterase type 3, found in high concentrations in cardiomyocytes and smooth muscle cells, and they may activate a sodium-dependent calcium channel. The end result is an increase in intracellular cAMP and calcium, with the physiological effect being an improvement in diastolic myocardial function, and for this reason these agents are felt to be positive lusiotropes. Clinically, they are used as positive inotropes, given by continuous intravenous infusion following a loading dose, with their catecholamine-independent mechanism of action making them theoretically attractive as inotropic support of choice in patients with potential β_1-adrenoreceptor down-regulation.

Vasodilators

Afterload reducing vasodilators act via vascular smooth muscle relaxation. Vascular dilatation is mediated by both nitric oxide (NO) and non-NO-based mechanisms, NO being a powerful, locally acting vascular smooth muscle relaxant. Among commonly used vasodilators in haemodynamically unstable patients, both sodium nitroprusside and glyceryl trinitrate (nitroglycerine) function as NO donors. Numerous other non-NO donor vasodilating agents are available, with hydralazine, clonidine, and inhibitors of the renin-angiotensin system being the most commonly employed non-NO-based vasodilators in patients with cardiovascular instability.

A simple approach to the pharmacotherapy of circulatory shock

Loss of vasomotor tone requires both fluid resuscitation to achieve the increased vascular volume needed to restore an effective pressure gradient for venous return, and increased α-adrenergic tone via sympathomimetic agents to restore arterial and venous vasomotor tone. Targets for resuscitation are an Svo_2 greater than 70% with a MAP greater than 60 mmHg. Impaired contractility requires afterload reduction, as tolerated, up to a decrease in MAP to approximately 70 mmHg, targeting pulmonary artery occlusion ('wedge') pressure less than 18 mmHg, and Svo_2 greater than 70%. In sepsis, Svo_2 is usually elevated following fluid resuscitation, hence resuscitation targets usually focus on reaching elevated levels of Do_2 (e.g. >450 ml/min per m^2). In states of RV failure, maintaining a MAP greater than pulmonary arterial pressure is essential to minimize RV myocardial ischaemia. Regrettably, the only prospective clinical trials documenting benefit from such resuscitation strategies were applied early in the course of sepsis or in high-risk surgical patients. However, it makes physiological sense to prevent organ ischaemia by maintaining blood flow, hence strategies such as those described above seem warranted in the absence of clinical trial evidence.

Further reading

Bland RD, *et al.* (1985). Hemodynamic and oxygen transport patterns in surviving and nonsurviving postoperative patients. *Crit Care Med*, **13**, 85–90.

Bellomo R, *et al.* (2000). Low-dose dopamine in patients with early renal dysfunction: a placebo-controlled randomised trial. Australian and New Zealand Intensive Care Society (ANZICS) Clinical Trials Group. *Lancet*, **356**, 2139–2143.

Cohn JN, *et al.* (1974). Right ventricular infarction: clinical and hemodynamic features. *Am J Cardiol*, **33**, 209–14.

Dorin RI, Kearns PJ (1988). High output circulatory failure in acute adrenal insufficiency. *Crit Care Med*, **16**, 296–7.

Forrester JS, *et al.* (1976). Medical therapy of acute myocardial infarction by application of hemodynamic subsets. *N Engl J Med*, **295**, 1356–62.

Heyland DK, *et al.* (1996). Maximizing oxygen delivery in critically ill patients: a methodologic appraisal of the evidence. *Crit Care Med*, **24**, 517–524.

Kandel G, Aberman A (1983). Mixed venous oxygen saturation. Its role in the assessment of the critically ill patient. *Arch Intern Med*, **143**, 1400–2.

Kern JW, Shoemaker WC (2002). Meta-analysis of hemodynamic optimization in high-risk patients. *Crit Care Med*, **30**, 1686–92.

Kumar A, *et al.* (2004). Pulmonary artery occlusion pressure and central venous pressure fail to predict ventricular filling volume, cardiac performance, or the response to volume infusion in normal subjects. *Crit Care Med*, **32**, 691–9.

Leier CV, *et al.* (1978). Comparative systemic and regional hemodynamic effects of dopamine and dobutamine in patients with cardiomyopathic heart failure. *Circulation*, **58**, 466–75.

Michard F, *et al.* (2000). Relation between respiratory changes in arterial pulse pressure and fluid responsiveness in septic patients with acute circulatory failure. *Am J Respir Crit Care Med*, **162**, 134–8.

Michard F, Teboul JL (2002). Predicting fluid responsiveness in ICU patients: a critical analysis of the evidence. *Chest*, **121**, 2000–8.

Monnet X, *et al.* (2006). Response to leg raising predicts fluid responsiveness during spontaneous breathing or with arrhythmia. *Crit Care Med*, **34**, 1402–7.

Nakagawa Y, *et al.* (1998). Sublingual capnometry for diagnosis and quantitation of circulatory shock. *Am J Respir Crit Care Med*, **157**, 1838–43.

Rivers E, *et al.* (2001). Early goal-directed therapy in the treatment of severe sepsis and septic shock. *N Engl J Med*, **345**, 1368–77.

Ross J Jr, Peterson KL (1973). On the assessment of cardiac inotropic state. *Circulation*, **47**, 435–8.

Ross J (1976). Afterload mismatch and preload reserve. *Prog Cardiovasc Dis*, **18**, 255–270.

Scheidt S, Ascheim R, Killip T 3rd (1970). Shock after acute myocardial infraction: A clinical and hemodynamic profile. *Am J Cardiol*, **26**, 556–64.

Shenkin HA, *et al.* (1944). On the diagnosis of hemorrhage in man: a study in volunteers bled large amounts. *Am J Med Sci*, **208**, 421–36.

Suga H, Sugawa K (1974). Instantaneous pressure–volume relationships and their ratio in the excised supported canine left ventricle. *Cir Res*, **35**, 117–26.

Tang W, *et al.* (1994). Gastric intramural PCO_2 as a monitor of perfusion failure during hemorrhagic and anaphylactic shock. *J Appl Physiol*, **76**, 572–77.

Thijs LG, Groenveld ABJ (1988). Peripheral circulation in septic shock. *Appl Cardiopulm Pathophysiol*, **2**, 203–14.

Weil MH, Shubin H (1968). Shock following acute myocardium infarction: Current understanding of hemodynamic mechanisms. *Prog Cardiovasc Dis*, **11**, 1–17.

Acute respiratory failure

Susannah Leaver and Timothy Evans

Essentials

Acute respiratory failure

Acute respiratory failure is defined clinically by hypoxaemia (Pa_{O_2} <8 kPa, normal range 10–13.3 kPa) with (type 2) or without (type 1) hypercapnia (Pa_{CO_2} >6.5 kPa). It is one of the most common problems afflicting the severely ill patient and often necessitates intensive care unit admission.

Clinical context—critical illness may be manifest solely as respiratory insufficiency, especially in patients with covert infection. Acute respiratory failure frequently coexists with other organ system failures in the critically ill, and delayed recognition of the condition has been shown to affect outcome adversely.

Clinical features—the signs of critical illness tend to be similar whatever the precipitating cause and are manifest in failure of the respiratory, cardiovascular, and neurological systems. The airway, breathing, circulation, disability, and exposure (ABCDE) approach to clinical assessment is advocated. Respiratory rate should normally be 12 to 20 breaths per minute: a higher or increasing rate is a 'hard' sign of critical illness. Full and repeated physical examination may be required to elucidate the cause of acute respiratory failure.

Investigation—pulse oximetry allows the continuous noninvasive monitoring of arterial oxygen saturation and is useful in all clinical settings. Arterial blood gas (ABG) analysis confirms the type and severity of acute respiratory failure. A full range of imaging modalities, particularly including computed tomography and echocardiography, may be required for diagnosis.

Management—the main steps in treating acute respiratory failure are:

(1) Establishing and securing the airway (if compromised)—this may require (1) endotracheal intubation—evaluating the need for this is a task that should be undertaken only by those experienced in the technique (usually an anaesthetist); the decision to intubate is based on a number of factors including (a) inability to maintain an airway, (b) exhaustion, (c) deteriorating physiological parameters despite the provision of adequate therapy, (d) reversibility of underlying condition; (2) tracheostomy—this may be indicated (and beneficial) early in the course of

acute respiratory failure in patients likely to require prolonged ventilatory support, but respiratory arrest consequent upon tracheostomy blockage with sputum or blood, although rare, is well documented and preventable.

(2) Increasing Fi_{O_2} to treat hypoxaemia—oxygen can be administered by a variety of different methods depending on the required oxygen concentration.

(3) Instituting mechanical ventilation (invasive or noninvasive) as necessary to treat impaired oxygenation and hypercapnia—noninvasive positive pressure ventilation involves the delivery of mechanically generated breaths via a tight-fitting nasal or full face mask. In patients receiving mechanical ventilation, the optimum mode depends in part upon the nature of the underlying illness, particularly the presence or absence of pulmonary parenchymal or airway pathology, the phase of the illness (acute or chronic), and the aims of support at the time it is applied.

(4) Identifying and managing the precipitating condition.

(5) Discontinuing and withdrawing support in stages ('weaning') as the underlying condition improves.

Acute lung injury and acute respiratory distress syndrome (ARDS)

Acute lung injury and ARDS are characterized by intense inflammatory reactions in the alveolar space. There are three identifiable phases: (1) exudative, characterized by increased pulmonary capillary permeability; (2) inflammatory, in which alveolar neutrophilia predominates; (3) fibroproliferative or reparative, during which inflammation gradually resolves, giving way to increased collagen deposition. These conditions complicate a wide variety of serious medical and surgical conditions, not all of which involve the lung directly.

Diagnosis—this requires:

(1) An appropriate clinical setting, with one or more recognized risk factors.

(2) New, bilateral, diffuse, patchy, or homogenous pulmonary infiltrates on chest radiography.

(3) No clinical evidence of heart failure, fluid overload, or chronic lung disease.

(4) Pao_2:Fio_2 ratio of less than 40 kPa (for acute lung injury) or <26.6 kPa (for ARDS).

Investigations—these are aimed at defining the extent of lung injury and elucidating the precipitating cause. Computed tomography (CT), if practical, may be useful in guiding therapy and detecting complications.

Management and prognosis—aside from other standard supportive measures, low tidal volume ('protective') ventilation has been shown to improve outcome. Overall mortality of patients with ARDS is in the range 25 to 40%, but higher in some subgroups (e.g. sepsis) than others (e.g. trauma). Survivors of ARDS may have persistent functional disability and require long-term follow-up and support.

Acute respiratory failure

Definition and epidemiology

Respiratory failure is defined by reduced arterial oxygen tension (Pao_2), with or without elevated levels of carbon dioxide ($Paco_2$), and is one of the most common problems necessitating intensive care unit (ICU) admission. Traditionally, it has been classified according to rapidity of onset (acute and chronic), and into hypoxaemic and hypoxaemic/hypercapnic subtypes. Chronic respiratory failure is discussed in Chapter 18.15.

Type 1 (hypoxic or acute hypoxaemic) respiratory failure is the most common cause of acute respiratory failure and is defined by hypoxaemia (Pao_2 <8 kPa, normal range 10–13.3 kPa) with a normal or low $Paco_2$ (normal range 4.8–6.1 kPa). It is attributable to a failure of gas exchange due to lung parenchymal damage and/or intrapulmonary shunting in which alveoli are perfused but not ventilated; extrapulmonary shunt may also occur (e.g. in patients with cyanotic heart disease). Common causes are shown in Table 17.5.1.

Type 2 (ventilatory or hypercapnic) respiratory failure is characterized by hypercarbia ($Paco_2$ >6.5 kPa) associated with hypoxaemia (Pao_2 <8 kPa) and is associated with a failure of alveolar ventilation through reduced minute ventilation, an inability to overcome an increased resistance to ventilation, or an increase in anatomical or physiological dead space. Common causes are shown in Table 17.5.1.

Although the above definitions are useful, they should not be used in isolation to dictate clinical management. Thus, in practice, patients may progress from type 1 to type 2 respiratory failure as the precipitating condition evolves. Moreover, either type of respiratory failure may complicate a wide variety of pathologies. The incidence, prevalence, and attributable mortality is therefore difficult to determine, particularly as acute respiratory failure often coexists with other organ system failures in the critically ill. Nevertheless, recent studies suggest an incidence in the order of 77.6 to 88.6 cases per 100 000 population per year, with an associated mortality rate of approximately 40%. While mortality for acute respiratory failure alone is probably better than this, death rates increase with each additional organ failure.

Clinical approach

History and examination

Acute respiratory failure can be caused by extrapulmonary as well as pulmonary causes. Clinical evaluation must therefore not be restricted to the respiratory system. Early identification of the deteriorating patient is essential, as delayed recognition and therapeutic intervention have both been shown to affect outcome adversely.

Prompt (and where necessary repeated) evaluation should commence where possible with the acquisition of a detailed history and physical examination. The signs of critical illness tend to be similar whatever the precipitating cause and are manifest in failure of the respiratory, cardiovascular, and neurological systems. Abnormal physiological signs are frequently encountered in patients cared for in general wards, and their charting and recognition is often inadequate. Medical early warning scoring systems and critical care outreach teams have been developed to address this deficiency, as have courses designed to educate more junior health care workers in relevant clinical skills, but there is no substitution for appropriate experience.

Clearly, if the patient has suffered a respiratory or cardiac arrest, or is in extremis, resuscitation and stabilization should be initiated immediately. The airway, breathing, circulation, disability, and exposure (ABCDE) approach is advocated, and is incorporated into the Resuscitation Council (UK) Guidelines. All clinicians practising at any level should be competent in providing life support of this type.

Alternatively, critical illness may be manifest solely as respiratory insufficiency. In these circumstances, the history should help to elicit the cause of the clinical deterioration. Thus, cough productive of green sputum in association with systemic disturbance suggests pneumonia; central chest pain and breathlessness in a patient with known cardiac disease is indicative of pulmonary oedema; a history of underlying chronic respiratory insufficiency such as chronic obstructive pulmonary disease (COPD) or asthma, with worsening breathlessness and wheeze, suggests an acute exacerbation of these conditions; and respiratory distress in patients with sepsis, trauma, multiple blood transfusions, or pancreatitis may be caused by incipient acute lung injury or acute respiratory distress syndrome (ARDS). Respiratory symptoms may also be a nonspecific indication of increased respiratory demand from a nonpulmonary source (e.g. in diabetic ketoacidosis, poisoning, acute renal failure).

Clinical examination should quantify the signs of respiratory distress (Table 17.5.2). The respiratory rate should normally be 12 to 20 breaths per minute, and a higher or increasing rate is a 'hard' sign of critical illness and a warning that the patient may deteriorate suddenly. The depth of each breath should be assessed, and whether chest expansion is bilateral and symmetrical. Reduced expansion and breath sounds with tracheal shift to the contralateral side are indicative of pneumothorax, and the presence of bronchial breathing of pneumonia. An inability to lie flat with pink frothy sputum and bilateral crackles is suggestive of pulmonary oedema. However, clinical examination may be unhelpful and clinical signs absent in conditions such as pulmonary thromboembolism or

Table 17.5.1 Causes of acute respiratory failure

Type of cause	Type 1 acute respiratory failure—PaO_2 <8 kPa (60 mmHg)	Type 2 acute respiratory failure—PaO_2 <8 kPa with $PaCO_2$ >6.5 kPa (50 mmHg)
Acute lung diseases	Pneumonia Acute asthma Pulmonary oedema Acute lung injury/acute respiratory distress syndrome Pneumothorax Lobar collapse Pulmonary contusion (blunt chest trauma) Aspiration Pleural effusion	Acute severe asthma Depression of respiratory drive, e.g. drug overdose (narcotic drugs) Upper airway obstruction, e.g. foreign body
Chronic lung diseases	Chronic obstructive pulmonary disease Pulmonary fibrosis Interstitial lung disease Lymphangitis carcinomatosis Pneumoconiosis Bronchiectasis Granulomatous lung diseases	Chronic obstructive pulmonary disease
Pulmonary vascular diseases	Pulmonary embolism Right-left shunts Pulmonary arterial hypertension Fat embolism	
Neuromuscular diseases		Myasthenia gravis Polyneuropathy Poliomyelitis Acute neuropathies, e.g. Guillain–Barré Primary muscle disorders, e.g. muscular dystrophy Primary alveolar hypoventilation Obesity hypoventilation syndrome Brainstem and cervical cord injury
Skeletal disorders		Chest wall deformities, e.g. kyphoscoliosis, ankylosing spondylitis Flail chest injury
Other		Exhaustion from any cause of type 1 respiratory failure

Table 17.5.2 Signs of respiratory distress and hypercapnia

General clinical signs of respiratory distress	Indicators of hypercapnia
Inability to speak in full sentences	Warm peripheries
Cyanosis	Bounding pulse
Sweating	CO_2 retention flap
Obstructed airway/stridor	Somnolence/lethargy/confusion
Tachycardia/bradycardia/arrhythmias	Decreased consciousness
Respiratory rate >25/min or <8/min	Headache
Use of accessory muscles of respiration	Asterixis
Intercostal recession	
Pulsus paradoxus	
Restlessness/agitation	
Asynchronous respiration	
Inability to lie flat	
Paradoxical respiration	

and haemoglobin levels. ABGs should be repeated following any intervention to assess improvement, which may require repeated arterial puncture or insertion of an indwelling catheter. Oximetry is an invaluable aid to monitoring (see below). Box 17.5.1 provides a stepwise approach to interpreting ABGs in patients with acute respiratory failure.

> **Box 17.5.1** Interpretation of arterial blood gases in acute respiratory failure
>
> Steps in interpreting arterial blood gas results:
>
> 1 Confirm presence of respiratory failure: is PaO_2 <8 kPa on room air?
> 2 What is the $PaCO_2$? Does the patient have type 1 or type 2 respiratory failure?
> 3 Is the A-a PO_2 gradient high (normal 2.6–8.7 kPa, 20–65 mmHg)?
> 4 If normal/low A-a gradient, is hypoxaemia due to hypoventilation?
> 5 If high A-a gradient, is hypoxaemia secondary to V/Q mismatch (e.g. chronic obstructive pulmonary disease, acute severe asthma, pulmonary embolism or shunt)?
> 6 If hypoxia improves with 100% oxygen then V/Q mismatch is likely.
> 7 If hypoxia does not correct with oxygen, respiratory failure is due to shunt (alveolar perfusion without ventilation).
>
> A-a gradient (PAO_2–PaO_2), alveolar–arterial gradient; PAO_2, alveolar partial pressure of oxygen, obtained from the alveolar gas equation; $PaCO_2$, partial pressure of carbon dioxide in arterial blood; PaO_2, partial pressure of oxygen in arterial blood, obtained from arterial blood gases; V/Q, ventilation/perfusion.

the incipient onset of acute lung injury. This is particularly so in patients in whom respiratory insufficiency is a secondary manifestation of pathology elsewhere.

Clinical investigations
Arterial blood gas analysis
Arterial blood gas (ABG) analysis confirms the type and severity of acute respiratory failure, with some ABG analysers providing additional valuable information concerning electrolyte, lactate,

Table 17.5.3 Blood tests often used in the assessment of patients with acute respiratory failure

Investigation	Utility
Full blood count	Anaemia contributes to tissue hypoxia; polycythaemia is indicative of chronic hypoxaemia.
Coagulation screen	Altered in disseminated intravascular coagulation.
Electrolytes, renal function, liver blood tests, C-reactive protein	Guide the clinician to associated complications, underlying causes, and premorbid conditions.
Phosphate and magnesium	Low levels aggravate respiratory failure.
Serum amylase	Pancreatitis is a common cause of acute lung injury/ARDS.
Thyroid function tests	Hypothyroidism is a rare cause of hypoventilation.
Creatine kinase and Troponin I	Can confirm or exclude recent myocardial infarction. A high creatine kinase with a normal troponin may indicate myositis.

ARDS, acute respiratory distress syndrome.

Blood tests

Haematological and biochemical indices can provide diagnostic information (Table 17.5.3).

Screening for infection

A full infection screen should be dispatched immediately. This should include samples for blood, sputum, and urine culture, especially if signs of sepsis, severe sepsis, or septic shock are present. Requests for typical and atypical (e.g. viral, legionella, mycoplasma) organisms should be made if clinically appropriate. Depending upon the immune status of the patient and the presence of underlying pathologies (e.g. malignancy, immunosuppression), evidence of tuberculous, and fungal infections should be sought. *Pneumocystis carinii* infection may induce type 1 respiratory failure.

Chest radiograph

A chest radiograph is essential in any patient with acute respiratory failure. It may be normal in patients with COPD or asthma, or following pulmonary thromboembolism. By contrast, areas of localized increased density (pneumonia, or pulmonary embolism with infarction), diffuse bilateral alveolar type shadowing (cardiogenic pulmonary oedema, acute lung injury/ARDS, diffuse pneumonia), or a pneumothorax may be visible.

Chest radiography is also mandatory following placement or repositioning of central venous catheters, endotracheal tubes, nasogastric tubes, and pleural drains. A daily chest radiograph is recommended in critically ill patients admitted to ICU.

Ultrasonography

If a pleural collection is suspected clinically or following plain chest radiography, then a diagnostic or therapeutic tap can be performed under ultrasonic guidance. Removal of moderate quantities of pleural fluid should improve ventilation, perfusion mismatch, oxygenation, and pulmonary compliance.

Computed tomography (CT)

Thoracic CT, especially high resolution and contrast-enhanced, can reveal pathologies not detected by a plain chest radiograph, such as pulmonary embolus, abscess cavity, parenchymal infiltrates, or pleural effusions. Transporting critically ill patients to and from the CT scanner is not without risk, but has been shown to identify at least one new significant finding resulting in a change in management in up to 30% of patients. Nonpulmonary causes of acute respiratory failure may also be revealed by CT examination of extrapulmonary sites such as abdomen or brain.

Electrocardiography and echocardiography

An ECG is necessary to identify arrhythmias and reveal evidence of cardiac ischaemia. Echocardiography (transthoracic, and particularly transoesophageal) is helpful in excluding cardiac causes for acute respiratory failure and may help to differentiate between pulmonary oedema and acute lung injury/ARDS.

Fibreoptic bronchoscopy

Fibreoptic bronchoscopy with directed bronchoalveolar lavage is useful for obtaining samples for microbiological and cytological examination. It may be indicated therapeutically for the alleviation of endobronchial obstruction, or for localizing sources of bleeding or a site of trauma. However, bronchoscopy should only be performed once the patient is stabilized and the airway secured, the only exception being when a bronchoscope is required to aid a difficult endotracheal intubation.

Respiratory monitoring
Arterial oxygen saturation (Sao_2)/pulse oximetry

A pulse oximeter can be attached to the finger or earlobe and allows the continuous noninvasive monitoring of arterial oxygen saturation by spectrophotometric analysis of the relative proportions of oxygenated and deoxygenated haemoglobin. This is useful in all clinical settings, especially the ward, during transfers, and in ICU, reducing the need for regular arterial blood gas analysis.

Oxygenation is usually regarded as acceptable if the Sao_2 is above 90%. A sudden drop in arterial oxygen saturation should prompt an immediate and full re-evaluation of the patient. However, it should be remembered that pulse oximetry is unreliable in a number of circumstances, especially if there is poor peripheral perfusion, nail polish has been applied, or if there is excessive movement or high ambient light. It does not measure arterial carbon dioxide levels and is unusable in patients with certain haemoglobinopathies (e.g. glucose-6-dehydrogenase (G6PD) deficiency).

Indwelling arterial catheter

Insertion of an arterial line not only provides invasive blood pressure monitoring, but permits repeated arterial blood gas analysis.

Estimation of lung function

In the mechanically ventilated patient (invasive or noninvasive) the efficiency of gas exchange can be quantified by the alveolar-arterial (A-a) Po_2 gradient or the Pao_2/fractional inspired oxygen concentration (Fio_2) ratio. Alveolar ventilation can be estimated through arterial and end-tidal CO_2 analysis. Most machines used to apply ventilatory support via an endotracheal tube provide breath by breath quantification of tidal volume, respiratory rate, minute volume (the product of tidal volume and respiratory rate), airway pressure and compliance. The latter is an index of the pressure-volume relationship of the respiratory system (elasticity) and is high when the lungs are distensible (e.g. in emphysema) and low when they are stiff (e.g. in acute lung injury/ARDS).

Compliance may also be adversely influenced by chest wall or abdominal pathology.

In self-ventilating patients, serial measurements of peak expiratory flow rate (PEFR) may be useful to assess therapeutic response (e.g. in asthmatics). Serial estimations of vital capacity are a useful indicator of deterioration in patients with neuromuscular problems involving the respiratory muscles, such as Guillain–Barré syndrome.

Capnography

A continuous measurement of exhaled carbon dioxide concentration mirrors $Paco_2$ and is therefore a useful indicator of alveolar ventilation in patients without significant airflow limitation. Portable machines are available and should always be used at endotracheal intubation, or when continuous capnography is unavailable.

Management

Once identified, the main steps in treating acute respiratory failure are:

+ Establishing and securing the airway (if compromised)

+ Increasing Fio_2 to treat hypoxaemia

+ Instituting mechanical ventilation (invasive or noninvasive) as necessary to treat impaired oxygenation and hypercapnia

+ Identifying and managing the precipitating condition

+ Discontinuing and withdrawing support in stages ('weaning') as the underlying condition improves

Airway management

Ensuring the patient has a patent airway and adequate oxygen supply is a therapeutic priority in all circumstances. Simple techniques such as head positioning (jaw thrust or head tilt) and removal of obstructions (e.g. dentures, secretions in the oropharynx) may alleviate the problem. However, insertion of a nasopharyngeal or oropharyngeal airway, which lifts the tongue off the posterior pharynx, and the application of positive-pressure ventilation using an Ambu or other type of self-inflating bag valve mask apparatus may be necessary to ensure adequate ventilation.

Continuing respiratory support can be delivered by a number of devices, including face masks, to increase Fio_2, and intermittent positive-pressure ventilation (IPPV) administered noninvasively (via nasal or full face mask) or invasively (via endotracheal tube or tracheostomy) to improve gas exchange and augment alveolar ventilation.

Endotracheal intubation

Evaluating the need for endotracheal intubation is a task that should be undertaken only by those experienced in the technique (usually an anaesthetist). The decision to intubate is based on a number of factors including:

+ Inability to maintain an airway—endotracheal intubation is mandatory in patients with a Glasgow Coma Score of 8 or less

+ Exhaustion—elective intubation is infinitely preferable to an emergency procedure, the latter being associated with increased morbidity and mortality

+ Deteriorating physiological parameters (specifically arterial gas tensions, acid base status, and respiratory rate) despite the provision of adequate therapy

+ Reversibility of underlying condition—intubation and mechanical ventilation are not therapeutic interventions and supporting

respiration in this manner may be inappropriate in patients with terminal illness or irreversible pathology

General indications for endotracheal intubation are shown in Box 17.5.2 and complications listed in Table 17.5.4. The equipment, sedative and neuromuscular blocking agents required, and the exact techniques employed are beyond the scope of this chapter.

Tracheostomy

Tracheostomy is a useful intervention in patients who require airway protection and toilet, or prolonged periods of assisted ventilation. A tracheostomy is better tolerated and more comfortable than prolonged endotracheal intubation and thereby permits sedation to be decreased. Resistance to airflow is reduced and dead space diminished, thereby aiding weaning. Tracheostomies facilitate communication, oral nutrition, removal of secretions, and prevent the nasal, laryngeal, and pharyngeal complications associated with endotracheal intubation.

The timing of insertion of a tracheostomy remains controversial and was the subject of a multicentre trial in the United Kingdom (2007). However, meta-analysis of the small number of trials performed to date indicates a reduced duration of ventilation and shorter ICU length of stay among patients who have undergone tracheostomy early (i.e. within 7 days of endotracheal intubation). The procedure can be performed surgically or (in the ICU setting) percutaneously, using a Seldinger technique with bronchoscopic guidance. Although tracheostomies are associated with fewer complications than endotracheal intubation, those that do develop can be more serious (Table 17.5.5). As with endotracheal tubes, cuff pressure should be measured regularly and maintained between 24 to 30 mmH_2O (usually at 25 mmH_2O). Table 17.5.6 shows the different types of tracheostomy that are available.

Box 17.5.2 Indications for endotracheal intubation and mechanical ventilation

+ Protection of airway from gastric aspiration and secretions in an obtunded patient (Glasgow Coma Score <8)

+ Airway obstruction

+ Apnoea with cardiopulmonary or respiratory arrest

+ Inadequate oxygenation (Pao_2 <8 kPa or saturation <90%) despite Fio_2 >0.6 and the use of CPAP

+ Hypercapnia with associated impaired conscious level, acidosis (pH <7.25), or risk of raised intracranial pressure

+ To control and remove excess bronchial secretions

+ Exhaustion (to remove the work of breathing)

+ Respiratory rate >35 or <10 breaths/minute (normal range 10–20)

+ Vital capacity <15 ml/kg (normal 65–75), <1 litre or <30% predicted (especially in a patient with neuromuscular disease)

+ Tidal volume <5 ml/kg (normal range 5–7)

+ Inadequate inspiratory force <25 cm H_2O (normal 75–100)

CPAP, continuous positive airway pressure; Fio_2, inspired oxygen concentration; Pao_2, arterial partial pressure of oxygen.

Table 17.5.4 Complications associated with endotracheal intubation

Immediate	Upper airway and nasal trauma
	Dental damage
	Oropharyngeal laceration
	Laceration or haematoma of vocal cords
	Tracheal laceration
	Hypoxia secondary to oesophageal intubation
	Intubation of right main bronchus
	Aspiration of gastric contents
Early	Leaks around the endotracheal tube
	Displacement of endotracheal tube
	Endotracheal tube obstruction
Prolonged	Sinusitis
	Tracheal necrosis
	Tracheal stenosis
	Tracheomalacia
	Glottic oedema
	Ventilator associated pneumonia
	Ventilator induced lung injury

Table 17.5.5 Complications associated with tracheostomy

Timing	Complication
Immediate	Haemorrhage
	Death
	Hypoxia and respiratory distress
	Tube misplacement, formation of a false lumen
	Pneumothorax and pneumomediastinum secondary to tube misplacement
	Subcutaneous emphysema
	Cuff leak
	Damage to posterior tracheal membrane
Intermediate	Occlusion secondary to build-up of secretions
	Stomal colonization and infection
	Haemorrhage secondary to erosion of the anterior tracheal wall or innominate artery
	Tracheal ulceration and necrosis secondary to excessive cuff pressure
	Tracheo-oesophageal fistula as a result erosion of the tracheal cartilage
	Pneumonia
Late	Tracheal necrosis and stenosis
	Tracheitis
	Tracheo-oesophageal fistula
	Overgranulation of the tissue surrounding the trachea

Table 17.5.6 Types of tracheostomy

Type of tracheostomy	Characteristic	Comments
Single lumen	No inner tube	
Double lumen	Inner and outer tube	The double lumen permits removal of the inner tube for cleaning. The inner tube can be replaced with a fenestrated one for weaning
Cuffed	Has a cuff at the distal end to provide a seal around the trachea	Provides a seal for mechanical ventilation and prevents aspiration of gastric contents
Uncuffed		Rarely used in ICU. Used in long-term patients in the community, where the advantages are that (1) if a blockage occurs the patient can breathe around the tube, (2) the patient can talk, and (3) they cause less trauma
Fenestrated	The inner tube has a small opening	Fenestrated tubes facilitate normal breathing, weaning, and talking
Unfenestrated	The inner tube has no small opening	
Adjustable flange tracheostomy tube		Supports tracheostomy and prevents displacement. Used in patients with structural abnormalities such as kyphoscoliosis or obesity
Mini-tracheostomy	Small (3.5–4 mm diameter) and uncuffed	Used in patients who have been successfully weaned but require regular suctioning for sputum clearance. These patients may have an ineffective cough or neurological impairment

Management of tracheostomies in the non-ICU setting Tracheostomies are employed increasingly in patients cared for on general medical and surgical wards. Respiratory arrest consequent upon tracheostomy blockage with sputum or blood, although rare, is well documented and preventable. Emergency equipment must be immediately available and should include a new tracheostomy tube; one the size of that *in situ*, and one a size smaller. Patients with tracheostomies on the general ward require care delivered by an experienced multidisciplinary team including physiotherapists, dieticians, speech and language therapists, and doctors. Ideally, patients should have a double lumen tracheostomy *in situ*, which permits removal and cleaning of the inner sleeve.

Tracheostomies should be suctioned regularly in patients with excess bronchial secretions. When suctioning a tracheostomy, a nonfenestrated inner tube must be in place. Tracheostomies should be changed by an experienced practitioner (often using local anaesthetic and over a catheter or guide) every 4 to 6 weeks according to the manufacturers' instructions. If a tracheostomy falls out, high flow oxygen should be administered over the nose and mouth. If the stoma has been fashioned for more than 7 days and a track has clearly been established, then the tube can usually be reinserted immediately. If the tracheostomy is less than 7 days old, reinsertion

Table 17.5.7 Oxygen delivery systems

Method of delivery	FiO$_2$ achieved	Type of patient
Nasal cannula (1–2 litres/min)	0.24–0.30	Stable patients
Venturi mask	0.24–0.50	Type 2 respiratory failure and COPD
Partial rebreathing mask	0.60–0.80	Acute type 1 respiratory failure, e.g. pneumonia, asthma, and acute pulmonary oedema
Nonrebreathing reservoir mask	Up to 0.90	Severely hypoxic patients
Anaesthetic face mask or endotracheal tube	Up to 1.0	Patients requiring intubation

COPD, chronic obstructive pulmonary disease; FiO$_2$, inspired oxygen concentration.
Modified from Warrell DA, *et al.* (eds) (2003). *Oxford Textbook of Medicine*, 4th edition. Oxford University Press.

into a false track is possible and should not be attempted by the inexperienced. Following reinsertion, the position of the tube must be confirmed by chest radiography.

If a patient with a tracheostomy *in situ* shows signs of respiratory distress or desaturates, high flow oxygen should be administered, the tracheostomy suctioned, and/or the inner tube removed. If it remains blocked, the tracheostomy should be removed and the patient ventilated with a bag valve mask until expert help arrives. If the tracheostomy is patent, an alternative cause of respiratory distress must be sought.

Oxygen therapy

Oxygen is administered by a variety of different methods depending on the required oxygen concentration (Table 17.5.7). Systems used for the delivery of oxygen can be broadly classified into fixed and variable performance devices. The flow rate of gas supplied, the volume of the mask itself, and the presence of holes or other entrainment systems determines into which category the device fits.

Fixed performance devices

These are designed to provide a constant and predictable inspired oxygen concentration, irrespective of the patient's ventilatory pattern.

Table 17.5.8 Different modes of ventilation and mechanical respiratory support

Mode	Description	Trigger mechanism	Advantages	Disadvantages
CMV/IPPV	The ventilator will deliver a preset number of mandatory pressure or volume controlled breaths	Ventilator	Full control of ventilation Useful for initial control of ventilation and in patients with poor respiratory drive or cardiac instability	No spontaneous breaths Patient-ventilator dyssynchrony May require heavy sedation ± neuromuscular blockade
Assist control	Volume controlled The patient can trigger a breath resulting in a machine-delivered preset tidal volume. If the patient is apnoeic the ventilator will trigger	Patient or ventilator	Work of breathing requirement small A minimum minute volume is guaranteed	Can lead to high respiratory rate and therefore hypocapnia and respiratory alkalosis
SIMV	Combination of spontaneous ventilation (pressure supported) and mandatory machine-triggered (tidal volume) ventilation	Patient or ventilator	Guaranteed minimum minute volume Avoids breath stacking Useful mode for weaning by gradual reduction of mandatory breaths Enables avoidance of heavy sedation or paralysis	Dyssynchrony Increased work of breathing
PSV/ASB	The ventilator augments the patient's spontaneous breaths with a preset positive pressure	Patient	Useful for weaning by gradually reducing pressure support	Under and overventilation is possible Dyssynchrony
BIPAP	The ventilator cycles between two pressures and the patient can breathe spontaneously at any point	Patient or ventilator	Useful for weaning Less sedation required	Tidal volume not constant
PEEP	Continuous positive pressure in expiration Used in conjunction with other modes of ventilation	Depends on ventilation mode selected	Allows recruitment of alveoli, thus improving oxygenation Lungs work above the lower inflection point thus improving work of breathing	May reduce cardiac output by reducing venous return Increases risk of barotrauma
CPAP	Continuous positive pressure throughout respiratory cycle		Prevents reduction in functional residual capacity and associated collapse of lung units Used in weaning Can be used noninvasively in patients with type 1 respiratory failure	Mask CPAP discourages coughing and may increase risk of aspiration

ASB, assisted spontaneous breathing; CMV, controlled mechanical ventilation; CPAP, continuous positive airway pressure; IPPV, intermittent positive-pressure ventilation; PSV, pressure-support ventilation; SIMV, synchronized intermittent mandatory ventilation; BIPAP, biphasic positive airway pressure; PEEP, positive end-expiratory pressure.

Oxygen is passed through a jet in the mask, which entrains air through ports in the side. The total flow rate of gas to the mask should exceed the peak inspiratory flow rate of the patient at rest. Examples of fixed performance devices include the Venturi, Hudson, and MC masks.

Variable performance devices

These provide an inspired oxygen concentration (Fio_2) which varies according to the gas flow rate and patient's ventilatory pattern. Most patients require only a modest increase in Fio_2 to overcome the combined effects of mild hypoventilation, diffusion hypoxia, and some degree of ventilation/perfusion mismatch. In these circumstances an Fio_2 of 0.3 is usually adequate, which is achieved by supplying a flow rate of 4 litres/min to any of the variable performance devices. However, in patients with COPD and/or type 2 respiratory failure ventilatory drive is largely stimulated by hypoxaemia. If this is relieved by the administration of oxygen in an uncontrolled fashion (e.g. applying a large increase in Fio_2 via a variable performance device), then arterial oxygen tension rises and respiratory drive is depressed. This leads to reduced entrainment of room air, an increase in the proportion of oxygen inhaled, and respiratory drive is further reduced.

In rare circumstances a high Fio_2 is needed. Large capacity systems are required to achieve this. Modern devices therefore have an added reservoir bag and large effective dead space, with the capacity for significant CO_2 storage. Nevertheless, using these masks, an Fio_2 up to 85% can be achieved using oxygen flows of 10 litres/min or greater. However, considerable CO_2 rebreathing occurs if the oxygen supply fails or is reduced. Rebreathing can be eliminated and delivered Fio_2 increased still further if unidirectional valves are added. However, high inspired oxygen concentrations administered for prolonged periods can cause direct cellular toxicity and resorption atelectasis and should be avoided where possible.

Mechanical ventilation

The primary aim of mechanical ventilation is to support adequate gas exchange, while minimizing side effects. In the modern ICU, microprocessor controlled mechanical ventilators are employed to supply intermittent positive-pressure ventilation (IPPV). During inspiration the machine generates and delivers a flow of gas of preset Fio_2 into the lungs, cycling to expiration after a specified tidal volume has been delivered (volume cycling), or more commonly after a given time period has elapsed (time cycling), or when a certain pressure is reached within the respiratory circuit (pressure cycling). Customarily, the nature of the breath supplied can be modified by adjusting the flow rate with which the gas is delivered.

Modes of mechanical ventilation (Table 17.5.8)

The optimal mode of ventilation depends in part upon the nature of the underlying illness, particularly the presence or absence of pulmonary parenchymal or airway pathology, the phase of the illness (acute or chronic), and the aims of support at the time it is applied (e.g. delivery of IPPV or weaning). Volume-cycled modes are unforgiving of low compliance and have largely been discarded. Time-cycled modes permit the use of an inspiratory breath hold or plateau pressure, thereby facilitating gas exchange, and can be used to shorten inspiration and prolong expiration, which is desirable in patients with significant airflow limitation. Pressure-cycling modes involve the cyclical provision of a preset inspiratory pressure and positive end-expiratory pressure (PEEP), the tidal volume delivered being dependent upon airway resistance, lung compliance, and the set inspiratory time. During inspiration, the ventilator delivers the preset pressure and sustains it for a given inspiratory time before cycling into expiration. Pressure modes facilitate alveolar recruitment and reduce lung injury by limiting peak inspiratory pressure.

Positive end-expiratory pressure (PEEP)

PEEP prevents the baseline airway pressure returning to atmospheric (0 cmH_2O on the ventilator manometer) at end expiration. This prevents alveolar collapse, thereby increasing functional residual capacity and compliance. In addition, recruitment of atelectatic alveoli is encouraged, and V/Q mismatch reduced. Lymphatic drainage may be stimulated, decreasing alveolar oedema and further improving oxygenation. PEEP is applied in conjunction with other modes of ventilation. Its main disadvantage is that peak and mean inspiratory pressures are raised, thereby reducing venous return and increasing right ventricular afterload and therefore impairing cardiac output.

Complications of mechanical ventilation

These are summarized in Table 17.5.9.

Noninvasive ventilation (NIV)

Noninvasive positive pressure ventilation involves the delivery of mechanically generated breaths via a tight-fitting nasal or full face mask. Most modern systems deliver gas to preset inspiratory (IPAP) and expiratory (EPAP) positive airway pressures. Other terms used for NIV include noninvasive pressure support ventilation (NIPSV), nasal/noninvasive intermittent positive pressure ventilation (NIPPV), and bilevel positive pressure ventilation or BIPAP, a specific bilevel ventilatory mode. Continuous positive airway pressure (CPAP) is sometime incorporated under the general term noninvasive ventilation as it can also be delivered via a nasal or full face mask. NIV also incorporates negative pressure ventilation such as jacket (cuirass) ventilators which are now rarely used.

Noninvasive ventilation has been successfully used in the management of patients with chronic hypercapnic respiratory failure secondary to neuromuscular disease, in those with chest wall deformities, and in patients with impaired central respiratory drive. It has also been used successfully in the support of patients with acute lung injury.

In the acute setting, the evidence base supporting the use of NIV is most complete in patients with acute exacerbations of COPD who do not require immediate endotracheal intubation. Following ICU admission, NIV significantly reduces the need for intubation (26% in NIV group vs 64% in standard group) and thus the associated complications. Length of stay and inpatient mortality are both reduced. A similar study has supported the use of NIV on medical wards in patients with COPD with mild to moderate acidosis. Other benefits of NIV include the facilitation of ventilation 'breaks' for food and drugs, easier communication, earlier mobilization, more cooperation with physiotherapy, and cough preservation.

A trial of NIV can therefore be advocated in patients with acute exacerbations of COPD who have a persistent respiratory acidosis (pH <7.35) despite controlled oxygen therapy and maximal medical treatment. Prior to its institution, however, a decision should be made as to whether the patient will proceed to endotracheal intubation if deterioration should occur. In some patients, endotracheal intubation is not appropriate and NIV is employed as a 'ceiling' therapy. It can be delivered on general medical wards if staff have received

Table 17.5.9 Complications associated with mechanical ventilation

System affected	Complication	Comment
Cardiac	Reduced cardiac output	Positive pressure ventilation increases intrathoracic pressure, causing a reduction in venous return and thus stroke volume and cardiac output
Renal	Reduced renal perfusion Salt and water retention (especially when associated with PEEP)	As a result of a reduced cardiac output Due to increased ADH secretion, reduced renal blood flow, and a reduction in antinatriuretic peptide secretion
Respiratory	Ventilator induced lung injury Pneumothorax Pneumomediastinum Pneumopericardium Subcutaneous emphysema Ventilator-associated pneumonia	Due to ventilation with high tidal volumes resulting in overdistension of the alveoli Due to barotrauma Early recognition and prompt management of a tension pneumothorax is essential. This is nosocomial pneumonia developing more than 48 h postintubation. It is partly due to microaspiration of gastric contents or nasopharyngeal secretions and is associated with increased mortality
Gastrointestinal	Abdominal distension and ileus Stress ulceration	Also associated with the use of opiates The most common cause of gastrointestinal bleeding in ICU. Associated with an increased mortality when compared to patients without bleeding
Neurological	Critical illness myopathy and polyneuropathy	Attributed to steroid and paralysing agents and associated with the systemic inflammatory response syndrome
Others	Oxygen toxicity Ventilator failure or disconnection	High inspired oxygen concentrations can cause reabsorption atelectasis and direct cellular toxicity. It is usual clinical practice to decrease the inspired oxygen concentration to <60% where possible Alarms must be in place to alert the clinicians of ventilator failure or disconnection. A bag valve mask for manual ventilation and oxygen should be available at each bed space

appropriate training, and provided that monitoring with continuous pulse oximetry and regular arterial blood gas analysis is available. The benefit to patients with more severe acidosis (pH <7.25) is less clear and NIV should be administered on ICU where facilities for endotracheal intubation are readily available. See Chapters 18.8 and 18.15 for further discussion of the management of patients with COPD and chronic respiratory failure respectively.

The evidence base concerning the benefits of NIV is less strong for patients with acute respiratory failure secondary to restrictive lung disease, cystic fibrosis/bronchiectasis, acute lung injury, trauma, and postoperatively. It is probably reasonable to attempt a trial of NIV for hypoxaemic respiratory failure in such cases, but preferably in the ICU setting if the patient is a candidate for endotracheal intubation. If there is no significant improvement in pH, $Paco_2$ and respiratory rate after 1 to 2 h of NIV, the trial is likely to fail and invasive ventilation must be considered. NIV is not routinely recommended for the treatment of acute exacerbations of asthma.

NIV has also been shown to be of benefit in some groups of patients to aid weaning (see below).

Box 17.5.3 and Table 17.5.10 show the contraindications and complications of NIV.

Continuous positive airway pressure (CPAP)

CPAP can be supplied either via an endotracheal tube or to a conscious patient via a tightly fitting face mask. It is generated either using a bellows/pressure device, or through a flow generator. Gas must be delivered at a sufficient flow rate to ensure that airway pressure does not fall below zero during inspiration, with a positive end-expiratory pressure valve fitted to the system.

CPAP can be used in a trial of spontaneous ventilation at the end of weaning from mechanical ventilation. It may also be given noninvasively via a face mask in patients with hypoxic (type 1) respiratory failure. In patients with cardiogenic pulmonary oedema that remain hypoxic despite medical therapy, CPAP has been shown to reduce intubation rates, with a trend towards reduced mortality.

Weaning from mechanical ventilation

Patients who have received only a few days of mechanical ventilation should not require weaning and a trial of spontaneous breathing via the endotracheal tube using an open 'T piece' or similar circuit can be used to predict those that are likely to be extubated successfully. Generally, patients can be extubated once they are fully alert and able to protect their airway, their underlying pathology has improved or resolved, and their respiratory muscle strength is adequate for normal respiration.

Box 17.5.3 Contraindications to noninvasive ventilation

- Reduced Glasgow Coma Score/inability to protect airway
- Confusion/agitation
- Life-threatening hypoxaemia
- Vomiting
- Recent facial, upper airway, or upper gastrointestinal surgery
- Fixed upper airway obstruction
- Facial abnormalities, e.g. trauma or burns
- Bowel obstruction
- Excessive secretions
- Haemodynamic instability
- Undrained pneumothorax

Table 17.5.10 Limitations of noninvasive ventilation

Limitations	Comment
Mask leak and discomfort	Can be minimized by correct mask fitting: numerous, different sized, full face and nasal masks are available
Nasal bridge ulceration	Protective barrier dressings can be used to reduce this
Gastric dilatation and vomiting	A nasogastric tube should be inserted, although this may increase leak
Lack of airway protection	If a patient is unable to protect their airway, an endotracheal tube should be inserted
No endotracheal suction	Patients often require regular physiotherapy
Exact FiO_2 delivered unknown	Oxygen is entrained proximally in the circuit or directly into the mask. Pulse oximetry and ABGs are used to guide oxygen enrichment
Exact tidal volume and minute volume delivered unknown	Due to leak

ABG, arterial blood gas; FiO_2, inspired oxygen concentration.

Table 17.5.11 Causes of acute lung injury and acute respiratory distress syndrome (ARDS)

Pulmonary causes	Nonpulmonary causes
Pneumonia	Sepsis
Aspiration of gastric contents	Severe trauma
Inhalational injury	Cardiopulmonary bypass
Hypoxia/reperfusion injury	Massive transfusion
Fat emboli	Drug overdose
Pulmonary contusion	Acute pancreatitis
Near drowning	

Weaning is the term used to describe the gradual reduction and withdrawal of ventilatory support, during which the work of breathing is transferred back to the patient. Prolonged mechanical ventilation is associated with increased morbidity and mortality and increases the risk of weaning failure. Weaning involves the gradual increase in the amount of time the patient is breathing spontaneously, while gradually decreasing the level of ventilatory support. Modes of ventilation used in weaning include synchronized intermittent mandatory ventilation (SIMV), BIPAP, assisted spontaneous breathing (pressure support), and CPAP. If a patient is thought to require a long period of ventilation a tracheostomy may be inserted. In patients with COPD, noninvasive ventilation can be used to continue weaning following extubation: this has been shown to reduce weaning time, shorten ICU length of stay, reduce nosocomial pneumonia, and improve 60-day survival rates.

Although a number of tests and indices are sometimes used to assess whether a patient will be able to breathe spontaneously or not, ultimately the decision on the speed of weaning and time of extubation/decannulation will be based on clinical experience and judgment (see also Box 17.5.4).

Acute lung injury and acute respiratory distress syndrome (ARDS)

Definition

Acute lung injury and its extreme manifestation, ARDS, complicate a wide variety of serious medical and surgical conditions, not all of which involve the lung directly (Table 17.5.11). Both are defined by refractory hypoxaemia associated with lung inflammation and increased pulmonary vascular permeability. The first widely accepted radiological and physiological criteria were developed by an American-European Consensus Conference (AECC) (Box 17.5.5), which recognized acute lung injury and ARDS as separate but related states on a continuum of pulmonary damage. The emergence of these criteria greatly facilitated the design of clinical investigations in permitting direct comparisons between patient groups with widely differing underlying pathologies to be enrolled in trials of putative therapeutic interventions. However, the current definitions take no account of the prognostic significance of the precipitating condition, fail to specify the ventilatory strategy to be used when the presence and severity of hypoxaemia are established, and make no recommendation concerning the

Box 17.5.4 Steps for ventilatory weaning and decannulation of tracheostomy

1 Gradually reduce mechanical ventilation
2 Try spontaneous breathing with tracheostomy cuff down
3 Increase periods of time with cuff down
4 Occlude tracheostomy with finger to ensure adequate airflow through patient's nose and mouth
5 Try speaking valve—ensure fenestrated inner tube and cuff is down
6 Once the patient can tolerate 4 h or more with the speaking valve *in situ*, try capping tracheostomy
7 If the patient can manage with the tracheostomy capped for more than 4 h, has a good cough, is able to expectorate, and is stable on <0.4 FiO_2, then decannulate

Box 17.5.5 Definitions of acute lung injury and acute respiratory distress syndrome (ARDS)

- Appropriate clinical setting with one or more recognized risk factors (Table 17.5.11)
- New, bilateral, diffuse, patchy, or homogenous pulmonary infiltrates on chest radiograph
- No clinical evidence of heart failure, fluid overload, or chronic lung disease (pulmonary artery occlusion pressure, PAOP <18 mmHg)
- PaO_2:FiO_2 ratio of <40 kPa (for acute lung injury) or <26.6 kPa (for ARDS)

FiO_2, inspired oxygen concentration; PaO_2, arterial partial pressure of oxygen; PAOP, pulmonary artery occlusion pressure.

interpretation of chest radiographs. The Consensus Conference therefore met again in October 2000 to address these concerns in revised criteria, although revised criteria have yet (2009) to emerge.

Epidemiology

Incidence

Susceptibility to acute lung injury/ARDS is determined in part by the nature of the underlying condition (Table 17.5.11). Thus, of patients with sepsis, severe sepsis, and septic shock, some 40 to 60% develop associated acute lung injury, regardless of the anatomical site of infection. By contrast, only 16% develop acute lung injury following trauma. Genetic polymorphisms in the expression of genes encoding specific pathophysiological pathways which increase susceptibility have been demonstrated.

Early estimates of the overall incidence of ARDS varied from 1.5 to 75 cases per 100 000 population. In Europe, the most recent epidemiological data found acute lung injury/ARDS defining criteria were met in 15.8% of patients requiring ICU admission through acute respiratory failure of all causes, with 16.1% requiring mechanical ventilation. Of those who developed acute lung injury/ARDS, 65.4% of cases fulfilled the relevant criteria early in ICU admission and the remainder did so within a median of 3 days. Of those who developed acute lung injury within the first 24 h, 54.4% evolved to ARDS. By contrast, only 18.4% of patients with established ARDS had preceding acute lung injury.

In North America, 17.9 and 13.5 cases of acute lung injury and ARDS have been identified respectively per 100 000 population, but a prospective, population-based cohort study in 21 hospitals over 14 months also using Consensus Conference criteria for acute lung injury found a much higher crude incidence of the condition (78.9 per 100 000 population). The incidence increased with age (16 per 100 000 for patients 15–19 years; 306 per 100 000 for those aged 75–84). Overall, this study suggested there are around 190 000 cases of acute lung injury per year in the United States of America, with 74 500 deaths and some 3.6 million hospital days taken up by such patients.

Morbidity and mortality

Death rates attributable to acute lung injury/ARDS are difficult to interpret in that prognosis is determined in part by the nature of the precipitating illness. Thus, the mortality associated with lung injury complicating the sepsis syndromes is typically higher (40–60%) than that with trauma (14%), or following surgery necessitating cardiopulmonary bypass (15%). Early publications thereby reinforced the emerging concept that ARDS might represent merely the pulmonary manifestation of a panendothelial insult, to which the lungs were specifically susceptible. This impression was supported by the finding that most patients with the established syndrome did not die as a direct result of respiratory insufficiency, but rather succumbed to multiple organ dysfunction. Despite this, an improvement in outcome has been reported in recent years; one study reporting a reduction in mortality from 66% to 34% over the years 1990 to 1997. Recent controlled trials of putative therapeutic interventions in patients with acute lung injury have identified mortality rates of 25–40% in the control arms.

Survivors of ARDS have persistent functional disability 1 year after discharge from the intensive care unit. Most patients have extrapulmonary conditions, with muscle wasting and weakness being most prominent.

Pathophysiology

Acute lung injury and ARDS are characterized by intense inflammatory reactions in the alveolar space. Cytokines and chemokines are released by native fibroblasts, epithelial cells and alveolar macrophages, triggering endothelial cell activation and neutrophil recruitment. These secrete cytokines and chemokines to further up-regulate the proinflammatory stimulus, and release highly reactive oxygen species, which together with destructive enzymes such as myeloperoxidase are cytotoxic. Lower levels of reactive oxygen species modulate cell signalling moieties relevant to the proinflammatory pathway. These mechanisms are manifest in three identifiable phases. The exudative is characterized by increased pulmonary capillary permeability with leakage of a protein-rich exudate from the pulmonary vasculature into the interstitium and alveoli. Around 7 days later, the inflammatory phase ensues, in which alveolar neutrophilia predominates. Finally, in patients who survive, a fibroproliferative or reparative phase has been described: this commences after 10 to 14 days, during which inflammation gradually resolves, giving way to increased collagen deposition. Rarely, progressive fibrosis occurs.

The refractory hypoxaemia that characterizes both acute lung injury and ARDS is attributable to atelectasis of lung units. Dysregulation of pulmonary vascular tone due to endothelial dysfunction is manifest in impaired hypoxic pulmonary vasoconstriction and increased pulmonary vascular resistance, the development of which is associated with a poor prognosis. Rarely, right heart failure may develop. The distribution of pulmonary blood flow relative to alveolar ventilation has been the subject of recent research and is of relevance therapeutically in the context of agents designed to improve ventilation perfusion (V/Q) matching (e.g. inhaled nitric oxide, prone positioning) and optimize mechanical ventilation (e.g. by using the most appropriate levels of positive end expiratory pressure, PEEP).

Reduced lung compliance is also a hallmark of the syndrome. Some have speculated that lung dysfunction may vary in patients with ARDS according to whether the precipitating insult directly (ARDSp) or indirectly (ARDSexp) involves the lung. Mechanics (elastance, intra abdominal pressure, end expiratory lung volume) measured during varying levels of PEEP together with computed tomography (CT) have indicated a differing recruitment response, more suggestive of consolidation in ARDSp patients, and oedema/collapse in those in the ARDSexp category.

Investigations

Initial investigations should be aimed at defining the extent of lung injury, and elucidating the precipitating cause. Subsequent investigations detect complications and guide therapy. Imaging may prove to be particularly helpful, with CT of the thorax increasingly used in patients with acute lung injury and ARDS because it has far greater sensitivity for detecting pneumothoraces, pleural collections, or pulmonary infiltrates than plain chest radiography. As well as detecting such complications, CT has also contributed to the understanding of the pathophysiology of ARDS by demonstrating patchy involvement of lung parenchyma rather than the homogenous appearance seen on chest radiographs. Typically, areas of dense opacification are apparent in dependent ung regions, with ground glass shadowing elsewhere (Fig. 17.5.1).

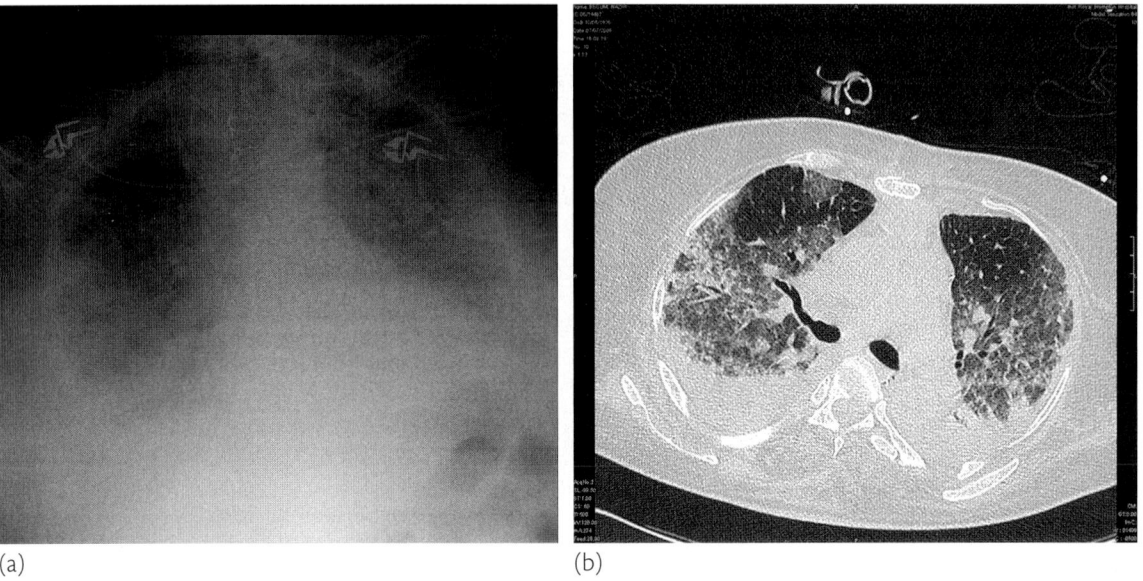

(a)   (b)

Fig. 17.5.1 Plain chest radiograph (a) and CT (b) of patient with ARDS. Note greater detail provided by CT and dependent distribution of consolidation.

Attempts have been made to use CT to predict responsiveness to interventions, one study correlating a response to inhaled nitric oxide with CT evidence of alveolar recruitment following increased PEEP (see above). Fibreoptic bronchoscopy is often used to obtain microbiological samples to rule out infection. Analysis of bronchoalveolar lavage fluid can also provide information concerning neutrophil infiltration and cytokine levels, which may have prognostic implications.

Management

Treatment of both the precipitating condition and complications of supportive management such as barotrauma and nosocomial infection are essential in managing these patients. A suitable management protocol is shown in Fig. 17.5.2.

General supportive measures
Nutrition

Adequate nutrition introduced early in the clinical course is now regarded as crucial to the management of patients with acute lung injury/ARDS. Wherever possible this should be administered via the enteral route, and the use of prokinetic drugs, avoidance of agents that impair gastric emptying (e.g. dopamine), and the use of postpyloric feeding tubes can all help achieve this aim.

Recent research has suggested that feeds rich in certain fatty acids and antioxidants may be of benefit in ARDS, presumably via changes in the host immune response. Eicosapentaenoic acid modulates production of proinflammatory eicosanoids, and γ-linoleic acid may suppress production of leukotrienes while itself being metabolized to prostaglandin E_1. A recent randomized

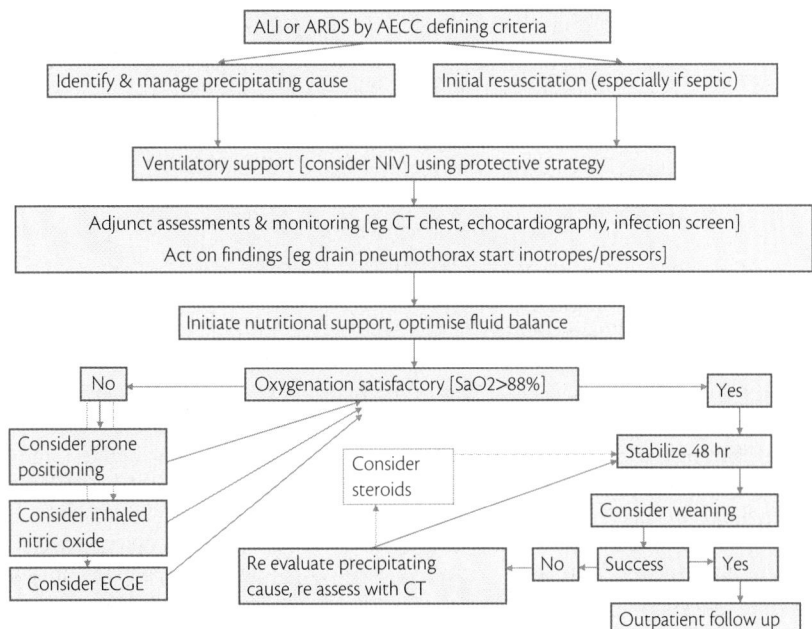

Fig. 17.5.2 Suggested protocol for management of patients with acute lung injury.

controlled trial of eicosapentaenoic acid/γ-linoleic acid supplemented feeds in patients with ARDS has shown improvements in oxygenation and shorter periods of ventilation and ICU stay: further investigation is required.

Fluid management

Pulmonary oedema in acute lung injury/ARDS is caused by increased pulmonary vascular permeability in the face of apparently normal pulmonary capillary pressure. Several studies have shown an association between a persistent positive fluid balance and poor outcome in ARDS, but it is not clear whether this represents administration of unnecessary fluid or greater haemodynamic instability in a group with a pre-existing poor prognosis. However, in a recent study of the safety and efficacy of 'fluid conservative' vs 'fluid liberal' management strategies, applying interventions based on measurements of central venous or pulmonary artery occlusion pressures made at least every 4 h, the primary endpoint (death at 60 days) did not differ between strategies. There were, however, advantages in ventilator free, and organ failure free (cardiovascular and central nervous system) days in favour of the fluid restricted group.

Mechanical ventilation

The lung protection approach

Most patients with ARDS require mechanical ventilatory support to maintain adequate gas exchange. Whilst some studies have indicated that satisfactory oxygenation can be achieved in some patients by using nasally administered positive pressure ventilation, most cases require endotracheal intubation. Unfortunately, it is now apparent that traditional strategies of ventilation applied to these patients may have contributed to the propagation of lung injury. Excessive stretching of the lung parenchyma together with cyclical opening and closing of damaged lung units is thought to generate proinflammatory mediators which then exacerbate pulmonary damage, and if disseminated into the systemic circulation also contribute to the development of distant organ failure to which many patients succumb. As a result, ventilatory strategies now aim to limit the shear forces applied to the lung parenchyma, and reduce the cyclical recruitment and derecruitment of alveolar units. Thus, tidal volumes are set at lower levels than have traditionally been thought necessary, the so-called protective approach. This reduces CO_2 clearance, often resulting in a respiratory acidosis. A large multicentre trial in the United States of America demonstrated a convincing reduction in mortality (from 40% to 31% p=0.007) associated with this approach (using tidal volumes of 6 ml/kg) compared to conventional (12 ml/kg) ventilation.

Positive end-expiratory pressure

High levels of positive end-expiratory pressure (PEEP) can also be used to ensure recruitment and retention of damaged lung units. Customarily, PEEP is increased transiently in a stepwise manner to high levels (e.g. 35–40 cmH$_2$O) before a similar graded reduction to a maintenance level above the lower inflection point of the pressure-volume curve. CT tomograms taken during such manoeuvres have demonstrated recruitment of atelectatic regions, especially in dorsal areas of the lung, which remain inflated after the PEEP is reduced, with an associated improvement in gas exchange. However, while higher PEEP may result in better oxygenation and possibly less ventilator-associated lung injury, circulatory depression and overdistension of recruitable lung units may also occur.

The relationship between potentially recruitable lung (indicated by CT) and effects of PEEP has been explored in patients with acute lung injury and appropriate controls (healthy patients with unilateral pneumonia). Those patients with greater recruitability had greater calculated lung weight, poorer oxygenation and respiratory system compliance, higher dead space, and higher rates of death. Thus, in this patient population the percentage of recruitable lung is variable, but strongly associated with level of PEEP. Despite such knowledge, the application of varying levels of PEEP in clinical trials has not influenced outcome favourably. When patients with acute lung injury were randomized to low or high levels of PEEP using preset Fio$_2$/PEEP (levels achieved in the two groups were 8.3 and 13.2 cmH$_2$O respectively), none of the study endpoints (mortality, days of unassisted breathing, inflammatory markers) differed between the two groups.

Prone positioning

Mechanical ventilation in the prone position is frequently employed in the management of patients with ARDS, around 60% of whom respond to this manoeuvre with significant improvements in gas exchange that may persist even after they are returned to the supine position. Since response cannot be predicted, a trial period is often used to identify those patients who are likely to benefit. While a large (>300 patients) study carried out in Italy demonstrated no survival benefit in response to at least 6 h prone ventilation per day, more prolonged 'proning' (e.g. 17 h per day) applied early to patients with more severe lung injury may reduce mortality.

High frequency ventilation

High frequency ventilation (HFV) employs rapid respiratory rates (>4 times those used in conventional techniques). Tidal volumes are reduced, and are often smaller than the anatomical dead space. The two modes of HFV most widely used are high frequency jet ventilation (HFJV) and high frequency oscillatory ventilation (HFOV).

HFJV involves the intermittent delivery of high pressure gas jets into the endotracheal tube, but optimal gas warming and humidification are difficult to achieve, which leads to problems with airway secretions and debris that, when coupled with a reliance on passive expiration, can lead to air trapping. HFOV involves the delivery of a continuous distending pressure to the endotracheal tube, which is then modified by the movement of a vibrating loudspeaker. Humidification and warming of the fresh gas flow are easier to achieve, and an active expiratory phase leads to less gas trapping. The only randomized controlled trial of HFJV in patients with severe acute respiratory failure was unable to show a significant improvement in gas exchange or a survival benefit. However, recent evidence suggesting that low tidal volumes reduce ventilator associated lung injury, and that high levels of continuous airway pressure (PEEP) improve recruitment and retention of lung units, has renewed interest in HFV (especially HFOV) as an appropriate mode of ventilation in ARDS.

Extracorporeal gas exchange

Extracorporeal gas exchange (ECGE) is performed using a variety of techniques (e.g. venoarterial bypass) and can be used in the absence of conventional forms of ventilation as the sole mechanism of gas exchange, or may be coupled to mechanical ventilation (where its principal function is to enhance CO_2 clearance). Two randomized controlled trials of extracorporeal membrane oxygenation have failed to reveal a survival advantage, but a third recently completed study found a 16% survival benefit without severe disability among patients transferred to an ECMO centre compared to those receiving conventional ventilatory support. Increased understanding about the most appropriate way to ventilate patients with severe ARDS is likely to lead to this technique being used less frequently in the future.

Nonventilatory adjuncts to gas exchange
Nitric oxide
Nitric oxide (NO) is an endogenous vasodilator which can be given by inhalation at concentrations of up to 20 parts per million. It has been shown to improve oxygenation in patients with acute lung injury and ARDS through effects on ventilation/perfusion matching, and to decrease pulmonary vascular resistance. However, only a proportion of patients with ARDS benefit from inhaled nitric oxide (iNO), and randomized controlled trials of iNO in acute lung injury and ARDS have failed to show an improvement in mortality or a reduction in the duration of mechanical ventilation. Moreover, improvements in oxygenation are only transient, disappearing after 24 h of iNO therapy. Prostacyclin (PGI_2) is another endogenous vasodilator that may have beneficial effects in ARDS. Like iNO it is thought to redistribute pulmonary blood flow to ventilated lung units, thus improving ventilation/perfusion matching. A sequential trial of iNO and PGI_2 in patients with ARDS showed the two treatments to have identical effects on oxygenation and shunt flow, but as PGI_2 is easier to monitor and deliver than iNO, it is frequently used in its place.

Surfactant administration
Surfactant supplementation has proved effective in neonatal respiratory distress syndrome, and surfactant deficiency and dysfunction has been demonstrated in adult patients with ARDS. However, a number of randomized controlled trials have failed to demonstrate an effect in adults on mortality, or length of ventilation, or ICU stay. A recent small trial has shown a survival benefit following use of bovine surfactant, but further large-scale trials are necessary.

Other pharmaceutical interventions
ARDS (and potentially acute lung injury) has considerable clinical and fiscal significance. Many investigations have been performed to evaluate the potential of both supportive and pharmacotherapeutic interventions, most of which were designed to reduce cellular and mediator-driven inflammation. Although evaluated in large, randomized, placebo-controlled trials, all have failed to show a survival benefit. The most significant of these are described.

Corticosteroids
Steroids have been used to treat ARDS since its first description in the 1960s. However, several multicentre trials in the 1980s failed to show a beneficial role for steroids either in the prevention of ARDS in at-risk groups, or in the treatment of established ARDS. Indeed, recent meta-analyses have concluded that steroids do not improve and may worsen mortality in sepsis—a major group at risk of ARDS. However, despite this evidence, there has been a recent resurgence in enthusiasm for the use of steroids in the late (fibroproliferative) phase of ARDS. Early controlled data that appeared to support such therapy randomized patients on day 7 of ARDS to receive methylprednisolone or placebo for a further 32 days. A much larger randomized, double-blind trial compared corticosteroids to placebo in severe, late phase ARDS (7–14 days). There were two objectives; firstly, to determine if the administration

of corticosteroids (methylprednisolone) in severe late phase ARDS would reduce mortality and morbidity; and secondly, to evaluate the effects of steroids on markers of inflammation and fibroproliferation. Methylprednisolone increased the number of ventilator-free and shock-free days during the first 28 days in association with an improvement in oxygenation, respiratory system compliance, and blood pressure, with fewer days of vasopressor therapy. There was no increase in the rate of infectious complications, but steroid therapy was associated with a higher rate of neuromuscular weakness. These results do not support the routine use of steroids for persistent ARDS despite the improvement in cardiopulmonary physiology. In addition, starting methylprednisolone therapy more than 2 weeks after the onset of ARDS might have increased the risk of death.

Antioxidants
Oxidative stress is thought to be central to the pathogenesis of ARDS. Alveolar macrophages and recruited activated neutrophils release highly reactive oxygen species which cause injury through interactions with proteins, lipids, and DNA. It is thought that excessive production of reactive oxygen species in acute lung injury and ARDS overwhelms the endogenous antioxidant systems that normally regulate redox state within the lung. Attempts have therefore been made to introduce antioxidants to redress this balance, in particular using N-acetylcysteine, but none has shown a survival benefit or a reproducible effect on pulmonary physiology.

Anti-inflammatory agents
Ketoconazole is an imidazole used primarily for its antifungal effects, but which also has immune modulating functions which may be of benefit in preventing the development of ARDS. Although a large multicentre trial showed that ketoconazole had no effect on mortality or duration of ventilation in patients with established acute lung injury or ARDS, two smaller studies in critically ill surgical patients demonstrated a significant reduction in the incidence of ARDS.

Further reading
Abel SJ, et al. (1998). Reduced mortality in association with the acute respiratory distress syndrome (ARDS). Thorax, 53, 292–4.
Acute Respiratory Distress Syndrome Network (2000). Ventilation with lower tidal volumes as compared with traditional tidal volumes for acute lung injury and the acute respiratory distress syndrome. The Acute Respiratory Distress Syndrome Network. N Engl J Med, 342, 1301–8.
American College of Radiology (2006). ACR Practice Guidelines for the performance of pediatric and adult portable (mobile unit) chest radiography. http://www.acr.org.
Bekemeyer WB, et al. (1985). Efficacy of chest radiography in a respiratory intensive care unit. A prospective study. Chest, 88, 691–6.
Bernard GR, et al. (1994). The American-European Consensus Conference on ARDS. Definitions, mechanisms, relevant outcomes, and clinical trial coordination. Am J Respir Crit Care Med, 149, 818–24.
British Thoracic Society Standards of Care Committee (2002). Non-invasive ventilation in acute respiratory failure. Thorax, 57, 192–211.
Brochard L, et al. (1995). Noninvasive ventilation for acute exacerbations of chronic obstructive pulmonary disease. N Engl J Med, 333, 817–22.
Brun-Buisson C, et al. (2004). Epidemiology and outcome of acute lung injury in European intensive care units. Results from the ALIVE study. Intensive Care Med, 30, 51–61.
Cook DJ, et al. (1994). Risk factors for gastrointestinal bleeding in critically ill patients. Canadian Critical Care Trials Group. N Engl J Med, 330, 377–81.

Cook DJ, *et al.* (2001). The attributable mortality and length of intensive care unit stay of critically important gastrointestinal bleeding in critically ill patients. Canadian Critical Care Trials Group. *Crit Care*, **5**, 368–75.

Craven DE (2006). Preventing ventilator-associated pneumonia in adults: sowing seeds of change. *Chest*, **130**, 251–60.

Dakin J, Griffiths M (2002). The pulmonary physician in critical care 1: pulmonary investigations for acute respiratory failure. Thorax, **57**, 79–85.

Davidson AC (2002). The pulmonary physician in critical care. 11: critical care management of respiratory failure resulting from COPD. *Thorax*, **57**, 1079–84.

Gattinoni L, *et al.* (2001). Effect of prone positioning on the survival of patients with acute respiratory failure. *N Engl J Med*, **345**, 568–73.

Goldstone J (2002). The pulmonary physician in critical care. 10: difficult weaning. *Thorax*, **57**, 986–91.

Greenbaum DM, Marschall KE (1982). The value of routine daily chest X-rays in intubated patients in the medical intensive care unit. *Crit Care Med*, **10**, 29–30.

Griffiths J, *et al.* (2005). Systematic review and meta-analysis of studies of the timing of tracheostomy in adult patients undergoing artificial ventilation. *BMJ*, **330**, 1243–46.

Griffiths MJ, Evans TW (2005). Inhaled nitric oxide therapy in adults. *N Engl J Med*, **353**, 2683–95.

Herridge MS (2003). One-year outcomes in survivors of the acute respiratory distress syndrome. *N Engl J Med*, **348**, 683–93.

Isakow W, Kollef MH (2006). Preventing ventilator-associated pneumonia: an evidence-based approach of modifiable risk factors. *Semin Respir Crit Care Med*, **27**, 5–17.

Jackson R, Carley S (2001). Towards evidence based emergency medicine: best BETs from the Manchester Royal Infirmary. CPAP in acute left ventricular failure. *Emerg Med J*, **18**, 63–4.

Lewandowski K (2003). Contributions to epidemiology of acute respiratory failure. *Crit Care*, **7**, 288–90.

Miller WT Jr, Tino G, Friedburg JS (1998). Thoracic CT in the intensive care unit: assessment of clinical usefulness. *Radiology*, **209**, 491–8.

National Heart, Lung, and Blood Institute Acute Respiratory Distress Syndrome (ARDS) Clinical Trials Network, *et al.* (2006). Pulmonary-artery versus central venous catheter to guide treatment of acute lung injury. *N Engl J Med*, **354**, 2213–24.

National Heart, Lung, and Blood Institute Acute Respiratory Distress Syndrome (ARDS) Clinical Trials Network, *et al.* (2006). Comparison of two fluid-management strategies in acute lung injury. *N Engl J Med*, **354**, 2564–75.

Nava S, *et al.* (1998). Non-invasive mechanical ventilation in the weaning of patients with respiratory failure due to chronic obstructive pulmonary disease A randomized, controlled trial. *Ann Intern Med*, **128**, 721–8.

Pang D, *et al.* (1998). The effect of positive pressure airway support on mortality and the need for intubation in cardiogenic pulmonary edema: a systematic review. *Chest*, **114**, 1185–92.

Peek GJ, *et al.* (2009). Efficacy and economic assessment of conventional ventilatory support versus extracorporeal membrane oxygenation for severe adult respiratory failure (CESAR): a multicentre randomised controlled trial. *Lancet*, **374**(9698), 1351–63.

Plant PK, Owen JL, Elliott MW (2000). Early use of non-invasive ventilation for acute exacerbations of chronic obstructive pulmonary disease on general respiratory wards: a multicentre randomised controlled trial. *Lancet*, **355**, 1931–5.

Resuscitation Council (UK). *Resuscitation Guidelines 2005*. http://www.resus.org.uk/pages/guide.htm.

Reynolds SF, Heffner J (2005). Airway management of the critically ill patient: rapid-sequence intubation. *Chest*, **127**, 1397–412.

Rivers E, *et al.* (2001). Early goal-directed therapy in the treatment of severe sepsis and septic shock. *N Engl J Med*, **345**, 1368–77.

Steinberg KP, *et al.* (2006). Efficacy and safety of corticosteroids for persistent acute respiratory distress syndrome. *N Engl J Med*, **354**, 1671–84.

Spragg RG, *et al.* (2004). Effect of recombinant surfactant protein C-based surfactant on the acute respiratory distress syndrome. *N Engl J Med*, **351**, 884–92.

Suntharalingam G, *et al.* (2001). Influence of direct and indirect etiology on acute outcome and 6-month functional recovery in acute respiratory distress syndrome. *Crit Care Med*, **29**, 562–6.

Taylor RW, *et al.* (2004). Low dose inhaled nitric oxide in patients with acute lung injury: a randomized controlled trial. *JAMA*, **291**, 1603–9.

Tobin MJ (2001). Advances in mechanical ventilation. *N Engl J Med*, **344**, 1986–96.

TracMan Trial Office, Kadoorie Centre for Critical Care, John Radcliffe Hospital, Oxford. *TracMan Tracheostomy management in Critical Care*. http://www.tracman.org.uk

Wyncoll D, Evans TW (1999). Acute respiratory distress syndrome. *Lancet*, **354**, 497–501.

Management of raised intracranial pressure

David K. Menon

Essentials

Normal intracranial pressure (ICP) is between 5 and 15 mmHg in supine subjects. Intracranial hypertension (ICP >20 mmHg) is common in many central nervous system diseases and in fatal cases is often the immediate cause of death.

Aetiology and pathogenesis—increases in intracranial volume and hence—given the rigid skull—ICP may be the consequence of (1) brain oedema, (2) increased cerebral blood volume, (3) hydrocephalus, and (4) space-occupying lesions. Brain perfusion depends on the difference between mean arterial pressure and ICP, termed cerebral perfusion pressure (CPP). The normal brain autoregulates cerebral blood flow down to a lower limit of CPP of about 50 mmHg in healthy subjects, and perhaps 60 to 70 mmHg in disease. CPP reduction to below these values results in cerebral ischaemia.

Clinical features—the cardinal symptom of intracranial hypertension is headache, which may be accompanied by vomiting, visual disturbance, and alterations in mental function or conscious state.

Papilloedema is the classical sign, but may be absent. Severe elevation of ICP can result in bradycardia and hypertension (Cushing's response), abnormalities of breathing (Cheyne–Stokes respiration, central neurogenic hyperventilation, 'ataxia of breathing'), and various forms of cerebral herniation.

Investigation—if clinical features suggest intracranial hypertension, a lumbar puncture must be preceded by CT imaging, and avoided if the basal cisterns are effaced by cerebral oedema.

Management—this involves (1) ensuring normoxia and normocapnia (Pao_2 >11 kPa, $Paco_2$ 4.5–5 kPa), with tracheal intubation and ventilatory support where required; (2) treating precipitating factors such as fits, pyrexia, and electrolyte abnormalities; (3) treating raised ICP with mannitol, dexamethasone (for tumours), hyperventilation (if pupillary dilatation/clinical picture merits); and (4) monitoring ICP if appropriate (e.g. trauma).

Introduction

The normal intracranial pressure (ICP), measured at the level of Monro's foramen, is between 5 and 15 mmHg in supine subjects. Intracranial hypertension (ICP >20 mmHg) is a common accompaniment of many central nervous system (CNS) diseases. In many of these situations intracranial hypertension is the most important cause of symptoms and modulator of outcome, and in fatal cases is often the immediate cause of death.

Pathophysiology

The cranial cavity contains brain (80%), blood (10%), and cerebrospinal fluid (CSF; 10%). These incompressible contents are bounded by a rigid skull with a fixed capacity. Consequently, an increase in volume of any of these contents, or the presence of any space-occupying pathology, results in an increase in ICP unless one of the other constituents can be displaced or its volume decreased (Fig. 17.6.1). This principle is referred to as the Monro–Kellie doctrine. Increases in intracranial volume may be the consequence of:

◆ Brain oedema, which may have different pathogenic mechanisms:

  • Cytotoxic oedema occurs as a result of cell swelling, most commonly due to ischaemic energy depletion and rises in intracellular Na^+ and water.

  • Vasogenic oedema results from an increased permeability of the blood–brain barrier with an expansion of the extracellular fluid compartment.

  • Interstitial oedema occurs in the context of hydrocephalus, where increased intraventricular CSF pressures result in permeation of CSF into adjacent brain, typically in the frontal periventricular regions.

◆ Vascular engorgement that results from increased cerebral blood volume. This may be due to the vasodilatation that accompanies normal or abnormal (e.g. epileptiform) neuronal activity. In other situations vasodilatation may be due to loss of

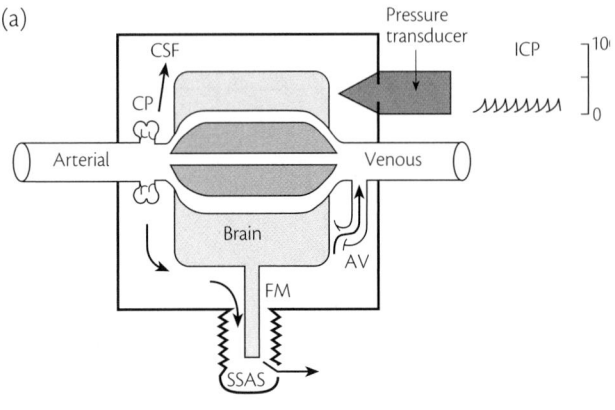

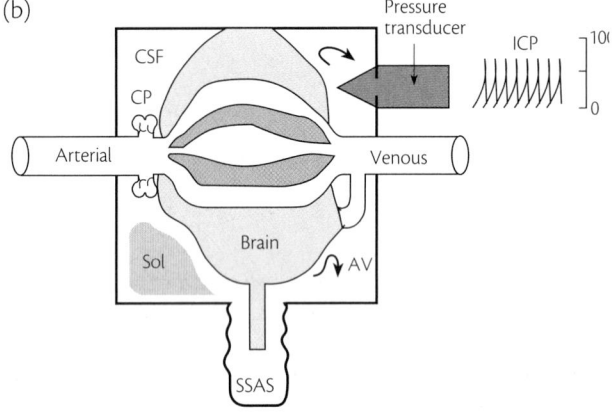

Fig. 17.6.1 Schematic diagram showing intracranial contents in the normal brain (a) and with elevated intracranial pressure (b). Note that cerebrospinal fluid (CSF) is produced by the choroid plexus (CP), circulates freely, passing through the foramen magnum (FM) into the spinal subarachnoid space (SSAS), before absorption by arachnoid villi (AV) in the cerebral venous sinuses. Increases in ICP may be due to brain oedema, vascular engorgement, space-occupying lesions (SOL), or impaired CSF circulation or absorption. Compensatory mechanisms include translocation of CSF to the SSAS, and compression of cerebral vascular beds. The ICP trace shows a higher mean value, and the inability of the noncompliant brain to cope with increased blood during each systole results in an increased pulsatility of the ICP waveform.

vasoregulation, either due to disease (vasoparalysis), or due the effect of potent physiological (carbon dioxide) or pharmacological (nitrates and other nitric oxide donors) cerebral vasodilators.

◆ Hydrocephalus, which may be noncommunicating (where an obstruction prevents the ventricular system communicating with the subarachnoid space), or communicating (where there is a defect in CSF reabsorption).

◆ Space-occupying lesions (SOL), which may be either chronic (e.g. intracranial tumours) or acute (e.g. intracranial haematomas associated with trauma).

Temporal patterns of ICP change

Initial increases in intracranial volume are buffered by displacement or reduction in volume of other contents. Thus, cerebral oedema may result in compression of the ventricles, with translocation of CSF to the spinal subarachnoid space, and compression of cerebral vasculature. Over longer time periods, normal brain may be compressed and CSF production diminished. The relationship between intracranial volume (ICV) and ICP is

commonly depicted as a hyperbolic curve, with an initial flat part during which compensatory mechanisms are effective, a knee which represents their progressive exhaustion, and a steep phase when even small increases in intracranial volume produce large increases in ICP. However, the extent and efficiency with which these mechanisms buffer increases in volume depend on the speed of progression of disease. Given these considerations, it is more appropriate to depict the evolution of pathophysiology as a family of curves, with variable rates of progression (Fig. 17.6.2). It is important to make three further points in this context:

◆ First, a precipitating factor may suddenly increase the speed of progression of a relatively slow pathophysiological process, and be the proximate cause of symptomatic decompensation.

◆ Secondly, acute changes in cerebrovascular physiology are an important cause of such deterioration. Both hypoxia and hypercarbia can cause cerebral vasodilatation and elevate ICP. While severe hypertension may result in cerebral oedema, it is far more common to find that relatively minor reductions in mean arterial pressure compromise cerebral perfusion and trigger reflex vasodilatation and secondary increases in ICP. Such haemodynamic instability may be the underlying cause of phasic increases in ICP (Fig. 17.6.3).

◆ Finally, since patients with significant intracranial hypertension operate on the steep part of the ICV/ICP curve, even small decreases in intracranial volume (e.g. a 5 ml decrease in cerebral blood volume produced by mild hyperventilation) can have gratifyingly large effects on ICP.

Why treat intracranial hypertension?

Brain perfusion depends on the difference between mean arterial pressure (MAP) and ICP, termed cerebral perfusion pressure (CPP). While the normal brain autoregulates cerebral blood flow across a large range of CPP values, the lower limit of such autoregulation is about 50 mmHg in healthy subjects, and may be significantly higher (60–70 mmHg) in disease. CPP reduction below the lower limit of autoregulation results in cerebral ischaemia, and even minor reductions in CPP may trigger reflex vasodilatation and increase ICP in a noncompliant intracranial cavity. Such cerebral ischaemia is important in its own right. Therefore,

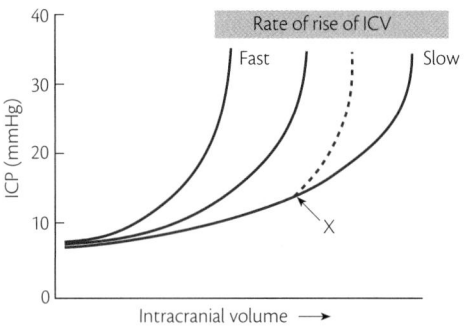

Fig. 17.6.2 Intracranial volume/pressure curves. Increases in ICV are initially buffered by compensatory mechanisms, but eventually result in ICP elevation. The ability to buffer ICV increases depends on the speed at which pathology develops. Gradually progressive increases in ICV (such as those produced by a slow growing tumour) may be well compensated, until a precipitating factor (e.g. the development of hydrocephalus, denoted by X in the diagram) shifts the relationship to a steeper curve.

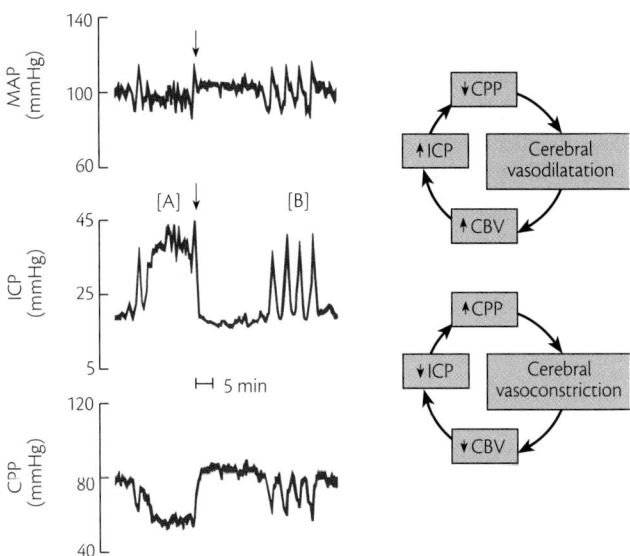

Fig. 17.6.3 Intracranial pressure (ICP) traces show phasic variations which may last several minutes (Lundberg A waves; (A)) or may be more transient (Lundberg B waves; (B)). ICP elevations are often initiated by reductions in mean arterial pressure (MAP), which trigger compensatory vasodilatation and increase cerebral blood volume (CBV) and ICP. This vicious cycle may be terminated by spontaneous hypertension associated with a Cushing's response (arrow in MAP and ICP traces), or by therapeutic elevation of MAP, which triggers compensatory cerebral vasoconstriction and reductions in ICP. Note that a period of stable MAP greater than 100 mmHg is associated with a low, stable ICP.
(Modified from Rosner MJ (1993). Pathophysiology and management of increased intracranial pressure. In: Andrews BT (ed) *Neurosurgical intensive care*, p. 75. McGraw-Hill, New York.)

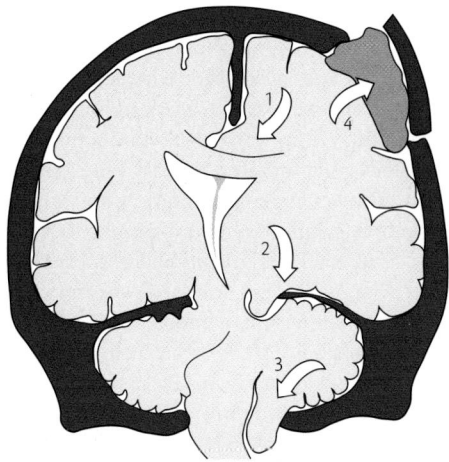

Fig. 17.6.4 Cerebral herniation may be (1) subfalcine (beneath the falx cerebri), (2) transtentorial (through the tentorial hiatus with compression of the midbrain and posterior cerebral artery), (3) tonsillar (where the cerebellar tonsils herniate through the foramen magnum and compress the lower brainstem upper cervical cord), or (4) transcalvarial (through a traumatic or surgical defect in the roof of the cranial cavity).
(Modified from Fishman RA (1975). Brain edema. *New Engl J Med*, **293**, 706–11.)

for instance, intracranial hypertension may be the direct cause of neurocognitive deficits in survivors of head injury.

An expanding focal mass can generate pressure gradients within the intracranial cavity, and the resulting displacement of brain against rigid structures, and protrusion (herniation) of brain through narrow openings between intracranial compartments can press on vital structures and result in death (Fig. 17.6.4).

Prolonged intracranial hypertension may result in permanent damage to critical structures. Thus, benign intracranial hypertension rarely results in herniation syndromes, but if left untreated, frequently results in optic atrophy.

Diagnosis

Symptoms

The symptoms that accompany ICP elevation can be nonspecific and insensitive. The cardinal feature of intracranial hypertension is headache, which may be described as severe ('worst ever') and explosive in onset in the setting of intracranial haemorrhage. The headache of intracranial tumour is often progressive, worst on awakening (possibly due to ICP elevations associated with the supine position and $Paco_2$ elevation in sleep), and is exacerbated by coughing and straining. However, it may be indistinguishable from common tension headache, and dangerous intracranial hypertension may occur without headache.

The headache is often accompanied by vomiting, which is classically described as projectile and not preceded by nausea. Visual disturbances are often reported, which may be attributable to optic or oculomotor nerve compression (with accompanying visual failure or

diplopia, respectively). Alterations in mental function or conscious state may be observed, ranging from impaired concentration, through increased irritability, impaired cognition and memory, and altered personality, to increased somnolence and deep coma.

Signs

While papilloedema is the classical sign associated with ICP elevation, it is not seen with acute intracranial hypertension, and may be absent even with large intracranial masses. Pressure on cranial nerves may result in weakness of ocular movement. The abducens nerve is often involved in such a process due its long intracranial course, and the resultant diplopia provides the classical example of a false localizing sign. Lesions that irritate the posterior fossa dura can produce neck stiffness.

Progressive rises in ICP result in bradycardia and hypertension, which constitute the Cushing's response and signify stimulation of brainstem autonomic nuclei. Worsening brain stem compression and/or ischaemia result progressively in Cheyne–Stokes respiration, central neurogenic hyperventilation, and irregular respiratory patterns ('ataxia of breathing'). Both neurogenic pulmonary oedema and the adult respiratory distress syndrome have been associated with intracranial hypertension.

Severe elevation of ICP may result in herniation of the temporal lobe through the tentorial notch (Fig. 17.6.4). This produces clinical features due to pressure on the ipsilateral oculomotor nerve (ipsilateral pupillary dilatation), pyramidal tract (contralateral weakness), and brainstem (Cushing's response and abnormal respiratory patterns followed by circulatory collapse and respiratory arrest). The posterior cerebral artery is frequently compressed by the herniating temporal lobe, and successful resuscitation from threatened or early transtentorial herniation may leave a patient with an ipsilateral occipital infarction.

Imaging

The most informative standard imaging in patients with intracranial hypertension is computed tomography (CT), which may reveal subarachnoid or intracerebral blood, contusions, or a tumour.In addition, cerebral oedema may be manifest by loss of sulci, compression of the third and lateral ventricles, and effacement of the perimesencephalic and suprasellar cisterns. Unilateral lesions may result in midline shift (which can occur without pupillary asymmetry), compression of the ipsilateral lateral ventricle, and in some cases dilatation of the contralateral ventricle due to obstruction of Monro's foramen. It is important to recognize that overt ventricular dilatation may be absent when hydrocephalus coexists with cerebral oedema. Indeed, the presence of normal sized ventricles in the context of intracranial hypertension (demonstrated by ICP monitoring) should suggest the possibility of coexisting hydrocephalus and trigger the consideration of CSF drainage as a means of therapy.

MRI may provide better definition of underlying pathology, particularly in the posterior fossa, and its multiplanar capability may provide a better appreciation of the extent of space-occupying lesions. Modern imaging methods can also detect patients who may have relatively normal ICP, but are at high risk of severe intracranial hypertension. For example, patients with a middle cerebral artery (MCA) territory infarction are at high risk of severe brain swelling if more than 50% of the MCA territory is hypodense.

Lumbar puncture

A lumbar puncture offers the opportunity to directly measure CSF pressure, and can be the defining investigation in meningitis, subarachnoid haemorrhage, or benign intracranial hypertension. However, in the context of clinical features that suggest intracranial hypertension, a lumbar puncture must be preceded by CT, and avoided if the basal cisterns are effaced by cerebral oedema.

Removal of CSF from the lumbar subarachnoid space under these circumstances can markedly increase the pressure differential between the infratentorial and supratentorial compartments, or the intracranial and spinal compartments, and precipitate transtentorial or cerebellar herniation, respectively.

Monitoring intracranial pressure

The clinical evaluation of intracranial hypertension is difficult due to its nonspecific clinical picture and phasic variations. Management may therefore be greatly facilitated by direct monitoring of ICP using intraparenchymal or ventricular monitoring devices. Such monitoring is mandatory in severe intracranial hypertension and in sedated or deeply unconscious patients, in whom changes in clinical signs do not provide an alternative means of assessing progress and response to therapy.

Strategies for therapy

Management focuses on four areas, which are described below.

Monitoring progression of disease and response to therapy

Monitoring will depend on the clinical context. Repeated clinical examination with regular charting of the Glasgow Coma Scale may suffice in many cases. Patients with benign intracranial hypertension may require regular visual field assessment, while those with head injury, intracranial haemorrhage, or severe cerebral oedema may benefit from direct ICP monitoring. The value of ICP monitoring may be substantially enhanced by the use of other monitoring modalities such as jugular bulb oximetry.

Table 17.6.1 Treatment of intracranial hypertension

CPP augmentation by increasing MAP	Maintenance of CPP >60–70 mmHg prevents ischaemia, and further increases (90–100 mmHg) may reduce ICP by autoregulatory cerebral vasoconstriction. Efficacy demonstrated in head injury
Corticosteroids	Reduce vasogenic oedema by restoring BBB integrity. Particularly effective in peritumoural oedema and benign intracranial hypertension. No outcome benefit in trauma. Prophylactic use may reduce incidence of hydrocephalus and other sequelae in tuberculous and acute bacterial meningitis
Diuretics	Furosemide used to potentiate mannitol. Acetazolamide and thiazide diuretics used in benign intracranial hypertension
Osmotic agents	Mannitol is effective in emergencies and can be used repeatedly if effective and plasma osmolality ≤325 mOsm/litre. Hypertonic NaCl (3–30%) may reduce ICP when mannitol is ineffective and tends to cause less problems with major fluid shifts. Hyperosmotic agents may be less effective when there is widespread disruption of the blood–brain barrier
Reduction of cerebral blood volume	Sedation and treatment of epilepsy can produce reductions in CBF and CBV that are coupled to reduction of neuronal metabolism Hyperventilation has been commonly used to reduce CBV by inducing cerebral vasoconstriction, but can produce critical reductions in CBF. Needs to be used with care and with monitoring of cerebral oxygenation (usually with jugular bulb oximetry)
Hypothermia	Mild to moderate hypothermia (33–36 °C) may be directly neuroprotective, but this benefit remains unproven except following cardiac arrest. It is clearly effective at controlling refractory intracranial hypertension by multiple mechanisms, including metabolic suppression and anti-inflammatory effects, but clear outcome benefits have not been demonstrated
CSF drainage	Ventriculostomy provides emergency drainage of CSF in trauma, acute hydrocephalus (subarachnoid haemorrhage, tumours) Ventriculoperitoneal, ventriculoatrial, and lumboperitoneal shunts provide chronic CSF diversion in idiopathic or secondary hydrocephalus Endoscopic third ventriculostomy provides communication between ventricular and cisternal CSF in noncommunicating hydrocephalus. May remove the need for shunts and the associated risk of shunt malfunction and sepsis
Surgical decompression	Trials are underway of decompressive craniectomy for refractory intracranial hypertension in head injury. Decompressive craniectomy improves survival, and probably functional outcome, in 'malignant' MCA stroke with severe cerebral oedema. Optic nerve decompression may prevent visual deterioration in benign intracranial hypertension

BBB, blood–brain barrier; CBF, cerebral blood flow; CBV, cerebral blood volume; CPP, cerebral perfusion pressure; CSF, cerebrospinal fluid; ICP, intracranial pressure; MAP, mean arterial pressure; MCA, middle cerebral artery.

Maintenance of stable physiology and removal of precipitating factors

Hyponatraemia and low plasma osmolality will tend to worsen cerebral oedema by favouring water entry into the brain, and should be vigorously corrected. Maintenance of cerebral perfusion pressure with fluid resuscitation and vasoactive agents will prevent cerebral ischaemia. Comatose patients should have arterial blood gas levels measured, and intubation and ventilatory support provided if airway protection is required or gas exchange is impaired (see Chapter 17.5). While hyperventilation has been widely used to control ICP in the past, there is increasing concern regarding the induction of critical cerebral ischaemia by hypocapnic vasoconstriction. Current recommendations suggest that near normal $Paco_2$ levels (4.5–5 kPa) should be maintained, with moderate hyperventilation ($Paco_2$ 4.0–4.5 kPa) guided by jugular bulb oximetry and reserved for control of acute episodes of severe intracranial hypertension. Attention should also be paid to treating epilepsy and significant pyrexia, both of which can precipitate rises in ICP, and to discontinuing or reversing the action of drugs such as opioids, which may be responsible for physiological derangements that precipitate ICP elevation.

Treatment of the underlying condition

Early neurosurgical evaluation and operative therapy may be life-saving if a patient has an acute intracranial haematoma, a large tumour, or established hydrocephalus. Specific antimicrobial therapy may be required for meningitis, encephalitis, or brain abscess. Systemic hypertension commonly accompanies intracranial hypertension, and should generally not be treated because it may be needed to preserve cerebral perfusion. If therapy is needed for extreme hypertension or for hypertensive encephalopathy, then it is best to avoid nitric oxide donors such as nitrates, which can cause cerebral vasodilatation and further increase ICP.

Specific treatment of intracranial hypertension

Several therapies can be used to reduce intracranial pressure, and their application will depend on the cause and severity of

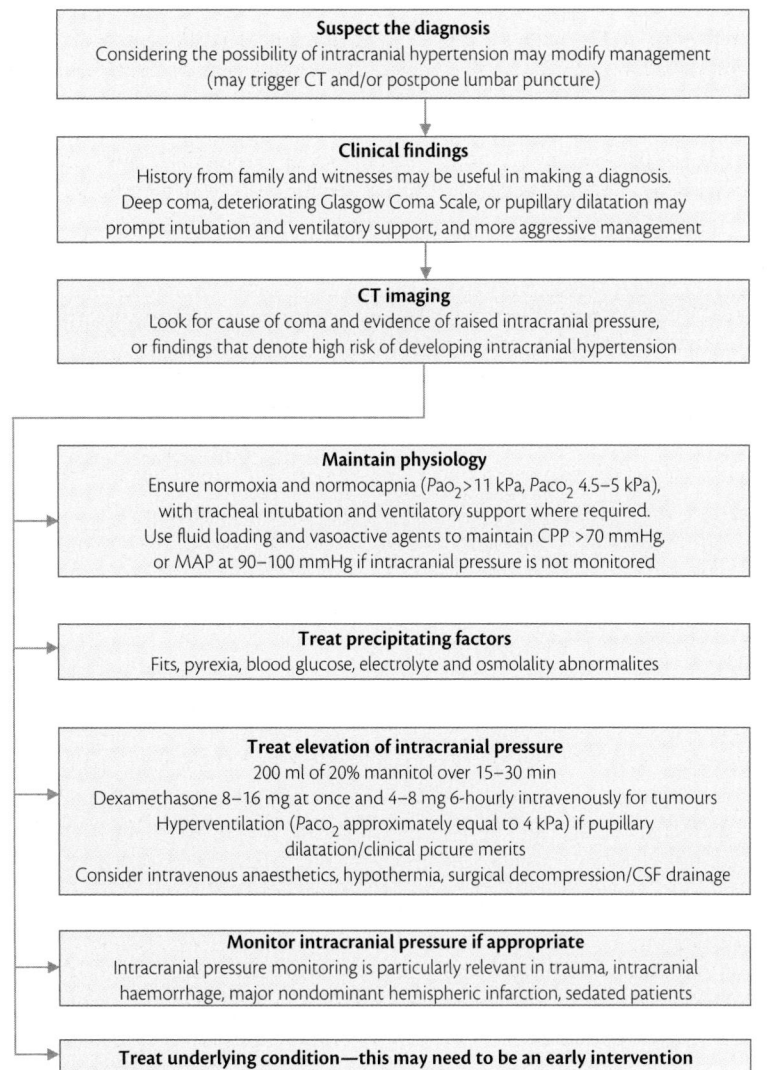

Fig. 17.6.5 Management of the unconscious patient with intracranial hypertension. CPP, cerebral perfusion pressure; MAP, mean arterial pressure.

ICP elevation. Commonly used interventions and their indications are outlined in Table17.6.1, but it must be pointed out that few of these have been assessed by good quality outcome studies. Treatment pathways for the emergency management of an unconscious patient with suspected intracranial hypertension are outlined in Fig. 17.6.5.

Further reading

Brain Trauma Foundation. *Guidelines for the treatment of severe head injury.* http://www.braintrauma.org/site/PageServer?pagename=Guidelines.

Hofmeijer J, *et al.* (2009). Surgical decompression for space-occupying cerebral infarction (the Hemicraniectomy After Middle Cerebral Artery infarction with Life-threatening Edema Trial [HAMLET]): a multicentre, open, randomised trial. *Lancet Neurol*, **8**, 326–333.

Menon DK (2000). Cerebral circulation. In: Priebe H-J, Skarvan K (eds) *Cardiovascular physiology*, pp. 240–277. BMJ Books, London.

Plum F, Posner JB (eds) (1992). *Diagnosis of stupor and coma*, 3rd edition. F.A. Davis Company, Philadelphia.

Reilly PL (2005). Management of intracranial pressure and cerebral perfusion pressure. In: Reilly PL, Bullock R (eds) *Head injury*, pp. 331–355. Hodder Arnold, London.

Roberts I, Schierhout G, Alderson P (1998). Absence of evidence for the effectiveness of five interventions routinely used in the intensive care management of severe head injury: a systematic review. *J Neurol Neurosurg Psychiatr*, **65**, 729–33.

Sahuquillo J, Arikan F (2006). Decompressive craniectomy for the treatment of refractory high intracranial pressure in traumatic brain injury. *Cochrane Database Syst Rev*, **1**, CD003983.

Salmond CH, *et al.* (2005). Cognitive sequelae of head injury: involvement of basal forebrain and associated structures. *Brain*, **128**, 189–200.

Skau M, *et al.* (2006). What is new about idiopathic intracranial hypertension? An updated review of mechanism and treatment. *Cephalalgia*, **26**, 384–99.

van de Beek D, *et al.* (2006). Community-acquired bacterial meningitis in adults. *N Engl J Med*, **354**, 44–53.

Sedation and analgesia in the critically ill

Gilbert Park and Maire P. Shelly

Essentials

Nearly all critically ill patients need analgesia, anxiolysis, hypnosis, or measures to help them tolerate their tracheal tube. Although making the patient unconscious may appear the easiest way to achieve this, it is fraught with hazards.

Pain relief and tube tolerance—these are the first priority, and usually involves giving opioids. Morphine, which has both analgesic and sedative effects, is the opioid against which others are judged. Remifentanil is a relatively new agent that has properties useful in critically ill patients: fast onset of action, a predictable short half-life (10–21 min), and it is broken down by a nonspecific enzyme system present in plasma such that accumulation does not occur, and the drug wears off rapidly, even after prolonged infusions and in renal or hepatic failure.

Hypnosis—the agents most commonly used are (1) the benzodiazepine midazolam, which accumulates in liver failure, and in renal failure the accumulation of a metabolic product can cause prolonged sedation or coma; and (2) the anaesthetic agent propofol, which does not accumulate to a significant extent in hepatic or renal failure.

Agitation, delirium, and confusion—these are some of the most difficult problems to deal with in the critically ill patient and may need to be controlled with drugs such as clonidine, or haloperidol. In addition to pharmacological restraint there is increasing interest in the use of physical restraint.

Introduction

Sedation and analgesia are used to increase patient comfort by minimizing the pain and anxiety produced by illness and its treatment. Factors contributing to patient discomfort are shown in Fig. 17.7.1.

Although this chapter concentrates on the use of drugs to make patients comfortable, it is important to realize that a few kind words or an explanation of what is going on, as well as ensuring that simple physical things such as a full bladder or bowel have been corrected, may have a dramatic effect. If this fails then sedation may be needed. The term sedation covers a broad range of conscious states, from almost wide awake to deeply unresponsive. Although 'sleep' (really 'coma') induced by drugs is often thought to be kind and safe, there is increasing evidence that this is not so. Box 17.7.1 shows some of the adverse effects that coma can have.

The relief of pain is an obvious and essential part of being comfortable; indeed, it is the primary need of most critically ill patients along with tolerance of a tracheal tube. The analgesic needs of patients can be met with regular bolus doses of analgesic titrated against repeated assessment of the pain, or by continuous infusion of an ultrashort acting opioid such as remifentanil.

The use of the latter method of analgesia has been associated with a reduced need for mechanical ventilation and a shorter period in the intensive care unit (ICU).

The role of hypnosis is more complex. Many patients who have the discomfort of the tracheal tube and pain removed do not need hypnosis and can be awake. Hypnosis may be needed in some patients for a variety of reasons, including:

◆ reducing anxiety caused by fear, inability to communicate, loss of control, or unfamiliar environment

◆ allowing patients to tolerate treatment, such as stopping them from pulling out various tubes and monitoring lines

◆ allowing patterns of ventilation to be imposed that will not synchronize with the patient's own breathing

◆ preventing awareness when neuromuscular paralysis is used

◆ minimizing distress during uncomfortable procedures

◆ allowing sleep

◆ controlling seizures

The indications for neuromuscular relaxation in the critically ill are listed below, with the use of muscle relaxants otherwise avoided.

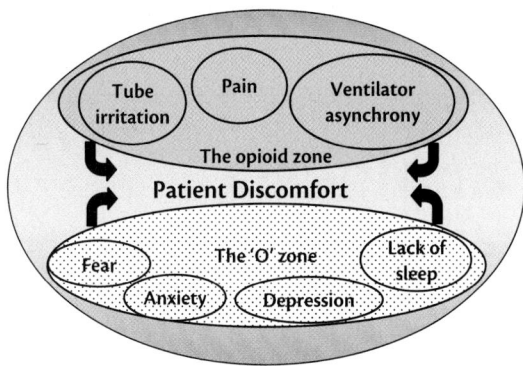

Fig. 17.7.1 Factors contributing to patient discomfort and their treatment. Some of the areas of discomfort experienced by critically ill patients. Those in the Opioid zone can be best relieved using opioids, often in relatively high doses. The remaining patients in the 'O' (Other) zone need some thought about which drug is best. Propofol is good for hypnosis, benzodiazepines for anxiety.

Box 17.7.1 Adverse effects of coma

- Increased morbidity, length of stay, and mechanical ventilation
- Immobility increases risk of pressure sores, deep vein thrombosis etc.
- Inability to communicate with relatives and carers
- Difficulty in diagnosis
- Inability to assess comfort
- Unable to cooperate with carers
  - Needs several nurses to turn patient (risk of injury to nurses, increased rate of line loss)
  - Physiotherapy passive rather than active
- Because of the increased memory loss, there may be an increased risk of traumatic psychological injury

---

- Acute respiratory distress syndrome (ARDS)—paralysis allows the patient to tolerate unusual ventilatory modes, e.g. reverse ratio ventilation
- Raised intracranial pressure—paralysis prevents coughing and straining
- Status asthmaticus—paralysis may reduce risks of barotrauma to lungs

The intravenous route is used almost exclusively for the administration of analgesic and hypnotic drugs in the critically ill, as it is faster and more reliable than other routes. Drugs can be given either as repeated bolus doses, or as a continuous infusion. Although a continuous infusion has the advantage of avoiding peaks and troughs associated with boluses, there is also an increased risk of inadvertent overdose or accumulation.

Hazards of sedation and analgesia

Although seeing a patient 'asleep' may make carers think they are being kind, it is important to remember that the use of drugs for sedation and analgesia involves risks to the patient. These include:

- oversedation, or a prolonged sedative effect caused by poor elimination in the critically ill
- hypotension/myocardial depression, possibly resulting in the unnecessary use of inotropes
- antitussive effects leading to failure to clear pulmonary secretions once the trachea is extubated
- hypoventilation, delaying weaning
- immobility, perhaps increasing the risk of deep vein thrombosis and pulmonary embolism
- toxic effects due to accumulation of hypnotic/analgesic agents or their metabolites
- expense, both of the drugs and their adverse effects

There are many reasons why the behaviour of drugs administered to the critically ill patient may be abnormal. These include:

- hepatic failure, leading to poor metabolism or biliary excretion of the drug

- renal failure, leading to decreased excretion of the drug or its metabolites; haemofiltration/dialysis may have unpredictable effects on clearance of the drug or its metabolites
- altered plasma protein levels (e.g. albumin and α_1-glycoprotein) may alter free (active) drug levels
- volume of distribution may be affected by oedema, ascites, or hyper/hypovolaemia
- interactions between drugs
- solvent toxicity

The risks of using drugs can be minimized by knowledge of their routes of breakdown and excretion. Agents that are unlikely to accumulate should be chosen when possible. Drugs with more than one site of metabolism are preferred, or those which can undergo non-organ-based breakdown. The risk of accumulation of a hypnotic and analgesic drug can be reduced by stopping it every 24 h whenever possible, and letting the patient recover from its effects. If the patient wakes or becomes restless, the drug can be restarted knowing that accumulation has not occurred.

To avoid under or oversedation requires some assessment of drug effects. However, because of the many components that are involved in sedation, there is no simple method. Although work is progressing on physical methods of assessing the level of sedation (e.g. spectral analysis of electroencephalogram waveforms), the most commonly used methods rely on bedside observations. A scoring system comprising several different elements is used (Fig. 17.7.2). The key to avoiding under or oversedation is regular assessment of the patient and adjustment of analgesia and hypnosis accordingly.

Psychological disturbances

The combination of severe illness, the intensive care environment, and drugs usually prevent patients from sleeping normally. Deprivation of sleep, especially if prolonged, combined with the fear of dying may make some patients psychotic. Close attention to environment (e.g. normal day/night light levels, clocks, noise etc.) may help. Drugs may be of some benefit, but can cause prolonged sedation or 'daytime hangover'. If the patient has a prolonged

Date/time							
Agitated							
Awake							
Roused by voice							
Roused by tracheal suction							
Unrousable							
Paralysed							
Asleep							
Pain—Yes/No							
Comfortable on ventilator —Yes/No							

Fig. 17.7.2 The Addenbrooke's Sedation Score. This allows monitoring not just of coma, but also of pain, ventilator tolerance, and sleep.

recovery phase then depression is common. Antidepressants are rarely of value and can have toxic effects. The effect of hypnotic drugs on cognitive recovery after critical care can be substantial.

Drug treatment

Two main types of drugs are used for sedation and analgesia in the critically ill: those principally analgesic and those mostly hypnotic. Before using drugs, causes of pain and agitation such as a full bladder or rectum should be excluded. Where possible, a sympathetic explanation of the reasons why the patient is in intensive care and what is happening should be given.

Analgesic drugs

Opioid drugs remain the mainstay of analgesic treatment in the critically ill, and morphine is the most common choice. Some properties of the opioid drugs used in the critically ill are listed in Table 17.7.1.

Morphine

Morphine is a cheap and effective analgesic agent and is the opioid against which others are judged. It has both analgesic and sedative effects, although an excessive dose would be required to produce adequate sedation by its use alone. It is often given with a benzodiazepine,

such as midazolam, to achieve analgesia and sedation. It is the standard agent for use in patient- and nurse-controlled syringe pumps. Morphine is metabolized in the liver, forming two major metabolites—morphine-3-glucuronide and morphine-6-glucuronide, both of which are active, the latter being a potent analgesic, while the former is thought to be antianalgesic.

Pethidine (meperidine)

Pethidine is a synthetic compound and was originally developed as an anticholinergic agent. It does tend to cause anticholinergic effects, such as dry mouth, blurred vision, and tachycardia. It is claimed that pethidine induces less constriction of the biliary sphincter than morphine, and perhaps the only indication for its use is in patients with biliary pathology. It is metabolized in the liver to form norpethidine, pethidinic acid, and pethidine-N-oxide. These metabolites are excreted by the kidneys, and in renal failure significant amounts of norpethidine may accumulate, leading to grand mal convulsions.

Fentanyl

Fentanyl is approximately 100 times as potent as morphine, and has a rapid onset of action (3 min). In low doses its analgesic effect ends after about 20 min by its rapid redistribution around the body. With larger doses, tissues may become saturated and drug action is prolonged, termination depending on the slow process of N-demethylation in the liver. The major metabolite, norfentanyl, is excreted by the kidneys, and its accumulation may cause toxic delirium in patients with renal failure. Accumulation of fentanyl itself may occur in hepatic failure, causing prolonged effect. Fentanyl has a potent apnoeic effect, and in large doses it can produce muscle rigidity, particularly of the chest wall.

Alfentanil

Alfentanil is approximately 10 to 20 times as potent as morphine and has a very fast onset time (1 min). Its effects are short-lived (approximately 10–15 min), ending by redistribution to tissues. Because of this, alfentanil is not widely used in patient-controlled syringe pumps, and it is administered by continuous infusion. Elimination takes place almost exclusively in the liver. It can accumulate in hepatic failure, cirrhosis, or when hepatic enzyme inhibitors such as cimetidine or fluconazole are used.

Remifentanil

Remifentanil is a relatively new agent that has properties useful in critically ill patients. It has a fast onset of action and a predictable, very short half-life (10–21 min). Remifentanil has an ester linkage within its structure, which is broken down by a nonspecific, nonsaturable enzyme system present in plasma. This breakdown pathway means that accumulation does not occur, and the drug wears off rapidly, even after prolonged infusions and in renal or hepatic failure. Remifentanil must be given by constant infusion, indeed the effects wear off so rapidly that even small delays, such as the time taken to make up a new syringe, can leave the patient without analgesia.

Hypnotic agents

The agents most commonly used for hypnosis are the benzodiazepine midazolam and the anaesthetic agent propofol. These, and other agents commonly used for sedation in the ICU, are described below.

Table 17.7.1 Properties of opioid drugs

Opioid	Speed of onset of action	Suitable[a] for PCAS/ NCAS	Liable to accumulate in hepatic failure	Liable to accumulate in renal failure
Morphine	Slow	Yes	Yes	Yes
Diamorphine	Moderate	Yes	Yes	Yes
Pethidine	Moderate	Yes	Yes	Yes
Fentanyl	Fast	Yes	Yes	Yes
Alfentanil	Very fast	No[a]	Yes	No
Remifentanil	Very fast	No[a]	No	No

PCAS, patient-controlled analgesia system; NCAS, Nurse-controlled analgesia system.
[a]Except with special supervision.

Midazolam

Midazolam is a water-soluble benzodiazepine, which can be given peripherally without causing thrombophlebitis or pain. Like all benzodiazepines it has sedative, amnesic, anxiolytic, and anticonvulsive properties. It has a rapid onset, short half-life (approximately 2 h), and is commonly used in combination with morphine in order to achieve both analgesia and sedation. It is primarily metabolized by the liver, and accumulation occurs in liver failure. The (phase I) metabolic product, 1'-hydroxymidazolam has around 10% of the activity of the parent drug. In renal failure, accumulation of 1'-hydroxymidazolam glucuronide (the phase II metabolic product) can cause prolonged sedation or coma.

Lorazepam

Lorazepam has been used as an alternative to midazolam. It undergoes metabolism only by glucuronidation to render it water-soluble, making it less likely for the parent drug to accumulate. It is dissolved in propylene glycol. Its adverse psychological effects are increasingly recognized.

Diazepam

Diazepam is rarely used in the critically ill, having been replaced by midazolam. It has a much longer duration of action and has many metabolites with significant activity of their own. This increases the risk of accumulation.

Propofol

Propofol (2,6-diisopropylphenol) was introduced as an anaesthetic agent, but is widely used as a hypnotic in the critically ill as a continuous infusion. Emergence from sedation is rapid and without hangover effect. Hypotension associated with propofol use (caused by a reduction in cardiac output and vasodilation) is common in the critically ill and is dose related. Propofol is a respiratory depressant, and prolonged apnoea can occur after bolus doses. Although metabolized primarily in the liver, extrahepatic breakdown does occur. There are no significantly active metabolites and propofol does not accumulate in hepatic or renal failure to a significant extent. However, because it is formulated in soya bean extract, prolonged infusion (more than 48 h) can lead to hyperlipidaemia.

Dexmedetomidine

Dexmedetomidine is not available in the United Kingdom and most of Europe, but is widely used elsewhere. It is a potent, highly selective α_2-adrenoceptor agonist. It has sedative, anxiolytic, amnesic, and sympatholytic effects. In addition, it reduces requirements for opioid analgesia. These effects are mediated centrally at postsynaptic α_2-receptors. In contrast to the agents already discussed, dexmedetomidine does not cause respiratory depression and exhibits remarkable cardiovascular stability.

Thiopentone

The intravenous anaesthetic agent thiopentone retains certain specialized indications, e.g. use in status epilepticus or to reduce raised intracerebral pressure. It has a half-life of 11 h, and prolonged infusion (i.e. >24 h) is usually associated with extremely prolonged action.

Combinations of agents

The combination of opioids and benzodiazepine does reduce the doses of both that are required, increasing efficacy and reducing toxicity.

Sedative drugs often act via differing mechanisms and so have slightly different actions. This difference can be used to advantage: e.g. propofol is mostly a hypnotic, while midazolam is a good anxiolytic and amnesic agent as well as producing hypnosis; in combination they are synergistic.

Analgesic and hypnotic antagonists

When accumulation of a drug or its metabolite is suspected as the cause of prolonged sedation, the diagnosis can be confirmed with the use of antagonists. Naloxone will quickly (but temporarily) reverse the effects of opioids, while flumazenil is a benzodiazepine antagonist. Their use is not recommended in patients suffering from head injury. Large doses of either antagonist given quickly can produce sudden arousal, causing agitation. When using naloxone, the sudden reversal of analgesia can cause a massive outpouring of catecholamines and precipitate arrhythmias.

Regional and epidural anaesthesia

For analgesia after certain surgical procedures or trauma, regional and epidural techniques can be extremely effective. Lumbar or thoracic epidurals can prevent hypoventilation and diaphragmatic splinting caused by pain after abdominal or thoracic procedures and fractured ribs, while avoiding the side effects of high-dose opioids. The problem of correct placement of regional blocks in critically ill patients is a considerable one, and complications (such as pneumothorax after intercostal block) must be carefully considered. Epidural analgesia, although desirable, may be contraindicated in the critically ill patient because of coagulopathy or sepsis.

Management of agitation, delirium, and confusion

Agitation, delirium, and confusion are some of the most difficult problems to deal with in the critically ill patient. Rapid, especially sudden, stopping of both therapeutic and recreational drugs (including alcohol and nicotine) may cause an acute abstinence syndrome. Prolonged use of analgesic and hypnotic drugs will also result in this problem when they are stopped, and any severe illness may also contribute to the problem. Gradually stopping drugs, and perhaps the use of substitute substances such as nicotine patches, may reduce this.

Once the patient has become agitated, delirious, or confused, they may need to be controlled with drugs such as clonidine, or haloperidol. Clonidine is a less selective α-agonist than dexmedetomidine and thought to act by competitively binding opioid catecholaminergic receptors. The maximum intravenous dose is 200 μg/h, and the oral dose 100 μg increasing to 200 μg 8-hourly. Haloperidol is a butyrophenone tranquillizer: the usual dose is 5 to 10 mg, with an onset of action 30 to 60 min after intravenous administration. Bolus doses of haloperidol and clonidine give better outcomes than continuous infusion.

Physical vs pharmacological restraint

There is considerable variation in the use of physical rather than pharmacological restraint in different countries. Part of this may be cultural: physicians and nurses accustomed to using physical restraints have little difficulty in doing so, whereas others feel it is inappropriate, and some regard it as unethical and find it difficult to use at all. However, with proper guidelines that address the ethical problems, the use of restraints such as boxing gloves and restrictive ties may offer the patient safety by preventing accidental removal of tubes and catheters while avoiding the toxicity of drugs.

Further reading

Carrupt PA, *et al.* (1991). Morphine 6-glucuronide and morphine 3-glucuronide as molecular chameleons with unexpected lipophilicity. *J Med Chem*, **34**, 1272–5.

Jacobi J, *et al.* (2002). Clinical practice guidelines for the sustained use of sedatives and analgesics in the critically ill adult. *Crit Care Med*, **30**, 119–41.

Park G, *et al.* (2007). A comparison of hypnotic and analgesic based sedation in a general intensive care unit. *Br J Anaesth*, **98**, 76–82.

Park GR (1996). Molecular mechanisms of drug metabolism in the critically ill. *Br J Anaesth*, 77, 32–49.

Schulte-Tamburen AM, *et al.* (1999). Comparison of five sedation scoring systems by means of auditory evoked potentials. *Intensive Care Med*, **25**, 377–82.

Trivedi M, Shelly M, Park G (2009). Advances in patient comfort: awake, delirious, or restrained. *Br J Anaesth*, **103**, 2–5.

Discontinuing treatment of the critically ill patient

M.J. Lindop

Essentials

A patient may have made an advance directive before the moment of decision about life-prolonging treatments, and their view is paramount. However, many patients have not made such a directive, and in this circumstance the responsibility for such decisions remains with the doctor.

Most people agree that prolongation of life itself is not necessarily a benefit: it is only valuable if that life is of adequate quality. Continuing aggressive treatment of a patient who is severely ill may not be kind or sensible.

Depending on the clinical situation, it may be appropriate to decide not to escalate treatment, not to attempt cardiopulmonary resuscitation in the event of circulatory arrest, or to withdraw treatment. Key points in management in such circumstances are:

(1) early anticipation of possible outcomes

(2) continuing review of whether treatments remain beneficial

(3) establishment of local guidelines for limiting or withdrawing treatment

(4) good communication with the patient (where possible), family, and health team

(5) clear documentation of decisions

Once a decision to withdraw treatment is made, then a drug or a feeding regimen can simply be stopped, and an intermittent therapy such as haemofiltration can be omitted. Terminal weaning is a protocol that allows death with dignity as mechanical ventilation is discontinued without causing distress to the patient or the family and carers.

The nature of the problem

A long-standing dilemma for doctors has been to judge the appropriateness of further treatment for patients who are already gravely ill. There has commonly been a reluctance to embark on major treatment, such as mechanical ventilation, for fear that it will be more difficult to withdraw this treatment than to avoid its introduction in the first place. Decisions are made on a constantly changing background—the views of society on the ethics of medical management, and the efficacy of new medical techniques are two prime factors. Admission for intensive care is no longer barred to patients on grounds of age alone.

Who is the patient without hope?

The public finds increasing difficulty with the concept that death is inevitable. There can be great pressure to prolong life for its own sake. Sometimes this is because the family has not had time to come to terms with the inevitability of a death. Most people would define an adequate quality of life as requiring:

◆ an ability to interact with others

◆ an awareness of his or her own existence, with a pleasure in the fact of that existence; and

◆ an ability to achieve some purposeful or self-directed action, or some self-set goal.

Where it is possible to know the patient's own wishes and values, it may be possible to infer whether he or she would consider life-prolonging treatment to be beneficial.

How certain is the outcome of a medical treatment?

Many treatments in intensive care will prolong life (mechanical ventilation or haemofiltration) but may not have a high likelihood of allowing complete recovery. Many scoring systems, such as APACHE (Acute Physiology, Age, and Chronic Health Evaluation), and later APACHE II and III, have been developed to describe the severity of initial illness and have had some success in predicting hospital mortality for large sample groups. However, they have proved of little value in making decisions on individual patients.

Is the decision to withdraw treatment different from the decision not to institute therapy?

Although it is emotionally easier for the doctor to avoid embarking on treatment than to withdraw it once started, there are no legal or moral differences between these options. The patient will never have the chance of benefit if a treatment is untried. It must be remembered, however, that prolongation of life itself is not necessarily a benefit, unless it is associated with the aforementioned qualities. If no benefit can be foreseen, then a treatment should be withdrawn, and knowing that it is possible to withdraw a treatment can give the confidence to embark on that treatment where its outcome is uncertain.

Ways of tackling the problem

How is the decision to withhold or to withdraw treatment made?

The patient

Some patients, such as those with particular types of advanced neurological disease, will be able to participate in decision-making. This may be in the form of an advance directive made before the moment of decision about life-prolonging treatment. In this situation the patient's view is paramount and limits the need for further discussion, but it is important that a full account of treatment options and their implications is given, and that the patient is judged to understand the issues involved. The challenge for the physician is to embark on these discussions: they must not be avoided, but must take place at a time that has been chosen with the advice of family and nursing staff.

The family

Much time may need to be spent with the family to gain information about the quality of previous lifestyle, and the likelihood that the patient will see life-prolonging treatment as a benefit. They should understand and support any discontinuation of treatment, but should not be asked to make the decision to stop treatment, or be put in a position where they think that they are being asked to do so. This is rarely a problem if full discussions have taken place throughout the course of the illness. In rare instances, families can have complex structures such that it will be clear that they are not able to put the interest of the patient first. In this situation further discussions may be required, and the help of social workers and religious advisers can be useful in orchestrating dialogue. Neither the next of kin nor those with enduring power of attorney have any legal right to determine treatment. This responsibility remains with the doctor assisted by the health care team, and—very rarely—by the courts of law. However, the requirements (in the United Kingdom) of the Mental Capacity Act 2005 and the Mental Health Act 2007 may make assistance from the hospital's legal advisors necessary where the discussion with the family is in any way not straightforward.

The medical, nursing, and paramedical team

Much important information can be gained by talking to the patient's own doctor (general practitioner). Nurses caring for a patient over a prolonged period will also be able to provide further useful information and should be consulted. Several physicians may have cared for patients with complex problems, and in an intensive care unit (ICU) there will be a team of consultants: a formal arrangement should be made to consult all these doctors in the process of making decisions, and their opinions should be carefully documented. Their help will be needed to answer the essential questions:

1 Is the diagnosis secure? Are further investigations required before a decision can be made?

2 Is the benefit of further treatment to the patient clear?

3 Is the invasiveness and discomfort of any treatment justified in the circumstances?

How can treatment be withdrawn?

Once a decision is made, then a drug or a feeding regimen can simply be stopped, and an intermittent therapy such as haemofiltration can be omitted. However, patients who are mechanically ventilated need more careful management. Despite the discussions about terminal weaning of patients in the 1980s, a survey of critical care physicians in 1994 revealed widespread disparity of practice.

Terminal weaning is a protocol that allows death with dignity as mechanical ventilation is discontinued without causing distress to the patient or the family and carers. This is conducted as follows:

1 Stop vasoactive and antibiotic drugs.

2 Stop any paralysing drugs.

3 Continue sedatives and analgesics to avoid distress.

4 Continue physiological monitoring and recording of observations and medical actions.

5 Change the mode of ventilation to synchronized intermittent mandatory ventilation (SIMV), which allows the patient to breathe but superimposes a defined number of breaths per minute.

6 Halve the SIMV rate every 30 min until less than 6, and then discontinue SIMV.

7 Use morphine to control dyspnoea and benzodiazepines to control restlessness.

8 If breathing has become stable, allow the patient to breathe spontaneously, and consider lying the patient on the side for extubation.

9 Usually the patient will have died by this stage, but sometimes adequate respiration is established. Death usually follows shortly, but it may be necessary to transfer them to a general ward area for basic care, although this can be very disruptive for the family and should be avoided if at all possible.

Decisions not to escalate treatment and not to resuscitate a patient

Careful discussions as described above, which should be clearly documented in the medical notes, are a prerequisite of making decisions not to escalate treatment, or not to resuscitate a patient. The decisions must be reviewed each day by the consultant in charge of the patient to ensure their continuing relevance.

Do not escalate

If further complications supervene it can be decided that new treatment is unlikely to give the patient real benefit. A 'do not escalate' order is made so that no therapies will be added. Typically, it may be decided not to increase the inotrope dose, not to use haemofiltration, not to transfuse blood or blood products, or not to implement or to increase ventilatory support. In summary, the current level of treatment continues while the patient continues to show a beneficial response.

Do not resuscitate

In similar circumstances it may be appropriate to decide that in the event of unexpected circulatory arrest no resuscitation will be attempted. If the documentation is not clear, a resuscitation attempt will be necessary and this can be very distressing to the family at the bedside if it seems inappropriate. Where circulatory arrest has occurred as a result of a drug administration error, a tension pneumothorax, or a complication of therapy, it may be appropriate that a limited (5 min) attempt at resuscitation is made despite the existence of a 'do not resuscitate' order, but this is contentious.

Does basic care include provision of fluids and nutrition?

Basic care provides warmth, shelter, hygiene, and comfort to the patient by relieving pain and distress. It includes the regular offer of oral fluid and nutrition. Fluid and nutrition provided 'artificially' by intravenous infusion, or by tube (whether nasogastric or percutaneous endoscopic gastrostomy—PEG), is considered a form of treatment and as such can be withdrawn (although, in the specific instance of the persistent vegetative state in England and Wales, review by a court of law is needed).

Case report

An 80-year-old patient with many severe chronic health problems is admitted with acute abdominal pain and shock. A laparotomy is required to establish the diagnosis. The patient may be admitted to an ICU for stabilization prior to surgery.

- Scenario 1—The bowel is extensively infarcted with no hope of survival. The patient is extubated at the end of surgery, and is allowed to die peacefully with appropriate analgesia and sedation, perhaps in the postanaesthesia care unit or the general ward.

- Scenario 2—There is extensive peritoneal sepsis that could respond to definitive surgery and antibiotic therapy. The patient is admitted to an ICU where monitoring and initial treatment is aggressive. Limits are set beyond which treatment will not escalate. These may be a maximum dose of adrenaline of, say, 0.25 μg/kg per min, no haemofiltration in the event of renal failure, and no resuscitation and no continuing mechanical ventilation after 48 h if there has been no improvement.

Further reading

Faber-Langendoen K (1994). The clinical management of dying patients receiving mechanical ventilation. *Chest*, **106**, 880–8.

General Medical Council (2006). *Withholding and withdrawing life-prolonging treatments: Good practice in decision-making.* http://www.gmc-uk.org/guidance/current/library/witholding_lifeprolonging_guidance.asp.

Grenvik A (1983). 'Terminal weaning'; discontinuance of life-support therapy in the terminally ill patient. *Crit Care Med*, **11**, 394–5.

Knaus WA, *et al.* (1991). The APACHE III prognostic system. Risk prediction of hospital mortality for critically ill hospitalized adults. *Chest* **100**, 1619–36.

Brainstem death and organ donation

M.J. Lindop

Essentials

Brain death in the United States of America is defined as the 'irreversible cessation of all functions of the entire brain, including the brainstem...that are clinically ascertainable'; in the United Kingdom the definition focuses on brainstem function. Half of those who fulfil the necessary clinical criteria will have a cardiac arrest despite intensive treatment within 24 h, and this happens to almost all within 72 h.

Organ donation when brainstem death occurs is well known to the public. In the United Kingdom, under the Human Tissue Act 2004, any known wishes of the patient relating to organ donation are considered paramount.

There are three essential components to the clinical testing of brainstem function prior to the declaration of brainstem death.

(1) Preconditions—the diagnosis must confirm irreversible damage; the patient must be in unresponsive coma.

(2) Exclusions—reversible causes of coma must be excluded, in particular drug activity, metabolic/endocrine causes, and hypothermia.

(3) Clinical criteria—testing must show absence of brainstem reflexes and of spontaneous respiration.

If the patient is brainstem dead and will become an organ donor, the focus of management becomes the care of the potential donor organs.

Introduction

The statement by the Conference of Medical Royal Colleges and their Faculties in 1976 led to the establishment of the concept of brainstem death in British practice. Similar procedures took place in many other countries, such as The President's Guidelines in the United States of America in 1981. Although the motive was to clarify the practice of organ donation for transplantation, the concept has proved useful in determining appropriate care for many patients in intensive care who are certainly not suitable as organ donors.

The concept of brainstem death

Brain death in the United States of America is defined as the 'irreversible cessation of all functions of the entire brain, including the brainstem ... that are clinically ascertainable'. In the United Kingdom, the focus has been on brainstem function since it is argued that, in the absence of brainstem function, there will be no activity of the reticular formation and the capacity for consciousness is lost. Deep unconsciousness results from damage bilaterally to a circumscribed area in the tegmentum of the mesencephalon and the rostral pons. In the determination of brainstem death, there is no testing of the function of other areas of the brain, such

as electroencephalography of the cerebral cortex. The diagnosis can be made on clinical signs alone, and half of those who fulfil the necessary clinical criteria will have a cardiac arrest despite intensive treatment within 24 h, and this happens to almost all within 72 h.

Managing the patient who is potentially brainstem dead (Fig. 17.9.1)

The patient with severe brain damage will be unconscious and on a ventilator. There will have been neurological testing to chart progress, showing that it is likely that the clinical signs of brainstem death will be present. The admitting consultant or the intensive care consultant should see the family to discuss the severity of the brain damage and explain that there will be formal clinical testing of brainstem reflexes that will determine whether there is any prospect of recovering consciousness. A timetable for this testing should be proposed, with the interview being an opportunity to discuss the option for organ donation with the family.

Organ donation when brainstem death occurs is well known to the public, and often the family will be the first to raise the matter. In the United Kingdom, there is no legal obligation for the doctor to raise the subject, but many families will feel cheated if they have had no chance to offer organ donation: they commonly

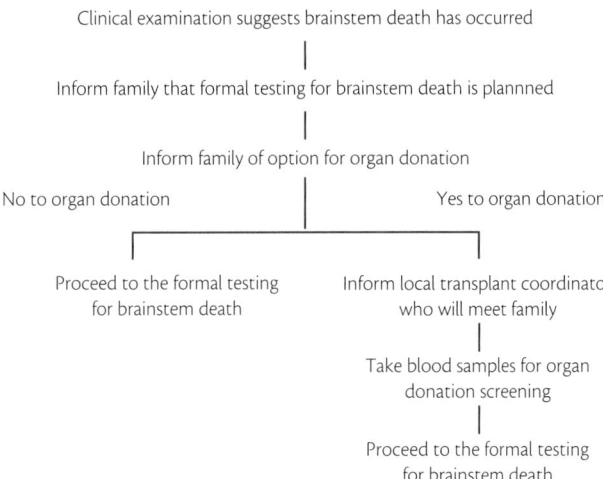

Fig. 17.9.1 Management of brainstem death.

feel comfort when donation is seen as the only good that can come out of the disaster of an unexpected death. A transplant coordinator will be available to meet the family and discuss the process of organ donation, and this is the time to check whether the patient fulfils the criteria for acting as an organ donor. In the United Kingdom, under the Human Tissue Act 2004, any known wishes of the patient relating to organ donation are considered paramount, and this can now be reviewed within a clearly defined framework. The family may influence which organs should be available for donation, but they may not influence or make conditions regarding the choice of recipient.

Diagnosis of brainstem death

Planning the tests (Fig. 17.9.2)

In the United Kingdom, the diagnosis must be confirmed by two medical practitioners that are competent in neurological examination and have been registered with the General Medical Council for more than 5 years. At least one should be a consultant, and neither can be a member of the transplant team. They can conduct the tests either separately or jointly. A second testing is done at a later time to remove the risk of observer error. The interval between the tests is not fixed, but is usually between 1 and 6 h based on clinical judgement that will reassure all those concerned with the care of the patient that there has been a measured assessment. The legal time of death is the completion of the first set of tests that reveals no brainstem function. The declaration of death and, if organs will not be donated, the stopping of the ventilator take place after the second testing. Most intensive care units (ICU) now have a pro forma which guides the process of testing.

Performance of the tests

There are three essential components to the clinical testing of brainstem function prior to the declaration of brainstem death—preconditions, exclusions, and clinical criteria.

Preconditions

1 The diagnosis must give an aetiology that confirms that the damage is irreversible.

2 The patient must be in unresponsive coma, though spinal reflexes do not exclude the diagnosis.

Exclusions

Reversible causes of coma must be excluded with certainty.

1 Drug activity, such as narcotics, muscle relaxants, or hypnotics. Due attention must be made to the possibility of prolonged action from previous overdosage, or from metabolism that could be impaired by hepatic or renal failure.

2 Metabolic or endocrine causes of coma—such as hypoglycaemia, hyperglycaemia, hyponatraemia, hepatic failure, uraemia, myxoedema, or Reye's syndrome.

3 Hypothermia—there is no fixed recommendation, but testing should be done at higher than 35°C.

Clinical criteria

These tests show absence of brainstem reflexes and of spontaneous respiration. It is helpful to remember them by relating them to the relevant cranial nerves.

1 No pupillary response to light (II, III).

2 Absent corneal reflexes (V, VII).

3 Absent vestibulo-ocular reflex (VIII)—no nystagmus with installation of 20 ml of cold fluid into the unblocked ears.

4 No motor response within cranial nerve distribution with pain stimulus to face, trunk, or limbs. No limb response to painful pressure over supraorbital notch (V, VII).

5 Absent gag reflex (IX).

6 Absent cough reflex (X).

7 Absence of spontaneous respiration—the apnoea test. At the beginning of reflex testing, the ventilator should be set to deliver 100% oxygen for more than 10 min to denitrogenate the lungs.

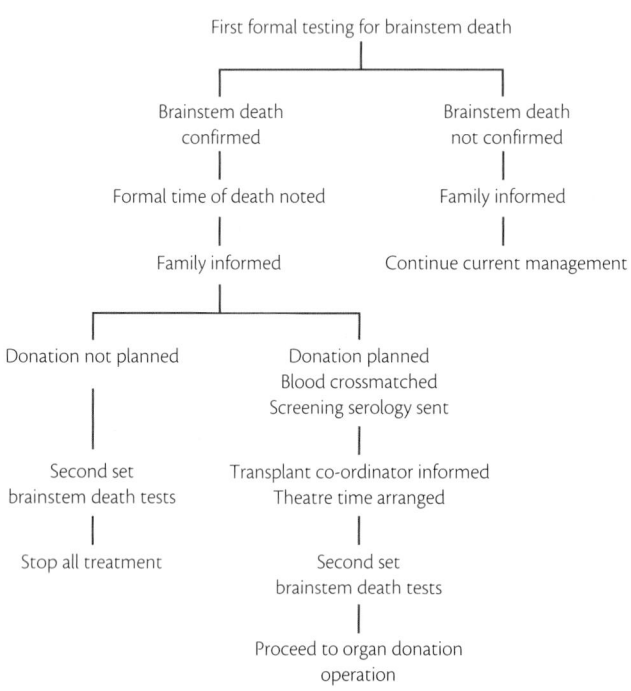

Fig. 17.9.2 Organization of brainstem death testing after first family interviews.

An arterial blood gas sample may be taken. The patient is disconnected from the ventilator and oxygen is insufflated via a catheter into the tracheal tube. Although less than 1 litre/min is absorbed, a flow of 6 litre/min is usually recommended. In apnoea, the $Paco_2$ rises at between 0.5 and 1 kPa/min. Careful observation of the patient for respiratory movements during the disconnection continues until arterial blood gas analysis shows that the $Paco_2$ has risen to more than 7 kPa (just over 50 mmHg). Oxygenation is usually well maintained. An alternative arrangement is to connect the patient to an anaesthetic breathing circuit with a reservoir bag. Respiratory movements may be seen more easily by movement of the bag than by observing the chest, but small cardiac pulsations can be transmitted by the airway and these can be mistaken for breathing activity by inexperienced staff. The patient is usually reconnected to the ventilator once the target $Paco_2$ is reached if this is the first testing, or if organ donation is planned.

The patient who is brainstem dead and will not become an organ donor

After the completion of the apnoea test in the second testing, the oxygen catheter is removed from the tracheal tube, the patient is not reconnected to the ventilator, and death is pronounced. The heart will stop over the next 15 min.

The patient who is brainstem dead and will become an organ donor

Acceptability as an organ donor

Transplant coordinators are informed that the tests have now been completed and have confirmed brainstem death, following which they will ensure that the criteria in Table 17.9.1 are met.

Clinical management of the organ donor on the ICU

The management of the patient now changes dramatically. Previously, all therapy has been directed at maintaining cerebral perfusion to preserve brain function. Now the emphasis changes to focus on care of the potential donor organs, and the donor operation is arranged as soon as possible. The common problems of the organ donor are hypotension, cardiac arrhythmias, diabetes insipidus, pulmonary oedema, and disseminated intravascular coagulation.

Cardiovascular problems

Cardiovascular instability is the most common problem in the organ donor. Brainstem death leads to high catecholamine levels that may increase heart rate, blood pressure, cardiac output, and systemic vascular resistance. Widespread myocardial ischaemic damage can occur associated with defective oxidative metabolism. These changes in autonomic tone, combined with myocardial ischaemia and metabolic and electrolyte instability, all lead to a high incidence of cardiac rhythm disturbance. The ECG may show atrial and ventricular arrhythmias, atrioventricular conduction blocks, and widespread ST segment and T wave changes. An initial hypertensive phase is followed by hypotension in 80% of patients, the common causes of which are shown in Box 17.9.1. Direct arterial and central venous pressure monitoring are essential, and a pulmonary

Table 17.9.1 Criteria for organ donation

1		General	
	a	Age up to 75—upper age limit varies with organ	
	b	Brainstem death is confirmed	
	c	Currently on a ventilator	
	d	No known malignant disease, unless group 1 primary brain tumour (Council of Europe Consensus Document 1997)	
	e	No systemic sepsis	
	f	No known social or medical high risk factors for HIV	
2		**Registration with the United Kingdom Transplant Support Services Authority (UKTSSA)**	
3		**Consent from the coroner or procurator fiscal may be required because of the circumstances of the death, but is not specifically required for organ donation. Nevertheless, the coroner or fiscal is usually informed about a death leading to organ donation**	
4		**Family confirmation that contraindications to transplantation do not exist. The donor should not:**	
	a	have been positive for HIV, hepatitis B, or C	
	b	have been treated for haemophilia or clotting disorders	
	c	have injected themselves with drugs	
	d	have had sexual relationships with special risk of virus transmission	
	e	have had Creutzfeldt–Jakcob disease (CJD), nor be related to a sufferer of CJD, nor have had any neurological disease of unknown cause	
	f	have had malaria, rabies, or tuberculosis	
	g	have had a previous malignant disease	

artery catheter may prove useful to assess preload and to estimate cardiac output and systemic vascular resistance. Targets for management are: (1) mean arterial pressure at least 70 mmHg; (2) central venous pressure about 10 mmHg; and (3) urine output at least 1 ml/kg per h.

Intravascular volume depletion should be treated with blood or colloid, with urinary losses replaced with appropriate electrolyte solutions—nasogastric water or intravenous 5% dextrose in uncontrolled diabetes insipidus. Likely electrolyte imbalance such as hypokalaemia must be sought by regular blood electrolyte measurements. Anti-arrhythmic drugs, inotropic agents, and vasopressors may be required, but inotropes and vasopressors should be used as sparingly as possible since the direct action of large doses will threaten perfusion and function of the donor organs. Their use should only be considered when cardiac output studies confirm an indication; e.g. when a profound fall in systemic vascular resistance with high cardiac output may justify use of noradrenaline in a small dose of 0.02 µg/kg per min. Some protocols use dopamine at 2 µg/kg per min routinely to improve renal, mesenteric, and coronary blood flow. Dopexamine at 1 µg/kg per min may give similar benefit. Use of a hormone replacement regimen may improve cardiovascular stability (see below).

Box 17.9.1 Causes of hypotension in brainstem death

- Hypovolaemia
  - Drug- or hyperglycaemia-induced diuresis
  - Diabetes insipidus
  - Previous therapeutic fluid restriction
  - Blood loss
- Peripheral vasodilatation from loss of vasomotor tone
- Myocardial depression
  - Subendocardial ischaemic damage, even in previously healthy hearts
  - Impaired oxidative metabolism and low energy stores from hormonal changes
  - Previous contusion (or tamponade)
  - Acute electrolyte disturbances

Tight control of fluid balance is important as overload can impair organ function, particularly in lung transplantation.

Endocrine problems

Pituitary damage leads to failure of endocrine homeostasis. Triiodothyronine (T_3) and thyroxine (T_4) levels fall. Loss of ADH leads to diabetes insipidus in up to 65% of donors: Table 17.9.3 shows the characteristics of this condition. Cortisol production may fall, but this does not seem to correlate with cardiovascular changes. Blood sugar control is often defective and an insulin infusion is commonly required.

The routine use of endocrine supplements is not established. Animal studies show no correlation between hormone deficiencies and cardiovascular instability, but endocrine supplements should be used where there is significant cardiovascular instability with substantial inotrope requirements. A suitable regimen is: (1) triiodothyronine as a 4 µg bolus followed by infusion of 3 µg/h; (2) desmopressin or vasopressin (see Table 17.9.2); (3) insulin, continuous infusion of 1 to 10 unit/h titrated to keep blood sugar at 6–8 mmol/litre; and (4) hydrocortisone supplements at 100 mg every 2 h (there is no risk of toxicity during the short period prior to donation).

Respiratory problems

The organ donor commonly has some pulmonary dysfunction. Possible causes are pneumonia, aspiration of gastric contents,

Table 17.9.2 Diabetes insipidus

Urine flow > 4 ml/kg per h
Urine osmolality < 300 mosmol/kg
Urine sodium < 10 mmol/litre
Treatment to achieve urine flow of 1 ml/kg per h:
desmopressin as a 1–4 µg intravenous bolus (up to hourly)
or vasopressin at 2 units/h by continuous infusion

neurogenic pulmonary oedema, and direct contusion. Controlled ventilation should be used to achieve $Paco_2$ in the normal range (4.5–5.5 kPa) to avoid hypocapnic reduction of peripheral oxygenation and disruption of regional blood flows, with sufficient oxygen given to achieve a Pao_2 of 11 to 13 kPa. A large tidal volume (12–15 ml/kg) delivered at a low ventilatory rate promotes gas exchange and reduces atelectasis. Modest positive end-expiratory pressure (PEEP), about 5 cmH$_2$O, is useful, but higher levels may impair cardiac output and hepatic and renal blood flow.

'Neurogenic' pulmonary oedema occurs in about 20% of donors. The causes of this are not known and there is no specific therapy. The usual approach is to monitor the circulation closely and endeavour to optimize left ventricular function. PEEP often helps, but even at high levels (up to 15 or 20 cmH$_2$O) is not always effective.

Unless there is pulmonary oedema, regular tracheal toilet to prevent accumulation of secretions and atelectasis is important. If PEEP is being used, then tracheal suction should be used sparingly and via a closed system. Strict asepsis must be maintained as lungs that may be implanted into a recipient will become prone to infection.

Coagulation abnormalities

Disseminated intravascular coagulation can be precipitated in 30% of donors by release of tissue thromboplastin, fibrinolytic substances, and plasminogen activators in severe head injury. Characteristic changes are thrombocytopenia with fall in fibrinogen levels and the appearance of D-dimer fibrin degradation products. Effective haemostasis is needed during the donor operation to reduce blood loss and maintain cardiovascular stability. Fresh frozen plasma and platelets should be given to correct the deficiencies. Antifibrinolytics such as ε-aminocaproic acid must be avoided in case they provoke microvascular thrombosis in donor organs.

Temperature control

Temperature regulation is impaired. Heat production falls with low metabolic rate and muscle inactivity, and vasodilatation promotes heat loss. Cooling can lead to impaired oxygen delivery to tissues, aggravation of cardiac arrhythmias, increased diuresis, and impaired platelet function. There should be active warming (to higher than 35 °C) by limitation of exposure to the environment, warming blankets, fluid warming, and proper humidification of inspired gases.

Clinical management of the organ donor operation

The operation lasts 3 to 6 h. Four units of blood should be cross-matched to compensate for blood loss. Although anaesthesia is not required, an anaesthetist or a specially trained medical technician will be required to supervise cardiovascular monitoring and maintenance of a stable circulation. Reflex hypertension can be a problem: small doses of vasodilating isoflurane or intravenous vasodilators are often required.

Further reading

Anon (1976). Diagnosis of brain death. Statement issued by the honorary secretary of the Conference of Medical Royal Colleges and their Faculties in the United Kingdom on 11 October 1976. *Br Med J*, **ii**, 1187–8.

Chase TN, Moretti L, Prensky AL (1968). Clinical and electroencephalographic manifestations of vascular lesions of the pons. *Neurology*, **18**, 357–68.

Council of Europe (1997). *Standardisation of organ donor screening to prevent transmission of neoplastic diseases*. Council of Europe.

Intensive Care Society Working Group on Organ and Tissue Donation. *Chapter 5. Clinical management of the potential heartbeating organ donor*. http://www.uktransplant.org.uk/ukt/about_transplants/donor_care/policy_documents/ICS_guidelines_for_adult_organ_and_tissue_donation_chapter_5(nov2004).pdf

Mackersie RC, Bronsther OL, Shackford SR (1991). Organ procurement in patients with fatal head injuries. The fate of the potential donor. *Ann Surg*, **213**, 143–50.

Mollaret P, Bertrand I, Mollaret H (1959). Coma dépassé et nécroses nerveuses centrales massives. *Rev Neurol (Paris)*, **101**, 116–39.

Wheeldon DR, *et al.* (1993). Transplantation of unsuitable organs? *Transplant Proc*, **25**, 3014–5.

SECTION 18

Respiratory disorders

Structure and function

Contents

18.1.1 The upper respiratory tract

J.R. Stradling and S.E. Craig

Essentials

The upper respiratory tract extends from the anterior nares to the larynx and comprises (1) the nose—with main function as first-line defence against problems with incoming air, acting as a coarse particle filter and a conditioner (temperature and humidity) of the air, and with the sense of smell helping to detect noxious substances that are best avoided. (2) The pharynx—this has to be a rigid tube when used for breathing, but during swallowing it has to be a collapsed tube capable of peristalsis, a combination of functions which is achieved by complex innervation and musculature. Subepithelial collections of lymphoid tissue in the pharynx are ideally suited to process inhaled and swallowed antigens. (3) The larynx—this has three important functions: communication, protection of the airway, and dynamic control of lung volume.

The nose

Anterior nares

The anterior nares, which include the nasal valve just inside the nose, are usually the narrowest part of the respiratory tract and account for about 40% to 50% of the total respiratory resistance. In normal subjects the resistance in the lower airways is small (<25%) compared with the larynx and nose. This anterior nasal resistance is actively controlled by the levator alae nasi and procerus muscles,

which flare the nostrils, and the compressor naris muscle, which narrows the nasal valve further. During mild exercise these muscles (combined with sympathetic nasal mucosal vasoconstriction) can halve the nasal resistance and allow minute ventilations up to 30 litres/min before conversion to oral breathing is necessary. These muscles receive a phasic inspiratory signal, to brace open the nares with each breath, just in advance of diaphragmatic activity.

Occasionally, owing to deformity of the anterior nasal cartilages, the anterior nares are very narrow and limit inspiration, particularly during sleep when the dilator muscle activity is reduced. This is one of the rarer causes of snoring that is amenable to treatment.

Turbinates

The main function of the nose is as first-line defence against problems with the incoming air. In this respect it acts as a coarse particle filter and a conditioner (temperature and humidity) of the air, and helps the sense of smell to detect noxious substances that are best avoided. The turbinates in the nose present a surface on to which large inhaled particles, such as pollen grains and house dust mite faecal particles, will be retained, with the potential for an allergic response producing allergic rhinitis. Debris arriving on the mucosal surfaces is wafted backwards to be swallowed eventually. Without this so-called 'mucociliary carpet' there is decreased resistance to infections (usually a generalized respiratory problem and not just in the nose), with pooling of mucopurulent material and recurrent sinus infections. This mucociliary function can be tested by placing a saccharine tablet on the anterior floor of the nasal cavity and timing the period that elapses before it can be tasted in the oral cavity. The normal interval is about 15 to 20 min, but with ciliary defects this can extend to an hour or more.

Vascular supply

The turbinates fill such a large proportion of the nasal cavity that minor swelling produces large changes in nasal airflow resistance (Fig. 18.1.1.1). There are several rich vascular beds at different depths in the nasal mucosa, providing a large surface area to warm and humidify incoming air. These are supplied by the sphenopalatine branch of the maxillary artery, with venous drainage passing back into the cavernous sinus around the carotid artery. The volume of fluid in these vascular beds is controlled via the vidian nerve, which contains sympathetic vasoconstrictor and parasympathetic

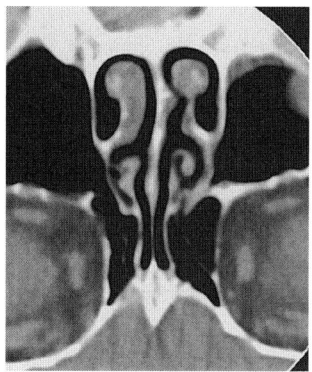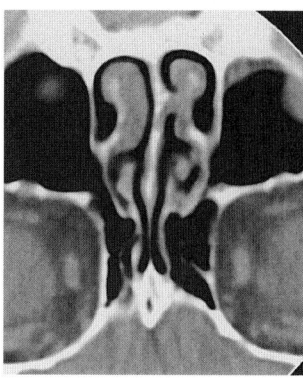

Fig. 18.1.1.1 Coronal sections of human maxillary sinuses and the turbinates in the nose. The view in the panel on the left is taken after ephedrine drops and shows mucosal shrinkage. The consequent small increase in the size of the lumina was attended by a large increase in maximum nasal airflow. (Courtesy of Dr F Gleeson).

vasodilator fibres acting on both arterioles and venules. The overall blood flow and total volume of blood in the sinusoids determine the degree of mucosal congestion, which undergoes a cyclical reciprocal change across the two sides of the nose over 2 to 4 h, hence as the mucosa on one side is congesting that on the other side is shrinking. This cycle, usually only obvious to individuals with already narrowed nasal passages (when blockage can occur intermittently), can be interrupted by a reflex mediated by pressure on the side of the thorax or in the axilla. Thus, in the decubitus position, the upper nostril becomes clearer and the lower more congested, with the two sides swapping within a minute or two of turning on to the other side. The purpose of this nasal cycle is not known, but using the upper rather than the lower nostril when lying on one's side may lessen the chance of inhaling particulate matter. In addition to this effect there is a general increase in nasal congestion on lying down due to a hydrostatic rise in capillary pressure.

The volume of fluid needed to humidify the incoming air is considerable, but is reduced by condensation of some of this moisture back on to the cooler nasal mucosa during exhalation. Of course, this conditioning is lost during oral breathing, which has important implications for exercise-induced asthma, which is due to cooling and drying of intrathoracic airways.

Secretory function and sensory innervation

Nasal secretions come mainly from submucosal glands that are stimulated by parasympathetic (cholinergic) fibres. There is some evidence that sympathetic activity can also stimulate secretions, but of higher viscosity.

The sensory fibres from the nose travel in the maxillary nerve (mainly the ophthalmic branch) and are the afferent limb of some interesting reflexes. Airflow is sensed and can itself influence breathing pattern. Nerves containing substance P in the epithelium seem to be responsible for sensations leading to sneezing. Sneezing is like coughing in that an explosive expiration is generated in an attempt to expel foreign matter. Coughing involves closure of the larynx until pressure builds up, whereas sneezing involves closure of the pharynx. Unlike coughing, sneezing is never voluntary. Sensory fibres from much of the upper airway, nose and face are also involved in the diving reflex. This reflex is of great importance to diving mammals, when the combination of facial stimulation

by cold water, apnoea and hypoxaemia produce intense peripheral, splanchnic, renal, and muscular vasoconstriction. This diverts blood to the brain and conserves oxygen (producing a heart–lung–brain circulation that prolongs diving time), with the rise in blood pressure limited by a marked vagally induced bradycardia. This vestigial reflex in humans can be utilized in the control of some cardiac arrhythmias, when a brisk increase in vagal tone can be produced by applying ice-cold water to the face.

Nasal irritation can lead to either bronchoconstriction or bronchodilation. The bronchoconstriction can be prevented by atropine and is presumably vagally mediated. This reflex may be important in provoking bronchospasm in some asthmatics. Negative pressure in the nasal cavities can also be sensed, producing a reflex increase in upper airway dilator action (see the following section on the pharynx).

Olfaction depends on recognition of molecules by mucosal receptors at the very top of the nose. These olfactory cells have central axons that pass through multiple tiny holes in the skull (cribriform plate) to the brain. At this point they are very vulnerable to shearing forces during a blow to the head, leading to anosmia (loss of ability to smell).

The pharynx

Anatomical divisions

The pharynx is divided into the nasopharynx, oropharynx, and laryngopharynx or hypopharynx—behind the soft palate, the back of the oral cavity down to the tip of the epiglottis, and the tip of the epiglottis down to the cricoid cartilage, respectively. Thus the top end is level with the base of the skull and the bottom end is about level with the sixth cervical vertebra, giving an overall length of about 12 cm. When being used for breathing, the pharynx has to be a rigid tube (like the trachea), but during swallowing it has to be a collapsed tube capable of peristalsis (like the oesophagus). This combination of functions is achieved by having a muscular tube that can constrict to propel food, but also has external muscles whose function is to brace open the pharynx when required.

Pharyngeal muscles

Fig. 18.1.1.2 shows the enormous complexity of the pharyngeal musculature, supplied mainly by the hypoglossal nerve (XII). The pharyngeal constrictors (superior, middle, and lower) are the main peristaltic muscles; the lower part of the inferior constrictor also functions as a sphincter to the top of the oesophagus, preventing air entry during inspiration. Most of the other pharyngeal muscles work in concert to hold open the pharynx. For example, the genioglossus pulls forward the tongue, the geniohyoid together with the strap muscles (sternothyroid, thyrohyoid, etc.) pulls forward the hyoid (enlarging the oropharynx), and the stylopharyngeus probably pulls sideways on the lateral pharyngeal walls. The palatopharyngeus will hold open the pharynx if supported by the levator palati, but will also pull forward the palate to open the nasopharynx. The upper pharyngeal muscles (tensor palati and levator palati) also close off the nasal cavity during swallowing to prevent regurgitation of fluids into the nose. To prevent aspiration, closure of the larynx and the false cords above is coordinated with swallowing. Some of these actions require sensory information about the exact location and consistency of any food being swallowed, carried via the glossopharyngeal and vagus nerves (IX and X). Sensory branches

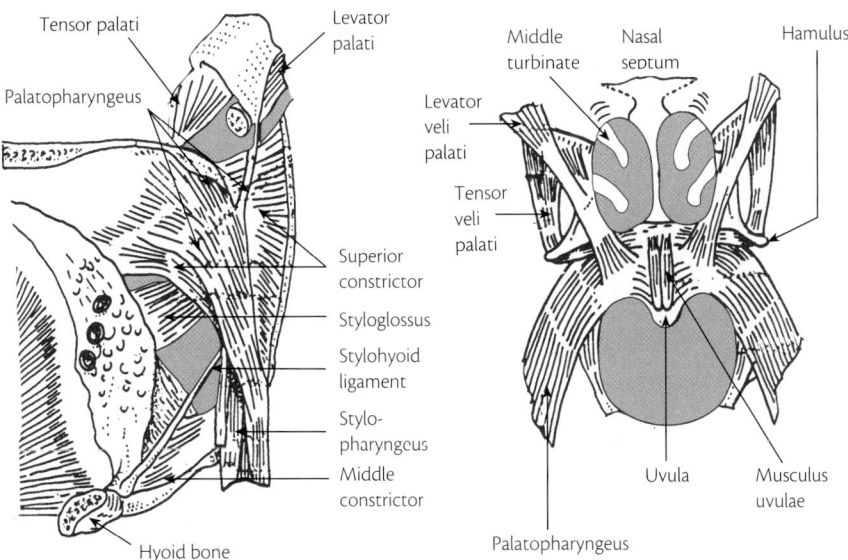

Fig. 18.1.1.2 Two views of the pharyngeal muscles: from inside the pharynx looking laterally (left panel), and from high up on the posterior pharyngeal wall looking anteriorly (right panel). These muscles act in concert and the physical effect of their contraction depends on which other muscles are simultaneously activated.

of these nerves also supply the ear, which explains why pharyngeal lesions may present with pain in the ear.

Given the complexities of pharyngeal function, it is not surprising that severe swallowing difficulties with aspiration of food and drink are often seen following cerebrovascular accidents in the brainstem involving the control of pharyngeal muscles and sensory pathways.

Powerful mechanisms maintain patency of the pharyngeal airway during breathing. As with the alae nasi, the pharyngeal dilator muscles receive a respiratory input in time with diaphragm activation. The diaphragm receives a gradually increasing level of phrenic activity to overcome elastic recoil as tidal volume increases, whereas the pharyngeal activation follows more of a 'square wave'. This makes teleogical sense, since the collapsing force is dependent on inspiratory flow and this is roughly constant throughout inspiration. Dilator activity increases if pharyngeal patency is threatened. Fig. 18.1.1.3 shows the reflex increase in genioglossus tone in response to a fall in intrapharyngeal pressure that will pull in the pharyngeal walls, which is thought to be mediated by 'distortion' receptors of some kind. Snoring occurs when the pharynx narrows enough to vibrate, and there is some evidence that this vibration itself can also activate pharyngeal dilators, thus warding off full collapse. The factors predisposing to pharyngeal collapse during sleep are discussed in Chapter 18.5.2.

Lymphoid tissue

Waldeyer's ring of lymphoid tissue, comprising the adenoids, the palatine tonsils, and the lingual tonsils (back of tongue), is situated in the pharynx. These subepithelial collections of lymphoid tissue are ideally suited to process inhaled and swallowed antigens. Unfortunately, if they hypertrophy too much in response to recurrent infections, they are also positioned such that they obstruct the airway, particularly in small children. This is usually first apparent during sleep, but may become severe enough to provoke inspiratory stridor, even while awake. Adenoidal enlargement, by blocking nasal airflow, will force mouth breathing which, if it occurs early enough (perhaps <18 months of age), retards development of the lower jaw (the so-called 'adenoidal facies'). This probably leads to overcrowding of the teeth and a narrower retroglossal space (further discussed in Chapter 18.5.2).

The larynx

The larynx (Fig. 18.1.1.4) has three important functions: communication, protection of the airway, and dynamic control of lung volume.

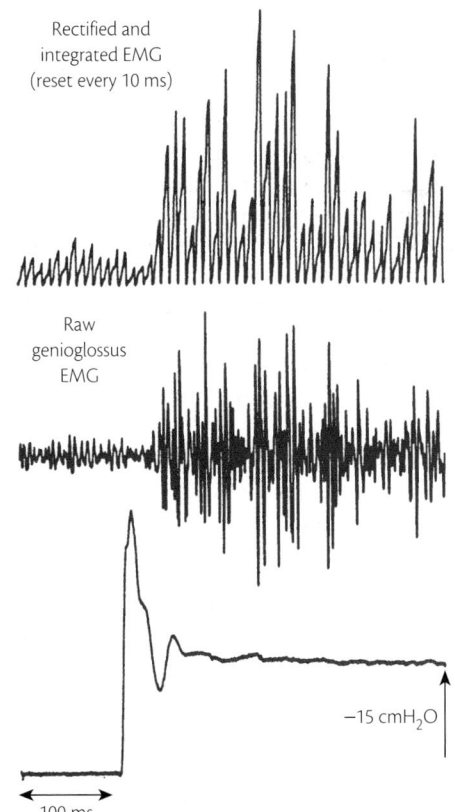

Fig. 18.1.1.3 Response of the genioglossus muscle in a conscious human to a sudden fall in intrapharyngeal pressure. The time delay (about 50 ms) is too short to be due to a cortical response and is presumably a spinal cord reflex.
(From Horner RL (1991). Evidence for reflex upper airway dilator muscle activation by sudden negative airway pressure in man. J Physiol, 436, 15–29, with permission of Wiley-Blackwell.)

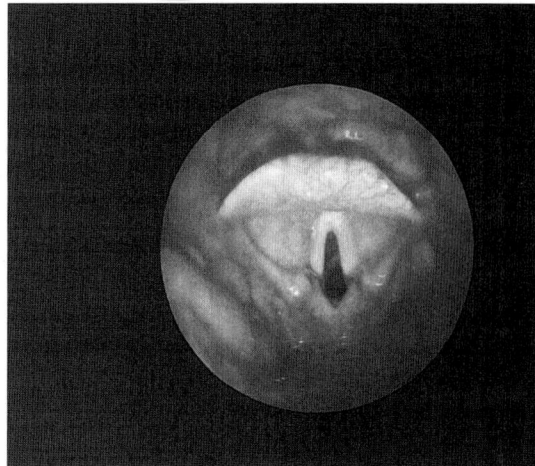

Fig. 18.1.1.4 Bronchoscopic view of the larynx from above. The top of the picture is the anterior.
(Courtesy of Dr P Stradling.)

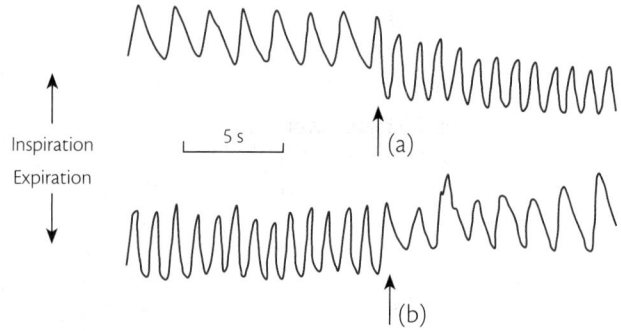

Fig. 18.1.1.5 Recorder tracings in a dog with atelectasis showing the effect of switching from upper airway to tracheostomy breathing (arrow at a) and from tracheostomy to upper airway breathing (arrow at b). The signal from an inductive plethysmograph measuring movement of both the ribcage and abdomen which represents lung expansion and contraction.

Communication and neuromuscular function

A few of the intrinsic and extrinsic muscles of the larynx (e.g. crico-thyroid, posterior cricoarytenoid) open (abduct) or brace the vocal cords, whereas most (e.g. thyroarytenoid, transverse, and oblique arytenoids) close (adduct) the cords. The recurrent laryngeal nerve (from the vagus) supplies all the muscles apart from the cricothy-roid (supplied from the superior laryngeal nerve, which is also a branch of the vagus). The left recurrent laryngeal nerve comes off the vagus and passes under the aortic arch before running up close to the thyroid gland to the larynx. This means it can be damaged by a tumour at the left hilum and surgically during a thyroidectomy. The right recurrent laryngeal nerve passes under the right subcla-vian artery, where it can be damaged by a right-sided apical lung tumour.

Recurrent laryngeal nerve paralysis

Complete paralysis of the recurrent laryngeal nerve gives perma-nent hoarseness of the voice, and the affected cord assumes a posi-tion midway between full abduction and adduction. The cord is floppy and can be moved passively very easily, being 'sucked' towards the midline during inspiration and blown open during expiration. The unparalysed cord may eventually compensate to some degree and move nearer the paralysed cord, improving the voice. If paralysis of the recurrent laryngeal nerve is incomplete, the affected cord may take up the adducted position, presumably because fibres running to the abductors are damaged first. When there is bilateral damage to the recurrent laryngeal nerves, loss of adequate abduction causes inspiratory stridor as the cords are passively drawn together.

Protection of the airway

As mentioned earlier, there are reflexes initiated by supralaryngeal sensory fibres (mainly via the internal branch of the superior laryn-geal nerve) to protect the airway. Fluid or food landing on or near the vocal cords will provoke coughing and/or laryngeal closure. During sleep, irritation of the cords tends to produce apnoea and laryngeal adduction, and coughing occurs only when wakefulness supervenes.

Dynamic control of lung volume

One of the less well-known functions of the larynx is to brake expiratory flow and thereby control lung volume. In some species, and in neonates, laryngeal expiratory braking is very important, acting rather like positive end-expiratory pressure to maintain end-expiratory lung volume above the passive functional residual capacity, thus preventing atelectasis. In adults there is no good evidence that the rate of expiration is under active laryngeal control, but this mechanism may come into action during respira-tory illnesses (such as pneumonia), especially if there is marked hypoxaemia. If the upper airway is bypassed, for instance by tra-cheostomy or intubation, then other mechanisms come into play to maintain end-expiratory lung volume, such as postinspiratory contraction of the diaphragm (thus delaying expiration) and short-ening of expiratory time (thus starting inspiration again before lung volume has fallen too far). Fig. 18.1.1.5 is from a tracheot-omized dog with areas of atelectasis. This shows how once laryn-geal braking is denied to the animal, expiration proceeds faster, lung volume falls, and expiratory time is shortened to produce tachypnoea. This reflex was not present when the areas of atelectasis had resolved. The clinical correlate of this is sometimes seen as an expiratory grunt in babies who have a respiratory illness. Intubation may worsen gas exchange in this situation unless positive end-expiratory pressure is also applied.

Further reading

Brouillette RT, Thach BT (1979). A neuromuscular mechanism maintaining extrathoracic airway patency. *J Appl Physiol*, **46**, 722–9.

Gautier H (1973). Control of the duration of expiration. *Resp Physiol*, **18**, 205–21.

Horner RL (1991). Evidence for reflex upper airway dilator muscle activation by sudden negative airway pressure in man. *J Physiol*, **436**, 15–29.

Matthew OP, Sant 'Ambrogio GS (1988). Respiratory function of the upper airway. In: *Lung biology in health and disease*, Vol. 35. Marcel Dekker, New York.

Remmers JE, Bartlett D (1977). Reflex control of expiratory airflow and duration. *J Appl Physiol*, **42**, 80–7.

18.1.2 Airways and alveoli

Peter D. Wagner

Essentials

The lung is the organ of gas exchange, providing the means of transferring oxygen (O_2) from the air to the blood by passive diffusion for subsequent distribution to the tissues, and of similarly removing metabolically produced carbon dioxide (CO_2) from the blood, which is then exhaled to the atmosphere.

A large area of contact between alveolar gas and capillary blood is required to ensure sufficient gas flux across the blood–gas barrier to meet metabolic demand: the lungs contain about 300 million very small (radius $c.$ 150 μm) alveoli.

After the mainstem bronchi have arisen from the trachea, the airways continue an essentially dichotomous branching pattern until the alveoli are reached. Successive branching of connected conducting pipes to the 16th generation yields in the order of 50 000 to 100 000 airways (called terminal bronchioles), each of which supplies a functional lung unit comprising a further 7 generations of divisions (3 divisions of respiratory bronchioles, then alveolar ducts, finally alveoli).

The lungs are enclosed within the thoracic cavity. Inspiration is driven by contraction of the intercostal muscles and the diaphragm, which expands the ribcage in both anteroposterior and lateral dimensions, such that the pressure inside the thoracic cavity but external to the lungs is reduced to below that of the air, which is thereby drawn in. Expiration to return lung volume to functional residual capacity after inspiration can occur by elastic recoil.

Lung diseases of many types commonly affect each of the steps involved in gas exchange, and the clinical consequences can usually be readily understood if the structure–function relationships are known.

The organ of gas exchange

The lung is the organ of gas exchange, providing the means of transferring oxygen (O_2) from the air to the blood for subsequent distribution to the tissues. At the same time it enables removal of metabolically produced carbon dioxide (CO_2) from the blood, which is then exhaled to the atmosphere. Not just in health, but also in lung disease, the volumes of O_2 taken up and CO_2 removed by the lung per minute must equal the rate of O_2 consumption and CO_2 production by the whole body.

The lung will also exchange any other gas that is presented to it, but the principles involved—passive diffusion—mirror those for O_2 and CO_2. Quantitative but not qualitative differences occur in how such gases (e.g. anaesthetic agents, carbon monoxide, toxic gases inhaled by accident) are handled by the lung. These differences stem from the means by which any particular gas is transported in the blood; whether in simple physical solution alone, or also in some chemical combination with molecules such as haemoglobin.

The principles are similar for gas uptake into blood and elimination from the blood. In fact, because gas exchange occurs by passive diffusion, whether a gas is taken up from the air into the blood or eliminated from the blood into the air depends simply on the partial pressures of the gas on each side of the blood–gas barrier, the 0.3 μm thick tissue layer separating alveolar gas from pulmonary capillary blood.

For transfer of a gas from the environment to the blood to occur, the gas in question must first be brought to the alveolar blood–gas barrier by the process of ventilation. Diffusion across this barrier then occurs at a rate proportional to (1) the alveolar surface area available and (2) the partial pressure difference between alveoli and blood, and inversely proportional to the thickness of the barrier, in concordance with the rules of simple passive diffusion. The gas molecules, now present dissolved physically in plasma, also distribute into the red cells. Depending on the gas, chemical associations may occur—with haemoglobin in the case of O_2, CO_2, carbon monoxide (CO), and nitric oxide (NO), and through transformation to bicarbonate ion for CO_2. The last element of the exchange process now occurs—the transport of the gas in blood pumped by the heart through the systemic circulation to the tissues of the body.

This chapter focuses on the first two of these three steps in gas exchange—ventilation and diffusion. A separate chapter deals with the third step—the pulmonary circulation (see Chapter 16.15.1). The structural basis of ventilation and diffusion, and the associated functional consequences, will be presented with particular emphasis on implications for disease. Lung diseases of many types commonly affect each of the steps involved in gas exchange, and the clinical consequences can usually be readily understood if the structure–function relationships are known.

Basic airway and alveolar design

In essence, the lung is a balloon undergoing cyclical inflation and deflation (ventilation, or tidal breathing) around some partially inflated state; the main anatomical elements are shown in Fig. 18.1.2.1. The gas-filled interior of the balloon corresponds to the alveolar gas spaces of the lung. The thin wall of the balloon may be likened to the blood–gas barrier, with the pulmonary capillary network imagined as covering the balloon's surface, separated from the interior (alveolar) gas by the elastic material making up the balloon's wall. The lung is inflated through the trachea with each inspiration, thus bringing fresh air (21% O_2, no CO_2) to the alveoli. This fresh gas is rapidly mixed with resident gas already present. This resident gas is partially depleted of O_2 by ongoing diffusion of O_2 into the capillaries, whilst at the same time CO_2 is evolved into the gas from the capillary blood. Each inflation, by bringing fresh air into the alveoli, slightly increases alveolar Po_2 and decreases alveolar Pco_2. Each deflation moves some of this alveolar gas back to the environment. This rids the lung of some CO_2, but also removes some O_2, albeit at lower concentrations than in room air. In normal quiet breathing, alveolar O_2 concentration averages about 16% over a respiratory cycle, whereas that of CO_2 is about 5%, and a long-term steady-state of gas exchange is achieved.

Because the process of gas exchange depends on simple, passive diffusion, a large area of contact between alveolar gas and capillary blood is required to ensure sufficient gas flux across the blood–gas barrier to meet metabolic demand. The balloon analogy, while useful as an initial concept, thus exhibits a major difference from how

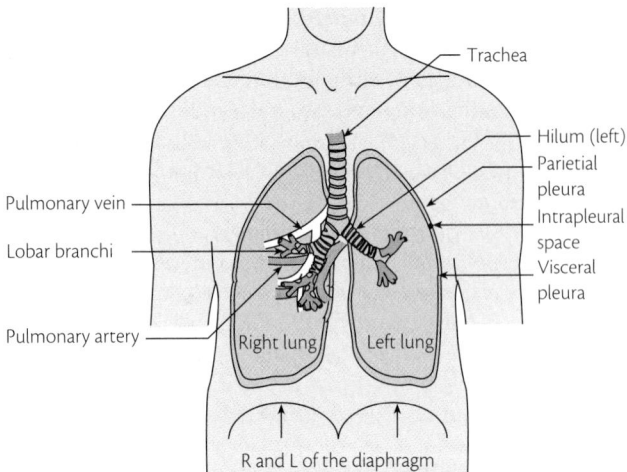

Fig. 18.1.2.1 The right and left lungs are separately encased within the thorax, and each is covered by a visceral pleural membrane. This is continuous with the parietal pleural membrane which lines the interior thoracic cavity, and the thin fluid-filled space between the visceral and parietal pleuras constitutes the intrapleural space. The hila of the two lungs contain the mainstem bronchi, and accompanying pulmonary arteries and veins. The mainstem bronchi join at the carina to form the trachea. The pulmonary arteries emanate from the right ventricle; the pulmonary veins empty into the left atrium. Within the lungs, the airways and blood vessels continue branching for approximately 20 generations. The major muscle of inspiration, the diaphragm, consists of two domes upon which the right and left lungs sit, and which separate the thoracic and abdominal contents.

the real lung is configured. The real lung has its total gas volume constituted not as a single balloon-like gas chamber, but as a very large number (about 300 million) of very small, almost spherical, balloons or alveoli(radius, r, $c.150\,\mu$m). Since the volume (V) of a sphere is $V = (4/3) \times \pi \times r^3$, while its surface area (A) is $A = 4 \times \pi \times r^2$, dividing a lung of a given volume (given because the lung must fit within the thoracic cage) into many small alveoli allows a much larger total surface area than if the lung were indeed a single large chamber. Given that a typical value for V is 4000 ml, a single sphere of this volume would have a radius of about 10 cm and a surface area of about 1200 cm^2, whereas 300 million alveoli, each with a radius of 150 μm have the same total volume but have a total surface area of about 800 000 cm^2, which approximates the area of a tennis court. Given the laws of diffusion, maximal pulmonary O_2 exchange would be insufficient for life were the lung a single chamber.

The lungs inside the thoracic cavity

As with a balloon, the lung cannot inflate itself (although, as an elastic structure, once inflated it is capable of unassisted deflation just like a balloon). Inflation requires creation of a pressure difference between the outside and inside of the lung, pressure being higher inside. This may be accomplished in one of only two ways. One is by positive pressure inflation, typical of most clinical ventilators that are connected to the trachea and produce inflation by mechanically increasing intratracheal airway pressure. Spontaneous breathing throughout normal life does not happen in this way, and so the only possibility of normally achieving lung inflation is by the second option—that of decreasing the pressure around the lungs below that of the surrounding air. This is accomplished by encasing

the lungs within the closed thoracic cavity, and having the muscles in the wall of this cavity (the intercostal muscles and the diaphragm) contract when inflation is desired. Contraction of these muscles moves the diaphragm caudally and expands the ribcage in both anteroposterior and lateral dimensions. As a result, the pressure inside the thoracic cavity but external to the lungs (i.e. within the intrapleural space) is reduced to below that of the air. Since the alveolar tissue is extremely thin and easily deformable, the pressure within the alveolar gas spaces is also reduced to below that of the air, and thus inflation occurs as a result of a hydrostatic pressure gradient from the mouth to the alveoli.

Inflation in the course of normal tidal breathing usually commences from a state of partial lung inflation that reflects that particular volume of the lung at which its own elastic recoil tendency to collapse is exactly balanced by the opposite, natural tendency of the ribcage to expand outwards. This volume is known as the functional residual capacity (FRC) and because it reflects recoil balance between lung and chest wall, it is the only volume which can be maintained without muscular effort. Thus, to either inhale above FRC or to exhale below FRC requires respiratory muscle contraction, but the return to FRC from either higher or lower volumes can be passive, stored elastic energy provided by respiratory muscle contraction from the preceding active volume change being used to reverse the transpulmonary pressure difference and enable gas flow from the alveoli to the mouth.

Clinical significance

Elastic properties and lung volume

If the elastic properties of either the lungs or the chest wall are altered by disease, FRC will change. Should the lungs become less elastic, typically seen in emphysema due to disorganization of the elastin and collagen fibres making up much of the alveolar wall structure, the tendency for the lung to collapse is less, and the lung/chest wall recoil balance shifts to a higher lung volume, thus increasing FRC. By contrast, diseases characterized by proliferation of alveolar wall elements—collagen in particular—renders the lung more elastic and thus collapsible, shifting FRC to lower values. These changes in FRC may be used to aid in diagnosis and in following the natural history and response to treatment of such diseases, since FRC is readily measured in the pulmonary function laboratory by either plethysmography or helium dilution methods. Changes in FRC also have important implications for lung function, discussed later in this chapter.

Whilst FRC is a key volume upon which to focus, the lung can normally be inflated to well above FRC, and also deflated to considerably below FRC. At maximal inflation, lung volume is referred to as the total lung capacity (TLC), while at maximal deflation, lung volume is called the residual volume (RV). Of major significance, RV is well above zero volume. As will be apparent, if all alveoli could be fully emptied of gas, they would be very difficult to reinflate to allow resumption of gas exchange, due to surface tension. The difference between TLC and RV is called the vital capacity (VC). As with FRC, each of these volumes is readily measured during routine pulmonary function testing, and together they provide a simple yet informative profile useful in characterizing many lung diseases and their progress. Unlike some physiological variables such as arterial pH or haemoglobin concentration, all of the above volumes depend to a major extent on body size. They also depend to a lesser degree on gender (smaller in females), age (deterioration with ageing), bodily habitus (often smaller in the obese), and ethnicity. Many tables of normal values have been published, and interpretation must allow for all of the determinants mentioned above.

Trachea, main bronchi, and pleura

For all 300 million alveoli to participate in the gas exchange process, each must be connected to the environment by an air pathway. The analogy now changes from a balloon to a tree. Imagining an upside-down tree, the main trunk represents the trachea, the single common airway segment through which inhaled and exhaled gas from all alveoli must pass. The upper end of the trachea begins at the lower margin of the larynx. The trachea lies anteriorly in the neck and chest, passing caudally in the midline retrosternally to the level of about the sternal attachment of the second rib. There it divides into left and right mainstem bronchi, each smaller and shorter than the trachea. These two airways angle caudally and laterally within the upper mediastinum to enter the left and right lungs at the left and right hilar regions, respectively, and they divide into the lobar bronchi, three on the right to feed the right upper, middle, and lower lobes, and two on the left to feed the two left lobes, upper and lower.

Note that the two hilar regions are the only normal points of actual connection of the left and right lungs to any thoracic structures, and also contain the large pulmonary arteries and veins, lymphatics, and nerves. The entire remaining lungs, while opposed against the chest wall, are not connected to it and are able to slide easily over the inner chest wall surface. This inner surface is covered by the parietal pleural membrane, and the outer surface of the lungs is similarly covered by the visceral pleural membrane. These two pleural membranes are joined at the hilar regions to form a fully enclosed sac that separates the lung and chest wall. The left and right pleural sacs do not communicate with each other, and normally contain only a very thin layer of plasma-like fluid and no gas at all. This arrangement may be pictured by imagining a sealed, but empty, plastic sandwich bag from which all air has been expelled and which contains a very small volume of water. If one's right hand is balled into a fist and invaginates this bilayered bag against the cupped left hand, we have the analogy to the right (or left) lung and chest wall. The balled right fist is the lung; the right wrist and forearm represent the hilar structures. The cupped left hand is the chest wall, and the two layers of the closed sandwich bag form the pleural membranes.

Clinical significance

Mainstem bronchial branching angles

The mainstem bronchial branching from the trachea is not quite symmetrical. The right mainstem bronchus continues caudally a little more directly in line with the trachea above it than does the left, which angles laterally more sharply. As a result, accidentally inhaled foreign bodies more frequently lodge in the right than left lungs. For similar reasons, advancing an endotracheal tube too deeply may cause it to lodge in the right mainstem bronchus rather than where intended—the trachea. This will result in lack of ventilation of the left lung, and if not recognized, hypoxaemia from continued perfusion of this unventilated lung with venous blood, and ultimately left lung collapse (over minutes to hours).

The intrapleural space and pneumothorax

The pressure within the pleural space (i.e. between visceral and parietal pleural surfaces) is normally subatmospheric because of the above-mentioned counterbalancing inward lung and outward chest wall recoil forces. This prevents lung collapse. Disruption of either the visceral or parietal pleura (i.e. pneumothorax) allows air to enter the pleural space, increasing the intrapleural pressure back to atmospheric. This results in collapse of the lung, with abolition of ventilation even if chest wall muscle contraction continues. Gas exchange therefore ceases, with life threatened. In humans, since the right and left lungs are encased in separate pleural sacs, if one side suffers pneumothorax, gas exchange can usually be maintained by the other.

Pneumothorax can occur from rupture of lung surface alveoli in predisposed individuals, or from chest wall trauma in anyone. Whether the source of the intrapleural air is alveolar gas as in the former case or room air in the latter makes no difference. However, depending on conditions, intrapleural air pressure may actually rise above that of room air. This situation, the tension pneumothorax, can arise whenever air enters the pleural space via a valve-like mechanism, when the patient's respiratory effort or that of a mechanical ventilator can lead to intrapleural pressure rising well above atmospheric. The lung collapses, but the (increasingly desperate) respiratory effort or mechanical ventilator keeps pumping air into the pleural space via the torn lung surface. This is a true emergency requiring immediate needle puncture of the chest wall of the affected side to relieve the built-up pressure. If this is not done, the high intrathoracic pressure compresses and distorts the mediastinum and vena cavae, impeding venous return. Both pulmonary gas exchange and the circulation fail, and death follows rapidly.

Mediastinal shifts

The separation of the right from left pleural spaces provides for lateral movement of the mediastinum should there be a difference in mechanical properties of the right and left lungs or their associated pleural spaces or chest wall structures. For example, fibrosis of the right lung, or alternatively its collapse from complete airway obstruction, will reduce the volume of intrathoracic contents and therefore pressure on that side, and mediastinal contents will shift towards the right, visible on chest radiography. In fact, the trachea may also be shifted from its normal midline location in this direction, evident on clinical examination of tracheal position just above the suprasternal notch. Conversely, a pleural effusion on the right or a right pneumothorax (see below) may raise intrathoracic pressure above that on the left, and have the opposite effects on mediastinal and tracheal position.

The bronchi and bronchioles

After the mainstem bronchi have arisen from the trachea, the airways continue an essentially dichotomous branching pattern until the alveoli are reached. Thus, successive branching yields in the order of 50 000 to 100 000 airways (called terminal bronchioles) that constitute the 16th generation ($2^{16} = 65\,536$). The entire collection of airways from the trachea to these last bronchioles before alveoli begin forms a system of connected conducting pipes needed to deliver gas between the alveoli and the environment during ventilation (Fig. 18.1.2.2).

As with the branching of a tree, both the diameter and the length of each successive branch fall. The trachea typically is 12 cm long

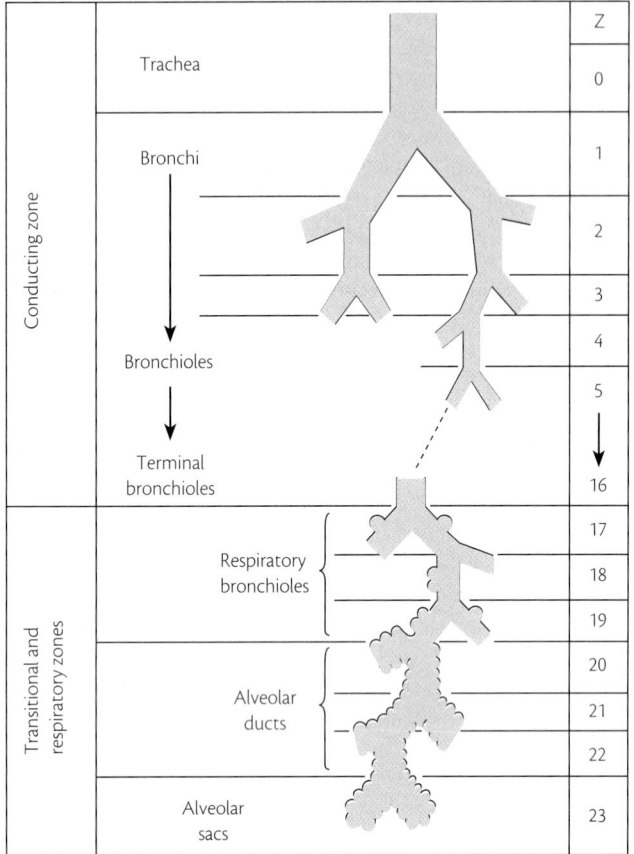

(a)

(b)

Fig. 18.1.2.2 (a) This shows a stylized model of the branching of the airways from trachea to alveoli, encompassing some 23 generations of branching. The first 16 generations contain no alveoli and are purely conducting airways, but the next 7 generations contain progressively more alveoli in the airway walls and serve the dual purpose of conducting air to the alveolar sacs and also providing gas exchange. (b) Total cross-sectional area of each generation shown in (a). This is obtained by multiplying the average cross-sectional area of a single airway by the number of airways in the particular generation. Cross-sectional area is small throughout the conducting zone (first 16 generations), but then increases exponentially in the respiratory zone. The implications are that the forward velocity of inspired gas falls dramatically in the respiratory zone such that diffusion becomes the faster mode of molecular movement. In addition, this diagram implies that during flow between the mouth and alveoli, most of the airway resistance resides in the first 15 generations.
(Adapted from Weibel ER (1984). *Pathway for oxygen: structure and function in the mammalian respiratory system*. Harvard University Press, Cambridge, MA, with permission.)

and 2 cm in diameter. By contrast, the typical terminal bronchiole is just 1 to 2 mm long and 0.6 mm in diameter. Airflow is normally mostly laminar (except for that in the upper airways) and therefore is governed by Poiseuille's law of fluid dynamics. The essence of this law is that resistance to airflow depends inversely on the fourth power of the airway radius, but varies only in direct proportion to airway length. As airways become both narrower and shorter with increasing branching, it is evident that resistance of a single airway increases dramatically because of the dominating effect of the fourth power of the radius. However, if one asks how the entire system behaves by plotting how airway pressure must fall from trachea to generation 16, e.g. during steady inspiratory flow, one must allow for the fact that all airways of any single generation are arranged in parallel with one another. Because branching is essentially dichotomous, there are twice as many airways in any given generation as in the one before. Thus, total airway resistance of any one generation is diminished in proportion to the exponentially increasing number of airways as branching continues. This actually overcomes the fourth power disadvantage of Poiseuille's law, such that most of the pressure drop, or put another way, most of the system airway resistance, is associated with the first few generations despite their large individual airway size.

Another way to understand this somewhat counterintuitive result is to consider the sum total of the cross-sectional areas of all airways in a single generation. This is of course the area of a typical airway multiplied by the number of airways in that generation. That number is low for the first few generations, but then rises dramatically because of the exponentially increasing number of airways in each generation. Airway resistance of a generation therefore falls from the first few generations to the terminal bronchioles. The summed total volume of gas contained within all 16 generations of these conducting airways is only about 150 ml despite their prodigious number.

Clinical significance

Dead space

The interposition of airways between the mouth and the alveoli creates a volume of gas (*c.* 150 ml as mentioned) called the anatomical dead space. The gas in this dead space simply passes back and forth during inspiration and expiration without contributing to gas exchange since the conducting airways contain no alveoli in their walls. It constitutes a penalty since it adds an obligatory 150 ml volume requirement to every breath taken. This is of no importance in health, but in patients with severe lung disease such as chronic obstructive lung disease or fibrosis, the energy cost of overcoming either high resistance in obstructed airways or low compliance of fibrotic lung tissue, and of thus mounting adequate ventilation, may be greatly increased. Then, the need to breathe some 150 ml more per breath than actually required for alveolar gas exchange can be clinically important as a factor contributing to respiratory failure. Recognition of this has led to the use of transtracheal insufflation of air, which permits the anatomical dead space of at least the upper airways to be circumvented and reduces the ventilation necessary for any given activity.

Particle deposition

Ventilation involves breathing some 6 to 10 litres of air every minute of our lives. Air contains much particulate matter of very small size.

Depending on particle size, rate of gas flow in the airways, and airway geometry, such particles may move harmlessly in and out with the next breath or they may be deposited somewhere on the epithelial surface in the bronchial tree. To the extent that they do deposit and are chemically or physically harmful to tissue, they can be responsible for disease. Pneumoconioses, chronic obstructive pulmonary disease, bacterial and viral infections, asthma, and other diseases may all be initiated and/or affected by such mechanisms. The dividing airway structure described above combines everdiminishing individual airway diameter with ever-diminishing gas velocity (due to increasing summed cross-sectional airway area of all airways in a generation) as branching continues. As airways narrow and flow velocity falls, the chance of airborne particles being deposited on airway walls increases. It is for this reason that coal dust, for example, settles mostly in the terminal bronchiolar region deep within the branching system. Thus, the basic nature of gas exchange, demanding the branching network of airways described, leads to intrinsic vulnerability to disease from airborne particulate matter.

Mucociliary function

As seen commonly in evolutionary responses to deleterious phenomena, a protective system has been developed to mitigate the consequences of particle deposition in the airways. This is the mucociliary apparatus. It has several components. There are submucosal glands in the walls of the conducting airways that secrete mucus into the airway lumen when stimulated by irritant signals. These glands are supported by other secretory cells in the epithelium of the airways such as goblet cells. The epithelial cells that line the entire conducting airway system are ciliated, and they function in a coordinated manner, beating rhythmically to move the secreted mucus upward from smaller to larger airways. The primary purpose of the mucus is to trap inhaled particulates before they can reach and damage the airway and lung tissues themselves. This upwardly transported mucus is clinically evident as sputum.

The volumes of sputum produced normally are so small as to be unnoticeable, and are usually swallowed. However, inhalation of toxic irritants, infectious agents, and other particles will rapidly increase the volume of sputum to noticeable levels, and chronic airway inflammation from, for example, cigarette smoking will produce chronically increased amounts of mucus that give rise to the syndrome of chronic bronchitis. It is especially noteworthy that in asthma, not only is the volume of mucus increased, probably from airway inflammation, but its composition is altered, rendering it much more tenacious and difficult to eliminate by the ciliary system. Mucus thus accumulates in the airway lumina, particularly those of the smaller conducting bronchioles, creating mucus plugs that cause obstruction to airflow and marked reduction in ventilation of alveoli lying distal to them. When this occurs, asthma is often refractory to usual pharmacological therapy, and patients dying from asthma universally exhibit widespread airway mucus plugging.

Dynamic airway compression

Another intrinsic physiological problem of the branching airway system within the chest is related to the mechanical nature of respiration—the need for inflating and deflating the lung by altering the pressure around it—combined with the fact that the airways are not rigid tubes. The airways are thus susceptible to expansion and compression (and therefore to collapse) on inspiration and

expiration, respectively. The intrapleural pressure may be transmitted to the conducting airways, and while reduction in this pressure on inspiration will only distend the airways, allowing air to flow more freely, opposite effects during expiration may not be innocuous. Passive expiration—i.e. expiration fuelled only by the elastic energy stored in the lung tissue from the previous inspiration, without active expiratory muscle effort—does not compress the airways because the intrapleural pressure remains subatmospheric. However, active expiratory muscle contraction, as occurs during a forced expiratory manoeuvre and during heavy exercise, leads to compression of the airways because intrapleural pressure is raised to above atmospheric. In fact, the greater the expiratory effort made, the greater the increase in intrapleural pressure and the degree of airway compression. Because of this, flow rates during forced expiration cannot be increased by making a greater muscular effort: any greater driving pressure for expiratory flow is balanced by the increased resistance resulting from more compression. As a result, even in normal subjects, expiratory flow of air under these conditions is limited by this phenomenon, known as dynamic compression, which is illustrated in Fig. 18.1.2.3.

The loss of elastic recoil in emphysema, mentioned above in the context of its effects on FRC, also has a major influence on dynamic compression. The airways are much more susceptible to

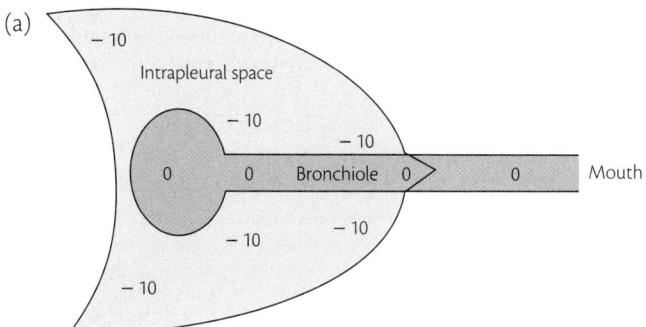

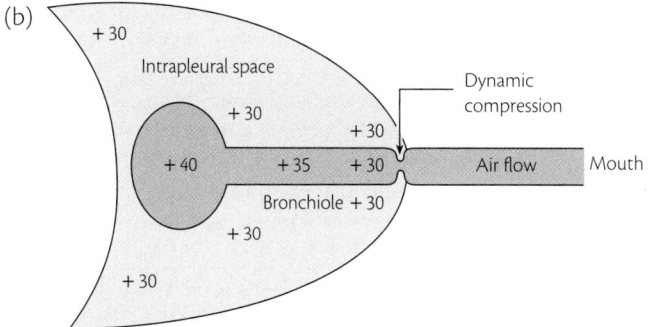

Fig. 18.1.2.3 Diagram to explain dynamic compression during expiration. (a) This depicts intrapleural, alveolar, and airway pressures while breath holding with an open glottis at total lung capacity. Due to lung elasticity, intrapleural pressure is negative (-10 cmH$_2$O), but because of breath holding there is no flow, and pressure in the airways and alveoli equals that at the mouth, 0 cmH$_2$O. Immediately after commencing a forced expiration from total lung capacity (b), intrapleural pressure is high due to expiratory muscle contraction ($+30$ cmH$_2$O). Alveolar pressure is even higher due to 10 cmH$_2$O of lung elastic recoil pressure. However, due to flow resistance, pressure falls from $+40$ gradually to $+30$ as shown. At this point, intrapleural pressure equals intraluminal pressure and immediately downstream dynamic compression occurs as airway pressure falls even further and is now less than intrapleural pressure.

dynamic compression (discussed below), such that even breathing at rest with just small increases in intrapleural pressure from active expiratory muscle contraction may be subject to flow limitation by this mechanism. When this problem is compounded by the separate phenomenon of increased airway luminal mucus from chronic inflammation induced by cigarette smoking, it is easy to understand how chronic obstructive lung disease (emphysema and chronic bronchitis) has airway obstruction as its major disturbance.

In the consideration of dynamic compression it is important to note that the alveoli are not physically independent of one another or of the conducting airways, which run within the lung parenchyma from the lobar bronchi all the way out to the terminal bronchioles. The alveoli share walls in their mutual attachments, and the alveoli beside any intrapulmonary conducting airway are physically connected to the outside of that airway wall. A good analogy for how the alveolar parenchyma is configured comes from examining the cut surface of a sponge where the myriad air cells are surrounded by thin tissue walls. Every wall serves two adjacent air cells, and the overall structure is solid (rather than like the leaves of the tree which are physically independent of each other even while being connected to the same dividing network of branches). The net result of this matrix of alveolar and airway connections is that when the lung is inflated, the elastic tension in the parenchyma exerts radial traction on the conducting airways, increasingly so as the lung is further inflated. This stiffens the airway walls and acts to oppose dynamic compression during active expiration. That maximal expiratory flows are greater at high than low lung volumes is explained by the greater radial traction at high volumes as the alveoli are stretched more.

The walls of the larger conducting airways (the trachea and first few generations of bronchi) are reinforced with cartilage rings that further help to counter the forces favouring dynamic compression. However, the smaller conducting airways do not enjoy this protection, and it is in the smaller airways that dynamic compression usually has its major effects.

Airway smooth muscle

All generations of conducting airways contain smooth muscle cells. When stimulated to contract, their concentric arrangement leads to reduction in airway lumen size, and airway obstruction results. While not a significant effect in normal individuals, patients with asthma have hyperresponsive airway smooth muscle that contracts in response to the inflammatory reaction usually present in the asthmatic airway walls. This is a major mechanism of airway obstruction in asthma, and is the basis of the mainstay therapy in this disease—bronchodilators. For reasons that remain unclear, smooth muscle contraction does not occur to the same degree in all airways of the asthmatic lung: there are different degrees of obstruction both with respect to airway generation number and among airways of a given generation. Ventilation of alveoli is thus very uneven, with many alveoli being very poorly supplied with air, yet others well-supplied. Gas exchange becomes inefficient as a result, and arterial hypoxaemia is seen.

Airway smooth muscle also contracts when local CO_2 concentrations fall. This happens commonly in pulmonary thromboembolism, when vascular obstruction results in focal areas of hypoperfusion that remain relatively overventilated, such that their local alveolar CO_2 tension falls. This, possibly in concert with bronchoactive inflammatory mediators released in association with the embolic event, can produce local airway smooth muscle contraction and airway obstruction. This might tend to better matching of local ventilation with blood flow, but the benefit is generally small, and local bronchoconstriction can manifest as wheezing, which should not be mistaken for asthma.

Dynamic tests of airflow

All of the consequences of the branched structure of the airways and their interconnectedness need to be integrated if one is to understand common pulmonary function tests. How the 'static' lung volumes (FRC, TLC, VC, and RV) are affected by changes in elastic recoil are discussed above, but such measures form only a part of standard pulmonary function testing. Usually included are 'dynamic' tests that measure expiratory and inspiratory gas flow rates, conventionally during manoeuvres wherein the patient is asked to make a maximal inspiratory or expiratory muscle effort. These are discussed in Chapter 18.3.1.

Distribution of ventilation

The extremely large number of very small respiratory bronchioles creates an environment in which alveoli distal to each bronchiole become susceptible to impaired ventilation. Small intrinsic or pathological reductions in airway diameter of such bronchioles can impair distal ventilation substantially. When the effects of variation in mucus secretion, bronchial smooth muscle tone, and radial traction are added to this inherently vulnerable system, it is surprising that the distribution of ventilation to the 300 million alveoli is as uniform as it is. Were it not, there would probably be considerable hypoxaemia, even in health. This topic is discussed further below.

The parenchyma distal to the terminal bronchioles

The terminal bronchioles (16th generation airways) are the final divisions of the wholly conducting airways. They are completely lined with ciliated epithelium, and function primarily as simple conduits for gas, linking the air around us to the alveoli where gas exchange occurs. The next few divisions of the airways result in transitional airways called respiratory bronchioles, so named because they serve a dual role—as continued gas conduits and as the first locations for gas exchange. Respiratory bronchioles are partly lined with ciliated epithelium, but also have small alveolar outpouchings opening directly into the airway lumen. With continued branching of these bronchioles, more and more of the luminal surface is given to the alveolar outpouchings, and less and less to ciliated epithelium. After about three generations of respiratory bronchioles, the airways, whilst still essentially tubular in shape, are made up entirely of alveolar tissue capable of gas exchange, and are called alveolar ducts. These alveolar ducts branch even further into collections of alveoli whose distal end is blind, known as alveolar sacs, the end of the line of the airway branching system. A diagram of the functional lung unit is shown in Fig. 18.1.2.4. With some 7 orders (or division points) of branching between the terminal bronchioles and the final alveoli, together with 16 orders of branching in the conducting airway segment, the whole airway tree consists of about 23 orders or branch points. Because, after the final branch point, the alveolar sacs are blind, the process of ventilation must

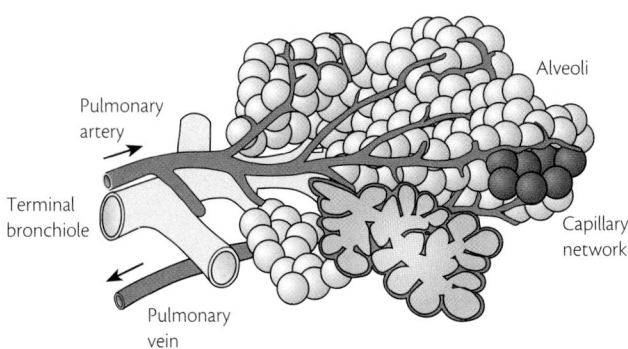

Fig. 18.1.2.4 Diagram of the functional lung unit. The collection of alveoli and associated pulmonary arteries and veins distal to the terminal bronchiole constitutes a functionally homogeneous unit of gas exchange. Mixing of gas amongst alveoli and of blood in the capillary networks of the alveoli in the unit is sufficiently rapid that gas concentrations are in effect uniform throughout. This unit, also called the acinus, corresponds approximately to generations 17 to 23 of Fig. 18.1.2.2.

occur as a tidal (back and forth) event, alternately adding air to, and removing alveolar gas from, each alveolus with each breath.

The transport of gas in either direction between the trachea and the last conducting airway takes place principally by convective flow, much as water flowing in a pipe depends on the pressure difference between the two ends of the pipe and the flow resistance of the pipe. Since flow is mostly laminar, velocity profiles are largely parabolic, flow being highest in the centre of the lumen and lowest at the airway wall, just as is the velocity profile across a quietly flowing river. There are, however, minor additional influences of diffusive movement at the interface between the convective front of each inspiration and residual gas from the previous breath. These interactions, and eddies that develop at each branch point, may assist gas mixing, but their effects are physiologically small. Of much more significance is the fact that the total luminal cross-sectional area of each generation increases exponentially as the airways divide. Since total volumetric flow of gas is the same in each generation, average gas velocity falls reciprocally with the increase in area.

By the time inspired gas reaches the first alveoli, forward velocity has dropped to such a low level that random, thermally fuelled molecular motion (i.e. diffusion) becomes a more important mechanism of gas transport than convection. The small size of the alveoli, about 150 μm in radius, means that diffusive mixing of each new breath with gas resident in the alveoli from prior breaths is nearly instantaneous. Although careful physiological studies can show that low-molecular-weight gases mix slightly faster than those of high molecular weight, this turns out to be of essentially no quantitative significance to gas exchange. Even in emphysema, where many alveolar spaces are enlarged, there is evidence that diffusive mixing in alveolar gas is functionally complete and does not pose a gas exchange threat.

Of more concern for gas exchange is whether all alveoli receive a similar share of each breath. It was pointed out above that the intrinsic structure of the lungs makes it vulnerable to ventilatory inequality, and that this has the potential to disrupt gas exchange. Indeed, recent studies of the structural influence on gas distribution reveal that there are sometimes substantial differences in the ventilation of different alveoli. One property of the system that lessens the negative effects of such inhomogeneity on gas exchange is the finding that individual alveoli do not maintain gas exchange

differences from closely adjacent alveoli. In fact, a fairly large number of connected alveoli are normally able to function as a single homogeneous unit of gas exchange. This is no doubt due partly to the rapid diffusive movement of molecules throughout the alveolar gas mentioned above, but it is also facilitated by the rich capillary network lying in the wall of each alveolus. The density of capillaries is so great that should flow fall in one, its neighbour can seamlessly take over its gas exchange role without any resultant inefficiency. It turns out that the functional unit of gas exchange, known as the acinus, corresponds approximately to all the alveoli distal to the last terminal bronchiole.

Clinical significance

The functional lung unit

Pathological events, in either the alveoli or the capillaries, occurring at a scale smaller than that of the functional lung unit will not *per se* have much impact on gas exchange. Thus, a large number of tiny pulmonary emboli each lodging in one capillary of different functional lung units will not impair gas exchange function, whilst a single large embolus of the same total mass obstructing one much larger vessel may. However, if enough microvessels within functional units become obstructed, their summed effects may become considerable.

Surface tension and mechanical instability of the lung

Another consequence of the branched nature of the lungs resulting in so many very small alveoli is inherent mechanical instability. The alveolar wall, where it interfaces with alveolar gas, forms a roughly spherical air–liquid interface. In this context, the alveoli may be likened to a mass of soap bubbles lying together. All air–liquid interfaces are subject to surface tension, which in this case will act to minimize the surface area of each bubble. For an enclosed bubble, this tension increases the pressure inside the bubble, with the relationship between the tension and the interior pressure given by the law of Laplace: pressure = 2 × surface tension/radius. Thus, pressure inside a small bubble exceeds that inside a larger bubble, and if two such unequal bubbles are in contact and their interiors become connected, the small bubble will collapse into the larger. This process of bubble accretion may continue until the many small soap bubbles have collapsed into a single large one. Based on the opening premise of this chapter, if small alveoli had this tendency to collapse into larger neighbours due to surface tension effects, the end result would be disaster for gas exchange. There would be massive alveolar collapse, and with loss of surface area, sufficient O_2 exchange to support metabolic needs would not be possible. Only if all alveoli were identical in both size and surface tension would this problem be avoided, but when 300 million alveoli exist, it is impossible to imagine them all being identical, and indeed they are not.

The lung avoids this dilemma through two quite separate but complementary mechanisms of stabilization. The first, already mentioned above in a different context, is the interconnected nature of the whole alveolar structure. Any tendency for one alveolus to collapse would have to increase the tension on all its immediately connected neighbours. This tension from surrounding alveoli will automatically serve to splint open the alveolus in question, thus opposing its tendency to collapse. This concept, termed alveolar interdependence, is felt to be of considerable importance in maintaining alveolar stability. The second mechanism is the presence of phospholipid molecules that reduce surface tension in the alveolar air–liquid interface. Termed surfactant, and produced in conjunction with proteins from alveolar type II epithelial cells lying free in the alveolar spaces against alveolar walls, this material reduces surface tension severalfold (Fig. 18.1.2.5). Thus, the surface tension of the alveolar lining fluid is only about 10 mN/m whereas that of water is some 75 mN/m. Moreover, probably due to molecular realignment of surfactant molecules, surface tension is even lower when lung volume is reduced. Based on the law of Laplace given above, this can be seen to be even more advantageous for evening out surface tension differences among alveoli of different size.

Surfactant is thought to have another crucial role that promotes efficient gas exchange between alveolar gas and capillary blood. Given that adjacent alveoli share a common wall, the tendency for surface reduction in each alveolus will create a force that tends to reduce the interstitial tissue pressure around capillaries in the alveolar wall between the adjacent alveoli. From the Starling relationship that governs water escape out of capillaries in any tissue (based on the transcapillary differences in both hydrostatic and oncotic pressures), reducing pressure around the capillary will lead to increased water escape into the alveolar wall. This could have several deleterious consequences. First, the affected alveolar walls would become stiffer and harder to inflate, tending to reduce lung volume. Second, the tissue separating gas from capillary

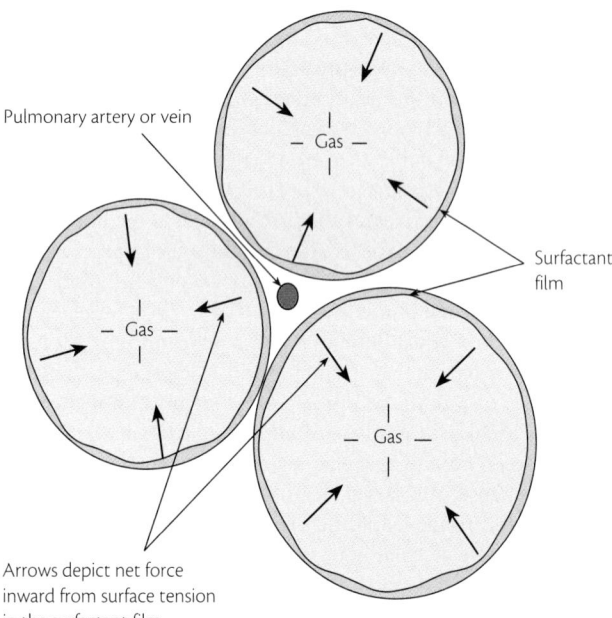

Arrows depict net force inward from surface tension in the surfactant film

Fig. 18.1.2.5 Diagram to indicate potential effects of surface tension on lung structure and function. Three gas-filled alveoli are shown, each lined by a thin film of surfactant. A pulmonary artery or vein is shown in the corner formed where the three alveoli come together. Arrows show the net inward force produced by surface tension, tending to reduce alveolar gas volume and promote atelectasis. In addition, the pressure in the perivascular space around the corner vessel shown will be reduced by these inward surface forces, increasing the pressure difference from inside to outside the vessel lumen and thereby promoting fluid movement from plasma to interstitial space. The presence of surfactant reduces the magnitude of surface tension forces and therefore stabilizes the alveoli against atelectasis and reduces the transmural pressure difference, attenuating transvascular fluid movement.

blood would become thicker, directly impairing diffusive transport between gas and blood. Third, this water would find its way into the pulmonary lymphatics, which begin in the alveolar interstitium and run along the large airways and vessels to the hilar regions, before exiting the lungs and emptying into the superior vena cava. Extra water frequently accumulates in the peribronchial and perivascular spaces and results in their partial compression, reducing distal ventilation and/or blood flow of subtended alveoli, causing maldistribution of either or both, and rendering gas exchange inefficient. The presence of surfactant is thought to reduce the rate of transcapillary water exchange, and therefore to contribute to efficient gas exchange.

Clinical significance

Impaired surfactant activity

When surfactant is not present, when its rate of renewal is insufficient, or when it is inactivated rapidly, pathological changes can be severe. Best known is the infant respiratory distress syndrome, occurring in otherwise normal premature infants born before the late-maturing surfactant system is functional. Without exogenous surfactant replacement therapy the condition may be fatal because of alveolar collapse and pulmonary oedema. Surfactant activity is also compromised in the adult respiratory distress syndrome and may compound the disturbances of pulmonary function arising from the primary cause of the pulmonary disease.

Gravity and lung function

Causes of potential unequal distribution of ventilation or blood flow to the alveoli extend beyond those associated with the intrinsic branching structure of the lungs discussed above. In particular, the presence of gravity influences lung function because key components of the lungs have significant weight. The weight of the parenchyma itself, plus the blood within the alveolar capillaries, feeding arteries and draining veins, together cause the lungs to sag toward the diaphragm in the upright lung sitting at FRC. The upper pole of the lungs is still applied to the parietal pleural surface of the chest wall—there is no pleural airspace created by this gravitational stress. Rather, the rest of the lung is displaced caudally, sagging much like a heavy sweater pegged to a clothes line. As expected, this creates stress in the alveolar walls, more in the uppermost than lowermost alveoli. A good analogy is the toy Slinky—a coiled spring that when hanging vertically under its own weight shows wider separation between adjacent coils at its top than at its bottom. Correspondingly, the uppermost alveoli in the upright lung are larger than the lowermost alveoli. The lowermost alveoli are thus more compliant—that is, able to be further inflated more per unit transpulmonary pressure—than the uppermost alveoli, because the latter are stretched almost to their limit. Accordingly, normal ventilation from FRC results in greater ventilation of the lung bases than of the lung apices. Much the same effect is seen for blood flow: apical blood flow is less than that at the base of the upright lung. In this case it is the weight of the blood itself that is responsible: perfusion depends on pulmonary arterial pressure, which falls linearly with height up the lung.

The apex to base differences in perfusion exceed those of ventilation, such that the ratio of ventilation to blood flow is higher at the apex than at the base. The local ventilation/perfusion ($\dot{V}_A/\dot{Q}$) ratio determines local alveolar Po_2 and Pco_2, Po_2 increasing and Pco_2

falling as the $\dot{V}_A/\dot{Q}$ ratio increases. Thus, Po_2 at the apex is higher, and Pco_2 lower than at the base. If the $\dot{V}_A/\dot{Q}$ ratio everywhere was the same, so too would be Po_2 and Pco_2, and the exchange of O_2 and CO_2 would be maximally efficient. However, the presence of a range of $\dot{V}_A/\dot{Q}$ ratios (no matter what its cause) results in gas exchange inefficiency and arterial hypoxaemia.

Clinical significance

Effects of gravity on lung function in disease

Although gravity creates $\dot{V}_A/\dot{Q}$ maldistribution, common disease processes are in large part randomly distributed in the lungs, and their effects on $\dot{V}_A/\dot{Q}$ matching are generally much greater than those of gravity. Thus, whilst the effect of gravity on arterial Po_2 is barely measurable, $\dot{V}_A/\dot{Q}$ mismatching based on nongravitational influences in many diseases leads to profound gas exchange disturbances. However, the presence of gravity must not be discounted in several disease states.

Emphysema, and even the normal ageing process, often causes tissue breakdown in the apical lung regions, probably because, as in the Slinky analogy, the alveolar wall stresses are largest there. When mechanical failure occurs, it is most likely to happen in the regions of greatest stress, and as a result the alveolar wall breakdown so typical of emphysema, and to a much lesser extent normal ageing, is often exaggerated in the apices. An important gravitational influence occurs in patients in intensive care with severe lung disease. In any body position, both blood flow and alveolar fluid collection tend to be concentrated in dependent regions (e.g. posteriorly in the supine patient). Those regions with high blood flow may also have little or no ventilation if their alveoli are filled with fluid and cell debris. The blood flowing through such regions can therefore pick up little or no O_2, and hypoxaemia may be severe. This has led some intensive care staff to rotate their patients from supine to lateral to prone and back. The argument being that the gravitational influences on blood flow are essentially instantaneous, whilst those on alveolar fluid collection may take hours to respond to body positional changes. Thus, for a time after rotating a patient, the dependent region may enjoy high flow but not yet be fluid filled and thus still be well ventilated. Gas exchange is therefore enhanced, and arterial hypoxaemia is mitigated. Such behaviour may also explain positional influences on gas exchange in patients with unilateral lung disease such as pneumonia, effusion, or atelectasis.

Further reading

Crystal R, West JB (1997). *The lung: scientific foundations*. Raven Press, New York.

Weibel ER (1963). *Morphometry of human lung*. Springer-Verlag, Berlin.

Weibel ER (1984). *Pathway for oxygen: structure and function in the mammalian respiratory system*. Harvard University Press, Cambridge, MA.

West JB (2004). *Respiratory physiology, the essentials*, 7th edition. Williams & Wilkins, Baltimore, MD.

The clinical presentation of respiratory disease

Julian Hopkin

Essentials

Respiratory disease can present in many ways, with variations attributable to many factors. The clinical presentation directs diagnostic hypothesis making, the choice of diagnostically discriminating investigations, and the most appropriate management. If a detailed history is not taken, the patient not observed carefully and examined diligently, and the information from these sources is not analysed correctly, then inappropriate investigation and management is likely.

History—common symptoms of respiratory disease are breathlessness, cough, haemoptysis, and pleuritic chest pain, details of which can point to particular diagnoses. An account of environmental exposures at work and home, and of family history, is critically important in some cases.

Clinical examination—this begins with assessment of general features: physical findings outside the chest can be vital in diagnosis. Accurate monitoring and documentation of respiratory rate, pulse rate, and temperature are essential in the acute setting. Immediate pointers to respiratory disorder are repeated cough, wheeze or stridor, painful breathing, laboured or ineffective breathing, or cyanosis, but it is crucial to remember that respiratory failure can present as a torpid or drowsy state without clear respiratory distress. Observation of the chest, followed by palpation, percussion, and auscultation must be performed systematically, and the physician who practices these skills regularly will be better at them than the one who does not. In chronic respiratory disease, where breathlessness and disability are to be assessed, walking with the patient and observing exercise tolerance and distress (and pulse oximetry) can provide valuable information.

Introduction

The clinical presentation of respiratory disease is protean, with many diseases of different respiratory structures presenting in both common and rare ways. The presentation varies according to many factors—heterogeneity of disease under one diagnostic banner, the natural vagaries of one disease, comorbidities, age and family and social circumstances, and personality traits such as timidity or stoicism. The proper assessment of the clinical presentation therefore needs care and thought.

The clinical presentation directs diagnostic hypothesis making, the choice of diagnostically discriminating investigations, and ultimately the most appropriate management. The combination of the clinical presentation and its careful assessment usually provides the crucial signal as to the seriousness or threat of an acute disorder, and the impact of disease on life and its quality likely to be caused by a chronic problem. The information from a carefully conducted clinical review—the detailed history and careful examination and observation of the patient on exercise as well as at rest as appropriate—often provides a more complete view of the condition and its impact than the sum of body scans, and detailed molecular and physiological investigations. These diverse methodologies are of course complementary in good clinical practice, where at the point of

management the patient's investigations need to be interpreted in the context of the clinical picture.

Symptoms

Breathlessness

Breathlessness is the cardinal feature of many respiratory diseases (Table 18.2.1). The detailed characteristics of this breathlessness and accompanying symptoms often vary according to the specific respiratory disease. Without sufficient care, breathlessness due to respiratory disease may be readily confused with breathlessness due to cardiovascular disease of diverse origin. Anaemia and hyperthyroidism may also be the basis of breathlessness.

Breathlessness—an awareness of difficulty with breathing—is a complex physiological phenomenon. Its perception is cerebral, with two principal components relevant to most breathless patients, both of which depend on integration of information. The first allows the perception of breathlessness, and the second allows gauging of its distressfulness. In the first component, the interconnecting neural pathways allow comparison between the volume of motor neurone output to drive respiration, and the volume of sensory input recording the ventilatory effects achieved in stretching of the lung, thoracic respiratory muscles, and chest wall.

Table 18.2.1 Some causes of breathlessness in patients presenting to a medical admissions unit

Cause	Example
Upper airway obstruction	Anaphylaxis Inhaled foreign body
Airways disease	Acute exacerbation of asthma Acute exacerbation of chronic obstructive pulmonary disease
Lung disease	Infective—pneumonia Inflammatory parenchymal disease, e.g. extrinsic allergic alveolitis Acute presentation of malignancy, e.g. pulmonary/lobar collapse in bronchial carcinoma, lymphangitis carcinomatosa
Pulmonary oedema	Left ventricular failure Adult respiratory distress syndrome (ARDS) in sepsis Inhalation of gastric contents Inhalation of noxious industrial gases Narcotics abuse Renal failure
Pulmonary embolism	
Pneumothorax	
Pleural effusion	

A discrepancy—where the motor output (representing effort) exceeds the sensory input from thoracic structures (the result achieved)—is perceived as breathlessness. In the second component, further connecting intracerebral neurones allow for this perception of breathlessness to be emotionally interpreted with regards to its degree of distressfulness.

This model offers an understanding of how diverse disorders of the bronchi (limiting airflow) and of the lung parenchyma, pleura and chest wall (limiting distension) cause breathlessness. It also offers an understanding of how two patients, for instance with chronic obstructive pulmonary disease, can have the same derangement of lung function and blood gas measurements, but suffer very different degrees of distress due to their breathlessness and different degrees of impact on their lives. Such variability in emotional apprehension of breathlessness is important to recognize. It can valuably influence the deployment of rehabilitation programmes, or perhaps cognitive behavioural therapy, in the patient with chronic distressing breathlessness.

This model of breathlessness places circulating oxygen and carbon dioxide levels as key drivers to respiration, but not as dominant sensory inputs for the perception of breathlessness. Hence, increasing inspired oxygen (FiO_2) can be envisaged to ease breathlessness in many patients by diminishing respiratory motor output.

The character of breathlessness, as related in the history, may provide clear diagnostic pointers. Most asthmatics clearly describe episodic breathlessness, with a feeling of chest tightness with audible wheeze, and regular early morning (c.04.00–06.00 h) worsening. Many can relate some episodes to exposures to extrinsic triggers, e.g. cats, perfumes, cigarette smoke, or occupational agents, such as flour in bakers. In chronic obstructive pulmonary disease, the typical picture is progressive exertional breathlessness over many months or years, punctuated by exacerbations of this breathlessness during

bouts of winter-season, virus-initiated bronchitis, with cough and purulent sputum. Progressive breathlessness, with strict limitation of exercise, is often a feature of fibrosing alveolitis and related disorders of the pulmonary parenchyma. Progressive breathlessness over days and weeks, where the symptoms by night and in bed are worse than the day, and where there are repeated awakenings from sleep by breathlessness, and relief from sitting up, suggest heart failure. Pneumothorax often presents as truly abrupt onset of breathlessness with or without pleural pain.

The character of the breathlessness is often less decisive than in the examples given above, and it is only the complete clinical picture (with the full history and clinical examination) and the chest radiograph that advances the diagnostic possibilities, and then further investigations that clarify the diagnosis. For example, most physicians are only too familiar with variable presentation of pulmonary embolism across a clinical spectrum of breathlessness syndromes, fleeting pleuritic pain, and sudden circulatory arrest. Moreover, there is always the potential for diagnostic confusion between the rare manifestation of a common disease (pulmonary oedema due to malaria in the pregnant female), the occasional respiratory manifestation of a multisystem disease (e.g. lupus pneumonitis, or infection in the immunosuppressed), the usual manifestation of a relatively rare respiratory disease (bronchiolitis obliterans organizing pneumonia), or an idiosyncratic reaction to a medication such as pulmonary eosinophilia syndrome (see later).

It should also be noted that breathlessness is not always a prominent presenting symptom in cases of respiratory failure. In respiratory failure due to progressive neuromuscular disorder, chest wall deformity and severe obesity, fatigue and morning headaches due to CO_2 retention may dominate the clinical picture.

All of this plainly recommends a thorough clinical approach by the physician, and caution over the use of oversimplified or streamlined diagnostic approaches that can emerge from clinical guidelines.

Cough

The cough reflex is triggered by irritant and chemical receptors, predominantly of the upper respiratory tract and large airways, and cough can be the principal manifestation of many acute and chronic lung diseases, but also of other disorders (Table 18.2.2).

Viral upper respiratory tract infection is the commonest cause of acute onset cough with or without sputum. This can take some two to three weeks to subside fully in the otherwise healthy. In asthma, chronic obstructive pulmonary disease, and bronchiectasis, such viral infections may be accompanied by significant decline in airflow function, with breathlessness and wheeze, or respiratory failure.

Cough of acute onset due to inhalation of foreign body is relatively rare, but needs consideration and investigation by bronchoscopy in adults as well as children when there is stridor (see below) or localized inspiratory wheeze in the chest, when dry cough persists unabated, or when the chest radiograph shows asymmetric lung field volumes. A foreign body may inflate or deflate a lung or lobe, dependent on the mechanics of the obstruction.

Chronic cough, with little or no sputum, can often be due to gastro-oesophageal reflux disease (GORD), paranasal sinus disease, or common medications such as angiotensin converting enzyme inhibitors or angiotensin receptor antagonists used for hypertension or cardiac failure. Other features of the history should provide

Table 18.2.2 Some causes of mainly dry cough

Cause	Example
Upper airway	Upper respiratory tract infection Paranasal sinus disease Inhaled foreign body Upper respiratory tract tumour
Airways disease	Asthma, cough variant asthma
Lung disease	Pneumonia (some) Bronchial carcinoma or adenoma Inflammatory parenchymal lung disease, e.g. sarcoidosis, fibrosing alveolitis, extrinsic allergic alveolitis Inhalation of noxious fumes or gases
Gastro-oesophageal reflux	
Medications	ACE inhibitors
Functional	

ACE, angiotensin converting enzyme.

Table 18.2.3 Causes of haemoptysis

Cause	Example
Infection	Tuberculosis, bronchiectasis, pneumonia, lung abscess, acute purulent bronchitis, aspergilloma, other locally endemic fungal diseases (coccidioidomycosis)
Tumour	Bronchial carcinoma, bronchial adenoma, pulmonary or bronchial metastases, Kaposi's sarcoma in AIDS
Vascular	Pulmonary embolism, left ventricular failure, mitral stenosis, pulmonary or bronchial arteriovenous malformation
Immune/inflammatory disorder	Systemic vasculitis (e.g. Wegener's granulomatosis, systemic lupus), Goodpasture's syndrome, lung transplant rejection (capillaritis)
Other	Idiopathic pulmonary haemosiderosis, pulmonary contusion or laceration (accidental trauma), inhaled foreign body, bronchial, pulmonary, or pleural medical or surgical procedures, bleeding diathesis including therapeutic anticoagulation

useful pointers to sinus disease (past history of sinus surgery, post-nasal drip, nasal blockage or periodic facial discomfort or fullness) or GORD (episodic 'heartburn', regurgitation of food or acid into the mouth, morning sore throats).

Long-standing cough (of many years' duration) is usually due to tobacco smokers' chronic bronchitis or bronchiectasis. Milder forms of bronchiectasis—with only periodic purulent sputum production, sparse pulmonary crackles, and absent finger clubbing—need high resolution CT scanning of the thorax to be recognized.

Asthma is now a common cause of chronic or periodic cough, and in some instances this symptom overshadows wheeze ('cough variant asthma'). Most cases have demonstrable labile airways function on serial peak expiratory flow rate recordings; in others the diagnosis may require bronchoscopic biopsy to demonstrate the eosinophilic bronchitis typical of asthma.

Cough of some weeks' or months' duration, with or without sputum production, can signify important infectious or neoplastic disease. Tuberculosis must be addressed by chest radiograph and microscopy and culture of any sputum since clinical examination of the lungs is rarely useful (except in advanced cases). Likewise, the clinical features of surgically curable carcinoma of the bronchus are not reliable, and the diagnosis should be addressed in smokers with changed cough by CT scanning of the thorax and bronchoscopy.

Other infections, such as lung abscess due to various bacterial infections or fungal infections with localized endemicity (e.g. coccidioidomycosis and paracoccididioidomycosis in the Americas) need the same approach as for tuberculosis above, supplemented as appropriate by serology for certain mycoses, CT scanning, or bronchoscopic samplings for microscopy and culture.

Cough, despite the predominance of airways receptors in its production, can be an important and distressing feature of parenchymal lung disease such as fibrosing alveolitis, when opioids may provide the most useful relief. Cough may feature in pleural effusion or pneumothorax, perhaps because of the bronchial distortion caused.

A prominently productive cough usually suggests bronchial disorder, such as bronchiectasis or others as above. Parenchymal lung disease may also cause prominently productive cough, as in alveolar cell carcinoma or tuberculosis. Experienced clinicians recognize that pneumonia may occur without cough and often without sputum, and where the clinical picture is dominated by systemic disturbance (fever, chills, anorexia, or confusion in the elderly), with or without other respiratory symptoms such as pleuritic pain or breathlessness. In some pneumonias, e.g. pneumocystis in the immunosuppressed, breathlessness is regularly the cardinal respiratory symptom.

Haemoptysis

Haemoptysis is a frightening symptom, hence presentation to the physician is often rapid. Careful enquiry will almost always exclude epistaxis or haematemesis. There a number of important causes (Table 18.2.3).

Haemoptysis can occur in simple bouts of acute infective bronchitis, especially in some young smokers, when cessation of smoking is often needed to end the bleeding. Haemoptysis is a well-recognized feature of pneumonia, as may occur for instance with pneumococcal or klebsiella infection. Haemoptysis, often periodic and coinciding with infective exacerbation, is a common feature of bronchiectasis. Though the bleeding can be relatively profuse, it almost invariably subsides spontaneously and quickly with antibiotic treatment. Haemoptysis is an important presenting feature of carcinoma of the bronchus, tuberculosis, or pulmonary embolism—when the quantity of blood *per se* may not be impressive.

If haemoptysis occurs without clinical features of acute bronchial or pulmonary infection, clinical review needs to be followed by definitive investigation. CT scanning of the lungs, with adjunctive CT pulmonary angiography (CTPA), will prove or exclude pulmonary embolism; it will give some clear indication whether carcinoma or tuberculosis are likely, indicating the need for proceeding to bronchoscopy or microscopy for mycobacteria in sputum. The CT and CTPA can also identify or suggest other rarer diagnoses such as pulmonary arteriovenous malformation, or some forms of pulmonary vasculitis (e.g. Wegener's granulomatosis, where pulmonary nodules with or without cavitation may be shown). Diagnosis of Goodpasture's syndrome or lupus depends on clinical suspicion, and serology for antiglomerular basement membrane (anti-GBM) and antinuclear autoantibodies.

In massive haemoptysis, resuscitation and treatment may run concurrently with or precede definitive investigation. Bronchoscopy can localize the bleed and allow the application of topical epinephrine as a vasoconstrictor and limiter of bleeding, or of balloon tamponade. This is ideally performed with a rigid bronchoscope under general anaesthesia. Preventing blood from flooding the unaffected lung is crucial and can be secured by double tracheal intubation and ventilation. Most episodes stabilize. If not, radiological therapeutic embolization of a bronchial artery or arteriovenous pulmonary malformation can be performed as appropriate or, *in extremis*, surgical resection of the bleeding lobe.

Chest pain

Pleuritic pain—with its sharp, 'catching' character and exacerbation on breathing—can arise from any irritation of the parietal pleura. Most often that irritation arises from lung disease with extension to the pleura, most commonly with infection, infarction, and tumour. Pleural disorder can also occur without significant lung disorder, for instance due to infection (e.g. from subdiaphragmatic or blood-borne spread), asbestos (inflammatory effusions and mesothelioma), tumour (e.g. metastatic from breast or other cancer), serositis (in lupus or rheumatoid disease), or in trauma (fractured rib, pneumothorax and its tube drainage).

Pleuritic pain, with audible pleural rubs on auscultation (Table 18.2.4), occurs with or without the presence of pleural fluid. By contrast, pleural effusions as a result of transudation from oedematous lungs in heart failure produce neither pleuritic pain nor audible rub; hence their presence under such circumstances suggests compounding disorder, such as pulmonary embolism and infarction.

Pleuritic pain needs to be distinguished from chest wall pain due to injury of ribs; or associated muscles from unusual use, trauma, or forceful repeated coughing. Such chest wall pain can cause diagnostic confusion, particularly in patients with asthma and chronic obstructive pulmonary disease, due to their coughing. The absence

of audible pleural rub and of pleural effusion, together with marked localized tenderness on palpation at the site of the pain, suggests chest wall disorder.

In Bornholm's disease (epidemic pleurodynia due to coxsachievirus strains B1–5) there is pleuritic-type pain with accompanying malaise and fever and marked local chest tenderness, but normally no audible rub.

Chest pain of a nonpleuritic type is not often a feature of lung disease. Exceptions are when bronchial carcinoma invades sensitive tissues in the thorax to cause a dull but often severe pain, and sarcoidosis, where inexplicable fleeting chest pains often occur.

Other symptoms

Respiratory disease may also present with non-thoracic symptoms, and the dominant features vary: daytime sleepiness is the vital feature in obstructive sleep apnoea, and is assessed by Epworth Score; drowsiness, headache, and fatigue may dominate in respiratory failure; anorexia and weight loss in bronchial carcinoma or tuberculosis; chills and prostration in pneumonia; fever and sweatiness in thoracic empyema; seizure and hyponatraemia in inappropriate ADH syndrome; neuromuscular disorder in bronchial carcinoma. The physician must be alert to such diverse possibilities.

Other features of the history

In order to address the potential causes of pulmonary disease, the physician may need to take a full and detailed history, not just of the presenting complaint but also of the patient's background.

Evidence for inherited disease may emerge from the family history. Affected siblings with premature emphysema due to α_1-antitrypsin or with cystic fibrosis exemplify autosomal recessive disease. Dominant inheritance, but with variable penetration of disease, can sometimes be traced in deep vein thrombosis and pulmonary embolism. One example of such inherited thrombophilia is resistance of coagulation factor V to protein C inhibition (factor V Leiden). Atopic asthma with rhinitis and eczema is a common polygenic clinical complex which can show familial aggregation.

It is important to consider environmental respiratory disease due to behaviour and exposures at work and home. Such factors include: contact with others with respiratory infection (e.g. tuberculosis, mycoplasma, influenza); place of residence or travel predisposing to acquisition of infections such as coccidioidomycosis and legionella; the presence at home of pet animals (e.g. cats and dogs) which can trigger asthmatic reactions or underlie extrinsic allergic alveolitis or hypersensitivity pneumonitis (e.g. psittacines or pigeons). It is also especially important to consider occupational disease. Asbestos causes inflammatory effusions, mesothelioma, pulmonary fibrosis, and carcinoma of the bronchus. Coal and stone mining cause pneumoconiosis and silicosis. A number of inorganic agents (e.g. isocyanates, acid anhydrides) and organic agents (e.g. bread flour, antibiotics) can cause occupational asthma. Acute isocyanate exposures can cause pulmonary oedema. Spores from thermophilic bacteria and fungi on vegetable matter are an important agricultural cause of extrinsic allergic alveolitis (e.g. farmer's lung). Industrial accidents include inhalation of noxious gases and fumes.

Drug use—medical and illicit—is an important cause of lung disease. β-Adrenergic blockers exacerbate asthma, sometimes catastrophically. Aspirin and nonsteroidal inflammatory drugs can cause asthma and rhinitis in susceptible individuals, where variant

Table 18.2.4 Some causes of pleuritic pain with rub

Cause	Example
Infection	Acute pneumonia. Empyema—various, including spread from hepatic amoebiasis Tuberculosis
Tumour	Mesothelioma Spread from bronchial carcinoma Other metastatic disease
Pulmonary embolism with infarction	
Pneumothorax	(Before and after tube drainage)
Immune/inflammatory disorder	Rheumatoid disease Lupus
Fractured rib	
Asbestos	(Inflammatory)

prostaglandin metabolism may underlie the reaction. Drugs (e.g. dapsone, isoniazid), as well as parasitic worms, can cause pulmonary eosinophilia syndromes. Various drugs used in cancer programmes or immunosuppressive or anti-inflammatory regimens (e.g. busulphan, methotrexate) can cause diffuse alveolitis, or can predispose to both pathogenic and opportunistic pulmonary infections (e.g. prolonged high-dosage corticosteroids and pneumocystis, infliximab and tuberculosis). Illicit drugs must also be considered. They may cause injury directly (e.g. opiates producing pulmonary oedema, and various sedatives causing respiratory failure), or by association (e.g. intravenous drug abuse with dirty needles causing lung abscess by haematogenous spread, or acquisition of the AIDS syndrome to be complicated by pneumocystis pneumonia).

The dangers of cigarette smoking have been only too well documented. It can have devastating results on respiratory health—chronic bronchitis, episodic purulent bronchitis, progressively disabling chronic obstructive pulmonary disease, and bronchial carcinoma.

Clinical examination

General features

General features are especially important in the clinical examination of a patient who has, or might have, a respiratory disorder, and they are noticeable from the start of the clinical review in the clinic or medical admissions unit. In the latter, accurate monitoring and documentation of respiratory rate, pulse rate, and temperature are essential.

Serious disease may be reflected by an expression of anguish, especially when it is acute, or of dejection when it has progressed inexorably over some time. However, mortal disease can also present unobtrusively.

Immediate pointers to respiratory disorder, whatever its origin, are repeated cough, wheeze, or stridor, painful breathing, laboured or ineffective breathing, or evident cyanosis.

Stridor and pattern of breathing

Stridor, a creaking or musical sound on inspiration (see below), is a key pointer to upper airway obstruction. It may signify life-threatening acute disease, such as haemophilus epiglottitis in the child, inhalation of a foreign body, or laryngeal oedema in anaphylaxis. It may also signal more insidious disease, such as cancers of diverse origin (e.g. tracheobronchial, larynx, thyroid, lymphoma) that obstruct or compress the upper airway.

Fast, deep breathing is consistent with severe pneumonia, other inflammatory parenchymal lung disease (diverse alveolitides), pulmonary embolism, or pulmonary oedema. Such rapid and deep breathing can also be observed as a response to severe acidosis (e.g. diabetic ketoacidosis, or renal failure), when the patient does not complain of breathlessness and when there is no hypoxaemia (Kussmaul breathing). Waxing and waning of respiratory rate and volume, and including spells of apnoea, can occur in severe heart failure, in neurological disease, or at high altitude (Cheyne-Stokes breathing). The disordered ventilation of obstructive sleep apnoea is not seen in the medical admissions unit or clinic but can be well documented by overnight camera recording in special sleep units.

In chronic obstructive pulmonary disease and asthma, laboured breathing at high lung volumes (with an inflated thorax), and with respiratory rate limited by prolonged expiration, is typical.

A patient's insistence on sitting upright is a regular feature of heart failure with pulmonary oedema (limiting dependent alveolar oedema to the lower zones of the lungs) or severe asthma or chronic obstructive pulmonary disease (gaining mechanical advantage by fixing the upper thorax with rigid arms clutching the bedside). By contrast, many patients with pulmonary embolism and inflammatory lung disease (pneumonia, fibrosing alveolitis, or other interstitial disorder) seem ready to lie fairly flat on their back or side.

Cyanosis

Cyanosis is a blue discoloration of the skin (especially nail beds, ear lobes, and lips) and mucous membranes of the mouth which is seen when the absolute quantity of reduced haemoglobin in capillaries is about 3 g/dl. Hypoxaemia is the most important and frequent cause, when the resulting cyanosis can often only be detected when haemoglobin–O_2 saturation decreases to 85%. Moreover, polycythaemia and anaemia respectively increase and decrease the likelihood of visible cyanosis for any degree of hypoxaemia. Thick or pigmented skin makes cyanosis harder to detect, hence important degrees of hypoxaemia can occur without clinically detectable cyanosis, emphasizing the value of simple pulse oximetry in the medical admissions unit and ward.

Cyanosis can be observed in other states. One occasional cause is methaemoglobinaemia, due to oxidation of haemoglobin by extrinsic oxidants such as nitrites used medically or illicitly, or due to inherited haemoglobin M or deficiency of methaemoglobin reductase. With high levels of methaemoglobinaemia the reduced haemoglobin binds oxygen poorly and can lead to symptoms of hypoxaemia, with fatigue and dizziness, which can be treated by intravenous methylene blue (depending on cause).

Cyanosis of the peripheries alone, when oral mucous membranes remain pink, can occur in states of peripheral vascular shutdown, as in poor cardiac output or extremes of cold. In such states, the partial pressure of arterial oxygen, Pao_2, is normal.

Impairment of cerebral function

Just as significant hypoxaemia can occur without evident cyanosis, it is important to realize that respiratory failure can present as a torpid or drowsy state, and without clear respiratory distress—as in severe chronic obstructive pulmonary disease, asthma, sedative overdose, brain stem disorders and encephalitis, neuromuscular disorder, and extreme obesity. Hence, arterial blood gases are a vital investigation in the torpid or drowsy patient—providing vital information on possible respiratory failure or metabolic acidosis.

Cerebral disturbance as the presenting feature in respiratory failure is one important example of unexpected presentation; for others, see the Symptoms section above.

Special examples of extrapulmonary features

A thorough clinical examination is required in all but the simplest clinical cases to thoroughly assess the severity of lung disease and to observe vital clues to causation, of which the following are some examples:-

Skin and subcutaneous tissues

Urticaria in anaphylaxis; erythema nodosum in acute sarcoidosis; painful purpura in systemic vasculitis; telangiectases as the cutaneous counterpart to arteriovenous malformations in the lung; the flushed or pallid face of sepsis; venous engorgement of the upper thorax, face, and arms in superior vena cava obstruction; distended, crackling subcutaneous tissue over the upper thorax and neck in pneumothorax; finger clubbing in bronchial carcinoma; pulmonary suppuration (bronchiectasis, lung abscess, or empyema of some duration), or diffuse pulmonary fibrosis; scarred veins of forearms in illicit drug abuse (causing lung abscess, AIDS and respiratory infections); facial skin lesions in paracoccidioidomycosis.

Skeleton and muscles

Kyphoscoliosis as the basis of respiratory failure; immobile stiff neck and back of ankylosing spondylitis as the basis for progressive upper lobe fibrosis; stiff and deformed joints of the hand in rheumatoid disease as the basis for pulmonary nodules, fibrosing alveolitis, and pleural effusion; muscle wasting and weakness from motor neurone disease as the basis of respiratory failure; diplopia and muscle fatigability of myasthenia as the basis for respiratory failure; abdominal in-drawing on inspiration denoting diaphragmatic palsy (e.g. neuropathy in lupus, the inherited myopathy of Pompe's disease).

Heart and cardiovasular system

Third heart sound and resting tachycardia of left ventricular failure as the cause of pulmonary oedema, also underlying aortic stenosis or sustained hypertension; mitral stenosis causing pulmonary venous hypertension, breathlessness and haemoptysis; loud $P2$ and parasternal heave of pulmonary arterial hypertension (e.g. chronic primary lung disease, chronic pulmonary embolism); signs of deep vein thrombosis as the origin for pulmonary embolus.

Exercising the patient

In chronic respiratory disease, where breathlessness and disability are to be assessed, walking with the patient and observing exercise tolerance and distress can provide particularly valuable information. This can be supplemented by recording the haemoglobin–oxygen saturation by simple pulse oximetry before, during, and after some modest exercise in the clinic room.

Signs in the chest

Observation, palpation and percussion

Observation of respiration, and its importance, has already been described. Poor expansion of one hemithorax usually points to ipsilateral pneumonia, lung collapse, pleural effusion, or pneumothorax. In trauma, it may suggest a foreign body in a major bronchus, haemothorax or pneumothorax, or be due to multiple rib fractures. In the latter a flail segment of thorax, drawn in on inspiration, may be found.

Palpation is often valuable in resolving the origin of pains in and about the thorax. Their origin may be declared by local tenderness, such as in marked local chest wall tenderness due to rib fracture or cough trauma (see above), or in spinal tenderness with thoracic dermatome hypoaesthesia or hyperaesthesia due to thoracic vertebral disc collapse.

Percussion is a simple but valuable clinical technique, at its best in defining a region of intense thoracic dullness, and indicating a pleural effusion, haemothorax, or empyema. It can also suggest, with variable accuracy, the presence of pneumothorax with resonant percussion note, or lobar collapse or consolidation with dull percussion note.

Auscultation

Auscultation by stethoscope remains an excellent clinical method for the astute physician. Noting the intensity of breath sounds over the lung is the first and very valuable test. These may be globally reduced in chronic obstructive pulmonary disease and severe asthma. Regions of quiet sounds are important and can denote partial bronchial obstruction of the bronchus to the region (when no other signs may be found), an underlying large bulla in emphysema, or pulmonary collapse, or pleural effusion. In such instances, transmitted voice sounds (the patient saying 'ninety nine') are also reduced.

A change in the character of the breath sounds over a region of lung to a tubular quality—'bronchial breath sounds'—is accompanied by increased transmission of voice sounds. It usually signifies a region of pulmonary consolidation due to pneumonia where the bronchus is patent. Occasionally, bronchial breathing can be heard over the upper regions of pleural effusions, when it does not necessarily imply underlying consolidation, or over small areas of lung in gross pulmonary oedema or fibrosing alveolitis.

Added sounds (adventitial sounds) are important diagnostically but have suffered from different names, definitions, and distinctions at different times and in different countries.

Stridor is indicative of upper airway compression or obstruction (see above) and is heard during inspiration. It has a continuous quality (duration more than 80 milliseconds, and often longer), is creaking or musical, and is often better heard by ear at the patient's mouth than by stethoscope.

Pleural rubs have a grating sound and are generally heard to and fro with inspiration and expiration. They result from friction between disordered pleural surfaces (see Symptoms, above); accompanying effusions into the pleural space do not abolish them, since some areas of disordered visceral and parietal pleura remain in contact. Their audibility by stethoscope auscultation can vary hour by hour or day by day through the course of disease. Hence repeated auscultation may vital to their first identification. Important causes include pneumonia, pulmonary infarction (when they may be heard bilaterally), empyema, mesothelioma or secondary tumour, and inflammatory effusions due to asbestos or rheumatoid disease (Table 18.2.4).

Wheezes are continuous, musical, often rather whistling sounds (always>80 ms, and usually >250 ms in duration) that derive from partially obstructed and vibrating lower airways. They are usually heard in expiration, when these airways are subject to dynamic compression, in which case expiration is often prolonged. They are typical of asthma but also often occur in chronic obstructive pulmonary disease, bronchiectasis, and in viral infections of the bronchi in infants. Short high-pitched wheezes may also sometimes be heard on inspiration in asthma.

Crackles, or crepitations, are shorter discontinuous sounds (<20 ms) whose anatomical origin is principally the airspaces and smallest conducting airways of the lung parenchyma. They are to be distinguished from the rattles of mucus in airways cleared by coughing, and from the basal crackles sometimes heard in inpatients on early morning ward rounds and which clear after one or two deep breaths.

Many clinicians are content to recognize persistent pulmonary crackles as indicators of disorder of the air spaces and smallest conducting airways, as indicated above, using parallel information from the history and other physical and radiographic signs to determine the diagnosis. Others believe that the duration of crackles in milliseconds and their position in inspiration (early to late) are more specific diagnostically. This author inclines to the first method.

Table 18.2.5 Some causes of obstructive and restrictive ventilatory disorder

Cause	Example
Obstructive	Asthma
	Chronic obstructive pulmonary disease of smokers
	Chronic obstructive pulmonary disease of α_1-antitrypsin deficiency
	Bronchiectasis, including cystic fibrosis
	Reactive airways disease syndrome (RADS)
Restrictive	Cryptogenic fibrosing alveolitis
	Other alveolitides—rheumatoid disease, drugs (e.g. methotrexate), extrinsic allergic alveolitis
	Sarcoidosis (can show mixed restrictive/obstructive pattern)
	Obesity
	Kyphoscoliosis
	Neuromuscular disorders (e.g. motor neuron disease, poliomyelitis)

Rather indistinct crackles in early inspiration can sometimes be heard at the lung bases in chronic obstructive pulmonary disease. Coarse crackles (of longer duration, close to 20 ms) are usual in bronchiectasis. Mid-range duration crackles occur in pulmonary oedema, pneumonia, and other various segmental parenchymal lung diseases, and they are not reliably distinguishable. Many cases of fibrosing alveolitis (but not all) feature distinctively late and very fine crackles (<10 ms), which can be overlooked by the unwary. In some severe cases of fibrosing alveolitis and adult respiratory distress syndrome (ARDS), short musical sounds on inspiration (squawks), can accompany the crackles.

Initial investigations

It should be recognized that a number of important lung diseases do not produce auscultatory pulmonary signs. In some this relates to their early phase (e.g. bronchial carcinoma); in others it typifies the diseases through their course (e.g. sarcoidosis, diverse nodular lung diseases as opposed to diffuse or segmental disorders, some diffuse pneumonias such as pneumocystis, and tuberculosis). Findings on clinical examination can be unreliable in small to moderate pneumothorax and in pulmonary embolism.

A plain posteroanterior (PA) chest radiograph is an essential adjunct to early diagnostic assessment in the medical admissions unit or specialist chest clinic, but note that practice varies; in rural and poor global settings, for instance, microscopy of sputum for mycobacteria is used efficiently instead of radiology in the detection of endemic tuberculosis.

In the medical admissions unit, pulse oximetry and (in most cases) arterial blood gas analysis (see deceptive clinical features of respiratory failure above) are also an essential adjunct to the clinical assessment of respiratory disorder. A haemoglobin–oxygen saturation lower than 94% signifies clinically significant hypoxaemia. As an exception carbon monoxide poisoning—causing tissue hypoxaemia—shows normal pulse oximetry.

Peak expiratory flow measurement is an essential adjunct in acute asthma. In the clinic, well-conducted but simple spirometry provides an excellent and objective assessment of diverse obstructive and restrictive respiratory disorders (Table 18.2.5). The key measurements are the forced expiratory volume in one second and the forced vital capacity (FEV_1 and FVC), relating these carefully to predicted values according to age, gender, height and ethnic origin. Repeated spirometry also provides the basis for assessing objectively the response to treatments. See Chapter 18.3.1 for further discussion.

Further reading

Fishman AP (ed.) (2008). *Fishman's pulmonary diseases and disorders*, 4th edition. McGraw-Hill, New York.

Von Leupoldt A, *et al.* (2009). Dyyspnoea and pain share emotion related brain network. *Neuroimage*, **48**, 200–6.

Vyshedskiy A, *et al.* (2005). Transmission of crackles in patients with interstitial fibrosis, heart failure and pneumonia. *Chest*, **128**, 1468–74.

Clinical investigation of respiratory disorders

Contents

18.3.1 **Respiratory function tests**

G.J. Gibson

Essentials

Respiratory function tests are used in diagnosis, assessment and prognosis and in monitoring the effects of treatment of various respiratory conditions. Their use as a diagnostic tool is in recognizing patterns of abnormality which characterize particular types of disease; more often they are used to quantify the severity of functional disturbance or to locate the likely anatomical site(s) of disease (airways, alveoli, or chest wall).

The commonly applied tests are most conveniently classified as (1) tests of respiratory mechanics, (2) carbon monoxide uptake, (3) arterial blood gases and acid–base balance, and (4) exercise.

Tests of respiratory mechanics

Spirometers record the volume of air that is displaced from the lungs in tidal breathing or with forced inspiratory and expiratory manoeuvres. This allows measurement of the tidal volume (V_T), inspiratory capacity (IC), forced expiratory volume in 1 s (FEV_1) and vital capacity (VC). Residual volume (RV) remains in the lungs after full expiration. Total lung capacity (TLC) represents the volume of air in the lungs after full inspiration—the sum of VC and RV.

RV cannot be measured by spirometric methods: inert gas dilution and whole-body plethysmography are the two main clinical methods used for the measurement of absolute lung volume.

Forced expiratory tests are simple to perform, do not require complex equipment, and are relatively independent of the effort applied by the patient.

The characteristic feature of diffuse airway obstruction is slowing of the rate of expiration, so that the ratio of FEV_1 to FVC (or FEV_1 to VC) is reduced, which defines an 'obstructive' ventilatory defect. In the alternative 'restrictive' pattern of ventilatory function TLC is reduced and both FEV_1 and VC are reduced in approximate proportion.

Measurement of FEV_1 and VC is not sensitive to localized narrowing of the central airway: air flow during forced expiration and inspiration should be examined as maximum flow–volume curves if this is suspected.

Measurements of respiratory muscle function are indicated in evaluation of patients with various neuromuscular diseases.

Carbon monoxide uptake

Carbon monoxide (CO) diffusing capacity ($D_L CO$) or transfer factor ($T_L CO$) is widely used as a simple test of the integrity of the alveolar capillary membrane and the overall gas exchanging function of the lungs.

Arterial blood gases and acid–base balance

The primary measurements made by modern blood gas analysers are the arterial partial pressures of oxygen (Pao_2) and carbon dioxide ($Paco_2$), and hydrogen ion concentration $[H^+]$ or pH.

A reduction in Pao_2 can occur by various mechanisms, but in disease the commonest is mismatching of alveolar ventilation ($\dot{V}_A$) and perfusion ($\dot{Q}$).

Respiratory failure is defined in terms of the arterial blood gas tensions as a reduction in Pao_2 below 8 kPa (60 mmHg) at sea level, either without ('type I') or with ('type II', 'ventilatory failure') CO_2 retention.

The ratio of Pao_2/F_iO_2 is widely used in assessment of patients with severe problems of oxygenation: in acute lung injury a value greater than 300 (Pa_{O_2} in mmHg, $F_{I}O_2$ as a fraction) indicates relatively mild hypoxaemia, whilst a value of less than 100 represents very severe disturbance of gas exchange.

Abnormal acid–base disturbances are traditionally classified as one of four types: respiratory acidosis and respiratory alkalosis—where the primary disturbance is reduced or increased CO_2 excretion respectively—and metabolic acidosis and metabolic alkalosis—where the primary disturbance is increased or decreased [H^+] respectively. A mixed picture is frequently seen.

The likely cause(s) of metabolic acidosis are usefully classified in terms of the 'anion gap', which is calculated simply by subtracting the concentrations of the most abundant anions in blood (chloride and bicarbonate) from the most abundant cations (sodium and potassium).

Exercise

Exercise tests can be useful in evaluating the symptom of breathlessness, in the assessment of disability, and in determining the likely factors limiting performance.

Introduction

Respiratory function tests are used in diagnosis, assessment and prognosis and in monitoring the effects of treatment of various respiratory conditions. In the diagnosis of specific diseases, respiratory function tests —like functional tests of other organs—inevitably have limitations. Their use as a diagnostic tool is in recognizing patterns of abnormality which characterize particular types of disease. More often they are used to quantify the severity of functional disturbance or to locate the likely anatomical site(s) of disease (airways, alveoli, or chest wall). The commonly applied tests are most conveniently classified as (1) tests of respiratory mechanics, (2) carbon monoxide uptake, (3) arterial blood gases and acid–base balance, and (4) exercise. Measurements made during sleep are described elsewhere (see Chapter 18.5.2).

Tests of respiratory mechanics

Mechanics of breathing

The volume of air in the lungs at the end of tidal expiration at rest (functional residual capacity—FRC) represents the 'neutral' volume of the thorax, i.e. the volume pertaining when the respiratory muscles are inactive (as also during anaesthesia with muscle paralysis). Expansion of the lungs above FRC is achieved by contraction of the inspiratory muscles (predominantly the diaphragm), while normal resting tidal expiration is essentially passive, with the driving force provided by elastic recoil of the lungs. The main expiratory muscles are those of the abdominal wall; their contraction increases abdominal pressure which is transmitted to the thorax. In health these muscles become active when ventilation is increased markedly, as on exercise, or during coughing, when a high intrathoracic pressure aids the clearance of airway secretions.

Measurements of ventilation

Measurements of tidal breathing (tidal volume, respiratory frequency) are rarely made in the resting awake subject, other than recording respiratory rate as part of clinical examination.

Measurement of ventilation is, however, of importance in patients receiving ventilatory support (such as in intensive care units), during detailed exercise testing, and during sleep investigations. During exercise testing, ventilation is usually obtained by electrical integration of airflow measured at the mouth, but this approach is impracticable for prolonged monitoring (such as during sleep) and the application of a mouthpiece and nose clip may itself disturb the pattern of resting breathing. Less intrusive methods of varying complexity are available, based on measuring external movement of the chest wall (ribcage and abdomen). Most are at best semiquantitative. They include the traditional mercury/rubber tube stethograph (measuring chest circumference), magnetometers (diameter) and the inductance plethysmograph (cross-sectional area). To obtain an estimate of ventilation, measurements of both ribcage and abdominal motion are required, together with an appropriate calibration procedure using a spirometer. The most recent and most complex technique of optoplethysmography uses a number of small reflectors on the chest and abdomen, illuminated by infrared light, with the reflected signals captured and processed electronically to allow three-dimensional reconstruction of dynamic chest wall volume, e.g. during exercise testing.

Elastic properties of the lungs

In principle the mechanical function of the respiratory system can be characterized by the compliance ('stiffness') of the lungs and chest wall and the resistance of the airway. In practice, however, none of these is commonly measured directly in clinical testing. For measurement of pulmonary compliance the pressure required to distend the lungs is obtained by recording oesophageal pressure, which equates to pleural pressure. In clinical investigation, the elastic properties of the lungs are usually inferred from measurements of lung volumes, because lungs which are unusually stiff and poorly compliant (as in pulmonary fibrosis) are usually shrunken and reduced in volume, while lungs with abnormally high compliance (as in emphysema) are easily distensible and are associated with increased total lung capacity. The traditional subdivisions of lung volume are illustrated in Fig. 18.3.1.1 and the changes seen in disease in Fig. 18.3.1.2.

Airway resistance

Direct measurement of airway resistance requires estimation of the pressure difference along the airway, between the alveoli and mouth. The various techniques available for estimating alveolar pressure include oesophageal pressure monitoring, body plethysmography, and transient interruption of airflow. With the latter (interruption) method, mouth pressure during transient occlusion is assumed to equal the alveolar pressure immediately prior to occlusion. As this requires little cooperation from the subject it is used more often in paediatric than adult practice. The plethysmographic method can be combined with measurement of lung volumes (see below). It requires the subject to make gentle panting efforts both with and without an occlusion at the mouth, while seated in a body plethysmograph.

Airway resistance varies with lung volume, falling as volume increases due to an expanding effect of more negative pleural pressure and the increased tension in the lung tissue surrounding the intrapulmonary airways. Resistance (R_{AW}) is often expressed as its reciprocal, conductance (G_{AW}), which in turn can be divided by the lung volume at which it is measured (specific airway

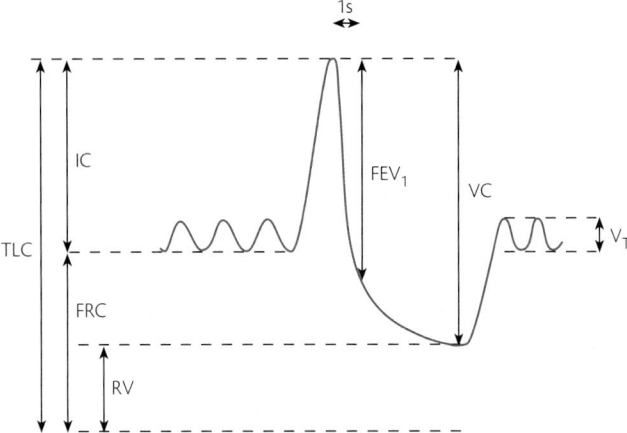

Fig. 18.3.1.1 Subdivisions of lung volume illustrated by spirometric recording of volume against time during tidal breathing for three breaths, followed by maximal inspiration and then maximal forced expiration, before returning to tidal breathing in a normal subject. FEV_1, forced expiratory volume in 1s; FRC, functional residual capacity; IC, inspiratory capacity; RV, residual volume; TLC, total lung capacity; VC, vital capacity; V_T, tidal volume. Note that TLC = FRC + IC = VC + RV.

conductance, SG_{AW}) to allow for variations in volume. Resistance is dominated by the narrowest part of the airway, which in the normal subject is the upper airway (trachea and larynx). Although more peripheral airways are smaller individually, the great increase in their number with sequential branching creates a much larger overall cross-sectional area. Since chronic airway disease usually has its greatest impact on peripheral airways, plethysmographic measurements of airway resistance are not sensitive to the earlier stages of disease.

An alternative method for evaluating airway resistance is by forced oscillation, which involves superimposition of a small oscillating

pressure at the mouth during tidal breathing; the resulting pressure and flow information is used to calculate airway resistance.

In practice airway function is more commonly assessed by tests based on forced expiration (see below).

Measurements of lung volume

A spirometer records only the air which can be displaced from the lungs and not their absolute volume, because the unmeasured residual volume (RV) remains in the lungs after full expiration. The maximum volume expired after a full inspiration (or inspired after a full expiration) is known as the vital capacity (VC), and the total lung capacity (TLC) represents the volume of air in the lungs after full inspiration—the sum of VC and RV (Fig. 18.3.1.1). Two main clinical methods are used for measurement of absolute lung volume—inert gas dilution and whole-body plethysmography.

Inert gas dilution

The subject breathes a gas mixture containing an inert marker gas, usually helium, from a closed circuit. The helium equilibrates gradually with the gas in the lungs so that its concentration falls progressively and stabilizes once mixing is complete. In a healthy individual this occurs in 5 to 10 min, but equilibration is much slower due to uneven ventilation but in patients with diffuse airway disease, such as asthma or chronic obstructive pulmonary disease, equilibration and the endpoint may be much less definite. The lung volume measured is that in the lungs when the subject was connected to the circuit (usually FRC). After disconnection from the rebreathing circuit the subject inspires fully and the volume inspired (inspiratory capacity, IC) added to FRC gives TLC (Fig. 18.3.1.1). Uneven distribution of the inspired gas and poor mixing in the lungs result in underestimation of lung volumes in patients with moderate or severe airway disease.

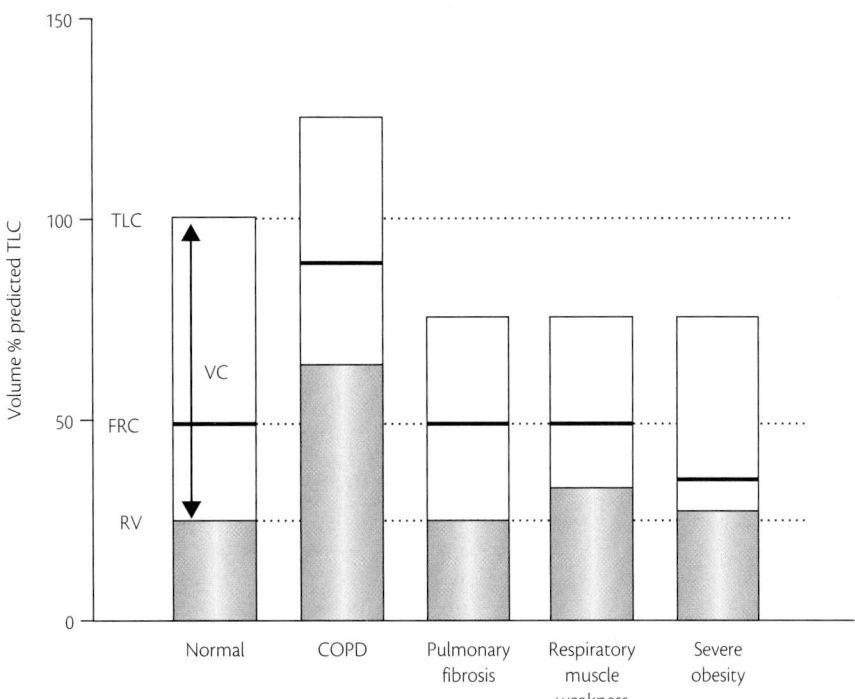

Fig. 18.3.1.2 Pattern of lung volumes in disease. Overall height of bars represents total lung capacity (TLC) as % predicted; shaded areas show relative sizes of residual volume (RV); horizontal solid line shows functional residual capacity (FRC); vital capacity (VC) is represented by open bars. Dotted lines refer to normal TLC, FRC, and RV.

Whole-body plethysmography

The subject sits within a large airtight rigid chamber and makes gentle breathing efforts against a shutter, which closes the airway at the mouth. According to Boyle's law (pressure × volume = a constant), as intrathoracic pressure falls during an inspiratory effort, the air in the lungs is rarefied and lung volume increases by a small amount. This, in turn, causes the pressure in the plethysmograph to increase. The converse occurs during expiratory efforts and the thoracic gas volume can be calculated from the pressure changes recorded. Total lung capacity and residual volume are then derived by full inspiration and expiration immediately on opening the shutter. This method measures the volume of any air spaces within or without the lung that share pressure changes during breathing efforts, hence poorly ventilated areas of lung (or even those totally unventilated, such as a bulla) are included.

Abnormalities of lung volumes

An increase in TLC occurs in most patients with symptomatic diffuse airway obstruction. A large increase is characteristic of emphysema, but is not specific for this condition. Increases are also seen in asthma, even in relative remission. A pathological reduction in TLC occurs in several conditions (Table 18.3.1.1), not only lung diseases such as pulmonary fibrosis, but also extrapulmonary conditions affecting the pleura, thoracic skeleton, or respiratory muscles, conditions which—along with severe obesity—all potentially impede full lung expansion (Fig. 18.3.1.2).

Patients with airway disease develop marked increases in RV and FRC, and the latter (or more strictly, the end expiratory lung volume) increases further on exercise, a phenomenon known as dynamic hyperinflation. This is a useful adaptation for such patients in that breathing over a higher tidal volume range allows ventilation to increase on exertion. However, maintaining higher lung volumes requires more work by the inspiratory muscles, and hyperinflation contributes significantly to the dyspnoea which such patients develop on exertion. The extent of dynamic hyperinflation can be assessed by measuring inspiratory capacity during exercise by having the subject inspire periodically to full inflation and then return to tidal breathing.

Tests of forced expiration

Spirometry

The strengths of forced expiratory tests include the simplicity of both the manoeuvre and equipment required, and also the relative independence of the measurements of the effort applied by the patient.

Table 18.3.1.1 Common causes of reduced total lung capacity

Intrapulmonary	Surgical resection of lobes/lung
	Pulmonary collapse
	Consolidation
	Pulmonary oedema
	Interstitial fibrosis
Extrapulmonary	Pleural effusion
	Pleural thickening
	Pneumothorax
	Ribcage deformity, e.g. scoliosis
	Respiratory muscle weakness
	Gross obesity

Forced expiratory tests are effort-dependent to the extent that a preceding full inspiration is required, but during forced expiration the larger intrathoracic airways are subject to dynamic compression by the surrounding pleural pressure. The net result is that, provided a modest effort is applied, increasing the effort merely compresses the airway further and produces no increase in flow. This effort independence is more marked as forced expiration proceeds, and is also more marked in patients with airway obstruction than in healthy subjects.

Maximum expiratory flow is most dependent on effort at higher lung volumes (i.e. closer to full inflation). As peak expiratory flow (PEF) is attained very rapidly at the start of forced expiration, it is therefore more effort-dependent than the forced expiratory volume in 1 s (FEV_1), which effectively integrates flow over a large proportion of the expired volume. PEF is measurable with a simple peak flow meter and is used by patients, particularly those with asthma, to monitor respiratory function at home.

The most commonly used index of mechanical function of the lungs is the 1 s forced expiratory volume (FEV_1)—the volume expired forcefully in 1 s following complete inspiration (Fig. 18.3.1.1). This is usually obtained together with the forced vital capacity (FVC), the maximum volume expired during a forced expiration. In healthy subjects the FVC is effectively the same as VC, but in patients with airway disease the FVC is often appreciably less than the true ('relaxed') VC obtained if the subject is encouraged to expire completely without excessive initial effort.

The characteristic feature of diffuse airway obstruction is slowing of the rate of expiration so that the ratio of FEV_1 to FVC (or FEV_1 to VC) is reduced. This defines an 'obstructive' ventilatory defect. In the alternative 'restrictive' pattern of ventilatory function, both FEV_1 and FVC are reduced in approximate proportion but, strictly, a restrictive defect implies that TLC is reduced so cannot be diagnosed confidently by spirometry alone.

Although in patients with diffuse airway obstruction the FVC and VC are reduced—at least in those with symptomatic disease—the reduction is proportionally less than that in FEV_1. The ratio of FEV_1 to (F)VC indicates the presence of airway obstruction but it is a poor guide to severity, which is better assessed by comparing the FEV_1 alone with its predicted value. An obstructive spirometric pattern is seen in asthma, chronic obstructive pulmonary disease, and widespread bronchiectasis, while a restrictive ventilatory pattern is seen in numerous conditions (Table 18.3.1.1).

A further feature of diffuse airway obstruction is an increase in RV and in the ratio RV/TLC, but the latter is less specific than a reduced FEV_1/VC ratio as it also occurs in some patients with cardiac disease or respiratory muscle weakness. With dual pathology, combined obstructive (low FEV_1/VC) and restrictive (low TLC) defects are often found. Sometimes TLC may be within the normal range due to opposing influences with, for example, lung fibrosis tending to reduce it and airway obstruction to increase it.

Maximum flow–volume curves

Measurement of FEV_1 and VC is the best way of identifying the diffuse airway narrowing of chronic obstructive pulmonary disease or asthma, but is less sensitive to localized narrowing of the central airway. If the latter is suspected, it is particularly helpful to visualize air flow obtained during forced expiration (and also inspiration) as maximum flow–volume curves, which relate instantaneous flow to volume expired and inspired (Fig. 18.3.1.3).

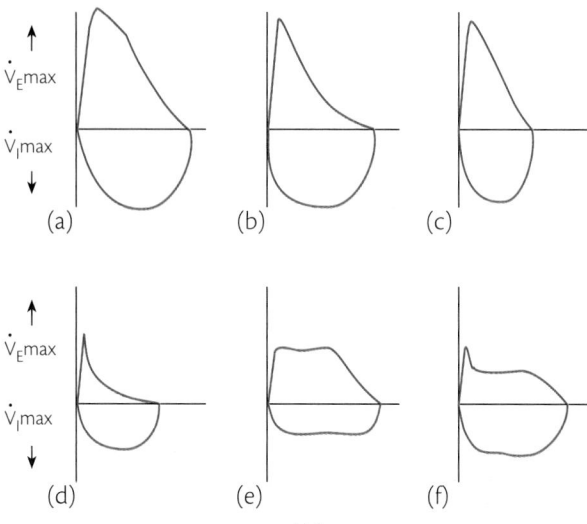

Fig. 18.3.1.3 Schematic maximum expiratory and inspiratory flow–volume curves in: (a) normal young adult; (b) normal older adult; (c) patient with pulmonary fibrosis and reduced FVC; (d) patient with moderately severe chronic obstructive pulmonary disease showing overall reduction in maximal flow but particularly in $\dot{V}_E$ max, at lower lung volumes; (e) patient with subglottic (extrathoracic) tracheal stenosis showing markedly reduced $\dot{V}_I$ max at all volumes and reduced $\dot{V}_E$ max at higher volumes; (f) patient with central intrathoracic (carinal) tracheal narrowing showing similar plateau of flow to (e) but greater reduction of $\dot{V}_E$ max than of $\dot{V}_I$ max.

Expiration

The expiratory curve has a characteristic shape, with an early peak equivalent to the PEF obtained with a peak flow meter. Maximum expiratory flow then declines progressively as volume is expired. In young healthy subjects (Fig. 18.3.1.3a), the descending limb of the curve approximates a straight line, whilst in older normal subjects (Fig. 18.3.1.3b), maximum expiratory flow is less, particularly at lower lung volumes, and the curve becomes concave to the volume axis. In patients with diffuse intrathoracic airway obstruction (such as chronic obstructive pulmonary disease or asthma) the pattern is qualitatively similar to that of ageing, but greatly exaggerated, with expiratory flow reduced more markedly as lung volume declines (Fig. 18.3.1.3d). The shape of the flow–volume curve does not distinguish between different causes of diffuse airway narrowing and so cannot allow the distinction of asthma from chronic obstructive pulmonary disease or emphysema. In principle, measurements of maximum expiratory flow in the latter part of forced expiration should be more sensitive to milder degrees of airway narrowing. In practice, however, use of indices such as maximum flow after 75% of the FVC has been expired (FEF$_{75}$) has proved disappointing because the very wide normal range seriously reduces its discriminating power. Another widely used measurement is the average maximum flow over the middle two quarters of expiration (FEF$_{25-75}$, formerly known as maximum mid-expiratory flow—MMEF). Again, however, the value of this index is seriously compromised by its wide variation in the healthy population and also by its dependence on VC, such that reductions are seen with both obstructive and restrictive ventilatory defects.

The 'plateau' of maximum expiratory flow seen with upper airway obstruction has implications for the shape of the more commonly recorded forced expiratory spirogram. Since, on the spirogram (volume vs time) flow is represented by the gradient of the curve, a plateau on the flow–volume curve implies a 'straight' (rectilinear) spirogram over the same volume range. Such an appearance should therefore raise the possibility of narrowing of the central airway rather than the more common diffuse airway obstruction seen with asthma and chronic obstructive pulmonary disease (Fig. 18.3.1.4).

Inspiration

The maximum inspiratory flow–volume curve has a more symmetrical appearance than the expiratory curve. In patients with diffuse airway narrowing there is an overall reduction in maximum inspiratory flow, but little change in shape (Fig. 18.3.1.3d). In patients with a restrictive ventilatory defect caused, for example, by pulmonary fibrosis, the volume displaced (FVC) is reduced but absolute flows are little affected (Fig. 18.3.1.3c).

Characteristic features are seen in patients with localized narrowing of the central airway, with the pattern depending on whether the narrowing is extra- or intrathoracic. Extrathoracic narrowing (Fig. 18.3.1.3e), such as occurs with subglottic tracheal stenosis or upper tracheal tumours, has a relatively greater effect on inspiratory than expiratory flow (which corresponds to the predominantly inspiratory timing of the stridor of upper airway narrowing). Maximum expiratory flow is also affected, but unlike chronic obstructive pulmonary disease or asthma the effects are most marked at higher lung volumes, often producing a virtual 'plateau' of expiratory flow in the first part of forced expiration. If the central airway is narrowed within the thorax (e.g. lower trachea or carina) a similar plateau of expiratory flow, often with a small initial peak, may be seen, but maximum inspiratory flow is relatively less affected (Fig. 18.3.1.3f).

These patterns can be quantified in terms of various ratios, such as that of maximum expiratory to inspiratory flow at 50% of VC, or the ratio of PEF (markedly reduced with upper airway obstruction) to FEV$_1$ (proportionally less reduced). Such derived indices should be interpreted in light of the overall shape of the curves.

Respiratory muscle function

Forcible static inspiratory and expiratory efforts against a closed airway allow measurement of maximum expiratory and inspiratory pressures (P_E max, P_I max). In general, the expiratory

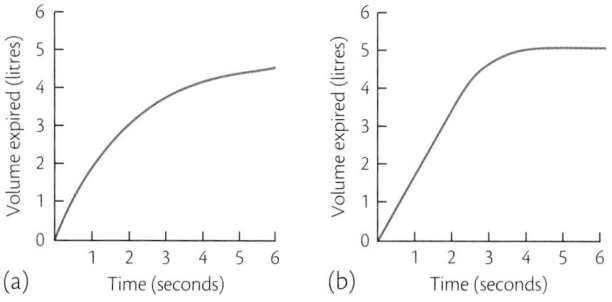

Fig. 18.3.1.4 Schematic spirograms of two patients with airway obstruction and similar FEV$_1$. (a) Diffuse intrathoracic airway narrowing (chronic obstructive pulmonary disease or asthma). Note that forced expiration is continuing after 6 s. (b) Upper airway narrowing with 'straight' spirogram which corresponds to plateau of flow in earlier part of expiration in Fig. 18.3.1.3e.

(predominantly abdominal) muscles perform most effectively at high lung volumes and the inspiratory muscles (predominantly the diaphragm) at lower volumes. P_E max is therefore usually measured after full inspiration and P_I max at FRC or RV. Unfortunately, the normal ranges for these tests are wide and some patients find difficulty in performing the manoeuvres, which are by definition completely effort-dependent. Alternatively, inspiratory muscle strength can be assessed during a forceful sniff, with the pressure measured in the nose via an occluded nostril. Many (though not all) patients find this easier than performing maximum static inspiratory manoeuvres, so that the maximal sniff technique may give more reproducible results. Many laboratories ask patients to perform both and report the numerically greater result.

These measurements all assess the global strength of the inspiratory or expiratory muscles. More specific information on diaphragmatic function requires measurement of transdiaphragmatic pressure using pressure-sensing devices in both oesophagus and stomach—a specialized investigation available in only a few centres. A simple indirect index of disproportionate diaphragmatic weakness or paralysis is a large (>25%) reduction in VC in the supine compared with the erect posture. However, isolated bilateral diaphragmatic paralysis or severe weakness is very uncommon and most patients with respiratory muscle weakness have disease affecting all the muscles. Causes include not only primary neuromuscular diseases such as myopathies, muscular dystrophies, motor neuron disease, and myasthenia gravis, but also drug treatment (corticosteroids), several endocrine and connective tissue disorders, and cachexia from whatever cause. Respiratory muscle weakness is often an important factor preventing weaning from assisted ventilation.

Measurements of respiratory muscle function are indicated in evaluation of patients with various neuromuscular diseases. They are also helpful in confirming or excluding muscle problems in those with otherwise unexplained dyspnoea and in patients with a restrictive ventilatory defect in whom the cause of the lung volume reduction is not apparent on clinical and radiographic grounds. Interpretation may be complicated in patients with airway obstruction (such as chronic obstructive pulmonary disease or asthma) because the associated hyperinflation of the lungs itself impairs inspiratory muscle function. Maximum expiratory pressure is not affected by hyperinflation, however, and can be used as a guide to the presence of true muscle weakness in this situation.

Carbon monoxide uptake

Carbon monoxide (CO) diffusing capacity ($D_L$co) or transfer factor ($T_L$co) is widely used as a simple test of the integrity of the alveolar capillary membrane and the overall gas exchanging function of the lungs. It has good sensitivity but poor specificity, as impairment can result from several pathological processes (Table 18.3.1.2).

In the commonest method, the subject inspires fully a gas mixture containing a very low concentration of CO and the rate of uptake of gas is measured during breath holding for 10 s. The most important determining factor in most conditions is the effective surface area of alveoli available for gas exchange. Consequently $D_L$co is reduced, for example, after resection of lung, but also with widespread emphysema, in which normal-sized alveoli are replaced by much larger air spaces, with a consequently greatly diminished area. $D_L$co is also reduced when there is loss of the 'effective' alveolar

Table 18.3.1.2 Common causes of reduced carbon monoxide diffusing capacity (transfer factor, $T_L$co)

Pulmonary diseases	COPD/emphysema[a]
	Asthma (with severe airway obstruction)
	Pneumonectomy
	Pulmonary fibrosis[a]
	Sarcoidosis
	Pulmonary vascular disease[a]
Cardiac diseases	Pulmonary oedema[a]
	Mitral valve disease[a]
	Congenital right to left shunts[a]
Systemic diseases	Anaemia[a]
	Renal failure[a]
	Hepatic cirrhosis[a]
	Rheumatoid disease
	Systemic sclerosis[a]
	Systemic lupus[a]

COPD, chronic obstructive pulmonary disease.
[a]Kco usually also reduced.

volume (V_A) in which the test gas is distributed. The latter is measured simultaneously from the dilution of helium which is also included in the inspired gas. The 'effective' V_A is reduced if there is maldistribution of ventilation as this causes some alveoli to receive little or none of the inspired gas. Other factors affecting the $D_L$co include the haemoglobin concentration and disease involving the pulmonary capillaries.

The transfer coefficient (Kco), which is obtained along with $D_L$co, represents the uptake of CO per litre of 'effective' alveolar volume, that is, Kco = $D_L$co/V_A. Kco is typically normal or increased after lung resection, when both $D_L$co and V_A are reduced. It is usually normal (or sometimes mildly increased) in asthma, where any reduction in $D_L$co is due only to maldistribution of ventilation secondary to airway narrowing. By contrast, $D_L$co is reduced in widespread emphysema not only due to maldistribution of inspired gas, but also because even in the relatively better ventilated parts of the lung the gas exchanging surface area is diminished, hence Kco is also reduced. Some of the diseases associated with low $D_L$co and Kco are listed in Table 18.3.1.2.

In some conditions Kco and, less commonly, $D_L$co may be high (Table 18.3.1.3). Both increase with an increase in red blood cells in the lungs due to increased capillary blood volume, alveolar haemorrhage, or polycythaemia. Kco is also increased if, at full inflation, the density of pulmonary capillaries per unit alveolar volume is greater than normal. This occurs most commonly in patients with extrapulmonary volume restriction (e.g. muscle weakness), when the density of pulmonary capillaries is unusually high in relation to the (restricted) TLC at which the measurement is made.

Interpretation of respiratory function tests
Reference values

The results of respiratory function tests should be compared with reference values obtained in an appropriate healthy population. The major factors determining the results of most tests in the normal population are sex, age, body size (usually defined by height)

Table 18.3.1.3 Conditions producing increased carbon monoxide diffusing capacity

	↑$D_L$co	↑Kco
Asthma	Sometimes	+
Pneumonectomy	–	+
Extrapulmonary restriction		
Pleural disease	–	+
Ribcage deformity	–	+
Respiratory muscle weakness	–	+
Obesity	–	+
Left-to right-shunts	+	+
Polycythaemia	+	+
Lung haemorrhage	+[a]	+[a]

[a] May be an increase from an initially reduced value (e.g. Goodpasture's syndrome).

and ethnicity. A variety of sources of reference values is available (see 'Further reading') and, increasingly, prediction equations are being developed for countries and ethnic groups hitherto poorly represented. Choice of the most appropriate equation(s) for a local population or a specific individual may not be straightforward; the problems are discussed extensively in the references quoted. The counsel of perfection is to compare results with those obtained in a large number of the local healthy population of the same ethnicity, but often this is not possible. An alternative is to use whichever equation(s) give results similar to those obtained in healthy subjects studied by the same operator or in the same laboratory. Good recent reference equations relevant to residents of North America are available (at least for spirometric and related measurements) from the third National Health and Nutrition Examination Survey (NHANES III). No equivalent large data sets are available in Europe and many laboratories still use the 'summary equations' derived by combining the results of many different series and published by the European Respiratory Society (ERS) in 1993, although these are no longer endorsed officially by the ERS in their latest (2005) recommendations.

Normal or abnormal?

After standardizing for the variables mentioned above, most lung function measurements are distributed normally in the healthy population. Classification of 'normal' or 'abnormal' is best done in terms of the number of standardized residuals by which a given measurement deviates from the mean predicted value (z score). With this approach a z score ranging from –2 to +2 encompasses 95% of a normally distributed population and –1.645 to +1.645 encompasses 90%. In general, when evaluating the results of respiratory function tests, the need is to identify a unidirectional abnormality, e.g. a low, rather than high, FEV_1. It is therefore conventional to regard z values outside the 90% confidence intervals as 'abnormal'. Thus, a z value more negative than –1.645 represents the lower 5th percentile of the normal range, i.e. only 1 in 20 of the healthy population would be expected to have a result below this value. The choice of this level is of course a compromise between sensitivity and specificity and should not be regarded as an absolute 'cut-off' which will accurately classify every individual.

The test results should be examined for internal consistency and interpreted in the light of the clinical and radiographic information available. A number of characteristic patterns of abnormality of spirometry, lung volumes, and CO diffusing capacity are recognized (Table 18.3.1.4).

Arterial blood gases

The primary measurements made by modern blood gas analysers are the arterial partial pressures of oxygen (Pao_2) and carbon dioxide ($Paco_2$), and hydrogen ion concentration [H^+] or pH. The alternative, commonly used, method of assessing oxygenation is by pulse oximetry, which estimates arterial oxygen saturation (Sao_2). An oximeter has the advantage of allowing continuous monitoring, but it provides no information on $Paco_2$. Easy to use transcutaneous electrodes for estimating $Paco_2$ are becoming more widely available, but experience is limited to date.

Haemoglobin–oxygen dissociation curve

The general relation between the oxygen partial pressure in blood and haemoglobin saturation is defined by the oxygen–haemoglobin dissociation curve (Fig. 18.3.1.5). Its position is influenced by the prevailing pH, temperature, and Pco_2 as well as by the concentration of 2,3-diphosphoglycerate (2,3-DPG) in red cells. Approximate values for normal arterial and resting mixed venous Po_2 and saturation are shown in Fig. 18.3.1.5. A clinically useful 'landmark' is a saturation of 90% which, with a normally positioned curve, represents a Po_2 of approximately 8 kPa (60 mmHg). Also shown in Fig. 18.3.1.5 is the P_{50}, i.e. the Po_2 at a saturation of 50%, which for normal adult haemoglobin is approximately 3.5 kPa (27 mmHg). This is measured

Table 18.3.1.4 Common patterns of abnormal lung volumes and carbon monoxide diffusing capacity

Condition	FEV_1	VC	FEV_1/VC	RV	TLC	$D_L$co	Kco
COPD/emphysema	↓↓	↓	↓	↑↑	↑	↓↓	↓
Asthma	↓↓	↓	↓	↑↑	↑	→	→ or ↑
Interstitial lung disease	↓	↓	→	→	↓	↓↓	↓ or →
Extrapulmonary volume restriction	↓	↓	→	↑ or →	↓	→	↑
Pulmonary vascular disease	→	→	→	→	→	↓↓	↓↓
Combined pathology (e.g. COPD + interstitial fibrosis)	↓↓	↓	↓	↑ or →	→ or ↓	↓↓	↓↓

COPD, chronic obstructive pulmonary disease.
→, normal; ↓, moderately reduced; ↓↓, markedly reduced.

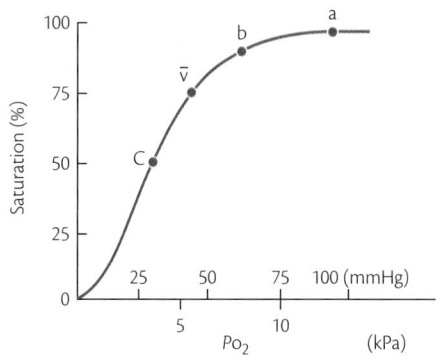

Fig. 18.3.1.5 Normal haemoglobin–oxygen dissociation curve relating saturation to Po_2. Point a represents normal arterial values (Po_2 90 mmHg, 12 kPa; Sao_2 98%) and v̄ normal resting mixed venous values ($P\bar{v}o_2$ 40 mmHg, 5.3 kPa; Sao_2 75%). Also shown are the Po_2 (c.60 mmHg, 8 kPa) corresponding to 90% saturation (point b) and the P_{50} (point c), i.e. Po_2 corresponding to 50% saturation (c.27 mmHg, 3.5 kPa).

in vitro and used to characterize abnormal haemoglobin molecules associated with increased (low P_{50}) or decreased (high P_{50}) affinity for oxygen.

Ventilation–perfusion mismatching

A reduction in Pao_2 can occur by various mechanisms (Table 18.3.1.5). In disease, the commonest is mismatching of alveolar ventilation ($\dot{V}_A$) and perfusion ($\dot{Q}$). Even in healthy lungs, distribution of both ventilation and perfusion is uneven, due mainly to gravity. In disease, these relatively small effects are outweighed by unevenly distributed pathological changes affecting the distribution of ventilation or perfusion or both. Alveoli with greater than average $\dot{V}_A/\dot{Q}$ have higher than average local Po_2 and lower Pco_2, i.e. closer to those of inspired air. Conversely, alveoli with lower than average $\dot{V}_A/\dot{Q}$ have lower Po_2 and higher Pco_2, i.e. closer to the values in mixed venous (pulmonary arterial) blood. Within a single alveolus, complete equilibration of local gas tensions usually occurs, but in different pulmonary capillaries the gas tensions essentially reflect those of the alveoli which they subtend. For CO_2 the effects of high $\dot{V}_A/\dot{Q}$ and low $\dot{V}_A/\dot{Q}$ areas on the final arterial Pco_2 approximately cancel out, so that the arterial Pco_2 is close to the average value in all the capillaries draining the alveoli. With oxygen, however, blood draining alveoli with high $\dot{V}_A/\dot{Q}$ (and therefore relatively high local Po_2) cannot compensate for the areas with low $\dot{V}_A/\dot{Q}$ (and low Po_2). This arises mainly because of the

Table 18.3.1.5 Mechanisms of arterial hypoxaemia

Mechanism	Cause
Low inspired Po_2	Altitude (including air travel)
Hypoventilation	Neuromuscular diseases
	Drugs depressing ventilatory drive
$\dot{V}_A/\dot{Q}$ mismatching	All pulmonary diseases
Anatomical shunt	Intracardiac right-to-left shunt
	Pulmonary arteriovenous malformations
Limitation of oxygen diffusion	Pulmonary fibrosis (on exercise)

shape of the oxygen dissociation curve: the relatively flat upper part of the curve implies that increasing Po_2 adds very little to oxygen saturation or concentration (content). Consequently, mixed pulmonary venous (and therefore systemic arterial) blood has an appreciably lower Po_2 than would be found in mixed alveolar air.

An approximate assessment of the overall effects of $\dot{V}_A/\dot{Q}$ mismatching on arterial oxygenation and Pao_2 is given by calculation of the alveolar to arterial oxygen pressure gradient ($P(A-a)o_2 = PAo_2 - Pao_2$). This requires estimation of the average alveolar Po_2 (PAo_2), which depends on the inspired Po_2 (P_Io_2) and the average alveolar Pco_2 ($PAco_2$). For the reasons discussed above, alveolar and arterial Pco_2 (unlike Po_2) are virtually the same and the alveolar Po_2 is given approximately by:

$$PAo_2 = P_Io_2 - Paco_2/0.8 \qquad \text{(Equation 18.3.1.1)}$$

The P_Io_2 breathing room air at sea level (moistened and warmed to body temperature) is 20 kPa (150 mmHg). In normal young subjects the upper limit for $P(A-a)o_2$ is about 2 kPa (15 mmHg). It increases with age and in healthy subjects aged 60 to 70 years may be as high as 4.7 kPa (35 mmHg). Unfortunately, interpretation of the $P(A-a)o_2$ is complicated by the fact that its relation to the severity of $\dot{V}_A/\dot{Q}$ mismatching is not constant. For a given degree of $\dot{V}_A/\dot{Q}$ mismatching, the $P(A-a)o_2$ increases as the alveolar Po_2 increases. It therefore increases if the inspired oxygen is increased or if $Paco_2$ falls (see Equation 18.3.1.1).

Alternative indices which relate more predictably to the severity of $\dot{V}_A/\dot{Q}$ mismatching are the ratios of arterial to alveolar Po_2 (a/A Po_2), and of arterial Po_2 to the inspired oxygen fractional concentration (Pao_2/F_Io_2). The former is normally greater than 0.75 and changes little as F_Io_2 increases, whereas the more traditional $P(A-a)o_2$ difference increases. The ratio of Pao_2/F_Io_2 is widely used in assessment of patients with severe problems of oxygenation. For example, in acute lung injury a value greater than 300 (Pao_2 in mmHg, F_Io_2 as a fraction) indicates relatively mild hypoxaemia, whilst a value of less than 100 represents very severe disturbance of gas exchange.

Estimation of 'anatomical' shunt

The dependence of $P(A-a)o_2$ on inspired oxygen is exemplified by the effects of breathing pure oxygen. This is sometimes used as a test for the presence of anatomical right to left shunting, since the effects of $\dot{V}_A/\dot{Q}$ mismatching on Pao_2 are effectively eliminated by breathing pure oxygen: even in diseased lungs, nitrogen is gradually 'washed out' of all the alveoli and the only remaining cause of arterial hypoxaemia is the anatomical shunt via channels which bypass the lungs, or through the capillaries supplying any alveoli that are totally unventilated. Although prolonged breathing of 100% oxygen encourages alveolar atelectasis which would exaggerate the shunt, in practice the technique is often helpful in investigating the causes of hypoxaemia. The usually quoted normal upper limit for the 'anatomical' shunt measured in this way is 5% of the cardiac output. In terms of the Pao_2, a value greater than 500 mmHg (>73 kPa) is usually achieved.

Respiratory failure

Respiratory failure is defined in terms of the arterial blood gas tensions as a reduction in Pao_2 below 8 kPa (60 mmHg) at sea level, either without ('type I') or with ('type II') CO_2 retention. Hypercapnic (type II) respiratory failure is also known as ventilatory failure. The causes of type I respiratory failure are legion and include virtually all diseases which can affect the alveoli or the airways, either primarily or secondarily (e.g. cardiac failure). Hypercapnic (type II) respiratory failure is most commonly due to severe chronic airway disease. Less often it results from reduced ventilation as, for example, with severe respiratory muscle weakness or scoliosis. The mechanisms of elevation of Pa_{CO_2} in type II respiratory failure are twofold. Sustained 'pure' hypoventilation—reduction in overall ventilation resulting in hypercapnia—is rare. It is seen with inadequate performance of the respiratory 'bellows', e.g. in neuromuscular disease, or because of reduced drive to breathe in the unconscious subject. Much more commonly, as in chronic airway disease, the 'effective' alveolar ventilation is reduced as a consequence of mismatching of ventilation and perfusion. In this situation there is often a considerable amount of ineffectual or wasted ventilation ('physiological dead space') and consequently in such patients the total ventilation is often greater than normal, even in the presence of hypercapnia.

Acid–base balance

The carriage of CO_2 by the blood and its excretion by the lungs constitute one of the two homeostatic mechanisms for regulating the acid–base status of the body. Because of the ease with which CO_2 excretion can normally be increased, the lungs are able to adjust acid–base balance much more rapidly than the kidneys.

The carbonic acid association/dissociation equation is:

$$CO_2 + H_2O \Leftrightarrow H_2CO_3 \Leftrightarrow H^+ + HCO_3^- \qquad \text{Equation (18.3.1.2)}$$

This defines the chemical relation between the three variables, Pco_2, hydrogen ion concentration $[H^+]$, and bicarbonate concentration $[HCO_3^-]$. If two are measured, the third is readily calculated. Hydrogen ion concentration is usually expressed as pH, its negative logarithm (to the base 10). This has the dubious advantage of expressing a very small numerical value as a more easily accessible number, but the pH scale is deceptive as it obscures the fact that the hydrogen ion concentration in blood and the changes seen in disease are exquisitely small in comparison to other commonly measured ions. Thus, a normal arterial pH of 7.4 represents $[H^+]$ of 40×10^{-9} mol/litre (i.e. approximately 1 millionth the concentration of other ions, which are usually expressed in units of 10^{-3} mol/litre). Doubling $[H^+]$ to 80×10^{-9} mol/litre or halving it to 20×10^{-9} mol/litre are equivalent to reducing pH to 7.1 or increasing it to 7.7 respectively (since the $\log_{10}$ of 2 is $c.0.3$, and pH is the negative $\log_{10}$ of $[H^+]$, 0.3 is simply subtracted from, or added to, the normal value of 7.4 if $[H^+]$ is multiplied or divided by 2).

Abnormal acid–base disturbances are traditionally classified in terms of these variables as four types (Table 18.3.1.6 and Fig. 18.3.1.6), but combined disturbances are frequently seen. The commoner causes of each are given in Table 18.3.1.7.

Respiratory acidosis and alkalosis

In respiratory acidosis the prime event is accumulation of CO_2 due to inadequate or ineffective ventilation. This causes the equilibrium of Equation 18.3.1.2 to shift to the right, generating hydrogen and bicarbonate ions. The immediate increase in bicarbonate concentration is dictated by this chemical relationship and not by the physiological response, which occurs later. The vast majority of hydrogen ions produced are buffered by proteins and the increase in $[HCO_3^-]$ (measured in 10^{-3} mol/litre) is actually very much greater than the measured increase in hydrogen ion concentration

Table 18.3.1.6 Types of acid–base disturbance

Arterial	$[H^+]$	pH	Pa_{CO_2}	$[HCO_3^-]$
Respiratory acidosis:				
Acute	↑↑	↓↓	↑	↑
Chronic	↑	↓	↑	↑↑
Respiratory alkalosis	↓	↑	↓	↓
Metabolic acidosis	↑	↓	↓	↓
Metabolic alkalosis	↓	↑	↑ or →	↑

→, normal; ↓, moderately reduced; ↓↓, markedly reduced; ↑, moderately increased; ↑↑, markedly increased.

(10^{-9} mol/litre). Conventionally the effects of acute respiratory acidosis are distinguished from the chronic respiratory acidosis, which results after several hours or days. This follows renal retention of even more bicarbonate, which in turn tends to correct the pH towards normal (Table 18.3.1.6).

In respiratory alkalosis the primary event is increased CO_2 excretion resulting from hyperventilation, so that both $[HCO_3^-]$ and $[H^+]$ fall (pH rises), but, again, most of the change in $[H^+]$ is buffered.

Metabolic acidosis and alkalosis

In metabolic acidosis $[H^+]$ rises (pH falls) and $[HCO_3^-]$ falls. The physiological response is so rapid that acute and chronic phases are

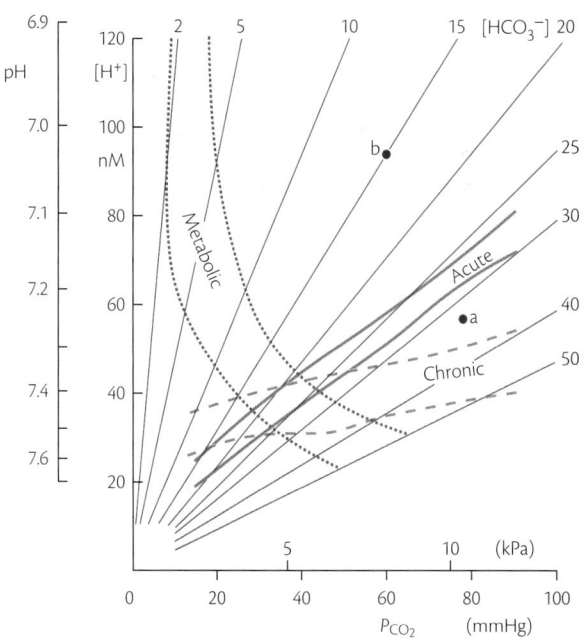

Fig. 18.3.1.6 Relations of pH and $[H^+]$ to Pco_2 in acid–base disorders. Bands indicate the expected ranges in uncomplicated respiratory (acute and chronic) and metabolic disorders. Isopleths represent corresponding estimates of arterial $[HCO_3^-]$ ($\times 10^{-3}$ mol/litre). Values outside these bands indicate intermediate or combined disturbances. For example: patient a with an acute exacerbation of chronic obstructive pulmonary disease has an 'acute-on-chronic' respiratory acidosis (Pa_{CO_2} 10.6 kPa, pH 7.24, $[H^+]$ 58×10^{-9} mol/litre, $[HCO_3^-]$ 34×10^{-3} mol/litre); patient b with both respiratory and circulatory failure has a combined respiratory and metabolic acidosis (Pa_{CO_2} 8 kPa, pH 7.04, $[H^+]$ 95×10^{-9} mol/litre $[HCO_3^-]$ 15×10^{-3} mol/litre).

Table 18.3.1.7 Commoner causes of acid–base disturbance

Disturbance and site of disease	Cause
Respiratory acidosis	
Cerebral	Drugs (sedatives, hypnotics, anaesthetics)
	Raised intracranial pressure
	Primary alveolar hypoventilation (very rare)
Spinal cord	Trauma
Motor neurons	Motor neuron disease, poliomyelitis
Peripheral nerves	Guillain–Barré syndrome, etc.
Motor endplate	Myasthenia gravis, neuromuscular blocking agents
Respiratory muscles	Myopathies, dystrophies etc.
Ribcage	Scoliosis, trauma, thoracoplasty
Lung parenchyma	ARDS, pulmonary oedema (severe), interstitial fibrosis (very advanced)
Airways	COPD, asthma (severe), upper airway obstruction (very severe)
Respiratory alkalosis	
Cerebral	Anxiety, central neurogenic hyperventilation (very rare), drugs (aspirin)
Pulmonary	Pulmonary fibrosis etc., pneumonia, pulmonary embolism, asthma, pulmonary oedema
Iatrogenic	Mechanical overventilation
Metabolic acidosis	
Increased anion gap	Ketoacidosis, uraemia, lactic acidosis, drugs (aspirin), poisons (ethylene glycol)
Normal anion gap	Renal tubular acidosis, severe diarrhoea
Metabolic alkalosis	
Severe vomiting	Pyloric stenosis, etc.
Iatrogenic	Diuretics, corticosteroids, bicarbonate infusion

ARDS, acute respiratory distress syndrome; COPD, chronic obstructive pulmonary disease.

not distinguishable. Any tendency for $Paco_2$ to rise (equilibrium of Equation 18.3.1.2 shifted to the left) is more than offset by the increased drive to breathe resulting from production of acid, and the measured effect is a reduction in $Paco_2$. The likely cause(s) of metabolic acidosis are usefully classified in terms of the 'anion gap', which is calculated simply by subtracting the concentrations of the most abundant anions in blood (chloride and bicarbonate) from the most abundant cations (sodium and potassium). The difference represents other anions (mostly protein and inorganic phosphate) normally present in blood. An increase above the normal anion gap therefore implies an excess of other anions associated with metabolic acidosis (e.g. lactate, ketoacids).

In metabolic alkalosis there is an increase in $[HCO_3^-]$ and a reduction in $[H^+]$ (pH increases). The measured result is somewhat variable due to opposing influences: any increase in $Paco_2$ tends to stimulate breathing, but the reduced acidity tends to inhibit it. In subjects with healthy lungs, the net effect is often maintenance of $Paco_2$ in the high normal range, unless the alkalosis is profound (e.g. as seen with vomiting due to pyloric stenosis and severe depletion of acid). However, in patients with chronic airway disease and

pre-existing or incipient hypercapnia, an increase in $Paco_2$ occurs more readily. This is particularly relevant to patients with chronic obstructive pulmonary disease receiving treatment with diuretics and corticosteroids, both of which tend to produce a metabolic alkalosis.

Other acid–base indices

Several other indices of acid–base status have their advocates. Standard bicarbonate, base excess and deficit, and total buffer base are often derived when blood gases are measured by automated equipment. They are obtained by titration of the blood *in vitro* to specified standard values of pH and/or Pco_2. They are open to the objection that the results differ from those which would be obtained if the same titration could be performed *in vivo*, where the extracellular fluid, and not just the blood, participates in buffering. Indices such as standard bicarbonate and base excess are used mainly to distinguish 'respiratory' and 'metabolic' components of an acid–base disturbance, but in this context the 'metabolic' component includes renal compensation for a primary respiratory disturbance. Consequently, in a respiratory acidosis, an increased standard bicarbonate indicates some degree of chronicity. Conversely, the severity of acidaemia in a hypercapnic patient is a useful practical index of the 'acute' component of an acute-on-chronic respiratory acidosis and is widely used, for example, when deciding on the need for noninvasive ventilation.

Another simple and frequently available index of acid–base status is the venous 'bicarbonate' (strictly total CO_2 content), which is often obtained routinely when electrolytes are measured. A raised value is seen with primary metabolic alkalosis, but in patients with respiratory disease it may also be a useful clue to unsuspected ventilatory failure.

'Strong ion' approach

The analysis of acid–base balance presented above is oversimplified. A more comprehensive (but more complex) approach based on the principles of physical chemistry was proposed by Stewart and subsequently developed by others. This focuses on the factors that independently determine $[H^+]$, reducing the emphasis on $[HCO_3^-]$, which is shown to be itself a dependent variable. According to this analysis, the independent variables controlling acid–base balance are three: the Pco_2, the 'strong ion difference' (SID), and the total weak acid concentration (a weak acid is one which is partly dissociated rather than completely ionized). SID is the difference between the charge of the strong (completely dissociated) cations and anions in plasma, which in effect boils down to $[Na^+] + [K^+] - [Cl^-]$. A higher value of SID reduces acidity (higher pH). The weak acids in blood are predominantly proteins, particularly albumin, with a small contribution from inorganic phosphate.

This approach defines six rather than four primary acid–base disorders. Respiratory disturbances remain as before, but metabolic acidosis and alkalosis can each be either of two types, resulting from increases or decreases either in SID or total weak acid concentration. Decreasing SID or increasing [weak acid] produces acidosis, while increasing SID or decreasing [weak acid] produces alkalosis.

In practice the strong ion approach is of most value in understanding complex metabolic disturbances, as commonly occur in patients receiving intensive care. In particular it highlights the important role of albumin concentration: since albumin is a weak acid, a reduction in its concentration has an alkalinizing effect, such that a metabolic acidosis resulting from a reduction in SID may be underestimated or concealed in patients with hypoalbuminaemia. Again, it is well recognized that infusion of large volumes of normal saline can result in an acidosis: in terms of the strong ion theory this is readily explicable as due to a reduction in plasma SID as plasma $[Cl^-]$ increases relatively more than $[Na^+]$. An important determinant of SID is renal function, in particular the regulatory effect of the kidneys on plasma chloride concentration. Thus, in 'renal compensation' for a respiratory acidosis, the strong ion approach emphasizes increased excretion of chloride (rather than retention of bicarbonate); this increases plasma SID and therefore reduces acidaemia.

Exercise testing

Exercise tests can be useful in evaluating the symptom of breathlessness, in the assessment of disability, and in determining the likely factors limiting performance.

In healthy subjects during progressive exercise, ventilation and cardiac output increase with oxygen consumption. Oxygen uptake ($\dot{V}o_2$) increases with work rate, but at higher levels of exercise anaerobic respiration increases with generation of lactic acid. Initially, CO_2 production is proportional to oxygen consumption until increasing anaerobic metabolism results in disproportionate production of CO_2. Measurement of an 'anaerobic threshold' during progressive exercise is favoured by some investigators, but the criteria used for its identification are not universally agreed.

In a healthy subject, the maximum oxygen consumption (maximum aerobic capacity) is determined by the ability of the circulation to supply oxygen to exercising muscle, rather than by the maximum ventilation which can be achieved. In patients with lung disease, however, the maximum attainable ventilation is reduced, approximately in proportion to the abnormality of pulmonary mechanics. This may then determine exercise capacity, although circulatory factors and deconditioning also contribute in many patients and dominate in some.

Exercise tests vary considerably in complexity and in the number and types of measurements made. Simple self-paced tests of walking distance, most commonly in 6 min, aim to mimic the real life situation and are widely used for global assessment of disability. However, such tests are insensitive to mild disease and there is a significant learning effect, as well as dependence on motivation and encouragement. An alternative simple test is the shuttle walk test in which the subject increases his walking speed each minute; this gives more reproducible results than the 6-min walk and is more akin to laboratory-based tests of maximum performance.

More formal testing involves controlled exercise on a bicycle ergometer or treadmill. Usually the workload is increased progressively by a constant amount, with periods of 1 to 3 min at each level. Measurements include heart rate, ventilation, gas exchange ($\dot{V}o_2$ and $\dot{V}co_2$), and oxygen saturation by pulse oximetry. The level of breathlessness at each workload in an incremental test can be assessed using simple self-rating scales (visual analogue scale or Borg scale). The subject exercises at increasing loads until no longer able to continue because of discomfort, or until stopped by the investigator. The maximum oxygen consumption (symptom limited $\dot{V}o_2$ max) is a useful indicator of overall exercise capacity. Comparison of the maximum ventilation and heart rate at the end of progressive exercise with those predicted from spirometric measurements and age, respectively, gives some indication of the likely factor(s) limiting performance. If, for example, a patient achieves the predicted maximum heart rate during a progressive test (as is seen in normal subjects), it is reasonable to conclude that the limit to further exercise is set by the cardiovascular system. In most respiratory diseases, patients cease exercise with a lower heart rate, as more often the limit is set by the maximum ventilation achievable. Arterial oxygen desaturation is seen in some (but not all) patients with advanced chronic obstructive pulmonary disease, and also in those with interstitial lung disease and pulmonary vascular disease; this can be helpful in predicting patients likely to benefit from the use of ambulatory oxygen.

The identification of exercise-induced asthma has rather different requirements. During exercise, most subjects with asthma show bronchodilatation; in those who develop exercise-induced asthma, bronchoconstriction develops after exercise. Of course many patients with asthma become unduly breathless during exercise, but in most this is due to the increased work of breathing associated with a degree of pre-exercise airway obstruction or to deconditioning, rather than to exercise-induced bronchoconstriction. The intensity of exercise necessary to provoke asthma is relatively high and, for this reason, exercise-induced asthma is relevant mainly to children and young adults. Optimally it is demonstrated after exercising for at least 5 min at a constant rate, chosen to increase ventilation to around 50% maximal or to increase heart rate to around 80% maximal. FEV_1 or peak flow should be measured beforehand and for up to 30 min afterwards.

Miscellaneous tests

Analysis of expired air has traditionally been limited to oxygen and carbon dioxide, but recently attention has turned to other gases which are present in very low concentrations. The concentration of exhaled carbon monoxide has been used for some years as a guide to its inhalation and as a valuable method for confirming nonsmoking claims. The measurement can now be made very simply with a portable analyser. Breath carbon monoxide is also increased in nonsmoking subjects with asthma, where it appears to be released as a result of airway inflammation. In similar fashion, expired nitric oxide concentration is increased as a consequence of airway inflammation and it has been proposed as a non-invasive way of assessing airway inflammation and its treatment, particularly in those with asthma. Care needs to be taken to avoid contamination of expired air from the bronchial tree with that from the nose and nasal sinuses, which contain higher concentrations of NO.

Further reading

American Thoracic Society/European Respiratory Society (2002). ATS/ERS statement on respiratory muscle testing. *Am J Respir Crit Care Med*, **166**, 518–624.

Gibson GJ (2009). *Clinical Tests of Respiratory Function*, 3rd edition. Hodder Arnold, London.

Hughes JMB (2009). *Physiology and Practice of Pulmonary Function. Association for Respiratory Technology and Physiology*, Boldmere, UK.

Kharitonov S, Alving K, Barnes PJ (1997). ERS Task Force Report: Exhaled and nasal nitric oxide measurements: recommendations. *Eur Respir J*, **10**, 1683–93.

MacIntyre N, *et al.* (2005). Standardisation of the single breath determination of carbon monoxide uptake in the lung. *Eur Respir J*, **26**, 720–5.

Miller MR, *et al.* (2005). General considerations for lung function testing. *Eur Respir J*, **26**, 153–61.

Miller MR, *et al.* (2005). Standardisation of spirometry. *Eur Respir J*, **26**, 319–38.

Pellegrino R, *et al* (2005). Interpretative strategies for lung function tests. *Eur Respir J*, **26**, 948–68.

Roca J, Whipp BJ (eds) (1997). Clinical exercise testing. *Eur Respir Monogr*, **2**(6).

Sirker AA, *et al.* (2002). Acid–base physiology: the 'traditional' and the 'modern' approaches. *Anaesthesia*, **57**, 348–56.

Wanger J, *et al.* (2005). Standardisation of the measurement of lung volumes. *Eur Respir J*, **26**, 511–22.

West JB, Wagner PD (1997). Ventilation–perfusion relationships. In: Crystal RG, West JB (eds) *The lung: scientific foundations*, 2nd edition, pp. 1693–709. Lippincott-Raven, Philadelphia.

Sources of normal reference values

Cerveri I, *et al.* (1995). Reference values of arterial oxygen tension in middle-aged and elderly. *Am J Respir Crit Care Med*, **152**, 934–41.

Cotes JE, Chinn DJ, Miller MR (2006). *Lung function*, 6th edition. Blackwell, Oxford.

European Respiratory Society (1993). Standardised lung function testing. *Eur Respir J*, **6**(Suppl 16).

Hankinson JL, Odenkrantz JR, Fedan KB (1999). Spirometric reference values from a sample of the general U.S. population. *Am J Respir Crit Care Med*, **159**, 179–87.

Jones NL, Summers E, Killian KJ (1989). Influence of age and stature on exercise capacity during incremental cycle ergometry in men and women. *Am Rev Respir Dis*, **140**, 1373–80.

18.3.2 Thoracic imaging

Susan J. Copley and David M. Hansell

Essentials

Radiographic findings should always be interpreted in conjunction with the clinical picture.

Chest radiography—this remains the commonest technique in the investigation of suspected thoracic disease. Advantages are cost, availability, and a significantly lower radiation dose than CT, but even with optimal technique nearly one-third of the lungs are partially obscured by the overlying mediastinum, diaphragm, and ribs.

CT—is more sensitive and specific than chest radiography in a range of pulmonary disorders, including airways disease and diffuse interstitial lung disease. In the latter condition high-resolution CT images of the lung correlate closely with the microscopic appearances of pathological specimens and are a substantial improvement over chest radiography in terms of sensitivity, specificity and diagnostic accuracy. In many centres spiral CT has supplanted ventilation–perfusion radionuclide imaging in the investigation of patients with suspected pulmonary embolism.

Ventilation/perfusion radionuclide scanning—is the commonest radionuclide study of the lungs and is most frequently used to confirm or exclude the diagnosis of suspected pulmonary embolism.

Positron emission tomography (PET) and CT/PET—usually employed with the isotope ^{18}F-fluorodeoxyglucose (FDG) and increasingly available for investigation and staging of lung cancer.

Ultrasonography—the use of this technique in the chest is limited because high-frequency sound waves do not traverse normally aerated lung, but fluid can be readily detected and the main use of ultrasound is for the localization of small or loculated pleural effusions.

MRI—imaging of the mediastinum by CT scanning and MRI are comparable, but MR images of the lungs are currently markedly inferior to those obtained by CT because of their very low water (and therefore proton) content.

Introduction

Despite recent technological advances, chest radiography remains the cornerstone of thoracic imaging. The chest radiograph is justifiably regarded as an integral part of the examination of the patient in respiratory medicine. Because of the wealth of information available from chest radiography, careful interpretation of the chest radiograph remains a necessary clinical skill. Advances in cross-sectional imaging have had a great impact in improving the diagnosis of thoracic pathology, not only for the assessment of mediastinal disease but also in the evaluation of patients with suspected diffuse lung disease. Nevertheless, a chest radiograph should always be obtained and looked at carefully before submitting a patient to more sophisticated imaging techniques. In the case of CT the expense and radiation burden are important considerations.

Techniques in thoracic imaging

Chest radiography

The first chest radiograph was taken over 100 years ago and chest radiography is now the most frequently requested radiological investigation worldwide. The technique has changed surprisingly little over the years, although digital technology has recently been used to overcome some of the shortcomings of conventional film-based radiography.

Technical considerations

An ideal chest radiograph is taken with the patient standing erect, suspending respiration at total lung capacity and with the X-ray beam traversing the thorax from back to front (the posteroanterior (PA) or frontal view). Because of the wide range of densities within the chest (soft tissues of the mediastinum through to aerated lung), perfect exposure of every part of the chest radiograph is impossible. The resulting suboptimal exposure of the denser part of the chest can be partially overcome with a high kilovoltage technique (120 to 150 kVp). With this technique there is greater penetration of the mediastinum, which improves visualization of the trachea and main bronchi. However, a disadvantage of high-kilovoltage radiography is the relatively poor demonstration of calcified structures so that rib fractures and calcified pulmonary nodules or pleural plaques are less conspicuous. Even with optimal technique, nearly one-third of the lungs is partially obscured by the overlying mediastinum, diaphragm, and ribs.

Automatic exposure devices have been developed to expose optimally the various parts of the chest. One such is phosphor plate computed radiography which uses digital technology; this is ultimately expected to replace conventional film radiography and has already done so in most centres in resource-rich countries. A phosphor plate is handled in a conventional cassette (which does not contain film) and is exposed in the normal way. The energy of the incident X-ray beam is stored as a latent image. The phosphor plate is then scanned with a laser beam and the light emitted from the excited latent image is detected by a photomultiplier. Thereafter this signal is processed in digital form. The digital image may either be viewed on a television monitor or laser-printed on to film. The advantage of phosphor plate computed radiography is that it can retrieve an image of diagnostic quality from an imperfect exposure which would result in a nondiagnostic conventional film radiograph. Manipulation or post-processing of the digital image, e.g. 'edge enhancement', aids the detection of linear structures such as the edge of a pneumothorax or central venous catheters. With the advent of picture archiving and communication systems (PACS) that enable storage and transfer of digital images, many radiology departments are now 'filmless', with images available to view simultaneously on monitors throughout the hospital.

Standard radiographic views of the chest

The posteroanterior (PA) projection is the standard view (see Fig. 18.3.2.11a). The patient is positioned with the anterior chest wall against the film cassette and the arms are abducted to rotate the scapulae away from the posterior chest. Chest films in the anteroposterior (AP) projection are usually taken when the patient is too ill to stand for a formal PA radiograph. A consequence of this view is that the heart is magnified because it lies further from the film. Moreover, the shorter distance from X-ray tube to film, which is inevitable when a portable AP radiograph is taken, causes further magnification that must be taken into account when assessing the heart size on an AP chest radiograph.

The lateral radiograph is obtained by placing the patient at right angles to the film cassette. The lateral projection provides the third dimension and helps to determine the site of a lesion identified on the PA projection, although it is surprising how often an opacity clearly seen on the PA radiograph is invisible on the lateral radiograph. As well as allowing accurate localization of lesions, the lateral radiograph may reveal abnormalities that lie behind the heart or diaphragm.

Over the years a number of supplementary projections have been developed to provide information about areas that are not easily seen on the standard PA and lateral radiograph. With the advent of cross-sectional imaging, notably CT, many of these extra views have become obsolete. However, even with access to CT, some of these views supply extra anatomical detail readily and inexpensively. The lateral decubitus projection is sometimes useful for the demonstration of small pleural effusions, for which view the patient lies on their side (suspected effusion downwards). However, ultrasonography is increasingly being used as a reliable technique for demonstrating small pleural effusions. Other supplementary projections, e.g. apical and lordotic views, used to improve visualization of the lung at the extreme apices, are now less commonly performed: CT is much more effective at showing pathology in these difficult areas.

Ultrasonography

High-frequency sound waves do not traverse air and are completely reflected at interfaces between soft tissue and air. The use of this technique in the chest is therefore limited because of normally aerated lung. However, fluid can be readily detected, and the main use of ultrasound examination is for the localization of small or loculated pleural effusions (Fig. 18.3.2.1). Furthermore, ultrasonography can differentiate between pleural fluid and pleural thickening in cases where radiography cannot make this distinction.

Ultrasonography is also an extremely useful technique for guiding percutaneous needle biopsy of masses arising from the chest wall or pleura, or peripheral pulmonary masses or consolidation, and for aiding the accurate placement of a chest drain within a pleural collection.

CT

CT depends on the same basic principle as conventional radiography, namely the differential absorption of X-rays by tissues of disparate densities, although CT has much greater sensitivity to differences in attenuation of X-rays by various tissues. A CT machine consists of an X-ray source and an array of detectors that surround the patient. The X-ray source rotates around the patient and the resulting attenuated beam is measured by the detectors. The signals from the detectors are used to construct an image by a mathematical technique. The reconstructed images are transverse (axial) cross-sections of the patient and are viewed as if from the feet end of the patient (i.e. on the image, the patient's right side is to the viewer's left). Each CT section is a matrix of three-dimensional elements (voxels) containing a measurement of X-ray attenuation, arbitrarily expressed as Hounsfield units (HU): water measures 0 HU and air −1000 HU (so that lung parenchyma are approximately −600 HU), fat is 80 HU, soft tissue 40 to 80 HU and bone 800 HU. If a voxel is completely occupied by a tissue of uniform density (most frequently the case with narrow sections), then the HU will be truly representative of that tissue. If the section

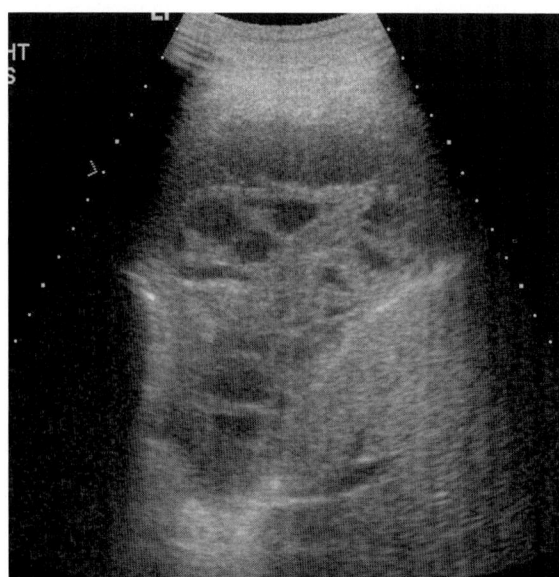

Fig. 18.3.2.1 Ultrasonography showing an empyema. Thick fibrinous septations traverse the pleural space. The diaphragm and liver are seen on the right of the image.

contains tissues of two different densities (more likely with thicker sections), e.g. half lung and half dome of diaphragm, then the attenuation value will be a weighted average of the two components—the so-called 'partial volume' effect.

The cross-sectional nature of CT means that it can accurately localize lesions seen on only one view on chest radiography. The superior contrast resolution of CT gives exquisite detail of the various components of mediastinal anatomy (e.g. lymph nodes and vessels) and density differences (e.g. calcifications within a pulmonary nodule). Different image settings are needed to view the soft tissue structures of the mediastinum and the aerated lung parenchyma respectively (Fig. 18.3.2.2).

Spiral (helical) CT

The principle of spiral CT involves continuous rotation of the X-ray beam and detectors around the patient while the table moves into the gantry. Markedly reduced scan times are possible with this technique, allowing the entire thorax to be imaged in a single breath-hold. An examination of sufficient diagnostic quality can be obtained in dyspnoeic patients and young children during quiet respiration. Another advance has been the development of multidetector CT (MDCT), where multiple rows of detectors rotate around the patient acquiring volumetric data, allowing even further reduced scan times—hence most modern helical CT scanners are also termed 'volumetric'.

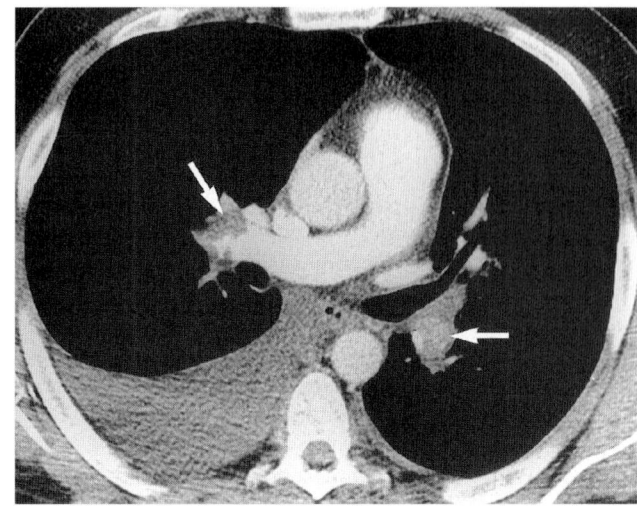

Fig. 18.3.2.3 CT of a patient with acute bilateral pulmonary emboli. Filling defects in contrast media opacification are seen within the right main pulmonary artery and the left interlobar pulmonary artery (arrows). Note the right-sided pleural effusion.

The technique allows accurate timing of an intravenous injection of contrast medium for optimum opacification e.g. of the pulmonary arteries, enabling pulmonary emboli to be detected (Fig. 18.3.2.3). In many centres spiral CT has supplanted ventilation/perfusion (*V/Q*) radionuclide imaging in the investigation of patients with suspected pulmonary embolism and, with optimum technique, accuracy approaches that of pulmonary arteriography for the diagnosis of central, lobar and segmental pulmonary emboli, although radiation dose and availability remain important considerations. The technique is most useful in patients with coexisting lung disease which would result in an inconclusive *V/Q* radionuclide study.

Computer software can perform multiplanar two- and three-dimensional image reconstructions of volumetric data sets, including views of the bronchial tree which can aid interventional techniques such as bronchial stent placement (Fig. 18.3.2.4). With the advent of MDCT and the use of ECG gating, evaluation of structures such

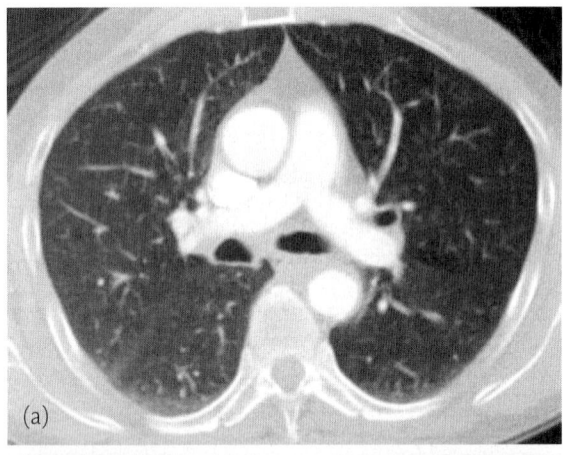

(a)

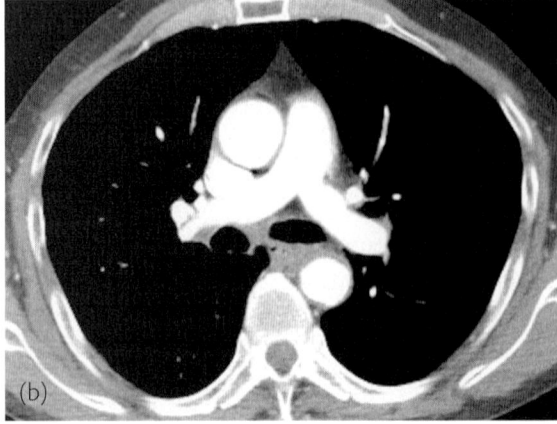

(b)

Fig. 18.3.2.2 CT section through the mid-thorax. The window settings have been adjusted to show details of (a) the lungs and (b) the soft tissues of the mediastinum.

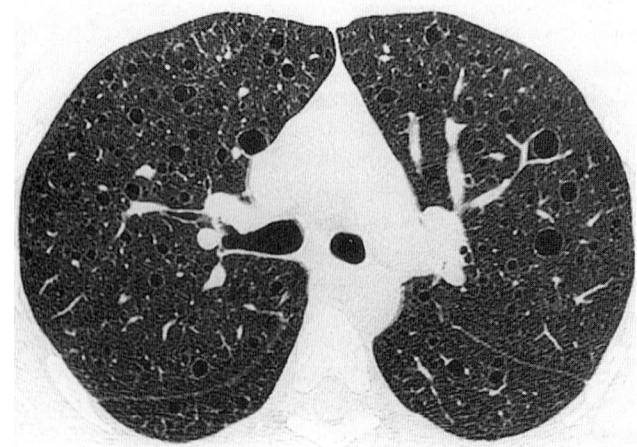

Fig. 18.3.2.4 High-resolution CT of a patient with lymphangioleiomyomatosis showing thin-walled cysts throughout the lungs. These cysts were not apparent on chest radiography.

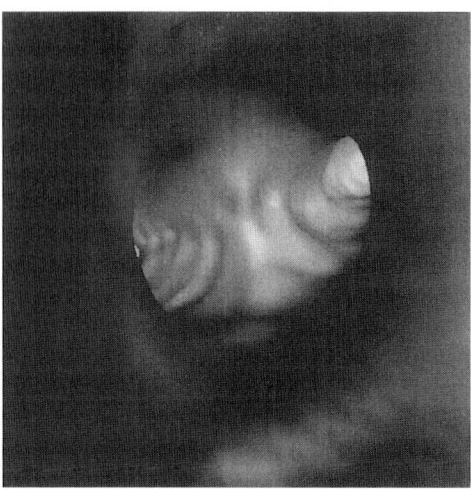

Fig. 18.3.2.5 Reconstructed three-dimensional image from spiral CT showing the carina and the right and left main bronchi viewed from above.

as coronary arteries is increasingly feasible due to reduction in motion artefact and increased spatial resolution.

High-resolution CT

High-resolution CT uses very thin sections (1–3 mm) and a high spatial frequency reconstruction algorithm to produce highly detailed sections of the lung parenchyma. Both conventional and spiral CT scanners can produce thin sections, and the terms 'spiral CT' and 'high-resolution CT' should not be confused. Submillimetre structures can be resolved with this technique, allowing the subtle and sometimes complex morphology of interstitial lung diseases to be shown with great clarity (Fig. 18.3.2.5). Since the mid 1980s the development of high-resolution CT has changed the radiological approach to the diagnosis of diffuse lung disease. High-resolution CT images of the lung correlate closely with the macroscopic appearances of pathological specimens, and high-resolution CT represents a substantial improvement over chest radiography in terms of sensitivity, specificity, and diagnostic accuracy. Furthermore, CT samples a far greater volume of lung than even the most generous lung biopsy, making it less prone to sampling errors.

High-resolution CT has also been shown to provide useful information regarding prognosis and response to treatment in some diffuse lung diseases. Nevertheless, despite the increased confidence with which a specific diagnosis of diffuse lung disease can be made with high-resolution CT, open lung biopsy is still required to achieve a definitive histological diagnosis in difficult cases. The extent of diffuse lung disease can be precisely estimated on high-resolution CT and, when a biopsy is indicated, the distribution of disease will indicate whether a transbronchial biopsy or an open lung biopsy is more likely to obtain a representative specimen.

The disadvantages of CT are its relatively high cost and high radiation exposure to the patient, particularly in comparison with chest radiography. For these reasons, CT should not be regarded as a routine investigation and examinations should always be tailored to solve questions not answered by less sophisticated investigations. The commonest indications for thoracic CT are summarized in Box 18.3.2.1.

MRI

The physical principles of MRI are very different from those governing CT. An MR image is obtained by placing the subject in a strong magnetic field that polarizes some of the ubiquitous hydrogen protons (which can be thought of as behaving like randomly orientated bar magnets) in the body so that they have the same alignment. The application of radio-frequency wave pulses of specified lengths and repetition (pulse sequences) displaces the protons and some of this transmitted energy is absorbed by them. With the cessation of the radio-frequency pulse, the protons return to their initial alignment and in so doing they emit, as a weak signal, some of the energy they have absorbed; this signal is received and then amplified and handled in digital form and is subsequently reconstructed into an image.

The advantages of MRI include the improved contrast resolution between different soft tissues compared with CT (Fig. 18.3.2.6), and the use of special sequences which give functional information, e.g. the velocity of blood flow. An important advantage of MRI is the lack of any known hazard to the patient, in contrast to CT with its small attendant risk from ionizing radiation. Disadvantages of MRI include the long scan time (although this is continually being shortened), reduced spatial resolution compared with CT, the inability to image calcium, reduced acceptability to patients because of the claustrophobic bore of the magnet, and important contraindications such as permanent cardiac pacemaker devices and ferromagnetic intraocular foreign bodies.

In many respects the imaging of the mediastinum by CT and MRI are comparable. However, MR images of the lungs are currently markedly inferior to CT because of their very low water (and therefore proton) content, meaning that the signal produced by normal lung is small and not visualized by conventional sequences. However, the relatively recent introduction of hyperpolarized gases, including helium-3, has enabled evaluation of pulmonary function; the use of such agents by inhalation is largely still a research tool, but may provide valuable insights into pulmonary ventilation and small airways function in the future.

Radionuclide imaging

V/Q radionuclide scanning is an effective noninvasive method of providing both anatomical and physiological information about

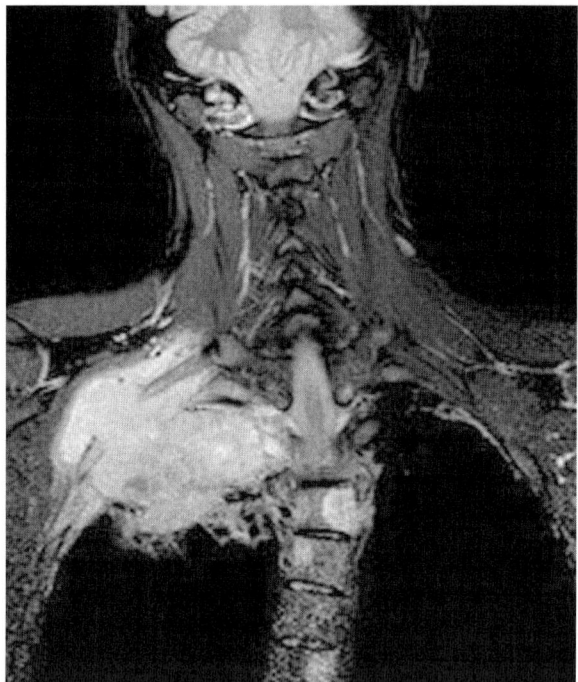

Fig. 18.3.2.6 MRI (T_2-weighted coronal section) showing the relationship of an apical bronchial carcinoma (Pancoast tumour) to the chest wall and adjacent mediastinum. Note the multiple high signal (bright) areas within the vertebral bodies consistent with bony metastases.

the lung. It is the commonest radionuclide study of the lungs and is most frequently used to confirm or exclude the diagnosis of suspected pulmonary embolism.

Regional pulmonary capillary perfusion can be assessed following the intravenous injection of a bolus of particles that have been labelled with technetium-99m. The minute particles are microspheres or macroaggregates of human albumin (15–70 μm in diameter). These particles are evenly dispersed by the time they reach the pulmonary circulation and they become temporarily lodged in a very small fraction (<0.5%) of the precapillary arterioles and capillaries of the lungs. There is a small theoretical risk of compromising the pulmonary vascular bed in patients with severe pulmonary hypertension, although this is not an absolute contraindication to the examination. The distribution of γ-ray emission from the technetium-labelled particles is directly proportional to the regional pulmonary flow and a significant defect in perfusion is usually readily detected. However, it is important to appreciate that such defects may be due to a variety of conditions other than pulmonary embolism, including any cause of hypoxic vasoconstriction such as an area of subsegmental collapse or a space-occupying lesion not supplied by the pulmonary circulation. However, in these cases the affected area of lung will be neither ventilated nor perfused, whereas in acute pulmonary embolism there is no corresponding defect of ventilation. Thus, to improve the specificity of the diagnosis of pulmonary embolism, ventilation scintigraphy is usually performed at the same time as perfusion scanning.

Evaluation of ventilation of the lungs depends on filling the distal air spaces with a γ-ray-emitting radionuclide. The radionuclides suitable for inhalation are the inert gases xenon-133 and krypton-81m, or a technetium-99m aerosol (Technegas). Although krypton-81m gives the highest-quality images, Technegas is being increasingly

used because of its ready availability. The characteristic abnormality of pulmonary embolism is the so-called 'mismatched defect' in which a regional defect in perfusion is not matched by a defect in ventilation (Fig. 18.3.2.7a, b). However, the picture in pulmonary embolism may not always be clear-cut, particularly when pulmonary infarction has occurred, at which time there will be a matched defect of both ventilation and perfusion.

Because of the importance of establishing a correct diagnosis of pulmonary embolism, *V/Q* scans should always be interpreted in the light of current chest radiographs and clinical information. Even then a proportion of *V/Q* scans remain indeterminate, hence the increasing use of CT angiography. However, due to the decreased radiation burden, *V/Q* scanning remains a reasonable first-line investigation in young patients with no pre-existing lung disease and a low pretest probability for pulmonary embolism.

Positron emission tomography

Positron emission tomography (PET) relies on tissue uptake of radio-isotopes that decay by positron emission. Detectors located around the patient map the site of origin of the two resultant photons emitted at 180° from each other. The most widely used isotope for the detection of pulmonary malignancy is ^{18}F-fluoro-deoxyglucose (FDG), a D-glucose analogue. The increased uptake

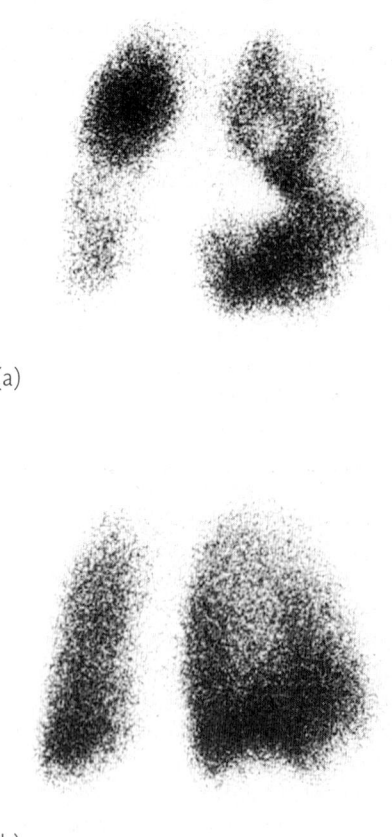

(a)

(b)

Fig. 18.3.2.7 A *V/Q* radionuclide study (oblique views). The perfusion scan (a) shows a defect in the left mid-zone which is not matched on the corresponding view of the ventilation scan (b). The so-called mismatched defect is characteristic of a pulmonary embolus.

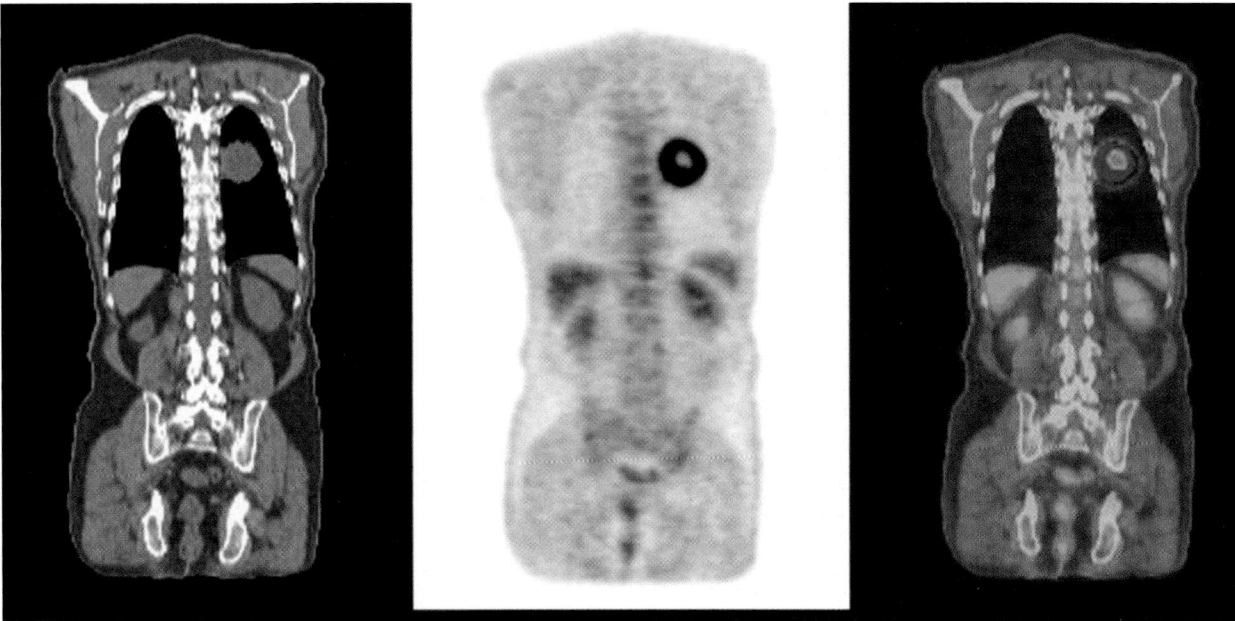

Fig. 18.3.2.8 CT/PET image showing increased uptake of ^{18}F-fluorodeoxyglucose (FDG) in the left lung corresponding to a primary bronchial carcinoma. The image on the left is the coronal MDCT image, the central image is the coronal PET, and the image on the right is the coregistered CT/PET. Note the central necrosis resulting in central photopenia, also the physiological uptake of tracer in the liver, spleen, kidneys, and bladder.
(Courtesy of Dr Z Win, Hammersmith Hospital, London.)

and retention of glucose by malignant cells allows differentiation of benign from malignant pulmonary masses, detection of lymph node involvement by tumour, and identification of distant metastases. Limitations of the technique include false positive results caused by granulomatous infection and acute inflammation, and false-negative results with certain tumours (e.g. bronchioloalveolar carcinomas and carcinoid tumours). Small (<1 cm diameter) malignant lesions may also give false negative results.

CT/PET is a more recent development where a helical CT is performed simultaneously with PET and the images then coregistered (Fig. 18.3.2.8). The fusion of CT images (which give good anatomical resolution) with PET images (which provide functional data) may be an advantage in the staging of thoracic malignancies including lung carcinoma and mesothelioma.

Pulmonary and bronchial arteriography; superior vena cavography

The 'gold standard' for identifying emboli within the pulmonary arteries has traditionally been pulmonary arteriography (Fig. 18.3.2.9), which requires the catheterization of an antecubital, jugular, or femoral vein and guidance of the catheter through the right heart under fluoroscopic control. Although the complication rate is low, it is a time-consuming procedure that requires an experienced angiographer. The technique allows embolization of pulmonary arteriovenous malformations with multiple metallic coils—a specialized technique available in certain centres.

The bronchial arteries that supply the airways become hypertrophied in chronic inflammatory pulmonary disease, notably bronchiectasis. Rupture of these vessels can cause severe and life-threatening haemoptysis. The bronchial arteries are selectively catheterized by the passage of a catheter via the femoral artery and aorta. Having identified the abnormally hypertrophied bronchial arteries (Fig. 18.3.2.10), they can be therapeutically embolized. This technique is usually successful in abating a massive haemoptysis in patients not able to undergo immediate surgical treatment.

Superior vena cavography is usually performed to evaluate the exact site of narrowing in patients with symptoms of obstruction of the superior vena cava; it is not generally required to confirm the diagnosis, which is usually evident from the clinical signs alone. Patients with symptoms of superior vena cava obstruction—most frequently due to neoplastic involvement of mediastinal lymph nodes—may be successfully palliated by radiotherapy or the insertion of an expandable metallic wire stent at the site of the narrowing.

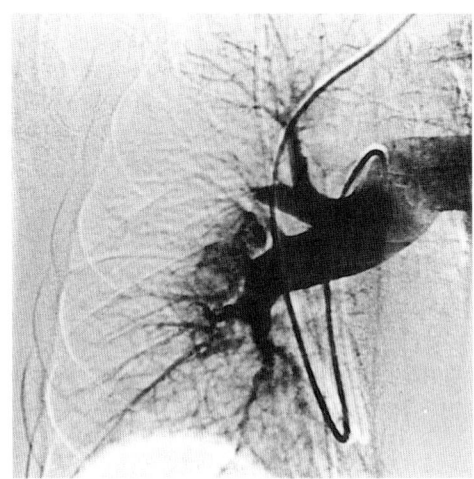

Fig. 18.3.2.9 A digital subtraction pulmonary arteriogram showing abrupt termination of the vessels supplying the right upper lobe caused by a pulmonary embolus.

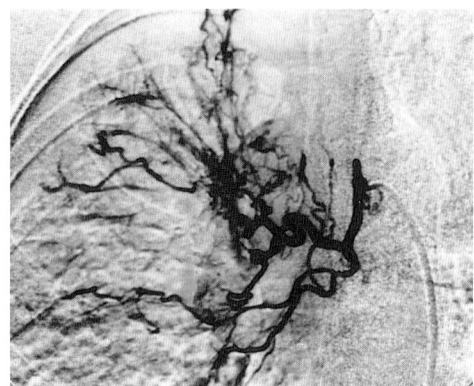

Fig. 18.3.2.10 Abnormally hypertrophied bronchial arteries supplying the right upper lobe shown on a selective digital subtraction bronchial arteriogram. The patient had cystic fibrosis and had had a massive haemoptysis; these bronchial arteries were subsequently embolized.

Percutaneous lung biopsy

Percutaneous needle biopsy of a pulmonary lesion or mediastinal mass is usually performed in patients in whom a bronchoscopic biopsy has failed to produce a histological specimen or if a thoracotomy to resect the lesion is deemed inappropriate. It should not be regarded as a routine procedure in the investigation of all solitary pulmonary nodules and should only be performed after considering the risks to the patient and whether the information forthcoming from the procedure will direct management.

Many different types of needles have been developed and the frequency of complications, mainly pneumothorax and haemoptysis, is in part related to the diameter of the needle and the depth of the lesion. Percutaneous biopsy is performed under local anaesthesia with either CT or ultrasound guidance if the mass abuts the pleura. Contraindications to the procedure include any patient with poor respiratory reserve who is unable to withstand a pneumothorax and pulmonary arterial hypertension.

Radiofrequency ablation

Radiofrequency ablation, which employs a small electrode that produces radio-frequency waves, is a relatively new technique usually performed under CT guidance to treat either primary or secondary lung tumours using thermal energy. The common indications are small primary lung tumours in a patient too unwell to undergo thoracotomy, debulking of large primary tumours, and treatment of small numbers of pulmonary metastases. Complications are similar to those of percutaneous lung biopsy.

Normal radiographic anatomy

The mediastinum

On a PA chest radiograph (see Fig. 18.3.2.11a) the mediastinal structures are superimposed on one another and thus cannot be distinguished individually. The mediastinum is conventionally divided into superior, anterior, middle and posterior compartments: the practical use of these arbitrary divisions is that specific mediastinal pathologies show a definite predilection for individual compartments (e.g. a superior mediastinal mass is most frequently due to intrathoracic extension of the thyroid gland, a middle mediastinal mass is usually due to enlarged lymph nodes). However, it

should be borne in mind that the position of a mass within one of these compartments is no guarantee of a specific diagnosis, nor do these boundaries preclude disease from spreading from one compartment to the next.

Because only the outline of the mediastinum and the air-containing trachea and bronchi are clearly seen on a PA chest radiograph, the mediastinal anatomy will be considered in more detail in the description of CT anatomy. On a chest radiograph, the right superior mediastinal border is formed by the right brachiocephalic vein and superior vena cava. The mediastinal border to the left of the trachea above the aortic arch represents the sum of the left carotid and left subclavian arteries together with the left brachiocephalic and jugular veins. The left cardiac border comprises the left atrial

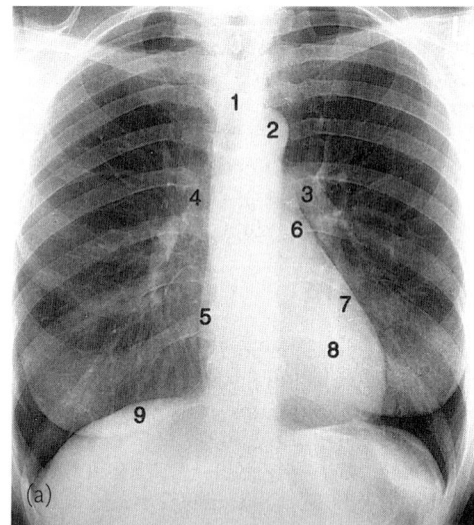

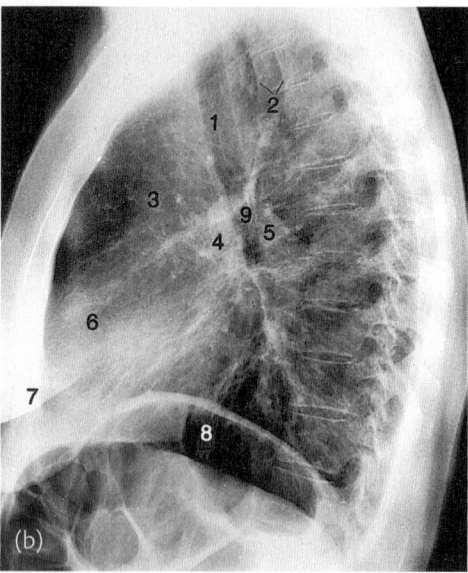

Fig. 18.3.2.11 Normal radiographic anatomy on (a) pa and (b) lateral chest radiographs. (a) 1, trachea; 2, aortic arch; 3, left main pulmonary artery; 4, right main pulmonary artery; 5, right atrial border; 6, left atrial appendage; 7, left ventricular border; 8, right ventricle; 9, right dome of diaphragm; 10, costophrenic angle; 11, breast shadow. (b) 1, trachea; 2, scapulae; 3, anterior aortic arch; 4, right pulmonary artery; 5, left pulmonary artery; 6, right ventricle; 7, breast shadows; 8, gastric bubble under the left hemidiaphragm; 9, left main bronchus.

appendage which merges inferiorly with the left ventricle. The cardiac silhouette is always sharply outlined: any blurring of the border denotes replacement of the aerated lung, usually by collapse or consolidation, in the immediately adjacent lung (see 'Silhouette sign' in 'Common radiological signs of disease').

The density of the cardiac shadow to the left and right of the vertebral column should be identical and any difference signals pulmonary pathology (e.g. consolidation in a lower lobe). A density with a convex lateral border is often seen through the right heart border on a well-penetrated film: this apparent mass is due to the confluence of the pulmonary veins as it enters the left atrium and is of no pathological significance.

The trachea and main bronchi are visible through the upper and middle mediastinum. The trachea is rarely straight and is often to the right of the mid-line at its mid-point. In elderly patients, the trachea may appear dramatically displaced by a dilated aortic arch. The angle of the carina is usually somewhat less than 80°. Splaying of the carina is a sign of gross disease, either in the form of massive subcarinal lymphadenopathy, or a markedly enlarged left atrium. A more sensitive sign of a subcarinal mass is obliteration of the azygo-oesophageal line which is usually visible on a well-penetrated chest radiograph. The origins of the lobar bronchi, where they are projected over the mediastinal shadow, can usually be made out but the segmental bronchi within the lungs are not generally seen on plain radiography.

The hilar structures

The hilar shadows on a chest radiograph are a complex summation of the pulmonary arteries and veins with virtually no contribution from the overlying bronchial walls or normal-sized lymph nodes. The hila are approximately the same size and the left hilum always lies between 0.5 cm and 1.5 cm above the level of the right hilum. The size and shape of the hila in normal individuals show remarkable variation so that subtle abnormalities are difficult to detect. At least as important as an abnormal contour in detecting a mass at the hilum, is a discrepancy in density between the two hila: both hilar shadows, at equivalent points, will be of equal density and a mass at the hilum (or an intrapulmonary mass projected over the hilum) will be evident as increased density of that hilum.

The pulmonary fissures, vessels, and bronchi

The lobes of each lung are surrounded by visceral pleura: the upper and lower lobes of the left lung are separated by the major (or oblique) fissure. The upper, middle, and lower lobes of the right lung are separated by the major (or oblique) and minor (horizontal or transverse) fissures. The minor fissure is visible in about 60% of normal PA chest radiographs. In normal individuals, this fissure runs horizontally and any deviation from this course represents loss of volume of a lobe. The major fissures are inconstantly identifiable on lateral radiographs. Other fissures are occasionally seen; e.g. in the left lung a minor fissure can occur which separates the lingula from the remainder of the upper lobe.

All of the branching structures seen within the lungs on a chest radiograph represent either pulmonary arteries or veins. The larger pulmonary vessels can be traced back to the hila and mediastinum. The pulmonary veins can sometimes be differentiated from the pulmonary arteries: the superior pulmonary veins have a distinctly vertical course, but in practice it is often impossible to distinguish arteries from veins in the outer two-thirds of the lung. On a chest radiograph taken in the erect position, there is a gradual increase in the diameter of the vessels, at equidistant points from the hilum, travelling from lung apex to base; this is a gravity-dependent effect and is abolished if the patient is supine or in cardiac failure.

The lobes of the lung are divided into segments, each of which is supplied by its own segmental bronchi. The walls of the segmental bronchi are rarely seen on the chest radiograph, except when lying parallel with the X-ray beam, when they are seen end-on as ring shadows measuring up to 8 mm in diameter.

The diaphragm and thoracic cage

The interface between aerated lung and the domes of the diaphragm is sharp and in general the highest point of each dome is medial to the midclavicular line. The right dome of the diaphragm is higher than the left by up to 2 cm in the erect position unless the left dome is temporarily elevated by air in the stomach. Laterally, the diaphragm dips steeply downwards to form an acute angle with the chest wall. Filling in or blunting of these costophrenic angles usually represents pleural disease, either pleural thickening or an effusion.

Localized humps on the dome of the diaphragm are common and represent minor weaknesses or defects of the diaphragm. Similarly, interposition of the colon in front of the right lobe of the liver is a frequently seen normal variant.

Deformities of the thoracic cage may cause distortion of the normal mediastinum and so simulate disease. One of the commonest deformities is pectus excavatum which, by compressing the heart between the depressed sternum and vertebral column, causes displacement of the apparently enlarged heart to the left and causes blurring of the right heart border.

High-kilovoltage chest radiographs often allow the vertebral bodies to be seen through the cardiac shadow. However, with this technique the ribs, and particularly their posterior parts, are often rendered invisible.

Anatomy on the lateral chest radiograph

It is useful to become accustomed to viewing a lateral film (Fig. 18.3.2.11b) in the same orientation, whether it is a right or left lateral projection. Familiarity with the same orientation improves the viewer's ability to detect deviations from normal.

The trachea is angled slightly posteriorly as it runs towards the carina, and the posterior wall of the trachea is always visible as a fine stripe. Furthermore, the posterior walls of the right main bronchus and the right intermediate bronchus are outlined by air and are also seen as a continuous stripe on the lateral radiograph. The spines of the scapulae are invariably seen running almost vertically in the upper part of the lateral radiograph and they should not be confused with intrathoracic structures. Further spurious shadows are formed by the soft tissues of the outstretched arms which are projected over the anterior and superior mediastinum. Although the carina is not visible on the lateral radiograph, the two transradiancies projected over the lower trachea represent the right main bronchus (superiorly) and the left main bronchus (inferiorly).

More lung is obscured by overlying structures on a lateral radiograph than on the PA view. The unobscured lung in the retrosternal and retrocardiac regions should be of the same transradiancy. Furthermore, as the eye travels down the dorsal spine, the viewer should be aware of a gradual increase in transradiancy. The loss of this phenomenon suggests the presence of disease in the posterobasal segments of the lower lobes (sometimes not visible on the frontal radiograph).

The two major fissures are seen as diagonal lines, often incomplete and of hair's breadth, running from the upper dorsal spine to the anterior surface of the diaphragm. Care must be taken not to confuse the obliquely running edges of ribs with fissures. The minor fissure extends horizontally from the mid-right major fissure. It is often not possible to distinguish the right from the left major fissures with confidence. Similarly, although the two hemidiaphragms may be identified individually (especially if the gastric bubble is visible under the left dome of the diaphragm), the distinction between the right and the left is often not possible. A helpful sign is the relative heights of the two domes: the dome furthest from the film is usually higher because of magnification.

The summation of both hila on the lateral radiograph generates a complex shadow. However, there are some generalizations which aid the interpretation of this difficult area. The right pulmonary artery lies anterior to the trachea and right main bronchus, whereas the left pulmonary artery hooks over the left main bronchus so that a large part of it lies posterior to the major bronchi. As a result, any mass identified on a PA and lateral radiograph that lies anterior to the left hilum or posterior to the right hilum is not vascular in origin and is most likely to represent enlarged hilar lymph nodes.

A band-like opacity is often seen along the lower third of the anterior chest wall behind the sternum. This represents a normal density and occurs because there is less aerated lung in contact with the chest wall because the space is occupied by the heart; it should not be confused with pleural disease.

Normal CT anatomy of the mediastinum

CT provides unique information about the anatomy of the mediastinum and is often used to provide further information about abnormalities which are seen merely as a deformity of the mediastinal contour on chest radiography. The normal structures that are always identified on a CT of the mediastinum are the blood vessels (which make up the bulk of the superior mediastinum), the major airways, the oesophagus and mediastinal fat. An appreciation of the relationship of these structures to each other is crucial for the correct interpretation of CT scans; four important levels are shown in Fig. 18.3.2.12.

Normal lymph nodes surrounded by fat may be identified throughout the mediastinum. Many schemes have been devised to map their precise locations but they can be broadly divided into (1) anterior mediastinal, (2) posterior mediastinal, and (3) tracheobronchial. The tracheobronchial can be further subdivided into the following regions: (1) right and left paratracheal, (2) subaortic, (3) pretracheal, and (4) subcarinal. It is important to appreciate that the absolute size of lymph nodes identified on CT (or by direct inspection at mediastinoscopy) should not be regarded as a foolproof criterion for significant disease, particularly in the context of lung cancer. Although markedly enlarged lymph nodes (>2 cm diameter) almost invariably signify important pathology, moderate enlargement of mediastinal lymph nodes may represent reactive hyperplasia of little clinical significance. Conversely, small volume lymph nodes or lymph nodes not identified by CT may sometimes contain micrometastases from a distant primary neoplasm.

The thymus gland occupies a large part of the anterior mediastinum in children. In adult life the remnants of the normal thymus are normally inconspicuous on CT.

Points in the interpretation of a chest radiograph

Even when there is an obvious radiographic abnormality, there is much to recommend a careful and systematic method in reviewing a chest radiograph. Such an approach will allow an appreciation of normal variations of anatomy to be built up with time. With increasing experience, an appreciation of deviation from normal appearances becomes more rapid and this leads quickly to a directed search for related abnormalities.

Before interpreting a chest radiograph, it is vital to establish whether there are any previous radiographs for comparison: the sequence and pattern of change is often as important as the identification of a radiographic abnormality. Information gained from preceding radiographs, particularly the lack of serial change, will often prevent needless further investigation. Demographic details, particularly the age and racial origin of the patient, should be noted since this information may increase the probability of a differential diagnosis which is based on the radiographic findings alone.

A quick check that the radiograph is of satisfactory quality includes an estimation of the radiographic exposure, depth of inspiration, and position of the patient. As a general rule, the intervertebral disc spaces of the entire dorsal spine should be visible on a correctly exposed radiograph; the midpoint of the right hemidiaphragm lies at the level of the anterior end of the sixth rib if the patient has taken a satisfactory breath in. The patient is axially rotated if the medial ends of the clavicles are not equidistant from the spinous process of the thoracic vertebral body at that level.

The order in which the structures on a chest radiograph are analysed is unimportant. A suggested sequence is to start with a scrutiny of the position of the trachea, of the mediastinal contour (which should be sharply outlined in its entirety), and then the position, outline, and density of the hilar shadows. Only then are the lungs examined, taking into account their size, the relative transradiancy of each zone, and the position of the horizontal fissure (and any other indirect signs of volume loss—see later section on lobar collapse). Pulmonary vessels are seen as far as the outer third of the lung and the number of vessels should be roughly symmetrical on the two sides. Next, the position and clarity of the hemidiaphragms should be noted, followed by an assessment of the ribs and soft tissues of the chest wall. Special care should be taken to look for pleural thickening along the lateral chest walls which may be easily overlooked.

Before saying that a chest radiograph is normal, it is worth reviewing areas that are either poorly demonstrated on chest radiography or often misinterpreted. These include: (1) the central mediastinum, where even a large mass may be barely visible on the PA view; (2) the areas behind the heart and hemidiaphragms; (3) the lung apices, often obscured by overlying clavicle and ribs; and (4) the lung and pleura just inside the chest wall.

Once a radiographic abnormality has been detected it should be considered in terms of gross pathology. Both the site and the radiographic characteristics of the lesion will allow the observer to produce, at the very least, a generic diagnosis. A precise (histopathological) diagnosis can only rarely be achieved from the

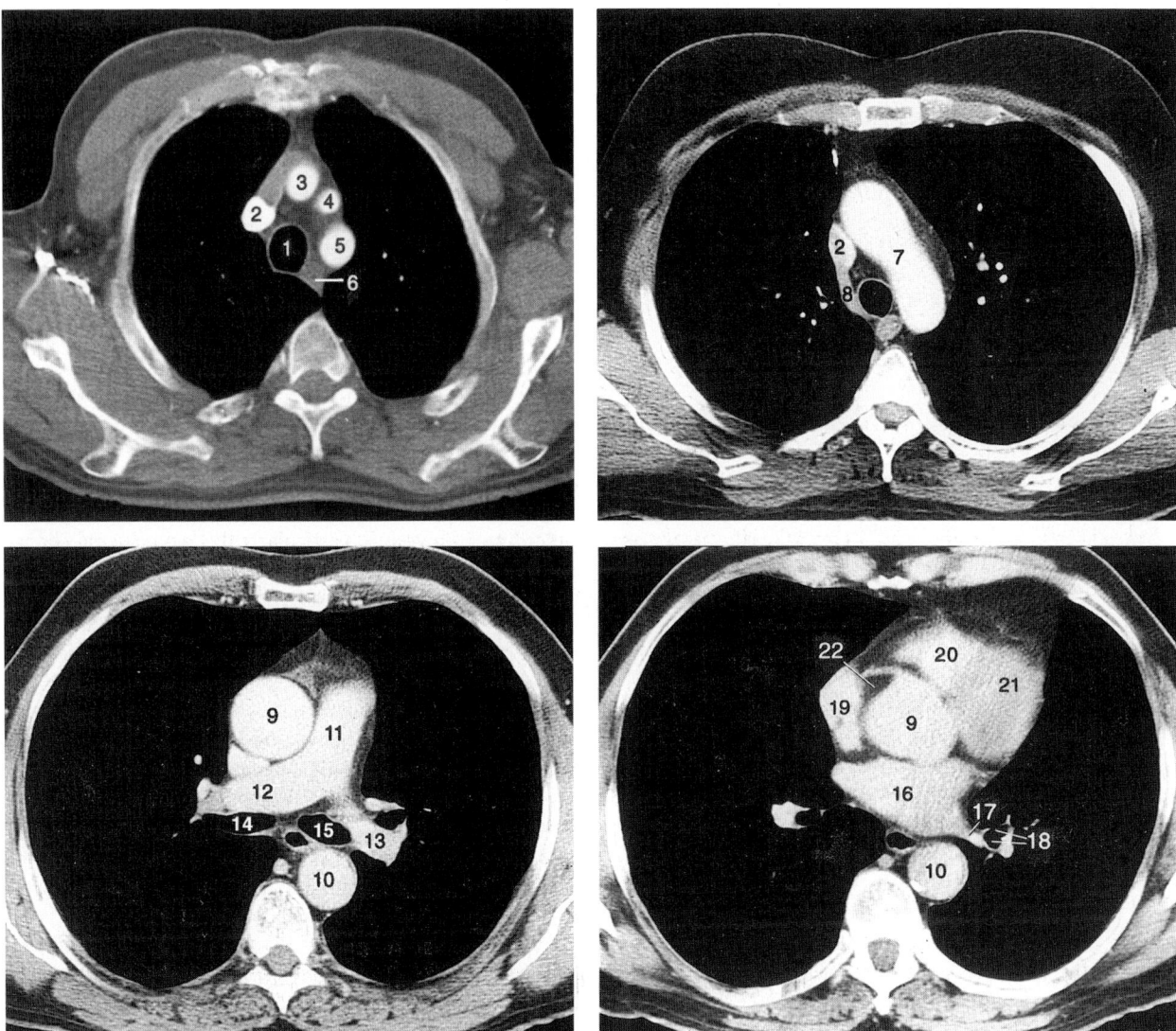

Fig. 18.3.2.12 CT with contrast enhancement to show the normal anatomy at four levels through the mediastinum. 1, trachea; 2, superior vena cava; 3, brachiocephalic artery; 4, left common carotid artery; 5, left subclavian artery; 6, oesophagus; 7, aortic arch; 8, azygos vein; 9, ascending aorta; 10, descending aorta; 11, main pulmonary artery; 12, right pulmonary artery; 13, left pulmonary artery; 14, right main bronchus; 15, left main bronchus; 16, left atrium; 17, left inferior pulmonary vein; 18, segmental bronchi of the left lower lobe; 19, right atrium; 20, right ventricular outflow; 21, left ventricle.

radiographic appearances alone without knowledge of the clinical context.

Common radiological signs of disease

Pulmonary consolidation

Consolidation is a pathological description of the state of the lungs when the normal air-filled spaces, distal to the bronchi, are occupied by the products of disease (e.g. water, pus, or blood). The most important radiographic signs of pulmonary consolidation are: (1) an area of increased opacification in the lungs which obscures the underlying blood vessels and has a poorly defined margin—unless it is bounded by a fissure; (2) an 'air bronchogram'; and (3) the 'silhouette sign' (Fig. 18.3.2.13). The air bronchogram is a distinctive and certain sign of intrapulmonary pathology and is seen as a radiolucent (grey) branching structure of the bronchi against a more opaque (white) background of airless lung. Although an air bronchogram is seen almost invariably in consolidation, lung which has become collapsed and airless—e.g. due to a large surrounding pleural effusion— may also show an air bronchogram. The silhouette sign is seen when the normally clear border of a structure is lost because the air-filled lung outlining the border is replaced by fluid or a mass. Recognition of this sign can help to localize the area of abnormality within the lungs; e.g. consolidation in the lingula will make the left heart border indistinct. As with the air bronchogram sign, the silhouette sign may be seen in either pulmonary consolidation or collapse—e.g. loss of a clear right heart border may be due to right middle lobe consolidation with or without lobar collapse; the common feature is loss of normal aeration of the affected lung. The causes of widespread pulmonary consolidation are numerous but may be broadly divided into five categories, as shown in Table 18.3.2.1.

Pulmonary collapse

This is the term used to describe loss of aeration and therefore inflation in part or all of a lung. Depending on the cause, collapse

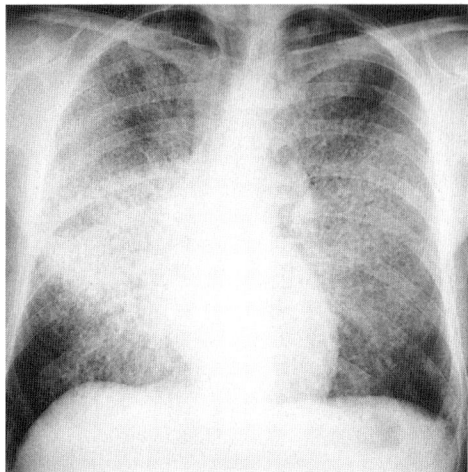

Fig. 18.3.2.13 Widespread pulmonary consolidation in a patient with alveolar proteinosis. The right heart border is obscured confirming that a large part of the consolidation is in the right middle lobe (the silhouette sign).

may occur at any level from small, subsegmental areas of lung through to an entire lung. Small areas of subsegmental collapse occur very commonly in debilitated and postoperative patients, where they are seen as linear, usually horizontal, opacities. At the other end of the spectrum, collapse of an entire lung, usually due to an endobronchial lesion or inhaled foreign body, has a dramatic radiographic appearance with complete opacification of the affected lung and loss of volume of that hemithorax. At the lobar level, the signs of collapse of an individual lobe are characteristic,

Table 18.3.2.1 Causes of widespread pulmonary consolidation

Pulmonary oedema	Cardiogenic/fluid overload
	Acute respiratory distress syndrome
	Inhalational injury (noxious gases)
	Drug abuse
	Neurogenic (raised intracranial pressure or head injury)
	Renal disease
	Traumatic (fat embolism)
Exudate	Infective consolidation
	Eosinophilic lung disease
	Collagen vascular disease
	Cryptogenic organizing pneumonia
	Radiation pneumonitis
Neoplasm	Bronchioloalveolar cell carcinoma
	Lymphoproliferative disorders
Blood	Contusion
	Infarction
	Idiopathic pulmonary haemorrhage (Goodpasture's syndrome)
Other	Alveolar proteinosis
	Sarcoidosis

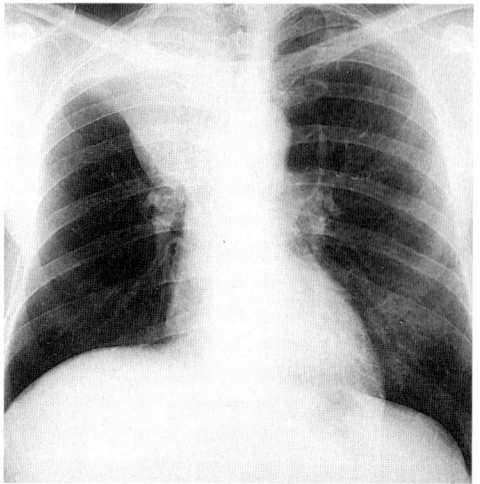

Fig. 18.3.2.14 Right upper lobe collapse.

but depending on the lobe, may be very subtle. Recognition of the collapse of individual lobes is important and these are described in detail.

Collapse of individual lobes
Right upper lobe
On the frontal radiograph there is elevation of the minor fissure and of the right hilum. If the collapse is complete the nonaerated lobe is seen as a density alongside the superior mediastinum (Fig. 18.3.2.14). On the lateral view the minor fissure moves upwards and the major fissure moves forwards. The retrosternal area becomes progressively more opaque and the anterior margin of the ascending aorta becomes obscured.

Right middle lobe
On the frontal radiograph the lateral part of the minor fissure moves down. There is blurring of the normally sharp right heart border and this may be a subtle abnormality which is easily overlooked (Fig. 18.3.2.15). On the lateral view, the minor fissure moves downwards and lower half of the major fissure moves forwards giving rise to a triangular shadow with its apex at the hilum and the base behind the lower sternum.

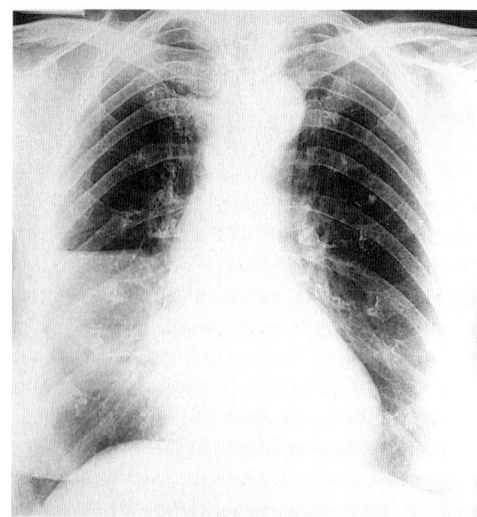

Fig. 18.3.2.15 Right middle lobe collapse.

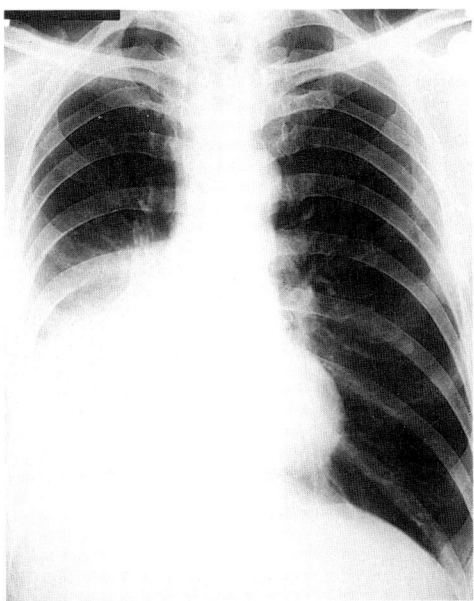

Fig. 18.3.2.16 Right lower lobe collapse.

Right lower lobe

There is an increase in density overlying and obscuring the medial portion of the right hemidiaphragm, and the right hilum is displaced inferiorly on the frontal radiograph (Fig. 18.3.2.16). In contrast to right middle lobe collapse, the right heart border usually remains sharply defined since this is in contact with the aerated right middle lobe. On the lateral view the major fissure moves backwards and downwards; with increasing collapse there is a loss of definition of the posterior part of the right hemidiaphragm as well as increased density overlying the lower dorsal vertebral column.

Left upper lobe

The main finding on the frontal radiograph is a veil-like increase in density, without a sharp margin (quite unlike right upper lobe collapse), spreading outwards and upwards from the elevated left hilum (Fig. 18.3.2.17). The outlines of the aortic knuckle, left hilum and left heart border become ill defined. As the collapse increases, the lobe moves centrally and the apical segment of the left lower lobe expands to fill the space left by the collapsed upper lobe—this is the cause of the relatively transradiant lung apex. With complete left upper lobe collapse, a sharp border may return to the aortic arch because it is surrounded by the hyperinflated apical segment of the lower lobe. On the lateral view the major fissure moves superiorly and anteriorly while remaining relatively vertical and roughly parallel to the anterior chest wall.

Left lower lobe

On the frontal radiograph there is a triangular density behind the heart with loss of the medial part of the left hemidiaphragm (Fig. 18.3.2.18), but even on a properly exposed radiograph it may be difficult to appreciate the collapsed lobe. Supplementary signs include inferior displacement of the left hilum, loss of volume and increased transradiancy of the left hemithorax. On the lateral view there is posterior displacement of the major fissure. As with right lower lobe collapse, there is increased density over the lower dorsal vertebral column and the posterior part of the left hemidiaphragm is effaced.

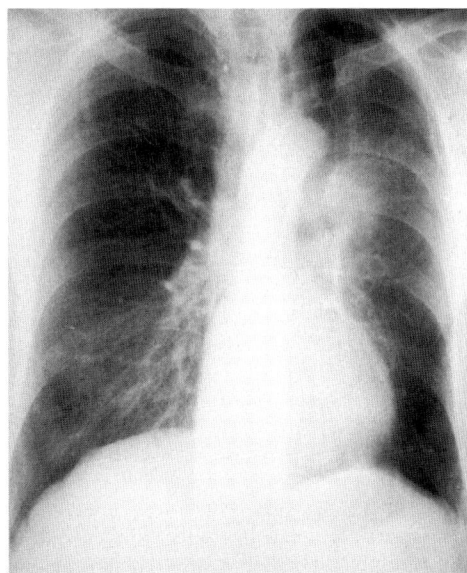

Fig. 18.3.2.17 Left upper lobe collapse.

Complete opacification (a 'white-out') of a hemithorax is generally due to either collapse of a lung or a large pleural effusion or tumour. Shift of the mediastinum to the affected side implies that volume loss, i.e. collapse of the lung, has occurred. In contrast, a pleural effusion or soft tissue mass which is large enough to cause complete opacification of a hemithorax will almost invariably displace the mediastinum away from the side of the opacified hemithorax. An important exception is an advanced mesothelioma which may encase one lung and 'freeze' the mediastinum and prevent contralateral mediastinal shift. Occasionally, when there is no obvious shift of the mediastinum, it is surprisingly difficult to differentiate between these two completely different causes of an opacified hemithorax. In these instances, ultrasonography and CT allow the distinction to be made with confidence and may give further information about the underlying disease.

Increased transradiancy of a hemithorax

There are many causes of increased transradiancy (darkening) of one lung. These may range from a loss of soft tissues of the chest wall (e.g. a mastectomy) through to reduced perfusion of one lung due to hypoxic vasoconstriction resulting from underventilation of

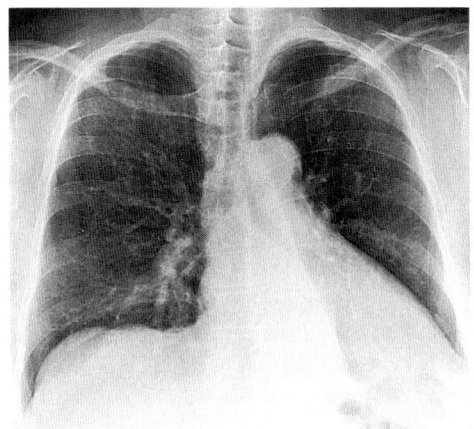

Fig. 18.3.2.18 Left lower lobe collapse.

Table 18.3.2.2 Causes of increased transradiancy of one hemithorax

Technical	Rotation of the patient
Chest wall	Loss of soft tissues, most commonly due to a mastectomy
Pneumothorax	Particularly in supine patients
Compensatory overinflation	Postlobectomy
	Overlooked lobar collapse (e.g. left lower lobe)
Reduced pulmonary perfusion	Hypoxic vasoconstriction due to underventilation caused by an inhaled foreign body or endobronchial tumour
	Following childhood viral infection (MacLeod's syndrome)
	Recurrent pulmonary emboli (rarely unilateral)

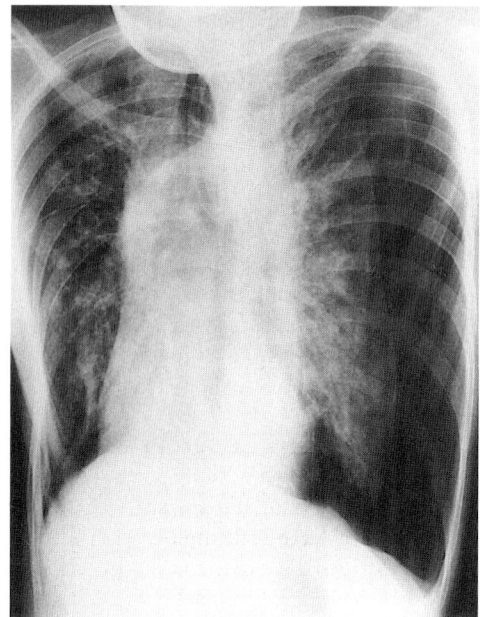

Fig. 18.3.2.19 A left-sided tension pneumothorax in a patient with cystic fibrosis. Note the mediastinal shift and straightening of the left hemidiaphragm.

the lung because of an inhaled foreign body or a tumour in a main bronchus. It is surprisingly easy to overlook this important radiographic abnormality, especially when the density difference between the two lungs is slight: a subtle discrepancy in density between the two hemithoraces is more readily appreciated by viewing the radiograph from a distance of at least 1.5 m. The commonest causes of a relatively transradiant hemithorax are shown in Table 18.3.2.2. Close scrutiny of the chest radiograph will usually indicate which one of the categories of causes is responsible for this radiographic sign. If there is any clinical suggestion that the cause of the increased transradiancy is due to an obstructing lesion in a central airway, a chest radiograph taken in full expiration will accentuate the increased transradiancy and will show that the lung fails to empty.

Once it has been established that the difference in density of the lungs is not due to a technical problem, e.g. rotation of the patient, points to look for are (1) loss of symmetry of the soft tissues of the chest wall, (2) discrepancy in the volumes and vascular pattern between the two lungs, and (3) a visceral pleural edge (denoting a pneumothorax). The identification of a pneumothorax on an erect chest radiograph is usually straightforward because of the appearance of the collapsed lung which is clearly demarcated by the fine edge of the visceral pleura. However, in the supine patient, such an edge is often not seen because air in the pleural space drifts anteriorly to the least dependent part of the chest. In this situation, a pneumothorax is only seen as a vague area of increased transradiancy over the lower zone of the chest. It is vital to recognize when the pressure of the air trapped in the pleural space exceeds alveolar pressure—a so-called tension pneumothorax. The typical signs are of contralateral mediastinal shift with straightening and flattening of the ipsilateral dome of the diaphragm (Fig. 18.3.2.19).

The pulmonary nodule/mass

Many pulmonary nodules or masses are discovered incidentally on a chest radiograph. Whenever possible, previous films should be obtained so that the growth rate of the lesion can be estimated. The growth rate is a more reliable indicator of the likely nature of a pulmonary mass than any one of its radiographic features: if a lesion doubles in volume (increases in diameter by c.25% on serial chest radiographs) in less than 1 week or more than 18 months, it is very unlikely to be malignant. The doubling time of most malignant lesions is between 1 and 6 months.

Over the years much importance has been attached to the radiological characteristics of a solitary pulmonary mass in an attempt to make the crucial distinction between benign and malignant lesions. With the possible exception of heavy calcification within the lesion (most commonly seen in ancient granulomas), no radiological appearance will reliably differentiate a benign from a malignant mass. Although generalizations can be made, e.g. that bronchial carcinomas have irregular and spiculated margins whereas benign lesions are more likely to have smooth outlines, in the individual patient it is not safe to rely on these radiographic features alone to make the distinction between a benign and malignant lesion.

After the discovery of a pulmonary mass on chest radiography, further imaging and other investigations of a patient will depend on the symptomatology, age, and smoking history of the patient. CT is valuable in evaluating extension of a central mass into the mediastinum (Fig. 18.3.2.20), for demonstrating the presence or absence of enlarged mediastinal lymph nodes which may, but do

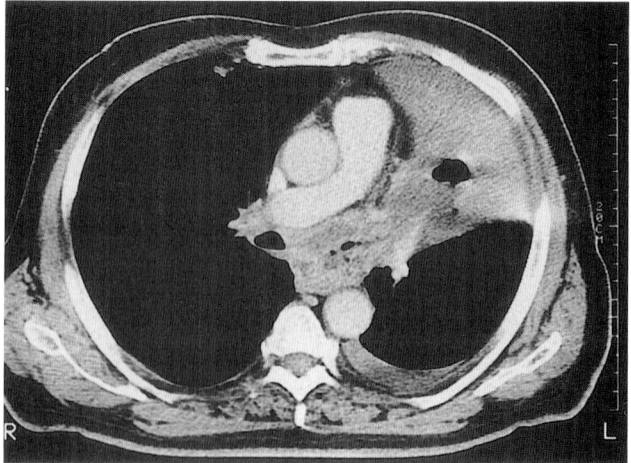

Fig. 18.3.2.20 CT of a central cavitating bronchial carcinoma showing direct extension of the tumour into the subcarinal region of the mediastinum.

not invariably, indicate local tumour spread, and for the detection of distant metastases, such as to the contralateral lung, adrenal glands, and liver. It is usually the overall pattern and extent of disease on a staging CT examination, rather than any single abnormality, which indicate whether a patient with bronchial carcinoma, who is otherwise fit, is likely to suitable for surgical resection. Local invasion of the chest wall by an adjacent bronchial carcinoma may not always be demonstrated by CT, and MRI may be useful because of its ability to image in different planes. When surgery is not indicated and a histological diagnosis is needed, percutaneous needle biopsy of central lesions can be safely performed under CT guidance. Similarly, smaller peripheral lesions that are not accessible by bronchoscopy may be biopsied, under CT or, if abutting the pleura, ultrasound guidance.

There has been recent interest in the use of CT for screening for lung cancer in high-risk groups of individuals, but as yet there is no clear improvement in outcome measures such as mortality, and the results of several large-scale multicentre trials are awaited. However, with the increased use of multidetector CT scanning in a range of conditions, many small (<1 cm) nodules are now detected 'incidentally'. Practical guidelines have been produced regarding the follow-up and management of such findings in both low-risk and high-risk individuals. Assessment of nodule volume with CT has been a useful adjunct to assessment of growth. Automatic pulmonary nodule detection using specially designed software packages may aid assessment of increasingly larger image data sets in the future, but at present these techniques are time-consuming and detect large numbers of false positives.

Cavitating pulmonary lesions

The radiological definition of cavitation is a lucency, representing air, within a mass or area of consolidation. The cavity may or may not contain a fluid level or an intracavitary body, and is surrounded by a wall of variable thickness. The two most likely diagnoses in an adult presenting with a cavitating pulmonary mass on chest radiography are bronchial carcinoma (central, large, and often squamous in type) (Fig. 18.3.2.21) or a lung abscess (usually peripheral and sometimes multiple). Cavitation is recognized in a variety of

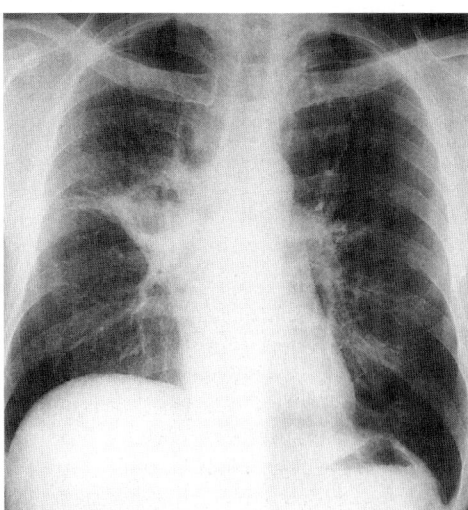

Fig. 18.3.2.21 Chest radiograph of a large cavitating squamous cell bronchial carcinoma adjacent to the right hilum. The right hemidiaphragm is raised because of phrenic nerve invasion by the tumour.

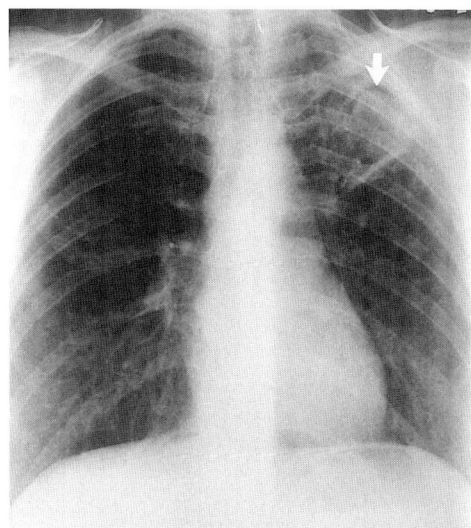

Fig. 18.3.2.22 An air crescent (arrow) around a fungus ball at the left apex. This had developed in a tuberculous fibrotic cavity.

bacterial pneumonias, particularly those due to tuberculosis, staphylococcus, anaerobes, and klebsiella. Less commonly, cavitation is seen within pulmonary infarcts and in areas of pulmonary contusion due to trauma. Long-standing cavities in lungs scarred by previous tuberculosis predispose to the formation of mycetomas; once these fungus balls occupy most of the cavity, a characteristic translucent 'air-crescent sign' may be seen between the upper surface of the fungus ball and the margin of the cavity on chest radiography (Fig. 18.3.2.22).

Multiple pulmonary nodules

Many conditions are characterized by multiple small pulmonary nodules. Only by combining the relevant clinical information with a precise description of the size and distribution of the nodules can the differential diagnosis be narrowed. In the United Kingdom, metastatic deposits are by far the commonest cause of multiple pulmonary nodules of varying sizes in an adult. In some parts of the southern United States of America, histoplasmosis is endemic and multiple granulomatous nodules are commoner than those due to disseminated malignancy. In the absence of a known malignancy and when clinical findings and laboratory investigations are inconclusive, biopsy of one of the nodules may be the only means of establishing a diagnosis.

A myriad of small nodules, less than 5 mm in diameter, produces a pattern that is often described as miliary (Fig. 18.3.2.23). A list of causes of miliary shadowing is given in Box 18.3.2.2. An important diagnosis to consider in any patient with this radiographic pattern is miliary tuberculosis. Other differential diagnoses in an asymptomatic patient with numerous pulmonary nodules include sarcoidosis, metastatic disease or, if there is a relevant occupational history, a pneumoconiosis. As always, comparison with previous radiographs will give invaluable information about the rate of progression and thus the likely nature of the pulmonary nodules. To a lesser extent the distribution of nodules is a consideration in refining the differential diagnosis of multiple pulmonary nodules: e.g. the small nodules of pulmonary sarcoidosis tend to be mid-zone and perihilar, whereas haematogenous metastases are generally of

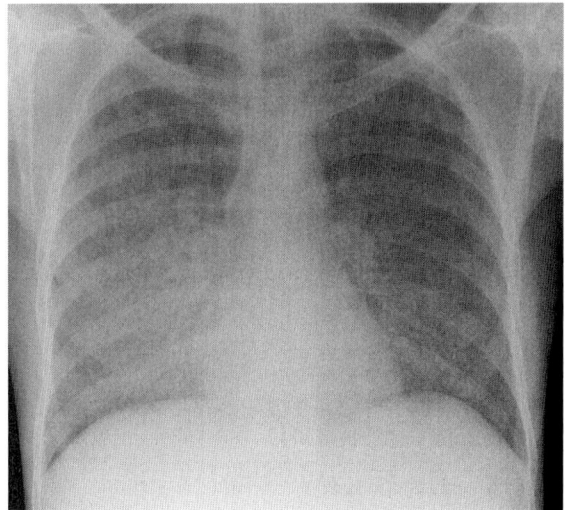

Fig. 18.3.2.23 Multiple small miliary pulmonary nodules in a patient with miliary tuberculosis.

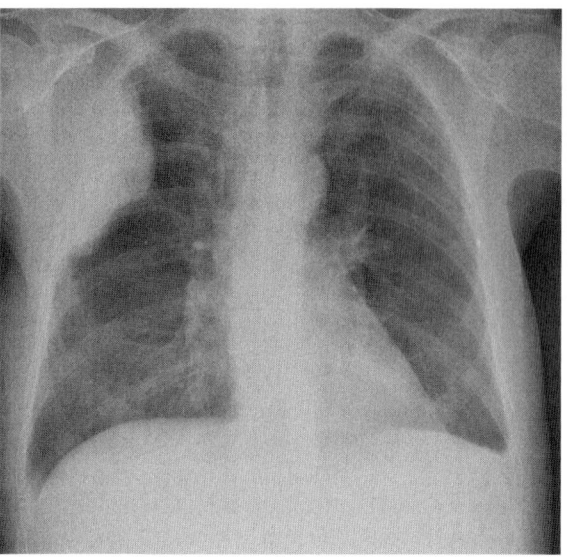

Fig. 18.3.2.24 A malignant chest-wall lesion resulting in rib destruction. Note the obtuse angle between the lesion and the pleural surface superiorly and inferiorly.

varying sizes and have a predilection for the lower lobes (probably because of increased blood flow to these regions).

The density of nodules sometimes provides conclusive evidence that the nodules are of benign aetiology—such as the heavily calcified nodules which are seen following histoplasmosis or chickenpox (varicella) pneumonia. The majority of multiple pulmonary nodules are of soft tissue density, and it may be extremely difficult to judge whether small nodules are of calcific or soft tissue density because their apparent density depends so critically on the radiographic technique used.

Numerous poorly defined, low-density nodules approximately 8 mm in diameter may be seen around areas of pulmonary consolidation. In other areas they may be confluent and so make up a larger poorly defined opacity; occasionally these nodules will be uniformly distributed throughout the lungs. At a pathological level these nodules correspond to individual acini which are full of the products of disease, such as pulmonary oedema, inflammatory exudates, or haemorrhage.

Radiological features of specific diseases

Pleural and chest wall disease

Because of the two-dimensional nature of a PA chest radiograph, abnormalities arising from the pleura or chest are often difficult

---

Box 18.3.2.2 Differential diagnosis of widespread fine nodular (0.5–3 mm diameter) shadowing

- Miliary tuberculosis
- Fungal diseases
- Metastatic disease
- Pneumoconiosis
- Sarcoidosis
- Extrinsic allergic alveolitis
- Idiopathic pulmonary haemorrhage

---

to assess. The appearance of a pleural mass on chest radiography depends on whether it is face on or tangential to the X-ray beam. Generally, a pleural mass will produce a rounded opacity with a sharp medial border and a less well-defined lateral margin, and an obtuse angle with the pleura. Although abnormality of an adjacent rib will usually indicate that an apparent 'pleural' mass is of chest wall origin (Fig. 18.3.2.24), the distinction between a pleural and chest wall mass often cannot be made from a chest radiograph alone.

With extensive pleural pathology it may be difficult to distinguish between a pleural effusion, chronic pleural thickening, or even a neoplasm of the pleura such as a mesothelioma. In such cases a lateral decubitus film will distinguish between pleural fluid or thickening by demonstrating redistribution of the shadowing if it is due to an effusion. Ultrasonography is also useful in identifying pleural fluid. CT will show even more precisely the site and extent of an abnormality which is apparently 'pleural' on a chest radiograph. Furthermore, CT will reveal subtle abnormalities not shown on a plain chest radiograph, such as flecks of calcification within the wall of a chronic empyema, or underlying rib abnormalities in the case of a neoplastic tumour. Similarly, masses arising from the chest wall that give the appearance of a 'pleural' mass, such as an intercostal neurofibroma or lipoma, are most accurately assessed by CT.

Chronic obstructive pulmonary disease (COPD)

Most patients with chronic obstructive airways disease show remarkably little radiographic abnormality despite often considerable symptoms. Of the two principal components falling under the heading chronic obstructive airways disease, emphysema can be detected on chest radiography when it is severe, whereas chronic bronchitis is a clinical diagnosis with no specific radiographic features.

Although emphysema is correctly regarded as a pathological diagnosis, the destruction of alveolar walls distal to the terminal bronchial results in certain radiographic features in more advanced cases: overinflation of the lungs causes flattening of the domes of the diaphragm, which may have a scalloped appearance; a lateral chest radiograph may show striking translucency of the enlarged retrosternal and retrocardiac regions. The pattern of the pulmonary vasculature is deranged, with the smooth tapering of the vessels replaced by an abrupt change in calibre from the larger proximal pulmonary arteries to spindly and attenuated peripheral vessels, giving a so-called pruned appearance. Depending on the aetiology of the emphysema, there may be an upper zone (e.g. smokers) or lower zone (e.g. α_1-antitrypsin deficiency) predominance; the relatively spared lung often shows a prominent vascular pattern due to blood diversion to these areas.

Bullous emphysema is characterized by cystic air spaces bounded by extremely thin walls. They may become extremely large and occupy a large part of the lung (Figs. 18.3.2.25a, b). A fluid level within a bulla represents either infection or haemorrhage. Another complication is a pneumothorax, which may be chronic and is sometimes difficult to distinguish from a large bulla.

CT is far more sensitive than chest radiography in the detection of emphysema and in some early cases will show evidence of emphysema before lung function tests become abnormal.

Bronchiectasis

Bronchiectasis, whatever the aetiology, is defined as damage to the bronchial wall causing irreversible dilatation of the bronchi. The diagnosis of bronchiectasis is rarely made with certainty from the chest radiograph alone, unless the disease is extensive and severe. On a chest radiograph the abnormal bronchi may be visible as either ring shadows and curvilinear shadows that represent thickened bronchial wall seen end-on, or as parallel thin lines or 'tramlines', particularly in the lower lobes; this latter sign can be very subtle and may be more obvious on the lateral chest radiograph. Other radiographic signs of bronchiectasis include round or oval nodular opacities, and sometimes band shadows representing grossly dilated fluid-filled bronchi.

High-resolution CT has supplanted bronchography (which was not without hazard) as the imaging technique of choice in investigation of patients with suspected bronchiectasis. Abnormally dilated and thickened bronchi are readily identified on high-resolution CT (Fig. 18.3.2.26); a normal bronchus is of approximately the same diameter as its accompanying pulmonary artery. In addition to allowing a confident diagnosis of bronchiectasis to be made, often in the face of a normal chest radiograph, high-resolution CT will show how many lobes are involved—an important consideration in deciding on medical or surgical management.

Chronic diffuse lung disease

Many conditions are characterized by diffuse shadowing of the lungs on a chest radiograph. The lung has few ways of responding to injury (capillary leak, cellular infiltration, or interstitial fibrosis) and the resulting spectrum of radiographic patterns is correspondingly limited. It is important that reproducible terms are used in the description of widespread pulmonary shadowing. Vague terms that may convey a pathological meaning (which in fact cannot be inferred from the gross signs of disease on a chest radiograph), e.g. 'inflammatory shadowing' should not be used. Instead, descriptions of the radiographic pattern should be limited to strictly morphological terms such as 'reticular'—a fine network, 'nodular'—small dots of a specified size, 'linear'—fine lines which are not vessels, 'ground-glass'—a greying-out of the lungs that makes the vascular markings

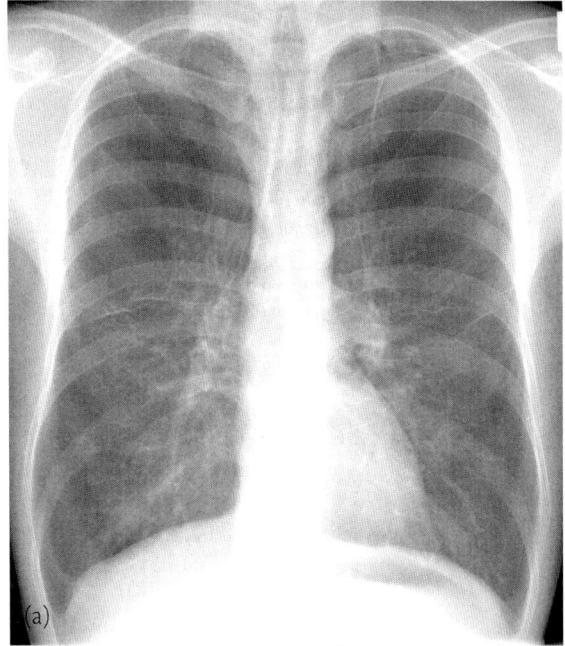

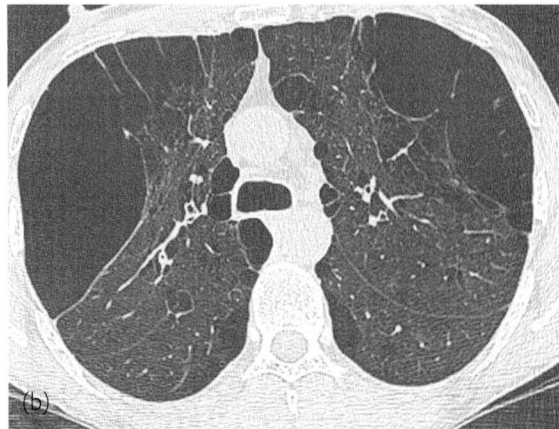

Fig. 18.3.2.25 The chest radiograph (a) and an axial CT section (b) in a patient with severe bullous emphysema. The absence of lung markings within the right upper zone makes it difficult to exclude a pneumothorax, however the CT demonstrates the multiple thin-walled bullae.

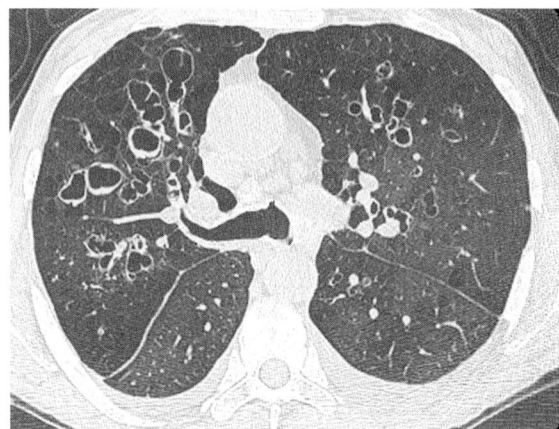

Fig. 18.3.2.26 Axial high-resolution CT section of a patient with allergic bronchopulmonary aspergillosis (ABPA) showing marked bilateral cystic bronchiectasis.

indistinct, and finally 'air-space shadowing' or 'consolidation'—opacification of the lungs in which an air bronchogram may be visible. These descriptors are more reproducible and are preferable to the wide range of imprecise and whimsical terms that have been coined in the past.

An analysis of the distribution of the disease is often at least as important as defining the radiographic pattern in reaching a differential diagnosis. This involves an assessment of whether the disease involves all parts of the lung uniformly, or whether there is a zonal predominance (upper, mid, or lower; central or peripheral). The perihilar, mid- and upper-zone distribution of the reticulonodular pattern in sarcoidosis is quite different from the lower-zone peripheral distribution of idiopathic pulmonary fibrosis; these differences in distribution are even more obvious on the cross-sectional images of CT. The differential diagnosis can be further refined by assimilating other radiographic abnormalities, such as the presence of pleural disease in the case of asbestosis, or enlarged hilar lymph nodes in the case of sarcoidosis or lymphangitis carcinomatosa.

Only when the radiographic findings of a patient with diffuse lung disease are taken in conjunction with the clinical features should a working diagnosis be attempted. Many pieces of information contribute to final diagnosis. In the context of diffuse lung disease, the chest radiograph should be considered as only one part of the clinical jigsaw since a specific diagnosis can rarely be achieved with complete confidence from the radiographic findings alone. In addition to the nonspecific appearances of many diffuse lung diseases, the sensitivity of chest radiography is less than ideal, with up to 15% of patients with biopsy-proven diffuse lung disease having a normal chest radiograph. Conversely, a less than ideally exposed chest radiograph, especially of an obese patient, may misleadingly raise the spectre of diffuse lung disease.

In the last two decades the development of high-resolution CT has changed the radiological approach to the diagnosis of diffuse lung disease, providing valuable prognostic insights that have substantially aided management of patients with diffuse interstitial lung disease. As stated previously, high-resolution CT images of the lung correlate closely with the macroscopic appearances of pathological specimens, can precisely estimate the extent of diffuse lung disease, and are less prone than biopsy to errors of sampling (although open lung biopsy is still required to achieve a definitive histological diagnosis in difficult cases). In addition, when a biopsy is indicated, the distribution of disease will indicate whether a transbronchial biopsy or an open lung biopsy is more likely to obtain a representative specimen.

Further reading

Austin JH, Stellman SD, Pearson GD (2001). Screening for lung cancer. *N Engl J Med*, **344**, 935.
Bruzzi JF, Munden RF (2006). PET/CT imaging of lung cancer. *J Thorac Imaging*, **21**, 137–6.
Engeler C (2001). Interpreting the chest radiograph. In: Grainger RG, Dixon AK and Allison DJ (eds) *Diagnostic radiology: a textbook of medical imaging*, 4th edition. Churchill Livingstone, Edinburgh.
Goodman LR (2007). *Felson's principles of chest roentgenology*, 3rd edition. W B Saunders, Philadelphia.
Hansell DM *et al.* (2008). Fleischner Society: Glossary of Terms for Thoracic Imaging. *Radiology*, **246**, 697–722.
Hansell DM, Lynch DA, McAdams HP, Bankier AA (2010). Imaging of Diseases of the Chest, 5th edition. Mosby Elsevier.

Heitzmann ER (1988). *The mediastinum: radiologic correlations with anatomy and pathology*, 2nd edition. Springer-Verlag, Berlin.
Ishii M, *et al.* (2005). Hyperpolarized helium-3 MR imaging of pulmonary function. *Radiol Clin North Am*, **43**, 235–46.
Lynch DA, *et al.* (2005). Idiopathic interstitial pneumonias: CT features. *Radiology*, **236**, 10–21.
MacMahon H, *et al*: Fleischner Society (2005). Guidelines for management of small pulmonary nodules detected on CT scans: a statement from the Fleischner Society. *Radiology*, **237**, 395–400.
Naidich DP *et al.* (2006). Computed tomography and magnetic resonance of the thorax, 4th edition. Lippincott Williams & Wilkins, Philadelphia.
Padley S and MacDonald SLS (2008). The Normal Chest. In: Grainger and Allison's Diagnostic Radiology: a textbook of medical imaging. Adam A and Dixon AK (eds), 5th edition. Elsevier Churchill Livingston, Philadelphia.
Proto AV, Speckman, JM (1979). *The left lateral radiograph of the chest. Medical radiography and photography*. Eastman Kodak Company, Rochester, NY.
Rémy-Jardin M, Rémy J (2001). *Spiral CT of the chest (medical radiology)*. Springer-Verlag, Berlin.
Webb RW, Müller NL, Naidich DP (2000). *High-resolution CT of the lung*, 3rd edition. Lippincott Williams & Wilkins, Philadelphia.
Wells AU (2003). High-resolution CT in the diagnosis of diffuse lung disease: a clinical perspective. *Semin Respir Crit Care Med*, **24**, 347–56.

18.3.3 Bronchoscopy, thoracoscopy, and tissue biopsy

Pallav L. Shah

Essentials

Bronchoscopy, thoracoscopy, and radiologically guided biopsy techniques provide different methods for visualizing and sampling thoracic lesions, the approach chosen in any particular case being based on a number of factors, including the anatomical location of abnormal areas, presence of coexisting pulmonary disease, presence of comorbidities, and local expertise. CT is useful in both selection and planning of the most appropriate sampling method.

Bronchoscopy

Bronchoscopy can be used for sampling central lesions, mediastinal lymph nodes, hilar lymph nodes, and—where magnetic navigation technology is available—peripheral nodules. Suspected lung cancer is the commonest indication.

Lung cancer—bronchoscopy is an essential tool in diagnosis and staging, when a combination of techniques such as bronchial washings, brushings, and biopsy improves diagnostic yield, as does review of CT imaging before the procedure. Any abnormal mediastinal lymph nodes should be sampled in the first instance by either transbronchial fine-needle aspiration (TBNA) or endobronchial ultrasound-guided TBNA. In the active palliation of lung cancer in patients with primary tumour or metastases involving the trachea or main bronchi, a variety of bronchoscopic techniques can be used to restore airway patency, including stenting in selected cases.

Diffuse lung disease and focal parenchymal infiltrates—bronchoalveolar lavage provides information on cellular processes involved, transbronchial lung biopsy on the pathological characteristics, and segmental lavage is a useful tool in patients with suspected respiratory infection.

Other indications—the role of therapeutic bronchoscopy is increasing with the development of new endoscopic treatments for respiratory diseases such as emphysema and asthma.

Thoracoscopy

Thoracoscopy allows visual inspection and direct sampling of pleural abnormalities, the commonest indications being (1) evaluation of an exudative pleural effusion when cytological analysis of aspirated fluid does not provide a conclusive diagnosis; and (2) in the treatment of a malignant pleural effusion, when a sclerosing agent such as talc can be evenly applied to the pleural surface, a technique which also has a role in the management of recurrent spontaneous pneumothorax.

Percutaneous biopsy

The role of 'blind' (unguided) pleural biopsy is diminishing as it has been superseded by either thoracoscopic or image-guided biopsy. Radiologically guided percutaneous biopsy is usually considered where cancer is suspected and there is no clear indication to proceed to surgical resection.

Introduction

Direct visualization of the airways by bronchoscopy has become an important tool in the diagnosis of respiratory disease since its introduction in Japan in 1966. The ability to visualize specific areas significantly improves diagnostic yield in comparison to blind procedures. Similarly, the diagnosis and treatment of pleural disease has improved significantly with the introduction of thoracoscopy, which allows the direct inspection of the pleural cavity. Tissue biopsy has also evolved, with more procedures now being performed with some form of image guidance.

Bronchoscopy

Bronchoscopy is an essential basic investigation for the respiratory physician. The first bronchoscopes were rigid instruments that were adapted from oesophagoscopes. The development of optical fibres enabled flexible bronchoscopes to be constructed, which significantly improved the utility of bronchoscopy, and today videobronchoscopes that provide high-quality images are used routinely.

Flexible bronchoscopy permits the visual inspection of the airways from the vocal cords, trachea, and endobronchial tree down to the subsegmental level. It also allows for a variety of samples to be easily obtained from the airways. The procedure is very safe and is performed as a day-case procedure, with local anaesthesia with or without short-acting intravenous sedation. Rigid bronchoscopy is still performed, primarily by thoracic surgeons and by some physicians for interventional procedures: the equipment has a greater intraluminal diameter than do flexible bronchoscopes and hence allows easier instrumentation, but at the expense of a more restricted field of view and the requirement for general anaesthesia.

Indications

The main indications for flexible bronchoscopy are listed in Table 18.3.3.1: suspected lung cancer is the commonest, followed by the assessment of pulmonary infiltrates for microbiological sampling. The role of therapeutic bronchoscopy is increasing with the development of new endoscopic treatments for respiratory diseases.

Contraindications

Informed consent from the patient or their representative is a prerequisite. The main contraindications for bronchoscopy are hypoxia that cannot be adequately corrected by oxygen supplementation, and a bleeding diathesis. However, even in these circumstances firm 'cut-offs' cannot be given—the risk-benefit must be evaluated on an individual patient basis. The procedure should only be performed by an individual with an appropriate level of experience, or under supervision by an experienced bronchoscopist. Adequate facilities for resuscitation, and the skills and equipment to deal with any potential complication, should be immediately available. Bronchoscopy staff should be trained and competent in dealing with problems such as respiratory failure,

Table 18.3.3.1 Indications for bronchoscopy

Investigation of symptoms	Haemoptysis
	Persistent cough
	Recurrent infection
Suspected neoplasia	Unexplained paralysis of vocal cords
	Stridor
	Localized monophonic wheeze
	Segmental or lobar collapse
	Unexplained paralysis of hemidiaphragm
	Suspicious sputum cytology
	Unexplained pleural effusion
	Mediastinal tissue—diagnosis and staging
	Assessing suitability for surgery
	Staging of lung cancer
Infection	Assessment of pulmonary infiltrates
	Identification of organisms
	Evaluation of airways if recurrent or persistent infection
Interstitial lung disease	Differential cell counts and cytology
	Transbronchial lung biopsy
Therapeutic	Clearance of airway secretions
	Recurrent plugging of patient on ventilators following lobar collapse
	Foreign body removal
	Palliation of neoplasm
	Endobronchial ablation of tumour
	Insertion of stents
	Bronchoscopic lung volume reduction
	Bronchial thermoplasty for asthma

cardiac arrhythmias, haemorrhage, and the requirement for intercostal drain insertion.

Equipment

The flexible bronchoscope is a flexible tube containing bundles of optical fibres that carry light to the distal end to illuminate the airways, and a further bundle to transmit the image back to the eyepiece. The distal end of the bronchoscope can be angled through 160° by a lever at the head of the scope. This, in combination with rotation of the scope, allows it to be manipulated during the examination of the airways. There is an instrument channel that allows procedures such as biopsies to be performed and which also functions as a suction channel. A variety of instruments are available, with the specification of the bronchoscope influencing its use—those with larger instrument channels are more suitable for interventional procedures, whereas smaller instruments allow more distal airways to be examined.

Modern videobronchoscopes have a charged couple device (CCD) chip at the distal end, which allows the image to be projected on to a monitor. The latest systems utilize high-definition TV technology and produce high-quality full-screen images, which significantly enhance diagnosis. There are also a number of hybrid devices that use fibre-optic bundles to carry light down and images back up towards the proximal portion of the bronchoscope. A CCD chip in the head of the scope allows the image to be transmitted onto a monitor, the image quality being determined by the number of optical fibres and the size of the CCD chip. These hybrid scopes have the advantage of having either a smaller external diameter or a much larger instrument channel than conventional videobronchoscopes.

An integrated bronchoscope with a linear array ultrasound probe at the distal end is now commercially available. Its primary use is to facilitate ultrasound-guided sampling of the mediastinum and it is discussed later in this chapter.

Disinfection

Bronchoscopes are cleaned and disinfected before and after the procedure. Particular care should be taken to clean the instrument channel and suction ports manually with a brush, as well as flushing the channel with sterile water. The instrument is then placed in a disinfection solution such as 2% alkaline glutaraldehyde (the commonest used), or phenyl or isopropyl alcohol, and automatic disinfection with 0.2% peracetic acid can also be used. In all cases the instruments should be soaked in the disinfectant solution for at least 20 min. Cross-infection has been observed with organisms such as environmental mycobacteria and pseudomonas species; processes must therefore be in place to document disinfection before use in each patient, and the serial number of the bronchoscope(s) used in individual patients should be recorded for tracing in the event of suspected cross-infection. In most cases of cross-infection, inadequate manual cleaning of bronchoscopes has been a factor. Biopsy forceps and needles are more invasive and hence need to be sterilized rather than simply disinfected.

The potential risk of infections with viruses and prions has driven the development of single-use disposable instruments, but the cost of single-use bronchoscopes would be prohibitive. The development of instruments that can be sterilized rather than disinfected is more realistic, but would still incur significant capital investment. Because there is a significant time delay for instruments that require sterilization (days, rather than the short time required for disinfection), more than 10 bronchoscopes would be required to maintain a clinical service.

Patient preparation

Patients need to provide informed consent before the procedure and should ideally be provided with written information in advance, with key aspects such as risks of the procedure and alternative approaches discussed prior to giving final consent. Bronchoscopy is usually performed as an outpatient procedure with conscious sedation, and patients should be advised not to eat or drink for at least 4 h beforehand. Box 18.3.3.1 provides a simple checklist for patient preparation.

All available imaging should be reviewed prior to bronchoscopy. Ideally, a recent CT scan should be available, as there is good evidence that review of such images before flexible bronchoscopy significantly improves the yield from the procedure. In one study, 171 patients being evaluated for suspected lung cancer were randomized: all had a CT scan performed before bronchoscopy, but in one group the scans were reviewed before the procedure, whereas in another (control) group they were not. The diagnostic yield of bronchoscopy was 73% in the former group compared to 54% in the latter and fewer investigations were required in the group where the CT scans were reviewed before bronchoscopy. This approach is therefore more cost-effective and this author advocates it for all patients undergoing assessment for possible lung cancer. It also allows additional staging procedures such as transbronchial needle aspiration to be performed at the same time as the initial diagnostic bronchoscopy.

A short-acting intravenous benzodiazepine such as intravenous midazolam or an opiate such as fentanyl or alfentanil may be used for sedation. Midazolam has the advantage of amnesic properties, whereas fentanyl and alfentanil have good antitussive properties. In some institutions a low-dose propofol infusion is used to induce and maintain sedation. Patients who have been given sedation should be advised not to drive or handle any machinery for at least

---

Box 18.3.3.1 Preparation for bronchoscopy

- Patient information—verbal and written information
- Informed consent
- Full blood count and clotting prior to transbronchial lung biopsy
- Baseline ECG if history of cardiac disease
- Spirometry if arterial oxygen saturation <95%
- Arterial blood gases if oxygen saturation <92%
- If the patient is to have any sedation, ensure that someone is going to accompany them home after the procedure
- Remind the patient that if they are sedated they will be unable to drive or operate machinery for at least 24 h
- Intravenous access
- Consider bronchodilators if evidence of bronchospasm
- Prophylactic antibiotics if asplenia, heart valve prosthesis, cardiac murmur, or history of endocarditis

24 h after the procedure. The procedure can be performed without any sedation, which should be considered in some individuals who become aggressive and uncontrollable following intravenous benzodiazepines. It is also an option in patients who cannot be accompanied for 24 h after the procedure.

Patients are monitored by continuous oximetry throughout the procedure. Those with pre-existing cardiac disease, or where hypoxia is not fully controlled by oxygen therapy, should also have ECG monitoring.

Basic procedure

Bronchoscopy can be performed with the patient semirecumbent and approached from the front, or alternatively the patient can be lying flat and approached from behind. The choice is determined by local practice and also the procedure that is being performed. Intubation can be performed through either the nose or the oropharynx. Again, local practice seems to influence the approach, but the external diameter of the bronchoscope and the procedure being undertaken should also be taken into account.

The oral pharynx is first anaesthetized with 4% lignocaine (lidocaine) for all procedures. The nasal passage is then anaesthetized with 2% lignocaine gel if a transnasal approach is used. With the nasal route, the bronchoscope is passed through the nares and nasopharynx under direct vision until the epiglottis is visualized. With the oral route, the patient is asked to gently bite onto a mouthguard and the bronchoscope is then placed through this mouthguard into the oropharynx to the level of the epiglottis.

The vocal cords should be visible from this level and their movement assessed, after which they are anaesthetized with 2 ml aliquots of 2% lignocaine. When the coughing subsides the scope is advanced through the widest part of the glottis, with care taken not to touch the vocal cords. The subglottic area of the trachea is very sensitive and patients initially feel as if they are choking. Further 2 ml aliquots of 2% lignocaine are administered in the trachea, carina, right main bronchus, and left main bronchus.

The trachea and endobronchial tree can be inspected down to the segmental areas (Fig. 18.3.3.1), the limiting factor being the size of the bronchoscope. The average bronchoscope with a 5 mm external

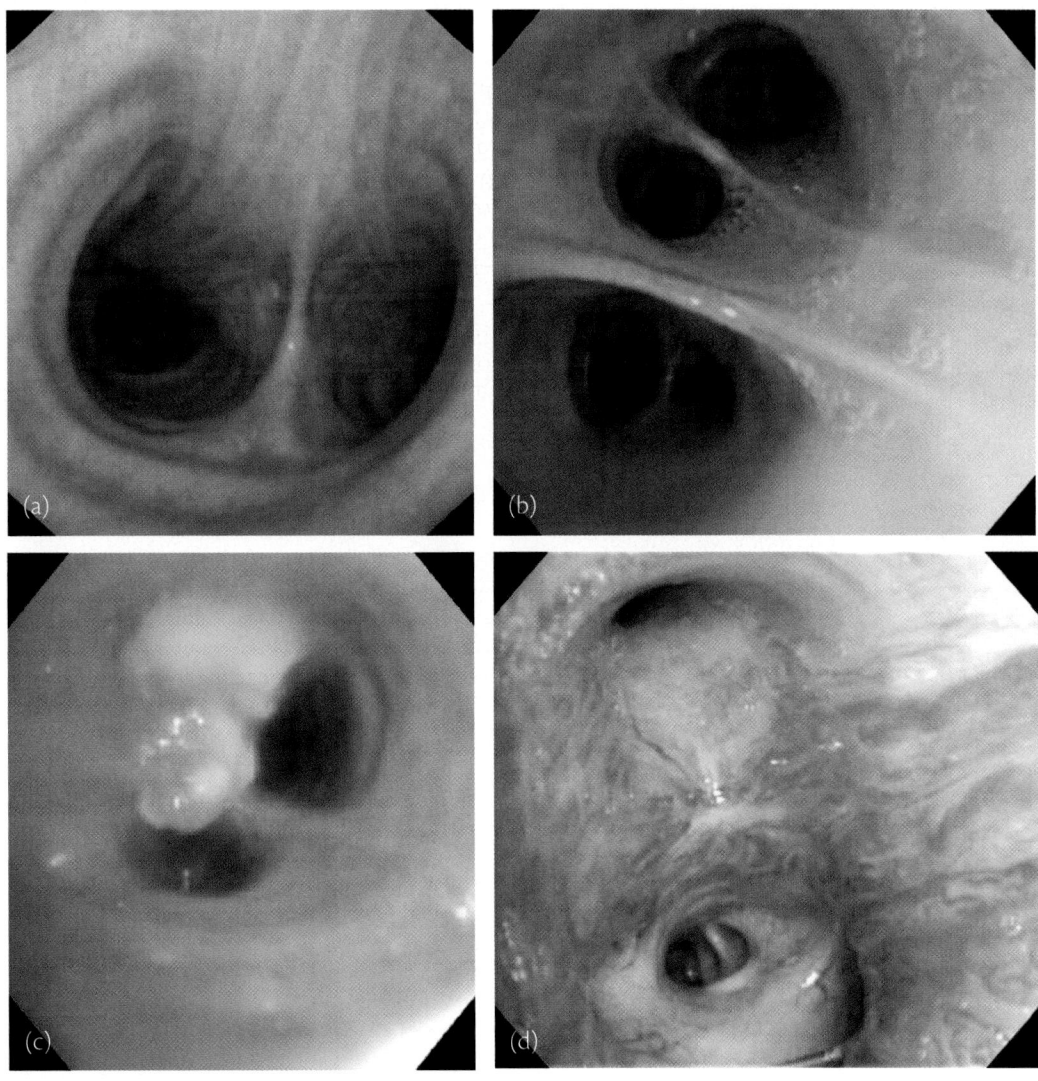

Fig. 18.3.3.1 The videobronchoscopic appearance of (a) the trachea and main bronchi; (b) segmental bronchi in the right lower lobe; (c) polypoid tumour arising from a bronchial segment; and (d) submucosal disease.

diameter can reach the second or third generation subsegments. The following can be assessed at bronchoscopy:

- Dynamic and fixed changes in airway calibre, including areas of extrinsic compression from enlarged lymph nodes or extrabronchial tumour masses

- Distortion of the airways due to traction from fibrotic or collapsed areas of lung

- The general appearance of the mucosa, with changes ranging from subtle abnormalities such as increased vascularity (Fig. 18.3.3.1d) and oedema through to gross tumour infiltration

Polypoid tumours involving the first or second generation subsegments should be easily identified at bronchoscopy (Fig. 18.3.3.1c). However, submucosal disease can be easily missed, and can range from subtle thickening of the airways through to small pearly nodules (may be present in tuberculosis or sarcoidosis). Small ulcers are also occasionally seen with tuberculosis or Wegener's granulomatosis. In Kaposi's sarcoma, cherry-red-like lesions are visible.

Basic techniques and sampling

Bronchial washings

Obtaining bronchial washings involves the instillation of 10 to 20 ml aliquots of 0.9% saline into a subsegment, as close as possible to the site of abnormality. The sensitivity is variable, being 48% (range 21–76%) in a recent review that evaluated 30 studies where the yield from the different bronchoscopic techniques was evaluated in at least 50 patients with suspected lung cancer.

Bronchial biopsies

Biopsy forceps can be inserted through the instrument channel of the bronchoscope and pinch biopsies obtained under direct vision, with several biopsies obtained to ensure that adequate tissue has been obtained for diagnosis. A higher yield can be obtained from endobronchial biopsies, with an overall sensitivity for lung cancer of 74% (range 48–97%), but where an exophytic tumour is visible the diagnostic yield should be at least 90%. The technique is generally very safe and the main complication is that of bleeding, particularly where vascular lesions are sampled, but this is rarely significant and can usually be controlled with conservative measures.

Bronchial brushings

A cytology brush can be used to scrape cells from the surface of any abnormal areas seen at bronchoscopy. These can then be either smeared onto a slide or rinsed in saline, according to local preference. In the meta-analysis described above the yield from bronchial brushings was 59% (range 23–93%). The main complication is minor bleeding, but there is a risk of a pneumothorax where a brush is advanced blindly beyond a subsegmental bronchus.

Transbronchial fine needle aspiration

In this technique a transbronchial fine needle is inserted through the mucosa and into a submucosal lesion beyond the endobronchial surface and a few cells are aspirated for cytological analysis. It has a sensitivity of around 56% (range 23–90%).

Transbronchial fine needle aspiration can also be used to sample lymph nodes and is particularly useful in the diagnosis and staging of lung cancer, with a recent CT scan of the thorax required for planning of the procedure. The needle is inserted through the instrument channel of the bronchoscope and then through the tracheal or bronchial surface at the position determined, as perpendicularly as possible (at least 45° angle) to the airway wall, with a jabbing motion, and with suction applied with a 20 ml syringe at the other end. The cells that are aspirated are sent off for cytological analysis. Occasionally a small piece of tissue is also obtained with this technique. The sensitivity of this technique in lung cancer is around 68% (range 45–85%). It provides both diagnostic and staging information, and is often the sole mode of diagnosis (25% of patients). The availability of rapid on-site cytological analysis significantly improves the diagnostic yield. However, a negative result does not exclude neoplastic disease and should be followed up by further investigations such as mediastinoscopy in appropriate cases.

Although it is possible to diagnose lymphoma with transbronchial fine needle aspiration, the samples obtained are predominantly cytological and do not provide the architectural information required to classify lymphomas. It is also a useful technique in the diagnosis of nonmalignant disease such as sarcoidosis and tuberculosis, but the sensitivity is lower.

Overall, transbronchial fine-needle aspiration is a very safe and effective technique: complications are rare, consisting of pneumothorax, pneumomediastinum, and bleeding (<0.01%).

Bronchoalveolar lavage

Bronchoalveolar lavage is a useful diagnostic test in the assessment of parenchymal lung disease. It enables sampling of the distal airways and alveolar spaces, and is particularly useful in the assessment of (1) diffuse drug induced interstitial lung disease, (2) parenchymal infiltrates, (3) pulmonary infiltrates in immunocompromised patients, and (4) assessment of occupational dust exposure.

The samples obtained provide information on the cellular composition of pulmonary infiltrates, types of infective organisms, and presence of particulate and acellular matter in the alveolar spaces (Table 18.3.3.2). Identification of specific bacteria, fungi, and acid-fast bacilli are diagnostic. Malignant cells may be identified in the lavage in patients with bronchoalveolar cell cancer, lymphangitis carcinomatosus, or diffuse metastatic disease. A milky lavage laden with amorphous periodic acid–Schiff positive staining cellular debris is diagnostic of pulmonary alveolar prognosis.

Bronchoalveolar lavage is performed by wedging the bronchoscope in the desired subsegment. In diffuse lung disease the right mid-lobe is the segment of choice as it drains well and hence provides the best yield; otherwise the optimal segment is selected on the basis of radiological findings. Once the bronchoscope is wedged, 30- to 60-ml aliquots of normal saline are instilled and aspirated back into a collecting bottle, either by gentle hand suction or with low-pressure suction. The total fluid instilled ranges from 100 to 250 ml, depending on the exact indication and local circumstances.

The main adverse effects of bronchoalveolar lavage are usually dyspnoea, wheezing, and transient fever. Many patients are hypoxic due to their underlying condition, and installation of significant volumes of saline can precipitate hypoxia and, in some cases, pulmonary oedema.

Transbronchial lung biopsy

Transbronchial lung biopsy is invaluable in the assessment of diffuse lung disease and in patients where there is localized parenchymal shadowing (at least of segmental distribution). It has a high diagnostic yield (>80%) in bronchocentric conditions such as sarcoidosis. It also has an important role in the diagnosis of

Table 18.3.3.2 Cellular composition of bronchoalveolar lavage according to disease aetiology

Lymphocytic cell composition	Sarcoidosis
	Extrinsic allergic alveolitis
	Hypersensitivity pneumonitis
	Connective tissue disease
	Tuberculosis
	Viral pneumonia
Neutrophilic cell composition	Idiopathic pulmonary fibrosis/usual interstitial pneumonia
	Desquamative interstitial pneumonitis
	Acute interstitial pneumonitis
	Acute respiratory distress syndrome
	Pneumonia
	Connective tissue disease
	Wegener's granulomatosis
	Cryptogenic organizing pneumonia/ obliterative bronchiolitis
Eosinophilic cell infiltrate	Eosinophilic pneumonia
	Churg–Strauss syndrome
	Allergic bronchopulmonary aspergillosis
	Drug-induced pneumonitis
Mixed picture	Cryptogenic organizing/obliterative bronchiolitis
	Connective tissue disease
	Nonspecific interstitial pneumonitis

lymphangitis carcinomatosis, disseminated malignancy, interstitial pneumonitis, and extrinsic allergic alveolitis.

The two main complications of transbronchial lung biopsy are haemorrhage and pneumothorax. The risk of the latter is 5 to10%, but a clinically significant pneumothorax requiring intervention occurs in about 1% of cases. The degree of bleeding is very variable, but blood loss of more than 250 ml is infrequent, and usually managed with aggressive suctioning of any blood combined with instillation of ice-cold saline and dilute adrenaline (1:100 000). Blocking balloons that occlude a lobar bronchus may be used to tamponade the bleeding, and blood transfusion may be required on rare occasions.

Advanced and research procedures

Endobronchial ultrasound-guided transbronchial needle aspiration

Endobronchial ultrasound was originally performed using a 20 MHz radial vascular mini-ultrasound probe enclosed in a water-filled balloon sheath. These ultrasound probes produce excellent images of the mediastinum and hilar structures, and can provide information on vascular invasion. They are able to identify the different bronchial layers from submucosa to adventitia and have the potential of determining if the mucosa has been breached by cancer and hence distinguish between carcinoma *in situ* and invasive carcinoma, but their value in a clinical setting is limited.

The development of a linear array ultrasound probe integrated into a videobronchoscope, which allows simultaneous ultrasound and conventional bronchoscopic imaging, has significantly improved the utility of ultrasound in bronchoscopy (Fig. 18.3.3.2). The probe can be applied against the tracheal wall and the mediastinum assessed for abnormal lymph nodes, which are visible as hypoechoeic lesions that can be distinguished from blood vessels using Doppler mode. A dedicated needle can be inserted through the instrument channel of the bronchoscope and transbronchial needle aspiration performed with real-time ultrasound imaging (Fig. 18.3.3.2). Abnormal lymph nodes as small as 5 mm in diameter can be sampled. Clinical experience suggests that the diagnostic yield is 85 to 90%, meaning that this technique has the promise of superseding mediastinoscopy in the staging of lung cancer.

Magnetic navigation

Magnetic positional tip technology can be integrated with CT scanning data to create a virtual CT scanner in the bronchoscopy suite. A spiral CT with reconstructions of between 1.5 and 3 mm is required, the data from which is used to create a virtual bronchoscopy model. Specific landmarks such as the primary and lobar carina are marked. At bronchoscopy, a catheter with a magnetic tracking device is inserted through the instrument channel and the catheter tip is positioned and calibrated with three to six points previously marked in the planning phase. The system then integrates the CT data with the bronchoscopy data and can be used to guide the catheter with the magnetic tracking device to the target lesion (Fig. 18.3.3.3). Once the target is reached, the tracking device is removed, the biopsy forceps or needle is inserted through the catheter, and appropriate samples are obtained for diagnosis.

The main benefit from this system is that it facilitates the biopsy of peripheral pulmonary lesions which measure more than 20 mm in size. The bronchoscopic route tends to be safer, with a lower incidence of complications such as pneumothoraces than percutaneous approaches. It may also improve the accuracy of transbronchial needle aspiration of mediastinal lymph nodes.

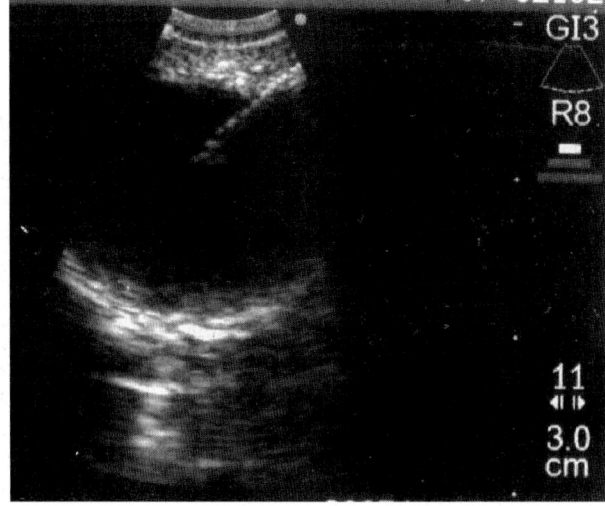

Fig. 18.3.3.2 An ultrasound image demonstrating a needle in a hypolucent ovoid lymph node during endobronchial ultrasound-guided transbronchial fine-needle aspiration.

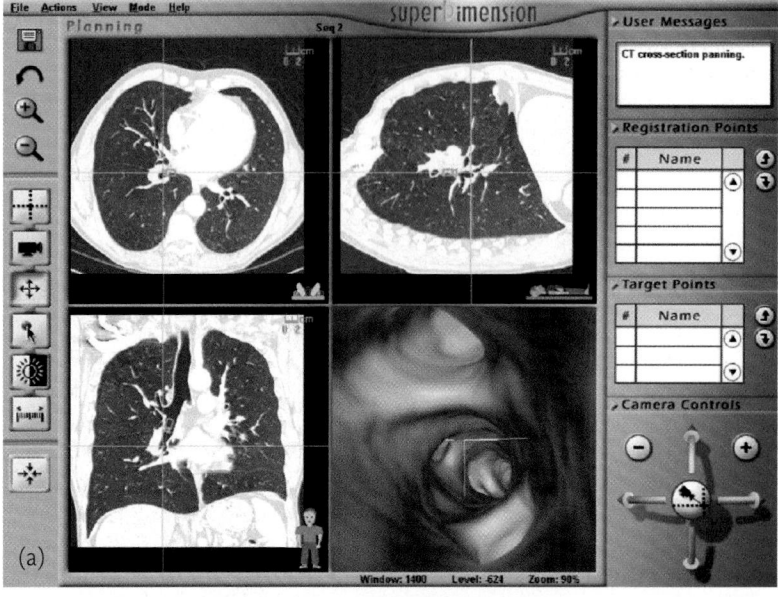

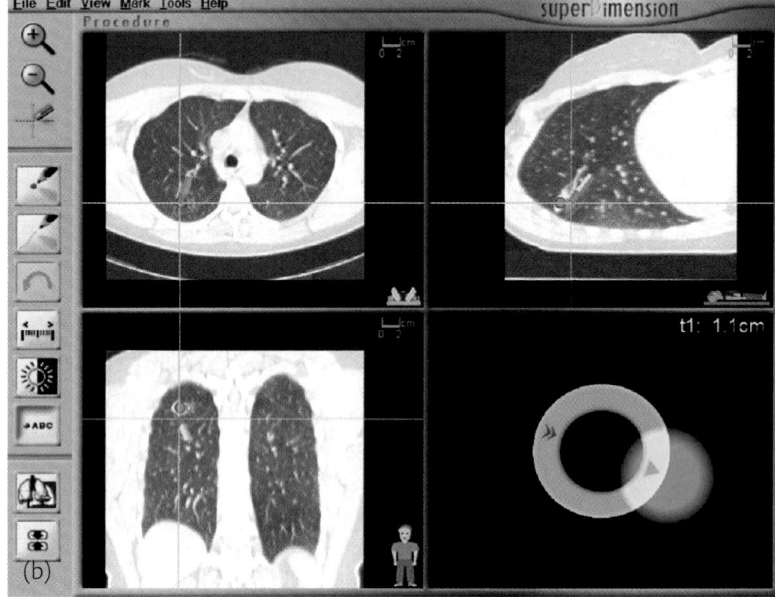

Fig. 18.3.3.3 Magnetic navigation-guided bronchoscopy: (a) screen shot during planning stage with virtual bronchoscopy and CT images; (b) screen shot of procedure stage which demonstrates the location of the magnetic tracker in relation to the target lesion.

Fluorescence bronchoscopy

Fluorescence bronchoscopy, currently a research tool, is directed to the early detection of lung cancer. It utilizes the finding that normal tissue emits a green fluorescence when illuminated by a light of blue wavelength, whereas dysplastic or cancerous tissue absorbs this fluorescence and appears reddish brown in colour. These changes are not visible to the unaided eye but can be visualized with the use of appropriate filters and image enhancement. Fluorescence bronchoscopy is significantly more sensitive at detecting severe dysplasia and carcinoma *in situ* than conventional white light bronchoscopy, but inflammatory lesions and metaplastic changes also appear abnormal; hence specificity is low and false-positive results are a limiting factor.

Diagnostic role of bronchoscopy in lung diseases

Lung cancer

Suspected lung cancer is one of the main indications for bronchoscopy, the value of which in the diagnosis of central lesions is self evident. Although the diagnostic rate is much lower in peripheral lesions, a variety of techniques such as bronchoalveolar lavage, fluoroscopic biopsy, and magnetic navigation-guided biopsy can improve this. Where there is mediastinal adenopathy, consideration should be given to sampling of these lymph nodes by transbronchial needle aspiration with, where available, endoscopic ultrasound guidance.

Diagnosis and staging should be evaluated simultaneously, with every effort made to sample mediastinal lymph nodes where they are enlarged (>10 mm in short axis on CT) or where there is increased uptake on a ^{18}F-fluorodeoxyglucose positron emission tomography (FDG-PET) scan.

Diffuse lung disease

Bronchoalveolar lavage and transbronchial lung biopsies in conjunction with high-resolution CT form the basis of diagnosis for diffuse lung disease. The cell morphology of the lavage fluid is useful in the diagnosis of specific conditions (Table 18.3.3.2): in sarcoidosis there is a lymphocytic infiltrate which may demonstrate a high CD4/CD8 ratio; a mixed lymphocytosis with CD8 predominance in the presence of foamy macrophages and plasma cells is suggestive of extrinsic allergic alveolitis; haemosiderin-laden macrophages are found in alveolar haemorrhage.

Respiratory infection

Bronchial lavage is useful in the diagnosis of respiratory infection when sputum cannot be obtained. It is usually reserved for patients who are failing to respond to empirical treatment, but has a vital role in the diagnosis of pulmonary infiltrates in those who are immunocompromised. Bronchial lavage allows optimal specimens to be collected for microscopy and culture before starting antituberculous chemotherapy in patients with suspected tuberculosis who are not smear positive on sputum samples.

Therapeutic role of bronchoscopy in lung diseases

Lung cancer

About 30% of patients with lung cancer present with advanced disease that involves the trachea or main bronchi. They develop symptoms such as breathlessness, cough, and haemoptysis, and are prone to recurrent pneumonia. Progressive symptoms of respiratory failure and recurrent endobronchial sepsis lead to death. Endobronchial metastases from other tumour sites have a similar effect.

Bronchoscopy can have an important palliative role in the treatment of tumours that are accessible via the bronchoscope. A number of techniques allow tumour debulking and restoration of airway patency, but these are generally underutilized and most patients only receive external beam radiation or chemotherapy. Tumours can be debulked by flexible bronchoscopy using electrocautery, argon plasma coagulation, neodymium YAG laser, photodynamic therapy, and cryotherapy, most of which can be performed on a day-case basis in the endoscopy suite under conscious sedation. Improving access to these techniques in the palliation of endobronchial malignancy should improve survival.

In selected patients debulking may need to be combined with the insertion of self-expanding metal stents, the key indication being where there is significant airway narrowing due to extrinsic compression by tumour, or where the airway structure has been destroyed by the cancer. In both situations a stent attempts to improve airway patency by exerting an outward radial force. Covered stents can also be used to seal off airway fistulas and also prevent tumour ingress into the airway. However, the use of airway stents is associated with important complications including displacement and endoluminal wall damage, mucus impaction, granuloma formation, reobstruction, infection, halitosis due to biofouling, haemoptysis, pain, cough, and stent fracture.

Emphysema

Dynamic airway collapse in emphysema in conjunction with bullous lung disease leads to significant air trapping, flattened diaphragms, impaired respiratory muscle dynamics and breathlessness. Lung volume reduction surgery has been shown to be effective in patients with upper lobe emphysema and poor baseline exercise tolerance. In selected patients bronchoscopic lung volume reduction can be performed with much lower morbidity and mortality than are associated with open surgical procedures. Two main devices are available: one is a valve that is placed in a segmental bronchus and allows air and secretions to drain, but prevents air from entering into that lung segment (Fig. 18.3.3.4a); the other is

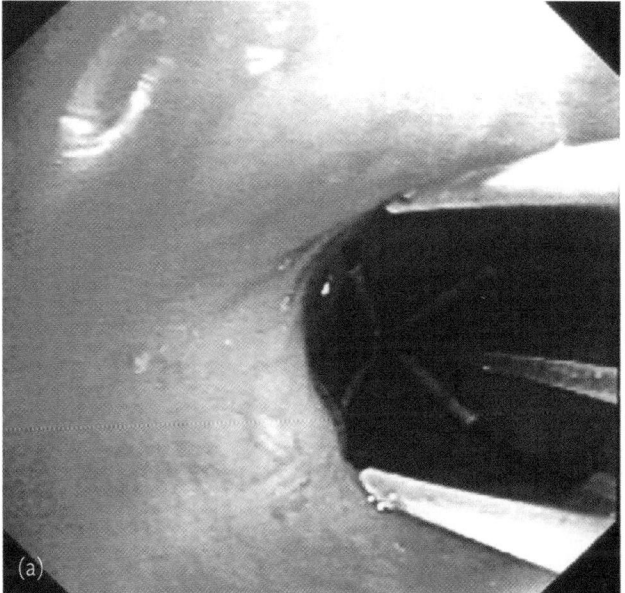

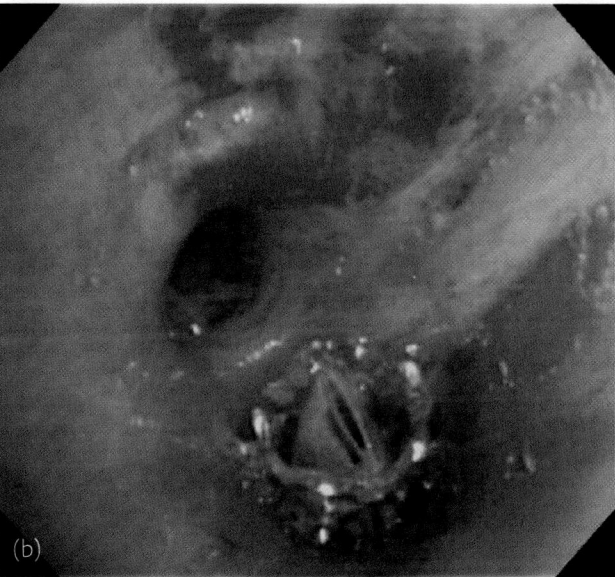

Fig. 18.3.3.4 (a) A catheter delivering thermal energy during bronchoscopy in an asthmatic patient (b) image of a valve in-situ in a patient undergoing bronchoscopic lung volume reduction.

an umbrella-like device (intrabronchial valve) that acts in a similar manner by blocking air from entering and allowing the drainage of secretions. Both methods are currently being used in clinical trials, with results thus far suggesting that segmental collapse is achieved in about 20% of patients, but improvements in exercise capacity and quality of life are observed in over one-third of patients treated.

A different approach, in which artificial airways are created between pockets of trapped gas and the segmental airways, has been developed for patients with homogenous emphysema. The technique identifies avascular areas in the airway with the use of Doppler ultrasound and employs a needle to create a hole measuring up to 5 mm in diameter, which is then maintained with a drug-eluting stent. These new airway passages allow trapped gas to escape and hence reduce lung volume. Preliminary reports suggest physiological improvements in lung volumes, exercise capacity and quality of life.

Asthma

Bronchial thermoplasty is a promising bronchoscopic treatment for asthma (Fig. 18.3.3.4b). The technique involves the application of thermal energy under direct vision to the wall of airways more than 3 mm in size, leading to a reduction in smooth muscle. Clinical studies have shown significant improvements in bronchial hyper-reactivity (as measured by methacholine challenge), spirometry, and asthma-related quality of life measures.

Thoracoscopy

Thoracoscopy is a simple invasive procedure which can safely be performed under local anaesthesia with or without conscious sedation. It provides excellent direct visualization of the pleural cavity.

Indications

The commonest indication for medical thoracoscopy is evaluation of an exudative pleural effusion when cytological analysis of aspirated fluid does not provide a conclusive diagnosis. It allows direct visualization of the pleura and targeted biopsies of any abnormal areas, and in experienced hands has a diagnostic sensitivity of 90 to 95%. It is also a key investigation in the assessment of patients with repeated pneumothoraces or a persistent air leak, and it is also used in some centres for the assessment of interstitial lung disease.

Contraindications

The main contraindication to thoracoscopy is absence of an adequate pleural space due to adhesions or previous surgery. Relative contraindications are a bleeding diathesis (INR >1.4), pulmonary hypertension, severe cardiac disease, or hypoxia. An uncontrolled cough or inability to lie still makes the procedure difficult and is another relative contraindication. However, as with bronchoscopy, the risk and benefits of the procedure should be evaluated for the individual patient.

Equipment

The basic equipment comprises of a rigid thoracoscope with a 9 or 11 mm diameter. These instruments have a variety of optics that allow straight and angled examination, and there are also integrated biopsy forceps with optics that allow accurate biopsy under direct vision. Other essential pieces of equipment include special needles (Verres or Deneke) for inducing an artificial pneumothorax in the absence of a pleural effusion. A gas insufflator is used to fill the pleural space with carbon dioxide or another gas to create a large enough space to facilitate inspection of the pleural cavity. The key precaution is to avoid inducing an artificial tension pneumothorax.

Sterilization

As thoracoscopy is an invasive procedure, it is not adequate to simply disinfect equipment as in bronchoscopy—all of the equipment used has to be sterilized by autoclaving.

Patient preparation and basic procedure

Patient preparation is as for flexible bronchoscopy. The procedure can be performed with local anaesthesia, with or without conscious sedation. Patients are fasted for at least 4 to 6 h beforehand, and oxygen saturation, ECG, and blood pressure are monitored during thoracoscopy. Aseptic conditions are required: operators should wash their hands thoroughly and use sterile gloves and gowns. The patient is usually placed in the lateral decubitus position and the entry site is cleaned with chlorhexidine, with appropriate sterile drapes placed around.

The access site is usually the 4th or 5th intercostal space in the midaxillary line, the exact entry port being influenced by the indication for the procedure and also guided by imaging such as CT or ultrasonography. The pleura is visualized and appears as a delicate, transparent, light-reflecting surface with a fine network of blood vessels within it. Any changes in its surface are recorded, varying from areas of increased vascularity or localized thickening to diffuse changes, and there may be obvious nodules or tumour deposits. An angle telescope is often used to inspect the far reaches of the thoracic cavity such as the apex, interlobar space, paravertebral gutter, and mediastinal surfaces.

Any fluid present can be sampled and sent for appropriate investigations, including cytology, and any areas of localized diffuse thickening may be biopsied. Whatever the visual findings, the parietal pleura should usually be biopsied, with care taken to obtain samples from the upper border of the ribs to avoid the neurovascular bundle that runs along the lower margin. It is possible to obtain visceral pleural biopsies and lung biopsies during thoracoscopy, but they carry a greater risk of bleeding and/or inducing a persistent air leak.

The main complications of thoracoscopy are bleeding and prolonged air leaks. Bleeding can usually be controlled by coagulation with either electrocautery or argon plasma photocoagulation. An intercostal drain should be placed whenever biopsy of the visceral pleura or lung has been performed. Serious but less common complications include secondary infection, mediastinal or subcutaneous emphysema, and air embolism. Re-expansion oedema is a theoretical risk, particularly in patients with long-standing effusions: this can be minimized with slow intercostal tube drainage and carefully managed re-expansion of the lung.

Therapeutic role of thoracoscopy

The most common therapeutic indication for thoracoscopy is in the treatment of a malignant pleural effusion. The procedure allows the even application of sclerosing agents such as talc on the pleural surface and is very successful in combination with tube drainage. Thoracoscopy also has a role in the management of spontaneous pneumothorax: small blebs may be identified and obliterated with argon plasma photocoagulation or electrocautery, usually combined with pleurodesis. It also has a therapeutic role in empyema and tuberculous pleuritis, where it can be used to break up adhesions and facilitate drainage of effusion.

Video-assisted thoracic surgery (VATS)

VATS is increasingly used in the management of patients with pleural disease (see Chapter 18.17) and also allows lung biopsy or resection in some patients in whom an open procedure would be high risk because of poor lung function. Under general anaesthesia the ipsilateral lung is collapsed with the use of a double lumen endotracheal tube, and a stab incision with adjacent instrument ports is made in the 6th or 7th intercostal space in the midaxillary line (Fig. 18.3.3.5). In other respects the technique is similar to standard thoracoscopy. Pulmonary tube drainage is required after

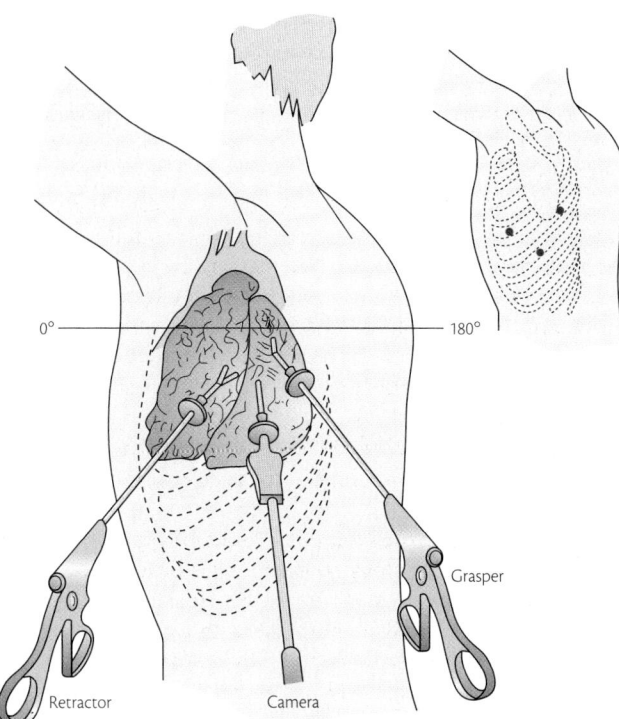

Fig. 18.3.3.5 The arrangement of ports for video-assisted thoracic surgery (VATS). The principal access is in the midaxillary line.

the procedure, but hospital stay is shorter than after standard surgical thoracotomy.

Percutaneous biopsy

Pleural biopsy

The use of 'blind' (unguided) pleural biopsy is diminishing: wherever possible, pleural biopsies should be performed with image guidance.

Traditionally, pleural biopsy was performed using an Abrams needle, which has three components: an outer trochar with a notch on its side near the distal tip, an inner cutting cannula that interlocks with the trochar, and a central stylette. A 5 mm incision is made in the skin surface and the whole unit is inserted carefully through the intercostal space just above a rib. The central stylette is withdrawn and the inner cannula is rotated anticlockwise and withdrawn slightly. Aspiration of pleural fluid confirms position in the pleural space. The Abrams needle is then angulated and slowly withdrawn to catch a small piece of pleura within the notch of the trochar, at which point the inner cannula is rotated and moved forwards to cut off and retain the specimen. There are a number of variants of the Abrams needle, such as the Cope needle and the Radja needle, but they all obtain a biopsy by tearing or shearing a piece of pleura.

The blind nature of the procedure and the shearing technique for obtaining a biopsy specimen result in a variable diagnostic yield and a complication rate of 15%, with more serious consequences in about 0.1% of procedures. These range from haemorrhage and pneumothorax to laceration of adjacent organs such as the liver, spleen, and kidneys.

Blind pleural biopsy has largely been superseded by CT or ultrasound-guided procedures, and wherever possible by thoracoscopy. The Tru-cut needle is favoured by many radiologists and

comprises an outer cutting column and an inner trochar that has a notch within which the biopsy material is collected.

Percutaneous lung biopsy

Percutaneous biopsies are primarily performed in the assessment of pulmonary nodules for suspected malignancy. They are a particularly important tool in the assessment of patients who are borderline candidates for surgery due to comorbidity or disease extent, but are less appropriate where a patient is operable and the nodule is considered highly likely to be cancer. Large masses may be more safely sampled with bronchoscopic techniques. Sampling of enlarged hilar or mediastinal lymph nodes should be considered as alternative sites for tissue biopsy and have the advantage of providing staging as well as diagnostic information.

The main contraindications to percutaneous lung biopsy are poor respiratory reserve (FEV_1 <1 litre) and bleeding diathesis (INR >1.4). Relative contraindications are extensive bullous emphysema, intractable cough, patients who are unable to lie still, pulmonary hypertension, and contralateral pneumonectomy.

Fine-needle aspirates can be used to diagnose malignancy but are very poor at firmly diagnosing benign conditions. The use of cutting needles, which obtain a core of tissue, provides greater diagnostic confidence. Under CT guidance the needle is placed so that when the needle tip is fired its distal position remains within the mass being sampled (Fig. 18.3.3.6), care being taken to avoid blood vessels, pulmonary fissures, bullae, and adjacent organs. The outer sheath is held in position after initial biopsy so that the procedure can be repeated and further samples obtained without the need to perform repeated needle punctures.

Pneumothoraces and haemorrhage are the two main complications of percutaneous biopsy, the frequency of which is influenced by the size, depth and position of the mass. The presence of parenchymal lung disease, particularly emphysema, also influences the incidence of pneumothoraces. Air embolism is a rare but serious complication and can occur if the needle lies within the pulmonary vein.

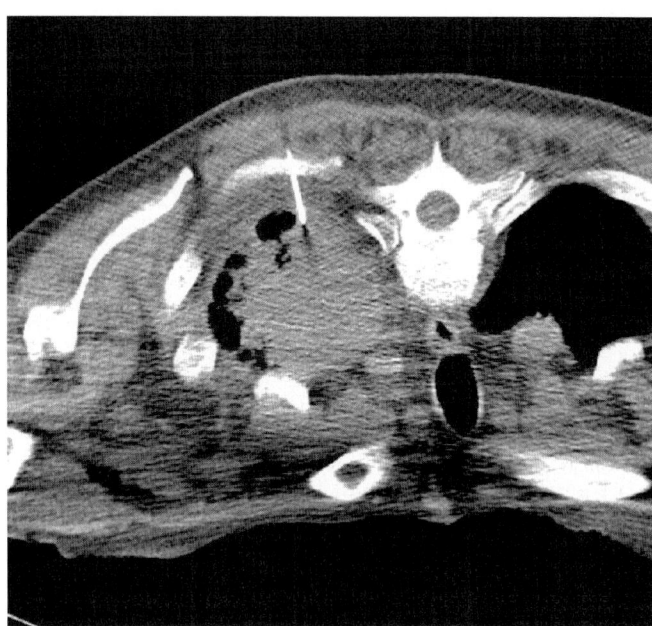

Fig. 18.3.3.6 CT-guided Tru-cut needle biopsy of a left upper lobe mass.

Further reading

Baaklini WA, *et al.* (2000). Diagnostic yield of fiberoptic bronchoscopy in evaluating solitary pulmonary nodules. *Chest*, **117**, 1049–54.

Bolliger CT, *et al.* (2006). Therapeutic bronchoscopy with immediate effect: laser, electrocautery, argon plasma coagulation and stents. *Eur Respir J*, **27**, 1258–71.

British Thoracic Society Bronchoscopy Guidelines Committee, a Subcommittee of the Standards of Care Committee of the British Thoracic Society (2001). British Thoracic Society guidelines on diagnostic flexible bronchoscopy. *Thorax*, **56** Suppl 1, i1–21.

Dasgupta A, *et al.* (1999). Utility of transbronchial needle aspiration in the diagnosis of endobronchial lesions. *Chest*, **115**, 1237–41.

Davenport RD (1990). Rapid on-site evaluation of transbronchial aspirates. *Chest*, **98**, 59–61.

Harrow EM, *et al.* (2000). The utility of transbronchial needle aspiration in the staging of bronchogenic carcinoma. *Am J Respir Crit Care Med*, **161** (2 Pt 1), 601–7.

Herth FJ, *et al.* (2006). Real-time endobronchial ultrasound guided transbronchial needle aspiration for sampling mediastinal lymph nodes. *Thorax*, **61**, 795–8.

Herth FJ, Eberhardt R, Ernst A (2006). The future of bronchoscopy in diagnosing, staging and treatment of lung cancer. *Respiration*, **73**, 399–409.

Krasnik M, *et al.* (2003). Preliminary experience with a new method of endoscopic transbronchial real-time ultrasound guided biopsy for diagnosis of mediastinal and hilar lesions. *Thorax*, **58**, 1083–6.

Kurimoto N, *et al.* (2004). Endobronchial ultrasonography using a guide sheath increases the ability to diagnose peripheral pulmonary lesions endoscopically. *Chest*, **126**, 959–65.

Lam WK, *et al.* (1983). Fibreoptic bronchoscopy in the diagnosis of bronchial cancer: comparison of washings, brushings and biopsies in central and peripheral tumours. *Clin Oncol*, **9**, 35–42.

Lam S, *et al.* (1998). Localization of bronchial intraepithelial neoplastic lesions by fluorescence bronchoscopy. *Chest*, **113**, 696–702.

Laroche C, *et al.* (2000). Role of computed tomographic scanning of the thorax prior to bronchoscopy in the investigation of suspected lung cancer. *Thorax*, **55**, 359–63.

Manhire A, *et al.* (2003). Guidelines for radiologically guided lung biopsy. *Thorax*, **58**, 920–36.

Prakash UB, Offord KP, Stubbs SE (1991). Bronchoscopy in North America: the ACCP Survey. *Chest*, **100**, 1668–75.

Reichenberger F, *et al.* (1999). The value of transbronchial needle aspiration in the diagnosis of peripheral pulmonary lesions. *Chest*, **116**, 704–8.

Schreiber G, McCrory DC (2003). Performance characteristics of different modalities for diagnosis of suspected lung cancer: summary of published evidence. *Chest*, **123** Suppl 1, 115S–128S.

Shah PL, *et al.* (2006). The role of transbronchial fine needle aspiration (TBNA) in an integrated care pathway for the assessment of patients with suspected lung cancer. *J Thoracic Oncol*, **1**, 324–7.

Tassi GF, Davies RJ, Noppen M (2006). Advanced techniques in medical thoracoscopy. *Eur Respir J*, **28**, 1051–9.

Vergnon JM, Huber RM, Moghissi K (2006). Place of cryotherapy, brachytherapy and photodynamic therapy in therapeutic bronchoscopy of lung cancers. *Eur Respir J*, **28**, 200–18.

Yasufuku K, *et al.* (2004). Real-time endobronchial ultrasound-guided transbronchial needle aspiration of mediastinal and hilar lymph nodes. *Chest*, **126**, 122–8.

Respiratory infection

Contents

18.4.1 Upper respiratory tract infections

P. Little

Essentials

Acute upper respiratory tract infections (URTIs) are the commonest reason for patients to seek medical advice in the United Kingdom.

Pharyngitis/tonsillitis—this is caused by both bacterial and viral organisms, with sore throat often accompanied by fever, headache, and other symptoms, with or without enlarged and tender cervical lymph nodes, tonsillar erythema, and exudate. Investigations are not generally performed or required. Antibiotics have modest benefit, so for patients who are not unwell systemically the physician should either not prescribe, or use a delayed prescribing approach, advising the patient to wait for several days before collecting or using their prescription. The antibiotic of choice is probably penicillin V, with a short acting macrolide the second-line agent. The benefits of tonsillectomy in preventing recurrent sore throat are modest.

Acute rhinitis—causes nasal congestion and rhinorrhoea, mild malaise, sneezing, sore throat, variable loss of taste and smell, and usually recovers within two weeks. Oral and topical decongestants can help symptoms; echinacea and antibiotics can provide modest benefit.

Acute sinusitis—usually defined as an infection that lasts for less than three weeks, is an uncommon complication of coryzal illness and pharyngitis. Diagnosis based on a clinical risk score is as sensitive and specific as any other method. The effectiveness of antibiotic or other treatments is questionable.

Introduction

Acute upper respiratory tract infections (URTIs) include acute pharyngitis/tonsillitis and acute rhinitis. Acute sinusitis, acute otitis media, and influenza also come under the umbrella of infections of the upper respiratory tract. Otitis media and influenza will be discussed elsewhere: this chapter concentrates on acute pharyngitis/tonsillitis, acute rhinitis, and acute sinusitis.

Acute URTIs are the commonest reason for patients to seek medical advice in the United Kingdom, and nearly all cases are managed in primary care. Respiratory tract infections are also the commonest reason for antibiotics to be prescribed, leading to serious concern that the inappropriate use of antibiotics for predominantly self-limiting conditions will foster the development of antibiotic resistance, with the danger that serious infections will become untreatable. Thus it is currently an international priority to discourage the use of antibiotics where there is poor evidence of their efficacy. The evidence for the effectiveness of treatments for URTI in this chapter comes from a search of the Cochrane Library databases of systematic reviews and randomized controlled trials.

Pharyngitis/tonsillitis

Clinical presentation

Pharyngitis is caused by both bacterial and viral organisms, and has been somewhat arbitrarily divided into nasopharyngitis (with nasal symptoms, i.e. rhinitis), and pharyngitis or tonsillopharyngitis (without nasal symptoms). Causal organisms include: group A β-haemolytic streptococcus; adenoviruses; influenza A and B; parainfluenza 1, 2, 3; Epstein–Barr virus (EBV); enteroviruses; *Mycoplasma pneumoniae*; and *Chlamydia pneumoniae*.

In addition to a sore throat, pharyngitis is often accompanied by fever, headache, nausea, vomiting, anorexia, and sometimes abdominal pain, with or without enlarged and tender cervical lymph nodes, tonsillar erythema and exudate. Scarlet fever has a characteristic 'scarlatiform' rash caused by group A β-haemolytic streptococcal exotoxins. Infectious mononucleosis due to EBV may present with or without exudative tonsillitis, cervical or general lymphadenopathy, palatal petechiae, splenomegaly, rhinitis, and cough.

Throat swabs, rapid tests, and clinical algorithms

Antibiotics can be targeted to those patients who have positive throat swabs for group A streptococcus, a positive rapid streptococcal test, or clinical characteristics associated with a positive throat swab (e.g. the Centor criteria of fever, tonsillar exudate, anterior cervical adenopathy, and absence of cough). However, the throat swab has limitations: in both unselected and clinically selected populations in primary care practice it is neither particularly sensitive nor specific when compared to a rise in antistreptolysin O titres (ASOT) or anti-DNAse B titres. A rise in ASOT or anti-DNAase B is probably a better indicator of serious infection and predicts complications, but these are not suitable for clinical diagnosis. The results of throat swabs take days to return to the clinic, and they greatly increase the costs of managing what is mostly a self-limiting condition. Furthermore, evidence suggests that in practice clinicians do not use the results, even of rapid tests, and that the overall accuracy of decision-making is little changed when they are used.

Attempts to derive algorithms or clinical decision rules based on the throat swab have the same limitations of validity as the throat swab itself. Although clinical scoring methods may provide a crude method of identifying patients at a higher risk of complications (see below), better evidence is needed of the effects of using such scoring methods in practice.

Treatment

Antibiotics for symptoms

The Cochrane review of the efficacy of antibiotics for the treatment of sore throat indicates that antibiotics have modest benefit in reducing the duration of symptoms—by approximately 16h for an illness lasting on average 8 days in total—and even less for trials which did not restrict selection according to the results of throat swabs. This marginal benefit of antibiotics in resolving symptoms suggests that, for patients who are not unwell systemically, the physician should either not prescribe, or use a delayed prescribing approach, advising the patient to wait for several days before collecting or using their prescription. Both these approaches have been shown in a large randomized controlled trial to be acceptable, to change attitudes and behaviour, and not to delay symptom resolution appreciably (Fig. 18.4.1.1).

In the context of a likely streptococcal infection, trial evidence suggests that delaying the prescription results in 20% fewer recurrences than the immediate prescriptions of antibiotics, presumably because antibiotics modify local or systemic immune mechanisms. Thus, any marginal symptomatic benefit from an immediate prescription of antibiotics for the current illness must be weighed against the disadvantage that the patient is more likely to suffer symptoms from a recurrence.

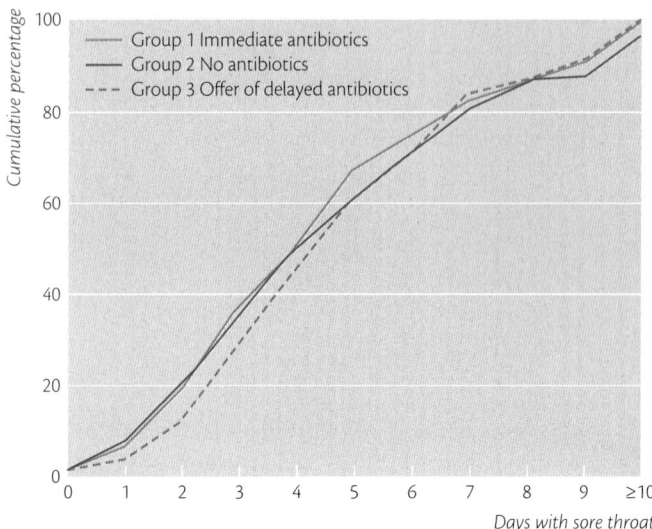

Fig. 18.4.1.1 A trial of three pragmatic antibiotic prescribing strategies: the graphs show the percentage of patients cured in the days following seeing the doctor. Reproduced from BMJ, Little *et al*, 314, 722–7, copyright 1997 with permission from BMJ Publishing Group Ltd.

Antibiotics to prevent complications

The Cochrane review of antibiotics for treating a sore throat supports the use of antibiotics to prevent complications, but the evidence is limited by both clinical importance and generalizability. For the commoner complications, e.g. otitis media, 200 people would have to be treated to prevent one case of a self-limiting illness: in other words, it is not important clinically. For the rarer complications—rheumatic fever and glomerulonephritis—the evidence is not generalizable; for instance, evidence of efficacy in rheumatic fever is based largely on trials where intramuscular penicillin was used in barracked military personnel after the Second World War. This evidence cannot be sensibly applied to modern settings where the attack rate is much lower and oral antibiotics are used. However, the benefits of antibiotics are likely to be greater in settings where complications are much more common.

The commonest complication of practical importance to health services is quinsy (peritonsillar abcess), but this is still relatively uncommon—about 1 in 400 following presentation in primary care with sore throat. The Cochrane systematic review, which demonstrates that antibiotics prevent quinsy, relies on data from patients with tonsillitis who were systemically unwell enough to be admitted to hospital shortly after the Second World War, when the prevalence of quinsy in untreated patients was very high (1 in 18). Clearly, this data cannot be extrapolated to patients presenting from modern populations who are not systemically unwell, treated with oral antibiotics, and where the prevalence of quinsy is much lower. Quinsy following sore throat is possibly slightly more common (1 in 60) in those who are unwell, with three out of four Centor criteria, most of whom have fever. Rigorously conducted placebo-controlled trials in patients with these criteria suggest quinsy may be prevented by oral penicillin, but in routine clinical practice, where compliance is not assessed, the preventive benefit of penicillin is not likely to be 100%, as reported in the trials where compliance was assured. There are limited routine data which suggest that many patients who develop quinsy after being seen in primary care do this despite being given penicillin. Whether using the clinical Centor criteria is better than the primary care physician's assessment of how unwell patients are is unclear: 20% of those considered 'not to be very unwell systemically' by the physician will still have three out of four of the Centor criteria, and we have limited data to assess whether the criteria predict the very few individuals who will develop quinsy. Thus, where the primary care physician judges the patient to be both systemically unwell and/or have three out of four of the Centor criteria, it would be reasonable to treat with penicillin, or at least discuss with patients the likely risks of nontreatment. There is some observational evidence to suggest that there has been no increase in admissions with quinsy since the uptake of the delayed-prescribing strategy in the United Kingdom.

Lemierre syndrome—a rare complication

This syndrome, caused by fusobacterium—an anaerobe that is part of normal throat flora—has been highlighted recently following a rise in reports between 1990 and 2000 to about 20 per year in the United Kingdom. A patient with pharyngitis does not improve, remains pyrexial, and develops pharyngeal swelling due to a local abscess. Internal jugular thrombosis or embolism to the lungs commonly occurs or is suspected, and in such cases prompt referral to hospital is needed. The condition responds to metronidazole, but—since the differential diagnosis is incipient quinsy—high-dose penicillin should also probably be given. All the isolates in recent case series have been sensitive to metronidazole, 2% resistant to penicillin, and 15% resistant to erythromycin. However, to encourage increased prescribing of antibiotics on the basis of an increase in Lemierre's syndrome is unwarranted: it would increase the dangers of both resistance and anaphylaxis—and anaphylaxis, although rare, is still commoner than Lemierre's syndrome.

Which antibiotic and for how long?

A systematic review has concluded that cephalosporins may provide some additional benefit to penicillin in streptococcal tonsillitis. However, there are several problems with advocating cephalosporin use as first-line agents: the extra benefit is small (85.8% vs 93.6% clinical cure); the trial data assume that the subgroup of patients with streptococcal infections has been identified, so the effect will be less in unselected patients; and whether cephalosporins provide additional benefit to a high dose of penicillin V is unclear. Thus penicillin is probably still the best first-choice antibiotic.

If an oral antibiotic is to be prescribed, then it is probably preferable to give a narrow-spectrum antibiotic (penicillin V) to minimize side effects and the risk of resistance developing. If penicillin V is used, there are arguments for using a large dose given the variable absorption (e.g. 2 g/day adults and 1 g/day children). A 10-day course will better eradicate streptococcus, but the clinical significance of this is unclear. Longer courses have the disadvantage of poorer compliance, and greater likelihood of antibiotic resistance developing in the long term. Twice-daily dosing of penicillin V compared with the same total dose over four doses per day may result in better compliance and better clinical/microbiological outcomes. Intramuscular injection of penicillin can be used, although in practice is rarely employed in the United Kingdom. Ampicillin will cause a rash in patients with infectious mononucleosis, so erythromycin is a suitable second-line agent among patients with penicillin allergy.

Treatment of patients with rheumatic fever

Patients who have had one attack of rheumatic fever are at a higher risk from new infections since they are likely to develop recurrent attacks of rheumatic fever and complications. Although most of the evidence for the prevention of rheumatic fever comes from old trials in unusual settings, it seems reasonable to treat patients with a past history who are at a high risk of recurrence and secondary complications, since what evidence there is suggests penicillin prevents rheumatic fever. (See Chapter 16.9.1 for further discussion of the issues involved.)

Other medical treatments

Treatment with aspirin in children is contraindicated because of the small but avoidable risk of Reye's syndrome. There are several trials of the use of nonsteroidal antiinflammatory drugs (NSAIDs) in providing effective relief of pain and fever in tonsillitis and pharyngitis. However, the limited trial evidence comparing them with standard treatment (paracetamol) does not clearly demonstrate their superiority. Limited trial data suggest that other useful analgesic adjuncts may include caffeine, and benzydamine hydrochloride gargle. There is also evidence from a systematic review that patients with more severe presentations who are receiving antibiotics may benefit from steroids. However, there is probably less benefit from oral steroids compared with parenteral preparations, and the effectiveness of steroids when no antibiotics are prescribed and in less severe presentations is unknown.

Recurrent attacks

Surgery

A Cochrane review has assessed the role of surgery for recurrent sore throat. The much-quoted Paradise trial, documented in the Cochrane review, assessed tonsillectomy for selected children with severe symptoms defined by the 'Paradise' criteria as meaning seven or more episodes of well-documented, clinically important and adequately treated throat infection in the preceding year, or five or more times per year for each of the preceding 2 years, or three or more times per year for each of the preceding 3 years. The study found approximately one less episode of throat infection rated as moderate or severe per child in the surgical group, but the trial was small and was criticized by the Cochrane review for imbalances of important baseline characteristics, although these are perhaps unlikely to affect the inferences. Other trial evidence has shown that for children with moderately frequent throat infections (on average three in the previous year) a wait-and-see approach results in acceptable symptom control, although those with more than three infections per year had some benefit from immediate operation—one fewer episode of sore throat. When discussing options with parents the modest benefits of surgery must be weighed against its disadvantages: tonsillectomy will result in considerable postoperative pain and some complications (4–7% requiring operative surgery for haemorrhage, or other significant symptoms such as severe nausea and dehydration).

Other treatments

There is preliminary trial evidence for the use of α-streptococci spray, immune stimulants, and pneumococcal vaccination, but further confirmation is required.

Nasal congestion and rhinorrhoea

Nasal symptoms are a common reason for attending the doctor. They may be due to a variety of causes—commonly acute viral infection (common cold), allergic rhinitis and sinusitis, vasomotor rhinitis and rhinitis medicamentosa, and less commonly atrophic rhinitis, hormonal rhinitis, and mechanical/obstructive rhinitis. Colds are responsible for significant morbidity: on average there are 0.4 episodes and 1.2 days of restricted activity per person per year for the common cold.

Acute rhinitis

Symptoms are acute nasal congestion and rhinorrhoea, mild malaise, sneezing, sore throat, variable loss of taste and smell, and usually last from 1 to 2 weeks unless sinusitis is present. Examination reveals a hyperaemic and oedematous mucosa, with or without purulent secretions.

Treatment

Symptomatic

Trial evidence supports the use of both oral and topical decongestants for the symptoms of rhinitis. Intranasal ipratropium bromide is also effective symptomatic treatment, but is only available (in the United Kingdom) on prescription. However, topical decongestants should probably not be used for more than a maximum of 7 days: rhinitis medicamentosa starts to develop at 10 days. Because of their moderate systemic effects, care should be taken with oral decongestants in patients with heart disease and hypertension. Saline drops are commonly advocated, but saline or medicated nose drops have been shown to be ineffective in trials in both children and adults. A Cochrane review suggests that steam may provide some relief of symptoms.

Antibiotics

The use of antibiotics for the common cold has been assessed in a Cochrane systematic review and shown to provide modest benefit.

Other

Reviews of trials indicate little benefit from antihistamines or zinc lozenges. A Cochrane review of the herb echinacea demonstrated positive results in most studies, but there was not enough evidence to recommend the use of a specific product.

Acute sinusitis

Diagnosis

Acute sinusitis, usually defined as an infection that lasts for less than 3 weeks, is an uncommon complication of coryzal illness and pharyngitis. There is no absolute standard against which symptoms and signs can be compared for accuracy of diagnosis: aspiration by sinus puncture is probably the definitive investigation, since it indicates the presence of infecting organisms, but for obvious reasons this is rarely performed, and contamination by commensal organisms can occur.

Four-view radiographs show acceptable agreement with aspiration and culture, although only moderate interobserver agreement. The United States Agency for Health Care and Policy Research has reviewed the diagnosis and treatment of sinusitis: combining all studies comparing sinus radiographs with sinus puncture demonstrated a sensitivity of 73% and specificity of 80%. A history of purulent nasal discharge, maxillary toothache, purulent secretions on examination, poor response to decongestants, and abnormal illumination of the sinuses, are all predictive of sinusitis defined using four-view radiographs as the standard: four or more

symptoms or signs giving a likelihood ratio of a positive test of 6. A problem with sinus illumination as a diagnostic tool in primary care is that it performs differently in different settings, probably due to operator sensitivity. There is preliminary evidence comparing symptoms with CT as the 'standard', which is justified since the presence of fluid and total opacification of the sinuses on CT predicts antibiotic response. Purulent rhinorrhoea, purulent secretion in the cavum nasae, a history of 'double sickening' (getting better, then getting worse again), and an erythrocyte sedimentation rate higher than 10 are predictive of a CT diagnosis of sinusitis—three of these features giving a likelihood ratio of a positive test of 1.8.

However, using a four-item clinical risk score—of purulent rhinorrhoea with unilateral predominance, local pain with unilateral predominance, bilateral purulent rhinorrhoea, and presence of pus in the nasal cavity—is as sensitive and specific as any other method in predicting the results of sinus puncture. Thus, for acute sinusitis, diagnostic tests are not currently indicated, and until valid nearpatient tests are available, clinical targeting probably performs as well as any other method.

Treatment

Antibiotics

A Cochrane review of all controlled trials suggests that the absolute benefit for symptom resolution is moderate, and must be balanced against the disadvantages of prescribing antibiotics. Furthermore, this review mostly includes trials where there was radiological confirmation—which is not appropriate for diagnosis in primary care—and does not include all the trials from primary care, which show moderate or no effect. An IPD (individual patient data) meta-analysis of trials using a clinical diagnosis documented a number needed to treat of 15 for all patients and 8 for those with purulence, and no greater benefit for those with symptoms for longer than a week. Thus both the effectiveness and cost-effectiveness of antibiotic treatment of acute sinusitis in primary care is questionable for most patients.

Other

Preliminary trial evidence shows that decongestants are unlikely to be helpful. There is limited evidence that antihistamines may be helpful for patients with a history of allergic rhinitis who develop sinusitis, and some evidence that proteolytics (e.g. bromelain) and mucolytics may help. There is mixed trial evidence for the benefit of topical steroids. Although trials of NSAIDs suggest they are helpful, they may not be significantly more effective than paracetamol.

Further reading

Systematic review of diagnosis of sore throat

Del Mar C (1992). Managing sore throat: a literature review. I: Making the diagnosis. *Med J Austral*, **156**, 572–5.

Antibiotics and recurrent sore throat, the 'medicalizing' effect of prescribing antibiotics, and the use of delayed prescriptions

Little PS, *et al.* (1997). An open randomised trial of prescribing strategies for sore throat. *BMJ*, **314**, 722–7.

Little PS, *et al.* (1997). Reattendance and complications in a randomised trial of prescribing strategies for sore throat: the medicalising effect of prescribing antibiotics. *BMJ*, **315**, 350–2.

Use of the 'Centor' criteria to target antibiotic prescribing for sore throat

Zwart S, *et al.* (2000). Penicillin for acute sore throat: randomised double blind trial of seven days versus three days treatment or placebo in adults. *BMJ*, **320**, 150–4.

Diagnosis and treatment of sinusitis

US Department of Health and Human Services (1999). *Evidence report/ technology assessment number 9: diagnosis and treatment of acute bacterial rhinosinusitis.* AHCPR, Rockville, MD.

Young J, *et al.* (2008). Antibiotics for adults with clinically diagnosed acute rhinosinusitis: a meta-analysis of individual patient data. *Lancet*, **371**, 908–14.

Diagnosis and management of rhinitis

Joint Task Force on Practice Parameters. (2008). The diagnosis and management of rhinitis: An updated practice parameter. *J Allergy Clin Immunol*, **122**, S1–S84.

Cochrane reviews

The Cochrane Library and Cochrane reviews can be accessed online at http://www.cochrane.org

18.4.2 Pneumonia in the normal host

John G. Bartlett

Essentials

Pneumonia is an acute or chronic infection involving the pulmonary parenchyma and is the most important infectious disease in terms of morbidity and mortality, which is 14% for patients who are hospitalized with community-acquired pneumonia.

Aetiology—most cases are caused by microbial pathogens, the commonest being *Streptococcus pneumoniae*, *Haemophilus influenzae*, *Mycoplasma pneumoniae*, *Chlamydia pneumoniae*, legionella, anaerobic bacteria, and viruses (influenza, parainfluenza, and respiratory syncytial virus). *Staphylococcus aureus* is an important superinfecting pathogen in influenza, and is the most common form of embolic pulmonary infection with injection-drug use and tricuspid valve endocarditis.

Prevention—the main preventive measures are influenza and *S. pneumoniae* vaccination, the best data for the latter being in favour of giving the protein conjugated vaccine to children under 2 years of age to protect both themselves and adults.

Clinical features—the classic presentation of pneumonia is with cough and fever, with variable sputum production, dyspnoea and pleurisy. Most patients have constitutional symptoms such as malaise, fatigue and asthenia, and many also have gastrointestinal symptoms. Clinical examination may reveal features indicative of the severity of respiratory compromise—appearance of exhaustion, use of accessory muscles, inability to talk in sentences, tachypnoea (or even more worryingly

when associated with exhaustion, a low respiratory rate), cyanosis—and (in some cases) of consolidation, in particular localized dullness to percussion and bronchial breathing. The 'CURB-65' score—based on compromised Consciousness, elevated blood Urea nitrogen, increased Respiratory rate, reduced Blood pressure and age over 65 years—is a useful predictor of severity and need for hospitalization.

Diagnosis—the key test to confirm the diagnosis of pneumonia is the chest radiograph, which will virtually always show an infiltrate. Most patients with symptoms of pneumonia and a negative chest radiograph have acute bronchitis. The use of laboratory studies for identifying pulmonary pathogens in pneumonia is controversial: even in studies with extensive use of diagnostic resources a likely aetiological agent is only detected in 40 to 60% of cases. Empirical therapy is generally advocated for outpatients; blood cultures (taken before the initiation of antibiotic treatment) and Gram stain and culture of expectorated sputum (if any) are recommended for inpatients. Rapid urinary antigen tests for legionella (which detect the subgroup responsible for 80% of cases) and *S. pneumoniae* are available. Pleural effusions should be sampled to exclude empyema.

Management—supportive treatment includes (as appropriate) intravenous fluids, supplementary oxygenation and ventilatory support. Antibiotics are the mainstay of therapy, with recommendations for empirical treatment of community-acquired pneumonia typically as follows (but local hospital protocols and policies may vary): (1) outpatients—doxycycline, or macrolide (erythromycin, clarithromycin, azithromycin), or fluoroquinolone (levofloxacin, moxifloxacin or other fluoroquinolone with enhanced activity against *S. pneumoniae*); (2) general hospital inpatients—β-lactam (cefotaxime, ceftriaxone) plus macrolide, or fluoroquinolone alone; (3) intensive care unit—β-lactam plus macrolide, or β-lactam plus fluoroquinolone; (4) special circumstances: aspiration pneumonia—clindamycin, or β-lactam-β-lactamase inhibitor; structural lung disease—include agent with activity against *Pseudomonas aeruginosa*.

Introduction

Pneumonia is an acute or chronic infection involving the pulmonary parenchyma. Most cases are caused by microbial pathogens, usually bacteria or viruses and less often fungi or parasites. Pneumonia may also refer to inflammation involving the pulmonary parenchyma due to nonmicrobial causes such as chemical pneumonia. Other modifying terms are used as follows: pneumonia may be acute, subacute, or chronic, depending on the duration of symptoms; it may be described as bronchopneumonia, consolidated (lobar) pneumonia, interstitial pneumonia, or necrotizing pneumonia based on changes seen on chest radiography; or it may be named after the putative agent, e.g. pneumococcal pneumonia, mycoplasma pneumonia, pneumocystis pneumonia, etc. Pneumonia is also identified by the place of acquisition, e.g. community-acquired, nursing home-acquired, or hospital-acquired. This chapter is restricted to community-acquired pneumonia in the adult immunocompetent host.

Aetiology

Although the list of microbes that can cause pneumonia is legion, only a relatively small number are frequent pathogens, e.g.

Table 18.4.2.1 Microbiology of community-acquired pneumonia

Microbial agent	British Thoracic Society[a] (%)	Meta-analysis[b] (%)
Bacteria		
Streptococcus pneumonia	60–75	65
Haemophilus influenza	5–5	12
Staphylococcus aureus	1–5	2
Gram-negative bacilli	Rare	1
Miscellaneous agents[c]	(Not included)	3
Atypical agents	–	12
Mycoplasma pneumoniae	(Not included)	1
Viral	8–16	3
No diagnosis	–	–

[a] Estimates based on analysis of 453 adults in a prospective study of community-acquired pneumonia in 25 British hospitals.

[b] Meta-analysis of 122 reports in the English language literature, 1966–1995; the analysis is restricted to 7079 cases in which a suspected pathogen was reported.

[c] Includes *Moraxella catarrhalis*, group A streptococcus, *Neisseria meningitides*, acinetobacter, *Coxiella burnetii*, and *Chlamyidia psittaci*.

Streptococcus pneumoniae, Haemophilus influenzae, Mycoplasma pneumoniae, Chlamydia pneumoniae, legionella, anaerobic bacteria, and viruses. Less common pathogens are *Moraxella catarrhalis, S. pyogenes*, acinetobacter, *C. psittaci, Coxiella burnetii, Neisseria meningitidis, Staphylococcus aureus*, and enteric Gram-negative rods. In most reported series, each of the latter group generally accounts for less than 1 to 2% of cases. The relative frequencies of different pathogens causing community-acquired pneumonia in two large studies are summarized in Table 18.4.2.1. However, important limitations of these studies should be acknowledged: all the cases in the review conducted by the British Thoracic Society were inpatients, as were the great majority of those reviewed in the meta-analysis. Most studies of pneumonia show that only 20 to 30% of patients are sufficiently sick to require hospitalization. Furthermore, nearly all studies, including those that use extensive diagnostic resources, only identify a likely aetiological agent in 40 to 60% of cases. This suggests that fastidious microbes are under-represented, that many cases of pneumonia may be caused by as yet unidentified organisms, and that current diagnostic testing is pretty poor.

Epidemiology

Pneumonia is the most important infectious disease in terms of morbidity and mortality. It is estimated that in the United States of America there are 4 million cases of pneumonia per year (45 000 deaths), and worldwide there are 4400 million cases per year (4 million deaths). In the United States of America, data suggest that between 20 and 30% of all patients with a diagnosis of pneumonia are hospitalized, and that the mortality rate for this subpopulation is about 14%. The crude death rate from influenza and pneumonia in the United States of America for 1994 was 31.8 deaths per 100 000 of the population; this represents a 59% increase over the 20 deaths per 100 000 recorded in 1979, suggesting that the frequency of lethal pneumonia in the United States of America is increasing. Those aged 65 or older accounted for 89% of the deaths in 1994, suggesting that increases in longevity account for most of this increase in mortality rate.

Those pathogens associated with specific epidemiological and underlying conditions are summarized in Table 18.4.2.2. When an

Table 18.4.2.2 Epidemiological conditions related to specific pathogens in patients with selected community-acquired pneumonia

Condition	Commonly encountered pathogens
Alcoholism	*Streptococcus pneumoniae*, anaerobes, Gram-negative bacilli
COPD/smoker	*S. pneumoniae, H. influenzae, Moraxella catarrhalis*, legionella
Nursing-home residency	*S. pneumoniae*, Gram-negative bacilli, *H. influenzae, Staphylococcus aureus*, anaerobes, *C. pneumoniae*
Poor dental hygiene	Anaerobes
Epidemic legionnaire's disease	Legionella
Exposure to bats or soil enriched with bird droppings	*Histoplasma capsulatum*
Exposure to birds	*Chlamydia psittaci*
Exposure to rabbits	*Francisella tularensis*
HIV infection	*S. pneumoniae, Pneumocystis jirovecii, H. influenzae, Mycobacterium tuberculosis*
Exposure to farm animals or parturient cats	*Coxiella burnetii* (Q fever)
Influenza active in community	Influenza, *S. pneumoniae, Staphylococcus aureus, S. pyogenes, H. influenzae*
Suspected large-volume aspiration	Anaerobes, chemical pneumonitis, obstruction
Structural lung disease (bronchiectasis, cystic fibrosis, etc.)	*P. aeruginosa, Burkholderia (Pseudomonas) cepacia*, or *Staphylococcus aureus*
Injection drug use	*Staphylococcus aureus*, anaerobes, tuberculosis, *S. pneumoniae*
Airway obstruction	Anaerobes

COPD, chronic obstructive pulmonary disease.

(From Bartlett JG, *et al.* (2000). Community-acquired pneumonia in adults: guidelines for management. *Clin Infect Dis*, **31**, 347–82.)

aetiological agent is identified, just three microbial agents account for most lethal cases of community-acquired pneumonia. Influenza accounts for an average of 20 000 deaths per year in the United States of America: the majority involve influenza A and occur in patients over 65 years of age, and most deaths are due to complications of influenza rather than influenza *per se*. The second common cause of lethal pneumonia is pneumococcal pneumonia; risk factors for a fatal outcome include bacteraemia, advanced age, and concurrent alcoholism. Legionella is the third agent, with associated mortality rates generally reported between 5 and 15% for patients with community-acquired infections.

Nearly all studies show that the risk of death with pneumonia is strongly associated with age extremes. Concurrent conditions that contribute to increased mortality rates include neoplastic disease, hepatic failure, congestive heart failure, cerebrovascular disease, and renal disease.

Pathogenesis

As with nearly all infectious diseases, the probability of disease depends on the virulence of the organism, the inoculum size, and

Table 18.4.2.3 Predominant mechanisms of pneumonia

Pathogen	Usual mechanisms
S. pneumoniae	Microaspiration
H. influenzae	Microaspiration
Gram-negative bacilli	Microaspiration
Anaerobic bacteria	Aspiration
Mycobacterium tuberculosis	Inhalation—patient source
Influenza	Inhalation—patient source
Legionella	Inhalation—environmental source
Aspergillus	Inhalation—environmental source
Pathogenic fungi	Inhalation—environmental source
Mycoplasma pneumoniae	Inhalation—patient source
Staphylococcus aureus	Embolic or inhalation or aspiration
Pneumocystis jirovecii	Endogenous in lung
Cytomegalovirus	Endogenous in host white cells

the status of host defences. The normal tracheobronchial tree and lung parenchyma are sterile below the level of the larynx, so that agents of pneumonia must reach this site from external or adjacent sources, usually either by aspiration or inhalation. Organisms may also reach the lung by haematogenous seeding, direct extension from infection in a contiguous structure, or by activation of dormant organisms in the lung. These mechanisms are pathogen-specific, as summarized in Table 18.4.2.3.

Most bacterial pneumonias are probably caused by aspiration, which is defined as the abnormal entry of endogenous secretions or exogenous substances into the lower airways. There is a problem here with semantics because most cases of pneumonia are probably due to aspiration as classically described, but 'aspiration pneumonia' probably accounts for only 5 to 10% of cases. The explanation is presumably quantitative—'aspiration' generally referring to the abnormal entry of relatively large volumes in patients who are so predisposed due to dysphagia or a compromised level of consciousness. The alternative form is presumed to be 'microaspiration', involving the aspiration of very small numbers of microbes, a process that commonly takes place in healthy patients during sleep and with no apparent sequelae.

Clinical features

The classic presentation of pneumonia is of a cough and fever with the variable presence of sputum production, dyspnoea, and pleurisy. Most patients have constitutional symptoms such as malaise, fatigue, and asthenia, and many also have gastrointestinal symptoms. Although patients with pneumonia usually possess these characteristic clinical features, there can be major differences in presentation based on the host and the aetiological agent, as summarized below.

Pneumococcal pneumonia

S. pneumoniae is nearly always the most commonly identified pathogen in patients hospitalized with community-acquired pneumonia. A meta-analysis of 122 reports of community-acquired pneumonia for the period 1966 to 1995 showed that *S. pneumoniae* accounted for 65% of all cases where a microbial pathogen was defined and 66% of all bacteraemic cases. Studies using transtracheal aspiration or transthoracic aspiration—methods that avoid the problem of expectorated sputum contamination—show the presence of *S. pneumoniae* in 50 to 80% of cases.

The classic presentation is of a previously healthy adult with an upper respiratory tract infection who then develops a rigor followed by fever, dyspnoea, pleurisy, and a cough that usually becomes productive of a purulent, blood-streaked, or 'rusty' sputum. However, most patients show variations in this pattern, including one of a more subtle onset. Moreover, atypical presentations are particularly common in elderly patients.

Clinical examination can reveal features indicative of the severity of respiratory compromise—appearance of exhaustion, use of accessory muscles, inability to talk in sentences, tachypnoea (or even more worryingly when associated with exhaustion, a low respiratory rate), cyanosis—and of consolidation, in particular localized dullness to percussion and bronchial breathing.

Chest radiography nearly always shows an infiltrate, and lobar consolidation specifically suggests this diagnosis (Fig. 18.4.2.1). A pleural effusion is present in about 25% of patients, but only 1 to 2% have an empyema. CT often shows lesions that are not apparent on chest radiographs.

Important observations over the past decade include the declining frequency of cases where this organism is identified, and the increasing resistance of *S. pneumoniae* to penicillin and a variety of other antibiotics. The declining frequency is commonly ascribed to a general decline in the quality of microbiological testing currently performed in cases of pneumonia in general, with greater dependence on rapid initiation of empirically selected antibiotics that are usually active against *S. pneumoniae*. Decreased antibiotic susceptibility is thought to reflect antibiotic abuse.

Poor prognostic findings in patients with pneumococcal pneumonia include advanced age, bacteraemia, alcoholism, and multiple lobe involvement.

The preferred antibiotics are amoxicillin for oral treatment and ceftriaxone or cefotaxime for parenteral treatment; penicillin-resistant strains may be treated with fluoroquinolones, vancomycin, or linezolid.

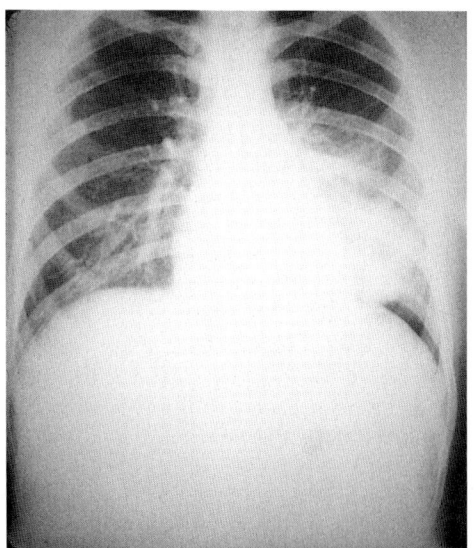

Fig. 18.4.2.1 Chest radiograph showing a left lower lobe pneumonia. Blood cultures grew *S. pneumoniae*.
Reproduced from BMJ, Little *et al*, 314, 722–7, copyright 1997 with permission from BMJ Publishing Group Ltd.

Haemophilus influenzae

This organism was originally described in 1892 by Pfeiffer who erroneously thought it was the agent of influenza; it was sometimes referred to as 'Pfeiffer's bacillus'. *H. influenzae* is always the second most common bacterial agent (behind *S. pneumoniae*) when an identified bacterial pathogen is found in community-acquired pneumonia. However, the diagnosis is difficult owing to problems with its recognition by direct Gram stain, the fastidious growth requirements of the organism, and interpretation—even when it is recovered—because it commonly colonizes the upper airways, leading to contamination of expectorated specimens. Type B *H. influenzae* is a well-established pathogen primarily in infants and young children, but is now a relatively rare cause of disease due to widespread use of *H. influenzae* (Hib) vaccine. *H. influenzae* strains causing pneumonia in adults are usually nontypable.

The clinical features are rather nonspecific and include fever, cough, purulent sputum, leucocytosis, and radiographic evidence of pneumonia—usually in a bronchopneumonic pattern, but it may occasionally be lobar. Patients with chronic obstructive lung disease often harbour *H. influenzae* in their lower airways and, allegedly, are prone to pneumonia caused by this organism, although supporting data for the association are not strong. Bacteraemia with *H. influenzae* in adults is infrequent. Most patients simply have a nonspecific pneumonia, with *H. influenzae* as the only potential pathogen identified in expectorated sputum.

About 30 to 45% of strains produce β-lactamase so that penicillin and amoxicillin are often ineffective. When *H. influenzae* is suspected or established the preferred agents are second- and third-generation cephalosporins, any combination of a β-lactam–β-lactamase inhibitor, azithromycin, or a fluoroquinolone.

Anaerobic bacteria

These organisms are the dominant components of the microbial flora in the upper airways and average 10^{12}/ml in the gingival crevice. Anaerobes are the major pathogens identified in aspiration pneumonia and its sequelae, lung abscess and empyema. The major pathogens in this group are peptostreptcocci, bacteroides (other than *Bacteroides fragilis*), prevotella, and *Fusobacterium nucleatum*.

The typical patient has gingival crevice disease combined with a predisposition for aspiration that is usually due to a suppressed level of consciousness or dysphasia. The clinical presentation is usually more subtle than that for pneumococcal pneumonia in that the infection evolves over a period of many days, weeks, or even months. Chest radiographs usually show infection in a dependent segment (usually the superior segments of the lower lobes or posterior segments of the upper lobes since these are dependent in the recumbent position), fever, sputum that is often putrid, and evidence of chronic disease with weight loss or anaemia. Putrid discharge is very characteristic and diagnostic of anaerobic bacterial infection (Fig. 18.4.2.2).

Aspiration pneumonia may also be due to chemical insults from gastric acid or other toxins, or may reflect the aspiration of foreign bodies or fluids (as in victims of drowning). However, the most common sequel to aspiration is bacterial infection involving the anaerobes that normally colonize the upper airways, and such bacteria account for 60 to 80% of cases of aspiration pneumonia, lung abscess, and, in many case series, empyemas. Although the bacterial aetiology can be identified from anaerobic cultures of uncontaminated specimens, these are generally not obtained except in the case of pleural fluid in the presence of empyema; even then the cultures are often falsely negative due to inadequate techniques used to recover oxygen-sensitive bacteria. Thus, the aetiological diagnosis is usually based on the clinical features—where key clues are the chronicity of the infection, associated conditions suggesting aspiration, tissue necrosis with abscess formation, or a bronchopleural fistula leading to empyema and/or putrid discharge.

The preferred drugs are clindamycin or a β-lactam–β-lactamase inhibitor.

Mycoplasma pneumoniae

This organism is one of the most common causes of lower airways infection in young adults, and it is now more frequently recognized in older adults. The original appellation was 'primary atypical

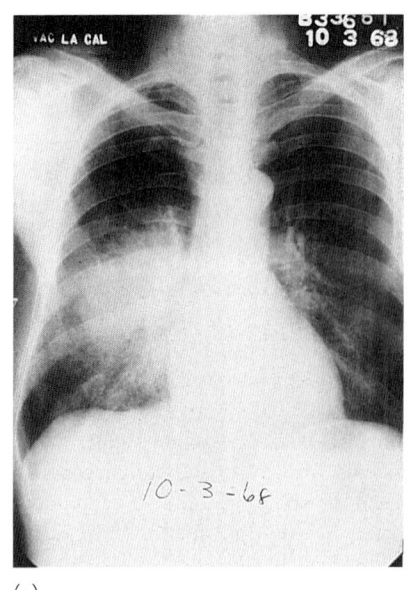
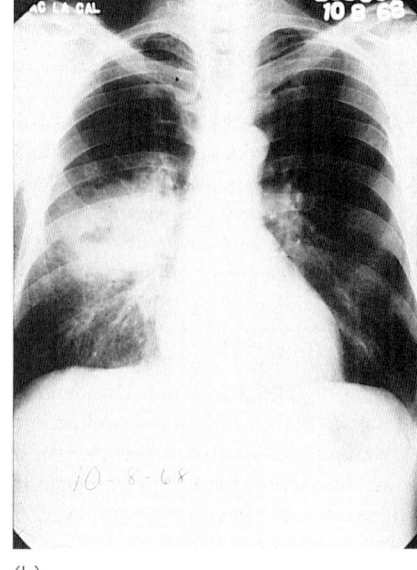

Fig. 18.4.2.2 (a) Consolidated pneumonia in the superior segment of the right lower lobe in a 56-year-old alcoholic. A transtracheal aspirate showed numerous anaerobic bacteria including *Prevotella melaninogenicus* and peptostreptococcus spp. (b) A follow-up radiograph 5 days later showing cavitation.

(a)   (b)

pneumonia', a term applied in the 1930s to a relatively benign form of pneumonia to distinguish it from pneumococcal pneumonia. Early work showed that it was associated with a serum factor that agglutinated erythrocytes in the cold; furthermore, Eaton reported that the infection was transmissible from person to person by intracheal inoculations. Thus, atypical pneumonia, cold-agglutinin pneumonia, and Eaton-agent pneumonia were found to be synonymous.

The typical patient is usually a young adult who experiences a respiratory tract infection accompanied by headache, myalgia, cough, and fever, and with a chest radiograph that shows bronchopneumonia. The cough is often nonproductive, but when sputum is obtained it is mucoid, shows predominantly mononuclear cells, and no dominant organism. A characteristic feature is the relatively high frequency of extrapulmonary complications such as rash, neurological syndromes (aseptic meningitis, encephalitis, neuropathies), myocarditis, pericarditis, and haemolytic anaemia. The diagnosis should be suspected in those patients with a relatively mild form of pneumonia, particularly in previously healthy young adults.

Most laboratories do not cultivate mycoplasma due to the effort needed to recover the organism, the long time required, and the ease of empirical treatment. Serological tests may be used, but their merits are disputed. Polymerase chain reaction (PCR) and other rapid diagnostic tests are under development.

With regard to treatment, the pathogen lacks a cell wall and hence is not susceptible to penicillin, cephalosporins, or other cell-wall active antibiotics. The usual therapeutic agents are macrolides (such as erythromycin, clarithromycin, or azithromycin) or doxycycline; fluoroquinolones are also active.

Chlamydia pneumoniae

This relatively recently identified pathogen is now thought to account for about 5 to 10% of all community-acquired cases of pneumonia, often in young adults who present in a fashion quite similar to that of patients with a mycoplasma pneumonia. *C. pneumoniae* continues to be regarded as a relatively benign agent of pneumonia: most patients have an upper airways infection with this organism, laryngitis is relatively common, bronchitis is less common, and pneumonitis is an infrequent complication. *C. pneumoniae* plays a role in exacerbations of asthma, and the organism was once thought to be involved in some chronic conditions such as cardiovascular disease, but more recent large controlled trials have not supported an association.

The diagnosis of chlamydia pneumonia is difficult. The organism is cultivated like a virus using tissue cultures, but few laboratories offer this test. Serology is difficult to interpret; the usual titres for IgM or serial changes with acute and convalescent sera are arbitrary. Like mycoplasma, this is an organism that is often suspected, infrequently proven, and easily treated empirically. A PCR test is expected soon.

The usual treatment is doxycycline, a macrolide (erythromycin, clarithromycin, or azithromycin), or a fluoroquinolone.

Legionella

Legionnaires' disease was originally described during the American Legion Convention in Philadelphia in 1976, with the putative agent reported the following year. Legionella cause two major syndromes: the pneumonic form or legionnaires' disease, referring to the American Legion Convention epidemic, and a benign influenza-like illness called 'Pontiac fever' in reference to an outbreak in 1967 in Pontiac, Michigan. Although legionnaires' disease is often grouped with mycoplasma and chlamydia infection as being an 'atypical pneumonia', it is a quite different pulmonary infection because it occurs primarily in older adults, is a serious and often lethal form of pneumonia, and most hospital laboratories have diagnostic resources to establish the aetiology. Legionnaires' disease is defined as pneumonia caused by any species of the genera legionella, but the great majority of cases are caused either by *Legionella pneumophila* (80 to 90% of cases) or *L. mcdadei* (5 to 10%). This disease may be epidemic or sporadic. Epidemics usually occur in buildings, especially hotels and hospitals, and they reflect legionella contamination of the potable water or cooling systems of air conditioners. Predisposing factors include exposure to environmental sources of legionella (there is no patient-to-patient transmission), age over 40 years, smoking, or reduced cell-mediated immune responses as with organ transplantation, cancer chemotherapy, or chronic corticosteroid usage; patients with AIDS do not seem to be uniquely susceptible.

There are no remarkable features of the clinical presentation, except that patients are almost invariably quite sick and may be critically ill. In addition to the typical symptoms of pneumonia with cough and dyspnoea, most present with a profound systemic illness with high fever and myalgias, often with gastrointestinal and neurological symptoms.

The diagnosis can be established with a urinary antigen assay for the detection of *L. pneumophila* serogroup I (which accounts for about 80% of cases), culture of respiratory secretions on selective media, or serology. All these tests are quite specific, but none are sufficiently sensitive to exclude the diagnosis when they are negative, and the urinary antigen assay is the only one that is easily done and gives results in a timely fashion.

The drugs of choice are fluoroquinolone, or a macrolide, or azithromycin, but mortality rate is generally reported to be 5 to 15% even with proper therapy.

Staphylococcus aureus

Staphylococcal pneumonia was classically described as a complication of influenza during the 1918 epidemic of 'Spanish flu'. This organism continues to be a potentially important superinfecting pathogen in influenza, and is the most common form of embolic pulmonary infection with injection drug use and tricuspid valve endocarditis. A relatively new form of *Staphyloccocus aureus* pneumonia involves strains with the Panton Valentine leukocidin (*PVL*) gene. These cases are most common in children or young adults with influenza, the clinical course is fulminant, often with pulmonary necrosis and leucopenia, and the mortality rate is high.

The organism can usually be recovered in blood cultures and in respiratory secretions. However, care must be exercised when interpreting respiratory secretion cultures that yield *Staphyloccocus aureus* since this may be a contaminant, and it is particularly common as a contaminant in those patients who have received previous antibiotic treatment.

The treatment should be based on *in vitro* susceptibility tests, usually an antistaphylococcal penicillin (flucloxacillin, oxacillin, or nafcillin), a first-generation cephalosporin (cefazolin), or vancomycin (for methicillin-resistant strains and for patients with severe penicillin allergy). The PVL-positive strains are usually methicillin-resistant and should be treated with vancomycin or linezolid.

Gram-negative bacilli

Klebsiella pneumoniae was originally described in 1882 by Friedlander, who believed it was the cause of pneumococcal pneumonia. This organism has continued to be a rare but important cause of community-acquired pneumonia, accounting for about 0.5 to 1.5% of all cases. The classic presentation of 'Friedlander's pneumonia' was a serious pneumonia in an alcoholic patient with a chest radiograph that showed upper lobe involvement and the 'bulging fissure sign' (indicating abscess formation) and sputum that resembled currant jelly. This form of klebsiella pulmonary infection is rarely encountered now, although klebsiella infection is occasionally implicated in community-acquired pneumonia.

Other Gram-negative bacilli may also cause pneumonia, but the frequency in immunocompetent hosts is very low. *Pseudomonas aeruginosa* is a rare pulmonary pathogen, but should be suspected when recovered in respiratory secretions from patients with specific predisposing conditions including structural lung disease, neutropenia, cystic fibrosis, or advanced AIDS. Gram-negative bacteria are commonly encountered in cultures of respiratory secretions in patients who have already started antibiotic treatment, when care must be exercised in interpretation because they are usually contaminants reflecting upper airway colonization.

Treatment should be based on *in vitro* sensitivity tests.

Viruses

Viral infections of the lower airways account for pneumonia in 10 to 15% of inpatients, and probably a substantially larger number of those managed as outpatients. The most frequent pathogens are influenza, parainfluenza, and respiratory syncytial virus (RSV). Influenza infections with bronchitis occur in epidemics, but influenza pneumonia is rare. More common in influenza patients with chest radiographs showing infiltrates is bacterial superinfection, most frequently with *S. pneumoniae* or *Staphylococcus aureus*; less common superinfecting pathogens in this setting are *N. meningiditis* and group A streptococcus. The diagnosis of influenza can be made by the combination of an established epidemic and typical influenza symptoms, especially fever. The alternative is to establish the presence of the organism by one of several rapid tests for influenza-A or influenza-B antigen that provide results that are available in about 20 min, have a sensitivity of about 70 to 80%, and excellent specificity (in epidemics).

Clinical features of influenza are generally well known and include cough, fever, purulent sputum, and myalgias. Patients with bacterial superinfections will usually have typical influenza-like symptoms, improve, and then deteriorate after 1 to 2 weeks.

Infections involving influenza A or B may be treated with the neuraminidase inhibitors zanamivir or oseltamivir. If given within 48 h of the onset of symptoms these reduce the duration of typical symptoms by 1 to 1.5 days. They are more effective in seriously ill patients and when given very early in the 48-h window. Amandidine and ramantidine are no longer commonly advocated for influenza due to high rates of resistance.

RSV has usually been considered a pathogen in children but is now recognized with increasing frequency in adults, especially older people. The diagnosis is easily established with a direct fluorescent mononoclonal antibody (DFA) stain of respiratory secretions in children, but this test is much less sensitive in adults. Ribavirin is active against RSV and is sometimes used by inhalation therapy in children, but the benefit of this treatment is debated.

Box 18.4.2.1 Recommended laboratory tests in suspected community-acquired pneumonia

Outpatients

- Sputum, Gram stain, and culture or sputum on heat-fixed slide for later reference (optimal)

Inpatients

- Chest radiography
- Blood culture
- Chemistry panel including glucose, sodium, liver function tests, renal function tests, electrolytes
- Blood gases or pulse oximetry
- HIV serology for patients aged 15–54 years (with informed consent)
- Gram stain and culture of expectorated sputum that is physician-procured, processed within 2–5 h of collection, and subjected to cytological screening as a contingency for culture
- Specialized tests for selected patients
  - Legionella: urinary antigen and/or legionella culture
  - Pneumococcus: urinary antigen
  - Acid-fast bacteria: sputum for acid-fast stain and culture, in triplicate
  - Pleural fluid pH, cell count, Gram stain, and culture

Laboratory diagnosis

Laboratory tests are used to establish the diagnosis, evaluate the severity, and identify the aetiological agent (Box 18.4.2.1).

Tests to establish the diagnosis and evaluate severity

Chest radiography

The chest radiograph is a pivotal test for the confirmation of pneumonia, it being impossible to make this diagnosis in the absence of a new infiltrate, with four possible exceptions: (1) dehydration, (2) neutropenia, (3) early in the course, or (4) pneumocystis pneumonia (PCP). None is common or verified, excepting PCP, which may show no infiltrate in up to 30% of cases. In all cases CT is more sensitive in detecting infiltrates and in defining pathology, and is indicated in unusual cases.

Most patients with symptoms of pneumonia and a negative chest radiograph have acute bronchitis, which is generally caused by viral pathogens that do not respond to antibiotic treatment. Thus, the importance of the chest radiograph is in confirming pneumonia, which is a critical feature in avoiding antibiotic abuse. Additional advantages of the chest radiograph are that it provides assistance in identifying the aetiological agent, establishes a baseline for subsequent evaluation, provides prognostic information, and permits the detection of underlying or associated conditions such as a neoplasm.

Other laboratory tests

The most useful additional laboratory tests to determine the severity of illness and need for hospitalization are evaluation of blood oxygenation with pulse oximetry or arterial blood gas determination, blood chemistries (glucose, blood urea nitrogen, and serum sodium levels), and a full blood count. Depending on context, patients who are hospitalized for pneumonia should generally undergo serological testing for HIV (after appropriate consent), since this is a common predisposing cause.

Studies to determine microbial aetiology

Laboratory studies for identifying pulmonary pathogens are among the most controversial issues in pneumonia management. Most physicians now have a nihilistic approach, concluding that microbial studies in cases of pneumonia are usually negative, are not cost-effective, and are largely unnecessary since empirical treatment is generally successful. The guidelines from the Infectious Diseases Society of America (IDSA) and the American Thoracic Society (ATS) emphasize the best indications for microbiological studies are for patients sufficiently sick to require hospitalization in an intensive care unit, cases where the cause is a pathogen not covered by standard empirically selected treatment, and for some specific agents that have important implications for prognosis and epidemiology such as legionellosis, *Staphylococcus aureus*, pandemic influenza, agents of bioterrorism, and Gram-negative bacilli (although several of these circumstances cannot be determined in advance of microbiological testing). However, it should be emphasized that Gram stain and culture of expectorated sputum is never 'wrong', especially if done with good quality control.

Although empirical therapy is generally advocated for outpatients, routine microbiological testing to identify the aetiological agent of pneumonia is generally recommended for inpatients. Such tests include blood cultures (from blood samples taken prior to the initiation of antibiotic treatment), which yield a pathogen in about 12% of cases. In general, the only additional test commonly performed to identify an aetiological agent is an expectorated sputum Gram stain and culture. Practice standards for this process include the following:

- The specimen should be obtained by deep cough and should be grossly purulent. It should be collected before antibiotic therapy, preferably in the presence of a physician or nurse.

- The specimen should be promptly transported to the laboratory for processing and incubation within 2 to 5 h.

- A qualified technician should select a purulent portion for Gram stain and culture.

- Cytological screening should be done under low-power magnification (×100) to determine cellular composition as a contingency for culture.

- The sample should be cultured using standard techniques, with results reported by semiquantitative assessment; most pathogens are recovered in moderate or heavy growth, indicating more than five colonies in the second streak.

- Interpretation should be based on the correlation of the Gram stain, semiquantitative culture results, and clinical observations.

The aetiological agent of pneumonia is considered to be clearly established if a likely pulmonary pathogen is recovered from an uncontaminated specimen such as blood culture, pleural fluid, transtracheal aspiration, or transthoracic aspirate. Alternatively, the very presence of a likely pathogen recovered from respiratory secretions is tantamount to a diagnosis; organisms in this category include legionella species, *Mycobacterium tuberculosis*, most viruses other than the herpesvirus group (influenza virus, respiratory syncytial virus, Hantavirus, parainfluenza virus, and adenovirus), and certain fungi (*Histoplasma capsulatum*, *Coccidioides immitis*, *Blastomyces dermatitidis*, and *Pneumocystis jirovecii*). Organisms such as *S. pneumoniae*, *M. catarrhalis*, *H. influenzae*, and *Staphylococcus aureus* may be pulmonary pathogens, but interpretation is problematic due to possible contamination with specimens from the upper airway flora. Organisms that virtually never represent pulmonary pathogens include *S. epidermidis*, enterococcus, neisseria other than *N. meningitidis*, candida, and Gram-positive bacilli other than nocardia or actinomyces.

Transtracheal aspiration was once a popular method of obtaining specimens from the lower airways that avoided upper airway contamination, but the technique requires a skilled clinician and is generally thought to be too invasive for routine use. Transthoracic aspiration has the same limitations, and furthermore seems to give a relatively large number of false-negative results. Bronchoscopy is an attractive method for obtaining respiratory secretions directly from the lower airways; however, the procedure is complicated by contamination with instrument passage through the upper airways so that routine cultures of bronchoscopic aspirates are no better than expectorated sputum. These results may be substantially improved with quantitative cultures of bronchoalveolar lavage specimens or quantitative brush specimens, but many laboratories do not offer this type of analysis, and many pulmonary services cannot provide the samples in a timely fashion.

Most hospital laboratories offer diagnostic tests for detecting legionella spp. using urinary antigen assay and culture. Urinary antigen testing is advocated because it is rapid, simply performed, and highly specific; disadvantages include the fact that it only detects *L. pneumophila* serogroup 1, although this accounts for 80% of cases. The alternative test for detecting legionella is culture, which has the advantage of detecting all species of legionella, but the disadvantage that it requires 3 days, requires specialized media, and is technically demanding. A new urinary antigen assay diagnostic test for *S. pneumoniae* can provide results within 3 h.

Most laboratories do not offer diagnostic tests to detect *M. pneumoniae* or *C. pneumoniae*, despite their presumed frequency. This reflects the lack of an acceptable test that is easily performed, provides adequate sensitivity and specificity, and can provide results in a timely fashion.

Treatment

Critical components of initial treatment may include intravenous hydration, oxygenation, and/or intubation and mechanical ventilatory support. Pleural effusions should be sampled to exclude empyema and, when the effusions are large, drained to improve oxygenation. Most authorities feel that expectorants, cough suppressants, and chest physiotherapy are of little value.

Antibiotic therapy

Antibiotics are the mainstay of therapy. Suggestions for specific agents according to microbial pathogen are summarized in Table 18.4.2.4. Most of these are relatively noncontroversial and demonstrate the advantage of establishing an aetiological agent. However, as noted above, no pathogen can be detected in 40 to 60% of cases despite arduous attempts to do so, and even when an agent is

Table 18.4.2.4 Treatment of pneumonia by pathogen

Agent	Preferred antimicrobial	Alternative antimicrobial
Streptococcus pneumoniae Penicillin-susceptible (MIC <2 µg/ml)[a]	Penicillin G Amoxicillin	Cephalosporins: cefazolin, cefuroxime, cefotaxime, ceftriaxone, cefepime Oral cephalosporins: cefpodoxime, cefprozil, cefuroxime Imipenem or meropenem Macrolides,[a] clindamycin Fluoroquinolones[b] Doxycycline Penicillins: ampicillin ± sulbactam, piperacillin ± tazobactam
Streptococcus pneumoniae Penicillin-resistant[c] (MIC >2 µg/ml)	Agents based on *in vitro* sensitivity tests, including: Cephalosporins (cefotaxime, ceftriaxone) Fluoroquinolone[b] Vancomycin	Linezolid
Haemophilus influenzae	Cephalosporin—2nd or 3rd generation β-lactam–β-lactamase inhibitors	Azithromycin Fluoroquinolone[b] Doxycycline Clarithromycin
Moraxella catarrhalis	Cephalosporin—2nd or 3rd generation Amoxicillin–clavulanate	Macrolides Fluoroquinolone[b] β-Lactam–β-lactamase inhibitors
Anaerobes	β-lactam–β-lactamase inhibitors Clindamycin	Carbapenem
Staphylococcus aureus[c] Methicillin-sensitive	Flucloxacillin/nafcillin/oxacillin ± rifampicin or gentamicin[c]	Cefazolin, cefuroxime Teicoplanin Vancomycin, clindamycin, TMP–SMX, fluoroquinolone[b]
Staphylococcus aureus[c] Methicillin-resistant	Vancomycin ± rifampicin or linezolid	Requires *in vitro* testing; linezolid, TMP–SMX
Enterobacteriaceae (coliforms: E. coli, klebsiella, proteus, enterobacter, etc.)[c]	Cephalosporin—3rd generation ± aminoglycoside Carbapenem	Aztreonam β-lactam–β-lactamase inhibitors Fluoroquinolone[b]
Pseudomonas aeruginosa[c]	Aminoglycoside + antipseudomonal β-lactam: ceftazidime, imipenem, meropenem, doripenem, piperacillin/ticarcillin, cefepime or aztreonam	Aminoglycoside + ciprofloxacin Ciprofloxacin + antipseudomonal β-lactam
Legionella	Macrolide[a] ± rifampicin Fluoroquinolone[b] (including ciprofloxacin)	Doxycycline ± rifampicin Azithromycin
Mycoplasma pneumoniae	Doxycycline Macrolide[a]	Fluoroquinolone[b]
Chlamydia pneumoniae	Doxycycline Macrolide[a]	Fluoroquinolone[b]
Chlamydia psittaci	Doxycycline	Erythromycin, fluoroquinolone
Nocardia spp.	TMP–SMX Sulphonamide ± minocycline or amikacin	Imipenem ± amikacin Doxycycline or minocycline
Coxiella burnetii (Q fever)	Tetracycline	Macrolide

Table 18.4.2.4 Treatment of pneumonia by pathogen

Agent	Preferred antimicrobial	Alternative antimicrobial
Influenza	Oseltamivir or zanamivir	
Hantavirus	Supportive care	

MIC, minimum inhibitory concentration; TMP–SMX, trimethoprim and sulfamethoxazole.

[a] Macrolide: erythromycin, clarithromycin, azithromycin, dirithromycin.

[b] Fluoroquinolone: levofloxacin, moxifloxacin, or other fluoroquinolone with enhanced activity against S. pneumoniae; ciprofloxacin is appropriate for legionella spp., C. pneumoniae, M. pneumoniae, fluoroquinolone-sensitive Staphylococcus aureus, and most Gram-negative bacilli.

[c] In vitro sensitivity tests are required for optimal treatment; for enterobacter the preferred antibiotics are the fluoroquinolones and carbapenems.

Note—choices should be modified on the basis of susceptibility test results and advice from local specialists.

found, this information is usually not available when initial therapeutic decisions are needed. For this reason, most patients are treated empirically, at least initially, whilst microbiological results are pending. Recommendations for empirical treatment are summarized in Table 18.4.2.5. These options are selected on the basis of predicted activity against the most likely pathogens and extensive clinical trials. Nevertheless, this is one of the most controversial areas in medicine based on concerns about antibiotic abuse, increasing resistance of S. pneumoniae to many antimicrobials, and sharp geographical differences in the rates of S. pneumoniae resistance.

Timing of antibiotic therapy

A retrospective trial of over 20 000 Medicare patients in the United States of America hospitalized with community-acquired pneumonia showed that mortality increased with a progressive delay in the time taken to initiate antibiotic therapy after patients had been evaluated. The increase in mortality became statistically significant when the delay exceeded 6 h. This observation is not surprising since pneumonia is a potentially lethal infection that usually responds to antibiotics, so any delay in treatment would be expected to have deleterious effects. As a result of these observations, many hospitals in the United States of America are now audited to determine their compliance with antibiotic recommendations according to ATS/IDSA guidelines and initiation of this treatment within 8 h of a patient's admission to the Emergency Department or hospital.

Table 18.4.2.5 Empirical treatment of community-acquired pneumonia

Outpatients	Amoxicillin, doxycycline, macrolide[a], or fluoroquinolone[b]
Inpatients	
General hospital	β-Lactam[c] + macrolide[a] or fluoroquinolone[b] alone
Intensive care unit	β-Lactam[c] + macrolide[a] or β-lactam[c] + fluoroquinolone[b]
Special circumstances	
Aspiration pneumonia	Clindamycin or β-lactam–β-lactamase inhibitor
Structural disease of lung	Treat with regimen that includes activity against P. aeruginosa

[a] Macrolide: erythromycin, clarithromycin, azithromycin.

[b] Fluoroquinolone: levofloxacin, gatifloxacin, moxifloxacin, or other fluoroquinolone with enhanced activity against S. pneumoniae.

[c] β-lactam: cefotaxime or ceftriaxone.

Note—always refer to local guidelines, which should take account of local prevalence of antibiotic-resistant pathogens, when these are available.

Monitoring response to therapy

Subjective responses are usually noted within 3 to 5 days of initiating treatment. Objective parameters to monitor include fever, oxygen saturation, peripheral leucocyte count, and changes on serial chest radiographs. The most carefully documented responses are mortality rates, time to defervescence, and duration of hospital stay. With regard to fever, the temperature in young adults with pneumococcal pneumonia usually drops within 2 to 3 days, whereas those with bacteraemic pneumococcal pneumonia (usually elderly patients) respond more slowly. Blood cultures in bacteraemic patients are usually negative within 24 to 48 h. Cultures of sputum will usually show eradication of bacterial pathogens within 24 to 48 h, a major exception being P. aeruginosa. Radiographic appearances are slow to improve and much less useful than clinical observations for evaluating response. Follow-up radiographs are generally not recommended, except for patients who are over 40 years of age or are smokers, and the suggested time to do this is 7 to 12 weeks after initiating treatment.

Patients who are initially treated with intravenous antibiotics can usually be changed to receive oral agents when they are able to take oral medications and show clinical improvement, such as a temperature below 38°C for 24 h, a respiratory rate of less than 24/min, and when the Po_2 has returned to normal.

Failure to respond

The major considerations in patients who fail to respond according to the guidelines noted above are:

- The disease is too far advanced at the time of treatment, or treatment is delayed for too long: this is most commonly seen with pneumonia caused by S. pneumoniae or legionella.

- The wrong antibiotic was selected: this is uncommon, but in our experience the most common exceptions are tuberculosis, pneumocystis pneumonia, and viral pneumonias.

- An inadequate antibiotic dosage is given.

- The wrong diagnosis is made: for example, there is a noninfectious disease such as pulmonary embolism with infarction, congestive failure, Wegener's granulomatosis, sarcoidosis, atelectasis, chemical pneumonitis, or bronchiolitis obliterans organizing pneumonia.

- The wrong microbial diagnosis is made.

- The patient may be debilitated, have a severe associated disease, or be immunosuppressed, or there may be other host inadequacies.

- There may be a complicated pneumonia with undrained empyema, metastatic site of infection (meningitis), or bronchial obstruction (foreign body, carcinoma).

- There may be a pulmonary superinfection: most patients in this category respond and then deteriorate with a new fever.
- There may be a complication of the antibiotic treatment such as an adverse drug reaction or antibiotic-associated colitis.

Prognosis

The overall mortality for patients who are hospitalized with community-acquired pneumonia, according to a meta-analysis of 122 reports, is 14%. Risk factors for lethal outcome were well described in the prepenicillin era, when extremes of age were probably the most important factor. Other risks included bacteraemia, the extent of changes on chest radiography, alcohol consumption, and the extent of leucocytosis. More recent studies have continued to show that these factors, especially age, are major risk factors for morbidity and mortality. Investigators from the Pneumonia Patient Outcomes Research Team (PORT) have developed a prediction rule using a cumulative point score obtained from five categories comprising 19 variables (Table 18.4.2.6). This prediction rule was applied retrospectively to 38 039 inpatients and showed a direct correlation between numerical score and mortality, the authors

Table 18.4.2.6 Prediction rule for outcome

(a) Scoring system

Variable	Points
Age	Male: age in years Female: age in years − 10
Nursing home	+10
Comorbidity	Neoplasm, +20 Liver disease, +20 Congestive failure, +10 Cerebrovascular disease, +10 Renal disease, +10
Physical examination	Altered mental status, +20 Respiratory rate >30/min, +20 SBP <90 mmHg, +20, temperature, <35°C or >40°C, +15 Pulse >125/min, +10
Laboratory	Arterial pH <7.35, +30 BUN >30 mg/dl (>5 mmol/litre), +20 Sodium <130 mEq/litre, + 20 Glucose >250 mg/dl (>15 mmol/litre), +10 Haematocrit <30%, +10 Arterial PO_2 <60 mmHg, +10 Pleural effusion, +10

(b) Risk class validation

Risk class	Points	No. patients	Mortality (%)	Recommended site of care
I	No predictors	3034	0.1	Outpatient
II	≤70	5778	0.6	Outpatient
III	71–90	6790	2.8	Outpatient or brief hospitalization
IV	91–130	13 104	8.2	Hospital
V	>130	9333	29.2	Hospital

BUN, blood urea nitrogen; SBP, systolic blood pressure.
Adapted with permission from Fine MJ et al. (1997). A prediction rule to identify low-risk patients with community-acquired pneumonia. New England Journal of Medicine 336, 243.

concluding that these factors predict outcome and can also be used to determine the need for hospitalization or the need for the intensive care unit.

An alternative metric that is simpler to remember and equally good for prediction is the six-point 'CURB-65' score, based on Confusion (impaired consciousness), elevated blood Urea nitrogen (>7 mmol/litre), increased Respiratory rate (>30/min), low systolic Blood pressure (<90 mmHg), low diastolic Blood pressure (<60 mmHg), and age over 65 years. In over 1000 prospectively studied patients with community-acquired pneumonia from three countries (United Kingdom, New Zealand, the Netherlands), the risk of mortality or need for intensive care admission was as follows: score 0, 0.7%; score 1, 3.2%; score 2, 13%; score 3, 17%; score 4, 41.5%; score 5, 57%. If the blood urea nitrogen level is not available and only the clinical parameters are considered (CRB-65), the risk of mortality for particular scores (out of a maximum of 5) was as follows: score 0, 1.2%; score 1, 5.3%; score 2, 12.2%; score 3, 32.9%; score 4, 18.2%. These data have led to recommendations from the British Thoracic Society that patients who have a CRB-65 score of 0 do not normally require hospitalization for clinical reasons; referral to and assessment in hospital should be considered for those with a score of 1 or (particularly) 2; and those with a score of 3 or more require urgent hospital admission (unless known to be terminally ill).

With regard to specific pathogens, the main agents of community-acquired pneumonia associated with high mortality rates are bacteraemic pneumococcal pneumonia and legionnaires' disease. Influenza is directly or indirectly implicated in 20 000 to 40 000 deaths per year in the United States of America, but primary influenza pneumonia is relatively rare and most of the influenza-associated deaths are of elderly patients who succumb to complications of influenza. It should also be noted that pneumonia is an extremely common terminal event in patients who die of other conditions, presumably because of aspiration in the terminal stages. Thus, pneumonia is a common autopsy finding when other medical conditions are actually the primary cause of death.

Prevention and control

The main preventive measures are influenza and *S. pneumoniae* vaccination. The components selected for the influenza vaccine each year are based on the anticipated strains for the forthcoming season, a prediction that has been quite accurate in 14 of the 16 influenza seasons from 1989/90 through 2006/07. Protective efficacy is generally 60 to 70% in the general population when there is a good match between the vaccine strains and the epidemic strain; it is less effective in elderly vaccinees, but those who develop influenza after vaccination usually have an attenuated course with significant reduction in mortality. The current recommendation is for vaccination between October and November of patients living in the northern hemisphere. Targeted populations are summarized in Box 18.4.2.2. Zanamivir and oseltamivir may be used to prevent influenza in unvaccinated patients who are so exposed. Amantidine and rimantidine are no longer recommended due to resistance.

The 23-valent vaccine for *S. pneumoniae* contains capsular polysaccharide from 23 serogroups that are responsible for 80 to 85% of bacteraemic pneumococcal infections. Studies of this vaccine suggest a 60% efficacy in preventing bacteraemic pneumococcal infection, but efficacy in reducing rates of community-acquired

People recommended for vaccination include:[a]

- Children aged 6 months until their 18th birthday
- Pregnant women
- People ≥50 years of age
- People of any age with certain chronic health conditions (such as asthma, diabetes, or heart disease)
- People who live in nursing homes and other long-term care facilities
- Household contacts of person at high risk for complications from influenza
- Household contacts and out-of-home caregivers of children <6 months of age
- Health care workers

People who should NOT be vaccinated include:

- People who have a severe allergy to chicken eggs
- People who have had a severe reaction to an influenza vaccination in the past
- People who develop Guillain–Barre syndrome within 6 weeks of getting an influenza vaccine
- People who have a moderate to severe illness with a fever (who should wait until they recover to get vaccinated)

[a] Based on their risk of complications from influenza or because they are in close contact with someone at higher risk of influenza complications. Recommendations of the Centers for Disease Control and Prevention, http://www.cdc.gov/flu/professionals/vaccination/vax-summary.htm, accessed 30 May 2008.

pneumonia or even pneumococcal pneumonia is not consistently shown. A more recently developed 7-valent protein-conjugated pneumococcal vaccine has the advantage of stimulating a good antibody response in children under 2 years of age. This has not been extensively tested in adults, but its use in children has resulted in a 50 to 80% decrease in rates of invasive pneumococcal infections in adults, the implication being that children less than 2 years are main vectors of pneumococcal infections (as they probably are for influenza).

Controversies

There are probably few diseases in medicine that have been better studied than pneumonia, but with such extraordinary controversy in management guidelines, including the utility of microbiology studies, the empirical selection of antibiotics, and the use of pneumococcal vaccine. Emergency of "replacement serotypes such as 19A has resulted in a new vaccine, Prevnar 13.

Studies of microbial aetiology

Culture and Gram stain of expectorated sputum is the time-honoured method for determining the microbiology of community-acquired pneumonia. Nevertheless, there is substantial controversy regarding the worth of this exercise and a wealth of

medical reports with highly divergent findings that simply fuel the debate. In general, the best results were achieved in the prepenicillin era, when sputum bacteriology was an art and many patients underwent transthoracic needle aspiration to be sure the pathogen was found, the reason being that the only available therapy was type-specific antisera for *S. pneumoniae*, hence treatment required retrieval of the specific strain. High-quality laboratory technology persisted through the mid-1980s, when the yield of *S. pneumoniae* in expectorated sputum samples for inpatients with community-acquired pneumonia was generally reported at 40 to 70%. More recent experience is much different, with the yield of *S. pneumoniae* in expectorated sputum by either Gram stain or culture being only 5 to 10% in most studies of large medical systems such as Medicare. Arguments favouring sputum microbiology are the benefits of pathogen-directed therapy that restrains antibiotic abuse, limits side effects, and reduces cost. In addition, this permits the identification of epidemiologically important organisms, knowledge of which provides the database for empirical therapy recommendations. Arguments against microbiological studies include the facts that this procedure, as currently performed in most laboratories, shows a low yield, the information is infrequently available when therapeutic decisions are made, empirical treatment is usually effective against the most common pathogens (Fig. 18.4.2.3), and—even if a pathogen is recovered—there is no good way to exclude the presence of a copathogen. Many authorities now feel molecular diagnostics will supplant traditional microbiology methods.

Antibiotic selection

The selection of antimicrobials is usually easy if the pathogen is known, but more difficult with empirical decisions when it is not. There are many 'trade-offs' with empiricism, including the consequence of promoting resistance, side effects, and cost. There is also controversy about the pathogens that need to be covered empirically, a major issue being whether or not it is necessary to treat 'atypical agents'.

Meta-analyses of proper trials show that β-lactams are as effective as regimens with activity against *Mycoplasma pneumoniae* and *C. pneumoniae*, although legionella is the exception. Thus, in many countries the standard for outpatient treatment is amoxicillin, and for the United States of America and some European countries it is doxycycline or a macrolide. Fluoroquinolones are highly effective against most treatable bacterial pathogens, but there is concern that excessive usage will lead to costs in the form of resistance and increased incidence of *C. difficile*. The ATS/IDSA 2007 guidelines recommend these agents only when penicillin-resistant *S. pneumoniae* is suspected, the major risks for which are antibiotic exposure within the previous 3 months, or patients with important comorbidities such as diabetes, chronic renal failure, or serious cardiopulmonary disease.

For hospitalized patients the ATS/IDSA recommendations are based on the Medicare database, which was analysed for mortality rates with different regimens for adults who are hospitalized for community-acquired pneumonia. These recommendations are (1) a fluoroquinolone (levofloxacin or moxifloxacin), or (2) a macrolide (usually azithromycin) combined with a cephalosporin (ceftriaxone or cefotaxime). These regimens reduced mortality in the analysis of over 14 000 Medicare patients by 36% and 24%, respectively.

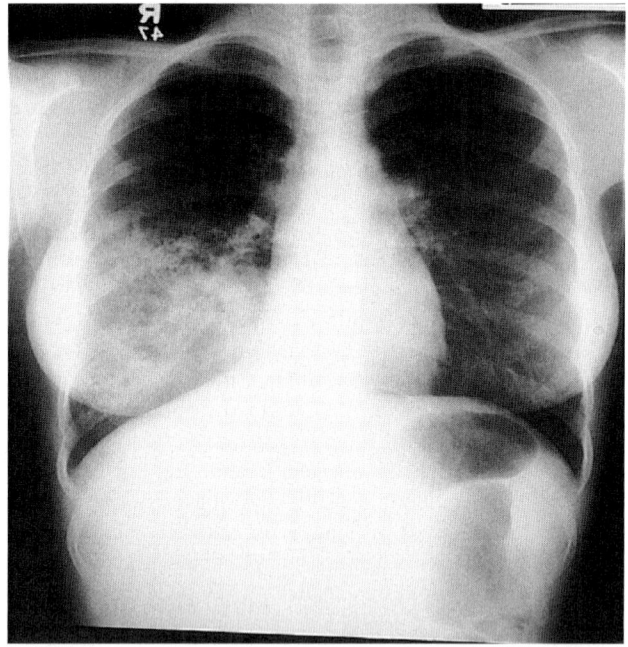

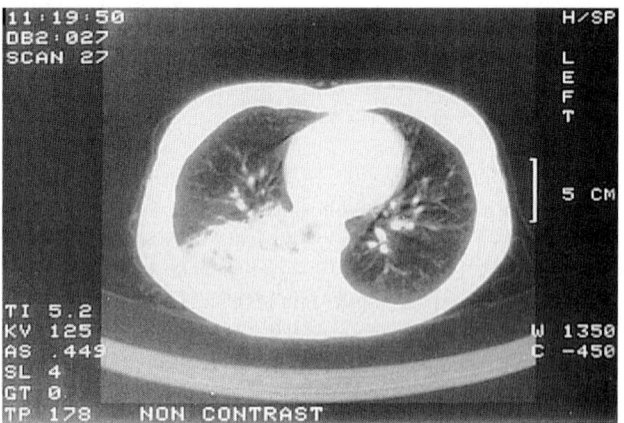

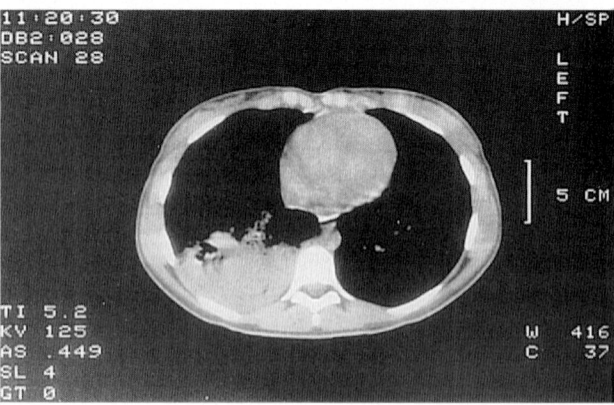

(a)

(b)

Fig. 18.4.2.3 Chest radiograph (a) and CT scan (b) showing pneumonitis in the right lower lobe of an 18-year-old college student. The patient responded to empirical antibiotic treatment.

Some of the controversies that have emerged include: the relative merits of β-lactams; the variable rates of β-lactam resistance by *S. pneumoniae*; the place of erythromycin in guidelines (based on price, tolerance, and activity vs legionella); the need to provide 'double coverage' (β-lactam plus a macrolide) in patients with pneumococcal bacteremia; the role of pathogen-directed therapy in the era of poor-quality microbiology; conclusiveness of the urinary antigen assay for *S. pneumoniae*; and the following important but often neglected exceptions to the recommendations:

- Influenza with suspected bacterial superinfection: in these cases the major pathogens are *S. pneumoniae* and *Staphylococcus aureus*, which need prioritization in antibiotic selection

- The immunocompromised patient, where the list of pathogens is legion and driven by multiple variables including characteristics of the immunological deficit

- Aspiration pneumonia, which may be bacterial, usually anaerobes and/or streptococci, or might be chemical or obstructive due to a foreign body

- 'Health care associated', with reference to people who are not in hospital but often have pneumonia that may be more similar to pathogens that cause nosocomial pneumonia (see Chapter 18.4.3) than those encountered in community-acquired pneumonia. This category includes patients in chronic care facilities, dialysis centres, and other extensions of the health care system

Pneumococcal vaccine

The polysaccharide vaccine has established merit in reducing pneumococcal bacteraemia, but most prospective randomized controlled trials have failed to show a significant benefit in terms of reducing the rates of pneumonia or rates of pneumococcal pneumonia. Most reports of a beneficial effect of vaccination have been based on statistical analyses of the serotype of patients with pneumococcal infection, which demonstrated higher rates of vaccine strains in unvaccinated patients. Even these studies failed to show a benefit in the highest risk group, namely the elderly and the immunosuppressed. The need for a pneumococcal vaccine is widely appreciated due to the extent of morbidity and mortality caused by *S. pneumoniae* and the increasing difficulty caused by resistance in treating these infections. Many authorities feel that the best solution to the dilemma is a better pneumococcal vaccine. The best data for benefit at present is widespread use of the protein-conjugated vaccine, such as Prevnar 13, given to children before 2 years of age to protect themselves and adults.

Further reading

Bartlett JG, Mundy L (1995). Community-acquired pneumonia. *N Engl J Med*, **333**, 1618–24.

Bartlett JG (2004). Diagnostic tests for etiologic agents of community-acquired pneumonia. *Infect Dis Clin North Am*, **18**, 809–27.

British Thoracic Society. *Guidelines for the management of adults with community-acquired pneumonia*. http://www.brit-thoracic.org.uk/ClinicalInformation/Pneumonia/tabid/106/Default.aspx (accessed 30 May 2007).

Calzada SR, *et al.* (2007). Empiric treatment in hospitalized community-acquired pneumonia. Impact on mortality, length of stay and re-admission. *Respir Med*, **101**, 1909–15.

Chen DK, *et al.* (1999). Decreased susceptibility of *Streptococcus pneumoniae* to fluoroquinolones in Canada. *N Engl J Med*, **341**, 233–9.

Lim WS, *et al.* (2003). Defining community-acquired pneumonia severity on presentation to hospital: an international derivation and validation study. *Thorax*, **58**, 377–82.

Marras TK, *et al.* (2000). Applying a prediction rule to identify low-risk patients with community-acquired pneumonia. *Chest*, **118**, 1339–43.

Marrie TJ, *et al.* (2000). A controlled trial of a critical pathway for treatment of community-acquired pneumonia. *JAMA*, **283**, 749–55.

Mandell LA, *et al.* (2007). Infectious Diseases Society of America/American Thoracic Society consensus guidelines on the management of community-acquired pneumonia in adults. *Clin Infect Dis*, **44** Suppl 2, S27–72.

Meehan TP, *et al.* (1997). Quality of care, process and outcomes in elderly patients with pneumonia. *JAMA*, **278**, 2080–4.

O'Brien WT Sr, *et al.* (2006). Clinical predictors of radiographic findings in patients with suspected community-acquired pneumonia: who needs a chest X-ray? *J Am Coll Radiol*, **3**, 703–6.

Oosterheert JJ, *et al.* (2003). How good is the evidence for the recommended empirical antimicrobial treatment of patients hospitalized because of community-acquired pneumonia? A systematic review. *J Antimicrob Chemother*, **52**, 555–63.

Renaud B, *et al.* (2007). Routine use of the Pneumonia Severity Index for guiding the site-of-treatment decision of patients with pneumonia in the emergency department: a multicenter, prospective, observational, controlled cohort study. *Clin Infect Dis*, **44**, 41–9.

18.4.3 Nosocomial pneumonia

John G. Bartlett

Essentials

Nosocomial pneumonia is generally defined as a new pulmonary infiltrate on chest radiography, combined with evidence of infection expressed as fever, purulent respiratory secretions and/or leucocytosis, with onset at least 72 h after admission. It is the most frequent lethal nosocomial infection (overall mortality 8 to 20%).

Aetiology—most cases are caused by Gram-negative bacteria (50–70%) or *Staphylococcus aureus* (20–30%). Gram-negative bacteria reach the lung by aspiration of gastric contents or by microaspiration of upper airway secretions, throat cultures revealing that 60 to 70% of patients on intensive care units are colonized by these organisms (compared to 2–3% of healthy people).

Prevention—the best proven methods of prevention are by nursing the patient in the semi-upright position to reduce the risk of aspiration, and hand washing between patients to prevent transmission of nosocomial pathogens.

Diagnosis—this is often straightforward: due to easy access to cultures from tracheal aspirates and the ease of growing likely pathogens.

Management—when empirical decisions are necessary in seriously ill patients, the favoured drugs directed against Gram-negative bacteria are ceftazidime, cefepime, imipenem/meropenem, doripenem, piperacillin/piperacillin–tazobactam, ticarcillin/ticarcillin–sulbactam, or ciprofloxacin. For *S. aureus*, vancomycin or linezolid is added.

Introduction

Nosocomial pneumonia is generally defined as a new pulmonary infiltrate on chest radiography, combined with evidence of infection expressed as fever, purulent respiratory secretions, and/or leucocytosis, with onset at least 72 h after admission, but despite the standard use of this definition, quantitative bronchoscopic specimens confirm an infection in only about half of the cases. Although these infections account for only about 15% of all nosocomial infections, they are the most frequent, lethal, nosocomial infection. The bacteriology and management are different from community-acquired infections of the lung (see Chapter 18.4.2).

Aetiology

Gram-negative bacteria account for 50 to 70% of cases; other pathogens include *Staphylococcus aureus* in 20 to 30% of cases; less common are anaerobic bacteria, *Haemophilus influenzae*, and *Streptococcus pneumoniae* (Table 18.4.3.1). Legionella accounts for about 1 to 2% of all nosocomial pneumonia, but the frequency may be much higher when it is epidemic or endemic within a hospital. Viruses are implicated in 10 to 20%—primarily influenza and respiratory syncytial virus and, in the immunocompromised host, cytomegalovirus. Tuberculosis is rare, but important to remember. Fungi are also rare, with the exception of aspergillus in selected immunocompromised patients.

Epidemiology

Most reports indicate that 0.5 to 1% of all hospitalized patients develop nosocomial pneumonia. The rates in intensive care units are generally higher, and among patients who are mechanically ventilated the rate is 6 to 20 times greater than for nonventilated patients. However, it should be noted that some of these incidence statistics are disputed due to the lack of precision in the diagnosis of nosocomial pneumonia. Other processes that may cause pulmonary infiltrates with variable presence of fever, purulent respiratory secretions, and/or leucocytosis include congestive heart failure, pulmonary embolism, atelectasis, adverse drug reactions, pulmonary haemorrhage, and the acute respiratory distress syndrome (ARDS).

The epidemiology of the pathogens in nosocomial pneumonia is highly variable. Some organisms become endemic, especially in intensive care units, the major pathogens in this setting being acinetobacter, extended-spectrum β-lactamase (ESBL)-producing

Table 18.4.3.1 Microbiology of nosocomial pneumonia

Microbe	Frequency (%)
Bacteria	80–90
Gram-negative bacteria	50–70
Staph. aureus	15–30
Anaerobic bacteria	10–30
Haemophilus influenzae	10–20
Streptococcus pneumoniae	10–20
Legionella	4
Viral	10–20
Fungi	<1

klebsiella, serratia, stenotrophamonas, pseudomonas, enterobacter, and methicillin-resistant *S. aureus* (MRSA). Another important nosocomial pathogen is legionella, which may cause outbreaks of legionnaire's disease in hospitals that can sometimes be traced to water supplies with distribution via air-conditioning cooling systems or shower heads. In these cases, the same species and serogroup found in the nosocomial cases should be found in the epidemiologically linked water supply. Aspergillosis may occur as epidemics among vulnerable patients with compromised cell-mediated immunity, neutropenia, or both. Influenza is highly contagious, and patients with influenza are commonly hospitalized, so it is now recommended that all patients with suspected influenza have confirmation of this diagnosis by rapid influenza testing, and the preference is for a single room when this is feasible.

Pathogenesis

The relatively high rates of pulmonary infections among patients who are hospitalized reflects (1) clustering of highly vulnerable patients; (2) patients rendered particularly vulnerable by violations of the integrity of the upper airways by intubation or tracheostomy; (3) many patients who are prone to aspiration due to compromised consciousness caused by associated medical conditions and anaesthesia; (4) patients rendered susceptible due to organ transplantation, cancer chemotherapy, and AIDS (Box 18.4.3.1).

As stated previously, the dominant pathogens in nosocomial pneumonia are Gram-negative bacteria, which reach the lung by aspiration of gastric contents or by microaspiration of upper airway secretions. The best explanation for this association between bacteriology and pathogenesis is the observation that patients with serious illness commonly have abnormal colonization of the upper airways by Gram-negative bacteria. Thus, throat cultures show that Gram-negative bacteria are found in only 2 to 3% of healthy persons, psychiatric patients, physicians, and medical students, whereas the rate of colonization in patients who are moderately ill is 30 to 40%, and in intensive care units the rate is 60 to 70%. These colonization rates are independent of antibiotic administration, but antibiotic exposure will increase the carrier rate even further. It can also be shown that buccal epithelial cells from patients who are seriously ill have enhanced attachment by Gram-negative

---

> **Box 18.4.3.1** Risks for nosocomial pneumonia
>
> ◆ Endotracheal intubation and tracheostomy-associated conditions
>
> • Age >70 years
>
> • Chronic lung disease
>
> • Poor nutritional status
>
> ◆ Risk of aspiration
>
> • Decreased consciousness
>
> • Intubation, tracheostomy, nasogastric intubation
>
> ◆ Thoracic or upper abdominal surgery
>
> ◆ Altered host defences
>
> • Immunosuppressive disorders

bacteria *in vitro*. The frequency of positive throat cultures for Gram-negative bacteria and the number that attach to respiratory cells are directly correlated with the severity of the associated disease. The usual mechanism of Gram-negative bacillary pneumonia in most hospitalized patients is aspiration of these organisms in the upper airways, or aspiration of these organisms from gastric contents after they are swallowed.

Pathogenesis of other organisms is quite different. Legionella, tuberculosis, influenza, and aspergillus are inhaled, the usual source being environmental (legionella or aspergillus) or another patient (influenza or tuberculosis).

Clinical features

The classic presentation for pneumonia is cough and fever, usually with purulent respiratory secretions. The diagnosis of pneumonia requires the demonstration of a pulmonary infiltrate on chest radiography. These same symptoms may be present in patients with acute bronchitis, which is virtually always a viral infection that does not merit antibacterial treatment. A notable exception is patients who have violation of the airways with endotracheal tubes or tracheostomies who may have 'febrile tracheobronchitis' due to bacterial infection, most frequently at the tip of the tube, the site of the cuff, or the site of insertion. As noted previously, many patients who satisfy the definition for nosocomial pneumonia based on a pulmonary infiltrate accompanied by fever and purulent respiratory secretions have alternative diagnoses when studied by reliable microbiological techniques using bronchoscopy with quantitative cultures of a bronchial-protected brush or bronchoalveolar lavage (BAL). The alternative noninfectious conditions in culture-negative cases include congestive heart failure, pulmonary embolism, atelectasis, bronchiolitis obliterans organizing pneumonia, etc.

Laboratory diagnosis

Tests to establish diagnosis and evaluate severity

The chest radiograph is critical for the confirmation of pneumonia. Major causes of false negative radiographs in the presence of nosocomial pneumonia are severe neutropenia and pneumonia caused by *P. jirovecii*. CT scans may reveal infiltrates that are not present on plain films, but it is not clear that this distinguishes a group that requires antibiotic treatment. Thus, the chest radiograph is generally viewed as adequately sensitive for detection of nosocomial pneumonia.

It is important to monitor blood gases to determine severity of illness and to monitor respiratory support.

Studies to determine microbial aetiology

Blood cultures are positive in 2 to 6% of patients with nosocomial pneumonia and clearly identify the causative agent. Some patients will have empyemas, and thoracentesis is necessary for both diagnosis and treatment. Again, this represents an uncontaminated source for culture, providing definitive evidence of the responsible pathogen. Empyema is an infrequent complication of nosocomial pneumonia, except in patients who have undergone thoracotomy who often have an empyema as a complication of chest tube placement.

Legionella, *Mycobacterium tuberculosis*, and respiratory viruses (influenza, parainfluenza, and respiratory syncytial virus) represent definitive pathogens when recovered in respiratory specimens since these organisms do not colonize the normal respiratory tract.

Most patients with nosocomial pneumonia do not have bacteraemia, empyema, or the pathogens that do not colonize the normal airway. In these cases, the physician must usually rely on routine bacterial cultures of respiratory secretions or resort to invasive diagnostic tests using bronchoscopy with quantitative cultures of BAL specimens or of the protected brush. Multiple studies have tested the validity of these techniques for distinguishing contaminants and pathogens. The results are somewhat variable, but often dependent on the precision of methodology. However, the use of these techniques has resulted in substantial controversy in the management of nosocomial pneumonia, especially in intensive care units where the stakes are high due to high rates of resistant pathogens and mortality. Arguments in favour of invasive diagnostic studies with bronchoscopy are the facts that the technology is well studied, about one-half of patients with suspected pneumonia have negative results and antibiotics can be avoided in this population, and the clear definition of pathogens permits pathogen-specific antibiotic treatment. Others argue that the invasive methods are unrealistic or unnecessary because routine semi-quantitative cultures of sputum or endotracheal aspirates are adequate semiquantitative cultures of tracheal aspirates are cheap, easy, and provide information that is equally valid.

Regardless of the method to obtain respiratory secretions for microbiological studies, it is usually beneficial to examine the specimen cytologically. Cultures should be reported with either quantitative or semiquantitative results. For quantitative results, the usual threshold for significance with the protected brush is 10^3/ml, and for BAL specimens it is usually 10^3 or 10^4/ml. With semiquantitative techniques, moderate or heavy growth usually indicates 'significant concentrations.' The main pathogens are summarized in Table 18.4.3.1: *S. epidermidis*, diphtheroids, *H. parainfluenzae*, enterococcus, and α-haemolytic streptococci are generally regarded as contaminants, regardless of concentrations. Anaerobic bacteria are frequently neglected pulmonary pathogens, but it is difficult to obtain specimens valid for anaerobic cultures, and many laboratories struggle with anaerobic microbiology even when the right specimens are obtained. The diagnosis of anaerobic pneumonia should be suspected when Gram stains show mixed bacteria, especially when there are morphotypes suggesting anaerobes, and specimens obtained by tracheal aspirate or bronchoscopy should be examined for these organisms. Putrid drainage always indicates anaerobic infection.

Treatment

The main management issues are antibiotic selection and respiratory support. The optimal method for selection of antibiotics is to base this decision on results of Gram stains and cultures (Table 18.4.3.2). When empirical decisions are necessary in seriously ill patients, agents are directed against Gram-negative bacteria, and the favoured drugs in this context are ceftazidime, cefepime, imipenem/meropenem, doripenem, piperacillin/piperacillin–tazobactam, ticarcillin/ticarcillin–sulbactam, or ciprofloxacin. For *S. aureus*, vancomycin is often added on the basis of Gram stain results or the perceived need to cover this pathogen. Some experts prefer linezolid for pneumonia involving MRSA, based on better lung penetration

Table 18.4.3.2 Treatment of nosocomial pneumonia

Pathogen	Antibiotic
Bacteria	
Gram-negative bacilli	
Pseudomonas aeruginosa[a]	Ceftazidime, imipenem, meropenem, doripenem, piperacillin/ticarcillin, cefepime or aztreonam, plus ciprofloxacin or an aminoglycoside
Xanthomonas[a]	Trimethoprim–sulfa
Enterobacteriaceae[a]	Cephalosporin (2nd or 3rd generation), β-lactam–β-lactamase inhibitor, aztreonam, imipenem, fluoroquinolone ± aminoglycoside
Anaerobes	Imipenem, β-lactam–β-lactamase inhibitor, clindamycin
Staphylococcus aureus[a]	Vancomycin or linezolid
Legionella	Gatifloxacin, levofloxacin, or azithromycin + rifampin
Viruses	
Influenza	Oseltamivir or zanamivir
Fungi	
Aspergillus	Voriconazole

[a] Need *in vitro* susceptibility data.

compared to vancomycin and limited clinical data favouring this drug.

Treatment for *Pseudomonas aeruginosa*, Acinetobacter, Klebsiella and other GNB are the predominant Gram-negative bacilli in nosocomial pneumonia in intensive care units, should be based on *in vitro* sensitivity tests. Anaerobic bacteria are well treated with imipenem/meropenem or any β-lactam–β-lactamase inhibitor; clindamycin can be used if these organisms are suspected and the alternatives are not used for other pathogens. The role of aminoglycosides in pulmonary infections involving Gram-negative bacilli is controversial due to the availability of effective less toxic alternatives. *S. aureus*, especially MRSA is also very important. The preferred antibiotics for MRSA in the lung are vancomycin or linezolide.

It should be emphasized that cultures of respiratory secretions obtained after the inception of antibiotic treatment have reduced validity. This observation emphasizes the importance of pretreatment cultures and caution with therapeutic decisions based on post-treatment cultures other than those of blood and pleural fluid.

Outcome

Nosocomial pneumonia is associated with a mortality rate reported at 8 to 20% for all cases. The mortality rate for infections acquired in the intensive care unit is 20 to 40%, with a mean of 25%. In the latter group the attributable mortality is 30 to 33%, meaning that associated conditions are the major factors in causing death.

Prevention

The frequency of nosocomial pneumonia and high mortality rate, especially in intensive care units, has prompted extensive studies of prevention. The methods that have withstood the test of time and have proven meritorious are the use of the semi-upright position to reduce the risk of aspiration, and hand washing between patients to prevent transmission of nosocomial pathogens.

The concern for patient positioning is based on marker studies showing that stomach contents are displaced to the lower respiratory tract with high frequency in patients in the recumbent position, and this can be easily corrected by use of an upright or semi-upright position. The assumption is that nosocomial pneumonia is frequently due to bacteria that reside in the stomach as a result of oral colonization.

Hand washing is a time-honoured method to reduce nosocomial infection that is commonly neglected by hospital personnel. It appears to be particularly important in the transmission of *S. aureus*, and is often important in organisms that are endemic or epidemic within hospital units such as acinetobacter, serratia, xanthomonas, pseudomonas, and enterobacter.

Other preventive measures are the use of orotracheal tubes instead of nasotracheal tubes, avoidance of intubation, maintenance of tube cuff pressure at more than 20 cm H_2O, and possibly the selective use of sulcrafate to reduce gastrointestinal bleeding.

A common practice in some intensive care units is 'selective decontamination' to interrupt the cycle of colonization of the colon by Gram-negative bacteria, followed by colonization of the upper airways by the same organisms, and then aspiration to cause pneumonia. The goal of selective decontamination is elimination or reduction in Gram-negative bacteria in the gastrointestinal tract with antibiotics that also preserve the anaerobic bacteria in the flora, since these are largely responsible for microbial population control in the colon. Drugs that are commonly used are oral preparations of polymyxin, aminoglycosides, aztreonam, trimethoprim–sulfamethoxazole, or cephalosporins. These are given orally with the expectation that they will have a substantial impact on the colonic flora, and they are sometimes also incorporated into paste formulations for application to the upper airways as well. Extensive trials with selective decontamination show that they achieve a substantial reduction in nosocomial pneumonia, but they do not seem to influence mortality due to this condition. Major concerns are the failure to reduce mortality rates, excessive costs of the regimens, and the perception of antibiotic abuse with encouragement of resistance.

Topical antibiotics have also been tested for utility in prophylaxis. The method is installation of drugs (usually polymyxin or aminoglycosides) through tracheostomies, endotracheal tubes, or by aerosolization. Extensive therapeutic trials with this tactic have shown that it is sometimes successful in interrupting epidemics due to susceptible bacteria, especially *P. aeruginosa*, but mortality rates have generally remained unchanged, and there is concern about the evolution of resistant bacteria. Topical antibiotics are generally not recommended, except for some patients with cystic fibrosis.

Interruption of epidemics involving legionella and aspergillus requires different tactics because these organisms are inhaled. For legionella and aspergillus, the goal is to eliminate the environmental source. Influenza is transmitted from person-to-person, so the goal is to eliminate this type of contact, which must include removal of health care workers with influenza from jobs that require patient contact. All hospital personnel should have influenza vaccine as a method to protect patients, and hospital personnel with jobs that require patient contact must be furloughed if they have suspected or established influenza.

Further reading

American Thoracic Society (2005). Hospital-acquired pneumonia in adults: diagnosis, assessment of severity, initial antimicrobial therapy and preventative strategies. A consensus statement. *Am J Respir Crit Care Med*, **171**, 388–416.

Canadian Critical Care Trials Group (2006). A randomized trial of diagnostic techniques for ventilator-associated pneumonia. *N Engl J Med*, **355**, 2619–30.

Fagon JY, *et al.* (1988). Detection of nosocomial lung infection in ventilated patients: use of a protected specimen brush and quantitative culture techniques in 147 patients. *Am Rev Respir Dis*, **138**, 110–16.

Fagon JY, *et al.* (1996). Nosocomial pneumonia and mortality among patients in intensive care units. *JAMA*, **275**, 866–9.

Fagon JY, *et al.* (2000). Invasive and noninvasive strategies for management of suspected ventilator-associated pneumonia. *Ann Intern Med*, **132**, 621–30.

Johanson WG, Pierce AK, Sanford JP (1969). Changing pharyngeal bacterial flora of hospitalized patients: emergence of Gram-negative bacilli. *N Engl J Med*, **281**, 1137–40.

Johanson WG Jr, Woods DE, Chaudhuri T (1979). Association of respiratory tract colonization with adherence of Gram-negative bacilli to epithelial cells. *J Infect Dis*, **139**, 667–73.

Morehead RS, Pinto SJ (2000). Ventilator-associated pneumonia. *Arch Intern Med*, **160**, 1926–36.

18.4.4 Pulmonary complications of HIV infection

Mark J. Rosen

Essentials

The lung is a frequent site of opportunistic infection in patients with HIV infection, and noninfectious pulmonary disorders associated with HIV infection and antiretroviral treatments are increasingly common. The severity of immunocompromise, with CD4+ lymphocyte count the most reliable surrogate, is the primary determinant of the risk of developing specific pulmonary disorders: early in the course of HIV these are similar to those seen in the general population; opportunistic infections occur with severe immunodeficiency, but with frequency reduced by prophylaxis.

Infectious diseases

Bacterial pneumonia—this is most commonly caused by *Streptococcus pneumoniae* and *Haemophilus influenzae*: diagnosis and treatment is substantially as for patients without HIV.

Pneumocystis jiroveci (formerly *P. carinii*)—pneumonia caused by this organism was the first opportunistic infection described in AIDS patients. Presentation is typically with a few weeks of fever and gradually increasing cough and breathlessness. The chest radiograph usually shows diffuse granular opacities. Diagnosis can be confirmed only by demonstrating organisms in a lung-derived specimen, either sputum induced by the inhalation of hypertonic saline solution, or by bronchoscopy. Trimethoprim–sulfamethoxazole is the preferred treatment (and also for prophylaxis), with steroids in more severe cases. Care in the intensive care unit with mechanical ventilation may be required and should not be denied on account of the diagnosis of HIV.

Other infections—tuberculosis often occurs before the development of opportunistic infections and may be difficult to diagnose, with cutaneous anergy making tuberculin skin tests of limited value. Pulmonary aspergillosis may develop in patients with advanced immunosuppression: invasive parenchymal infection is usually fatal; predominantly bronchial disease presents with dyspnoea and airway obstruction.

Neoplastic diseases

Kaposi's sarcoma (KS)—caused by human herpesvirus (HHV)-8, is the most common malignancy in individuals with HIV infection. The skin is the main site of involvement, but it may involve the airways, lungs tissue, mediastinal lymph nodes, and pleura. Lesions in the airways are usually asymptomatic, but can cause obstruction or haemoptysis. Parenchymal involvement is suggested by bronchial wall thickening, nodules, Kerley B lines and pleural effusion, especially in patients with cutaneous disease.

Other cancers—non-Hodgkin's B-cell lymphoma (NHL) and lung cancer are associated with HIV infection.

Other pulmonary conditions

Chronic bronchitis, bronchiectasis, and pulmonary hypertension are seen in patients with advanced HIV infection.

Immune reconstitution inflammatory syndrome (IRIS)—this is a diagnosis of exclusion when a patient with AIDS, on treatment with anti-HIV medications, develops symptoms consistent with an infectious or inflammatory condition while receiving antiretroviral therapy, with these symptoms not being explicable by a newly acquired infection, by the expected clinical course of the disease, or by the side effects of therapy. Treatment is symptomatic for most cases.

Introduction

The lung is a frequent site of opportunistic infection in immunocompromised patients, and noninfectious pulmonary disorders associated with HIV infection and antiretroviral treatments are increasingly common. Box 18.4.4.1 lists the infectious, neoplastic, and inflammatory diseases that occur in patients with HIV infection, and their typical radiographic patterns are summarized in Table 18.4.4.1.

The pulmonary disorders associated with HIV infection range from asymptomatic and mild abnormalities in pulmonary function to fulminating opportunistic infections. The initial approach to patients with suspected HIV-related pulmonary disorders is the same as for any other patient: the clinician will take a careful history, perform a physical examination and usually a chest radiograph, and determine whether or not to perform other diagnostic tests. The differential diagnosis will be influenced strongly by several factors that determine the risk of each specific HIV-associated lung disorder.

Risk factors for specific pulmonary disorders

Immune status

The severity of immunocompromise is the primary determinant of the risk of developing specific pulmonary disorders. Early in the course of HIV disease, when the immune system is relatively

---

Box 18.4.4.1 HIV-associated respiratory disorders

Bacterial pneumonia
- *Streptococcus pneumoniae*
- *Haemophilus influenzae*
- *Pseudomonas aeruginosa*
- *Staphylococcus aureus*
- *Moraxella catarrhalis*
- *Rhodococcus equi*
- *Mycobacterium tuberculosis*
- *Mycobacterium avium* complex (MAC)
- Other nontuberculous mycobacteria

Fungal infections
- *Pneumocystis jiroveci*
- *Cryptococcus neoformans*
- *Histoplasma capsulatum*
- *Aspergillus fumigatus*
- *Coccidioides immitis*
- *Blastomyces dermatitides*

Protozoal infections
- *Strongyloides stercoralis*
- *Toxoplasma gondii*

Viral infections
- Cytomegalovirus
- Adenovirus
- Herpes simplex

Malignancies
- Kaposi's sarcoma
- Non-Hodgkin's lymphoma
- Primary effusion lymphoma
- Carcinoma of the lung

Other disorders
- Sinusitis
- Bronchitis
- Bronchiectasis
- Emphysema
- Lymphocytic interstitial pneumonia
- Nonspecific interstitial pneumonia
- Cryptogenic organizing pneumonia
- Pulmonary arterial hypertension
- Immune reconstitution inflammatory syndrome

Table 18.4.4.1 Chest radiographic patterns and their common causes in HIV infection

Radiographic pattern	Causes
Focal infiltrates	Bacteria
	M. tuberculosis
	P. jiroveci
	Fungi
Diffuse infiltrates	P. jiroveci
	M. tuberculosis
	Kaposi's sarcoma
	Bacteria
	Fungi
	Cytomegalovirus
	Immune reconstitution
Diffuse nodules	Kaposi's sarcoma (large nodules)
	M. tuberculosis (miliary)
	Fungi (small nodules)
Pneumothorax	P. jiroveci
Mediastinal lymphadenopathy	M. tuberculosis
	M. avium complex
	Kaposi's sarcoma
	Lymphoma
	Fungi
	Immune reconstitution
Pleural effusion	Bacteria
	M. tuberculosis
	Kaposi's sarcoma
	Lymphoma (including primary effusion lymphoma)
	Cardiomyopathy
	Hypoproteinemia
	Immune reconstitution
Cavities	M tuberculosis (high CD4+)
	P. jiroveci (low CD4+)
	P. aeruginosa (low CD4+)
	R. equi
	Fungi

intact, respiratory disorders occur that are similar to those in the general population. Opportunistic infections occur only with severe immunodeficiency.

The CD4+ lymphocyte count is still the most reliable surrogate marker for immune function, the risk of opportunistic infection, and the risk of progression of HIV disease. Measurement of HIV activity (viral load) with serum HIV RNA is used routinely to assess the response to treatment with antiretroviral agents and to stratify patients by risk of the progression of disease, but is a less reliable predictor than CD4+ count in determining the risk of developing specific diseases.

Common respiratory problems like sinusitis and bronchitis may occur at any CD4+ lymphocyte count, and bacterial pneumonia and tuberculosis often occur before AIDS-defining opportunistic infections and neoplasms. With lower counts, different pulmonary infections occur with increasing frequency. Pneumocystis pneumonia (PCP) and other opportunistic infections tend to occur only with severe immunodeficiency (i.e. CD4+ count <200 cells/μl), and disseminated nontuberculous mycobacterioses, disseminated fungal infections, central nervous system toxoplasmosis, and cytomegalovirus (CMV) disease with even more severe immunocompromise.

Demographic factors

The increasing proportion of injection drug users in the HIV-infected population has been accompanied by the recognition that bacterial pneumonia is more common than PCP, and the risk of the development of bacterial pneumonia is significantly higher in injection drug users than in other persons with HIV infection.

Race and ethnicity may also influence the risk of bacterial pneumonia and tuberculosis developing, but these associations are confounded by differences in access to health care, the higher prevalence of tuberculosis in minority communities and underdeveloped countries, and the disproportionately high numbers of injection drug users who are black or Hispanic. Nevertheless, the risk of tuberculosis is higher in blacks and Hispanics than in whites, while whites have a higher risk of pneumocystis, HIV-associated malignancies, and CMV disease.

Residence

The place of residence strongly influences the risk of development of specific infections. The high incidence of PCP in the United States of America and Europe contrasts sharply with that in Africa, where it is much less common for reasons that remain unknown. The geographic distribution of endemic fungi is a strong determinant of the risk of those infections developing; for example, disseminated histoplasmosis and coccidioidomycosis are common in patients with AIDS who live in endemic areas. These infections may also occur as a reactivation disease after HIV-infected individuals move to other areas and immunocompromise develops.

Prophylaxis and active antiretroviral therapy

The risk of developing specific opportunistic infections declines with the use of prophylaxis. Even before the availability of combination active antiretroviral therapy (ART), the incidence of pneumocystis and tuberculosis, along with their attendant mortality rates, was declining, partly attributable to the use of prophylaxis by susceptible persons. Following the widespread use of ART, starting around 1996, the incidence of opportunistic infections and death among people infected with HIV declined dramatically because successful ART inhibits viral replication and restores immune function. However, immune reconstitution is associated with the development of other clinical syndromes, discussed later.

Infectious diseases

Bacterial pneumonia

HIV infection impairs humoral immunity through quantitative and functional defects in CD4+ lymphocytes, increasing the risk of developing bacterial infections, including sinusitis and pneumonia. These infections become more common as the CD4+ lymphocyte count declines. Injection drug users are at a higher risk than other groups, and neutropenia is an independent risk factor. Prophylaxis with trimethoprim-sulfamethoxazole appears to reduce the risk of bacterial pneumonia. Bacterial pneumonia may also accelerate the course of HIV disease, since it is an independent predictor of progression to AIDS and mortality.

Streptococcus pneumoniae and *Haemophilus influenzae* are the most frequent bacterial pathogens (Table 18.4.4.1). Pneumonia due to mycoplasma, legionella, and chlamydia is described, but seems to be relatively uncommon, especially in patients with severe immunosuppression. *Rhodococcus equi*, an aerobic Gram-positive acid-fast bacillus, may cause focal consolidation, endobronchial disease, and cavitation, usually in patients with advanced HIV disease. Pneumonia due to *Pseudomonas aeruginosa* may develop in patients with very low CD4+ lymphocyte counts (typically <50/µl), even in the absence of risk factors such as neutropenia, corticosteroid use, and hospital-acquired infection. *Nocardia asteroides* may cause nodules, consolidation, cavitation, pleural effusions, empyema, and intrathoracic lymphadenopathy in HIV-infected individuals.

The diagnosis and treatment of bacterial pneumonia in persons with HIV infection is in almost all respects the same as that for HIV-uninfected patients (see Chapter 18.4.2). Patients usually present with fever, chills, productive cough, and localized areas of consolidation on chest radiographs. While this clinical picture strongly suggests bacterial pneumonia, it may also occur with tuberculosis and fungal infection. Conversely, patients with bacterial pneumonia may have diffuse pulmonary opacities that resemble PCP.

Polyvalent pneumococcal vaccine is recommended for all HIV-infected people, although those with low CD4+ counts are less likely to mount an adequate antibody response. A vaccine against *H influenzae* type b (Hib) is available, but its use in patients with HIV infection is limited, since most infections are caused by strains that cannot be typed. Although influenza vaccine is also recommended, there are no data indicating that patients with HIV infection are at an increased risk of contracting influenza, or that the illness is more severe than in the general population.

Pneumocystis pneumonia (PCP)

Pneumonia caused by *Pneumocystis jiroveci* (formerly classified as *P. carinii*) was the first opportunistic infection described in AIDS patients, and has always been a major cause of illness and death. The term PCP has been used for decades, and rather than changing the terminology to 'PJP' to reflect the new nomenclature, there is consensus that PCP be used to refer to the term pneumocystis pneumonia.

Genomic analysis has revealed that *P. jiroveci*, once thought to be a parasite, is in fact a fungus that infects only humans, whereas *P. carinii* is pathogenic only in immunodeficient rats. The organism cannot be cultured reliably outside the lung, its source is still not identified, and hence the precise route of transmission is elusive.

Even though ART and effective prophylaxis for PCP have existed for years, this infection still occurs frequently for the following reasons: many patients do not know that they have HIV infection until an opportunistic infection develops; other patients know that they have HIV but are not receiving medical care; and some patients are receiving care and are not prescribed PCP prophylaxis or antiretrovirals. Adherence to complex regimens with intolerable side effects is often problematic, and the development of resistant strains of HIV is common. Patients may receive prophylaxis for PCP but be so profoundly immunocompromised that it is ineffective.

Clinical features

Patients with PCP usually present with fever and gradually increasing cough and dyspnea for a few weeks, but the disease sometimes presents as an acute illness with rapid deterioration over a few days. The chest radiograph usually shows diffuse granular opacities, which strongly suggest the diagnosis (Fig. 18.4.4.1). Some patients with PCP have nodular densities, lobar consolidation, or normal radiographic findings. Cystic abnormalities and spontaneous pneumothoraces in patients with known or suspected HIV infection are usually caused by PCP.

Adjunctive tests may support the diagnosis of PCP, but by themselves do not establish a diagnosis. This infection is unlikely in a patient who had a CD4+ cell count of more than 200 cells/µl in the preceding 2 months in the absence of other HIV-associated symptoms. Oxygen desaturation with exercise is a relatively sensitive and specific test in patients who are suspected to have PCP, but it is not diagnostic. About 90% of patients with PCP have an elevated serum lactate

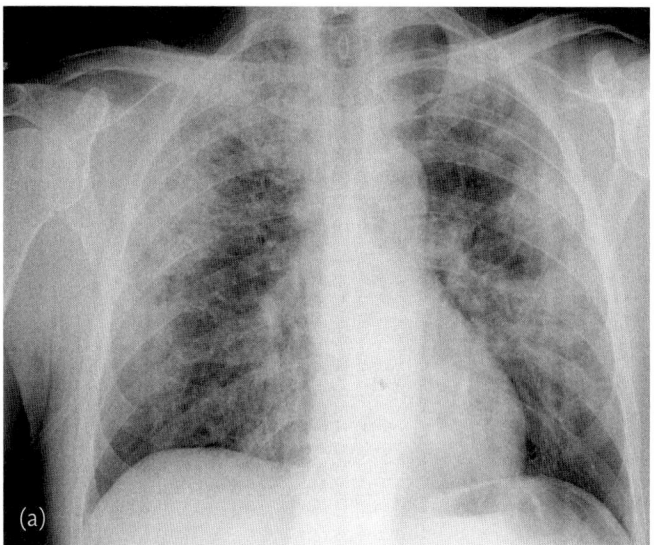

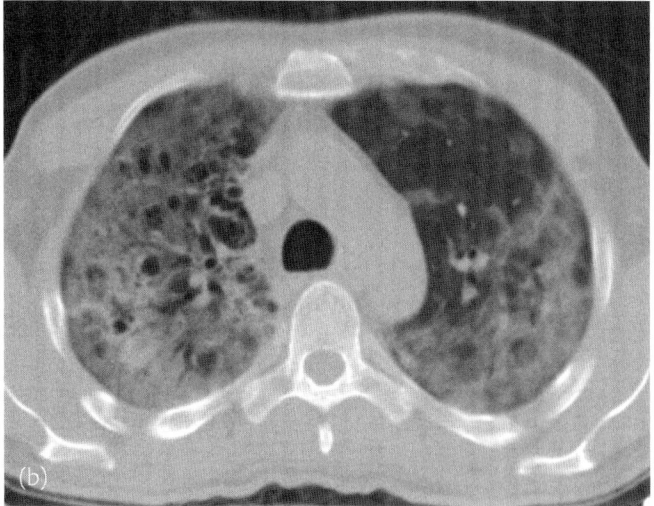

Fig. 18.4.4.1 (a) Chest radiograph of a patient with *P. jiroveci* pneumonia. Note the diffuse ground-glass opacities, most pronounced in the upper lobes. There are also poorly defined diffuse cystic changes, most pronounced in the right lower lung. (b) CT image of the chest of the same patient. There are diffuse areas of total lung opacification, as well large cysts.

dehydrogenase level, but this may occur with other pulmonary diseases, especially mycobacterial and fungal infections. Gallium-67 and Indium-111 lung scans are highly sensitive indicators of PCP, but isotope uptake also occurs in other pulmonary infections, so they are seldom useful in the diagnosis.

Microbiological diagnosis

Since *P. jiroveci* cannot be cultured *in vitro*, the diagnosis of PCP can be confirmed only by demonstrating organisms in a lung-derived specimen, either sputum induced by the inhalation of hypertonic saline solution, or obtained by bronchoscopy. Although establishing a diagnosis is not difficult, many clinicians treat patients with suspected PCP empirically, reserving bronchoscopy for those who do not respond to treatment. Bronchoalveolar lavage establishes the diagnosis in over 90% of cases, but some centres report that bronchoscopic lung biopsy increases the diagnostic yield not only for PCP, but also for other infections (especially *M. tuberculosis*) and noninfectious disorders. The optimal approach to the diagnosis of HIV-associated pulmonary disorders (including PCP) can be determined only by a prospective randomized clinical trial with outcome measures that include economic and survival analyses, but no trial has yet been performed, nor is such a trial likely as the incidence of these disorders is declining.

Treatment

Trimethoprim–sulfamethoxazole (TMP-SMX) is the preferred treatment for PCP in patients who have not had an adverse reaction to this drug, regardless of the severity of disease. It is consistently the most effective in comparative studies, and is also inexpensive and available in both oral and intravenous preparations. Patients with severe PCP who do not respond or are intolerant of this medication are usually given pentamidine, but this drug is associated with adverse reactions that are more serious than those associated with TMP-SMX. Trimetrexate–leucovorin is not as effective as TMP-SMX but is better tolerated than pentamidine. Mild to moderate PCP can be treated in the outpatient setting with dapsone/TMP, clindamycin/primaquine, or atovaquone. The optimal duration of treatment is unknown, but most clinicians treat for 14 to 21 days, followed by prophylaxis.

Respiratory failure caused by pneumocystis pneumonia

Animal models of PCP have shown that the clinical severity of infection correlates more closely with markers of inflammation than with the burden of organisms, suggesting that the immune response and its attendant inflammation account for the clinical manifestations of pneumonia. Respiratory compromise is associated with the presence of activated CD8+ cells and neutrophils in the lung, and corticosteroids are thought to attenuate these effects. The administration of corticosteroids at the start of antipneumocystis treatment reduces the likelihood of respiratory failure, the deterioration of oxygenation, and death in patients with moderate to severe pneumonia. Patients who are likely to benefit from therapy have a Pao_2 of less than 70 mmHg or an arterial-alveolar oxygen pressure difference of more than 35 mmHg. No benefits have been shown with less severe gas exchange abnormalities at the start of therapy, or in patients to whom corticosteroids were administered more than 72 h after antipneumocystis treatment was started. Adverse reactions to adjunctive corticosteroid therapy occur infrequently; life-threatening superinfections have been described, but they are uncommon. Patients in whom pulmonary symptoms with diffuse radiographic opacities develop shortly after apparently successful treatment of PCP should be evaluated for the presence of another opportunistic infection, especially CMV.

As the incidence of PCP declined in the last decade, fewer patients with PCP are admitted to the intensive care unit. Nevertheless, when the treatment of PCP is delayed or ineffective, hypoxaemic respiratory failure may develop. The clinical and radiographic features of severe PCP resemble those of the acute respiratory distress syndrome (ARDS), and the supportive treatment is similar, including intubation, mechanical ventilation, and the application of positive end-expiratory pressure. It is generally believed that patients who require mechanical ventilation for the treatment of PCP have a high mortality rate, possibly related to the lack of response to prophylaxis, antipneumocystis treatment, or adjunctive corticosteroid therapy. However, other studies found that 71% of these patients survived to hospital discharge, and the prospects for long-term survival following PCP are far more hopeful than earlier in the AIDS epidemic. However, the development of respiratory failure following several days of appropriate therapy for PCP, or of a pneumothorax while receiving mechanical ventilation, portend a poorer prognosis.

Prevention

Prophylaxis can be stopped safely in patients who achieve a sustained increase in CD4+ lymphocyte count to more than 200 cells/μl after starting ART. In those patients who have a suboptimal response to ART, lifelong antipneumocystis therapy is recommended for all HIV-infected patients with CD4+ cell counts lower than 200 cells/μl or for patients with HIV-related symptoms, including unexplained persistent fever (temperature >37.8°C or 100°F) for 2 weeks, oropharyngeal candidiasis that was unrelated to antibiotic or corticosteroid therapy, and unexplained weight loss. Prophylaxis with TMP-SMX is most effective but is associated with more adverse events requiring the discontinuation of therapy, and dapsone is generally used as second-line treatment. TMP-SMX has the additional advantages of being inexpensive and of preventing other infections, including cerebral toxoplasmosis and infection with some strains of pathogenic bacteria.

Tuberculosis

Modest reductions in cell-mediated immunity increase the risk of the reactivation of latent tuberculosis, and the risk increases as the CD4+ cell counts decline. In HIV-infected individuals, tuberculosis often occurs before the development of opportunistic infections, probably because *M. tuberculosis* is more virulent. In patients with mild immunodeficiency, the clinical presentation is similar to tuberculosis in HIV-negative patients. Atypical pulmonary presentations, including the presence of diffuse infiltrates, miliary patterns, intrathoracic lymphadenopathy, or normal chest radiograph findings occur more frequently in patients with advanced immunosuppression (Table 18.4.4.1). These patients also have a high incidence of extrapulmonary infection, including in the pleura, lymph nodes, gastrointestinal tract, bone marrow, and blood.

The diagnosis of tuberculosis may be difficult in HIV-infected individuals. Cutaneous anergy is more prevalent as CD4+ cell counts decline, making tuberculin skin tests less useful. Radiographic clues to the diagnosis include cavitation, hilar and mediastinal lymphadenopathy, and pleural effusions. When there is cavitation, acid-fast smears and cultures of sputum are usually positive. In patients who do not expectorate spontaneously, sputum may be induced with hypertonic saline solution. Bronchoscopy with bronchoalveolar lavage, transbronchial biopsy, and postbronchoscopy sputum is often diagnostic. Biopsy specimens enhance the immediate diagnostic yield of bronchoscopy in the diagnosis of pulmonary tuberculosis compared with analysis of bronchoalveolar lavage fluid alone.

Despite appropriate evaluation, acid-fast smears of sputum and bronchoscopic specimens may be negative, and cultures may not be positive for several weeks. Since early treatment of tuberculosis improves the outcome and reduces the transmission of the disease to others, initial empirical therapy is warranted for patients with radiographic abnormalities that are consistent with tuberculosis, unless another disorder is identified.

Aspergillosis

Life-threatening pulmonary aspergillosis may develop in patients with advanced immunosuppression. The following two common patterns of disease have been identified: an invasive parenchymal infection, which is usually fatal; and a predominantly bronchial disease presenting with dyspnea and airway obstruction. The classic risks for aspergillus infection—namely, prolonged neutropenia and treatment with high-dose corticosteroids—are often absent. Aspergillosis probably develops in patients with advanced AIDS because of defects in neutrophil or alveolar macrophage function. The CD4+ lymphocyte count is typically less than 30 cells/µl, and the prior use of corticosteroids and neutrophil counts of less than 500 cells/µl increase the risk. Disseminated disease is common, especially in the brain.

Clues to the diagnosis of invasive pulmonary aspergillosis include upper lobe disease with cavitation and haemoptysis. The diagnosis has traditionally required histological proof because aspergillus is ubiquitous, so its presence in nasopharyngeal secretions, sputum and bronchoalveolar lavage fluid may represent contamination or colonization. However, recent studies in patients with severe immunosuppression, including AIDS, indicate that the isolation of aspergillus in bronchoalveolar lavage fluid correlates strongly with histological proof of tissue invasion.

Neoplastic diseases

Kaposi's sarcoma

Kaposi's sarcoma (KS), caused by human herpesvirus (HHV-8), is the most common malignancy in persons with HIV infection. The skin is the major site of involvement, but visceral involvement with KS is common in advanced disease, and may involve the airways, lung tissue, mediastinal lymph nodes, and pleura. Patients with thoracic KS usually have obvious mucocutaneous lesions, but the lung may be the only site of disease in up to 15% of cases. The involvement of the airways, parenchyma, pleura, and intrathoracic lymph nodes causes a diverse range of symptoms and radiographic findings. Most patients with pulmonary KS that is diagnosed antemortem have cough, dyspnoea, and fever.

KS lesions in the airways are usually asymptomatic, but they sometimes cause obstruction or haemoptysis. The finding of typical lesions on inspection of the airways is usually considered to be diagnostic (Fig. 18.4.4.2), and achieving a histological diagnosis may be difficult because the yield of forceps biopsy is low. Furthermore, some authors believe that forceps biopsy of KS lesions carries significant risk of bleeding, but this is controversial.

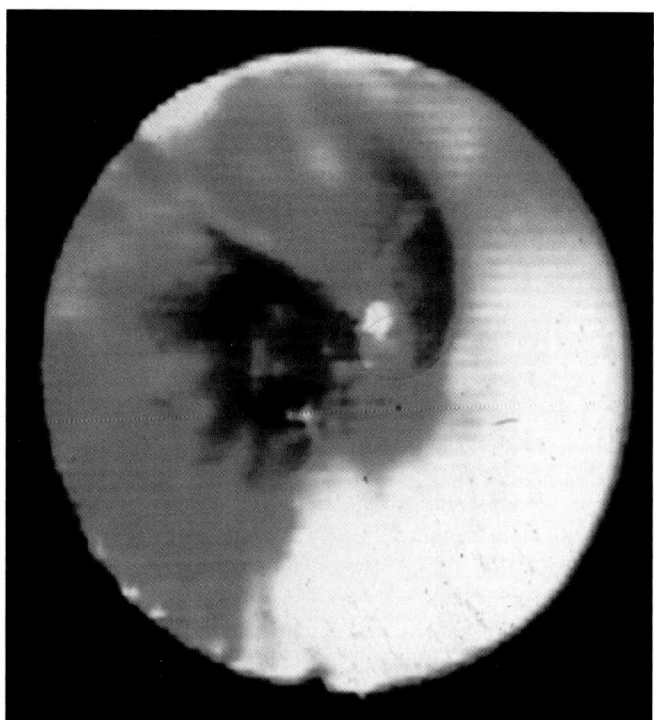

Fig. 18.4.2.2 Bronchoscopic appearance of Kaposi's sarcoma. The erythematous abnormality at branch points of large airways is typical of lung involvement with this neoplasm.

Parenchymal involvement with KS is suggested by bronchial wall thickening, nodules, Kerley B lines, and pleural effusion, especially in patients with cutaneous disease. Bronchoscopy can determine whether diffuse radiographic opacities are caused by KS or an opportunistic infection, but the yield of bronchoscopic lung biopsies in the diagnosis of KS is low, and even open-lung biopsy is nondiagnostic in about 10% of cases because of the focal distribution of the lesions. The diagnosis of pulmonary parenchymal KS is therefore usually inferred in patients with cutaneous disease, chest radiograph or CT findings that suggest this disorder, visual confirmation of airway lesions, and no evidence of opportunistic infection in bronchoalveolar lavage fluid or bronchoscopic lung biopsy specimens. Patients with parenchymal opacities who have typical lesions in the airways and no identified pulmonary infection are assumed to have parenchymal KS.

When KS involves the pleura, effusions are usually exudative and sanguinous, but cytological examination is nondiagnostic. Closed pleural biopsy specimens are rarely positive for KS due to the focal nature of the pleural lesions and the predominant involvement of the visceral pleura, rather than the parietal pleura. Since establishing a diagnosis therefore usually necessitates a thoracoscopic or open pleural biopsy, the presence of pleural involvement with KS is usually inferred in a patient with cutaneous disease and a serosanguinous effusion without a reasonable alternative explanation.

Lymphoma

Non-Hodgkin's B-cell lymphoma (NHL) is associated with HIV infection, and—unlike most other HIV-related disorders—continues to occur despite the use of highly active antiretroviral therapy (HAART). Although pulmonary involvement is usually clinically innocuous, the lung is a common site of extranodal disease. HIV-associated primary pulmonary lymphoma is most commonly a high-grade B-cell tumour occurring in the setting of advanced HIV infection.

If symptoms do occur, they tend to do so late in the course of HIV disease and simulate common opportunistic infections. Even in patients with an established diagnosis of lymphoma, lung involvement is usually a late feature of HIV disease that may present with lobar consolidation, nodules, reticular opacities, and masses. Airway involvement manifests as atelectasis.

The diagnosis is established by bronchoscopic or open biopsy; bronchoalveolar lavage has a very low diagnostic yield. In contrast to non-AIDS patients, mediastinal and hilar lymphadenopathy is generally not prominent in HIV-infected patients with NHL.

Pleural involvement is characterized by effusions and pleural thickening, with the diagnosis established by biopsy or cytological analyses of pleural fluid. Primary effusion lymphoma or body cavity lymphoma present with pleural, pericardial, or peritoneal growth of malignant lymphoma cells, usually in the absence of solid tumours. In almost all cases tumour DNA shows HHV-8, which is also the aetiological agent of KS (as previously described) and multicentric Castleman's disease, a dysplastic lymphoid disorder that may progress to plasmablastic lymphoma. The virus has a strong tropism for B-cells, and in some patients HHV-8-infected clones proliferate and transform into a large-cell 'liquid lymphoma' within serous cavities. In HIV-seropositive individuals the prognosis of primary effusion lymphoma is no better than in most other forms of lymphoma, and is probably worse.

Carcinoma of the lung

The incidence of lung cancer is increased in individuals with HIV infection, especially in the years following the use of combination ART as the standard of care. Although most populations with HIV infection are current or former smokers, their risk of developing lung cancer appears to be increased even when incidence ratios are adjusted for smoking. The prevalence of microsatellite alternations reflecting genomic instability occurs with greatly increased frequency in HIV-associated lung cancers, possibly playing a role in their pathogenesis.

Patients with lung cancer in the setting of HIV infection tend to be relatively young at presentation (mean age 45 years) and have mild or moderate immunosuppression. Similar to age-matched controls, 75 to 90% present with stage III or IV disease. Adenocarcinoma is the most common histological type, with its prognosis appearing to be worse in patients with HIV infection. The diagnostic and therapeutic approaches to HIV-associated lung cancer are the same as for other patients, although the efficacy and toxicity of chemotherapy and radiotherapy may be different.

Other pulmonary disorders

Airway disease

There is a propensity for the development of chronic bronchitis and bronchiectasis in patients with advanced HIV infection, even if they do not smoke. The CD4+ count is usually low (<100 cells/µl). Therapy with standard antimicrobial agents is usually effective, but symptoms are likely to recur, especially when *P. aeruginosa* is isolated from the sputum. The role and efficacy of therapy with bronchodilators and anti-inflammatory agents in HIV-associated airway disease have not been studied. HIV infection also appears to

accelerate the onset of smoking-related emphysema, possibly through cytotoxic lymphocyte activity.

Pulmonary hypertension

Pulmonary hypertension occurs more commonly in HIV-infected patients than in the general population and may eventually lead to cor pulmonale and death. HHV-8 (the aetiologic agent of KS) may be linked with pulmonary hypertension in patients without HIV infection, perhaps through the dysregulation of endothelial cell growth or growth-factor signalling. HIV-associated pulmonary hypertension appears to occur at all stages of HIV infection, and the approach to diagnosis and treatment is the same as that for idiopathic pulmonary arterial hypertension in HIV-uninfected persons (see Chapter 16.15.2).

Immune restoration syndromes

The effectiveness of HAART in restoring immune function has given rise to a new disorder, the immune reconstitution inflammatory syndrome (IRIS), which is defined as a paradoxical deterioration in clinical status that is attributable to the recovery of the immune system during HAART. When treatment with HAART is successful, the number of blood CD4+ lymphocytes increases, as does their activity. Increased immune function then leads to inflammation that may otherwise have been clinically silent, and to overt clinical illness.

The diagnostic criteria for IRIS include the diagnosis of AIDS, treatment with anti-HIV medications, symptoms consistent with an infectious or inflammatory condition that appear whilst receiving antiretroviral therapy, with these symptoms not being explicable by a newly acquired infection, by the expected clinical course of the disease, or by the side effects of therapy. 'Paradoxical worsening of tuberculosis' can manifest as fever with worsening or the emergence of cervical intrathoracic lymphadenopathy, pulmonary infiltrates, pleural effusions or other tuberculous lesions in patients shortly after starting HAART, which is associated with the restoration of cutaneous reactivity to skin test antigens. Respiratory failure caused by IRIS has been reported in several cases following introduction of HAART after the successful treatment of PCP. Other patients have had apparent exacerbations of disease after introduction of HAART following or during infection with *Mycobacterium avium* complex (MAC), cryptococcosis, CMV, herpes zoster, hepatitis B and C viruses, and the agent that causes progressive multifocal leukoencephalopathy.

IRIS is a diagnosis of exclusion suggested by a compatible clinical syndrome in a patient who is recovering from an infection and has begun receiving HAART in the preceding few months. The plasma HIV load and CD4+ lymphocyte counts are usually improved compared with previous measurements, but the circulating CD4+ count may be unchanged because these cells are compartmentalized to sites of active inflammation. Opportunistic infection is usually a diagnostic consideration, but in the absence of a severe illness and in the proper clinical setting, invasive procedures can usually be avoided and the patient observed. If bronchoscopy is performed, the mean CD4/CD8 ratio is significantly higher (0.54) than in HIV-infected patients who are undergoing bronchoscopy for other respiratory complaints (0.07). Most patients simply require palliative therapy for symptoms, such as antipyretic agents for fever. Systemic corticosteroids have been used successfully in the treatment of severe inflammatory disease causing significant end-organ damage.

Further reading

Centers for Disease Control and Prevention (2009). Guidelines for prevention and treatment of opportunistic infections in HIV-infected adults and adolescents. Recommendations from CDC, the National Institutes of Health, and the HIV Medicine Association of the Infectious Diseases Society of America. *MMWR*, **58**, No RR–4, 1–216.

Herida M, *et al.* (2003). Incidence of non-AIDS defining cancers before and during the highly active antiretroviral therapy era in a cohort of human immunodeficiency virus-infected patients. *J Clin Oncol*, **21**, 3447–53.

Hirschtick RE, *et al.* (1995). Bacterial pneumonia in patients infected with human immunodeficiency virus. *N Engl J Med*, **333**, 845–51.

Huang L, *et al.* (1996). Presentation of AIDS-related Kaposi's sarcoma diagnosed by bronchoscopy. *Am J Respir Crit Care Med*, **153**, 1385–90.

Huang L, *et al.* (2006). An official ATS workshop summary: recent advances and future directions in Pneumocystis pneumonia (PCP). *Proc Am Thorac Soc*, **3**, 655-664.

Lortholary O, *et al.* (1993). Invasive aspergillosis in patients with acquired immunodeficiency syndrome: report of 33 cases. *Am J Med*, **95**, 177–87.

Mehta NJ, *et al.* (2000). HIV-related pulmonary hypertension: analytic review of 131 cases. *Chest*, **118**, 1133–41.

Morris A, *et al.* (2004). Current epidemiology of *Pneumocystis* pneumonia. *Emerg Infect Dis*, **110**, 1713–20.

Narita M, *et al.* (1998). Paradoxical worsening of tuberculosis following antiretroviral therapy in patients with AIDS. *Am J Respir Crit Care Med*, **158**, 157–61.

National Institutes of Health-University of California Expert Panel for Corticosteroid as Adjunctive Therapy for Pneumocystis Pneumonia (1990). Consensus statement on the use of corticosteroid as adjunctive therapy for Pneumocystis pneumonia in the acquired immunodeficiency syndrome. *N Engl J Med*, **323**, 1500–4.

Rosen MJ (2005). Intensive care of patients with HIV infection: time to take another look. *J Intensive Care Med*, **20**, 312–15.

Sitbon O, Lascoux-Combe C, Delfraissy J-F (2008). Prevalence of HIV-related pulmonary arterial hypertension in the current antiretroviral therapy era. *Am J Respir Crit Care Med*, **177**, 108–13.

United Nations Programme on HIV/AIDS and World Health Organization (2006). AIDS Epidemic Update. http://www.who.int/hiv/mediacenter/2006_EpiUpdate_en.pdf. Accessed April 1, 2007.

Wallace JM, *et al.* (1993). Respiratory illness in persons with human immunodeficiency virus infection. *Am Rev Respir Dis*, **148**, 1523–9.

Wislez M, *et al.* (2001). Acute respiratory failure following HAART introduction in patients treated for *Pneumocystis* pneumonia. *Am J Respir Crit Care Med*, **164**, 847–51.

The upper respiratory tract

Contents

18.5.1 Upper airways obstruction

J.R. Stradling and S.E. Craig

Essentials

At resting levels of ventilation, the main airway can be reduced to a diameter of 3 mm or so before respiratory distress and stridor occur. Little more narrowing is required to precipitate complete asphyxia, hence when upper airways obstruction is suspected, assessment of severity, diagnosis, and treatment is a medical emergency.

Clinical features and diagnosis—recognizing the presence of upper airways obstruction requires a high degree of clinical suspicion: stridor or noisy breathing will initially only be heard on exercise, but will gradually appear at lower and lower levels of activity; a patient's complaint that the problem is 'somewhere in the neck' should be taken seriously.

Investigation—peak expiratory flow rate is reduced disproportionately to the forced expiratory volume in 1 s (FEV_1), but the best functional evidence of upper airways obstruction is obtained with a flow–volume loop, which shows a squared appearance.

Acute upper airway obstruction—this can be caused by aspiration, oedema (allergic, hereditary, and acquired angio-oedema, smoke inhalation), and infection (more commonly in children). The emergency treatment for aspiration is the Heimlich manoeuvre (abdominal thrust); allergic causes require intramuscular adrenaline (0.5 ml of 1:1000, and see Chapter 17.2 for details of the management of anaphylaxis). Intubation or emergency cricothyroidotomy (in rare cases) may be required.

Nonacute upper airway obstruction—this can be caused by tumours, tracheal stenosis (usually after intubation or tracheostomy), tracheal compression, various tracheal abnormalities, and laryngeal dysfunction. Spread of a primary bronchial carcinoma into the base of the trachea is probably the commonest cause. This unfortunately becomes a terminal event in many cases, when adequate sedation must be given to make the patient unaware that they are asphyxiating and choking to death.

Definition

The trachea and carina are usually included in discussions of upper airways obstruction because many of the conditions that can completely block off the main airway can affect the trachea, presenting in a similar way to those affecting the larynx and pharynx. For convenience, the causes of upper airways obstruction are divided into acute (within minutes or hours) and nonacute, although there is not quite such a clear distinction in clinical practice. Many of the causes of upper airways obstruction (particularly infection) are more common in children, but this chapter deals with the problem mainly from the perspective of an adults' physician.

At resting levels of minute ventilation, the main airway can be reduced to a diameter of 3 mm or so before respiratory distress and stridor occur. Little more narrowing is required to precipitate complete asphyxia, hence when upper airways obstruction is suspected, assessment of severity, diagnosis, and treatment is a medical emergency. The causes are listed in Table 18.5.1.1.

Diagnosis of the presence of upper airway obstruction

History

Diagnosis of the presence of upper airways obstruction requires a high degree of clinical suspicion. Not all that wheezes is asthma. If upper airways obstruction develops gradually, then it is most likely to be misdiagnosed as asthma or chronic airways obstruction, particularly if—for example—a carcinoma of the trachea coexists with chronic airways obstruction. This is not uncommon, since both are usually caused by smoking. Clues in the history will be a more

Table 18.5.1.1 Causes of upper airways obstruction

Acute	Nonacute
Inhaled foreign body	Tumours
Oedema	Tracheal stenosis
Allergy	Postintubation
Angio-oedema	Post-tracheostomy
Smoke burns	Tracheal compression
Infections	Tumour
Pharyngitis	Thyroid
Tonsillitis	Aneurysm
Epiglottitis	Tracheal abnormalities
Retropharyngeal abscess	Tracheomalacia
Croup	Tracheobronchiomegaly
	Tracheobronchopathia osteochondroplastica
	Recurrent laryngeal nerve palsy
	Laryngeal dysfunction

rapid onset than might be expected for chronic airways obstruction and no previous history of a similar problem. The progression is usually relentless, without fluctuations, although a course of steroids prescribed for 'asthma' may produce temporary tumour shrinkage. At first, stridor or noisy breathing will only be heard on exercise, but it will gradually appear at lower and lower levels of activity. Sometimes the patient is well aware that the blockage is 'somewhere in the neck' and such a complaint should be taken seriously, as should associated haemoptysis. A nonproductive cough is often present. A change in the voice in association with shortness of breath indicates the possibility of laryngeal obstruction. Upper airways obstruction is sometimes more symptomatic on lying down.

Examination

In pure upper airways obstruction, noisy breathing will localize to the airway and tends to be monophonic and stridulous, although stridor may be absent if there is a long segment of obstruction. The only sound at the periphery on auscultation of the chest will be the transmitted noise of the stridor. However, as mentioned above, some patients will have coincidental lower airways obstruction, which should not discourage further investigation of a suggestive history. If upper airways obstruction is extrathoracic, stridor will tend to be worse on inspiration, and the converse may be true when the lesion is intrathoracic. The reasons for this are discussed below.

Tests of lung function

Flow–volume loops

During a forced expiration from total lung volume down to residual volume there is a progressive fall in expiratory flow rate. This is largely due to the fact that the airways become narrower as the lungs become smaller, and this progressively restricts maximum flow rate regardless of the effort made. This can be displayed graphically as a plot of expiratory flow against the volume exhaled

from total lung capacity down to residual volume, the so called 'flow–volume' plot or loop (Fig. 18.5.1.1a). This fall-off in maximal flow rates with falling lung volume is called 'volume dependence of flow'. However, if a fixed resistance is introduced (such as tracheal stenosis), then the maximal flow rate possible is independent of lung volume: high flow rates, usually seen at larger lung volumes, cannot be generated and, instead of the normal triangular appearance of the flow–volume plot, it has a squared appearance. At lower lung volumes the normal intrinsic airways resistance may again exceed the abnormal upper airways resistance so that the flow–volume plot may once again follow the normal path (Fig. 18.5.1.1a).

The normal inspiratory limb of the flow–volume loop is almost semicircular (Fig. 18.5.1.1b). This is because at residual volume the airways are small and limit flow; towards total lung capacity the inspiratory muscles are reaching their full contraction and power is falling off, hence maximum flows are achieved in the midrange of lung volume (Fig. 18.5.1.1b). Again, if upper airways obstruction is present, this pattern may be replaced by a squarer shape owing to the imposition of a lower maximum flow rate by the fixed resistance (Fig. 18.5.1.1b).

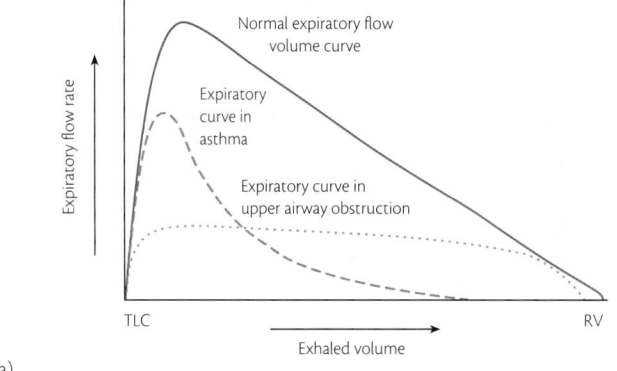

(a)

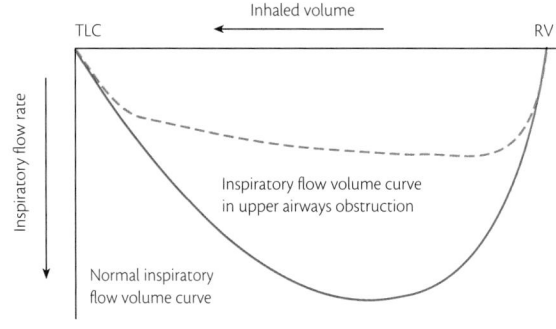

(b)

Fig. 18.5.1.1 (a) Expiratory flow–volume loop. The subject exhales with maximum effort from total lung capacity (TLC) until residual volume (RV) is reached. Normally, maximum flow (vertical axis) is reached early on and the flow falls almost linearly with lung volumes thereafter. In lower airways obstruction (e.g. asthma), all flows are reduced, but particularly at lower lung volumes. In upper airways obstruction, the maximum flow is clipped and roughly constant across most of the manoeuvre. (b) Inspiratory volume loop. The subject inhales maximally from residual volume (RV) up to total lung capacity (TLC). Normally, maximum flow is reached at about halfway when there is the best combination of airways size and muscle strength (see text). In upper airways obstruction, maximum flow is determined by the size of the remaining orifice and is roughly constant across the manoeuvre.

Comparison of the inspiratory and expiratory limbs of the flow–volume loop may give a clue as to the location of an upper airways obstruction. If the lesion is extrathoracic and has any variability to its lumen, it will tend to be narrowest during inspiration (walls sucked together) and widest during expiration (blown apart). Conversely, an intrathoracic lesion will tend to be squashed on expiration by the raised intrathoracic pressures, thus presenting a higher resistance than during inspiration when it will tend to be pulled open. Although in theory these statements are correct, in practice flow–volume loops are not always sufficiently characteristic to allow a confident diagnosis about the exact site and presence of an upper airways obstruction. They may be more useful as a tool to follow changes, such as in response to treatment.

Measurement of peak expiratory flow and spirometry

If the apparatus required to measure flow–volume plots or loops is not available, a peak expiratory flow (PEF) meter and spirometry plot may be useful. Because the fixed extra expiratory resistance clips the high flow rates predominantly, the PEF rate will be reduced disproportionately to the forced expiratory volume in 1 s (FEV_1) since FEV_1 is a measure over a longer time period, which includes lower flow rates because of the falling lung volume. This gives rise to a simple index of upper airways obstruction; FEV_1 (ml) divided by the PEF rate (litres/min). Normally the value will be less than 10, but as the PEF rate is preferentially clipped in upper airway obstruction (which does not happen when there is increased diffuse airways obstruction such as asthma) it may rise above 10. However, an index of less than 10 does not exclude upper airways obstruction because the lesion may not be rigid and, if it is intrathoracic, it may also narrow a little as lung volume falls.

Another spirometric clue to upper airway obstruction is the shape of the FEV_1 curve. Normally this is curved because flow rate falls with time, but it becomes straighter if flow rate is fixed (Fig. 18.5.1.2a).

Vocal cord paresis due to bilateral recurrent laryngeal nerve damage is often very much worse on inspiration. Simple spirometry can be diagnostic here. The expiratory tracing will be normal as the cords are blown apart. If the patient immediately inhales back from the spirometer (make sure that a new in-line filter is present first), then the inspiratory rate will be tortuously slow (Fig. 18.5.1.2b). The forced inspiratory volume in 1 s (FIV_1) will often be much smaller than the FEV_1, whereas normally the reverse is true (Fig. 18.5.1.2b).

For simple monitoring of progress of a patient with known upper airways obstruction on the ward, e.g. during treatment, sophisticated tests are not required, and measurement of the PEF rate is probably adequate for most purposes.

Specific causes of acute upper airway obstruction

Aspiration

Upper airways obstruction due to aspiration is usually due to the object lodging in the larynx, since this is the narrowest portion of the airway until two or three divisions down the bronchial tree. The usual culprit is a piece of food, and thus this condition has been colourfully called the 'café coronary'. The patient suddenly becomes distressed, is unable to talk, and apparently unable to breathe. He may point to his throat, trying to indicate the problem. Inspiration to provide the air necessary for a good expulsive cough

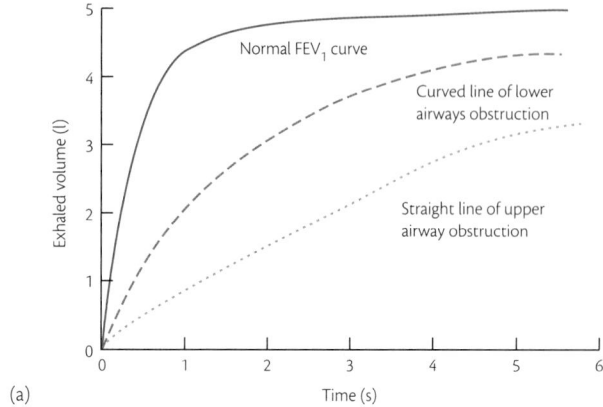

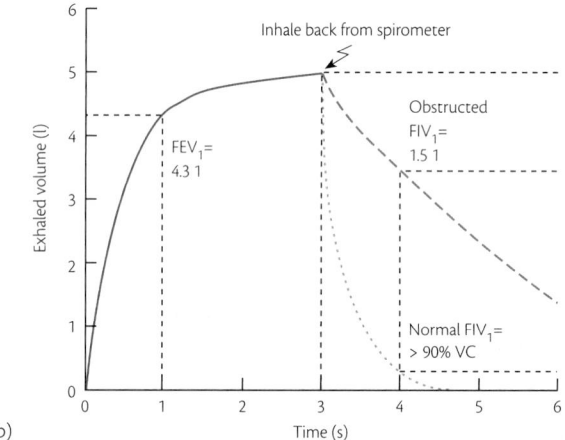

Fig. 18.5.1.2 (a) Curves of forced expiratory volume (FEV) against time. Normally exhalation is rapid, and more than 75% of the final volume (vital capacity (VC)) is exhaled in 1 s (FEV_1). In lower airways obstruction, flows are slower and thus less air is exhaled in 1 s; the line is still curved because flows are falling. In upper airways obstruction, because flows are roughly constant at a low level set by the remaining orifice, the line is nearly straight and FEV_1 is also low. (b) Following a forced exhalation manoeuvre into a spirometer, a forced inhalation can be made. Normally inspiration is fast and the forced inspiratory volume in 1 s (FIV_1) is almost the vital capacity (VC). If there is upper airways obstruction, particularly extrathoracic such as at the vocal cords, then inspiration will be very limited and FIV_1 will be small.

may not be possible. Indeed, lung volume may 'ratchet' down to residual volume.

The Heimlich manoeuvre (abdominal thrust) was invented for this circumstance and its principles should be taught to first-aid workers. If the patient is still upright, then the helper stands behind with his arms clasped around the upper abdomen. A very forceful pull, backwards and upwards, will drive the diaphragm upwards and should provide enough expired air to shift the aspirated food from the cords (Fig. 18.5.1.3). The manoeuvre can be repeated, of course, but a forceful first try is likely to be the most successful. If the Heimlich manoeuvre fails, then it may be possible to dislodge the lump of food with a finger once the patient has become unconscious. The only alternative is an emergency cricothyroidtomy, which requires a hole to be made in the cricothyroid membrane just below the Adam's apple of the thyroid cartilage and above the cricoid cartilage. Even a small hole (2 mm or so) will allow sufficient ventilation to keep the patient alive, and emergency cricothyroidotomies have been attempted with everything from penknives

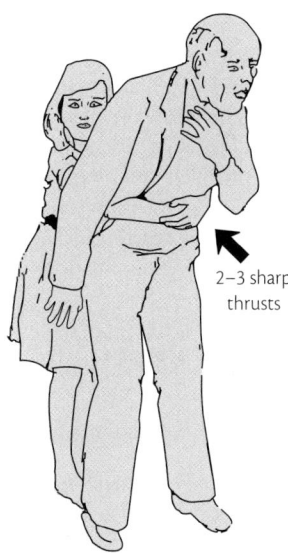

2–3 sharp
thrusts

Fig. 18.5.1.3 The Heimlich manoeuvre for the emergency treatment of acute pharyngeal or laryngeal obstruction due to a bolus of food. Two or three sharp thrusts in the direction of the arrow may cause the food to be ejected. (From Flenley DC (1990). *Respiratory medicine*. Baillière Tindall, London, with permission.)

to ball-point pens: special large-bore curved-needle kits are available for the purpose and are safer than an unskilled attempt at a tracheostomy.

Oedema

Acute oedema of the larynx or pharynx is usually either due to allergy (atopic or nonatopic), a hereditary abnormality in the complement pathway, or inhalation of noxious gases.

Allergic oedema

Episodes of upper airways and facial oedema sometimes have no known cause and appear without warning. Usually, however, there will be an atopic history with a specific allergy, a prior history of hay fever, and the oral allergy syndrome with tingling in the lips and tongue after certain fruits and nuts. Whereas oral ingestion of allergens rarely progresses to IgE-mediated anaphylaxis with life-threatening upper airway obstruction (the offending proteins are broken down before absorption, exceptions being certain nuts, fish, and egg), insect stings can do so as they are directly injected. Some apparently allergic reactions are not based on atopy and IgE, but may occur through IgG mechanisms, direct activation of other inflammatory pathways, or ingestion of vasodilator substances. For example, histamine and toxic histamine-like breakdown products from 'spoiled' scombroid fish (e.g. tuna) can cause airway oedema, but general flushing, urticaria, diarrhoea, and hypotension are usually present.

Treatment of these allergic causes of upper airways obstruction consists of intramuscular adrenaline (epinephrine) (1 ml of 1:1000), with antihistamines and steroids (see Chapter 17.2 on acute anaphylaxis). Aerosolized adrenaline may also be useful, using 10 ml of 1:10 000 in an ordinary nebulizer.

Hereditary and acquired angio-oedema

Nonallergic hereditary and acquired angio-oedema are due to deficiency of plasma C1 inhibitor, which regulates the enzyme activating the first component of the complement pathway. This deficiency allows abnormal increase in activity of the whole pathway, leading to consumption and lowering of C4 and C2 levels and production of vasoactive products such as bradykinin that are probably responsible for the resulting oedema.

Hereditary angio-oedema (OMIM 106100) is due to mutations in the C1 inhibitor gene (chromosome 11), causing either type I disease (85%, in which there are low levels of normal protein) or type II (15%, in which there are normal levels of dysfunctional mutant protein). It is transmitted as an autosomal dominant trait and typically presents in childhood or adolescence in patients who are normally well with no other underlying diseases.

Attacks may be precipitated by local trauma such as tooth extraction and are usually in one of three sites: subcutaneous tissues (face, limbs, genitals) most commonly, abdominal organs (which may mimic a surgical emergency with vomiting and colicky abdominal pain) in 25% of cases, and larynx, which may lead to laryngeal oedema (70% lifetime incidence). The episodes often worsen over 12 to 24 h, with resolution within 72 h. Importantly, there is absence of urticaria and pruritus such as is seen with allergic oedema.

Diagnosis hinges on the clinical presentation, a positive family history (although new mutations do occur), and low levels of C4 and C1 inhibitor. If there are normal levels of C1 inhibitor and low C4 then type II hereditary angio-oedema should be suspected and functional studies requested.

A similar syndrome occurs in about 0.1 to 1% (depending on ethnic origin) of patients taking angiotension converting enzyme (ACE) inhibitors (and less frequently with angiotensin receptor blockers), usually soon after starting therapy. Death from laryngeal oedema has been reported, but the exact mechanism of this is not fully understood. Nonetheless, it is sensible to recommend that ACE inhibitors should not be used in patients with a history of angio-oedema and C1 inhibitor deficiency.

Acquired angio-oedema presents in later life, usually after age 40, and is also classified into two forms: type I is associated with lymphoproliferative or other malignant diseases, and type II is due to autoantibodies directed against the C1 inhibitor molecule. C4 and C1 inhibitor levels are low. Symptoms and attacks are similar to hereditary angio-oedema, except there is no family history. Transient depressions of C1 inhibitor have been associated with viral infections.

Any acute attack that involves the airway is potentially life threatening. Management should be initially directed at protecting the airway with early intubation, or emergency cricothyroidotomy in rare cases. If the diagnosis is known, then C1 inhibitor concentrate (not available in the United States of America) should be given during an acute attack although very large doses are frequently needed for those with an acquired defect. Fresh frozen plasma has been reported to work sometimes, but it contains larger amounts of the substrates C4 and C2, which might theoretically provoke worsening oedema.

Abdominal attacks should have analgesia and intravenous fluids as well as C1 inhibitor concentrate in severe cases. Milder abdominal attacks and cutaneous swelling respond to tranexamic acid or may resolve spontaneously.

Attenuated androgens, e.g. danazol, raise C1 inhibitor levels within a few weeks, probably by increasing hepatic synthesis, and can usually prevent attacks in hereditary angio-oedema. Acquired angio-oedema generally fails to respond to this treatment, but can be treated prophylactically with antifibrinolytic agents. If episodes such as tooth extractions are triggers, then C1 inhibitor can be given beforehand.

Smoke inhalation

Inhalation of hot smoke can burn the upper airways and contributes significantly to deaths due to fires. Upper airways obstruction due to heat injury and mucosal swelling usually develops within 24 h of exposure, but stenosis due to scarring can develop later. A hoarse voice, stridor, severe conjunctivitis, burnt nasal hairs, and falling peak flow all suggest significant upper airways damage. Bronchoscopy is then the best tool to establish whether there is significant oedema or mucosal ulceration obstructing the airways.

Management usually consists of simple measures such as elevating the head of the bed and inhaling cool moist air with added oxygen. If peak flow continues to fall, then transfer to an intensive care unit and bronchoscopy with the capability to perform an intubation, guided by direct vision, is the correct approach.

Infections

Upper airway infections rarely cause obstruction in adults, but can do so in infants and young children. Presentation with upper airways obstruction can be dramatic, but prodromal symptoms usually occur. Streptococcal pharyngitis, tonsillitis, and retropharyngeal abscesses are amongst the most important. Croup (due to respiratory syncytial, parainfluenza, and other viruses) is very common, with narrowing of the subglottic trachea, sometimes with a thick purulent coating over the larynx and trachea. Treatment consists of cool mist and supplemental oxygen, with careful monitoring of upper airways function.

Although again more common in children, acute epiglottitis, usually due to *Haemophilus influenzae*, can affect adults. Pyrexia, drooling, hoarse voice, difficulty in breathing, intense sore throat, and stridor are the usual presenting symptoms. Compared with croup, there is generally a faster onset and course. The diagnosis may be missed initially, but a lateral neck radiograph can show swelling of the epiglottis (Fig. 18.5.1.4). Attempts to examine the back of the throat may precipitate further obstruction, particularly

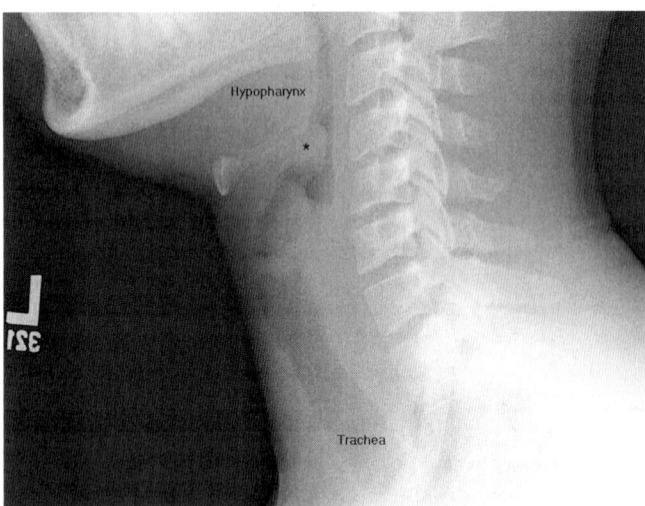

Fig. 18.5.1.4 Lateral neck radiograph of a patient with epiglottitis. Note the swollen epiglottis overlying the glottis marked with a *.
With permission from MedPix. Card 3605 and original contributor Dr. David M.Delonga.

in children, and even tipping the head back for a lateral neck radiograph can provoke complete obstruction and be disastrous. Thus, if there is evidence of breathing difficulty with stridor and the clinical diagnosis is epiglottitis, then the correct management for children is immediate transfer to intensive care and intubation for 48 to 72 h whilst the infection is controlled by amoxicillin or chloramphenicol. In adults, close monitoring in intensive care is probably adequate and prophylactic intubation is not routinely practised. Widespread vaccination against *H. influenzae* is making this problem increasingly rare.

Nonacute causes of upper airway obstruction

Tumours

Laryngeal, and less commonly tracheal, tumours are usually seen in smokers. The dominant cell type is squamous. Spread of a primary bronchial carcinoma into the base of the trachea is probably the commonest cause of upper airways obstruction in respiratory practice.

Laryngeal tumours nearly always present with hoarseness, or voice change, and cough. Large airways tumours are commonly not diagnosed until far advanced. This is because they mimic lower airways obstruction, as mentioned earlier, and chest radiography is often normal. Tumours may also respond to asthma therapy, showing temporary shrinkage with steroids, which may further mask the real diagnosis.

If history, examination, and lung function tests suggest upper airways obstruction, then some form of imaging is required. CT is the least invasive approach and therefore least likely to disturb the airway and make matters worse, but will not provide histology. Plain films (posteroanterior and lateral) may show tracheal narrowing, but can be very deceptive. Direct visualization is usually necessary for diagnosis and biopsy.

There is disagreement as to whether fibreoptic or rigid bronchoscopy should be the investigation of first choice. Rigid bronchoscopy requires anaesthesia and sometimes this precipitates acute obstruction, when the bronchoscope then has to be passed quickly and forced through the obstructing tumour. This 'core-out' can reduce tumour bulk, with control of haemorrhage possible under direct vision, and improvement in the airway may buy time while other treatments such as radiotherapy are employed. Flexible fibre-optic bronchoscopy may be possible without disturbing the tumour, although coughing and increased secretions can precipitate complete occlusion. In theory cocaine (a vasoconstrictor) would be preferable to lignocaine as a local anaesthetic, and direct application of adrenaline may help as an initial emergency treatment. If stenosis reduces tracheal diameter to less than 4 mm or so, it is best left alone during flexible bronchoscopy and should certainly not be biopsied (Fig. 18.5.1.5). In cases that are likely to be difficult, it can be helpful to pass an endotracheal tube over the flexible bronchoscope before it is introduced. This allows a guided intubation in an emergency, using the bronchoscope as a guide wire.

Aside from intubation or tracheostomy (when appropriate), emergency treatment of tumours compromising the upper airway consists of dexamethasone (12 mg daily), nebulized adrenaline (10 ml of 1:10 000 up to six times daily), humidification of inspired air, and breathing heliox (21% oxygen in helium). Improvement in the airway may then be achieved by treatment of the tumour with

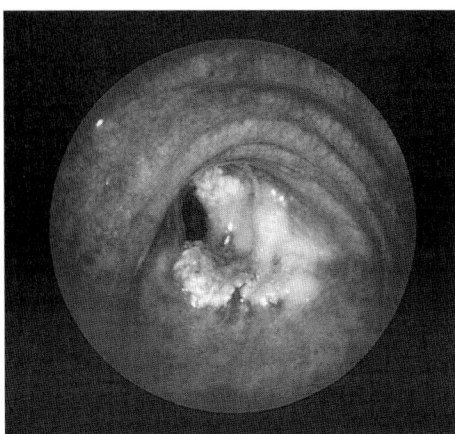

Fig. 18.5.1.5 Bronchoscopic view of a tracheal carcinoma blocking most of the lumen.
By courtesy of Dr.P.Stradling.

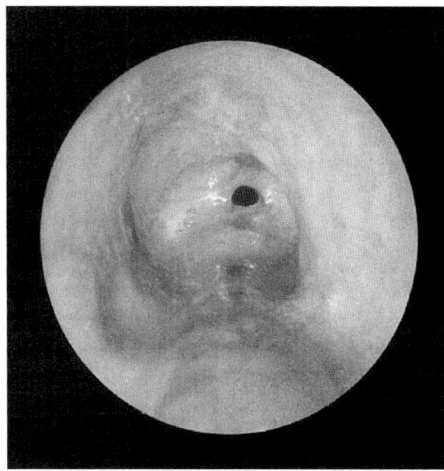

Fig. 18.5.1.6 Bronchoscopic view of post-tracheostomy tracheal stricture. The remaining hole is about 2 to 3 mm in diameter.
By courtesy of Dr.P.Stradling.

chemotherapy or radiotherapy. Sometimes, however, these can initially provoke swelling of the tumour, so that steroids are usually prescribed first, with emergency treatments kept close to hand (heliox, adrenaline). If these therapies do not help, then palliation can be achieved with the use of bronchoscopically guided laser therapy or cryotherapy, which either burn or freeze away tumour tissue with a low incidence of serious haemorrhage. Laser therapy is a laborious procedure, currently only available in a few specialist centres. Cryotherapy is quicker, safer, and can be performed down a flexible bronchoscope. However, these techniques are only of use with intraluminal tumours and cannot be applied when the narrowing is due to external compression. Another approach is the use of silicone or metal endobronchial stents, some of which can be inserted via a flexible bronchoscope, although others require surgery. They are particularly useful when external compression is present, and can produce dramatic resolution of symptoms. It is rarely appropriate to 'debulk' a malignant tumour at thoracotomy in an attempt to improve large airway patency.

Upper airways obstruction from tumour unfortunately becomes a terminal event in many cases. Adequate sedation must be given to make the patient unaware that they are asphyxiating and choking to death.

Some rare, nonmalignant tumours can obstruct the trachea, and rarely granulomatous conditions such as sarcoid and Wegener's granulomatosis may mimic tumour.

Tracheal stenosis

Tracheal stenosis usually develops following prolonged intubation, or after a tracheostomy has been allowed to close following tube removal (Fig. 18.5.1.6). This scarring may appear some time after the initiating event. Again, radiology or bronchoscopy will usually confirm the diagnosis, already strongly suspected from the history. Temporary relief may be obtained by dilating the stricture at rigid bronchoscopy. Definitive treatment involves resection of the stenosed portion and reanastomosis.

Tracheal compression

Tracheal compression (Fig. 18.5.1.7) may be due to malignant or nonmalignant conditions. External compression by malignant tumour (primary or secondary) has been covered in the previous section.

Nonmalignant causes include thyroid enlargement, aortic aneurysm, sclerosing mediastinitis, mediastinal neurofibroma, and Castleman's disease. If definitive treatment is not possible, then stenting the airway is the only option available. When thyroid enlargement leads to tracheal obstruction, surgical removal may not solve the problem completely. Prolonged pressure on the trachea can lead to tracheomalacia, so that the tracheal wall collapses when unsupported by the thyroid. Temporary use of an endotracheal stent is then appropriate.

Tracheal abnormalities

Tracheomalacia may be secondary to prolonged external compression (see above) or a primary abnormality that presents in childhood. It is essentially a weakness or deficiency of the supporting cartilages. It is sometimes seen secondary to a long history of chronic airways obstruction. Normally the anteroposterior diameter of the trachea decreases by up to about 10% during a cough. In tracheomalacia,

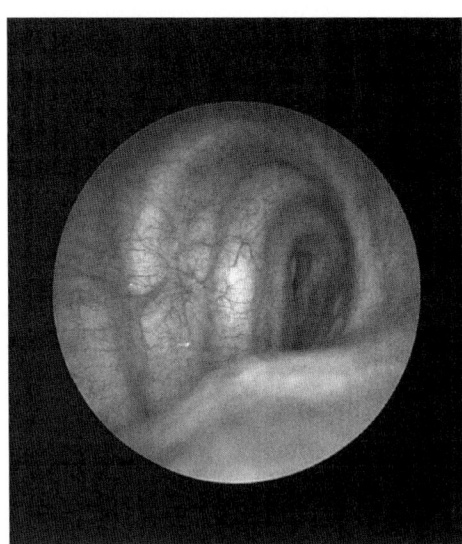

Fig. 18.5.1.7 Bronchoscopic view of external tracheal compression by right-sided paratracheal malignant nodes.
By courtesy of Dr.P. Stradling.

collapse during coughing is over 50% and is sometimes complete. The symptoms of this are usually stridor, shortness of breath, and paroxysms of coughing. In addition, inefficient coughing can lead to recurrent pneumonia and bronchiectasis. Unacceptable nocturnal cough in this condition can respond to nasal continuous positive airway pressure (NCPAP), as used in obstructive sleep apnoea (see Chapter 18.5.1.2).

A 'scabbard trachea' is said to be present when the lateral dimensions of the trachea are significantly narrower than the anteroposterior dimensions. This deformity, usually present along the whole intrathoracic trachea, is normally associated with chronic airways obstruction. It rarely causes severe upper airways obstruction and on a plain chest radiograph there is obvious tracheal ring calcification.

Tracheobronchiomegaly (or Mounier–Kuhn disease) is probably an inherited structural abnormality of the trachea presenting in adult life as apparent chronic airways obstruction. The trachea is dilated from the larynx to the second- or third-generation airways. There is atrophy of both cartilage and muscle. It is usually misdiagnosed as chronic airways obstruction, but the presence of prolonged but ineffectual coughing and harsh upper airway sounds should lead to lung function tests which then show evidence of an expiratory (intrathoracic) upper airway resistance. Radiological examination will show the dilated airways.

Tracheobronchopathia osteochondroplastica is a very rare condition characterized by cartilaginous and bony excrescences growing into the large airway lumina. This can lead to significant upper airways obstruction, but is more often a post-mortem finding which is unsuspected in life.

Relapsing polychondritis is an autoimmune systemic disorder affecting cartilage all over the body (ribs, trachea, ear lobes, nose, joints) and may be associated with systemic lupus erythematosus, Wegener's granulomatosis, and cryptogenic liver cirrhosis. Large-airways involvement is a frequent cause of death in this condition. There is irregular narrowing of the trachea and main airways, with flaccidity of the tissues sometimes allowing marked collapse on expiration. The diagnosis can be hard to make: involvement of other cartilaginous sites is the critical feature to look for. The condition is often difficult to treat. Aside from local surgical or stenting procedures, steroids and other immunosuppressive therapies are usually given.

Laryngeal dysfunction

Damage to one recurrent laryngeal nerve usually causes a weak voice that improves a little with time as the opposite cord 'learns' to compensate by moving slightly across the midline to improve apposition. If the recurrent laryngeal nerve is invaded or compressed (usually by tumour at the left hilum), differential effects on laryngeal abductors and adductors may be seen, e.g. unopposed adduction may occur prior to complete paralysis.

Bilateral recurrent laryngeal nerve paralysis produces flaccid cords that lie passively midway between full abduction and adduction. Abduction is very poor, such that rapid inspiration will draw the cords together and produce stridor, thus limiting exercise tolerance. Inspiratory stridor may initially be present only during sleep, when a general decrease in muscle tone reduces any residual laryngeal abductor activity. Although this may be labelled as snoring, careful questioning of a witness will identify whether snoring or the machinery-like screech of inspiratory stridor is present (particularly if the physician can imitate the two noises!).

The usual clinical history is of voice change following thyroidectomy some years before. This may have been quite subtle, such as difficulty in singing, but with speech relatively unaffected. Nocturnal stridor and reduction in exercise tolerance then develop over a period of years. Eventually the obstruction at night can be sufficient to produce obstructive apnoea and respiratory failure. These events may be due to involvement of the previously damaged recurrent laryngeal nerves in scarring at the thyroidectomy site. Sometimes bilateral paralysis can occur for no apparent reason, and it is assumed that the aetiology is similar to Bell's palsy or the diaphragmatic palsy of neuralgic amyotrophy. A very rare differential diagnosis is an Arnold–Chiari malformation causing brainstem compression and presenting with sleep-related stridor in association with ventilatory failure.

Laryngeal surgery could prevent inspiratory cord closure, but would do so at the expense of the voice. Thus a tracheostomy with a speaking tube is the usual approach. However, if night-time obstruction is the main problem (with sleep disruption and daytime sleepiness), NCPAP will usually keep the cords apart during sleep.

Damage to the superior laryngeal nerves supplying the cricothyroid (a vocal cord tensor) causes only a weak voice. Speech is still possible, because the main adductors still function.

Apart from laryngeal paralysis, laryngeal destructive conditions such as rheumatoid arthritis can lead to poor abduction with inspiratory stridor, particularly at night. In Parkinson's disease with autonomic involvement (Shy–Drager syndrome) or more generalized brain atrophy (multisystem atrophy) there can be a fairly specific wasting of the laryngeal abductors. This also presents with inspiratory stridor (or apnoea) at night and can progress to respiratory failure and sudden nocturnal death.

Functional laryngeal abnormalities can occur, with narrowing during inspiration and/or expiration. These may be due to psychological problems, but the syndrome blends with reflex laryngeal dysfunction in patients with asthma. Expiratory laryngeal wheezing can occur in response to emotional pressure, even in well-controlled asthma, and in this situation the laryngeal component of the increased airways resistance can be considerable. Inhalations of histamine can sometimes mimic this, which might therefore be due to a reflex originating from afferent receptors. Why this should happen is not clear, but it may be activation of the laryngeal braking mechanism to help raise functional residual capacity. There is some evidence that techniques used by speech therapists can help with this problem. A similar problem, with easily provoked inspiratory laryngeal stridor, may follow an upper respiratory tract infection and persist for several weeks.

Further reading

Bowen T, *et al.* (2004). Canadian 2003 international consensus algorithm for the diagnosis, therapy, and management of hereditary angioedema. *J Allergy Clin Immunol*, **114**, 629–37.

Empey DW (1972). Assessment of upper airways obstruction. *Br Med J*, **iii**, 503–5.

Flenley DC (1990). *Respiratory medicine*. Baillière Tindall, London.

Fraser RG, *et al.* (1990). *Diagnosis of diseases of the chest*, Vol. 3. W B Saunders, Philadelphia.

Goldman J, Muers M (1991). Vocal cord dysfunction and wheezing. *Thorax*, **46**, 401–4.

Valsecchi R, *et al.* (1997). Autoimmune C1 inhibitor deficiency and angio-oedema. *Dermatology*, **195**, 169–72.

18.5.2 Sleep-related disorders of breathing

J.R. Stradling and S.E. Craig

Essentials

Obstructive sleep apnoea (OSA) and other sleep-related breathing problems significantly impair the functioning of about 0.5 to 1% of the population and are becoming increasingly common.

Obstructive sleep apnoea

OSA in adults is commoner in men than women (3–5:1) and usually caused by obesity (BMI typically >30 kg/m^2) and fat deposits in the neck area (typically collar size of 17 inches (43 cm) or more). This external loading can be fended off during wakefulness but not during sleep, when the withdrawal of postural muscle tone allows the pharyngeal dilators to be overwhelmed, leading to excessive narrowing or collapse of the airway, with consequent apnoea. The most important consequence of sleep-induced upper airway narrowing is sleep fragmentation.

Clinical features—there is a continuum from light intermittent snoring through to severe, all-night, OSA. The main symptom of OSA is daytime hypersomnolence, which correlates broadly with the degree of sleep disruption. Other common symptoms are loud snoring, restless or unrefreshing sleep, observed apnoeas, nocturia, and apparent personality change.

Diagnosis—it is important to ask the correct questions to assess sleepiness; a well validated and simple way to do this being with the Epworth Sleepiness Scale, in which the patient is asked to state how likely they are to doze off or fall asleep in a number of ordinary situations, e.g. sitting and reading. Patients scoring higher than normal generally merit further investigation in the form of some type of sleep study to (1) assess sleep fragmentation, (2) establish if a respiratory problem is responsible, and (3) decide if upper airway obstruction is the primary cause. Classical OSA, observed with a simple commercially available monitoring system, causes a snoring–silence–snoring pattern of sleep (from room microphone) together with body movements (from video) and oscillations in the pulse and SaO_2 (from oximeter). Full polysomnography can provide much further information, but is not generally required in straightforward cases.

Management—mild symptoms may resolve with simple treatments and advice as follows: (1) learn to sleep on your side and avoid sleeping on your back, (2) no alcohol after 18.00 h, (3) no sedatives, (4) lose weight, (5) stop smoking, (6) keep the nose as clear as possible. However, if OSA and symptoms are severe, there is only one fully effective therapy—nasal continuous positive airway pressure (NCPAP): this involves wearing a small mask over the nose while asleep, with the air pressure kept at a fixed level above atmospheric (usually about 10 cmH$_2$O) by a pump, sufficient to splint open the pharynx and resist collapse, allowing unobstructed breathing and undisturbed sleep.

Prognosis—many patients with OSA have visceral obesity and the metabolic syndrome (hypertension, insulin resistance,

hyperlipidaemia), and their vascular mortality is higher than average. However, there is no controlled interventional data to support the routine use of NCPAP to reduce vascular risk in patients with OSA who would not otherwise want to use the treatment for relief of daytime sleepiness.

Sleep-induced hypoventilation and central sleep apnoea

Aetiology—breathing during sleep may decrease because of a reduction in central output to the respiratory muscles, which can be caused by (1) absent ventilatory drive—Ondine's curse, caused by congenital abnormality, brainstem damage, or blunting secondary to lung disease; (2) unstable ventilatory drive—at sleep onset, with hypoxaemia, altitude, heart failure; (3) REM-related oscillations—neuromuscular diseases, chest-wall abnormalities, and chronic airways obstruction; (4) reflex central apnoea—when pharyngeal collapse inhibits inspiration.

Clinical features—some of the central apnoeas disturb sleep and present with daytime sleepiness, such that they can be confused with OSA, whereas others tend to present with symptoms of respiratory failure, such as morning headaches with confusion, cyanosis, and ankle oedema.

Management—without treatment the chronic ventilatory failure associated with some neurological disorders (e.g. acid maltase deficiency, postpoliomyelitis syndrome, motor neuron disease, Duchenne dystrophy) usually progresses rapidly to death. Supporting breathing overnight can fully reverse ventilatory failure, and the response to treatment can be dramatic, with resolution of all symptoms, restoration of normal blood gases, and addition of decades of active life.

Introduction

This chapter discusses the disorders of breathing that appear, or markedly deteriorate, only during sleep. Obstructive sleep apnoea (OSA) and sleep-related problems in general are becoming increasingly common, especially as they are often related to obesity. OSA is the third most common serious respiratory disorder (after asthma and chronic obstructive pulmonary disease (COPD)) and is thought to significantly impair the functioning of about 0.5 to 1% of the population. Most general hospitals will have some form of sleep monitoring system for the diagnosis of sleep apnoea syndromes, although tertiary centres tend to provide most of the treatment. The diversity of symptoms produced by these disorders means that all physicians need to have an understanding of them and are likely to come across many cases during their professional life.

Normal physiology of breathing during sleep (Table 18.5.2.1)

Sleep can be divided into two very different states. The dominant sleep stage is non-rapid eye movement (NREM) sleep (Figs. 18.5.2.1 and 18.5.2.2). This phase of sleep, which is preferentially reclaimed following sleep deprivation, appears to be when the brain shuts down, and is necessary for maximum daytime alertness and continuing cognitive function. NREM sleep shows a continuum from

Table 18.5.2.1 Sleep and breathing

	NREM	REM
Electroencephalogram	Progressively slower frequency and higher amplitude	Similar to the awake pattern
Eye movements	Initially slow and pendular, then none	Bursts of rapid binocular movements
Postural muscle tone	Reduced from wakefulness	Very much reduced or absent
Factors controlling breathing	Loss of wakefulness input	Cortical over-riding and apparent reduction in responses to classical stimuli
	Brainstem and classical stimuli dominate, but reduced compared with wakefulness	
Arousal response	Small deteriorations in PaO_2 and $PaCO_2$, with the consequent ventilatory response, are required for arousal	Larger changes in PaO_2 and $PaCO_2$ required before arousal occurs
Potential effect on breathing	Rise in pharyngeal resistance	Further rise in pharyngeal resistance
	Fall in minute ventilation	Loss of use of accessory muscles of respiration
	Fall in PaO_2	Further falls in PaO_2 tolerated longer before rescued by arousal

NREM, non-rapid eye movement: REM, rapid eye movement.

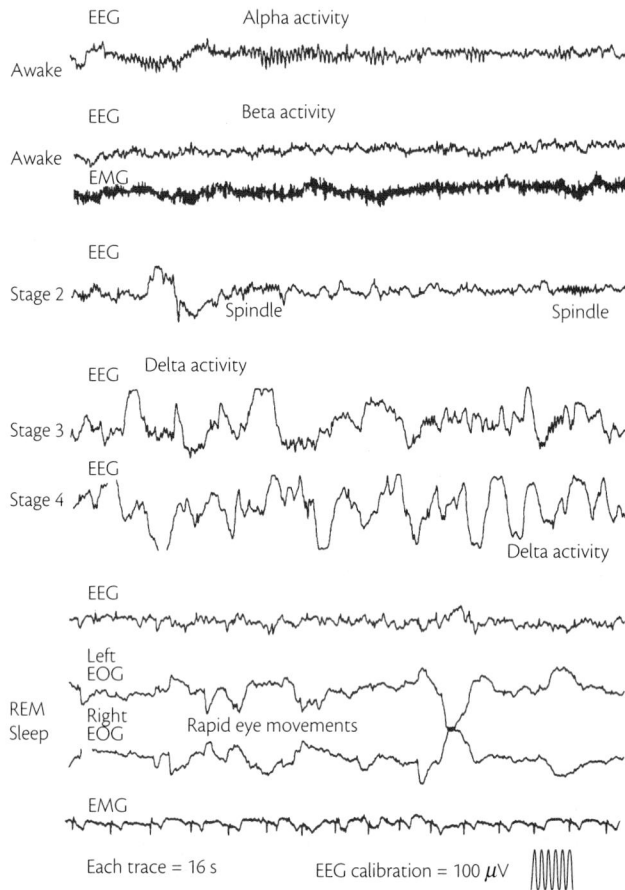

Fig. 18.5.2.1 Examples of electrical brain activity (EEG), eye movements (EOG), and chin muscle tone (EMG) during wakefulness and the different sleep stages.

drowsy down to very deep sleep, arbitrarily subdivided into stages 1, 2, 3, and 4. The awake electroencephalogram (EEG) is characterized by low-voltage, high-frequency activity, with the only dominant frequency being the so-called alpha activity (*c.*10 Hz), present when the eyes are closed. As sleep supervenes, the alpha activity disappears, overall EEG frequency falls, muscle tone (usually measured from a chin electromyogram (EMG)) falls, and the eyes begin to roll from side to side. This transition phase is called stage 1. Stage 2 is defined by the appearance of K complexes (isolated slow waves) and sleep spindles (bursts of *c.*13 Hz activity). As sleep deepens further, increasing amounts of large, slow waves (*c.*1 Hz) appear. These stages are called 3 and 4, or slow-wave sleep.

The other main phase of sleep is rapid eye movement (REM) sleep or dreaming sleep. This stage is characterized by a return of the EEG to a pattern resembling wakefulness. The EMG tone falls to very low levels and there are bursts of rapid eye movements, mainly from side to side, under closed eyelids. Effectively the cortex is 'awake' again, processing randomly activated images and able to integrate outside noises or other stimuli into complex dreams. The fall in EMG tone is because the rest of the body's muscles have been 'cut off' from the brain and paralysed, hence the fall in EMG tone. This paralysis (or atonia) is under active control from Jouvet's centre in the pons that hyperpolarizes the lower motor neurons via inhibitory reticulospinal pathways. Cats in whom this centre has been destroyed no longer show atonia during REM sleep, and as a consequence they may get up and walk around

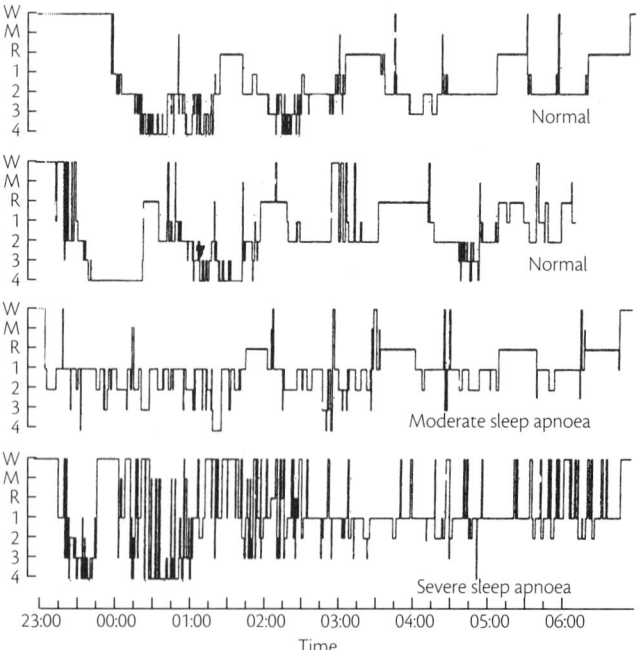

Fig. 18.5.2.2 Examples of all-night hypnograms (based on 20-s epochs) in two normal subjects and two patients with sleep apnoea. Note the reduced deep sleep (stages 3 and 4) in the patients, but no indication that they are waking up hundreds of times a night. W, awake; M, movement (awake); R, REM sleep; 1 to 4, stages 1, 2, 3, 4 of non-REM sleep.

or appear to chase phantom birds, presumably reflecting their dream content. The function of this atonia centre may therefore be to prevent the dreaming brain from influencing the rest of the body. Paralysis during REM sleep occurs dominantly in muscles that normally have a tonic postural activity; thus the diaphragm is spared, although pharyngeal, intercostal, and accessory muscles are all affected to differing extents.

The normal pattern of the oscillation between NREM and REM sleep is shown in Fig. 18.5.2.2. This 'hypnogram', as it is called, is constructed by classifying successive 20- or 30-s epochs from tracings of EEG, EMG, and eye movement data into either awake, movement, REM sleep, or stages 1 to 4; thus about 1000 epochs are obtained from a night's sleep.

During wakefulness breathing is influenced by a variety of pathways, some conscious and voluntary, others entirely automatic and involuntary. Classic responses to hypoxia, hypercapnia, and vagal afferents (integrated in the brainstem) can be overruled by cortical signals to subserve functions such as talking. These two types of control are separate and can be damaged separately by disease processes. The presence of wakefulness itself provides an input to the respiratory centre, almost equivalent to the amount of ventilation seen at rest. Thus, following a period of hyperventilation, a normal subject will go on breathing at just below normal levels, despite hypocapnia and hyperoxia, until the CO_2 level rises and normal ventilation is re-established. This is not true during NREM sleep, when hypocapnia will produce apnoea until the $Paco_2$ rises back to a critical threshold level.

Another component of wakefulness is the high muscle tone that holds the body in the required posture. This 'awake' input into the anterior horn cells means that other inputs, such as those from the respiratory centre, can further activate muscles, including the intercostals and pharyngeal. The withdrawal of this 'awake' tone with the onset of sleep means that a certain respiratory centre output to the relevant anterior horn cells is less able to raise membrane potentials to firing threshold, such that respiratory muscle activity falls with sleep onset, minute volume typically reduces by about 10 to 15%, and $Paco_2$ rises by 3 to 8 mmHg. Reduction of pharyngeal muscle tone narrows the lumen, and thus there is normally a rise in upper airway resistance. This reduction in ventilation has trivial effect on the arterial oxygen saturation (Sao_2) in the normal circumstance when Sao_2 is on the flat part of the haemoglobin dissociation curve, but dramatic falls in saturation will be apparent when Sao_2 starts below 92%, the steep part of the curve, such as is seen in patients with COPD. If ventilatory responses to carbon dioxide or hypoxia are measured during NREM sleep, the slopes are flatter and right shifted, indicating a reduced overall sensitivity. Exactly why this occurs is not known, but reduced tone of the respiratory muscles, the withdrawal of awake drive, increased upper airway resistance, and (probably) true reduction in central sensitivity to CO_2 or $[H^+]$, could all contribute. If, as a consequence of respiratory disease, compensatory mechanisms are already employed to cope with the extra work of breathing (sternomastoids, scalenes), then these seem to be particularly reduced during sleep as well.

During REM sleep, overall ventilation stays much the same as in NREM sleep, but the breath-to-breath variability increases considerably, sometimes with apnoeas during the actual periods of eye movements, and compensatory increases in between. Sensitivities to CO_2 and hypoxia were originally thought to be further reduced, but they are hard to measure in the presence of spontaneously variable

breathing and more recent evidence suggests that the response to CO_2 may not be as suppressed as previously thought. What is far more important is the atonia of postural muscles. The hyperpolarization of the anterior horn cells greatly reduces the efficacy of respiratory signals to the intercostal, accessory, and pharyngeal muscles. This will not matter in a normal subject with an efficient diaphragm and an uncompromised pharynx. However, if the subject is dependent on muscles other than the diaphragm to maintain breathing, or has a narrow, compromised pharynx, then REM sleep may powerfully interfere with ventilation with consequent hypoxaemia and hypercapnia.

Also of relevance to breathing during REM sleep are the reduced arousal responses to respiratory stimuli compared with non-REM sleep. The arousal responses to some ventilatory stimuli (hypoxia, hypercapnia, extra resistive load) are believed to be mediated mainly by the perception of the ventilatory effort made in response, rather than the specific ventilatory stimulus itself. If a ventilatory response to hypoxia is measured during REM sleep, then the subject will usually tolerate a much lower Sao_2 before arousing, compared to NREM sleep. Furthermore, if the drive to sleep is high, such as after sleep deprivation, arousal will be delayed still further.

It can be seen from the above that, although sleep is not a problem for those with normal respiratory systems, once abnormalities are present there is potential for a damaging interaction between sleep and breathing, particularly during REM sleep.

Obstructive sleep apnoea

Definition

Sleep apnoea was first properly documented in neurophysiological sleep laboratories using techniques that had been developed for the investigation of conditions such as insomnia, narcolepsy, and depression. It was realized that hundreds of episodes of breath cessation, or apnoea, usually due to upper airway obstruction with associated snoring, were related to marked sleep disturbance. As simple oronasal flow detectors were used, the critical event was defined as an episode of apnoea. An arbitrary definition was made, due to ease of measurement, and breath cessation for longer than 10 s became an official apnoea. Early work suggested that normal, young people rarely had more than about 30 apnoeas per night, so that the standard definition of 'sleep apnoea syndrome' became more than 35 apnoeas per night, or more than 5 per hour of sleep, each lasting for 10 s or longer. This definition has existed long beyond its clinical usefulness: it is quite clear that recurrent partial obstruction to the upper airway can fragment sleep just as severely with no actual apnoeas or hypopnoeas developing at all. A more pragmatic and clinically useful definition of the syndrome might now be 'sleep disruption due to a respiratory problem engendered by sleep itself, sufficient to cause symptoms when awake'. Usually this is upper airway incompetence during sleep (obstructive sleep apnoea), but may also be due to problems of respiratory drive (central sleep apnoea, periodic breathing or Cheyne–Stokes breathing). As the pathogenesis of sleep apnoea is explained, this shift in emphasis, with the inclusion of symptoms, will become clear.

Aetiology (Box 18.5.2.1)

The upper pharyngeal airway has to serve two functions, swallowing and breathing, which require different design features. When used for swallowing the pharynx has to behave like the oesophagus,

Box 18.5.2.1 Causes of obstructive sleep apnoea

- ◆ Anatomical
  - · Central (neck) obesity
  - · Micro- or retrognathia
  - · Maxillary underdevelopment (e.g. cranial dysostoses, such as Apert's and Treacher Collins syndromes)
  - · Pharyngeal encroachment (e.g. tonsillar hypertrophy, acromegaly, tumours, mucopolysaccharidoses, oedema)
- ◆ Neuromuscular
  - · Bulbar palsies
  - · Neurological degenerative disorders (e.g. multisystem atrophy)
  - · Myopathies (e.g. Duchenne dystrophy)
- ◆ Other provoking factors
  - · Alcohol
  - · Sedative drugs
  - · Sleep deprivation
  - · Increased nasal resistance
  - · Hypothyroidism
  - · Acromegaly

and when used for breathing it has to remain an open tube like the trachea. These dual functions are achieved by having a floppy and collapsible muscular tube that is also capable of being held rigidly open by dilator muscles. The muscles responsible for this dilator function are discussed in the section on the structure and function of the upper respiratory tract (see Chapter 18.1.1). All these muscles have reduced activation during sleep, so that some pharyngeal narrowing occurs normally. There are, then, additional factors that determine whether this reduction leads to significant upper airflow obstruction in a particular individual. There are various theories as to these additional factors. Firstly, there may be abnormalities of the activation of the pharyngeal dilator muscles, perhaps due to defective or unstable central control. Secondly, there may be anatomical abnormalities that allow significant obstruction to occur even with the normal sleep-related reduction in muscle tone.

Neuromuscular function

Early investigations of EMG activity in pharyngeal muscles found reductions in tone with sleep during obstructive apnoeas. However, it was very difficult to show that these reductions were truly abnormal. It is now accepted that there is in fact an increase in activity of these muscles, both awake and asleep, in response to factors provoking pharyngeal collapse. In some patients with primary neuromuscular problems (from brainstem lesions to myopathies) there can be associated obstructive sleep apnoea, and pharyngeal muscle involvement seems a probable explanation. However, this is uncommon and most patients with obstructive sleep apnoea do not show evidence of any other neuromuscular problems.

During inspiration, pharyngeal dilator activity has to be synchronized with diaphragmatic activity and be adequate to overcome negative intrapharyngeal pressure. It has been suggested that a lack of coordination between diaphragmatic and pharyngeal activation may allow the pharynx to collapse as a secondary phenomenon. For example, normal subjects breathing against an inspiratory resistance can be made to have a few obstructive apnoeas by artificially inducing periodic breathing during sleep. The gradual return of respiratory drive, following the nadir of ventilation, seems to activate the diaphragm first, leaving the pharynx unbraced. The presence of an inspiratory resistance then 'challenges' the pharynx and allows collapse for a few breaths before pharyngeal tone returns and restores patency.

Although instability of respiratory control during sleep has been postulated as a cause of obstructive sleep apnoea, following treatment with nasal continuous positive airway pressure therapy (see later) there is very rarely evidence of a premorbid underlying respiratory instability, nor does altering respiratory drive have a useful effect. More convincing is the suggestion that there may be failure of normal reflex protective mechanisms in the pharynx, whereby receptors in the pharynx detect falls in pressure that distort the airway and provoke protective increases in pharyngeal dilator tone (see Section 18.1.1). Snoring itself may also be one of the stimuli that activate this dilator reflex, and it is conceivable that interruption of this reflex arc can occur, perhaps through years of pharyngeal trauma from snoring, mucosal oedema, or toxic agents such as cigarette smoke and alcohol.

Anatomical causes

Anatomical abnormalities influence pharyngeal function in a variety of ways. Simple encroachment of the pharyngeal lumen, e.g. with tonsillar hypertrophy, means that the normal fall in pharyngeal dilator tone with sleep can lead to critical narrowing and obstruction. Alternatively, there are abnormalities which 'load' the upper airway, requiring increased dilator muscle action that is then lost during sleep (e.g. high nasal resistance or increased external compression from neck obesity). Finally, there may be mechanical problems such that muscular activity fails to dilate the pharyngeal lumen effectively.

There are many case reports of obvious anatomical abnormalities provoking obstructive sleep apnoea, e.g. tonsillar hypertrophy, pharyngeal oedema, tumours, acromegaly, mucopolysaccharidoses, and mandibular or maxillary underdevelopment. These reports show that pharyngeal narrowing (asymptomatic while awake) can provoke obstructive sleep apnoea, but such diagnoses represent only a small proportion of cases.

Most patients with obstructive sleep apnoea are overweight. In many clinics the average body mass index (BMI) is well over 30 kg/m², equivalent to being about 30% overweight, e.g. 95 kg (15 stone) at a height of 1.78 m (5 ft 10 in). Weight loss can certainly cure obstructive sleep apnoea, and all studies identifying risk factors have found obesity to be dominant, accounting for up to 40% of the variance in severity.

Most groups have found neck circumference to be a better predictor of severity of obstructive sleep apnoea than obesity itself, suggesting that it is neck obesity and external pharyngeal loading that is important (Fig. 18.5.2.3). Animal studies have shown that only a small amount of extra external pressure over the pharynx is required to collapse it during sleep, and recent imaging studies have suggested that there are quite small amounts of extra fat on either side of the pharynx in patients with obstructive sleep apnoea,

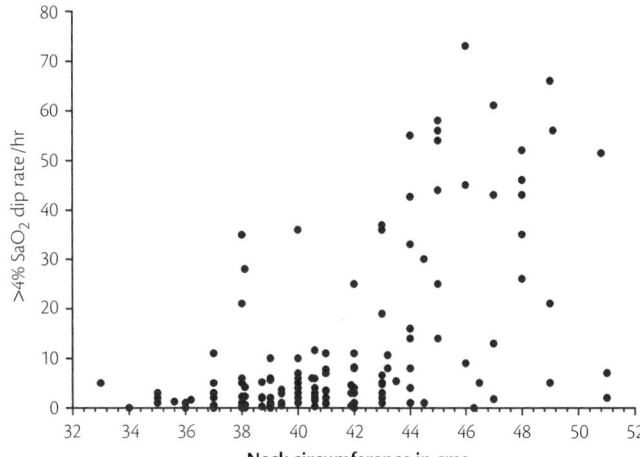

Fig. 18.5.2.3 Correlation between sleep apnoea (number of >4% dips/h during sleep) vs neck circumference in 124 sleep clinic patients. Increasing severity is usually associated with increasing neck circumference.

together with larger amounts subcutaneously. Fig. 18.5.2.3 also shows that it is possible to have a very large neck but not have sleep apnoea; these patients were loud snorers and on average significantly younger that the rest, and it is likely that they will develop sleep apnoea as they get older.

Although general obesity is related to neck obesity, the overall correlation is only about 0.75. This is because fat distribution varies considerably between individuals. The 'female' distribution tends to be in the lower body and the 'male' distribution is more central, hence a man who is not particularly overweight can have a large neck.

As mentioned earlier, there is evidence that some of the upper airway dilator muscles (e.g. genioglossus) of obese patients with obstructive sleep apnoea are actually working harder than normal, perhaps as compensation for the added external loading from neck obesity. Compensations by the respiratory system for other types of extra loading have been shown to be much less active during sleep.

In summary, the evidence overall suggests that most obstructive sleep apnoea in adults is due to loading of the upper airway caused by obesity and fat deposits in the neck area. This external loading can be fended off during wakefulness but not during sleep, when the withdrawal of postural muscle tone allows the pharyngeal dilators to be overwhelmed, leading to excessive narrowing or collapse of the airway, with consequent apnoea.

However, not all adult sleep apnoea can be explained by obesity or intrapharyngeal anatomical abnormalities. The significance of marked retro- or micrognathia for obstructive sleep apnoea was recognized early on, particularly in children (Pierre–Robin syndrome). Careful cephalometric studies of facial and skull morphology have revealed that some patients with obstructive sleep apnoea have longer faces, retropositioning of the mandible (measured as a more acute angle between the sella to nasion and nasion to supramentale planes), a downward movement of the hyoid, elongation of the soft palate, and a narrower anteroposterior distance behind the tongue. Some, or all, of these changes may be secondary to many years of sleep apnoea rather than part of the cause, but the retropositioning of the mandible may be contributory, and surgery or dental devices to advance the mandible may be

helpful in carefully selected cases. In Fig. 18.5.2.3 it will be noted that not all the patients with significant sleep apnoea had large necks, and it is these patients who had retrognathia.

Retropositioning of the mandible may be a legacy from childhood. There is good evidence that facial development is altered by nasal blockage and mouth breathing very early in life (the so-called 'adenoidal facies'). One feature of this is mandibular retropositioning, and the mandible can return to its normal position following early adenoidectomy and resumption of nasal breathing. One theory is that mandibular underdevelopment is a risk factor for OSA that—if severe—may be adequate to provoke disease on its own, with lesser degrees acting synergistically with other causes, such as tonsillar hypertrophy in children and upper-body obesity in adults.

Other factors provoking obstructive sleep apnoea

Alcohol is a potent reducer of muscle tone and can further reduce pharyngeal dilator muscle tone during sleep. It is well known that alcohol worsens snoring, but it can also convert snoring to full apnoea. Other sedatives, such as benzodiazepines, barbiturates, and opiates, can do the same, and this has important consequences for anaesthesia in such patients. Sleep deprivation itself can reduce upper airway muscle tone during subsequent sleep, provoking a vicious circle, whereby apnoea causes sleep disruption, causing worsening apnoea.

Hyperarousability may contribute to OSA. Many people have significant increases in upper airway resistance with sleep onset, with or without snoring. After a short period of hypoventilation, stable ventilation is achieved with an increase in inspiratory muscle activity without sleep disturbance. However, if arousal is provoked before stability is achieved, then a cycle of sleep fragmentation may develop. Thus, increased arousability in conjunction with increased upper airway resistance may cause symptomatic sleep disordered breathing in a subgroup of patients, but the prevalence of this variant of OSA is unknown.

Nasal blockage can contribute to the tendency of the pharynx to collapse by lowering intrapharyngeal pressure. If extra effort has to be made to inspire through a high nasal resistance, there will be a greater vacuum effect in the pharynx, increasing its tendency to collapse. Once collapse occurs, flow ceases, pharyngeal pressure returns to atmospheric, the lumen opens, and the cycle repeats. This certainly leads to snoring, but may no longer be very important when there is full apnoea. However, nasal obstruction may contribute in the long term to sleep apnoea by damaging the pharynx through years of snoring, making it more collapsible, but improving nasal patency rarely cures obstructive sleep apnoea.

Hypothyroidism is associated with obstructive sleep apnoea, but the mechanism is not clear. It may be through weight gain, or tissue or fluid deposition in the pharynx, or a low thyroxine level may interfere directly with muscle function.

Immediate consequences of sleep apnoea

Upper airway narrowing, sometimes with complete apnoea, usually commences as sleep passes from awake to stage 2. Once significant obstruction occurs there will be increasing respiratory effort to try and overcome it. The length of such events is highly variable, ranging from only a few seconds to well over 1 min. At some point arousal occurs, with an improvement in upper airway resistance, resolution of any asphyxia, and then a return to sleep, whereupon the cycle repeats (Figs. 18.5.2.4–6). Hypoxaemia and

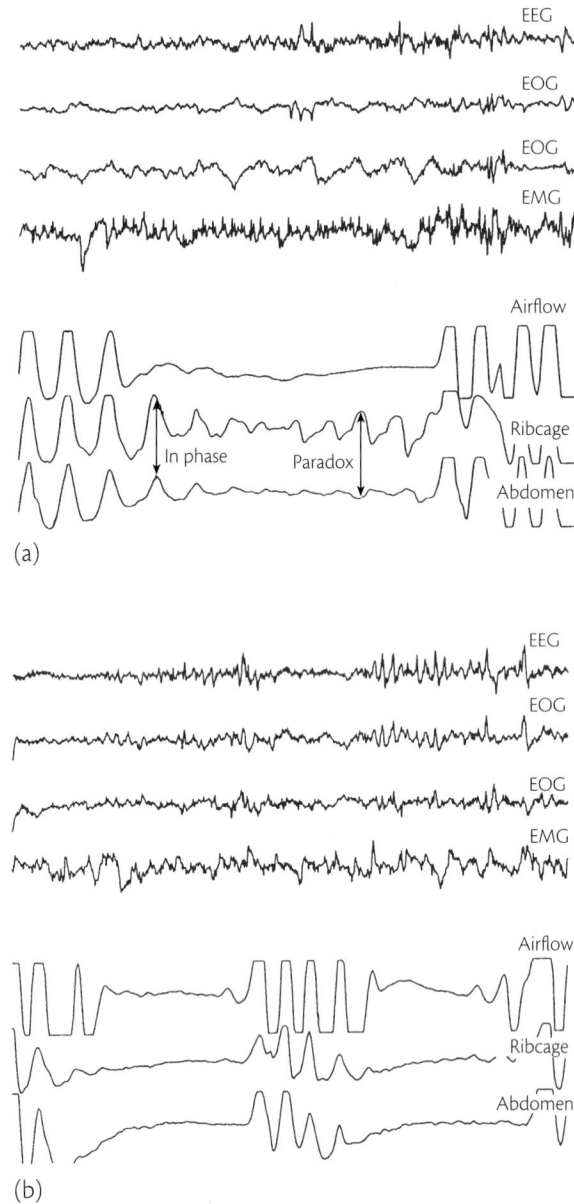

Fig. 18.5.2.4 Obstructive (a) and central (b) apnoeas (16-s traces): (a) airflow ceases, but ribcage and abdominal movements persist and become paradoxical; (b) ribcage and abdominal movements cease as well as airflow.

mild hypercapnia usually accompany these periods of obstructed breathing. If there is complete apnoea, the rate of fall of Sao_2 will depend mainly on the amount of oxygen stored in the lungs. This depends on the functional residual capacity since apnoeas occur at end expiration, preventing inspiration. The length of the apnoea also determines how low the Sao_2 will fall, and varies considerably between patients. The consequences of such hypoxaemia and hypercapnia are not clear: the blood gas derangements are transient and may do little harm, unless they are severe and there is (e.g.) ischaemic heart disease.

Hypoxaemia was believed to play an important part in the arousal response that saves the patient from continuing asphyxia. In animal models, removal of the carotid body abolishes significant ventilatory response to hypoxaemia during sleep and there is no arousal. Giving extra added oxygen does prolong apnoeas to a small extent and delay arousal. However, recent evidence suggests that the main arousal stimulus is the actual respiratory effort being made in response to asphyxia, rather than the asphyxia *per se*. Normal subjects tend to wake when they have to make respiratory efforts about three times above the normal (10–20 cmH$_2$O pleural pressure swings). This degree of effort is easily reached in obstructive sleep apnoea, when pressures down to –80 cmH$_2$O can be recorded during the frustrated inspiratory efforts. Such pressures can also be reached by heavy snorers, even if they do not develop hypoxaemia, and this can also lead to arousals.

In terms of symptoms, the most important consequence of sleep-induced upper airway narrowing is sleep fragmentation. The original methodology of sleep analysis, using coarse 30-s epochs to stage sleep, effectively glossed over the multitude of transient arousals that are the main consequence of obstructive sleep apnoea. Superficially, a sleep hypnogram in a moderately severe case (see Fig. 18.5.2.2) could look almost normal despite hundreds of arousals. The importance of trying to measure these has recently been appreciated, and there are a variety of techniques to measure, or infer, these arousals. However, the level of sleep disruption (e.g. number and degree of arousals) necessary to cause daytime symptoms is not known. There is a clear, but variable, relationship between increasing sleep disruption and deteriorating daytime function, but there is no clear cut off between normality and abnormality.

In addition to blood gas disturbances and sleep disruption, there are many other consequences of obstructive sleep apnoea. During the apnoea there is activation of the diving reflex that produces bradycardia and arteriolar vasoconstriction in muscles, particularly when there is associated hypoxaemia. Upon arousal there is a sudden pulse rate and blood pressure rise, probably due to general activation of the vascular sympathetic nervous system as part of the arousal process itself. During the actual frustrated inspiratory efforts, blood pressure falls with each reduction in intrathoracic pressure (pulsus paradoxus) and, in conjunction with the blood pressure rise on arousal, produces a very characteristic trace (Fig. 18.5.2.5). As well as increased nocturnal catecholamine secretion in patients with obstructive sleep apnoea, there is also a suppression of growth hormone and possibly testosterone levels. There is marked polyuria during sleep (a reversal of the normal relative oliguria), but the mechanism is not clear. It may be related to the recurrent arousals, or to increased natriuretic peptide (ANP and BNP) production following cardiac chamber distension due to the large inspiratory efforts. There is some recent evidence that OSA may provoke atrial fibrillation, but whether this is via increased sympathetic activity or perhaps atrial distension is not known.

It will be clear from this account that there are areas of uncertainty regarding definition and measurement of some aspects of sleep apnoea. We discussed earlier that original definitions centred on the actual obstructive event. There has now been a shift towards trying to look more closely at the most important result—sleep fragmentation. This is particularly necessary now we know that 10-s apnoeas are not the only result of upper airway narrowing during sleep that can provoke multiple arousals and daytime sleepiness. Since heavy snorers can have considerable sleep fragmentation without significant falls in Sao_2, examining blood gas abnormalities (e.g. with an oximeter) is not always good enough either. The implications for this in terms of investigations are discussed later. A considerable amount of effort is being put into establishing which variable that can be measured during a sleep study best defines

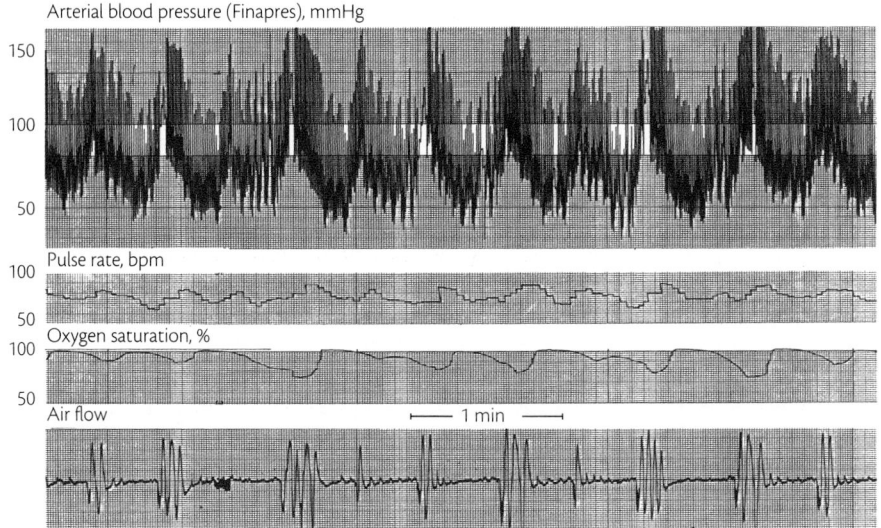

Fig. 18.5.2.5 A 5-min tracing from a patient with obstructive sleep apnoea. The rises in blood pressure (top trace) and heart rate (second trace) coincide with the cessation of each apnoea and an arousal. During each apnoea (evident from the bottom airflow trace) each frustrated inspiratory effort is accompanied by a fall in blood pressure (pulsus paradoxus).

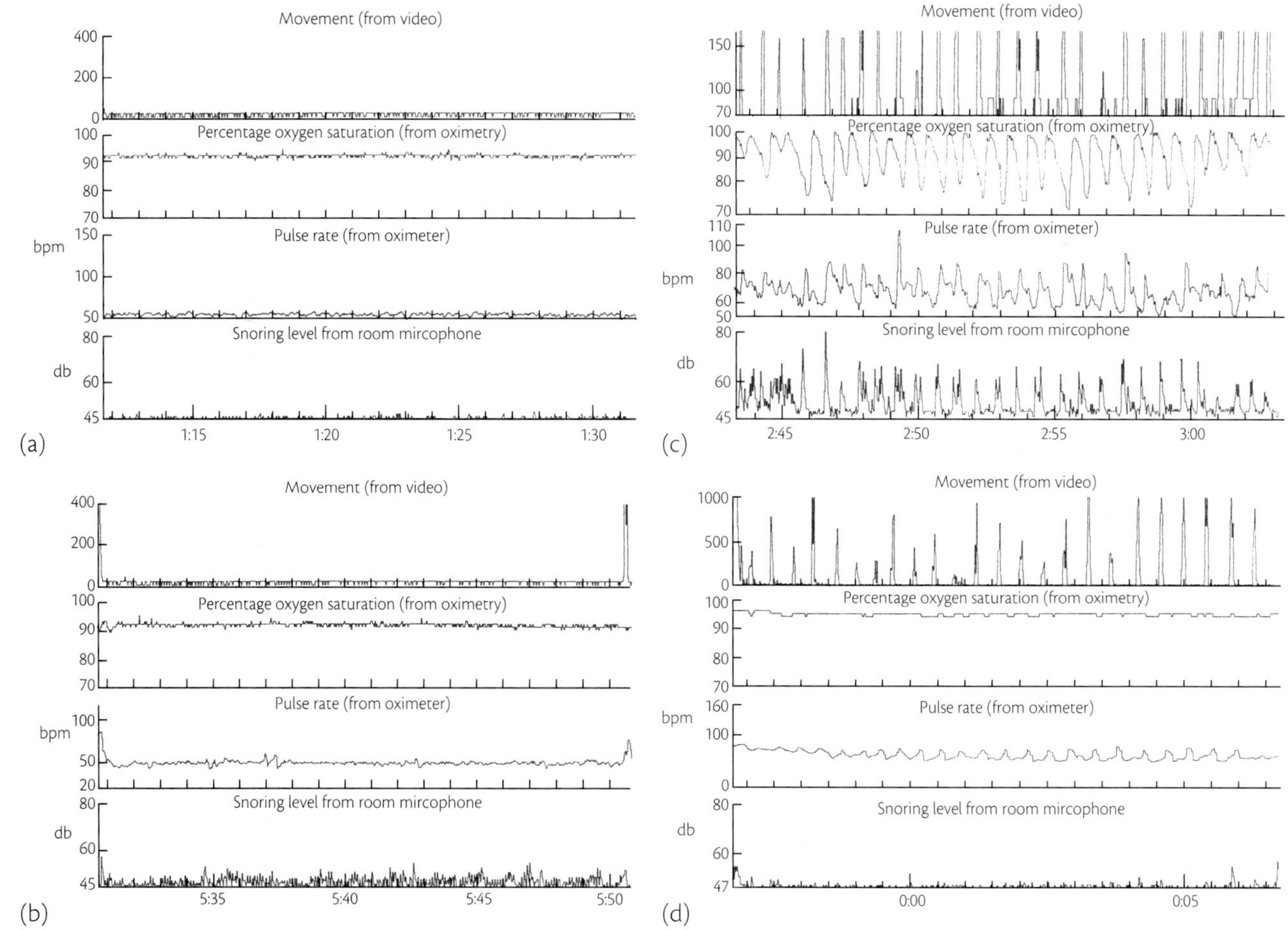

Fig. 18.5.2.6 Short sleep tracings of body movement, SaO$_2$, pulse rate, and snoring level in four different subjects. (a) Normal subject (no fluctuations in any signals), 20 min. (b) Patient with continual low level snoring and almost no arousals, 20 min. (c) Patient with classical obstructive apnoeas, evident from the snoring–silence–snoring pattern together with movements and oscillations in the pulse and SaO$_2$, 20 min. (d) Patient with periodic movements of the legs during sleep, recurrent arousal (oscillations in pulse and body movements), but no evidence of a respiratory cause (no snoring or SaO$_2$ dips), 10 min. A video recording of the whole night is always available and can be viewed when the exact cause of abnormal signals is not immediately obvious.

the severity of the disorder. At present there is no clear answer, although there is good evidence that simple approaches are at least as good as the more complex approaches often used, but different approaches to diagnosis and management remain.

Symptoms and presentation

The main symptom of obstructive sleep apnoea is daytime hypersomnolence, and this correlates broadly with the degree of sleep disruption. Early in the development of the disorder the daytime sleepiness is little more than often experienced by normal people after a few disturbed nights. While occupied, the individual has little difficulty in concentrating and staying awake, but once activities become more boring, unwanted sleepiness intervenes. Initially this may be viewed as normal, such as falling asleep in front of the television every evening. As the sleep disruption worsens there will be interference with an increasing number of activities. Of particular importance is sleepiness while driving. Sleepiness can be devastating, particularly on long motorway journeys after dark, when sensory stimulation is low. Initially there will be lane wandering, with sudden arousal and correction. Accidents involving driving off the road, or driving into vehicles in front, are more common in patients with obstructive sleep apnoea and reduce with treatment. Sleepiness also impinges greatly on work performance and home life. The patient will develop a reputation for slothfulness and lack of interest.

It is important to ask the correct questions to assess sleepiness. It is not the same as tiredness, which is a lack of energy or desire to get up and do anything, without a desire to sleep. Because of the insidious onset of obstructive sleep apnoea, any sleepiness may be regarded as normal by the patient, and thus situational questions need to be asked such as, 'How often do you have to pull off the road while driving owing to sleepiness?' rather than just 'Are you sleepy?' A well validated and simple way to do this is with the Epworth Sleepiness Scale (Fig. 18.5.2.7). Objective sleepiness can be assessed by measuring how long the patient takes to fall asleep when asked to stay awake, lying down in a quiet room on a number of occasions across the day. This is useful for research purposes but only occasionally adds to the clinical management of such patients. A list of other symptoms seen in obstructive sleep apnoea is given in Box 18.5.2.2. It is sad to say, but the corrosive effect of sleepiness on all aspects of a patient's life has often been present for years before someone (usually not a doctor) tumbles to the diagnosis.

A typical case history would be that of a middle-aged man complaining of increasing daytime sleepiness. It is usually some specific event that prompts initial consultation, such as falling asleep while driving or operating machinery, or during an important business meeting. There will be a long history of gradually worsening snoring with apnoeas, possibly witnessed by the spouse, who will probably have moved out of the bedroom because of the noise. There is likely to have been a weight gain over the last few years with a BMI of greater than $30\,kg/m^2$ and a collar size of 17 in (43 cm) or more. There is sometimes a history of fairly high alcohol intake and smoking. On examination there may be nasal stuffiness, evidence of a small lower jaw (such as teeth crowding or several extractions for this problem), and a small pharynx with mucosal bogginess and wrinkling. Of course, it should be stressed that not all these features are likely to be present in one individual.

Part of the history and examination of patients with possible obstructive sleep apnoea should be directed towards precipitating factors such as hypothyroidism and acromegaly. Other diagnoses

EPWORTH SLEEPINESS SCALE

Name: ....   Hospital number ....

Date: .... Your age (Yrs) ....   Your sex (Male = M/Female = F) ....

How likely are you to doze off or fall asleep in the situations described in the box below, in contrast to feeling tired?

This refers to your usual way of life in recent times.

Even if you haven't done some of these things recently try to work out how they would have affected you.

Use the following scale to choose the *most appropriate number* for each situation:-

   0 = would *never* doze
   1 = *Slight* chance of dozing
   2 = *Moderate* chance of dozing
   3 = *High* chance of dozing

Situation	Chance of dozing
Sitting and reading	
Watching TV	
Sitting, inactive in a public place (eg a theatre or a meeting)	
As a passenger in a car for an hour without a break	
Lying down to rest in the afternoon when circumstances permit	
Sitting and talking to someone	
Sitting quietly after a lunch without alcohol	
In a car, while stopped for a few minutes in the traffic	

Thank you for your cooperation

Fig. 18.5.2.7 Questionnaire scale to assess subjective sleepiness. The scores for each answer (0–3) are summed to give a range from 0 (no sleepiness at all) to 24 (maximally sleepy). The upper limit of normal is about 9, and most patients with symptomatic obstructive sleep apnoea are in the middle teens.

such as mucopolysaccharidosis, pharyngeal tumours, tonsillar hypertrophy, neurological disorders, and significant retrognathia will be more obvious. There should be a higher index of suspicion for causes other than obesity when the neck circumference is not raised.

Diagnosis

Following the history and examination, further outpatient tests may be appropriate, e.g. thyroxine or growth hormone estimations. Blood gases and simple lung function tests may be necessary if associated diurnal respiratory failure is suspected. A raised haemoglobin may also signify diurnal respiratory failure, as will a raised venous bicarbonate. A raised $Paco_2$ should suggest the possibility of lower airways obstruction (so-called 'overlap syndrome') because patients with 'pure' OSA rarely have hypercapnia when awake: an additional factor(s) such as COPD or morbid obesity usually needs to be present. Obstructive sleep apnoea tends to go with findings that constitute the so-called 'metabolic syndrome',

Box 18.5.2.2 Symptoms of obstructive sleep apnoea

◆ Most common (>60%)
  · Loud snoring
  · Excessive daytime sleepiness
  · Restless sleep
  · Unrefreshing sleep
  · Nocturia
  · Apparent personality changes
  · Witnessed apnoeas
◆ Less common (10–60%)
  · Choking or shortness of breath sensations at night
  · Reduced libido
  · Nocturnal sweating
  · Morning headaches
◆ Rare (10%)
  · Enuresis
  · Complaint of recurrent arousals and insomnia
  · Nocturnal cough
  · Symptomatic oesophageal reflux

i.e. hypertension, central obesity, raised triglyceride levels, reduced HDL cholesterol, and insulin resistance/raised fasting plasma glucose. Blood pressure, fasting blood sugar, and lipids should therefore be measured as part of good care and opportunistic screening.

Unless the presenting problem turns out not to be sleep related, some form of sleep study will be required. In the past, the usual procedure was to employ full polysomnography, which measured sleep state and respiratory variables (see Figs. 18.5.2.2 and 18.5.2.4). However, this investigation and its analysis is expensive and time consuming, particularly if all recurrent arousals are documented. The primary requirements are to (1) assess sleep fragmentation, (2) establish if a respiratory problem is responsible, and (3) decide if upper airway obstruction is the primary cause. Full polysomnography, properly interpreted, will usually allow this, with the EEG and EMG giving good information on sleep disruption, and aspects of respiration deduced from ribcage/abdominal movement transducers, oronasal airflow, and snoring and continuous oximeter recordings. However, there is considerable signal redundancy in such recordings, and the essential derivatives—sleep disruption and ventilation—can be assessed in much simpler ways (see Fig. 18.5.2.6). In view of this, most clinical respiratory sleep laboratories have abandoned routine, conventional polysomnography because of its unnecessary expense.

Sleep fragmentation can be inferred from a variety of signals. The most sensitive appears to be autonomic markers of brainstem activation, such as blood pressure and pulse rate rises. In addition, since most abnormal respiratory events will end in some form of arousal, counting body movements provides some guide to the degree of sleep fragmentation, and may be most predictive of daytime symptoms. Upper airway obstruction can be inferred from

snoring, a particular inspiratory pattern on a nasal flow tracing (flow limitation), paradoxical ribcage/abdominal movements, and from pulsus paradoxus visible on a beat-to-beat blood pressure tracing (now easily obtainable non-invasively, Fig. 18.5.2.5). Many simple, commercial monitoring systems can be used to record these signals and to assess the extent of the sleep fragmentation and whether upper airways obstruction is the likely cause. Recent work suggests that these simpler measures can predict sleepiness in obstructive sleep apnoea, and its response to treatment, at least as well as EEG-based approaches, which are clearly not the 'gold standard' they were once thought to be. The attention paid to each signal, and perhaps the exact sleep study system used, will depend to some extent on the condition under investigation. Fig. 18.5.2.6 shows data provided by the system in routine use in our laboratory, designed primarily to identify obstructive sleep apnoea and its variants, but it will also identify central sleep apnoea (see below) and nonrespiratory problems such as periodic movements of the legs during sleep.

Because of the imprecise relationship between the number of abnormalities on a sleep study and the severity of symptoms, trying to count them precisely is pointless, particularly given that there can be considerable night to night variation. Hence, the reporting of sleep studies tends to be more qualitative than previously, with divisions simply into mild, moderate, and severe. These bandings are sometimes arbitrarily allocated on the basis of event rates, with 5 to 15 respiratory events per hour being mild, 15 to 30 moderate, and more than 30 severe—the aim simply being to see if there is an adequate and understandable explanation for the patient's symptoms, and assess the severity of any problem.

Differential diagnosis

Obstructive sleep apnoea syndrome (i.e. the combination of sleep apnoea plus symptoms) should be relatively easy to diagnose in a patient who snores, has witnessed apnoeas, is sleepy, and has a compatible abnormal sleep study. However, there are alternative diagnoses that should be considered, from either the history or sleep study.

Periodic leg movements during sleep

Sleep fragmentation leading to daytime somnolence can be due to periodic leg movements during sleep which lead to multiple arousals during NREM sleep. These leg movements are common in older people and may not provoke symptoms, but they can cause excessive daytime sleepiness if they provoke significant recurrent arousals over an extended period of time, with such patients usually having restless leg syndrome when awake, particularly in the evening. Periodic leg movements during sleep usually occurs in isolation but can be associated with renal impairment (especially if on dialysis), low ferritin level, peripheral neuropathy, and previous sciatica. It is easily diagnosed by sleep study (see Fig. 18.5.2.6d) and, if sufficiently symptomatic, treated with dopaminergic agonists.

Narcolepsy

Narcolepsy is due to destruction of orexin (also known as hypocretin) neurons in the hypothalamus that are involved in the maintenance of wakefulness and muscle tone. This destruction is thought to be immunological, and there is a very strong association with HLA DQB1 0602 subtype (>95% compared to 30% in the general population). The condition will present to sleep physicians, although snoring and witnessed apnoeas are not usual features. Vivid disturbing dreams (particularly at sleep onset), sleep paralysis, uncontrollable somnolence, and cataplexy (loss of muscle tone/falling in response to strong emotion or laughter) should suggest the diagnosis. There may be a family history. The patient should be HLA typed, with absence of the relevant HLA type strongly refuting the diagnosis. The history, rather than a sleep study, is the mainstay of diagnosis, although recognition of early onset REM sleep during daytime naps is sometimes helpful. Where available, measurement of orexin in cerebrospinal fluid is being used by some to help with diagnosis. Specialist referral is required for diagnosis and management: narcolepsy is a lifelong condition with significant ramifications for employment and driving. See Chapter 24.5.2 for further discussion.

Multisystem atrophy

Multisystem atrophy (Shy–Drager syndrome) can present to sleep clinics with apparent snoring and sleep fragmentation. In fact the 'snoring' is due to laryngeal abductor weakness and laryngeal closure during sleep, with stridulous inspiratory obstruction. It is important to distinguish this stridor from the usual pharyngeal snoring of OSA because these patients can suddenly die from nocturnal respiratory arrest. They can be successfully treated with standard CPAP therapy (see 'Treatment', below).

Patients with multisystem atrophy and Parkinson's disease may also occasionally present with REM sleep behaviour disorder. This strange phenomenon is due to loss of the atonia normally present during REM sleep, which allows extensive movements while dreaming that appear to match the dream content. The patient may become aggressive and sometimes attack the sleeping partner. It is due to damage to Jouvet's centre in the pons (responsible for the normal atonia) and is strongly associated with the development of multisystem atrophy, often occurring many years later. It usually responds to clonazepam, which generally reduces muscular tone.

Other causes of excessive daytime sleepiness are listed in Box 18.5.2.3 but do not have apnoeic episodes on sleep study; and see Chapter 24.5.3 for further discussion.

Sleep study misinterpretation

Central sleep apnoeas (see below) can occasionally be difficult to distinguish from obstructive sleep apnoeas as the patient may have a few obstructed breaths at the end of the apnoea cycle, which are secondary to the central apnoea. Conversely, patients who are morbidly obese or with inspiratory muscle weakness may have such small chest-wall movements against the upper airway obstruction that they are misinterpreted as having central apnoeic events.

Overlap syndromes

It is also important to realize that OSA may coexist with other respiratory disorders that can have an additive effect, leading to profound respiratory failure. The term 'overlap syndrome' was originally coined to refer to the combination of chronic obstructive pulmonary disease and OSA, but morbid obesity can interact with both of these conditions so that the term is often now used to describe mixtures of these three provokers of ventilatory failure. When obesity alone provokes ventilatory failure then the term 'obesity hypoventilation syndrome' (previously Pickwickian syndrome) is used.

Treatment

Once it is established that the patient's symptoms are likely to be due to sleep disruption from sleep-induced upper airway obstruction, then therapy has to be tailored to symptom severity.

Box 18.5.2.3 Causes of excessive daytime sleepiness

- ◆ Most common
  - Depression
  - Lifestyle, e.g. alcohol (reduces slow wave sleep and leads to rebound alertness and insomnia, can also worsen OSA), shift work, caffeine, poor sleep hygiene.
  - Drugs, e.g. β blockers, antidepressants, sedatives, major tranquillizers
- ◆ Less common
  - Periodic limb movements during sleep
  - Narcolepsy
  - Hypothalamic damage following severe head injury or cranial irradiation
  - Postinfectious, e.g. Epstein–Barr virus
  - Neurological disorders such as Parkinson's disease, multisystem atrophy, myotonic dystrophy, previous CVA
- ◆ Other
  - Idiopathic
  - Blind insomnia/sleepiness

CVA, cerebrovascular accident.

Advice and simple treatments

Mild symptoms may resolve with simple treatments and advice (Box 18.5.2.4). Weight loss is undoubtedly effective, but often very difficult to achieve. If sleep disruption only occurs while the individual is supine, when upper airway obstruction tends to be worst, then learning to lie on one's side may be helpful. Stopping sedatives and evening alcohol can help. Initial enthusiasm for the tricyclic antidepressants has waned, although they may slightly improve mild cases. They are believed to work through REM sleep suppression and by improving upper airway tone. No other drug has shown any consistent effect.

Nasal continuous positive airway pressure

If the sleep apnoea and symptoms are severe, there is only one fully effective therapy—nasal continuous positive airway pressure (NCPAP). This treatment involves wearing a small mask (Fig. 18.5.2.8) over the nose while asleep, with the air pressure kept at a fixed level above atmospheric by a pump. Pressures in the region of

---

Box 18.5.2.4 Advice for patients with snoring, or mild to moderate obstructive sleep apnoea usually due to postural dependence

- ◆ Learn to sleep on your side and avoid sleeping on your back
- ◆ No alcohol after 18.00 h
- ◆ No sedatives
- ◆ Lose weight
- ◆ Stop smoking
- ◆ Keep the nose as clear as possible

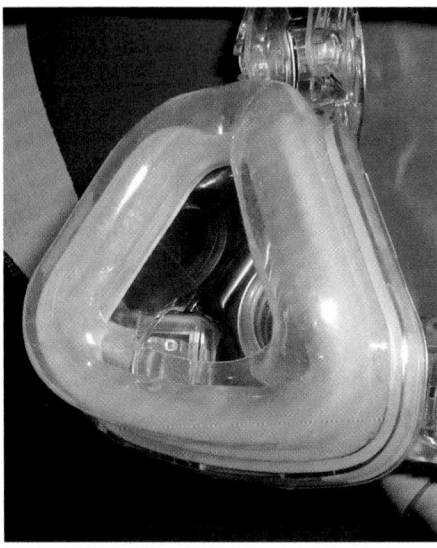

Fig. 18.5.2.8 A soft silicone nasal mask and its headgear, used in the treatment of obstructive sleep apnoea.

10 cmH$_2$O are enough to splint open the pharynx and resist collapse, allowing unobstructed breathing and undisturbed sleep (Fig. 18.5.2.9). The exact pressure required can be established in a number of ways. The response is dramatic, in terms of both physiology and daytime symptoms, which resolve rapidly even after one night of treatment. There are several randomized placebo-controlled trials and a recent Cochrane review proving beyond doubt the large symptomatic benefit. The unpleasantness and unaesthetic appearance of this treatment initially repel patients, but once the benefits have been experienced, acceptance is high, and indeed the compliance has been shown to be better than that with asthma therapy or antihypertensives. Off-the-shelf systems, with comfortable soft masks, are now available for home use at about £300 each. Such equipment will last for many years (with regular mask replacements) and represents extraordinary value for money given the enormous improvement in quality of life that it produces. NCPAP machines that automatically hunt, moment to moment, the pressure required by the patient to overcome their obstructive sleep apnoea are available. These can be used either to establish the fixed pressure subsequently required by the patient, or as the long-term machine at home, but there is no evidence that their extra expense is justified except in patients requiring higher pressures.

Experienced sleep clinics put much effort into helping patients to become established on NCPAP, through attentive education and comfort-improving measures such as humidification. Once established on NCPAP, patients with obstructive sleep apnoea are likely to require it for life unless they can lose a significant amount of weight.

Surgical and other treatments

Weight loss may only be achieved through gastric surgery, such as silastic ring gastroplasty to reduce food consumption.

Another surgical treatment is uvulopalatopharyngoplasty, which consists of removing part of the soft palate and any residual tonsils, and 'tightening up' the side walls of the pharynx. Although it can reduce snoring, its success rate at treating obstructive sleep apnoea is not good, and a recent Cochrane review has confirmed its lack of efficacy. Attempts to select patients who might respond has had very limited success, although thin patients with large soft palates,

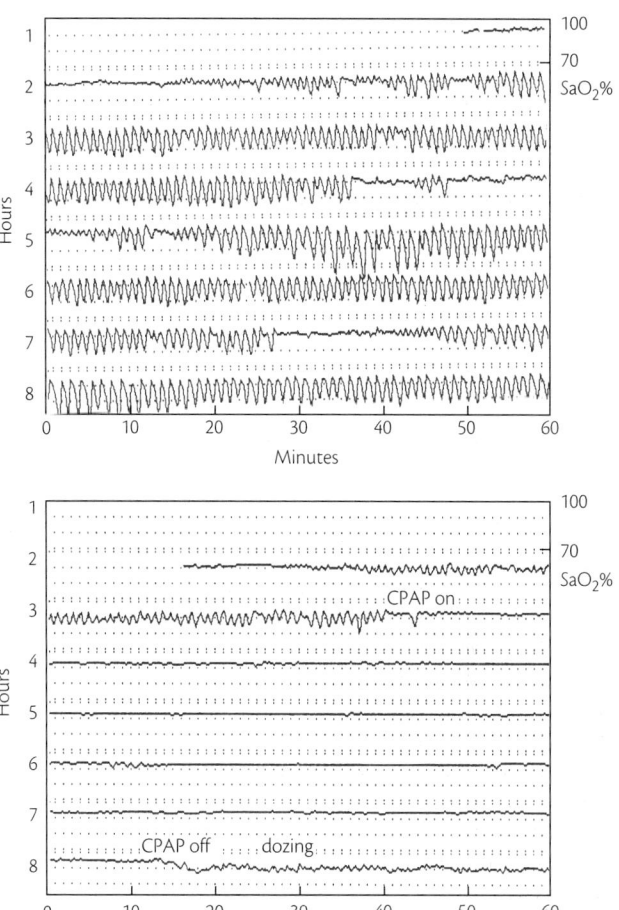

Fig. 18.5.2.9 Two all-night oximetry tracings from a patient with obstructive sleep apnoea, before treatment and during his first night on nasal CPAP. Each tracing starts top left and finishes bottom right. Each tracing is continuous for 8 h with the vertical axis for each individual line scaled 70–100% SaO$_2$.

residual tonsils, and milder disease probably do best. By contrast, there is good evidence that tonsillectomy is effective in children with OSA and large tonsils.

Other operative techniques involving advancement of the mandible (and sometimes the maxilla) may be appropriate in highly selected cases. Tracheostomy was the first therapy ever tried and was (of course) very effective: it may still be appropriate in occasional patients.

A newer approach has been the use of mandibular advancement devices, worn in the mouth at night (Fig. 18.5.2.10). These hold the lower jaw closed and forward, thus increasing the space behind the tongue and hence pharyngeal volume. They have undergone extensive trials in a variety of situations, but matters are complicated by the plethora of such devices available. The current conclusion is that they do work, but less so as the severity of the obstructive sleep apnoea (and usually therefore the obesity) increase. Their main use seems to be in the control of unacceptable snoring, mild OSA, or as an alternative to NCPAP for short periods, or when NCPAP cannot be tolerated despite maximal support.

Epidemiology

Given the difficulties over definition, the prevalence of symptomatic obstructive sleep apnoea is hard to establish, and will depend

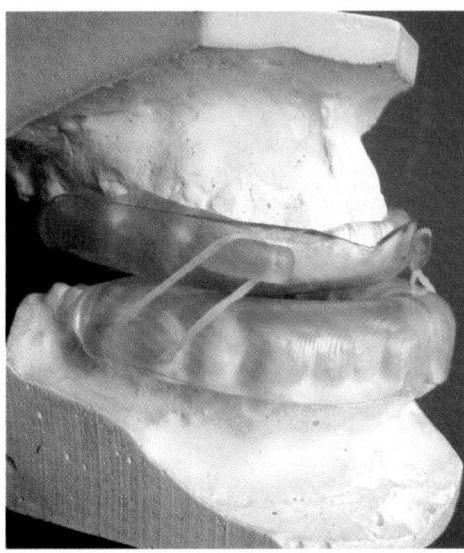

Fig. 18.5.2.10 Example of a mandibular advancement device, worn in the mouth at night. These hold the lower jaw forward and closed, thus increasing pharyngeal dimensions. They are used extensively for the control of snoring but are not very effective in anything more severe than mild obstructive sleep apnoea.

on where an arbitrary cut-off is placed. In an early study, about 0.3% of men aged 35 to 65 years clearly had severe, symptomatic obstructive sleep apnoea, requiring nasal continuous positive airway pressure (NCPAP) therapy and were responsive to such treatment. However, about 5% had more than five dips of more than 4% Sao_2 per hour, one suggested threshold for normality; most of these subjects were not obviously symptomatic and would not have wanted a treatment such as NCPAP. Overall in this study, sleepiness correlated with snoring, and more sleepiness seemed to be due to snoring than classical sleep apnoea. Other studies in Israel, the United States of America, and Italy have found prevalences of 'significant' sleep apnoea in the 0.5 to 2% range.

Predictors of sleep apnoea in these prevalence studies have been obesity, snoring, age, self-reported sleepiness, and alcohol consumption. Snoring is more common in men than in women, and obstructive sleep apnoea syndrome itself is about three to five times more common in men. The prevalence in women probably increases after the menopause with redistribution of body fat to a more male-like, upper body, distribution. Rapidly increasing levels of obesity in many countries means that the prevalence of OSA is increasing.

If these prevalence studies are correct, then obstructive sleep apnoea is the third most common serious respiratory disease after asthma and COPD. Sleep apnoea is now the commonest reason for referral in some respiratory units.

Prognosis and long-term complications

Many patients with OSA are of the physiognomy to have associated visceral obesity and the metabolic syndrome (hypertension, insulin resistance, hyperlipidaemia). The vascular mortality in these patients is in general higher than average, their 10-year vascular event rate being approximately 36%. However, it is not clear whether OSA is a further independent vascular risk factor, or merely associated. This is important because many sleep units still treat patients mainly on the basis of their daytime symptoms, usually excessive sleepiness, and not to reduce future vascular risk.

To do so would greatly increase the requirement for nasal CPAP, perhaps three- or fourfold based on epidemiological studies of sleep-study-defined OSA, rather than OSA syndrome (with symptoms).

There are plausible hypotheses for a causative link between OSA and vascular disease. With the arousal after each apnoea or hypopnoea, there is a surge in blood pressure, often by over 50 mmHg. Overnight blood pressure levels do not fall normally, itself an adverse vascular risk factor, and there is good evidence of raised daytime blood pressure in patients with OSA syndrome. Nasal CPAP treatment not only abolishes the nocturnal blood pressure surges, but also reduces the daytime blood pressure (Fig. 18.5.2.11).

Uncontrolled work has suggested increased oxidative stress, increased coagulability, increased inflammatory markers, and increased cholesterol levels as possible mechanisms for increased vascular damage. Cross-sectional studies have shown an association between OSA and hypertension, stroke, and other vascular events,

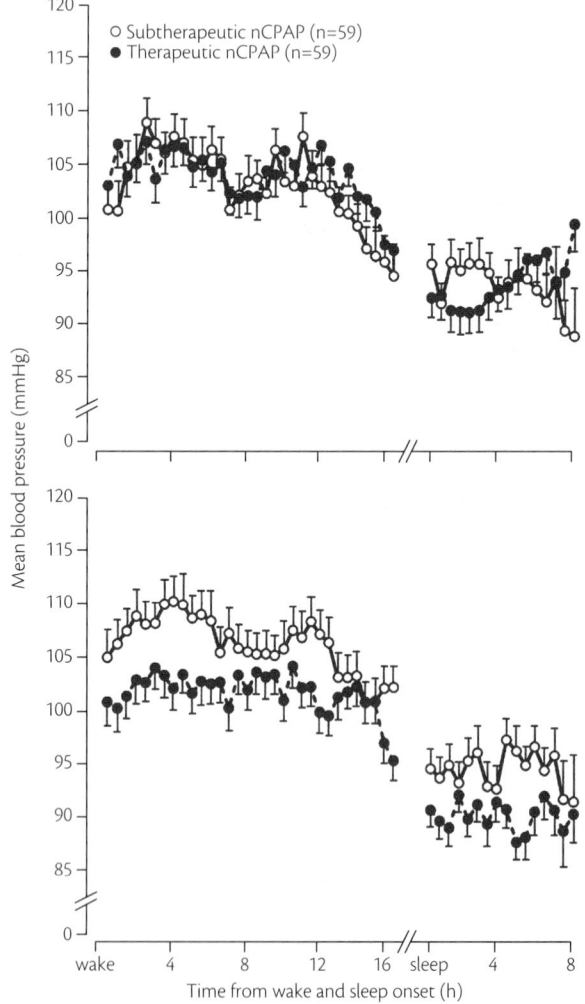

Fig. 18.5.2.11 Mean ambulatory blood pressure profile in two groups of patients with OSA- a control group (given subtherapeutic CPAP, °) and a treatment group (given therapeutic CPAP, •). The top panel shows the two groups' profiles before any treatment, confirming that they had similar blood pressure profiles. The bottom panel shows the groups after treatment, showing that the group given therapeutic CPAP had a lower mean blood pressure profile. Reproduced from Pepperell *et al.* Lancet. 2001; 359:204–210 with permission from Elsevier.

but despite trying to control for confounders such as visceral obesity it is impossible to be sure that any residual effects of OSA are not due to a further confounder, or one inadequately controlled for. For example, surface measurements of central obesity (waist, or waist/hip ratio) are poor measures of true visceral obesity, and OSA is particularly present in those with visceral obesity.

Uncontrolled interventional studies have strongly suggested that treatment of OSA reduces vascular events compared to untreated control patients (Fig. 18.5.2.12). Other studies have shown that noncompliant patients in general are clearly different from compliant ones, with considerably higher vascular mortality, perhaps due to poor compliance with a range of other healthy activities and medications. As yet there are no controlled interventional long-term morbidity and mortality studies of nasal CPAP for OSA, hence there is no evidence-based justification for routine use of nasal CPAP to reduce vascular risk in patients with OSA who would not otherwise want to use nasal CPAP for relief of daytime sleepiness.

Driving regulations and obstructive sleep apnoea

There have been some recent high-profile cases of fatal road traffic accidents caused by drivers falling asleep at the wheel, some of which have led to prison sentences. This has highlighted the issue for patients with OSA who are up to seven times more likely to have a road traffic accident than controls, although this higher incidence is probably only present at the more severe end of the spectrum. In the United Kingdom the law says that drivers are responsible for their vigilance while driving and should not drive when sleepy for whatever reason. OSA syndrome (i.e. with symptoms) is a notifiable illness, and such patients should inform the Driver and Vehicle Licensing Agency (DVLA). Licences will only be revoked if there is continuing sleepiness, thus once on treatment full licensing is possible, hence a professional diagnosis and confirmation of response to treatment is required. Uncontrolled evidence shows normal road traffic accident rates following treatment, and work using driving simulators has confirmed the beneficial effect of nasal CPAP.

Treatment costs for OSA would be covered, several times over, by the costs incurred by avoidable road traffic accidents amongst patients with this condition. In addition, undiagnosed patients with OSA have increased general health costs in the years leading up to their diagnosis, which fall afterwards.

Sleep-induced hypoventilation and central sleep apnoea

Breathing during sleep may decrease, not because of upper airway obstruction, but because of a reduction in central output to the respiratory muscles—so-called central, rather than obstructive, apnoea, or hypoventilation (see Fig. 18.5.2.4). There are many causes for central sleep apnoea or hypoventilation: Table 18.5.2.2 shows one way of classifying them. Some of the central apnoeas disturb sleep and present with daytime sleepiness, whereas others tend to present with symptoms of respiratory failure, such as morning headaches with confusion, cyanosis, and ankle oedema.

Absent ventilatory drive

Brainstem abnormalities may damage the areas responsible for automatic chemical control of ventilation. While awake, the wakefulness-related ventilatory drive may be adequate to maintain Pao_2 and $Paco_2$ levels, but on falling asleep the drive falls or even disappears, with marked hypoventilation (or apnoea) and hypoxaemia. Arousal is then necessary to restore the blood gases. This failure of brainstem automatic control (known as Ondine's curse) can be congenital, or may be acquired as the result of a stroke, infection, surgical damage, multiple sclerosis, or compression by a tumour or syrinx. Congenital causes have been shown to be due to a variety of different genetic abnormalities associated with the development and differentiation of neural crest tissue.

Reduction of chemical drive can occur as a secondary problem when ventilation is reduced by mechanical problems such as chronic airways obstruction or weak respiratory muscles. It appears that chronic underventilation can lead to blunting of

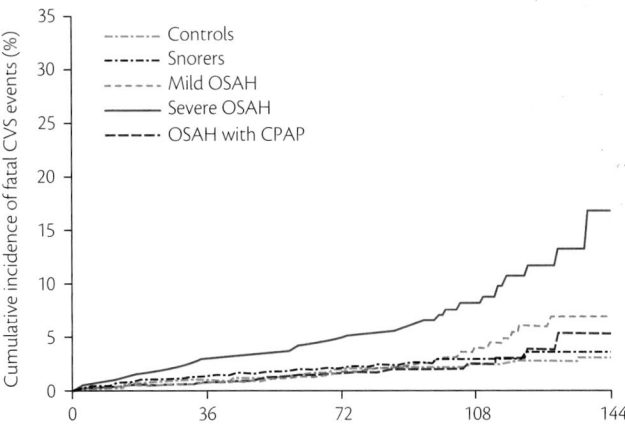

Fig. 18.5.2.12 12-year follow-up (in months) of patients with varying degrees of OSA, showing cardiovascular events in various groups of patients and controls. The group with severe untreated OSA (OSAH) did badly compared to a treated group (OSAH with CPAP), those with mild OSAH, snorers and normal controls. However, this was an uncontrolled study in which patients either chose or declined to be treated, which may have led to bias.
Reproduced from Marin et al Lancet 2005; 365:1046–53, with permission from Elsevier.

Table 18.5.2.2 Types of central sleep apnoea

Type	Examples	Daytime arterial CO_2 level
Absent or reduced ventilatory drive (Ondine's curse)	Brainstem damage or congenital abnormality	Raised
	Acquired blunting, e.g. secondary to lung disease	
Unstable respiratory drive	Sleep onset, hypoxaemia, altitude, heart failure	Normal or low
REM-related oscillations	Normal in REM sleep	Normal or raised
	Due to neuromuscular disorders and respiratory muscle weakness.	
Reflex central apnoea	Pharyngeal collapse inhibits inspiration	Normal
Apparent central apnoea (wrongly diagnosed)	Respiratory muscle weakness or gross obesity cause chest wall movement transducers to fail to demonstrate any ventilatory effort during obstructive apnoeas	Normal or raised

ventilatory drive, perhaps through alteration in acid–base buffering in the brainstem, and can also be associated with marked falls in ventilation during sleep.

Unstable ventilatory drive

The wakefulness-related ventilatory drive stabilizes ventilation and prevents it from falling below a certain level. If reasons for ventilatory instability exist then, by removing this stabilizing effect, sleep will allow periodic respiration to develop and be maintained. The usual provoker of instability is an increased gain in the ventilatory response to a stimulus, usually hypoxia or hypercapnia. Control theory shows that increasing the gain in any feedback system causes instability through overshoot and undershoot. A good example is the effect of altitude hypoxaemia on newly arrived lowlanders. While awake the breathing is driven by hypoxia, but also limited by the hypocapnic alkalosis. When sleep occurs, and drive is therefore reduced, hypoventilation ensues until the rise in $PaCO_2$ and fall in PaO_2 restarts ventilation. Often this leads to sufficient hyperpnoea to arouse the individual who now has extra hypoxia, which steepens the CO_2 response line and, along with the return of wakefulness drive, produces marked overshoot of ventilation. On returning to sleep with much improved $PaCO_2$ and PaO_2, hypopnoea or apnoea recurs, and the cycle is perpetuated. Thus, periodic breathing with recurrent arousals is very common at altitude, with the expected daytime consequence of sleepiness and complaints of insomnia. Acetazolamide produces a metabolic acidosis and increases the ventilation at a given $PaCO_2$, the hypoxaemia is relieved, and thus the ventilatory response to CO_2 becomes less steep. Both these factors restore stability and reduce periodic respiration.

In left ventricular failure there is also extra ventilatory drive, mainly due to stimulation of interstitial lung receptors (J-receptors) by the raised left atrial and pulmonary venous pressure. In conjunction with the longer circulation time seen in heart failure, this also provokes instability with waxing and waning of the ventilation. This periodic breathing, or Cheyne–Stokes respiration, is quite common in heart failure and, through sleep disruption, produces daytime sleepiness and complaints of nocturnal dyspnoea (Fig. 18.5.2.13). The patient is usually aware that on arousal the dyspnoea disappears within a few seconds, unlike the paroxysmal nocturnal dyspnoea of pulmonary oedema which usually takes at least 15 min or so to abate following getting out of bed. Treatment with overnight oxygen, acetazolamide or benzodiazepines can sometimes reduce the periodicity and improve both sleep quality

and symptoms. There has been some recent interest in NCPAP as a treatment for left ventricular failure and periodic breathing. However, a recent randomized controlled trial showed no benefit on mortality in patients with dominantly Cheyne–Stokes respiration, although there is good evidence of benefit to cardiac function from treating obstructive sleep apnoea in patients with left ventricular failure.

Instability of respiratory control can also occur in normal subjects in the early stages of sleep, or if sleep is disturbed for other reasons. This is because sleep depth is oscillating back and forth between drowsy wakefulness and light sleep, with the ventilatory drive oscillating as well.

REM sleep apnoeas

During normal REM sleep the phasic bursts of eye movements are associated with transient falls in ventilation, and even the occurrence of apnoeas. The ribcage muscles are affected most, but diaphragmatic excursion can also fall. Such periodicities are entirely normal.

As discussed earlier, the REM sleep inhibition of most muscles (apart from the diaphragm) can greatly reduce overall ventilation when the accessory muscles of respiration are needed for breathing. Thus on entering REM sleep there can be profound falls in ventilation and SaO_2 in patients with neuromuscular diseases, chest-wall abnormalities, and chronic airways obstruction.

Generalized neuromuscular diseases tend to involve the respiratory muscles in concert with other muscles. However in some disorders the respiratory muscles (and particularly the diaphragm) may be involved very early on, at a time when other muscles are virtually normal. A particular example of this is adult-type acid maltase deficiency, where patients may present in respiratory failure while still able to walk normally. REM-sleep-related hypoxaemia may be the first sign that there are problems, and it is not known whether this actually accelerates the onset of eventual diurnal respiratory failure, or is merely a marker that respiratory failure will soon follow. Sometimes there may be associated upper airway obstruction during REM sleep, leading to even larger falls in SaO_2. Overnight oximetry studies will indicate the degree of hypoxaemia but will not establish if there is additional upper airway obstruction.

There has been great interest in the REM-sleep-related hypoxaemia seen in chronic airways obstruction. It was thought possible that these hypoxic episodes might be the reason why some patients developed respiratory failure but others did not. However,

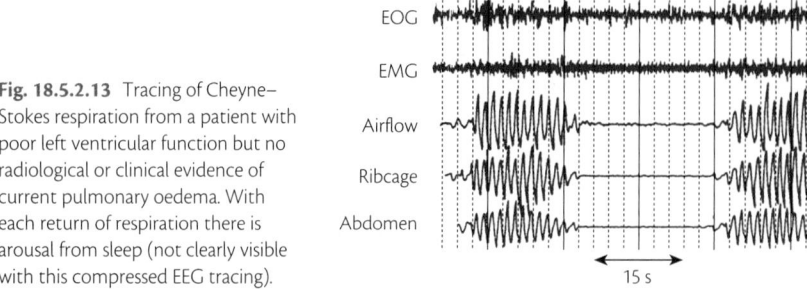

Fig. 18.5.2.13 Tracing of Cheyne–Stokes respiration from a patient with poor left ventricular function but no radiological or clinical evidence of current pulmonary oedema. With each return of respiration there is arousal from sleep (not clearly visible with this compressed EEG tracing).

it appears that REM sleep hypoventilation and a fall in Pao_2 is fairly universal in this group of patients. If the patient is initially well oxygenated and on the flat part of the haemoglobin dissociation curve, the fall in Sao_2 (which is usually what is monitored) is not particularly dramatic; however, if the patient is initially poorly oxygenated and on the steep part of the curve, similar hypoventilation will produce dramatic falls in Sao_2. As yet there is no evidence that these REM sleep falls in Sao_2 contribute to the morbidity and mortality of patients with chronic airflow obstruction, although some centres have shown that overnight oxygen therapy reduces arousals, thus improving sleep quality. The main problem is that the falls in Sao_2 can look superficially like obstructive sleep apnoea, leading to an erroneous diagnosis and the inappropriate use of NCPAP.

Reflex apnoea

Central respiratory output can be modified by a number of reflexes from receptors in the upper airway. There is a reflex from the pharynx that inhibits inspiratory flow when the pharynx is being sucked in and collapsed, which makes teleological sense as a slowing of inspiratory flow would reduce the tendency to collapse. There are some patients with pharyngeal collapse who, instead of struggling to inspire against the blocked airway, simply stop breathing until they finally arouse, presumably due to the fall in Pao_2 and rise in $Paco_2$ itself. This then appears as a central apnoea, despite the aetiology being pharyngeal collapse, with the problem tending to happen when the patient is supine, with snoring or ordinary obstructive apnoeas when decubitus. Evidence that superficial receptors are responsible comes from the observation that inspiratory attempts return if the pharynx is anaesthetized. These patients usually present with histories typical of obstructive sleep apnoea, respond to NCPAP, and should be managed in the same way.

Apparent central apnoea

The diagnosis of central apnoea depends on demonstrating the absence of respiratory effort when airflow at the nose and mouth stops. Surface measurements of ribcage and abdominal movement are sometimes employed as evidence of continuing respiratory effort, but in two circumstances—marked obesity and muscular weakness—the surface transducers may fail to register that inspiratory efforts are still being made (although more sensitive measures of inspiratory effort, such as oesophageal pressure tracings, will usually do so). Obesity lessens the sensitivity of surface transducers, and with muscle weakness the inspiratory muscles may not be able to move the chest wall detectably against a closed upper airway. In severe OSA with diurnal ventilatory failure, the same situation may develop where inspiratory effort is so reduced that a misdiagnosis of central apnoea is made. Such cases of apparently pure obesity—hypoventilation then subsequently turn out be OSA. This is usually revealed when ventilatory failure has been reversed by a period of overnight ventilation, and the sleep study repeated later, when the upper airway obstruction and frustrated inspiratory efforts become obvious.

Overnight ventilation for central sleep apnoea or hypoventilation

The chronic ventilatory failure associated with some neurological disorders (e.g. acid maltase deficiency, postpoliomyelitis syndrome, motor neuron disease, Duchenne dystrophy) usually progresses rapidly to death, even when quality of life is otherwise very good. The same is true of chest-wall restrictive disorders such as scoliosis, as well as the ventilatory failure that can develop many years after extensive thoracoplasty. However, supporting breathing overnight can fully reverse ventilatory failure, and the response to treatment can be dramatic, with resolution of all symptoms and restoration of normal blood gases, even when off the ventilator during the day.

The mechanism by which supporting breathing at night corrects ventilatory failure is not clear, but there are various possibilities. Firstly, it may simply be that the respiratory muscles are rested so that they can respond better to the demands of the respiratory centre during the day. Secondly, it may be that improving blood gases at night and preventing the marked REM sleep deteriorations leads to resetting of the respiratory centre back towards normal, thus reversing an acquired blunting of drive. Tricyclic antidepressants such as protriptyline can virtually abolish REM sleep periods and their associated hypoxaemia and have been shown to improve daytime blood gases temporarily, suggesting that simply abolishing these periods of particular hypoxia can help. Thirdly, by increasing chest-wall and lung excursion (tidal volumes on the ventilator can be in excess of the voluntary vital capacity) overall respiratory compliance may improve, allowing the muscles to work more efficiently. Whatever the explanation, there is no doubt that this is a life-saving therapy that in certain conditions can add decades of active life.

Most of the original techniques to support ventilation overnight evolved from positive-pressure ventilation developed during the polio epidemics in the early 1950s, and the subsequent use of the iron lung that was developed to support these poliomyelitis victims long term. Evacuating the air from around the chest expands the lungs, recreating the normal way of breathing. A range of devices involving airtight jackets and shells over the chest were developed, but required much attention to detail and often individual, tailor-made systems. Efficacy was also limited by an unfortunate specific complication that resulted from the abolition of spontaneous ventilatory drive to the diaphragm and pharyngeal muscles, namely upper airway collapse during the mechanical inspiratory phase due to an unbraced airway. The recent development of comfortable nasal and face masks has revolutionized the overnight ventilation of these patients. Positive pressure ventilation can be used via a face mask, or sometimes via the nasal masks used for NCPAP (see Fig. 18.5.2.8). Although there are still many problems to be overcome when establishing patients on such equipment (particularly mask comfort and air leaks through the mouth when using nasal masks), the systems can be bought off the shelf ready to use (current cost c.£1500). Most units now use positive-pressure ventilation in preference to negative-pressure systems.

Electrical pacing of the diaphragm is occasionally used for supporting ventilation in conditions where the phrenic nerve and diaphragm are intact and the problem is central. This involves the implantation of bilateral phrenic electrodes and induction coils under the skin that are activated by external induction coils.

Further reading

Gastaut H, Tassinari CA, Duron B (1966). Polygraphic study of the episodic diurnal and nocturnal (hypnic and respiratory) manifestations of the Pickwick syndrome. *Brain Res*, **2**, 167–86.

Guilleminault C, Stoohs R, Duncan S (1991). Snoring (1). Daytime sleepiness in regular heavy snorers. *Chest*, **99**, 40–8.

Jenkinson C, *et al.* (1999). Randomised prospective parallel trial of therapeutic nasal continuous positive airway pressure (NCPAP) against sub-therapeutic NCPAP for obstructive sleep apnoea. *Lancet*, **353**, 2100–5.

Remmers JE, *et al.* (1978). Pathogenesis of upper airway occlusion during sleep. *J Appl Physiol*, **44**, 931–8.

Robinson G, Davies Rjo, Stradling Jr (2004). Obstructive sleep apnoea and hypertension. *Thorax*, **59**, 1089–94.

Stradling JR, Davies RJO (2004). Obstructive sleep apnoea, definitions, epidemiology and natural history. *Thorax*, **59**, 73–78.

Sullivan CE, *et al.* (1981). Reversal of obstructive sleep apnoea by continuous positive airway pressure applied through the nares. *Lancet*, **i**, 862–5.

Weiss JW, *et al.* (1996). Hemodynamic consequences of obstructive sleep apnea. *Sleep*, **19**, 388–97.

Allergic rhinitis

Stephen R. Durham and Hesham Saleh

Essentials

Allergic rhinitis affects more than 20% of the population of Westernized countries and has a significant impact on quality of life and school/work performance.

Aetiology and clinical features—important environmental factors include tree and grass pollens (seasonal allergic rhinitis); house dust mite and domestic pets, most often cats (perennial allergic rhinitis); and a variety of occupational exposures (occupational rhinitis). Many genetic loci confer susceptibility. Immediate symptoms (itching, sneezing, and watery nasal discharge) occur as a consequence of allergen cross-linking adjacent IgE molecules on the surface of mast cells in the nasal mucosa, resulting in the release of histamine and tryptase, and the generation of bradykinin.

Diagnosis and classification—diagnosis is usually straightforward and based on the history, examination and (when indicated) the results of skin prick tests and/or serum allergen-specific IgE levels. Classification is according to the severity and duration of symptoms as defined by ARIA (Allergic Rhinitis and its Impact on Asthma) guidelines, which describe four categories of disease: (1) mild intermittent, (2) moderate/severe intermittent, (3) mild persistent, and (4) moderate/severe persistent. Differential diagnosis and management of more complex cases are helped by flexible or rigid nasal endoscopy and CT of the nose and paranasal sinuses.

Management—allergen avoidance, topical intranasal corticosteroids, and nonsedating oral antihistamines are the mainstay of treatment and are effective and safe. Treatment failure often results from poor compliance or inadequate technique in use of nasal sprays. Allergen injection immunotherapy, which has been shown to induce long-term disease remission, is indicated in patients with severe seasonal allergic rhinitis who fail to respond to usual measures. Rhinitis is often accompanied by significant comorbidities that include conjunctivitis, sinusitis, otitis media, and bronchial asthma: these require separate recognition and treatment.

Introduction

Rhinitis means inflammation of the nasal mucosa: in clinical terms it may be defined as symptoms of nasal itching, sneezing, discharge, or blockage, that occur for more than 1 h on most days.

The lining of the nose and paranasal sinuses is in continuity with the lower respiratory tract such that diseases of the upper and lower airways frequently coexist. The World Health Organization position paper 'Allergic Rhinitis and its Impact on Asthma' (ARIA) recognized this association and provided a classification of the disease based on the severity and duration of symptoms as a basis for the modern management of allergic rhinitis. In this section a historical perspective and the aetiology, epidemiology, and pathogenesis of allergic rhinitis are described, followed by practical guidelines for the diagnosis and management of the condition. Finally, immunotherapy (desensitization), including novel approaches are discussed.

Historical perspective

The term 'hay fever' was originally coined by John Bostock in 1819. It is a misnomer, since the disease is not caused by hay and there is no fever. Nonetheless, the term highlighted the seasonality of the disease 'being associated with the effluvium of hay' and the association of severe hay fever with constitutional upset. William Gordon in 1829 referred to "the aroma emitted by the flowers of grass...", whereas Elliotson in 1831 considered "... it [hay fever] to depend upon the flower of grass and probably the pollen". Charles Blackley, a physician in Manchester, referred in 1873 to hay fever (catarrhus aestivus) as "an aristocratic disease ... rarely, if ever, met with but among the educated", and measured pollen counts in the air and related them to the intensity of hay fever symptoms. He also reproduced the disease in himself by experimental challenge with grass pollen, a technique still widely used today to investigate pathogenesis and to test novel treatment approaches. In 1911 Noon and

Freeman published their classic paper on desensitization for hay fever, and William Frankland, who was a student of Freeman at St Mary's Hospital, London, published the first randomized controlled trial of desensitization for hay fever in the same journal in 1958 and continues to practice allergy in 2010.

Aetiology

Environmental factors

Seasonal allergic rhinitis

Pollens of importance include tree pollens in the spring and grass pollens during the summer (Fig. 18.6.1). Weed pollens and mould spores predominate in the latter part of the summer and early autumn. Grass pollen counts above $50/m^3$ are considered high and are the threshold level at which most hay fever sufferers experience symptoms.

Perennial allergic rhinitis

By far the commonest cause of perennial allergic symptoms are house dust mites (*Dermatophagoides pteronyssinus*, *D. farinae*, and *Euroglyphus maynei*). These are found in almost every home, where they live in the dust that accumulates in carpets, bedding, fabrics, and furniture. They live on shed human skin scales and thrive in temperatures of between 15 and 20°C and a relative humidity of 45 to 65%, conditions which are typical of many modern centrally heated homes. The major allergen of the house dust mite (Der p1) is a digestive enzyme (a cysteine protease) present in the gut and excreted in high concentrations in the mite faeces.

Domestic pets are the second important cause of perennial allergy, relevant in up to 40% of children with asthma and/or rhinitis. The major allergen (Fel d1) is a salivary protein that is preened on to the fur and released on very small particles (<2.5 μm diameter) which remain airborne for many hours, explaining why a sensitized person can experience symptoms almost immediately upon entering a home containing a cat, without being directly exposed to the animal. Dog allergens are less well characterized (Can f1). Cockroaches have been described as a cause of perennial allergic symptoms, particularly in inner-city areas.

Food allergy is unusual as a cause of rhinitis in the absence of other organ involvement. However, rhinitis may be one component of IgE-mediated food-induced symptoms commonly due to egg, milk, and nuts in children and to nuts, fish, shellfish, and fruit in adults. Preservatives such as tartrazine, benzoates, and sulphites may provoke symptoms of rhinitis. Important drugs that can trigger rhinitis include β-blockers, aspirin, and (occasionally) angiotensin converting enzyme (ACE) inhibitors.

Occupational rhinitis

Occupational rhinitis refers to rhinitis caused by an agent inhaled in the workplace. Like other causes of seasonal and perennial rhinitis, occupational rhinitis may also be associated with bronchial asthma. Occupations at risk include laboratory animal workers (rats, guinea pigs, mice), bakers (flour, grain mites), agricultural workers (cows, pollens, fungal spores), electronic solderers (colophony), and health workers and other users of rubber gloves (latex).

Genetic influences

Atopy (the predisposition to develop allergic disorders as defined by a positive skin prick test or raised IgE antibody level to one or more common allergens) and allergic diseases such as hay fever and asthma occur as a complex interaction between genetic and environmental factors. Twin studies in which a higher concordance rate of atopy and allergic diseases is found in monozygotic twins compared to dizygotic twins provides unequivocal evidence of genetic influences.

Candidate gene approaches (which study a narrow region of the genome around a suspected gene with highly polymorphic markers) have been difficult to interpret because of variability in the definition of clinical phenotypes within atopy and allergy. Nonetheless, multiple genetic loci have been identified, including the high-affinity IgE receptor β-chain (localized on chromosome 11q), and the interleukins IL-4, IL-3, IL-5, IL-9, IL-13, the β-glucocorticoid receptor, and leukotriene C4 (LTC4) synthase (all colocalized to chromosome 5q). All of these genes have biological functions consistent with a role in pathogenesis of allergic disorders.

With the completion of the Human Genome Project, the more usual approach now and in future will be to list all of the genes localized to the chromosomal region where a linkage marker has been identified. For example, a recent study identified strong linkage between asthma and bronchial hyperresponsiveness with the gene for ADAM-33, a cell surface protease that is part of the matrix metalloproteinase family, considered important in remodelling responses in the basement membrane to damaged epithelium and airway smooth muscle.

Epidemiology

Recent estimates based on community surveys in western Europe have suggested that more than 20% of the population have perennial

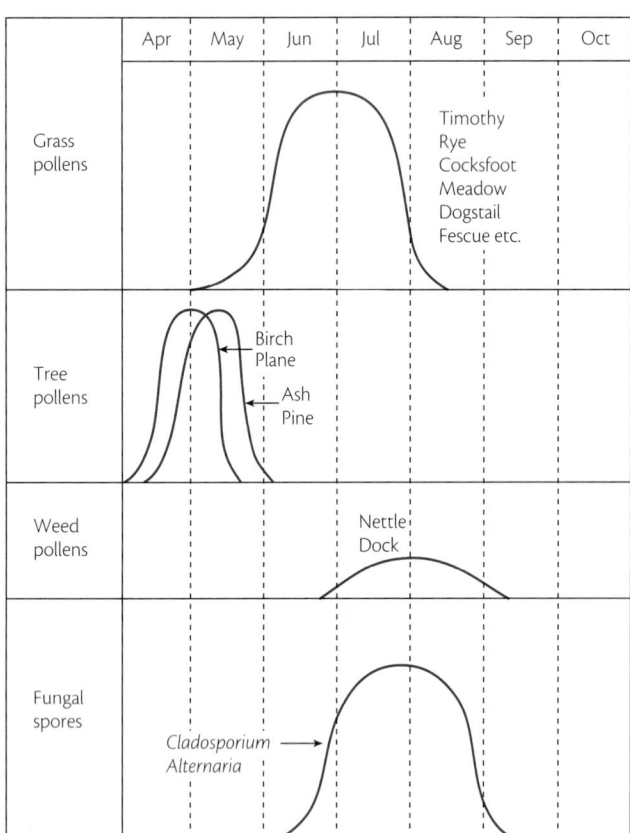

Fig. 18.6.1 Calendar of common seasonal aeroallergens.
(By courtesy of Professor A B Kay, Imperial College School of Medicine, London.)

and/or seasonal allergic rhinitis. The burden that this places on medical services is increasing: in the United Kingdom in 1955–56 there were 5.1 consultations with general practitioners for hay fever per 1000 population per year; in 1981–82 this had increased to 19.8. A recent telephone-based community survey in 6 European countries gave an estimated mean prevalence of allergic rhinitis of 23%.

The increased prevalence of hay fever in countries with a 'Westernized' lifestyle, together with the known increased prevalence associated with small sibships, has given rise to the 'hygiene hypothesis' which implies that reduced exposure to bacterial pathogens may be the basis of the modern epidemic of allergic disorders. These observations tie in with Blackley's recognition of hay fever as a disease more common in the privileged classes over 130 years ago.

Pathogenesis

Immediate symptoms of allergic rhinitis occur as a consequence of allergen cross-linking adjacent IgE molecules on the surface of mast cells in the nasal mucosa (in Coombs' classification, type I, immediate hypersensitivity). This results in the release of granule-derived mediators, including histamine and tryptase, and the generation of bradykinin. IgE-dependent activation of mast cells also results in the release of newly formed membrane-associated mediators derived from arachidonic acid associated with the membrane lipid, including LTC4, LTD4, LTE4 and prostaglandin D_2.

In patients with allergic rhinitis, eosinophils, basophils, and T lymphocytes are prominent in biopsies of the nasal mucosa. The mechanisms of selective localization of inflammatory/effector cells to allergic tissue sites is currently under investigation: the chemokine receptors (CCR3 and CCR4) and their ligands—eotaxin monocyte derived chemokine (MDC) and thymocyte associated and released chemokine (TARC)—may be particularly important, thereby representing a potential target for therapy. Cytokines released predominantly from T lymphocytes—but also from mast cells, eosinophils and other cell types—are known to be critically important in allergic inflammation. The biological properties of Th2 cytokines are also consistent with their involvement in allergic rhinitis, and increases in cells expressing these cytokines have been detected in the nasal mucosa during the 'late' nasal responses that occur in sensitized subjects between 6 and 24 h following experimental nasal provocation with allergen. Allergen-immunotherapy has been shown to alter the Th2/Th1 balance in favour of Th1 responses, and a distinct population of antigen-specific regulatory T cells are also detectable following immunotherapy. These down-regulate Th2 responses directly by mechanisms involving cell–cell contact and by production of the inhibitory cytokines IL-10 and TGFβ (Fig. 18.6.2).

Clinical diagnosis

The diagnosis of allergic rhinitis is usually straightforward (Fig. 18.6.3), but the differential diagnosis should be considered in every case: frequently more than one cause coexists.

History

A careful history is essential both to establish the diagnosis of rhinitis and to assess the severity of symptoms. An allergic aetiology is suggested by dominant itching, sneezing, and watery nasal discharge. Associated eye or chest symptoms (asthma) also point to an allergic cause, and a history of potential allergic triggers should always be sought. However, in addition to provoking immediate nasal

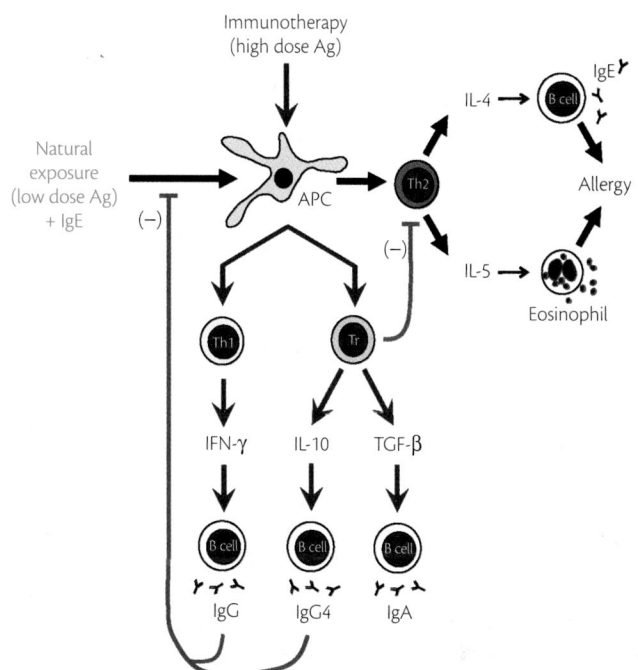

Fig. 18.6.2 Pathogenesis of allergic rhinitis and influence of treatment. Th2 cells are predominantly T lymphocytes, although mast cells, basophils, and eosinophils represent alternative sources of Th2-type cytokines. Topical corticosteroids down-regulate the production of Th2-type cytokines from T lymphocytes and other cells. Allergen immunotherapy acts by immune-deviation of Th2 responses in favour of Th1 responses and/or by inducing a population of antigen-specific T regulatory cells. Both mechanisms may act directly to down-regulate Th2 responses and indirectly by inducing 'protective' antibody responses. APC, antigen presenting cell; IFN, interferon; Ig, immunoglobulin; IL, interleukin; TGF, transforming growth factor; T_r, regulatory T cell.

symptoms, allergen may also cause late symptoms several hours after exposure, and these may not be recognized as being related.

A history of potential allergic triggers includes enquiry into the seasonality of symptoms and whether symptoms are work-related (i.e. do they occur at work or in the evening following work, with improvement at weekends and during holiday periods). The home environment, including the presence of domestic pets, birds, fitted carpets, central heating, and the use of blankets on beds should be established. A personal or family history of atopy is extremely common in patients with allergic rhinitis.

There are many alternative causes of rhinitic symptoms. It is common for there to be more than one cause, and important to consider the differential diagnosis (Box 18.6.1). The presence of facial pain, fever, systemic upset, and mucopurulent discharge suggests infection. Nasal obstruction, which alternates with the nasal cycle, is common to both allergic and infective causes. Nasal crusting and/or bleeding may occur in granulomatous disorders, atrophic rhinitis, or (rarely) tumours (particularly if associated with persistent unilateral symptoms). Impaired taste and/or smell may occur with many forms of rhinitis, but is particularly common with nasal polyposis and may occasionally follow trauma (olfactory nerve damage).

The presence of infertility and recurrent respiratory infections (including bronchiectasis) should raise the possibility of mucus abnormalities (Young's syndrome or cystic fibrosis) or ciliary dysfunction (primary ciliary dyskinesia, Kartagener's syndrome). Recurrent respiratory infections or a history of chronic rhinosinusitis should

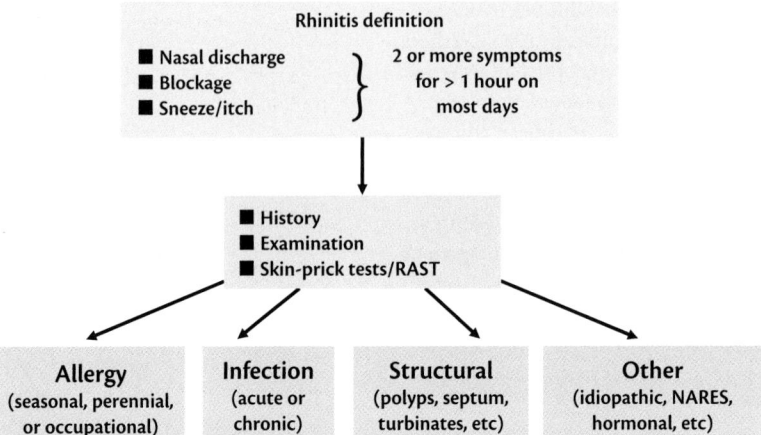

Fig. 18.6.3 Diagnostic approach to patients presenting with nasal symptoms. A careful history, clinical examination, and skin prick tests and/or measurement of serum allergen-specific IgE (RAST or ELISA) should be performed in every case. More than one cause may be present. 'Other' causes include hormonal (pregnancy, premenstrual), drugs (aspirin, β-blockers, ACE inhibitors, cocaine abuse, and atrophic, postsurgical, and ageing). Idiopathic rhinitis refers to nasal hyper-reactivity of unknown cause, manifest as an exaggerated response to nonspecific stimuli such as changes in temperature, tobacco smoke, domestic sprays, etc. The differential diagnosis includes vasculitis (Churg–Strauss syndrome), granulomatous conditions (Wegener's, sarcoidosis), atrophy (old age, surgical), and—rarely—tumours of the nose and paranasal sinuses.

also raise the possibility of immune deficiency disorders including hypogammaglobulinaemia and AIDS.

Hormonal imbalance (premenstrual symptoms, pregnancy, hypothyroidism, or acromegaly) may be associated with rhinitis. A history of trauma or previous nasal surgery should be sought.

Enquiry regarding associated chest disease is important. Rhinitis and asthma frequently coexist and recognition and appropriate treatment of rhinitis may improve asthma control. Similarly, allergic conjunctivitis may be particularly bothersome in patients with seasonal disease and requires recognition and treatment. The efficacy, frequency, and regularity of previous treatments should also be considered, as should the patient's perception of possible side effects of treatment, a frequently missed cause of poor compliance.

Examination

Local examination may be performed with a head mirror and speculum or an auroscope. Allergic rhinitis is accompanied by a pale bluish 'boggy' appearance of the nasal mucosa only if the patient has current symptoms. A red inflamed appearance with pus suggests an infective cause. A granular appearance with fine pale nodules is diagnostic of sarcoidosis. Enlarged turbinates may be confused with polyps by the unwary. If doubt exists, further examination with a rigid and/or flexible endoscope should be performed. The identification of structural abnormalities such as polyps, deflected nasal septum, or enlarged turbinates is important: surgical treatment may be indicated (a major advance being the development of minimally invasive endoscopic sinus surgery).

Examination of the nose should also include tests of smell and examination of the ears, eyes, mouth, and throat. Examination of the chest and a general examination should be performed when indicated in view of the common association of nasal disease with lower respiratory and systemic conditions.

Investigations

Skin prick tests

In the presence of a clear history, particularly of seasonal hay fever symptoms, skin prick testing is not essential. However, skin prick tests are useful for several reasons (Box 18.6.2). They should only be interpreted in conjunction with the clinical history, and not performed when the patient is taking antihistamines, if 'dermographism' (wealing in response to pressure) is present, or in the presence of severe eczema. In these circumstances measurement of

---

Box 18.6.1 Causes of rhinitis

◆ Allergic
  · Seasonal (tree or grass pollens)
  · Perennial (house dust mite, domestic pets)
  · Occupational (latex, laboratory animals, antibiotics, etc.)
◆ Nonallergic
  · Infective (acute, chronic)
  · Autonomic
  · Hormonal (premenstrual, pregnancy, hypothyroidism)
  · Drugs (aspirin, β-blockers)
  · Mucociliary abnormalities (Kartagener's, Young's syndromes)
  · Immunodeficiency syndromes (congenital and acquired, including HIV)
  · Atrophic
  · Idiopathic
◆ Differential diagnosis
  · Structural (polyps, deflected nasal septum, etc.)
  · Connective tissue disorders
  · Granulomatous disorders (sarcoid, Wegener's)
  · Tumours (benign, malignant)
  · Cerebrospinal fluid rhinorrhoea (secondary to trauma or surgery)

Box 18.6.2 Advantages of skin prick tests

- They diagnose atopy—the underlying predisposition to develop allergic disorders
- They provide helpful supportive evidence (positive or negative) for the clinical history
- They are essential when potentially expensive and time-consuming environmental control measures, the removal of a family pet, or a change of occupation are involved
- They have educational value, providing a clear illustration to the patient and reinforcing verbal advice

Box 18.6.3 Treatment of allergic rhinitis

- Allergen avoidance (house dust mite, animal danders, occupational causes)
- Nonsedative antihistamines, either alone or in combination with topical corticosteroids
- Topical corticosteroids; check technique and place emphasis on regular use even when symptoms are absent
- Sodium cromoglicate or nedocromil is useful for allergic eye symptoms
- Immunotherapy is helpful in pollen-sensitive patients unresponsive to the above measures
- If the patient fails to respond, review the diagnosis and treat any associated conditions (e.g. antibiotics for infection, surgery for structural problems)

serum IgE antibodies by radioallergosorbent test (RAST) or enzyme-linked immunosorbent assay (ELISA) is indicated.

A useful basic skin prick testing kit should include the following:

- a positive control (histamine 10 mg/ml)
- a negative control (allergen diluent solution)
- house dust mite (*D. pteronyssinus*)
- grass pollen
- cat fur
- *Aspergillus fumigatus*

Skin prick tests should be performed with a sterile 23-gauge needle or lancet, which is lightly inserted through the epidermis without inducing bleeding. Responses are recorded as the mean weal diameter at 15 min, a positive test being defined as a weal diameter 3 mm or more greater than that of the negative control test.

Treatment

Treatment for allergic rhinitis involves the avoidance of provoking allergens where possible and the use of topical corticosteroids and H_1 selective antihistamines. Allergen immunotherapy has a place in patients who do not respond to these measures. The approach is summarized in Box 18.6.3 and summarized in relation to the ARIA classification (Fig. 18.6.4), which emphasize that rhinitis and asthma are associated and that patients with one condition often also have the other.

Allergen avoidance

It is impossible to avoid pollens, although sensible advice includes wearing sunglasses and keeping car windows tightly shut. All windows should be kept closed, particularly in high buildings. Walking in parks and wide open spaces should be avoided, particularly during the late afternoon or evening when pollen counts are highest. A holiday by the sea or abroad during the peak pollen season may be helpful.

House dust mite control and avoidance measures should be considered in sensitive individuals with disease. Although some success has been achieved in children, the value of mite avoidance measures in adults, such as a single intervention with mite-proof bedding, has been questioned. Further studies involving more effective and multiple interventions are needed, including—in addition to covers for the pillow, duvet and mattress—restriction of soft toys, which should be washable, changing to hardwood, vinyl, or cork flooring,

and thorough vacuum cleaning and damp-dusting at least once weekly. There is no firm evidence to recommend the additional use of air conditioners, air ionizers, or acaricides.

Where animal exposure is relevant, there is frequent resistance to advice to remove a family pet. However, patients can be advised to avoid replacing animals, to confine them to the kitchen or outdoors where possible, and to avoid contact with them or with contaminated clothing.

Pharmacotherapy

The availability of potent specific histamine H_1 receptor antagonists with a low potential for anticholinergic side effects and a low sedative profile has been a major advance. Antihistamines are particularly effective for sneezing, itching, and rhinorrhoea, but unlike topical corticosteroids they have less effect on nasal blockage. They are also effective for eye and throat symptoms.

A rare but important complication of older antihistamines, including terfenadine and astemizole, is prolongation of the QT interval on the ECG. This only occurs when doses in excess of those recommended are employed, or in the presence of hepatic impairment or concomitant use of ketoconazole or erythromycin, both of which modify the hepatic metabolism of terfenadine. Modern antihistamines including acrivastine, loratadine, desloratidine, cetirizine, L-cetirizine, fexofenadine, and mizolastine are effective

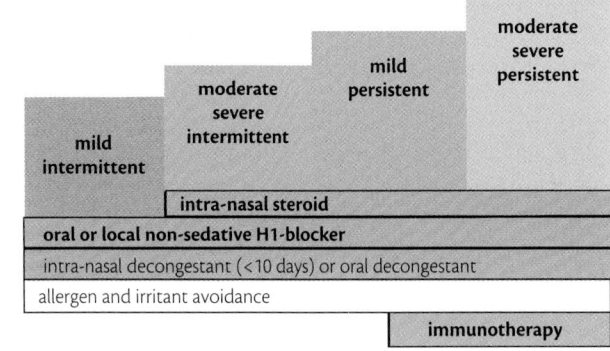

Fig. 18.6.4 A stepwise approach to management of allergic rhinitis. Classification of rhinitis according to ARIA guidelines.

H_1 antihistamines with an extremely low (or absent) potential for cardiac side effects. H_1-selective antihistamines can also be given as a topical nasal spray (levocabastine, azelastine). Antihistamines should be avoided when possible during pregnancy, particularly during the first trimester. If antihistamines are considered essential then recent guidelines from the United States Food and Drug Administration include the use of loratidine and cetirizine.

Topical corticosteroids are highly effective in most hay fever sufferers, with preparations including beclomethasone, budesonide, fluticasone, triamcinolone, and mometasone. Aqueous formulations are better tolerated and have a better local distribution in the nose. Treatment should begin before the hay fever season for maximal effect, and the importance of regular treatment, even when symptoms are absent, should be emphasized. Side effects are minor. Systemic effects are virtually absent at conventional doses, but caution should be exercised in children, particularly those receiving additional corticosteroids by other routes (e.g. for associated asthma and/or eczema).

The topical anticholinergic agent ipratropium bromide is a potent inhibitor of glandular secretion and may be effective where watery nasal discharge is the dominant symptom, uncontrolled by the measures described above.

Sodium cromogliycate is available as a topical nasal spray for use four times daily. It is less effective than topical corticosteroids. Topical cromoglicate eye drops are effective for allergic eye symptoms in most patients. Topical nedocromil sodium eye drops have the advantage of a longer duration of action, allowing twice daily administration.

In the few patients whose symptoms are not otherwise controlled, there is a place for a short course of prednisolone (20 mg daily for 5 days). This approach may unblock the nose, thereby improving access for topical corticosteroids, which may then be more effective.

Topical decongestants (oxymetazoline) are effective in treating nasal blockage, although they should only be used for short periods (no more than 2 weeks) in view of the risk of tachyphylaxis and rebound persistent nasal blockage (so-called rhinitis medicamentosa).

Allergen immunotherapy

Immunotherapy (desensitization) is an alternative treatment option in patients with severe summer hay fever unresponsive to topical corticosteroids and antihistamines, and in those reluctant to take long-term medication. This involves the subcutaneous injection of increasing concentrations of allergen (standardized pollen extract) at weekly intervals for 6 to 12 weeks, followed by monthly injections of a maintenance dose for 3 to 5 years. It should only be given by those who are properly trained, with adrenaline (epinephrine) and facilities for cardiopulmonary resuscitation immediately available, and patients should be kept under medical observation for at least 60 min following injections.

Recent controlled studies have confirmed the efficacy of immunotherapy, particularly for patients with summer hay fever induced by grass pollen. It is less effective in those with perennial rhinitis and asthma, where the disease is frequently heterogeneous with multiple allergic sensitivities and/or other causes of ongoing symptoms. The risk/benefit ratio is less favourable in patients with chronic bronchial asthma, in whom the risks of systemic adverse reactions are greater. Recent data suggests that pollen immunotherapy may confer long-term benefits including prolonged disease remission, prevention of onset of new sensitizations and—in one controlled trial—a threefold reduction in the risk of progression of rhinitis to asthma in children with pollen-induced rhinitis that persisted for 10 years after initiating treatment. The data suggest that allergen immunotherapy, unlike pharmacotherapy, has the potential to modify the course of the disease (see proposed mechanisms in Fig. 18.6.2).

Recent data support the sublingual route as an effective and safe form of immunotherapy suitable for home use, although the initial prescription and first dose should be administered by physicians trained in the diagnosis and treatment of allergic disorders. However, whether sublingual immunotherapy is as effective as the injection route or confers long-term benefits is not known. Recent studies suggest that daily use of grass pollen sublingual tablets may be as effective as the injection route and also confer long-term benefit.

Future prospects for immunotherapy include the use of adjuvants (lipopolysaccharide derivatives, bacterial CpG-containing DNA oligonucleotides) combined with conventional allergen extracts for subcutaneous immunotherapy, and the use of recombinant natural allergens and their mutated hypoallergenic variants. Low-molecular-weight allergen peptides have the potential to modify human T-cell responses with clinical benefit without the potential for IgE cross-linking and attendant risk of serious IgE-mediated side-effects. All of these approaches are currently at the stage of phase II–III clinical trials, their aim being to improve safety while preserving efficacy and long-term benefits.

Further reading

Durham SR (2008). Sublingual immunotherapy: what have we learnt from the 'Big Trials', *Curr Opin Allergy Clin Immunol*, **8**, 577–84.

Durham SR *et al.* (2010). Long-term clinical efficacy in grass pollen-induced rhinoconjunctivitis after treatment with SQ-standardized grass allergy immunotherapy tablet. *J Allergy Clin Immunol*, (in press).

James LK, Durham SR. (2008). Update on mechanisms of allergen injection immunotherapy, *Clin Exp Allergy*, **38**, 1074–88.

Till SJ, *et al.* (2004). Mechanisms of immunotherapy. *J Allergy Clin Immunol*, **113**, 1025–34.

18.7

Asthma

A.J. Newman Taylor and Paul Cullinan

Essentials

Asthma is a chronic inflammatory disease of the bronchial airways that is characterized pathologically by a desquamative eosinophilic bronchitis and clinically by reversible airway narrowing and increased airway responsiveness to nonspecific provocative stimuli. The condition is common, frequently disabling, and can cause death. In the Western world it now affects more than 10% of children and more than 5% of adults, and in England and Wales it is the cause of more than 100 000 hospital admissions and is the certified cause of death of 1500 to 2000 people each year.

Asthma triggers

The risk of developing asthma is increased in atopic individuals, and in asthmatics natural allergen exposure induces asthma and airway hyper-responsiveness. Viral infections, most commonly with rhinoviruses, cause 80 to 85% of exacerbations of asthma in children and 50 to 75% in adults.

Occupational asthma—agents inhaled at work can be the primary cause (induce) or can exacerbate (provoke) asthma. Such occupational asthma may be due to inhalation of irritant chemicals ('irritant induced asthma') or substances that induce an allergic reaction ('hypersensitivity induced asthma').

Drugs—some can exacerbate asthma, with β-blockers and nonsteroidal anti-inflammatory drugs (NSAIDs) being the most important.

Clinical features

History—symptoms are nonspecific, typically shortness of breath, wheezing, chest tightness and cough. They are usually variable in severity over short periods of time, but can be persistent, and are typically worse at night. Because occupational causes are potentially avoidable, all cases of asthma that have occurred or recurred in adult life should be questioned about symptomatic improvement when away from work, and, if present, enquiry made about potential causes of asthma in the workplace.

Clinical examination—outside the context of an acute exacerbation (see below), the physical signs of mild or moderate asthma may be limited to expiratory wheezes audible over the lungs. Because of the variable nature of airway narrowing some patients have normal lung sounds, but this would not be expected in those with persistent symptomatic asthma.

Diagnosis

Asthma needs to be differentiated from localized airways obstruction, other causes of generalized airways obstruction, and other causes of intermittent breathlessness.

Demonstration of airflow limitation—asthma is most typically diagnosed by the demonstration that this varies spontaneously over short periods of time, or improves after inhalation of a short acting β-agonist or, over a more prolonged period of time, use of a corticosteroid either by inhalation or by mouth. The most clinically useful measurements of airflow limitation are (1) forced expiratory volume in 1 s (FEV_1), which may be expressed as a proportion of the forced vital capacity (FVC) as $FEV_1/FVC\%$, and (2) peak expiratory flow rate (PEF).

Occupational asthma—(1) in irritant-induced asthma the association of the onset of asthma with inhalation of a toxic chemical is usually clear; (2) in hypersensitivity-induced asthma the diagnosis depends on (a) exposure to a sensitizing agent at work; (b) a characteristic history of onset of asthma after an initial symptom-free period of exposure, with deterioration in symptoms during periods at work and improvements during absence from work; and (c) the results of objective investigations—lung function tests, immunological tests, and inhalation tests.

Classification—patients with asthma can be categorized, at any one time, by whether their symptoms are intermittent or persistent, and by the severity of their symptoms and underlying airway narrowing (measured by lung function tests).

Management—general aims

The aims of treating patients with intermittent or persistent asthma are to: (1) educate the patient about their disease and the objectives of its management; (2) minimize or eliminate asthma symptoms; (3) achieve best possible lung function and prevent an accelerated decline in lung function; (4) prevent exacerbations of asthma; (5) achieve these objectives with fewest drugs, keeping short-term and long-term adverse effects to a minimum.

The objectives for effective asthma control in individual patients are to: (1) allow normal daytime activities as well as the ability to enjoy physically demanding activities; (2) permit sleeping through night, without being awoken by respiratory symptoms; (3) achieve a situation where use of 'rescue' medication with inhaled β_2 agonists is needed less than once per day; (4) achieve normal or near normal PEF and FEV_1 with less than 20% variability between best and worst values; (5) to avoid drug side effects.

The 'stepped' approach to treatment

Education—there is clear evidence that patient education to enable adults to manage their asthma can reduce the frequency of unscheduled visits to general practitioners, hospital admissions, and time off work. The four important components of effective patient education are (1) information, (2) self-monitoring, (3) regular medical review, and (4) having a written action plan.

Avoidance of precipitants—the identification and, where feasible, the avoidance of relevant allergens at home or at work is an essential part of the management of asthma.

A 'stepped' approach to treatment is the basis of current guidelines for asthma management:

Step 1—mild intermittent asthma controlled by the use of an inhaled shorter-acting β_2-agonist (e.g. salbutamol or terbutaline) less than once a day. Requirement for more regular treatment implies the need for regular anti-inflammatory treatment (i.e. a higher step).

Step 2—mild persistent or intermittent asthma that is of sufficient frequency to require regular anti-inflammatory treatment. Treatment with an inhaled corticosteroid should be started at a dose of beclometasone 400 µg twice daily (or equivalent) in adults and continued for at least 3 months, before reducing the dose to the minimum required to maintain good control. Short-acting β_2-agonists are used as required for symptomatic relief.

Step 3—moderate persistent asthma that is not controlled by Step 1 and Step 2. The treatment of choice is the addition of a long-acting β_2-agonist. If it provides benefit but asthma remains inadequately controlled, the dose of inhaled corticosteroid should be doubled. If it provides no benefit it should be discontinued and the inhaled steroid dose doubled, and if this does not provide adequate control a trial of other treatments such as a slow-release theophylline or leukotriene antagonist should be instituted.

Step 4—asthma control remains poor despite the measures recommended in Step 3. Consideration should be given to further increasing the dose of the inhaled corticosteroid to the equivalent of beclometasone 2000 µg/day or to the addition of a fourth drug, e.g. slow-release theophylline, a leukotriene antagonist, or an oral β_2-agonist.

Step 5—failure to respond to combinations of Step 4 treatments requires the addition of an oral corticosteroid while continuing high-dose inhaled corticosteroid treatment.

Acute exacerbations of asthma

Asthma exacerbations are episodes of progressively worsening airway narrowing that can vary in severity from those that patients are able to manage themselves by following an agreed treatment plan, to severe attacks which at their most dramatic develop rapidly and become life threatening within minutes or hours.

Fatal or near fatal attacks—these are associated with (1) patients who have previously required hospital admission for severe asthma and who require regular oral steroid treatment; (2) failure to recognize severity of asthma by the patient; (3) failure to recognize the severity of asthma by the doctor; (4) undertreatment or inappropriate treatment, with failure to use oral corticosteroids in adequate doses early in an exacerbation probably being the single commonest remediable factor.

Clinical features—in acute severe asthma the patient is usually extremely short of breath, sitting up or leaning forward to use their accessory muscles of respiration, with impaired speech and increasingly prolonged expiration alternating with short inspiratory gasps. Tachycardia and pulsus paradoxus are often found. Airway narrowing may become sufficiently severe for no wheeze to be audible and gas exchange sufficiently impaired to cause detectable cyanosis, when the patient will be distressed, anxious, apprehensive and confused. Exhaustion ultimately leads to inadequate ventilation and a rising PCO_2, the two cardinal features that indicate the need for transfer to an intensive care unit in the event that assisted ventilation is required. A value of PEF of less than 50% of predicted or of the recent best value in an adult aged less than 50 years usually indicates severe asthma; a value of less than 33% indicates a potentially life-threatening attack.

Management—initial treatment of a severe attack of asthma should be with (1) oxygen (60% FiO_2); (2) β_2-agonist—nebulized salbutamol 2.5 to 5 mg or terbutaline 5 to 10 mg driven by oxygen; (3) steroid—oral prednisolone 30 to 60 mg or intravenous hydrocortisone 200 mg. If there is a poor response to initial treatment after 15 to 30 min, then (1) continue oxygen; (2) repeat nebulized salbutamol 5 mg after 15 min; (3) add ipatropium 0.5 mg to nebulized β_2-agonist; (4) give intravenous hydrocortisone 200 mg 4 hourly; (5) consider intravenous magnesium sulphate 1.2 to 2 g over 20 min.

Investigations—chest radiograph to exclude pneumothorax; arterial blood gases to assess oxygenation and ventilation; monitor serum K^+ (risk of hypokalaemia with high-dose β_2-agonist).

The patient *in extremis*—indications for transfer to intensive care and for consideration of intermittent positive-pressure ventilation (IPPV) are (1) hypoxia (PaO_2 <8 kPa) despite FiO_2 60%; (2) hypercapnoea ($PaCO_2$ > 6 kPa); (3) exhaustion with feeble respiration; (4) confusion or drowsiness; (5) unconsciousness; (6) respiratory arrest.

Introduction

Asthma is a chronic inflammatory disease of the bronchial airways that is characterized by a desquamative eosinophilic bronchitis (Fig. 18.7.1). The defining clinical characteristics of asthma—reversible airway narrowing and increased airway responsiveness to nonspecific provocative stimuli—are associated with an underlying chronic inflammatory process. Definitions of asthma which have focused on these clinical characteristics to distinguish it from diseases associated with predominantly irreversible airway narrowing have emphasized the intermittent nature of asthma rather than the persistence of the underlying inflammation, with potentially inappropriate implications for treatment.

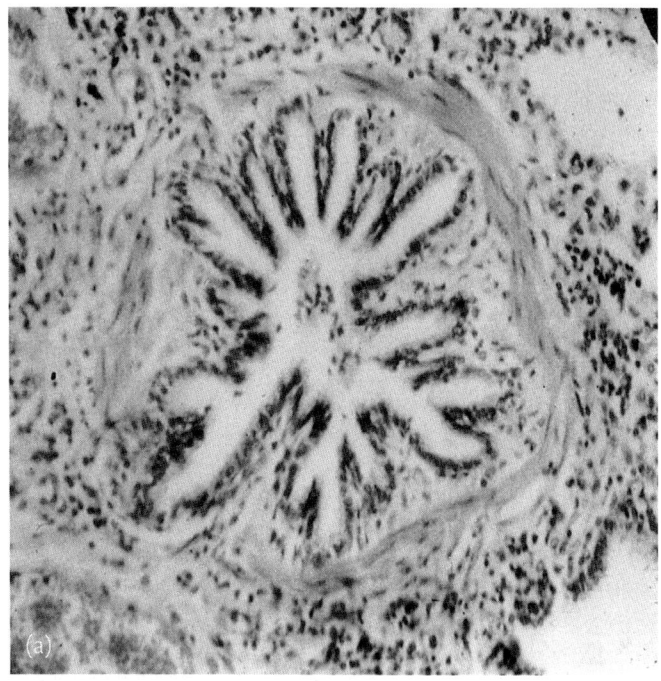

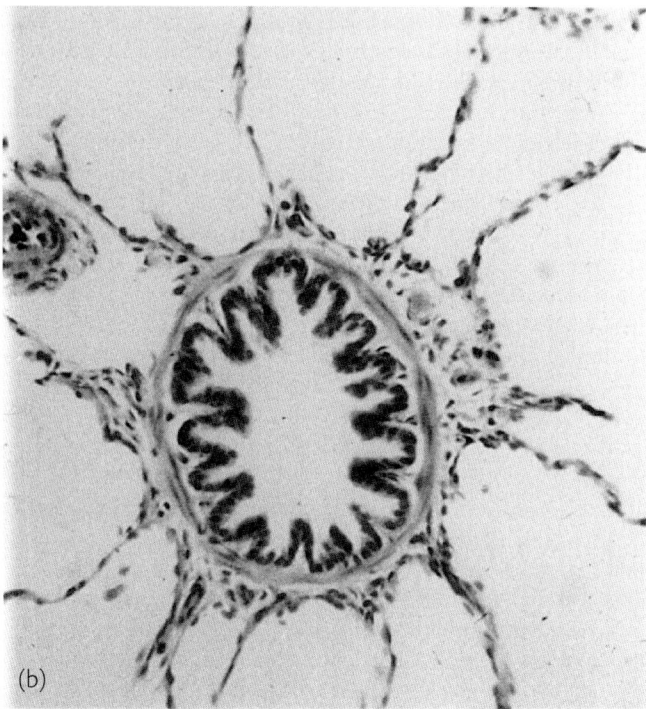

Fig. 18.7.1 The defining pathology of asthma: desquamative eosinophilic bronchitis (a) in comparison with normal histological appearances (b).

Pathophysiology

Airway hyper-responsiveness: inducers and provokers

The distinguishing abnormalities of lung function in bronchial asthma are (1) reversible airway narrowing, and (2) airway hyper-responsiveness to nonspecific provocative stimuli.

Airway responsiveness describes the ease with which acute airway narrowing can be provoked by a variety of stimuli. Nonspecific provocative stimuli include exercise, inhalation of cold dry air, inhaled respiratory irritants such as sulphur dioxide, and pharmacological agents such as histamine and methacholine (Table 18.7.1). Provocation of asthma by specific allergens can induce airway hyper-responsiveness to nonspecific stimuli. Patients with hyper-responsive airways require smaller doses of such stimuli to provoke acute airway narrowing. Inhaled nonspecific provocative stimuli such as histamine or methacholine incite airway narrowing that usually resolves within minutes; exercise provokes asthma within minutes which resolves within 1 h.

The degree of airway responsiveness can be expressed as the dose or concentration of the stimulus which provokes a specified fall in forced expiratory volume in 1 s (FEV_1)—commonly the dose or concentration of histamine or methacholine which provokes a 20% fall in FEV_1—PD_{20} or PC_{20}, histamine or methacholine.

Whereas provokers of asthma incite acute airway narrowing in individuals with hyper-responsive airways, inducers of asthma increase the magnitude of airway hyper-responsiveness and the clinical manifestations of asthma by increasing the severity of the underlying airway inflammation which can persist for days or weeks. The principal inducers of asthma are inhaled allergens, viral respiratory tract infections, and low-molecular-weight chemicals encountered at work (see Table 18.7.1).

Allergen inhalation tests are a good model of the airway response to an inducer and demonstrate the inter-relationship between airway inflammation, airway narrowing and airway hyper-responsiveness. Inhalation of an allergen by an individual allergic to it with asthma will provoke:

- an immediate fall in FEV_1 that develops within minutes and usually resolves spontaneously within 1 to 1.5 h

- a subsequent late fall in FEV_1 that develops in about 50% of cases 2 to 4 h or more after the inhalation test and persists for several hours, on occasions for days

Table 18.7.1 Inducers and provokers of asthma

Inducers of asthma		
Allergens		Increased airway inflammation
Viral respiratory tract infections	→	Increased airway responsiveness
Low molecular weight chemicals		Increased severity of asthma
Provokers of asthma		
Exercise		
Cold dry air		
Respiratory irritants (e.g. sulphur dioxide)	→	Acute transient airway narrowing in individuals with hyperresponsive airways
Histamine		
Methacholine		

The recognition that asthma is a chronic inflammatory disease implies that, in addition to identifying and avoiding inducing causes, such as domestic pets and occupational sensitizers, disease control is likely also to require long-term anti-inflammatory treatment. Appreciation of the inflammatory nature of asthma has also led to recognition of the associated injury and damage to the airway wall—airway remodelling—which may lead to irreversible loss of function.

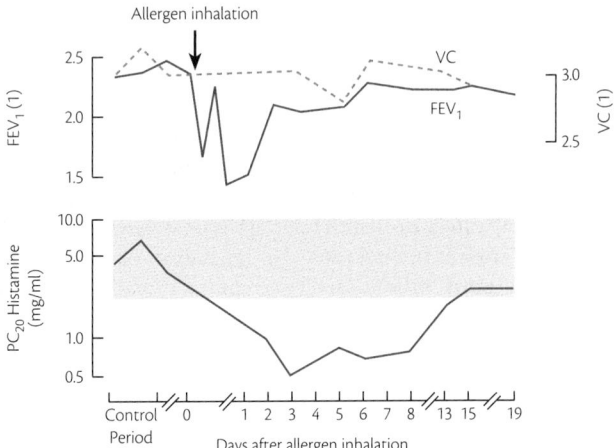

Fig. 18.7.2 Increased airway responsiveness associated with late asthmatic reaction provoked by inhalation of ragweed pollen.

◆ an increase in airway responsiveness, usually associated with the late fall in FEV_1, which is frequently of longer duration than the late FEV_1 fall

The immediate fall in FEV_1 is IgE dependent and due to airway smooth muscle contraction and airway wall oedema provoked by mediators, such as histamine, released from mast cells resident in the airways. It is not associated with an increase in airway responsiveness. The late fall in FEV_1 is the outcome of recruitment to the airways of inflammatory cells, particularly Th2 lymphocytes and eosinophils, reducing airway calibre. It is associated with an increase in airway responsiveness (manifest as a reduction in PC_{20}) which can persist, with associated increased diurnal variation in airway calibre, for several days after resolution of airway narrowing (Fig. 18.7.2).

Airway inflammation

Because asthma is an inflammatory disease of the airways, markers of airway inflammation have been sought both for diagnostic purposes and as a guide to the effectiveness of treatment. Two particular indices have been investigated: sputum eosinophil count and exhaled nitric oxide (NO) concentration. An increase in sputum eosinophil count (>2% or >3% total cell count in sputum) is an indicator of reversible airway narrowing and is associated with corticosteroid responsiveness. Management of asthma with the additional intention of decreasing sputum eosinophil counts to normal has been shown to reduce the frequency of asthma exacerbations. In addition, some patients may present with cough and sputum, without evidence of reversible airway narrowing, with an increased eosinophil count in sputum, responsive to inhaled corticosteroids—chronic eosinophilic bronchitis.

NO concentration in exhaled breath (F_ENO) is increased in patients with asthma, correlates with sputum eosinophilia, particularly in steroid-naive patients, and is reduced by treatment with inhaled corticosteroids. Unfortunately the range of F_ENO in the normal population overlaps with the range in patients with asthma, and F_ENO is a less good discriminator between normals and asthmatics than sputum eosinophilia. In one population-based study F_ENO greater than 50 ppb was a specific (96% specificity) but insensitive (20% sensitivity) test for asthma, and to date F_ENO has proved less successful than sputum eosinophilia as a biomarker to monitor the severity of asthma and its response to treatment.

Asthma triggers

Atopy and allergy

Atopy is defined as the production of specific IgE antibody to common inhalant allergens, such as grass pollen, house dust mite, and cat. Atopy may be identified by the presence of immediate skin prick test responses (or of specific IgE in serum) to extracts of common inhalant allergens and has a prevalence of some 40% in the adult population of the United Kingdom.

The risk of developing asthma as well as eczema and hay fever is increased in atopic individuals. In a random population sample in the south-western United States of America a close relationship was found at all ages between skin test responses to local inhalant allergens and the prevalence of asthma and allergic rhinitis. Similarly, in Canadian university students the prevalence of airway hyper-responsiveness to inhaled histamine correlated significantly with the degree of atopy.

In asthmatics, natural allergen exposure induces asthma and airway hyper-responsiveness. In a study of hospital admissions during seven years in Canadian cities, admission rates correlated with increases in levels of aeroallergens, including grasses, trees, weeds, and moulds, with an interaction with ozone levels. Both the severity of asthma and airway responsiveness are increased in asthmatic patients allergic to ragweed pollen during the season. Similarly, avoidance of relevant allergen exposure is associated with an improvement or resolution of asthmatic symptoms, improved lung function, and decreased airway responsiveness. Patients with asthma allergic to house dust mite have shown considerable symptomatic and objective improvement when avoiding house dust mite for several months at altitude in Davos in the Swiss Alps, also for several weeks in a London hospital. In the south-eastern United States of America asthma deaths in patients allergic to the mould *Alternaria alternata* increased during the months of the year when alternaria spore counts were highest.

Although there is clear evidence that in asthmatics natural exposure to allergens to which they are allergic can provoke asthma (and avoidance can improve it), the influence of allergen exposure on the development of asthma is less clear. Studies comparing populations born and living in different environments and climates, and therefore exposed to different allergens in childhood, demonstrate allergy and associated disease in relation to allergens present in the particular environment. For example, children born and living in Marseilles, on the Mediterranean coast of France (humid and at sea level, encouraging the growth of house dust mite) were compared with those in Briançon, the highest town in the French Alps (not conducive to the growth of house dust mite, but encouraging to the growth of many wind-pollinated plants). Allergy to house dust mite was found to be considerably more prevalent in Marseilles than in Briançon, whereas allergy to pollens was considerably more prevalent in Briançon than Marseilles. The prevalence of asthma was similar in both environments, although the associated allergies differed. The introduction of a new allergen into an environment can cause the development of allergy and asthma, particularly among adults. Unloading soya beans in Barcelona harbour caused 'epidemic days', when the number of hospital admissions with asthma increased several fold. The 'epidemic days' continued for 7 years before the cause was identified. Filters placed on the silos to prevent the release and dissemination of soya bean during unloading resolved the problem.

Respiratory virus infections

Acute exacerbations of asthma, commonly recognized as an increase in respiratory symptoms of sufficient severity for a patient to seek medical attention, are major causes of ill health, death, and costs, accounting for some 50% of total asthma related costs. Respiratory virus infections have long been suspected to be the major cause of exacerbations of asthma, but it is only with the development and use of the polymerase chain reaction (PCR) in controlled studies that the true proportion of virus-induced asthma exacerbations, in both children and adults, has become clear. There is now consistent evidence that 80 to 85% of exacerbations of asthma in children and 50 to 75% of exacerbations in adults are caused by viral infections, of which the great majority are attributable to rhinoviruses. Exacerbations of asthma provoked by respiratory infections are often severe, can be prolonged, and are associated with increased airway responsiveness. Peak flow measurements in schoolchildren have been shown to remain abnormal for several weeks after a respiratory tract infection.

In schoolchildren the peaks of respiratory infections and asthma admissions both occur at the start of the school year. In Canada hospital admissions for asthma in school-age children during a 13-year period consistently peaked in September during the third week after return to school after the summer vacation. Similar but lower peaks in preschool children and adults followed on average 2 and 6 days after the peak for schoolage children, suggesting these acted as the vectors of transmission to their families. Aeroallergen levels are also high in Canada during the summer months and in September during the weeks following return to school and during the peak period for asthma admissions to hospital.

A number of studies have suggested that asthma exacerbations occur particularly in atopic children infected with rhinovirus concurrently exposed to relevant allergens. In one study in the United Kingdom of children aged between 3 and 17 years the risk of admission to hospital with asthma was markedly increased in children with detectable virus infection with allergen-specific IgE and heavily exposed to the sensitizing allergen, as compared to age- and sex-matched children with stable asthma or admitted to hospital with nonrespiratory disease. Virus infection, allergen, or sensitization alone, were not associated with increased risk in this study. In another study in the United States of America of children aged between 2 and 16 years, the strongest risk factors for wheezing requiring emergency care were RT-PCR evidence of rhinovirus together with atopy or eosinophilic inflammation in nasal secretions. These observations demonstrate the importance of viral infection, particularly rhinovirus infection, in exacerbations of asthma in children and adults. In addition, in children at least, virus-induced exacerbations of asthma occur particularly in the context of exposure to a relevant allergen and eosinophilic inflammation.

Recent studies have found evidence of impaired innate immunity in airway epithelial cells in patients with asthma: interferon production is deficient, and the magnitude of deficiency is related to the severity of asthma exacerbations. There is also evidence that infection with *Chlamydia pneumoniae* may play a role in asthma exacerbations, with one study showing a reduction in the severity and duration of asthma exacerbations in a randomized controlled trial in those treated with the antibiotic telithromycin as compared to placebo.

Occupation

Agents inhaled at work can be the primary cause (induce) or can exacerbate (provoke) asthma. Asthma whose primary cause is an agent inhaled at work is called 'occupational asthma' to distinguish it from 'work-exacerbated' asthma. Occupational asthma can be (1) 'irritant-induced asthma', caused by the inhalation of an irritant chemical in toxic concentrations, also known less felicitously as reactive airways dysfunction syndrome (RADS), or (2) 'hypersensitivity-induced asthma', the outcome of an acquired hypersensitivity (allergic) reaction to an inhaled protein or chemical. Irritant-induced occupational asthma can follow the inhalation, in sufficient concentration, of a toxic soluble chemical such as sulphur dioxide, chlorine, or ammonia. The number of described causes of hypersensitivity-induced occupational asthma is now legion, but a relatively small number cause most cases. These include chemical sensitizers such as isocyanates, complex platinum salts, and colophony fume, and proteins such as flour, enzymes used in baking and detergent manufacture, latex. and laboratory animal urine proteins (Table 18.7.2).

It is estimated from a national reporting scheme that in the United Kingdom some 2500 new cases of occupational asthma occur each year. An American Thoracic Society systematic review found that 15% of new or relapsed cases of asthma in adult life are attributable to an occupational exposure, suggesting that about 1 in 7 cases of new or relapsed asthma in adult life are potentially preventable.

Work can exacerbate asthma in several different ways, usually as a consequence of airway hyper-responsiveness, e.g. exposure to irritant chemicals such as sulphur dioxide or dust particles, inhalation of cold air in refrigerators or outdoors, or exertion, particularly in an irritant environment. One-third of patients with asthma report worsening of their symptoms at work.

Drugs

Relatively few drugs exacerbate asthma, β-blockers and nonsteroidal anti-inflammatory drugs (NSAIDs) being the most important. Although ACE inhibitors may cause cough, and occasionally rhinitis and angio-oedema, they have not been associated with the provocation of asthma and are therefore not contraindicated in asthma.

β-Blockers

Precipitation or worsening of asthma was first reported with propanolol, but subsequently found to occur with all nonselective β-adrenoceptor antagonists. This reaction to β-blockers implies adrenergic bronchodilator tone in asthmatic airways. The severity of the airway narrowing provoked by β-blockers is not predictable, nor is it closely related to the severity of airway hyper-responsiveness. The dose provoking asthma can be low: severe asthma can be precipitated by timolol eye drops, a nonselective β-blocker used to treat glaucoma. Selective $β_1$-antagonists, such as atenolol, acebutalol, and metoprolol, provoke less severe reactions than nonselective β-blockers such as propanolol.

Although the fall in lung function provoked by a β-blocker can be reversed by an inhaled $β_2$-agonist, patients with asthma should avoid β-blockers—including $β_1$-selective antagonists—because of the unpredictable and potentially serious consequences of a severe asthmatic reaction, and alternative drugs should be used for treatment of hypertension and angina.

Table 18.7.2 Selected causes of hypersensitivity-induced occupational asthma by occupational group: high- and low-molecular-mass agents

Occupation	Agent(s)
High molecular mass	
Baking and milling	Flour (wheat, barley, rye, oat, soya), fungal α-amylase, egg proteins, milk proteins, storage mites
Research science, animal handling, laboratory work	Small animal proteins (urine, dander, serum): rats, mice, guinea-pigs, ferrets etc. insect proteins: cockroach, locust, housefly, fruit fly, gypsy moth, mealworm etc. other animal proteins: latex
'Biological' detergent powder manufacture	Detergent enzymes (protease, amylase, lipase, cellulase)
Food processing (nonbaking/milling)	Linseed, green coffee bean, castor bean, tea dust, tobacco leaf, rosehip, shellfish proteins, fish proteins, milk proteins, egg proteins, cocoa proteins, proteolytic enzymes
Nursing, dentistry, other health care work	Latex
Farming and other agriculture	Storage mites, mealworms, spider mite, poultry mite, cow dander, cow β-lactoglobulin, pig urine, mink urine, insect larvae, poultry feathers, honeybee dust, silkworm larvae, fruit, vegetable and flower pollens, fungi, grain dust, spider mite, vine weevil
Floristry, botany	Pollens, *Ficus elastica*, gypsophila
Low molecular mass	
Spray painting	Hexamethylene diisocyanate, toluene diisocyanate, dimethylethanolamine, other amines
Welding, soldering, electronic assembly	Colophony fume, stainless steel welding fume, aminoethylethanolamine, cyanoacrylates, toluene diisocyanate, persulphate salts
Woodwork	Hardwood dusts (western red cedar, iroko, aprican maple, mahogany, mansonia, obeche, etc.)
Chemical processing	Azodicarbonamide, phthalic anhydride, trimellitic anhydride, maleic anhydride, hexavalent chromium
Plastics manufacture and processing	Diphenylmethane diisocyanate, toluene diisocyanate, monomer acrylates, various amines
Food processing (nonbaking/milling)	Chloramine-t, metabisulphite
Hairdressing	Persulphate salts, henna
Textile/fabric work	Reactive dyes, gum acacia
pharmaceutical manufacture, pharmacy	Psyllium, ispaghula, methyldopa, penicillins, cephalosporins, tetracycline, sulphathiazole, spiramycin, isoniazid, piperazine, cimetidine, dichloramine, ipecacuanha, bromelain, morphine and other opiates
Nursing, dentistry, other health care work	Glutaraldehyde, formaldehyde, monomer acrylates, antibiotics, psyllium, hexachlorophene, pancreatic extracts, N-acetylcysteine
Metal refining	Complex platinum salts, hexavalent chromium, nickel, vanadium, furfuryl alcohol

Aspirin and nonsteroidal inflammatory drugs (NSAIDs)

Aspirin and other NSAIDs, which inhibit cyclooxygenase 1 (COX1), can provoke severe attacks of asthma in some 10% of adults with asthma, more frequently in women than men. Aspirin-induced asthma (AIA) may be part of a well-recognized association of aspirin intolerance, asthma, and rhinitis with nasal polyps (Samter's triad) that is characterized by severe mucosal eosinophilic inflammation of the nose and airways. The onset is usually in the third or fourth decade, with chronic nasal congestion, discharge, and nasal polypi. Subsequently asthma and AIA develop, when ingestion of aspirin or an NSAID typically provokes acute severe asthma within 1 h, accompanied by profuse nasal discharge, periorbital oedema, conjunctival injection, in some cases with flushing of the head and neck and, on occasions, vomiting and diarrhoea. AIA can provoke life-threatening asthma resistant to bronchodilators: in one survey, 25% of 145 patients requiring mechanical ventilation for acute severe asthma had AIA.

Despite avoidance of aspirin and NSAIDs, severe asthma and rhinitis with nasal polyps usually persist, associated with raised blood eosinophil count and intense eosinophil infiltration of the nasal and airway mucosa. The most plausible explanation of AIA is that it occurs as a consequence of specific inhibition in respiratory cells of intracellular COX enzymes. NSAIDs with anti-COX activity provoke asthma in patients with AIA; NSAIDs which do not inhibit COX activity do not provoke asthma; the potency of NSAIDs to inhibit COX correlates with their ability to provoke

asthma in AIA individuals; and cross-tolerance to NSAIDs that inhibit COX occurs after desensitization to aspirin. Cross-tolerance involving such chemically distinct moieties argues strongly against AIA being an immunological reaction.

The intense tissue eosinophilia associated with AIA is accompanied by overproduction of cysteinylleukotrienes, which are important mediators of nasal inflammation and asthma. These are continuously synthesized in AIA patients, even in the absence of aspirin ingestion, are released into nasal and bronchial secretions, and can be collected in urine, and COX inhibition is associated with their release. Aspirin provoked nasal and asthmatic reactions are attenuated by leukotriene antagonists, both cysteinyl leukotriene receptor antagonists (zafirlukast, montelukast, and pranlukast) and 5-lipoxygenase inhibitors (zileuton).

Patients with AIA should avoid all aspirin-containing products and other analgesics or anti-inflammatories that inhibit COX (Table 18.7.3). Patients with AIA can usually, although not always, take paracetamol. Selective inhibitors of COX-2, celecoxib and rofecoxib, while potentially safe in AIA are associated with an increased frequency of cardiovascular events, and rofecoxib has been withdrawn.

Tolerance to aspirin and NSAIDs can be induced in patients with AIA by the ingestion of increasing doses of aspirin over 2 to 3 days, until 400 to 650 mg aspirin can be tolerated. Daily doses of between 80 and 325 mg aspirin can maintain tolerance, allowing aspirin and other COX inhibitors to be taken safely. A dose of aspirin of

Table 18.7.3 NSAIDs that cross-react with aspirin in respiratory reactions

Type of COX inhibitor	NSAID
Inhibitors of both COX-1 and COX-2[a]	Piroxicam
	Indomethacin
	Sulindac
	Tolmetin
	Ibuprofen
	Naproxen
	Naproxen sodium
	Fenoprofen
	Meclofenamate
	Mefenamic acid
	Flurbiprofen
	Difluniusal
	Ketoprofen
	Diclofenac
	Ketoralac
	Etodolac
	Nabumetone
Poor inhibitors of COX-1 and COX-2[b]	Oxaprozin
	Paracetamol (acetaminophen)
	Salsalate
Selective inhibitors of COX-2[c]	Celecoxib
	Rifecoxib (now withdrawn)

[a] On first exposure to the drug, cross-reactions with low provoking doses.
[b] A small percentage of patients with AIA cross- react with high dose of these drugs
[c] In theory should not cross-react.

650 mg twice daily can provide improvement in asthma and particularly in nasal inflammation. One report has suggested that regular aspirin treatment after sinus surgery for polypectomy may delay recurrence of nasal polyps, on average by 6 years. However, aspirin desensitization requires daily maintenance of high-dose aspirin that may not be well tolerated. Furthermore, omission of aspirin for 2 to 3 days can result in complete loss of tolerance, in which case the initial desensitization protocol needs to be repeated. It is also not clear whether aspirin desensitization has the potential to modify the long-term course of asthma. For these reasons, aspirin desensitization has not been widely adopted.

Prevalence

Asthma is a common disease. It is frequently disabling, and—uncommonly—can cause death. In the Western world it now has an estimated prevalence of more than 10% in children and more than 5% in adults. It is the cause of more than 100 000 hospital admissions and is the certified cause of death of some 1500 to 2000 people in England and Wales each year.

The prevalence of asthma has markedly increased in the Western world, most obviously but not exclusively in children. Studies of disease frequency in the last half of the 20th century suggest a doubling

in asthma prevalence in developed nations every 15 years. More recent evidence suggests that in some countries the increase in both children and adults has slowed or plateaued. There have been similar trends in the prevalence of specific IgE sensitization to common aeroallergens. Although in part changes in prevalence may reflect a greater awareness of and tendency to diagnose asthma, repeat cross-sectional studies of children in the United Kingdom, using identical methods of ascertainment at different time points, have shown a definite increase. A study of Aberdeen schoolchildren found the prevalence of wheeze and of diagnosed asthma had increased 2.5-fold in the 25 years between 1964 and 1989. A similar study in South Wales at two time points 15 years apart found a history of reported asthma to have doubled from 6 to 12%, and also reported similar increases of reported hay fever and eczema and of the proportion of children in whom exercise provoked asthma. A third study of the same population in 1998 found a further increase in asthma symptoms but a decrease in exercise-provoked bronchoconstriction, possibly reflecting more frequent use of effective treatments by asthmatic children.

Comparison of the prevalence of asthma in different parts of the world suggests that the high prevalence in the Western world is associated with urbanization and material prosperity, and comparisons between countries are reflected in comparisons within countries. A study of school children in Zimbabwe found asthma to be uncommon in those living in a rural area, more common in poor urban dwellers, and most common in the affluent urban dwellers, equally in black and white, in Harare. In Europe the reunification of Germany allowed comparison of the prevalence of asthma and associated conditions in cities in former East and West Germany. The prevalence of asthma, hay fever, eczema, and atopy (identified as immediate skin test responses to common inhalant allergens) was greater in school-age children living in the West German city of Munich than in the East German cities of Leipzig and Halle. Interestingly, the prevalence of atopy (particularly skin test responses to pollens) and hay fever, but not asthma, subsequently increased in children living in reunified Germany who had lived the first 5 years of their lives in Leipzig. Other intranational studies of European populations suggest stark differences in disease prevalence between urban and rural communities, even where these are geographically close.

Many explanations have been advanced to explain these observations. These include increased indoor allergen exposure (particularly house dust mite and cat), increased exposure to vehicle exhaust pollution, increased tobacco smoking by women of childbearing age, changing diet, and reduced infection rates in childhood. Of these, outdoor air pollution has until recently grabbed most public attention, although there is no substantive evidence in its support: the prevalence of asthma in urban parts of the United Kingdom is no greater (and possibly less) than in rural parts, including Skye, where measured levels of air pollutants are the lowest in United Kingdom. Similarly, there is little evidence that the increased prevalence of asthma and other atopic disease has been caused by increased indoor allergen exposure or tobacco smoking, although the increase in asthma has been paralleled by an increase in cigarette smoking by women of childbearing age. Several dietary explanations have also been advanced, including increased salt and reduced antioxidant intake.

The most plausible explanation for increased prevalence of atopy and asthma advanced to date is that it is a consequence of reduced levels of microbial exposure during childhood. The evidence is both indirect and direct, although not yet conclusive. The most consistent observation, providing indirect evidence, is of an inverse relationship between family size and/or birth order and the risk of atopy and hay fever, a pattern that is evident in populations born almost a century ago. This has been interpreted as being consistent with the age at which a child encounters microbial agents having a decisive influence on the development of atopy and associated diseases: children in large families and those with older sibs are more likely to encounter infections earlier in life, reducing their risk of becoming atopic. More directly, several studies, most of them in European populations, have shown a relationship between growing up on a farm and a reduced risk of developing atopy, hay fever, and asthma, and the effects may persist into adult life. If a farm childhood confers protection then it remains unclear which exposure(s) may be responsible; unpasteurized milk, pig farming, haymaking, and endotoxin in domestic dust have all been proposed, but none as yet confirmed.

Prognosis

Knowledge of the outcome of asthma has been hindered by the lack of a clear workable definition of asthma, which includes all cases (sensitive) and excludes noncases (specific), and by the relative paucity of longitudinal data on well-defined community cohorts including a representative group of cases of asthma and not limited to those coming to medical attention. Nonetheless there is now sufficient information to allow a reasonable view of the outcome of the disease.

The relationship between wheezing in preschool children and asthma in school-age children has been clarified by a number of overlapping studies. Wheezing and cough in children aged less than 2 to 3 years is common and typically associated with viral respiratory infections. In one study in the United States of America, wheezing episodes in children aged less than 2 years were primarily associated with respiratory syncytial virus (RSV) infection (as opposed to rhinovirus infection in children aged >2 years). The important risk factors for wheezing in children aged less than 2 to 3 years are reduced lung function at birth, prematurity or low birth weight, and maternal smoking during pregnancy, which both reduces lung function and alters the baby's immune responses. The prognosis for such children is good, with remission in most by school age and normal lung function in adult life. 'Wheezy bronchitis' in preschool years does not occur more frequently in school-age children with asthma, whose risk factors are different, suggesting the two disorders are independent. The peak prevalence of asthma occurs between the ages of 5 and 10 years, and is associated with eczema in infancy and evidence of sensitization to common inhalant allergens (identified either by skin test responses or by increased total IgE).

The outcome for children who develop asthma has been the subject of several general practice and hospital-based reports, which of necessity will describe the prognosis of more severe cases. The outcome for cases identified in random population samples has been reported from Australia and the United Kingdom. The Australian study found that risk of asthma persisting at ages 21 and 28 years was associated with the frequency of wheezing at ages 7 and 14 years. Children who wheezed infrequently in childhood and adolescence were least likely to have continuing asthma as young adults: more than one-half of those with asthma before the age of 7 years that had remitted by the age of 14 years remained symptom free aged 21 years. However, less than 20% of those with persistent symptoms in childhood were symptom free in adolescence, and frequent attacks in this group continued to the age of 28 years. Some two-thirds of those without symptoms in adolescence remained free of asthma at the age of 28 years. The United Kingdom study described the incidence of wheezing from birth to age 33 years. The incidence of wheezy illness at all ages was related to a history of eczema and hay fever. One-quarter of children with a history of asthma or wheezy bronchitis by the age of 7 years continued to have symptoms when aged 33 years. Asthma developing in adult life was strongly associated with cigarette smoking and a history of hay fever.

In both the United Kingdom and Australian studies, asthma recurred in adult life after a period of remission in adolescence. More than one-half of those in the United Kingdom study who had wheezed before the age of 7 years and reported wheezing aged 33 years had been free of symptoms for 7 years between the age of 16 to 23 years. Similarly, in the Australian study wheezing had recurred in 30% of those who were free of wheezing aged 21 years. In both studies asthma recurred in some individuals with mild symptoms in childhood that were frequently not recalled, and who would otherwise have been labelled as having 'adult-onset' asthma.

Clinical manifestations

The symptoms of asthma are nonspecific: shortness of breath, wheezing, chest tightness, and cough. These are manifestations of airway narrowing, which is usually variable in severity over short periods of time, but can be persistent, and of airway hyper-responsiveness. Asthma as the cause of these symptoms is suggested by the variability in their severity and distinguished by their periodicity (e.g. daily, weekly, monthly, or seasonal), their provocation by specific (e.g. allergen) and nonspecific stimuli, and their reversibility with bronchodilators or corticosteroids.

Patients with asthma can be categorized, at any one time, by whether their symptoms are intermittent or persistent, and by the severity of their symptoms and underlying airway narrowing (measured by lung function tests). It is important to appreciate that even those with mild intermittent asthma can develop severe exacerbations given an appropriate stimulus.

- Mild intermittent asthma—symptoms less than weekly with normal or near normal lung function between episodes

- Mild persistent asthma—symptoms more than weekly but less than daily with normal, or near normal, lung function between episodes

- Moderate persistent asthma—daily symptoms with mild to moderate airflow limitation

- Severe persistent asthma—daily symptoms that interfere with normal activities, frequent nocturnal waking and moderate to severe airflow limitation

It is also helpful to distinguish chronic and acute asthma: chronic asthma is asthma requiring maintenance treatment; acute asthma is an exacerbation of underlying asthma requiring additional treatment.

Symptoms

Symptoms of asthma are typically worse at night, waking the affected individual on occasion several times in the early hours of the morning and on first waking in the morning, when chest tightness may be the dominant symptom. Asthmatic symptoms may also be provoked by nonspecific stimuli such as exercise and cold air, and by specific allergens such as domestic animals, particularly cats. In patients allergic to pollens or moulds, asthmatic symptoms occur or worsen during the relevant season (in the United Kingdom tree pollen in the late spring, grass pollen in May and June, and mould spores in the late summer months). In patients with asthma induced by occupational sensitizers, symptoms characteristically increase in severity during the working week and improve when away from work on holidays of 1 week or more, if not at weekends.

Because occupational causes of asthma are potentially avoidable, all cases of asthma that have occurred or recurred in adult life should be questioned about symptomatic improvement when away from work, and if this is present enquiry should be made about potential causes of asthma in the workplace. The onset of symptoms occurs after a latent interval usually of months or years from the onset of exposure. By contrast, irritant-induced occupational asthma follows a single identifiable exposure to an irritant chemical in toxic concentrations causing irritation of eyes, nose, and airways of sufficient severity for the individual to seek medical advice within 24 h of the incident.

Respiratory viral infections that occur predominantly in the autumn and winter months are the most important precipitating causes of exacerbations of asthma. In some women asthma has a monthly periodicity, becoming increasingly severe during the days before menstruation and improving with its onset.

Although breathlessness and wheeze are often considered the most characteristic symptoms of asthma, cough can be the dominant and, on occasions, the only symptom of asthma. Nocturnal cough particularly suggests asthma, although in community studies isolated nocturnal cough has been found to be a poor predictor of asthma. 'Cough-variant asthma' is occasionally seen in adults in whom cough and eosinophil-rich sputum are the only manifestations of the disease.

The characteristic symptoms of asthma are manifestations of variable airway narrowing and airway hyper-responsiveness. Patients with chronic severe asthma have more persistent airway narrowing, are limited in their day-to-day activities by breathlessness, and may have less symptomatic evidence of spontaneous variability of airway narrowing, although they can be awoken by asthma at night as well as having symptoms provoked by inhalation of cold air or by laughter.

Patients with acute severe asthma are usually distressed by severe shortness of breath with wheezing, and are unable to sleep or to complete sentences in one breath because of the severity of the airway narrowing.

Signs

The physical signs of mild or moderate asthma may be limited to expiratory wheezes audible over the lungs. Because of the variable nature of the airway narrowing some patients have normal lung sounds, although expiratory wheezes are to be anticipated in patients with persistent symptomatic asthma. Patients with chronic persistent asthma can develop hyperinflated lungs.

In acute severe asthma patients are usually extremely short of breath, sitting up or leaning forward using their accessory muscles of respiration. Characteristically, with increasingly severe airway narrowing increasingly prolonged expiration alternates with short inspiratory gasps, impairing speech. Tachycardia and pulsus paradoxus (an exaggeration of the normal fall in systolic blood pressure on inspiration to >10 mmHg) often accompany acute severe asthma, but pulsus paradoxus is not a reliable indicator of severity (because it depends on respiratory effort and is therefore not seen in the patient who is exhausted, and may be near death). Airway narrowing may become sufficiently severe for no wheeze to be audible and gas exchange sufficiently impaired to cause detectable cyanosis. Patients with asthma of this severity are usually distressed, anxious, apprehensive and can be confused because of hypoxia. Exhaustion ultimately leads to inadequate ventilation and a rising $P\text{co}_2$, the two cardinal features that indicate the need for transfer to an intensive care unit in the event that assisted ventilation is required.

Diagnosis

Although asthma is now defined by characteristic pathological changes in the airways, it is usually identified by its pathophysiological manifestations, variable or reversible airway narrowing and airway hyper-responsiveness. In some patients the presence of eosinophils in sputum or a raised eosinophil count in the blood can be a valuable diagnostic pointer.

Most typically, asthma is diagnosed by the demonstration of airflow limitation that varies spontaneously over short periods of time, or which reverses after inhalation of a short-acting β-agonist or, over a more prolonged period of time, use of a corticosteroid either by inhalation or by mouth. In a few patients provocation tests using exercise or pharmacological agents such as histamine or methacholine can be valuable. Inhalation tests with the specific agent may be indicated in suspected cases of occupational asthma, but inhalation tests with common inhalant allergens are rarely indicated in clinical practice.

Airflow limitation

The most clinically useful measurements of airflow limitation are (1) FEV_1, which may be expressed as a proportion of the forced vital capacity (FVC) as $FEV_1/FVC\%$; and (2) peak expiratory flow rate (PEF). Both tests require the patient to provide a reproducible maximal forced expiratory manoeuvre using tested and validated equipment. FEV_1 has the advantage of a visible tracing of the expelled volume of air over time that allows the observer to determine whether reproducible maximal forced expiratory manoeuvres have been made. PEF does not provide this opportunity. Peak flow meters, used to measure PEF, continue to be used more often than spirometers to measure FEV_1 for home use, and they can be used regularly by patients to provide them with an assessment of their lung function and indication of the need for further treatment at an early stage. Whether abnormality of FEV_1 and PEF should be expressed in absolute or proportional terms remains undecided. Expression as an absolute difference from the average value anticipated for an individual of given age, gender, and height has more physiological validity, but most lung function laboratories in United Kingdom continue to define values of FEV_1 or PEF of 20% or more below the mean predicted value as abnormal (see Chapter 18.3.1).

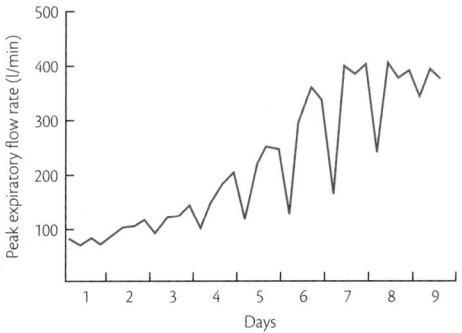

Fig. 18.7.3 Circadian rhythm in peak expiratory flow rate in a patient with asthma recovering from an acute attack.

Variability and reversibility

Serial measurements of PEF in most (although not all) patients with asthma show spontaneous variability. The most characteristic pattern is of a circadian variation with airflow limitation, most severe on waking in the morning (and during the night if awoken) and with improvement occurring during the morning after waking (Fig. 18.7.3). A small circadian variation in PEF or FEV_1 is seen in normal individuals; in asthma a difference of 20% or more between the highest and lowest values may be found.

Other patterns of variation in severity of airflow limitation may be imposed on the circadian pattern, such as falls in PEF provoked by exercise, exposure to an allergen or occupational sensitizer, which resolve after avoidance of the stimulus. While variations of 20% or more in FEV_1 or PEF are commonly regarded as indicating asthma, in patients with severe airflow limitation and an FEV_1 of 1 litre, 20% variability equates to 200 ml, a level of spontaneous variation observed in nonasthmatics.

The most commonly used means to identify asthma in clinical practice is an improvement in airflow limitation, identified by FEV_1 or PEF, 15 to 20 min after inhalation of bronchodilator, usually a short-acting β-agonist such as salbutamol 200 μg: improvement in FEV_1 or PEF of 20% or more is generally regarded as evidence of asthma. However, it is important to appreciate that the absence of a significant improvement in lung function after inhalation of bronchodilator does not exclude a diagnosis of asthma (i.e. it is a more specific than sensitive test). Rapid reversibility of airflow limitation is more readily seen in young adults with mild or moderate asthma than in more elderly patients with more severe airflow limitation. Reversibility cannot be tested in a patient whose lung function is normal at the time of testing.

Expressing changes in airflow as a proportion of baseline will exaggerate the degree of improvement in those with a low initial FEV_1 or PEF. A 20% increase in FEV_1 in a patient with a baseline FEV_1 of 4 litres is 800 ml, but only 200 ml in a patient whose baseline FEV_1 is 1 litre. Studies of short-term (20 min) variability in FEV_1 in patients with airflow limitation have found that the increase in FEV_1 needed to exclude natural variability with 95% confidence was 160 ml. This value did not differ significantly from the value in normal individuals, in whom an absolute increase in FEV_1 of 190 ml was needed to exclude a chance increase with 95% confidence. Both in normal individuals and in those with an airflow limitation, expression of variability as an absolute difference was similar at all levels of FEV_1, whereas when expressed as a percentage change, the degree of variability decreased with

increasing FEV_1. This means that selecting a specific percentage change in FEV_1 (or PEF) to define asthma will necessarily include a greater proportion of patients with lower prebronchodilator FEV_1: patients with a higher baseline FEV_1 need to achieve a greater absolute increase to fulfil the defined criterion. Expression of variability as an absolute change has more biological and statistical validity: an increase of more than 200 ml in FEV_1 has a probability of less than 5% of occurring by chance. However, as with expression of lung function, it is unlikely that the use of results based on absolute values, although biologically more valid, will be adopted. It should be appreciated, however, that in patients with a low FEV_1 a 20% increase in FEV_1 may have occurred by chance, and in those with a high FEV_1 an increase of more than 200 ml is unlikely to have occurred by chance.

In some patients with asthma, particularly those with severe airflow limitation, inhalation of a short-acting bronchodilator does not provide significant improvement in FEV_1 or PEF. In these circumstances the diagnosis of asthma and differentiation from less reversible causes of airflow limitation such as chronic bronchitis and emphysema can be made with a 'trial' of treatment with corticosteroids. Significant improvement in airflow limitation both implies a diagnosis of asthma and demonstrates that corticosteroids (inhaled or oral) are effective treatment. However, corticosteroids can also improve exercise tolerance by enhancing mood and outlook, and the benefit of a trial of steroids therefore has to be judged by its effect on lung function. Although there is no formally agreed protocol for a steroid trial, a generally acceptable trial would be oral prednisolone taken in a dose of 0.6 mg/kg, (e.g. 40 mg/day in a 70-kg man) for 3 weeks, with measurement of lung function made on at least two separate occasions, once before and once at the end of the trial. Symptomatic improvement with an increase in FEV_1 or PEF of 20% or more during the trial is generally considered as evidence of asthma and an indication for treatment with corticosteroids, inhaled or oral.

Tests of airway hyper-responsiveness

Airway hyper-responsiveness—an exaggerated response to nonspecific provocative stimuli—is a cardinal feature of asthma. Tests of airway responsiveness to exercise and to inhaled histamine or methacholine, which can provoke acute airway narrowing in a dose-dependent fashion, can be of value in the diagnosis of asthma, particularly in patients with symptoms suggestive of asthma but in whom lung function when measured is normal or, if abnormal, shows no reversibility with inhaled bronchodilators. These tests are required in only a few patients, and each has its limitations: exercise testing can be insensitive (i.e. false negatives), and tests of airway reactivity to inhaled histamine or methacholine nonspecific (i.e. false positives), although the provocation of a 20% fall in FEV_1 by histamine 4 mg/ml or less (or equivalent) occurs uncommonly in nonasthmatic patients.

In general, normal airway responsiveness to exercise, histamine, or methacholine makes a diagnosis of current asthma very unlikely, whereas an abnormal test is diagnostically less helpful.

Exercise testing

Acute airway narrowing provoked by exercise is a common feature of asthma, particularly in children. To test for exercise provoked asthma requires continuous exertion for 6 min. This is most conveniently undertaken in a lung function laboratory by running on a treadmill or exercising on a cycle ergometer, although free running is more likely to provoke an asthmatic reaction. Measurements are made of FEV_1 or PEFR during 5 min before and for 30 min at intervals of 5 min after the test. A normal individual will have a less than 5% increase in FEV_1 or PEFR during and a less than 10% fall after exercise. Depending on the level of baseline, patients with asthma can have a greater than 5% increase during exercise and greater than 10% fall from pretest value after exercise. Exercise is a valid and reproducible test for asthma, but particularly when undertaken by methods other than free running, can have false negatives. It has, however, proved less reliable in community studies, with a significant false-positive rate.

Airway reactivity to inhaled histamine or methacholine

Acute airway narrowing can be provoked in a dose-dependent manner by the inhalation of increasing doses of a bronchoconstrictor, of which histamine or methacholine are the most commonly used. The test as described by Cockcroft *et al.* consists of tidal breathing of doubling doses of histamine, with measurement of FEV_1 6 min after each inhaled dose. The percentage change in FEV_1 from a post-saline baseline after each concentration of inhaled (histamine) can be plotted, with the test terminated when either a 20% or greater fall in FEV_1 is provoked or the maximum concentration (usually 16 or 32 mg/ml) is reached. The level of airway reactivity is usually expressed as the concentration of histamine that provokes a 20% fall in FEV_1 (PC_{20} histamine), which can be identified by linear interpolation: the lower the PC_{20}, the more reactive the airways. The test is usually repeatable within one doubling dose, but may not be consistent in any individual, PC_{20} falling for instance after exposure to allergen or occupational sensitizer.

In population studies the major determinants of airway reactivity have been atopy (in older children and young adults) and smoking in older adults (probably reflecting reduced FEV_1). Airway responsiveness can be increased in atopic children with rhinitis and in healthy adults after a viral respiratory tract infection. Evidence of measurable airway reactivity is therefore not necessarily evidence of asthma. However, it is uncommon for nonasthmatic individuals to have a PC_{20} for histamine or methacholine of less than 8 mg/ml.

Measurement of airway reactivity to histamine or methacholine is more sensitive than exercise testing, although a less specific test for asthma. Like exercise testing its value in clinical practice is primarily in symptomatic patients with normal or near normal FEV_1, without evidence of spontaneous variability or reversibility. A negative test in a symptomatic patient suggests that current asthma is unlikely to be the cause of their symptoms.

Diagnosis of occupational asthma

The diagnosis of occupational asthma should be considered in any adult who develops asthma or whose asthma has deteriorated in working life. In the case of irritant-induced asthma the association of the onset of asthma with inhalation of a toxic chemical is usually clear. The association of asthma caused by a specific hypersensitivity reaction is often less apparent, and the diagnosis is based on the following:

• Exposure to a sensitizing agent at work

• A characteristic history of onset of asthma after an initial symptom-free period of exposure; and deterioration in symptoms during periods at work and improvements during absence from work

• The results of objective investigations: lung function tests, immunological tests, and inhalation tests

Lung function tests

The most commonly used criterion for diagnosing asthma—improvement in airflow limitation (FEV_1 or PEF) after inhalation of bronchodilator—is often not present in cases of occupational asthma because lung function may be normal when the patient is seen away from work and, if present, does not identify a work relationship. The measure of lung function most commonly used to identify work related asthma is serial self-recorded PEF. A patient with suspected occupational asthma is asked to record their PEF at intervals of 2 to 3 h for a month from waking to sleeping, and at night if awoken, both during periods at and absences from work. The results can be summarized in a graphical display that records the best, worst, and average values for each day, allowing comparison of PEF during days at work with days away from work (Fig. 18.7.4). The diagnostic value of the test depends on the reproducibility of the patients' forced expiratory manoeuvres and their honesty and compliance. Concurrent treatment can influence the results, particularly when treatment is systematically increased during periods at work and reduced during absences from work, hence when possible treatment should be kept constant during the period of testing, and at a minimum any changes should be recorded.

Comparisons with the results of inhalation testing as the 'gold standard' have shown that serial self-recorded PEF measurements are a sensitive and specific index of work-related asthma. The major diagnostic difficulties are in patients with evidence of asthma on PEF records without a work relationship, of whom a proportion are eventually shown to have occupational asthma, the commonest reason for such 'false-negative' responses being insufficient time away from work for significant improvement to have occurred.

Immunological tests

The presence of specific IgE antibody, identified either by immediate skin test response to a soluble protein extract or a hapten–protein conjugate, or by immunoassay in serum, is evidence of sensitization to a specific agent. Specific IgE can be identified in most, if not all, protein causes of occupational asthma, and in a small number of low-molecular-weight chemical causes of asthma, notably complex platinum salts, acid anhydrides, and reactive dyes. No reliable immunological test has been developed for sensitivity to other important causes of asthma such as isocyanates and colophony. The diagnostic value of a positive test has been formally examined for few of the causes of occupational asthma, and in these cases has been found to be significantly associated with asthma caused by both proteins and low-molecular-weight chemicals inhaled at work.

Specific inhalation testing

The objective of an inhalation test is to expose the individual under single-blind conditions to the putative cause of their asthma in circumstances that resemble as closely as possible the conditions of exposure at work. The different test methods used depend upon the physical state of the test material, which can be water soluble (most proteins) and inhaled in solution, a volatile organic liquid inhaled as a vapour, or a dust. Any change in lung function, both in airways calibre (usually measured as FEV_1 or PEF) and in airways

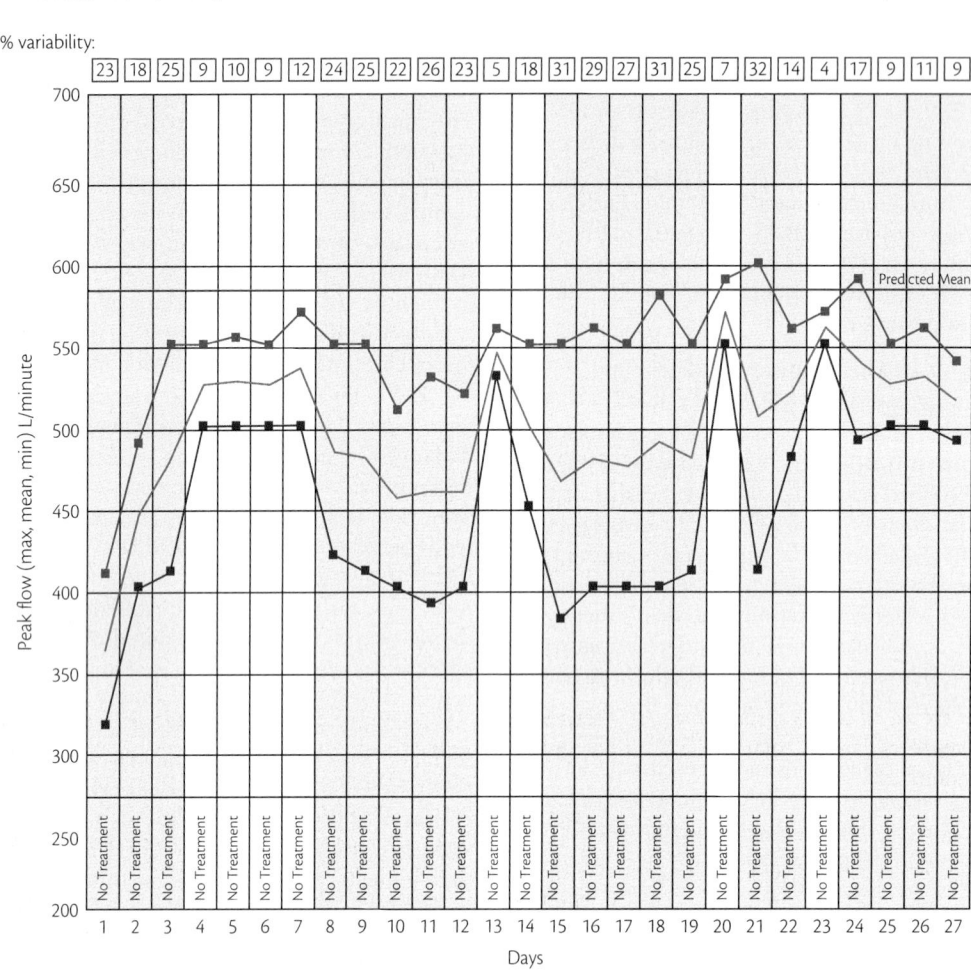

Fig. 18.7.4 The 27-day serial peak flow record of a baker with occupational asthma from fungal alpha amylase. On each day, represented by a column, the average, maximum, and minimum peak flow measurements are plotted. Blue columns are work days. The boxed figures at the top of each day are measures of diurnal variation (percentage).

responsiveness to inhaled histamine or methacholine (measured as PC_{20}), is compared with results on appropriate control days. The patterns of airways response provoked by specific inhalation tests have been distinguished by their time of onset and duration (Fig. 18.7.5). Immediate asthmatic responses occur within minutes of the test exposure and usually resolve spontaneously within 1 to 2 h. Late asthmatic responses develop 1 h or more after the test exposure and can persist for 24 to 36 h. Late asthmatic (but usually not immediate) responses are accompanied by an increase in non-specific airways responsiveness 3 h and, less reliably, 24 h after the test inhalation. An immediate response followed by a late response has been called a dual response.

Inhalation testing allows the investigation of specific causes of asthma in individuals exposed to them. Provided that the agent being tested is not a nonspecific mucosal irritant and does not provoke an immediate asthmatic response in patients with hyper-responsive airways—such as sulphur dioxide, histamine, or exercise—the provocation of an asthmatic response by an occupational agent implies that it is a cause of asthma. This causal relationship is strengthened if the agent reproducibly provokes a late asthmatic response and increases nonspecific airways responsiveness.

There are four major indications for inhalation testing in the diagnosis of occupational asthma:

♦ Where the diagnosis or cause of occupational asthma remains in doubt after other investigations, including serial PEF and immunological tests (where applicable), have been completed

♦ Where the agent considered responsible for causing asthma has not previously been reliably shown to do so

♦ Where an individual with occupational asthma is exposed at work to more than one potential cause, which cannot be distinguished by other means, and where such a distinction is going to be clinically and occupationally helpful

♦ Where asthma is of such severity that further uncontrolled exposure at work is unjustifiable

Inhalation tests should be undertaken only for clinical purposes to provide information important for future management advice: conducting them solely for medicolegal purposes is not justified.

The diagnosis of occupational asthma requires differentiation from work-exacerbated asthma, which is incidental asthma aggravated by nonspecific provocative stimuli encountered at work such

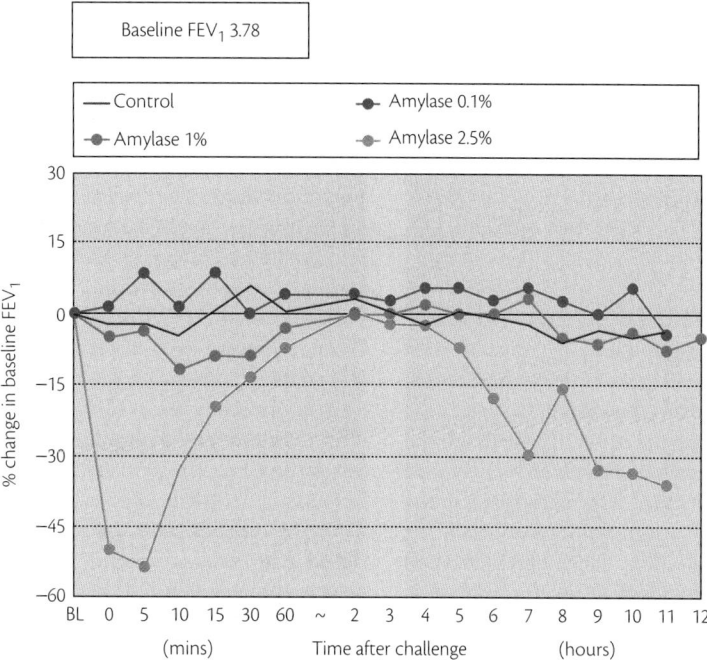

Baseline FEV$_1$ 3.78

— Control   ● Amylase 0.1%
● Amylase 1%   ● Amylase 2.5%

Fig. 18.7.5 Specific inhalation test demonstrating dual asthmatic response in baker with occupational asthma from fungal α-amylase.

as sulphur dioxide, exercise, or cold air, also from other causes of similar respiratory symptoms, in particular chronic airflow limitation and hyperventilation.

Particular causes of occupational asthma

Occupational asthma is a prescribed disease for 'employed earners' and includes asthma caused by exposure to any one of a number of specified agents as well as 'any other sensitizing agent inhaled at work'.

One condition worthy of note that should probably be considered as a form of occupational asthma is byssinosis, which in the United Kingdom most commonly occurs in cotton mill workers after 20 to 25 years of exposure to cotton dust. It is characterized by chest tightness on the first day of the working week, which usually develops 3 to 4 h after the start of a work shift and typically improves on subsequent working days despite continuing exposure. Proportion of cotton textile workers with byssinosis develop COPD, with chronic airflow limitation.

Imaging

Imaging of the chest is not commonly of diagnostic value in asthma but can be important in identifying its complications. In patients in whom asthma develops over the age of 30 years the chest radiograph is usually normal, but about one-quarter of children and one-fifth of adults show changes of hyperinflation. These changes include a low diaphragm (below the sixth intercostal space anteriorly) and an increased retrosternal space. In some children with chronic persistent asthma the length of the lung becomes greater than the width of the thorax, with the posterior ends of the ribs becoming more horizontal. A commonly observed radiographic sign in asthma is of thickened bronchial walls due to eosinophilic infiltration of the airways: these are visible on the chest radiograph as parallel lines ('tram lines'), or as a thick-walled ring shadow when seen end on.

The complications of asthma include pneumothorax, pneumomediastinum, pulmonary collapse, and eosinophilic pneumonia. The physical signs of pneumothorax can be difficult to discern in asthmatic attack, but its detection can be life saving. Pneumomediastinum is of less clinical importance. Plugging of the airways by mucus characteristically occurs in allergic bronchopulmonary aspergillosis (ABPA), but can occur in asthmatic patients without ABPA: in both it can cause atelectasis, which is usually lobar or segmental.

ABPA causes fleeting nonsegmental areas of consolidation that are characteristically perihilar, accompanied by a moderate blood eosinophilia ($1-1.5 \times 10^9$/litre). Less commonly, lobar or segmental atelectasis is caused by mucus impaction. With progression the disease characteristically causes bronchiectasis that is predominantly proximal, visible both on the chest radiograph and CT scan, and upper lobe fibrosis.

Eosinophilic pneumonia is characterized by consolidation on the chest radiograph accompanied by a raised blood eosinophil count. This can be a manifestation of several conditions, including ABPA, helminth infections, and drug reactions, as well as being of unknown cause—acute and chronic eosinophilic pneumonia (see Chapter 18.14.2). Of these, ABPA and chronic eosinophilic pneumonia (which can be a manifestation of Churg–Strauss syndrome—allergic granulomatosis, see Chapters 18.11.5 and 18.14.5) are the most common causes of eosinophilic pneumonia in patients with asthma.

Chronic eosinophilic pneumonia causes fleeting consolidation that is characteristically peripheral in distribution, either in localized areas or more widespread (the 'photographic negative' of pulmonary oedema). The blood eosinophil count is usually considerably more elevated than in ABPA. If seen as a manifestation of Churg–Strauss syndrome, a granulomatous vasculitis that develops in patients with rhinitis and asthma, then other features can include pleural and pericardial effusions, congestive cardiomyopathy and mononeuritis multiplex. Abnormalities on the chest radiograph include enlargement of the heart, because of pericardial or myocardial disease, and consolidation due to chronic eosinophilic pneumonia.

Differential diagnosis

Asthma needs to be differentiated from localized airways obstruction, other causes of generalized airways obstruction, and other causes of intermittent breathlessness.

Localized airways obstruction

Upper airways obstruction of the larynx or trachea causes a monophonic inspiratory wheeze (stridor) audible over the trachea, with a characteristic abnormality of the flow volume loop showing decreased inspiratory flow rate. Wheezing in a child can be caused by an inhaled foreign body (classically a peanut), which should be suspected particularly if wheeze develops suddenly in a child who is previously healthy. The chest radiograph may show the foreign body if opaque, or distal atelectasis, consolidation or air trapping on an expiratory film (which may not be possible to obtain in small children), but it can be normal and—if foreign body inhalation is suspected—bronchoscopy should be undertaken to identify and remove it or to exclude the possibility. In adults localized airway narrowing is more likely to be due to a tumour, benign or malignant, which may occasionally cause a unilateral monophonic wheeze. The tumour may be visible on the chest radiograph, but definite diagnosis will require bronchoscopy and biopsy.

Generalized airways obstruction

The main causes of generalized airways obstruction from which asthma needs to be distinguished are chronic bronchitis and emphysema (COPD), although in some cases these may coexist with asthma. Other causes such as obliterative bronchiolitis are less common. In general, chronic bronchitis and emphysema (COPD) cause breathlessness that increases slowly in severity over years and only uncommonly causes breathlessness before the age of 40 years. Nocturnal waking by respiratory symptoms is uncommon in chronic bronchitis and emphysema (COPD), although not universal in asthma. Chronic severe asthma responsive to corticosteroids, but without significant reversibility to inhaled bronchodilators, may have similar radiographic and spirometric abnormalities. In both the lungs may be hyperinflated on the chest radiograph, but in asthma—unlike emphysema—there is no associated loss of vascular markings.

Lung function tests in both asthma and emphysema can show airflow limitation with reduced FEV_1, reduced FEV_1/FVC ratio, and hyperinflated lungs with increased total lung capacity. However, while factor transfer (T_Lco) and gas transfer coefficient (Kco) are reduced in emphysema, in asthma Kco is normal or increased.

Differentiation from chronic bronchitis can be difficult because, like asthma, there is no loss of vascular markings on the chest radiograph or reduction of Kco. Sputum (and blood) eosinophilia, if present, can suggest asthma, but differentiation in these circumstances often depends on the outcome of a trial of steroids.

In young children asthma needs to be differentiated from wheezing episodes associated with viral respiratory tract infections, and in children and adolescents from cystic fibrosis. Cystic fibrosis is suggested by a disproportionate production of (usually discoloured) sputum, weight loss, and an abnormal chest radiograph. The presence of staphylococci in sputum and the development of nasal polyps in childhood are very suggestive of cystic fibrosis. Other causes of chronic suppurative lung disease in children, such as primary ciliary dyskinesia (PCD) and severe combined immunodeficiency (SCID), may also need to be excluded.

Other causes of intermittent breathlessness

The most important causes of intermittent breathlessness from which asthma should be differentiated are left ventricular failure, pulmonary emboli, extrinsic allergic alveolitis, hyperventilation, and vocal cord dysfunction.

Left heart failure sufficient to cause breathlessness will usually be apparent on clinical examination, and the chest radiograph and echocardiogram are likely to be abnormal, as is the ECG. The heart is clinically and radiographically enlarged with the exception of pulmonary venous hypertension caused by mitral stenosis. Inspiratory crackles are usually audible at the lung bases, and jugular venous pressure may be elevated. In addition to an enlarged heart the chest radiograph may show upper lobe venous distension, Kerley 'B' lines and pleural effusion. Echocardiography will usually show evidence of left ventricular disease, or in the case of mitral stenosis left atrial enlargement. However, identification of the cause of breathlessness can be difficult when left heart failure is provoked by an intermittent arrhythmia.

Pulmonary embolism causes breathlessness that can occasionally be associated with wheezing. The diagnosis is suggested by associated pleuritic pain and haemoptysis. The diagnosis is usually made by imaging with a ventilation–perfusion scan or spiral CT scan. A normal ventilation–perfusion scan makes all but the smallest emboli unlikely, although interpretation can be difficult in patients with widespread ventilatory disease. A normal spiral CT scan excludes pulmonary emboli to subsegmental level. The chest radiograph and CT scan (lung windows) may show pleural-based 'humpback' opacities and pleural effusion.

Extrinsic allergic alveolitis

Extrinsic allergic alveolitis (EAA) can provoke recurrent episodes of breathlessness that characteristically develop 4 to 8 h after exposure to the cause (usually mouldy hay or birds—pigeons or budgerigars). Breathlessness in EAA is usually not accompanied by wheeze but with fever, influenza-like symptoms, and a neutrophil leucocytosis. The chest radiograph often shows widespread nodular or ground-glass shadowing, the CT scan discrete areas of ground-glass opacification. Lung function tests show a proportionate reduction in FEV_1 and FVC that may be accompanied by a reduced T_Lco and Kco. For further discussion see Chapter 18.14.4.

Hyperventilation

Episodes of hyperventilation may be difficult to distinguish symptomatically from asthma, and in some cases complicate asthma, which can be very confusing. The diagnosis should be suspected in a patient who complains of breathlessness that occurs without identifiable cause (e.g. while sitting reading), may be associated with pins and needles in the fingers and dizziness (attributable to hypocapnoea), and does not disturb sleep, although hyperventilation may inhibit the onset of sleep. The symptoms complained of can often be reproduced by a short period of voluntary overbreathing: 20 deep breaths are usually sufficient. Various explanations for the tendency of some patients to hyperventilate have been suggested, but none are convincing. However, it is important to recognize that asthma is characteristically a variable condition and a diagnosis of hyperventilation should not be made solely on the basis of absent physical signs or normal lung function at the time of consultation, but on the characteristics described above.

Vocal cord dysfunction

Vocal cord dysfunction is easily misdiagnosed as asthma and may coexist with asthma. In vocal cord dysfunction wheezing is caused by adduction of the anterior two-thirds of the vocal cords, and does not occur during sleep. The diagnosis if best made by direct examination of the cords during an attack, which shows characteristic paradoxical vocal cord adduction on inspiration. Other helpful pointers include poorly reproducible spirometry and flow–volume curves (particularly during the inspiratory phase), and a disproportionate reduction in FEV_1 compared to other effort-independent measures of airflow obstruction, such as specific airways conductance as determined by whole-body plethysmography. Management can be difficult, but recognition of this not uncommon condition allows high dose oral corticosteroid treatment for 'uncontrolled asthma' to be avoided.

Hyperventilation and vocal cord dysfunction can each occur in patients with underlying asthma, frequently in association with underlying psychosocial problems. A critical point can be to determine the relevant life events associated in time with the onset of deterioration in a patient often with previously well controlled asthma. The inciting event may have occurred several years previously, e.g. bereavement, family upheaval, etc., and require specific probing in the history. Vocal cord dysfunction is more common in women and in those engaged in health care provision.

The objectives of treatment

The objectives of treating patients with intermittent or persistent asthma are to:

- Educate the patient about their disease and the objectives of its management

- Minimize or eliminate asthma symptoms

- Achieve best possible lung function and prevent an accelerated decline in lung function

- Prevent exacerbations of asthma

- Achieve these objectives with fewest drugs, keeping short-term and long-term adverse effects to a minimum

These objectives are most likely to be achieved by treatment that reduces airway inflammation, either by avoidance of its inducing cause or by drugs with anti-inflammatory activity. The risk of side effects of asthma treatment should be appreciated and minimized, and patients' concerns about the potential side effects of long-term treatment recognized and relevant information provided to them.

A number of recent studies have compared the level of asthma control, particularly with regard to the frequency of exacerbations and duration of freedom from an exacerbation, in patients with asthma whose management was based on usual clinical criteria (symptom severity, lung function, and bronchodilator requirements), with management based on a measure of airway inflammation, usually sputum eosinophilia but also exhaled NO (F_ENO). In general these studies have shown that using indices of airway inflammation to guide treatment reduced the frequency of exacerbations and duration of exacerbation free interval without an increase in the need for corticosteroid treatment. In one study of 74 patients with moderate or severe asthma followed up for 1 year after random allocation to management by BTS guidelines or by maintenance of sputum eosinophils to less than 3%, there were significant fewer exacerbations (35 vs 109) and hospital admissions (1 vs 6) in the group managed by maintaining sputum eosinophils lessthan 3% (Fig. 18.7.6). In a second similar study the exacerbation frequency was reduced overall by one-half, and by two-thirds in those with moderate or severe asthma, in patients whose management was controlled on the basis of maintaining sputum eosinophils less than 2% as compared to usual clinical indices of symptoms, lung function and bronchodilator requirement. In a similar comparison study maintaining F_ENO <15ppb was associated with a nonsignificant reduction in exacerbations by 50% in the year of follow-up, and a reduction by 40% in overall corticosteroid dosage as compared to a group managed on usual clinical criteria.

These studies indicate the value of using an index of airway inflammation (at present better demonstrated for sputum eosinophils than for F_ENO) as a guide to clinical management (particularly dosage of

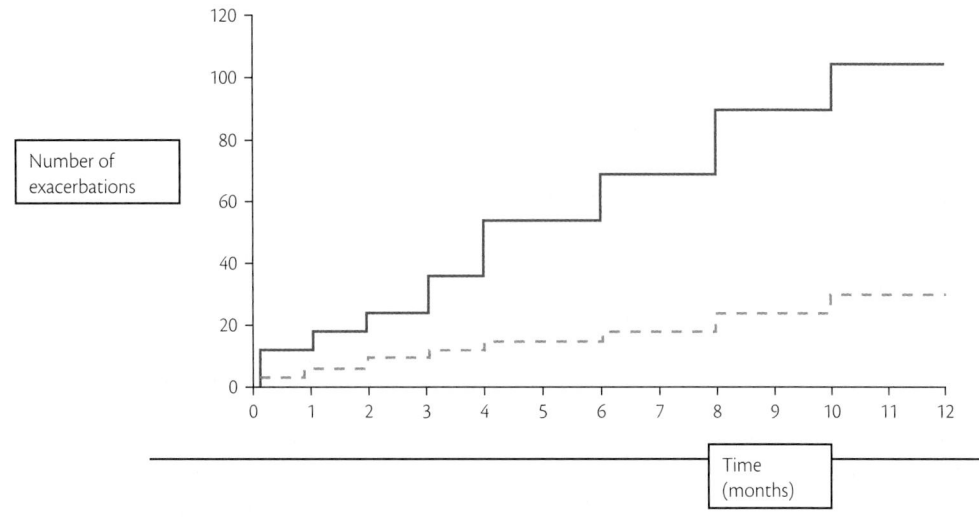

Fig. 18.7.6 Cumulative frequency of asthma exacerbations in BTS management (solid line) vs sputum management group (dashed line) (see text for details). (From Green RH, *et al.* (2002). Asthma exacerbations and sputum eosinophil counts: a randomized controlled trial. *Lancet*, **360**, 1715–21.)

inhaled corticosteroid) of patients with moderate and severe asthma. However, these are not currently widely used in clinical practice, and if they are introduced decisions will need to be guided by them in addition to—not instead of—the current indices of symptom severity, lung function, and bronchodilator requirements.

Treatment selection

Randomized controlled trials of asthma treatments have determined the benefit of different treatment interventions in patients with asthma of varying severity. This information has provided a secure basis for deciding which treatment is likely to be most effective in individual patients, with broadening of the indications for the use of inhaled corticosteroids being of particular importance, and has informed the published guidelines for asthma management in the United Kingdom, the United States of America, and elsewhere.

The objectives for effective asthma control in individual patients are to:

◆ Allow normal daytime activities (e.g. going to work or to school) as well as the ability to enjoy physically demanding activities (e.g. sport)

◆ Permit sleeping through night, without being awoken by respiratory symptoms

◆ Achieve a situation where use of 'rescue' medication with inhaled β_2-agonists is needed less than once per day.

◆ Achieve normal or near normal PEF and FEV_1 with less than 20% variability between best and worst values.

◆ Avoid drug side effects

Asthma, except where caused by a dominant and avoidable agent (e.g. a domestic pet or an occupational sensitizer) is not curable, but current treatment offers the great majority of patients the opportunity to enjoy a normal life. In most cases asthma is mild: in one community survey only 15% of patients had persistent asthma of moderate severity (Step 3 BTS Guidelines or worse—see below), but some 5% of patients have severe asthma that responds poorly to conventional treatment. These patients suffer most both from their disease and from the side effects its treatment, and are at highest risk from hospitalization and death from asthma.

Patient education

There is now clear evidence from a systematic review and additional randomized controlled trials for patient education to enable adults to manage their asthma. In comparison to usual care it has been shown that this can reduce the frequency of unscheduled visits to general practitioners, hospital admissions, and time off work. The four important components of effective patient education are:

◆ Information—provision of information about asthma and its management

◆ Self monitoring—regular assessment by the patient of symptoms, or peak expiratory flow rate, or both

◆ Regular medical review—assessment of asthma control, severity, and treatment

◆ Written action plan (Box 18.7.1): an individualized written plan to allow self-management of asthma exacerbations that is informed by the severity and treatment of the patients' asthma and includes

---

Box 18.7.1 Components of written asthma plan

◆ When to increase treatment
  · Symptoms v PEF
  · PEF % predicted vs personal best
  · Number of action points based on % best PEF
◆ How to increase treatment
  · Increased inhaled corticosteroids
  · Oral corticosteroid
  · Combination
◆ For how long
  · Duration of treatment increase
◆ When to call for help

(After Gibson PG, Powell H (2004). Written action plans for asthma: an evidence based review of key components. *Thorax*, **59**, 94–9.)

---

four essential components: (1) information about when to increase treatment, (2) how to increase treatment, (3) the duration of treatment increase, and (4) when to cease self-treatment and seek medical help

Treatments to prevent or avoid asthma

Allergen avoidance

The identification and, where feasible, the avoidance of relevant allergens at home or at work is an essential part of the management of asthma. It enables patients to recognize important causes of their asthma and take responsibility for their avoidance. Allergen avoidance should be regarded as complementary to drug treatment of asthma, with the advantage in some cases (where a single allergen is the dominant cause) of providing a cure with avoidance of the potential side effects of drugs. Complete avoidance of exposure to house dust mite, domestic pets, and occupational causes of asthma have been associated with marked improvement in respiratory symptoms, lung function, and airway hyper-responsiveness. Avoidance of exposure to the house dust mite, *Dermatophagoides pteronyssinus*, by spending several months in the Alps or in a hospital, has been shown to provide symptomatic and functional improvement. However, house dust mites are ubiquitous in many environments, including much of the United States of America, the United Kingdom, and Europe, and elimination of mites from the home sufficient to reduce exposure to the relevant allergens (e.g. Der p1) to concentrations that do not continue to induce airway inflammation can be difficult. The issue with house dust mite avoidance is therefore the feasibility of securing an effective intervention, and the utility of routine advice for implementation of house dust mite avoidance strategies in mite-sensitive adult asthma has been questioned following the results of a recent large randomized controlled trial of a single intervention of mite-proof bedding for 12 months, which failed to improve symptoms or PEF rates or reduce asthma medication requirements. Given that effective mite avoidance is both expensive and time-consuming, more trials involving multiple interventions are needed. Data in favour of mite avoidance is more convincing in mite-allergic asthmatic children than in adults.

Avoidance of exposure is most clearly indicated and usually most feasible when the cause of asthma is an agent inhaled at work. Removal of a pet from the home, particularly a cat, is most effective when accompanied by thorough cleaning and washing of the house to remove residual allergen, which can otherwise persist in concentrations sufficient to provoke asthma for many months.

Occupational asthma

Occupational asthma offers a rare opportunity to cure a patient of their disease. In almost all cases of hypersensitivity-induced asthma there is considerable and often complete resolution of symptoms and accompanying bronchial hyper-responsiveness once exposure to the causative agent has ceased. However, occupational asthma, whatever its cause, may become chronic and persist for several years, if not indefinitely, even after avoidance of exposure to the causative agent. The only important determinant of chronicity identified to date has been the duration of symptomatic exposure to the initiating cause after the onset of asthma: those who remain exposed to the cause are more likely to develop chronic asthma. Any improvement after avoidance of exposure seems to occur in the first 2 years, subsequently reaching a plateau. There is little evidence that pharmacological treatments affect the rate or extent of recovery.

Patients who develop 'hypersensitivity-induced' occupational asthma in whom a specific cause is identified should be advised to avoid further exposure to that cause. In this way the risk of developing chronic asthma and airways hyper-responsiveness is diminished, and the likelihood of significant improvement or cure is enhanced.

Avoidance of further exposure may be achieved by relocation within the same workplace, but frequently requires a change of job or occupation. This requires sensitive handling, and liaison with the occupational health service (if there is one) is essential. However, in some cases a change of job may be impossible for social or financial reasons. In the short term individuals who are unable to avoid further exposure altogether should be advised to minimize it by attention to their work practices and consideration of adequate respiratory protection, the choice of suitable protective equipment being a matter for an expert. It is probably helpful to institute treatment with an inhaled corticosteroid; antihistamines and sometimes sodium cromoglicate may also be useful, especially where there is predictable and only occasional exposure, such as in some jobs involving animal contact. However, it should be emphasized that such measures are temporary, and in the long term means should be sought to avoid exposure to the cause of asthma.

When an individual does remain exposed to the cause of their asthma, either directly or indirectly, the effectiveness of relocation or of respiratory protection needs to be monitored. This can be done conveniently by serial self-recordings of PEF to determine whether or not asthma is continuing and, if so, whether it is work related.

It is a rule of thumb that if there is one employee with occupational asthma, then there is likely to be one or more others in the same place of work. A confirmed 'index' diagnosis should therefore prompt a wider investigation, with detailed consideration of exposures in the workplace. In many countries employers (sometimes physicians) are required to notify new cases of occupational asthma to a central authority, instigating a formal, external inspection of the workplace with recommendations for the prevention of any further cases.

These processes have had some notable success in preventing new cases of occupational asthma. Examples include asthma arising from enzymes in the detergent manufacturing industry, from latex (gloves) in health care workers, from laboratory animal proteins in the pharmaceutical industry, and from diisocyanates in a variety of settings. Other common causes of occupational asthma—in particular those associated with commercial baking—have been more intractable.

Immunotherapy

Allergen immunotherapy involves the provision of gradually increasing doses of allergen subcutaneously to promote immunological tolerance to future environmental exposures to the specific allergen. This fell into disrepute some 20 to 30 years ago because of reports of anaphylactic reactions, and in a few cases death, following allergen injection. More recent studies have demonstrated its efficacy and safety, particularly in seasonal allergic rhinitis with or without peak seasonal wheezing, where there is clear evidence of efficacy and long-term benefits that may persist for years following its discontinuation. However, subcutaneous immunotherapy should only be undertaken under direct medical observation and supervision, with immediate access to resuscitation facilities.

A recent Cochrane review has shown that allergen immunotherapy is effective in reducing asthma symptoms as compared to placebo, reducing the need for asthma medication and, where measured, improving airway hyper-responsiveness. The most consistent evidence of benefit was found for pollen and mite allergens. However, the risks of systemic side effects of treatment are increased in patients with bronchial asthma, and immunotherapy has been shown to be ineffective for asthma in patients with multiple allergies. Thus, although immunotherapy for seasonal allergic rhinitis with or without asthma is recommended in patients who fail to respond to usual medication, in view of the increased risks and less benefit, asthma remains a relative contra-indication for immunotherapy, at least in the United Kingdom. Exceptions may include asthmatics whose disease is clearly related to a single allergen (with associated elevated allergen-specific IgE), and where the allergen cannot be avoided, such as occupational exposure to cats in veterinary practitioners.

Drug treatments for asthma

The drugs primarily used to treat asthma are the progeny of cortisol and adrenaline (epinephrine): selective β_2-agonists, both short and long acting, and lipid-soluble topically active inhaled corticosteroids; these drugs accounting for nearly 90% of prescriptions for asthma in the United Kingdom. Other drugs sometimes used in the treatment of asthma include sodium cromoglicate and nedocromil sodium amongst the prophylactic agents, and ipratropium bromide and theophyllines amongst the bronchodilators.

The core treatments for mild and moderately severe persistent asthma are inhaled corticosteroids and inhaled β_2-agonists. Other treatments are added when these alone are not sufficient to provide control. Leukotriene receptor antagonists and 5-lipoxygenase inhibitors have been introduced recently; their place in the treatment of asthma continues to be evaluated.

Corticosteroids

Corticosteroids are the most effective treatment for asthma. Systemic corticosteroids were introduced for the treatment of asthma in the 1950s, but their use was limited by serious unwanted side effects, which stimulated research into the development of equally effective but safer alternatives. The introduction of topically active corticosteroids—administered by inhalation and free of the systemic side effects of oral corticosteroids at therapeutically effective doses—revolutionized the treatment of asthma.

Corticosteroids suppress airway inflammation, with improvement in airway hyperresponsiveness, lung function and associated respiratory symptoms. Although their mechanism of action continues to be debated, they inhibit the formation of cytokines relevant to asthmatic inflammation, such as interleukins IL-4, IL-5, IL-13 and GM-CSF, by lymphocytes and macrophages by inhibition of transcription of cytokine genes. While suppressing inflammation they do not, however, cure the disease: to be effective they must be taken continuously.

Oral corticosteroids

Oral corticosteroids—prednisolone and prednisone—are rapidly absorbed from the gut, achieving peak plasma levels at 1–2 h. Prednisone is biologically inactive but rapidly and completely converted in the liver to the active form, prednisolone, which has a plasma half-life of around 2–3 h. Some 20% of prednisolone is inactivated in the liver by conjugation by first-pass metabolism, leaving 80% of the oral dose bioavailable. Hepatic enzyme inducers such as rifampicin, barbiturates, and phenytoin can reduce the half-life of prednisolone by 50%. To counter the consequent reduction in anti-inflammatory activity the dose of oral prednisolone should be doubled in patients concurrently receiving these treatments. Drugs, such as itraconazole, reduce the rate of metabolism of corticosteroids, both oral and inhaled, increasing its blood level for a given dose.

Oral corticosteroids effect detectable improvement in airflow limitation in patients with asthma within 6–12 h of administration. In cases of severe asthma maximum improvement can take several days, probably reflecting the time to reverse the inflammatory changes in the airways.

The early use of oral corticosteroids in the treatment of asthma was severely limited by the high risk of unwanted effects, including osteoporosis, hypertension, diabetes mellitus, cataract formation, adrenal suppression, and (in children) growth suppression. The introduction in the 1970s of inhaled corticosteroids allowed local anti-inflammatory activity without limiting systemic side effects.

Inhaled corticosteroids

Inhaled corticosteroids are highly lipophilic and rapidly enter cells within the airways. They combine high topical potency with low systemic bioavailablilty of the swallowed dose and rapid metabolic clearance of any corticosteroid reaching the systemic circulation, conferring a high benefit:risk ratio. Although 80% to 90% of an inhaled dose from a metered dose inhaler is deposited in the oropharynx, swallowed, and absorbed, more than 80% of beclometasone, 90% of budesonide, and 99% of fluticasone is inactivated by first-pass metabolism in the liver. The 10 to 20% of the inhaled dose deposited in the airways is also absorbed from the lungs and misses first-pass metabolism, as does medication deposited in the oropharynx. For fluticasone and budesonide, devices that increase lung deposition (such as large-volume spacer and Turbohaler) therefore increase the dose available for systemic absorption.

Three inhaled corticosteroids are generally available at present: beclometasone diproprionate, budesonide, and fluticasone diproprionate. Beclometasone and budesonide are equipotent; fluticasone

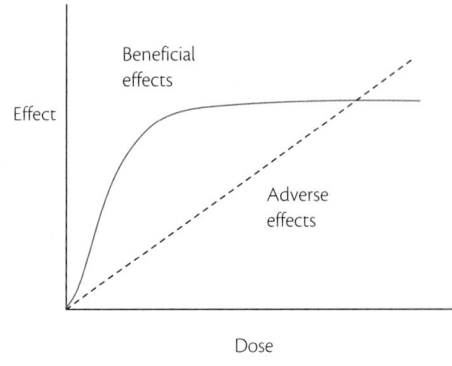

Fig. 18.7.7 Schematic dose–response curve for beneficial and adverse effects of inhaled corticosteroids. The beneficial effects are seen at lower doses and plateau. The adverse effects increase progressively with increasing dose.

is twice as potent, requiring half the dose to achieve the same benefit as beclometasone and budesonide. Ciclesonide, a new inhaled corticosteroid, is of equivalent potency to beclometasone; a second new inhaled corticosteroid, mometasone, is twice as potent as budesonide.

Inhaled corticosteroids have a dose–response relationship for both efficacy and adverse effects: in general most therapeutic benefit is obtained at low to moderate doses; further increases in dosage provide small increases in benefit but a steep rise in the incidence of adverse effects (Fig. 18.7.7).

The clinical effects and side effects of inhaled corticosteroids have been the subject of considerable clinical investigation. Systematic reviews of randomized controlled trials and additional randomized controlled trials of 393 adults and adolescents with mild, persistent asthma have shown that low-dose inhaled corticosteroids improve symptoms and lung function and reduce the need for as-needed inhaled bronchodilators as compared with placebo. In addition, a number of randomized controlled trials have shown that low-dose inhaled corticosteroids reduce the frequency of exacerbations in this group of patients. The OPTIMA trial, which compared inhaled budesonide 200 µg/day with placebo in 700 patients with mild persistent asthma who had not previously taken corticosteroids, found a significant reduction in exacerbation frequency in the budesonide group as compared to placebo (0.77 vs 0.29 exacerbations/year). The consistently shown benefits of inhaled corticosteroids in mild persistent asthma mean that these are the treatments of choice in this group of patients.

Inhaled corticosteroids are also effective in school-age children with mild and moderate persistent asthma. The START trial compared low-dose inhaled budesonide with placebo on the progression of asthma in adults and children (aged 5–11 years) with newly diagnosed mild persistent asthma as measured by time to first severe exacerbation requiring hospital treatment and decline in postbronchodilator FEV_1. By 3 years the frequency of exacerbations (6% vs 3%) and need for added treatment with inhaled corticosteroids (50% vs 30%) was greater in the placebo than the budesonide group.

Local side effects of inhaled corticosteroids

The severe adverse effects of systemic steroids and the widening indications for the use of inhaled corticosteroids have led to close scrutiny of their side effects. Oropharyngeal candidiasis (thrush) and dysphonia are well recognized and dose dependent. Oropharyngeal candidiasis occurs in about 5% of patients but can be problem, particularly in older people. The risk of its development can be reduced by the use of a large volume spacer and rinsing the mouth out after each inhaled dose. Dysphonia is the commonest side effect of inhaled steroids, occurring in at least one-third of patients. It can cause particular problems for public speakers and professional singers. It is believed to be due to a myopathy of the laryngeal muscles and reverses when treatment is stopped. Inhaled corticosteroids do not cause atrophy of the airway epithelium after 10 years of treatment and are not associated with an increased risk of pulmonary infection, including tuberculosis.

Systemic side effects of inhaled corticosteroids

Concern about systemic side effects of inhaled steroids stems from the need for their regular use for prolonged periods, of several years or decades, in both adults and children. Because many patients who take inhaled corticosteroids also require oral corticosteroids, distinguishing the adverse systemic effects of inhaled corticosteroids can be difficult.

Three important risks of inhaled corticosteroids that have been the subject of recent concern are osteoporosis in adults, and growth suppression and acute adrenal failure in children at the time of intercurrent infection. Studies that have addressed these outcomes are limited by their relatively short duration as compared to the length of time for which the treatment is usually taken in routine clinical practice.

In general, systematic reviews have found that inhaled corticosteroids are associated with a reduction in bone mineral density related to cumulative dose. In addition there is evidence for an increased risk of hip fracture in older people: a population-based case–control study using the United Kingdom General Practice Research Database comparing inhaled corticosteroid use between 16 341 cases of hip fracture and 29 889 control patients matched for age (mean 79 years), sex, and general practice found that the risk of hip fracture was increased by some 25% in those who had taken inhaled corticosteroids, and by some 20% after adjustment for use of oral corticosteroids.

Both asthma and oral corticosteroids can impair growth in children. Several short-term studies in growth during a 1-year period have found evidence for growth retardation of approximately 1.5 cm/year in children taking inhaled beclometasone 400 μg/day. However, a recent prospective study of children with asthma, followed up for an average of 9.2 years, taking budesonide in a mean daily dose of 412 μg, found the children to attain their expected adult height.

Several studies have found a dose-related reduction in adrenal cortisol secretion with increasing doses of inhaled corticosteroids. In comparison to the effect of oral prednisolone, 1 mg inhaled budesonide was equivalent to between 3 and 8.7 mg prednisolone, and 1 mg fluticasone to about 8.5 mg prednisolone. A number of cases of acute adrenal failure were recently reported in patients in United Kingdom taking inhaled corticosteroids. The risk of adrenal failure is also increased in patients taking itraconazole for ABPA, which inhibits hepatic corticosteroid metabolism.

The evidence for side effects caused by inhaled corticosteroids, particularly osteoporosis and adrenal suppression, is now sufficient to imply that the lowest dose of inhaled corticosteroid that is clinically effective should be prescribed in both children and adults, and particularly in patients taking topical corticosteroids by other routes (e.g. nose or skin), and the dose tapered to the minimum necessary when symptomatic and functional improvement

is achieved. However, in general current evidence indicates that inhaled corticosteroids do not cause important side effects in doses of beclometasone and budesonide of up to 400 μg/day in children and 800 μg/day in adults. The side effects that may occur at higher doses—more with beclometasone than with budesonide or fluticasone—can be reduced by the use of a spacer with metered-dose inhalers, and by rinsing the mouth after inhalation of a dry powder inhaler, which should be recommended when doses of 400 μg per day or more in children and 800 μg per day or more in adults are prescribed.

β_2-Adrenoreceptor agonists

The β-agonists are sympathomimetic amines that include catecholamines, both naturally occurring (adrenaline, noradrenaline, and dopamine) and synthetic (isoprenaline), and noncatecholamines, both short acting (e.g. salbutamol and terbutaline) and long acting (salmeterol and formoterol). Catecholamines have been replaced in the treatment of asthma by β_2-selective noncatecholamines. Noncatecholamines have a longer half-life than catecholamines because they are not subject to catecholamine uptake mechanisms and not broken down by catechol-O-methyl transferase (COMT). This means that the duration of bronchodilatation after inhalation of noncatecholamines is longer, salbutamol and terbutaline persisting for 3 to 6 h and salmeterol and formoterol for up to 12 h.

The actions of β-agonists in asthma are the result of stimulation of β-adrenoreceptors that are located in the airways, on airway epithelium, submucosal glands, airway and vascular smooth muscle. β-Receptors in the airways are entirely β_2, with the exception of some β_1 receptors on submucosal glands. β_2-Agonists can influence airways function through several mechanisms: relaxation of bronchial smooth muscle by direct effect on β_2 receptors; inhibition of mast cell mediator release; and enhanced mucociliary clearance.

Inhalation of a β_2-agonist by a patient with asthma increases airway calibre and reduces airway hyper-responsiveness. β_2-Agonists also cause tachycardia and increased cardiac output, systemic vasodilatation, and increased muscle blood flow. The tachycardia and increased cardiac output are the results of both stimulation of cardiac β adrenoreceptors and a reflex response to peripheral vasodilation. In addition, β_2-agonists cause tremor and have metabolic effects, of which hypokalaemia is probably the only one of clinical importance.

Inhaled selective, short-acting β_2-agonists reverse mild acute airway narrowing and are sufficient treatment, alone, for mild intermittent asthma causing occasional symptoms (Step 1 of the BTS guidelines: Table 18.7.4).

Studies in patients with asthma not taking inhaled corticosteroids comparing regular with as-needed inhaled β_2-agonists have shown that regular treatment confers no benefit over as needed inhalation and can have adverse consequences. An randomized controlled trial in 255 patients with mild intermittent asthma, comparing salbutamol taken as needed with regular treatment, found no difference at 16 weeks in respiratory symptoms, airway function, or frequency of exacerbations. However, those taking regular salbutamol took more salbutamol, showed more variability in peak flow rates, and had increased airway responsiveness to inhaled methacholine. Short-acting β_2-agonists should, in general, be reserved to provide reversal of acute airway narrowing, taken as-needed, and prior to exercise in patients with exercise-provoked asthma, except in cases of severe asthma not controlled with maximal

Table 18.7.4 Steps in the management of chronic asthma

Steps	Asthma severity	Treatment
Step 1	Mild intermittent	Short acting β_2 agonist as required
Step 2	Mild persistent	Low-dose ICS (BDP or BUD <800 μg/day, FP <500 μg/day, or DSG or nedocromil sodium plus short-acting β_2-agonist as required.
Step 3	Moderate persistent	High-dose ICS (BDP or BUD > 800 μg/day or FP > 500 μg/day OR low-dose ICS (as for Step 2) plus long acting β_2-agonist OR plus slow-release theophyllines plus short-acting β_2-agonist as required
Step 4	Severe persistent	High-dose ICS (as for Step 3) plus regular bronchodilator, e.g. long-acting β_2-agonist or slow-release theophylline or inhaled antimuscarinic or long-acting oral β_2-agonists or high-dose inhaled β_2-agonists
Step 5	'Difficult' (not responsive to maximal inhaled treatment)	Regular oral corticosteroids (in single daily dose) plus high-dose ICS and (as for Steps 3 and 4) long-acting bronchodilators (as for Step 4) and inhaled bronchodilators as required

BDP, beclomethasone; BUD, budesonide; DSG, deoxyspergualin; FP, fluticasone; ICS, inhaled corticosteroids.

doses of inhaled corticosteroids and additional long acting β_2-agonist (Step 4 of the BTS guidelines), when regular inhaled short-acting β_2-agonists can be added.

Two epidemics of asthma deaths, the first in the 1960s in six countries following the introduction of isoprenaline forte, the second in the mid 1970s in New Zealand after the introduction of fenoterol, led to concerns about the safety of inhaled β-agonists. Case–control studies have also identified an association between asthma deaths and overuse of inhaled β_2-agonists. However, it is difficult to distinguish cause and effect from confounding in these studies: overuse of β_2-agonists to treat frequent symptoms is more likely to occur in patients with severe uncontrolled asthma who

are at high risk of a fatal attack. The evidence for cause and effect in asthma epidemics is stronger: the increased death rates that followed the introduction of the particular inhaled β-agonists fell rapidly after recognition of the association and no other plausible explanation has been advanced. Isoprenaline is a nonselective β-agonist and fenoterol is less selective than salbutamol and terbutaline. Both drugs were marketed in high dose and are cardiotoxic in the presence of hypoxia, hence the two epidemics may have been due to the acute cardiac effects of β-agonists inhaled in high dose by hypoxic patients with acute severe asthma. The evidence that selective β_2-agonists formulated in lower doses have a similar cardiotoxic effect and cause asthma deaths outside these epidemics is limited to associations in case–control studies, from which it is not possible to infer cause and effect. However, a small effect can be difficult to detect and, as pointed out by Tattersfield, if a fatal arrhythmia occurred in 1 in 8000 patients treated with β-agonists each year this would account for 50% of asthma deaths in patients under 65 years, but its detection would require observation of many thousands of patients.

A systematic review and additional randomized controlled trials have shown that the addition of long-acting β_2-agonists (LABAs) improved respiratory symptoms and lung function with reduced requirement for 'rescue medication' as compared to doubling the dose of inhaled corticosteroid in patients with asthma poorly controlled by inhaled corticosteroids alone. The OPTIMA study investigated the addition of the LABA formoterol to the inhaled corticosteroid budesonide in patients with mild persistent asthma. In 700 patients with mild persistent asthma who had not previously used inhaled corticosteroids, the frequency of exacerbations was reduced in those taking budesonide 200 μg alone as compared with placebo (0.77 vs 0.29 exacerbations per patient per year). The addition of formoterol provided no further benefit in this group of patients with mild persistent asthma. In contrast, the addition of formoterol in patients with moderate persistent asthma already using inhaled corticosteroids provided significant benefit in exacerbation frequency, indicating that combination treatment is indicated in patients with moderate persistent asthma insufficiently controlled by low doses of inhaled corticosteroids (Fig. 18.7.8).

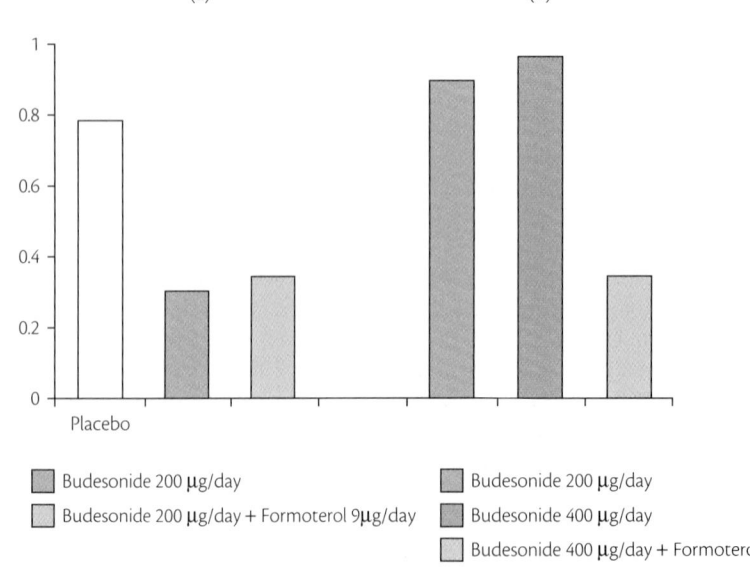

Fig. 18.7.8 Frequency of exacerbations—the OPTIMA Study. (a) In mild asthma frequency is reduced in patients taking budesonide 200 μg/day as compared to placebo, but there is no additional benefit from additional formoterol 9 μg/day. (b) In moderate asthma frequency is reduced in patients taking budesonide 400 μg/day and formoterol 9 μg/day as compared to budesonide 200 μg/day and budesonide 400 μg/day. (After O'Byrne P, *et al.* (2001). Low dose inhaled budesonide and formoterol in mild persistent asthma. The OPTIMA Randomised Trial. *Am J Respir Crit Care Med*, **164**, 1392–7.)

(a)   (b)

Placebo
■ Budesonide 200 μg/day
■ Budesonide 200 μg/day + Formoterol 9μg/day
■ Budesonide 200 μg/day
■ Budesonide 400 μg/day
■ Budesonide 400 μg/day + Formoterol 9μg/day

LABAs are intended for regular use with 12-h duration of action. Of the two currently used, salmeterol has a slower onset of action than formoterol. One systematic review and a number of additional randomized controlled trials have shown that in patients with moderately severe asthma, not controlled by low-dose inhaled corticosteroids, the addition of a LABA improved symptoms and lung function and reduced the need for rescue medication as compared to increasing the dose of inhaled corticosteroid. Several randomized controlled trials have shown that the addition of a LABA to an inhaled corticosteroid improved lung function as compared to the addition of a leukotriene antagonist. However, treatment with LABAs (both salmeterol and formoterol) has been associated with an increased frequency of exacerbations of asthma requiring hospitalization, of life-threatening exacerbations in both adults and children, and of asthma-related deaths. The SMART study, which followed more than 26 000 participants for 6 months, found a fourfold increase in the risk of asthma-related deaths in those taking salmeterol, which equated to 2 asthma-related deaths per 1000 patient years of salmeterol usage. Those most at risk of asthma-related deaths were African Americans, which might reflect an increase in asthma severity in this population and a high proportion taking salmeterol without an inhaled corticosteroid. A recent meta-analysis of the results from 19 trials with 33 826 participants found, as compared to placebo, a 2.6-fold increased risk of exacerbations requiring hospitalization, a 1.7-fold increased risk of life-threatening exacerbations; the risk of asthma-related deaths was also significantly increased. Furthermore, the risk for asthma exacerbations requiring hospitalization was increased twofold in patients taking salmeterol with concomitant inhaled corticosteroids.

To put these findings into context, the addition of a LABA to low-dose inhaled corticosteroids in patients with moderately severe asthma has been shown to provide greater improvement in symptoms and lung function than doubling the dose of inhaled corticosteroid. What is clearly important is not to prescribe a LABA without a concurrent inhaled cortico steroid, not to add a LABA unnecessarily in a patient with mild asthma adequately controlled on low-dose inhaled corticosteroids, and to discontinue a LABA in those patients with moderately severe asthma in whom it is not providing benefit.

Methylxanthines

Theophylline is the pharmacologically active methylxanthine most usually employed in clinical medicine, because of its greater bronchodilator activity, less erratic absorption and longer half-life than other methylxanthines. More predictable theophylline absorption can be obtained by slow-release formulations, and the addition of ethylene diamine to theophylline (aminophylline) provides the increased solubility required for intravenous administration. Nonetheless, theophylline has a relatively narrow 'therapeutic window' for a safe and effective dose, with wide differences between individuals in its metabolism, which can also be adversely affected by several extrinsic factors to cause clinically important side effects (Table 18.7.5). The most common side effects are 'caffeine-like' anorexia, nausea, and vomiting, followed by headache and insomnia. It increases the force and rate of heart contraction and causes vasodilatation, and in toxic doses it can cause arrhythmias that may be fatal. It is also a central nervous system stimulant causing increased alertness and—in toxic doses—confusion, irritability, and fits.

Theophylline relaxes bronchial smooth muscle and, like β-agonists, is a functional antagonist that causes bronchial muscle

Table 18.7.5 Factors influencing the half-life of theophylline

Increase half-life	Decrease half-life
Liver disease	Cigarette smoking
Heart failure	Alcohol
Virus infection	
Drugs	
Cimetidine	Rifampicin
Erythromycin	Barbiturates
Clarithromycin	Phenytoin
Ciprofloxacin	Carbamazepine
Oral contraceptives	

relaxation irrespective of the constrictor stimulus. Its action was previously thought to be mediated via phosphodiesterase inhibition increasing intracellular cAMP, but the intracellular concentration of theophylline necessary to achieve this is some 20 times greater than its therapeutic plasma levels. More recently, anti-inflammatory activity in 'sub-therapeutic' concentrations (i.e. <10 µg/ml) has been suggested as a possible mechanism of action in asthma.

Theophylline is metabolized to inactive products by cytochrome P450-dependent pathways in the liver. The variation between individuals is large and the half-life for theophylline can vary between 4 and 24 h. This may in part reflect the wide range of exogenous factors that influence hepatic metabolism of the drug. The half-life of theophylline is increased by several drugs—cimetidine (but not ranitidine), erythromycin, ciprofloxacin, and oral contraceptives—and decreased by rifampicin, barbiturates, and carbamazepine (see Table 18.7.5).

Bronchodilatation increases linearly with increase in serum theophylline concentration. Toxic effects show a similar linear relationship, but at higher concentrations, although there are considerable differences between individuals in the serum concentration at which side effects occur. Serum concentrations of between 10 and 20 µg/ml combine substantial bronchodilatation with a low risk of side effects. Safe, effective theophylline treatment requires monitoring of plasma concentration at the start of treatment to ensure a concentration within the therapeutic window, and subsequently to ensure its maintenance. This can be measured by immunoassay: in patients on regular, twice daily, maintenance treatment the difference between peak and trough levels is usually between 5 and 10 µg/ml, although greater in smokers, who may require three times daily treatment.

Theophyllines are now most commonly used as an additional treatment in patients whose asthma is inadequately controlled by inhaled corticosteroids. Comparison in a randomized controlled trial of budesonide 400 µg twice daily and theophylline (250 or 375 mg twice daily) with budesonide 800 µg twice daily for 3 months in 62 patients, whose asthma was not controlled by the lower dose of inhaled steroid, found the combination of low-dose inhaled corticosteroid and theophylline provided the greater improvement in lung function, peak flow variability, and β_2-agonist use. In those receiving it, median theophylline concentration was 8.7 µg/ml, and the additive effect was similar to that provided by inhaled salmeterol, suggesting that oral theophylline at doses lower than the conventional therapeutic dose can be an appropriate alternative to the addition of inhaled salmeterol where this does not provide adequate control at Stage 3 of the BTS guidelines.

Sodium cromoglicate

Sodium cromoglicate is a bischromone that has prophylactic but not bronchodilator activity in asthma. Originally available as a dry powder (mixed with lactose), it is now also formulated as a metered-dose inhaler and as a nebulizer solution. In inhalation tests it inhibits asthmatic reactions provoked by inhaled allergen, by exercise, and by other provocative stimuli including sulphur dioxide and adenosine, although it is less effective in a dose of 20 mg than salbutamol 200 μg in preventing asthma provoked by exercise. The major benefit of sodium cromoglicate is its safety, but it is less effective than inhaled corticosteroids and its use is now generally reserved for children with mild asthma, taken immediately prior to exercise to prevent exercise-induced asthma.

Nedocromil sodium

Nedocromil sodium has a similar activity profile to sodium cromoglicate. It is available as a metered-dose inhaler, needing to be taken four times a day. Its activity is equivalent to low-dose inhaled corticosteroid and it can be used either in place of inhaled corticosteroid or to reduce the dose of inhaled corticosteroid. Both sodium cromoglicate and nedocromil sodium are alternatives to inhaled corticosteroids in Step 2 of the BTS guidelines and may be tried when inhaled corticosteroids cause unacceptable hoarseness of the voice, as can occur occasionally.

Antileukotrienes

Antileukotrienes are new classes of anti-inflammatory drugs that inhibit leukotriene synthesis (5-lipoxygenase inhibitors) or antagonize leukotriene receptors (leukotriene receptor antagonists). The 5-lipoxygenase inhibitor zileuton inhibits the conversion of arachidonic acid into 5-hydroperoxyeicosatetraenoic acid (5-HPETE) prior to its transformation into cysteinyl-leukotriene A_4. The leukotriene receptor antagonists (montelukast, pranlukast, and zafirlukast) block the receptors for the cysteinyl-leukotrienes C_4, D_4, and E_4.

Anti-leukotrienes are used in the treatment of asthma as either single or combined therapy with inhaled corticosteroids. In general, systematic reviews of their efficacy as single therapy suggest they are safe but less effective than inhaled corticosteroids in preventing asthma exacerbations. Beclometasone 400 μg/day and fluticasone 200 μg/day are superior in efficacy to montelukast 10 mg/day and zafirlukast 20 mg twice daily. However, in patients whose asthma is not sufficiently controlled with beclometasone 400–800 μg/day (or equivalent) the addition of a leukotriene antagonist in usual doses has been found to provide some improvement in asthma control, but although the addition of a leukotriene antagonist may be an alternative to doubling the dose of inhaled corticosteroids, in adults with moderate persistent asthma both are less effective than the addition of a long-acting β_2-agonist in improving asthma control.

Antileukotrienes are generally safe at usual licensed doses, but increasing the licensed dose two- to fourfold—although associated with increased efficacy—is not recommended because of the two- to fourfold increased risk of abnormal liver function tests. Churg–Strauss syndrome has now been reported with all marketed antileukotrienes, with one systematic review identifying 22 cases in patients taking antileukotrienes, but the total number of patients taking antileukotrienes in whom these cases occurred was not stated.

The 'stepped' approach to the treatment of asthma

The purpose of treatment of asthma varies in different patients, from the reversal of occasional mild symptoms to the restoration of normal life in a patient with severe disabling ill health. Treatment needs vary greatly between different patients, which is reflected in the 'stepped' approach to treatment that is the basis of current guidelines for asthma management, including the British Thoracic Society (BTS) and Scottish Intercollegiate Guidelines Network (SIGN) guidelines that are regularly updated. In the stepped approach, asthma severity is defined by the treatment step needed to achieve and maintain good control (see Table 18.7.4).

Inhaled corticosteroids form the mainstay of maintenance treatment for most patients, the initial dose being that considered on clinical grounds the dose most likely to control the disease. Inhaled β_2-agonists are used primarily for symptomatic relief. There is good evidence that regular treatment with short-acting β_2-agonists alone is less effective than regular inhaled corticosteroids and provides less good control of asthma, both symptomatically and of lung function.

Steps 1 to 5 of the BTS guidelines identify the treatment requirements for asthma of increasing severity (see Table 18.7.4). Failure to achieve treatment targets at any step implies the need to increase treatment to a step that provides good control.

◆ Step 1—patients with mild intermittent asthma whose asthma is controlled by the use of an inhaled shorter-acting β_2-agonist (e.g. salbutamol or terbutaline) less than once a day. Requirement for more regular treatment implies the need for regular anti-inflammatory treatment (i.e. a higher step).

◆ Step 2—patients with mild persistent or intermittent asthma that is of sufficient frequency to require regular anti-inflammatory treatment. Inhaled corticosteroids are the most effective and commonly used anti-inflammatory drugs. Treatment with an inhaled corticosteroid should be started at a dose of beclometasone 400 μg twice daily (or equivalent) in adults and 200 μg twice daily in children. This dose should be continued for at least 3 months, the period when most benefit of the inhaled steroid is obtained, before reducing the dose to the minimum required to maintain good control. This can be achieved by reducing the dose by 25 to 50% every 1 to 3 months. Short-acting β_2-agonists are used as required for symptomatic relief.

◆ Step 3—patients with moderate persistent asthma whose disease, despite adherence to treatment and correct inhaler technique, is not controlled. The treatment of choice is the addition of a LABA, which should be continued if it provides good asthma control. If it provides benefit, but asthma remains inadequately controlled, the dose of inhaled corticosteroid should be doubled (e.g. beclometasone 400 to 800 μg/day). If the LABA provides no benefit, then it should be discontinued and the inhaled steroid dose doubled, and if this does not provide adequate control a trial of other treatments such as a slow-release theophylline or leukotriene antagonist should be instituted.

◆ Step 4—if asthma control remains poor despite the measures recommended in Step 3, consideration should be given to increasing further the dose of the inhaled corticosteroid to the equivalent of beclometasone 2000 µg/day, or to the addition of a fourth drug, e.g. slow-release theophylline, a leukotriene antagonist, or an oral β₂-agonist.

◆ Step 5—patients who fail to respond to these combinations of Step 4 treatments will require the addition of an oral corticosteroid while continuing high-dose inhaled corticosteroid treatment. The dose of oral corticosteroid should be the lowest to provide adequate control, which is an important decision that should be made in consultation with a respiratory physician. Patients who require oral corticosteroids for longer than 3 months or need frequent courses of oral corticosteroids are at risk of systemic side effects including hypertension, diabetes mellitus, and osteoporosis. A long-acting bisphosphonate should be prescribed for those taking oral corticosteroids for more than 3 months, with their bone mineral density monitored regularly. Children should have their growth monitored and eyes regularly examined for cataracts. There is no reliable evidence for a steroid-sparing effect in the treatment of asthma for immunosuppressants such as methotrexate and gold, and inconsistent evidence for ciclosporin.

Most cases of asthma in the community are mild—Steps 1 and 2 of the BTS guidelines; 'difficult' asthma, requiring treatment equivalent to Step 5, constitutes less than 5% of cases. A community study of five large general practices in South Nottinghamshire, England (a population of 38 865) found a prevalence of asthma of 9%, with a peak of 17% in 10 to 14-year-olds, falling to less than 6% in adults aged more than 70 years. Most patients with diagnosed asthma were either not receiving treatment (8%) or receiving treatment equivalent to Steps 1 and 2 (76%); 11% were on Step 3 and some 5% on Steps 4 and 5. The authors endeavoured to assess the effectiveness of asthma treatment in this population by measuring the proportion of patients who during a 1-year period required oral corticosteroid courses or were prescribed 10 or more short acting β₂-agonist inhalers: 12.5% patients not taking them regularly had been prescribed one or more courses of oral corticosteroids, 1.6% on three or more occasions; 13.6% patients had been prescribed 10 or more short-acting β₂-agonist inhalers; both outcomes were increasingly more frequent in patients on Steps 3 or higher of the BTS guidelines. However, because only a few patients (15%) were in these categories, more than one-half of the patients who required either oral corticosteroids or 10 or more β₂-agonist inhalers were on Steps 1 or 2, indicating continuing significant morbidity among some cases of asthma receiving either low dose or no anti-inflammatory treatment.

Difficult asthma

Difficult asthma is asthma that is not controlled by maximum doses of inhaled treatment, including inhaled corticosteroids in doses of beclometasone of up to 2000 µg/day (or equivalent) with additional treatment such as long-acting β₂-agonists. It is uncommon, probably less than 5% of asthmatics, but important. The severity of disease and associated disability is considerable: the risks of near fatal and fatal asthma are high, and the adverse consequences of treatment are severe and worthwhile only if these are demonstrably effective.

Box 18.7.2 Difficult asthma—why is it failing to respond?

1 Does patient have asthma?
◆ Is there evidence of significant response to bronchodilators/steroids?
◆ Have other relatively common causes of similar symptoms been excluded?
  · COPD (irreversible airflow limitation)
  · Localized obstruction
  · Left heart failure
  · Pulmonary thromboembolic disease
  · Vocal cord dysfunction
◆ Have other relatively uncommon causes of similar symptoms been excluded?
  · Vasculitis—Churg–Strauss syndrome

2 Is prescribed treatment reaching the airways?
◆ Is patient taking the treatment (inhaled and oral)
◆ Is inhaler technique satisfactory?

3 Are there any unrecognized provoking factors?
◆ Domestic allergens—particularly cats
◆ Occupational agents
◆ Drugs—e.g. aspirin, NSAIDs, β-blockers
◆ Upper airway disease—rhinitis/sinusitis
◆ Gastro-oesophageal reflux

4 Does the patient have a particular type of difficult asthma?
◆ Unstable asthma:
  · Nocturnal asthma
  · Premenstrual asthma
  · Brittle asthma—type I, type II
◆ Corticosteroid-dependent asthma
◆ Corticosteroid-resistant asthma

5 Are there significant psychological and social factors?

Failure to respond to maximal inhaled treatment can result from several causes (Box 18.7.2). It is clearly important to confirm the diagnosis of asthma and ensure the patient is taking the asthma treatment prescribed: misdiagnosis and poor compliance with medication represent a significant proportion of patients with 'difficult asthma'. The conditions most easily mistaken for asthma were considered earlier in this chapter (see 'Differential diagnosis'). Demonstration of spontaneous variability or reversibility of airflow limitation is important to avoid treatment of irreversible airflow limitation, due either to localized obstruction or to chronic obstructive pulmonary disease (COPD) with ever-increasing doses of oral corticosteroids. Assessment of reversibility may require a formal steroid trial of oral prednisolone 30–40 mg taken each morning for 1 month to determine whether this provides significant improvement in airway function.

Having confirmed the diagnosis of asthma, it is important to ensure good inhaler technique and adherence to prescribed treatment, failure to take treatment properly being a common reason for failure to respond. This may reflect lack of understanding that preventive treatment needs to be taken regularly and not 'as needed', or poor inhaler technique. Patients may take preventive treatment irregularly because, unlike short-acting β_2-agonists, it does not provide immediate symptomatic relief. Others may be inappropriately concerned about potential side effects or resent the need to take regular inhaled treatment. In patients taking oral corticosteroids blood eosinophil count is markedly reduced and often reported as 0. Failure to take prednisone can be confirmed by demonstrating its absence in serum. A blood eosinophil count above 0.3×10^9/litre in a patient prescribed oral steroid suggests that this drug is not to being taken regularly, or alternatively that another disease—particularly Churg–Strauss syndrome—may accompany the asthma.

One study, using a computerized timing device in a dry powder inhaler, found only 18% of patients took inhaled steroids as prescribed. However, in routine clinical practice adherence to inhaled treatment is difficult to monitor. Poor treatment adherence may be suspected as a cause of difficult asthma in patients whose asthma improves when treatment, although unchanged, is supervised. Patient understanding of the effectiveness of regular treatment may also be reinforced by this means.

Unidentified provoking factors include allergens, commonly domestic pets (in particular cats), whose allergens can be present in sufficient concentrations to cause asthma for several months after the animals have left the home. Sensitizing agents encountered at work can also cause asthma that is poorly controlled by inhaled treatment. Early identification and avoidance of the cause is important to minimize the risk of development of chronic asthma. Aspirin, NSAIDs, and β-blockers can also be important provoking factors.

Rhinitis commonly accompanies asthma, and its treatment can be associated with improvement in asthma and airway hyperresponsiveness. The explanation for this association is unclear but may be a consequence of inflammatory mediators in postnasal drip increasing airway responsiveness and provoking cough. Similarly, gastro-oesophageal reflux can provoke cough and worsen asthma, and a trial with a proton pump inhibitor such as omeprazole should be instituted when this is suspected to an exacerbating factor, although objective improvement in asthma with such treatment is uncommon.

Uncommonly asthma may be a manifestation of systemic disease, particularly a systemic vasculitis—Churg–Strauss syndrome—when asthma, which can be difficult to control, is accompanied by a high blood eosinophil count (usually >1.5×10^9/litre). Other manifestations include eosinophilic pneumonia, pleural and pericardial effusions, and mononeuritis multiplex. Effective treatment requires high dose oral corticosteroids and in some cases other immunosuppressant treatment.

Nocturnal asthma can persist in some patients despite treatment with inhaled corticosteroids that provides good daytime control. This may be improved by the addition of a long-acting β_2-agonist or slow-release theophylline.

Premenstrual deterioration of asthma is not uncommon, and in some women can be severe and unresponsive to corticosteroid treatment. Characteristically symptoms increase and PEF falls 2 to 5 days before the menstrual period, improving with the onset of menstruation that coincides with the fall in progesterone secretion and increase in oestrogen:progesterone ratio. Some patients are improved by treatment with intramuscular, but not oral, progestogen during the week before menstruation. Patients with severe premenstrual exacerbations can require hospital admission, in some cases ventilation, and may only be improved by surgical removal of the ovaries. There is also now the option of inducing a short-term chemical menopause with GnRH analogues prior to surgery.

Brittle asthma is characterized by widely varying peak flow rates uncontrolled by maximum inhaled treatment. Two patterns have been distinguished: type I, where there is persistent chaotic daily variability in peak flow (usually >40% diurnal variation in PEF> 50% of time), and type II, where there are sporadic sudden falls in PEF against a background of usually well-controlled asthma with normal or near normal lung function.

Treatment of brittle asthma of both types is difficult. Type I brittle asthma, not responding to inhaled long-acting β_2-agonists or regular nebulized β_2-agonists, can be improved by subcutaneous terbutaline administered via an insulin infusion pump, usually in a dose of between 3 and 12 mg in 24 h. Treatment is limited by side effects, of which the most important is muscle cramp associated with increased levels of serum creatinine kinase. Type II brittle asthma requires immediately available treatment for what can be catastrophic falls in peak flow. The speed of onset of attacks requires immediately injected bronchodilator. Such patients should have preloaded adrenaline syringes (e.g. Epi-pen) available at all times and wear a medical ID bracelet (e.g. MedicAlert). Potential provoking factors, such as foods, should be sought and avoided.

In a very few patients asthma is only controlled with continuous oral corticosteroids, often in high doses, reduction in dose being followed by worsening of asthma. The term 'corticosteroid-dependent asthma' has been used for such patients. They differ from corticosteroid-resistant asthma in their response to oral corticosteroids, patients with corticosteroid-resistant asthma showing no response to oral corticosteroids even in high dose, although they do show spontaneous variability of peak flow and reversibility with inhaled bronchodilators. Corticosteroid-resistant asthma is very uncommon, estimated at between 1 in 1000 and 1 in 10 000 patients, and it probably forms the end of a spectrum of resistance to the anti-inflammatory activity of corticosteroids to which corticosteroid-dependent asthma also belongs. Treatment of corticosteroid-resistant asthma is difficult, but should include stopping oral corticosteroids—which still cause side effects—and relying on other forms of treatment, including long-acting β_2-agonists.

Several treatments including methotrexate, gold, and ciclosporin have been evaluated in the treatment of asthma. In general these have not provided robust evidence of benefit in patients with severe asthma. In addition, two monoclonal antibodies—anti TNFα (etanercept) and anti IgE (omalizumab)—have been shown to provide benefit in patients with severe asthma in early trials. Their possible place in the treatment of these 2 agents is still being evaluated.

Acute exacerbations of asthma

Asthma exacerbations are episodes of progressively worsening airway narrowing associated with increasing shortness of breath, cough, wheezing, and chest tightness, or some combination of these.

They can vary in severity from episodes in which patients are able to manage themselves by following an agreed treatment plan, to severe and potentially life-threatening episodes that require medical attention and hospital admission. Severe attacks can vary in their speed of onset from deterioration over days to episodes that progress rapidly and can become life threatening within minutes or hours. In about one-half of cases of fatal asthma the attack lasted more than 24 h, in one-quarter less than 1 h.

Fatal or near fatal attacks of asthma are associated with:

♦ Patients who have previously required hospital admission for severe asthma and who require regular oral steroid treatment

♦ Failure to recognize severity of asthma by the patient: those with long-standing asthma can become accustomed to their symptoms and not appreciate an important increase in their severity that may persist for days or weeks, sometimes associated with psychosocial problems and poor adherence to treatment

♦ Failure to recognize the severity of asthma by the doctor, the risk of which can be minimized by making appropriate objective measurements of respiratory, heart, and peak flow rates to assess severity

♦ Undertreatment or inappropriate treatment: failure to use oral corticosteroids in adequate doses early in an exacerbation is probably the single commonest remediable factor; the use of sedatives or anxiolytics to reduce the anxiety or agitation that can often accompany acute severe asthma is absolutely contraindicated

Many of these problems can be overcome by improved patient understanding, allowing them to have control over their illness supported by a jointly agreed management plan.

Moderate exacerbations

Exacerbations of asthma with increased symptoms, both during the daytime and at night, frequently follow a viral infection or allergen exposure in allergic individuals (or both), or a reduction in anti-inflammatory treatment. The increase in symptoms, associated with deterioration in peak flow, is often treated adequately by the patient increasing the frequency of inhaled short-acting bronchodilators, doubling the dose of inhaled steroids, or taking a short course of oral steroids. Several studies have shown that early treatment with oral corticosteroids taken at the start of an acute exacerbation reduces the need for hospital admission, the frequency of relapse, and the need for β_2-agonists. One recent overview of 7 randomized controlled trials in 320 patients found that systemic corticosteroids, taken at the onset of an acute exacerbation, reduced hospital admissions in both children and adults by 65% in the first week compared with placebo, an effect maintained for 21 days. No difference was observed between the use of oral and intramuscular corticosteroids. Oral corticosteroids continued for a short period after hospital discharge reduce the risk of early relapse, which occurs in some 10 to 15% of patients following discharge after emergency treatment. A Cochrane review of seven trials comparing oral corticosteroid treatment with placebo following discharge found a two-thirds reduction in relapse rate in those taking oral corticosteroids and a reduced need for β_2-agonists at 1 and at 3 weeks after discharge.

Severe exacerbations

Acute severe asthma is a potentially life-threatening increase in the severity of asthma that can develop over minutes, hours, or days, and which has often failed to respond to conventional inhaled bronchodilator treatment. It is usually the outcome of airways increasingly narrowed by the consequences of chronic inflammation to cause increasing resistance to airflow identified as a reduction in PEF and FEV_1, hyperinflated lungs, ventilation–perfusion inequality, and hypoxia, which is the most serious consequence of severe asthma. Initially these stimulate alveolar hyperventilation with a reduction in P_{CO_2}, but—with increasing airway narrowing and exhaustion—arterial pO_2 continues to fall while arterial P_{CO_2} rises to normal, and subsequently increases steeply with the development of alveolar hypoventilation. In general, P_{CO_2} rises into the normal range when FEV_1 is some 25% and PEF 30% of predicted normal values.

The clinical features of importance in identifying acute severe asthma and assessing its severity are shown in Box 18.7.3. Patients are usually extremely breathless and unable to complete sentences in one breath. A rapid respiratory rate and heart rate are good markers of severity of asthma and hypoxia. Although anxiety and increased use of β_2-agonists can increase heart rate, a rapid heart rate should not be ignored by attributing it to these factors. An objective measure of airflow should be obtained because the severity of limitation is difficult to assess clinically. Although PEF is an effort-dependent measurement it is usually possible to obtain a reading from patients with severe asthma: a value of less than 50% of predicted or of the recent best value in an adult aged less than 50 years usually indicates severe asthma; a value of less than 33% indicates a potentially life-threatening attack.

Arterial blood gas analysis should be made in adults seen in hospital as an important guide to the severity of asthma; children can often be managed safely by measurement of Sao_2 alone. Most patients admitted to hospital with acute severe asthma are hypoxic, of whom about one-third will have Po_2 <8 kPa (60 mmHg). P_{CO_2} is reduced in patients with moderately severe asthma, but with increasingly severe airways obstruction and fatigue P_{CO_2} falls and

---

Box 18.7.3 Acute severe asthma: assessment of severity

Features of acute severe asthma

♦ Unable to complete sentences in one breath

♦ Respiration rate >25 breaths/min

♦ Pulse rate >110 beats/min

♦ Peak expiratory flow rate <50% predicted or best

Life-threatening features

♦ PEF <33% predicted or best

♦ Silent chest

♦ Bradycardia or hypotension

♦ Exhaustion, confusion, or coma

Markers of life-threatening attack

♦ Normal (5–6 kPa or 36–44 mmHg) or high P_{CO_2}

♦ Severe hypoxia: Po_2 <8 kPa (60 mmHg)

♦ Low pH or high $[H^+]$

subsequently rises in parallel with a falling P_{O_2}. A normal P_{CO_2} in a hypoxic patient with acute severe asthma indicates impending hypoventilation, with a rapidly increasing P_{CO_2}, falling P_{O_2}, acidosis, narcosis, and death.

Management

The aims of the treatment of acute severe asthma are to reverse the hypoxia, airflow limitation and airway inflammation with oxygen, bronchodilators, and corticosteroids (Box 18.7.4).

Oxygen

Oxygen relieves the hypoxia present in most patients with acute severe asthma. High concentrations of inspired oxygen are safe in patients with asthma, and certainly in those aged less than 50 years; a high Pa_{CO_2} in acute severe asthma reflects fatigue and the severity of airways obstruction and is not a contraindication for a high concentration of inspired oxygen. Oxygen can be administered by nasal cannulae or by face mask in high concentrations (usually F_{IO_2} between 40 and 60%). The aim is to increase Sa_{O_2} to above 92% or Pa_{O_2} to above 9 kPa (80 mmHg).

Bronchodilators

The purpose of bronchodilator treatment in acute severe asthma is to reverse the airway narrowing due to smooth muscle contraction, before the onset of the anti-inflammatory action of corticosteroids that usually takes 6 to 12 h from administration.

Box 18.7.4 Treatment of acute severe asthma

Initial treatment

- Oxygen (60% F_{IO_2})
- Nebulized salbutamol 2.5–5 mg or terbutaline 5–10 mg (driven by oxygen via nebulizer)
- Oral prednisolone 30–60 mg or intravenous hydrocortisone 200 mg

If poor response to initial treatment after 15–30 min

- Continue oxygen
- Repeat nebulized salbutamol 5 mg after 15 min
- Add ipatropium 0.5 mg to nebulized β-agonist
- Intravenous hydrocortisone 200 mg 4 hourly
- Consider intravenous magnesium sulphate 1.2–2 g over 20 min
- Investigations:
  - Chest radiograph to exclude pneumothorax
  - Monitor serum K⁺ (risk of hypokalaemia with high-dose β-agonist)
- Consider intravenous salbutamol (see text)
- Consider intravenous aminophylline (see text)

If poor response within 1 h

- Admit to intensive care for possible intubation and ventilation

---

Inhaled bronchodilators

Inhaled high-dose β₂-agonists (salbutamol, terbutaline) administered by spacer or nebulizer are used as initial treatment. The benefit of a nebulizer is that it allows inhalation of bronchodilator to be driven by a high flow of oxygen, which can be important in severe and life-threatening asthma as β₂-agonists may increase ventilation–perfusion inequality and consequent arterial hypoxia, hence β₂-agonists should not be administered without oxygen to those who are hypoxic. Nebulized salbutamol (5 mg) or terbutaline (10 mg) driven by 6 litres/min oxygen can be given safely by trained ambulance crews during transfer to hospital. However, nebulizers are inefficient and widely variable in their performance, which has led to the suggestion that large volume spacers be used as alternative delivery systems. In adults and children with severe but not life-threatening asthma, inhalation of β₂-agonist by nebulizer has not been found to provide additional bronchodilatation as compared to inhalation of a metered dose inhaler via a spacer, and the latter is associated with fewer side effects. However, it should be appreciated that the studies on which these observations are based are of patients with moderately severe asthma who did not require hospital admission. Spacers do not easily allow concurrent administration of oxygen and require patient cooperation, which can be difficult in severely breathless patients.

Intravenous bronchodilators

The intravenous bronchodilators used in clinical practice are β₂-agonists and theophylline. The theoretical advantage of giving β₂-agonists intravenously rather than by inhalation is access to peripheral airways so narrowed that they cannot be reached by inhalation, although inhaled salbutamol is rapidly absorbed from the lungs, reaching a peak concentration within 10 min of inhalation. The major disadvantage of intravenous β₂ agonists, in comparison to inhalation, is the greater frequency of systemic side effects. However, the key clinical question is whether intravenous β₂-agonists provide additional improvement in bronchodilator response to inhaled β₂-agonists and corticosteroids. In adults with acute asthma, intravenous salbutamol 12 µg/min taken 4 hourly after an initial dose of nebulized salbutamol 5 mg and intravenous hydrocortisone provided greater bronchodilation as compared to three further doses of nebulized salbutamol given during 2 h, although the patients receiving intravenous salbutamol had a greater increase in heart rate. Similarly, in a study of children with acute severe asthma, the addition of salbutamol (15 µg/kg) in a 10-min infusion to nebulized salbutamol and intravenous hydrocortisone was associated with a reduced period of need for inhaled salbutamol, a decreased requirement for oxygen, and earlier discharge from the Emergency Department.

The use of intravenous aminophylline in the treatment of asthma has decreased with the recognition that it does not provide additional benefit to repeated or continuous nebulized β₂-agonist bronchodilators in the initial hours of emergency treatment. This, together with its narrow therapeutic window, need for drug monitoring, and interactions with other drugs, has led to its replacement as first-line bronchodilator treatment of asthma by inhaled β₂-agonists. However, it is recommended as additional therapy for patients not responding to initial treatment with inhaled β₂-agonists and corticosteroids and as initial treatment in the very severely ill patient with a normal or high P_{CO_2}. In patients who have not been taking theophylline prior to admission, a loading dose of 5 mg/kg body weight over 20 min should be followed by a maintenance dose of 0.5 mg/kg body weight per hour until a serum level of 10 to 20 µg/litre is obtained. The loading dose should be omitted in those currently taking theophyllines, in whom the serum concentration should be measured. The infusion rate should be decreased in patients with liver or heart failure, or in those taking cimetidine, macrolide antibiotics (erythromycin, clarithromycin) or ciprofloxacin. Toxic side effects are increasingly common in patients whose serum level exceeds 25 µg/litre, ranging from gastrointestinal symptoms to fits and cardiac arrhythmias.

Antimuscarinics

The purpose of antimuscarinic treatment is to reverse airway narrowing caused by increased vagal tone that is not responsive to high-dose inhaled β_2 agonists. Several studies have suggested the addition of a nebulized antimuscarinic provides additional benefit in the treatment of acute severe asthma, both in children and in adults. A Cochrane review in children found that multiple doses of ipatropium bromide in addition to a β_2-agonist significantly increased FEV_1 and reduced the risk of hospital admission in comparison to a β_2-agonist alone in moderate and severe exacerbations of asthma. A Cochrane review of similar combination therapy in adults found consistent evidence for similar improvements in FEV_1 and reduction in hospital admissions. Systematic reviews have confirmed the benefits of using inhaled ipatropium bromide in combination with a β_2-agonist in the treatment of patients with moderate to severe acute asthma.

Magnesium

Systematic reviews have shown that intravenous magnesium sulphate is a safe and effective treatment in patients with exacerbations of severe asthma. A Cochrane review found that in severe asthma the addition of magnesium sulphate to a β_2-agonist and intravenous corticosteroids improved lung function and reduced the need for hospitalization, without causing adverse effects.

Corticosteroids

Systemic corticosteroids are given in acute severe asthma to reverse the underlying airway inflammation, such anti-inflammatory action requiring 6 to 12 h from administration for demonstrable bronchodilatation to occur. Within 1 h of their administration, steroids may also reverse β_2 receptor desensitization induced by regular β_2 inhalation.

The value of corticosteroid treatment in acute severe asthma was first demonstrated in a randomized controlled trial in 1956 and has since been generally accepted. Corticosteroids are usually given by intravenous administration, but other than in life-threatening asthma and in patients vomiting or unable to swallow, there is no demonstrable advantage of intravenous over oral administration. When indicated, intravenous doses initially of 200 mg hydrocortisone 4 to 6 hourly can be followed by oral prednisolone in a dose of 40 to 60 mg/day. The duration of treatment with oral prednisolone will depend on the severity of and rate of recovery from the acute episode. In general, oral prednisolone should be continued until resolution of the acute episode with return to usual daytime activities, resolution of nocturnal symptoms, and PEF within 80% of the patient's predicted or best values. Short courses of oral corticosteroids (taken for <2 weeks) do not need to be tapered provided patients are taking an appropriate dose of inhaled corticosteroid. Although some studies in patients with relatively mild exacerbations of asthma (PEF >60% predicted or best) have suggested that

> **Box 18.7.5** Acute severe asthma
>
> #### Indications for intensive care
> - Hypoxia (Pao_2 <8 kPa) despite Fio_2 60%
> - Hypercapnoea ($Paco_2$ > 6 kPa)
> - Exhaustion with feeble respiration
> - Confusion or drowsiness
> - Unconsciousness
> - Respiratory arrest
>
> #### Indications for intermittent positive-pressure ventilation (IPPV)
> - Hypoxia (Pao_2 <8 kPa) despite 60% Fio_2
> - Increasing hypercapnoea
> - Drowsiness or unconsciousness
> - Respiratory arrest

high-dose inhaled steroids are an effective alternative to oral corticosteroids, these results should not to extrapolated to acute severe asthma where the recommended guideline is that all patients should be given systemic corticosteroid treatment.

Intensive care and intermittent positive pressure ventilation

Most attacks of acute severe asthma respond to treatment with high inspired oxygen, systemic corticosteroids and inhaled β_2-agonists. However, this treatment is insufficient in a few cases, which require intensive care and—on occasion—intermittent positive-pressure ventilation (IPPV). This need arises in two particular situations: patients who have a catastrophic hyperacute attack, and those whose asthma progressively increases in severity despite maximal bronchodilator and corticosteroid treatment. The indications for intensive care and IPPV are given in Box 18.7.5. Patients with increasing drowsiness or who lose consciousness with hypoxia and worsening hypercapnoea require IPPV, as do those who suffer a respiratory arrest. However, because of the high inflation pressures needed to overcome the high airway resistance and hyperinflated lungs and chest wall, IPPV in acute severe asthma can be difficult and hazardous. High inflation pressures can cause barotrauma with pneumomediastinum and, on occasion, pneumothorax. In addition, up to one-third of patients develop clinically significant hypotension, requiring inotropic support.

Further reading

Barnes PB (1998). Current issues for establishing inhaled corticosteroids as the anti-inflammatory agents of choice in asthma. *J Allergy Clin Immunol*, **101**, 5427–33.

Barnes PJ, Pederson S, Busse WW (1998). Efficiency and safety of inhaled corticosteroids. *Am J Rsp Crit Care Med*, **157**, 551–3.

Berry MA, *et al.* (2006). Evidence of role of tumour necrosis factor α in refractory asthma. *N Engl J Med*, **354**, 697–708.

Drazen JM, Israel E, Boushey HA *et al.* (1996). Comparison of regularly scheduled with as needed use of albuterol in mild asthma. Asthma clinical research network. *New Eng J Med*, **335**, 841–7.

Evans DJ, *et al.* (1997). A comparison of low dose inhaled budesonide plus theophylline and high dose inhaled budesonide for moderate asthma. *New Engl J Med*, **337**, 1412–18.

Garbelt JF, *et al.* (1997). Nebulised salbutamol with and without ipratropium bromide in the treatment of acute asthma. *J Allergy Clin Immunol*, **100**, 165–70.

Gibson PG, Powell H (2004). Written action plans for asthma: an evidence based review of key components. *Thorax*, **59**, 94–9.

Green RH, *et al.* (2002). Asthma exacerbations and sputum eosinophil counts: a randomised controlled trial. *Lancet*, **360**, 1715–21.

Greening AP, *et al.* (1994). Added salmeterol versus higher dose corticosteroid in asthma patients with symptoms on existing inhaled corticosteroid. *Lancet*, **344**, 219–24.

Haahtela T, *et al.* (1991). Comparison of a β_2 agonist terbutaline with an inhaled corticosteroid budesonide in newly detected asthma. *New Engl J Med*, **325**, 388–92.

Haahtela T, *et al.* (1994). Effects of reducing or discontinuing inhaled budesonide in patients with mild asthma. *New Engl J Med*, **331**, 700–5.

Jayaram L, *et al.* (2006). Determining asthma treatment by monitoring sputum cell counts: effect on exacerbations. *Eur Respir J*, **27**, 483–94.

Lipworth B (1999). Systemic adverse effects of inhaled corticosteroid therapy. A systematic review and meta-analysis. *Arch Intern Med*, **159**, 941–55.

Mallia P, Johnston S (2006). How viral infections cause exacerbations of airway disease. *Chest*, **130**, 1203–10.

Marquette CH, *et al.* (1992). A 6 year follow up study 145 asthmatic patients who underwent mechanical ventilation for near-fatal attack of asthma. *Am Rev Respir Dis*, **146**, 76–81.

Mortimer KJ, Tattersfield AE (2005). Benefit versus risk for oral inhaled and nasal glucocorticosteroids. *Immunol Allergy Clin North Am*, **25**, 523–39.

Nicholson PJ, *et al.* (2005). Evidence based guidelines for the prevention, identification, and management of occupational asthma. *Occup Environ Med*, **62**, 290–9.

Nowak D (2006). Management of asthma with anti-immunoglobulin E: a review of clinical trials of omalizumab. *Respir Med*, **100**, 1907–17.

O'Byrne P, *et al.* (2001). Low dose inhaled budesonide and formoterol in mild persistent asthma. The OPTIMA Randomised Trial. *Am J Respir Crit Care Med*, **164**, 1392–7.

Pauwels RA, *et al.* (1997). Effect of inhaled formoterol and budesonide on exacerbations of asthma. *New Engl J Med*, **337**, 1405–11.

Pauwels RA, *et al.* (2003). Early intervention with budesonide in mild persistent asthma: a randomised double-blind trial. *Lancet*, **361**, 1071–6.

Tattersfield AE, Postma DS, Barnes PJ (1999). Exacerbations of asthma. A descriptive study of 425 severe exacerbations. *Am J Respir Crit Care Med*, **160**, 594–9.

Todd GRG, *et al.* (2003). Survey of adrenal crisis associated with inhaled corticosteroids in the United Kingdom. *Arch Dis Child*, **87**, 457–61.

Walsh LJ, *et al.* (1999). Morbidity from asthma in relation to regular treatment: a community based study. *Thorax*, **54**, 296–300.

Woolcock AJ, *et al.* (1996). Comparison of addition of salmeterol to inhaled steroids with doubling of the dose of inhaled steroids. *Am J Respir Crit Care Med*, **153**, 1481–8.

Chronic obstructive pulmonary disease

William MacNee

Essentials

Chronic obstructive pulmonary disease (COPD) is a group of diseases—chronic bronchitis, small-airway disease (obstructive bronchiolitis), and emphysema. These should be considered in patients over the age of 35 who have (1) exposure to risk factors, usually tobacco smoke; (2) a history of chronic progressive symptoms—cough, wheeze, and/or breathlessness; (3) airflow limitation that is not fully reversible, confirmed by spirometry. They are slowly progressive conditions characterized by airflow limitation that is largely irreversible and which produce considerable morbidity and mortality: COPD is the sixth commonest cause of death worldwide.

Definition

Chronic bronchitis—defined clinically as the presence of a chronic productive cough on most days for 3 months, in each of two consecutive years, in a patient in whom other causes of chronic cough have been excluded.

Emphysema—defined pathologically as abnormal, permanent enlargement of the distal air spaces, distal to the terminal bronchioles, accompanied by destruction of their walls and without obvious fibrosis.

Aetiology

Cigarette smoking—this is the single most important identifiable aetiological factor, with at least 10 to 20% of smokers developing clinically significant disease. The greater the total tobacco exposure, the greater the risk of developing COPD, although about 10% of cases occur in patients who have never smoked.

Genetic factors—there is significant familial risk for developing airflow limitation in smoking siblings of patients with severe COPD, but apart from α_1-antitrypsin deficiency other functional genetic variances which may influence the development of COPD have not been proven.

Pathology and pathophysiology

Pathology—this is complex, with changes affecting both large and small airways and the alveolar compartment. (1) Chronic bronchitis—hypersecretion of mucus is associated with an increase in the volume of the submucosal glands, and an increase in the number and a change in the distribution of goblet cells in the surface epithelium. (2) Obstructive bronchiolitis or small-airways disease—this results from inflammation, squamous cell metaplasia and/or fibrosis in airways less than 2 mm in diameter; bronchiolitis is present in the peripheral airways at an early stage of the disease, with changes in inflammatory response as the disease progresses that are thought to represent innate and adaptive immune responses to long-term exposure to noxious particles and gases. (3) Emphysema—two main types are recognized: (a) centriacinar (or centrilobular) emphysema, in which enlarged air spaces are initially clustered around the terminal bronchiole; and (b) panacinar (or panlobular) emphysema, where the enlarged air spaces are distributed throughout the acinar unit.

Pathophysiology—the characteristic finding in COPD is a decrease in maximum expiratory flow, which can be reduced by two factors—(1) loss of lung elasticity, and (2) an increase in airways resistance in small and/or large airways. There is no consensus on whether the fixed airway obstruction in COPD is largely due to inflammation and scarring in the small airways, resulting in narrowing of the airway lumen, or to loss of support for the airways due to loss of alveolar walls, as in emphysema. Ventilation–perfusion (V/Q) mismatching is the main cause of impaired gas exchange. A combination of pulmonary over-inflation and malnutrition, resulting in muscle weakness, reduces the capacity of the respiratory muscles in patients with severe COPD.

Clinical features

History—details of current smoking status and number of pack years smoked (pack years = number of cigarettes smoked/day × number of years smoked/20) are essential, as are those of previous and present occupations, particularly exposure to dusts and chemicals. Breathlessness can be assessed on the Medical Research Council and Borg Visual Analogue scales.

Examination—signs of airflow limitation may not be present until there is significant impairment of lung function, but the breathing pattern in COPD is often characteristic, with a prolonged expiratory phase, and there may be signs of overinflation of the chest.

Investigation

Spirometry—this is the most robust test of airflow limitation in patients with COPD. A post-bronchodilator FEV_1 less than 80% predicted, together with a forced expiratory volume in 1s/forced vital capacity (FEV_1/FVC) ratio less than 0.70, confirms the presence of airflow limitation that is not fully reversible and is a diagnostic criterion for COPD. Depending largely on the degree of impairment of FEV_1, the severity of COPD can be graded (Global Initiative for Obstructive Lung Disease, GOLD) as mild, moderate, severe, or very severe. The rate of decline of the FEV_1 can be used to assess susceptibility in cigarette smokers and progression of disease.

Lung function tests—static lung volumes such as total lung capacity (TLC), residual volume (RV), and functional residual capacity (FRC) are measured to assess the degree of overinflation and gas trapping. Dynamic overinflation occurs particularly during exercise and may be an important determinant of breathlessness in patients with COPD.

Arterial blood gases—these are needed to confirm the degree of hypoxaemia and hypercapnia in stable patients with an FEV_1 less than 50% predicted, or those with clinical signs of respiratory or right heart failure.

Exercise testing—the 6-min walk is most commonly employed, but is only useful in patients with moderately severe COPD (FEV_1 <1.5 litres) who would be expected to have an exercise tolerance of less than 600 m in 6 min.

Imaging—(1) posterior–anterior chest radiograph—findings are not specific for COPD; there may be no abnormalities, even in patients with very appreciable disability; emphysema produces signs of overinflation (low flat diaphragm, increased retrosternal air space, obtuse costophrenic angle), vascular changes (reduction in size and number of pulmonary vessels, vessel distortion, and areas of transradiency), and bullae. (2) CT scanning—a variety of techniques (visual assessment of low-density areas; CT lung density methods) can be used to quantitate emphysema and bullous disease.

Other tests—α_1-antitrypsin levels and phenotype should be measured in all patients under the age of 45 years, and in those with a family history of emphysema at an early age.

Prevention

Cessation of cigarette smoking—this is the single most important issue, and the 'five As' of smoking cessation should form a routine component of health care delivery: (1) Ask about tobacco use; (2) Advise quitting smoking; (3) Assess willingness to make an attempt; (4) Assist in quit attempt; and (5) Arrange follow-up.

Management

Stable COPD—treatment depends on severity. (1) Mild disease—active reduction of risk factors (e.g. stopping smoking, influenza vaccination); add short-acting bronchodilator as needed. (2) Moderate disease—add regular treatment with one or more long acting bronchodilators when needed; add pulmonary rehabilitation. (3) Severe disease—add inhaled glucocorticosteroids if repeated exacerbations. (4) Very severe disease—add long-term oxygen if chronic respiratory failure; consider surgical treatments.

Acute exacerbations—most of these can be managed in the community, but severe exacerbations require admission to hospital for (1) oxygen therapy to achieve PaO_2 greater than 8 kPa (60 mmHg) or SaO_2 >90%, without inducing significant CO_2 retention; (2) nebulized bronchodilators; (3) antibiotics—if two of the following are present, (a) increase in dyspnoea, (b) increase in sputum volume, and (c) increase in sputum purulence; (4) corticosteroids—prednisolone 30 to 40 mg daily for 7 to 14 days; and (5) ventilatory support—usually noninvasive, if required and if appropriate.

Surgical treatments—(1) bullae—the only treatment possible for large bullae is surgical obliteration, which may allow re-expansion of adjacent compressed lung. Best results are obtained in younger patients with mild symptoms, large bullae, relatively well-preserved pulmonary function, and normal surrounding lung: patients with small bullae, FEV_1 less than 1 litre, or hypercapnia, tend to do badly. (2) lung volume reduction surgery—this aims to reduce the volume of overinflated emphysematous lung by 20 to 30%: it can be recommended only in very carefully selected patients. (3) Lung transplantation—should be considered in selected patients with very advanced COPD.

Definition

Chronic obstructive pulmonary disease (COPD) is not truly a disease, rather it is a group of diseases—chronic bronchitis, small-airway disease (obstructive bronchiolitis), and emphysema. The airflow limitation characteristic of COPD results from small-airway disease (obstructive bronchiolitis) and destruction of the lung parenchyma (emphysema), with the relative contributions of these conditions to the airflow limitation varying between individuals.

Chronic bronchitis is defined clinically as the presence of a chronic productive cough on most days for 3 months, in each of two consecutive years, in a patient in whom other causes of chronic cough have been excluded. Chronic bronchitis can be classified into three forms: simple bronchitis, defined as mucus hypersecretion; chronic or recurrent mucopurulent bronchitis in the presence of persistent or intermittent mucopurulent sputum; and chronic obstructive bronchitis when chronic sputum production is associated with airflow obstruction. Cough and sputum production may precede the development of airflow limitation, but some patients develop airflow limitation without cough and sputum production.

Emphysema is defined as abnormal, permanent enlargement of the distal air spaces, distal to the terminal bronchioles, accompanied by destruction of their walls and without obvious fibrosis. As with chronic bronchitis, the definition of emphysema does not require the presence of airflow limitation: it has pathological definition.

Obstructive bronchiolitis or small-airways disease results from inflammation, squamous cell metaplasia, and/or fibrosis in airways less than 2 mm in diameter. These changes are amongst the earliest to appear in cigarette smokers but are difficult to detect by physiological measurements. Although relatively little is known of the natural history of this condition, it is considered to contribute increasingly to the airflow limitation in COPD as the disease progresses.

The relative contribution made by airway abnormalities or distal air space enlargement to the airflow limitation in an individual patient with COPD is difficult to determine. Thus the term COPD was introduced in the early 1960s to describe patients with largely irreversible airflow limitation, due to a combination of airways disease and emphysema, without defining the contribution of these conditions to the airways obstruction.

In their statement on the Standards for Diagnosis and Care of Patients with COPD, the American Thoracic Society/European Respiratory Society defined COPD as

a preventable and treatable disease characterized by airflow limitation that is not fully reversible. The airflow limitation is usually progressive and is associated with an abnormal inflammatory response of the lungs to noxious particles or gases, primarily caused by cigarette smoking.

Furthermore the systemic effects of COPD are emphasized such that "although COPD affects the lungs, it also produces significant systemic consequences". The recent Global Initiative for Obstructive Lung Disease (GOLD) has a very similar definition, emphasizing again that the pulmonary component—airflow limitation—is associated with an abnormal inflammatory response in the lungs to noxious particles or gases, and that there are significant extrapulmonary effects of COPD which may contribute to the severity in individual patients.

In clinical practice a diagnosis of COPD should be considered in patients over the age of 35 who have:

◆ exposure to risk factors, usually tobacco smoke (although occupational dust and chemicals, and exposure to smoke from home cooking and heating fuel should also be considered)

◆ a history of chronic progressive symptoms (cough, wheeze, and/or breathlessness)

◆ airflow limitation, confirmed by performing spirometry.

◆ post-bronchodilator forced expiratory volume in 1 s/forced vital capacity ratio (FEV_1/FVC) less than 0.70 and FEV_1 less than 80% predicted (which confirms the presence of airflow limitation that is not fully reversible)

The term COPD excludes a number of specific causes of chronic airways obstruction, such as cystic fibrosis, bronchiectasis, and bronchiolitis obliterans (e.g. associated with lung transplantation or chemical inhalation). However, a substantial problem in defining COPD is the difficulty of differentiating this condition from asthma, particularly the persistent airways obstruction of older chronic asthma sufferers that is often difficult or even impossible to distinguish clinically from that in COPD. Furthermore, many patients with COPD show some reversibility of their airflow limitation with bronchodilators. COPD can coexist with asthma, and individuals with asthma who are exposed to noxious particles and gases such as cigarette smoke can also develop fixed airflow limitation. In addition, there is evidence from epidemiological studies that long-standing chronic asthma can itself lead to fixed airflow limitation.

The underlying chronic airway inflammation is different in COPD and asthma (Fig. 18.8.1), but some patients with COPD have features of the asthmatic inflammatory pattern such as increased eosinophils in the airways. Thus, although asthma can usually be distinguished from COPD, in some individuals with chronic symptoms and a degree of fixed airflow limitation it is

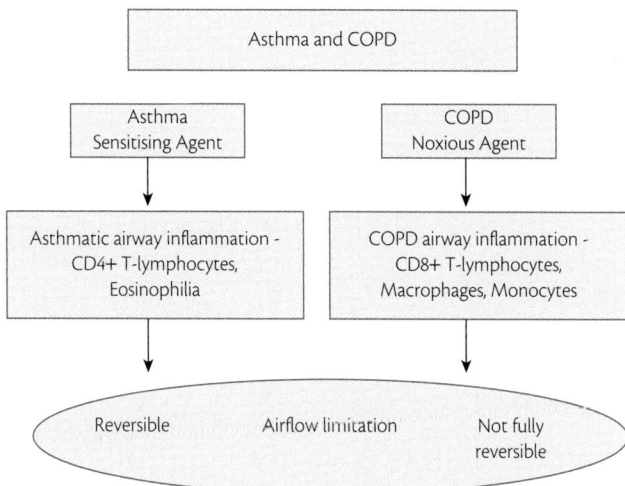

Fig. 18.8.1 Characteristics of the airflow limitation of asthma and COPD. (From GOLD Guidelines - http://www.goldcopd.com/GuidelineList) Global strategy for the diagnosis, management, and prevention of Chronic Obstructive Pulmonary Disease, Updated 2008, figure 1-4 Asthma and COPD.

difficult to differentiate these two diseases. In such cases a history of heavy cigarette smoking, evidence of emphysema by imaging techniques, decreased diffusing capacity for carbon monoxide, and chronic hypoxaemia favour a diagnosis of COPD. However, population studies suggest that chronic airflow limitation can occur in up to 10% of individuals aged 40 years or older who are lifelong nonsmokers; the reason(s) for this is unknown.

Aetiology

The risk of developing COPD depends on interaction between genes and environment (Table 18.8.1): cigarette smoking results in COPD in an individual as a result of an interaction of the environmental exposure with other factors such as a genetic predisposition or failure of lung growth and development.

Environmental factors

Tobacco smoke

Cigarette smoking is the single most important identifiable aetiological factor in COPD. The often quoted figure of 10 to 20% of smokers who develop clinically significant COPD is now known to be an underestimate. In general, the greater the total tobacco exposure, the greater the risk of developing COPD, thus the age of starting to smoke, total pack years, and current smoking status are predictive of COPD mortality. However, for any exposure there are clearly individual variations in susceptibility to the effects of tobacco smoke (Fig. 18.8.2). Although smoking is the dominant

Table 18.8.1 Risk factors for COPD

Host factors	Exposure factors
Genetic factors (α_1-antitrypsin deficiency)	Smoking
Gender	Occupational dust and chemicals
Airway hyper-reactivity and asthma	Recurrent bronchopulmonary infections
	Diet
	Lung growth

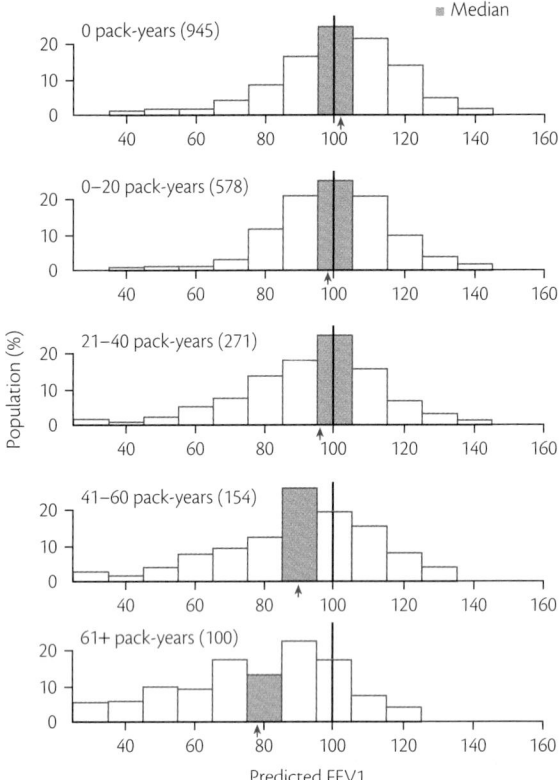

Fig. 18.8.2 Effect of increasing cigarette smoke consumption on FEV_1. Although the mean FEV_1 falls as smoking consumption increases there is a wide variation in this effect, which suggests variable susceptibility to the effects of tobacco smoke. Adapted from Burrows et al. Am J Respir Crit Care Med 1977;115:195–205. © American Thoracic Society

risk factor, COPD does occur in nonsmokers, with about 10% of cases occurring in those who have never smoked.

The most important evidence linking smoking and mortality from COPD comes from a study of 40 000 medical practitioners in the United Kingdom who recorded their smoking habits. In male doctors, mortality from chronic bronchitis fell between 1953 and 1967 by 24%, compared with a fall of only 4% in other men in the United Kingdom of the same age. This difference was attributed to the decrease in smoking in doctors, compared with an overall increase in smoking in the general population.

Cigarette smokers have higher prevalence of respiratory symptoms and lung function abnormalities, a greater annual rate of decline in FEV_1, and a greater mortality rate than nonsmokers. COPD morbidity and mortality rates are greater in pipe and cigar smokers than in nonsmokers, although their rates are lower than those for cigarette smokers.

Passive smoking

There is a trend to an increased relative risk of the development of respiratory symptoms and chronic airflow limitation from passive smoking (also known as environmental tobacco smoke). Cumulative lifetime exposure to environmental tobacco smoke during childhood is inversely associated with peak levels of FEV_1 in adulthood. Smoking during pregnancy is associated with low birth weight, and smoking by either parent is associated with an increased incidence of respiratory illnesses in the first 3 years of life, suggesting an effect on the immune system.

Outdoor air pollution

The introduction of 'clean air' legislation in many countries led to a reduction in smoke and sulphur dioxide levels during the 1960s, which produced less discernible peaks of pollution related to morbidity and mortality in comparison with the 1950s. More recent studies show an association between respiratory symptoms, general practitioner consultations, and hospital admissions in patients with airways diseases at levels of particulate air pollution below $100\,\mu g/m^3$, these currently being experienced in many urban areas in Europe. Furthermore, levels of particulate air pollution are associated with deaths from all causes, particularly cardiorespiratory. There are also clear associations between the levels of outdoor pollution, especially particulate air pollution, and exacerbations of COPD. Longitudinal studies have also shown evidence of an effect of outdoor air pollution on decline in lung function.

Although there have been associations between exacerbations of airways diseases and photochemical air pollutants, such as nitrogen dioxide and ozone, these association has been largely confined to patients with asthma.

Indoor air pollution

Indoor air pollution, e.g. from the use of biomass fuel for cooking in poorly ventilated dwellings in low-income countries, is associated with the development of COPD, particularly in women, and accounts for the high prevalence of COPD among nonsmoking women in low-income countries.

Chronic bronchopulmonary infection

Studies in the 1960s and 1970s in men with chronic bronchitis demonstrated that prophylactic antibiotics to prevent recurrent infective exacerbations did not slow the decline in lung function. However, acute bronchopulmonary infection was associated with an acute decline in lung function that may persist for several weeks, but which usually recovered completely. More recent data in a population of COPD patients has challenged this view and suggested that recurrent exacerbations of COPD may accelerate the decline in FEV_1.

Cough and sputum production between the ages of 20 and 36 years is more commonly reported in those with a history of chest illness in childhood, and a history of severe respiratory infections in childhood is also associated with reduced lung function in adulthood. The association between childhood respiratory illness and lung function impairment in adulthood is probably multifactorial. Several factors such as low economic status, greater exposure to passive smoking, poor diet and housing, and residence in areas of high pollution may all contribute to this finding.

Occupation

It is generally accepted that there is a causal link between occupational dust exposure—including organic and inorganic dusts, chemical agents, and fumes—and the development of mucus hypersecretion. Cigarette smoking is a confounding factor, since the prevalence of smoking remains disproportionately high in many workers who are exposed to dusts. Longitudinal studies on workforces exposed to dusts show an association between dust exposure and a more rapid decline in FEV_1 and increased mortality. It has been estimated that occupational exposures account for 10 to 20% of either symptoms or lung function impairment consistent with COPD.

The accumulating evidence for an association between coal dust exposure and the development of COPD led to the establishment of COPD as a disease that is considered for compensation in miners in the United Kingdom. A small but significant effect of exposure to welding fumes on the development of COPD has been shown in a study of shipyard workers, and workers exposed to cadmium have an increased risk of emphysema.

Diet

One study of British adults has shown that there is a correlation between consumption of fresh fruit in the diet and ventilatory function, a relationship that held both in smokers and in those who had never smoked. Dietary factors, particularly a low intake of vitamin C and low plasma levels of ascorbic acid, were related to a diagnosis of bronchitis in the United States National Health and Nutrition Examination Survey.

Socioeconomic factors

The risk of developing COPD is inversely related to socioeconomic status. This may reflect exposures to indoor/outdoor air pollutants, poor housing, poor diet, or other factors related to low socioeconomic status.

Host factors

Genetic factors

There is significant familial risk of the development of airflow limitation in smoking siblings of patients with severe COPD, suggesting a genetic susceptibility. Genetic association studies have suggested that a variety of genes are linked to the development of COPD, including microsomal epoxide hydrolase-1, tumour necrosis factor (TNF) and transforming growth factor β (TGFβ). Genetic linkage analysis has also suggested several regions of the genome that are likely to contain COPD susceptibility genes, including chromosome 2q. However, the results of these studies have been inconsistent when studied in different populations, hence apart from α_1-antitrypsin deficiency (see 'Pathogenesis', below) other functional genetic variances which may influence the development of COPD have not been proven.

Gender

The role of gender as a risk factor in COPD remains unclear. Historical studies have shown that COPD prevalence and mortality is greater among men than among women. However, recent studies now show that in developed countries the prevalence of COPD is now almost equal in men and women, which probably reflects the changing patterns of tobacco smoking. There are some studies suggesting that women are more susceptible to the effects of tobacco smoke than men, but the question of gender as a risk factor for COPD has not been entirely resolved.

Atopy and airway hyperresponsiveness

In the 1960s Dutch workers proposed that smokers with chronic, largely irreversible airways obstruction and subjects with asthma shared a common constitutional predisposition to allergy, airway hyperresponsiveness, and eosinophilia—the 'Dutch hypothesis'. Numerous studies have shown that smokers tend to have higher levels of IgE and higher blood eosinophil counts than nonsmokers, but the levels are not as high as those in individuals with asthma. Studies in middle-aged smokers with a degree of impairment of lung function show a positive correlation between accelerated decline in FEV_1 and increased airway responsiveness to either methacholine or histamine. However, atopic status, as defined by positive skin tests, does not differ between smokers and those who have never smoked, and whether airway hyper-responsiveness is a cause or consequence of COPD is still a matter of debate.

Factors acting in gestation

Several recent studies have suggested that mortality from chronic respiratory diseases and adult ventilatory function correlate inversely with birth weight and weight at 1 year of age. Thus, impaired growth *in utero* may be a risk factor for the development of chronic respiratory diseases. Any factor which adversely effects lung growth during gestation will potentially increase an individual's risk of developing COPD.

Other considerations

Chronic mucous hypersecretion

Population studies of respiratory symptoms show a much higher prevalence of cough and sputum production among smokers than among nonsmokers. A survey in urban and rural populations in the United Kingdom found that a history of chronic bronchitis was present in 17.6% of men aged 55 to 64 who were heavy smokers, 0.9% of light smokers, and 4.4% of ex-smokers, but was absent in nonsmokers. Smoking cessation produces cessation of the sputum production in 90% of cases. Pipe and cigar smokers have a much lower prevalence of chronic bronchitis and less impairment of respiratory function, which may reflect lower rates of smoke inhalation in pipe and cigar smokers.

The 'British hypothesis' suggested that chronic airflow limitation resulted from the development of chronic mucus hypersecretion as a result of recurrent bronchial infection. This hypothesis was tested in the landmark studies of Fletcher and Peto in working men in London followed up between 1961 and 1969, which showed that smoking accelerated the decline in FEV_1 but failed to show a correlation between the degree of mucus hypersecretion and an accelerated decline in FEV_1 or mortality. By contrast, mortality was strongly related to the development of low FEV_1. However, more recent data from a study of 15 000 adults from the general population in Copenhagen, followed up between 1976 and 1994, suggested that increased mucus secretion was not such an innocent phenomenon since it was associated with increased risk of hospital admission and accelerated decline in FEV_1. Moreover, as the FEV_1 decreased, the association between mucus secretion and mortality became stronger. Differences in the degree of airflow limitation between the populations in these two studies may explain the different findings.

Epidemiology

COPD is a major cause of morbidity and mortality worldwide, with its prevalence projected to increase in the next few decades. The diagnosis is significantly under-reported, with existing information on the burden of COPD varying with differences in the methodology of survey, diagnostic criteria, and analysis of the data. The methods which have been used in surveys include spirometry with or without bronchodilator, questionnaires of the prevalence of respiratory symptoms, and self-reported doctor diagnosis for COPD or equivalent condition.

Prevalence

Prevalence based on self-reporting of a doctor diagnosis of COPD provides the lowest estimates, indicating that less than 6% of the population have the condition, which is likely to reflect under-recognition or underdiagnosis of COPD. By contrast, prevalence surveys using spirometry have estimated that up to 25% of adults aged 40 and older may have airflow limitation.

The symptom of cough and sputum production has been extensively studied in general population surveys over the last 40 years. In these studies, usually in middle-aged men, the prevalence of chronic cough and sputum production ranges between 15 and 53%, with a lower prevalence of between 8 and 22% in women, with prevalence being greater in urban than in rural areas. A study in the late 1980s showed a decline in the prevalence of chronic cough and phlegm in middle-aged men to 15 to 20%, with little change in women.

Prevalence studies of COPD based on spirometry have produced different estimates depending on the measurement used. Defining irreversible airflow limitation as a fixed post-bronchodilator FEV_1/FVC ratio less than 0.70 can lead to an underdiagnosis in younger adults and an overdiagnosis in those over the age of 50 years. A survey in the United Kingdom in 1987 of a representative sample of 2484 men and 3063 women in the age range 18 to 64 years showed that 10% of men and 11% of women had an FEV_1 that was more than 2 standard deviations below their predicted values. The numbers increased with age, particularly in smokers, with 18% of current male smokers (and 14% of women) aged 40 to 65 years having an FEV_1 more than 2 standard deviations below normal, compared with 7 and 6% of male and female nonsmokers, respectively. A further study from Manchester found nonreversible airflow limitation in 11% of adults aged over 45 years, of whom 65% had not had a diagnosis of COPD. In the United States of America the prevalence of airflow limitation with an FEV_1 less than 80% of predicted was 6.8%, with 1.5% of the population having more severe disease (FEV_1 <35% predicted), and again 40% of those with airflow limitation had not been diagnosed as having COPD.

In England and Wales some 900 000 people have a diagnosis of COPD—although because of underdiagnosis the true number is likely to be closer to 1.5 million. The mean age at diagnosis in the United Kingdom is 67 years, with prevalence increasing with age, more common in men than in women, and associated with socio-economic deprivation.

The prevalence of diagnosed COPD has increased in the United Kingdom in women from 0.8% in 1990 to 1.4% in 1997, but did not change over the same period in men (Fig. 18.8.3). Similar trends

are found in the United States of America, probably reflecting differences in smoking habits in men and women. National surveys of consultations in British general practices have shown a modest decline in the number of middle-aged men consulting their doctor with symptoms suggestive of COPD and a slight increase among middle-aged women, but these trends are confounded by changes over the years in the application of the diagnostic labels for this condition, particularly the overlap between COPD and asthma.

Studies from the Latin American Project for the Investigation of Obstructive Lung Disease (PLATINO) found in five major Latin American cities (each in a different country) that the prevalence of mild COPD, as assessed by post-bronchodilator FEV_1, increased steeply with age, with the highest prevalence in those over the age of 60 years, but there was a wide variation between the cities.

Morbidity/use of health resources

COPD places an enormous burden on health care resources, including physician visits, Emergency Department visits, and hospitalizations. An estimate of the annual workload in primary and secondary care attributable to COPD and its associated conditions in an average United Kingdom health district is shown in Table 18.8.2. The economic costs of COPD are more than twice those of asthma, and the effect on quality of life is considerable, particularly in those with frequent exacerbations. It has been calculated that airways diseases (chronic bronchitis and emphysema, COPD, and asthma) account for 24.4 million lost working days per year in the United Kingdom, which represents 9% of all certified sickness absence among men, and 3.5% of the total among women. Respiratory diseases in the United Kingdom rank as the third commonest cause of days of certified incapacity, with COPD accounting for 56% of these days lost in males and 24% in females. Emergency admissions for exacerbations of COPD have risen by 50% in recent years: in 2002–3 there were 110 000 hospital admissions for this reason in England, representing 8% of all emergency admissions. The burden in primary care is even greater (Table 18.8.2). Direct costs to the United Kingdom National Health Service for COPD are estimated to be £819 million per year, with 54% of these due to hospital admissions and 19% due to drug treatment.

The European Respiratory Society White Book provides data on the mean number of consultations for major respiratory diseases across 19 western European countries, in most of which consultations for COPD equate with the number for consultations for asthma, pneumonia, lung cancer, and tuberculosis combined. In the United States of America in 2000 there were 8 million physician

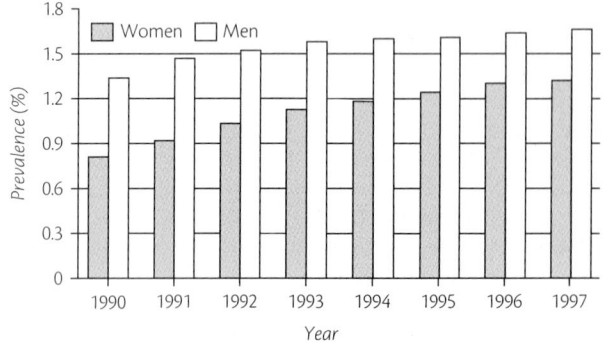

Fig. 18.8.3 Prevalence of diagnosed COPD in United Kingdom men and women during 1990–7.

Table 18.8.2 Estimated annual health service workload due to chronic respiratory disease in an average United Kingdom health district serving 250 000 people

	Hospital admissions	Inpatient bed-days	General practice consultations
Chronic bronchitis	100	1 500	4 400
Emphysema and COPD	240	3 300	2 700
Asthma	410	1 800	11 900
Total	750	6 600	19 000

Modified from Anderson H, et al. (1994). *Epidemiologically based needs assessment: lower respiratory disease*. Department of Health, London.

office/hospital outpatient visits for COPD, 1.5 million Emergency Department visits and 673 000 hospitalizations.

The morbidity burden of disease can also be estimated by calculating years of living with disability (yld). The Global Burden of Disease Study estimates that COPD results in 1.68 yld/1000 population, representing 1.8% of all years of living with disability, with a greater burden in men than in women.

In developed countries exacerbations of COPD account for the greatest burden on the health care system. In the European Union total direct costs of respiratory diseases have been calculated to be around 6% of the total health care budget, with COPD accounting for 56% (38.6 billion euros) of this figure. In the United States of America in 2002 direct costs of COPD were around $18 billion and indirect costs around $14 billion. There is a direct relationship between the cost of care for COPD and the severity of the condition.

Mortality

COPD is the fourth leading cause of death in the United States of America and Europe and will become the third leading cause of death worldwide by 2020 as a result of the increase in smoking in the developing world. There are large international variations in the death rate for COPD, which cannot be entirely explained by differences in diagnostic patterns, labels, or by differences in smoking habits (Fig. 18.8.4). COPD is often a contributory factor to the cause of death, hence figures from death certification underestimate mortality from the condition, most of which occurs in those over 65 years. In the United Kingdom in 2003, 26 000 people (14 000 men, 12 000 women) died of COPD, representing 4.9% of all deaths (5.4% male, 4.2% female). Within the United Kingdom, age-adjusted death rates from chronic respiratory diseases vary by a factor of 5 to 10 in different geographical locations, with mortality tending to be higher in urban areas than in rural areas.

Mortality from COPD in the United Kingdom has fallen in men but risen in women over the last 25 years, except in the group over 75 years of age. In American women the decline in mortality that was recorded until 1975 has increased substantially between 1980 and 2000, from 20.1 to 56.7 per 100 000, whereas the increase in men has been more modest, from 73.0 to 82.6 per 100 000. These trends presumably relate to the later time of the peak prevalence of cigarette smoking in women compared with men.

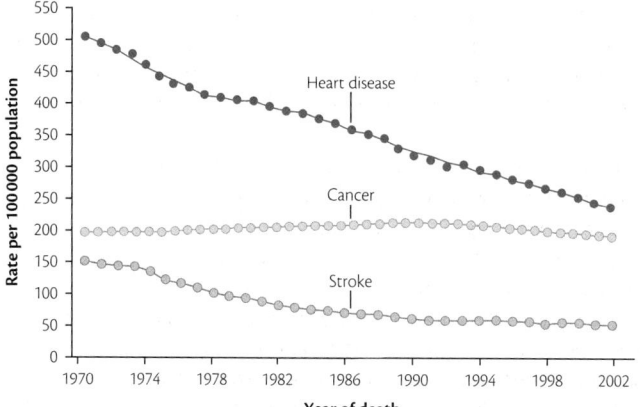

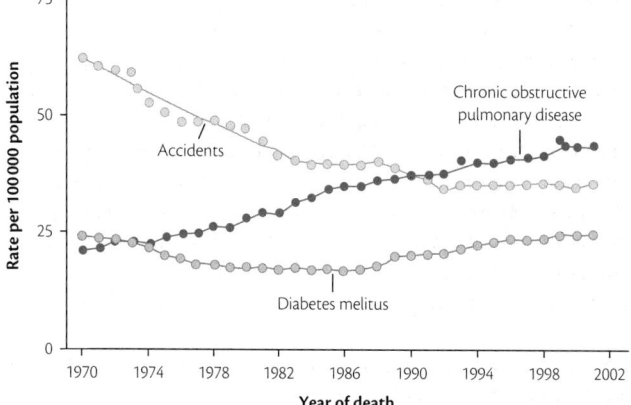

Fig. 18.8.5 Trends in age-standardized death rates for the six leading causes of death in the United States 1970–2002.

The Global Burden of Disease Study has projected that COPD, which ranked sixth as a cause of death in 1990, will become the third leading cause of death by 2020. This will largely result from the epidemic of smoking, particularly in lower income countries, and more of the population living longer. Trends in death rates for COPD appear to be rising in the United States of America but falling in Europe; the reason for this is as yet unexplained (Fig. 18.8.5).

Natural history and prognosis

COPD is generally a progressive disease, particularly if the patient's exposure to noxious agents continues. However, the natural history of COPD is variable, not all individuals following the same course. Stopping exposure to noxious agents such as cigarette smoke may result in some improvement in lung function and may slow or halt progression of the disease.

Severe airways obstruction occurs in susceptible smokers as a result of years of an accelerated decline in FEV_1. In nonsmokers the FEV_1 declines at a rate of 20 to 30 ml/year (Fig. 18.8.6); this occurs at a faster rate in smokers, reported changes in FEV_1 in patients with COPD being more than 50 ml/year. Fletcher and colleagues found a relationship between the initial level of FEV_1 and the annual rate of decline in FEV_1 over a follow-up period of 8 years in working men in London. From these data they suggested that susceptible cigarette smokers could be identified in early middle age by a reduction in the FEV_1. They also suggested that there

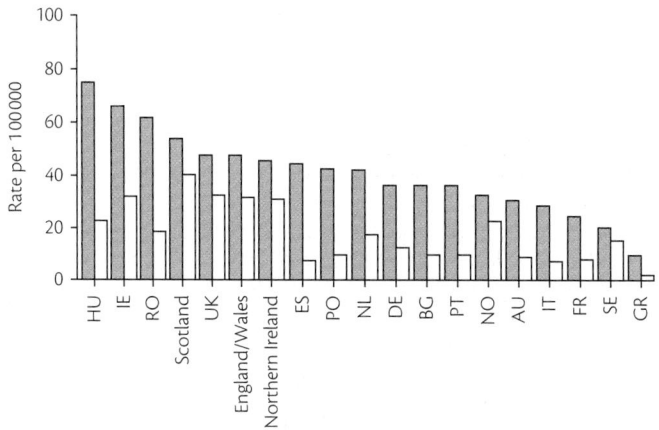

Fig. 18.8.4 Age-adjusted death rates for chronic obstructive pulmonary disease for males (blue bars) and females (open bars) in 19 European countries. (From Stang P et al. (2000). Chest, **117**; Suppl 2: 354A–9S, with permission.)

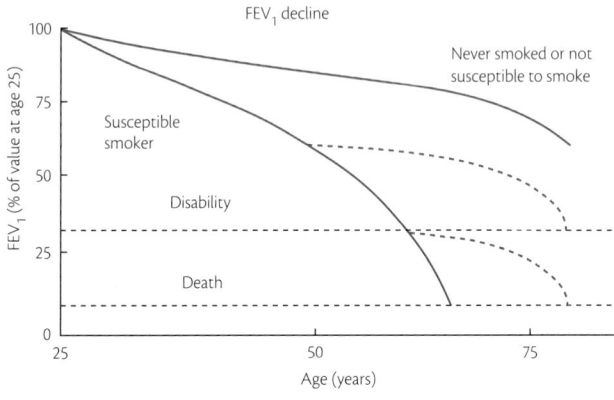

Fig. 18.8.6 The effect of age on airflow obstruction in normal subjects and susceptible cigarette smokers. Cessation of smoking (dotted curved lines) returns the rate of decline to normal.

was a tracking effect, whereby individuals in the highest or lowest FEV_1 percentiles remained in the same percentiles over subsequent years. Support for the tracking effect comes from a study of 2718 working men whose pulmonary function was assessed in the 1950s and subsequently followed up over 20 years. In those whose initial FEV_1 was more than 2 standard deviations below predicted values, the risk of death from chronic airways obstruction was 50 times greater than those whose initial FEV_1 was above average. There is a tendency for annual rates of decline in FEV_1 to be slower in advanced than in mild disease.

It is increasingly recognized that COPD may have its origins in impaired growth of lung function in childhood caused by recurrent infections or exposure to tobacco smoke. This abnormal growth combined with a shortened plateau phase in teenage smokers increases the risk of COPD (Fig. 18.8.7).

The strongest predictors of survival in patients with COPD are age and baseline FEV_1. Less than 50% of patients whose FEV_1 has fallen to 30% of predicted are alive 5 years later, and there is an

even stronger relationship between survival and the post- (rather than pre-) bronchodilator FEV_1. Other unfavourable prognostic factors include severe hypoxaemia, raised pulmonary arterial pressure, low carbon monoxide transfer, and weight loss, which become apparent in patients with severe disease. Factors favouring improved survival are stopping smoking and a large bronchodilator response. A reduced FEV_1 is also an important additional risk factor for lung cancer, independent of age or cigarette smoking.

Pathology

The pathological changes in the lungs in patients with COPD are complex: they occur in both the large and small airways, and in the alveolar compartment (Box 18.8.1). The relative contributions that the pathological changes in the airways and those of emphysema make to airways obstruction have been the subject of considerable study. In general, pathological changes correlate rather poorly with both clinical and functional patterns of the disease. As a result there is still no clear consensus on whether the fixed airway obstruction in COPD is largely due to inflammation and scarring in the small airways, resulting in narrowing of the airway lumen, or to loss of support for the airways due to loss of alveolar walls, as in emphysema.

Although the pathology of COPD is complex, it can be simplified by considering separately the three sites described above in which pathological changes could produce a clinical pattern of largely fixed airways obstruction in smokers. However, the clinicopathological picture is complicated by the fact that these three entities, or any combination of the three, may exist in an individual patient, leading to the clinical and pathophysiological heterogeneity seen in patients with COPD.

Some believe that chronic asthma should be included as part of the spectrum of COPD, but although the clinical and physiological presentation of chronic asthma can be indistinguishable from that of COPD, the pathological changes are distinct from those in most cases of COPD, although the histological features of COPD in the 10% of cases who are nonsmokers have not yet been studied in detail.

COPD is characterized by poorly reversible airflow obstruction and an abnormal inflammatory response in the lungs. This latter feature represents innate and adaptive immune responses to long-term exposure to noxious particles and gases, particularly cigarette smoke. All cigarette smokers will develop an inflammatory response in their lungs, but those who develop COPD have an enhanced or abnormal response to inhaling toxic agents. This amplified response may result in mucous hypersecretion (chronic bronchitis), tissue destruction (emphysema), and destruction of normal repair and defence mechanisms, causing small-airway inflammation and eventual fibrosis (bronchiolitis). These pathological changes result in increased resistance to airflow in the small conducting airways, increased compliance of the lungs, leading to air trapping and progressive airflow limitation—all of which are characteristic features of COPD.

Chronic bronchitis

The pathological basis of the hypersecretion of mucus in chronic bronchitis is an increase in the volume of the submucosal glands, and an increase in the number and a change in the distribution of goblet cells in the surface epithelium. Submucosal mucus glands are confined to the bronchi, decreasing in number and in size in the smaller, more peripheral bronchi, and not present in the bronchioles.

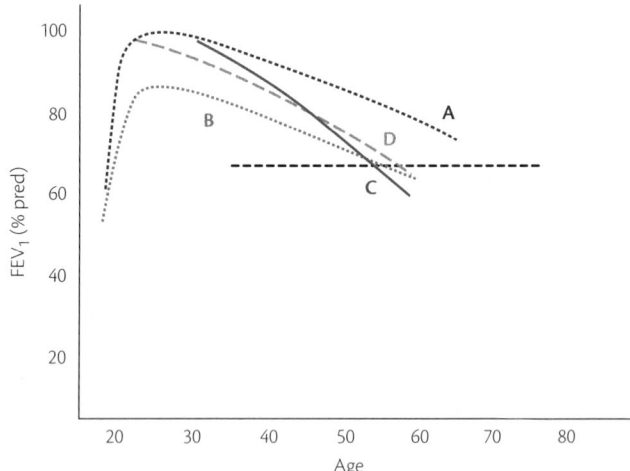

Fig. 18.8.7 Line A shows the normal course of FEV_1 over time. The result of impaired growth of lung function is shown as line B. Lines C and D represent an accelerated decline and a shortened plateau phase respectively.
From ERS/ATS Guidelines—http://www.ersnet.org

Box 18.8.1 Pathological changes in COPD

Proximal airways (trachea and cartilaginous airways >2 mm diameter)

- Submucosal bronchial gland enlargement, glands and goblet cell metaplasia—resulting in excessive mucus production or chronic bronchitis; cellular infiltrates (neutrophils, lymphocytes) also occur in bronchial glands

- Increased macrophages, CD8+ T lymphocytes (cytotoxic T cells); few neutrophils or eosinophils, but neutrophils increase as the disease progresses

- Airway wall changes include squamous metaplasia of the airway epithelium, ciliary dysfunction, and increased smooth muscle and connective tissue

Peripheral airways (noncartilaginous airways <2 mm internal diameter)

- Bronchiolitis is present at an early stage of the disease. Luminal and inflammatory exudates that are increased in inflammatory response; exudates correlate with the disease severity

- Pathological extension of goblet cells and squamous metaplasia in peripheral airways

- Increased macrophages, T lymphocytes, CD8+ > CD4+, increased B lymphocytes, lymphoid follicles, fibroblasts; few neutrophils or eosinophils

- Peribronchial fibrosis and airways narrowing as the disease progresses

Parenchyma (respiratory bronchioles and alveoli)

- Emphysema-defined as abnormal enlargement of air spaces distal to terminal bronchioles

- Alveolar wall destruction, apoptosis of epithelial and endothelial cells

- Centrilobular emphysema—dilatation and destruction of respiratory bronchioles; commonly seen in smokers; predominant in upper zones

- Panacinar emphysema—destruction of the whole of the acinus; commonly seen in α_1-antitrypsin deficiency; more common in the lower lung zones

- Microscopic emphysema in the early stages of the disease, progressing to macroscopic lesions or bullae (defined as an emphysematous space >1 cm diameter)

- Increased macrophages, CD8+ T lymphocytes

Pulmonary vasculature

- Increased thickening of the intima; endothelial dysfunction early in the course of the disease

- Increased vascular smooth muscle occurs later

- Increased macrophages and T lymphocytes

- Collagen deposition, emphysematous destruction of the capillary bed, in later stages.

- Structural changes eventually lead to pulmonary hypertension and right ventricular dysfunction (cor pulmonale)

In chronic bronchitis there is mucus gland hypertrophy in the larger bronchi with infiltration of the glands with inflammatory cells (Fig. 18.8.8).

In healthy subjects who have never smoked, goblet cells are predominantly seen in the proximal airways and decrease in number in more distal airways, being absent normally in the terminal or respiratory bronchioles. By contrast, in smokers, goblet cells not only increase in number but extend more peripherally, hence mucus is produced in greater quantities in peripheral airways where the mucociliary escalator is less developed. Mucociliary function is also decreased in smokers.

The use of bronchoscopy to obtain airway cells by bronchoalveolar lavage and bronchial tissue samples by biopsy has added new insights into the role of inflammation in COPD. Bronchial biopsy studies confirm those in resected lung tissue, which show bronchial wall inflammation in this condition (Box 18.8.2). As in asthma, bronchial biopsies in patients with chronic bronchitis reveal that activated T lymphocytes are prominent in the proximal airway walls. However, in contrast to asthma, macrophages also feature, and the CD8 suppressor T-lymphocyte subset (rather than CD4) predominates. Increased numbers of neutrophils are present, particularly in the glands, which become even more prominent as the disease progresses.

Bronchial biopsies from limited studies in patients during exacerbations of chronic bronchitis show increased numbers of eosinophils in the bronchial walls, although their numbers are small compared with exacerbations of asthma and—unlike those in asthma—these cells do not appear to have degranulated.

Bronchoalveolar lavage, or more recently studies of spontaneously produced or induced sputum, has shown increased intraluminal air space inflammation in patients with chronic bronchitis, with or without airways obstruction, with predominantly neutrophils and macrophages in the bronchoalveolar lavage studies. There is also evidence that air space inflammation in patients with chronic bronchitis persists following smoking cessation if the production of sputum persists.

These studies of sputum and bronchial biopsies in chronic bronchitis have mainly sampled the proximal airways, but recent studies suggest that inflammatory changes present in the large airways may reflect those in the small airways, and perhaps even in the alveolar walls.

Emphysema

Emphysema is defined as enlargement of the airways distal to the terminal bronchioles, due to destruction of their walls without obvious fibrosis. Two major types are recognized, according to the distribution of enlarged air spaces within the acinar unit, the acinus being that part of the lung parenchyma supplied by a single terminal bronchiole:

- centriacinar (or centrilobular) emphysema, in which enlarged air spaces are initially clustered around the terminal bronchiole

- panacinar (or panlobular) emphysema, where the enlarged air spaces are distributed throughout the acinar unit

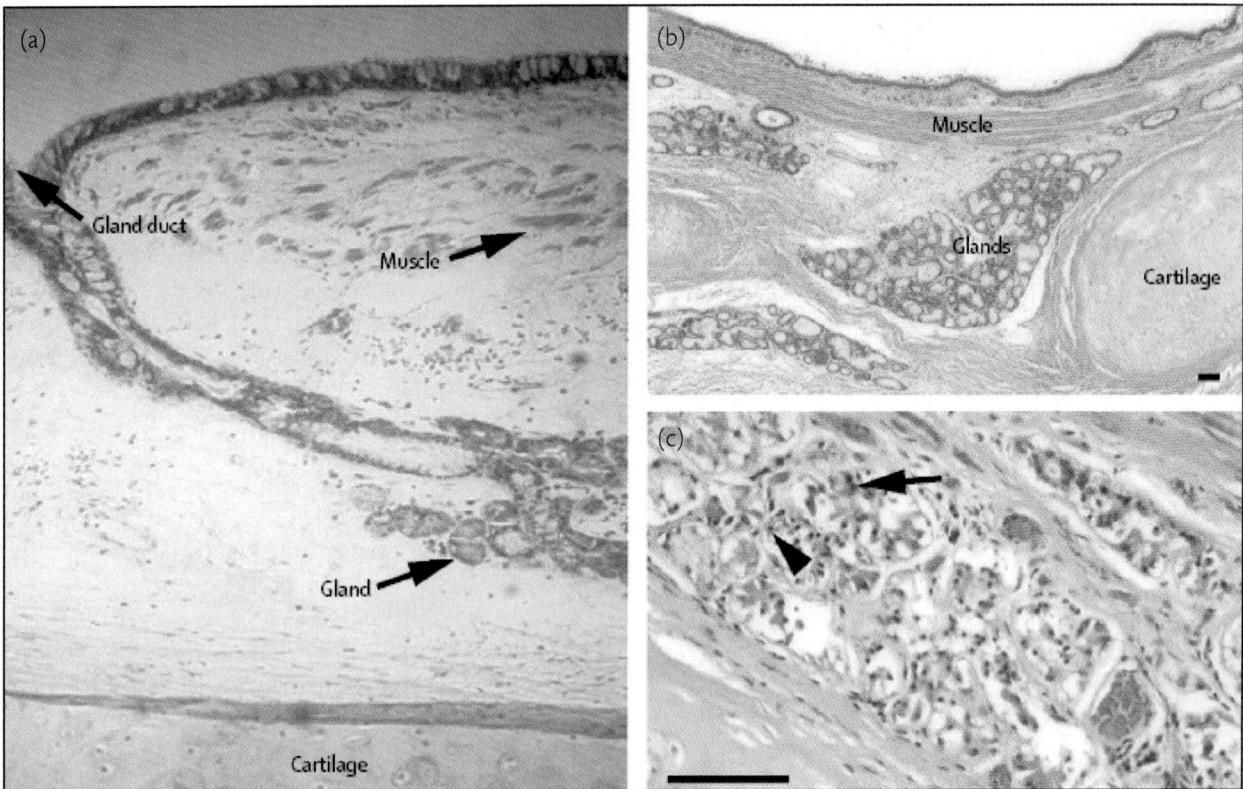

Fig. 18.8.8 Pathological changes of the central airways in COPD. A central bronchus from the lungs of a cigarette smoker with normal lung function (A) shows small amounts of muscle present in subepithelium and small epithelial glands. In a patient with chronic bronchitis (B) the muscle appears as a thick bundle and the bronchial glands are enlarged. At a higher magnification (C) these glands show evidence of a chronic inflammatory process involving polymorphonuclear leucocytes (arrow head) and mononuclear cells, including plasma cells (arrow).
Reproduced from the GOLD Workshop Report with the kind permission of Professor James C Hogg.

Centriacinar emphysema is more common in the upper zones of the upper and lower lobes and is the common type in COPD: panacinar emphysema may be found anywhere in the lungs, but is more prominent at the bases, and is associated with α_1-antitrypsin deficiency. Both types of emphysema can occur alone or in combination in a patient with COPD. There is still debate over whether centriacinar and panacinar emphysema represent different disease processes, and hence have different aetiologies, or whether panacinar emphysema is a progression from centriacinar emphysema. There is a clearer association between centriacinar emphysema and cigarette smoking than with panacinar emphysema. Smokers with centriacinar emphysema have more small-airways disease than those patients with predominantly panacinar emphysema.

Periacinar (or paraseptal or distal acinar) emphysema describes enlarged air spaces along the edge of the acinar unit, but only where it abuts against a fixed structure such as the pleura or a vessel. This is less common and usually of little clinical significance, except when extensive in a subpleural position when it may be associated with pneumothorax. Scar and irregular emphysema are terms sometimes used to describe enlarged air spaces around the margins of a scar, unrelated to the structure of the acinus, but this lesion is excluded from the current definition of emphysema.

In the early stages of the disease, emphysematous lesions are microscopic (<1 mm diameter); they may progress to macroscopic lesions or bullae. A bullae is an area of emphysema that has locally overdistended; conventionally to more than 1 cm in size. Bullous disease can also occur in the absence of COPD.

Normal bronchioles and small bronchi are supported by attachments to the outer aspect of their walls of adjacent alveolar walls, an arrangement which maintains the tubular integrity of the airways. It has been suggested that loss of these attachments in emphysema may lead to distortion and irregularity of airways, which results in airflow limitation (Fig. 18.8.9).

Box 18.8.2 Inflammation and inflammatory cells in COPD

◆ Neutrophils—increase in sputum and distal air spaces in smokers, with a further increase in COPD related to disease severity. These are important in the secretion and release of proteases

◆ Macrophages—increase in number in airways, lung parenchyma and in bronchoalveolar lavage fluid. These produce increased inflammatory mediators and proteases

◆ T lymphocytes—increase in the peripheral airways and within lymphoid follicles, possibly as a response to chronic infection of the airways. Both CD4 and CD8 cells increase in airways and in lung parenchyma, with an increase in CD8:CD4 ratio. There is an increase in TH1 and TC1 cells that produce interferon-γ. CD8+ cells may be cytotoxic, causing alveolar wall destruction

◆ Eosinophils—increase in airways walls, with increased eosinophil proteins in sputum, in some exacerbations of the disease.

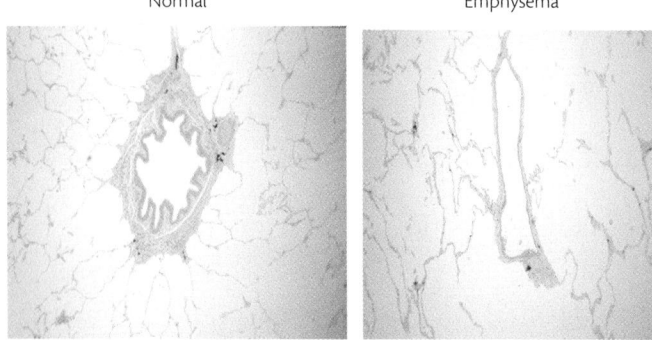

Normal   Emphysema

Fig. 18.8.9 Pathological changes in emphysema. Cross-section of a normal small peripheral bronchiole, showing a circular outline supported by adjacent alveolar walls (left panel). A small bronchiole at the same magnification in a patient with very early macroscopic emphysema: the loss of alveolar supporting walls results in an elliptical airway (right panel).

The inflammatory cell profile in the alveolar walls and the air spaces is similar to that described in the airways and persists throughout the course of the disease, even after smoking cessation. Absence of fibrosis is a prerequisite in the most recent definition of emphysema, but fibrosis occurs in the terminal or respiratory bronchioles as part of a respiratory bronchiolitis in COPD patients. Furthermore, there is an increase in collagen in the lung parenchyma in smokers compared with nonsmokers.

Bronchiolitis/small-airways disease

Hogg, Macklem, and Thurlbeck introduced the concept of 'small-airways disease' in studies using a retrograde catheter in which they showed that the increased flow resistance in the lungs in patients with COPD largely occurred in the small airways (<2 mm diameter) at the periphery of the lungs. Inflammation in the small airways is among the earliest changes to be found in asymptomatic cigarette smokers and considerable changes in these airways can occur without giving rise to symptoms or alterations in spirometry. Several pathological changes are found in small airways (Fig. 18.8.10), including inflammatory infiltrate in the airway wall, mucus and cells in the lumen, goblet cell hyperplasia, fibrosis in the airway wall, squamous-cell metaplasia, mucosal ulceration, increased amount of muscle, and pigmentation.

Bronchiolitis is present in the peripheral airways at an early stage of the disease. The inflammatory cells in the airway wall and air spaces are similar to those in the larger airways. Recent studies using resected lung specimens, and those obtained during lung volume reduction surgery, have shown changes in inflammatory response as the disease progresses (Figs. 18.8.11 and 18.8.12). These changes are thought to represent innate and adaptive immune responses to long-term exposure to noxious particles and gases. A further feature, recently described is the later stages of the disease, is the presence of an increase in B lymphocytes and lymphoid follicles around the bronchioles. The cause of these changes is not known, but it is possible that they represent an autoimmune or a adaptive immune response to chronic lower respiratory infection (see below). As the disease progresses there is fibrosis and increased deposition of collagen in the small-airway wall (Fig. 18.8.10).

Pulmonary vasculature

Pathological changes in the pulmonary vasculature occur early in the course of the disease. The initial changes are characterized by thickening of the vessel wall and endothelial dysfunction. These are followed by increased vascular smooth muscle and infiltration of the vessel walls by inflammatory cells, including macrophages and CD8+ lymphocytes. In the later stages of the disease there is collagen deposition and emphysematous destruction of the capillary bed in the alveolar walls. These structural changes eventually lead to pulmonary hypertension and right ventricular dysfunction (cor pulmonale).

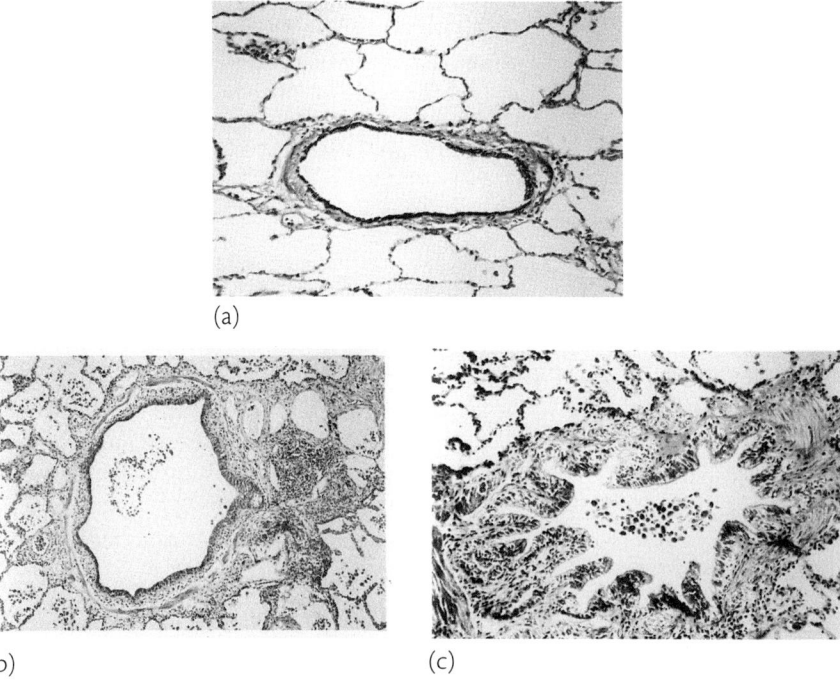

(a)

(b)   (c)

Fig. 18.8.10 Histological sections of peripheral airways. (A) Section from a cigarette smoker with normal lung function, showing a nearly normal airway. (B) Section from a patient with small-airways disease, showing inflammatory exudate in the wall and lumen of the airway. (C) A more advanced case of small-airways disease, with reduced lumen, structural reorganization of the airway wall, increased smooth muscle, and deposition of peribronchiolar connective tissue.
Images reproduced with the kind permission of Professor James C Hogg, University of British Columbia

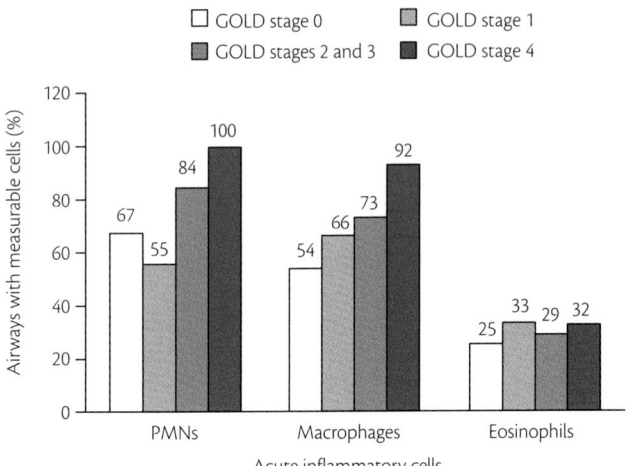

Fig. 18.8.11 The extent of the airway inflammatory response, as measured by the percentage of the airways containing polymorphonuclear neutrophils (PMNs), macrophages and eosinophils, among patients in each GOLD stage of COPD. Reproduced with permission from Kyle RA, Prevalence of Monoclonal Gammopathy of Undetermined Significance. New England Journal of Medicine 354(13):1362–9. Copyright © 2006 Massachusetts Medical Society. All rights reserved.

Pathogenesis

Inflammation is present in the lungs of all smokers and is thought to be a normal protective response to inhaled toxins, amplified in patients who develop COPD. The precise mechanisms of this amplification are not really understood, but the abnormal inflammatory response in COPD leads to tissue destruction, impairment of defence mechanisms that limit such destruction, and impairment of the repair mechanisms. In general the inflammatory and structural changes in the airways increase with disease severity and persist even after smoking cessation. However, in addition to inflammation, two other processes are central to the pathogenesis of COPD, namely an imbalance between proteases and antiproteases, and imbalance between oxidants and antioxidants (oxidative stress) in the lungs (Fig. 18.8.13).

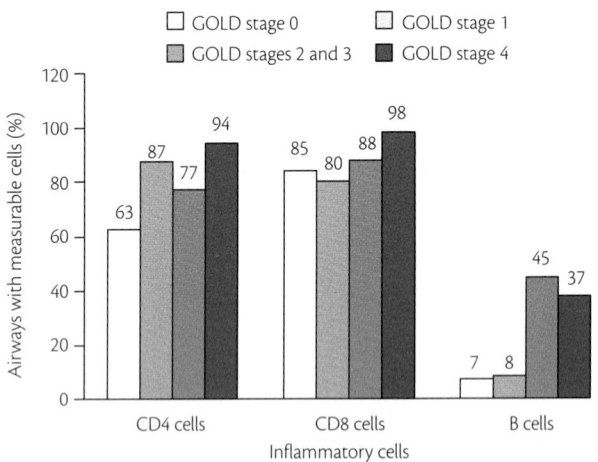

Fig. 18.8.12 The extent of the airway inflammatory response, as measured by the percentage of the airways containing CD4 cells, CD8 cells, and B cells, among patients in each GOLD stage of COPD.
(From Hogg JC, et al. (2004). The nature of small-airway obstruction in chronic obstructive pulmonary disease. N Engl J Med, **350**, 2645–53, with permission.)

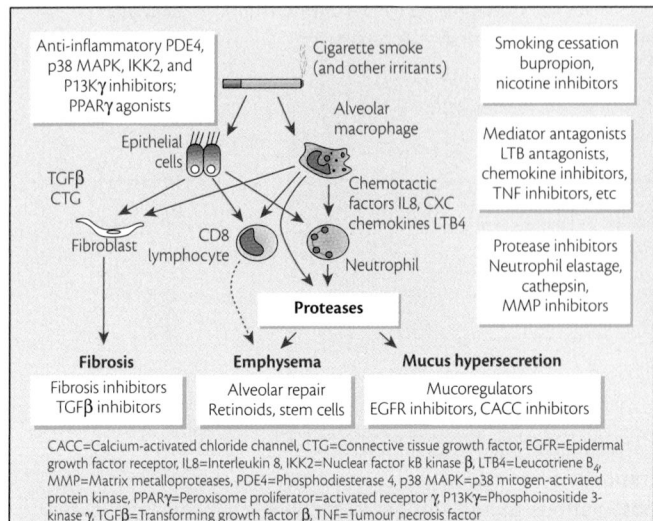

Fig. 18.8.13 Inflammatory mechanisms with possible therapeutic interventions in COPD. Cigarette smoke activates macrophages and epithelial cells to release chemotactic factors that recruit neutrophils and CD8+ T lymphocytes from the circulation. These cells release factors that activate fibroblasts, resulting in abnormal repair processes and bronchiolar fibrosis. An imbalance between proteases (released from neutrophils and macrophages) and antiproteases leads to alveolar wall destruction (emphysema). Proteases also cause the release of mucus. An increased oxidant burden, resulting from smoke inhalation or release of oxidants from inflammatory leucocytes, causes epithelial and other cells to release chemotactic factors, inactivate antiproteases, and directly injure alveolar walls and cause mucus secretion.
From GOLD Guidelines—http://www.goldcopd.com/GuidelineList

Inflammatory cells and mediators

The inflammatory cellular response which characterises COPD consists of increased numbers of neutrophils, macrophages, and T lymphocytes (CD8 more than CD4) in the lungs (see Box 18.8.2). These inflammatory cells are activated to release a variety of cytokines and mediators that participate in the disease process, with the inflammatory pattern in COPD being markedly different from that seen in patients with asthma (Fig. 18.8.1).

A wide range of inflammatory mediators have been shown to be increased in COPD and to amplify the inflammatory process (Box 18.8.3).

Box 18.8.3 Inflammatory mediators in COPD

- Leucotriene B$_4$—a neutrophil and T-cell chemoattractant that is produced by macrophages, neutrophils, and epithelial cells

- Chemotactic factors—e.g. the CXC chemokines IL-8 and growth-related oncogene α—produced by macrophages and epithelial cells; attract cells from the circulation and amplify proinflammatory responses

- Proinflammatory cytokines—e.g. TNFα, IL-1β, IL-6

- Growth factors—e.g. TGFβ—which may cause fibrosis in the airways either directly or through release of another cytokine, connective tissue growth factor

Table 18.8.3 Proteases and antiproteases involved in COPD

Protease	Antiprotease
Serine proteinases	α_1-antitrypsin
Neutrophil elastase	α_1-antitrypsin
Cathepsin G	Secretory leukoprotease inhibitor
Proteinase 3	Elafin
Cysteine proteinases (cathepsins B, K, L, S)	Cystatins
Matrix metalloproteinases (MMP-8, MMP-9, MMP-12)	Tissue inhibitor of MMP (TIMP1–4)

Table 18.8.4 α_1-Antitrypsin phenotypes: frequency in United Kingdom population, concentration of serum α_1-protease inhibitor, and the risk for emphysema

Phenotype	Frequency (%)	Average concentration (g/litre)	Risk factor for emphysema
MM	86	2	No
MS	9	1.6	No
MZ	3	1.2	No
SS	0.25	1.2	No
SZ	0.2	0.8	Yes
ZZ	0.03	0.4	Yes

Protease/antiprotease imbalance

Important to understanding the pathogenesis of COPD were the observations of an association between α_1-antitrypsin deficiency and the development of early-onset emphysema, and the development of emphysema following instillation of the proteolytic enzyme papain into rat lungs. These two important observations form the basis of the protease/antiprotease hypothesis of the pathogenesis of emphysema, which states that under normal circumstances the release of proteolytic enzymes from inflammatory cells that migrate to the lungs to fight infection does not cause lung damage because of inactivation of these proteolytic enzymes by an excess of inhibitors. However, in conditions of excessive enzyme load, or where there is an absolute or a functional deficiency of antiproteases, an imbalance develops between proteases and antiproteases in favour of proteases, leading to uncontrolled enzyme activity and degradation of lung connective tissue in alveolar walls, resulting in emphysema (Table 18.8.3).

α_1-Antitrypsin/α_1-protease inhibitor

α_1-Antitrypsin is a polymorphic glycoprotein that is responsible for most of the antiprotease activity in the serum. It is a potent inhibitor of serine proteases, with greatest affinity for the enzyme neutrophil elastase. It is synthesized in the liver and increases from its usual plasma concentration of about 2 g/litre as part of the acute phase response. The activity of the protein is critically dependent on the methionine–serine sequence at its active site.

Laurell and Eriksson in 1963 were the first to describe the association between α_1-antitrypsin deficiency and the development of early-onset emphysema, and that the abnormality was transmitted as an autosomal recessive. Since the discovery of the deficiency, over 75 biochemical variants have been described relating to their electrophoretic properties, giving rise to the phase inhibitor (Pi) nomenclature. The average α_1-antitrypsin plasma levels for the more common phenotypes are shown in Table 18.8.4. Aside from causing emphysema, the Z deficiency state (PiZZ) is associated with periodic acid–Schiff (PAS)-positive inclusion bodies in the liver, which represent accumulations of α_1-antitrypsin protein. Although liver and mononuclear cells from PiZZ patients can manufacture normal amounts of messenger RNA, and the protein can be translated, there is little secretion of the protein. It is now recognized that the Z α_1-antitrypsin gene is normal except for a single point mutation, resulting from substitution of a glycine nucleotide for adenine in the DNA sequence that codes for the amino acid at position 342 in the protein molecule. This results in spontaneous polymerization of the protein, with large polymers of α_1-antitrypsin accumulating in the liver and unable to pass through the endoplasmic reticulum.

A deficiency in antitrypsin levels, particularly the inability to increase levels in the acute phase response, leads to unrestrained proteolytic damage to lung tissue leading to emphysema, which develops at an earlier age than in the common variety of emphysema in COPD. Cigarette smoking is a cofactor in the development of emphysema in α_1-antitrypsin deficient patients, probably as a result of oxidation and hence inactivation of the remaining functional α_1-antitrypsin by oxidants in cigarette smokes.

In the United States of America, screening of adult blood donors identified a 1 in 2700 prevalence of PiZZ subjects, most of whom had normal spirometry. Around 1 in 5000 children in the United Kingdom are born with the homozygous deficiency (PiZZ). However, the number of subjects identified with disease is much less than predicted from the known prevalence of the deficiency, hence it is by no means inevitable that all individuals with a homozygous deficiency develop respiratory disease. Indeed, a few PiZZ individuals live beyond their sixth decade and escape the development of progressive airways obstruction. Prospective follow-up of PiZZ subjects has shown an accelerated decline in FEV_1, but with large variation between individuals and the development of predominantly panlobular emphysema. Life expectancy of subjects deficient in α_1-protease inhibitor is significantly reduced, especially if they smoke.

Oxidative stress

The oxidative burden is increased in COPD as a result of oxidants from cigarette smoke and reactive oxygen and nitrogen species released from inflammatory cells. There may also be a reduction in endogenous antioxidant responses. Both of these contribute to oxidant–antioxidant imbalance and hence oxidative stress, many markers of which are increased in stable COPD and further increased in exacerbations of disease. Oxidative stress can lead to inactivation of antiproteases, stimulation of mucus production, and activation of proinflammatory genes. Amplification of inflammation can result from oxidative stress enhanced transcription factor activation (such as NF-κB) by oxidants, and may also result from a decrease in histone deacetylase activity in lung cells of patients with COPD with consequent increased gene expression of inflammatory mediators.

Pathophysiology

The pathogenic mechanisms described above produce the pathological changes found in COPD, which in turn result in the physiological abnormalities—mucus hypersecretion and ciliary dysfunction, airflow limitation and hyperinflation, gas exchange abnormalities, pulmonary hypertension, and systemic effects.

Mucus hypersecretion and ciliary dysfunction

Mucus hypersecretion results in a chronic productive cough—chronic bronchitis. Chronic bronchitis is not necessarily associated with airflow limitation, and conversely not all patients with COPD have chronic productive cough. Mucus hypersecretion is due to squamous metaplasia, increased numbers of goblet cells, and increased size of bronchial submucosal glands in response to chronic irritation by noxious particles and gases, usually cigarette smoke. Ciliary dysfunction results from squamous metaplasia of epithelial cells and results in abnormal function of the mucociliary escalator and thus difficulty expectorating sputum.

Airflow limitation and hyperinflation

The characteristic physiological abnormality in COPD is a decrease in maximum expiratory flow, which can be reduced by two factors: loss of lung elasticity and an increase in airways resistance in small and/or large airways.

In healthy young subjects significant airway closure only occurs below functional residual capacity (FRC), but enhanced airway closure at higher lung volumes occurs in the early stages of COPD. The closing volume in healthy young nonsmokers is about 5 to 10% of the vital capacity (VC), rising to 25 to 35% of VC in old age. Compared with nonsmokers, young asymptomatic adult smokers have an increase in closing volume.

The main site of airflow limitation in COPD occurs in the small conducting airways (<2 mm diameter) and results from inflammation and inflammatory exudates and narrowing caused by airway remodelling, features which correlate with the reduction in FEV_1. Other contributing factors to airflow limitation include loss of the lung elastic recoil (due to the destruction of alveolar walls) and the destruction of alveolar support (from alveolar attachments). The consequent airway obstruction results in progressive trapping of air during expiration, resulting in hyperinflation at rest and dynamic hyperinflation during exercise. Lung hyperinflation reduces the inspiratory capacity and thus functional residual capacity increases, particularly during exercise. These features are thought to occur early in the course of the disease and result in the breathlessness and limited exercise capacity that is typical of COPD. Bronchodilators reduce air trapping and thus decrease lung volumes, thereby improving symptoms and exercise capacity (Fig. 18.8.14).

Tests of overall lung mechanics such as the FEV_1 and airways resistance are usually abnormal in patients with COPD when breathlessness develops. Residual volume, FRC, and (in some cases) TLC increase. Maximum expiratory flow–volume curves (MEFV) show a characteristic convexity towards the volume axis, initially with preservation of peak expiratory flow (Fig. 18.8.15).

The uneven distribution of ventilation in advanced COPD causes a reduction in 'ventilated' lung volume and thus the carbon monoxide transfer factor ($T_L$co) is almost always reduced, although the $T_L$co normalized to ventilated alveolar volume (Kco) may remain relatively well preserved in those without emphysema.

The characteristic changes in the static pressure/volume (P/V) curve of the lungs in COPD are an increase in static compliance and a reduction in static transpulmonary pressure at a standard lung volume (Fig. 18.8.16) resulting from emphysema.

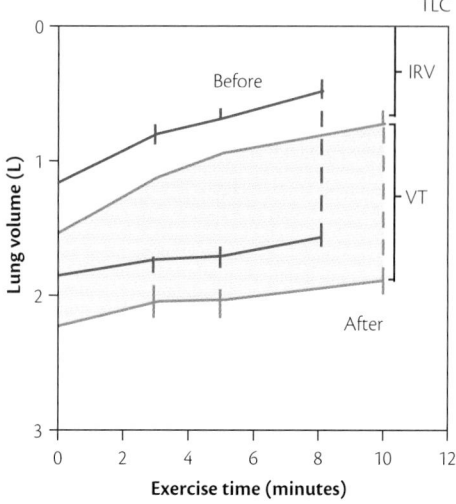

Fig. 18.8.14 Changes in operational lung volumes are shown as ventilation increases with exercise in a constant load cycle exercise in patients before and one hour after receiving nebulized ipratropium bromide. In response to ipratropium FEV_1 increased by 7% predicted, FVC by 10%, inspiratory capacity (IC) by 14%, and the patient's endurance time by 32%. Increased IC, which is an index of reduced resting lung hyperinflation, best reflected the improvements in exercise endurance and dyspnoea. IRV, inspiratory residual volume; V_T, tidal volume (V_T). IC=IRV+V_T.
O'Donnell DE, Lam M, Webb KA. Spirometric correlates of improvement in exercise performance after anticholinergic therapy in chronic obstructive pulmonary disease. Am J Respir Crit Care Med 1999; 160: 542–549.

Loss of lung elastic recoil pressure is also important in terms of airways obstruction, particularly in those with severe emphysema, as a result of a reduction in the distending force on all intrathoracic airways. Dynamic expiratory compression of the airways is enhanced by loss of lung recoil, by atrophic changes in the airways, and loss of support from the surrounding alveolar walls, allowing flow limitation at lower driving pressures and flows.

Gas exchange abnormalities

Ventilation–perfusion (V/Q) mismatching is the main cause of impaired gas exchange in the lungs in COPD. Other causes such as

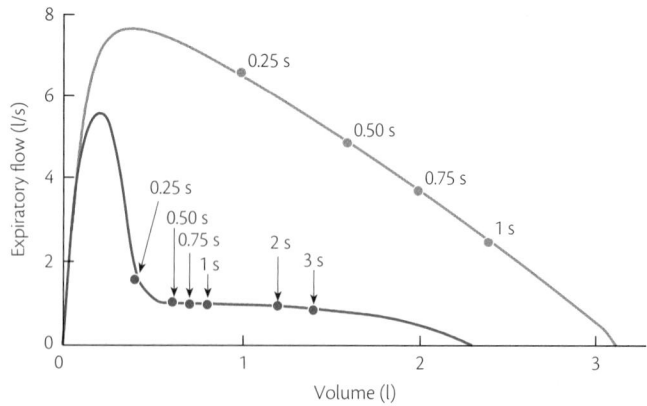

Fig. 18.8.15 Maximum flow–volume curves in a healthy subject (FEV_1 2.4 litres) and a subject with COPD and airways obstruction (FEV_1 0.8 litres). The development of convexity of the expiratory curve in mild obstruction is characteristic, as is the relative preservation of peak expiratory flow in the patient with COPD. Timepoints in second(s) are plotted on the flow volume curves.

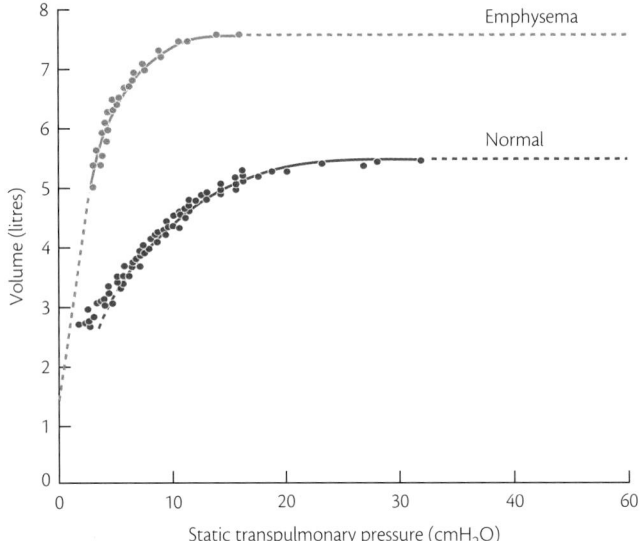

Fig. 18.8.16 Static expiratory pressure–volume curves of lungs in a subject with severe emphysema compared with a normal subject. The broken lines represent extrapolation of the curve—to infinite pressure and to the volume axis at zero pressure.

alveolar hypoventilation, impaired alveolar–capillary diffusion to oxygen, and increased shunt are of much less importance. In general, gas exchange worsens as the disease progresses. The distribution of ventilation is very uneven in patients with COPD. Several mechanisms result in a reduction of blood flow, including local destruction of vessels in alveolar walls as a result of emphysema, hypoxic vasoconstriction in areas of severe alveolar hypoxaemia, and passive vascular obstruction as a result of increased alveolar pressure and distension. These factors result in V/Q imbalance, which together with impaired ventilatory muscle function in severe disease lead to reduced ventilation and CO_2 retention.

Impaired respiratory muscle function

In patients with severe COPD a combination of pulmonary overinflation and malnutrition, resulting in muscle weakness, reduces the capacity of the respiratory muscles to generate pressure over the range of tidal breathing. In addition the load against which the respiratory muscles need to act is increased due to the increase in airways resistance. Overinflation of the lungs leads to shortening and flattening of the diaphragm, thus impairing its ability to lower pleural pressure. During quiet tidal breathing in normal subjects, expiration is largely passive and depends on the elastic recoil of the lungs and the chest wall. Patients with COPD increasingly need to use their rib cage muscles and inspiratory accessory muscles, such as the sternomastoids, even during quiet breathing. During exercise, this pattern may be even more distorted and result in paradoxical motion of the rib cage.

Patients with COPD have impaired global function of the respiratory muscles, e.g. reduced maximum inspiratory mouth pressures, although these measurements are very effort dependent. Diaphragmatic function, as assessed during inspiration by measurement of transdiaphragmatic pressure using balloon-tipped catheters with small transducers placed in the oesophagus and stomach, is reduced in patients with COPD.

Pulmonary hypertension

Pulmonary arterial hypertension occurs late in the course of COPD with the development of hypoxaemia (Pao_2 <8 kPa) and usually also hypercapnia. The contributing factors include pulmonary arterial constriction (as a result of hypoxia), endothelial dysfunction and destruction of the pulmonary capiliary bed. Structural changes in the pulmonary arterioles result in persistent pulmonary hypertension: this is usually of a mild to moderate degree in COPD, but is associated with the development of right ventricular enlargement and dysfunction (cor pulmonale) and poor prognosis. Further details can be found in Chapter 18.15.

Systemic effects of COPD

Although primarily a disease of the lungs, it is increasingly recognised that COPD—particularly if severe—results in important systemic features that may affect morbidity, also that it is associated with a variety of comorbid conditions (Box 18.8.4). Weight loss is associated with a poor prognosis. Increased systemic inflammatory mediators such as TNFα, interleukin (IL)-6, and oxygen free radicals may mediate some of these systemic effects.

Pathophysiology of exacerbations

Exacerbations of COPD are associated with a further increase in the inflammatory response in the lungs, with increased predominantly neutrophilic inflammation and—in some mild exacerbations—the presence of increased numbers of eosinophils. This increased inflammatory response can be triggered by infection with bacteria, viruses or environmental pollutants. Exacerbations are associated with increased concentrations of mediators such as TNFα, LTB$_4$, and IL-8 in the airways and increased markers of oxidative stress.

In mild exacerbations airflow limitation is unchanged or only slightly increased. Severe exacerbations are associated with worsening of pulmonary gas exchange due to increased inequality between ventilation/perfusion and respiratory muscle fatigue.

Box 18.8.4 Systemic features and comorbidities of COPD

Systemic features

- Cachexia—loss of fat-free mass
- Skeletal muscle wasting: apoptosis, disuse atrophy
- Increased risk of cardiovascular disease: associated with increased CRP
- Normochromic normocytic anaemia
- Osteoporosis

Comorbidities

- Respiratory infection
- Lung cancer
- Myocardial infarction, angina
- Depression
- Diabetes

CRP, C-reactive protein.

The worsening *V/Q* mismatch results from airway inflammation, oedema, mucus hypersecretion, and bronchial constriction, effects which also reduce ventilation and cause hypoxic vasoconstriction of pulmonary arterioles that in turn impairs perfusion.

Respiratory muscle fatigue and alveolar hypoventilation can contribute to hypoxaemia, hypercapnia, and respiratory acidosis and lead to severe respiratory failure and death. Hypoxia and respiratory acidosis can induce pulmonary vasoconstriction to increase the load on the right ventricle, which together with renal and hormonal changes can result in peripheral oedema.

Clinical history

A diagnosis of COPD should be considered in anyone over 35 years who complains of symptoms of breathlessness, chronic cough, sputum production, frequent respiratory infections, an impaired exercise tolerance, and/or a history of exposure to risk factors for the disease. The diagnosis should be confirmed by objective evidence on spirometry of airflow limitation which is not fully reversible (post-bronchodilator FEV_1 <80% predicted, FEV_1/FVC <0.70).

Symptoms

Patients with COPD characteristically complain of breathlessness on exertion, sometimes accompanied by wheeze and cough, which is often, but not invariably, productive. Breathlessness is the symptom that commonly causes the patient to seek medical attention and is usually the most disabling problem. Patients often date the onset of their illness to an acute exacerbation of cough with sputum production that leaves them with a degree of chronic breathlessness. However, close questioning will usually reveal the presence of a 'smoker's cough', with the production of small amounts of mucoid sputum (usually <60 ml/day), often predominating in the morning, for many years.

A smoking history of at least 20 pack years is usual before symptoms develop, commonly in the fifth decade, following which there is progression through the clinical stages of mild, moderate, and severe disease. Breathlessness, usually first noticed on climbing hills or stairs, or hurrying on level ground, heralds the development of moderate impairment of airway function, and patients may adapt their breathing pattern and their behaviour to minimize the sensation of breathlessness. The perception of breathlessness varies greatly for individuals with the same impairment of ventilatory capacity, but is usually present on minimal exertion when the FEV_1 has fallen to 35% or less of the predicted values. Severe breathlessness is often affected by changes in temperature and occupational exposure to dust and fumes. Some patients have severe orthopnoea, relieved by leaning forward, whereas others find greatest ease when lying flat. Breathlessness can be assessed on the Medical Research Council and Borg Visual Analogue scales (Tables 18.8.5 and 18.8.6).

A productive cough occurs in up to 50% of cigarette smokers and may precede the onset of breathlessness. Many patients dismiss this as simply a 'smoker's cough'. The frequency of nocturnal cough does not appear to be increased in stable COPD. Paroxysms of coughing in the presence of severe airway obstruction generate high intrathoracic pressures, which can produce syncope and cough fractures of the ribs. Wheeze is common, but not specific to COPD, since it is due to turbulent airflow in large airways from any cause.

Table 18.8.5 The modified Borg scale for assessing breathlessness

Scale	Severity experienced by patient
0	Nothing at all
0.5	Very, very slight (just noticeable)
1	Very slight
2	Slight (light)
3	Moderate
4	Somewhat severe
5	Severe (heavy)
6	
7	Very severe
8	
9	Very, very severe (almost maximal)
10	Maximal

Patients in whom a diagnosis of COPD is being considered should also be asked about the following symptoms: effort intolerance, fatigue, nocturnal wakening, weight loss, occupational hazards, occupational history, ankle swelling, family history of COPD or other chronic respiratory disease, chest pain, and haemoptysis.

In addition, as part of their overall assessment, they should be asked about current drug treatment, frequency of exacerbations, previous hospitalization, days missed from work, social and family support, symptoms of anxiety and depression, and comorbidities.

Chest pain is common in patients with COPD, but is often unrelated to the disease itself and may be due to underlying ischaemic heart disease or gastro-oesophageal reflux, which are commonly associated with the condition. Chest tightness is a common complaint during exacerbations of breathlessness, particularly during exercise, and this is sometimes difficult to distinguish from ischaemic cardiac pain. Pleuritic chest pain may suggest an intercurrent pneumothorax, pneumonia, or pulmonary infarction. Haemoptysis can be associated with purulent sputum and may be due to inflammation or infection. However, this symptom should be treated seriously and the need for investigations for bronchial carcinoma should be considered.

Weight loss and anorexia are features of severe COPD and thought to result from both decreased calorie intake and hypermetabolism.

Table 18.8.6 The modified MRC dyspnoea scale for assessing breathlessness

Grade	Degree of breathlessness related to activities
0	Not troubled by breathlessness except on strenuous exercise
1	Short of breath when hurrying or walking up a sight hill
2	Walks slower than contemporaries on the level because of breathlessness, or has to stop tor breath when walking at own pace
3	Stops for breath after walking about 100 m or after a few minutes on the level
4	Too breathless to leave the house, or breathless when dressing or undressing
5	Breathless at rest

Psychiatric morbidity, particularly depression, is common in patients with severe COPD, reflecting social isolation and the chronicity of the disease. Sleep quality is impaired in advanced COPD, which may contribute to impaired neuropsychiatric performance.

Smoking and occupational history

A history of current smoking status and number of pack years smoked (pack years = number of cigarettes smoked/day × number of years smoked/20) is important in patients with COPD because the disease is rare in lifelong nonsmokers. In general there is a dose–response relationship between the number of cigarettes smoked and the level of the FEV_1, but there is huge individual variation reflecting variation in the susceptibility to cigarette smoke.

Patients should be questioned about previous and present occupations, particularly exposure to dusts and chemicals. Occupational exposure to dusts has an additive effect with smoking on the decline in lung function, as has been shown in coal miners, where both smoking and years of dust exposure contribute to the decline in FEV_1, although the contribution of smoking is three times as great as that of the dust exposure.

Differential diagnosis

COPD needs to be distinguished from other causes of breathlessness, asthma being the most difficult differential diagnosis (Table 18.8.7).

Clinical examination

It must be recognized that signs of airflow limitation may not be present until there is significant impairment of lung function, and because of the heterogeneity of COPD, patients may show a range of signs. Physical signs in patients with COPD are not specific and depend on the degree of airflow limitation and lung overinflation, but their sensitivity to detect or exclude moderately severe COPD is poor, and the absence of physical signs does not exclude the diagnosis.

General inspection

Tachypnoea may be present at rest in patients with severe COPD, and prolonged forced expiratory time (>5 s) can be a useful indicator of airway obstruction. The breathing pattern in COPD is often characteristic, with a prolonged expiratory phase, and some patients adopting pursed-lipped breathing on expiration, which reduces expiratory airway collapse. Use of the accessory muscles of respiration, particularly the sternomastoids, is often seen in advanced disease, and these patients often adopt the position of leaning forward, supporting themselves with their arms to fix the shoulder girdle, allowing the use of the pectorals and the latissimus dorsi to increase chest-wall movement.

In advanced disease cyanosis may be present, indicating hypoxaemia, but this is a fairly subjective sign and may be diminished by anaemia or accentuated by polycythaemia. The flapping tremor associated with hypercapnia is neither sensitive nor specific, and papilloedema associated with severe hypercapnia is rarely seen.

Tar-stained fingers emphasize the smoking habit. Finger clubbing is not a feature of COPD and should suggest the possibility of complicating bronchial neoplasm or bronchiectasis. Weight loss may be apparent in advanced disease, as well as a reduction in muscle mass. Body mass index should be recorded (BMI = weight (kg)/height (m)^2), with BMI <21 kg/m^2 categorized as underweight, 21–25 kg/m^2 as normal, 25–30 kg/m^2 as overweight, and ≥30 kg/m^2 as obese.

Examination of the chest

In the later stages of COPD the chest is often barrel-shaped with a kyphosis and an apparent increased anterior–posterior diameter, horizontal ribs, prominence of the sternal angle, and a wide subcostal angle. Due to the elevation of the sternum the distance between the suprasternal notch and the cricoid cartilage (normally three fingerbreadths) may be reduced. These are all signs of overinflation. An inspiratory tracheal tug may be detected, which has been attributed to the contraction of the low, flat diaphragm. The horizontal position of the diaphragm also acts to pull in the lower ribs during inspiration—Hoover's sign. Widening of the xiphisternal angle and abdominal protuberance occur, the latter due to forward displacement of the abdominal contents, giving the appearance of apparent weight gain. Increased intrathoracic pressure swings may result in inspiratory indrawing of the suprasternal and supraclavicular fossas and of the intercostal muscles.

On percussion of the chest there is decreased hepatic and cardiac dullness, indicating overinflation, a useful sign of gross overinflation being the absence of a dull percussion note, normally due to the underlying heart, over the lower end of the sternum.

Breath sounds may have a prolonged expiratory phase, or may be uniformly diminished, particularly in the advanced stages of the disease. Wheeze may be present on both inspiration and expiration, but is not an invariable clinical sign. Crackles may be heard, particularly at the lung bases, but are usually scanty and vary with coughing.

Cardiovascular examination

The presence of emphysema or overinflation of the chest produces difficulty in localizing the apex beat and reduces the cardiac dullness.

Characteristic signs indicating the presence or consequences of pulmonary arterial hypertension may be detected in advanced cases. The heave of right ventricular hypertrophy may be palpable at the lower left sternal edge. Heart sounds are generally soft, but in pulmonary hypertension the pulmonary component of the second heart sound may be exaggerated in the second left intercostal space, and a gallop rhythm may be detectable, with a third sound

Table 18.8.7 Differences between COPD and asthma

	COPD	Asthma
Age	>35 years	Any age
Cough	Persistent and productive	Intermittent and nonproductive
Smoking	Almost invariable	Possible
Breathlessness	Progressive and persistent	Intermittent and variable
Nocturnal symptoms	Uncommon unless in severe disease	Common
Family history	Uncommon unless family members also smoke	Common
Concomitant eczema or allergic rhinitis	Possible	Common

audible in the fourth intercostal space to the left of the sternum. The jugular venous pressure can be difficult to estimate in patients with COPD as it swings widely with respiration and is difficult to discern if there is prominent accessory muscle activity. However, when the right heart is compromised (cor pulmonale) there may be evidence of functional tricuspid incompetence, producing a prominent 'v' wave in the jugular venous pulse, a pansystolic murmur at the left sternal edge, and a tender and pulsatile liver. The liver may also be palpable below the right costal margin as a result of overinflation of the lungs. Pitting peripheral oedema may also be present as a result of fluid retention.

Peripheral vasodilatation accompanies hypercapnia, producing warm peripheries with a high-volume pulse.

Investigation of respiratory function and exercise capacity

The most important disturbance of respiratory function in COPD is the obstruction to forced expiratory airflow. The degree of airflow obstruction cannot be predicted from the symptoms and signs, hence an assessment of the degree and the progression of airflow limitation should be made in all patients who may have COPD. At an early stage of the disease conventional spirometry may reveal no abnormality, since the earliest changes in COPD affect the alveolar walls and small airways, producing a modest increase in peripheral airway resistance that is not reflected in spirometric measurements. Tests of small-airway function, such as the frequency dependency of compliance and closing volume, may be abnormal. These tests are difficult to perform, have high coefficients of variation, and are only valid when lung elastic recoil is normal and there is no increase in large airway resistance: they are therefore not recommended in normal clinical practice.

Spirometry

Spirometry is the most robust test of airflow limitation in patients with COPD. It is important that the techniques used meet published standards: the tests are effort dependent and it is therefore important to ensure that maximum effort has been achieved. The reproducibility the FEV_1 should vary by less than 170 ml between manoeuvres.

To avoid the effect of airway collapse in patients with COPD during forced expiration, it is suggested that VC should be estimated by a slow or relaxed measurement, which allows patients to exhale at their own pace. The slow VC is often 0.5 litres greater than the FVC. It is important that a volume plateau is reached when performing the FEV_1, which can take 15 s or more in patients with severe airways obstruction: if this manoeuvre is not carried out the FVC can be underestimated.

Spirometric measurements are evaluated by comparison of the results with appropriate reference values based on age, height, sex, and race. The presence of a post-bronchodilator FEV_1 less than 80% predicted, together with a FEV_1/FVC ratio less than 0.70, confirms the presence of airflow limitation that is not fully reversible (Fig. 18.8.17) and is a diagnostic criterion for COPD. The FEV_1 as a percentage of the predicted value can be used to assess the severity of the disease (Table 18.8.8), although the FEV_1 does not fully capture the impact of COPD on patients' functional capabilities. The rate of decline of the FEV_1 can be used to assess susceptibility in cigarette smokers and progression of disease.

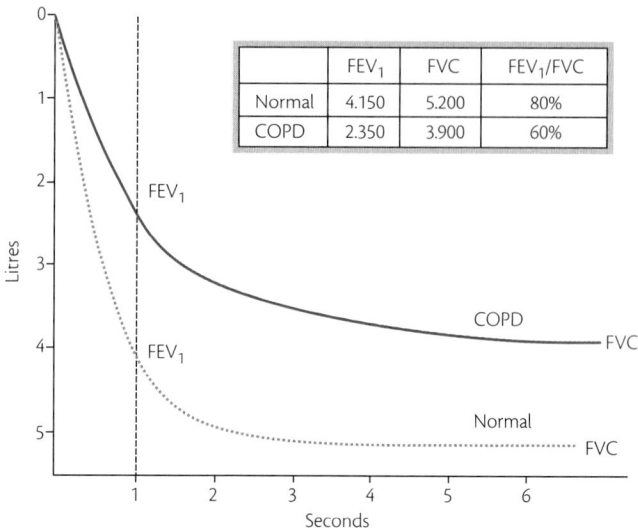

	FEV_1	FVC	FEV_1/FVC
Normal	4.150	5.200	80%
COPD	2.350	3.900	60%

Fig. 18.8.17 Forced expiratory volume measurements in a patient with COPD and a person with normal lung function.
http://www.goldcopd.com/GuidelineList Pocketguide to COPD diagnosis, management and prevention. A Guide for Healthcare Professionals. Updated 2008 Figure 2. Normal spirogram and spirogram Typical of Patients with Mild to Moderate COPD

Reversibility testing

Testing for reversibility with bronchodilators can be performed in patients with COPD to help distinguish those patients with marked reversibility who have underlying asthma, also because the post-bronchodilator FEV_1 is the best predictor of survival. There is, however, no agreement on a standardized method of assessing reversibility, which is usually recorded as change in FEV_1 or peak expiratory flow, although there may be changes in other lung volumes (such as inspiratory capacity) after bronchodilators. This may explain why symptoms improve in some patients following a bronchodilator without change in spirometry, also why small changes (e.g. <400 ml) in FEV_1 which occur in COPD following a bronchodilator do not reliably predict the patients' response to treatment. Different degrees of bronchial smooth muscle constriction can lead to different classification of reversibility status depending on the day of testing. Thus, when airway smooth muscle tone is higher, and thus FEV_1 is lower, a response to bronchodilators may be more likely to be achieved than when muscle tone is lower and FEV_1 is higher. Recognition of this underlies a move away from testing bronchodilator reversibility in all patients with COPD, but in some cases—particularly where the diagnosis of

Table 18.8.8 Disease severity in COPD

Severity	NICE		GOLD	
	FEV_1	FEV_1/FVC	FEV_1	FEV_1/FVC
Stage 1: Mild	50–80% pred	<70%	≥80% pred	<70%
Stage 2: Moderate	30–49% pred	<70%	50–79% pred	<70%
Stage 3: Severe	<30% pred	<70%	30–49% pred	<70%
Stage 4: Very severe			<30% pred	<70% or <50% pred *plus* chronic respiratory failure

Pred, predicted; NICE - National Institute for Health and Clinical Excellence; GOLD - Global Initiative for Chronic Obstructive Lung Disease.

Box 18.8.5 Suggested protocol for reversibility testing in COPD

- Improvement in FEV_1 by ≥15% and 200 ml 20 min after 400 µg salbutamol by metered dose inhaler or 2.5 mg nebulized salbutamol
- Improvement in FEV_1 by ≥15% and 200 ml after 30 mg prednisolone for 2 weeks

---

asthma is being considered e.g. in a patients with atypical history—then bronchodilator and/or glucocorticoid steroid reversibility testing can be performed. A suggested protocol is shown in Box 18.8.5.

Whether all patients with symptomatic COPD should have a formal assessment of steroid reversibility remains controversial. The commonest regimen is the administration of 30 mg of prednisolone for 2 weeks (Table 18.8.13). Those patients who have previously shown a response to nebulized bronchodilators are more likely to show a response to steroids, but it is not possible to predict the response to corticosteroids in an individual patient. An alternative approach is to assess the response to inhaled steroids, usually over a 6-week period, measuring the FEV_1 before and after the average of the first 5 days and the last 5 days measurements of peak expiratory flow.

Flow volume loops

Expiratory flows at 75% or 50% of vital capacity have been used as a measure of airflow limitation. These measurements are less reproducible than spirometry, such that values must fall to below 50% of predicted to be regarded as abnormal. Flows at lung volumes less than 50% of vital capacity were previously considered to be an indicator of small-airways function, but probably provide no more clinically useful information than measurements of FEV_1.

Peak expiratory flow

Peak expiratory flow can either be read directly from the flow volume loop or measured with a handheld peak flow meter; the latter are relatively easy to use and are particularly useful in subjects with asthma for revealing variations in serial measurements, although

in COPD the variations are often within the error of the measurement. The peak expiratory flow may underestimate the degree of airflow obstruction in COPD (Figs. 18.8.15 and 18.8.18).

Lung volumes

Static lung volumes such as total lung capacity (TLC), residual volume (RV), and functional residual capacity (FRC) are measured in patients with COPD to assess the degree of overinflation and gas trapping. Dynamic overinflation occurs particularly during exercise and may be an important determinant of the symptom of breathlessness.

The standard method of measuring static lung volumes, using the helium dilution technique during rebreathing, may underestimate lung volumes in COPD, particularly in those patients with bullous disease where the inspired helium does not have time to equilibrate properly in the air spaces. Body plethysmography uses Boyle's law to calculate lung volumes from changes in mouth and plethysmographic pressures. This technique measures trapped air within the thorax, including poorly ventilated areas, and therefore gives higher readings for lung volumes than the helium dilution technique.

Gas transfer for carbon monoxide ($T_L$co)

A low $T_L$co is present in many patients with COPD. Although there is a relationship between the $T_L$co and the extent of emphysema, the severity of the emphysema in an individual patient cannot be predicted from the $T_L$co, nor is a low $T_L$co specific for emphysema. The commonly used method is the single-breath technique, which uses alveolar volume calculated from helium dilution during the single-breath test. This will underestimate alveolar volume in patients with severe COPD, producing a lower value for the $T_L$co.

Arterial blood gases

Arterial blood gases are needed to confirm the degree of hypoxaemia and hypercapnia in patients with COPD. This test is usually performed in stable patients with an FEV_1 less than 50% predicted or in those with clinical signs suggestive of respiratory failure or right heart failure. Respiratory failure is indicated by a Pao_2 less

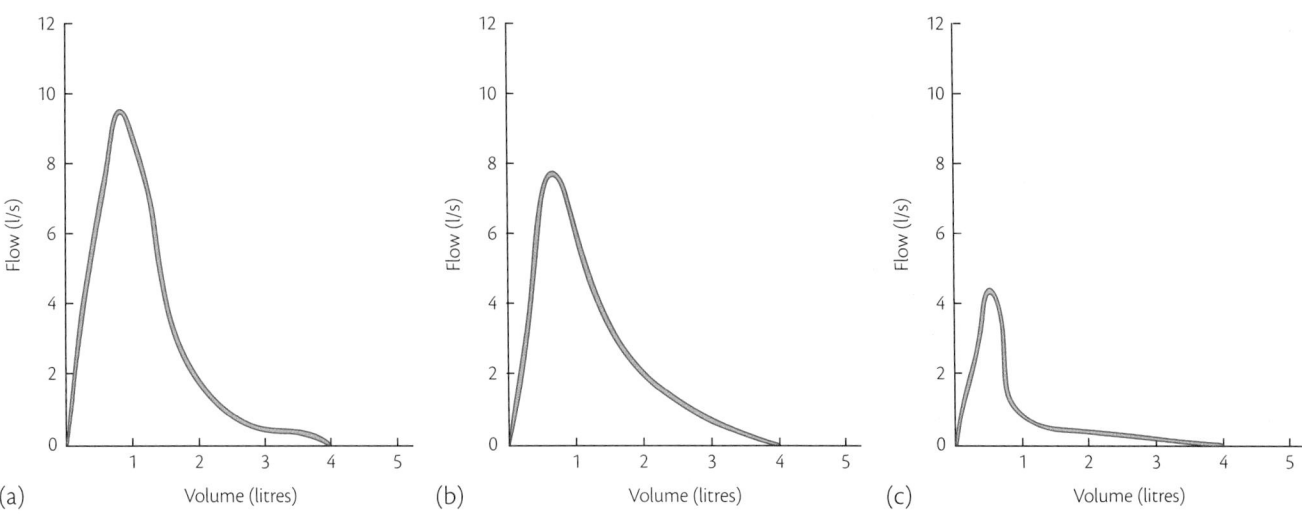

Fig. 18.8.18 Examples of flow–volume curves in (a) mild obstruction, (b) moderate obstruction, and (c) severe obstruction.

than 8 kPa (60 mmHg) (hypoxaemic or type 1 respiratory failure) with or without $Paco_2$ greater than 6.5 kPa (50 mmHg) or with raised $Paco_2$ (hypercapnic or type 2 respiratory failure), while breathing air.

It is always essential to record the inspired oxygen concentration when reporting blood gases. It is also important to note that it may take at least 30 min for a change in inspired oxygen concentration to have its full effect on the Pao_2 because of long time constants for alveolar gas equilibration in COPD, particularly during exacerbations.

Pulse oximetry is increasingly used to measure the level of oxygenation, but should not replace an assessment of blood gas tensions, since measurements of $Paco_2$ are often required. Pulse oximetry can be used to screen for hypoxaemia, with patients with a resting oxygen saturation of less than 92% having measurements of arterial blood gases.

Acid–base status can also be assessed from the arterial pH (hydrogen ion concentration) and the bicarbonate. Increases in $Paco_2$, which can occur rapidly, can be compensated by renal conservation of bicarbonate ions, which is a relatively slow process. Acid–base status, particularly mixed respiratory and metabolic disturbances, can be characterized by plotting values on an acid–base diagram (Fig. 18.8.19).

Exercise tests

Exercise increases oxygen consumption and CO_2 production from skeletal muscle. Patients with COPD have the same oxygen consumption for a given workload as normal subjects, but because their dead-space ventilation is higher, a larger minute ventilation is needed to maintain a constant CO_2 level. Since in many patients expiratory airflow is limited within the tidal volume range, the only

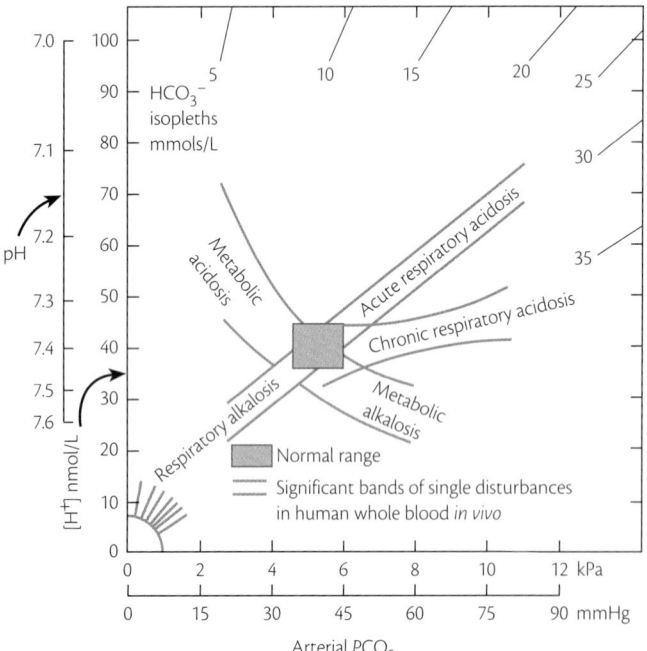

Fig. 18.8.19 A nonlogarithmic acid–base diagram derived from the measured acid-base status of patients within the five abnormal bands illustrated and of normal subjects (hatched box). This plot of CO_2 tension against hydrogen ion concentration (pH) allows the likely acid–base disturbance and calculated bicarbonate value (obtained from the relevant isopleth) to be rapidly determined, whilst changes during treatment can be plotted serially for each patient. Reprinted with permission from Elsevier (The Lancet, 1971;l:961–965).

way to increase minute ventilation is to increase inspiratory flow and/or shift the end-expiratory position. Both of these manoeuvres are problematic in patients with COPD and require more work from already compromised inspiratory muscles, or result in progressive overinflation, which increases both the work of breathing and symptoms. Metabolic acidosis develops at lower work rates in patients with severe COPD. In patients with COPD, progressive cycle exercise is limited by dyspnoea in 40% and by leg fatigue in 25%, probably reflecting general debility. The following three forms of exercise test can be performed.

Progressive symptom-limited exercise

In this test the patient is encouraged to maintain exercise, on a treadmill or a cycle, until symptoms prevent them from continuing. A maximum test is usually defined as a heart rate of greater than 85% predicted or ventilation greater than 90% predicted. The results are useful to assess whether coexisting cardiac or psychological factors contribute to exercise limitation.

Self-paced exercise

These tests are easy to perform. The 6-min walk is the most commonly used test and has a coefficient of variation of around 8%. However, it is only useful in patients with moderately severe COPD (FEV_1 <1.5 litres) who would be expected to have an exercise tolerance of less than 600 m in 6 min. There is a weak relationship between walking distance and FEV_1.

The incremental shuttle walk test is an alternative self-paced exercise test and involves walking at an ever faster speed around cones placed 10 m apart. Increased speed is encouraged by the use of an audio signal. It is in essence a symptom-limited maximal performance test.

Steady-state exercise

This involves exercise at a sustainable percentage of maximum capacity for 3 to 6 min, during which blood gases are measured, enabling calculation of dead space:tidal volume ratio (V_D/V_T) and shunt. This assessment is seldom required in patients with COPD.

Tests of respiratory muscle function

The usual tests of respiratory muscle function in COPD are maximum mouth pressures. The maximum inspiratory pressure is impaired, usually because of hyperinflation or abnormal mechanics of breathing. By contrast, a reduction in the maximum expiratory pressure can be attributed to muscle weakness. These tests can be useful in cases where breathlessness or hypercapnia is not fully explained by other lung function testing and peripheral muscle weakness suspected.

Sleep studies

Hypoxaemia occurs during sleep, particularly rapid eye movement (REM) sleep, in patients with COPD. However, measurement of nocturnal hypoxaemia does not provide any further prognostic or clinically useful information in the assessment of patients with COPD, unless coexisting sleep apnoea syndrome is suspected.

The predictive value of combinations of tests

A combination of variables can give a more detailed indication of disease severity that any single parameter. The BODE index—which is a composite score of BMI, airways obstruction, dyspnoea,

Table 18.8.9 The body mass index, airflow obstruction, dyspnoea, and exercise capacity (BODE) index in COPD

Variable	Points on BODE index			
	0	1	2	3
FEV$_1$ (% predicted)	≥65	50–64	36–49	≤35
Distance (m) walked in 6 min	≥350	250–349	150–249	≤149
MRC dyspnoea scale	0–1	2	3	4
Body mass index	≥21	≤21		

The hazard ratio for death from any cause increases by 1.34 and for respiratory death increases by 1.62 for every point increase on the BODE score.

and exercise—appears to be a better predictor of subsequent survival than any single component (Table 18.8.9).

Other routine tests

A full blood count may reveal the anaemia of chronic disease which occurs in COPD. Polycythemia may be present: this is present but uncommon in patients with severe COPD, but important to recognize since it predisposes to vascular events. It should be suspected when the haematocrit is greater than 47% in women and 52% in men, and/or the haemoglobin is greater than 16 g/dl in women and 18 g/dl in men, provided other causes of spurious polycythaemia, due to decreased plasma volume, such as caused by dehydration or diuretics, can be excluded.

α$_1$-Antitrypsin levels and phenotype should be measured in all patients under the age of 45 years, and in those with a family history of emphysema at an early age.

There is no indication for measuring blood biochemistry routinely in patients with clinically stable COPD. Similarly, routine electrocardiography is not required in the assessment of patients with COPD and is an insensitive technique in the diagnosis of cor pulmonale.

Imaging
Plain chest radiography

The features on a plain posterior–anterior chest radiograph are not specific for COPD and are usually those of severe emphysema. There may be no abnormalities, even in patients with very appreciable disability. Bronchial wall thickening, shown as parallel line opacities on a plain chest radiograph, has been described, but this finding may relate to coincidental bronchiectasis. The most reliable radiographic signs of emphysema can be divided into those due to overinflation, vascular changes, and bullae.

Overinflation of the lungs results in the following:

◆ There is a low flattened diaphragm (Fig. 18.8.20) such that the border of the diaphragm in the midclavicular line is at or below the anterior end of the sixth rib. In a flattened diaphragm the maximum perpendicular height from a line drawn between the costal and cardiophrenic angles to the border of the diaphragm is less than 1.5 cm.

◆ An increased retrosternal air space occurs when the horizontal distance from the anterior surface of the aorta to the sternum exceeds 4.5 cm on the lateral film at a point 3 cm below the manubrium.

◆ There is an obtuse costophrenic angle on the posterior–anterior or lateral chest radiograph.

◆ The inferior margin of the retrosternal air space is 3 cm or less from the anterior aspect of the diaphragm.

The vascular changes associated with emphysema result from loss of alveolar walls and appear as:

◆ a reduction in size and number of pulmonary vessels, particularly at the periphery of the lung

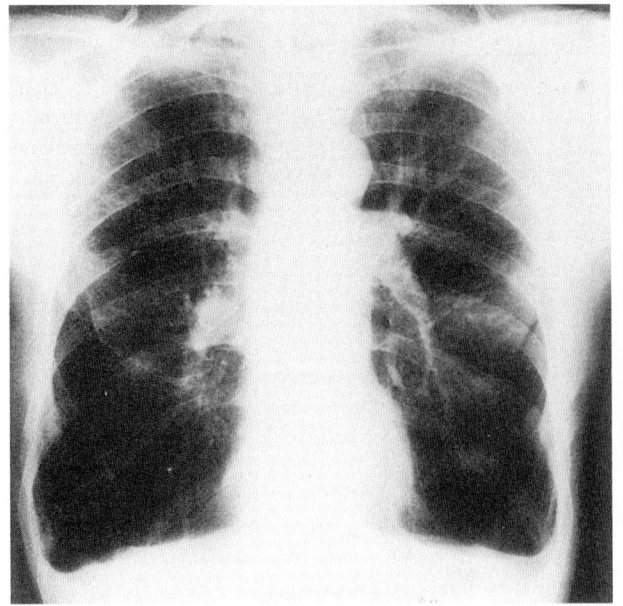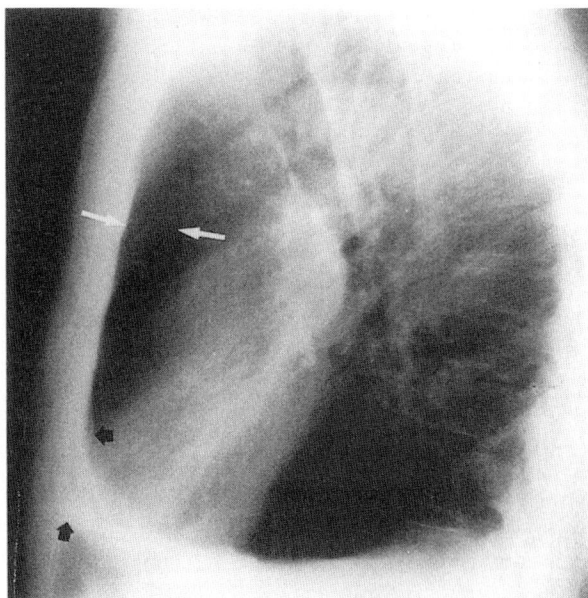

Fig. 18.8.20 PA and lateral chest radiographs showing generalized emphysema. On the PA radiograph the diaphragm is low (below the anterior ends of the seventh ribs) and flat, the lower zones are transradient because of oligaemia, and there are obtuse costophrenic angles. On the lateral chest radiograph the diaphragm is mildly inverted and the retrosternal transradiency is wide (white arrows) and inferiorly it closely approaches the diaphragm (black arrows).

- vessel distortion, producing increased branching angles, excess straightening, or bowing of vessels

- areas of transradiency

A general increased transradiency may be due to an overexposed chest radiograph. Focal areas of transradiency surrounded by hairline walls represent bullae. These may be multiple, as part of a generalized emphysematous process, or localized. An 'increase in lung markings' rather than areas of increased transradiency has often been described in patients with COPD: the cause of these changes is unknown, but may at least be contributed to by nonvascular linear opacities due to scarring.

The accuracy of diagnosing emphysema on the plain chest radiograph increases with severity of the condition, being 50 to 80% in patients with moderate to severe disease. However, the sensitivity has been reported as being as low as 24% in patients with mild to moderate disease. However, despite this a plain chest radiograph is useful at the time of diagnosis to help exclude alternative diagnoses and to establish the presence of significant comorbidities.

CT

CT imaging has been used since the early 1980s to detect and quantify emphysema. Studies using CT can be divided into those that use visual assessment of low-density areas of the CT scan, which can be either semiquantitative or quantitative, and those that use CT lung density to quantify areas of low X-ray attenuation. These studies roughly divide into those that measure macroscopic or microscopic emphysema, respectively.

A visual assessment of emphysema on CT scan (Fig. 18.8.21) reveals:

- areas of low attenuation without obvious margins or walls

- attenuation and pruning of the vascular tree

- abnormal vascular configurations

The sign that correlates best with areas of macroscopic emphysema is an area of low attenuation. However, visual assessment of the extent of macroscopic emphysema by CT scanning is insensitive, subjective, and has a high intra- and interobserver variability. Thus, CT scanning generally tends to underestimate the severity of the disease, with centrilobular lesions smaller than 5 mm particularly likely to be missed.

It is possible using high-resolution CT to distinguish the various types of emphysema, particularly when the changes are not severe, depending on the distribution of the lesions.

A more quantitative approach of assessing macroscopic emphysema is by highlighting pixels within the lung fields in a predetermined low-density range, between −910 and −1000 Hounsfield units, the so-called 'density mask' technique. The choice of the density range is fairly arbitrary, but a good correlation has been shown between pathological emphysema scores and CT 'density mask' score, although areas of mild emphysema may still be missed. Microscopic emphysema can be quantified by measuring CT lung density, which is expressed on a linear scale in Hounsfield units (water = 0; air = −1000). In this range, CT lung density is a direct measure of physical density and is determined by the relative mix of air, blood, and interstitial fluid in tissue. Thus, as emphysema develops, a decrease in alveolar surface area would occur as alveolar walls are lost, associated with an increase in distal air space

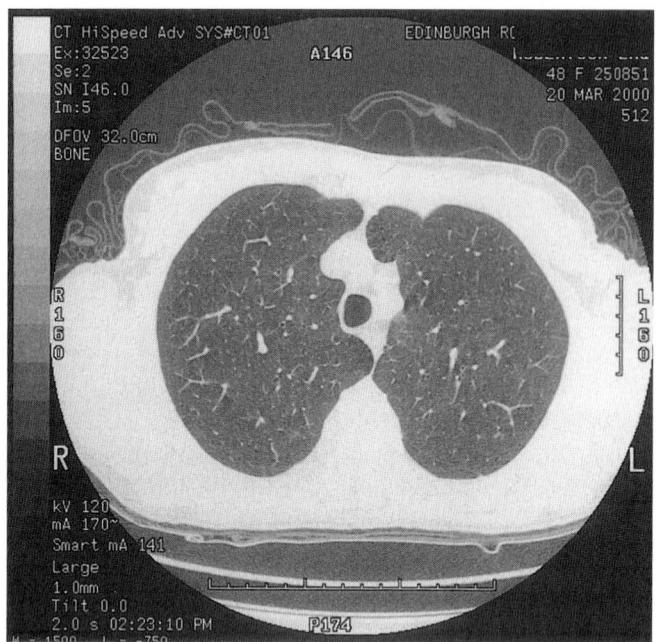

(a)

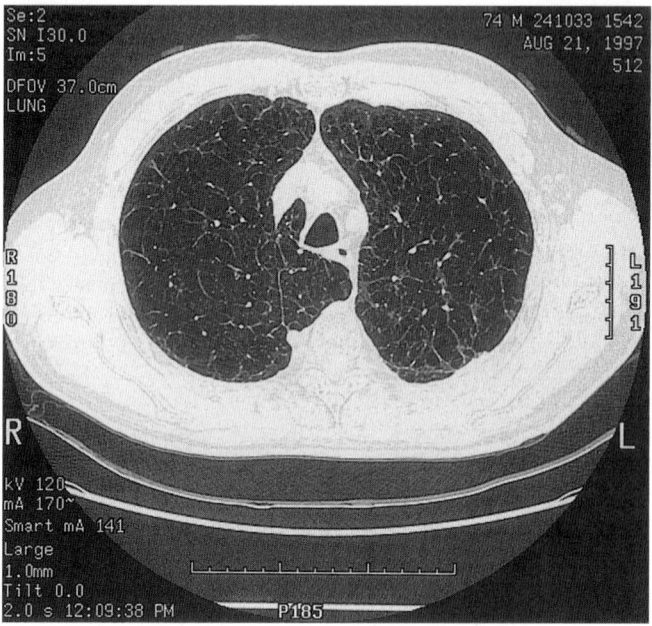

(b)

Fig. 18.8.21 High-resolution CT scan of (a) normal lung, (b) panacinar emphysema.

size, which would decrease lung CT density in association with a decrease in lung function.

More studies are required before CT lung density can be used as a standardized technique to quantify microscopic emphysema. It is particularly important to define the range of normality, and to standardize the calibration of CT scanners and the lung volume at which scans should be performed. However, at present, CT is the most sensitive and specific imaging technique for assessing emphysema in life and can detect mild emphysema in symptomatic patients with a normal chest radiograph. CT can also be useful in detecting the distribution of emphysema during assessment for lung volume reduction surgery, in the detection of bullous disease, and in some cases of diagnostic doubt.

Imaging in patients with pulmonary hypertension/cor pulmonale

Right ventricular hypertrophy or enlargement produces nonspecific cardiac enlargement on the plain chest radiograph, the most widely used measurement to assess the presence of pulmonary hypertension being the width of the right descending pulmonary artery, measured just below the right hilum, where the borders of the artery are delineated against air in the lungs laterally and the right mainstem bronchus medially. The upper limit of the normal range of the width of the artery in this area is taken as 16 mm in men and 15 mm in women. Other studies have suggested an upper limit of normal ranging between 16 and 20 mm, which gives a sensitivity of detecting a pulmonary arterial pressure greater than 20 mmHg of 68 to 95%, with a specificity of 65 to 88%. Although these measurements can be used to detect the presence or absence of pulmonary arterial hypertension, they cannot accurately predict the level of the pulmonary arterial pressure, and can therefore only be used as a screening test.

Echocardiography can be used to assess the level of pulmonary arterial pressure in patients with COPD, although overinflation in such patients makes assessment by echocardiography difficult. Right heart catheterization remains the 'gold standard' for measurement of pulmonary arterial pressure but is rarely required in the assessment of patients with COPD.

Prevention of COPD

Since tobacco smoking is the major aetiological factor in COPD the disease is theoretically preventable, with cessation of cigarette smoking is the single most important way of affecting the outcome. Other important aetiological factors such as atmospheric pollution are also preventable. In the United Kingdom around 31% of men and 29% of women are current cigarette smokers, and around 80 to 90% of patients with COPD have been regular smokers at sometime in their life. At least 90% of smokers are aware of the adverse health effects of cigarette smoking, 70% wish to give up the habit, and most of these have made a serious attempt to quit. However, only 40% of regular smokers have succeeded in quitting cigarette smoking by age 60. Nicotine in tobacco smoke is addictive, and regular smokers who reduce or cease their nicotine intake experience the characteristic withdrawal syndrome resulting from nicotine craving, manifest as anxiety, lack of concentration, irritability, restlessness, and increased appetite. Nicotine addiction develops rapidly and withdrawal symptoms can be shown to occur even in adolescent smokers, hence a critical preventive measure is to reduce the number of children starting smoking.

Smoking cessation

Smoking cessation reduces the subsequent decline in lung function (see Fig. 18.8.6) and is the single most important step that can be taken to prevent the progression of the disease. This is particularly true during the early stages of COPD, where both symptoms and lung function may improve. In advanced disease, quitting smoking may not improve pulmonary function, but symptoms such as cough may still improve. The implications for their future health should be discussed with every patient who smokes.

Box 18.8.6 The five As of smoking cessation

These should form a routine component of health care delivery

- **Ask** about tobacco use
- **Advise** quitting smoking
- **Assess** willingness to make an attempt
- **Assist** in quit attempt
- **Arrange** follow-up

Advice should be given in a nonjudgemental and empathetic manner. It should be emphasized that stopping smoking is not easy and that several attempts may be required to achieve long-term success. It is most important to determine whether patients are motivated to stop and, if so, to support a quit attempt as soon as possible. If patients are not motivated, the reasons for not quitting should be explored and they should be encouraged to consider quitting in the future. Brief advice on smoking cessation is shown in Box 18.8.6.

Asking about smoking habit in every patient may have a positive reinforcing effect against starting smoking in nonsmokers. The reported success rates of smoking cessation interventions come mainly from studies conducted in a primary care setting, and vary between 10 and 30%. A recent review of the literature suggests that in those who request extra help to stop smoking, and when this is given in the form of nicotine replacement or even contact with a support group, the success rate can be up to 25%.

Although it would seem logical, as in other addictions, to suggest a reduction in nicotine levels by a gradual reduction in the number of cigarettes smoked, so as to reduce the severity of withdrawal symptoms, it has been shown that patients who gradually cut down the number of cigarettes smoked tend to inhale more to maintain their usual blood nicotine levels. It has also been shown that those who are unable to quit abruptly are not successful in reducing their consumption of cigarettes over the long term.

The intensity of the strategy employed in a cessation programme should depend on the motivation of the patient to give up smoking. There is no difference in the success rates in unselected smokers between regimens involving brief intervention and those with more prolonged intervention, whereas it is clear that those who are motivated to attend smoking cessation clinics have a better chance of long-term cessation than those who have a brief intervention by the general practitioner. It is therefore better to put time and effort only into those patients who are motivated to give up, and offer only a brief intervention in those with less motivation.

It is important that patients are given a clear strategy for smoking cessation and that the success rates are measured by corroboration with carbon monoxide measurements in breath, or urinary cotinine levels. Meta-analysis of randomized controlled trials of nicotine gum found a clear benefit in terms of abstinence rates at 1 year (23% vs 13%) in a smoking cessation clinic, but no effect in a general practice setting (11% vs 12%). Similar abstinence rates at 1 year have been quoted in a general hospital study in the United Kingdom.

Nicotine skin patches allow a slow infusion of nicotine, which creates plasma nicotine levels up to half of those produced by smoking. Trials carried out with nicotine patches indicate that similar success rates to nicotine chewing gum can be achieved. Recent studies using the antidepressant drug bupropion have also shown quit rates similar to those of nicotine replacement therapy in smokers. The nicotine receptor partial agonist varenicline has also shown good quit rates.

Management of stable COPD

The ideal goals of treatment for COPD are to:

* relieve symptoms
* improve exercise tolerance
* improve health status
* prevent disease progression
* prevent and treat complications
* prevent and treat exacerbations
* reduce mortality

It is important that these goals are reached with minimal side effects from treatment, and it is important to acknowledge that none of the existing medications for COPD has been shown to modify the long-term decline in lung function that characterizes the disease. However, treatments have been shown to reduce symptoms, improve exercise tolerance, improve quality of life, and reduce exacerbation rates. In general, treatment tends to be cumulative, with increasing medications required as the disease progresses. Individuals differ in their response to treatment, and in the side effects they report, hence careful monitoring is required to balance improvement with treatment and the unacceptable side effects of commonly used drugs and formulations (Table 18.8.10).

Therapy at each stage of COPD is summarized in Fig. 18.8.22, with details of specific treatments discussed below.

Bronchodilators

Bronchodilator therapy is the cornerstone of treatment to reduce symptoms and increase exercise tolerance in patients with COPD. By contrast with bronchial asthma, the effects are small in patients with COPD, due to structural changes within the airways. The principal bronchodilators—β_2-agonists, anticholinergic drugs, and theophylline derivatives—relax airway smooth muscle as their primary action and hence decrease airway resistance (Fig. 18.8.23). However, these drugs may also reduce overinflation of the lungs, allowing the lungs to empty more completely. It should be emphasized that relatively small changes in airway dimensions can have major effects on respiratory mechanics, which may be translated into improvement in symptoms and exercise capacity, but regular bronchodilator use does not modify the decline in lung function in COPD.

β-Agonists

The major action of β-agonists is to relax airway smooth muscle by stimulating β-adrenergic receptors, which increase cAMP. Inhaled β_2-agonists are preferred to oral preparations because they are as efficacious in much smaller doses and have fewer side effects. They have a relatively rapid onset of action and are therefore used for symptomatic relief, and they can also increase exercise tolerance in patients with COPD. The effects of short-acting β-agonist last for 4 to 6 h. There is no evidence that the response to a β-agonist diminishes with

time and patients with COPD should be told to take them as required, although those with severe disease may prefer to take regular doses three to four times daily to obtain symptomatic relief.

Long-acting β_2-agonists (such as salmeterol and formoterol) have duration of action of at least 12 h due to their prolonged receptor occupancy and can be given twice daily. Formoterol has a more rapid onset of action than salmeterol. In randomized placebo-controlled studies long-acting β-agonists have been shown to improve symptoms and quality of life, producing a small improvement in spirometry without any significant change in exercise capacity. A Cochrane Systemic Review of trials of long acting β-agonists failed to show a consistent effect on exacerbation rates in patients with COPD.

Side effects of treatment with β-agonists include tachycardia and the potential to precipitate cardiac rhythm disturbances in susceptible patients, although this is uncommon with inhaled therapy. However, this can be troublesome in some cases, particularly older patients treated with high doses of β-agonist, and hypokalaemia can occur, particularly if treatment is combined with thiazide diuretics. These effects show tachyphylaxis, unlike the bronchodilator actions. Small reductions in Pao_2 have been shown to occur after administration of short and long-acting β-agonist, but these are of doubtful clinical significance. Despite previous concerns, studies have shown no associations between β-agonist use and accelerated loss of lung function or increased mortality in COPD. There is little evidence to support the use of sustained-release oral β_2-agonists in patients with COPD.

Anticholinergics

Anticholinergic drugs block the effect of acetycholine on muscarinic receptors. Like β_2-agonists, short-acting anticholinergics (e.g. ipratropium and oxitropium) affect both central and peripheral airways and also reduce FRC. They take 30 to 60 min to reach peak effect in most patients with COPD, which is slower than β_2-agonists, but they act for longer (6–10 h). Optimal bronchodilatation occurs with 80 μg of ipratropium and 200 μg of oxitropium bromide, with studies comparing these treatments suggesting no difference in the peak or duration of bronchodilatation. Thus 80 μg of ipratropium should be used in patients with COPD, rather than the customary 40 μg, to produce maximum effect.

Tiotropium bromide is an anticholinergic agent that has a longer time course of action than ipratropium, showing effects over 24 h, and thus can be given once daily. It has been shown to improve symptoms, decrease lung overinflation, and decrease exacerbation rates in patients with COPD.

Theophyllines

Theophyllines, or methylxanthine derivatives, produce a modest bronchodilator effect in patients with COPD. There is still controversy over their exact mode of action: they may act as nonselective phosphodiesterase inhibitors, producing bronchodilatation by increasing cAMP, but they have a range of other proposed actions, including anti-inflammatory and to improve inspiratory muscle function, although the clinical significance of these effects is disputed (Box 18.8.7).

The effect of theophyllines on symptoms and on exercise tolerance is variable and often occurs at the top of the therapeutic range. Long-term treatment with theophyllines is limited to the oral route, resulting in a slower onset of action compared with inhaled bronchodilators. Improvement in the phamacokinetics of

Table 18.8.10 Common formulations of drugs used in COPD

Drug	Inhaler (μg)	Solution for nebulizer (mg/ml)	Oral	Vials for injection (mg)	Duration of action (h)
β2-Agonists					
Short-acting					
Fenoterol	100, 200 (MDI)	1	0.05% (syrup)		4–6
Salbutamol	100, 200 (MDI and DPI)	5	5 mg (pill) 0.024% (syrup)	0.1, 0.5	4–6
Terbutaline	400, 500 (DPI)	–	2.5, 5 (pill)	0.2, 0.25	4–6
Long-acting					
Formoterol	4.5–12 (MDI and DPI)				12+
Salmeterol	25–50 (MDI and DPI)				12+
Anticholinergics					
Short-acting					
Ipratropium bromide	20, 40 (MDI)	0.25–0.5			6–8
Oxitropium bromide	100 (MDI)	1.5			7–9
Long-acting					
Tiotropium	18 (DPI)				24+
Combination short-acting β2-agonists plus anticholinergic in one inhaler					
Fenoterol/ipratropium	200/80 (MDI)	1.25/0.5			6–8
Salbutamol/ipratropium	75/15	0.75/4.5			6–8
Methylxanthines					
Aminophylline			200–600 mg (pill)	240 mg	Variable up to 24
Theophylline (SR)			100–600 mg (pill)		Variable up to 24
Inhaled glucocorticosteroids					
Beclomethasone	50–400 (MDI and DPI)	0.2–0.4			
Budesonide	100, 200, 400 (DPI)	0.20, 0.25, 0.5			
Fluticasone	50–500 (MDI and DPI)				
Triamcinolene	100 (MDI)	40		40	
Combination long-acting β₂-agonists plus glucocorticosteroids in one inhaler					
Formoterol/budesonide	4.5/160, 9/320 (DPI)				
Salmeterol/fluticasone	50/100, 250, 500 (DPI) 25/50, 125, 250 (MDI)				
Systemic glucocorticosteroid					
Prednisone			5–60 mg (pill)		
Methylprednisolone			4, 8, 16 mg (pill)		

DPI, dry powder device; MDI, metered-dose inhaler.

oral theophyllines has occurred with the production of long-acting formulations.

The bronchodilator action of theophyllines is relatively limited in patients with COPD, and exercise tolerance changes little with theophylline treatment. Any improvement in exercise tolerance has been thought to result from an effect on respiratory muscles, which may reflect a fall in trapped gas volume.

Theophyllines have a narrow therapeutic index and patients often experience side-effects within the therapeutic range (Box 18.8.8). Other factors that are common in COPD—such as smoking, hypoxaemia, antibiotics and infection (Table 18.8.11)—all alter

theophylline clearance and make the control of theophylline dosage difficult, requiring measurement of plasma theophylline levels (therapeutic levels 10–20 mg/litre, 55–110 μm). The possible beneficial effects of theophyllines have to be balanced against their potential side effects and the fact that a similar benefit may be achievable with inhaled bronchodilators, hence theophyllines are reserved for patients in whom other treatments have failed to control symptoms adequately.

Selective phosphodiesterase-4-inhibitors (roflumolast, cilomolast) have recently been developed: these may retain the beneficial properties of theophylline whilst avoiding unwanted side effects.

Therapy at Each Stage of COPD*

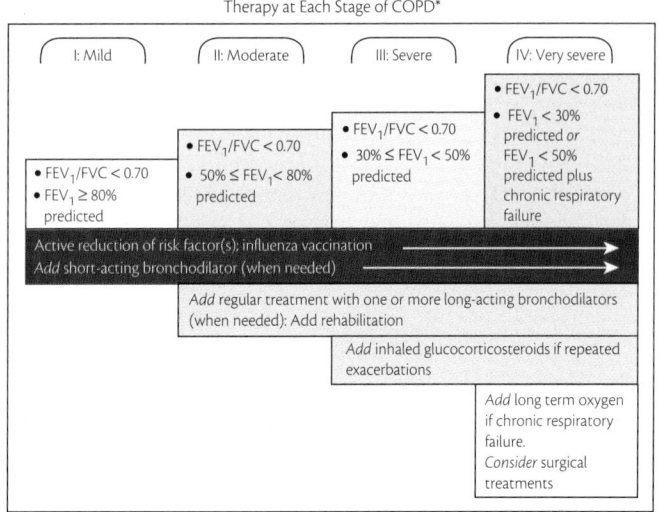

I: Mild	II: Moderate	III: Severe	IV: Very severe
• $FEV_1/FVC < 0.70$ • $FEV_1 \geq 80\%$ predicted	• $FEV_1/FVC < 0.70$ • $50\% \leq FEV_1 < 80\%$ predicted	• $FEV_1/FVC < 0.70$ • $30\% \leq FEV_1 < 50\%$ predicted	• $FEV_1/FVC < 0.70$ • $FEV_1 < 30\%$ predicted or $FEV_1 < 50\%$ predicted plus chronic respiratory failure

Active reduction of risk factor(s); influenza vaccination
Add short-acting bronchodilator (when needed)

Add regular treatment with one or more long-acting bronchodilators (when needed): Add rehabilitation

Add inhaled glucocorticosteroids if repeated exacerbations

Add long term oxygen if chronic respiratory failure. *Consider* surgical treatments

Postbronchodilator FEV_1 is recommended for the diagnosis and assessment of severity of COPD.

Fig. 18.8.22 Therapy at each stage of COPD.
From GOLD Guidelines—http://www.goldcopd.com/GuidelineList Pocketguide to COPD diagnosis, management and prevention. A Guide for Healthcare Professionals. Updated 2008 Figure 6: Therapy at each stage of COPD

Combination therapy

Studies of combination therapy are difficult to assess because of problems of suboptimal dosing. Some suggest that drug combinations such as salbutamol and ipratropium, or salbutamol and theophyllines, produce improvement in lung function, exercise tolerance, and health status. It is unclear whether higher doses of one bronchodilator could have achieved a similar effect. Thus, combinations of bronchodilator drugs should only be used if single drugs have been tried and have failed to give adequate symptomatic relief, and combination therapy should only be continued if there is good subjective or objective benefit.

Drug delivery devices

Compliance with inhaled treatment is poor. In the Lung Health Study the overall compliance with therapy was 65%. Since many patients with COPD are elderly, the difficulties encountered with

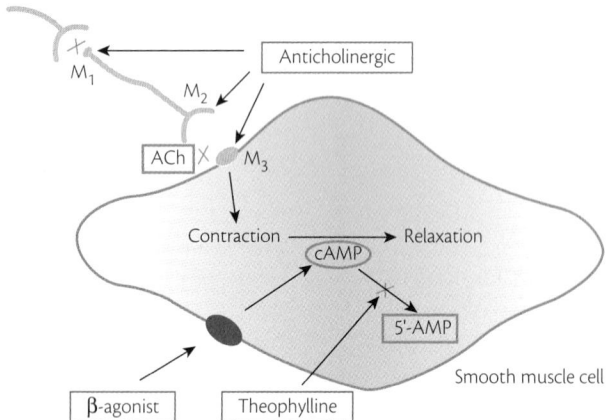

Fig. 18.8.23 Mechanisms of action of bronchodilators. Anticholinergics block muscarinic receptors so that acetylcholine is unable to act upon them; β-agonists increase levels of cAMP; theophylline blocks conversion of cAMP to 5′-AMP. M1, M2, and M3 are three distinct types of muscarinic cholinergic receptors. ACh, acetylcholine.

standard metered dose inhalers (MDI) are exaggerated. These problems can often be overcome by dry powdered formulations or by a spacer device. However, patients with severe COPD are only able to achieve low inspiratory flow rates, and rates as low as 40 litre/min may cause failure of the one-way valve in a spacer device to open.

Home nebulizer therapy

There is controversy over the use of home nebulizer therapy in patients with stable COPD. Using endpoints such as spirometry and exercise tests, it has been shown that nebulized salbutamol is no more effective in patients with COPD than lower doses of the same drug given through a spacer device. However, patients appear to prefer nebulized bronchodilator therapy. This may be because the total dose of the drug delivered by nebulizer therapy is higher, and the facial cooling that occurs with the nebulized solution may itself have an effect on dyspnoea, independent of any effect on airway calibre.

Acute improvement in spirometry with nebulized bronchodilator therapy does not necessarily predict a long-term response, and only a few patients are likely to obtain benefit from high-dose

---

Box 18.8.7 Potential mechanisms of action of theophylline in COPD

• Unselective phosphodiesterase inhibition leading to an increase in cAMP and hence smooth muscle relaxation and airway dilation

• Reduction of diaphragmatic muscle fatigue

• Increased mucociliary clearance

• Respiratory centre stimulation

• Inhibition of neutrophilic inflammation

• Depression of inflammatory gene expression by activation of histone deactylases

• Inhibition of cytokines and other inflammatory cell mediators

• Potentiation of antiinflammatory effects of inhaled corticosteroids

• Potentiation of bronchodilator effects of β_2-agonists

Box 18.8.8 Adverse effects of theophylline

• Nausea and vomiting

• Hypokalaemia

• Abdominal pain

• Headache

• Diarrhoea

• Irritability and insomnia

• Tachycardia

• Seizures

• Cardiac arrhythmias

Table 18.8.11 Factors affecting plasma theophylline concentration

Increased concentration (reduced plasma clearance)	Reduced concentration (increased plasma clearance)
Heart failure	Cigarette smoking
Advanced age	Chronic alcoholism
Liver cirrhosis	Rifampicin
Erythromycin	Phenytoin
Clarithromycin	Lithium
Ciprofloxacin	Carbamazepine
Verapamil	

bronchodilator therapy. Patients should only be supplied with a nebulizer if they have been fully assessed by a respiratory physician who is able to assess the risk/cost benefit. This assessment should include ensuring that optimal use is made of a simple metered dose inhaler or dry powdered device, and that some assessment is made of the patient's response to nebulizer therapy, including a home trial with peak expiratory flow measurements. Dosage regimen must be tailored to individual patient's needs and side effects monitored.

Corticosteroids

The chronic inflammation that occurs in the large and small airways provides a rationale for the use of corticosteroids in COPD. However, the use of corticosteroids in this condition remains contentious, particularly the prediction of which patients will respond.

Oral corticosteroids

A subgroup of patients respond, with a meta-analysis of trials of oral corticosteroids indicating that a significant improvement in FEV_1 (>15% and >200 ml improvement) occurs in 10 to 20% of patients with clinically stable COPD. However, there are no reliable predictors of which patients will respond, and the response to high doses of oral prednisolone in short-term studies does not necessarily predict continued FEV_1 response to long-term inhaled steroids.

Significant side effects may occur with long-term treatment with systemic corticosteroids, in particular steroid myopathy which can contribute to muscle weakness and respiratory failure in patients with advanced COPD. Thus, based on the lack of good evidence of benefit and the potential for side effects, this treatment cannot be recommended for stable COPD.

Inhaled corticosteroids

Four large controlled trials of the effects of a range of doses of inhaled corticosteroids in patients with COPD have failed to show an effect on disease modification as measured by the rate of decline in FEV_1. However, one study in patients with moderate to severe COPD given fluticasone (1000 µg/day) showed a significant benefit in health status and a reduction in exacerbation rates by 25%. The effect was largely seen in those patients with more severe disease (FEV_1 <50% predicted). A reanalysis of pooled data from several long-term studies of inhaled glucocorticoids in COPD has suggested that this treatment may reduce all-cause mortality, but this conclusion requires confirmation in prospective studies.

The side-effect profile of inhaled corticosteroids has been assessed in clinical trials. A few studies have shown an increased incidence of skin bruising in a small percentage of COPD patients, and one long-term study has shown an effect of budesonide on bone density and fracture rate. A further study using triamcinolone acetonide was also associated with decreased bone density, but the clinical relevance of these findings requires further study.

Based on the results of these large-scale trials there appears to be no effect of inhaled corticosteroids on the decline in FEV_1 in mild to moderate COPD. However, there may be an effect on health status and exacerbation rates in moderate/severe COPD. Inhaled corticosteroids may therefore be of benefit to patients with moderate to severe COPD (FEV_1 <50% predicted) who have frequent exacerbations (two or more per year).

Combination treatment with an inhaled corticosteroid and long-acting β-agonist appears to be more effective in reducing symptoms and exacerbations than the individual components. A recent study has also suggested there may be a reduction in mortality with such combination treatment.

Other agents

Vaccines

Influenza vaccination can reduce mortality from influenza in patients with COPD by around 50%. Vaccines containing killed or inactivated viruses are recommended, with the vaccine given once each year, adjusted to be effective against the appropriate strains.

Streptococcal pneumonia is the commonest cause of community-acquired pneumonia, and pneumococcal vaccination is recommended for patients with COPD aged 65 years and older. It is also recommended for those under 65 years of age who have severe disease (FEV_1 <40% predicted), in whom it has been shown to reduce the incidence of community-acquired pneumonia.

Antibiotics

The use of continuous prophylactic antibiotics has not been shown to have any significant effect on the frequency of exacerbations of COPD, hence there is no evidence to support their use.

Mucolytic agents (carbocisteine, mecysteine hydrochloride)

A number of long-term studies have shown some benefit from the regular use of mucolytic therapy in reducing frequency of exacerbations. Although the results of these studies are controversial and the benefits are relatively small, these agents can be tried in patients who have difficulty expectorating sputum or with frequent exacerbations. The mucolytic and antioxidant N-acetylcysteine has been reported in small studies to reduce exacerbation frequency, but a large randomized controlled trial found no effect on the frequency of exacerbations, except in patients who were not treated with inhaled corticosteroids. More data is required before this drug can be recommended as treatment.

Antitussives

Cough can be a troublesome symptom in patients with COPD, but has a significant protective role. Regular use of antitussive therapy is not recommended in stable COPD.

Vasodilators and other drugs

The rationale for the use of vasodilators is based on the relationship between pulmonary arterial pressure and mortality in COPD. Numerous studies of various vasodilators show that most produce small or no change in pulmonary arterial pressure, but are associated with worsening *V/Q* mismatching and therefore worsening gas exchange, hence there is no indication for vasodilators in COPD.

There is no evidence for the use of anti-inflammatory drugs such as sodium cromoglicate, nedocromil sodium, or antihistamines in patients with COPD.

Oxygen therapy

The only treatment that improves the long-term prognosis in patients with COPD is long-term domiciliary oxygen therapy, given for at least 15 h/day, as shown by two multicentre trials, the Medical Research Council (MRC) trial in the United Kingdom and the Nocturnal Oxygen Therapy Trial (NOTT) in the United States of America. The MRC trial of oxygen for 15 h/day showed an increase in 5-year survival from 25 to 41% (compared with no oxygen). The NOTT trial demonstrated the continuous use of oxygen therapy, with a mean use of 17.5 h/day, was beneficial in terms of survival, whereas use for only 12 h/day conferred no benefit.

The reasons for the improvement in survival with oxygen therapy in patients with COPD are still uncertain, but are not clearly related to improvements in pulmonary haemodynamics. In the MRC trial there was no significant improvement in pulmonary arterial pressure following oxygen therapy, but the increase of 3 mmHg/year in pulmonary arterial pressure in the control group did not occur in those who were treated. Overnight oxygen therapy, which abolishes nocturnal desaturation, also decreases pulmonary arterial pressure. However, since the changes in pulmonary haemodynamics produced by long-term oxygen therapy are small, it seems unlikely that these have a major influence on survival.

In addition to the improvement in survival, a number of studies have examined other effects of supplementary oxygen therapy. The impact on breathlessness remains unclear, but several studies have shown that oxygen therapy can lead to an improvement in exercise endurance in patients with COPD, associated with a reduction in ventilation at a given submaximal work rate, and an improvement in walking distance and in ability to perform daily activities.

Assessment of patients taking part in the NOTT study showed that they have marked disturbances in mood and quality of life: after 6 months of oxygen therapy, 42% showed evidence of an improvement in cognitive function, but little change in mood or quality of life. As in all studies of patients with COPD, the FEV_1 is the strongest predictor of survival in patients receiving long-term oxygen therapy, but this treatment does not influence the decline in FEV_1.

Long-term oxygen therapy has been shown to affect the polycythaemia that occurs in patients with chronic hypoxaemia, by reducing both the haematocrit and the red-cell mass, but the clinical relevance of these haematological changes remains unclear.

There are three forms of domiciliary supplemental oxygen therapy:

- long-term controlled oxygen therapy for at least 15 h/day in patients with chronic respiratory failure
- ambulatory oxygen therapy for exercise-related hypoxaemia
- short-burst oxygen therapy—a palliative treatment for the temporary relief of breathlessness

Controlled oxygen is typically delivered by means of nasal prongs, or by mask in patients who are intolerant of nasal cannulas

because of local irritation and dermatitis, although patient compliance with masks is generally less than with nasal prongs. Oxygen can also be delivered by the transtracheal route in patients in whom there is refractory hypoxaemia: this can reduce the resting flow rate requirements by 25 to 50% compared with nasal prongs, resulting in considerable financial savings, particularly if liquid oxygen is the supply mode. However, there are complications, including the formation of mucus balls in 25% of cases, cough, infection, and catheter dislodgement. Reservoir devices have also been developed to reduce total oxygen requirement and cost: these work on the basis that the reservoir fills during the patient's exhalation and supplies oxygen only during inspiration. Continued cigarette smoking should be a relative contraindication to long-term oxygen therapy.

Long-term oxygen therapy

The criteria for the prescription of long-term oxygen therapy are based on the clinical parameters of those patients with COPD who showed an improved survival in the two controlled trials of long-term oxygen therapy. Central to the prescription criteria is the demonstration of significant hypoxaemia in a patient with COPD breathing room air, measured when clinically stable. Long-term oxygen therapy should be considered in COPD patients with:

- low Pao_2 (<7.3 kPa, 55 mmHg), with or without hypercapnia, measured during a period of clinical stability, *or*
- Pao_2 between 7.3 kPa (55 mmHg) and 8.0 kPa (60 mmHg) if there is evidence of pulmonary hypertension, polycythemia (haematocrit >55%) or peripheral oedema

In the United States of America, long-term oxygen therapy can be prescribed based on pulse oximetry (Sao_2 ≤88%). In the United Kingdom it is usually prescribed in the form of oxygen concentrators; liquid oxygen, providing a more portable delivery system, is available in other countries. Adherence to the criteria for the prescription of long-term oxygen therapy is less than optimal in around 40% of patients. Data from the NOTT study showed that 43% of patients who were initially shown to fit the criteria for long-term oxygen therapy were no longer eligible when reassessed 4 weeks later. It is therefore essential that clinical stability is demonstrated, with no exacerbation of COPD for at least 4 weeks, before a decision is made to prescribe long-term oxygen therapy, and that other treatments such as bronchodilators and inhaled steroids are optimized before prescription. Furthermore, reassessment is recommended to ensure that the patient remains significantly hypoxaemic and still fits the criteria for long-term oxygen therapy and to ensure that adequate oxygenation is achieved while breathing oxygen.

On oxygen therapy a Pao_2 of 8 kPa is desirable, and this can usually be achieved by nasal prongs at flow rates between 1 and 3 litre/min. Precipitation of increasing hypercapnia by long-term oxygen therapy is seldom a problem in clinically stable patients. Long-term oxygen therapy should be prescribed for at least 15 h/day and continuously during sleeping hours, which prevents episodes of oxygen desaturation at night and improves sleep quality.

A supply of portable oxygen cylinders should be provided that will allow the patient to leave their home and to exercise without significant desaturation. Oxygen flow rates may have to be increased during exercise to maintain adequate oxygenation.

Ambulatory oxygen

A number of studies have shown that delivering oxygen during exercise can increase the duration of exercise endurance and/or reduce the intensity of exercise induced breathlessness, which is associated with a reduction in the rate at which dynamic hyperinflation occurs in exercise. These changes occur whether or not patients are hypoxaemic at rest and can result in improved health status.

There are no good randomized control trials of the use of ambulatory oxygen. Present guidelines suggest that it should be prescribed to patients with COPD who are receiving long-term oxygen therapy, depending on their activity. To allow patients to travel outside the home, ambulatory oxygen should generally be given at the same flow rate as for long-term oxygen. In those who are active, assessment should be made to evaluate the oxygen flow rate necessary to correct exercise induced desaturation.

Patients with mild hypoxaemia (Pao_2 >7.3 kPa) who are not on long-term oxygen, and those who show a desaturation on exercise (a fall in Sao_2 of 4% to a value of <90%), should have a formal assessment for ambulatory oxygen which should take the form of a 6-min walk or shuttle walking test performed without oxygen. Ambulatory oxygen should only be prescribed if there is evidence of exercise desaturation that is corrected by the proposed device and who show improvement in exercise tolerance, although this recommendation is controversial.

Short-burst oxygen therapy to reduce breathlessness

Many patients on maximum drug therapy for COPD remain breathless on exercise, which has led to the use of oxygen to minimize the sensation of breathless. Studies of oxygen used in this way have failed to show any consistent effect on either breathlessness or the rate of recovery from breathlessness, but have shown a reduction in the degree of dynamic hyperinflation during recovery from exercise. The use of short-burst oxygen therapy remains controversial.

Oxygen during air travel

Commercial aircraft cabins are pressurized to the equivalent of an altitude of no greater than 2600 m, producing a cabin oxygen tension of around 100 mmHg (equivalent to breathing 15% oxygen at sea level). Worsening hypoxaemia may exacerbate the symptoms of breathlessness, particularly in patients who are already hypoxaemic with a Pao_2 less than 8 kPa, and this will worsen with minimal exercise.

Patients whose oxygen saturations are ≥95% or whose resting Pao_2 at sea level is great than 9.3 kPa (70 mmHg) are likely to be safe to fly without supplemental oxygen.

Patients whose oxygen saturation is less than 92% at rest should have in-flight oxygen prescribed, including all those already on home oxygen therapy. The airline should be contacted by letter by the patient's respiratory physician, recommending the use of oxygen: most will provide oxygen throughout the flight.

Patients who have saturations between 92 and 95% can desaturate profoundly at altitude and can be offered a hypoxic challenge test in a lung function laboratory. Those who fly should ideally be able to maintain an in-flight Pao_2 of at least 6.7 kPa (50 mmHg). In those whose Pao_2 remains above 7.4 kPa (>55 mmHg), oxygen should not be required. In those in whom Pao_2 falls below 6.6 kPa it is generally accepted that in-flight oxygen should be prescribed at a rate of 2 litres/min. In the remainder it is a matter of clinical judgement as to whether the prescription of oxygen is required.

Ventilatory support

Non-invasive ventilatory support has been used extensively in exacerbations of COPD, but there is no good evidence to support the use of noninvasive intermittent positive pressure ventilation (NIPPV) in patients with stable COPD and respiratory failure. Randomized controlled trials have failed to show a definite survival advantage or benefit to quality of life. However, a combination of NIPPV with long-term oxygen therapy may be of some use in selected patients with pronounced daytime hypercapnia.

Pulmonary rehabilitation

Pulmonary rehabilitation has been defined as a 'multidisciplinary programme of care for patients with chronic respiratory impairment that is individually tailored and designed to optimize physical and social performance and autonomy'. This is particularly important in the moderate to severe stages of COPD, when breathlessness may result in avoidance of activity and result in deconditioning of the skeletal muscles, which in turn leads to increasing disability, social isolation, and depression. This compounds the problem of dyspnoea and lack of fitness, with a vicious circle ensuing that leads to increasing dependency, disability, and worsening quality of life (Fig. 18.8.24). The aim of pulmonary rehabilitation is to break this vicious circle of increasing inactivity, breathlessness and physical deconditioning, and improve exercise capacity and functional status. There is now a large body of evidence that this approach is effective for patients with COPD, with benefits as summarized in Box 18.8.9. These effects are achieved with little impact on pulmonary function measurements.

Pulmonary rehabilitation programmes should be tailored to each individual patient's needs, addressing their individual symptoms, functional limitation, knowledge of the disease, emotional disturbance, cognitive and psychosocial function, and nutritional needs. This involves a multidisciplinary team which varies between

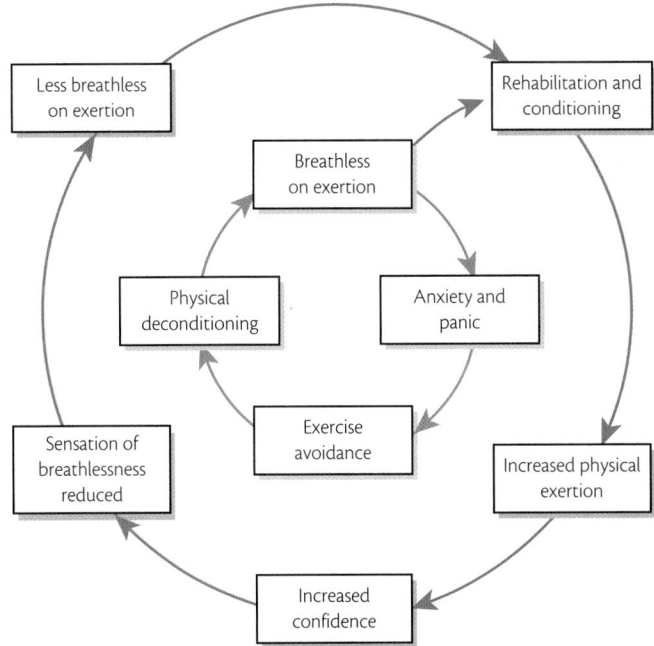

Fig. 18.8.24 The vicious circle of deconditioning and inactivity that occurs in COPD, and the effect of pulmonary rehabilitation.

Box 18.8.9 The benefits of pulmonary rehabilitation in COPD

- Reduces intensity of breathlessness on exercise
- Improves exercise tolerance
- Improves health related quality of life
- Reduces the number of days admitted to hospital
- Reduces anxiety and depression associated with COPD

programmes but includes physicians, nurses, respiratory therapists, physiotherapists, occupational therapists, psychologists, dietitians, and social workers. Pulmonary rehabilitation should be considered in all patients with symptoms of breathlessness or other symptoms, e.g. decreased exercise tolerance or restrictions of activities, or impaired health status, because of their disease. There are no specific inclusion criteria that indicate the need for pulmonary rehabilitation, but the following should be considered when choosing patients. Firstly, functional status—the approach is beneficial in patients with a wide range of disability, but those who are severely disabled (e.g. chair bound) are unlikely to respond even to home rehabilitation programmes. Secondly, severity of breathlessness—assessing breathlessness using the MRC questionnaire can be helpful in selecting patients likely to benefit from rehabilitation: those with MRC grade 5 dyspnoea may not benefit. Thirdly, motivation and smoking status—there is no evidence that smokers benefit less than nonsmokers, but many believe that inclusion of smokers in a rehabilitation programme should be conditional on their participation in a smoking cessation programme. Fourthly, the presence of comorbid conditions—some patients may not be suitable for pulmonary rehabilitation, such as those with disabling arthritis or other conditions that put them at risk during exercise, e.g. unstable angina.

There are several components to a comprehensive pulmonary rehabilitation programme including exercise training, education, psychosocial and behavioural intervention, nutritional therapy, and determination of outcome, the latter most typically being assessed by impact on breathlessness, exercise tolerance, and health status.

Exercise training

Exercise training is a key component of pulmonary rehabilitation to recondition skeletal muscles and improve exercise endurance. It is generally undertaken in two forms: endurance or aerobic training, and strength training.

Endurance training involves training of large muscles in a programme that usually involves 30-min sessions at an intensity of at least 50% of maximal oxygen consumption. Leg training is the normal mode of endurance training, with most programmes including exercise sessions of at least 30 min, two to five times a week, for 6 to 12 weeks. Bicycle ergometry and treadmill exercise are both suitable aerobic activities. A number of physiological variables, such as maximum oxygen consumption, maximum heart rate, and maximum work performed can be measured. A less complex approach can be taken utilizing a self-paced walking test, e.g. a 6-min walking distance or shuttle walking tests.

Strength training can be used to supplement endurance training, usually involves training of peripheral muscles, and is of proven benefit. The role of respiratory muscle training in pulmonary rehabilitation is still controversial and has produced equivocal results in patients with COPD.

Patients at all stages of COPD appear to benefit from exercise training programmes, which can be shown to improve exercise tolerance and reduce symptoms of breathlessness and fatigue. These benefits may be sustained even after a single pulmonary rehabilitation programme if exercise training is maintained at home.

Education

Although education is generally regarded as an important component of the management of any chronic disease, it has been relatively poorly studied in patients with COPD. It has been shown that education alone does not improve exercise performance and lung function, but it may improve skills and ability to cope with illness and health status, and is an integral and important component of a comprehensive pulmonary rehabilitation programme. Components which should be covered as part of patient education are shown in Box 18.8.10, and educational programmes also incorporate breathing strategies, such as pursed-lip and diaphragmatic breathing, and energy conservation.

Psychosocial and behavioural intervention

Anxiety and depression are common in a chronic disease such as COPD and should be treated. Difficulties in coping are relatively common and contribute to morbidity. Psychosocial and behavioural intervention, as part of a pulmonary rehabilitation programme, may include educational sessions or support groups that are directed at problems such as stress management, or instruction in progressive muscle relaxation and panic control. Involvement of family members or friends in pulmonary rehabilitation support groups may be useful.

Nutritional therapy

Weight loss and muscle wasting in COPD have an important effect on symptoms, disability and prognosis, independent of the degree of airflow limitation. Depletion of fat-free mass has been reported in around 20% of stable outpatients with the condition. Although weight loss is generally accompanied by a significant loss of fat-free mass, muscle wasting may occur even in patients with COPD whose weight is stable. Weight loss and muscle wasting have several consequences: impairment of skeletal muscle strength and

Box 18.8.10 Patient education in COPD

For all patients
- Information and advice should be given about reducing risk factors

For patients with mild/severe disease
- Information about the nature of COPD
- Instruction how to use inhalers and other treatments
- Pecognition and treatment of exacerbations
- Strategies for minimizing breathlessness

For patients with very severe COPD
- Information about complications
- Information about oxygen treatment
- Advance directives and end of life decisions

exercise capacity, reduced diaphragm muscle mass and reduced diaphragmatic contractility, and decreased health status.

Several studies have now shown that weight loss or being underweight is an independent risk factor for mortality in COPD, hence screening for nutritional status is recommended as part of the assessment of patients with the condition and usually involves measurement of the BMI and of weight change, the criteria to defined weight loss being more than 10% in the past 6 months or more than 5% in the last month. Nutritional intervention should be considered for those who have BMI less than $21 \, kg/m^2$ or involuntary weight loss as defined above.

Nutritional supplementation should initially consist of adapting the patient's dietary habits and the administration energy-dense supplements. The latter should be given in divided quantities during the day to avoid loss of appetite and adverse effects on metabolic and ventilatory efforts resulting from a high caloric load. However, meta-analysis of studies of dietary supplementation concluded that the beneficial effects of nutritional therapy are limited, also that increasing energy intake in patients with severe COPD is difficult to achieve. In advanced COPD combining nutritional supplementation with an anabolic stimulus, such as exercise, to optimize function should be considered. Weight gain can be achieved under these circumstances and has been shown to decrease mortality, independently of FEV_1.

Although being underweight is bad, being obese is not good. Obese patients with COPD are more likely to have greater impairment of activity and a greater degree of breathlessness than patients of normal weight: they should be encouraged to lose weight while participating in regular exercise.

Surgery in the patient with COPD

Patients with COPD have a 2.7 to 4.7-fold increase of postoperative pulmonary complications. Although there are no absolute contraindications for surgery, preoperative evaluation must carefully weigh the benefits and risks, with the latter depending upon the indications for surgery, the surgical procedure, the type of anaesthesia, and the degree of respiratory impairment.

Postoperative complication rates in patients with COPD are dependent on the region of the body in which surgery is performed. In general, the further the procedure from the diaphragm the lower the risk, with abdominal and cardiovascular surgery clearly presenting major risks.

A careful history, physical examination, and assessment of functional capacity should be made prior to any operation. Patients who have a diagnosis of COPD or who have symptoms or risk factors for COPD should have preoperative spirometry, with analysis of arterial blood gases in patients with moderate to severe COPD (FEV_1 <50% predicted). Smoking cessation at least 4 to 6 weeks preoperatively and optimizing lung function can decrease postoperative complications.

Lung resection has an adverse effect on lung function, with thoracoscopic lung resection less invasive and better tolerated than open thoracotomy. Lobectomy produces an approximately 10% reduction in FVC at 6 months after surgery. Pneumonectomy usually causes a permanent reduction of about 30% in lung function and can have significant consequences in patients with COPD. The risk of postoperative respiratory failure is highest in patients undergoing pneumonectomy with a preoperative FEV_1 less than 2 litres or 50% predicted and/or a $T_L co$ less than 50% predicted.

Further assessment of lung function and exercise capacity is required in such cases to determine suitability for surgery.

Management of acute exacerbations of COPD

Exacerbations of COPD are characterized by a sustained worsening of respiratory symptoms (breathlessness, cough, and/or sputum production) that are acute in onset and beyond the normal day-to-day symptom variations. They usually require the patient to seek medical help or alter treatment. Other common symptoms of exacerbations are chest tightness, malaise, and reduced exercise tolerance.

Exacerbations in COPD occur on a background of established disease and are amongst the commonest acute respiratory problems presenting to both primary and secondary care. They account for up to 10% of all medical admissions to hospitals in the United Kingdom. Patients with frequent exacerbations have an accelerated decline in lung function, impaired quality of life, and restricted daily activities. As the disease becomes more severe, the frequency of exacerbations also increases, and—particularly if severe— they affect prognosis, with all cause mortality up to 49% 3 years after hospitalization for an exacerbation of COPD. The mortality of patients admitted for COPD with hypercapnic respiratory failure is around 10%, and long-term outlook is poor, with mortality reaching 40% at one year for those needing ventilatory support.

Prevention, early detection, and prompt treatment of exacerbations have an important impact on clinical progression and improving quality of life in patients with COPD. Exacerbations of COPD are mainly caused by viruses, bacteria, or environmental pollutants, although the precise cause remains unknown in many cases.

Assessment of severity

Determining the severity of an exacerbation depends on assessing the patient's medical history before the exacerbation, including pre-existing comorbidities, together with presenting symptoms, physical examination, and arterial blood gas measurements. When available, prior blood gas measurements are useful for comparison with those during the acute episode.

Spirometry and peak flow measurements are difficult in patients who are acutely ill such that their accuracy is reduced, hence they are not routinely recommended. Pulse oximetry can be used to evaluate oxygen saturation and the need for supplementary oxygen therapy. The diagnosis and management of respiratory failure in COPD is dealt with in Chapter 18.15.

It is important to obtain a chest radiograph during any severe acute exacerbation, in particular to identify some of the possible alternative diagnoses (Box 18.8.11). Pulmonary embolism can be particularly difficult to diagnose during an exacerbation of COPD, particularly when this is advanced. Low systolic blood pressure and an inability to increase Pao_2 above 8 kPa despite high flow oxygen may suggest embolic disease, and if there are strong indications that pulmonary embolism has occurred it is best to treat this along with the exacerbation. A full blood count is rarely informative in an exacerbation of COPD.

Most exacerbations of COPD can be managed in the community. The factors which influence the need for hospital management are shown in Box 18.8.12.

Box 18.8.11 Differential diagnosis of an exacerbation of COPD

- Exacerbation of asthma
- Pulmonary embolism
- Bronchopneumonia
- Bronchial carcinoma
- Bronchietasis
- Pneumothorax
- Upper airways obstruction
- Pulmonary oedema

Oxygen therapy

Oxygen therapy is essential in the management of patients with severe exacerbations of COPD who are admitted to hospital. It should be given to achieve adequate levels of oxygenation (Pao_2 >8 kPa (60 mmHg), or Sao_2 >90%). Patients with respiratory failure should be given controlled oxygen therapy (24–28%) through a venturi mask, or 1 to 2 litres by nasal prongs. Once oxygen is started gases should be checked 30 to 60 min later to ensure satisfactory oxygenation without CO_2 retention or acidosis. Treatment of respiratory failure is discussed in Chapter 18.15.

Bronchodilators

Nebulized bronchodilators should be given as soon as possible to patients with acute exacerbations of COPD, and at 4- to 6-hourly intervals thereafter, or more frequently if required. It is important to ensure that patients do not become hypoxic during such treatment by being denied oxygen treatment, but also that excessive oxygen does not lead to narcosis with a significant rise in $Paco_2$, which is a particular risk in those with an elevated initial $Paco_2$. When this is likely a balance can be achieved by driving the nebulizer with compressed air and simultaneously delivering oxygen by nasal prongs at 1 to 2 litre/min during nebulization.

β-Agonists (salbutamol 2.5–5 mg, or terbutaline 5–10 mg) or an anticholinergic drug (ipratropium bromide 0.5 mg) are commonly used. No difference has been shown between these drugs given alone or in combination in nebulized form in acute exacerbations

---

Box 18.8.12 Factors likely to require that an exacerbation of COPD is treated in hospital

- Marked increase in intensity of symptoms, such as sudden development of resting dyspnoea
- Severe underlying COPD
- Failure of exacerbation to respond to initial medical treatment
- Significant comorbidities
- Frequent exacerbations
- Newly occurring arrhythmias
- Diagnostic uncertainty
- Insufficient home support

---

of COPD. Several studies have shown no difference in the degree of bronchodilatation achieved when the same dose of bronchodilator is given by a metered dose inhaler, with or without a spacer device, or via a nebulizer, even in patients with an acute exacerbation of airways obstruction. However, patients with respiratory failure have been excluded from these studies and hence nebulized bronchodilators are still recommended, but in most cases these should only be necessary for 24 to 48 h and a change to a metered dose inhaler, or a dry powder device, should be made 24 to 48 h before discharge. A response to a nebulized bronchodilator in an acute exacerbation does not imply long-term benefit and assessment for a home nebulizer should be made when the patient is in a stable condition (see previous discussion).

If a patient is not responding to nebulized bronchodilators during an exacerbation, then intravenous methylxanthines may be considered. However, a small randomized placebo-controlled trial of intravenous aminophylline showed no differences in spirometry, arterial blood gases, or the sensation of dyspnoea between the aminophylline and placebo groups over a period of 72 h following admission with exacerbation of COPD. Thus, the prescription of theophyllines has no clear role in management of acute exacerbations of COPD and the possible benefits should be weighed against the side effects, particularly in patients with COPD who have hypoxaemia, infection, and are receiving antibiotics, all of which can affect theophylline clearance. Thus the dose must be carefully individualized and the serum level maintained within a narrow therapeutic range (10–20 mg/litre), the usual loading dose being 6 mg/kg of aminophylline, with a maintenance dosage of 0.5 mg/kg per hour.

Antibiotics

Infection is a common precipitating feature in exacerbations of COPD, although only 50% of patients with severe exacerbations with associated respiratory failure will have a positive sputum culture for a bacterium. The commonest organisms are *Haemophilus influenzae*, *Streptococcus pneumoniae*, and *Moraxella catarrhalis*. However, patients with COPD are often chronically colonized with common bacterial pathogens, hence culture of one of these organisms during an acute exacerbation does not necessarily imply that this organism is responsible for the exacerbation. Viral infections have been shown to be responsible for up to 30% of all exacerbations.

There is limited information from controlled trials on the effects of antibiotics in exacerbations of COPD. In a trial of 173 patients with 362 exacerbations of COPD, patients received either a 10-day course of sulphamethoxazole, amoxicillin, doxycycline, or placebo: relief of symptoms within 21 days was achieved in 68% of the antibiotic-treated group and in 55% of those given placebo. Peak expiratory flow recovered faster with antibiotics, but the differences were small, and treatment failures were twice as common with placebo. The difference in successful outcome between antibiotic and placebo were significant if two of the following symptoms were present—increase in dyspnoea, increase in sputum volume, and increase in sputum purulence—hence antibiotics are recommended if two of these are present.

In view of the limited range of bacteria present in the sputum of patients with exacerbations of COPD, broad-spectrum antibiotics such as amoxycillin at a dose of 250 mg three times daily, or clarithromycin 250 to 500 mg twice daily (as an alternative in patients with penicillin allergy) are recommended. However, prescription of antibiotics should take into account local bacteriological sensitivity patterns, particularly the prevalence of β-lactamase-positive *H. influenzae*, which is around 20% in most areas, and *M. catarralis*, of which 90% are β-lactamase positive. If the patient is known to have had β-lactamase-positive organisms previously in sputum, or fails to respond to amoxicillin, then co-amoxiclav should be considered. Antibiotics should be given orally unless there is a specific indication for intravenous treatment.

Corticosteroids

There are several controlled trials showing benefit of oral corticosteroids in patients with acute exacerbations of COPD. A placebo-controlled study in hospital patients without hypercapnic respiratory failure showed improvement in FEV_1 and reduction in days in hospital in those treated with 30 mg prednisolone daily. A further study of exacerbations treated with prednisolone in the community also showed a positive result. The beneficial effects are small, but the usual regimen is 30–40 mg prednisolone daily for 7–14 days, with no additional benefit for longer courses. The lowest dose that produces benefit is not known. It is important to instruct the patients to discontinue oral corticosteroids after a short course, and to be aware of potential side effects. Those taking oral corticosteroids for less than 3 weeks do not usually need to taper off the dose.

Respiratory stimulants

Since the introduction of noninvasive ventilation the use of respiratory stimulants such as doxapram has become far less common for hypercapnic respiratory failure. If noninvasive ventilation is contraindicated or not immediately available, then doxapram can be used by continuous infusion, but its use may be limited by adverse side effects such as agitation, tachycardia, confusion and hallucinations. Noninvasive ventilation is now standard therapy for hypercapnic respiratory failure in exacerbations of COPD, as discussed in Chapter 18.15.

Diuretics

In patients with fluid retention as a result of respiratory failure and cor pulmonale, diuretics should be used with great care. Grossly swollen legs significantly limit a patient's mobility and can be painful, such that some relief is required, but overdiuresis has the potential to reduce right ventricular end-diastolic volume considerably and hence cardiac output.

Anticoagulants

Pulmonary emboli are probably under-recognized in patients with severe COPD, when they are difficult to diagnose. If *V/Q* scans are performed they will often reveal abnormalities, leading to false-positive reports of pulmonary thromboembolic disease, hence CT pulmonary angiography is the investigation of choice. Prophylactic subcutaneous low-molecular-weight heparin is usually given to patients with exacerbations of COPD, particularly those who have respiratory failure.

Physiotherapy

There is very little evidence to support the use of physiotherapy to improve expectoration in patients with acute exacerbations of COPD, although some studies suggest that there is some benefit for those producing large amounts of sputum.

Surgical treatments for COPD

Bullous emphysema

Exertional dyspnoea is the usual presenting feature in patients with bullous disease, although a single bullae of moderate size is unlikely to produce symptoms when the remaining lung is normal. Bullae may present as a chance finding on a chest radiograph or as a pneumothorax, and they may compress adjacent more normal areas of lung. Occasionally they become infected, in which case there may be a fluid level, sometimes with surrounding consolidation. Such infection may result in closure of the bronchial connection, shrinkage, or even obliteration of the bullae.

Respiratory function tests may be nonspecific and simply reflect COPD. Almost always there is some degree of airway obstruction, which may result from concomitant diffuse emphysema or airways disease, or as a result of the loss of lung elastic recoil that accompanies large bullae. Overinflation is typically present, but is underestimated if measured by the helium dilution technique rather than by plethysmography. Gas exchange is usually impaired as shown by a reduced $T_L$co. The Kco may reflect the quality of the nonbullous lung if the bullae are nonventilating, which may be helpful in making a decision concerning surgery.

The only treatment possible for large bullae is surgical obliteration, which may allow re-expansion of adjacent compressed lung. The principal indication is progressive dyspnoea, but in those with airflow limitation it has been difficult to determine which patients will benefit from bullectomy. Many techniques have been used in the past to assess suitability for the procedure, such as bronchography and pulmonary angiography, which have now been replaced by CT scanning. A critical feature is the quality of the nonbullous lung: airflow limitation is determined by the degree of emphysema in the nonbullous lung rather than the extent of the bullous disease. Quantitative perfusion lung scanning may demonstrate retained perfusion in collapsed peribullous lung, which may improve after operation. Patients with small bullae (<1 litre or <50% of the hemithorax), with an FEV_1 of less than 1 litre, or with hypercapnia, carry a high risk of a poor response to surgery.

The aims of surgery are to obliterate the bullous space and restore the elastic integrity of the lung. Several techniques have been described, including excision, plication, marsupialization, and intracavity drainage. Most operations are performed by a conventional lateral thoracotomy, but superficial bullae have also recently been dealt with using thoracoscopic and laser techniques. The perioperative mortality in published series ranges from 0 to 20% in patients with a wide range of disability and hence operative risk. The best functional results are obtained in younger patients with mild symptoms, large bullae, relatively well-preserved pulmonary function, and normal surrounding lung. Studies of the long-term follow-up of patients after surgery indicate that giant bullae do not recur.

Lung volume reduction surgery

The rationale for the technique of lung volume reduction surgery is to reduce the volume of overinflated emphysematous lung by 20 to 30% by removing emphysematous lung.

The National Emphysema Treatment Trial (NETT), which involved 1200 patients, compared lung volume reduction surgery (LVRS) with medical treatment and showed that after 4.3 years patients with upper lobe emphysema and low post-rehabilitation exercise capacity who had received surgery had a greater survival rate than similar patients who received medical therapy (54% vs 39.7%). Patients who received LVRS also experienced greater improvements spirometry, lung volumes, exercise tolerance, breathlessness, and health-related quality of life. The advantages of surgery compared with medical treatment were less significant among patients who had different distributions of emphysema or a high exercise capacity. However, the trial data also suggests that spirometric lung function returns towards preoperative baseline levels, with consequent worsening breathlessness over a period of time. Hence, although there are positive results of multicentre trials in a selected group of patients, LRVS is an expensive treatment and can be recommended in only very carefully selected patients.

Lung transplantation

Lung transplantation, which is discussed in Chapter 18.16, should be considered in selected patients with very advanced COPD. This has been shown to improve quality of life and functional capacity, although review of studies has indicated that it does not confer survival benefit on patients with endstage emphysema after 2 years.

Further reading

Agusti AG, et al. (2003). Systemic effects of chronic obstructive pulmonary disease. Eur Respir J, 21, 347–60.

Anto JM, et al. (2001). Epidemiology of chronic obstructive pulmonary disease. Eur Respir J, 17, 982–94.

Barnes PJ. (2000). Chronic obstructive pulmonary disease. N Engl J Med, 343, 269–80.

Calverley PMA, et al. (eds) (2003). Chronic obstructive pulmonary disease. Arnold, London.

Celli BR, MacNee W (2004). Standards for the diagnosis and treatment of patients with COPD. Eur Respir J, 23, 841–5.

Celli BR, et al. (2004). The body-mass index, airflow obstruction, dyspnea, and exercise capacity index in chronic obstructive pulmonary disease. N Engl J Med, 350, 1005–12.

Glenny R, et al. (2000). Gas exchange in health: rest, exercise, and aging. In: Roca J, Rodriguez-Roisin R, Wagner PD (eds) Pulmonary and peripheral gas exchange in health and disease, pp. 121–48. Marcel Dekker, New York.

Global Initiative for Chronic Obstructive Pulmonary Disease Workshop Report. http://www.goldcopd.com (accessed August 2008).

Hogg JC, Senior RM. (2002). Chronic obstructive pulmonary disease. II. Pathology and biochemistry of emphysema. Thorax, 57, 830–4.

Hogg JC, et al. (2004). The nature of small-airway obstruction in chronic obstructive pulmonary disease. N Engl J Med, 350, 2645–53.

Jeffery PK (1999). Differences and similarities between chronic obstructive pulmonary disease and asthma. Clin Exp Allergy, 29, 14–26.

MacNee W (2001). Oxidants/antioxidants and chronic obstructive pulmonary disease: pathogenesis to therapy. Novartis Foundation Symp, 234, 169–88.

MacNee W (2005). Pathogenesis of chronic obstructive pulmonary disease. Proc Am Thorac Soc, 2, 258–66.

MacNee W, Calverley PMA. (2003). Chronic obstructive pulmonary disease 7: Management of COPD. Thorax, 58, 261–5.

National Emphysema Treatment Trial Research Group. (2003). A randomized trial comparing lung-volume reduction surgery with medical therapy for severe emphysema. N Engl J Med, 348, 2059–73.

NICE (2004). Chronic obstructive pulmonary disease: management of chronic obstructive pulmonary disease in adults in primary and secondary care., February. National Institute for Health and Clinical Excellence, London.

O'Donnel DE (2002). Assessment and management of dyspnea in chronic obstructive pulmonary disease. In: Similowski T, Whitelaw WA, Derenne JP (eds) Clinical management of chronic obstructive pulmonary disease, pp. 113–70. Marcel Dekker, New York.

Pauwels RA, et al. (2001). Global strategy for the diagnosis, management, and prevention of chronic obstructive pulmonary disease. NHLBI/WHO Global Initiative for Chronic Obstructive Pulmonary Disease (GOLD) Workshop summary. Am J Respir Crit Care Med, 163, 1256–76.

Voelkel N, MacNee W (eds) (2002). Chronic obstructive pulmonary disease. B C Decker, Hamilton, Canada.

Saetta M, et al. (2001). Cellular and structural bases of chronic obstructive pulmonary disease. Am J Respir Crit Care Med, 163, 1304–9.

Schols AMWJ, et al. (1993). Prevalence and characteristics of nutritional depletion in patients with stable COPD eligible for pulmonary rehabilitation. Am Rev Respir Dis, 147, 1151–6.

Vestbo J, et al. (1996). Association of chronic mucus hypersecretion with FEV_1 decline and COPD morbidity. Am J Respir Crit Care Med, 153, 1530–5.

Wouters EFM (2000). Muscle weakness in chronic obstructive pulmonary disease. Eur Respir Rev, 10, 349–53.

Bronchiectasis

D. Bilton

Essentials

Bronchiectatic lung contains permanently dilated subsegmental airways that are inflamed, tortuous, and often partially or totally obstructed with secretions. It arises as a result of the combination of an infectious insult with associated impaired clearance mechanisms: local obstruction and infection distal to the obstruction are both required. Causes include developmental defects, immune deficiency, mucociliary clearance defects and mechanical obstruction, but in many cases (40–60%) the cause is unknown.

Clinical features—bronchiectasis should be suspected when there is a history of persistent cough productive of mucopurulent or purulent sputum throughout the year. About 80% of patients have upper respiratory tract symptoms (postnasal drip, chronic sinus sepsis, recurrent ear infections). Clinical examination is often normal, although 'classical' severe cases show finger clubbing and widespread coarse crackles.

Investigation—the 'gold standard' for diagnosis is high-resolution CT of the chest, which reveals abnormal thick-walled and dilated bronchi. The chest radiograph is normal in at least 50% of cases, but abnormal thickened and dilated bronchi may produce tramline opacities and ring shadows. Investigations to determine the underlying cause will be determined by clinical suspicion but may include testing for cystic fibrosis, immunoglobulins, bronchoscopy, nasal nitric oxide, nasal brushing/biopsy, and tests for allergic bronchopulmonary aspergillosis. Disease status is assessed by high-resolution CT, lung function tests, sputum culture, and measurement of inflammatory markers.

Management—involves the treatment of the specific underlying cause (when possible) and treatment of the bronchiectasis itself, with the most important elements being sputum clearance by physiotherapy and antimicrobials, which need to be given in high dose, often by the nebulized or parenteral routes, and with careful assessment of response in each individual patient. Surgery can be a curative for patients with single lobe, focal bronchiectasis secondary to bronchial obstruction, and lobar resection may also be indicated for otherwise uncontrollable bleeding, or if it is felt that a particular lobe is acting as a 'sump' of infection which prevents good control of symptoms with medical therapy. Lung transplantation may be appropriate in carefully selected cases.

Introduction

The definition of bronchiectasis is based on morbid anatomy described first by Laennec as abnormal chronic dilatation of the bronchi. The word itself is from the Greek *bronchion* (windpipe or tube) and *ektasis* (stretched out or extension). In 1819 Laennec described the condition in an infant who died following whooping cough, but by 1891 it was recognized in a textbook of medicine that bronchiectasis was 'not a separate disease' but 'a result of various affectations of the bronchi'. Thus bronchiectasis is not a precise diagnosis but the final pathology of a number of causes which may require their own specific treatment. The 'gold standard' for diagnosis today is the presence of abnormal thick-walled and dilated bronchi on high-resolution CT in a patient with a persistent cough productive of sputum.

Epidemiology

Since the diagnosis of bronchiectasis depends on the cardinal feature of abnormal chronic dilation of one or more bronchi, it is likely that people with chronic sputum production previously not investigated by bronchography or CT may have been mislabelled as 'bronchitic', leading to an underestimate of the true prevalence of bronchiectasis in the population. Estimates in the United Kingdom up to 1953 varied from 0.77 to 1.3 per 1000 population, but it seems that following the introduction of antibiotic therapy for pulmonary infection, the control of TB, and effective vaccination for whooping cough and measles, that the prevalence of bronchiectasis in the United Kingdom—at least of the more severe type—has fallen, as judged by a reduction in hospital admissions and deaths. The disease does, however, represent a significant problem, even in developed countries. A recent study based on health care claims in the United States of America suggested an estimated prevalence ranging from 4.2 per 100 000 persons aged 18 to 34, to 271.8 per 100 000 among those aged 75 years and older. Prevalence was higher in women than men at all ages.

Recent CT studies of patients with so-called 'chronic bronchitis' suggest that rather than declining, this disorder may simply be underdiagnosed, but only the development of noninvasive imaging applied to large community surveys will tell us the true prevalence. In less developed countries, where antibiotics are less readily available, socioeconomic conditions are poor, and the prevalence of both tuberculosis and HIV infection are high, bronchiectasis is regarded as a common problem.

Pathology

Macroscopic inspection of bronchiectatic lung reveals permanent dilatation of subsegmental airways, which are inflamed, tortuous, and often partially or totally obstructed with secretions. The process also includes bronchioles, and at end stage there may be marked fibrosis of small airways.

In allergic bronchopulmonary aspergillosis (ABPA) the changes are predominantly in proximal airways, and bronchiectasis caused by cystic fibrosis, post-tuberculosis, or ABPA is likely to be more marked in the upper lobes. There is a spectrum of disease ranging from cylindrical, where there is uniform dilatation, to saccular, where there may be gross terminal dilatation of the bronchi (saccules or cyst). An intermediate form is termed varicose bronchiectasis.

Microscopic features

The overall appearance is of chronic inflammation in the bronchial wall, with inflammatory cells and mucus in the lumen. Neutrophils are the dominant cell population in the bronchial lumen, with mainly mononuclear cells in the bronchial wall. There is characteristic destruction of the elastin layer of the bronchial wall with a variable amount of fibrosis. The label follicular is applied when, as part of extensive mural inflammation, there is lymphoid follicle formation, which may in subepithelial sites cause finger like projections blocking the bronchial lumen.

Aetiology and pathogenesis

There is a broad spectrum of causes and underlying conditions associated with bronchiectasis: these are summarized in Table 18.9.1.

The pathogenesis of bronchiectasis requires the combination of an infectious insult with associated impaired clearance mechanisms that may result from local obstruction, impaired local structural defences, or defective immune defences. Experimental animal models support the theory that local obstruction and infection distal to the obstruction are both required in order to produce bronchiectasis. Furthermore the infection is required to be active, with damage to the airway wall then occurring as a result of direct microbial insult or the secondary effects of the host inflammatory response. It has been proposed that a 'vicious cycle' explains the development of bronchiectasis in a predisposed individual given a trigger insult (Fig. 18.9.1). Neutrophil elastase is thought to play a key role. Neutrophils are recruited as part of the natural defences, but the inflammation is not self limiting and in patients with bronchiectasis neutrophils persist in the airway secretions, with free neutrophil elastase activity usually present. Elastase, a neutrophil-derived serine proteinase, is known to inhibit ciliary beating, damage epithelia, act as a mucus secretagogue, and inhibit opsonophagocytosis via cleavage of immunoglobulins. All these actions contribute to persistence of bacteria in the respiratory tract and long-term tissue damage.

Fig. 18.9.1 clearly demonstrates that however a patient enters the pathway, e.g. in primary ciliary dyskinesia, which inhibits

Table 18.9.1 Causes of bronchiectasis and associated conditions

Type of cause	Examples
Developmental defects	Deficiency of bronchial wall (= Williams–Campbell syndrome)
	Structural:
	Pulmonary sequestration
	Tracheobronchomegaly (= Mounier–Kuhn syndrome)
	Biochemical:
	α_1-Antitrypsin deficiency
Immune deficiency	Primary:
	Panhypogammaglobulinaemia,
	Selective immunoglobulin deficiency
	Secondary:
	HIV infection
	Malignancy (chronic lymphocytic leukaemia)
Excessive immune response	Allergic bronchopulmonary aspergillosis
	Post lung transplantation
Mucociliary clearance defects	Primary ciliary dyskinesia
	Cystic fibrosis
	Young's syndrome
Toxic insult	Aspiration of gastric contents.
	Inhalation of toxic gases or chemicals, e.g. ammonia
Mechanical obstruction	Intrinsic—tumour or foreign body
	Extrinsic—e.g. tubercular lymph node
Postinfective	*Bordetella pertussis*
	Measles
	Tuberculosis
Associated conditions	Chronic rhinosinusitis
	Rheumatoid arthritis
	Inflammatory bowel disease (ulcerative colitis, Crohn's disease)
	Coeliac disease
	Yellow nail syndrome
	Connective tissue disorders and vasculitides
Idiopathic	

mucociliary clearance, or with immunoglobulin deficiency, which favours persistence of microbes in the bronchial tree, the vicious cycle becomes self perpetuating with the final outcome of airway damage.

Developmental defects

The congenital forms of bronchiectasis frequently show deficiency of the elements of bronchial wall which are necessary to prevent collapse and hence 'obstruction' of the airway. In Williams–Campbell syndrome there is deficiency of the bronchial cartilage. The Mounier–Kuhn syndrome or tracheobronchomegaly is the 'adult equivalent' of congenital deficiency of bronchial cartilage.

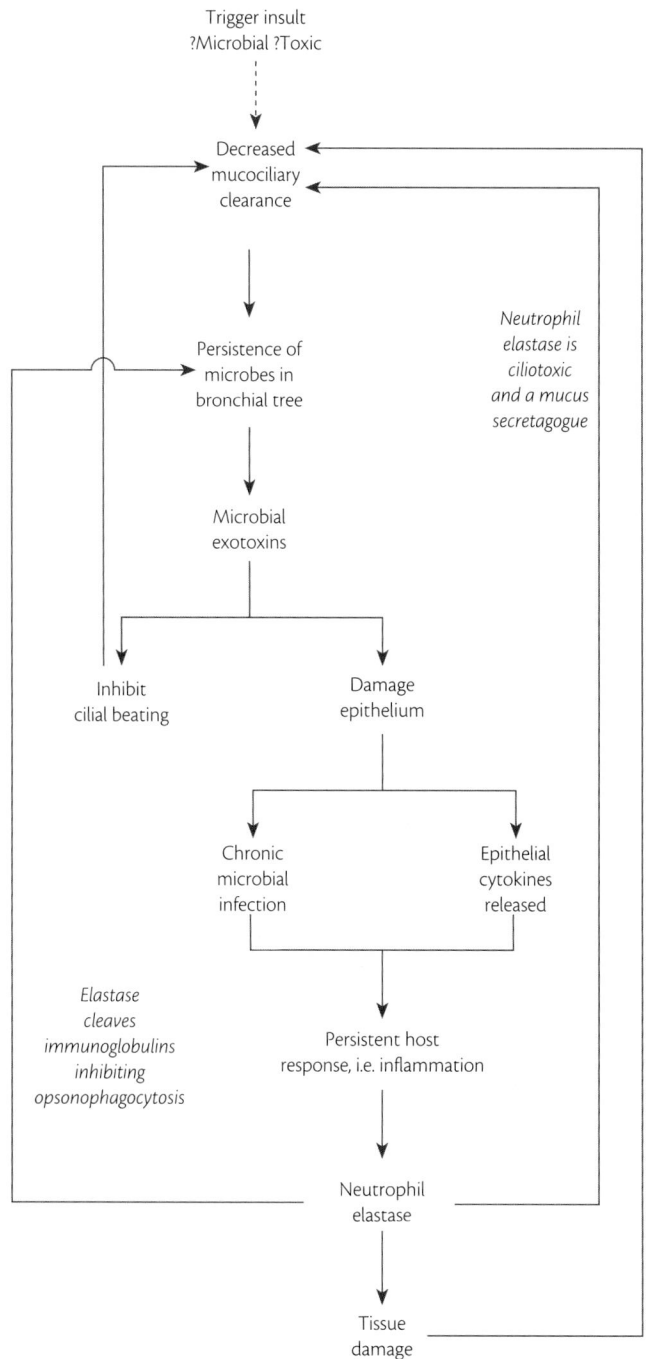

Fig. 18.9.1 The vicious cycle of infection and inflammation leading to progressive tissue damage in bronchiectasis.

Pulmonary sequestration predisposes to bronchiectasis because of decreased pulmonary clearance of the affected segment.

Immune deficiency

Immune deficiency is an important cause of bronchiectasis because treatment with immunoglobulins, where appropriate, will correct the defect and should prevent progression of the condition.

Childhood bronchiectasis should trigger an extensive assessment of phagocytic and cellular immune defences. X-linked hypogammaglobulinaemia, a rare disorder, presents early in life, with bronchiectasis a frequent complication if untreated. Adult-onset acquired panhypogammaglobulinaemia frequently presents with recurrent respiratory infection and is complicated by bronchiectasis if untreated. Selective immunoglobulin deficiencies of IgG and IgM, and IgG subclass deficiencies are also treatable causes of bronchiectasis.

The importance of functional antibody deficiencies in the presence of normal immunoglobulin levels has been recognized as a risk factor for recurrent respiratory tract infections and development of bronchiectasis. In subjects with low levels of specific antibodies it is advisable to evaluate the antibody response to both the *Haemophilus influenzae* type b conjugate vaccine as well as pneumococcal vaccine. Failure to mount and maintain adequate responses to antigen challenge may be associated with bronchiectasis and represent a risk for more severe disease. Patients with functional antibody deficiency and normal immunoglobulin levels can be managed with antibiotic therapy but may require immunoglobulin therapy if there is evidence of disease progression despite best antibiotic therapy.

Immune defects may be secondary to malignancy or be related to treatment with immunosuppressive agents. In addition, bronchiectasis is now a recognized complication of HIV disease.

Excessive immune response

Fig. 18.9.1 illustrates the damage that may occur as a result of the host response to chronic airway infection. ABPA is a condition in which the excessive reaction to a 'noninfecting' organism seems to be the main factor in producing the associated characteristic proximal upper-lobe bronchiectasis. The appearance of obliterative bronchiolitis and subsequent bronchiectasis in lung transplant rejection further highlights the role of a damaging immune response in the development of the condition.

Disorders of mucociliary clearance

Cystic fibrosis provides the archetypal model of a genetic predisposition for the development of bronchiectasis. In this disorder (described in Chapter 18.10) there is dysfunction of the cystic fibrosis transmembrane regulator (CFTR), a transmembrane chloride channel and ion transport regulatory protein. The resulting abnormal salt and water transport across respiratory epithelia predisposes to respiratory infection and the effects of the vicious cycle are clearly demonstrated as a structurally normal lung suffers progressive airway damage and the development of bronchiectasis.

In primary ciliary dyskinesia (PCD) ineffective ciliary function impairs mucociliary clearance, leading to mucus retention and recurrent infections in the paranasal sinuses, middle ear, and lungs, with progression to bronchiectasis. It is an inherited disorder, mostly in an autosomal recessive pattern, with an estimated incidence of 1 in 15 000 to 1 in 30 000 births. The diagnosis is made on electron microscopic appearance, which indicates the component of the cilia affected. Nasal nitric oxide concentrations are extremely low in PCD and provide a useful screening test to identify patients for further investigation with nasal brush biopsy to examine of ciliary beat frequency and ultrastructural analysis with transmission electron microscopy. In the largest subgroup of this syndrome, in which electron microscopic appearances were originally described, the cilia were found to lack dynein arms, the structure responsible for movement of cilia or spermatozoa. Subsequently it has been appreciated that a range of components of the cilia are affected, but the link between the ultrastructural changes and the genetic defects have been difficult to unravel because defects in any of the 250 proteins that constitute a cilium could potentially result in disease. However, we are now a step nearer genetic testing as the gene that encodes the human intermediate dynein, *DNAI1*, has been shown to exhibit recessively inherited mutations in some PCD families. Furthermore, mutations in *DNAH5*, the gene encoding a heavy chain of the outer dynein arm, have been shown in almost one-half of PCD subjects that have defects of this dynein arm.

The intriguing observation that about 50% of all subjects with immotile cilia syndrome have situs invervus is true for most subgroups, apart from those who have absent cilia or those whose main characteristic is lack of the two central microtubules. When ciliary dyskinesia is associated with abnormal situs the condition is called Kartagener's syndrome after the paediatrician who described four patients with the association of dextrocardia, sinusitis, and bronchiectasis in 1933.

Young's syndrome seems to represent an acquired defect of mucociliary clearance in which obstructive azospermia is associated with sinusitis and broncheictasis. The condition may occur after successful parentage and may be associated with mercury poisoning from 'tooth powders' used in infancy (Pink's disease). Secondary ciliary dyskinesia refers to the situation in which cilia are intrinsically normal but ciliary beating is reduced because of toxic damage from neutrophil or bacterial products. Tobacco smoke and other environmental pollutants have also been implicated in reducing ciliary beat frequency.

Toxic insult

In some patients, e.g. fire victims, there is a clear history of an inhalation accident or exposure to hot gases. Aspiration of gastric contents is another important cause of bronchiectasis, in that treatment to prevent aspiration will prevent further airway damage.

Mechanical obstruction

Bronchiectasis confined to a single lobe may be the result of a local mechanical obstruction either in the lumen (intrinsic), e.g. tumour or foreign body, or originating outside the lumen (extrinsic), e.g. from lymph node enlargement from tuberculosis or tumour.

Postinfective

The true incidence of postinfective bronchiectasis is difficult to confirm, as studies are retrospective, relying on histories obtained 'second hand' from parents. The microorganisms known to cause infection likely to progress to bronchiectasis are *Bordetella pertussis*, measles virus, adenoviruses, *Trypanosoma cruzi*, and *Mycobacterium tuberculosis*.

As mentioned above, the pattern of bronchiectasis has changed since the introduction of vaccinations and widespread availability of antibiotics in the developed world. The gross saccular bronchiectasis associated with severe repeated childhood respiratory infections in the preantibiotic era has been superseded by a population with cylindrical bronchiectasis, which may be associated with a childhood history of a chesty cough, a long period of remission of symptoms through teens and twenties, followed by the onset of symptoms of cough productive of purulent sputum and/or sinusitis in the third or fourth decade of life. Some of these patients may report a childhood episode of whooping cough or measles, but it is more useful not to label them as postinfective unless symptoms have been persistent, without remission since childhood.

Associated conditions

The association of rheumatoid arthritis with bronchiectasis is well recognized. Treatment needs to achieve the right balance of immunosuppression, which helps the underlying inflammatory disease process, but may impair antimicrobial defences. The association between inflammatory bowel disease and bronchiectasis highlights the usefulness of immunosuppression, as some patients with both conditions report an improvement in chest symptoms when they take systemic corticosteroids for flares of inflammatory bowel symptoms. Indeed, corticosteroid therapy is beneficial in bronchiectasis associated with ulcerative colitis.

Idiopathic

Even in specialist bronchiectasis clinics, the underlying cause of bronchiectasis remains unknown in 40 to 60% of patients, who are currently labelled as having 'idiopathic' disease.

Clinical features

History

Bronchiectasis should be suspected when there is a history of persistent cough productive of mucopurulent or purulent sputum throughout the year. Patients have often been treated for recurrent chest infections and labelled as 'bronchitic', often despite the absence of a smoking history. Patients presenting in adulthood often recall a 'chesty cough' or 'wheezy bronchitis' associated with upper respiratory tract infections in childhood. They then report a complete resolution of symptoms in teens and early adult life but return of symptoms after a viral trigger.

Early in the disease patients may produce mucoid sputum until they suffer an exacerbation associated with viral upper respiratory tract infection, when the sputum becomes purulent. Exacerbations may be associated with pleuritic chest pain, haemoptysis, and fever, and patients may also become wheezy.

About 80% of patients with bronchiectasis have upper respiratory tract symptoms, with postnasal drip being the most common. About 30% have chronic sinus sepsis, with fewer having recurrent ear infections, although the latter are almost invariably present in ciliary dyskinesia. Patients with bronchiectasis also suffer from undue tiredness, which many find more troublesome than the productive cough.

Examination

'Classical' severe cases of bronchiectasis seen in the preantibiotic era or in less developed countries are associated with obvious clinical signs including finger clubbing and widespread coarse crackles. Nowadays it is much more likely for clinical examination to be normal: the absence of clubbing or lung crackles does not exclude bronchiectasis.

Pulmonary function tests often show airflow obstruction, but mild restriction is also recognized, particularly in patients with loss of volume in a single lobe.

Investigation and diagnosis

Radiological imaging

The gold standard for the diagnosis of bronchiectasis is thin-section high-resolution CT of the chest, which has replaced the

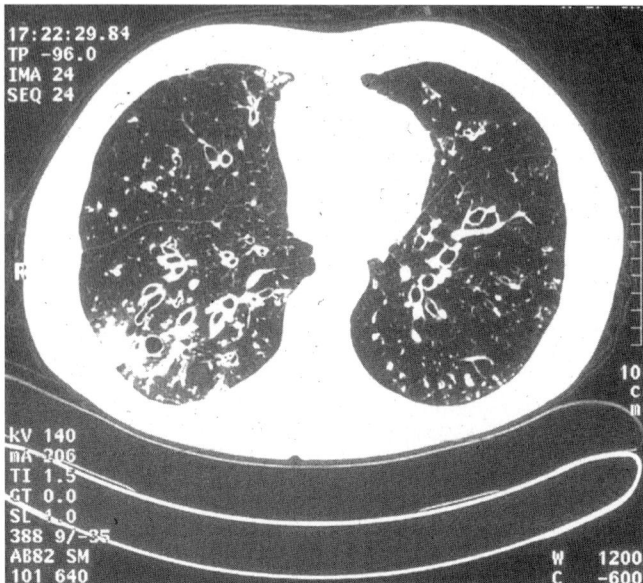

Fig. 18.9.2 A CT scan of a patient with bronchiectasis showing many characteristic 'signet ring' signs.

Table 18.9.2 Investigations to assess current disease status

Investigation	Purpose
High-resolution CT	Assess extent of bronchiectasis—single or multilobular involvement?
Lung function tests	To assess extent of loss of airway function Include assessment of reversibility to β_2 agonists and anticholinergic agents
Sputum culture	To assess colonizing microorganisms, including culture for acid-fast bacilli and aspergillus
Haematology	Differential white count, ESR, and CRP

CRP, C-reactive protein; ESR, erythrocyte sedimentation rate.

more invasive investigation of bronchography. The diagnostic criteria for bronchiectasis on high-resolution CT depend on the findings of both dilatation and thickening of the affected bronchi. Dilatation is present if the internal diameter of the bronchus is greater than the diameter of its accompanying pulmonary artery. The classic appearance of a cross-section of a thick-walled dilated bronchus next to the accompanying pulmonary artery is the 'signet ring', as shown in Fig. 18.9.2. Bronchial dilatation is also recognized when airways are seen in longitudinal section on CT and there is a failure of tapering as the bronchus courses towards the periphery.

There is a morphological spectrum of bronchiectasis, with cylindrical broncheictasis forming one group, cystic or saccular broncheictasis at the other end of the spectrum, and an intermediate group termed varicose broncheictasis also recognized. The CT appearances are well described: in cylindrical bronchiectasis there is uniform dilatation of the bronchi as they extend towards the periphery; cystic bronchiectasis is recognized by rings representing the markedly dilated bronchi, which may be clustered together and may contain air fluid levels; varicose bronchiectasis produces a beaded appearance, best shown when bronchi are imaged in the plane of the scan.

In addition to defining the extent of bronchiectasis, CT scanning may suggest the need for bronchoscopy, e.g. if there is a bronchial obstruction, possibly due to foreign body or tumour.

The chest radiograph is normal in at least 50% of patients with CT or bronchographic evidence of bronchiectasis. If the chest radiograph is abnormal, the findings relate to abnormal thickened and dilated bronchi which produce tramline opacities and ring shadows. Retained mucus may be manifest as tubular opacities, and there may be associated volume loss of the affected lobe.

Determining the state of disease

Once high-resolution CT has proven the presence of bronchiectasis, investigations are directed at defining the current status of the disease and then at attempting to define an underlying cause. Table 18.9.2 highlights the minimum required to assess the current disease status.

Examination of a sputum specimen is crucial, it being important to document the character of the sputum, i.e. mucoid or purulent, and to determine the colonizing organism. The typical colonizing organisms are nontypeable *Haemophilus influenzae*, *Moraxella catarrhalis*, *Streptococcus pneumoniae*, and *Pseudomonas aeruginosa*. *H. influenzae* is the most common (40–60%). *P. aeruginosa* is usually associated with worsening symptoms and more severe lung disease. As patient's sputum microbiology may alter over time it is helpful to obtain repeated samples to ensure that an appropriate antibiotic management plan is in place.

Measurement of inflammatory markers allows an assessment of the patient's current 'inflammatory burden'. Patients may come to accept persistent purulent sputum over a period of time and not complain of being particularly unwell, in which case a raised erythrocyte sedimentation rate and/or C-reactive protein would weight the argument in favour of early antibiotic intervention.

Determining the cause of disease

Table 18.9.3 outlines the investigations required to tie down a cause of broncheictasis, some of which will then require specific treatment, e.g. immunodeficiency. It is important to recognize that ABPA is a treatable cause of bronchiectasis, with corticosteroid treatment producing major improvements in symptoms and well being, restoring lung function, and preventing the development of further bronchiectasis. Similarly, the appreciation that chronic aspiration is the precipitant of lung damage leads to appropriate therapeutic manoeuvres aimed at prevention of further damage.

Opportunistic mycobacteria in bronchiectasis

Primary infection with the *Mycobacterium avium* complex is a recognized cause of bronchiectasis, particularly in white women over 60 years of age. In contrast to reported families suffering from disseminated opportunistic mycobacterial infection, this has not been shown to be associated with mutations in the interferon-γ receptor pathway, but the possibility remains that these patients have a defect in processing of intracellular pathogens that has yet to be identified.

Infection with the opportunistic (sometimes called nontuberculous) mycobacteria can also complicate pre-existing bronchiectasis. It is therefore important to obtain cultures for acid-fast bacilli at first assessment and when there is deterioration in clinical status.

Table 18.9.3 Investigations to assess underlying causes of bronchiectasis

Investigation	Purpose
Bronchoscopy	If CT suggests bronchial obstruction—to establish whether tumour or foreign body
Saccharin test	As screening test of nasal mucociliary clearance
Nasal brushing/biopsy	To establish ciliary beat frequency and obtain EM appearances of cilia
Nasal nitric oxide	As evidence of primary ciliary dyskinesia
Seminal analysis	If primary ciliary dyskinesia or CF is suspected
CF genetics and sweat test	To exclude CF
Immunoglobulins and IgG subclasses, vaccine responses to Pneumovax, Hib, tetanus, and flu	To identify immunodeficiency
Barium swallow ± oesophageal physiology studies	If aspiration is suspected
α_1-Antitrypsin measurement	To identify α_1-antitrypsin deficiency
Autoantibody screen	To identify associated connective tissue disorders or vasculitis
Aspergillus skin testing and IgE and RAST to aspergillus	To identify ABPA

ABPA, allergic bronchopulmonary aspergillosis; CF, cystic fibrosis; EM, electron microscopy, Hib, *Haemophilus influenzae* B; RAST, radioallergosorbant test.

Cystic fibrosis/bronchiectasis overlap

The diagnosis of cystic fibrosis should be considered in any patient with unexplained bronchiectasis, but particularly in the presence of upper lobe bronchiectasis or colonization with *Staphylococcus aureus* and *P. aeruginosa*, and also in the presence of aspergillus and nontuberculous mycobacteria. Male infertility and a family history are useful pointers when present, but a normal sweat test does not exclude the diagnosis, in particular in mutations which produce mild disease. The diagnostic label of atypical cystic fibrosis has been coined to describe patients with mild nonclassic cystic fibrosis: where there is diagnostic doubt the patient should be referred to a specialist cystic fibrosis centre for further investigations (see Chapter 18.10).

Management

The principles of management of bronchiectasis are outlined in Box 18.9.1. The medical approach is two-pronged, with close attention given to treating any underlying cause while also treating the established bronchiectasis.

Sputum clearance

As mucociliary clearance is reduced in bronchiectasis, it seems sensible to aid sputum clearance by employing physiotherapy. This does not simply prevent mucus retention but also allows a patient to expectorate sputum at a chosen convenient time, rather than coughing throughout the day or night. There are no controlled trials to prove or disprove its usefulness in terms of disease modification or survival.

Box 18.9.1 Principles of management of bronchiectasis

- Medical treatment specific to the determined cause of bronchiectasis (if available)
- Medical treatment for bronchiectasis:
  - Sputum clearance
  - Physiotherapy
  - Mucolytic therapy
  - Antimicrobial therapy
  - Chronic prophylactic therapy
  - Acute exacerbation
  - Anti-inflammatory therapy
  - Bronchodilator therapy
- Surgical treatment:
  - Resection of 'single' lobe bronchiectasis
  - Lung transplantation for endstage disease

The use of mucolytics in bronchiectasis is controversial: the success of recombinant human DNase in cystic fibrosis was not repeated in patients with bronchiectasis not due to cystic fibrosis, with those treated showing an accelerated decline in lung function and an increase in exacerbations.

New approaches currently under investigation to enhance mucociliary clearance in bronchiectasis include the use of nebulized hypertonic saline and inhalation of dry powdered mannitol.

Antimicrobial therapy

There are two approaches to the use of antimicrobial therapy in bronchiectasis: one involves the treatment of acute exacerbations; the other is based on the 'vicious cycle' hypothesis, suggesting that chronic targeted antimicrobial therapy should reduce bacterial numbers, thereby reducing the host response and hence reducing the potential for further lung damage. Whilst the latter approach has theoretical merits it has not been proved in randomized controlled trials. The modern approach to antimicrobial treatment in bronchiectasis has been derived from regimens used in cystic fibrosis which have yielded impressive improvements in survival (see Chapter 18.10).

Developing an antibiotic regime for treatment of bronchiectasis depends on knowledge of a patient's colonizing organism, but several principles apply regardless of the bacterial species. First, high doses are often required to penetrate scarred, thickened bronchial walls, and the tenacious secretions act as a physical barrier to reduce antibiotic penetration to the microbes while harbouring drug-inactivating enzymes such as β-lactamases. Secondly, to avoid a high oral dose of an antibiotic, which may result in unacceptable side effects, the nebulized or parenteral route is often employed to achieve high levels of drug in the bronchial wall and secretions. Thirdly, to determine the best treatment regimen for a patient it is worth assessing their initial response to an agent appropriate for the colonizing organism, in particular the rapidity of return of purulent sputum. If purulent sputum becomes mucoid after a 14-day course of oral antibiotics and remains mucoid until the next viral trigger, then one is likely to recommend 'exacerbation

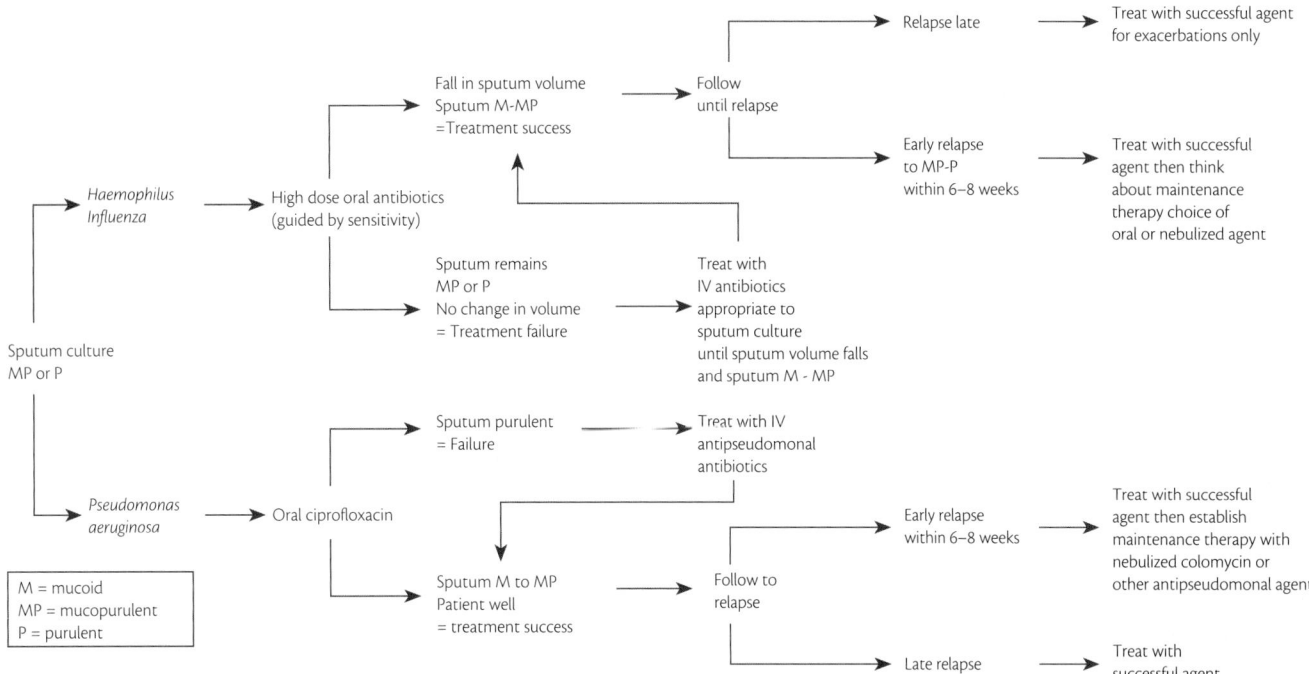

Fig. 18.9.3 Guide to therapy for patients with bronchiectasis.

only' treatment. By contrast, if sputum returns to purulent within a few days of treatment finishing, it is likely that chronic suppressive therapy will be required.

Figure 18.9.3 suggests a plan for developing a regimen for a patient depending on the characteristics of their sputum and the colonizing organism.

Bronchodilator therapy

Patients with bronchiectasis may have a restrictive or an obstructive picture. Some patients will have significant reversibility, hence it is worth assessing each individual for their response to β_2-agonists and anticholinergic agents.

Anti-inflammatory therapy

The 'vicious cycle' hypothesis suggests that the addition of anti-inflammatory therapy to antibiotics should be of benefit. Trials of oral corticosteroids have shown significant benefit in terms of lung function in cystic fibrosis. Short-term trials of inhaled corticosteroids have been carried out in bronchiectasis, but the evidence for long-term use is limited and further trials are required. There is a suggestion that patients chronically infected with *P. aeruginosa* may be more likely to benefit from inhaled corticosteroids in terms of reduction in sputum volume and exacerbation frequency, and it is worth noting that where there is reversible airflow obstruction a trial of steroids is warranted. If there is a documented improvement in lung function after a 2-week course of oral steroids, then one is justified in introducing inhaled steroids.

Monitoring response to treatment

As each patient requires a tailored management plan, it is critical that both the patient and physician agree defined criteria for assessing response. Clearly lung function produces an objective measure of response to corticosteroids, but the introduction of antibiotics may not alter lung function to a great degree, although it does

improve sputum colour, volume, and consistency, and there may be improvement in general well-being. Diary cards documenting these parameters have proved helpful, and studies have confirmed the validity of grading sputum colour as a marker of the microbial and inflammatory load in these patients. This approach also facilitates patient education and self-management plans.

Surgery

Surgery is the only 'curative' treatment for a select group of patients and should be carefully considered. In particular, for single-lobe, focal bronchiectasis secondary to bronchial obstruction, surgery removes the need for lifelong medical therapy. However, it is important that patients undergo careful assessment regarding the distribution of bronchiectasis and the possibility of underlying causes which would predispose to disease progression. Surgery is unlikely to produce a cure if bronchiectasis is present in several lobes, and lobar resection is then indicated only if there is uncontrolled bleeding unresponsive to bronchial artery embolization, or if it is felt—after a failure of aggressive antimicrobial therapy—that a particular lobe is acting as a 'sump' of infection which prevents good control of symptoms with medical therapy.

Lung transplantation

Lung transplantation provides an effective treatment for endstage bronchiectasis, providing that an underlying cause has been carefully assessed and treated and is unlikely to jeopardize the transplanted organs; e.g. patients with immunoglobulin deficiencies are not discounted from transplant assessment provided they are receiving adequate immunoglobulin replacement therapy.

Complications

The most common complication to precipitate hospital admission in patients with bronchiectasis is infective exacerbation, which may be associated with pleuritic chest pain and minor haemoptysis. Massive haemoptysis is rare nowadays, but is managed by bronchial artery embolization. Metastatic spread of infection rarely occurs in the developed world with good control of pulmonary infection with antibiotics, and for similar reasons empyema is now very rare. Amyloidosis is described as a 'classic' complication of bronchiectasis, but is now extremely rare in the United Kingdom. Arthropathy is a complication of bronchiectasis which seems to flare in association with the chest disease, and antimicrobial treatment will often result in remission of joint pain. Some patients may suffer vasculitic skin lesions in association with flares of bronchiectasis.

Prognosis

It was reported in 1940 that 70% of 400 patients with bronchiectasis were dead before the age of 40. The situation is clearly different now, as in the developed world we do not see the florid postinfective saccular type of bronchiectasis, but more commonly see patients presenting in their fourth and fifth decade of life with symptoms developing after a trigger illness and CT findings of cylindrical bronchiectasis. In 1981a study following 116 patients for 14 years revealed that only 20% of patients treated medically and 17% of surgically treated patients died at a mean age of 53 years. A Finnish study published in 1997 used the national hospital discharge register to identify patients with newly diagnosed bronchiectasis from 1982 to 1986, comparing them with 842 age- and sex-matched patients with chrnoic obstructive pulmonary disease (COPD) and asthma discharged at the same time. Over a 10-year follow-up the prognosis for those with bronchiectasis was better that that for patients with COPD but poorer than that those with asthma. Bronchiectasis was the main cause of death in 13% of patients with the condition.

Future developments

Further studies are required to identify the main factors which affect prognosis. For example, chronic colonization with *P. aeruginosa* may be a bad prognostic factor, but this may be negated by aggressive antimicrobial therapy, hence study of homogenous groups of patients (with respect to aetiology and colonizing organisms) should help assess various management regimens with regard to their effect on decline in lung function and survival.

It is likely that a careful search for genetic factors which affect lung defences will yield new causes of bronchiectasis and allow the current so called 'idiopathic' group to be assigned a cause.

The role of the macrolide antibiotics as immunomodulators in chronic airway inflammation and infection, with well-defined benefits in cystic fibrosis, has led to preliminary studies in bronchiectasis which suggest that large trials are warranted.

Further reading

Angrill J, *et al.* (2002). Bacterial colonisation in patients with bronchiectasis. *Thorax*, **57**, 15–19.

Barker AF (2002). Bronchiectasis. *N Engl J Med*, **346**, 1383–93.

Crockett AJ, *et al.* (2000). Mucolytics for bronchiectasis. *Cochrane Database Syst Rev*, **2**, pCD001289.

Davies G, *et al.* (2006). The effect of *Pseudomonas aeruginosa* on pulmonary function in patients with bronchiectasis. *Eur Respir J*, **28**, 974–9.

Fowler SJ, *et al.* (2006). Nontuberculous mycobacteria in bronchiectasis: prevalence and patient characteristics. *Eur Respir J*, **26**, 1204–10.

Hornef N, *et al.* (2006). DNAH5 mutations are a common cause of primary ciliary dyskinesia with outer dyneinarm defects. *Am J Respir Crit Care Med*, **174**, 120–6.

Jones AP, Rowe BH (2000). Bronchopulmonary hygiene physical therapy for chronic obstructive pulmonary disease and bronchiectasis. *Cochrane Database Syst Rev*, **2**, pCD00045.

Kolbe J, Wells A, Ram FS (2000). Inhaled steroids for bronchiectasis. *Cochrane Database Syst Rev*, **2**, pCD000996.

Noone PG, *et al.* (2004). Primary ciliary dyskinesia. *Am J Respir Crit Care Med*, **169**, 459–67.

Pasteur MC, *et al.* (2000). An investigation into causative factors in patients with bronchiectasis. *Am J Respir Crit Care Med*, **162**, 1277–84.

Vendrell M, *et al.* (2005). Antibody production deficiency with normal IgG levels in bronchiectasis of unknown etiology. *Chest*, **127**, 197–204.

Weycker D, *et al.* (2005). Prevalence and economic burden of bronchiectasis. *Clin Pulm Med*, **12**, 205–9.

Zariwala MA, *et al.* (2006). Mutations of DNAI1 in primary ciliary dyskinesia. *Am J Respir Crit Care Med*, **174**, 858–66.

Cystic fibrosis

Andrew Bush and Caroline Elston

Essentials

Cystic Fibrosis (CF) is a recessively inherited disease caused by mutations in the cystic fibrosis gene, located on the long arm of chromosome 7, which codes for a membrane protein—the cystic fibrosis transmembrane regulator protein (CFTR)—that is a chloride channel. Around 1300 CF mutations have been identified, with the ΔF508 mutation being the most common (70% of CF chromosomes in the European population). Birth incidence varies with country of origin from 1 in 2000 to 1 in 100 000.

Pathophysiology—the mutant CFTR fails to transport chloride ions normally, and there is secondary impairment of sodium, bicarbonate, and water transport. This leads to dehydration of pancreatic secretions, eventually leading to pancreatic failure, and in the lungs to increased fluid absorption from the airway lumen and reduction in the depth of the film of airway surface liquid (the 'low volume hypothesis'), with impairment of ciliary function, mucus stasis, and thus chronic infection and inflammation.

Clinical features—most cases of CF are diagnosed in early childhood by newborn screening, or, with the classical clinical picture of pancreatic insufficiency and suppurative lung disease, but patients with milder genetic mutations may present in late childhood or adulthood. Other pulmonary manifestations include haemoptysis, pneumothorax, allergic bronchopulmonary aspergillosis (ABPA), and atypical mycobacterial infection. Patients presenting in adult life are often clinically pancreatic sufficient, or they present with other conditions that are also associated with CF gene mutations, e.g. azoospermia, idiopathic pancreatitis.

Diagnosis—this is usually established by the sweat test (pilocarpine iontophoresis or macroduct collection) revealing a high sweat chloride concentration, although increasingly the diagnosis is likely to be made by newborn screening (heel prick blood samples tested for immunoreactive trypsin and by PCR for common CF mutations).

Prognosis—pulmonary infection and inflammation account for most CF-associated morbidity and mortality. The lungs become transiently infected in early childhood and ultimately chronically infected, typically with *Staphylococcus aureus* and *Haemophilus influenzae*, and subsequently with *Pseudomonas aeruginosa*, which is associated with a worse prognosis. Chronic infection and inflammation lead to bronchiectasis, progressive airflow obstruction, and ultimately death from respiratory failure, although outcome has improved dramatically over the past 20 years such that estimated survival for a child born with CF in the late 1990s is 40 to 50 years.

Management of respiratory disease—airway clearance with regular physiotherapy is an integral part of routine management. Antibiotic treatment is initially directed at preventing chronic infection. Prophylactic nebulized antibiotic therapy (colomycin, tobramycin) is beneficial once patients become chronically infected with Pseudomonas. Mucolytic agents are often indicated. Azithromycin, a macrolide antibiotic that appears to modulate inflammation in CF by an ill-understood mechanism, is used increasingly.

Management of other features—(1) Pancreatic insufficiency is associated with malabsorption and requires pancreatic enzyme replacement therapy and a high-energy diet in most patients. (2) Distal intestinal obstruction syndrome—severe constipation sometimes leading to bowel obstruction with faecal material in the distal ileum and associated abdominal pain—is relatively common. (3) Diabetes—this occurs in up to 30% of patients, with the incidence increasing with age; a high-energy diet should be maintained, with insulin doses adjusted accordingly. (4) Liver function—mild abnormalities are common, with disease progression to cirrhosis in around 5% of patients. (5) Fertility—nearly all men with CF are infertile, but most women with CF can conceive normally. (6) Osteoporosis—low bone mineral density is found in 60% of patients.

Definition

Cystic fibrosis (CF) is a recessively inherited disease caused by mutations in the cystic fibrosis gene located on the long arm of chromosome 7. The classical clinical picture is a combination of pancreatic insufficiency, suppurative lung disease, and high sweat chloride concentration, presenting in early childhood and progressing to early death from respiratory failure. However, genetic analysis has identified many patients with less severe disease, and the clinical spectrum of CF has been expanded by recognition of mutations in association with other conditions, including azoospermia, allergic bronchopulmonary aspergillosis, and idiopathic pancreatitis. Carriers are usually healthy.

The genetic defect

The CF gene codes for a 168-kDa membrane protein, the CF transmembrane regulator protein (CFTR). CFTR is an ATP-responsive chloride channel, but it also influences other cellular functions such as sodium transport across the respiratory epithelium, cell-surface glycoprotein composition, and normal antibacterial defences, at least 20 functions in all having been described. The protein is expressed in organs involved in CF disease—lungs, pancreas, sweat glands, etc.—but also in some places that do not seem to be affected clinically, such as the choroid plexus, heart, and renal tubules.

More than 1300 disease-related mutations of the CF gene have been described. These have been classified according to their impact at a cellular level: type 1, no protein; type 2, disordered trafficking, with intracellular destruction of CFTR; type 3, defective regulation; type 4, defective channel function; type 5, reduced protein synthesis. A sixth class is reduced half life of CFTR at the apical cell membrane, due to increased breakdown. The understanding of these abnormalities is valuable as a basis for the design of new potentially corrective treatments, as illustrated in Fig. 18.10.1.

Most mutations are very rare; the commonest in European populations is ΔF508, which is found on 70% of affected chromosomes, with some variation across Europe. Most genetic laboratories restrict routine testing to the commonest 30 mutations which together account for over 90% of mutations within a given population. Genotype–phenotype correlations have shown linkage of so-called severe mutations, such as ΔF508, to pancreatic insufficiency and a tendency to more severe lung disease, while mild mutations go with pancreatic sufficiency and a tendency to less severe lung disease. However, in general, the correlation between genotype and the severity of lung disease is poor. Virtually all disease-associated mutations are linked with congenital absence of the vas deferens, resulting in infertility in more than 98% of men with CF, while rarer mutations are linked with isolated male infertility with no other evidence of CF disease.

Pathogenesis

Sweat duct

The primary secretion of the sweat duct is normal in volume and electrolyte concentration. However, as this secretion passes along the sweat duct mutant CFTR fails to absorb chloride ions, which therefore remain in the lumen and secondary impairment of sodium absorption. The resultant sweat has high concentrations of both sodium and chloride, which is useful for diagnosis and can lead to salt depletion in hot weather.

Pancreas

The synthesis and secretion of pancreatic enzymes in the acinus is normal, but disordered ion transport—primarily of chloride and secondarily of bicarbonate—results in relative dehydration of pancreatic secretions. This in turn leads to low flow and stagnation of secretions in the pancreatic ducts with subsequent autodigestion. The clinical consequences are that low volumes of bicarbonate-depleted pancreatic secretions reach the duodenum, with consequent malabsorption and progressive destruction of the pancreas with cyst formation. Although the islet cells are relatively unaffected at first, they too are progressively destroyed, leading to insulin deficiency.

Biliary tract

Intrahepatic biliary secretions are probably normal in CF, but disordered electrolyte transport across the bile duct results in reduced water movement into the lumen. The bile is therefore concentrated and its volume depleted, leading to plugging and chronic local damage. This eventually causes biliary cirrhosis and associated extrahepatic biliary stenoses. There are secondary changes in bile acids. Other factors may also be important, including human leucocyte antigen (HLA) haplotype, and the effect of modifier genes.

Gut

Gastric secretions have decreased volume with increased viscosity and sodium concentration. The chloride transport defect similarly leads to altered fluid movement across large and small intestine. These changes are worsened by the addition of dehydrated biliary and pancreatic secretions, as well as by alterations in the osmotic load in the lumen secondary to pancreatic exocrine failure. The resulting deficiency of intraluminal water contributes to meconium ileus in neonates and the distal intestinal obstruction syndrome in adults.

Respiratory tract

The epithelium in the nose, paranasal sinuses, and intrapulmonary conducting airways is disordered in CF, but alveolar function is normal. Defective chloride transport is associated with increased sodium absorption from the lumen. This leads to the net surface electrical charge being altered from a normal of −20 mV to about −40 mV, which can be used for diagnosis. However, the link between the absence or impaired function of CFTR and lung disease is not clear. Perhaps the most likely explanation—the 'low volume hypothesis'—is that uncontrolled sodium and hence water absorption from the lumen leads to a reduction in the depth of the

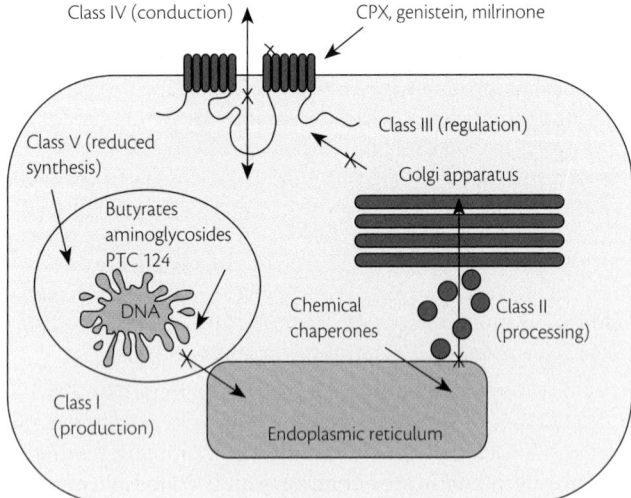

Fig. 18.10.1 Five categories of cystic fibrosis mutation with possible corrective treatments.
(From Rosenstein BJ, Zeitlin PL (1998). Seminar on cystic fibrosis. *Lancet*, **351**, 278, with permission.)

film of airway surface liquid, with impairment of ciliary function, mucus stasis and thus chronic infection and inflammation. Less plausible is the 'high salt hypothesis', which argues that local antibacterial defences—including lactoferrin, lysozyme, and the cationic antibacterial peptides such as the β-defensins—may be impaired by local changes in salt concentration. Other, not necessarily mutually exclusive explanations include that bacterial adherence to epithelial cells is increased by changes in cell surface glycoproteins; and that there is reduced binding of microorganisms to CFTR and thus impaired internalization and clearance by the epithelial cells. The net effect is to promote chronic bacterial infection, and to reduce bacterial clearance, with subsequent inflammatory lung damage.

One consequence of chronic bacterial infection of the lower respiratory tract is an exuberant neutrophilic inflammatory response involving especially interleukin-8 (IL-8) and neutrophil elastase. The combination of elastase and other inflammatory mediators, while initially providing a useful antibacterial defence, is thought to contribute to lung damage and speed the progression of bronchiectasis and small airway narrowing. This has lead to the seemingly somewhat paradoxical concept of using prednisolone to reduce inflammation in the setting of chronic bacterial infection.

Heterozygote advantage

The high frequency of the carrier state in European populations (1 in 25) has led to a number of suggested advantages for the carrier, none of which are proven. These range from reduced susceptibility to infections such as cholera (reduced gut chloride secretion) and typhoid (reduced ingestion of bacteria by gut epithelium) to increased fertility among CF carriers. As yet, no carrier advantage has been proven.

Epidemiology

Genotype

The prevalence and distribution of the more than 1300 disease-related mutations in the CF gene vary with ethnic origin. ΔF508 is commonest in northern European populations, accounting for 82% of CF chromosomes in Denmark but only 32% in Turkey. The W1282X mutation is common in Ashkanazi Jews (48% of CF chromosomes) but rare in other populations. All disease-associated mutations are rare in African and almost unknown in Chinese populations.

Phenotype

Birth incidence varies with country of origin from 1 in 2000 to 1 in 100 000, as listed in Table 18.10.1. Prevalence figures are few and less reliable. CF is likely to be underdiagnosed in the developing world because early childhood malnutrition, diarrhoea, and chest infections are so common in children with no underlying disease. There are at least 7000 people in the United Kingdom and 30 000 in the United States of America with CF, and these numbers are increasing along with life expectancy. Soon, there will be more adults than children with CF.

Survival

From 1938 to 1960, most children with CF died before the age of 10. Since 1968, the first-year mortality (chiefly from meconium ileus) has fallen from 18% to virtually zero, and survival curves are linear

Table 18.10.1 Frequency of cystic fibrosis in different populations

Country	Incidence	Calculated carrier frequency
United Kingdom	1:2500	1:25
Turkey	1:3000	1:27
United States of America	1:2000–1:4000	1:22–1:32
Israel	1:5000	1:35
Italy	1:15 000	1:60
African Americans	1:17 000	1:65
Finland	1:40 000	1:100
China	?1:100 000	?1:160

thereafter, showing progressive improvement over succeeding decades (Fig. 18.10.2). In 1986, the median survival was 25 years and in 1999 about 30 years. Cohort survival analysis shows continuing improvement, and estimated survival for a child born with CF in the late 1990s is 40 to 50 years. Age-specific mortality rates for females are a little worse than for males, although this difference is narrowing and the world record longevity for both sexes is now over 70 years.

Microbiology

People with CF have no detectable immune deficiency and, except for the respiratory tract, have no increased susceptibility to infection. The lungs show evidence of transient infection and inflammation very early in childhood and thereafter become chronically infected, characteristically by *Staphylococcus aureus* and *Haemophilus influenzae*, followed some years later by *Pseudomonas aeruginosa*. Many other organisms have been implicated, especially in advanced disease, including the different genomovars of *Burkholderia cepacia*, *Alcaligenes*, *Achromobacter*, and *Stenotrophomonas maltophilia*. Methicillin-resistant *S. aureus* (MRSA) is becoming an increasing problem. *Aspergillus fumigatus* is frequently isolated, but is associated with allergic rather than invasive disease, although this is not necessarily a benign organism. Atypical mycobacteria are increasingly found, in particular in those with milder disease and *S. aureus* rather than *P. aeruginosa* infection.

Viral, chlamydial, pneumococcal, and other respiratory infections are not more common or severe in CF, but the consequences of these infections may be more important in the damaged and permanently infected CF lung.

The microbiology of the nose and sinuses is the same as for the lung, but the clinical consequences are usually less important.

Staphylococcus aureus

This is the commonest colonizing organism in childhood, with a prevalence of over 50% in children aged under 9. The predilection of *S. aureus* for CF lungs has been ascribed to high electrolyte content of airway surface liquid or enhanced retention in the airways. No phage type predominates and the organism usually remains sensitive to flucloxacillin in spite of prolonged antibiotic treatment. Resistance to tetracycline or erythromycin is relatively common, but multiple antibiotic resistance is rare, although MRSA, both hospital and community acquired, is becoming an increasing problem. The prevalence of staphylococcal colonization falls in adult life when *P. aeruginosa* predominates.

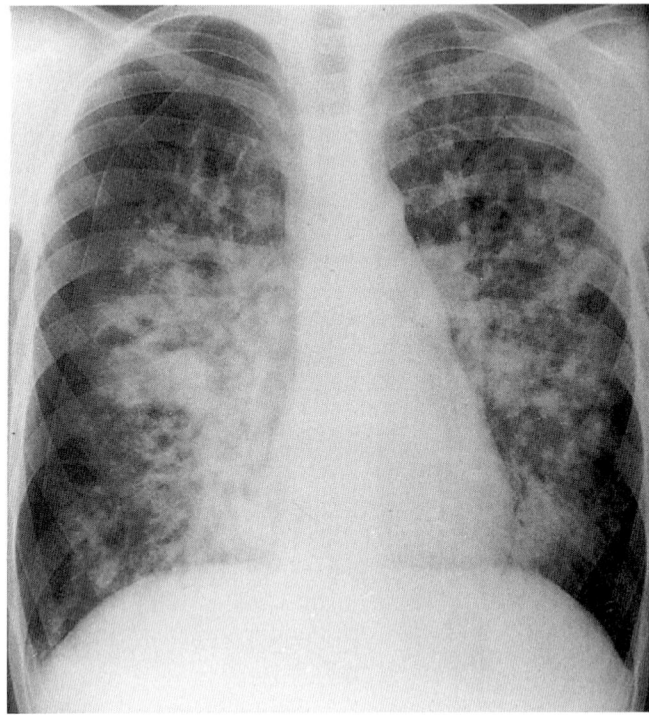

(a)

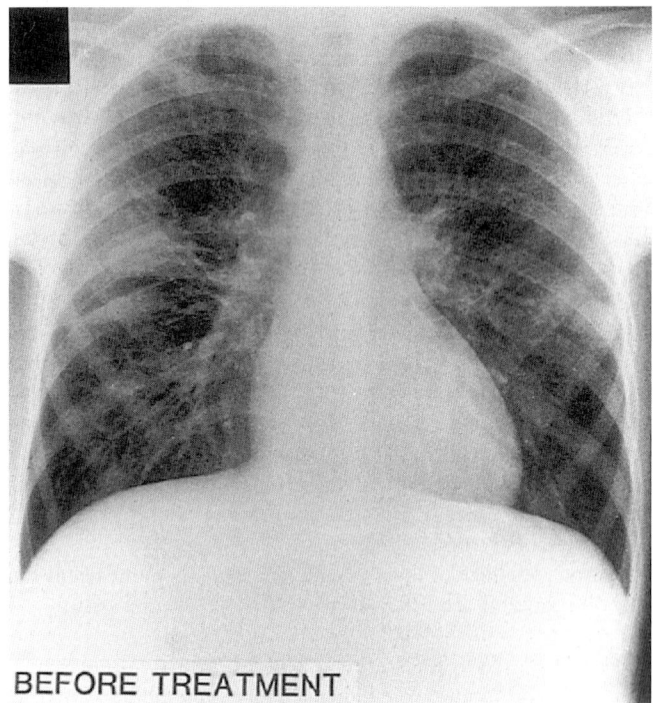

BEFORE TREATMENT

(b)

Fig. 18.10.2 (a) The typical chest radiograph appearances of advanced cystic fibrosis lung disease. There is also a right pneumothorax. (b) The chest radiograph in an adolescent child with cystic fibrosis complicated by allergic bronchopulmonary aspergillosis. Note the wedge-shaped shadow in the right mid zone.

Pseudomonas aeruginosa

This is the commonest infecting organism after the age of 10 years, with reported prevalence varying between 40 and 80%. Enhanced adherence to CF airways promotes infection, but prior antibiotic treatment—in particular if cephalosporin prophylaxis is employed—may play a part. No particular strain predominates, but siblings with CF often carry the same type, and environmental sources have been identified in CF centres, dentistry equipment, hydrotherapy pools, and nebulizers. After some months or years of infection, *P. aeruginosa* produces mucoid alginate as a protective biofilm and the organisms live in mucoid microcolonies. This mucoid variant is associated with a worse prognosis and greater antibiotic resistance. Most infecting strains of *P. aeruginosa* are sensitive to antibiotics at first, but over the years and in association with antibiotic treatment they develop multiple resistance to most antibiotics (except colomycin). There is increasing concern about epidemic strains of *P. aeruginosa*, which may spread through clinics and carry a worse prognosis. This has resulted in increased emphasis on infection control precautions.

Haemophilus influenzae

Noncapsulated *H. influenzae* is a relatively frequent infecting organism, with prevalence of up to 30%, although it may not be isolated due to overgrowth of staphylococcus or pseudomonas. Antibiotic resistance is seldom a problem.

Burkholderia cepacia complex

There are at least 9 different families ('genomovars') of this organism. Genomovar III (*B. cenocepacia*) is the most resistant and virulent organism, but other genomovars are not necessarily benign. The overall prevalence of this organism is low, at 3 to 5%, but it poses a particular problem due to cross-infection, and some forms can cause rapid deterioration in patients previously only mildly affected. More usual is chronic asymptomatic carriage or progressive deterioration in the late stage of lung disease. Multiple antibiotic resistance is characteristic.

Diagnosis

The vast majority of patients (>98%) with CF can be diagnosed by a sweat test. The occasional patient, particularly with a mutation giving rise to a mild or atypical clinical phenotype, may require more sophisticated testing. However, the major difficulty is usually not in confirming the diagnosis, but in thinking of it in an appropriate context (below, and Table 18.10.2). Increasingly, the diagnosis will be made by newborn screening (below). Conversely, false-positive diagnoses are not rare, and a new referral of a patient with CF to the adult clinic should prompt a full review of the diagnosis.

Presenting features

The various age-related problems that can lead to a diagnosis of CF are given in Table 18.10.2. Paediatric presentations are relevant to adult life in that if an adult with atypical respiratory disease turns out to have a family history of a child with CF or an illness shown in Table 18.10.2, then CF should be considered in the adult. The new diagnosis of CF in a younger relative will also prompt cascade screening (below), usually aiming to discover carriers, but occasionally someone with a clinically mild CF phenotype is discovered.

Table 18.10.2 Presentation of cystic fibrosis by age group

Age group	Presenting complaint
Antenatal	Chorionic villus sampling
	Ultrasound diagnosis of bowel perforation[a]
	Fetal hyperechogenic bowel[b]
At or soon after birth	Bowel obstruction (meconium ileus[a], bowel atresia)
	Haemorrhagic disease of the newborn
	Prolonged jaundice
	Screening (population based or previous affected sibling)
Infancy and childhood	Recurrent respiratory infections
	Diarrhoea and failure to thrive[c]
	Rectal prolapse[d]
	Nasal polyps[e]
	Acute pancreatitis
	Portal hypertension and variceal haemorrhage[f]
	Pseudo-Bartter's syndrome, electrolyte abnormality
	Hypoproteinaemia and oedema
	Screening as a result of cystic fibrosis diagnosis in a sibling/relative
Adolescence and adult life	Recurrent respiratory infections
	Atypical asthma
	Bronchiectasis
	Male infertility (congenital bilateral absence of the vas deferens)
	Electrolyte disturbance/heat exhaustion
	Atypical mycobacterial infection
	Acute pancreatitis
	Screening as a result of diagnosis in affected relative
	Portal hypertension and variceal haemorrhage

[a] Note that meconium ileus may be seen in pancreatic sufficient infants with CF, as well as rarely in those without the disease.
[b] Most fetuses with hyperechogenic bowel are normal; around 6% have a trisomy, and 4% CF.
[c] Note that up to 15% may be pancreatic sufficient, at least at diagnosis; thriving does not exclude CF.
[d] One in six cases of rectal prolapse is due to CF, if obvious anatomical abnormalities are excluded.
[e] Unlike in adults, where aspirin-sensitive asthma is commonly associated with polyps, children with polyps almost invariably have CF.
[f] Presentation with hepatocellular failure is very rare.

The United States Cystic Fibrosis Foundation Registry data show that as many as 10% of CF patients are not diagnosed until adult life.

Less than 5% pancreatic function is necessary for normal digestive function, and those presenting with CF in adult life are often clinically pancreatic sufficient. The main presentation is with respiratory problems, usually recurrent lower respiratory infections with chronic sputum production. Some patients have a prior diagnosis of bronchiectasis, atypical asthma, nasal polyposis, acute pancreatitis, nontuberculous mycobacterial infection, or allergic bronchopulmonary aspergillosis. A new CF diagnosis has been described even in adults in their seventh decade. Depletion of sodium, chloride, and potassium due to excessive sweating, and secondary renal chloride retention, may result in presentation with dehydration and heat exhaustion in an otherwise apparently completely fit adult.

Another important mode of presentation is male infertility due to azoospermia because of congenital bilateral absence of the vas deferens (CABVD). There are different forms of this condition: (1) in association with congenital malformations of the upper urinary tract, in which case there is no increased incidence of CF mutations; (2) as part of classical CF; and (3) as a truly isolated *forme fruste* of CF, with only a single CF mutation and ion transport abnormalities overlapping with, but different from, true CF.

Portal hypertension secondary to macronodular cirrhosis in adult life may also be the first presentation of CF.

There is considerable debate as to the status of adults with single organ manifestations characteristic of, but not confined to, CF—e.g. idiopathic pancreatitis or allergic bronchopulmonary aspergillosis. Some series report a higher than expected incidence of CF mutations, and the occasional unsuspected CF compound heterozygote. In practice, although CF should be excluded as far as possible by appropriate investigations in the patient with a possible single-organ disease, most will not have the traditional clinical CF disease as it is currently defined.

Sweat testing

The test must be performed by someone who is experienced in conducting it. Techniques include the classical pilocarpine iontophoresis of Gibson and Cooke, and more recently the macroduct collection. For the diagnosis to be established, tests should be performed in duplicate. The normal concentrations of sweat sodium and chloride increase with age. To diagnose CF in a child, the sweat chloride concentration should be greater than 60 mmol/litre, and the sweat sodium concentration less than that of chloride. A sweat chloride of less than 40 mmol/litre is normal in older children and adults, and intermediate concentrations are equivocal. However, there are undoubted cases of CF with normal sweat electrolytes, and the sweat test should always be interpreted in the light of the whole clinical picture. If the sweat test is equivocal, consider repeating it the day after giving fludrocortisone 3 mg/m^2 for 2 days. In CF patients, sweat electrolyte concentrations fail to suppress into the normal range. There are a few rare conditions that also cause elevation in sweat electrolyte concentration, but these are rarely a serious diagnostic consideration in practice (Box 18.10.1).

Nasal electrical potential difference

The abnormal potential difference across mucosal surfaces can be measured by passing a soft catheter under the inferior turbinate, referencing it to an electrode placed on abraded skin of the forearm. Normal values are −10 to −30 mV and the CF range is −34 to −60 mV. The test is unreliable if the patient has an upper respiratory tract infection. The diagnosis can be further refined by perfusing the nose with solutions of amiloride to block sodium transport, and isoprenaline/low chloride to stimulate CFTR. Nasal potentials require extensive experience if results are to be accurate.

Ion transport can be measured directly from intestinal biopsies in an Ussing chamber, but in most centres this remains a research technique only.

Cystic fibrosis genotype

More than 1300 different mutations causing CF have been reported. Testing for all of them is not currently practical in most centres,

Box 18.10.1 Conditions characterized by elevated sweat electrolyte concentrations; in most cases, confusion with cystic fibrosis is very unlikely

- Cystic fibrosis
- Untreated adrenal insufficiency
- Type 1 glycogen storage disease
- Nephrogenic diabetes insipidus
- Malnutrition
- Panhypopituitarism
- Acquired immunodeficiency syndrome
- Artefact (incorrectly performed sweat test, eczema)
- Fucoscidosis
- Hypothyroidism
- Ectodermal dysplasia
- Mucopolysaccharidosis

although complete sequencing of the CFTR gene is increasingly performed. It is essential to distinguish disease producing mutations from harmless polymorphisms. Thus DNA analysis can confirm the diagnosis if two mutations are found, but not exclude it. Linkage analysis can be used for antenatal diagnosis if a couple have already had an affected child, even if the actual mutations are not known.

Other investigations

In doubtful cases, evidence of subclinical organ dysfunction may be sought. Pancreatic dysfunction may be manifest by low stool elastase, elevation in 3-day faecal fat excretion, or abnormal results of pancreatic stimulation tests. CT scan of the chest or bronchoscopy may be used to discover minor bronchiectatic changes or infection with typical CF organisms. Azoospermia is strongly supportive of the diagnosis of CF. But note, however, that it is important not to place too much diagnostic weight on clinically minor changes.

Summary

The diagnosis of CF is usually easy to confirm with a properly performed sweat test. There remain a few atypical cases which defy a firm diagnosis. In that event, clinical organ dysfunction should be treated appropriately, and the patient followed up very carefully: often time will clarify the diagnosis.

Screening

Screening tests can be used to make an early diagnosis of CF in populations in order for treatment to be instituted before irreversible organ damage occurs, and to detect CF carriers to allow antenatal diagnosis and the option of termination of affected pregnancies. In both areas there is controversy as to the indications and methods to be used. Currently neither is routinely available everywhere in the United Kingdom, but universal screening is now offered everywhere in the United Kingdom.

Methods

In the past, crude tests on meconium have been used, but these lacked accuracy and have been superseded by tests carried out on the routine heel-prick blood sample collected from all babies in the first few days of life. These include estimation of immunoreactive trypsin, often combined with polymerase chain reaction (PCR) methods for one or more common abnormal genes, or pancreatitis-related protein. Routine neonatal screening in the United Kingdom is with both immunoreactive trypsin and PCR. Pancreatitis-related protein screening may perform equally well, and obviates the need for genetic testing, which may be an advantage in some cultures.

Carrier screening is by PCR for several of the common CF genes on a blood or mouthwash sample. In principle, this sort of screening may be offered to relatives of known CF patients (cascade screening), by written invitation to the general population, or opportunistically at routine antenatal clinic visits or the GP surgery. It is generally considered that carrier testing at birth will not be useful because of the time lag between obtaining and utilizing the information.

Outcome

The evidence for the value of screening for the disease has come from a number of retrospective trials, all showing benefit, but with the disadvantage of using historical controls. There has been one prospective randomized trial of neonatal screening from Wisconsin (United States of America) in which 650 341 babies were screened. Of those in whom the diagnosis of CF was made, in 56 the diagnosis was communicated to the parents, and in 40 the diagnosis was suppressed until it emerged on clinical grounds. There were small but clear-cut nutritional benefits in the group in which the screening diagnosis was communicated, persisting to 10 years of age. Furthermore, there were subtle neurocognitive defects detectable in the nonscreened population, who had the lowest fat-soluble vitamin levels at 10 years of age. The nutritional benefits were clearest early in life, at the time when growth is at its most rapid.

In general, carrier screening is poorly taken up when done by invitation, and at antenatal clinics it may be difficult to obtain a sample from the putative father. Cascade screening is generally better utilized, and should be offered at the time of making a new diagnosis.

Summary

Any screening test has false positives, which engender unnecessary anxiety, and false negatives, which may result in complacency. The balance of evidence is clearly in favour of neonatal screening so that early treatment can be given, and antenatal diagnosis offered for future pregnancies. The anxiety about false positives seems transient and deemed by the parents to be an acceptable price for subsequent reassurance. Carrier screening other than by cascade is more difficult, and, unless combined with wider public education, is unlikely to have a major impact. It should be noted that when universal screening becomes established, it will become increasingly rare to make a new diagnosis clinically. However, some mild patients will inevitably be missed on screening and present late, hence it will be important to remember the possibility of a new case of CF, even in a screened population.

Respiratory management

Most of the morbidity and mortality of CF is due to respiratory disease. Much of the treatment is therefore devoted to preventing chronic infection and inflammation, which lead to bronchiectasis, progressive airflow obstruction, cor pulmonale, and ultimately death. As with many aspects of the treatment of CF, there is a dearth of good randomized controlled trials.

Typical physical findings are finger clubbing and cough with purulent sputum, together with crackles and occasional wheezes, chiefly in the upper lobes. Clinical scoring systems include the comprehensive Schwachman and simpler Taussig scores. The chest radiograph shows thickened bronchial walls and small areas of consolidation which start in the upper lobes and may progress to involve the whole lung (Fig. 18.10.2a). A variety of radiographic scoring systems have been proposed, e.g. Crispin–Norman or Brasfield scores. Lung function tests show obstruction with relatively well preserved gas transfer. The forced expiratory volume in 1 s (FEV_1) is conventionally used to assess the extent and progression of lung disease. Exercise tolerance and arterial blood gases are well maintained until there is extensive lung damage, when hypoxaemic respiratory failure supervenes. CO_2 retention occurs late.

Antimicrobials

Oral antibiotics

The use of prophylactic antistaphylococcal antibiotics is controversial: most would use continuous twice-daily oral flucloxacillin if there is evidence of chronic infection. Minor exacerbations of respiratory symptoms in the patient not colonized with *P. aeruginosa* should be treated with a 1-month course of a high-dose antibiotic that will cover *S. aureus* and *H. influenza*.

Ciprofloxacin is used at the time of first isolation of *P. aeruginosa*, combined with nebulized antibiotics (below) to try to prevent chronic infection: the duration of therapy is controversial. Ciprofloxacin is also used to cover exacerbations of symptoms in the patient chronically infected with *P. aeruginosa*, but ciprofloxacin resistance soon becomes common.

Nebulized antibiotics

Nebulized colomycin combined with oral ciprofloxacin is indicated at the time of first isolation of *P. aeruginosa*. This approach has been shown in a randomized trial to delay chronic infection. However, the combination of oral, intravenous, and nebulized antibiotics that is most effective in preventing the progression from first isolation to chronic infection has not been established. Once *P. aeruginosa* infection is established, randomized controlled trials have shown benefit from long-term nebulized antibiotics. In Europe, colomycin is the drug most often used. In the United States of America, nebulized tobramycin is preferred. No medium-term comparison of the two has been reported. Occasional patients bronchoconstrict with nebulized antibiotics: a test dose should therefore be given, with spirometry measured before and afterwards, and if necessary pretreatment with a bronchodilator prescribed. There are ongoing trials of newer antibiotics, and also studies to determine the best protocols.

Intravenous antibiotics

Infective exacerbations not responding to oral antibiotics, particularly those of *P. aeruginosa*, are usually treated with a combination of an intravenous aminoglycoside and a semisynthetic antipseudomonal penicillin or cephalosporin. These are frequently given at home. A large randomized controlled trial has established that once-daily tobramycin is equally efficacious and at least as safe as three times daily treatment. Drug metabolism in the CF patient is very different from normals and other patient groups. Some centres recommend 3-monthly courses of intravenous antibiotics, irrespective of symptoms, for all CF patients chronically infected with *P. aeruginosa*. A randomized trial in the United Kingdom, although underpowered, did not support this approach. However, the threshold for giving intravenous antibiotics has become low, with very few clinicians waiting until the patient has developed several new symptoms.

Particular issues related to infection

Cross-infection

Fear of nosocomial acquisition of resistant organisms is widespread in the CF community. The apparent increase in prevalence of *P. aeruginosa* in specialized clinics probably reflects more assiduous bacterial culture techniques. However, most centres advocate separate clinics for CF patients with and without *P. aeruginosa*. Strict cohorting has also been advocated with regard to more resistant organisms, in particular *B. cenocepacia*.

Sensible guidelines should be applied to all CF patients: these include diligent handwashing, no sharing of physiotherapy equipment, and the use of single cubicles for inpatients with difficult organisms. Communal physiotherapy and keep-fit sessions should be discouraged, and there is no doubt that conferences for CF patients can result in transmission of infection. Careful microbiological surveillance is essential, and special measures may be needed if there is a true epidemic strain within a particular clinic.

Viral infections

Viral infections, trivial in themselves, have been implicated in causing transient reduction in airway defences and an increased risk of *P. aeruginosa* acquisition. Most physicians would at least give oral antibiotics (as above) to cover viral exacerbations. Annual influenza immunization is advisable.

Atypical mycobacteria

These organisms may be harmless commensals. Unlike *M. tuberculosis*, evidence of tissue invasion is generally held to be required to diagnose infection, but this evidence cannot often be sought in CF and decisions as to whether to treat are difficult. Evidence from autopsy studies suggests that atypical mycobacteria should be treated only if they are repeatedly found in sputum. CT scanning may be helpful in reaching a decision as to whether to treat, with indications for treatment being deterioration in clinical state and CT appearances in a patient with repeated positive isolates. *M. abscessus* seems to carry a particularly poor prognosis.

Aspergillus, including allergic bronchopulmonary aspergillosis

Evidence of exposure to *A. fumigatus* is common in CF (e.g. positive skin prick test, RAST, IgG precipitins, and sputum culture). It is becoming clearer that this organism, even in the absence of allergic bronchopulmonary aspergillosis (ABPA, see Chapter 18.14.2), may not be as benign as was once thought. The prevalence of ABPA is disputed, but probably around 10%, although the major diagnostic criteria for this condition are also common features of otherwise uncomplicated CF. Sophisticated immunological testing has been used to try to refine the diagnosis, but an abrupt four-fold rise in total IgE, often in association with IgG precipitins to aspergillus, is the simplest and most reliable investigation. By contrast to typical infective exacerbations of CF, large fleeting radiographic shadows are typical (Fig. 18.10.2b). Treatment is with oral corticosteroids; the roles of itraconazole and voriconazole are controversial, but they are increasingly used.

Other methods of treatment

Airway clearance

Chest physiotherapy should be performed twice daily as a routine, increasing at times of infective exacerbation. Different groups advocate different techniques, e.g. active cycle of breathing, autogenic drainage, and mechanical devices, such as the positive expiratory pressure (PEP) mask, flutter, and external oscillation jacket. There are no good comparisons between these approaches, and none has emerged as best. It is probably best to offer a choice of techniques to the patient. Physical exercise such as swimming supplements but should not replace formal airway clearance sessions.

Alteration in mucus properties

Human recombinant DNase *in vitro* reduces sputum viscosity. In the largest randomized controlled trial in the CF literature, once-daily nebulized human recombinant DNase resulted in small but sustained improvement in lung function and reduction in infective exacerbations. However, individual responses are very variable, and the treatment is expensive. A carefully monitored $n = 1$ trial is recommended before starting long-term therapy.

Two trials of hypertonic saline have shown minimal improvement in lung function, but the second trial, which was the only one powered for this purpose, showed a significant reduction in infective exacerbations. The burden of two extra nebulized treatments must be considered if this is to be prescribed.

Oxygen and other respiratory support

By analogy with the Medical Research Council and Nocturnal Oxygen Treatment Trial (NOTT) trials of oxygen in chronic obstructive pulmonary disease (see Chapters 18.10 and 18.15), one would anticipate that long-term oxygen would be beneficial to the chronically hypoxic CF patient. The only trial of this approach was underpowered and thus inconclusive. Oxygen is usually prescribed for symptoms, and for patients with chronic hypoxia irrespective of symptoms. Nasal ventilation may used during acute deteriorations, and as a useful short-term expedient while transplantation is awaited. It may usefully palliate symptoms during terminal care.

Bronchodilatation

Bronchial hyper-reactivity is common. Troublesome wheeze may need treatment with short-acting bronchodilators. However, β_2-agonists may cause paradoxical bronchoconstriction, and should be used cautiously. Long-acting β_2-agonists should only be given if there is clear-cut evidence of benefit. Persistent recurrent wheeze, particularly in the atopic CF patient, may be treated with inhaled or oral corticosteroids.

Anti-inflammatory therapy

The pathogenesis of CF lung disease includes an exuberant neutrophil-mediated inflammatory response which, via the release of neutrophil elastase and other mediators, may cause much of the tissue damage in the airways. Early in the course of the disease it is unclear whether infection is a prerequisite for inflammation, or if CF is intrinsically proinflammatory. However, in established CF airway disease, both are present. This has lead to the seemingly paradoxical proposal that patients with chronic bronchopulmonary sepsis should be iatrogenically immunosuppressed. Various approaches have been tried, although none is in wide clinical use.

Oral corticosteroids

Usage in severe airway obstruction and allergic bronchopulmonary aspergillosis are discussed above. Long-term routine use was assessed in a multicentre, double-blind trial comparing prednisolone 2 mg/kg on alternate days, 1 mg/kg on alternate days, and placebo. This showed: (1) no benefit, except in patients infected with *P. aeruginosa*; (2) sustained improvement in lung function in colonized patients; (3) unacceptable side effects (growth failure, cataract, glucose intolerance), necessitating stopping the higher dose after 2 years and the lower dose after 4 years. Although regular alternate-day steroids may be considered for up to 2 years in some patients, their routine use cannot be justified.

Inhaled corticosteroids

Since oral steroids are beneficial, but at the cost of unacceptable side effects, it would seem logical to use long-term inhaled corticosteroids. However, a recent study showed no detrimental effects if inhaled corticosteroids were withdrawn from a large group of CF patients, although an observational database review suggested some benefit, most would consider that they should not be a routine part of treatment. If they are used, consideration should be given to stepping down the dose at every clinic visit, analogous to the treatment of asthma.

Ibuprofen

A multicentre, double-blind, placebo-controlled trial of ibuprofen showed a slowing of the rate of decline of lung function, particularly in young patients. However, ibuprofen is not widely used. A second, underpowered study showed better forced vital capacity (FVC) but not FEV1, on ibuprofen. This may be because: (1) not all age groups benefited; (2) there are theoretical reasons for believing that lower doses may actually be harmful, meaning that ibuprofen levels need to be measured and a high dose given; and (3) if intravenous aminoglycosides have to be administered for an acute exacerbation of chest disease, there is a significant risk of nephrotoxicity.

Macrolide antibiotics

These are included in this section because modulation of inflammation is their likeliest mode of action. They were first used in a CF-like illness, diffuse panbronchiolitis, prevalent in middle-aged people in East Asia. Diffuse panbronchiolitis is characterized by chronic airway infection with mucoid strains of *P. aeruginosa*, the hallmark of CF. It was shown serendipitously that treatment with low-dose erythromycin reduced the 10-year mortality from 90% to less than 10%. Subsequently, four randomized controlled trials have demonstrated benefit of azithromycin in CF, and this treatment is used increasingly. Macrolides have multiple actions on the immune system and growth factors *in vitro*, but their precise mechanism of action in CF has not been determined.

Other anti-inflammatory approaches

Although anti-inflammatory defences are normal in CF, they are overwhelmed by the burden of neutrophil elastase. Boosting the natural defences (α_1-antitrypsin, secretory leukoprotease inhibitor) by nebulizer has been the subject of small and inconclusive trials; α_1-antitrypsin therapy has been shown to be ineffective in a large trial; a trial of a leukotriene B_4 receptor antagonist was halted because of increased infective exacerbations in the active treatment arm, underscoring the fact that immune modulation may not always be beneficial.

There are anecdotal reports of the successful use of methotrexate, ciclosporin, and intravenous immunoglobulin in CF, particularly in those with severe, nonbronchiectatic airflow obstruction. There are no large trials of these approaches.

Particular respiratory complications

Haemoptysis

Blood streaking of sputum is common in CF and requires no special treatment. Massive haemoptysis is variously defined, usually as the expectoration of more than 250 ml of blood in 24 h, and is a frightening emergency which requires active management. It is usually a complication of severe lung disease, and the source is from hypertrophied bronchial arteries. The patient should be admitted, given antipseudomonal intravenous antibiotics, and any clotting abnormalities corrected. Careful chest physiotherapy should be continued. Tranexamic acid and vasopressin are sometimes used to try to control haemorrhage. If bleeding does not settle, or recurs, then bronchial artery embolism should be considered. All sizeable bronchial arteries should be occluded. Preoperative bronchoscopy does not influence management, and often fails to define the side of bleeding. The major risk of embolization is inadvertent occlusion of a major spinal artery, resulting in paraplegia. Lobectomy is rarely necessary, and carries a high risk in these patients, who are often very compromised.

Pneumothorax

This is usually a complication of late-stage lung disease. Small pneumothoraces may require no special measures; moderate or large pneumothoraces are initially treated with tube drainage. Careful physiotherapy must be continued, and intravenous antibiotics given. If there is a continued air leak, pleurodesis should be undertaken. However, it is important to consult with the local transplant service before doing this, because aggressive pleurectomy is seen by some to be a contraindication to subsequent transplantation.

Upper airway disease

Nasal polyps are seen in up to 50% of adults with CF. Treatment is with nasal steroids in the first instance. If medical management fails, surgical polypectomy is indicated, but 50% will require a second procedure within 2 years. Abnormal sinus radiographs are universal, but symptomatic sinusitis relatively rare. If present, sinusitis should be treated medically with prolonged antibiotics, nasal steroids, and possibly decongestants in the first instance; surgery is rarely required. Rarely, surgery is needed for mucocoele of the frontal sinuses.

Gastrointestinal management

Pancreatic insufficiency needs to be treated in 85% of cases; meconium ileus or distal intestinal obstruction syndrome affects up to 30%; symptomatic liver disease occurs in about 5%, but in general the gastrointestinal manifestations of CF are less important than the lung disease. For a few patients, however, they are the dominant problem.

Pancreatic insufficiency

This is usually present from birth, with low levels of bicarbonate and lipolytic and proteolytic enzymes in pancreatic secretions. Those with clinical pancreatic sufficiency secrete low but adequate levels of enzymes. Some develop pancreatic insufficiency later in life. The usual presentations are neonatal meconium ileus (which is occasionally seen in pancreatic-sufficient CF patients, and normal babies) or failure to thrive with associated steatorrhoea and malnutrition. Consequences can include anaemia, vitamin deficiency, and occasionally oedema; complications include rectal prolapse, intussusception, volvulus, and distant intestinal obstruction.

The diagnosis is confirmed by estimation of human faecal elastase (which can be used even if the patient has been started on pancreatic enzymes), demonstration of unsplit fat globules in the stool, or increased faecal fat on a 2- or 3-day stool collection. Formal testing of pancreatic function is seldom required.

Treatment with pancreatic enzyme and vitamin supplementation is usually straightforward and successful. Enteric-coated enzyme preparations are taken before meals and the quantity adjusted to achieve normal stools. Most adults need four to eight capsules with main meals and two to four with snacks, and learn to adjust the dose according to the fat content of the meal. The commonest cause of failure is poor compliance, although occasionally lactose intolerance, inflammatory bowel disease, coeliac disease, or bowel infection/infestation may coexist. A few patients need to take H_2 blockers, proton pump inhibitors, or antacids to achieve better control of symptoms. Large-bowel strictures have developed in some patients (usually children) taking high-strength enzyme preparations, probably as a toxic effect of the coating rather than the enzymes themselves.

Nutrition

Vitamin supplementation should be given to all patients to cover fat-soluble vitamin deficiency. Multivitamin tablets contain vitamins A and D, but vitamin E needs to be given separately to maintain adequate intake. The diet should otherwise be normal, with a high calorie intake, usually 130% of recommended daily allowance. However, a recent study suggested that oral high-calorie supplements are often ineffective, and patients unable to maintain weight in spite of optimal dietary advice can be helped by enteral feeding, which is better tolerated by gastrostomy than by a nasogastric tube in the long term.

Distal intestinal obstruction syndrome

Constipation and a loaded colon are relatively common in CF and usually respond to modification of the diet, pancreatic supplements, and a high fluid and roughage intake; occasionally lactulose and/or a macrogol laxative (e.g. Movicol) is helpful. Severe constipation merges into the distal intestinal obstruction syndrome with pain, palpable faecal masses, and complete obstruction with faecal material in the distal ileum or ascending colon. The cause is multifactorial with imbalance of pancreatic enzymes and diet, disturbed fluid and electrolyte transport, faecal dehydration, and abnormal intestinal mobility all playing a part.

Patients present with chronic intermittent pain or episodes of complete obstruction. Although the differential diagnosis is wide and includes common conditions such as appendicitis, most patients improve with medical treatment and surgery should be avoided unless there is clear evidence of another diagnosis. Treatment with a balanced intestinal lavage solution, 500 to 1000 ml/h by nasogastric tube, usually moves the faecal blockage within 4 to 6 h. Alternatives are gastrograffin by mouth or enema, or oral N-acetylcysteine. Occasionally, removal of inspissated faeces at colonoscopy is needed.

Other gastrointestinal complications

Pancreatitis is rare but should be excluded in cases of abdominal pain. It usually affects those who are clinically pancreatic sufficient. Treatment is conventional, with special attention to pulmonary infections, because the pain of pancreatitis may interfere with physiotherapy.

Gastro-oesophageal reflux is common, sometimes with overt vomiting, and may be associated with coughing, physiotherapy, and bronchodilators which may relax the oesophageal sphincter. Aspiration of stomach contents is seldom a clinical problem. Although peptic ulcer disease might be expected in view of the low pancreatic bicarbonate secretion, there is only one report of an increased frequency of ulceration. *Helicobacter pylori* infection is uncommon, perhaps because of antibiotic treatment.

Lactose intolerance, coeliac disease, and inflammatory bowel disease occur with slightly increased frequency in the CF population, but symptoms may be misattributed to CF and diagnosis therefore delayed. Both giardiasis and *Clostridium difficile* gut infection have been reported as being more frequent in CF, but these are not common clinical problems.

Liver disease

Liver disease causes problems in 5% and death in 2% of people with CF, but abnormal liver function tests are very common and up to 50% have biliary cirrhosis demonstrable at autopsy. With increasing survival, liver disease may become more important.

Although liver enlargement and jaundice occasionally occur in early childhood, liver disease is usually signalled by hepatosplenomegaly or abnormal liver function on routine testing. Decompensation with jaundice, ascites, or encephalopathy are rare and occur late. Variceal bleeding only occurs in a minority of those with established chronic liver disease, but may be the presenting symptom of CF itself, or of liver disease in a patient known to have CF. Minor or modest elevations of aminotransferase, γ-glutamyl transpepdidase, or alkaline phosphatase levels are very common but do not correlate with established liver disease unless the enzyme levels are greater than four times normal. Routine ultrasonography detects fatty change or multilobular cirrhosis: the finding of portal vein dilatation, splenomegaly, or collateral vessels indicating portal hypertension. Cholangiography is occasionally needed for diagnosis of gallstones: this may reveal irregularities of the intrahepatic ducts, suggesting chronic liver disease, and significant strictures of the common bile duct may also be seen. Liver biopsy is seldom needed.

No treatment has been shown to modify the course of chronic liver disease in CF, although clinical and biochemical improvements have been shown following treatment with ursodeoxycholic acid. This bile acid stimulates bile flow, may protect the hepatocyte from toxicity of bile acids, and is helpful in primary biliary cirrhosis. Many hepatologists therefore recommend its use in CF.

Jaundice must be investigated to exclude drug hepatotoxicity or treatable obstructive cause, but is otherwise a late event with poor prognosis. Variceal bleeding is treated with injection sclerotherapy or banding ligation, and in the short term balloon tamponade or vasoconstrictor drugs may buy a little time. Surgical treatment is hazardous due to lung disease and in a few patients the insertion of a transjugular intrahepatic portal systemic shunt may be an alternative. Prophylactic treatment of varices has not been shown to help and

may be detrimental. Ascites and encephalopathy are rare and are usually preterminal events to be managed conventionally.

In most cases of complicated chronic liver disease, management is made more difficult by the presence of lung infection that must be aggressively treated. Respiratory failure may develop concurrently. When this occurs, intubation and ventilation are seldom successful.

Diabetes

Glucose intolerance in CF increases with age, being rare under 10 years, affecting 14% by 15 years, and over 65% at 25 years. By this age 32% are frankly diabetic. Even when glucose tolerance is normal, reduced insulin secretion is frequent, and should be sought in a patient who is deteriorating on conventional treatment. This is caused by gradual and progressive loss of β cell mass in line with pancreatic fibrosis. Peripheral insulin sensitivity is usually normal and autoimmune factors are not involved.

Diagnosis is based on conventional World Health Organization (WHO) recommendations. Many recommend annual oral glucose tolerance tests, but screening for diabetes in a CF clinic is sometimes done by measurement of HbA1c (not a useful screening tool), together with random or fasting blood sugar levels. Diabetes is usually diagnosed at such screening, but a few patients present with weight loss and increased frequency and severity of chest infections, although polyuria and polydipsia occasionally develop first. It has been suggested that the onset of diabetes is a marker of general deterioration, but many patients return to their previous level of health when diabetes is controlled. Oral hypoglycaemic agents may provide control in a few patients for a limited time, but most clinics have now discarded them: insulin replacement is usually necessary. Control of blood sugar is relatively simple, with flexible use of short- and long-acting insulins. The usual dietary recommendation is to maintain an energy intake of 150% of normal with frequent balanced meals, with adjustment of insulin to fit. Ketoacidosis and insulin resistance are almost unknown.

Early microangiopathy has been shown in CF patients with diabetes, but retinopathy, neuropathy, and nephropathy are very rare. This may be in part due to the mildness of the diabetes, but is likely to become more common as survival improves. Nevertheless, CF patients with diabetes tend to have excess morbidity and slightly increased rate of decline in weight and lung function.

Other organ systems

Reproduction

Almost all men with CF have obstructive azoospermia with otherwise normal sexual function. This is due to absence of the vas deferens, and although there are no sperm in the ejaculate (which is usually of reduced volume) there is normal spermatogenesis and Leydig cell function. Counselling about infertility should be done well before the time of puberty, and certainly before permanent relationships develop. Most men opt to confirm the azoospermia by a sperm count. *In vitro* fertilization using aspirated sperm has been successful and there are now many CF fathers.

Early reports of reduced fertility in women with CF have not been confirmed and most can conceive normally. The child must carry one mutation from the mother: the risk of CF in the baby is therefore 1 in 50 in white populations, with a carrier frequency of 1 in 25. Counselling and paternal genotyping allows reassurance for most CF pregnancies and identifies a 1 in 2 risk when the father is a carrier. Successful pregnancies have been completed by many hundreds of CF women, but women with severe lung disease may not be able to complete a pregnancy safely, the risks rising with impaired lung function and especially when the FEV_1 is less than 30% predicted. Children born have been healthy, without an increased frequency of birth defects despite the mothers' extensive drug treatment. Lactation is normal.

Vaginal candidiasis secondary to antibiotic treatment is relatively common in CF. Stress incontinence is particularly distressing, and may interfere with coughing, physiotherapy, and normal sexual relationships. Sexual behaviour in both genders may be inhibited by low weight, delayed puberty, cough, sputum, haemoptysis, breathlessness, and indwelling catheters, but most people adapt well and persistent problems are few.

Skin and joints

Clubbing is almost universal in those with significant lung disease, and regresses after successful lung transplantation. Hypertrophic osteoarthropathy is rare. Episodic arthritis, predominantly affecting the large joints, is quite common and associated with chest infections. Erosive arthritis is rare. Pain responds to nonsteroidal anti-inflammatory drugs (NSAIDs), and steroids or immunosuppression are seldom needed. Systemic vasculitis has occasionally been reported but is surprisingly rare considering the extent of immune activation, the frequency of circulating immune complexes, and the number of drugs taken.

Kidneys

Glomerulonephritis has been reported but is probably no more frequent than in the normal population. Acute tubular necrosis is rare and usually associated with higher than recommended aminoglycoside levels or the additional prescription of NSAIDs. Very large numbers of aminoglycoside treatments are associated with progressive decrements in renal function; some patients have had over 100 courses. Renal stones are commoner in CF, probably due to excess oxalate absorption secondary to altered bowel bacterial flora. Systemic amyloidosis has occasionally been reported secondary to prolonged pulmonary infection.

Central nervous system

Acute ototoxicity occasionally results from aminoglycoside treatment but is not seen when serum levels are well controlled, but there does seem to be a cumulative effect from repeated aminoglycoside courses. Cerebral abscess rarely complicates lung sepsis. Vitamin E deficiency leads to a cerebellar syndrome combined with peripheral neuropathy.

Osteoporosis

Reduced bone mineral density is common in CF, with prevalence among adults of up to 60%. This is partly due to general malnutrition as well as vitamin D malabsorption, but relative immobility is sometimes a factor. Other factors may include delayed puberty and hypogonadism, the effect of the systemic inflammatory response, immobility, inhaled and oral steroid therapy, and vitamin K deficiency. An increased rate of fractures has been reported, and rib fractures from coughing can interfere with adequate physiotherapy. Vertebral compression fractures are fortunately rare. Regular bone mineral density measurements are recommended with extra vitamin D and calcium

supplementation when low. Bisphosphonates can cause bone pain when given intravenously. Oral preparations can be used, and trials are ongoing to determine the optimal timing of treatment. Prevention is by encouraging a high dairy intake, weight-bearing exercise, and probably supplementation with vitamin K.

Management of respiratory failure

Recurrent and persistent chest infection leads to progressive decline in lung function with eventual respiratory failure in most patients, although in about 2% the liver fails first. At this stage the issues of transplantation should be addressed. If a patient wishes to explore the possibility of transplantation, then preoperative work-up, counselling, surgical assessment, and placement on the waiting list should take place 2 years before the predicted date of death. Others may opt for palliative care.

Lung transplantation (see also Chapter 18.16)

Selection criteria are listed in Table 18.10.3. The timing of assessment is judged on the level and rate of decline of lung function, arterial blood gases, and the frequency and severity of chest infections. Patients on the waiting list must be managed optimally to maintain lung function and nutrition, often with gastrostomy feeding. Noninvasive ventilatory support can provide a bridge to transplantation for patients with progressive respiratory failure, but intubation and conventional ventilation are not recommended. Donor organs are scarce and at least 50% of listed CF patients never receive a transplant. The results for lung transplantation are the same as for other lung diseases, with a survival of 70% at 1 year and 50% at 3 years. Recently, living donor lobar transplantation has been offered to CF patients, with comparable results. Liver transplantation is appropriate for the occasional patient dying of liver failure with relatively good lung function: survival at 1 year is 40%.

Terminal care

The timing of the decision to switch to palliative care is difficult and should be made in conjunction with the patient and relatives. The most distressing symptoms are cough, sputum retention, breathlessness, and exhaustion. Small doses of morphine are usually well tolerated and only seldom worsen respiratory failure.

The CF team

As with many chronic diseases, the purely medical care of CF is relatively straightforward. Proper holistic care requires a team approach,

Table 18.10.3 Selection criteria for lung transplantation

Indications	Severe respiratory failure in spite of optimal treatment
	Severely impaired quality of life
	Patient positively wants a transplant
Strong contraindications	Active aspergillus or mycobacterial infection
	Noncompliance with treatment
	Other end-organ failure
	Gross malnutrition
Relative contraindications	Preoperative ventilation
	Previous thoracic surgery
	Chemical pleurodesis

and without such a team, care will be second rate. Typically, the core of the team is formed by a specialist nurse, a physiotherapist, a dietitian, a psychologist, and a social worker, together with a specialist doctor. It is unrealistic to expect every hospital to provide this, and hence close contact with a tertiary centre is advisable. Many of the physical issues (airway clearance, nutritional management) have been discussed above. Equally important are many of the psychological problems springing from the presence of a chronic disease.

The normal process of adolescence includes rebelling and breaking free of parental care. In those with CF this may never have been achieved, because the parents have wanted to keep control of treatment regimens, and have been reluctant to allow independence. Although paediatric clinics should have established a pattern of the adolescent coming into the consulting room alone, frequently this does not happen, and the adult physician is often confronted with parents who resent the idea that their now grown-up child should be seen on their own. Conversely, the consequences of a full-blown adolescent revolt (no treatment done, abuse of cigarettes, alcohol, soft and hard drugs, and high-risk sexual behaviour) may be particularly catastrophic in the patient with CF. The authors know of no easy answer to adolescence and its aftermath.

Knowledge of fertility issues is notoriously poor amongst adult men with CF: these may need to be tackled tactfully. The issues surrounding pregnancy in the woman with CF, who may herself be severely breathless, but desperately wishing for a child, also require sensitive handling.

Further education and employment are also difficult issues in the setting of chronic physical disability, but skilled help may allow patients with CF to maximize their potential. A fuller account of the many and complex psychosocial issues surrounding care can be found elsewhere, but appreciation of these issues is just as important as knowing the correct management of the physical problems of CF.

Future prospects

The growth in basic scientific understanding of CF will lead to a number of new treatments directed at the mutant CFTR gene or protein. These include gene therapy, which has already reached preliminary clinical trials, protein replacement therapy, and drug therapy to correct the molecular defect (as illustrated in Fig. 18.10.1). Research into correction of the disordered electrophysiology with sodium channel blockers, such as amiloride, or promoters of chloride transport, such as UTP, is already well advanced. There is, therefore, a real prospect of new fundamental treatments to prevent the development of CF disease and lead to improved health, prolonged survival, and reduction in lifelong supportive therapy.

Further reading

Brennan AL, *et al.* (2004). Clinical importance of cystic fibrosis-related diabetes. *J Cyst Fibros*, **3**, 209–22.

Chmiel JF, Berger M, Konstan MW. (2002). The role of inflammation in the pathophysiology of cystic fibrosis lung disease. *Clin Rev Allergy Immunol*, **23**, 5–27.

Cohn JA, *et al.* (1998). Relations between mutations of the cystic fibrosis gene and idiopathic pancreatitis. *N Engl J Med*, **339**, 653–8.

Colombo C, *et al.* (2006). Liver disease in cystic fibrosis. *J Pediatr Gastroenterol Nutr*, **43** Suppl 1, S49–55.

Cystic Fibrosis Genotype–Phenotype Consortium (1993). Correlation between genotype and phenotype in patients with cystic fibrosis. *N Engl J Med*, **329**, 1308–13.

De Boeck K, *et al.* (2006). Cystic fibrosis: terminology and diagnostic algorithms. *Thorax*, **61**, 627–35.

Eigen H, *et al.* (1995). A multicenter study of alternate-day prednisone therapy in patients with cystic fibrosis. *J Pediatr*, **126**, 515–23.

Elkins MR, *et al.* (2006). A controlled trial of long-term inhaled hypertonic saline in patients with cystic fibrosis. *New Engl J Med*, **354**, 229–40.

Farrell PM, *et al.* (1997). Nutritional benefits of neonatal screening for cystic fibrosis. *N Engl J Med*, **337**, 963–9.

Flume PA, *et al.* (2005). Pneumothorax in cystic fibrosis. *Chest*, **128**, 720–8.

Flume PA, *et al.* (2005). Massive hemoptysis in cystic fibrosis. *Chest*, **128**, 729–38.

Frederiksen B, Koch C, Hoiby N (1997). Antibiotic treatment of initial colonization with *Pseudomonas aeruginosa* postpones chronic infection and prevents deterioration of pulmonary function in cystic fibrosis. *Pediatr Pulmonol*, **23**, 330–5.

Fuchs HJ, *et al.* (1994). Effect of aerosolized recombinant human DNase on exacerbations of respiratory symptoms and on pulmonary function in patients with cystic fibrosis. *N Engl J Med*, **331**, 637–42.

Gibson RL, Burns JL, Ramsey BW (2003). Pathophysiology and management of pulmonary infections in cystic fibrosis. *Am J Respir Crit Care Med*, **168**, 918–51.

Griesenbach U, Geddes DM, Alton EWFW (2006). Gene therapy progress and prospects: cystic fibrosis. *Gene Ther*, **13**, 1061–7.

Hodson ME, Geddes DM, Bush A (eds) (2007). *Cystic fibrosis*. Chapman & Hall, London.

Konstan MW, *et al.* (1995). Effect of high-dose ibuprofen in patients with cystic fibrosis. *N Engl J Med*, **332**, 848–54.

Liou TG, Woo MS, Cahill BC (2006). Lung transplantation for cystic fibrosis. *Curr Opin Pulm Med*, **12**, 459–63.

Marchant JL, Warner JO, Bush A (1994). Rise in total IgE as an indicator of allergic broncho-pulmonary aspergillosis in cystic fibrosis. *Thorax*, **49**, 1002–5.

McMullen AH, et al. (2006). Impact of pregnancy on women with cystic fibrosis. *Chest*, **129**, 706–11.

Middleton PG, Geddes DM, Alton EWFW (1994). Protocols for in vivo measurement of the ion transport defects in cystic fibrosis nasal epithelium. *Eur Respir J*, **7**, 2050–6.

Mukhopadhyay S, *et al.* (1996). Nebulised antipseudomonal antibiotic therapy in cystic fibrosis: a meta-analysis of benefits and risks. *Thorax*, **51**, 364–8.

Ramsey BW, *et al.* (1999). Intermittent administration of inhaled tobramycin in patients with cystic fibrosis. *N Engl J Med*, **340**, 23–30.

Rao S, Grigg J (2006). New insights into pulmonary inflammation in cystic fibrosis. *Arch Dis Child*, **91**, 786–8.

Ratjen F (2006). Treatment of early *Pseudomonas aeruginosa* infection in patients with cystic fibrosis. *Curr Opin Pulm Med*, **12**, 428–32.

Ratjen F, Doring G (2003). Cystic fibrosis. *Lancet*, **361**, 681–9.

Robertson MB, Choe KA, Joseph PM (2006). Review of the abdominal manifestations of cystic fibrosis in the adult patient. *Radiographics*, **26**, 679–90.

Rosenstein BJ, Cutting GR, for the Cystic Fibrosis Foundation Consensus Panel (1998). The diagnosis of cystic fibrosis: a consensus statement. *J Pediatr*, **132**, 589–95.

Rowe SM, Miller S, Sorscher EJ (2005). Cystic fibrosis. *N Engl J Med*, **352**, 1992–2001.

Saiman L (2004). The use of macrolide antibiotics in patients with cystic fibrosis. *Curr Opin Pulm Med*, **10**, 515–23.

Shidrawi RG, *et al.* (2002). Emergency colonoscopy for distal intestinal obstruction syndrome in cystic fibrosis patients. *Gut*, **51**, 285–6.

Smyth A (2005). Prophylactic antibiotics in cystic fibrosis: a conviction without evidence? *Pediatr Pulmonol*, **40**, 471–6.

Wallis C, *et al.* (1997). Stool elastase as a diagnostic test for pancreatic function in children with cystic fibrosis. *Lancet*, **350**, 1001.

Welsh MJ, Smith AE (1993). Molecular mechanisms of CFTR chloride channel dysfunction in cystic fibrosis. *Cell*, **73**, 1251–4.

Diffuse parenchymal lung diseases

Contents

18.11.1 Diffuse parenchymal lung disease: an introduction

A.U. Wells

Essentials

The nomenclature of diffuse parenchymal lung disease has caused a great deal of confusion, with use of complicated histopathological terms not always corresponding exactly to clinico-radiological entities.

'Cryptogenic fibrosing alveolitis'—Hamman and Rich first described a presentation of rapidly progressive fatal diffuse parenchymal lung disease in which the cardinal histological features were interstitial inflammation and fibrosis. A typical clinical picture was defined, consisting of progressive dyspnoea, bilateral predominantly basal crackles on auscultation, reticulonodular predominantly basal abnormalities on chest radiography, and a restrictive ventilatory defect on lung function testing. This clinical entity was termed 'cryptogenic fibrosing alveolitis' (CFA) or 'idiopathic pulmonary fibrosis', but it has become clear that the outcome associated with this presentation—termed the 'CFA clinical syndrome'—is highly heterogeneous.

Diffuse parenchymal lung diseases can be subdivided into five major groupings: (1) idiopathic interstitial pneumonias; (2) diseases associated with systemic conditions, including rheumatological disease; (3) diseases caused by environmental triggers or drug ingestion; (4) granulomatous diseases; and (5) other diffuse lung diseases.

Idiopathic interstitial pneumonias

Classification—this is based on recognition of clinical, radiological, and histopathological patterns, as opposed to the purely histopathological terminology. The following are recognized: (1) usual interstitial pneumonia (UIP); (2) nonspecific interstitial pneumonia (NSIP); (3) desquamative interstitial pneumonia (DIP); (4) respiratory bronchiolitis–interstitial lung disease (RBILD); (5) diffuse alveolar damage (DAD); (6) lymphocytic interstitial pneumonia (LIP); and (7) cryptogenic organizing pneumonia.

Diagnosis—is complicated by the large number of disorders grouped within the diffuse parenchymal lung diseases. A systematic diagnostic algorithm, based upon careful clinical evaluation and a logical sequence of tests, is essential. This approach can be broken down into two phases: (1) clinical history, clinical examination, chest radiography, pulmonary function tests, and selective blood tests; and (2) high-resolution CT, bronchoalveolar lavage (in some cases), and lung biopsy (in a few cases).

Clinical patterns of disease—the chronic diffuse parenchymal lung diseases can be broadly subclassified into five patterns of longitudinal disease behaviour, based upon cause, severity, the relative degree of inflammation and fibrosis, and observed change in the short term. Each clinical pattern is associated with a separate approach to management:

1 Self-limited inflammation—usually caused by an extrinsic agent, usually responds to withdrawal of an offending agent, and other therapy is unnecessary.

2 Stable fibrotic disease—most commonly encountered in sarcoidosis, following drug-induced lung disease, and in patients with formerly active rheumatological disorders. Treatment is not

required, but monitoring of serial pulmonary function tests is needed.

3 Major inflammation, with or without supervening fibrosis—often a feature of drug-induced lung disease, and also of some patients with cryptogenic organizing pneumonia, DIP, hypersensitivity pneumonitis, sarcoidosis, and aggressive inflammatory disease in rheumatological disease. Treatment with corticosteroids is usual, initially at high dosage.

4 Slowly progressive fibrotic disease, in which stabilization is a realistic goal—frequently seen in sarcoidosis, hypersensitivity pneumonitis, rheumatological conditions, and in many patients with fibrotic NSIP. Aggressive initial treatment is usually warranted to ensure optimal control of disease activity. Long-term therapy is often required.

5 Inexorably progressive fibrotic disease—the hallmark of IPF, but an IPF-like course is sometimes observed in idiopathic fibrotic NSIP, rheumatological disease, and in a few patients with chronic hypersensitivity pneumonitis. Long-term treatment may slow disease progression, but initial high-dose therapy achieves nothing in known IPF and may cause unnecessary drug toxicity.

Definition

The nomenclature of diffuse parenchymal lung disease has caused a great deal of confusion. There have been too many complicated histopathological terms, not always corresponding exactly to clinico-radiological entities. The free use of synonymous terms—e.g. extrinsic allergic alveolitis and hypersensitivity pneumonitis; idiopathic pulmonary fibrosis (IPF) and cryptogenic fibrosing alveolitis (CFA)—has added to difficulties faced by general and respiratory physicians in coming to terms with a difficult group of idiopathic diseases. Before the recent reclassification of the idiopathic interstitial pneumonias, the use by clinicians of the 'umbrella term' CFA/IPF to group idiopathic diseases with a common clinical presentation was an understandable attempt to simplify terminology. However, attempts to lump disorders together according to their clinical presentation contributed to imprecision in defining individual diseases.

Diffuse parenchymal lung disease was formerly known as interstitial lung disease. The change of terminology reflects the fact that disease processes involve the lung parenchyma, but also in many cases the air-space components of the acini. Infective pneumonias, pulmonary oedema, and some malignancies involve the acinar regions of the lung but are not, by convention, grouped with the diffuse parenchymal lung diseases, although they may present with similar clinical and radiological findings and should be considered in the formulation of a differential diagnosis.

Specific diseases are considered in subsequent chapters. In this introduction, a broad approach to the classification of the diffuse lung diseases and their diagnosis and investigation is discussed.

Classification

Diffuse parenchymal lung diseases can be subdivided into five major groupings:

1 idiopathic interstitial pneumonias

2 diseases associated with systemic conditions, including rheumatological disease

3 diseases caused by environmental triggers or drug ingestion

4 granulomatous diseases

5 other diffuse lung diseases

In most patients with environmentally induced and drug-induced lung disease, granulomatous lung disease, or lung disease complicating systemic disease, the cause and thus the diagnosis is immediately apparent, or is rapidly disclosed by standard investigations detailed below. By contrast, diagnosis is less straightforward when a cause is not immediately apparent. By definition, most patients can be categorized as having one of the idiopathic interstitial pneumonias, discussed in detail in the remainder of this chapter. Box 18.11.1.1 lists diseases of known and unknown cause falling within the broad headings above, and disorders that present more acutely are shown in Box 18.11.1.2.

Idiopathic interstitial pneumonias

The diseases grouped as the 'idiopathic interstitial pneumonias' give rise to particular confusion, largely because terms used to describe histopathological patterns have been used interchangeably but inaccurately with disease 'labels'. In 1944, Hamman and Rich first described a presentation of rapidly progressive fatal disease, in which the cardinal histological features were interstitial inflammation and fibrosis. It subsequently became clear that chronic insidiously progressive fibrosing disease was much more common. A typical clinical picture was defined, consisting of progressive dyspnoea, bilateral predominantly basal crackles on auscultation, reticulonodular predominantly basal abnormalities on chest radiography, and a restrictive ventilatory defect on lung function testing. This clinical entity was termed 'cryptogenic fibrosing alveolitis' or 'idiopathic pulmonary fibrosis'. However, it became clear that the outcome associated with this presentation, hereafter termed the 'CFA clinical syndrome', was highly heterogeneous. Although most patients progressed inexorably to a fatal outcome, usually within 3 to 4 years, a more insidious course was seen in a significant minority, and in 10 to 15% of cases there was a response to corticosteroid therapy and, usually, a good long-term outcome.

Histological patterns of disease encountered in the CFA clinical syndrome were first classified by Liebow in 1975 as usual interstitial pneumonia (UIP), desquamative interstitial pneumonia (DIP), bronchiolitis obliterans with UIP, lymphocytic interstitial pneumonia (LIP), and giant-cell interstitial pneumonia. However, it subsequently became clear that these patterns of disease were also present outside an idiopathic setting. The most frequent, UIP, was occasionally found in connective tissue disease, drug-induced lung disease, and chronic hypersensitivity pneumonitis, and LIP was most commonly associated with rheumatological disease and, more recently, AIDS-related disease. Giant-cell interstitial pneumonia was seldom idiopathic but was caused by exposure to hard metals (cobalt, tungsten carbide, titanium salts). It also became apparent that the historical histological pattern of UIP did, in fact, encompass separate patterns of UIP and nonspecific interstitial pneumonia (NSIP), which denoted a better outcome.

These considerations led to a revision of Liebow's classification. The interstitial pneumonias of known cause were removed (although smoking-related disorders were retained). The revised

Box 18.11.1.1 Diffuse parenchymal lung diseases

Associated with systemic diseases

◆ Rheumatological:

- Systemic sclerosis, rheumatoid arthritis, polymyositis/dermatomyositis, systemic lupus erythematosus, Sjögren's syndrome, ankylosing spondylitis

◆ Vasculitis:

- Wegener's granulomatosis, Churg–Strauss granulomatosis, microscopic polyangiitis, pulmonary–renal syndrome (including Goodpasture's syndrome), capillaritis, Behçet's syndrome

◆ Vascular:

- Primary pulmonary hypertension, idiopathic pulmonary haemosiderosis, pulmonary veno-occlusive disease, antiphospholipid syndrome

Diseases caused by environmental triggers or drug ingestion

◆ Hypersensitivity pneumonitis: fungal, bacterial, avian, chemical

◆ Fibrogenic inorganic dusts: asbestosis, silica, hard metal alloy-beryllium, coal, aluminium

◆ Therapeutic agents,[a] illicit drugs, radiation, pesticides, oxygen and other inhaled gases

Granulomatous diseases

◆ Sarcoidosis, hypersensitivity pneumonitis, berylliosis, Langerhans' cell histiocytosis, Wegener's granulomatosis, Churg–Strauss syndrome, lymphomatoid granulomatosis, bronchocentric granulomatosis

Idiopathic interstitial pneumonias

◆ Idiopathic pulmonary fibrosis, nonspecific interstitial pneumonia, desquamative interstitial pneumonia, respiratory bronchiolitis–interstitial lung disease, acute interstitial pneumonia, cryptogenic organizing pneumonia, lymphocytic interstitial pneumonia

Other diffuse lung diseases

◆ Inherited disorders: tuberous sclerosis, neurofibromatosis, Hermansky–Pudlak syndrome, lipid storage disorders, familial idiopathic pulmonary fibrosis

◆ Pulmonary eosinophilia: known causes (fungi, parasites, drugs), acute idiopathic, chronic idiopathic

◆ Lymphangioleiomyomatosis

◆ Alveolar proteinosis

◆ Alveolar microlithiasis

◆ Amyloidosis

◆ Chronic aspiration

[a] See http://pneumotox.com for full listing.

Box 18.11.1.2 Acute presentations of diffuse parenchymal lung disease: differential diagnosis

Primary diffuse parenchymal lung disorders

◆ Acute interstitial pneumonia

◆ Acute exacerbations of idiopathic pulmonary fibrosis

◆ Diffuse alveolar haemorrhage due to vasculitis or coagulopathy

◆ Fulminant cryptogenic and secondary organizing pneumonia

◆ Acute pneumonitis due to rheumatological disease

◆ Hypersensitivity pneumonitis

◆ Acute pulmonary eosinophilia

◆ Drug-induced lung disease

Mimics of diffuse parenchymal lung disease

◆ Left ventricular failure

◆ Other causes of pulmonary oedema, including mitral stenosis

◆ Lung manifestation of uraemia

◆ Infection, especially opportunistic with pneumocystis

◆ Extensive, rapidly progressive metastatic malignancy

classification, constructed by a nomenclature committee of the American Thoracic Society and European Respiratory Society (ATS/ERS), included UIP, NSIP, DIP, respiratory bronchiolitis–interstitial lung disease (RBILD), diffuse alveolar damage (DAD), LIP, and cryptogenic organizing pneumonia (Table 18.11.1.1). In this classification, disease nomenclature incorporates clinical, radiological, and histopathological patterns, as opposed to the purely histopathological terminology used previously. The pattern of UIP and the associated clinical disorder, idiopathic pulmonary fibrosis, is discussed separately in Chapter 18.11.2: the term 'cryptogenic fibrosisng alveolitis' is now synonymous with IPF, requiring an underlying histological pattern of UIP or compatible high-resolution CT appearances, and should not be confused with the nonspecific CFA clinical syndrome. Cryptogenic organizing pneumonia is covered in Chapter 18.11.3. The other idiopathic interstitial pneumonias, all commonly presenting with the CFA clinical syndrome, are reviewed briefly below.

Table 18.11.1.1 American Thoracic Society/European Respiratory Society nomenclature of idiopathic interstitial pneumonias

Clinical diagnosis	Pathological pattern
Cryptogenic fibrosing alveolitis (idiopathic pulmonary fibrosis)	Usual interstitial pneumonia
Desquamative interstitial pneumonia (alternative name: alveolar macrophage pneumonia)	Desquamative interstitial pneumonia
Respiratory bronchiolitis–interstitial lung disease	Respiratory bronchiolitis– interstitial lung disease
Acute interstitial pneumonia	Diffuse alveolar damage
Cryptogenic organizing pneumonia	Organizing pneumonia
Lymphocytic interstitial pneumonia	Lymphocytic interstitial pneumonia

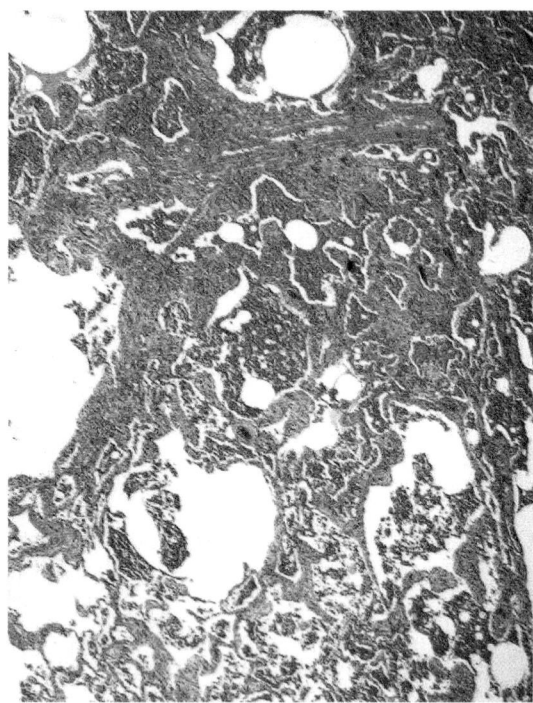

Fig. 18.11.1.1 A case of desquamative interstitial pneumonia (DIP) with typical appearances of macrophage filling of alveolar spaces diffusely within pulmonary acini. There is also mild interstitial fibrosis and focal background emphysema, in keeping with the association between DIP and cigarette smoking.

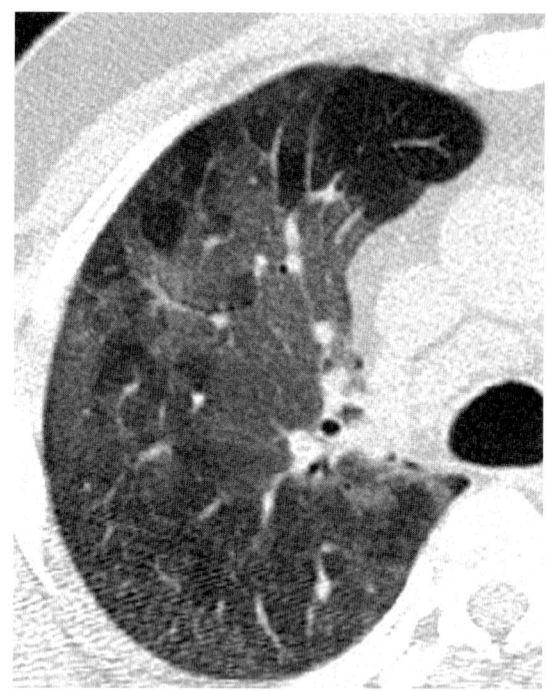

Fig. 18.11.1.2 High-resolution CT appearances in a patient with histologically proven desquamative interstitial pneumonia (DIP). There is extensive ground-glass attenuation with no traction bronchiectasis or admixed reticular abnormalities. Although typical of DIP, these appearances are nonspecific but denote a high likelihood of reversible inflammatory disease.

Desquamative interstitial pneumonia

The cardinal histological feature is diffuse accumulation of alveolar macrophages in airspaces in a uniform pattern, variably associated with minor interstitial inflammation and fibrosis (Fig. 18.11.1.1). DIP is almost exclusively found in smokers and is now a rare disorder. Typical high-resolution CT appearances comprise patchy ground-glass attenuation which is often extensive (Fig. 18.11.1.2). The disease presents with the features of the CFA clinical syndrome but, unlike IPF and NSIP, a response to corticosteroids is usual (although not invariable) and the treated outcome is usually good.

Respiratory bronchiolitis–interstitial lung disease

As in DIP, the histological features of RBILD are dominated by the presence of pigmented macrophages, but unlike DIP these accumulate in the air spaces around the bronchioles (respiratory bronchiolitis) (Fig. 18.11.1.3), often with associated peribronchiolar interstitial inflammation and fibrosis. The most frequent high-resolution CT findings are bronchial wall thickening, poorly defined centrilobular nodules, and patchy ground-glass attenuation. RBILD is found only in current or former smokers, and in many patients there is overlap in histological features between RBILD and DIP. The histological appearances in RBILD are identical to those of asymptomatic respiratory bronchiolitis, which is always present in current smokers. The distinction between RBILD and respiratory bronchiolitis is based upon disease severity, as defined by symptoms, the severity of lung function impairment, and the extent of disease on high-resolution CT. RBILD is diagnosed when a clinically significant diffuse lung disease is considered to be present. The disorder usually has a good outcome and often regresses with

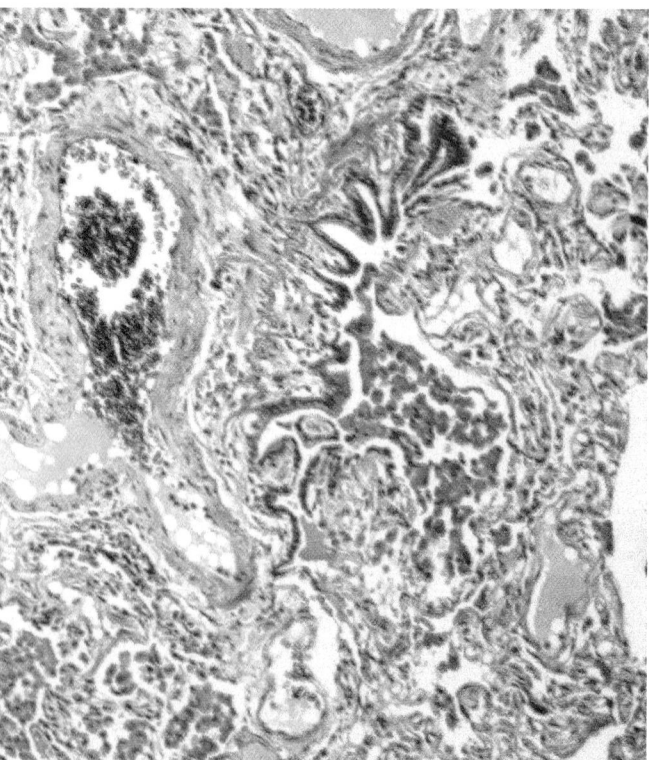

Fig. 18.11.1.3 Biopsy from a patient with respiratory bronchiolitis-associated interstitial lung disease showing macrophages with similar histological appearances to those of desquamative interstitial pneumonia (see Fig. 18.11.1.1), but the aggregation is centred on bronchioles where there is also a mild chronic inflammatory cell infiltrate within the airway walls.

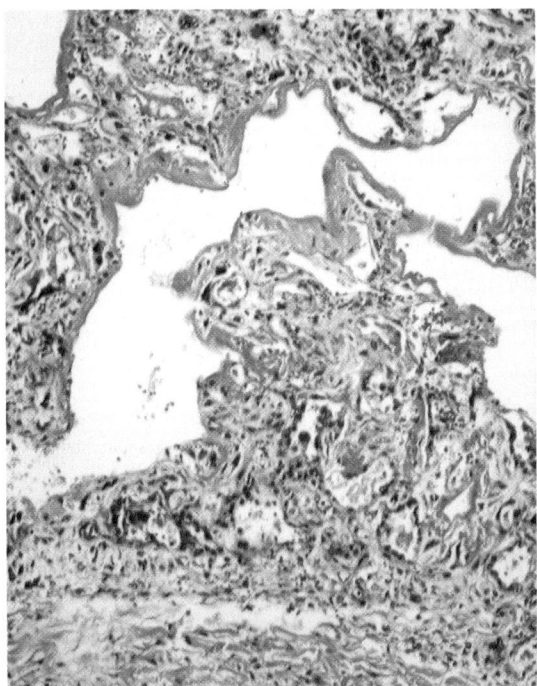

Fig. 18.11.1.4 A case of acute interstitial pneumonia (AIP) showing the exudative phase of diffuse alveolar damage with hyaline membranes lining alveolar walls, indicating AIP when present in an idiopathic setting.

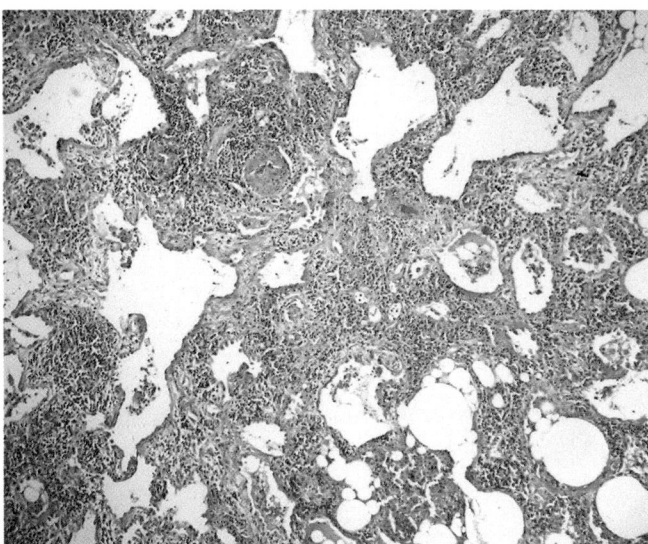

Fig. 18.11.1.5 A case of lymphoid interstitial pneumonia (LIP) showing dense interstitial chronic inflammation diffusely involving the alveolar parenchyma, in this case associated with minimal interstitial fibrosis.

smoking cessation, but (on the basis of limited data) corticosteroid therapy is seldom efficacious.

Acute interstitial pneumonia

Diffuse alveolar damage is rare but seen in the adult respiratory distress syndrome and in acute interstitial pneumonia (AIP, commonly viewed as idiopathic adult respiratory distress syndrome, ARDS). Diffuse alveolar damage is characterized by hyaline membranes lining damaged alveoli (Fig. 18.11.1.4) and buds of organization in the alveoli of those acini that have been damaged and are undergoing the healing process. There is widespread ground-glass consolidation, often with traction bronchiectasis, and dependent consolidation on high-resolution CT. AIP probably equates to the Hamman–Rich syndrome and is fatal in 80 to 90% of cases. Although high-dose corticosteroid therapy and immunosuppressive agents are commonly given, there is no evidence that treatment influences outcome in most cases.

Lymphocytic interstitial pneumonia

The histopathological pattern of LIP is most commonly found in patients with rheumatological disease and in immunodeficiency syndromes, but can also occur as an idiopathic disorder. The histological findings consist of diffuse interstitial lymphocytic infiltration (Fig. 18.11.1.5), variably associated with follicular bronchiolitis. The high-resolution CT features consist of patchy and sometimes extensive ground-glass attenuation with a variable nodular component. Corticosteroid and immunosuppressive therapy is effective in over 50% of cases.

Nonspecific interstitial pneumonia

NSIP is the least satisfactory entity amongst the idiopathic interstitial pneumonias. Histologically, there is variable interstitial inflammation

and fibrosis but, unlike UIP—the pattern with which it is most likely to be confused—disease is uniform throughout biopsy specimens, both in severity and in the age of fibrosis (Fig. 18.11.1.6). Fibroblastic foci, the cardinal finding in UIP, are absent or sparse. The radiological and clinical manifestations of NSIP are diverse. In a few cases inflammation predominates and the treated outcome is uniformly good, but in most patients with fibrotic NSIP, fibrosis is as at least as prominent as inflammation. Certain clinico-radiological profiles are increasingly recognized in NSIP. Most commonly patients present with the CFA clinical syndrome, the basal distribution of disease on high-resolution CT is similar to that of IPF, but unlike IPF there is prominent ground-glass attenuation and no

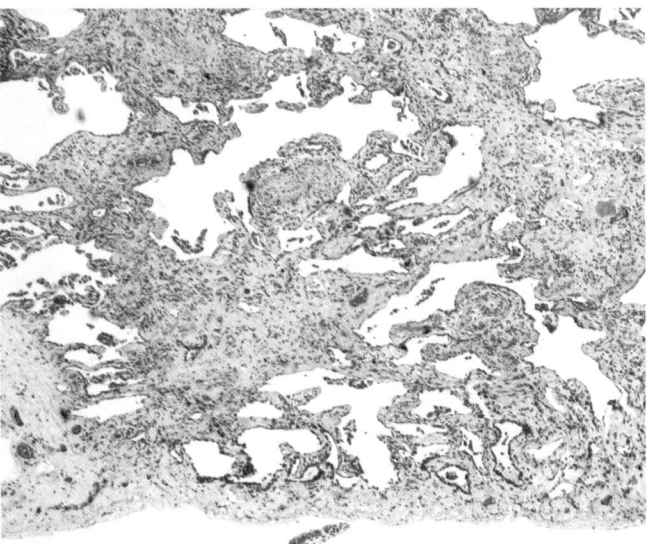

Fig. 18.11.1.6 A case of fibrotic nonspecific interstitial pneumonia showing established interstitial fibrosis with a moderate degree of associated chronic inflammation. In areas of affected lung the features appear homogeneous and diffuse, unlike appearances in usual interstitial pneumonia (see Chapter 18.11.2), and fibroblastic foci are not present.

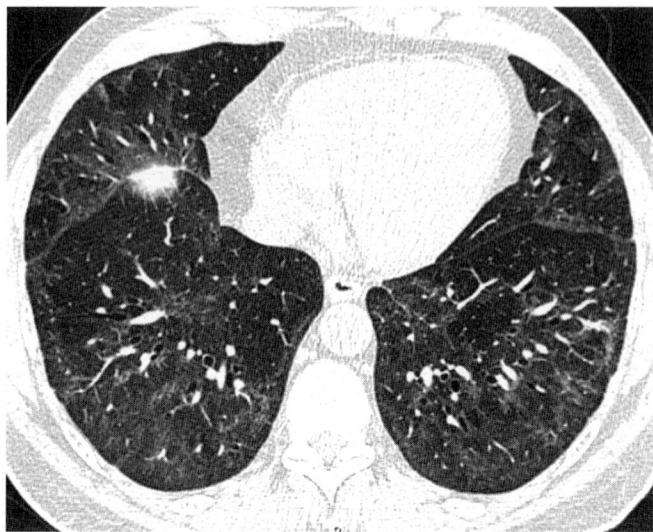

Fig. 18.11.1.7 High-resolution CT appearances of the lower lung zone in a patient with biopsy-proven fibrotic nonspecific interstitial pneumonia. There is widespread ground-glass attenuation with mild traction bronchiectasis and, in some regions, a subtle admixed reticular element, resulting in a sense of increased texture within abnormal lung.

honeycombing (Fig. 18.11.1.7). A similar profile is typically present in pulmonary fibrosis associated with systemic sclerosis. In a second large subgroup, predominating in reports from South Korea and Japan, the clinical and radiological features resemble organizing pneumonia with fibrosis and there is a prominent lymphocytosis on bronchoalveolar lavage. Another group of patients are likely to have a form of hypersensitivity pneumonitis, based upon exposure histories and high-resolution CT features, despite the absence of granulomas in biopsy tissue. Corticosteroid and immunsosuppressive therapy are often effective in producing regression or stabilization of disease, but in a few cases, largely confined to those presenting with the CFA clinical syndrome, there is inexorable progression to a fatal outcome despite treatment.

Diagnostic approach

Diagnosis is complicated by the large number of disorders grouped within the diffuse parenchymal lung diseases. A systematic diagnostic algorithm, based upon careful clinical evaluation and a logical sequence of tests, is essential. This approach can be broken down into in two phases, as shown in Box 18.11.1.3.

Clinical history

In most patients, the presentation is insidious dyspnoea, variably accompanied by cough which is usually nonproductive. The duration of dyspnoea is diagnostically important: an acute presentation narrows the differential diagnosis considerably (see Box 18.11.1.2).

Wheeze is a useful discriminatory symptom, as the presence of an airway-centred component informs the differential diagnosis. Disorders with variable but sometimes prominent wheeze include extrinsic allergic alveolitis, sarcoidosis, lymphangioleiomyomatosis, and Langerhans' cell histiocytosis. Other less frequent respiratory symptoms are also diagnostically useful. Pleuritic chest discomfort often occurs in the rheumatological diseases and occasionally in drug-induced disease, but never in idiopathic pulmonary fibrosis or extrinsic allergic alveolitis. Haemoptysis, which may be trivial

---

> **Box 18.11.1.3** Diagnostic algorithm for diffuse parenchymal lung diseases
>
> **Phase 1**
> 1 Clinical history
> 2 Clinical examination
> 3 Chest radiography
> 4 Pulmonary function tests
> 5 Selective blood tests
>
> **Phase 2**
> 1 High resolution CT
> 2 bronchoalveolar lavage
> 3 Lung biopsy

even when haemorrhage is severe, may be indicative of diffuse alveolar haemorrhage due to capillaritis, occurring in a number of disorders. A history of pneumothorax should prompt suspicion of cystic lung disease, especially Langerhans' cell histiocytosis and lymphangioleiomyomatosis.

The patient's previous medical history may provide crucial information, including diagnoses of rheumatological disease or other relevant systemic diseases (including vasculitis). Even when no previous systemic diagnosis has been made, the nature of preceding systemic symptoms may point strongly to a hitherto undiagnosed rheumatological disorder. Knowledge of underlying cardiac and malignant disease is also essential as cardiac failure and disseminated malignancy may both simulate diffuse parenchymal lung disease, clinically and radiologically. A detailed list of medications serves to alert the clinician to the possibility of drug-induced lung disease. The agents most frequently responsible include nitrofurantoin, methotrexate and bleomycin, but a long list of other drugs occasionally cause lung disease. The comprehensive website http://pneumotox.com provides a rapid and fruitful means of checking possible pulmonary toxicities.

The occupational history should include all occupations from leaving school onwards: diseases caused by some exposures (including asbestos exposure) manifest decades later. Environmental conditions in which pneumoconioses most commonly arise include sawing, grinding, and drilling. Hypersensitivity pneumonitis arises from the inhalation of organic dusts including fungal contaminates of hay (as in farmer's lung) and avian proteins found on the bloom and in the excreta of domestic birds. Many other organic antigens can give rise to hypersensitivity pneumonitis, with over 200 causes now recognized.

Other relevant historical information includes foreign travel, which may raise the possibility of parasitic infection as an explanation of pulmonary eosinophilia. A history of cigarette smoking identifies a predisposition to Langerhans' cell histiocytosis, DIP, and RBILD, and is also a risk factor for exacerbations of pulmonary vasculitis. Paradoxically, smoking appears to protect against the development of sarcoidosis and hypersensitivity pneumonitis.

Clinical examination

Digital clubbing is common in IPF and NSIP, not infrequent in hypersensitivity pneumonitis, but unusual in the other diffuse parenchymal lung diseases. Predominantly basal fine end-inspiratory crackles are a cardinal feature of the CFA clinical syndrome, are expected in IPF, and variably present in the other idiopathic interstitial pneumonias. Sporadic crackles are heard in many diffuse parenchymal lung diseases, but are seldom present in sarcoidosis. Expiratory wheeze is indicative of airway disease. Inspiratory squawks are strongly predictive of hypersensitivity pneumonitis or obliterative bronchiolitis. In advanced disease, clinical evidence of secondary pulmonary hypertension should be sought, as oxygen supplementation may have a pivotal role in management.

Relevant systemic findings include ocular disease (in sarcoidosis or vasculitis), skin disease (in sarcoidosis or rheumatological disease), musculoskeletal signs (in rheumatological disease), and neurological abnormalities (mononeuritis multiplex in sarcoidosisis, rheumatological disease and vasculitis; a wide variety of central and peripheral signs in sarcoidosis).

Chest radiography

Chest radiography was formerly a central part of the diagnostic evaluation of diffuse parenchymal lung disease. Although high-resolution CT has now supplanted chest radiography in routine diagnosis, the chest radiograph continues to provide useful information.

Radiographic findings suggestive of pulmonary fibrosis are a required feature of the CFA clinical syndrome. Patients with fibrosing lung diseases tend have reduced lung volumes. If other clinical features are indicative of IPF, normal-sized or large lungs on chest radiography are suggestive of the coexistence of emphysema and pulmonary fibrosis, a frequent association in cigarette smokers with IPF. Large or normal-sized lungs on chest radiography, in association with nodular or reticular shadowing, also occur in Langerhans' cell histiocytosis, lymphangioleiomyomatosis (a disorder involving smooth muscle proliferation arising in premenopausal women), and the closely related disorder tuberous sclerosis. Idiopathic bronchiectasis or cystic fibrosis, with increased radiographic volumes due to hyperinflation, can also be mistaken radiologically for diffuse parenchymal lung disease, although the clinical profile of chronic purulent sputum production is usually discriminatory.

The distribution of disease is often helpful. Primary fibrosing disorders, including IPF, fibrotic NSIP, pulmonary fibrosis in rheumatological disease, and asbestosis, produce predominantly basal reticular or reticulonodular abnormalities, which may also be overtly peripheral when disease is not advanced. By contrast, granulomatous disorders, including sarcoidosis and hypersensitivity pneumonitis (as well as tuberculosis and allergic bronchopulmonary asbestosis) most often have a predominantly upper and mid zone distribution. In the correct clinical setting, chest radiographic findings typical of sarcoidosis (predominantly upper zone fibrotic change, variably associated with lymphadenopathy and hilar retraction towards the apices) often suffice for a confident diagnosis.

The size and shape of abnormalities is sometimes diagnostically useful, although this aspect of radiological evaluation has largely been supplanted by high-resolution CT. Shadows of more than 5 mm in diameter are often present in Wegener's granulomatosis, lymphoma, and other malignancies. Cavitating nodules are a frequent feature in Wegener's granulomatosis, but necrotizing carcinomas and multiple staphylococcal abscesses should also be considered. The presence of nodules of differing size and shape is strongly suggestive of metastatic malignancy. An alveolar filling

pattern, consisting of widespread confluent shadowing, usually denotes the presence of life-threatening disease. The differential diagnosis includes pulmonary oedema (due to left ventricular failure or mitral stenosis), diffuse alveolar haemorrhage, uraemia, drug-induced lung disease (and other forms of diffuse alveolar damage), infection (especially opportunistic infection in immunosuppressed patients), and alveolar proteinosis. When widespread confluent shadowing is chronic, alveolar cell carcinoma, lymphoma, and pulmonary eosinophilia should also be considered.

Inspection of previous chest radiographs is often highly revealing, especially in the patient presenting with multifocal consolidation. Waxing and waning of consolidation effectively excludes malignant disease and is strongly suggestive of immunologically mediated disorders, including cryptogenic organizing pneumonia, vasculitis, and pulmonary eosinophilia. Fixed consolidation may occur in all of these disorders but should also prompt suspicion of lymphoma, alveolar cell carcinoma and chronic infection.

Pleural thickening, with or without effusion, occurs commonly in rheumatological disease, rheumatoid arthritis, and systemic lupus erythematosus. Pleural abnormalities also occur commonly in asbestosis, Churg–Strauss syndrome, and Wegener's granulomatosis. The presence of pleural disease should always prompt consideration of a second disease process, including malignancy, heart failure, tuberculosis, pulmonary embolism, and drug-induced lung disease. Pleural involvement is not a feature of uncomplicated hypersensitivity pneumonitis or IPF and is seldom present in the other idiopathic interstitial pneumonias, although occasionally encountered in sarcoidosis and cryptogenic organizing pneumonia.

Symmetrical hilar lymphadenopathy is usually indicative of sarcoidosis, but tuberculosis, lymphoma, and other malignancies should always be considered, especially if the changes are unilateral. Lymphadenopathy is seldom visible on chest radiography in other diffuse lung diseases, with the exception of silicosis. Hilar calcification occurs in sarcoidosis, silicosis, and tuberculosis.

Pulmonary function testing

In most patients with diffuse parenchymal lung disease, there is a restrictive ventilatory defect with reduced gas transfer ($D_L$co). Arterial oxygen tensions (Pao_2) are normal or mildly reduced until disease is advanced, although the alveolar-arterial oxygen gradient is often widened in associated with $Paco_2$ levels that are at the lower end of the normal range. In early disease, maximal exercise testing may unmask abnormalities or, when normal, may reassure the clinician that the disease is not clinically significant. In IPF, maximal exercise testing typically leads to a fall in the Pao_2 and widening of the alveolar–arterial oxygen gradient (A–a gradient), reflecting ventilation–perfusion mismatch and, at maximal exercise, impairment of diffusion. The anatomical dead space to tidal volume ratio (V_D/V_T) normal falls on exercise in the healthy individual but is unchanged or increases in restrictive lung disease. Striking rises in the V_D/V_T ratio are strongly suggestive of disproportionate pulmonary vascular limitation.

A mixed (restrictive–obstructive) ventilatory defect is seen in disorders in which airway involvement is associated with diffuse parenchymal lung disease. This ventilatory pattern most commonly occurs in hypersensitivity pneumonitis, sarcoidosis, and rheumatological disorders. The coexistence of pulmonary fibrosis and emphysema, usually found in cigarette smokers with IPF or fibrotic NSIP, may also give rise to a mixed ventilatory defect, but more commonly there is spurious preservation of lung volumes and a disproportionate reduction in $D_L$co.

Blood tests

Routine haematological and biochemical tests have little discriminatory value in the diffuse lung diseases. A peripheral blood eosinophilia ($>1.5 \times 10^9$/litre) is a prerequisite for diagnosis of Churg–Strauss vasculitis and may also be indicative of pulmonary eosinophilia (although not always present in that disorder). An increased level of serum angiotensin converting enzyme (ACE) is a helpful ancillary diagnostic finding in some patients with sarcoidosis and may also confirm ongoing disease activity. Routine immunoglobulin estimation may disclose hypogammaglobulinaemia in undiagnosed granulomatous disorders, but has no diagnostic value in other diffuse lung disorders.

Autoantibody testing is an essential part of routine evaluation. The presence of a positive antinuclear antibody, with specific extractable nuclear antigen profiles, or rheumatoid factor, may disclose an occult systemic rheumatological condition. The autoantibody profile is sometimes indicative of the likely pattern of pulmonary involvement. In systemic sclerosis the anti-DNA topoisomerase autoantibody is often associated with clinically significant pulmonary fibrosis, whereas the anticentromere antibody is linked to pulmonary vascular disease. Anti-t-RNA synthetase autoantibodies occur when polymyositis is associated with diffuse parenchymal lung disease. Other common associations include anti-Sm in systemic lupus erythematosus, SS-A and SS-B in Sjögren's syndrome, and the anti-RNP autoantibody in mixed connective tissue disease. Mild increases in antinuclear antibody and rheumatoid factor titres are commonly found in IPF and idiopathic fibrotic NSIP but appear to have no clinical significance. Increased antineutrophil cytoplasmic antibodies (ANCA) with a cytoplasmic pattern are strongly suggestive of Wegener's granulomatosis or microscopic polyangiitis: the perinuclear (P-ANCA) pattern is less discriminatory.

The presence of specific precipitins to organic antigens is often diagnostically useful in hypersensitivity pneumonitis. However, positive precipitins are not diagnostic in isolation, confirming only the presence of immunological recognition. Avian precipitins, for example, are often present in healthy pigeon breeders. Moreover, the absence of precipitins does not exclude a diagnosis of hypersensitivity pneumonitis: avian proteins causing disease in an individual may be species specific or even specific to a single bird.

High-resolution CT

High-resolution CT provides a three-dimensional anatomical reconstruction of both lungs, with careful evaluation of the distribution and pattern of disease resulting in improved diagnostic accuracy compared to chest radiography. A number of high-resolution CT patterns can now be viewed as pathognomonic of particular diseases (Box 18.11.1.4), and high-resolution CT is often diagnostic in other patients when the findings are integrated with clinical information. A detailed review of the rapidly enlarging high-resolution CT literature lies beyond the scope of this chapter and the reader is referred to sources listed in the 'Further reading' section.

High-resolution CT is much more sensitive than chest radiography, leading to the earlier diagnosis of limited disease. While this is sometimes highly advantageous, the sensitivity of high-resolution CT can cause problems. The detection of limited abnormalities in

> **Box 18.11.1.4** Diffuse parenchymal lung disease with characteristic high-resolution CT features
>
> - Cryptogenic fibrosing alveolitis
> - Extrinsic allergic alveolitis
> - Sarcoidosis
> - Langerhans' cell histiocytosis
> - Lymphangioleiomyomatosis
> - Alveolar proteinosis

cigarette smokers, or when high-resolution CT is used as a screening tool in rheumatological disorders, sometimes leads to difficulty in assigning clinical significance to the findings. In this context pulmonary function tests have a pivotal role, but they are sometimes difficult to interpret when functional impairment is minor, due to the wide normal range: an FVC 75% of predicted can equally represent a minor fall or a major reduction from premorbid values of 80% and 120% of predicted, respectively. Absence of oxygen desaturation on maximal exercise testing is especially helpful in this scenario in excluding clinically significant disease.

A simple high-resolution CT diagnostic algorithm can be usefully be applied to apparently idiopathic diffuse lung disease. Confirmation of fibrosing disease is readily demonstrated by the presence of reticular abnormalities, anatomical distortion or, when ground-glass attenuation predominates, traction bronchiectasis. The essential preliminary question is whether high-resolution CT appearances are typical of IPF (i.e. predominantly basal reticular abnormalities, with or without honeycombing, with little ground-glass attenuation). If not, it is appropriate to look for the high-resolution CT features of fibrotic NSIP, sarcoidosis, hypersensitivity pneumonitis, and organizing pneumonia with fibrosis, disorders which—along with IPF—account for up to 95% of diagnoses in apparently idiopathic disease. When high-resolution CT appearances are not typical of one of these disorders and disease is progressive, IPF with atypical high-resolution CT features is the most frequent diagnosis made at surgical biopsy.

High-resolution CT imaging has a number of other advantages. Even when the high-resolution CT diagnosis is uncertain, signs of fibrosis often make it clear that disease is irreversible. The identification of reversible disease is less straightforward. Prominent ground-glass attenuation often denotes inflammation, but only when there is no admixed reticular pattern or traction bronchiectasis. High-resolution CT is also invaluable in allowing the thoracic surgeon to select optimal sites for biopsy, by which means the full range of morphological abnormalities and disease severity can be sampled. Serial high-resolution CT is sometimes useful in monitoring changes in disease severity, especially when pulmonary function trends are inconclusive, although it should be used for this purpose only in order to cast light on clinically important questions and not performed rigidly by protocol.

Finally, high-resolution CT is often revealing when disease processes are admixed. In rheumatological disorders and in smoking-related disease, patterns of functional impairment are often complex and an assessment of the extent of interstitial disease allows a better understanding of the presence and likely functional impact of emphysema and airway disease. The complications of diffuse lung disease are often disclosed by high-resolution CT. Lung malignancy is increased in prevalence in fibrosing lung disease but can sometimes be difficult to detect on chest radiography when interstitial fibrosis is extensive. Infection is also sometimes masked by extensive disease, and this applies especially to aspergillomas which tend to develop in fibrobullous sarcoidosis.

Bronchoalveolar lavage (BAL)

When first employed, it was hoped that BAL might replace diagnostic surgical biopsy or provide accurate prognostic information, and that serial BAL might disclose important changes in disease activity. These expectations were eventually shown to be baseless and the role of BAL has now been downgraded. However, BAL has an ancillary diagnostic role in diffuse lung diseases and is also sometimes helpful in excluding infection. Granulomatous and drug-induced lung diseases are characterized by an excess of lymphocytes with or without granulocytes. The presence of a BAL lymphocytosis is occasionally pivotal in alerting the clinician to the possibility that a fibrosing process may be due to hypersensitivity pneumonitis or sarcoidosis. BAL can also be diagnostic in some rare lung disorders, including alveolar proteinosis (milky effluent; PAS-positive material), Langerhans' cell histiocytosis (increased numbers of Langerhans' cells identified by CD1a staining), alveolar haemorrhage (iron-laden macrophages) and hard metal lung disease (bizarre multinuclear giant cells). By contrast, a BAL neutrophilia is an expected finding when pulmonary fibrosis is moderately extensive and has little diagnostic value. It appears increasing likely, based on recent data, that the observed linkage between disease progression and a BAL neutrophilia in rheumatological disease reflects the presence of more severe disease, which is itself more likely to progress.

BAL is an essential part of the diagnostic algorithm in patients presenting acutely with widespread interstitial abnormalities. Diffuse alveolar haemorrhage does not always manifest with haemoptysis but is readily disclosed by BAL. In patients receiving immunosuppressive drugs, increased treatment may be urgently required in the hope of reversing disease progression, but acute decompensation due to opportunistic infection can be confidently excluded only with BAL.

Lung biopsy

Assessment of a surgical biopsy offers the important advantage that further investigation is unlikely to clarify the situation and a final diagnosis must now be made, integrating all clinical, radiological, and histological information. A confident diagnosis leads to more confident management, with a more accurate evaluation of the balance of risk and benefit with suggested treatments. Clinicians are better able to inform the patient of the likely natural history and treated course of disease. However, in many patients a firm diagnosis can be made from clinical and high-resolution CT data such that a surgical biopsy is redundant, and in other cases a biopsy is contraindicated by the severity of disease, major comorbidity, or the wishes of the patient.

Transbronchial biopsies are used to diagnose some airway-centred disorders. In sarcoidosis and lymphangitis carcinomatosis the histological appearances are sufficiently characteristic to allow a confident diagnosis to be made from very small biopsy specimens. However, for most diffuse lung diseases, including the idiopathic interstitial pneumonias, the overall pattern of disease

cannot be meaningfully evaluated without a larger surgical biopsy. The acquisition of biopsies from more than one lobar site increases the likelihood of obtaining representative tissue. The limited thoracotomy approach used historically has now been largely supplanted by video-assisted thoracoscopic surgical procedures, which are less invasive, provide equivalently sized samples, and are associated with less morbidity.

The morbidity and mortality associated with diagnostic surgical biopsy are low provided that pulmonary reserve is adequate. However, postoperative mortality increases significantly when disease is extensive and approached 15% in one IPF series in which the average level of functional impairment were severe. Thus, if the $D_L$co level is less than 30% of predicted, a surgical biopsy should be performed only if considered indispensable. The histological diagnosis is, in any case, less prognostically useful in advanced disease. Mortality is very similar in IPF and fibrotic NSIP when $D_L$co levels are less than 35%, despite striking differences in survival when disease is less severe.

Key clinical issues

Integrated diagnosis

Although a surgical biopsy was once viewed as definitive in diffuse parenchymal lung disease, it is now widely accepted that all clinical, radiological, and histopathological data must be integrated into the final diagnosis. The limitations of a purely histological diagnosis are now better understood. 'Sampling error' consists of the acquisition of nonrepresentative tissue, e.g. in some patients with IPF there are lung regions with the histological appearances of fibrotic NSIP, but this finding has no prognostic significance. Sampling error can be minimized by ensuring that large samples are taken, by sampling more than one site, and by selecting the sites of biopsy to sample the full range of disease morphology and severity based on high-resolution CT appearances. However, diagnostic variation between pathologists remains problematic, with less agreement than documented with many clinically useful tests. Moreover, in some cases there is 'appropriate' interobserver variation, reflecting the fact that histological appearances occasionally lie intermediate between classical entities. To complicate matters further, the diagnostic significance of a histological pattern is critically dependent upon the clinical context. For example, UIP is the required histological pattern in IPF but has a better outcome when occurring in patients with rheumatological disorders, drug-induced lung disease, or hypersensitivity pneumonitis.

The 'gold standard' for diagnosis of diffuse parenchymal lung disease is now a multidisciplinary diagnosis, with participation by clinicians, radiologists, and—when applicable—histopatholologists. As a useful rule of thumb, in nonbiopsied cases the clinical and high-resolution CT evaluation is, on average, equally influential, and careful clinical assessment should not be curtailed because of the ready availability of high-resolution CT. In patients undergoing surgical biopsy, clinical and high-resolution CT findings are usually inconclusive and the histological features tend to carry the most diagnostic weight. However, it is accepted that the final diagnosis will differ from the histological diagnosis in a few patients when all available information is integrated.

Principles of management

The chronic diffuse parenchymal lung diseases can be broadly subclassified into five patterns of longitudinal disease behaviour, based upon cause, severity, the relative degree of inflammation and fibrosis, and observed change in the short term. Each clinical pattern is associated with a separate approach to management.

The schema below is proposed to capture key thought processes and to serve as a rationale for treatment and monitoring decisions. The idiopathic interstitial pneumonias can each be broadly assigned to one clinical pattern or another. In many cases the pattern of disease behaviour is evident at presentation, but in other instances careful short-term observation is highly informative.

1 Self-limited inflammation

This is usually caused by an extrinsic agent (as in drug-induced disease, hypersensitivity penumonitis, and RBILD), but may also be idiopathic as in a subset of patients with sarcoidosis. Disease usually responds to withdrawal of an offending agent, therapy is often unnecessary, and monitoring consists of confirming that disease has regressed.

2 Stable fibrotic disease

This is most commonly encountered in sarcoidosis, following drug-induced lung disease, and in patients with formerly active rheumatological disorders. Treatment is not required but monitoring is needed to ensure that disease is truly stable, usually with serial pulmonary function tests until a long-term 'track record' of disease stability has been established.

3 Major inflammation, with or without supervening fibrosis

This is often a feature of drug-induced lung disease, and this category also applies to some patients with cryptogenic organizing pneumonia, DIP, hypersensitivity pneumonitis, sarcoidosis, and aggressive inflammatory disease in rheumatological disease. High-dose therapy is usual, often with corticosteroids, and the short term response is quantified, often at 4 to 6 weeks. Once inflammation is controlled and the residual level of functional impairment has been quantified, treatment is gradually reduced with monitoring centred around serial pulmonary function tests, usually at 3- to 4-monthly intervals. In this way, the minimum dose of immunosuppression required to maintain control of disease is established.

4 Slowly progressive fibrotic disease, in which stabilization is a realistic goal

This is frequently seen in sarcoidosis, hypersensitivity pneumonitis, rheumatological conditions, and in many patients with fibrotic NSIP. In this scenario long-term therapy is often required, and long-term monitoring with serial pulmonary function tests—often at increasing time intervals—is needed to ensure that stabilization has been achieved and maintained. Aggressive initial treatment is usually warranted to ensure optimal control of disease activity.

5 Inexorably progressive fibrotic disease

This is the hallmark of IPF, but an IPF-like course is sometimes observed in idiopathic fibrotic NSIP, rheumatological disease, and in a small subset of patients with chronic hypersensitivity pneumonitis. Long term treatment may slow disease progression, as suggested by a recent trial of anti-oxidant therapy in IPF. However, in known IPF, initial high-dose therapy achieves nothing and may cause unnecessary drug toxicity. The early realization that fibrotic disease is relentlessly progressive, either because IPF is diagnosed or because disease continues to progress despite treatment, is especially important when lung transplantation is realistic. Monitoring is performed to quantify disease progression, usually at three to four monthly intervals.

When should a surgical biopsy be performed?

A broad classification of disease behaviour also serves as a rationalization of when to recommend diagnostic surgical biopsy. This is usually warranted, disease severity and comorbidity permitting, when the underlying diagnosis is uncertain and the clinician is unable to assign likely disease behaviour such that management is difficult. However, if the diagnosis is uncertain but the pattern of disease behaviour is already clear, a diagnostic biopsy is much less likely to inform management. For example, when it is already known from previous investigations that fibrotic abnormalities are long-standing and wholly stable, a histological diagnosis is unlikely to change management.

When considering whether or not to recommend biopsy, it is useful to construct scenarios in which long-term management may differ significantly depending upon histological findings. It is important to reach an early decision. The empirical approach of initiating treatment, with recourse to biopsy if the response is unsatisfactory, has serious flaws. Modification of the histological appearances by treatment may make diagnosis more difficult and, more importantly, deterioration during the interim period may make the biopsy more hazardous, as well as increasing the likelihood of side effects to treatment, including postoperative infection and impaired wound healing. Thus, if biopsy is to be performed, the best time is shortly after presentation before treatment is instituted.

Further reading

ATS/ERS (2000). International consensus statement. Idiopathic pulmonary fibrosis: diagnosis and treatment. *Am J Respir Crit Care Med*, **161**, 646–64.

ATS/ERS (2002). International multidisciplinary consensus classification of the idiopathic interstitial pneumonias. *Am J Respir Crit Care Med*, **165**, 277–304.

BAL Co-operative Group Steering Committee (1990). Bronchoalveolar lavage constituents in healthy individuals, idiopathic pulmonary fibrosis, and selected comparison groups. *Am Rev Respir Dis*, **141**, S169–202.

Bjoraker JA, *et al.* (1998). Prognostic significance of histopathologic subsets in idiopathic pulmonary fibrosis. *Am J Respir Crit Care Med*, **157**, 199–203.

Desai SR, Wells AU (2007). Imaging. In: Costabel U, du Bois RM, Egan JJ (eds) *Diffuse parenchymal lung disease*, pp. 29–43. Karger, Basel.

Flaherty KR, *et al.* (2004). Idiopathic interstitial pneumonia. What is the effect of a multi-disciplinary approach to diagnosis? *Am J Respir Crit Care Med*, **170**, 904–10.

Flaherty KR, *et al.* (2001). Histologic variability in usual and nonspecific interstitial pneumonias. *Am J Respir Crit Care Med*, **164**, 1722–7.

Katzenstein AL, Myers JL (1998). Idiopathic pulmonary fibrosis: clinical relevance of pathologic classification. *Am J Respir Crit Care Med*, **157**, 1301–15.

Liebow AA (1975). Definition and classification of interstitial pneumonias in human pathology. In: Basset F, Georges R (eds) *Progress in respiration research*, pp. 1–33. Karger, New York.

Muller NL, Colby TV (1997). Idiopathic interstitial pneumonias: high-resolution CT and histologic findings. *Radiographics*, **17**, 1016–22.

Nicholson AG, *et al.* (2004). Inter-observer variation between pathologists in diffuse parenchymal lung disease. *Thorax*, **59**, 500–5.

Nicholson AG, *et al.* (2000). The prognostic significance of the histologic pattern of interstitial pneumonia in patients presenting with the clinical entity of cryptogenic fibrosing alveolitis. *Am J Respir Crit Care Med*, **162**, 2213–17.

Wells AU (2003). High resolution computed tomography in the diagnosis of diffuse lung disease: a clinical perspective. *Semin Respir Crit Care Med*, **24**, 347–56.

Wells AU (2004). Histopathologic diagnosis in diffuse lung disease: an ailing gold standard. *Am J Respir Crit Care Med*, **170**, 828–9.

Wells AU, Hansell DM, Nicholson AG (2007). What is this thing called CFA? *Thorax*, **62**, 3–4.

Website

Pneumotox On Line. *The Drug-Induced Lung Diseases*. http://pneumotox.com/

18.11.2 Idiopathic pulmonary fibrosis

A.U. Wells, A.G. Nicholson, and N. Hirani

Essentials

The synonymous terms idiopathic pulmonary fibrosis (IPF) and cryptogenic fibrosing alveolitis (CFA) refer to a relentlessly progressive fibrotic lung disorder that is the underlying diagnosis in over one-half of patients presenting with typical clinical features of the 'CFA clinical syndrome' (see Chapter 18.11.1). Incidence is about 10 to 15 per 100 000, men are more often affected than women, and it most commonly presents in the seventh and eighth decades. Aetiology remains uncertain.

Clinical features—typical presentation is with progressive exertional dyspnoea, without wheeze, and a nonproductive cough. Digital clubbing is present in over 50% of patients. Very fine end-inspiratory crackles are usually heard bilaterally at the lung bases and become widespread in advanced disease. Central cyanosis and clinical evidence of pulmonary hypertension are late features.

Diagnosis—this requires a surgical biopsy revealing a usual interstitial pneumonia (UIP) histological pattern in association with (1) the absence of other known causes of interstitial lung disease, (2) a restrictive lung function profile, and (3) compatible features on chest radiography or high-resolution CT scans. Diagnosis in the absence of a surgical biopsy requires (1) the absence of other known causes of interstitial lung disease, (2) a restrictive lung function profile, (3) high-resolution CT appearances of predominantly basal reticular abnormalities with honeycombing and little or no ground-glass attenuation, and (4) no features of an alternative diagnosis in transbronchial lung biopsy or bronchoalveolar lavage; together with at least three of the following: (a) age over 50 years, (b) insidious unexplained exertional dyspnoea, (c) duration of illness exceeds 3 months, and (d) predominantly basal or widespread crackles on auscultation of the chest.

Differential diagnosis—the distinction between IPF and fibrotic nonspecific interstitial pneumonia (NSIP) (discussed in Chapter 18.11.1) poses particular difficulty and is crucial because of their very different prognoses: the 5-year survival is 10 to 15% in IPF compared to over 60% in fibrotic NSIP.

Management—in definite IPF there is little evidence that traditional treatment regimens have a major impact on outcome. The use of antioxidant (*N*-acetylcysteine) and low-dose steroid therapy (prednisolone 10 mg/day), with or without an immunosuppressive agent (azathioprine), appears reasonable and is the therapeutic approach preferred by the authors, and the routine use of such a regimen can be justified when a diagnosis of fibrotic NSIP is possible. In 10 to 15% of patients with IPF there is an accelerated deterioration over several weeks that often leads rapidly to a fatal outcome: intravenous high-dose corticosteroids together with intravenous cyclophosphamide are often used in this circumstance.

Introduction

The disorder previously known as fibrosing alveolitis, first described in 1907, was increasingly recognized following the description of a small group of patients with rapidly progressive fatal disease, grouped as the Hamman–Rich syndrome. Until late in the 20th century, a stereotypical clinical presentation of idiopathic interstitial lung disease was termed idiopathic pulmonary fibrosis (IPF) or cryptogenic fibrosing alveolitis (CFA), and a number of histological patterns were unified under this term. However, it became increasingly clear that the clinical presentation of IPF/CFA ('CFA clinical syndrome') was shared by a number of diseases, including predominantly inflammatory and predominantly fibrotic disorders, now known collectively as the idiopathic interstitial pneumonias. Their separation is essentially pragmatic, being justified by large differences in treated outcome. The classification proposed by an American Thoracic Society/European Respiratory Society (ATS/ ERS) nomenclature committee is now widely accepted and can be readily applied to routine practice, with increasing recognition of characteristic patterns of disease on high-resolution CT. Histological evaluation is reserved for a minority of patients in whom accurate management cannot be based on clinical and high-resolution CT findings alone. The synonymous terms IPF and CFA now refer to a relentlessly progressive fibrotic disorder, associated with a histological pattern of usual interstitial pneumonia (UIP) or typical high-resolution CT and clinical features in nonbiopsied cases.

The CFA clinical syndrome is discussed in more detail in Chapter 18.11.1. The remainder of this chapter is devoted to IPF. Epidemiological and aetiological data are briefly reviewed and the clinical picture is summarized. Key clinical issues are then discussed, including diagnosis, prognostic evaluation, routine monitoring and treatment.

Epidemiology and aetiology

IPF is the underlying diagnosis in over one-half of patients presenting with typical clinical features of the CFA clinical syndrome, hence the epidemiology is necessarily that of the CFA clinical syndrome as epidemiological studies cannot be confined to younger patients undergoing a surgical biopsy.

The CFA clinical syndrome may develop at any time but most commonly presents in the seventh and eighth decades: in childhood, it has a largely benign outcome and is not associated with UIP. The syndrome has a slight male predilection and exhibits considerable geographical variation. The incidence and prevalence have risen steadily in recent decades, with the incidence now about 10–15 per 100 000, based on evaluation of death certificates and registry studies in the United States of America, the United Kingdom, and elsewhere. A recent study, using case definitions more reliably indicative of IPF, has suggested an incidence of 5 to 10 per 100 000.

The aetiology remains uncertain, but a single cause appears unlikely, even in patients with biopsy-proven IPF. Case–control studies of the CFA clinical syndrome have consistently identified an association with smoking, although the strength of the association has diminished in recent years as smoking itself has become less prevalent. A number of viruses, including especially the Epstein–Barr virus, have been proposed as trigger factors, but data are contradictory. Occupational exposure to metal dusts and wood fires has also been implicated in controlled evaluations. Thus, it appears that a number of airborne insults may trigger the CFA clinical syndrome, in keeping with the prominent lung epithelial damage observed in IPF in particular and in the idiopathic interstitial pneumonias in general.

Genetic factors have been widely evaluated but remain obscure. In 10% of patients with IPF there is a family history of a pulmonary fibrotic disorder, but although IPF is the most frequent disorder, other idiopathic interstitial pneumonias may develop in family members, suggesting a general predisposition to pulmonary fibrotic disease. Recent data have suggested that smoking and advancing age are the cardinal risk factors for the development of familial disease. The Hermansky–Pudlak syndrome is a rare genetically transmitted pulmonary fibrotic disorder characterized by oculocutaneous albinism and abnormal platelets.

Diagnostic criteria

The diagnostic criteria for IPF, stated by the ATS/ERS nomenclature committee, are now widely accepted.

At surgical biopsy, a usual interstitial pneumonia (UIP) histological pattern is required in association with:

- the absence of other known causes of interstitial lung disease (drug toxicity, occupational or environmental exposures, rheumatological disorders)

- a restrictive lung function profile (reduced vital capacity (VC) often with an increased FEV_1/FVC ratio) or an isolated reduction in the carbon monoxide diffusing capacity ($D_L$co))

- compatible features on chest radiography or high resolution CT

In patients not undergoing a surgical lung biopsy, diagnostic criteria are more rigorous (Box 18.11.2.1).

It should be appreciated that a requirement for bronchoscopy is unrealistic in many elderly patients and in those with advanced disease and major respiratory limitation. In these contexts, a diagnosis of IPF may be made without bronchoscopic support.

Histological features and pathogene sis

In UIP, the histological pattern underlying IPF (Fig. 18.11.2.1), temporal and spatial heterogeneity of disease is the cardinal feature. Normal lung is seen adjacent to regions of fibrosis, with enlarged cystic air-spaces (honeycomb lung) and areas of milder interstitial fibrosis. A patchy chronic inflammatory cell infiltrate is variably present. Subepithelial foci of proliferating fibroblasts ('fibroblastic foci') are a characteristic feature: these occur occasionally and

---

Box 18.11.2.1 IPF: diagnostic criteria

All major criteria and at least three of the four minor criteria are required.

Major criteria

- Absence of other known causes of interstitial lung disease (drug toxicity, occupational or environmental exposures, rheumatological disorders)

- A restrictive lung function profile (reduced vital capacity (VC) often with an increased FEV_1/FVC ratio) or an isolated reduction in the carbon monoxide diffusing capacity ($D_L$co))

- High-resolution CT appearances of predominantly basal reticular abnormalities with honeycombing and little or no ground-glass attenuation

- No features of an alternative diagnosis in transbronchial lung biopsy (granulomas) or bronchoalveolar lavage (an excess of lymphocytes)

Minor criteria

- Age >50 years

- Insidious unexplained exertional dyspnoea

- Duration of illness >3 months

- Predominantly basal or widespread crackles on auscultation of the chest

---

sparsely in nonspecific interstitial pneumonia (NSIP) but are not seen in other idiopathic interstitial pneumonias.

Historically it was believed that inflammation was the key pathogenetic process, preceding and leading to fibrotic disease, but this view has been largely abandoned (although inflammation may be an ancillary pathogenetic feature). Corticosteroid and immunosuppressive therapy, effective in primary inflammatory disorders, has at best a minor beneficial effect in slowing disease progression. There is increasing evidence that IPF has an epithelial fibrotic pathogenesis, with initial epithelial damage leading to the formation of fibroblastic foci and subsequently to more widespread thickening of the connective tissue matrix in advanced disease. Thus, IPF can be conceptualized as a disorder of abnormal wound healing. In established disease, lung injury—an immunological and inflammatory response—and fibrogenesis appear to occur in parallel. It is not known whether a single key mechanism is pivotal in pathogenesis. Oxidant–antioxidant imbalance and the release of damaging enzymes from inflammatory cells appear to amplify injury, but a wide variety of biological mechanisms interact in the lungs of patients with IPF, with up-regulation of tumour necrosis factor α (TNFα) and chemokines (interleukin (IL)-8, and growth factors, especially transforming growth factor β (TGFβ) and connective tissue growth factor), and activation of the coagulation cascade, known to promote fibrogenesis. However, it is not clear whether these mechanisms are primarily pathogenetic or represent physiological responses to some upstream abnormality. The profusion of fibroblastic foci and serum levels of protein markers of epithelial damage have both been linked to mortality and disease progression.

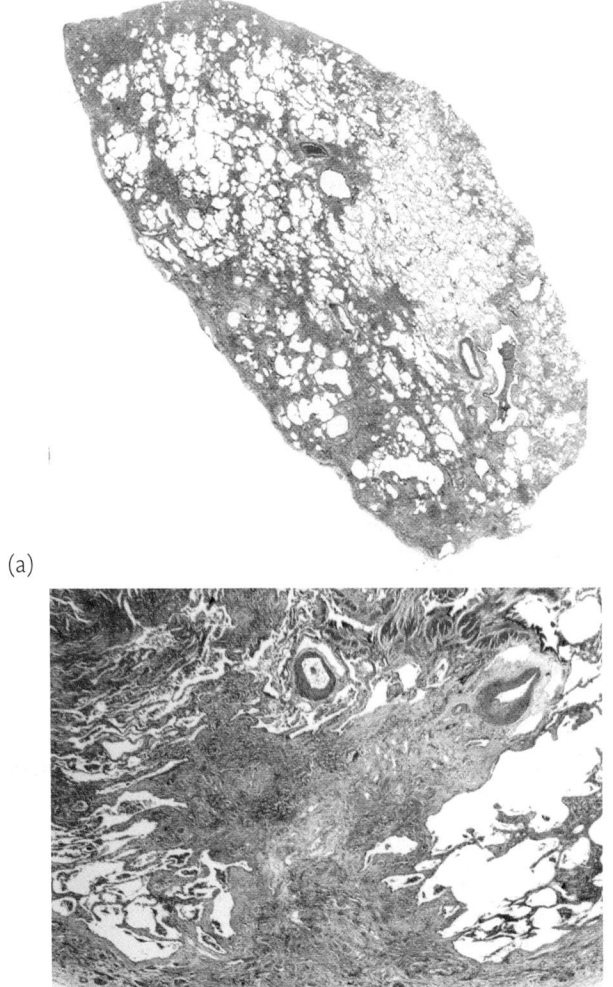

(a)

(b)

Fig. 18.11.2.1 (A) Surgical lung biopsy from a patient with idiopathic pulmonary fibrosis showing a patchy established fibrosis with a predominantly subpleural distribution. (B) At high power there is a mild degree of associated nonspecific chronic inflammation with fibroblastic foci in continuity with the established fibrosis. Note the relatively sharp demarcation between normal and abnormal parenchyma.

Presentation and features on investigation

Clinical features

The typical presentation is progressive exertional dyspnoea without wheeze and a nonproductive cough, although sputum production is present in few patients. Haemoptysis should prompt investigation for lung malignancy, which is approximately 10-fold more prevalent in IPF after the smoking history has been taken into account. Chest discomfort, fatigue, and weight loss are occasional features. Digital clubbing is present in over 50% of patients and has been an adverse prognostic determinant in some series. On auscultation, very fine end-inspiratory crackles are typically heard bilaterally at the lung bases and become widespread in advanced disease. Central cyanosis and clinical evidence of pulmonary hypertension, with or without right ventricular failure, are late features. Evidence of rheumatological disease, which is generally indicative of a much better outcome, should be sought from the history and examination.

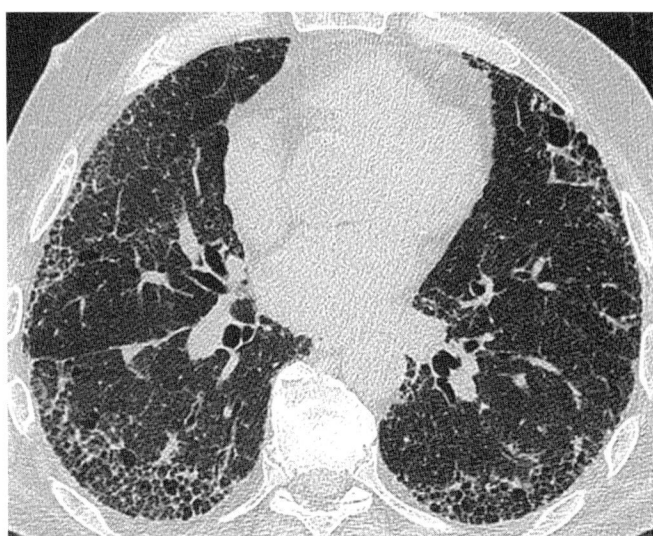

Fig. 18.11.2.2 High-resolution CT scan of a patient with biopsy-proven idiopathic pulmonary fibrosis (IPF). Appearances are typical of IPF with a subpleural distribution of microcystic and macrocystic honeycomb change.

Chest radiography

The chest radiograph typically shows small lung volumes and predominantly peripheral and basal reticulonodular shadowing, with obscuration of the heart borders and diaphragms in advanced disease and overt honeycombing in 10% of cases. However, this profile is very nonspecific, occuring in fibrotic NSIP, asbestosis, rheumatological disorders, and other fibrotic processes. Lymphadenopathy or pleural disease should suggest an alternative diagnosis or a concurrent pathological process. The heart may appear to be enlarged in the absence of cardiovascular disease as a result of reduced intrathoracic volume.

High-resolution CT

High-resolution CT appearances are virtually pathognomonic in up to 70% of patients (Fig. 18.11.2.2). The disease is predominantly posterobasal and peripheral, becoming widespread in advanced disease, and consists of a reticular pattern, with or without honeycombing, and a minor component of ground-glass attenuation, usually indicative of fine fibrosis (rather than inflammation). It should be stressed that high-resolution CT appearances are atypical in at least 30% of cases, with the most frequent variant consisting of prominent ground-glass attenuation admixed with a fine reticular pattern and associated with traction bronchiectasis, which is an appearance also suggestive of NSIP (Fig. 18.11.2.3). However, IPF is also diagnosed (i.e. a histological pattern of UIP at biopsy) in occasional patients with markedly atypical high-resolution CT appearances (Fig. 18.11.2.4). Reactive mediastinal lymphadenopathy is usual on high-resolution CT and is not indicative of a coexisting disease process unless also present on chest radiography. In early disease, prone high-resolution CT sections may be required to distinguish abnormal appearances from normal increases in density due to gravity-related increases in perfusion in dependent areas.

Other imaging modalities

Ventilation–perfusion scans show ventilation mismatch due to vascular ablation in areas of cystic lung, which typically continue to

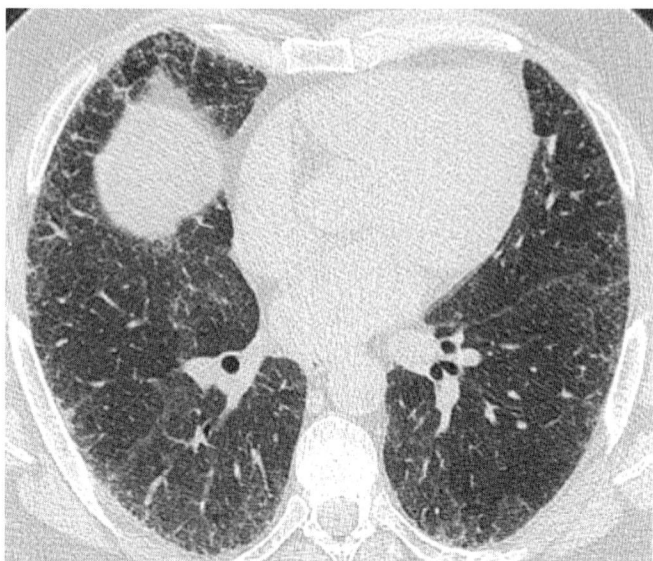

Fig. 18.11.2.3 High-resolution CT scan of a patient with biopsy-proven idiopathic pulmonary fibrosis (IPF) showing abnormalities that overlap in appearance with those seen in nonspecific interstitial pneumonia. Disease is predominantly sub-pleural but consists of a mixture of ground-glass attenuation and fine reticular abnormalities, without honeycombing. This appearance is seen in a significant minority of patients with IPF.

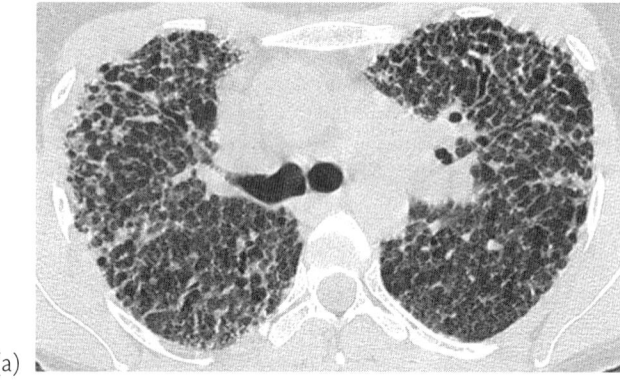

(a)

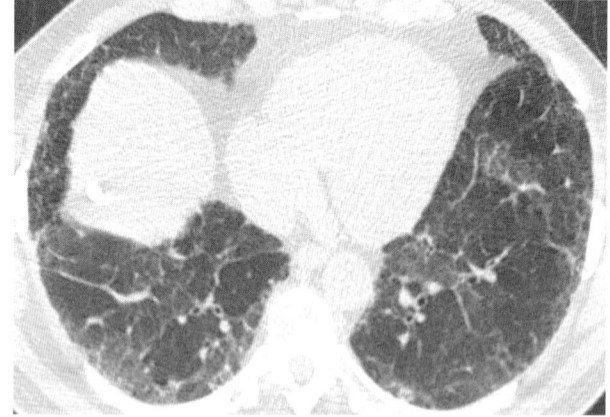

(b)

Fig. 18.11.2.4 High-resolution CT scans in patients with biopsy-proven idiopathic pulmonary fibrosis (IPF). In both cases high-resolution CT appearances are markedly atypical, with no features indicative of IPF or of any other form of idiopathic interstitial pneumonia. IPF should always be suspected when disease is inexorably progressive and high-resolution CT appearances are difficult to classify.

ventilate normally. These appearances simulate pulmonary thromboembolism and probably account for a widespread misperception that pulmonary embolism is a frequent complication of IPF. CT pulmonary angiography is required when pulmonary embolism is suspected, especially when $D_L$co levels are disproportionately reduced, but is usually negative in this context.

Gallium scanning almost invariably reveals abnormal signal, as in other forms of pulmonary fibrosis associated with macrophage activation, but does not contribute usefully to prognostic evaluation or management. Rapid clearance from the lung of inhaled technetium-99m diethylinetriamine pentacetate (DTPA) may be indicative of a more progressive course, but rapid clearance is also seen in healthy smokers and the test has no established role in routine management.

Lung function tests

Lung function tests reveal a restrictive ventilatory defect, as shown by reductions in vital capacity, total lung capacity, residual volume and pulmonary compliance. However, the wide range of normal premorbid lung volumes sometimes results in apparent normality (when lung volumes have fallen from the upper to the lower end of the normal range). Thus, measures of gas transfer, especially $D_L$co levels, may be reduced in isolation in early disease. Adjustment of $D_L$co for reduced alveolar volume (Kco) has been advocated as a more specific index of interstitial fibrosis, but Kco levels are disproportionately reduced by coexistent emphysema, which is present in over 30% of IPF patients. The combination of emphysema and IPF may result in spurious preservation of lung volumes, even in advanced disease, and disproportionate reduction in $D_L$co levels. Overall, the severity of disease is most accurately captured by $D_L$co levels, which correlate best with the extent of IPF as judged by high-resolution CT.

In early disease arterial gases may be normal, but mild arterial hypoxia with widening of the alveolar-arterial gradient and normal or low Paco_2 levels are usual. Severe hypoxia is a late feature and increased Paco_2 levels occur in terminal disease.

Blood tests

Blood tests contribute little to the management of IPF, except in rare cases in which an unsuspected underlying cause is identified. Mild increases in the erythrocyte sedimentation rate, serum immunoglobulins, rheumatoid factor and antinuclear antibodies are frequent, and secondary polycythaemia may occur in severe disease. A high neutrophil count may be indicative of infection but a moderate increase is also seen in association with corticosteroid therapy. However, striking increases in autoantibodies may be indicative of a hitherto undiagnosed rheumatological disorder. Precipitin tests against fungal and avian antigens should be performed when there is suggestive exposure history because chronic extrinsic allergic alveolitis occasionally presents with the CFA clinical syndrome, high-resolution CT appearances suggestive of IPF, and a pattern of UIP at surgical biopsy.

Bronchoalveolar lavage

Bronchoalveolar lavage is a useful ancillary diagnostic test when a surgical biopsy is not performed. Typically, there is an increase in total cell counts with an excess of neutrophils and/or eosinophils. A mild lymphocytosis is not infrequent, but striking rises in lymphocyte counts are not generally a feature of IPF and suggest an alternative disorder such as NSIP, extrinsic allergic alveolitis, fibrotic sarcoidosis, cryptogenic organizing pneumonia complicated by interstitial fibrosis, or drug-induced lung disease. Bronchoalveolar lavage is occasionally useful in excluding opportunistic infection in treated patients.

Surgical lung biopsy

A surgical lung biopsy is the histological diagnostic procedure of choice. Video-assisted thoracoscopic biopsy is the most widely used procedure, but minithoracotomy is occasionally required in advanced disease. It is strongly recommended that at least two sites are biopsied, with high-resolution CT findings taken into account to ensure that the full spectrum of morphological abnormalities is sampled and to avoid areas of endstage disease which seldom yield diagnostic tissue. The diagnosis of IPF and other idiopathic interstitial pneumonias cannot be based upon appearances at transbronchial biopsy: larger biopsies are required to determine whether abnormalities are spatially heterogeneous or truly homogeneous (as in NSIP), a crucial discriminatory diagnostic feature.

Echocardiography

Based upon recent reports of a high prevalence of pulmonary hypertension in IPF, routine echocardiography is warranted at presentation and in patients subsequently developing disproportionate hypoxia or a selective serial reduction in $D_L$co. In some patients with IPF the development of pulmonary hypertension is a feature of endstage disease, but in other cases early pulmonary hypertension occurs, not associated with major functional impairment due to interstitial lung disease.

Diagnosis

Once suspected in the symptomatic patient, IPF is usually easy to detect using lung function tests and chest radiography, but in early disease high-resolution CT may be required to confirm or exclude interstitial lung disease. However (as discussed earlier), clinical, chest radiographic and physiological features are highly nonspecific in discriminating between individual idiopathic interstitial pneumonias, and high-resolution CT plays a crucial role in this regard. High-resolution CT appearances are diagnostic in an appropriate clinical setting in most patients with IPF, hence it is seldom necessary to confirm the diagnosis at surgical biopsy, especially when a typical course of relentless progression is already apparent. However, in a few patients diagnostic imprecision leads to major prognostic uncertainties and inaccurate management and a diagnostic biopsy is warranted. Thus, biopsy should not be performed by protocol in all cases but should be reserved for situations in which it appears realistic that clinician perceptions of best management, including treatment and the approach to monitoring, might change significantly with additional information.

In less typical cases the findings at bronchoalveolar lavage may play an important ancillary role in excluding alternative disorders such as extrinsic allergic alveolitis and respiratory bronchiolitis with associated interstitial lung disease (characterized by a striking lymphocytosis and a marked increase in pigmented macrophages respectively).

It should be stressed that the distinction between IPF and fibrotic NSIP (discussed in Chapter 18.11.1), based on clinical and high-resolution CT features, poses particular difficulty. Even when high-resolution CT appearances are considered typical for NSIP, there is a significant likelihood that a surgical biopsy will disclose a pattern of UIP, indicative of a worse outcome. In difficult cases, it is essential to review the diagnosis in a multidisciplinary meeting, with the reconciliation of clinical and radiological features, in order to confirm that a diagnostic surgical biopsy is truly required. This decision is often difficult when IPF is likely, because of patient age (typically advanced), disease severity, and the presence of comorbidity, especially cardiovascular disease. The threshold for performing a biopsy is increased in patients aged over 70 years and when $D_L$co levels are less than 35% of predicted, both factors being associated with a significant increase in morbidity and very occasional fatalities following biopsy.

It is also important that histological findings are no longer viewed as a diagnostic 'gold standard' in interstitial lung disease, although usually more diagnostically influential than clinical and high-resolution CT features when the diagnosis is uncertain. A multidisciplinary diagnosis, made by negotiation between clinicians, radiologists, and pathologists, is now considered optimal. A histological pattern other than UIP is considered to exclude IPF, with one important caveat: 'sampling error' (i.e. a biopsy taken from a non-representative site) should be kept in mind when high-resolution CT findings and the subsequent clinical course are strongly suggestive of IPF. Conversely, when UIP is disclosed at biopsy, the final consensus diagnosis sometimes differs from the histological diagnosis. This applies especially to patients with clinical evidence of extrinsic allergic alveolitis or a rheumatological disorder.

Prognosis

Accurate diagnosis is central to prognostic evaluation. The 5-year survival is approximately 10 to 15% in IPF, as compared to over 60% in fibrotic NSIP, and over 90% in patients with predominantly inflammatory idiopathic interstitial pneumonias. In established IPF a number of adverse prognostic factors have been identified (summarized in Table 18.11.2.1).

Table 18.11.2.1 Features associated with a worse outcome in idiopathic pulmonary fibrosis, with evidence graded as possible but uncertain (±), definite and moderately useful in routine practice (+), or definite and highly predictive (++)

Features associated with a worse outcome	Grade of evidence
Increasing age	++
Male gender	±
Former or current smoking	±
High profusion of fibroblastic foci at biopsy	+
Prominent honeycombing on high-resolution CT	++
Presence of pulmonary hypertension	++
Moderate impairment of lung function	+
Resting hypoxia	++
Major desaturation on maximal exercise testing	+
Major desaturation during a 6-min walk test	++
Increasing dyspnoea	+
Serial decline in FVC or $D_L$co	++

Increasing age has consistently been an adverse prognostic determinant, although it is not clear whether disease is on average more progressive in older people, or—as seems more likely—comorbidity (cardiac disease and malignancy) is largely responsible for an adverse outcome. Disease severity at presentation is a crucial consideration. Increased mortality is associated with severe functional impairment, with $D_L$co levels providing the most accurate guidance to likely outcome amongst lung function tests performed at rest. A composite physiological index, containing $D_L$co, FVC, and FEV_1 levels, has recently been shown to predict survival more accurately than any single lung function test in isolation. Severe resting hypoxia is indicative of a very poor outcome.

Maximal exercise testing is advocated as a superior prognostic determinant by some authorities but, in reality, there are no convincing data establishing that maximal exercise data are superior to $D_L$co levels in this regard. However, desaturation below 88% during a 6-min walk test has consistently identified IPF patients with a much worse outcome in several series. It is not yet clear whether desaturation during exercise is primarily linked to incipient pulmonary hypertension, but the presence of moderate to severe pulmonary hypertension is indicative of a very poor outcome.

Mortality and a more progressive course have both been linked to a higher profusion of fibroblastic foci at surgical biopsy in IPF, but this finding has yet to be applied to routine practice. High-resolution CT features have also been linked to outcome, with prominent honeycombing associated with a high short-term mortality, although this finding may partially reflect an association between severe honeycombing and extensive disease. Patients with biopsy-proven IPF and high-resolution CT appearances suggestive of NSIP have a better treated outcome than patients with high-resolution CT appearances typical of IPF.

Smoking status may also be important. The provocative observation that current smokers have a higher survival than former smokers or non-smokers is likely to represent merely a "healthy smoker effect". However, recent analyses have suggested that lifelong non-smokers have a better survival in IPF than current and former smokers.

Serial observations are more prognostically accurate than observations made at a single point in time in patients with IPF. Changes in FVC over time have consistently predicted mortality more reliably than baseline data, and serial $D_L$co trends have been similarly predictive in some but not all reports. The distinction between stability and significant decline at 12 months is particularly useful. Once this information is known the histological diagnosis provides no additional prognostic information in mixed patient populations with UIP or fibrotic NSIP.

Routine monitoring

Lung function tests have traditionally been used to identify treatment responsiveness (in inflammatory disorders) and deterioration (in IPF and other fibrotic disorders). However, measurement variation is a major limitation which requires the use of thresholds for 'significant change'. A 10% change from baseline FVC levels, or a 15% change from baseline $D_L$co levels, is required to identify definite regression or progression of disease: the greater measurement variation in $D_L$co may explain the fact that serial FVC trends are more predictive of longer-term outcome than serial $D_L$co trends. However, the interpretation of serial lung function testing must be modified in some contexts. Concurrent emphysema often has a major confounding effect, with spurious preservation of FVC levels but a disproportionate reduction in $D_L$co (reduced in both disorders), in which case a selective serial decline in $D_L$co levels may be seen with no change in FVC despite significant progression of disease. A selective reduction in $D_L$co may also be indicative of incipient pulmonary hypertension. Thus, serial lung function trends must be integrated with clinical, high-resolution CT and—when indicated—echocardiographic information.

A marginal reduction in lung function indices (a 5–10% change in FVC levels, a 10–15% change in $D_L$co levels) commonly causes difficulties for clinicians. These changes may indicate true disease progression in some patients, but lie within the measurement variation of lung function tests. Symptomatic change is sometimes a useful guide in this difficult scenario, but is sometimes misleading. Exertional dyspnoea may increase because of disease progression, loss of fitness, comorbidity, or weight gain and myopathy due to corticosteroid therapy. Serial high-resolution CT is sometimes informative, with clear evidence of disease progression in the context of marginal lung function decline. However, serial high-resolution CT should be reserved for situations in which the demonstration of disease progression is likely to influence management: it is difficult to assign significance to minor change on high-resolution CT in the absence of lung function deterioration.

Detailed lung function tests are often impracticable in advanced disease with increasing hypoxia, when serial tests tend to be less informative than observations of changes in oxygen saturation (in the steep component of the oxygen dissociation curve).

In IPF the intensity of monitoring is critically dependent upon the therapeutic goal. Regular monitoring at 3- to 4-monthly intervals is especially important in patients receiving treatment, especially novel therapies, and when referral for lung transplantation is contemplated. In other cases, in which no change in therapy is contemplated, less frequent monitoring may be appropriate. However, the importance of best supportive care, including the correct use of oxygen in advanced disease, justifies continued monitoring in the long term.

Treatment

Treatment in IPF can be broadly subdivided into treatment of definite IPF and treatment of patients in whom IPF is likely but fibrotic NSIP is a realistic differential diagnosis. This distinction is important because in definite IPF it may be possible to slow decline in some cases, but long-term stability is very seldom observed. By contrast, prevention of disease progression is a realistic therapeutic aim in fibrotic NSIP, justifying vigorous treatment.

Treatment decisions should be made before the development of limiting dyspnoea, which is indicative of the loss of pulmonary reserve and—usually—a reduction in $D_L$co to less than 50% predicted. The outcome is better when disease is less severe and when there is less honeycombing, considerations that are especially important when IPF and fibrotic NSIP are both possible, the outcome being better in NSIP except when disease is severe (at which point mortality is high and differs little between the two disorders). To delay therapy until disease is advanced, in the belief that IPF is the likelier diagnosis, is to risk the loss of an important window of opportunity in fibrotic NSIP.

Loss of lung function due to fibrosis is irreversible and thus improvement in lung function is seldom seen with treatment in IPF.

It is essential to focus on the prevention of disease progression as a valid primary aim, underlining the importance of initiating therapy before severe lung function impairment has developed. Too often stability without improvement is incorrectly taken to indicate failure of therapy, both by the patient and by medical colleagues not used to treating fibrotic lung disease.

Definite IPF

In definite IPF there is little evidence that traditional treatment regimens have a major impact on outcome. Corticosteroid therapy, often in association with other immunosuppressive treatment, has been widely used, although not based on prospective, placebo-controlled, randomized trials. In the absence of a definitive evidence base, the ATS/ERS consensus committee made a weak recommendation in 2000, supporting the use of a combination of low-dose prednisolone (such as 10 mg daily) and azathioprine (2.5 mg/kg per day up to a maximum dose of 150 mg/day). During the first month a test dose of azathioprine (50 mg/day) is usual, with weekly full blood count monitoring to avoid enhanced bone-marrow toxicity due to the rare methyltransferase deficiency. A change to full dosage is made at four weeks, with full blood counts and liver function tests performed 6- to 8-weekly thereafter. Other traditional IPF treatments, including high-dose prednisolone and cyclophosphamide, have been largely discredited due to unacceptable toxicity without a worthwhile therapeutic benefit. Colchicine and ciclosporin have also been used to treat IPF, without evidence of efficacy.

More recently, attention has turned to number of antifibrotic agents, many of which are currently under study. Pirfenidone, a pleiotrophic agent with antifibrotic, anti-inflammatory and antioxidant activity, appears promising, based on early evidence of a reduction in the rate of decline of FVC levels, but is not yet available for routine use and requires further study. IPF patients receiving antioxidant therapy, consisting of N-acetylcysteine (600 mg three times a day), given in combination with low-dose prednisolone and azathioprine (at doses detailed above), were recently shown to have a significant reduction in decline of FVC and $D_L$co over 12 months, compared with patients receiving prednisolone and azathioprine alone. It is not clear whether this benefit was due to antioxidant therapy in isolation or represented synergism between the three agents. Pending further data, the use of antioxidant and low-dose steroid therapy, with or without an immunosuppressive agent, appears reasonable and is the therapeutic approach preferred by the authors. However, the lack of definitive evidence should be freely acknowledged, the patient should be encouraged to take part in decision making, and a firm decision by the patient to decline therapy in definite IPF should be supported (although most patients prefer a trial of treatment).

IPF and fibrotic NSIP both possible

There is often diagnostic uncertainty in routine practice in nonbiopsied patients. A realistic differential diagnosis of NSIP is important, even when IPF is more probable, because long-term stability has been observed in over 50% of NSIP cases with treatment (steroid therapy, alone or in combination with an immunosuppressive agent). The routine use of low-dose prednisolone and azathioprine at doses suggested for IPF (detailed above) can be justified when a diagnosis of fibrotic NSIP is possible. However, progression of disease despite treatment in the next 6 to 12 months is associated with an equally poor outcome, whether the histological diagnosis is NSIP or UIP. Thus, if significant deterioration occurs despite treatment, a therapeutic approach as for IPF becomes appropriate, with acceptance of a lower likelihood of arresting further decline, and a lower threshold for reducing treatment for reasons of toxicity.

Acute exacerbations of IPF

In 10 to 15% of patients there is an accelerated deterioration occurring over several weeks and often leading rapidly to a fatal outcome. The pathogenesis of this phenomenon is not well understood and it is important to exclude supervening infection, heart failure and thromboembolism. If an acute exacerbation of IPF is diagnosed, intravenous corticosteroids (e.g. 1 g/day methylprednisolone for 3 days) together with intravenous cyclophosphamide (600 mg/m^2 as a single dose, repeated at roughly 2-week intervals if blood counts are satisfactory) are often used, although no controlled treatment data exist. Noninvasive ventilation is sometimes useful, but mechanical ventilation should be avoided because of its uniformly poor outcome.

Transplantation

Single lung transplantation is now the preferred procedure. As in other endstage lung diseases a 3-year survival rate of over 50% can be achieved, but a worse outcome is seen in severely deconditioned patients and those over the age of 65. The rapidly progressive nature of IPF, compared to other chronic lung diseases, demands the early referral of suitable cases to a transplantation centre, ideally before $D_L$co levels fall below 30% of predicted normal.

Supportive therapy

Supportive therapy is central to the management of advanced disease. Supplemental oxygen can be provided in the home through oxygen concentrators, and in some patients ambulatory oxygen (in small oxygen cylinders) may be beneficial in improving exercise tolerance. The prompt treatment of complications, including infection and heart failure (sometimes triggered by hypoxia), is also important. In terminal disease small doses of opiates alleviate the distressing severe dyspnoea associated with striking reductions in lung compliance.

It is difficult for patients and family members to come to terms with the chronic, relentlessly progressive nature of IPF. The input of medical and nonmedical health care professionals is indispensable to optimal supportive management: social workers, physiotherapists, and occupational therapists all have important roles to play. Rehabilitation programmes may benefit some patients, although less likely to be useful in preterminal disease.

Further reading

ATS/ERS International Consensus Statement. (2000). Idiopathic pulmonary fibrosis: diagnosis and treatment. International consensus statement. *Am J Respir Crit Care Med*, **161**, 646–64.

Azuma A, *et al.* (2005). Double-blind, placebo-controlled trial of pirfenidone in patients with idiopathic pulmonary fibrosis. *Am J Respir Crit Care Med*, **171**, 1040–7.

Carrington CB, Gaensler EA, Coutu RE (1978). Natural history and treated course of usual and desquamative interstitial pneumonia. *N Engl J Med*, **298**, 801–9.

Collard HR, *et al.* (2003). Changes in clinical and physiologic variables predict survival in idiopathic pulmonary fibrosis. *Am J Respir Crit Care Med*, **168**, 538–42.

Demedts M, *et al.* (2005). High-dose acetylcysteine in idiopathic pulmonary fibrosis. *N Engl J Med*, **353**, 2229–42.

Flaherty KR, *et al.* (2003). Radiological versus histological diagnosis in UIP and NSIP: survival implications. *Thorax*, **58**, 143–8.

Flaherty KR, *et al.* (2003). Prognostic implications of physiologic and radiographic changes in idiopathic interstitial pneumonia. *Am J Respir Crit Care Med*, **168**, 543–8.

Flaherty KR, *et al.* (2004). Idiopathic interstitial pneumonia: what is the effect of a multidisciplinary approach to diagnosis? *Am J Respir Crit Care Med*, **170**, 904–10.

Gay SE, *et al.* (1998). Idiopathic pulmonary fibrosis: predicting response to therapy and survival. *Am J Respir Crit Care Med*, **157**, 1063–72.

Hunninghake GW, *et al.* (2001). Utility of a lung biopsy for the diagnosis of idiopathic pulmonary fibrosis. *Am J Respir Crit Care Med*, **164**, 193–6.

Katzenstein AL, Myers JL (1998). Idiopathic pulmonary fibrosis: clinical relevance of pathologic classification (review). *Am J Respir Crit Care Med*, **157**, 1301–15.

King TE, Tooze JA, Schwarz MI, Brown KR, Cherniack RM. Predicting survival in idiopathic pulmonary fibrosis: scoring system and survival model. *Am J Respir Crit Care Med* 2001, **164**, 1171–81.

King TE, Jr., *et al.* (2001). Idiopathic pulmonary fibrosis: relationship between histopathologic features and mortality. *Am J Respir Crit Care Med*, **164**, 1025–32.

Lama VN, *et al.* (2003). Prognostic value of desaturation during a six-minute walk test in idiopathic interstitial pneumonia. *Am J Respir Crit Care Med*, **168**, 1084–90.

Latsi PI, *et al.* (2003). Fibrotic idiopathic interstitial pneumonia: the prognostic value of longitudinal functional trends. *Am J Respir Crit Care Med*, **168**, 531–7.

Mogulkoc M, *et al.* (2001). Pulmonary function in idiopathic pulmonary fibrosis and referral for lung transplantation. *Am J Respir Crit Care Med*, 2001, **164**, 103–8.

Raghu G, *et al.* (2006). Incidence and prevalence of idiopathic pulmonary fibrosis. *Am J Respir Crit Care Med*, **174**, 810–16.

Steele MP, *et al.* (2005). Clinical and pathologic features of familial interstitial pneumonia. *Am J Respir Crit Care Med*, **172**, 1146–52.

Selman M, King TE, Pardo A (2001). Idiopathic pulmonary fibrosis: prevailing and evolving hypotheses about its pathogenesis and implications for therapy (review). *Ann Intern Med*, **134**, 136–51.

Wells AU, *et al.* (2003). Idiopathic pulmonary fibrosis: a composite physiologic index derived from disease extent observed on computed tomography. *Am J Respir Crit Care Med*, **167**, 962–9.

18.11.3 Bronchiolitis obliterans and cryptogenic organizing pneumonia

A.U. Wells and Nicholas K. Harrison

Essentials

The nomenclature of the bronchiolitides is complicated by the interchangeable use of pathological and clinical descriptions and a diversity of classification systems. The four primary histological patterns are (1) organizing pneumonia (also termed proliferative bronchiolitis and bronchiolitis obliterans organizing pneumonia); (2) bronchiolitis obliterans (also termed obliterative bronchiolitis

and constrictive bronchiolitis); (3) follicular bronchiolitis; and (4) diffuse panbronchiolitis.

Organizing pneumonia—the most characteristic abnormality is a filling of alveoli with granulation tissue and buds of loose collagen and connective tissue matrix cells with a uniform appearance. Presentation is typically subacute with nonproductive or minimally productive cough, insidious dyspnoea, and systemic symptoms including malaise, fever or chills, weight loss, and myalgia. Clinical signs are nonspecific. The chest radiograph most commonly shows patchy bilateral peripheral consolidation, which is often basal, and serial radiographs often show migration of infiltrates. High-resolution CT most often shows focal subpleural consolidation, with or without air bronchograms. Corticosteroid therapy is usually effective, with other immunosuppressive agents given to fulminant cases or those that do not respond. Prognosis is usually good, with overall mortality less than 5%.

Bronchiolitis obliterans—results from progressive obliteration of the terminal bronchioles with connective tissue matrix, which is cryptogenic in most cases. The usual presentation is with progressive breathlessness and the most characteristic physical finding is of inspiratory 'squawks', which are reliably indicative of small airway disease. High-resolution CT is often diagnostic, revealing focal areas of decreased attenuation representing regional gas-trapping and associated hypoperfusion, termed 'mosaic attenuation' or 'mosaic perfusion'. The disease is not responsive to treatment, but in cases of diagnostic uncertainty it is usual to institute a trial of corticosteroids.

Follicular bronchiolitis—results from polyclonal hyperplasia of lymphoid follicles with formation of germinal centres within the bronchiolar walls. Patients usually present with progressive breathlessness, cough, and symptoms of recurrent respiratory infection. high-resolution CT invariably reveals centrilobular nodules less than 3 mm in diameter. Prognosis is generally good.

Diffuse panbronchiolitis—is characterized by bronchiolocentric inflammation, lymphoid hyperplasia, and an accumulation of interstitial foam cells in the lungs. Patients (most typically Japanese) present with subacute symptoms of cough productive of purulent sputum, dyspnoea, and sometimes weight loss. Survival has been transformed by the use of long-term, low-dose erythromycin therapy.

Introduction

The bronchioles are airways without cartilaginous support and include the terminal bronchioles and the respiratory bronchioles which lead to the alveolar ducts. The nomenclature of the bronchiolitides is complicated by the interchangeable use of pathological and clinical descriptions and a diversity of classification systems. The four primary histological patterns are organizing pneumonia (also termed proliferative bronchiolitis and bronchiolitis obliterans organizing pneumonia), bronchiolitis obliterans (also termed obliterative bronchiolitis and constrictive bronchiolitis), follicular bronchiolitis, and diffuse panbronchiolitis. All four disorders may ablate or obstruct the bronchioles. Organizing pneumonia and bronchiolitis obliterans may be associated with other disease processes (Table 18.11.3.1). The terminological similarity between bronchiolitis obliterans and an unrelated acinar disorder, bronchiolitis obliterans organizing pneumonia (BOOP), causes particular

Table 18.11.3.1 Causes of bronchiolitis obliterans and organizing pneumonia

Cause	Bronchiolitis obliterans	Organizing pneumonia
Infection	Viral, mycoplasma	Viral, bacterial, fungal, parasites
Rheumatological disease	Especially rheumatoid arthritis,	Especially dermato/polymyositis, rheumatoid arthritis
Transplantation	Bone marrow, heart/lung, lung	Bone marrow, lung
Drugs	E.g. penicillamine	E.g. amiodarone, sulphasalazine, gold, minocycline
Other	Toxicity from inhaled gases, smoke	Radiotherapy Malignant haematological disorders Immunodeficiency syndromes
Cryptogenic	Cryptogenic	Cryptogenic

confusion as the terms are commonly but incorrectly regarded as synonymous. Because of this widespread confusion bronchiolitis obliterans and BOOP are covered in the remainder of this chapter, also follicular bronchiolitis and diffuse panbronchiolitis, although BOOP is properly an idiopathic interstitial pneumonia, as recently reclassified by an American Thoracic Society/European Respiratory Society nomenclature committee.

The term 'cryptogenic organizing pneumonia' is preferable to BOOP, but it is likely that both terms will continue to appear in the medical literature for the foreseeable future. Cryptogenic organizing pneumonia/BOOP also involves the bronchioles, but these are not truly obliterated and instead are filled with loose intraluminal fibrous tissue. The clinical presentation, radiological features, physiological features and responsiveness to treatment differ radically between bronchiolitis obliterans and cryptogenic organizing pneumonia (Table 18.11.3.2). Essentially, bronchiolitis obliterans is an irreversible disorder of small airways whereas cryptogenic organizing pneumonia is a largely reversible disorder of the lung interstitium.

Bronchiolitis obliterans

In common with other forms of bronchiolitis, bronchiolitis obliterans is associated with a number of triggers but is cryptogenic in most cases. A viral pathogenesis is often proposed based on the fact that the disease often presents following an apparent respiratory

Table 18.11.3.2 Contrasting features of bronchiolitis obliterans and organizing pneumonia

	Bronchiolitis obliterans	Organizing pneumonia
Histology	Obliteration of bronchioles	Bronchioles filled with loose fibrous tissue
Chest radiography	Hyperinflation	Consolidation
High-resolution CT	Mosaic attenuation	Consolidation, with occasional reticular elements
Pulmonary function tests	Airflow obstruction	Restrictive defect
Response to therapy	Invariably poor	Good in most cases

infection, but this is unproven. Occasionally, bronchiolitis obliterans precedes the development of an overt rheumatological disorder.

The disease results from progressive obliteration of the terminal bronchioles with connective tissue matrix. In early reports it was found to progress relentlessly to a fatal outcome. With the advent of CT and the detection of less advanced disease, it is now clear that the natural history is highly variable. Although inexorable progression occurs in some patients, especially those with rheumatological disease, an indolent course is probably more frequent, and some patients who appear to develop the disease after a severe viral insult do not progress even when there is severe airflow obstruction.

Histopathology

The terminal bronchioles are predominantly affected, with variable involvement of the proximal respiratory bronchioles. There is fibrotic obliteration of the airway lumen with an occasional inflammatory component, especially in rheumatological disease (Fig. 18.11.3.1). Diagnostic appearances may be lost in advanced disease as a result of airway occlusion by dense connective tissue matrix, which may render the airways invisible.

Clinical features

The usual presentation is with progressive breathlessness. Wheeze and a sensation of chest tightness are occasionally present as nonspecific consequences (respectively) of constriction of small airways and hyperinflation. Nonproductive cough is frequent, but haemoptysis is not a feature. On examination an expiratory wheeze is occasionally heard, but the more characteristic finding is of inspiratory 'squawks', which are reliably indicative of small-airway disease. There may be subtle evidence of rheumatological disease, especially rheumatoid arthritis.

Investigations

Imaging

Chest radiography is normal until disease is advanced. The typical findings are nonspecific, consisting of large lung fields with variable loss of vascular markings but no interstitial abnormalities.

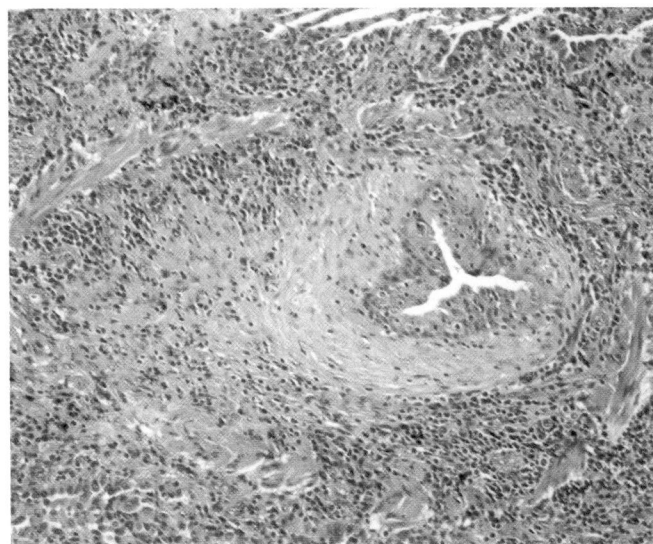

Fig. 18.11.3.1 A case of bronchiolitis obliterans showing virtual occlusion of the bronchiole by a mixture of fibrosis and a chronic inflammatory cell infiltrate that includes scattered eosinophils.

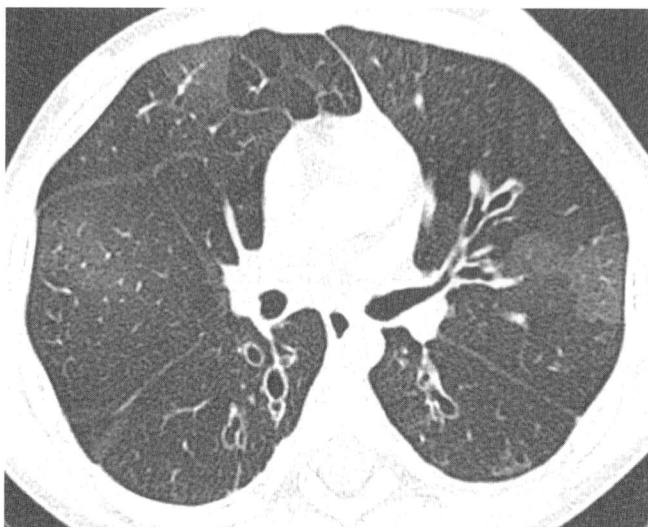

Fig. 18.11.3.2 High-resolution CT scan in a patient with severe bronchiolitis obliterans. There is extensive decreased attenuation, indicative of severe gas trapping, with small areas of increased density representing normal interstitium. There is also severe bronchiectasis, a frequent ancillary finding in advanced bronchiolitis obliterans.

High-resolution CT is often diagnostic (Fig. 18.11.3.2). There are focal areas of decreased attenuation representing regional gas-trapping and associated hypoperfusion, termed 'mosaic attenuation' or 'mosaic perfusion'. Such an appearance is occasionally present in pulmonary vascular disease, but mosaicism on CT is enhanced on expiration in bronchiolitis obliterans as density contrasts due to regional gas-trapping are exaggerated. Bronchiectasis and bronchial wall thickening are usually present, hence it is sometimes difficult to distinguish bronchiolitis obliterans from bronchiectasis (in which 'mosaic attenuation' indicative of small-airways involvement is generally present).

Lung function tests

Lung function tests show fixed airflow obstruction with an increase in residual volume and total lung capacity. Preservation of the total gas transfer for carbon monoxide ($D_L$co), except when the forced expiratory volume is 1 s (FEV$_1$) is less than 1 litre, is a useful ancillary feature distinguishing between intrinsic airway disease and emphysema. The gas transfer index (total gas transfer corrected for alveolar volume) is preserved even when airflow obstruction is severe. Arterial gases at rest remain normal until disease is advanced.

Other investigations

Blood tests show no diagnostic features except when autoantibodies are indicative of unsuspected rheumatological disease. In mild to moderate disease bronchoalveolar lavage shows a characteristic neutrophilia, and absence of eosinophilia may help to distinguish between bronchiolitis obliterans and refractory asthma. Lavage should not be performed in advanced disease as it may cause respiratory decompensation.

Differential diagnosis

The chronic airflow obstruction of bronchiolitis obliterans is indistinguishable from the chronic airflow obstruction seen in emphysema, bronchiectasis, in some patients with asthma, and in bronchiolitis obliterans complicating other disorders. The diagnosis can generally be made with confidence by reconciling patterns of functional impairment with high-resolution CT appearances. Preserved gas transfer distinguishes intrinsic airways disease from emphysema. The appearances on high-resolution CT are often diagnostic of small-airways disease and help exclude emphysema as a cause of airflow obstruction. The auscultatory finding of inspiratory 'squawks' is also strongly indicative of the diagnosis. In early disease the clinical and radiological features may overlap with those of bronchiectasis, but the obstructive defect tends to be much more severe in bronchiolitis obliterans. A surgical biopsy is seldom required to make the diagnosis and is contraindicated in severe airflow obstruction.

Treatment

The disease is not responsive to treatment. In cases of diagnostic uncertainty it is usual to institute a trial of corticosteroids (e.g. prednisolone 40 mg/day for 4 weeks). A significant objective response, based on an improvement in lung function tests, is suggestive of an alternative bronchiolar disorder. Following any response the corticosteroid dosage should be tapered and the minimum maintenance dose should be established. Inhaled steroid therapy and long-acting β_2-adrenoceptor agents such as salmeterol or eformoterol are occasionally efficacious in this context. However, in irreversible disease there is no proven role for long-term corticosteroid or immunosuppressive therapy.

Supportive measures play a crucial role. Patients with bronchiolitis obliterans have difficulty in clearing infective secretions, and in indolent disease prolonged infection may be associated with irreversible worsening of the functional defect. A policy of early antimicrobial therapy for respiratory infection is essential. Enrolment in a pulmonary rehabilitation programme is appropriate in advanced disease. For younger patients with inexorably progressive disease, lung transplantation is the only treatment known to improve life expectancy. There is no evidence that post-transplantation obliterative bronchiolitis, the most common lethal complication of lung transplantation, is more prevalent in patients transplanted for bronchiolitis obliterans.

Organizing pneumonia

Introduction

Organizing pneumonia is a disorder of unknown cause originally described as a clinicopathological entity by Davidson in 1983. Epler and colleagues described a larger series of patients with similar clinical and histological abnormalities which they referred to as 'bronchiolitis obliterans organizing pneumonia' (BOOP) in 1985. Cryptogenic organizing pneumonia is the preferred term because it better describes the clinical and pathological findings, which are those of an acinar rather than an airway disease, and because the term BOOP is often confused with bronchiolitis obliterans.

Organizing pneumonia can be associated with a number of other disorders (listed in Table 18.11.3.1) and is then called 'secondary organizing pneumonia'. The clinical features of cryptogenic and secondary disease are very similar, but the distinction is important because the prognosis of secondary disease is often worse.

Histopathology

The most characteristic abnormality is a filling of alveoli with granulation tissue and buds of loose collagen and connective tissue

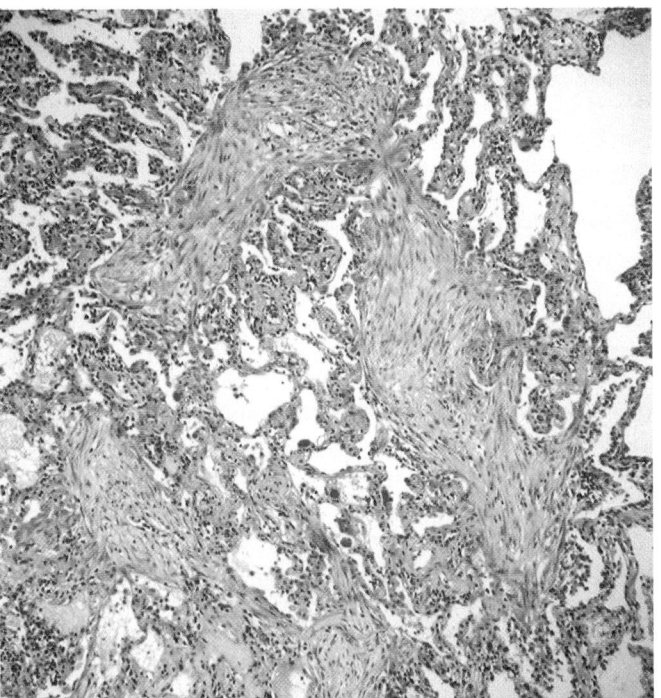

Fig. 18.11.3.3 A case of organizing pneumonia showing intra-alveolar buds of granulation tissue, the typical features of cryptogenic organizing pneumonia when identified in an idiopathic setting.

matrix cells with a uniform appearance (Fig. 18.11.3.3). Fibroblasts are embedded in a myxoid matrix containing a variable infiltrate of inflammatory cells forming characteristic polypoid masses known as Masson bodies or 'bourgeons conjunctifs'. The distribution is peribronchial, and airways distal to the terminal bronchiole are also involved. There is variable surrounding chronic inflammation. Supervening interstitial fibrosis, an occasional feature, usually has a pattern of nonspecific interstitial pneumonia.

Clinical features

The incidence and prevalence are unknown. The disease most commonly presents in the sixth and seventh decade, but the age range (20–80 years) is wide. In young adults, underlying rheumatological disease should be suspected. There is no gender predilection. Most patients are non- or ex-smokers.

Presentation is typically subacute with nonproductive or minimally productive cough, insidious dyspnoea, and systemic symptoms including malaise, fever or chills, weight loss and myalgia. Wheeze and haemoptysis are rare. Symptoms usually develop over several months and may be preceded by a suspected respiratory tract infection. Rarely, the condition may present as a fulminating illness with acute respiratory failure, and by contrast the disorder can present (5–20% of cases) as an incidental radiological abnormality in an asymptomatic patient, most typically a solitary pulmonary nodule, usually in the upper lobes.

Clinical signs are nonspecific: focal or more widespread crackles are usually, but not always, present. Digital clubbing does not occur. Systemic abnormalities suggestive of rheumatological disease are often subtle and easily overlooked.

Investigations

Imaging

The chest radiograph most commonly shows patchy bilateral peripheral consolidation, which is often basal. Serial radiographs often show migration of infiltrates, a useful diagnostic feature. Extensive reticulonodular abnormalities predominate in occasional cases with extensive supervening interstitial fibrosis. Presentation with a solitary pulmonary nodule is sometimes termed 'unifocal organizing pneumonia'. Pleural abnormalities are rare.

High-resolution CT scans most often show focal subpleural consolidation, with or without air bronchograms (Fig. 18.11.3.4). Ground-glass attenuation is commonly present and sometimes predominates, especially in patients with immune deficiency. Other occasional abnormalities include small (<10 mm) nodules along the bronchovascular bundles, larger nodules, and peripheral reticular abnormalities, denoting supervening fibrosis. The most frequent atypical variant consists of consolidation surrounding bronchovascular bundles, often associated with fibrotic abnormalities and more prevalent in organizing pneumonia complicating polymyositis/dermatomyositis.

Lung function tests

Lung function tests show a restrictive ventilatory defect without coexisting airflow obstruction, and reduced gas transfer. Disproportionate hypoxia may occur due to shunting through dilated vessels within consolidated lung even in apparently limited disease.

Other tests

Blood tests show nonspecific inflammatory changes, including a markedly raised ESR, raised C-reactive protein, and peripheral blood neutrophilia. Increased autoantibody titres, including antinuclear antibodies, rheumatoid factor, and extractable nuclear antigens, may disclose underlying rheumatological disease that is not clinically overt.

Bronchoalveolar lavage

Abnormalities in bronchoalveolar lavage fluid are nonspecific. However, the usual cell profile of a lymphocytosis (with a low CD4:CD8 ratio) associated with foamy macrophages reduces the

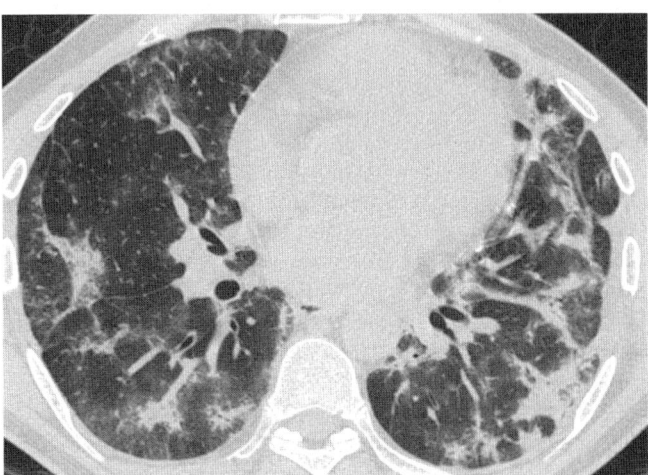

Fig. 18.11.3.4 High-resolution CT scan in a patient with organizing pneumonia. There is bilateral multifocal consolidation which is most prominent subpleurally.

likelihood of bacterial infection, vasculitis or solid cell malignancy. A neutrophilia and/or eosinophilia is not infrequent, and a prominent neutrophilia is reported in patients who progress to extensive fibrosis. Mast cells and plasma cells are occasionally present.

Differential diagnosis

If serial imaging demonstrates that infiltrates are migratory, alternative immunologically mediated abnormalities should be considered, including eosinophilic pneumonia, vasculitis (especially Churg–Strauss vasculitis and Wegener's granulomatosis) and allergic bronchopulmonary aspergillosis. However, fixed consolidation is seen in many patients with cryptogenic organizing pneumonia and in other cases imaging has not been performed before presentation. In this context the differential diagnosis includes infection, alveolar cell carcinoma and other solid malignancies, lymphoma, and alveolar proteinosis. Lung cancer is the usual differential diagnosis in cases that present as a solitary pulmonary mass.

When the clinical and radiological features are typical, the diagnosis may be made if the histological features of organizing pneumonia are evident on a transbronchial biopsy. A bronchoalveolar lavage should also be performed, both to exclude infection and because a compatible cellular profile provides useful diagnostic support, especially when transbronchial biopsies are inconclusive. In some cases, a surgical biopsy is required and this should be of sufficient size to ensure that organizing pneumonia is the main histological finding and not secondary to another pathological process such as infection, vasculitis or malignancy. It should be stressed that areas of organizing pneumonia may be seen at biopsy in infection, vasculitis, eosinophilic pneumonia and malignancy. Thus 'sampling error' at transbronchial biopsy occasionally leads to misdiagnosis and the diagnosis should always be reconsidered when the presentation or disease course are atypical. Moreover, histological appearances do not distinguish between cryptogenic disease and secondary organizing pneumonia.

Treatment

There are no controlled studies of treatment, but corticosteroid therapy is usually efficacious, with complete remission in over 60% in published series and a partial response in most of the remaining cases. Response is often rapid, with symptomatic improvement reported within days, although chest radiographic and pulmonary function responses tend to be slower, sometimes requiring up to 3 months of treatment. It is essential that alternative diagnoses be considered in cases that fail to respond.

Until recently initial treatment has generally consisted of oral prednisolone at a dose of 0.75 mg/kg per day, with intravenous methyl prednisolone sometimes used at doses of 500–1000 mg daily for three days in severe disease, followed by prednisolone at 20 mg daily with further reductions tailored according to the clinical course. However, no single recommendation covers all patients and regimens should be adjusted according to initial disease severity and the rapidity and degree of responsiveness. Good response rates were seen in one series with much lower corticosteroid doses (prednisolone 0.75 mg/kg for 4 weeks; 0.5 mg/kg for 4 weeks; 20 mg daily for 4 weeks; 10 mg daily for 6 weeks; 5 mg daily for 6 weeks), relapse rates were not excessive, and the long-term outcome was not adversely affected by rapid withdrawal of prednisolone prior to relapse. Rigorous adherence to traditional regimens in patients with limited disease or a good initial response may therefore result in steroid overtreatment.

Disease which is refractory to corticosteroids may respond to immunosuppressive therapy, such as azathioprine or cyclophosphamide (given orally or intravenously). However, in other cases nonresponsiveness indicates supervening interstitial fibrosis, seen more often in secondary organizing pneumonia, especially that of drug-induced or rheumatological disease. Treatment goals must be adjusted accordingly: once an organizing pneumonia component has been suppressed, prevention of disease progression may become the main therapeutic goal.

Acute fulminating organizing pneumonia rarely presents as the adult respiratory distress syndrome (ARDS), but with typical organizing pneumonia at biopsy or autopsy. Mechanical ventilation is often required. Such patients are treated with high doses of corticosteroids, with cyclophosphamide most commonly added in those who fail to respond. Rapid progression to death may occur and the overall mortality rate in this group exceeds 50%.

Prognosis

In typical cryptogenic organizing pneumonia the prognosis is usually good, with an overall mortality of less than 5%. Relapses occur in up to 60% of cases as corticosteroids are reduced or stopped, but such relapses respond well to reinstitution of high-dose treatment. A few cases have a poor outcome, with adverse prognostic determinants including a reticular imaging pattern suggestive of pulmonary fibrosis, a prominent neutrophilia or lack of lymphocytosis on bronchoalveolar lavage, associated connective tissue disease, and histological features of interstitial fibrosis with architectural remodelling of lung parenchyma. Treatment is usually effective in preventing progression of supervening pulmonary fibrosis, but in occasional cases the disease progresses inexorably to a fatal outcome. This is seen more commonly in organizing pneumonia occurring secondary to other disorders, which had a 5-year survival of only 44% in one series.

Unifocal organizing pneumonia presenting as a solitary pulmonary nodule has a uniformly good outcome, with no reported recurrences. The diagnosis is usually made following resection for suspected malignancy.

Follicular bronchiolitis

Follicular bronchiolitis results from polyclonal hyperplasia of lymphoid follicles with formation of germinal centres within the bronchiolar walls. These cause airway obstruction by encroaching upon or obliterating the bronchiolar lumen. Follicular bronchiolitis may occur as an isolated or primary phenomenon, but more commonly arises secondary to a number of other conditions such as chronic aspiration or infection (bronchiectasis, cystic fibrosis, lung abscess), tumours, and immune deficiencies including HIV. It is also frequently associated with collagen vascular diseases such as rheumatoid arthritis, systemic sclerosis, and Sjögren's syndrome. When a secondary phenomenon, its clinical presence may be masked by concomitant bronchial or alveolar disease.

Patients usually present with progressive breathlessness, cough, and symptoms of recurrent respiratory infection. They usually have inspiratory crackles, but no finger clubbing. The chest radiograph shows diffuse small nodular or reticulonodular infiltrates but may be normal. High-resolution CT invariably reveals centrilobular nodules less than 3 mm diameter. Peribronchial and subpleural nodules may also occur and patchy, nonsegmental ground-glass opacification is common. Lung function tests may show a restrictive, obstructive, or mixed pattern. Diagnosis of primary follicular bronchiolitis often requires a surgical lung biopsy.

Treatment involves optimum management of any underlying condition. Primary follicular bronchiolitis usually improves with corticosteroids, but other immunosuppressive agents such as azathioprine or methotrexate may be required. The prognosis is generally good, although in younger patients the disease may progress.

Diffuse panbronchiolitis

Diffuse panbronchiolitis is a chronic obstructive pulmonary disease of unknown aetiology that was first described in 1969. The pathological features are a triad of bronchiolocentric inflammation, lymphoid hyperplasia, and an accumulation of interstitial foam cells in the walls of respiratory bronchioles, adjacent alveolar ducts and alveoli. There may also be luminal collection of neutrophils, but the typical concentric submucosal fibrosis of obliterative bronchiolitis is not a feature.

Diffuse panbronchiolitis is relatively common in Asia, particularly amongst the Japanese and to a lesser extent Chinese and Koreans, although occasional cases have also been described in Europe and the United States of America. In Japan it is associated with HLA Bw54, an antigen unique to east Asian ethnic groups, whilst in Korea the association appears to be with HLA A11. This suggests the gene or genes conferring susceptibility lie in the class 1 region between the *HLA-A* and *HLA-B* loci. Any age may be affected, but the mean is around 50 years, and most patients have never smoked. There is a male preponderance of over 2:1. There have been reports of diffuse panbronchiolitis complicating ulcerative colitis and adult T-cell leukaemia.

Patients present with subacute symptoms of cough productive of purulent sputum, dyspnoea, and sometimes weight loss. Up to 75% have chronic sinusitis, which often predates chest symptoms. On auscultation there are widespread coarse crackles and wheeze, but finger clubbing is unusual.

Common features on chest radiography are ill-defined nodules up to 5 mm in diameter, symmetrically distributed and most prominent in the lung bases. There may also be hyperinflation and in the later stages changes of bronchiectasis become evident. On high-resolution CT centrilobular nodules are evident, often with distal branching structures giving a 'tree in bud' appearance. Thickened, ectatic bronchioles are also seen, and in more advanced disease there is bronchiectasis and air trapping. Pulmonary function tests show an obstructive or mixed picture, and transfer factor is normal or sometimes reduced. Most patients show resting hypoxaemia. Laboratory investigations are nonspecific, but there may be elevated IgA, IgG, and cold agglutinins, and low titres of rheumatoid factor and antinuclear antibodies. In early disease sputum cultures grow *Haemophilus influenzae* or *Steptococcus pneumoniae*, but later *Pseudomonas aeruginosa* predominates. Diagnostic lung biopsy is rarely necessary in countries where the prevalence is high, but may be required elsewhere in the world where the condition is rare.

Without treatment patients with diffuse panbronchiolitis run a deteriorating course punctuated by episodic superinfections and have 50% mortality at 5 years. However, survival has been transformed by the use of long-term, low dose erythromycin therapy (400–600 mg daily), which improves lung function and CT appearances and extends 10-year survival to 90%. This improved survival is independent of the presence of *Pseudomonas* infection, suggesting that macrolide therapy works by an anti-inflammatory effect.

Further reading

Cordier J-F (2000). Organising pneumonia. *Thorax*, **55**, 318–28.

du Bois RM, Geddes DM (1991). Obliterative bronchiolitis, cryptogenic organizing pneumonitis and bronchiolitis obliterans organizing pneumonia: three names for two different conditions. *Eur Respir J*, **4**, 774–5.

Epler GR, et al. (1985). Bronchiolitis obliterans organizing pneumonia. *N Engl J Med*, **312**, 152–8.

Howling SJ, et al. (1999). Follicular bronchiolitis: thin-section CT and histologic findings. *Radiology*, **212**, 637–42.

Keicho N, et al. (1998). Contribution of HLA genes to genetic predisposition in diffuse panbronchiolitis. *Am J Respir Crit Care Med*, **158**, 846–50.

Kudoh S, et al. (1998). Improved survival in patients with diffuse panbronchiolitis treated with low-dose erythromycin. *Am J Respir Crit Care Med*, **157**, 1829–32.

Lazor R, et al. (2000). Cryptogenic organizing pneumonia: characteristics of relapses in a series of 48 patients. *Am J Respir Crit Care Med*, **162**, 571–7.

Lohr RH, Boland BJ, Douglas WW (1997). Organizing pneumonia. Features and prognosis of cryptogenic, secondary and focal variants. *Arch Intern Med*, **157**, 1323–9.

Muller NL, Miller RR (1995). Diseases of the bronchioles: CT and histopathologic findings. *Radiology*, **196**, 3–12.

Myers JL, Colby TV (1993). Pathologic manifestations of bronchiolitis, constrictive bronchiolitis, cryptogenic organizing pneumonia, and diffuse panbronchiolitis. *Clin Chest Med*, **14**, 611–12.

Ryu JH (2006). Classification and approach to bronchiolar diseases. *Curr Opin Pulmon Dis*, **12**, 145–51.

Wells AU (2001). Cryptogenic organizing pneumonia. *Semin Resp Crit Care Med*, **22**, 449–59.

Worthy SA, et al. (1997). Mosaic attenuation pattern on thin-section CT scans of the lung: differentiation among infiltrative lung, airway, and vascular diseases as a cause. *Radiology*, **205**, 465–70.

18.11.4 The lung in autoimmune rheumatic disorders

A.U. Wells and H.R. Branley

Essentials

Lung complications occur in all rheumatological disorders, but their frequency and type vary strikingly between different systemic diseases. Greater routine use of high-resolution CT and echocardiography means that interstitial lung disease and pulmonary vascular disease are increasingly recognized, which can create clinical difficulty in distinguishing between subclinical involvement and significant disease.

Particular autoimmune disorders

Systemic sclerosis—pulmonary function is abnormal in up to 90% of cases. Lung disease usually consists of nonspecific interstitial pneumonia (NSIP) and is present on chest radiography at some stage in most patients. Both isolated pulmonary vascular disease and secondary pulmonary hypertension occur. Lung cancer is increased in prevalence. Lung and pulmonary vascular disease are now the main cause of morbidity and mortality.

Polymyositis/dermatomyositis—interstitial lung disease, usually with organizing pneumonia or NSIP, is the commonest pulmonary complication. Aspiration pneumonia is a frequent feature of advanced disease and a common cause of death.

Rheumatoid arthritis—is associated with a wide range of pleuro-pulmonary complications including interstitial lung disease (with usual interstitial pneumonia and NSIP of equal prevalence), organizing pneumonia, bronchiolitis obliterans, bronchiectasis, pleural effusion, pulmonary vasculitis (rarely), and pulmonary rheumatoid nodules.

Sjögren's syndrome—interstitial lung disease takes the form of fibrotic NSIP or lymphocytic interstitial pneumonia. Tracheobronchial disease can be in the form of loss of mucus secretion in the trachea (xerotrachea), bronchi and bronchioles, or (less frequently) lymphocytic bronchiolitis.

Systemic lupus erythematosus—clinically significant interstitial lung disease affects about 10% of patients, with NSIP the usual form. Acute lupus pneumonitis is an uncommon life-threatening disorder. Diffuse alveolar hemorrhage due to capillaritis can occur. The 'shrinking lung syndrome' is thought to be due to respiratory muscle weakness. Pulmonary hypertension is increasing recognized. Pleural disease is common, affecting 50% of patients at some time.

Management

Is treatment required on account of lung disease?—it is critical that high-resolution CT findings and lung function tests are reconciled, with clear definition of all complications and deconstruction of the functional defect. Most clinicians regard $D_L\text{CO}$ levels below 65% of predicted normal as indicative of clinically significant disease. Maximal exercise testing is often useful in marginal cases, when careful monitoring with regular repetition of pulmonary function tests is wise.

Introduction of treatment for lung disease—the threshold for introducing therapy is reduced by three considerations: (1) the risk of progression of lung disease appears to be greatest early in the course of systemic disease; (2) severe functional impairment has consistently been associated with a higher mortality because it is indicative of a previously progressive course and an increased likelihood of future disease progression, also because loss of pulmonary reserve implies that the symptomatic consequences of a further preventable loss of lung function may be substantial; and (3) observed disease progression is a major indication for treatment.

Therapeutic options—when inflammatory disease predominates, as in organizing pneumonia or lymphocytic interstitial pneumonia, it is appropriate to treat with high-dose steroid therapy, or with intense immunosuppressive therapy in refractory cases. Treatment decisions are less straightforward in predominantly fibrotic disease.

Introduction

Lung complications occur in all rheumatological disorders, but their frequency and type vary strikingly between different systemic diseases. With greater routine use of high-resolution CT and echocardiography, interstitial lung disease and pulmonary vascular disease are increasingly recognized, although the detection of limited abnormalities poses difficulties for clinicians who must now distinguish between subclinical involvement and clinically significant disease. The presence or absence of exertional dyspnoea is often misleading as musculoskeletal limitation may mask respiratory symptoms or, alternatively, may cause exercise intolerance without lung pathology, due to the increased work associated with inefficient locomotion. Furthermore, interstitial lung disease precedes the onset of systemic disease in some cases, although typical autoantibody profiles are often diagnostic.

The range of lung histological patterns in rheumatological disease mirrors that seen in the idiopathic interstitial pneumonias, but processes are frequently admixed, with interstitial disease commonly associated with prominent lymphoid follicles (Fig. 18.11.4.1) or pleural thickening (Fig. 18.11.4.2). Nonspecific interstitial pneumonia (NSIP), usual interstitial pneumonia (UIP), and organizing pneumonia are the most frequent findings, with lymphocytic interstitial pneumonia, acute interstitial pneumonia, and smoking-related disorders (desquamative interstitial pneumonia, respiratory bronchiolitis with associated interstitial lung disease) occurring in occasional cases. However, unlike the idiopathic interstitial pneumonias (see Chapters 18.11.1 and 18.11.2), NSIP is the most frequent pattern, especially in systemic sclerosis and polymyositis/dermatomyositis, partly accounting for the better prognosis consistently reported in lung involvement in rheumatological disorders compared to idiopathic disease in which UIP predominates. However, even in rheumatoid arthritis, in which UIP and NSIP are approximately equally prevalent, the outcome is usually better than in idiopathic fibrotic interstitial pneumonia for reasons that are not well understood.

The clinical features of lung disease in particular rheumatological disorders will now be discussed, followed by consideration of key problems and treatments.

Systemic sclerosis

The diagnostic criteria for systemic sclerosis are detailed in Chapter 19.11.3. Pulmonary involvement (Table 18.11.4.1), whether due to lung or pulmonary vascular disease, is now the major source of morbidity and mortality.

Interstitial lung disease

Lung disease, which consists of NSIP in most cases (Fig. 18.11.4.3), occasionally precedes systemic symptoms. Exertional dyspnoea (reported by over 50% of patients at some stage of disease) is the commonest presenting feature. Nonproductive cough is less frequent and pleuritic chest pain is uncommon. Digital clubbing is rare and should raise the suspicion of underlying malignancy. Fine, predominantly basal 'Velcro' crackles are present. Raynaud's phenomenon is a useful clue to the underlying systemic diagnosis, which—in limited disease—is confirmed by capillaroscopy, digital thermography, strongly positive antinuclear antibodies and, in most cases, the presence of the Scl 70 anti-DNA topoisomerase autoantibody.

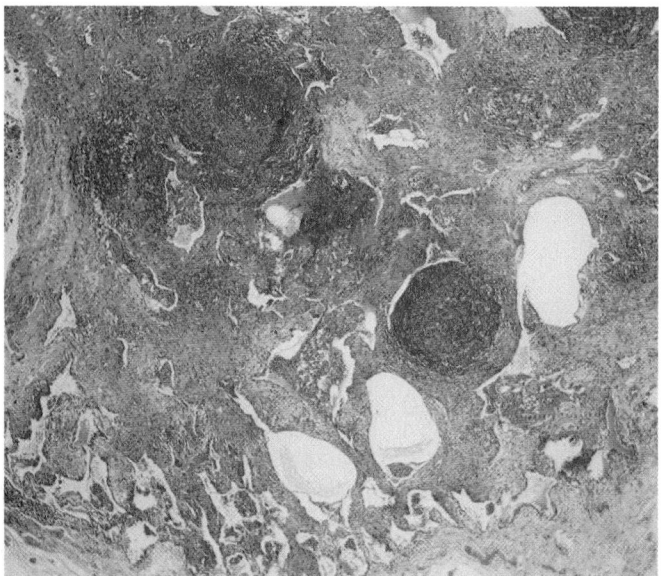

Fig. 18.11.4.1 A case of rheumatoid arthritis involving the lung, with diffuse interstitial fibrosis (fibrotic nonspecific interstitial pneumonia) and prominent lymphoid follicles (reactive germinal centres): an association that is typical of rheumatoid lung.

Interstitial lung disease is present on chest radiography at some stage in most patients and may be associated with oesophageal dilatation. Lung function is abnormal in up to 90% of cases, but reduction in carbon monoxide diffusing capacity ($D_L$co), the most frequent functional defect, does not in isolation discriminate between interstitial lung disease and pulmonary vasculopathy. Bronchoalveolar lavage is often performed to exclude underlying infection and as a guide to prognosis (with a neutrophilia linked to a poor outcome), although this remains contentious. In NSIP and UIP, granulocytes and lymphocytes are often present in excess, whereas a lymphocytosis is the rule in organizing pneumonia, with a granulocytosis usually indicative of supervening fibrosis.

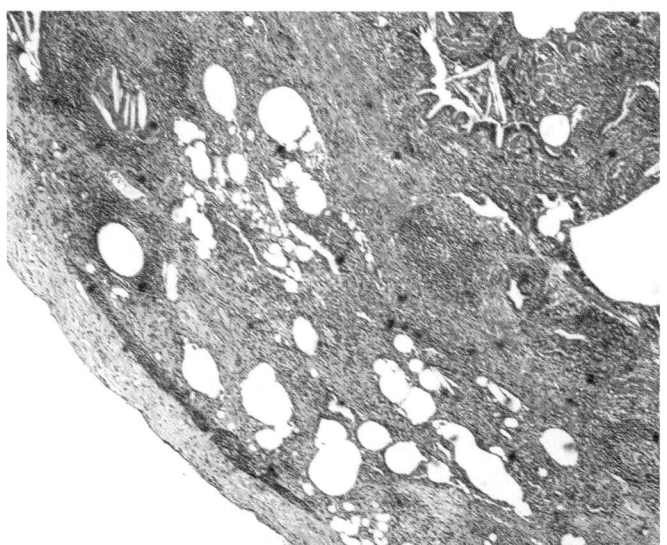

Fig. 18.11.4.2 A case of systemic lupus erythematosis showing thickening of the visceral pleura in association with fibrotic nonspecific interstitial pneumonia.

Pulmonary vascular disease

Both isolated pulmonary vascular disease and secondary pulmonary hypertension (complicating extensive interstitial lung disease) occur. Isolated pulmonary vascular disease takes the form of concentric fibrosis, with ablation of arteriolar intima and media but no vasculitic element. This mainly complicates limited systemic sclerosis (including the CREST syndrome—calcinosis, Raynaud's phenomenon, esophageal dysmotility, sclerodactyly, telangiectasiae) and is typically associated with the anticentromere autoantibody. There is usually no evidence of interstitial lung disease on chest radiography, high-resolution CT, or bronchoalveolar lavage, and lung function tests generally show an isolated fall in $D_L$co or a disproportionate reduction in $D_L$co in patients with coexisting lung involvement. Doppler echocardiography is often diagnostic and is widely used as a screening test, but is insensitive in early disease because of the large reserve in the pulmonary vascular bed. Isolated pulmonary vascular disease is a common cause of mortality and is partly responsible for the very poor prognosis associated with marked reduction in $D_L$co in clinical series.

Other pulmonary complications

Lung cancer is increased in prevalence, even in nonsmokers, with adenocarcinoma more frequent than other histological subtypes. Extrapulmonic restriction due to severe cutaneous involvement is an extremely rare finding. Pleural disease and organizing pneumonia have been reported occasionally. Despite the fact that oesophageal dysfunction is common, aspiration pneumonia seldom occurs.

Polymyositis/dermatomyositis

Diagnostic criteria for polymyositis and dermatomyositis are described in Chapter 19.11.7. Pulmonary disease (Table 18.11.4.1), occurring in up to 60% of patients, is the most frequent cause of death.

Interstitial lung disease

Interstitial lung disease is the commonest pulmonary complication of polymyositis/dermatomyositis. Although the presentation is usually with organizing pneumonia or NSIP, a rapidly progressive form of acute pneumonitis occurs more frequently than in other rheumatological disorders. Lung disease (usually organizing pneumonia) precedes systemic disease in up to one-third of patients. Pulmonary capillaritis resulting in haemoptysis has occasionally been reported. Exertional dyspnoea is a common presenting symptom and orthopnoea is occasionally prominent, especially when myopathy is severe. Cough is a frequent feature, especially in organizing pneumonia, but is seldom severe. Haemoptysis and pleuritic chest pain are rare. In fibrotic disease, fine basal 'Velcro' crackles are usual, and these are variably present in organizing pneumonia. Organizing pneumonia is often obvious on chest radiography, but high-resolution CT is frequently required to demonstrate the characteristic combination of patchy consolidation and fibrotic disease (a peripheral reticular pattern). Lung function tests usually show a restrictive ventilatory defect with a reduction in $D_L$co. When reduced lung volumes are associated with preservation of $D_L$co and an increase in the gas transfer index (Kco), extrapulmonic restriction due to respiratory muscle weakness should be suspected. Bronchoalveolar lavage is useful in discriminating between infection and autoimmune organizing pneumonia,

Table 18.11.4.1 Pulmonary complications in autoimmune rheumatic disorders, with the range in prevalence, from rare (±) to frequent (+++), indicated semiquantitatively

	Rheumatoid arthritis	Systemic sclerosis	Polymyositis/ dermatomyositis	Systemic lupus erythematosus	Sjögren's syndrome
Fibrotic lung disease	++	+++	++	+	+
Organizing pneumonia	++	±	++	±	±
Lymphocytic interstitial pneumonitis	±		±	±	++
Constrictive (obliterative) bronchiolitis	+		±	±	
Bronchiectasis	++			±	±
Pleural disease	+++	±	±	+++	±
Respiratory muscle weakness		±	++	++	
Pulmonary hypertension		+++	+	++	±
Diffuse alveolar haemorrhage		±	±	+	

especially when immunosuppressive therapy has previously been instituted for systemic disease, but has little value in prognostic evaluation. Autoantibodies to aminoacyl-tRNA synthetases, especially Jo-1 (antihistidyl tRNA synthetase) are often present when prominent inflammatory myopathy coexists with diffuse lung disease, but are found in less than 5% of patients without diffuse lung disease. Testing for Jo-1 autoantibodies is a useful screening procedure in patients with aggressive or relapsing idiopathic organizing pneumonia, especially when there is supervening lung fibrosis.

Other pulmonary manifestations

Aspiration pneumonia, a very frequent feature of advanced disease and a common cause of death, should also be considered in earlier disease if there is upper airway/pharyngeal muscle weakness, especially when the dependent lung regions are selectively involved. Respiratory muscle weakness, occurring in up to 5% of patients, may occasionally lead to hypercapnic respiratory failure but requires muscle function testing for confirmation in milder cases. Mild pulmonary hypertension is increasingly recognized, although

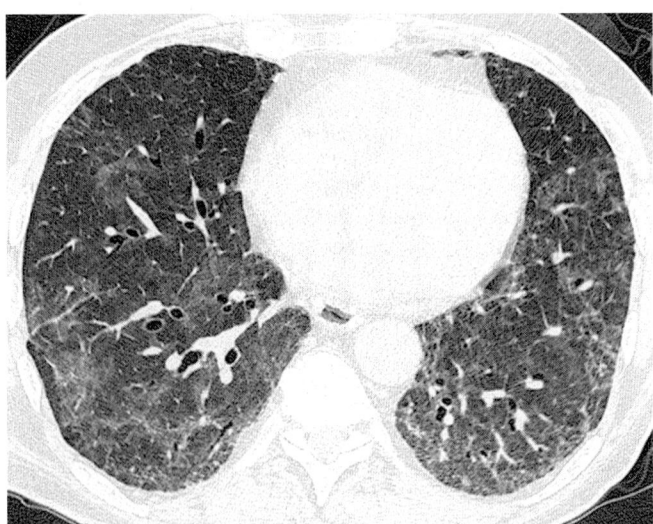

Fig. 18.11.4.3 High-resolution CT scan in a patient with systemic sclerosis. There is prominent ground-glass attenuation, admixed with fine reticular abnormalities: these appearances are typical of nonspecific interstitial pneumonia.

the exact prevalence is uncertain, but vascular involvement is generally self-limited.

Rheumatoid arthritis

Diagnostic criteria for rheumatoid arthritis are detailed in Chapter 19.5. Pleuropulmonary complications (Table 18.11.4.1) are more variable than in other rheumatological disorders.

Interstitial lung disease

Interstitial lung disease has a male predominance (male:female 3:1) and is associated with high titres of rheumatoid factor, the presence of rheumatoid nodules, a history of smoking, and HLA B8 and HLA Dw3 positivity. Although there are discrepant findings in a number of series, it appears that UIP and NSIP are approximately equal in prevalence, with organizing pneumonia less frequent. Interstitial lung disease precedes the onset of systemic disease in about 15% of cases.

Exertional dyspnoea is the most frequent presenting symptom, with nonproductive cough also common, especially in patients with sicca symptoms. Bilateral, predominantly basal 'Velcro' crackles are usual and digital clubbing is more prevalent than in other rheumatological diseases. Radiologically overt interstitial lung disease, usually with a basal predominance, was present in less than 5% of cases in three large chest radiographic series. High-resolution CT often shows limited interstitial abnormalities when chest radiographs are normal, although the significance of 'subclinical' disease has yet to be ascertained. In established disease, a restrictive ventilatory defect is associated with reduced $D_L$co levels, but an isolated reduction of $D_L$co is seen in up to 40% of unselected rheumatoid arthritis patients. As in other rheumatological disorders, bronchoalveolar lavage may be very useful when opportunistic infection is suspected, but it has limited routine value when disease is overtly fibrotic.

Organizing pneumonia

Organizing pneumonia more commonly mimics infectious pneumonia in rheumatoid arthritis than in polymyositis/dermatomyositis. Cough and exertional dyspnoea are commonly accompanied by fever and weight loss. There is multifocal consolidation on chest radiography and high-resolution CT. Lung function tests show a restrictive defect and reduced $D_L$co, often associated with disproportionate hypoxia due to shunting through consolidated lung. A lymphocytosis is usual on bronchalveolar lavage, with a granulocytosis usually indicative of underlying fibrotic disease. Transbronchial or surgical lung biopsy reveals acini filled with loose connective tissue and a variable inflammatory infiltrate. Organizing pneumonia responds well to corticosteroid therapy in most cases.

Bronchiolitis obliterans

This rare but often lethal bronchiolar disorder usually presents with exertional dyspnoea, often with a component of wheeze and nonproductive cough. The breath sounds are usually quiet, with inspiratory 'squawks' a very specific sign of small-airways disease. The chest radiograph is normal or shows hyperinflation. high-resolution CT shows a 'mosaic' pattern which is more obvious on expiratory images and represents regional gas trapping. In most cases the lung function defect is obstructive, although there is occasionally a mixed obstructive/restrictive pattern. Measures of gas transfer ($D_L$co and Kco) are preserved provided the forced expiratory volume in 1 s (FEV_1) exceeds 1 litre. Preservation of gas transfer is especially useful in discriminating between obliterative bronchiolitis and emphysema, in which both $D_L$co and Kco are significantly reduced. Bronchiolitis obliterans is characterized histologically by fibrous destruction and ablation of the terminal bronchiolar wall by granulation tissue. Although a fatal outcome was almost invariable in early reports, the increasing use of high-resolution CT has disclosed many patients with milder disease in whom the course is often indolent.

An association with the use of penicillamine was postulated in the first descriptions of obliterative bronchiolitis 20 to 30 years ago. Based on subsequent case reports and small series this is probably a true association, but it should be stressed that more cases of obliterative bronchiolitis are seen in patients with rheumatoid arthritis who have not used penicillamine than in those who have.

Bronchiectasis

Bronchiectasis is more prevalent in rheumatoid arthritis than in other rheumatological diseases. From a definitive literature review of 289 rheumatoid arthritis patients with associated bronchiectasis reported since 1928, it is clear that the condition precedes the onset of systemic disease in some cases. Before the routine use of high-resolution CT bronchiectasis was generally diagnosed in patients presenting with chronic purulent sputum production. However, it is increasingly apparent that asymptomatic ('dry') bronchiectasis is extremely common, being present on high-resolution CT in 30% of 50 rheumatoid arthritis patients with normal chest radiographs on prospective evaluation. The high-resolution CT overlap between bronchiectasis and obliterative bronchiolitis should be stressed. Bronchiectasis and a 'mosaic' pattern may coexist in both disorders, and bronchiectasis is often present in rheumatoid arthritis patients with interstitial lung disease.

Pleural disease

Pleural involvement is present at autopsy in about 50% of cases, but only 20% of patients experience pleuritic pain at some stage and most pleural effusions are found incidentally on chest radiography. Clinically overt pleural effusions occur in less than 5% of patients, usually in males, but evidence of pre-existing pleural disease is found on screening chest radiography in up to 20%. Pleural disease has been linked to the presence of rheumatoid nodules but not to more severe systemic disease. Symptoms are confined to a minority of cases and generally consist of pleuritic pain and prominent fever, often necessitating the exclusion of empyema. Effusions may occasionally develop acutely in association with pericarditis or exacerbations of arthritis. Dyspnoea may result from pulmonary compression when effusions are large, especially when there is underlying interstitial lung disease. The fluid is exudative, with a low glucose level, a low pH, and usually a predominant lymphocytosis. The most frequent histological finding is replacement of the normal mesothelial cell covering by a pseudostratified layer of epithelioid cells, with focal multinucleated giant cells and regular small papillae containing branching capillaries, but no necrosis or granulomata. These findings are pathognomonic for rheumatoid pleuritis when present, but histological appearances are often nonspecific. Some cases respond well to corticosteroid therapy, but more often remission is at best partial.

Pulmonary vasculitis

Pulmonary vasculitis is a surprisingly uncommon complication of rheumatoid arthritis given the relatively high prevalence of systemic vasculitis in the disease. However, it is likely that pulmonary vasculitis is not detected in many cases as the diagnosis is often elusive and requires a surgical lung biopsy. Diffuse alveolar haemorrhage has been reported in a handful of cases.

Pulmonary rheumatoid nodules

These are present on chest radiography in less than 1% of patients and are usually associated with subcutaneous rheumatoid nodules. Caplan's syndrome consists of the association of pulmonary nodules, especially cavitating nodules, with coal miner's pneumoconiosis. Single nodules in cigarette smokers often require histological confirmation of the diagnosis (by means of percutaneous needle or surgical biopsy) as malignancy cannot be excluded noninvasively. Nodules may fluctuate in size, waxing and waning with variations in underlying rheumatoid activity, and can reach 5–10 cm in diameter. Usually nodules are asymptomatic and found incidentally on chest radiography, but occasionally nodules cavitate or rupture, giving rise to haemoptyis, or pneumothoax when subpleural. Multiple nodules occasionally occur, with respiratory failure a reported complication of intense nodular infiltration.

Other pulmonary manifestations

Nonproductive cough due to secondary Sjögren's syndrome is not uncommon in rheumatoid arthritis and may result from either impaction of viscid secretions within small airways or from a lymphocytic bronchiolitis, often associated with enlargement of lymphoid follicles. Full-blown follicular bronchiolitis is a rare disorder (see Chapter 18.11.3), in which reticulonodular chest radiographic appearances are often suggestive of interstitial lung disease and lung function tests may be restrictive or obstructive. Unlike obliterative bronchiolitis, follicular bronchiolitis often responds to corticosteroid therapy. Lymphocytic interstitial pneumonia is a rare benign lymphoproliferative disorder which may be limited or extensive, presents as an interstitial lung disease, and is variably responsive to corticosteroids. Lower respiratory tract infection is increased in frequency in rheumatoid arthritis, especially in advanced disease. Bronchopneumonia is a common terminal event, accounting for 15 to 20% of deaths.

Sjögren's syndrome

The diagnostic criteria for Sjögren's syndrome are detailed in Chapter 19.11.6. There is evidence of pulmonary abnormalities (Table 18.11.4.1) in about one-quarter of cases, but disease is usually self-limited and seldom progresses to severe disability or death.

Interstitial lung disease

Parenchymal disease, once thought to consist exclusively of lymphocytic infiltration (lymphocytic interstitial pneumonia) based on historical series, occurs in up to 10% of patients. However, it is increasingly recognized that clinically significant disease more often consists of fibrotic NSIP (with UIP very seldom reported). Interstitial lung disease is often asymptomatic but may declare itself with cough or exertional dyspnoea. The findings are nonspecific, consisting of crackles on auscultation, reticular or reticulonodular abnormalities on chest radiography, and a restrictive ventilatory defect associated with a reduction in $D_L$co. This presentation is common to lymphocytic interstitial pneumonia and fibrotic disease, but high-resolution CT often discriminates usefully between these processes. Ground-glass attenuation is prominent in both disorders, but fibrotic NSIP is characterized by coexisting admixed reticular abnormalities and traction bronchiectasis. Lymphocytic interstial pneumonitis not infrequently evolved to lymphoma in older series, but it is possible that in some cases modern diagnostic technqiues would have established that lymphoma was present throughout. Extrapulmonary lymphoma is also increased in prevalence in Sjögren's syndrome and is probably as frequent as pulmonary lymphoma. Lymphoma often mimics organizing pneumonia, which has occasionally been reported in Sjögren's syndrome.

Tracheobronchial disease

Tracheobronchial disease may take two forms. The more frequent disorder consists of loss of mucus secretion in the trachea (xerotrachea), bronchi, and bronchioles. Xerotrachea occurs in up to 25% of patients with primary Sjögren's syndrome in older series, but may be less prevalent with the increasing recognition of milder variants of the syndrome. The histological picture consists of atrophy of tracheobronchial mucous glands, with or without a lymphoplasmocytic infiltrate. Less frequently, airway disease is due to a lymphocytic bronchiolitis, and occasionally there is considerable enlargement of lymphoid follicles (follicular bronchiolitis). Both xerotrachea and lymphocytic bronchiolitis present with an unremitting dry cough. Endobronchial inflammation is often obvious at bronchoscopy and there is an increased prevalence of bronchial hyper-responsiveness, reported in 40 to 60% of patients with Sjögren's syndrome, and studies of airflow at low lung volumes in unselected patients disclose a high prevalence of small-airway disease. The increased viscidity of secretions results in a high prevalence of secondary infection and in some patients the predominant feature is recurrent episodes of bronchopneumonia. Lymphocytic bronchiolitis usually responds to oral or inhaled corticosteroid therapy, but the increased risk of oral candidiasis in Sjögren's syndrome needs to be kept in mind. Xerotrachea responds variably to nebulized saline.

Systemic lupus erythematosus

The diagnostic criteria for systemic lupus erythematosus (SLE) are detailed in Chapter 19.11.2. Pleuropulmonary manifestations are listed in Table 18.11.4.1.

Diffuse lung disease

Although limited interstitial fibrosis is found at autopsy in up to 70% of patients, it is likely that this represents postinflammatory sequelae in most cases. Clinically significant interstitial lung disease is present in less than 5% of patients at the onset of systemic disease, and develops in a further 5% during follow-up. The clinical presentation closely resembles that of interstitial lung disease in other rheumatological disorders and typically includes dyspnoea, cough, predominantly basal crackles, a restrictive lung function defect or isolated reduction in $D_L$co, and predominantly basal reticulonodular abnormalities on chest radiography. There are no definitive reports of typical high-resolution CT appearances, although there is a high prevalence of limited sub-clinical interstitial abnormalities. The most common histological pattern is NSIP, although UIP has also been reported (Fig. 18.11.4.2).

Acute lupus pneumonitis is an uncommon life-threatening disorder, seen in less than 2% of patients, but with a mortality rate despite treatment of up to 50% once respiratory failure has developed. It may resemble organizing pneumonia, which is very infrequent in SLE. It is believed by some that acute lupus pneumonitis represents an aberrant immunological response to infection, facilitated by the intrinsic immune defect of the systemic disease.

Extrapulmonary restriction

Extrapulmonary restriction in SLE takes the form of the 'shrinking lung syndrome', consisting of a marked reduction in lung volume on chest radiography in association with a restrictive functional defect, preservation of $D_L$co, and a marked increase in Kco. The lung interstitium is normal and the disorder is thought to represent respiratory muscle weakness, especially diaphragmatic weakness. The syndrome is usually self limited, although producing severe exercise limitation in more advanced cases. Improvements have been reported with corticosteroid or immunosuppresssive therapy, but these appear to be unpredictable and there is no other efficacious treatment.

Diffuse alveolar hemorrhage

Diffuse alveolar hemorrhage due to capillaritis occurs more frequently than in other rheumatological conditions but is rare in SLE. Typically, patients present with subacute or acute dyspnoea and extensive infiltrates on chest radiography. Haemoptysis is occasionally torrential but is more often minimal or absent, even when there is extensive intra-alveolar hemorrhage. The presentation is similar to those of acute lupus pneumonitis and opportunistic infection, especially in the absence of haemoptysis. The diagnosis is best made by bronchoalveolar lavage, when increasingly heavy blood-staining is typical as the distal airways are lavaged in cases without overt endobronchial haemorrhage. Diffuse alveolar haemorrhage is life-threatening with a mortality of up to 50% in patients with respiratory failure. There are no definitive treatment data, but empirical treatments have included intravenous corticosteroid therapy, intravenous cyclophosphamide and plasmapheresis.

Pulmonary hypertension

Pulmonary hypertension, once regarded as rare, is encountered with increasing frequency. In early reports, largely containing patients with severe disease, the 2-year mortality approached 50%. However, with the increasing use of echocardiography, subclinical pulmonary vascular abnormalities are detected in 10% of patients.

In some cases associated with Raynaud's phenomenon it appears that vasoconstriction with secondary irreversible damage is the dominant pathophysiological mechanism. In other cases vasculitis predominates, and this may respond strikingly to corticosteroid therapy or intravenous cyclophosphamide, even in advanced disease. Thromboembolism or microthrombosis in small intrapulmonary arterioles also occur in many cases, especially when antiphospholipid antibodies are present. It is often impossible to determine which mechanism predominates as surgical biopsy is contraindicated by severe pulmonary hypertension. Treatment is empirical, consisting of immunosuppression, anticoagulation, and vasodilator agents such as bosentan.

Pleural disease

Pleural disease is common in SLE. There is clinical or radiographic evidence of pleural involvement in 20% of patients at the onset of systemic disease, and at least 50% have overt pleural involvement at some time. Pleural disease is often detected on incidental chest radiography in asymptomatic patients, but in other cases pleuritic pain is recurrent or intractable. The pleural fluid is usually serosanguinous and exudative, with a high neutrophil content in patients with pleurisy, but a predominant lymphocytosis is the rule in chronic disease and in some cases effusions are hemorrhagic. Corticosteroid therapy is usually much more efficacious than in rheumatoid arthritis.

Relapsing polychondritis

Relapsing polychondritis is described in Chapter 18.5.1. Respiratory involvement accounts for about 10% of deaths and takes the form of obstruction of the glottis, trachea, and bronchi, leading to airway stricture, collapse, and distal infection. Pulmonary vasculitis is common but often subclinical, and pulmonary hypertension is rare. Parenchymal disease seldom occurs in isolated relapsing polychondritis, but many other autoimmune conditions, including most rheumatological disorders, are associated with relapsing polychondritis and may be complicated by interstitial lung disease. Lung function tests typically show severe airflow obstruction due to airway collapse, with reduced maximal inspiratory and expiratory flow representing extrathoracic and intrathoracic airway involvement respectively. Airway abnormalities are prominent on chest radiography, with bronchiectasis and bronchial wall thickening evident on high-resolution CT. Bronchoscopy has been reported to trigger fatal airway obstruction and should be undertaken with caution. The diagnosis may be made using dynamic CT scanning showing collapse of the larger airways on inspiratory manoeuvres. However, definitive diagnosis requires biopsy, which often shows characteristic features in extrapulmonary cartilaginous areas. Immunosuppression is sometimes effective in preventing disease progression, and mechanical stenting may be life-saving in advanced destructive disease.

Ankylosing spondylitis

Ankylosing spondylitis is described in Chapter 19.6. Interstitial lung disease is a rare complication, identified on chest radiography in less than 2% of cases, although subclinical interstitial abnormalities are highly prevalent on high-resolution CT, including fibrotic abnormalities and paraseptal emphysema. Fibrobullous lung disease is largely or entirely confined to the upper zones and is usually symmetrical. Fibrotic abnormalities may be more extensive in

occasional patients with severe long-standing spinal disease. Interstitial lung disease does not respond to corticosteroid therapy and immunosuppressive therapy has no recognized role and may predispose to chronic infection. Cavities tend to develop within distorted fibrotic apical tissue and are often colonized by mycobacteria or fungi, especially *Aspergillus fumigatus*. Life-threatening haemoptysis is an occasional complication of intracavitary mycetoma formation. Bronchial artery embolization is sometimes effective, but surgical resection of a mycetoma is generally held to be contraindicated and carries a high mortality, due to postoperative bronchopleural fistula formation and empyema.

Extrapulmonary restriction is more frequent than interstitial lung disease and results from immobilization of the chest wall due to fusion of the costovertebral joints. This complication is often asymptomatic and the lung function defect is mild, perhaps because the diaphragm is able to compensate for chest wall immobility. Exercise tolerance is seldom impaired, provided that an active lifestyle is maintained. Chest-wall fixation increases in prevalence and severity in long-standing disease and does not respond to anti-inflammatory treatment. Management is confined to spinal extension exercises and the maintenance of general fitness with exercise programmes.

Mixed connective tissue disease

In this syndrome there are variable features of SLE, systemic sclerosis, and polymyositis/dermatomyositis in association with high titres of autoantibody directed against the extractable nuclear antigen U1-RNP. However, the diagnosis is often elusive because clinical features evolve as disease progresses and individual criteria may be ephemeral. Pulmonary involvement encompasses the full spectrum of disease seen in systemic sclerosis, polymyositis/dermatomyositis, and SLE, the three most frequent disorders being pleural effusions, interstitial lung disease, and pulmonary hypertension. Pleuritic pain is reported by up to 40% of patients but effusions are typically small and generally remit spontaneously. Interstitial lung disease is even more prevalent and usually mimics the interstitial fibrosis of systemic sclerosis: organizing pneumonia is surprisingly infrequent and, when present, is generally self-limited. Pulmonary vascular disease is well recognized and is occasionally fatal: reported mechanisms include, most commonly, vasoconstriction in association with arteriolar obliteration, as in systemic sclerosis, but also pulmonary vasculitis and pulmonary thromboembolism. Other rare pulmonary complications are those of the dominant rheumatological picture and include respiratory muscle weakness, severe diffuse alveolar haemorrhage, aspiration pneumonia due to pharyngeal dysfunction, and opportunistic infection in patients receiving immunosuppressive therapy. The investigation and management of pulmonary complications is as for the individual rheumatological diseases. Long-term outcome has not been quantified with any precision.

Key clinical problems in interstitial lung disease in patients with rheumatological disorders

Detection of disease

The reported prevalence of interstitial lung disease is critically dependent on which diagnostic modality is used. Rheumatoid arthritis patients without overt lung involvement were found to have interstitial fibrosis in almost one-half of cases in an early biopsy study, yet abnormalities are present on chest radiography in less than 5%. Chest radiography is now known to be insensitive and symptoms are often misleading.

There is an increasing tendency to screen patients with rheumatoid arthritis, systemic sclerosis, and polymyositis/dermatomyositis for interstitial lung disease as lung involvement is most prevalent in these disorders. However, lung function tests are often difficult to interpret, as minor abnormalities, especially isolated reductions in $D_L$co, occur in most patients. Moreover, even normal lung function tests may be misleading: the normal range is wide and may conceal substantial loss of lung function in some cases. Bronchoalveolar lavage was once widely advocated as a means of detecting underlying alveolitis, but abnormalities are present in most patients with systemic sclerosis, ankylosing spondylitis, and Sjögren's syndrome, and are probably equally prevalent in the other rheumatological diseases. Subclinical alveolitis has never been shown to evolve into clinically significant interstitial lung disease and hence this use of bronchoalveolar lavage is largely discredited. High-resolution CT is the most sensitive and reliable means of detecting interstitial lung disease but should probably be reserved for patients with symptoms, chest radiographic abnormalities, or lung function impairment.

Determination of clinically significant disease

The advent of high-resolution CT has undoubtedly helped clinicians greatly in identifying interstitial lung disease, but has led to a separate problem: the identification of limited subclinical abnormalities. Severe interstitial fibrosis is rare in Sjögren's syndrome, SLE, and ankylosing spondylitis, but high-resolution CT abnormalities are present in many patients. In unselected patients with rheumatoid arthritis, interstitial lung disease is evident in 25% of cases, but clinically overt pulmonary fibrosis develops in less than 10%. It is inappropriate to base treatment decisions on high-resolution CT findings in isolation, but the interpretation of lung function tests is often complicated by the coexistence of interstitial lung disease and other processes, especially pulmonary vascular disease and pleural disease.

High-resolution CT findings and lung function tests must be reconciled, with a clear definition of all complications and deconstruction of the functional defect. In this way, the degree of functional impairment ascribable to parenchymal lung disease can usually be approximately apportioned. Except in patients with a severe restrictive ventilatory defect, $D_L$co levels provide the best overall guide to disease severity. Although there is no exact consensus, most clinicians regard $D_L$co levels below 65% of predicted normal as indicative of clinically significant disease. In marginal cases, maximal exercise testing is often useful, as respiratory symptoms may be shown to result from musculoskeletal limitation (i.e. there is no desaturation or widening of the alveolar–arterial oxygen gradient at the limits of exercise). However, there is lingering doubt as to whether abnormalities are clinically significant in many cases and in this situation there is no substitute for careful monitoring, with regular repetition of pulmonary function tests if treatment is not instituted immediately.

Prognostic evaluation and when to treat

The decision as to whether to start treatment is often a very close call. Many patients have intrinsically stable disease and hence the introduction of immunosuppressive therapy in attempt to prevent disease progression is often unnecessary and may result in avoidable drug toxicity. Accurate prognostic evaluation is essential, with treatment ideally reserved for patients at higher risk of progression, but this goal is not straightforward. It is important that the few patients with predominantly inflammatory disease be identified, with a view to therapy aimed at reversing disease and restoring lung function. high-resolution CT plays a significant role in this regard: patients with organizing pneumonia and other forms of inflammatory cell infiltration are readily identifiable from characteristic high-resolution CT patterns. However, most patients have underlying irreversible interstitial fibrosis, most commonly taking the form of fibrotic NSIP. The pattern of disease at surgical biopsy can be an invaluable aide to management in the idiopathic interstitial pneumonias, but has little to offer in this respect in the rheumatological disorders, in which the distinction between NSIP and UIP seems to be less important (except, possibly, in rheumatoid arthritis). The morphological definition of interstitial fibrosis using high-resolution CT has yet to lead to reliable therapeutic recommendations. The presence of a bronchoalveolar lavage neutrophilia in systemic sclerosis is held by some to indicate a worse outcome, but this is not universally accepted as it may merely indicate that disease is extensive and fibrotic.

Given the above, treatment must be based on general principles. The threshold for introducing therapy is reduced by the following three considerations:

- The risk of progression of lung disease appears to be greatest early in the course of systemic disease. In systemic sclerosis this has long been recognized, with the risk of deterioration being highest in the first 4 years. In polymyositis/dermatomyositis acute life-threatening progression of disease is much more prevalent in the first year, especially when lung disease precedes systemic disease. The same principle applies to other rheumatological disorders, although there is a paucity of data.

- Severe functional impairment has consistently been associated with a higher mortality in clinical series of rheumatological disorders. This is best documented in systemic sclerosis, with severe reduction in $D_L$co and severe lung restriction both being malignant prognostic determinants. The severity of disease becomes an increasingly important therapeutic consideration as $D_L$co levels fall below 60% of predicted normal values. Severe disease requires treatment for two reasons. (1) it is indicative of a previously progressive course and an increased likelihood of future disease progression. (2) Loss of pulmonary reserve implies that the symptomatic consequences of a further preventable loss of lung function may be substantial.

- Observed disease progression is a major indication for treatment, even when the systemic disease is long-standing and the functional defect is mild to moderate. In systemic sclerosis, decline in gas transfer over 1 to 3 years is associated with a substantially increase in mortality, although it is sometimes necessary to confirm progression of lung disease (as opposed to worsening of pulmonary vascular disease) using serial high-resolution CT scanning. This is especially the case when the reduction in gas transfer is disproportionate.

Treatment

The treatment of interstitial lung disease in rheumatological disorders has until recently been largely empirical. When inflammatory disease predominates, as in organizing pneumonia or lymphocytic interstitial pneumonia, it is appropriate to treat for a therapeutic response with high-dose steroid therapy, or intense immunosuppressive therapy in refractory cases. Following a response it has been usual to gradually reduce treatment to establish the minimum dose required to prevent relapse, and in many patients with organizing pneumonia it is eventually possible to withdraw treatment altogether, although continuation of careful monitoring is advisable in the long term. There is now ample evidence from a number of clinical series that this approach works well in most patients with polymyositis/dermatomyositis, with corticosteroid monotherapy often highly efficacious.

Treatment decisions are less straightforward in predominantly fibrotic disease. Controlled evaluations are confined to systemic sclerosis. A recent placebo-controlled trial of oral cyclophosphamide therapy has shown a definite treatment effect, although the inclusion of many patients with mild disease makes it difficult to draw conclusions on its clinical significance. Intravenous cyclophosphamide, given at monthly intervals, is less toxic and may be equally efficacious, based on the amplitude of the treatment effect in a placebo-controlled evaluation (although the study was underpowered). In both studies the greater part of the effect was prevention of disease progression, with regression of disease relatively infrequent. Based on these findings, which appear to validate an immunosuppressive approach, the use of other agents such as azathioprine and mycophenolate mofetil is likely to continue, usually in combination with low dose corticosteroid therapy. It should be stressed that high-dose corticosteroid therapy is associated with a greatly increased risk of renal crisis in systemic sclerosis and is strongly contraindicated in that disease.

The same broad principles are applicable in rheumatological disorders other than polymyositis/dermatomyositis and systemic sclerosis, but data remain sparse.

Further reading

Bouros D, et al. (2002). Histopathological subsets of fibrosing alveolitis in patients with systemic sclerosis and their relationship to outcome. *Am J Respir Crit Care Med*, **165**, 1581–6.

Cervera R, et al. (1993). Systemic lupus erythematosus: clinical and immunologic patterns of disease expression in a cohort of 1000 patients. The European working party on systemic lupus erythematosus. *Medicine*, **72**, 113–24.

DeMarco PJ, et al. (2002). Predictors and outcomes of scleroderma renal crisis: the high-dose versus low-dose D-penicillamine in early diffuse systemic sclerosis trial. *Arthritis Rheum*, **46**, 2983–9.

du Bois RM, Wells AU (2000). Pulmonary involvement of connective tissue disease. In: Murray JF, Nadel JA (eds) *Respiratory medicine*, pp. 1691–715. W B Saunders, Philadelphia.

Friedman AW, Targoff IN, Arnett FC (1996). Interstitial lung disease with autoantibodies against aminoacyl-tRNA synthetases in the absence of clinically apparent myositis. *Semin Arthritis Rheum*, **26**, 459–67.

Haupt HM, Moore GW, Hutchins G (1981). The lung in systemic lupus erythematosus. Analysis of the pathologic changes in 120 patients. *Am J Med*, **71**, 791–8.

Hoyles RK, Wells AU (2007). Pulmonary fibrosis in collagen vascular diseases. In: Costabel U, du Bois RM, Egan JJ (eds) *Diffuse parenchymal lung disease*, pp. 185–96. Karger, Basel.

Hoyles RK, et al. (2006). A multicenter, prospective, randomized, double-blind, placebo-controlled trial of corticosteroids and intravenous cyclophosphamide followed by oral azathioprine for the treatment of pulmonary fibrosis in scleroderma. *Arthritis Rheum*, **54**, 3962–70.

Hyland RH, et al. (1983). A systematic controlled study of pulmonary abnormalities in rheumatoid arthritis. *J Rheumatol*, **10**, 395–405.

King TE (1998). Connective tissue disease. In: Schwarz MI, King TE (eds) *Interstitial lung disease*, pp. 645–84. BC Decker, Hamilton, Canada.

Latsi PI, Wells AU (2005). Evaluation and management of alveolitis and interstitial lung disease in scleroderma. *Curr Opin Rheumatol*, **15**, 748–55.

Marie I, et al. (1998). Pulmonary involvement in polymyositis and dermatomyositis. *J Rheumatol*, **25**, 1336–43.

Nicholson AG, Colby TV, Wells AU (2002). Histopathological approach to patterns of interstitial pneumonia in patients with connective tissue disorders. *Sarcoidosis Vasc Diffuse Lung Dis*, **19**, 10–17.

Papiris SA, et al. (1999). Lung involvement in primary Sjögren's syndrome is mainly related to the small airways disease. *Ann Rheum Dis*, **58**, 61–4.

Tanoue LT (1998). Pulmonary manifestations of rheumatoid arthritis. *Clin Chest Med*, **19**, 667–85.

Tashkin DP, et al. (2006). Cyclophosphamide versus placebo in scleroderma lung disease. *N Engl J Med*, **354**, 2655–66.

Wells AU, et al. (1994). Fibrosing alveolitis associated with systemic sclerosis has a better prognosis than lone cryptogenic fibrosing alveolitis. *Am J Respir Crit Care Med*, **149**, 1583–90.

18.11.5 The lung in vasculitis

A.U. Wells and Roland M. du Bois

Essentials

Lung involvement in vasculitic disease can manifest in two ways: (1) Diffuse alveolar haemorrhage—presenting features include fever, weight loss, and other systemic symptoms in association with cough, breathlessness, and clinical signs suggestive of pneumonia. Haemoptysis may be present but is not invariable. A fall in haemoglobin over a day or longer is diagnostically useful. Bronchoalveolar lavage is usually diagnostic. (2) Other pulmonary vasculopathies—present with breathlessness on exertion. Investigation reveals isolated reduction in gas transfer (carbon monoxide diffusing capacity, D_LCO), with or without pulmonary hypertension.

Churg–Strauss syndrome—a prodromal phase of rhinitis with nasal polyps generally precedes the eventual development of treatment-resistant late-onset asthma that is followed, often years later, by vasculitic manifestations. Chest radiography shows patchy lung infiltration in up to 80% of patients: pulmonary nodules and pleural involvement can also occur. First-line treatment is with steroids, with cyclophosphamide added for severe disease.

Wegener's granulomatosis—chronic rhinitis, sinusitis, or mastoiditis is typically followed by progression to generalized disease over months to years, with lower respiratory tract involvement in 65 to 85% often manifesting with cough, which may be purulent, and less frequently with haemoptysis. The main lung manifestations are with pulmonary nodules (one or more, which can cavitate), localized or diffuse infiltrates, alveolar haemorrhage that may be part of a pulmonary–renal syndrome, and large and small airway disease. Standard first-line treatment for the induction of remission is with prednisolone and cyclophosphamide, with the latter switched to azathioprine for maintenance treatment. Co-trimoxazole is effective for localized but not systemic disease. Rituximab therapy seems promising for disease that is refractory to standard treatments.

Other vasculitides—microscopic polyangiitis can present with diffuse alveolar haemorrhage, which can have a poor prognosis, and other primary systemic vasculitides occasionally present with respiratory features.

Introduction

It is useful to subdivide pulmonary vasculitides into primary systemic or secondary, and to differentiate them from nonvasculitic disorders that can affect the pulmonary circulation, listed in Table 18.11.5.1. The secondary and non-vasculitic diseases are discussed in other chapters: Table 18.11.5.2 summarizes the primary vasculitides, indicating those in which the lung is involved.

Clinical manifestations of pulmonary vasculitis

Lung involvement in vasculitic disease can manifest as:

♦ diffuse alveolar haemorrhage

♦ an isolated reduction in gas transfer (carbon monoxide diffusing capacity, $D_L co$), with or without pulmonary hypertension.

Other features of the underlying or associated disease may be present, and the pulmonary disorder may present as part of a pulmonary–renal syndrome, of which Goodpasture's disease (see Chapter 21.8.7) is the best-known example.

Diffuse alveolar haemorrhage

The presenting features of diffuse alveolar haemorrhage include fever, weight loss, and other systemic symptoms in association with cough, breathlessness and clinical signs suggestive of pneumonia. A history of previous haemoptysis is sometimes helpful, but in other cases diffuse alveolar haemorrhage presents acutely. Chest radiography shows consolidation, typically resolving within a matter of days, unlike the usual time-course in infective pneumonia. High-resolution CT may reveal an extensive ground-glass appearance, denoting partial alveolar filling. A fall in haemoglobin over a day or longer is diagnostically useful, and chronic iron-deficiency anaemia can arise from low-grade haemorrhage over a lengthy period.

Bronchoalveolar lavage is usually diagnostic in the absence of haemoptysis, revealing overt blood staining in sequential lavage in the acute presentation, or the presence of numerous macrophages containing iron, identified by Perl's stain, in chronic disease. The gas transfer corrected for alveolar volume ($K co$) is elevated in acute haemorrhage, but only if measured within 36 h, seriously limiting the diagnostic yield. Investigations listed in Box 18.11.5.1 should be performed if alveolar haemorrhage is suspected. Diffuse pulmonary haemorrhage occurring without identifiable cause or association is known as idiopathic pulmonary haemosiderosis (see Chapter 18.14.1).

Table 18.11.5.1 Pulmonary vascular disease

Vasculitic	Nonvasculitic
Primary systemic	Thromboembolic
Secondary	Primary pulmonary hypertension
Rheumatological	Secondary pulmonary hypertension
Pulmonary–renal	Systemic sclerosis
Behçet's syndrome	Idiopathic pulmonary haemosiderosis
Chronic infection	Arteriovenous malformations
Lymphoma	
Drugs	
Penicillamine	
Hydralazine	
Propylthiouracil	
Nitrofurantoin	

Isolated gas transfer deficit with or without pulmonary hypertension

Pulmonary vasculopathies other than alveolar haemorrhage present with breathlessness on exertion. Clinical examination of the respiratory system and routine lung imaging are normal. Lung function tests show preservation of lung volumes with an isolated reduction of $D_L co$. In severe pulmonary vascular disease pulmonary hypertension may be clinically overt, and in other cases it is detected by echocardiography, especially if tricuspid regurgitation allows Doppler estimation of pulmonary artery pressures. Vasculopathies other than vasculitis should be considered in this clinical context, including ablative vasculopathies (as in systemic sclerosis and primary pulmonary hypertension) and coagulopathies leading to thromboembolism or intrapulmonary microvascular thrombosis (see Chapter 16.15.2).

The following sections discuss lung involvement in specific vasculitic disorders, followed by discussion of key clinical problems, prognosis, and treatment.

Table 18.11.5.2 Chapel Hill International Consensus nomenclature of systemic vasculitis (1992)

	Lung disease
Large vessel	
Giant-cell arteritis	Rare
Takayasu's arteritis	Frequent
Medium-size vessel	
Polyarteritis nodosa	Rare
Kawasaki disease	No
Small vessel (medium-size vessel involvement may be present)	
Wegener's granulomatosis	Frequent
Churg–Strauss syndrome	Frequent
Microscopic polyangiitis	Frequent
Henoch–Schönlein purpura	No
Essential cryoglobulinaemia	No

Box 18.11.5.1 Investigations to be considered if pulmonary haemorrhage is suspected

- Imaging
  - Chest radiography with or without high-resolution CT
- Lung function tests
  - Kco
- Renal function
  - Urine dipstick testing and microscopy for proteinuria, haematuria, and cellular casts; estimation of renal function; consider renal biopsy (if evidence of nephritis)
- Immunology
  - Antineutrophil cytoplasmic antibodies (ANCA), antiglomerular basement membrane (anti-GBM) antibodies, immune complexes, rheumatoid factor, antinuclear antibodies (ANA), antiphospholipid antibodies
- Bronchoalveolar lavage
  - Iron-laden macrophages
- Biopsy
  - Renal
  - Skin
  - Lung (surgical)

Churg–Strauss syndrome

First described by Churg and Strauss in 1951, this rare condition has an estimated annual incidence of approximately 3 per million and mostly affects adults aged 30 to 50 (although the reported age range is 7–74 years). There is no strong gender predilection. Typically, asthma and eosinophilia are associated with the characteristic histological findings (Fig. 18.11.5.1), consisting of profuse eosinophilic infiltration, extravascular granulomatous inflammation, and necrotizing arteritis affecting small to medium-sized vessels. There is little information about geographical variation.

Aetiology and pathogenesis

The underlying pathogenetic mechanism is generally considered to be an eosinophilic granulomatous response to a foreign antigen, akin to the eosinophilic granulomatosis seen in schistosomiasis. In support of this hypothesis, immunological stimuli (vaccination or immunotherapy) have been reported to trigger the disease, although the pauci-immune nature of the histopathology has yet to be explained. The introduction of antileukotriene therapy for asthma has been associated with an increased incidence of Churg–Strauss syndrome, but it remains unclear whether the drug triggers the onset of disease. It is also possible that reduction or withdrawal of corticosteroids with better control of asthma unmasks the condition in some cases, although some individuals who have never received corticosteroids have developed the syndrome with the introduction of an antileukotriene agent.

Antineutrophil cytoplasmic antibodies (ANCA), first described in 1982, are frequently present in systemic vasculitides involving small and medium sized vessels, including Churg–Strauss syndrome,

Wegener's granulomatosis and microscopic polyangiitis. ANCA are directed against cytoplasmic antigens in polymorphonuclear leucocytes and monocytes and are subcategorized according to their immunofluorescent staining pattern as C (cytoplasmic), P (perinuclear), or A (atypical). The pathogenetic significance of ANCA is unclear, but ANCA receptors on the surface of neutrophils are up-regulated at disease sites, and ANCA can also interact with endothelial cells to cause injury and coagulation. All ANCA patterns have been reported in Churg-Strauss syndrome, but P-ANCA occur most frequently, usually directed against myeloperoxidase (MPO) and only very infrequently against proteinase 3 (PR3).

Clinical presentation

Two sets of diagnostic criteria have been used: Lanham's criteria and the criteria of the American College of Rheumatology. In addition to systemic features such as fever and weight loss, Lanham defined the disease as requiring:

1 asthma

2 eosinophilia greater than 1.5×10^9/litre in the peripheral blood

3 evidence of systemic vasculitis in two or more organs other than the lung

The American College of Rheumatology definition requires the satisfaction of at least four of the following six criteria:

1 the presence of asthma

2 eosinophilia greater than 10% in the peripheral blood

3 evidence of a neuropathy in a vasculitic pattern (e.g. mononeuritis multiplex)

4 transient pulmonary infiltrates

5 a history of sinus disease

6 evidence of extravascular eosinophilia on biopsy

In most patients asthma precedes vasculitic manifestations, often by years, although these features develop simultaneously in up to 20% of cases. Typically the prodromal phase consists of rhinitis with nasal polyps, which often lasts for years before the eventual development of late-onset asthma that is generally resistant to treatment. The second phase is characterized by eosinophilia in the peripheral blood and tissues and often follows a relapsing and remitting course. The final phase, systemic vasculitis, often follows the onset of the second phase by several years and is immediately preceded by improvement in asthma. This pattern of evolution of disease is more than 95% specific and sensitive for Churg–Strauss syndrome. Table 18.11.5.3 lists the major pulmonary manifestations. Pulmonary infiltrates are much more common than pulmonary nodules and, in contrast to Wegener's granulomatosis, cavitation of nodules in extremely rare. Respiratory failure and status asthmaticus account for 10% of deaths.

Other organ involvement

Skin lesions

These are seen in about 60% of patients, generally manifesting as palpable purpura or subcutaneous nodules. Skin infarcts also occur.

Cardiac involvement

The heart may be involved diffusely, producing congestive cardiac failure or restrictive cardiomyopathy. Eosinophilic myocarditis is

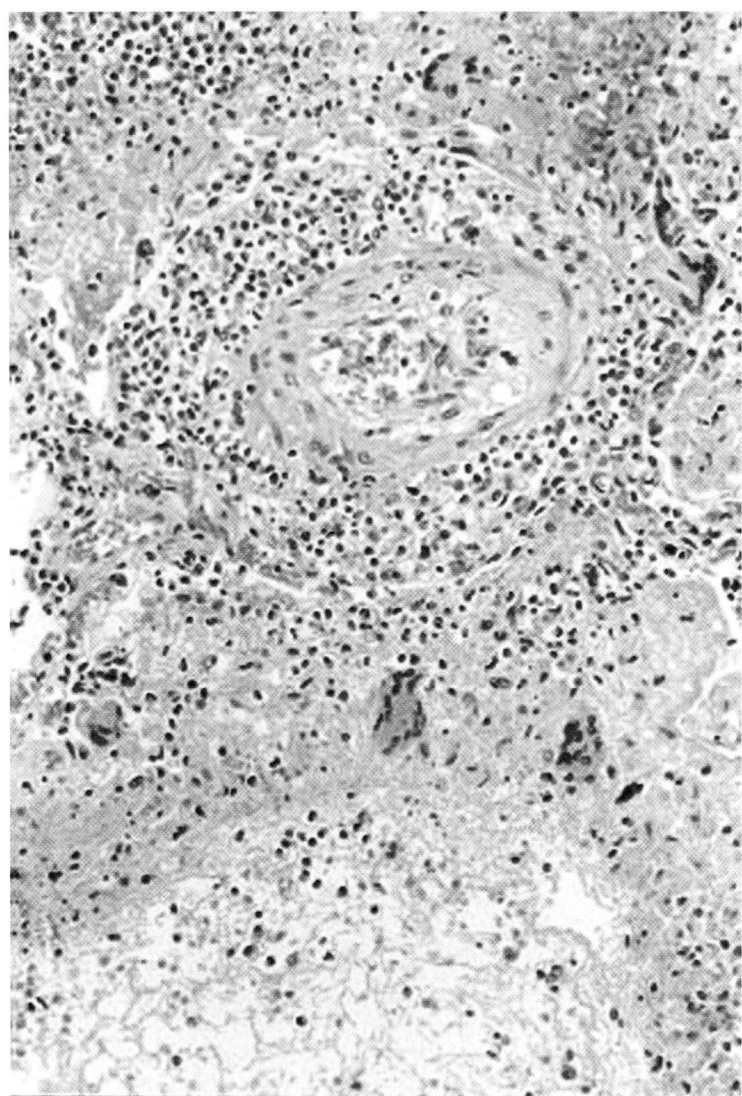

Fig. 18.11.5.1 A case of Churg–Strauss syndrome showing a pulmonary artery surrounded by granulomatous inflammation and a florid mixed inflammatory cell infiltrate that includes abundant eosinophils.

present in up to 50% of cases, with coronary artery vasculitis and pericardial effusions much less frequent. Cardiac disease is the most common cause of death.

Renal disease

This is much less common than in Wegener's granulomatosis or microscopic polyangiitis, but the histopathology is very similar, consisting of a focal segmental necrotizing glomerulonephritis. Renal disease is generally mild, but endstage renal failure is reported.

Central nervous system

Mononeuritis multiplex is the most common manifestation, occurring in up to 75% of patients. Cranial nerve involvement is less common, but cerebrovascular disease may occur.

Gastrointestinal involvement

Vasculitis of the mesenteric vessels may produce bowel abnormalities, including perforation, and less commonly eosinophilic infiltration may cause obstruction.

Musculoskeletal system

Arthritis is relatively common, as are myalgias.

Investigation

Chest radiography shows patchy lung infiltration in up to 80% of patients and pleural disease is present in up to 50%. High-resolution CT is much more sensitive than chest radiography, although the full spectrum of abnormalities has yet to be defined. The most frequent findings are patchy ground-glass infiltration and patchy consolidation. An extensive ground-glass appearance is usual in patients which alveolar haemorrhage due to capillaritis, whereas consolidation is more suggestive of granuloma formation in association with involvement of medium-sized vessels.

There is a peripheral blood eosinophilia, matched by a marked eosinophilia on bronchoalveolar lavage. The diagnostic role of ANCA continues to be debated. ANCA, usually P-ANCA, are present in up to two-thirds of patients, but in some series their prevalence is much lower and P-ANCA also occur in many other nonvasculitic autoimmune and infectious conditions. Thus, the presence of P-ANCA is no more than a useful ancillary finding, increasing the diagnostic likelihood, and the absence of P-ANCA should not materially influence the diagnostic algorithm.

The classical triad at lung biopsy consists of necrotizing angiitis, granulomas, and tissue eosinophilia (Fig. 18.11.5.1). Giant cells

Table 18.11.5.3 Distinguishing thoracic features in primary vasculitis

	Churg–Strauss syndrome	Wegener's granulomatosis	Microscopic polyangiitis
Subglottic stenosis		+	+
Multiple nodules	+	+	
Solitary nodules		+	
Cavities		+	
Localized infiltrates		+	+
Transient infiltrates	+		+
Pleural involvement	+	+	
Cardiac involvement	+		

Adapted from Specks U (1998). Pulmonary vasculitis. In: Schwarz MI, King TE Jr (eds) *Interstitial lung disease*, pp. 507–34. B C Dekker, Hamilton, Canada.

and fibrinoid necrosis are present. However, it is not uncommon for histological appearances to be indeterminate, with the presence of some but not all of the characteristic features, and in some cases there is overlap with the histopathological appearances of Wegener's granulomatosis or microscopic polyangiitis. Surgical biopsies have a much higher diagnostic yield than transbronchial biopsies, which seldom disclose vasculitis.

Wegener's granulomatosis

The systemic features of Wegener's granulomatosis are described in Chapter 21.10.2. This condition, the third most prevalent systemic vasculitis (after giant cell arteritis and vasculitis in rheumatoid arthritis), occurs throughout the world with an annual incidence of 3 to 11 per million, depending upon the geographic region. It mainly affects adults aged 30 to 50 (although it may occur in any age group), and there is no gender predilection. The histological abnormalities consist of granulomatous inflammation associated with necrotizing vasculitis, affecting small to medium-sized vessels (Fig. 18.11.5.2). Lung involvement occurs at some stage of disease in up to 85% of

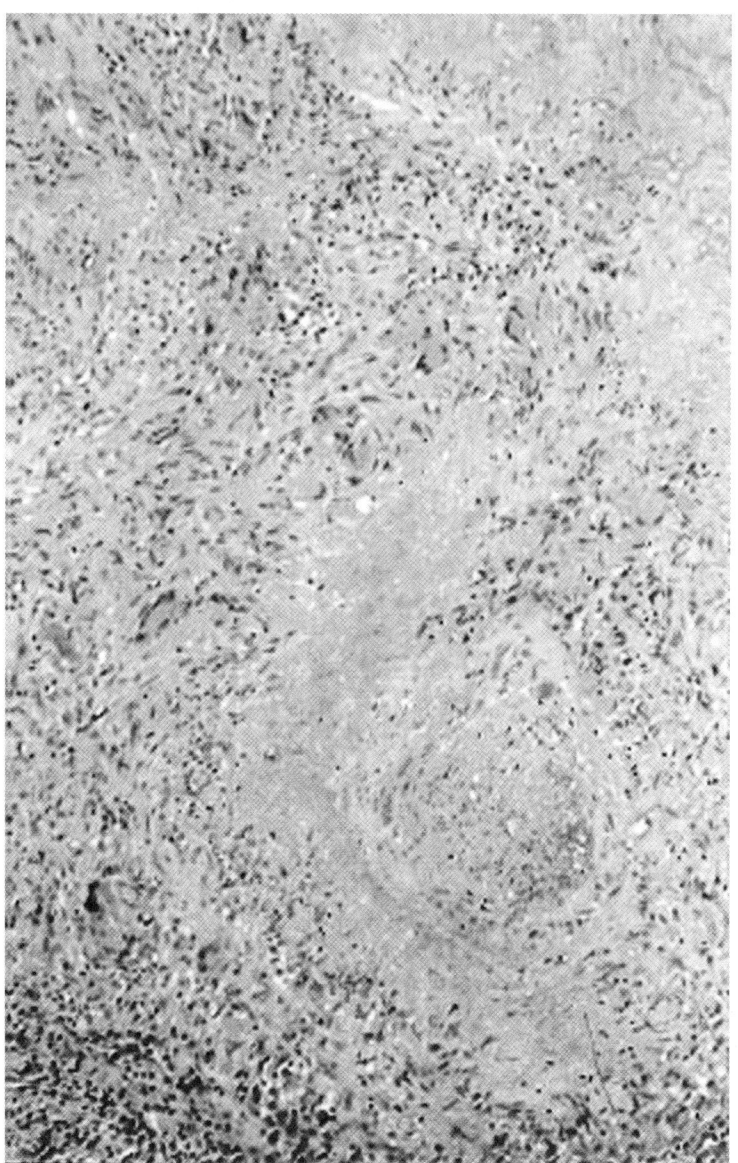

Fig. 18.11.5.2 A case of Wegener's granulomatosis showing an area of geographic necrosis around a partly destroyed pulmonary vessel. This focus is surrounded by chronic inflammation and fibrosis, within which there is granulomatous inflammation with the giant cells showing a somewhat pyramidal morphology.

cases; upper respiratory tract and renal involvement (due to necrotizing glomerulonephritis) are frequent.

Aetiology and pathogenesis

Studies of possible genetic associations have yielded conflicting results, with linkage to HLA DR1 or HLA DR2 in some but not all populations. The importance of environmental factors is equally uncertain. Case–control studies have suggested that exposure to silica or silicone might be pathogenetic in some cases. ANCA-positive vasculitis mimicking Wegener's granulomatosis has been induced by propylthiouracil, hydralazine, and penicillamine, possibly by modifying MPO and thereby creating an antigenic stimulus. However, the most suggestive data relate to infection, especially with *Staphylococcus aureus*. Chronic nasal carriage of *S. aureus* is substantially more prevalent in Wegener's granulomatosis than in control populations, and it has been suggested that staphylococcal acid phosphatase might be antigenic in susceptible individuals. An immunostimulatory role for *S. aureus* B-cell superantigens has also been proposed. The partial efficacy of prophylactic trimethoprim–sulfamethoxazole in reducing both infection and the likelihood of relapse of Wegener's granulomatosis provides further indirect support for an infectious pathogenesis.

Pathogenetic concepts are complicated by the histological spectrum of disease, ranging from prominent granulomatous lesions, associated with a lymphocytosis on bronchoalveolar lavage, to fulminant necrotizing vasculitis, in which a bronchoalveolar lavage neutrophilia is the rule. The genesis of granulomata is not well understood, but there is strong indirect evidence that neutrophils play a key role in initiating vasculitis. PR3 is the main target antigen for C-ANCA, which is found in about 90% of patients with generalized Wegener's granulomatosis (as compared to 50% of patients with localized disease). As in other ANCA-positive vasculitides, there is *in vitro* and animal model evidence to suggest that PR3-ANCA might interact with primed neutrophils, leading to neutrophil degranulation and thus to endothelial damage and further neutrophil recruitment.

Pulmonary presentation

Involvement of the upper and/or lower respiratory tract is the presenting feature in 90% of cases. Disease usually evolves in two phases. Initially there is chronic rhinitis, sinusitis, or mastoiditis, after which most patients progress to generalized disease over months to years, with lower respiratory tract involvement in 65 to 85% often manifesting with cough, which may be purulent, and less frequently with haemoptysis due to diffuse alveolar haemorrhage. Systemic symptoms, including fever and weight loss, are frequent in generalized disease, along with variable involvement of other organs as described in Chapter 21.10.2. Lung involvement is asymptomatic in about one-third of cases, with the main lung manifestations being (see Table 18.11.5.3):

- one or more nodules, which can cavitate (Fig. 18.11.5.3a)
- localized or diffuse infiltrates (Fig. 18.11.5.3b)
- alveolar haemorrhage that may be part of a pulmonary–renal syndrome
- large and small airway disease

Investigations

As in other vasculitides, classical features are not always present at biopsy, with many patients having only one or two of the three

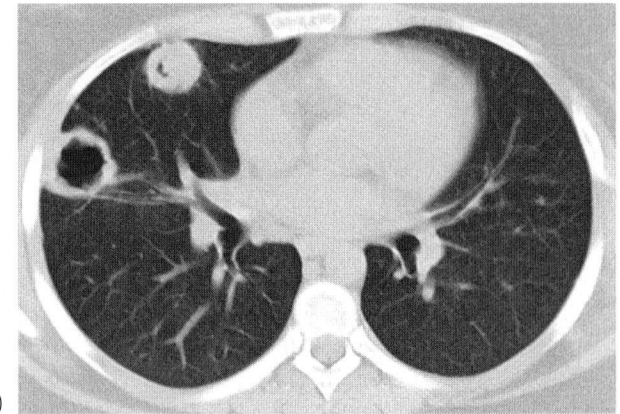
(a)

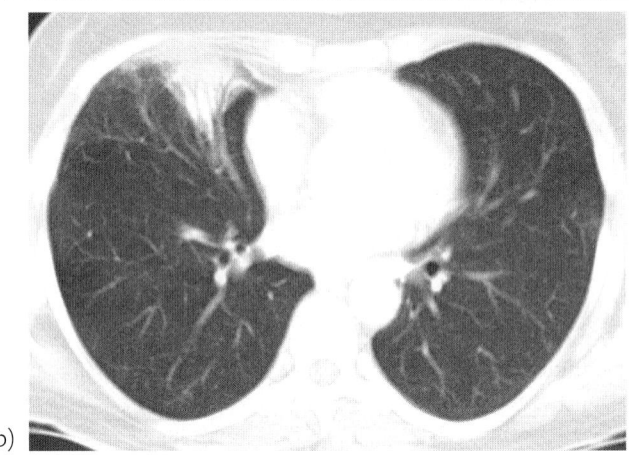
(b)

Fig. 18.11.5.3 Wegener's granulomatosis most often presents radiologically. CT scans may reveal one or more nodules, which can cavitate (a), or localized (b) or diffuse infiltrates.

cardinal histological features (granuloma, necrosis, vasculitis). If a lung biopsy is required, surgical biopsy is preferred, transbronchial biopsies having a much lower diagnostic yield, especially when not targeted to areas with overt abnormalities on chest radiography or high-resolution CT. In advanced pulmonary disease the hazards of biopsy should prompt a search for an alternative biopsy site, including the kidney, skin, and skeletal muscles. Endoscopic nasal biopsy appearances are most often nonspecific, although positive features in a few cases provide a definitive diagnosis. Irrespective of the biopsy site, suggestive appearances may be diagnostic when combined with clinical and serological information even when diagnostic histological features are absent.

The two main patterns on chest radiography and high-resolution CT are nodules and consolidation, with pleural effusions an occasional finding. High-resolution CT offers the important advantage of better definition of nodule cavitation, a key diagnostic feature, and may also disclose abnormalities of the large intrathoracic and extrathoracic airways, including subglottic stenosis, stenosis of large airways, and bronchiectasis. Subglottic stenosis is present in up to 25% of cases and can develop without concomitant systemic disease activity.

Fibre-optic bronchoscopy may show tracheobronchitis, including ulceration and 'cobblestoning' of the mucosa, or airway stenosis. Bronchoalveolar lavage fluid contains an excess of neutrophils and usually of eosinophils (with diffuse infiltrates) or lymphocytes (more interstitial disease), but is most useful in excluding alveolar haemorrhage or infection, including opportunistic infection in treated patients.

Haematological and biochemical investigations reflect the inflammatory process. The diagnosis should never be based upon C-ANCA positivity in isolation because these are also found in other contexts, including other vasculitides, chronic bacterial infections and cryoglobulinaemia.

Microscopic polyangiitis

The main description of microscopic polyangiitis occurs elsewhere (see Chapter 21.10.2), but this necrotizing vasculitis affects small to medium-sized vessels, with few or no immune complex deposits, and lung disease occurs in 35 to 55% of cases.

Pulmonary presentation

The major presentation in the lung (Table 18.11.5.3) is diffuse alveolar haemorrhage, which can have a poor prognosis. Pulmonary capillaritis may be associated with evidence of disease outside the lung, particularly necrotizing glomerulonephritis, mononeuritis multiplex, and skin lesions.

It is often difficult to distinguish microscopic polyangiitis from Wegener's granulomatosis clinically. The key histological distinction is the absence of granulomas, which are characteristically present in Wegener's. Renal biopsies can be identical in the two conditions. Microscopic polyangiitis also needs to be distinguished from polyarteritis nodosa that, by definition, only affects arteries, rarely arterioles, and never small vessels. Renal vasculitis with microaneurysm formation occurs in polyarteritis nodosa but not microscopic polyangiitis, and diffuse alveolar haemorrhage does not occur in polyarteritis nodosa.

Other diseases

Other primary systemic vasculitides occasionally present with respiratory features.

Takayasu's arteritis

This arteritis affects predominantly the aorta and its main branches but involves the pulmonary arteries in up to 50% of patients, presenting with pulmonary vascular occlusion.

Giant-cell arteritis

There is rarely objective evidence of lung involvement, but 25% of patients with giant-cell arteritis have cough, hoarseness, and sore throat at presentation.

The other systemic vasculitides that feature in the Chapel Hill International consensus nomenclature, but which rarely if ever present with lung disease, are Henoch–Schönlein purpura and essential cryoglobulinaemia.

Behçet's disease

This occurs predominantly in Mediterranean countries and can produce pulmonary vascular inflammation affecting all sizes of vessels and resulting in pulmonary arterial aneurysms, arterial and venous thrombosis, pulmonary infarcts, and pulmonary haemorrhage. It is crucial to differentiate haemorrhage from thrombosis because of the treatment implications.

Pulmonary veno-occlusive disease

This is a disorder of unknown cause that manifests with progressive occlusion of the postcapillary venules, resulting in features similar to those of pulmonary oedema. There is no known effective treatment. Differentiation from cardiogenic causes of raised pulmonary venous pressure must be made.

Lymphomatoid granulomatosis

This has been included historically within the category of pulmonary vasculitis but is now believed to be a lymphoproliferative disease.

Key clinical problems in vasculitis

Diagnosis

Ideally, typical histological appearances should be present, and when they are not present the requisite number of clinical criteria should be met. However, formal diagnostic criteria are merely a basis for diagnostic negotiation in many cases. Classification systems fail to capture the entire spectrum of vasculitic disease, with many patients having features overlapping between diagnostic entities. With the advent of ANCA antibodies, *formes frustes* of full blown vasculitic syndromes are increasingly diagnosed, with transient or no fulfilment of full diagnostic criteria in many instances. Even in cases satisfying diagnostic criteria, the clinical heterogeneity of the vasculitic syndromes is notorious, it often being stated that no two patients are alike.

An appreciation of these difficulties informs the clinician of the need for a versatile diagnostic approach. When vasculitis is suspected but full clinical criteria are not satisfied, a histological diagnosis should generally be sought, targeted to involved organs. Failure to capture typical appearances at biopsy does not necessarily exclude a diagnosis of vasculitis as vasculitic processes may be patchy and nonspecific inflammatory change may be evident: this applies especially to upper airway biopsies in patients with Wegener's granulomatosis. An empirical diagnosis of a vasculitic syndrome must sometimes be made, and in these cases—which tend to foment a great deal of insecurity in patients and clinicians alike—it is essential to do everything possible to exclude the most frequent differential diagnoses, namely infection and malignancy.

When formal diagnostic criteria for a vasculitic syndrome are not fulfilled and empirical treatment is required, the general approach—including initial treatment and monitoring—should be as for the vasculitic syndrome most closely resembling the particular clinical presentation of the patient. When the diagnosis is uncertain the initial treatment should be definitive because a satisfactory response provides useful ancillary diagnostic support ('diagnosis by therapeutic challenge'): a tentative initial therapeutic approach often merely serves to prolong diagnostic uncertainty.

Prognosis

The outcome of the more frequent vasculitic syndromes was poor when they were first described but has improved strikingly, as best illustrated by the mortality of Wegener's granulomatosis: the mean survival of 5 months in early reports has now been transformed, with complete initial remission in 75% of cases, increasing further with the recent use of rituximab. However, long-term follow-up continues to be needed in Wegener's granulomatosis (with relapse occurring in 50–70% of cases) and in other vasculitides despite these improvements.

The improvement in prognosis in Wegener's granulomatosis, also seen in Churg–Strauss syndrome, in part reflects the increasing use of immunosuppressive agents in combination with corticosteroid therapy. However, the increasing detection of milder disease, including patients with limited involvement, has also undoubtedly improved average outcome. Localized Wegener's granulomatosis has a better outcome than disease with multiorgan involvement. The prognosis of Churg–Strauss syndrome is generally good for those with isolated intrathoracic disease (5-year survival 88%), but worsens with two or more extrapulmonary complications (5-year survival 54%), particularly with proteinuria more than 1 g/day, renal insufficiency (creatinine >140 μmol/litre), cardiomyopathy, gastrointestinal disease, or central nervous system involvement.

The causes of death in vasculitis can be broadly subdivided into sepsis (as a complication of treatment) and disease progression. In Wegener's granulomatosis death from progressive disease is most commonly due to renal failure or lung involvement. In Churg–Strauss syndrome the main cause of death is cardiac disease, followed by renal failure, cerebrovascular involvement, and gastrointestinal disease, with lung disease accounting for 10% of deaths.

Treatment

Wegener's granulomatosis

Intense immunosuppression is used to induce remission, followed by less intense maintenance therapy. First-line treatment for the induction of remission should consist either of oral cyclophosphamide (2.0 mg/kg per day) or intravenous cyclophosphamide (600 mg/m², at intervals dependent on disease severity). These are equally successful in inducing remission, but intravenous therapy tends to be much less toxic, although possibly associated with a higher likelihood of relapse. The particular toxicities of concern are haemorrhagic cystitis and subsequent malignancy, both of which are seen with prolonged oral treatment. However, irrespective of the mode of administration, these complications justify an early change to alternative treatments once remission has been induced in all forms of vasculitis, with standard maintenance treatment being azathioprine (2.0 mg/kg per day).

In the absence of major organ involvement, methotrexate (0.3 mg/kg per week) may be as effective as daily oral cyclophosphamide in the induction of remission, but relapse is more likely following the cessation of treatment at 12 months, suggesting that methotrexate therapy should be extended beyond 12 months if used instead of cyclophosphamide.

Low-dose corticosteroid therapy is generally used in combination with immunosuppressive agents. High-dose corticosteroids are less frequently used than formerly (in combination with cyclophosphamide) to induce remission, but a combination of cyclophosphamide and intravenous methyl prednisolone should be considered in life-threatening disease.

Co-trimoxazole has been efficacious in Wegener's granulomatosis for localized upper respiratory tract or minor lower respiratory tract disease, but is not recommended for aggressive systemic disease, although it may have an ancillary role in maintaining remission. Intravenous immunoglobulin and antithymocyte globulin have been used with variable success in resistant disease, but rituximab therapy has provided the most promising recent data in patients with Wegener's granulomatosis that is refractory to standard treatments.

Churg–Strauss syndrome

Initial treatment depends upon severity of presentation and the organs involved. In isolated pulmonary disease the first-line treatment is oral prednisolone (1 mg/kg per day, up to 60 mg/day) or—in more severe disease such as alveolar haemorrhage—intravenous methylprednisolone (up to 1 g/day on three successive days). Response is usually good. Cyclophosphamide is added in life-threatening disease, either orally or intravenously at doses used in Wegener's granulomatosis. Evidence for other immunosuppressive agents (azathioprine, methotrexate, mycophenolate mofetil) is inconclusive.

There is no evidence that plasma exchange has a routine place in Churg–Strauss syndrome or other pauci-immune pulmonary vasculitides. Prophylactic co-trimoxazole (trimethoprim 160 mg/sulphamethoxazole 800 mg) three times a week is often used when prolonged intense immunosuppression is needed, to reduce the risk of *Pneumocystis jirovecii* opportunistic infection.

Further reading

Conron M, Beynon HLC (2000). Churg–Strauss syndrome. In: du Bois RM, Tattersfield A (eds) *Thorax Rare Disease Series. Thorax*, **55**, 870–7.

Guillevin L, *et al.* (1996). Prognostic factors in polyarteritis nodosa and Churg–Strauss syndrome. A prospective study in 342 patients. *Medicine*, **75**, 17–28.

Jayne D, *et al.* (2003). A randomized trial of maintenance therapy for vasculitis associated with antineutrophil cytoplasmic autoantibodies. *New Engl J Med*, **349**, 36–44.

Jennette JC, *et al.* (1994). Nomenclature of systemic vasculitides. Proposal of an International consensus conference. *Arthritis Rheum*, **37**, 187–92.

Keogh KA, *et al.* (2006). Rituximab for refractory Wegener's granulomatosis: report of a prospective, open-label pilot trial. *Am J Respir Crit Care Med*, **173**, 180–7.

Lanham JG, *et al.* (1984). Systemic vasculitis with asthma and eosinophilia: the clinical approach to the Churg–Strauss syndrome. *Medicine (Baltimore)*, **63**, 65–81.

Lhote F, Guillevin L (1998). Polyarteritis nodosa, microscopic polyangiitis and Churg–Strauss syndrome. *Semin Respir Crit Care Med*, **19**, 27–46.

Specks U (1998). Pulmonary vasculitis. In: Schwarz MI, King TE Jr (eds) *Interstitial lung disease*, pp. 507–34. B C Dekker, Hamilton, Canada.

Sarcoidosis

Robert P. Baughman and Elyse E. Lower

Essentials

Sarcoidosis is a disease of unknown cause that is characterized by the presence of noncaseating granulomas in at least two organs. It can present in a wide variety of ways. Differential diagnosis is most commonly from tuberculosis or lymphoma.

Clinical features

Respiratory involvement—described in more than 90% of patients and staged according to the chest radiograph appearance: Stage 1, hilar adenopathy alone; stage 2, adenopathy and parenchymal disease; stage 3, parenchymal disease alone; and stage 4, fibrosis. Such staging predicts outcome (resolution in 2–3 years—stage 1, 90%; stage 3, 30%) but not the degree of extrapulmonary disease. Pulmonary function studies typically demonstrate a restrictive pattern.

Skin involvement—the second most commonly affected organ: manifestations include hyperpigmentation; hypopigmentation; keloid reaction; waxy, maculopapular lesions, which when present on face are called lupus pernio and diagnostic of sarcoidosis; erythema nodosum.

Other organ involvement: eye—uveitis and lacrimal glands; neurological—cranial nerves (especially VII), central nervous system (lymphocytic meningitis, hypothalamic involvement) and peripheral nerves; liver—abnormal liver function tests in 50%; hypercalcaemia/hypercalciuria; heart—involvement is rare but can be serious with arrhythmic death.

Acute vs chronic disease—acute disease (which lasts for <2 years) is associated with erythema nodosum, hilar adenopathy, anterior uveitis and cranial nerve VII paralysis. Chronic disease includes such manifestations as lupus pernio, stage 4 chest radiograph, posterior uveitis, urolithiasis, and bone cysts.

Investigations and management

Investigations—those of particular note include: (1) serum angiotensin converting enzyme (ACE) levels—elevated in 60% of patients with acute and one-third of those with chronic disease; (2) bronchoalveolar lavage—revealing increased lymphocytes, especially an increased CD4:CD8 ratio; (3) transbronchial biopsy—noncaseating granulomas found in greater than 60% of stage 1 and 80% of stage 2 or 3 disease; (4) gallium scan—uptake in the parotid and conjunctiva (the 'panda' sign) and/or in the hilar nodes (the 'lambda' sign) are fairly characteristic and useful confirmation of diagnosis in difficult cases.

Management—there is no single treatment for all patients with sarcoidosis. Key issues are to determine (1) whether the patient requires treatment, this usually being based on symptoms, and then (2) the extent of symptomatic disease, and (3) whether this is acute or chronic. First line treatment is usually with corticosteroids, often prednisolone 20 to 40 mg/day (initial dosage, followed by gradual reduction) if topical administration is not possible, although it is not universally accepted that steroids change the course of the disease. If the dose of steroid cannot be reduced to an acceptable level, or if the patient is not responding, then other agents (e.g. chloroquine/hydroxychloroquine, methotrexate, leflunomide, infliximab) are added.

Prognosis—most patients with sarcoidosis will experience disease resolution within 2 to 5 years; about 25% will develop residual fibrosis in the lungs or elsewhere; in a few the disease will become chronic and persist for more than 5 years. Most series from referral centres report 5% disease-related mortality, usually from respiratory failure.

Introduction

Sarcoidosis was first recognized in 1869 by Jonathan Hutchinson, who treated a man with skin lesions that appeared unrelated to tuberculosis. Over the next few decades most case reports of sarcoidosis described patients with skin lesions, and pathological information was scarce since the disease is often self limiting.

Schaumann in Sweden was one of the first to recognize the multiorgan features of the disease combined with common pathological feature: his original thesis was written in 1914, but not published until 1936.

After the Second World War the use of routine screening chest radiographs identified patients with asymptomatic abnormalities.

Lofgren described a group with erythema nodosum, uveitis, and hilar adenopathy. Others began to appreciate the unique aspects of sarcoidosis compared to tuberculosis. Interestingly, as tuberculosis becomes less frequent in a country, sarcoidosis becomes more obvious, which may reflect the observation that sarcoidosis is a disease of industrial nations and temperate climates, although several groups have reported series of patients with sarcoidosis in India, Thailand, and China.

Pulmonary sarcoidosis can be evaluated by chest radiography, with Scadding in Scotland and Wurm in Germany independently developing a staging system based on the chest radiograph pattern that has become a useful method of describing the extent of and characterizing lung involvement, and which also provides prognostic information.

Newer radiological techniques have been evaluated in sarcoidosis. The chest CT scan provides more detailed information regarding adenopathy, but has not replaced the prognostic information available from the chest radiograph. Gallium scanning will reveal increased uptake in areas of inflammation such as lung and mediastinum. MRI and positron emission tomography (PET) scanning have brought new methods for evaluating extrapulmonary disease.

Bronchoalveolar lavage provides a sample of lower airway secretions, with lavage findings from patients with sarcoidosis being distinctly different from those without disease, this window into the lung providing insights into the true inflammatory response of the lung.

Aetiology

The cause of sarcoidosis remains obscure, one hypothesis being that it is an inflammatory response to an environmental agent (including infection) which occurs in a susceptible host, susceptibility being determined by genetic predisposition.

Several potential infectious agents have been proposed as causes of sarcoidosis. The granulomatous reaction reminds many of tuberculosis, and much effort has been made to identify a mycobacterial cause of sarcoidosis. Several studies using polymerase chain reaction (PCR) and similar molecular biological techniques have been employed, but there is still no convincing evidence that *Mycobacterium tuberculosis* causes most cases of the condition, which may lead to an occasional case of sarcoid-like reaction. Other mycobacteria have been identified in some cases, and

cell-wall-deficient mycobacteria have been grown from the blood of patients with sarcoidosis. However, a controlled trial failed to demonstrate a difference in the incidence of cell-wall-deficient mycobacteria between sarcoidosis patients and controls. Another potential pathogen is *Propiniobacter acnes*.

Epidemiology

Sarcoidosis is a worldwide disease. It has been reported to have a higher prevalence in Scandinavian countries and in Ireland. Table 18.12.1 summarizes the relative frequency of sarcoidosis per 100 000 population around the world. In the United States of America, a higher incidence of sarcoidosis has been reported in African-Americans.

The disease presentation differs in different parts of the world, with Table 18.12.1 listing some of the more frequent patterns seen in various ethnic groups. For example, lupus pernio is common among African-Americans and West Indians who have migrated to the United Kingdom, whereas erythema nodosum is common among Scandinavians. Cardiac disease has been reported at a higher frequency in Japanese sarcoidosis patients than for other groups.

There is evidence that there is a link between genetic predisposition and environmental exposure, but genetic studies regarding the cause of sarcoidosis are hindered whilst the cause remains unknown. However, once a patient has sarcoidosis it is clear that genetic background may affect clinical outcome, e.g. most patients who present with Löfgren's syndrome (erythema nodosum and hilar adenopathy) resolve their disease within a few years, and about 10% have chronic disease; resolution occurs in almost everyone with the human leucocyte antigen (HLA) alleles DRB1*0301/DQB1*0201, but only 55% of those without.

Several occupations have been associated with sarcoidosis, including health care workers, firefighters, and seamen aboard aircraft carriers. In a detailed study of exposures of over 700 patients with recently diagnosed sarcoidosis compared to unaffected age-, race-, and sex-matched controls from the same geographic area, those with sarcoidosis were more likely to have been exposed to mouldy environments or insecticides, although one-half of them had no known exposure to these factors.

Occupational exposures can lead to reactions mimicking sarcoidosis. Beryllium—a metal used in certain industries (ceramics, nuclear processing, dental)—can cause a reaction in the lung and

Table 18.12.1 Sarcoidosis around the world

	Scandinavia	Ireland	Japan	USA		West Indies
				African-American	White	
Prevalence per 100 000	1200	213	20	90	20	180
Female predominant	No	Yes	No	Yes	No	No
Erythema nodosum	+3	+3	Rare	Rare	+2	Rare
Lupus pernio	Rare	Rare	Rare	+1	Rare	+1
Hypercalcaemia	+3	+2	Rare	Rare	+2	Rare
Cardiac	Rare	Rare	+3	+1	+1	+1
Neurological	+1	+1	+1	+1	+1	+1
Hypergammaglobulinaemia	+1	+1	+1	+4	Rare	+1

Rare, < 1%; +1, 1–5%; +2, 5–10%; +3, 10–30%; +4 >30%.

skin indistinguishable from sarcoidosis. Besides clinical history, the distinguishing feature about berylliosis is the lymphocyte's sensitivity to beryllium salts, and the lymphocyte stimulation test of blood, or the more sensitive bronchoalveolar lavage, is a reliable way of detecting which patients are reacting to the metal.

None of the infectious, occupational, and environmental exposures encompass all cases of sarcoidosis, one possible explanation being that the condition is a common reaction to several agents.

Pathogenesis

Sarcoidosis is defined by its immunological reaction, the granuloma. Original immunological studies stressed a lack of systemic immune response by the sarcoidosis patient, including anergy, which is a common feature of active sarcoidosis. A reduction in circulating leucocytes, especially lymphocytes, is an important feature of the disease.

In the 1970s, new techniques helped us understand sarcoidosis better. The most important tool introduced at the time was bronchoalveolar lavage, which provided a sampling of the inflammatory cells in the lower respiratory tract. Alveolar macrophages are the usual resident inflammatory cell retrieved by lavage, with lymphocytes and neutrophils much less frequent in normal lavage fluid. The T lymphocyte is usually increased in the lavage fluid from patients with active sarcoidosis: these are often T helper/inducer lymphocytes (CD-4+), and the ratio of CD4/CD8 lymphocytes is increased from that normally found in the blood, often to greater than 3.5. T lymphocytes can mount either a Th1 or Th2 response, the Th1 response being associated with granuloma formation, whereas Th2

is associated with an eosinophilic response and fibrosis. The initial response of sarcoidosis follows a Th1 pattern, with lymphocytes releasing interleukin (IL)-2 spontaneously, and γ-interferon being released by lymphocytes and macrophages. Increase in IL-12 and reduced levels of IL-10 have also been described, both consistent with a Th1 response. The resolution of sarcoidosis has also been studied with serial lavages: the T lymphocytes remain elevated for some time, but the proportion of CD4 to CD8 decreases to the ratio found in blood (0.8–2.2), and the amount of cytokines released also decreases. This normalization of the inflammatory response has been shown to occur during treatment of sarcoidosis with corticosteroids or methotrexate.

The alveolar macrophage is also activated in sarcoidosis. Increased levels of IL-1, tumour necrosis factor (TNF) and oxygen free radicals are released by macrophages retrieved by bronchoalveolar lavage. For those patients with chronic disease, the macrophages and other resident cells may continue to release proinflammatory cytokines, especially TNF, which has become a target for some therapies. Alveolar macrophages from patients may also begin releasing profibrotic factors such as IL-8 and endothelin.

Clinical features

Patients with sarcoidosis may have a variety of presentations. Commonly affected organs include the lung, skin, and eyes. Less commonly the liver, heart, and brain are affected by the disease. Individual organ involvement can be proven by a biopsy showing noncaseating granuloma; organ involvement is presumed if certain criteria are met. Table 18.12.2 lists some of the criteria suggested

Table 18.12.2 Organ involvement in patients with biopsy-confirmed sarcoidosis[a]

Organ	Definite	Probable
Lung	Positive biopsy of lung Chest radiograph characteristic for sarcoidosis (hilar adenopathy. diffuse infiltrates, or upper lobe fibrosis) Pulmonary function tests showing restriction	Lymphocytic alveolitis by bronchoalveolar lavage Any other pulmonary infiltrate Isolated reduction of D_LCO (carbon monoxide transfer factor)
Skin	Positive biopsy of skin Lupus pernio Erythema nodosum Annular lesion	Macular/papular lesion New nodules (including subcutaneous)
Eyes	Positive biopsy of eye Lacrimal gland swelling Uveitis Optic neuritis	Blindness
Liver	Positive biopsy of liver Liver function tests >3 times normal	Compatible CT scan Elevated alkaline phophatase
Neurological	Positive biopsy of nerve tissue MRI with gadolinium uptake in meninges, brainstem, or mass lesion Cerebrospinal fluid with increased lymphocytes or protein Diabetes insipidus Cranial nerve VII paralysis Other cranial nerve dysfunction	Other abnormalities on MRI Unexplained neuropathy Positive electromyogram
Cardiac	Positive cardiac biopsy Treatment responsive cardiomyopathy ECG showing intraventricular or nodal block Positive gallium scan of heart	Cardiomyopathy or ventricular arrythmias and no other cardiac problems Positive thallium scan

D_LCO, carbon monoxide transfer factor.
[a] Patients with documented sarcoidosis and no other explanation for organ specific abnormality.

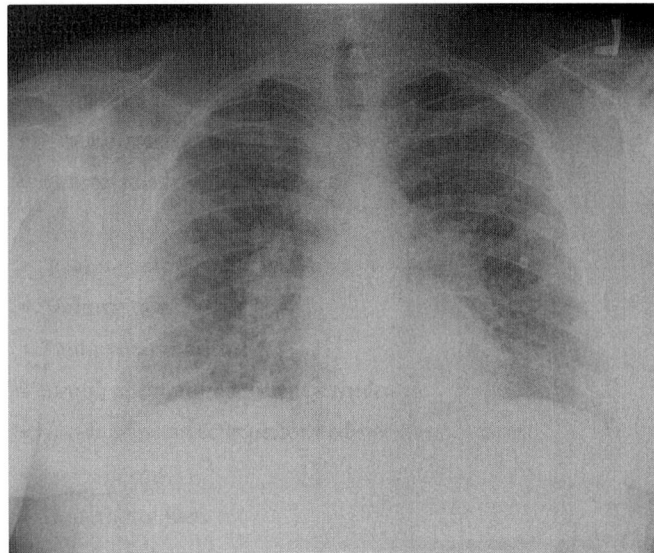

Fig. 18.12.1 Chest radiograph showing stage 2 involvement with sarcoidosis. Enlarged hilar lymph nodes and lung infiltrates are seen.

for definite or probable organ involvement for some of the more commonly affected organs in sarcoidosis.

Respiratory involvement has been described in more than 90% of patients, including both the lymph nodes and the lung parenchyma. Scadding and Wurm independently described stages of the chest radiograph, the commonly used stages being: stage 1, hilar adenopathy alone; stage 2, adenopathy and parenchymal disease (Fig. 18.12.1); stage 3, parenchymal disease alone; and stage 4, fibrosis. The interstitial disease usually has a diffuse reticulonodular appearance, but confluent patches of disease (alveolar sarcoidosis) have been described. Fibrotic changes due to sarcoidosis are usually in the upper lobe, with retraction. The staging system

has proved useful both in standardizing the reports of pulmonary level of involvement, also as a prognostic measure. Patients with stage 1 disease have a 90% rate of resolution within 2 to 3 years, whereas stage 3 patients possess only a 30% chance of resolution. However, 'staging' by chest radiograph appearance does not predict the degree of extrapulmonary disease, hence the choice of the term 'stage' is unfortunate, although it is so standard that it will not be easily replaced.

Table 18.12.3 lists the other diseases to be considered in the differential diagnosis based on the chest radiographic pattern. The presence of mediastinal adenopathy alone (stage 1 disease) is certainly consistent with lymphoma or metastatic cancer, although it has been pointed out that symmetrical bilateral adenopathy with right paratracheal adenopathy in an asymptomatic individual is almost always sarcoidosis. Asymmetrical adenopathy raises the question of lymphoma, and a tissue diagnosis is usually required. For patients with diffuse infiltrates, adenopathy points one toward sarcoidosis. However, several other conditions may have some adenopathy, including hypersensitivity pneumonitis and idiopathic pulmonary fibrosis.

The use of the CT scan has changed the evaluation of many interstitial lung diseases, when the larger the adenopathy, the more likely the patient has sarcoidosis (Fig. 18.12.2). Nodularity may be more obvious on high-resolution CT than on plain chest radiography, and peribronchial thickening is often seen in the upper lobe in sarcoidosis (Fig. 18.12.3). The CT scan is also useful in patients with more advanced disease, since it can identify honeycombing, traction bronchiectasis, and superimposed mycetomas (Fig. 18.12.4). It must, however, be appreciated that increased adenopathy is much more frequently recognized on CT scan than on chest radiographs, making the staging system only applicable for plain radiography. But if the CT scan identifies adenopathy in a patient with possible extrapulmonary sarcoidosis, then this may help in deciding where to proceed to obtain a tissue diagnosis (e.g. brain biopsy vs mediastinoscopy).

Table 18.12.3 Differential diagnosis of sarcoidosis according to the stage on chest radiography

	Stage 1	Stage 2	Stage 3	Stage 4
Pattern	Hilar adenopathy	Adenopathy plus lung infiltrates	Lung infiltrates alone	Fibrosis
Diseases that can commonly cause similar appearances on chest radiography	Tuberculosis Lymphoma Enlarged pulmonary arteries Metastatic carcinoma Histoplasmosis	Lymphangitic carcinoma *Pneumocystis jirovecii* *Pneumoconiosis* Histoplasmosis Berylliosis	Lymphangitic carcinoma *Pneumocystis jirovecii* Pneumoconiosis Histoplasmosis Idiopathic pulmonary fibrosis Berylliosis Hypersensitivity pneumonitis Bronchoalveolar cell carcinoma Pneumonia Congestive heart failure Collagen vascular disease associated lung disease Eosinophilic granuloma	Lymphangitic carcinoma Pneumoconiosis Histoplasmosis Idiopathic pulmonary fibrosis Berylliosis Hypersensitivity pneumonitis Bronchoalveolar cell carcinoma Pneumonia Congestive heart failure Collagen vascular disease associated lung disease Eosinophillic granuloma
Diseases that can rarely cause similar appearances on chest radiography	Leukaemia Infectious monocleosis	Alveolar proteinosis Idiopathic hemosiderosis α_1-Antitrypsin disease Bronchoalveolar cell carcinoma	Sjögren's syndrome Haemosiderosis Alveolar proteinosis	Sjögren's syndrome Haemosiderosis Alveolar proteinosis

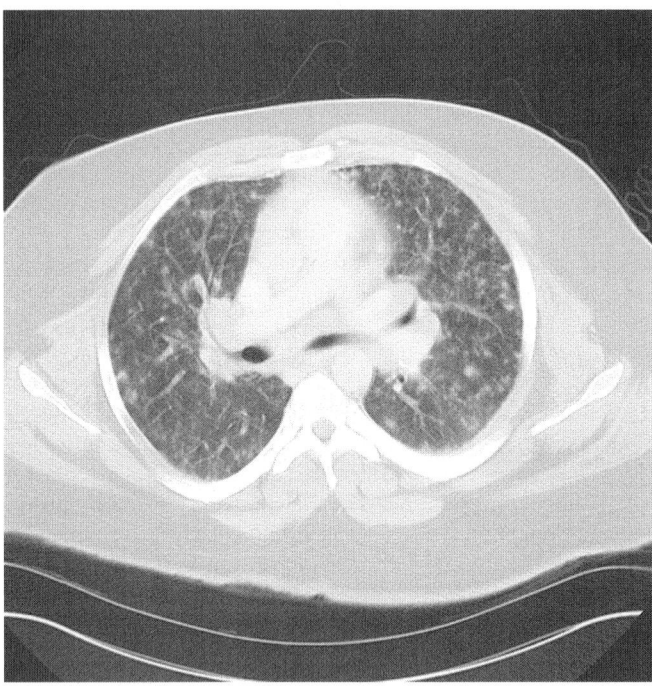

Fig. 18.12.2 High-resolution CT scan of the chest demonstrating both interstitial infiltrate as well as significant hilar adenopathy in sarcoidosis.

Pulmonary function studies in patients with sarcoidosis classically demonstrate a restrictive pattern, with reduction of lung volumes. The transfer factor is usually reduced out of proportion to the loss of lung volume, as one would expect in an interstitial lung disease. In advanced cases, the oxygen level will be reduced, especially during exercise. Obstructive disease can also occur due to airway involvement by sarcoidosis or associated with cough, a common complaint in sarcoidosis.

The skin is the second most commonly affected organ in sarcoidosis. Hyperpigmentation, hypopigmentation, and keloid reaction may demonstrate granulomas on biopsy, but their appearance is not always specific. Waxy, maculopapular lesions, which occur on the extremities, back, and face, are usually raised with most less than 2 cm in diameter. When the lesions occur on the face, especially on the cheeks and nose, they are called lupus pernio (Fig. 18.12.5).

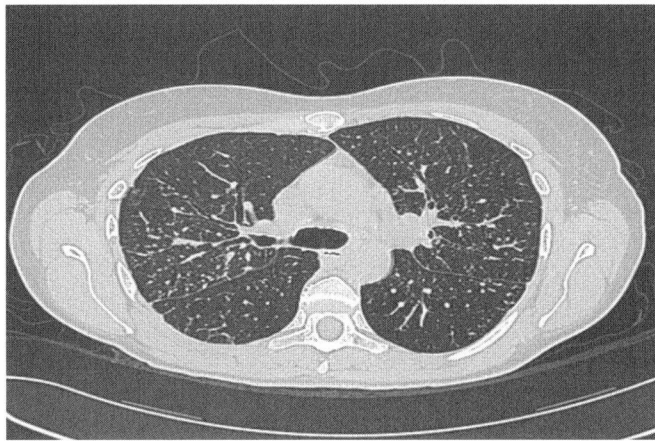

Fig. 18.12.3 High-resolution CT scan of the chest demonstrating peribronchial thickening, which is more prominent in the right lung.

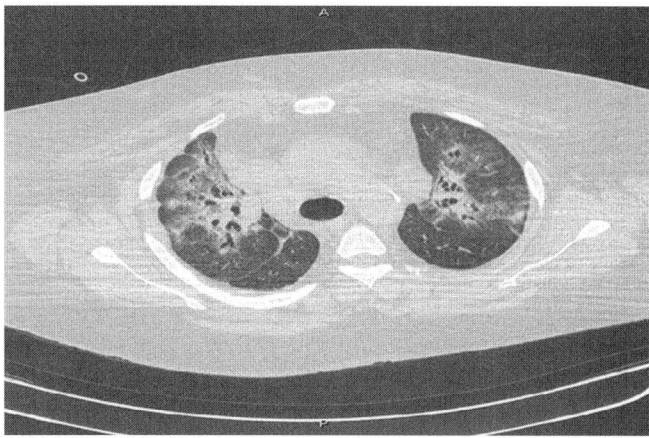

Fig. 18.12.4 High-resolution CT scan of the chest from the upper lobe area, which is more commonly affected in sarcoidosis, demonstrating fibrotic changes including traction bronchiectasis and honeycombing.

Erythema nodosum—red nodular lesions on the extremities—usually involves the legs. The constellation of erythema nodosum, arthritis (in the ankles), and hilar adenopathy is referred to as Löfgren's syndrome, which as noted above usually has a good prognosis. Interestingly, the skin lesions from erythema nodosum do not contain granulomas, but are thought to be due to circulating immune complexes from the disease.

The eye can be affected in more than 20% of patients with sarcoidosis. The most common findings are uveitis and lacrimal gland involvement. Anterior uveitis is often self limiting and can be treated topically, but posterior uveitis is a more chronic form of the disease and may require injections of corticosteroids or systemic therapy. Sicca (dry eyes) and glaucoma are long-term complications which are encountered in patients often years after other sarcoidosis symptoms have resolved. They are consequences of the fibrotic changes in the lacrimal glands and eye and do not respond to anti-inflammatory therapy. Optic nerve involvement can be seen with sarcoidosis, with idiopathic disease and multiple sclerosis being

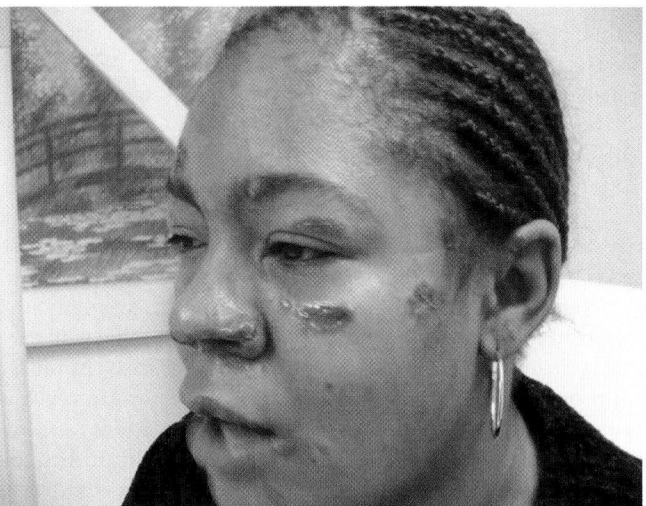

Fig. 18.12.5 Lupus pernio due to sarcoidosis. The plaque-like lesions can be seen on forehead and both cheeks; the nasal area is also affected and can be associated with sinusitis, as it was in this case.
Reproduced with permission.

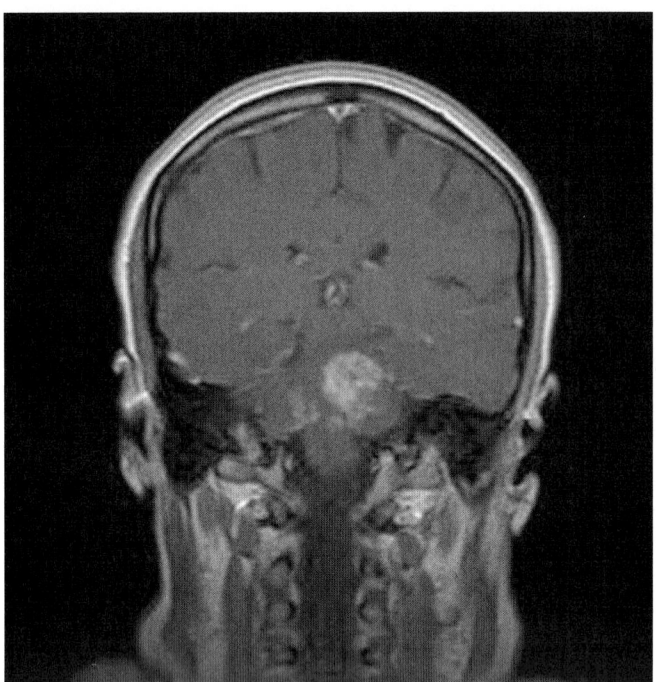

Fig. 18.12.6 Brain MRI with gadolinium contrast. There is uptake in multiple areas (white areas) indicating inflammatory lesions within the brain due to neurosarcoidosis.

the other major causes of this sight-threatening complication. Retinal disease has also been reported. Blindness from sarcoidosis is fortunately rare, and it is usually a consequence of untreated uveitis, retinitis, or optic neuritis.

Neurological disease from sarcoidosis can affect the cranial nerves, central nervous system (CNS), and peripheral nerves. Cranial nerve involvement, especially of the nerve VII, is a common complaint in neurosarcoidosis. CNS lesions can lead to a lymphocytic meningitis. Hypothalamic involvement is a characteristic pattern, with diabetes insipidus as a resulting complaint. Contrast-enhanced MRI is the most sensitive method for detecting CNS disease (Fig. 18.12.6). The lumbar puncture is complementary, with increased protein and lymphocytes often seen in active disease. Detection of angiotensin converting enzyme (ACE) in the spinal fluid is suggestive but not diagnostic of neurosarcoidosis.

Liver and spleen involvement may be found in over one-half of patients with sarcoidosis, but symptomatic disease occurs in less than 10% of cases. Liver function tests are often elevated, especially the alkaline phosphatase, suggesting an obstructive pattern. Hyperbilirubinemia is relatively rare, but implies extensive disease and is usually an indication for therapy. Massive splenomegaly can occur, and occasionally splenectomy is performed to avoid rupture.

Hypercalcaemia and hypercalciuria can be seen with sarcoidosis. One mechanism is the granuloma converting 25-hydroxyvitamin D_3 to the biologically active form 1,25-dihydroxyvitamin D_3, which is also increased by sunlight exposure. In the Unites States of America, hypercalcemia is far more common in whites than in African-Americans. Because of the effect of increased calcium absorption, urolithiasis may be also seen in patients with sarcoidosis.

A less common but serious complication of sarcoidosis is cardiac involvement. Direct involvement of the heart can lead to arrythmias such as heart block and ventricular ectopy, which can lead to sudden death. Once the problem is recognized, the use of an implanted defibrillator may reduce the risk of death. Cardiomyopathy is also seen, and cardiac sarcoidosis should be considered in a young patient who presents with unexpected heart failure. Endomyocardial biopsy rarely makes a diagnosis because the granulomas are patchy. The technetium scan showing nonsegmental fixed defects is the most sensitive test. Gallium uptake of the heart is more specific than thallium scan.

Sarcoidosis granulomas can involve virtually any organ of the body. Rare manifestations of sarcoidosis include bone cysts, usually in the distal portion of the fingers, sinus invasion, pleural disease, breast disease, and ovarian or testicular masses.

Fatigue is a major complaint of over half of patients with sarcoidosis. This may be related to sleep apnoea, which occurs in about one-third of patients with the condition, although other factors may also be involved.

The multiorgan involvement of sarcoidosis distinguishes it from other diseases, with lymphoma and tuberculosis the two that are most often considered in the differential diagnosis. Table 18.12.4 summarizes the common features in all three of these diseases and points out features that can be used to separate them.

Pathology

The noncaseating granuloma is the characteristic pathological feature of sarcoidosis. The centre of the granuloma includes macrophages and giant cells which are of the Langerhans' type and can contain more than 10 nuclei. This core of cells is surrounded by lymphocytes. Immunohistochemical studies have shown that the lymphocytes present two rings of cell types: the larger component is the CD4 lymphocyte, while the outer ring usually includes CD8 lymphocytes. The granulomas tend to be well formed, and in lung biopsies they are often well demarcated from normal tissue. The central area will occasionally contain a Schaumann body, which is formed of crystallized material (calcium phosphate) and different in appearance from the foreign bodies or caseation that can be seen in other granulomatous diseases. Occasionally the granuloma will have a necrotic area, but most are bland.

Table 18.12.4 Comparison of features of sarcoidosis, tuberculosis, and lymphoma

Feature	Sarcoidosis	Tuberculosis	Hodgkin's lymphoma
Bilateral hilar adenopathy	Very common	Rare, except in HIV patients	Common
Skin lesions	Common	Rare	Rare
Lupus pernio	Diagnostic	None	None
Erythema nodosum	Common	Rare	Very rare
Hypercalcemia	Can occur	Very rare	Rare
Eye disease	Common	Rare	Very rare
Pleural disease	Very rare	Common	Common
Cranial nerve VII paralysis	Common	Very rare	Very rare
Elevated ACE	Very common	Rare	None
Tuberculin skin test	Anergic	Positive	Anergic
BAL lymphocytes	Very common	Common	Very rare

ACE, angiotensin converting enzyme; BAL, bronchoalveolar lavage.

The diagnosis of sarcoidosis is always one of exclusion, but the finding of noncaseating granulomas in two or more organs is—for practical purposes—considered diagnostic. Cultures and special stains for tuberculosis and deep-seated fungal infections should be taken to rule out infection as the cause of granulomas. Close examination should also be made for foreign bodies and malignancy, both of which could lead to a grnaulomatous reaction.

Investigation

Serum ACE levels

In 1976, Lieberman reported that serum ACE was elevated in the blood of some patients with sarcoidosis, and it has subsequently become clear that this can also occur in a few other conditions. Only 60% of patients with acute sarcoidosis and less than one-third of patients with chronic disease will have elevated levels of ACE. Patients with infectious granulomatous diseases such as tuberculosis, histoplasmosis, and coccidiomycosis occasionally have an elevated ACE level. Mild elevations have also been reported in diabetes mellitus and osteoarthritis, and high levels have been detected in Gaucher's disease, leprosy, and hyperthyroidism. ACE levels are usually lower than normal in patients with Hodgkin's lymphoma, and because ACE is measured using a biological assay, patients on ACE inhibitors have low functional levels. In sarcoidosis the ACE level will decrease in response to treatment or disease resolution with time. It has been proposed as a marker for disease activity, but corticosteroids independently suppress ACE levels, and reducing the dose of corticosteroids may lead to a rise in ACE level without a clinical worsening of disease.

There is a genetic polymorphism for ACE, with an insertion (I) or deletion (D) of a nonsense DNA fragment. ACE levels are higher in DD patients, which needs to be considered when interpreting the serum ACE level, but there appears to be no difference in the distribution of the alleles in patients with sarcoidosis versus the general population.

Serum lysozyme is also elevated in the same way as ACE. Unfortunately, it is elevated in a smaller number of patients with sarcoidosis. Most clinicians will only determine ACE levels.

Tests of the lung

Bronchoalveolar lavage findings have proved to be fairly characteristic in sarcoidosis. The finding of increased lymphocytes, especially an increased CD4:CD8 ratio, has been interpreted by some groups as enough evidence to make a diagnosis of sarcoidosis, and lavage findings may be considered sufficient in a patient with a compatible clinical history and no evidence for infection or malignancy. A more definitive answer from bronchoscopy includes a transbronchial biopsy showing noncaseating granulomas. In over 60% of patients with a stage 1 chest radiograph the biopsy should be positive, rising to 80% in patients with stage 2 or 3 disease. Transbronchial needle aspiration can sample mediastinal and hilar lymph nodes, but unfortunately incomplete sampling of the lymph node in a granulomatous response to malignancy can occur. Mediastinoscopy and video assisted thoracoscopy provide minimally invasive methods to obtain more tissue and are usually definitive.

Imaging

Aside from chest radiography and CT scanning, which have already been discussed, gallium and PET scans can demonstrate active inflammation in lymph nodes and other active areas in sarcoidosis. However, the uptake is nonspecific and the level of uptake can be the same as seen with malignancy. This can lead to confusion in patients undergoing PET scan for possible lymphoma, when the activity will be the same for both sarcoidosis and lymphoma. In the gallium scan, which is the older-established procedure, uptake in the parotid and conjunctiva (the 'panda' sign), and uptake in the hilar nodes (the 'lambda' sign), are fairly characteristic for sarcoidosis and are useful confirmation in difficult cases.

Other tests

The Kviem–Siltzbach agent is a suspension of spleen tissue from a patient with confirmed sarcoidosis. Six weeks after an intradermal injection of the agent, the site is inspected for a reaction, which will occur in over 60% of patients with acute sarcoidosis. On biospy the reaction will show noncaseating granuloma, consistent with sarcoidosis. Properly prepared Kviem–Siltzbach agent has a less than 1 in 500 chance of causing a false positive, however, because of the difficulties in preparing the agent and concerns regarding transmission of an infectious agent, the test is rarely used except in centres with a well-established reagent.

Other laboratory tests may support the diagnosis of sarcoidosis or the level of disease activity. For example, the sedimentation rate and C-reactive protein can be elevated in sarcoidosis and may be useful for disease monitoring, but in over half of patients these inflammatory markers are normal, hence they are neither specific nor sensitive diagnostic tests.

Serum calcium is elevated in 10% of patients with sarcoidosis and is supportive of the diagnosis, but hypercalcaemia can be seen in other conditions which mimic the condition, such as malignancy. Hypercalcaemia due to sarcoidosis should be associated with a normal to low serum phosphate. Renal failure may occur in those with significant hypercalcaemia, which is usually reversible with treatment of the hypercalcaemia.

Hypergammaglobulinemia is also a feature of sarcoidosis, with activated T lymphocytes in the lung capable of stimulating circulating peripheral blood B cells to produce the polyclonal gammaglobulin response found in the condition. Serological markers for some diseases may be falsely elevated as a result of this nonspecific reaction, including antifungal and antinuclear antibodies. The hypergammaglobulinemia is more common in African-Americans than in whites.

As stated previously, liver involvement occurs in over one-half of patients with sarcoidosis, although in some cases there is no serum chemistry test indicating involvement. However, most patients with liver involvement will have elevated serum enzymes, and usually the pattern is obstructive with a rise in the serum alkaline phosphatase. In some patients an elevation of the transaminases is seen. Elevation of the serum bilirubin is less frequent and associated with more extensive liver involvement. Rarely, lymphadenopathy at the porta hepatis can lead to biliary obstruction.

Haematological abnormalities are common in sarcoidosis. Lymphopenia is frequently seen, and is probably due to sequestration of the lymphocytes into the area of inflammation, such as the lung. Anaemia has been reported in about 20% of cases: the mechanism is multifactorial, including a high proportion with iron deficiency. Other causes include direct bone marrow invasion by granulomas and suppression of the bone marrow by cytokines such as IL-2.

Treatment

The natural course of sarcoidosis is unclear because corticosteroids are normally used to treat symptomatic patients. The prognosis is often good for the patient with no symptoms on presentation, with spontaneous resolution of the disease often occurring within a year or two of diagnosis. However, the disease can also take a chronic form, with symptoms for many years.

The concept of acute disease, which lasts for less than 2 years, vs chronic disease has been a useful method of discussing patients, especially in terms of therapy. Table 18.12.5 lists several factors associated with resolution within 2 to 5 years, as well as those predicting chronic disease. Acute disease is associated with erythema nodosum, hilar adenopathy, anterior uveitis, and paralysis of cranial nerve VII. Chronic disease includes such manifestations as lupus pernio, stage 4 chest radiograph, posterior uveitis, urolithiasis, and bone cysts. Most chronic disease is controllable by therapy, but there are refractory patients. Mortality from sarcoidosis occurs, but is less than 5% in most series, with the most common causes of death being from lung, cardiac and neurological disease refractory to therapy.

The main indication for therapy in sarcoidosis is symptoms, although hypercalcaemia should be treated even if the patient is asymptomatic. An eye examination should be performed in all patients with sarcoidosis: uveitis may be misdiagnosed as sicca (dry eyes), but the former will require anti-inflammatory agents, whilst the latter will only need a wetting agent.

Corticosteroids

If possible, treatment should be topical. Corticosteroid topical creams and eye drops are effective if the inflammation is superficial. The effectiveness of inhaled steroids is less clear cut. The higher-potency steroids such as budesonide appear to have a role in reducing the dosage of systemic corticosteroids, and randomized trials have indicated a role for this drug as maintenance therapy for a patient who has received systemic therapy for 3 months to induce a remission.

It is not clear whether corticosteroids change the natural course of the disease. Early randomized trials found no difference in the long term outcome of patients who received corticosteroids versus controls. A British Thoracic Society randomized study demonstrated a small benefit for corticosteroids over placebo for patients with persistent, but not severe disease. However, in this study—as in most of the early studies—patients with symptomatic

disease were excluded and always treated with corticosteroids, which could lead to a limit in the observed response to therapy.

Several groups have looked at the need for treatment and the duration of therapy. The genetic background of these groups varies, from mostly white northern European decent, where 60% never required systemic therapy, to African-Americans, where 70% were treated. In general, about one-half of sarcoidosis patients will require systemic therapy for their disease, and after 2 to 5 years, 18–53% of the patients could not be withdrawn from therapy. In patients who were tapered off corticosteroids, one group found that 80% eventually relapsed and required reinstitution of therapy. The differences in rate of continued therapy and relapse between the centres could be due to either the genetic background of the patients or the bias of the treating physicians. Interestingly, two studies demonstrated that if the patient did not require initial systemic therapy, there was a less than 10% chance that they would require treatment after 2 to 5 years.

The toxicities of corticosteroids are well known. These include weight gain, diabetes mellitus, hypertension, and mood swings, and with prolonged use avascular necrosis and osteopenia are significant problems. Some patients with sarcoidosis will have lost weight as part of their disease, but the weight gain with treatment often surpasses the amount of weight lost. The longer a patient is on corticosteroids, the more problematic, and unfortunately most patients will require more than a year of treatment.

Several alternatives to systemic corticosteroids have been proposed over the years. These are summarized and compared to corticosteroids in Table 18.12.6, which includes the usual doses, commonly encountered toxicities, an estimate of response rate, and the usual indications for use.

Other agents

The commonly prescribed antimalarial agents chloroquine and hydroxychloroquine possess anti-inflammatory activity, with the major toxicities being eye and gastrointestinal. Hydroxychloroquine has been associated with less eye toxicity and therefore it is more frequently prescribed, although some experts feel chloroquine is a more effective agent. The drugs concentrate in the skin and have been most efficacious for skin disease and hypercalcaemia: they are less successful for treating pulmonary disease.

Methotrexate is an antimetabolite chemotherapy used for various solid tumours. In a double-blind randomized placebo-controlled trial of acute pulmonary sarcoidosis it was found to be steroid sparing, but required 6 months to be effective. The response rate for chronic sarcoidosis is 60 to 80% and methotrexate is usually used in this context. Most patients who respond can be treated with methotrexate alone, but about 20% of patients will require low-dose corticosteroids in addition. The usual dose is 10 to 15 mg orally each week, which may need to be adjusted for toxicity. We have successfully treated patients with doses as small as 2.5 mg of methotrexate a week. Acute toxicity, including mucositis and nausea, can be minimized with supplements of folic acid at 1 mg/day. Leucopenia can also occur, but is usually insignificant unless the patient is already leucopenic from sarcoidosis or the patient has renal insufficiency. The long-term toxicity of methotrexate can include hypersensitivity pneumonitis and cirrhosis, the latter being a concern because 50% of chronic patients will have sarcoidosis granulomas in a liver biopsy, hence we recommend liver biopsies every 2 years for patients requiring prolonged treatment with methotrexate.

Table 18.12.5 Features predictive of the clinical course of sarcoidosis

Organ	Acute	Chronic
Chest radiograph	Stage 1	Stage 4
Skin	Erythema nodosum	Lupus pernio
Eyes	Anterior uveitis	Posterior uveitis Pars planitis
Joint involvement		Bone cysts
Calcium metabolism	Hypercalcaemia	Urolithiasis
Cardiac		Cardiomyopathy
Neurological	Cranial nerve VII palsy	Central nervous system mass
Sinus		Sinus involvement

Table 18.12.6 Treatments for sarcoidosis

Drug	Dosage	Efficacy (%)	Toxicity	Usage
Prednisone/Prednisolone	5–40 mg/day	90	Weight gain Diabetes Hypertension Osteoporosis Psychiatric	Acute Chronic Refractory
Hydroxychloroquine	200–400 mg/day	30–50[a]	Gastrointestinal Retinal	Acute Chronic
Methotrexate	10–25 mg once a week	60–80	Haematological Gastrointestinal Lung Hepatic Mutagenic	Chronic Refractory
Leflunomide	10–20 mg/day	60–80	Haematological Gastrointestinal Hepatic Mutagenic	Chronic Refractory
Azathioprine	50–200 mg/day	50–80	Haematological Gastrointestinal Carcinogenic Mutagenic	Chronic Refractory
Pentoxifylline	400 mg three times a day	50	Gastrointestinal	Acute
Cyclophosphamide	50–150 mg/day orally, 500–2000 mg every 2 weeks IV	80	Gastrointestinal Haematological Carcinogenic Bladder Teratogenic	Chronic Refractory
Thalidomide	50–100 mg/day	80[a]	Teratogenic Somnolence Peripheral neuropathy	Chronic Refractory
Infliximab	3–5 mg/kg IV initially, 2 weeks later, then every 4–8 weeks	90	Allergic reactions Infections Worsening heart failure Probable carcinogen	Refractory

IV, intravenous

[a] Refers to efficacy for skin manifestations of sarcoidosis: other manifestations respond less well.

Leflunomide is an antimetabolite similar to methotrexate but with less pulmonary and gastrointestinal toxicity. It appears to be as effective as methotrexate and has also been given in combination with methotrexate, when the two drugs appear to be synergistic.

Azathioprine has been used as an immunosuppressant for solid organ transplant patients and patients with idiopathic pulmonary fibrosis for many years. However, its use in sarcoidosis has been more sporadic, and it is usually reserved for chronic cases.

Other drugs have been used for refractory sarcoidosis. Cyclophosphamide, a cytotoxic agent used in the treatment of many vasculitic diseases, has been reported as very useful in neurological and cardiac sarcoidosis, but it has more gastrointestinal, haematological, and bladder toxicity than methotrexate or azathioprine. Ciclosporin has been used with limited success in some neurological cases, but a randomized trial failed to show additional benefit over corticosteroids alone in patients with pulmonary sarcoidosis.

Persistent release of TNF by alveolar macrophages is a feature of patients with chronic sarcoidosis, hence the effects of drugs that block TNF release or action have been studied. These include corticosteroids, methotrexate, and azathioprine, which have been discussed previously. Others include pentoxifylline, which inhibits alveolar macrophage release of TNF, and can provide benefit in some cases of acute sarcoidosis, although associated with significant gastrointestinal toxicity which has limited its use. Thalidomide also has significant anti-TNF activity and is effective at treating chronic, severe skin lesions including lupus pernio, but the drug has severe teratogenic potential such that close monitoring is required, and it also causes hypersomnolence, constipation, and a peripheral neuropathy. The treatment of eye or pulmonary eye disease often requires high doses of thalidomide, hence the risk–benefit ratio limits use of the drug to skin disease.

Biological agents directed against TNF have been developed for various inflammatory diseases such as rheumatoid arthritis, Crohn's disease, and psoriasis. These include infliximab, which is a monoclonal antibody that binds TNF, and etanerecept, a TNF receptor antagonist. Numerous case reports and case series have demonstrated a rapid and sometimes dramatic response to infliximab in refractory cases of sarcoidosis. In a double-blind placebo-controlled randomized trial of infliximab for chronic pulmonary sarcoidosis, infliximab was found effective in further improving the vital capacity of those patients already on at least 10 mg prednisone and/or cytotoxic agents, with the study demonstrating a larger effect of therapy for those with more severe disease. The TNF receptor antagonist etanerecept has been less successful in treating sarcoidosis: in pulmonary and ocular disease less than one-third of patients improved on therapy, and one-third became worse during treatment. The difference in efficacy between infliximab and etanercept has also been noted in Crohn's disease, where infliximab is also the biological agent of choice. The differences between agents may be due to mechanism of action or peak dose of the drug (infliximab is given intravenously, etanerecept subcutaneously). Infliximab binds TNF on the cell surface, whereas etanerecept blocks soluble TNF. The interaction on the cell surface can affect the transmembrane TNF effect, and the binding has also been associated with inducing apoptosis that would lead to reduction of the number of inflammatory cells releasing TNF and other proinflammatory cytokines.

The biological agents are associated with significant toxicities and cost. Among the class toxicities are the allergic reactions, increased rate of infection, worsening of pre-existing congestive heart failure, and potential carcinogenic effects. Compared to etanercept, infliximab is associated with a higher rate of reactivation of tuberculosis, which may be a reflection of its superior antigranulomatous properties. Overall, because of the potential severe toxicities, infliximab use appears limited to refractory cases.

Strategy

There is no single treatment for all patients with sarcoidosis. The first step is to determine whether the patient requires treatment, the decision to treat usually being based on the patient's symptoms. The clinician needs to determine the extent of the symptomatic disease and whether the disease is acute or chronic. Asymptomatic or minimally symptomatic patients with hypercalcaemia, cardiac, or central nervous system disease may require therapy to prevent life-threatening complications. The use of systemic therapy usually means corticosteroids first. If the patient is able to be successfully treated with corticosteroids, the dose is gradually reduced to minimize toxicity. If the dose cannot be reduced to an acceptable level, or if the patient is not responding to corticosteroids, then steroid sparing agents should be added. For most of these the onset of action is 6 months or more, hence the clinician should not hesitate to add these drugs early into therapy if the patient has evidence for chronic disease (Table 18.12.5) or recurrent symptoms whenever steroids are withdrawn.

Prognosis

Most patients with sarcoidosis will experience disease resolution within 2 to 5 years; about 25% will develop residual fibrosis in the lungs or elsewhere; in a few the disease will become chronic and persist for more than 5 years. For the chronic patient, treatment can usually palliate symptoms, but organ failure—including eye, liver, cardiac, or respiratory—can occur as a result of disease. Most series from referral centres report 5% disease related mortality, with 1% probably the rate in nonselected patients. The most common cause for sarcoid-related death is respiratory failure, with cardiac, neurological, and liver disease as other causes. Respiratory failure leading to death can be predicted from pulmonary function

tests, e.g. one study found no patient with a vital capacity of more than 1.5 litres died from respiratory failure, whereas one-third of those with vital capacity persistently less than 1 litre died of this complication. In patients with severe restriction the best predictor of death was presence of pulmonary hypertension and evidence of right heart failure (as associated with an elevated right atrial pressure). Organ transplantation has been successfully performed in sarcoidosis patients: although sarcoidosis lesions can occur in the new organ, organ failure due to sarcoidosis is unlikely.

Particular complications

As stated above, endstage lung disease is the most common problem for patients with severe sarcoidosis, with fibrotic disease leading to cor pulmonale and respiratory distress. In addition, cavitary lesions can lead to bronchiectasis or become colonized with aspergillus. Aspergillomas can cause haemoptysis, which can be fatal, and treatment is difficult because most patients are not good surgical candidates: embolization has been used for life-threatening bleeding.

In studies of patients who are persistently dyspnoeic due to sarcoidosis, up to 50% have pulmonary hypertension. Factors associated with this are stage 3 or 4 chest radiograph, hypoxia, and reduced $D_L$co. A right heart catheterization is an important part of their evaluation because they may have coincident left ventricular disease. In case reports of patients with sarcoidosis associated pulmonary arterial hypertension, both epoprostenol and bosanten have been reported as useful, working independently of any anti-inflammatory drugs used to treat the underlying condition.

Steroid-induced osteopenia is a significant problem with long-term corticosteroid therapy. Patients are often not treated initially with calcium supplements because of the risk of hypercalcaemia, but calcium supplementation should be considered if a patient requires long-term systemic steroids, with monitoring serum calcium during therapy usually sufficient to avoid complications. The use of nasal calcitonin or biphosphonates should also be considered if the patient requires prolonged therapy.

Cardiac sarcoidosis can lead to sudden death, hence arrythmias must be evaluated in patients with sarcoidosis. Continuous electrocardiographic monitoring is useful to identify episodes, and we use electrophysiological studies in patients with symptomatic arrythmias to determine their source. Treatment of the sarcoidosis alone may be insufficient to control rhythm disturbances in patients with ventricular arrythmias: an implanted defibrillator may be required, particularly for those with refractory ventricular tachyarrthymias.

Areas of uncertainty/controversy

Some clinicians have proposed the use of bronchoalveolar lavage as the exclusive diagnostic test for sarcoidosis: this is based on the rationale that, in the appropriate clinical setting, findings of increased lymphocytes and a CD4:CD8 ratio greater than 3.5 represents a granulomatous process. In patients with cultures negative for tuberculosis and fungal infection, sarcoidosis is most likely and no further diagnostic testing may be needed. However, the percentage of patients with increased lymphocytes and CD4:CD8 ratio varies from centre to centre: in our institution at least 50% will meet these criteria, but the use of bronchoalveolar lavage does not provide an absolute diagnosis of sarcoidosis. As previously noted, transbronchial needle aspirate may also be useful in making a diagnosis, but the finding of a granuloma does not assure the diagnosis.

The use of corticosteroids for the treatment of sarcoidosis remains controversial. In the patient with minimal symptoms, treatment can be withheld or topical. If the disease spontaneously resolves, no therapy is indicated. However, if the patient becomes symptomatic, corticosteroids will probably be useful. The best treatment of the patient with persistent, mild disease is unclear: the British Thoracic Society study suggests that these patients should receive corticosteroids; others argue that the differences are small and do not justify treatment.

Possible future developments

The cause of sarcoidosis remains unknown. Newer molecular biological techniques may provide further insight into a causative agent and/or an underlying genetic predisposition for the disease, and study of causality may provide better answers to other questions in the disease process as well.

The patient with chronic disease represents a disproportionate number of cases with increased morbidity and need for medical services, and the use of corticosteroids alone is not adequate for many of these. Research is still required into whether other agents are truly steroid sparing and associated with improved clinical outcome, and pulmonary arterial hypertension and its treatment has to be studied in these chronic cases.

The quality of life of patients with sarcoidosis is affected by both the disease and its treatment. Corticosteroids may cause more problems than benefit, and steroid sparing drugs also have their toxicity. Fatigue is a major complaint for the patient and not well treated by our current drugs: new agents such as modafinil and methylphenidate are being developed to treat fatigue and may be applicable in sarcoidosis.

Further reading

Baughman RP, et al. (2006). Infliximab therapy in patients with chronic sarcoidosis and pulmonary involvement. *Am J Respir Crit Care Med*, **174**, 795–802.

Baughman RP, du Bois RM, Lower EE (2003). Sarcoidosis. *Lancet*, **361**, 1111–18.

Baughman RP, et al. (2001). Clinical characteristics of patients in a case control study of sarcoidosis. *Am J Respir Crit Care Med*, **164**, 1885–9.

Hunninghake GW, et al. (1999). ATS/ERS/WASOG statement on sarcoidosis. American Thoracic Society/European Respiratory Society/World Association of Sarcoidosis and other Granulomatous Disorders. *Sarcoidosis Vasc Diffuse Lung Dis*, **16**, 149–73.

Song Z, et al. (2005). Mycobacterial catalase-peroxidase is a tissue antigen and target of the adaptive immune response in systemic sarcoidosis. *J Exp Med*, **201**, 755–67.

Sulica R, et al. (2005). Distinctive clinical, radiographic, and functional characteristics of patients with sarcoidosis-related pulmonary hypertension. *Chest*, **128**, 1483–9.

18.13

Pneumoconioses

A. Seaton

Essentials

Pneumoconiosis describes a diffuse reaction in the lung, usually fibrotic, following exposure to mineral dust, usually in the workplace. In many cases epidemiological studies have shown an exposure–response relationship between the total mass of respirable dust to which workers have been exposed and their risks of developing disease, which form the basis of regulations specifying permitted levels of exposure. Lung damage occurs when dusts are inhalable to acinar level and when they cannot be cleared by lung macrophages. There is a very large number of causes, for some of which workers with exposure are entitled to compensation in some countries.

Coal-worker's pneumoconiosis—caused by inhalation of coal-mine dust. Now uncommon in the United Kingdom and other Western countries, but in China the disease is widespread and in India it afflicts about 1 to 2% of the workforce. Characterized pathologically by the presence of multiple centriacinar and interlobular foci of dust, inflammatory cells, macrophages, and reticulin or collagen—the coal macule. Simple pneumoconiosis, which causes no symptoms or physical signs, is diagnosed when small discrete nodules are visible on the chest radiograph. Complicated pneumoconiosis, or progressive massive fibrosis, is present when one or more of these lesions is greater than 1 cm in diameter: this usually progresses, causing a mixture of lung restriction and airflow obstruction, and sometimes leading to cor pulmonale and death.

Silicosis—caused by inhalation of crystalline silicon dioxide, usually in the form of quartz. Silicotic lungs show fibrous pleural adhesions, enlarged lymph nodes that contain fibrotic nodules, often calcified, and grey nodules throughout the lung with a typical whorled appearance when cut across. Causes a spectrum of presentations, ranging from acute silicosis (very rare), which leads to death within months, to slowly progressive lung fibrosis, to asymptomatic radiological abnormalities. Liable to be complicated by tuberculosis and lung cancer.

Asbestosis—exposure to fibres of asbestos can cause a range of respiratory conditions including benign pleural plaques, acute effusion, diffuse fibrosis (asbestosis) and mesothelioma (see Chapter 18.19.3). Asbestosis occurs only in people working regularly with asbestos for years and not in those with occasional or incidental exposure. Disease is usually progressive, with radiological appearances identical to that in most cases of cryptogenic pulmonary fibrosis—predominantly basal and peripheral irregular linear shadowing, progressing to honeycombing. The risk of lung carcinoma is related to asbestos exposure, interacting multiplicatively with smoking.

Other causes of pneumoconiosis—these include talc, kaolin, Fuller's earth, mica, fibrous erionite, berylliosis.

Introduction

Most lung diseases are caused or provoked at least in part by the inhalation of harmful material. A wide range of lung conditions, including cancer (exposure to asbestos, radon daughters in mines, polycyclic aromatic hydrocarbons, nickel refining, chloromethyl ethers), pneumonia (legionnaire's disease in hospitals), asthma (flour, wood dust, isocyanates, epoxy resins), allergic alveolitis (farmer's lung, malt worker's lung), and toxic pneumonitis (silo filler's disease, chlorine poisoning, cadmium poisoning), may occur as a result of workplace exposure. The condition is called a pneumoconiosis when exposure to mineral dust in the workplace results in a diffuse, usually fibrotic, reaction in the lung acinus.

The distinction between tuberculosis and a specific effect of dust in the causation of respiratory disease was made in the mid 19th century. By this time silicosis, often complicated by tuberculosis, was widespread amongst metal miners, tunnellers, potters, and cutlers. The Industrial Revolution stimulated the need for coal, and the production of this fuel resulted in increasing numbers of sufferers from coal-worker's pneumoconiosis. This in turn was not distinguished from silicosis until the late 1940s, and in some countries the two conditions are still referred to by the one name.

In the United Kingdom, and generally in the West, dust controls in mines and decline of traditional industries have both resulted in a reduction in the numbers of workers suffering from these two diseases. As this has happened, interest has been drawn to the possibility that exposure to mineral dusts may have a role in the aetiology of chronic obstructive pulmonary disease (COPD), and this link has been established in the case of coal dust. By contrast, industrialization of developing countries has stimulated the need for indigenous coal and minerals, and in China, South America, and India several million workers are employed in mining, often in conditions that ensure a high incidence of pneumoconiosis. At the same time, the rise of the asbestos and chemical industries has added new problems for society in weighing the benefits of the product against the cost in terms of human morbidity. Fortunately, these problems are potentially soluble by application of preventive measures, as emphasized in the following sections.

Coal-worker's pneumoconiosis

Coal-worker's pneumoconiosis is caused by inhalation of coal-mine dust, a complex mixture of coal, kaolin, mica, silica, and other clay minerals. It is now uncommon in the United Kingdom, and good dust control together with reduction in the mining industry means that the disease may disappear in the next few years. Nevertheless, the strategic importance of coal as a long-term source of fuel supply and as a chemical feedstock means that it will continue to be needed, and any relaxation of dust control in mines for any reason will be followed by the reappearance of pneumoconiosis. Other Western countries have also seen a reduction in the incidence of coal-worker's pneumoconiosis, but in China the disease is widespread and in India it afflicts about 1 to 2% of the current coal industry workforce of 800 000.

Aetiology and pathology

The pathogenicity of coal dust differs in different regions. If lung damage is to occur, the dust must be inhalable to acinar level within the lung, hence the particles must have aerodynamic characteristics that make them equivalent to a sphere of unit density between 0.5 and 7 μm in diameter. Once inhaled, the particles must be able to overcome the lung's defences. Some, containing a high proportion of quartz (crystalline silicon dioxide), are toxic to macrophages and cause their disruption after phagocytosis. Such particles are cleared predominantly to the lymph nodes, where they remain and set up a fibrotic reaction that ultimately destroys the node. However, some remain in the peribronchiolar and perivascular parts of the acinus, where whorled fibrosis occurs leading to the typical silicotic nodule. The mechanisms of quartz-induced fibrosis are discussed further in the silicosis section below. However, since most coal dust contains relatively little quartz and is not particularly toxic to macrophages *in vitro*, some other explanation for its harmfulness must be sought. *In vivo* studies in rats have shown that inhalation of relatively low concentrations of coal dust, comparable with those occurring in United Kingdom mines in the recent past, cause inhibition of macrophage migration and provoke an inflammatory response, mediated by interleukin 1 (IL-1) and tumour necrosis factor (TNF) among others, resulting in the release of elastase and the degradation of fibronectin. It seems likely that *in vivo* these toxic effects on macrophages are fundamental to the pathological processes in coal-worker's pneumoconiosis, including the concomitant centriacinar emphysema.

The total amount of dust inhaled is also a critical factor in the development of pneumoconiosis. Epidemiological studies have

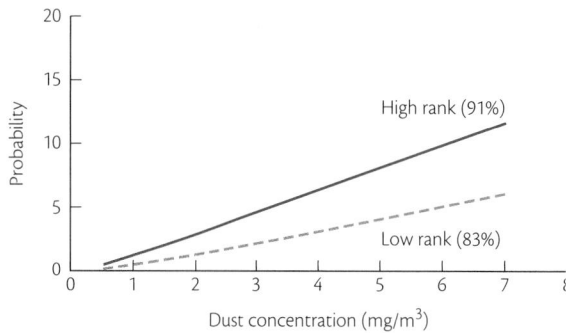

Fig. 18.13.1 Relationship between risk of category 2 or 3 radiological simple pneumoconiosis and daily exposure over a working lifetime to different concentrations of coal dust. The greater risk in association with exposure to dust from coals of higher combustibility (rank) should be noted.

shown clear relationships between cumulative dust exposure and radiological evidence of disease. However, this is not straightforward, as some coal dusts are clearly more toxic than others, and it is not always possible to characterize this toxicity by the relative mineralogical composition of the coal dust. There is evidence that the different minerals in coal dust interact and that some clays may reduce its overall toxicity, perhaps by blocking the surface activity of the toxic fraction. As a general rule, the higher the combustibility (rank) of the coal, the more likely is its dust to cause pneumoconiosis (Fig. 18.13.1).

Pathologically, coal-worker's pneumoconiosis is characterized by the presence of multiple centriacinar and interlobular foci of dust, inflammatory cells, macrophages, and reticulin or collagen—the coal macule (Fig. 18.13.2). In miners exposed to relatively high proportions of quartz, the lesions have a greater resemblance to the silicotic nodule. The presence of small, discrete nodules is known as simple pneumoconiosis, and when sufficient numbers of these lesions are present they become visible on the chest radiograph. Complicated pneumoconiosis, or progressive massive fibrosis, is present by definition when one or more of these lesions is more than 1 cm in diameter (Fig. 18.13.3). This occurs either by aggregation of several, usually collagenous, smaller nodules, or by a more diffuse accumulation of dust associated with dead cells and ischaemic

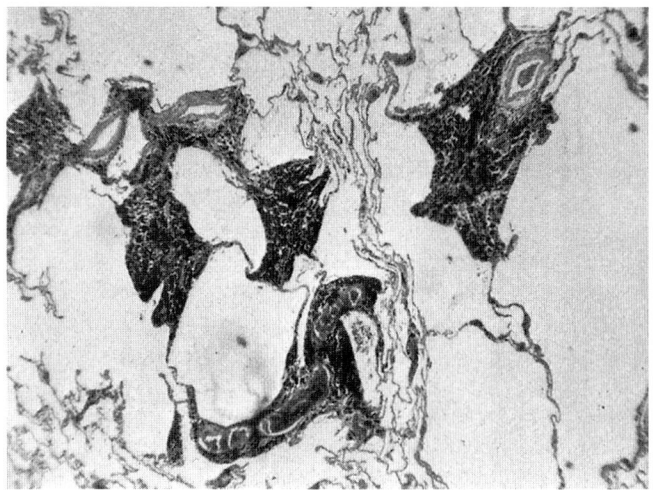

Fig. 18.13.2 Simple coal macules, showing accumulations of dust and cells around centre of lobule with associated emphysema.

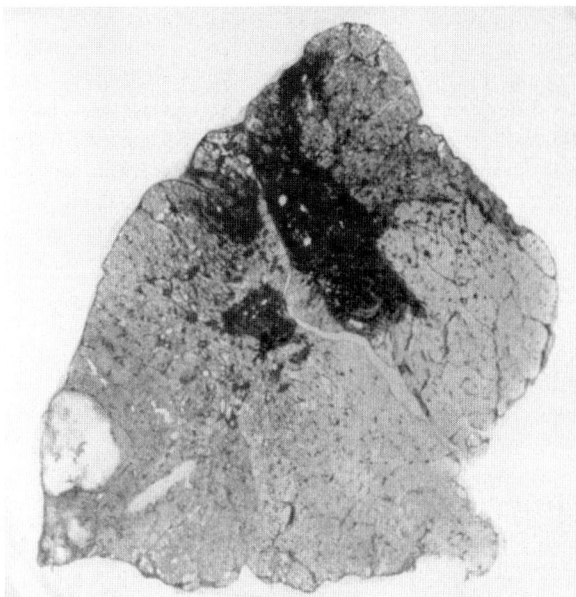

Fig. 18.13.3 Whole-lung section of a coal miner's lung showing progressive massive fibrosis.

necrosis of lung tissue. The former mechanism is less common and occurs particularly in relation to relatively high quartz exposures, while the latter seems more frequent with exposure to high-carbon dusts. With either type, and with intermediate types, there is a tendency for the lesions to grow and to be associated with surrounding bullous emphysema, ultimately being responsible for destruction of large volumes of the lung.

The aetiology of progressive massive fibrosis is not completely understood. It is more common in the upper lung zones and in taller men, suggesting a relationship to failure of lung clearance. High-carbon or high-quartz dusts are particularly liable to cause the condition, and the higher the dust exposure, the greater is the risk (Fig. 18.13.4). Tuberculous infection is no longer an important factor in the developed world, although it may have been in the past. The rheumatoid diathesis is responsible for initiating a rare type of progressive massive fibrosis (Caplan's syndrome), but this is not an important factor overall. For further discussion of the aetiology of progressive massive fibrosis, see the section on silicosis below.

Clinical features

The people most at risk of coal-worker's pneumoconiosis are those working in the dustiest areas, such as face-workers cutting coal,

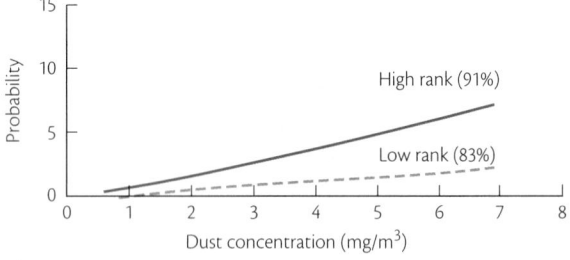

Fig. 18.13.4 Relationship between risk of progressive massive fibrosis and exposure to dust over a working lifetime. Again, greater risk in association with exposure to dust from coals of higher combustibility (rank) should be noted.

drilling for shot-firing, developing headings, and drilling bolts into the roof to prevent it falling. Open-cast miners rarely work in such dusty surroundings, except in hot dry countries such as India where loading operations may be extremely dusty. Simple coal-worker's pneumoconiosis causes no symptoms or physical signs, nor any important physiological abnormality. This fact is of importance because it means that symptoms of respiratory disease in a miner with this condition are due to some other cause, such as bronchitis, heart failure, or asthma, which may be treatable. Radiological progression or regression of simple pneumoconiosis occurs only very rarely after dust exposure ceases, apparent regression sometimes being associated with the development of emphysema.

The danger associated with simple pneumoconiosis is that it predisposes to progressive massive fibrosis, a risk directly related to the profusion of simple pneumoconiosis on the radiograph. Progressive massive fibrosis may occur during working life or appear for the first time after (sometimes many years after) dust exposure ceases, even when there is no apparent simple pneumoconiosis on the radiograph. Progressive massive fibrosis usually progresses and causes a mixture of restriction of lung volume and, owing to associated emphysema, airflow obstruction. Ultimately it may lead to cor pulmonale and death, but the rate of progression is very variable. In general, the earlier progressive massive fibrosis develops in a person's life, the more rapidly progressive and thus the greater a threat to health it is.

The patient with progressive massive fibrosis may complain of shortness of breath and symptoms of cor pulmonale. An unusual but pathognomonic symptom is melanoptysis—the expectoration of the black contents of a cavitated lesion. Haemoptysis and finger clubbing suggest lung cancer and should not be attributed to pneumoconiosis. Abnormal signs in the chest, if present, relate to the presence of bullae, although lobar collapse can occur very rarely.

Coal-worker's pneumoconiosis is not associated with an increased risk of tuberculosis or lung cancer, although obviously these diseases can occur in coal miners in endemic areas and should be suspected if unusual progression of radiological changes occurs. The association between pneumoconiosis and emphysema has been controversial, but there is now clear evidence of a parallel association between dust exposure and two effects—pneumoconiosis and airflow obstruction. The more dust that a miner has been exposed to, the greater are his risks of pneumoconiosis on the one hand, and productive cough, reduction in forced expiratory volume in 1 s (FEV_1), and presence of centriacinar emphysema on the other. Of course, the latter risks are also related to cigarette smoking, and the effect of dust exposure is additive to this.

The radiological lesions in simple pneumoconiosis are predominantly rounded opacities between 1 and 5 mm in diameter, although small irregular and linear opacities and Kerley B lines are frequently present also. The round opacities tend to be more profuse in the upper and middle zones, whereas the irregular lesions predominate in the lower zone (Fig. 18.13.5). Progressive massive fibrosis almost always starts in an upper zone, gradually increasing in size until it may occupy up to one-third of the lung. Such lesions are frequently multiple, often shaped like short fat sausages, with their outer border curved with the chest wall and separated from the pleura by bullous emphysema (Fig. 18.13.6). Calcification is not a feature, but cavitation may occur. Caplan's syndrome is the name given to the combination of rheumatoid disease and several round nodules (usually 1–5 cm in diameter) in the lungs of

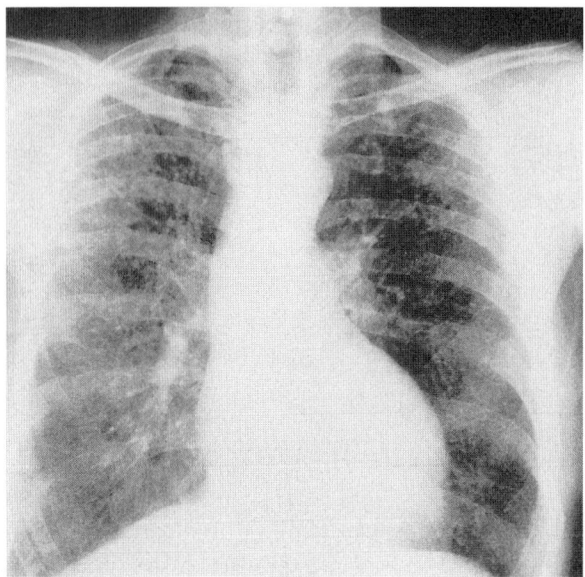

Fig. 18.13.5 Radiograph of a coal miner showing small round lesions of simple pneumoconiosis. Some irregular shadows are also present in the lower zones.

a coal miner. The lesions have a rheumatoid histology and rarely cause any serious pulmonary impairment; they often cavitate and disappear. The radiological features of all pneumoconioses are properly described in terms of a set of standard radiographs produced by the International Labour Organization, and use of these standards is mandatory for epidemiological studies.

Prevention and management

Epidemiological studies have shown an exposure–response relationship between the total mass of respirable coal dust to which miners have been exposed and their risks of developing simple pneumoconiosis. This has allowed standards to be set for coal-mine dust levels that have resulted in falls in the prevalence of the disease in coal mines in the West. Their success depends on regular monitoring of the respirable dust by gravimetric sampler, constant attention to dust suppression by ventilation, and the use of water at

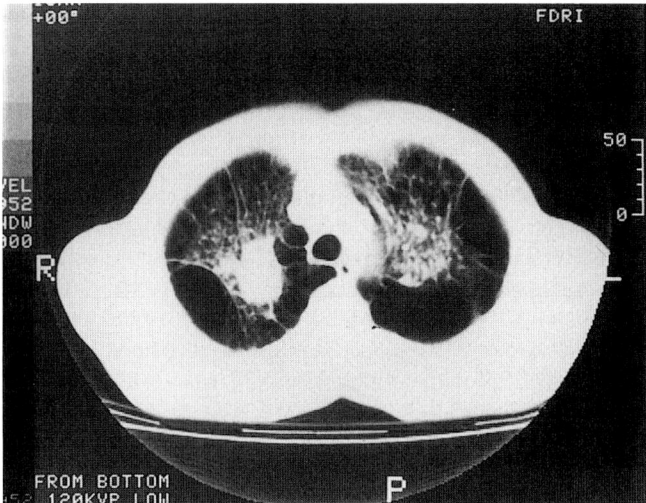

Fig. 18.13.6 CT scan of miner, showing central progressive massive fibrosis and surrounding bullous emphysema.

points of dust production, together with regular radiography of the workforce to detect early signs of dust retention. The incidence of progressive massive fibrosis is largely controlled by preventing miners from contracting simple pneumoconiosis, and working conditions in British mines are currently such that this disease is now very rare indeed. The present United Kingdom standard is $7\,mg/m^3$, measured in the air returning from the coalface.

If a miner develops simple pneumoconiosis late in his career, no action normally needs to be taken, apart from (in the United Kingdom) advising him to apply to the Respiratory Diseases Board via the Benefits Agency for assessment of disablement and possible benefit payments. A younger man, with several years of further dust exposure ahead, should be advised to work in an area of approved low dust conditions. In the United Kingdom this advice should be given by the employer's occupational health service. Men with more than the earliest stages of radiological change are entitled to disablement benefits from the Benefits Agency, the value of these depending on the extent of disability. Since simple pneumoconiosis *per se* does not disable, these benefits are often small. Payment of benefits for airflow obstruction as an associated effect of coal dust exposure are also made in the United Kingdom if the miner has worked underground for a minimum of 20 years and his FEV_1 is 1 litre below that predicted. The presence of associated radiological change is not necessary. Following a legal judgement in the United Kingdom, civil compensation through the government is now available for individuals with symptoms of chronic bronchitis or with airflow obstruction, and such workers should be referred to their trade union for advice.

Silicosis

Silicosis is a fibrotic disease of the lungs due to inhalation of crystalline silicon dioxide, usually in the form of quartz. Such a disease has occurred in metal miners and masons since ancient times, but assumed particular importance in the cutlery and pottery trades in the 19th century. Silicosis may affect anyone involved in quarrying, carving, mining, tunnelling, grinding, or sandblasting, if the dust generated contains quartz. In the United Kingdom the traditional trades that caused the disease (pottery, cutlery, flint knapping, sandblasting, tin and iron mining, and slate quarrying) have either introduced safe substitute materials or have declined, so that true silicosis is now quite rare. Between 50 and 60 cases are diagnosed in the United Kingdom each year, usually in the production of slate or granite, among miners cutting through rock, and in fettlers in foundries. However, the author has seen a series of severe cases in British workers who had been employed in circumstances where the risks had been forgotten or were being ignored, and there is no doubt that the disease still occurs even in advanced industrial societies.

Aetiology and pathology

Crystalline silica in the Earth's crust is usually quartz, although other forms such as crystobalite and tridymite occur occasionally. All are extremely toxic to macrophages. Quartz seems to be most toxic when freshly fractured, suggesting that surface properties are important in toxicity. This concept is supported by experimental evidence that various clay minerals and other chemicals that occlude the surface reduce the toxicity of inhaled quartz when inhaled simultaneously in mixtures of dust. The quartz content of dust from different types of stone may vary considerably, from some sandstones which are 100% quartz to shales and slates which may contain less than 10%.

Inhaled particles of quartz small enough (generally <7 μm aerodynamic diameter) to reach the acinus are engulfed by macrophages and cause disruption of the phagosome, probably by peroxidation of membrane lipids. Before macrophage death, other reactions occur leading to release of inflammatory mediators, including IL-1, various growth factors, TNF, and fibronectin, largely from interstitial rather than alveolar macrophages. Silica is probably transported across the alveolar epithelium by migrating macrophages and by endocytosis by type 1 alveolar cells, and it is clear from the distribution of pathological lesions that quartz is transported widely in the lung via lymphatics, much of it ultimately being deposited in hilar nodes, which it destroys. This destruction of the nodes is very likely to be responsible for blockage of the exit route for further inhaled dust, and therefore for its retention in the lung and the development of progressive massive fibrosis or—rarely—accelerated or even acute silicosis.

Macroscopic inspection of silicotic lungs shows fibrous pleural adhesions, enlarged lymph nodes that contain fibrotic nodules, often calcified, and grey nodules throughout the lung. These nodules vary from a few millimetres to several centimetres in diameter and are more profuse in the upper zones (Fig. 18.13.7). They may rarely be calcified, and they have a typical whorled appearance when cut across (Fig. 18.13.8). The largest lesions consist of many such nodules that have become confluent, and—as in coal-worker's pneumoconiosis—this progressive massive fibrosis may undergo ischaemic necrosis and cavitate. Under the microscope the silicotic nodule consists of concentric layers of collagen surrounded by a zone of doubly refractile silica particles, macrophages, and fibroblasts.

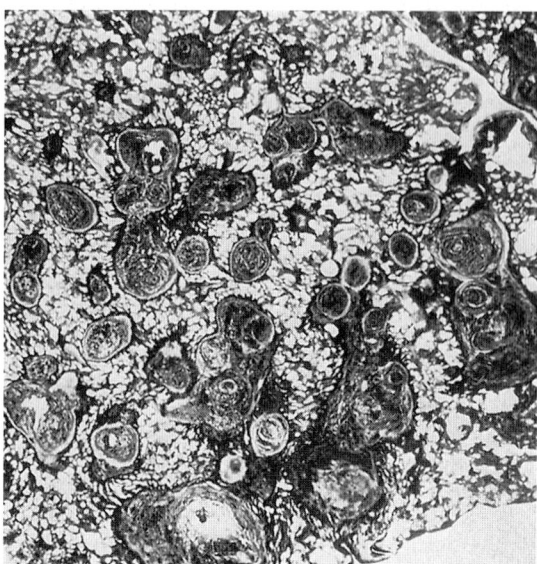

Fig. 18.13.8 Silicotic nodules, showing the typical whorled appearance.

The nodule may contain the remnants of the respiratory bronchiole and arteriole, destroyed by fibrosis. The mechanisms responsible are destruction of macrophages leading to inflammation and laying down of collagen, release of the quartz, further macrophage attraction, and repetition of the cycle. This presumably occurs first in nodes on the drainage pathway, and as these become progressively blocked the process is repeated in the lung. As the quartz never gets removed thereafter, the process continues indefinitely and severity of disease depends on the mass inhaled and retained.

Macroscopically, acute silicosis appears like pulmonary oedema. Under the microscope the alveoli are filled with eosinophilic fluid and the alveolar walls contain plasma cells, lymphocytes, fibroblasts, and silica. In the author's experience this condition first requires hilar node destruction by the inhaled quartz.

Clinical features

Silicosis presents a spectrum of clinical disease depending on the circumstances in which it is contracted. The most severe, acute silicosis, may be acquired after mere months of very heavy exposure, such as may occur in sandblasting without respiratory protection. These patients become intensely breathless and die within months (Fig. 18.13.9). The radiograph shows appearances resembling pulmonary oedema. Less heavy exposure causes progressively less dramatic symptoms, ranging from a progressive upper lobe fibrosis with slowly increasing exertional dyspnoea over several years (accelerated silicosis) to radiographic nodular change similar to coal-worker's pneumoconiosis unassociated with any symptoms or physical signs. The latter type of silicosis is the most common, and is usually associated with exposure to dust containing 10 to 30% silica over a prolonged period. Simple nodular silicosis differs from coal-worker's pneumoconiosis in that the lesions tend to be larger (3–5 mm) and that it is progressive even after dust exposure ceases. Lesions increase in size and become more profuse. Moreover, extensive simple silicosis may be associated with some restriction of lung volumes. Simple silicosis rarely seems to be associated with emphysema, unlike coal-worker's pneumoconiosis, but silicotic progressive massive fibrosis is commonly associated with bullous disease. Curiously, it has only recently been recognized

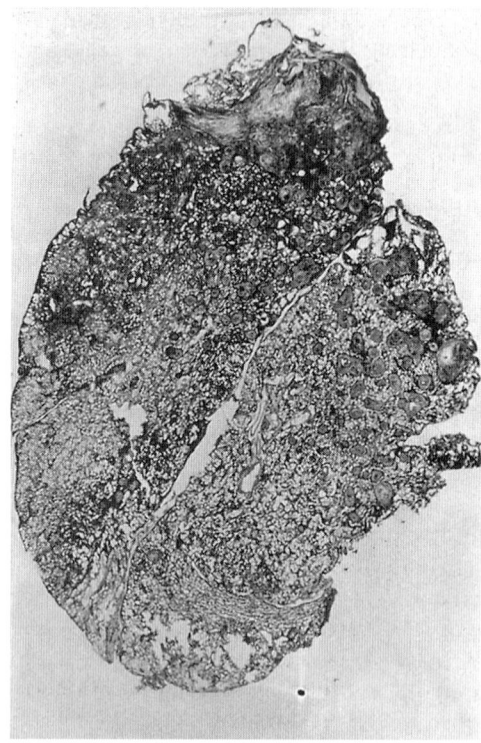

Fig. 18.13.7 Whole-lung section from a coal miner whose work had been predominantly in hard rock, showing silicotic nodules in upper parts of upper and lower lobes.

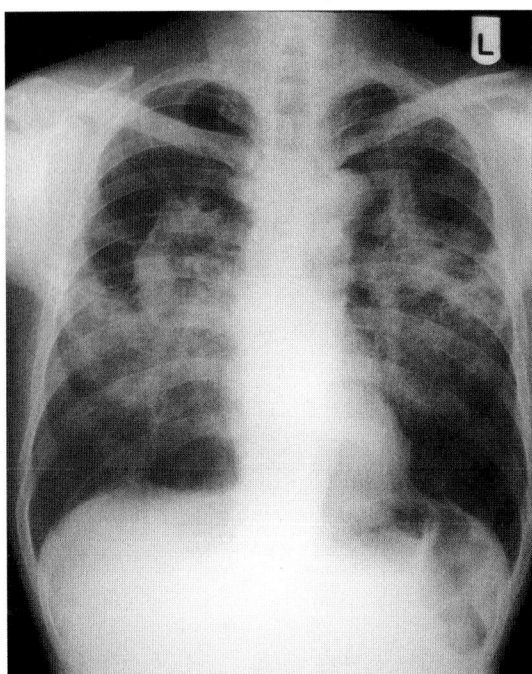

Fig. 18.13.9 Radiograph of a stonemason with intense exposure to quartz over 5 years following a prolonged period of low exposure, showing massive fibrosis and a pneumonia-like pattern of bilateral consolidation that led to his death from respiratory failure.

that acute enlargement of hilar nodes mimicking sarcoidosis may be an early feature of silicosis (Fig. 18.13.10). Accelerated silicosis and progressive massive fibrosis cause lung restriction and lead to cor pulmonale and cardiorespiratory failure.

Apart from evidence of cardiac failure or distortion of lung architecture by extreme degrees of massive fibrosis, physical signs are not prominent. Clubbing and crackles are not seen. Diagnosis depends on a history of exposure and the radiographic appearances. The most characteristic of these are nodules between 3 and 5 mm in diameter, predominantly in the upper zones, and eggshell calcification in the hilar nodes (Fig. 18.13.11). The latter is virtually a pathognomonic feature, only occurring otherwise (very rarely) in sarcoidosis.

All forms of silicosis are liable to be complicated by tuberculosis, usually due to reactivation of a quiescent lesion, and other mycobacterial diseases (*Mycobacterium kansasii* and *Mycobacterium avium-intracellulare*) also occur more frequently than would be expected. There is a weak association between silicosis and lung cancer, even when exposures to cigarette smoke and other occupational carcinogens have been accounted for. The evidence is sufficient for lung cancer to have been recognized as an occupational disease in patients with silicosis in the United Kingdom. Pneumothorax is also an occasional complication of silicosis, as it is of any disease associated with lung fibrosis.

Subjects with silicosis, particularly of the accelerated type, seem to be at increased risk of the development of autoantibodies and of rheumatoid disease, scleroderma, and systemic lupus erythematosus; these conditions have been described in about 10% of patients with silicosis in some series. Focal glomerulonephritis has also been described: the cause of this is unknown, but it is speculated that it may be a consequence of a direct toxic effect of quartz particles being excreted through the nephron.

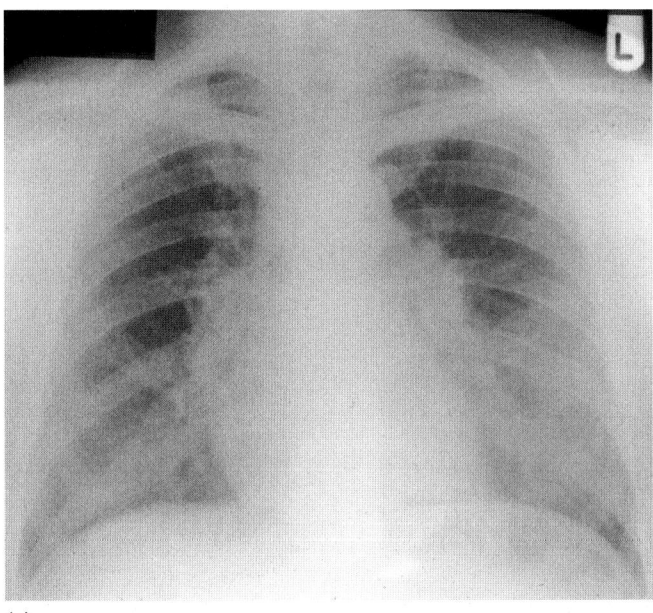

(a)

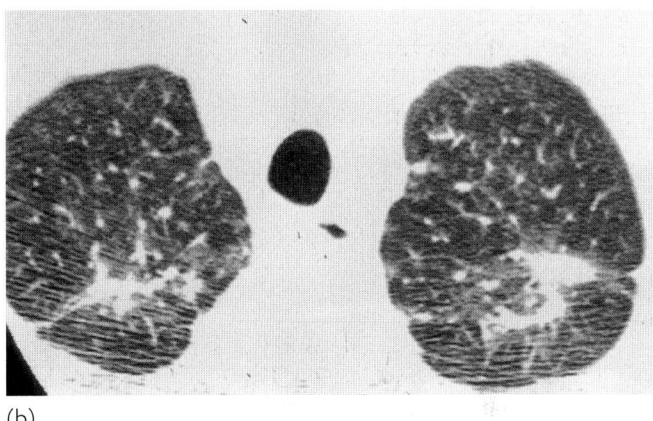

(b)

Fig. 18.13.10 (a) Radiograph of apprentice stonemason after 5 years of exposure to high concentrations of quartz, showing bilateral hilar node enlargement thought initially to be due to sarcoidosis. (b) CT scan of the same man 5 years later, with no further dust exposure, showing the development of massive fibrosis.

Prevention and management

The epidemiological evidence suggests that workers exposed to levels of respirable silica in excess of 1 mg/m³ have a high risk of silicosis, and that a risk may still exist even at levels of around 0.1 mg/m³. The United Kingdom maximum exposure limit is 0.1 mg/m³, and industry is obliged to keep exposures of workers below this level as far as practicable by appropriate ventilation, extraction, and other dust-suppression measures. For historic reasons, quartz exposures in coal mining are controlled by total dust levels rather than the silica component of the dust. If higher levels are inevitable, workers should wear appropriate respiratory protection, although this must be regarded as a second-best and potentially risky procedure. A worker who has developed the disease should be prevented from working with silica again. The only medical management necessary is regular sputum examination for tubercle bacilli, as tuberculosis accelerates the lung damage but responds normally to chemotherapy. Acute silicosis would

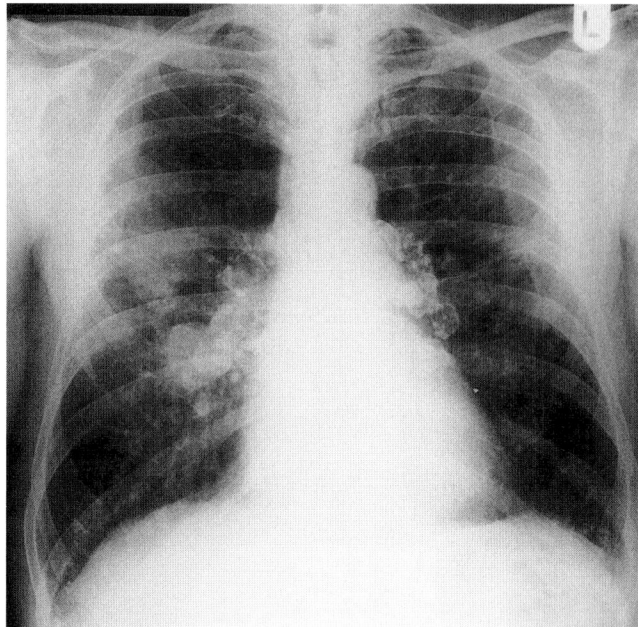

Fig. 18.13.11 Radiograph of a hard-rock miner, showing massive fibrosis in right mid zone and eggshell calcification of hilar nodes.

nowadays be an indication for consideration of transplantation. In the United Kingdom, workers with silicosis (whether or not complicated by lung cancer) should apply to the Respiratory Diseases Board of the Benefits Agency for industrial injuries benefits.

Asbestosis

Asbestosis is pulmonary fibrosis caused by exposure to fibres of asbestos. It was originally described at the end of the 19th century and its importance as an occupational disease was recognized in epidemiological studies in the 1930s. However, in the 1st century AD, Pliny recorded that the weavers of wicks for the lamps of the vestal virgins wore masks for respiratory protection, and so some recognition of its hazards may go back to antiquity.

Asbestos is mined principally in Canada, South Africa, and the former Soviet Union. It is a generic term for a group of fibrous silicates, the most important being chrysotile (white), crocidolite (blue), and amosite (brown). Chrysotile has a serpentine configuration and breaks up into microfibrils, while the other types (amphiboles) are straight and less liable to longitudinal fracture (Fig. 18.13.12). All types are resistant to physical and chemical destruction, which gives them their commercial value in fireproofing, insulation, reinforcement of cement, weaving into cloth, bonding in brake linings and plastics, and so on. The asbestos is obtained by crushing the rock to release the fibres, which are then carded and transported in nonporous bags to the user industry.

Asbestos causes several separate pleuropulmonary lesions. The commonest are benign pleural plaques, but acute effusion and diffuse fibrosis also occur. Mesothelioma, discussed in Chapter 18.19.3, is the most important. It now occurs in about 2500 people in the United Kingdom annually, and the incidence is predicted to rise further in relation to exposures some 30 years previously. It is most frequent in people who have worked in construction, ship repair, and such trades as electrician, plumber, and insulator, where regular direct or indirect exposure to asbestos has occurred.

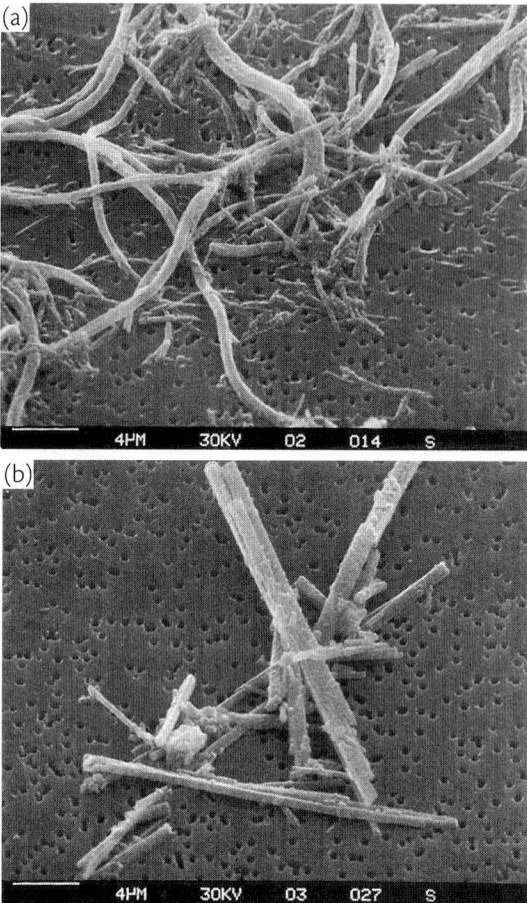

Fig. 18.13.12 Scanning electron micrographs of (a) chrysotile and (b) amosite on Millipore filters. The curly configuration and microfibrils of chrysotile should be noted. Scale bar, 4 μm.

The pulmonary disease asbestosis occurs in about 100 people annually in the United Kingdom; all have worked regularly with asbestos for many years. Risk of lung carcinoma is also related to asbestos exposure, interacting multiplicatively with smoking. All these risks appear to have been greater with exposure to amphiboles than with exposure to chrysotile, but most workers (except in specific mining/production industries) have usually been exposed to a mixture of the different types.

Aetiology and pathology

The harmful asbestos fibres are those less than 3 μm in transverse diameter and more than 10 μm in length, which are sufficiently narrow to be inhaled to the acinus, yet too long to be removed by macrophages. Their toxicity depends on their dimensions and their persistence in lung tissue once inhaled. All types of asbestos of these dimensions can cause fibrosis and carcinoma when inhaled by rats. Moreover, injection of any asbestos type (and indeed many fibres other than asbestos) into the peritoneum of rats causes mesothelioma in a dose-related manner. The lower risk of mesothelioma in association with pure chrysotile exposure in humans is related to this fibre's curly configuration, which reduces the number penetrating to the acinus, and its propensity to break up into minute short fibrils that can eventually be removed from the lung by the action of macrophages. As with coal and silica, the fibrogenicity of asbestos is probably related to damage to macrophages, which are unable to cope with fibres much longer than themselves, and the liberation of substances that activate fibroblasts to produce collagen. Among the substances shown to result from experimental challenge of rats with asbestos are TNF and macrophage- and platelet-derived growth factors (GM-CSF and PDGF).

The macroscopic appearance of an asbestotic lung is of grey fibrosis, more marked peripherally and in the lower zones. In severe cases the fibrosis appears like a honeycomb. Yellow shiny parietal pleural plaques are also usually seen in the thoracic cavity, although these frequently also occur in the absence of pulmonary fibrosis. Microscopically there is diffuse alveolar wall fibrosis with minimal cellular infiltrate or desquamation of type 2 pneumocytes, initially around the centre of the acinus and later spreading to destroy the acinar structure, leading to the appearance of honeycombing. Larger asbestos fibres may be seen coated with a protein–ferritin complex (the asbestos or ferruginous bodies), whilst smaller fibres remain uncoated but may still just be visible with the light microscope (Fig. 18.13.13). However, for every fibre visible by light microscopy, several hundred uncoated fine fibres can always be found on electron microscopy. Pleural plaques have the appearance of basket-weave collagen, and fibres are almost never seen within them.

Clinical features

Asbestosis occurs in people exposed regularly over years to airborne asbestos as a result of the material being used or removed, and not as a result of occasional exposure. It is more likely to be seen in trades involving the application or removal of asbestos in lagging and insulation than in asbestos mining, preparation, or weaving, where control of fibre levels is more careful. The disease may first become apparent and progress after exposure has ceased.

The symptoms are shortness of breath, initially on exertion, and dry cough. Repetitive end-inspiratory basal crackles commonly precede symptoms, and finger clubbing may occur later. The disease is usually progressive, the speed of progression being related to the dose of asbestos to which the lungs have been subjected, and results in increasing disability and death from cardiorespiratory failure. However, in cases of late-onset asbestosis, usually reflecting relatively low doses over a very prolonged period, progression is slow and sometimes imperceptible, an important feature in differentiation from cryptogenic fibrosis. Forty to fifty per cent of

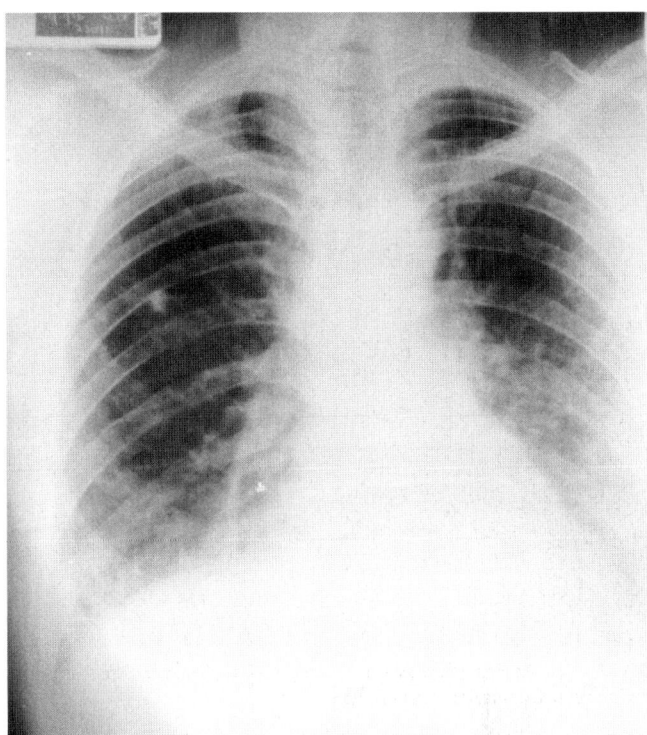

Fig. 18.13.14 Radiograph of a thermal insulator (lagger) with asbestosis. The irregular basal and middle zone fibrosis should be noted. A calcified TB focus is present in the right upper zone.

smokers with asbestosis die of bronchial carcinoma, but there is no increased risk of tuberculosis.

The radiological appearance of asbestosis is identical to that in most cases of cryptogenic pulmonary fibrosis — predominantly basal and peripheral irregular linear shadowing, progressing to honeycombing (Fig. 18.13.14). The presence of pleural plaques, which frequently calcify, is an indication of asbestos exposure and may help in the differential diagnosis (Fig. 18.13.15). In advanced asbestosis the fibrosis obscures the cardiac border, giving a shaggy appearance. The radiological appearances are best described by comparison with the International Labour Organization standard radiographs. CT scans are useful in differentiating asbestosis from diffuse pleural fibrosis, which may mimic it clinically and radiologically (Fig. 18.13.16).

Asbestosis causes a restrictive pattern of lung function, with reduced volumes and transfer factor. These measurements are the most suitable for screening for the disease and following its progress. Pulmonary compliance is reduced in relation to the extent of the fibrosis, and arterial oxygen desaturation occurs in the later stages.

Pleural plaques cause no symptoms and are usually a coincidental finding on chest radiography. Diffuse bilateral pleural thickening, often calcified, which can cause breathlessness and restricted lung volumes, occurs infrequently. Inspiratory crackles may be heard over this in the absence of significant asbestosis. Benign pleural effusion may occur very uncommonly, developing within the first two decades after exposure as a transient haemorrhagic effusion and diagnosed by the exclusion of infective and malignant causes. There is no evidence that any of these benign disorders predisposes to pleural mesothelioma, the risk of which relates to the prior extent of asbestos exposure.

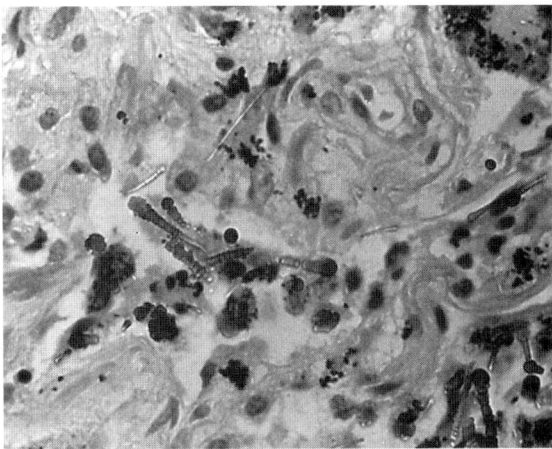

Fig. 18.13.13 Histological appearance of asbestosis, with interstitial fibrosis, asbestos bodies, and several uncoated fibres.

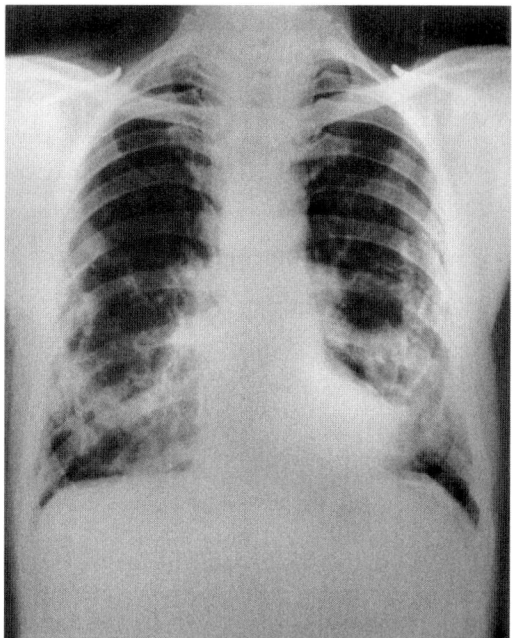

Fig. 18.13.15 Radiograph of a lagger, showing extensive calcified pleural plaques.

Differential diagnosis

The differentiation of asbestosis from other causes of pulmonary fibrosis is important from the points of view of prognosis and of management, including giving advice on compensation issues. The *sine qua non* for diagnosis of asbestosis is an adequate history of exposure, in terms of both intensity and duration. Short exposures, less than daily over several years, do not cause the disease under conditions likely to pertain nowadays in the Western world. Thus, a patient who has had only occasional or incidental exposure to asbestos will not develop disease, but given an appropriate history, the presence of symmetrically distributed fibrosis on chest radiography can be taken to indicate asbestosis. Difficulty arises when someone who has pulmonary fibrosis also gives a history of occasional or apparently light exposure. In such circumstances, the

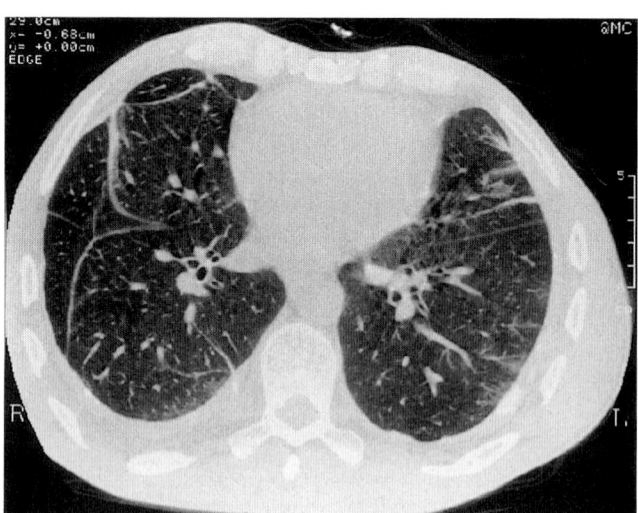

Fig. 18.13.16 CT scan of a lagger, showing bilateral pleural fibrosis with areas of calcification and fibrous strands extending into peripheral lung. This does not imply the same functional effects or prognosis as asbestosis.

distribution of the fibrosis on high-resolution CT scanning and the natural history of the condition may provide help. Late-onset asbestosis is a relatively slowly progressive condition, whereas cryptogenic fibrosis of the usual sort ('usual interstitial pneumonitis', UIP) tends to progress downhill inexorably (see Chapter 18.11.2). UIP is also characterized by a more irregular distribution of fibrosis on high-resolution CT, both in space and in maturity of the lesions, which may range from alveolar filling to advanced honeycombing in the same subject. Such appearances are extremely unlikely to occur in true asbestosis. However, it is apparent that in some cases the appearances of the two conditions are very similar on CT and differentiation relies on a careful assessment of likely exposure by someone experienced in such techniques.

Prevention and management

The prevention of asbestosis, as of other pneumoconioses, depends on reducing the exposure of individuals to fibre levels that have been shown to be insufficient to cause the disease in a lifetime of exposure. Unfortunately, the difficulties of making valid measurements of airborne fibres and the uncertainties attached to the early diagnosis of asbestosis have prevented the formulation of really reliable evidence on which to base a standard. The present British standard for chrysotile of 0.3 respirable fibres/ml has been based on work that suggests such levels would, when breathed over a working lifetime, result in asbestosis in fewer than 1% of those exposed. The corresponding standard for amphiboles is 0.2 fibres/ml. However, it should be noted that these concentrations do not take account of what is the much more serious risk of mesothelioma, and for this reason use of the mineral is now banned in the United Kingdom. It should also be noted that a concentration 0.1 fibres/ml sounds small until it is realized that it represents 100 fibres/litre, or many hundreds of thousands of fibres inhaled over a working day. The need for a material with the properties of asbestos has meant that many industries have now introduced other fibrous or crystalline minerals in its place. The potential of such new materials to cause similar diseases depends on their fibre dimensions, solubility in tissue, and the concentrations achieved in the workplace air. It is important that they should be handled with appropriate care by industry.

Regular medical and radiological examination of asbestos workers is essential for the early detection of asbestosis, and there is some evidence that removal of the worker from exposure at this stage is associated with slower progression. Workers should also be advised not to smoke, in view of the interaction between cigarettes and asbestos in causing lung cancer. Once asbestosis is suspected, the workers in the United Kingdom should apply to the Benefits Agency for assessment for industrial injuries benefit. Diffuse pleural fibrosis also attracts benefits, as does lung cancer in the presence of asbestosis or pleural fibrosis, but pleural plaques do not.

Risks of asbestos-related disease in the nonoccupationally exposed population

Much anxiety has been engendered amongst the general public by media interest in asbestos, and doctors may find themselves being asked about, e.g., the risks to children of asbestos wall panelling in houses or asbestos inserts in ironing boards. In general it can be stated that asbestosis occurs only in people working regularly with asbestos for years. However, this has included, at least in the past, wives washing the dusty clothes of asbestos workers and people who have lived or worked near polluting asbestos factories.

Occasional or incidental exposure to asbestos can be dismissed as a cause of asbestosis. Similarly, lung cancer risks seem to be significantly increased only with the doses of asbestos that lead to asbestosis, and individuals who do not smoke and who only have asbestos fittings in their houses can be reassured that their risks of this disease are negligible. However, mesothelioma, although also dose-related, occurs after smaller exposures and it is well established that a sufficient dose of crocidolite or amosite can be inhaled in a period of intense exposure of a few months. Of the 1500 cases occurring in the United Kingdom each year, almost all individuals give a history of having worked in a trade known to have been associated with asbestos use and have large numbers of fibres in their lungs, suggesting that employment rather than incidental exposure has been responsible. Small and occasional exposures to asbestos are highly unlikely to entail an important risk, but if regular exposures are thought to be occurring in the domestic or general environment, steps should be taken to eliminate them.

Other pneumoconioses

Several silicates apart from asbestos are of commercial importance, and some of these have been shown to cause pneumoconiosis. Talc (hydrated magnesium silicate) is mined as soapstone in the United States of America, China, and the Pyrenees. It is milled and has many uses including in cosmetics, the rubber industry, paints, ceramics, and pharmaceuticals. Kaolin (hydrated aluminium silicate) is quarried in south-west England, Georgia (United States of America), Japan, Egypt, Germany, and the Czech lands. It is used mainly in the manufacture of ceramics, paper and paint, and in pharmaceuticals. Fuller's earth (calcium montmorillonite) is an absorbent clay quarried in England, the United States of America, and Germany. It was originally used in fulling or removing grease from wool, and is now used in oil refining and bonding foundry moulds. Mica is a complex aluminium silicate occurring in two forms, muscovite and phlogopite. Muscovite is mined in the United States of America and India and used in fire-resistant windows and the manufacture of paper and paint. Phlogopite, mined in Canada, is used in the electrical industry because of its resistance to heat and electricity.

Two widely used silicate materials—cement and vitreous fibres—are not established as causes of pulmonary disease. Although cement exposure has occasionally been reported to be associated with pneumoconiosis, the evidence for this is flimsy. It is often mixed with asbestos, and asbestosis may occur in its production. Artificial vitreous fibres (glass wool and rock wool) have not so far been shown to cause pulmonary fibrosis or neoplasia in humans exposed to them, although mesothelioma has been produced by intraperitoneal injection in rats.

Talc pneumoconiosis

Talc is commonly contaminated with tremolite, a non-commercially-exploited amphibole asbestos, and with silica. It has been difficult to disentangle the effects of these components. The disease appears clinically to resemble asbestosis, with finger clubbing and basal crackles, although radiological descriptions emphasize lesions predominantly in the middle zones with nodular as well as reticular components. Progressive massive fibrosis has been described.

Talc has also been shown to be associated with pulmonary disease in a number of other circumstances. Bronchoconstriction may occur in children exposed to high concentrations, and drug users may have granulomatous reactions in the lungs as a result of either intravenous injection or inhalation of ground-up tablets. Fortunately, the widespread use of talc for producing pleurodesis has not been shown to be associated with the later development of mesothelioma, because the cosmetic grades of talc used are not contaminated with tremolite.

Kaolin pneumoconiosis

Kaolin causes a pneumoconiosis similar to coal-worker's pneumoconiosis with small, discrete nodular lesions initially and a tendency to produce massive fibrosis. It has been described in workers involved in the drying and milling processes in the production of china clay. Kaolin may also have been the component of the dust responsible for pneumoconiosis in the now defunct Scottish shale oil industry. There is no evidence linking kaolin pneumoconiosis with carcinoma or tuberculosis.

Fuller's earth pneumoconiosis

This condition has been described in workers extracting this clay mineral. It is a benign nodular pneumoconiosis similar in pathological and radiological appearance to simple coal-worker's pneumoconiosis; progressive massive fibrosis has not been described.

Mica pneumoconiosis

A few reports of radiological change in those exposed to ground mica have been recorded, but there is no recent publication describing pathological or clinical features.

Fibrous erionite

Exposure to this fibrous hydrated aluminium silicate has occurred in certain areas of Turkey and probably elsewhere in the Middle East. The populations of several villages have been exposed for many generations, as they used local erionite rock as stucco and whitewash in their homes. Pleural plaques, pulmonary fibrosis, and both lung cancer and mesothelioma were endemic in these villages. Fibrous erionite has no general commercial use, but this episode illustrates the potential dangers of inhaling fine fibrous material, whether asbestos or some other mineral.

Berylliosis

Beryllium is a metal that is used in alloys for the nuclear industry and in the production of X-ray tubes. It was used in ceramics, metallic alloys, and fluorescent lights until its toxicity was recognized and it was replaced by other materials. It is mined as an ore mostly in South America and extracted by chemical processes.

Beryllium is highly toxic when inhaled, and may also cause granulomatous ulcers on contact with the skin. Inhalation of high concentrations causes an acute pneumonitis and tracheobronchitis, which can be fatal. Chronic berylliosis, which may occur as a sequel to acute exposure, usually follows more prolonged exposure to lower levels. It is not common in the United Kingdom, where no more than about 50 cases have been diagnosed, but it has been recorded much more frequently in the United States of America. Reported cases have occurred in beryllium workers, in wives exposed to dust from their husbands' clothes, and in people living near the factories.

The patient with chronic berylliosis presents with cough and shortness of breath. The features mimic those of sarcoidosis: bilateral pulmonary mottling with upper lobe fibrosis is the usual radiographic feature initially, with bilateral hilar lymphadenopathy being

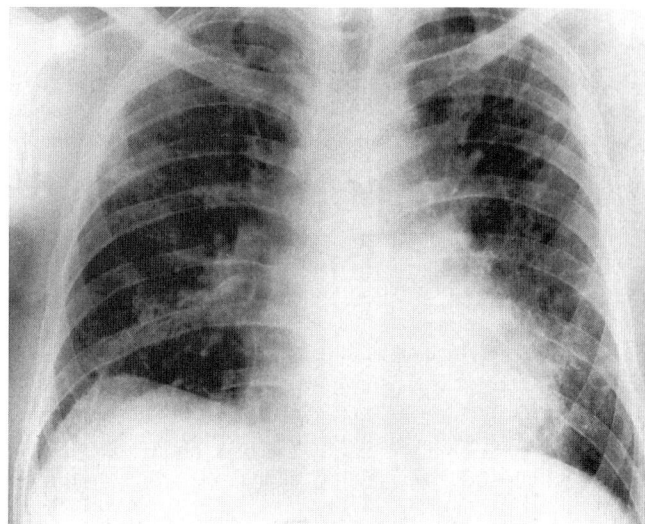

Fig. 18.13.17 Radiograph of a beryllium refinery worker, showing the diffuse fibrosis of berylliosis.

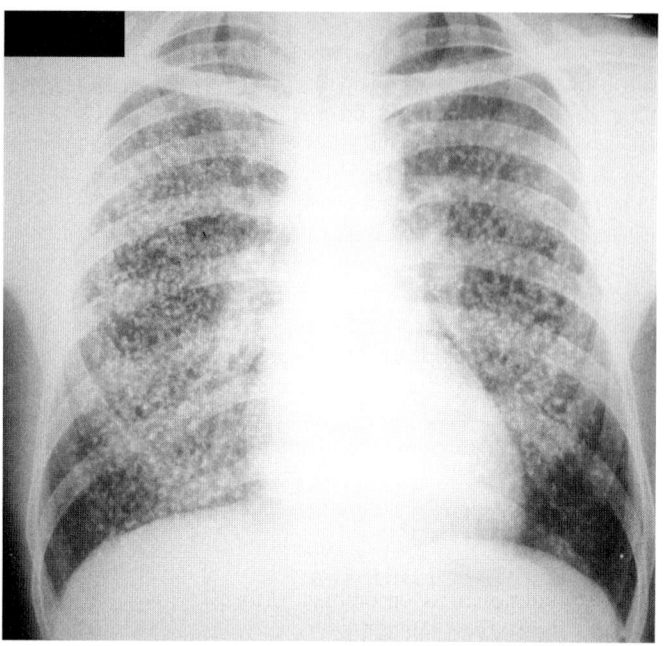

Fig. 18.13.18 Radiograph of a worker exposed to tin oxide fume in refining. He was completely symptom-free and had normal lung function.

less common. The disease typically progresses to diffuse fibrosis (Fig. 18.13.17), but the rate of progression is very variable. The functional lesion is a restrictive pattern with a low transfer factor. The progress of the disease can be controlled with corticosteroid therapy, but this needs to be continued indefinitely in most cases.

The pathological lesion is identical to that of sarcoidosis, with non-caseating granulomas and varying amounts of interstitial fibrosis. The diagnosis is made on the basis of a history of exposure, compatible clinical and histological features, a negative Kveim test (when performed), and a positive beryllium lymphocyte stimulation test. A skin-patch test is inadvisable as it can cause sensitization.

Berylliosis is prevented by keeping exposures below the threshold limit value ($2 \, ng/m^3$), although as it is a hypersensitivity disease even this will not prevent all cases, and there is debate as to whether sensitization may occur as a result of skin contact and transmission of the particles through the skin. Efficient respiratory and skin protection should also be provided for workers in these industries.

Less common pneumoconioses

Many other pneumoconioses have been described, although most are very rare and relatively benign. Haematite lung, occurring in iron ore miners, used to be seen in Cumbria in the United Kingdom; it is a fibrotic reaction to a mixed dust containing silica and iron. Radiographically it resembles silicosis and pathologically differs from it only in that the lungs are coloured red. There was an increased risk of lung cancer, probably due to radiation in the mines. Closely related to haematite lung is siderosis, a benign iron oxide pneumoconiosis occurring in welders and other workers in iron foundries. The radiological lesions often regress after exposure ceases. Barium processing and tin refining may be associated with the development of dramatic radiological nodular shadowing—baritosis and stannosis, respectively. These are also benign conditions, the radiological appearances reflecting radio-opaque dust in macrophages (Fig. 18.13.18).

Pneumoconiosis associated with diffuse lung fibrosis has been described in work with aluminium oxide (Shaver's disease) and tungsten carbide (hard metal disease). This latter condition, which is probably a hypersensitivity reaction to cobalt in cooling liquids, may also present with features of asthma or allergic alveolitis. A pneumoconiosis resembling that in coal miners has been described in workers with graphite and other forms of carbon, and in shale miners. A benign pneumoconiosis, consisting of simple accumulations of dust and macrophages with minimal nodular radiological shadowing, has also been described in workers producing polyvinyl chloride.

Further reading

Buchanan D, Miller BG, Soutar CA (2003). Quantitative relations between exposure to respirable quartz and risk of silicosis. *Occup Environ Med*, **60**, 159–64.

Henderson VL, Enterline PE (1979). Asbestos exposure: factors associated with excess cancer and respiratory disease mortality. *Ann N Y Acad Sci*, **330**, 117–26.

Hurley JF, *et al.* (1982). Coalworkers' simple pneumoconiosis and exposure to dust at 10 British coalmines. *Br J Indust Med*, **39**, 120–7.

International Labour Organization (1980). *Guidelines for the use of ILO international classification of radiographs of pneumoconioses.* Occupational Safety and Health Series No. 22 (rev. 87), International Labour Organization, Geneva.

Marine WM, Gurr D, Jacobsen M (1988). Clinically important respiratory effects of dust exposure and smoking in British coal miners. *Am Rev Respir Dis*, **137**, 106–12.

Morgan WKC, Seaton A (1995). *Occupational lung diseases*, 3rd edition. W B Saunders, Philadelphia.

Mossman BT, *et al.* (1990). Asbestos: scientific developments and implications for public policy. *Science*, **247**, 294–301.

Peto J, *et al.* (1995). Continuing increase in mesothelioma mortality in Britain. *Lancet*, **345**, 535–9.

Seaton A (1990). Coalmining, emphysema and compensation. *Br J Indust Med*, **47**, 433–5.

Seaton A (1998). The new prescription: industrial injuries benefit for smokers? *Thorax*, **53**, 335–6.

Seaton A, Cherrie JW (1998). Quartz exposure and severe silicosis: a role for the hilar nodes. *Occup Environ Med*, **55**, 383–6.

Seaton A, *et al.* (1991). Accelerated silicosis in Scottish stonemasons. *Lancet*, **337**, 341–4.

18.14

Miscellaneous conditions

Contents

18.14.1 Pulmonary haemorrhagic disorders

D.J. Hendrick and G.P. Spickett

Essentials

There are many causes of bleeding within the lung and haemoptysis, but the term 'pulmonary haemorrhagic disorder' applies only to diffuse bleeding from pulmonary alveolar capillaries. The condition is characterized by haemoptysis (not invariable), breathlessness, diffuse air space shadowing on the chest radiograph, anaemia (normochromic normocytic if acute, iron deficient with chronicity), and elevated carbon monoxide gas transfer (T_LCO).

Goodpasture's disease—diffuse pulmonary haemorrhage and glomerulonephritis with linear deposition of antibodies along the glomerular basement membrane (anti-GBM antibodies). Renal failure is a much commoner threat to survival than lung haemorrhage, but in some cases (almost invariably smokers) the latter can be life threatening. Treatment is supportive (artificial ventilation occasionally necessary) and with steroids, other immunosuppressants (cyclophosphamide) and plasmapheresis.

Idiopathic pulmonary haemosiderosis—a rare disorder of unknown cause with recurrent alveolar bleeding. Chest imaging shows the nonspecific appearances of intra-alveolar blood, which usually clears spontaneously over 1 to 3 weeks, but with chronicity diffuse pulmonary fibrosis with honeycombing may supervene. Treatment is supportive.

Other causes—pulmonary haemorrhage may occur with or complicate a wide variety of disorders with vasculitic, immunological, infective, vascular, haemostatic, toxic, or unknown origins.

Introduction

Bleeding within the lung and subsequent haemoptysis is common in clinical practice and may be the consequence of many unrelated disorders. The term 'pulmonary haemorrhagic disorder' is properly applied only to the particular circumstances of bleeding arising diffusely from pulmonary alveolar capillaries. A preferable and more explicit diagnostic term is therefore pulmonary capillary (or alveolar) haemorrhage, which is not a disease entity of itself, merely a clinical feature of several diseases, but it is a defining characteristic of two, Goodpasture's syndrome and idiopathic pulmonary haemosiderosis.

Although the lung can accommodate only small quantities of blood in the major airways without threatening life from asphyxiation, it can sequester surprisingly large amounts (litres) at alveolar level. This has a curious effect, unique among diffuse parenchymal diseases of the lung and of considerable diagnostic value; the carbon monoxide gas transfer ($T_L$co) is raised significantly above normal. Not only are physiologically useful red cells within the alveolar capillaries able to absorb the inhaled carbon monoxide, but so too are those lost from the circulation into the alveolar spaces.

Pulmonary capillary haemorrhage is thus characterized by haemoptysis, breathlessness, diffuse air space shadowing on the chest radiograph (Fig. 18.14.1.1), anaemia (normochromic normocytic if acute, iron deficient with chronicity), and an elevated $T_L$co (see Chapter 18.3.1). The extravasated red cells are not readily expectorated, although enough generally escape to cause haemoptysis, and so haemosiderin accumulates within alveolar macrophages as the red cells and their debris are engulfed. The diagnosis of pulmonary capillary haemorrhage is largely confirmed when haemosiderin-laden macrophages are identified in sputum (and there is no localized site of bleeding). If sputum is not expectorated or haemoptysis is absent, minimal, or otherwise explained, then bronchoalveolar lavage and/or lung biopsy are often necessary to establish the diagnosis. An alternative approach is CT or MRI, which may alone provide convincing evidence of blood sited diffusely within the alveoli.

Although diffuse alveolar capillary haemorrhage may characterize or complicate a wide variety of specific diseases or disease settings, the direct effects of the haemorrhage itself are not influenced by

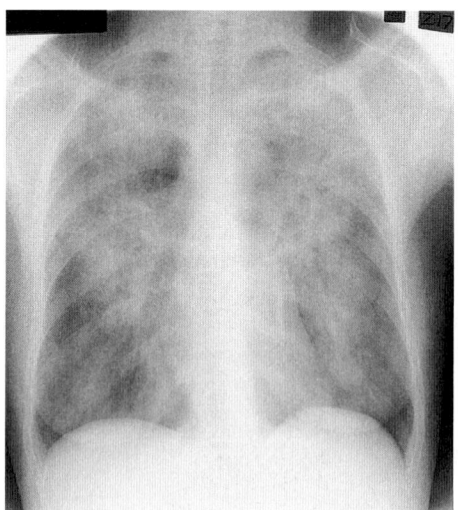

Fig. 18.14.1.1 Radiograph showing gross alveolar shadowing following severe pulmonary haemorrhage in a 60-year-old man with systemic vasculitis.

the cause, nor are the means by which it can be recognized. There may, nevertheless, be substantial differences at presentation from case to case according to severity and chronicity.

Goodpasture's syndrome

Goodpasture described a man with pulmonary haemorrhage and renal failure from glomerulonephritis. A number of conditions can cause such a 'pulmonary–renal syndrome', the best-characterized of which (although almost certainly not the illness suffered by the patient in the original report) is now termed Goodpasture's disease. This consists of diffuse pulmonary haemorrhage and glomerulonephritis with linear deposition of antibodies along the glomerular basement membrane (anti-GBM antibodies), 90% of which are directed against the α-3 chain of type IV collagen. Increased susceptibility is associated with HLA DRB11 501 and DRB11 502 alleles, while protection is associated with HLA DR1 and DR7.

Clinical features

In general, glomerulonephritis proves to be a much commoner threat to survival than lung haemorrhage, and the diagnosis of Goodpasture's disease is reached more conveniently from kidney rather than lung biopsy, together with serological testing for anti-GBM antibodies. In some cases, however, lung disease dominates the clinical picture. Most such patients are male smokers; some have recent exposure to volatile hydrocarbons, and case reports have additionally identified recent exposure to chlorine and smoked cocaine. This suggests that—when there is susceptibility—inhaled toxic agents enhance pulmonary endothelial damage and thus allow the initiation of autoimmunity or the ready access of existing autoantibody to basement membrane. The usual respiratory presentation is with cough, breathlessness, and haemoptysis, which is intermittent and ranges from occasional streaks to massive fatal bleeding. Systemic symptoms of fever, joint pains, or weight loss occur occasionally but are unusual. The chest radiograph shows patchy or diffuse shadowing due to intra-alveolar blood, usually resolving over the course of 2 weeks unless there is further bleeding. At the time of bleeding there may be arterial hypoxaemia and reduced lung volumes. Serial measurement of $T_L$co can be used to monitor progression. Prolonged bleeding may lead to iron-deficiency anaemia. Renal function may be normal initially and then deteriorate over days to weeks.

Treatment and prognosis

Supportive treatment may be required during acute bleeding, and artificial ventilation is occasionally necessary. Steroids, other immunosuppressant drugs (cyclophosphamide in particular), and plasmapheresis may all be used to control renal disease and are additionally helpful in treating pulmonary haemorrhage. Patients should not smoke (there are case reports of even a single cigarette leading to catastrophic recurrence of haemorrhage), and should avoid hydrocarbon exposure. Prognosis generally depends more on the renal effects than the pulmonary effects. For further discussion see Chapter 21.8.7.

Idiopathic pulmonary haemosiderosis

This is a rare disorder of children and young adults in which there is recurrent alveolar bleeding in the absence of kidney disease. The alveolar blood may provoke a fibrogenic stimulus and the development of diffuse pulmonary fibrosis. Anti-GBM antibody has not been detected, and the electron microscopic appearance of the basement membrane shows no consistent abnormality. Recent studies suggest that many cases may be a consequence of vasculitis at the pulmonary capillary level (pauci-immune pulmonary capillaritis). This is associated inconsistently with P-ANCA activity.

Although termed 'idiopathic', the condition is associated with premature birth and an increasing number of environmental exposures. One such that has incited particular interest is to the stachybotrys mould, which may contaminate wet or damp accommodation, and which releases a particularly potent toxin with haemorrhagic properties. This is now thought to cause some childhood cases, perhaps in synergy with environmental tobacco smoke. Associations with rheumatoid arthritis, cow's milk allergy, and coeliac disease are also recognized (and long-term survivors have an increased incidence of autoimmune disease), but the association with coeliac disease might be a consequence of cow's milk allergy also rather than gluten intolerance. A number of other environmental causes have been suggested, but the stronger the evidence for their causal roles, the less appropriate is the diagnostic rubric of 'idiopathic' pulmonary haemosiderosis, hence these are identified below under the heading 'other causes'.

Clinical features

Recurrent alveolar haemorrhage is generally manifested by cough with haemoptysis and breathlessness, but haemoptysis is not invariably present, and in children a failure to thrive may be prominent together with the effects of severe chronic iron-deficiency anaemia. Severe acute bleeds are more common in childhood and may be life threatening. Physical examination is unhelpful. The chest radiograph and CT scan show the nonspecific appearances of intra-alveolar blood, which usually clears spontaneously over 1 to 3 weeks. With chronicity the appearances of diffuse pulmonary fibrosis with honeycombing may supervene. Lung function tests then show a progressive loss of volume and reduction of gas transfer, but an unexplained obstructive pulmonary defect occurs occasionally.

Treatment and prognosis

Supportive treatment is the same as for Goodpasture's syndrome. In addition, there are case reports recording responses to the avoidance of milk and gluten, and to the use of immunosuppressive agents including corticosteroids and cyclophosphamide. Some patients recover spontaneously with or without residual pulmonary damage.

Other causes of diffuse alveolar haemorrhage

Although diffuse alveolar haemorrhage is not a principal or defining feature of disorders other than Goodpasture's syndrome and idiopathic pulmonary haemosiderosis, it may occur with or complicate a wide variety of disorders with vasculitic, immunological, infective, vascular, haemostatic, toxic, or unknown origins. In many of the cases that have been reported a contributory role could have been played by several different disorders, their complications, and their various treatments.

Vasculitic disorders occasionally cause prominent diffuse alveolar haemorrhage, particularly Wegener's granulomatosis and microscopic polyangiitis. These may simulate Goodpasture's disease closely, since they commonly cause necrotizing glomerulonephritis. Wegener's granulomatosis is distinguished from Goodpasture's syndrome clinically by the common involvement of upper respiratory tract structures, histologically by granulomatous vasculitis, and immunologically by circulating anti-neutrophil cytoplasmic antibodies (ANCA) that are of the cytoplasmic type (C-ANCA) and are directed against proteinase-3 in about 90% of cases. By contrast, microscopic polyangiitis does not typically involve the upper respiratory tract, its vasculitis is not granulomatous, and its anti-neutrophil cytoplasmic antibodies are perinuclear (P-ANCA), directed against the myeloperoxidase of neutrophil cytoplasmic granules. Other vasculitic disorders involving the lung are very rare causes of diffuse alveolar haemorrhage, but include Churg–Strauss syndrome, polyarteritis nodosa, Henoch–Schönlein purpura, and Takayasu arteritis. Diffuse capillary haemorrhage from fulminant vasculitic disease of whatever cause carries a grave prognosis, with mortality of 25 to 50%.

Diffuse alveolar haemorrhage may also arise as an unusual respiratory feature of several nonvasculitic immunological disorders. Most prominent is systemic lupus erythematosus, in which lupus anticoagulant, thrombcytopenia and active nephritis may all play a role, but there are also reports of diffuse alveolar haemorrhage complicating the primary antiphospholipid antibody syndrome, IgA nephropathy, idiopathic membranous nephropathy, scleroderma, renal and bone marrow transplantation, and chronic active hepatitis.

Other reports have implicated lymphangioleiomyomatosis, hymenopteran stings and snake bites, moulds other than stachybotrys and their mycotoxins, infections (AIDS, invasive aspergillosis, dengue fever, cytomegalovirus, leptospirosis, stenotrophomonas, group A streptococci, strongyloidiasis, varicella), familial Mediterranean fever, cardiopulmonary bypass, cold injury, occupational exposure to tri- and pyromellitic anhydride, lymphangiography contrast media, and several medications (amiodarone, azathioprine, carbimazole, nitrofurantoin, mitomycin C, D-penicillamine, rituximab, sirolimus, surfactant therapy, valproate), with many of these conditions involving disseminated intravascular coagulation. The list is completed by causes of chronic pulmonary venous congestion (mitral stenosis, chronic left ventricular failure, pulmonary veno-occlusive disease), certain congenital anomalies of the heart, malignant hypertension, and disorders (or medications) that disrupt bleeding and coagulation mechanisms (thrombocytopenia, leukaemia, thrombinolytic therapy, platelet glycoprotein IIb/IIIa inhibitor, anticoagulant poisoning, clopidogrel, factor V deficiency). Combinations of such factors are commonly found in individual cases, and it may be that important interactions occur, without which the probability of diffuse haemorrhage is remote. Although capillary stress from high pressure gradients is thought to be a major factor underlying diffuse pulmonary haemorrhage in exercising horses (and camels), it appears a rare or unheard cause in most other species, but the use of negative-pressure ventilation in humans has been reported to have a similar effect.

Further reading

Albelda SM, et al. (1985). Diffuse pulmonary hemorrhage: a review and classification. *Radiology*, **154**, 289–97.
Anonymous (2000). From the Centers for Disease Control and Prevention. Update: pulmonary hemorrhage/hemosiderosis among infants—Cleveland, Ohio, 1993–1996. *JAMA*, **283**, 1951–3.

Bosch X, Guilabert A, Font J (2006). Antineutrophil cytoplasmic antibodies. *Lancet*, **368**, 404–18.

Collard HR, Schwarz MI (2004). Diffuse alveolar hemorrhage. *Clin Chest Med*, **25**, 583–92.

Hudson BG, *et al.* (2003). Alport's syndrome, Goodpasture's syndrome, and type IV collagen. *N Engl J Med*, **348**, 2543–56.

Ioachimescu OC, Sieber S, Kotch A (2004). Idiopathic pulmonary haemosiderosis revisited. *Eur Respir J*, **24**, 162–70.

Jara LJ, Vera-Lastra O, Calleja MC (2003). Pulmonary-renal vasculitic disorders: differential diagnosis and management. *Curr Rheumatol Rep*, **5**, 107–15.

Pacheco A, *et al.* (1991). Long term follow-up of adult idiopathic pulmonary hemosiderosis. *Chest*, **99**, 1525–6.

Schwarz MI, Brown KK (2000). Small vessel vasculitis of the lung. *Thorax*, **55**, 502–10.

Semple D, *et al.* (2005). Clinical review: Vasculitis on the intensive care unit-part 1: diagnosis. *Crit Care*, **9**, 92–7.

Specks U (2001). Diffuse alveolar hemorrhage syndromes. *Curr Opin Rheumatol*, **13**, 12–17.

18.14.2 Eosinophilic pneumonia

D.J. Hendrick and G.P. Spickett

Essentials

Eosinophilic pneumonia occurs when alveolar spaces are consolidated because of eosinophil inflammation/infiltration, usually with an accompanying eosinophilia of peripheral blood. The diagnosis should be considered when infiltrates on a chest radiograph, often migratory, are associated with blood eosinophilia, and confirmed by demonstrating an excess of eosinophils in bronchoalveolar lavage fluid.

Aetiology—before concluding that the cause is 'idiopathic', the following must be considered: (1) parasitic infestation; (2) adverse drug reaction; (3) asthma; (4) allergic bronchopulmonary mycosis; (5) vasculitis; (6) hypereosinophilic syndrome; and (7) other disorders known to be associated with eosinophilic pneumonia.

Acute eosinophilic pneumonia (Löffler's syndrome)—transitory migratory pulmonary shadows associated with modest peripheral eosinophilia in patients with a mild self-limiting illness. Patients are often atopic. May be an allergic reaction to blood-borne parasites (particularly *Ascaris lumbricoides*) or drugs.

Chronic eosinophilic pneumonia—pulmonary shadows, typically peripheral, persist for more than 1 month and are often associated with systemic symptoms (particularly fever). May result in diffuse fibrosis or fixed airway obstruction, or both.

Eosinophilic pneumonia with asthma—may be associated with fungal hypersensitivity (commonly *Aspergillus fumigatus*, i.e allergic bronchopulmonary aspergillosis) or Churg–Strauss syndrome (a vasculitic and granulomatous disorder).

Tropical eosinophilia—due to migrating larvae of filarial worms (*Wucheria bancrofti, Brugia malayi*). Chronic cases may develop pulmonary fibrosis.

Hypereosinophilic syndrome—when eosinophilic pneumonia (and infiltrative eosinophilic disorders of other organs) is not comfortably classified by any other diagnostic category. Two mechanisms may explain many cases: (1) a genetic deletion creating a protein with tyrosine kinase activity that affects myeloid differentiation (responds to imatinib); (2) a lymphocytic variant where an abnormal clone of T-cells releases 'eosinophilic' cytokines.

Causal factors need to be treated, but eosinophilic pneumonia otherwise often responds well to corticosteroid medication.

Introduction

Eosinophilic pneumonia occurs when alveolar spaces are consolidated because of eosinophil inflammation/infiltration. This does not imply that there is microbial infection, and most commonly there is not. There is characteristically an accompanying eosinophilia of peripheral blood ($>0.45 \times 10^9$/litre), hence the alternative terms 'pulmonary eosinophilia' and 'pulmonary infiltration with eosinophilia' (PIE syndrome). Eosinophilic pneumonia is the preferred term, since eosinophilia of peripheral blood may be present coincidently when eosinophils are not relevant to a pulmonary infiltrate, and conversely true eosinophilic pneumonia is occasionally not associated with blood eosinophilia. To avoid further confusion, note that eosinophilic pneumonia is unrelated to eosinophilic granuloma: this is a disorder of histiocytic Langerhans' (dendritic) cells and is not characterized by eosinophil infiltration of the alveolar spaces. Eosinophilic pneumonia is uncommon. It may occur at any time in life, but is rare in children and adolescents.

The plethora of diagnostic terms is exceeded by the multitude of causes, and evenly matched by suggested systems of classification. In essence they reflect the following features of eosinophilic pneumonia:

♦ It may arise acutely and resolve quickly over a matter of days—acute eosinophilic pneumonia, Löffler's syndrome, simple pulmonary eosinophilia.

♦ It may arise gradually and persist for many months, leading sometimes to pulmonary fibrosis or fixed airway obstruction—chronic eosinophilic pneumonia, prolonged pulmonary eosinophilia.

♦ Its morbidity may vary over a wide range, from negligible to severely disabling and life-threatening.

♦ It may be a consequence of allergy, particularly to blood-borne parasites (tropical eosinophilia), inhaled moulds (allergic bronchopulmonary mycosis), or other common environmental allergens.

♦ It is often due to drugs, whether through allergy, idiosyncrasy, or toxicity.

♦ It is often associated with asthma—asthmatic eosinophilia.

♦ It may be associated with pulmonary vasculitis—Churg–Strauss syndrome, Wegener's granulomatosis, microscopic polyangiitis.

♦ It may be a component of the hypereosinophilic syndrome.

♦ It may be associated with a variety of other distinct disease entities, including the adult respiratory distress syndrome, rheumatoid disease, Hodgkin's disease, hypogammaglobulinaemia, leprosy, T-cell lymphoma, sarcoidosis, shock.

♦ It may seem to be idiopathic.

Since there is often overlap, there is limited benefit from using any classification system: the important issue is to identify potentially remediable causes.

Diagnosis

In practice the finding of blood eosinophilia in association with a radiographic pulmonary infiltrate provides a valuable clue that pneumonia of infectious origin may not be the diagnosis. Eosinophilic pneumonia is not likely to respond to conventional antibiotic medication, hence a blood eosinophil count should be obtained if an apparent pneumonia fails to respond to antibiotics. Remember, however, that blood eosinophilia may be masked if a patient is receiving steroid medication. Once suspected, eosinophilic pneumonia is most conveniently confirmed by demonstrating an excess of eosinophils in bronchoalveolar lavage fluid (eosinophils generally account for 2–25% of the cells) in the absence of pathogenic microorganisms. Sometimes sputum alone is sufficient, whether expectorated spontaneously or induced. Alternatively, an excess of alveolar eosinophils is revealed in lung biopsy tissue. Not surprisingly, the use of CT scanning in subjects with confirmed eosinophilic pneumonia has shown that episodes of recurrent pulmonary infiltration occur more frequently than can be detected from plain chest radiographs. As different segments of lung become involved the infiltrates may characteristically 'migrate' from one to another.

Once eosinophilic pneumonia is confirmed, a variety of possible causes should be considered before it is assumed to be idiopathic in origin and before empirical treatment with corticosteroids is administered. Look for evidence of:

- parasitic infestation
- administration of drugs
- asthma
- allergic bronchopulmonary mycosis (particularly aspergillosis)
- other manifestations of vasculitis
- other manifestations of the hypereosinophilic syndrome
- other disorders known to be associated with eosinophilic pneumonia

Treatment

Eosinophilic pneumonia often responds well to corticosteroid medication, though treatment may need to be prolonged (6 months or more) in the chronic forms of the disorder. The importance of identifying whether it is associated with the causal factors listed above lies with the additional need to treat these also. Otherwise eosinophilic pneumonia may not respond adequately to steroid therapy and the associated diseases may produce other manifestations.

Particular varieties of eosinophilic pneumonia

Acute eosinophilic pneumonia (Löffler's syndrome, simple pulmonary eosinophilia)

The essential features are transitory migratory pulmonary shadows associated with modest peripheral eosinophilia in patients with a mild self-limiting illness. Some cases are asymptomatic and discovered incidentally. Most patients present with cough, sometimes with oddly yellowish sputum containing an abundance of eosinophils, and a few have general malaise and a mild fever. The pulmonary shadows reflect fan-shaped areas of consolidation, often peripheral and sometimes rather nodular, which last a few days only and appear haphazardly in various lobes, seldom following a truly segmental pattern. In some cases they are single and in others they are multiple. The peripheral eosinophilia is obvious but rarely gross; a differential of more than 20 per cent in a modestly raised total white cell count is unusual and more often the absolute eosinophil count ranges between 1×10^9 and 2×10^9/litre (normal <0.45 × 10^9/litre).

Patients are often atopic and may have other manifestations of an atopic diathesis such as asthma, urticaria, and angio-oedema. Allergy has been shown since Löffler's original description to play an important role, and cases can be seen to fall into two broad aetiological groups with a third miscellaneous group of unexplained aetiology.

In the first group, eosinophilic pneumonia represents an allergic reaction to bloodborne parasites migrating through the lung, particularly larvae of *Ascaris lumbricoides*: occasionally *A. suum*. Ancylostoma, strongyloides, taenia, trichinella, and trichuris species provide further examples.

Drugs form the second major aetiological group. Löffler's syndrome is described after administration of aspirin, calcium stearate (oral antihistamine additive), imipramine, penicillin, *p*-aminosalicylic acid, and sulphonamides (including the antimalarial combination of sulphadiazine and pyrimethamine, Fansidar). It may also occur with nitrofurantoin (although this can also give a diffuse reticulonodular radiological picture and is a cause of the more chronic type of eosinophilic pneumonia), toxic smoke (and possibly tobacco smoke), and lymphangiography contrast medium.

Successful management requires the eradication of any parasites or the cessation of relevant medication, as well as the administration (if necessary) of oral corticosteroids.

Tropical eosinophilia

Eosinophilic pneumonia in tropical climates is often a consequence of migrating larvae of the filarial worms *Wucheria bancrofti* and *Brugia malayi*. The effects are fundamentally similar to those of Löffler's syndrome, but tend to be more persistent and more serious, are more often associated with asthma, and may be associated with systemic symptoms of weight loss, persistent fever, and lymphadenopathy. Also the peripheral eosinophil count tends to be greater than in Löffler's syndrome (>3 × 10^9/litre), and the total serum IgE level is markedly elevated. With chronicity, pulmonary fibrosis is characteristic. A cure is to be expected with antifilariasis medication (e.g. diethylcarbamazine).

Chronic eosinophilic pneumonia (prolonged pulmonary eosinophilia)

Eosinophilic pneumonia persisting for more than a month is distinguished from the more transitory Löffler's syndrome, although its clinical characteristics are fundamentally similar. As with eosinophilic pneumonia associated with tropical filariasis, it tends to be more persistent and more serious than Löffler's syndrome (it is sometimes life threatening), and to be associated with systemic symptoms (particularly fever), progressive pulmonary fibrosis, and fixed airway obstruction. It may last for several months and be associated additionally with eosinophilic pleural effusion, focal skin lesions, atopic manifestations such as rhinitis, sinusitis and angio-oedema, hepatosplenomegaly, and even hepatic necrosis. The pulmonary disease is often extensive, and may cause hypoxaemia as well as dyspnoea. A curious peripheral radiographic distribution of infiltrates, dubbed a 'negative photographic image of pulmonary oedema', is particularly suggestive of chronic eosinophilic pneumonia but occurs in only a few cases. The radiological abnormalities tend to recur and last for weeks or months, and like the shadows of Löffler's syndrome may vary in site during the course of the illness.

Chronic eosinophilic pneumonia is more commonly idiopathic than Löffler's syndrome, but may also be a consequence of parasite infestation (e.g. tropical filariasis) or drug hypersensitivity. Case reports have identified aminoglutethimide, BCG vaccination, bicalutamide, captopril, chlorpropamide, clarithromycin, clomipramine, dapsone, diflunisal, ethambutol, ibuprofen, meloxicam, mesalazine, minocycline, nitrofurantoin, perindopril, progesterone, sertraline, sotalol, sulphonamides, trimethoprim, and venlafaxine as possible causes. Peripheral blood eosinophilia is less consistent with chronic compared with acute forms of eosinophilic pneumonia, although is often of greater level (>1 × 10^9/litre).

When a definitive cause is identified, appropriate specific management should follow, but often no cause is evident and oral corticosteroid therapy should be given. Responses are often dramatic, but recurrences are common if treatment is discontinued within 6 to 12 months. There may be a persistent mixed obstructive and restrictive loss of ventilatory function, and radiographic evidence of persistent pulmonary fibrosis.

Eosinophilic pneumonia with asthma

Eosinophilic pneumonia is commonly associated with asthma, even in the absence of parasite infestation or drug hypersensitivity. In a study of 53 cases, asthma preceded eosinophilic pneumonia in about half, and then worsened; in the remainder it arose by similar proportion either contemporaneously or within about 2 years. Two particular associations with asthma are noteworthy.

Allergic bronchopulmonary mycosis

When fungal hypersensitivity develops in atopic subjects with asthma, additional manifestations may occur in the lung: these include eosinophilic pneumonia, mucoid impaction, bronchiectasis, and pulmonary fibrosis. The ensuing syndrome of allergic bronchopulmonary mycosis occurs most commonly with *Aspergillus fumigatus*, though has been reported with other aspergillus, candida, curvularia, and helminthosporium species. It accounts for most cases of eosinophilic pneumonia with asthma in the United Kingdom and is best considered a complication of atopic asthma, appearing to result from airway colonization by the relevant mould. The mechanism, however, is clearly one of hypersensitivity, not infection/invasion, and both IgE and IgG antibodies are necessary to support its diagnosis.

In acute phases there is patchy obstruction of bronchi with inspissated mucus that, if expectorated, appears as brown rubbery lumps in the sputum (plugs). Fungal hyphae may be recovered from them, indicating that fungal growth has occurred within the airway. This impaction of mucus in one or more bronchi leads to patchy atelectasis within (or of) segments (even lobes), and is often associated with eosinophilic pneumonia. The radiographic appearances are of fleeting pulmonary infiltrates (Fig. 18.14.2.1).

The condition usually responds well to corticosteroids, a useful diagnostic feature being the expectoration of plugs during this

period of resolution. In the medium term the involved bronchi (generally proximal) may become bronchiectatic, leading in turn to the characteristic features of bronchiectasis (productive cough, intermittent haemoptysis). In the longer term, pulmonary fibrosis may ensue, particularly in the upper lobes and apices, so that the radiographic appearances resemble tuberculosis. If mucoid impaction and/or eosinophilic pneumonia become superimposed, the radiographic appearances may simulate active tuberculosis very closely. Suspicion of tuberculosis in an individual with atopic asthma should always prompt consideration of allergic bronchopulmonary mycosis.

Churg–Strauss syndrome

A much rarer association of eosinophilic pneumonia with asthma is that involving Churg–Strauss syndrome, a vasculitic and granulomatous disorder that commonly involves lungs, gut, peripheral nerves, skin, and kidneys, and occasionally heart. It is characterized typically by asthma, eosinophilic pneumonia, and very high

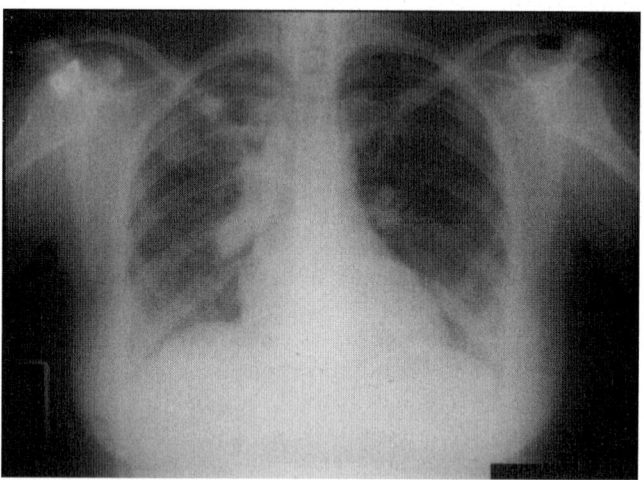

(a)

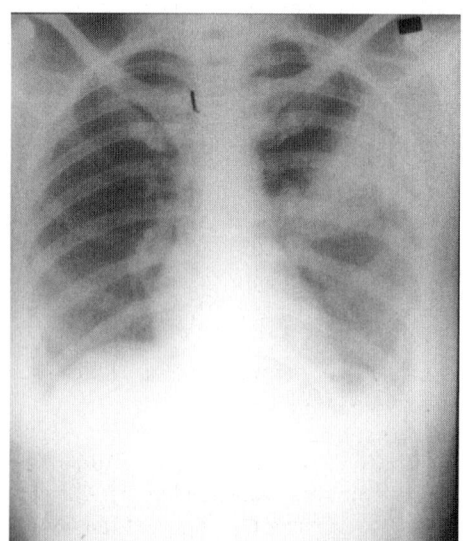

(b)

Fig. 18.14.2.1 Allergic bronchopulmonary aspergillosis: two radiographs taken 6 months apart from a woman with asthma, peripheral eosinophilia, and high titres of IgE and precipitating IgG antibodies to *Aspergillus fumigatus*.

numbers of circulating eosinophils ($>5 \times 10^9$/litre), but the pulmonary manifestations may additionally include haemorrhage and haemoptysis. Serological investigation may also demonstrate raised serum levels of IgE and eosinophil cationic protein, P-ANCA (perinuclear antineutrophil cytoplasmic antibodies) with myeloperoxidase activity (in most cases), and C-ANCA with proteinase-3 specificity (in a few cases). Autoantibodies against eosinophil granule enzymes have also been described. Pathologically there is vasculitis of small arteries and veins with necrotizing extravascular granulomas. Biopsy tissue is needed to confirm the diagnosis, and may be diagnostic even in the prevasculitic phase if there is characteristic eosinophilic infiltration of involved tissue.

Although Churg–Strauss syndrome is idiopathic in most cases, a few appear to be a consequence of drug hypersensitivity. A recent example of particular interest has been allergic granulomatosis and angiitis (the nomenclature of Churg and Strauss) complicating the use for asthma of oral leukotriene receptor antagonists. It has been suggested, however, that the drugs themselves do not cause the disease, but merely lead to it being uncovered as the beneficial effect of leukotriene receptor antagonism allows a reduction (or withdrawal) of chronic steroid therapy.

Hypereosinophilic syndrome

The hypereosinophilic syndrome completes what might be described as a spectrum of overlapping disorders. Over recent decades it has come to encompass what remains when eosinophilic pneumonia (and infiltrative eosinophilic disorders of other organs) is not comfortably classified by any of the diagnostic categories discussed above. Although in consequence it is likely to be heterogeneous in nature, a number of features are characteristic, leading Chusid and colleagues in 1975 to define the hypereosinophilic syndrome as idiopathic if there is blood eosinophilia exceeding 1.5×10^9/litre for at least 6 months, no identifiable cause after extensive investigation, and end organ damage/dysfunction associated with eosinophil infiltration. The heart, skin, and nervous system are the most common targets: the lungs are not commonly involved, hence the idiopathic hypereosinophilic syndrome (IHES) is a particularly rare cause of eosinophilic pneumonia.

Recent advances in molecular biology have produced an interesting insight into pathogenesis, and two distinct mechanisms seem likely to explain many if not most cases. One involves an interstitial deletion on chromosome 4 that produces a 'fusion' gene from the adjacent segments, the new gene encoding a protein with tyrosine kinase activity that affects early myeloid differentiation. These findings are closely associated with eosinophilic leukaemia, and the emerging treatment of choice for this myeloid variant of IHES (m-IHES) is imatinib, an effective chemotherapeutic agent for chronic myeloid leukaemia which antagonizes tyrosine kinase. Whether imatinib will reduce the substantial risk of premature death from cardiac involvement or the development of acute myeloid leukaemia remains to be seen.

The other variant is lymphocytic (l-IHES), where an abnormal clone of T cells, whether malignant or benign, releases 'eosinophilic' cytokines, principally interleukin 5 (IL-5) which stimulate bone marrow generation and inhibit peripheral destruction. This condition is less likely to cause end-organ dysfunction and is often readily controlled with corticosteroids. The emergent treatment of interest here is with anti-IL-5 monoclonal antibodies. The prognosis is generally more favourable, but there is a risk of lymphoma.

Further reading

Al-Alawi A, Ryan CF, Flint JD (2005). Aspergillus-related lung disease. *Can Respir J*, **12**, 377–87.

Muller NL, Allen J (2006). Acute eosinophilic pneumonia. *Semin Resp Crit Care Med*, **27**, 142–7.

Bosch X, Guilabert A, Font J (2006). Antineutrophil cytoplasmic antibodies. *Lancet*, **368**, 404–18.

Churg A (2001). Recent advances in the diagnosis of Churg-Strauss syndrome. *Modern Pathol*, **14**, 1284–93.

Cottin V, Cordier JF (2005). Eosinophilic pneumonias. *Allergy*, **60**, 841–57.

DuMouchel W, et al. (2004). Association of asthma therapy and Churg-Strauss syndrome: an analysis of postmarketing surveillance data. *Clin Therapeut*, **26**, 1092–1104.

Keogh KA, Specks U (2006). Churg-Strauss syndrome: update on clinical, laboratory and therapeutic aspects. *Sarcoidosis Vasc Diffuse Lung Dis*, **23**, 3–12.

Marchand E, Cordier (2006). Idiopathic chronic eosinophilic pneumonia. *Semin Respir Crit Care Med*, **27**, 134–41.

Oermann CM, et al. (2000). Pulmonary infiltrates with eosinophilia syndromes in children. *J Pediatr*, **136**, 351–8.

Ong RK, Doyle RL (1998). Tropical pulmonary eosinophilia. *Chest*, **113**, 1673–9.

Roufosse F, Cogan E, Goldman M (2004). Recent advances in pathogenesis and management of hypereosinophilic syndromes. *Allergy*, **59**, 673–89.

18.14.3 Lymphocytic infiltrations of the lung

D.J. Hendrick

Essentials

Many disorders are associated with lymphocytic infiltration of the lung, but there is a spectrum of conditions in which such infiltration is the chief focus of attention, ranging from benign (e.g. lymphocytic interstitial pneumonia) to malignant (e.g. lymphoma).

Lymphocytic interstitial pneumonia—characterized by diffuse infiltration of the lung interstitium and alveolar walls with small mature lymphocytes, immunoblasts, and plasma cells. May be idiopathic or associated with other disease (autoimmune, HIV infection, Epstein–Barr virus infection) or drug hypersensitivity. Radiographic features are of diffuse interstitial shadowing. Open biopsy is generally required for definitive diagnosis. Usually progresses slowly. May respond to corticosteroids.

Lymphomas—apparent 'primary' lymphomas of the lung generally fall into three categories: (1) lymphomatoid granulomatosis—systemic symptoms usually dominant, pulmonary lesions usually discrete and nodular, cure requires cytotoxic therapy for lymphoma; (2) low-grade B-cell non-Hodgkin's lymphoma—the commonest primary lymphoma affecting the lung parenchyma, usually arises from mucosa-associated lymphoid tissue (MALT) of the bronchi, presents with one or more pulmonary nodules, systemic symptoms unusual; and (3) high-grade B-cell non-Hodgkin's lymphoma—commonly occurs in association with immunosuppression (AIDS, organ transplantation), likely to have respiratory and systemic symptoms.

Introduction

Lymphocytic infiltration of the lung is associated with a number of disorders. It is often a 'nonspecific' finding rather than the defining characteristic of a particular disease entity, and it is an expected feature of several respiratory diseases. Examples include extrinsic allergic alveolitis, flock worker's lung, bronchiolitis obliterans with organizing pneumonia, and nonspecific interstitial pneumonia. It is a feature particularly of sarcoidosis and Wegener's granulomatosis—disorders dependent on granulomatous and vasculitic inflammation. All are described separately in other chapters. They occupy the middle ground of an overlapping spectrum. The topics of this chapter are the few and uncommon disorders which lie at the ends of this spectrum and for which lymphocytic infiltration of the lung is the chief focus of attention. The benign end of the spectrum is represented by lymphocytic interstitial pneumonia; the malignant end by lymphoma.

Apparent progression from lymphocytic interstitial pneumonia to granulomatous and vasculitic inflammation, or from granulomatous and vasculitic inflammation to lymphoma, is not uncommon, but it is not always clear whether individuals affected in this way truly progress from one disease to another. They might, alternatively, have a single disease whose early manifestations are similar to (and mistaken for) those of less serious neighbours in the disease spectrum.

Dominant lymphocytic infiltration is, nevertheless, a convenient definitive feature from which to consider the diseases that are described in this chapter. There is often paraprotein production, implying that a lymphocyte clone is involved. Depending on severity, these disorders are characterized clinically by cough (usually dry) and progressive undue exertional breathlessness, but systemic features of fever, malaise, and weight loss may also be prominent. Clubbing is not common, but there are frequently inspiratory crackles at the lung bases. The chest radiograph shows a diffuse interstitial pattern or patchy 'pneumonic' (i.e. air space) infiltrates with the more benign disorders, but nodular shadows at the more malignant end of the disease spectrum. Lung function tests show a nonspecific pattern of ventilatory restriction with impaired parenchymal function.

Lymphocytic interstitial pneumonia (pneumonitis)

At the most benign end of the spectrum, lymphocytic (or lymphoid) interstitial pneumonia is characterized by diffuse infiltration of the lung interstitium and alveolar walls with small mature lymphocytes, immunoblasts (activated lymphocytes), and plasma cells. Occasionally plasma cells dominate the lymphoid cell infiltrate, and in these circumstances the term plasma cell interstitial pneumonia is preferred.

Lymphocytic pulmonary infiltration may occur in isolation without obvious cause (idiopathic lymphocytic interstitial pneumonia); it may also be a consequence of underlying pulmonary or systemic disease, such as HIV or Epstein–Barr virus (EBV) infection, drug hypersensitivity (sometimes toxicity), Castleman's disease (giant follicular lymph node hyperplasia), and a variety of autoimmune disorders, of which Sjögren's syndrome, rheumatoid disease, and systemic lupus erythematosus are most prominent. It may also be a consequence of a graft-vs-host reaction, and of common variable immunodeficiency—a primary antibody deficiency syndrome. When it occurs in children with AIDS it is thought to be largely a consequence of EBV infection. Recently it has been described in Japan as a consequence of ingested herbal medicine (ou-gon).

The infiltrating lymphocytes show various levels of activation, and excess circulating immunoglobulins (usually IgM), whether monoclonal or polyclonal, are commonly observed. Occasionally there is hypo- rather than hypergammaglobulinaemia. When plasma cells rather than lymphocytes are dominant, the immunoglobulins are much less likely to be of the IgM class, though later complications may still include Waldenstrom's macroglobulinaemia or multiple myeloma. Bronchoalveolar lavage shows an excess of CD8+ T cells when lymphocytic interstitial pneumonia is associated with HIV, whilst in Sjögren's syndrome the recovered lymphocytes are of the CD4+ phenotype. The lymphocytic response appears to depend on an excess expression of interleukins IL-6 and IL-18.

The radiographic features, best seen with high-resolution CT scans, are those of diffuse interstitial shadowing similar to cryptogenic fibrosing alveolitis, or (less commonly) air space filling. Cysts are often present, the mechanism being uncertain, and occasionally there are large nodules (>10 mm diameter). Effusion is not characteristic. The overall appearances are not specific, and since the disorder is rare, open biopsy is generally required for definitive diagnosis. It is seen in both sexes, usually in middle age, though children are sometimes affected. Slow progression is characteristic, though lymphocytic interstitial pneumonia is rather more responsive to corticosteroid or other immunosuppressive therapy than is cryptogenic fibrosing alveolitis, and it sometimes remits spontaneously. There may, however, be complicating (even fatal) sepsis. The ultimate prognosis depends most on that of any underlying disease.

A prospective study in Denver over 14 years usefully identified 15 cases. Women were more often affected than men (11:4), and the age at presentation ranged from 17 to 78 years (mean 47). Only three cases proved to be idiopathic. Of the remainder, most were associated with Sjögren's syndrome (8) or other autoimmune disorders (3). One patient had variable immunodeficiency with dysproteinaemia. Three patients died because of progressive lung disease during the surveillance period—one of the three with 'idiopathic' disease, one of the eight with Sjögren's syndrome, and the one with rheumatoid disease. Lymphoma was not observed.

Lymphoma

All lymphoma types may present with intrathoracic disease, and all may involve the thorax later if they present elsewhere. Lymph nodes, lymphatics, lung parenchyma, and pleura may all become infiltrated, but the patterns vary between tumour types. A comprehensive review is beyond the scope of this chapter, and the reader is referred to Chapter 22.4.3 for fuller details. Non-Hodgkin's lymphoma is more common than Hodgkin's disease and tends to affect an older population. Its thoracic manifestations are similar to those of Hodgkin's disease, but it is the more likely malignant 'complication' of the other lymphocytic pulmonary infiltrations identified in this section. It also has a greater tendency to be disseminated at presentation and to have more 'high-grade' features histologically and clinically. To the chest physician the distinction of Hodgkin's disease and low-grade non-Hodgkin's lymphoma from high-grade non-Hodgkin's lymphoma is of particular value, since the former are often curable, or at least highly responsive to treatment.

When malignant clonal proliferation of lymphoid cells involves the lung parenchyma, other organs are usually infiltrated already. In only a small proportion of extranodal forms of lymphoma is the lung involved alone (or first), and these represent less than 1% of primary lung tumours. Apparent 'primary' lymphomas of the lung generally fall into the categories of lymphomatoid granulomatosis, low-grade B-cell lymphoma, and high-grade B-cell lymphoma, which are non-Hodgkin's lymphomas. Primary pulmonary plasmacytoma is extremely uncommon, and it is similarly uncommon for Hodgkin's disease to affect the lung parenchyma in isolation. However, both Hodgkin's disease and non-Hodgkin's lymphoma not uncommonly involve the lung in their advanced and widely disseminated stages.

Lymphomatoid granulomatosis (angiocentric lymphoma)

Most authorities now regard lymphomatoid granulomatosis as a lymphoma. Its typical histological appearances of granuloma formation and prominent infiltration of blood vessel walls have, until recently, suggested a more benign site on the spectrum of lymphocytic infiltration of the lung, with close similarity to Wegener's granulomatosis. The infiltrating cells comprise a mixture of lymphocytes, plasma cells, histiocytes, and atypical lymphoid cells. The latter are derived from B lymphocytes and appear to be clonal and malignant. A favoured hypothesis is that they arise because of EBV infection, but activated T cells are also prominent in focal lesions. Proliferation and vascular infiltration were initially assumed to cause luminal obstruction followed by ischaemic necrosis, but there are now doubts whether true granuloma formation and true vasculitis actually occur. As a consequence it has been proposed that angiocentric lymphoma is a more appropriate descriptive term.

The disease is very uncommon in childhood but occurs throughout adult life with a slight predilection for males. A total of 500 to 600 cases have been reported. It may arise on a background of an immunocompromised state. The lungs are almost invariably affected, but skin, central nervous system, and renal involvement is frequently seen, and there is often peripheral neuropathy. The disease is typically multifocal, affecting several organs and simulating disseminated carcinoma, but lymph nodes, bone marrow, liver, and spleen are characteristically spared. Pulmonary lesions are usually discrete and nodular, whether single or multiple, but may vary in size from less than 1 cm in diameter to several centimetres. Occasionally outlines are irregular and indistinct, suggesting patchy consolidation. Cavitation may suggest infection or simulate the radiographic appearances of Wegener's granulomatosis.

Symptoms are commonly dominated by systemic upset (fever, malaise, and weight loss), but respiratory involvement is likely to cause cough (sometimes with haemoptysis), undue breathlessness or even respiratory failure. The involvement of other organs may provide valuable diagnostic insight, but biopsy is necessary for definitive diagnosis. Temporary improvement sometimes follows treatment with corticosteroids alone, but a realistic chance of cure requires cytotoxic therapy for lymphoma.

Low-grade B-cell lymphoma

Low grade B-cell non-Hodgkin's lymphomas account for most primary lymphomas affecting the lung parenchyma. They generally arise in middle aged or elderly adults from mucosa-associated lymphoid tissue (MALT) of the bronchi, and they possibly depend on a prolonged period of antigenic stimulation and/or high B-cell turnover—hence their association with autoimmune disorders. They usually produce several parenchymal nodules with diameters ranging up to a few centimetres, but progression is slow, and the multifocal nature of the disorder may only be revealed by CT scanning. Many cases present at an asymptomatic stage, with one or more masses discovered by chance on a chest radiograph. A tendency to spread outside the bronchi and pulmonary vessels but within the bronchovascular bundles may leave the airway patent and so produce air bronchograms within the tumorous opacities. In a few cases there is a diffuse nodular infiltration.

When there are symptoms, these are usually respiratory. They include cough, haemoptysis, chest pain, and occasionally breathlessness. Systemic upset is uncommon. Bronchoalveolar lavage, transbronchial biopsy, or fine needle aspiration may be sufficient to demonstrate a B-cell clone and to evaluate the grade of activity, thereby avoiding a need for video-assisted or open lung biopsy. With appropriate treatment, median survival exceeds 10 years, and more than 80% of affected subjects survive 5 years.

High-grade B-cell lymphoma

High grade B-cell non-Hodgkin's lymphomas account for 10 to 20% of primary lymphomas affecting the lung parenchyma. They commonly occur in association with life-threatening immunosuppression, particularly with AIDS or the management of organ transplants, with these associated problems playing a major role in determining prognosis. Treatment may otherwise produce survival for several years, but the outlook is much less favourable than with low-grade disease.

The more aggressive nature of high-grade disease is reflected by the greater likelihood of respiratory and systemic symptoms. These may result from either multifocal involvement, similar to that shown with lymphomatoid granulomatosis, or from the local effects of single tumour masses (atelectasis and pleural effusion). Any associated disease may provide additional clinical features.

Treatment

Chemotherapeutic regimens for the treatment of lymphoma continue to develop rapidly and have properly become the responsibility of specialist haemato-oncologists. Chemotherapy is, of course, attended by the familiar risks of bone marrow suppression and an immunocompromised state. Such risks are particularly noteworthy when lymphoma involves the lung since many of the chemotherapeutic agents can themselves cause interstitial lung disease—including lymphocytic infiltration. The supervising physician may consequently face a classic diagnostic dilemma when, after an initial satisfactory remission, the patient's radiographs show pulmonary shadows consistent with infection, drug hypersensitivity/toxicity, or recurrent lymphomatous infiltration. A prompt and accurate diagnosis is essential since each possibility requires fundamentally different management. The diagnostic possibities may develop together in any combination, and infection may be with more than one microorganism. Expectorated secretions may provide adequate evidence of infection to justify a trial of antibiotic therapy (perhaps with the use of the polymerase chain reaction to amplify fragments of genetically specific microbial material), but if immediate progress is unsatisfactory, fibre-optic bronchoscopy with lavage and/or transbronchial biopsy is generally needed. A multidisciplinary approach to management is essential, involving chest physicians, radiologists, microbiologists, and histopathologists under the expertise of supervising oncologists or haematologists.

Further reading

Cadranel J, Wislez M, Antoine M (2002). Primary pulmonary lymphoma. *Eur Respir J*, **20**, 750–62.

Cha SI, Fessler MB, Cool CD, Schwarz MI, Brown KK (2006). Lymphoid interstitial pneumonia: clinical features, associations and prognosis. *Eur Respir J*, **28**, 364–9.

Chilosi M, Zinzani PL, Poletti V (2005). Lymphoproliferative lung disorders. *Semin Respir Crit Care Med*, **26**, 490–501.

Donnelly TJ, Tuder RM, Vendegna TR (1998). A 48-year-old woman with peripheral neuropathy, hypercalcaemia, and pulmonary infiltrates. *Chest*, **114**, 1205–9.

Glickstein M, *et al.* (1986). Non lymphomatous lymphoid disorders of the lung. *Am J Roentgenol*, **147**, 227–37.

Guinee DR, *et al.* (1998). Proliferation and cellular phenotype in lymphomatoid granulomatosis: implications of a higher proliferation index in B cells. *Am J Surg Pathol*, **22**, 1093–100.

Haque AK, *et al.* (1998). Pulmonary lymphomatoid granulomatosis in acquired immunodeficiency syndrome: lesions with Epstein–Barr virus. *Modern Pathol*, **11**, 347–56.

Honda O, *et al.* (1999). Differential diagnosis of lymphocytic interstitial pneumonia and malignant lymphoma on high-resolution CT. *Am J Roentgenol*, **173**, 71–4.

Liebow AA (1973). Pulmonary angiitis and granulomatosis. *Am Rev Respir Dis*, **108**, 1–18.

Wannesson L, Cavalli F, Zucca E (2005). Primary pulmonary lymphoma: current status. *Clin Lymphoma Myeloma*, **6**, 220–7.

18.14.4 **Extrinsic allergic alveolitis**

D.J. Hendrick and G.P. Spickett

Essentials

Extrinsic allergic alveolitis is an uncommon inflammatory disorder of the lungs that results from hypersensitivity responses to inhaled environmental agents. Most varieties are occupational in origin, but sporadic cases arise in domestic settings or from recreational activities. Causal agents chiefly comprise allergenic microbial spores that contaminate stored vegetable produce (e.g. farmer's lung caused by *Saccharopolyspora rectivirgula*, previously known as *Micropolyspora faeni*, and *Thermoactinomyces vulgaris*) or reservoirs of water, but a number of animal proteins (particularly those present in feather bloom, e.g. pigeon fancier's lung) and a few reactive chemicals are also inducers.

Pathology—acute disease is characterized by a nonspecific diffuse pneumonitis with inflammatory cellular infiltration of the bronchioles, alveoli, and interstitium; subacute disease by the formation of epithelioid noncaseating granulomas; and chronic disease by fibrosis, particularly in the upper lobes.

Acute disease—following a sensitizing period of exposure, which may vary from weeks to years, the affected subject experiences repeated episodes of an influenza-like illness accompanied by cough and undue breathlessness some hours (usually 3–9) after commencing exposure to the relevant organic dust. Fever and basal crackles are the main physical signs. Most patients recover fully from each acute exacerbation within a day or so, and if the cause is recognized and further exposure avoided there is little risk of persisting pulmonary dysfunction.

Chronic disease—typically seen following long-standing low-level antigenic exposure, e.g. in the person who keeps a single budgerigar (parakeet) in the home. Presents less dramatically than acute disease with increasing shortness of breath, but without systemic upset except for weight loss in some cases. Clinical features are similar to those of other varieties of pulmonary fibrosis, but clubbing is uncommon. Permanent fibrotic lung damage can eventually lead to hypoxaemia, pulmonary hypertension, right heart failure, and death.

Investigation—is directed towards the lungs, the relevant exposure, and determination of hypersensitivity. (1) Lungs—in acute disease the chest radiograph may be normal or show a ground-glass appearance; in subacute disease small reticular opacities may be seen; in chronic disease there is fibrosis. CT provides better images, but no single feature or pattern is pathognomonic. Lung function studies show a restrictive pattern. (2) Determination of relevant exposure—in many cases the history alone is sufficient, but industrial hygiene measurements made from personal samplers may be required when the disease is suspected in an environment not previously incriminated. (3) Determination of hypersensitivity—demonstration of a serum IgG antibody response to the inducing organic dust is unsatisfactory for 'confirming' hypersensitivity because it correlates with exposure better than disease, but a negative test generally excludes the diagnosis. Some form of inhalation challenge test may be necessary when there is diagnostic doubt.

Management—requires that the diagnosis is secure, and then centres on reducing any further exposure to a minimum. There is debate as to whether the use of corticosteroids for acute episodes confers any long-term benefit. In acute disease cessation of exposure usually leads to complete resolution and in chronic cases usually prevents further progression. Persistent exposure can lead to progressive and permanent fibrotic damage in some cases, but not in all.

Historical perspective

Farmer's lung is often regarded as the prototype of the alveolar, bronchiolar, and interstitial disorders that result from hypersensitivity to inhaled organic dusts. These occur worldwide and are known collectively by the term 'extrinsic allergic alveolitis' (or simply allergic alveolitis), although it is recognized that the underlying inflammatory response occurs diffusely throughout the gas-exchanging tissues and is not confined to the alveoli. For this reason many prefer the term 'hypersensitivity pneumonitis'. These disorders were not clearly distinguished from asthma until 1932 when Campbell published his celebrated report describing three affected English farm workers, the appellation 'farmer's lung' being suggested in 1944. However, the disease had been recognized in Iceland in the 19th century, and probably contributed to the occupational ailments of grain workers so graphically described by Ramazzini in the 18th century.

Part of the eminence of farmer's lung itself stems from its industrial importance, and part from its historical role in the understanding of extrinsic allergic alveolitis. Its relation to the inhalation of dust from mouldy hay, straw, or grain had been recognized from the outset, but it was not until 1961, when Pepys and colleagues demonstrated the presence of precipitins to antigens of mouldy hay in patients suffering from the disease, that the idea of an allergic aetiology gained general acceptance. These and other investigators showed that the main sources of antigen were contaminating thermophilic actinomycetes, particularly *Saccharopolyspora rectivirgula* (then known as *Micropolyspora faeni*) and *Thermoactinomyces vulgaris*. These thermophilic microbes (which are bacteria, not fungi) colonize fermenting damp vegetable produce as it heats up. When it eventually dries, a respirable dust laden with antigenic microbial spores is left. Symptoms are consequently most common during winters following wet summer harvests, when hay or grain is used for feeding stock, and astonishing numbers of spores (thousands of millions per cubic metre) are released into the air.

For deposition of the dust to occur predominantly in the gas-exchanging tissues, particle size must be largely confined to the range 0.5 to 5 μm. This encompasses the diameters of many antigenic bacterial and fungal spores, and a large number of microbial species are now recognized as causes of extrinsic allergic alveolitis. In addition, the disease has been described following respiratory exposure to a variety of antigens derived from animal, vegetable, and even chemical sources, both in the workplace and in the home. It may also occur because of allergy to ingested agents, chiefly medications, but only inhalant causes will be addressed in this chapter. Drug-induced examples of the disease are discussed in Chapter 18.14.13.

Aetiology, pathology, and pathogenesis

Aetiology

Table 18.14.4.1 lists the various agents, principally organic proteins, reported to cause extrinsic allergic alveolitis. Most are encountered in working environments and so the disease is usually occupational, but some are encountered in the home or during recreation. Intriguing recent reports have additionally incriminated sources of exposure within the community at large—local pigeons and migrating Canada geese. Most causal agents are microorganisms that are found contaminating a variety of vegetable products, buildings, or equipment, but some are derived directly from animal or vegetable sources, and a few are reactive chemicals. The latter are thought to act as haptens, combining with body proteins to produce larger and now antigenic molecules. Although the microorganisms associated with the more celebrated disorders—farmer's lung, mushroom worker's lung, and bagassosis—are usually thermophilic, most causing extrinsic allergic alveolitis are not. Even with mouldy hay and farmer's lung there is evidence that nonthermophilic organisms (e.g. aspergillus) may occasionally be involved.

Some microbial contamination may occur during growth of the vegetable host, but most of the antigenic load is usually acquired after harvest. Prolonged storage under damp conditions increases the risk of extrinsic allergic alveolitis substantially, and drying to reduce the water content below 30% greatly lessens the risks. Farmer's lung and bagassosis are not therefore primary disorders of hay/grain or sugar cane harvest. They usually arise months or even years later, when the stored product is used or moved. In the interim, moulding is likely to have involved a series of different microorganisms that colonize the forage material sequentially. As the exothermic process increases the ambient temperature, so thermophilic microbes come to dominate.

Inevitably there are situations where contamination arises with a number of different microbes, and affected subjects show antibodies to several of them. Unless time-consuming inhalation challenge tests are carried out with extracts of the individual microbial species, it is not possible to identify a single responsible agent in a given case or cases, and it is conceivable that several could be relevant in these circumstances. This is a characteristic feature of contaminated water reservoirs in humidifiers and air conditioners, and a great variety of agents have been suggested as possible causes of humidifier lung, including bacteria, mycobacteria, fungi, protozoa (amoebae), and metazoa (nematode debris). Some authors prefer to distinguish extrinsic allergic alveolitis attributable in such circumstances to microorganisms growing in cool or cold water (humidifier lung) from that arising from heated water (ventilation pneumonitis). Additional sources of causal organisms include hot tubs and saunas, containing both thermophilic and nonthermophilic organisms (including nontuberculous mycobacteria), and water-based metal-working fluids. The latter, often contaminated with oil, are recycled during use to lubricate and cool rotating or cutting equipment in the metal-working industry, and may therefore be dispersed as respirable aerosols. The chief microbial contaminants are generally environmental nontuberculous mycobacteria or fungi, but a variety of other organisms may be involved. Although granulomatous responses might be expected from mycobacterial infection, the mechanism of the diffuse pneumonitis resulting from mycobacterial contamination of metal-working fluids (and hot tubs) does seem to depend on hypersensitivity alone.

Hypersensitivity is also presumed to explain the unusual and rare form of diffuse alveolitis associated with cobalt and tungsten (or cobalt and diamond dust)—the constituents of 'hard metal' cutting and sharpening tools. It is unusual because of characteristic giant, multinucleated, scavenger macrophages within the alveolar spaces, and because no microbial contaminants are involved; it is rare because of the small population of workers with relevant exposure. Alternative diagnostic labels are 'hard metal disease' and 'giant cell interstitial pneumonia'.

Curiously, contamination with multiple microbial species does not seem to be a feature of Japanese summer-type pneumonitis, which arises seasonally in the hot and humid regions in the south and west of Japan and neighbouring countries. This is the result of the excessive growth of trichosporon (or, occasionally, *Cryptococcus albidus*) in poorly ventilated homes. Mould contamination of domestic environments (e.g. cellars, ultrasonic nebulizers, steam irons, oil heaters, air conditioners) in other regions is recognized to cause extrinsic allergic alveolitis far less frequently, but there are many convincing case reports of domestic causes.

Pathology

There has been little opportunity to characterize the acute form of extrinsic allergic alveolitis histologically in humans because biopsies are very rarely taken within 24 to 48 h of a provoking exposure, and because death leading to autopsy is even less common.

Table 18.14.4.1 Agents reported to cause extrinsic allergic alveolitis

Agent	Source	Appellation (if any)
Microorganisms		
Acinetobacter iwoffii	Metal-working fluid	Machine worker's lung
Alternaria	Paper-mill wood pulp	Wood pulp worker's lung
Aspergillus sp.	Farm produce, maize (corn)	Farmer's lung
Aspergillus clavatus	Whisky maltings	Malt worker's lung
Aspergillus fumigatus	Vegetable compost, cork	Farmer's lung, suberosis
Aspergillus versicolor	Dog bedding (straw)	Dog house disease
Aureobasidium pullulans	Redwood/domestic cellar	Sequoiosis
Bacillus subtilis	Wood/cleaning preparations	
Candida albicans	Heated swimming pool	
Cephalosporium	Sewage	Sewage worker's lung
Cryptococcus albidus	Asian homes in humid summers	Summer-type hypersensitivity pneumonitis
Cryptostroma corticale	Maple	Maple bark stripper's lung
Debaryomyces hansenii	Home ultrasonic nebulizer	
Eurotium sp.	Metal-working fluid	Machine worker's lung
Fusarium sp.	Metal-working fluid/home	Machine worker's lung
Graphium	Redwood	Sequoiosis
Grifola fondosa	Maitake mushrooms	Mushroom worker's lung
Humicola fuscoatra	Domestic home	
Hypsizigus marmoreus	Mushrooms	Mushroom worker's lung
Lentinus edodes	Mushrooms	Mushroom worker's lung
Lycoperdon	Puffballs	Lycoperdonosis
Lyophyllum aggregatum	Mushrooms	Mushroom worker's lung
Merulius lacrymans	Domestic wood	
Mucor stolonifer	Paprika	Paprika splitter's lung
Mycobacterium sp.	Metal-working fluid	Machine worker's lung
Paeccilomyces sp. (*nivea/variotii*)	Hardwood, oil heater	
Penicillium camembertii[a]	Salami production	
P. casei	Cheese	Cheese washer's lung
P. chrysogenum/cyclopium	Domestic wood	
P. citrinum	Enoki mushroom cultivation	
P. frequentens	Cork	Suberosis
P. nalgiovense	Pork sausage mould	
P. verucosum	Gorganzola cheese	
Pezizia domiciliana	Flooded basement	El Niño lung
Pleurotus osteatus/ergngi	Mushrooms	Mushroom worker's lung
Pseudomonas fluorescens	Metal-working fluid	Machine worker's lung
Rhodotorula sp.	Ultrasonic humidifier	
Saccharomonspora viridis	Logging plant	
Sphingbacterium spiritivorum	Domestic steam iron	
Sporobolomyces	Horse barn straw	
Streptomyces albus	Soil/peat	
Thermophilic actinomycetes (*Saccharopolyspora rectivirgula*, *Thermoactinomyces sacchari/vulgaris*)	Hay/straw/grain/mushroom compost/bagasse/heated water/domestic cellar/esparto grass	Farmer's lung Mushroom worker's lung Bagassosis Esparto plasterer's lung
Trichosporon cutaneum/ovoides	Asian homes in humid summers	Summer-type hypersensitivity pneumonitis
Miscellaneous bacteria/mycobacteria/fungi/amoebae/nematode debris	Air conditioners/humidifiers/tap water/showers/heated pools,saunas,tubs/metal fluids	Humidifier lung Ventilation pneumonitis Sauner taker's lung
Unknown	Roof thatch	New Guinea lung

Table 18.14.4.1 (*Cont'd*) Agents reported to cause extrinsic allergic alveolitis

Agent	Source	Appellation (if any)
Animals		
Arthropods (*Sitophilus granarius*)	Grain dust	Wheat weevil disease
Birds	?Feather bloom/?excreta	Bird fancier's lung
Fish	Fish meal	Fish meal worker's lung
Mammal pituitary (cattle, pig)	Pituitary extracts	Pituitary snuff taker's lung
Mammal hair	Fur	Furrier's lung
Mollusc shell	Nacre-button manufacture	
Urine (rodents)	Urinary protein	Rodent handler's lung
Vegetation		
Cabreuva	Wood dust	
Coffee	Coffee bean dust	Coffee worker's lung
Esparto grass[b]	Plaster	Esparto plasterer's lung
Amorphophalus konjak	Konjak flour	Konnyaku maker's lung
Peat moss[c]	Peat moss packaging plant	
Shimeji[d]	Shimeji cultivators	
Tiger nut	Tiger nut dust	
Wood (*Gonystylus bacanus*)	Wood dust	Wood worker's lung
Chemicals		
Bordeaux mixture (fungicide)	Vineyards	Vineyard sprayer's lung
Cobalt dissolved in solvents	Tungsten carbide grinding	
Diphenyl methane diisocyanate	Plastics industry	
Hexamethylene diisocyanate	Plastics industry	
Methyl methacrylate	Dentistry	
Pauli's reagent	Laboratory	
Phthalic (or trimellitic) anhydride	Epoxy polyester powder paint	
Pyrethrum	Insecticide spray	
Tetrachloroethylene	Dry cleaning	
Toluene diisocyanate	Plastics industry	
Triglycidyl isocyanate	Plastics industry	
Trimellitic anhydride	Plastics industry	
Vanadium catalyst	Maleic anhydride manufacture	
Miscellaneous		
Hijikia fusiforme (algae)	Konjak flour	Konnyaku maker's lung
Pet fish food		

[a] Alternative possible causes, *Penicillium notatum, Aspergillus fumigatus*.

[b] Possibly due to microbial contamination (*Aspergillus* sp.).

[c] Possibly due to microbial contamination (*Monocillium* sp., *Penicillium citreonigrum*).

[d] Possibly due to microbial contamination (*Cladosporium sphaerospermum, Penicillium frequentens*, or *Scopulariopsis* sp.).

Initially there is a nonspecific diffuse pneumonitis with inflammatory cellular infiltration of the bronchioles, alveoli, and interstitium, accompanied by oedema and luminal exudation. With ongoing exposure, whether continuous or intermittent, the more familiar appearances of the subacute forms of extrinsic allergic alveolitis evolve. The most characteristic feature is the formation of epithelioid noncaseating granulomas. These are generally less well formed than in sarcoidosis, less profuse, and often evanescent. They can be recognized within 3 weeks of the initiating exposure, and generally resolve within 6 to 12 months. In parallel, fibrosis evolves alongside cellular infiltration of the interstitium with histiocytes, lymphocytes, and plasma cells. Macrophages with foamy cytoplasm may be prominent in the alveolar spaces, and organization of the inflammatory exudate may lead to intra-alveolar fibrosis. Obstruction or obliteration of bronchioles is common. Foreign-body giant cells may reflect the dependence of extrinsic allergic alveolitis on antigens derived from inhaled foreign material, as does a peribronchial predominance of the inflammatory response. Vasculitis is notable by its absence. The typical histological appearance of subacute extrinsic allergic alveolitis is illustrated in Fig. 18.14.4.1.

Progressive, widespread, and irreversible fibrosis may occur with continued exposure, leading to disruption of the normal architecture of the lung. In advanced cases honeycombing may develop. Granulomas are no longer characteristic and the overall appearances

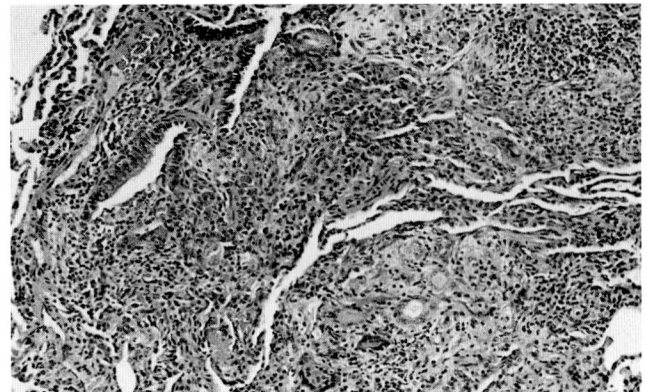

Fig. 18.14.4.1 Histological appearance: subacute disease. There is bronchocentric interstitial fibrosis and chronic inflammation, with poorly formed interstitial granulomas including giant cells. (Haematoxylin and eosin stain at medium magnification.)
(Courtesy of Dr T Ashcroft.)

may differ little from other causes of progressive interstitial pulmonary fibrosis. With extrinsic allergic alveolitis, however, there may be disproportionate fibrosis of the upper lobes.

Pathogenesis

Immune mechanisms

An outline of the possible immunopathology of extrinsic allergic alveolitis through acute, subacute, and chronic phases is illustrated in Figs. 18.14.4.2 and 18.14.4.3. The presumption that complexes of antigen and complement-activating antibodies are primarily responsible for extrinsic allergic alveolitis is now largely discarded. The evidence for deposition of immune complexes is not convincing, and neither IgG nor IgM antibodies are uniformly demonstrated in the sera of affected subjects unless sensitive detection techniques such as the enzyme-linked immunosorbent assay (ELISA) or radioimmunoassays are used. More importantly, these antibodies are frequently found in subjects who are similarly exposed but clinically unaffected, irrespective of the method of detection. A closer association of disease with the IgG4 antibody subclass has been suggested, but the significance of this is not yet apparent. It is clear, however, that vasculitis—a cardinal feature of the experimental Arthus reaction—is not a characteristic; the inflammatory reaction is dominantly lymphocytic or mononuclear rather than polymorphonuclear, although a transitory polymorphonuclear leucocyte response is typical immediately following exposure. Lung tissue is most commonly examined during subacute phases of the disease, at which time a noncaseating granulomatous response suggesting cell-mediated hypersensitivity is the usual finding.

It could be argued that these histological appearances merely represent a healing reaction, but the consistent finding of an acute T-lymphocyte response in fluid obtained at bronchoalveolar lavage supports the current consensus that cell-mediated hypersensitivity plays the dominant pathogenic role in extrinsic allergic alveolitis. The results from animal models of the disease are consistent with this, disease being transferred from animal to animal only with sensitized T lymphocytes. This is not to say that other mechanisms play no role, nor that all inflammatory diseases of the gas-exchanging tissues induced by organic dusts share a common mechanism. Indeed, the onset of symptoms within a few hours of exposure, coupled with polymorphonuclear leucocytosis in bronchoalveolar lavage fluid and peripheral blood, favours the participation of an additional (perhaps priming) immunological or toxic process, and B-lymphocyte aggregates have been noted in transbronchial biopsies obtained during the acute phase. Components of a number of organic dusts associated with extrinsic allergic alveolitis are known to activate complement by the alternative pathway and this, with or without humoral hypersensitivity, might also prove to be relevant.

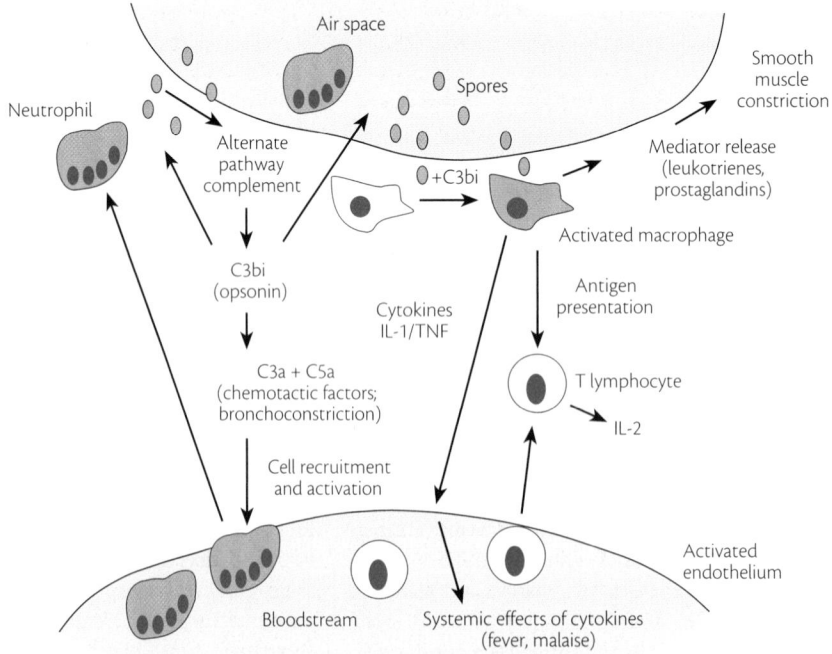

Fig. 18.14.4.2 Possible immunopathogenesis: acute phase.

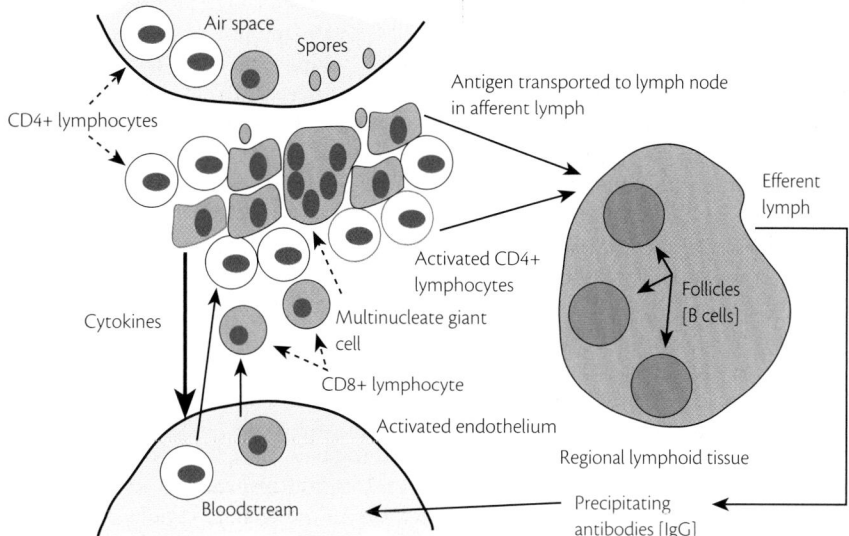

Fig. 18.14.4.3 Possible immunopathogenesis: subacute/chronic phase.

Bronchoalveolar lavage in similarly exposed subjects has shown excess numbers of T lymphocytes, whether they were clinically affected or not, although the proportions of T-cell subpopulations has varied according to disease activity and the circumstances of exposure. Most investigators have detected a relative excess of CD8+ T cells in exposed but asymptomatic subjects, thereby 'inverting' the normal CD4+ to CD8+ ratio. The balance appears to be less disturbed in those with disease, and in one sequential study the ratio changed from 0.43 to 1.47 with disease progression. In an intriguing study of an animal model of extrinsic allergic alveolitis, monkeys that developed characteristic reactions to inhalation challenge showed a helper CD4+ cell lymphocytosis in bronchoalveolar fluid and a relative deficiency of suppressor CD8+ cells, compared with the monkeys giving no clinical reaction who showed responses with both CD4+ and CD8+ cells. When the nonreactors were challenged again after low doses of whole-body irradiation had impaired suppressor- more than helper-cell function, characteristic reactions were noted. These observations suggest that a relative impairment of suppressor-cell function, or of its activation following antigenic exposure, is fundamental to the development of extrinsic allergic alveolitis—a situation that has interesting parallels with sarcoidosis. It is also interesting that lymphopenia in peripheral blood is a typical feature of acute exacerbations of the disease, the T lymphocytes migrating from blood to lungs within hours of the provoking exposure. It is small wonder that studies of systemic and local immune responses have given discordant results, and clear that continuing research should address both aspects of the immune response.

It is known that different antigenic determinants from a given inducing microbial source may lead to different immunological responses, and it seems likely that cytotoxic activity and released cytokines (e.g. interleukin (IL)-6 and tumour necrosis factor α (TNFα)) play some role, possibly by activating the vascular endothelium and thereby recruiting and activating further macrophages and inflammatory cells. In experimental models interferon-γ has been shown to play a major role (an excess of interferon-γ-producing T cells is present in the lungs), and IL-10 ameliorates the disease. There are also increased levels of IL-12 and IL-18, and these cytokines contribute to T-cell polarization towards a Th1-type response. IL-8, a chemotactic factor for neutrophils, and monocyte chemotactic protein-1 (MCP-1) are both elevated in some types of the disease, perhaps accounting for the increase in macrophage and neutrophil recruitment and activation. Serum levels of IL-6 and intercellular adhesion molecule 1 (ICAM-1) are also raised. Bronchoalveolar lavage has also shown that natural killer (NK) cells (CD57+) and mast cells may be prominent additional players in pathogenesis, and there is evidence that the capacity of macrophages to present antigen is enhanced by viral infection and diminished by cigarette smoking. The latter is known to decrease the severity of clinical symptoms as well as the immunological abnormalities.

Cytokines, possibly together with anaphylotoxins from the degradation of complement components (C4, C3, C5), are likely to be responsible for the systemic influenza-like symptoms that are so characteristic of the acute form of extrinsic allergic alveolitis. These symptoms are indistinguishable from those of grain fever in grain workers, 'Monday fever' in cotton workers, humidifier fever in subjects exposed to microbially contaminated humidifiers, and metal fume fever in welders. In these situations the febrile disorder is not characteristically associated with clinical alveolitis, raising the possibility that its occurrence with the acute form of extrinsic allergic alveolitis is an independent phenomenon, not an integral part of extrinsic allergic alveolitis itself. In favour of this hypothesis has been the finding of high levels of endotoxin from Gram-negative bacteria (which are known to provoke these symptoms) in grain dust, cotton dust, contaminated humidifiers, and many of the 'mouldy' vegetable dusts that cause extrinsic allergic alveolitis. However, neither metal fume nor several other causative agents of extrinsic allergic alveolitis are likely to be contaminated with endotoxin, and so endotoxin-induced release of inflammatory mediators is not an entirely satisfactory explanation. For example, inhalation provocation tests with uncontaminated bird serum in subjects with bird fancier's lung reproduce both alveolar and influenza-like responses. Evidently the influenza-like response is an integral feature of the acute form of extrinsic allergic alveolitis, but it is relatively nonspecific and can occur in many other situations.

Extrinsic allergic alveolitis occurs in families only sporadically, and few associations with HLA phenotypes have been demonstrated.

However, a number of studies have suggested associations between HLA D alleles and pigeon fancier's lung and Japanese summer-type hypersensitivity pneumonitis. This genetic background is associated with a high production of TNFα, and these alleles may exert effects on immune suppression, offering one mechanism by which a genetic predisposition could play a role in the development of extrinsic allergic alveolitis. It has also been suggested that an acute inflammatory episode (from viral infection or the inhalation of microbial toxins or chemicals) may be necessary to disrupt the normal defence equilibrium of surface membrane and local immune responses, thereby permitting antigen to be presented in a fashion that leads to hypersensitivity. Undue 'leakiness' of the alveolar membrane can be demonstrated by an increased clearance of inhaled 99Tcm-DTPA, and this has been reported in both the early and continuing phases of extrinsic allergic alveolitis.

Relation to smoking

The disruptive effect of smoking on the alveolar membrane does not appear to augment the risk for extrinsic allergic alveolitis or to increase its severity: in fact the reverse is true. Although smoking enhances acute phase reactions and IgE production, it diminishes IgA, IgG, and IgM antibody responses, increases circulating CD8+ T-lymphocyte numbers, and probably reduces the incidence and severity of extrinsic allergic alveolitis. However, smokers without IgG antibodies are particularly liable to find their respiratory symptoms attributed to other diseases, and so this negative association between extrinsic allergic alveolitis and smoking may have been exaggerated. That it is real is supported by evidence that smoking may also reduce the risk for other T-cell-mediated immunological disorders such as sarcoidosis, ulcerative colitis, and some types of occupational asthma (generally those associated with low-molecular-weight chemicals). The key cell in a complex series of interactions is probably the alveolar macrophage, which is critical in presenting antigen to CD4+ T lymphocytes and so to activating cellular immune mechanisms. Although smoking increases macrophage numbers and their metabolic activity, the activated cells show impairment of both the expression of surface major histocompatibility (MHC) class 2 antigens and the production or release of IL-1 and inflammatory mediators derived from arachidonic acid metabolism (leukotriene B$_4$, prostaglandin E$_2$, thromboxane B$_2$). It is also argued that the increased macrophage numbers down-regulate pulmonary immune responses in a purely nonspecific fashion by impairing antigen access to more effective blood monocytes.

Relation to coeliac disease

Reports that cryptogenic fibrosing alveolitis (now known, depending on histological characteristics, as 'usual interstitial pneumonia' and 'nonspecific interstitial pneumonia') and extrinsic allergic alveolitis (and particularly bird fancier's lung) might be associated with coeliac disease led to the interesting hypothesis that in some cases absorbed food antigens from the disrupted bowel mucosa might play a role in the pathogenesis of the lung disorder; i.e. the lung disorder might be a 'metastatic' complication of the bowel disease. Alternatively, systemic hypersensitivity to a common inhaled and ingested avian antigen might give rise to similar immune reactions and diseases in the relevant target organs. The avian IgG antibody response seen in coeliac disease is, however, distinct from that associated with bird fancier's lung and seems to be a response to dietary egg. It is not related to environmental exposure to birds but does correlate with the activity of the bowel disorder.

Subsequent experience suggests a much less strong association between these bowel and lung disorders that, if real, is probably a consequence of their dependence on similar immunological mechanisms and host susceptibility to them. The association is not sufficiently strong that the one disorder should stimulate investigation for the other.

Epidemiology

Extrinsic allergic alveolitis is an uncommon but not rare disease, but its comparative scarcity limits epidemiological knowledge, as does the use of different methods of investigation. For every case of extrinsic allergic alveolitis there may be 100 cases of 'extrinsic allergic' asthma, but there is even greater geographical variation than with asthma, reflecting the much larger dependence of extrinsic allergic alveolitis on occupational causes and climate. As a consequence, its incidence and its principal causes vary considerably from country to country, and from region to region.

Incidence

Experience over 3 years with the Surveillance of Work-related and Occupational Respiratory Disease (SWORD) project indicated that extrinsic allergic alveolitis of occupational origin accounted for 2% of occupational lung diseases in the United Kingdom. Asthma, the most common, accounted for 26%. This does, of course, ignore extrinsic allergic alveolitis of nonoccupational origin, which is much less easily assessed. It also disguises the absolute risk, since few workers encounter relevant occupational exposures. Almost 50% of reported cases involved farmers or farm workers, followed by 15% affecting workers in material, metal, or electrical processing trades. Among the farmers, the average incidence was 41 per million per year, though this approached 100 in some regions, and has been estimated at 3000 in Quebec, Canada. However, the estimated incidences are crude and must vary considerably according to the prevailing weather. They may be compared with 200 to 700 per million per year among working groups at greatest risk of developing occupational asthma in the United Kingdom. Contaminating microorganisms underlie over 50% of the cases of extrinsic allergic alveolitis reported to SWORD, followed in order of importance by animal antigens in 6% and chemicals in 5%. In 27% of reports a suspected agent was not specified.

Prevalence

Figures for prevalence are more readily available than those for incidence, and demonstrate quite marked national differences. In developed countries, humidifier lung is being recognized with increasing frequency both in the workplace and in the home, and remarkable prevalences of 15 to 70% have been suggested in populations from contaminated offices in North America. Bird fancier's lung may be more prevalent at present over the whole of the United Kingdom, simply because of the great popularity of keeping budgerigars (known as parakeets in North America) and pigeons. Budgerigars are kept in some 12% of British homes, and it has been estimated that 0.5 to 7.5% of the population involved are likely to have extrinsic allergic alveolitis as a consequence, albeit mildly in most cases. Pigeon keeping is 40 times less common, and the measured prevalence of pigeon fancier's lung among pigeon keepers has been a good deal more varied (0–21%). This may reflect both true differences between groups of pigeon breeders as exposure levels vary, for instance, according to number of birds, duration of exposure, loft ventilation, and cleaning habits, and artefactual differences arising as a result of selection bias and variable compliance. The avian antigen responsible and its precise source have yet to be identified, but bloom from the feathers containing oil, saliva, and secretory IgA is currently favoured over dust emanating from dried droppings.

In areas of high rainfall where 'traditional' farming methods are used, the prevalence of farmer's lung may reach 10%. This is likely to be the commonest cause of extrinsic allergic alveolitis in developing countries. In developed countries, where modern farming methods are used, prevalences rarely exceed 2 to 3% and are usually a good deal less. Furthermore, the farming population at risk represents a mere 1 to 2% of the population at large, although there are marked regional variations. Even smaller populations are employed making whisky from germinating barley (maltings), raising mushrooms on a variety of antigenic composts, or handling bagasse (the fibrous stem that remains when sugar is extracted from sugar cane), but within some of these populations extrinsic allergic alveolitis was a common problem until excessive exposure levels were controlled. Extrinsic allergic alveolitis associated with animals other than birds is extremely uncommon, as is the case with chemical-induced extrinsic allergic alveolitis.

In Japan, the seasonal summer growth of *T. cutaneum* in the home is by far the commonest cause of extrinsic allergic alveolitis where the remarkable 'summer-type hypersensitivity pneumonitis' accounts for about 75% of all cases of extrinsic allergic alveolitis. It is approximately 10 times as common as farmer's lung and 20 times as common as bird fancier's lung.

The important risk of extrinsic allergic alveolitis from metal-working fluids varies substantially according to the degree and nature of microbial contamination, and the ease with which aerosols of the fluids are released into the working environment. Up to one-third of exposed occupational populations have become affected.

Prevention

Once extrinsic allergic alveolitis is recognized in one individual, the environment concerned should be assessed for the risk it poses to others. In many circumstances this will be well known already, and exposure levels will be within the range considered acceptable. In others, neither the risk nor the precise causative agent (nor its level of exposure) will be known, and in such unfamiliar circumstances there may be a need to survey the exposed population at risk. Questionnaires and serological tests are most convenient for this, at least as a screening procedure. When large populations are involved, comprehensive investigation is sensible before major modifications are considered to the working environment.

Modifications can always be made to the environment to lessen the level of exposure, but their extent will be limited by expense and should be justified by need. Dry storage and adequate ventilation are the two most important factors when vegetable produce is involved, and in some farming areas there is benefit in drying produce artificially after harvest. An alternative is some form of 'pickling', so that the produce is preserved chemically. With silage, for example, newly cut grass is kept under impervious covering in relatively sealed conditions. Initial enzymic and moulding processes use up available oxygen, and produce aldehydes and other

preservative chemicals. These create nearly anaerobic conditions and protect the produce until it is used. Similarly, hay may be sealed in plastic bags, or grain or bagasse may be treated with propionic acid.

When ventilation and humidification systems are themselves responsible for extrinsic allergic alveolitis, major mechanical alterations may be necessary and the methods of humidification and temperature control may need to be changed. The crucial need is to reduce the ease with which normal airborne microbial contaminants are able to proliferate in stagnant, reservoir, collections of water. For this there may be a role for 'biocide' sterilizing agents, but these are also likely to become airborne and respirable and so must have low intrinsic toxicity and sensitizing potency. For one such biocide (isothiazolinone) there have been reports of occupational dermatitis and asthma, though not of extrinsic allergic alveolitis.

An industrial need for rapid air changes coupled with close control of humidity and temperature poses formidable problems. The use of recirculated filtered air is the most economical, but effective filters are expensive and can become contaminated themselves, increasing rather than decreasing the load of respirable microbial antigens. The use of heat exchangers minimizes the cost of temperature control if contaminated exhaust air is not recirculated, but does not conserve water.

Clinical features

Acute extrinsic allergic alveolitis

The acute form of extrinsic allergic alveolitis is the most easily recognized because symptoms are often distressing and incapacitating and have a high degree of specificity. Following a sensitizing period of exposure, which may vary from weeks to years, the affected subject experiences repeated episodes of an influenza-like illness accompanied by cough and undue breathlessness some hours (usually 3–9 h) after commencing exposure to the relevant organic dust. The systemic influenza-like symptoms generally dominate those that are respiratory, and the affected subject complains most of malaise, fever, chills, widespread aches and pains (particularly headache), anorexia, and tiredness. They are unlikely to feel like exercising and may well put themselves to bed, therefore remaining unaware of undue shortness of breath, though likely to develop a dry cough without wheeze and to have some difficulty taking deep, satisfying breaths. Occasionally there is an asthmatic or bronchitic response and wheezing or productive cough becomes an additional feature.

Despite the delay in onset after exposure begins, affected subjects soon learn to associate symptoms with the causative environment, especially if they follow a period away from the causal exposure. Recognition is particularly easy for groups such as farmers and pigeon fanciers for whom these risks are well known. However, in some cases there may be a tendency to deny such a relationship for fear of compromising the ability to pursue a livelihood or hobby, and the clinical history may appear much less convincing than it should.

The severity and duration of symptoms depend critically on exposure dose and individual susceptibility. With low levels of acute exposure, symptoms are mild and persist for a few hours only. When occupation is responsible, the affected worker may feel unwell only at home during the following evening or night, and be fully recovered by the next morning, hence obscuring the relevance of the workplace. When severe responses follow particularly heavy exposures the relation of the one to the other will be more obvious, and complete remission may require several days or even weeks.

In exceptionally severe cases, life-threatening respiratory failure may develop and emergency admission to hospital becomes necessary. Death is not unknown. Respiratory distress at rest with fever and gravity-dependent crackles are the main physical signs, with breathing being fast but shallow. Clubbing is very rarely seen. Hypoxaemia is typically accompanied by hypocapnia, and the chest radiograph shows a diffuse alveolar filling and interstitial pattern. Supplemental oxygen may be required, and in rare cases there may be a brief need for mechanical ventilatory support. Spontaneous recovery can be expected to begin within 12 to 24h, and can be accelerated with corticosteroids.

Most subjects recover fully from each acute exacerbation, and if the cause is recognized and further exposure avoided there is little risk of persisting pulmonary dysfunction. However, it is not always realistic to expect affected individuals to avoid further exposure, particularly among farming communities, and there is some risk that continuing exposure and repeated acute exacerbations will eventually lead to permanent impairment of lung function.

Chronic extrinsic allergic alveolitis

In some patients extrinsic allergic alveolitis presents in a much less dramatic but potentially more serious way. Exercise tolerance is gradually lost due to shortness of breath, but without systemic upset aside from (in some cases only) prominent loss of weight. This is the result of diffuse pulmonary fibrosis, which has often been progressing for years before the individual seeks advice: the slower the progression, the longer the delay and the greater the likely degree of permanent fibrotic damage. Eventually hypoxaemia and pulmonary hypertension may supervene, and the right heart fails. There are no acute exacerbations, and each day and each month is much like any other. The clinical features are similar to those of other varieties of pulmonary fibrosis, although clubbing is uncommon, and it may prove extremely difficult to distinguish this form of extrinsic allergic alveolitis from usual interstitial pneumonia, nonspecific interstitial pneumonia, sarcoidosis, or other slowly progressive forms of pulmonary fibrosis. There may also be asthmatic or bronchitic symptoms, but these are best regarded as independent airway manifestations of hypersensitivity to the causal agent.

The chronic form of extrinsic allergic alveolitis is typically seen in the person who keeps a single budgerigar in the home. The level of antigenic exposure to avian dust is comparatively trivial compared with that of the farm worker forking bales of heavily contaminated hay in a poorly ventilated barn, but it is encountered almost continuously, particularly if the affected individual is housebound. Differing exposure patterns are largely responsible for these distinct forms of extrinsic allergic alveolitis, although differences in host responsiveness exert an important additional influence, hence there may consequently be considerable variability in clinical features among individuals affected by the same source of antigenic exposure.

Recent reports have suggested that farmer's lung may additionally be complicated by emphysema, even in never-smokers, although this has not so far been recognized to contribute to the natural history of other types of extrinsic allergic alveolitis. Of possible relevance has been the additional recognition from high-resolution CT

that extrinsic allergic alveolitis is associated in a few cases with thin walled cysts together (unsurprisingly) with evidence of bronchiolar obstruction.

Intermediate forms

The acute and chronic forms of extrinsic allergic alveolitis represent the extremes of a continuous spectrum. Individual cases are distributed widely over this spectrum, hence it can be argued that few fall comfortably into one extreme form or the other and that the classification into 'acute' or 'chronic' has limited practical value. It is important to recognize the marked clinical variability that may occur between cases, and the changes that may occur within cases with the passage of time. The fact that the acute form of extrinsic allergic alveolitis can be produced by inhalation provocation tests in subjects with the chronic form of the disease emphasizes the major role that dose exerts in determining the clinical nature of the response that occurs. Depending on exposure dose and host responsiveness, affected subjects will come to lie at different points on the spectrum at different times. It is possible for acute exacerbations to occur in subjects manifesting predominantly the chronic form of the disease, and for a limited degree of recovery to follow cessation of exposure.

Differential diagnosis

Acute extrinsic allergic alveolitis is not the only disorder characterized by systemic influenza-like symptoms and respiratory distress to follow an unusually heavy exposure to microbially contaminated vegetable produce. In 1986 an international symposium considered a further disorder that occurs within hours of heavy respiratory exposure to dusts containing fungal toxins, especially those released on decapping silos. It is the result of direct toxicity rather than hypersensitivity and the term 'organic dust toxic syndrome' was recommended to describe it. Its effects are usually mild and self-limiting, but severe respiratory embarrassment can occur and there is a small risk of ongoing, and potentially fatal, fungal invasion of the lungs. This risk could be enhanced if corticosteroid treatment is given, and death has occurred in subjects who appear to have been fully immunocompetent. Not only does organic dust toxic syndrome occur in circumstances which favour the occurrence of extrinsic allergic alveolitis (particularly silos and swine/poultry confinement buildings), but its clinical features have much in common with extrinsic allergic alveolitis, and to a lesser extent with nitrogen dioxide toxicity, which may also affect silo workers. Indeed, there is so much overlap that it can be very difficult indeed to distinguish one disorder from the others (Table 18.14.4.2).

The acute form of extrinsic allergic alveolitis can only be the result of an acute and recent (a matter of hours) exposure to the relevant causal antigen. This limits the opportunity for diagnostic error, although the circumstances of an unusually heavy exposure may be subtle. For example, a pigeon fancier might spend rather less time than usual with his birds, but much more time than usual in the more hazardous dusty car he uses regularly to transport racing birds for training exercises.

Just as acute and heavy exposures to organic dusts may cause disorders other than extrinsic allergic alveolitis, they may also be quite irrelevant and purely coincidental to the acute respiratory disorder with which the patient presents. Consequently the differential diagnosis should include consideration of other acute disorders

Table 18.14.4.2 Characteristics of nitrogen dioxide toxicity (silo filler's disease), organic dust toxic syndrome, and acute farmer's lung

	Nitrogen dioxide toxicity	Organic dust toxic syndrome	Acute farmer's lung
Susceptibility in smokers	Unknown	Unknown	Decreased
Relation to time of harvest	Days	Months to years	Months to years
Microbial decomposition of harvest product	Little	Marked	Variable
Confined exposure space	+++	+	+
Previous episodes	–	+	++
Symptoms			
Dry cough	++	++	++
Breathlessness	++	++	++
Wheeze	–	–	–
Systemic upset	+	+	++
Signs			
Basal crackles	+	+	+
Fever	+	+	+
Time of onset after beginning exposure	1–10 h	1–10 h	1–10 h
Duration	Hours to days	Hours to days	Hours to days
Investigations			
Leucocytosis	+	+	+
Radiograph–small irregular opacities, alveolar shadows	+	±	+
Restricted ventilation	+	±	+
Reduced gas transfer	+	±	+
Hypoxaemia	+	±	+
Fungi from secretions/biopsy	–	++	+
Methaemoglobinaemia	+	–	–
Serum precipitins	–	–	+ (?– in smokers)
Response to steroids	+	–	++
Life threatening	Not uncommonly	Rarely	Rarely

of the lung parenchyma and interstitium, such as infections, other immunological disorders, drug reactions, and even paraquat poisoning, which sometimes occurs accidentally in farm workers. In bird keepers the diagnosis of viral, mycoplasmal, and chlamydial infection may itself be confounded by false-positive microbial antibody tests. This is the result of pre-existing avian antibodies cross-reacting with egg protein in the microbial cultures used to provide the test agents.

When subacute or chronic forms of extrinsic allergic alveolitis are encountered, the differential diagnosis lies with other diffuse infiltrative and fibrotic disorders of the lung. Those most frequently resembling extrinsic allergic alveolitis include usual interstitial pneumonia, nonspecific interstitial pneumonia, sarcoidosis, pneumoconiosis, tuberculosis, and metastatic cancer, although a huge variety of less common disorders may also need to be considered.

Clinical investigation

Establishing a diagnosis of extrinsic allergic alveolitis involves three areas of investigation: the lungs, the exposure, and the evidence for hypersensitivity.

Pulmonary

In many cases extrinsic allergic alveolitis is first suspected after the presence of diffuse alveolitis or progressive pulmonary fibrosis is established. With the acute form of the disease the chest radiograph commonly shows no abnormality unless symptoms are moderately severe. When the radiograph is abnormal, there is a widespread ground-glass appearance or an alveolar filling pattern, particularly in the lower and mid-zones. This may resolve within a mere 24 to 48 h once exposure has ceased. In more subacute forms small reticular opacities, simulating asbestosis, are seen within the same distribution: these may persist for several weeks despite cessation of exposure and, if exposure continues, honeycombing may develop. Occasionally a more nodular pattern occurs. In contrast to the distribution of acute and subacute radiological abnormalities, the upper zones are predominantly affected by the irreversible fibrotic process that characterizes the chronic form of disease. This may simulate sarcoidosis or even tuberculosis, and may lead to considerable shrinkage and distortion. In practice, the radiographic appearances vary considerably from patient to patient and correlate poorly with the clinical severity of the disease.

CT provides a much clearer picture of the type of radiographic abnormality and of its extent, particularly when thin-section high-resolution techniques are used, but no single feature or pattern is pathognomonic (Fig. 18.14.4.4). Again, investigation within hours of exposure has been limited and experience is largely confined to patients with subacute and chronic disease. Increased ground-glass density of the lung parenchyma is the most prominent finding in the subacute form, followed almost equally by reticular or nodular infiltration, more uniform involvement of the lung fields being demonstrated than is obvious from plain radiographs. At end expiration a mosaic pattern is characteristic, reflecting patchy bronchiolar involvement and the different degrees by which residual gas can be expelled from distal lobules. The attenuated areas may then be normal, the translucent areas indicating gas retention. Lymph node enlargement and/or pleural involvement are not characteristic. With chronic forms, the CT scan shows a similar pattern of fibrosis and disruption to the plain radiograph, but again is considerably more sensitive.

Lung function studies vary according to severity and recent activity. As with asthma, they may be unremarkable in the acute form of the disease when there has been little recent exposure. When lung function is impaired, the pattern suggests parenchymal and interstitial disease but is otherwise nonspecific. There is impaired carbon monoxide gas transfer (diminished $T_{L}co$ and K_{co}) with restricted ventilation (i.e. forced vital capacity (FVC) is diminished as much as forced expiratory volume in 1 s (FEV_1) or more so, with respect to predicted values), decreased compliance, and (in more severe cases) arterial hypoxaemia and hypocapnia, particularly

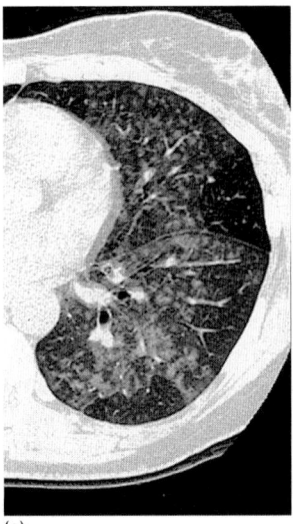 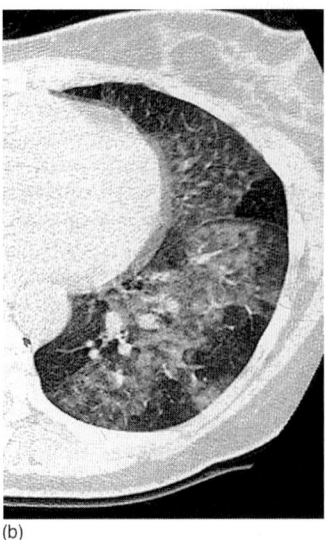

(a) (b)

Fig. 18.14.4.4 (a) CT scan of a woman aged 44 years who had never smoked whose lung biopsy showed the typical appearances of subacute extrinsic allergic alveolitis. She kept two budgerigars in her home and had serum precipitins to avian antigens. The scan shows marked ground glass attenuation of the lung parenchyma, which is nodular in some areas due to characteristic peribronchiolar (and centrilobular) foci. In other areas there is increased translucency because of bronchiolar obstruction and air trapping. Both the ground glass attenuation and the increases in translucency are exaggerated in the expiratory film (b), giving a 'mosaic' pattern. She recovered fully after the birds left her home.

on exercise. Although total lung capacity is reduced, residual volume is often increased, suggesting air trapping as a result of bronchiolar involvement. Occasionally there is also obstruction of the large airways, but this implies a coincidental asthmatic or bronchitic effect. Serial measurements of lung function may be particularly useful in demonstrating that impairment is closely related to the relevant exposure.

Bronchoscopy is useful in demonstrating that there is no macroscopic abnormality, apart from the occasional presence of mucosal inflammation, and bronchoalveolar lavage fluid may usefully show that no microbial growth occurs on culture. If lavage fluid, or induced sputum, is obtained within a matter of hours of exposure, a polymorphonuclear leucocyte response may dominate, simulating usual interstitial pneumonia, but this is followed by an accumulation of lymphocytes over the following 24 to 48 h. In the subacute and chronic forms of the disease, T lymphocytes represent 10 to 20% or more of recovered cells, although the absolute numbers of macrophages are generally increased also. This characteristic cellular picture is not specific for extrinsic allergic alveolitis, but it strongly supports the diagnosis if other suggestive features are present. Other inflammatory granulomatous disorders, such as sarcoidosis and tuberculosis, hypersensitivity reactions to drugs, and a number of rare lymphoid infiltrative disorders are also associated with a lymphocytosis in lavage fluid, but in practice sarcoidosis is generally the most plausible alternative diagnosis.

In sarcoidosis, B-lymphocyte numbers are decreased and the excess T lymphocytes are typically CD4+ helper cells, with the CD4+ to CD8+ ratio normally exceeding 1 and so exaggerated. By contrast, the ratio is typically reversed in extrinsic allergic alveolitis, CD8+ cells outnumbering CD4+ cells, and B-lymphocyte numbers are not decreased. Lymphocyte markers may therefore help distinguish

sarcoidosis from extrinsic allergic alveolitis. Unfortunately, the pattern favouring extrinsic allergic alveolitis does not distinguish so readily between subjects with exposure and symptoms and those with exposure but no symptoms. Both T-cell types show increased numbers if there is exposure, and the number of CD8+ cells tends to show a relatively greater, not lesser, increase in asymptomatic subjects, as described above. The absolute value of the CD4+ to CD8+ ratio therefore provides limited diagnostic benefit in identifying active disease, but this is rarely a relevant issue outside a research setting. A number of cytokines can also be recovered from the lavage fluid, but these are of research rather than diagnostic interest.

Inflammatory activity may also be detected by measurements of exhaled nitric oxide. Although different patterns over the period of exhalation in relation to different speeds of exhalation may allow a parenchymal source to be distinguished from an airway source, the procedure has no diagnostic specificity for alveolar responses that are allergic in origin. It may, however, be more useful as a monitoring tool by showing that particular periods of exposure are associated with pulmonary inflammatory responses. Transbronchial or video-assisted thoracoscopic lung biopsy may occasionally be indicated when other diagnostic procedures do not distinguish extrinsic allergic alveolitis from other diffuse infiltrative or fibrotic disorders of the lung. Biopsy is more likely to be needed in the subacute or chronic forms of the disease when hypersensitivity is less obvious, or acutely when there has been an unduly heavy exposure to microbial spores and there is suspicion of microbial invasion.

Environmental exposure

In many cases the history alone provides the evidence of relevant exposure, but this is not always reliable and an independent account of the exposures involved can be invaluable. Ideally, industrial hygiene measurements are made (particularly from personal samplers) so that respirable agents can be recognized and quantified, and microbiological techniques are used to identify specific microbial contaminants. These are sophisticated investigations and usually indicated only when extrinsic allergic alveolitis is first suspected in an environment not previously associated with the disease, particularly in industries where many individuals may be at risk and where modification of the plant and its respirable environment may be a costly matter.

Hypersensitivity

The demonstration of a serum IgG antibody response to the inducing organic dust is the most widely used method of 'confirming' hypersensitivity (saliva may be used more conveniently in children), but this has proved to be unsatisfactory. Although affected subjects tend to have higher antibody levels than those who are exposed but unaffected, the antibody response tends to correlate more closely with exposure than with disease. If the more sensitive ELISA is used, rather than the traditional Ouchterlony double-gel diffusion test, even higher rates of false-positive results are obtained. In practice the absence of an IgG precipitin response is extremely uncommon in subjects eventually proved to have extrinsic allergic alveolitis, providing they are nonsmokers. This is of considerable value in that a negative test generally excludes the diagnosis. The limited value of a positive test is to be expected in view of the current belief that cellular, not humoral, immunity provides the principal mechanism underlying the disease. It is unfortunate that practicable tests for cellular hypersensitivity are not readily available.

When the diagnosis remains in doubt, some form of inhalation challenge test may be necessary. The simplest method involves comparison of experimental periods spent away from the suspected causative environment with similar periods of continuing exposure. The acute form of the disease is likely to be recognized in this way, though the procedure can be time consuming and there may be practical problems of compliance. When a definitive diagnosis is particularly important, laboratory-based inhalation challenge tests can be used. These employ a variety of techniques, ranging from nebulizing soluble extracts to recreating natural environmental exposures in an exposure chamber. The influenza-like component of positive reactions is often uncomfortable, and if excessive doses are administered these tests can be hazardous. Furthermore, objective evidence for positive reactions may be difficult to obtain from conventional lung function tests, hence tests of this nature should be restricted to centres with special expertise. Personal experience of evaluating objective changes in body temperature, circulating neutrophil and lymphocyte numbers, forced vital capacity, and exercise studies from 144 inhalation challenge tests is summarized in Table 18.14.4.3. Together they provide high specificity and high sensitivity. Auscultation, chest radiography, measurements of gas transfer, and arterial blood gas analyses are often too insensitive to provide useful diagnostic information.

Criteria for diagnosis

In the hope of avoiding a need for biopsy or other invasive investigation, the United States-led Hypersensitivity Pneumonitis Study Group recently concluded that five features across these three domains, plus weight loss, are generally sufficient to make a diagnosis: recurrent (relevant) symptoms, inspiratory crackles, exposure to a recognized inducer, symptoms arising within 4–8 h of exposure onset, and precipitating antibodies to the putative causal agent.

Management

Management of the individual first demands that the diagnosis is secure and then centres on reducing any further exposure to a minimum. There is no place for desensitization. Ideally, the affected individual changes the relevant working, domestic, or recreational environment completely, but this may mean a profound loss in income or great expense, and is often unrealistic. Nor is it fully justified on purely medical grounds, since continued exposure does not lead inevitably to progressive disease.

The affected individuals who continue to work in the occupation responsible for their disease can often reduce their exposure substantially by changing the pattern of their particular duties. An alternative is the use of industrial respirators, which filter out 98 to 99% of respirable dust from the ambient air. These are especially valuable when exposures are intermittent and short, but may be uncomfortably hot when worn for long periods or when there is heavy work, and so compliance with their use may be poor.

Whatever course is followed, continuing exposure should be accompanied by regular medical surveillance. If there is no progression, it is reasonable for some exposure to continue. When there is progressive disease, exposure should cease. This may involve a loss of earnings and may entitle the affected worker to compensation. Rarely, the individual with progressive disease will refuse to change their occupation or hobby, and the physician must weigh the possible advantages of long-term, or pulsed, corticosteroid therapy against the risks. An additional medication, pentoxifylline, is currently under investigation, since it interferes with a number of macrophage functions of probable relevance and diminishes macrophage release of TNFα and IL-10.

Compensation of industrial causes

In the United Kingdom, industrial injuries legislation provides compensation from central government for disability in employees (but not employers) from extrinsic allergic alveolitis of occupational origin. The level of disability, and hence compensation, is assessed following examination by a 'medical board'. State benefits are limited to a maximum figure, which is adjusted from time to time according to inflation. Acceptance of state compensation in the United Kingdom no longer debars the recipient from seeking redress additionally in the civil courts, which is the primary mechanism of compensation in many countries.

Prognosis

No further exposure

As with occupational asthma the risk of continuing active disease following cessation of exposure increases with duration of the exposure period. With the acute form of extrinsic allergic alveolitis the exposure period is generally short and the disorder usually resolves without sequelae once the diagnosis is made and exposure ceases, but serial bronchoalveolar lavage and clearance studies suggest continuing inflammation and membrane leakiness for periods up to 15 years. The significance of this is unclear since the subjects involved generally remained asymptomatic and gave normal results on radiographic and lung function studies. Cessation of exposure in the more chronic cases has a less obvious beneficial effect, but usually prevents further progression.

Continuing exposure

There is greater concern when exposure continues. This may lead not only to recurrent acute attacks but to progressive and permanent fibrotic damage—i.e. to the chronic form of the disease. While concern for the risk of progressive fibrosis is undoubtedly justified, and while the chronic form of the disease certainly carries a greater risk of long-term morbidity or mortality, chronic disease occurs in

Table 18.14.4.3 Diagnostic features of positive inhalation challenge tests

Diagnostic changes within 36 h of challenge exposure	Sensitivity (%)
Increase in body temperature to >37.2° C	78
Increase in circulating neutrophils by ≥2.5 × 10^9/litre	68
Decrease in circulating lymphocytes by ≥0.5 × 10^9/litre, with lymphopenia (<1.5 × 10^9/litre)	52
Decrease in forced vital capacity by ≥15%	48
Increase in exercise minute volume by ≥15%	85
Increase in exercise respiratory frequency by ≥25%	64

The data were taken from a series of 144 antigen and control challenge tests in 31 subjects. Diagnostic endpoints were chosen to produce specificities of approximately 95% after mean changes associated with positive challenge tests were shown to be highly significant. When each monitoring parameter was given a score of 1 for a significant result, a total score of 2/6 or more was associated with a specificity of 100% and a sensitivity of 78% for the 144 challenge tests.

only a minority of affected subjects. A 2- to 40-year follow-up survey of 92 farm workers presenting with acute farmer's lung showed that while most continued to live on farms, only some developed radiographic evidence of pulmonary fibrosis (39%) or impairment of carbon monoxide gas transfer (30%), but as many as 28% gave histories of chronic productive cough and 25% had airway obstruction. A similar 10-year outcome has been reported in pigeon fanciers with acute extrinsic allergic alveolitis; again, most elected to continue their antigenic exposures despite medical advice to the contrary.

Therefore, in some cases—perhaps most—important protective mechanisms emerge that lead to tolerance of the effects of further acute exposures, or at least prevent the development of damaging fibrosis. A history of similar increasing tolerance is occasionally noted with occupational asthma, and tolerance not progressive disease is the rule rather than the exception in most animal models of extrinsic allergic alveolitis. However, with both asthma and extrinsic allergic alveolitis some affected subjects give clear accounts of increased responsiveness to a given level of exposure months or years after initial antigen exclusion, which suggests that protective mechanisms may be downgraded more quickly than the causal mechanisms.

As with sarcoidosis, there is debate as to whether the use of corticosteroids for acute episodes confers any long-term benefit. The answer is not clear, but one recent investigation failed to demonstrate any long-term functional differences between groups randomized to treatment with corticosteroids or placebo for the initial acute episode of farmer's lung. Although the corticosteroid group recovered more quickly from the acute episode, there was the suspicion, already voiced by other investigators, that early steroid therapy carries a greater risk of long-term recurrence. It is possible that the initial response to steroids encouraged less care over subsequent exposures. Alternatively, steroid therapy may have induced a different equilibrium between immunological responses, perhaps interfering disproportionately with the development of protective mechanisms.

Further reading

Anonymous (2002). From the Centers for Diseases Control and Prevention. Respiratory illness in workers exposed to metalworking fluid contaminated with nontuberculous mycobacteria—Ohio, 2001. *JAMA*, **287**, 3073–4.

Bourke SJ, et al. (2001). Hypersensitivity pneumonitis: current concepts. *Eur Respira J*, **32** (Suppl), 81–92.

Braun SR, et al. (1979). Farmer's lung disease: long-term clinical and physiologic outcome. *Am Rev Respir Dis*, **119**, 185–91.

Churg A, et al. (2006). Chronic hypersensitivity pneumonitis. *Am J Surg Pathol*, **30**, 201–8.

Cormier Y, et al. (2000). High-resolution computed tomographic characteristics in acute farmer's lung and in its follow-up. *Eur Respir J*, **16**, 56–60.

Erkinjuntti-Pekkanen R, Rytkonen H, Kokkarinen JI, Tukiainen HO, Partanen K, Terho EO (1998). *American Journal of Respiratory & Critical Care Medicine*, **158**, 662–5.

Fink JN, et al. (2005). Needs and opportunities for research in hypersensitivity pneumonitis. *Am J Respir Crit Care Med*, **171**, 792–8.

Franquet T, et al. (2003). Lung cysts in subacute hypersensitivity pneumonitis. *J ComputAssist Tomogr*, **27**, 475–8.

Grammar LC (1999). Occupational allergic alveolitis. *Ann Allergy Asthma Immunol*, **83**, 602–6.

Hendrick DJ, Faux JA, Marshall R (1978). Budgerigar fancier's lung: the commonest variety of allergic alveolitis in Britain. *Br Med J*, **ii**, 81–4.

Hendrick DJ, et al. (1980). Positive 'alveolar' responses to antigen inhalation provocation tests: their validity and recognition. *Thorax*, **35**, 415–27.

Ismail T, McSharry C, Boyd G (2006). Extrinsic allergic alveolitis. *Respirology*, **11**, 262–8.

Kreiss K, Cox-Ganser J (1997). Metalworking fluid-associated hypersensitivity pneumonitis: a workshop summary. *Am J Indust Med*, **32**, 423–32.

Lacasse Y, et al. (2003). Clinical diagnosis of hypersensitivity pneumonitis. *Am J Respir Crit Care Med*, **168**, 661–70.

Martinez FJ, Keane MP (2006). Update in diffuse parenchymal lung diseases 2005. *Am J Respir Crit Care Med*, **173**, 1066–71.

Meredith SK, Taylor VM, McDonald JC (1991). Occupational respiratory disease in the United Kingdom 1989: a report to the British Thoracic Society and the Society of Occupational Medicine by the SWORD project group. *Br J Indust Med*, **48**, 292–8.

Patel AM, Ryu JH, Reed CE (2001). Hypersensitivity pneumonitis: current concepts and future questions. *J Allergy Clin Immunol*, **108**, 661–70.

Pepys J, et al. (1963). Farmer's lung. Thermophilic actinomycetes as a source of 'farmer's lung hay' antigens. *Lancet*, **ii**, 607–11.

Yoshizawa Y, et al. (1999). Chronic hypersensitivity pneumonitis in Japan: a nationwide epidemiologic survey. *J Allergy Clin Immunol*, **103**, 315–20.

18.14.5 Pulmonary Langerhans' cell histiocytosis

S.J. Bourke and D.J. Hendrick

Essentials

Pulmonary Langerhans' cell histiocytosis is characterized by a reactive monoclonal proliferation of activated histiocytes in the distal bronchioles. It presents, nearly always in smokers, with cough, breathlessness, and (sometimes) systemic symptoms. Pneumothorax (sometimes bilateral) is a common complication. Chest radiography typically shows micronodules, reticulation, and small cysts, with fibrosis in advanced cases. Patients must stop smoking. About 25% of cases resolve, 50% stabilize, and 25% lose lung function. Corticosteroids and/or cytotoxic drugs are usually given for progressive disease, but the benefits are unclear.

Pulmonary Langerhans' cell histiocytosis (LCH) is a rare disease characterized by a reactive monoclonal proliferation of activated histiocytes in the distal bronchioles resulting in inflammatory nodules, cyst formation, and fibrosis. Langerhans' cells are a particular type of histiocyte derived from dendritic cells in the bone marrow. They normally migrate in the blood to the squamous epithelium of the skin, lungs, gastrointestinal, and female genital tract, where they are involved in antigen presentation to T cells. Abnormal proliferation of histiocytes is also the pathological basis for acute disseminated LCH (Letterer–Siwe disease) and multifocal LCH (Hand–Schüller–Christian disease)—disorders which produce a spectrum of distinct clinical features. For general discussion of LCH and other disorders of histiocytes, see Chapter 22.4.7.

In adult pulmonary LCH the clinical manifestations are usually confined to the lungs, but in 10 to 15% of cases lesions are also present in bone, skin, lymph nodes, and the posterior pituitary (potentially causing diabetes insipidus). It affects about one in 560 000 adults, with an equal male to female ratio and a peak age of onset between 20 and 40 years. There is a striking association with smoking, likely—probably along with other factors—to play a causal role; 97 to 100% of patients have smoked cigarettes. Cough and breathlessness are the most common symptoms, and about one-third of patients have systemic symptoms such as fever or weight loss. Pneumothorax follows rupture of lung cysts, occurs in about 25% of patients, and may be recurrent, with LCH providing an explanation for the rare but catastrophic event of spontaneous bilateral pneumothorax. About 25% of patients have no symptoms.

The chest radiograph typically shows micronodules, reticulation, and small cysts in the mid and upper zones symmetrically with sparing of the costophrenic angles; the lung volumes are often normal or increased, in contrast with many other fibrotic lung diseases. High-resolution CT (Fig. 18.14.5.1) characteristically shows multiple centrilobular nodules with cavitation, progressing to cyst formation and fibrosis in later stage disease. Pulmonary physiological tests often show a mixture of airways obstruction, air trapping with elevated residual volume, and impaired diffusing capacity for carbon monoxide. Typical clinical and CT features may be sufficient for diagnosis, but video-assisted thoracoscopic lung biopsy is sometimes required. The characteristic histopathology features are mitotically active Langerhans' cells forming nodules and granulomas with a surrounding inflammatory cell infiltrate of lymphocytes, macrophages, and eosinophils (hence the previous diagnostic labels of eosinophilic granuloma and Langerhans' cell granulomatosis). Langerhans' cells are identified by immunostaining of the CD1a membrane antigens or the S100 intracellular protein, and by electron microscopy showing Birbeck granules—rods of tennis racket-shaped structures unfolding from the cell membrane. In advanced disease, fibrosis and honeycombing predominate. Biopsies often show features of other smoking-related diseases such as desquamative interstitial pneumonia, obstructive bronchiolitis, and emphysema. Langerhans' cells can also be identified in bronchoalveolar lavage fluid, but this is neither sensitive nor specific in diagnosing the disease.

Because pulmonary LCH varies greatly in its clinical course, management has to be individualized for the particular patient. Treatment is supportive rather than specific. Smoking cessation is crucial. About 25% of cases resolve, 50% stabilize, and 25% progress with loss of lung function. Corticosteroid therapy is usually given for progressive disease, but the benefits are unclear. Cytotoxic drugs such as vinblastine, cyclophosphamide and cladribine have been used in multisystem histiocytosis, but their role in pulmonary LCH is uncertain. Pleurodesis or pleurectomy may be needed for recurrent pneumothoraces and, in view of the risk of bilateral (and rapidly fatal) pneumothorax, is best considered sooner rather than later. Lung transplantation is the main option for patients with advanced disease, although recurrence in the transplanted lungs has been described.

Further reading

Caminati A, Harari S (2006). Smoking-related interstitial pneumonias and pulmonary Langerhans cell histiocytosis. *Proc Am Thorac Soc*, **3**, 299–306.

Tatevossian R, *et al.* (2006). Adults with Langerhans cell histiocytosis—orphans with an orphan disease. *Clin Med*, **6**, 404–8.

Tazi A (2006). Adult pulmonary Langerhans cell histiocytosis. *Eur Respir J*, **27**, 1272–85.

Websites

Histiocytosis Association of America. http://www.histio.org [Links to other sites worldwide.]

Histiocytosis Research Trust (UK). http://www.hrtrust.org/web/guest/about

18.14.6 Lymphangioleiomyomatosis

S.J. Bourke and D.J. Hendrick

Essentials

Lymphangioleiomyomatosis is caused by mutations (usually sporadic, sometimes in tuberous sclerosis) of the *TSC1* or *TSC2* genes and results in cystic destruction of the lungs, with CT features being sufficiently characteristic to establish the diagnosis in many cases. Two-thirds of patients suffer pneumothoraces. Hormonal therapy with progesterone or tamoxifen is usually given for progressive disease; medical or surgical pleurodesis is advisable; lung transplantation is the main option for advanced disease.

Lymphangioleiomyomatosis (LAM) is a rare disease in which lymphatics ('lymph'), blood vessels ('angio'), and airways are infiltrated by proliferating smooth muscle cells ('leiomyo'), resulting in cystic destruction of the lungs, pneumothoraces, chylous effusions, and haemorrhage. It can occur as a sporadic disorder or in association with tuberous sclerosis. Both sporadic and tuberous sclerosis-associated LAM result from mutations of the tumour suppressor genes *TSC1* (encoding hamartin) and *TSC2* (encoding tuberin). Hamartin and tuberin form a cytoplasmic complex and so inhibit the protein mTOR

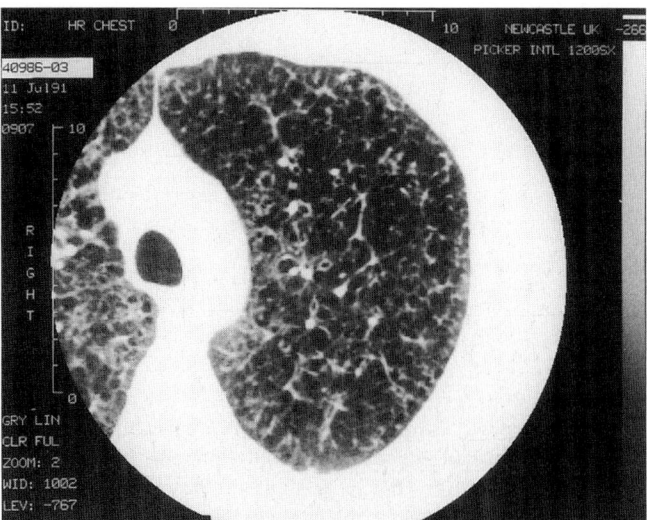

Fig. 18.14.5.1 High-resolution CT of a 45-year-old smoking man with biopsy-proven Langerhans' cell histiocytosis, showing centrilobular nodules, cysts and reticulation.

which stimulates cell proliferation. Sporadic LAM occurs exclusively in women, predominantly between the menarche and the menopause. Exceptionally rare cases of LAM have been reported in men with tuberous sclerosis, but the disease is almost confined to women. This suggests that the proliferation of LAM cells depends on female sex hormones, and oestrogen and progesterone receptors have been found in some LAM cells.

Sporadic LAM is due to somatic (noninherited) mutations in the *TSC1* and *TSC2* genes and occurs in about 2 in a million women. It accounts for most of the patients who seek medical attention for LAM, despite tuberous sclerosis being the more common disorder (about 1 woman in 6000 is affected). The discordance reflects the low proportion of women with tuberous sclerosis who have symptoms from LAM and seek attention because of them; nevertheless, as many as 40% of adult women with tuberous sclerosis have been shown to have features of LAM on high-resolution CT. Tuberous sclerosis results from a germ-line mutation of the *TSC1* and *TSC2* genes and is an autosomal dominant inherited disorder (OMIM 191 100) whose manifestations include epilepsy, learning difficulties, skin lesions (angiofibromas, shagreen patches), and hamartomas in the brain, kidneys, and other organs (see Chapters 24.17 and 24.17.1).

Pneumothorax occurs in about two-thirds of patients with LAM and is a common mode of presentation. Other manifestations include breathlessness from progressive parenchymal involvement, cough, haemoptysis, and chest pain. Involvement of the thoracic duct may result in chylous pleural effusions and ascites. Other abdominal features include renal angiomyolipomas, cystic lymphatic masses, and lymphadenopathy. Renal angiomyolipomas are present in about 50% of patients: they rarely cause symptoms, but bleeding may require treatment by embolization or surgical resection.

The chest radiograph typically shows diffuse small cysts with reticulonodular shadowing, but normal or increased lung volumes. Lung function tests usually show progressive airways obstruction and reduced gas transfer. The CT features are sufficiently characteristic to establish the diagnosis in many cases, with well-defined cystic airspaces with thin walls distributed throughout both lungs (Fig. 18.14.6.1), and more widespread use of CT imaging is detecting

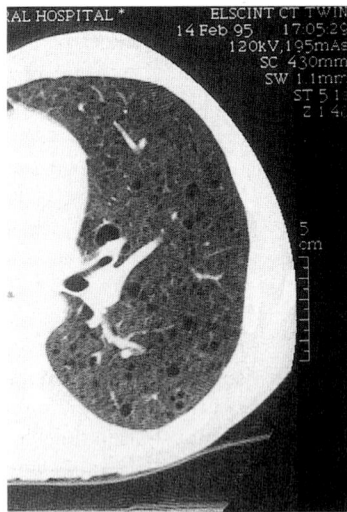

Fig. 18.14.6.1 CT scan of a 37-year-old woman with pulmonary lymphangioleiomyomatosis and tuberous sclerosis. She had experienced sequential spontaneous pneumothoraces affecting each side. The scan shows multiple thin-walled cysts throughout the lung.

milder cases in an extended spectrum of patients including some postmenopausal women. Lung biopsy may be needed where there is doubt about the diagnosis, revealing abnormal infiltration by smooth muscle cells which can be identified by immunohistochemical staining for the HMB45 (human melanoma black) antigen. Aspirated pleural fluid may show diagnostic clusters of immature muscle cells.

Hormonal therapy with progesterone or tamoxifen is usually given to patients with progressive disease: there are reports of benefit, but clear evidence of effectiveness is lacking. Pneumothorax is common and likely to recur such that medical or surgical pleurodesis is advisable. Lung transplantation is the main option for patients with advanced LAM, but recurrence of the disease due to migration of LAM cells to the donor lung has been reported. Rapamycin (sirolimus), like the hamartin–tuberin cytoplasmic complex, inhibits the protein mTOR and is being tested in clinical trials as a specific treatment targeted against the cellular mechanisms causing LAM. The clinical course of LAM is variable, with about 70% survival 10 years after diagnosis. Although some patients with LAM have had uncomplicated pregnancies, the hormonal changes of pregnancy pose a risk of disease progression.

Further reading

Bissler JJ, *et al.* (2008). Sirolimus for angiomyolipoma in tuberose sclerosis complex or lymphangioleiomyomatosis. *N Engl J Med*, **358**,140–51.
Johnson SR (2006). Lymphangioleiomyomatosis. *Eur Respir J*, **27**, 1056–65.
Ryu JH, *et al.* (2006). The NHLBI lymphangioleiomyomatosis registry. *Am J Respir Crit Care Med*, **173**, 105–11.

Websites

LAM Action. *Working for patients with lymphangioleiomyomatosis.* http://www.lamaction.org/
The LAM Foundation. *A breath of hope.* http://lam.uc.edu [Provides links to other LAM sites worldwide.]

18.14.7 Pulmonary alveolar proteinosis

D.J. Hendrick

Essentials

Pulmonary alveolar proteinosis is caused by failure, usually due to autoimmune antibodies, of GM-CSF to stimulate surfactant catabolism by alveolar macrophages. Presentation is with progressive shortness of breath, or with pneumonic illness due to superimposed infection. Chest radiography characteristically shows a picture simulating pulmonary oedema. Bronchoalveolar lavage or lung biopsy demonstrates alveolar secretions that are strongly PAS-positive but contain no organisms and no excessive cellular response. In 30 to 50% of cases the disease improves spontaneously or fails to progress. When intervention is necessary the most effective measure is physical removal of secretions by whole-lung bronchoalveolar lavage. GM-CSF has been given to a few patients, with half seeming to respond. Eradication of infection may be difficult when opportunistic organisms are involved. Survival is about 70% at 10 years.

Introduction

First described in 1958, pulmonary alveolar proteinosis is a rare (400–500 reported cases) but interesting disorder that exerts its primary effects in the alveolar spaces. Over a period ranging from months to years they become filled with an amorphous, largely cell-free, lipoproteinaceous material (surfactant) that is not readily expectorated. Inflammation, fibrosis, and destruction of alveolar architecture are conspicuously absent. There are two major consequences. First, depending on the number of alveoli involved, the lungs become stiff, ventilatory function becomes restricted, and shunting occurs at the alveolar–capillary level, causing hypoxaemia. The outcome is breathlessness, reduced exercise tolerance, cough, and in some cases death from respiratory failure. Secondly, and a not uncommon cause of death, is secondary infection. The responsible organisms are generally those that are associated with intracellular infection and impaired T-lymphocyte function, nocardia being particularly prominent. In many cases, however, extensive involvement does not occur, there being little or no progression, or even spontaneous remission. Epidemiological data are scarce but estimates suggest a world-wide prevalence of the order 2 to 5 per million, and an annual incidence of about 0.4 per million. All age groups may be involved, and smoking probably enhances the risk. This may explain why men are affected more commonly than women. Whole-lung lavage offers effective primary treatment, but is not always necessary.

Aetiology, genetics, and pathogenesis

Despite the small number of cases, the explosive advance of molecular biology over recent years has resolved most of the enigmas of this curious disease. The lipoproteinaceous material (chiefly the phospholipid dipalmitoyl phosphatidylcholine) filling the alveolar spaces is normally derived from surfactant secreted by the type II pneumocytes. It stains strongly with periodic acid–Schiff (PAS) and eosin. It also contains structures resembling tubular myelin, which are derived from lamellar bodies of the type II pneumocytes. The abnormality lies with the subsequent clearance of this material. Three distinct mechanisms have been recognized to explain this, which have been uncovered largely by chance because a strain of laboratory mice, bred to be deficient for the haemopoietic cytokine growth factor GM-CSF, unexpectedly developed pulmonary alveolar proteinosis.

Most human cases (>90%) result from an acquired failure of GM-CSF to stimulate surfactant catabolism by the alveolar macrophages. To date no abnormality has been discovered in affected subjects of GM-CSF itself, or of its monocyte/macrophage receptors, but systemic neutralizing antibodies to GM-CSF are generally found that imply an autoimmune cause for this 'acquired' form of the disease. These antibodies are extremely uncommon in unaffected subjects unless other autoimmune disorders are present.

A few cases of pulmonary alveolar proteinosis are recognized soon after birth, and often within families already affected by the disease, most resulting from genetic aberrations (autosomal recessive) that lead to abnormalities of the surfactant proteins or of the GM-CSF receptors.

The remaining cases are deemed 'secondary' because they appear to arise as complications of other diseases. Most celebrated is acute silicosis (silicoproteinosis or silicolipoproteinosis), which arises within months of massive exposure to respirable crystalline silica—both in the unfortunate worker exposed without adequate respiratory protection and in experimental animal models. This is relentlessly progressive. Less commonly aluminium dust may be responsible, and there have been reports implicating titanium and insecticides. The exposures are assumed to overwhelm macrophage function, much as silica additionally impairs macrophage handling of tubercle bacilli. For further discussion, see Chapter 18.13. 'Secondary' pulmonary alveolar proteinosis may also complicate certain haematological disorders (usually malignant and often after the use of cytotoxic agents) and immune disorders (e.g. immunodeficiency, rheumatoid disease, IgA nephropathy).

Clinical features

The patient usually presents with progressive shortness of breath due to the disease itself, or with a pneumonic illness due to superimposed infection. Occasionally the disease is without symptoms and first recognized from the appearances of an incidental chest radiograph. Cough is common but is usually nonproductive unless there is infection. Low-grade fever, weight loss, haemoptysis, and pleuritic pain occur infrequently, and some authors report an initial febrile incident. There may be crackles and even clubbing in advanced stages, and fever becomes typical when infection supervenes. When nocardia is not responsible for this, aspergillus, blastomyces, candida, coccidioides, cryptococcus, cytomegalovirus, histoplasma, HIV, mucor, mycobacteria, pneumocystis, streptomyces, and viruses are the most common culprits.

Clinical investigation and criteria for diagnosis

The chest radiograph characteristically shows an alveolar filling pattern, which radiates from the hila and simulates pulmonary oedema. There is no associated evidence of heart failure, however, and the appearances may be patchy and asymmetrical. Diffuse pulmonary fibrosis is very rare unless provoked by complicating infection. A micronodular infiltration is occasionally seen, particularly in children, but lymphadenopathy is usually absent. CT scanning, particularly with high resolution, shows the nonspecific features of air-space filling (ground-glass attenuation) and commonly a patchiness which distinguishes affected from unaffected lobules. There may also be septal thickening and hence the 'crazy paving' appearance typical of combined alveolar and interstitial disease.

Pneumonia or aspiration is often suspected initially, but the cough produces little or no sputum and no organisms are isolated if the disease remains uncomplicated. White gelatinous material is expectorated occasionally, and bronchoalveolar lavage fluid is typically milky in colour. Gallium scanning may be useful in showing negligible pulmonary uptake, in contrast to the findings in pneumonia, and in established disease a positive scan may be invaluable in suggesting the development of superimposed infection.

The key to the diagnosis of uncomplicated pulmonary alveolar proteinosis rests with the demonstration that the alveolar secretions are strongly PAS-positive but contain no organisms and no excessive cellular response. Indeed, the macrophages appear to be deficient in numbers as well as function, although they are engorged (foamy) with ingested surfactant. Biochemical and immunochemical tests may show that phospholipids and specific surfactant proteins are present in excess. Identification of lamellar

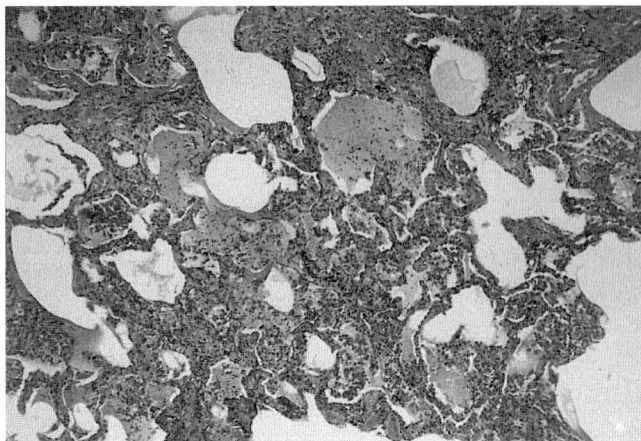

Fig. 18.14.7.1 Pulmonary alveolar proteinosis arising acutely following massive exposure to silica. Some alveoli are filled with a noninflammatory proteinaceous exudate, characteristic of pulmonary alveolar proteinosis. The lung interstitium shows fibrosis and inflammation which can be attributed to acute silicosis (haematoxylin and eosin, medium magnification).
(Courtesy of Dr D E Banks.)

bodies or their debris by electron microscopy is particularly useful. These may be found within macrophages or pneumocytes, or may lie free within secretions. Occasionally the sputum provides diagnostic material. More commonly, bronchoalveolar lavage or lung biopsy is required, though the former should suffice since PAS-positive amorphous globules demonstrated by cytological smears have high diagnostic specificity. The characteristic histological features are shown in Fig. 18.14.7.1.

Raised serum levels of surfactant proteins and lactic dehydrogenase (LDH) from pulmonary epithelial cells are to be expected, but these occur in a number of other diffuse disorders of the lung and so are of no value in diagnosis. However, serum levels of LDH and the mucin-like glycoprotein KL-6 (which is released from type II pneumocytes) tend to correlate with disease activity and may be useful markers for monitoring disease progression or responses to treatment.

Treatment

No appreciable disability develops in one-third to one-half of cases and the disease improves spontaneously (in about 8%) or fails to progress. When intervention proves to be necessary, the most effective measure is physical removal of secretions by whole-lung bronchoalveolar lavage. This is usually performed under general anaesthesia using a double-lumen endotracheal tube. Lavage is repeatedly carried out on one lung with a total of 20 to 50 litres of warm sterile buffered saline while the other is mechanically ventilated. The procedure is then reversed so that the other lung is treated. The practice of adding heparin and acetylcysteine to the lavage fluid has not been shown to be beneficial, but chest percussion during the procedure does seem to enhance the yield. When severe respiratory failure has already supervened despite ventilatory support, cardiopulmonary bypass has been used successfully to maintain gas exchange during the lavage procedure. An alternative is sequential lobar lavage using a fibre-optic bronchoscope and a cuffed catheter. Further lavage is usually necessary every few weeks or months, but the activity of the disease may lessen and the need

for frequent treatment may diminish. A useful description of the technical procedure was published by Shah and colleagues in 2000 (see 'Further reading').

GM-CSF has been used additionally and experimentally for 'acquired' pulmonary alveolar proteinosis in a few patients over the last few years. It can be administered subcutaneously or by aerosol and has proved modestly effective despite the usual presence of neutralizing antibodies. Meaningful responses were observed in about one-half of 20 treated patients in one study.

The risk of premature death in most series has been low, but a considerable threat to life is associated with complicating infection. This should be recognized and treated promptly. An accelerated clinical course together with the development of fever, increased (and productive) cough, malaise, evidence of systemic illness, and the radiographic demonstration of cavitation or pleural effusion all provide pointers to its development. Blood cultures together with smear and culture studies of sputum may identify the organism or organisms responsible, but often bronchoscopy with brushings and diagnostic lavage is needed. Sometimes a biopsy procedure is considered necessary, particularly when the underlying presence of alveolar proteinosis is not clearly established. The eradication of infection may prove to be difficult when opportunistic organisms are involved, perhaps reflecting the underlying impairment of macrophage function. It has therefore been argued that regular bronchoalveolar lavage, even in the absence of impaired exercise tolerance, may provide valuable prophylaxis against this vulnerability to infection. A recent study demonstrated improved macrophage function following lavage, which slowly diminished over 18 months as clinical relapse occurred. If the argument is followed fully, lavage may also play a role in eradicating the acute infection.

Prognosis

Seymour and Presneill reviewed 343 published cases and found survival rates of 79% (2 years), 75% (5 years), and 68% (10 years). Of the 69 deaths, 60 were attributed to pulmonary alveolar proteinosis—47 (72%) from respiratory failure, 12 (18%) from complicating infection, and one (2%) from cardiac arrest during lavage. The actuarial 5-year disease-specific survival rate for patients diagnosed during life was 88%. Of those dying within 5 years, more than 80% did so during the first year after diagnosis. Thereafter there was a significantly reduced risk of mortality. The risk of death was not significantly different between men and women, or between smokers and nonsmokers, but it was greater (unsurprisingly) among the older patients, and much greater among the few children. Successive birth cohorts showed substantially improved survival rates, reflecting the increasing proportions diagnosed during life and the more widespread use of effective treatment.

Further reading

Goldstein LS, *et al.* (1998). Pulmonary alveolar proteinosis: clinical features and outcomes. *Chest*, **114**, 1357–62.

Greenhill SR, Kotton DN. (2009). Pulmonary alveolar proteinosis: a bench-to-bedside story of granulocyte-macrophage colony stimulating factor dysfunction. *Chest*, **136**, 571–77.

Inoue Y, Trapnell BC, Tazawa R, *et al.* (2008). Characteristics of a large cohort of patients with autoimmune pulmonary alveolar proteinosis in Japan. *AJRCCM*, **177**, 752–62.

Ioachimescu OC, Lavuru MS (2006). Pulmonary alveolar proteinosis. *Chron Respir Dis*, **3**, 149–59.

Mazzone P, Thomassen MJ, Kavuru M (2001). Our new understanding of pulmonary alveolar proteinosis: what an internist needs to know. *Cleveland Clin J Med*, **68**, 977–93.

Mikami T, *et al.* (1997). Pulmonary alveolar proteinosis: diagnosis using routinely processed smears of bronchoalveolar lavage fluid. *J Clin Pathol*, **50**, 981–4.

Seymour JF, Presneill JJ (2002). State of the art: pulmonary alveolar proteinosis. Progress in the first 44 years. *Am J Respir Crit Care Med*, **166**, 215–35.

Shah PL, *et al.* (2000). Pulmonary alveolar proteinosis: clinical aspects and current concepts on pathogenesis. *Thorax*, **55**, 67–77.

Tanaka N, *et al.* (1999). Lungs of patients with idiopathic pulmonary alveolar proteinosis express a factor which neutralizes granulocyte-macrophage stimulating factor. *FEBS Lett*, **442**, 246–50.

Trapnell BC, Whitsett JA, Nakata K (2003). Mechanisms of disease: pulmonary alveolar proteinosis. *N Engl J Med*, **349**, 2527–39.

Wang BM, *et al.* (1997). Diagnosing pulmonary alveolar proteinosis: a review and an update. *Chest*, **111**, 460–6.

18.14.8 Pulmonary amyloidosis

D.J. Hendrick

Essentials

Amyloidosis rarely affects the lungs, but when it does, primary (AL) disease usually produces benign masses of amyloid tissue in the central airways or the parenchyma, and secondary (AA) disease typically causes diffuse infiltration of alveolar walls and interstitium. Laryngotracheobronchial deposits sometimes require resection if they are causing obstruction; parenchymal lung nodules rarely need to be removed, providing their histological nature is not in doubt; the prognosis of diffuse alveolar–interstitial disease is poor.

Introduction

Amyloidosis—discussed in Chapter 12.12.3—is a consequence of the deposition of insoluble proteins in extracellular sites. Clinically important involvement of the lungs is extremely uncommon. When primary (AL) amyloidosis affects the lungs, it usually does so in a patchy, localized manner, producing benign masses of amyloid tissue in the central airways or the parenchyma. The parenchymal masses rarely cause symptoms (or need treatment), but masses arising in and around central airway mucosa often cause disabling, even life-threatening, obstruction. They can generally be controlled endoscopically with laser therapy or piecemeal excision. By contrast, secondary (AA) amyloidosis typically causes diffuse infiltration of alveolar walls and interstitium (and occasionally pulmonary vasculature). This restricts ventilation and impairs oxygen transfer, and may progress to cause death unless lung transplantation is available. The matter is complicated because AL amyloidosis may atypically infiltrate alveoli and interstitium diffusely like AA amyloidosis, and because there are additional inherited forms of amyloidosis. Most of the latter pose no threat to the lung, but

familial Mediterranean fever may lead to secondary AA amyloidosis and to its typical alveolar–interstitial effects.

Clinical features

Those affected are usually middle-aged or elderly, and the sexes are equally represented. Hilar or mediastinal lymphadenopathy is rarely demonstrated on plain chest radiographs, but mild nodal enlargement is commonly seen on CT scanning. The pleura are rarely involved, but recurrent pleural effusion may occur. Although symptomatic pulmonary involvement is uncommon, there is usually microscopic evidence of diffuse pulmonary infiltration whenever there is symptomatic disease resulting from infiltration of any organ. Most cases of symptomatic pulmonary disease are caused by primary (AL) amyloid.

The following clinical varieties of pulmonary amyloidosis, in descending order of epidemiological importance, are the most clearly recognized. Localized disease is almost invariably due to deposition of AL protein and is essentially benign in nature, although it is often a consequence of malignant myeloma.

Localized laryngotracheobronchial disease

Discrete and often multiple masses of amyloid protein enlarge in the walls of the airways or the peribronchial tissues, causing cough, obstruction, and sometimes bleeding. Obstruction of airways may lead to wheeze, stridor, breathlessness, atelectasis and infection, and may eventually give rise to bronchiectasis. Central lesions may pose particular difficulty for intubation and the administration of anaesthesia. When a single lesion is involved it may simulate the effects of a bronchial adenoma, appearing as a polypoid mass on endoscopic inspection.

Localized parenchymal nodule(s)

Discrete nodules or masses, which may be single or multiple and may occasionally reach the size of a tennis ball, are seen within the lung parenchyma on the chest radiograph. They rarely cause symptoms or disrupt lung function and may eventually calcify, cavitate, or even ossify. They are likely to simulate bronchial neoplasms if single and so be resected; if multiple they often entice biopsy, although in the future it may be that CT and MRI scanning will offer a useful means of distinguishing amyloid tissue from tumour and thus prevent the need for this. Biopsy in one unusual case (that of an HIV-positive intravenous drug abuser) showed AA rather than AL protein, but there was focal birefringency and a foreign body giant-cell reaction reflecting deposition of the carrier material of the illicit drug and implying that focal inflammation within the lung may occasionally lead to localized 'secondary' amyloid deposition.

Diffuse alveolar–interstitial disease

Amyloid is deposited diffusely throughout the alveolar walls and interstitium of the lung, and may be the consequence of either AL or AA protein deposition (Figs. 18.14.8.1 and 18.14.8.2). Systemic symptoms of tiredness, malaise and weight loss are common. There is progressive breathlessness (often a consequence of concomitant cardiac involvement) and dry cough. Scattered crackles are characteristic and there may be pleural effusions. Prognosis is poor, with respiratory failure supervening as ventilation becomes increasingly restricted and gas transfer impaired, although death more commonly results from cardiac or renal involvement.

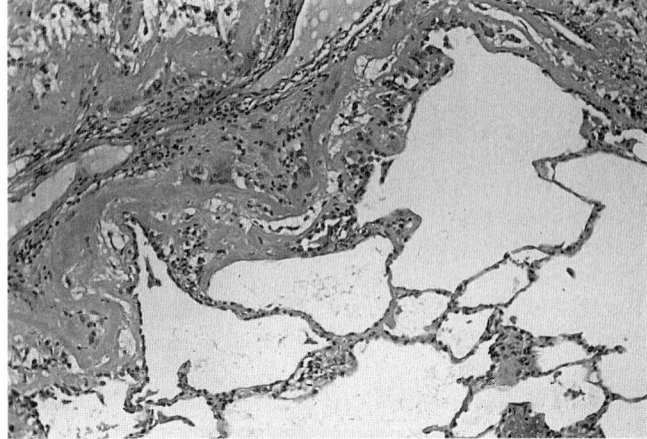

Fig. 18.14.8.1 Alveolar-interstitial type amyloidosis of the lung. Staining with haematoxylin and eosin (medium magnification) reveals interstitial deposits of hyaline eosinophilic material with a foreign body type giant cell response in adjacent tissue. This is an almost unique feature of amyloidosis affecting the lung. By courtesy of Dr T. Ashcroft.

Other manifestations

Histological examination may also show evidence of amyloid infiltration of the pulmonary vasculature. This is usually of no clinical consequence, but has been reported to cause pulmonary hypertension and undue bleeding after biopsy, although other reports suggest that biopsy, particularly transbronchial biopsy, is generally both safe and effective. Another rare effect of amyloidosis on respiratory function is enlargement of the tongue, which can cause or exacerbate obstructive sleep apnoea.

Treatment and prognosis

For discussion of the treatment of systemic amyloidosis, which is often unrewarding but now includes the possibility of autologous stem cell transplantation for the AL type, see Chapter 12.12.3. Ultimately, organ transplantation may become the only hope of survival, and this is sometimes carried out when renal failure or cardiac failure is the only immediate threat to life and the patient

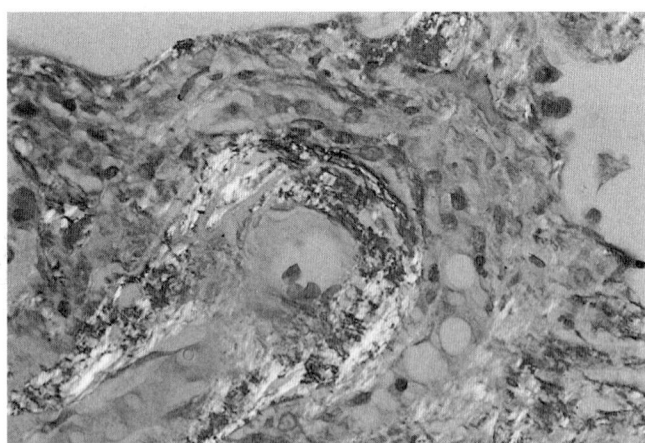

Fig. 18.14.8.2 Alveolar-interstitial type amyloidosis of the lung. Staining with Congo red stain under polarized light (high magnification) demonstrates the characteristic dichroic birefringence. By courtesy of Dr T. Ashcroft.

does not have a significant amyloid burden elsewhere. Very few cases of lung transplantation have been reported, hence the risk of recurrent disease in the transplant is unclear: median survival was only 16 months for 35 subjects reported from the Mayo Clinic with systemic AL amyloidosis.

With local forms of the disease, the outlook is a good deal brighter. Progression may be slow and the disease may become quiescent. Laryngotracheobronchial deposits can sometimes be resected or depleted piecemeal endoscopically, perhaps using laser therapy, but there is some risk of serious bleeding from this. Corticosteroids have been reported to have a beneficial effect when there is critical airway stenosis. Parenchymal nodules in the lung rarely need to be removed, providing their histological nature is not in doubt. Three recently described cases showed no meaningful morbidity over a period of observation lasting more than 5 year.

Further reading

Miyamoto T, *et al.* (1999). Monoclonality of infiltrating plasma cells in primary pulmonary nodular amyloidosis: detection with polymerase chain reaction. *J Clin Pathol*, **52**, 464–7.

Pickford HA, Swensen SJ, Utz JP (1997). Thoracic cross-sectional imaging of amyloidosis. *Am J Roentgenol*, **168**, 353–5.

Shah SP, *et al.* (1998). Nodular amyloidosis of the lung from intravenous drug abuse: an uncommon cause of multiple pulmonary nodules. *South Med J*, **91**, 402–4.

Shiue ST, McNally DP (1988). Pulmonary hypertension from prominent vascular involvement in diffuse amyloidosis. *Arch Intern Med*, **148**, 687–9.

Suzuki H, *et al.* (2006). Three cases of the nodular pulmonary amyloidosis with a longterm observation. *Intern Med*, **45**, 283–6.

Utz JP, Swensen SJ, Gertz MA. Pulmonary amyloidosis. The Mayo Clinic experience from 1980 to 1993. *Ann Intern Med*, **124**, 407–13.

18.14.9 Lipoid (lipid) pneumonia

D.J. Hendrick

Essentials

Lipids that accumulate within airways and alveolae are difficult to remove and may lead to an inflammatory response. Exogenous lipid can be aspirated in those with impaired swallowing mechanisms who take or are given agents such as olive oil or paraffin, or can be inhaled from oil aerosols/mists. Endogenous lipid can (rarely) be deposited when chronic inflammation accompanies some cause of localized bronchial obstruction. Presentation is with a chronic 'pneumonic' illness or asymptomatic radiographic abnormality, when appearances may closely simulate bronchial carcinoma. Demonstration of lipid material within pulmonary secretions or alveolar macrophages obtained from sputum or bronchoalveolar lavage is diagnostic. If treatment is needed, therapeutic bronchoalveolar lavage may remove substantial quantities of lipid from the alveoli; episodes of secondary bacterial infection require antibiotic treatment.

Exogenous lipoid pneumonia

When exogenous mineral or vegetable lipids are deposited in the lung, they usually prove to be relatively inert but difficult to remove. Lung lipases have little effect, and the macrophages are slow to transport the free or emulsified material into the lymphatics. The result is often a chronic low-grade inflammatory response that may lead to secondary infection and/or local fibrosis. Animal lipids are more readily degraded by lung lipases, releasing irritating fatty acids and causing a brisk and more widespread pneumonitis. The latter may also occur if lipid material is inhaled in large quantities.

Aetiology

Aspiration of mineral or vegetable oil is not common in the population at large but is seen not infrequently within certain subgroups, particularly those with impaired swallowing mechanisms, in whom lipoid pneumonia should be suspected whenever a 'pneumonic' illness is slow to resolve or is recurrent. Most affected are the very young and the old, and the regular nasal instillation of vegetable oils (e.g. olive oil) or paraffin to relieve nasal congestion, or their ingestion to relieve constipation, are often responsible. A portion of any nasal dose is likely to enter the trachea, as may part of an ingested dose if the individual then reclines in bed or has any disturbance of swallowing. The critical point is that paraffin and many vegetable oils are not irritating to the tracheal mucosa, so coughing is rarely excited and aspiration occurs without immediate sequelae.

Reluctant children forced to swallow cod liver oil are said to have encountered similar risks during the 1940s and 1950s, a period when paraffin was commonly used at all ages to relieve constipation. Patients fed by nasogastric tube are particularly vulnerable, as are those fed regularly with high-lipid diets (e.g. with milk fat or ghee). Embolic lipoid pneumonia may also occur because of intravenous infusion, whether accidental or wilful, and because of industrial accidents which forcibly inject mineral oil into peripheral tissues.

Adults with unimpaired swallowing are affected only sporadically. Shipwrecked sailors have occasionally aspirated floating oil, and lipoid pneumonia has been recognized in workers and firefighters exposed to oil mists and burning fats. The potential risk from oil aerosols has been highlighted in the automotive industry and other industries using metal working fluids for coolant and lubrication purposes, though such exposures may more commonly produce the clinical picture of extrinsic allergic alveolitis (especially if the fluids are contaminated by mycobacteria or fungi). Aspirated petroleum products such as kerosene (paraffin) may be absorbed from the lung and give rise to toxic responses in other organs (particularly the heart), and this may prove to be life threatening. Less unwilling inhalers of mineral oil and vaseline have been the blackfat tobacco smokers and chewers of Guyana, who obtain more satisfaction when these additives are mixed to native tobacco leaf. A distinctive geographical picture of progressive and often fatal pulmonary fibrosis complicates this habit in some 20% of blackfat users, but has not been observed among nonsmoking residents.

Clinical features

If there is little or no pulmonary response to aspiration of oil, there may be no symptoms, and the affected subject presents by chance with an abnormal chest radiograph. In about 50% of cases there is a chronic 'pneumonic' illness with productive cough, low-grade fever, and (occasionally) haemoptysis. Often there is a cyclical course with intermittent symptoms. Repeated aspiration may lead to fibrotic shrinkage of the affected segment or segments (usually in the lower lobes or the middle lobe), bronchiectasis, or persistent consolidation. The radiographic appearances may closely simulate bronchial carcinoma, and many resections have been carried out for this reason, sometimes revealing a characteristic granulomatous mass (paraffinoma). When more substantial quantities are aspirated the radiographic abnormalities are necessarily more diffuse, and when the lipid material is more reactive an acute 'pneumonic' illness occurs.

The key to diagnosis is the demonstration of lipid material within pulmonary secretions or alveolar macrophages, whether obtained from sputum or bronchoalveolar lavage. If lung tissue is resected or a biopsy is taken, there may be fibrosis, evidence of chronic inflammation, and foreign body granulomas/giant cells in addition to lipid material retained within alveoli and macrophages (Fig. 18.14.9.1).

CT may allow the identification of lipid material by its low density (similar to body fat, −150/130 to −80/60 Hounsfield units, compared with +50 to +150 units for solid tumours) and also show patchy areas of ground-glass attenuation and interstitial thickening, thereby producing a 'crazy paving' pattern. This may be seen more readily with high resolution scans, which may additionally show interspersed poorly defined small nodules.

Prevention and treatment

Prophylactic management centres on minimizing any tendency to aspiration associated with impaired swallowing, and in persuading the misuser (or abuser) of vegetable and mineral oils to adopt alternative habits. Once aspiration has occurred there may be a role for therapeutic bronchoalveolar lavage, which may remove substantial quantities of lipid from the alveoli. During episodes of secondary bacterial infection there is an obvious role for antibiotics, and when there is acute inflammation corticosteroids are sometimes used.

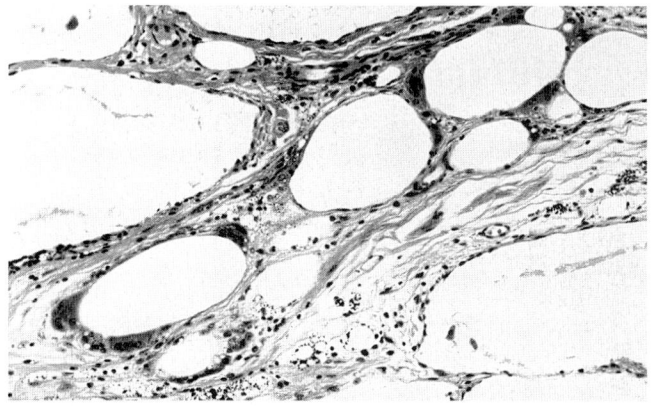

Fig. 18.14.9.1 Section of lung showing exogenous lipoid pneumonia due to aspirated paraffin. There is interstitial fibrosis containing oil vacuoles which are enclosed within multinucleated giant cells (haematoxylin and eosin stain, medium magnification).
By courtesy of Dr T. Ashcroft.

Endogenous lipoid pneumonia

The body may itself produce and retain lipid (mainly cholesterol) within the lungs, though this is not a common phenomenon. Endogenous lipid is most commonly deposited when chronic inflammation accompanies bronchiectasis, bronchial carcinoma, or some other cause of persisting localized bronchial obstruction, and appears to depend on cigarette smoking. The lipid will also be ingested by macrophages and may be recovered in the sputum, hence sputum macrophages laden with lipid are not pathognomonic of aspiration from an exogenous source, although chemical tests can distinguish the two varieties and histological examination of affected lung does not show a granulomatous response to endogenous lipid. The radiological appearances are of a persisting pneumonia, which may stimulate resection for fear a carcinoma is present. Endogenous lipoid pneumonia in a more diffuse form has been associated with the use of amiodarone in patients dying with adult respiratory distress syndrome (ARDS).

Further reading

Anonymous (1999). Case records of the Massachusetts General Hospital. Weekly clinicopathological exercises. Case 33–1999. A 57-year-old woman with a pulmonary mass. *N Engl J Med*, **341**, 1379–85.

Carby M, Smith SR (2000). A hazard of paint spraying. *Lancet*, **355**, 11.

Cohen MA, Galbut B, Kerdel FA (2003). Exogenous lipoid pneumonia caused by facial application of petrolatum. *J Am Acad Dermatol*, **49**, 1128–30.

Gondouin A, et al. (1996). Exogenous lipoid pneumonia: a retrospective multicentre study. *Eur Respir J*, **9**, 1463–9.

Lee JS, et al. (1999). Exogenous lipoid pneumonia: high-resolution CT findings. *Eur Radiol*, **9**, 287–91.

Miller GJ, et al. (1971). The lipoid pneumonia of blackfat tobacco smokers in Guyana. *Q J Med*, **40**, 457–70.

Oldenburger D, et al. (1972). Inhalation lipid pneumonia from burning fats. *JAMA*, **222**, 1288–9.

Segev D, et al. (1999). Kerosene-induced severe acute respiratory failure in near drowning: reports on four cases and review of the literature. *Crit Care Med*, **27**, 1437–40.

Silverman JF, et al. (1989). Bronchoalveolar lavage in the diagnosis of lipid pneumonia. *Diagn Cytopathol*, **5**, 3–8.

18.14.10 Pulmonary alveolar microlithiasis

D.J. Hendrick

Essentials

Pulmonary alveolar microlithiasis is caused by mutations of the type IIb sodium phosphate cotransporter gene, which by an unknown mechanism leads to the accretion of calcified microliths in the lungs. Almost invariably the patient is symptom free when the diagnosis is made after a chest radiograph is taken incidentally (or during family screening) and reveals profuse small calcified nodules. Patients usually survive 10–20 years from diagnosis, lung transplantation being the only effective treatment in severe cases.

Introduction

Pulmonary alveolar microlithiasis is a very rare disorder, with less than 600 cases reported since its initial description in 1918. It is remarkable for a number of unusual if not unique features. Tiny calcified concretions, 0.05 to 5 mm in size, concentrically laminated, form progressively in the alveolar spaces, usually with some degree of interstitial fibrosis. As their profusion slowly increases, they produce a striking 'whiteout' appearance on the chest radiograph as the border of one intensely radio-opaque microlith overlaps that of another, even if the two are not immediately adjacent. Progression commonly leads to death from respiratory failure, but only after a decade or two. There is a strong tendency for cases to occur within families, reflecting the genetic cause. There is no effective means of therapy apart from transplantation.

Aetiology, genetics, pathogenesis, and pathology

The clustering of cases within families is most consistent with autosomal recessive inheritance, and a study in 2006 indicates that the disease arises from mutations of the type IIb sodium phosphate cotransporter gene on chromosome 4. This will doubtless stimulate further elucidation of the causal mechanisms, and advantage may be taken of the serendipidous discovery that a strain of laboratory mice (mutant nackt mice) appears to develop the disease.

No abnormality of calcium metabolism has been demonstrated, and analytical studies—including X-ray energy spectroscopy and microscopic infrared spectroscopy—have shown no evidence of mineral dust deposition. Nor is there evidence of an initiating infection. Heavily calcified alveolar microliths have also been noted complicating mitral stenosis. These are thought to arise from the organization of chronic alveolar exudates, raising the possibility that in the presence of impaired phosphate transport any alveolar exudate might lead to the production of calcified microliths. They are characteristically rounded or oval in alveolar microlithiasis, but are irregular and bosselated with mitral stenosis. Both types show massive calcification, and both may be associated with bone formation (hydroxyapatite) and interstitial fibrosis.

Epidemiology

In 2004 Mariotta and colleagues reviewed all 576 published cases. Most had arisen in Europe (43%) or Asia (41%), and overall one-third (but 44% amongst 48 Italian cases) had positive family histories. The disease usually presents in middle age, but any age may be involved and both sexes are equally represented.

Clinical features

Almost invariably the patient is symptom free when an initial film is taken for incidental reasons, and there may be wonder that this can be possible when the radiograph is grossly abnormal. This is a consequence of there being no associated cellular, exudative, fibrotic, or vascular disruption of normal physiological processes in the early stages of the disease. Physical signs are conspicuous by their absence for most of the long course of the disease, although crackles, clubbing (even hypertrophic pulmonary osteoarthropathy) and signs of respiratory failure may be observed ultimately as the

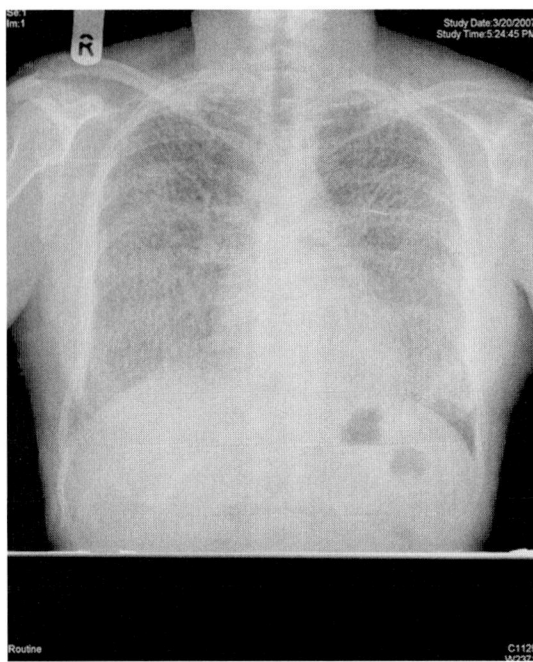

Fig. 18.14.10.1 A chest radiograph showing typical appearances of pulmonary alveolar microlithiasis with micronodular calcific densities seen throughout the lungs.
http://www.ispub.com/ostia/index.php?xmlFilePath=journals/ijpm/vol9n1/pam.xml

alveolar spaces are progressively filled with microliths and fibrosis of the interstitium advances. Shunting occurs at alveolar–capillary level causing hypoxaemia, and the bronchial circulation contributes increasingly to pulmonary venous return. In some cases subpleural cysts give rise to spontaneous pneumothoraces, and pleural adhesions may become prominent.

Although death supervened rapidly in the reported cases of two newborn infants, survival of 10 to 20 years is characteristic, and may be much longer. In most symptomatic cases there is slowly progressive breathlessness with dry cough. Haemoptysis and chest pain occur occasionally. The lungs stiffen, ventilation becomes restricted, and gas transfer is impaired. Eventually respiratory failure and cor pulmonale supervene. At death, extensive areas of the chest radiograph show a dense 'whiteout' appearance due to the considerable accumulation of calcium, the lungs are difficult to cut, and they sink in water.

Clinical investigation

The radiographic appearances of profuse, small, calcified nodules are almost diagnostic, particularly in moderately advanced cases when the dense 'whiteout' picture is seen but symptoms are still absent or unimpressive (Fig. 18.14.10.1). Early cases are occasionally simulated by sarcoidosis or healed chicken pox pneumonia. Biopsy, bronchoalveolar lavage, or expectorated sputum should provide diagnostic material (the microliths themselves), in less advanced cases (the microliths themselves), but with transbronchial biopsy it may prove difficult to close the forceps and extract them through the fibre-optic bronchoscope. Initially the chest radiograph shows a mere haziness of the lower zones, and CT may be invaluable in demonstrating the nodular shadows and their calcific nature. It may also confirm an early predominance for the basal and posterior segments. High-resolution images may also demonstrate the presence of interstitial fibrosis. As the profusion and size of the calcified concretions increase, the lung fields become diffusely and densely opaque. Measurement of lung function during the asymptomatic stage reveals little or no abnormality, the affected subject remaining well for many years.

Treatment and prognosis

Corticosteroids, calcium chelating agents, bisphosphonates, and bronchoalveolar lavage have not proved to be effective therapies, and treatment is merely supportive in the absence of lung transplantation. A detailed description of a 37-year-old man presenting in respiratory failure recorded severe hypoxia and pulmonary hypertension. Considerable intrapulmonary shunting was demonstrated, which was greatly improved by nasal continuous positive airway pressure, but not by conventional supplemental oxygen therapy. This presumably reflects the dominant effect of the disease in restricting alveolar ventilation over impairing gas diffusion. Although lung transplantation experience is necessarily limited in such a rare disorder, it clearly provides the most optimistic outlook for advanced disease. Survival otherwise is of the order 10–20 years from disease recognition.

Further reading

Barbolini G, Rossi G, Bisetti A (2002). Pulmonary alveolar microlithiasis. *N Engl J Med*, **247**, 69–70.

Castellana G, *et al.* (2002). Pulmonary alveolar microlithiasis: clinical features, evolution of the phenotype, and review of the literature. *Am J Med Gen*, **111**, 220–4.

Corut A, *et al.* (2006). Mutations in SLC34A2 cause pulmonary alveolar microlithiasis and are possibly associated with testicular microlithiasis. *Am J Hum Genet*, **79**, 650–6.

Freiberg DB, *et al.* (1992). Improvement in gas exchange with nasal continuous positive airway pressure in pulmonary alveolar microlithiasis. *Am Rev Resp Dis*, **145**, 1215–16.

Helbich TH, *et al.* (1997). Pulmonary alveolar microlithiasis in children: radiographic and high-resolution CT findings. *Am J Roentgenol*, **168**, 63–5.

Mariotta S, *et al.* (2004). Pulmonary alveolar microlithiasis: report on 576 cases published in the literature. *Sarcoid Vascul Diffuse Lung Dis*, **21**, 173–81.

Starost MF, Benavides F, Conti CJ (2002). A variant of pulmonary alveolar microlithiasis in nackt mice. *Vet Pathol*, **39**, 390–2.

Weinstein DS (1999). Pulmonary sarcoidosis: calcified micronodular pattern simulating pulmonary alveolar microlithiasis. *J Thorac Imaging*, **14**, 218–20.

Yesner R (2003). Pulmonary alveolar microlithiasis revisited. *N Engl J Med*, **348**, 84–5.

18.14.11 Toxic gases and aerosols

D.J. Hendrick

Essentials

Acute exposure—the effects of noxious gases or aerosols on the airways and lungs are determined by (1) their solubility in water, with those that are highly soluble having their main effect on the lining of the upper respiratory tract and those with lower solubility mainly affecting the lungs, and (2) the dose of exposure, with overwhelming exposures having adverse effects throughout the respiratory tract.

Clinical features—acute effects are usually the result of industrial or farming accidents and comprise (1) acute upper airway toxicity—caused by highly soluble gases (e.g. ammonia, sulphur dioxide); laryngeal oedema may be severe enough to cause airflow obstruction and require intubation; (2) acute tracheobronchitis—usually caused by less soluble gases at less pungent levels of exposure (e.g. chlorine); full recovery is expected if the patient survives, but some are left with the reactive airways dysfunction syndrome; (3) acute pneumonitis—caused by gases of low solubility (e.g. nitrogen dioxide—silo filler's disease); produces acute pneumonitis and pulmonary oedema some hours after exposure; (4) asphyxiation—some inhaled gases, most commonly CO_2 and methane, have no toxic effects but may cause death through asphyxiation by displacing oxygen from inhaled air.

Management—this is essentially supportive. While ensuring the safety of potential rescuers, prompt removal from the source of exposure (and from any toxic agent that contaminates clothing and/or lies on the skin) is followed by attention to airway patency, oxygenation and swift transportation to specialized emergency care.

Subacute exposure—working exposures over weeks/months to a few chemical agents are recognized to cause a variety of additional airway and interstitial effects.

Introduction

Noxious airborne substances may be delivered to the respiratory tract as gases (including vapours, i.e. substances that at ambient temperature and pressure are normally liquid, occasionally solid) or aerosols (i.e. particulates). The effects of noxious gases are determined mainly by their solubility in water; those with high solubility are largely dissolved in the secretions lining the upper respiratory tract, those with low solubilities penetrate to the gas-exchanging tissues and exert their dominant effects there. However, with overwhelming exposures adverse effects will occur at all levels of the respiratory tract, and dose becomes a more important determinant of outcome than solubility.

Particulates that are dispersed in air (aerosols) may be solid (dusts) or liquid (mists), and may carry toxic chemicals through surface adsorption or solution, even if the carrier agent itself is harmless. If the particles are large (diameter >10 µm), they become trapped chiefly in the nose, throat, or major airways. If they are small (diameter <5 µm), they are deemed 'respirable' and may readily penetrate deeply to become retained in the gas-exchanging tissue and (through macrophage transport) the lung interstitium. Fume and smoke are important examples of toxic aerosols. Fume is a dispersion of fine (readily respirable) particles that form as vaporized material (usually metal) condenses at ambient temperature and oxidizes. Smoke is an aerosol of solid combustion products; it is often mixed with toxic gases and/or fume.

Many adverse effects may follow the inhalation of toxic gases and aerosols. Most are manifested in the lung itself, but some are manifested in other organs after the lung provides a route for absorption (e.g. poisoning from carbon monoxide or hydrogen cyanide, which are described in Chapter 9.1). Not only do the respiratory effects occur at different levels, but they may appear at different times. It is useful, therefore, to consider acute, subacute, and chronic effects separately, and to recognize that some are dominantly airway effects while others are dominantly parenchymal effects. The chronic effects, such as chronic bronchitis, emphysema, pneumoconiosis, pleural thickening, and lung cancer, generally require months or years of exposure, and arise only after a latency of 10 to 20 years or more. Although 'toxic' or 'irritant' in nature, rather than a consequence of allergy or infection, they are usually considered separately from disorders attributable to 'toxic gases and aerosols', and so are described in other chapters.

In general, the acute effects of toxic gases and aerosols are the result of industrial or farming accidents, since the potential for toxic exposure is rare outside occupational environments. However, train or tanker crashes have occasionally caused the rupture of chemical containers and the release of toxic gases into non-occupational environments, and the tragic events at Bhopal (India) in 1984 illustrate the alarming potential for an industrial accident to have profound effects well beyond the workplace. At the opposite extreme of a wide clinical spectrum, a brief exposure to a toxic agent (even one of high potency) may cause no more than mild transitory mucosal irritation. These accidental circumstances of exposure contrast importantly with those of continuous 'subacute' exposure over weeks or months to a handful of notable occupational agents. These may cause slowly evolving toxic effects over the same time course, leading to profound respiratory disability, even death, and they deserve mention despite their rarity.

The topic of 'inhalant injury' to the respiratory tract is a substantial one: this section provides no more than a brief overview and the reader is advised to consult more specialized and comprehensive texts when called upon to manage particular examples. A particularly useful Internet source for constantly updated information is http://toxnet.nlm.nih.gov/

Acute toxic injury to the respiratory tract

Acute upper airway toxicity

If toxic gases of high solubility (e.g. ammonia, hydrogen chloride, or sulphur dioxide) are involved, or aerosols comprising particles of large average diameter, the adverse effects will dominate in the upper respiratory tract and large airways. Laryngeal oedema, severe enough to cause airflow obstruction and require intubation, is the most important effect, but oedema is to be expected also in the conjunctivae, nose, mouth, and throat, together with inflammatory secretions, even bleeding. One breath is usually sufficient to provoke an immediate withdrawal from further exposure, if this is possible, and so protects against further damage.

Acute tracheobronchitis

If withdrawal from exposure is not possible, or less soluble gases are involved at less pungent levels of exposure (e.g. chlorine), there will be greater penetration beyond the larynx and an acute tracheo-bronchitis results. This too may become life threatening, and may predispose to secondary infection. If the patient survives, full recovery is the rule, but a few are left with asthma that persists for weeks, months, or even indefinitely. Such an outcome has been called the reactive airways dysfunction syndrome.

Acute pneumonitis

Gases of low solubility (e.g. oxides of nitrogen, ozone, or phosgene) penetrate readily to the gas-exchanging tissues. In the absence of immediate toxicity to the upper respiratory tract they may be encountered in an increasing cumulative and hence dangerous dose. The outcome is an acute pneumonitis and pulmonary oedema some hours later, and is exemplified by nitrogen dioxide toxicity.

When grain is stored in silos (or silage is preserved under impervious coverings) microbial contamination leads to the release of nitrogen dioxide along with other toxic gases (principally aldehydes) and asphyxiants (CO_2, methane), and to the removal of oxygen. Such processes have the beneficial effect of 'pickling' and preserving the vegetable produce, but they create a dangerous environment for the unwary farm worker, who is typically exposed when the silo is decapped. Moulding vegetable produce can also provoke an allergic or toxic pneumonitis (acute farmer's lung or organic dust toxic syndrome, respectively) that require differentiation from nitrogen dioxide toxicity (see Chapter 18.14.4). Nitrogen dioxide toxicity can also occur when welding is carried out in poorly ventilated sites, and with the combustion of nitrogen-containing substances, such as nitrocellulose, with one notorious incident involving a fire of stored radiographs.

A curious observation with nitrogen dioxide toxicity has been a recurrent episode of pulmonary oedema 1 to 3 weeks after the initial exposure. The explanation is not clear, though possibly represents the well-recognized complication of adult respiratory distress syndrome (ARDS) that may follow any cause of toxic pneumonitis. The prophylactic use of oral steroid is said to reduce this risk. Once ARDS occurs, additional risks of pneumothorax and secondary infection arise, sometimes with fatal result. Otherwise recovery is usually full, though rarely bronchiolitis obliterans (or bronchiolitis obliterans with organizing pneumonia) complicates the picture (see Chapter 18.11.3).

Illustrative causal agents

Fire smoke

Smoke from fires is a complex mixture of gases and particulates released during combustion and pyrolysis. Its nature can vary greatly with the severity of the fire, the availability of oxygen, and the nature of the burning materials. It may contain toxic concentrations of carbon monoxide, hydrogen cyanide, ammonia, sulphur dioxide, chlorine, phosgene, nitrogen dioxide, aldehydes, and other gases, together with particulates derived from the burning material that are contaminated with surface absorbed gases. Thus, its effects may be diverse; they include suffocation and metabolic poisoning as well as direct toxic injury throughout the respiratory tract. If fat or oil is involved, a lipoid pneumonia may result, particularly if combustion (or explosion) leads to oil nebulization.

Metal fume fever

Metal fume fever is an acute and self-limiting febrile illness that characteristically occurs after unusually heavy exposures to metal fume, and recurs on re-exposure after a brief absence from work. It closely simulates other occupational fevers, such as Monday fever in cotton workers (see byssinosis, Chapter 18.7), polymer fever in chemical workers, and the fevers associated with humidifier lung and allergic alveolitis (see Chapter 18.14.4). It can occur on the first day of exposure. It results from alveolar deposition of very fine particulate metal oxides (fumes) produced in processes such as welding, burning (oxyacetylene cutting) and smelting of metal, particularly (but not exclusively) zinc, copper, and magnesium. Within some 6h of exposure, there is thirst, a metallic taste in the mouth, cough, tightness in the chest, and chills, with fever, head-ache, myalgia, and leucocytosis. Resolution follows within 24h without permanent sequelae. This benign course is dramatically distinguished from that associated with heavy exposure to fume released specifically from heating cadmium, an anticorrosive metal used in electroplating and the production of alloys. Cadmium fumes may be encountered during extraction, soldering, burning, and welding in poorly ventilated conditions, and may lead to an acute toxic reaction in both lungs and kidneys with high mortality.

Simple asphyxiants

Some inhaled gases have no toxic effects but may severely threaten life through asphyxiation by displacing oxygen from inhaled air. Most common are CO_2 and methane, which replace oxygen when vegetable produce decomposes through microbial contamination. A less common source is the slow combustion of coal in disused mines or cellars. Oxygen-deficient air in working mines (black-damp) has been long recognized as a cause of asphyxiation in miners, but careful monitoring and high levels of ventilation provide effective prevention. Occasionally, however, disused mines accumulate blackdamp during periods of high barometric pressure, only to release the asphyxiant gas when the barometric pressure falls. Most escapes harmlessly to the atmosphere from mine shafts, but some may be trapped in the ground under impervious layers of rock or clay. This may find an escape route through faults in the strata and so be emitted at high flow rates into surface buildings, with cellars that breach a layer of clay in coal-mining areas sometimes providing a particularly dangerous environment for the unsuspecting. Decaying vegetable matter in the soil may also provide the mechanism for CO_2 to replace oxygen, and entry of this oxygen-deficient air into wells during periods of low barometric pressure has also led to asphyxiation of those climbing into them.

Treatment

The management of toxic and asphyxiant insults is essentially supportive. Prompt removal from the source of exposure (and from any toxic agent that contaminates clothing and/or lies on the skin) is followed by attention to airway patency, oxygenation, and swift transportation to specialized emergency care. Rarely there may be an indication for the administration of specific antidotes, e.g. with cyanide poisoning (nitrites and sodium thiosulphate) or methaemoglobinaemia (methylene blue). Such treatment may be life saving, hence it is essential to learn the chemical nature of any accidentally released gases or aerosols, and to seek specialist advice and/or consult specialist literature. Note, however, that smoke inhalation victims may sometimes be poisoned by cyanide and have methaemoglobinaemia, and there is some danger in these circumstances that methylene blue could liberate cyanide that is bound relatively safely to methaemoglobin. It is also essential to consider the safety of potential rescuers.

Because of the risk of laryngeal obstruction or pulmonary oedema following toxic insults, a minimum period of 24 h of hospital care is needed for subjects presenting with hoarseness, stridor, wheeze, or hypoxaemia, and those with a history indicative of heavy exposure to a poorly soluble toxic gas. Humidified air, oxygen supplementation, and bronchodilators may be required. Bronchoscopy may be needed to remove excessive secretions and clear the airway. Laryngeal obstruction demands intubation, and tracheostomy may be necessary if there is extensive upper airway inflammation. Severe pulmonary oedema should be managed as for the adult respiratory distress syndrome (ARDS) (see Chapter 17.5). The role of corticosteroids in limiting inflammation is unclear; these drugs add to the risk of secondary infection and may interfere with normal reparative processes, but they do appear to prevent the development of late pulmonary oedema after nitrogen dioxide exposure.

Finally, there is a need to review the circumstances surrounding any potentially life-threatening case. What is the risk of a further event, and how best can this be minimized? Is a formal risk assessment document needed?

Subacute toxic injury to the respiratory tract

'Normal', rather than accidental, working exposures to a few chemical agents over a matter of weeks or months have been recognized over recent years to pose unusual and unexpected risks of toxic airway and interstitial effects. These could be described as bronchiolitis and pneumonitis, some cases within an affected population being centred more in the smaller airways, others more in the lung parenchyma. Some have satisfied the diagnostic criteria for bronchiolitis obliterans organizing pneumonia (BOOP).

The Ardystil syndrome, first reported in 1992, resulted from the use of sprayed printing dyes in certain textile factories (one being the Ardystil factory in Valencia, Spain). Affected individuals from a dozen or so factories developed BOOP or progressive pulmonary fibrosis, and several died. The key factors proved to be a polyamideamine substitution for polyurea in the pigment carrier Acramin, and its application by a water-based spray. The polyurea formulation had previously been used widely and safely, but only by topical (not spray) application.

Also in 1992, BOOP and fixed airway obstruction was reported to occur with surprising frequency in groups of popcorn workers, and again it proved to be life threatening. The causal agent was traced to airborne flavouring materials, and principally to a chemical with a butter-like flavour, 2,3-butanedione (diacetyl).

A number of reports from 1995 similarly incriminated 'nylon flocking' as a potent and life-threatening cause of nonspecific pneumonitis (which may be prominently lymphocytic), BOOP, or progressive pulmonary fibrosis. The key factor here was the use of rotary rather than guillotine cutters, which caused the nylon fibres to fragment and melt, and so produce particles of respirable size.

This subacute development of a spectrum of progressive disorders encompassing obstructive bronchiolitis, BOOP, pneumonitis, and pulmonary fibrosis caused surprise because the clinical picture differed considerably from that which had been associated traditionally with environmental and occupational disorders of

the lung. There are, however, other examples which illustrate that toxic environmental and occupational agents from diverse sources may produce, subacutely, devastating effects at the small airway/gas exchanging level of the lungs. Lung toxicity from ingested agents is beyond the remit of this section, but the reader should recognize that bronchiolar disease and interstitial fibrosis may follow not only the ingestion of paraquat (see Chapter 9.1), mineral oil (which, in one notorious incident, contaminated cooking oil), and a variety of drugs (see Chapter 18.14.13), but the ingestion, because of its perceived anorectic properties, of extracts from the Asian shrub *Sauropus androgenus*. More relevant to inhaled toxic agents are acid anhydrides, trimellitic anhydride and pyromellitic dianhydride, which uniquely in the occupational setting (plastics industry) may cause diffuse pulmonary haemorrhage as well as interstitial fibrosis.

Further reading

Ainslie G (1993). Inhalational injuries produced by smoke and nitrogen dioxide. *Respir Med*, **87**, 169–74.

Brooks SM, Weiss MA, Bernstein IL (1985). Reactive airways dysfunction syndrome (RADS). Persistent asthma syndrome after high level irritant exposures. *Chest*, **88**, 376–84.

Kern DG, *et al.* (2000). Flock worker's lung: broadening the spectrum of clinicopathology, narrowing the spectrum of suspected etiologies. *Chest*, **117**, 251–9.

Gelpi E, *et al.* (2002). The Spanish toxic oil syndrome 20 years after its onset: a multidisciplinary review of scientific knowledge. *Environ Health Perspect*, **110**, 457–64.

Kreiss K, *et al.* (2002). Clinical bronchiolitis obliterans in workers at a microwave-popcorn plant. *N Engl J Med*, **347**, 330–8.

Moya C, Anto JM, Taylor AJ (1994). Outbreak of organising pneumonia in textile printing sprayers. Collaborative Group for the Study of Toxicity in Textile Aerographic Factories. *Lancet*, **344**, 498–502.

Nemery B (2002). Toxic pneumonitis: chemical agents. In: Hendrick DJ, *et al.* (eds) *Occupational disorders of the lung: their recognition, management, and prevention*, pp. 93–103. W B Saunders, London.

Schwartz DA (2002). Toxic tracheitis, bronchitis, and bronchiolitis. In: Hendrick DJ, *et al.* (eds) *Occupational disorders of the lung: their recognition, management, and prevention*, pp. 93–103. W B Saunders, London.

Smith TJ, Petty TL, Ridding JC (1976). Pulmonary effects of exposure to airborne cadmium. *Am Rev Respir Dis*, **114**, 161.

Website

National Library of Medicine. *Toxnet toxicology data network.* http://toxnet.nlm.nih.gov/

18.14.12 **Radiation pneumonitis**

S.J. Bourke and D.J. Hendrick

Essentials

The lungs can be injured by radiation used in cancer treatment, with the rapidly dividing endothelial cells and type II pneumocytes most affected. Immediate injury is followed by an inflammatory response and at a later stage by fibrosis. Chest radiography reveals asymptomatic changes in about 50% of patients after radiotherapy.

Acute radiation pneumonitis presents with cough, breathlessness and fever about 2 months after exposure; corticosteroids are usually effective in relieving symptoms but do not prevent the subsequent development of fibrosis. Fibrosis typically develops about 6 months later, may progress for 6 to 24 months, but has usually stabilized by 2 years. Prevention depends on refining techniques for giving radiotherapy.

Introduction

The lungs are vulnerable to injury from radiation used in the treatment of cancers of the lung, breast, oesophagus, spine, thymus, and lymph glands, and when whole-body irradiation is given in preparation for bone marrow transplantation. Radiation causes direct injury to cells and DNA within the field of radiotherapy, giving rise to pneumonitis and/or fibrosis. The induction of reactive oxygen species and the initiation of cytokine-mediated inflammatory responses result sporadically in more diffuse radiation lung injury involving areas of the lung outwith the radiotherapy field. Acute radiation pneumonitis is characterized by interstitial inflammation occurring up to 4 months after radiotherapy and then resolving over a matter of weeks or months. Radiation fibrosis, which can occur without preceding pneumonitis, develops about 6 months after radiotherapy and may progress over 6 to 24 months: it does not resolve, but usually stabilizes by 2 years.

Pathogenesis

Factors which influence the development of radiation pneumonitis and fibrosis include the volume of lung irradiated, the total radiation dose administered, and the dose rate and fractionation. Concomitant use of chemotherapeutic drugs such as bleomycin, doxorubicin, methotrexate, and cyclophosphamide can aggravate radiation lung injury. Furthermore, when chemotherapy is given after radiotherapy, 'recall pneumonitis' may develop in the areas of lung previously irradiated. Tamoxifen has been shown to enhance lung injury in patients receiving radiotherapy for breast cancer, which may be due to increased release of transforming growth factor β (TGFβ). Corticosteroid withdrawal may also precipitate radiation pneumonitis, and there is increased risk with pre-existing lung fibrosis or current lung infection.

Absorption of radiation by lung tissues accelerates electrons, generating ion pairs and reactive oxygen species which damage DNA and produce chemical and biological effects in cells. Rapidly dividing cells, such as endothelial cells and type II pneumocytes, are most affected. The earliest changes involve injury to small vessels with thrombosis, increased permeability, and exudation of protein-rich fluid into the alveoli. Epithelial injury results in sloughing of cells, hyaline membrane formation and proliferation of type II pneumocytes. Inflammatory cells accumulate in the alveolar walls, followed at a later stage by fibroblasts. Increased plasma concentrations of TGFβ and intercellular adhesion molecule (ICAM)-1 correlate with an increased incidence of radiation pneumonitis. ICAM-1 stimulates the accumulation of inflammatory cells, whereas TGFβ stimulates fibroblast proliferation and induces synthesis of collagen, and genetic polymorphisms that result in high production of TGFβ are associated with more severe radiation fibrosis. Cellular expression of CD95 and CD95-ligand

are increased after radiotherapy, and these receptors are involved in the induction of apoptosis, inflammatory cytokine responses, and the attraction of inflammatory cells. These immunologically mediated responses are not confined to the radiotherapy field.

Clinical features

Asymptomatic changes are detectable on a chest radiograph in about 50% of patients after radiotherapy. Characteristically there is an area of opacification that does not show a segmental or lobar distribution: it crosses the normal anatomical structures and is demarcated by a sharp margin corresponding to the limits of the radiotherapy field (Fig. 18.14.12.1). Air bronchograms are often present and there is usually a loss of volume.

Symptoms occur in about 5 to 15% of patients, depending on the treatment regimen used, with the onset of cough, breathlessness, and fever about 2 months after radiotherapy. Pre-existing lung disease may increase the clinical impact of radiation pneumonitis, but symptoms often resolve spontaneously. Fibrosis may result in permanent loss of lung function, with a reduction in total lung capacity and carbon monoxide transfer factor associated with chronic breathlessness. This typically develops about 6 months after radiotherapy and may progress for 6 to 24 months, but has usually stabilized by 2 years.

CT is more sensitive than the chest radiograph in detecting radiation-induced changes such as ground-glass shadowing, septal thickening, and fibrosis, and is useful in differentiating radiation injury from tumour recurrence or infection.

Severe acute reactions to radiotherapy are rare but can occasionally result in respiratory failure and the acute respiratory distress syndrome (ARDS). Patterns of injury that involve the lungs more diffusely are well recognized. Bilateral lymphocytic alveolitis is often present after unilateral radiotherapy in patients with breast cancer, while positron emission tomography (PET) has shown increased metabolic activity in nonirradiated areas of the lung in patients who have had radiotherapy for lung cancer. Diffuse bronchiolitis obliterans organizing

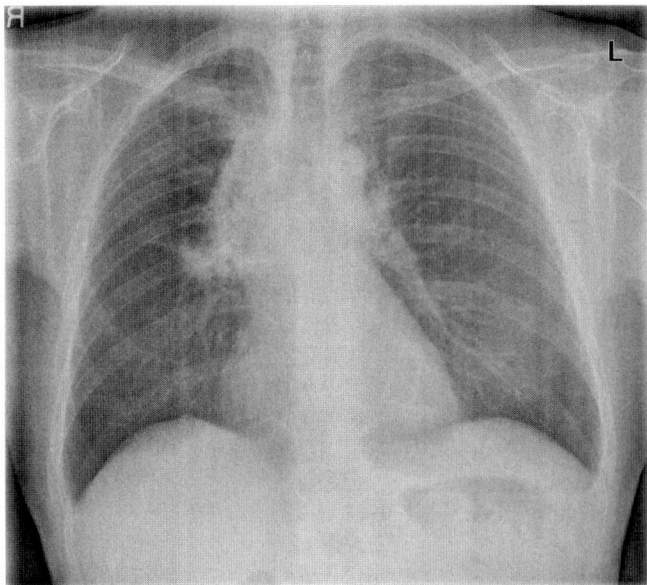

Fig. 18.14.12.1 Chest radiograph showing radiation-induced fibrosis, particularly in the right upper zone. Note the sharply demarcated edge to the fibrosis, which does not conform to any normal anatomical structure.

pneumonia and chronic eosinophilic pneumonia have also been reported in patients with breast cancer treated by radiotherapy. Other short-term risks of chest radiotherapy relate to pneumothorax, pleural reactions, and rib fractures, and in the long term there is an increased risk of lung cancer.

Treatment

Most cases of radiation pneumonitis are subclinical or cause only minor symptoms that do not require treatment. In more severe cases corticosteroids are usually effective in relieving symptoms during the acute phase, but they do not prevent the subsequent development of fibrosis. Typically, prednisolone 40 to 60 mg daily is given until there is clinical improvement, at which stage the dose is tapered whilst watching for signs of recrudescence of the pneumonitis. Prevention of radiation-induced lung injury is particularly focused on refining techniques which increase the radiation dose delivered to the cancer and reduce exposure of normal lung. Radiotherapy lung injury has been reduced in animal models by the administration of agents such as amifostine, captopril, pentoxifylline, and manganese superoxide dismatase, but a clinical role for these agents has not been established.

Further reading

Cottin V, *et al.* (2004). Chronic eosinophilic pneumonia after radiation therapy for breast cancer. *Eur Respir J*, **23**, 9–13.

Crestani B, *et al.* (1998). Bronchiolitis obliterans organizing pneumonia syndrome primed by radiation therapy to the breast. *Am J Respir Crit Care Med*, **158**, 1929–35.

Heinzelmann F, *et al.* (2006). Irradiation-induced pneumonitis mediated by the CD95/CD95-ligand system. *J Natl Cancer Inst*, **98**, 1248–51.

Hesham A, *et al.* (2005). Positron emission tomography demonstrates radiation-induced changes to non irradiated lungs in lung cancer patients treated with radiation and chemotherapy. *Chest*, **128**, 1448–52.

Hill RP (2005). Radiation effects on the respiratory system. *Br J Radiol*, **27** (Suppl), 75–81.

Martin C (1999). Bilateral lymphocytic alveolitis: a common reaction after unilateral thoracic irradiation. *Eur Respir J*, **13**, 727–32.

Movsas B (1997). Pulmonary radiation injury. *Chest*, **111**, 1061–75.

Neugut AI, *et al.* (1994). Increased risk of lung cancer after breast cancer radiation therapy in cigarette smokers. *Cancer*, **73**, 1615–20.

Rowinsky EK, Abeloff MD, Wharam MD (1985). Spontaneous pneumothorax following thoracic irradiation. *Chest*, **88**, 703–6.

18.14.13 Drug-induced lung disease

S.J. Bourke and D.J. Hendrick

Essentials

Drug-induced lung disease is common and needs to be considered in the differential diagnosis of many respiratory conditions. The nature and timing of events often provide an important clue and are sometimes sufficiently characteristic for drug-induced lung disease to be diagnosed with confidence, with resolution of symptoms

on drug cessation providing invaluable supportive evidence. Well-recognized adverse drug effects are listed in formularies and drug data sheets, but it is often helpful to consult a constantly updated website: http://www.pneumotox.com is highly recommended.

Direct drug effects may arise through toxic, pharmacological, allergic, or idiosyncratic mechanisms, and there may also be indirect effects, e.g. a predisposition to lung infection from cytotoxic and immunosuppressive therapies. From a clinical perspective adverse effects may be classified according to the induced disorder and/or the site of involvement.

Asthma—the most common airway disorder to be induced or exacerbated by drugs; may be produced by a predictable effect related to the drug's pharmacological properties (e.g. β-adrenergic antagonists) or as an idiosyncratic reaction (e.g. aspirin).

Cough—a well-recognized side effect of treatment with angiotensin-converting enzyme (ACE) inhibitors.

Alveolar/interstitial reactions—comprise three main categories: (1) alveolar capillary leakage, e.g. hydrochlorothiazide; (2) alveolar/interstitial inflammation and/or fibrosis, e.g. bleomycin, amiodarone; and (3) pulmonary eosinophilia, e.g. sulphonamides.

Pulmonary vasculature—venous thromboembolism, e.g. oral contraceptive pill; pulmonary hypertension, e.g. aminorex (now withdrawn), fenfluramine.

Pleura and mediastinum—lymphadenopathy, e.g. phenytoin; pleural effusion, e.g. procainamide; oculomucocutaneous syndrome, e.g. practolol; fibrosis, e.g. methysergide.

Introduction

Drug-induced lung disease is common. It needs to be considered in the differential diagnosis of many respiratory conditions and in prescribing drugs for the treatment of diseases in all areas of clinical practice. Direct effects may arise through toxic, pharmacological, allergic, or idiosyncratic mechanisms, although often the precise mechanism is unknown. There may also be indirect effects, e.g. a predisposition to lung infection from cytotoxic and immunosuppressive therapies and the development of respiratory failure from sedation. Some causes of drug-induced lung disease have now been eradicated (e.g. aminorex pulmonary hypertension) as the causative drug is no longer prescribed. For others, the risks are now so well established that the potential for lung toxicity is considered in the risk–benefit assessment of prescribing (e.g. methotrexate, amiodarone, bleomycin) and the patient is informed of the risks and monitored for the adverse effects. It is for newly introduced drugs that particular vigilance is required: adverse effects must be identified as speedily as possible (e.g. leflunonide, infliximab), early recognition of problems being critical both for the affected individual, so that drug cessation is prompt and the adverse effect is minimized, and also to prevent others coming to harm.

The first step in diagnosis is to consider the possibility that any clinical presentation might be drug-induced. The nature and timing of the events often provide important clues. In some circumstances they are sufficiently characteristic that drug-induced lung disease can be diagnosed with confidence, with subsequent resolution of symptoms on drug cessation providing invaluable supportive evidence. Reintroduction of the drug is rarely indicated unless it is essential in the management of the underlying disease (not uncommon in treating tuberculosis) or there is doubt about the diagnosis of an adverse drug effect. The exclusion of an alternative cause of any clinical events is an important step, with the diagnostic approach adapted to the circumstances of the clinical problem, the likelihood of an adverse drug effect, the possibility of an alternative diagnosis, and the need for a definitive diagnosis to guide management decisions. For example, a patient may develop breathlessness and show diffuse infiltrates on chest radiography when taking immunosuppressive drugs for a connective tissue disease or chemotherapeutic agents for cancer. The clinical features could be due to an adverse drug effect on the lungs, infection, lung involvement by the underlying disease, or the development of coincidental lung disease. Management in these circumstances depends crucially upon accurate diagnosis, hence invasive tests such as bronchoscopy, bronchoalveolar lavage, and lung biopsy are likely be indicated.

Although well-recognized adverse drug effects are listed in formularies and drug data sheets, the field of drug-induced lung disease is continuously evolving, and it is often helpful to consult a constantly updated website: http://www.pneumotox.com is highly recommended. It is also important to report possible adverse drug reactions to appropriate local authorities, such as the Committee on Safety of Medicines in the United Kingdom, who may also be able to provide invaluable information to aid the management of individual cases.

The clinical spectrum of drug-induced lung disease is diverse and complex: adverse effects may be classified according the induced disorder and/or the site of involvement (e.g. airways, alveoli/interstitium, pulmonary vasculature, mediastinum, and pleura).

Airways

Asthma

The most common airway disorder to be induced or exacerbated iatrogenically by drugs is asthma. In theory, drugs (like other environmental agents) may produce asthmatic symptoms either by elevating the patient's pre-existing level of airway responsiveness into the asthma range, or by acting as a specific or nonspecific stimulus when airway responsiveness already lies within that range. By the first mechanism, the drug acts as a cause of asthma (an asthma inducer); by the second it acts as a cause of asthmatic reactions (an asthma trigger). Some drugs doubtless act through both mechanisms. The mechanism is of limited consequence in the drug setting (though not in the occupational/environmental setting), since treatment cessation and future avoidance is the way forward in both circumstances. If, nevertheless, a given drug is known to be a potential trigger but not an inducer, concern over its use need arise only for individuals who are already asthmatic.

In practice, airway obstruction provoked by drugs usually presents as an exacerbation of pre-existing asthma. In some cases asthma is not recognized until it is 'uncovered' by the adverse effect of a drug, but in these instances clues to its pre-existence are usually elicited when the appropriate history is taken. Drugs that exacerbate symptoms in subjects with pre-existing asthma may conveniently be classified as those that produce a more or less predictable effect, related to their pharmacological properties, and those which produce bronchoconstriction due to an idiosyncratic effect (Table 18.14.13.1).

Table 18.14.13.1 Drugs that may cause or exacerbate asthma

Pharmacological effects
Cholinergic agents (e.g. carbachol, pilocarpine)
Cholinesterase inhibitors (e.g. pyridostigmine)
Prostaglandin F
Histamine-releasing agents (e.g. curare derivatives)
β-Sympathetic antagonists
ACE inhibitors (cough without asthma more common)

Sensitizing and idiosyncratic effects
Oral
Aspirin and other NSAIDs
Tartrazine-containing preparations
Nitrofurantoin (alveolar reaction more common)
Carbamazepine
Propafenone
Parenteral
Penicillin
Iron–dextran complex
Aminophylline
Hydrocortisone sodium succinate
N-Acetylcysteine
Inhaled
Nebulized pentamidine
Nebulized colistin
Eye drops
NSAIDs

ACE, angiotensin-converting enzyme; NSAIDs, non-steroidal anti-inflammatory drugs.

Less commonly, asthma develops *de novo*, probably because immunological hypersensitivity has developed.

Asthmatic symptoms can also be a consequence of the particular formulation of a drug or its method of delivery. For example, nebulized solutions of low osmolality can trigger asthmatic reactions if there is a high level of airway responsiveness. This appears to have been the main mechanism of bronchoconstriction induced paradoxically by nebulized ipratropium bromide, and since the drug was reformulated in isotonic solution the problem has largely disappeared. A further cause of bronchconstriction from nebulized drugs has been the presence of certain preservatives or stabilizers (e.g. benzalkonium chloride, edetate disodium) in the excipient solution, with the effect particularly unexpected if the administered drug is used for asthma.

Cholinergic drugs, such as carbachol, occasionally produce bronchoconstriction when given systemically, and in very sensitive asthmatic patients exacerbations have occurred after use of pilocarpine as eye drops. An inhaled anticholinergic agent would seem a logical approach to this problem and has been shown to be effective in reversing occasional untoward effects of cholinesterase inhibitors in asthmatic patients with myasthenia gravis. The bronchoconstrictor prostaglandin $F_{2\alpha}$, if used to induce abortion, may be hazardous in asthmatic patients. The occurrence of bronchoconstriction after thiopentone, opiates, and muscle relaxants (tubocurarine, suxamethonium, and pancuronium) is probably due to their capacity to release histamine.

A more common problem is worsening of airway obstruction by β-adrenergic antagonists. Although these have become increasingly selective to avoid β₂-antagonism, none is completely specific for $β_1$-receptors. Of the β-blockers currently available, sotalol and metoprolol seem to have the least adverse effects on airway function, but many patients with asthma will show a reduction in forced expiratory volume in 1 s (FEV_1) or peak flow on therapeutic doses of these agents—occasionally a dangerous reduction. β-Blockers should consequently be avoided in patients with clear-cut asthma, but the situation with chronic airway obstruction is less clear. Adverse reactions in such patients are less common and usually less severe. They possibly reflect the coincidental presence of mild asthma anyway, rather than a true adverse effect on chronic obstructive pulmonary disease (COPD) attributable to emphysema or obstructive bronchiolitis. Although the adverse effects of oral or systemic β-blockers are well recognized, those of ophthalmic preparations are easily overlooked. Timolol, which is used commonly in eye drops for the treatment of glaucoma, is a potent nonselective β-blocker. Its use has frequently been associated with worsening asthma. The ophthalmic formulation of a newer β-blocker, betaxolol, appears to be less dangerous, but should be avoided in patients with asthma unless no suitable alternative is available.

The mechanism by which drugs lead to asthmatic symptoms when there is no obvious pharmacological effect is often unclear, though immunological sensitization and idiosyncrasy are likely to provide the main pathways. The most dramatic presentation of drug-related asthma is as part of an acute anaphylactic reaction, and penicillin and intravenously administered iron–dextran are particularly noteworthy among the causal agents. Other drug hypersensitivity reactions that include asthma among the manifestations are often associated with blood eosinophilia and/or eosinophilic pneumonia (see Chapter 18.14.5).

Immunological hypersensitivity is presumed to underlie most causes of occupational asthma, some of which involve pharmaceutical agents. Most prominent are certain antibiotics (e.g. cephalosporins, isoniazid, penicillins, piperazine, spiramycin, tetracycline,), the H_2-receptor antagonist cimetidine, the laxative psyllium (ispaghula), pancreatic enzymes, and certain hormones (ACTH, gonadotropin, pituitary snuff). If an individual sensitized by inhalation in the workplace subsequently uses the relevant drug therapeutically, the potential arises for an asthmatic reaction (Fig. 18.14.13.1). The medical history, when symptoms suggest asthma, should always include details of occupation and medication, and if the patient has ever worked in the pharmaceutical industry the possibility of occupationally induced hypersensitivity to a current medication should be considered.

Idiosyncrasy probably underlies many asthmatic symptoms related to medication and is the likely explanation for exacerbations following use of intravenous N-acetylcysteine in paracetamol poisoning, use of which requires caution in asthmatic patients. Idiosyncrasy more obviously underlies asthmatic reactions to aspirin and other nonsteroidal anti-inflammatory drugs (NSAIDs). Exacerbation of asthma after ingestion of aspirin was described as long ago as 1910, but its precise mechanism remains elusive. Most patients who are sensitive to aspirin also react to other NSAIDs, their widely differing chemical structures making an immunological hypersensitivity reaction unlikely. As with cholinergic drugs and β-blockers, asthmatic reactions to NSAIDs may rarely follow ocular administration, and so eye drops deserve careful attention when asthma worsens unexpectedly.

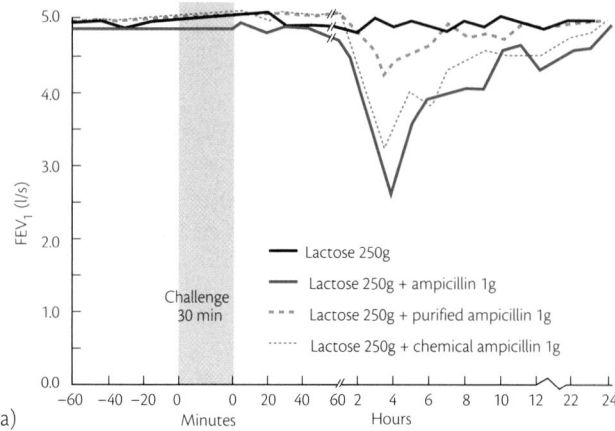

(a)

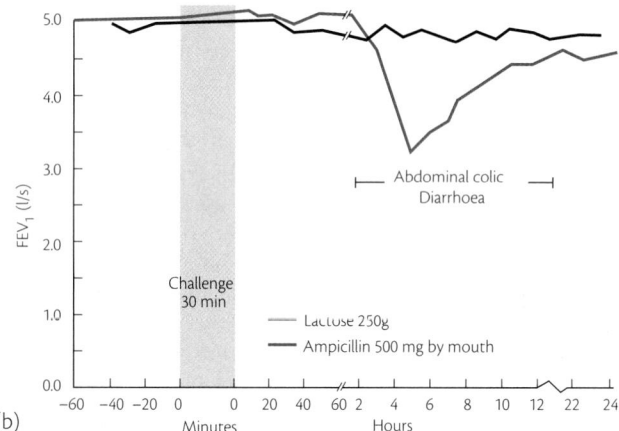

(b)

Fig. 18.14.13.1 Results of inhalation and ingestion challenge tests with ampicillin. The inhalation test confirmed that the patient had become sensitized to ampicillin as a consequence of respiratory exposure at work, and the ingestion test showed that asthmatic reactions would be provoked also by oral ingestion at therapeutic dose levels.
(Data taken from Davies RJ, Hendrick DJ, Pepys J (1974). Asthma due to inhaled chemical agents: ampicillin, benzyl penicillin, 6-amino-penicillanic acid and related substances. *Clin Allergy*, **4**, 227–47.)

NSAIDs are inhibitors of prostaglandin synthesis via the cyclooxygenase pathway, and it is presumed that their adverse effects are mediated in this way. It is possible that metabolism of arachidonic acid is diverted to the production of bronchoconstrictor leukotrienes, but why a few patients with asthma should be affected is not clear (hence the idiosyncrasy). Asthmatic deaths have been reported with both aspirin and indomethacin. Of the commonly used analgesic agents, paracetamol is the least likely to provoke a significant response, although occasional adverse reactions are well documented. A further interesting feature is that aspirin-sensitive individuals can be made tolerant to further aspirin by ingesting graded doses over a couple of days. This state of tolerance can then be maintained by daily treatment with aspirin, but sensitivity returns within a few days of discontinuing regular treatment. Any attempt at inducing tolerance in this way requires very careful supervision.

Many patients with analgesic-induced asthma are also sensitive to the azo dye tartrazine (and often to alcoholic beverages). Tartrazine has hitherto been a commonly used colouring agent in medications (particularly those coloured orange or red) and foodstuffs, and since it is an approved food and drug additive its presence is not always declared and the extent of the problems it may cause is not clear. In the past tartrazine was present, ironically, in some medications used to treat asthma, but most pharmaceutical companies no longer use it in their formulations. Other dyes may, however, have similar adverse effects and some of these still occur in drug formulations. Patients with aspirin and tartrazine sensitivity may also develop troublesome nasal polyposis as well as asthma. Such patients may benefit from a diet low in salicylates and free of azo dyes, in addition to strict avoidance of NSAIDs.

The potential exacerbation of asthma by drugs used to treat it presents a special dilemma, as a drug effect may be difficult to dissociate from spontaneous deterioration. There are well-documented reports of worsening asthma after intravenous hydrocortisone. This is a particular problem in asthmatic patients who also show adverse reactions to aspirin and NSAIDs. The sensitivity to hydrocortisone of these individuals does not extend to other steroids; it appears to be related to the succinate moiety of the hydrocortisone sodium succinate molecule, as it is not seen with the alternative phosphate salt.

The uses of nebulized pentamidine for treatment or prophylaxis of pneumocystis infection in patients with HIV infection and nebulized colistin for treatment of pseudomonal lung infection in bronchiectasis have been associated with bronchoconstriction in many individuals. The mechanism is unclear. Although patients with asthma show larger responses, others with no previous evidence of asthma may also be affected. The adverse effect may be inhibited by prior use of a nebulized bronchodilator, an approach that has become standard in many centres.

Cough

Cough in the absence of asthma is a well-recognized side effect of treatment with angiotensin-converting enzyme (ACE) inhibitors. It develops in 10 to 20% of individuals so treated and is an effect of the class of drug rather than of specific agents. The cough is nonproductive. There appears to be a weak relation to dose, such that dose reduction may result in some improvement, but in many individuals the symptom remains sufficiently troublesome to necessitate drug withdrawal. Deterioration of pre-existing asthma has also been reported occasionally, but features of asthma are not present in most individuals with cough related to ACE inhibition. The mechanism is unclear; ACE catalyses not only the conversion of angiotensin I to angiotension II, but also the breakdown of bradykinin and substance P. Since these agents are cough stimulants, their accumulation offers a possible mechanism for this adverse effect. The cough disappears on withdrawal of the drug.

Alveoli and the lung interstitium

Alveolar/interstitial reactions to drugs range from acute noncardiogenic pulmonary oedema (e.g. from cremaphor, the agent used to provide soluble ciclosporin for intravenous use) or the acute respiratory distress syndrome (ARDS) at one extreme (i.e. causes of alveolar capillary leakage), to insidiously developing pulmonary fibrosis at the other. They are conveniently considered under three main categories: alveolar capillary leakage, alveolar/interstitial inflammation and/or fibrosis, and pulmonary eosinophilia (Table 18.14.12.2). Some overlap is inevitable: inflammatory reactions (whether toxic or allergic) may cause capillary leakage and hence radiographic air space filling; allergic reactions may or may not be characterized by inflammation and eosinophil infiltration.

Table 18.14.13.2 Alveolar reactions

Alveolar capillary leakage

Cytosine arabinoside
Hydrochlorothiazide
Low-molecular-weight dextran
Naloxone
Salicylates
Tocolytic agents (e.g. isoxsuprine, ritodrine, terbutaline)

Alveolar/interstitial inflammation and/or fibrosis

Tocainide
Leflunomide
Antiretroviral therapy
Infliximab
Leflunomide
Antiretroviral therapy
Infliximab
Cytotoxic agents
   Azathioprine
   Bleomycin
   Busulphan
   Carmustine (BCNU)
   Chlorambucil
   Cyclophosphamide
   Cytosine arabinoside
   Lomustine (CCNU)
   Melphalan
   6-Mercaptopurine
   Mitomycin C

Pulmonary eosinophilia

Aspirin
Carbamazepine
Chlorpropamide
Chlorpromazine
Gold salts*
Imipramine
Methotrexate*
Naproxen
Nitrofurantoin*
Penicillamine*
Penicillins
Phenytoin
Procarbazine*
Sulphasalazine
Sulphonamides
Tetracycline

*Eosinophilia not consistent.

Alveolar capillary leakage

Of the drugs that may produce ARDS, hydrochlorothiazide and salicylates are the commonest. The reaction to hydrochlorothiazide is idiosyncratic and not shared with other thiazide drugs. In the case of salicylates, there is a clearer relation to dose, with reactions usually occurring with frank overdose (as also occurs with opiates) or—occasionally—with chronic high-level ingestion. Infused β_2-adrenergic agonists are sometimes used as uterine relaxants (tocolytics) to inhibit premature labour, with several—in particular isoxsuprine, ritodrine, and terbutaline—having been associated with florid pulmonary oedema. This reaction is occasionally life threatening and caution is required over the rate of infusion.

Alveolar/interstitial inflammation and/or fibrosis

Several drugs produce widespread alveolar damage ('pneumonitis' or 'alveolitis') which may or may not be followed by fibrosis. Patients present acutely with cough, fever, shortness of breath, and occasionally systemic upset. Alternatively, there is slowly progressive fibrosis with gradually worsening dyspnoea and widespread shadowing on the chest radiograph. The mechanisms of such reactions are uncertain, but may include toxicity, hypersensitivity, and possibly idiosyncrasy. With some drugs—including bleomycin, carmustine, amiodarone, and nitrofurantoin—there a relation to dose or duration of treatment. Evidence in cases of nitrofurantoin- and bleomycin-induced pneumonitis suggests a role for the production of toxic oxygen radicals in the lungs, perhaps providing a link with the known pulmonary toxicity of oxygen itself and the synergistic adverse effects of high oxygen concentrations and some cytotoxic agents.

Much interest has centred on the cardiac antiarrhythmic drug amiodarone. It has been estimated that about 6% of patients taking 400 mg or more per day for 2 months or more will develop overt pulmonary toxicity, and there have been several well-documented cases involving smaller doses. The mechanisms may include both immunologically mediated and direct toxic effects. Histologically the lung shows features of chronic inflammation together with interstitial and intra-alveolar fibrosis (Fig. 18.14.13.2). Characteristic 'foamy' macrophages are seen, but they are not specific for serious toxic reactions as they are also demonstrable in most patients taking the drug without adverse clinical effects. Occasionally the histological picture is of cryptogenic organizing pneumonia. Symptoms include progressive dyspnoea, a troublesome cough, and (occasionally) pleuritic chest pain. Radiographic appearances are varied: most frequently there is a diffuse nodular or alveolar filling pattern, sometimes with upper lobe predominance (Fig. 18.14.13.3); occasionally a pleural effusion is present.

The differential diagnoses of amiodarone pulmonary toxicity in patients likely to be taking this drug include left ventricular failure and pneumonia. Further investigation, including estimation of left ventricular function and lung biopsy, is often necessary. Bronchoalveolar lavage in some (but not all) patients shows a lymphocytic pattern. This investigation is also of value for the exclusion of infection, but the finding of 'foamy' macrophages in lavage fluid is insufficient to confirm the diagnosis. If amiodarone lung toxicity is suspected, cessation of treatment is desirable, but the very long half-life of drug metabolites (many weeks) means that elimination is very slow. Corticosteroids probably suppress the reaction and sometimes allow treatment to be continued or recommenced in cases of 'malignant' arrhythmia unresponsive to other agents.

Cryptogenic organizing pneumonia is a rare manifestation of drug-induced lung disease, but is increasingly recognized in complex settings where drug therapy may have played a dominant or contributory role. In addition to amiodarone, associations have been reported with carbamazepine, nitrofurantoin, phenytoin, sotalol, tacrolimus, ticlopidine, and a number of herbal medications. One of particular interest is a presumed (but unproven) anorectic agent derived from the leaf of *Sauropus androgynus*, an Asian shrub of the Euphoriaceae family. In a remarkable period of a few months,

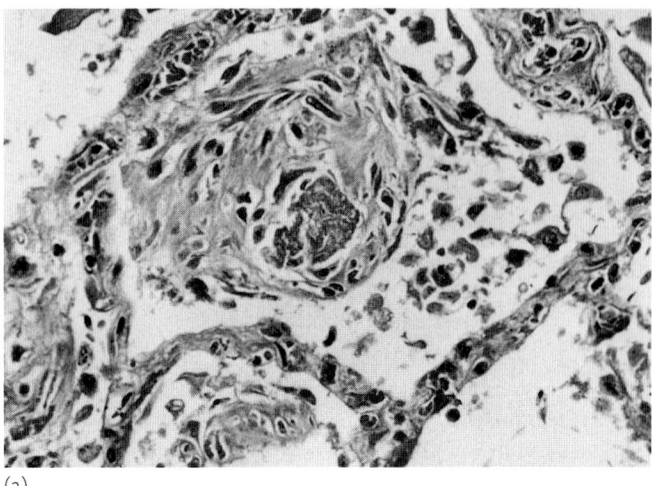

(a)

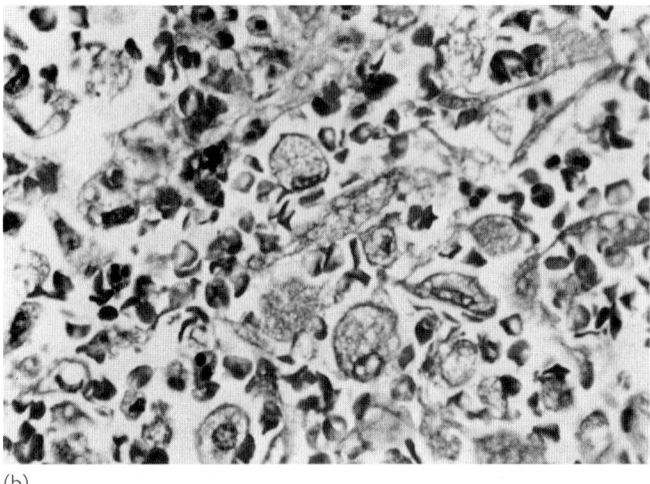

(b)

Fig. 18.14.13.2 Histological specimen of the lung of a patient who died from amiodarone pulmonary toxicity, showing (a) alveolar wall thickening and organizing intra-alveolar exudates; and (b) the alveolar exudate with characteristic 'foamy' macrophages, seen at higher magnification.
Adams *et al.* (1986). *Quarterly Journal of Medicine* 59, 449–71.

more than 60 people who had ingested juice containing uncooked leaf extract of *S. androgynus* presented to hospital in Taiwan with progressive undue breathlessness: in 23 the breathlessness was severe; plain radiographs were essentially normal, but CT scanning and biopsies demonstrated organizing pneumonia with (in a few cases) bronchiectasis in the segmental and subsegmental bronchi; responses to corticosteroid therapy were poor.

Cytotoxic and immunosuppressive drugs pose an increasing problem for the lung parenchyma, with most reported to cause pulmonary complications. Bleomycin causes problems most frequently, followed by busulphan and methotrexate. Cyclophosphamide and azathioprine are the most widely used drugs in this group, because of their roles in nonmalignant disease, but produce adverse pulmonary reactions only occasionally. In most cases it is not clear whether the effects are due to direct toxicity or to hypersensitivity. With bleomycin, however, toxicity is dose-related, occurring more commonly at cumulative doses greater than 300 000 units.

The recorded frequency of adverse reactions varies with the means by which they are detected, with fibrosis occurring in 5 to

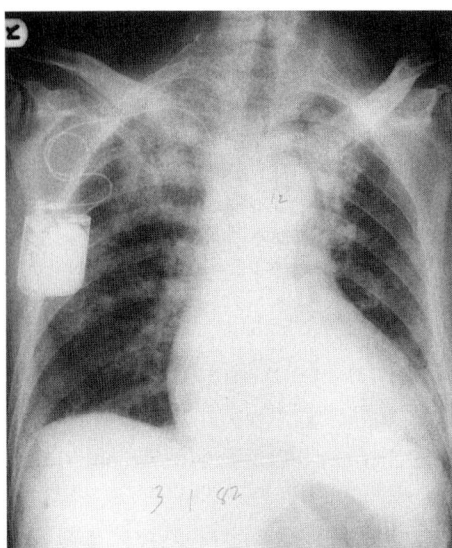

Fig. 18.14.13.3 Chest radiograph of a patient with amiodarone pulmonary toxicity showing confluent alveolar shadowing in both upper lobes. (From Adams PC, Gibson GJ, Morley AR et al. (1986) Amiodarone pulmonary toxicity: clinical and subclinical features. *Quarterly Journal Medicine*, **59**, 449–71.)

10% of patients treated with busulphan on clinical and functional criteria, but a much higher proportion on the basis of pathological and cytological evidence. Similarly, the increasing use of CT scanning shows an appreciably higher prevalence than found in surveys that employ plain chest radiography. The frequency of overt lung involvement may also be related to length of survival, as determined by the primary disease. With busulphan, the interval between starting treatment and the appearance of toxic effects can be as long as 4 years, and in some cases the lung changes appear to progress after the drug has been discontinued. With carmustine (BCNU), pulmonary fibrosis may first be recognized several years after treatment has finished. Other factors that may increase the toxicity of a given drug include advanced patient age, and synergism with other drugs, lung radiation, or the subsequent inhalation of high concentrations of oxygen.

Histologically, most cytotoxic drugs produce evidence of diffuse alveolar damage with destruction of lining cells, formation of hyaline membranes, and variable degrees of inflammatory infiltration and fibrosis. Fibrosis is particularly common with busulphan and bleomycin, but rare with methotrexate. With methotrexate and procarbazine (and very occasionally with bleomycin) there may be blood and tissue eosinophilia, and correspondingly a good therapeutic response to steroids.

Pulmonary eosinophilia

Eosinophilic reactions in the lung include conditions that would be classified as Löffler's syndrome, simple or prolonged pulmonary eosinophilia, and eosinophilic pneumonia (see Chapter 18.14.2). Tissue eosinophilia is a more consistent feature than peripheral blood eosinophilia. Historically, sulphonamides have been the drugs most frequently reported to cause pulmonary eosinophilia, and such a reaction has even occurred to a sulphonamide-containing vaginal cream. Sulphonamide sensitivity may also explain some of the reactions to sulphasalazine and to chlorpropamide, which is chemically related. The pulmonary eosinophilia recorded with aspirin appears to be distinct from aspirin-induced asthma.

Nitrofurantoin may produce an acute pulmonary eosinophilic reaction in addition to more insidious fibrosis.

The roles of gold salts and penicillamine in eosinophilic reactions have been a matter of some debate, but the evidence suggests that both are involved. It seems unlikely, however, that drugs are responsible for many of the cases of fibrosing alveolitis associated with rheumatoid arthritis. Penicillamine has been incriminated in two other types of adverse pulmonary reaction: (1) pulmonary haemorrhage (Goodpasture's syndrome) when used in high doses for the treatment of Wilson's disease, and (2) obliterative bronchiolitis in patients treated for rheumatoid arthritis. The evidence that penicillamine is responsible (rather than rheumatoid disease itself) is not conclusive.

The clinical severity of eosinophilic reactions is very variable, ranging from a transient and asymptomatic radiographic opacity to a severe eosinophilic pneumonia with dyspnoea, cough, fever, and hypoxaemia. Concomitant asthma is not uncommon. The chest radiograph shows fluffy opacities, frequently with peripheral or predominantly upper-lobe distribution. The prognosis is usually good: the changes often subside spontaneously on withdrawal of the drug, while in more severely ill patients there is usually a dramatic improvement on instituting treatment with corticosteroids. Although repeated exposure to the offending agents continues to produce reactions, the severity of these may progressively decrease.

Adverse effects of new drugs

New adverse effects emerge as new drug therapies are introduced. Leflunomide is a newer immunomodulatory drug used in the treatment of rheumatoid arthritis. It was initially thought to have less adverse effects on the lung than methotrexate, but there have now been several reports of its association with severe acute interstitial pneumonitis. Colestyramine or activated charcoal can be used to aid elimination.

Tumour necrosis factor α (TNFα) inhibitors (infliximab, etanercept, adalimumab) are being used increasingly in the treatment of rheumatoid arthritis and inflammatory bowel disease. Increased susceptibility to respiratory infections, and to tuberculosis in particular, is an important adverse effect of these drugs, and reports are also accruing of interstitial pneumonitis with these agents.

A granulomatous lung disease, mimicking sarcoidosis, has been described after instituting highly active antiretroviral therapy with protease inhibitors in patients with HIV infection. This pattern of lung disease seems to be related to immune reconstitution with enhanced lymphoproliferative responses rather than to any infective organism.

Pulmonary vasculature

Pulmonary thromboembolism related to use of the contraceptive pill is well established; its frequency correlates with the oestrogen content and has been reduced since the introduction of low-oestrogen preparations (see Chapter 14.19).

The statistical association between pulmonary hypertension and the use of the anorectic agent aminorex in Switzerland, Germany and Austria in the 1960s was of great interest, and an epidemic of pulmonary hypertension subsided when the drug was withdrawn. No similar rise was seen in countries that did not introduce this agent. Occasional cases of pulmonary hypertension have been reported

Table 18.14.13.3 Drugs associated with pleural reactions

Drug-induced lupus	Procainamide, gold, hydralazine, isoniazid, penicillamine, sulphonamides
Oculomucocutaneous syndrome	Practolol
Isolated	Methysergide, bromocriptine, methotrexate, dantrolene, acebutalol

also in patients taking fenfluramine and various amphetamine-like drugs (see Chapter 16.15.2).

Pulmonary veno-occlusive disease has been reported after carmustine (BCNU), mitomycin, and bleomycin.

Analgesics given during labour have been implicated in the development of pulmonary hypertension in the newborn; drugs such as aspirin, indomethacin, and naproxen delay premature labour but, by their inhibitory effects on prostaglandin synthesis, may also cause constriction of the ductus arteriosus leading to pulmonary hypertension *in utero*. This persists into the postpartum period and causes respiratory distress.

Pleura and mediastinum

Hilar and mediastinal adenopathy are occasionally seen as part of the generalized lymphadenopathy produced by the anticonvulsant phenytoin, and mediastinal lipomatosis has been reported in patients receiving large doses of corticosteroids.

Drugs that have been associated with pleural reactions (effusion or fibrous thickening) are shown in Table 18.14.13.3. Several have been reported to produce a syndrome like systemic lupus erythematosus (SLE): the antiarrhythmic procainamide is most often implicated, but other agents include gold, hydralazine, isoniazid, penicillamine, and sulphonamides. The main respiratory target of this syndrome is the pleura, but (as with pleural disease induced by methysergide and bromocriptine) there is often some fibrosis of underlying lung.

Practolol, a now obsolete selective β-sympathetic antagonist, produced a characteristic 'oculomucocutaneous' syndrome. This differed from drug-induced SLE in that autoantibodies to histones were not usually present, and ocular symptoms (not usually a feature of drug-induced SLE) were common. Pleural effusions and subsequent pleural thickening occurred in association with characteristic corneal ulceration, discoid rash, and fibrinous peritonitis. Affected patients sometimes developed effusions months or years after discontinuing the drug, and in some the chronic changes led to significant respiratory disability. Other β-sympathetic antagonists, in particular acebutolol, have been reported occasionally to cause an alveolar or pleural reaction, but it seems unlikely that other β-blockers are associated with the full-blown oculomucocutaneous syndrome.

Methysergide, which is used in treatment of the carcinoid syndrome and occasionally for migraine, may induce mediastinal or pleural fibrosis with or without retroperitoneal fibrosis. Improvement follows early withdrawal of the drug. Bromocriptine has some structural similarities to methysergide and may also produce chronic pleural effusions and thickening. The pleural fluid characteristically contains a high proportion of lymphocytes. The frequency of this reaction is uncertain, but it may be relatively common. Methotrexate has been associated with pleurisy, independent of its alveolar effects. The smooth-muscle relaxant dantrolene, used for relief of spasticity, has been reported to produce an unusual type of pleurisy with effusion in which pleural fluid and blood eosinophilia are prominent. There is no evidence of any parenchymal abnormality, and although the changes gradually resolve on withdrawing the drug some residual pleural fibrosis may remain.

Complications of radiographic and other procedures

Lipoid pneumonia may follow bronchography with oily media, with an oleogranulomatous reaction that can progress to fibrosis and may sometimes produce a localized mass simulating a neoplasm. Similar reactions can follow aspiration of oily medicines (e.g. laxatives) into the lungs (see Chapter 18.14.9)

Lymphangiographic media that drain through the thoracic duct and so into the venous circulation can enter and impact in the pulmonary circulation. This is often symptomless, but may cause dyspnoea and cough with the expectoration of fat globules or haemoptysis. Occasional deaths have been recorded. The chest radiograph characteristically shows a fine stippling.

Pleural effusion and (less commonly) mediastinitis can occur following endoscopic sclerotherapy of oesophageal varices: the symptoms usually subside within a few days.

Further reading

British Thoracic Society Standards of Care Committee. (2005). BTS recommendations for assessing risk and for managing *Mycobacterium tuberculosis* infection and disease in patients due to start anti-TNF-α treatment. *Thorax*, **60**, 800–5.

Camus P, et al. (2001). Drug-induced infiltrative lung disease. *Eur Respir J*, **18**, 93–100s.

Camus P, Gibson GJ (2003). Iatrogenic respiratory disease. In: Gibson GJ, et al. (eds) *Respiratory medicine*, 3rd edition, pp. 764–806. W B Saunders, London.

Davies RJ, Hendrick DJ, Pepys J (1974). Asthma due to inhaled chemical agents: ampicillin, benzyl penicillin, 6-amino-penicillanic acid and related substances. *Clin Allergy*, **4**, 227–47.

De Vuyst P, Pfitzenmeyer P, Camus P (1997). Asbestos, ergot drugs and the pleura. *Eur Respir J*, **10**, 2695–8.

Foucher P, et al. (1997). Drugs that may injure the respiratory system. *Eur Respir J*, **10**, 265–79.

Lai R-S, et al. (1996). Outbreak of bronchiolitis obliterans associated with consumption of *Sauropus androgynus*. *Lancet*, **348**, 83–5.

Naccache JM, et al. (1999). Sarcoid-like pulmonary disorder in human immunodeficiency virus-infected patients receiving antiretroviral therapy. *Am J Respir Crit Care Med*, **159**, 2009–13.

Pneumotox. *Drug-induced lung diseases*. http://www.pneumotox.com

Sczeklik A, Picado C (2003). Aspirin-induced asthma. *Eur Respir Monogr*, **23**, 239–48.

Simonneau G, et al. (1998). Primary pulmonary hypertension associated with use of fenfluamine derivatives. *Chest*, **114**, 195–9s.

Chronic respiratory failure

P.M.A. Calverley

Essentials

Chronic respiratory failure describes a clinical state when the arterial Po_2 breathing air is less than 8.0 kPa, which may or may not be associated with hypercapnia (defined as Pco_2 more than 6.0 kPa (45 mmHg)). Four processes cause arterial hypoxaemia due to inefficient pulmonary gas exchange—ventilation–perfusion (V/Q) mismatch, hypoventilation, diffusion limitation, and true shunt, with the most important of these being V/Q mismatching. The arterial CO_2 is increased by inadequate alveolar ventilation and/or V/Q abnormality.

A wide range of disorders can cause chronic respiratory failure, with the commonest being chronic obstructive pulmonary disease (COPD), interstitial lung diseases, chest wall and neuromuscular diseases, obstructive sleep apnoea, and morbid obesity.

Diagnosis—the detection of mild/moderate hypoxaemia rests on an awareness of the possibility rather than any specific clinical finding. Central cyanosis may be apparent when there is an increase in the reduced circulating haemoglobin to approximately 5 g/dl, but this is an unreliable clinical sign. Measurement of arterial blood gases is required, preferably when the patient is breathing air.

Management—the treatment of stable chronic respiratory failure involves: (1) making a firm diagnosis; (2) correction of the underlying disorder (when possible); (3) increasing the inspired oxygen concentration; and (4) increasing alveolar ventilation. The benefits of regular oxygen treatment on breathlessness are marginal and there are no data to suggest that the severity or subsequent progression of breathlessness is influenced by chronic oxygen treatment. Regular 'continuous' treatment with oxygen of patients with COPD and stable hypoxaemia (Pao_2 <7.3 kPa (55 mmHg)) prolongs life. Noninvasive nasal positive-pressure ventilation (NIPPV) has generally superseded other methods of providing chronic mechanical ventilatory support, but the patient–mask interface remains a significant problem in some cases.

Introduction

Although respiration is ultimately a biochemical process involving the generation of ATP, the term 'respiratory failure' is used more loosely to describe the failure of gas exchange within the lung to maintain arterial blood gas homeostasis. Defining normal blood gas tensions is harder than it may appear initially, as Pao_2 falls with age and the extent of this is debated. The most commonly applied formula to describe this is:

$$Pao_2 \text{ (kPa)} = 13.86 - [0.036 \times age(years)]$$

Thus a Pao_2 of 10.6 kPa may be abnormal in a man of 24 years but a 'normal' value in a woman of 80. Subnormal levels of arterial oxygenation are described as hypoxaemia, whereas arterial CO_2 tensions, which do not show similar age dependence, are considered to be hypercapnic when they exceed 6.0 kPa (45 mmHg).

Respiratory failure is defined primarily in terms of hypoxaemia and is arbitrarily considered to be present when the arterial Po_2 (at sea level) is less than 8.0 kPa (60 mmHg). It need not be accompanied by hypercapnia, but when this develops it leads to acidosis due to the accumulation of carbonic acid by the Henderson–Hasselbalch equilibrium. If the acidosis is not rapidly progressive, and in the presence of intact renal compensatory mechanisms that generate bicarbonate ions, it becomes 'chronic'—a compensated state where the arterial pH returns to normal.

In summary, chronic respiratory failure describes a clinical state when the arterial Po_2 breathing air is less than 8.0 kPa, which may or may not be associated with hypercapnia, but is accompanied by a normal arterial pH and has been present for several days or more. This definition emphasizes the physiological determinants of gas exchange that characterize the problem.

Unlike other forms of organ system failure, such as cardiac or hepatic failure, the clinical symptoms and signs of chronic respiratory failure are relatively undramatic, but its development is equally significant, both as a marker of disease progression and in producing serious complications beyond those normally seen with the underlying disease. This chapter reviews the causes, clinical features, and assessment of chronic respiratory failure as well as specific means of treatment. However, to do so logically requires some understanding of the principles underlying the development of this condition, as well as the factors relevant to the selection of the threshold values used in defining this state.

Physiological determinants of blood gas tensions

In health there is a predictable fall in the partial pressure of oxygen from that in the room air to that in mixed venous blood. This reflects the effect of diluting room air with resident gas in the alveoli, the efficiency of pulmonary oxygen exchange, and the consumption of oxygen by metabolizing tissues. Conversely, there is a predictable increase in the amount of CO_2 added to the circulation and subsequently removed from the lungs during expiration. This simple system is reliant on a range of physical processes that differ somewhat for oxygen and CO_2. Within the lungs gas transport is largely by convective bulk transport, and in the alveoli by diffusion. In the blood oxygen combines with haemoglobin, which augments transportation to the tissues where diffusion is the final process involved. By contrast, CO_2 transport begins with diffusion from relatively high tissue concentrations and is buffered in solution in the blood. This complex mechanism can be deranged in a number of predictable ways that are discussed below.

In the last 30 years the analysis of pulmonary gas exchange has been revolutionized by the use of the complex multiple inert gas elimination techniques in research laboratories around the world. This gives a relatively complete description of the distribution of gas exchange abnormalities within the lungs. However, for an understanding of the general principles involved in disease states the traditional three-compartment model is easier to follow. This assumes that alveolar air within the lungs is either ideally matched to pulmonary arterial blood flow within the pulmonary capillary bed or is totally mismatched, meaning that either the ventilation–perfusion (V/Q) ratio is unity (ventilation without perfusion—physiological dead space, V_D) or zero (perfusion without ventilation—shunt effect). The physiological dead space includes a component due to dilution of the resident gas in the airways, the anatomical dead space, while the shunt fraction incorporates the very small amount of cardiac output (<1%) not passing through the pulmonary capillary bed.

Hypoxaemia

The principal mechanisms leading to arterial hypoxaemia are shown in Table 18.15.1. Individuals resident at altitude, e.g. in the

high Andes or Himalayas, experience significantly lower inspired oxygen tensions than those at sea level and in these circumstances even individuals with normal lungs can develop clinically significant hypoxaemia, especially during sleep. Even minor degrees of respiratory impairment in these circumstances can produce dramatic changes in blood gas tensions and the early onset of cor pulmonale. Conversely, people with established hypoxaemia at sea level can occasionally experience worsening symptoms when travelling by air, where cabin pressurization is 75% of atmospheric. However, in clinical practice, this is relatively infrequent.

Four processes cause arterial hypoxaemia due to inefficient pulmonary gas exchange:

- *V/Q* mismatch
- hypoventilation
- diffusion limitation
- true shunt

Much the most important of these is *V/Q* mismatching. In many diseases where minute ventilation is increased, the additional inspired gas is distributed to well-perfused areas of the lungs, but when the opposite occurs and perfusion exceeds effective ventilation (low *V/Q* states), arterial Pao_2 falls. At first this might seem surprising as most diseases associated with *V/Q* imbalance are of patchy distribution and compensation from areas of high *V/Q* ratios might be expected. However, this does not occur because of an important feature of the oxyhaemoglobin dissociation curve (Fig. 18.15.1), whose sigmoid shape means that well-perfused parts of the lung cannot increase the arterial oxygen saturation of the blood leaving them beyond 100%, hence the saturation of the pulmonary venous blood must fall if low *V/Q* areas are present.

The second important mechanism contributing to arterial hypoxaemia is alveolar hypoventilation, where the supply of fresh oxygen is globally reduced because of generally inadequate minute ventilation. This process often coexists with *V/Q* mismatching and tends to exacerbate it. In some situations, such as during exercise, total minute ventilation may lie within the normal range but can

Table 18.15.1 Determinants of a reduced arterial oxygen tension

Inspired oxygen concentration	Reduced at altitude and iatrogenically
Pulmonary factors	
V/Q mismatching	
Alveolar hypoventilation	
Diffusion limitation	
Arteriovenous shunts	
Extrapulmonary factors	
Increased oxygen uptake	Reduced mixed venous Po_2
Low cardiac output	Reduced mixed venous Po_2
Reduced pulmonary capillary transit time	Reduced end-capillary Po_2

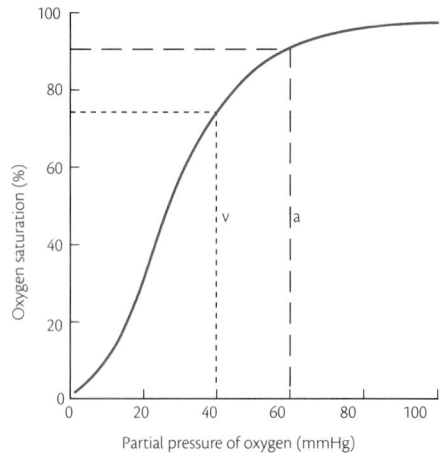

Fig. 18.15.1 The haemoglobin–oxygen dissociation curve. a, Partial pressure of oxygen of 8 kPa (60 mmHg), which is the definition of arterial hypoxia. v, partial pressure of oxygen of 5.3 kPa (40 mmHg), which is typical of mixed venous blood. Note that once the Pao_2 falls below 8 kPa small further falls dramatically decrease the arterial oxygen saturation.

still be inappropriately low for the subject's metabolic requirements, thereby leading to hypoxaemia.

Anatomical shunting and diffusion limitation are less important mechanisms for hypoxia. The former occurs predominantly with intrapulmonary arteriovenous malformations. Congenital cardiac anomalies such as ventricular septal defects with reversed flow are often lumped in with this problem, although technically they are extrapulmonary in origin. The failure to increase Pao_2 to more than 40 kPa (300 mmHg), even when exposed to 100% oxygen, is diagnostic. Diffusion limitation has gone in and out of fashion as an explanation for arterial hypoxaemia. It was initially believed to be important in many diseases, the assumption being that passive diffusion of oxygen was reduced to the point where equilibration with haemoglobin during red-cell transit of the pulmonary capillaries was incomplete. Detailed studies with modern techniques of gas exchange analysis have shown that this is seldom the case, except for small falls in arterial oxygen tension at maximum levels of performance in elderly athletes. Recent data suggest that diffusion limitation contributes to some of the resting and most of the exercise-induced hypoxaemia in some forms of interstitial lung disease.

Although it is not the sole explanation of arterial hypoxaemia, the degree of hypoxaemia can be worsened when the mixed venous arterial oxygen tension is significantly reduced as occurs in low cardiac output states or conditions where peripheral oxygen consumption is increased.

Hypercapnia

Analysis of the pulmonary causes for changes in arterial CO_2 tension is much simpler, the relevant relationship being:

$$Paco_2 = K \times Vco_2 / V_A$$

where Vco_2 is the CO_2 production by the body, V_A is the alveolar ventilation, and K is a constant.

It is easy to see that inadequate alveolar ventilation, due to either low total alveolar ventilation or an inability to increase V_A in response to an increase in metabolic CO_2 production, will increase the arterial CO_2. Alveolar ventilation is influenced by a range of factors, reflecting the balance of the intrinsic capacity of the ventilatory pump and the demands placed on it (Fig. 18.15.2).

The second important mechanism for hypercapnia is V/Q abnormality, although here the important component is the increased

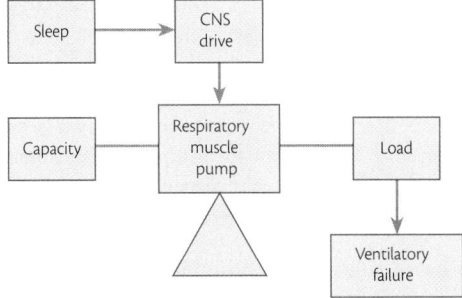

Fig. 18.15.2 Alveolar ventilation reflects the balance of the intrinsic capacity of the ventilatory pump and the demands placed on it. A reduced respiratory drive, particularly during sleep, reduces alveolar ventilation but does not produce significant hypercapnia.

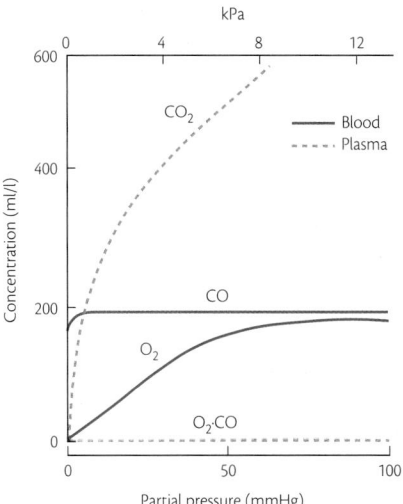

Fig. 18.15.3 Concentration of oxygen (O_2), carbon monoxide (CO), and carbon dioxide (CO_2) in blood and plasma at differing partial pressures of these gases.

physiological dead space. This can be seen by a rearrangement of the equation above to:

$$Paco_2 = K \times Vco_2 / V(1 - V_D/V_T)$$

where V_D/V_T is the ratio of the physiological dead space to the tidal volume and V is the total minute ventilation.

An increase in V_D occurring when V/Q ratios are high can lead to an increase in CO_2 tension. Rather surprisingly, low V/Q units are much less important in producing CO_2 retention than they are in producing hypoxia since CO_2 transport from the blood to the alveolar gas is linear (Fig. 18.15.3). This means that in areas of normal V/Q ratios an increase in overall minute ventilation will increase CO_2 elimination and compensate for the CO_2 that is not excreted from areas of reduced perfusion.

In most cases of chronic respiratory failure with CO_2 retention, both of these processes operate and the patient is unable to sustain the high overall levels of ventilation needed to maintain CO_2 tension within the normal range. An important compensatory mechanism in the trade-off between the increased chemical drive to breathing and the mechanical limitations on ventilation is the breathing pattern. In both chronic obstructive and restrictive lung disease a rapid shallow breathing pattern is adopted to minimize respiratory discomfort whilst maintaining minute ventilation. However, the relative fall in tidal volume further worsens the V_D/V_T ratio and can itself contribute to CO_2 retention. Some of these problems are resolved when the buffering capacity of the blood rises as compensation for respiratory acidosis occurs.

Special circumstances

As already noted, residence at altitude and exercise pose particular problems for gas exchange and may induce temporary respiratory failure. There is now a wealth of data indicating that similar changes can occur during sleep. All healthy people show an approximately 15% reduction in minute ventilation in the transition from wakefulness to stable non-rapid eye movement (REM) sleep, and this may be greater still in phasic REM sleep. The ventilatory responses to both hypoxia and hypercapnia decline as sleep deepens and upper airway resistance rises, especially in those who snore. Despite this the blood gas tensions vary little in health during sleep, but dramatic abnormalities can develop during periods of repetitive upper airway obstruction (see Chapter 18.5.2) or when coexisting neuromuscular weakness leads to excessive dependence on muscle groups whose activity declines with sleep (see below). Persistent nocturnal hypoxaemia can 'feed forwards' to contribute to daytime hypoxaemia in patients with otherwise normal lungs by its adaptive effect on chemoreceptor responsiveness. This occurs in a few people with obstructive sleep apnoea but its relevance to most patients with this disease is debatable, usually being noted when there is coexisting severe obesity (see below).

Gas transport to the tissues

Oxygen delivered to the tissues depends on the oxygen saturation of arterial blood (Sao_2), the haemoglobin concentration (Hb), and the cardiac output (C.O.), related as follows:

$$\text{Oxygen delivery } (Do_2) = \text{C.O.} \times (\text{Hb} \times 1.34) \times (Sao_2/100)$$

This is influenced only indirectly by the effectiveness of gas exchange. Since oxygen delivery is the clinically relevant outcome of oxygenation, decisions about when and how much to intervene therapeutically will be influenced by this variable. Small changes in saturation become clinically more important in individuals with impaired cardiac function and/or reduced haemoglobin concentration, and a higher Sao_2 should be maintained. In general, there is little to be gained by increasing Sao_2 to the high 90s, especially as this may cause secondary CO_2 retention in some diseases. As is clear from Fig. 18.15.1, desaturations below 90% only occur when the arterial oxygen tension is below 8.0 kPa (60 mmHg) and this is also influenced by a number of other factors that determine the position of the dissociation curve (see Table 18.15.2). This provides the rationale for the choice of 8.0 kPa as the cut-off point for the onset of respiratory failure.

Causes of chronic respiratory failure

The principal causes of chronic respiratory failure are summarized in Box 18.15.1, with the commonest causes discussed below.

Chronic airflow limitation

This term covers the most important cause of chronic respiratory failure, chronic obstructive pulmonary disease (COPD), but is also relevant to diseases such as chronic bronchial asthma, which is now excluded from the definition of COPD, and bronchiectasis, where airflow obstruction is a frequent finding as the disease advances.

Table 18.15.2 Important facts about the oxygen dissociation curve

Pao_2 = 100 (13.3), Sao_2 = 97.5%	Arterial blood values
Pao_2 = 80 (10.7), Sao_2 = 96%	Lower limit of normal
Pao_2 = 60 (8.0), Sao_2 = 89%	Dissociation curve changes shape
Pao_2 = 40 (5.3), Sao_2 = 75%	Mixed venous blood, or severe arterial hypoxaemia
Increased temperature, Pco_2, acidosis, 2,3-DPG shifts the curve to the right and vice versa	Reduces O_2 uptake from pulmonary venous blood but increases O_2 delivery in the tissues

2,3-DPG, 2,3-diphosphoglycerate in red cells; Sao_2, arterial oxygen saturation.
Figures for Pao_2 are mmHg (kPa).

In all these cases there is a reduction in the forced expiratory volume in 1 s (FEV_1) to forced vital capacity (FVC) ratio below 70% and a reduction in the FEV_1, which is commonly below 35% predicted before chronic respiratory failure is noted clinically.

In chronic airflow limitation hypoxaemia is the earliest abnormality and largely due to V/Q mismatching. Attempts at relating these changes to structural patterns of airway and alveolar disease in COPD have proved unsuccessful. As lung mechanics worsen (commonly when FEV_1 falls below 1.5 litres or 35% of the predicted value), arterial CO_2 increases. This has been related to the development of inspiratory threshold loading (PEEPi) with the onset of chronic hyperinflation, but the degree of CO_2 retention varies between subjects suggesting that individual variations in chemoresponsiveness/perception of ventilatory load contribute to this process. There is no predictable relationship between the severity of impaired lung mechanics below the thresholds indicated and the degree of hypoxaemia or hypercapnia, and many patients who maintain arterial CO_2 tensions within the normal range develop acute CO_2 retention during exacerbations of their disease. These changes can be relatively short lived and the hypercapnia resolves by the time of discharge. Coexisting left ventricular impairment reduces cardiac output and increases venous admixture, which can cause severe hypercapnia and acidosis, which none the less respond rapidly to appropriate treatment.

Patients with COPD in association with persistent hypercapnic respiratory failure have a worse prognosis than those with intermittent hypercapnia during exacerbations (Fig. 18.15.4). The pattern in chronic asthma and bronchiectasis appears similar to COPD, indicating that lung mechanics rather than individual pathology dictates the severity of the gas exchange disorder.

Interstitial lung disease

Despite the wide range of primary pathologies covered by the term 'interstitial lung disease', they present with a relatively stereotyped physiological picture. A restrictive physiological disorder (FEV_1/FVC >75% with a reduced absolute FEV_1 and FVC) is usual, although patients with sarcoidosis commonly show airways involvement and can present with severe airflow limitation or a mixed physiological pattern. Near normal spirometry can be seen with significant exercise limitation and exercise-induced oxygen desaturation in some patients where COPD and interstitial lung disease coexist. Typically, resting gas exchange is relatively preserved in interstitial lung disease until late in the course, whereas exercise-induced desaturation is an early finding, often seen when spirometric changes are unimpressive. Studies using the multiple inert gas technique have described a bimodal pattern of V/Q distribution, with some areas of lung having normal V/Q relationships and others relatively little ventilation (increased physiological shunting), a situation which worsens during exercise. A small number of patients with severe interstitial lung disease develop CO_2 retention and cor pulmonale in the terminal phase of their illness. The physiological mechanisms underlying this are poorly studied but are probably similar to those in COPD.

Chest wall and neuromuscular disease

Here the underlying lung structure and potential for gas exchange are unimpaired, but the ability to maintain adequate alveolar ventilation is reduced. This can be due to increased chest wall stiffness as in kyphoscoliosis, or reduced inspiratory muscle force as in

---

Box 18.15.1 Causes of chronic hypoxaemia alone or with hypercapnia

With normal or low P_{aO_2}

Pulmonary diseases

- Obstructive ventilatory disorders
  - COPD
  - Chronic asthma
- Mixed ventilatory disorders
  - Bronchiectasis
  - Sequelae of tuberculosis
- Interstitial lung disorders
  - Idiopathic pulmonary fibrosis
  - Pneumoconiosis
  - Sarcoidosis
  - Extrinsic allergic alveolitis
- Pulmonary vascular diseases
  - Pulmonary vascular hypertension
  - Chronic pulmonary thrombosis
  - Arteriovenous malformations

Nonpulmonary diseases

- Severe heart failure
- Hepatopulmonary syndrome

With hypercapnia

Pulmonary diseases

- Obstructive ventilatory disorders
  - COPD

- Mixed ventilatory disorders
  - Bronchiectasis
  - Sequelae of tuberculosis

Nonpulmonary diseases

- Dysfunction of respiratory centres
- Primary alveolar hypoventilation
- Obesity hypoventilation syndrome
- Depressant drugs
- Myxoedema
- Lesion of brainstem
- Neuromuscular diseases
  - Poliomyelitis
  - Amyotrophic lateral sclerosis
  - Myasthenia gravis
  - Muscular dystrophies, polymyositis
- Chest wall deformities
  - Kyphoscoliosis
  - Ankylosing spondylitis
  - Chest trauma
  - Thoracoplasty
- Pleural thickening
- Obstruction of upper respiratory tract

COPD, chronic obstructive pulmonary disease.

---

neuromuscular disease. In this latter group the reduction in maximum inspiratory pressure can be global, such as in Duchenne muscular dystrophy, or more specific, such as isolated diaphragmatic weakness, where gas exchange abnormalities may only be present during specific sleep stages. Significant abnormalities of gas exchange at rest only occur with advanced disease and not in every patient. Alveolar hypoventilation is the dominant mechanism of both hypoxaemia and hypercapnia, although secondary changes such as pulmonary microatelectasis may contribute an element of V/Q mismatching. Assessing exercise hypoxaemia is difficult in these patients due to their generalized muscle weakness. However, sleep-related oxygen desaturation, particularly during REM sleep when the inspiratory system is most dependent on diaphragm function, is a common finding in patients with mild daytime hypoxaemia due to chest wall problems or neuromuscular diseases. Occasionally these changes are dramatic, but in boys with muscular dystrophy the presence of transient hypoxaemic episodes was no better guide to prognosis than was measurement of the vital capacity (Fig. 18.15.5). Arterial CO_2 tensions often lie in the high normal range, daytime hypercapnia only being seen in advanced disease.

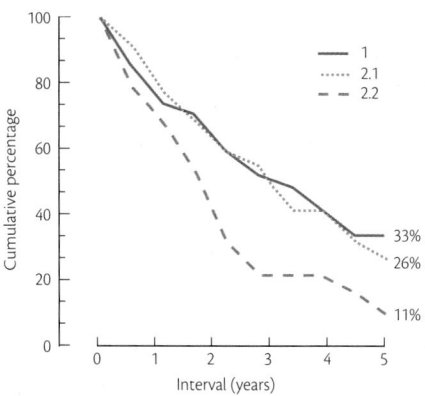

Fig. 18.15.4 Survival after index admission in three groups of patients with COPD who had similar initial spirometry. Group 1 never exhibited CO_2 retention; group 2.1 retained CO_2 during the admission but this resolved; group 2.2 had persistent arterial hypercapnia.
(Based on data from Costello R, *et al.* (1997). Reversible hypercapnia in chronic obstructive pulmonary disease: a distinct pattern of respiratory failure with a favorable prognosis. *Am J Med*, **102**, 239–44.)

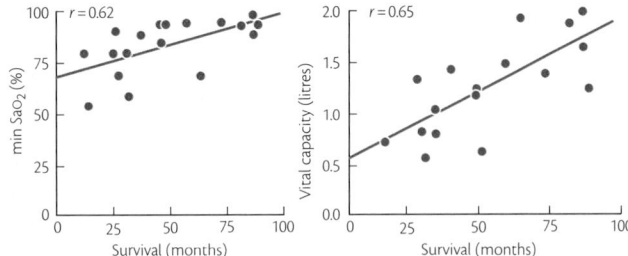

Fig. 18.15.5 Survival of boys with respiratory failure due to neuromuscular disease plotted against minimum arterial oxygen saturation recorded during sleep and vital capacity.
(Based on data from Phillips MF, *et al.* (1999). Nocturnal oxygenation and prognosis in Duchenne muscular dystrophy. *Am J Respir Crit Care Med*, **160**, 198–202.)

As obesity becomes more prevalent in developed countries, so the incidence of the 'obesity–hypoventilation' syndrome rises. This condition is characterized by waking hypercapnia and mild hypoxemia in the absence of factors known to cause CO_2 retention. Overnight polysomnography shows marked and sustained hypoventilation with a rise in the CO_2 retention throughout the night. A significant number of these patients have coexisting obstructive sleep apnoea with repetitive upper airway obstructions, which worsens both their hypoxemia and sleep disruption. However, the arterial oxygen tension before sleeping may still be low, with a waking saturation below 90% as a result of closure of the dependent airways during tidal breathing and a consequent worsening of the *V/Q* relationships.

Nonpulmonary disorders

Patients with stable congestive cardiac failure often show mild reductions in Pao_2 and a normal or low $Paco_2$ due to premature airway closure secondary to pulmonary oedema. Some patients with severe liver cirrhosis develop the so-called hepatopulmonary syndrome, with otherwise unexplained hypoxaemia due to *V/Q* mismatching and true anatomical shunting through arteriovenous communications in the pulmonary circulation.

Morbidly obese individuals can develop hypoxaemia and hypercapnia due to profound nocturnal hypoventilation and chemoreceptor resetting. Rather more common are the problems of patients with severe obstructive sleep apnoea who develop daytime hypoxaemia and hypercapnia secondary to recurrent nocturnal upper airway obstruction and oxygen desaturation. Careful review of these 'Pickwickian' patients often shows coexisting hypothyroidism or obstructive lung disease, and this diagnosis should be suspected in any patient with COPD with significant respiratory failure and an FEV_1 greater than 1.5 litres. Correction of the sleep apnoea by nasal continuous positive airway pressure can produce significant improvement in daytime blood gases, but in most patients with obstructive sleep apnoea no significant abnormalities of waking gas exchange are seen.

Pulmonary vascular disease

This is an uncommon cause of hypoxaemia, and at the time of diagnosis CO_2 retention is rare. Rather variable changes in D_Lco are reported, but as pulmonary hypertension becomes more advanced, exercise and resting hypoxaemia develops, a significant component being secondary to the reduced cardiac output and increase in mixed venous oxygen tension.

Assessment of chronic respiratory failure

The diagnosis of mild/moderate hypoxaemia rests on an awareness of the possibility rather than any specific clinical finding. Impairment of concentration and memory can be demonstrated when the arterial Po_2 is below 8.0 kPa, but these features are extremely nonspecific. Although tempting to ascribe to hypoxaemia, the principal cause of breathlessness in these patients is usually the underlying disease. Reduction of peripheral chemoreceptor activity by supplementary oxygen can be beneficial, but this is usually secondary to a fall in minute ventilation rather that to any specific 'dyspnogenic' effect of hypoxia itself.

Hypercapnia is equally nonspecific, with headache the most commonly attributed symptom. There are no good data to support this in compensated respiratory failure, although a generalized degree of vasodilatation is seen in some patients with CO_2 retention, which may be accompanied by a large-volume pulse and warm peripheral extremities.

On examination, central cyanosis may be apparent as a bluish discoloration of the mucous membranes associated with an increase in the reduced circulating haemoglobin to approximately 5 g/dl, but this is an unreliable clinical sign in some ethnic groups and in the presence of artificial illumination. Chronic hypoxaemia can lead to secondary polycythaemia due to increased renal secretion of erythropoietin. This is usually seen when the patient is also a heavy smoker. The resulting increase in haemoglobin concentration contributes to a ruddy complexion, which increases the ability to detect cyanosis clinically. When right heart failure develops the jugular venous pressure may be elevated, and ankle swelling develops as CO_2 retention worsens.

The principal diagnostic steps are listed in Box 18.15.2. Measurement of arterial blood gases, preferably breathing air, is the most reliable way of diagnosing chronic respiratory failure. If a sample is taken when a patient is breathing supplementary oxygen, it is essential to record at what inspired concentration: without this information the Pao_2 simply cannot be interpreted sensibly. Patients with chronic airflow limitation treated with bronchodilators nebulized in oxygen may show unexpectedly high Pao_2 for some time after this treatment. Noninvasive measurement of arterial oxygen saturation using pulse oximetry can be used to screen individuals at risk of chronic respiratory failure and to monitor patients in hospital or overnight, but it is no substitute for assessing blood gas tensions to make the diagnosis correctly.

Box 18.15.2 Diagnostic steps in detecting respiratory failure

1 Consider the possibility—see Box 18.15.1

2 Look for central cyanosis and other clinical signs

3 If the probability is high or unanticipated signs are present, measure arterial blood gases while breathing air

4 If it is not possible to measure arterial blood gases on air, note the inspired oxygen concentration

5 Blood gas tensions can change with the clinical state of the patient and measurements need to be repeated when this happens

6 Noninvasive pulse oximetry is useful for monitoring progress but cannot diagnose hypercapnia or its acidosis

Treatment of chronic respiratory failure

Managing stable chronic respiratory failure involves several steps:

1 Making a firm diagnosis

2 Correcting the underlying disorder (when possible)

3 Increasing the inspired oxygen concentration

4 Increasing alveolar ventilation

Making a firm diagnosis

This is essential for rational management. It is important to remember that more than one process may contribute to the development of chronic respiratory failure; e.g. poor left ventricular function due to cardiac disease and COPD together. The relative importance of each factor should be determined.

Correction of the underlying disorder

In general, treatment of the primary pathology improves both V/Q relationships and hence oxygenation, and respiratory system mechanics, which increases ventilatory capacity and lowers the $Paco_2$. In patients with COPD this usually involves administration of inhaled bronchodilators and corticosteroids (see Chapter 18.8), but marked improvement is the exception rather than the rule in patients where chronic respiratory failure has developed. Medical therapy tends to be ineffective by the time chronic respiratory failure has developed in interstitial lung disease and the neuromuscular disorders.

Specific pulmonary vasodilator treatment has been used to treat pulmonary hypertension, with most evidence of improvement seen after infusion of prostacyclin in primary pulmonary hypertension. Attempts to improve gas exchange in secondary pulmonary hypertension by the use of inhaled nitric oxide, a specific pulmonary arterial vasodilator, have been disappointing and resting gas exchange has usually deteriorated rather than improved after this treatment.

Unfortunately there is no specific treatment for most neuromuscular diseases or the abnormalities of the thoracic skeleton which produce chronic respiratory failure. Dramatic weight loss after bariatric surgery is possible in patients with obesity–hypoventilation, but this treatment can be hazardous, particularly in subjects with deranged waking gas exchange, and most reports of improvement after surgery remain anecdotal rather than systematic.

Increasing the inspired oxygen concentration

Hypoxaemia secondary to V/Q mismatch or global hypoventilation is relatively easily corrected by supplementary oxygen. In chronic airflow limitation and especially COPD, where respiratory time constants for gas exchange are long, it may take 30 min before a new steady state is reached when breathing relatively low concentrations of oxygen. Monitoring of blood gases should be adjusted accordingly.

In the chronic stable state, treatment with oxygen is given to prevent or reverse the chronic consequences of hypoxaemia. The benefits of regular oxygen treatment on breathlessness are marginal and there are no data to suggest that the severity or subsequent progression of breathlessness is influenced by chronic oxygen treatment. Almost all data about oxygen therapy in chronic respiratory failure are based on observations in hypoxaemic COPD, treatment in other conditions being offered by analogy with this more common problem.

Two well-performed randomized clinical trials have shown that regular treatment of patients with COPD and stable hypoxaemia (Pao_2 <55 mmHg) prolongs life (Fig. 18.15.6a). These data suggest that patients using more oxygen (the 'continuous' limb of the Nocturnal Oxygen Therapy Trial Group) do better than either the United Kingdom Medical Research Council treatment group or the North American patients using oxygen only at night. A more recent Polish study found no benefit when patients with COPD with a Pao_2 of 7.3 to 8.8 kPa were treated with oxygen at home for 15 h/day (Fig. 18.15.6b), emphasizing that chronic oxygen therapy is only of value when the oxygen saturation falls below 90%.

These studies showed that progression of secondary pulmonary hypertension can be halted by regular oxygen treatment and secondary polycythaemia can be corrected. However, secondary polycythaemia in COPD is influenced by the amount of carboxyhaemoglobin from cigarettes, and patients who continue to smoke do not show a fall in red-cell mass or packed cell volumes with oxygen treatment. Neuropsychological effects of chronic hypoxaemia have been described and may be improved by regular oxygen treatment, although the evidence for this is limited.

Giving oxygen during exercise increases performance and particularly endurance in patients with COPD who are relatively normoxaemic, as well as those with resting hypoxaemia. Again carbon monoxide from cigarette smoking reduces this response, and whether oxygen desaturation during exercise is necessary for the benefit to occur has not been conclusively established, although

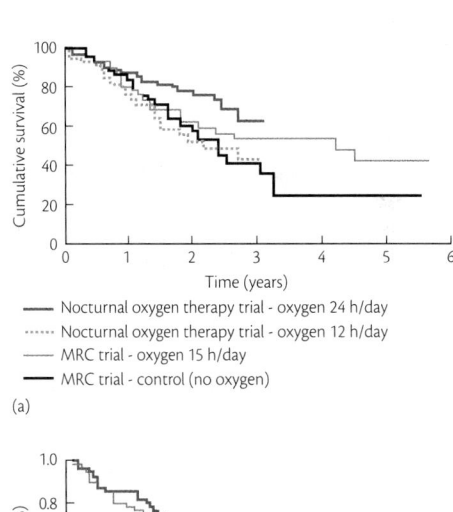

(a)

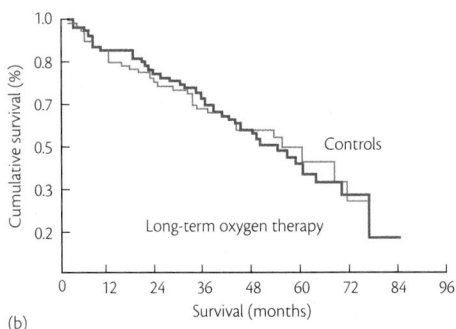

(b)

Fig. 18.15.6 The effect of regular domiciliary oxygen on survival in COPD. Panel (a) combines data from the MRC and NIH oxygen trial in the United States of America: survival was greatest in those receiving oxygen for 24 h/day. Panel (b) is based on the study of Gorecka *et al.* for COPD patients with a Pao_2 between 7.3 and 8.5 kPa who were treated with oxygen or normal medical therapy: there was no survival benefit in the oxygen treated group, confirming the importance of the 7.3-kPa threshold in selecting patients for this therapy.

it is used as a reimbursement criterion for portable oxygen in North America.

Oxygen concentrators are the most cost-effective way of delivering oxygen for near-continuous use. These devices have proved reliable and safe; they use the ability of zeolite cells to separate nitrogen from room air and so generate an oxygen-enriched inspirate. Liquid oxygen has the advantage of allowing relatively easy refilling of portable oxygen units for use during exercise. Oxygen masks are the most accurate way of delivering oxygen, with a range of inspired concentrations (24, 28, 35%) available. However, these are easily dislodged during sleep, and plastic nasal prongs with a long extension pipe offer an easier system for use in the home. Occasional patients, especially those with severe interstitial lung disease, may have difficulties obtaining a Pao_2 greater than 8.0 kPa with these systems. Transtracheal oxygen delivery may have a role here, but early enthusiasm for this has been tempered by problems with cannula occlusion, infection, and bleeding. A variety of oxygen-conserving devices that deliver oxygen only during inspiration have been developed which increase the time between refills of portable oxygen equipment as well as having financial advantages in some health care systems.

Improving alveolar ventilation

Mechanical

This is a potentially valuable way of reducing arterial CO_2 in disorders like COPD and can increase arterial oxygen tension as well, especially in conditions such as neuromuscular disease where hypoventilation predominates. The use of tank respirators in neuromuscular weakness has now been superseded by the development of noninvasive nasal positive-pressure ventilation (NIPPV), which is normally only needed at night. This therapy is used increasingly in the management of acute-on-chronic respiratory failure in patients where the primary problem is ventilatory without coexisting pneumonia/acute lung injury. Its chronic use arose from the belief that respiratory muscle fatigue was an important cause of CO_2 retention in COPD and the empirical observation that gas exchange and survival were better in patients with kyphoscoliosis treated with night-time cuirass ventilation. Newer studies have shown that respiratory muscle function is well preserved in COPD when allowance is made for the muscle shortening secondary to pulmonary hyperinflation. Several trials of NIPPV in stable hypoxaemic but normacapnic COPD have reported relatively unimpressive results. By contrast, NIPPV mainly given at night improved blood gases in patients with hypercapnic COPD, as well as leading to benefits in health status. No good randomized trial of this therapy has yet been reported and the role of NIPPV in the treatment of hypercapnic COPD is still controversial.

By contrast, significant symptomatic and blood gas improvements have been demonstrated in patients with kyphoscoliosis, but again no randomized clinical trial data are available. At present, it appears unlikely that trials will be set up, given the significant and sustained symptomatic benefits seen clinically. The only study to report prospective data on muscular dystrophy found no effect of regular NIPPV on survival in normocapnic patients, but use of this therapy as supportive treatment in the terminal phases of advanced muscular dystrophy appears to be associated with prolonged survival. A carefully constructed randomized control trial has shown improvements in survival and quality of life with NIPPV in those patients with motor neuron disease who are free from bulbar problems. However, it is always important in the face of progressive disease such as muscular dystrophy or motor neuron disease that the patient should be fully informed of the complications of NIPPV and the fact that it is unlikely to influence the underlying progression of the condition. Provided a good dialogue between patient, carer, and physician is established, then reasonable decisions about the use of this ethically difficult treatment are still possible.

Although volume-cycled ventilation was initially preferred, most patients are now managed with a bilevel pressure-cycled patient-triggered device. This may have some advantages in obstructive lung disease, where small amounts of PEEP can be added to reduce static PEEPi. Adequate peak inspiratory pressure generation, preferably in excess of 20 cmH$_2$O, is needed in both COPD and kyphoscoliosis, where total respiratory system compliance is reduced. The patient–mask interface remains a major problem, especially for those with unusual craniofacial structure where getting a comfortable mask fit without excessive tightness can be difficult. Progress should be assessed by regular blood gas measurements, and overnight monitoring of oxygenation and CO_2 tensions is useful at the start of therapy. Patience and trained respiratory therapists are the best way of ensuring long-term compliance with treatment.

Chronically ventilator dependent patients

In most patients with chronic respiratory failure who require ventilatory support the instigation of this treatment is a considered decision as part of the patient's ongoing management. However, for a few, chronic ventilation becomes necessary when they have presented with an acute life-threatening illness which has led to ventilatory support in the intensive care unit. Many of these patients would have previously succumbed from diseases with a poor initial prognosis, e.g. adult respiratory distress syndrome, but now survive to leave the intensive care unit, and inevitably some do not recover the level of lung function or independence which they had experienced before hospitalization. There is no universally agreed definition for this' ventilator dependence', but a patient who requires at least 6 h/day of ventilatory support for 21 or more days meets the most widely used operational approach. Patients of this type raise important ethical, logistical, and economic issues, but it is possible to offer them a good quality of life and a reasonable prognosis if they are cared for by appropriately trained staff in specialized units. In this setting many patients can be transferred from tracheostomy-dependent ventilation to NIPPV with a significant improvement in personal well-being and the options for community care. Given the continuing developments in critical care medicine, an increase in the number of patients with chronic respiratory failure who meet these criteria appears likely.

Specific pharmacological therapy

Although mechanical ventilatory support is effective, it is also cumbersome, uncomfortable, and restricting; hence a drug treatment for chronic respiratory failure would be invaluable. Although medroxyprogestrone acetate has nonspecific ventilatory stimulant effects and can produce small falls in CO_2 tension in patients with COPD, its oestrogen-like side effects limit its use. Methylxanthines like theophylline have some chemoreceptor stimulant effects, but are mainly of use for their bronchodilator and anti-inflammatory properties. Almitrine bismethylate is an interesting specific peripheral chemoreceptor stimulant drug, which also modifies intrapulmonary V/Q matching and increases arterial oxygen while reducing

CO_2 tensions in patients with resting hypoxaemia. These properties have led to its use in parts of Europe, but it is associated with the development of peripheral neuropathy and possibly increasing pulmonary artery pressure during exercise, which has limited its more widespread application.

Despite the attractions of a pharmacological approach, concerns over the precipitation of inspiratory muscle fatigue and the recognition that, in most diseases, the central drive to breathe is already high, mean that treatment with respiratory stimulant therapy is likely to have only limited clinical application.

Further reading

Anonymous (1980). Continuous or nocturnal oxygen therapy in hypoxemic chronic obstructive lung disease: a clinical trial. Nocturnal Oxygen Therapy Trial Group. *Ann Intern Med*, **93**, 391–8.

Anonymous (1981). Long term domiciliary oxygen therapy in chronic hypoxic cor pulmonale complicating chronic bronchitis and emphysema. Report of the Medical Research Council Working Party. *Lancet*, **i**, 681–6.

Bourke SC, *et al.* (2006). Effects of non-invasive ventilation on survival and quality of life in patients with amyotrophic lateral sclerosis: a randomized control trial. *Lancet Neurol*, **2**, 40–7.

Calverley PM, Leggett RJ, Flenley DC (1981). Carbon monoxide and exercise tolerance in chronic bronchitis and emphysema. *BMJ*, **283**, 878–80.

Calverley PM, *et al.* (1982). Cigarette smoking and secondary polycythemia in hypoxic cor pulmonale. *Am Rev Respir Dis*, **125**, 507–10.

Costello R, *et al.* (1997). Reversible hypercapnia in chronic obstructive pulmonary disease: a distinct pattern of respiratory failure with a favorable prognosis. *Am J Med*, **102**, 239–44.

Gorecka D, *et al.* (1997). Effect of long-term oxygen therapy on survival in patients with chronic obstructive pulmonary disease with moderate hypoxaemia. *Thorax*, **52**, 674–9.

Haluszka J, *et al.* (1990). Intrinsic PEEP and arterial P_{CO_2} in stable patients with chronic obstructive pulmonary disease. *Am Rev Respir Dis*, **141**, 1194–7.

MacIntyre NR, *et al.* (2005). The management of patients requiring prolonged mechanical ventilation: report of a NAMDRC concensus conference. *Chest*, **128**, 3937–54.

Meecham JD, *et al.* (1995). Nasal pressure support ventilation plus oxygen compared with oxygen therapy alone in hypercapnic COPD. *Am J Respir CritCare Med*, **152**, 538–44.

Olson AL, Zwillich C (2005). The obesity hypoventilation syndrome. *Am J Med*, **118**, 948–56.

Phillips MF, *et al.* (1999). Nocturnal oxygenation and prognosis in Duchenne muscular dystrophy. *Am J Respir Crit Care Med*, **160**, 198–202.

Raphael JC, *et al.* (1994). Randomised trial of preventive nasal ventilation in Duchenne muscular dystrophy. French Multicentre Cooperative Group on Home Mechanical Ventilation Assistance in Duchenne de Boulogne Muscular Dystrophy. *Lancet*, **343**, 1600–4.

Rodriguez-Roisin R (2003). Pulmonary gas exchange. In: Gibson GJ, *et al.* (eds) *Respiratory medicine*, 3rd edition, pp. 130–46, W B Saunders, London.

Lung transplantation

K. McNeil

Essentials

Lung transplantation offers the only therapeutic option for many patients with a variety of endstage pulmonary and cardiopulmonary diseases, but organs are scarce and the major challenge facing lung transplantation (as with all solid organ transplants) is the critical shortage of donor organs.

Recipient selection—emphysema/chronic obstructive pulmonary disease (COPD), cystic fibrosis, idiopathic pulmonary fibrosis, and pulmonary vascular disease are the main disease groups referred for lung transplantation. Most patients are listed for transplantation when their survival is estimated to be less than 2 years without a transplant. Exclusion criteria include malignancy (excluding localized skin malignancies) within the last 2 years, inability to cooperate or comply with medical therapy/instruction, recent substance addiction, active or noncurable extrapulmonary infection, significant chest wall/spinal deformity, and significant extrathoracic organ dysfunction.

Donor selection—most organs come from cadaveric donors who have sustained brainstem death, are free of systemic infection and disease, and who have satisfactory lung function (arterial oxygen level ≥35 kPa (300 mmHg) on 100% inspired O_2, with airways free of purulent secretions, and chest radiograph free of consolidation). Increasingly however, more liberal acceptance criteria are being applied along with the use of lungs from non-heart beating donors, in an attempt to overcome the critical shortage of donor lungs. Donor/recipient matching is on the basis of ABO blood group, as in blood transfusion practice, and size.

Transplant (surgical) procedure—three types of transplant are performed: (1) single lung transplantation, (2) bilateral sequential single or double lung transplantation (required for septic lung diseases and preferred for younger patients with COPD), and (3) heart–lung transplantation (required for Eisenmenger's syndrome).

Immediate post-transplantation management—important issues are early extubation, fluid (crystalloid) restriction and diuresis, early mobilization, ensuring adequate nutrition, and prevention of infection (with antibacterial, antifungal, antipneumocystis, and anticytomegalovirus prophylaxis).

Immunosuppression—most centres employ a combination of an induction regimen based on either (antithymocyte globulin (ATG) or interleukin-2 receptor (IL-2R) blocker) followed by triple therapy with a calcineurin inhibitor (ciclosporin or tacrolimus), a lymphocyte proliferation inhibitor (azathioprine or mycophenolate), and a corticosteroid (usually prednisolone).

Longer-term management—the incidence of acute rejection and infection are highest in the first 3 months. Acute rejection is diagnosed via transbronchial biopsy and defined by perivascular lymphocytic infiltrates of varying severity, graded from minimal (grade 1) to severe (grade 4): it is usually treated with intravenous methyprednisolone. Chronic rejection is defined histologically by airway fibrosis with/without accompanying vascular sclerosis (obliterative bronchiolitis). The bronchiolitis obliterans syndrome is defined clinically and graded by a fall in the forced expiratory volume in 1s (FEV_1), as measured from the patient's baseline (best achieved after transplantation). This condition is the main cause of death in long-term survivors of lung transplantation, with complicating infection the most common terminal event. Gastro-oesophageal reflux contributes significantly to both acute and chronic allograft dysfunction and is likely to be a major contributor to the development and progression of the bronchiolitis obliterans syndrome, hence there should be a low threshold for investigation with oesophageal pH monitoring, and an equally low threshold for laparoscopic fundoplication if significant reflux is demonstrated. Solid organ and lymphoid malignancies affect up to 4% of recipients.

Prognosis—survival figures of 80 to 90% at 1 year and 50 to 60% at 5 years are achievable for all types of lung transplant and underlying disease categories. Many patients are able to return to work and live a near normal life. Several female recipients have undergone normal pregnancies without complications.

Introduction

For many patients with endstage lung disease the only prospect for survival and improved quality of life is through a successful lung transplant. The first (heart–)lung transplant was performed in 1981, and since then over 30 000 pulmonary transplants have been reported to the registry of the International Society for Heart and Lung Transplantation (ISHLT). This number, however, falls considerably short of the number of patients with advanced lung disease who might benefit from lung transplantation, and the major challenge facing lung transplantation (as with all solid organ transplants) is the critical shortage of donor organs. Increasing pressure on waiting lists has translated into much more liberal donor acceptance criteria (including the use of non-heart beating donors) with donors over the age of 45 now becoming the norm rather than the exception. Despite this apparent reduction in donor quality, survival following lung transplantation has improved to the point where a first-time lung or heart–lung transplant recipient has a 50 to 60% chance of surviving for 5 years or more.

Infection remains the most significant problem encountered by the lung transplant recipient at any time. The lung allograft is unique within solid organ transplants in that it is in direct contact with the external environment. This directly and continuously exposes the allograft to potential infections and allergens, which in turn predisposes the allograft to many of the numerous problems encountered both early and late after transplantation.

Obliterative bronchiolitis (OB) remains the most significant challenge faced by lung transplant recipients and lung transplant physicians in the long term, with most deaths after the first year attributable to this complication. However, the impact of OB is lessening, and recipients are enjoying improved quality of life for many years.

The transplant process

The transplant process as a whole is an amalgamation of six separate steps—recipient selection, donor selection, donor/recipient matching, the transplant (surgical) procedure, immediate post-transplantation care, and longer-term monitoring. Each of these steps is critical in its own right: a compromise in any one of these areas can spell disaster for the overall outcome.

Lung transplantation is also unique amongst solid organ transplants in that there are different transplant options available (single lung, bilateral lung, and combined heart–lung), with the choice of procedure determined primarily by the recipient's underlying disease process.

Recipient selection

Most pulmonary diseases can be considered for transplantation, with emphysema/chronic obstructive pulmonary disease (COPD, including α_1-antitrypsin deficiency), cystic fibrosis, idiopathic pulmonary fibrosis, and pulmonary vascular disease (idiopathic pulmonary arterial hypertension (iPAH) and Eisenmenger's syndrome) being the main disease groups referred for lung transplantation.

Disease (or the major impact of any disease process) should be confined to the thorax, although in carefully selected patients some systemic diseases with predominantly pulmonary manifestations (scleroderma, sarcoidosis, etc.) can be transplanted successfully. There are also limited opportunities (largely dictated by donor organ availability and allocation policies) for combined organ transplantation, such as heart–lung–liver transplantation in patients with cystic fibrosis.

Most patients are listed for transplantation when their survival is estimated to be less than 2 years without a transplant. The prognosis of patients with cystic fibrosis, idiopathic pulmonary arterial hypertension, and cryptogenic fibrosing alveolitis can be estimated within this sort of time frame. In patients with Eisenmenger's syndrome and emphysema however, survival on the waiting list is less predictable, and in some cases can be as good if not better than following a transplant: transplantation in this setting is performed primarily for quality-of-life issues. Box 18.16.1 summarizes the specific disease referral recommendations, based on guidelines published by the ISHLT.

Contraindications to transplantation are based on the experience gained in this field over the last 20 years and are well defined. Lung transplantation is a complex undertaking, associated with significant mortality and the potential for significant morbidity, and patients with a bigger burden of disease (including age) simply do not fare as well after a lung transplant as younger and (in relative terms) fitter patients. Most contraindications are relative and are considered in the context of the patient's overall status and expected outcome. Patients are generally considered up to 65 years of age, but many units have an upper limit of 60 years in view of a shortage of donors and poorer outcomes in the older recipient group. As noted above, selected patients with coexisting advanced kidney or liver disease can be considered for combined thoracic and abdominal organ transplant procedures.

'Absolute' exclusion criteria for transplantation are confined to malignancy (excluding localized cutaneous malignancies) within the last 2 years, untreatable psychiatric conditions or social issues associated with an inability to cooperate or comply with medical therapy/instruction, recent (within 6 months) substance addiction, active or noncurable extrapulmonary infection, significant chest wall/spinal deformity, and significant extrathoracic organ dysfunction (with the exceptions noted above).

A number of diseases for which lung transplantation is applicable can recur after transplantation, including sarcoidosis and some hard metal pneumoconioses, pulmonary lymphangioleiomyomatosis, histiocytosis, and desquamative interstitial pneumonitis. As a general rule, recurrence of these conditions does not significantly affect the transplant outcome, but on occasions they do cause diagnostic dilemmas. Cystic fibrosis does not directly affect lung allografts (which do not carry the genetic abnormality), and idiopathic pulmonary arterial hypertension has not been documented to recur after transplantation.

Donor selection

The vast majority of lung allografts are procured from cadaveric donors who have sustained brainstem death. A small number of living related lung transplants are performed, and a small (but likely to increase) number of transplants from deceased cardiac (non-heart beating) donors. The following details refer primarily to donors sustaining brainstem death, but the principles applying to the selection of a lung allograft from any type of donor are the same.

All donors should be free of systemic infection or disease. The allograft is assessed on the basis of function (gas exchange and compliance) and appearance (macroscopic, bronchoscopic, and radiographic). In heart–lung transplantation, cardiac function is assessed via haemodynamic performance based on systemic arterial and venous pressures, urine output and occasionally via Swann–Ganz catheterization. The heart is also inspected macroscopically

---

Box 18.16.1 Disease-specific indications for lung transplantation (based on ISHLT guidelines)

Patients with the following characteristics should be considered for *referral* for transplant assessment.

Obstructive lung disease

- BODE index of 5–7
- FEV_1 <25% predicted
- Diffusing capacity of the lung for carbon monoxide ($D_L$co) <20%
- Homogenous emphysema
- Respiratory failure
- Cor pulmonale

Cystic fibrosis

The following parameters are associated with 20% 2-year survival on the waiting list, and ideally patients will be referred for assessment before reaching them:

- FEV_1 <25% predicted
- Respiratory failure
- Severely reduced exercise capacity—≤500 m on a 12-min walk or equivalent
- Compromised nutrition—BMI ≤16

In addition, early referral should be considered for:

- Adolescent females with rapidly declining lung function
- Patients with increasingly frequent and difficult infective exacerbations
- Patients with recurrent severe haemoptysis
- Patients with multiple antibiotic resistant organisms

Idiopathic pulmonary arterial hypertension

- WHO functional class III or IV
- Requirement for increasing doses of prostacyclin

The following parameters are associated with a median survival of only 12 months and/or an overall survival of < 20% at 3 years and are also indications for referral:

- Mean right atrial pressure >15 mmHg
- Mixed venous oxygen saturation <60%
- Cardiac index <2.0 litres/min per m^2
- 6-min walk test <350 m

Eisenmenger's syndrome

- Severely compromised quality of life
- Refractory right heart failure
- Frequent presyncopal or syncopal events
- Poorly controlled arrhythmia

Eisenmenger's syndrome patients with complex lesions and/or repairs tend to benefit from transplantation in their third decade: those with 'simple' lesions such as VSD and PDA tend to come to transplantation later, in their fourth decade.

Idiopathic pulmonary fibrosis

These patients often deteriorate rapidly, with no effective treatment and up to a 50% death rate on the waiting list after only 12 months. Consequently, they should *all* be referred early. Gas transfer values <60% predicted are indicative of advanced disease.

PDA, patent ductus arteriousus; VSD, ventricular septal defect.

---

to assess contractility and the appearance of the coronary arteries. If indicated (and available), coronary angiography and/or echocardiography may be performed, but these investigations are not routinely available at every donor hospital.

Lung donors are generally under 55 years of age, although because of the critical shortage of donor organs there is an increasing trend to accept organs from donors older than this if function (as assessed above) is acceptable. Older donors are more prone to early graft dysfunction, and this is particularly the case in combination with longer ischaemic times. Unlike the situation in heart transplantation, there are limited options for improving lung allograft function in the donor prior to retrieval. Nonetheless, it is important to optimize lung allograft function by employing ventilator strategies that minimize barotrauma, perform active airway clearance to prevent accumulation of secretions and basal collapse, and use cautious fluid resuscitation of the donor to avoid pulmonary oedema.

A potential lung allograft will generally be considered acceptable if, just before retrieval, the arterial oxygen level is at least 300 mmHg (35 kPa) on 100% inspired O_2, airways are free of purulent secretions, and a chest radiograph is free of consolidation. However, suitability is always considered in the light of donor age, projected ischaemic time, and condition of the potential recipient.

Donor/recipient matching

Matching the donor organ with a suitable recipient is done simply on the basis of ABO blood group, with the same principles of ABO matching applying in solid organ transplantation as in blood transfusion practice, and size (based on total lung capacity). Perfect size matching is rarely achieved because recipients will have either a restricted or hyperinflated chest cavity reflecting their underlying disease process (e.g. pulmonary fibrosis and emphysema respectively). Size-matching algorithms are largely based on the experience of the lung transplant team, who need to take into account measured and predicted total lung capacity (TLC) of the recipient, predicted TLC of the donor, and the type of transplant being performed (single or bilateral lung transplant). As a general rule, oversizing should be avoided as the resultant lung compression and atelectasis predisposes to postoperative infection.

Surgery

Management of the donor, allograft preservation, and surgical retrieval of allograft(s) are outside the scope of this chapter (but for information, see Further Reading).

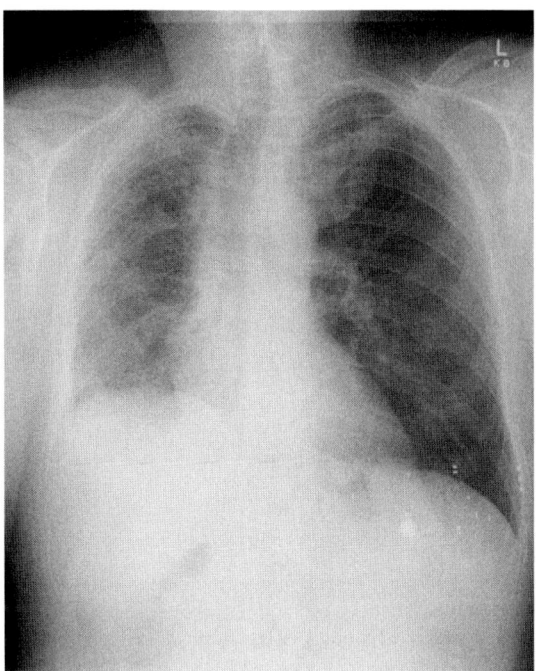

Fig. 18.16.1 Chest radiograph of a patient with a left single lung transplant for pulmonary fibrosis. Note the hyperinflation of the allograft.

There are three basic options available when replacing diseased lung tissue—single lung transplantation, bilateral sequential single lung (or double lung) transplantation, and heart–lung transplantation. The choice of procedure is determined by the recipient's underlying disease process, by the expected outcome of the procedure in terms of survival and functional result, and on occasions by surgical preference. The commonest disease indications for bilateral lung transplantation have been cystic fibrosis (30%) and COPD/emphysema (24%), and for single lung transplantation, COPD/emphysema (53%) and idiopathic pulmonary fibrosis (26%). However, it is now recognized that bilateral sequential single lung transplantation is superior to single lung transplantation in terms of both long-term survival and functional status for recipients with emphysema/COPD. Thus, for younger patients with emphysema/COPD (including α_1-antitrypsin

deficiency), bilateral lung replacement is now the preferred transplant option.

Septic lung diseases such as cystic fibrosis and bronchiectasis require the replacement of both lungs (either bilateral lung transplantation or heart–lung transplantation). Diseases such as Eisenmenger's syndrome that involve both the heart and lungs mandate combined heart–lung replacement. Some centres/surgeons also prefer heart–lung transplantation for idiopathic pulmonary arterial hypertension, which avoids issues in the immediate post-transplantation period with a severely dysfunctional right ventricle, and in cystic fibrosis, where the option for domino heart transplantation maximizes organ utilization (the heart from the heart–lung transplant recipient is used for a patient requiring a heart transplant).

Single lung transplantation can be applied to most other diseases but is most effectively used in patients with pulmonary fibrosis (Fig. 18.16.1). In this situation the underlying restrictive lung disease allows hyperinflation of the allograft, and as a consequence these recipients will often achieve near-normal spirometry despite only receiving a single lung. Older patients with emphysema will also benefit significantly from single lung transplantation because longer-term functional requirements in this group are not as demanding as those in younger individuals.

Bilateral lung transplantation is performed as two sequential single lung transplantations and can be done via a sternotomy, a bilateral thoracotomy, or a 'clamshell' incision which involves a bilateral thoracotomy with transection of the lower sternum (Fig. 18.16.2). Heart–lung transplantation mandates cardiopulmonary bypass and is performed via a sternotomy or clamshell approach. Bilateral sequential single lung transplantation can be performed with or without cardiopulmonary bypass dependent on the underlying disease (e.g. severe pulmonary hypertension almost always requires cardiopulmonary bypass), and surgical/anaesthetic preference.

A number of surgical principles are essential for a successful outcome from any form of lung transplantation. Careful and unhurried dissection minimizes intra- and postoperative bleeding, and avoids damage to mediastinal (phrenic, vagus, and recurrent laryngeal) nerves. Careful implantation reduces the chances of vascular or airway anastamotic complications after transplantation. Technical complications, which are virtually all avoidable, are responsible for 8.4% of the early deaths reported in the ISHLT registry.

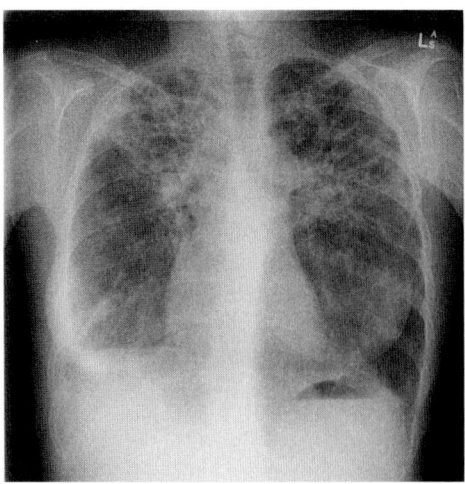
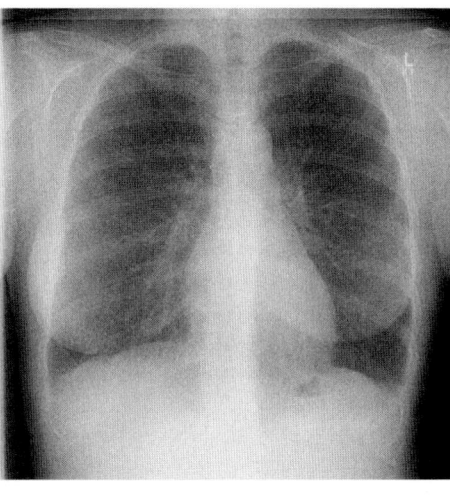

Fig. 18.16.2 Chest radiographs taken before (left panel) and after (right panel) bilateral sequential single lung transplant in a patient with cystic fibrosis.

Implantation and reperfusion should ideally be achieved within 6 h because shorter ischaemic times are generally associated with better immediate and short-term results (particularly when older donors are utilized) as there is less propensity for development of ischaemia/reperfusion injury (see below). Likewise, controlled reperfusion of the allograft(s) using low pressures over a prolonged (≥10 min) period is also associated with reduced risk of severe reperfusion injury and therefore improved early allograft function and outcome.

Postoperative care

The 24 to 48 h after reperfusion of the allograft(s) are critical for minimizing early complications and setting the scene for a good long-term result. Immediate postoperative care is aimed specifically at reducing the impact of the ischaemia/reperfusion injury that is sustained by all lung allografts to some degree, and is the underlying cause of primary lung allograft dysfunction, which is reported in the ISHLT registry to be the major cause (28.4%) of death within 30 days of transplantation. The pathophysiology of this process involves injury to and consequent dysfunction of the pulmonary vascular endothelium, resulting in a breakdown of the normal alveolar–capillary endothelial barrier, the endothelial injury itself being perpetuated by ventilator-induced barotrauma and infection. This manifests as leakage of fluid into alveoli (pulmonary oedema) and impaired gas exchange and is essentially a form of acute lung injury, which in its severest form results in diffuse alveolar damage with all its consequences. Severe pulmonary oedema can be precipitated by injudicious fluid management, even in cases where the initially injury is only mild. Severe injury inevitably results in prolonged mechanical ventilatory support with the increased risk of more infection and barotrauma, thus perpetuating the injury and potentially leading to irreversible damage to the allograft. Any bleeding requiring resuscitative fluid efforts inevitably results in severe pulmonary oedema, the requirement for increased ventilatory support, which again will be associated with the aforementioned problems, hence all efforts should be made to ensure haemostasis at the conclusion of the transplant procedure.

With careful management most cases of severe ischaemia/reperfusion injury will resolve over a few days. There is no specific treatment, although there are promising early reports of the use of exogenous surfactant therapy (instilled into distal airways via a fibre-optic bronchoscope). Nitric oxide can improve gas exchange and thus reduce ventilation pressures, but as yet has not been shown to alter outcomes.

In addition to ischaemia/reperfusion injury, the other major cause of postoperative morbidity and mortality is noncytomegalovirus (CMV) infection (predominantly bacterial), which accounts for 21% of reported 30-day mortality.

Key issues in early postoperative management are as follows.

Early extubation

Extubation is possible within 12 h of the procedure in most patients, and in many cases much earlier than this, which permits active coughing and clearance of secretions, the institution of enteral nutrition, and the early commencement of rehabilitation.

Fluid (crystalloid) restriction and diuresis

This minimizes the development of pulmonary oedema, thus optimizing gas exchange and enabling early extubation. Colloid solutions are used for haemodynamic requirements, with vigorous diuresis achieved by regular administration of a loop diuretic (furosemide). Diuresis (removal of water) should not be discontinued simply because colloid is required to maintain filling pressures, and total input of oral fluids and intravenous crystalloid (combined) should be rigorously restricted to 1500 ml/24 h (or thereabouts) in association with vigorous diuresis for at least the first 48 h.

Early mobilization

Patients with endstage lung disease are usually debilitated and it is important they are mobilized and commence rehabilitation as early as possible. This prevents complications such as basal atelectasis and deep venous thrombosis, improves appetite and promotes sleep. Most patients are able to sit out of bed within 24 h and can participate in a gymnasium programme by day 3. Adequate analgesia is imperative for effective rehabilitation at this early stage, with epidural anaesthesia very effective for pain control following thoracotomy or clamshell incisions.

Nutrition

Patients with endstage lung disease are usually nutritionally compromised and an adequate calorie intake is necessary to overcome the severe catabolism stimulated by surgery. Enteral feeding can usually be started within 24 h (either orally or via a nasogastric tube), but parenteral nutrition should be considered if the gut is not functioning.

One issue that has been increasingly recognized as a potential cause of early allograft dysfunction is gastro-oesophageal reflux. This can be a particular problem in patients with cystic fibrosis, and can be exacerbated by mediastinal nerve injury (usually reversible) sustained during the transplant procedure. The problem is discussed in more detail below.

Prevention of infection

Bacterial infection remains the most significant problem encountered in the perioperative period and is responsible for most deaths during the first 30 days. It is a significant factor in the exacerbation of ischaemia/reperfusion injury and acute lung injury, and is the final common pathway of death in most cases affected by this problem. The organisms encountered are usually recipient derived, hence antibiotic prophylaxis (started immediately before transplantation) is tailored according to the recipient's known or likely microbiology and administered until the patient is mobile, all drains have been removed, and respiratory secretions are clear. Antibiotics are chosen to cover *Pseudomonas aeruginosa* and *Staphylococcus aureus* in cystic fibrosis and other septic lung diseases, and patients with these conditions will usually have well-documented microbiology, antibiotic sensitivity, and drug allergy data available to aid in the choice. In other patients, community-acquired respiratory pathogens (pneumococcus, haemophilus, etc) and *Staphylococcus aureus* are targeted. Many units administer vancomycin to cover the transplantation procedure and subsequent 48 h until MRSA cultures are confirmed negative. However, despite the availability of effective antibiotics it should be stressed again that the most effective strategy for prevention of bacterial infection after transplantation is early extubation and mobilization.

Oropharyngeal candidiasis is common after transplantation and is effectively controlled with topical nyststin or amphotericin: routine systemic prophylaxis against candida is not generally necessary.

Aspergillus is the commonest cause of invasive fungal disease in the early postoperative period, and in single and bilateral lung

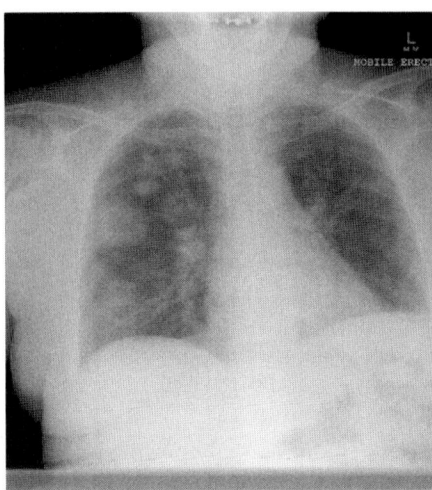
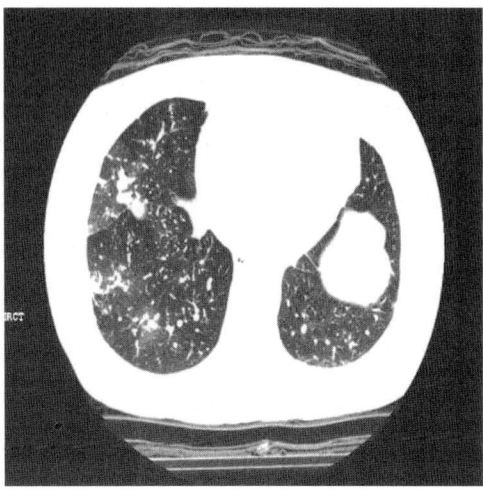

Fig. 18.16.3 Chest radiograph and CT showing invasive aspergillosis after bilateral lung transplant.

transplantation the ischaemic airways render patients at particular risk of developing this infection and related complications. They are at increased risk if exposed to high aspergillus loads, such as can occur in the setting of hospital building work (Figs. 18.16.3 and 18.16.4). Nebulized amphotericin prophylaxis given for the first month after transplantation is effective in reducing aspergillus-related problems. Prophylaxis with itraconazole or voriconazole is dependent on local policy and experience. Documented aspergillus infection is treated with either liposomal amphotericin B or voriconazole, with caspofungin used if these agents are ineffective or not tolerated. Widespread invasive disease may require combination therapy.

Viral infections (specifically herpesviruses) tend to occur later in the recovery period, but prophylaxis must be administered from the early stages to be effective. Ganciclovir is very effective in reducing both the incidence and severity of CMV-related illness. There is no consensus on the optimal prophylaxis regimen, but most units opt for a combination of intravenous followed by oral therapy for 1 to 3 months. The newer oral formulation of ganciclovir (valganciclovir) is well absorbed and achieves equivalent blood concentrations to intravenous therapy. Herpes simplex virus (HSV), which most commonly causes mucocutaneous infection and occasionally lower airway infection, is also effectively covered by ganciclovir.

Co-trimoxazole prophylaxis is effective in preventing both pneumocystis infection and toxoplasma reactivation. Standard therapy is 480 mg daily or 960 mg three times a week. Therapy is usually continued for 12 months or until corticosteroid doses have been reduced to those required for physiological replacement. Nebulized pentamidine (300 mg/month) is an effective alternative for those who cannot take co-trimoxazole.

Immunosuppression

Three phases of immunosuppression are used in lung transplantation—induction, consolidation, and maintenance. Although the

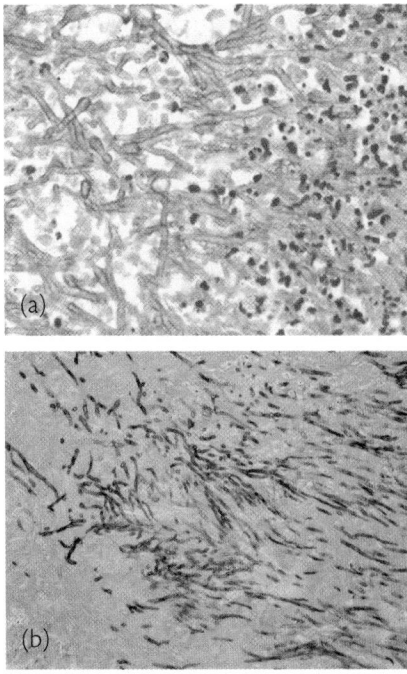
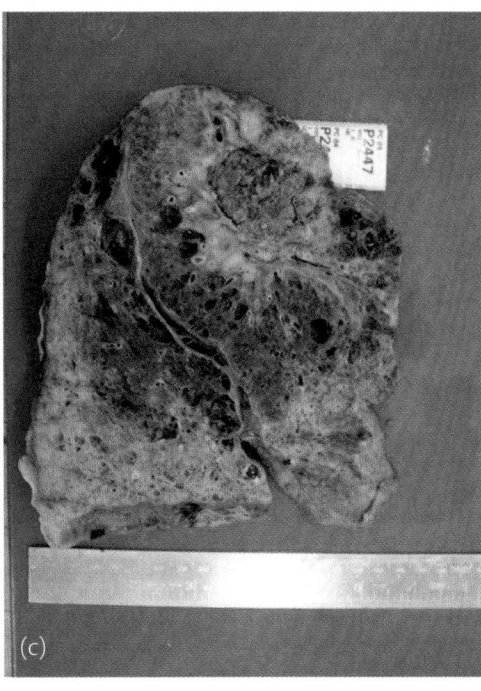

Fig. 18.16.4 (a) Hyphae of aspergillus seen in sputum. (b) Hyphae of aspergillus seen within a heart valve in a case of aspergillus endocarditis after bilateral sequential single lung transplant. (c) Aspergilloma in the upper lobe of an explanted lung.

details of the exact combinations and doses of agents used vary from unit to unit, the principles are similar.

Most regimens employ a combination of three agents—a calcineurin inhibitor (CNI—ciclosporin or tacrolimus), a lymphocyte proliferation inhibitor (azathioprine or mycophenolate), and a corticosteroid (usually prednisolone). Induction therapy, given either immediately before or after transplantation, is used variably in lung transplantation according to individual unit protocols and/or individual patient requirements. There is no consistent or conclusive evidence that induction with any agent is associated with better or worse outcomes compared with no induction therapy, but data from the ISHLT registry in 2006 showed for the first time a small favourable impact of induction therapy on long-term survival (conditional on 14-day survival) in lung transplant recipients. Other benefits such as the ability to introduce CNI therapy more slowly in patients with renal dysfunction, and a reduction in the number of episodes of acute rejection, have also been reported.

Induction agents

Induction agents commonly used are antithymocyte globulin (ATG) and interleukin-2 receptor (IL-2R) blockers. ATG is a polyclonal immunoglobulin directed at T lymphocytes. Use of this agent for 3 to 7 days is associated with profound depletion of circulating T cells and nonspecific immunomodulatory effects which appear to affect B-cell functions, although there is no direct B-cell depleting action. Use of ATG is associated with an increased incidence of side effects, the most important being infection and malignancy, but these are much reduced with shorter (3-day) and less intense courses such that the risk of infection at 1 year and malignancy at 10 years is no different from a cohort who received no induction therapy.

Monoclonal antibodies directed at IL-2R are increasingly being used for induction in lung transplantation, with evidence for this practice being extrapolated from other solid organ (particularly kidney) models or taken from small clinical series. IL-2 is an important signalling molecule leading to the proliferation of activated T cells, hence blocking this signal is very effective at reducing T-cell alloreactivity. The safety and side-effect profile of these agents (either dacluzimab or basiliximab) appears to be excellent, and apart from the cost and need for intravenous administration, there seems to be little disadvantage to the use of this class of drugs.

Calcineurin inhibitors (CNIs)

CNIs are the cornerstone of immunosuppressive regimens in all solid organ transplants: they work by preventing IL-2 production by T cells. Ciclosporin and tacrolimus are the two agents used from this class of drugs. Although they have similar immunosuppressive efficacy, there are several important differences in side-effect profiles which dictate use of one or other agent in individual patients. Ciclosporin causes upregulation of TGF-β production and as such contributes to the growth of tissue in general. This can result in cosmetic issues with hirsutism and gum hypertrophy, and overgrowth of nasal polyps, particularly in patients with cystic fibrosis. For this reason, tacrolimus (which does not have these effects) is often substituted for ciclosporin at the onset of bronchiolitis obliterans syndrome in an attempt to reduce airway scarring (see below). Tacrolimus is diabetogenic, whereas ciclosporin is not. Both agents list nephrotoxicity, hypertension, and dyslipidaemia amongst their extensive side effect profiles.

Antiproliferative agents

These agents act to directly suppress lymphocyte proliferation at the bone marrow level. Azathioprine is a purine analogue, converted to 6-mercaptopurine in the liver. It inhibits the early stages of purine metabolism as well as blocking several enzyme systems, leading to a reduction in the synthesis of nucleic acids. Its major side effects are bone marrow suppression and gastrointestinal (including liver) toxicity. Mycophenolate mofetil (MMF) is an inhibitor of IMPDH and works in a similar fashion to azathioprine, interfering with de novo DNA synthesis. Major side effects are also gastrointestinal toxicity and bone marrow suppression. Mycophenolate may have additional clinical benefits in transplantation as it has a potent anti-B cell effect, including inhibition of the Epstein–Barr virus (EBV)-driven B-cell replication responsible for post-transplantation lymphoproliferative disorders. Furthermore, in heart transplantation the use of MMF in standard immunosuppressive regimens has been shown to be associated with a significantly lower risk of developing malignancy in general.

Corticosteroids

Corticosteroids have a number of effects on the immune system, disrupting a variety of signalling and transcription pathways. This results in a nonspecific anti-inflammatory response, with a predominantly lympholytic action when used in high doses. Prednisolone is most commonly used, either in small oral doses in combination with a CNI and an antimetabolite as part of a triple maintenance regimen, or in high doses as intravenous methylprednisolone as part of the transplant induction regimen or for treatment of episodes of acute rejection or nonspecific allograft dysfunction (e.g. organizing pneumonia).

Newer agents

Newer immunosuppressive agents in clinical use include the mTOR (mammalian Target Of Rapamycin) inhibitors sirolimus and everolimus. These drugs are structurally similar to tacrolimus (all are macrolide antibiotics) but work downstream of CNIs, interfering with the T-cell response to IL-2 signalling by preventing the progression of the T cell from the G1 to the S phase of the cell cycle. They also have a powerful antiproliferative action and are generally not used immediately after transplantation because of their adverse effect on wound healing (including airway anastamoses). Other major side effects include oral ulceration, skin rash, haematological (thrombocytopaenia, anaemia), disturbances and dyslipidaemia. Experience with these agents in lung transplantation is limited: thus far they have mainly been used in bronchiolitis obliterans syndrome because of their antiproliferative effects, and also as CNI-sparing agents in cases of significant renal impairment. However, caution should be exercised if these agents are used for the latter indication: some (but not all) trials in kidney and heart transplantation, and anecdotal reports in lung transplantation, have highlighted an unacceptably high rate of acute rejection when mTOR inhibitors have been used without any adjunctive CNI therapy.

Longer term monitoring

The incidence of acute rejection and infection is highest in the first 3 months. Acute rejection episodes are uncommon after 6 months unless immunosuppression strategies are changed (either intentionally or through noncompliance), but infection remains an ever-present threat.

Baseline lung function is usually established by 6 to 9 months after transplantation, this level being used to define bronchiolitis obliterans syndrome, discussed in detail below, which is the greatest threat to long-term survival and quality of life faced by lung transplant recipients.

The thrust of long-term management is to maintain allograft function and to minimize the side effects of immunosuppression. As a general principle, immunosuppression should be gradually reduced, but dose adjustments of all agents must be tailored to individual requirements, balancing the need to prevent acute rejection against reduction of adverse effects.

As time from the transplant increases, outpatient visits occur less frequently. Monitoring of symptoms, chest radiography, and spirometry are the basis of allograft surveillance. Small handheld spirometers enable daily home monitoring of lung function, with a 10% or greater fall in the forced expiratory volume in 1 s (FEV_1) prompting review and investigation of the cause.

Bronchoscopy and transbronchial biopsy are performed in the event of allograft dysfunction. Acute rejection and infection cannot be distinguished clinically and may occur simultaneously, hence histopathological confirmation of the cause(s) of dysfunction is highly desirable. Some units perform regular surveillance transbronchial biopsies, but there is no evidence that this improves long-term outcome.

Specific complications

Many of the complications experienced by lung transplant recipients are common to all forms of solid organ transplantation and relate to immunosuppressive drug side effects, including the increased risk of infection. The following discussion focuses on issues specific to lung transplantation.

Rejection

As in all solid organ transplantation, the lung allograft is at risk of both acute and so-called 'chronic' rejection. These are defined not by their timing of occurrence after transplantation but by their histopathology and/or clinical presentation. Acute rejection can occur at any time after transplantation and is directly related to the efficacy of the immunosuppression strategy used. Chronic rejection can occur early (in the first year after transplantation), but is more commonly seen after 2 to 3 years. The two processes can coexist. Histopathological criteria for the diagnosis and grading of rejection have been published by the ISHLT.

Hyperacute (antibody-mediated) rejection

This is a very rare cause of primary graft failure in lung transplantation. It is caused by preformed anti-HLA antibodies in the recipient, which activate complement, leading to rapid destruction of the allograft. Plasma exchange, intravenous immunoglobulin and specific anti-B cell therapies such as intravenous cyclophosphamide and rituxamb are used in this scenario.

Acute rejection

This is diagnosed via transbronchial biopsy and defined by perivascular lymphocytic infiltrates of varying severity, graded from minimal (grade 1) to severe (grade 4). It is conventionally treated with intravenous methyprednisolone (typically 0.5–1 g daily for 3 days), followed by an oral taper from 1 mg/kg per day back to the maintenance dose, which is effective in most cases. Steroid resistant acute rejection is usually treated with adjunctive ATG, and if moderate to severe acute rejection occurs on two or more occasions it is now usual practice to change the background immunosuppression by either substituting tacrolimus for ciclosporin, or mycophenolate for azathioprine (or both), and/or adding an mTOR inhibitor. There are no firm data to support this strategy, but most lung transplant physicians have now adopted this approach.

Chronic rejection

In lung transplantation the term 'chronic rejection' is used to denote the presence of obliterative bronchiolitis, which is a pathological entity defined histologically by airway fibrosis with or without accompanying vascular sclerosis. However, the term is something of a misnomer in lung transplantation, as both alloimmune and nonalloimmune processes may result in fibrotic obliteration of the airway lumen. The term 'chronic allograft dysfunction' is therefore preferred.

The fibroproliferative scarring characteristic of obliterative bronchiolitis leads to either total or subtotal obliteration of the affected airway. This translates clinically into fixed airflow obstruction of varying severity, which can be easily measured, providing a useful noninvasive marker of the both the presence and severity of the condition. The bronchiolitis obliterans syndrome (BOS) is defined and graded by a fall in FEV_1, as measured from baseline, defined as the average of the two best FEV_1 measurements achieved after transplantation, taken at least 1 month apart (Table 18.16.1). No reversible cause of the fall in lung function should be present. A classification of BOS incorporating a pre-BOS stage has been proposed, however the clinical utility of this newer system has not been validated. It has been confirmed in a number of large series that bronchiolitis obliterans syndrome accurately reflects the presence and severity of obliterative bronchiolitis, and it is widely used in clinical practice for this purpose.

Recurrent and/or severe acute rejection remains the strongest risk factor for the development of obliterative bronchiolitis. Of nonalloimmune factors, gastro-oesophageal reflux has emerged as a major player in the aetiology and progression of this condition (see below), with infection of any type being the main determinant of natural history and prognosis following the acquisition of bronchiolitis obliterans syndrome. Obliterative bronchiolitis is the main cause of death in long-term survivors of lung transplantation, with complicating infection the most common terminal event.

There are no controlled trials to guide treatment of bronchiolitis obliterans syndrome. In some cases the disease arrests spontaneously. Augmented immunosuppression is rarely effective (although usually tried) and increases the risk of infection. Most experienced centres change immunosuppression early in the disease process, focusing on antiproliferative strategies, with the substitution of

Table 18.16.1 Classification of bronchiolitis obliterans syndrome

Baseline	Average of two best FEV_1 measurements achieved post-transplantation, taken at least 1 month apart
Bronchiolitis obliterans syndrome	
Grade 0	FEV_1 >80% baseline
Grade 1	FEV_1 66–79% baseline
Grade 2	FEV_1 51–65% baseline
Grade 3	FEV_1 <50% basline

tacrolimus for ciclosporin and the use of mycophenolate and mTOR inhibitors. It is common practice to reduce immunosuppression in an attempt to minimize the impact of infections if the disease progresses despite these changes.

Malignancy

Solid organ and lymphoid malignancies occur at an increased frequency in lung transplantation, affecting up to 4% of recipients. Lymphoproliferative disorders are related to EBV-driven B-cell proliferation and to the intensity of immunosuppression, and in a small number of cases to primary EBV infection in EBV-naive recipients. In lung transplantation most cases of lymphoproliferative disorder are focused in the allograft, with most occurring in the first 12 to 18 months after transplantation. Patients are usually treated with a 1- to 2-month trial of (val)aciclovir in conjunction with dramatically reduced background immunosuppression,which involves (say) cutting ciclosporin levels by 30 to 50%, stopping azathioprine, and reducing prednisolone to less than 10 mg/day. Chemotherapy is indicated for those who do not respond, or if histology demonstrates lymphoma from the outset. There are no evidence-based data to support these recommendations, which are based on clinical experience only. The prognosis of these disorders is surprisingly good, especially if confined to a single organ system, but patients diagnosed with advanced disease invariably have a poor outcome. The role of mycophenolate (which inhibits EBV-driven B-cell replication) in reducing the incidence of these disorders is yet to be determined, although a study of a large number of heart transplants showed a significant reduction in the incidence of malignancy in general for recipients receiving mycophenolate as part of their standard immunosuppressive regimen.

Occasionally, despite thorough donor screening, a lung malignancy will be transplanted into the recipient. Inevitably this will lead to the development of clinically significant disease, although surprisingly this may not occur for many years.

Airway complications

The bronchial anastamosis is devoid of its normal bronchial arterial supply and therefore prone to the development of problems relating to ischaemia and subsequent scarring (Fig. 18.16.5). These range from asymptomatic narrowing (often related to size mismatching of the donor and recipient airway) to severe stenosis requiring intervention, and occasionally to dehiscence and death. Most units experience an airway complication rate of between 5 and 10%. Bronchial artery revascularization procedures are time consuming, technically demanding, and not widely performed.

Bronchial stenoses are effectively treated with dilatation and stenting, which is optimally performed after the early inflammation related to ischaemia and infection has resolved (Fig. 18.16.6).

Heart–lung transplantation is rarely associated with airway complications as the tracheal anastamosis has a collateral blood supply derived from the coronary arteries and is therefore not ischaemic.

Gastro-oesophageal reflux

This problem, which has undoubtedly been under-recognized, is now known to contribute significantly to both acute and chronic allograft dysfunction and is likely to be a major contributor to the development and progression of bronchiolitis obliterans syndrome. It can be diagnosed if transbronchial biopsy specimens reveal food matter or highly positive Oil Red O staining, and suspected if there are recurrent acute episodes of allograft dysfunction, particularly if associated with organizing pneumonia. The condition is often asymptomatic in lung transplant recipients because of the widespread use of proton pump inhibitors. It is a particular problem in the patient with cystic fibrosis, and in any patient sustaining mediastinal nerve injury at the time of transplant. There should be a low threshold for investigation with oesophageal pH monitoring, and an equally low threshold for laparoscopic fundoplication if significant reflux is demonstrated.

Outcome

Many studies have shown that lung transplantation confers significant survival and quality-of-life benefits. Survival figures of 80 to 90% at 1 year and 50 to 60% at 5 years are achievable for all types of lung transplant and underlying disease categories.

The main contributor to mortality in the first 12 months is infection (predominantly bacterial). Acute rejection rarely causes death directly. Obliterative bronchiolitis is the main factor determining long-term survival in most lung transplant recipients. Coronary occlusive disease affecting the cardiac allograft in a heart–lung transplant occurs predominantly in the setting of this complication, and it is the airway disease that dominates the clinical picture long term in all forms of lung transplantation.

Survival is usually associated with markedly improved lung function that translates into improved functional capacity. As long as lung function is maintained (implying an absence of bronchiolitis obliterans syndrome), quality and quantity of life are maintained. Many patients are able to return to work and live a near normal life. Several female recipients have undergone normal pregnancies without complications.

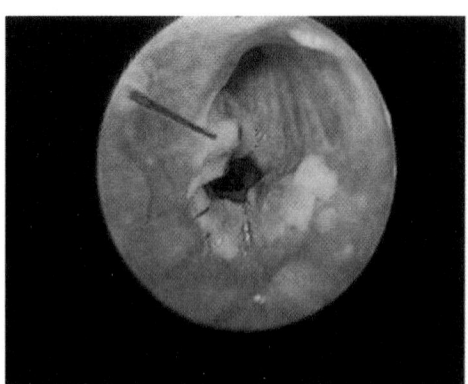
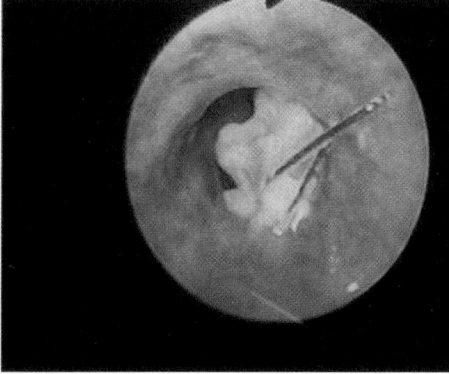

Fig. 18.16.5 Appearance at 2 weeks of bronchial anastomosis with mucosal slough secondary to ischaemia: this airway would be expected to heal well.

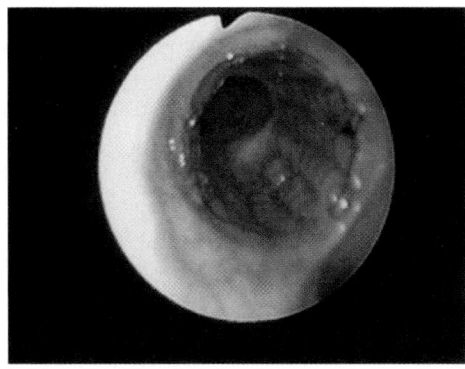 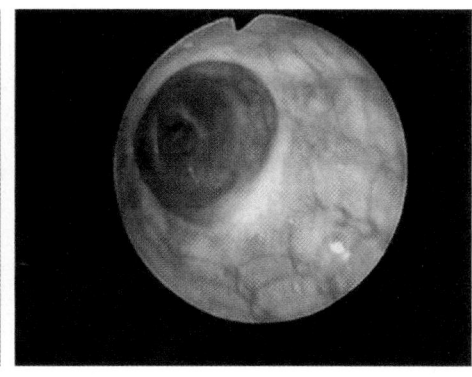

Fig. 18.16.6 An expanding metal 'ultraflex' stent in a bilateral sequential single lung transplant recipient.

Further reading

Barr ML, *et al.* (1998). Recipient and donor outcomes in living related and unrelated lobar transplantation. *Transplant Proc*, **30**, 915–22.

Boehler A, Estenne M (2003). Post-transplant bronchiolitis obliterans. *Eur Respir J*, **22**, 1007–18.

Charman SC, *et al.* (2002). Assessment of survival benefit after lung transplantation by patient diagnosis. *J Heart Lung Transplant*, **21**, 226–32.

Christie JD, *et al.* (*2005*). ISHLT Working Group on Primary Lung Graft Dysfunction Parts I—VI. Report of the ISHLT Working Group on Primary Lung Graft Dysfunction. *J Heart Lung Transplant*, **24**, 1451–500.

Dennis CM, *et al.* (1993). Heart–lung transplantation for end-stage respiratory disease in patients with cystic fibrosis at Papworth Hospital. *J Heart Lung Transplant*, **12**, 893–902.

Dennis CM, *et al.* (1996). Heart–lung–liver transplantation. *J Heart Lung Transplant*, **15**, 536–8.

Heng D, *et al.* (1998). Bronchiolitis obliterans syndrome: incidence, natural history, prognosis, and risk factors. *J Heart Lung Transplant*, **17**, 1255–63.

Herrera JM, *et al.* (2001). Airway complications after lung transplantation: treatment and long-term outcome. *Ann Thorac Surg*, **71**, 989–93 (discussion 993–4).

Higgins R, *et al.* (1994). Airway stenosis after lung transplantation: management with expanding metal stents. *J Heart Lung Transplant*, **13**, 774–8.

Hopkins PM (2006). Pharmacological manipulation of the rejection response. *Methods Mol Biol*, **333**, 375–400.

Jackson CH, *et al.* (2002). Acute and chronic onset of bronchiolitis obliterans syndrome (bronchiolitis obliterans syndrome): are they different entities? *J Heart Lung Transplant*, **21**, 658–66.

Jonas M, Oduro A (1997). Management of the multi-organ donor. In: Higgins RSD, *et al.* (eds) *The multi-organ donor. Selection and management*, pp. 123–9. Blackwell Scientific Publications, Oxford.

McNeil K, Dennis CM (1998). Heart–lung transplantation: intensive care. In: Klinck JR, Lindop MJ (eds) *Anaesthesia and intensive care for organ transplantation*, pp. 115–20. Chapman & Hall, London.

McNeil K, Wallwork J (1997). Principles of lung allocation. In: Collins GM, *et al.* (eds) *Procurement, preservation and allocation of vascularised organs*, pp. 223–6. Kluwer, Dordrecht.

Orens JB, *et al.* (2006). International guidelines for the selection of lung transplant candidates—a consensus report from the Pulmonary Scientific Council of the International Society for Heart and Lung Transplantation. *J Heart Lung Transplant*, **25**, 745–55**.**

Sharples LD, *et al.* (2002). Risk factors for bronchiolitis obliterans: a systematic review of recent publications. *J Heart Lung Transplant*, **21**, 271–81.

Studer SM, *et al.* (2004). Lung transplant outcomes: a review of survival, graft function, physiology, health-related quality of life and cost-effectiveness. *Eur Respir J*, **24**, 674–85.

Trulock EP, *et al.* (2006). Registry of the International Society for Heart and Lung Transplantation: Twenty-third Official Adult Lung and Heart–Lung Transplantation Report. *J Heart and Lung Transplant*, **25**, 869–92.

Yeatman M, *et al.* (1996). Lung transplantation in patients with systemic diseases: an eleven year experience at Papworth Hospital. *J Heart Lung Transplant*, **15**, 144–9.

Yousem SA, *et al.* (1996). Revision of the 1990 working formulation for the classification of pulmonary allograft rejection: Lung Rejection Study Group. *J Heart Lung Transplant*, **15**, 1–15.

Pleural diseases

Robert J.O. Davies, Fergus V. Gleeson, and Y.C. Gary Lee

Essentials

Pleural effusion—general considerations

This is a common clinical problem which can complicate a range of lung and systemic diseases. Most cases can be diagnosed by pleural fluid analysis and pleural biopsy, with a pleural fluid protein level of less than 27 g/litre reliably identifying a transudate and greater than 35 g/litre an exudate, with Light's criteria applied in indeterminate cases. These state that a pleural effusion is an exudate if any of the following are present: (1) pleural fluid to serum protein ratio greater than 0.5; (2) pleural fluid lactate dehydrogenase (LDH) greater than two-thirds of the upper limit of normal serum LDH; (3) pleural fluid to serum LDH ratio greater than 0.6.

Aetiology—common causes of a transudative effusion are heart failure, liver cirrhosis, and hypoalbuminaemia; common causes of an exudative effusion are malignancy, empyema/parapneumonic effusion, and tuberculosis.

Diagnosis—a low pH and low glucose are found in pleural fluid caused by very inflammatory processes, most commonly pleural infection. A single cytological test of pleural fluid for malignant cells is about 40% sensitive for malignancy, with a second sample increasing sensitivity to about 60%. Where cytology is negative, image-guided pleural cutting needle biopsy or thoracoscopy are the most sensitive techniques to identify malignancy (c.80%) and are superior to closed pleural biopsy (c.45%). For the diagnosis of tuberculosis the choice of diagnostic methodology is more finely balanced (closed biopsy c.80% sensitive vs thoracoscopy c.100%). Where an effusion remains undiagnosed, specifically treatable conditions such as pulmonary embolism and tuberculosis should be reconsidered.

Pleural effusion—particular diseases

Pyogenic pleural infection—community-acquired infection is usually due to *Streptococci* (50% of cases, including *milleri* group, and *pneumoniae*), enterobacteria, anaerobes, and *Staphylococci*; hospital-acquired infection is most commonly due to *Staphylococcus aureus* (50% of cases, of which most are methicillin-resistant (MRSA)), enterobacteria, or enterococci. Clinical features can range from fulminant sepsis to an indolent presentation with weight loss. Diagnosis depends on sampling pleural fluid to identify purulence, the presence of bacteria or low pleural pH/glucose. Treatment depends on effective chest tube drainage, appropriate antimicrobials (for at least 3 weeks), adequate nutrition, and prompt thoracic surgical drainage where clinical recovery is delayed. Mortality is greater than 20%. Recent trials are suggesting a possible role for adjuvant pleural drainage therapy delivered through the chest tube.

Tuberculous pleural effusion and empyema—hypersensitivity tuberculous pleurisy is due to a delayed hypersensitivity reaction to mycobacteria in the pleural space, occurs in cases of primary infection, and is associated with a low pleural mycobacterial load. Diagnosis is often dependent on pleural histology revealing granulomas. Tuberculous empyema is caused by rupture of cavitating tuberculosis into the pleural space and usually involves coinfection with mycobacteria and pyogenic bacteria (due to inoculation of the pleural space from the infected lung tissue). Treatment is as for tuberculosis elsewhere. Corticosteroids may have an adjuvant role in hastening pleural fluid reabsorption. Antibiotics for pyogenic bacteria are required in addition to antituberculous treatment in tuberculous empyema.

Chylothorax and pseudochylothorax—white pleural fluid has three common causes, with diagnosis established by lipid analysis of pleural fluid: (1) true chylothorax—due to leaking of chyle from a damaged thoracic duct, which usually caused by lymphoma, other cancers and trauma (including surgery); treatment is of the underlying disease where possible, and talc pleurodesis or thoracic duct repair for fluid control; nutrition is a high priority; (2) pseudochylothorax—due to chronic pleural inflammation; and (3) atypical empyema.

Haemothorax—this condition, most commonly caused by chest trauma or iatrogenically, is distinguished from heavily blood stained pleural effusion by the pleural fluid haematocrit being greater than 0.5 of that in blood. Traumatic haemothorax is not detectable on a presentation chest radiograph in 20% of cases, when it subsequently evolves over a few days. Initial treatment is by large bore chest tube drainage. About 20% of patients require surgery (video-assisted thoracoscopic surgery, or thoracotomy) to control blood loss, repair organ injury, and evacuate the blood. Failure to evacuate a large haemothorax can lead to late extensive pleural fibrosis ('fibrothorax').

Benign asbestos-induced pleural disease

The commonest benign asbestos-induced pleural disease is pleural plaque. These are fibrotic and sometimes calcified pleural thickenings on the lateral chest wall and the dome of the diaphragm that have no clinical significance. Diffuse pleural fibrosis is less common and occurs due to asbestos-mediated pleural inflammation, sometimes following benign asbestos pleural effusion. There is no specific treatment and care is supportive. When visceral pleural thickening causes the lung to enfold it forms a characteristic lesion known as 'rounded atelectasis'.

Pneumothorax

Pneumothoraces, defined as air in the pleural space, are classified as traumatic (including iatrogenic) or spontaneous, with the latter being primary (where the lung is largely normal) or secondary (where the pneumothorax is due to an underlying lung disease, most commonly chronic obstructive pulmonary disease). The diagnosis is usually established by visualization of a lung edge—a pleural line—on the chest radiograph. Treatment involves removing air from the pleural cavity and preventing recurrence.

Primary pneumothorax—associated with smoking, tall stature, and the presence of macroscopic subpleural apical lung blebs; generally a benign disease; usually treated conservatively. Supplementary oxygen can be given (where the patient is an inpatient) to hasten reabsorption. Aspiration is recommended for pneumothorax of greater than 15% of hemithorax volume, with chest tube drainage required if this fails. Recurs in 40% of cases, with video-assisted thoracic surgery typically recommended to prevent recurrence in patients who have had three events. All should be advised to stop smoking.

Secondary pneumothorax—diagnosis can be difficult if the chest radiograph is very abnormal due to the underlying lung disease; CT is used in this setting. Most patients require chest tube drainage and recurrence prevention.

Tension pneumothorax—a rare but important variant of pneumothorax where a 'flap valve' mechanism at the visceral pleural surface results in the development of increasing positive pressure in the pleural space. Diagnosis is based on the clinical features of a large pneumothorax with mediastinal shift away from the affected side, cardiovascular compromise, and severe progressive dyspnoea. Treated by urgent thoracic decompression, followed by placement of a chest tube.

Pleural effusion

Pleural effusion is common, with an incidence of greater than 0.3% of the population each year. It can complicate a range of lung and systemic diseases, hence establishing the cause can be challenging.

Aetiology

Normal physiology of pleural fluid

The pleural cavity is lined by a monolayer of predominantly mesothelial cells. These are metabolically active and capable of synthesizing numerous inflammatory mediators in response to stimuli, which regulate biological responses within the pleural cavity.

The normal pleural cavity contains a very small volume of fluid for lubrication ($c.0.13 \pm 0.06$ ml/kg body mass, per pleural cavity). This is mostly filtered from the systemic blood supply to the intercostal arterial circulation of the parietal pleura, with biochemical composition resembling that of other interstitial fluids. The bronchial circulation of the visceral pleura is unlikely to contribute significantly as the visceral pleura is thick and the microvascular pressure for fluid filtration in the bronchial circulation is low. Fluid filters between mesothelial cells and into the pleural space according to the net hydrostatic–oncotic pressure gradient, and some molecules can be actively transported through the mesothelial cells. The drainage capacity of the pleura can increase up to 30-fold, hence significant impairment of pleural fluid reabsorption is usually needed for disease to produce a pleural effusion.

Formation of pleural effusion

Pleural fluid accumulates when the rate of pleural fluid formation exceeds the rate of pleural fluid removal due to a combination of intravascular pressures (positive driving pressure), increased pleural fluid protein levels (pleural oncotic pressure), and decreased intrapleural pressure (e.g. due to lung collapse). Changes in pressure gradients produce a transudate with a low protein concentration, and changes in vascular permeability produce an exudate with a high protein level. Inflammatory cellular debris and pleural fluid protein increase oncotic pressure, further promoting fluid collection.

Fluid may also enter the pleural cavity by leaking from other structures. Abdominal fluid (ascites or peritoneal dialysis fluid) may cross the diaphragm, chyle (chylothorax) can enter from a ruptured thoracic duct, blood (haemothorax) from a blood vessel or, rarely, urine (urinothorax) from the kidney or bile (bilothorax) from the biliary tract.

The most common cause of decreased pleural fluid absorption is obstruction of the lymphatics draining the parietal pleura due to inflammation (e.g. empyema or tuberculosis) or parietal pleural malignancy.

Physiological consequences of a pleural effusion

A rise in pleural pressure usually accompanies the accumulation of pleural effusion that increases thoracic cavity size. The degree of dyspnoea induced by a pleural effusion is related to the effect of this on the diaphragm. If the diaphragm is domed and is functioning normally, dyspnoea is mild and worsens as the diaphragm flattens or inverts. High pleural pressures due to a large effusion can impair cardiac function by reducing venous return. In animals, right ventricular diastolic collapse begins when mean pleural pressure is increased about 5 mmHg, and cardiac output falls about 30% if mean pleural pressure reaches 15 mmHg.

Investigation of an undiagnosed pleural effusion

The aim when investigating a patient with a pleural effusion is to reach an accurate diagnosis with as few invasive pleural procedures as possible, thus reducing pain, the risk of infection, the risk of pleural fluid loculation and septation (making later fluid control difficult), and the frequency of chest wall tumour invasion in

Table 18.17.1 The causes of transudative and exudative pleural effusions

Transudative effusion	Exudative effusion
Common	
Heart failure	Malignancy
Liver cirrhosis	Empyema/parapneumonic effusion
Hypoalbuminaemia	Tuberculosis
Peritoneal dialysis	
Uncommon	
Hypothyroidism	Pulmonary infarction
Nephrotic syndrome	Rheumatoid arthritis
Mitral stenosis	Autoimmune disease
Pulmonary embolism	Benign asbestos effusion
	Pancreatitis
	Post-myocardial infarction syndrome
Rare	
Constrictive pericarditis	Yellow nail syndrome
Urinothorax	Drugs (see Box 18.17.1)
Superior vena cava obstruction	Fungal infections
Ovarian hyperstimulation	
Meigs' syndrome	

Box 18.17.1 Drugs particularly associated with pleural effusion

- Cabergoline
- Pergolide
- Amiodarone
- Nitrofurantoin
- Phenytoin
- Methotrexate

---

patients who ultimately prove to have malignant pleural mesothelioma, which is increasing in incidence in the United Kingdom.

Establishing a diagnosis begins with history and examination (Table 18.17.1), particularly seeking any history of asbestos or tuberculosis exposure, evidence of malignancy, and a drug history (Box 18.17.1). Clinical assessment can often reliably identify the causes of transudative effusions and, in the context of manifest heart failure, these effusions do not need to be sampled unless there are atypical features or they fail to respond to therapy.

The clinical history and examination are supplemented by an erect, plain chest radiograph (Fig. 18.17.1). Characteristically an effusion forms a basal opacity, drawn into a fluid meniscus by surface tension, and the costophrenic angle is lost, which helps differentiate pleural fluid from dense lung consolidation. The radiograph may also demonstrate pleural calcification, due to benign asbestos related pleural plaques, or previous chronic pleural inflammation (particularly tuberculous treated with an artificial pneumothorax, or a chronic bacterial empyema, Fig. 18.17.2). Failure of the pleural fluid to form a typical basal opacity suggests loculation of the fluid, which occurs in exudative effusions, particularly those that are heavily inflamed (see section on 'Pyogenic pleural infection', below). In patients imaged supine, free-flowing pleural fluid lies posteriorly, and is seen as a hazy opacity of one hemithorax (Fig. 18.17.1).

Pleural fluid analysis

The first investigation of an undiagnosed pleural effusion should be a small volume pleural fluid aspiration through a fine bore (c.21G) needle, under ultrasound guidance if the effusion is small. In a very large symptomatic effusion, 1 to 2 litres of fluid may be removed to reduce breathlessness, but the thorax should not be drained dry to allow informative CT (see below).

The odour and colour of pleural fluid should be noted. Bloodstained pleural fluid suggests malignancy, tuberculosis, pulmonary infarction, benign asbestos effusion, or post-cardiac surgery syndrome. Milky pleural fluid suggests a chylothorax, pseudochylothorax (see later in this chapter), or atypical empyema. Foul-smelling fluid suggests anaerobic pleural infection, and pleural fluid that smells like urine suggests urinothorax.

Fluid should be sent for estimation of protein and lactate dehydrogenase (LDH) concentrations (to differentiate pleural transudates and exudates); cytological assessment for malignant cells, and dominant cell type (>80% lymphocytes suggest tuberculosis or lymphoma); and pH, glucose, Gram smear for bacteria, and microbial culture (for pleural infection).

Transudative and exudative effusions

Few patients with a low-protein and LDH (transudative) effusion have an active pleural disease, with most being managed by treating the underlying disorder. High-protein and LDH (exudative) effusions usually have specific pleural pathologies. Differentiating these two groups is clinically helpful, although diagnostic confusion can occur, e.g. some patients with both pleural cancer and heart failure have a transudative pleural effusion, and patients with heart failure treated with diuretic therapy may have moderately raised pleural fluid protein levels.

Transudative and exudative effusions are usually differentiated using 'Light's criteria'. A pleural effusion is an exudate if it satisfies any of the following criteria:

- Pleural fluid to serum protein ratio >0.5
- Pleural fluid LDH > 2/3 of the upper limit of normal serum LDH
- Pleural fluid to serum LDH ratio >0.6

In routine clinical practice a pleural fluid protein level of less than 27 g/litre reliably identifies a transudate and over 35 g/litre an exudate, with Light's criteria applied in indeterminate cases. Analysing pleural protein and LDH concentrations as continuous variables improves their diagnostic accuracy slightly, but the traditional simple threshold criteria are generally robust in clinical practice.

Pleural fluid cytology for malignant cells

Overall, about 40% of patients with malignant pleural disease will have a positive diagnosis established by a single cytological test of pleural fluid. This is increased if both cell blocks and smears are prepared. A further 20% are identified by a second fluid sample, but a third examination adds little. The sensitivity of pleural cytology depends on tumour cell type. Malignant mesothelioma is particularly difficult to diagnose with cytology, and only about 30% of cases are positive. Immunocytochemistry improves the accuracy of diagnosis of the cell type: epithelial membrane antigen (EMA) is widely used to confirm epithelial malignancy, and the markers

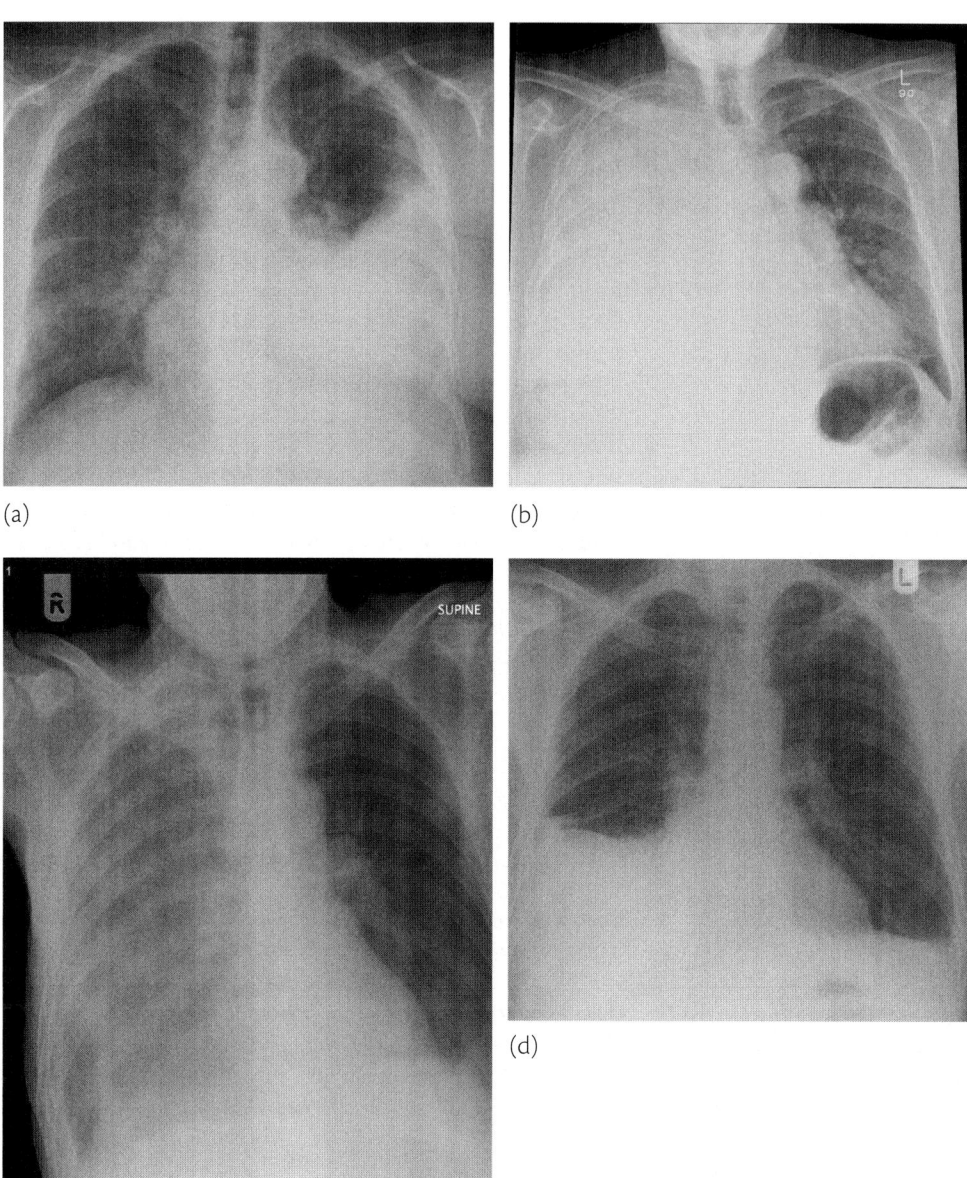

(a)

(b)

(c)

(d)

Fig. 18.17.1 Chest radiograph appearances of a free-flowing left pleural effusion imaged erect (a); a massive right pleural effusion with mediastinal shift (b); and a pleural effusion radiographed supine (c) and erect (d) in the same patient.

for CEA, B72.3, Leu-M1, calretinin and cytokeratin 5/6 help distinguish adenocarcinoma from mesothelioma.

The diagnosis of pleural infection

Pleural fluid Gram's smear for bacteria and microbial culture is performed in all cases of exudative pleural effusion. Inoculation of pleural fluid into culture medium bottles (widely used for blood cultures) may improve the sensitivity of bacterial culture, but 40% of cases of pleural infection are negative by standard culture techniques. The use of genetic bacterial identification techniques reduces this false-negative rate, with pleural fluid biochemical indices used to identify the residual cases.

Intense pleural inflammation reduces pleural fluid pH as lactate is produced by leucocyte and bacterial metabolism. A pleural fluid pH of less than 7.2 (measured on a heparinized pleural fluid sample with a blood gas analyser), in association with a clinical presentation suggestive of pleural infection, is a clinically robust diagnostic test that predicts the need for pleural effusion drainage, as well as antibiotic therapy, hence measurement of pleural fluid pH should be routine in the assessment of all nonpurulent pleural effusions. The interpretation of a pleural acidosis should always consider the differential diagnosis of other less common diseases that cause intense pleural inflammation and so lower pleural pH, particularly rheumatoid disease, oesophageal perforation (which is causing pleural infection), and advanced malignancy.

The inflammatory processes that produce pleural acidosis also reduce pleural fluid glucose as it is consumed by metabolically active cells and bacteria, and raise the pleural LDH level as this is released from apoptotic leucocytes. Quantifying these indices are alternative ways of identifying intense pleural inflammation, but in practice they add little to the measurement of pleural fluid pH alone.

Other pleural fluid analyses to diagnose exudative pleural effusion

A pleural fluid amylase level is useful for diagnosing the cause of exudative pleural effusion associated with pancreatitis, which can sometimes occur without abdominal pain. Isoenzyme analysis

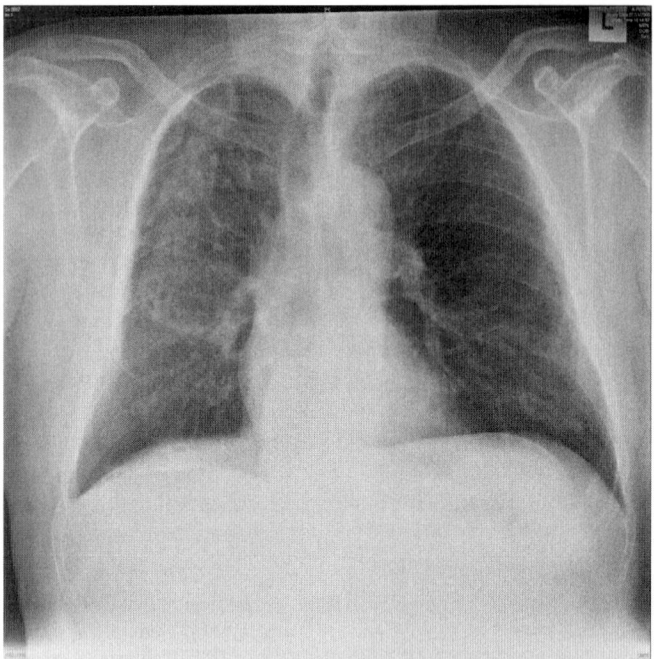

Fig. 18.17.2 Right pleural calcification following treatment of tuberculosis with an artificial pneumothorax in the prechemotherapy era.

shows that the amylase is pancreatic in origin. Oesophageal perforation allows amylase of salivary origin to enter the pleural space, and identification of this can suggest an oesophageal leak. Some adenocarcinomas also secrete amylase (usually salivary) and so amylase rich effusions are seen in some cases of carcinoma.

Measurements of pleural fluid triglyceride, lipid profiles, and cholesterol levels are valuable in the differential diagnosis of chylo/pseudochylothorax. Adenosine deaminase levels are raised in pleural tuberculosis, which is diagnostically valuable where the clinical probability of tuberculous pleural infection is high (e.g. in a highly lymphocytic effusion in a patient from a tuberculosis endemic area), but its diagnostic accuracy is limited in areas with a low tuberculosis prevalence because it is elevated by other pleural inflammatory conditions. The demonstration of a pleural fluid to serum creatinine ratio greater than 1 is diagnostic of the rare

syndrome of urinothorax, where urine has extravasated from an obstructed kidney through the retroperitoneal space and into the pleural cavity.

Pleural imaging
CT and MRI
Three-dimensional imaging is very helpful in the differential diagnosis of pleural effusion. CT and MRI are equally effective in defining pleural anatomy, though CT is favoured for cost and convenience reasons. MRI is preferred where minimizing radiation dosage is particularly important (e.g. a young woman with benign disease, to avoid irradiating breast tissue).

CT technique is important to achieve effective delineation of pleural abnormality. Images should be gathered with pleural fluid *in situ* and following intravenous contrast administration. The contrast medium should be allowed time to enter the tissue phase (60–90 s after injection), to allow for the enhancement of abnormal parietal pleural tissue which is then easily seen against the lower attenuation pleural fluid (Fig. 18.17.3). Pleural thickening which is nodular, extends onto the mediastinal pleural surface, or is >1 cm in thickness is suggestive of malignant disease, and CT scan approaches 100% specificity for malignancy where all these criteria are fulfilled.

Positron emission tomography (PET) scanning is sensitive for pleural malignancy but of limited specificity as it cannot differentiate tumour from pleural inflammation (including the effects of pleurodesis). PET scanning predicts survival in malignant mesothelioma.

Ultrasound examination
Pleural ultrasonography is simple, safe, and increasingly performed at the bedside by appropriately trained respiratory physicians (Fig. 18.17.4). After an unsuccessful 'blind' pleural fluid sample, ultrasound-guided aspiration yields fluid in more than 95% of cases and reduces the risk of lung or organ trauma. Patients with effusions that are small or appear loculated on the chest radiograph should have pleural fluid sampling performed under ultrasound guidance. Pleural fluid that appears septated on ultrasound is consistently exudative, although free-flowing effusions can be transudates or exudates. Nodularity of the pleura or diaphragm, which is suggestive of malignancy, can also be identified.

Fig. 18.17.3 Identification of malignant pleural tumour by CT scanning. Imaging was performed in the same patient without contrast administration (a) and 90 s after the administration of intravenous contrast to allow it to enter the 'tissue phase' (b). Parietal pleural thickening (due to pleural malignancy) which was invisible on the unenhanced images is clearly seen following contrast enhancement (arrow).

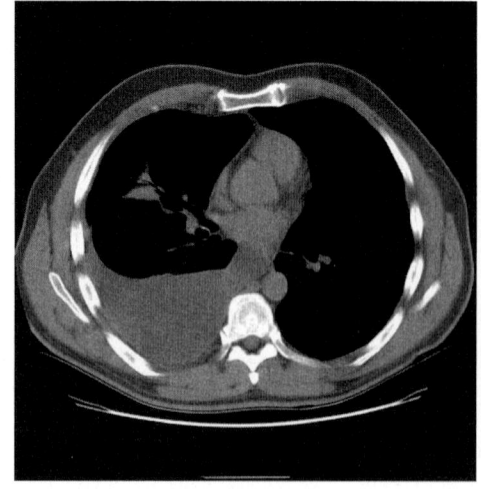 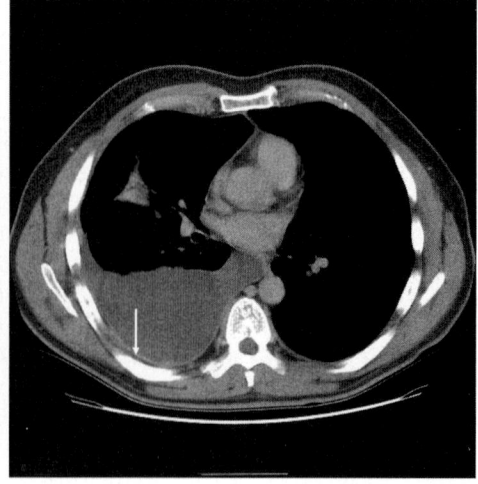

(a) (b)

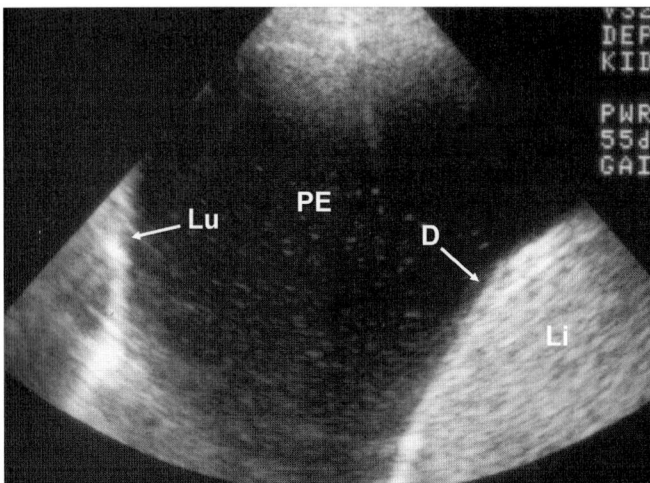

Fig. 18.17.4 The appearances of a free-flowing right pleural effusion on ultrasound. The large echo free space is the pleural effusion (PE). The diaphragm (D), liver (Li) and lung (Lu) are shown.

Pleural biopsy

Pleural malignancy

Exudative pleural effusions where pleural fluid analysis has not yielded a diagnosis usually require the sampling of pleural tissue to make a specific diagnosis, particularly of malignancy, tuberculosis, and some rarer conditions such as amyloidosis and sarcoidosis. There are three common approaches to gaining this tissue: thoracoscopy (under general or local anaesthesia), image-guided pleural biopsy (where pleural thickening has been shown on contrast-enhanced CT), or blind closed pleural biopsy (using an Abrams biopsy needle).

For malignant pleural disease, both thoracoscopic and image-guided cutting needle biopsy of pleural tissue are at least 80% sensitive, which is superior to the sensitivity of closed pleural biopsy. Image-guided pleural biopsy and thoracoscopy have similar diagnostic sensitivities, but thoracoscopy allows pleurodesis to control recurrent pleural fluid, hence thoracoscopy is preferred where fluid control is required.

The histological differential diagnosis of malignant pleural mesothelioma from reactive mesothelium and metastatic carcinoma by morphological examination is not reliable: accurate diagnosis often relies on a panel of immunohistochemical markers. Where the eventual diagnosis is malignant pleural mesothelioma, three fractions of radiotherapy to the sites of biopsies is recommended to reduce the risk of tumour invasion into biopsy sites.

Tuberculosis

The choice of biopsy method is more finely balanced when possible tuberculosis is the indication for the procedure. Closed (Abrams) pleural biopsy with acid-fast bacillus staining and culture of a biopsy sample for mycobacteria is diagnostic of tuberculosis in about 80% of cases when histological appearances and mycobacterial culture results are combined. This is less sensitive than thoracoscopic pleural biopsy, which is nearly 100% sensitive, although the diagnostic advantage to thoracoscopy is smaller than it is in malignant disease.

Other specific causes of exudative pleural effusion

Rheumatoid arthritis

Pleural involvement occurs in about 5% of patients with rheumatoid arthritis. This is more common in men and characteristically painless (unlike systemic lupus erythematosus; see below). Effusions are characteristically heavily inflamed exudates, with the pleural fluid usually having a low pH and glucose level, and a high LDH level, mirroring pleural infection. A normal pleural fluid glucose level is strongly against the diagnosis of rheumatoid disease. Cholesterol accumulates in a chronic rheumatoid effusion and may crystallize to produce a pseudochylothorax.

Systemic lupus erythematosus (SLE)

Up to 50% of patients with SLE have pleural disease at some time. This may be a 'dry pleurisy' with pleural rubs, or an exudative pleural effusion which is often small. SLE pleurisy is often painful and the fluid does not have the low pH/glucose and high LDH features of severe inflammation (cf. rheumatoid disease, above). A low pH/glucose effusion in a patient with SLE should raise the possibility of bacterial or mycobacterial infection. The presence of 'LE' cells in pleural fluid is diagnostic of SLE.

Pulmonary embolism

Small pleural effusions are present in up to 40% of cases of pulmonary embolism. These effusions have no specific diagnostic features, but it is uncommon for them to be large. Physicians must maintain a high index of suspicion for this diagnosis and should pursue appropriate diagnostic tests as required.

Benign asbestos pleural effusion

This is a diagnosis of exclusion when an exudative and often blood-stained effusion occurs in a patient with asbestos exposure (which can be within the preceding 10 years) and no other cause is found after full investigation, including pleural histology and prolonged follow-up (to exclude malignancy). The risk of benign asbestos effusion is asbestos exposure dose-dependent but can occasionally occur after minimal exposure. It usually resolves in less than 6 months but may precede the development of diffuse pleural thickening.

Persisting but undiagnosed pleural effusion

About 15% of exudative pleural effusions remain undiagnosed after careful investigation and about 15% of these will eventually prove to have a malignant cause. In cases of undiagnosed effusion, those diagnoses where there is specific therapy to prevent significant morbidity/mortality should be reconsidered. CT pulmonary angiography for pulmonary embolism and immunological testing for tuberculosis are particularly worthy of consideration.

Pyogenic pleural infection

Pleural empyema was probably described by the ancient Egyptian clinician Imhotep, but its first clear description was by Hippocrates in 500 BC. It affects about 65 000 people each year in the United States of America and the United Kingdom (combined) and carries a mortality rate of over 20%, with another 15% of patients requiring thoracic surgical drainage of their pleural infection.

Bacteriology and prognosis

The bacteriology of pleural infection is varied, with notable differences between community- and hospital-acquired infection (Fig. 18.17.5). Hospital-acquired infection is characterized by a greater proportion of antibiotic-resistant organisms, most commonly due to *Staphylococcus aureus* (representing 50% of cases, of which nearly three-quarters are methicillin-resistant (MRSA)), enterobacteria, or enterococci.

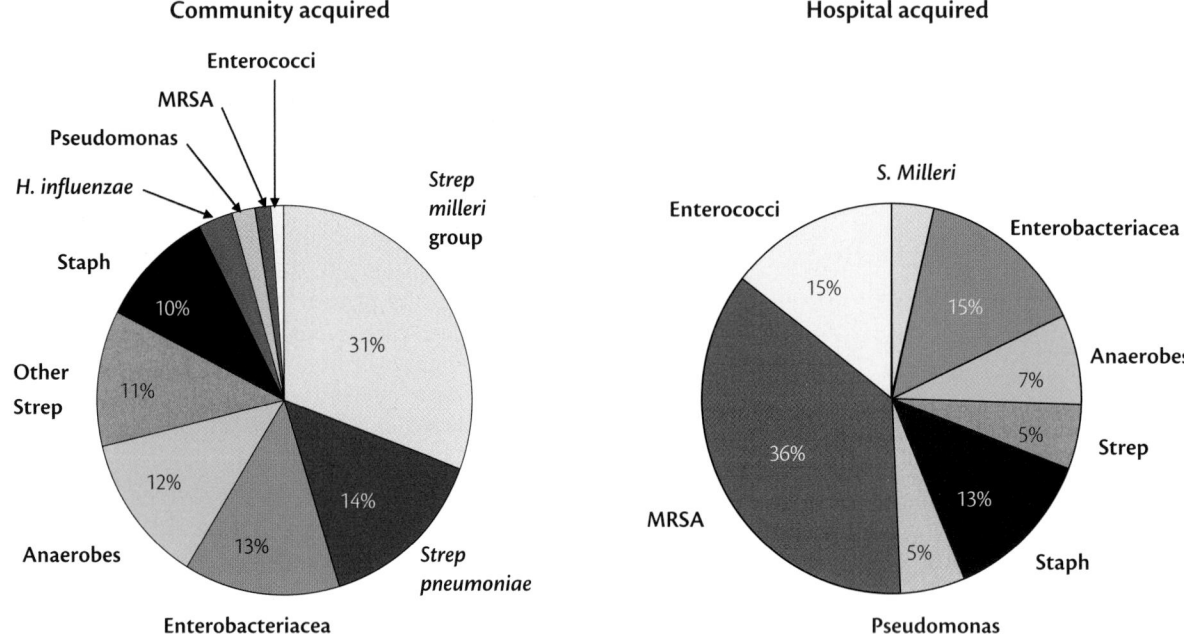

Fig. 18.17.5 Pie charts showing the proportions of different bacterial classes in community-acquired and hospital-acquired pleural infection.

Mortality is substantially higher in patients with hospital-acquired pleural infection and in patients with infections due to staphylococci, mixtures of aerobic bacteria, or enterobacteria. Patients with streptococcal infection (of any genus) or infections with anaerobic bacteria have a better survival (Fig. 19.17.6).

Aetiology

Pleural infection is believed to develop in most cases as a complication of parenchymal lung infection (which may or may not form a clinically manifest pneumonia), but may also complicate trauma or iatrogenic procedures that infect the pleural cavity. Risk factors for the development of pleural infection include diabetes mellitus, alcohol abuse, gastro-oesophageal reflux, and intravenous drug abuse. Anaerobic infection may be associated particularly with aspiration and poor dental hygiene. Pleural infection is also rarely described following bronchial obstruction due to tumour or foreign body (Fig. 18.1.7.7). About one-third of patients with pleural infection do not have any identifiable risk factors.

Pathogenesis

The development of empyema involves a progression from a sterile, simple parapneumonic effusion to a complicated parapneumonic effusion characterized by bacterial invasion, fibrin, and (later) collagen deposition within the pleural space. The initial formation of a sterile effusion ('exudative' stage) is mediated by an increase in vascular permeability following leucocyte migration into the pleural space and the production of proinflammatory cytokines. The pleural mesothelial cell plays an active role in this process: it is capable of phagocytosis and nitric oxide production, expresses adhesion molecules which facilitate migration of neutrophils and mononuclear cells into the pleural cavity, and releases proinflammatory cytokines including interleukin-8 (IL-8) and tumour necrosis factor α (TNFα). Such an effusion will resolve with antibiotic treatment alone if it is not secondarily infected. Bacterial migration into

the fluid to produce secondary infection produces the pleural infection syndrome, and requires drainage for resolution.

At this stage there is activation of the coagulation system with inhibition of fibrinolysis (the 'fibrinopurulent' stage). Bacterial metabolism and phagocytic activity in the pleural space lead to lactic acid production and increased glucose consumption, resulting in the characteristic biochemical features of pleural infection: a reduced pleural fluid pH (<7.2), reduced glucose (<1 mmol (35 mg/dl)) and elevated LDH (>1000 IU/litre). The production of fibrin forms septations in the pleural cavity which impede fluid drainage (Fig. 18.17.8), and ongoing infection eventually leads to the accumulation of pus in the pleural space (empyema).

After a variable time interval, pleural infection enters an 'organizing' stage characterized by fibroblast proliferation and the development of a solid fibrous pleural peel. This inhibits lung re-expansion and usually necessitates surgical thoracotomy and decortication. The clinical treatment of pleural infection aims to drain the infected fluid and to control infection with antibiotics before the fibrotic process becomes too advanced.

Clinical features

Pleural infection commonly presents with fever, cough, chest pain, breathlessness, and physical signs of a pleural effusion on examination. Patients may also present in a more indolent manner, with nonspecific symptoms such as weight loss, and the diagnosis can be missed if it is not actively considered in this setting. Analysis of the pleural fluid is essential in any patient with a pleural effusion and a history consistent with pleural infection. The finding of frankly purulent pleural fluid and/or the presence of organisms on pleural fluid Gram stain or culture is diagnostic of pleural infection and necessitates chest tube drainage, and as stated above pleural fluid of low pH and/or low glucose in the appropriate clinical setting is highly suggestive of pleural infection and also an indication for chest tube drainage.

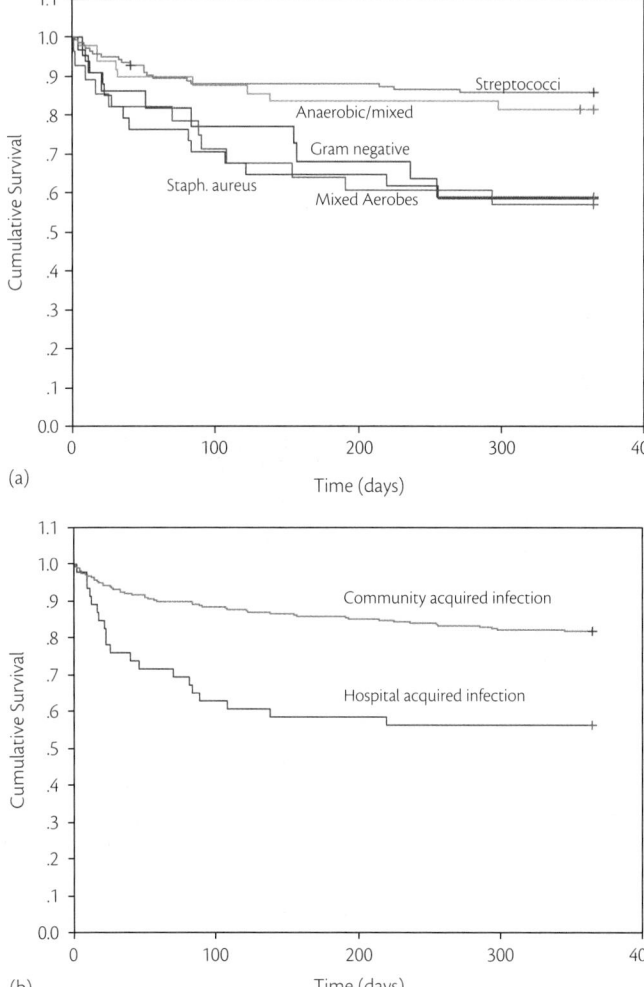

(a)

(b)

Fig. 18.17.6 Survival curves for different classes of bacterial pleural infection in 270 culture-positive cases of pleural infection (a), and hospital-acquired vs community-acquired infection (b).

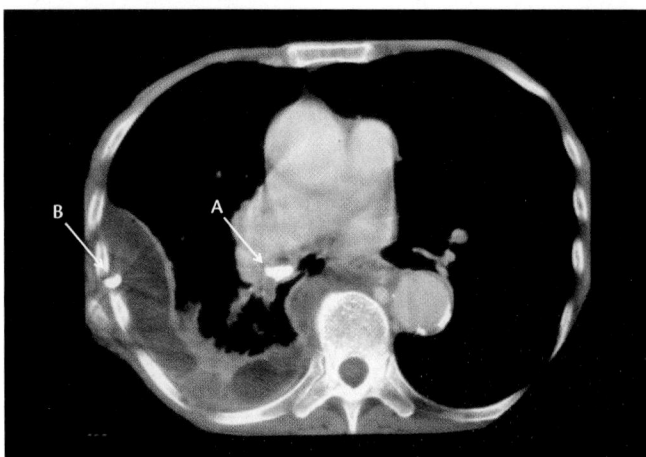

Fig. 18.17.7 Thoracic CT scan showing an empyema complicating an aspirated foreign body (marked A). This was piece of lamb chop bone later removed at bronchoscopy. A chest drain is also seen (marked B).

Culture of pleural fluid provides a bacteriological diagnosis in about 60% of cases. Blood cultures are positive in few cases, but in these patients they are often the only diagnostic microbiological test, and their routine use is therefore recommended. The amplification of bacterial DNA can provide a bacterial diagnosis in cases that are negative on standard culture.

The chest radiographic appearance is variable, but typically shows a loculated pleural effusion (Fig. 18.17.9). The appearance may be rounded and mass-like, and can be confused with pleural or lung malignancy. Ultrasound scanning typically shows a septated echogenic effusion (Fig. 18.17.8) and is beneficial in guiding aspiration of small or loculated pleural effusions. The severity of infection and fluid purulence can vary between separate locules (Fig. 18.17.10). On contrast-enhanced CT, pleural infection is characteristically manifest by a thickened, enhancing pleura with increased attenuation of extrapleural subcostal fat. The enhanced pleural thickening 'splits' around the empyema, which helps its radiographic differentiation from subpleural lung abscess.

Management

The key components of the treatment of complicated parapneumonic effusion and empyema are the use of appropriate antibiotics, provision of nutritional support, and drainage of infected pleural fluid. These are highlighted in care guidelines from the British Thoracic Society.

Initial empirical antibiotic treatment should be administered intravenously and target the likely organisms based on location of acquisition of infection (Fig. 18.17.5). Community-acquired empyema requires antibiotics for penicillin-sensitive Gram-positive bacteria, staphylococci, and anaerobic bacteria. Hospital-acquired empyema requires treatment for both Gram-positive and Gram-negative organisms, many of which are extensively resistant to antibiotics: the regimen should treat MRSA, multiresistant coliforms, and anaerobic infections.

Antibiotic choices should be modified when the results of blood and pleural fluid cultures and sensitivities are available; coexisting anaerobic organisms are frequently resistant to culture, however, and additional empirical anaerobic cover should be considered. Narrow-spectrum antipneumococcal antibiotics can be used when *Streptococcus pneumoniae* has been confidently identified, as other unidentified pathogens are rare in this group. The optimal duration of antibiotic treatment is unknown, although is likely to be at least 3 weeks.

Patients with pleural infection have chronic sepsis and are often malnourished. A low serum albumin is associated with a poor prognosis. Many patients benefit from supplementary nasogastric feeding, and parenteral nutrition is sometimes required.

Indications for chest tube drainage are frankly purulent pleural fluid, identification of organisms on pleural fluid Gram stain or culture, or pleural fluid pH less than 7.2 in the clinical setting of a pneumonic illness. The optimal chest tube size remains controversial; small-bore (12–14 French) drains are adequate for most cases, and regular saline flushes and use of suction helps prevent their occlusion. Infected pleural fluid frequently becomes loculated, and the administration of intrapleural fibrinolytic agents to dissolve fibrinous adhesions has previously been advocated. However, recent multicentre trials showed that this intervention is ineffective and the routine use of single agent intrapleural fibrinolytics is no longer recommended. Interestingly the preliminary results of a recent

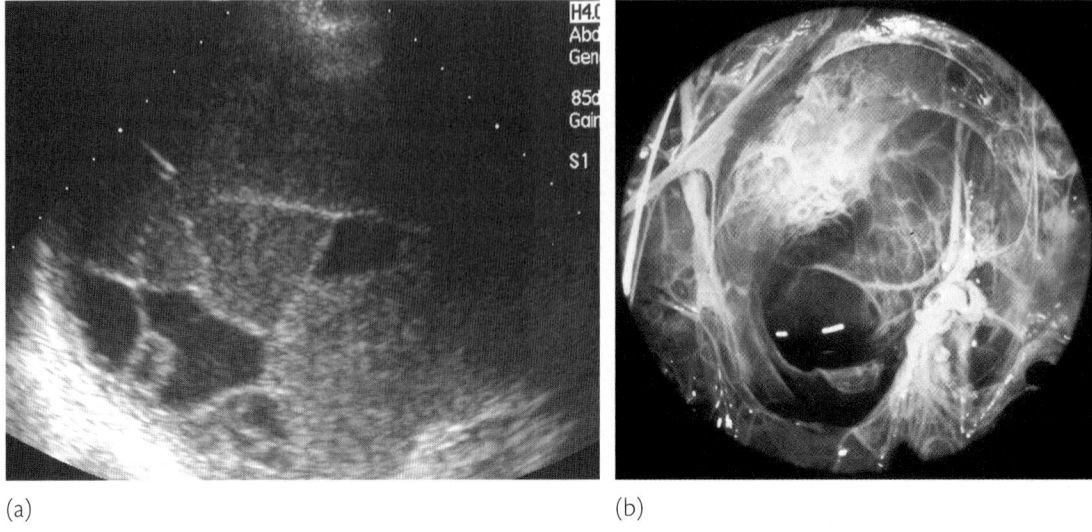

(a)   (b)

Fig. 18.17.8 Fibrinous septations due to pleural infection shown on ultrasonography (a) and directly observed at thoracoscopy (panel b).

trial suggest that combination intrapleural fibrinolytic and DNAse therapy improves drainage and clinical outcome and such adjuvant pleural therapy may find a role in care in the next few years.

Approximately 15% of patients with pleural infection fail to improve with chest tube drainage and antibiotics, and require prompt surgical drainage of infected fluid. Surgical approaches for empyema include video-assisted thoracoscopic surgery (VATS), thoracotomy and decortication, and rib resection with open thoracic drainage. VATS allows the disruption of pleural adhesions and the drainage of pleural fluid without a thoracotomy incision and is the surgical intervention of choice for early stages of disease. Thoracotomy and decortication are indicated for the treatment of empyema in the 'organizing' stage, where the visceral pleura is thickened. Rib resection with open thoracic drainage may be performed under local anaesthesia, and is used in patients who are unable to tolerate general anaesthesia.

Once the infection has been effectively controlled, extensive radiological abnormalities will improve without further intervention over many months, and even striking radiographic features are not an indication for surgery in a well patient whose infection has been controlled (Fig. 18.17.11).

Tuberculous pleural effusion and empyema

The general treatment of tuberculosis is discussed in detail elsewhere (see Chapter 7.6.25). There are two tuberculous pleural effusion syndromes. Most cases are due to a delayed hypersensitivity reaction to mycobacteria in the pleural space and occur in cases of primary infection. They are characterized by a low mycobacterial load and the pleural fluid is rarely smear-positive for acid-fast bacilli. More rarely, a true tuberculous empyema develops, usually in patients with cavitating lung disease and a direct communication between the lung parenchyma and the pleural space. In these cases, the pleural fluid is purulent and smear-positive for acid-fast bacilli, and there is often coinfection with pyogenic bacteria.

Clinical features

Hypersensitivity-mediated tuberculous pleural effusions may be asymptomatic, or present with weight loss, chest pain or fever.

They are exudates and the pleural fluid glucose is often moderately depressed (c.50% of blood glucose). Cytological analysis reveals a highly cellular fluid, dominated (>80%) by lymphocytes: mycobacteria are only infrequently seen on direct stains of pleural fluid or grown in culture of pleural fluid. The diagnosis is usually inferred from the finding of granulomas on pleural biopsy in the appropriate clinical setting (Fig. 18.17.12A), but it is important to remember that the typical granulomas are lost in patients who are immunosuppressed (e.g. HIV infection) (Fig. 18.17.12C). Pleural biopsy using an Abrams closed biopsy technique identifies about 80% of cases when the results of both histology for granulomas and culture for tuberculosis are available; the larger biopsies achieved by thoracoscopy (often under local anaesthesia) are more diagnostically accurate, approaching 100% sensitivity.

The diagnostic value of pleural fluid biochemical markers such as adenosine deaminase (ADA) is affected by both the local

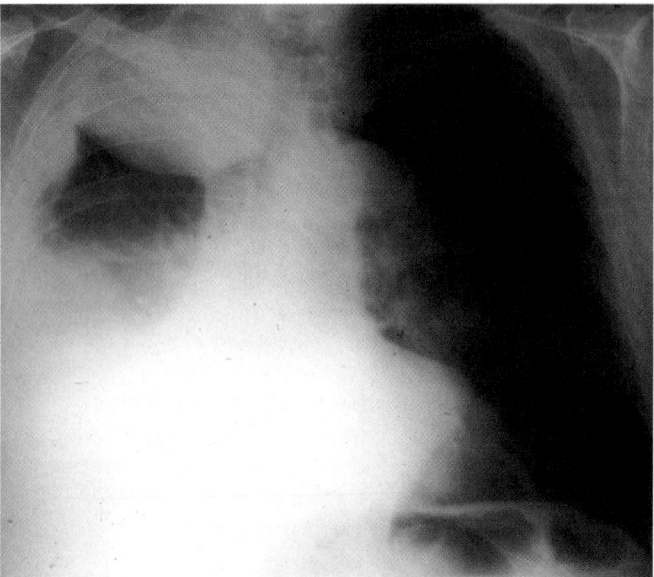

Fig. 18.17.9 Chest radiograph showing a typical pleural infection with a severely loculated pleural effusion, which mimics a lung mass.

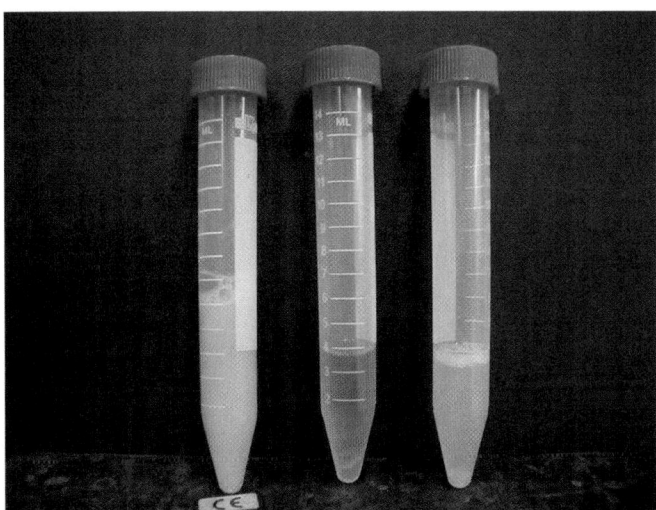

Fig. 18.17.10 Pleural fluid samples obtained from locules with varying echogenicity on ultrasound in a case of pyogenic bacterial pleural infection. Those with greater echogenicity contain fluid of greater purulence, thus emphasizing that the pleural inflammatory process is not uniform.

prevalence of tuberculosis and the likelihood of an alternative diagnosis. Pleural fluid ADA levels are high in conditions such as infection and malignancy as well as in pleural tuberculosis, but a raised ADA value is highly sensitive and specific in areas where tuberculosis is prevalent, especially in young patients in whom empyema has been excluded.

Treatment

Most tuberculous effusions resolve without specific anti-TB treatment, but left untreated over 50% of these patients will develop active tuberculosis (usually pulmonary) within the next 5 years. Treatment is therefore given primarily to prevent recurrent disease.

The treatment of hypersensitivity-mediated tuberculous pleural effusion requires the same antimicrobial regimen as used for pulmonary tuberculosis (see Chapter 7.6.25). The use of adjuvant

corticosteroids does not alter the long-term outcome, but may be symptomatically helpful by hastening pleural fluid absorption.

In tuberculous empyema, where infection with pyogenic bacteria as well as *Mycobacterium tuberculosis* has occurred, antibiotics appropriate for the pyogenic bacteria are also required. These patients may have a persisting pyopneumothorax due to rupture of a tuberculous cavity into the pleural space. Treatment may require surgical resection of tuberculous cavities, but such surgery is difficult.

Chylothorax and pseudochylothorax

Pleural fluid that is white or milky in colour and does not clear with centrifugation almost always has a high lipid content. This occurs when chyle enters the pleural space following disruption of the thoracic duct (a true chylothorax), or large amounts of cholesterol or lecithin–globulin complexes accumulate in a long-standing inflammatory effusion (a pseudochylothorax).

Chylothorax

Pathophysiology

About 2 litres of chyle is created daily, carrying dietary fat in the form of chylomicrons and rich in T lymphocytes. This travels in the thoracic duct, which usually passes through the aortic hiatus of the diaphragm on the right, crosses between the T4 and T6 vertebrae to the left, and then continues cephalad on the left side of the oesophagus. A true chylothorax forms when the thoracic duct is disrupted, either before or after it crosses the midline, tending to produce right-sided and left-sided chylothoraces respectively.

Aetiology

Over 50% of chylothoraces are due to tumours, of which 75% are lymphomas (Fig. 18.17.13). Trauma, most often a surgical procedure, is the second most common cause, with oesophagectomy complicated by chylothorax in 1 to 4% of cases. In the paediatric setting, chylothorax is common after surgical repair of congenital diaphragmatic hernia and is usually left sided.

Penetrating injuries of the neck or thorax, and nonpenetrating trauma with spine hyperextension or vertebral fracture, can cause thoracic duct damage. Rupture after weightlifting, severe coughing

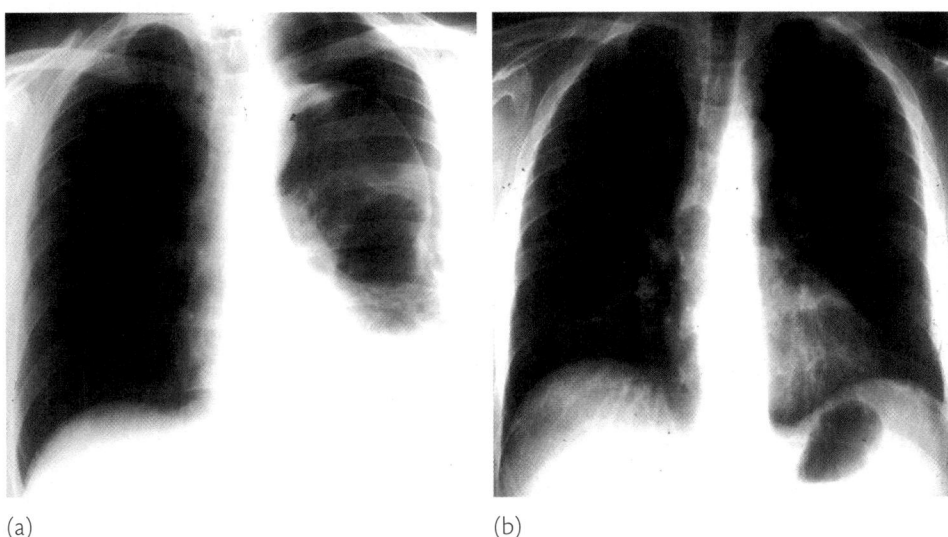

(a)   (b)

Fig. 18.17.11 Chest radiographs in a patient with a left lung that has not re-expanded due to visceral pleural thickening following drainage and treatment of a pleural infection (a). The patient was clinically well and the radiographic changes resolved spontaneously over 3 months (b).

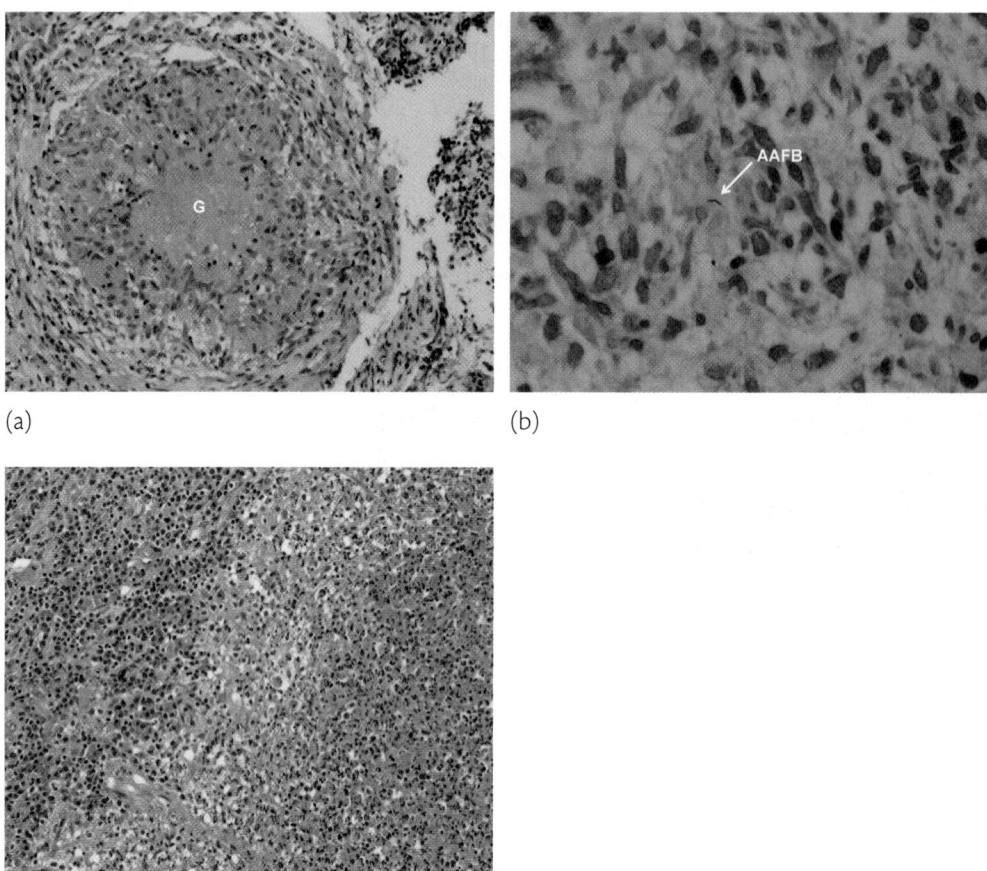

Fig. 18.17.12 Histological appearances of pleural biopsies in patients with tuberculosis. The appearance in an immunocompetent patient (a) shows a typical caseating granuloma (G). Panel b shows staining for acid- and alcohol-fast bacilli (AAFB) and demonstrates *Mycobacterium tuberculosis* (later confirmed by culture). The appearance in a patient with immunosuppression due to HIV disease (c) shows no granulomas.

or vomiting, childbirth, and vigorous stretching while yawning are also occasionally reported. Chylothorax can follow chylous ascites. Pulmonary lymphangioleiomyomatosis is the most common other cause of chylothorax and this is discussed in Chapter 18.14.6. Other precipitants include intestinal lymphangiectasis, yellow nail syndrome, superior vena caval or subclavian vein thrombosis/obstruction, filariasis, lymph node enlargement, mediastinal fibrosis, lymphangitis of the thoracic duct, tuberous sclerosis, amyloidosis and Gorham's syndrome (disappearing bone disease; massive osteolysis).

Clinical features

The clinical features are those of a pleural effusion, but chest pain and fever are rare as chyle is not irritant. In traumatic chylothorax, effusion onset is typically delayed for 2 to 10 days: during this time chyle may accumulate in the posterior mediastinum as a 'chyloma'—sometimes visible on the chest radiograph—which resolves when it ruptures into the pleural space. The main threat to life with chylothorax is malnutrition if the chyle is drained externally, as the daily loss of 1500 to 2500 ml of fluid containing substantial amounts of protein, fats, electrolytes, and lymphocytes rapidly makes a patient malnourished and immunocompromised.

Diagnosis

Diagnosis is usually easy from the distinctive white, odourless, milky appearance of aspirated pleural fluid (Fig. 18.17.14), although it may appear bloody, turbid, or clear yellow. The usual differential diagnoses are empyema fluid and pseudochylothorax. In empyema,

the milky appearance is from suspended white blood cells and debris, which sediment on centrifugation. In pseudochylothorax, the lipids are cholesterol crystals or lecithin-globulin complexes rather than chylomicrons (Fig. 18.17.15).

Biochemical assessment of the pleural fluid is key to accurate diagnosis. Patients who have a true chylothorax usually have a pleural fluid triglyceride level above 110 mg/dl (1.24 mmol/litre), a ratio of pleural fluid to serum triglyceride of greater than 1.0, and a ratio of the pleural fluid to serum cholesterol of less than 1.0. The demonstration of chylomicrons on pleural fluid lipoprotein electrophoresis is diagnostic of a chylothorax. Fasting may significantly reduce the triglyceride level in the pleural fluid and lead to a false-negative result, hence fluid sampling after a high-fat meal is helpful if diagnostic doubt persists.

CT scanning of the chest should be obtained in all patients with nontraumatic chylothorax to look for thoracic and abdominal lymphadenopathy suggestive of lymphoma (Fig. 18.17.13). In young women the appearance on CT scanning of cystic lung disease may indicate lymphangioleiomyomatosis. Unlike most other pleural effusions, examination of the pleura is not usually diagnostic, and pleural biopsy or thoracoscopy is usually only indicated for fluid control.

Treatment

Treatment aims to correct the underlying disease, maintain nutrition, reduce the flow of chyle, relieve dyspnoea, and (sometimes)

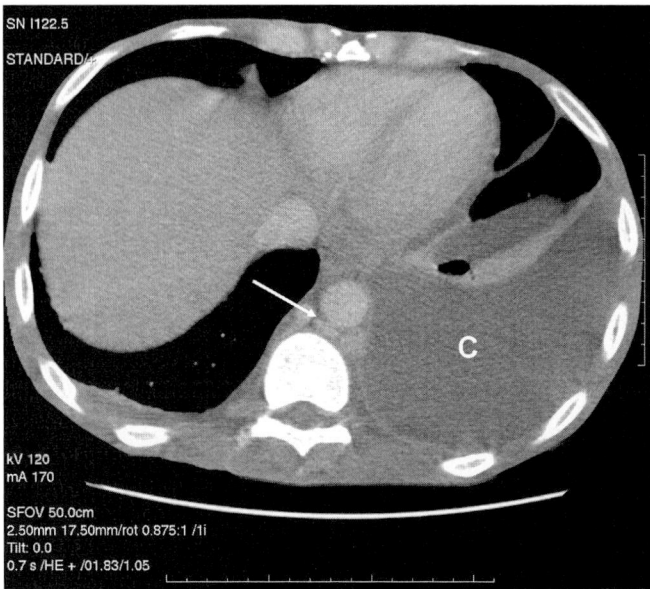

Fig. 18.17.13 A case of chylothorax (C) where the thoracic duct has been ruptured by enlarged mediastinal lymph nodes (arrowed).

close the thoracic duct defect. Malnutrition and a compromised immunological status can quickly follow chest tube drainage through loss of large amounts of protein, fat, electrolytes, and lymphocytes. This means that definitive control of the effusion is required before the patient becomes too debilitated. Spontaneous closure of a thoracic duct leak may follow reduction of the flow of chyle by parenteral feeding or use of a low-fat diet rich in medium-chain triglycerides that are absorbed directly into the blood, but this diet is often difficult to tolerate as it tastes unpleasant. Octreotide, a somatostatin analogue, may be effective in hastening the closure of a thoracic duct leak: the mechanism of its action is not clear but may be through reduced intestinal fat absorption and increased faecal fat excretion.

If the cause is lymphoma or metastatic carcinoma, a chylothorax often responds to effective chemotherapy or mediastinal radiotherapy. Pleuroperitoneal shunts can be used if a chylothorax fails to settle, which avoids malnourishment and immunodeficiency since lymph is not removed from the body.

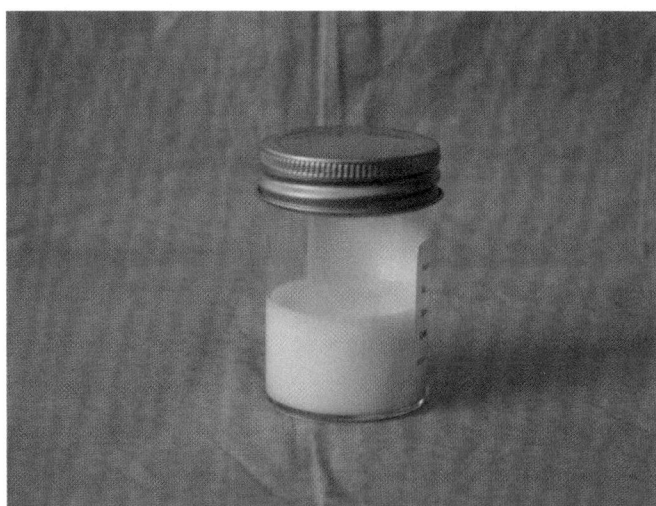

Fig. 18.17.14 Typical milky pleural fluid from a true chylothorax.

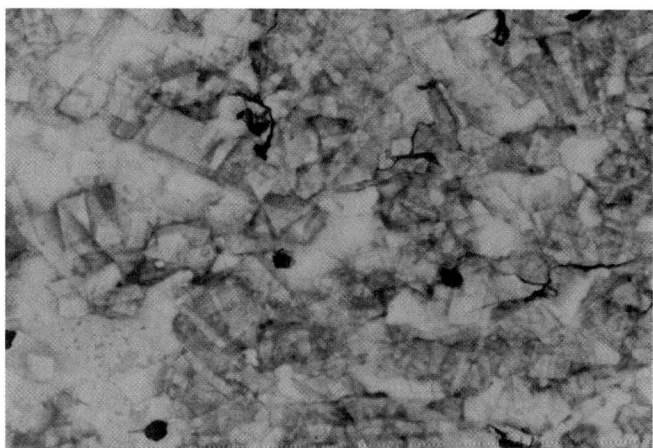

Fig. 18.17.15 Microscopy of pleural fluid from a pseudochylothorax showing multiple cholesterol crystals (Giemsa stain with birefringence).

In traumatic chylothorax, the defect in the thoracic duct often closes spontaneously. The volume of fluid drainage (more or less than c.400 ml/day) seems to predict the likelihood of such resolution. Thoracoscopic talc pleurodesis is often effective when conservative therapy fails. Lymphatic embolization of the thoracic duct from the abdomen can decrease fluid flow.

Surgical intervention involves thoracic duct ligation at video assisted thoracoscopic surgery or thorocotomy. The site of the leak may be identified preoperatively by lymphangiography, and identification of the duct at surgery can be facilitated by preoperative drinking of cream. Laparoscopic ligation of the abdominal thoracic duct has also been successful.

Pseudochylothorax

Pseudochylothorax is less common than chylothorax. The fluid is turbid due to high levels of cholesterol or lecithin–globulin complexes (Fig. 18.17.15). Pathogenesis remains unknown, but most patients with pseudochylothorax have marked pleural thickening and a chronic pleural effusion and it is hypothesized that inflammation increases filtration of cholesterol into pleural fluid and/or cholesterol is liberated from degenerative inflammatory red and white blood cells within the effusion. The thickened pleura may also inhibit the exit of cholesterol from the pleural space. Pseudochylothorax is most frequently attributable to tuberculous (54%) or rheumatoid (10%) pleurisy. The clinical picture is of a stable chronic effusion, although in some cases the effusion gradually enlarges with time.

Haemothorax

Haemothorax is blood in the pleural space, defined as a pleural fluid haematocrit of more than 50% that of blood. A heavily blood-stained pleural effusion often has a haematocrit of under 5%, hence a haematocrit should be performed whenever haemothorax is suspected.

Traumatic haemothorax

Traumatic haemothorax should be suspected following any chest trauma, whether penetrating or not. It often develops in the first few days after trauma, is not detectable on 25% of presentation chest radiographs, and in patients with multiple or displaced rib fractures late haemothorax may occur up to a week after presentation. Thoracic CT identifies all cases, and bedside ultrasonography has similar diagnostic sensitivity. The condition is a potential surgical emergency and should be managed by a thoracic/trauma surgeon.

Traumatic haemothorax is treated with an immediate large-bore chest tube for blood evacuation. This can stop the bleeding if this is from pleural lacerations by bringing the two pleural surfaces together, and allows quantification of continued bleeding. Blood lost from haemothorax can be autotransfused if necessary, and early effective evacuation of haemothorax may decrease the frequency of late thoracic contraction due to pleural scarring ('fibrothorax').

About 20% of patients with haemothorax require surgical intervention for suspected cardiac tamponade, vascular injury, pleural contamination, debridement of devitalized tissue, chest wounds, major bronchial air leaks, or continued pleural haemorrhage. Post-traumatic haemothorax was managed exclusively by thoracotomy, but advances in VATS have made this minimally invasive technique the procedure of choice in many centres, with thoracotomy reserved for massive haemorrhage. There are no precise criteria for the amount of pleural bleeding that should mandate surgery, and each case must be managed on its merits, but surgical intervention is likely to be required if bleeding is more than 200 ml/h and shows no signs of slowing.

The four main pleural complications of traumatic hemothorax are the retention of clotted blood in the pleural space, pleural infection, pleural effusion, and fibrothorax. Most patients with small to moderate amounts of clotted blood remaining in their pleural space have no residual pleural abnormalities even if no intervention is undertaken, but evacuation is recommended if more than 30% of the hemithorax is occupied by clotted blood. In a randomized trial, VATS was more effective than thoracostomy tube drainage, reducing the duration of hospital stay and chest tube drainage. Intrapleural administration of fibrinolytic agents to improve clot drainage may be safe in haemothorax, but there have been no comparative studies to confirm these agents are efficacious and safe in this setting.

Empyema occurs in 1 to 4% of cases and should be suspected in the febrile patient. The administration of prophylactic antibiotics at presentation reduces the incidence of pleural infection in randomized trials. The treatment of empyema complicating haemothorax is similar to that of other pleural infections.

Iatrogenic haemothorax

The incidence of iatrogenic haemothorax is highest after thoracic surgery, perforation of a central vein or artery by a percutaneous

catheter, or aortic leak after translumbar aortography. Other common procedures that are rarely associated with such bleeding include thoracentesis, pleural biopsy (Fig. 18.17.16), chest tube insertion, percutaneous lung aspiration or biopsy, transbronchial biopsy, endoscopic oesophageal variceal therapy, and cardiopulmonary resuscitation. Management is similar to traumatic haemothorax.

Nontraumatic haemothorax

Non-traumatic haemothoraces are uncommon, but most frequently follow malignant pleural disease or anticoagulation (particularly for pulmonary embolism). Rarer causes include abnormal blood vessels (subpleural arteriovenous malformations, aneurysm of the aorta or pulmonary artery, patent ductus arteriosus, coarctation of the aorta), bleeding disorders (hemophilia, thrombocytopenia), spontaneous pneumothorax, bronchopulmonary sequestration, thoracic endometriosis, chickenpox pneumonia, and intrathoracic extramedullary hematopoiesis. Rarely, neurofibromatosis can cause haemothorax from aneurysmal changes in large arteries or from dysplastic changes in small vessels. Blood can accumulate in the pleural space from abdominal pathology (e.g. rupture of a splenic artery aneurysm through the diaphragm, pancreatic pseudocysts, and rupture of hepatocellular carcinoma). The cause of some spontaneous haemothoraces remains unknown despite thoracotomy.

Benign asbestos-induced pleural diseases

Asbestos is a family of hydrated silicate fibres subdivided into curly (serpentine) and needlelike (amphibole) types. Crysotile is the main serpentine form; amphiboles include crocidolite (blue asbestos), amosite (brown asbestos), anthophyllite, tremolite, and actinolite. Most benign asbestos-induced pleural diseases are due to occupational exposure, although environmental exposure causes disease in some high-prevalence asbestos areas such as central and southeast Turkey, north-west Greece, and Finland. The benign asbestos pleural diseases comprise pleural plaques, benign asbestos pleurisy, diffuse pleural thickening, and rounded atelectasis.

Pathogenesis

The pathogenesis of benign asbestos-induced pleural disease is poorly understood. The route by which asbestos fibres transfer to the pleura after inhalation is unclear. Fibre burden studies have shown higher fibre numbers in lymph nodes and pleural plaques than in lung parenchyma, and it is likely that at least some fibres are cleared from the lung parenchyma to the lymph nodes and pleura through

Fig. 18.17.16 Haemothorax due to laceration of an intercostal artery during chest drain insertion. The CT (a) shows acute haemorrhage (H) into a pleural effusion that was already present (E). The angiogram (b) shows acute haemorrhage (H) from intercostal artery, which was halted by intercostal embolization.

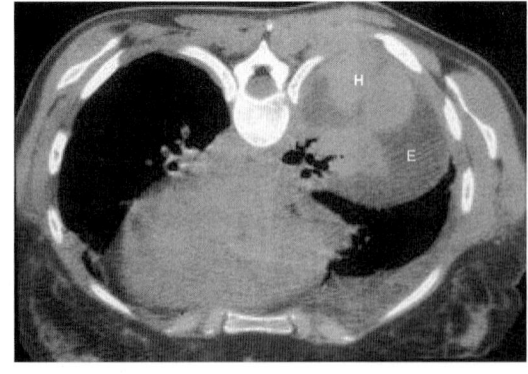
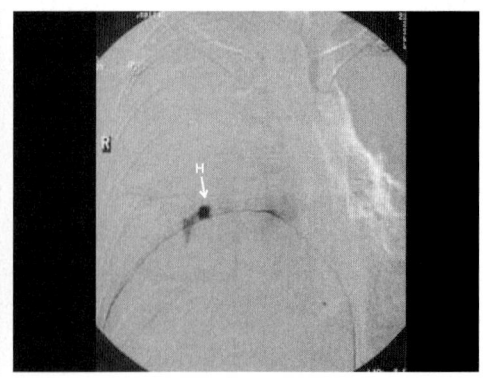

(a)　　　　(b)

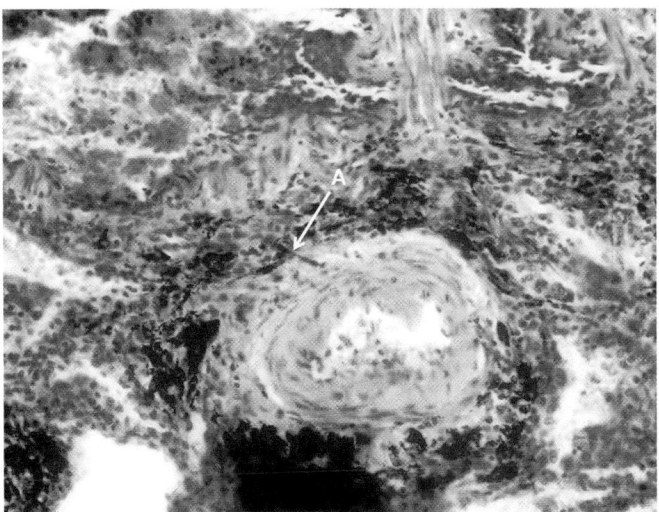

Fig. 18.17.17 An asbestos body where an asbestos fibre (A, arrowed) has become encased in iron-rich material.

lymphatic spread. Amphiboles fibres in particular are associated with 'black spots' of anthracotic deposit near lymphatic vessels.

Fibre toxicity may be related to a number of factors, including fibre length and diameter, chemical properties such as iron content and surface charge, and durability. Long, thin fibres (e.g. crocidolite) are especially carcinogenic and clear more slowly from the lung, although the exact relationship of different fibre types to benign and malignant pleural diseases is still debated. The iron content of asbestos bodies (Fig. 18.17.17) may influence reactive oxygen species generation, causing pleuropulmonary toxicity.

A primary mechanism of asbestos fibre induced injury is pleural inflammation. Fibres induce intrapleural IL-8 production from pleural mesothelial cells which causes a neutrophil influx that precedes the development of pleural plaques. A prolonged macrophage influx follows, probably due to monocyte chemoattractant protein-1 (MCP-1), TNFα, or IL-1β production. The mechanisms that cause pleural fibrosis and plaque formation following this inflammation are not clearly understood.

Clinical manifestations

Benign asbestos-related pleural plaques

Circumscribed pleural plaques are the most common manifestation of asbestos exposure and comprise discrete areas of white or yellow thickening on the parietal pleura with a raised 'beaded' edge visible at thoracoscopy (Fig. 18.17.18). They are frequently bilateral and occur particularly on the posterolateral chest wall between the fifth and eighth ribs overlying the internal rib surfaces. They also occur on the dome of the diaphragm and over the mediastinal pleura. Histologically they are acellular, with a 'basket-weave' pattern of hyalinized collagen strands, covered by a single layer of normal mesothelial cells on the pleural surface (Fig. 18.17.18).

Pleural plaques typically develop 20 to 30 years after asbestos exposure. They affect up to 50% of exposed workers, with incidence relating to exposure dose, although the extent of plaques within an individual case is not dose related. There are no convincingly demonstrated lung function consequences of pleural plaques, but they may be weakly associated with coronary artery disease risk. Pleural plaques do not have any potential for malignant transformation and clinical management consists of patient reassurance.

Diffuse, benign asbestos-induced pleural thickening

Diffuse pleural thickening consists of extensive fibrosis of the visceral pleura, with areas of adhesion with the parietal pleura and consequent obliteration of the pleural space. It is arbitrarily defined as extending over more than 25% of the hemithorax on the chest radiograph, or more than 8 cm craniocaudally and 5 cm laterally on thoracic CT. Unlike pleural plaques, the margins of the fibrosis are ill defined. It frequently involves the costophrenic angles, apices, and interlobar fissures. Diffuse fibrosis sometimes follows benign asbestos related pleural effusion.

Diffuse pleural thickening may be asymptomatic or cause breathlessness. Chest pain, when present, causes clinical uncertainty as it places malignant pleural mesothelioma (see Chapter 18.19.3) in the differential diagnosis. Pleural thickening is usually slowly progressive and may cause significant lung function impairment, especially if the costophrenic angle is involved. Hypercapnic ventilatory failure can (rarely) develop. Surgical decortication is generally ineffective in providing clinical or functional improvement.

Rounded atelectasis

Rounded atelectasis (also known as folded lung, Blesovsky syndrome, or shrinking pleuritis with atelectasis) develops as contracting visceral pleural fibrosis rolls and ensnares the underlying lung. This results in the distinctive radiological appearance of a rounded or oval pleural-based mass 2.5 to 5 cm in diameter, with bands of contracted and atelectactic lung radiating out in a whirling fashion (known as 'comet tails') on chest radiograph or thoracic CT (Fig. 18.17.19).

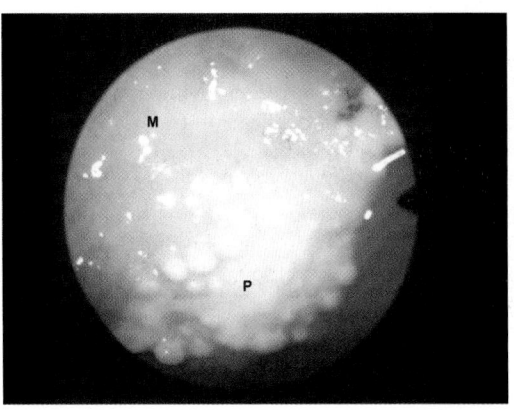

(a)

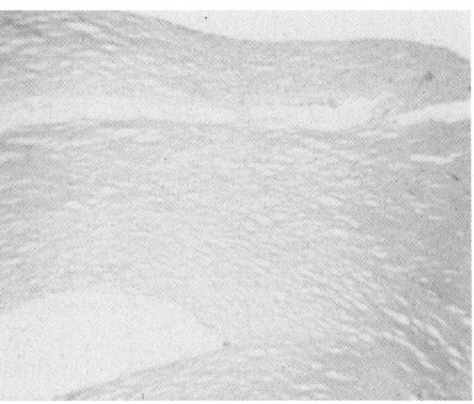

(b)

Fig. 18.17.18 (a) A pleural plaque (marked P) seen at local anaesthetic thoracoscopy. The raised 'beaded' edge of the plaque is clearly seen. Malignant pleural mesothelioma is also present in this case, with tumour tissue seen infiltrating superiorly to the plaque (marked m). (b) shows the typical histological appearance of benign pleural plaque.

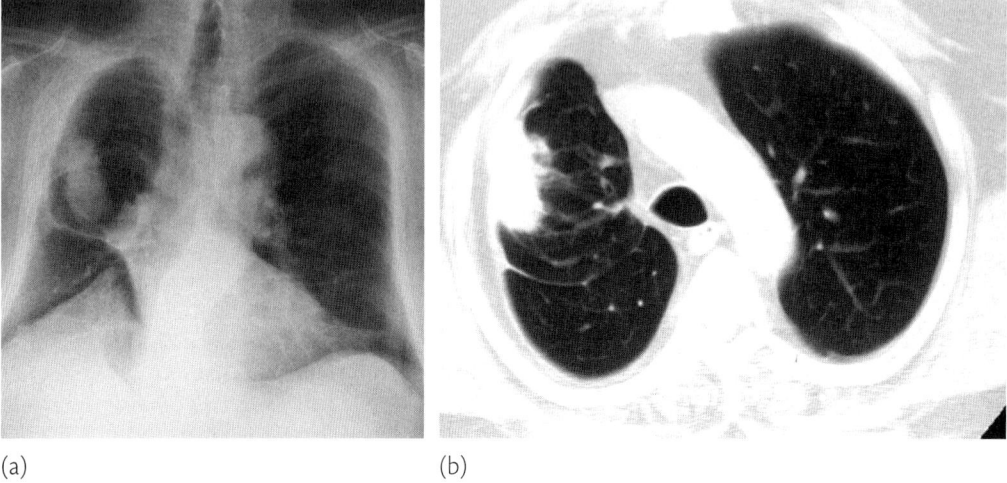

(a)   (b)

Fig. 18.17.19 (a) Chest radiograph and (b) CT showing 'rounded atelectasis' where visceral pleural fibrosis has contracted to enfold the underlying lung. Characteristic 'comet tails' are seen in the lung parenchyma.

Rounded atelectasis is typically asymptomatic and stable or only slowly progressive. Specific therapy is rarely required. Serious complications such as obstructive pneumonia and local pulmonary artery thrombosis are rare. Surgical decortication often results in reduced lung volumes and is not generally recommended.

Pneumothorax

Pneumothorax is defined as air in the pleural space and is subclassified as spontaneous (occurring without preceding trauma or other obvious precipitant) or traumatic (following direct or indirect trauma to the chest). Iatrogenic pneumothorax is a traumatic pneumothorax following a diagnostic or therapeutic procedure.

Spontaneous pneumothoraces are divided into primary or secondary. Primary pneumothorax occurs in an otherwise healthy person where the lung has no underlying disease other than the minor pathologies specifically associated with primary pneumothorax. Secondary pneumothorax complicates an underlying lung disease, most commonly chronic obstructive pulmonary disease (COPD).

Pathophysiology

During normal tidal breathing the pleural pressure is continuously negative with respect to alveolar/atmospheric pressure. When a communication develops between the lung and pleural space (or outside atmosphere via a chest wall injury), then air flows into the pleural space until this negative pressure equilibrates or the airways in the collapsing lung occlude to prevent further alveolar gas escape via the airway. This 'air trapping' occurs earlier in patients with COPD. The removal of negative pleural pressure also causes the chest wall to 'spring out' due to loss of the recoil pressure across the chest wall (by about 8% of vital capacity), hence the overall volume of the hemithorax increases.

Primary spontaneous pneumothorax

Incidence

The annual incidence of pneumothorax is about 24 per 100 000 for men and 9.8 per 100 000 for women. About 50% of these are primary pneumothoraces.

Aetiology

Primary spontaneous pneumothorax is statistically associated with macroscopic subpleural apical lung blebs, which can be found in 75% of patients with pneumothorax at thoracoscopy. The pathogenesis of these subpleural blebs is unclear: they have been attributed to congenital abnormalities, inflammation of the bronchioles, and disturbances of the collateral ventilation. How frequently they are directly aetiological for pneumothorax is also debated: air leaks are rarely directly from a bleb (which is often inflated at thoracoscopy), and there are more extensive subpleural and pleural anatomical changes in the areas around for blebs that may frequently be the site of the air leak.

Primary pneumothorax is strongly associated with smoking: over 80% of patients are smokers, and there is a dose–response relationship between the amount of smoking and pneumothorax risk. In men, the relative risk of pneumothorax is 7 times increased in light smokers; 21 times in moderate smokers; and 100+ times in heavy smokers.

Patients with primary pneumothorax tend to be taller and thinner than control subjects. An increased chest height may contribute to the formation of apical anatomical changes as pleural pressure falls by about 0.20 cm H_2O/cm vertical lung height, hence pleural pressure is more negative at the apex of the lung in tall than in short people.

Primary pneumothorax has a genetic component, with some families exhibiting an autosomal dominant inheritance with incomplete penetrance. Birt–Hogg–Dube syndrome (OMIM 135150) is an autosomal dominant syndrome which includes spontaneous pneumothorax (25% of patients), benign skin tumours and renal tumours. Pneumothorax also occurs with increased frequency in Marfan's syndrome (OMIM 154700), although the fibrillin gene (causal of Marfan's syndrome) is not the explanation of primary pneumothorax in those families with dominant inheritance where it has been studied. Pneumothorax is also increased in frequency in homocystinuria.

Clinical features

The peak age for primary pneumothorax is the early 20s and the condition is rare after age 40. Pneumothoraces usually develop at rest.

Dyspnoea and ipsilateral chest pain are the main symptoms, and about 66% of patients have both. Ipsilateral Horner's syndrome is a rare complication—probably through mediastinal shift causing traction on the sympathetic ganglia.

Physical examination is usually normal, with the exception of moderate tachycardia. Pneumothorax can cause electrocardiographic changes, including shift of the frontal QRS axis, diminution of precordial R wave, precordial T-wave inversion and a prominent R wave in V2, mimicking posterior myocardial infarction.

Tension pneumothorax

Tension pneumothorax is a rare but important variant of pneumothorax where a 'flap valve' mechanism at the visceral pleural surface results in the development of increasing positive pressure in the pleural space. This causes progressive mediastinal shift away from the side of the pneumothorax, and ultimately impedes venous return to the heart—causing hypotension, shock and collapse.

The diagnosis of tension pneumothorax is based on the clinical features of a large pneumothorax with mediastinal shift away from the affected side, cardiovascular compromise, and severe progressive dyspnoea. The pulse rate exceeds 140 beats/min, and hypotension, cyanosis, or electromechanical dissociation may occur. On examination the side of the chest affected is enlarged, moves less during the respiratory cycle, and the trachea may be shifted toward the contralateral side. Tactile fremitus is absent, the percussion note is hyperresonant, and the breath sounds are absent or reduced on the affected side. The liver may be shifted inferiorly with a right-sided pneumothorax.

The demonstration by chest radiograph of modest deviation of the mediastinum away from the site of pneumothorax and depression of diaphragm ipsilateral to the pneumothorax are not, in the absence of the characteristic clinical features, sufficient to diagnose tension pneumothorax. These changes are common features of an uncomplicated pneumothorax and are due to expansion of the thoracic cavity following the loss of elastic lung recoil pressure.

The treatment of tension pneumothorax requires urgent thoracic decompression, followed by chest tube placement (see Chapter 33.2).

Diagnosis of uncomplicated pneumothorax

The diagnosis is established by visualization of a lung edge—a pleural line—on the chest radiograph (Fig. 18.17.20). Other radiographs are rarely needed, though a lateral decubitus film may help. About 15% of radiographs showing a primary pneumothorax also show a small pleural effusion causing a fluid level. This pleural fluid is usually eosinophilic on cytology. Rarely, spontaneous pneumothorax causes brisk pleural bleeding from a torn pleural adhesion, with urgent surgery often required to stop this.

The volumes of the lung and the hemithorax are roughly proportional to the cube of their diameters. Estimating the size of a pneumothorax therefore requires the measurement of the horizontal diameter of the lung and chest wall and the use of the formula:

$$\% \text{ pneumothorax volume} = 100 \times [1 - (\text{lung diameter}^3/\text{hemithorax diameter}^3)]$$

Treatment

Treatment aims to empty the pleural space of air and decrease the likelihood of recurrence. Treatment strategies should remember that primary pneumothorax is mainly a nuisance and rarely life-threatening. Detailed care guidelines have been produced by the British Thoracic Society and the American College of Chest Physicians.

Simple observation while awaiting spontaneous reabsorption of pneumothorax is appropriate for patients with few/no symptoms and small pneumothoraces. Increased inspired oxygen concentrations hasten reabsorption of such pneumothoraces, provided the lung air leak has ceased and reabsorbed gas is not replenished. This is due to the effect of supplemental oxygen on the nitrogen pressure gradient from the pleural space into the capillaries and alveolar space: it decreases the partial pressure of nitrogen in the alveolar space and in the blood (by increasing alveolar P_{O_2} and therefore inevitably decreasing alveolar P_{N_2}), which increases the gradient in P_{N_2} between the pneumothorax and venous blood and the alveolar space, and thereby hastens pneumothorax reabsorption.

Pneumothorax aspiration aims to reduce the volume of a closed pneumothorax (Fig. 18.17.20), reducing the time to final pneumothorax resolution, and is recommended for patients with a

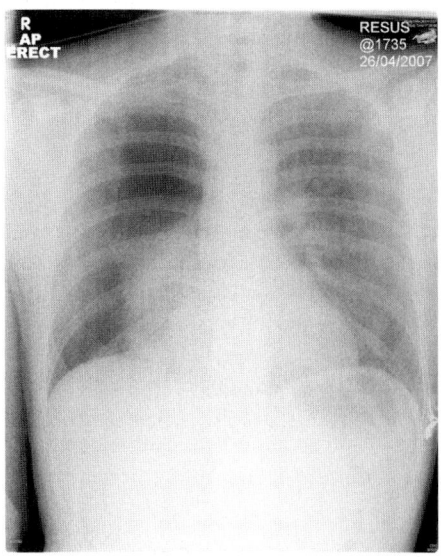

(a)

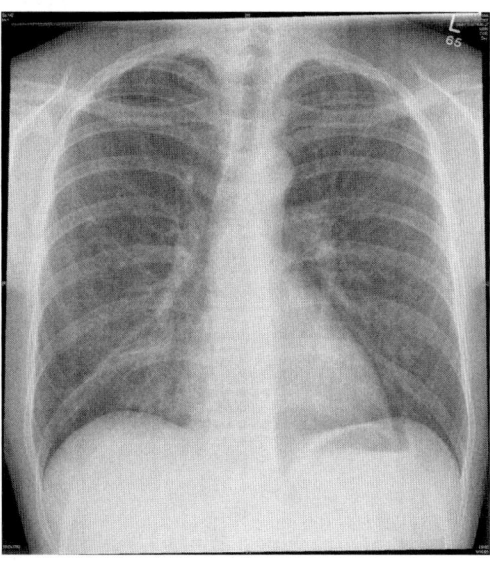

(b)

Fig. 18.17.20 Chest radiographs showing a primary spontaneous pneumothorax before (a) and after (b) successful pleural aspiration.

pneumothorax of over 15% of hemithorax volume. A small catheter (c.16 G) is inserted either into the second anterior intercostal space at the midclavicular line, or into the posterior chest second, third or fourth intercostal space medial to the scapula (see Chapter 33.2), after local anaesthesia. An alternative site is selected if the pneumothorax is loculated or adhesions are present. A three-way stopcock and a 60-ml syringe are attached to the catheter. Air is manually withdrawn until no more can be aspirated. If the volume of air aspirated is more than 4 litres, it is assumed that there is a continuing air leak and aspiration is abandoned.

A technique similar to simple pneumothorax aspiration is used to gently decompress a true tension pneumothorax before chest tube insertion, with air allowed to pass freely through the catheter to reduce pleural pressure to atmospheric.

Most patients with primary pneumothorax can be managed with simple aspiration on an outpatient basis (Fig. 18.17.20). Even where lung expansion does not follow aspiration, a patient with few/and no symptoms who is stable after a few hours can be managed without chest tube drainage and the pneumothorax will resolve with time. Chest tube drainage is indicated whenever conservative therapy is inappropriate, with lung expansion following for most patients in less than 5 days. Relatively small tubes (12–16F) appear to be as effective as larger tubes, and are less painful.

Prognosis

About 40% of patients who have had a primary pneumothorax without subsequent treatment to prevent recurrence will have a further episode on the same side, mostly within 1 year, and about 15% will develop pneumothorax on the contralateral side. Once a patient has had one recurrence, further episodes occur in over 50%, hence surgical recurrence prevention is performed in most patients who have had three events. Recurrence is more likely in patients who are tall and do not cease smoking. There is no relationship between the number of lung blebs on CT or the appearance of the lung at thorocotomy and the risk of recurrence.

Prevention of recurrence

VATS is the mainstay of recurrence prevention for primary pneumothorax. The procedure consists of a pleurodesis (by pleural abrasion or talc administration), variably combined with excision of apical blebs. The recurrence rate is less than 5% with either approach, but it is not clear whether apical bleb excision improves outcome and randomized trials are needed in this area. Open thorocotomy may be marginally more effective, but its higher morbidity and longer inpatient stays mean that video assisted thoracoscopic surgery is preferred. Chest tube drainage with installation of a pleurodesis agent such as talc slurry or doxycycline reduces the recurrence rate to about 25%: this is clearly inferior to surgery, which is therefore the preferred option.

Air travel after pneumothorax

Guidelines suggest that air travel should be avoided for 6 weeks after recovery from a pneumothorax. Commercial aircraft are not pressurized to atmospheric pressure and thus a pneumothorax may expand, causing breathlessness or chest pain at altitude. If a chest tube attached to an underwater seal is *in situ* in any known pneumothorax, the expanding pleural air can escape and so this is not a specific contraindication to all flight (e.g. for air ambulance transfer). If the pneumothorax develops during flight, its size will be similar to a pneumothorax developing at ground level, and if the air leak has closed, it will become smaller during aircraft descent.

Secondary spontaneous pneumothorax

Secondary spontaneous pneumothorax is defined as occurring due to an underlying lung disease and is more severe than primary pneumothorax as the patient has reduced underlying pulmonary reserve. The comorbidity also complicates management, and the natural history of any leaks from pathological lung differs from that from normal lung. The incidence of secondary pneumothorax is similar to that of primary pneumothorax. An estimated 15 000 new cases occur annually in the United States of America. Men aged over 75 years have the highest incidence of pneumothorax, at 60 in 100 000 per year.

Aetiology

COPD is the most common underlying disease, although almost every lung disease has been associated with pneumothorax: in 505 cases, 348 had COPD, 93 tumours, 26 sarcoidosis, 9 tuberculosis, 16 other pulmonary infections, and 13 other diseases. The incidence of pneumothorax increases with severity of COPD. *Pneumocystis jiroveci* infection complicating AIDS is a well-recognized cause. About 12.5% of patients with cystic fibrosis experience pneumothorax, which is also common in lymphangioleiomyomatosis (see Chapter 18.14.6) and pulmonary Langerhans' cell histiocytosis (see Chapter 18.14.5).

Clinical features

Symptoms are more severe than in primary pneumothorax due to underlying lung disease. Dyspnoea (sometimes life-threatening) is almost always present, and reported mortality rates vary from 1 to 10%. The possibility of pneumothorax should be considered in every patient with COPD who suddenly deteriorates, particularly if there is associated chest pain. Physical examination is rarely helpful and a chest radiograph is required for diagnosis. It is sometimes difficult to see the lung edge ('pleural line') on such radiographs because the emphysematous lung is hyperlucent, and large, thin-walled, air containing emphysematous bullae can mimic pneumothorax. With a large bulla, the apparent pleural line is usually concave towards the lateral chest wall as it represents the medial border of the bulla, whereas the pleural line with a pneumothorax is usually orientated convexly towards the lateral chest wall. Since chest drain insertion into a lung bulla mistaken for a pneumothorax in a patient with COPD who is already very ill can be disastrous, thoracic CT should be used to clarify the diagnosis before chest tube insertion where there is uncertainty. The diagnosis can be particularly difficult where air in the subcutaneous tissues further obscures the radiographic features (Fig. 18.17.21).

Treatment

Prompt treatment and effective recurrence prevention are higher priorities in secondary than in primary pneumothorax as patients are more symptomatic, have an appreciable mortality before treatment, and a higher recurrence rate (45% over 3–5 years). Most patients should have tube drainage as the evacuation of even small secondary pneumothoraces can lead to rapid improvement in symptoms.

The prognosis after tube drainage is also worse than in primary pneumothorax. The median duration of drainage for a secondary pneumothorax due to COPD is 5 days, compared with 1 day for primary pneumothorax, and about 20% of patients with secondary pneumothorax have a prolonged air leak lasting for more than 7 days.

Prevention

Video-assisted thoracoscopic pleurodesis has a recurrence rate of about 5%, compared to 20% after chest-tube-based chemical

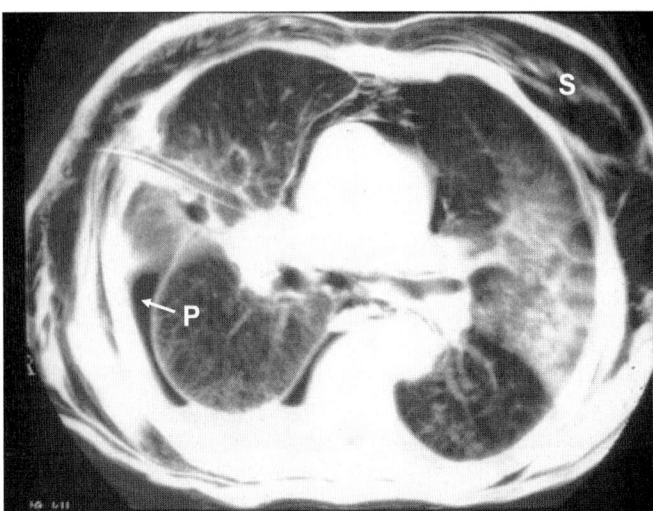

Fig. 18.17.21 CT showing a complex secondary pneumothorax (P). This was difficult to assess by plain radiography as subcutaneous air (S) obscured the radiographic features. A chest tube that lies in the interlobar fissure is seen.

pleurodesis, and should be the treatment of choice where possible. If the patient is not fit for anaesthesia, then pleurodesis with talc slurry or doxy/tetracycline is appropriate.

For patients who may require lung transplantation for their primary lung disease, recurrence prevention is still possible without transplantation being rendered impossible, but it is recommended that the surgical teams who will be involved in later transplantation are involved in such recurrence prevention.

Iatrogenic pneumothorax

Iatrogenic pneumothorax is probably more common than all other types combined and is becoming commoner with the increased use of interventional thoracic procedures including transbronchial biopsy, percutaneous lung biopsy, central venous catheterization, and assisted ventilation at high levels of pressure. About 25% of patients develop pneumothorax after transthoracic needle aspiration of lung, with rates being highest if the patient has COPD or a lesion deep within the lung.

During mechanical ventilation about 4% of patients develop a pneumothorax, which is more frequent if the patient has aspiration pneumonia, is ventilated with high positive end-expiratory or inflation pressures (particularly in adult respiratory distress syndrome), the right main bronchus is intubated, or the patient has COPD.

Diagnosis and treatment

The diagnosis is established by appropriate clinical suspicion in a high-risk patient, combined with a chest radiograph. Treatment differs from spontaneous pneumothorax in that recurrence prevention is not needed as the underlying lung is normal, hence air evacuation is the sole aim of treatment. If the patient has few/no symptoms, is not artificially ventilated, and the pneumothorax occupies less than 15% of the hemithorax, simple observation with the administration of supplemental oxygen is appropriate. Simple aspiration or chest-tube drainag e is appropriate if the patient has significant symptoms or the pneumothorax is large.

The patient with an iatrogenic pneumothorax secondary to assisted mechanical ventilation should always receive chest-tube drainage to avoid the development of a tension pneumothorax

due to the positive inspiratory pressures generated by the ventilator driving air into the pleural space. Sometimes this mechanism produces an air leak so large that a high percentage of the total inspired volume exits via the chest tube. This usually still provides effective ventilation, as the drained gases have a similar CO_2 content to exhaled air.

Traumatic pneumothorax

The incidence of a pneumothorax after blunt trauma depends on the severity of the injury, but is high and exceeds 35% in some series. With penetrating chest trauma the mechanism of pneumothorax is simply air entry through the wound or via the visceral pleura from injury to the lung. With nonpenetrating trauma a pneumothorax may develop if the visceral pleura is lacerated by a rib fracture or dislocation, but in most cases there are no associated rib fractures and it is thought that sudden chest compression increases alveolar pressures and causes alveolar rupture. Air then enters the interstitial space and dissects towards either the visceral pleura or the mediastinum, with a pneumothorax developing when the visceral or mediastinal pleura ruptures and allows air to enter the pleural space.

Diagnosis and treatment

The diagnosis is made by chest radiograph or CT, with 40% of pneumothoraces demonstrated on the initial chest radiograph being clinically unexpected. Thoracic ultrasonography, performed at the bedside, is also a sensitive diagnostic technique, but is inaccurate in subjects with COPD.

Most traumatic pneumothoraces are treated with chest-tube drainage, although an occult or small pneumothorax can be managed conservatively if assisted ventilation is not needed. After chest-tube drainage the lung usually expands within 24 h.

Traumatic pneumothorax is occasionally the presenting feature of rupture of the trachea or a major bronchus (usually after anterior or lateral fracture of some of the first three ribs). Most of these patients also have haemoptysis. Bronchoscopy should be performed when this diagnosis is suspected, with rapid surgical repair of any defect identified.

Traumatic rupture of the oesophagus is another uncommon but important differential diagnosis presenting as pneumothorax. Hydropneumothorax is usual in this situation. The measurement of pleural fluid amylase (due to the entry of amylase rich saliva into the pleural space) reliably identifies this problem.

Catamenial pneumothorax

Catamenial pneumothorax is pneumothorax occurring in conjunction with menstruation, with patients typically having about five episodes before the relationship with the menstrual cycle is recognized. Respiratory symptoms usually develop within 24 to 48 h of the onset of menstrual flow. Most pneumothoraces are right sided, but left sided and bilateral examples are reported.

The aetiology of catamenial pneumothorax is not clear: possibilities include air gaining access to the peritoneal cavity during menstruation, and then entering the pleural cavity via a diaphragm defect, or pleural or diaphragmatic endometriosis. In a series of eight cases undergoing particularly careful thoracoscopy, diaphragmatic abnormalities were present in all—diaphragmatic defects and endometriosis in four, a diaphragmatic defect alone in one, and diaphragmatic endometriosis alone in three. It has been hypothesized that diaphragmatic endometriosis may undergo cyclical necrosis, leading to a diaphragmatic defect.

The treatment of catamenial pneumothorax targets any endometriosis, but this is effective in only about 50% of patients. Direct pneumothorax recurrence prevention is similar to standard care, with additional therapies such as stapling of blebs and closure of diaphragmatic defects.

Re-expansion pulmonary oedema

Unilateral pulmonary oedema (re-expansion pulmonary oedema) occurs when the lung is rapidly reinflated after a period of collapse due to a pneumothorax or pleural effusion. The phenomenon is uncommon and only very rarely fatal, and its clinical frequency is far lower than the frequency with which it is discussed. There were 3 cases in the Veterans Administration cooperative study of more than 500 spontaneous pneumothoraces.

Aetiology

The oedema fluid has a high protein content, hence it is due to increased capillary leakiness rather than increased hydrostatic pressure. Possible mechanisms include damage caused by mechanical stresses applied to the lung during re-expansion, or ischaemia/reperfusion injury due to oxygen free radicals. Oxygen-scavenging compounds such as dimethylthiourea, catalase, or superoxide dismutase partially inhibit neutrophilic infiltration of re-expansion pulmonary oedema, but do not substantially decrease the amount of oedema itself. In experimental animals, re-expansion oedema only occurs if the lung has been collapsed for several days and is re-expanded rapidly: this fits the clinical picture where the pneumothorax or effusion has usually been present for more than 3 days.

Clinical features

Re-expansion and oedema causes coughing and chest tightness during or immediately after lung re-expansion. Symptoms may progress for 12 to 24h, with chest radiographs showing ipsilateral pulmonary oedema that may rarely progress to involved contralateral lung. If the patient does not die within the first 48h, recovery is usually complete. Treatment is supportive, with administration of supplemental oxygen, diuretics, intubation, and mechanical ventilation if needed.

Prevention

The risk of re-expansion oedema is probably reduced if lung inflation is gentle, hence a chest tube for pneumothorax should be attached to an underwater seal drainage without suction to allow gradual lung re-expansion. During drainage of a pleural effusion, the procedure should be terminated if the patient develops chest tightness or persistent coughing. Arbitrary maximal volumes for a single thoracentesis are often suggested to reduce the risk of re-expansion oedema, but there is no direct evidence to substantiate this strategy.

Further reading

Pleural effusion

Diacon AH, et al. (2003). Diagnostic tools in tuberculous pleurisy: a direct comparative study. *Eur Respir J*, **22**, 589–91.
Heffner JE, Highland K, Brown LK (2003). A meta-analysis derivation of continuous likelihood ratios for diagnosing pleural fluid exudates. *Am J Respir Crit Care Med*, **167**, 1591–9.

Leung AN, Muller NL, Miller RR (1990). CT in differential diagnosis of diffuse pleural disease. *AJR Am J Roentgenol*, **154**, 3–92.
Light RW, et al. (1972). Pleural effusions: the diagnostic separation of transudates and exudates. *Ann Intern Med*, **77**, 507–13.
Maskell NA, Gleeson FV, Davies RJO (2003). Standard pleural biopsy versus CT-guided cutting-needle biopsy for diagnosis of malignant disease in pleural effusions: a randomised controlled trial. *Lancet*, **361**, 1326–30.
Maskell NA, Butland RJ (2003). The British Thoracic Society guidelines for the investigation of a unilateral pleural effusion in adults. *Thorax*, **58**, 8–17.

Pyogenic pleural infection

Colice GL, et al. (2000). Medical and surgical treatment of parapneumonic effusions: an evidence-based guideline. *Chest*, **118**, 4–71.
Davies CWH, Gleeson FV, Davies RJO (2003). The British Thoracic Society Guidelines for the management of pleural infection. *Thorax*, **58**, 18–28.
Heffner JE, et al. (1995). Pleural fluid chemical analysis in parapneumonic effusions. A meta-analysis. *Am J Respir Crit Care Med*, **151**, 1700–8.
Maskell NA, et al. (2005). UK controlled trial of intrapleural streptokinase for pleural infection. *N Engl J Med*, **352**, 865–74.
Maskell NA, et al. (2006). The bacteriology of pleural infection by genetic and standard methods and its mortality significance. *Am J Respir Crit Care Med*, **174**, 817–23.

Tuberculous pleural effusion and empyema

Baumann MH, et al. (2007). Pleural tuberculosis in the United States: incidence and drug resistance. *Chest*, **131**, 1125–32.
Diacon AH, et al. (2003). Diagnostic tools in tuberculous pleurisy: a direct comparative study. *Eur Respir J*, **22**, 589–91.
Gopi A, et al. (2007). Diagnosis and treatment of tuberculous pleural effusion in 2006. *Chest*, **131**, 880–9.

Chylothorax and pseudochylothorax

Light RW and Lee YCG (2005). Pneumothorax, chylothorax, hemothorax and fibrothorax. In: Murray J, et al. (eds) *Textbook of respiratory diseases*, 4th edition, pp. 1961–88. W B Saunders, Philadelphia.

Haemothorax

Maxwell RA, et al. (2004). Use of presumptive antibiotics following tube thoracostomy for traumatic hemopneumothorax in the prevention of empyema and pneumoni—a multi-center trial. *J Trauma*, **57**, 742–8.

Benign asbestos-induced pleural disease

Chapman SJ, et al. (2003). Benign asbestos pleural diseases. *Curr Opin Pulm Med*, **9**, 266–71.

Pneumothorax

Baumann MH, et al. (2001). Management of spontaneous pneumothorax: an American College of Chest Physicians Delphi consensus statement. *Chest*, **119**, 590–602.
Henry M, et al. (2003). British Thoracic Society guidelines for the management of spontaneous pneumothorax. *Thorax*, **58** Suppl 2, **ii**, 39–52.
Noppen M, et al. (2002). Manual aspiration versus chest tube drainage in first episodes of primary spontaneous pneumothorax: a multicenter, prospective, randomized pilot study. *Am J Respir Crit Care Med*, **165**, 1240–4.
Noppen M, et al. (2006). Fluorescein-enhanced autofluorescence thoracoscopy in patients with primary spontaneous pneumothorax and normal subjects. *Am J Respir Crit Care Med*, **174**, 26–30.
Tschopp JM, et al. (2006). Management of spontaneous pneumothorax: state of the art. *Eur Respir J*, **28**, 637–50.

Disorders of the thoracic cage and diaphragm

John M. Shneerson

Essentials

Disorders of the thoracic skeleton—these can lead to a severe restrictive ventilatory defect, the risk of respiratory failure being highest with (1) scoliosis—particularly if the following characteristics are present: early onset, severe angulation, high in the thorax, respiratory muscle weakness, low vital capacity; (2) kyphosis—but only if of very sharp angulation (gibbus), most commonly seen following tuberculous osteomyelitis; and (3) after thoracoplasty—historically performed as treatment for pulmonary tuberculosis.

Diaphragmatic weakness—unilateral paralysis rarely causes symptoms unless there is coexisting lung disease or weakness of other respiratory muscles. Bilateral weakness usually presents as orthopnoea, which (by contrast to orthopnoea in cardiac failure) is relieved promptly by sitting up, and on examination the abdomen moves paradoxically inwards as the diaphragm ascends during inspiration. Vital capacity in the sitting position is about 50% of that predicted and may fall by a further 50% when supine. Diaphragmatic screening or ultrasound examination reveals paradoxical diaphragmatic movement during sniffing.

Respiratory failure—this occurs initially during sleep, when the respiratory drive is reduced and the work of breathing is increased, and then in wakefulness. Pulmonary hypertension and right heart failure often develop once the arterial Pco_2 is elevated during the day. Arterial blood gases and quality of life can both be readily improved with noninvasive ventilation, usually using a nasal or face mask. Survival in most skeletal disorders after starting ventilation is around 80 to 90% at 1 year, 75% at 3 years and 50% at 5 to 10 years.

Other clinical features—some conditions of the thoracic cage, particularly pectus excavatum and the straight back syndrome, can cause cardiac problems due primarily to distortion of the heart and major vessels. Ankylosing spondylitis leads to apical bullae, pleural thickening/effusions, and cricoarytenoid arthritis, but rarely causes respiratory failure.

Introduction

Skeletal disorders of the thorax are an important group of conditions that frequently impair ventilation. They are often associated with respiratory muscle weakness due to neuromuscular disorders, which are described elsewhere. Most of these conditions restrict the development and/or the expansion of the lungs so that alveolar ventilation rather than intrapulmonary gas exchange is primarily impaired.

Disorders of the spine

Scoliosis

Scoliosis is defined as a lateral curvature of the spine, but it is invariably also associated with rotation of the vertebral bodies (Fig. 18.18.1). This results in an unstable lordosis rather than a kyphosis, and hence the frequently used term kyphoscoliosis is inaccurate. A mild degree of scoliosis is very common. Angles of curvature of 5° or 10° have been used to define when it becomes pathological, but these are arbitrary figures. Postural scoliosis can be distinguished from a structural scoliosis by its temporary nature and because it disappears on bending forward.

The age of onset and natural history of scoliosis vary according to its cause (Box 18.18.1). When it is due to a neuromuscular disorder ('paralytic' scoliosis) it usually arises during childhood or adolescence, or in poliomyelitis within about 2 years of the acute infection. Typically, the curve has a long C shape and may be severe. The scoliosis is due to asymmetrical weakness of the axial muscles causing the spine to rotate and move to one side. Weakness of chest wall muscles is almost invariable, occurs in a pattern which is characteristic of each disorder, and may have a profound influence on the clinical features.

When the scoliosis is due to a congenital abnormality, such as a hemivertebra or a segmentation defect, it usually becomes apparent early in childhood. The scoliosis of neurofibromatosis and Marfan's syndrome is probably due to an abnormality of connective tissue. Scoliosis due to pleural or pulmonary disease is less common than in the past, now that chronic infections are less frequent and more successfully treated.

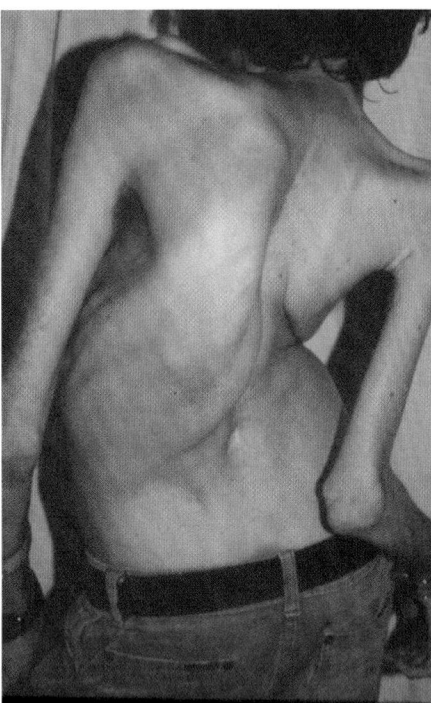

Fig. 18.18.1 Scoliosis following poliomyelitis.

The commonest type is adolescent idiopathic scoliosis, where the spinal deformity develops at the time of the pubertal growth spurt. It is around four times as common in girls as in boys, and the convexity of the deformity is on the right in 80% of cases. The scoliosis may continue to worsen slightly even after growth of the spine stops. An infantile form of idiopathic scoliosis is less common

---

Box 18.18.1 Causes of scoliosis

◆ Idiopathic
  · Infantile, adolescent
◆ Osteopathic
  · Congenital (e.g. hemivertebrae)
  · Thoracoplasty
◆ Neuromuscular
  · Syringomyelia
  · Friedreich's ataxia
  · Poliomyelitis
  · Duchenne's muscular dystrophy
◆ Connective tissue disorders
  · Marfan's syndrome
  · Neurofibromatosis
  · Osteogenesis imperfecta
◆ Pleuropulmonary
  · Empyema
  · Pneumonectomy
  · Unilateral lung fibrosis

---

and can progress to a severe deformity, although it often resolves spontaneously.

Pathophysiology

The most important immediate consequence of scoliosis is the respiratory abnormality, a direct result being that the compliance of the chest wall is reduced. This is more marked in older people, possibly owing to degenerative changes in the costovertebral joints. The compliance of the lungs is also reduced, largely because of their small volume. In addition, the distortion of the ribcage puts the inspiratory muscles at a mechanical disadvantage; those on the side of the convexity of the scoliosis are shortened and those on the side of the concavity lengthened. The vital capacity falls when changing from the sitting to the supine position, implying that diaphragmatic function is impaired. A restrictive defect and reduction of the maximum inspiratory and expiratory pressures develops even in the absence of any muscle weakness, but is more marked if this is present.

In adults with severe scoliosis, exercise capacity is linked to the degree of reduction of the vital capacity and the forced expiratory volume in 1 s (FEV_1). On exercise the tidal volume increases initially and then remains constant, while respiratory rate rises as exercise becomes more intense. Ventilation at any given oxygen uptake is greater than normal, and maximal exercise ventilation, which limits exercise capability, is often severely curtailed. The cardiac output may increase normally during exercise, but pulmonary artery pressure rises rapidly, and its rate of increase is linearly related to oxygen uptake and inversely related to the vital capacity.

In mild scoliosis, the arterial blood gases are often normal, but the first abnormality is a fall in the partial pressure of oxygen (Po_2). This is due to suboptimal ventilation and perfusion matching, particularly at the bases of the lungs. Even when the anatomical distortion of the two lungs is gross, there is usually rather less difference in function between the two lungs than might be expected.

Acute ventilatory failure may be precipitated by e.g. a chest infection or asthma, but chronic hypoventilation initially occurs during sleep. Sleep is associated with loss of the voluntary respiratory drive and a reduction in the reflex drive in response to hypoxia, hypercapnia, and other stimuli. Within each stage of non-rapid eye movement (NREM) sleep the respiratory pattern is regular, but it varies as NREM sleep moves from one stage to another. Central apnoeas may appear and the arterial Pco_2 rises slightly despite a reduction in metabolic rate. In rapid eye movement (REM) sleep the respiratory drive overall is less than during NREM sleep, and it is much more variable from moment to moment. Muscle activity is reduced, and whereas in NREM sleep this affects all the respiratory muscles to an equal extent, in REM sleep diaphragmatic activity is selectively retained. Relaxation of the other respiratory muscles is more intense than during NREM sleep and loss of activity in the upper airway dilator muscles increases the upper airway resistance and the work of the chest wall muscles.

These changes during sleep are particularly important in scoliosis, where the diaphragm is attached to an asymmetrical ribcage and the respiratory pump often has little reserve. The effects of sleep are accentuated when the scoliosis is the result of neuromuscular disorders because the presence of muscle weakness in addition to the skeletal deformity reduces tidal volume and increases respiratory frequency, leading to alveolar hypoventilation. Arousals initially occur in REM sleep, which becomes fragmented, and at a later stage in NREM sleep, with loss particularly of stages 3 and 4. Sleep fragmentation itself reduces the respiratory drive and impairs the strength and probably the endurance of the respiratory muscles, promoting a vicious circle in which there are progressively more respiratory-induced arousals and deterioration in respiratory drive and muscle function. Central apnoeas and hypopnoeas develop; hypercapnia then appears during wakefulness as well as in sleep.

Chronic hypercapnia during the day is uncommon in childhood and is determined in patients with scoliosis by the following:

- Age of onset—if the scoliosis appears before the age of about 8 years it may prevent normal alveolar multiplication so that the lungs fail to develop fully. The capillary surface area is reduced and there is an increased risk of developing respiratory and right heart failure later in life. The later onset of adolescent idiopathic scoliosis is probably the main reason why these complications only rarely occur in this condition.

- Level of the scoliosis—in general, the higher the curve in the thoracic spine, the more marked are the cardiac and respiratory problems. Thoracolumbar or lumbar scoliosis has virtually no effect on respiration.

- Severity of scoliosis—the angle of scoliosis is closely related to the reduction in lung volume. This association is seen with the residual volume, total lung capacity and functional residual capacity, as well as with vital capacity, except in patients with neuromuscular disorders where the changes in lung volumes are due to the weakness of the respiratory muscles as well as the degree of deformity. The changes in lung volumes become significant when the angle of scoliosis is greater than about 100°.

- Presence of muscle weakness—the functioning of the respiratory muscles is impaired in scoliosis, and any further loss of strength or endurance due to neuromuscular disorders may precipitate respiratory failure. Conversely, respiratory function often worsens in neuromuscular disorders when scoliosis develops as the strength of the axial muscle becomes asymmetrical.

- Small lung volumes—respiratory failure usually occurs when lung volumes have been reduced to a degree such that vital capacity is less than 1.0 to 1.5 l.

Hypoxia causes pulmonary vasoconstriction, which increases the pulmonary vascular resistance and leads to pulmonary hypertension, but the rate of rise of pulmonary artery pressure during exercise correlates with the degree of restriction of lung volumes rather than arterial Po_2. Right ventricular and atrial hypertrophy develop if hypoxia is prolonged. Significant pulmonary hypertension is rarely seen unless the arterial Po_2 is less than about 8 kPa, and pulmonary hypertension by itself rarely causes right heart failure, hence the exact mechanisms underlying these right-sided cardiac changes are uncertain. The increase in sympathetic activity and circulating catecholamines associated with hypoxia cause renal vasoconstriction and a reduction in renal blood flow. This activates the renin–angiotensin–aldosterone system, leading to sodium and water retention. Hypercapnia is associated with an increase in renal tubular hydrogen ion excretion with sodium reabsorption in exchange for hydrogen. This leads to fluid retention, which is accentuated by an increase in antidiuretic hormone (ADH) secretion. Hypercapnia probably also increases capillary permeability, which contributes to the appearance of oedema.

Polycythaemia occasionally occurs as a result of erythropoietin release from the kidneys in response to hypoxia. This adaptive mechanism increases the oxygen carrying capacity of the blood, but also raises blood viscosity, increasing the work of the right and left ventricles and predisposing to arterial and venous thrombosis.

Symptoms and physical signs

The earliest symptom of scoliosis is usually a change in the appearance of the patient, such as asymmetry of the shoulders or prominence of the posterior rib hump. Backache is a late and uncommon symptom. With mild curvatures there may be no respiratory symptoms, but mild shortness of breath on exertion is common and a change in this often signifies the development of complications such as respiratory failure. Orthopnoea suggests that diaphragmatic function is impaired. When respiratory failure develops, fatigue, ankle swelling, and even syncope may indicate that pulmonary hypertension and right heart failure are present. Frequent awakenings during sleep, associated with excessive daytime somnolence, indicate sleep fragmentation due to apnoeas and hypopnoeas, and are important symptoms that warn of impending respiratory failure.

Physical examination may reveal the cause of the scoliosis, such as Marfan's syndrome or neurofibromatosis, and other congenital abnormalities. Any associated muscle weakness or congenital heart disease may be apparent. Ribcage expansion may be predominantly lateral or anterior, or achieved by extension of the spine. In some subjects, chest expansion is mainly oblique because of the rotation of the spine, and some areas of the chest wall may move paradoxically. Accessory muscle action is usually prominent. The presence of central cyanosis indicates that the arterial oxygen saturation is below around 80%. Signs of hypercapnia may also be present, including tachycardia, large volume pulse, peripheral venous dilatation, papilloedema, a flapping tremor, reduction in tendon reflexes, small pupils and—if severe—confusion and coma ('CO_2 narcosis').

Investigations

The severity of scoliosis can be demonstrated radiologically, but chest radiography is often unhelpful in thoracic scoliosis because rotation of the spine obscures much of the lung fields. This can be overcome by obtaining an oblique view of the chest which, by aligning the spine behind the heart, simulates a posteroanterior view. Lung function testing reveals a restrictive defect with reduction in all lung volumes, although the change in residual volume is least marked such that the ratio of residual volume to total lung capacity is increased. Kco is raised, as in other chest wall disorders that cause a restrictive defect and in which the lung tissue is normal. Maximum inspiratory and expiratory pressures and transdiaphragmatic pressure are reduced. Chest wall and lung compliance are less than normal, and exercise tolerance is impaired. Arterial blood gas analysis reveals a slightly low Pco_2 in mildly affected subjects, but later in the course of disease a rise in Pco_2 and a proportional fall in Po_2 develop. Sleep studies show a variable degree of hypoxia and hypercapnia which are usually most marked in REM sleep. Electrocardiography and echocardiography may be required to establish if pulmonary hypertension or congenital heart disease is present and identify precise abnormalities.

Prognosis

The prognosis in adolescent idiopathic scoliosis is virtually normal, but life expectancy is reduced in many of the other forms of scoliosis.

This is particularly so in scoliosis of early onset, when it is both severe and high in the thorax and associated with respiratory muscle weakness, low vital capacity, and abnormal blood gases.

In most patients the cause of death is either cardiac or respiratory. Pneumonia and respiratory failure are particularly common in neuromuscular disorders, but hypoxic dysrhythmias during sleep are probably responsible for some deaths. Congenital heart defects, which have an increased prevalence in those with scoliosis, particularly when this is due to a congenital abnormality or of the idiopathic type, also contribute to mortality.

Treatment

Mild scoliosis does not need any specific treatment. The prognosis is normal and there is minimal respiratory deficit. However, as the scoliosis becomes more severe, spinal fusion or a costectomy, in which the parts of the ribs comprising the posterior hump are removed, may be of cosmetic value. Spinal fusion may also be required to prevent progression of the scoliosis, to stabilize the spine, particularly in neuromuscular disorders, and in selected cases to try to improve cardiac or respiratory function or to prevent its deterioration.

The value of spinal fusion to prevent cardiorespiratory deterioration in adolescent idiopathic scoliosis is still under debate. Many studies of respiratory function before and after surgery have shown remarkably little change in lung volumes, blood gases, or exercise ability. However, in some patients with muscle weakness, particularly Duchenne's muscular dystrophy, the rate of fall of the vital capacity can be slowed considerably, and it can even be improved in patients who have had poliomyelitis. However, despite these short-term improvements, there have been no studies which indicate whether or not spinal fusion performed in childhood or adolescence prevents respiratory failure from appearing later in life.

If respiratory failure does develop, any acute illness—most commonly an infection or bronchial asthma—that has precipitated it should be actively treated. Noninvasive ventilation or endotracheal intubation and ventilation may be required during the acute illness. If the latter is needed, the patient is then weaned from this either completely or on to a noninvasive method of long-term respiratory support.

Chronic ventilatory failure usually responds to long-term mechanical respiratory support. Administration of oxygen at night and/or during the day may be dangerous because of the risk of hypercapnia. Nasal or face mask positive pressure ventilation is the treatment of choice, but a negative-pressure system, such as a cuirass or jacket, is an alternative. Noninvasive ventilation is usually only required during sleep, but some patients benefit from 1 or 2 h treatment during the day as well. A tracheostomy is rarely required to provide ventilatory support, but in complex neuromuscular disorders it may be indicated to bypass upper airway obstruction, e.g. due to vocal cord adduction, or to gain access to the tracheobronchial tree to aspirate secretions, or to protect the airway from aspiration of material from the pharynx.

Noninvasive ventilatory support at night can improve the quality of sleep, breathlessness on exertion, daytime sleepiness, and early morning headaches. Activities of daily living may be carried out more easily and the number of visits required by general practitioners and the quantity of drugs prescribed can be reduced. Sleep architecture, daytime arterial blood gases and nocturnal oxygen saturation, and transcutaneous P_{CO_2} can all be improved. Survival once treatment

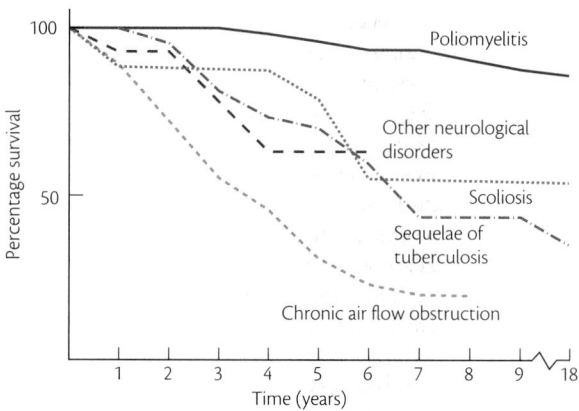

Fig. 18.18.2 Actuarial survival during treatment with ventilatory assistance for respiratory failure.
(Reproduced from Shneerson JM (1988). *Disorders of ventilation*, Blackwell, Oxford.)

has been instituted is around 75 to 85% at 5 years and 60% at 10 years (Fig. 18.18.2).

Kyphosis

Exaggeration of the normal thoracic kyphosis is most commonly due to osteoporosis and is not usually associated with any significant changes in respiratory function. The exception to this is when a very sharp kyphosis (gibbus) develops, usually caused by tuberculous osteomyelitis of the spine (Pott's disease), although other conditions such as radiotherapy can cause a similar picture.

The spine becomes rigid in the region of the gibbus, and when tuberculosis is the cause the costovertebral joints also become ankylosed and limit the expansion of the ribcage. A restrictive defect in which the total lung capacity is reduced more than the residual volume is characteristic, but respiratory problems are uncommon unless the gibbus is high in the thoracic spine and develops in early childhood. This is probably because in this circumstance the thoracic deformity prevents the normal development of the lungs in a similar way to early-onset scoliosis. Hypoxia and hypercapnia appear during sleep before they become apparent during wakefulness, but may be severe. Pulmonary hypertension and right heart failure frequently develop once chronic hypercapnia has become established.

Slight breathlessness on exertion is common in the presence of a gibbus, but is rare in other types of kyphosis. Physical examination reveals the spinal deformity and limitation of ribcage expansion.

The posteroanterior chest radiograph shows superimposition of the spinal deformity on the lung fields and heart, which makes it difficult to interpret. The extent and severity of the kyphosis is usually well seen on a lateral projection. The typical changes in lung volumes have been described above. The arterial P_{O_2} and P_{CO_2} are usually normal, and—as in scoliosis—the earliest abnormalities are revealed by sleep studies.

Treatment of acute tuberculous infection with chemotherapy often prevents a gibbus from developing. Once it has been established and respiratory failure has developed, the only effective treatment is long-term respiratory support. This is best provided noninvasively by a nasal positive-pressure ventilator, rather than a negative-pressure system, because the sharp kyphosis makes it difficult to lie in the supine position required for negative-pressure ventilation.

Straight-back syndrome

In this disorder the normal thoracic kyphosis is absent or greatly reduced. This may result in a mild restrictive ventilatory defect, but cardiac problems are more prominent. The heart and great vessels may be compressed between the anterior ribcage and the spine, with results similar to those seen in pectus excavatum. The right ventricular outflow tract or pulmonary artery may be narrowed, causing a systolic murmur, and occasionally right ventricular filling is impaired.

Ankylosing spondylitis

The initial manifestation of ankylosing spondylitis is usually painful inflammation of the sacroiliac joints, but this may spread to affect almost any joint including the intervertebral, costovertebral, manubriosternal, costochondral, and chondrosternal joints. When the inflammatory phase of the disease subsides, the joints become ankylosed and the spinal ligaments calcify.

The effect of ankylosing spondylitis on the thorax is that the ribcage becomes rigid. There is little spinal mobility, and a pronounced kyphosis often develops. The changes in lung volumes are characteristic in that, unlike all other skeletal disorders affecting the thorax, functional residual capacity increases. This is because the ribcage becomes fixed at its own relaxation volume, which is greater than the normal functional residual capacity that is influenced by the inward pull of the elastic recoil of the lungs. Total lung capacity and vital capacity are slightly reduced, and residual volume often increases.

The immobility of the ribcage leads to atrophy of the intercostal muscles and both maximal inspiratory and expiratory pressures are reduced. However, there is no impairment of diaphragmatic or abdominal muscle function, and this largely compensates for the restriction of ribcage expansion. The ventilatory responses to exercise are virtually normal and exercise is usually limited by musculoskeletal and circulatory rather than respiratory factors. Respiratory failure is extremely uncommon in ankylosing spondylitis, probably as a result of the normal diaphragmatic function, unless another complication develops, which may be one of the following:

- Air flow obstruction—cricoarytenoid arthritis is a feature of ankylosing spondylitis and may present with stridor, hoarseness of the voice, breathlessness, obstructive sleep apnoeas, or respiratory failure.

- Pleural thickening and effusion—these rare complications of ankylosing spondylitis may precipitate respiratory failure.

- Aspiration pneumonia—oesophageal motility is often impaired in ankylosing spondylitis and aspiration pneumonia may develop.

- Bullas—apical fibrobullous lung disease is a feature of ankylosing spondylitis and may be complicated by opportunist infections such as *Aspergillus fumigatus* or saprophytic mycobacteria, and occasionally by pulmonary tuberculosis.

- Abdominal surgery—this restricts diaphragmatic function on which adequate respiration depends. Conversely, thoracic surgery has relatively little effect on respiration because of the small contribution that ribcage expansion plays.

Chest pain during sudden movements such as coughing and laughing is common if the active phase of inflammation affects the thorax. These symptoms, which originate in either the joints or the muscles, become less prominent as the disease advances. Breathlessness and other respiratory symptoms are uncommon. Cricoarytenoid arthritis may occasionally present with hoarseness, stridor or breathlessness, and extensive fibrobullous disease may also cause breathlessness.

The most obvious physical sign related to the chest is restriction of ribcage movement associated with prominent accessory muscle activity and abdominal respiratory movements.

Chest radiography may show calcification of the paraspinal ligaments (bamboo spine) and reveal evidence of complications of ankylosing spondylitis such as pleural thickening, aspiration pneumonia, and apical fibrobullous disease. The changes in lung volumes have been described above. Chest wall compliance is reduced but lung compliance is normal. The Kco is increased and arterial blood gases are normal during both rest and exertion.

Physiotherapy and nonsteroidal anti-inflammatory drugs may improve vital capacity and chest expansion, particularly in the early phase of the disease or during acute exacerbations.

Disorders of the sternum and ribs

Congenital abnormalities

Congenital abnormalities of the ribs and sternum rarely cause any important respiratory problems. Multiple congenital rib abnormalities may occasionally lead to paradoxical movement of the chest wall or impair diaphragmatic function if they occur in the region of its insertion. Severe congenital defects of the sternum (e.g. agenesis or a bifid sternum) are rare, but may require surgery in the neonatal period in order to stabilize the anterior chest wall.

Pectus excavatum

Pectus excavatum is a depression deformity of the sternum that is often present at birth but may worsen during the adolescent growth spurt. It is occasionally familial and may be associated with other abnormalities such as the straight-back syndrome or scoliosis. It appears to result either from an increased inward pull on the sternum by the sternal diaphragmatic fibres or from an abnormally compliant chest wall.

Transient paradoxical movement of the sternum during respiration is seen in neonates, particularly in the presence of upper airway obstruction or pneumonia. The sternal depression may become permanent even if the cause, such as enlarged tonsils, resolves completely.

In adults pectus excavatum rarely causes any symptoms. Lung volumes are normal or only slightly diminished, and chest wall mobility appears to be normal. Arterial blood gases are normal both at rest and during exercise. Right ventricular filling can be impaired if the heart is compressed between the depressed sternum and the spine, and compression of the pulmonary outflow tract may cause a systolic murmur. These problems are most marked in the erect position and during exercise. Occasionally atrial dysrrhythmias develop, and opening of a patent foramen ovale induced by hyperventilation may lead to a right-to-left shunt and arterial hypoxaemia.

Surgery is sometimes indicated for cosmetic reasons, although the result can be disappointing. It has little or no effect on the mild restrictive defect or exercise ability, except in the rare situation when right ventricular filling is impaired or atrial dysrrhythmias have developed.

Pectus carinatum

Pectus carinatum is a protrusion deformity of the sternum in which the chest is often narrowed transversely. It becomes most marked during the pubertal growth spurt, although it may be present from birth and is occasionally associated with severe childhood asthma or ventricular septal defects. It is probably the result of excessive growth of the ribs or costal cartilages, and if this is asymmetrical the sternum becomes oblique.

The respiratory consequences of pectus carinatum have hardly been investigated. Chest pain may arise at the insertions of the intercostal muscles anteriorly, or in the costal cartilages and anterior ribs. Lung volumes appear to be normal. Surgery is indicated only for cosmetic reasons and not in order to improve respiratory function or exercise ability.

Asphyxiating thoracic dystrophy (Jeune's disease)

Asphyxiating thoracic dystrophy is a generalized disorder of cartilage in which radiological changes are most prominent in the pelvis, phalanges, and other limb bones. Like the other long bones, the ribs are shortened so that the ribcage becomes narrowed. Lung development may be impaired as a result, and respiratory failure often appears during infancy or childhood. Surgical reconstruction of the ribcage with splitting of the sternum to enable lung growth to occur has been largely unsuccessful.

Acquired abnormalities

Flail chest

A flail chest is one in which multiple rib fractures cause paradoxical movement of the chest wall during respiration. It may be associated with other injuries, such as rupture of the aortic arch or spleen, and with fractures of the skull and long bones. It is frequently associated with pulmonary contusion, pneumothorax, or haemothorax.

Surgical stabilization of the chest wall is rarely required. Sufficient analgesia to enable the patient to cough adequately may be all that is needed in less severe cases, as long as the paradoxical movement does not impair alveolar ventilation. Positive-pressure ventilation can achieve 'pneumatic splinting' of the flail segment if the problem is more severe. The effectiveness of this has not been definitely established, but it appears that positive end-expiratory pressure or continuous positive airway pressure is beneficial by preventing any negative pressure swings within the pleura.

Thoracoplasty

The operation of thoracoplasty was developed for the treatment of pulmonary tuberculosis, when varying lengths of up to 11 ribs were removed in order to collapse the chest on the affected side (Fig. 18.18.3). This treatment has been superseded by antituberculous chemotherapy, but is still occasionally required to treat chronic infections, particularly when there is a problem in obliterating the pleural space after pulmonary resection. It is estimated that as many as 30 000 operations were carried out in the United Kingdom between 1951 and 1960: some of these patients still survive, and increasing numbers are being seen by chest physicians because of the late complications of the surgical procedure.

The consequences of thoracoplasty on respiratory function have been hard to elucidate because they are often combined with the effects of the underlying lung disease for which the surgery was carried out, and those of other treatments such as lung resection.

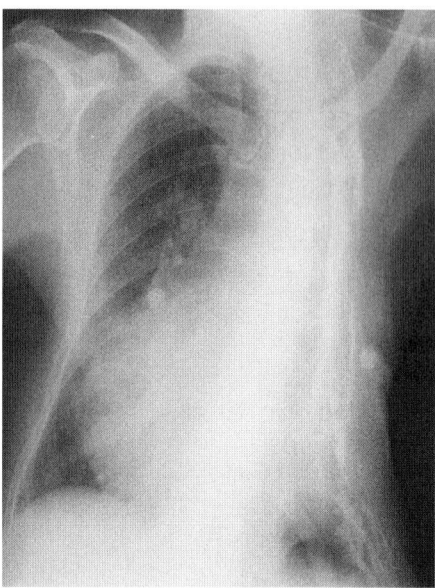

Fig. 18.18.3 Chest radiograph showing effects of thoracoplasty.

However, the removal of the ribs has the direct result of flattening the chest and reducing the volume of the thorax. The normal movements of the ribcage may be impaired and paradoxical movement at the site of the thoracoplasty is common. The compliance of the chest wall is reduced, and it may fall further because the small range of movements of the costovertebral joints after surgery probably induces soft tissue changes which further limit the mobility of these joints. Chest wall compliance is also reduced by the almost invariable development of a thoracic scoliosis. This is convex to the side of the thoracoplasty and may progress for several years after the surgery. The severity of the scoliosis correlates with the number of ribs removed, but also depends on the details of the surgical technique.

Respiratory muscle function is impaired by a thoracoplasty. The intercostal and shoulder girdle muscles are directly damaged by the surgery, and distortion of the ribcage and the development of a scoliosis put the inspiratory muscles at an additional mechanical disadvantage. Diaphragmatic excursion is reduced, particularly on the side of the thoracoplasty, but also occasionally contralaterally.

The combination of reduced chest wall compliance and impaired respiratory muscle function accounts for the restrictive defect. All lung volumes are reduced, and in general the severity of the restrictive defect is proportional to the number of ribs that have been resected. A rapid respiratory rate with a small tidal volume is the characteristic respiratory pattern, particularly during exertion. Exercise is limited by ventilatory factors rather than by the cardiovascular system. Chronic air flow obstruction, which may be due to either tuberculous endobronchitis or the effects of tobacco smoking, may be significant in some patients, resulting in a progressive fall in exercise ability and contributing to the development of respiratory failure.

Ventilation and perfusion of the lung on the side of the thoracoplasty are usually reduced equally, hence the arterial Po_2 often remains virtually normal. The function of the contralateral lung is much more important in determining the blood gases. Hypoxaemia usually first appears during sleep, as in scoliosis, and may be associated with hypercapnia. The presence of daytime hypercapnia correlates with the reduction in maximal inspiratory and transdiaphragmatic pressures.

The symptoms of patients with a thoracoplasty are similar to those with a scoliosis, but recurrence of pulmonary tuberculosis should be suspected and investigated if a productive cough develops. Right heart failure often develops insidiously, either when respiratory failure appears or subsequently. It may be manifested by progressively worsening ankle swelling and fatigue. Physical examination reveals a thoracotomy scar and a flattened area of chest in the region of the thoracoplasty which may move paradoxically. Accessory muscle activity, particularly on the side of the thoracoplasty, is often marked.

The chest radiograph shows the extent of the thoracoplasty, other features which indicate the site and extent of previous tuberculous infection, and the sequelae of treatment such as a previous phrenic nerve crush or an artificial pneumothorax, which often causes extensive, calcified pleural thickening. The characteristic physiological defect is restrictive, but airflow obstruction may also be significant. Maximum inspiratory and expiratory pressures and transdiaphragmatic pressures are reduced. Most patients are mildly hypoxic, but later in the clinical course the arterial $P\text{CO}_2$ may rise, particularly during sleep.

Life expectancy is reduced after a thoracoplasty for pulmonary tuberculosis, with death occurring particularly from respiratory but also from cardiac causes. These complications are related to the extent of the tuberculosis and to whether or not an artificial pneumothorax was induced on the contralateral side to the thoracoplasty, since this often leads to pleural thickening and may indicate extensive tuberculous damage of the underlying lung. Respiratory failure can develop quite suddenly after a long period of stability, even when an acute illness such as a chest infection is not responsible.

Conventional treatment of airflow obstruction with (for instance) bronchodilators may be effective, and right heart failure may respond to diuretics and angiotensin-converting enzyme (ACE) inhibitors.

Chronic ventilatory failure usually responds well to nocturnal, noninvasive respiratory support. A few patients can be managed adequately with oxygen during the day and/or at night as long as the $P\text{CO}_2$ remains normal or only slightly raised. When respiratory support is required, nasal positive-pressure ventilation or (occasionally) a negative-pressure system such as a cuirass or jacket used at night is usually effective. Some patients gradually require more intensive support, so that treatment is needed during the day as well as at night. This deterioration may be due to progressive worsening of small airway obstruction or respiratory muscle function, or to a fall in oxygen delivery to the tissues caused by a deteriorating cardiac output associated with advancing pulmonary hypertension. Survival at 1 year is around 90%, at 3 years 75–85%, and at 5 years 50–65%.

Disorders of the diaphragm

Aetiology

Diaphragmatic paralysis or paresis may be due to lesions affecting the diaphragm itself or the phrenic nerve, its nucleus, or higher control centres or pathways. The most common causes of diaphragmatic weakness are shown in Table 18.18.1. Often no cause is found in unilateral weakness, which is then presumed to be due to a cryptogenic phrenic neuropathy, either as part of a widespread peripheral neuropathy or isolated to the phrenic nerves.

Table 18.18.1 Main causes of diaphragmatic weakness

Unilateral	Bilateral
Congenital (e.g. agenesis, eventration)	Trauma
Trauma	High cervical cord lesions
Adjacent mass (e.g. neoplasm, aneurysm)	Motor neuron disease
Herpes zoster	Poliomyelitis
Poliomyelitis	Peripheral neuropathy
Peripheral neuropathy	Acute idiopathic polyneuropathy
Neuralgic amyotrophy	Myopathies
Open-heart surgery	Muscular dystrophies

Pathophysiology

Unilateral weakness of the diaphragm causes it to move upwards (paradoxically) into the thorax during inspiration, instead of descending. This decreases the tidal volume and the mechanical efficiency of breathing. It is worse in the supine position when the weight of the abdominal contents pushes the paralysed diaphragm further into the thorax and decreases the functional residual capacity. The diaphragm is splinted in an expiratory position so that it moves relatively little even though it is paralysed. When the subject lies on one side, the lower half of the diaphragm behaves in this way if it is paralysed, but if the upper half is paralysed it moves paradoxically.

The loss of inspiratory muscle strength is partially compensated by recruitment of intercostal and accessory muscles, but the maximum inspiratory and transdiaphragmatic pressures are reduced. The vital capacity in the upright position is approximately 20 to 25% less than normal, and a further fall of about 15% occurs when lying supine. There are similar changes in the total lung capacity and functional residual capacity; residual volume is unchanged and expiratory muscle strength is largely preserved.

The distribution of ventilation and perfusion is affected by unilateral diaphragm weakness. Ventilation is slightly diminished, particularly at the base on the side of the diaphragmatic paralysis in the sitting position, but this is more marked when supine. Similar changes occur with perfusion on a regional basis, but ventilation–perfusion matching is impaired and hypoxia results. Hypercapnia does not occur during wakefulness or sleep.

The physiological abnormalities seen with bilateral diaphragmatic weakness in adults are much more marked than in unilateral diaphragmatic disorders. The diaphragm moves paradoxically during inspiration and expiration, and intrapleural pressure changes are transmitted across it so that abdominal pressure falls during inspiration and the anterior abdominal wall moves paradoxically. The maximum transdiaphragmatic pressure falls in proportion to the degree of diaphragm weakness, and since the diaphragm is the main inspiratory muscle, the maximum inspiratory pressure is correspondingly reduced. The vital capacity in the sitting position is about 50% of that predicted and may fall by a further 50% when supine, the influence of the supine position being greater than with unilateral diaphragmatic weakness because the weight of the abdominal contents pushes both halves of the diaphragm into the thorax. Ventilation is particularly reduced at the bases in the supine position, with less change in perfusion so that the arterial $P\text{O}_2$ falls. This postural change is partly responsible for the hypoxia that has been observed during sleep, but the rapid respiratory rate, small tidal volume, and short inspiratory time contribute to this and to hypercapnia.

Symptoms and physical signs

Unilateral diaphragmatic paralysis in adults rarely causes symptoms unless there is coexisting pulmonary disease or weakness of other respiratory muscles. In contrast, bilateral weakness can cause severe breathlessness. This may occur during exertion, but a specific feature is orthopnoea: this occurs within a few seconds of lying flat and is relieved promptly by sitting up, in contrast to left ventricular failure and nocturnal asthma with which it is frequently confused. Breathlessness may also occur when standing in water, since the passive inspiratory descent of the diaphragm due to gravity is prevented by the raised extra-abdominal pressure.

The physical signs of unilateral diaphragm weakness can be subtle. Dullness to percussion over the lower part of the thorax may be present, and the level of dullness may rise paradoxically on the paralysed side during inspiration. The normal inspiratory outward movement of the abdomen may be reduced or absent on the side of diaphragmatic paralysis, and expansion of the lower chest may lag behind the normal expansion of the other side.

The physical signs of bilateral diaphragmatic paralysis are much more obvious. Orthopnoea is usually readily apparent, and the abdomen moves paradoxically inwards as the diaphragm ascends during inspiration. A maximum transdiaphragmatic pressure of less than 30 cmH$_2$O is necessary for this sign to be detected. The accessory muscles are active, particularly in the supine position. The quality of sleep is often poor and as a result excessive daytime somnolence may be a problem. Bilateral, basal dullness due to the high diaphragms is characteristic, but can be mimicked by bilateral pleural effusions.

Investigations

In unilateral diaphragmatic paralysis the chest radiograph shows whether the affected diaphragm is elevated and usually reveals any adjacent mass that may be responsible. Both the diaphragms are raised if there is bilateral paralysis, and there is often some basal linear shadowing due to subsegmental lung collapse. Diaphragmatic screening or ultrasound examination reveals that the diaphragm moves paradoxically, particularly during sniffing, a test which should be carried out in the supine position with a weight on the abdomen. These precautions prevent abdominal muscle contraction during expiration from mimicking diaphragmatic activity by reducing the end expiratory volume below functional residual capacity, so that inspiration then occurs through the elastic recoil of the lungs and chest wall. In the upright position, the effect of gravity on the abdominal contents can lead to inspiration without any diaphragmatic activity.

A low vital capacity, which falls further in the supine position, is the hallmark of diaphragmatic weakness, particularly when this is severe and bilateral. All lung volumes are reduced except for the residual volume since expiratory muscle strength is largely preserved. Maximum inspiratory pressure is also reduced, but diaphragmatic weakness can be more specifically diagnosed by estimating the transdiaphragmatic pressure. This can be carried out by asking the patient to sniff or to take a maximum inspiratory effort, or by magnetic or percutaneous electrical stimulation of the phrenic nerve in the neck. Care is required to carry out these investigations using a standardized method in order to obtain repeatable results.

The function of the phrenic nerve can also be estimated by measuring its conduction time: this is normally less than about 9.5 ms, but is prolonged if the nerves are diseased.

The arterial P_{O_2} is characteristically slightly reduced, with a normal P_{CO_2} during the daytime and in sleep as long as pulmonary function is normal and there is no other muscle weakness. If either of these is present, however, bilateral diaphragmatic weakness can cause hypercapnia with profound hypoxia during sleep.

Treatment

Plication for hemidiaphragmatic paralysis is rarely required in adults unless coexistent pulmonary disease is severe enough to cause breathlessness. Bilateral plication is not effective and mechanical respiratory support is often required if there is bilateral weakness. Treatment with nasal positive-pressure ventilation or a negative-pressure ventilator, such as a cuirass or jacket, is usually required, although rocking beds have also been found to be effective in the past. Ventilatory support is usually needed only at night and until the function of the diaphragm or phrenic nerve improves. Phrenic nerve pacemakers are only indicated when diaphragmatic weakness is due to lesions above the phrenic nerve nucleus in C3 to C5 or C6. The commonest cause of this is a high cervical spinal cord injury. Breathlessness on exertion often remains a problem, but may lessen as other inspiratory muscles partially compensate for diaphragmatic weakness.

Further reading

Bredin CP (1989). Pulmonary function in long-term survivors of thoracoplasty. *Chest*, **95**, 18–20.

Budweiser S, *et al.* (2006). Impact of ventilation parameters and duration of ventilator use on non-invasive home ventilation in restrictive thoracic disorders. *Respiration*, **73**, 488–94.

Dolmage TE, Avendano MA, Goldstein RS (1992). Respiratory function during wakefulness and sleep among survivors of respiratory and non-respiratory poliomyelitis. *Eur Resp J*, **5**, 864–70.

Franssen MJAM, *et al.* (1986). Lung function in patients with ankylosing spondylitis. A study of the influence of disease activity and treatment with non-steroidal antiinflammatory drugs. *J Rheumatol*, **13**, 936–40.

Gibson GJ (1989). Diaphragmatic paresis: pathophysiology, clinical features, and investigations. *Thorax*, **44**, 960–70.

Haller JA Jr, *et al.* (1996). Chest wall constriction after too extensive and too early operations for pectus excavatum. *Ann Thorac Surg*, **61**, 1618–25.

Kafer ER (1975). Idiopathic scoliosis. Mechanical properties of the respiratory system and the ventilatory response to carbon dioxide. *J Clin Invest*, **55**, 1153–63.

Kinnear WJM, *et al.* (1988). The effects of one year of nocturnal cuirass-assisted ventilation in chest wall disease. *Eur Resp J*, **1**, 204–6.

Laroche CM, Moxham J, Green M (1989). Respiratory muscle weakness and fatigue. *Q J Med*, **NS 71**, 373–97.

Lindahl T (1954). Spirometric and bronchospirometric studies in five-rib thoracoplasties. *Thorax*, **9**, 285–90.

Midgren B, *et al.* (1988). Nocturnal hypoxaemia in severe scoliosis. *Br J Dis Chest*, **82**, 226–36.

Mier-Jedrzejowicz A, *et al.* (1988). Assessment of diaphragm weakness. *Am Rev Resp Dis*, **137**, 877–83.

Newsom-Davis J, *et al.* (1976). Diaphragm function and alveolar hypoventilation. *Q J Med*, **145**, 87–100.

Pehrsson K, Bake B, Larsson S, Nachemson A (1991). Lung function in adult idiopathic scoliosis: a 20 year follow up. *Thorax*, **46**, 474–8.

Phillips MS, *et al.* (1989). Exercise responses in patients treated for pulmonary tuberculosis by thoracoplasty. *Thorax*, **44**, 268–74.

Ras GJ, *et al.* (1994). Respiratory manifestations of rigid spine syndrome. *Am J Resp Crit Care Med*, **150**, 540–6.

Romagnoli I, *et al.* (2004). Chest wall kinematics and respiratory muscle action in ankylosing spondylitis patients. *Eur Respir J*, **24**, 453–60.

Sawicka EH, Branthwaite MA, Spencer GT (1983). Respiratory failure after thoracoplasty: treatment by intermittent negative-pressure ventilation. *Thorax*, **28**, 433–5.

Shneerson JM (1978). The cardiorespiratory response to exercise in thoracic scoliosis. *Thorax*, **33**, 457–63.

Shneerson J (1998). Sleep in neuromuscular thoracic cage disorders. *Eur Resp Monogr*, **10**, 324–44.

Shneerson JM (2004). Respiratory failure in tuberculosis: a modern perspective. *Clin Med*, **4**, 72–6.

Shneerson JM, Simonds AK (2002). Noninvasive ventilation for chest wall and neuromuscular disorders. *Eur Respir J*, **20**, 480–7.

Smith IE, *et al.* (1996). Kyphosis secondary to tuberculous osteomyelitis as a cause of ventilatory failure: Clinical features, mechanisms and management. *Chest*, **110**, 1105–10.

Tzelepis GE, McCool FD, Hoppin FG Jr (1989). Chest wall distortion in patients with flail chest. *Am Rev Resp Dis*, **140**, 31–7.

18.19

Malignant diseases

Contents

18.19.1 Lung cancer

S.G. Spiro

Essentials

Lung cancer remains the commonest killing cancer in both men and women in the developed world, and is increasingly common in developing countries, although as a result of decreased tobacco consumption in Western countries there has been a considerable reduction in the incidence amongst men over the last 20 years, and a slowing down in incidence in women over the last few years. Nevertheless, lung cancer in women is commoner than breast cancer in some Western countries. There are several important industrial associations with lung cancer, in particular asbestos, but tobacco remains by far the most important cause.

Pathology—there are four main cell types of lung cancer, of which adeno-, squamous and large cell varieties comprise non-small-cell lung cancer (NSCLC), with the more aggressive type—small cell—being regarded as a separate entity from the point of view of staging and treatment.

Clinical features—there are no particular presenting features that strongly suggest a new lung cancer, hence it is a disease

that often presents late and with widespread metastatic disease. Symptoms and signs can be subdivided into (1) intrapulmonary symptoms—cough (most commonly), haemoptysis (most dramatically), wheeze, chest discomfort, and breathlessness (rare as a presenting feature); (2) extrapulmonary, intrathoracic symptoms and signs—Horner's syndrome, vocal cord paralysis, superior vena caval obstruction, dysphagia; (3) extrathoracic, metastatic manifestations—30% of patients present with symptoms due to distant metastases, the most common sites being bones, liver, adrenal glands, brain and spinal cord, lymph nodes, and skin; and (4) paramalignant syndromes—syndrome of inappropriate secretion of antidiuretic hormone, ectopic ACTH syndrome, hypercalcaemia, neuromyopathies, finger clubbing, and hypertrophic pulmonary osteoarthropathy.

Incidental findings and screening—about 5% of lung cancers are found by chance on a chest radiograph performed for reason other than suspicion of cancer, and these tend to have a better prognosis. Screening of high-risk groups for lung cancer with low-dose spiral CT is attracting interest and randomized trials are recruiting, but data as to whether mortality is reduced will not be available for at least 2 years.

Clinical staging—accurate clinical staging is paramount for treatment decisions, especially for NSCLC, which may be resectable. Following a chest radiograph, a CT of the thorax and upper abdomen should be performed. Biopsy of the primary tumour (via a bronchoscope for centrally situated lesions or by percutaneous image-guided needle, depending on best access) or of a metastasis is required, the latter providing a diagnosis and staging information at the same time. PET scanning, which depends on the uptake of a glucose analogue (fluorodeoxyglucose, FDG) by active tumour and its metastases, is recommended as the final staging test in those patients where resection or another curative treatment is contemplated.

Prognosis and management—(1) NSCLC— 'curative' treatment by surgical resection can be applied to 5 to 10% of all cases, of whom about 25% survive at 5 years. Radical radiotherapy cures very few with locally advanced disease, although better results are claimed with the addition of chemotherapy. In patients with advanced NSCLC and good performance status, survival at 1 year is 15 to 20% with supportive care, with chemotherapy adding about 5 months to the untreated median survival with an improvement in quality of life. (2) Small-cell tumours—life expectancy of those with untreated disease is about 3.5 months for limited disease and 6 weeks for extensive disease. Chemotherapy remains the cornerstone of treatment: modern regimens would be expected to achieve a complete response rate (i.e. disappearance of all measurable disease) in 40 to 50% of cases and a partial response rate (>50% reduction in tumour bulk) in a further 40%. Patients achieving a complete response after chemotherapy should have prophylactic cranial irradiation.

Management of complications—some complications of lung cancer require specific measures to alleviate symptoms: (1) vocal cord paralysis may be helped by injection of Teflon into the affected cord; (2) obstruction of the upper airway causing stridor, or of the lower major airways, is usually treated initially with radiotherapy; (3) malignant pleural effusion is treated with talc pleurodesis; (4) dexamethasone may control the symptoms of brain metastasis and, if so, this should be consolidated with radiotherapy.

The multidisciplinary team—the importance of the combined support to the patient and the family given by the family doctor, palliative care medical and nursing staff, and hospice organizations, and the hospital team cannot be overemphasized.

General epidemiology

Lung cancer is the most common malignant disease in the Western world. It has shown the greatest relative and absolute rise in mortality of any tumour this century in England and Wales, and particularly in Scotland. It causes 38 000 deaths per year in England and Wales, with 80% of these occurring in men. In the European Union there are 1.35 million deaths per year in men (the highest death rate from any tumour), and in women in 1995 it accounted for 24% of all female cancer deaths. In the United States of America it has been increasing in incidence by up to 10% per year since the 1930s, but over the last decade this trend has levelled off, particularly in men. Nevertheless, about 120 000 American men die of lung cancer each year, the figure for women being 34 000, similar to that for breast cancer. However, whereas the age-adjusted incidence in women increased by 4.1% per year between 1973 and 1994, between 1990 and 1994 the annual incidence rose by only 0.2%.

Age-standardized mortality rates for cancer show that in western Europe lung cancer in men was by far the commonest cause of death. Belgium has the highest mortality (77.16 deaths per 100 000 population) with Scotland (75.9) second, and England and Wales (60.9) fifth. The figures for central and eastern Europe are worse in that the death rates for lung cancer are rising exponentially, particularly in men—75.8/100 000 in the Czech Republic, 74.0 in Hungary, 69.4 in Poland, and 68.7 in Slovakia. For women, Scotland has the highest incidence (27.2, equal to the rate of breast cancer in Scottish women), with England and Wales (20.4) third. Age-adjusted lung cancer death rates in eastern Europe are still considerably less than in western European countries, ranging from 14.4 in Hungary to 6.8 in Slovakia. Perhaps the worst epidemic is in China, where 0.8 million men died in the year 2000 from smoking-related diseases. Of all deaths attributed to tobacco in China, 15% were due to lung cancer.

Aetiological factors

Tobacco

In every country, the increase in mortality from lung cancer has appeared to coincide with an increase in tobacco usage, particularly cigarette smoking, after what seemed to be an appropriate latent interval. Prospective studies, among which the long-term study of British doctors was particularly informative, confirmed the increased risk of death from lung cancer from any tobacco use, but most specifically that of cigarettes. There was a strong dose–response relationship with the number of cigarettes smoked, illustrated in Table 18.19.1.1. The most important variable in smoking intensity is the number of cigarettes smoked, but other variables include the depth of inhalation, number of puffs, butt length, use of a filter, and the type of tobacco smoked. Further evidence that the relationship was causal came from a study which documented reduction in mortality after stopping smoking: 15 years after cessation the risk of death fell from 15.8 times to twice that in nonsmokers, equivalent to 11% of that pertaining in those who continued to smoke. Stopping smoking before the age of 40 years greatly reduces the risk of developing smoking-related diseases.

Globally, there has been a huge change in cigarette consumption. Between 1970 and 1985 the overall world consumption rose by 7% while there was a drop of 25% and 9% in consumption in the United Kingdom and the United States of America, respectively. This is due to huge increases in Asia (22%), Latin America (24%), and Africa (42%). The current epidemic of smoking in China lags behind Western society by 20 years. Thus, in China in 1996 the average number of cigarettes smoked per adult male was 11 per day, a figure that that peaked in the West at 10 a day in 1980. Nearly one-third of the world's smokers reside in China, who reported 1.3 million new cases of lung cancer in 2003.

Another disturbing trend is the increasing incidence among women. More women in developed nations will die of lung cancer than breast cancer. Due to historical smoking patterns the incidence rates of lung cancer in women are not declining, because smoking rates have not yet started to decline, as they have in men. Currently far more men than women are dying of this disease, but

Table 18.19.1.1 Death rate from lung cancer in males by smoking habits when last asked (British doctors' study)

Tobacco use category	Death rate (age standardized per 100 000)
Nonsmokers	10
Ex-smokers	43
Continuing smokers	
Any tobacco	104
Pipe and/or cigar only	58
Mixed	82
Cigarette smokers only	140
Number smoked per day	
1–14	78
15–24	127
25 or more	251

the gap is relentlessly closing. With regard to socioeconomic status, lung cancer is likelier to occur in the poor and less educated, which is a widespread pattern around the world. Primary prevention and smoking cessation must be directed at these groups.

Passive smoking

Evidence that passive smoking predisposes to lung cancer is far from certain. Approximately 15% of lung cancers occur in non-smokers, and 5% of these have been attributed to passive smoking. However, the perceived risk to those working in smoke-filled environments has lead to a ban on smoking in public places in an increasing number of countries.

Occupation

People who develop lung cancer as a result of their occupation are a small but important group. The association with asbestos is now firmly established, various studies having identified that those exposed are at 4.9 to 7.3 times greater risk than those who are not. This risk is much enhanced if the asbestos industry worker smokes cigarettes; one study estimating this at 93 times higher than for nonsmokers not exposed to asbestos.

Exposure to radioactive isotopes, mainly radon daughters, is associated with a higher risk of lung cancer and occurs among various groups of miners, particularly those involved in extraction of pitchblende and uranium. Polycyclic aromatic hydrocarbons are believed to be responsible for the increased risk in workers in gas and coke ovens and in foundry workers. Workers in nickel refining, chromate manufacture, and the arsenical industry are also exposed to a higher risk of lung cancer. The amount of lung cancer caused by occupational exposure may well have been underestimated in the past, and a summary of the importance industrial products and processes involved is shown in Box 18.19.1.1.

Box 18.19 1.1 Industrial products and processes known to cause or suspected of causing lung cancer

- Fibre exposure (asbestos)
- Nickel refining
- Aluminium industry
- Arsenic and arsenic compounds
- Benzoyl chloride
- Beryllium
- Cadmium
- Chloromethyl ether
- Chromates
- The electronics industry
- Irradiation
- Soots, tar, oils
- Mustard gas

Reproduced from Coggon D, Acheson ED (1983), with permission.

Air pollution

The decline in male mortality is occurring earlier than would be expected from changes in smoking habits. The high mortality figures in the United Kingdom and Germany compared with France and Italy, for example, seem likely to be due in part to heavy industry and coal burning. Analysis by county in the United States of America shows an association between lung cancer deaths and counties with chemical, petroleum, ship-building, and paper industries. Legislation for cleaner air has caused both environmental and occupational pollution to fall dramatically in the past 30 years, and this has preceded changes in smoking habits.

Pathology

A detailed understanding of the natural history, pathology, and pathogenesis of bronchial carcinoma is becoming increasingly important as the assessment, management, and prognosis of the disease depends largely upon the cell type and the presence or absence of metastases at the time of presentation. It has been estimated that about seven-eighths of a tumour's life will have passed when it is diagnosed, and that the vast majority will be disseminated at the time of diagnosis.

Bronchogenic carcinomas seem to arise most commonly in segmental and subsegmental bronchi in response to repetitive carcinogenic stimuli or inflammation and irritation. The mucosal lining is most susceptible to injury at the bifurcation of bronchial structures. Dysplasia is followed by carcinoma *in situ*, when the entire thickness of the mucosa may be replaced by proliferating neoplastic cells. These changes may be strictly localized or multicentric, and are thought to be a field cancerization effect, sometimes causing synchronous primaries. Tumour infiltration follows loss of the basal membrane. The precise origins of small-cell carcinomas remain an enigma, and those of adenocarcinomas are not precisely defined. The latter may arise from the mucosal lining or from the submucosal bronchial mucous glands. A significant number of lung tumours arise in the periphery of the lung, perhaps three-quarters of adenocarcinomas and large-cell anaplastic malignancies, one-third of squamous (or epidermoid) carcinomas, and one-fifth of small-cell carcinomas.

Adenocarcinoma has become the commonest cell type; it is more prevalent in eastern Asia and the United States of America where approximately 50% of new lung cancers are adenocarcinomas. Squamous-cell lung cancer still accounts for up to one-half of new cases in Europe and one-third in eastern Asia and the United States. There has been a slow decline in the prevalence of small-cell lung cancers to 15–20% of new diagnoses, with 10–15% of the less easily differentiable large-cell tumours comprising the rest. Adeno-, squamous-, and large-cell tumours are grouped as non-small-cell lung cancers (NSCLC) as their staging and treatment is similar. From studies of growth rates of radiologically measurable primary tumours, adenocarcinomas have a volume-doubling time of 90–120 days, squamous-cell 60 days and small-cell 30 days, making this last cell type extremely aggressive.

Squamous (epidermoid) carcinoma

These tumours are composed predominantly of flattened to polygonal neoplastic cells that tend to stratify, form intercellular bridges, and elaborate keratin. About 60% present as obstructive lesions in lobar and main-stem bronchi. The tumours tend to be bulky and to produce intraluminar granular or polypoid masses, hence distal pneumonia and abscess formation are common, and cavitation is seen in about 10%. The cells are usually well differentiated, but in some cases differentiation is poor and the appearances are those of predominantly anaplastic cells, frequently arranged in the classical pattern of stratifying sheets.

Small-cell anaplastic carcinoma

This is now recognized as a pathologically and clinically distinct form of lung cancer. The tumour is composed of neoplastic cells with dark oval to round spindled nuclei and scanty, indistinct cytoplasm arranged in ribbons, nests and sheets. The cells tend to crush easily on biopsy, and extensive areas may be necrotic. This type of tumour presents as a proximal lesion in 75% of cases and may arise anywhere in the tracheobronchial tree and rapidly invade vessels and lymph nodes, disseminating widely even before symptoms arise from the primary tumour. More than one-half of the patients have extensive, advanced disease at presentation. The cells secrete peptides which cause clinical syndromes in 10% of cases.

Adenocarcinoma

This tumour forms acinar or granular structures, having prominent papillary processes, and may be mucin-provoking. About 70% appear to originate peripherally in the lung and they are frequently fairly circumscribed. The initial presentation is a pleural effusion in about 10% of cases. If related to bronchi, they tend to cuff and stenose the lumen. They occasionally arise in old tuberculous scars.

Large-cell carcinoma

These tumours, which have been described as an unclassified category, include all tumours that show no evidence of maturation or differentiation. They are composed of pleomorphic cells with variable enlarged nuclei, prominent nucleoli and nuclear inclusions, and abundant cytoplasm, and they are mucin-producing in many instances. The tumours tend to be bulky and are often necrotic. They are frequently peripheral, invade locally and disseminate widely, with about one-half of patients having disseminated disease on presentation. Although these tumours are highly malignant and undifferentiated, the cure rate after surgery is surprisingly high, but radiotherapy is ineffective in controlling the disease. Large-cell carcinoma is a smoking-related disease in more than 90% of patients.

Bronchioloalveolar carcinoma

There has been considerable controversy as to whether this tumour, which has the least association with tobacco smoking, arises from alveolar or bronchial epithelium, but derivation from the alveolar type II cell has been suggested. The tumour tends to spread as cuboidal or columnar 'epithelium' along the lining of the alveoli, with single or multiple rows of cells and often papillary formation. There is production of a large amount of mucus in 20% of cases, and it is believed that malignant cells shed into the mucus may carry over into the contralateral lung. The tumour can spread within a lobe and occupy it fully. Sometimes, however, the tumour is multicentric in origin, and diffuse nodular lesions are to be found on radiographic examination. Invasion of neighbouring tissue and lymph nodes is common, but extrathoracic spread is unusual. There is some resemblance to metastases from adenocarcinomas emanating from other organs, which sometimes leads to confusion. The tumour tends to grow along alveolar septae as a framework, and it may be difficult to distinguish from metastatic tumours from colon, breast, or pancreas.

Carcinoid tumours

Carcinoid tumours are described in Chapter 15.9.

Genetics and biology

Genetic influences may play a role in the development of lung cancers, particularly in patients under 50. In one study, lung cancers were attributable to a mendelian dominant inheritance pattern in 27% of patients under 50, but only 9% of those over 70.

The *ras* family of oncogenes (H, K, and N) was the first to be described in association with lung cancer. Mutations of *ras* genes occur in 20 to 40% of NSCLC, especially adenocarcinomas, and the presence of K-*ras* mutations is linked with significantly shortened survival.

Lung cancer cells not only show mutations that activate dominant cellular proto-oncogenes, but also genetic mechanisms that inactivate recessive tumour suppressors. The commonest abnormality is a deletion in the short arm of chromosome 3, which is found in over 90% of small-cell lung cancer and 50% of NSCLC patients. Other sites of loss of heterozygosity include 11p, 13q, and 17p. Tumour suppressor genes have been identified in inherited cancers, mainly in studies of familial retinoblastoma. Mutations in *TP53* occur in 75% of small-cell lung cancer and 50% of NSCLC. The gene is located on the short arm of chromosome 13q14, and it is thought that it may normally protect cells against accumulation of mutations. Depletions and mutations of *TP53* are linked with metastatic disease. Alterations of p53 protein have been found in early bronchial neoplasia, and may be a useful marker for the early detection of lung cancer. Other markers, including heterogenous nuclear ribonuclear protein A2/B1 overexpression in sputum, may allow earlier detection of tumours.

Several monoclonal antibodies have been generated against lung-cancer-associated antigens. Thirty-six monoclonal antibodies raised against small-cell lung cancer have been grouped into eight clusters. No antigen is specific for small-cell lung cancer. Antibodies belonging to the major cluster (cluster 1) are directed against the neural-cell adhesion molecule (NCAM), but the nature of the other antigens remains unclear. Studies of both small-cell and NSCLC cell lines show that NCAM secretion is associated with a neuroendocrine phenotype irrespective of the histological type of lung cancer. Monoclonal antibodies may have a therapeutic value when coupled with a radionuclide or a toxin. Radiolabelled antibodies can be used to detect minimal disease in bone marrow aspirates or biopsy specimens.

The growth factors bombesin/gastrin-releasing peptide, insulin-like growth factor 1 (IGF-1), and transferrin stimulate can all stimulate tumour growth. There is much interest in attempts to retard or disrupt these processes.

Recent interest in the expression of the epidermal growth factor receptor (EGFR) tyrosine kinase in lung cancers has demonstrated it to be up-regulated in 70% of squamous-cell cancers and 50% of adenocarcinomas. This has led to trials with the small-molecule inhibitors gefitinib and erlotinib. A few patients have substantial responses to these drugs, with molecular analysis revealing that specific mutations within the regulatory domains predict such sensitivity. Amplification of the gene provides additional predictive information. EGFR mutations occur largely in adenocarcinoma and are more prevalent in Asians.

Clinical features

Lung cancers present late in their natural history. In general, death will occur when a tumour load reaches 1 kg, which is equivalent to 40 volume doubling times, yet halfway through the lifespan of a lung cancer—20 volume doublings—it is only 1 mm in diameter (Fig. 18.19.1.1). It becomes visible on a chest radiograph at about 1 cm and the typical size at presentation with symptoms or signs is 3–4 cm. CT and PET will identify lesions as nodules when they are considerably smaller, but most incidentally discovered nodules tend to be benign, making investigation problematic.

The clinical features of lung cancer are very variable: they can be respiratory, but all too often they are constitutional and attributable to metastatic disease. In one series of 678 consecutive patients only 27% presented with symptoms related to the primary tumour. Most had either nonspecific symptoms, including anorexia, weight loss, and fatigue (27%), or specific symptoms of metastatic disease (32%). However, in about 5% of patients the presentation is a radiographic abnormality found by chance on routine examination (Fig. 18.19.1.2). These patients tend to have a better prognosis (18% 5-year survival) than those with symptoms related to the primary tumour (12% 5-year survival). There is usually a considerable time delay between the patient noticing a symptom and presenting to a primary care physician, which varies in different studies from 4 months to 2 years, with the specific exception of haemoptysis, when the mean delay from first symptom to first visit is much shorter at about 43 days (range 0–256 days). There may also be a delay between first presentation to a physician and the realization that there may be a lung cancer present. One study identified a delay of 56 days (range 0–477 days). This is understandable in the context that an average primary care physician (in the United Kingdom) sees a new lung cancer only every 9 months or so, and

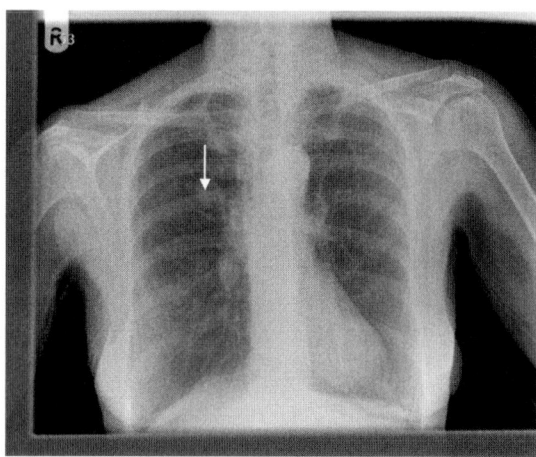

Fig. 18.19.1.2 Chest radiograph showing a chance finding of a right upper lobe mass (arrow) with a bulky right hilum.

in a Dutch study of patients presenting with cough (11 092 separate patient encounters), lung cancer was not listed as a separate entity amongst the 20 most common eventual causes.

Clinical symptoms and sign of lung cancer can be subdivided into those arising from the lung itself; from the extrapulmonary intrathoracic structures; extrathoracic metastases; and from endocrine, metabolic, and neurological (paramalignant) syndromes (Table 18.19.1.2).

Intrapulmonary symptoms

Cough is the most common initial presenting symptom, but because it is a symptom of so many respiratory disorders, the possibility of tumour may be overlooked and cough may be attributed to some other cause, particularly in smokers who have had chronic bronchitis for many years. Patients with a persistent cough should have a chest radiograph, particularly if they are smokers over 40 years of age (Figs. 18.19.1.3–18.19.1.7). A change in the cough habit is significant and also requires investigation. If the trachea or main bronchi are involved, the cough may be harsh in character and may be accompanied by wheezing or stridor. If cough is manifestly ineffective, with its explosive ability lost, involvement of the recurrent laryngeal nerve should be suspected.

Expectoration of sputum may be due to irritation of the tumour in a major airway or to infection occurring distal to partial bronchial obstruction. The value of sputum cytology in diagnosis is described below.

Haemoptysis, which is the sole presenting symptom in about 5% of cases and occurs at some stage in the disease in 50% of patients, is a symptom not easily ignored by patient or physician. The degree varies from streaking of the sputum with blood to larger amounts, but massive haemoptysis (>200 ml) is rare, except as a terminal event when the tumour may erode a large pulmonary blood vessel. The most significant description given by patients is that of coughing up blood every morning for several days in succession.

Wheeze may be observed in a few patients. Localized persistent wheeze, often volunteered to come from one side of the chest, even after coughing is a significant observation indicating obstruction of a larger or central airway (Fig. 18.19.1.7).

Stridor is a feature that is poorly recognized and often confused with wheeze. It is due to narrowing of the glottis, trachea, or

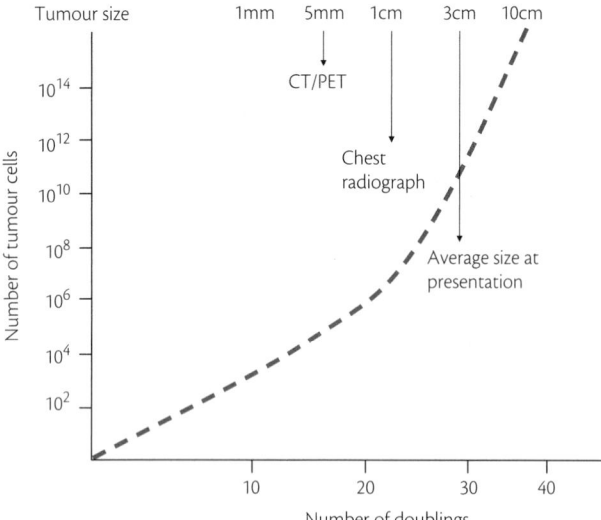

Fig. 18.19.1.1 The lung cancer growth curve and ability to detect a tumour during its natural history.

Table 18.19.1.2 The presentation of lung cancer (frequency (%) of commoner symptoms/signs indicated)

Chest symptoms	Mediastinal involvement	Chest radiographic abnormalities	Paramalignant syndromes	Extrathoracic metastases
Haemoptysis (6–35)	Superior vena caval obstruction (0–4)	Peripheral nodule	Hypercalcaemia (0–10)	Bone pain (6–25)
Cough (8–75)	Left recurrent laryngeal nerve palsy (0–10)	Lobar/lung collapse	SIADH (0–50)	Neurological
Wheeze (0–10)	Diaphragmatic palsy (0–5)	Cavitating mass	SIACTH (0–5)	Jaundice
Stridor (0–2)	Pericardial effusion	Abnormal hilum	HPOA/clubbing (0–20)	Skin nodules
Pain (20–50)	Dysphagia	Pleural effusion	Lambert–Eaton syndrome (0–3)	Lymphadenopathy
Dyspnoea (3–60)		Lymphangitis	Cerebellar dysfunction	Weight loss (0–68)
		Bone lesion	Neuropathies	Lethargy (0–10)
		Wide mediastinum		

SIACTH, syndrome of inappropriate ACTH; SIADH, syndrome of inappropriate antidiuretic hormone; HPOA, hypertrophic pulmonary osteoarthropathy.

major bronchi, and is best heard after the patient coughs and then breathes in deeply with the mouth open.

Dyspnoea is a presenting symptom in only a few patients. As the disease progresses dyspnoea is inevitable, being proportional to the amount of lung involved, either directly by tumour replacement or indirectly by endobronchial disease causing airway narrowing or obstruction. Progressive breathlessness is also a feature of malignant pleural and, rarely, pericardial effusion, superior vena caval obstruction, and lymphangitis carcinomatosis.

Chest discomfort is a common symptom, occurring in up to 40% of patients at diagnosis. The discomfort is often of an ill-defined nature and may be described in terms of intermittent aching somewhere in the chest. Definite pleural pain may occur in the presence of infection, but invasion of the pleura by tumour is often painless. However, invasion of the ribs or vertebrae causes continuous, gnawing, localized pain (Fig. 18.19.1.8). A tumour in the superior pulmonary sulcus (Pancoast tumour) can cause progressive constant pain in the shoulder, upper anterior chest, or interscapular region, soon spreading to the arm once the brachial plexus is invaded. Other symptoms of this type of tumour include weakness and atrophy of the muscles of the hand, Horner's syndrome, hoarseness, and spinal cord compression at levels D1 and D2.

Fever, chills, and night sweats may occur due to chest infection, but fever may very rarely be present in rapidly progressive tumours

without evidence of infection, particularly if there are hepatic metastases.

Extrapulmonary, intrathoracic symptoms

Invasion of adjacent, mainly mediastinal, structures can give rise to certain specific clinical features. Involvement of the last cervical and first thoracic segment of the sympathetic trunk by cancer produces Horner's syndrome. Malignant infiltration of the recurrent laryngeal nerve—almost always the left branch because of its course adjacent to the left hilum—gives rise to vocal cord paralysis. The right recurrent laryngeal nerve is occasionally affected in the base of the neck. Recurrent aspiration pneumonias may follow vocal cord paralysis.

Extension of the tumour with invasion or compression of the superior vena cava or by paratracheal lymphadenopathy results in the characteristic features of superior vena caval obstruction—awareness of tightness of the collar, fullness of the head, and suffusion of the face (particularly after bending down), blackouts, breathlessness, and engorgement of veins with a downward venous

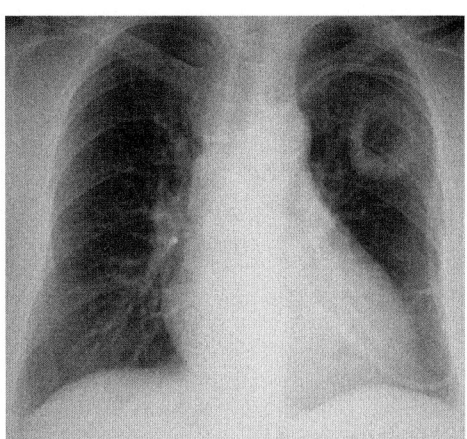

Fig. 18.19.1.3 Cavitating squamous-cell lung cancer.

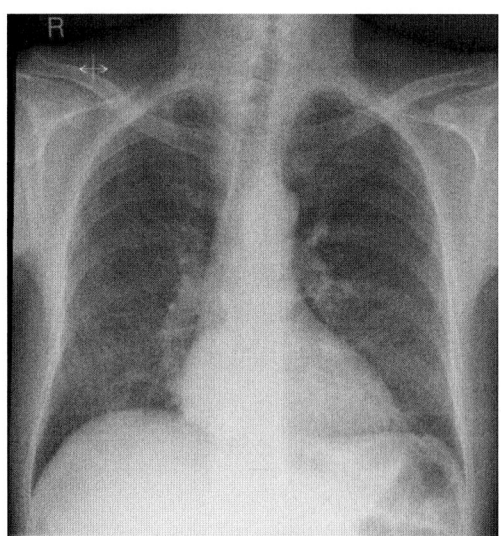

Fig. 18.19.1.4 Chest radiograph showing a tumour in the right lower lobe behind the heart causing a double shadow for right heart border.

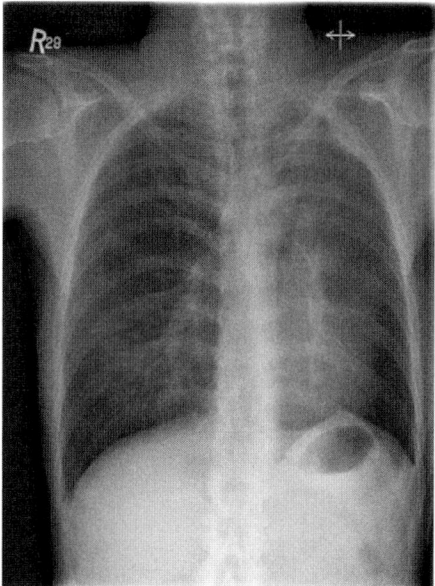

Fig. 18.19.1.5 Chest radiograph showing a collapsed left upper lobe due to proximal tumour.

flow in the neck, the upper half of the thorax, and arms, often accompanied by oedema of the face.

Dysphagia is due to compression of the oesophagus from without by tumour metastases in subcarinal lymph nodes and only rarely to direct invasion. Cardiac and pericardial metastases usually occur late in the disease and are manifested clinically by tachycardia, arrhythmias, pericardial effusion, and breathlessness. Invasion of the phrenic nerve results in elevation and paralysis of a hemidiaphragm.

Involvement of the ribs, spine, and pleura are extrathoracic manifestations. Very rarely bronchogenic carcinoma causes spontaneous pneumothorax. It must not be forgotten that spread of tumour to the other lung may occur, or that synchronous primaries may coexist.

Extrathoracic metastatic symptoms

About 30% of patients present with symptoms due to distant metastases, the most common sites being bones, liver, adrenal glands, brain and spinal cord, lymph nodes, and skin (Figs. 18.19.1.8–18.19.1.11). Metastases to nodes are frequent and should be sought with great care, particularly those in the scalene area, which are usually the first to be involved. The best position for examination for these is from behind with the patient seated relaxed in a chair. The side affected usually corresponds to the side of the lung lesion, the exception being that tumours from the left lower lobe may metastasize to the nodes in the right scalene area. Involvement of the nodes in the floor of the supraclavicular fossa is equally common.

Bony metastases are common, particularly in small-cell tumours, and occur predominantly in the skull, ribs, vertebrae, humeri, and femora. They cause pain as a presenting symptom in up to 25% of patients. Early involvement may be detected by a rise in alkaline phosphatase of bony origin, isotope scanning, or biopsy. Conventional skeletal surveys are often unhelpful and misleading.

Liver secondaries are common and may be silent, although a rise in liver enzymes, particularly alkaline phosphatase of liver origin, may be an early sign. CT scans and ultrasonography may detect

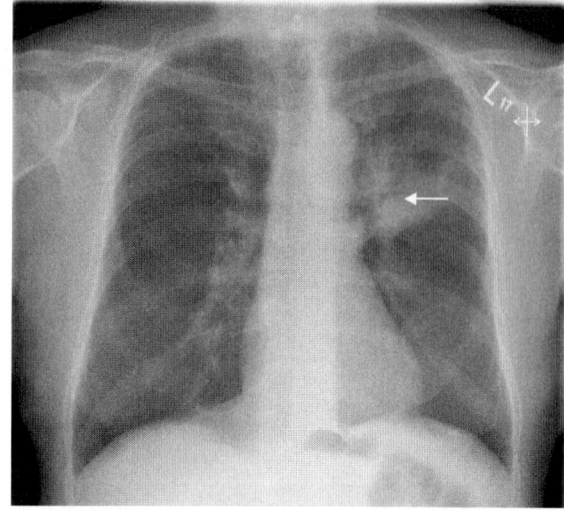

(a)

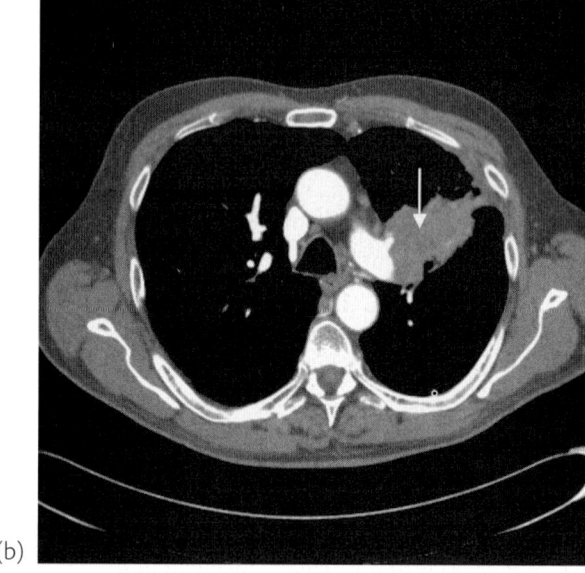

(b)

Fig. 18.19.1.6 (a) Chest radiograph showing an ill-defined parenchymal mass (arrow) in the left upper lobe; (b): CT scan of the chest of the same patient as in (a), confirming a large central mass (arrow) encasing the left upper lobe bronchus.

involvement in a liver which is not clinically enlarged, but as the metastases develop the liver becomes grossly enlarged with an irregular outline.

Metastases to the brain may account for the presenting symptom in lung cancer in 4% of patients and may be encountered at some time in the illness in 30% (Fig. 18.19.1.10). The symptoms simulate those of any expanding brain tumour.

The adrenal glands are involved in 15 to 20% of patients, rarely producing symptoms. The skin should be examined for the presence of the typical, slightly bluish, umbilicated lesions of tumour spread. Subcutaneous metastases may be found at almost any site (Fig. 18.19.1.11).

It is recommended that organ-specific scans are only conducted in patients with organ-specific symptoms, or with general symptoms such as weight loss or malaise. Lack of energy and, more particularly, loss of interest in normal pursuits are symptoms of great importance; a sense of vague ill health commonly occurs.

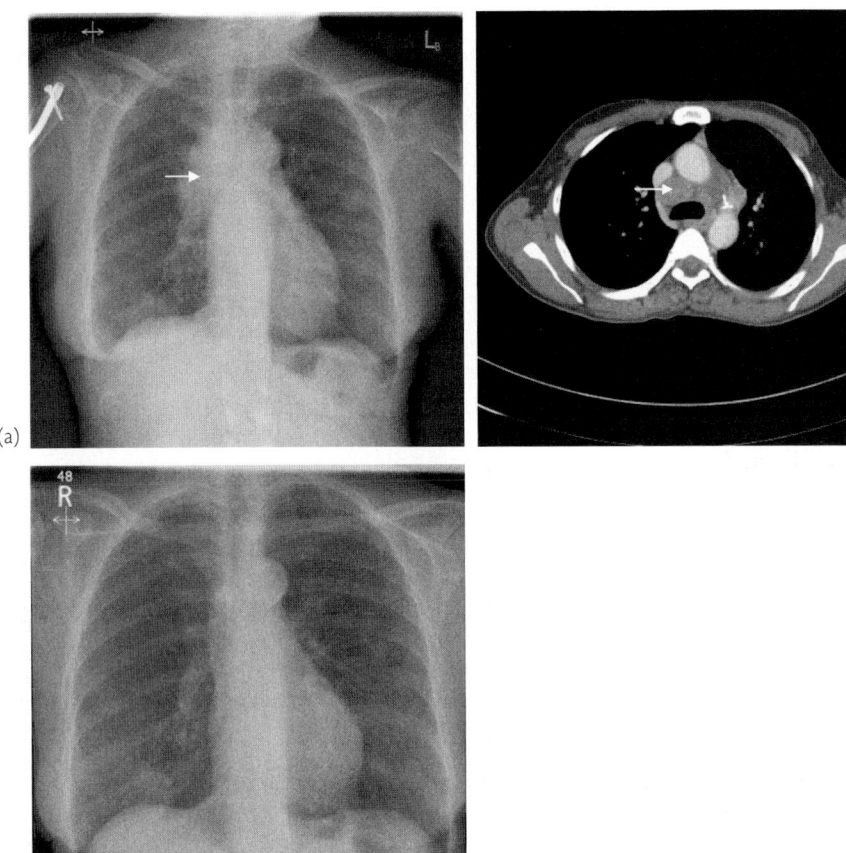

Fig. 18.19.1.7 (a) Chest radiograph showing a right upper lobe tumour causing wheeze with bulky right paratracheal nodes (arrow); (b) CT scan of the chest of the same patient as in (a), showing grossly enlarged mediastinal pretracheal lymph nodes (arrow); (c) chest radiograph of the same patient as in (a), showing complete response after two courses of chemotherapy.

Paramalignant syndromes

Endocrine and metabolic manifestations

Many of the unusual manifestations of malignant disease are the result of endocrine and metabolic manifestations of the cancer itself. Cancer cells appear to be able to synthesize polypeptides that mimic virtually all the hormones produced by conventional endocrine organs—hence the term 'ectopic hormones'. From time to time the clinical features resulting from ectopic hormone secretion precede those of the pulmonary tumour, emphasizing the importance of a high index of suspicion in such circumstances.

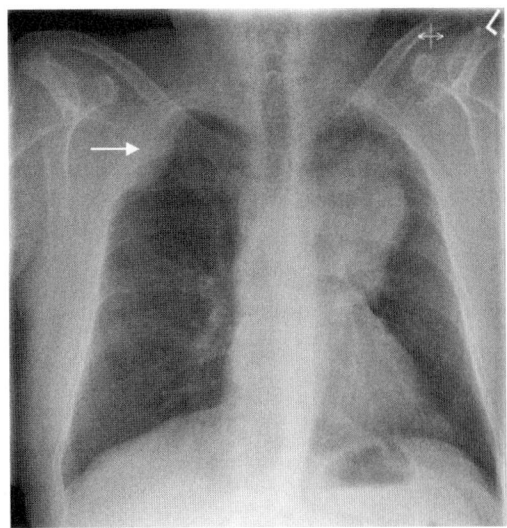

Fig. 18.19.1.8 Chest radiograph showing a large left upper lobe mass with a right rib metastasis (arrow) causing pain, which was the reason for presentation in this case.

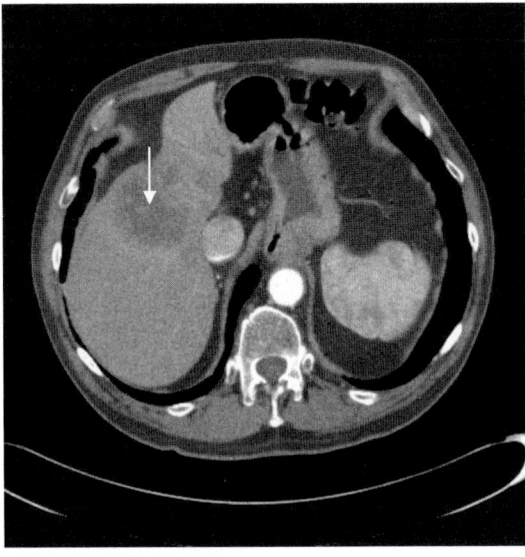

Fig. 18.19.1.9 CT scan of the upper abdomen of the same patient as shown in Fig. 18.19.1.6, revealing a large necrotic liver metastasis (arrow).

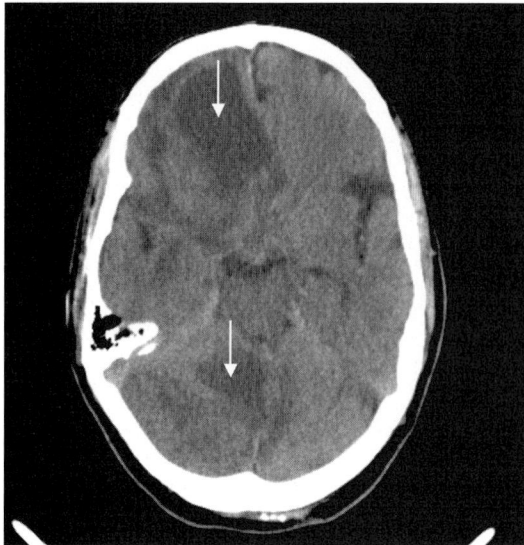

Fig. 18.19.1.10 CT scan of the brain in patient presenting with vagueness. Note marked cerebral oedema around metastases (arrows), and midline shift.

Ectopic hormone measurement cannot, however, be used for screening purposes. These syndromes can occur in up to 10% of patients with lung cancer.

Syndrome of inappropriate secretion of antidiuretic hormone (SIADH)

The continued secretion of vasopressin (ADH) in excess of the body's needs leads to retention of water in both the intracellular and extracellular compartments. The cerebral oedema resulting from water intoxication can cause drowsiness, lethargy, irritability, mental confusion, and disorientation, with fits and coma being the most profound features. Peripheral oedema is remarkably rare. The patient is usually asymptomatic until the sodium falls below 120 mmol/litre, when the hyponatraemia is dilutional in type with a low serum osmolality. Urine osmolality usually exceeds 300 mosmol/kg. The commonest cancer causing this syndrome is small-cell lung cancer, where it is clinically obvious in 1 to 5% of cases, with subclinical involvement detectable by a water-loading test in more than 50%. Restriction of fluid to a daily intake of 700 to 1000 ml may redress the hyponatraemia, but demethylchlortetracycline (demeclocycline) 600 to 1200 mg daily is often highly effective, making water restriction

unnecessary. The syndrome resolves promptly (within 3 weeks) with combination cytotoxic chemotherapy in 80% of patients with small-cell lung cancer, but commonly recurs at, or predicts, relapse.

Ectopic ACTH syndrome

Secretion of an adrenocorticotrophic substance by a small-cell carcinoma or bronchial carcinoid leads to bilateral adrenal hyperplasia and to secretion of large amounts of cortisol. The onset of symptoms may be so acute that death may occur within a few weeks, when the typical features of Cushing's syndrome do not have time to develop. However, it is a common paramalignant syndrome and increased levels of ACTH may be detectable in up to 50% of patients with small-cell lung cancer, with Cushing's itself described in 1 to 5% of these patients. The chief clinical features are thirst and polyuria, oedema, pigmentation, and hypokalaemia. Hypertension and profound myopathy may also be present. Serum cortisol is often grossly elevated, with loss of the normal diurnal rhythm; the level is not suppressed by dexamethasone; and hypokalaemic alkalosis can be severe, with plasma potassium less than 3.0 mmol/litre and bicarbonate more than 30 mmol/litre. Drugs which block adrenocortical steroid biosynthesis may produce partial and reversible medical adrenalectomy, and metyrapone in doses from 250 mg thee times daily to 1 g four times daily may cause temporary relief of symptoms. Removal of the tumour, if practicable, will cause remission, particularly if the cause is a carcinoid tumour. Small-cell lung cancers with this syndrome seem to respond poorly to chemotherapy.

Hypercalcaemia

Hypercalcaemia may be associated with ectopic secretion of parathormone by squamous-cell cancers but is more commonly due directly to the presence of multiple bone metastases. The primary tumour may also produce a cAMP-stimulating factor or a prostaglandin causing hypercalcaemia. A protein with parathormone-like activity has been purified from lung cancer cell lines. Increased bone resorption as the explanation for hypercalcaemia has been attributed to the parathormone like protein released from cancer cells. The incidence in patients with lung cancer ranges from 2 to 6% at presentation, to 8 to 12% during the course of the disease. Hypercalcaemia is unlikely to cause symptoms unless the serum calcium exceeds 2.8 mmol/litre, and levels much higher than this are sometimes encountered. The main clinical features are nausea,

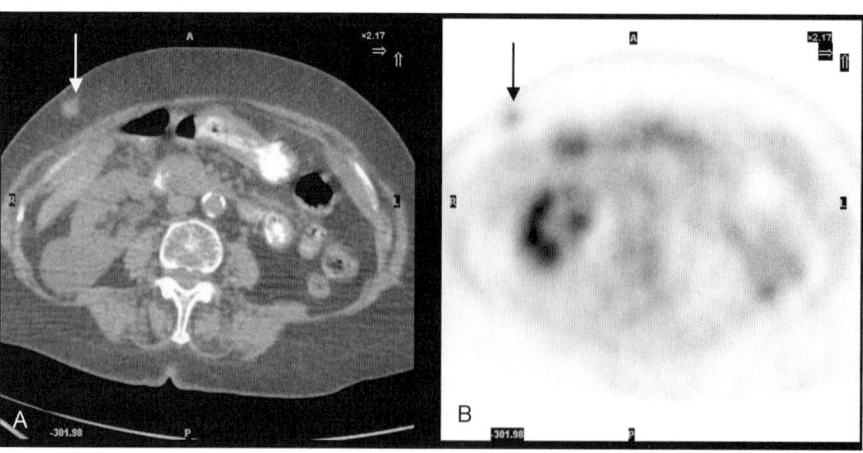

Fig. 18.19.1.11 CT (A) and PET (B) scan of the abdomen showing a solitary mass in the right anterior abdominal wall (arrows) in a patient with a lung tumour. The mass is PET positive.

vomiting, abdominal pain and constipation, polyuria, thirst and dehydration, muscular weakness, psychosis, drowsiness, and eventually coma. Immediate treatment is to relieve fluid depletion, and large volumes of intravenous saline (up to 5 litres in 24 h) may be required. Intravenous bisphosphonates followed by oral maintenance therapy is now the treatment of choice.

Gynaecomastia

Swelling of the breasts, which may be painful, occurs mainly in the subareolar area, and there may be atrophy of the testes. The association is chiefly with large-cell carcinomas. Increased gonadatropin production is the cause.

Other endocrine manifestations

Hyperthyroidism is a rare feature, but neither goitre nor eye signs are prominent. Spontaneous hypoglycaemia, the masculinizing syndrome in young women, and hyperglycaemia are very rarely encountered. Pigmentation associated with α- and β-melanocyte-stimulating hormone may occur.

Neuromyopathies

A variety of poorly understood neurological syndromes can occur with lung cancer. The diagnosis of a paramalignant neurological syndrome should only be made once other causes including electrolyte imbalance, metastatic disease, cerebral and spinal vascular disease, infection, and toxicity from associated treatment have been eliminated. The main neurological syndromes include the Lambert–Eaton myasthenic syndrome (LEMS), limbic encephalopathy, polyneuropathy, cerebellar degeneration, retinopathy, and autonomic neuropathy. LEMS is the most widely recognized of these disorders and presents with gradual onset of proximal limb weakness, more noticeable in the legs than the arms. Difficulty in swallowing and dryness of the mouth are common, although diplopia is rare. The symptoms may be worse in the mornings and improve as the day progresses. Physical examination will confirm weakness and loss of tendon jerks, but the latter can be restored for a few minutes by performing tasks of repetitive forced contractions (post-tetanic potentiation).

Neurological paramalignancies are associated almost exclusively with small-cell lung cancers, affecting up to 4% of cases. Recent studies of consecutive new patients with small-cell lung cancer reported LEMS in 1.6%, polyneuropathy in <1%, subacute cerebellar degeneration in <1%, and limbic encephalitis in <1%. The severity of the syndromes is not related to tumour bulk and seems to occur more frequently in patients with limited disease; in some a primary tumour is not detected before death, despite disabling symptoms.

Nearly all the neurological paramalignant syndromes are associated with the presence of type 1 antineuronal nuclear antibodies (ANNA-1), also known as anti-Hu antibodies. Small-cell lung cancers express Hu antigen and up to 20% of these patients have detectable circulating levels of anti-Hu antibodies, although not all will develop paramalignant disorders.

The response of these syndromes to effective chemotherapy of the underlying tumour is variable. Improvement is uncommon with motor or sensory neuropathies, or with cerebellar degeneration. However, LEMS can be associated with a better overall prognosis, and the condition responds to specific therapy with 4-aminopyridine which appears to potentiate the release of acetylcholine at the nerve receptor end plate.

Finger clubbing and hypertrophic pulmonary osteoarthropathy

Finger clubbing accompanies a variety of intrathoracic disorders. Gross clubbing is readily recognizable; its early presence may best be demonstrated by the ability to rock the nail on its abnormally spongy bed; the nail fold angle will become obliterated as increased transverse curvature of the nail develops. Clubbing of the toes can be present but is less pronounced.

Hypertrophic pulmonary osteoarthropathy (HPOA), which is a systemic disorder, may be preceded by finger clubbing alone. It consists of a painful symmetrical arthropathy, usually of the ankles, knees, and wrists, and periosteal new bone formation in the distal limb long bones. Associated finger clubbing can be gross. Clubbing and HPOA can be associated with any cell type of lung cancer, but mostly with squamous and adeno, and very rarely with small cell types. The typical radiographic appearances are shown in Fig. 18.19.1.12. The affected areas are hot and painful and sometimes oedematous, making walking difficult. Removal of the tumour is followed by immediate regression, but symptoms recur if the tumour recurs.

Clubbing is much more common than HPOA, occurring in up to 25% of patients presenting with lung cancer. It seems to be commoner in women than men, and in NSCLC compared to small-cell, while HPOA is seen in <5% of patients with NSCLC.

Miscellaneous

The haematological effects of lung cancer are normally nonspecific. Normocytic normochromic anaemia is the most common finding. Leucoerythroblastic anaemia denotes bone marrow infiltration and is particularly likely in small-cell lung cancer. Venous thrombosis and thrombophlebitis due to hypercoagulability are common

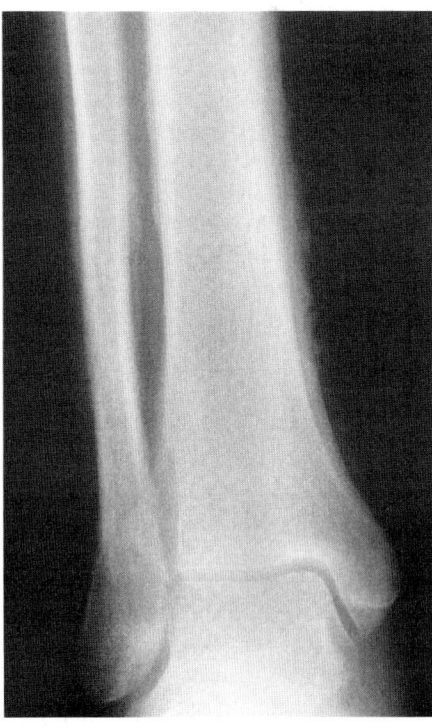

Fig. 18.19.1.12 Radiograph of the ankle showing new periosteal growth due to hypertrophic pulmonary osteopathy.

complications of malignancy and may precede the detection of the underlying cancer; recurrent migratory phlebitis resistant to anti-coagulation is an ominous feature. Marantic endocarditis is extremely rare, as are skin rashes such as acanthosis nigricans, dermatomyositis, hypertrichosis languinosa, and erythema gyratum repens. Rarely, the nephrotic syndrome due to membranous glomerulonephritis is encountered.

Investigations and staging

The investigations used to make the diagnosis and assess the stage of lung cancer will vary according to the presentation, the cell type, and the age and general condition of the patient.

The rapid doubling time of small-cell lung cancer causes it to disseminate widely, and at diagnosis it is very rarely considered operable. However, the slower doubling times for squamous-cell cancers and adenocarcinomas, together with the relatively lesser tendency for the former to disseminate, makes surgery the best option whenever possible for the NSCLCs. A precise anatomical staging classification was first applied to lung cancer in 1973 and immediately demonstrated that the prognosis of NSCLC depended strongly on the extent (or stage) of the disease, and the introduction of the TNM staging system (T describing the primary tumour, N the extent of regional lymph node involvement, and M the absence or presence of metastases) encouraged an ordered assessment of investigations and selection of cases for surgery. On the basis of this experience, the system was modified in 1997 and again in 2009 using a much more extensive data set from centres around the world, and survival data is now based on more than 100 000 cases (Table 18.19.1.3 and Table 18.19.1.4).

The following investigations form the basis for the diagnosis and staging of patients with lung cancer.

Radiological assessment

The value of the chest radiograph in the diagnosis and management of pulmonary neoplasm needs no emphasis (see Figs. 18.19.1.2–18.19.1.8). No initial examination is complete without a lateral radiograph, although many investigators move directly to a CT scan of the thorax and upper abdomen when faced with the likelihood of a new lung cancer.

The finding of a normal radiograph of the chest does not exclude bronchial carcinoma, as patients presenting with haemoptysis and a normal chest radiograph are sometimes found to have a central tumour on bronchoscopy. The rounded or ovoid shadow of a peripheral tumour is described in greater detail below; these are sometimes cavitated. The common appearance of a tumour arising from the main central airways (70% of all cases) is enlargement of one or other hilum. Even experienced observers sometimes have difficulty in deciding whether or not a hilar shadow is enlarged, and if there is any suspicion, investigation by CT and/or bronchoscopy should be pursued. Consolidation and collapse distal to the tumour may have occurred by the time that the patient presents, with the tumour itself often being obscured in the process. Collapse of the left lower lobe is often hard to identify, as is a tumour situated behind the heart (see Fig. 18.19.1.4). Apically located masses or superior sulcus tumours (Pancoast tumours) may be misdiagnosed as pleural caps, and often have a long history of pain in the distribution of the brachial nerve roots. Loss of the head of the first, second, or third rib is not unusual.

The mediastinum may be widened by enlarged nodes. Involvement of the phrenic nerve may lead to paralysis and elevation of the hemidiaphragm, which then moves paradoxically on sniffing. Tumour spreading to the pleura causes effusion, but such an abnormality may be secondary to infection beyond obstruction caused by a central tumour. The ribs and spine should be carefully examined for the presence of metastasis (see Fig. 18.19.1.8). Spread of tumour from mediastinal nodes peripherally along the lymphatics gives the appearance characteristic of lymphangitis carcinomatosa—bilateral hilar enlargement with streaky shadows fanning out into the lung fields on either side. Rarely, localized obstructive emphysema may be observed.

Sputum cytology

Cytological examination of sputum is a very useful noninvasive test for the diagnosis of malignant pulmonary disease. The positive incidence on a single sample is lower with tumours less than 2 cm in diameter (40%) and higher with larger masses (60%). Central tumour yields a higher proportion of positive results than peripheral lesions. The yield increases according to the number of specimens examined, and three consecutive morning specimens should be submitted in the first instance. The yield rose to 85% with four samples in a study of those in whom a diagnosis of lung cancer was made.

CT

Thoracic CT imaging is extremely important in the staging of lung cancer. It can identify the site, size, and extension of the primary tumour far more clearly than a conventional chest radiograph. It also frequently identifies mediastinal lymphadenopathy when posteroanterior and lateral chest radiographs fail to show any abnormality. It will also identify silent metastatic disease in the liver, adrenal glands and in abdominal lymph nodes. It is recommended that a CT is performed prior to considering bronchoscopy as the primary lesion may be shown to be poorly accessible to the bronchoscope and may be easier to sample by CT controlled transthoracic biopsy. The CT scan may also identify mediastinal involvement which can be directly sampled by bronchoscopic or ultrasound-guided techniques, or direct sampling towards an abdominal metastasis. These would both provide a diagnosis and also help stage the disease from a single procedure.

Mediastinal lymphadenopathy on CT is arbitrarily taken to be pathological if the glands are more than 10 mm in transverse diameter. However, previous infective conditions such as tuberculosis or an associated distal pneumonia can cause appearances indistinguishable from malignant enlargement. Thus, positive CT scans of the mediastinum must be confirmed by mediastinal lymph node biopsy to confirm tumour involvement. This is important because nearly 40% of lymph nodes deemed enlarged on CT criteria are found not to contain cancer when they are sampled, either by biopsy or at the time of surgery.

Another advantage of CT is its ability to detect tumour invasion of the surrounding pleura and chest wall, although its ability to assess invasion of the mediastinum itself is poor and should not be used as a criterion of unresectability.

Bronchoscopy

Bronchoscopy, which is described in detail in Chapter 18.3.3, is frequently the definitive diagnostic method in lung cancer. About 70%

Table 18.19.1.3 International Association for the Study of Lung Cancer staging project: TNM classification

cTNM clinical classification	
Primary tumour (T-factor)	
TX	Primary tumour cannot be assessed, or tumour proven by the presence of malignant cells in sputum or bronchial washings but not visualised by imaging or bronohoscopy
TO	No evidence of primary tumour
Tis	Carcinoma *in situ*
T1	Tumour <3 cm in greatest dimension, surrounded by lung or visceral pleura, without bronchoscopic evidence of invasion more proximal than the lobar bronchus (*i.e.* not in the main bronchus)
T1a	Tumour <2 cm in greatest dimension
T1b	Tumour:>2 cm but not >3 cm in greatest dimension
T2	Tumour >3 cm but not >7 cm; or tumour with *any* of the following features:
	Involves main bronchus, >2 cm distal to the carina
	Invades visceral pleura
	Associated with atelectasis or obstructive pneumonitis that extends to the hilar region but does not involve the entire lung
T2a	Tumour >3 cm but not >5 cm in greatest dimension
T2b	Tumour >5 cm but not >7 cm in greatest dimension
T3	Tumour more than 7 cm or one that directly invades any of the following: chest wall (including superior sulcus tumours), diaphragm, phrenic nerve, mediastinal pleura, parietal pericardium; or tumour in the main bronchus less than 2 cm distal to the carina but without involvement of the carina; or associated atelectasis or obstructive pneumonitis of the entire lung or separate tumour nodule(s) in the same lobe
T4	Tumour of any size that invades any of the following: mediastinum, heart, great vessels, trachea, recurrent laryngeal nerve, oesophagus, vertebral body, carina; separate tumour nodule(s) in a different ipsilateral lobe
Regional lymph nodes (N-factor)	
NX	Regional lymph nodes cannot be assessed
NO	No regional lymph node metastasis
N1	Metastasis in ipsilateral peribronchial and/or ipsilateral hilar lymph nodes and intrapulmonary nodes, including involvement by direct extension
N2	Metastasis in ipsilateral mediastinal and/or subcarinal lymph node(s)
N3	Metastasis in contralateral mediastinal, contralateral hilar, ipsilateral or contralateral scalene, or supraclavicular lymph node(s)
Distant metastasis (M-factor)	
MX	Distant metastasis cannot be assessed
MO	No distant metastasis
M1	Distant metastasis
M1a	Separate tumour nodule(s) in a contralateral lobe; tumour with pleural nodules or malignant pleural (or pericardial) effusion
M1b	Distant metastasis

of all lung cancers arise in a main bronchus, lobar, first-, or second-generation airways, and will be visible and within biopsy or cytological brush range. Bronchoscopy also yields valuable information regarding suitability for surgical resection. Attempts to resect are ill advised if the main carina is obviously involved, or unequivocally broad with splaying of the main bronchi and immobility on respiration, or where there is involvement of the trachea, unless confined to the right lateral wall. Histological confirmation is now obtainable in 85 to 90% of bronchoscopically visible lesions, and three or more biopsies of a visible endobronchial lesion should approach 95% accuracy. Endobronchial biopsies provide the highest sensitivity, followed by brushings and then washings.

Transbronchial and transoesophageal biopsy

Historically the mediastinum has been staged and malignant involvement of mediastinal nodes has been confirmed by surgical sampling by mediastinoscopy (for right paratracheal and subcarinal nodes) and/or anterior mediastinotomy for left-sided nodes. Although these techniques remain the 'gold standard', they have been to some extent replaced by minimally invasive techniques including transbronchial needle aspiration (TBNA) and transoesophageal endoscopic ultrasound (EUS), fine-needle aspiration, or biopsy. The use of TBNA in staging lung cancer is reported to be moderately sensitive and highly specific in diagnosing spread to mediastinal nodes accessible through the bronchial wall at

Table 18.19.1.4 International Association for the Study of Lung Cancer staging project: stage grouping

Occult carcinoma	TX N0 M0
Stage 0	Tis N0 M0
Stage IA	T1a, b N0 M0
Stage IB	T2a N0 M0
Stage IIA	T1a, b N1 M0
	T2a N1 M0
	T2b N0 M0
Stage IIB	T2b N1 M0
	T3 N0 M0
Stage IIIA	T1, T2 N2 M0
	T3 N1, N2 M0
	T4 N0, N1 M0
Stage IIIB	T4 N2 M0
	Any T N3 M0
Stage IV	Any T Any N M1

fibre-optic bronchoscopy, in particular the paratracheal nodes and those around the carina. Often involvement of these structures causes widening of the carina, making targeting easy. The sensitivity can be improved by using an ultrasound-guided endoscope, allowing better identification of an abnormal node which can then be sampled under direct ultrasound vision. A recent meta analysis showed the sensitivity of blind TBNA in NSCLC was between 39 and 78%, but depended greatly on the prevalence of cancer in the lymph nodes. The specificity was 99%.

Use of the EUS technique via the oesophagus also has a high yield. It is currently performed by gastroenterologists and will sample nodes in the posterior mediastinum or the subaortic fossa, and also within the abdomen. When used as both a diagnostic tool and as a staging method, the yield is high and the specificity 100%.

Transbronchial biopsy of the lung parenchyma via the fibre-optic bronchoscope is now rarely used for peripheral tumours as direct sampling under CT or ultrasound control has superseded this technique. It remains useful for more diffuse lesions such as may be seen in adenocarcinoma, bronchoalveolar-cell carcinoma, and lymphangitis carcinomatosis.

Percutaneous needle biopsy

Percutaneous needle biopsy of an intrapulmonary mass may be carried out using a variety of cutting needles to obtain a core of tissue for both histology and cytology. The procedure can be performed under fluoroscopic, CT, or ultrasound control, but is best avoided in patients with poor respiratory function or with bleeding diatheses. Positive yields as high as 90% have been reported, with biopsy samples having a higher and more specific yield than cytological aspirates. It is a useful diagnostic method in patients for whom exploratory thoracotomy may be hazardous, or in attempts to determine whether a solid mass is a primary, secondary, or benign tumour. Pneumothorax occurs following about 25% of procedures, with some 2 to 4% requiring a chest drain. Small haemoptyses are a common complication.

Thoracoscopy

Visualization of the parietal and visceral pleura plays an important part in the diagnosis of effusions and pleural tumours. Biopsy of lesions can be carried out under direct vision, and absence of pleural tumour is important in decisions about resectability of a lung tumour. Thoracoscopy is inadvisable in the absence of effusion or pneumothorax, and is unsatisfactory in the presence of empyema or gross haemothorax. However, in otherwise operable tumours with a pleural effusion that is not bloodstained and without positive cytology or pleural biopsy, thoracoscopy may be a useful next step in determining operability. Video-assisted thoracoscopy (VATS) has extended this technique and will also permit inspection and sampling of suspicious mediastinal lymph nodes.

Positron emission tomography (PET) scanning

PET scanning, which depends on the uptake of a glucose analogue (fluorodeoxyglucose, FDG) by active tumour and its metastases, has gained wide acceptance as a test with much better characteristics than CT, especially for the mediastinum. It is now recommended as the final staging test in those where resection or another curative treatment is contemplated. Furthermore, the intensity of uptake of the FDG isotope reflects the aggression of the tumour: the higher the uptake, the likelier the disease is to spread and do badly following surgery. Because uptake of the PET isotope in malignant structures is based on tumour activity and not (as with CT) just lymph node size, its routine use as a preoperative staging tool has been shown to save about 20% of all thoracotomies, which (if proceeded with) would have been futile and noncurative. However, PET scanning has a 10% false-positive rate, due to coexisting infection or inflammation, and a positive area of uptake should always be confirmed by sampling if that abnormal area would directly affect a management decision. A new generation of combined CT/PET scanners will provide the advantages of both techniques and outperform either test alone.

Lung function testing

The ability to climb one flight of stairs without breathlessness has been claimed to be a very good indication of fitness for resection, but formal evaluation of lung function is essential in all patients for whom surgery is being considered. Simple spirometry is usually adequate if the forced expiratory volume in 1 s (FEV_1) and forced vital capacity (FVC) are greater than 70% of predicted normal. If either value is less than 70% predicted, the gas transfer needs to be also 70% of predicted for the subject to withstand a pneumonectomy. If it is less, then differential lung function needs assessing using a ventilation perfusion scan to calculate the quality of performance of the remaining lung tissues. Simple formulae are available to predict the post operative lung function from these scans with reasonable accuracy. However, if the predictions are borderline for the resection intended, then an exercise test should be performed to calculate the maximum oxygen uptake and surgery only performed if this is more than 15 ml/kg per min. In general, the risks are greater for a pneumonectomy and worse for a right-sided operation. The surgeon needs to be given clear advice as to how extensive a resection an individual patient can tolerate safely, without becoming a respiratory cripple as a result of a curative pulmonary resection.

Other investigations

In general, the ability to identify small metastatic deposits is as unsatisfactory for lung carcinomas as for other solid tumours. The available techniques are relatively crude, and this partially explains the high extrathoracic relapse rate following so-called 'curative' resections for NSCLC. In patients with no symptoms other than those caused by their primary tumour, imaging scans of brain, liver, and bones are unhelpful if there is no clinical evidence of neurological, hepatic, or bony disease and normal biochemistry. CT brain scans have a high accuracy in detailing cerebral metastases in patients with neurological symptoms. In patients with a palpable liver and/or abnormal liver function tests, a liver CT scan or ultrasonography should be performed. CT scan of the upper abdomen identifies abnormalities of one or both adrenal glands in up to 10% of patients considered for surgery, and fine-needle aspiration of the adrenal gland should be performed if this remains the only contraindication to pulmonary resection. Bone scans have a high false-positive rate due to Paget's disease, active arthritis, healing fractures, renal disease, and hyperparathyroidism. However, a bone scan should be ordered in patients with bone pain, local tenderness, or nonspecific symptoms of weight loss or malaise.

Biopsy or cytological aspiration of enlarged lymph nodes and skin metastases should be carried out whenever indicated. Indeed, some studies have shown that routine ultrasound scans of the scalene nodes and the supraclavicular fossae in subjects whose CT shows mediastinal nodal enlargement, will have identifiable nodes containing tumour in 30% of cases with ultrasound-guided fine-needle aspiration of the neck region. If an isolated hepatic or bony lesion identified with isotope or CT scanning appears to be the only contraindication to surgery, then this should be biopsied under radiological control.

Staging

The staging algorithm investigations for NSCLC are summarized in Fig. 18.19.1.13. The final procedure before thoracotomy, or other localized treatment such as radical radiotherapy, is assessment of the mediastinum, since this may be involved in up to 50% of patients with a peripheral, poorly differentiated tumour and in a much greater percentage of central lesions. If CT shows no other obvious site of disease and a PET scan only confirms uptake in the primary tumour and at no other distant site, then the surgeon can proceed directly to thoracotomy. If the CT and/or PET scan is abnormal at a distant site, or is not available, then mediastinal exploration should be performed by whatever technique is applicable. Increasingly this is by TBNA or EUS, proceeding to mediastinoscopy only if suspicious areas are not confirmed by these techniques. Similarly, isolated suspicious lesions in the liver, adrenal glands, etc should be biopsied as they both stage as inoperable and provide the cell-type diagnosis. Most patients with extrathoracic metastases will have abnormal nodes within their mediastinum.

Treatment and prognosis of NSCLC

Surgery

Surgery remains the single modality most likely to be curative in NSCLC. Before surgery the patient should have been carefully staged (Fig. 18.19.1.13), and the chances of long-term survival will

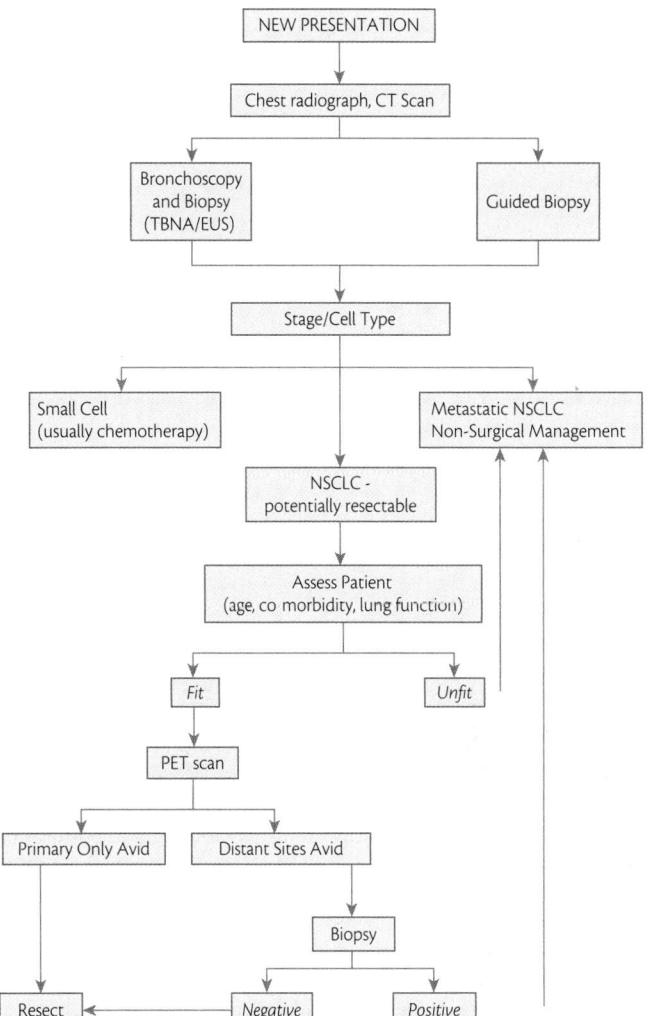

Fig. 18.19.1.13 Staging algorithm for non-small-cell lung cancer.

be greatly influenced by this. All patients with stage IIIB disease (Table 18.19.1.4) should not undergo thoracotomy, but those with stage I, II, and some with IIIA disease can be considered for resection. In general, patients with squamous-cell carcinomas have higher 5- and 10-year survival rates than those with adenocarcinoma and large-cell carcinomas, and the more differentiated the tumour the better is the prognosis. Table 18.19.1.5 summarizes survival data at 5 years for preoperatively staged NSCLC. Clearly, small peripheral lesions with no nodal disease (stage IA) fare best (up to 70% survival at 5 years), but the survival rate decreases with both size of tumour and increasing involvement of hilar and mediastinal nodes. The 5-year survival curves for a more recent series of 3211 patients from Norway, operated upon between 1993 and 2002, are shown in Fig. 18.19.1.14 for survival by pathological stage and for extent of resection. Essentially the survival data is similar to that for a decade previously as used by Mountain in the setting of the updated TNM classification although it may change with the new, 2009, classification (Table 18.19.1.5).

About 15% of all patients who present with NSCLC eventually come to thoracotomy. Most of the others are excluded almost immediately because of clinically evident metastatic disease, radiological or bronchoscopic evidence of inoperability, general

Table 18.19.1.5 Cumulative percentage surviving 5 years and median survival by clinical and surgical TNM subsets

TNM subset	Stage	Clinical			Surgical		
		No.	Percentage surviving	Median survival (months)	No.	Percentage surviving	Median survival (months)
T1 N0 M0	IA	591	61.9	60	429	68.5	60
T2 N0 M0	IB	1012	35.8	26	436	59.0	60
T1 N1 M0	IIA	19	33.6	20	67	54.1	60
T2 N1 M0	IIB	176	22.7	17	250	40.0	29
T3 N0 M0	IIB	221	7.6	8	57	44.2	26
T3 N1 M0	IIIA	71	7.7	8	29	17.6	16
Any N2 M0	IIIA	497	4.9	11	168	28.8	22

(From Mountain CF (1997). Revisions in the international system for staging lung cancer. Chest, **111**, 1710–17.)

frailty and/or significant associated other illnesses, or inadequate lung function. Of those having a 'curative' resection, the overall survival rate at 5 years is approximately 25% and at 10 years it is 16 to 18%. Death from local or distant recurrence of the tumour is equally probable, highlighting the inadequacies of current staging techniques. However, the careful application of the TNM system and the advent of more sophisticated scanning equipment such as PET may lead to improvement.

Only very rarely is there an indication for palliative surgery, and resection should not be considered in the presence of intrathoracic or distant metastasis.

Advanced age is not a contraindication to surgery. About 45% of new patients with lung cancer are over 70 years of age and these individuals appear to tolerate lobectomy as well as younger patients, although the mortality for pneumonectomy (8–10%) is double that of those under 70. There is no evidence that tumours grow more slowly in elderly people, hence the disease is as likely to be the terminal event in older as in younger patients and resection should be encouraged in patients who are fit. Smokers should be persuaded to stop smoking before thoracotomy because continued smoking increases perioperative complications.

Video-assisted thoracoscopic resection of peripheral masses is currently reserved for those with inadequate lung function for lobectomy, as hilar and mediastinal node evaluation and dissection is not always possible. However, these lung sparing procedures may be more suitable for elderly subjects. The cure rates for segmentectomy by VATS is less good than by open thoracotomy and lobectomy with lymph node dissection.

Radiotherapy

Patients who are excluded from surgery because of adverse prognostic factors, advanced stage of tumour, or other coincidental disease constitute the largest group treated with radiotherapy. Although the usual aim of radiotherapy will be palliative, there will be a small group of patients in whom more aggressive therapy will be used in the hope of cure, or at least long-term survival, particularly in those who have refused surgery. Radiotherapy for lung cancer is limited by the comparative radiosensitivity of three critical normal tissues likely to be included in the radiation beam: normal lung, spinal cord, and the heart, each of which has a specific tolerance dose. Increased radiation dose leads to greater killing of tumour cells but may produce unwanted damage to normal cells. Radiation dose must be expressed not only in terms of total dose but also numbers of fractions and overall time. There is no clear evidence for an optimum radical (curative) radiation dose, but doses of 60 Gy (6000 rad) in 5 to 6 weeks are commonly given, with higher doses becoming more commonplace as the accuracy of dose delivery improves with the use of CT scanners, and even PET

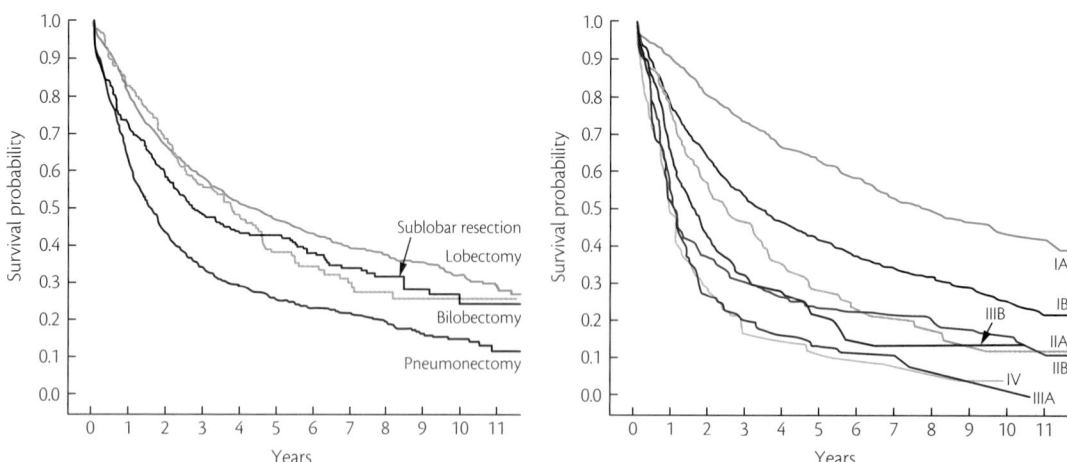

Fig. 18.19.1.14 Left panel: Kaplan–Meier survival curves according to surgical procedure for patients resected for lung cancer diagnosed between 1993 and 2002 in Norway. Right panel: same population showing survival by stage.
(from *Thorax* 2006; **61**, 40, with permission.)

scanners, to set the fields, and confocal techniques allowing normal tissues to be increasingly spared.

Alternative to surgery

In some patients with a technically resectable tumour there may be medical contraindications for resection or the patient may refuse surgery. In general, the results of radical radiotherapy in these patients are inferior to the 5-year survival following surgery. The best result for radiotherapy was a 5-year survival rate of 22% for peripheral squamous-cell cancers, but other series record a 5-year survival rate of 6%.

Preoperative and/or postoperative radiotherapy

Preoperative radiotherapy has been given in a few uncontrolled studies, but there is no evidence that this approach improves survival. Two recent meta-analyses have shown no benefit from postoperative radiotherapy for stage I and II disease, and it is not clear whether or not it has any value in stage IIIA disease with nodal involvement, but benefit is likely to be small and it is not recommended.

Radical radiotherapy for locally advanced, inoperable disease

In otherwise fit patients with small-volume intrathoracic disease which is not resectable, usually because of mediastinal involvement, it is common practice to attempt to cure with radiotherapy. Results with daily single fractions are disappointing, even with doses of up to 60 Gy, with 5-year survival rates ranging from 5 to 17%.

Recently, continuous hyperfractionated accelerated radiotherapy (CHART), with a fraction every 8 h for 12 consecutive days to a total of 54 Gy, has been compared to conventional daily radiotherapy in NSCLC. CHART gave an absolute improvement in 2-year survival from 20% to 29%, with the greatest benefit (14% absolute improvement) in squamous-cell cancers. This appears a real advance in the provision of radiotherapy for locally advanced, inoperable tumours, but it has not proved to be a feasible technique for busy radiotherapy departments. A similar approach with no treatment at week-ends (CHARTWELL) may be as useful and seems to be effective.

Studies of combining radiotherapy with concurrent or sequential courses of chemotherapy have been compared to radiotherapy alone and shown a survival benefit. It also appears that concurrent chemotherapy may be better than the two treatment modalities given consecutively, although the toxicity for the concurrent approach is higher. Chemoradiotherapy is now regarded as the approach of choice for locally advanced, inoperable NSCLC.

Palliation

Radiotherapy can provide excellent palliation for many symptoms, with two of the most distressing, haemoptysis and cough, controlled in up to 80% of cases. Administration of two fractions (each of 8.5 Gy, 1 week apart) appears adequate. Dyspnoea from bronchial obstruction and dysphagia are relieved in most cases. The syndrome of superior vena caval obstruction is relieved in about 80% of sufferers, but usually requires a more conventional course of five to ten fractions of radiotherapy. Pain from bone secondaries can be relieved in more than 50% by a single fraction of 8 Gy, often given at the same time as a clinic visit. Brain metastases generally respond poorly to radiotherapy. A 48-h trial of dexamethasone, 4 mg orally four times daily, is recommended as initial management. If a worthwhile response follows the resolution of the oedema

surrounding the metastases, then radiotherapy will consolidate this gain, after which steroids should be rapidly withdrawn. Spinal cord compression is a relatively common occurrence associated with vertebral body metastatic disease. Pain and bony tenderness often precede it and may be helpful in localizing the lesion. Responses to radiotherapy are usually incomplete and disappointing, often because of interruption of the vascular supply to the spinal cord by the tumour.

Chemotherapy

Several cytotoxic agents show activity against NSCLC, but much less frequently or dramatically than with small-cell tumours. However, combination chemotherapy can achieve impressive response rates; partial responses in 50% of patients with locally advanced disease and in 35% of those with advanced extrathoracic disease have been reported. The most active regimens include two agents: cisplatin or carboplatin, and gemcitabine or paclitaxel or vinorelbine. These 'third-generation' drugs have replaced the more toxic and often harder to give agents such as ifosfamide, mitomycin, or vindesine. A meta-analysis of 53 randomized controlled studies in which patients received or did not receive chemotherapy in addition to surgery, radiotherapy, or to best supportive care was published in 1995. This suggested a 5% advantage for the addition of chemotherapy to surgery (confidence intervals −1 to 7%), a smaller nonsignificant advantage for the addition of chemotherapy to radiotherapy, and—in those with advanced disease—a 10% improvement in survival at 1 year for the addition of chemotherapy to best supportive care. Subsequent trials of adjuvant chemotherapy following successful surgery versus no further treatment have confirmed a 5.2% increase in the 5-year postsurgery survival with the addition of chemotherapy, and patients should be offered this choice.

In advanced disease, which will affect up to 90% of all cases of NSCLC, chemotherapy only confers a survival advantage of 6 to 8 weeks compared to best supportive care alone, making evaluation of effects on quality of life important. A large trial of second-generation cytotoxic chemotherapy vs best supportive care showed no disadvantage in global health scores with chemotherapy, and modern third-generation combinations have been shown to improve quality of life, at least while the patient is responding and in remission. There is no particular regimen that stands out, but chemotherapy in advanced disease for patients with a good performance status will increase the median survival by 4 to 6 months and the 1-year survival from 18% untreated to 35 to 40%.

With chemotherapy on a plateau for NSCLC, new data is emerging on so-called targeted therapy. As described previously, mutations in EGFR have been identified in lung cancer, and overexpression of EGFR and its ligands in NSCLC has made it a target for treatment. Two oral inhibitors of EGFR, gefitinib and erlotinib, have been studied in detail, mainly in patients with advanced disease. Studies assessing different doses of gefitinib in patients previously treated and relapsed after chemotherapy showed tumour activity, responses and improvements in quality of life. However, a trial of gefitinib vs placebo in patients who had relapsed following chemotherapy showed only trends to better survival with the active treatment, although a similar trial of erlotinib did show both a survival advantage (2 months) and an improvement in quality of life in previously treated patients with advanced relapsed disease. Neither gefitinib nor erlotinib has been shown to be of added value when given at the start of treatment, concurrently with chemotherapy. The best responses in patients with pretreated advanced disease have been in women, of Asian origin, never smokers, and with adenocarcinoma. Other targeted therapies are in preparation and this approach may become of increasing value in the future.

Treatment and prognosis of small-cell lung cancer

Small-cell lung cancer is separated from the other types of lung cancer because of its very different biological and clinical features. It has an explosive growth pattern, such that the TNM staging classification makes no impact on prognosis or survival, almost certainly because careful staging puts most patients into the inoperable category. However, simple staging has some prognostic impact and those with limited disease (tumour confined to one hemithorax and the ipsilateral supraclavicular fossa) fare better than those with extensive disease (involvement of any site outside the hemithorax). The life expectancy of those with untreated small-cell lung cancer is about 3.5 months for limited disease and 6 weeks for extensive disease.

Prognostic factors

Multivariate analyses of large patient populations show that routine biochemical values such as serum sodium, albumin, and alkaline phosphatase allow separation of prognostic subgroups. In addition, performance status and extent of disease are important influences. For instance a good performance status and normal biochemical values (i.e. a good prognostic category) has a 2-year survival rate of 20%, yet a correspondingly low performance status with one or more abnormal biochemical parameters (poor prognosis) has virtually no 2-year survivors (Fig. 18.19.1.15). Women tend to do better than men and those under 60 better than those over 60 years of age. These factors are helpful both for stratification within clinical studies and for identifying those patients likely to do well with chemotherapy and those for whom intensive potentially toxic chemotherapy would appear inappropriate. Survival beyond 5 years (cure) is achieved in 4 to 12% of patients with limited disease and in hardly anyone with extensive disease at diagnosis. Most studies of long-term survival report late deaths due to other cancers, including NSCLCs in up to 30% of these long-term survivors.

Surgery

Very occasionally patient with small-cell lung cancer can be surgically cured, usually those presenting with a peripheral tumour and no evidence of local spread or metastasis despite extensive staging investigations. These patients are rare, but nevertheless have a 5-year survival rate in the region of 30 to 40%.

Radiotherapy

Radiotherapy has an important role in palliation of symptoms that may develop after relapse following chemotherapy. Chest irradiation also significantly decreases the rate of recurrence at the primary tumour site and in the mediastinum. A total dose of 40 to 50 Gy is usually given. Two meta-analyses on the value of adding radiotherapy to chemotherapy have shown a 5% advantage at 3 years for the addition of radiotherapy. The optimal timing of radiotherapy in relation to chemotherapy is not clear, and studies looking at giving

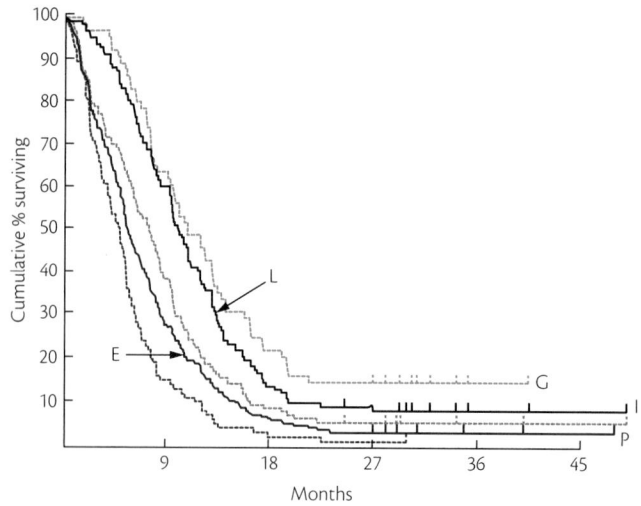

Fig. 18.19.1.15 Survival in small-cell lung cancer by prognostic factors (G, good; Im intermediate; P, poor) compared to full staging (L, limited; E, extensive disease).

it early (within the first 30 days of starting chemotherapy) or late (at the end of chemotherapy) have been inconclusive, but the most important factor in efficacy seems to be ensuring the prescribed chemotherapy is achieved. In several studies the additional toxicity of radiotherapy has prevented planned chemotherapy, with disadvantageous effects on survival.

Cranial irradiation

Cranial metastases are common, with 10% of patients in remission developing them as their first site of relapse. Prophylactic cranial irradiation given at the end of chemotherapy will delay the presentation of cerebral metastases and also reduce their overall incidence. This is important, as the development of cerebral disease is associated with severe morbidity, often making it difficult for the sufferer to live at home. A meta-analysis looking at the effects of prophylactic cranial irradiation on survival showed that the cumulative incidence of brain relapse was halved and the risk of death reduced by 16%, with this survival benefit being maintained after 6 years, hence it is now recommended that patients achieving a complete response after chemotherapy should have prophylactic cranial irradiation.

Chemotherapy

Small-cell lung cancer is much more sensitive to cytotoxic chemotherapy than the NSCLC tumours, with a much higher response rate for several cytotoxic drugs. In the late 1970s there was a very rapid improvement in median survival, and subsequent studies using combinations of three and four drugs brought longer response times, but responses have subsequently reached a plateau. Nevertheless, with modern combination cytotoxic treatment, which is usually given as an outpatient procedure every 3 weeks, the median survival has been extended to 14 to 18 months for limited disease and to 9 to 12 months for extensive disease. Most combinations include etoposide, cisplatin or carboplatin, cyclophosphamide, doxorubicin, and vincristine. There is no outstanding regimen, although etoposide and carboplatin is favoured by most. Modern regimens would be expected to achieve a complete response rate (i.e. disappearance of all measurable disease) in 40 to 50% of cases and a partial response rate (>50% reduction in tumour bulk) in a further 40%, giving a total response rate of 80 to 85%. All these regimens have side effects: most patients will experience some nausea and vomiting, and life-threatening septicaemia occurs in 1 to 4%, but treatment-related deaths are uncommon.

Much effort has been applied during the last 25 years to improve the median and long-term survival of patients with small-cell lung cancer, without any notable success. In general, those patients likely to do better are those who present with limited disease and a good performance status. Patients with extensive disease tend to have a universally bad prognosis and very few survive beyond 2 years. However, some metastatic sites (bone and bone marrow) are not as sinister as others (brain or liver), and the occasional patient with extensive disease does well with chemotherapy, but in general treatment is offered in this circumstance for palliation and not in the hope of cure. Studies assessing the quality of life in patients presenting with small-cell lung cancer have shown that over 70% have important symptoms such as weight loss, malaise, bone pain, dyspnoea, and haemoptysis. Most of these patients have extensive disease, but after 3 months of chemotherapy symptoms can be relieved in 60 to 70% of sufferers, making chemotherapy worthwhile, with symptomatic benefits far outweighing the potential side-effects. Ten per cent of small-cell lung cancer patients present with superior vena caval obstruction: this responds as well as any presentation to chemotherapy.

Intensity of treatment

Intensifying the dosage or the frequency of administration of cytotoxic agents has been thoroughly explored without real benefit on median survival. Small advantages are occasionally seen, but these have to be balanced by the increased toxicity resulting from a more aggressive approach. Attempts to overcome or delay the emergence of cell resistance to chemotherapy have involved alternating combinations of drugs, but these more complicated regimens have not been rewarding either. Similarly, the use of colony growth stimulation factors to allow higher or more frequent doses of drugs has not added to survival. Other studies with very high dose schedules and bone marrow harvesting and reinfusion have been unsuccessful.

Duration of treatment

Toxicity of chemotherapy increases with the number of courses given. It is now apparent that most of the tumour response to chemotherapy occurs within the first two or three cycles. Studies attempting to minimize the duration of chemotherapy without adversely affecting survival have shown that six courses of combination chemotherapy is optimal (with a course every 3 weeks), with no benefit from maintenance regimens.

General management of patients with lung cancer

There are certain complications which require specific measures to alleviate symptoms.

Patients who seem likely to survive for 6 months or more and who have vocal cord paralysis are considerably helped by an injection of PTFE (Teflon) into the affected cord, which restores voice production in a high percentage of cases and reduces the risk of aspiration.

Obstruction of the upper airway causing stridor, or of the lower major airways, is usually treated initially with radiotherapy.

Should this complication recur or be unsuitable for radiotherapy, then it can sometimes be treated by laser photocoagulation administered either via a fibre-optic bronchoscope or under general anaesthetic via a rigid instrument. This is most suitable as a palliative treatment in central tumours occluding large airways: removal of considerable quantities of tumour can be achieved in a single treatment session with the rigid instrument. Trials are in progress assessing the additional benefits of endobronchial radiotherapy (brachytherapy) using iridium or caesium wires delivered via the fibre-optic bronchoscope. This procedure irradiates endobronchial tumour to a circumferential depth of about 1 cm, and will often produce a further remission. It is used where further external-beam radiotherapy cannot be given because of the risk of exceeding normal tissue tolerance. Infection distal to tumour requires antibiotic therapy and, where appropriate, oxygen therapy and bronchodilators. Severe, recurrent haemoptysis may be controlled by radiotherapy or laser.

Malignant pleural effusion recurs after aspiration unless the pleural space is obliterated. Chemical pleurodesis can be induced by intrapleural instillation of a number of agents, or by the more invasive procedure of talc pleurodesis. However, the increasing availability of VATS makes a talc pleurodesis preferable in all reasonably fit patients who can undergo a general anaesthetic (see Chapter 18.17). In general a pleurodesis is recommended early in management, before embarking on chemotherapy in NSCLC. In small-cell lung cancer it is worthwhile to give chemotherapy first as it is likely to gain control.

Dexamethasone, 4 to 16 mg orally daily, may control the symptoms of brain metastasis and, if so, this should be consolidated with radiotherapy to prevent severe steroid-induced myopathy, especially in patients who show a good symptomatic response to the steroids.

Prednisolone, 20 mg orally daily, is often used to improve the sense of well-being, as are blood transfusion or hyperalimentation.

Palliative care is described in Chapter 31.1, but the importance of the combined support to the patient and the family given by the family doctor, palliative care medical and nursing staff, hospice organizations, and the hospital team cannot be overemphasized.

Prevention and screening

Lung cancer is a preventable disease which in 80% of cases is due to smoking, particularly of cigarettes. Strenuous efforts must be made to persuade people not to start smoking, to establish more effective methods of enabling people to stop, and to promote further research into effective health education. The promotion of cigarettes with low tar, nicotine, and carbon monoxide contents may have made a small contribution to prevention, but low-tar cigarettes are not a substitute for giving up smoking. Penal taxation by governments may help, as will smoke-free public places.

The identification of occupational hazards and implementation of appropriate measures to safeguard the health of employees are clearly important preventive measures, even although the number at risk is very small.

Screening of normal but high-risk populations with chest radiography and/or sputum cytology has been shown to have no effect on the mortality from lung cancer, even though more cancers are discovered. However, new studies of various populations using low-dose spiral CT have identified lung cancers in 1.4 to 2.7% of subjects in prevalence screens, the great majority having stage I disease, which is about 4 to 6 times what one would pick up by chest radiography. The older the subjects screened, the greater the smoking history and the presence of airways obstruction, the higher the incidence of occult lung cancers. As yet there are no randomized controlled trials of low-dose CT vs a control group to assess the effect of this modality on mortality, but at least one large study of 50 000 individuals has closed to recruitment. However, although low-dose CT may be a possible method of identifying lung cancers early, it has its problems and limitations. It will only pick up peripheral tumours, i.e. adenocarcinomas in the lung parenchyma, and not central, mainly squamous tumours. Small-cell cancers appear to grow too rapidly to be found by screening and will present with symptoms. Depending on where in the world the study is performed, many subjects will be found to have benign nodules that require follow up according to radiological algorithms which require repeated scans. The incidence of nodules varies from 15 to 40%, which is a potentially huge burden for imaging departments. Clearly, if low dose CT is found to identify stage I tumours and studies show an improvement in mortality, then this expensive technique will have to be considered as part of the preventive approach to smokers and ex-smokers who are fit enough to be likely to survive for 5 years or more, making screening in them worthwhile.

Other primary lung tumours

The slow-growing intrabronchial lesions previously grouped under the heading of bronchial adenoma have now been reclassified into bronchial carcinoids, adenoid cystic tumours, and mucoepidermoid tumours. They are not related to cigarette smoking, and tend to be diagnosed at a younger age than carcinoma of the bronchus.

True bronchial adenomas derived from bronchial glands are rare. These tumours were once thought to be benign, but they are potentially and often frankly malignant, being capable not only of destructive local growth but also of metastasis to regional lymph nodes in about one-third of patients, and to distant organs, particularly liver and brain, in about 10%. They are occasionally located in the trachea.

The most common symptoms of bronchial carcinoids are cough, haemoptysis, and recurrent pneumonia, although not infrequently the lesion is discovered on routine radiographic examination before symptoms develop. In the few cases that have extensive liver secondaries, there may be the classical symptom pattern of intermittent cyanotic flushings, intestinal cramps and diarrhoea, bronchoconstriction, and cardiovascular lesions. The radiographic appearances are those of a solitary nodule, pulmonary collapse, or obstructive hyperinflation. As most of the tumours occur in main stem or proximal portions of lobar bronchi, bronchoscopy is usually the definitive diagnostic measure. The tumour appears as a white or pink polypoid or lobulated mass, with the bronchial mucosa appearing to be intact. Biopsy may be followed by brisk haemoptysis.

Surgical resection is the treatment of choice. In the absence of regional spread or distant metastases 5-year survival prospects are excellent, but if there is involvement of regional nodes, survival rates fall to 70%. Some aggressive carcinoid tumours carry a much worse prognosis. The mechanism and management of the general symptoms of the carcinoid syndrome are described in Chapter 15.9.

Further reading

Ahrendt SA, et al. (1999). Molecular detection of tumor cells in bronchoalveolar lavage fluid from patients with early stage lung cancer. *J Natl Cancer Inst*, **91**, 332–9.

American Thoracic Society and European Respiratory Society (1997). Pretreatment evaluation of non-small-cell lung cancer. *Am J Respir Crit Care Med*, **156**, 320–32.

Auperin A, et al. (1999). Prophylactic cranial irradiation for patients with small cell lung cancer in complete remission. Prophylactic Cranial Irradiation Overview Collaborative Group. *N Engl J Med*, **341**, 476–84.

Beckles MA, et al. (2003). The physiological evaluation of patients with lung cancer being considered for surgery. *Chest*, **123**, 105–14S.

British Thoracic Society, Society of Cardiothoracic Surgeons of GB, Ireland Working Party (2001). Guidelines on the selection of patients with lung cancer for surgery. *Thorax*, **56**, 89–106.

Brown JS, et al. (1996). Age and the treatment of lung cancer. *Thorax*, **51**, 564–8.

Bruske-Hohlfeld I, et al. (2000). Occupational lung cancer risk for men in Germany: results from a proband case-control study. *Am J Epidemiol*, **151**, 384–95.

Carney DN (1992). Biology of small-cell lung cancer. *Lancet*, **339**, 843–6.

Depierre A, et al. (2002). Preoperative chemotherapy followed by surgery compared with primary surgery in resectable Stage I (except T1N0), II and IIIa non-small-cell lung cancer. *J Clin Oncol*, **20**, 247–53.

Doll R, Peto R (1976). Mortality in relation to smoking: 20 years' observations on male British doctors. *Br Med J*, **ii**, 1525–36.

Fountana RS, et al. (1984). Early lung cancer detection: results of the initial (prevalence) radiologic and cytologic screening in the Mayo Clinic Study. *Am Rev Respir Dis*, **130**, 561–5.

Fritscher-Ravens A, et al. (2000). Role of transesophageal endosonography-guided fine-needle aspiration in the diagnosis of lung cancer. *Chest*, **117**, 339–45.

Furuse K, et al. (1999). Phase III study of concurrent versus sequential thoracic radiotherapy in combination with mitomycin, vindesine, and cisplatin in unresectable Stage III non-small-cell lung cancer. *J Clin Oncol*, **17**, 2692–9.

Goldstraw P, Crowley J, on behalf of the IASLC International Staging Project. (2006). The International Association for the Study of Lung Cancer international staging project on lung cancer. *J Thorac Oncol*, **1**, 281–6.

Goldstraw P, Crowley J, Chansky K et al. (2007). The IASLC Lung Cancer Staging Project: proposals for the revision of the TNM stage groupings in the forthcoming (seventh) edition of the TNM Classification of malignant tumours. *J Thorac Oncol*, **2**, 706–14.

Grant D, Edwards D, Goldstraw P (1988). Computed tomography of the brain, chest, and abdomen in the preoperative assessment of non-small-cell lung cancer. *Thorax*, **43**, 883–6.

Henschke CI, et al. (1999). Early lung cancer detection project: overall design and baseline screening. *Lancet*, **354**, 99–105.

Holty JE, Kuschner WG, Gould MK (2005). Accuracy of transbronchial needle aspiration for mediastinal staging of non-small-cell lung cancer: a meta-analysis. *Thorax*, **60**, 949–55.

Izbicki JR, et al. (1992). Accuracy of computed tomographic scan and surgical assessment for staging of bronchial carcinoma. A prospective study. *J Thorac Cardiovasc Surg*, **104**, 413–20.

Kaneko M, et al. (1996). Peripheral lung cancer: screening and detection with low-dose spiral CT versus radiography. *Radiology*, **201**, 798–802.

Kaplan DK (1992). Mediastinal lymph node metastases in lung cancer: is size a valid criterion. *Thorax*, **47**, 332–3.

Landreneau RJ, et al. (1992). Thoracoscopic resection of 85 pulmonary lesions. *Ann Thorac Surg*, **54**, 415–19.

Laroche C, et al. (2000). Role of computed tomographic scanning of the thorax prior to bronchoscopy in the investigation of suspected lung cancer. *Thorax*, **55**, 359–63.

Mountain CF (1997). Revisions in the international system for staging lung cancer. *Chest*, **111**, 1710–17.

Muers MF, Round CE (1993). Palliation of symptoms in non-small-cell lung cancer. *Thorax*, **48**, 339–43.

Non-Small-Cell Lung Cancer Collaborative Group (1995). Chemotherapy in non-small-cell lung cancer: a meta-analysis using updated data on individual patients from 52 randomised clinical trials. *BMJ*, **311**, 899–909.

Pandey M, Mathew A, Nair MK (1999). Global perspective of tobacco habits and lung cancer. A lesson for third world countries. *Eur J Cancer Prev*, **8**, 271–9.

Pignon JP, *et al.* (1992). A meta-analysis of thoracic radiotherapy for small cell lung cancer. *N Engl J Med*, **327**, 1618–24.

Pless-Mulloli T, *et al.* (1998). Lung cancer, proximity to industry, and poverty in northeast England. *Environ Health Perspect*, **106**, 189–96.

PORT Meta-analysis Trialists Group (1998). Postoperative radiotherapy in non-small-cell lung cancer: systematic review and meta-analysis of individual patient data from nine randomised controlled trials. *Lancet*, **352**, 257–63.

Reed CE, *et al.* (2003). Results of the American College of Surgeons Oncology Group Z0050 trial: the utility of positron emission tomography in staging potentially operable non-small-cell lung cancer. *J Thorac Cardiovasc Surg*, **126**, 1943–51.

Ries LAG, *et al.* (1995). *Cancer statistics review: 1973–1993.* US Government Printing Office, Bethesda, MD.

Saunders M, *et al.* on behalf of the CHART Steering Committee (1997). Continuous hyperfractionated accelerated radiotherapy (CHART) versus conventional radiotherapy in non-small-cell lung cancer: a randomised multicentre trial. *Lancet*, **350**, 161–5.

Scagliotti GV (1995). Symptoms and signs and staging of lung cancer. In: Spiro SG (ed.) *Carcinoma of the lung*, European Respiratory Monograph, Vol. 1, No. 1, pp. 91–137. European Respiratory Society Journals, Sheffield.

Schiller JS, *et al.* (2002). Comparison of four chemotherapy regimens for advanced non-small-cell lung cancer. *N Engl J Med*, **346**, 92–8.

Shepherd RA, *et al.* (2005). Erlotinib in previously treated non-small-cell lung cancer. *N Engl J Med*, **353**, 123–32.

Shigematsu H, Gazdar AF (2006). Somatic mutations of epidermal growth factor receptor signaling pathway in lung cancers. *Int J Cancer*, **118**, 257–62.

Silvestri G, Pritchard R, Welch HG (1998). Preferences for chemotherapy in patients with advanced non-small-cell lung cancer: descriptive study based on scripted interviews. *BMJ*, **317**, 771–5.

Silvestri GA, *et al.* (2003). The noninvasive staging of non-small-cell lung cancer: the guidelines. *Chest*, **123**, 147–56s.

Sobue T, *et al.* (2002). Screening for lung cancer with low-dose helical computerd tomography: anti-lung cancer association project. *J Clin Oncol*, **20**, 911–20.

Souhami RL, *et al.* (1985). Prognostic significance of laboratory parameters measured at diagnosis in small cell carcinoma of the lung. *Cancer Res*, **45**, 2878–82.

Spiro SG, Goldstraw P (1984). The staging of lung cancer. *Thorax*, **39**, 401–7.

Spiro SG, *et al.* (2004). Chemotherapy versus supportive care in advanced non-small-cell lung cancer: improved survival without detriment to quality of life. *Thorax*, **59**, 828–36.

Spiro SG, *et al.* (2006). Early compared with late radiotherapy in combined modality treatment for limited-disease small-cell lung cancer: A London Lung Cancer Group multicenter randomized clinical trial and meta-analysis. *J Clin Oncol*, **24**, 3823–30.

Strand T-E, *et al.* (2006). Survival after resection for primary lung cancer: a population based study of 3211 resected patients. *Thorax*, **61**, 710–15.

Thatcher N, *et al.* (1995). Chemotherapy in non-small-cell lung cancer. *Ann Oncol*, **6** (Suppl. 1), S83–95.

Thatcher N, *et al.* (2005). Gefitinib plus best supportive care in previously treated patients with refractory advanced non-small-cell lung cancer:

results from a randomised, placebo-controlled, multicentre study (Iressa Survival Evaluation in Lung Cancer). *Lancet*, **366**, 1527–37.

Tockman MS, *et al.* (1997). Prospective detection of preclinical lung cancer: results from two studies of heterogeneous nuclear riboprotein A2/B1 over-expression. *Clin Cancer Res*, **3**, 2237–46.

Van Tinteren H, *et al.* (2002). Effectiveness of positron emission tomography in the preoperative assessment of patients with suspected non-small-cell lung cancer: the PLUS Multicentre Randomised Trial. *Lancet*, **359**, 1388–93.

Wallace MD, *et al.* (2001). Endoscopic ultrasound-guided fine needle aspiration for staging patients with carcinoma of the lung. *Ann Thorac Surg*, **72**, 1861–7.

Wells FC, Kendall SWH (1992). Thoracoscopy: the dawn of a new age. *Resp Med*, **86**, 365–6.

18.19.2 Pulmonary metastases

S.G. Spiro

Essentials

Malignant metastasis to the lung is common. It may present as a solitary enlarging nodule, as multiple nodules ranging enormously in size and number, or with diffuse lymphatic involvement. Diagnosis can usually be secured by percutaneous CT-guided biopsy. Surgical excision may prolong survival or result in cure in rare cases.

Malignant metastasis to the lung is common because of the lung's rich blood supply, and may present as a solitary enlarging nodule, as multiple nodules, or with diffuse lymphatic involvement.

About 10% of all round pulmonary lesions are metastases, but some 70% of round lesions in patients with a known malignancy. Colorectal cancer is reported to be the commonest tumour of origin. Diagnosis can usually be secured by percutaneous CT-guided biopsy. In rare cases, surgical excision may prolong survival or result in cure, depending on the state of the primary tumour and the likelihood of other occult metastases.

Multiple metastases range enormously in size and number, from 'cannon balls'—which are the commonest appearance—to multiple lesions of varying size, and then to miliary shadowing, which may be accompanied by hilar lymphadenopathy or pleural effusion. Breast, colon, renal, melanoma, and lung primaries are probably the commonest underlying tumours, but other tumours amenable to chemotherapy occur, such as testicular cancer, choriocarcinoma, and also sarcomas. Diagnosis may be achieved by cytology or histology on various samples from the pleura or lung and can occasionally be made from cytology of expectorated or induced sputum. Tumours that are suitable for chemotherapy (e.g. choriocarcinoma) or endocrine manipulation (e.g. breast) need to be recognized. Solitary or multiple Kaposi's sarcoma is a feature of AIDS and can involve the bronchi and pleura as well as lung tissue.

Resection remains the treatment of choice and good prognostic factors include the time from treatment of the primary tumour to the development of lung metastases, the fewer the number, the

Table 18.19.2.1 5-year survival following resection of pulmonary metastases according to primary tumour type

Tumour type	5-year survival (%)
Soft tissue sarcoma	25
Osteogenic sarcoma	20–40
Colon/rectal carcinoma	8–37
Renal cell carcinoma	13–50
Breast carcinoma	14–49
Head/neck carcinoma	40–50
Melanoma	25

absence of extrapulmonary metastases, and the longer the tumour doubling time. The most favourable group are younger patients with a good performance status, with sarcomas who present with few lesions a year or more after successful treatment of the primary disease. Survival following surgical excision is summarized in Table 18.19.2.1.

Further reading

Mountain CF, McMurtrey MJ, Hermes KE (1984). Surgery for pulmonary metastasis: a 20 year experience. *Ann Thorac Surg*, **38**, 323–30.

Regal AM, *et al.* (1985). Median sternotomy for metastatic lung lesions in 131 patients. *Cancer*, **55**, 1334–9.

Rusch VW (1995). Pulmonary metastatectomy: current indications. *Chest*, **107** (Suppl 6), 322–31S.

Stewart JR, *et al.* (1992). Twenty years' experience with pulmonary metastasectomy. *Am Surg*, **58**, 100–3.

Van Geel AN, *et al.* (1996). Surgical treatment of lung metastases: the European organization for Research and Treatment of Cancer—Soft Tissue and Bone Sarcoma Group study of 255 patients. *Cancer*, **77**, 675–82.

18.19.3 Pleural tumours

Robert J.O. Davies and Y.C. Gary Lee

Essentials

Benign tumours are rare in the pleural cavity, with solitary fibrous tumour of the pleura, the most frequent of these rarities.

Malignant pleural tumours are common and can arise from the pleura (most commonly mesothelioma) or as metastases from extrapleural malignancies (especially lung and breast cancer). They typically present with breathlessness, chest pain, and pleural effusion. Diagnosis requires histocytological confirmation of malignant cells from pleural fluid and/or histological biopsies.

Mesothelioma—most cases are due to asbestos exposure, characteristically after a latent period of more than 20 years, with risk related to the duration and intensity of asbestos exposure and the fibre type (needle-like amphiboles are worst). The condition is incurable, with overall median survival being about 9 months. Care involves

pain control, pleurodesis to prevent fluid re-accumulation, chemotherapy with multitargeted antifolate agents in combination with cisplatin, and radiotherapy for symptom palliation. Pemetrexed and raltitrexed, novel multitargeted antifolate agents used in combination with cisplatin, may be useful in selected cases.

Metastatic pleural malignancy—a tumour that has spread to the pleura is incurable in most cases. Treatment of primary tumours that are highly responsive to chemotherapy (e.g. lymphoma or small cell carcinoma) may control pleural effusion. However, in the majority of patients pleural fluid is not controlled without specific treatment and recurs after simple aspiration. Provided the patient's life expectancy is more than three months, these patients should have pleurodesis (adherence of the pleural membranes). Where this fails, repeated pleurodesis with a different pleurodesis agent, implantation of a chronic indwelling catheter, pleuro-peritoneal shunting, serial therapeutic thoracentesis, or surgical pleurodesis should be considered.

Benign pleural tumours

Benign tumours are relatively rare in the pleural cavity, with solitary fibrous tumour of the pleura the most frequent of these rarities. Asbestos pleural thickening (e.g. plaques and round atelectasis) are discussed elsewhere (see Chapter 18.17). Extrapleural fat can occasionally mimic malignant pleural thickening, especially in obese patients. Pleural lipoma is a rare entity of little clinical significance.

Solitary fibrous tumour of the pleura (SFTP)

This is a rare disease accounting for less than 5% of all pleural tumours. It has also been called 'localized fibrous mesothelioma', 'benign mesothelioma' or 'pleural fibroma'. The aetiology is unknown, but there is no established relationship with asbestos or tobacco exposure. It affects both sexes equally and can affect patients of all ages. The tumour arises from mesenchymal cells, usually from the visceral pleura.

Symptoms and effusions are uncommon. Cough, chest pain, or dyspnoea is relatively mild, even if present. Hypertrophic pulmonary osteoarthropathy affects around 20% of patients, and intermittent hypoglycaemia due to tumour secreted insulin-like growth factor is reported. SFTPs are often huge when discovered (>10 cm in 50% of cases in one series—Fig. 18.19.3.1) and can be pedunculated (more common) or sessile. CT scanning usually reveals a well-encapsulated, lobulated mass showing heterogeneous attenuation, but there are no pathognomonic findings on imaging. The condition is usually amendable to surgery, which thereby serves diagnostic and therapeutic purposes.

Most SFTPs (c.80%) are benign with good long-term prognosis after resection. Malignant SFTPs do occur, the diagnosis usually being based on histological findings (hypercellular clusters, high mitotic activity, and infiltrations) but not on clinical or radiological findings. Recurrence after resection occurs at a rate of 2 to 8% in benign SFTPs, but up to 63% in malignant variants, and patients with malignant sessile SFTPs have a 30% mortality at 2 years. The role of neoadjuvant or postoperative chemotherapy has not been established.

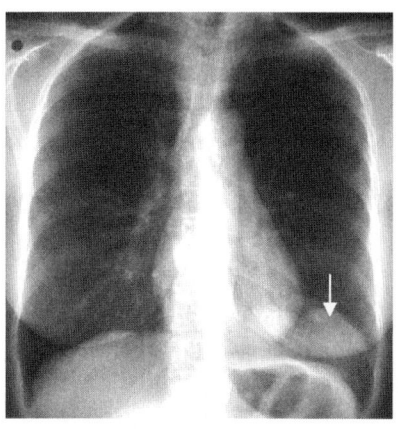
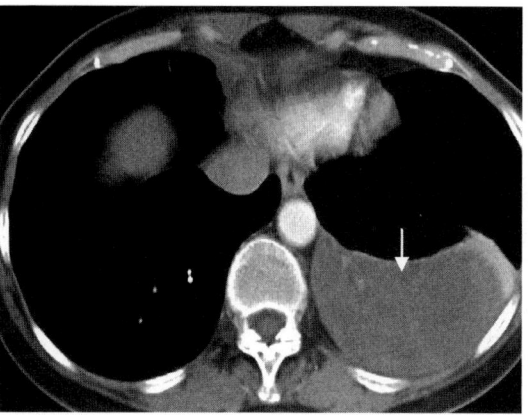

Fig. 18.19.3.1 A chest radiograph and thoracic CT scan showing a solitary fibrous tumour of the pleura at the left base (arrows). After surgical resection, histological examination showed malignant change in the centre of the tumour.

Malignant pleural tumours

Malignant pleural effusion affects about 660 patients per million population annually, with a malignant aetiology found in some 50% of patients presenting with exudative effusions. Malignant tumours involving the pleura can arise as a primary tumour from the pleura (of which mesothelioma accounts for the vast majority) or as metastases from extrapleural tumours to the pleura. Relatively little research has been performed on the best management for malignant effusions, and a recent worldwide survey of 859 respiratory specialists identified marked differences in clinical practice.

Malignant pleural mesothelioma

The incidence of mesothelioma is rising substantially, leading to a global epidemic. Up to 250 000 deaths from mesothelioma are expected in western Europe alone over the next three decades.

Most mesotheliomas are due to asbestos exposure, characteristically after a long latent period (>20 years in 96% of patients). As asbestos mining and its global uses are still increasing, especially in countries where regulation is poor, mesothelioma will remain a significant world health issue.

Most (>90%) of mesothelioma arises from the pleura, occasionally from the peritoneum, and rarely from the pericardium and tunica vaginalis of the testis.

Aetiology

Asbestos exposure

The risk of mesothelioma is related to the duration and intensity of asbestos exposure and the fibre type. Workers involved in the mining and processing of asbestos, and those using end-products of asbestos for insulation (e.g. plumbers and builders), are at obvious risk of developing mesothelioma, but family members of asbestos workers are also at increased risk from asbestos fibres brought home on work clothes.

The risk of developing mesothelioma depends on the physical characteristics of the inhaled asbestos fibres. Needle-like amphibole fibres (e.g. crocidolite (blue asbestos), amosite (brown asbestos), anthophyllite, tremolite, and actinolite) are eliminated slowly from the lungs (half-life >7 years) and carry the highest risk. Serpentine fibres (e.g. chrysotile (white asbestos)) are cleared more rapidly as they are curly, more soluble, prone to fragment, and are less oncogenic than amphiboles.

The oncogenic mechanism of asbestos is not fully understood, but involves DNA damage, alteration of cell-cycle check points, chromosomal rearrangement/loss, altered expression of cytokine mediators, and dysregulation of apoptosis pathways.

There are currently no means to identify which people exposed to asbestos are likely to develop mesothelioma. However, recent research efforts have identified screening tests for early mesothelioma, such as serum-soluble mesothelin levels. Mesothelin has sufficient sensitivity and specificity to be clinically useful.

Nonasbestos causes

Erionite, a naturally occurring mineral found mainly in Turkey, induces pleuropulmonary diseases similar to asbestos and including mesothelioma. Mesothelioma is not linked with prior thoracic irradiation (e.g. for Hodgkin's lymphoma), or with smoking. Simian virus 40 (SV40) can induce pleural, peritoneal, and pericardial mesotheliomas in experimental animals, but epidemiological studies do not support a link with mesothelioma development in humans, and recent studies show that the apparent presence of SV40 in clinical mesothelioma tissues was due to laboratory contamination. No definite cause can be identified in up to 20% of patients with mesothelioma.

Pathology

Mesothelioma grows as a diffuse spreading sheet along the pleura, with encasement of the underlying lung (Figs. 18.19.3.2 and 18.19.3.3).

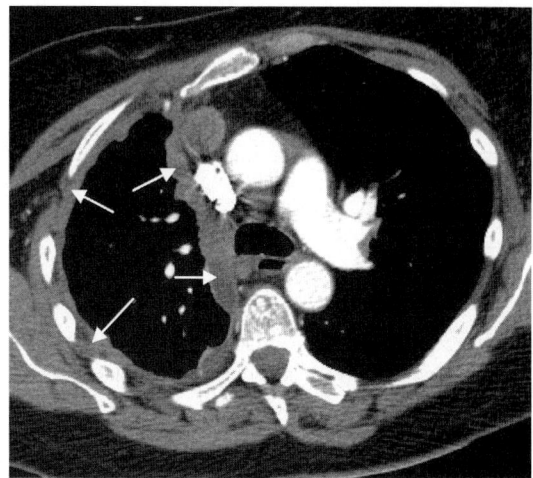

Fig. 18.19.3.2 A patient with advanced right pleural mesothelioma: CT scan showed a thick rind of tumour encasing the lung (arrows). with resultant shrinking of the ipsilateral hemithorax.

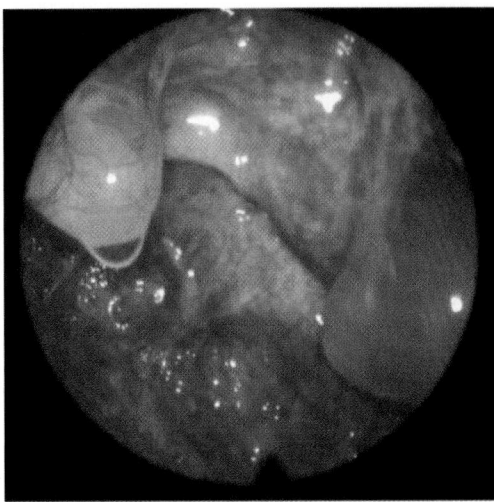

Fig. 18.19.3.3 Thoracoscopic view of pleural mesothelioma on the parietal pleural surface.

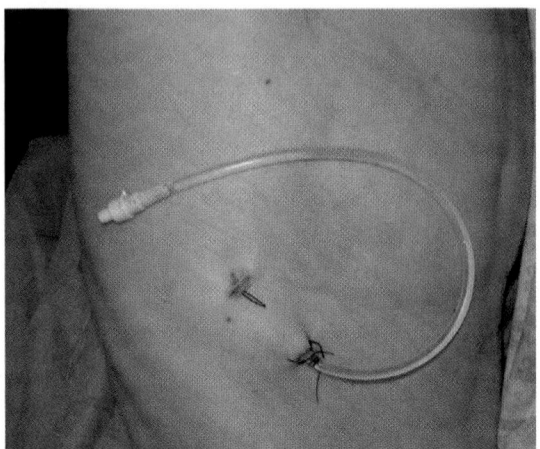

Fig. 18.19.3.4 An indwelling pleural catheter in a patient with recurrent pleural effusions.

This process may be preceded by an *in situ* phase. As mesothelioma progresses it can infiltrate surrounding structures including the ipsilateral lung, chest wall, mediastinum, and later the contralateral pleural cavity and peritoneum. The gross appearance is often indistinguishable from pleural metastatic carcinoma. Spread to regional lymph nodes is common, but clinically significant distant metastases are infrequent, although at autopsy one-half to two-thirds of patients have distant metastases that had been clinically asymptomatic.

The common histological subtypes of malignant mesothelioma are epithelioid (60% of cases), sarcomatoid (10%), and biphasic with components of both (30%). Median survival is worse in patients with the sarcomatoid variant (7 months) than in the epithelioid type (14 months). Desmoplastic mesothelioma is a rare (<1%) variant that histologically mimics benign fibrous tissue.

Clinical features and diagnosis

Most (95%) patients develop a pleural effusion at some time, hence the most common presentations are dyspnoea and/or chest pain (from tumour invasion). About 30% of patients have weight loss and lethargy at presentation. Less commonly, involvement of other (mainly intrathoracic) structures may result in dysphagia, Horner's syndrome, spinal cord compression, superior vena cava obstruction or pericardial effusion. Distant metastases, eg cerebral involvement, are late events.

The diagnosis of pleural mesothelioma usually arises from the investigation of undiagnosed pleural effusion (see Chapter 18.17).

Prognosis

Overall median survival for malignant pleural mesothelioma is about 9 months, but occasionally patients with mesothelioma pursue an indolent course and survivals of over 10 years have been reported. Improved survival is associated with good performance status and epithelioid histology.

There are several staging systems (e.g. Buchart system and International Mesothelioma Interest Group classification), and early-stage disease (e.g. limited to parietal pleura) carries better prognosis. Disease response in research settings are usually monitored by the modified RECIST criteria.

Treatment

Mesothelioma is incurable. It spreads along serosal surfaces infiltrating underlying structures, hence complete surgical resection is not feasible. Radiotherapy has been tried with curative intent, but the disease area to be covered is too large and the resulting irradiation toxicity (to the underlying heart, liver, etc) is intolerable. Intensity-modulated radiotherapy is under investigation. Mesothelioma is relatively resistant to common chemotherapeutic agents and drug penetration to the pleura and underlying tissues is variable.

Effective management should therefore aim to improve quality of life and prolong survival. The use of a multidisciplinary palliative care team experienced in mesothelioma is recommended, as the clinical course of mesothelioma differs from other solitary tumours. Patients often pursue legal claims for compensation, which can create significant additional stress in what is often an already desperate situation.

Pain control

Most patients eventually experience pain and dyspnoea, and early use of opioids is required. Radiotherapy is effective for localized pain (e.g. from bone erosion) and needle tract metastases, and can palliate invasion of the oesophagus, superior vena cava, and spinal cord. Invasive pain control techniques with indwelling epidural catheters and spinal cordotomy are sometimes needed.

Pleural fluid control

Recurrent effusions (and dyspnoea) are a key problem for most patients with mesothelioma. Pleurodesis is usually effective in preventing fluid reaccumulation and should be performed early (see below) because it is ineffective when tumour has encased the visceral pleura, preventing lung expansion ('trapped lung') and prohibiting apposition of the pleural surfaces. In this situation, and in patients with failed repeated talc pleurodesis, an indwelling tunnelled pleural catheter may be useful for domiciliary pleural fluid drainage (Fig. 18.19.3.4).

Radiotherapy

Radiotherapy has an established role in symptom palliation, with about 60 to 80% of patients experiencing improvement in specific tumour-related complications, although it does not prolong survival.

Mesothelioma invades about 40% of the sites of pleural procedures. Prophylactic radiotherapy (21 Gy in three fractions) is probably effective at preventing such tumour invasion, though the results of (small) clinical trials are somewhat variable in this regard. All efforts should be taken to minimize the number of pleural procedures in patients with possible mesothelioma to minimize the frequency of unpleasant chest wall tumour invasion. The current consensus view is that prophylactic radiotherapy should be given to larger bore chest puncture sites such as chest drain/thoracoscopy insertion sites.

Chemotherapy
Pemetrexed and raltitrexed, novel multitargeted antifolate agents used in combination with cisplatin, have shown activity against mesothelioma, prolonging survival by about 3 months and improve tumour symptoms, and are now standard therapies in most countries.

Multimodality treatment
Radical surgery (e.g. extrapleural pneumonectomy) to provide tumour cytoreduction has been attempted in combination with adjuvant radiotherapy and chemotherapy. This involves surgical resection of the entire lung, parietal pleura, pericardium, diaphragm, and mediastinal lymph nodes, but it has not shown any convincing benefits and carries significant mortality (5–10% from surgery alone) and morbidity (>25% life-threatening complications). Quality of life is significantly impaired for at least the first 6 months after surgery, which are otherwise the best months in the remaining lifespan of the patient. Survivals after multimodality therapy are skewed by selection bias and no evidence suggests it provides benefits over untreated patients matched for disease stage. A randomized clinical trial to define the role of this approach is under way, but currently surgery or multimodality therapy is not established as standard care.

Metastatic pleural malignancy

Most malignant tumours can spread to the pleura, and these patients often present with dyspnoea caused by pleural effusion. Most malignant effusions arise from metastatic carcinomas, especially lung,

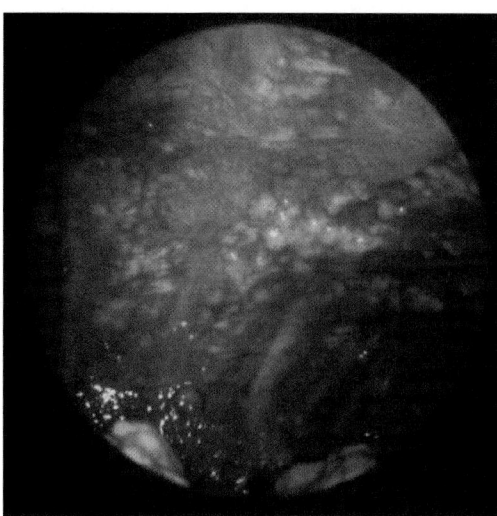

Fig. 18.19.3.5 Thoracoscopy showing scattered tumour from metastatic breast carcinoma on the parietal pleural surface.

breast (Fig. 18.19.3.5) and ovarian primaries, and lymphoma. Adenocarcinoma from unknown primary source also occurs.

Metastatic malignant disease may follow direct spread or haematogenous embolization of tumour to the peripheral lung parenchyma, followed by visceral pleural invasion. The parietal pleura is assumed to be secondarily affected by shedding of malignant cells from the visceral pleura, or from tumour migration via adhesions, although despite this accepted hypothesis tumour bulk on the parietal pleura is often more impressive than that on the visceral membrane during thoracoscopic examination. Pleural involvement from direct cancer invasion (e.g. from breast cancer) or haematogenous spread can occur.

Malignant effusions develop primarily as a result of increased vascular permeability and resulting plasma leakage. Reduced pleural fluid outflow, secondary to tumour blockage of parietal pleural stomata and/or the downstream lymphatic drainage pathways, also contributes.

Clinical features
Dyspnoea is the most common presenting symptom and is a particular feature of large effusions that invert the diaphragm due to mass loading. Small malignant effusions are usually asymptomatic, and underlying lung disease (e.g. lymphangitis, airway obstruction, comorbid chronic obstructive pulmonary disease, or pulmonary embolus) or the presence of a 'trapped lung' or extrapulmonary causes (e.g. pericardial effusion) should be suspected when such patients are breathless.

Pleuritic pain is common and implies malignant infiltration of the parietal pleura, as the visceral pleura is devoid of pain sensation.

Diagnosis
The diagnosis of malignant pleural metastases should be made by histological or cytological assessment of pleural fluid or pleural tissue samples (see Chapter 18.17). Clinical assessment, radiological appearances (e.g. on CT or PET) or tumour marker measurements cannot provide a definitive diagnosis. It is important to obtain a histocytological diagnosis of the type of malignancy (e.g. between mesothelioma and metastatic carcinoma): this alters treatment strategies and has prognostic implications.

Management
A tumour that has spread to the pleura is incurable in most cases. Surgery and radiotherapy are unable to eradicate pleural metastases. In patients whose primary tumour is highly responsive to chemotherapy (e.g. lymphoma or small cell carcinoma), treatment may control the pleural effusion. For subjects with less responsive tumours, the standard strategy is to create pleurodesis—the adherence of the parietal and visceral pleura—either surgically or by introducing a chemical agent. This can be achieved in about 70% of cases, although reported success rates vary markedly with the agents employed, clinical methods, and definitions of success. No clinical or biochemical markers reliably predict the outcome of pleurodesis in individual patients, but a low pleural fluid pH (<7.20) or glucose (<1 mmol/litre) often reflects a higher tumour load and is associated with a lower pleurodesis success rate and shorter survivals.

Many breathless patients with a malignant effusion do not gain significant benefit after pleural fluid drainage: pleurodesis should be considered only in those who do. The presence of a trapped lung is a relative contraindication to pleurodesis as poor apposition of the pleural surfaces will render pleurodesis ineffective.

Pleurodesis should be reserved for patients with good short-term prognosis (arbitrarily defined as expected survival >3 months), with prediction of this typically made by assessment of performance status, e.g. Karnofsky Performance Score (KPS). In one study of patients with malignant effusions a KPS of 70 or more was associated with a median survival of 395 days, compared to 34 days with KPS less than 30.

There are no controlled studies that define the best timing of pleurodesis, with most physicians recommending the procedure when the patient has had at least one episode of fluid recurrence. An alternative approach is to attempt pleurodesis of large effusions when they first present, as the recurrence rate is high (>70%) and early pleurodesis, before trapped lung ensues, may be more successful. This strategy avoids some episodes of unpleasant dyspnoea as fluid recurs.

Methods of pleurodesis

Chemical pleurodesis agents produce adherence of the pleural surfaces by provoking acute pleural injury, which results in pleural inflammation. If the inflammatory process is sufficiently intense, chronic inflammation and fibrosis ensues, resulting in pleural adhesions and eventual obliteration of the pleural cavity (successful pleurodesis). This process is often painful, as the parietal pleura is heavily infiltrated by sensory nerves. It is probable that the more intense the induced pleural inflammation, the higher the likelihood of success, but at the expense of producing more pain and distress to the patient.

Technical aspects of pleurodesis

Pleurodesis can be performed by various surgical means (e.g. abrasion of the pleura or pleurectomy), but most patients with malignant effusions are frail and not suitable for general anaesthesia, hence a thoracoscopic approach is preferred to thoracotomy. Alternatively, pleurodesis agents can be delivered intrapleurally via a chest tube when complete lung re-expansion is confirmed on radiographs following drainage of effusions.

The most commonly used agent worldwide is talc, followed by tetracycline/doxycycline, and bleomycin, though other agents (e.g. iodoprovidone, silver nitrate, and picibanil (OK432)) have also been employed. A meta-analysis of 11 studies showed that talc is superior in efficacy to tetracycline and bleomycin.

Talc can be delivered via a chest tube (as a slurry) or insufflated (as a poudrage) during thoracoscopy; whether the latter is more effective remains controversial. Two published randomized trials have compared the two and shown no significant differences in their primary endpoints, but post-hoc analyses of a recent trial showed that in a subgroup of patients with lung and breast cancers whose lung could fully re-expand, there was a higher success rate using talc poudrage. If a patient undergoes thoracoscopy for diagnostic purposes, talc poudrage can be performed at the same setting, but pleurodesis can be performed by either talc slurry or poudrage, depending on availability, in patients with an established diagnosis.

Pain is the most common side effect of pleurodesis, and narcotic analgesics and/or conscious sedation (e.g. midazolam) should be used where possible. Rotation of the patient does not improve the success rates of pleurodesis.

In animal studies, systemic corticosteroids and heparin can significantly reduce effective pleurodesis by inhibiting pleural inflammation and the coagulation cascade respectively. Whether these data can be extrapolated to humans is unknown, but the use of steroids and anticoagulants should be reduced or discontinued at the time of pleurodesis if possible.

Talc pleurodesis toxicity

Talc can induce fever and pain, which usually subsides within 72 h. Systemic absorption of talc particles and embolization to distant organs have also been reported. Recent studies have shown that preparations containing a large proportion of small talc particles (<10 μm) can cause marked systemic and pulmonary inflammation with resultant hypoxaemia, presumably from systemic absorption of small talc particles. Talc-related adult respiratory distress syndrome (ARDS) occurred in 6% of patients and caused the death of 2.3% in a study of 484 patients. Talc-related ARDS can occur with either talc poudrage or slurry, and with doses from 2 to 10 g, but no cases of the condition were observed in a longitudinal study of over 550 patients in which a graded talc preparation was used (with median particle size >20 μm)—though even in this study patients had a higher oxygen requirement after the pleurodesis and seven subjects developed pulmonary infiltrate after talc administration.

Recurrent pleural effusions

For patients where pleurodesis fails, another attempt with a different agent, implantation of a chronic indwelling catheter, pleuroperitoneal shunting, serial therapeutic thoracentesis, or a surgical pleurodesis are possible. Repeated thoracenteses combined with narcotics and oxygen are appropriate when a very short life expectancy (<6 weeks) is likely. For other patients, repeated pleurodesis or permanent pleural drainage (indwelling catheter or pleuroperitoneal shunt) are better, although a pleuroperitoneal shunt is contraindicated in the presence of ascites. Indwelling small-bore catheters are now available for ambulatory drainage, allowing patients to perform fluid drainage when symptoms arise (Fig. 18.19.3.4). The adverse event rate with prolonged use of these catheters is not yet fully defined, but infection, catheter blockage and catheter tract metastases can occur, as can spontaneous pleurodesis in up to 50% of patients.

Possible future developments

Current treatments for malignant pleural effusion are crude, but this is an area where clinical advances in the next few years are likely. The development of novel pleurodesis agents that stimulate controlled pleural inflammation (such as Tol like receptor agonists), or may induce fibrosis without pleural inflammation, e.g. tumour growth factor-β (TGFβ), may allow effective pleurodesis without the adverse events associated with talc use. Alternatively, direct inhibition of pleural fluid accumulation (via manipulation of vascular permeability mediators, such as anti-vascular endothelial growth factor antibodies) may become possible. These approaches are all currently in clinical trials. A randomized trial is under way to compare ambulatory drainage with indwelling catheters vs conventional pleurodesis as the first line therapy.

Further reading

Boutin C, et al. (1993). Thoracoscopy in pleural malignant mesothelioma: a prospective study of 188 consecutive patients. Part 2: Prognosis and staging. Cancer, 72, 394–404.

Boutin C, Rey F, Viallat JR (1995). Prevention of malignant seeding after invasive diagnostic procedures in patients with pleural mesothelioma. A randomized trial of radiotherapy. *Chest*, **108**, 754–8.

Dresler CM, *et al.* (2005). Phase III intergroup study of talc poudrage vs talc slurry sclerosis for malignant pleural effusion. *Chest*, **127**, 909–15.

Lee YCG, Light RW (2004). Management of malignant pleural effusions. *Respirology*, **9**, 148–56.

Lee YCG, *et al.* (2002). In: Hendrick DJ, *et al.* (eds) Malignant mesothelioma. In: *Occupational disorder of the lung. Recognition, management and prevention*, pp. 359–79. W B Saunders, London.

Lee YCG, *et al.* (2003). Pleurodesis practice for malignant pleural effusions in five English speaking countries: survey of pulmonologists. *Chest*, **124**, 2229–38.

Nowak AK (2005). CT, RECIST, and malignant pleural mesothelioma. *Lung Cancer*, **49** (Suppl 1), S37–40.

Peto J, *et al.* (1999). The European mesothelioma epidemic. *Br J Cancer*, **79**, 666–72.

Putnam JBJ, *et al.* (2000). Outpatient management of malignant pleural effusion by a chronic indwelling pleural catheter. *Ann Thorac Surg*, **69**, 369–75.

Robinson BWS, *et al.* (2003). Mesothelin-family proteins and diagnosis of mesothelioma. *Lancet*, **362**, 1612–16.

Robinson LA (2006). Solitary fibrous tumor of the pleura. *Cancer Control*, **13**, 264–9.

Rusch VW (1996). A proposed new international TNM staging system for malignant pleural mesothelioma from the International Mesothelioma Interest Group. *Lung Cancer*, **14**, 1–12.

Shinto RA, *et al.* (1988). Does therapeutic thoracentesis improve the exercise capacity of patients with pleural effusion? *Am Rev Respir Dis*, **135**, A244.

Spugnini EP, *et al.* (2006). Human malignant mesothelioma: Molecular mechanisms of pathogenesis and progression. *Int J Biol Cell Biol*, **38**, 2000–4.

Sugarbaker DJ, *et al.* (1999). Resection margins, extrapleural nodal status, and cell type determine postoperative long-term survival in trimodality therapy of malignant pleural mesothelioma: Results in 183 patients. *J Thorac Cardiovasc Surg*, **117**, 54–65.

Vogelzang NJ, *et al.* (2003). Phase III study of pemetrexed in combination with cisplatin versus cisplatin alone in patients with malignant pleural mesothelioma. *J Clin Oncol*, **21**, 2636–44.

West SD, Lee YCG (2006). Current management of malignant pleural mesothelioma. *Clin Chest Med*, **27**, 335–54.

18.19.4 **Mediastinal cysts and tumours**

Malcolm K. Benson and Robert J.O. Davies

Essentials

Mediastinal masses are most conveniently categorized by their anatomical site in the anterior, middle, or posterior mediastinum. Most present as a radiographic abnormality alone, or in association with symptoms arising from local compression of the numerous mediastinal structures. Nonspecific constitutional symptoms such as fever or weight loss are more likely with malignant tumours such as lymphomas or thymomas.

Anterior mediastinal masses are commonly caused by thymic tumours (including thymic lymphoma), germ-cell tumours, and thyroid masses. Thymomas are often benign, but they can be locally invasive, and can be associated with paraneoplastic phenomena, with myasthenia gravis in 30%.

Middle mediastinal masses—most commonly caused by lymph node enlargement (e.g. secondary to carcinoma, lymphoma, sarcoidosis, tuberculosis, histoplasmosis), bronchogenic carcinomas, and cysts arising from mediastinal structures such as the pericardium, bronchi, and oesophagus. Giant follicular lymph node hyperplasia (Castleman's disease) is a rare condition that can present with symptoms due to local pressure or systemic symptoms, with some progressing to frank malignancy.

Posterior mediastinal masses—most commonly these are neurogenic tumours; if benign they tend to be asymptomatic, whilst if malignant they cause pressure effects.

Introduction and anatomy

The mediastinum encompasses all the intrathoracic structures with the exclusion of the lungs and pleura. The superior boundary is the thoracic inlet represented by a plane at the level of the first rib. The inferior boundary is the diaphragm. The mediastinum has traditionally been subdivided into a number of compartments: a superior and inferior compartment, with the latter being subdivided into anterior, middle, and posterior divisions. In fact there are no true anatomical boundaries, and structures in the superior mediastinum are contiguous with those inferiorly, hence a more logical subdivision is simply into anterior, middle, and posterior compartments (Figs. 18.19.4.1 and 18.19.4.2). Such a division helps to compartmentalize what is a complex anatomy and give some guide to the most likely pathology occurring in any particular area.

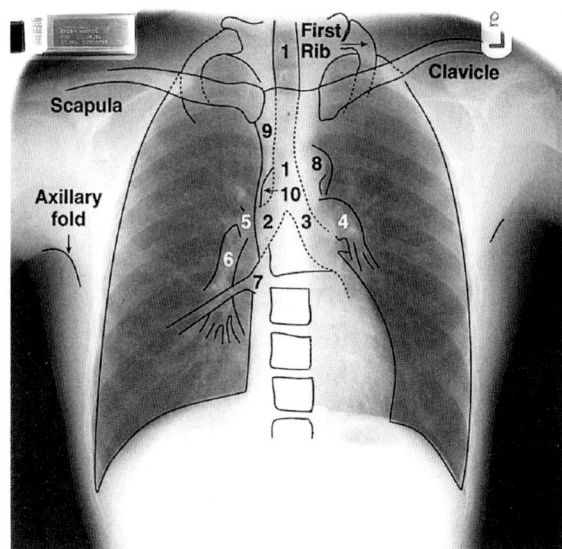

Fig. 18.19.4.1 Posteroanterior chest radiograph with diagrammatic overlay to illustrate normal mediastinal structures: (1) trachea, (2) right main bronchus, (3) left main bronchus, (4) left main pulmonary artery, (5) right upper lobe pulmonary vein, (6) right interlobular artery, (7) right lower and middle lobe vein, (8) aortic knuckle, (9) superior vena cava, (10) azygous vein.

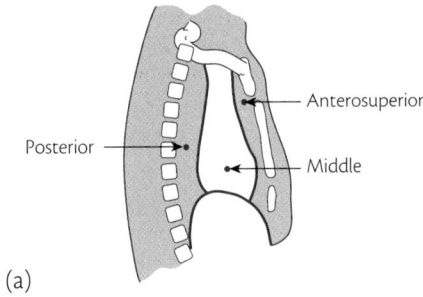

(a)

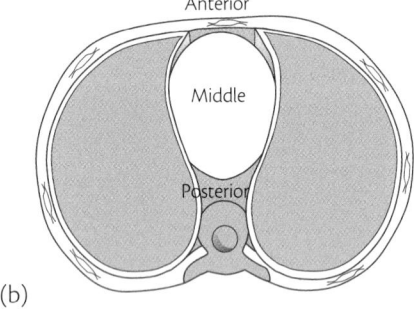

(b)

Fig. 18.19.4.2 A schematic representation of the mediastinal compartments: (a) lateral projection showing division into anterior (or anterosuperior), middle and posterior compartments, (b) cross-sectional depiction.

Detailed knowledge of normal mediastinal anatomy is a prerequisite to the interpretation of both normal and abnormal chest radiographs. It is not within the remit of this chapter to describe the anatomy in detail, but the major structures can be identified on CT scan.

The anterior mediastinum is bounded anteriorly by the sternum and posteriorly by the pericardium, aorta and brachiocephalic vessels. It contains the remnant of the thymus gland, branches of the internal mammary artery, veins, and associated lymph nodes.

The middle mediastinum contains the pericardium, ascending aorta and aortic arch, the vena cavae, the brachiocephalic vessels, and the pulmonary arteries and veins. It also encompasses the trachea and major bronchi with their associated lymph nodes, the phrenic nerves, and the vagus nerve.

The posterior mediastinum is bounded anteriorly by the pericardium, laterally by the mediastinal pleura, and posteriorly by the vertebral bodies. It also includes structures in the paravertebral gutter. It contains the descending thoracic aorta, oesophagus, azygos veins, thoracic duct, lymph nodes, and autonomic nerves.

Lymph nodes are present in all three compartments, and knowledge of their anatomical relationships, together with sites of drainage, is helpful in interpreting an abnormal chest radiograph with mediastinal enlargement. The most important group of visceral nodes lie in the middle mediastinum and are predominantly subcarinal and paratracheal. Bronchopulmonary or hilar nodes are numerous but not visible radiographically unless pathologically enlarged.

Clinical investigation

Radiological assessment

Most mediastinal cysts and tumours present as a radiographic abnormality alone, or in association with symptoms arising from the numerous mediastinal structures. Any such radiographic abnormality usually warrants investigation. CT provides accurate localization of mediastinal masses, can define their relationship to and displacement of normal structures, and may be able to define lines of demarcation, particularly if there is adjacent fatty tissue. It is not ideal for determining the composition of any particular mass, although it can demonstrate heterogeneity or the presence of calcification. Contrast enhancement can be used to identify vascularity. MRI has relatively little to offer in addition to information obtained from CT scan, with the one exception being the assessment of spinal tumours.

Biopsy techniques

Fine-needle aspiration biopsy is the usual method for investigating pulmonary masses but is of more limited use in assessing those in the mediastinum. The presence of a cyst can be confirmed by aspiration of clear fluid. Anterior mediastinal masses can easily be approached percutaneously, although cytological examination alone may be insufficient. Anterior mediastinotomy allows open biopsy of such lesions. Neural tumours arising in the posterior mediastinum usually require surgical resection and there is little to be gained by preceding this with fine-needle aspiration.

Mediastinoscopy is performed through an incision in the neck and allows inspection of structures surrounding the superior vena cava and trachea as far as the carina. It is particularly useful in obtaining lymph node biopsies prior to possible surgery for lung cancer. Bronchoscopy is of limited value when evaluating mediastinal masses, except when there is a suspicion of a bronchial neoplasm or possible lymphadenopathy due to sarcoidosis.

Clinical features

It is not surprising that the diversity of anatomical structures in the mediastinum is reflected by an equally diverse range of neoplastic, developmental and inflammatory masses (Box 18.19.4.1). Although clinical symptoms and signs may give diagnostic clues, many mediastinal masses—particularly those that are benign—are asymptomatic and usually detected on routine chest radiography.

Mediastinal masses in children are more likely to be malignant than those in adults. There have been a large number of studies documenting the relative frequency of different causes of primary mediastinal tumours and cysts, with neurogenic tumours and thymic tumours being the commonest (c.20% each), followed by lymphoma, reduplication cysts, germ-cell tumours, and thyroid masses.

Nonspecific constitutional symptoms such as fever or weight loss are more likely to occur with malignant tumours such as lymphomas or thymomas. The commonest symptoms are cough and chest pain, arising as a consequence of distortion of the normal mediastinal anatomy. Compression of vital structures can also result in specific symptoms, thus tracheal or bronchial compression leads to breathlessness with stridor or wheeze; oesophageal narrowing results in dysphagia; superior vena caval compression produces the characteristic features of facial and periorbital oedema, chemosis, and distended veins; involvement of the recurrent laryngeal nerve results in hoarseness and a bovine cough (usually resulting from a malignant tumour, but also occurring with benign lesion such as aneurysms of the aortic arch); involvement of the sympathetic chain as it emerges in the upper mediastinum (also likely to be due to malignant infiltration) results in characteristic features of

Anterior compartment

♦ Thyroid
  · Goitre
  · Carcinoma
♦ Thymus
  · Thymoma
  · Hyperplasia
  · Cyst
  · Lymphoma
♦ Germ-cell tumours
  · Dermoid cyst
  · Seminoma
  · Teratoma
♦ Parathyroid adenoma

Middle compartment

♦ Pericardium
  · cysts
♦ Vascular
  · Aneurysm
  · Anomalous vessels
♦ Bronchogenic cysts
♦ Lymph nodes[a]
  · Sarcoidosis
  · Infections (tuberculosis)
  · Lymphoma
  · Metastatic cancer
  · Castleman's disease

Posterior compartment

♦ Oesophagus
  · Gastroenteric cyst
  · Leimyoma
♦ Vascular
  · Aneurysm
♦ Neural tumours
  · Neurilemmoma
  · Neurofibroma
  · Malignant shwannoma
  · Ganglioneuroma
  · Neuroblastoma
  · Phaechromocytoma

[a]May be present in more than one compartment.

Horner's syndrome with enophthalmos, miosis, ptosis, and unilateral facial anhidrosis; compression of intercostal nerves may produce neuralgia; and intraspinal extension of tumours lead to long tract signs.

Anterior mediastinal masses

Thymus

The normal thymus is located in the superior portion of the anterior mediastinum. Its main function is the production of T lymphocytes. Radiographically, the normal thymus can only be seen in childhood and regression occurs during adolescence. Enlargement of the thymus is the commonest single cause of an anterior mediastinal mass, which can be due to the development of a thymoma, thymic hyperplasia or a thymic cyst. The thymus can also be the site of involvement by lymphoma, particularly Hodgkin's disease.

Thymomas

These are due to neoplastic proliferation of the thymus gland and can present at any age, peak incidence being in middle age. They are often benign, but can behave in a malignant fashion with invasion of adjacent structures and the occurrence of distant metastases. Localized symptoms of chest pain and cough are more common with malignant disease. Systemic symptoms occurring in association with thymic tumours are of particular interest: myasthenia gravis is the commonest, affecting 30% of patients; other rare associations include red-cell aplasia, hypogammaglobulinaemia, systemic lupus erythematosus, and polymyositis.

Most thymomas are slow-growing lobulated masses which are well encapsulated. In such cases surgical resection can be expected to result in a cure. Local invasion is less common but often precludes complete resection and recurrence is the rule. In these patients therapy is palliative and consists of a combination of surgical debulking, radiotherapy, and chemotherapy.

Thymic cysts

These are uncommon. They can be unilocular or multilocular and usually contain straw-coloured fluid. Most patients are asymptomatic, but since cystic change can occur in some thymomas and in Hodgkin's disease, thorough cytological examination of the cyst's contents and wall must be carried out to exclude malignant disease.

Thymic lymphoma

This is fairly common, particularly in patients with Hodgkin's disease, when the histological picture is usually of the nodular sclerosing variety. The presence of other mediastinal or hilar nodes should alert the clinician to the possibility of a lymphoma.

Germ-cell tumours

This group of neoplasms includes tumours that are identical to certain testicular and ovarian neoplasms and are thought to be derived from primitive germ cells that have migrated to the mediastinum during oncogenesis.

Benign teratomas (dermoid cysts)

These consist of a disorganized mixture of ectodermal, mesodermal, and endodermal tissues which can include skin, hair, cartilage, bone, epithelium, and neural tissue. They often contain cystic areas, with the CT appearances giving a strong clue to the diagnosis.

Unless there is a major contraindication to surgery, they should be excised to prevent further expansion and to exclude malignant change.

Malignant germ-cell tumours

These are classically divided into seminomas and teratomas, although biopsy often reveals a spectrum of malignant tissue. Nonseminomatous germ-cell tumours (malignant teratoma) can range from well differentiated to trophoblastic, and they are often associated with elevated serum levels of β-human chorionic gonadotropin (hCG) and α-fetoprotein (AFP), which can be used both diagnostically and to monitor response to treatment. Seminomas tend to be nonsecretory. Both types of tumour are highly malignant and invade adjacent mediastinal structures. They are not curable by surgery, but both are responsive to chemotherapy using cisplatin-based regimes. Response rates are high (up to 70%), but cure rates are lower than they are with testicular germ cell tumour.

Thyroid masses

Retrosternal extension of an enlarged thyroid is one the commoner causes of a mass in the superior mediastinum. Most are multinodular benign goitres that arise in the neck and extend into the mediastinum through the thoracic inlet. They may contain cystic areas, sometimes with haemorrhage and areas of calcification. Radiographically, they have a sharply defined and often lobulated outline. Whilst they rarely cause symptoms, compression of the trachea at the thoracic inlet can result in respiratory distress and is an indication for surgical resection.

Thyroid cancer may also involve the mediastinum, either by direct extension or by metastases to intrathoracic nodes.

Middle mediastinal masses

Lymphadenopathy

Enlarged lymph nodes are not confined the middle mediastinum, although this is the commonest site of intrathoracic lymphadenopathy. Reactive changes occur in association with many pulmonary infections, but in the most cases the nodes are not grossly enlarged and may be undetected on plain chest radiograph. Gross lymphadenopathy is a feature of carcinoma and lymphoma, with sarcoidosis, tuberculosis, and histoplasmosis being other causes.

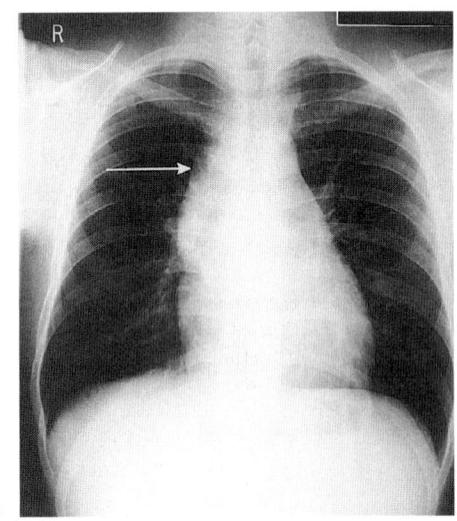

(a)

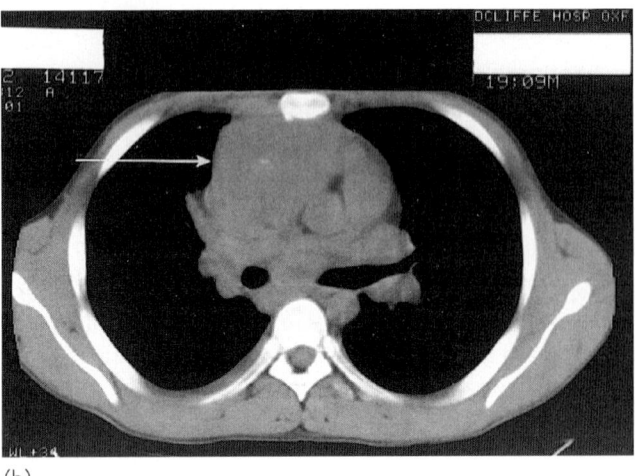

(b)

Fig. 18.19.4.3 Chest radiograph and CT scan showing a large anterior mediastinal mass (arrows) which on histology showed features of Castleman's disease.

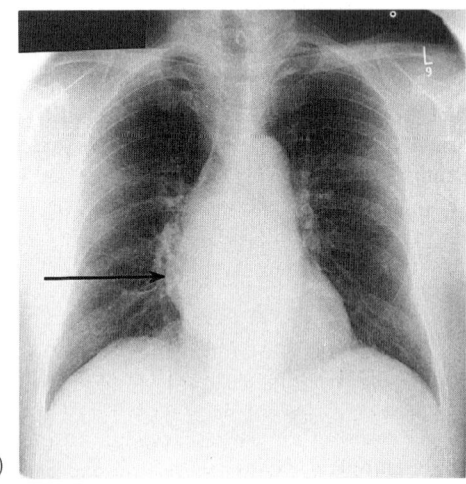

(a)

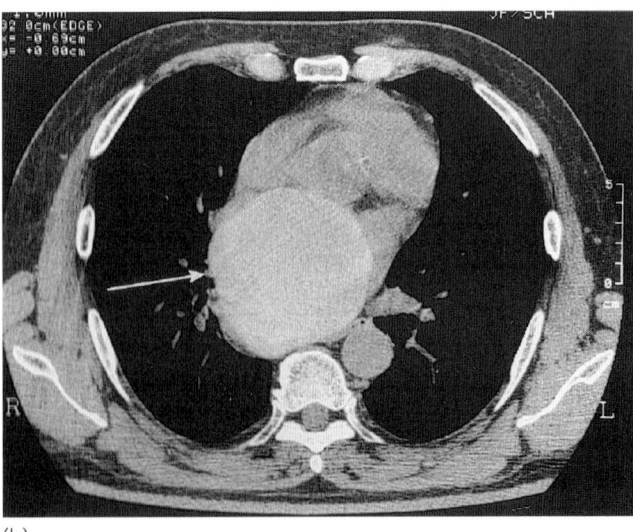

(b)

Fig. 18.19.4.4 Chest radiograph and CT scan showing a large mass in the mediastinum (arrows) due to a bronchogenic cyst that had been present for 20 years. It was removed when compression of the oesophagus resulted in dysphagia.

Giant follicular lymph node hyperplasia (Castleman's disease)

This is a rare condition of unknown aetiology. It is not clear whether it represents a focus of lymphoid hyperplasia or has an infectious origin. The lesion consists of a vascular tumour with satellite lymphadenopathy. Two histological subgroups are described: (1) a more common hyaline vascular picture with lymphoid follicles and penetrating capillaries, and (2) a plasma cell type characterized by sheets of plasma cells between germinal centres. Both types can result in symptoms from local pressure, but the plasma cell type also causes systemic symptoms with fever, anaemia and weight loss. There are no diagnostic radiographic features: the picture is simply one of a solitary mass (Fig. 18.19.4.3), with the diagnosis usually being made after surgical resection or biopsy. The condition is usually benign, but a few patients with multicentric disease have progressive hyperplasia, recurrent infections and subsequently develop a frank malignant tumour.

Mediastinal cysts

Cysts within the mediastinum are a relatively common cause of a mediastinal mass. They can arise in association with the pericardium, bronchi, gut or thoracic duct. Most patients are asymptomatic.

Pericardial cysts

These develop embryologically in relationship to the pericardium, although direct communication with the pericardial sac is rare. Radiographically they appear as smooth, clear, demarcated densities which can be mistaken for a pericardial fat pad or a hernia through the foramen of Morgagni. Aspiration reveals clear fluid. Surgical excision is not recommended.

Bronchogenic cysts

These arise in association with the major airways, are lined by respiratory epithelium, and they may contain inspissated mucus (Fig. 18.19.4.4). Local pressure on the trachea or bronchi can result in cough or wheezing. Occasionally the cysts communicate with the trachea and, when this is the case, there is an increased tendency to recurrent infections. Surgical excision is recommended, particularly if there are associated symptoms.

Reduplication cysts may also be associated with the oesophagus and can be lined by gastric or oesophageal mucosa.

Posterior mediastinal masses

Oesophageal lesions and aneurysms of the descending thoracic aorta can both result in abnormal shadows in the posterior mediastinum. Tumours, particularly those found in the paravertebral gutters, are likely to be neural in origin. Benign tumours tend to be asymptomatic, whilst malignant tumours cause pressure effects. Occasionally, spinal cord compression results from direct extension into the intravertebral foramen. Tumours arising from peripheral nerve cell sheath include neurilemmoma (schwannoma) and neurofibroma, also their malignant counterparts. Tumours of the autonomic chain include ganglioneuroma and neuroblastoma.

A neurilemmoma is the commonest neural tumour arising in the mediastinum. These are more common in middle age and can extend into the intravertebral foramen, producing a dumbbell appearance. Radiographically they can erode adjacent bone, hence CT scanning or MRI should be undertaken prior to surgical excision.

Neurofibromata are also common. They may be solitary, with clinical and radiological features very similar to those of a neurilemmoma, but many patients will have more generalized neurofibromatosis. Surgical resection is recommended, partly because of the small risk of developing malignant neurosarcoma, which has a poor prognosis.

Ganglioneuroma arise from the autonomic plexus and are usually perispinal in position. Associated endocrine symptoms include hypertension, flushing, sweating and diarrhoea. These tumours are often very large before they become clinically apparent. Prognosis is good after surgical resection.

Ganglioneuroblastoma and neuroblastoma represent the malignant end of the spectrum and are predominantly tumours of infants and children. Neuroblastoma in particular is highly invasive, with metastatic spread often established by the time of presentation.

Further reading

Adkins RB, Maples MD, Ainsworth J (1994). Primary malignant mediastinal tumours. *Ann Thorac Surg*, **38**, 648–59.

Bower RJ, Kiesewetter WB (1977). Mediastinal masses in infants and children. *Arch Surg*, **112**, 1003–9.

Davies RD Jnr, Oldham HM Jnr, Sabiston DC Jnr (1987). Primary cysts and neoplasms of the mediastinum: recent changes in clinical presentation, methods of diagnosis, management and results. *Ann Thorac Surg*, **44**, 229–35.

Hejna M, Haberl I, Raderer M (1999). Non surgical management of malignant thymoma. *Cancer*, **85**, 1871–84.

Morrissey B, *et al.* (1993). Percutaneous needle biopsy of the mediastinum: review of 94 procedures. *Thorax*, **48**, 632–7.

Shields TW, Reynolds M (1988). Neurogenic tumours of the thorax. *Surg Clin North Am*, **68**, 645–68.

Thomas CR Jnr, Wright CD, Loehrer PJ Snr (1999). Thymoma: state of the art. *J Clin Oncol*, **17**, 2280–9.

SECTION 19

Rheumatological disorders

Structure and function: joints and connective tissue

Tim E. Cawston

Essentials

The joint is a discrete unit that consists of cartilage, bone, tendon, and ligaments. Tendon consists of a matrix mainly made of collagen; bone consists of a mineralized collagen matrix; and cartilage is made up of collagens, proteoglycans, and specialized glycoproteins. Many studies have focused on single tissues of the joint, rather than regarding the joint as an organ made up of cartilage, bone, tendon, and muscle: future studies would benefit from an integrated approach.

All of the tissues in a joint are actively synthesized and degraded by the resident connective-tissue cells, such that there is a balance between matrix synthesis and degradation in adult tissues. Different classes of proteinase play a part in connective tissue turnover: active proteinases can cleave matrix protein during resorption, but the proteinase that predominates varies between different tissues and diseases. The matrix metalloproteinases (MMPs) are potent enzymes that degrade connective tissue and are inhibited by tissue inhibitors of metalloproteinases (TIMPs), the balance between active MMPs and TIMPs determining the extent of degradation in many tissues. Cysteine proteinases are responsible for the breakdown of collagen in bone. Various cytokines and growth factors, alone or in combination, can promote or inhibit matrix synthesis and stimulate proteinase production and matrix destruction. Growth factor combinations can be used in conjunction with artificial matrices to promote the repair of cartilage defects in large joints in some circumstances.

Introduction

Skeletal structures provide stable support for all multicellular organisms and are vital where mobility is also required. The normal human body contains 187 joints, with the crucial components including tensile connectors, flexible interfaces, and unique lubricating tissues. The function of the articular joint is to transmit force from one bone to another, giving movement and mobility to the rigid bony skeleton. Bones are linked by ligaments, muscles, and tendons, and the articular cartilage provides a deformable elastic tissue that helps distribute load evenly to the underlying bone, while allowing easy movement between two smooth and almost frictionless opposing surfaces.

All structures of the joint respond to mechanical forces. Without motion *in utero* joints do not develop normally, and disuse after birth leads to thinning and atrophy of the articular cartilage, which loses its matrix and mechanical properties. High usage leads to hypertrophy and an increase in mechanical strength. Many of the changes in the joint after prolonged periods of chronic disease may reflect the adapted responses to altered patterns of load distribution in the joint, as well as the more direct effects of the disease processes themselves. Thus the structures of the joint are not static and are in a constant dynamic state of adaptation and response, even in adults.

The joint as an organ

Many previous studies have focused on single tissues of the joint, rather than regarding the joint as an organ made up of cartilage, bone, tendon, and muscle. For example, in osteoarthritis many studies have considered this as a disease predominantly of cartilage, with any changes in other tissues being assumed to be secondary. However, recent data using MRI show early changes in the surrounding tendons and ligaments that appear to precede cartilage lesions. Laxity within such surrounding tendons could alter the distribution of mechanical load and so lead to altered stress being placed on areas of cartilage within the joint that are less adapted to withstand load. Other studies have considered that the cartilage changes are secondary to a thickening of the subchondral bone, such that this underlying bone is less able to absorb and distribute mechanical load, putting high stress on the cartilage above, which then subsequently breaks down. The research focus on single tissues has often been to the detriment of progress: future studies would benefit from an integrated approach.

Cartilage

From the age of Hippocrates to the present age it is universally allowed that ulcerated cartilage is a troublesome thing and that when destroyed it is not recovered.

(Hunter, 1743)

Articular cartilage is a unique tissue containing relatively few cells, called chondrocytes, embedded in an extensive extracellular matrix; it has no basement membrane, and no innervation or blood supply. It relies on the diffusion of nutrients from synovial blood vessels into the tissue to maintain the healthy function of chondrocytes.

Cartilage is able to withstand compressive loads, a physical property directly related to the structure and precise organization of the matrix macromolecules. Both fibrillar and nonfibrillar components have an important impact on the properties of the tissue. Cartilage contains predominantly type II collagen, and these triple helical, rod-shaped molecules aggregate in staggered arrays to form cross-linked fibres, giving connective tissues strength and rigidity. Type IX and type XI collagen molecules are found respectively in the centre and at the surface of these type II fibrils (Table 19.1.1). Fine collagen fibres run parallel at the surface of the joint, but in deeper layers they are less well organized and become perpendicular to the surface in the deeper zones. These collagen fibres give the tissue shape and form and contribute to its tensile properties. Entrapped within the collagen fibrils are the proteoglycans, predominantly aggrecan, which consist of a core protein containing three globular domains interspersed with heavily glycosylated and sulfated linear polypeptide. In the presence of hyaluronan these form highly charged aggregates that attract water into the tissue and so allow cartilage to resist compression.

In normal adult cartilage, cartilage chondrocytes synthesize the matrix components and maintain a steady state in which the extent of matrix synthesis equals that of degradation. Any change in this steady state affects the functional integrity of the cartilage. During growth and development the synthesis of matrix components in connective tissues exceeds degradation, and in various diseases a reduction in matrix synthesis and an increase in the rate of degradation occurs, leading to a net loss of tissue matrix.

Proteoglycans within the cartilage matrix are readily cleaved but can be rapidly resynthesized. The mechanisms of turnover include the synthesis, secretion, and assembly of proteoglycan aggregates by chondrocytes, followed by degradation within the extracellular space; both processes are carefully coordinated by the chondrocytes. There is a constant level of aggrecan breakdown and new synthesis. The breakdown of aggrecan involves proteolytic cleavage at a precise and susceptible site between the first and second globular

Table 19.1.1 Collagens found in joint tissues

Class I, fibril-forming	Type I	Major constituent of bone, tendon, and ligament
	Type II	Major constituent of cartilage
	Type III	Minor component of bone, tendon; major constituent of blood vessel wall
Class 2, 300 nm, triple helix	Type XI	At core of type II fibrils
Class 3, short helix molecules	Type VI	Concentrated around chondrocytes
	Type IX	In cartilage on surface of type II fibrils and around chondrocytes
	Type X	In deep calcified zone cartilage (high in growth plate)

domain to release a large fragment containing the carbohydrate side chains from the aggregate, which then diffuses from the matrix. At least two aggrecanases have been identified, belonging to the 'a disintegrin and metalloproteinase with thromombospondin motifs' (ADAMTS) family of proteinases (see below).

The primary cause of cartilage and bone breakdown in normal turnover and in the arthritides involves elevated levels of active proteinases, secreted from a variety of cells, which degrade collagen and aggrecan. These tissue-degrading enzymes are vital for normal physiological processes such as embryonic development, growth, and tissue remodelling, in which the extracellular matrix must be degraded and tissue remodelled (see 'Proteolytic pathways of connective tissue breakdown', below). In disease the sources of these proteinases vary: in osteoarthritis the proteinases produced by chondrocytes play a major role; by contrast, in a highly inflamed rheumatoid joint the proteinases produced by chondrocytes, synovial cells, and inflammatory cells all contribute to the loss of tissue matrix.

Joint tissues are capable of repair: but although aggrecan can be readily resynthesized, the replacement of collagen that has been destroyed is more difficult. Various growth factors and cytokines present in the joint are able to upregulate matrix synthesis, and these factors have been studied to determine if cartilage and bone defects can be repaired *in vivo*.

Skeletal growth and the growth plate

The series of events required for bone elongation and patterning is highly regulated and coordinated. Cartilage formation begins during embryonic development, as early as 6 weeks, with the condensation and differentiation of mesenchymal cells into chondrocytes to form the key elements of the skeleton. After its formation, the central portion of the cartilage rudiment calcifies and blood vessels form, leading to the formation of a bony diaphysis capped at each end by a cartilaginous epiphysis. Later a secondary centre of ossification develops in each epiphysis, dividing the region of major cartilage growth from the cartilage that forms the articular surface of the joint. The transverse plate of cartilage between the diaphysis and epiphysis remains as the site of growth during development, but this calcifies and becomes inactive at skeletal maturity, usually between 14 and 18 years.

Chondrocytes originating at the growth plate are initially proliferative and organized in short columnar rows, between which they secrete type II collagen. As the chondrocytes progress away from the growth plate they stop proliferating and become prehypertropic. Finally, hypertropic cells—expressing predominantly type X collagen—mineralize the cartilage matrix (Fig. 19.1.1). The hypertrophic chondrocytes then undergo apoptosis and blood vessels invade the newly formed cartilaginous matrix, this vascularization being the step required for replacement of the soft tissue with trabecular bone. Osteoclast precursors originating from haemopoietic stem cells migrate, together with endothelial cells, into the mineralized cartilage, where they fuse to form large multinucleated osteoclast cells. These dissolve bone mineral and degrade the matrix. Osteoblasts are then recruited to the sites of resorption to lay down trabecular bone. In this aspect, endochondral ossification can be said to be unique, in that it involves the remodelling and replacement of a template tissue (cartilage) with a distinct permanent tissue (bone). The growth plate is thus a dynamic structure, with proliferating chondrocytes at its leading edge and depositing bone at its trailing edge, to which effect the genes that control progression of cellular phenotype are highly regulated across the growth plate (Fig. 19.1.1).

The regulation of longitudinal growth at the growth plate is controlled through the interaction of circulating systemic hormones and locally produced peptide growth factors, which can trigger changes in gene expression by growth-plate chondrocytes. Several cytokine families have been identified as key players in the regulation of limb formation, including fibroblast growth factors, bone morphogenic proteins, parathyroid hormone and Indian Hedgehog, with their action involving both Sox and Runx transcription factor family members (Fig. 19.1.1). In addition to being responsible for long bone growth, endochondral ossification is a process that also occurs in fracture healing and in osteophyte formation.

Given the complexity of limb growth and patterning it is not surprising that disturbances to the order of events or lack of specific genes within the process of limb bud development or endochondral ossification can cause severe skeletal abnormalities. Both the composition of the extracellular matrix and the distribution, division and response to external factors such as growth factors and cytokines of chondrocytes change with age (Box 19.1.1): these give clues as to why this tissue is susceptible to damage with increasing age.

Bone

Bone is a metabolically active tissue that is constantly formed and removed throughout life. The processes are carefully coordinated by bone cells, which respond to a variety of external factors, includ-

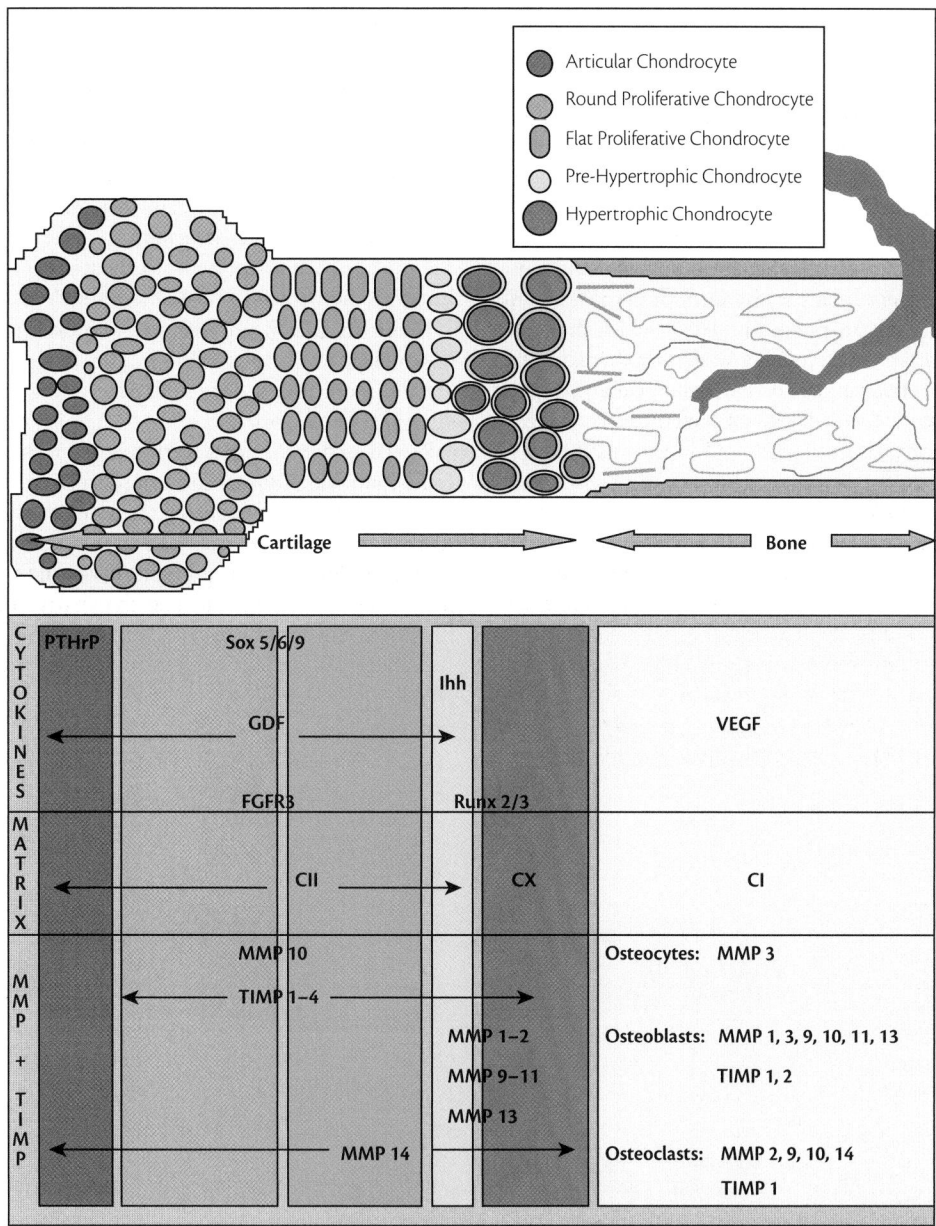

Fig. 19.1.1 Schematic representation of gene expression in a mouse long bone at a late stage of fetal development. See text for explanation. C, collagen; FGFR, fibroblast growth factor receptor; GDF, growth and differentiation factor; IHH, Indian hedgehog; PTHLH, parathyroid hormone-like hormone; Runx, runt transcription factor family; Sox, SRY-related transcription factor family; MMP, matrix metalloproteinase; TIMP, tissue inhibitor of metalloproteinases; VEGF, vascular endothelial growth factor.

ing genetic, mechanical, hormonal, and nutritional, and a large number of growth factors and cytokines. The cells contained in bone belong to three types: osteoblasts, osteocytes, and osteoclasts. These are all contained within a highly mineralized matrix of type I collagen and other specialized proteins, such as osteocalcin, osteonectin and proteoglycan. The mineral is present mainly as a mixture of calcium and phosphate in the form of hydroxyapatite. There are two anatomical types of bone: trabecular and cortical. In trabecular bone there are more metabolically active surfaces at which the basic multicellular units act on the surface of trabecular bone, whereas these multicellular units operate through resorbing channels in cortical bone.

The cells of bone are central to its active metabolism. Osteoclasts are haemopoietic in origin, formed following the activation of macrophage-like mononuclear cells, and are responsible for the resorption of bone. Many bone hormones and cytokines regulate osteoclasts, with two very important factors recognized: osteoclast differentiation factor (ODF, or RANKL) and macrophage colony stimulating factor (M-CSF) (Fig. 19.1.2). ODF is produced by osteoblasts and binds to a receptor on the osteoclast called RANK, causing a rapid differentiation of osteoclast precursor cells, increased activity, and reduced apoptosis. Osteoblasts also produce a decoy ligand, osteoprotegerin (OPG), which binds to ODF (RANKL) and blocks its activity. Osteoblast formation and activity are controlled by the amount of OPG and ODF, and many of the activities of the osteoclast depend on the osteoblast.

Osteocytes are formed from osteoblasts that become isolated in bone and surrounded by matrix: they communicate with each other through extended cellular processes that link cells, allowing them to respond to stimuli such as changes in mechanical forces.

In childhood more bone is formed than is resorbed, whereas in the young adult these two processes are balanced, and the bone mass is constant. In later life more resorption than formation leads to diseases such as osteoporosis. Bone is also destroyed in rheumatoid arthritis, with both the metalloproteinases and cysteine proteinases involved. Osteoblasts respond to parathyroid hormone and other agents that induce bone resorption, such as interleukin 1(IL-1) and tumour necrosis factor-α (TNFα), by increasing the secretion of metalloproteinases to remove the osteoid layer on the bone surface. Osteoclast precursors then adhere to the exposed bone surface, differentiate, and form a low pH microenvironment beneath their lower surface. This removes mineral, and lysosomal proteinases then resorb the exposed matrix (Fig. 19.1.2) (see 'Proteolytic pathways of connective-tissue breakdown', below).

The synovium

Synovial tissue is a connective tissue bound by the fibrous joint capsule on one side and the joint space on the other. The synovium has a major role in facilitating metabolic exchange, and its capillary network is particularly rich at the intimal surface of the synovium. The synovium is considerably more vascular than the capsule, ligaments, tendons, and other structures supporting the joint. Most of

Fig. 19.1.2 Control of bone formation and removal. Various hormones, vitamins, cytokines, and growth factors are required to allow the maturation of the osteoclast or the osteoblast. Osteoblasts produce matrix metalloproteinases (MMPs) that remove the surface of bone and allow osteoclasts to adhere. The osteoclasts form a ruffled border on their lower surface and secrete hydrogen ions and cathepsin K to remove mineral and collagen. Some MMPs are also involved as the pH rises following the movement of the osteoclast away from the resorption pit. Osteoblasts then populate the resorption pits and new bone is laid down.

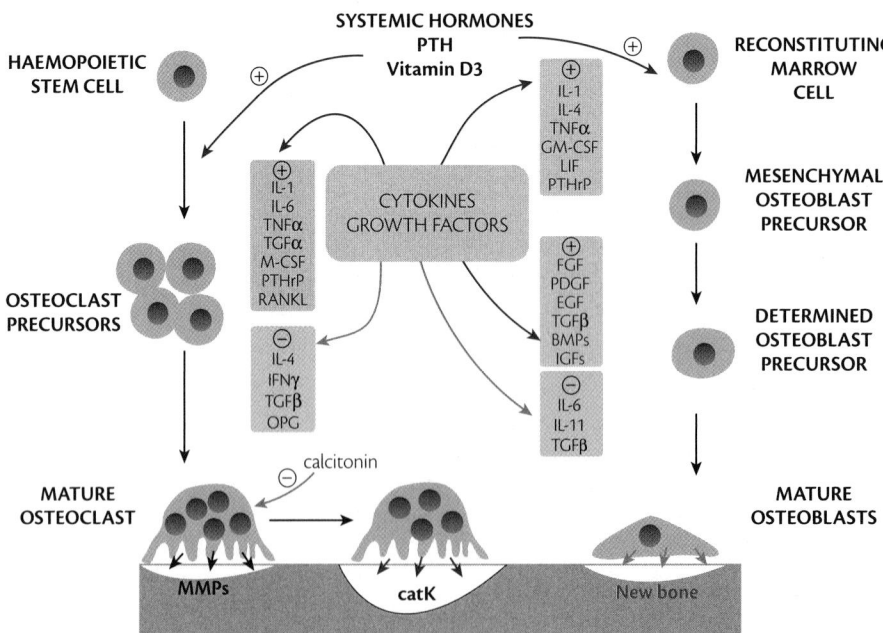

this tissue is relatively sparsely populated by cells, apart from a discontinuous layer of cells at the surface, commonly called the synovial membrane.

The intimal cells form a thin, discontinuous layer, and the whole synovium is bathed in synovial fluid, as there is no basement membrane beneath these cells. In some areas the cells may be three or four cells deep, and these are recognized as being of two types. The first, type A, is characterized by a prominent Golgi apparatus, numerous vesicles and vacuoles, many filopodia, and numerous mitochondria that are thought to be derived from tissue macrophages. The second, type B, contain a prominent endoplasmic reticulum and a few large vacuoles, and resemble a classical fibroblast derived from mesenchyme. These cells produce the components of synovial fluid, which is present in small quantities: the human knee joint contains only 1 to 4 ml of fluid, which is an ultrafiltrate of plasma, with specialized components secreted by the synoviocytes. The most important of these components is hyaluronan, a linear repeating disaccharide with a high molecular weight that is most responsible for the unique viscoelastic properties of the fluid. Other proteins are also present, such as lubrican, which is a glycoprotein that acts as a highly efficient lubricant.

The production of synovial fluid is very important for chondrocyte nutrition. As the cartilage surface is deformed under load, waste is expelled from the tissue, and when the load is removed and the tissue returns to its original shape, nutrients are drawn into the tissue.

In chronic inflammation, a wide variety of morphological changes occur in the joint. The synovial cell layer becomes thickened (six to eight cells deep) as the synoviocytes proliferate with an increase in cell size; there is thus both hyperplasia and hypertrophy. Underneath the synovial cell layer there is a large increase in the number of lymphocytes and macrophages. The lymphocytes accumulate around the postcapillary venules and sometimes organize into structures that resemble lymphoid follicles, with plasma cells at the margins. Large numbers of macrophages are scattered widely through the underlying tissue: these are thought to migrate to the synovial cell layer to replace the type A cells. Inflammation in the synovium has not been thought to be important in osteoarthritis, but there is growing recognition that in some osteoarthritic joints there is evidence of an inflammatory component.

Tendon and ligaments

Tensile connective tissues play important roles within the joint, with ligaments preventing inappropriate movement and tendons facilitating active joint motion. Every ligament links bone to bone; tendons also insert into muscle. Both ligaments and tendons are strong, dense bundles of parallel type I collagen fibres, and they insert into bone at anatomical sites known as entheses. At these and other wrap-around sites, the collagenous fibres include a protective fibrocartilaginous matrix that includes proteoglycan to protect the tissue when it is subjected to compressive forces.

Many of the problems associated with tendons and ligaments occur at the entheses. These highly specialized structures contain both fibrocartilage and hyaline cartilage elements and provide routes for the vascularization of the tissues. Enthesopathy is the central lesion of the seronegative spondyloarthropathies (see Chapter 19.6). It has been proposed that tissues under tension may be protected, such that it is harder to mount an inflammatory reaction within these sites to prevent destruction of important

tensile structures. Tendons often run through sheaths to eliminate any point of friction.

Proteolytic pathways of connective tissue breakdown

The extracellular matrix proteins found in connective tissues are broken down by different proteolytic pathways. Five main classes of proteinases are classified according to the chemical group that participates in the hydrolysis of peptide bonds (Fig. 19.1.3). Cysteine and aspartic proteinases are predominantly active at acidic pH and act intracellularly; threonine proteinases (the proteasome being the best characterized) also act intracellularly at near-neutral pH; the serine and metalloproteinases, active at neutral pH, mostly act extracellularly. Other enzymes, such as elastase, are released when neutrophils are stimulated. Some enzymes, such as furin, may not participate in the proteolysis of matrix proteins, but they activate proenzymes that then degrade the matrix. Membrane-bound proteinases are associated with cytokine processing, receptor shedding and the removal of proteins that are responsible for cell–cell or cell–matrix interactions.

All these classes of proteinases play a part in the turnover of connective tissues, and one proteinase pathway may precede another. The pathway that predominates varies with different resorptive situations and often involves complex interactions between different cell types. The osteoid layer in bone is removed by osteoblast metalloproteinases before the attachment of osteoclasts, which then secrete predominantly cysteine proteinases such as cathepsin K that degrade bone matrix after the removal of mineral. An intricate series of interactions occur in the rheumatoid joint between T cells, macrophages, synovial fibroblasts and chondrocytes, all resulting in the secretion of different proteinases. In septic arthritis neutrophils release both serine and metalloproteinases that exceed the local concentration of inhibitors, resulting in rapid removal of the cartilage matrix from the joint cavity.

The matrix metalloproteinase (MMP) family, when activated and acting collectively, can degrade all the components of the extracellular matrix. MMPs are zinc-dependent endopeptidases: all contain common domains and are secreted as latent (inactive) proenzymes, with proteolytic loss of a propeptide leading to activation. MMPs are divided into four main groups, called the

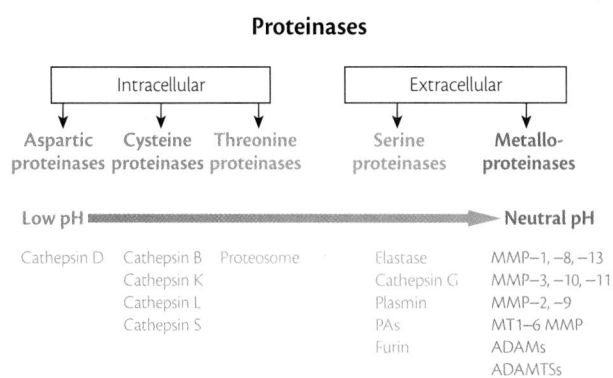

Fig. 19.1.3 Five classes of proteinases are known. Aspartic, cysteine, and threonine proteinases act at acidic pH and generally act intracellularly; the metallo and serine proteinases act at neutral pH, mainly extracellularly. Examples are shown for each class.

stromelysins, collagenases, gelatinases, and MT-MMPs. Once activated, the collagenases (MMP-1, -8, -13) cleave fibrillar collagens at a single site, producing three-quarter- and one-quarter-sized fragments.

The metalloproteinases are carefully controlled, via a number of critical steps, including synthesis and secretion, activation of the proenzymes, and inhibition of the active enzymes (Fig. 19.1.4). There is an increase in levels of different MMPs in rheumatoid synovial fluid, in conditioned culture media from diseased connective tissues and cells, in synovial tissue at the cartilage–pannus junction of rheumatoid joints, in osteoarthritic cartilage, and in animal models of arthritis. These proteinases are therefore implicated both in the normal turnover of connective tissue matrix that occurs during growth and development, and in pathological destruction of joint tissue. In osteoarthritis both the rate of matrix synthesis and breakdown are increased, leading to the formation of excess matrix in some regions (osteophytes), with focal loss of matrix in other areas.

Two additional families of proteinases that are closely related to MMPs are also implicated in cartilage biology, particularly in relation to proteoglycan turnover. ADAMs (a disintegrin and metalloproteinases) are usually membrane-anchored proteinases with diverse functions conferred by the addition of different protein domains. Some members are associated with the cleavage and release of cell-surface proteins; for example, ADAM17 is known for its ability to release TNFα from the cell surface. ADAM10, ADAM12, and ADAM15 are also found within cartilage. ADAMTS family members are distinguished from the ADAMs in that they lack some domains but have additional thrombospondin (TS)-1-like domains, predominantly at the C-terminus, which mediate interactions with the extracellular matrix. Several members of this family are aggrecanases, including ADAMTS4 and ADAMTS5, which can cleave cartilage proteoglycan in disease. Many of the ADAM and ADAMTS family members are inhibited by TIMP3, which effectively blocks aggrecan release from cartilage in *in vitro* studies.

Cathepsins B and L cleave collagen types II, IX, and XI and destroy cross-linked collagen matrix at low pH. Osteoclasts also produce the cysteine proteinase cathepsin K, which cleaves type I collagen at the N-terminal end of the triple helix. This enzyme plays a key role in the degradation of bone collagen, and its expression correlates with bone resorption. Bone resorption is impaired in situations in which cathepsin K is deficient. Cathepsin K is also produced by synovial fibroblasts and is thought to contribute to synovium-initiated bone destruction in the rheumatoid joint.

Model systems of breakdown and repair

Although IL-1 and TNFα are sometimes able to initiate cartilage collagen resorption alone, when these cytokines are combined with oncostatin M (OSM), a rapid and reproducible release of collagen is found in bovine and porcine cartilage. Human cartilage also responds to this combination of cytokines. Synthetic MMP inhibitors, as well as TIMP1 and TIMP2, are able to prevent this release, strongly implicating the collagenolytic MMPs in this process; chondrocytes are known to synthesize collagenase-1, -2, and -3.

Considerable progress is being made in understanding the mechanisms of cartilage repair. Defects found in diseased or damaged cartilage can be repaired in model systems after the delivery of agents that will stimulate chondrocytes to synthesize new matrix. Various methods have been used, including: (1) the isolation of autologous chondrocytes or stem cells that are grown and differentiated in culture and then implanted into defects at high density; (2) the grafting of cartilage into large defects; and (3) the filling of defects with various natural or synthetic polymers, with the addition of growth factors to encourage the migration of chondrocytes into the defect and the subsequent synthesis of matrix components. These techniques are currently only applicable to discrete injuries in younger patients; they are not yet applicable to the repair of larger areas of damaged cartilage in patients with osteoarthritis.

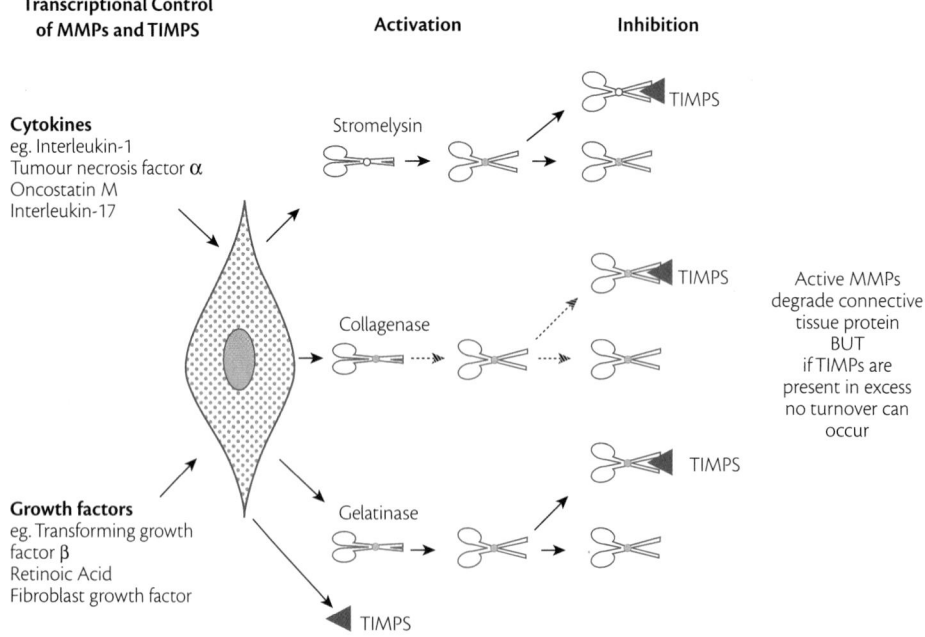

Fig. 19.1.4 Control of matrix metalloproteinases. Control occurs at three levels: regulation, activation, and inhibition. Various cytokines and growth factors can up-regulate or down-regulate the production of matrix metalloproteinases (MMPs) and tissue inhibitor of metalloproteinases (TIMPs), thus influencing the potential for tissue resorption to occur. MMPs are produced as proenzymes that have to be activated proteolytically. Tissue resorption takes place when the level of active MMPs exceeds the level of available TIMPs.

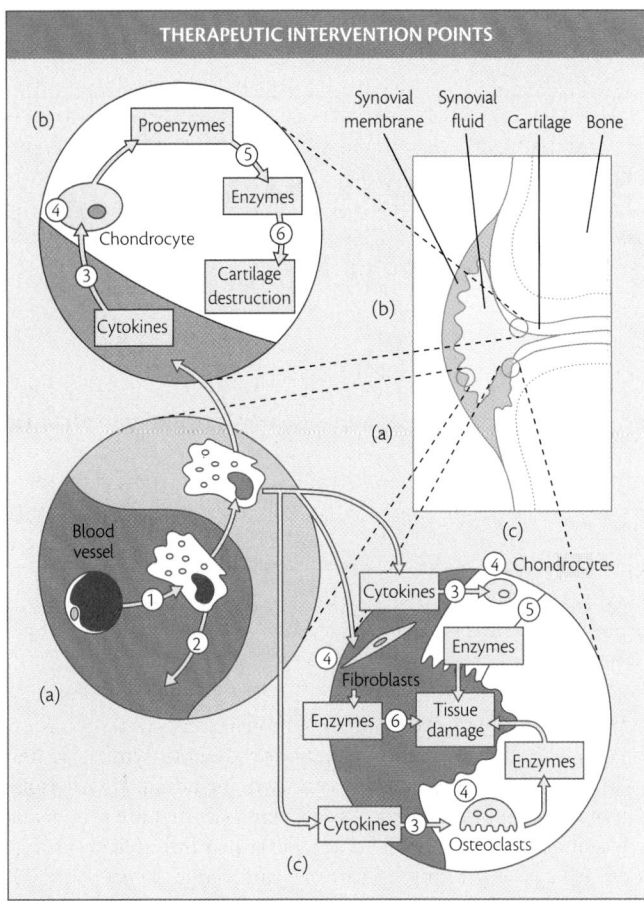

Fig. 19.1.5 Therapeutic intervention points that could block tissue damage. There are a number of points at which the cellular mechanisms involved in tissue damage could be blocked to prevent connective-tissue destruction. These include: (a) (1) blocking entry of inflammatory cells; (2) removal of inflammatory cells from the joint; (b) (3) blocking or mimicking cytokine/growth factor action; (4) blocking inflammatory intracellular signalling pathways involved in the production of proteinases; (5) preventing proteinase activation; (6) direct inhibition of destructive proteinases involved in bone and cartilage loss; (c) within the joint mixtures of cytokines stimulate chondrocytes, synovial fibroblasts, osteoclasts, T cells, and macrophages, leading to the destruction of bone and cartilage.

Future therapeutic options to prevent joint destruction

Many approaches have been used to prevent joint destruction. These include preventing inflammatory cells entering the joint, removing inflammatory cells from the joint, blocking cytokine action, blocking signalling pathways, and preventing activation of proteinases or blocking their action with inhibitors (Fig. 19.1.5).

The success of the anti-TNF therapies in the treatment of rheumatoid arthritis, particularly in relation to the prevention of joint destruction, has raised the standard in terms of future therapeutic options. Small-molecule drugs that also block TNF action are under development: these include inhibitors of proteinases that release TNF from the surface of cells, inhibitors of signalling pathways involved in the production of TNF, and small molecules that

block binding to the receptor. Therapies are also being tested that target other cytokines, such as IL-6 and OSM.

Other targets include the use of synthetic proteinase inhibitors that block joint destruction, but here the future prospects are uncertain. Compounds that inhibit MMPs are the most studied, with the aim of treatment being to shift the balance away from matrix degradation to prevent the loss of connective tissue matrix without leading to excess synthesis. Despite favourable results in the treatment of some cancers, trials of compounds that inhibit the collagenases in patients with rheumatoid arthritis have not been successful, although some studies treating patients with osteoarthritis show promise. It may be necessary to combine different proteinase inhibitors, either in sequence or with other agents that target different but specific steps in the pathogenesis, before the chronic cycle of joint destruction found in these diseases can be broken.

Further reading

Aigner T, *et al*. (2004). Functional genomics of osteoarthritis: on the way to evaluate disease hypotheses. *Clin Orthop Relat Res*, **427**, S138–43.

Burrage PS, Mix KS, Brinckerhoff CE (2006). Matrix metalloproteinases: role in arthritis. *Front Biosci*, **11**, 529–43.

Canty EG, Kadler KE (2005). Procollagen trafficking, processing and fibrillogenesis. *J Cell Sci*, **118**, 1341–53.

Cawston TE, Wilson AJ (2006). Understanding the role of tissue degrading enzymes and their inhibitors in development and disease. *Best Pract Res Clin Rheumatol*, **20**, 983–1002.

Eyre DR, Weis MA, Wu JJ (2006). Articular cartilage collagen: an irreplaceable framework? *Eur Cell Mater* **12**, 57–63.

Firestein GA (2003). Evolving concepts of rheumatoid arthritis. *Nature*, **423**, 356–61.

Goldring S (2003). Inflammatory mediators as essential elements in bone remodelling. *Calcif Tissue Int*, **73**, 97–100.

Hunter W (1995). On the structure and disease of articulating cartilages. 1743. *Clin Orthop Relat Res*, **317**, 3–6.

Karouzakis E, *et al*. (2006). Molecular and cellular basis of rheumatoid joint destruction. *Immuno Lett*, **106**, 8–13.

Malemud CJ (2006). Matrix metalloproteinases: role in skeletal development and growth plate disorders. *Front Biosci*, **11**, 1702–15.

Mundy GR, *et al*. (1995). The effects of cytokines and growth factors on osteoblastic cells. *Bone*, **17**, 71S–75S.

Nagase H, Visse R, Murphy G (2006). Structure and function of matrix metalloproteinases and TIMPs. *Cardiovasc Res*, **69**, 562–73.

Raisz LG (2005). Pathogenesis of osteoporosis: concepts, conflicts and prospects. *J Clin Invest*, **115**, 3318–25.

Riley G (2004). The pathogenesis of tendinopathy: a molecular perspective. *Rheumatology*, **43**, 131–42.

Roughley PJ (2006). The structure and function of cartilage proteoglycans. *Eur Cell Mater*, **12**, 92–101.

Sandell LJ, Hering T, Heinegard D (2007). Cell biology, biochemistry and molecular and cell biology of articular cartilage in osteoarthritis. In: Moskowitz, RW (ed.) *Osteoarthritis*, 4th edition. Lippincott, Williams & Wilkins, Philadelphia, PA.

Stanton H, *et al*. (2005). ADAMTS5 is the major aggrecanase in mouse cartilage in vivo and in vitro. *Nature*, **434**, 648–52.

Van den Berg WB (2002). Pathophysiology of osteoarthritis. *Joint Bone Spine*, **67**, 555–6.

19.2

Clinical presentation and diagnosis of rheumatic disease

Anthony S. Russell and Robert Ferrari

Essentials

Most rheumatological diagnoses are made through effective history taking and physical examination rather than investigation.

Systemic symptoms, such as weight loss, anorexia, and fever, point to systemic diseases such as rheumatoid arthritis, other polyarthritides, systemic lupus erythematosus, polymyalgia, and vasculitides. Swelling of joints is a symptom commonly reported by patients with no objective evidence of this on examination. Inflammatory arthropathies should not be diagnosed unless the physician is able to identify objective swelling, if necessary by arranging a prompt review during an active episode. Diagnostic criteria for the systemic rheumatic diseases are useful in directing the history taking to verify a suspected diagnosis.

Investigations are best used to confirm a strongly suspected diagnosis, already made on the basis of history and examination, not as a screening tool for rheumatic disease.

Introduction

'Medicine is a first-rate profession for a second-rate intellect.' Although we may not fully agree with that statement from a first-class iconclast (George Bernard Shaw), we do agree that with experience it is possible to discipline the mind to follow routine pathways to arrive at a correct diagnosis and therefore a valid treatment plan. In modern medicine, rheumatologists are almost unique in relying heavily on the patient's history and physical examination before applying a relatively restricted number of valid tests to clarify the diagnosis.

Pitfalls occur at every stage of the diagnostic process. The first trap is the referral note or phone call from the primary care physician, conveying their impression of the case, plus laboratory results which may or may not be of relevance. This information is obviously important but must never be blindly accepted as fact. After all, the patient has been referred for a second opinion, which should be truly unbiased and not merely an automatic repetition of the views of the referring doctor. For example: 'This man has refractory gout that is not responding to treatment and his uric acid level is high. Allopurinol has not helped him and after 5 days he still cannot walk because of pain and swelling in his right foot.' The referring physician's clinical assumption that the patient has gout may be incorrect, and the plasma uric acid level could well be irrelevant. Furthermore, if the clinical assumption is correct, then the treatment is inappropriate. Therefore, while at no time hinting to the patient that aspersions are being cast on the referring physician's assumptions, the physician reviewing the case must start from the very beginning, taking a careful history. This should include any previous or family history of such attacks, a general history for systemic disease, or any cause for secondary gout. There should be a comprehensive physical examination, commencing with inspection of the affected part. The correct diagnostic process can be laid out as in the algorithm (a term we use for expediency) for monarticular arthritis, but note that algorithms can be initiated only at some distance down the diagnostic pathway (Fig. 19.2.1).

General approach

The diagnostic process begins with the referral consultation note, followed by observation of the patient as they come in: their gait, demeanour, attire, and whether they are alone or accompanied. These, together with the presenting complaint and the initial features of the history, allow the development of an intuitive approach, in which the physician attempts to define aspects of the disorder and to arrive at a diagnosis (Table 19.2.1). The subsequent interview and examination are used to provide feedback and to support or refute these intuitive diagnoses, some observations necessitating a complete rethink of the process. Sometimes this rethink may relate to results of investigation or the development of new clinical features. Central to this diagnostic process is the classification into systemic rheumatological problems, localized—usually structural—problems, or functional somatic syndromes—perhaps best thought of as biopsychosocial disorders, an ungainly term, but one which emphasizes that biological, psychiatric, and social factors are all important. Although there is obvious overlap between these categories, we believe it provides a useful framework for proceeding, partly because it allows for a positive diagnostic and

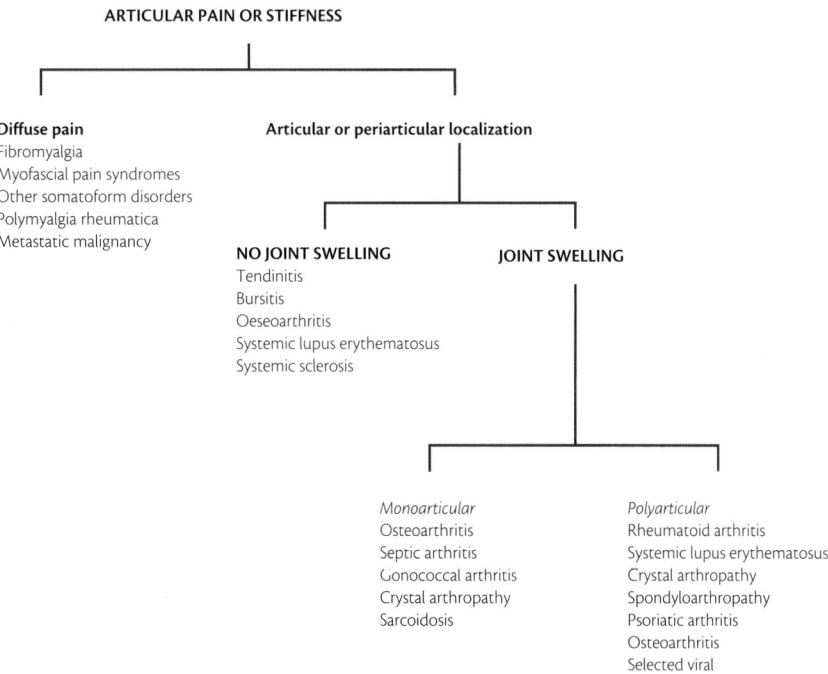

Fig. 19.2.1 An algorithm for rheumatology diagnosis.

therapeutic approach to this latter group, rather than simply regarding them as a group of patients for which other diagnoses need to be excluded.

Some physicians feel insecure in a rheumatological diagnosis because of a lack of confidence in their rheumatological examination. This is unfortunate, because although the examination will provide important information, the principal diagnostic pointers come from a good history. The initial interview also provides a useful way of getting to know the patient and their environment. It is important, by open-ended questioning, to find out not only the details of the problem(s), but what the patient's fears and perceptions are, and—especially in a chronic disorder—what led them or their physician to seek a consultation at this time. This format

Table 19.2.1 Preconsultation intuitive observations (note that intuitive diagnoses must be constantly subject to reflection and reassessment)

Clinical problem	Possible diagnosis
Painful foot in an elderly lady on diuretics	Gout
Young, sexually active; hot swollen joint	Gonococcal arthritis
Headache with diffuse aches and pains in an elderly person	Polymyalgia rheumatica
Antinuclear antibody-positive, but no symptoms	Referring physician's dilemma, not the patients
On allopurinol with a high uric acid, but no arthritis	Not gout
Postpubertal male with low back pain	Ankylosing spondylitis
Woman, 6 weeks postpartum; small joint arthritis	Rubella vaccination; rheumatoid arthritis
Woman describing excruciating pain (like red hot pokers)	Fibromyalgia/somatoform disorders

also allows the patient to become at ease, and make them confident that you are truly listening. Specific directed questions are also of importance, both to elicit less frequent complaints, for example photosensitivity, xerophthalmia, and recurrent miscarriage, and to elaborate on misleading terms. Thus, patients often describe 'hip pain', meaning pain in the buttocks, rarely due to hip disease, and 'weakness' possibly reflecting true neuromuscular disease, but more commonly reflecting pain, e.g. in the shoulders or hip, or simply exhaustion or fatigue. These distinctions are crucial (Table 19.2.2).

One of the key questions in rheumatology is 'Where is the pain?', but it must be followed up with 'And do you have pain anywhere else?'. Sometimes the answer to this, eventually, is 'all over', which by itself is very suggestive of a chronic pain syndrome. Instruments such as a pain diagram, where the patient is asked to shade in areas that are painful, and also to indicate their intensity, may present a vivid pictorial representation of this. We find these useful, particularly for demonstrating the diagnostic value of this response.

When confronted with the patient who 'hurts all over', the next set of questions will often readily yield the diagnosis. The patient with diffuse pain should be asked to list all their other symptoms: a lengthy list indicates fibromyalgia or another functional somatic syndrome, and hearing extreme descriptions of individual symptoms is the next best clue. Indeed, after this, examination confirming lack of joint swelling and the presence of tender points provides ready and simple confirmation of the diagnosis, avoiding unnecessary consideration of other conditions in most cases. By contrast, when the patient fails to give a lengthy list of other symptoms, the less common causes of diffuse (poorly localized) pain should be sought. Be wary of those who complain of weight loss: this is rarely one of the long list of symptoms of patients with fibromyalgia and its presence in someone suspected of having fibromyalgia mandates a complete history and emphasis on the physical examination to look for another process. Conditions to be carefully considered in

Table 19.2.2 Misinterpreted physical signs/symptoms

Sign	Misinterpretation	Correct interpretation
Muscle tenderness	Myositis	Muscle tenderness
Tenderness on sacroiliac joint palpation	Sacroiliitis	Probably mechanical back dysfunction
Adson's manoeuvre*	Thoracic outlet root compression	Probably not clinically relevant (as frequently normal)
Positive Tinel's sign†	Carpal tunnel compression	Too non-specific and insensitive to be relied on
'Hip' pain	Hip disease	Buttock pain reflecting a back problem, or lateral hip reflecting trochanteric bursitis
'Weakness'	Neuromuscular disease	Pain and/or fatigue
'Numbness'	Sensory deficit	Paraesthesiae which may be referred
Arm pain	Local lesion	Pain referred to the deltoid from shoulder or cervical spine

*Adson's manoeuvre: the patient inhales, extends the neck fully, and turns the head to the side being examined. A positive test is a reduction in the radial pulse, plus a reproduction of the patient's symptoms.
†Tinel's sign: percussion of the median nerve at the flexor reticanculum produces paraesthesiae in the hand, particularly in the median nerve distribution.

this context include polymyalgia rheumatica and metastatic bone disease (see below).

Systemic disorders

Systemic disorders include rheumatoid arthritis, other polyarthritides, systemic lupus erythematosus, polymyalgia, vasculitides, etc. Pointers to this type of disorder are malaise, anorexia, weight loss, rashes, fever, and multifocal symptoms including a description of actual joint swelling or persistent sensory or motor deficits. Rheumatoid arthritis may begin as a monarticular problem, and although there are ways—even here—to approach a probable diagnosis, it may require more prolonged observation to establish this with certainty, obviously coupled with empirical management of symptoms. Even though the systemic disorders are typically widespread, they are multifocal—that is a widespread focal problem in different joints. By contrast, pain 'all over' or 'from my head to my toes' suggests fibromyalgia, as indicated previously.

Patients' observations and descriptions of joint swelling are often unreliable and are particularly frequent, for example, in fibromyalgia, where—by definition—it does not occur (unless there is a second disease process going on). There is little point in going through all the diagnostic questions about rheumatoid arthritis and risk factors for gout in a patient who has never had documented swelling. However, if swelling is present on examination, then a further list of questions is aimed at making a specific diagnosis. This means that in practice it is not uncommon for rheumatologists to immediately examine the hands if the patient says that they hurt, and on seeing swelling return to diagnostic questions about the polyarthritides to expand on a presumptive diagnosis, e.g. of rheumatoid arthritis.

Inflammatory arthritides are usually associated with morning stiffness of over 30 min, and the patterns of joint involvement

Table 19.2.3 Patterns of arthritis

Migratory	Rheumatic fever
	Gonococcal arthritis
Additive	Rheumatoid arthritis
	Psoriatic arthritis
	Chronic polyarticular gout
Intermittent	Palindromic arthritis
	Crystal synovitis
	Familial Mediterranean fever
	Early SLE/rheumatoid arthritis, etc.
	Arthritis of inflammatory bowel disease

SLE, systemic lupus erythematosus.

(Table 19.2.3) and acuteness of presentation may help indicate the likely diagnosis (Fig. 19.2.1). Specific questions directed to associated disorders are important, for example bowel disturbance, rectal bleeding, urethritis, mucosal lesions, conjunctivitis, psoriasis, etc.

Ensure that 'sun sensitivity' is not fatigue, headache, or cholinergic urticaria, but a true photosensitivity. Vague circulatory changes and cold hands are so common that this is of no help. A diagnosis of Raynaud's requires an extension of this to include at least pallor, usually followed by reactive hyperemia, but even this may occur in 5% of people without other disease. Always remember to question the validity of previous diagnoses: who made them, and on what grounds?

An important diagnosis in the over-55 age group is polymyalgia rheumatica. Patients may report fatigue and sometimes weight loss. Here the problems are located especially around the limb girdles and are associated with marked morning stiffness and sometimes systemic features. The erythrocyte sedimentation rate is virtually always substantially elevated, although this is very nonspecific. Commonly the examination may be normal, and muscle tenderness is uncommon. In younger individuals with similar symptoms a somatoform disorder is more likely. Myositis itself is not usually painful, and weakness is the predominant complaint, as it is for myopathies. Metastatic bone disease is less common than polymyalgia rheumatica. Patients with this condition usually have weight loss and fatigue as well as nocturnal 'bone pain', symptoms which should lead to enquiry about any previous malignancies and risk factors for malignancy.

Although in one sense a focal problem, a patient with a single, hot, swollen joint is best considered as having a systemic disorder. The crucial issue here is to decide whether or not the joint is infected. Because of the risk of infection, the same initial decision process is involved in a patient with known rheumatoid arthritis who has an acute monarticular flare. If examination confirms an acute synovitis, i.e. not merely tenderness or a periarticular lesion such as cellulitis or erythema nodosum, then joint aspiration and fluid analysis and culture are the most important investigative procedures to be undertaken. Elements of the history are helpful, for example the development 2 to 5 days postoperatively of pain and swelling in the hallux points to gout, and in the knee or wrist to pseudogout. If gonococcus is a possibility, then, as culture of joint fluid may be negative, cultures from other sites are equally important. However, the most important point is to remember that even in seemingly classical situations, aspiration remains advisable to achieve a definitive diagnosis.

So-called 'diagnostic criteria' are generally designed not for diagnosis of the individual patient but for classification of groups of patients, for example for studies or reports. They are, however, useful in providing an aide-memoire to direct questions regarding specific features. Thus the symmetric arthritis of rheumatoid arthritis, the photosensitivity and serositis of systemic lupus erythematosus, the widespread pain above and below the waist of fibromyalgia, the lack of important pain in myositis, the good response of spondylitis to therapy with nonsteroidal anti-inflammatory drugs, etc. are all reinforced as important points to record.

Focal disorders

In a focal disorder, the patient presents with pain or other symptoms in one area, although there may be some radiation or spread. For such disorders it is important to know the relevant anatomy and patterns of pain referral. Some of these are listed in Table 19.2.4, together with diagnostic pointers. To recognize meralgia paraesthetica, for example, one has to know of the existence and supply of the lateral cutaneous nerve of the thigh. A diagnosis of tendonitis should not be made unless it is associated with the name of the specific tendon or—if diffuse—with a systemic disease such as rheumatoid arthritis that can induce this. Too often it is an inappropriate attempt at diagnostic specificity in the presence of vague symptoms; diffuse pain and tenderness are often better considered under the functional section below.

Focal problems can be divided into truly articular and periarticular disorders. It must be remembered that they can be early manifestations of a systemic disease—see Table 19.2.5—which illustrates why an inflammatory lesion is best regarded *ab initio* as a systemic problem.

Table 19.2.4 Clinical pointers in syndromes where pain is poorly localized (other, better localized syndromes, for example calcaneal bursitis, plantar fasciitis, infrapatellar bursitis, should be immediately apparent on examination of the painful area)

Diagnosis	Clinical pointer
Periarticular shoulder pain	Referred to deltoid insertion (e.g. rotator cuff disease)
Tennis and golfer's elbow	Diffuse forearm pain on gripping
Carpal tunnel	Nocturnal paraesthesiae, often diffuse
Digital flexor tenosynovitis	Triggering and/or finger pain on gripping (pulp-pinch sign positive)
DeQuervain's tenosynovitis	Positive Finkelstein test*
Mechanical back pain	Tenderness over gluteals and sacroiliac ligaments frequent
Trochanteric bursitis	Nocturnal pain when lying on that side; focal point tenderness
Hip arthritis	Usually groin and outer thigh pain, occasionally elsewhere
Anserine bursitis	Often nocturnal medial knee pain if knees are touching; localized tenderness

*Finkelstein's test: the thumb is placed in the palm and the fingers flexed over it. Passive ulnar deviation of the wrist stretches the tendons and reproduces pain if positive.

Table 19.2.5 Primarily non-rheumatic illnesses presenting in the rheumatology clinic

Symptom/sign	Illness
Weight loss/bone pain	Multiple myeloma
Carpal tunnel syndrome	Acromegaly, hypothyroidism, amyloid
Bone pain	Secondary tumour
Stiffness and difficulty in walking	Parkinson's disease
Chronic synovitis with bowel problems	Inflammatory bowel disease
Stiff fingers, shoulder pain	Diabetic cheiroarthropathy
Ankle swelling/arthritis	Sarcoidosis
Wrist synovitis	CPPD disease/haemochromatosis

CPPD, calcium pyrophosphate deposition.

Diffuse muscle pains are common. In older people, in which radiological changes of osteoarthritis, particularly of the spine, are frequent, the pains may inappropriately be attributed to 'widespread osteoarthritis'. In general this is a diagnosis to be avoided. It does occur, for example in haemochromatosis, epiphyseal dysplasias, etc., but should be confirmed by clear-cut joint tenderness and decreased range of movement. However, elderly people may accumulate a number of focal disorders, e.g. unilateral osteoarthritis of the knee, a frozen shoulder on the right, postural cervical pain, and an osteoporotic fracture of the dorsal spine, the combination of which may simulate a systemic disease.

Functional somatic syndromes

Functional somatic syndromes are common in rheumatological practice and are often badly managed because physicians tend to focus on organic disease. We are much more likely to be chagrined at missing the rare secondary deposit as a cause of thigh pain than by initially failing to recognize a patient whose somatic symptoms reflect depression or other emotional distress. We are subject to WHIMS (the 'what have I missed syndrome') that encourages repeated and fruitless investigation in this group to eventually arrive at a diagnosis by exclusion.

It is possible and beneficial to make the diagnosis after a good history and examination. Common symptoms are fatigue, weakness, sleeping difficulties, headache, muscle aches, joint pains (plus a description of swelling), paraesthesias, problems with memory and concentration, gastrointestinal symptoms including nausea, and alternating constipation and diarrhoea, and even irritable bladder. Such symptoms have been termed idioms of distress and may be presented with a characteristic hyperbole. Thus, the pain is 'excruciating' like 'red hot pokers in the back—you know' (as if this were an everyday experience for physicians). Apart from this, excruciating pain is seen with fractures, septic/crystal arthritis, or nerve involvement. Patients with rheumatoid arthritis or osteoarthritis, however severe, do not normally use this terminology.

Patients with a functional somatic syndrome may also have arrived at a diagnostic label for their illness: repetitive strain injury, chronic whiplash, side effects of silicone breast implants, candida hypersensitivity, and Gulf War syndrome, to name but a few.

We would also include fibromyalgia, chronic fatigue, irritable bowel syndrome, and others. It is possible, as has been suggested, that fibromyalgia (for example) may represent a central disorder of pain perception, perhaps associated with altered levels of substance P or nerve growth factor. We are unconvinced, but in any event this could be equally true of individuals with depression, with dysfunctional personalities, etc., and does not affect the overall approach to these disorders, among which there is considerable symptomatic overlap. All of these symptoms are common in the healthy population, and it may be more fruitful to ask oneself why the patient has presented to a physician, and at this time, rather than why they have headaches or fatigue in the first place. See Chapter 26.5.3 for further discussion.

Examination

The ability to detect joint swelling is important, but we are referring to obvious changes—if they are merely 'possible' or subtle, then rely more on the history for diagnostic pointers. A distinction between bony swelling and soft tissue/effusion is important and will often be of diagnostic significance.

Contrary to common belief, evident warmth of a joint (or redness) is unusual and points to infection or crystal synovitis. The knee is normally somewhat cooler than the thigh or foreleg, and a lack of this coolness may actually be a sign that an observed knee swelling is inflammatory.

Careful palpation should allow one to distinguish between joint line tenderness, seen in arthritis, tenderness between joints, as in an acute flexor tendonitis, periarticular tenderness, for example in lateral epicondylitis, and diffuse muscle tenderness, seen in some patients with local or generalized fibromyalgia (and very, very rarely in myositis).

The tender points found in fibromyalgia and many other somatoform diagnoses reflect a lowered pain threshold, and it has been suggested that they can be thought of as a 'sed(imentation) rate for emotional distress'. They may provide diagnostic reassurance to the physician, as other aspects of the examination are negative. In particular, joint swelling does not occur—although it is frequently referred to and described by the patient. The physician's observations are important here, because if swollen joints are found, then some disease process is going on that may also need assessment, perhaps in addition to fibromyalgia.

With some exceptions, physical signs in rheumatology have not yet been subjected to assessments of their validity or positive predictive value. Thus, the stress tests for sacroiliac inflammation, while often described, are of no value. Tinel's sign (parasthesia in the distribution of the median nerve when the clinician taps on the distal wrist crease over the median nerve) and Phalen's sign (sustained palmar flexion of the wrist to 90° for 60 s induces finger paraesthesia) have become modified and integrated into an approach to improve their use in the diagnosis of carpal tunnel compression. Adson's manoeuvre is also of little value (a test for thoracic outlet syndrome in which the right or left radial pulse is palpated and disappears if the patient's head is rotated to the left or right on deep inspiration). Palpation of tender muscle bands is subject to great intra- and interobserver error, and the relevance of tender trapezius or gluteal muscles in the diagnosis of postural/mechanical neck and back pain, although clinically probable, remains unproven. Even the classic limitation of straight leg raising

has a relatively poor sensitivity and specificity. Crossed straight-leg raising appears quite specific, but is relatively insensitive. A great deal still needs to be done here.

Investigations

As physicians, we are trained to request tests to help throw light on, and perhaps confirm, a diagnosis. We very commonly use them inappropriately. Thus the idea of a 'rheumatology screen', so popular with some physicians, is entirely inappropriate. There are far, far more healthy people who have a positive test for rheumatoid factor, antinuclear antibodies, or HLA B27 than there are those with significant disease. Thus, for any test to be useful diagnostically, a Bayesian approach considering the pretest probability of diagnosis is crucial, or to put it simply, the result must be taken in context. If the outcome, positive or negative, cannot affect the diagnostic probability, then the test should not normally be ordered. Otherwise, we subject the patient to unnecessary tests and often, when the results are positive, unreasonable anxiety that may take months and a specialty consultation to assuage. This does not include tests done for reasons other than diagnosis, for example to establish a baseline before treatment, or to obtain prognostic information, etc.

Diagnostic tests are sometimes ordered for the false reassurance a negative result provides in the presence of an insecure history and/or physical examination. Unfortunately, a false positive may occur and can be disastrous. Particular caution is therefore advised in ordering tests, or further consultations, to reassure the patient, especially those with a somatoform disorder. Negative findings generally fail to reassure, and indeed may heighten anxieties: a negative test is interpreted as puzzling and means that the problem is not yet solved. Similarly, if treatment, such as rest, does not improve the situation, the implication is that the disorder is too bad, not that the treatment was inappropriate. In fibromyalgia, for example, acknowledging and legitimizing the patient's distress and complaints is important. But although the patient may want a diagnostic label, and this seems reasonable, labelling has been shown to increase disability and labels should not be applied that can be used to validate the 'sick role', i.e. they must come with reassurance and explanation. This reassurance will only be perceived as helpful rather than dismissive if the physician has initially taken care to legitimize and accept the validity of the complaints. The goal of treatment becomes the recognition and management of factors increasing symptoms and the focus on coping and improving functional status rather than curing 'the disease'. See Chapter 26.5.3 for further discussion.

Treatment

For many rheumatic diseases, therapy has advanced enormously in the past 20 years, but the patient will not benefit if the correct diagnosis is not made. Thus, gout should rarely be an active problem with allopurinol, but patients are frequently still admitted to hospital for antibiotics because the correct diagnostic approach of synovial fluid aspiration has not been performed, or because the fluid has been allowed to clot so that crystals are not seen, or because crystals were not looked for, etc. The therapies for rheumatoid arthritis and ankylosing spondylitis, for example, have all progressed, but not to the stage of a cure. Thus, rheumatologists spend a lot of time informing and educating patients. Many of these educational endeavours, when put to the test, have been shown not merely to convey retained information, but to actually alter behaviour and outcomes. It is always rewarding if we can 'fix' a problem, for example by prescribing antimalarials for palindromic arthritis, but all too often the additional role of the rheumatologist is supportive—to inform, to reassure where possible, and to provide continued advice and encouragement.

Further reading

Barsky AJ, Borus JF (1999). Functional somatic syndromes. *Ann Intern Med*, **130**, 910–21.

Deyo RA, Rainville J, Kent DL (1992). What can the history and physical examination tell us about low back pain? *JAMA*, **268**, 760–5.

Grimes DA, Schulz KF (2005). Refining clinical diagnosis with likelihood ratios. *Lancet*, **365**, 1500–5.

Straus SE (1999). Bridging the Gulf War syndrome. *Lancet*, **353**, 162–3.

Clinical investigation

Michael Doherty and Peter C. Lanyon

Essentials

Laboratory and imaging markers are an adjunct to competent clinical assessment and should not be used as a substitute. Tests should only be ordered if the results will alter diagnosis, prognosis, or clinical management.

Synovial fluid examination—this is the key investigation to confirm the diagnosis of either acute crystal or septic arthritis. Fluid can usually be obtained by direct aspiration from any peripheral joint, or alternatively under ultrasound guidance. The identification of crystals requires compensated polarized light microscopy.

Plain radiographs—these remain the single most useful imaging technique, enabling the detection of soft-tissue swelling, changes in bone density, and cartilage and bone erosion or remodelling, which in conjunction with the pattern of joint sites involved can aid confirmation of diagnosis and assessment of disease extent. The cardinal radiological features of rheumatoid arthritis are osteopenia and cartilage/bone erosion: the features of osteoarthritis are preserved bone density, joint-space narrowing, osteophyte formation, and bone cysts.

Other imaging techniques—(1) MRI provides additional benefit with plain radiographs in the assessment of the anatomy and biochemistry of soft tissues as well as bone; (2) ultrasound is emerging as an effective bedside technique for detecting joint effusions (particularly at clinically occult sites) and to assess joint erosions and neovascularity.

Blood tests—(1) inflammatory markers: C-reactive protein is the single most useful measure of the acute phase response, having greater reproducibility and greater sensitivity to change than the ESR; (2) specific antibodies: antibodies to cyclic citrullinated peptides are a novel marker associated with rheumatoid arthritis, with similar sensitivity to rheumatoid factor but higher specificity for distinguishing between rheumatoid arthritis and other rheumatic diseases; antibodies detected against nuclear components (ANAs) have high sensitivity for connective-tissue diseases (e.g. systemic lupus erythematosus) but low specificity, and hence a positive result does not confirm the diagnosis unless appropriate clinical features are present. Compared with ANA, antibodies to extractable nuclear antigens have higher specificity and associate with patterns of system involvement within the same disease.

Introduction

Disease markers are pathological or physiological characteristics of an individual that assist in determining the diagnosis, the current activity of disease, or the expected prognosis of the condition in that individual (Fig. 19.3.1). Some markers relate to just one of these elements; others may relate to two, or occasionally all three.

Clinical markers are derived from enquiry and examination of the patient. For many common rheumatic disorders, clinical assessment alone gives sufficient information for patient diagnosis and management. In some situations, however, particularly with inflammatory, metabolic, or multisystem disease, a search for additional investigational markers may be warranted. It is important to emphasize that the requirement for and selection of investigations, as well as their subsequent interpretation, is principally determined by the clinical assessment. Investigations are an adjunct, never a substitute, for competent clinical assessment.

There is no place for a battery of screening tests. Investigational markers may include:

◆ laboratory markers (biochemical, haematological, microbiological, histological) sought through investigation of body fluids and tissues

◆ structural and physiological markers, mainly assessed by imaging (radiography, scintigraphy, MRI, ultrasonography)

◆ genetic disease susceptibility and prognostic markers—these hold promise for the future but at present have clinical application only to rare monogenic disorders

When considering any investigation, the following deliberations are pertinent.

◆ 'Is this the most appropriate investigation to answer the clinical question?' This may depend on various factors, e.g. the sensitivity and specificity of the marker being sought, its predictive value (which takes into account disease prevalence as well as the

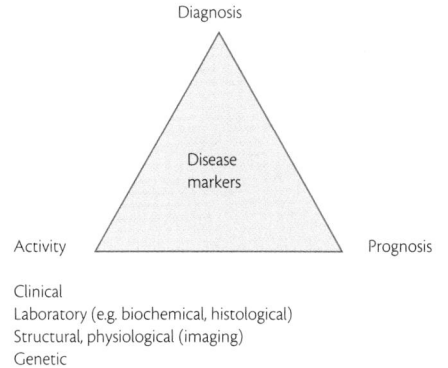

Fig. 19.3.1 Markers may be used for diagnosis, assessment of disease activity, or prognosis.

Diagnosis

Disease markers

Activity   Prognosis

Clinical
Laboratory (e.g. biochemical, histological)
Structural, physiological (imaging)
Genetic

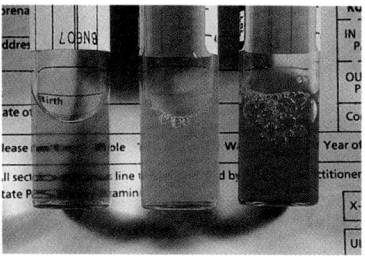

Fig. 19.3.2 Different macroscopic appearances of synovial fluids: (a) on the left, clear straw-coloured fluid from an osteoarthritic knee (easy to read writing behind it); (b) less viscous, turbid (high cell count) 'inflammatory' fluid from a rheumatoid knee; and (c) uniform bloodstaining (haemarthrosis) due to acute pseudogout.

sensitivity and specificity), the cost and availability of the investigation, and the pros and cons of invasive vs noninvasive tests.

◆ 'Will the result of this test alter the diagnosis or clinical management of the patient?' It is easy to initiate more investigations than are really required.

◆ 'Will I be able to interpret and act on the results of this test?' Tests should only be ordered if the implications of either a normal or abnormal result are understood.

In common rheumatological practice the investigations that are of most use in diagnosis are synovial fluid analysis and the plain radiograph. Confirmation of clinically assessed inflammatory disease activity and its response to treatment is mainly by full blood count and either direct or indirect measures of the acute phase response. These investigations are therefore given special prominence in this chapter: the usefulness of other investigations will be discussed in the context of specific clinical scenarios.

Synovial fluid analysis

This is the key investigation to confirm the diagnosis of the two curable rheumatic diseases—septic arthritis and gout. Other crystal-associated arthropathies and intra-articular bleeding are also diagnosed in this way. Synovial fluid analysis is thus the pivotal investigation for an acute monoarthritis, especially with overlying erythema.

Synovial fluid can be obtained from almost any peripheral joint, with only a small volume required for diagnostic purposes. Aspiration of large joints should be no more uncomfortable than venepuncture. The patient should be informed of the purpose and nature of the procedure and positioned on a couch in a comfortable and relaxed position, with full exposure of the relevant joint. The risk of introducing sepsis is negligible, as long as sterile equipment and the same sensible precautions used for venepuncture are employed.

Macroscopic appearance

Normal synovial fluid is present in small volume, contains very few cells, is clear, colourless to pale yellow, and has high viscosity due to macromolecular hyaluronan (Fig. 19.3.2). In general, with increasing joint inflammation the volume increases, the total cell count and proportion of neutrophils rises (causing turbidity), and the viscosity lowers (due to degradation of hyaluronan

by protease). However, there is such overlap between arthropathies that these features are of little diagnostic value. Frank pus or pyarthrosis due to very high neutrophil counts should always lead to exclusion of sepsis, but can occur with any florid synovitis such as acute crystal synovitis or rheumatoid. High concentrations of urate or cholesterol crystals may result in white synovial fluid—joint 'milk'.

Nonuniform bloodstaining of synovial fluid is common and reflects inconsequential needle trauma to synovial vessels. Uniform bloodstaining (haemarthrosis) most commonly occurs in association with florid synovitis but may also result from a bleeding diathesis, trauma, or pigmented villonodular synovitis. A lipid layer floating above bloodstained fluid is diagnostic of intra-articular fracture.

Gram stain and culture

Synovial fluid should be sent for urgent Gram stain and culture if sepsis is suspected. Placement in blood culture bottles in addition to a sterile universal container increases positive yields, especially of anaerobes. If gonococcal sepsis or uncommon organisms are suspected, especially in immunocompromised patients, it is advisable to discuss this with the microbiologist so that the optimal cultures can be established and molecular techniques of antigen detection used if appropriate. Although a positive result on Gram staining is found in over 50% of cases of adult septic arthritis (predominantly *Staphylococcus aureus*), a negative result does not exclude infection. If there is a strong clinical suspicion of sepsis, the patient should be given intravenous antibiotics pending the results of synovial fluid, blood, and other culture results.

Crystal identification

Accurate identification of common synovial fluid crystals requires a compensated polarized light microscope and an experienced observer. Monosodium urate and calcium pyrophosphate crystals may be seen by ordinary light microscopy, but confident identification resides in their light characteristics as well as their morphology. Analysis is best performed on fresh unrefrigerated synovial fluid taken into a plain container to avoid problems of crystal dissolution, postaspiration crystallization, and artefacts from tube additives. If only a few drops are obtained, these should be placed straight onto a clean microscope slide and a second slide or coverslip placed on top. Even with an apparently 'dry tap' it is worth expelling the contents of the needle on to a slide: a very small amount of fluid is sometimes obtained and may be diagnostic.

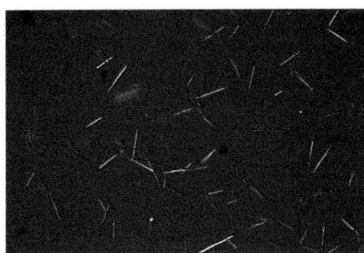

Fig. 19.3.3 Monosodium urate crystals viewed by compensated polarized light microscopy (×400) showing bright birefringence (negative sign) and needle-shaped morphology.

Urate crystals are long and needle shaped and show a strong intensity with negative birefringence (Fig. 19.3.3). Pyrophosphate crystals are smaller, rhomboid in shape, usually less numerous than urate, and have weak intensity and positive birefringence (Fig. 19.3.4).

Although usually identified in the setting of acute synovitis, crystals are also often present in fluid aspirated from the joint after the attack has settled. Aspiration of an asymptomatic first metatarsophalangeal joint (gout) or knee (gout, pseudogout) may therefore permit confirmation of a suspected diagnosis. This is particularly important in gout because of the possible implications of life-long hypouricaemic therapy. The diagnosis can also be made by analysis of a tophus aspirate.

Plain radiography

In conjunction with a full history and examination, plain radiography remains the single most useful imaging technique for assessment of rheumatic disease. Although a radiograph is a static record of predominantly past events, it can demonstrate visually alterations that reflect the underlying pathological processes of rheumatic disease, e.g. cartilage and bone erosion, bone remodelling, calcification. The abnormalities that may be seen on a plain film include:

♦ soft-tissue swelling—seen as altered skin contours and displaced fat planes and intracapsular fat pads (fat appears dark on a radiograph)

♦ decreased or increased bone density (localized or generalized) (Table 19.3.1)

♦ joint erosion (nonproliferative or proliferative marginal erosion, central erosion)

Fig. 19.3.4 Calcium pyrophosphate crystals viewed by polarized light microscopy (×400) showing weak birefringence (positive sign), scant numbers, and a predominantly rhomboid morphology. These are clearly more difficult to detect than urate crystals.

Table 19.3.1 Some causes of changes in bone density

Causes of increased bone density	Causes of decreased bone density
Generalized/multiple regional	
Myelofibrosis	Osteoporosis
Osteopetrosis	Myeloma, leukaemia
	Osteomalacia, rickets
	Hyperparathyroidism
	Vitamin C deficiency
	Osteogenesis imperfecta
Localized	
Paget's disease (with altered trabecular pattern and radiolucent areas)	Inflammatory arthritis (juxtaarticular)
Metastases (especially prostate, breast)	Infection
Osteoid osteoma (sometimes with a central radiolucency)	Algodystrophy (regional) Extreme disuse
Bone islands	

♦ joint-space narrowing (osteoarthritis—focal; inflammatory arthritis—generalized)

♦ new bone formation (osteophyte, enthesophyte, syndesmophyte)

♦ periosteal reaction (Table 19.3.2)

♦ calcification (cartilage (chondrocalcinosis), synovium, capsule, ligament, tendon, muscle, fat, vascular, skin)

♦ bone cysts and radiolucent lesions (Box 19.3.1)

♦ intra-articular osteochondral bodies

♦ deformity

Although most of these abnormalities taken individually have low specificity, various combinations of some of these features, together with their targeting of certain joint sites (Fig. 19.3.5), result in characteristic patterns of abnormality and distribution that have high diagnostic specificity. The distribution of joint involvement, of course, is usually apparent following clinical assessment of the patient, and joints to be investigated by radiography will usually be selected on this basis. However, an important exception is seronegative spondyloarthropathy, in which sacroiliac involvement is often asymptomatic and is difficult to detect clinically. When this condition is suspected, an anteroposterior view of the pelvis and a lateral thoracolumbar spine view (i.e. two films)

Table 19.3.2 Some causes of periosteal reaction

Localized	Infection
	Trauma
	Tumour
Multiple sites	Hypertrophic osteoarthropathy
	Seronegative spondyloarthropathy
	Scurvy

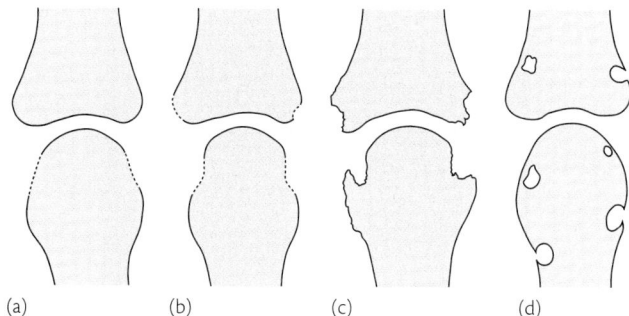

Fig. 19.3.6 Diagram of metacarpophalangeal joint showing (a) early dot-dash erosion, (b) the later definite nonproliferative erosion of rheumatoid arthritis, (c) the proliferative erosion of psoriatic arthritis, and (d) the intra- and extracapsular pressure erosions of gout.

are usually sufficient to show sacroiliitis and syndesmophytes if these are present.

Radiographs should be selected to answer specific questions. For example, to address the question of whether a patient with chronic inflammatory polyarthritis affecting hands, elbows, neck, knees, and ankles has erosive disease typical of rheumatoid, posteroanterior views of hands and feet (i.e. two films), but not radiographs of all symptomatic joints, are appropriate. This is because rheumatoid erosions appear first in wrists and the small joints of hands and feet, and may first affect the metatarsophalangeal joints, even if they are relatively asymptomatic. However, if the degree of structural damage in one large joint is a principal cause for concern, then a radiograph of that particular joint should obviously be taken. For most joints a single (two-dimensional) view is sufficient (e.g. anteroposterior view of pelvis, posteroanterior view of both hands, posteroanterior view of both feet), although two views are required for some (e.g. posteroanterior standing view of both knees, plus individual lateral or bilateral skyline patellofemoral view). Thus selection of radiographs will often differ for purposes of diagnosis or disease assessment.

Erosions

An important hallmark of inflammatory arthropathies is cartilage and bone erosion. Intracapsular bone erosion first occurs at the 'bare areas' of the joint margin (marginal erosion) where bone is exposed directly to inflammatory synovium without the protection of overlying cartilage. Loss of the sharp cortical line, the 'dot-dash' appearance, is the first radiographic sign that precedes more definite scalloping of the bony contour (Fig. 19.3.6). Cartilage erosion also commences at the joint margin and slowly works centrally,

resulting in relatively late loss of interosseous distance or 'joint space'.

Both rheumatoid disease and the seronegative spondyloarthropathies (especially psoriatic and chronic reactive arthritis) cause marginal erosions. In rheumatoid disease, however, the aggressive synovitis overwhelms any reparative response, presenting a very atrophic appearance ('nonproliferative erosions') (Figs. 19.3.6 and 19.3.7) with no new bone or periosteal reaction and only juxta-articular osteopenia (a sign of inflammation) and soft-tissue swelling as accompanying early radiographic features. By contrast, the seronegative spondyloarthropathies are characterized by a degree of low-grade inflammation that permits some reparative response. Such inflammation results in a tendency to fibrosis, calcification, and ossification. Marginal erosions in these arthropathies are therefore commonly accompanied by fluffy new bone formation ('proliferative erosions') (Figs. 19.3.6 and 19.3.8) with normal or

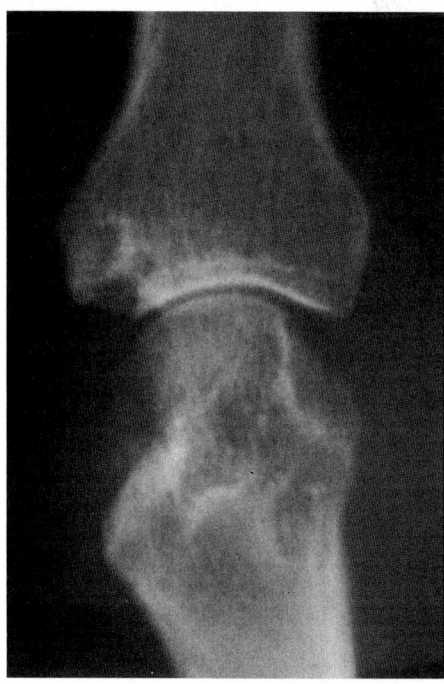

Fig. 19.3.7 Radiograph of metacarpophalangeal joint showing late nonproliferative marginal erosions of rheumatoid arthritis, more obvious proximally than distally (reflecting the more proximal than distal distribution of synovium in small finger joints) and eventual global loss of cartilage.

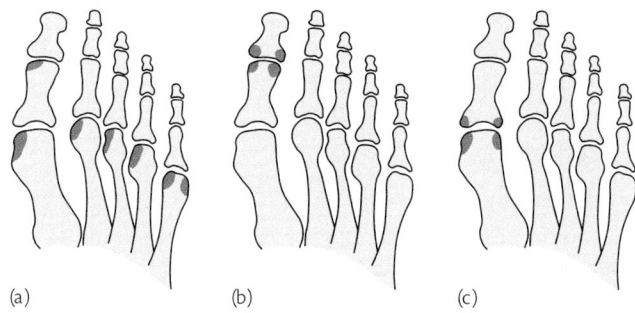

(a)   (b)   (c)

Fig. 19.3.5 Diagram to show different target sites of involvement in the forefoot for (a) rheumatoid arthritis, (b) psoriatic arthritis, and (c) osteoarthritis.

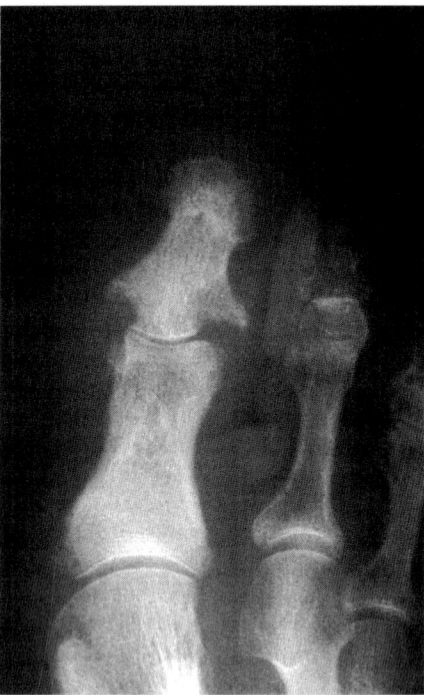

Fig. 19.3.8 Radiograph of the hallux showing proliferative erosions and cartilage loss of the interphalangeal joint, and associated increased bone density (ivory phalanx) typical of psoriatic arthropathy.

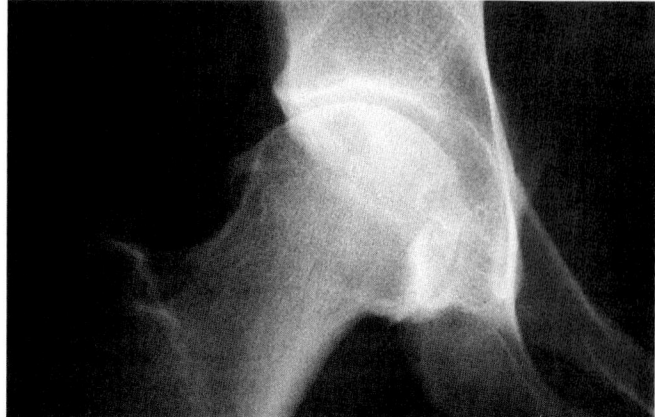

Fig. 19.3.9 Radiograph of the hip to show changes of osteoarthritis, specifically superior joint-space narrowing, subchondral sclerosis, marginal osteophyte, and cysts.

increased periosteal and bone density rather than osteopenia. The fact that different joints are targeted in these conditions, and the common accompanying involvement of entheses—fibrous insertions of tendons, ligaments, or capsule into bone—further assists differentiation in most cases.

In early septic arthritis the radiograph is often normal, apart from osteopenia and soft-tissue swelling, for 1 to 2 weeks. However, erosion proceeds rapidly and results in generalized loss of joint space with loss of cortical integrity centrally (central erosion) as well as marginally. In chronic gout, bony defects develop slowly as massive crystal concretions (tophi) causing pressure necrosis to surrounding bone; such pressure erosions (Fig. 19.3.6) occur at extracapsular as well as intracapsular sites and are unaccompanied by osteopenia.

Osteoarthritis

The features of osteoarthritis, by far the most common joint disease, are highly characteristic and contrast with those of inflammatory arthropathy. The two cardinal features are narrowing of the joint space and osteophytes. By contrast to inflammatory arthropathies, joint-space narrowing is focal rather than widespread within the joint, mainly targeting the maximum load-bearing region (Fig. 19.3.9). Bony osteophyte is most noticeable at the margins of the joint but also occurs centrally and as periosteal osteophyte ('buttressing') at sites such as the femoral neck. Subchondral sclerosis, or increased density of bone is also common, principally below the site of maximal narrowing. Additional features include subchondral 'cysts', osteochondral ('loose') bodies within the synovium, and an increased association with chondrocalcinosis. In contrast to inflammatory arthritis, the bone density is normal or increased and marginal erosions are not a feature.

Calcification

Calcification can affect any locomotor tissue. Calcification of fibro- and hyaline cartilage (chondrocalcinosis) is most commonly due to calcium pyrophosphate crystals, less commonly to apatite or other basic calcium phosphates. This can occur as an isolated phenomenon (mainly age associated, rarely as a result of metabolic or familial disease predisposition) or in association with structural changes of osteoarthritis (chronic pyrophosphate arthropathy). Less commonly pyrophosphate crystals also cause calcification of the synovium and capsule, and linear tendon calcification (mainly hip adductors, Achilles, triceps).

Periarticular calcification is usually apatite. Isolated periarticular calcification mainly affects central sites such as the shoulder (supraspinatus tendons) or hip (abductor tendons), appearing as single dense concretions with rounded contours, as opposed to the linear calcification of pyrophosphate. Shedding of these crystal deposits can result in severe, self-limiting inflammation (acute calcific periarthritis) with reduction or loss of the radiographic calcification.

Spotty, multiple calcification of soft tissues (calcinosis) mainly targets peripheral and intermediate sites such as the finger pulps, wrists and forearms and is a feature of connective tissue disease, most commonly CREST syndrome (calcinosis, Raynaud's, oesophageal dysmotility, sclerodactyly, telangiectasia). Calcinosis requires distinction from small blood vessel calcification, which has a thin, meandering tramline appearance (and is increased in diabetes and chronic renal failure), sesamoids, and solitary dense calcified phleboliths. Myositis ossificans is rare and appears as dense sheets of calcification mainly at proximal sites such as the hip. Fine reticular or linear calcification of subcutaneous fat and muscle may follow young onset dermatomyositis.

Other imaging

Arthrography

Injection of positive (iodinated) or negative (air) contrast, or a combination of both, can help delineate the soft tissue outline of a joint or other tissue space (for example bursa). The main use of plain film arthrography is at the knee to demonstrate a ruptured popliteal (Baker's) cyst as a cause of calf pain and swelling, although in many centres this has been superseded by ultrasonography or MRI, which provide better anatomical assessment.

Scintigraphy

Scintigraphy is a cheap, readily available technique that delivers only a very small amount of radiation. It involves gamma camera imaging following an intravenous injection of radioisotope, usually technetium-99m diphosphonate. Early 'flow' images obtained immediately postinjection, or a little later when the isotope is in the soft tissues ('blood pool' phase), reflect vascularity and will show, for example, the increased perfusion of inflamed synovium, Pagetic bone, or hypervascular primary or secondary bone tumour (Fig. 19.3.10). 'Delayed' images, taken a few hours after injection, indicate bone remodelling due to localization of the diphosphonate to sites of active bone turnover. Although nonspecific and lacking high spatial resolution, the major advantage of scintigraphy is its high sensitivity for detecting important bone and joint pathology that may not be apparent on plain radiographs. It is particularly useful, following a normal or inconclusive plain radiograph of the presenting painful region, as the second imaging investigation to detect the following:

◆ bone metastases (at the presenting site and at clinically occult sites)

◆ bone or joint sepsis (at the presenting site and at clinically occult sites)

◆ early osteonecrosis (at the presenting site and at clinically occult sites)

◆ stress fracture

◆ reflex sympathetic dystrophy (algodystrophy)

◆ hypertrophic osteoarthropathy

Scintigraphy is also useful in delineating the extent and current activity of Paget's disease of bone.

CT

This can give detailed information on anatomy, especially of bone, allowing three-dimensional visualization of structures such as the spinal canal and facet joints. Its principal use is therefore in assessing

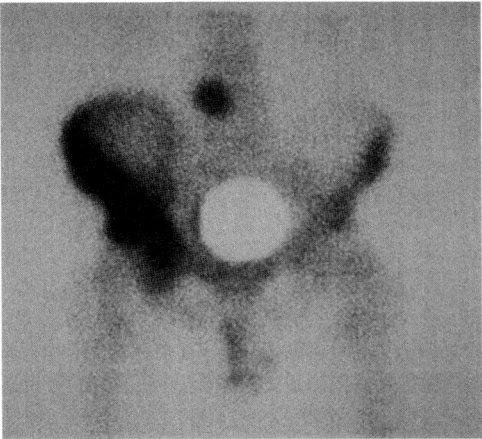

Fig. 19.3.10 Bone scan demonstrating secondary deposits of prostate cancer. The presenting painful lesion was in the right hemipelvis and the plain pelvic radiograph was normal. The spinal lesion (and two others not shown on this photograph) were asymptomatic.

areas of complex anatomy such as the spine or pelvis, where plain radiographs may be inadequate (e.g. to investigate stenosis of the spinal canal). Drawbacks, however, include limited soft-tissue resolution and exposure to a considerable radiation dose; in many situations it is has now been superseded by MRI.

MRI

The ability of MRI to image the anatomy and biochemistry of soft tissue as well as bone means that it provides detailed information not only on structure but also on the pathophysiology of all locomotor tissues. Further advantages include its capacity for multiplanar imaging (for example coronal, axial, sagittal, oblique) and its safety, without radiation exposure. The physics of MRI is complex. When a patient is placed in the magnetic field of the scanner the protons in the body align along the central axis of the field. Application of a radiofrequency pulse, or sequence, causes the protons to spin in phase with each other. When the pulse is stopped the protons return to random spinning and dephase. As they do so they emit a signal that is converted to an image by computer manipulation. In general, T_1-weighted short sequences are useful for defining anatomy, and T_2-weighted long sequences are useful for assessing pathology. Other sequences are selected for special purposes, e.g. the short tau inversion recovery sequence, is used to image marrow as it suppresses fat and makes the marrow appear dark. MRI, with or without enhancement with gadolinium, is particularly useful in detecting and assessing the following:

◆ early osteonecrosis (at the presenting site and the contralateral clinically occult site)

◆ intervertebral disc disease, root entrapment, and spinal cord compression

◆ osteoarticular and soft-tissue sepsis

◆ osteoarticular and soft-tissue malignancy

◆ internal mechanical derangement of joints (particularly the knee)

◆ assessment of soft-tissue and periarticular pathology (e.g. early synovitis, rotator cuff tears, bursitis, tenosynovitis)

The choice between three-phase scintigraphy and MRI for detection of conditions such as early osteonecrosis, where both have excellent sensitivity (scintigraphy 90%, MRI 100%), will depend on practical issues such as ease of access, musculoskeletal reporting expertise, and local cost.

Ultrasonography

This is a safe, accessible technique that can be used at the bedside and is increasingly used to detect synovitis/effusions at both clinically occult joints (e.g. hip) and small peripheral joints (e.g. proximal interphalyngeal joints) when there is clinical uncertainty. It can also be used to assess for neovascularity and erosions, and hence is important in assessing response to treatment. Ultrasound examination is also very useful to assess soft-tissue changes such as popliteal cysts, or Achilles tendon pathology, and can also be used to guide intra-articular and soft-tissue injection.

Blood tests for inflammation and systemic disease

The full blood count, ESR, and C-reactive protein may show changes that indicate the presence of inflammation somewhere in the body. These changes are very sensitive but are nonspecific: they are mainly used as a semiquantitative measure to complement the clinical assessment of inflammatory disease and its response to treatment.

The systemic response to injury that results in these changes is summarized in Fig. 19.3.11. At any site of injury or inflammation, macrophages and monocytes release soluble intercellular signalling polypeptides (cytokines) including interleukin 1, interleukin 6, and tumour necrosis factor-α. Some of these enter the systemic circulation and exert effects on the hypothalamus, bone marrow, and liver. These combined systemic effects are called the acute phase response, even though they accompany chronic as well as acute inflammation. Interleukin 6 is the main cytokine to influence the liver, causing increased production of certain acute phase proteins (including fibrinogen and C-reactive protein) and decreased production of other negative acute phase reactants (such as albumin and transferrin).

Much of the acute phase response is beneficial for body defence and adaptation to injury, especially for dealing with the two major complications of injury that threaten life: haemorrhage and sepsis. For example, the thrombocytosis and increased serum levels of clotting factors facilitate haemostasis; neutrophilia and the increased serum levels of complement, immunoglobulin, and C-reactive protein (an opsonin) combat infection; and the anaemia and low serum transferrin levels result in diminished delivery of iron to bacteria and parasites.

Of all the acute phase proteins, C-reactive protein shows the greatest shift from very low to very high levels, varying over a several-hundred-fold range in concentration. C-reactive protein also closely mirrors the current degree of inflammation, rising rapidly at its onset and falling as inflammation subsides, such that it is therefore the single most useful direct measure of the acute phase response. Interestingly, some rheumatic diseases—specifically lupus, systemic

sclerosis, and dermatomyositis—associate with only modest or no elevation of C-reactive protein, despite unequivocal pathological evidence of inflammation and tissue damage. The reason for this remains unclear, but patients with such disease are capable of mounting a typical acute phase response, e.g. in response to infection. In a patient with lupus or scleroderma, gross elevation of C-reactive protein should therefore suggest an incidental cause such as sepsis. Some clinical features of active systemic lupus and infection overlap; hence in this situation the C-reactive protein can prove a useful test.

The ESR is a long-established indirect measure of the acute phase response. It mainly reflects the degree of rouleaux formation. Normally our circulating erythrocytes do not clump together because of the net balance of three electrical forces (Fig. 19.3.12), namely weak attractant van der Waal's forces resulting from red cells being bodies; a strong repellent net negative surface charge, or zeta potential, due mainly to membrane sialic acid residues; and an attractant dielectric constant resulting from the charge characteristics of the plasma constituents.

In health the zeta potential far exceeds the sum of the two attractant forces, so that erythrocytes electrostatically repel each other and remain single. However, during the acute phase response the change in plasma protein concentrations leads to an increase in dielectric constant. Fibrinogen is particularly important in this respect. Although its increase in concentration is relatively modest, fibrinogen is a very asymmetric molecule that exerts a major electrical charge effect. The resulting increase in dielectric constant is sufficient to overcome the zeta potential so that rouleaux form more readily. Rouleaux have a higher ratio of mass per surface area and so sediment faster than single red cells, which is the property measured in the ESR. In the Westergren test system a 200 mm capillary tube is filled with the patient's blood. After 1 h the clearance of red cells from the top is measured. If there is little rouleaux formation, the discrete red cells sediment only slowly and the clearance is small (<5–10 mm). However, if there is significant rouleaux

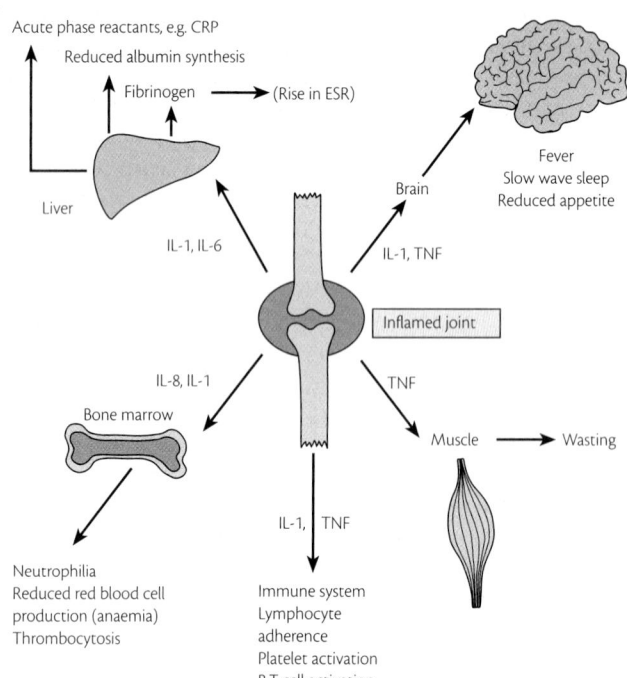

Fig. 19.3.11 Diagram to show the important elements of the acute phase response.

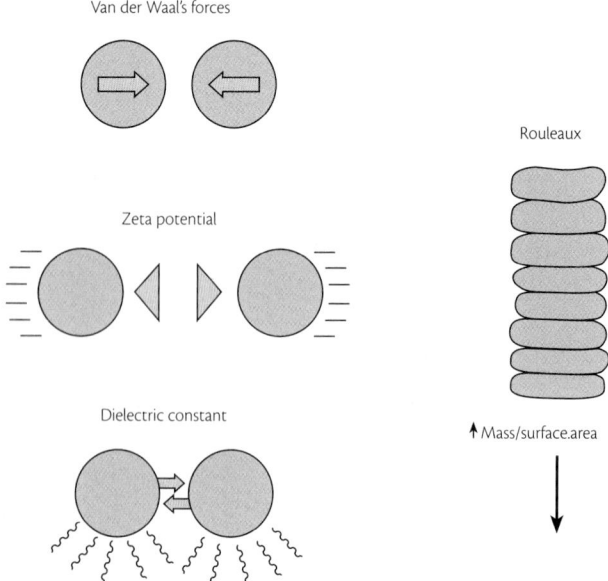

Fig. 19.3.12 Diagram showing the balance of three electrical forces that influence clumping of erythrocytes. Rouleaux sediment faster than individual erythrocytes.

formation, the clearance is greater and the ESR in the first hour is elevated. Therefore, in a patient with an acute phase response, the ESR and C-reactive protein are both elevated, with the ESR lagging behind the C-reactive protein in terms of speed of change.

It is important to recognize, however, that the ESR may be elevated for reasons other than the acute phase response. Immunoglobulins are very symmetrical molecules, and their modest increase in concentration during the acute phase response has relatively little effect, compared with fibrinogen, on the dielectric constant. However, large increases in immunoglobulin concentration (e.g. in multiple myeloma or associated with autoimmune diseases such as Sjögren's syndrome) will increase the dielectric constant and lead to rouleaux formation. In this situation, the patient may have a high ESR but normal or relatively low C-reactive protein. Such discordance between the ESR and C-reactive protein should lead to consideration of hypergammaglobulinaemia and myeloproliferative disease and to direct measurement of serum immunoglobulins and paraprotein electrophoresis.

In addition to the changes reflecting an acute phase response, the full blood count may show other alterations that are nonspecific in themselves but which, taken in the context of the clinical features, may be characteristic of certain rheumatic diseases or their complications (Fig. 19.3.13). For example, neutrophilia may be seen in systemic vasculitis and neutropenia in lupus. Furthermore, many of the slow-acting drugs used to control chronic inflammation have toxicity on the bone marrow, such that the full blood count is often included in the routine monitoring of such treatment.

Taken together, therefore, the full blood count, ESR, and C-reactive protein can be a useful complement of tests in the major rheumatic diseases, to:

◆ assess inflammatory disease activity
◆ assess response to disease-suppressing treatment
◆ detect certain disease complications
◆ screen for drug toxicity

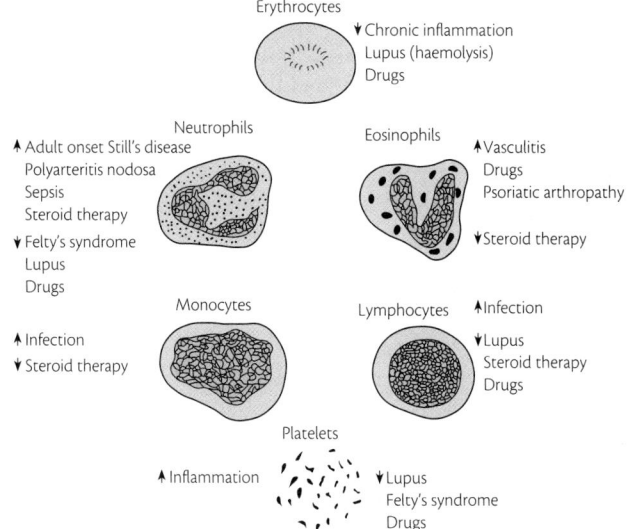

Fig. 19.3.13 Diagram showing some of the nonspecific changes that may occur in individual elements of the full blood count in patients with systemic rheumatic disease.

However, it is important to appreciate that although an elevated acute phase response is consistent with inflammatory rheumatic disease, it is nonspecific; also that the degree of elevation is often proportional to the amount or 'burden' of inflammatory tissue—e.g. isolated small joint synovitis in rheumatoid arthritis may not be sufficient to cause a detectable acute phase response, but this does not mean that inflammatory disease is not present.

Immunological tests

There are an increasing number of autoantibodies that can be detected in a serum sample by clinical laboratory services. Production of some of these is a common, age-related phenomenon that may be exaggerated by the presence of chronic inflammation. The isolated presence of some autoantibodies therefore has low diagnostic specificity and may not imply the presence of any disease at all. If present in high concentrations, however, their disease specificity usually increases; hence it is always important to know how much antibody is present (the titre or concentration in units), rather than just whether it is detectable. The titre of some autoantibodies (e.g. antineutrophil cytoplasmic antibody (ANCA)) may be used to monitor the activity of the associated disease and predict relapse risk after treatment; only a few antibodies (e.g. anti-dsDNA) have high diagnostic specificity. Again, the correct choice and interpretation of tests will depend on detailed knowledge of the patient. There are different detection and assay systems for many of these autoantibodies: close liaison with the local immunology service is required.

Rheumatoid factor

The definition of a rheumatoid factor is an antibody directed against a specific region of the Fc (crystallizable) fragment of human IgG. The antibody itself may be of any immunoglobulin class, although IgM anti-IgG is the rheumatoid factor that is most commonly measured in the first instance. One of the traditional methods used to detect IgM rheumatoid factor is to coat latex beads with human IgG. If the patient's serum is then added to the test system the pentameric IgM antibody binds to the IgG, causing the latex particles to flocculate, producing a positive latex fixation test. The amount the patient's serum must be diluted before this flocculation is lost is then determined; the higher this 'titre' the higher the concentration of antibody present. Although 'rheumatoid factor' was so named because it was first detected in the sera of patients with rheumatoid arthritis, it also occurs in association with a variety of other conditions, as well as in some normal adults (Box 19.3.2). It thus has low diagnostic specificity, particularly in older people, and is not a 'test for rheumatoid arthritis'. In terms of sensitivity, it is present in most patients with erosive rheumatoid disease but may only appear after many months or years of disease, once the diagnosis is beyond dispute. It is therefore of little value in making a diagnosis of rheumatoid arthritis, being neither sufficient nor necessary: rheumatoid arthritis is predominately a clinical diagnosis, based on detecting the presence of synovitis (capsular swelling, joint line tenderness, stress pain). However, if present in high titre at the onset of rheumatoid arthritis it associates with a poorer prognosis. IgG rheumatoid factor has greater specificity for major rheumatic disease, but the above caveats still remain. One situation in which a negative rheumatoid factor is of diagnostic significance is in a patient with arthritis and nodules. As a general

---

Box 19.3.2 Associations with a positive rheumatoid factor

- Rheumatoid arthritis (about 75%)
- Lupus, scleroderma, Sjögren's syndrome, dermatomyositis
- Chronic infection:
  - Bacterial endocarditis
  - Viruses (rubella, cytomegalovirus, infectious mononucleosis)
  - Parasites
- Neoplasms—after irradiation or chemotherapy
- Hyperglobulinaemic states:
  - Hypergammaglobulinaemic purpura
  - Cryoglobulinaemia
  - Chronic liver disease

Note that normal subjects can be seropositive.

Box 19.3.3 Associations with a positive antinuclear antibody

- Systemic lupus erythematosus
- Rheumatoid arthritis
- Sjögren's syndrome
- Polymyositis
- Polyarteritis nodosa
- Juvenile idiopathic arthritis
- Chronic active hepatitis
- Autoimmune thyroid disease
- Myaesthenia gravis
- Extensive burns

Note that normal subjects may be ANA positive.

---

rule all patients with nodular rheumatoid are seropositive (as are those patients who have extra-articular disease manifestations), so that in this situation other causes of 'arthritis plus nodules' must be considered—e.g. tophaceous gout or hypercholesterolaemia.

Anti-CCP antibodies

A highly specific autoantibody system has recently been described in rheumatoid arthritis in which antibodies are detected against modified arginine (citrullinated) residues. The detection of antibodies to cyclic citrullinated peptides (anti-CCPs) is a relatively new test, with good diagnostic properties (sensitivities 65–80%, specificities 89–98%), although at the moment widespread use is limited by much greater cost than rheumatoid factor. It can, however, be positive in patients who are negative for rheumatoid factor, and this is one of the clinical scenarios in which the test is most useful. Anti-CCP positivity in the setting of a patient with possible early inflammatory arthritis has prognostic significance, as it is strongly associated with progression to persistent rheumatoid disease, higher inflammatory markers and greater erosive change. Unlike rheumatoid factor, anti-CCP status is unlikely to be influenced by age, the presence of other autoimmune diseases, infection, or smoking, and therefore has a much lower false positivity rate.

Antinuclear antibody

An antinuclear antibody (ANA) is any autoantibody directed against one or more components of the nucleus. The standard method of detection is immunofluorescence microscopy after serum has been applied to a nucleated tissue substrate, usually either rodent liver, kidney, or a human cell line (e.g. HEp-2). Four main patterns of staining are reported. As with rheumatoid factor, the higher the titre of ANA the greater its significance, but a high titre does not necessarily imply more severe disease. The specificity and sensitivity also vary according to the antigen preparation used in the test system, but tests are not universally standardized and (again) liaison with the laboratory is important in order to determine the cut-off titre that is considered to be 'abnormal'. The many causes of a positive antinuclear antibody are outlined in Box 19.3.3.

The commonest reason to undertake an ANA test is in a patient with suspected lupus. For lupus, the ANA has high sensitivity (97–100%), but because the specificity is very low (10–40%), a positive result does not make the diagnosis; by contrast, a negative ANA virtually excludes it.

If a screening serum antinuclear antibody test is positive, most laboratories will then attempt to determine the specific antigenic determinants. Some of these determinants are soluble and can be extracted from the nucleus, hence 'extractable nuclear antigens' (ENAs), although many of the antigen–antibody specificities in human disease remain to be discovered. Compared with the antinuclear antibody, antibodies against specific nuclear antigens have higher specificity for certain diagnoses or for certain patterns of system involvement within the same disease. For example, antinuclear antibody directed against double-stranded DNA is highly specific for lupus but present in only a minority of patients—usually those who have more severe disease, with a greater likelihood of renal involvement, in whom the diagnosis is usually already clear. Antibodies to Sm antigen occur almost exclusively in lupus and are associated with a higher risk of renal disease. Antitopoisomerase 1 and anticentromere antibodies are found in diffuse cutaneous and limited cutaneous systemic sclerosis, respectively. Antibodies to Ro antigen occur predominantly in Sjögren's syndrome (often in combination with anti-La) and in lupus and are associated with a high frequency of photosensitive rashes and a risk of neonatal heart block. Antibodies to ribonucleoprotein (RNP) are found in lupus but are often associated with the presence of overlap connective tissue disorders that may have features of scleroderma, myositis, and rheumatoid arthritis.

The antiphospholipid syndrome (secondary APS), defined by the occurrence of arterial and venous thromboses, recurrent fetal losses, and thrombocytopenia in the presence of antiphospholipid antibodies, occurs in lupus and other autoimmune diseases and also in subjects with no other underlying disease (primary APS). Antiphospholipid antibodies can be detected in assays for anticardiolipin antibodies (predominantly directed against β2 glycoprotein 1) and in phospholipid-dependent coagulation studies to detect lupus anticoagulants (prolonged activated partial thromboplastin time (APTT) which fails to correct with the addition of normal serum). Antiphospholipid antibodies also occur in a wide variety of rheumatic, infectious (bacterial, viral, protozoal) and malignant conditions, and can also be drug induced, but in these situations they are not usually associated with thromboses.

Further information on these tests can be found in Chapters 14.14 and 19.11.2.

Tests for specific clinical situations

Chronic inflammatory disease at a single site

Patients with unexplained inflammatory disease at a single locomotor site (monoarthritis, bursitis, tenosynovitis, osteitis) should be considered for biopsy. The timing for this will vary according to how florid the lesion appears, but in general this should be undertaken for any undiagnosed lesion that has persisted for 6 months. The reason is to determine or exclude specific disease that can only be diagnosed by this means (Box 19.3.4). Although these conditions are uncommon or rare, they require a specific treatment approach, rather than a continuing empirical symptomatic one. The commonest site for unexplained inflammatory monoarthritis is the knee, followed by the wrist and small hand joints. Arthroscopic biopsy is ideally used for larger joints (for additional information from direct visualization and guided biopsy), open biopsy for smaller joints and periarticular lesions. Tissue should be examined histologically and sent for culture, including mycobacteria. Apart from the specific conditions in Box 19.3.4, histopathology has no role in the diagnosis or management of most common rheumatic disease.

Investigation of suspected muscle disease

There are three principal investigations for the diagnosis and monitoring of muscle disease: serum creatine kinase, electromyography, and muscle histology. None are 100% sensitive, hence each may be normal despite abnormality detected by one or both of the others. Although creatine kinase is the most indirect measure, it is readily available and commonly measured in the first instance. It is important to realize that elevation of the creatine kinase may result from a variety of causes (Box 19.3.5), and certain racial groups (e.g. Afro-Caribbean) have higher 'normal range' values. Electromyography or muscle biopsy will be undertaken next, the choice depending on local availability and expertise. How much information on diagnosis and disease activity has been gained from the first two tests will then often determine whether the third is also undertaken. The one used for subsequent monitoring of disease activity will be that which was most helpful in confirming the diagnosis.

> **Box 19.3.4** Causes of chronic single-site synovitis
>
> - Foreign body (e.g. plant thorn)
> - Infection, including tuberculosis, fungi
> - Sarcoidosis
> - Amyloidosis
> - Pigmented villonodular synovitis
> - Synovial chondromatosis
> - Synovial sarcoma

> **Box 19.3.5** Causes of elevation of serum creatine kinase
>
> - Inflammatory myositis ± vasculitis
> - Muscular dystrophy
> - Motor neuron disease
> - Alcohol, drugs
> - Trauma, strenuous exercise
> - Myocardial infarction
> - Hypothyroidism, metabolic myopathy
>
> Note that rhabdomyolysis is associated with massive elevation of serum creatine kinase.

Electromyography measures the action potentials produced at rest and during voluntary contraction. Normal muscle is electrically silent at rest. On slight contraction motor-unit potentials of 500 to 1000 μV in amplitude and 4 to 8 ms in duration are recorded. On maximal contraction, as many motor units as possible are recruited and an interference pattern develops. With inflammatory polymyositis the electromyography may show a diagnostic triad of:

- spontaneous fibrillation
- short-duration action potentials in a polyphasic disorganized outline
- repetitive bouts of high-voltage oscillations produced by contact of diseased muscle with the needle

Muscle histology can readily be obtained from a needle muscle biopsy sample. This is a relatively simple procedure requiring a local anaesthetic, small skin incision (no stitches required), an appropriate muscle biopsy needle, and no subsequent limitation of activity: it can easily be repeated serially for subsequent monitoring of response to treatment. The quadriceps is usually chosen, although the deltoid or other muscles can also be biopsied this way. The two or more small cores of tissue obtained need to be transported rapidly to the laboratory and correctly orientated before freezing and sectioning. Immunohistochemical staining in conjunction with plain histology gives considerable information concerning primary and secondary muscle and neuromuscular disease. Although open biopsy will yield more tissue than needle biopsy, only a small amount of muscle is actually required and serial open biopsy is clearly problematic.

If both EMG and biopsy prove negative in a patient who is strongly suspected to have muscle disease, MRI is useful to document where muscle abnormality/oedema is present in order to guide further biopsies.

For further discussion of the investigation of muscle disease, see Chapter 24.24.4.

Investigation of suspected vasculitis

The presenting features of vasculitis are usually those of vessel wall inflammation leading to ischaemia in the affected organ (e.g. upper airway, kidney, peripheral nerve, abdomen, skin), in combination with the nonspecific systemic effects of inflammation (malaise, weight loss, night sweats). These symptoms can also be produced both by severe infection and by malignancy, and in view of this—and

Table 19.3.3 Investigations to perform in multiple regional pain

Investigation	Condition
ESR/CRP	Systemic inflammation
Creatine kinase	Myositis
Antinuclear antibody	Lupus
Calcium	Parathryoid disease, osteomalacia
Thyroid function tests	Thyroid disease

CRP, C-reactive protein.

the potential toxicity of appropriate treatment—further investigation is always required. In terms of laboratory tests, simple measures such as a urine dipstick test and microscopy should not be overlooked, as the prognosis of many of these diseases is dictated by renal involvement.

ANCAs, initially detected in patients with glomerulonephritis, are antibodies directed against enzymes present in neutrophil granules. Two main patterns of immunofluorescence are detected: cytoplasmic and perinuclear. Most c-ANCAs and p-ANCAs are specific for the neutrophil enzymes proteinase 3 and myeloperoxidase, respectively. These two patterns associate with particular disease manifestations, e.g. c-ANCA with Wegener's granulomatosis and p-ANCA with microscopic polyangiitis. However, positive ANCAs occur in a variety of other settings, including malignancy and infections (bacterial and HIV) as well as other autoimmune diseases (inflammatory bowel disease, rheumatoid arthritis, lupus, pulmonary fibrosis). Equally, some patients with definite systemic vasculitis are ANCA negative, and thus diagnosis of these conditions should not be made or refuted on the ANCA test alone. Other supporting evidence should be obtained whenever possible by biopsy of an appropriate organ (nose, kidney, muscle, skin).

For further information see Chapter 20.10.2.

Investigation of multiple regional pain

In most patients who present with widespread musculoskeletal pain, the diagnosis is made from clinical examination alone, e.g. widespread rheumatoid disease. In some cases, however, there may be little to detect on clinical examination to explain the widespread pain. In most cases the diagnosis will be fibromyalgia. This is confirmed clinically by the appropriate symptoms (e.g. widespread pain, nonrestorative sleep, marked fatigue, 'tension' headache, 'irritable bowel' symptoms, anxiety and depression, poor memory and concentration, urinary frequency) and the presence of widespread hyperalgesic tender sites and negative control sites (see Chapters 19.2 and 26.5.3). However, a number of other conditions may present similarly with multiple regional symptoms and few, if any, physical findings. In this situation, a limited screen (Table 19.3.3) is justified to detect conditions for which there are specific treatments.

Further reading

Avouac J, Gossec L, Dougados M (2006). Diagnostic and predictive value of anti-cyclic citrullinated protein antibodies in rheumatoid arthritis: a systematic literature review. *Ann Rheum Dis*, **65**, 845–51.

Bosch X, Guilabert A, Font J (2006). Antineutrophil cytoplasmic antibodies. *Lancet*, **368**, 404–18.

Brower A (1997). *Arthritis in black and white*, 2nd edition. WB Saunders, Philadelphia, PA.

Gabay C, Kushner L (1999). Acute-phase proteins and other systemic responses to inflammation. *New Engl J Med*, **340**, 448–54.

McCarty DJ (1997). Synovial fluid. In: Coopman WJ (ed.) *Arthritis and allied conditions*, 13th edition, pp. 81–102. Williams and Wilkins, Maryland.

Wakefield R, Brown A, O'Connor PJ, Emery P (2003). Power Doppler sonography: improving disease activity assessment in inflammatory musculoskeletal disease. *Arthritis Rheum*, **48**, 285–8.

Back pain and regional disorders

Simon Carette

Essentials

Low back pain

Over 70% of people in industrialized countries suffer from low back pain at some time, and it is one of the leading reasons for visits to physicians. Risk factors include heavy physical work, smoking, stress, depression, and job dissatisfaction. In more than 90% of cases the exact anatomical source of back pain cannot be determined, and the preferred diagnostic label is 'nonspecific low back pain'.

'Red flags' is the term used for the presence on history of any of the following: age over 50, fever, weight loss, significant trauma, previous history of neoplasia, use of corticosteroids, drug or alcohol abuse, neurological symptoms and signs, night pain, morning stiffness, and the persistence of pain after 1 month of conservative therapy. Such red flags suggest the possibility of serious disorders, e.g. neoplasia, infection, or inflammatory spinal disease.

Investigation and management: investigation should be restricted to patients with red flags, with MRI the best imaging modality for the diagnosis of lumbar disorders. In the absence of red flags, patients with acute low back pain should be reassured and encouraged to remain active: simple analgesics, nonsteroidal anti-inflammatory drugs (NSAIDs), muscle relaxants, and spinal manipulation may help for pain relief.

The early recognition of psychosocial risk factors, or 'yellow flags', is important to identify patients who are at higher risk of progressing towards chronic low back pain. Cognitive behavioural therapy, supervised exercise therapy, brief educational interventions, multidisciplinary treatment, and short courses of manipulation/mobilization can each be recommended in patients with nonspecific chronic low back pain, but the condition is often refractory.

Other regional disorders

Neck pain—the clinical approach should follow the same principles as described for low back pain.

Regional musculoskeletal pain disorders—painful conditions affecting a specific region of the body are extremely common. Various pains have been described affecting the shoulder, elbow, wrist and hand, hip, knee, ankle, and foot regions. Most of these can usually be identified by a careful history and directed physical examination. The principles of management include temporary rest, analgesics or NSAIDs, local corticosteroid injections, thermal modalities, orthotics, and graded flexibility and strengthening exercises.

Low back pain

Low back pain is one of the commonest symptoms and was the fifth leading reason for all visits to doctors' surgeries in the United States of America in 1990. Between 60 and 80% of adults suffer from at least one episode of back pain during their lifetime. Acute back pain is usually self-limiting, and most sufferers do not seek medical advice. Of those who do, more than 90% are back to work within 2 months, independent of the treatment received, including those in whom the acute episode results from a work-related injury for which compensation might be available. The 5 to 10% of patients who remain disabled after this time are a difficult therapeutic challenge, owing to the influence of psychological and social factors on the continuation of pain. These few patients are responsible for more than 75% of the total costs of low back pain

to society, estimated to be between 1 and 2% of the gross national product in most industrialized countries.

Significant risk factors for the occurrence of back pain include older age, heavy labour (in particular jobs requiring lifting in an awkward position), lower education and income, smoking, high birth rate (in males), and obesity. Twin studies suggest that genetic factors have an important influence on the lifetime prevalence of back pain, with heritability ranging from 52 to 68%. Long-distance driving and whole-body vibration such as experienced by truck drivers are well-known risk factors for disc herniation. Previous episodes of back pain are strong predictors of recurrence. A number of psychosocial risk factors, or so-called 'yellow flags', predict poor outcomes. These include beliefs that back pain is harmful or potentially severely disabling, resulting in fear/avoidance behaviour and reduced activity levels, excessive reliance on aids and appliances, depressed mood, withdrawal from social interaction, and job dissatisfaction.

Many structures of the back, including the muscles, ligaments, discs, bones and zygapophyseal and sacroiliac joints are innervated and can therefore be a source of pain. However, in more than 90% of patients presenting with low back pain it is extremely difficult—if not impossible—to identify precisely the anatomical source of the pain on the basis of history and physical examination. These patients should be diagnosed as suffering from 'nonspecific low back pain'. A host of clinical entities such as muscle strain, degenerative disc disease, facet syndrome, myofascial pain syndrome, segmental instability, minor intervertebral displacement, iliolumbar syndrome, piriformis syndrome, etc. have been described within this broad category based on the localization of pain and tenderness, reproduction of symptoms by specific manoeuvres, radiological features, or pathophysiological hypotheses. Unfortunately, the signs and manoeuvres described for each of these clinical syndromes lack sensitivity and specificity and are not reproducible, even by experienced clinicians. Moreover, the claim that any of these entities is responsible for the pain in a given patient can very rarely be validated. For example, it is hazardous to ascribe pain to degenerative disc disease or zygapophyseal joint osteoarthritis when it has been shown that individuals with similar radiological changes can be completely asymptomatic. The only way to determine if the discs or zygapophyseal or sacroiliac joints are the source of pain in a given patient is through injection studies done under stringent, controlled conditions (see below).

Clinical approach to the diagnosis of low back pain

In evaluating a patient presenting with low back pain, the physician should not try to differentiate between the various elusive entities responsible for nonspecific back pain, but rather should focus on determining if the patient needs emergency surgery, has sciatica with signs of nerve root compression, or has an underlying medical cause of back pain (infectious, inflammatory, metabolic, tumoural or visceral) (Table 19.4.1).

Is this a surgical emergency?

Cauda equina syndrome and an expanding vascular aneurysm are two extremely rare but important conditions to recognize, because both are surgical emergencies. In the first instance, the patient will usually present with low back and/or buttock pain, associated with bilateral sciatica, neurological symptoms in the lower extremities, and urinary and/or bowel incontinence. Physical examination may show bilateral weakness, sensory losses, saddle anaesthesia, decreased reflexes in the legs, and decreased rectal tone. Diagnostic procedures (MRI, CT, or myelogram) should be performed on an emergency basis if bowel and bladder control are to be preserved. Central disc herniation is the most common cause of the syndrome, followed by tumours and epidural abscesses.

An aortic aneurysm can be responsible for a dull, gnawing back pain due to direct compression of the aneurysm on the lumbar vertebrae. They are typically seen in elderly patients, especially white men, and physical examination may reveal a pulsating abdominal mass and decreased pulses in the legs. Diagnosis is most important because rupture or dissection of the aneurysm is often fatal, the patient presenting with sudden, excruciating, tearing abdominal

Table 19.4.1 Causes of back pain

Surgical emergencies	Cauda equina syndrome (disc, tumour mass, abscess)
	Aortic aneurysm (ruptured, dissected)
Sciatica with neurological signs	Ruptured intervertebral disc
	Spinal stenosis (the neurological examination is often normal)
	Spinal cord tumours (extradural, intradural–extramedullary/intramedullary)
Medical conditions	
Neoplastic	Benign: osteoid osteoma
	Malignant: primary (multiple myeloma), secondary (metastasis)
Infectious	Acute: pyogenic discitis, osteomyelitis
	Chronic: tuberculosis
Inflammatory	Ankylosing spondylitis
	Psoriatic arthritis
	Reactive arthritis
	Inflammatory bowel diseases
Metabolic	Osteoporosis (with fractures)
	Osteomalacia
	Paget's disease of bone
Visceral	Pelvic organs (endometriosis, prostatitis)
	Renal disease (pyelonephritis, renal colic)
	Gastrointestinal (pancreatitis)
	Aortic aneurysm
Nonspecific low back pain	Muscle
	Ligaments
	Discs
	Zygapophyseal joints
	Sacroiliac joints
	Spondylolisthesis

or back pain radiating to the groin, buttocks, or thighs along with haemodynamic compromise (hypotension, tachycardia, and shock). Up to 30% of ruptured aneurysms are initially misdiagnosed. Preventive surgery (before rupture or dissection) is the optimal treatment.

Does the patient have sciatica and/or neurological signs?

Sciatica can be defined as pain radiating below the knee. It is a rare symptom, being reported by only 1% of patients with back pain, but its presence is usually associated with an identifiable aetiology. It typically results from compression of the spinal nerve originating between L4 and L5 (L5 nerve root) and/or L5 and S1 (S1 nerve root) by a herniated disc, bone, or a combination of the two (spinal stenosis). Tumours, infections, or epidural haemorrhage can very rarely produce similar symptoms and signs. The pain in a patient with a herniated disc tends to be aggravated by prolonged sitting as well as any manoeuvre that increases intrathecal pressure, such as sneezing, coughing, or defecation. It is often associated with paraesthesias and weakness in the distribution of the involved nerve.

Patients with spinal stenosis are usually older and typically complain of pain and/or paraesthesias in one or both buttocks, thighs, and/or legs that develop on standing or walking and are relieved by 15 to 20 min rest (neurological claudication). These patients often walk with the trunk flexed, as extension aggravates their symptoms by worsening nerve impingement. The neurological examination is most often normal or shows nonspecific abnormalities, such as reduced or absent ankle reflexes. Differentiating neurological from vascular claudication can be difficult, as both problems occur in the same age category, but pain from vascular claudication is typically relieved faster with rest than that of neurological claudication.

Does the patient have an underlying medical cause for their back pain?

The history is by far the most important diagnostic step in the search for potential medical causes of low back pain. A number of clues or 'red flags' should be looked for systematically. These include the presence of fever, chills, night sweats, weight loss, and nocturnal pain, which should direct the clinician towards the possibility of neoplasia or infection. An insidious onset of back pain accompanied by significant early morning stiffness in a young patient suggests a spondyloarthropathy and should prompt the clinician to enquire about the family history and undertake a detailed review of the ocular (conjunctivitis, iritis), cutaneous (psoriasis, mouth ulcers, balanitis, keratoderma blennorrhagica), gastrointestinal (diarrhoea, haematochezia, abdominal pain), genitourinary (urethritis), and musculoskeletal (peripheral arthritis, dactylitis, enthesitis, heel pain) systems. Risk factors for neoplasia (previous or current history of malignancy), infection (history of tuberculosis, AIDS, intravenous drug abuse, or recent genitourinary procedures), and metabolic bone diseases (previous fractures, menopause, corticosteroid intake, history of anorexia nervosa) should also be sought in patients suspected of having a medical problem underlying their back pain.

What are the key signs to look for in the physical examination?

A good examination of the lumbar spine and relevant nerves can be accomplished in less than 3 min if it is done systematically (Table 19.4.2). A full physical examination must be completed in patients suspected of having a medical cause for their back pain. The diagnostic utility of the many physical manoeuvres described to identify zygapophyseal and sacroiliac joint pain has been refuted when validated against diagnostic blocks with local anaesthetic. Waddell has described a number of nonorganic physical signs (Box 19.4.1): psychological factors or secondary gains may be involved when a patient has three or more of these.

Who should be investigated and how?

There is a general agreement that the initial assessment should focus on the detection of 'red flags' suggestive of a medical aetiology, and that the vast majority of patients with back pain do not need any investigations. Recommendations for ordering a plain radiograph in a patient presenting with back pain include the following: age over 50, fever, weight loss, significant trauma,

Table 19.4.2 Physical examination of the patient with back pain

Patient standing	Posture (protruding abdomen, hyperlordosis, loss of lordosis, scoliosis)
	Spinal motion (flexion–extension–lateral flexion)
	Walking on heels (L4–L5) and toes (S1)
	Squatting (L2–L3–L4)
Patient sitting	Straight leg-raising test (tripod sign)
	Knee (L4) and ankle (S1) reflexes
Patient supine	Abdominal examination (mass, bruit)
	Vascular examination
	Sensory examination:
	L4: anteromedial knee and leg
	L5: lateral leg, web space between first and second toes
	S1: lateral aspect of the foot, heel
	Motor examination (if abnormalities are noted in the standing position):
	L4: quadriceps
	L5: dorsiflexion of first toe
	S1: plantar flexion of foot and toes
	Hip examination
Patient prone	Palpation (spinous processes, paraspinal muscles)
	Sensory examination:
	S2–S4: saddle anaesthesia
	Motor examination:
	S1: contraction of gluteus maximus
	Femoral stretch test (L2 to L4)
	Sphincter tone

Box 19.4.1 Waddel's tests for functional low back pain

- Tenderness to superficial touch
- Simulation tests[a]
  - Axial loading
  - Spinal rotation in one plane
- Distraction tests
  - Inconsistent results on confirmatory testing
- Regional disturbances
  - Abnormalities not following neuroanatomical structures
- Overreaction
  - Disproportionate verbalization

[a]A positive test results in aggravation of low back pain.

previous history of neoplasia, use of corticosteroids, drug or alcohol abuse, neurological symptoms and signs (particularly if widespread), night pain, morning stiffness (in which case a pelvic rather than a lumbar radiograph is recommended to detect sacroiliitis), and the persistence of pain after 1 month of conservative therapy.

All other tests should be restricted to patients in whom a medical aetiology is suspected from the history and physical examination, and patients with abnormalities on neurological examination who do not improve with conservative management. Ordering blood tests and imaging in any other situation can not be justified, as not only are these tests unhelpful but they contribute significantly to medical costs. In addition, as many as 25 to 50% of asymptomatic individuals have been shown to have abnormalities such as disc herniation on CT and MRI.

The erythrocyte sedimentation rate (ESR) is the most useful blood test in patients suspected of having spinal infection, as it is elevated in up to 80% of cases. Neutrophilia and anaemia are also commonly seen in patients with neoplasia and infection. Laboratory evaluation of patients with osteoporosis and/or pathological fractures should include serum calcium, phosphate and alkaline phosphatase, as well as serum and urine immunoelectrophoresis (to detect myeloma), particularly if the ESR is elevated.

MRI is the imaging modality of choice for the diagnosis of lumbar disorders. It provides a unique noninvasive means of studying the spine and is unsurpassed for imaging soft tissues. It is particularly helpful in the evaluation of spinal cord tumours, as well as infections of the spine, including discitis and epidural and paraspinal abscesses. CT is superior to MRI for the evaluation of bony structures and therefore is a good choice for spinal stenosis, particularly when combined with myelography. Plain myelography is rarely used today, except in patients who have contraindications to MRI or CT (claustrophobia in particular). The diagnostic accuracy of MRI, plain CT and CT myelography is comparable for the assessment of nerve root compression due to disc herniation. Although MRI is noninvasive and involves no radiation to the patient, the much lower cost of plain CT makes it an excellent choice in this context. CT-guided percutaneous biopsy is commonly used to obtain histological material from patients with tumour mass or infection.

As mentioned previously, injection studies done under fluoroscopic guidance are the only means of diagnosing back pain of discal, zygapophyseal, or sacroiliac joint origin. When normal discs are injected with contrast material, the individual does not experience pain. A provocative discography should be considered positive only if the injection reproduces the patient's pain and no pain is experienced during the injection of adjacent discs. In a recent report, 40% of patients with chronic low back pain attending a large specialist spinal centre satisfied this strict definition and demonstrated a radial fissure on CT. Similarly, between 10 and 15% report a significant improvement in their pain when their zygapophyseal joints or their sacroiliac joints are injected with a local anaesthetic, but not with isotonic saline. Taken together, these figures suggest that the anatomical source of pain can be established in as many as 70% of patients with nonspecific back pain by using these invasive techniques. However, the impact of this approach on patient management is unclear, as no specific treatment has yet been demonstrated to be effective for these conditions.

Radionuclide bone scintigraphy with technetium-99m is helpful in conditions characterized by increased bone turnover. These include bone metastases, fracture, Paget's disease, and infections. Gallium-67 binds to polymorphonuclear leucocytes and can be helpful in the evaluation of vertebral osteomyelitis and sacroiliac septic arthritis. Typically, bone scans are negative in patients with multiple myeloma, which is characterized by lytic lesions.

Neurophysiological studies are rarely indicated, except in patients in whom it is difficult to distinguish between a neuropathy, radiculopathy, or plexopathy. Fibrillations in the paraspinous muscles are the most common and earliest findings seen in radiculopathy. Their presence indicates a lesion proximal to the vertebral foramen and excludes a plexopathy.

How are patients with low back pain best managed?

Surgical emergencies

As mentioned earlier, cauda equina syndrome and a ruptured vascular aneurysm are the only two conditions that must be managed surgically on an emergency basis.

Sciatica and neurological deficits

About 90% of patients with a herniated lumbar disc will improve significantly with limited rest, analgesics and anti-inflammatory drugs. The role of epidural steroids remains unclear: they may afford short-term improvement in leg pain, but they do not reduce the need for surgery. Indications for surgery include persistent disabling buttock and/or leg pain despite 2 to 3 months of conservative management, and/or severe or progressive worsening neurological deficit while on treatment. Surgery may also be indicated in patients with neurological claudication due to spinal stenosis, but only after all attempts with conservative management have failed. Patients with spinal stenosis who are more incapacitated by back pain than by neurological claudication should probably not be operated on, because surgery is rarely effective and may even worsen back pain.

Medical back pain

Primary and secondary tumours of the spine can be treated by surgery, radiotherapy, or chemotherapy, whereas antibiotics with or without surgical drainage are the treatment for discitis and osteomyelitis. Postural exercises and nonsteroidal anti-inflammatory drugs (NSAIDs) remain the cornerstone of treatment for patients with spondyloarthropathies. Sulfasalazine and methotrexate are helpful for the peripheral arthritis associated with these conditions, but they have no role in the treatment of the spinal disease. Biological agents—including etanercept, infliximab, and adalimumab—are the drugs of choice in patients with spinal disease associated with spondyloarthropathies who fail NSAIDs. The treatment of metabolic bone diseases is discussed in Chapters 20.1 and 20.4.

Nonspecific low back pain

A number of systematic reviews of randomized controlled trials of the most common interventions have been published and form the basis of the recommendations found in the many national guidelines published in the past two decades. The European guidelines for the management of low back pain are the most recently published (2006). They were developed with the main objectives of improving prevention and management of acute and chronic nonspecific low back pain.

Patients with acute back pain should be reassured and advised to stay active and continue normal daily activities, including work if possible. If necessary, medications for pain relief, including paracetamol and NSAIDs, should be prescribed and preferably taken at regular intervals. A short course of muscle relaxants to reduce pain may be tried in patients failing paracetamol or NSAIDs, and referral for spinal manipulation should be considered in patients failing to return to normal activities. Exercise therapy is ineffective in the acute phase but should be recommended for prevention of recurrence.

An important objective in managing acute low back pain is to reduce the likelihood of patients progressing to chronicity, not least because there are only a few modalities that have been shown to be beneficial in chronic back pain. The early identification of psychosocial risk factors, or 'yellow flags', should lead to appropriate cognitive and behavioural management in an attempt to influence positively some of these factors, although evidence of the effectiveness of this approach or of other psychosocial interventions at this stage is currently lacking.

In patients with chronic low back pain, cognitive behavioural therapy, supervised exercise therapy, brief educational interventions and multidisciplinary (biopsychosocial) treatment can each be recommended, and so can the short-term use of NSAIDs and weak opioids for pain relief. Noradrenergic or noradrenergic–serotoninergic antidepressants, muscle relaxants and capsicum plasters may also be considered for pain relief. Invasive treatments, including acupuncture, epidural corticosteroids, intra-articular steroid injections and local facet nerve blocks, intradiscal injections, and prolotherapy are not recommended. Surgery should be considered only in carefully selected patients with a maximum of two level degenerative disc disease who have failed 2 years of all previously recommended treatments.

Neck pain

Neck pain is a very common symptom. In a recent large epidemiological survey from Norway, 34.4% of adult respondents reported troublesome neck pain in the previous year, with 13.8% reporting pain lasting more than 6 months. As for low back pain, neck pain can rarely be attributed to a specific anatomical source, and most patients presenting with this symptom should be diagnosed as suffering from 'nonspecific neck pain' or 'cervical spinal pain of unknown origin', rather than applying nonvalidated diagnostic labels. Trauma, in particular acceleration–deceleration (whiplash) injuries, increasing age, lower education, and psychosocial factors are the most common risk factors associated with the development of neck pain.

The clinical approach to the patient with neck pain should follow the same principles as described for low back pain. Signs of nerve root and/or spinal cord compression should always be looked for, particularly in patients complaining of associated pain, numbness, or weakness in their arms or legs. Older patients with cervical spinal stenosis due to severe osteoarthritis may present with wasting and lower motor neuron weakness in the arms or hands and spastic weakness and sensory disturbance in the legs.

A number of diseases of the pharynx (pharyngitis, retropharyngeal abscess), larynx (laryngitis), trachea (tracheitis), thyroid (acute thyroiditis), lymph nodes (lymphadenitis), carotids (carotidynia), lungs (Pancoast tumour), heart (myocardial infarction), pericardium (pericarditis), aorta (dissecting aneurysm), and diaphragm (subphrenic abscess) can refer pain to the neck and should be considered.

These conditions will usually have other clinical manifestations to alert the physician to the proper diagnosis. The neoplastic, infectious, inflammatory, and metabolic conditions enumerated in Table 19.4.1 can also affect the cervical spine. In addition, rheumatoid arthritis and diffuse idiopathic skeletal hyperostosis should be considered in the differential diagnosis, as both can involve the cervical spine and cause spinal cord compression.

A special task force proposed a classification of cervical disorders associated with whiplash injury that takes into account both the severity and duration of symptoms (Table 19.4.3). Although specifically designed to address problems related to whiplash injuries, it can be very useful in classifying and guiding management of patients presenting with nonspecific neck pain unrelated to trauma.

Investigation of patients with neck pain—who and how?

Guidelines are only available for patients presenting with whiplash injuries. Patients with grade I whiplash-associated disorder do not usually require radiographic evaluation. Those with grade II to IV whiplash-associated disorder need a baseline radiological examination consisting of plain films with anteroposterior, lateral, and open-mouth views. Radiographs are usually unhelpful in patients with nonspecific neck pain. Degenerative changes in the discs and zygapophyseal joints increase with age and do not correlate with symptoms of neck pain. CT is helpful for evaluating the bony structures of the neck, but it must be combined with myelography to adequately visualize the neural tissues. MRI is therefore preferred in most cases with spinal cord or nerve root compromise. Fifty per cent of patients with chronic neck pain after motor vehicle accidents respond to diagnostic zygapophyseal joint injection, suggesting that these joints are responsible for their pain.

Management of patients with neck pain

Most treatments recommended for the management of patients with neck pain have not been evaluated in a scientifically rigorous manner. Those that have been have shown very little, if any, evidence of efficacy. These include soft cervical collars, zygapophyseal joint injections and acupuncture. Patients with acute neck pain should be encouraged to maintain their usual level of activity. There is evidence that non-narcotic analgesics, NSAIDs, mobilization, and manipulation are effective, whereas the promotion of rest

Table 19.4.3 Classification of whiplash-associated disorders

Grade	Clinical presentation
I	Neck complaint of pain, stiffness, or tenderness only; no physical signs
II	Neck complaint and musculoskeletal signs[a]
III	Neck complaint and neurological signs[b]
IV	Neck complaint and fracture or dislocation

Acute, less than 4 days and 4 to 21 days; subacute, 22 to 45 days and 46 to 180 days; chronic, more than 180 days.
Symptoms and disorders that can manifest in all grades include deafness, dizziness, tinnitus, headache, memory loss, dysphagia, and temporomandibular joint pain.
[a] Musculoskeletal signs include decreased range of motion and point tenderness.
[b] Neurological signs include decreased or absent deep tendon reflexes, weakness, and sensory deficits. Adapted from Spitzer et al. Scientific monograph of the Quebec Task Force on Whiplash-Associated Disorders (WAD): Redefining "whiplash" and its management. Spine 1995. 20 (supp) pS1–73. With permission from Lippincott Williams and Wilkins.

Table 19.4.4 Regional pain disorders

Diagnosis	Epidemiology	Clinical symptoms	Physical examination	Associations	Investigations	Treatment
Shoulder region						
Rotator cuff tendinitis	Any age	Pain maximum in the deltoid region; increased at night and by specific movements	Painful arc of abduction 60–120 degrees. Full passive movements; pain aggravated by resisted movement of the involved tendon. Positive impingement signs	DM, repetitive movements	Radiograph in chronic cases may show cysts and sclerosis of greater tuberosity	NSAIDs, steroid injection, physio
Calcific tendinitis	Age 20–60	Acute severe pain on the tip of the shoulder	Limitation of both active and passive movements by pain. Occasional swelling when bursa involved		Calcification on radiograph	Rest in sling, NSAIDs, ?steroid injection
Adhesive capsulitis	Age > 40	Diffuse pain in the shoulder area. Progressive restriction of movements	Limitation of both active and passive movements in all directions (external rotation-abduction internal rotation)	DM, MI stroke, thyroid and pulmonary diseases	Arthrography	NSAIDs, steroid injection, physiotherapy, ?distension
Bicipital tendinitis	Very rare in isolation	Pain anterior aspect of the shoulder and deltoid region	Speed's* and Yerganson's† manoeuvres non-specific	Rotator cuff tendinitis	None	NSAIDs, steroid injection
Rotator cuff rupture	Age > 40	Sudden pain deltoid area	Weakness of abduction if complete tear		US, arthrography, MRI	Surgery if acute and patient <65, NSAIDs physio otherwise
Elbow region						
Lateral epicondylitis	Age 40–60	Pain lateral epicondyle; may spread up and down the arm	Tenderness lateral epicondyle; increased by resisted extension of the wrist	Over use		NSAIDs, physio, steroid injection
Medial epicondylitis	15 times rarer than lateral epicondylitis	Pain medial epicondyle	Tenderness medial epicondyle; increased by resisted flexion of the wrist	Over use		NSAIDs, physio, steroid injection
Olecranon bursitis		Swelling ± pain olecranon bursa	Swelling ± erythema ± tenderness	Trauma, RA, gout	Bursal aspiration: cell count, Gram stain, culture, crystals	NSAIDs, steroid injection, antibiotics if septic
Wrist and hand region						
DeQuervain tenosynovitis	Women, age 30–50	Pain radial aspect of wrist and thumb base during pinching	Tenderness ± swelling abd.pollongus. Finkelstein manoeuvre‡ +			NSAIDs, splinting, steroid injection
Trigger finger	Any age	Pain palm of hand; snapping finger	Tenderness ± swelling ± nodule flexor tendon	Diabetes, RA		NSAIDs, steroid injection
Dupuytren's contracture	Males, age 40–80	Flexion contracture of 4th and 5th fingers	Thickening palmar aponeurosis	Alcohol, liver disease, DM		?Steroid injection

Hip region

Trochanteric bursitis	Women, age 40–70	Pain lateral aspect of hip and thigh; worse at night; increased by lateral decubitus	Tenderness greater trochanter	Hip OA, obesity		NSAIDs, steroid injection

Knee region

Prepatellar bursitis	Women	Swelling ± pain anterior aspect of knee	Tenderness greater trochanter	Kneeling	Synovial fluid aspiration	NSAIDs, steroid injection
Patello-femoral syndrome	Age 15–40	Pain anterior knee, increased in stairs and by squatting	Tenderness patella ± patellofemoral crepitus			?NSAIDs, exercises
Anserine bursitis	Women, age 40–60	Pain medial aspect upper tibia	Tenderness medial aspect of tibia	Knee OA, obesity		Rest, NSAIDs, steroid injection
Popliteal cyst	Any age	Pain, stiffness, swelling posterior knee	Swelling posterior knee. Leg swelling if rupture	Inflammatory arthritis		Steroid injection

Ankle and feet

Achilles tendinitis	Age 20–50	Pain over Achilles tendon	Tenderness ± swelling ± crepitus over Achilles tendon	Spondylarthrcpathies		Rest, NSAIDs
Plantar fasciitis		Pain plantar aspect foot	Tenderness heel, increased by passive flexion of the toes	Spondylarthrcpathies		Orthotics; weight reduction; steroid injection
Morton's neuroma	Women, age 40–60	Burning pain interdigital clefts increased by walking	Tenderness interdigital cleft; rarely sensory alteration, cleft 4th toe	Pes planus, pes cavus, tight shoes		Proper shoes, surgery

*Speed's manoeuvre: the examiner resists shoulder forward flexion while the patient's arm is held in extension and supination. A positive test causes pain in the bicipital groove.
†Yergason's test: the patient's elbow is flexed to 90 degrees and the forearm pronated. The examiner resists the patient's attempts to flex and supinate the forearm. A positive test causes pain in the bicipital groove.
‡Finkelstein's manoeuvre: the patient's thumb is flexed inside the fingers and the wrist is passively deviated in an ulnar direction. A positive test results ir pain over the abductor pollicis longus and extensor pollicis brevis tendons at the wrist.

Abbreviations: DM, diabetes mellitus; NSAIDs, non-steroidal anti-inflammatory drugs; physio, physiotherapy; MI, myocardial infarction; US, ultrasonography; MRI, magnetic resonance imaging; RA, rheumatoid arthritis; OA, osteoarthritis.
Adapted from Spitzer et al. Scientific monograph of the Quebec Task Force on Whiplash-Associated Disorders (WAD): Redefining "whiplash" and its management. Spine 1995. 20 (supp) pS1–73. With permission from Lippincott Williams and Wilkins.

NB: For internet usage, a link must be included to the LWW website: http://lww.com

and soft collars tends to prolong disability. Surgery is indicated only for patients with severe radiculopathy not responsive to 6 to 12 weeks of conservative management.

There is no consensus as to how best to manage patients with chronic neck pain.

Regional pain disorders

Regional musculoskeletal pain disorders, defined as painful conditions in a specific region of the body, are extremely common. A number of clinical entities have been described for the shoulder, elbow, wrist and hand, hip, knee, ankle, and foot regions (Table 19.4.4). Most of these can usually be identified by a careful history and directed physical examination, although recent research indicates that interobserver diagnostic agreement is only moderate for the conditions related to the shoulder region, particularly in patients complaining of severe or chronic pain, and those with bilateral involvement. Investigations are not usually required for the diagnosis of most regional pain disorders.

In a patient presenting with regional pain, one should aim to determine whether the pain has its origin in the bones and joints, periarticular soft tissues (tendons, bursa, and fascia), nerve roots and peripheral nerves, or blood vessels, or if it is referred from distant musculoskeletal or visceral structures. Lesions of the periarticular soft tissues account for most causes of regional pain disorders. Plain radiographs are helpful in delineating soft tissue calcification that may or may not be related to the pain presented by the patient. Ultrasonography and MRI are of equal value in confirming a diagnosis of tendon rupture in the shoulder, knee, or ankle regions.

The principles of management include temporary rest, analgesics or NSAIDs, local corticosteroid injections, thermal modalities, orthotics, and graded flexibility and strengthening exercises.

Diffuse musculoskeletal pain

Between 8 and 10% of adults report suffering from chronic diffuse musculoskeletal pain, and about half of these satisfy the classification criteria for fibromyalgia. The aetiology of fibromyalgia is unknown, but recent data indicate that psychological distress is a strong predictor of the development of this condition. Although the pain is felt primarily in the muscles, the muscles show no histological or metabolic abnormalities other than those associated with physical deconditioning. Management that includes patient education, cognitive-behavioural approaches, regular aerobic training, and low-dose tricyclic agents generally provides benefit only to few patients. For further discussion see Chapters 19.2 and 26.5.3.

Further reading

Airaksinen O, et al. (2006). Chapter 4. European guidelines for the management of chronic nonspecific low back pain. *Eur Spine J*, **15** (Suppl. 2), S192–300.

Burton AK, et al. (2006). Chapter 2. European guidelines for prevention in low back pain. *Eur Spine J*, **15** (Suppl. 2), S136–68.

Carette S, Fehlings MG (2005). Cervical radiculopathy. *New Engl J Med*, **353**, 392–9.

Gupta A, et al. (2006). The role of psychosocial factors in predicting the onset of chronic widespread pain: results from a prospective population-based study. *Rheumatology*, **46**, 666–71.

Linton SJ, Halldén K (1998). Can we screen for problematic back pain? A screening questionnaire for predicting outcome in acute and subacute back pain. *Clin J Pain*, **14**, 209–15.

Loney PL, Stratford PW (1999). The prevalence of low back pain in adults: a methodological review of the literature. *Phys Ther*, **79**, 384–96.

MacGregor AJ, et al. (2004). Structural, psychological, and genetic influences on low back and neck pain: a study of adult female twins. *Arthritis Rheum*, **51**, 160–7.

Mease P (2005). Fibromyalgia syndrome: review of clinical presentation, pathogenesis, outcome measures and treatment. *J Rheumatol Suppl* **75**, 6–21.

Manek NJ, MacGregor AJ (2005). Epidemiology of back disorders: prevalence, risk factors, and prognosis. *Curr Opin Rheumatol*, **17**, 134–40.

Schwarzer AC, et al. (1994). The relative contributions of the disc and zygapophyseal joint in chronic low back pain. *Spine*, **19**, 801–6.

Schwarzer AC, et al. (1995). The prevalence and clinical features of internal disc disruption in patients with chronic low back pain. *Spine* **20**, 1878–83.

Schwarzer AC, Aprill CN, Bogduk N (1995). The sacroiliac joint in chronic low back pain. *Spine* **20**, 31–7.

Spitzer WO et al. (1995). Scientific monograph of the Quebec Task Force on Whiplash-associated Disorders: redefining 'whiplash' and its management. *Spine* **20** (Suppl. 8), S1–73.

Van Tulder M, et al. (2006). Chapter 3. European guidelines for the management of acute nonspecific low back pain in primary care. *Eur Spine J*, **15** (Suppl 2), S169–91.

Winters ME, Kluetz P, Zilberstein J (2006). Back pain emergencies. *Med Clin North Am*, **90**, 505–23.

19.5

Rheumatoid arthritis

Ravinder Nath Maini

Essentials

Rheumatoid arthritis is a common, painful, and disabling disease affecting 0.8 to 1.0% of the adult population worldwide, with a female:male ratio of 3:1.

Clinical features

The predominant feature of the disease is a deforming and destructive polyarthritis, with (less commonly) extra-articular manifestations such as subcutaneous nodule formation, serositis, vasculitis, fibrosing alveolitis, amyloidosis, and Felty's syndrome. Patients also exhibit systemic features of inflammation, including fatigue, anaemia, weight loss, a raised ESR, and elevated concentrations of acute phase proteins.

Severe disease is associated with comorbidities including cardiovascular disease, serious infections, and B-cell lymphomas; although iatrogenic factors are contributory factors to some or all of these, there is good evidence that endogenous mechanisms involved in rheumatoid disease also play an important part. Severe disease is a cause of premature death.

Aetiology, pathogenesis, and diagnosis

Aetiology is multifactorial, with a role for genetic factors, such as HLA DR genes coding a pentapeptide sequence in the antigen-binding region, and PTDN22, a signalling molecule in T cells. Genetic factors interact with environmental and host factors, including smoking and sex hormones, and initiate a biological response to an unidentified trigger that results in the recruitment of cells derived from the bone marrow into the joints and other sites of disease, where a chronic immune-inflammatory reaction ensues. Production by B cells of autoantibodies, such as rheumatoid factors and antibodies to citrullinated peptides, as well as interactions between activated T cells and monocyte-macrophages and synoviocytes mediated by cell contact and cytokines, sustain and amplify the inflammatory reaction. Invasion and enzymatic degradation of cartilage by synoviocytes and of bone by osteoclasts follows and leads to irreversible structural damage and joint failure.

Diagnostic features include: (1) the presence for at least 6 weeks of an observable symmetrical, soft tissue swelling of three or more joints, which usually include metacarpophalangeal, interphalangeal, or wrist joints; (2) stiffness of joints in the morning for more than 1h; (3) subcutaneous nodules; (4) the presence of IgM rheumatoid factor and/or anticitrullinated protein antibody (ACPA); and (5) radiographic erosions and/or osteopenia of bones in the hand. Diagnostic specificity increases with the presence of increasing numbers of these features.

Prognosis and management

The disease follows a relentless progressive course of variable trajectory in individual patients if untreated. Symptoms, signs, laboratory tests, and imaging are used to monitor inflammatory disease activity, damage to joints, and extra-articular disease.

Mild disease—is treated with judicious use of analgesics and nonsteroidal anti-inflammatory drugs (NSAIDs). Corticosteroid injections into individual affected joints, tendon sheaths, and bursas for persistent swelling, tenderness, or loss of normal range of movement can be very effective.

Moderate or severe disease—this occurs when there is an unremitting pattern of polyarthritis with evidence of significant functional impairment and joint damage in early stages of presentation. In these circumstances, the aim of drug treatment is to achieve rapid control of disease activity and, if possible, remission. This usually requires simultaneous or sequential use of NSAIDs, disease-modifying antirheumatic drugs (DMARDs), corticosteroids, and biological therapies.

(1) NSAIDs are used at optimal doses for control of pain and stiffness, with naproxen, low-dose celecoxib, and low-dose ibuprofen being relatively free of cardiovascular risk. These alleviate symptoms and signs of inflammation but have no effect on preventing structural damage.

(2) DMARDs should be used in all patients with moderate or severe disease. The two most commonly employed are sulfasalazine and methotrexate, the latter being the drug of choice in most centres because of its efficacy and superior effect in the long term. Methotrexate can be used alone or concomitantly with other traditional DMARDs or anti-tumour necrosis factor (anti-TNF) drugs.

(3) Corticosteroids are required in practice in over 50% of patients with moderate or severe disease. If continuing long-term use appears necessary, the aim should be to reduce the dose to the equivalent of 5 to 7.5 mg of prednisolone daily by more aggressive use of DMARDs or instigation of anti-TNF therapy.

(4) Biological monoclonal antibody and recombinant protein drugs that have proved efficacious in rheumatoid arthritis include: (a) three anti-TNF drugs (two monoclonal antibodies, infliximab and adalimumab, and etanercept, a TNF receptor fused to Fc IgG); (b) an interleukin-1 receptor antagonist (anakinra); (c) an anti-CD20 B-cell-depleting monoclonal antibody (rituximab); and (d) CTLA4-Ig, a receptor-fusion-FcIgG recombinant protein (abatacept). Anti-TNF therapy should ideally be instituted as soon as it becomes apparent that remission or near-remission is not induced by the best use of traditional DMARDs in the early stages of an established diagnosis, but cost constraints or safety concerns may limit the institution of this therapeutic approach.

Systemic rheumatoid vasculitis is potentially a life-threatening complication: therapy with high-dose corticosteroids and cyclophosphamide is favoured by many specialists.

Long-term outcome: with a holistic approach, judicious use of drugs and nonpharmacological measures such as patient education, physiotherapy, aids, appliances, and surgical treatment, mobility and pain-free quality of life can be maintained in most patients for many years. Effective control of disease prevents progressive disability, comorbidity, and premature death. The goal of reliable cure of disease has not yet been achieved.

Historical background

The first clinical description of rheumatoid arthritis (RA) in the medical literature is generally accorded to Landry-Beavais (1800), although Garrod was the first to use the term in his book published in 1859. Whether RA existed in western Europe in ancient times is debated by scholars of medical history: descriptions of chronic deforming arthritis suggestive of RA in classical writings of Galen and others have, for example, been ascribed to chronic polyarticular gout. The suggestion has been made that RA was imported to Europe after the discovery of the New World in the 15th century, where it pre-existed, as evidenced by examination of clusters of archaic Amerindian skeletal remains. The possibility that RA spread from the New World in modern times is not only of historical interest but has also led to speculation suggesting the importance of environmental factors in its causation.

The concept of RA as a disease entity continues to evolve with advances in knowledge of the multiple causes of chronic inflammatory joint diseases. Thus, improved microbiological, immunological, and epidemiological methods have led to a reclassification of certain forms of chronic arthritis, which in the past may have been labelled as RA. These include arthritis caused by infections, such as rubella, parvovirus, and borrelia (Lyme disease), or resulting from biological responses to nonviable products of microorganisms (reactive arthritis) such as yersinia, salmonella, and chlamydia. Diseases of uncertain aetiology, e.g. the spondyloarthropathies, sarcoidosis, and chronic arthritis associated with systemic lupus erythematosus (SLE), primary Sjögren's syndrome, and other connective tissue diseases, have all been recognized as distinct from RA in the relatively recent past.

Definition

RA is a chronic systemic inflammatory disorder characterized by deforming symmetrical polyarthritis of varying extent and severity, associated with synovitis of joint and tendon sheaths, articular cartilage loss, erosion of juxta-articular bone, osteopenia, and—in most patients—the presence of IgM rheumatoid factor and/or anticitrullinated protein antibodies (ACPAs) in the blood. In some patients systemic and extra-articular features may be observed during the course of the disease, and rarely before joint disease. These include anaemia, weight loss, vasculitis, serositis, mononeuritis multiplex, interstitial inflammation in lungs and exocrine salivary and lacrimal glands, as well as nodules in subcutaneous, pulmonary, and scleral tissues.

The American College of Rheumatology (ACR) has developed and revised criteria for the classification of RA based on a hospital population of patients with established active disease (Box 19.5.1). These criteria distinguish active RA from other forms of inflammatory arthritis, with a diagnostic sensitivity and specificity of about 90%. However, they are of less value in prevalence studies, which should include patients with inactive RA.

The classification criteria are too restrictive to diagnose RA reliably early in its presentation, as not all the required features may be present at this stage. Moreover, a few patients presenting with polyarthritis may later differentiate into other disease types or follow a self-limiting course.

Box 19.5.1 American College of Rheumatology criteria for the classification of rheumatoid arthritis

Criteria 1 to 4 of at least 6 weeks' duration. Rheumatoid arthritis is defined by the presence of four or more criteria.

1 Morning stiffness in and around joints for at least 1 h

2 Soft tissue swelling of three or more joints observed by a physician

3 Swelling (arthritis) of proximal interphalangeal, metacarpophalangeal, or wrist joints

4 Symmetrical swelling of joints

5 Subcutaneous rheumatoid nodules

6 Presence of IgM rheumatoid factor in abnormal amounts

7 Radiographic erosions and/or periarticular osteopenia in hand and/or wrist joints

From Arnett FC, *et al.* (1988). The American Rheumatism Association 1987 revised criteria for the classification of rheumatoid arthritis. *Arthritis Rheum*, **31**, 315–34. © 1988. Reprinted with permission of John Wiley and Sons Inc.

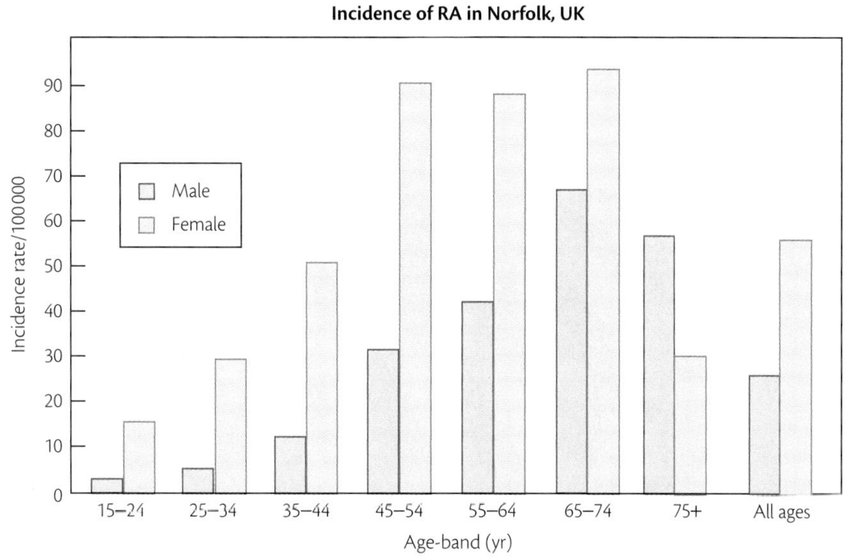

Incidence of RA in Norfolk, UK

Fig. 19.5.1 Age-specific incidence applying modified ACR criteria for rheumatoid arthritis in a United Kingdom population registered in 1990 in whom multiple assessments were made over a 5-year period. Any one of seven criteria may be positive only once during this period. Data from: Wiles N et al. (1999) Arthritis and Rheumatism 42, 1339–46, with permission.

Epidemiology

Criteria and methods for diagnosis of RA have varied in different epidemiological studies: some have been based on retrospective analysis of hospital records and others on prospective observation of patients attending hospitals where clinical examination, rheumatoid factor tests, and radiography have been employed. However, in recent years the more widespread use of ACR criteria, including a version with a modified format for use in population studies, has introduced a measure of standardization.

Given the inherent variability in the methodology employed, it is not surprising that estimates of the incidence of RA in the United States of America and Europe vary. In a study in the United Kingdom the incidence was 54 per 100 000 in women and 24.5 per 100 000 in men. The incidence increases sharply from the age of 18 to a maximum in women over the age of 45, and in men continues to rise into the seventh decade (Fig. 19.5.1). A declining trend in the incidence of RA among women has been observed in recent years.

The prevalence of RA has been consistently assessed as being between 0.8 and 1.1% of the adult population in cross-sectional studies in the United States of America and western Europe, with a female:male ratio of 3:1 and higher prevalence rates in older people. Lower rates of 0.2 to 0.3% have been reported in China and Japan. The prevalence of RA among the black population is low in rural South Africa (c.0.2%) and it is virtually nonexistent in parts of Nigeria. By contrast, prevalence rates of almost 1% have been observed in black populations in urban South Africa and in the United States of America. A strikingly high prevalence rate of over 5% has been noted among certain American Indian tribes in the United States of America, e.g. the Pima and Chippewa Indians. Differences in both genetic and environmental factors are likely to impact on these variations in incidence and prevalence rates, as are differing access to medical facilities, population age structures, and mortality.

Aetiology

Genetic factors

The initiating cause of RA remains unknown. A prevalence of 12 to 15% in genetically identical (monozygotic) twins observed in Finland and the United Kingdom, compared with 4% in nonidentical (dizygotic) twins, and between 0.5 to 1% in the general population, strongly favours multigenic influences. It also argues for an environmental trigger. Genetic factors are estimated to contribute around 60% of the liability to disease.

Genotyping confirms an association between the occurrence of RA and allelic polymorphisms of genes on the short arm of chromosome 6 that code for a hypervariable region of the β chain of HLA DR molecules. The critical expressed pentapeptide sequence (glutamine–arginine or lysine–arginine–alanine–alanine) of amino acid residues 70 to 74 has been located to the helical wall of the antigen-binding cleft of the HLA DR β chain by molecular structural studies (Fig. 19.5.2). This pentapeptide region is also referred to as the 'shared epitope' because of its detection by a specific monoclonal antibody. The sequence is present, e.g., on HLA DR4 subtypes Dw4 and Dw14, and HLA DR1 subtype Dw1, coded by DRB1*0401, *0404, and *0101 genes, respectively. The shared sequence and corresponding allelic genes have been detected in a frequency of up to 90% in patients with RA of western European descent. Their association with RA supports the hypothesis that these particular HLA DR molecules present antigens to T-cell receptors and activate pathogenic reactions.

By contrast, HLA DR4 subtypes, of which Dw10 and Dw13 are examples (coded by DRB1*0402 and *0403 genes, respectively), are negatively associated with RA. These subtypes are characterized by a substitution of the basic amino acids glutamine and arginine in positions 70 and 71 by acidic amino acids aspartic and glutamic acid. These alterations are sufficient to alter the specificity of binding such that a different set of antigens binds to the HLA cleft. Another possibility is that specific shared epitope sequences influence T-cell receptor interactions with the HLA-DR β chain α-helix independently of peptide. It is proposed that under these circumstances, signals delivered to T cells lead to the activation of regulatory pathways that elicit a protective response.

It is suggested that major histocompatibility (MHC) genes exert a major influence in the genetic component of susceptibility to RA. However, the presence of DRB1*04 susceptibility genes also correlates with seropositive, erosive, and extra-articular disease. Homozygosity for DRB1*0401 or DRB1*0404, or when they are

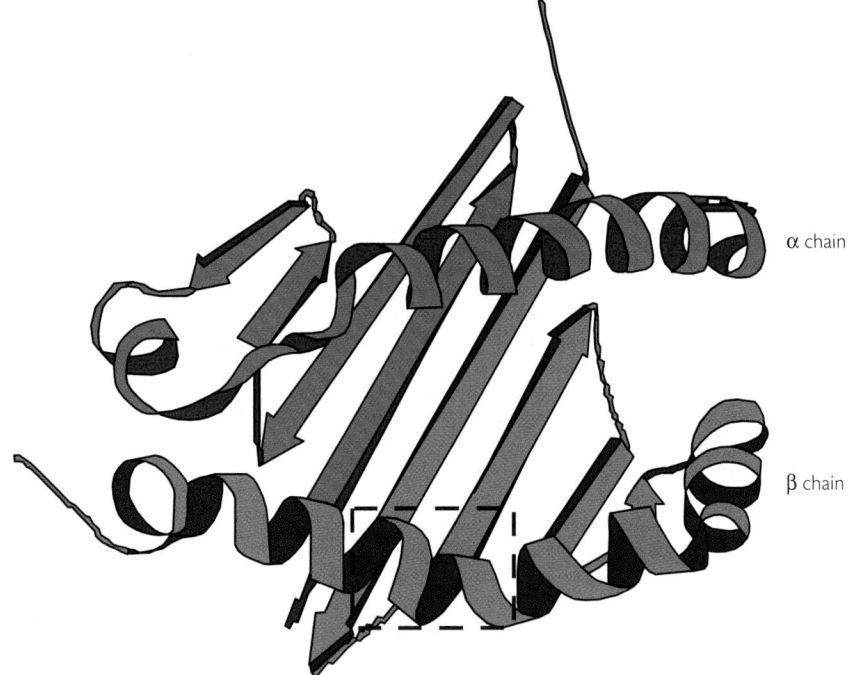

α chain

β chain

Fig. 19.5.2 Ribbon diagram of HLA class II molecule, demonstrating the antigen-binding cleft. The floor consists of a β pleated sheet and the walls are helical structures. The rectangle delineates the hypervariable region of the β chain containing the shared epitope (amino acid residues 70–74).

combined with each other or with *DRB1*0101* (as compound homozygotes), appears to correlate with more severe disease. These data have been interpreted as indicating that the shared epitope-encoding genes may be more useful as markers of disease severity in established RA, rather than as markers of disease susceptibility.

It is intriguing to note that the *HLA DRB1* allele **0405*—coding the shared epitope in a different HLA DR4, Dw15 subtype—is increased in Japanese patients, whereas the *DRB1*1402* gene coding HLA DR6, Dw16 is increased in Yakima American Indians. However, other population studies, e.g. in black Americans with RA, show no increase in frequency of the gene coding the shared epitope, thus casting some doubt on the hypothesis that it is an essential aetiological factor.

Recent studies have sought positive or negative correlations between susceptibility or disease severity and non-HLA gene polymorphisms detected by genome-wide screens and single nucleotide sequencing. Associations with polymorphic alleles of candidate genes have been described, and a single nucleotide polymorphism (SNP) of a protein tyrosine phosphatase-22 (*PTPN22*) gene has now been confirmed in several studies as being associated with rheumatoid-factor-positive RA. PTPN22 is expressed by haemopoietic cells and encodes a cytoplasmic signalling tyrosine phosphatase in T cells, thus supporting the concept that the gene product may be implicated in T-cell-mediated pathogenesis of RA. SNPs of cytokines and receptors that positively or negatively regulate inflammation, such as the promoter region of tumour necrosis factor α (TNFα) and its type II receptor, interleukin 10 (IL-10), and IL-4 receptor (IL-4R) have also been described in severe subtypes of RA but need confirmation. In Japanese but not in white populations, an increased susceptibility to RA is associated with genetic polymorphism of peptidylarginine deiminase-14 (PAD14), an enzyme that citrullinates proteins. This is of interest, as antibodies to citrullinated proteins occur in RA patients with high specificity.

Environmental factors

Infectious agents such as rubella, parvovirus B19, and Epstein–Barr virus (EBV) have been implicated in initiating rheumatoid disease. One study, for example, described the parvovirus B19 antigen VP-1 as being expressed in active lesions in synovium with RA, but not in osteoarthritis or controls. An increase in EBV-viral DNA load and isolation of rubella virus or sequences has been described in synovial cells from rheumatoid patients. In other studies, EBV-specific or rubella-specific lymphocytes have been detected in joints with RA. However, the arthritis caused by such known infections is almost always sporadic and self-limiting, and the clustering of new cases that one might expect if RA was an infectious disease caused by an unknown virus has not been reported. Moreover, corroboration of claims by independent studies is still lacking; hence these theories of causation remain speculative.

In attempts to define a role for environmental factors in the aetiology of RA, epidemiological studies have sought differences in the incidence or prevalence of the disease in genetically similar populations exposed to urbanization, different socioeconomic conditions, lifestyles, and known industrial noxious agents. Some differences have been found in genetically homogeneous populations exposed to urbanization, as well as exposure to silica dust, organic solvents, and mineral oils. A gene–environment interaction is strongly suggested by a study from Sweden showing that the risk of RA with smoking is associated with the occurrence of rheumatoid factors and antibodies to citrullinated proteins in the presence of the HLA DR shared epitope. However, the link between smoking and the shared epitope did not extend to the presence of rheumatoid factor in the absence of antibodies to citrullinated proteins. It is therefore proposed that the HLA DR shared-epitope gene, in a dose-dependent manner, primarily determines risk in ACPA-positive, but not antibody-negative, RA.

It is possible that a decline in the incidence of RA among women noted in Rochester, United States of America, in the period 1950 to

1975, and in a general practice register in the United Kingdom in the decade following 1976, are indicative of a change in environmental pressures or in lifestyle.

Host factors

A number of observations implicate sex hormones and prolactin in susceptibility to, or protection from, RA. Thus nulliparous females have a higher incidence of RA and the highest female:male predominance occurs in the premenopausal period (see Fig 19.5.1). Exposure to the oral contraceptive pill confers a level of protection and postpones the onset of RA. Pregnancy is associated with suppression of disease, and the incidence of RA is increased following parturition and during lactation. Testosterone levels are reported to be low in men with RA, and the incidence of disease increases with advancing age when levels of male sex hormones are on the decline. Interconnections between the hypothalmic–pituitary axis, hormones, and cytokines have been described, suggesting possible mechanisms whereby these may influence the evolution of RA.

Pathology

Joints

The rheumatoid disease process in the joints is characterized by synovitis, an inflammatory effusion and cellular exudate into the joint space, and by damage to tendons, ligaments, cartilage, and bone in and around articulating surfaces of the joint. Long tendons with sheaths lined by synovial membrane—such as in the palms, wrists, ankles, and feet—may also be involved by the inflammatory process and cause malfunction due to damage, rupture, and fibrosis.

In health the synovial membrane (the intima) is a film of one or two cells lining the capsule and its circumferential attachment to the periosteum at the cartilage–bone junction of the joint (Fig. 19.5.3). The normal synovial membrane consists of type A and B cells, without a basement membrane and lying on a bed of loose connective tissue and a network of small blood vessels (the subintima). Type A cells have morphological and phenotypic features of macrophages. Type B cells are of mesenchymal

origin and share many, but not all, of the phenotypic features of typical tissue fibroblasts and are hence referred to as fibroblast-liken synoviocytes.

In established RA the synovial membrane typically becomes enormously thickened and assumes a villous appearance. The diseased tissue now consists of an intima that is several (2–10) cell layers deep and coated by a film of fibrin. Type A cells predominate over type B cells and tend to lie in the more superficial part of the intima. The sublining layer (subintima) is also greatly expanded by newly formed blood vessels and infiltrating activated mononuclear cells, including T lymphocytes, lymphoblasts, B cells, plasma cells, monocytes, macrophages, dendritic cells, synoviocytes, and mesenchymal stem cells (Fig. 19.5.3). The cellular infiltrate usually has a recognizable architecture, comprising perivascular aggregates of CD4+ T cells (Fig. 19.5.4a). Interaggregate areas show a mixed inflammatory cell population, including dendritic cells and macrophages expressing HLA class II, CD8+ T cells, activated B cells, and plasma cells. The aggregates may be organized into prominent lymphoid follicles, some of which display germinal centre formation.

The surface of the thickened synovial membrane is bathed in an inflammatory synovial fluid containing a predominance of polymorphonuclear cells, but also CD4+ and CD8+ lymphocytes, dendritic cells, macrophages, and synoviocytes. The synovial fluid is rich in proinflammatory cytokines and immune complexes containing rheumatoid factor. It is a site of local complement consumption, resulting in low haemolytic complement activity, low C3 and C4, and increased complement breakdown products.

The destructive lesion in the joint typically occurs at the circumferential attachment of the joint capsule, just below and adjacent to the articular cartilage and subchondral bone. Here the intima of the adjacent hypertrophic synovial membrane creeps over the cartilage, and hypoxic tissue rich in newly formed blood vessels, macrophages, osteoclasts and synoviocytes (termed pannus) invades and destroys variable parts of articular cartilage and subchondral bone. The cells at the cartilage–pannus junction are synoviocytes and macrophages, whereas the pannus invading subchondral bone is enriched in osteoclasts. The connective tissue matrix of cartilage adjacent to pannus tissue becomes depleted of proteoglycans and

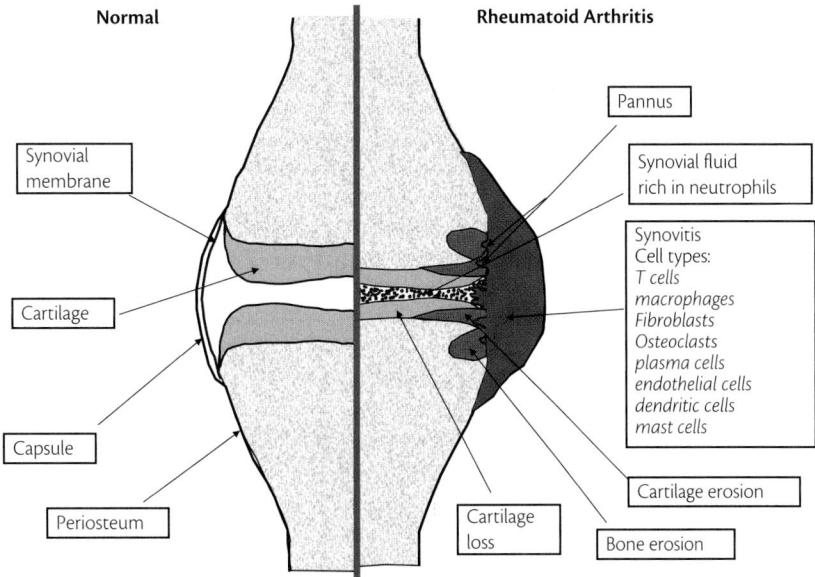

Fig. 19.5.3 The pathology of rheumatoid arthritis: normal joint (left) and rheumatoid joint (right).

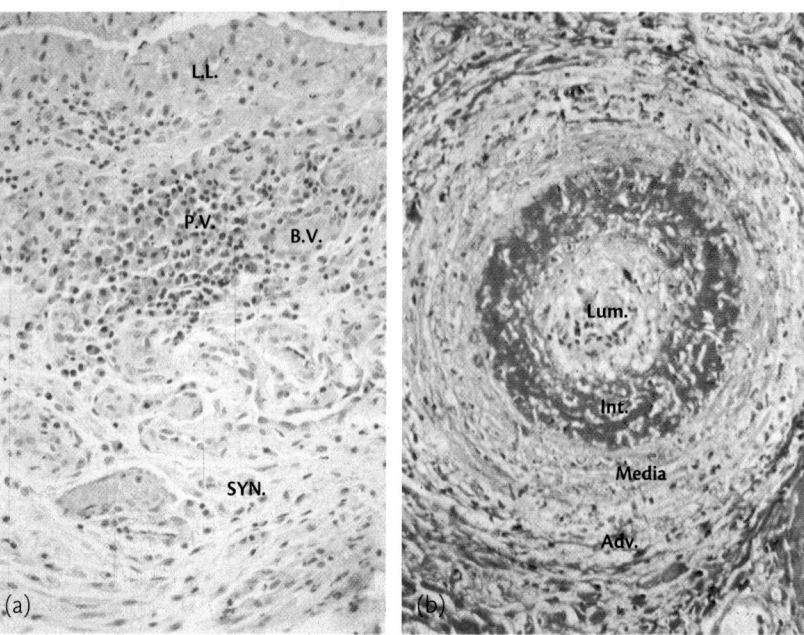

Fig. 19.5.4 Histology of rheumatoid arthritis: (a) rheumatoid arthritis synovitis (haematoxylin and eosin staining). (b) Small vessel arteritis. Arterial wall shows a thrombosed vessel with intimal hyperplasia, destruction of internal elastic lamina, and mononuclear cell infiltration of media and perivascular tissue (methylene blue and safranine staining). See also Fig. 19.5.1. Adv., adventitial tissue; BV, blood vessel; Int., Intima; LL, lining layer; Lum., lumen; PV, perivascular aggregate of lymphocytes and macrophages; SYN, synoviocytes.

collagen type II as a result of enzymatic degradation and lack of regeneration. A number of enzymes responsible for degradation of cartilage matrix have been demonstrated in the rheumatoid joint, including the collagen-degrading matrix metalloproteinases I, III, and XIII, neutrophil-derived cathepsins L and D, and collagenase, as well as aggrecanase, which degrades proteoglycans (see Chapter 19.1 for further discussion). The matrix in which chondrocytes are embedded becomes depleted, with loss of chondrocyte numbers, suggesting that matrix degeneration is secondary to degradative effects mediated by both pannus and chondrocyte activity and cell death. Bone erosion is mainly mediated by activated osteoclasts. Enzymatic degradation of bone matrix beneath the microenvironment of osteoclasts is implicated in the evolution of bone erosions. There may also be an ineffective reparative response in the later stages of disease, as suggested by the presence of fibrous tissue replacing areas of destroyed cartilage and bone in joints removed at surgery.

Extra-articular disease

Extra-articular features associated with RA include four types of tissue pathology: (1) diseased arterial walls, (2) the formation of extravascular nodules consisting of fibrotic lymphocyte–macrophage granulomas, (3) chronic inflammation of pleuro-pericardial surfaces, and (4) chronic immune inflammatory reactions in organs such as the lungs and salivary glands.

Two types of pathology are described in lesions involving arterial walls. The first is a bland fibro-intimal hyperplasia, without obvious inflammatory changes, resulting in vascular occlusion. This is typically observed in digital vessels of patients with longstanding disease and is associated with collateral blood vessel formation. It correlates with a history of benign, intermittent nailfold infarcts that develop in winter months. By contrast, the second type of lesion has polyarteritic pathology and is observed in patients with rheumatoid systemic vasculitis and a poor prognosis. Medium-sized and small arteries of the limbs, peripheral nerves, and organs are involved, but renal vessels are spared. Histopathological examination of involved vessels reveals lymphocytic, histiocytic, and

inflammatory cell infiltration of the medial and perivascular area, disruption of the internal elastic lamina by fibrinoid necrosis, and proliferation of the vessel wall intima with intravascular thrombosis and occlusion (Fig. 19.5.4b).

Extravascular nodule formation in areas subject to pressure or friction, such as the elbow, is the characteristic granulomatous lesion of RA. Nodules have a central core of fibrinoid eosinophilic material surrounded by a palisade of histiocytes, occasional giant cells, and an outer layer of lymphocytes, fibroblasts, and fibrous tissue. Extravascular granulomatous inflammation, with or without nodule formation, has also been documented on the surface of the pleura, pericardium, sclera, and endocardial valves. As is the case with systemic vasculitis and Felty's syndrome, the occurrence of nodules correlates with seropositive disease and the carriage of *HLA DRB1*04* alleles. Notable among organ-based chronic inflammatory diseases are fibrosing alveolitis and/or bronchiolitis, and salivary gland exocrinopathy (secondary Sjögren's syndrome).

Pathogenesis

Although the initiating cause of RA remains uncertain, there has been considerable progress in understanding the cellular and molecular mechanisms involved in chronic immune hyperreactivity, inflammation, and tissue damage (Fig. 19.5.5). The immune-inflammatory reaction is characterized by expression of cytokines, adhesion molecules and chemokines that result in recruitment of lymphoid and inflammatory cells. These recruited cells interact with each other and local resident cells via cytokines and contact-mediated interactions, resulting in chronic inflammation and tissue damage.

B cells and autoantibodies

The discovery of rheumatoid factor in the blood of patients with rheumatism over half a century ago led to the immunological hypothesis of disease pathogenesis. As rheumatoid factor is an autoantibody directed against epitopes on the constant domains

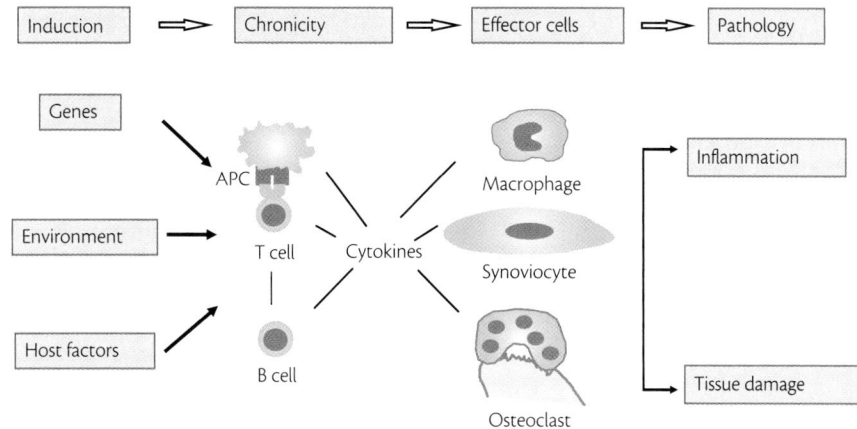

Fig. 19.5.5 In this simplified diagram the role of cytokines in coordinating four steps in the aetiopathogenesis of rheumatoid arthritis are shown: (a) the induction phase involving interactions among genetic, environmental, and host factors; (b) the chronicity phase dependent upon immunological reactions; and (c) the effector phase of pathology mediated by macrophages, synoviocytes, and osteoclasts, which leads to (d) pathology, namely inflammation and tissue damage.

of the Fc portion of IgG1, the concept that RA is an autoimmune disease gained credibility. However, IgM rheumatoid factor occurs in a variety of other diseases in the absence of joint pathology. In the case of RA, rheumatoid factor complexes are present in synovial fluids, and IgG-producing B cells, whose rearranged immunoglobulin gene sequences implicate antigen stimulation, are present in inflamed synovium. B cells in rheumatoid joints also synthesize antibodies to some cartilage components such as collagen type II, but these are not disease specific.

By contrast, recent research has shown a highly disease-specific antibody directed against citrullinated peptides in the serum of patients and some experimental models of RA. The presence of such IgG ACPAs has been detected in healthy individuals several years before the onset of symptoms of RA and correlates with a severe disease course. Antibodies also play a crucial role in an experimentally produced, genetically modified, strain of KBN T-cell receptor transgenic mice, which develop antibodies to glucose-6-phosphatase and a rheumatoid-like disease. This disease can be transferred by the antibody to healthy mice, requiring complement and mast cells for its expression. The presence of antibodies to glucose-6-phosphatase in RA has been reported in one study, but subsequent studies failed to show diagnostic sensitivity and specificity of classical significance.

It seems possible that autoantibodies could interact with complement and Fc receptors expressed on cells in the rheumatoid joint and so contribute to inflammation. Alternative hypotheses include a role for B cells as producers of pathogenic cytokines and as cells that present antigens to T cells. The proven therapeutic efficacy of a B-cell-depleting monoclonal antibody supports a role for B cells in the pathogenesis of RA.

T cells

The predominance of CD4+ T cells in proximity to antigen-presenting cells in the rheumatoid joint suggests their involvement in perpetuating the immune response. This is also supported by the association of RA with HLA class II genes and the beneficial response to T-cell-directed therapies (lymphophoresis, ciclosporin, and the biological drug CTLA4-Ig, abatacept, which blocks interactions between antigen-presenting cells and T cells). In animal models, rheumatoid-like disease can be induced by immunizing with collagens and proteoglycans restricted to cartilage, administered with mycobacterial adjuvant. These cartilage antigens and citrullinated peptides such as fibrinogen and α-enolase that are

present in inflamed joints are candidate autoantigens under current investigation in RA.

An alternative proposal envisages that disease is initiated as a result of molecular mimicry between epitopes on antigens present on infectious agents and autoantigens. Molecular mimicry, by a phenomenon known as epitope spreading, overcomes tolerance mechanisms and results in autoimmunity. Candidate exogenous antigens proposed include *Escherichia coli* bacterial heat shock protein DNAj and EBV gp110 envelope protein, which share a peptide sequence with the HLA DR shared epitope.

The predominant CD4+ T cells in joints appear to be of the Th1 type, bearing memory and activation markers such as CD45 RO+, CD45B dim+, VLA-4+, CD69+, and HLA class II+. However, whether these T cells are activated by a dominant antigen is debated, as they show variable T-cell receptor oligoclonality and antigen specificity. Moreover, T cells in joints do not proliferate but increase in number by recruitment and accumulation.

Recent data have highlighted a deficiency in a naturally occurring subset of CD4+ T cells that regulate the effector function of CD4+ T cells *in vitro*. This regulatory T-cell subset (Tregs) shows a characteristic phenotype and is CD4+, CD25^{bright}, and FOXP3^{+ve}. Tregs not only regulate responses to exogenous, potentially pathogenic antigens, but also promote self-tolerance to autoantigens, thereby preventing autoimmune disease. Treg function has been found to be defective in RA. As the abnormal function of T cells can be replicated *in vitro* by exposure to TNFα, it has been postulated that T cells in RA are conditioned by TNFα to promote T-cell-mediated inflammation. Other cytokines such as IL-15 and IL-6 produced in excess, and IL-10 produced in insufficient quantity, may also promote the loss of homeostasis of the immune-inflammatory reaction. Cell membrane contact between macrophages and cytokine-activated T cells may also be a key event in driving production of the pivotal cytokine TNFα (see below).

Cytokines

Cytokines are protein messenger molecules that transmit signals from one cell to another by binding to specific receptors on the surface of cell membranes. Their activity is usually restricted to adjacent cells in the local milieu. Cytokines are normally produced and exported as soluble molecules into the fluid phase, although some cytokines, such as TNFα, are also active as molecules displayed on the surface of the producer cells. Expression of mRNA and protein of a large number of cytokines is reported in rheumatoid synovial tissue, and these molecules regulate a diverse range of functions relevant to an understanding of the pathogenesis and clinical features of rheumatoid disease. Both pro- and anti-inflammatory cytokines, chemokines, and mitogenic factors are produced, but proinflammatory mediators predominate during active phases of disease.

Of the proinflammatory cytokines, TNFα, IL-1, and IL-6 are of key importance in the pathogenesis of inflammation in RA (Fig. 19.5.6). Experimental evidence *in vitro* and in animal models suggests that they are intimately involved in activation of the cytokine network, leucocyte recruitment and activation, the local immune response, angiogenesis, and fibroblast proliferation in joints. IL-1 and TNFα also regulate production of a number of mediators of connective tissue damage by synoviocytes, including matrix metalloproteinases and prostaglandins. Furthermore, these cytokines in combination with the cytokines monocyte colony stimulating factor (M-CSF) and receptor activator of NF-κβ ligand (RANKL), activate osteoclasts that are implicated in bone damage.

TNFα is produced mainly by type A cells of the macrophage lineage in the intima, subintima, and cartilage–pannus junction. The p55- and p75-TNF receptors are coexpressed by cells in the vicinity. The hypothesis that TNFα is a dominant proinflammatory mediator in the cytokine disequilibrium observed in the rheumatoid synovium has gained considerable support. In particular, TNFα regulates production of IL-1 and together these two cytokines orchestrate rheumatoid inflammation and damage. The identification of TNFα as a molecular target for therapy has been validated by clinical trials of biological inhibitors of TNFα—a monoclonal chimeric and a human anti-TNF antibody, as well as a soluble TNF receptor-IgG Fc fusion protein—that bind to TNFα, thereby neutralizing its activity. The IL-1 antagonist, human recombinant

IL-1 receptor antagonist (IL-1RA), is relatively less effective, but its efficacy supports a role for IL-1 in disease pathogenesis.

The importance of TNFα as a mediator of rheumatoid disease is also supported by a number of observations on blood and joint tissues in clinical studies. For example, following treatment with infliximab, a monoclonal anti-TNFα antibody, there is a: reduction in the expression of adhesion molecules and chemokines involved in the recruitment of immune inflammatory cells (Fig. 19.5.7); reduction in angiogenesis; reduction in the production of proinflammatory cytokines; and an inhibition of molecular and cellular pathways of cartilage and bone destruction.

Many other cytokines and chemokines have been described in rheumatoid joints and implicated in the pathogenesis of disease, and interventional studies have proved to be a powerful tool for investigating their role in disease. In clinical trials in RA, blockade of IL-6 and IL-15 has shown promise, supporting their proinflammatory role. Many other cytokines expressed in disease may be implicated, but because of overlapping function with other cytokines they may be redundant in this respect. Thus far the blockade of chemokines, e.g. MCP-1 and IL-8, by biological agents has not proved successful, and similarly the administration of anti-inflammatory cytokines such as human-recombinant IL-4, IL-10, and IL-11 in clinical trials has proved to be ineffective at the doses used.

Clinical features

Presentation

The onset of RA is frequently insidious, and the principal symptoms are pain and stiffness, mainly of peripheral joints, with associated swelling. Prolonged stiffness of joints on waking and following inactivity is usual and may last an hour or more. There is progressive decline in physical function and ability to perform daily activities. Fatigue and lethargy are common and there may also be low-grade fever and weight loss. Symptoms are persistent in affected joints, although there may be some day-to-day variation in severity. As the disease evolves, further joints may become involved and some may remit, but ultimately the distribution of arthritis becomes permanently established.

Other patterns of disease presentation are also recognized. Up to one-third of patients present with an explosive or subacute onset of arthritis, leading to severe immobility. In a minority of patients a migratory polyarthritis flitting from joint to joint is observed. This is referred to as palindromic rheumatism and may be a recurring pattern over months before chronic polyarthritis becomes established. About 10% of patients present with features of the syndrome of polymyalgia rheumatica, characterized by prominent limb-girdle pain, stiffness, and painful movement of the neck, shoulders, and hips. Persistent inflammatory arthritis of a single joint such as the knee, wrist, ankle, shoulder, or hip may be the only rheumatological symptom and can antedate the onset of polyarthritis by months or years.

In some patients bilateral diffuse swelling of the fingers and hands may be a presenting complaint, often associated with symptoms of carpal tunnel syndrome. Synovitis of tendon sheaths of the dorsal extensors of the wrist and of flexor tendons in the palm and wrist may be present with concurrent joint signs, but may also occur as a prominent clinical feature in the absence of polyarthritis. Swelling of the ankles with pitting oedema is commonly seen in

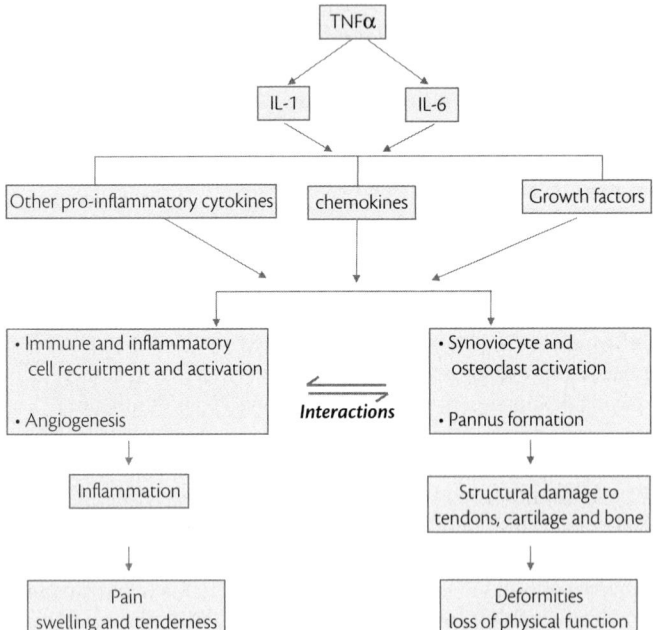

Fig. 19.5.6 The role of tumour necrosis factor-α in the pathogenesis of inflammation and structural damage to tendons and bone in rheumatoid arthritis.

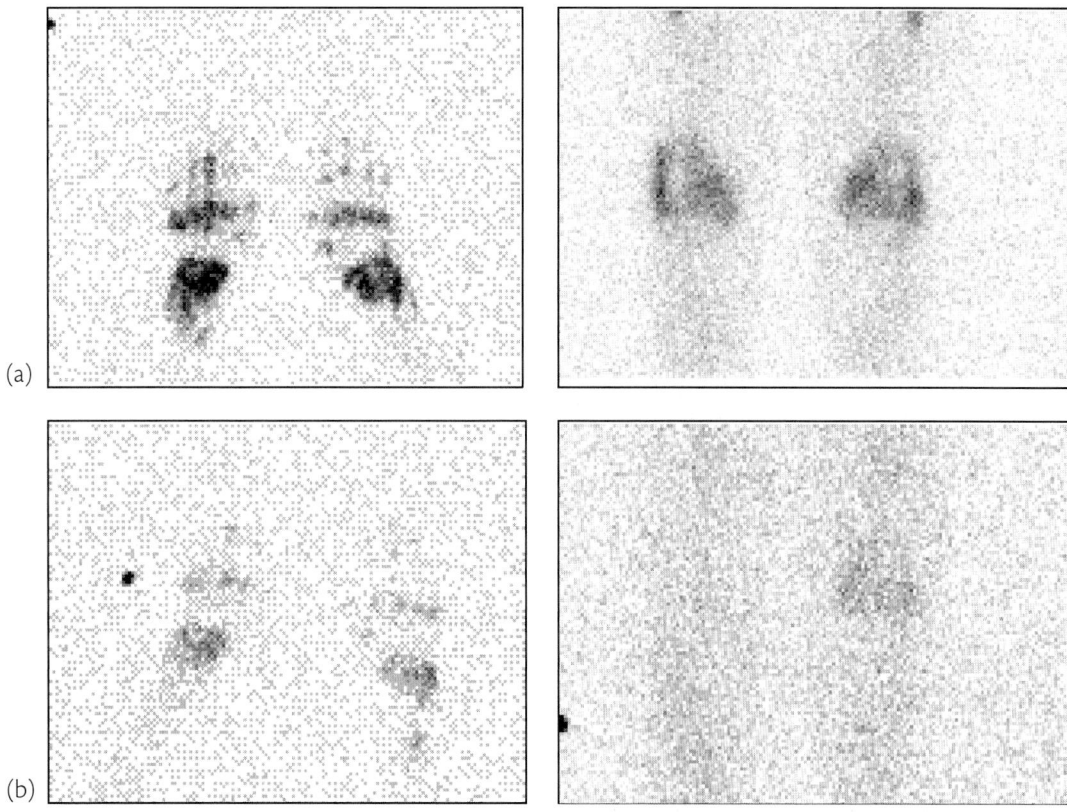

Fig. 19.5.7 Gamma camera images of the hands and knees of a patient with rheumatoid arthritis. Images were taken 22 h after a bolus injection of autologous radiolabelled (indium-111) granulocytes (a) before and (b) after a single 10 mg/kg intravenous bolus of anti-TNFα antibody (infliximab). There was a reduction in signal after treatment. From Taylor PC, Peters AM, Paleolog E, Chapman PT, Elliott MJ, McCloskey R, Feldmann M, Maini RN. Reduction of chemokine levels and leukocyte traffic to joints by tumor necrosis factor alpha blockade in patients with rheumatoid arthritis. *Arthritis and Rheumatism* 43 (2000), pp38–47. Copyright 2000. Reprinted with permission of John Wiley and Sons Inc.

active RA. Lymphoedema of the forearm or lower limb is observed less frequently.

Rarely, the initial manifestations of RA are confined to extra-articular disease. Examples include subcutaneous nodules, one or more nodules in the thorax presenting as pulmonary lesions on a chest radiograph, pleurisy with pleural effusion, pericarditis, episcleritis, and vasculitis.

Joint distribution

The expression of RA shows interindividual variation with respect to the anatomical sites and numbers of involved joints. For example, some patients have mainly small joints affected, whereas others show simultaneous involvement of small and large joints. The hip and shoulder joints may be spared in some, while in others they bear the brunt of the disease. The actual numbers of diseased joints can vary from three or four to over fifty. Diseased neck joints may be asymptomatic until, in the late stages, neurological complications alert the physician to subluxation of the cervical spine or the atlantoaxial joint.

In over 80 to 90% of patients, one or more of the metacarpophalangeal and proximal interphalangeal joints of the hand and the metatarsophalangeal joints are involved. Other frequently involved sites include the wrists, glenohumeral joints of the shoulders, knees, and the elbow joints, followed by the midtarsal, acromioclavicular, interfacetal, and atlantoaxial joints of the cervical spine and hip joints. The temporomandibular, sternoclavicular, and cricoarytenoid joints are involved in about one-third of patients.

Symmetrical involvement of the joints is usual, but joint damage and deformity may be asymmetrical and related to overuse or traumatic injury. Conversely, neurological paralysis of a limb results in joint protection.

In addition to involvement of diarthrodial joints, the rheumatoid process frequently involves tendon sheaths of hands, wrists, shoulders, and ankles.

Features of joint disease

Hands and wrists

In active rheumatoid disease, soft tissue swelling and tenderness of metacarpophalangeal and proximal interphalangeal joints is observed (Fig. 19.5.8). Thickening and nodularity of flexor tendons in the palms may be palpable and tenosynovitis can be a cause of 'triggering' of the fingers. Wasting of the interossei is prominent and fist closure restricted. Flexor tendonitis and wrist synovitis may be associated with signs and symptoms of median nerve compression (carpal tunnel syndrome).

Ulnar deviation and volar subluxation of the digits and wrists may develop later. Other recognized deformities include boutonnière (buttonhole) flexion deformity of the proximal interphalangeal joint and 'swan-neck' deformities of fingers due to hyperextension of the proximal interphalangeal joint and flexion at the distal interphalangeal joint.

Diffuse synovial swelling may be pronounced at the dorsal aspect of the wrist and the ulnar styloid may become dorsally subluxed. The carpus may drift in a volar direction such that supination of

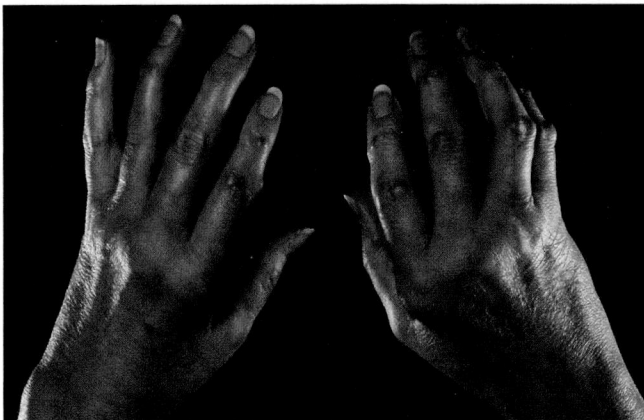

Fig. 19.5.8 The hands of a person suffering from rheumatoid arthritis. Features to note include symmetrical soft tissue swelling of the second and third metacarpophalangeal joints, early swan-neck deformity of the left ring finger, ulnar deviation at the metacarpophalangeal joints, and wasting of the small muscles of the hand. In addition, several small rheumatoid nodules are present. (See also Fig. 19.5.2.)

the hand is restricted. In this late stage, the extensor tendons appear stretched across a shrunken carpus ('the bowstring' sign). Extensor tendons may occasionally rupture, most commonly affecting the little or ring fingers.

Nail fold and fingertip infarcts and splinter haemorrhages indicate digital vascular occlusive disease. Palmar erythema is common but not specific for RA.

Elbows and shoulders
Physical signs in early stages include swelling, limitation of movement, and inability to flex or extend the elbow. Later, pronation and supination are restricted, and the head of the proximal radioulnar joint may dislocate. Olecranon bursitis and subcutaneous nodules around the elbow are common. In the shoulder, aside from glenohumeral joint synovitis, there may be accompanying subacromial bursitis and rotator and biceps tendon involvement.

The neck
Rheumatoid involvement of the apophyseal joints of the neck can cause pain, stiffness, and restricted movement. Loss of stability in the spine may occur at several levels and be associated with symptoms and signs of radicular or cord compression. Subluxation of the atlantoaxial joint diagnosed by plain radiography or MRI occurs in 6% of the rheumatoid population and up to 30% of patients who are admitted to hospital. It may be asymptomatic, but when severe tends to occur in patients who also suffer from severe generalized disease and advanced disability, and is a recognized cause of quadriplegia and sudden death.

The knees
Involvement of the knees is common, and chronically active synovitis is associated with irreversible destruction and rapid deterioration in functional capacity. In early stages especially, high pressure in the knee joint on active flexion, e.g. during squatting, can lead to joint rupture and leakage of inflammatory fluid into the calf. This complication simulates signs and symptoms of a calf deep vein thrombosis: it can be diagnosed by arthrography using contrast medium, or by ultrasonography of the knee. A chronic effusion in the knee joint may also be associated with a posterior popliteal (Baker's) cyst and occasionally this extends into the medial aspect of the calf.

Ankles and feet
Inflammation of the metatarsophalangeal joints is common and results in subluxation of the metatarsal heads and, ultimately, claw- or hammer-toe deformities. The soft-tissue pad that is normally positioned underneath the metatarsal heads becomes displaced such that the heads of the metatarsal bones become painful to walk on. Patients may describe this as feeling as if they were walking on marbles or stones. Involvement of the tarsal and subtalar joints may result in flattening of the arches of the foot and valgus deformity of the hindfoot. These deformities cause difficulties with footwear, and where shoes rub the feet there is a tendency for callosities to form.

Hips
The hips are less often involved, but there may be erosions in severe cases with remodelling of the acetabulum (protrusio acetabuli). There may also be secondary degenerative disease at the hip.

Extra-articular disease
Nodules
Nodules occur in 25 to 30% of patients with RA and are associated with seropositive disease. Common sites for subcutaneous nodules include the elbow, ischial tuberosity, heel, and dorsum of fingers. Multiple, small, rapidly evolving nodules can occur in those on methotrexate treatment (Fig. 19.5.8). Nodules in the pleura may present as single or multiple round shadows on a routine chest radiograph.

Systemic vasculitis
Rheumatoid vasculitis occurs in patients with seropositive and nodular disease. It presents with a severe systemic illness characterized by fever and weight loss. Associated clinical features are consequent upon occlusion of medium- to small-sized arteries. These include Raynaud's phenomenon, nail fold and digital infarcts, and gangrene, skin ulceration, mononeuritis multiplex, scleromalacia perforans, and occlusion of arteries to visceral organs. The latter include coronary, pulmonary, coeliac axis, and cerebral vessels. In some patients vasculitis may present as a skin rash associated with necrotizing polyangiitis of small cutaneous blood vessels.

Fibrosing alveolitis and obliterative bronchiolitis
Physiological abnormalities in lung function tests indicative of airways and interstitial disease may be present without symptoms. In some patients with RA, more frequently men than women, dyspnoea of insidious onset, physical signs, characteristic lung function abnormalities, a chest radiograph, and high-resolution CT may reveal characteristic features of chronic fibrosing alveolitis. More rarely, acute pneumonitis may be the presenting feature, with rapid deterioration and development of respiratory failure. Patients with fibrosing alveolitis are usually seropositive, have a high frequency of antinuclear antibodies, and may also exhibit evidence of multisystem disease, including vasculitis.

Obliterative bronchiolitis can be associated with RA. It is usually rapidly progressive, but some patients follow a chronic protracted course that may respond to corticosteroid and immunosuppressive therapy. See Chapter 18.11.4 for further discussion.

Serositis
Evidence of previous pericardial and pleural inflammation is common at autopsy and may be discovered by imaging techniques

in asymptomatic patients. Both may present with clinical symptoms, generally following a benign course with resolution associated with disease-modifying antirheumatoid drugs (DMARDs) or corticosteroid therapy. Rare cases of constrictive pericarditis have been reported. Typically, pleural effusions are exudates with a high protein content and cellular exudate enriched in lymphocytes, but also containing polymorphonuclear cells and macrophages. A low level of complement activity relative to blood concentrations and a low glucose concentration (usually <1.4 mmol/litre) is of diagnostic value.

Eye complications

Scleritis, episcleritis, scleromalacia perforans, corneal melt, and keratoconjunctivitis sicca have all been described and need evaluation and treatment by a specialist.

Amyloidosis

Secondary amyloidosis due to deposition of amyloid AA fibrils in blood vessels and parenchyma of kidneys, liver, spleen, and gastrointestinal tract has been described in the tissues of 10 to 15% of patients examined at autopsy, or in the blood vessels in the submucosa of rectal and gingival biopsies. Proteinuria, nephrotic syndrome, or renal failure are less common and have a poor prognosis unless detected and treated before irreversible renal failure has occurred.

Osteoporosis

Juxta-articular osteoporosis is a common feature of radiographs of affected joints and is related to local disease activity. However, decreased bone mineral density of the spine and pelvis has been described in patients with active severe RA. This is likely to reflect the response of bone metabolism to prostaglandins and catabolic cytokines such as IL-6, IL-11, and the receptor for activation of NF-$\kappa\beta$ (RANK) ligand, which increase osteoclast activity. This is distinct from immobility-associated or corticosteroid-induced osteoporosis, although these factors may be additive in individual patients. It has been suggested that increased mobility following low-dose prednisolone may be beneficial and reverse, rather than aggravate, corticosteroid-induced osteopenia.

Felty's syndrome

Felty's syndrome is characterized by a combination of seropositive RA, neutropenia, and splenomegaly. Lymphadenopathy, leg ulcers, and nodular hyperplasia of the liver have been described. Patients with severe neutropenia are liable to bacterial infections. Some patients also develop anaemia and thrombocytopenia. In a variant of Felty's syndrome, an expansion of large granular lymphocytes is found in the blood: these are cytotoxic CD8+ lymphocytes and may present as clonally expanded cell populations.

Cardiac disease

Myocardial disease due to diffuse fibrosis or granulomatous lesions is recognized in RA, although the more frequently recognized association is with coronary artery disease. Systemic vasculitis may also involve coronary vessels. Aortic incompetence due to valvular thickening and nodule formation or dilation of the ascending aorta have been described.

Neurological complications

A number of compression neuropathies may occur in RA. These include compression of the median nerve at the wrist, the ulnar nerve and posterior interosseous branch of the radial nerve at the elbow, and posterior tibial nerve at the level of the knee or ankle. It is important to recognize and confirm these neuropathies by nerve conduction studies, as surgical decompression usually cures symptoms.

A mild, symmetrical, sensory peripheral neuropathy involving the hands and legs in a 'glove and stocking' distribution also occurs in RA. This is distinct from the rarer and more severe sensorimotor mononeuritis multiplex associated with wrist and foot drop and usually due to vasculitis of vasa nervora, when other features of a systemic vasculitis and extra-articular disease may be present. In some patients, however, no vascular pathology is demonstrable and the cause of axonal degeneration is not understood.

Rheumatoid involvement of the transverse ligament and odontoid process of the atlantoaxial joint may lead to posterior subluxation or upward movement of the odontoid and cause cervical cord compression. Cord compression may also occur because of rheumatoid damage at lower levels of the cervical spine. Compression is a recognized cause of tetraparesis and sudden death. Surgical stabilization of the neck can be successful but cannot always be recommended in patients with associated severe disability and poor health status.

Infections

Patients with RA are susceptible to local and systemic bacterial, and opportunistic infections. Infections of joints, respiratory and urinary tracts, skin ulcers, and septicaemia are all described, and infections are one of the causes of increased mortality in the condition. Endogenous disease-related and iatrogenic immunosuppressive mechanisms are thought to play an important part. Neutropenia compromises host defence in Felty's syndrome.

Cancer

The incidence of lymphoproliferative disease, mainly B-cell lymphoma, is significantly increased in RA. In a case–control retrospective study from Sweden in an era when cytotoxic agents were not in use, the risk of lymphomas was increased several fold in patients with severe inflammatory disease. Confounding variables such as smoking are thought to play a part in the increased risk of lung cancer reported in some studies.

Clinical course

Disease activity

The course of the disease activity fluctuates over time, partly due to the endogenous mechanisms of disease and partly as a result of effective therapy. Recurring periods of weeks or months of exacerbation of symptoms, described as 'flares', alternate with periods of relative quiescence of disease. In about 10 to 20% of patients the disease continues unabated throughout.

The key clinical features of disease activity in RA are pain, fatigue, stiffness of joints on waking, swelling, tenderness of joints on palpation, restriction of joint motion, and loss of physical functional capacity (see below). Joint deformities become apparent as the disease progresses. Symptoms are assessed by taking a history in descriptive terms, but also by attempting to quantify their severity by a visual analogue scale. These measurements have been incorporated into various criteria for assessment of disease activity, remission, and response to therapy, developed and validated e.g. by the ACR and the European League Against Rheumatism (ELAR).

Swelling of joints caused by synovial thickening may be detected by palpation as a 'spongy' or 'boggy' feel. Concomitant effusion can be demonstrated by fluctuation. In later stages of disease, subluxed surfaces of bones (such as the heads of metacarpals in the hands, the styloid of the ulna, and distal radius at the wrist) can give the appearance of bony swelling. Tenderness is elicited by digital pressure or squeezing of a joint. The classic signs of inflammation, such as redness and increased temperature overlying joints, are not usually prominent, although readily demonstrable by thermography. Active and passive movement of joints through their anatomical range of motion elicits restriction of movement associated with pain.

Functional capacity can be assessed by testing grip strengths using an inflatable bag attached to a sphygmomanometer, walking time over a standard distance, and by standard health assessment questionnaires (such as the Stanford questionnaire). In the early and mid stages, disease activity is the major determinant of impairment of physical function. The degree, quantity, and severity of pain is recorded as experienced by the patient, graded on a visual analogue scale of 1 to 10. The duration of morning stiffness is recorded in minutes. A 'global assessment' of disease activity on a visual analogue scale of 1 to 10 as judged by the patient and physician may also be used as a quantitative measurement of disease activity over time.

Structural damage

The rheumatoid disease process leads to structural damage to the cartilage, bone, and associated joint structures. Serial radiographs of the hands and feet are employed to assess structural damage to joints, with more sensitive techniques including ultrasonography and MRI employed for research studies. Damage is cumulative and irreversible and appears to be related to the severity of inflammatory activity over time. In later stages of disease, loss of normal joint architecture and mechanical derangement are the major cause of disability.

Prognosis

The longer-term health status of patients presenting to hospital clinics and in the community with recent-onset RA has been documented in a number of studies. Functional deterioration occurs rapidly, but the trajectory of the course of disease varies considerably in individual patients. In one hospital-based study, half were moderately disabled in 2 years and severely disabled by 10 years, with a severe impact on employability.

Patients with RA have a higher than expected prevalence of other serious illnesses and an increased mortality compared with the general population. Survival rates of about 50% at 5 years have been recorded in a subset of patients with severe polyarticular disease, poor functional status, or extra-articular disease (Fig. 19.5.9). RA itself may contribute to premature death in patients as a result of recognized extra-articular complications such as fibrosing alveolitis, vasculitis, secondary amyloidosis, cardiac disease, or transection of the cord due to cervical spinal subluxation. More frequently, death is the consequence of comorbid conditions, e.g. premature atheromatous coronary and cerebrovascular disease, predisposition to infections and lymphoproliferative diseases. Most of these complications and comorbidities are now considered to be a result of the systemic nature of molecular pathways involved in inflammation and a dysregulated immune response characteristic of

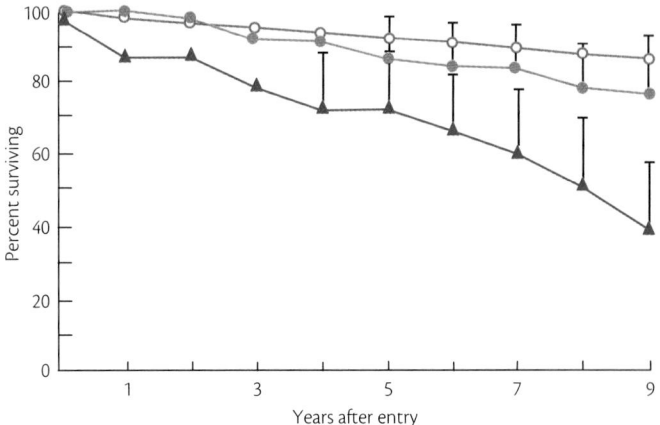

Fig. 19.5.9 Survival of female patients with rheumatoid arthritis attending hospital clinics compared with age-adjusted population data for England and Wales. ∘—∘, survival of whole population; •—• survival of female patients with rheumatoid arthritis and joint disease only (n = 38); ▲–▲ survival of patients with rheumatoid arthritis and extra-articular disease (n = 33). Bars represent 95% confidence limits.
Annals of the Rheumatic Diseases (1989) 48, 7 –13. Reproduced with permission from the BMJ Publishing Group.

the disease. Iatogenic causes also play an important role, e.g. causing gastrointestinal haemorrhage or perforation, renal failure, liver damage, and bone marrow suppression. However, treatment with DMARDs, especially methotrexate, is now recognized to improve the quality of life and life expectancy of rheumatoid patients.

Prognostic factors

A number of prognostic factors that herald rapid functional deterioration and premature death have been identified in cohorts of patients with RA. These include a large number of affected joints, a persistently raised level of acute phase proteins, detection of bony erosions on radiographs, lower socioeconomic status, early development of functional incapacity, a positive rheumatoid factor and ACPA tests, cryoglobulinaemia, and (in northern European patients) the presence of the *HLA DRB*04* genes. Their presence in combination is predictive of progressive, severe disease. However, on an individual patient basis the reliability and weighing attributed to each factor requires validation.

Remission

Criteria for defining remission have been developed by the ACR and ELAR. The former are very rigorous and require absence of specific symptoms and signs and a normal ESR for two consecutive months; the latter is a composite disease activity score, a continuous variable measurement, derived from a mathematical formula based on specified signs, symptoms, and ESR. These criteria do not give concordant results and have shortcomings, the former criteria being achieved by a smaller proportion of patients than the latter. They have been variably applied in epidemiological studies and clinical trials. However, there is general agreement that spontaneous remission of established disease is rare (<15% of patients). Drug-induced remission at single time points following therapeutic interventions is more common, being documented in up to about 50% patients, especially with early disease, but is not frequently long lasting. Progressive structural damage of joints has been observed despite remission by these criteria in some studies, suggesting that more sophisticated biomarkers and imaging techniques are required to define true disease remission.

Diagnosis and stages of disease

A diagnosis of RA is likely if three or more symmetrically distributed joints are found to be swollen and tender for more than 6 weeks in a patient with a positive rheumatoid factor and/or ACPA test and elevated ESR or serum concentration of C-reactive protein. However, not all these features are necessarily present at the early stages of disease, at which point arthritis is best termed 'undifferentiated'. The broad spectrum described in the 'presentation' section may cause considerable difficulty in making a definitive diagnosis.

With the passage of time, the emergence of other features, such as subcutaneous nodules, radiographic evidence of joint space narrowing, juxta-articular osteopenia, and bony erosions add further certainty to the diagnosis.

The ACR criteria in Box 19.5.1 may not be fulfilled for 6 to 12 months, by which time the pattern of joint involvement and a chronic disease course are usually evident. Prognostic factors declare themselves and the patient is regarded as having reached the stage of established disease.

Differential diagnosis

In patients with recent onset of symptoms of arthritis, the following disorders should be considered in the differential diagnosis.

Polyarthritis associated with connective tissue disease

Systemic lupus erythematosus (SLE) may present with chronic nondeforming polyarthritis, but features such as Raynaud's phenomenon, photosensitivity, rashes, alopecia, haemolytic anaemia, leucopenia, thrombocytopenia, and renal or neurological involvement are detectable sooner or later, and diagnostic antinuclear antibodies (anti-ds-DNA, anti-Sm and others) are present. Other connective tissue diseases such as systemic sclerosis, polymyositis, mixed connective tissue disease, 'overlap' syndromes, and primary Sjögren's syndrome may also present with marked polyarthralgia or polyarthritis that mimics RA. In many such patients, the presence of rheumatoid factor can further confuse the diagnosis. Careful clinical examination and measurement of marker autoantibodies directed against nuclear and cytoplasmic antigens will usually permit recognition of the underlying disorder. In some cases the diagnosis may only unfold after a period of weeks or months of a disorder best labelled 'undifferentiated connective tissue disease'.

Infection-related polyarthritis

The polyarthritis of rubella or other microbial agents, such as parvovirus B19 and *Borrelia burgdorferi*, and reactive arthritis associated with genitourinary or gastrointestinal infections can all cause diagnostic difficulty. A positive diagnosis is made by microbiological tests on relevant body fluids and serological tests for the detection of IgM antibodies or a rising titre of IgG antibodies to the suspected microorganism in sequential serum samples taken over 2 weeks.

Spondyloarthropathies

Peripheral joint disease can be seen in conjunction with ankylosing spondylitis, psoriasis, and inflammatory bowel disease.

Clinical examination of the spine, skin, and nails, radiological examination of the bowel using double-contrast enema or small bowel enema, endoscopy, and biopsy may reveal the underlying diagnosis. Many patients are HLA B27 positive.

Osteoarthritis

Osteoarthritis may present with inflammatory symptoms and signs but is readily distinguished by its different joint distribution (proximal and distal interphalangeal joints, carpometacarpal joints of the thumb) and radiographs that show joint space narrowing, subchondral new bone formation, osteophytes, and subchondral cysts. Where there is pre-existing osteoarthritis, the superimposition of RA can be difficult to distinguish.

Other conditions

In late middle-aged and elderly patients the clinical presentation of polyarticular chronic pyrophosphate arthropathy may be difficult to distinguish from RA. The former diagnosis may be suspected where there is an atypical distribution of synovitis together with periarticular complications. Chronic pyrophosphate arthropathy may be associated with a modest acute phase response and low-titre rheumatoid factor, but can usually be distinguished from RA on the basis of typical radiographic appearances and the finding of calcium pyrophosphate dihydrate (CPPD) crystals in synovial fluid aspirates. Rarely, RA and chronic pyrophosphate arthropathy may coexist.

Other diagnoses to be considered include hypermobility syndrome, polyarticular gout, psoriatic arthritis, haemochromatosis, sarcoidosis, sickle-cell disease, primary amyloidosis, and paraneoplastic disease.

Investigations

Laboratory tests

Laboratory studies are an integral part of the management of patients with RA and are employed for diagnosis, evaluation of prognosis, assessment of disease activity, response to therapy, and monitoring toxic effects of drugs. Only routinely used tests are considered here.

The measurement of IgM rheumatoid factors is useful in the early stages of assessment of a patient with suspected RA. In a patient with recent-onset polyarthritis, a positive rheumatoid factor is moderately specific for RA, but can also be observed in patients with other connective tissue diseases such as SLE and primary Sjögren's syndrome. A repeat test may be positive after an initial test is negative and is therefore necessary before a patient can be categorized as having seronegative RA. A significant titre of rheumatoid factor is associated with a poor prognosis and extra-articular disease.

The detection of IgG antibodies to citrullinated proteins (ACPAs) has been extensively validated as specific for rheumatoid disease and may be positive in the absence of rheumatoid factor. As routinely measured by a widely used enzyme-linked immunoassay (ELISA) 'kit' that detects antibodies to citrullinated synthetic peptides (anti-CCP), the sensitivity increases from around 50% in early disease to around 80% in established disease with more than 95% specificity.

Measurement of ESR (Westergren method) and serum C-reactive protein are extensively used. High values correlate with disease severity and a reduction is one criterion of response to therapy. Persistently elevated C-reactive protein concentrations correlate with deforming erosive disease.

Patients with active RA show haematological abnormalities as a consequence of disease-related mechanisms. A high level of disease activity is associated with a normocytic normochromic anaemia, polymorphonuclear leucocytosis, and thrombocytosis. An exception is Felty's syndrome, associated with neutropenia and thrombocytopenia. These abnormal values tend to return to normal as the inflammatory component of disease responds to therapy.

Active disease may also be associated with a raised serum alkaline phosphatase and a low serum albumin. Serum chemistry is otherwise normal. Serum immunoglobulin and complement C3 and C4 levels may be elevated.

Nonsteroidal anti-inflammatory drug (NSAID) therapy may cause microcytic iron-deficiency anaemia from blood loss from the gastrointestinal tract. A low serum ferritin level suggests iron deficiency, but this is not a reliable guide in cases of RA, as serum concentrations may be elevated as part of an acute phase response. Corticosteroids may be responsible for increased polymorphonuclear cell counts and decreased lymphocyte counts. Many DMARDs show dose-related bone marrow toxicity, and sulfasalazine, D-penicillamine, azathioprine, and gold can cause unexpected agranulocytosis as a result of hypersensitivity, unrelated to the dose administered.

Of the commonly used drugs, methotrexate, sulfasalazine, azathioprine, and leflunomide are hepatoxic and can cause elevation of liver enzymes and alkaline phosphatase. Repeated monitoring is advisable: persistent or highly raised values should prompt further investigation or discontinuation.

Imaging

Radiographs of hands and feet can be used to assess the presence and progression of cartilage loss and bone erosions (Fig. 19.5.10). Standardized measurements (the Larsen or Sharp scoring methods) have been devised to quantify these measures. Changes seen in the hands and feet correlate with radiological changes in other affected joints, showing a linear progression after the initial

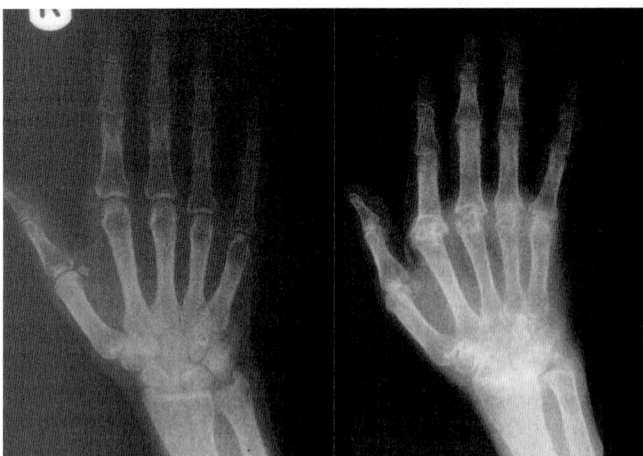

Fig. 19.5.10 Hand radiographs taken soon after symptom onset (left) and 12 years into established disease (right), showing extensive structural damage, especially in the metacarpophalangeal, interphalangeal, carpal, and wrist joints.

1 to 2 years. The erosion count correlates with physical function. Radiographs of affected joints are used for the assessment of integrity and damage. Flexion views of the cervical spine are suitable for demonstration of atlantoaxial subluxation and cervical instability. Arrest or retardation of radiographic change is considered to be a marker of good control of disease.

MRI and CT are valuable in assessing neck pathology and pressure on the cervical cord. MRI and high-frequency ultrasound examination are sensitive methods to evaluate synovitis and early change in cartilage and bone, but their place in routine management is not yet established. Dual emission X-ray absorptiometry (DEXA) scanning is in routine use for the assessment of bone mineral density.

Management

Aims of treatment

The aims of treatment are to:

◆ relieve symptoms and signs of disease and induce remission

◆ maintain normal physical function

◆ prevent structural damage to joints and associated structures

◆ restore and maintain quality of life that permits the pursuit of normal work, domestic, and social life

◆ reduce the comorbidity and increased mortality associated with the disease and therapies

◆ correct abnormal laboratory-based values of haemotopoietic function, acute phase proteins and other markers of disease process

General principles

Drug therapy

Considerable progress has been made in developing effective therapies for the rapid relief of symptoms and signs of disease. However, despite the best therapies in current use, the goals of durable drug-free remission halting structural damage and maintaining a normal quality of life, over the long term, have not yet been realized, although significant progress has been made. The realistic aims, therefore, are to maximize gains while minimizing toxicity of drugs (an optimum risk:benefit ratio) and to operate within the pharmacoeconomic constraints (cost–benefit and cost–utility) that apply in the setting in which the patient is being treated.

The costs of treatment of RA over the lifetime of a patient are considerable. Direct costs increase over the course of disease and include those of hospital admissions, drugs, surgery, aids, and appliances. Indirect costs include those arising from loss of economic productivity and earnings, unemployment and disability benefits, the cost of maintaining mobility, and domestic help and daily care for the severely disabled.

Once an individualized management plan has been instituted, response to therapy should be monitored to ensure efficacy, using quantifiable clinical and laboratory indices of inflammatory activity and impact on the progression of damage to joints. A lack of response to initial therapy should trigger a change in the management plan and consideration of alternative strategies at intervals of 3 to 6 months. A thorough knowledge of the scope and limitations of treatment modalities is essential in the art of management.

With aggressive and continuing use of disease-modifying chemical and biological therapeutic agents, it is possible to achieve low disease activity in most and maintain remission in some patients. As clinically defined low or absent disease activity correlates with retardation of joint damage, the long-term benefit of treatment is likely to be most marked in this early phase of disease.

Nonpharmacological measures and support

Other essential elements of the management include measures such as patient education; psychological and employment counselling; setting appropriate levels of rest and exercise; coping with tasks of daily living and maintaining mobility; access to splints, aids, and appliances for the disabled; and access to social and financial benefits. The provision of holistic care thus requires teamwork and coordination between the treating physician and other medical and healthcare professionals, including specialist nurses, physiotherapists, occupational therapists, and social workers. Fully involving patients in their management improves outcomes.

Bed rest and the use of resting splints may be helpful during the very acute stages of joint disease, but should always be accompanied by daily passive joint movements and appropriate isometric exercises to avoid contractures, muscle atrophy and osteoporosis, and to retain joint function. Exercise initiated under supervision and maintained by patients on a regular basis does not accelerate joint damage and is effective in diminishing pain and promoting a sense of well-being in those in whom fatigue is a major feature of active disease.

Dietary manipulation—including fasting and exclusion of certain foods and beverages, and a vegetarian diet—has enjoyed popularity and in some patients appears to be beneficial, but there is little evidence that most such diets are of durable value. Diets rich in fish oils and $\omega - 3$ fatty acids appear to be of some benefit. As excessive weight accelerates joint damage and increases the risk of complications when undergoing essential surgery, obese patients should be encouraged to lose weight.

Surgical treatment plays an important and essential role in relieving intractable symptoms and restoring loss of physical function and mobility caused by damage to joints, tendons, and associated soft tissues. It is also indicated in the treatment of secondary complications such as entrapment of peripheral nerves at the wrist and elbow and cervical cord compression due to instability of the cervical spine.

Maintenance of mobility requires attention to foot care, podiatry, comfortable shoes, a walking stick or elbow crutches, and specially adapted motor vehicles to get to work and for social purposes.

In the United Kingdom disabled people have certain privileges in employment and may qualify for disability allowances. Some may benefit from retraining for suitable work. The health care team needs to recognize that chronic illness and disability places increased pressure on spouses and family, who generally end up as carers of the patient with RA: support and counselling should therefore extend to them.

Management strategies

Mild disease

Mild disease may be defined as RA with limited joint involvement and low disease activity, and without markers of poor prognosis. Such patients will typically show most of the following features: involvement of less than six or seven individual joints and sparing of weightbearing joints; pain readily controlled with NSAIDs; less than 15 min of joint stiffness on waking or following inactivity; lack of extra-articular disease; minimally elevated ESR or concentration of C-reactive protein; negative rheumatoid factor test; a normal haematological profile; little or no impairment of physical function; and ability to undertake activities of daily living, maintaining employment, and enjoying nonstrenuous social and leisure activities. Radiographs of hands and feet show a lack of significant osteopenia, joint space narrowing, and bony erosions at baseline and annual follow-up. The disease course may be punctuated by self-limiting exacerbations of symptoms and signs. Patients with mild disease are only a small proportion of those referred to specialist clinics but are more numerous in the community and in the primary care setting.

Drug treatment involves judicious use of NSAIDs and analgesic drugs. Corticosteroid injections into individual affected joints, tendon sheaths, and bursas for persistent swelling, tenderness, or loss of normal range of movement can be very effective. Follow-up assessment is necessary to ensure that the disease has not evolved to a more severe pattern. DMARDs are indicated in those with recurrent or persistent symptoms and signs, deformities, or radiographic evidence of structural damage. Hydroxychloroquine or sulfasalazine are used initially. If the decision to embark on the use of DMARDs is made, the aims and management strategy are the same as for patients with moderate or severe disease.

Moderate or severe disease

Rheumatoid disease is defined as moderate or severe when it has evolved into an unremitting pattern of polyarthritis with evidence of significant functional impairment and joint damage in early stages of presentation. With increasing severity most of the following features are present: 10 to 30 swollen and tender joints; frequent involvement of proximal joints of the arms and legs; moderate to severe pain; inactivity and morning stiffness exceeding 1 h in duration; prominent fatigue; elevated ESR and/or C-reactive protein concentrations; low haemoglobin concentration, polymorphonuclear leucocytosis, and thrombocytosis; and positive rheumatoid factor test. Deformities of joints are apparent early in the course of disease and radiographs of hands, feet, and affected joints already show loss of joint space and subchondral erosions within 2 years of presentation. Such patients have significant impairment in daily activities and restricted ability to perform domestic and work-related tasks and to enjoy social and leisure activities.

The aim of drug treatment is to achieve rapid control of disease activity and, if possible, remission of disease. This usually requires simultaneous or sequential use of drugs belonging to different classes, e.g. NSAIDs, DMARDs, corticosteroids, and biological therapies, as discussed below.

So-called 'traditional' NSAIDs are used at optimal doses for control of pain and stiffness (see Table 19.5.1). Many physicians prefer to administer NSAIDs with a short half-life in slow-release preparations to be taken in the morning and before the patient retires to bed at night. In patients with a history of gastric intolerance, COX-2-selective NSAIDs may be preferable, or else the simultaneous use of a gastroprotective agent, most commonly a proton pump inhibitor. In addition, simple analgesics such as 0.5 to 1 g paracetamol every 6 h may be required for relief of pain. In clinical practice, a change of NSAIDs may be required to establish which of

Table 19.5.1 Current NSAIDs: dosage for rheumatoid arthritis in adults

COX inhibitor	Dose (mg)/24 h
COX-1/2 (nonselective)	
Ibuprofen	400–800, 3 times
Naproxen	250–500, twice
Diclofenac	25–50, 3 times or slow release 75 once or twice
Nabumetone	1000 at night; to 1000 twice
Fenoprofen	300–600, 3–4 times
Ketoprofen	50, 3–4 times
Indometacin	Slow release 75, once or twice or 25–50 morning and noon, and 50–100 at night
Piroxicam	10–30, once
Sulindac	200, twice
Tenoxicam	20, once
Flurbiprofen	50, 2–4 times Slow-release capsule 200, once
Diflunisal	250–500, twice
COX-2 selective (Cox 2>1)	
Meloxicam	7.5–15, once
Etodolac	300 twice or 600, slow release once
COX-2 specific	
Celecoxib	100–200, twice
Etoricoxib	90, once

COX, cyclooxygenase.

From Arnett FC *et al.* The American Rheumatism Association 1987 revised criteria for the classification of rheumatoid arthritis. *Arthritis and Rheumatism* 31 (1988), pp315–34. Copyright 1988. Reprinted with permission of John Wiley and Sons Inc.

the several NSAIDs available is most suited to an individual patient (see section on antirheumatic drugs for detailed discussion).

DMARDs should be used in all patients (see Table 19.5.2), the two most commonly employed being sulfasalazine and methotrexate, provided there are no contraindications. These are usually commenced as a single drug given in incremental doses over 3 to 4 months to the maximum recommended or tolerated dose. In most centres methotrexate is the drug of choice because of its efficacy and superior durability in the long term; indeed it has been described as the 'gold standard' drug. If a clearcut reduction in disease activity (or remission) is not observed with one of these drugs, then other DMARDs are added at this stage. Commonly used DMARD combinations include: methotrexate and hydroxychloroquine; methotrexate, sulfasalazine and hydroxychloroquine; and methotrexate and leflunomide or ciclosporin. The choice of therapy is ultimately determined by evaluation of risks of toxicity, efficacy, durability, and direct and indirect costs of treatment. There is no consensus on the most effective combination regimen. Meticulous monitoring for toxic effects is necessary.

In practice, over 50% of patients with moderate or severe disease require coadministration of corticosteroid therapy (see section on corticosteroids below). If continuing long-term use appears necessary, the aim should be to reduce the dose to the equivalent of 5 to 7.5 mg of prednisolone daily by more aggressive use of DMARDs, or instigation of anti-TNF therapy. By 2006, anti-TNF drugs, especially given concomitantly with methotrexate,

had become the standard of care in patients with continuing active disease despite prior exposure to DMARDs, one of which is methotrexate (for further information including safety issues see section on biological therapy below). The guidelines proposed by the National Institute of Health and Clinical Excellence (NICE) in the United Kingdom require high disease activity and nonresponsiveness to two DMARDs before anti-TNF biologicals can be prescribed. Anti-TNF drugs have become widely used, with an estimated 1 million patients exposed to them for a variety of indications, but mostly RA. High cost continues to restrict access to treatment with biologicals.

As 30 to 40% of patients do not respond to one of the three anti-TNF agents and develop resistance to therapy, switching to another (e.g. infliximab to etanercept or adalimumab or vice versa) appears to be effective in some patients. In patients with lack of efficacy or adverse events, anakinra has been used as an alternative in this setting. Two new biologicals, B-cell-depleting rituximab, or T-cell-activation-blocking abatacept (CTLA4-Ig), are efficacious in anti-TNF failures. However, the use of anakinra and abatacept simultaneously with anti-TNF biologicals does not improve outcomes and increases toxicity, hence their combined use is contraindicated. As the use of all biologicals is associated with adverse events, careful selection and monitoring of patients is mandatory (see section on biological therapy, below).

Treatment of extra-articular disease

Effective treatment of RA generally reduces the risk of developing severe extra-articular disease. Systemic rheumatoid vasculitis is potentially a life-threatening complication and may be aggravated by coincidental infection, such as through cutaneous ulcers. After due attention to confirming the diagnosis and excluding and treating infections with appropriate antimicrobial drugs, therapy with high-dose corticosteroids and cyclophosphamide is favoured by many specialists, although no randomized placebo-controlled trial data are available. One regimen recommends intravenous methylprednisolone at 1 g daily for 3 days, simultaneously with an initial single pulse of intravenous cyclophosphamide (10 to 15 mg/kg) in a fully hydrated patient to prevent bladder toxicity. Cyclophosphamide is repeated every 3 to 4 weeks, subject to a satisfactory clinical response or lack of toxicity, up to a total dose of 10 to 12 g in a cycle of treatment. Alternatively, oral cyclophosphamide at 2 mg/kg (maximum dose 150 mg daily) may be used. Oral high-dose prednisolone is continued until clinical response is observed or toxic effects occur, when it is rapidly tapered to a maintenance dose, generally about 15 mg daily. Similarly, cyclophosphamide is substituted by the less toxic azathioprine at 1.5 to 2 mg/kg daily or methotrexate at 15 mg/week.

Similar regimens have been used for severe fibrosing alveolitis and for severe scleritis and corneal melt in conjunction with local therapy. Occasional patients with Felty's syndrome and hypersplenism that do not respond to DMARDs benefit from splenectomy, and their neutropenia may respond to recombinant human granulocyte colony stimulating factor (G-CSF). Keratoconjunctivitis sicca and dry mouth due to secondary Sjögren's syndrome respond to local measures, including artificial tears, dental hygiene, and saliva substitute.

Effective treatment of RA with suppression of the acute phase response with DMARDs, corticosteroids, and anti-TNFα therapy prevents progression of secondary amyloidosis. In patients with

Table 19.5.2 DMARDs in adults[a,b]

Drug	Dose and comments	Contraindications	Some side effects[a]
Methotrexate	Oral 7.5 mg/week initially given as a single dose; usual dose 12.5–15 mg/week; increase up to 25 mg/week orally and try intramuscular route in unresponsive patients or in presence of gastrointestinal intolerance; folic acid 5 mg daily for 1–5 days/week improves tolerability	Pregnancy and planned conception (teratogenic), alcohol abuse, chronic liver disease, diabetes mellitus, moderate to severe chronic lung disease	Bone marrow suppression, hepatotoxicity, interstital pneumonitis, anorexia, nausea, stomatitis, vomiting, viral and opportunistic infections, possible increased risk of lymphoma
Sulphasalazine	Enteric-coated tablets 0.5 g once a day for initial week; thereafter 0.5 g increment in dose per week to total 2 g/day; maximum dose 3 g/day	Sulfonamide, salicylate allergy, glucose-6-phosphate dehydrogenase deficiency	Nausea, anorexia, rashes, blood dyscrasia (especially neutropenia), lupus-like syndrome, oligospermia on taking drug (reversible)
Hydroxychloroquine	200–400 mg in divided doses daily; maximum dose 6.5 mg/kg (not exceeding 400 mg/day); maintenance dose 200–400 mg daily	Glucose-6-phosphate dehydrogenase deficiency, retinal disease, psoriasis	Maculopathy; test visual acuity and fields, colour vision before commencing therapy; if abnormal, full ophthalmology examination required; patient to stop drug if any disturbance of vision noted. Annual check-ups advisable; discontinuation after 10 years recommended
or			
Chloroquine sulfate	(200 mg, equivalent to chloroquine phosphate 250 mg or chloroquine base 150 mg); daily dose of chloroquine base 150 mg, daily maximum 2.5 mg/kg	As above	
Injectable gold aurothiomalate	Deep intramuscular, upper/outer gluteal muscle; 10 mg test dose to check for hypersensitivity; 20–50 mg weekly according to tolerability and severity to a total of 1 g or until response is observed; maintenance dose 20–50 mg/month	Gold hypersensitivity, chronic liver and renal disease, psoriasis	Blood dyscrasias, aplastic anaemia, nephropathy, dermatitis
Azathioprine	Oral 1 to 3 mg/kg daily	Up to 1 in 200 of the population have hypersensitivity characterized by severe leucopenia on initial administration	Hepatitis, reversible dose-related bone marrow depression, possible increased risk of lymphoma
Ciclosporin	Oral initially 2–5 mg/kg up to 4 mg/kg provided serum creatinine is in normal range and does not increase more than 30% above baseline	Renal disease with compromised function hypertension	Nephrotoxicity, hirsurtism, hypertension, tremor
D-Penicillamine	Oral 250–1000 mg daily in divided doses starting at 125–250 mg initially	Penicillin hypersensitivity	Taste loss, thrombocytopenia and other dyscrasias, nephropathy, myaesthenia gravis, rashes
Leflunomide	Initial loading dose 100 mg orally, once daily for 3 days, followed by maintenance dose 10–20 mg daily	Pregnancy (teratogenic), planned conception; long half-life (several months): cholestyramine accelerates clearance	Increases serum concentrations of drugs metabolized by CYPZC9, including NSAIDs; diarrhoea, alopecia, hepatotoxicity, and (rarely) bone marrow suppression

[a]Refer to institutional, and or/national, and/or British Society for Rheumatology Drug Monitoring Guidelines (National guidelines for monitoring second-line drugs, July 2000, http://www.rheumatology.org.uk/resources/guidelines/guidelines_archive.aspx)

[b]For other contraindications and details consult product literature before use.

British Society for Rheumatology Drug Monitoring Guidelines (National guidelines for monitoring second line drugs, July 2000, www.rheumatology.org/guidelines/clinicalguidelines

a continuing acute phase response despite the standard DMARD therapy, treatment with chlorambucil is reported to be of some benefit. Imaging of radionuclide-labelled serum amyloid P protein in the spleen and kidneys may be used to monitor treatment.

Antirheumatic drugs: clinical trials, mechanism of action, and use in the clinic

NSAIDs

NSAIDs are widely used for treating symptoms of inflammation and pain in RA and do not modify the progression of structural damage. They act by inhibiting the enzymes COX-1 and/or COX-2, which convert lipid substrates in cells to prostanoids. Tissues such as the gastric and duodenal mucosa express COX-1, which in the gastroduodenal mucosa regulates the production of prostaglandins, including PGE_2, that exert a protective effect on its integrity by reducing acid secretion and increasing the secretion of mucus and bicarbonate. COX-2 is mainly induced by proinflammatory cytokines in synovial tissue cells and monocytes at sites of inflammation, stimulating production of inflammatory prostaglandins—hence it was thought that COX-2 might be an ideal anti-inflammatory drug target for treating RA.

Aspirin blocks COX-1 activity and is an effective anti-inflammatory drug in high doses, but it is a well-recognized cause of gastric bleeding. Many of the previous generation of NSAIDs, such as indometacin, diclofenac, and high-dose ibuprofen, which inhibit both

COX-1 and -2 activity, exert an anti-inflammatory effect by inhibiting the production of inflammatory mediators. However, they compromise the gastroprotective effect of COX-1, and traditional NSAIDs—apart perhaps from naproxen—do not significantly inhibit the prothrombic platelet COX-1 activity and synthesis of thromboxane A_2 (which is inhibited by low-dose aspirin).

With regard to specific COX-2 inhibitors, based on laboratory experiments, it is suggested that they might suppress the production of prostacyclin by endothelial cells. As prostacyclin plays a protective role as a vasodilator and regulator of blood pressure and cardiac function, blockade of COX-2 could theoretically leave unopposed the action of COX-1-induced platelet aggregation, potentially promoting hypertension and cardiovascular thrombotic complications (see below).

The traditional NSAIDS are responsible for admission to hospital of over 1% of patients with RA per year for complications such as peptic ulceration, gastric haemorrhage, and perforation, and account for a twofold increase in death over expected rates. It is claimed that the least gastrotoxic are ibuprofen and nabumetone, with naproxen and diclofenac carrying intermediate risk, followed by drugs with a high risk, such as fenoprofen, ketoprofen, indometacin, piroxicam, and azapropazone. It is claimed that drugs such as meloxicam that act by greater selective inhibition of COX-2 and thus spare COX-1 also have fewer gastropathic effects (see Table 19.5.1 for drugs and dose ranges).

For patients who develop dyspepsia and/or NSAID-induced gastropathy, or elderly patients who have a high risk of gastroduodenal side effects, concomitant administration of prostaglandin analogues (such as misoprostol) or proton pump inhibitors (such as omeprazole or lansoprazole) is recommended, and NSAIDs are best avoided for patients with a history of peptic ulcers. Eradication of *Helicobacter pylori* infection results in long-term healing of preexisting gastric and duodenal ulcers, but whether it decreases dyspepsia or ulceration caused by NSAIDs is uncertain.

The highly selective or specific inhibitors of COX-2, including celecoxib, rofecoxib, valdecoxib, and etoricoxib, possess no significant COX-1 inhibitory activity at anti-inflammatory therapeutic doses. Clinical trials have demonstrated their improved safety profile in respect to endoscopically detectable gastroduodenal ulcers, upper gastrointestinal haemorrhage, and perforation when compared with conventional NSAIDs. However, rofecoxib was withdrawn in 2004 by the manufacturer after a trial for the prevention of adenomatous polyps demonstrated a twofold increase in cardiovascular complications at a dose of 25 mg daily. Similar concerns were raised in regard to celocoxib 400 mg twice daily in the same preventive setting, but at lower doses it appeared to have an acceptable risk (similar to naproxen) for cardiovascular thrombotic events. Valedocoxib was withdrawn following reports of serious adverse events in 2005.

Although the adverse risk profiles of individual drugs continues to be debated, meta-analyses of controlled and observational trials has confirmed that all COX-2 inhibitors have increased risk of thrombotic cardiovascular complications, such as myocardial infarction and stroke, most marked for rofecoxib at normal doses and at high dose for celocoxib. Meta-analyses of observational studies have also demonstrated that traditional NSAIDS such as diclofenac, indometacin, and (probably) meloxicam also carry an increased cardiovascular risk, whereas naproxen does not appear to increase or decrease this risk. Based on these observations,

naproxen, low-dose celecoxib, and low-dose ibuprofen emerge as relatively free of cardiovascular risk. Regulatory authorities advise use for short periods and careful monitoring for longer-term use of all NSAIDs, and specifically advise against the use of COX-2 inhibitors in patients with ischaemic heart disease or cerebrovascular disease. Evidence from meta-analysis supports the view that the same advice is appropriate for high doses of traditional NSAIDs.

All NSAIDs can cause fluid retention and oedema by a renin–angiotensin-dependent mechanism that may also aggravate congestive cardiac failure and systemic hypertension. Patients with impaired renal function, cirrhosis of the liver, and decreased plasma volume from any cause are at risk from developing NSAID-induced renal toxicity. It is claimed that sulindac may be safer than other NSAIDs in patients with renal failure.

NSAIDs, especially indometacin, may cause central nervous system side effects such as headache, dizziness, anxiety, disorientation, and drowsiness. Use of NSAIDs may aggravate asthma and cause hypersensitivity reactions, and they may rarely be associated with aseptic meningitis. Blood dyscrasias and an increase in serum concentration of liver enzymes and alkaline phosphatase are described. Drug interactions may decrease the efficacy of some concomitantly prescribed therapies—e.g. antihypertensives and lithium—and potentiate the effects of others—e.g. anticoagulants, antiepileptics, and oral hypoglycaemics. NSAIDs decrease the excretion of methotrexate but do not appear to increase its toxicity in the dose range used to treat RA. They also increase plasma concentrations of ciclosporin and tacrolimus (FK-506) and hence may increase the risk of renal toxicity.

DMARDs

DMARDs modify the trajectory of progressive structural damage and disability and are the cornerstone of drug therapy for RA (Table 19.5.2). They are also classified as slow-acting antirheumatoid drugs (SAARDs) because of the lag period of some weeks before their anti-inflammatory effect becomes apparent. Drugs in this category include: the antimalarials hydroxychloroquine or chloroquine sulfate; sulfasalazine; weekly low-dose oral or parenterally administered methotrexate; weekly injections of gold aurothiomalate or gold aurothioglucose; leflunomide; ciclosporin; azathioprine; and D-penicillamine.

Drugs such as gold, antimalarials, and methotrexate were introduced for use in RA by serendipity. Others such as azathioprine, ciclosporin, and lefluomide were developed as immunosuppressive agents for preventing transplant rejections and subsequently used to curb the aberrant immunological response in RA. The mechanism of action of these drugs in RA is complex and still incompletely understood. Inhibitory effects on inflammatory pathways, immune responses, and cell activation have been described in experimental systems and clinical studies.

Clinical trials have demonstrated superior efficacy of all these drugs over placebo in controlling symptoms and signs in patients previously treated with only NSAIDs in early and established RA. In addition, sulfasalazine, methotrexate, and leflunomide retard progression of structural damage, as assessed by serial radiographs of the hands and feet in controlled trials lasting 6 to 12 months compared with placebo.

A meta-analysis of clinical trials of commonly used DMARDs, usually given to patients stabilized on NSAIDS and—in many instances—low-dose corticosteroid therapy, has been analysed for efficacy and toxicity relative to each other and to placebo treatment. Methotrexate and sulfasalazine have the best and equal efficacy in the short term compared with placebo. The antimalarials (hydroxychloroquine and chloroquine) and azathioprine appear to be less efficacious in this analysis. However, the toxicity profile shows a different rank order: antimalarials are least toxic, followed by methotrexate and sulfasalazine in an intermediate range, with injectable gold, azathioprine, and D-penicillamine at the most toxic end of the spectrum. Methotrexate and sulfasalazine emerge with the best balance between efficacy and toxicity, and injectable gold and D-pencillamine are now rarely used. Leflunomide was introduced recently and not included in this meta-analysis, but its efficacy and toxicity profile is similar to that of methotrexate and sulfasalazine.

Conclusions from short-term randomized clinical trials do not reflect the effectiveness of DMARDs in controlling disease activity in the longer term. Incomplete responses, relapses, and adverse events are common and account for discontinuation of antimalarials, gold salts, D-penicillamine, sulfasalazine, and azathioprine in most patients in 1 to 3 years. By contrast, responses to methotrexate appear to be more durable in follow-up studies of large cohorts of patients with RA, with about 50% continuing therapy at 5 years. Data on long-term effectiveness, tolerability, and toxicity of leflunomide are not yet available.

Combinations of DMARDs have been used in the expectation that their different modes of action might provide added efficacy. Differing approaches have been used: e.g. sequential change from one DMARD to another; add-on of DMARDS, referred to as 'step-up'; commencing with a combination from the start with phased withdrawal of all except one ('step-down'); and long-term continuing combinations of two or more DMARDS (in parallel). A meta-analysis showed that there was only marginal benefit at the doses and combinations used before 1994, especially in the reduction of number of tender joints, with increased toxicity when compared with single agents. However, several subsequent randomized controlled trials have demonstrated significantly improved efficacy of combination therapy, without increased toxicity: some examples of such trials are given below.

In a Finnish study on patients with disease of less than 2 years' duration, the introduction of a combination of sulfasalazine, methotrexate, hydroxychloquine, and oral prednisolone not only controlled symptoms better but, at the end of 2 years, had induced remission in 37% compared with 21% of patients on monotherapy with sulfasalazine (initially) or methotrexate alone, plus prednisolone in two-thirds of patients. There was greater retardation of joint damage and a better quality of life in the combination than in the monotherapy group.

In a North American trial lasting 2 years, a combination of oral methotrexate (7.5 to 17.5 mg/week), sulfasalazine (0.5 g twice daily) and hydroxychloroquine (200 mg twice daily) showed superior control of symptoms and signs compared with methotrexate alone or a combination of sulfasalazine and hydroxychloroquine. Patients enrolled in this trial with advanced disease had already failed to respond to DMARD monotherapy.

In a Dutch study, a combination of sulfasalazine 2 g/day, methotrexate 7.5 mg per week for 40 weeks, and prednisolone in a dose of 60 mg daily for 6 weeks, rapidly tapered to 7.5 mg per day and withdrawn at 28 weeks, was compared with monotherapy with sulfasalazine 2 g/day. Clinical responses were better in the combination

therapy group at 1 year, and markedly so for the first 28 weeks. In a follow-up study during which patients received similar exposure to DMARDs, the rate of radiographically assessed join damage remained slower in the group initially treated with combination of high-dose corticosteroid and DMARDs.

In a British trial, an intensive therapy group was compared with a group receiving routine care from specialist physicians. The intensively treated group was seen every month and, according to protocol if disease was active, therapy escalated with maximum tolerated doses of sulfasalazine followed by addition of corticosteroids and methotrexate, or variously of ciclosporin or leflunomide or sodium aurothiomalate. Routinely treated patients mostly received DMARD monotherapy and intra-articular corticosteroid. At 18 months the intensively treated groups had superior outcomes in all measurements of disease activity, with higher remission levels and control of structural radiographic damage than the group receiving routine care.

From these studies it may be concluded that if disease is not suppressed by monotherapy with methotrexate in maximum tolerated doses, then a combination of DMARDs with dose adjustments that achieve low disease activity is highly effective in a significant proportion of patients with moderate and severe RA.

Corticosteroids

Corticosteroids are potent anti-inflammatory agents and are most efficacious in treating symptoms and signs of RA and for amelioration of systemic features, but their use is limited by toxicity related to dose and duration of exposure. The circumstances in which use of corticosteroids has been established and those in which it is debated are described below.

In patients in whom loss of function and disease activity is restricted to a few joints, local corticosteroid therapy can be most effective. This indication may arise in those whose rheumatoid disease is limited to a few joints, or in patients with an incomplete response to NSAID and DMARD therapy. Several alternative corticosteroid preparations are available, the dose being dependent on the size of the joint. Depot methylprednisolone (dose range 4–40 mg) or triamcinolone acetonide (dose range 2.5–40 mg) are suitable alternatives. Repeat injections may be necessary, but more than three per joint per year should be avoided.

Corticosteroid administered orally in courses lasting a few weeks to months (such as prednisolone at 7.5–10 mg daily), or in the form of 'pulse therapy' (such as depot methylprednisolone at 80–120 mg by intramuscular injection), is a suitable adjunctive therapy in patients in whom the benefit of DMARDs is not yet established. Longer-term, more or less indefinite, treatment with low-dose prednisolone is necessary in patients with moderate to severe disease, especially if associated with refractory anaemia that is not controlled with currently used antirheumatoid drugs. Long-term low-dose prednisolone retards the progression of rheumatoid bone erosions in radiographs of hands and feet and, hence it is claimed, deterioration of physical function. Whether this benefit is outweighed by the side effects and morbidity of corticosteroid therapy is debatable. Higher doses of corticosteroids are indicated in the treatment of severe extra-articular disease.

Prevention of corticosteroid-induced osteoporosis and reduction in risk of fractures requires adequate prophylaxis with calcium and vitamin D intake (e.g. daily intake of 1000 mg of calcium and 800 IU of vitamin D). In susceptible patients, or those on doses

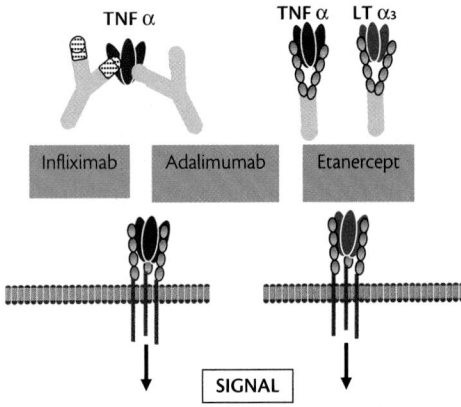

Fig. 19.5.11 Anti-TNFα-specific chimaeric (infliximab) and human (adalimumab) monoclonal antibodies bind to TNFα with high affinity. p75 soluble receptor TNF linked to Fc IgG (etanercept) binds to both TNFα and lymphotoxin (also known as TNFβ). The binding to TNF inhibits binding to TNF receptors and intracellular signalling that leads to the expression of inflammatory and tissue destructive responses in rheumatoid arthritis.

exceeding the equivalent of 7.5 mg of prednisolone daily, measurement of bone mineral density is used to identify and monitor management. Bisphosphonates may be required in addition to calcium and vitamin D, and hormone replacement therapy is recommended in perimenopausal women.

Biological therapies

Biological monoclonal antibody and recombinant protein drugs that have proved efficacious in double-blind randomized controlled clinical trials include three anti-TNF drugs—two monoclonal antibodies, infliximab and adalimumab, and etanercept, a TNF-receptor

fused to Fc IgG—which are the most widely used biologicals, and other biologicals, namely anakinra, an IL-1 receptor antagonist; rituximab, an anti-CD20 B-cell-depleting monoclonal antibody; and abatacept (CTLA4-Ig), a receptor-fusion-FcIgG recombinant protein. More biological drugs for the treatment of rheumatoid arthritis are emerging, including 2 additional anti-TNF blocking agents (golimumab, a fully human monoclonal antibody and certolizumab, a PEGylated Fab' fragment of a humanized anti-TNF monoclonal antibody) and tocilizumab, a monoclonal antibody which inhibits binding of IL-6 to its receptor.

Anti-TNF biologicals

Despite good initial responses to currently available DMARD treatments, about 40 to 50% of hospital patients eventually show continuing disease activity and progressive disability. A TNF-receptor-FcIgG recombinant protein (etanercept) and a chimeric monoclonal antibody specific for TNF (infliximab), followed by a humanized monoclonal antibody (adalimumab), were in the first group of biologicals to be shown to be beneficial for the treatment of RA in this setting. All three (and the newer anti-TNF drugs) inhibit the binding of TNFα to its cell surface receptors, thereby inhibiting its immune and inflammatory action (Fig. 19.5.11). Although there are some differences in their biological properties *in vitro*, their efficacy in placebo-controlled randomized clinical trials and observational studies is similar.

Symptoms and signs are rapidly alleviated in approximately 60 to 70% of patients (examples shown in Fig. 19.5.12) in clinical trials and confirmed by large single and multicentre observational studies. Attempts to identify the nonresponders by clinical characteristics or biomarkers have not been successful thus far. Continuing therapy is needed by those who do respond, with relapse following withdrawal except in early stages of disease (see below).

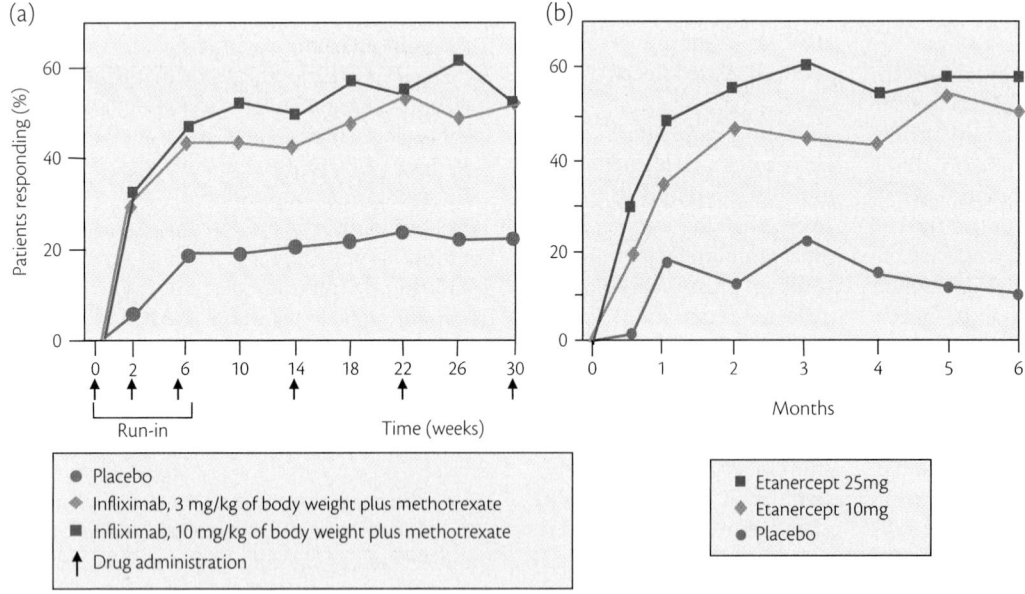

Fig. 19.5.12 Anti-TNF therapy. (a) Efficacy of combination of infliximab and methotrexate compared with methotrexate and placebo. Percentage of patients achieving a clinical response of a 20% change from baseline as defined by the American College of Rheumatology 20 (ACR20) criteria. Patients were treated with methotrexate (10 to 35 mg/week) and either placebo, 3, or 10 mg/kg infliximab administered intravenously at time points indicated, in a patient group unresponsive to DMARDs with active disease despite methotrexate therapy (Maini *et al.* 1999). (b) Efficacy of etanercept compared with placebo. ACR 20 results in patients treated with two doses of etanercept or placebo injections administered subcutaneously twice weekly over a 6-month period in a population unresponsive to DMARDs.
Reproduced from Moreland LW, Schiff MF, Baumgartner SW, et al: Etanercept therapy in rheumatoid arthritis. Ann Intern Med 1999 (16th March), 130:478–486. Fig 2. http://www.annals.org/cgi/reprint/130/6/478.

Infliximab is given intravenously at a dose of 3 mg/kg over 1 h every 8 weeks in combination with methotrexate therapy once a week. Etanercept is given at a dose of 25 mg subcutaneously twice weekly or 50 mg weekly, and adalimumab 40 mg subcutaneously weekly or fortnightly, both of these drugs being efficacious as monotherapy or in combination with methotrexate. Further details, including contraindications and some side effects, are shown in Table 19.5.3.

In patients with long-standing disease and a high level of disease activity despite DMARD and methotrexate therapy, in whom DMARDs are discontinued, randomized controlled trials have demonstrated that anti-TNF drugs are efficacious as monotherapy in approximately 70% of patients. The concomitant addition of anti-TNF drugs to methotrexate shows more marked efficacy in the control of signs, symptoms, and especially structural damage, when compared with continuing methotrexate or initiating monotherapy with the anti-TNF drugs. Improvement in quality of life measurements and work employability is well documented.

In early disease and in methotrexate naïve patients, infliximab and methotrexate given concomitantly is more effective than methotrexate alone. Similarly, etanercept or adalimumab and concomitant methotrexate is more effective than methotrexate, etanercept, or adalimumab alone.

In two observational studies in early RA it was shown that following induction therapy with a combination of infliximab and methotrexate for 6 to 9 months, anti-TNF drug-free remission could be maintained in around 50% of patients on methotrexate alone for up to 3 years, which has possible pharmacoeconomic benefits.

Notable additional features of therapy with anti-TNF drugs in combination with methotrexate include radiographic changes suggestive of the healing of structural damage in some patients. A subanalysis of trials with infliximab or etanercept plus methotrexate given concomitantly also demonstrates inhibition of radiographically assessed structural damage, even in patients with no improvement in clinical signs of inflammatory disease, suggesting that this combination, unlike methotrexate monotherapy, uncouples mechanisms of inflammation and tissue damage.

Durable responses in the responder population have been demonstrated in several observational studies from single or multiple centres for 2 to over 5 years. An increase in the dose of the anti-TNF drugs may be necessary to maintain efficacy. In patients with loss of efficacy following dose adjustments (secondary nonresponders), switching to a different anti-TNF biological may be efficacious.

Anti-TNF biologicals are generally well tolerated, but concerns have been raised from reported adverse events in controlled clinical trials of serious infections, increased incidence of antinuclear antibodies, infrequent drug-induced lupus, and an increased incidence of B-cell lymphomas and cancer.

Post-marketing surveillance of adverse events has confirmed the occurrence of rare but significant numbers of cases of sepsis, tuberculosis, and fungal and opportunistic infections. These infections are compatible with the consequences of blockade of the postulated role of TNF in host defence mechanisms. Based on these reports, regulatory authorities in the United States of America and Europe have advised that anti-TNF therapy is contraindicated

Table 19.5.3 Biological therapies for rheumatoid arthritis

Drug	Description	Dose/comments	Contraindications	Side effects
Anti-TNFα				
Adalimumab	Fully human IgG1 monoclonal antibody	40 mg SC alternate weeks; given with methotrexate; may be used as monotherapy	Infection, especially *Mycobacterium tuberculosis*, cancer, heart failure, SLE, demyelinating disease, e.g. MS	Unusual infections, diarrhoea, constipation, vomiting, gastritis rash
Etanercept	TNF receptor-Fc-IgG1 fusion protein	25 mg SC twice weekly or 50 mg SC once weekly, alone or with methotrexate	Infection, cancer, heart failure, SLE, demyelinating disease, e.g. MS	Vomiting/oesophagitis, cholecycystitis, hypotension/hypertension, lymphadenopathy
Infliximab	Mouse/human chimaeric IgG1 monoclonal antibody	3 mg/kg IV, repeated at 2 weeks and 6 weeks after initial infusion, then maintenance 8 weekly; given with methotrexate	Infection, especially *Mycobacterium tuberculosis*, cancer, heart failure, SLE, demyelinating disease, e.g. MS	Dyspepsia, diarrhoea, constipation, hepatitis, cholecystitis, flushing, bradycardia, arrhythmias, rash
Anti-IL-1				
Anakinra	Recombinant nonglycosylated synthetic human form of the IL-1RA protein	100 mg/day SC	Neutropenia, documented hypersensitivity to *E. coli* derivatives	Neutropenia, injection site reaction, headache, infections
B-cell depletion				
Rituximab	Chimeric mouse/human monoclonal antibody against CD20+ B cells	1 g IV, day 1 and day 15; given with methotrexate	Known hypersensitivity to murine products	Hypersensitivity reaction to first infusion, fever, chills, angioedema, nausea, pruritis, rash, infusion reaction
Blockade of CD28 on T cells				
Abatacept	Human recombinant CTLA-4 IgG fusion protein	500 mg–1 g IV (depending on body weight), repeated at 2 weeks and then every 4 weeks after initial administration	Cancer, infections	Headache, nasopharyngitis, dizziness, cough, hypertension, rash

CTLA-4, cytotoxic T-lymphocyte-associated antigen 4; IL-1RA, interleukin 1 receptor antagonist; IV, intravenously; MS, multiple sclerosis; SC, subcutaneously; SLE, systemic lupus erythematosus.
Data from the British Society for Rheumatology Drug Monitoring Guidelines (National guidelines for monitoring second line drugs, July 2000)

in the presence of active serious infections and latent untreated tuberculosis, and screening for latent tuberculosis and prophylactic antituberculosis therapy has markedly reduced complication with this infection. Other rare adverse events have included the occurrence of B-cell lymphomas, demyelinating syndromes (hence it is advisable not to treat patients with a history of multiple sclerosis), lupus syndrome, and bone marrow depression. Based on reports of an unexpected number of deaths observed in a phase II clinical trial of infliximab in the treatment of severe congestive cardiac failure, use of anti-TNF biologicals is not advisable for the treatment of patients with RA in moderate or severe congestive cardiac failure.

Prospective and retrospective studies of control populations of rheumatoid patients that have not been exposed to biologicals have demonstrated that in an aging rheumatoid population the incidence of infections, lymphomas, other cancers, myocardial infarction, and strokes is higher than the normal population. When these confounding variables are taken into consideration in analysing large databases in Europe and North America, the conclusions have been at variance from those described above. Thus it is suggested that aside from opportunistic infections, the incidence of life-threatening infections, lymphomas, cancers (apart from skin cancers), and cardiovascular comorbidity appears not to be increased in anti-TNF-treated patients. However, at least in respect of infections, these findings may reflect the exclusion from treatment of patients who are susceptible to comorbidity such as infections, and to early detection and treatment of potentially serious infections.

Provided suitable screening and monitoring practices are in place, the benefit of anti-TNF therapy exceeds harm and is indicated for the treatment of moderate to severe RA with persistent disease activity despite best available standard therapy. Ideally, anti-TNF therapy should be instituted as soon as it becomes apparent that remission or near-remission is not induced by the best use of traditional DMARDs in the early stages of an established diagnosis, but cost constraints or safety concerns may limit the institution of this therapeutic approach.

Other biologicals

Recombinant human IL-1RA (anakinra) binds to IL-1 receptor, thereby inhibiting access of IL-1 to the receptor and initiating an IL-1-mediated proinflammatory response. In RA the endogenous production of IL-1RA is very significantly increased simultaneously with overproduction of IL-1, but insufficient to inhibit the action of excess amount of IL-1. To be clinically effective in fully inhibiting the action of IL-1, almost full engagement of IL-1 receptors by anakinra is required, and even daily administration may not achieve this goal, because anakinra is very rapidly cleared from the circulation.

In randomized controlled trials, anakinra is effective vs placebo in reducing signs, symptoms, and progressive radiographically assessed structural damage in rheumatoid patients who have failed traditional DMARDs. In clinical trials the coadministration of anakinra in patients with active disease despite methotrexate is similarly efficacious. Its use in early RA has not been demonstrated.

Anakinra is administered at a dose of 100 mg daily by subcutaneous injection. Injection site reactions occur in most patients, and severe infections have been described, although not activation of tuberculosis as seen with anti-TNF drugs. However, it is unclear whether infections occur in a higher incidence than in a matched-control population of rheumatoid patients, and postmarketing databases are not as extensive as those for anti-TNF

drugs. The combined use of anakinra and etanercept showed no additional efficacy, but was associated with increase in serious infections, hence combination of anti-TNF drugs and anakinra is not recommended. It is not definitively established whether anakinra is effective in anti-TNF failures, but it has been used clinically in this setting. Anakinra is licensed for use alone or in combination in the United States of America, but only in combination with methotrexate in the European Union. According to NICE guidelines in the United Kingdom, it may only be prescribed as part of an experimental protocol.

Rituximab, a chimeric monoclonal antibody that depletes B cells, has been licensed since 1997 for the treatment of B-cell lymphomas. It binds to mature B cells and activated B cells (plasmacytoid cells) but not plasma cells. In RA, randomized placebo-controlled trials have demonstrated efficacy of rituximab in patients who have failed on DMARD and anti-TNF therapy. Combination therapy with methotrexate is more effective than monotherapy, and is administered as a course of two infusions of rituximab at a dose of 1 g separated by 2 weeks with corticosteroid co-administration (see Table 19.5.3).

Rituximab administration is associated with a loss of circulating B cells for several months and a reduction in rheumatoid factor levels, but no significant reduction in circulating immunoglobulin concentrations. Relapse in disease usually occurs after about 6 months, and there is limited experience thus far of the long-term efficacy and safety of repeat therapy. Infusion reactions occur, especially with the first infusion. Severe infections are described and it is recommended that if vaccination against influenza or pneumococcal pneumonia is deemed necessary, these should be given before commencing rituximab therapy.

Abatacept, a recombinant protein, consists of the extracellular domain of cytotoxic T-lymphocyte antigen 4 (CTLA4) linked to the Fc portion of IgG1. Abatacept binds to CD80 and CD86 on antigen-presenting cells, thereby preventing their ability to bind to CD 28 on T cells. The engagement of CD28 is the second signal that a T cell requires for activation in addition to the signal delivered by antigen–HLA complex via the T-cell receptor. It is proposed that in RA abatacept terminates the activation of T cells and subsequent pathology, e.g. as mediated by proinflammatory cytokines.

Abatacept administered as monotherapy and in combination with methotrexate is efficacious in patients who have failed DMARD and anti-TNF therapy in randomized clinical trials. However, the co-administration of abatacept and anti-TNF biologicals or anakinra significantly increases serious infections without a corresponding increase in efficacy. Abatacept is administered by intravenous injection, and following initiating therapy at week 0 and at week 2 is given thereafter repeatedly every 4 weeks. It is envisaged that abatacept will offer a useful biological alternative in the group of patients with severe RA who fail to respond to anti-TNF agents. Its long-term efficacy, safety, and cost-effectiveness are not yet established.

Guidelines for the emerging class of biological drugs for the treatment of rheumatoid arthritis are being constantly updated, e.g. by The National Institute of Health and Clinical Excellence (NICE) in England and Wales.

Further reading

Anderson JJ, et al. (2000). Factors predicting response to treatment in rheumatoid arthritis: the importance of disease duration. *Arthritis Rheum*, **43**, 22–9.

Arnett FC, et al. (1988). The American Rheumatism Association 1987 revised criteria for the classification of rheumatoid arthritis. *Arthritis Rheum*, **31**, 315–34.

Boers M. et al. (1997). Randomised comparison of combined step-down prednisolone, methotrexate and sulphasalazine with sulphasalazine alone in early rheumatoid arthritis. *Lancet*, **350**, 309–18.

Bongartz T, et al. (2006). Anti-TNF antibody therapy in rheumatoid arthritis and the risk of serious infections and malignancies. *J Am Med Assoc*, **295**, 2275–85.

Breedveld F, et al. (2006). The PREMIER study. A multicentre, randomized, double-blind clinical trial of combination therapy with adalimumab plus methotrexate versus methotrexate alone or adalimumbab alone in patients with early, aggressive rheumatoid arthritis who had not had previous methotrexate treatment. *Arthritis Rheum*, **54**, 26–37.

Brennan M, et al. (2006). Comparing rates of dyspepsia with coxibs vs NSAID and PPI: a meta-analysis. *Am J Med*, **119**, 448.

Brooks P, et al. (1999). Interpreting the clinical significance of the differential inhibition of cyclooxygenase-1 and cyclooxygenase-2. *Rheumatology*, **38**, 779–88.

Chakravarty K, McDonald H, Pullar T, et al. (2008). BSR/BHPR guideline for disease-modifying anti-rheumatic drug (DMARD) therapy in consultation with the British Association of Dermatologists. *Rheumatology* (Oxford), **47**(6), 924–5.

Choi HK, et al. (2002). Methotrexate and mortality in patients with rheumatoid arthritis: a prospective study. *Lancet*, **359**, 1173–7.

Cohen SB, et al. (2006). Rituximab for rheumatoid arthritis refractory to anti-tumor necrosis factor therapy: results of a multicentre, randomized, double-blind, placebo-controlled, phase III trial evaluating primary efficacy and safety at twenty-four weeks. *Arthritis Rheum*, **54**, 2793–806.

Emery P (2006). Treatment of rheumatoid arthritis. *Br Med J*, **332**, 152–5.

Erhardt CC, et al. (1989). Factors predicting a poor life prognosis in rheumatoid arthritis: an eight year prospective study. *Ann Rheum Dis*, **48**, 7–13.

Feldmann M, Brennan FM, Maini RN (1996). Role of cytokines in rheumatoid arthritis. *Annu Rev Immunol*, **14**, 397–440.

Feldmann M, Maini RN (2001) Anti-TNF alpha therapy of rheumatoid arthritis: what have we learned? *Annu Rev Immunol*, **19**, 163–96.

Feldmann M. Maini RN (2003). TNF defined as a therapeutic target for rheumatoid arthritis and other autoimmune diseases. *Nat Med*, **9**, 1245–50.

Felson DT, Anderson JJ, Meenan RF (1994). The efficacy and toxicity of combination therapy in rheumatoid arthritis: a metaanalysis. *Arthritis Rheum*, **37**, 487–91.

Felson DT, et al. (1995). American College of Rheumatology preliminary definition of improvement in rheumatoid arthritis. *Arthritis Rheum*, **38**, 727–35.

Fries JF, Spitz PW, Young DY (1982). The dimensions of health outcomes: the health assessment questionnaire, disability and pain scales. *J Rheumatol*, **9**, 789–93.

Furst DE (2000). Aggressive strategies for treating aggressive rheumatoid arthritis: has the case been proven? *Lancet* **356**, 183–4.

Furst DE, et al. (2006). Updated consensus statement on biological agents for treatment of rheumatic diseases, 2006. *Ann Rheum Dis*, **65** Suppl 3, iii2–15.

Gardner DL (1992). Rheumatoid arthritis: cell and tissue pathology. In: Gardner DL, (ed.) *Pathological basis of the connective tissue diseases*, pp. 444–526. Edward Arnold, London.

Genovese MC, et al. (2005). Abatacept for rheumatoid arthritis refractory to tumor necrosis factor alpha inhibition. *New Engl J Med*, **353**, 1114–23.

Goekoop-Ruiterman, et al. (2005). Clinical and radiographic outcomes of four different treatment strategies in patients with early rheumatoid arthritis (the BeSt study). *Arthritis Rheum*, **52**, 3381–90.

Graham DJ (2006). COX-II inhibitors, other NSAIDs, and cardiovascular risk. The seduction of common sense. *J Am Med Assoc*, **296**, 1653–6.

Gregersen PK, Silver J, Winchester RJ (1987). The shared epitope hypothesis. An approach to understanding the molecular genetics of susceptibility to rheumatoid arthritis. *Arthritis Rheum*, **30**, 1205–13.

Griffiths ID (2004). Extra-articular features of rheumatic diseases. In: Isenberg DA, Maddison PJ, Woo P, Glass DN, Breedveld F (eds) *Oxford textbook of rheumatology*, 3rd edition, pp. 110–7. Oxford University Press, Oxford.

Grigor C, et al. (2004). Effect of a treatment strategy of tight control for rheumatoid arthritis (the TICORA study): a single-blind randomised controlled trial. *Lancet*, **364**, 263–9.

Kearney RM, et al. (2006). Do selective cyclo-oxygenase-2 and traditional non-steroidal anti-inflammatory drugs increase the risk of atherothrombosis? Meta-analsysis of randomized trials. *BMJ*, **332**, 1302–8.

Kirwan JR (1995). The effect of glucocorticoids on joint destruction in rheumatoid arthritis. The Arthritis and Rheumatism Council Low-Dose Glucocorticoid Study Group. *New Engl J Med*, **333**, 142–6.

Klareskog L, et al. (2004). Therapeutic effect of the combination of etanercept and methotrexate compared with each treatment alone in patients with rheumatoid arthritis: double-blind randomised controlled trial. *Lancet*, **363**, 675–81.

Klareskog L, et al. (2006). Smoking may trigger HLA-DR (SE)-restricted immune reactions to autoantigens modified by citrullination. *Arthritis Rheum*, **54**, 38–46.

Lawrence JS (1970). Rheumatoid arthritis: nature or nurture? *Ann Rheum Dis*, **29**, 357–69.

Maetzel A, et al. (2000). Meta-analysis of treatment termination rates among rheumatoid arthritis patients receiving disease-modifying anti-rheumatic drugs. *Rheumatology*, **39**, 975–81.

Maini RN, Feldmann M (2002). How does infliximab work in rheumatoid arthritis? *Arthritis Res*, **4** Suppl 2, S22–8.

Maini RN, et al. (1998). Therapeutic efficacy of multiple intravenous infusions of anti-tumor necrosis factor α monoclonal antibody combined with low-dose weekly methotrexate in rheumatoid arthritis. *Arthritis Rheum*, **41**, 1552–63.

Maini RN, et al. (1999). Randomised phase III trial of infliximab (Chimeric anti-TNFα monoclonal antibody) versus placebo in rheumatoid arthritis patients receiving concomitant methotrexate. *Lancet* **354**, 1932–9.

Mangge H, Hermann J, Schauenstein K (1999). Diet and rheumatoid arthritis—a review. *Scand J Rheumatol*, **28**, 201–9.

Moreland LE, et al. (1999). Etanercept therapy in rheumatoid arthritis. *Ann Intern Med*, **130**, 478–86.

National Institute of Clinical Excellence. Guidelines on the use of biological therapies in rheumatoid arthritis. Completed appraisals of etanercept, infliximab, adalimumab; rituximab; and abatacept http://www.nice.org.uk/TA36/TA130/TA126/TA141

O'Dell JR, et al. (2004). Therapeutic strategies for rheumatoid arthritis. *New Engl J Med*, **350**, 2591–602.

Osiri M, et al. (2003). Leflunomide for treating rheumatoid arthritis. *Cochrane Database Syst Rev*, **1**, CD002047.

Pinals RS, et al. (1981). Preliminary criteria for clinical remission in rheumatoid arthritis. *Arthritis Rheum*, **24**, 1305–15.

Pincus T, Callahan LF (1993). What is the natural history of rheumatoid arthritis? *Rheum Dis Clin North Am*, **19**, 123–51.

Prevoo MLL, et al. (1995). Modified disease activity scores that include twenty-eight-joint counts development and validation in a prospective longitudinal study of patients with rheumatoid arthritis. *Arthritis Rheum*, **38**, 44–8.

Scott DL, et al. (2000). The links between joint damage and disability in rheumatoid arthritis. *Rheumatology*, **39**, 122–32.

Short CL (1974). The antiquity of rheumatoid arthritis. *Arthritis Rheum*, **17**, 193–205.

Silman AJ, Pearson JE. (2002). Epidemiology and genetics of rheumatoid arthritis. *Arthritis Research and Therapy*. **4** Suppl 3, S265–72.

Smolen JS, Aletaha D, Keystone E. (2005). Superior efficacy of combination therapy for rheumatoid arthritis. Fact or fiction? *Arthritis Rheum*, **52**, 2975–83.

Suarez-Almazor ME, *et al.* (1998). Methotrexate for treating rheumatoid arthritis. *Cochrane Database Syst Rev*, **1**, CD000957.

Symmons DPM, Silman AJ (2006). What determines the evolution of early undifferentiated arthritis and rheumatoid arthritis? An update for the Norfolk arthritis register. *Arthritis Res Ther*, **8**, 214–20.

Visser H, *et al.* (2002). How to diagnose rheumatoid arthritis early. A prediction model for persistent (erosive) arthritis. *Arthritis Rheum*, **46**, 357–65.

Warner TD, Mitchell JA (2004). Cyclooxygenases: new forms, new inhibitors, and lessons from the clinic. *FASEB J*, **18**, 790–804.

Weinblatt ME, *et al.* (1994). Methotrexate in rheumatoid arthritis. *Arthritis Rheum*, **37**, 1492–8.

Wiles N, *et al.* (1999). Estimating the incidence of rheumatoid arthritis. Trying to hit a moving target? *Arthritis Rheum*, **42**, 1339–46.

Young A, *et al.* (2000). How does functional disability in early rheumatoid arthritis (RA) affect patients and their lives? Results of 5 years of follow-up in 732 patients from the early rheumatoid arthritis study (ERAS). *Rheumatology*, **39**, 603–11.

Ankylosing spondylitis, other spondyloarthritides, and related conditions

J. Braun and J. Sieper

Essentials

The spondyloarthritides are a group of inflammatory rheumatic diseases with predominant involvement of axial and peripheral joints and entheses, together with other characteristic clinical features, including inflammatory back pain, sacroiliitis, peripheral arthritis (mainly in the legs), enthesitis, dactylitis, preceding infection of the urogenital/gastrointestinal tract, psoriatic skin lesions, Crohn-like gut lesions, anterior uveitis, and a family history of Spondyloarthritis. They are the second most frequent inflammatory rheumatic diseases after rheumatoid arthritis.

Five subsets can be distinguished on clinical grounds: (1) ankylosing spondylitis; (2) reactive (spondylo)arthritis/Reiter's syndrome (see Chapter 19.8); (3) psoriatic (spondylo)arthritis; (4) (spondylo) arthritis associated with inflammatory bowel diseases; and (5) undifferentiated spondyloarthritis. Prevalence in any population correlates roughly with that of HLA B27, but the relevance of this to pathogenesis is not known. Another more recent approach is to differentiate the SpA on the basis of the predominant clinical manifestation: predominant axial and/or peripheral SpA.

Ankylosing spondylitis

Diagnosis requires one of three clinical criteria—(1) inflammatory back pain; (2) limitation of spinal movement in three planes; or (3) deterioration of chest expansion—and radiological sacroiliac joint changes (bilateral grade 2 or unilateral grade 3/4). Sacroiliac radiographs may be normal in early disease when dynamic MRI of the sacroiliac joints can be helpful in providing objective evidence of sacroiliitis in clinically suspicious cases.

Age of onset is commonly in the twenties, with male:female ratio of 2:1. Early in the course of disease there may be no limitation of spinal movement or chest expansion, but as it progresses there is restriction of lateral flexion, forward flexion, and extension.

Treatment options include acute anti-inflammatory therapy with nonsteroidal anti-inflammatory drugs (NSAIDs) and local corticosteroids, disease-modifying drugs (DMARDs: sulfasalazine and methotrexate) and biologicals (anti-tumour necrosis factor), together with physiotherapy. There is no cure.

Psoriatic arthritis

Psoriasis precedes joint disease in most cases, but there is poor correlation between onset, severity and activity of psoriatic skin lesions and arthritis. More than 80% of patients with psoriatic arthritis have nail dystrophy.

The most characteristic features are dactylitis and osteoproliferative changes in radiographs of peripheral joints. The CASPAR criteria, which are both sensitive and specific, require established inflammatory articular disease with at least three points from the following features: (1) current psoriasis (score 2); (2) a history of psoriasis (unless current psoriasis); (3) a family history of psoriasis (unless current psoriasis or history of psoriasis); (4) dactylitis; (5) juxta-articular new bone formation; (6) rheumatoid factor negativity; and (7) nail dystrophy.

Many patients improve with the use of NSAIDs and intra-articular steroids, especially in the case of large joint involvement or flexor tenosynovitis. Those who do not improve need to be treated with DMARDs (sulfasalazine, methotrexate).

Arthritis associated with inflammatory bowel disease

Similar to the other spondyloarthritides, the arthritis is mostly asymmetric and predominantly affects the legs. Flaring of gut symptoms is often associated with arthritis. Treatment with NSAIDs may be effective for arthritis and spondylitis but can exacerbate bowel disease: there are few data on the use of DMARDs.

Undifferentiated spondyloarthritis

Diagnosis requires inflammatory back pain and/or peripheral arthritis of the legs (usually asymmetrical) and at least one other of the following characteristic features in addition: (1) enthesitis; (2) a positive family history for spondyloarthritis; (3) psoriasis; or (4) inflammatory bowel disease. Dactylitis, anterior uveitis, and HLA B27 may also be used for making a diagnosis of undifferentiated spondyloarthritis. Nonspecific therapy is as for other arthritides. Sulfasalazine may be useful for peripheral and axial symptoms, but very few therapeutic trials with DMARDs have been performed.

SAPHO syndrome

There are no evaluated diagnostic criteria for SAPHO syndrome (synovitis, acne, pustulosis palmaris et plantaris, hyperostosis, and osteitis): most convincing clinically is the combination of a classi-cal skin symptom—such as pustolosis or significant acne—with a characteristic joint or bone lesion—such as arthritis of the sterno-clavicular joint, osteitis, or hyperostosis in the anterior chest wall. Analgesics, NSAIDs, and intra-articular steroids are usually effective.

Introduction and definitions

The spondyloarthritides are a heterogenous group of inflammatory rheumatic diseases with predominant involvement of axial and peripheral joints and entheses. In addition to these, the spondyloarthritides share other characteristic clinical features, e.g. anterior uveitis, psoriasis and colitis with Crohn-like gut lesions. Clinical symptoms in subsets of spondyloarthritides can overlap, e.g. psoriatic skin lesions in reactive arthritis, especially the subform Reiter's syndrome, and patients can move from one subset to another, for example from undifferentiated spondyloarthritis to ankylosing spondylitis.

The various names that have been and are still used for the spondyloarthritides include seronegative spondarthropathies, spondarthritis, spondylarthropathy, and Spondyloarthritis. Importantly, the term spondyloarthritis means a category of inter-related rheumatic disease, it does not only mean axial involvement, as the asymmetric pattern of involvement of mainly the legs by oligoarthritis and enthesitis is also typical. The prefix seronega-tive, referring to the general absence of rheumatoid factors in the spondyloarthritides, is historical and redundant. The term spondyloarthritis is now generally preferred.

The spondyloarthritides are not 'modern' diseases, with ankylosing spondylitis first having been described in 1649 (Table 19.6.1).

Epidemiology

The mean age at onset is 20 to 30 years, with just a slight preponderance of men in most subsets of spondyloarthritis. Next to rheumatoid arthritis, the spondyloarthritides are the most frequent inflammatory rheumatic diseases (Table 19.6.2), with ankylosing spondylitis, psoriatic spondyloarthritis, and undifferentiated spondyloarthritis being the most common subsets. The overall prevalence of spondyloarthritides in patients presenting with back pain to general practitioners' surgeries in the United Kingdom has been estimated at 5%.

The spondyloarthritides are associated with the major histocompatability complex class I antigen HLA B27, and the prevalence of spondyloarthritides in any population correlates roughly with that of HLA B27. The magnitude of association differs between the subsets (Table 19.6.3): it has been mainly shown for ankylosing spondylitis, but in Inuit populations Reiter's syndrome is more frequent.

Pathogenesis

The overall influence of genes in the pathogenesis of ankylosing spondylitis has been estimated to be 80 to 90%, leaving only 10 to 20% to other causative factors, such as environmental influences. *HLA B27* is responsible for about one-third of the total genetic load: 32 subtypes are now recognized by polymerase chain reaction technology, three of which are not associated with ankylosing spondylitis, or are associated less strongly. There is weaker association of ankylosing spondylitis with *HLA B60* and *HLA DR1*, the interleukin 1 (*IL1*) gene cluster, and possibly also tumour necrosis factor α (TNFα) polymorphisms. Recently, ERAP-1, IL-23R and IL-1 polymorphism have also been genetically associated with ankylosing spondylitis.

The relevance of HLA B27 to disease pathogenesis is not known: several models have been proposed to explain tissue tropism, the aberrant immune response to certain bacteria, and the HLA B27 association of the spondyloarthritides (Table 19.6.4).

The classical arthritogenic peptide model is backed by the demonstration of HLA B27-restricted CD8+ T-cell clones in the synovial fluid of patients with reactive arthritis. Immunodominant peptide motifs and peptides have been described, but their pathogenetic relevance is not yet clear. Lipopolysaccharide and RNA of bacteria associated with reactive arthritis and a CD4+ T-cell response directed against bacterial antigens have been detected in reactive arthritis, but it is not clear whether this immune response is beneficial or arthritogenic. At the humoral and the cellular level, molecular mimicry (partial sequence homologies at the protein and DNA level) between bacterial antigens and self structures has been described, mainly of the HLA B27 molecule. It also seems

Table 19.6.1 First historical descriptions of spondyloarthritis

Spondyloarthritis	Moll/Wright 1974, ESSG 1991
Ankylosing spondylitis	Connors 1649, Brodie 1888
Reactive arthritis/Reiter's syndrome	Reiter 1916, Ahonen 1973
Psoriatic arthritis	Wright 1959
Arthritis associated with inflammatory bowel diseases	Bargen 1930
Enthesitis	Niepel 1961
HLA B27 association	Brewerton, Schlosstein 1973
Undifferentiated Spondyloarthritis	Khan/van der Linden 1990

ESSG, European Spondylarthropathy Study Group.

Table 19.6.2 Prevalence of spondyloarthritis

Disease	Prevalence
Spondyloarthritis	0.6–2.0%
Ankylosing spondylitis	0.2–1.4%
Undifferentiated Spondyloarthritis	0.2–0.7%
Reactive arthritis	0.01%
Psoriasis	1.0–3.0%
Psoriatic arthritis	0.3%
Arthritis associated with inflammatory bowel disease	0.001%

Table 19.6.3 HLA B27 association of the spondyloarthritis. Note that the prevalence of spondyloarthritis (mainly of the first four listed above) relates to the prevalence of HLA B27 in different populations, which is as shown in the second table

Spondyloarthritis	HLA B27 prevalence
Ankylosing spondylitis	85–95%
Reactive arthritis	30–80%
Reiter's syndrome	60–90%
Psoriatic arthritis:	
Peripheral arthritis	10–30%
Axial involvement	40–60%
Arthritis associated with inflammatory bowel diseases	
Peripheral arthritis	10–30%
Axial involvement	40–60%
Undifferentiated Spondyloarthritis	50–70%
Population	**HLA B27 prevalence**
Native Americans	6–50%
Inuit	15–25%
North Europeans	10–25%
Middle Europeans	6–9%
North Americans	6–8%
South Europeans	4–6%
Africans	1–5%

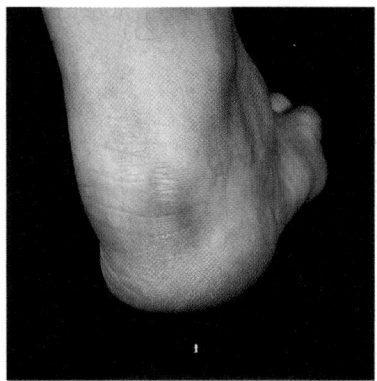

Fig. 19.6.1 Enthesitis at the insertion of the Achilles tendon in a patient with reactive arthritis.

possible that patients with HLA B27+ spondyloarthritis have deficient immune reactivity, e.g. diminished ability to secrete TNFα, or a synovial Th2 response (secretion of too little interferon-γ, too much IL-4, IL-10), making elimination of bacteria difficult. Presentation of HLA B27-derived peptides themselves by HLA class II molecules, or even by HLA class I molecules, has been proposed as an explanation of the association of HLA B27 with disease.

The 'HLA-B27 misfolding hypothesis' suggests that HLA B27 has a tendency to misfold in the endoplasmic reticulum, it being a particular feature of HLA B27 that newly synthesized HLA B*2705 molecules fold and associate with β$_2$-microglobulin (β(2)m) more slowly than other MHC class I molecules. As a consequence of this misfolding, free HLA B27 heavy chains (HC) can form abnormal HC homodimers, which, as β(2)m-free HLA B27 homodimers and multimers, are expressed at the cell surface of leucocytes, dendritic, and other cells with the possible function of antigen presentation.

Table 19.6.4 Spondyloarthritis—pathogenetic models

Model	Mechanism
Arthritogenic peptide model	Bacterial protein processed/ presented by B27 to CD8+ T cells
Deficient immune response	Failure of B27+ cells to properly present and eliminate bacteria
Molecular mimicry	Similarity of bacterial and self structures, possibly resulting in autoimmunity
Autoimmunity	Self structures such as B27-derived peptides presented by class I or II molecules

Clinical features

The characteristic clinical features of the spondyloarthritides (see Figs. 19.6.1–19.6.3) are listed in Table 19.6.5.

Diagnosis

Five subsets of spondyloarthritis can be distinguished on clinical grounds: ankylosing spondylitis; reactive (spondylo)arthritis/Reiter's syndrome; psoriatic (spondylo)arthritis; (spondylo)arthritis associated with inflammatory bowel diseases; and undifferentiated spondyloarthritis (Box 19.6.1).

Diagnostic criteria for spondyloarthritides are shown in Table 19.6.6. Inflammatory back pain is one of the main clinical criteria used to make a diagnosis. To classify a patient younger than 45 with chronic back pain (defined as being present for more than 3 months) requires two of the following four criteria to be present: morning stiffness; relief by exercise but not by rest; waking up in the second half of the night because of pain; and alternating buttock pain. Other features of possible relevance include the initially deep localization, a good response to nonsteroidal anti-inflammatory drugs (NSAIDs), other clinical signs of spondyloarthritis (enthesitis, arthritis, anterior uveitis, family history), elevated acute phase reactants (C-reactive protein, ESR), and the presence of HLA B27.

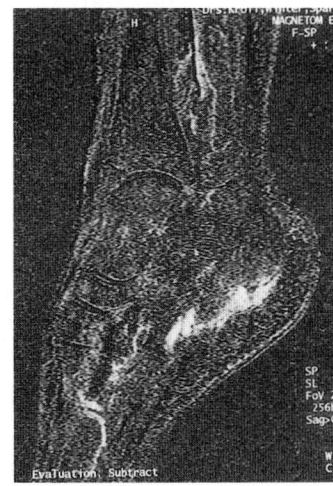

Fig. 19.6.2 MRI showing inflammation of the plantar fascia in a patient with undifferentiated spondyloarthritis.

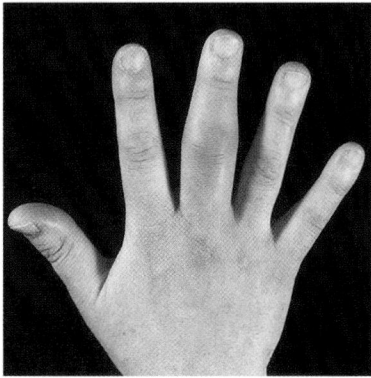

Fig. 19.6.3 Dactylitis of the third finger of the right hand in a patient with undifferentiated spondyloarthritis.

Box 19.6.1 ASAS Classification Criteria for axial SpA

In patients with ≥3 months back pain and age at onset <45 years
Sacroiliitis on imaging plus ≥1 SpA feature, or HLA-B27 plus ≥2 other SpA features
SpA features

  IBP

  arthritis

  enthesitis heel

  uveitis

  dactylitis

  psoriasis

  Crohn's/colitis

  good response to NSAIDs

  family history for SpA

  HLA-B27

  elevated CRP

To make a diagnosis of ankylosing spondylitis, HLA B27 contributes most, whereas elevated acute phase reactants contribute relatively little. Note, however, that HLA B27 alone can never make a diagnosis, but it does increase the probability of an underlying spondyloarthritis by about tenfold. Likelihood ratios have also been calculated for the other items. In combination with the leading symptom of chronic or inflammatory back pain, HLA B27 is of value to screen for patients with spondyloarthritis in a primary care setting.

Differential diagnosis

The most important, because most frequent, differential diagnosis is nonspecific low back pain, especially if it exceeds 3 months duration in a patient younger than 45 years. The leading clinical symptom of inflammatory back pain may be associated with pain radiating from the lower back to the thighs. Hence an important initial differential diagnosis is sciatica, but this usually has an acute onset. In inflammatory back pain, radiation is more often bilateral than unilateral, rarely extends below the knees, almost never into the foot, and is not associated with paraesthesia, although cough impulse pain may be present. Diagnostic procedures for the detection of disc herniation by MRI or CT can be misleading, as disc prolapses are found in as many as 30% of normal individuals.

Diffuse idiopathic skeletal hyperostosis (DISH) or Forestier's disease, an often-severe radiographic spondylosis, can be difficult to distinguish from longstanding ankylosing spondylitis. The appearance and localization of the spondylophytes helps to differentiate DISH from syndesmophytes and ankylosing spondylitis. Scoliosis is not usually a marked feature of ankylosing spondylitis.

Table 19.6.5 Characteristic clinical features of spondyloarthritis

Clinical feature	Details
Inflammatory back pain	
Sacroiliitis	
Peripheral arthritis	Affects predominantly but not exclusively the lower limbs; it is often asymmetric but may also involve both knees or ankles
Enthesitis	Inflammation at the insertion sites of tendons and ligaments to bone (Figs. 19.6.1 and 19.6.2).
Dactylitis	Inflammatory involvement of a whole finger or toe (Fig. 19.6.3) with tendovaginitis and arthritis (sausage digit).
Preceding infection in the urogenital/enteral tract	
Psoriatic skin lesions	
Crohn-like gut lesions	
Anterior uveitis	
Family history of Spondyloarthritis	

Table 19.6.6 Diagnostic criteria for spondyloarthritis (1991 European Spondylarthropathy Study Group criteria)

Major criteria
Inflammatory back pain
Oligoarthritis (asymmetric) of the lower limbs
Minor criteria
Enthesitis
Alternating buttock pain
Preceding symptomatic infection
Psoriasis
Crohn-like gut lesions
Family history
Radiographic sacroiliitis

To make the diagnosis requires the presence of one major and one minor criterion.
Note that dactylitis, uveitis and HLA B27 are not included in these criteria. The peripheral arthritis does not have to be asymmetric, although it often is; both knees or ankles might well be involved. Inflammatory back pain is mostly due to sacroiliitis but can also be caused by enthesitis.

Table 19.6.7 Differential diagnosis of sacroiliitis

Spondyloarthritis

Reactive arthritis

Psoriatic arthritis

Arthritis associated with inflammatory bowel disease

Undifferentiated Spondyloarthritis

SAPHO syndrome

Other rheumatic diseases

Rheumatoid arthritis

Systemic lupus erythematosus

Sjögren's syndrome

Gout

Osteoarthritis

Paget's disease

Hyper/hypoparathyroidism

Non-rheumatic diseases

Septic sacroiliitis

Acute (staphylococci, steptococci, others)

Chronic (tuberculosis, brucellosis)

Malignancies (lymphoma, metastasis)

Sacroiliitis occurs in a number of other rheumatic and infectious diseases, as shown in Table 19.6.7. The differential diagnosis of peripheral arthritis of the legs includes Lyme disease, sarcoidosis (Löfgren's syndrome), gout, and undifferentiated oligoarthritis. The differential diagnosis of enthesitis includes epicondylitis and fibromyalgia, and that of dactylitis is erysipela and infection.

Prognosis

There are no good studies, but the following seem to be poor prognostic factors: hip arthritis, limitation of lumbar spine movements, dactylitis, oligoarthritis, young age at onset (<16 years), poor efficacy of NSAIDs, an ESR of more than 30 mm in the first hour, and already the presence of syndesmophytes.

Ankylosing spondylitis

Ankylosing spondylitis is a chronic inflammatory rheumatic disease that mainly affects the axial skeleton, starting in the sacroiliac joints and often progressing to the spine, but peripheral joints, enthesial structures, the anterior uvea, and the aorta can also become affected.

The diagnosis is made on the basis of significant radiological changes in the sacroiliac joints and the spine, the typical clinical history of inflammatory back pain and stiffness, and evidence of limited spinal movement and/or chest expansion on physical examination.

Epidemiology

The age of onset is commonly in the twenties, but ankylosing spondylitis can begin in childhood, or considerably later (at age >50). The men:female ratio is about 2:1. About 90% of white patients with ankylosing spondylitis are positive for HLA B27, the risk of developing this condition being increased tenfold in HLA B27-positive individuals. If a first-degree relative or dizygotic twin is affected, the risk is 25 to 30%, rising to 50 to 60% in monozygotic twins. Reactive arthritis, psoriasis, and inflammatory bowel disease are additional, partly independent, risk factors.

Immunopathology and pathogenesis

The leading features of ankylosing spondylitis are spinal inflammation and ankylosis, but their cause is unknown. The association of ankylosing spondylitis with bacterial infections is a lot less clear than in reactive arthritis. Antibodies to *Klebsiella pneumoniae* are more frequently detected in patients with ankylosing spondylitis than in healthy controls, but similarly often in patients with Crohn's disease and first-degree relatives of those with ankylosing spondylitis. This finding is probably explained by increased gut permeability, and its predominant clinical association is with peripheral (not axial) arthritis.

The sacroiliac joint is the structure most frequently involved in the initial phase of disease. If biopsy is performed, T cells and macrophages are seen to be the predominant infiltrating cells, with CD4+ and CD8+ T cells both present. The reason for this tropism is unclear. The fact that sacroiliac and spinal joints are affected in diseases caused by mycobacteria and other microbes may argue for a pathogen-triggered pathogenesis in ankylosing spondylitis, but bacteria associated with reactive arthritis have not been detected in the sacroiliac joints.

Clinical features

The most common initial symptom is inflammatory back pain, commonly in the lower back and the buttocks. Early in the course of disease there may be no limitation of spinal movement or chest expansion. As it progresses, there is restriction of lateral flexion, forward flexion, and extension. There is often a flattening of the lumbar lordosis, or an inability to reverse this on forward flexion. With more advanced disease a thoracic kyphosis develops, with concomitant restriction of thoracic rotation and chest expansion due to inflammation and ankylosis of the costovertebral and costotransverse joints. In severe cases movements of the cervical spine are also restricted in all planes, with dramatic limitation of lateral flexion. The combination of cervical stiffness and severe thoracic kyphosis can lead to difficulties with forward vision. An example of a young patient with severe progressive disease is shown in Fig. 19.6.4. Severe spinal disease is more frequent in men than in women. There is no evidence that pregnancy has a significant impact on the course of the disease.

Peripheral joint involvement occurs in 30 to 50% of cases at some time, with about 20 to 30% of patients having acute peripheral arthritis of the legs, often with joint effusions as the first symptom, this being especially marked in children. This situation is difficult to differentiate from reactive arthritis. Joint involvement is usually oligoarticular and often asymmetrical. The joints most often involved are the knees, ankles, hips, shoulders, wrists, temporomandibular joints, sternoclavicular joints, manubriosternal joints, costovertebral joints, zygapophyseal joints, and symphysis pubis. Small joints are rarely affected.

Enthesitis occurs at the heel at the insertion of the Achilles tendon (Fig. 19.6.1) and the plantar fascia (Fig. 19.6.2), and at the iliac crests, the ischial tuberosities, the greater trochanters, and other

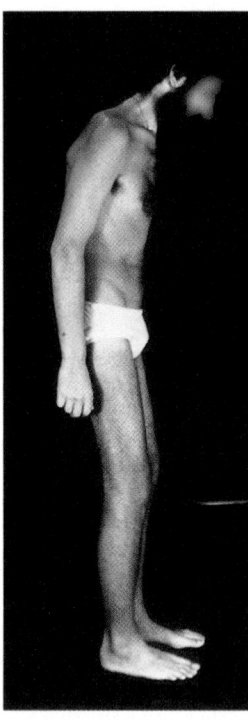

Fig. 19.6.4 Thirty-year-old man with rapidly progressive ankylosing spondylitis (disease of 5 years' duration).

sites. The diagnosis is often difficult if no swelling is apparent, in which case ultrasound can be revealing. Dactylitis of fingers and toes is uncommon in ankylosing spondylitis, being seen most often in psoriatic arthritis.

Physical examination of the spine and thoracic cage
The physical examination is important in the evaluation of patients with ankylosing spondylitis—in particular to quantitate flexibility of the spine and thoracic cage. The following measurements are useful, but it should be stressed that the values expected of normal individuals are dependent on age and physical training.

- Anterior and lateral spinal mobility (Schober test):
  - Ventral—with the patient standing upright, a horizontal line is drawn across the lumbar spine connecting the two posterior superior iliac spines. Marks are made in the midline over the spine 10 cm cranial (original version) and 5 cm caudal (modified version) to the horizontal line. The patient then bends with legs straight and the distance is measured again. It normally increases by more than 3 cm, and in younger people by more than 5 cm. The measure is age dependent.
  - Lateral—the distance between the tip of the longest finger and the floor is measured in the upright position. This is repeated when the patient tries to flex laterally towards the ground as far as possible, normally moving by more than 10 cm.

- Chest expansion—the circumference of the thorax is measured in the fourth intercostal space after maximal inspiration and expiration. It normally alters by more than 3 cm, in younger people by more than 5 cm: again the measure is age dependent. In patients with ankylosing spondylitis it indicates involvement of the costovertebral joints.

- Occiput/wall distance—in the upright position the patient leans backwards against a wall. The distance between occiput and wall is measured: there is no gap (0 cm) in most young patients; in patients with ankylosing spondylitis it usually indicates hyperkyphosis of the thoracic spine.

- Chin/sternum distance—the chin is maximally bent towards the sternum, and should normally be able to touch it.

- Cervical rotation—the head is rotated to the left and right sides, with the angles of rotation measured (normally >50°).

- Intermalleolar distance—the patient tries to stand with their feet together and also to spread their legs maximally: the malleoli should normally touch and the distance of the spread feet usually exceeds 1 m. This measure is dependent on age, training, and the degree of osteoarthritis of the hip.

Physical examination for extra-articular organ involvement
Acute anterior uveitis can occur at any time in the course of disease and is seen in 20 to 30% of patients. It is typically unilateral, but either eye may be affected in separate episodes. Recurrent attacks are common. Aortic regurgitation secondary to aortitis occurs in about 1 to 2% of patients with ankylosing spondylitis, most frequently in advanced disease, and may be associated with atrioventricular block. Probably on the basis of a restrictive pulmonary defect due to limited chest expansion, apical pulmonary fibrosis occurs in no more than 1% of patients, especially those with advanced disease. Cauda equina syndrome caused by arachnoid cysts may complicate severe longstanding disease, with resultant disturbance of the bladder and bowel function. Lumbar diverticulae may be demonstrated by MRI.

Diagnosis
The 1984 modified New York criteria for ankylosing spondylitis are shown in Table 19.6.8. There is a significant diagnostic delay in women (8 years) and in men (5 years), the most probable reason being that back pain is a very frequent complaint, and that primary care and general physicians are often not trained to distinguish inflammatory from other causes of back pain, such that referral for specialist opinion is delayed.

Laboratory and radiological features
The ESR and the C-reactive protein are raised in 30 to 50% of patients, with moderate correlation to overall disease activity.

Table 19.6.8 Diagnostic criteria for ankylosing spondylitis

Clinical parameters
Inflammatory back pain
Limitation of spinal movement in three planes
Deterioration of chest expansion

Radiological parameters
Sacroiliac joint changes of at least:
Bilateral grade 2
Unilateral grade 3 or 4

Note that other Spondyloarthritis-like symptoms and syndesmophytes are not part of these criteria. For a definite diagnosis of ankylosing spondylitis, the radiological criterion is essential and one clinical criterion required. If only clinical symptoms and findings are present, a diagnosis of probable ankylosing spondylitis may be made.

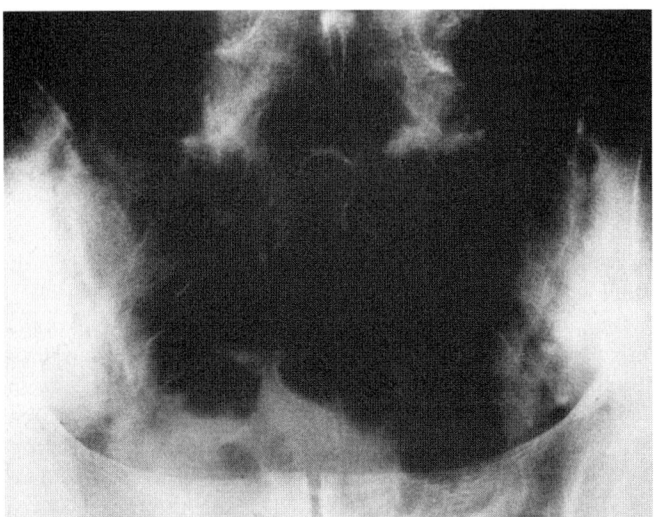

Fig. 19.6.5 Radiographic sacroiliitis (stage IV in both joints) in a 28-year-old man with ankylosing spondylitis.

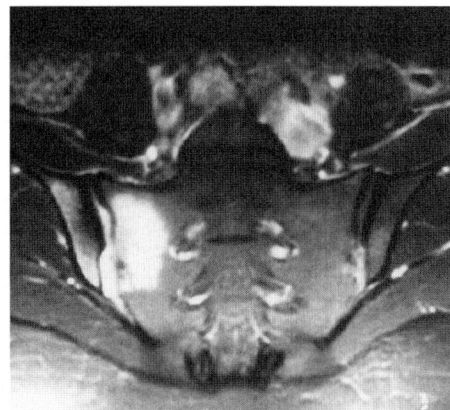

Fig. 19.6.6 Dynamic MRI showing right-sided active sacroiliitis.

Less commonly, serum IgA levels are raised. Mild to severe normochromic normocytic anaemia occurs in about 10 to 20% of patients.

Sacroiliac radiography

Dependent on stage, severity, and duration of disease, there are sacroiliac joint abnormalities in almost all patients. The radiological changes are graded from 0 (normal), to I (minimal changes), II (sclerosis, some erosions), III (severe erosions, pseudodilatation of joint space, limited ankylosis), and IV (ankylosis) (Fig. 19.6.5). They are crucial for the diagnosis of ankylosing spondylitis and for the differentiation from undifferentiated spondyloarthritis, but it must be noted that significant inter- and intraobserver variability has been reported—particularly concerning grades I and II—which creates diagnostic problems and confusion. Sclerosis, joint space narrowing, and even synchondrosis occur in healthy elderly individuals. Oblique and other special views are generally not significantly better than normal anteroposterior pelvic radiographs, but can be helpful in a few cases.

Sacroiliac MRI and CT

In early ankylosing spondylitis sacroiliac radiographs may be normal, and in clinically suspicious cases dynamic MRI of the sacroiliac joints can be helpful in providing objective evidence of sacroiliitis (see 'Undifferentiated Spondyloarthritis'). Active inflammation can be demonstrated by enhancement after application of a contrast agent (gadolinium DTPA) or by special magnetic resonance sequences, such as short tau inversion recovery (STIR) or other fat saturation techniques that optimize the visualization of oedematous areas (Fig. 19.6.6). CT of the sacroiliac joints is superior to normal radiographs for documenting bony changes such as erosions and ankylosis. The sacroiliac joint is accessible to biopsy under CT guidance.

Spinal radiography

The characteristic spinal lesion, mostly occurring in more advanced disease, is the syndesmophyte—a bony proliferation originating from an inflammatory area at the ligamentous/discal attachment to the vertebral edge. This early ankylotic structure predominantly grows cranially to fuse with the next vertebral body and has to be distinguished from the spondylophyte, which mainly grows laterally and typically indicates degenerative vertebral disease.

In ankylosing spondylitis the earliest spinal lesions are frequently in the lower thoracic and upper lumbar spine, sometimes preceded by squaring of the vertebrae seen on lateral films. The zygapophyseal joints are frequently involved at all stages. Anterior spondylitis is indicated by lateral spinal radiographs showing hypersclerotic corners (Romanus lesion, Fig. 19.6.7). Spondylodiscitis (Anderson lesion) is revealed by erosion of the disc and vertebra with a hypersclerotic lining. In later stages new bone formation and calcification of ligaments occurs, eventually leading to bridging syndesmophytes and the characteristic 'bamboo spine' (Fig. 19.6.8).

Spinal MRI

Early spinal inflammation (spondylitis, spondylodiscitis) can be detected by dynamic MRI, which can be useful for localizing inflammation in the spine in the early stages when plain radiographs are normal.

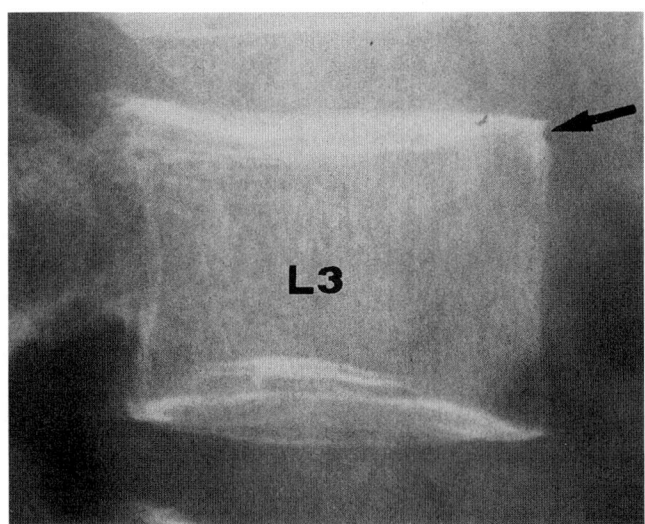

Fig. 19.6.7 Radiographic anterior spondylitis (arrow) in a 42-year-old man with ankylosing spondylitis.

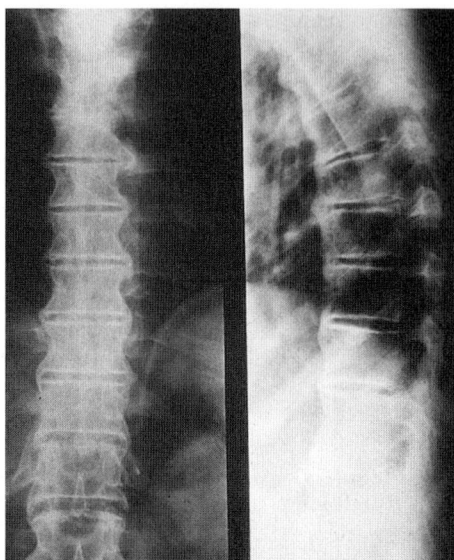

Fig. 19.6.8 Spinal radiograph showing classical bamboo spine.

Treatment

Although there is no cure for ankylosing spondylitis, several treatments are available. The main therapeutic options are:

◆ Acute anti-inflammatory therapy—NSAIDs and local corticosteroids; systemic corticosteroids are not recommended

◆ Disease-modifying therapy—sulfasalazine for peripheral arthritis and possibly in early disease stages; methotrexate has limited value for peripheral arthritic is clearly not useful for axial conditions. There is no evidence for the use of leflunomide, gold, or hydroxychloroquine

◆ Antiresorptive therapy—bisphosphonates (disodium pamidronate) may have some value in selected patients

◆ Biologicals—anti-TNF therapy (infliximab, adalimumab, etanercept, golimumab)

NSAIDs are better than analgesics and can be used in combination with them. Diclofenac (50–150 mg), meloxicam (7.5–15 mg), acemetacin and indometacin (50–150 mg) are frequently given. Thalidomide and phenylbutazone are reserved for severe cases when other agents have failed. The more novel COX-2 selective coxibs (celecoxib 100–200 mg, etoricoxib 90–120 mg) are also useful. The main risk of NSAIDs is gastrointestinal side effects: 25% of patients suffer these, ranging from dyspepsia to peptic ulceration and (rarely) bleeding, perforation, and death. It is important to identify patients at risk and to provide them with proper information about possible symptoms, and prophylactic therapy with proton pump inhibitors is indicated in those at particularly high risk (older age, history of ulcer, disability, comorbidity). As most NSAIDs may be associated with a slightly increased incidence of cardiovascular events over time, the individual risk profile of the patient also has to be taken into account. This might be of special clinical relevance, as patients with ankylosing spondylitis may have increased cardiovascular risk because of persistent inflammation.

Most patients with ankylosing spondylitis do not respond to small doses of corticosteroids. Transient high-dose steroid treatment has been tried in extreme cases with additional symptoms of inflammatory bowel disease. In our experience, women and HLA B27-negative ankylosing spondylitis patients are most likely to respond to low-dose corticosteroid therapy.

Sulfasalazine is given in a dosage of 2 to 3 g/day, when effects may be seen after 2 to 4 months. The influence on peripheral joint disease is more significant than for axial symptoms, but this may be due to the preferential study of patients with longstanding disease. Sulfasalazine is mainly indicated for patients with early, active disease.

The anti-TNFα antibodies infliximab (in a dosage of 5 mg/kg intravenously every 6 to 8 weeks after an initial induction phase at weeks 0, 2, and 6), which has also been found to be effective in Crohn's disease and rheumatoid arthritis, and adalimumab (40 mg subcutaneously every 2 weeks) and golimumab 50 mg s.c/month have been shown in randomized placebo-controlled trials to have significant clinical efficacy in patients with persistently active ankylosing spondylitis. The TNF receptor antagonist etanercept (50 mg subcutaneously weekly, given either in one or two dosages) has similar clinical efficacy for musculoskeletal symptoms but seems to be less effective or without effect for gut, skin, and eye symptoms associated with spondyloarthritis.

The aim of physiotherapy is to maintain and enhance function by improving mobility and muscle strength. Patients affected by spinal stiffness should have physiotherapy on a regular daily basis. Hip replacement is indicated for those with severe hip involvement, and osteotomy can be indicated in cases where visual problems are due to severe kyphosis.

Prognosis

The established myth is that 'patients with ankylosing spondylitis generally do well'. However, one-third are severely disabled and experience intense pain and impairment of health comparable to those with rheumatoid arthritis. Ankylosing spondylitis does not burn out: disease activity and pain are independent of its duration. As the disease usually starts in the second or third decade of life, patients with ankylosing spondylitis typically suffer its effects for many years. Mortality may be slightly increased, possible causes of premature death being amyloidosis, NSAID gastropathy (ulcers, bleeding), vertebral fractures, and cardiac or respiratory complications.

Reactive arthritis/Reiter's syndrome

For further information see Chapter 19.8.

Undifferentiated spondyloarthritis

Definition

The term undifferentiated spondyloarthritis (uSpA) was introduced and defined by the European Spondylarthropathy Study Group (ESSG) in 1991. Terms such as incomplete Reiter's syndrome, syndrome of enthesopathy and arthritis, HLA B27-positive oligoarthritis (and others) had been used previously. Patients with uSpA have the typical clinical features of spondyloarthritides but do not fit into any of the other defined categories. The fact that patients with a clinical picture of peripheral oligoarthritis but without spinal symptoms are also classified/diagnosed with uSpA by the ESSG criteria can be confusing in some cases, and uSpA may represent an early form of another spondyloarthritis subset (most often ankylosing spondylitis), or be a genuine spondyloarthritis subset of its own. The new ASAS criteria for SpA cover axial and peripheral SpA, especially axial SpA is a possible predecessor of ankylosing spondylitis, since at least 50% of the patients develop ankylosing spondylitis.

Epidemiology

The prevalence of uSpA is not known precisely, but the frequency is not much less than that of psoriatic arthritis, and it is commoner in men. About 70% of patients are HLA B27-positive. In some contrast to other spondyloarthritides, late-onset disease has been reported.

Clinical features

The main clinical features are inflammatory back pain, asymmetric peripheral arthritis, predominantly of the lower limbs, enthesitis, dactylitis, and anterior uveitis.

Diagnosis

The diagnosis of uSpA requires inflammatory back pain and/or peripheral arthritis of the lower limbs and at least one other characteristic feature in addition—enthesitis, a positive family history for spondyloarthritis, psoriasis, or inflammatory bowel disease. Dactylitis, anterior uveitis, and HLA B27 are not part of the ESSG Group criteria, but are part of Amor's criteria, and may also be used for making a diagnosis of uSpA. It has recently been argued that at least three to four of these parameters should be positive before a diagnosis can be made. Radiographs are not essential for a diagnosis, but in clinically suspicious cases MRI of the sacroiliac joints can be helpful in providing objective evidence of sacroiliitis.

The differential diagnosis of asymmetric peripheral arthritis of the lower limbs in spondyloarthritis comprises Lyme disease, sarcoidosis, gout, osteoarthritis, atypical rheumatoid arthritis, and connective tissue diseases and other rarer conditions.

Treatment

Nonspecific therapy with NSAIDs, intra-articular steroid injections, transient immobilization, ice packs, and physiotherapy is similar to that of other arthritides. Sulfasalazine may have some efficacy for peripheral and axial symptoms, but very few therapeutic trials with disease-modifying agents have been performed in uSpA. TNF blockers are probably as effective as in established ankylosing spondylitis.

Prognosis

The long-term prognosis in uSpA is uncertain: in about 50% of cases a transition to ankylosing spondylitis has been reported, which may occur over several years.

Psoriatic arthritis

Definition

All kinds of arthritis occurring in association with psoriasis can be regarded as psoriatic arthritis, but it is clear that there can be considerable variability in arthritic manifestation. Many patients can be classified as having a spondyloarthritis, but some are affected in a manner more closely resembling rheumatoid arthritis, and there are other unique forms such as arthritis mutilans. Different forms of psoriasis may be associated with a somewhat different form of arthritis.

Epidemiology

Psoriasis is common, with prevalence between 1 and 3% of the population. Arthritic symptoms occur in 20 to 40% of these patients, with the axial skeleton affected in 15 to 25%, such that the overall prevalence of psoriatic arthritis is somewhere around 0.1 to 0.3%. The peak age of onset of psoriatic arthritis is between 20 and 40 years: juvenile disease is rare. Both sexes are equally affected, but women more frequently get polyarthritis and men more often have spinal involvement.

Pathogenesis

Familial aggregation and high concordance rates in monozygotic (70%) compared with dizygotic twins (20%) suggest that there are important genetic factors in psoriasis and psoriatic arthritis. About 30% of patients give a clear history of affected first-degree relatives. The genetic impact is thought to be multifactorial. Psoriasis is associated with *HLA B13*, *B17*, *B37*, and *HLA DR7*, the strongest association being with Cw6 (RR = 24). HLA associations of psoriatic arthritis are with *HLA B38* and *B39* (peripheral arthritis), with *HLA DR4* (symmetric polyarthritis) and *HLA B27* (spondylitis).

The importance of HLA genetic linkage may lie in determination of the immunological response to particular antigens, and there has been much interest in the possible role of streptococcal infection. A proliferative response of skin and synovial T cells to streptococcal antigens has been detected in psoriatic arthritis, but also in rheumatoid arthritis, and the (immuno)histology is similar in the two conditions, although some differences have been described.

Koebner's phenomenon is described in psoriasis, when plaques arise at sites of skin injury, scratches, and scars, but the role of trauma in psoriatic arthritis is not clear. Drugs can exacerbate and trigger psoriasis: most well known are β-blockers, antimalarials, and lithium, and withdrawal of corticosteroids can induce a skin flare, but the relevance of these factors to psoriatic arthritis is uncertain.

Clinical features

The most characteristic features of psoriatic arthritis are dactylitis and osteoproliferative changes in radiographs of peripheral joints. The pattern of axial involvement is somewhat different from that in ankylosing spondylitis, and in contrast to rheumatoid arthritis, patients with psoriatic arthritis may have involvement of the distal

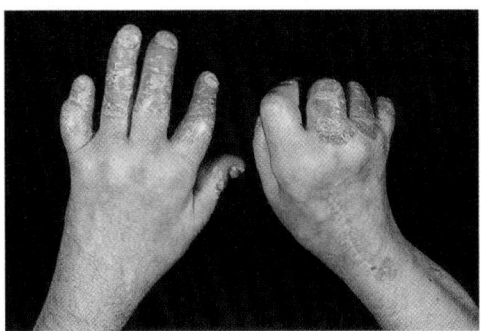

Fig. 19.6.9 Severe psoriatic arthritis (arthritis mutilans).

interphalangeal joints. It is possible that psoriatic arthritis can occur without skin involvement.

Psoriatic arthritis has been divided into five subgroups: distal interphalangeal (overlapping, most common); asymmetrical (Spondyloarthritis-like); symmetrical (rheumatoid arthritis-like); mutilans (unique, rare; see Fig. 19.6.9); and spinal (ankylosing spondylitis-like). It must be stressed, however, that these subgroups are not clearcut. In one study the initial classification pattern changed when patients were evaluated over a period of 8 years: finally only two categories remained—peripheral disease without axial involvement (70%), and axial involvement with or without peripheral arthritis (30%). The latter was correlated with duration of the disease and magnitude of joint involvement. Erosions were found in 70% of the patients.

Psoriasis precedes joint disease in most cases (70–80%); both occur simultaneously in 15%; and in about 10% arthritis comes first. There is poor correlation between onset, severity, and activity of psoriatic skin lesions and arthritis. More than 80% of patients with psoriatic arthritis have nail dystrophy, whereas this is the case in only 20% of those with uncomplicated skin disease. Nail dystrophy, ranging from some to many nail pits and horizontal (not longitudinal) ridging to onycholysis, occurs most often in those with distal interphalangeal involvement. In some patients the involvement of interphalangeal joints and nails is closely correlated, with both appearing on the same finger(s). Acute anterior uveitis occurs mainly in those with radiological sacroiliitis and ankylosing spondylitis.

Different types of psoriatic skin involvement lead to different types of arthropathy. Most frequent is the common psoriasis vulgaris, but a type of skin disease that frequently affects the palms of the hands and soles of the feet with many psoriatic plaques is also seen: pustolosis palmaris et plantaris. This type is associated with the SAPHO syndrome (see below), which is related to the spondyloarthritis but has unique features that justify the designation as a separate subset of these disorders.

A severe form of psoriatic arthritis can occur in HIV-infected patients, although is not clear whether HIV increases the overall prevalence of psoriatic arthritis. Severe peripheral enthesitis (predominantly of the heel) and dactylitis are characteristic. Knee arthritis can be rapidly destructive. Axial inflammation is less frequent.

There is an overlap between psoriatic arthritis and reactive arthritis in the form of keratoderma blennorrhagica—a desquamating psoriasis-like lesion mostly occurring on the soles of the feet in patients with Reiter's syndrome.

Psoriatic arthritis often improves during pregnancy. There is no adverse effect of the disease on mother or child.

Diagnosis

Scaling erythematous papules and plaques on the scalp and extensor aspects of the extremities, often surmounted by a silvery white micaceous scale that is easily removed, are suggestive of psoriasis. Elbows and knees are often affected. The diagnosis of psoriatic arthritis is based on the presence of these characteristic skin lesions, which are not always obvious. Less accessible areas such as the navel, perineum, and scalp need to be examined carefully. The patient should be asked whether they have a family history of psoriasis or psoriatic arthritis.

As psoriasis is a frequent disease, it must be remembered that a patient with psoriasis can have an attack of gout or another form of arthritis. The diagnosis of psoriatic arthritis should be considered

in those without skin lesions if there is distal interphalangeal joint involvement, dactylitis, the involvement of a whole finger or toe, tendon sheaths and bone of an affected limb, and/or typical radiographic changes.

The CASPAR (Classification criteria for psoriatic arthritis) criteria consisted of established inflammatory articular disease with at least three points from the following features: current psoriasis (assigned a score of 2; all other features are assigned a score of 1), a history of psoriasis (unless current psoriasis is present), a family history of psoriasis (unless current psoriasis is present or there is a history of psoriasis), dactylitis, juxta-articular new bone formation, rheumatoid factor negativity, and nail dystrophy. These criteria are sensitive (0.914) and specific (0.987).

Laboratory and radiological features

Acute phase reactants are often raised. HLA determinations including HLA B27 do not provide diagnostic help in those with psoriatic arthritis, but in HLA B27-negative patients who appear to have ankylosing spondylitis, psoriasis (and inflammatory bowel disease) should always be sought. The presence of rheumatoid factor does not formally exclude a diagnosis of psoriatic arthritis, there being a background prevalence of rheumatoid factor positivity, but a positive result should always make the physician consider the diagnosis carefully.

The distribution of radiological changes reflects clinical involvement, with the interphalangeal joints involved earlier than larger joints. A characteristic lesion in advanced cases is the so-called pencil-in-cup deformity (Fig. 19.6.10), which evolves by resorption of the distal end of a phalanx or metacarpal with uniform deep erosion of the end of the corresponding distal phalanx. In some cases the joints can be completely destroyed and invisible on the radiograph.

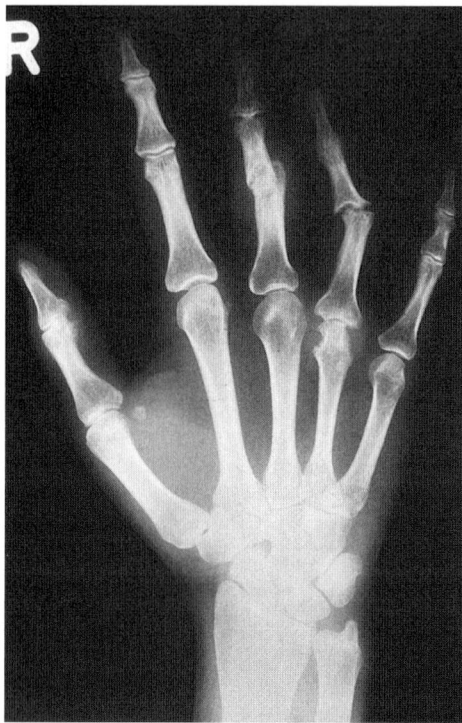

Fig. 19.6.10 Radiograph of a hand showing destructive psoriatic arthritis.

Radiological grounds for thinking the diagnosis more likely to be psoriatic arthritis than rheumatoid arthritis are distal interphalangeal joint involvement, asymmetric joint involvement, marginal erosions with adjacent bone proliferation (whiskering), osteolysis, periostitis, proliferative new bone formation, and ankylosis. Radiological sacroiliitis is a finding in 20 to 40% of patients. The axial disease in psoriatic arthritis can be indistinguishable from that in primary ankylosing spondylitis, but in psoriatic arthritis the following are more likely: asymmetrical sacroiliitis; less zygapophyseal joint involvement; fewer, coarser, and asymmetric syndesmophytes; and bony bridging that is more often than not asymmetrical. Psoriatic arthritis syndesmophytes can be indistinguishable from spondylophytes typical of DISH (Forestier's disease).

When scintigraphy is used to detect the extent and localization of arthritis, an increased uptake of the isotope technetium-99 can frequently be detected in the sternoclavicular and manubriosternal joints, but this is not necessarily associated with clinical symptoms.

Treatment

Many patients improve with the use of NSAIDs and intra-articular steroids, especially in the case of large joint involvement or flexor tenosynovitis. However, 20 to 40% of patients will not improve and need to be treated with disease-modifying antirheumatic drugs (DMARDs). Sulfasalazine 2 to 3 g daily is often effective against arthritis. Methotrexate 7.5 to 25 mg orally or subcutaneously weekly is also good for arthritis, and even better for the skin. Intramuscular gold and azathioprine can be tried. Antimalarials and penicillamine are not used; the former may exacerbate psoriasis. Ciclosporin is given in severe cases. There is limited information on the use of combination therapy. Systemic corticosteroids are limited to extreme cases of arthritis: psoriasis usually flares when they are withdrawn.

Local skin therapy has no effect on joint symptoms. Etretinate is not clearly beneficial for arthritis and may cause arthralgias and many other adverse reactions. The role of physiotherapy is similar to that in other spondyloarthritides, and there are no special considerations for surgical intervention in psoriatic arthritis, apart from the fact that the presence of florid skin lesions close to a joint is a relative contraindication to surgery.

Prognosis

Severe psoriasis can lead to significant disability. There are only limited data from long-term studies in psoriatic arthritis, but in cross-sectional studies 10 to 20% of patients with psoriatic arthritis are in a poor functional class, and the HLA antigens HLA B27, HLA B39, and DQw3 have been associated with such an outcome.

Arthritis associated with inflammatory bowel disease

Definition

An arthropathy with various clinical symptoms occurring in association with Crohn's disease and ulcerative colitis is termed arthritis associated with inflammatory bowel disease. Other forms of arthropathy occurring in association with enteropathy are Whipple's disease, and arthritis after intestinal bypass surgery.

Epidemiology

A relationship between gut and joint disease was postulated in 1922 when Smith treated arthritis patients with segmental bowel surgery. Bargen and Hench in 1929 and 1935 described arthritis in association with ulcerative colitis and Crohn's disease. Moll and Wright included arthritis associated with inflammatory bowel disease in the concept of spondyloarthritis in 1973. Mielants and Veys described Crohn's-like gut lesions in all subsets of spondyloarthritis in 1984.

The prevalence of Crohn's disease and ulcerative colitis is between 0.05 and 0.1% of the population, generally higher in white and Jewish people. The peak occurrence of both diseases is between 15 and 35 years, but it may appear in every decade of life; both sexes are equally involved. Arthritis associated with inflammatory bowel disease occurs in 10 to 30% of patients with inflammatory bowel disease, in general more frequently in Crohn's disease than in ulcerative colitis, and more often in patients with colonic involvement and in those with extensive bowel disease.

There is a genetic predisposition for inflammatory bowel disease with documented familial aggregation for both Crohn's disease and ulcerative colitis. The association with HLA B16, HLA B18, and HLA B62 is not strong. The peripheral arthritis of inflammatory bowel disease is only weakly associated with HLA B27, but axial inflammation is more strongly associated with it (50%). The patient with inflammatory bowel disease who is HLA B27-positive is at high risk of developing spondylitis. The relative frequency of sacroiliitis and ankylosing spondylitis in inflammatory bowel diseases varies between 2 and 20% or more, partly depending on the sensitivity of the diagnostic imaging procedure. Only 4% of patients with ankylosing spondylitis develop overt inflammatory bowel disease, whereas 60% have microscopically detectable Crohn-like gut lesions.

Pathogenesis

The pathogenesis of inflammatory bowel disease and arthritis associated with inflammatory bowel disease is not known. One hypothesis is of an aberrant immune response to gut bacteria, with gut inflammation leading to increased permeability, allowing bacteria to cross the mucosal border and get access to joints. There is some evidence from the HLA B27 transgenic rat model that gut and joints are closely linked: susceptible rats get both colitis and arthritis once they have left a germ-free environment.

Clinical features

Patients with ulcerative colitis and Crohn's disease typically present with bloody diarrhoea and abdominal pain, and in severe cases with fever, weight loss, and fatigue. For further details of gastrointestinal and other nonrheumatological presentations, and criteria for diagnosis, see Chapters 15.11 and 15.12.

As with the other spondyloarthritides, the arthritis is mostly asymmetric and predominantly affects the legs. The arthritis is migratory, often transient, but tends to recur. It does not frequently become chronic but may be associated with erosive disease in some patients. Flaring of gut symptoms is often associated with arthritis, especially in ulcerative colitis. Patients experience significantly fewer joint symptoms after colectomy.

Two types of arthropathy were distinguished in a study of almost 1500 patients with inflammatory bowel disease, essentially on the basis of the number of joints involved and (importantly) without knowledge of spinal radiographs. Pauciarticular disease (type I, fewer than five joints involved) affected 3.6% of patients with ulcerative colitis and 6% of those with Crohn's disease and was acute and self-limiting, with episodes lasting 4 to 5 weeks, in 83 and 79% of the cases. Polyarticular disease (type II, five or more joints) affected 2.5% of patients with ulcerative colitis and 4% of those with Crohn's disease and was associated with persistent symptoms in 87 and 89% of the cases.

The onset of peripheral arthritis is associated with exacerbations of colitis, but there is no link between enteric and spinal symptoms. Acute anterior uveitis occurs in 10% of patients with inflammatory bowel disease. It is associated with axial involvement and with HLA B27. The type of uveitis is somewhat different in inflammatory bowel diseases to that in other spondyloarthritides: posterior uveitis and scleritis may occur. The most common skin lesion in arthritis associated with inflammatory bowel disease is erythema nodosum, occurring in association with exacerbation of enteritis.

Diagnosis

Most arthritic symptoms occurring in patients with inflammatory bowel disease can generally be attributed to spondyloarthritides. However, as in psoriasis, patients can have more than one disease (osteoarthritis, etc.). As many as 50 to 60% of all patients with ankylosing spondylitis have gut lesions resembling those in Crohn's disease, but most are asymptomatic. Clinically apparent ankylosing spondylitis often precedes Crohn-like symptoms. This spectrum of diseases clearly and typically belongs to the spectrum of spondyloarthritides. The differentiation (if needed) will rarely cause problems, as one disease is usually predominant. Along with psoriasis, inflammatory bowel disease should always be looked for in HLA B27-negative patients who appear to have ankylosing spondylitis.

Treatment

Treatment of inflammatory bowel disease is always the first consideration and will probably influence peripheral arthritis. Treatment with NSAIDs may be effective for arthritis and spondylitis but can exacerbate bowel disease. There are few data on the use of DMARDs. Sulfasalazine is effective in ulcerative colitis and other spondyloarthritides and may accordingly be used in arthritis associated with inflammatory bowel disease. Azathioprine is effective in Crohn's disease and can be tried to treat severe and chronic joint disease. Corticosteroids are the therapy of choice in acute inflammatory bowel disease and will generally help arthritis, but they should not be used for mild and transient joint symptoms. As stated above, NSAIDs tend to exacerbate gut symptoms, but etoricoxib did not cause more flares than placebo (both *c.*10%) in one controlled study.

Prognosis

The prognosis of arthritis associated with inflammatory bowel disease is generally good. Joint destruction is a rare event. Patients may have ankylosing spondylitis at presentation of inflammatory bowel disease, or develop this later.

SAPHO syndrome

Definition

French workers proposed SAPHO (synovitis, acne, pustolosis palmaris et plantaris, hyperostosis, and osteitis) as a unifying diagnosis for several idiopathic bone and skin diseases, thereby combining over 50 different terms published in the literature (including pustulotic arthro-osteitis, chronic multifocal osteomyelitis, Tietze syndrome (German), and acquired hyperostosis syndrome). Their description of the common symptoms and overlapping features of this heterogenous group of rheumatic joint, bone, and skin diseases has led to better recognition of the relatively rare condition.

There is an argument that SAPHO simply represents a subset of psoriatic arthropathy; also that it might not really belong to the spondyloarthritides at all, because only 43% of patients with SAPHO fulfilled the European Spondylarthropathy Study Group criteria, and only 1 in 19 was HLA B27-positive in one follow-up study. However, there are some clear similarities.

Pathogenesis

The pathogenesis of SAPHO syndrome is unclear. Some authors think that it is similar to that of reactive arthritis. *Propionibacterium acnes*, which can induce arthritis in animals, has been detected in acne lesions and grown from osteitic lesions in some cases. However, cultures are negative in the vast majority of cases, and antibiotics are ineffective.

Diagnosis

There are no evaluated diagnostic criteria for SAPHO. Most convincing clinically is the combination of a classical skin symptom—such as pustolosis or significant acne (acne conglobata and acne fulminans or hidradenitis suppurativa)—with a characteristic joint or bone lesion such as arthritis of the sternoclavicular joint, osteitis, or hyperostosis in the anterior chest wall.

Diagnosis is important to avoid unnecessary biopsy procedures, but can be very difficult, especially in those without typical skin lesions. The most important differential diagnoses are bacterial osteomyelitis and malignancy. The pattern of joints affected differs from other rheumatic diseases: the sternoclavicular joint (Figs. 19.6.11 and 19.6.12), the clavicle, the ribs, and the mandible are frequently involved by arthritis, osteitis, and/or hyperostosis. Sacroiliitis, mostly unilateral, occurs in one-third of patients.

Treatment

Analgesics, NSAIDs, and intra-articular steroids are usually effective. In severe cases systemic corticosteroids should be considered.

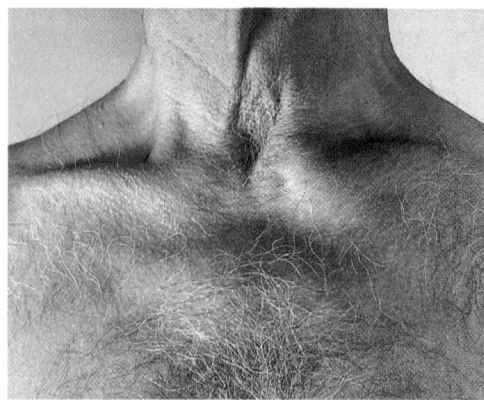

Fig. 19.6.11 Arthritis/hyperostosis of the left sternoclavicular joint in a 52-year-old man with SAPHO syndrome.

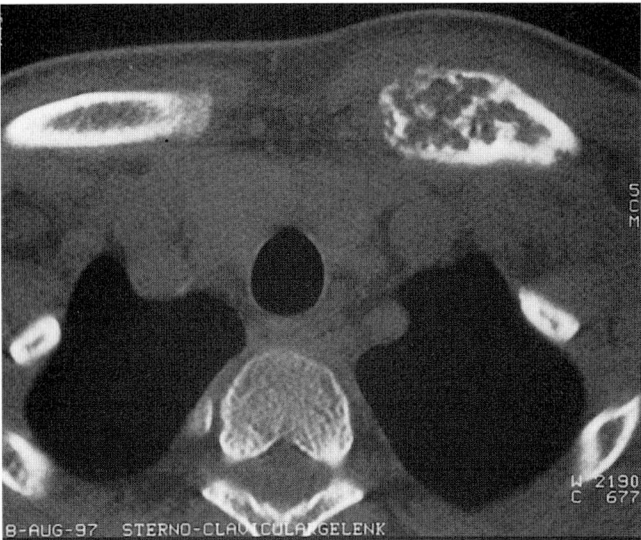

Fig. 19.6.12 CT showing severe osteitis of the left sternoclavicular joint in a 35-year-old woman with SAPHO syndrome.

Immunosuppressive agents can be added if the steroid dose cannot be tapered to less than 10 mg/day (of prednisolone, or equivalent). Sulfasalazine, azathioprine, and methotrexate have been tried successfully in some cases. Radiation therapy can also be effective in refractory cases. No controlled studies have been performed. Patients with refractory disease might also respond to treatment with TNF blockers.

Prognosis

The course of disease is very variable. Initially, occurrence of several flares per year is common. Further progress is usually favourable, but complications such as axillary vein and C8 compression can occur. Some patients may develop ankylosis and a few progress into ankylosing spondylitis.

Other enteric arthropathies

Whipple's disease

Whipple's disease is a rare systemic disease that usually involves the small intestine (see Chapter 15.10.6). The associated arthritis is often symmetric and polyarticular, and may antedate the intestinal complaints by years. It is not usually destructive. Axial involvement occurs but is not typical.

Arthritis associated with coeliac disease

For a description of coeliac disease (gluten-sensitive enteropathy) see Chapter 15.10.3. The joint manifestations show a striking response to a gluten-free diet, which strongly suggests a causal relationship. The pattern of arthritis is very variable, and overt bowel symptoms are absent in half of cases, making diagnosis difficult. The lumbar spine, hips, knees, shoulders, elbows, wrists, and ankles are most frequently affected, often symmetrically. The arthritis is not destructive. HLA B8 and DR3 are frequently found. The pathogenesis is unclear.

Arthropathies associated with collagenous colitis

Collagenous colitis is a chronic diarrhoeal disease characterized by a normal or near-normal mucosa endoscopically and a thick subepithelial collagen layer. More than half of patients with this disorder have some form of arthritis and use NSAIDs regularly.

Arthropathies associated with intestinal bypass surgery

Arthritis has been reported in 5 to 50% of patients in the first 3 years after jejunoileal bypass surgery. A symmetric peripheral polyarthritis involves the knees, wrists, metacarpophalangeal and metatarsophalangeal joints, elbows, proximal interphalangeal joints, and ankles and is usually nondestructive. Almost half of those affected also have vesicopustular skin lesions. No specific HLA association has been found, but two previously healthy HLA B27-positive patients developed spondylitis. Bacterial overgrowth of the blind loop is critical for pathogenesis.

Further reading

General

Amor B, et al. (1994). Predictive factors for the long-term outcome of spondyloarthropathies. *J Rheumatol*, **21**, 1883–7.

Braun J, et al. (1998). Prevalence of spondylarthropathies in HLA-B27 positive and negative blood donors. *Arthritis Rheum*, **41**, 58–67.

Braun J, Bollow M, Sieper J (1998). Radiologic diagnosis and pathology of the spondyloarthropathies. *Rheum Dis Clin North Am*, **24**, 697–735.

Brebam M, Hacquard-Bouder C, Falgarone G (2004). Animal models of HLA-B27-associated diseases. *Curr Mol Med*, **4**, 31–40.

Calin A, et al. (1977). Clinical history as a screening test for ankylosing spondylitis. *J Am Med Assoc*, **237**, 2613–14.

Dougados M, et al. (1991). The European Spondylarthropathy Study Group preliminary criteria for the classification of spondylarthropathy. *Arthritis Rheum*, **34**, 1218–27.

Khan MA, van der Linden SM (1990). A wider spectrum of spondyloarthropathies. *Semin Arthritis Rheum*, **20**, 107–13.

Moll JM, et al. (1974). Associations between ankylosing spondylitis, psoriatic arthritis, Reiter's disease, the intestinal arthropathies, and Behcet's syndrome. *Medicine (Baltimore)*, **53**, 343–64.

Sieper J, Braun J (1995). Pathogenesis of spondylarthropathies. Persistent bacterial antigen, autoimmunity, or both? *Arthritis Rheum*, **38**, 1547–54.

Ankylosing spondylitis

Bollow M, et al. (2000). Quantitative analysis of sacroiliac biopsies in spondyloarthopathies: T cells and macrophages predominate in early and active sacroiliitis–cellularity correlates with the degree of enhancement detected by magnetic resonance imaging. *Ann Rheum Dis*, **59**, 135–40.

Braun J, Seiper J (2007). Ankylosing spondylitis. *Lancet*, **369**, 1379–90.

Brophy S, et al. (2002). The natural history of ankylosing spondylitis as defined by radiological progression. *J Rheumatol*, **29**, 1236–43.

Gorman JD, Sack KE, Davis JC Jr (2002). Treatment of ankylosing spondylitis by inhibition of tumor necrosis factor alpha. *N Engl J Med*, **346**, 1349–56.

Gran JT, Skomsvoll JF (1997). The outcome of ankylosing spondylitis: a study of 100 patients. *Br J Rheumatol*, **36**, 766–71.

McGonagle D, et al. (1998). Characteristic magnetic resonance imaging entheseal changes of knee synovitis in spondylarthropathy. *Arthritis Rheum*, **41**, 694–700.

McLeod C, et al. (2007). Adalimumab, etanercept and infliximab for the treatment of anklosing spondylitis: a systematic review and economic evaluation. *Health Technol Assess* **11**, 1–158, iii–iv.

Rudwaleit M, Metter A, Listing J, et al. (2006). Inflammatory back pain in ankylosing spondylitis: a reassessment of the clinical history for application as classification and diagnostic criteria. *Arthritis Rheum*, **54**, 569–78.

Zink A, *et al.* (2000). Disability and handicap in rheumatoid arthritis and ankylosing spondylitis—results from the German rheumatological database. *J Rheumatol*, **27**, 613–22.

Undifferentiated spondyloarthritis

Gomariz EM, *et al.* (2002). The potential of ESSG Spondyloarthritis classification criteria as a diagnostic aid in rheumatological practice. *J Rheumatol*, **29**, 326–30.

Olivieri I, *et al.* (2001). Ankylosing spondylitis and undifferentiated spondyloarthropathies: a clinical review and description of a disease subset with older age at onset. *Curr Opin Rheumatol*, **13**, 280–4.

Zeidler H, Mau W, Khan A (1992). Undifferentiated spondyloarthropathies. *Rheum Dis Clin North Am*, **18**, 187–202.

Psoriatic arthritis

Gladman DD (1998). Psoriatic arthritis. *Rheum Dis Clin North Am*, **24**, 829–44.

Helliwell P, *et al.* (1991). A re-evaluation of the osteoarticular manifestations of psoriasis. *Br J Rheumatol*, **30**, 339–45.

Helliwell PS (2004). Relationship of psoriatic arthritis with the other spondyloarthropathies. *Curr Opin Rheumatol*, **16**, 344–9.

Marsal S, *et al.* (1999). Clinical, radiographic and HLA associations as markers for different patterns of psoriatic arthritis. *Rheumatology*, **38**, 332–7.

Reece RJ, *et al.* (1999). Distinct vascular patterns of early synovitis in psoriatic, reactive and rheumatoid arthritis. *Arthritis Rheum*, **42**, 1481–4.

Richter Cohen M, *et al.* (1999). Baseline relationships between psoriasis and psoriatic arthritis: analysis of 221 patients with active psoriatic arthritis. *J Rheumatol*, **26**, 1752–6.

Taylor W, *et al.* (2006). Classification criteria for psoriatic arthritis: development of new criteria from a large international study. *Arthritis Rheum*, **54**, 2665–73.

Arthritis associated with inflammatory bowel disease

Leirisalo-Repo M, *et al.* (1994). High frequency of silent inflammatory bowel disease in spondyloarthropathy. *Arthritis Rheum*, **37**, 23–35.

Mielants H, *et al.* (1996). Course of gut inflammation in spondylarthropathies and therapeutic consequences. *Baillière's Best Pract Res Clin Rheumatol*, **10**, 147–64.

Orchard TR, Jewell DP (1999). The importance of ileocaecal integrity in the arthritic complications of Crohn's disease. *Inflamm Bowel Dis*, **5**, 92–7.

Orchard TR, Wordsworth BP, Jewell DP (1998). Peripheral arthropathies in inflammatory bowel disease: their articular distribution and natural history. *Gut*, **42**, 387–91.

Taurog J, *et al.* (1994). The germfree state prevents the development of gut and joint inflammatory disease in HLA B27 transgenic rats. *J Exp Med*, **180**, 2359–64.

SAPHO syndrome

Boutin RD, Resnick D (1998). The SAPHO syndrome: an evolving concept for unifying several idiopathic disorders of bone and skin. *Am J Rheumatol*, **170**, 585–91.

Kahn MF, Khan MA (1994). The SAPHO syndrome. *Baillière's Best Pract Res Clin Rheumatol*, **8**, 333–62.

Koehler H, *et al.* (1975). Sterno-kosto-klavikuläre Hyperostose. *Deutsche Medizinische Wochenschrift*, **100**, 1519–23.

Maugars Y, *et al.* (1995). SAPHO syndrome: a followup study of 19 cases with special emphasis on enthesis involvement. *J Rheumatol*, **22**, 2135–41.

Moll C, *et al.* (2008). Ilium osteitis as the main manifestation of the SAPHO syndrome: response to infliximab therapy and review of the literature. *Semin Arthritis Rheum*, **37**, 299–306.

Sonozaki H, *et al.* (1981). Clinical features of 39 patients with pustolotic arthroosteitis. *Ann Rheum Dis*, **40**, 547–53.

Other enteric arthropathies

Fleming JL, Wiesner RH, Shorter RG (1988). Whipple's disease: clinical, biochemical and histopathological features and assessment of treatment in 29 patients. *Mayo Clin Proc*, **63**, 539–51.

Goff JS, *et al.* (1997). Collagenous colitis: histopathology and clinical course. *Am J Gastroenterol*, **92**, 57–60.

Pinals RS (1986). Arthritis associated with gluten-sensitive arthropathy. *J Rheumatol*, **13**, 201–4.

Stein HE, *et al.* (1981). The intestinal bypass arthritis-dermatitis syndrome. *Arthritis Rheum*, **24**, 684–90.

Pyogenic arthritis

Anthony R. Berendt

Essentials

Acute pyogenic arthritis may be primary (by haematogenous spread) or secondary (to trauma, surgery, or arthrocentesis). Organisms that cause primary septic arthritis are usually aggressive pathogens: *Staphylococcus aureus* (most commonly), streptococci, salmonella species (especially in African children) and Gram-negative organisms (neonates and older people). The causes of secondary and chronic septic arthritis are more diverse, including lower-grade pathogens from skin, mycobacteria, and fungi.

Clinical presentation—patients with acute pyogenic arthritis typically present with fever and an acutely painful joint that is swollen (effusion), warm to the touch, tender on palpation, and painful—frequently exquisitely so—on active or passive movement. The host response appears to reduce the risk of bacteraemia and death, but at the cost of joint damage. If not fatal through septicaemia, untreated septic arthritis generally causes joint destruction or fusion, sometimes with sinus formation and persistent infection. Chronic native joint septic arthritis presents in more indolent fashion with a mono- or polyarthropathy.

Diagnosis, management and prognosis—the diagnosis of pyogenic arthritis is established by isolation of a recognized pathogen from samples of synovium or synovial fluid obtained through biopsy or aspiration. After obtaining blood cultures and (whenever possible) synovial fluid, acute pyogenic arthritis should be treated promptly with intravenous antibiotics active against aerobic Gram-positive cocci and, where appropriate, Gram-negative organisms. Two or three weeks of antibiotic treatment is usually given in uncomplicated cases. Urgent consultation with an orthopaedic surgeon is recommended: arthroscopic washout is usually recommended, although some cases can be managed by joint aspiration once or twice daily until clinical response is evident. If acute native joint infection is treated promptly, the prognosis is good. Many patients make a complete recovery, but joint damage is highly likely when the diagnosis is made late. Outcomes are less favourable in prosthetic joint infection.

Introduction

Pyogenic arthritis, which may be acute or chronic, describes infection and resulting inflammation in a joint, native or prosthetic. It should not be confused with postinfectious (reactive) arthritis (discussed in Chapter 19.8). As with other musculoskeletal infections (see Chapter 20.3), failings in diagnosis or management may have long-term functional consequences, and clinicians should therefore know when to consider the diagnosis and obtain expert help.

Aetiology, pathogenesis, and pathophysiology

Acute pyogenic arthritis may be primary (by haematogenous spread) or secondary (to trauma, surgery, or arthrocentesis). Organisms that cause primary septic arthritis are usually aggressive pathogens capable of causing a bacteraemia, seeding a joint, and multiplying within it—hence they are also common causes of septicaemia. *Staphylococcus aureus* dominates in most circumstances, but streptococci are also important, salmonella species have been found to be important causes in African children, and Gram-negative organisms are more common in neonates and older people. The causes of secondary and chronic septic arthritis are more diverse. In prosthetic joints they also include lower-grade pathogens from skin. In native joints, mycobacteria and fungi are seen as causes of chronic septic arthritis alongside all the causes of acute infection when this has not been cured. Table 20.3.1 shows the common pathogens involved in both pyogenic arthritis and osteomyelitis.

In primary septic arthritis, organisms exit the bloodstream to access the joint. In the case of *S. aureus*, invasion of endothelial cells can occur through interactions between bacterial fibronectin-binding proteins and cell surface-associated fibronectin. This triggers integrin-dependent uptake of bacteria and may be a key first step in seeding of sites of metastatic infection during bacteraemia.

S. aureus releases a number of toxins and proteases thought to affect host defences. It also expresses numerous cell-wall-associated adhesins that mediate attachment of bacteria to the matrix proteins associated with cell surfaces, cartilage, and bone.

Animal models demonstrate that T-cell dependent inflammation plays a central role in damage to articular cartilage following an acute inflammatory response. In these models immunomodulation (e.g. with corticosteroids) can substantially reduce arthritis, but at the expense of host survival if antibiotic therapy is not also given. Thus the host response appears to reduce the risk of bacteraemia and death, but at the cost of joint damage. If not fatal through septicaemia, untreated septic arthritis generally causes joint destruction or fusion, sometimes with sinus formation and persistent infection (see Fig. 19.7.1) through the involvement of bone and dead cartilage as foci.

In a prosthetic joint, the presence of foreign material impairs local antibacterial defences. As with dead bone in chronic osteomyelitis (see Chapter 20.3), the bacteria adhere to inanimate material (in this case, plastic or metal) to produce a community called a biofilm. In this state they become relatively resistant to the action of antibiotics and to phagocytic killing. Ineffective but chronic inflammation causes pain and triggers bone loss at the interface with the infected implant or its associated bone cement, with subsequent mechanical loosening, pain, and failure of the joint.

Epidemiology

The incidence of pyogenic arthritis has been estimated at 7 in 100 000 in northern industrialized nations: the incidence is highest in children and older people, and more common in males, but there are large worldwide variations, with a chance of 1 in 1000 that a child in Malawi will develop the condition in the first 5 years of life. The increased incidence in older people probably reflects a higher prevalence of potential sources of bacteraemia, such as urinary tract infection, skin ulceration, pneumonia, and hospitalization with intravenous and/or urinary catheterization. Infection complicates some 0.5 to 2% of total joint replacements, but the true prevalence of prosthetic joint infection is unknown, and there is evidence of variation in rates between centres.

Prevention and control

There are no proven means of preventing primary pyogenic arthritis. Secondary cases can be prevented by meticulous attention to infection control measures whenever a joint is aspirated or operated on, and by thorough cleaning, debridement, and antibiotic treatment when a joint is contaminated through trauma. Prevention of prosthetic joint infection is optimized by fastidious sterile technique, ultrafiltered laminar air flow, and prophylactic antibiotics. The evidence that secondary prophylaxis is necessary or beneficial for patients with prosthetic joints *in situ* who are undergoing medical or dental procedures is not of high quality; some expert bodies recommend prophylaxis should accompany dental procedures occurring within 1 to 2 years of implantation of a prosthetic joint.

Clinical features

Patients typically present with fever and an acutely painful joint. The joints adjoining the long bones are most commonly affected (knee, hip, shoulder, elbow, wrist, and ankle). There may be bacteraemia (in some series in up to 70% of cases), causing prostration, vomiting, or hypotension. Infants localize pain poorly and commonly present refusing to use the affected limb. Adults may be unable to localize pain if a sternoclavicular, acromioclavicular, sternocostal, or manubriosternal joint is involved. Infection in these locations often presents as atypical chest wall pain. Sacroiliac joint infection causes buttock or low back pain and may mimic hip or spine pathology.

Clinical examination reveals a joint that is swollen, warm to the touch, tender on palpation, and painful, frequently exquisitely so, on active or passive movement. This presentation should be considered as infection until proven otherwise. To minimize pain, the patient will often nurse the joint in a neutral position. A joint effusion is usually present and this may be accompanied by synovitis, depending on the duration of the history. Erythema is not usually prominent and if present, may signal the presence of bursitis, cellulitis, or a more superficial abscess.

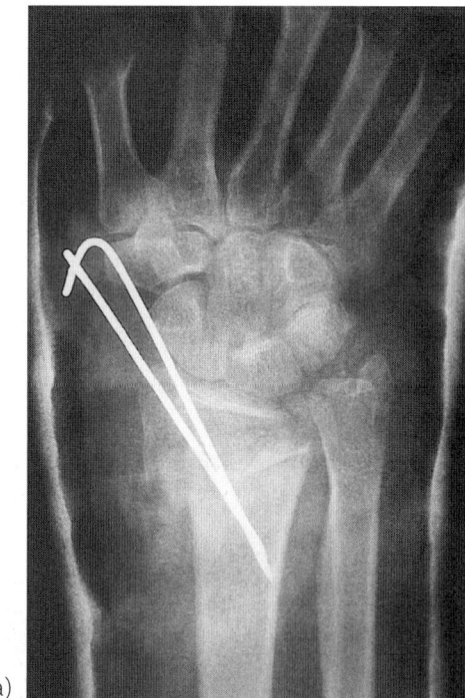

(a)

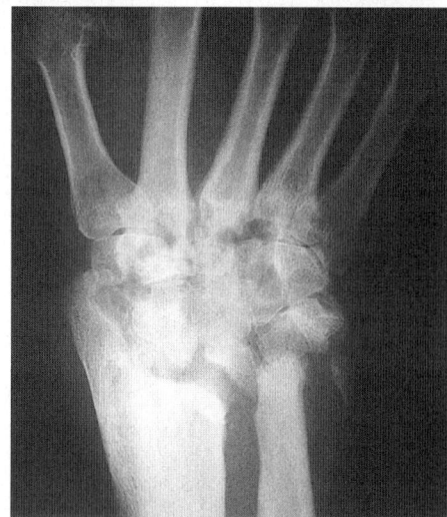

(b)

Fig. 19.7.1 (a) A Colles' fracture fixed with percutaneous K wires. (b) A few months later, after *S. aureus* infection associated with the K wires has led to septic arthritis in the wrist, the wrist joint is completely destroyed and the bones dead and osteomyelitic.

The pain of acute pyogenic arthritis generally resolves within the first 1 to 2 weeks of successful treatment, but stiffness and swelling usually persist for very much longer.

Chronic native joint septic arthritis presents in more indolent fashion with a mono- or polyarthropathy and a variable degree of joint destruction. There may be systemic features or evidence of involvement of other organ systems (for example, but not always, in tuberculosis). There may be strong epidemiological clues to exposure to unusual pathogens through the travel or occupational history, or there may be a history suggestive of an earlier acute septic arthritis. Patients with peripheral neuropathy may present with an obvious chronic septic arthritis underlying a neuropathic ulcer that has penetrated to the joint.

Prosthetic joint infection may present as an acute wound infection, a periarticular abscess, an acute arthritis, or loosening of the implant (as progressive and chronic pain). A sinus discharging in or near the operative scar represents infection of the prosthesis until proved otherwise. Loosening of an implant within a few years of primary surgery should raise the suspicion of infection unless there is an obvious mechanical problem.

Differential diagnosis

Septic arthritis must be distinguished from other acute or chronic monoarthropathies: notably gout, pyrophosphate arthropathy, and haemarthrosis. Rheumatoid and reactive arthritis can initially present with involvement of only a single joint. Infection is most commonly monoarticular, but multiple joints can be involved. Polyarticular infection may be mistaken for a flare in the underlying disease in a patient with known inflammatory arthritis. Trauma to the joint involving vegetable material, such as thorns, may introduce infection, but the organic matter can also lead to a very aggressive sterile inflammatory arthritis. In the case of a prosthetic joint, the differential is from superficial wound infection, haemarthrosis, periprosthetic fracture or dislocation, and aseptic loosening.

Clinical investigation

The criterion for diagnosis of pyogenic arthritis is the isolation of a recognized pathogen from samples of synovium or synovial fluid obtained through biopsy or aspiration. Infected synovial fluid is generally turbid or purulent. It should be sent for Gram stain, semiquantitative or quantitative white cell count, examination under polarized light for pyrophosphate or uric acid crystals, and culture. If tuberculosis, brucellosis, or fungi are suspected, the laboratory should be advised so that the sample can be appropriately processed. If *Neisseria gonorrhoeae* is suspected, urethral, endocervical, throat, and rectal swabs should also be obtained for microscopy and culture.

Blood cultures should always be obtained in suspected acute infection. The white cell count, C-reactive protein, and ESR are usually raised, but can also be elevated during flares of inflammatory arthritis or acute crystal arthropathy. Their value is probably greatest in following the response to treatment. Measurement of serum uric acid may be elevated in gout, but cannot be used to establish or refute this diagnosis. Serological tests may be of retrospective value in diagnosing *Borrelia burgdorferi* (Lyme disease), and brucella. Detection of microbial nucleic acid in joints remains a research technique, but this is likely to change as technologies become increasingly robust.

Plain radiographs can show fracture, effusion, chondrocalcinosis, bone destruction, or loss of joint space. An effusion may be seen acutely, but bony changes appear over at least 10 to 14 days. If seen at presentation they either indicate chronic infection or represent underlying arthropathy. A radiograph at presentation provides a useful baseline for subsequent comparisons. The role of CT or MRI is to demonstrate or exclude surgical disease in the joint or neighbouring bone (Fig. 19.7.2). Ultrasonography may assist in this and in distinguishing between effusion and synovitis, allowing diagnostic samples to be obtained more reliably.

Criteria for diagnosis

Consensus criteria for diagnosing infection have not been agreed. The isolation of microbes from joint fluid, capsule, or synovium is pathognomonic of infection as long as contamination of the specimen(s) can be ruled out. Cellular pathology is a valuable confirmatory test, with synovial fluid containing polymorphs and the synovium showing an acute inflammatory response with a fibrinous exudate on its surface, which may be ulcerated. A chronic synovitis may develop, with a lymphocytic and mononuclear infiltrate. Tissue from infected prosthetic joints shows a polymorph infiltrate accompanied by chronic inflammatory changes representing a reaction to foreign materials. Where low-grade or fastidious pathogens are suspected, multiple independent specimens can increase diagnostic yield and help to distinguish contamination of samples from true infection.

Treatment

Acute septic arthritis poses a threat to the joint and is a musculoskeletal (orthopaedic or rheumatological) emergency. Treatment should

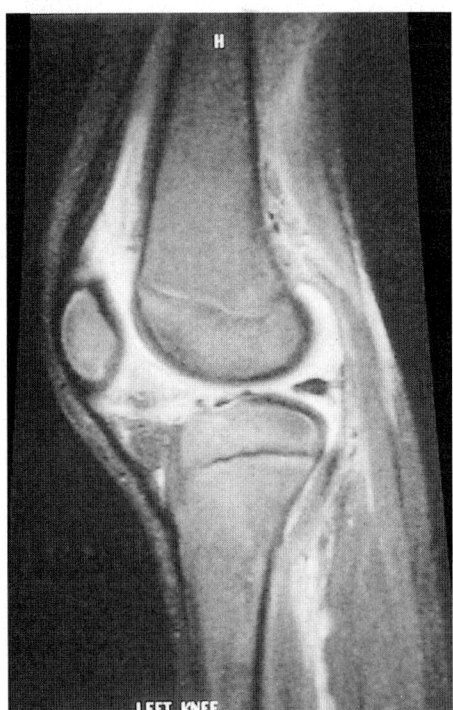

Fig. 19.7.2 MRI scan showing marked synovitis, but no osteomyelitis, in a 10-year-old with group A streptococcal infection of the knee.

generally be in an inpatient hospital setting. Patients with suspected chronic septic arthritis may initially be managed on an outpatient basis, but most eventually require surgical intervention.

After obtaining blood cultures and (whenever possible) synovial fluid, acute pyogenic arthritis should be treated promptly with intravenous antibiotics active against aerobic Gram-positive cocci and, where appropriate, Gram-negative organisms. Suitable regimens include a high-dose semisynthetic antistaphylococcal penicillin (flucloxacillin, dicloxacillin, or nafcillin), with or without an aminoglycoside; a β-lactam–β-lactamase combination (amoxicillin–clavulanate or ampicillin–sulbactam); or cefuroxime (or another antistaphylococcal cephalosporin). Patients allergic to β-lactams, or with risk factors for methicillin-resistant *S. aureus* (MRSA), should receive vancomycin, usually with an aminoglycoside, until culture results are obtained. The specific choice of empirical regimen should be determined with microbiological input based on local sensitivity patterns. Definitive treatment regimens should be based on culture results.

Urgent consultation with an orthopaedic surgeon is advised. Arthroscopic washout has largely replaced arthrotomy, reducing morbidity. Surgery can sometimes be avoided altogether by aspiration once or twice daily until clinical response is evident, but may still be needed if there is clinical deterioration or failure to settle within 5 days. If the joint is accessible this strategy can be applied to children or adults, particularly when anaesthesia is thought to carry high risks, e.g. in the patient with multiple comorbidities. Whether delaying surgery in this way gives worse outcomes than immediate washout is unknown. There is broad consensus on the need for prompt surgery on the hip, where the capsular vessels are reflected up the neck of the femur and are vulnerable to thrombosis, which causes avascular necrosis of the femoral head. If this occurs, joint destruction, with or without chronic infection of the dead bone, is inevitable. In the shoulder, despite the similar anatomy, it is not clear if arthrotomy or washout is superior to aspiration.

The optimal duration and mode of administration of antibiotics is unknown. In uncomplicated infection, 2 to 3 weeks is probably adequate, depending on the pathogen (2 weeks for streptococci, 3 weeks for *S. aureus* and aerobic Gram-negative rods). In children it is possible to convert to oral therapy within 48 to 72 h of defervescence, provided that there has been a rapid clinical response. This strategy requires the organism to be sensitive to a reliably bioavailable oral antibiotic, the parents or carers to understand clearly the importance of adhering to the antibiotic regimen, and the clinician to monitor clinical progress carefully. Some authorities treat adults with an oral regimen provided that similar criteria are met, whereas others prefer intravenous antibiotics when there has been accompanying bacteraemia or where there are concerns about bony involvement, absorption of oral antibiotic, or adherence to the treatment regimen. Many patients are suitable for outpatient intravenous antibiotic therapy, provided this is properly organized and supervised. Longer courses of treatment are indicated if there have been complications, slow resolution, or suspected involvement of underlying bone.

Chronic septic arthritis has generally led to joint destruction, with death of cartilage and involvement of underlying bone, by the time the patient presents. The condition is thus usually a form of chronic osteomyelitis (see Chapter 20.3). Surgical debridement is generally necessary to control infection, and staged arthrodesis or joint replacement—after an infection-free interval— the most frequent reconstructive strategy. Surgery to remove or to attempt to salvage the joint is also the rule in prosthetic joint infection, although for a few patients a decision not to operate may be the option with the least associated morbidity. Antibiotic treatment is usually prolonged in chronic or prosthetic joint infection, and may be long term where a decision is made to attempt to suppress, rather than cure, the infection.

Prognosis

If diagnosed and treated promptly, the prognosis of acute native joint infection is good, with many patients making a complete recovery. Conversely, joint damage is highly likely when the diagnosis is made late, for which reason clinical guidelines have been produced to aid appropriate early management. Infection in young children may lead to disturbance of the growth plate around the infected joint, causing deformity. Mortality is low in uncomplicated septic arthritis, higher when it is complicated by *S. aureus* bacteraemia (up to 20%), and highest in polyarticular disease (50%). Recurrence is uncommon and generally indicates a persisting surgical focus in the joint.

Outcomes are less favourable in prosthetic joint infection. Salvage of the original infected prosthesis can be achieved in 30 to 70% of cases where the prosthesis is retained. Infection can be eradicated in up to 90% of cases with revision surgery, but with very much poorer results expected when revision surgery for infection is itself complicated by further infection. This and the need for expert surgical and microbiological input, as well as the considerable comorbidity such patients often have, makes the management of infected prosthetic joints a formidable challenge best undertaken by, or with the support of, a specialist multidisciplinary team in a major centre.

Chronic infections have significant effects on quality of life through pain, poor function, and general debility. This is most prolonged and severe in prosthetic joint infection, which may culminate in amputation if sufficiently persistent or recurrent to cause major bone and soft tissue loss. For these reasons, while patients with acute infection may experience some psychosocial issues in adjusting to their abrupt change in functional ability and to uncertainties over the extent of functional recovery, patients with chronic infections usually have more obvious difficulties, especially when there is a nosocomial cause for their problems.

Areas of uncertainty or controversy

Numerous aspects of treatment await clarification in prospective studies, including the relative merits of arthrotomy, arthroscopic washout, or repeated aspiration; the optimal duration and route of administration of antibiotics; and the possible benefit of adjunctive steroids to modify destructive inflammatory responses in native joint infection.

Likely future developments

The dominance of staphylococci as a cause of septic arthritis makes likely a continuing increase in the prevalence of infections due to methicillin-resistant organisms. In some centres this is already driving changes in empirical treatment regimens and in the choices for definitive therapy. Molecular methods of diagnosis will yield a greater understanding of the range of causative pathogens, particularly in previously culture-negative cases and in prosthetic joint infections, and are likely to become standardized tools. It remains to be seen whether trends in rising antimicrobial resistance and rising numbers of elderly patients at risk of native and prosthetic joint infection will be balanced or overcome by improvements in surgical technique, coordinated programmes to reduce healthcare-associated infections, and investigational compounds that might reduce the ability of bacteria to adhere to implants. Septic arthritis is expected to remain a diagnostic and therapeutic challenge for some time to come.

Further reading

Berendt AR (1999). Infections of prosthetic joints and related problems. In: Armstrong D, Cohen J (eds). *Infectious diseases*, pp. 2.44.1–2.44.6. Mosby, London.

Berendt T, Byren I (2004). Bone and joint infection. *Clin Med*, **4**, 510–8.

Christodoulou C, Gordon P, Coakley G (2006). Polyarticular septic arthritis. *BMJ*, **333**, 1107–8.

Coakley G, *et al.* on behalf of the British Society for Rheumatology Standards GaAWG (2006). BSR & BHPR, BOA, RCGP and BSAC guidelines for management of the hot swollen joint in adults. *Rheumatology*, **45**, 1039–41.

Courtney P, Doherty M (2009). Joint aspiration and injection and synovial fluid analysis. *Best Pract Res Clin Rheumatol*, **23**, 161–92.

Girdlestone GR (1943). Acute pyogenic arthritis of the hip: an operation giving free access and effective drainage. *Lancet* **1**, 419. [Reprinted in *Clin Orthop*, **170**, 3–7 (1982)]

Kaandorp C. *et al.* (1997). The outcome of bacterial arthritis: a prospective community-based study. *Arthritis Rheum*, **40**, 884–92.

Kang SN, Sanghera T, Mangwani J, *et al.* (2009). The management of septic arthritis in children: systematic review of the English language literature. *J Bone Joint Surg Br*, **91**, 1127–33.

Kaplan SL (2009). Challenges in the evaluation and management of bone and joint infections and the role of new antibiotics for gram positive infections. *Adv Exp Med Biol*, **634**, 111–20.

Lavy CB, Thyoka M, Pitani AD (2005). Clinical features and microbiology in 204 cases of septic arthritis in Malawian children. *J Bone Joint Surg Br*, **87**, 1545–8.

Lowy FD (1998). *Staphylococcus aureus* infections. *New Engl J Med*, **339**, 520–9.

Mathews CJ, *et al.* (2007). Management of septic arthritis: a systematic review. *Ann Rheum Dis*, **66**, 440–5.

Stengel D, *et al.* (2001). Systematic review and meta-analysis of antibiotic therapy for bone and joint infections. *Lancet Infect Dis*, **1**, 175–88.

Syrogiannopoulos GA, Nelson JD (1988). Duration of antimicrobial therapy for acute suppurative osteoarticular infections. *Lancet*, **ii**, 37–40.

Reactive arthritis

J.S. Hill Gaston

Essentials

Reactive arthritis is a subset of postinfectious arthritis in which infection, usually of the gastrointestinal or genitourinary tracts, leads to inflammatory arthritis. Following infection, organisms or their components find their way to joints, where they provoke inflammatory immune responses. Whether the responses cross-react with self antigens is unclear; arthritis may be maintained by persistent infection. The disease commonly has specific extra-articular features not seen in other forms of postinfectious arthritis, and is genetically and pathologically a form of spondyloarthritis (see Chapter 19.6).

Clinical presentation—an acute oligoarthritis of weight-bearing joints is a common finding in secondary care, whereas community cases show mild polyarthritis. In addition to synovitis, enthesopathy is common, and extra-articular features include conjunctivitis, keratoderma, balanitis, and mouth ulcers. Urethritis can be reactive and does not necessarily indicate genitourinary infection.

Diagnosis—this depends on a careful history to determine whether there has been preceding infection, followed by examination for enthesopathy and extra-articular features in addition to joint involvement. Definitive proof requires demonstration of recent infection by a triggering organism, using serological, culture, and nucleic acid amplification techniques. In some cases, when the nature of the triggering infection cannot be established, patients may be classified as having undifferentiated spondyloarthritis (see Chapter 19.6).

Management—treatment is with symptomatic measures—nonsteroidal anti-inflammatory drugs, intra-articular steroids, and physiotherapy suffice in most cases. Severe, relapsing, or persistent disease may require methotrexate or sulfasalazine. Little evidence supports prolonged treatment with antibiotics, although chlamydial infection requires conventional short-term treatment.

Introduction and historical perspective

The term 'reactive arthritis' was introduced in 1969 by Aho in Finland, where the combination of a high prevalence of HLA B27 and gastrointestinal yersinia infection afforded opportunities for studying the disease. However, the condition was first recognized in the 18th and 19th centuries as an arthritis that followed dysentery or venereal disease, and there were descriptions by Hans Reiter and other contemporaries of the disease among troops affected by dysentery in the trenches of the First World War. The term 'Reiter's disease' has been used extensively since that time, but should now be abandoned for several reasons: Reiter was not the first to describe the disease; he erroneously attributed it to spirochaetal infection; and the triad that makes up Reiter's disease—arthritis, conjunctivitis, and urethritis/cervicitis—is not a clinically meaningful subgroup within reactive arthritis. The incorrect assumption that a patient with Reiter's triad has sexually acquired reactive arthritis is particularly unhelpful.

Definition

The term 'reactive arthritis' is sometimes used rather loosely to cover any form of arthritis that follows infection, and then includes postviral arthritides, rheumatic fever, Lyme disease, and other forms of arthritis that do not generally share clinical features. This usage is not appropriate, and the term 'postinfectious arthritis' is much preferred, with this all-embracing term subdivided into different clinical syndromes, one of which is reactive arthritis (Box 19.8.1). Defined in this way, reactive arthritis is seen as one of the seronegative spondyloarthritides (ankylosing spondylitis, psoriatic arthritis, arthritis associated with inflammatory bowel disease, undifferentiated spondyloarthritis), sharing clinical and immunogenetic features with those diseases. Other postinfectious arthropathies lack these common features.

In the absence of agreed and validated diagnostic or classification criteria for reactive arthritis, Box 19.8.2 presents a useful working classification of those patients who could reasonably be considered to have reactive arthritis. This takes as its starting point the classical pattern of arthritis and typical extra-articular features (Box 19.8.3) that are commonly seen after infection by five organisms—salmonella, yersinia, campylobacter, *Shigella flexneri*, and *Chlamydia trachomatis*. The same clinical syndrome (i.e. arthritis and extra-articular signs) is also seen, but more rarely, following various other infections, especially of the gastrointestinal tract, e.g. by *Clostridium difficile*; but genitourinary infection with

---

Box 19.8.1 Postinfectious arthritis

- Postviral arthritis, e.g. parvovirus
- Poststreptococcal arthritis
- Rheumatic fever
  - Arthritis alone
  - Post-neisseria arthritis
- Lyme disease
- Whipple's disease
- Reactive arthritis

Box 19.8.3 Extra-articular features and their occurrence in other forms of spondyloarthritis

- Eyes
  - Conjunctivitis
  - Uveitis (ankylosing spondylitis and inflammatory bowel disease)
- Skin and mucous membranes
  - Oral ulceration
  - Circinate balanitis
  - Keratoderma blennorrhagica (psoriasis)
  - Nail dystrophy (psoriasis)
  - Erythema nodosum (inflammatory bowel disease)
- Cardiac
  - Aortitis (ankylosing spondylitis)
  - Conduction defects (ankylosing spondylitis)

---

ureaplasma and respiratory infection with *Chlamydia pneumoniae* can probably also act as triggers of reactive arthritis. The other large group of patients is those who have asymmetric oligoarthritis without extra-articular features, but with definite laboratory evidence of preceding infection by one of the five major reactive arthritis-associated bacteria.

Laboratory diagnosis of infection is given priority over symptoms as a classification criterion because infection may be clinically silent. Chlamydia is notorious for this, particularly in women, whilst in yersinia infection arthritis is inversely correlated with the severity of gastrointestinal symptoms. Positively identifying the triggering infection often poses practical problems. Patients in whom arthritis develops (with or without extra-articular signs) after symptomatic episodes of gastrointestinal or genitourinary infection are therefore usually regarded as having reactive arthritis, even when no triggering organism can be identified, although the diagnosis is inevitably less secure in these cases. Improvement in methods for diagnosing preceding infection should decrease the size of this group, and may show reactive arthritis to be the commonest cause of acute inflammatory oligo- or monoarthritis in young adults.

Box 19.8.2 Working definition of reactive arthritis

- Classical clinical features:
  - Asymmetric oligoarthritis, legs predominate
  - Enthesitis
  - Extra-articular signs
  - **and** proven infection by salmonella, campylobacter, yersinia, shigella, or *Chlamydia trachomatis* (whether symptomatic or not)
- Classical clinical features **and** proven infection by other organisms (e.g. *Clostridium difficile*, *Mycobacterium bovis* BCG)
- Any acute inflammatory arthritis (including monoarthritis) **and** proven infection by reactive arthritis-associated bacteria
- Classical clinical features **and** preceding diarrhoea or urethritis/cervicitis, infection not proven

---

Epidemiology

Community studies in Scandinavia, where *HLA B27* is present in around 12% of the population (compared with 6–7% elsewhere in Europe), have suggested an incidence of 40 to 50 cases/million for each of the endemic organisms (chlamydia, campylobacter). The lower figure of 1.3/million for shigella probably represents a similar incidence to other organisms, as almost all cases were acquired by travellers. Incidence has also been studied in single outbreaks of food poisoning, in which the proportion of infected patients developing arthritis can be accurately assessed. However, in such studies the proportion who develop reactive arthritis varies widely (0–21%). By contrast, careful population studies of campylobacter infection have shown a high incidence (7–16%) of musculoskeletal symptoms not severe enough to require secondary care. The influence of *HLA B27* on incidence is important: 60 to 80% of patients with reactive arthritis presenting to rheumatology clinics are positive for *HLA B27*, whereas among those with mild disease the figure drops to 30% or lower. *HLA B27* seems to be associated mainly with the severity and persistence of arthritis, rather than its incidence.

Pathogenesis

There is considerable evidence that organisms reach the joints following infection of the gut or genitourinary tract. They may arrive intact, when they can be detected using the polymerase chain reaction (PCR), or as antigenic material (proteins, lipopolysaccharide) that can be demonstrated in synovial macrophages and polymorphs using organism-specific antibodies. This process can continue for months or even years, suggesting that some of the infections, e.g. yersinia, persist such that antigens/organisms continue to reach the joint. Elevated and persistent titres of IgA antibody to these organisms in reactive arthritis compared with uncomplicated infection also favour the idea of persistence. A clear distinction between septic and postinfectious arthritis is no longer possible, as viable organisms can be detected in the joint in various forms of postinfectious arthritis, including Lyme disease and reactive arthritis. However, an important distinction is that in postinfectious arthritis the organisms in synovium or synovial fluid are noncultivable (although viable), and antibiotics generally do not influence the course of disease (see below).

Within the joint, cellular immune responses to the bacteria responsible for triggering reactive arthritis are readily detected, particularly responses by CD4+ helper T lymphocytes, but also CD8+ T cells. Interestingly, although the association with HLA B27 is often taken to imply that CD8+ T cells are the principal effector cells in the disease, HIV-positive patients with reactive arthritis present during stage I infection, when numbers of CD4+ T cells are less depressed. By contrast, arthritis can be relatively quiescent in full-blown AIDS. Both CD4+ and CD8+ lymphocytes produce proinflammatory cytokines such as interferon-γ and interleukin 17 that can drive joint inflammation by secondary effects on synoviocytes.

How does HLA B27 influence the course of reactive arthritis—particularly its severity and persistence? It has been proposed that infection generates a B27-restricted response by CD8+ T cells to a bacterial peptide that cross-reacts with a component of the joint, i.e. infection triggers autoimmunity by 'molecular mimicry'. However, no such autoimmune response has yet been demonstrated. Alternatively, HLA B27 may adversely affect the efficiency with which the immune system clears the triggering organism. In this case disease does not require autoimmunity but is primarily driven by persistent bacterial antigens. Lastly, HLA B27 might affect the immune response to the triggering organism qualitatively, e.g. by allowing hyper-responsiveness to particular antigens, or biasing the immune response in favour of the production of proinflammatory cytokines.

Clinical features

Preceding illness

A history of urethritis (dysuria or discharge) and diarrhoea must be sought specifically, as patients do not automatically link these occurrences with their arthritis. The interval between infection and arthritis is variable but not usually more than 3 weeks. By the time a rheumatologist is consulted, many weeks may have passed and the triggering illness forgotten, particularly if symptoms were mild. Note that urethritis may be triggered by gastrointestinal infection: minimally symptomatic gastrointestinal infection and prominent urethritis may cause diagnostic confusion if this possibility is forgotten.

Arthritis

The classical clinical picture in reactive arthritis is an asymmetric oligoarthritis (generally fewer than six joints), predominantly affecting the legs (Box 19.8.4). However, any joint can be affected, and some patients have monoarthritis only. Affected joints are often hot and markedly swollen, with septic arthritis and crystal-induced arthritis being the most likely differential diagnoses. Dactylitis, similar to that seen in psoriatic arthritis, also occurs. Many patients describe low back or buttock pain, suggesting involvement of the sacroiliac joint. Arthritis is usually at its worst early in the course of the disease, but new sites can be affected after several months and relapses are not uncommon, even in those in whom disease eventually settles completely. The presence of enthesitis (inflammation of ligamentous and tendinous insertions) in addition to arthritis is

> **Box 19.8.4** Pattern of joint involvement in reactive arthritis
>
> ◆ Oligo- or monoarthritis
> - Asymmetric
> - Predominantly legs
> ◆ Coexisting enthesitis or reactive enthesopathy alone
> ◆ Sacroiliac joint involvement
> ◆ Inflammatory back pain
> ◆ Polyarthritis (mild)

helpful diagnostically, with plantar fasciitis and involvement of the Achilles tendon insertion the commonest sites.

The features described above are commonly seen in secondary care, but the milder cases detected in community surveys commonly have polyarthritis, whereas some have only inflammatory back pain or an enthesopathy such as reactive tendonitis.

Extra-articular features

In acute severe disease patients have constitutional symptoms of malaise, fatigue, and fever. More useful diagnostically are the specific extra-articular signs listed in Table 19.8.3 and illustrated in Figs. 19.8.1, 19.8.2, and 19.8.3. The fact that these extra-articular features are common to other forms of spondyloarthritis greatly strengthens the case for including reactive arthritis in this disease family, and for defining reactive arthritis as a distinct postinfectious syndrome.

Extra-articular features are more common in those with severe joint involvement. Conjunctivitis is often transient and no longer present by the time the patient presents. More persistent eye inflammation or painful eyes should raise the question of an acute anterior uveitis rather than a simple conjunctivitis and prompt full

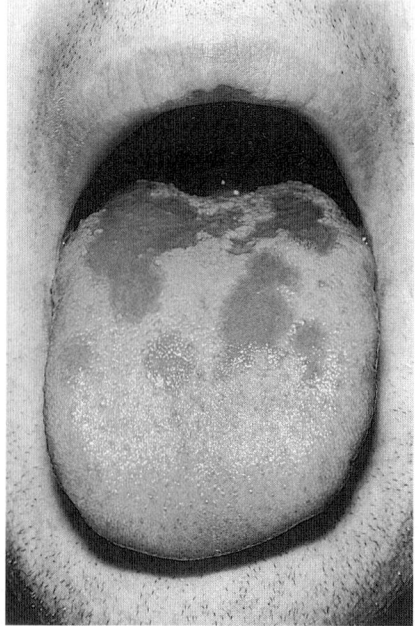

Fig. 19.8.1 Ulceration of the tongue in reactive arthritis.
Courtesy of Dr CJ Eastwood.

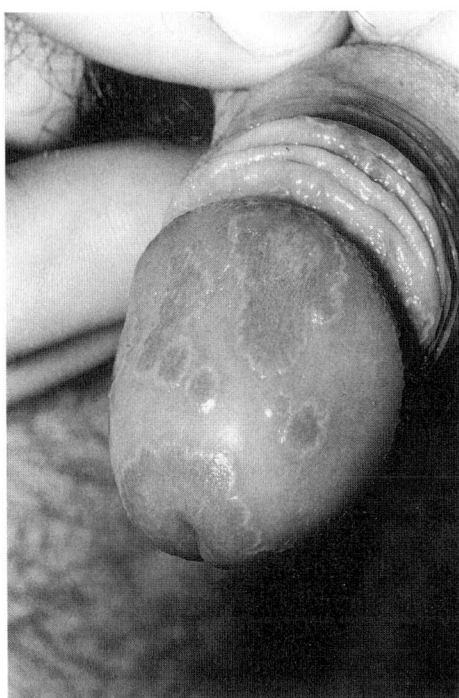

Fig. 19.8.2 Circinate balanitis in reactive arthritis.
Courtesy of Dr CJ Eastwood.

ophthalmological assessment. Circinate balanitis is usually asymptomatic and needs to be specifically sought in uncircumcised males. Oral ulceration is usually asymptomatic. Keratoderma blennorrhagica is histologically identical to psoriasis; it is most commonly seen on the soles of the feet, but can also involve the hands or trunk, and psoriaform nail changes are also seen. Erythema nodosum is associated with yersinia infection, but is otherwise uncommon in reactive arthritis. Aortitis and cardiac conduction disorders are rare.

Differential diagnosis

The differential diagnosis of reactive arthritis is summarized in Box 19.8.5. The principal concerns in acute disease are septic arthritis, crystal arthropathies, and other forms of postinfectious arthritis such as Lyme disease, poststreptococcal arthritis, or gonococcal arthritis. In chronic disease it may be difficult to distinguish reactive arthritis from other forms of spondyloarthritis, especially in those with inflammatory bowel disease, and many patients in whom no infectious trigger can be implicated can be classified as having an undifferentiated spondyloarthritis.

Laboratory features

General

The principal aims of investigation are to exclude important differential diagnoses and to identify the triggering organism. Abnormalities in the early stages, when arthritis is most active, are those of a pronounced acute inflammatory response—raised ESR and C-reactive protein, the latter often very marked (>100 mg/litre). Rheumatoid factor and antinuclear antibodies are absent. Positive antineutrophil cytoplasmic antibodies have been described, but the antibodies are not directed against proteinase-3 or myeloperoxidase and the test is not diagnostically useful. Septic arthritis and crystal arthropathies are best excluded by aspiration of synovial fluid followed by culture and microscopy. Blood cultures should be performed and serum urate checked. A chest radiograph may reveal hilar lymphadenopathy, suggesting the diagnosis of sarcoidosis, although yersinia can cause both reactive arthritis and a sarcoid-like illness. Throat swab and antibodies to streptococcal antigens may point to poststreptoccocal arthritis, which does not share extra-articular features with reactive arthritis. In endemic areas, Lyme disease should be considered and antibodies to *Borrelia burgdorferi* measured.

Microbiological

Stool should be cultured for pathogens associated with reactive arthritis, although cultures are often negative after gastrointestinal

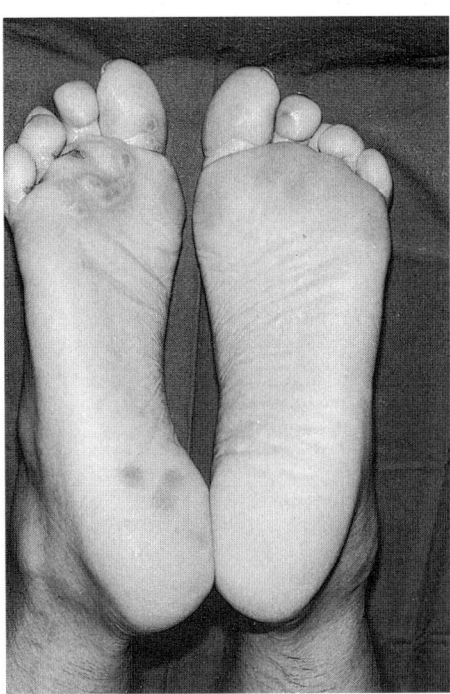

Fig. 19.8.3 Keratoderma blennorrhagica in reactive arthritis.
Courtesy of Dr CJ Eastwood.

Box 19.8.5 Differential diagnosis of reactive arthritis

- Septic arthritis
- Postinfectious arthritis
  - Lyme disease
  - Poststreptococcal or neisseria infection
  - Viral arthritis
- Crystal arthropathies
- Other forms of spondyloarthritis
- Behçet's
- Sarcoidosis
- Trauma, sports injury

symptoms have settled—despite the recent evidence that persistent infection contributes to pathogenesis. Chlamydia infection must be sought in sexually active patients with new partners, particularly when there is no history of gastroenteritis. Formal referral to a department of genitourinary medicine is often helpful. Patients are not infrequently infected with both chlamydia and gonococcus. This can cause confusion, but gonococcal arthritis differs from reactive arthritis with its characteristic rash and absence of classical extra-articular features. Chlamydia can be cultured from urethral or cervical swabs or from urine, and chlamydia antigens can be demonstrated by enzyme-linked immunosorbent assay techniques or by direct immunofluorescence tests. The latter are highly sensitive, in principle able to detect one organism per smear, but require skilled technicians. PCR techniques achieve similar sensitivity and can be applied to urine specimens, which is useful in patients understandably reluctant to undergo urethral and vaginal instrumentation in the investigation of their arthritis.

Spondyloarthritis in the context of HIV infection also needs to be considered, although this is rare in developed countries. By contrast, many cases of reactive arthritis, often related to dysentery, have recently emerged among the HIV-infected population in sub-Saharan Africa, where the disease was previously unknown. HIV testing should be considered, particularly in patients with unusually severe disease and relevant risk factors.

Immunological

When the triggering organism cannot be demonstrated directly, infection can be inferred on the basis of immune responses. However, this evidence needs to be interpreted cautiously, as in many cases the findings simply imply immunological memory for the organism in question and do not demonstrate a clear relationship between infection and arthritis. For enteric pathogens, specific IgM antibodies may be demonstrated and these, along with IgG, form the basis of the agglutination tests that are widely used. Rising IgG titres may also be helpful. However, when patients present several months into their illness, IgM may no longer be evident and IgG titres stable. In these circumstances high and persistent IgA titres to organisms such as salmonella and yersinia may be useful. Serological diagnosis of chlamydia infection is particularly difficult because of high community levels of infection with *Chlamydia pneumoniae*, an organism that shares several highly conserved antigens with *Chlamydia trachomatis*.

Lastly, cellular immune responses to triggering organisms can be demonstrated, particularly in the synovial fluid. Again, these demonstrate only T-cell memory for the organism and do not demonstrate causality—patients with, e.g., rheumatoid arthritis and incidental salmonella infection will have salmonella-specific T cells in their synovial fluid. Such tests are currently used in research rather than diagnostically.

Radiological

Radiological investigations are not diagnostically helpful in the acute stages of disease, with soft tissue swelling and occasionally periarticular osteoporosis at affected joints being the only abnormalities. Radionuclide scintigraphy can demonstrate acute sacroiliitis and may show the full extent of acute synovitis and enthesitis, but is not usually required for clinical management. Radiological changes are confined to the few patients with persistent disease (>1 year duration), with the principal features being erosion of affected joints, including the sacroiliac, and new bone formation manifested as periostitis of metatarsal and metacarpal bones and 'enthesophytes', such as plantar spurs. In the spine paravertebral ossification can be seen in the lumbar region: this is asymmetric and differs from the classical changes of ankylosing spondylitis. Erosive changes are also seen at sites of enthesitis such as the calcaneum.

Treatment

Evidence-based therapies for reactive arthritis are lacking, and consensus opinion is the current guide. In the acute phase, affected joints should be rested until they improve substantially. This often needs emphasizing to young, active patients involved in sports, and alternative forms of exercise should be considered. Physiotherapy and advice on exercise is helpful, with quadriceps function needing particular attention in view of the frequent involvement of the knees. Synovial effusions should be aspirated and, when septic arthritis has been excluded, will respond well to injection with long-acting corticosteroids. If chlamydia infection is established or thought likely, patients require conventional treatment with short-term antibiotics, but there is little evidence that this has any effect on the progress of reactive arthritis. Enteric infections do not require antibiotics in their own right, and the arthritis does not respond to antibiotics (see below). Uveitis requires formal ophthalmological assessment and treatment with local steroids.

There are two major unresolved treatment issues in reactive arthritis. Firstly, the place of disease-modifying drugs: sulfasalazine and methotrexate are useful in other forms of spondyloarthritis, and on this basis have been used in reactive arthritis, but without controlled trials confined to this condition (because the disease is often self-limiting, controlled trials of second-line agents are difficult to perform). The second issue is whether long-term antibiotics confer any benefit. In a controlled trial in 1991, a subset of patients with evidence of chlamydia infection benefited from prolonged lymecycline, but subsequent trials using ciprofloxacin and azithromycin have been negative. It may be that organisms in the joint, being in an uncultivable state, are also not susceptible to antibiotics, most of which affect bacterial cell division. A very recent (2009) trial suggests that a combination of rifampicin and doxycycline or azithromycin may be useful in chronic reactive arthritis.

Psychological and quality of life issues

Reactive arthritis commonly affects young fit adults who have not previously experienced any form of prolonged illness or disability. The danger is that the rheumatologist, all too used to the relatively gloomy prognosis of rheumatoid arthritis, may treat reactive arthritis, where there is a high likelihood of complete resolution of disease, too lightly. Patients need to be given a realistic prognosis, i.e. that symptoms may well persist at some level for 6 to 12 months, although in the latter stages these are usually very mild compared with those experienced in the first 4 to 8 weeks. Exacerbations during this time are not uncommon and do not imply that the disease will not eventually resolve. The chances of the patient developing chronic arthritis are less than 10%. Patients benefit from continuing psychological and clinical support throughout the course of their illness, with rapid access to joint aspiration and intra-articular steroid injection when there is recurrent joint swelling.

Areas of uncertainty

Current uncertainties concern classification criteria and management strategies. Both may be resolved by developing more secure diagnostic techniques for identifying the triggering infection. Improved treatment is likely to come from either (1) additional evidence about the importance of persistent infection and how to eliminate it, or (2) discovery of the immune responses responsible for maintaining joint inflammation, whether these are directed against a bacterial antigen or an autoantigen. If a target antigen can be identified, specific immunomodulation strategies would become relevant.

Reactive arthritis differs from other forms of inflammatory arthritis in having a clearly defined onset and being triggered by known infectious agents. Genetic influences that result in a minority of infected individuals developing arthritis are being investigated. These include *HLA B27*, but it is likely that other genes are also involved. Genome screening now being applied to ankylosing spondylitis may throw up candidates that also play a role in reactive arthritis.

Further reading

Reviews of pathogenesis

Gaston JSH (2000). Immunological basis of chlamydia induced reactive arthritis. *Sex Transm Infect*, **76**, 156–61.
Sieper J, Braun J (1995). Pathogenesis of spondylarthropathies: persistent bacterial antigen, autoimmunity, or both? *Arthritis Rheum*, **38**, 1547–54.

Incidence following enteric infection

Fendler C, *et al.* (2001). Frequency of triggering bacteria in patients with reactive arthritis and undifferentiated oligoarthritis and the relative importance of the tests used for diagnosis. *Ann Rheum Dis*, **60**, 337–43.
Gaston JSH (2005). Shigella induced reactive arthritis. *Ann Rheum Dis*, **64**, 517–8.
Hannu T, *et al.* (2002). Campylobacter-triggered reactive arthritis: a population-based study. *Rheumatology (Oxford)* **41**, 312–8.
Hannu T, *et al.* (2005). Reactive arthritis attributable to *Shigella* infection: a clinical and epidemiological nation-wide study. *Ann Rheum Dis*, **64**, 594–8.

Evidence that bacteria or bacterial antigens reach the joint in reactive arthritis

Gaston JSH, Cox C, Granfors K (1999). Clinical and experimental evidence for persistent *Yersinia* infection in reactive arthritis. *Arthritis Rheum*, **42**, 2239–42.

Gerard HC, *et al.* (1998). Synovial *Chlamydia trachomatis* in patients with reactive arthritis/Reiter's syndrome are viable but show aberrant gene expression. *J Rheumatol*, **25**, 734–42.
Granfors K, *et al.* (1989). Yersinia antigens in synovial fluid cells from patients with reactive arthritis. *New Engl J Med*, **320**, 216–21.
Granfors K, *et al.* (1990). Salmonella lipopolysaccharide in synovial cells from patients with reactive arthritis. *Lancet*, **335**, 685–8.

Immune responses in reactive arthritis

Gaston JSH, *et al.* (1989). Synovial T lymphocyte recognition of organisms that trigger reactive arthritis. *Clin Exp Immunol*, **76**, 348–53.
Granfors K, Toivanen A (1986). IgA-anti-yersinia antibodies in yersinia-triggered reactive arthritis. *Ann Rheum Dis*, **45**, 561–5.
Hermann E, *et al.* (1993). HLA-B27-restricted CD8 T-cells derived from synovial fluids of patients with reactive arthritis and ankylosing spondylitis. *Lancet*, **342**, 646–50.

Reactive arthritis and other spondyloarthritis in HIV infection

Njobvu P, McGill P (2005). Human immunodeficiency virus related reactive arthritis in Zambia. *J Rheumatol*, **32**, 1299–304.

Treatment in reactive arthritis

Dougados M, *et al.* (1995). Sulfasalazine in the treatment of spondylarthropathy: a randomized, multicenter, double-blind, placebo-controlled study. *Arthritis Rheum*, **38**, 618–27.
Kvien TK, Gaston JSH, *et al.* (2004). Three month treatment of reactive arthritis with azithromycin: a EULAR double blind, placebo controlled study. *Ann Rheum Dis*, **63**, 1113–9.
Lauhio A, *et al.* (1991). Double-blind, placebo-controlled study of three-month treatment with lymecycline in reactive arthritis with special reference to chlamydia arthritis. *Arthritis Rheum*, **34**, 6–14.
Sieper J, *et al.* (1999). No benefit of long-term ciprofloxacin treatment in patients with reactive arthritis and undifferentiated oligoarthritis—a three-month, multicenter, double-blind, randomized, placebo-controlled study. *Arthritis Rheum*, **42**, 1386–96.
Wakefield D, *et al.* (1999). Ciprofloxacin treatment does not influence course or relapse rate of reactive arthritis and anterior uveitis. *Arthritis Rheum*, **42**, 1894–7.
Yli-Kerttula T, *et al.* (2000). Effect of a three month course of ciprofloxacin on the outcome of reactive arthritis. *Ann Rheum Dis*, **59**, 565–70.
Yli-Kerttula T, *et al.* (2003). Effect of a three month course of ciprofloxacin on the late prognosis of reactive arthritis. *Ann Rheum Dis*, **62**, 880–4.

Osteoarthritis

Paul H. Brion and Kenneth C. Kalunian

Essentials

Osteoarthritis is the commonest form of arthritis, detectable radiographically in 80% of patients over the age of 55 and accounting for more dependency in walking and stair-climbing than any other disease. In clinical practice it is defined by the presence of joint symptoms (pain, aching, stiffness) plus evidence of structural change (including crepitus on active joint motion, bony enlargement, radiographic changes of joint space narrowing or osteophytes).

Aetiology and pathogenesis

Risk factors include being female, increasing age, obesity, family history of osteoarthritis (particularly for the hand), increased bone density, trauma, and certain occupational exposures (particularly for the knee). Early onset severe osteoarthritis has been linked to an autosomal dominant mutation in the type 2 procollagen gene (COL2A1), and mutations in other genes may also be important. There are many causes of secondary osteoarthritis, including congenital/developmental abnormalities, trauma, and metabolic and endocrine conditions.

Osteoarthritis results from an imbalance in catabolic and anabolic processes that lead to progressive cartilage damage and destruction. Early stages are characterized by increased water content and cartilage swelling, followed by fragmentation. Reparative processes, involving the formation of fibrocartilage in place of hyaline cartilage, may initially lead to joint stabilization, but ultimately contribute to disease progression by exposing subchondral bone to increased forces. Sclerosis and osteophyte formation develop.

Clinical features

Idiopathic osteoarthritis commonly involves the hands, hips, knees, and spine. Mild to moderate pain is the predominant symptom, increasing with joint use and at the end of the day, and generally improved with rest and moderation of activity. Physical examination reveals tenderness to palpation, bony thickening (osteophyte formation), small effusions, and crepitus. Specific joint findings in the hand are bony enlargement of the proximal interphalangeal joints (Bouchard's nodes) and the distal interphalangeal joints (Heberden's nodes), and a 'squared' appearance of the lateral aspect of the hand owing to involvement of the first carpometacarpal joint.

Radiographic findings include asymmetry, joint space narrowing, subchondral sclerosis, subchondral cysts, and (the hallmark) osteophytes.

Management

Treatment modalities for all forms of osteoarthritis are limited. Weight loss is effective but difficult to achieve and maintain. Physical therapy and exercise have been demonstrated to improve functional outcome and pain scores in clinical trials. Paracetamol (acetaminophen) is superior to placebo but less efficacious than nonsteroidal anti-inflammatory drugs (NSAIDs) in relieving pain. NSAIDs have been a cornerstone of treatment for many years, but recently their use has diminished because of reports of serious cardiovascular adverse effects. Intra-articular corticosteroids may be effective, but injections should be limited to three to four per year in any given joint to minimize the risk of complications.

Physical aids—a joint that is unstable and painful can be made more stable and less painful by appropriate aids. Walking sticks can be very effective; wheelchairs and other appliances may make it possible for patients to maintain their independence.

Surgical intervention—this is generally reserved for patients who have failed conservative management, including analgesics, physiotherapy, and intra-articular injection. Options include synovectomy, repair of meniscal tears, realignment osteotomy, and total joint replacement (the only known 'cure' for osteoarthritis).

Other proposed treatments—irrigation of osteoarthritic joints has been used as a method of relieving joint pain, but remains controversial. Intra-articular injections of hyaluronic acid preparations have become popular in recent years, but any effect is likely to be small. Many patients feel that glucosamine salts and chondroitin sulphate improve symptoms, but recent data from large randomized clinical trials do not support these claims.

Introduction

Osteoarthritis is the commonest form of arthritis, detectable radiographically in 80% of patients over the age of 55. Symptomatic osteoarthritis of the knee (pain with radiographic abnormalities) was noted in 6.1% of adults aged 30 and over in the Framingham Study, with comparable frequency in the United Kingdom. Approximately 20.7 million people in the United States of America have physician-diagnosed osteoarthritis, and although some of these may be asymptomatic, many have significant pain and disability, with one study finding that osteoarthritis accounts for 12.3% of all those with limitation of activity. The prevalence of osteoarthritis is likely to increase, paralleling the increase in the absolute and relative number of people who are over 65 years of age. The social impact of this disease is enormous, accounting for more dependency in walking and stair climbing than any other disease. The estimated annual cost associated with osteoarthritis in the United States of America is $15.5 billion in 1994 dollars, which approaches 1% of the gross national product, with more than 50% of the costs due to work loss.

Definition

Osteoarthritis has been defined by the American College of Rheumatology (ACR) as:

> a heterogeneous group of conditions that lead to joint symptoms and signs which are associated with defective integrity of articular cartilage, in addition to related changes in the underlying bone at the joint margins.
>
> Source: Altman R, Asch E, Bloch D, *et al.* (1986) The American College of Rheumatology criteria for the classification and reporting of osteoarthritis of the knee. *Arthritis Rheum*, **29**, 1039–49.

There are alternative definitions, including those based on symptoms, physical findings, and radiographic and arthroscopic findings. The presence of joint symptoms plus evidence of structural change generally defines clinical osteoarthritis, whereas many studies use radiographic assessment alone as the primary means of identifying the condition. Most clinical investigators use the Kellgren and Lawrence scale for grading osteoarthritis of the knee, which defines osteoarthritis on the basis of osteophytes, the presence of which relates well with the presence of knee symptoms. The American College of Rheumatology has developed classification criteria for the presence of osteoarthritis based on

Table 19.9.1 American College of Rheumatology clinical criteria for the classification of osteoarthritis of the hand

Hand pain, aching, or stiffness with three of the following four:
Hard tissue enlargement of two or more of ten selected joints
Fewer than three swollen MCP joints
Hard tissue enlargement of two or more DIP joints
Deformity of one or more of ten selected hand joints

♦ Selected joints are the second and third DIP joints, the second and third proximal interphalangeal joints and the first CMC joint of both hands
♦ Hand osteoarthritis is readily diagnosed by clinical criteria alone. There are no recommended lab and/or radiographic classification criteria
♦ Sensitivity = 94%, specificity = 87%

Table 19.9.2 American College of Rheumatology clinical, laboratory, and radiographic criteria for the classification of osteoarthritis of the hip

Hip pain for most days in the previous month with two of the following three features:
Femoral and/or acetabular osteophytes on radiograph
Erythrocyte sedimentation rate > 20 mm/h
Joint space narrowing on radiograph

♦ Clinical and lab criteria alone yield poor results. Only clinical with lab and radiographic criteria are recommended
Sensitivity = 89%, specificity = 91%

the joint involved (Tables 19.9.1–19.9.3): these are based on clinical criteria alone, clinical and laboratory criteria, and clinical plus radiographic criteria. Initially, only the clinical and radiographic criteria were validated; more recently, Wu and colleagues have validated the clinical classification criteria.

Table 19.9.3 Criteria for the classification of osteoarthritis of the knee

Clinical criteria*
Knee pain for most days of previous month with three of the following six:
Age > 50 years
Morning stiffness < 30 min duration
Crepitus on active joint motion
Bony enlargement on examination
Bony tenderness on examination
No palpable warmth
Clinical and laboratory criteria†
Knee pain for most days of previous month with five of the following nine:
Age > 50 years
Morning stiffness < 30 min duration
Crepitus on active joint motion
Bony enlargement on examination
Bony tenderness
No palpable warmth
Westergren ESR < 40 mm/h
RF titre < 1:40
Synovial fluid suggestive of osteoarthritis§
Clinical, laboratory, and radiographic criteria‡
Knee pain for most days of the previous month with osteophytes on the radiograph with one of the following three:
Age > 50 years
Morning stiffness < 30 min
Crepitus on active joint motion

*Sensitivity = 95%, specificity = 69%.
†Sensitivity = 92%, specificity = 75%.
‡Sensitivity = 91%, specificity = 86%.
§Synovial fluid suggestive of osteoarthritis has a clear colour, viscous fluid, and a white cell count of less than 2000/mm³.
ESR, erythrocyte sedimentation rate; RF, rheumatoid factor.

Risk factors and epidemiology

There are many risk factors for the development of osteoarthritis of the knee, including being female, increasing age, obesity, family history, increased bone density, trauma, and certain occupational exposures (Table 19.9.4).

Age, sex, and race

Age is the strongest associated risk factor for the development of osteoarthritis in many studies. The National Health and Nutrition Examination Survey found a prevalence of osteoarthritis of only 0.1% in people aged 25 to 34 years, compared with over 80% in those aged 55 to 64 years. This increased incidence occurs in osteoarthritis of the hands, back, hip, and knees.

Sex differences in osteoarthritis are complicated. There is an overall higher prevalence in women, in whom the disease more often involves multiple joints. However, before the age of 50 years there is a higher prevalence and incidence in men, whereas after 50 years the reverse applies, with increasing female predominance as age increases. There is a plateau or decline in both sexes by the age of 80 years. The sex- and age-related differences in prevalence parallel the effect of postmenopausal oestrogen deficiency in increasing the risk of osteoarthritis. Other probable factors that help explain the increase in the incidence and prevalence of osteoarthritis with age include a decreased responsiveness of chondrocytes to growth factors that stimulate repair, an increase in the laxity of ligamentous structures, and a decrease in proprioceptive responses.

Racial differences in osteoarthritis of the hip are conflicting, but the higher relative weight of African–American women may predispose them to higher rates of osteoarthritis of the knee. There are few data available for other racial differences in osteoarthritis of the knee among the population of the United States of America.

Table 19.9.4 Risk factors and protective factors for osteoarthritis

Risk factors for osteoarthritis
Age
Obesity
Female gender
Family history
Prior trauma
Congenital abnormality
African-American race
Increased bone density
Quadriceps weakness
Occupation (e.g. farming)
Competitive level sports
Protective factors for osteoarthritis
Osteoporosis
Oestrogen replacement therapy
Vitamin C
Vitamin E
Vitamin D

Genetic factors

Several studies have confirmed that inheritance is a risk factor for osteoarthritis, with conventional twin and nontwin sibling, population, and modern molecular studies implicating genetic factors in the development of the condition. Most cases of osteoarthritis of the hand are inherited; the percentage for osteoarthritis of the knee is smaller, perhaps because this often develops more as a result of repeated mechanical insults. Individuals are at higher risk of developing osteoarthritis if their parents had it, especially if the parental disease was polyarticular or had its onset in middle age or earlier. Inheritance may be more important among women than men. Numerous extended families with high rates of early onset severe osteoarthritis have been characterized in which the condition has been linked to an autosomal dominant mutation in type II procollagen; using linkage analysis, two reports on three unrelated families showed co-inheritance of generalized osteoarthritis with specific alleles of a type II procollagen gene (*COL2A1*) on chromosome 12. Mutations in genes other than *COL2A1* may also be important, such as genes encoding minor collagen types and extracellular matrix protein. The gene for asporin, a matrix protein, appears to be a promising candidate; an allele that increases the number of aspartic acid residues in one portion of the asporin molecule associates with knee osteoarthritis in a Japanese population, and asporin produced from this allele appears to suppress transforming growth factor β (TGFβ)-stimulated synthesis of the major articular cartilage structural proteins, type II collagen and aggrecan, by cultured chondrocytes.

Obesity

Several longitudinal studies suggest that increased weight is a risk factor for the development of osteoarthritis of the knee, and that overweight patients with established osteoarthritis of the knee are at greater risk of developing progressive disease compared with those who are not overweight. The associations between obesity and osteoarthritis of the knee are significantly greater for women than men and are not affected by adjustments for concurrent diseases. Data from the Chingford Study showed that patients in the highest weight tertile had an odds ratio of 6.17 for radiographic osteoarthritis of the knee compared with the lowest weight tertile. For every two-unit increase in body mass index (BMI) ($c.5$ kg), the odds ratio for radiographic osteoarthritis of the knee increased by 1.36. A follow-up study of incident osteoarthritis of the knee in women with unilateral disease found the tertile with the highest BMI had a relative risk of 4.69 for developing osteoarthritis in the contralateral knee compared with patients in the lowest BMI tertile. There are similar findings for osteoarthritis of the hand and hip, but the association is less robust; a recent study noted a significant association between BMI and total hip arthroplasty for osteoarthritis in a cohort of over 1 million Norwegian men and women. The importance of obesity cannot be understated, as this may be a modifiable risk factor. An obvious possible mechanism for the effect of obesity on osteoarthritis of the knee is increased force across the weight-bearing joint, which induces cartilage breakdown by altered walking mechanics, but obesity may also have effects through metabolic intermediaries.

Oestrogen deficiency

Oestrogen deficiency has been implicated as a risk factor for the development of osteoarthritis, as evidenced by the high incidence of osteoarthritis after the menopause. Several studies suggest that oestrogen replacement therapy reduces the risk of osteoarthritis of the hip and knee. Both the Study of Osteoporotic Fractures and the Framingham Study have reported a strong inverse relationship between oestrogen replacement therapy and osteoarthritis among those taking long-term oestrogen replacement therapy.

Reactive oxygen species

Reactive oxygen species have been implicated in the development of osteoarthritis, and antioxidants may prevent or delay the onset of the condition. In the Framingham Study, those in the lowest tertile of vitamin C intake had a threefold greater risk of progression of osteoarthritis of the knee, joint space loss, and onset of knee pain compared with subjects with a higher intake. However, the effects of β-carotene and vitamin E against disease progression were inconsistent. No effect of serum 25-hydroxyvitamin D was seen on incident osteoarthritis, but among subjects with radiographic osteoarthritis at baseline, those who were in the lowest tertile of serum 25-hydroxyvitamin D had a higher rate of radiographic progression compared with those in the highest tertile. There is conflicting evidence related to the association of specific polymorphisms of vitamin D receptor and oestrogen receptor genes and a predisposition for osteoarthritis; however, no association between these polymorphisms and osteoarthritis was seen in a well-designed case–control study.

Local biomechanical factors

Local biomechanical factors such as caused by hip dislocation, congenital dysplasia, trauma or repetitive joint use are risk factors for osteoarthritis. In animal models, a change in biomechanics that occurs after injury leads to increased shear stress on local areas of cartilage, possibly causing osteoarthritis. In humans, traumatic injury to joints is a common cause of osteoarthritis, and Kellgren and Lawrence found that a history of previous trauma could be elicited in about 40% of men and 20% of women aged 55 to 64 years with osteoarthritis of the knee. In the Framingham Study, men with a history of major trauma to the knee had a fivefold increased risk of osteoarthritis of the knee, and women with a similar history had a greater than threefold increased risk. Trauma that causes damage to a cruciate ligament and/or a meniscus has been associated with subsequent development of osteoarthritis of the knee, perhaps through concurrent damage to articular cartilage. With regard to repetitive use, occupations that require kneeling and squatting are associated with a higher prevalence of osteoarthritis of the knee, but heavy physical work is less consistently associated. The level of physical activity increases the risk of developing osteoarthritis. In the Framingham Study, physical activity (generally consisting of walking and gardening in this population) was found to correlate directly with the risk of developing radiographic osteoarthritis of the knee in elderly subjects followed for 8 years. Those with high levels of these activities had a threefold increase in the risk of osteoarthritis compared with sedentary controls. Elite athletes have higher rates of incidence of osteoarthritis of weight-bearing joints compared with controls, probably because athletic activities often involve both increased risk of injury and repetitive use.

Quadriceps weakness has been associated with radiographic osteoarthritis of the knee. Muscular strength may be required to stabilize the knee, distribute force, or lessen the effect of an impact load, and maintenance of muscular strength may be important in decreasing the incidence of osteoarthritis of the knee and its progression and disability due to established disease. Proprioceptive sensation, which declines with age, is impaired in elderly patients with osteoarthritis of the knee, suggesting that poor proprioception may contribute to functional impairment in these patients.

Protective factors

The incidence of osteoarthritis is lower in the setting of osteoporosis: bone density in patients with osteoarthritis is greater than in age-matched controls, even at sites distant from the affected joints. Most studies linking osteoarthritis with high bone density are cross-sectional. Although osteoarthritis and high bone density are both linked to obesity, the association of osteoarthritis with high bone density is independent of BMI. It has been suggested that osteophyte formation rather than cartilage loss is linked to high bone density, which suggests the presence of a circulating bone growth factor in those with osteophytes; possibilities include insulin-like growth factor type 1 (IGF-1), platelet-derived growth factor (PDGF), fibroblast growth factor (FGF), TGFβ, and colony-stimulating factor (CSF).

Pathogenesis and pathological features

The pathogenesis of osteoarthritis remains controversial. Once thought of as a normal consequence of ageing, the complex nature of this disease is only now being understood. Current theories suggest that osteoarthritis results from an imbalance in catabolic and anabolic processes that lead to progressive cartilage damage and destruction. Increased catabolism may be the result of acute injuries such as an acute meniscal tear or of chronic microtraumatic events. Initially, anabolic processes such as proteoglycan synthesis maintain balance with catabolic processes, and damage to cartilage is repaired. However, with time and age, anabolic processes decline and progressive cartilage damage ensues.

Histological changes in osteoarthritis are complex. Early stages are characterized by increased water content and cartilage swelling, and this swollen cartilage is believed to be more susceptible to injury and may lead to fragmentation of the articular surface. Fragmented cartilage is less able to withstand biomechanical insults, resulting in further deterioration. Chondrocytes become activated and proinflammatory cytokines such as interleukin 1 (IL-1) and tumour necrosis factor α (TNFα) are synthesized. These cytokines increase the synthesis of degradative proteases such as collagenase, gelatinase, and stromelysin. As cartilage destruction progresses, proteoglycan content becomes reduced and it becomes thinned and fragmented.

Reparative processes may initially lead to joint stabilization, but ultimately contribute to progression of the disease. Fibrocartilage may be synthesized in response to loss of the more durable hyaline cartilage, temporarily improving joint mechanics and protecting the subchondral bone. However, fibrocartilage is less able to withstand mechanical loading, exposing the subchondral bone to increased force relative to that when covered by hyaline cartilage. Subchondral bony changes, such as sclerosis and osteophyte formation, develop.

The gross pathological findings of osteoarthritis include cartilage loss and reactive bone formation. Cartilage loss occurs primarily in areas of joint loading and may be related to repetitive mechanical insults. Cartilage loss may be best visualized arthroscopically, when findings include cartilage softening, fibrillation, and thinning. Areas of complete cartilage loss may be seen. More commonly, the clinician will recognize these findings as radiographic joint space narrowing. Similarly, bony changes may be seen on pathological specimens or arthroscopically, including osteophyte projections and subchondral bone visualized through denuded cartilage. The classic radiographic bony changes include osteophyte formation and subchondral bony sclerosis and cysts.

The pathological abnormalities of osteoarthritis can also extend to juxta-articular bone marrow. Recent MRI studies have demonstrated bone marrow abnormalities that correlate with the presence of relatively increased bone mineral density, although the significance of this finding from the perspective of pathogenesis is uncertain.

Clinical features

Precise definition of clinical osteoarthritis has remained elusive, as radiographic findings and symptoms may diverge. In addition, osteoarthritis may be categorized by the joint area involved or as being idiopathic or secondary to other disorders. An essential element to diagnosis of osteoarthritis is the correct attribution of symptoms to the affected joint. Initial evaluation of soft tissue abnormalities such as bursitis, tendinitis, and ligamentous strain should be performed. In addition, consideration of neurological or underlying bone abnormalities should be entertained when appropriate.

A thorough history and physical examination should be performed to evaluate for secondary forms of osteoarthritis. These include developmental, mechanical, or biochemical abnormalities known to increase the risk for osteoarthritis (Table 19.9.5). These forms tend to present earlier in life (e.g. congenital hip abnormality),

in atypical joints (e.g. calcium hydroxyapatite), or as more inflammatory in nature (e.g. calcium pyrophosphate deposition disease).

Idiopathic osteoarthritis may occur localized to one body area or as a more generalized disease. Common areas of involvement include the hands, hips, knees, and spine. Less commonly, osteoarthritis involves the shoulders, wrists, ankles, feet, and jaw.

Pain is the predominant symptom of osteoarthritis, usually mild to moderate in nature and increasing with joint use and at the end of the day. Pain is generally improved with rest and moderation of activity. Severe disease may cause pain at rest or at night. The source of pain may be the underlying bone, the joint capsule, or surrounding structures. Cartilage is avascular and without nerves and not itself a source of pain.

Stiffness may occur but is generally limited to less than 30 min in duration (gelling phenomenon). It is typical in the morning or after any prolonged rest (theatre sign). Effusions may occur, but warmth and soft tissue swelling is rare and suggests another diagnosis.

Physical examination reveals tenderness to palpation, bony thickening (osteophyte formation), small effusions, and crepitus. Specific joint findings also occur. Typical in the hand are bony enlargement of the proximal interphalangeal joints (Bouchard's nodes) and the distal interphalangeal joints (Heberden's nodes). The first carpometacarpal joint may be involved, causing a 'squared' appearance of the lateral aspect of the hand (in anatomical position) (Fig. 19.9.1). Involvement of the foot yields bunions, and of the knee pronounced valgus and varus deformities, Baker's cyst, or locking, suggesting meniscal damage. Early hip findings include limited internal and external rotation. Back findings include pain: true osteoarthritis occurs at the apophyseal joints; degenerative disc disease and diffuse idiopathic skeletal hyperostosis are distinct entities.

In an effort to standardize the diagnosis of osteoarthritis, the American College of Rheumatology formed a subcommittee to define osteoarthritis of the knee, hip, and hand. Clinical, laboratory, and radiographic findings were evaluated by an expert panel and statistical analysis to yield classification criteria with acceptable sensitivity and specificity values. These instruments should be used with caution in individual patients but provide a framework for analysis (see Tables 19.9.1–19.9.3).

Table 19.9.5 Secondary causes of osteoarthritis

Type of cause	Clinical condition	
Congenital/ developmental	Localized diseases	Perthes' disease Congenital hip dislocation Slipped femoral epiphysis
	Mechanical factors	Valgus/varus deformity Hypermobility syndromes
	Bone dysplasias	Epiphyseal dysplasia
Metabolic	Haemochromatosis Ochronosis (alkaptonuria) Wilson's disease Gaucher's disease	
Endocrine	Acromegaly Hyperparathyroidism Diabetes mellitus Hypothyroidism	
Other	Neuropathic (Charcot joints) Trauma (acute or chronic) Calcium deposition diseases (pseudogout) Other bone and joint diseases Endemic (Kashin–Bek) Haemoglobinopathies	

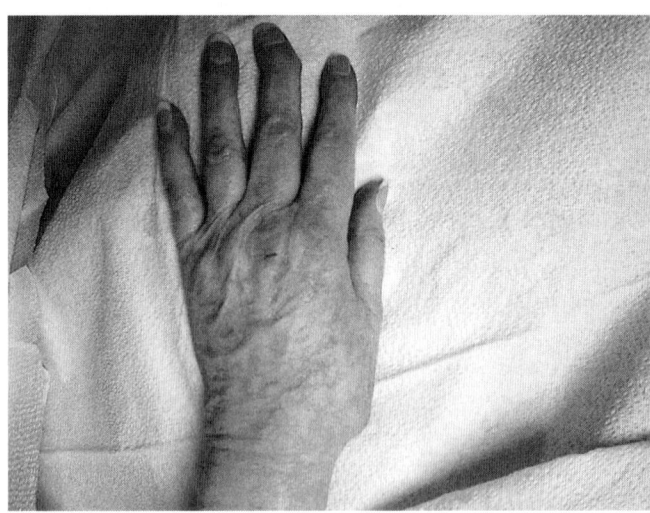

Fig. 19.9.1 Osteoarthritis of the hand. Note squaring of first carpometacarpal (CMC) joint and evidence of a Heberden's node on the third distal interphalangeal joint.

Common clinical mimics of osteoarthritis include rheumatoid arthritis, calcium pyrophosphate deposition disease, and infectious monoarticular arthritis.

Hand osteoarthritis may be confused with rheumatoid arthritis, as both cause pain and visible swelling. Less commonly hip or knee arthritis may present as diagnostic challenges. Hand osteoarthritis typically involves the proximal interphalangeal and the distal interphalangeal joints; the 'swelling' is not true swelling but hard, bony thickening due to osteophyte formation; and stiffness is limited. By contrast, rheumatoid arthritis typically involves the proximal interphalangeal, metacarpophalangeal, and carpal joints, sparing the distal interphalangeals. True swelling occurs and is soft with palpation. Multiple joints are involved, symptoms of systemic inflammation occur, and rheumatoid factor is usually positive. In rheumatoid arthritis radiographs demonstrate symmetric joint space narrowing, bony erosions, minimal sclerosis, and minimal osteophyte formation.

Calcium pyrophosphate deposition disease is difficult to differentiate from idiopathic osteoarthritis because the two may coexist. Typical distributions for this disease include the knees, wrist, shoulder, and metacarpophalangeals. Patients may have more prolonged stiffness and pain, and swelling may occur. Radiographs with evidence of chondrocalcinosis strongly suggest calcium pyrophosphate deposition disease, but the presence of crystals on arthrocentesis is the gold standard for diagnosis.

Infectious monoarthritis can occasionally mimic osteoarthritis. The distinction is more difficult with subacute infections, such as fungal or mycobacterial infections. If there is clinical suspicion, radiographs and arthrocentesis should be performed.

Investigation

Laboratory tests, if performed, reveal normal sedimentation rates and noninflammatory synovial fluid. Radiographic findings include asymmetry, joint space narrowing, subchondral sclerosis, subchondral cysts, and (the hallmark) osteophytes (Figs. 19.9.2–19.9.5).

Treatment

Treatment modalities for all forms of osteoarthritis, listed in Table 19.9.6, remain limited. Traditional therapies include analgesics, NSAIDs, intra-articular corticosteroid injections, intra-articular hyaluronic acid injections, topical agents, tidal lavage, arthroscopic irrigation, and total joint replacement. With the exception of joint replacement, none of these therapies address the underlying problem of cartilage damage. Newer therapies include weight loss and exercise, both of which have been difficult to maintain over long periods of time. Emerging therapies such as tetracycline, cytokine modulators, and inhibitors of metalloproteinases may potentially alter the progression of osteoarthritis. Nutrition supplements such as glucosamine, chondroitin sulphate, soybean, and avocado products have been reported to provide better long-term analgesia than NSAIDs, and some of these agents may alter the progression of osteoarthritis and repair cartilage damage.

Weight loss

Weight loss, although effective, is difficult to achieve and maintain, but a weight loss of 4.5 kg (10 lb) over 10 years may decrease the risk of developing contralateral knee osteoarthritis by 50%.

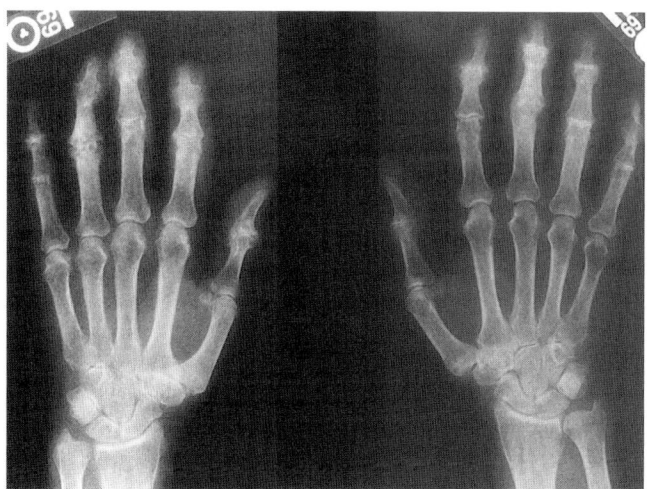

Fig. 19.9.2 Typical radiographic changes of osteoarthritis of the hand. Note abnormalities in the distal interphalangeal joints and proximal interphalangeal joints, as well as at the base of the thumb (carpometacarpal). There is loss of joint space, bony sclerosis, and the presence of osteophytes: the bony changes seen in the distal interphalangeal and proximal interphalangeal joints would manifest as Bouchard's and Heberden's nodes on clinical examination.

Studies demonstrating improvement in disease outcome are more controversial. However, given potential benefits in osteoarthritis as well as the additional health benefits of a normal BMI, obese patients should be encouraged to lose weight.

Exercise and psychosocial support

Physical therapy and exercise are advocated in osteoarthritis for a variety of reasons. Improvements in flexibility and muscle strength may decrease joint loading, preventing further damage, and they have been demonstrated to improve functional outcome and pain scores in clinical trials. In addition, they provide a sense of self-determination, an adjunct for weight loss, improve depressive symptoms, and decrease patient disability. Obstacles include

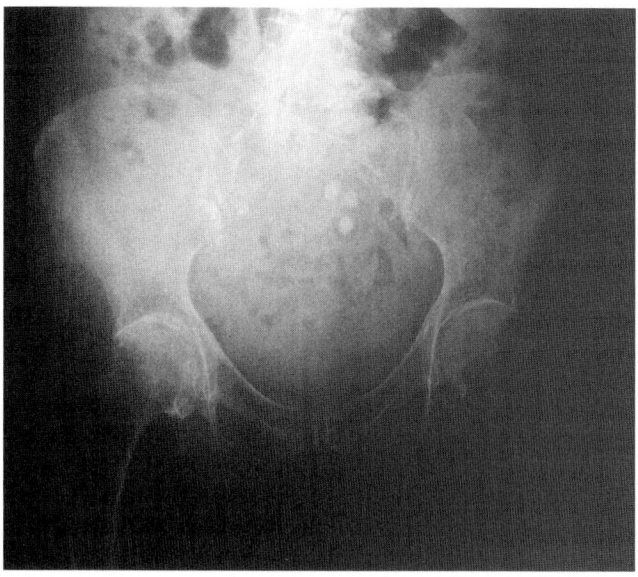

Fig. 19.9.3 Hip radiograph demonstrating osteoarthritis. Note joint space narrowing and sclerosis.

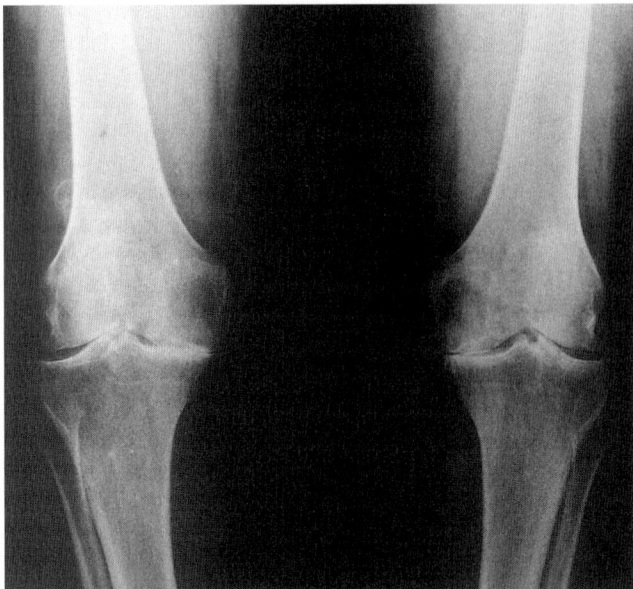

Fig. 19.9.4 Bilateral knee osteoarthritis. Note the asymmetric joint space narrowing, bony sclerosis, and the presence of osteophytes.

expense and the lack of motivation to continue exercising after a programme has been completed.

The role of psychosocial support may be significant. Telephone helplines providing contact and education have been demonstrated to improve pain and functional status. Education and support improve feelings of frustration, minimize dependency, and improve coping mechanisms.

Simple analgesics

A recent meta-analysis of 10 randomized clinical trials found that paracetamol (acetaminophen) is superior to placebo but less efficacious than NSAIDs in relieving pain due to osteoarthritis, but the lower relative risk of complications has favoured the use of this

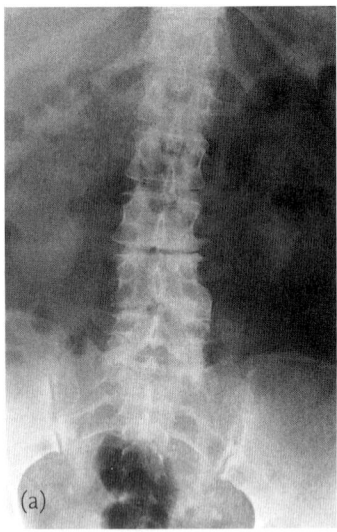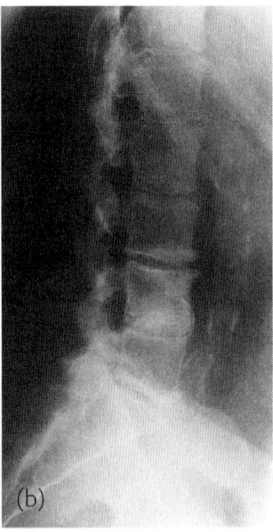

Fig. 19.9.5 Lumbar spine arthritis (a) and (b). Note the changes of degenerative disc disease as narrowing, and the presence of large osteophytes. Although often called osteoarthritis these changes are not true osteoarthritis, which occurs at the facet joints. Sclerosis is seen in the inferior facet joints.

Table 19.9.6 Therapies for osteoarthritis

Non-pharmacological
Weight loss
Physical therapy
Exercise
Aids/appliances
Pharmacological
Acetominophen/paracetamol
Non-selective NSAIDs
Cox-2 selective NSAIDs
Narcotic analgesics
Other analgesics
Intra-articular corticosteroids
Intra-articular hyaluronic acid
Surgical
Joint lavage
Meniscectomy
Synovectomy
Realignment osteotomy
Total joint replacement
Potential therapies
Glucosamine salts
Chondroitin sulphate
Tetracyclines
Diacerin
Avocado/soybean
Unsaponifiables

drug over NSAIDs, especially in older populations. Typical daily doses of paracetamol are 4 g (3 g in elderly patients), but this drug may be associated with liver problems and interactions with other drugs such as warfarin. Narcotic analgesics are generally avoided because of potential complications, including constipation, sedation, addiction, and impairment of balance.

NSAIDs

NSAIDs have been a cornerstone of osteoarthritis treatment for many years, but recently their use has diminished as a treatment for osteoarthritis because of reports of serious cardiovascular adverse effects. The selective cyclooxygenase-2 (COX-2) inhibitors (e.g. celecoxib and etoricoxib), which appear to be similarly efficacious to the traditional nonselective NSAIDs for the relief of pain associated with osteoarthritis but with less associated gastroduodenal toxicity and antiplatelet effects compared with nonselective NSAIDs, were the first NSAIDs reported to be associated with increased risks of cardiovascular adverse events. These reports led to the withdrawal of two agents, rofecoxib and valdecoxib, from the market, and subsequent claims of serious cardiovascular adverse events with nonselective NSAIDs has led to mandated warnings of the potential of cardiovascular effects with all NSAIDs, including nonselective and COX-2 inhibitors. Besides their association with peptic ulcer disease and antiplatelet effects, nonselective NSAIDs less commonly cause rash, hepatic dysfunction, and central nervous system effects.

Corticosteroids

Intra-articular corticosteroids may be effective in decreasing joint pain associated with osteoarthritis. Dosage varies depending on patient body size, comorbidity, and the joint involved. They have multiple side effects, including risk of infection, bleeding, and (possibly) cartilage damage. To minimize the risk of complications, injections should be limited to three to four per year in any given joint.

Hyaluronic acid

The use of hyaluronic acid preparations (e.g. Hyalgan, Synvisc) has become popular in recent years. These agents are reported to increase viscosity of synovial fluid by replacing depleted hyaluronic acid (which occurs in osteoarthritis), and one meta-analysis concluded that hyaluronic acid injections were superior to intra-articular saline injections, but the effect was relatively small. A subsequent meta-analysis noted statistically significant improvements in rest pain between 2 and 6 weeks after hyaluronic acid injections compared with placebo injections. In a trial comparing hyaluronic acid to NSAIDs, there were similar effects in those receiving injections and those receiving naproxen, but a reanalysis of the data using an intention-to-treat basis suggested that there were no differences between the hyaluronic acid and placebo groups at either 12 or 26 weeks of treatment.

Joint lavage

Irrigation of osteoarthritic joints has been proposed as a method of relieving joint pain by removing debris or inflammatory cytokines, but remains controversial. Livesley compared arthroscopic irrigation with physiotherapy and found that the arthroscopic group experienced significant improvement in pain that was sustained over 12 months. Ike and colleagues compared medical management plus joint lavage without arthroscopy with medical management alone in a multicentre, randomized prospective study: significant improvements in pain and stiffness occurred in the group receiving irrigation. Ravaud and colleagues evaluated the efficacy of joint lavage and intra-articular steroid injection in osteoarthritis of the knee. Patients who underwent joint lavage had improved significantly at 6 months; those given only corticosteroids had early improvement but no long-term benefit. Kalunian and colleagues studied the effectiveness of visually guided arthroscopic irrigation in early osteoarthritis of the knee unresponsive to conservative management. Patients received 3 litre or minimal (<250 ml) arthroscopic irrigation, the former having an effect on pain as measured on two rating scales. In a hypothesis-generating post-hoc analysis of the effect of positively birefringent intra-articular crystals, patients with and without intra-articular crystals had statistically significant improvements in pain assessments at 12 months; patients with crystals had statistically greater improvements in pain. Moseley et al. conducted a randomized, placebo-controlled, double-blind trial comparing arthroscopic debridement, arthroscopic lavage, and placebo surgery as treatment modalities for osteoarthritis of the knee. Placebo surgery consisted of skin incisions and simulated debridement without insertion of an arthroscope. At no point did either of the intervention groups report less pain or

better function than the placebo group, but this study did not examine the effects of associated crystals or inflammation on outcome.

Surgery

Surgical intervention is generally reserved for patients who have failed conservative management, including analgesics, physiotherapy, and intra-articular injection. Prescribed treatments include synovectomy, repair of meniscal tears, realignment osteotomy, and total joint replacement. Total joint replacement removes the affected structure and is the only known 'cure' for osteoarthritis to date, providing marked pain relief and functional improvement.

Aids and appliances

A joint that is unstable and painful can be made more stable and less painful by appropriate aids. Wheelchairs and other appliances may make it possible for a patient to maintain their independence. Walking sticks can be very effective, and for a painful hip or knee should be held in the contralateral hand to transfer weight from the affected joint. If the main problem is instability, the stick should be held in the hand that inspires most confidence. Splinting to correct instability, correction of valgus or varus deformity at the knee or ankle, use of a rocker sole to ease hallux rigidus pain, or a heel raise if the legs are of unequal length, can all allow significant reduction of symptoms, as can the simple recommendation of shoes with good shock-absorbing soles. These simple and apparently mundane issues should not be ignored by the physician.

Other therapies

Glucosamine and chondroitin sulphate

Many patients with osteoarthritis feel that glucosamine salts and chondroitin sulphate improve symptoms; however, recent data from large randomized clinical trials do not support these claims, and there is little data to suggest that these supplements repair cartilage damage.

Glucosamine, an aminomonosaccharide, is present in almost all human tissues, but particularly in articular cartilage, where it is an intermediate substrate in the synthesis of glycosaminoglycan and proteoglycans. Exogenous glucosamine salts significantly enhance chondrocyte synthesis of glycosaminoglycans, collagen, and DNA. Both glucosamine hydrochloride and glucosamine sulphate are rapidly absorbed after oral administration and are not toxic, even at high oral doses. Chondroitin sulphate is a long-chain polymer of a repeating disaccharide. It is the predominant glycosaminoglycan found in articular cartilage and differs from glucosamine in that it stimulates glycosaminoglycan and proteoglycan synthesis by both extracellular and intracellular mechanisms, whereas glucosamine utilizes only intracellular mechanisms. By virtue of its long chains, chondroitin sulphate competitively inhibits enzymes that degrade proteoglycans, and this may be its mechanism of action, with increased availability of substrates for formation of articular matrix another possibility. It is 70% absorbed after oral ingestion, with affinity for synovial fluid and articular cartilage.

A meta-analysis of 20 controlled trials of glucosamine sulphate, which included 2570 patients with osteoarthritis, was reported in 2005. When results of all these trials were considered, a significant improvement with glucosamine sulphate was noted; however, when the analysis of efficacy was restricted to the eight studies that were adequately blinded, there was no significant benefit of glucosamine for pain or function. In a large, multicentre study that compared glucosamine hydrochloride, chondroitin sulphate, the combination of the two supplements, celecoxib, and placebo, glucosamine hydrochloride either used alone or in combination with chondroitin sulphate was not more effective in relieving pain or improving function than placebo. In this study, there were no significant differences in pain relief in those receiving chondroitin sulphate alone compared to the placebo group. In an exploratory subgroup analysis, a possible benefit of the combination of glucosamine hydrochloride and chondroitin sulphate was suggested for patients with osteoarthritis of the knee who had moderate to severe pain.

Tetracyclines, IL-1 antagonists, and collagenase inhibitors

Tetracyclines have been demonstrated to inactivate matrix metalloproteinases, such as collagenase, stromolysin, and gelatinase. Dog models using doxycycline reduce the incidence of osteoarthritis. In a large, multicentre study in which obese women with symptomatic and radiographically apparent unilateral knee osteoarthritis were treated with either doxycycline or placebo for 30 months, the rate of joint space narrowing was significantly less in those treated with doxycycline compared with the placebo group, but there were no significant differences between the two groups in reduction of knee pain.

Other agents demonstrating efficacy in osteoarthritis include use of diacerein and avocado/soybean extracts. Diacerein is an oral agent with analgesic properties, hypothesized to have an effect in osteoarthritis by inhibiting synthesis and activity of IL-1 and demonstrating cartilage preservation in an animal model. Human studies have demonstrated improvements in pain and function in hip osteoarthritis, as well as an NSAID-sparing effect. Similarly, avocado and soybean unsaponifiables are believed to exert their effects through IL-1. Clinical studies have demonstrated an NSAID-sparing effect and improvement in functional index and pain.

Cipemastat (Ro 32-335, Trocade) is an orally active collagenase inhibitor that has demonstrated chondroprotection by radiographic criteria in a mouse osteoarthritis model. Bay 129566 is a stromelysin-1 (MMP-3) inhibitor that demonstrated efficacy in both dog and guinea pig menisectomy models. Further studies of these compounds are needed. Future strategies for chondroprotection include manipulation of tumour necrosis factor, nitrous oxide, and insulin-like growth factor.

Further reading

Altman R, et al. (1986). Development of criteria in the classification and reporting of osteoarthritis: classification of the knee. *Arthritis Rheum*, **29**, 1039–49.

Anderson J, Felson DT (1988). Factors associated with osteoarthritis of the knee in the First National Health and Nutrition Examination Survey (HANES 1). *Am J Epidemiol*, **128**, 179–89.

Arrich J, et al. (2005). Intra-articular hyaluronic acid for the treatment of osteoarthritis of the knee: systemic review and meta-analysis. *CMAJ*, **172**, 1039–43.

Brandt KD, et al. (2005). Effects of doxycycline on progression of osteoarthritis: results of a randomized, placebo-controlled, double-blind study. *Arthritis Rheum*, **52**, 1956–9.

Clegg DO, et al. (2006). Glucosamine, chondroitin, and two in combination for painful knee osteoarthritis. *New Engl J Med*, **354**, 795–808.

Davis MA, et al. (1988). Sex differences in osteoarthritis of the knee: the role of obesity. *Am J Epidemiol*, **127**, 1019–30.

Drovanti A, Bignamini AA, Rovati AL (1980). Therapeutic activity of oral glucosamine sulfate in osteoarthritis: a placebo-controlled double-blind investigation. *Clin Ther*, **3**, 260–72.

Ettinger WH Jr., et al. (1997). A randomized trial comparing aerobic exercise and resistance exercise with a health education program in older adults with knee osteoarthritis: the Fitness Arthritis and Seniors Trial (FAST). *J Am Med Assoc*, **277**, 25–31.

Felson DT, et al. (1991). Occupational physical demands, knee bending and knee osteoarthritis: results from the Framingham study. *J Rheumatol*, **18**, 1587–92.

Felson DT, Zhang Y (1998). An update on the epidemiology of knee and hip osteoarthritis with a view to prevention. *Arthritis Rheum*, **41**, 1343–55.

Felson DT, et al. (1997). Risk factors for incident radiographic knee osteoarthritis in the elderly. *Arthritis Rheum*, **40**, 728–33.

Felson DT, et al. (2002). Hyaluronate sodium injections for osteoarthritis: hope, hype, and hard truths. *Arch Intern Med*, **162**, 245–7.

Flugsrud GB, et al. (2006). The impact of body mass index on later total hip arthroplasty for primary osteoarthritis: a cohort study in 1.2 million persons. *Arthritis Rheum*, **54**, 802–7.

Hannan MT, et al. (1991). Occupational physical demands, knee bending and knee osteoarthritis: results from the Framingham Study. *J Rheumatol*, **18**, 1587–92.

Hart DJ, Spector TD (1993). The relationship of obesity, fat distribution and osteoarthritis in women in the general population. The Chingford Study. *J Rheumatol*, **20**, 331–5.

Kalunian KC, et al. (2000). Visually-guided irrigation in patients with early knee osteoarthritis: a multicenter, randomized, controlled trial. *Osteoarthritis Cartilage*, **8**, 412–8.

Kellgren JH, Lawrence JS (1957). Radiographic assessment of osteoarthritis. *Ann Rheum Dis*, **16**, 494–502.

Kelsey JL, Hochberg MC (1988). Epidemiology of chronic musculoskeletal disorders. *Annu Rev Public Health*, **9**, 379–401.

Kizawa H, et al. (2005). An aspartic acid repeat polymorphism in asporin inhibits chondrogenesis and increases susceptibility to osteoarthritis. *Nat Genet*, **37**, 138–44.

Kujala UM, et al. (1995). Knee osteoarthritis in former runners, soccer players, weight lifters and shooters. *Arthritis Rheum*, **38**, 539–46.

LaPlante MP (1988). *Data on disability from the National Health Interview Survey (1983-5). An InfoUse Report.* National Institute of Disability and Rehabilitation, Washington, DC.

Lo GH, et al. (2003). Intra-articular hyaluronic acid in treatment of knee osteoarthritis: a meta-analysis. *J Am Med Assoc*, **290**, 3115–21.

Lo GH, et al. (2005). Bone marrow lesions in the knee are associated with increased local bone density. *Arthritis Rheum*, **52**, 2814–21.

Loughlin J, et al. (2000). Association analysis of the vitamin D receptor gene, the type I collagen gene COL1A1, and the estrogen receptor gene in idiopathic osteoarthritis. *J Rheumatol*, **27**, 779–84.

Morreale P, et al. (1996). Comparison of the antiinflammatory efficacy of chondroitin sulfate and diclofenac sodium in patients with knee osteoarthritis. *J Rheumatol*, **23**, 1385–91.

Moseley JB, et al. (2002). A controlled trial of arthroscopic surgery for osteoarthritis of the knee. *New Engl J Med*, **347**, 81–8.

Oliveria SA, et al. (1995). Incidence of symptomatic hand, hip and knee osteoarthritis among patients in a health maintenance organization, *Arthritis Rheum*, **38**, 1134–41.

Setnikar I, Pacinic MA, Revel L (1991). Antiarthritic effects of glucosamine sulfate studied on animal models. *Arzeimitte-Forshung*, **41**, 542–5.

Towheed TE, et al. (2005). Glucosamine therapy for treating osteoarthritis. *Cochrane Database Syst Rev*, CD002946.

Wu CW, et al. Validation of American College of Rheumatology classification criteria for knee osteoarthritis using arthroscopically defined cartilage damage scores. *Semin Arthritis Rheum*, **35**, 197-201.

Zhang W, et al. (2004). Does paracetamol (acetaminophen) reduce the pain of osteoarthritis? A meta-analysis of randomized controlled trials. *Ann Rheum Dis*, **63**, 901–7.

19.10

Crystal-related arthropathies

Edward Roddy and Michael Doherty

Essentials

Many crystals have been associated with arthropathies or periarticular syndromes: only monosodium urate monohydrate (gout), calcium pyrophosphate dehydrate (pseudogout, chondro-calcinosis), and basic calcium phosphates (mainly hydroxyapatite) are common.

Crystals implicated in joint disease are stable, hard particles that exert biological effects via surface-active (activation of humoral and cell-derived mediators, interaction with cell membranes) and mechanical properties. In general, smaller particle size, marked surface irregularity, and high negative surface charge correlate with inflammatory potential.

Gout

Aetiology and pathogenesis—gout is caused by the formation of monosodium urate crystals, and the primary risk factor for its development is hyperuricaemia. It is common (prevalence 0.5–1.4%, rising with age). Risk factors for primary gout include being male, hypertension, obesity, insulin resistance, metabolic syndrome, excess alcohol consumption (especially beer), and a diet rich in purines. These act primarily by reducing efficient elimination of uric acid via the kidney. Important risk factors for secondary gout are diuretic therapy, chronic renal impairment, and osteoarthritis.

Clinical features—four clinical phases are recognized. (1) Asymptomatic hyperuricaemia—the risk of developing gout increases with the degree of hyperuricaemia, but around 95% of hyperuricaemic patients remain asymptomatic throughout life. (2) Acute gout—in almost all initial episodes a single peripheral joint is involved, with the first metatarsophalangeal joint (podagra) the site of the first attack in 50% of patients. Other common sites are the midtarsal joints, ankle, knee, small hand joints, wrist, and elbow. The pain is often described as 'the worst ever experienced'. The joint and surrounding tissues are swollen, hot, red, shiny, and extremely tender. (3) Intercritical gout—after resolution of the first attack there is a variable time period before the second, but this usually occurs within 1 year and chronic symptoms usually develop within 10 years. (4) Chronic tophaceous gout—large crystal deposits (tophi) produce irregular firm nodules and chronic joint damage. Gout is associated with renal disease—uric acid stones (10–25% of patients) and chronic urate nephropathy (endstage renal failure occurs in up to 25% of cases of untreated chronic tophaceous gout).

Diagnosis—proof of gout requires the identification of mono-sodium urate crystals on polarized light microscopy of aspirates from synovial fluid or tophus (strongly birefringent, negative sign). Although gout is strongly associated with hyperuricaemia, serum urate is frequently normal during an acute attack, and hyperuricae-mia *per se* is not a diagnostic test for gout.

Management—treatment of an acute attack aims to reduce inflam-mation: options include nonsteroidal anti-inflammatory drugs, low-dose colchicine, joint aspiration, intra-articular (occasion-ally systemic) steroids, and ice packs. Alteration of uric acid levels is avoided until the attack has resolved. Long-term management involves lifestyle modification advice and urate-lowering therapy. Encouragement concerning weight loss and restriction of the con-sumption of alcohol (especially beer) and purine-rich foods should be offered to all appropriate patients with primary gout. Urate-lowering therapy should be titrated with the aim of lowering the serum urate well below 360 μmol/litre (6 mg/dl)—the physiological saturation point for urate crystal formation. Allopurinol, a xan-thine oxidase inhibitor, is the usual drug of choice. The uricosurics probenecid and sulfinpyrazone are rarely used, but benzbromarone, a potent uricosuric, is now increasingly used in parts of Europe.

Pyrophosphate arthropathy

Deposition of calcium pyrophosphate dihydrate crystals in articular cartilage can be seen on radiographs in 4.5% of adults over the age of 40. It is almost always of unknown cause (sporadic/idiopathic, associated with osteoarthritis), but can be associated with meta-bolic disease (hyperparathyroidism, haemochromatosis, hypophos-phatasia, hypomagnesaemia) or be hereditary.

Clinical features, diagnosis and management—the following are com-mon presentations. (1) Acute synovitis (pseudogout)—one of the commonest causes of acute monoarthritis in older people. A typical attack develops rapidly (6–24 h)—usually in the knee—with severe pain, stiffness and swelling, and a florid synovitis on examination.

Fluid aspirated from the joint is often turbid or bloodstained with an elevated cell count, and polarized light microscopy reveals calcium pyrophosphate crystals (weakly birefringent, positive sign). Local therapy is preferred with ice packs and aspiration (combined with intra-articular steroid in florid cases). (2) Chronic pyrophosphate arthropathy—a common condition that affects mainly elderly women and targets the same large and medium-sized joints as pseudogout. Presentation is with chronic pain, stiffness, and functional impairment, with or without superimposed acute attacks. Affected joints show signs of osteoarthritis with varying degrees

Introduction

Diversity and terminology

Many crystals have been associated with acute synovitis, chronic arthropathy, or periarticular syndromes (Box 19.10.1). In practice only monosodium urate monohydrate, calcium pyrophosphate dihydrate, and basic calcium phosphates (mainly hydroxyapatite) are commonly encountered.

The taxonomy of these conditions is not universally agreed. Difficulties arise from our poor understanding of pathogenesis, historical extrapolation from gout to other crystal-related conditions, and multiple terms for the same clinical syndrome. Possible relationships between crystals and disease are outlined in Fig. 19.10.1. A 'crystal deposition disease' is defined as a pathological condition associated with mineral deposits that contribute directly

---

Box 19.10.1 Crystalline particles associated with joint disease

Intrinsic

- Monosodium urate monohydrate
- Calcium pyrophosphate dihydrate (monoclinic, triclinic)
- Calcium phosphates
  - Basic—hydroxyapatite, octacalcium phosphate, tricalcium phosphate
  - Acidic—brushite, monetite
- Calcium oxalate
- Lipids
- Cholesterol
- Lipid liquid crystals
- Charcot–Leyden (phospholipase) crystals
- Cystine
- Xanthine, hypoxanthine
- Protein precipitates (e.g. cryoglobulins)

Extrinsic

- Synthetic corticosteroids
- Plant thorns (semicrystalloid cellulose), especially blackthorn, rose, dried palm fronds
- Sea urchin spines (crystalline calcium carbonate)
- Methylmethacrylate

---

of synovitis. There is no specific therapy and treatment of any underlying metabolic disease does not influence outcome, which is generally good. (3) Asymptomatic incidental radiographic finding.

Apatite-associated syndromes

Apatites, or basic calcium phosphates, are the usual minerals deposited in extraskeletal tissues, e.g. in arterial walls or tuberculous lesions. Apatite deposition in the supraspinatus tendon is a not uncommon incidental finding, occasionally resulting in severe acute inflammation (acute calcific periarthritis).

to the pathology. This is probably the situation for all manifestations of gout, for acute syndromes associated with calcium pyrophosphate dihydrate, and for acute apatite periarthritis. However, the role of nonurate crystals in chronic arthropathy is unclear and confounded by the following observations:

- Most crystals lack disease specificity and occur in a variety of clinical settings, often unaccompanied by symptoms or other abnormality.
- Crystal deposition may coexist with other rheumatic disease, most commonly osteoarthritis, and often follows, rather than precedes, articular damage.
- Combined deposition of several crystal species is common (mixed crystal deposition).

For descriptive purposes, confusion may be avoided by specifying the crystal, the site of involvement, and the clinical syndrome (e.g. chronic urate olecranon bursitis, acute pyrophosphate arthritis of the knee).

Crystal deposition and clearance

Many factors determine crystal formation and dissolution (Fig. 19.10.2). High solute concentrations alone are often insufficient to initiate crystal formation, and the presence of nucleating factors that aid initial particle formation and the balance of growth-promoting and inhibitory factors are probably more important. Little is known of such tissue factors, although they may in part explain:

- the characteristic, limited distribution of different crystals
- the frequency of mixed crystal deposition (via epitaxial nucleation and growth of one crystal on another)
- nonspecific predisposition to crystal formation in osteoarthritic tissues (via accompanying alterations in proteoglycan, collagen, and lipid)

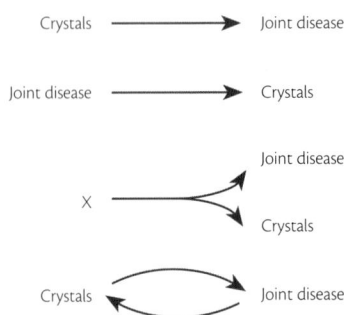

Fig. 19.10.1 Possible relationships between crystals and joint disease.

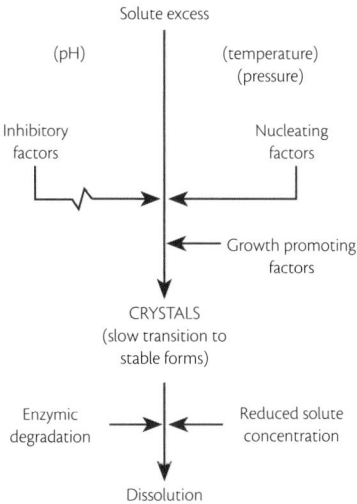

Fig. 19.10.2 Factors affecting crystal formation.

Formation of crystals *in vivo* is a dynamic process, although usually slow. At any time the crystal load will depend on the rate of formation, the rate of dissolution, and trafficking of crystals away from their site of formation (via shedding from preformed deposits with secondary uptake by synovial and other cells).

Crystal-induced inflammation and tissue damage

Crystals implicated in joint disease are stable, hard particles that exert biological effects via surface-active and mechanical properties. With respect to acute inflammation, they are all markedly phlogistic agents in a wide range of *in vitro* and *in vivo* systems. Surface-active interaction has been demonstrated with:

◆ humoral mediators, e.g. complement activation via classical and alternative pathways, activation of Hageman factor

◆ cell-derived mediators, e.g. superoxide production and release of lysozymes, chemotactic factor, and lipoxygenase-derived products of arachidonic acid by neutrophils, release of interleukin 1 (IL-1), IL-6, and tumour necrosis factor (TNF) by monocytes and synoviocytes

◆ cell membranes, e.g. membranolysis of lysosomes, erythrocytes, and neutrophils, non-lytic platelet and neutrophil secretory responses

In general, monosodium urate monohydrate is the most inflammatory, followed by calcium pyrophosphate dihydrate, then apatite and the less common crystals. In general, smaller particle size, marked surface irregularity, and high negative surface charge correlate with inflammatory potential. Some surface effects result from direct crystal contact, but others are mediated via adsorbed protein, particularly immunoglobulin. Although adsorbed IgG may enhance inflammation, most other protein binding is inhibitory.

Less is known of chronic crystal-induced tissue damage. Postulated effects include persistent synovial inflammation, altered cell metabolism (ingested calcium crystals may stimulate mitogenesis, fibrosis, and calcium-related cellular effects), and deleterious mechanical effects from large deposits. Evidence for activation of inflammatory mediators in chronic crystal-associated synovitis is lacking, although a chronic 'granulomatous' reaction often occurs around large accretions. The physicochemical effects of hard, highly charged crystals embedded within cartilage, or occurring as wear particles at the surface, are largely unknown.

Gout

Monosodium urate monohydrate crystals are undoubted causal agents in gout, which arises following supersaturation of body tissues with monosodium urate. Subsequently the deposition of crystals in previously normal tissues may elicit acute inflammation and eventual tissue damage. Their effective removal halts progression and results in cure. In these respects, gout is a true crystal deposition disease.

The incidence of gout varies in populations from 6.2 to 18.0 per 10 000 patient-years, with an overall prevalence of 5.2 to 14.0 per 1000. Prevalence rises with age and there is strong predominance in men (ranging from 3.6:1 to 8:1), particularly under 65 years of age. Untreated gout evolves slowly through four clinical phases: asymptomatic hyperuricaemia, acute gout, intercritical gout, and chronic tophaceous gout.

Clinical features

Asymptomatic hyperuricaemia

Hyperuricaemia is the primary risk factor for the development of gout and arises from either overproduction or renal underexcretion of uric acid, or a combination of both (see Chapter 12.4). Although hyperuricaemia and gout are strongly linked, they are not synonymous. Around 95% of hyperuricaemic subjects remain asymptomatic throughout life. The risk of developing gout increases with the degree of hyperuricaemia. However, even in patients with the highest levels of serum urate (>540 μmol/litre (9.0 mg/dl)) annual incidence is less than 5%, emphasizing the importance of local tissue factors in crystal nucleation/growth. How many hyperuricaemic patients have occult monosodium urate monohydrate deposits is unknown.

Monosodium urate monohydrate crystals preferentially deposit in peripheral connective tissues in and around synovial joints. Deposits occur first in articular cartilage, most commonly the first metatarsophalangeal and small joints of the feet, developing later in synovium, capsule, and periarticular soft tissues. Crystals probably take months if not years to grow *in vivo* to detectable size, implying a long asymptomatic phase. Absence of inflammation during this period may relate to low crystal yield, positioning within hypovascular tissues, or inhibitory protein coating.

Acute attacks

The classical attack

In almost all initial episodes, a single peripheral joint is involved. The first metatarsophalangeal joint (podagra) is the site of the first attack in 50% of patients and is affected at some point in over 70%. This may relate to the common occurrence of osteoarthritis at this joint. Other common sites are the midtarsal joints, ankle, knee, small hand joints, wrist, and elbow. The axial skeleton and large central joints are rarely involved and never as the first site.

Attacks often wake the patient in the early morning with localized irritation and aching. Within just a few hours the joint and surrounding tissues are swollen, hot, red, shiny, and extremely painful. The patient cannot bear even bedclothes to touch the joint and it is often described as 'the worst pain ever experienced'. Inflammation is maximal within 24 h and is often associated with pyrexia and malaise. Examination reveals florid synovitis and swelling, extreme tenderness, and overlying erythema. If left untreated, the attack resolves spontaneously over 5 to 15 days, often with pruritus and desquamation of overlying skin.

Although many attacks occur spontaneously, some situations encourage shedding of preformed monosodium urate monohydrate crystals and triggering of acute attacks. Suggested mechanisms include mechanical loosening (local trauma), partial dissolution and reduction of crystal size (initiation of hypouricaemic treatment, reduction in uric acid levels as part of the acute phase response), and local increase in cytokines that encourage inflammatory responses to crystals and facilitate crystal escape via alterations in cartilage matrix (intercurrent illness, surgery). Although some triggers (alcohol, dietary excess) increase local urate levels, acute crystallization is considered unlikely.

Atypical attacks

Acute attacks may manifest as tenosynovitis, bursitis, or cellulitis. Many patients describe mild episodes of discomfort without swelling lasting a day or so (petite attacks). Ten per cent of all typical attacks involve more than one joint. Sometimes acute gout, by triggering the acute phase response, provokes migratory attacks in other joints over subsequent days (cluster attacks). Polyarticular attacks are rare, usually occurring after a long history of recurrent attacks: marked systemic upset, fever, and confusion may dominate the clinical picture.

Intercritical periods

Following the resolution of the first attack, a variable time period elapses before the next attack occurs. The asymptomatic interval between attacks is called the intercritical period. Some patients never have a second attack; in others the next episode occurs after many years; in most, however, a second attack occurs within 1 year. With time, the frequency and severity of attacks and number of sites involved increases, and attacks are more often pauci- or polyarticular. Eventually, recurrent attacks and continuing monosodium urate monohydrate deposition cause joint damage and chronic pain. The interval between the first attack and development of chronic symptoms is variable, but averages about 10 years. The principal determinant is the serum uric acid—the higher it is, the earlier and more extensive the development of joint damage and tophaceous deposits.

Chronic tophaceous gout

Large crystal deposits (tophi) produce irregular firm nodules, principally around extensor surfaces of fingers, hands, the ulnar surface of the forearms, olecranon bursae, Achilles tendons, first metatarsophalangeal joints, and the cartilaginous helix of the ear. Marked asymmetry, both locally and between sides, is particularly characteristic (Fig. 19.10.3). Monosodium urate monohydrate crystals beneath the skin may show a white-yellow 'chalky' discolouration (Fig. 19.10.4). If untreated, tophi can enlarge into gross knobbly swellings that may ulcerate, discharging white and gritty material that causes local inflammation (erythema, pus) even in the absence of secondary infection. If extensive, tophi may rarely involve the eyelids, tongue, larynx, or heart (causing conduction defects and valvular dysfunction).

Joints most commonly involved with signs of damage (restricted movement, crepitus, deformity) and varying degrees of synovitis are the first metatarsophalangeal joints, midfoot, small finger joints,

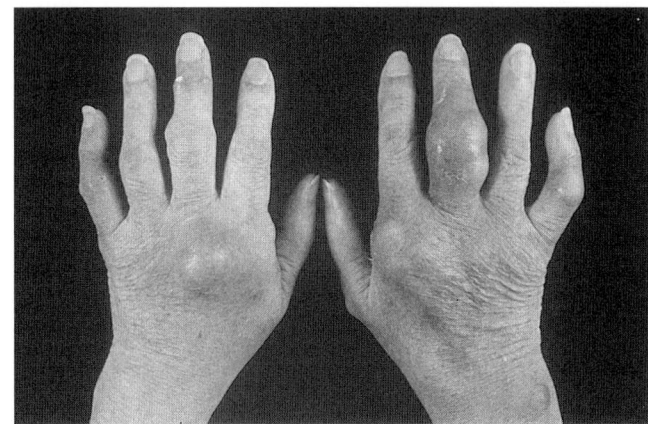

Fig. 19.10.3 Chronic tophaceous gout affecting the hands. Note the eccentric nature of the tophi and the asymmetry between sides.

and wrists. As with tophi, joint involvement is usually asymmetrical. Occasionally gross destruction may occur in feet and hands, and less commonly other sites. Acute attacks may become less of a feature as chronic symptoms become established. If untreated, the combination of extensive joint destruction and large tophi may cause grotesque deformities, particularly of hands and feet. Ankylosis is a rare late event. Although axial involvement is rare, even in late stages, gouty involvement of hips, shoulders, spine and sacroiliac joints, and spinal cord compression by tophi, are all reported.

Classification

Gout is traditionally classified into primary and secondary, with different clinical patterns and separate risk factors and associations

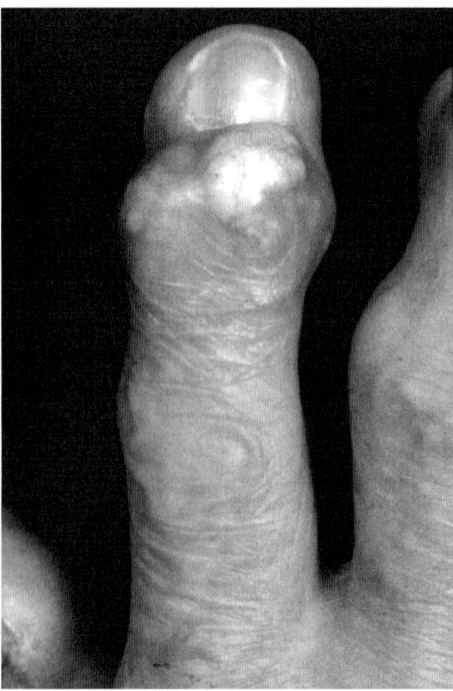

Fig. 19.10.4 Diuretic-induced gout in an elderly woman, showing tophaceous deposition on preexisting nodal osteoarthritis; the white monosodium urate monohydrate crystals are clearly visible beneath the skin.

Table 19.10.1 Primary and secondary gout: clinical features

Clinical feature	Primary gout	Secondary gout
Sex	Males >> females	Males = females
Age	Middle-age	Elderly
Acute attacks	Common	May be less common
Distribution	Lower limb >> upper limb	Lower limb = upper limb
Tophi	Develop late	Develop early

described for each (Tables 19.10.1 and 19.10.2). Primary gout characteristically affects men, with an age of onset between 30 and 60 years of age and a predeliction for the legs, particularly the first metatarsophalangeal joint. Presentation is with acute attacks, and untreated disease progresses to chronic tophaceous gout. Over 75% of patients with primary gout are underexcretors of uric acid. A family history of gout is common due to an inherited isolated renal lesion that reduces fractional urate clearance. Fewer than 10% are overproducers of uric acid. The cause usually remains unclear, although a very few have an inherited purine enzyme defect (see Chapter 12.4).

Secondary gout, by contrast, mainly presents in older individuals (>65 years) and shows a more equal gender distribution and equal involvement of the arm and leg peripheral joints. Acute attacks are said to be less frequent and tophi may be the initial manifestation.

Primary gout

Primary gout associates strongly with metabolic syndrome and obesity, type IV hyperlipidaemia, hypertension, and insulin resistance. Hypertension and obesity are independent risk factors for the

Table 19.10.2 Primary and secondary gout: clinical associations and accompanying screening tests

Clinical association		Screening test
Primary gout	Male	
	Family history	
	Metabolic syndrome	
	Hypertension	Blood pressure monitoring
	Hyperlipidaemia	Fasting lipids
	Insulin resistance	Fasting plasma glucose
	Obesity	
	Alcohol	MCV, liver function tests
	Purine-rich foods	
Secondary gout	Diuretics	
	Chronic renal failure	Creatinine (eGFR)
	Lead poisoning (rare)	
	Osteoarthritis	
	Ciclosporin (rare)	
	Myeloproliferative disorders (rare)	FBC, ESR

e GFR, estimated glomerular filtration rate; FBC, full blood count; MCV, mean cell volume.

development of gout; hypertensive microvascular renal damage leads to hyperuricaemia and, in obese patients, insulin resistance and hyperinsulinaemia impair renal urate excretion. The association of primary gout with these common cardiovascular risk factors, not surprisingly, translates into an important association between primary gout and cardiovascular disease. Excessive consumption of alcohol and purine-rich foods are also independent risk factors for primary gout. Beer drinking confers the greatest risk, attributable in part to its high guanosine content, followed by spirits, with wine conferring only slight risk. The 19th century association with port is partly explained by storage of wines in lead-lined casks and the addition of lead to sweeten the port: lead inhibits uric acid excretion and also promotes nucleation of monosodium urate monohydrate. Saturnine gout still occurs in individuals who drink alcohol distilled or stored in lead-contaminated containers ('moonshine'). Purine-rich foods, e.g. meat and seafood, are associated with increased risk of gout, whereas consumption of dairy products is protective.

Secondary gout

The most important risk factors for secondary gout are diuretic therapy and chronic renal impairment. Diuretics are an independent risk factor for the development of gout, even after adjustment for hypertension. Renal tubular organic anion transporters have recently been identified, through which diuretics exert their hyperuricaemic effect. Other drugs may predispose to gout, such as low-dose aspirin and ciclosporin, although the urate-enhancing effect of low-dose aspirin is not thought to be of clinical significance when compared with its cardiovascular benefits in this high-risk group. More widespread organ transplantation and use of ciclosporin as an immunosuppressant have resulted in transplant-associated gout becoming a challenging problem in secondary care. Secondary gout is also associated with osteoarthritis, with both acute attacks of gout and tophi occurring at Heberden's and Bouchard's nodes in elderly women (Fig. 19.10.4).

There is a strong negative association between gout and rheumatoid arthritis. This remains unexplained, but probably reflects impaired nucleation/growth of monosodium urate monohydrate crystals rather than masking of monosodium urate monohydrate crystal-induced inflammation (e.g. by crystal coating with rheumatoid factors). A less strong negative association is also reported between rheumatoid arthritis and calcium pyrophosphate crystal deposition.

Gout and renal disease

Urolithiasis

Uric acid stones account for 5 to 10% of all stones in the United Kingdom and the United States of America, and up to 40% in Israel. A history of renal colic can be obtained in 10 to 25% of patients with gout, the important aetiological factors being low urinary pH, low urinary volume, and high urinary uric acid concentration. High urinary concentrations occur in overproducers of uric acid, if renal urate clearance is increased (uricosuric drugs, defects in tubular reabsorption), and in situations of dehydration with lowering of urinary pH (diarrhoea, ileostomy). Gouty patients also have an increased incidence of calcium-containing stones, particularly calcium oxalate, with no detectable uric acid nidus.

Acute uric acid nephropathy describes rapid precipitation of uric acid crystals in renal collecting ducts with secondary acute obstructive renal failure. This event correlates with the amount of uric acid excreted rather than the level of hyperuricaemia. Strongly acid urine, which reduces uric acid solubility, potentiates the problem. The condition occurs in ill, dehydrated patients with lymphoma or malignancy subjected to aggressive chemotherapy without adequate prophylactic treatment (with allopurinol and/or recombinant uricase). It also occurs in gouty patients with markedly accelerated purine synthesis, e.g. following excessive exercise or epileptic seizures, when again the condition is largely avoidable by appropriate hydration, urinary alkalinization, and allopurinol prophylaxis.

Chronic urate nephropathy

Widespread monosodium urate monohydrate deposition in the interstitium of the medulla and pyramids results in crystal-induced inflammation with surrounding giant-cell reaction and fibrosis, affecting in particular the tubular epithelium of the loop of Henle and juxtaposed interstitial tissues. Subsequent changes include glomerular hyalinization and hypertrophy of the intima and media of arterioles. Hypertensive damage, tubular obstruction, and secondary pyelonephritis may all complicate this picture. Albuminuria and inability to concentrate the urine maximally are early clinical manifestations. Progressive renal disease is an important complication of untreated chronic tophaceous gout, endstage renal failure occurring in up to 25% of cases.

Calcium oxalate or phosphate crystals may deposit in the renal parenchyma in advanced renal disease of any cause, but are predominantly cortical in location (compared with the medullary site of monosodium urate monohydrate).

The association between parenchymal disease and less severe gout remains controversial, being confounded in men by frequent accompanying obesity, hypertension, and drug therapy. The minor progression of renal insufficiency that occurs in most gouty patients, however, is probably largely age related, and life expectancy is not reduced.

Differential diagnosis

Acute attacks

Sepsis and other crystal-associated synovitis are the main considerations. However, the rapidity of onset of severe symptoms that plateau within 12 to 24h is highly characteristic of crystal inflammation; sepsis presents more slowly and is progressive. Gout and sepsis may coexist, as may monosodium urate monohydrate and calcium pyrophosphate dihydrate deposition (particularly in elderly patients). Examination of aspirated fluid for both crystals and sepsis (Gram stain, culture) is the only sure way of obtaining the correct diagnosis. A wider search for sepsis may be indicated (e.g. blood and urine cultures), particularly in those who are ill. With less classic attacks, other conditions that may be considered include psoriatic and acute Reiter's arthropathy, acute sarcoid arthropathy, traumatic arthritis, palindromic rheumatism, and exacerbation of osteoarthritis. A search for synovial fluid crystals should be undertaken in all patients with unexplained inflammatory arthritis.

Chronic tophaceous gout

Other causes of arthritis and periarticular swellings/nodules that require differentiation are rheumatoid arthritis, generalized nodal osteoarthritis, xanthomatosis with arthropathy, and multicentric reticulohistiocytosis. Gout is usually less symmetrical in distribution than these conditions and, except for xanthomatosis, acute attacks are not a feature. Nodal osteoarthritis, of course, may coexist with gout. Aspiration (joint fluid, nodules) and plain radiographs readily facilitate correct diagnosis.

Clinical investigation

The history and signs of classical acute or chronic tophaceous gout are highly characteristic, and with a raised serum urate a strong presumptive diagnosis is readily made. However, definitive confirmation requires demonstration of monosodium urate monohydrate crystals by compensated polarized light microscopy of fluid from a gouty joint, bursa, or tophus. Synovial fluid in acute attacks is typically turbid with diminished viscosity and greatly elevated cell count (>90% neutrophils). Chronic gouty fluid is more variable, but occasionally appears white owing to the high crystal load. Only a few drops collected directly on to a slide are required for crystal identification. Monosodium urate monohydrate crystals are seen readily as strongly birefringent (negative sign), needle-shaped crystals, 5 to 20μm in length, within cells or occurring freely in fluid. In tophaceous material they occur as dense, tightly packed sheets. During intercritical periods, aspiration of an asymptomatic first metatarsophalangeal joint or knee often permits confirmation of the diagnosis by revealing monosodium urate monohydrate crystals.

Measurement of the serum urate level is an important investigation, both to confirm the presence of hyperuricaemia and monitor response to treatment. Urate is a negative acute phase reactant, and hence urate levels are frequently lowered during an acute attack of gout. If the serum urate is found to be within the 'normal range' during a suspected acute attack it should be repeated during the intercritical period.

In primary gout in a young patient, determination of undersecretion or overproduction of uric acid is best undertaken by measuring total urinary excretion on a low-purine diet, but a quick guide is given by the uric acid/creatinine ratio estimated on a single urine sample (normally <0.5). In young overproducers, a purine enzyme defect becomes more likely and should be sought. Assessment of renal function (creatinine, urea, electrolytes, urine testing) should always be undertaken (Table 19.10.2). Given the association of primary gout with cardiovascular disease and the metabolic syndrome, measurement of fasting lipoprotein concentrations and glucose should be made in all patients with primary gout. An intercritical full blood count and measurement of ESR/viscosity should detect any underlying chronic myeloproliferative disease. During acute attacks a marked acute phase response (high ESR, neutrophil leucocytosis, thrombocytosis, elevated C-reactive protein) is usual; modest elevations of ESR may also accompany chronic gout.

Radiographs supplement the clinical assessment of structural damage but can also aid diagnosis. In early disease they are usually normal. During acute gout, nonspecific soft tissue swelling (rarely juxta-articular osteopenia) may be evident. After repeated attacks, and in chronic disease, joint space narrowing, sclerosis, cysts, and osteophytes (that is, the changes of osteoarthritis) become more frequent in feet and hands. Gouty 'erosions' are a less common but more specific abnormality, occurring as para-articular 'punched-out' bone defects with well-demarcated sclerotic margins, overhanging hooks of bone, and retained bone density (Fig. 19.10.5). They are typically asymmetric, eccentric lesions positioned away

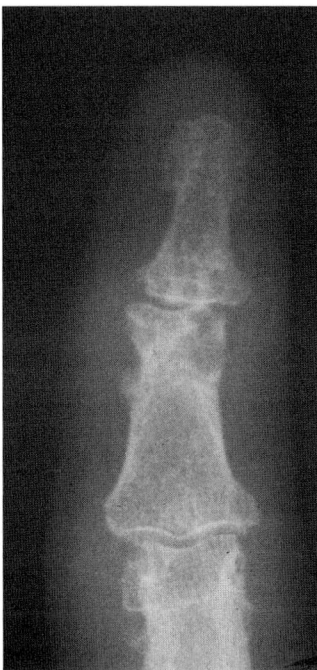

Fig. 19.10.5 Characteristic radiographic changes of established gout in a finger: joint space loss and cystic change at the distal interphalangeal joint, 'pressure erosions' with overhanging bony 'hooks' at both interphalangeal joints, and eccentric soft tissue swelling at the proximal joint.

from the 'bare area' of the joint, contrasting with more symmetrical, ill-defined marginal erosions (with osteopenia) of rheumatoid arthritis. Tophi appear as eccentric soft tissue swellings, occasionally with patchy calcification due to epitaxial growth of apatite. In late disease, severe destructive change with osteopenia may occur, and distinction from rheumatoid arthritis or other conditions becomes more difficult.

Treatment

Acute gout

The treatment aim is pain relief by reducing inflammation and intra-articular hypertension. Alteration of uric acid levels is avoided until the attack has resolved, as initiation of hypouricaemic drugs may prolong the attack and important information concerning lifelong treatment is best delivered when the patient has fully recovered from their painful episode.

Rapid symptom relief may be obtained with a quick-acting nonsteroidal anti-inflammatory drug (NSAID), given in full dosage. Indometacin has traditionally been considered to be the NSAID of choice but, given its frequent renal, gut, and nervous system side effects, is less preferable to other NSAIDs, e.g. diclofenac or naproxen. In the presence of risk factors for gastrointestinal toxicity (e.g. old age) a gastroprotective agent (a proton pump inhibitor or misoprostol) should be coadministered with a traditional NSAID, or alternatively a selective inhibitor of cyclooxygenase-2 (COX-2), such as etoricoxib can be given, although long-term use should be cautioned by the adverse cardiovascular profile of both COX-2 selective agents and primary gout.

Oral colchicine is rapidly effective within a few hours. At the doses described in the British National Formulary (1 mg immediately, followed by 0.5 mg every 2–3 h until symptoms abate), diarrhoea,

nausea, and abdominal cramps are very common, causing the patient 'to run before he can walk'. Low-dose colchicine, e.g. 0.5 mg two or three times daily, is widely used with both symptomatic benefit and less toxicity and is a useful alternative if NSAIDs are contraindicated. Intravenous colchicine, however, is particularly toxic and should never be used. Although previously used as a 'diagnostic test', the efficacy of colchicine is not specific to gout: it also ameliorates other crystal-associated syndromes.

Joint aspiration often provides immediate relief by reducing intra-articular hypertension, and in difficult cases joint lavage may terminate an attack. Intra-articular steroid is useful for large joints such as the knee. When NSAIDs or colchicine are contraindicated or unsuccessful, intra-articular steroid or oral prednisolone (20 mg/day) can be effective, and for troublesome polyarticular attacks there is support for the use of parenteral steroid. Application of ice locally to an affected joint also provides symptomatic relief.

Long-term management

Once any acute attack has resolved, long-term strategies need consideration. Gout is potentially curable. Treatment may involve both considering and eliminating modifiable factors that cause hyperuricaemia, and utilizing hypouricaemic drugs. Management of gout may therefore require alteration in lifestyle and chronic medication: patient compliance and motivation, which depend on appropriate education and counselling, are essential for success.

Modification of provoking factors

Lifestyle modification is a key component of the management of primary gout. In particular, obesity, excess alcohol consumption, and a high-purine diet are independent risk factors that are amenable to modification. Advice concerning weight loss and restriction of the consumption of alcohol (especially beer) and purine-rich foods should be offered to all patients with primary gout where appropriate.

In diuretic-induced gout, the diuretic should be discontinued or the dose reduced whenever possible, and this may be all that is required. However, this cannot often be achieved where the indication for the diuretic is cardiac failure rather than hypertension, and pharmacological measures are necessary.

Urate-lowering drug therapy

Indications for urate lowering therapy are:

* recurrent, troublesome acute attacks

* presence of tophi

* bone or cartilage damage on radiographs

* coexistent renal disease, uric acid urolithiasis

* very high uric acid levels (particularly with overproduction and hyperexcretion)

The aim of urate-lowering therapy is the reduction and maintenance of serum urate well below 360 μmol/litre (6 mg/dl), which is below the physiological saturation threshold of urate within the serum (approximately 380 μmol/litre (6.4 mg/dl)). The lowering of urate below this level reduces the frequency of acute attacks and crystal load. Allopurinol, a xanthine oxidase inhibitor, is the usual drug of choice, permitting flexible tailoring of dose to reduce urate levels below the solubility limit. Allopurinol is usually started at the relatively low dose of 100 mg daily. The serum urate should then be checked at regular intervals (e.g. monthly) and, if tolerated, the dose of allopurinol increased in 100 mg increments up to a maximum dose of 900 mg daily until the serum urate lies well below 360 µmol/litre (6 mg/dl). In patients with renal insufficiency, particularly older people, excretion of the active metabolite oxipurinol is delayed, and hence dose escalation should be more cautious. Treatment should be lifelong.

The uricosurics probenecid (0.5–1.0 g twice a day) and sulfinpyrazone (100 mg three or four times daily), which prevent proximal tubular reabsorption of urate, are rarely used. They are alternatives to allopurinol in patients with normal renal function but are contraindicated in those with renal impairment, urolithiasis, or gross overproduction of uric acid (due to reduced efficacy and risk of worsening renal function). Benzbromarone, a potent uricosuric, is now increasingly used in parts of Europe, and is the one uricosuric that can be used in patients with mild to moderate renal impairment. Its availability, however, is limited, owing to reports of occasional severe hepatotoxicity (possibly limited to Japanese patients).

Losartan, an angiotension-II receptor antagonist, and fenofibrate have mild uricosuric properties that may prove useful in patients with hypertension and/or hyperlipidaemia in addition to gout. Losartan is therefore a logical alternative antihypertensive agent in diuretic-induced gout.

Acute attacks may be provoked during the first few months of hypouricaemic treatment, especially if initiation is with higher doses (e.g. 300 mg allopurinol). Prophylactic colchicine (0.5 mg twice a day) or a standard dose of NSAID given for the first 2 to 3 months of treatment largely avoids 'breakthrough' attacks. With any uricosuric, high fluid intake and urine alkalinization in the early weeks of treatment are recommended to avoid deposition of uric acid within the kidney.

Serious side effects are unusual with any hypouricaemic drugs. Rare problems include toxic epidermal necrolysis, interstitial nephritis and vasculitis (allopurinol hypersensitivity syndrome), nephrotic syndrome (probenecid), and hepatitis and marrow suppression (both drugs). Important interactions with allopurinol occur with coumarin anticoagulants (due to hepatic microsomal enzyme inhibition) and purine analogues (such as azathioprine) that are inactivated by xanthine oxidase. Associated hypertension should be treated, but preferably not with diuretics, which elevate serum urate and may provoke acute attacks.

New urate-lowering agents are in development. Febuxostat, a nonpurine-based xanthine oxidase inhibitor, has been shown to produce greater reductions in serum urate levels than allopurinol 300 mg daily, with apparently less toxicity. Recombinant uricase, currently licensed for the prevention of tumour-lysis syndrome, produces significant reductions in serum urate levels in patients unresponsive to, or intolerant of, allopurinol.

Pyrophosphate arthropathy

Deposition of calcium pyrophosphate dihydrate crystals ($Ca_2P_2O_7.2H_2O$) in articular cartilage is a common age-related phenomenon. Calcium pyrophosphate dihydrate crystals preferentially deposit within fibrocartilage and are the most common cause of cartilage calcification (chondrocalcinosis).

Calcium pyrophosphate dihydrate deposition may occur in otherwise normal cartilage or associate with structural change and clinical arthropathy—'arthropathy'. A causal role for calcium pyrophosphate dihydrate crystals in acute inflammation is accepted, but their role in chronic arthropathy is unclear. The strong association/overlap with osteoarthritis has led some to consider pyrophosphate arthropathy not as a crystal deposition disease but as a subset of osteoarthritis, with calcium pyrophosphate dihydrate a 'process' marker associating with a hypertrophic bone response.

Radiographic chondrocalcinosis has an age-adjusted standardized prevalence of 4.5% in adults over age 40, its prevalence at the knee rising to about 20% in those over age 80. There is an equal sex distribution. Community studies have confirmed an association with osteoarthritis at the knee (age, sex-adjusted odds ratio 2.0), but this is largely through an association with osteophyte rather than joint space narrowing. The age-standardized prevalence of osteoarthritis plus chondrocalcinosis (i.e. pyrophosphate arthropathy) in the United Kingdom in people older than 40 is 2.40%.

Clinical features

Common presentations are acute synovitis, chronic arthritis, or as an asymptomatic incidental radiographic finding. Other presentations are rare.

Acute synovitis (pseudogout)

This is one of the commonest causes of acute monoarthritis in older people. Attacks may occur as isolated events or be superimposed upon a background of chronic joint symptoms. Most attacks occur spontaneously, but provoking factors include intercurrent illness, surgery, and local trauma. Although any joint may be involved, the knee is by far the commonest site, followed by the wrist, shoulder, and ankle. Concurrent attacks in several joints are uncommon and polyarticular attacks rare.

The typical attack develops rapidly with severe pain, stiffness, and swelling, becoming maximal within just 6 to 24 h of onset. Examination reveals a very tender joint with signs of florid synovitis (increased warmth, tense effusion, restricted movement with stress pain) and often overlying erythema. Fever is common, and elderly patients may appear unwell or mildly confused, especially when more than one joint is involved. Attacks are self-limiting, usually resolving within 1 to 3 weeks. The identical clinical presentation of such attacks to gout is the reason for the term 'pseudogout'.

Chronic pyrophosphate arthropathy

This common condition affects mainly elderly women and targets the same large and medium-sized joints as pseudogout. Knees are the usual and most severely affected joint. Presentation is with chronic pain, stiffness, and functional impairment, with or without superimposed acute attacks. Symptoms usually relate to just a few joints, although examination often reveals more widespread joint involvement. Affected joints show signs of osteoarthritis (crepitus, bony swelling, restricted movement) with varying degrees of synovitis (often most marked at the knee, radiocarpal, or glenohumeral joint). Knees typically show abnormality of two or three compartments; valgus or varus deformity may occur.

Although symptoms and signs are those of osteoarthritis, chronic pyrophosphate arthropathy may often be distinguished from uncomplicated osteoarthritis by:

- the joint distribution—in osteoarthritis wrist, glenohumeral, ankle, elbow, and midtarsal involvement is less common

- the often marked inflammatory component

- superimposition of acute attacks

The outcome for chronic pyrophosphate arthropathy is generally good, most patients running a relatively benign course, particularly with respect to small and medium-sized joints. If progression occurs, it is usually slow and related to knees, hips, or shoulders. Severe, rapidly progressive, destructive arthropathy occasionally develops at these sites. This is virtually confined to very elderly women and is associated with severe pain, recurrent haemarthrosis (shoulder, knee), and occasional joint leakage.

Incidental finding

As with osteoarthritis, clinical or radiographic evidence of pyrophosphate arthropathy and chondrocalcinosis are not uncommon incidental findings in older people, and may confound the cause of regional pain if a thorough history and examination are not undertaken.

Uncommon presentations

Acute tendinitis (triceps, Achilles), tenosynovitis (hand flexors, extensors), and bursitis (olecranon, infrapatellar, retrocalcaneal) occur uncommonly, usually in patients with widespread calcium pyrophosphate dihydrate crystals. Median and ulnar nerve compression at the wrist may accompany flexor tenosynovitis. Rare tophaceous deposits of calcium pyrophosphate dihydrate usually present as solitary lesions in areas of chondroid metaplasia (usually benign cartilage tumours).

Classification and associations

Calcium pyrophosphate dihydrate deposition is traditionally classified as: being hereditary; associated with metabolic disease; or sporadic/idiopathic (by far the commonest, associated with osteoarthritis).

Familial predisposition

This is reported from many countries and different ethnic groups. Two clinical phenotypes occur: early onset (third to fourth decade) florid polyarticular chondrocalcinosis with variable severity of accompanying arthropathy; and late onset (sixth to seventh decade) oligoarticular chondrocalcinosis (mainly knee) with arthritis resembling sporadic disease. The pattern of inheritance varies, although autosomal dominance is usual. Two chromosomal locations have been identified in kindreds with young-onset chondrocalcinosis: *CCAL1* on chromosome 8 (associating with severe structural arthritis), and *CCAL2* on chromosome 5 (mainly associating with isolated polyarticular chondrocalcinosis). The responsible gene at *CCAL2* encodes the multipass transmembrane transporter protein ANKH (ankylosis human) that regulates passage of intracellular inorganic pyrophosphate to the extracelluler space. Mutations in ANKH in British, French and American kindreds result in greatly increased exit of pyrophosphate from chondrocytes, sufficient to exceed the saturation point for calcium pyrophosphate crystal formation. Other mechanisms may operate in other families. For example, histological studies in Japanese and Swedish families suggest a primary abnormality in cartilage matrix that promotes calcium pyrophosphate dihydrate crystal nucleation and growth.

Metabolic disease associations

Inorganic pyrophosphate is a by-product of many biosynthetic reactions, with a turnover of several kilograms per day. Most extracellular inorganic pyrophosphate derives from breakdown of extracellular ATP via the action of the NTP pyrophosphatase plasma cell membrane glycoprotein-1 (PC-1). Normally this

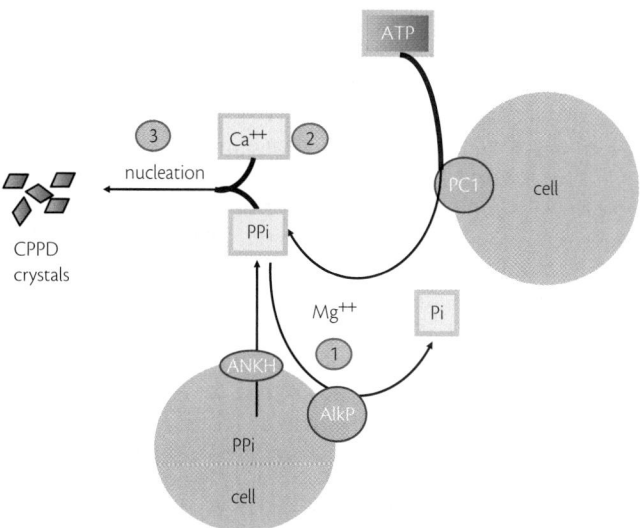

Fig. 19.10.6 Simplified scheme of extracellular pyrophosphate metabolism, showing putative sites of interaction by metabolic diseases. Hyperparathyroidism, 1,2; haemochromatosis, 1,3; hypophosphatasia, 1; Wilson's disease, 1,3; and hypomagnesaemia, 1. Alk P, alkaline phosphatise; ANKH, ankylosis human protein; ATP, adenosine triphosphate; CPPD, calcium pyrophosphate dehydrate; Mg^{++}, magnesium; PC1, plasma cell glycoprotein-1; PPi, pyrophosphate.

extracellular pyrophosphate is rapidly converted to orthophosphate by pyrophosphatases (particularly alkaline phosphatase) (Fig. 19.10.6). A number of metabolic diseases associate with deposition of calcium pyrophosphate dihydrate (Table 19.10.3), their association being rationalized through putative effects on metabolism of inorganic pyrophosphate. Suggested mechanisms include:

- reduced breakdown of inorganic pyrophosphate by alkaline phosphatase, owing to (1) reduced levels, (2) inhibitory ions (calcium, iron, copper), or (3) impaired complexing with magnesium

Table 19.10.3 Metabolic diseases associated with calcium pyrophosphate dihydrate (CPPD) crystal deposition

	Chondrocalcinosis	Pseudogout	Chronic CPPD arthropathy
Definite associations			
Hyperparathyroidism	+	+	−
Haemochromatosis	+	+	+
Hypophosphatasia	+	+	−
Hypomagnesaemia	+	+	−
Possible associations			
Hypothyroidism	+	−	−
Gout	+	+	−
X-linked hypophosphataemic rickets	+	+	+
Familial hypocalciuric hypercalcaemia	+	−	−
Wilson's disease	+	−	−
Ochronosis	+	−	−
Acromegaly	+	−	−

- enhanced nucleation by iron or copper
- increased calcium concentration

Osteoarthritis and joint insult

Several observations support a relationship between osteoarthritis and deposition of calcium pyrophosphate crystals, the latter often following rather than preceding joint damage. However, a negative association exists between deposition of calcium pyrophosphate dihydrate and rheumatoid arthritis, with atypical radiographic features in coexistent disease (retained bone density; marked osteophyte, cyst, and bone remodelling) suggesting that the primary association of calcium pyrophosphate dihydrate is with hypertrophic tissue response/osteoarthritis and not joint damage *per se*. The explanation for this association probably relates to changes both in pyrophosphate metabolism and in tissue factors that encourage crystal formation. Levels of inorganic pyrophosphate in synovial fluid are increased in pyrophosphate arthropathy, osteoarthritis, and in metabolic diseases that predispose to chondrocalcinosis, but are lower than normal in rheumatoid arthritis. Calcium pyrophosphate crystals form in pericellular sites and associate with lipid, proteoglycan depletion, and adjacent hypertrophic chondrocytes containing lipid granules. It is therefore possible that reduction of inhibitors (such as proteoglycan) and increase in promotors (such as lipid) may combine to copromote calcium pyrophosphate dihydrate formation in metabolically active osteoarthritic tissue that associates with high levels of extracellular pyrophosphate.

Investigations and diagnosis

Critical investigations are synovial fluid analysis and plain radiographs. In pseudogout aspirated fluid is often turbid or bloodstained with an elevated cell count (>90% neutrophils). Compensated polarized microscopy reveals calcium pyrophosphate crystals as weakly birefringent (positive sign) rhomboids or rods, about 2 to 10 µm long. Calcium pyrophosphate crystals are less readily identified and often less numerous than those of monosodium urate; examination of a spun deposit may increase detection.

Radiographic aspects relate both to calcification and arthropathy. Chondrocalcinosis signifies extensive deposition and is not always evident: it mainly affects fibrocartilage (particularly knee menisci, wrist triangular cartilage, symphysis pubis), and less commonly hyaline cartilage (Fig. 19.10.7). Although occasionally monoarticular, it usually affects several sites. Calcification of capsule, synovium, and tendons is less common. Chondrocalcinosis and calcification may increase or decrease with time, diminishing chondrocalcinosis often accompanying crystal shedding or cartilage loss.

Changes of arthropathy are those of osteoarthritis: cartilage loss, sclerosis, cysts, and osteophytes. However, characteristics that suggest pyrophosphate include:

- distribution between and within joints that is atypical of osteoarthritis (e.g. glenohumeral disease; isolated or predominant patellofemoral or radiocarpal involvement)
- prominence of osteophytes and cysts
- prominent osteochondral bodies

Such combined features may present a distinctive 'hypertrophic' appearance even in the absence of chondrocalcinosis (Fig. 19.10.8).

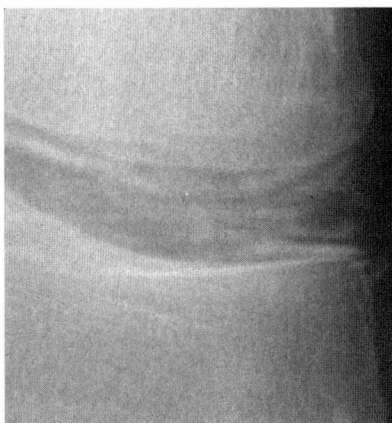

Fig. 19.10.7 Radiographic chondrocalcinosis of the knee affecting meniscal fibrocartilage (central, triangular) and hyaline cartilage (linear, parallel to bone).

Marked cartilage and bone attrition with fragmentation and loose osseous bodies may resemble a Charcot joint in destructive arthropathy.

Metabolic predisposition is rare and routine screening of all patients is unrewarding. Nevertheless, arthritis associated with calcium pyrophosphate crystals may be the presenting feature of metabolic or familial disease, and a search is warranted in early onset chondrocalcinosis or pseudogout (<55 years), florid polyarticular chondrocalcinosis, or presence of additional clinical or radiographic clues. A reasonable screen would include serum calcium, alkaline phosphatase, magnesium, ferritin, and liver function.

Differential diagnosis

The principal differential diagnosis for pseudogout is sepsis or gout, both of which may coexist with calcium pyrophosphate deposition. Gram stain and culture of joint fluid should be undertaken even when calcium pyrophosphate (and/or monosodium urate)

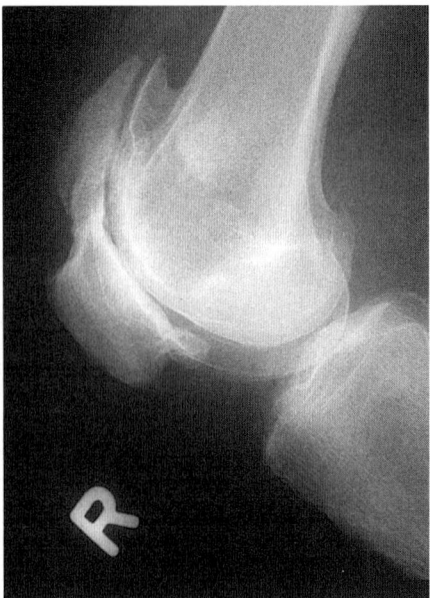

Fig. 19.10.8 Lateral knee radiograph showing predominant patellofemoral involvement by 'hypertrophic' osteoarthritis characteristic of pyrophosphate arthropathy.

crystals are identified. Marked bloodstaining may lead to consideration of other causes of haemarthrosis, especially a bleeding disorder or subchondral fracture.

Chronic pyrophosphate arthropathy is usually readily distinguished from rheumatoid arthritis by the synovial fluid and radiographic findings, the infrequency of severe systemic upset, absence of extra-articular features, and an acute phase response that is only modest. Proximal stiffness due to glenohumeral involvement may suggest polymyalgia rheumatica, although clinical examination and near normal ESR should exclude the diagnosis. Destructive pyrophosphate arthropathy may simulate a neuropathic joint, although such joints are severely symptomatic and neurological abnormality is absent.

Treatment

Pseudogout

As pseudogout usually affects only one or a few joints in elderly patients, local therapy is preferred. Aspiration alone often relieves symptoms, but should be combined with intra-articular steroid in florid cases. Local ice packs are safe and often helpful. With respect to systemic treatments, paracetamol is safe but opioids and oral NSAIDs should be used with caution in the older people (coprescription of a proton pump inhibitor or misoprostol with an NSAID is indicated in those over 65; alternatively, the short-term use of a selective COX-2 inhibitor may be considered). Joint lavage is reserved for troublesome steroid-resistant cases. Colchicine is effective but rarely warranted. Triggering illness (e.g. chest infection) will require appropriate treatment. Rapid mobilization should be instituted once the synovitis is settling.

Chronic pyrophosphate arthropathy

Unlike gout, there is no specific therapy, and treatment of any underlying metabolic disease does not influence outcome. Treatment aims are to reduce symptoms and maintain or improve function. This may include education of the patient in appropriate use of the affected joints, reduction in obesity, improvement of muscle strength, use of a stick or other walking aid, and surgery for severe disease. Chronic synovitis may be improved by intermittent steroid injection or intra-articular radiocolloid (yttrium-90). As with pseudogout, symptomatic drugs are to be used with caution in older patients; simple analgesics are generally preferable to NSAIDs.

Other crystal-related disorders

Apatite-associated syndromes

Hydroxyapatite is the principal bone mineral. Apatites or basic calcium phosphates (partially carbonate-substituted hydroxyapatite, octacalcium phosphate, tricalcium phosphate (rarely)) are the usual minerals to deposit in extraskeletal tissues (e.g. tuberculous lesions, arteries).

The [calcium × phosphate] product must be kept high to maintain skeletal integrity. Specific cellular mechanisms activate calcification where appropriate (e.g. matrix vesicles in growing cartilage), whereas other mechanisms (such as pyrophosphate and aggregated proteoglycan) inhibit calcification elsewhere. In general, abnormal calcification results from:

- elevation of the [calcium × phosphate] product, causing widespread metastatic calcification

- alteration in the balance between inhibitory and promoting tissue factors, resulting in local dystrophic calcification.

In rheumatic diseases, abnormal deposition of basic calcium phosphates may occur in periarticular tissues (particularly tendon), hyaline cartilage, in association with osteoarthritis, or subcutaneous tissues and muscle, principally in connective tissue diseases.

Apatite crystals are too small (5–500 nm) to be seen by light microscopy, but particles may aggregate to form spherulites that are visible on microscopy. Confirmation of basic calcium phosphates requires sophisticated analytical techniques, and most clinical diagnoses are presumptive, based on radiographic calcification or nonspecific staining of joint fluid or histological material.

Acute calcific periarthritis

Apatite deposition in the supraspinatus tendon (Fig. 19.10.9) is a relatively common incidental finding (about 7% of adults). It occasionally results in severe acute inflammation of the subacromial bursa, periarticular tissues, or joint itself. Periarticular sites around the greater hip trochanter, the foot, or the hand are less commonly affected.

Acute episodes may follow local trauma or occur spontaneously. Within a few hours pain and tenderness are often extreme and the area appears swollen, hot, and red. Modest systemic upset and fever are common. Sepsis is usually considered first, but the diagnosis is made following demonstration of radiographic calcification. If the lesion is aspirated, thick white fluid containing many apatite aggregates may be obtained. The condition usually resolves spontaneously over 1 to 3 weeks, often accompanied by radiographic dispersal of modestly sized calcifications (crystal shedding). NSAIDs ameliorate symptoms, and the attack can be abbreviated by aspiration and injection of steroid. Large deposits may cause mechanical impingement and blocking of movement and require surgical removal. Calcific periarthritis rarely results from metabolic abnormality (renal failure, hyperparathyroidism, hypophosphatasia) and measurements of serum calcium, alkaline phosphatase, and creatinine are usually normal. Rare families are predisposed to calcific periarthritis at multiple sites despite no evidence of altered calcium phosphate product.

Osteoarthritis and apatite-associated destructive arthritis

Modest amounts of basic calcium phosphates are commonly found in synovial fluid from osteoarthritic joints, in isolation or with calcium pyrophosphate dihydrate (mixed crystal deposition).

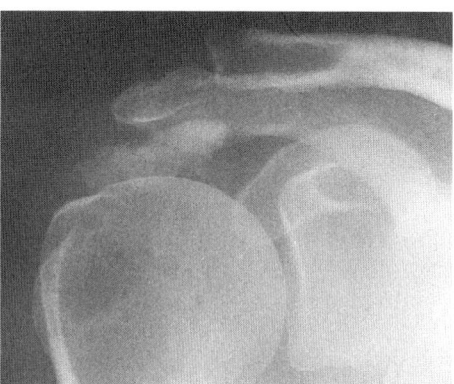

Fig. 19.10.9 Shoulder radiograph showing florid supraspinatus tendon calcification (calcific periarthritis).

Whether apatite plays any part in inflammatory exacerbations or associates with severity or progression of osteoarthritis remains uncertain.

The uncommon condition 'apatite-associated destructive arthritis' is often considered a subset of osteoarthritis. It is virtually confined to elderly women and affects the hip, shoulder (Milwaukee shoulder), or knee. It has the general appearance of severe large joint osteoarthritis but is particularly characterized by: rapid progression, often leading to severe pain and disability within a few months of onset; development of marked instability; large, cool effusions; and an atrophic radiographic appearance with marked cartilage and bone attrition and little osteophyte or bone remodelling.

Aspirated fluid has normal viscosity and a low cell count but contains large amounts of apatite aggregates, seen readily on light microscopy following nonspecific calcium staining (Alizarin Red, acidic pH). The differential diagnosis may include sepsis (excluded by synovial fluid culture), late avascular necrosis, or neuropathic joint. The pathogenesis of this condition remains unclear. Although apatite particles could contribute to tissue damage by stimulating release of collagenase and other proteolytic enzymes from synovial cells, it is most likely that the apatite is noncontributory and principally reflects the severity of subchondral bone attrition. The outcome is poor and usually requires surgical intervention.

Other apatite syndromes

Deposition of very large tophaceous periarticular apatite (tumoural calcinosis) may occur in patients with chronic renal failure managed by dialysis. Apatite has also been incriminated in the occasional erosive interphalangeal arthropathy seen in such patients.

Other crystals

Cholesterol

Cholesterol crystals may induce acute synovitis, acute tenosynovitis, and chronic xanthomatous tendinitis in hypercholesterolaemic subjects. Cholesterol and other lipid crystals may also occur as a nonspecific finding in chronic synovitis, most commonly due to rheumatoid arthritis. In this situation the lipid probably derives from cellular debris and its pathogenic significance is uncertain.

Oxalate

Oxalate crystals have been incriminated in acute and chronic articular and periarticular syndromes occurring in association with either primary familial oxalosis (types I and II) or secondary oxalosis (Chapter 12.10). Chronic renal failure managed with dialysis is the commonest cause of secondary oxalosis, particularly if ascorbic acid supplementation has been given. Acute symmetrical interphalangeal and metacarpophalangeal arthritis, with or without tenosynovitis, and digital calcific deposits are the usual manifestation. Large joint involvement, chondrocalcinosis, and tophaceous periarticular masses are less common. Calcium oxalate crystals may also cause life-threatening organ involvement, with peripheral vascular insufficiency and digital necrosis, cardiomyopathy, peripheral neuropathy, and aplastic anaemia. There is no effective treatment.

Extrinsic crystals

These rare causes of locomotor problems. Acute flares following intra-articular injection of corticosteroids are uncommon but may represent iatrogenic crystal-induced inflammation. Penetrating injuries involving plant thorns and sea-urchin spines may cause acute and chronic inflammatory synovitis, periostitis, or periarticular lesions that only resolve following surgical removal of the crystalline material.

Further reading

Bieber JD, Terkeltaub RA (2004). Gout—on the brink of novel therapeutic options for an ancient disease. *Arthritis Rheum*, **50**, 2400–14.

Choi HK, Mount DB, Reginato AM (2005). Pathogenesis of gout. *Ann Intern Med*, **143**, 499–516.

Doherty M, Dieppe PA (1986). Crystal deposition disease in the elderly. *Clin Rheum Dis*, **12**, 97–116.

Emmerson BT (1996). The management of gout. *New Engl J Med*, **334**, 445–51.

McCarty DJ (1988). Crystalline deposition diseases. *Rheum Dis Clin North Am*, **14**, 2.

Reginato A, Kurnik B (1989). Calcium oxalate and other crystals associated with kidney diseases and arthritis. *Semin Arthritis Rheum*, **18**, 198–224.

Rosenthal AK (1998). Calcium crystal-associated arthritides. *Curr Opin Rheumatol*, **10**, 273–7.

Rott KT, Agudelo CA (2003). Gout. *J Am Med Assoc*, **289**, 2857–60.

Underwood M (2006). Diagnosis and management of gout. *Br Med J*, **332**, 1315–19.

Zhang W, *et al.* (2006). EULAR evidence based recommendations for gout—part I diagnosis: report of a task force of the Standing Committee for International Clinical Studies Including Therapeutics (ESCISIT). *Ann Rheum Dis*, **65**, 1301–11.

Zhang W, *et al.* (2006). EULAR evidence based recommendations for gout—part II management: report of a task force of the Standing Committee for International Clinical Studies Including Therapeutics (ESCISIT). *Ann Rheum Dis*, **65**, 1312–24.

Autoimmune rheumatic disorders and vasculitides

Contents

19.11.1 Introduction

I.P. Giles and David A. Isenberg

Essentials

About 1 in 20 people develop an autoimmune disease, many of which involve the musculoskeletal system. Young women are particularly at risk, but the development at any age of symptoms such as unexplained fever, rash, polyarthritis, Raynaud's phenomenon or mouth ulcers should encourage serological screening for autoimmune rheumatic or vasculitic disorder.

Aetiology and pathogenesis—common to all of the autoimmune rheumatic diseases is the phenomenon of production of autoantibodies by activated B cells. In the primary vasculitides, a pathogenic role has been proposed for antiendothelial cell antibodies and sensitized T cells, but undoubtedly the most important role is that of antineutrophil cytoplasmic antibodies (ANCA).

Diagnosis—detection of antinuclear antibodies or rheumatoid factor in high titre favours the diagnosis of an autoimmune rheumatic disease and should lead to a search for more specific autoantibodies, e.g. anti-dsDNA linked to lupus, anticyclic citrullinated peptides linked to rheumatoid arthritis, antineutrophil cytoplasmic antibodies (ANCA) linked to Wegener's granulomatosus and microscopic polyangiitis. Well-established and validated criteria have been set up for all the main autoimmune rheumatic diseases and vasculitides, but there is significant overlap between them. Physicians treating patients with these conditions need to be constantly aware of the possibility of organ involvement because prompt diagnosis and treatment may be necessary to prevent irreversible damage.

Definition and epidemiology

The autoimmune rheumatic diseases are a heterogeneous group of disorders characterized by clinical involvement of the joints, connective tissues, muscles, internal organs, Raynaud's phenomenon, and cutaneous manifestations. They include a broad clinical spectrum of disease, including systemic lupus erythematosus (SLE), rheumatoid arthritis, Sjögren's syndrome, scleroderma, dermatomyositis, polymyositis, antiphospholipid syndrome, and the vasculitides. This latter group of diseases all share inflammation and necrosis of blood vessels as cardinal features, and may be divided into primary (e.g. giant cell arteritis, Wegener's granulomatosis, polyarteritis nodosa, etc.), occurring in the absence of a recognized precipitating cause, or secondary to established disease (e.g. SLE or rheumatoid arthritis) or infection (e.g. hepatitis B, C, or HIV) (see Table 19.11.1.1). In general, autoimmune rheumatic diseases have a predilection for young women and share defects in immune regulation leading to the production of autoantibodies, activation of the complement system, and generation and deposition of immune complexes.

Autoimmune rheumatic diseases affect as many as 1 in 20 people. Some are rare, for example systemic sclerosis; others are common,

Table 19.11.1.1 Classification of systemic vasculitis

Dominant vessel involved	Primary	Secondary
Large arteries	Giant cell arteritis	Aortitis associated with RA
	Takayasu's arteritis	Infection (e.g. syphilis)
	Isolated CNS angiitis	
Medium arteries	Classical polyarteritis nodosa	Infection (e.g. hepatitis B)
	Kawasaki disease	
Small vessels and medium arteries	Wegener's granulomatosis[a]	Vasculitis secondary to RA, SLE, and SS
	Churg–Strauss syndrome[a]	Drugs
	Microscopic polyangiitis[a]	Infection (e.g. HIV)
Small vessels (leucocytoclastic)	Henoch–Schönlein purpura	Drugs[b]
	Essential mixed cryoglobulinaemia	Infection (e.g. hepatitis B,C)
	Cutaneous leucocytoclastic angiitis	

CNS, central nervous system; RA, rheumatoid arthritis; SLE, systemic lupus erythematosus; SS, Sjögren's syndrome.

[a]Diseases most commonly associated with ANCA (antimyeloperoxidase and antiproteinase 3 antibodies), a significant risk of renal involvement, and which are most responsive to immunosuppression with cyclophosphamide.

[b]E.g. sulphonamides, penicillins, thiazide diuretics, and many others.

rheumatoid arthritis affecting approximately 1% of the population (see Table 19.11.1.2). Some are severely debilitating or life-threatening illnesses, others produce minor symptoms that require little, if any, medical intervention.

The clinical spectrum

Each of the autoimmune rheumatic diseases is a distinct entity and can be clearly defined clinically, serologically, and in terms of treatment and prognosis. However, many patients with these diseases have nonspecific features of malaise, fever, and arthralgia, and about 30% of patients with lupus, myositis and Sjögren's have at least one other autoimmune rheumatic disease, there being much overlap in terms of multisystem involvement, as shown in Table 19.11.1.3. Organ-specific features, e.g. lung fibrosis, pericarditis, and less frequently glomerulonephritis, can all occur in several of the autoimmune rheumatic diseases and the presence of such a feature is not pathognomonic of an individual disease.

Table 19.11.1.2 Occurrence of major autoimmune rheumatic diseases in Western populations aged 15 years and over

Diseases	Annual incidence per 1000	Point prevalence per 1000
Rheumatoid arthritis	0.5	8.0
Systemic lupus erythematosus	0.05	0.4[a]
Polymyositis	0.005	0.08
Systemic sclerosis	0.01	0.1
Sjögren's syndrome	0.3	0.27

[a] There is a considerable variation according to ethnic origin, thus Afro-Caribbean women are five times as likely to get systemic lupus erythematosus as white women.

Table 19.11.1.3 The spectrum of the autoimmune rheumatic diseases

Disease	Major organ/system involvement	Principal immunological abnormalities
Rheumatoid arthritis	Joints, skin, eyes, lungs, heart, neurological, renal	Rheumatoid factor, IgM, G, or A, AB to CCP, central role for T and B cells
Systemic lupus erythematosus	Skin, joints, kidneys, brain, heart, lungs	AB to polynucleotides, histones, nucleosomes, ENA, PL, abnormalities in T and B cells and accessory cells
Poly-/dermatomyositis	Muscle, skin, blood vessels, lungs	Disease-specific AB (e.g. anti-Jo-1) and infiltrates of T cells in muscle
Scleroderma	Skin, gut, lungs, kidneys, heart, muscle	Disease-specific AB (e.g. anti-Scl-70, anticentromere, anti-PDGFR); T-cell and cytokine abnormalities
Primary antiphospholipid syndrome	Blood vessels any size, skin, pregnancy morbidity, neurological	AB to PL, β_2-GP1, and the lupus anticoagulant
Sjögren's syndrome	Exocrine glands, notably lacrimal and parotid	AB to ENA, SS A/Ro, SS B/La; major infiltrate of T cells in glands
Vasculitides (e.g. PAN, WG, CSS, MPA and GCA)	Skin, joints, muscles, lungs, central nervous system, kidneys, blood vessels of all sizes	Cellular infiltration of blood vessel walls; disease-related AB to c-ANCA or p-ANCA

AB, antibody; p-ANCA, perinuclear staining antineutrophil cytoplasmic antibody; c-ANCA, cytoplasmic staining antineutrophil cytoplasmic antibody; CSS, Churg–Strauss syndrome; ENA, extractable nuclear antigen; GCA, giant cell arteritis; MPA, microscopic polyangitis; PDGFR, platelet-derived growth factor receptor; PL, phospholipid; PAN, polyarteritis nodosa; SS, Sjögren's syndrome; WG, Wegeners granulomatosis; β2-GP1, β2-glycoprotein 1.

The clinical features of each patient must be considered together with the laboratory investigations, which should include an autoantibody profile. A preliminary 'autoimmune screen' includes a rheumatoid factor and antinuclear antibody test as a bare minimum, the results of which then guide the need for further autoantibody testing. Immunologically, rheumatoid factor remains the most important guide to establishing the diagnosis of rheumatoid arthritis (especially if the titre is greater than 1 in 320), although the American College of Rheumatology classification criteria for rheumatoid arthritis may still be fulfilled in the absence of rheumatoid factor. The antibody is of no value, however, in the monitoring of the disease. More recently antibodies to citrullinated peptides (anti-CCP) have been shown to be as sensitive and more specific for rheumatoid arthritis, and they may also be genuinely pathogenic.

The presence and pattern of staining of antinuclear antibody is a very useful guide to the presence of disease, as shown in Table 19.11.1.4, with the important proviso that an antinuclear antibody is present in low titre (up to 1 in 80) in about 1 to 2% of the normal population, and more frequently (up to 10%) in healthy people over the age of 75 years. Hence, its presence alone at low titres does not in itself justify the diagnosis of an autoimmune rheumatic disease: the whole clinical picture must be considered. In the case of the vasculitides, the antineutrophil cytoplasmic antibody (ANCA) should be regarded in the same manner as the antinuclear

Table 19.11.1.4 Antinuclear antibody use in diagnosis

Antinuclear antibody pattern	Other autoantibodies	Disease
Nuclear		
Homogenous	Chromatin, dsDNA	SLE
	Histone	DIL
Speckled	Sm, U1RNP	SLE
	Ro, La	SS, SCLE, CHB, NL
	High titre U1RNP	Overlap/UARD
Nucleolar		
Speckled	Scl-70, RNA Polymerase I	DcSSc
Homogenous	PM-Scl	SSc/PM overlap
Clumpy	U3RNP	DcSSc, PHT
Centromere	Anti-centromere	LcSSc

CHB, congenital heart block; DcSSc, diffuse cutaneous systemic sclerosis; DIL, drug-induced lupus; LcSSc, localized systemic sclerosis; NL, neonatal lupus; PHT, pulmonary hypertension; PM, polymyositis; SCLE, subacute cutaneous lupus; SLE, systemic lupus erythematosus; SS, Sjögren's syndrome.

antibody, but it should also be remembered that some autoantibodies may be found in more than one disease, such as anti-U1RNP (in SLE and undifferentiated autoimmune rheumatic disease), whilst others may be found in other diseases 'beyond' the autoimmune rheumatic diseases, such as perinuclear staining ANCA (p-ANCA), which is well recognized in patients with inflammatory bowel disease, some chronic infections, and malignancies.

Immunopathogenesis

Autoimmune rheumatic disorders

The precise aetiologies of the autoimmune rheumatic diseases remain unknown, but are undoubtedly complex. Inciting agents, such as infection, are involved, as are genetic susceptibility, hormonal factors, and both cellular and immune dysregulation.

Common to all of the autoimmune rheumatic diseases is the phenomenon of production of autoantibodies by activated B cells. Most of the pathogenic autoantibodies are of the IgG class and have undergone somatic mutation in their hypervariable regions, leading to a gradual increase in specificity and binding affinity of an antibody produced by a particular clone of cells. This latter finding is particularly true of anti-dsDNA antibodies in SLE and antiphospholipid antibodies in the antiphospholipid syndrome.

The origins of autoantibody production remain an enigma. Mechanisms that have been invoked include antigen-driven T helper cell responses, failure of efficient clearance of nuclear antigens which become surface expressed following cellular apoptosis, and epitope spreading. These might act alone, in combination with each other, or together with other factors. Each has been proposed to lead to increased B-cell activation. Impaired tolerance appears to be the central defect, and once this has occurred abnormal immunoregulation leads to persistence of the inappropriate self-directed immune response.

Cellular mechanisms also play a role in the development of autoimmunity in the autoimmune rheumatic diseases: T-cell dysfunction, impaired macrophage and natural killer cell cytotoxicity,

decreased clearance of immune complexes by the mononuclear phagocytic system, increase in the number of activated B cells, cytokine dysregulation, and up-regulation of adhesion molecules have all been reported.

Genetic factors are important, especially in the case of SLE, where there is a higher rate of concordance in monozygotic twins (25%) than dizygotic (3%). The best described of the genetic contributions to autoimmune rheumatic disease is the increased risk associated with particular human leucocyte antigen (HLA) class II molecules. The HLA DR4 (the Dw4 and Dw14 subtypes, notably the DR_1*0404 allele) and HLA DR1 (Dw1) are particularly associated with rheumatoid arthritis. These subtypes share a similarity of the amino acid sequence in the third hypervariable region of the DR_1 chain, the shared epitope that has been proposed as the underlying unit of susceptibility to rheumatoid arthritis. There are, however, conflicting data proposing that this epitope is better related to the severity of disease. In SLE, among white people, the haplotype A1 B8 DR3 is associated with an approximately tenfold increase in risk, although the primary link may be with the complement C4 null allele with which there is linkage disequilibrium.

HLA associations are not only seen with autoimmune rheumatic disease, but also with certain autoantibodies. Anti-Ro and La are strongly correlated with HLA DR3 and DQ, an association that is stronger than that seen with the disease in which these autoantibodies are most frequently encountered (SLE and Sjögren's syndrome).

Vasculitides

HLA class I and class II associations are seen throughout the primary vasculitides, whereas infectious agents and circulating immune complexes are pathogenic in the secondary vasculitides. In the primary vasculitides a pathogenic role has been proposed for antiendothelial cell antibodies and sensitized T cells, but undoubtedly the most important role is that of ANCA. Immunofluoresence studies have localized the antigen to the cytoplasm of granulocytes in the azurophilic granules, and two patterns of staining are seen: cytoplasmic ANCA (c-ANCA), of which 90% of sera recognize proteinase 3; and perinuclear staining ANCA (p-ANCA) that is directed against myeloperoxidase in 70% of patients with p-ANCA vasculitis. A positive c-ANCA is strongly associated with Wegener's granulomatosis, although 10% of these patients may be p-ANCA positive, whilst antimyeloperoxidase antibodies occur in necrotizing glomerulonephritis (65%), Churg–Strauss syndrome (60%), and microscopic polyangiitis (45%).

Clinical features

As mentioned previously, the presentation of an autoimmune rheumatic disease may be variable and nonspecific, with fatigue and arthralgia frequently the major features. In this instance, systemic review should enquire for the presence of alopecia, mouth ulcers, Raynaud's phenomenon, rash, sicca symptoms, and lymphadenopathy. The presence of these would lend an autoimmune flavour to the illness, but not necessarily help to make a precise diagnosis. The history should also seek a possible trigger such as a preceding infection, drugs (for example hydralazine, isoniazid, procainamide in drug-induced lupus), or environmental exposure to chemicals, as may be seen in scleroderma-like illnesses. A family history must pay particular attention to the presence, not only of other autoimmune rheumatic diseases, but also other autoimmune diseases such as diabetes, pernicious anaemia, and thyroid disease, which are often found in association with the autoimmune rheumatic diseases.

The protean clinical manifestations mean that an autoimmune rheumatic disease may present not only to a rheumatologist but to many other specialists, including those in nephrology, dermatology, and less commonly neurology, cardiology, haematology, or even obstetrics, in the case of recurrent miscarriages in the antiphospholipid syndrome.

In many cases it is not possible to make a precise diagnosis on the first encounter with a patient. In those with mild disease, symptomatic relief can be obtained with a nonsteroidal anti-inflammatory drug (NSAID), whilst the results of baseline investigations and an 'immunological screen' of antinuclear antibody and rheumatoid factor are awaited. It is worth noting, however, that there is increasing emphasis on trying to make the diagnosis of rheumatoid arthritis promptly, so that a disease-modifying drug can be used as early as possible, rather than waiting for the development of erosive, destructive joint disease.

Since the autoimmune rheumatic diseases are systemic disorders, it is always important to search for evidence of involvement of any of the major organ systems. Baseline investigations must therefore include urinalysis, a full blood count, simple blood tests of renal and liver function, measurement of serum inflammatory markers, an ECG, and a chest radiograph. The simple bedside test of urinalysis is particularly important: the finding of proteinuria and haematuria immediately identifies those who require renal investigation—often urgently—and whose prognosis may be chiefly determined by the extent of renal involvement.

Damage to major organ systems can be part of the presenting illness in a patient with an autoimmune rheumatic disease, but may also occur in a previously diagnosed patient with 'stable' disease. Myocardial infarction can occur as the result of a vasculitic illness, or accelerated atherosclerosis in SLE. Pericarditis can lead to tamponade (e.g. in SLE or rheumatoid arthritis), while myocarditis may induce complex arrhythmias or even heart failure (e.g. in SLE or polymyositis). Seizures or a disturbed level of consciousness can occur due to cerebral infarction or meningoencephalitis (e.g. in SLE, antiphospholipid syndrome, Wegener's granulomatosis). Rapidly progressive glomerulonephritis (SLE, Wegener's granulomatosis, microscopic polyangiitis) may be associated with pulmonary haemorrhage, while hypertension requires urgent treatment in scleroderma renal crisis. Pneumonitis or myositis due to SLE may be life threatening if not recognized and treated appropriately with adequate immunosuppression. Venous or arterial thromboses are likely to complicate the antiphospholipid syndrome, which in its primary form may be catastrophic and characterized by widespread microvascular disease with adult respiratory distress syndrome (ARDS), profound thrombocytopenia, and acute renal failure.

Physicians treating patients with autoimmune rheumatic diseases need to be constantly aware of the possibility of organ involvement, prompt diagnosis and treatment being necessary to prevent irreversible end organ damage. The immunosuppressive therapy used will be similar, regardless of the particular diagnosis.

Precise identification of an autoimmune rheumatic disease is reliant upon clinical and laboratory features, of which the presence of antinuclear antibody (and its pattern of staining), antibodies to extractable nuclear antigens, disease-specific antibodies, or ANCA are crucial. There are many instances where the disease may not be precisely labelled, and up to 20% of patients have features of several autoimmune rheumatic diseases, most commonly SLE/scleroderma and SLE/rheumatoid arthritis, or those who would be considered to have an undifferentiated autoimmune rheumatic disease. In the case of these latter diseases, treatment is guided according to disease features and the pattern of organ/system involvement.

Further reading

Bosch X, Guilabert A, Font J (2006). Antineutrophil cytoplasmic antibodies. *Lancet*, **368**, 404–18.

Giles I, Isenberg DA (2007). Antinuclear antibodies: an overview. In: Wallace DJ, Hahn BH (eds) *Dubois' lupus erythematosus*, 7th edition, Chapter 22. Lippincott Williams & Wilkins, Philadelphia.

Holers VM (2006). Are anti-cyclic citrullinated peptide antibodies pathogenic in rheumatoid arthritis. *Nat Clin Pract Rev*, **2**, 400–1.

Mok CC, Lau CS (2003). Pathogenesis of systemic lupus erythematosus. *J Clin Pathol*, **56**, 481–90.

Watts R, *et al.* (2007). Development and validation of a consensus methodology for the classification of the ANCA-associated vasculitides and polyarteritis nodosa for epidemiological studies. *Ann Rheum Dis*, **66**, 222–7.

19.11.2 **Systemic lupus erythematosus and related disorders**

Anisur Rahman and David A. Isenberg

Essentials

Systemic lupus erythematosus (SLE) is an autoimmune rheumatic disorder that can present with symptoms in almost any organ or system of the body. It is 10 to 20 times commoner in women than men, and commoner in Afro-Caribbeans than Asians than whites.

Aetiology is multifactorial, incorporating genetic, hormonal, and environmental elements. No single abnormality of the immune system can be considered responsible, pathogenesis depending on the interplay of a number of different factors, including autoantibodies, T lymphocytes, cytokines, the complement system, and apoptosis.

Clinical features

Common symptoms are constitutional (fatigue, anorexia), musculoskeletal (arthralgia/arthritis, myalgia), dermatological (alopecia, butterfly rash, vasculitic skin lesions, purpura), cardiopulmonary (breathlessness, pleurisy), and neurological (migraine, seizures, depression, psychosis).

Examination may show evidence of weight loss, low-grade fever, lymphadenopathy, arthritis (but rarely synovitis or deformity), skin rash, oral ulcers, dry eyes/mouth, pleural rub, and peripheral neuropathy (usually sensory).

Investigation and diagnosis

Investigation commonly reveals abnormalities in the following systems: (1) renal—proteinuria, microscopic haematuria, impaired glomerular filtration rate; (2) haematological—anaemia, leucopenia, lymphopenia, thrombocytopenia; and (3) cardiopulmonary—pulmonary function abnormalities.

The American College of Rheumatology classification criteria require four or more of the following to be present at some time: (1) malar rash; (2) discoid rash; (3) photosensitivity; (4) oral ulcers; (5) arthritis; (6) serositis; particular types of (7) renal, (8) neurological, and (9) haematological disorders; (10) immunological disorders (particular autoantibodies); and (11) raised titres of antinuclear antibody. In everyday practice, however, these requirements may be too stringent, and systemic lupus erythematosus should be suspected on the basis of typical clinical findings in one organ or tissue combined with the presence of appropriate autoantibodies. The antinuclear antibody assay is a sensitive (>95%) but not specific test for SLE, hence the absence of antinuclear antibody in a patient with suspected lupus raises serious doubt about the diagnosis. The presence of anti-dsDNA (and anti-Sm) antibodies is virtually specific for lupus. The most reliable measures of highly active disease are depletion of complement, and high anti-dsDNA levels.

Prognosis and management

SLE can kill (mortality c.10% at 10 years from diagnosis), but it may run a fairly indolent course in which an initial flare is followed by many years of low-grade activity. General treatment measures include (1) rest—as appropriate; (2) avoidance of overexposure to sunlight; (3) attention to modifiable cardiovascular risk factors—women with lupus between 35 and 45 years have a 50× increased risk of coronary disease; and (4) prophylaxis / treatment of osteoporosis—usually induced by steroid therapy.

Mild disease—patients whose disease activity is confined to arthralgia, tiredness, and/or mild rash can often be treated symptomatically, e.g. with simple analgesics and/or nonsteroidal anti-inflammatory agents (NSAIDs), with hydroxychloroquine added if these are not sufficient.

Treatment of flares of disease—corticosteroids and cytotoxic agents are used. A mild flare of arthralgia, myalgia, and general fatigue may be alleviated by a single intramuscular dose of corticosteroid. More severe flares of arthritis, pleuritis or pericarditis require oral prednisolone (20–40 mg daily). Renal flares require the most aggressive treatment, generally involving both corticosteroids (high-dose oral and/or intravenous pulse) and cyclophosphamide/mycophenolate mofetil. Biological therapies will be increasingly used in the future: B-cell depletion with the anti-CD20 chimeric reagent rituximab looks very promising, and trials are under way with many other agents.

Antiphospholipid antibody syndrome—immunosuppression is rarely useful and aspirin (150–300 mg daily) is recommended, with lifelong anticoagulation advised for those who have suffered recurrent thromboses or cerebral infarcts.

Pregnancy—SLE may be exacerbated during the pregnancy. Babies born to mothers with lupus are prone to the transient condition of neonatal lupus, also to heart block (particularly if the mother has anti-Ro and anti-La antibodies).

Introduction

Systemic lupus erythematosus (SLE) is an autoimmune rheumatic disorder that can present with symptoms in almost any organ or system of the body. Classification criteria that have been published by the American College of Rheumatology should be used to make the diagnosis. These are shown in Table 19.11.2.1 and demonstrate the wide variety of clinical and serological features that are associated with this condition. They provide a useful guide to the clinical features that should place the suspicion of SLE in the mind of a clinician. It is important not to be too dogmatic in searching for 'pathognomonic' features of the disease, e.g. although the characteristic butterfly rash over the face is perhaps the best-known sign of SLE, many patients will never develop such a rash.

Historical perspective

Although the term 'lupus' has been used for several hundred years, its meaning was vague until Cazerave and Clausit coined the term 'lupus erythematosus' in 1852, confining the condition to a skin rash affecting the face. The photosensitive nature of the rash (noted by Hutchinson in 1879) and the accompanying internal organ involvement (Kaposi in 1872) helped to frame the current usage of the term 'systemic lupus erythematosus' to define a multisystem disorder rather than a purely cutaneous condition. The development of the LE cell test (Hargreaves in 1948) and more importantly

Table 19.11.2.1 Criteria of the American College of Rheumatology for the classification of systemic lupus erytematosus*

1 Malar rash
2 Discoid rash
3 Photosensitivity
4 Oral ulcers
5 Arthritis
6 Serositis
  (a) Pleuritis or
  (b) Pericarditis
7 Renal disorder
  (a) Proteinuria > 0.5 g/24 h or 3+, persistently or
  (b) Cellular casts
8 Neurological disorder
  (a) Seizures or
  (b) Psychosis (having excluded other causes, e.g. drugs)
9 Haematological disorder
  (a) Haemolytic anaemia or
  (b) Leucopenia or < 4.0 ×10⁹/litre on two or more occasions
  (c) Lymphopenia or < 1.5 ×10⁹/litre on two or more occasions
  (d) Thrombocytopenia < 100 ×10⁹/litre
10 Immunological disorders
  (a) Raised antinative DNA antibody binding or
  (b) Anti-Sm antibody or
  (c) Positive finding of antiphospholipid antibodies
11 Antinuclear antibody in raised titre (in the absence of drugs known to be associated with drug-induced lupus)

*'…a person shall be said to have SLE if four or more of the 11 criteria are present, serially or simultaneously, during any interval of observation.' (Tan EM et al. (1982). The 1982 revised criteria for the classification of systemic lupus erythematosus. *Arthritis and Rheumatism* **25**, 1271–7.).

(and more specifically) the identification of anti-double-stranded (ds) DNA antibodies by four different laboratories (in 1957) facilitated the classification criteria by which SLE is now widely recognized.

Aetiology and pathology

The aetiology is multifactorial, incorporating genetic, hormonal, and environmental elements. The best-established genetic link is with the presence of null alleles of genes encoding early components of the complement cascade (C1q, C2, and C4). Over 90% of patients homozygous for C1q deficiency and 75% of those with C4 deficiency develop a lupus-like disease (similar clinical features but a relative paucity of antibodies). Major histocompatibility complex (MHC) genes, particularly *HLA A1*, *B8*, and *DR3*, have also been associated with the presence of lupus in family studies, although part of this association may be due to linkage disequilibrium with the *C4* and *C2* genes also present in that region of chromosome 6.

Hormones are likely to play a role in pathogenesis, because SLE is far more common in women than in men (see below). There is a relatively high incidence of the condition in Klinefelter's syndrome (males with the XXY karyotype), which is associated with abnormalities in oestrogen metabolism.

Viruses may be important in triggering the autoimmune dysfunction that leads to the production of pathogenic autoantibodies in SLE. Reactivation of BK polyomavirus infection, in particular, has been associated with the presence of antibodies to dsDNA in Norwegian studies. This association has not yet been confirmed in large populations.

Certain drugs induce a form of SLE that is generally characterized by the presence of antihistone rather than anti-dsDNA antibodies, a milder course of disease, and total remission when the causative drug is withdrawn. The most common drugs involved are isoniazid, procainamide, hydralazine, minocycline, penicillamine, and anticonvulsants.

No single abnormality of the immune system can be considered to be the sole cause of SLE. The pathogenesis of the disease depends on the interplay of a number of different factors, the relative importance of which may differ from one patient to another. These include autoantibodies, T lymphocytes, cytokines, the complement system, and apoptosis. Research to unravel this complex system of interrelated factors has been carried out by studying properties of cells and tissue components derived from patients with SLE and by studying mouse models of the condition.

Abnormalities of the immune system

B lymphocytes and autoantibodies

Autoantibodies are those that bind to antigens present within the tissues of the body itself. A wide variety of different autoantibodies has been described in SLE. Those most frequently reported are listed in Table 19.11.2.2.

Anti-dsDNA antibodies have been cited widely as possible causative agents in SLE, particularly in lupus glomerulonephritis. Raised titres of anti-dsDNA antibodies are found in 50 to 70% of patients with SLE, but hardly ever in healthy people or those with other diseases. Levels of these antibodies often rise and fall with disease activity, and deposits of anti-dsDNA antibodies occur in the glomeruli of patients with lupus nephritis. In experimental murine models of SLE, monoclonal anti-dsDNA antibodies can

Table 19.11.2.2 Major autoantibodies associated with systemic lupus erythematosus and their approximate prevalence in patients with the disease

Autoantibodies	Antigen/epitope	Approximate prevalence (%)
Intracellular		
DNA	dsDNA, (ssDNA)	50–70
Histone	H1, 2A, 2B, 3, 4	30–80
Sm	B/B', D, E, F, G	30 (Afro-Caribbean), ~ 10 (Caucasian)
U1RNP	A, C, 70 kDa ribonucleoprotein	20–35
rRNP	Three subunits: 38, 19, 17 kDa	5–15
Ro/SS-A	60, 52 kDa protein bound to cytoplasmic RNA (hY1–hY5)	10–15
La/SS-B	48 kDa protein bound to variety of RNA, U1RNA, hY RNA	10–15
Heat shock protein (hsp)	hsp 90	30
hnRNP	A2 protein (also known as RA-33)	30
Cell membrane		
Cardiolipin	Phospholipids	20–40
Neuronal antigen	Expressed on neuronal cell lines grown *in vitro*	70–90 (+CNS), ~ 10 (−CNS)
Lymphocyte	HLA component	~ 75 (IgM), ~ 45 (IgG)
Red cell	Non-Rh related	< 10
Platelet		< 10
Extracellular		
Rheumatoid factor	Fc region of IgG	~ 25
C1q	Complement component	20–45

be shown to deposit in the glomeruli and to be associated with proteinuria.

The titre of anti-dsDNA antibodies present in the bloodstream of patients with SLE can be a useful indicator of disease activity. It is increasingly clear, however, that not all anti-dsDNA antibodies are equally likely to be associated with tissue damage. Antibodies of the IgG isotype, which show specific high-affinity binding to dsDNA, generally show the closest association with disease activity in patients and the greatest ability to cause renal damage in experimental models.

Why are anti-dsDNA antibodies produced in patients with SLE?

Studies of monoclonal anti-dsDNA antibodies derived from patients or mice indicate that those that show the isotype and binding properties described above often show sequence characteristics suggestive of antigen-driven somatic mutation. This is the process whereby mutations accumulate in the expressed immunoglobulin gene sequences of a B lymphocyte under the influence of a particular antigen. The mutations are accumulated nonrandomly, such that the end-result is an increase in specificity and affinity of binding. This process is dependent on help from T lymphocytes and on the presence of an appropriate antigen. Naked mammalian DNA is, however, a poor immunogen in experimental animals, and the concentration of free DNA in the bloodstream is low even in patients with SLE. It is therefore believed that the antigen that stimulates production of high-affinity anti-dsDNA antibodies is probably a complex of DNA and protein. Nucleosomes derived from cell apoptosis (see below) may be the most important antigens involved in stimulating both T cells and B cells in SLE, although a role for viral DNA-binding proteins has also been suggested.

How do anti-dsDNA autoantibodies exert their pathogenic effects?

Deposition of IgG and complement in inflamed tissues such as kidney and skin is a consistent feature of active SLE. The pathogenic potential of autoantibodies in SLE (particularly IgG anti-dsDNA) may therefore rest on their ability to deposit in these tissues and to activate complement. Why are anti-dsDNA antibodies deposited in target tissues? Much of the work designed to answer this question has concentrated on autoantibodies in lupus nephritis. Originally, it was felt that DNA–anti-DNA immune complexes would form in the bloodstream and accumulate in glomeruli as the blood was filtered there. However, it has not been possible to demonstrate large quantities of such complexes in the blood of patients with SLE, although their clearance may well be abnormal due to complement deficiency. Anti-dsDNA antibodies may be targeted to the kidney due to cross-reaction with cell surface proteins there, or may deposit due to an interaction with histones and heparan sulphate. According to this latter model, anti-dsDNA antibodies bind to DNA in nucleosomes, and the positively charged histones in these nucleosomes bind to negatively charged heparan sulphate in the renal basement membrane.

Antiphospholipid antibodies

Between 20 and 30% of patients with SLE possess serum antiphospholipid antibodies. The origin of these antibodies may be similar to that of anti-dsDNA antibodies because monoclonal antiphospholipid antibodies from patients with SLE also show antigen-driven accumulations of somatic mutations. The antigen in this case may be phosphatidylserine on the outer surfaces of blebs derived from apoptotic cells.

Antiphospholipid (APL) antibodies may be present in healthy people or in those with infectious diseases such as syphilis, in which case they have no adverse effects. In patients with SLE, however, APL antibodies may cause arterial or venous thromboses or miscarriages. The combination of these clinical problems with the presence of APL antibodies defines the antiphospholipid syndrome (APS). APS may occur either in patients with other autoimmune diseases (particularly SLE), or alone in the absence of other disease (primary APS). Although it was previously thought that APL antibodies exerted their effects almost wholly through promotion of thrombus formation, it is now clear that they may have many other direct effects on platelets, monocytes, endothelial cells, and the trophoblast. The mechanism by which thrombosis is altered is not fully understood, but it has become clear that APL antibodies found in APS often bind to protein antigens associated with phospholipids rather than the phospholipids themselves. The most important of these proteins is β_2-glycoprotein 1, and a direct test for anti-β_2-glycoprotein 1 is an alternative diagnostic test for APS.

T lymphocytes

As the process of antigen-driven selection of mutations in B lymphocytes is dependent on help from helper T lymphocytes, it would be reasonable to suppose that antigen-specific T cells might also contribute to the pathogenesis of the disease. The isolation of T-cell clones reactive with DNA and/or DNA-binding proteins such as histones has been demonstrated from both patients with SLE and murine models of the disease. The clones frequently show specificity for histone epitopes that are cryptic (i.e. not exposed) in normal chromatin. These results reinforce the idea that the antigenic stimulus for production of pathogenic T cells and autoantibodies in SLE may be a DNA/histone complex rather than DNA alone.

Patients with SLE have decreased levels of the subset of T cells carrying the CD4 and CD45 Ro surface markers. This population may be involved in stimulation of suppressor T lymphocytes such that suppression in these patients is insufficient to prevent the production and survival of autoreactive B-lymphocyte and helper T-lymphocyte clones.

Apoptosis and complement

The links between apoptosis, complement, and lupus are complicated. MRL *lpr/lpr* mice are deficient in apoptosis because they lack the Fas protein that plays a major role in promoting this process. These mice develop a disease very similar to SLE, with death resulting from glomerulonephritis. One possible reason for this might be the failure of the immune system to delete by apoptosis autoreactive clones of T or B lymphocytes, which are then able to cause autoimmune disease. By contrast, humans with the equivalent genetic lesion to MRL *lpr/lpr* mice do not develop SLE, and other strains of mice show an accumulation of apoptotic debris within nephritic kidneys, which resemble those of SLE. A simple deficiency in apoptosis is therefore unlikely to be the underlying mechanism in SLE.

Apoptosis leads to the production of surface blebs of cellular material. These blebs include a number of the antigens to which autoantibodies develop in SLE, notably DNA and associated nuclear proteins and negatively charged phospholipids. A deficiency in the clearance of products of apoptosis has been demonstrated, which might allow the production of as wide a spectrum of autoantibodies as found in SLE. Removal of immune complexes containing such potentially antigenic material may be compromised in patients with SLE. Monocytes derived from such patients show reduced phagocytosis of cell debris *in vitro*. This process may be complement dependent, as people with homozygous C2 deficiency process immune complexes very differently from normal controls. Administration of fresh frozen plasma to such patients as a source of complement is successful in ameliorating the symptoms of SLE and in normalizing (albeit transiently) their processing of immune complexes.

C1q knockout mice develop a form of glomerulonephritis similar to that seen in SLE, and their kidneys are characterized by accumulations of apoptotic debris. In fact knockout mice deficient in both the classic and alternative pathways of complement develop this form of glomerulonephritis, showing that in this model the protective effects of complement outweigh its role as an effector of inflammation. Similarly, as noted earlier, humans homozygous for C1q deficiency develop a form of SLE with the frequent occurrence of nephritis.

Cytokines

Cytokines enhance the ability of cells to interact and are therefore critically important in abnormalities in both T- and B-cell functions seen in patients with lupus. Table 19.11.2.3 summarizes the major differences between the different subsets of T-helper (Th) cells in terms of their cytokine profiles and functions. The balance between cytokines from Th1 and Th2 cells is essential in determining the outcome of the immune response. Lupus might be expected to be a disease in which Th2 cells predominate, resulting in excessive help for B cells and overproduction of antibodies. In support of this notion, increased levels of interleukin 10 (IL-10) have been found in patients with lupus. This cytokine promotes secretion of antibodies by B lymphocytes but suppresses Th1 cells and thus impairs cell-mediated immunity, a characteristic feature of the disease. Both macrophage and natural killer cell-mediated cytotoxicity are frequently impaired in patients with lupus. Interferon-γ-induced enhancement of both types of cytotoxicity is also impaired, despite normal levels of interferon-γ production by lupus Th1 cells.

Accessory cells in lupus seem to produce insufficient amounts of IL-1 to provide the necessary activation signals for T cells. Both CD4+ and CD8+ T cells have been described as producing either normal or decreased amounts of IL-2 in response to exogenous antigens. Such a reduction is likely to have a profound effect on T-cell responses.

Interferon-α is increasingly recognized as playing a major role in the development of SLE. Levels of this cytokine are raised in patients with SLE, genetic studies show that interferon-related genes are risk factors for SLE, and gene expression studies show that such genes are activated in patients with the disease. Lupus in the NZB/NZW mouse model of lupus can be accelerated by the presence of interferon-α. Cytokines such as interferon-α and IL-10 are increasingly being considered as possible targets for future therapeutic agents in lupus.

Histopathology

The two tissues most often subjected to biopsy in SLE are the skin and kidneys.

Skin biopsies are chiefly carried out to facilitate the diagnosis of an atypical rash. If SLE is suspected, it is important to take a sample of apparently normal skin as well as skin from the rash. Both should show deposition of IgG and complement at the dermoepidermal junction (Fig. 19.11.2.1).

Renal biopsy may be performed to establish the diagnosis of SLE when this is not certain, e.g. in a patient with a poorly characterized multisystem disease with renal involvement. In a patient with known SLE it may be employed to help determine prognosis and decide on treatment when renal function is deteriorating, e.g. with the development of nephrotic syndrome and/or declining glomerular filtration rate (GFR). The glomerular pathology can be graded on a scale of I to V according to the World Health Organization criteria, and scores for activity and chronicity can be used to determine appropriate treatment and the risk of a progressive decline in renal function. The subject of renal pathology in SLE is considered further in Chapter 21.10.3.

Epidemiology

The incidence of SLE in the United Kingdom is about 4 cases/100 000 people per year. It occurs between 10 and 20 times more frequently in women than in men, and is more common in some ethnic groups. A study in Birmingham, United Kingdom gave the prevalence of SLE in women as 206 per 100 000 in people of African–Caribbean origin, 91 per 100 000 in those of Asian origin, and 36 per 100 000 in white people. These gender and racial differences are broadly consistent with those reported from studies in the United States of America and the Caribbean, although the reported prevalence of SLE in Africa is much lower.

Table 19.11.2.3 (a) Subsets of CD4+ T cells

	Function	Cytokines
T-helper 1 cell	Cell mediated immunity	IFN-γ, IL-10 (humans only), IL-12, TNF-α
T-helper 2 cell	B cell help	IL-4, IL-10

(b) Cytokine profiles in patients with active systemic lupus erythematosus

Cytokine	Serum level*	Spontaneous	Stimulation in vitro
IFN-γ	↑	Low	↓
TNF-α	↑ (or normal)	↓ (DR2, DQw1; ↑ nephritis), ↑ (DR3, 4; ↓ nephritis)	↓
IL-1	n.d.	↑ PBM production	↓ Monocyte production
IL-2	↑	Low	↓
IL-4	n.d.	Low	Low
IL-6	↑	↑	–
IL-10	↑ (or normal)	↑ (or normal)	Normal

*Serum levels of cytokines are difficult to interpret since these may be affected by soluble cytokine receptors which are shed from cells. Among the known shed receptors are those for IL-1, IL-2, IL-6, TNF-α, and IFN-γ. Soluble TNF-αR and IL-2R levels are increased in systemic lupus and correlate with disease activity and lupus nephritis.

Abbreviations: IFN-γ, interferon-γ; n.d. = not detected; PBM = peripheral blood mononuclear cell, TNF-α, tumour necrosis factor-α.

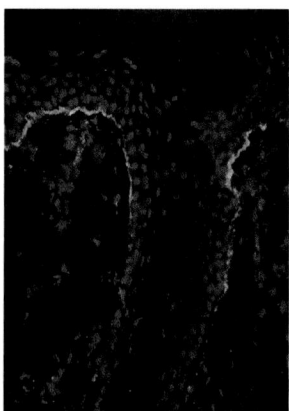

Fig. 19.11.2.1 Immunofluorescence microscopy showing deposition of IgG at the dermoepidermal junction in the skin of a patient with systemic lupus erythematosus (sometimes called the lupus band test).

Clinical features

SLE is a chronic condition punctuated by flares of acute activity. The overall severity of the disease in a particular patient depends on the nature and frequency of these flares and the long-term permanent damage that they cause.

The diverse clinical features of SLE mean that the disease may present to any of a number of different specialists, including rheumatologists, dermatologists, nephrologists, and general physicians. It is important to be aware of SLE as a possible diagnosis in any patient, especially a woman aged between 15 and 50, in whom a number of different organs are inflamed either simultaneously or sequentially. The frequency of occurrence of symptoms in various organs is shown in Table 19.11.2.4.

According to the diagnostic guidelines published by the American College of Rheumatology (see Table 19.11.2.1), SLE may be diagnosed where a patient meets at least 4 of the 11 criteria specified (though not necessarily at a single time). In everyday practice, however, these requirements may be too stringent, and SLE is often suspected on the basis of typical clinical findings in one organ or tissue combined with the presence of appropriate autoantibodies.

Constitutional symptoms

Patients with SLE find fatigue to be the most troublesome feature of the disease, excessive tiredness being both very common and difficult to treat. Hypothyroidism coexists in 5 to 10% of patients with SLE and so thyroid function tests should be performed in the fatigued patient. There is an ongoing debate as to whether fibromyalgia is a significant comorbid condition.

Weight loss and low-grade fever may both be indicative of disease activity. Lymphadenopathy is also recognized. The nodes may be markedly enlarged but show no diagnostic features on biopsy, which may nevertheless be necessary to exclude other conditions such as lymphoma.

Musculoskeletal involvement

Arthralgia/arthritis is the most common symptom in SLE, occurring in 90% of patients. This may be severe but is rarely associated with frank synovitis. Effusions may occur but the fluid shows no diagnostic features.

Erosive arthritis is uncommon, but up to 5% of patients may have an overlap syndrome with features of rheumatoid arthritis as well as SLE. These patients tend to have both serum rheumatoid factor and erosions.

When progressive deformity of the hands does occur in SLE, it is usually due to an aggressive tenosynovitis and tendon dysfunction rather than to joint damage. This leads to reversible subluxation of the joints, often known as Jaccoud's arthropathy (Fig. 19.11.2.2).

Development of hip pain in patients who have been treated with corticosteroids should raise the suspicion of avascular necrosis of the femoral head, which may be diagnosed on a plain radiograph or, in earlier stages, by MRI. Corticosteroids also promote osteoporosis, which can be diagnosed in the presymptomatic phase by bone density scanning, but may present with the acute pain of a vertebral fracture.

Myalgia is common and a true myositis may occur in 5% of cases. Corticosteroid-induced proximal myopathy may also be a problem where these drugs have been used for long periods.

Table 19.11.2.4 Cumulative prevalence of clinical features in patients with systemic lupus erythematosus

Clinical feature	Approximate cumulative prevalence (%)
Musculoskeletal	
Arthralgia/arthritis	90
Tenosynovitis	20
Myalgia	50
Myositis	5
Cardiopulmonary	
Shortness of breath	40
Pleurisy	35
Pleural effusion	25
Lupus pneumonitis	5
Interstitial fibrosis	5
Pulmonary function abnormalities	85
Cardiomegaly	20
Pericarditis	15
Cardiomyopathy	10
Myocardial infarction	5
Gastrointestinal	
Anorexia	40
Nausea	15
Vomiting	< 10
Diarrhoea	< 10
Ascites	< 10
Abdominal pain	30
Hepatomegaly	25
Splenomegaly	10
Renal	
Haematuria	10
Proteinuria	60
Casts	30
Serum albumin < 35 g/l	30
Serum creatinine > 125 µmol/l	30
Reduced 24-h creatinine clearance	35
Cerebral	
Depression	15
Psychosis	15
Seizures	20
Hemiplegia	10
Cranial nerve lesions	10
Cerebellar signs	5
Meningitis	1
Migraine	40

(Continued)

Table 19.11.2.4 *(Cont'd)* Cumulative prevalence of clinical features in patients with systemic lupus erythematosus

Clinical feature	Approximate cumulative prevalence (%)
Haematological	
Anaemia (iron deficiency)	30
Anaemia (of chronic disease)	75
Autoimmune haemolytic anaemia	15
Leucopenia	40
Lymphopenia	80
Thrombocytopenia	25
Circulating anticoagulants	15
Dermatological	
Butterfly rash	40
Erythematous maculopapular eruption	35
Discoid lupus	20
Relapsing nodular non-suppurative panniculitis	< 5
Vasculitic skin lesions	40
Livedo reticularis	20
Purpuric lesions	40
Alopecia	20–50

Cutaneous and mucosal involvement

Photosensitivity is very common, particularly in white female patients. Patients should be advised to avoid strong sunlight and to wear protective clothing and/or a high-factor sunblock.

The butterfly rash over the malar area of the face occurs in up to one-third of patients (Fig. 19.11.2.3). A number of other forms of cutaneous involvement can occur, although these are less specific for SLE. These include maculopapular rash, discoid lesions, alopecia, and nailfold infarcts. Scarring alopecia may be particularly distressing and difficult to treat (Fig. 19.11.2.4).

A variant of SLE in which cutaneous manifestations dominate is known as subacute cutaneous lupus. This condition is often associated with anti-Ro antibodies and may be exacerbated by smoking cigarettes.

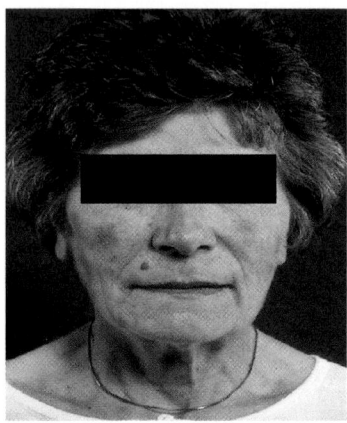

Fig. 19.11.2.3 Malar 'butterfly' rash.

APL antibodies are associated with a nonraised lattice-like rash concentrated particularly over the thighs and arms: livedo reticularis (Fig. 19.11.2.5).

Recurrent crops of oral ulcers are common enough to be recognized as one of the diagnostic criteria for SLE. About 20% of patients develop secondary Sjögren's syndrome; in this condition the dry eyes and mouth may respond to artificial tears and saliva.

Renal involvement

Glomerulonephritis is the most serious and potentially lethal manifestation of SLE. Its presence may be detected by the finding of haematuria and/or proteinuria on routine stick testing of the urine. It may present as the nephrotic syndrome or, less commonly, as a florid nephritis with haematuria, proteinuria, hypertension, and acute renal failure with red cell casts in the urine. The diagnosis and management of glomerulonephritis in SLE are more fully discussed in Chapter 21.10.3.

It is important to be aware of the possibility of glomerulonephritis in any patient with SLE (Fig. 19.11.2.6). Measurement of blood pressure and analysis of urine should be carried out at each consultation. Early diagnosis and treatment are invaluable in avoiding deterioration of renal function to the extent that dialysis or renal transplantation become necessary.

Patients with APS may develop a different type of renal lesion characterized by thrombi in small renal vessels rather than by glomerulonephritis. These patients develop hypertension and impairment of renal excretory function, detected as a fall in

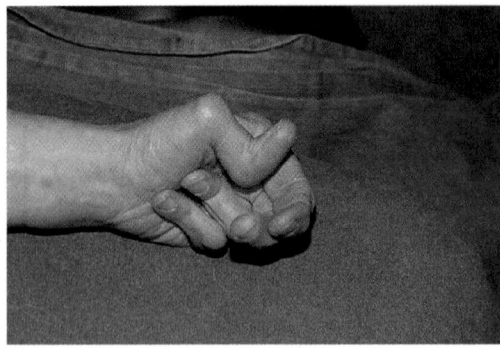

Fig. 19.11.2.2 Deforming Jaccoud's arthropathy.

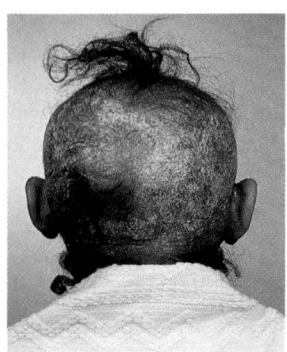

Fig. 19.11.2.4 Severe scarring alopecia.

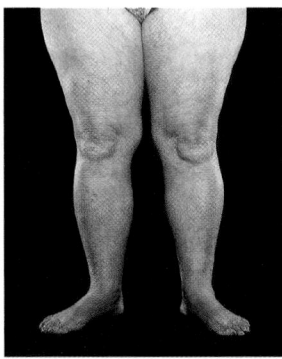

Fig. 19.11.2.5 Livedo reticularis.

estimated GFR (eGFR), rather than proteinuria, and are best managed by anticoagulation rather than immunosuppression.

Respiratory involvement

The most common form of respiratory involvement in SLE is pleuritis, manifesting either as pleuritic chest pain or as breathlessness caused by pleural effusion. The lung parenchyma is more rarely involved, but fibrosis can occur.

A patient with SLE may present with shortness of breath or chest pain for a number of reasons. Pulmonary emboli must be suspected in those with APL antibodies. Infections are common in immunosuppressed patients and rib fractures may occur, particularly in those rendered osteoporotic by treatment with corticosteroids.

The shrinking lung syndrome is characterized by reduced lung volumes and poor respiratory reserve in the face of a normal appearance of the lung parenchyma on CT. It is believed to arise from basal atelectasis in association with diaphragmatic dysfunction.

Cardiovascular involvement

The most common cardiac manifestation of SLE is pericarditis, which occurs in about 15% of patients. This generally presents with chest pain or an asymptomatic friction rub. Pericardial effusions may occur, but are rarely large enough to cause haemodynamic compromise.

Myocarditis and endocarditis are less common, though postmortem and echocardiographic studies suggest that both may occur without symptoms in a significant proportion of patients with SLE, e.g. the classic endocarditis described by Libman and Sacks is characterized by small vegetations that often do not cause murmurs or cardiac compromise, but which have been identified in up to 50% of patients with SLE post mortem.

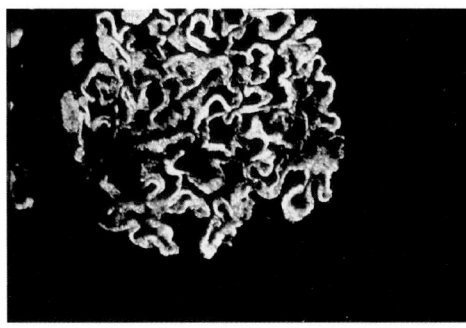

Fig. 19.11.2.6 Immunofluorescence microscopy showing deposition of IgG in the glomerulus of a patient with lupus nephritis.

It is increasingly recognized that atherosclerosis and its sequelae in the cerebral and cardiac circulations are more common in patients with SLE than in the general population. Women with lupus aged between 35 and 45 have a 50 times increased risk of coronary disease. This may be partially due to the use of corticosteroids, which raise serum cholesterol and can promote hypertension. Patients possessing APL antibodies are also at a higher risk of stroke or arterial thrombosis.

Raynaud's phenomenon occurs in about a third of patients with SLE, although it is not usually as severe as that seen in systemic sclerosis. Vasculitis presents with a skin rash or ulcers that may be very difficult to heal, but rarely affects the internal organs.

Gastrointestinal involvement

Similar to pleuritis, peritonitis may occur in patients with SLE and must be considered in the event of abdominal pain, while remembering that patients with lupus are not protected from more common causes of this condition, e.g. appendicitis.

Involvement of the liver and pancreas is recognized but uncommon. The term 'lupoid hepatitis' was previously used for a form of autoimmune hepatitis characterized by the presence of autoantibodies, but these patients do not generally have any form of SLE and the term is misleading. Minor enlargements of the liver and/or spleen occur in 10 to 25% of cases, but these are usually asymptomatic and require no treatment.

Neuropsychiatric involvement

SLE can affect the nervous system in many ways, so that the true incidence of neuropsychiatric involvement is difficult to quantify. Symptoms such as poor memory, change of personality, and depression or anxiety occur in many patients. It is difficult, however, to be sure whether these are caused by cerebral SLE or represent a reaction to the diagnosis and treatment of the disease.

More florid presentations such as psychotic episodes and convulsions are well recognized but rare. By contrast to the milder symptoms noted above, these manifestations generally call for immunosuppression.

Migraine occurs in up to 40% of patients with SLE, particularly in the presence of APL antibodies. Peripheral neuropathy can occur, and is usually sensory rather than motor. Cranial nerve palsies are less common, as is transverse myelitis (another feature linked to APL antibodies).

Ocular involvement can include episcleritis, conjunctivitis, and the presence of cytoid bodies (white patches on the retina). Patients treated with high-dose steroids may develop cataracts.

Haematological involvement

A normochromic normocytic anaemia is frequently seen in SLE, particularly during periods of high disease activity. Microcytic iron-deficiency anaemia may result from blood loss from gastritis and ulcers in patients treated with nonsteroidal anti-inflammatory drugs. Anaemia may also result from chronic renal failure in lupus nephritis.

A positive Coombs' test, signifying the presence of antibodies to red blood cells, is present in up to 20% of patients with SLE but does not always indicate haemolytic anaemia.

The presence of lymphopenia (less than 1.5×10^9/l) is common, occurring in up to 80% of patients. Neutropenia may occur secondary to the use of cytotoxic drugs such as azathioprine or cyclophosphamide.

Three different types of thrombocytopenia occur in SLE. The mildest form is characterized by stable platelet levels of between 50 and $100 \times 10^9/l$, is rarely symptomatic, and usually requires no treatment. Other patients develop an acute autoimmune thrombocytopenia with levels dropping rapidly below $10 \times 10^9/l$, but usually rising when treated with oral steroids. A third group of patients present with thrombocytopenia alone, are treated with steroids, intravenous immunoglobulins, rituximab, or (rarely these days) splenectomy, and some years later develop full-blown SLE. Thrombocytopenia is also one of the cardinal features of the APS and may be severe enough to necessitate splenectomy in that condition.

Other complicating disorders

About 30% of lupus patients have another autoimmune condition, including Sjögren's syndrome (the most common, affecting some 15 to 20% of patients with lupus), APS (10 to 15%), autoimmune thyroid disease (hyper- or hypothyroidism, 5 to 10%), and (less frequently) rheumatoid arthritis, myasthenia gravis, coeliac disease, diabetes, and pernicious anaemia.

Differential diagnosis

SLE is truly a chameleon of a disease. Its protean clinical manifestations mean that, theoretically, it should enter the differential diagnosis of virtually any unexplained symptom/feature. However, its predilection for women during the child-bearing years does restrict this potential diagnostic confusion significantly.

Among its general features, fever, weight loss, anorexia, and lymphadenopathy may easily be confused with a lymphoproliferative cancer, hence biopsy of a swollen lymph gland may often be required to be sure of the underlying problem. Polyarthralgia or polyarthritis in a young woman could be due to rheumatoid arthritis or lupus. As both rheumatoid factor and antinuclear antibodies can be found in both conditions, there is obvious room for confusion, but anti-CCP antibodies (rheumatoid) and anti-dsDNA antibodies (lupus) are more specific tests that can usually resolve the matter.

About 15% of patients presenting with 'idiopathic' thrombocytopenic purpura will eventually develop lupus. Unfortunately there are usually no clues at the onset to distinguish this 15% and very long-term follow-up may be needed.

Antibodies to Ro, La, Sm, RNP (ribonucleoprotein), and dsDNA may be detectable in the serum of patients who will develop lupus up to 10 years before the disease becomes clinically manifest, and rarely these antibodies are found in the healthy relatives of patients.

Occasionally lupus may present with isolated central nervous system (CNS) disease including convulsions, schizophrenic-like conditions, and neuropathies. As with many other clinical features, the most important consideration is to try to include systemic lupus in the differential diagnosis. The serological tests for it are widely available and will help to establish, quickly, the correct diagnosis.

Clinical investigation

Autoantibodies

The most commonly requested test to screen for SLE is the antinuclear antibody assay. A positive antinuclear antibody simply indicates that the patient's blood contains antibodies that will bind to the nuclei of a sample of cells used in the test. The test is a sensitive one because over 95% of patients with SLE are antinuclear antibody positive. Although a small group of patients do seem to have persistently antinuclear antibody-negative SLE, the absence of antinuclear antibody in a patient with suspected lupus raises serious doubt about the diagnosis.

The specificity of the antinuclear antibody test for SLE is not high. The titre of antibody represents the highest dilution of the patient's serum at which the test is still positive. Low-titre antinuclear antibody (1 in 10) is of little significance and may occur in healthy people. Higher titres (1 in 160 or more) are more worrying and are found in most patients with SLE and in patients with other autoimmune conditions including rheumatoid arthritis, systemic sclerosis, and Sjögren's syndrome. However, some people with high-titre antinuclear antibody may be followed in rheumatology clinics for years without developing a frank autoimmune disease.

The finding of a positive antinuclear antibody in a patient with symptoms suggestive of SLE should lead to a series of other autoantibody tests. These are listed in Table 19.11.2.2 together with the identity of the target antigen and the approximate prevalence of the antibodies.

Anti-dsDNA antibody levels are particularly useful. This test is virtually specific for SLE (as is the anti-Sm antibody), especially if the immunoglobulins are of the IgG isotype. The anti-dsDNA result is usually quantified and this value is often a measure of the activity of the disease, but there is a group of patients who have persistently high anti-dsDNA antibody levels but no clinically active disease (serologically active, clinically quiescent). Long-term follow-up suggests that many but not all of these patients will eventually flare. In one study, trial patients were treated with high-dose corticosteroids on the basis of anti-dsDNA levels alone. In comparison with a control group treated only when symptoms or signs also suggested disease activity, the trial group had less disease activity overall and fewer flares. However, frequent large doses of corticosteroids resulted in significant side effects and a number of participants dropped out of this arm of the trial. Anti-dsDNA should be used only as an adjunct to the clinical impression of disease activity when deciding on a treatment regimen.

Anti-Ro and anti-La antibodies are linked to concurrent Sjögren's syndrome. Mothers who have these antibodies have a higher incidence of neonatal lupus (see below) and should be advised about this before embarking on a pregnancy. Anti-Ro antibodies are also associated with photosensitivity.

There are no good antibody markers for the presence of disease of the CNS. Antibodies to ribosomal protein P were previously thought to have some value in the diagnosis of CNS lupus, but this has not been borne out by later results and the test is not available routinely in most laboratories. More recently, murine and clinical studies have suggested that antibodies to the N-Methyl-D-aspartate receptor (anti-NMDAR) may act on cerebral tissue to cause clinical features of CNS lupus, but this test is not used routinely in clinical practice.

APL antibodies can be recognized by one of two assays. The enzyme-linked immunosorbent assay for binding to cardiolipin distinguishes IgM and IgG isotypes. This is helpful because the level of IgG APL antibodies is a better predictor of clinical sequelae than that of IgM. APL antibodies can also be diagnosed by testing the clotting properties of the blood *in vitro* in the Russell's viper venom test. An abnormal result in this assay is reported as showing the presence of a lupus anticoagulant. It is quite possible for the anticardiolipin test to be positive while the lupus anticoagulant assay is negative or vice versa. If either is positive, the patient may be at risk of manifestations of the APS. Anti-β_2-glycoprotein 1 tests are now becoming available commercially, offering a third way of detecting APL antibodies.

Coombs' test and assays for antithyroid antibodies are often requested in patients with SLE, particularly those with coexisting anaemia or hypothyroidism.

Measures of disease activity and end-organ damage

Blood and urine tests

The most reliable measures of highly active disease are depletion of complement and high anti-dsDNA levels. The erythrocyte sedimentation rate (ESR) also tends to be increased in active disease, unlike the level of C-reactive protein (CRP). The combination of high ESR and normal CRP in a patient with a multisystem disorder should raise the suspicion of SLE, leading to appropriate autoantibody tests as described above. The CRP may, however, be raised in the presence of infection, serositis, or arthritis.

Complement components C3 and C4 are the most commonly measured, and both tend to fall in active SLE. A persistently very low level of either C3 or C4 (or a high level of their degradation products C3d or C4d), regardless of immunosuppressive therapy, may signify the presence of a homozygous complement deficiency disorder. Although such disorders are very rare, it is important to diagnose them because they respond better to infusions of fresh frozen plasma than to immunosuppression.

It is important to measure creatinine and electrolyte values regularly and to check the urine for proteinuria and/or haematuria. These measures ensure that renal involvement is diagnosed early. It must be remembered that substantial deterioration in renal function may occur before serum creatinine rises beyond the normal range, an issue emphasized by the now routine reporting of eGFR. If the patient can reliably perform a 24-h urinary collection, then creatinine clearance can provide a more precise estimate of GFR, but this, or radio-isotopic methods of measuring GFR, are rarely required in routine clinical practice. Persistent proteinuria on dipstick testing should be quantified by measuring the albumin/protein:creatinine ratio in a spot urinary sample (or with a 24-h urinary collection).

Liver function tests are usually normal in SLE (abnormal in less than 10% of patients), but a baseline value should be measured, particularly in cases where potentially hepatotoxic drugs such as azathioprine may be used. Thyroid function abnormalities, particularly hypothyroidism, are well recognized to coexist with SLE.

A full blood count should be measured regularly. Falling haemoglobin, white cell count, and platelet counts may all occur (see under Haematological involvement above). Anaemia in the presence of a positive Coombs' test may indicate haemolysis, which can be confirmed by requesting a blood film and serum haptoglobins.

Infections occur commonly in patients with SLE, particularly in those on high-dose immunosuppressants. Infection may not always be accompanied by high fever or leucocytosis, although CRP is usually raised. It is wise to carry out blood and urine cultures whenever even mild pyrexia is accompanied by a deterioration in health.

Imaging

Plain radiographs are rarely useful in SLE. There is no characteristic appearance in the joints, and chest radiographs are unlikely to show abnormalities except in the presence of infection or effusion.

Requests for more specialized imaging studies should be directed by the clinical findings, e.g. the presence of dyspnoea and abnormal respiratory function tests often necessitates a CT scan of the thorax, which is the investigation of choice for diagnosis of pulmonary fibrosis. Echocardiography is useful if pericardial effusion, myocarditis, or endocarditis is suspected clinically. Bone density scanning is becoming increasingly important, since patients with SLE are often at risk of osteoporosis due to the use of corticosteroids and reduced capacity for physical exercise during young adult life.

Criteria for diagnosis

Although strictly speaking classification and diagnostic criteria are not synonymous, the classification criteria discussed earlier, and shown in Table 19.11.2.1, are widely used for diagnostic purposes. Some unease with these criteria has been expressed, notably why 4 of the 11 features are confined to one organ system (mucocutaneous), and whether anti-nucleosome antibodies should be allowed as an alternative to anti-dsDNA antibodies. The Systemic Lupus International Collaborating Clinics group is reassessing the currently used classification criteria.

Treatment

SLE is a disease that still has the potential to kill. In many cases, however, the condition runs a fairly indolent course in which an initial flare is followed by many years of low-grade activity. General measures of value in the treatment of SLE are shown in Table 19.11.2.5.

In the pharmacological management of a patient with SLE, the clinician will typically seek to answer four 'classic' questions:

1 Can the patient be managed without immunosuppression?

2 If immunosuppression is needed, how should it best be started?

3 If immunosuppression is being used, is the current level of immunosuppression inadequate or excessive? How should it be increased or reduced?

4 Does the patient have any side effects from the drugs?

A fifth is increasingly being posed: would any of the new biologic treatments be of value?

Table 19.11.2.5 Treatment of lupus—general measures

1 Rest as appropriate; try to avoid stress
2 Avoid over-exposure to heat and sunlight. Use sun protection factor 15+ (30+ in United States) if in a sunny country; avoid exposing an arm on an open car window
3 Try to adhere to a low-fat diet and consider adding fish oil derivatives
4 Vaccination, for foreign travel etc., apart from 'live' vaccines in patients on immunosuppressives, is not contraindicated though the precise nature of the immune response differs from that in healthy individuals
5 Medium- or high-oestrogen contraceptive pills should be avoided—progesterone only or the lowest possible oestrogen pill (or other methods of contraception) are advised
6 The use of hormone replacement in the menopause remains controversial. Many patients do tolerate it without flaring, but not all

Is immunosuppression required?

Patients whose disease activity is confined to arthralgia, tiredness, and/or mild rash do not usually have greatly raised ESR or anti-dsDNA antibodies or reduced complement. These patients can often be treated symptomatically, e.g. with agents such as paracetamol and diclofenac to control joint pain.

Where such symptoms are more severe, the antimalarial agent hydroxychloroquine at a starting dose of 400 mg/day may be useful. This drug has less potential for retinal toxicity than the closely related chloroquine and is therefore preferred in SLE. It is often possible to reduce the dose to 200 mg/day after 3 months and gradually withdraw it thereafter. Regular blood tests are not required to monitor the effects of hydroxychloroquine, but there is a very small risk of retinopathy such that review by an ophthalmologist every 6 to 12 months is considered advisable in many units. The drug has the useful 'side effect' of lowering lipid levels.

Where the main symptoms in a patient with SLE are those of the APS immunosuppression is rarely useful. Aspirin at a dose of 150 to 300 mg daily is recommended for those with mild symptoms of the disease or who have other risk factors for thrombosis. Patients who have had recurrent thromboses or cerebral infarcts and who have serum APL antibodies should usually be treated with lifelong anticoagulation. This is a major commitment for a young patient and raises particular problems in pregnancy (discussed below).

Some patients require a low maintenance dose of oral steroids to control their symptoms even though laboratory indices do not indicate high activity of disease. A dose of 5 to 7.5 mg daily is typically used in such cases. Topical steroids may be useful where lupus activity is confined to the skin.

Judging the dose of immunosuppression

Corticosteroids and cytotoxic agents are used to treat flares of disease. A mild flare of arthralgia, myalgia, and general fatigue may be alleviated by a single intramuscular dose of a corticosteroid preparation such as prednisolone acetate (usually 50 to 125 mg are given).

More severe flares of arthritis, pleuritis, or pericarditis require oral prednisolone at a dose of 20 to 40 mg daily. This usually leads to a rapid improvement in symptoms, and the dose of prednisolone can then be reduced by 5 mg every 1 to 2 weeks until it reaches 5 mg/day. It may not be possible to withdraw the drug completely for several months.

Alternatively, a shorter course of corticosteroids can be given intravenously. A typical course would consist of 500 to 750 mg methylprednisolone given over 3 to 4 h on each of 3 successive days. This requires admission to hospital, making it less convenient than oral therapy, and it is generally reserved for those patients who are not responding to oral prednisolone or cannot tolerate that drug in high doses.

Autoimmune haemolytic anaemia requires higher doses (60–80 mg/day) of oral prednisolone, with the dose reduced in 5- to 10-mg increments according to the clinical response. Azathioprine may be required as a steroid-sparing agent and is used at a dose of 2.5 to 3 mg/kg per day.

Renal flares of SLE require the most aggressive treatment, generally involving both corticosteroids and cyclophosphamide. A number of regimens have been used, with debate continuing as to which is optimal. An 'older' regimen of high-dose oral prednisolone and 750 mg intravenous cyclophosphamide monthly for 6 months,

then 3 monthly for 2 years, has fallen into disrepute. Although reasonably effective, its side effects (especially infection and infertility) have led to the use of alternative regimens, including lower doses of intravenous cyclophosphamide (around 500 mg) for shorter periods of time and the use of oral mycophenolate mofetil (generally 2 to 3 g/day) instead of cyclophosphamide. Trial data suggest that mycophenolate is about as effective and has fewer serious side effects. In renal SLE it is critically important to control the patient's blood pressure. Angiotensin converting enzyme (ACE) inhibitors, α-adrenergic antagonists such as doxazosin, and calcium channel blockers such as nifedipine are the agents most commonly used.

The treatment of CNS lupus varies depending on the manifestation of cerebral dysfunction. Mild cases may respond to relatively small doses of oral steroids (up to 30 mg/day). More florid manifestations such as convulsions or major psychosis require treatment with appropriate anticonvulsants or antipsychotic drugs, higher-dose oral steroids (60 to 80 mg/day), and sometimes azathioprine or intravenous pulses of cyclophosphamide in similar doses to those used in renal SLE.

Does the patient have drug side effects?

The side effects of corticosteroids are well known. The most common early problems are weight gain, hirsutism, easy bruising, and insomnia. It is difficult to prevent them, except by using the lowest dose of steroid that is effective and reducing it as rapidly as possible while maintaining control of the disease.

Longer-term sequelae of corticosteroid use include increased susceptibility to infection, osteoporosis, avascular necrosis, and diabetes mellitus. The most rapid loss of bone in steroid-induced osteoporosis occurs within the first year of treatment, although doses of 7.5 mg/day or less of prednisolone are thought to have little effect on bone. At higher doses, it may be advisable to carry out a bone density scan and to give either calcium and vitamin D tablets or a bisphosphonate (either etidronate or alendronate is commonly used) as prophylaxis.

Cyclophosphamide causes alopecia, nausea, bladder toxicity, and gonadal dysfunction that may lead to infertility. The problem of infertility becomes more likely with increasing age, women over 30 given cyclophosphamide being at particular risk. Again, the best way to prevent such problems is to use as small a cumulative dose of the drug as is feasible. Bone marrow suppression may occur. During a programme of cyclophosphamide pulses the white blood cell count falls to a nadir 10 days after each pulse and should be measured at that time to decide whether the next pulse can be given safely. Nausea and vomiting during pulses may be so severe that antiemetics such as metoclopramide or granisetron are necessary.

Azathioprine also causes bone marrow suppression and can cause abnormalities of liver enzymes, which resolve once the drug is withdrawn.

Biologic therapies

We are entering an exciting era in which improved understanding of the causes of lupus is leading to newer therapeutic approaches. In particular B-cell depletion achieved by using 1 g on two occasions 2 weeks apart of the anti-CD20 chimaeric reagent rituximab (or in more severe cases using this with intravenous cyclophosphamide 750 mg twice and intravenous methylprednisolone 100 to 250 mg twice) looks very promising. The use of fully humanized anti-CD20 monoclonal antibodies is also being explored.

Recently double-blind controlled trials using an anti-CD22 reagent (epratuzumab) and a monoclonal antibody (belimumab) directed against the B cell activating factor BLyS have been reported to meet their end points. Other major trials of antibodies blocking other B cell activating factors (e.g. atacicept) and interferon alpha are ongoing but studies of a B cell toleragen (LJP-394) and CTLA4-Ig (which interferes with the stimulation of T cells by antigen-presenting cells) have failed to prove benefit so far.

SLE in pregnancy

SLE itself does not usually reduce the ability to conceive, although as described the drugs used to treat it, notably cyclophosphamide, may induce infertility due to gonadal failure. There is an increased risk of spontaneous abortion, particularly in the presence of high-titre APL antibodies. Pregnant mothers with a high APL antibody level and a history of previous miscarriage should be considered for anticoagulation until the birth of the baby. As warfarin is potentially teratogenic, heparin may be used from the second trimester until parturition.

Mothers often ask whether their children are likely to inherit SLE. Inheritance of the adult form of the disease is very rare (approximately 1% of all cases), although a transient illness termed 'neonatal lupus' can occur. The characteristics of this condition are rash, hepatitis, anaemia, and thrombocytopenia, which usually resolve by 8 months after birth, and inflammation of the cardiac conducting tissues that may lead to heart block in the fetus. The cardiac problem may be diagnosed by ultrasound scans of the fetal heart between 16 and 24 weeks' gestation. Treatment of the mother with 4 mg oral dexamethasone/day may prevent progression from incomplete to complete fetal heart block. If complete heart block occurs, the neonate may require a cardiac pacemaker. Interestingly, children born with neonatal lupus sometimes develop heart block later in life, with one reported case of this problem occurring at the age of 35.

The presence of maternal anti-Ro and anti-La antibodies predicts a higher risk of neonatal lupus. Where both are present the risk is approximately 2 to 5%. It is believed that the antibodies cross the placenta and bind to some component of the fetal cardiac tissue. Ro itself is expressed on the surface of cardiac myocytes at some point in fetal development and may be an important target for the antibodies. This may be why the fetal heart, but never the mother's heart, is affected by anti-Ro antibodies.

Although overall the risk of a flare during pregnancy is probably no greater than at other times, SLE may be exacerbated during the pregnancy. Corticosteroids may be used in moderate doses without affecting the fetus, but higher doses (over 30 mg) given for long periods can potentially cause fetal adrenal suppression. If lupus activity is such that these doses are required, the risk to the fetus of not treating the disease adequately should outweigh any risk from the drug.

Cyclophosphamide and methotrexate are contraindicated in pregnancy, although there have been many successful pregnancies in transplant recipients taking azathioprine without obvious increased risk of adverse effect. Use of hydroxychloroquine is not recommended by the manufacturers, but there is little evidence that it has adverse effects.

It may be difficult to distinguish pre-eclampsia from a flare of renal lupus. Both can cause hypertension and proteinuria, but in pre-eclampsia—unlike SLE—there are rarely urinary casts and levels of anti-dsDNA antibodies and complement are normal.

For further discussion of autoimmune rheumatic disorders in pregnancy see Chapter 14.14.

Occupational and psychological aspects of SLE

SLE typically presents in young people, especially women. The onset of a chronic, essentially incurable condition at a time of life when the patient is otherwise healthy and has many plans and responsibilities is an unexpected and unwelcome burden. Many concerns arise; in particular the outlook for fertility and the ability to care for children are substantial worries. In those cases where the use of high-dose corticosteroids and immunosuppressive agents is essential, detailed explanations of the benefits and risks of these treatments in both the short and the long term are necessary. Although a 10-year survival rate of 90% may appear reassuring, it is probably less so to a 25 year old who recognizes a 10% chance of dying by the age of 35.

In making the diagnosis of SLE, therefore, the doctor must consider the effect of this condition on the overall life of the patient as well as his or her individual organs. A sympathetic understanding of the anxieties associated with the diagnosis is vital.

Prognosis

Mortality from SLE has fallen significantly over the last half century. Whereas SLE was reported to have a 50% 5-year survival rate in the 1950s, 10-year survival rates rose to between 80 and 90% by the 1970s. Since then, survival rates have improved a little, but deaths from renal failure have become less common, while those from infection and cardiovascular disease have increased. Infection is generally associated with immunosuppressive therapy, highlighting the need for better and more accurately targeted methods of treating the underlying immunological abnormalities in this disease.

Morbidity from systemic lupus can be considerable. From the less serious, but troubling, severe fatigue to the necessity for renal dialysis, many aspects of lupus result in it having a big effect on quality of life. Analyses using the medical outcome survey, short form 36 (SF-36) quality-of-life index have shown that patients with lupus have impaired scores in every aspect of this index.

A damage index for lupus, derived by the Systemic Lupus International Collaborating Clinics (SLICC) group, has shown that within 10 years about two-thirds of patients have acquired permanent problems. Furthermore, early acquisition of damage—within 1 year of diagnosis—substantially increases the risk of mortality (fourfold) within 10 years.

Controversial areas and future prospects

We do not yet have a cure for SLE, or even a method of controlling the disease without the risk of significant side effects. The main sources of controversy concern attempts to develop new forms of treatment and to establish indices of disease activity that can be used to measure the effects of these treatments.

Plasma exchange and intravenous immunoglobulin therapy have been tried in SLE, particularly in renal crises. Overall, the results do not suggest that either form of treatment should be used routinely. New drugs such as rituximab and anti-IL-10 have been administered to relatively small numbers of patients. Some encouraging results have been reported, but it is too early to decide on the place of these agents in the management of the disease. It will be particularly interesting to determine whether biologic agents can be used sequentially, or even simultaneously.

There are now many different murine models of SLE. These differ in their clinical and serological characteristics and each represents at best a partial approximation to the human disease. This is important, because it is now possible to administer agents such as monoclonal anticytokine antibodies to these mice and to assess the effect on the disease process, but how far such studies can be used to predict which of these agents might be effective in humans remains unknown.

If new drugs or monoclonal antibodies are to be used in human SLE, it is necessary, given that mortality is now (thankfully) an uncommon end-point, to have recognized 'tools by which to judge the response to treatment'. A combination of a disease activity index, a damage index, a patient health perception index, a record of toxicity, and cost is required. Several global score disease activity indices, e.g. the systemic lupus activity measure (SLAM) and the European Community lupus activity measure (ECLAM) have been developed and provide a 'rough and ready' guide to activity. A more sophisticated approach based on the 'physician's intention to treat principle' has been derived by the British Isles Lupus Activity Group, providing an 'at a glance' review of activity in eight different organs or systems. A single damage index (the SLICC/ACR damage index) has been developed, which records a wide variety of potential permanent (present for at least 6 months) changes (e.g. avascular necrosis, myocardial infarction) that can occur in patients with lupus as part of the development of the disease. The medical outcome survey SF-36 provides a useful health perception index for patients with lupus. Although not designed specifically for this condition, it has been widely used in a number of ongoing drug trials, but it is likely that a more specific lupus quality-of-life index will be more widely used in future (three are being validated at present).

It is likely that the treatment of SLE in 10 years' time will be different from that given now. Basic science research is starting to identify the various strands of immune dysfunction at the core of this disease. At the same time, drug development is providing agents that are capable of selectively targeting single cell types or cytokines within the immune system. At least some of these agents are likely to be relevant to the dysfunctional mechanisms in SLE. In addition, clinicians are becoming more aware that conditions such as atherosclerosis and osteoporosis are common in patients with SLE. By increasing efforts to detect and control these associated conditions, as well as seeking to attack the underlying autoimmune disease, it should be possible to improve the lives of patients with SLE, even if a cure for the disease remains a distant prospect.

Further reading

Arbuckle MR, *et al.* (2003). Development of autoantibodies before the clinical onset of systemic lupus erythematosus. *N Engl J Med*, **349**, 1526–33.

Boumpas DT, *et al.* (1992). Controlled trial of methyl prednisolone versus two regimens of pulse cyclophosphamide in severe lupus nephritis. *Lancet*, **340**, 741–5.

Casciola-Rosen LA, Anhalt G, Rosen A (1994). Autoantigens targeted in systemic lupus erythematosus are clustered in two populations of surface structures on apoptotic keratinocytes. *J Exp Med*, **179**, 1317–30.

Cervera R, *et al.* (1993). Systemic lupus erythematosus—clinical and immunologic patterns of disease expression in a cohort of 1000 patients. *Medicine (Baltimore)*, **72**, 113–21.

Chan TM, *et al.* (2005). Long-term study of mycophenolate mofetil as continuous induction and maintenance treatment for diffuse proliferative nephritis. *J Am Soc Nephrol*, **16**, 1076–82.

Contreras G, *et al.* (2005). Sequential therapies for proliferative lupus nephritis. *N Engl J Med*, **350**, 971–8.

Datta SK, *et al.* (2005). T-helper cell intrinsic defects in lupus that break peripheral tolerance to nuclear antigens. *J Mol Med*, **83**, 267–78.

Goldblatt F, *et al.* (2005). New therapies for systemic lupus erythematosus. *Clin Exp Immunol*, **140**, 205–12.

Hahn BH (2003). Systemic lupus erythematosus and accelerated atherosclerosis. *N Engl J Med*, **349**, 2379–80.

Isenberg DA, *et al.* (2006). Systemic lupus erythematosus—2005 annus mirabilis. *Nature Clin Pract Rheum*, **2**, 145–52.

Isenberg DA, *et al.* (2007). 50 years of anti-dsDNA antibodies – are we approaching journey's end? *Rheumatology*, **46**, 1052–6.

Johnson AE, *et al.* (1995). The prevalence and incidence of systemic lupus erythematosus in Birmingham, England: relationship to ethnicity and country of birth. *Arthritis Rheum*, **38**, 551–8.

Kaliyaperumal A, *et al.* (2002) Naturally processed chromatin peptides reveal a major autoepitope that primes pathogenic T and B cells of lupus. *J Immunol*, **168**, 2530–7.

Khamashta MA, *et al.* (1995). The management of thrombosis in the antiphospholipid antibody syndrome. *N Engl J Med*, **332**, 993–7.

Koffler D, Schur PH, Kunkel HG (1967). Immunological studies concerning the nephritis of systemic lupus erythematosus. *J Exp Med*, **126**: 607–24.

Lu TY, Ng KP (2009). Cambridge G, Leandro MJ, Edwards JC, Ehrenstein MR, Isenberg DA. A retrospective seven-year analysis of the use of B cell depletion therapy in systemic lupus erythematosus at University College London Hospital: the first fifty patients. *Arthritis Rheum*, **61**, 482–7.

Manzi S, *et al.* (1997) Age-specific incidence rates of myocardial infarction and angina in women with systemic lupus erythematosus: comparison with the Framingham study. *Am J Epidemiol*, **145**, 408–15.

Okamura M, *et al.* (1993). Significance of enzyme linked immunosorbent assay (ELISA) for antibodies to double stranded and single stranded DNA in patients with lupus nephritis: correlation with severity of renal histology. *Ann Rheum Dis*, **52**, 14–20.

Rahman A (2004) Autoantibodies, lupus and the science of sabotage. *Rheumatology*, **43**, 1326–36.

Rahman A and Isenberg DA. (2008). Systemic Lupus Erythematosus. *New England Journal of Medicine*, **358**, 929–39.

Tan EM, *et al.* (1982). The 1982 revised criteria for the classification of systemic lupus erythematosus. *Arthritis Rheum*, **25**, 1271–7.

Walport MJ (1993). Inherited complement deficiency—clues to the physiological activity of complement *in vivo*. *Q J Med*, **86**, 355–8.

19.11.3 Systemic sclerosis

Christopher P. Denton and Carol M. Black

Essentials

The scleroderma spectrum of disorders includes a number of diseases that have Raynaud's phenomenon or skin sclerosis in common, comprising (1) limited cutaneous scleroderma; (2) systemic sclerosis (SSc)—the most important form of scleroderma—limited cutaneous SSc, diffuse cutaneous SSc, and overlap syndromes (with features of another autoimmune rheumatic disease, e.g. systemic lupus erythematosus); (3) Raynaud's phenomenon—autoimmune (with antinuclear or other SSc-associated antibodies) or primary. These conditions affect women four times as often as men, most often beginning in the fifth decade.

The cause of SSc is not known: current models suggest that (unknown) initiating events involve changes in the vasculature and immune system, with subsequent interplay between genetic, vascular, inflammatory, and fibrotic processes. Most patients carry a hallmark autoantibody: three generally (although not always) mutually exclusive reactivities are seen—anticentromere; antitopoisomerase-1 (anti-Scl 70); and anti-RNA polymerase III.

Clinical features

Limited cutaneous SSc—formerly termed 'CREST' (calcinosis circumscripta, Raynaud's, (o)esophagus, sclerodactyly, and telangiectasia), this condition accounts for 60% of cases of SSc. The onset of skin changes is gradual and often preceded by several years of worsening Raynaud's phenomenon; skin sclerosis is limited to the face, neck, and hands distal to the wrists. Telangiectasia and intracutaneous/subcutaneous calcification are common. Significant visceral disease is less frequent than in diffuse cutaneous SSc, affecting oesophagus (74%), lungs (pulmonary fibrosis 26%, pulmonary hypertension 21%), kidneys (8%), and heart (9%).

Diffuse cutaneous SSc—patients typically present over 1 to 3 years with widespread changes in skin texture, puffy oedematous extremities, generalized pruritus, and profound constitutional and inflammatory symptoms. Vasospastic symptoms are not usually prominent during the early stages. Presentation with headache, blurring of vision, and significant hypertension is a medical emergency, portending scleroderma renal crisis and requiring immediate action. Significant visceral disease is common, affecting oesophagus (60% of cases), lungs (pulmonary fibrosis 41%, pulmonary hypertension 17%), kidneys (18%), and heart (12%).

Management

Gastrointestinal symptoms—most patients with SSc have at least one gastrointestinal manifestation, usually oesophageal dysmotility and associated reflux oesophagitis that often responds dramatically to treatment with proton pump inhibitors.

Raynaud's phenomenon—is helped by hand warmers, protective clothing, and evening primrose oil, and may be helped by vasodilator drugs (e.g. oral calcium channel blockers, topical glyceryl trinitrate, and parenteral prostacyclin in severe cases).

Immunosuppressive and other treatments—it is believed that immunomodulatory strategies are most appropriate in the earlier stages of diffuse disease (1–3 years from onset). The most commonly used agents are steroids (particularly for fibrosing alveolitis), cyclophosphamide and (increasingly) mycophenolate mofetil, and intensive immunosuppression combined with autologous peripheral stem cell transplantation has been performed. Antifibrotic approaches might in theory be more appropriate in established cases, but none are proven effective.

Prognosis and complications

The most frequent cause of death related to systemic sclerosis is pulmonary disease, either fibrosing alveolitis (interstitial fibrosis) or pulmonary vascular disease.

Fibrosing alveolitis—serial lung function tests, including carbon monoxide diffusing capacity, are probably the most sensitive screening tools for this condition, with any abnormality pursued by high-resolution CT of the lungs, the appearances of which help predict response (or lack of it) to immunosuppressive treatment.

Pulmonary arterial hypertension—this is typically discovered during regular monitoring with pulmonary function tests (isolated reduction in carbon monoxide transfer factor, with preservation of lung volumes, is suggestive of the problem), ECG, and Doppler echocardiography. Milder cases are treated supportively with diuretics, oral anticoagulation, and (in some cases) digoxin. Patients with more severe disease are treated with oral endothelin receptor antagonists (e.g. bosentan, sitaxentan), switching to a phosphodiesterase V inhibitor (e.g. sildenafil) if there is no response. Advanced disease is treated with both of these agents in combination and/or inhaled or parenteral prostacyclin therapy, with lung transplantation appropriate for a very few cases.

Scleroderma renal crisis—this may be the first manifestation of SSc and typically presents with accelerated phase hypertension, acute renal impairment, and microangiopathic haemolysis. Treatment is with angiotensin converting enzyme (ACE) inhibitors, which have reduced mortality from over 75% to around 10%.

Prognosis—survival in SSc has improved to more than 80% at 5 years, even in the diffuse cutaneous subset. The therapeutic nihilism that was once prevalent is no longer appropriate—the disease should be regarded as often treatable, if not curable.

Introduction

The scleroderma spectrum of disorders includes a number of diseases with similar clinical and pathological features, which have Raynaud's phenomenon or skin sclerosis in common. They are clinically important because the systemic forms have the highest case-related mortality of any of the rheumatic diseases, and because of the particular difficulties encountered in their management. In the United Kingdom there are approximately 300 new cases of systemic sclerosis (SSc) per year and the population prevalence has been estimated to be 100 per million. Both these figures are significantly lower than estimates of disease frequency in the United States of America. Recent epidemiological survival analyses of patients with SSc suggest a reduction in mortality compared with earlier studies, but this may partly be accounted for by the greater awareness of milder forms of the disease. The disease most often develops in the fifth decade of life, and affects women approximately four times as often as men, with this ratio increasing during the child-bearing years.

Those disorders included within the scleroderma spectrum are described in Table 19.11.3.1. The term 'prescleroderma' can be applied to the subgroup of patients with autoimmune Raynaud's phenomenon who manifest an abnormal microcirculation and scleroderma hallmark autoantibodies (anticentromere antibodies, antitopoisomerase, or anti-RNA polymerase III).

Clinical features of localized scleroderma conditions are summarized in Table 19.11.3.2. The importance of distinguishing between these conditions and their subsets lies in the different clinical features, natural history, and patterns of visceral involvement that are characteristic of each subgroup.

There have been important developments in understanding the pathogenesis, clinical diversity, and management of the scleroderma spectrum disorders over the last few years. This progress

has occurred in parallel with improvements in the management of many of the organ-based complications of the condition.

Aetiology, genetics, pathogenesis, and pathology

Systemic sclerosis involves immunological, vascular, and connective tissue abnormalities. Models of pathogenesis focus on the importance of an initiating stimulus in a susceptible individual and subsequent amplification of pathogenic processes, leading to one of the different subsets of the disease. The initiating event is unknown: exposure to environmental agents (silica, organic solvents) has been proposed but not proven; there has been speculation that microchimaerism as a result of persistence of fetal T cells in the mother might initiate a graft-versus-host-like response, but this is not widely accepted.

Current models suggest that initiating events involve changes in the vasculature and immune system, with subsequent interplay of vascular, inflammatory, and fibrotic processes. It has been suggested that stimulatory autoantibodies against platelet-derived growth factor, which can activate collagen expression in fibroblasts, may be an important link between the immune system and fibrosis, but this is not certain. These are among a number of potentially important mediators of intercellular cross-talk that have been identified, which (hopefully) will ultimately suggest logical target factors or signalling pathways for therapeutic intervention. The culmination of these processes eventually leads to the establishment of a fibrogenic population of interstitial fibroblasts that produce increased amounts of extracellular matrix. Disruption of normal tissue architecture and secondary mechanisms such as ischaemia produce the pathological and clinical features.

Familial scleroderma is extremely rare, but it seems likely that there is a substantial, if complex, genetic component to the pathogenesis of SSc, which is likely to involve both severity and susceptibility loci. Twin data have failed to confirm a substantial inherited component, but some studies—e.g. of the Choctaw Native American tribe—have shown a very high incidence of diffuse SSc in some populations. Many studies have reported association between certain genetic polymorphisms and SSc or its complications, but very few have shown reproducibility in different populations. This reflects both the methodological challenge of such studies and the differences between genetic factors involved in different geographical or ethnic groups. Determination of the discrete patterns of organ involvement within and between disease subsets is not understood, although associations of class II major histocompatibility complex (MHC) haplotypes with particular autoantibodies suggest that genetic or immunological mechanisms may be important in the development of SSc hallmark reactivities. These associations, mainly within the MHC, are often robust across ethnic and geographical boundaries, in contrast to reported single nucleotide polymorphism associations.

The interplay between different cell types in the pathogenesis of SSc is summarized in Fig. 19.11.3.1. Many molecular intermediates have been shown to be expressed or function in an altered way in SSc. The pathology of tissue lesions in SSc is unified by vascular changes, including endothelial cell injury and proliferative changes in the vessel wall, with increased extracellular matrix deposition in the intima, media, and adventitia. Perivascular inflammatory infiltrates occur in the skin at an early stage, especially in diffuse

Table 19.11.3.1 The scleroderma spectrum of disorders

Localized cutaneous scleroderma	
Morphoea	
Localized	One or more skin lesions, often on truncal areas
Generalized	Widespread skin lesions can be reminiscent of diffuse cutaneous systemic sclerosis, but Raynaud's phenomenon is unusual, there is no visceral manifestations, and skin changes are less likely to be acral
Linear scleroderma	The most common form occurring in childhood. Skin changes follow a dermatomal distribution, especially on the limbs and lead to important secondary growth defects
En coup de sabre	Midline or parasagittal variant of linear scleroderma, which manifests in childhood and is often associated with defects in underlying fascial and skeletal structures
Systemic sclerosis	
Limited cutaneous systemic sclerosis	Skin sclerosis distal to the wrists (or ankles), over the face and neck
	Often longstanding Raynaud's phenomenon
Diffuse cutaneous systemic sclerosis	Truncal and acral skin involvement. Presence of tendon friction rubs. Onset of skin changes (puffy or hide-bound) within 1 year of onset of Raynaud's phenomenon
Overlap syndromes	Features of systemic sclerosis together with those of at least one other autoimmune rheumatic disease, e.g. SLE, RA, or polymyositis
Systemic sclerosis sine scleroderma	Vascular or fibrotic visceral features without skin sclerosis (less than 1% cases)
Raynaud's phenomenon	
Autoimmune Raynaud's phenomenon	Raynaud's phenomenon associated with antinuclear antibodies (or other SSc-associated autoimmune serology), usually also abnormal nailfold. capillaroscopy. Some patients later develop SSc
Primary Raynaud's phenomenon	Vasospastic symptoms with normal nailfold capillaroscopy and negative autoimmune serology and no other underlying medical/mechanical cause

RA, rheumatoid arthritis; SLE, systemic lupus erythematosus; SSc, systemic sclerosis.

Table 19.11.3.2 Localized scleroderma in adults and children

Pattern of disease	Clinical features	Treatment	Prognosis
Plaque morphoea	One or a few circumscribed sclerotic plaques with hypo- or hyperpigmentation and an inflamed violaceous border	Often unnecessary. Topical steroids or immunosuppression (e.g. tacrolimus) or phototherapy may be considered Serial measurement to assess progress	Good prognosis; lesions less active within 3 years but pigmentary changes often persist
Generalized morphoea	Widespread pruritic lesions, often symmetrical and following the distribution of superficial veins	Suppress inflammatory component using corticosteroids: in children oral doses up to 15 mg/day have been used. Intravenous infusions often effective Methotrexate or other immunosuppressive maintenance therapy often used, although benefit not proven in controlled trials. Vitamin D-containing creams may be useful Topical corticosteroids rarely helpful. PUVA has been used	Internal organ pathology very rare; Raynaud's phenomenon sometimes associated and antinuclear antibody present in 5% of cases. This does not necessarily imply systemic pathology Generally improves within 5 years of onset, although textural and pigmentary changes may persist
Linear scleroderma	Sclerotic areas occurring in a linear distribution often on limbs and asymmetrical; in childhood can lead to growth defect. MRI confirms the depth of lesions and associated musculoskeletal defects. Serial measurements of limb length and girth essential to monitor progression	Suppress inflammatory component using corticosteroids: in children oral doses up to 15 mg/day have been used. Intravenous infusions often effective Methotrexate or other immunosuppressive maintenance therapy often used, although benefit not proven in controlled trials. Vitamin D-containing creams may be useful Physiotherapy and appropriate regular exercise important to minimize growth defect in childhood-onset disease Surgical correction of limb defects may be considered when disease is inactive	Long-term effects of childhood-onset form are minimized by effective suppression of the inflammatory process and by good physiotherapy Ultimately the disease tends to resolve, but it can remain active for many years
En coup de sabre	Linear scleroderma affecting the face or scalp, often involving the underlying subcutaneous tissues, muscles, periosteum, and bone. Cerebral abnormalities also reported including intracranial calcification	Therapeutic options as for linear scleroderma; systemic treatment only for active inflammatory lesions	Scarring, growth defects and alopecia persist but the inflammatory component usually resolves

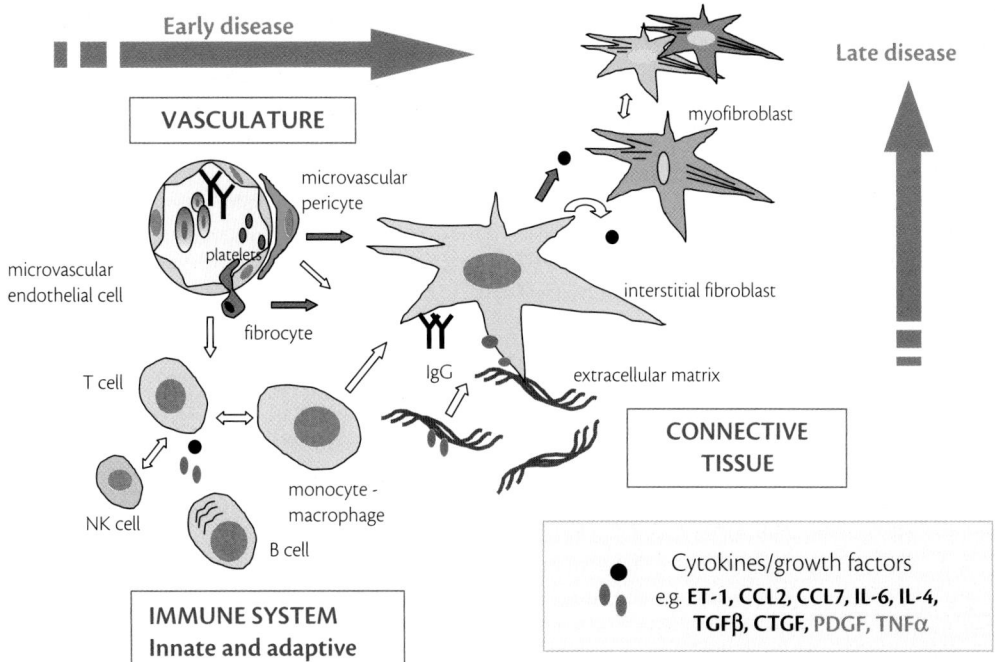

Fig. 19.11.3.1 Schematic summarizing the pathogenesis of scleroderma. Initial events in scleroderma focus on the microvasculature. Later inflammation occurs with involvement of the innate and adaptive immune systems. A mononuclear cell infiltrate around blood vessels is believed to facilitate activation of profibrotic pathways. In established disease there is a population of fibrogenic myofibroblasts within affected tissues that result in excessive extracellular matrix deposition.

cutaneous SSc, and there is destruction of specialized secondary structures and disruption of tissue architecture. In the skin, hair follicles are lost and exocrine glands become enmeshed in extracellular matrix, and there is loss of normal rête ridges. Some of these changes reverse at later stages, consistent with the clinical observation that skin involvement in SSc is not always progressive. Biopsy and postmortem studies consistently demonstrate increased fibrous connective tissue within many organs, including lung, heart, kidney, and bowel. Vascular changes in medium-sized arteries are similar in digital vasculopathy, pulmonary arterial hypertension (where they resemble idiopathic PAH) and sclerodermal renal crisis. This has led to speculation that interventions that are effective for one of these manifestations may also benefit other aspects of vasculopathy, but this remains to be confirmed in clinical practice.

Epidemiology

Systemic sclerosis is a sporadic disease that has a worldwide distribution and occurs in every ethnic group. No seasonal or geographical clustering of cases has been convincingly documented. The epidemiology of SSc has proven difficult to establish, reflecting the clinical diversity of the disease, absence of widely accepted criteria for diagnosis or classification, and the methodological challenges associated with population-based case ascertainment. Incidence estimates range from 9 cases to 19 cases per million per year, with prevalence rates ranging from 28 cases per million to as high as 253 cases per million in the United States of America, and 120 per million in the United Kingdom. Based on incidence and survival rates, it is estimated that there are 75 000 to 100 000 cases of SSc in the United States of America. The only community-based survey of SSc yielded a prevalence of 286 cases per million of the population. This study also suggested that SSc is not infrequently misdiagnosed, implying that its true prevalence may be higher than previously estimated. Similar to other connective tissue diseases, SSc is more frequent in women than in men, with the most common age of disease onset in the 30 to 50 years range.

Clinical features

Although thorough baseline and longitudinal investigation of patients with scleroderma spectrum disorders is central to their management, the diagnosis of scleroderma is essentially clinical. A number of other causes of skin sclerosis or poor peripheral circulation must be considered in the differential diagnosis (summarized in Box 19.11.3.1). Marked differences between the main subsets of SSc in the pattern and time course of clinical features allow most patients to be characterized into the appropriate subset.

Patients with diffuse, cutaneous SSc typically present over 1 to 3 years with widespread changes in skin texture, puffy oedematous extremities, generalized pruritis, and profound constitutional and inflammatory symptoms. Vasospastic symptoms are not usually prominent during the early stages, although within 18 months of their onset most patients will describe definite Raynaud's phenomenon. By contrast, the cutaneous and vasospastic symptoms of limited cutaneous SSc are very different. The onset of skin changes is more gradual, often preceded by several years of Raynaud's phenomenon, often becoming progressively more severe, with skin sclerosis limited to the face, neck, and hands distal to the wrists. The main differences between the subsets of SSc are summarized in Table 19.11.3.3.

Box 19.11.3.1 Differential diagnosis of scleroderma

Skin sclerosis
Infiltrative disorders
- Amyloidosis
- Scleromyxoedema
- Scleroderma of Buschke
- Lichen sclerosis et atrophicus

Metabolic disorders
- Myxoedema
- Porphyria cutanea tarda
- Congenital porphyrias
- Acromegaly
- Phenylketonuria

Inflammatory disorders
- Overlap connective tissue diseases
- Eosinophilic fasciitis
- Chronic graft-vs-host disease
- Sarcoidosis

Acral vasospasm
Raynaud's phenomenon
- Primary Raynaud's phenomenon
- Other autoimmune rheumatic disorders:
  - Systemic lupus erythematosus
  - Rheumatoid disease
  - Dermato-/polymyositis

Other vascular disease
- Haematological:
  - Cryoglobulinaemia
  - Cold-agglutinin disease
  - Hyperviscosity syndrome
- Systemic vasculitis
- Macrovascular disease

Raynaud's phenomenon

Raynaud's phenomenon is characterized by pallor, cyanosis, suffusion, and/or pain of the fingers in response to cold or stress. The same process can also affect the toes, ears, nose, or jaw. It is present in up to 15% of otherwise healthy individuals. About 1% of those showing the phenomenon develop a connective tissue disease. Other conditions associated with Raynaud's phenomenon include cervical rib, vibration white finger, hypothyroidism, and uraemia. Cold-induced peripheral vasospasm is present in most patients with SSc, although generally not in those with localized forms of scleroderma.

Table 19.11.3.3 Contrasting clinical features of the two main subsets of systemic sclerosis (SSc)

Diffuse cutaneous SSc (dcSSc)	Limited cutaneous SSc (lcSSc)
33% of patients	66% of patients
Inflammatory features more prominent at onset	Longstanding Raynaud's phenomenon
Raynaud's phenomenon may develop later	Skin changes: hands, face, neck
Skin sclerosis proximal to wrists/elbows and truncal areas	Compared with dcSSc, renal disease less frequent, isolated PHT, severe gut disease, and interstitial lung fibrosis (if antitopoisomerase-1 present)
Prominent pruritus and constitutional symptoms	Florid telangiectasis and calcinosis (especially anticentromere antibody positive)
Tendon friction rubs associated with progressive disease	Disease activity appears to remain fairly constant over many years, with prominent vasculopathy
Significant visceral disease more frequent than in lcSSc: renal, pulmonary fibrosis (secondary PHT), cardiac, gut	
Disease activity appears to be maximal in first 3 years from onset, then often plateaus and skin involvement may stabilize or improve	

Prevalence of organ-based complications in the main systemic sclerosis subsets[a]

Clinical feature	lcSSc (%)	dcSSc (%)	Overall (%)
Raynaud's phenomenon	99	98	99
Skeletal myopathy	11	23	15
Oesophageal	74	60	69
Other gastrointestinal	7	8	8
Cardiac	9	12	10
Pulmonary fibrosis	26	41	31
Pulmonary hypertension	21	17	20
Renal (overall)	8	18	12
Renal (crisis)	2	10	5

PHT, pulmonary hypertension.

[a] Data from patients attending The Royal Free Hospital Centre for Rheumatology.

It is important to distinguish between the primary and secondary forms of Raynaud's phenomenon. This is most reliably achieved by combining nailfold capillaroscopic assessment with autoantibody testing. Cases of primary Raynaud's phenomenon are often familial, typically with onset in the late teens or early adulthood, have normal or only minimally disrupted capillaroscopic architecture, and negative antinuclear antibody tests. Those who present with isolated Raynaud's phenomenon but later develop a connective tissue disease invariably have abnormal autoimmune serology and nailfold capillary studies before they develop associated clinical features. Patients who demonstrate antibodies, including hallmark specificities for lupus or SSc, may be designated as having autoimmune Raynaud's phenomenon.

Limited cutaneous systemic sclerosis

This was formerly termed 'CREST' (calcinosis circumscripta, Raynaud's, oesophagus, sclerodactyly, and telangiectasia) and is the most common form of SSc, accounting for over 60% of cases. Patients are usually women, aged between 30 and 50 years, with longstanding Raynaud's phenomenon.

Early in the disease there is nonpitting oedema of the fingers (sausage-shaped fingers), which—after several weeks or months—is gradually replaced by thickened and shiny skin. This is not usually so closely adherent to underlying structures that mobility is severely impaired, which is in sharp contrast to the findings in those with diffuse disease. Skin involvement does not spread proximally on to the trunk, but the face should be examined carefully for thin, tightly pursed lips, with furrowing and puckering of the surrounding skin, and microstomia. The most striking cutaneous finding is digital and facial telangiectasia caused by dilated capillary loops and venules (Fig. 19.11.3.2). Other evidence of structural vascular change is to be seen in the fingertips, where small areas of ischaemic necrosis or ulceration are common, often leaving pitting scars and pulp atrophy. Loss of the tufts of the terminal phalanges, confirmed on radiography, is also presumed to be due to ischaemia. Patients with limited cutaneous disease often develop intracutaneous and subcutaneous calcification. These deposits frequently occur in the fingers, particularly the digital pads, and in periarticular tissues such as the prepatellar area and olecranon bursa. The calcinotic masses vary in size and are often complicated by ulceration of the overlying skin, extrusion of calcific material, and secondary bacterial infection. Patients may complain of dyspepsia from reflux oesophagitis: this and other visceral complications are discussed in detail below.

Diffuse cutaneous systemic sclerosis

By contrast to limited cutaneous SSc, the onset of diffuse disease is often abrupt. It may present with widespread, symmetrical, sometimes itchy, painful swelling of the fingers, arms, feet, legs, and face. Rapid weight loss and constitutional symptoms of fatigue or weakness are frequent. If a patient with early disease presents with headache, blurring of vision, and significant hypertension, this is a medical emergency, portending hypertensive renal crisis and requiring immediate action (see below).

The clinical findings in diffuse scleroderma depend on the stage of the disease. At onset, examination of the skin will usually reveal cold, painful, swollen hands, with swelling and stiffness already extending to the arms, feet, lower legs, face, and trunk. This oedematous phase is usually replaced within a few months by one of induration, when the skin becomes tight, shiny, and bound to underlying structures. Pigmentary changes (hyperpigmentation or hypopigmentation)

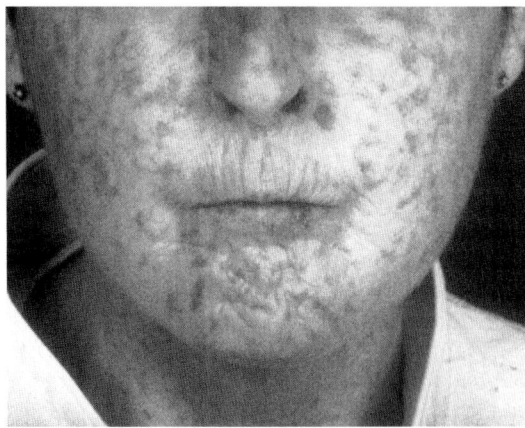

Fig. 19.11.3.2 This patient shows the typical facial features of limited cutaneous systemic sclerosis—microstomia, furrowing, and puckering of the skin around the mouth, beaking of the nose, and telangiectasia on the lips and face.

accompany skin thickening in many patients. Skin involvement in diffuse scleroderma is quite different from that in the limited form of the disease, and can be mapped semiquantitatively by measuring the degree and extent of cutaneous thickening at multiple sites, from which is derived a skin score. In diffuse scleroderma this score increases rapidly at first, often peaking after 1 to 3 years, and is accompanied by impaired mobility of tendons, joints, and muscles that is clinically all too apparent. Contractures and stretching of the skin over bony points often lead to painful ulcers that are slow to heal, particularly over the proximal interphalangeal joints, elbows, and ankle malleoli.

In its earliest stages, diffuse scleroderma can be confused with an acute inflammatory arthropathy, particularly if Raynaud's phenomenon is absent. The oedematous puffy skin is often accompanied by symmetrically stiff, painful joints (hands, feet, knees, ankles, and wrists), but the classic synovitis of rheumatoid arthritis is usually absent. The clinical sign of tendon friction rubs should carefully be sought in this group of patients: these have a distinctive leathery crepitus and can be elicited during joint movement over elbows, knees, fingers, wrists, and ankles. They frequently antedate a rapid increase in cutaneous involvement, or the onset of visceral disease. Signs of carpal tunnel syndrome may be present, due to flexor tenosynovitis at the wrist.

Mild muscle disease is common and can be detected on examination, but is not usually accompanied by an increase in plasma creatine kinase or inflammatory changes on muscle biopsy. It is generally nonprogressive. The few patients with florid changes of polymyositis are usually classified as having an overlap syndrome. As with limited disease, evidence of structural vascular damage—sometimes extensive—may be found in the nailfold capillaries and the digital pads.

Scleroderma sine scleroderma

These patients constitute less than 2% of those with SSc, but they are the most difficult group to recognize. They may or may not have Raynaud's phenomenon, but by definition they never have the skin changes of scleroderma; common presenting problems include oesophagitis, malabsorption, pseudo-obstruction, renal failure, cardiac arrhythmias, and interstitial lung disease.

Overlap syndromes

There are patients whose disease is not easy to define, having features overlapping with those of other connective tissue diseases. A variety of terms such as 'mixed connective tissue disease', 'undifferentiated connective tissue syndrome', and 'overlap syndromes' has emerged to describe such patients.

Whether or not mixed connective tissue disease is a true entity is controversial. Sharp and colleagues used the term in the 1970s to describe patients with some features of polymyositis, lupus, and scleroderma who ran a benign course with no pulmonary, cerebral, or renal involvement, and no vasculitis. They supposedly responded well to low-dose steroids, and could be identified by the presence of a high-titre antibody with specificity for a nuclear U1 ribonucleoprotein (RNP) antigen. However, the clinical features, laboratory tests, and response to therapy have all proved not to be specific, and these patients do not fulfil the definition of and diagnostic criteria for a single disease. Nor can they be sensibly described as having an 'overlap syndrome', assuming that this definition means the coexistence of two separate diseases. Nevertheless, over time,

many do develop major internal organ involvement and evolve into a defined connective tissue disease.

RNP antibodies can be found in patients with scleroderma or systemic lupus erythematosus. The typical patient with the overlap syndrome presents with Raynaud's phenomenon, puffy hands, arthralgia, myositis, abnormal oesophageal motility, and lymphadenopathy. Over a period of a few years the skin may become thickened, telangiectasia and calcinosis may appear, signs and symptoms of interstitial lung disease emerge, and the patient has developed scleroderma. Another patient with similar initial findings may develop alopecia, photosensitivity, mouth ulcers, renal disease, and antibodies to double-stranded (ds) DNA and have developed systemic lupus erythematosus. Other patients may develop a prominent destructive arthropathy reminiscent of rheumatoid disease.

Autoimmune serology

Most patients with scleroderma carry a hallmark autoantibody, and almost all have antinuclear reactivity, often with an antinucleolar pattern on Hep2 cells. Three generally (although not always) mutually exclusive reactivities are seen: anticentromere, antitopoisomerase-1 (anti-Scl 70), and anti-RNA polymerase III. Rarer specificities include fibrillarin (U3RNP), PM-Scl, and anti-Th/To. Each serologically defined group shows somewhat different clinical features, which is of some value in risk stratification for management. There are also well-established class II MHC associations with the various autoantibodies, although some differences in association occur in different racial groups. The reactivities and reported clinical associations of the autoantibodies associated with scleroderma are summarized in Table 19.11.3.4.

Studies using an immunoblotting technique, which is more sensitive than immunofluorescence, have demonstrated that the anticentromere antibody (the antigen actually resides in the kinetocore region of the chromosome) is predictive for the development of

Table 19.11.3.4 Clinical association of hallmark autoantibodies in systemic sclerosis

Reactivity	Target antigen	Frequency	Clinical association
Centromere	CENP proteins	60% lcSSc, 2% dcSSc	Limited skin sclerosis Severe gut disease. Isolated PAH
Scl-70	Topoisomerase-1	40% dcSSc, 15% lcSSc	Diffuse skin sclerosis Pulmonary fibrosis
RNAP	RNA polymerase III	25% dcSSc, 2% lcSSc	Diffuse skin sclerosis Hypertensive renal crisis
nRNP	U1-RNP	15% SSc	Overlap features of SLE, arthritis
PM-Scl	PM-Scl	l5% SSc	Myositis–systemic sclerosis overlap
U3-RNP	Fibrillarin	5% SSc	Isolated PAH cardiac involvement myositis Poor outcome in dcSSc
Th/To	Ribonucleoprotein	5% SSc	Associated with lung involvement in lcSSc including PAH

dcSSc, diffuse cutaneous systemic sclerosis; lcSSc, limited cutaneous systemic sclerosis; PAH, pulmonary arterial hypertension; RNP, ribonucleoprotein; SLE, systemic lupus erythematosus.

limited cutaneous disease (sensitivity 60%, specificity 98%), and Scl-70 (an antibody known to recognize the nuclear enzyme DNA topoisomerase I) for the diffuse subset (sensitivity 38%, specificity 100%). Other serum autoantibodies, notably those to nucleolar antigens, are also relatively specific for scleroderma, and the proportion of patients having one or more antibodies is over 80% of the total. Some of these antibodies have been shown to have correlations with class II MHC haplotypes.

Less specific serological abnormalities are also found in scleroderma and include hypergammaglobulinaemia, the presence of immune complexes, low concentrations of complement components, and a weakly positive rheumatoid factor. Antibodies to SSA/Ro and SSB/La are found in 50% of patients with scleroderma who also have Sjögren's syndrome, and are nearly always found in those with glandular lymphocytic infiltration rather than fibrosis.

Organ-based complications of systemic sclerosis

Despite the usefulness of an accurate subset classification of patients with SSc, management requires that an organ-based approach be taken once the subset has been assigned. This ensures that important complications, which occur with different frequencies in the different subsets, are not missed. The overall prevalence of the different complications is summarized in Table 19.11.3.4.

Vascular manifestations

Raynaud's phenomenon

Episodic acral vasospasm, precipitated by cold or emotional stress (Raynaud's phenomenon), is almost universally present in patients with SSc, although its prominence varies considerably between cases. The pathogenic mechanism is uncertain, but probably represents an imbalance between vasoconstrictor and vasodilator mechanisms in small blood vessels, or an exaggerated release of vasoconstrictor mediators in response to physiological levels of stimulation by cold or emotion.

Raynaud's phenomenon is common in otherwise healthy individuals, with some series estimating its prevalence to be up to 15% in women, with a much lower frequency in men. It may precede the onset of SSc, especially the limited cutaneous subset, by many years, whereas in diffuse cutaneous SSc it generally first becomes manifest around the time of the onset of other features of the disorder, or afterwards. Patients who have Raynaud's phenomenon in association with one of the hallmark autoantibodies of SSc, such as anticentromere or antitopoisomerase-1, will often develop other features of SSc, typically within 3 to 5 years, and so may represent a prescleroderma state, but they can also develop features of other autoimmune rheumatic disorders. Current approaches to the management of patients with Raynaud's phenomenon are summarized in Table 19.11.3.5.

Macrovascular disease

There have been several reports that macrovascular disease is increased in patients with SSc, and there is evidence of altered vessel biomechanical properties. This is plausible, given the number of common aetiopathogenic mechanisms between the processes of atherosclerosis and SSc, including endothelial-cell perturbation, activation, and damage, and subsequent fibroproliferation. Large-vessel disease has important implications for the organ-based

Table 19.11.3.5 Management of Raynaud's phenomenon

Treatment	Examples	Comments
Simple measures		
Non-drug	Hand warmers Protective clothing	Universally helpful; also useful to minimize cold exposure and ambient temperature changes in work environment
Pharmacological	Evening primrose oil Fish oil capsules Antioxidant vitamins	Evening primrose oil has been shown to be effective in controlled clinical trials Theoretical benefit due to increased synthesis of vasodilator prostanoids Potentially reduces oxidant stress which may contribute to Raynaud's phenomenon symptoms and pathology
Oral vasodilators		
Calcium channel blockers	Nifedipine Amlodipine Diltiazem	Variable and differential response to different agents. Slow titration of dose reduced the severity of side effects. Try each drug for at least 3 weeks if possible
Serotonin antagonists	Ketanserin Fluoxetine	Serotonin receptor antagonist: limited availability Serotonin reuptake inhibitor: readily available. Fewer vasodilatory side effects than calcium channel blockers. Depletes platelet 5HT levels
Angiotensin receptor blockers	Losartan	Well tolerated, potential remodelling by blocking fibrogenic effects of angiotensin II. ACEIs not effective in RP (QUINS trial)
Topical vasodilators	Topical nitrates	Shown to be effective in short-term use but systemic effects often cause headaches. New formulations under evaluation
Parenteral vasodilators	Prostacyclin analogues	Effective at healing ulcers and reducing severity and frequency of Raynaud's phenomenon attacks. Expensive and limited long-term duration of benefit. Most data for iloprost
Antibiotics	Flucloxacillin Erythromycin	Important adjunct to vasodilator therapy for secondary infection of digital ulcers. Prolonged treatment necessitated by poor tissue perfusion
Surgical procedures		
Lumbar sympathectomy Radical microarteriolysis Debridement, amputation	Chemical or surgical Division of adventitia of digital arteries. Sometimes termed digital sympathectomy Surgical or autoamputation	For severe lower limb Raynaud's phenomenon Useful treatment for individual critically ischaemic digits Surgery should be as conservative as possible to allow maximum possibility of spontaneous healing

5 HT, 5-hydroxytryptamine (serotonin); ACEI, angiotensin converting enzyme inhibitor.

complications of SSc such as renal disease, peripheral ischaemia, and bowel involvement. Some noninvasive studies have suggested the presence of flow abnormalities in large vessels in the cerebral and renal circulations in SSc. Extrapolating from the results of studies investigating cardiac and pulmonary blood flow variations attributable to vasomotor instability, it is certainly possible that episodic vasospasm is not restricted to the extremities in this disease.

Skin manifestations

Scleroderma means 'hard skin' and is the hallmark of the scleroderma spectrum disorders. The skin lesions of scleroderma differ between diffuse and limited cutaneous subsets, not only by their extent and distribution, but also by the greater tendency for there to be induration and oedema of affected tissues in diffuse cutaneous SSc, which may reflect a local release of cytokines or altered endothelial permeability. The inflammatory phase evolves into established fibrosis, sometimes leading to sheets of thickened skin or a hide-bound texture.

The skin sclerosis score (skin score) is a validated method for assessing the extent of skin involvement, and has been shown to predict survival and to correlate with some other disease features, e.g. a rapidly increasing skin score is associated with an increased occurrence of scleroderma renal crisis. Although baseline skin score associates with outcome in many SSc clinical trials, the relationship between skin extent and organ-based complications is less clear. The high frequency of severe pulmonary arterial hypertension in cases of limited cutaneous SSc exemplifies this. In diffuse cutaneous SSc many patients have their peak skin score within 12 to 18 months of disease onset (defined by first definite non-Raynaud's phenomenon manifestation of SSc), thus by the time they obtain specialist help such patients are often in a stable or improving phase of skin involvement, which has major implications in trying to assess treatment response in the skin.

Another common vascular manifestation of scleroderma is the development of local dilated loops of small blood vessels in the skin, termed 'telangiectasias'. These are often distressing for patients and may also cause problems from haemorrhage if they are at sites prone to trauma. Haemorrhage from mucosal telangiectasias is increasingly recognized as a clinical problem that may require local therapy if recurrent: gastrointestinal haemorrhage and epistaxis have both been reported. Men with facial telangiectasia may experience difficulties when shaving. Cosmetic camouflage techniques can be very effective in masking facial telangiectasia, and appropriate advice should be offered to all who might benefit. Pulsed dye laser treatment has also been used with some success.

Pulmonary disease

The most frequent cause of death related to SSc is pulmonary disease, which can take the form of interstitial fibrosis or pulmonary vascular disease. These two processes can coexist in patients with secondary pulmonary hypertension, a subgroup that should probably be considered separately from those with isolated pulmonary hypertension.

There has recently been substantial progress in the assessment of pulmonary disease in patients with SSc. This has refined diagnosis and classification, will almost certainly result in different treatment strategies for particular subsets of patients, and illustrates a general theme that the subsetting of organ-based complications

Table 19.11.3.6 Respiratory tract complications of systemic sclerosis

Lung disease	Pathology	Frequency	Clinical features	Investigation	Treatment
Pulmonary fibrosis	Predilection for lung bases. Inflammatory infiltrate precedes development of established fibrosis. At biopsy most patients show an NSIP histological pattern	Significant fibrosis in around 25% of SSc. Strongly associated with antitopoisomerase-1 autoantibody. Occurs in both major SSc subsets	Dry cough, exertional dyspnoea, bibasal crepitation. Finger clubbing uncommon	Restrictive pattern of PFT (low FVC and DlCO). HRCT and BAL most useful investigations. DTPA clearance accelerated. Thoracoscopic lung biopsy valuable in atypical cases	Recent studies suggest modest benefit from immunosuppression with cyclophosphamide or azathioprine. Other agents under evaluation
Pleural disease	Effusions and pleurisy uncommon except in overlap syndromes or renal crisis	Rare	Chest pain, dyspnoea	Chest radiograph	NSAIDs or low-dose prednisolone
Pneumothorax	Rupture of cyst into pleural cavity	Rare	Chest pain, dyspnoea	Chest radiograph	Intercostal drainage. Expansion may be poor, especially if lung fibrosis. Pleuradesis
Bronchiectasis	Suppurative inflammation of airways	Rare	Chronic productive cough	CT scan	Antibiotics, postural drainage
Lung carcinoma	Overall probably increased risk, especially scar type (alveolar cell)	Rare	Variable	Contiguous CT scan/ bronchoscopy. Biopsy	Dismal prognosis. Late diagnosis often due to associated lung pathology
Pulmonary arterial hypertension (PAH)	Isolated (no fibrosis) or associated with lung fibrosis. Some cases have secondary pulmonary hypertension	10–15% overall	Exertional breathlessness, chest pain, loud pulmonary P2, syncope, right heart failure	ECG, PFT (low DlCO preserved FVC in isolated PHT), Doppler echocardiography to estimate peak PAP. Right heart catheter definitive	Manage according to consensus recommendations (Galiè 2009). Oral endothelin receptor antagonists and selective phosphodiesterase inhibitors or inhaled and parenteral prostacyclin analogues according to clinical severity.

BAL, bronchoalveolar lavage; DlCO; CO diffusion coefficient; DTPA, diethylenetriaminepentaacetic acid; FVC, forced vital capacity; HRCT, high-resolution CT; NSAID, nonsteroidal anti-inflammatory drug; NSIP, non-specific interstitial pneumonia; PAP, pulmonary artery pressure; PFT, pulmonary function test PHT, pulmonary hypertension SSc, systemic sclerosis;

is becoming as important as the correct classification of major disease subsets. The investigation and treatment of the pulmonary manifestations of SSc are summarized in Table 19.11.3.6.

Fibrosing alveolitis

The initial events in the development of lung disease in patients with SSc appear to involve alveolar inflammation and subsequent epithelial and endothelial perturbation. Although all patients should be screened for this complication, it appears to affect only around 25% of those with limited cutaneous disease and up to 40% of those with the diffuse cutaneous form. It is strongly predicted by the presence of antitopoisomerase-1 autoantibodies, and also by associated MHC genotypes. Increased frequency also occurs in patients with anti-RNA polymerase III antibodies, but the presence of anticentromere antibodies is associated with a reduced risk. These tests are therefore of clinical value in planning the frequency and intensity of lung screening tests.

Technical developments have made the early detection of interstitial lung disease possible. Chest radiography is not sufficiently sensitive. Serial lung function tests including CO diffusing capacity are probably the most sensitive screening tool: a significant reduction from predicted values at baseline with a restrictive pattern, or a worsening of serial tests, warrants further testing with high-resolution CT of the lungs. Additional testing with bronchoalveolar lavage may be considered, but there is little evidence that this adds greatly to information obtained from high-resolution CT, although it remains a valuable research tool. Likewise, lung biopsy is generally not considered helpful in typical cases of SSc-associated lung fibrosis, although it remains important in cases that have atypical features, especially if an inflammatory pathology is suspected that may be steroid responsive. Tests of epithelial damage such as diethylenetriaminepentaacetic acid (DTPA) clearance scans or serum interleukin 6 (IL-6) levels have proved informative in research studies and may provide information that adds to that provided by lung function tests or high-resolution CT. Whether the combined use of these techniques and scans can provide earlier diagnosis and/or indices of progression remains to be determined.

The earliest detectable abnormality on CT is usually a narrow, often ill-defined, subpleural crescent of increased attenuation in the posterior segment of the lower lobe. Other early CT changes include an amorphous ground-glass pattern of parenchymal opacification, or a more reticular appearance (Fig. 19.11.3.3). The relative extent of each pattern is important because there is good correlation between these appearances and histological findings at open-lung biopsy; an inflammatory biopsy equates to an amorphous pattern and fibrosis to a reticular one, hence such information may reduce the need for an invasive biopsy.

DTPA scans, particularly serial studies, may become useful predictors of progression or improvement: a persistently abnormal DTPA scan is associated with a higher rate of decline in pulmonary function tests subsequently, whereas a reversion to normal clearance is associated with sustained improvement in pulmonary function.

These tests have obvious value for assessing the progress of the disease and are critically important in evaluating new treatments. Lung biopsy is still the 'gold standard' for establishing the diagnosis of fibrosing alveolitis, although it is required less often than previously. However, it is now recognized that histological and CT scan appearances allow further classification of SSc-associated fibrosing alveolitis into 'usual pattern interstitial pneumonia' (UIP) or 'nonspecific interstitial pneumonia' (NSIP). These have different

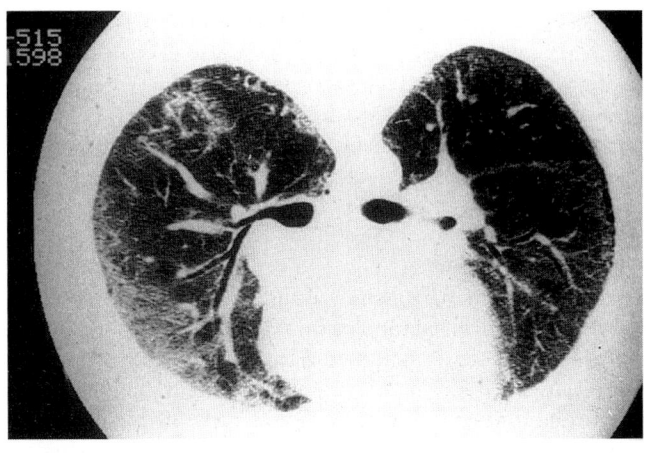

(a)

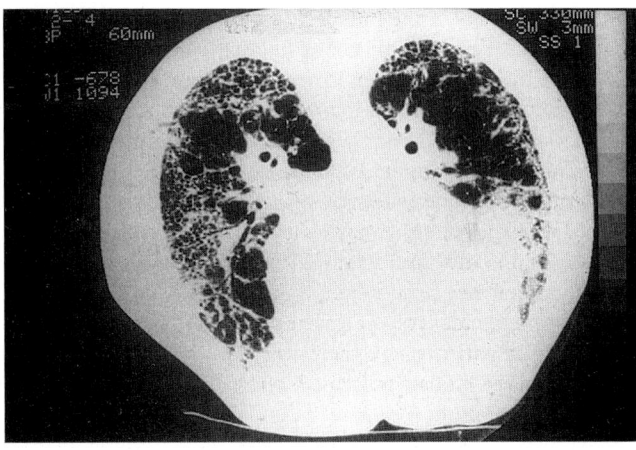

(b)

Fig. 19.11.3.3 (a) A thin-section CT scan illustrating the ground-glass appearance of early pulmonary involvement posteriorly. A chest radiograph taken at the same time was normal. (b) A thin-section CT scan illustrating extensive honeycomb shadowing and cystic air spaces involving both lower lobes. The chest radiographic appearances at the same time were of advanced interstitial lung disease (bibasilar reticulonodular shadowing).
Both images with grateful acknowledgement to Professors A. Wells, R. du Bois, and B. Strickland, Departments of Respiratory Medicine and Radiology, Royal Brompton National Heart and Lung Hospitals.

prognoses and probably require different treatment approaches. In general, the outcome for patients with SSc-associated fibrosing alveolitis is better than that for cryptogenic fibrosing alveolitis of equivalent extent. Most patients with active alveolitis receive immunomodulatory therapy, many studies having suggested that this is effective. However, formal prospective controlled trials are still needed to confirm this and to refine therapeutic regimens.

The mainstay of therapy for SSc-associated interstitial lung disease has long been corticosteroids or cyclophosphamide, given orally or as intermittent intravenous boluses. Two randomized controlled trials have recently been reported, both demonstrating a modest benefit for cyclophosphamide over placebo. Reports of treatment with mycophenolate mofetil have been encouraging; however, the place of immunosuppressive strategies remains uncertain and will require evaluation in randomized controlled trials.

In idiopathic pulmonary fibrosis, recent clinical trials of pirfenidone, etanercept, interferon-γ, and Mucodyne (acetylcysteine) have shown some efficacy. These agents are currently undergoing further evaluation, and it is likely that approaches to the management of lung fibrosis in SSc will be informed by such studies. Lung transplantation may be an option for selected cases of SSc with advanced pulmonary involvement.

The management of interstitial lung disease can be further complicated by the development of secondary pulmonary hypertension.

Pulmonary vascular disease

Pulmonary arterial hypertension (PAH), defined as an elevation in the mean pulmonary artery pressure of more than 25 mmHg at rest, occurs in both limited and diffuse cutaneous forms of SSc and is a leading cause of mortality. The outcome in SSc-associated pulmonary hypertension is considerably worse than that of idiopathic pulmonary hypertension, which may reflect comorbidity or differences in underlying pathogenic mechanisms. In patients with SSc, PAH is most commonly due to intrinsic fibroproliferative abnormalities in the pulmonary vasculature that are pathologically indistinguishable from idiopathic PAH. The second pattern of pulmonary hypertension in SSc occurs in association with pulmonary interstitial fibrosis and is driven by hypoxia as well as the destruction of the normal pulmonary vascular bed. Typical histological appearance of PAH can be found in lung biopsies from patients with SSc-associated lung fibrosis; indeed, it has been suggested that it is coexistent vasculopathy that determines outcome and survival in may cases of SSc-associated pulmonary fibrosis.

PAH may remain asymptomatic until quite advanced. Initial symptoms include exertional breathlessness, and less often chest pain or syncope. In patients with SSc, PAH is typically discovered during regular monitoring with pulmonary function tests, ECG, and Doppler echocardiography. An isolated reduction in CO transfer factor, with preservation of lung volumes, is suggestive of PAH. Definitive diagnosis requires exclusion of thromboembolic disease by ventilation:perfusion lung scan, spiral CT scan, or pulmonary angiography, and direct demonstration of a mean pulmonary artery pressure more than 25 mmHg at rest or more than 30 mmHg on exercise. There is a strong correlation between estimated peak pulmonary artery pressure determined by Doppler echocardiography and measurements at right heart catheterization, except when pulmonary artery pressures are in the range 30 to 50 mmHg. For this reason, cardiac catheterization is essential for the workup of patients with suspected PAH, right heart catheterization allowing the recognition of pulmonary venous hypertension and the precise determination of pulmonary vascular resistance, cardiac output (cardiac index), and pulmonary artery pressures. In addition to serial pulmonary function tests and Doppler echocardiography, determination of serum levels of the N-terminal pro-brain natriuretic peptide (BNP) may be helpful as a screening and monitoring tool for PAH in SSc. Indeed, the levels of serum BNP correlate with survival in patients with SSc-associated PAH.

PAH is historically associated with a grave prognosis, but substantial progress has been achieved with treatment in recent years, although pivotal trials of therapies have chiefly included patients with idiopathic PAH and only a relatively small number with SSc-associated PAH. Current focus is on early identification and determination of severity. World Health Organization/New York Heart Association (WHO/NYHA) functional classifications are useful for assessing the severity of PAH and for treatment decisions. Exercise capacity, commonly assessed by the distance walked in 6 min under standard conditions, has prognostic implications and is used for risk stratification.

Oral anticoagulation, spironolactone, and oxygen supplementation, when appropriate, are used as supportive therapy in PAH. Specific treatments for PAH are initiated only for relatively advanced disease (functional class III or IV), although earlier intervention may be advantageous and is under investigation. Options for class III PAH include oral endothelin-1 receptor blockade and 5′-phosphodiesterase inhibition. Alternative therapies include inhaled or subcutaneous prostacyclin analogues. Intravenous agents are generally reserved for patients with severe or advancing PAH.

Integration of these potential therapies in SSc-associated PAH is a substantial challenge. This is in part due to the difficult nature of PAH in SSc and also a reflection of the lack of high-quality evidence addressing such issues as combination therapy. Having confirmed the diagnosis of PAH, the degree of associated lung fibrosis is considered, it being possible that treatments for lung fibrosis such as immunosuppression may be appropriate. Milder cases of PAH in SSc (functional classes I and II) are treated supportively with diuretics, oral anticoagulation, and (in some cases) digoxin. When they reach functional class III patients are eligible for advanced therapy, current practice being to start treatment with an oral endothelin receptor antagonist (e.g. bosentan, sitaxentan), switching to a phosphodiesterase V inhibitor (e.g. sildenafil) if there is no response. Partial response, or response then deterioration, generally results in addition of sildenafil to endothelin receptor blockade, with further deterioration managed by adding inhaled iloprost or moving to parenteral prostacyclin therapy. These agents all have the potential for substantial complications, including line sepsis and catastrophic rebound pulmonary hypertension on interruption of the infusion. Cases with significant hypoxaemia benefit from supplemental oxygen.

In advanced PAH surgical intervention may be useful for symptom control (septostomy) or long-term benefit (single lung transplantation), but these approaches are suitable for only a few cases. Management of patients with SSc and coexistent PAH and pulmonary fibrosis is especially challenging, but they may respond to therapy for PAH, although outcome is poor.

Cardiac involvement

Postmortem studies have identified at least three patterns of myocardial involvement in SSc, with up to 50% of patients showing features of myocardial fibrosis. Other histological patterns of cardiac disease include contraction-band necrosis and, less frequently, inflammatory cardiomyopathy, the latter probably occurring most often in those with an inflammatory skeletal myopathy.

Noninvasive imaging techniques such as MRI or spiral CT scanning may allow myocardial fibrosis to be detected. Indirect clues of cardiac involvement may be deduced from ECG or echocardiographic studies, the investigation and management of the cardiac manifestations of SSc being summarized in Table 19.11.3.7.

Pericarditis is well recognized as a complication of SSc. It is seen particularly in the context of severe diffuse cutaneous disease and seems to be most frequently encountered in patients with an established or imminent sclerodermal renal crisis. Echocardiographic studies often reveal small, haemodynamically insignificant effusions in patients with scleroderma: around 17% of those with diffuse cutaneous and 4% of those with limited cutaneous disease. Therapeutic pericardiocentesis is only occasionally required, but

Table 19.11.3.7 Investigation and management of cardiac manifestations of systemic sclerosis

Cardiac complication	Pathology	Frequency (%)	Clinical features	Investigation	Treatment
Arrhythmias	Extrasystoles, paroxysmal tachyarrhythmias	30	Palpitations, syncope	ECG (including 24-h tape or telemetry); exercise stress test	Treat if haemodynamically significant
Conduction defects	Fibrosis of conduction tissue	15	Syncope, hypotension	ECG	Pacemaker may be required
Pericardial involvement	Pericarditis Pericardial effusion	10% clinically 35% at postmortem examination	Usually asymptomatic Haemodynamic effects rare	ECG, echocardiogram	Often none required Occasionally pericardiocentesis NSAIDs for pericarditis
Myocardial involvement	Myocarditis Myocardial fibrosis	Rare 30–50% dcSSc	Congestive cardiac failure, arrhythmias Congestive cardiac failure	ECG, echocardiogram, stress echocardiogram, cardiac enzymes (CK-MB), troponin levels, MUGA scan, MRI, or spiral CT may be discriminatory	Myocarditis treated with prednisolone. Cardiac failure managed with digoxin, ACEIs and diuretics, including spironolactone

CK-MB, creatine kinase myocardial-type; dcSSc, diffuse cutaneous systemic sclerosis; MUGA, multigated image acquisition (heart scan); NSAID, nonsteroidal anti-inflammatory drug.

pericardial effusion is associated with active progressive diffuse cutaneous disease.

Electrophysiological cardiac abnormalities are commonly seen in patients with scleroderma. Conduction defects are frequent, especially Q–Tc prolongation on the 12-lead ECG. Later, conduction tissue fibrosis may lead to varying degrees of heart block, including first- and second-degree block, or complete heart block necessitating pacemaker implantation. Bundle-branch blocks may reflect abnormalities in the conducting tissues or be complications of ventricular strain, hence right bundle-branch block may be seen in association with pulmonary hypertension, and left bundle-branch block may occur when there is left ventricular strain from hypertension or cardiac muscle disease. Paroxysmal arrhythmias are much more difficult to detect than conduction abnormalities and, in those with occult cardiac disease are probably an important cause of unexplained death in patients with SSc.

Renal disease

Several patterns of renal pathology are recognized in patients with scleroderma: all involve vascular abnormalities. The most clearly defined is the sclerodermal renal crisis, which describes the occurrence of acute renal failure in a patient with scleroderma, usually associated with accelerated hypertension (further compounding the renal pathology), and in whom no other cause for nephropathy is present. However, in addition to a sclerodermal renal crisis, many patients demonstrate less severe renal complications, probably associated with reduced renal blood flow and the consequent reduction in glomerular filtration rate (GFR). The mechanism of this slowly progressive form of chronic renal disease is unclear. A few patients develop significant glomerulonephritis.

Acute renal crisis

Sclerodermal renal crisis occurs in 10 to 15% of diffuse cutaneous SSc and 1 to 2% of limited cutaneous SSc cases during the course of the disease. Many cases occur within the first 12 months of disease, and in up to a quarter of patients with sclerodermal renal crisis the diagnosis of SSc is made at the time of the renal presentation. Typically, cases present with accelerated phase hypertension and progressive renal impairment. End-organ damage can result in encephalopathy with generalized seizures. Microangiopathic anaemia is common and disseminated intravascular coagulation sometimes develops.

Before the late 1970s, renal complications were a major cause of SSc associated death, largely due to the development of a sclerodermal renal crisis, which was almost always fatal. However, the routine use of angiotensin-converting enzyme inhibitors (ACEIs) has transformed outcome, with early case–control studies suggesting a fall in the 12-month mortality rate from 76% to less than 15%. It is less clear whether these drugs, or related agents such as angiotensin receptor blockers (ARBs), are effective in preventing or abrogating the effects of sclerodermal renal crisis: at present some units put all cases of early diffuse cutaneous SSc on ARBs or ACEIs, whereas others reserve treatment for those who develop features of sclerodermal renal crisis. It is possible that routine use is unhelpful and may even be detrimental. Certain drugs including ciclosporin and corticosteroids have been implicated as precipitants of sclerodermal renal crisis.

Our present approach to sclerodermal renal crisis is to admit all cases at diagnosis (based on new-onset accelerated phase hypertension with evidence of renal impairment, microangiopathic haemolysis, or significant end-organ damage in the context of SSc) and treat with ACEIs, increasing the dose every day to achieve a blood pressure reduction of 10 to 20 mmHg systolic per 24 h, even if there is continued deterioration in renal function, which can be followed by daily calculated estimated GFR (eGFR) or creatinine clearance. Patients are also routinely given continuous low-dose prostacyclin, which may help control blood pressure and has potentially beneficial effects on renal blood flow, endothelial cell function, and production of proinflammatory or profibrotic factors, although this treatment has not formally been proved effective. Additional antihypertensive agents may be useful, including combinations of ARBs and ACEIs or calcium channel blockers, nitrates (especially if there is pulmonary oedema), or other vasodilator agents such as doxazocin. However, vasodilatation may be associated with relative hypovolaemia, so care must be taken to monitor cardiac function closely. After control of blood pressure has been achieved, there is a good case for pursuing renal biopsy, which can confirm the diagnosis, provide prognostic information, and may occasionally reveal cases of SSc with inflammatory glomerular pathology that potentially require very different treatment to that for a classic sclerodermal renal crisis.

Although improved by the treatment described above, the outcome of a sclerodermal renal crisis remains inadequate.

About two-thirds of cases presenting to specialist centres will require renal replacement therapy, of which about half will eventually recover sufficiently to discontinue dialysis. This can occur up to 24 months after the crisis, so decisions about renal transplantation should be postponed until that time.

Chronic nephropathy

Patients who survive a sclerodermal renal crisis may develop similar but less florid proliferative changes in the interlobular and arcuate arteries. Even those who have never had a renal crisis may show reduplication of elastic fibres, sclerosed glomeruli, tubular atrophy, and interstitial fibrosis, presumably reflecting the chronic changes of scleroderma.

Glomerulonephritis

There are a few case reports of glomerulonephritis occurring in SSc, including a progressive crescentic glomerulonephritis in association with positive antimyeloperoxidase autoantibodies. More commonly, biopsy reveals coincident pathologies such as drug-induced injury or overlap syndromes with features of other connective tissue disorders such as systemic lupus erythematosus.

Gastrointestinal complications

Most patients with SSc exhibit at least one gastrointestinal manifestation, usually oesophageal dysmotility and associated reflux oesophagitis. These symptoms often respond dramatically to treatment with proton pump inhibitors. Involvement can also occur at other sites: these are described in Table 19.11.3.8, together with current management approaches for each complication.

Gastric involvement typically leads to slow gastric emptying and symptoms of postprandial fullness. This, together with sicca symptoms and difficulty swallowing, encourages poor nutritional intake and is a significant contributor to the weight loss observed in patients with this disease. The earliest feature of small bowel involvement is also dysmotility, leading to increased intestinal transit time, which together with a propensity to form wide-mouthed jejunal diverticula, leads to stagnation of the luminal contents and small intestinal bacterial overgrowth. This may in turn lead to bloating, flatulence, malabsorption, and chronic diarrhoea. Endstage involvement of the small bowel leads to profound malabsorption and malnutrition and is a significant cause of miserable scleroderma-associated death. Large-bowel manifestations include constipation and anorectal incontinence. Alternating constipation and diarrhoea is common and complicates management, which is generally empirical.

Musculoskeletal complications

Musculoskeletal features are almost universal in established SSc, although often relatively well tolerated. Arthralgia and stiffness are the most frequent symptoms. Most patients with diffuse disease experience muscle weakness, although prominent myositis is unusual. Flexion contractures of the interphalangeal joints are common and can be very debilitating. Surgical intervention can be valuable, but should focus on functional rather than cosmetic gain. Frank arthritis is uncommon and points towards an overlap syndrome. Other musculoskeletal manifestations include carpal tunnel syndrome, tendonitis (with friction rubs—most often in diffuse cutaneous disease), and the consequences of contractures—especially affecting the hands, but also more proximal joints in diffuse disease.

Table 19.11.3.8 Gastrointestinal tract manifestations of systemic sclerosis

Site	Disorder	Symptom	Investigation	Treatment
Mouth	Tight skin Dental caries Sicca syndrome	Cosmetic Toothache Dry mouth	None Dental radiograph Salivary gland biopsy	Facial exercises Dental treatment Artificial saliva
Oesophagus	Dysmobility/oesophageal spasm Reflux oesophagitis Stricture	Dysphagia Heartburn Dysphagia	Barium swallow Oesophageal scintigraphy Manometry Endoscopy	Proton pump inhibitors Minimize NSAID and calcium channel blocker use Elevate head of bed Avoid late meals
Stomach	Gastric paresis NSAID-related ulcer	Anorexia Nausea Early satiety	Endoscopy Scintigram Barium meal	Proton pump inhibitors Metoclopramide, Domperidone
Small bowel	Hypomotility Stasis Bacterial overgrowth Malnutrition Pseudo-obstruction Pneumatosis intestinalis	Weight loss Postprandial bloating Malabsorption Steatorrhoea Abdominal pain Distension Diarrhoea with blood; benign pneumoperitoneum	Barium follow-through MRI studies Hydrogen breath test Jejunal aspiration Faecal microscopy Plain abdominal radiograph Plain abdominal radiograph	Rotational antibiotics Erythromycin Domperidone, metoclopramide Oral nutritional supplements Percutaneous gastrostomy or jejunostomy if gastro-oesophageal disease severe Conservative management: 'drip and suck'
Large bowel	Hypomotility Colonic pseudodiverticula Pseudo-obstruction or volvulus (caecal/sigmoid)	Alternating constipation and diarrhoea Rare perforation Abdominal pain Distension	Barium enema Barium enema Plain abdominal radiograph	Dietary manipulation Stool expanders for constipation Loperamide for diarrhoea (resection as a last resort) Conservative management: 'drip and suck'
Anus	Sphincter involvement	Faecal incontinence	Rectal manometry Endoanal ultrasonography MRI	Protective measures Sacral nerve stimulation

Other organ involvement

Neurological involvement is uncommon, but in the late stages of limited cutaneous disease a small but significant proportion of patients develop unilateral or bilateral trigeminal neuralgia. Impotence is a problem for men, usually occurring 1 to 2 years after disease onset, thought to have a neurovascular cause, and is refractory to treatment. Dryness of the mucous membranes is common, leading to dyspareunia. Hypothyroidism occurs in as many as 50% of patients with SSc and is frequently missed: some patients have antithyroid antibodies, but lymphocytic infiltration in the gland is uncommon, fibrosis being the more typical finding.

Management

Disease management starts with diagnosis and classification: when faced with a patient with a scleroderma spectrum disorder the first consideration is to determine whether they have features of localized disease or SSc. The simplest discriminators are the presence of vascular symptoms, including Raynaud's phenomenon, and internal organ manifestations, of which the earliest is often reflux oesophagitis or dysphagia. Unfortunately both Raynaud's phenomenon and gastro-oesophageal reflux are common in otherwise healthy individuals. The pattern and distribution of skin involvement provide critical information about subset and classification: asymmetrical involvement and acral sparing are typical of localized scleroderma, whereas acral involvement is almost universal in systemic forms. Of the available laboratory investigations, autoantibody testing is perhaps the most useful, and provides additional information about likely subset and possible organ-based disease in SSc (see below). An additional clinical investigation that helps to discriminate primary Raynaud's phenomenon from early connective tissue disease is nailfold capillaroscopy. There are classic morphological changes in SSc, including capillary drop-out and dilatation, whereas capillaroscopy is usually entirely normal in cases of localized scleroderma.

One of the most improved areas of clinical understanding of the scleroderma spectrum of disorders has been the concept of risk stratification. This enables precious resources to be appropriately focused, so that patients at the highest risk of particular complications are thoroughly investigated. Subsetting and staging within subsets are the starting point. Associations with particular autoantibodies are helpful, as summarized in Table 19.11.3.4. Additional predictive power is provided by genetic markers, and this is likely to increase considerably over the next few years. In particular, functionally relevant single nucleotide polymorphisms, such as those in cytokine or growth-factor receptors, or other polymorphic markers, including immunogenetic ones, are likely to increase predictive power.

Unfortunately there has been relatively little progress in developing disease-modifying therapies for the most aggressive subset of patients, those with diffuse cutaneous SSc, which is at least in part a reflection of our relatively limited understanding of the pathogenesis of the condition. Effective therapies are likely to be directed against key processes or mediators, and may be different depending on the subset and stage of disease. In general, it is believed that immunomodulatory strategies are most appropriate in the earlier stages of diffuse disease (1 to 3 years from onset), whereas antifibrotic approaches would (if available) be more appropriate in established cases (Fig. 19.11.3.4). Current approaches to

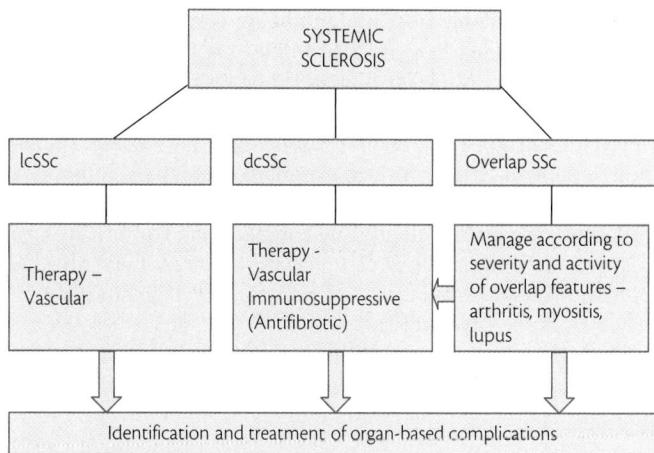

Fig. 19.11.3.4 Overview of the management strategy for patients with systemic sclerosis.

immunosuppressive treatment are summarized in Table 19.11.3.9. An induction–maintenance approach has been used in some centres. Although curative treatments are lacking, scleroderma spectrum disorders, and especially SSc, should be considered treatable, and strategies previously described in this chapter are available to treat all the diverse manifestations and complications of the condition. There are no proven antifibrotic therapies available at present.

Prognosis

As the clinical course of particular subsets of SSc can to a great extent be predicted, appropriate classification within the scleroderma

Table 19.11.3.9 Immunomodulatory strategies used in systemic sclerosis

Agent	Clinical trial data
Methotrexate	Two placebo-controlled trials suggest possible benefit for skin sclerosis, although this may not be clinically significant
Cyclophosphamide	Substantial uncontrolled evidence of efficacy for skin and lung disease. Recent placebo-controlled trials of oral or intravenous therapy are suggestive of limited benefit for lung fibrosis
Mycophenolate mofetil	Large experience in uncontrolled studies suggests that this drug is well tolerated and not inferior to other potent immunosuppressive agents. Small series point to benefit in lung fibrosis
Intensive immunosuppression with autologous peripheral stem cell transplantation	Ongoing studies in the USA and Europe. Registry data suggest that this approach is feasible, but superiority to other strategies of immunosuppression not yet demonstrated
Antithymocyte globulin (ATG)	Open study, 13 patients also treated with mycophenolate mofetil. Skin score improved
Oral tolerability to type I collagen	Favourable pilot data. A large study in the USA suggests possible improvement in skin score in late-stage disease
Ciclosporin	Open label data suggest improvement in skin score. Nephrotoxicity increases risk of renal crisis. Not generally used

spectrum is valuable in planning disease management. Patients with limited disease have an 'early phase' that lasts about 10 years, when the picture is usually dominated by vascular problems such as Raynaud's phenomenon, pitting scars, digital ulcers, and telangiectasias. Later there may be worsening of the vascular disease, both cutaneously and in the pulmonary circulation. Pulmonary interstitial disease, usually more indolent than that seen in the diffuse form, can also occur as a late complication. Gut involvement may worsen with time, and oesophageal strictures, malabsorption, pseudo-obstruction, and anal incontinence are all possible late and troublesome events in this subset.

During the early phase of diffuse disease (the first 5 years), the patient is fatigued and loses weight. Hypertensive renal crisis is a real risk, and rapid progression of pulmonary and cardiac disease may occur. Arthritis, myositis, and tendon involvement can be most marked at this time. After 5 years, considered to be the late stage of diffuse disease, the constitutional symptoms settle down, the skin and musculoskeletal problems have usually reached a plateau, and there is progression of existing visceral disease but a reduced risk of new organ involvement. These differences in the pattern and natural history influence evaluation and therapy.

There have been a number of studies of survival in the past 50 years, and the 5-year cumulative survival rate ranges from 34% to 73%. Even prolonged survival does not protect against an increased mortality risk, which continues for at least 15 years. Factors that adversely affect outcome are increasing age, being male, extent of skin involvement, and heart, lung, and renal disease. Most recent studies point to a substantial improvement in survival over the last 20 years: this is likely to be attributable to the treatment of renal crisis—previously almost invariably fatal—and perhaps to better detection and treatment of other major complications.

Likely developments over the next 5 to 10 years

There have been substantial advances in the assessment and management of SSc over the past 20 years and this is likely to continue. Over the past 5 years there have been prospective placebo-controlled clinical trials exploring safety and efficacy of established as well as novel therapies for SSc and its complications, with several of these studies suggesting clinical benefit. International collaboration in developing assessment tools and designing clinical trials makes further progress very likely over the next 5 years. Studies evaluating the benefit of immunoablation and autologous stem cell rescue are under way, which should define the potential for this very aggressive therapy in diffuse cutaneous SSc. Genetic markers and serological tests such as KL-6 for lung fibrosis and NT-proBNP for cardiac disease and pulmonary arterial hypertension may be combined to improve risk stratification for SSc cases, allowing investigation and treatment to be targeted to those cases most likely to benefit. The most appropriate way of combining therapies for PAH is being investigated. The therapeutic nihilism that was once prevalent in respect of SSc is no longer appropriate—this disease should be regarded as often treatable, if not curable.

Further reading

Allcock RJ, et al. (2004). A study of the prevalence of systemic sclerosis in northeast England. *Rheumatology (Oxford)*, **43**, 596–602.

Assassi S, Tan FK (2005). Genetics of scleroderma: update on single nucleotide polymorphism analysis and microarrays. *Curr Opin Rheumatol*, **17**, 761–7.

Baroni SS, et al. (2006). Stimulatory autoantibodies to the PDGF receptor in systemic sclerosis. *N Engl J Med*, **354**, 2667–76.

Bunn CC, Black CM (1999). Systemic sclerosis: an autoantibody mosaic. *Clin Exp Immunol*, **117**, 207–8.

Della Bella S, et al. (1997). Cytokine production in scleroderma patients: effects of therapy with either iloprost or nifedipine. *Clin Exp Rheumatol*, **15**, 135–41.

DeMarco PJ, et al. (2002). Predictors and outcomes of scleroderma renal crisis: the high-dose versus low-dose D-penicillamine in early diffuse systemic sclerosis trial. *Arthritis Rheum*, **46**, 2983–9.

Denton CP, Nihtyanova S (2007). Therapy of pulmonary arterial hypertension in systemic sclerosis: an update. *Curr Rheumatol Rep*, **9**, 158–64.

Denton CP, Black CM, Abraham DJ (2006). Mechanisms and consequences of fibrosis in systemic sclerosis. *Nat Clin Pract Rheumatol*, **2**, 134–44.

Denton CP, et al. (2006). Bosentan treatment for pulmonary arterial hypertension related to connective tissue disease: a subgroup analysis of the pivotal clinical trials and their open-label extensions. *Ann Rheum Dis*, **65**, 1336–40.

Desai SR, et al. (2004). CT features of lung disease in patients with systemic sclerosis: comparison with idiopathic pulmonary fibrosis and nonspecific interstitial pneumonia. *Radiology*, **232**, 560–7.

Feghali-Bostwick C, Medsger TA Jr, Wright TM (2003). Analysis of systemic sclerosis in twins reveals low concordance for disease and high concordance for the presence of antinuclear antibodies. *Arthritis Rheum*, **48**, 1956–63.

Galiè N, et al. (2009). Guidelines for the diagnosis and treatment of pulmonary hypertension. *Eur Respir J*, **34**, 1219–63.

Gendi NS, et al. (1995). HLA type as a predictor of mixed connective tissue disease differentiation. Ten-year clinical and immunogenetic follow-up of 46 patients. *Arthritis Rheum*, **38**, 259–66.

Goh NS, et al. (2008). Interstitial lung disease in systemic sclerosis: a simple staging system. *Am J Respir Crit Care Med*, **177**, 1248–54.

Hoyles RK, et al. (2006). A multicenter, prospective, randomized, double-blind, placebo-controlled trial of corticosteroids and intravenous cyclophosphamide followed by oral azathioprine for the treatment of pulmonary fibrosis in scleroderma. *Arthritis Rheum*, **54**, 3962–70.

Ioannidis JP, et al. (2005). Mortality in systemic sclerosis: an international meta-analysis of individual patient data. *Am J Med*, **118**, 2–10.

Maricq HR, et al. (1989). Prevalence of scleroderma spectrum disorders in the general population of South Carolina. *Arthritis Rheum*, **32**, 998–1006.

Mayes MD (2003). Scleroderma epidemiology. *Rheum Dis Clin North Am*, **29**, 239–54.

McNearney TA, et al. (2007). Pulmonary involvement in systemic sclerosis: Associations with genetic, serologic, sociodemographic, and behavioral factors. *Arthritis Rheum*, **57**, 318–26.

Mukerjee D, et al. (2003). Prevalence and outcome in systemic sclerosis associated pulmonary arterial hypertension: application of a registry approach. *Ann Rheum Dis*, **62**, 1088–93.

Nihtyanova SI, et al. (2007). Mycophenolate mofetil in diffuse cutaneous systemic sclerosis—a retrospective analysis. *Rheumatology (Oxford)*, **46**, 442–5.

Poormoghim H, et al. (2000). Systemic sclerosis sine scleroderma: demographic, clinical, and serologic features and survival in forty-eight patients. *Arthritis Rheum*, **43**, 444–51.

Schachna L, et al. (2006). Lung transplantation in scleroderma compared with idiopathic pulmonary fibrosis and idiopathic pulmonary arterial hypertension. *Arthritis Rheum*, **54**, 3954–61.

Scorza R, et al. (1997). Effect of iloprost infusion on the resistance index of renal vessels of patients with systemic sclerosis. *J Rheumatol*, **24**, 1944–8.

Shand L, et al. (2007). Relationship between change in skin score and disease outcome in diffuse cutaneous systemic sclerosis: application of a latent linear trajectory model. *Arthritis Rheum*, **56**, 2422–31.

Steen VD, *et al.* (1990). Outcome of renal crisis in systemic sclerosis: relation to availability of angiotensin converting enzyme (ACE) inhibitors. *Ann Intern Med*, **113**, 352–7.

Steen V, Medsger TA Jr (2003). Predictors of isolated pulmonary hypertension in patients with systemic sclerosis and limited cutaneous involvement. *Arthritis Rheum*, **48**, 516–22.

Steen VD, Medsger TA Jr (2007). Changes in causes of death in systemic sclerosis, 1972–2002. *Ann Rheum Dis*, **66**, 940–4.

Steen VD, Medsger TA Jr (1990). Epidemiology and natural history of systemic sclerosis. *Rheum Dis Clin North Am*, **16**, 1–10.

Tashkin DP, *et al.* (2006). Scleroderma Lung Study Research Group. Cyclophosphamide versus placebo in scleroderma lung disease. *N Engl J Med*, **354**, 2655–66.

Wells AU, *et al.* (1993). Clearance of inhaled ⁹⁹ᵐTc-DTPA predicts the clinical course of fibrosing alveolitis. *Eur Respir J*, **6**, 797–802.

Wells AU, *et al.* (1998). Bronchoalveolar lavage cellularity: lone cryptogenic fibrosing alveolitis compared with the fibrosing alveolitis of systemic sclerosis. *Am J Respir Crit Care Med*, **157**, 1474–82.

Williams MH, *et al.* (2006). Role of N-terminal brain natriuretic peptide (N-TproBNP) in scleroderma-associated pulmonary arterial hypertension. *Eur Heart J*, **27**, 1485–94.

Yanaba K, *et al.* (2003). Longitudinal analysis of serum KL-6 levels in patients with systemic sclerosis: association with the activity of pulmonary fibrosis. *Clin Exp Rheumatol*, **21**, 429–36.

19.11.4 Polymyalgia rheumatica and temporal arteritis

Jan Tore Gran

Essentials

Polymyalgia rheumatica and temporal arteritis are distinct but overlapping inflammatory conditions of unknown aetiology. They almost exclusively affect people over 50 years of age, women more than men (ratio 2–3:1), and particularly those of Nordic heritage.

Temporal arteritis is characterized by granulomatous inflammation that penetrates all layers of the wall of medium and (often) large muscular arteries, in particular the superficial temporal artery. Histological examination of tissues from patients with polymyalgia rheumatica shows nonspecific changes only. The term 'giant cell arteritis' is properly used only to describe patients with biopsy-proven arteritis.

Polymyalgia rheumatica

Clinical features—typical presentation is with symmetric limb girdle pain and/or stiffness, usually most pronounced in the morning or after rest, often associated with general constitutional symptoms, also with elevated levels of ESR and/or CRP. Peripheral arthritis occurs in one-quarter to one-third of patients.

Management—prednisolone at an initial dose of 15 mg/day is sufficient to suppress disease activity and provides significant relief in most patients. After remission is achieved, the dose is slowly reduced to a maintenance dose over the next few months and then continued for at least 12 months.

Temporal arteritis

Clinical features—the usual presentation is with headache (for which other causes are excluded), often followed by systemic symptoms—including malaise, weight loss, low-grade fever, loss of appetite, and night sweats—and in association with a significant acute phase response. Visual loss is a feared complication, most often caused by anterior ischaemic optic neuropathy. The temporal artery pulses are often reduced or absent, and there may be local tenderness.

Investigation—a temporal artery biopsy should be performed in all patients suspected of having temporal arteritis, but is not recommended in cases exhibiting no symptoms or signs of arteritis. Positive findings can be demonstrated even after 2 to 4 weeks of steroid therapy.

Management—prednisolone at an initial dose of 30 to 40 mg/day is recommended, increasing to 40 to 60 mg/day if there is no response. After remission is achieved, the dose is slowly reduced to a maintenance dose over the next few months, most patients needing treatment for several years. Visual disturbances can lead to permanent visual impairment and should be treated immediately with oral prednisolone at a dose of 60 to 80 mg/day.

The risk of developing arterial aneurysms is about 17 times greater than that of the general population, with aortic aneurysms causing death in 8% of patients.

Polymyalgia rheumatica

Typical presentation is with symmetrical limb girdle pain and/or stiffness, usually most pronounced in the morning or after rest, often associated with general constitutional symptoms, and also with elevated levels of the erythrocyte sedimentation rate (ESR) and/or C-reactive protein (CRP). Peripheral arthritis occurs in one-quarter to one-third of patients.

Prednisolone at an initial dose of 15 mg/day is sufficient to suppress disease activity and provides significant relief in most patients. After remission is achieved, the dose is slowly reduced to a maintenance dose over the next few months and then continued for at least 12 months.

Temporal arteritis

The usual presentation is with headache (for which other causes are excluded), often followed by systemic symptoms—including malaise, weight loss, low-grade fever, loss of appetite, and night sweats—and in association with a significant acute phase response. Visual loss is a feared complication, most often caused by anterior ischaemic optic neuropathy.

The temporal artery pulses are often reduced or absent, and there may be local tenderness.

A temporal artery biopsy should be performed in all patients suspected of having temporal arteritis, but is not recommended in cases exhibiting no symptoms or signs of arteritis. Positive findings can be demonstrated even after 2 to 4 weeks of steroid therapy.

Prednisolone at an initial dose of 30 to 40 mg/day is recommended, increasing to 40 to 60 mg/day if there is no response. After remission is achieved the dose is slowly reduced to a maintenance dose over the next few months, most patients needing treatment for several years.

Visual disturbances can lead to permanent visual impairment and should be treated immediately with oral prednisolone at a dose of 60 to 80 mg/day.

The risk of developing arterial aneurysms is about 17 times greater than that of the general population, with aortic aneurysms causing death in 8% of patients.

Historical perspective

The first evidence of polymyalgia rheumatica and temporal arteritis is probably to be found in a painting of Canon van der Paele by the Flemish artist Jan van Eyck (1385 to 1440). According to the minutes of the cathedral, the clergyman had significant problems in performing his duties because of morning stiffness and weakness, and the picture shows him to have a prominent temporal artery.

In 1890 Jonathan Hutchinson described temporal arteritis in an octogenarian whose inflamed arteries prevented the wearing of a hat; the term 'temporal arteritis' was introduced by Horton in the 1930s, who also provided a description of the histological appearance of the disease. The first description of polymyalgia rheumatica is usually attributed to Bruce in 1888.

Aetiology

The systemic features of polymyalgia rheumatica and temporal arteritis may suggest an infectious aetiology, but thorough investigations have not provided firm evidence to incriminate any specific microorganism as a causative agent. Whether or not there is a seasonal pattern in disease incidence is still debated. No particular environmental factor has been identified as an independent risk factor for contracting polymyalgia rheumatica or temporal arteritis.

Polymyalgia rheumatica and temporal arteritis are particularly prevalent among populations of Nordic descent, which may suggest genetically determined disease susceptibility. The finding of extremely low CD8+ T cells in both patients and healthy relatives also points to a genetic link, but studies of familial aggregation are sparse and no large-scale twin studies have yet been performed. It is generally agreed that there is an association of polymyalgia rheumatica with HLA DRB1*0401 and 0404, but not with regard to disease susceptibility in biopsy-proven temporal arteritis.

Pathology and immunology

Temporal arteritis is characterized by granulomatous inflammation, with cellular infiltrates of CD4+ T lymphocytes, macrophages, and giant cells penetrating all layers of the arterial wall. Tissue damage is mostly focused on the media and intima, as well as the elastic lamina, a structure preferentially found in medium-sized muscular arteries.

The adventitia, usually the only region penetrated by vasa vasorum, has emerged as the site of the initial immunological injury. The adventitial macrophages produce interleukin (IL)-1β and IL-6, while those invading the media produce matrix metalloproteases capable of destroying components of the arterial wall. After entering the arterial wall from the vasa vasorum of the adventitia, immunocompetent cells migrate through the media and thereafter focus on the periphery of the intima, where the elastic lamina is located. Giant cells tend to accumulate in the vicinity of destroyed

elastic tissue and are potent secretors of mediators such as matrix metalloproteases, platelet-derived growth factor, and vascular endothelial growth factor, the last promoting intimal proliferation that may be the main mechanism behind vessel obstruction in temporal arteritis. In temporal arteritis, the cellular infiltrates may thus be directed at specific antigens located in media and intima, conceivably in the elastic laminae separating the two layers, but what causes the elastic membrane to fragment initially and subsequently induce an immune response is yet to be determined.

The immunological and pathological processes involved in polymyalgia rheumatica are less well described. Histological examinations of synovial tissue from peripheral joints show nonspecific synovitis and biopsy specimens from striated muscle never reveal inflammatory changes.

Relationship between polymyalgia rheumatica and temporal arteritis

The discrepant clinical pictures of temporal arteritis and polymyalgia rheumatica may indicate two separate disease entities, while positron emission tomography (PET) scan findings of increased uptake of fluorodexoyglucose (FDG) in the thoracic vessels in most patients with polymyalgia rheumatica or temporal arteritis suggests a common vasculitic disorder. The reported incidence of biopsy-proven temporal arteritis among patients with pure polymyalgia rheumatica varies considerably—from 4% to 40%—which makes it difficult to reach an overall conclusion regarding the relationship between temporal arteritis and polymyalgia rheumatica.

Epidemiology

Polymyalgia rheumatica and temporal arteritis almost exclusively affect people aged over 50 years, the incidence rising until the 80s and declining thereafter. Women are affected more than men (ratio 2:1 to 3:1). Both conditions are more common in those of Nordic heritage than in other white populations, black populations, and Japanese individuals. In Scandinavian populations the annual incidence of biopsy-proven temporal arteritis is 22/100 000 to 29/100 000 in those aged over 50 (Table 19.11.4.1). The reported incidence of pure or isolated polymyalgia rheumatica varies considerably, depending on the methodology employed (Table 19.11.4.2), with studies of elderly individuals suggesting many missed diagnoses. The increase in incidence that has been reported recently may be due to a true increase in incidence, improved diagnosis, or increasing age of the general population.

Most studies conclude that the life expectancy of patients with polymyalgia rheumatica or temporal arteritis is almost identical to that of the general population. There is disagreement regarding the possibility of increased risk of cardiovascular diseases in patients with these conditions, but the risk of contracting arterial aneurysms is about 17 times greater than that of the general population, with aortic aneurysms causing death in 8% of patients. There is no increased risk of contracting malignant disease.

Clinical features

Pure or isolated polymyalgia rheumatica is the most common clinical presentation, occurring in 70 to 80% of cases, while isolated temporal arteritis accounts for 14 to 26%, and temporal arteritis

Table 19.11.4.1 Annual incidence of temporal arteritis per 100 000 inhabitants aged 50 years or older

Author	Year	Country	Incidence
Rajala	1969–89	Finland	7.2
Frantzen	1984–88	Finland	17.4–26.2
Baldursson	1984–90	Iceland	27.0
Nordborg	1990	Sweden	18.3
Petrusdottir	1999	Sweden	22.2
Gran	1987–94	Norway	24.8
Bengtsson	1973–75	Sweden	16.8–28.6
Huston	1950–59/1979–74	USA	5.1/17.4
Macado	1950–85	USA	17.0
Salvarani	1980–88	Italy	6.9
Sonnenblick	1980–91	Israel	10.2
Friedman	1960–64/1975–78	Israel	0.2/0.9
Gonzalez-Gay	1981–90	Spain	6.0
Barrier	1975–79	France	9.4
Jonasson	1964–77	Scotland	4.2
Smith	1983	USA	1.6

and polymyalgia rheumatica combined for only 4 to 5% of the total patient group.

Polymyalgia rheumatica

Patients may have a gradual, subacute, or acute disease onset. Although the disease may start asymmetrically and unilaterally, the classic clinical picture of general constitutional symptoms (malaise, fever, weight loss) and bilateral stiffness and pain of the shoulder and pelvic girdles, lower spine, and neck soon evolves. Stiffness often exceeds pain and is most pronounced in the morning or after rest.

Peripheral arthritis occurs in one-quarter to one-third of patients, most commonly in the knees (45%), metacarpophalangeal joints (40%), and wrists (40%). Mono- or oligoarticular disease is most frequent, with polyarthritis seen in less than 5% of cases. Using both MRI and ultrasonography, bilateral trochanteric

Table 19.11.4.2 Annual incidence of polymyalgia rheumatica per 100 000 population

Author	Year	Country	Age group	Incidence
Noltorp	1991	Sweden	All	33.6
Salvarani	1970–91	USA		52.5
Schaufelberger	1999	Sweden	All	17.1
			50+	49.7
Salvarani	1991	Italy	All	4.9?
			50+	12.7
Gran	1987–94	Norway	50+	96.3
Kyle	1985	England	65+?	400
Gonzalez-Gay	1999	Spain	50+	13.5?

bursitis is detected in 90% and synovitis of the hip in 45 to 85% of patients. Carpal tunnel syndrome is recorded in 14% of cases, and distal extremity swelling with pitting oedema in 1 to 12%. A diffuse swelling of the supraclavicular region can be seen, often called 'padding'.

Temporal arteritis

Headache is reported by the vast majority of patients. It is classically located to the temporal regions, but occipital, frontal, or general headache is often encountered. Constitutional symptoms frequently follow, including malaise, weight loss, low-grade fever, loss of appetite, and night sweats. Jaw claudication (pain during chewing), reduction or difficulty in jaw opening, and maxillary pain are not infrequent.

On examination the temporal artery pulses are often reduced or absent, and local tenderness may be present. In the absence of polymyalgia rheumatica, peripheral arthritis is an exceptional finding.

Ophthalmological features

Visual disturbances can be caused by anterior ischaemic optic neuropathy (90%), central retinal artery occlusion (10%), cilioretinal artery occlusion (10%), and/or posterior ischaemic optic neuropathy (4%).

Depending on the type of referral centre, they are seen in 3 to 60% of cases, while permanent visual loss occurs in 3 to 14%.

Visual disturbances such as partially obscured vision, visual field impairment, and diplopia usually develop early in the course of disease, and they may be the presenting clinical manifestation. All patients with biopsy-proven temporal arteritis should be carefully monitored for such complications, transient visual loss such as amaurosis fugax, transient blurring of vision, or diplopia often preceding permanent visual loss.

Cerebrovascular manifestations

Neurological manifestations of temporal arteritis most probably result from arteritis of the vasa vasorum of peripheral nerves or thromboembolic central nervous system (CNS) disease: inflammatory lesions are very rarely found beyond 5 mm after the artery's penetration of the dura. Neurological features, including visual disturbances, transient ischaemic attack, and stroke, develop in about 30% of patients with biopsy-proven temporal arteritis. Mononeuropathies, peripheral polyneuropathies of the arms and legs, vertebrobasilar ischaemia, hearing loss or tinnitus, and vestibular dysfunction may develop.

Miscellaneous manifestations

Scalp necrosis is a rare complication of temporal arteritis, manifesting with skin ulceration of the frontal, parietal, and/or temporal areas, most frequently bilaterally. It often starts before treatment with corticosteroids, and is significantly associated with visual disturbances. The outlook is good, with full healing being the rule. Tongue gangrene and hemianaesthesia of the tongue occasionally occur.

Cardiovascular and large artery manifestations.

About 80% of patients with giant cell arteritis have involvement of large vessels detectable by PET, which disappears in half of those rescanned at 3 months. Between a quarter and a fifth of patients develop aortic aneurysms or dissection. Most aneurysms develop in the ascending aorta, but abdominal aneurysms are also seen. They tend to be a late feature, occurring years after the onset of the disease, and even years after the completion of glucocorticosterid therapy. Yearly ultrasound screening of patients with giant cell arteritis for abdominal and thoracic aneurysms is likely to be cost-effective, there being no way of selecting those patients who are particularly prone to develop these problems. Coronary arteritis and cranial nerve involvement are very rarely diagnosed.

Stenosis of the superior branches of the aortic arch, especially the subclavian and axillary arteries, occurs in about 10 to 15% of patients. If lower limb arteritis occurs, it is usually bilateral, with rapidly progressive intermittent claudication of recent onset being the most common symptom.

Clinical investigation

A high ESR and CRP are recorded in the overwhelming majority of patients with temporal arteritis or polymyalgia rheumatica. The combination of normal values for both ESR and CRP is very rarely observed. Anaemia (of chronic disorder), leucocytosis, thrombocytosis, and increases in liver enzymes may be seen.

A temporal artery biopsy should be performed in all patients suspected of having temporal arteritis, but is not recommended in cases exhibiting no symptoms or signs of arteritis. In those who present predominantly with occipital or cervical symptoms, occipital artery biopsy can be a safe and effective diagnostic procedure. Traditionally, the recommended length of the biopsy should be 3 cm, but recent studies suggest that a reasonable sensitivity is obtained from biopsies of 0.5 to 1 cm. Most clinicians will recommend a second biopsy from the contralateral side if the first biopsy is negative, although the diagnostic yield of a second biopsy is low. Further sectioning of the biopsy is also often recommended in negative biopsies, but seldom reveals new positive findings. Prior corticosteroid treatment does not significantly hinder the correct interpretation of the biopsies: positive findings can be demonstrated even after 2 to 4 weeks of therapy.

The ultrasonographic finding of a hypoechoic halo around the lumen of the temporal arteries has been advocated as a method of making the diagnosis of temporal arteritis without the need for biopsy. However, the sensitivity is only 40% and specificity 79% for the diagnosis of biopsy-proven temporal arteritis. Negative ultrasonographic findings at the onset of disease may be because early adventitial inflammation does not produce the oedema that causes the halo effect. Ultrasonography should not therefore replace temporal artery biopsy for diagnosis, but it can serve as a means for identifying sites suitable for surgical biopsies.

PET does not detect metabolic signals within anatomical structures smaller than 4 to 5 mm, hence the method appears unsuitable for evaluation of small-vessel involvement, although it may be used to evaluate disease activity in large artery disease.

Diagnosis and classification criteria

In clinical practice, the diagnosis of polymyalgia rheumatica is made in patients aged 50 years and older, having symmetrical limb girdle pain and/or stiffness in addition to elevated levels of ESR and/or CRP. In clinical studies the Bird criteria of 1979 are preferred by most workers, exhibiting a sensitivity of 92% and a specificity of 75% for the diagnosis of polymyalgia rheumatica (Box 19.11.4.1).

The diagnosis of temporal arteritis in everyday clinical practice requires headache and/or systemic symptoms, age 50 years

---

> **Box 19.11.4.1**   Bird criteria for polymyalgia rheumatica
>
> ◆ Bilateral shoulder pain/stiffness
>
> ◆ Duration of onset <2 weeks
>
> ◆ Initial erythrocyte sedimentation rate >40 mm/h
>
> ◆ Morning stiffness >1 h
>
> ◆ Age >65 years
>
> ◆ Depression and/or weight loss
>
> ◆ Bilateral upper arm tenderness
>
> Probable polymyalgia rheumatica requires three or more positive criteria.

---

or older, histological proof of arteritis, a significant acute phase response, and exclusion of other causes of headache. In clinical studies the American College of Rheumatology (ACR) criteria of 1990 (Box 19.11.4.2) are usually preferred, and—as opposed to clinical diagnostic requirements—they do not require histological confirmation for diagnosis.

Differential diagnosis

The diagnosis of polymyalgia rheumatica is reached on clinical grounds, and after appropriate clinical and laboratory examinations to rule out other diseases (Box 19.11.4.3). Few diseases can be mistaken for what turns out to be biopsy-proven temporal arteritis. Vasculitis of the temporal arteries has been reported in polyarteritis nodosa, Churg–Strauss syndrome, microscopic polyangiitis, Wegener's granulomatosis, hepatitis B virus-related polyarteritis nodosa, hepatitis C virus-related cryoglobulinaemic vasculitis, and rheumatoid vasculitis, but the clinical features of these diseases distinguish them from temporal arteritis.

Treatment

The mainstay of therapy in polymyalgia rheumatica is the administration of oral glucocorticosteroids, although their mechanism of action is not thoroughly known. A low-dose regimen is preferred by most clinicians, side effects being more common in patients starting with doses exceeding 40 mg prednisolone/day and on high maintenance dosage. In pure or isolated polymyalgia rheumatica

---

> **Box 19.11.4.2**   American College of Rheumatology classification criteria for giant cell arteritis
>
> ◆ Age at onset 50 years or more
>
> ◆ New-onset headache or localized headache
>
> ◆ Tenderness or decreased pulsation in at least one of the temporal arteries
>
> ◆ Erythrocyte sedimentation rate 50 mm/h or more
>
> ◆ Abnormal artery biopsy with either mononuclear cell infiltrate or granulomatous inflammation (with giant cells)
>
> Giant cell arteritis requires at least three of the five criteria.

Box 19.11.4.3 Differential diagnoses of polymyalgia rheumatica

Rheumatological

- Old age at onset of rheumatoid arthritis
- Remitting seronegative symmetrical synovitis with pitting oedema
- Capsulitis of the shoulder ('frozen shoulder')
- Osteoarthritis
- Myositis
- Fibromyalgia

Bone disease

- Osteomalacia
- Osteoporosis
- Paget's disease

Infective

- Viral
- Other chronic infection, e.g. tuberculosis, endocarditis

Other

- Thyroiditis/hypothyroidism
- Multiple myeloma
- Parkinson's disease
- Myopathy associated with malignancy

an initial dose of prednisolone 15 mg/day is sufficient to suppress disease activity and provides significant relief in most patients. However, such a low starting dose may be associated with a significant risk of relapse and, if an adequate clinical response does not evolve within 36 h, 30 mg/day should be tried. The diagnosis must be re-evaluated if clinical response is still lacking, including screening for paraneoplastic myopathy. Nonsteroidal anti-inflammatory drugs (NSAIDs) offer little relief of symptoms and are rarely indicated in polymyalgia rheumatica.

When remission is achieved, the dose of steroid is slowly reduced to a maintenance dose over the next few months. This reduction is mainly guided by the patient's symptoms: monitoring of the ESR and CRP is often undertaken, but is not always reliable as a marker of response or likelihood of relapse. In one study, the mean daily maintenance dose of prednisolone during the first and second year was 5.7 mg and 4.3 mg, respectively.

In uncomplicated temporal arteritis a starting dose of prednisolone of 30 to 40 mg/day is recommended, but 40 to 60 mg/day should be tried if response is lacking. The dose is then slowly tapered to a maintenance dose, this being a mean of 6.6 mg/day and 4.1 mg/day during the first and second years for uncomplicated temporal arteritis in one study. If temporal arteritis is complicated by polymyalgia rheumatica, the maintenance dose is usually somewhat higher.

Most studies, but not all, have shown that most patients need treatment with corticosteroids for several years. In one prospective study the rate of steroid cessation after 2 years in polymyalgia rheumatica was 24%, in temporal arteritis 16%, and in temporal arteritis and polymyalgia rheumatica combined 5%. It is therefore not advisable to terminate corticosteroids in temporal arteritis before 2 years of treatment. In polymyalgia rheumatica, which is not associated with the complications that can affect patients with temporal arteritis, termination of therapy can be tried after 12 months, provided that complete remission has been obtained and the patient is only receiving a very low dose of corticosteroids. Appropriate prophylaxis against osteoporosis should be offered.

The effectiveness of alternate-day treatment with corticosteroids is doubtful, with as many as 35% of patients having to abandon treatment as a result of 'day-off' relapses. Deflazacort is preferred by some, but did not result in less bone loss than prednisone in one study. Methotrexate appears to be the drug of choice when additive treatment is warranted, but azathioprine can also be used. Trials with tumour necrosis factor α blockers have so far been disappointing.

It is not possible to identify reliably those patients who are prone to develop flare-ups, but these are best treated by increasing the dose of oral corticosteroids temporarily. Recurrences most often occur within the first 6 months after cessation of corticosteroids, with about half occurring within 1 month and nearly all within 1 year. Clinical experience suggests that, the slower the tapering of daily steroid dosage, the less the chance of recurrence.

Peripheral arthritis is best treated with NSAIDs or local injections of corticosteroids. In persistent peripheral arthritis, methotrexate and sulfasalazine should be considered.

Disease affecting the eye

Visual disturbances can lead to permanent visual impairment and should be treated immediately with oral prednisolone at a dose of 60 to 80 mg/day. The use of very high doses of steroid therapy, given intravenously, is probably not more effective than oral therapy in preventing visual deterioration.

In one study of patients with temporal arteritis the probability of loss of vision after 5 years of steroid therapy was 1%, and the chance of additional loss was 13% in patients who had a visual deficit at the time therapy was started. If treatment is instituted within 24 h from onset of symptoms, visual improvement is observed in about 60% of patients, compared with only 6% in cases where there is longer delay. If further visual deterioration occurs despite high doses of systemic corticosteroids, this almost invariably starts within 5 days of treatment. Some recommend the use of low-dose aspirin to prevent development of cerebrovascular disease.

Prognosis

Polymyalgia rheumatica and temporal arteritis are in general regarded as diseases with a favourable outcome, having a self-limited disease course, similar mortality rate to the general population, and no increased incidence of neoplasms. However, the quality of life and the coexistence of other diseases have been insufficiently studied. Similarly, it is difficult to differentiate between patients needing long-term versus short-term treatment, but patients with both polymyalgia rheumatica and temporal arteritis often run a protracted disease course.

Further reading

Bird HA, *et al.* (2005). A comparison of the sensitivity of diagnostic criteria for polymyalgia rheumatica. *Ann Rheum Dis*, **64**, 626–9.

Blockmans D, *et al.* (2006). Repetitive ^{18}F-fluorodeoxyglucose positron emission tomography in giant cell arteritis: a prospective study of 35 patients. *Arthritis Care Res*, **55**, 131–7.

Bongatz T, Matteson EL (2006). Large-vessel involvement in giant cell arteritis. *Curr Opin Rheumatol*, **18**, 10–7.

Cantini F, *et al.* (2000). Erythrocyte sedimentation rate and C-reactive protein in the evaluation of disease activity and severity in polymyalgia rheumatica: a prospective follow-up study. *Arthritis Rheum*, **30**, 17–24.

Caporali R, *et al.* (2004). Prednisone plus methotrexate for polymyalgia rheumatica: a randomized, double-blind, placebo-controlled trial. *Ann Intern Med*, **141**, 493–500.

Evans ME, O'Fallon M, Hunder GG (1995). Increased incidence of aneurysms and dissection in giant cell (temporal) arteritis. A population based study. *Ann Intern Med*, **122**, 502–7.

Gran JT (2002). Some thought about the etiopathogenesis of temporal arteritis. *Scand J Rheumatol*, **31**, 1–5.

Hayreh SS, Zimmerman B, Kardon RH (2002). Visual improvement with corticosteroid therapy in giant cell arteritis. Report of a large study and review of the literature. *Acta Ophthalmol Scand*, **80**, 353–67.

Hoffman GS, *et al.* (2002). A multicenter, randomized, double-blind, placebo-controlled trial of adjuvant methotrexate treatment for giant cell arteritis. *Arthritis Rheum*, **46**, 1309–18.

Hunder GG, Bloch DA, Michel BA (1990). The American College of Rheumatology 1990 criteria for the classification of giant cell arteritis. *Arthritis Rheum*, **33**, 1122–8.

Kremers HM, *et al.* (2005). Relapse in a population based cohort of patients with polymyalgia rheumatica. *J Rheumatol*, **32**, 65–73.

Liozon E, *et al.* (2001). Risk factors for visual loss in giant cell (temporal) arteritis: a prospective study of 174 patients. *Am J Med*, **111**, 211–17.

Mahr A, *et al.* (2006). Temporal artery biopsy for diagnosing giant cell arteritis: the longer, the better? *Ann Rheum Dis*, **65**, 826–8.

Myklebust G, Gran JT (1996). A prospective study of 287 patients with polymyalgia rheumatica and temporal arteritis: clinical and laboratory manifestations at onset of disease and at the time of diagnosis. *Br J Rheumatol*, **35**, 1161–8.

Myklebust G, Gran JT (2001). Prednisolone maintenance dose in relation to starting dose in the treatment of polymyalgia rheumatica and temporal arteritis. *Scand J Rheumatol*, **30**, 260–7.

Nordborg E, Nordborg C (2003). Giant cell arteritis: epidemiological clues to its pathogenesis and an update on its treatment. *Rheumatology*, **42**, 413–21.

Nordborg E, Nordborg C (2004). Giant cell arteritis: strategies in diagnosis and treatment. *Curr Opin Rheumatol*, **16**, 25–30.

Salvarani C, *et al.* (2002). Polymyalgia rheumatica and giant-cell arteritis. *N Engl J Med*, **347**, 261–71.

Schaufelberger C, Bengtsson BÅ, Andersson R (1999). Epidemiology and mortality in 220 patients with polymyalgia rheumatica. *Br J Rheumatol*, **34**, 261–4.

Spiera H, Davidson S (1982). Treatment of polymyalgia rheumatica. *Arthritis Rheum*, **25**, 120.

Weyand CM (2000). The pathogenesis of giant cell arteritis. *J Rheumatol*, **27**, 517–22.

Weyand CM, *et al.* (1999). Corticosteroid requirements in polymyalgia rheumatica. *Arch Intern Med*, **159**, 577–84.

19.11.5 Behçet's syndrome

Sebahattin Yurdakul, Izzet Fresko, and Hasan Yazici

Essentials

Behçet's syndrome is an inflammatory disorder of unknown aetiology that involves arteries and veins of all sizes. Most cases are from the countries around the Mediterranean basin, the Middle East and east Asia, with the highest prevalence in Turkey.

Clinical features—the disease typically presents in the second and third decades with recurrent oral ulcers (98% of cases), genital ulcers (85%), acneiform lesions (85%), pathergy reaction (60% in some countries), erythema nodosum (50%), uveitis (50%), arthritis (50%), thrombophlebitis (30%), and less commonly with arterial occlusion/aneurysm, central nervous system involvement or gastrointestinal lesions. A relapsing/remitting course is usual. Disease is more severe and mortality is higher in men. The diagnosis is clinical: laboratory findings are nonspecific—there is no specific diagnostic test for Behçet's syndrome.

Management and prognosis—elderly people, and women with mild mucocutaneous lesions, can be managed symptomatically. Young people and men need a more aggressive treatment approach, typically as follows (1) mucocutaneous lesions—can be helped by colchicine, thalidomide, and dapsone; (2) acute severe eye involvement—ciclosporin and anti-TNF agent or solo interferon is the first agent to use, often replaced by azathioprine to maintain remission; (3) thrombophlebitis—typically managed with aspirin and azathioprine; (4) severe vascular disease—cyclophosphamide and steroids is the preferred treatment, with steroids usually added initially; (5) parenchymal central nervous system disease—management remains problematic: steroids, immunosuppressives, interferon-α, and tumour necrosis factor α antagonists have all been tried. Major vessel disease and neurological involvement are the main causes of death. About 10–15% of male patients who have eye disease lose useful vision despite treatment.

Introduction

Hulusi Behçet, a Turkish dermatologist working in Istanbul, described three patients with oral and genital ulceration and uveitis with hypopyon in 1937; it soon became apparent that many other organ systems were involved and that the condition was a widespread vasculitis.

Aetiology, genetics, pathogenesis, and pathology

Behçet's syndrome is an inflammatory disorder of unknown aetiology. *HLA B51* is the genetic marker that has consistently been associated with the condition, but a whole-genome study has suggested that non-HLA loci may also be operative. A pathogenic role for the adaptive immune system is suggested by the strong T polarization, the presence of a cellular immune response, and interleukin (IL)-12 and interferon-γ in skin biopsy specimens of pathergy reactions (see below), and oligoclonal T-cell expansion induced by certain antigens. However, the lack of antigen specificity of the T-cell responses and the low levels of mannose-binding lectin are aspects that favour the role of the innate immune system. Most probably both systems are involved, but—although immuno-logical aberrations are seen—the syndrome has many clinical and laboratory features that differ from those of a classic autoimmune rheumatological disease, e.g. it is not usually associated with Sjögren's syndrome, autoantibodies, or particular MHC (major histocompatibility complex) class II alleles.

In considering the pathogenesis of Behçet's syndrome it might prove useful to consider particular variants of disease expression. One notable cluster of patients is those with acne and arthritis; another is those with superficial and deep vein thrombosis, and a propensity to dural sinus thrombi. These differing manifestations of what we now regard as Behçet's syndrome might indicate more than one disease mechanism.

Behçet's syndrome involves arteries and veins of all sizes, but there are some lesions where direct evidence of injury to the vessel wall cannot be demonstrated. Among these are the acne lesions of the skin, where histology is no different from ordinary acne, and, in the brain, where evidence for direct vessel wall injury is difficult to find. There is no specific cell type that dominates in vasculitic lesions and immune complex deposition can be seen only in some. Thrombophilic factors seem not to be the primary event in explaining the hypercoagulability of Behçet's syndrome: hypertriglyceridaemia might be a risk factor.

Epidemiology

Behçet's syndrome has a distinct geographical distribution, with most cases being from the countries around the Mediterranean basin, the Middle East, and east Asia. The prevalence ranges from $0.07/10^4$ in Spain to 8 to $42/10^4$ in Turkey. The Silk Route has been suggested as the mechanism through which an aetiological agent (genetic or environmental) was spread. It can affect every age group, but onset before puberty or after the sixth decade is relatively rare.

Clinical findings

Clinical manifestations are protean (Table 19.11.5.1) and the disease course is characterized by unpredictable periods of recurrences and remissions. Although skin and mucosal lesions are most common, the ocular, central nervous system (CNS), and large-vessel manifestations are more serious.

Mucocutaneous

Oral ulceration is generally the first, as well as the most frequent, manifestation of Behçet's syndrome. Smoking may decrease the frequency.

Genital ulcers cause pain and discomfort (Fig. 19.11.5.1), with the presence of genital scarring being quite useful for diagnosis. Urethritis is not observed, in contrast to that seen in Reiter's disease or sexually transmitted infections.

Papulopustular or acneiform lesions are usually indistinguishable from ordinary acne vulgaris, both in appearance and in histology. They are usually seen on the face, upper chest, and back,

Table 19.11.5.1 Clinical manifestations of Behçet's syndrome

Manifestation	Features
Recurrent oral ulcers (97–99%)	Usually the first and most recurrent manifestation Mostly minor ulcers; heal without scarring Usually indistinguishable in appearance and histology from recurrent aphthae
Genital ulcers (c.85%)	Mostly on the scrotum or both labiae Less frequent on the penis Large ulcers (>1 cm) heal with a scar
Papulopustular lesions (c.85%)	Indistinguishable from ordinary acne On face and back as well as unusual acne sites (extremities)
Erythema nodosum (c.50%)	Mostly on lower extremities Similar to primary erythema nodosum Confused with superficial thrombophlebitis.
Pathergy reaction (60%)	60–70% positivity in Turkey or Japan Rarely positive in northern Europe or the USA
Uveitis (c.50%)	Chronic, relapsing, bilateral panuveitis Hypopyon indicates a grave prognosis
Joints (50%)	Mono- or oligoarticular yet symmetrical Nondeforming, nonerosive, and self-limited Mostly knees, ankles, elbows, and wrists
Thrombophlebitis (30%)	Frequently superficial or deep veins of the legs Thromboembolism is rare
Arterial occlusion/aneurysm (c.4%)	Entire arterial tree Pulmonary artery aneurysms present with haemoptyses
CNS involvement (5–10%)	Parenchymal (80%) and dural sinus thrombi (20%) Peripheral neuropathy uncommon.
Gastrointestinal lesions (1–30%)	Rare in Turkey and 30% in Japan Mimicking inflammatory bowel diseases

but they can also affect sites not typically affected by acne vulgaris, such as the arms and legs. The lesions of erythema nodosum can be difficult to differentiate from superficial thrombophlebitis using the naked eye: ultrasound examination may obviate the need for a biopsy. Less common forms of skin lesions are papules, palpable purpura, skin ulcers, Sweet's syndrome, and pyoderma gangrenosum.

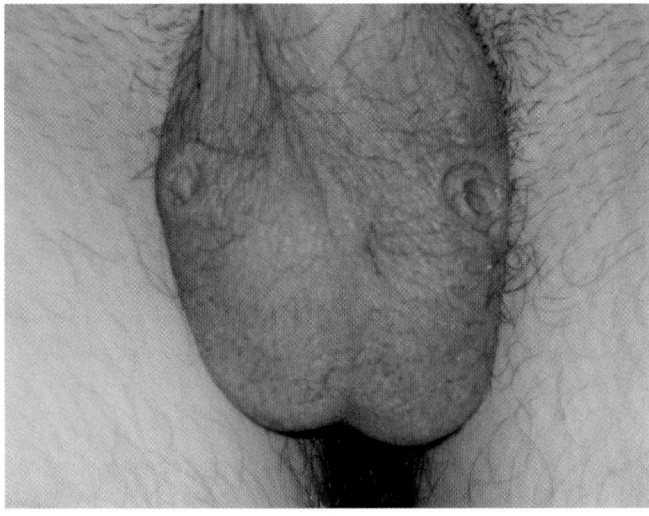

Fig. 19.11.5.1 Genital ulcers in a patient with Behçet's syndrome.

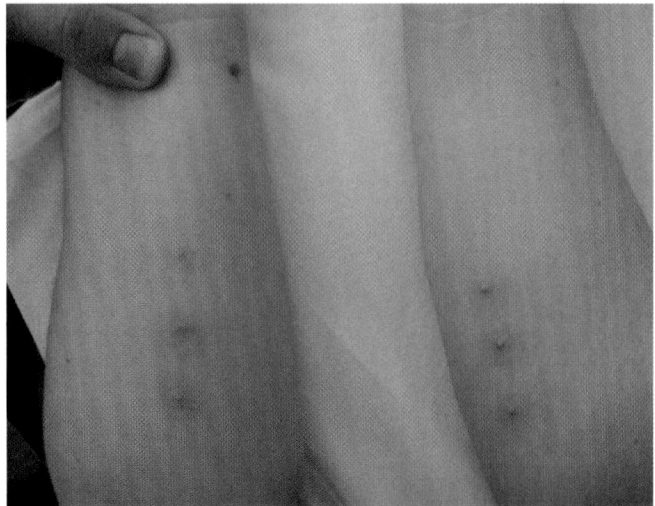

Fig. 19.11.5.2 The pathergy reaction induced by needle pricks to the forearms.

The pathergy phenomenon is defined as a nonspecific hyperreactivity to simple trauma. Typically, a papule or a pustule forms in 24 to 48 h after skin puncture with a needle (Fig. 19.11.5.2). This is quite specific for Behçet's syndrome, but although found in 60 to 70% of patients in Turkey or Japan, it is rarely observed in northern Europe or the United States of America. It can be observed in organs other than the skin, such as attacks of uveitis after eye surgery, synovitis after arthrocentesis, or development of an aneurysm after puncture of an artery. But moreover wound healing is normal.

Ocular

Eye involvement takes the form of a relapsing panuveitis that generally starts within the first 2 years of disease onset. It is more frequent (70%) and has a more severe course in men, and in young people (aged less than 25 years). Hypopyon uveitis, an intense inflammation in the anterior chamber that can be seen by the physician without any ophthalmological aids in 20% of patients with ocular disease, is associated with severe retinal disease.

Posterior uveal inflammation with retinal vasculitis causes retinal exudates, haemorrhages, venous thrombosis, papilloedema, and macular disease. Recurrent attacks of eye inflammation lead to structural changes such as synechiae and retinal scars, which are the main determinants of eye prognosis. Episcleritis, conjunctivitis, corneal ulcerations, and lid lesions are occasionally seen.

Musculoskeletal

Arthritis is mono- or oligoarticular, usually resolves in a few weeks, and is associated with acneiform lesions. A subgroup with acne and arthritis has increased enthesopathy when examined by ultrasonography. Chronic synovitis with erosions and deformity can be seen, but is rare. Back pain and sacroiliac joint involvement are not part of the clinical picture. Synovial fluid is commonly inflammatory, with a predominance of neutrophils, but it has a good mucin clot formation. Local myositis of the legs, or generalized similar to polymyositis, is infrequently seen, as is osteonecrosis.

Vascular

Behçet's syndrome involves both veins and arteries. Around a third of patients have thrombophlebitis, most frequently in the superficial or deep veins of the legs. Obstruction of the superior and/or inferior

vena cava (SVC and IVC) are less frequent, and occlusion of the suprahepatic veins (Budd–Chiari syndrome) is rare but carries a high mortality. Thromboembolism is rare, most probably due to the tight adherence of thrombi to the diseased vein.

The entire arterial tree can be affected by arterial aneurysms and/or occlusion: the abdominal aorta is the most frequent site, followed by the iliac, femoral, popliteal, carotid, and subclavian vessels. Pulmonary artery aneurysms are associated with thrombophlebitis of leg veins and IVC in 90% of patients. They present with haemoptyses, which can be fatal, with the typical finding on chest radiography being noncavitating single or multiple shadows (Fig. 19.11.5.3). CT scans confirm the diagnosis.

Neurological

Disease of the CNS is also more common and more severe in male patients. Most of those affected (80%) have parenchymal disease, which causes pyramidal, cerebellar, and sensory signs and symptoms, sphincter disturbances, and behavioural changes. The remaining 20% have nonparenchymal involvement in the form of intracranial hypertension due to dural sinus thrombosis presenting with headaches and papilloedema. Both types of involvement rarely occur in the same patient. Cerebrospinal fluid examination shows nonspecific findings, but a high protein or cell count implies a grave prognosis in the long run. Peripheral neuropathy, which is frequently seen in other vasculitides, is uncommon in Behçet's syndrome.

Gastrointestinal

Gastrointestinal involvement shows geographical variation, being rare among people who live in the Mediterranean countries although frequent among those in Japan. Mucosal ulceration, primarily in the ileum and colon, presents with colicky abdominal pain and diarrhoea that mimic inflammatory bowel diseases. It usually follows a fluctuating course, with exacerbations and remissions, and it tends to perforate.

Hepatic involvement is uncommon except for the rare Budd–Chiari syndrome. A slightly enlarged spleen can be found in men.

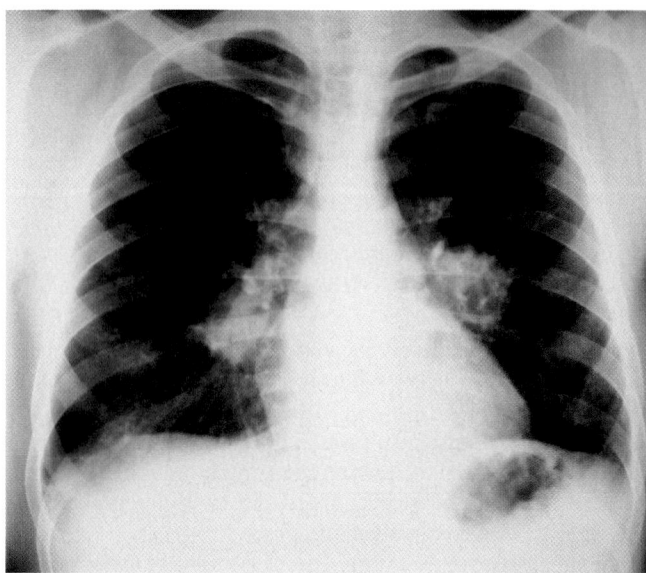

Fig. 19.11.5.3 Chest radiograph showing pulmonary artery aneurysms in a patient with Behçet's syndrome.

Cardiac

There have been sporadic reports of many types of conduction problem, valvular disease, and aortitis, as well as ventricular aneurysms and coronary vasculitis, and endomyocardial fibrosis with intracardiac thrombi. However, the overall frequency of cardiac disease was no different from that seen in controls in a prospective controlled study.

Other features

Renal involvement, seen infrequently, ranges from IgA nephropathy to rapidly progressive glomerulonephritis. Immune complexes are not usually found in the kidneys. Amyloidosis of the AA type occasionally occurs, as observed in other chronic inflammatory states, usually presenting in men with a nephrotic syndrome, which has a grave prognosis.

Epididymitis is a well-recognized feature, reported in up to 20% of cases. Voiding disturbances have also been described.

Differential diagnosis

The two conditions that most commonly cause problems in diagnosis are inflammatory bowel disease, especially Crohn's disease, and multiple sclerosis. Intestinal and especially ileocaecal ulcers are both observed in Crohn's disease and Behçet's syndrome, but fistulization and perianal ulcerations are rare in the latter. Furthermore, the eye inflammation of Behçet's syndrome is most often a panuveitis, compared with the anterior chamber disease seen in Crohn's disease. With regard to multiple sclerosis, optic neuritis is rare in Behçet's syndrome, and the characteristic MRI lesions of Behçet's syndrome are situated in the basal ganglia and diencephalon, whereas those in multiple sclerosis are usually seen as white matter lesions in the periventricular areas.

Clinical investigation

Laboratory findings are nonspecific. A mild anaemia of chronic disease and leucocytosis are seen in some patients. The erythrocyte sedimentation (ESR) rate and C-reactive protein (CRP) may be moderately elevated, and the latter may correlate with erythema nodosum and acute thrombophlebitis, although these inflammatory markers generally do not mirror clinical activity. Autoantibodies such as rheumatoid factors and antinuclear antibodies are absent and tests for antineutrophil cytoplasmic antibodies (ANCA) and anticardiolipin antibodies are usually negative.

Criteria for classification

In 1990 the International Study Group for Behçet's syndrome proposed a set of classification criteria that are sensitive (95%) and specific (98%) (Box 19.11.5.1).

Management

Treatment depends on the type and severity of symptoms, disease duration, and the age and sex of the patient. Those who are elderly, and women with mild mucocutaneous lesions, can be managed symptomatically, while young people and men need a more aggressive approach. A EULAR based recommendation concerning management has recently been published.

Controlled trials show that colchicine 1 to 2 mg/day is effective for genital ulcers, erythema nodosum, and arthritis in women. It is

> **Box 19.11.5.1** International Study Group Criteria for diagnosis of Behçet's disease
>
> - Recurrent oral ulceration (recurrent at least three times in one 12-month period)
>
> *plus* any two of the following findings:
>
> - Recurrent genital ulceration
> - Eye lesions
> - Skin lesions
> - Positive pathergy test
>
> Reprinted from The Lancet, 335, International Study Group for Behçet's Disease, Criteria for diagnosis of Behçet's disease , 1070-80, 1990, with permission from Elsevier

beneficial only for arthritis in males. Thalidomide at 100 mg/day is effective for orogenital ulceration, but its well-known adverse effects, in particular as a teratogen, hinder its more widespread use. Dapsone 100 mg/day is also beneficial in mucocutaneous lesions.

Azathioprine (2.5 mg/kg per day) helps preserve visual acuity in established eye disease and prevents the emergence of new eye disease. It also has salutary effects on oral–genital ulcers and arthritis, and its use early in the course of disease is associated with a more favourable outcome. A drawback is its slow onset of action—usually taking 4 to 6 months for full effect. Ciclosporin 3 to 5 mg/kg per day acts within weeks and is the first agent to use in acute and severe eye involvement. It decreases the frequency of mucocutaneous lesions as well. Adverse effects are hypertension, renal impairment, and neurotoxicity, which require close monitoring. Ciclosporin and azathioprine are frequently combined, with the former used to induce remission and the latter as a remission-maintaining agent.

Corticosteroids are widely used in managing Behçet's syndrome, but in the only controlled study methylprednisolone acetate (40 mg intramuscularly every 3 weeks) was useful only in controlling erythema nodosum lesions in women. Cyclophosphamide (2 to 2.5 mg/kg per day orally, or 500 to 1500 mg as monthly intravenous boluses) is the preferred treatment for severe vascular disease, with steroids usually added for the initial few months.

The management of the parenchymal type of CNS disease is problematic: steroids, immunosuppressives, interferon-α, and tumour necrosis factor (TNF)-α antagonists have all been tried. Dural sinus thrombosis is managed with brief courses of steroids.

Gastrointestinal involvement is initially managed by sulfasalazine at a dose of 2 to 6 g/day, but sometimes bowel resection is required.

There is debate about whether or not to use heparin or oral anticoagulants for the thrombophlebitis of Behçet's syndrome. As stated previously, pulmonary embolism is seldom observed, so antiplatelet drugs (i.e. aspirin) are probably sufficient. We also use azathioprine to generally suppress disease activity in the thrombophlebitis of Behçet's syndrome.

Surgical correction of peripheral arterial aneurysms is usually successful (in appropriate cases), with immunosuppressives given before surgical intervention to prevent recurrence. However, surgical correction of pulmonary arterial aneurysms should not be attempted because of high surgical mortality.

Data on α-interferon and the TNF-α blockers from open studies have shown that they are also beneficial in patients who are resistant to conventional treatments. Interferon-α (3 to 6 MU/day) was reported to cause a partial or complete response in patients with resistant posterior uveitis. Side effects such as flu-like symptoms were frequent and dose dependent. The TNF-α blocker infliximab 5 mg/ kg was useful in controlling severe and resistant uveitis, and other severe manifestations such as gastrointestinal and neurological Behçet's syndrome, but relapses were common after discontinuation. A double-blind, placebo-controlled study with the TNF-α blocker etanercept found it to be useful in controlling most mucocutaneous lesions of Behçet's syndrome when used at 25 mg twice a week for a period of 4 weeks.

Prognosis

Young men have the highest morbidity and mortality. Women have less severe disease than men. Major vessel disease and neurological involvement are the main causes of death. Eye inflammation and its greatest damage occur during the first 2 years. The disease tends to abate after 40 years of age, but CNS involvement and major vessel disease may have a late onset (5 to 10 years after diagnosis). Loss of useful vision ensues in about 10–15% of male patients with eye disease despite therapy.

Mortality attributable to Behçet's syndrome decreases with time after diagnosis, which is the opposite of the situation in rheumatoid arthritis and systemic lupus erythematosus. This may be due both to self-abating disease activity, and to the fact that atherosclerosis is not accelerated in Behçet's syndrome in the same way that it is in rheumatoid arthritis and systemic lupus erythematosus. A recent study of pulmonary arterial aneurysms has shown that the related mortality rate has decreased from 50% to around 20% in the last decade, due to either earlier recognition or more rational use of immunosuppressives.

Overall, the outlook for patients with eye disease and the mucocutaneous manifestations of Behçet's syndrome is considerably better than it was in the past, but management of CNS disease and thrombophilia/major vascular complications, including thrombotic events, remains problematic.

Further reading

Akman-Demir G, Serdaroglu P, Tasci B (1999). Clinical patterns of neurological involvement in Behcet's disease: evaluation of 200 patients. *Brain*, **122**, 2171–82.

Direskeneli H (2006). Autoimmunity vs. autoinflammation in Behcet's disease: do we oversimplify a complex disorder? *Rheumatology (Oxford)*, **45**, 1461–5.

Frassanito MA, *et al.* (1999). Th1 polarization of the immune response in Behcet's disease: a putative pathogenetic role of interleukin-12. *Arthritis Rheum*, **42**, 1967–74.

Gul A, *et al.* (2000). Familial aggregation of Behcet's disease in Turkey, *Ann Rheum Dis*, **59**, 622–5.

Hamuryudan V, *et al.* (1998). Thalidomide in the treatment of the mucocutaneous lesions of the Behçet syndrome. A randomized, double-blind, placebo-controlled trial. Ann Intern Med, **128**, 443–50.

Hatemi G, *et al.* (2009). Management of Behcet's disease: a systematic literature review for the European League Against Rheumatism: evidence based recommendations for the management of Behcet's disease. *Ann Rheum Dis*, **68**(10), 1528–34.

International Study Group for Behcet's disease (1990). Criteria for diagnosis of Behcet's disease. *Lancet*, **335**, 1078.

Kötter, *et al.* (2004). The use of interferon alfa in Behcet's disease: A review of the literature. *Semin Arthritis Rheum*, **33**, 320–35.

Kural-Seyahi E, *et al.* (2003). The long-term mortality and morbidity of Behçet syndrome: a 2-decade outcome survey of 387 patients followed at a dedicated center. *Medicine (Baltimore)*, **82**, 60–76.

Matsumoto T, *et al.* (1991). Vasculo-Behçet's disease: a pathologic study of eight cases. *Human Pathol*, **22**, 45–51.

Melikoglu M, *et al.* (2005). Short term trial of etanercept in Behcet's disease: a double blind, placebo controlled study. *J Rheumatol*, **32**, 98–105.

Melikoglu M, *et al.* (2006). Characterization of the divergent wound-healing responses occurring in the pathergy reaction and normal healthy volunteers. *J Immunol*, **177**, 6415–21.

Leiba M, *et al.* (2004). Thrombophilic factors are not the leading cause of thrombosis in Behçet's disease. *Ann Rheum Dis*, **63**, 1445–9.

Tugal-Tutkun I, *et al.* (2004). Uveitis in Behçet disease: an analysis of 880 patients. *Am J Ophthalmol*, **138**, 373–80.

Yazici H, *et al.* (2007). Behçet's syndrome; disease manifestations, management and advances in treatment. *Nat Clin Pract Rheumatol*, **3**(3), 148–55.

Yurdakul S, *et al.* (2001). A double-blind trial of colchicine in Behçet's syndrome. *Arthritis and Rheumatism*, **44**, 2686–92.

19.11.6 Sjögren's syndrome

Patrick J.W. Venables

Essentials

Sjögren's syndrome is characterized by inflammation and destruction of exocrine glands, particularly the salivary and lachrymal glands. Its cause is not known, but the condition may be primary, where the disease exists on its own, or secondary, where it is associated with other rheumatic diseases, most commonly rheumatoid arthritis. It affects women more than men (ratio 9:1) and is the second commonest autoimmune rheumatic disease (after rheumatoid arthritis), but in many patients remains undiagnosed because symptoms are mild.

Clinical features—presentation is typically with a gritty sensation in the eyes (or other ocular symptoms) and dryness of the mouth. Constitutional symptoms such as fatigue are common. Other systemic manifestations include Raynaud's phenomenon, purpura, arthralgia/arthritis, pleurisy, peripheral neuropathy, myelopathy, interstitial nephritis, and lymphoma.

Investigation and diagnosis—laboratory testing reveals raised immunoglobulin levels, rheumatoid factors of all isotypes (70% of cases), and autoantibodies against the cellular ribonucleoprotein antigens Ro (50–90%) and La (30–50%). Diagnosis should be based on the American/European Consensus criteria, which require the presence of four of the following six criteria: (1) ocular symptoms, (2) oral symptoms, (3) ocular signs, (4) oral signs, (5) positive labial biopsy, and (6) antibodies to Ro- and/or La (one or other of conditions 5 or 6 must be present).

Management—for most patients treatment is topical and symptomatic, with tear and saliva substitutes. Fatigue and arthralgia respond to hydroxychloroquine. Serious systemic complications are treated with steroids and cytotoxic drugs.

Introduction and historical perspective

Sjögren's syndrome was originally described in 1933 as a triad of dry eyes, dry mouth, and rheumatoid arthritis. It gained prominence as a rheumatic disease in 1966 with classification of primary and secondary Sjögren's syndrome. Its autoimmune nature was established in the 1970s when the autoantibodies to Ro and La were first described, although it was not until the 1990s that routine serological tests for these antibodies became widely available. A number of diagnostic criteria have been proposed over many years, but only the Consensus criteria of 2002 have attained widespread acceptance. Thus Sjögren's syndrome is a relatively 'new' disease in rheumatology, and is only recently being appreciated as a common multisystem disease that may present to other specialties.

Aetiology and pathology

The aetiology of Sjögren's syndrome is unknown, but is often considered to be an interaction between constitutional and environmental factors leading to autoimmunity. Primary Sjögren's syndrome is strongly associated with *HLA DR3*, and the linked genes *B8*, *DQ2*, and the *C4A* null gene. Candidates for triggering autoimmunity in Sjögren's syndrome are viruses that infect the salivary glands—including Epstein–Barr virus, cytomegalovirus, and human herpesvirus 6—all of which have been linked with the condition in some reports but not others. Retroviruses have also attracted interest because they infect and persist in cells of the immune system such as T cells and macrophages, and infect salivary gland epithelium, and Coxsackie viral sequences have been detected in salivary gland biopsies from Greek patients with Sjögren's syndrome, but these findings were not confirmed in a study from France. Thus, although viruses remain attractive candidates for a pathogenic role in Sjögren's syndrome, no particular agent has been consistently identified in independent studies.

The cardinal pathological features of Sjögren's syndrome are inflammation and destruction of salivary gland tissue. The inflammatory infiltrates consist of focal aggregates of lymphocytes, mainly CD4+ T cells, localized around ducts and acini. Scattered interstitial plasma cells are commonly found, although these are not disease specific and are also found in glands from healthy individuals. The destructive changes are predominantly duct dilatation, acinal atrophy, and interstitial fibrosis. However, these last findings have also been described in biopsies from people without Sjögren's syndrome, particularly in elderly people, and cannot be regarded as diagnostically specific.

The most striking feature of the systemic autoimmune response in Sjögren's syndrome is the marked activation of B cells which can lead to immunoglobulin levels of over three times the upper limit of the normal range. Rheumatoid factors of all isotypes are observed in blood in about 70% of patients, and their detection can lead to some patients with Sjögren's syndrome being misdiagnosed as having rheumatoid arthritis. The typical autoantibodies are those against the cellular ribonucleoprotein antigens Ro and La, named after the patients in whom the antibodies were originally described. Anti-Ro antibodies are more frequently detectable (50–90% of cases) than anti-La antibodies (30–50% of cases), but the latter are more diagnostically specific for primary Sjögren's syndrome. Two further potential autoantigens have also been described: fodrin, which is a cellular protein involved in apoptosis, and the muscarinic acetylcholine receptor, which is important in mediating parasympathetic stimulation of exocrine glands. A high degree of diagnostic sensitivity and specificity has been claimed for serum antibodies to both antigens in Sjögren's syndrome, but neither autoantibody system has yet been adopted for routine clinical use.

Clinical features

Sjögren's syndrome is nine times more common in women than in men and can develop at any age from 15 to 65. Recent epidemiological studies based on the 2002 Consensus criteria suggest a prevalence of 0.1 to 0.7% of the population, indicating that it is the second most common autoimmune rheumatic disease after rheumatoid arthritis, which affects 0.8 to 1%.

Patients with Sjögren's syndrome rarely complain of dry eyes, but rather a gritty sensation, soreness, photosensitivity, or intolerance of contact lenses. Excessive watering or deposits of dried mucus in the corner of the eye and recurrent attacks of conjunctivitis may occur in early disease. The dry mouth often manifests the 'cream cracker' sign, inability to swallow dry food without fluid, or waking up in the night to take sips of water. About half of those affected with the condition complain of intermittent or stable parotid swelling, which when excessively painful is often due to secondary bacterial infection. On examination, xerostomia can be detected as a diminished salivary pool, a dried fissured tongue, often complicated by angular stomatitis, and chronic oral candidiasis. The eyes may be reddened and roughened due to shallow erosions in the conjunctivae. Occasionally the front of the eye is eroded to reveal strands of underlying collagen, leading to the appearance of filamentary keratitis.

Other exocrine glands may be affected. Dry nasal passages and upper airways may lead to recurrent bouts of sinusitis, a dry cough, and (possibly) a higher than expected frequency of chest infections. Dry skin and dry hair are symptoms frequently elicited on direct questioning. About 30% of women with Sjögren's syndrome have diminished vaginal secretions and may present with dyspareunia. Involvement of the gastrointestinal tract leads to reflux oesophagitis or gastritis due to lack of protective mucus secretion, and some patients complain of constipation, which may be attributed to defective mucus in the colon and rectum. Rarely, pancreatic failure leading to a malabsorption syndrome may occur.

Recent studies have highlighted yet another complication, namely interstitial cystitis. It has been suggested that this is due to an autoimmune response to the muscarinic acetylcholine receptor which is extensively expressed in the bladder wall. There is no doubt about the clinical association, but the serological link awaits confirmation.

There is a higher than expected frequency of thyroid autoimmunity in those with Sjögren's syndrome; whether this is part of the same pathological process is debatable, but it is important to check thyroid function from time to time in patients with this condition.

Systemic manifestations

Sjögren's syndrome is a systemic disease: two-thirds of patients complain of fatigue, which according to several epidemiological studies is the single most important cause of disability. Occasionally weight loss and fever mimicking an occult malignancy may be the presenting symptoms, particularly in elderly people, in whom symptoms can be suggestive of polymyalgia rheumatica.

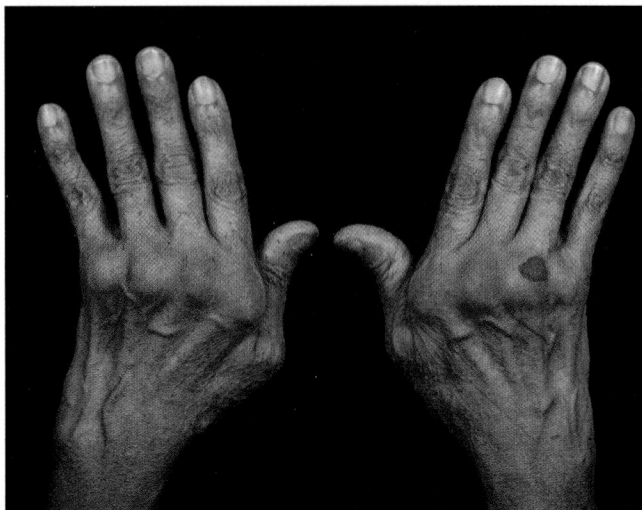

Fig. 19.11.6.1 Sjögren's arthropathy of the hands showing correctable deformities, in this case ulna deviation at the metacarpophalangeal joints and swan necking of the fingers. This is similar to the Jaccoud's-like arthropathy seen in systemic lupus erythematosus.

Raynaud's phenomenon occurs in about 50% of patients. Purpura affecting the lower legs is found in patients with very high IgG levels, but true vasculitis is uncommon. Other features include an arthritis that resembles the Jaccoud-like arthritis of systemic lupus erythematosus (Fig. 19.11.6.1). Polymyositis is a rare presentation.

Pleurisy occurs in about 40% of patients; abnormalities of pulmonary function are frequently described, but are rarely clinically significant.

A wide range of neurological presentations is recognized. Peripheral neuropathies are relatively common, an important but unusual type being mononeuritis multiplex mediated by vasculitis. Central nervous system (CNS) involvement can resemble multiple sclerosis, with a myelopathy leading to paraparesis being particularly characteristic and often termed 'Sjögren's syndrome myelopathy'. Although rare, occurring in less than 1% cases of Sjögren's syndrome, it is important to recognize the condition because it responds completely to treatment with steroids and cyclophosphamide.

Interstitial nephritis leading to renal tubular acidosis or nephrogenic diabetes insipidus occurs in about 30% of patients; these are usually subclinical but may lead to hypokalaemia, causing muscular weakness or (occasionally) nephrocalcinosis.

Lymphoma, almost always of B-cell lineage, is a characteristic but unusual feature. This occurs in about 5% of patients referred to specialist centres and is particularly likely in patients with high levels of immunoglobulins, autoantibodies, and cryoglobulins.

Women of child-bearing age are at increased risk of giving birth to babies with congenital heart block. Although rare, about 1 in 20 000 births, this complication is of great immunopathogenic interest as it is thought that damage to the developing conduction system is mediated by transplacental transfer of anti-Ro and anti-La antibodies.

In secondary Sjögren's syndrome the sicca symptoms are less severe than in primary disease. In rheumatoid arthritis with Sjögren's syndrome the patient tends to have more frequent extra-articular disease manifested as digital infarcts and subcutaneous ulcers. In systemic lupus erythematosus, those with Sjögren's syndrome have a lower frequency of renal disease and a relatively good prognosis.

Diagnosis

Keratoconjunctivitis sicca can be detected by Schirmer's test, tear break-up time, and rose Bengal staining, and xerostomia by a reduced parotid salivary flow rate and reduced uptake and clearance on isotope scans. However, it is important to remember that both salivary and lacrimal function decline with age and may be impaired in conditions other than Sjögren's syndrome. One cause of diagnostic confusion arises from treatment with drugs with anticholinergic side effects, the most frequent being the tricyclic antidepressants.

Biopsy and histology of the labial glands from behind the lower lip provides the most definitive diagnostic test. The area is anaesthetized with lidocaine containing adrenaline and an incision 1.5 cm long allows access to five to ten glands 2 to 4 mm in diameter that are removed by simple blunt dissection. A diagnosis of Sjögren's syndrome depends on finding foci of periductular infiltrates of at least 50 lymphocytes and/or plasma cells at a density of more than one focus/4 mm^2 (Fig. 19.11.6.2).

Most patients have a raised erythrocyte sedimentation rate (ESR) and a mild normocytic anaemia, with leucopenia in about 50% of cases. One of the most remarkable features of primary Sjögren's syndrome is a high level of IgG, which can be up to 50 g/l. Complement levels are usually normal, although C4 levels can sometimes be reduced because of the link between Sjögren's syndrome and the *C4A* null gene. Anti-La antibodies, although of relatively low sensitivity, are of great diagnostic help when present.

Rheumatoid factors, as measured by routine assays, occur in all forms of Sjögren's syndrome and their detection in primary disease is a common reason for misdiagnosing such patients as having rheumatoid arthritis. Antinuclear antibodies can also occur. Both rheumatoid factors and antinuclear antibodies, although not diagnostically specific, can help in distinguishing Sjögren's syndrome from nonautoimmune causes of sicca symptoms. Primary Sjögren's syndrome can be mimicked very closely by infection with HTLV-I (human T-lymphocytic virus I), HIV-1, and hepatitis C virus. All three diseases cause dry eyes and mouth, swelling of salivary glands, and biopsy changes very similar to those of primary Sjögren's syndrome. All are associated with hypergammaglobuli-

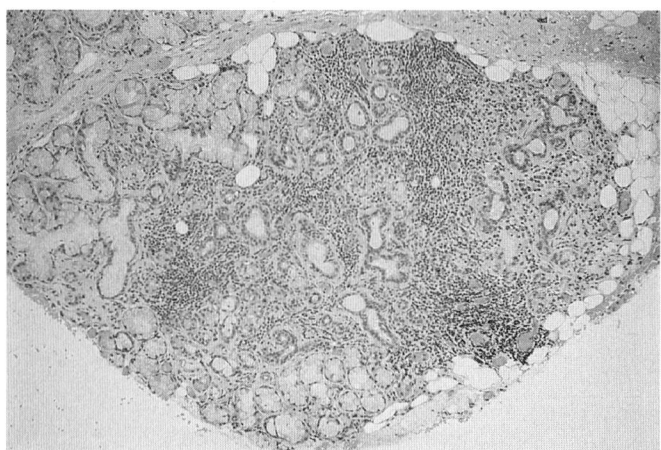

Fig. 19.11.6.2 Biopsy showing a lobule of minor salivary gland from a patient with Sjögren's syndrome. There is a focal inflammatory infiltrate surrounding blood vessels and ducts with the acini being relatively spared.

naemia, a raised ESR, and autoantibodies, although anti-Ro and anti-La are unusual. The only way to differentiate them with certainty is by specific serological testing. The Sjögren-like syndrome associated with HIV infection has been termed 'diffuse infiltrative lymphocytosis syndrome' and occurs in about 5% of HIV-positive individuals. Chronic fatigue syndrome is frequently mistaken for Sjögren's syndrome and vice versa (less frequently); a salivary gland biopsy usually clarifies the situation.

Diagnostic criteria

Diagnostic criteria are essential for the standardization of any research involving patient groups, particularly with a disease, or group of diseases, as heterogeneous as Sjögren's syndrome. In the case of Sjögren's syndrome such criteria are also useful in clinical practice. Currently used criteria depend on the demonstration of keratoconjunctivitis sicca, xerostomia, and a positive labial gland biopsy. The previously widely used 1993 'European' criteria, based on the results of a multicentre European study, have now been supplanted by the 2002 American/European Consensus criteria (Box 19.11.6.1). These are based on a short questionnaire about ocular and oral symptoms, with other criteria being ocular signs (by Schirmer's test or rose Bengal staining), lymphocytic infiltrates on lip biopsy, salivary gland involvement (decreased salivary flow

---

Box 19.11.6.1 The 2002 American/European Consensus criteria for the classification of Sjögren's syndrome

1 Ocular symptoms

A positive response to at least one of the three selected questions:
  a Have you had daily, persistent, troublesome dry eyes for more than 3 months?
  b Do you have a recurrent sensation of sand or gravel in the eyes?
  c Do you use tear substitutes more than three times a day?

2 Oral symptoms

A positive response to at least one of the three selected questions:
  a Have you had a daily feeling of dry mouth for more than 3 months?
  b Have you had recurrently or persistently swollen salivary glands as an adult?
  c Do you frequently drink liquids to aid in swallowing dry food?

3 Ocular signs

By Schirmer's test or rose Bengal staining.

4 Oral signs

Impaired unstimulated salivary flow rate.

5 Positive labial biopsy

6 Antibodies to Ro and/or La

The diagnosis of Sjögren's syndrome requires four out of the six criteria, which must include either (5) or (6).

Annals of Rheumatic diseases (2002) 61, 554–8. Reproduced with permission from the BMJ Publishing Group.

---

rate), and demonstration of serum Ro or La antibodies. Importantly, unlike the previous European criteria, these Consensus criteria must include either a positive biopsy or the presence of anti-Ro and/or anti-La antibodies.

Treatment

Most treatment in Sjögren's syndrome is topical and symptomatic. Simple measures can help preserve the integrity of the cornea as well as the gums and teeth, and are worth pursuing with enthusiasm, rather than with the negative attitude that some patients find in their physicians. Tear substitutes, such as hypromellose eye drops, are the mainstay of treatment for dry eyes, and it is generally worth trying several different types before settling on the most suitable preparation. Where thick mucus strands are a particular problem, topical acetylcysteine may help. Eye ointments, particularly at night, can help lubricate sticky eyes. Bacterial infection should be treated immediately with chloramphenicol ointment or drops. Some benefit can be achieved by preventing evaporation of tears by fitting side panels to spectacles. Temporary or permanent occlusion of the canaliculi or (rarely) tarsorrhaphy may help to retain tears within the conjunctival sac.

The dry mouth may be treated with saliva substitutes which are now available as convenient sprays. Pilocarpine tablets have shown promising results in recent controlled trials, but patients often seem to stop taking them after a few weeks or months because of cholinergic side effects such as palpitations, sweating, and abdominal cramps. Candidal infections are extremely common in Sjögren's syndrome and are often missed: they are best treated with prolonged courses of drugs such as fluconazole 50 mg daily for 10 days. Attention to dental hygiene may help to prevent the premature caries that is a common problem.

Hydroxychloroquine has established itself as a disease-modifying drug for patients with uncomplicated disease; it certainly helps with arthralgia and arthritis, lowers the ESR and immunoglobulin levels, may prevent bouts of purpura, and may help with fatigue. Fever, weight loss, parotid swelling, and interstitial cystitis often respond well to a low dose of steroids. Attempts to treat the underlying disease with steroids or cytotoxic drugs are generally thought ill-advised unless there are systemic complications. There is no convincing evidence that methotrexate has any useful role in management, and it is generally agreed that other second-line agents for rheumatoid arthritis such as gold or sulfasalazine are associated with a high frequency of side effects, which is one of the most important reasons for distinguishing between the arthritis of primary Sjögren's syndrome and that of rheumatoid arthritis. Serious systemic complications such as polymyositis, mononeuritis multiplex, or fibrosing alveolitis are treated with steroids and cytotoxic drugs.

Two published controlled trials of tumour necrosis factor (TNF)-α inhibitors have not shown benefit, which is perhaps not surprising because there is little evidence that TNFα is involved in the pathogenesis of glandular inflammation.

Prognosis

Sjögren's syndrome causes morbidity rather than mortality, with a few epidemiological studies suggesting that life expectancy is normal. Clinical experience suggests that the disease tends to remain relatively stable, unlike the catastrophic and unpredictable flares that characterize (for example) systemic lupus erythematosus. The main long-term complication that needs to be anticipated is lymphoma: several studies have shown that those with anti-Ro and anti-La antibodies, hypergammaglobulinaemia, hypocomplementaemia, and vasculitis are at highest risk, so such patients should be followed up on an annual basis in a specialized clinic. However, the relatively rare and potentially life-threatening complications such as lymphoma or CNS involvement appear to respond well to treatment.

Likely future developments

Polyclonal B-cell activation is a prominent feature of the disease. Trials of anti-CD20 are currently in progress, and trials involving monoclonal antibodies directed to other B-cell markers are now in the planning phase. Type 1 interferons are also thought to be important in Sjögren's syndrome and it has been suggested that inhibition of interferon-α might suppress exocrine inflammation, although paradoxically the use of low-dose interferon-α pastilles has been reported to increase salivary flow rate. One problem to be anticipated with such therapies is whether the cost of biologic agents can be justified for the treatment of what is usually a relatively mild disease.

Further reading

Alexander EL, *et al.* (1986). Primary Sjögren's syndrome with central nervous system dysfunction mimicking multiple sclerosis. *Ann Intern Med*, **104**, 323–30.

Bacman S, *et al.* (1996). Circulating antibodies against rat parotid gland M3 muscarinic receptors in primary Sjögren's syndrome. *Clin Exp Immunol*, **104**, 454–9.

Champey J, *et al.* (2006). Quality of life and psychological status in patients with primary Sjögren's syndrome and sicca symptoms without autoimmune features. *Arthritis Rheum*, **55**, 451–7.

Fox RI (2005). Sjögren's syndrome. *Lancet*, **366**, 321–31.

Haneji N *et al.* (1997). Identification of alpha-fodrin as a candidate autoantigen in primary Sjögren syndrome. *Science*, **276**, 604–7.

Harley JB *et al.* (1986). Gene interaction at HLA-DQ enhances autoantibody production in primary Sjögren's syndrome. *Science*, **232**, 1145–7.

Price EJ, Venables PJW (1995). Aetiopathogenesis of Sjögren's syndrome. *Semin Arthritis Rheum*, **25**, 117–33.

Thomas E, *et al.* (1998). Sjögren's syndrome: a community-based study of prevalence and impact. *Br J Rheumatol*, **37**, 1069–76.

Venables PJ (2006). Management of patients presenting with Sjögren's syndrome. *Best Pract Res Clin Rheumatol*, **20**, 791–807.

Vincent TL, *et al.* (2003). Sjögren's syndrome-associated myelopathy: response to immunosuppressive treatment. *Am J Med*, **114**, 145–8.

Vitali C, *et al.* (2002). Classification criteria for Sjögren's syndrome: a revised version of the European criteria proposed by the American–European Consensus Group. *Ann Rheum Dis*, **61**, 554–8.

19.11.7 Polymyositis and dermatomyositis

John H. Stone

Essentials

Polymyositis and dermatomyositis are two types of idiopathic inflammatory myopathy. The pathological findings in polymyositis suggest an HLA class I-restricted immune response mediated by cytotoxic T cells; dermatomyositis appears to be associated with humorally mediated destruction of muscle-associated microvasculature.

Clinical features—polymyositis is characterized by symmetrical painless proximal muscle weakness that develops slowly, usually over weeks to months, and typically associated with significant elevation of serum creatine kinase and other muscle enzymes. The pattern of muscle involvement in dermatomyositis is clinically indistinguishable from that of polymyositis, but with cutaneous manifestations including Gottron's sign, heliotrope rash, erythema, 'mechanic's hands', periungual abnormalities, and calcinosis cutis. Extra-muscular features include interstitial lung disease (30% of cases), aspiration pneumonia, and associated malignancy (polymyositis 9%, dermatomyositis 15%).

Investigation and diagnosis—disease is associated with 'myositis-specific' autoantibodies (30% of cases), of which there are three main types—antisynthetases, antisignal recognition particle (anti-SRP) antibodies, and anti-Mi-2 antibodies—and 'myositis-associated' autoantibodies. Particular autoantibodies are associated with particular disease phenotypes. The definitive test for establishing the diagnosis of inflammatory myopathy and excluding other causes of muscle weakness is muscle biopsy. Magnetic resonance imaging can demonstrate muscle involvement, be repeated as a method of evaluating response to therapy, and be useful in selecting a muscle group for biopsy.

Management and prognosis—treatment is with glucocorticoids, usually beginning with 1 mg/kg/day of prednisone. Second-line agents, usually azathioprine or methotrexate, are given to patients with aggressive disease. Biological agents are likely to be increasingly used in the future. The 5-year survival rate of patients with polymyositis or dermatomyositis is greater than 80%, but morbidity from both the diseases themselves and their treatments is high.

Introduction

Polymyositis and dermatomyositis are two major types of idiopathic inflammatory myopathy. Both diseases are associated with proximal muscle weakness, both may affect extramuscular organs such as the lungs and heart, and both are associated with features of autoimmunity, including autoantibody production. However, immunopathological evidence confirms that polymyositis and dermatomyositis are separate disorders. Although autoimmunity and systemic inflammation clearly contribute to both diseases, their aetiology remains unknown. A comparison of the principal features of these disorders is displayed in Table 19.11.7.1.

Historical perspective

The traditional classification of polymyositis and dermatomyositis proposed by Bohan and Peter distinguishes five subgroups of patients:

1 primary idiopathic polymyositis

2 primary idiopathic dermatomyositis

3 either disorder occurring in association with a malignancy

4 childhood dermatomyositis (or, more rarely, polymyositis)

5 overlap syndromes, in which polymyositis or dermatomyositis occur along with features of other autoimmune conditions such as systemic lupus erythematosus (SLE) or systemic sclerosis

In recent years, more detailed understanding of these diseases has permitted the refinement of the diagnostic classification, based on clinical, histopathological, and laboratory findings. Nevertheless, the original classification of Bohan and Peter remains useful for most clinical purposes.

Table 19.11.7.1 Principal features of polymyositis and dermatomyositis

	Polymyositis	Dermatomyositis
Typical patient	Any age	Any age
	Unusual in children	Juvenile form common
	Female and African–American predominance	Female and African–American predominance
Muscle groups affected	Proximal > distal	Proximal > distal
	Symmetrical	Symmetrical
CK elevation	40–50 times normal not unusual	40–50 times normal not unusual
		Weakness sometimes out of proportion to CK level
MSAs	Antisynthetase antibodies, anti-SRP	Antisynthetase antibodies, anti-Mi-2
Histopathology	Endomysial inflammation	Perivascular, interfascicular inflammation
	CD8+ cells invading non-necrotic muscle fibres, which bear HLA class I antigens	CD4+ predominance; complement membrane attack complex present; capillary obliteration; endothelial damage; perifascicular atrophy
Malignancy association	No	Yes
Other features	ILD Cardiac Malignancy	Skin ILD Cardiac Intramuscular calcification Vasculitis Malignancy

CK, creatine kinase; MSAs, myositis-specific antibodies; ILD, interstitial lung disease; SRP, signal recognition particle.

Pathology and pathophysiology

Polymyositis is characterized by an endomysial infiltrate containing large numbers of CD8+ T cells and foci of cytotoxic T cells and macrophages. The inflammatory infiltrate surrounds and invades non-necrotic muscle fibres. Both involved and uninvolved fibres express increased amounts of human leucocyte antigen (HLA) class I antigen, in contrast to normal muscle fibres which express neither class I nor class II antigens—hence the pathological findings in polymyositis suggest an HLA class I-restricted immune response mediated by cytotoxic T cells.

Muscle biopsies from patients with dermatomyositis contain increased numbers of CD4+ T cells and B lymphocytes. The inflammatory infiltrate in dermatomyositis is localized to perivascular regions, with capillary obliteration, fibrin thrombi, and endothelial cell damage all being hallmarks of the condition. The disease appears to be associated with humorally mediated destruction of muscle-associated microvasculature. The membrane attack complex, comprising complement components C5 to C9, is present within the blood vessels in early dermatomyositis, and focal capillary depletion is one of the earliest pathological changes. In addition to its vascular orientation, the inflammatory infiltrate in dermatomyositis centres on the interfascicular septa and around, rather than within, muscle fascicles. Even in the absence of inflammation, perifascicular atrophy is diagnostic of dermatomyositis.

Although dermatomyositis is clearly associated with a vasculopathy in which complement is involved, it is not known if the vasculopathy is mediated primarily by complement or if other pathophysiological events lead to the secondary deposition of complement proteins and other immune complexes.

Epidemiology

As defined clinically, both polymyositis and dermatomyositis have prevalence rates estimated to be one case per 100 000 in the general population. The diseases may afflict individuals of any age and either gender, but female cases outnumber male ones by a 2:1 ratio. Cases associated with malignancy are clustered among older patients with dermatomyositis, and seldom if ever occur among children.

Clinical features

Polymyositis

Polymyositis is characterized by symmetrical proximal muscle weakness that develops slowly, usually over weeks to months. Routine tasks that require proximal muscle strength, e.g. rising from a chair, climbing stairs, or performing overhead work, become increasingly challenging for the patient. In addition to weakness of the extremities, skeletal muscles at many sites are also susceptible to muscular inflammation. The upper third of the oesophagus, the muscles of neck flexion, the intercostal muscles, and the diaphragm may also be affected. Patients with severe neck flexor weakness secondary to polymyositis may be unable to lift their heads from the pillow. Hypercapnic respiratory failure sometimes results from weakness of the chest wall muscles and diaphragm. By contrast, polymyositis (and dermatomyositis) usually spares the muscles that mediate facial expression and extraocular movements, even in patients with profound weakness elsewhere. Similarly, handgrip strength and the ability to perform fine motor tasks usually remain preserved until advanced stages of the disease.

Prominent muscle pain and tenderness are atypical in the inflammatory myopathies and rarely constitute the chief complaint. Thus, 'painless weakness' is the usual presenting muscle symptom. Deep tendon reflexes and muscle bulk are preserved, except in cases of severe advanced disease. Fasciculations, a manifestation of denervation rather than myopathic injury, are not seen in polymyositis (and dermatomyositis). Similarly, sensory function remains normal even as muscle weakness progresses.

Endomysial inflammation leads to the release of muscle enzymes into the blood. Thus, polymyositis is usually characterized by striking elevations of serum creatine kinase, aldolase, lactate dehydrogenase, and aspartate aminotransferase.

Dermatomyositis

The pattern of muscle involvement in dermatomyositis is clinically indistinguishable from that of polymyositis, but in addition to inflammatory muscle disease, dermatomyositis has an array of characteristic cutaneous manifestations:

* Gottron's sign—an erythematous, scaly eruption confined to skin overlying the knuckles is pathognomonic of this disease (Fig. 19.11.7.1). Lesions identical to those of Gottron's sign may also occur over the extensor surfaces of many other joints, particularly the elbows and knees, when the lesions are termed 'Gottron's papules'.

* Heliotrope rash—a lilac discoloration of skin over the eyelids, often accompanied by eyelid oedema (Fig. 19.11.7.2).

* Erythema—cutaneous erythema may involve several sites in dermatomyositis, including the upper back and shoulders (the 'shawl sign'), the upper chest (in a 'V' distribution), and the face and hands. The erythema may appear over the malar region, mimicking SLE. Patients with dermatomyositis often manifest photosensitivity.

* 'Mechanic's hands'—roughened, cracked skin, particularly over the tips and lateral aspects of the fingers (Fig. 19.11.7.3), resulting in irregular, dirty-appearing lines on the fingers that cause the

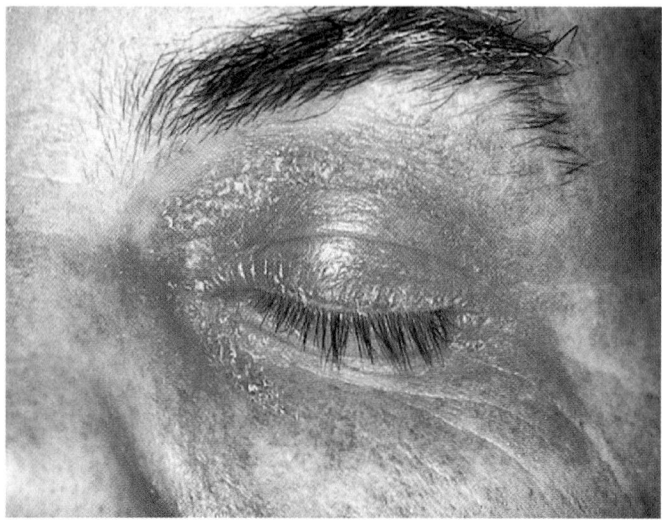

Fig. 19.11.7.2 Heliotrope rash: a lilac-coloured rash over the eyelids in dermatomyositis.
Reproduced from Gelber A, Nousari HC, Wigley FM (2000). Journal of Rheumatology 27,1542-5. With permission.

hands to resemble those of a manual labourer. Often found in association with the antisynthetase antibodies (see below).

* Periungual abnormalities—the capillary nailbeds in dermatomyositis (and polymyositis) may be erythematous and, in some cases, tender. Vascular changes observed in the nailbed resemble those found in other connective tissue diseases, e.g. systemic sclerosis and SLE. Abnormal capillary loops, visible to the naked eye, may alternate with areas of vascular dilatation and dropout (Fig. 19.11.7.4).

* Calcinosis cutis—the deposition of calcium within the skin, a finding known as calcinosis cutis, occurs commonly in juvenile dermatomyositis but is unusual in adults.

Amyopathic dermatomyositis (or 'dermatomyositis sine myositis') refers to a subset of dermatomyositis patients in which the classic skin features are apparent for months before muscle weakness

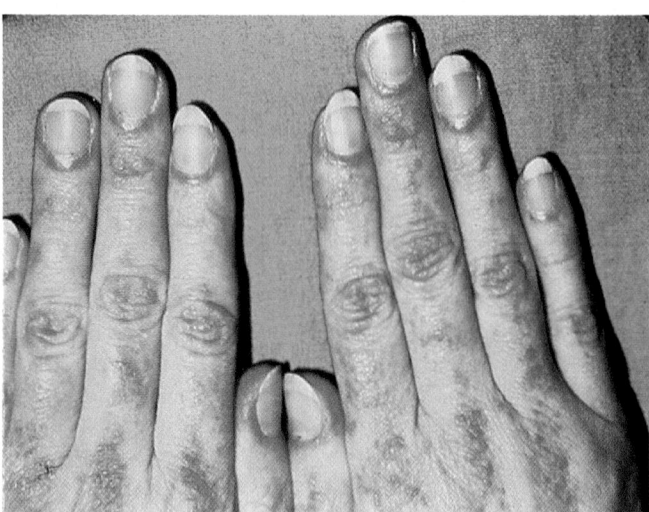

Fig. 19.11.7.1 Gottron's sign: scaly plaques over the dorsal surfaces of the knuckles in dermatomyositis.

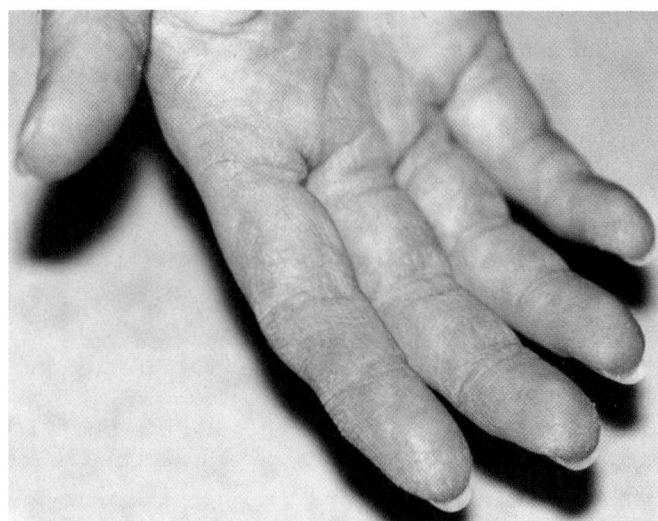

Fig. 19.11.7.3 'Mechanic's hands' in dermatomyositis.

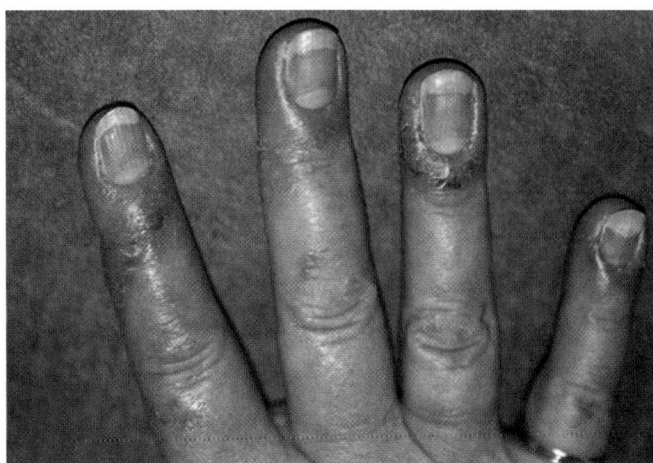

Fig. 19.11.7.4 Periungual abnormalities in dermatomyositis.

becomes evident. Most patients with amyopathic dermatomyositis eventually develop signs and symptoms of muscle disease. Clinically evident muscle dysfunction has been reported years after the development of skin changes consistent with dermatomyositis, and thorough clinical evaluation (including MRI studies) reveals subtle evidence of muscle dysfunction in many cases labelled as amyopathic dermatomyositis.

Extramuscular features

Lung

Weakness of the intercostal muscles and diaphragm occasionally leads to ventilatory failure in polymyositis or dermatomyositis. More commonly, however, patients have pulmonary involvement in the form of interstitial lung disease, a complication that occurs in up to 30% of cases. The pattern of pulmonary involvement in the inflammatory myopathies is typical of that which occurs in connective tissue disorders, namely interstitial fibrosis, predominantly at the lung bases. Pathological findings in such cases may reveal usual interstitial pneumonitis, nonspecific interstitial pneumonitis, diffuse alveolar damage, and bronchiolitis obliterans with organizing pneumonia.

High-resolution CT is very sensitive for detecting this type of pulmonary change. In the early stages of interstitial lung disease, the radiological findings correspond to an inflammatory alveolitis. The severity of interstitial lung disease in polymyositis and dermatomyositis ranges from asymptomatic radiological findings to a refractory process indistinguishable from idiopathic pulmonary fibrosis. Lung involvement is often, but not always, associated with antisynthetase antibodies (see below). Restrictive findings on pulmonary function testing are the rule.

Another common pulmonary complication of the inflammatory myopathies is aspiration pneumonia, caused by weakness of the hypopharynx and upper oesophagus.

Cardiac

Cardiac involvement in polymyositis or dermatomyositis is usually subclinical, and its prevalence is not known with certainty. When measured, creatine kinase-MB (CK-MB) isoenzyme levels are frequently elevated in the absence of overt cardiac symptoms. The most common reason for increased CK-MB levels in the inflammatory myopathies is that the fraction of the MB isoenzyme produced in regenerating skeletal muscle is increased. However, ECG may demonstrate nonspecific ST–T wave changes. Clinically evident myocarditis in polymyositis and dermatomyositis can rarely lead to cardiac failure or intractable, life-threatening arrhythmias.

Gastrointestinal

Dysphagia and nasopharyngeal regurgitation of food may result from oesophageal involvement, which when significant is a poor prognostic sign. Involvement of the gastrointestinal tract beyond the pharynx and oesophagus is particularly common in juvenile dermatomyositis (the childhood form). This complication is often mediated by vasculitis and may result in intestinal haemorrhage or perforation.

Malignancy

Some adults with polymyositis or dermatomyositis have underlying malignancies, usually carcinomas, the risk being estimated to be 9% for patients with polymyositis and 15% for those with dermatomyositis. Many types of malignancy are associated, including lung, oesophageal, breast, colon, and ovarian tumours. Among women with dermatomyositis, the risk of ovarian cancer may be 20 times greater than that of the general population. Most malignancies associated with polymyositis or dermatomyositis are diagnosed within the 2-year period before and after the development of myositis.

Patients diagnosed with primary polymyositis or dermatomyositis (children excepted) should undergo surveillance for a disease-associated malignancy, with screening based on careful histories, physical examinations, and the performance of a limited number of routine tests (e.g. CT of the chest). In addition, age-appropriate cancer screening such as mammography and flexible sigmoidoscopy should be performed. Unfocused 'fishing expeditions' are discouraged because they rarely benefit the patient and are costly.

Antisynthetase syndrome

About 30% of patients with polymyositis or dermatomyositis have a constellation of clinical findings termed 'the antisynthetase syndrome'. They have autoantibodies known as antisynthetase antibodies that are highly specific for polymyositis and dermatomyositis (see below), together with clinical features including constitutional symptoms (e.g. fever), Raynaud's phenomenon, mechanic's hands, arthritis, and interstitial lung disease.

Myositis-specific and myositis-associated autoantibodies

Patients with polymyositis and dermatomyositis may demonstrate both 'myositis-specific' autoantibodies and 'myositis-associated' autoantibodies. Whereas myositis-specific autoantibodies are unique to the inflammatory myopathies and provide information about patterns of organ system involvement and disease prognosis, myositis-associated autoantibodies may be found in a variety of other connective tissue diseases. A summary of autoantibodies associated with polymyositis and dermatomyositis is shown in Table 19.11.7.2.

Myositis-specific autoantibodies

About 30% of patients with polymyositis or dermatomyositis have myositis-specific autoantibodies, which are directed against a variety of nuclear or cytoplasmic antigens. Three major types of

Table 19.11.7.2 Overview of the most common myositis-specific autoantibodies

Autoantibody	Antigen	Frequency	Clinical association
Antisynthetase antibodies			
Anti-Jo-1	His-tRNA synthetase	<20%	Antisynthetase syndrome
Anti-PL-7	Thr-tRNA synthetase	2%	Antisynthetase syndrome
Anti-PL-12	Ala-tRNA synthetase	1%	Antisynthetase syndrome
Anti-EJ	Gly-tRNA synthetase	<4%	Antisynthetase syndrome
Anti-OJ	Ile-tRNA synthetase	1%	Antisynthetase syndrome
Anti-KS	Asp-tRNA synthetase	<1%	Antisynthetase syndrome
Other			
Anti-SRP	SRP complex	4%	Aggressive polymyositis
Anti-Mi-2	Nuclear helicase	10%	Classic dermatomyositis
Anti-hPMS-1	DNA mismatch-repair enzyme	7.5%	Poorly defined
Anti-CADM-140	Uncharacterized 140-kDa polypeptide	Unknown	Amyopathic dermatomyositis
Anti-p155	Uncharacterized 155-kDa protein	21% of dermatomyositis patients	Dermatomyositis and cancer

SRP, signal recognition particle.

myositis-specific autoantibodies have been identified: the antisynthetases, antisignal recognition particle antibodies (anti-SRP), and anti-Mi-2 antibodies. A variety of other myositis-specific autoantibodies have also been reported (Table 19.11.7.2). As a rule, individual patients generally develop only one type of these autoantibodies.

In contrast to patients with polymyositis or dermatomyositis that is not associated with cancer, those with an inflammatory myopathy related to a malignancy rarely have myositis-specific autoantibodies.

Antisynthetase autoantibodies

The antisynthetase antibodies are directed against aminoacyl-tRNA synthetases, enzymes that catalyse the attachment of specific amino acids to their cognate transfer or tRNAs. In the case of Jo-1, the most common type of myositis-specific autoantibody, the antibody is formed against antihistidyl-tRNA synthetase. Anti-Jo-1 antibodies inhibit the function of their target antigens *in vitro*. In addition to anti-Jo-1 antibodies, autoantibodies to several other aminoacyl-tRNA synthetase enzymes have been described, including autoantibodies to the OJ, EJ, KS, PL-7, and PL-12 antigens.

As described above, patients with antisynthetase antibodies often manifest a characteristic disease phenotype known as 'the antisynthetase syndrome'. This is characterized by relatively acute disease onset, the presence of constitutional symptoms

(e.g., fever), interstitial lung disease, Raynaud's phenomenon, arthritis, and 'mechanic's hands' (see Fig. 19.11.7.3). The presence of antisynthetase antibodies in a patient denotes a disease phenotype that usually responds to glucocorticoid treatment, but that is likely to persist, so patients with these antibodies may be candidates for early use of immunosuppressive agents in addition to glucocorticoids.

Not all patients with antisynthetase antibodies, or even those classified as having the antisynthetase syndrome, have all the manifestations of this syndrome. Some have relatively little myositis, with other features being more prominent, such as interstitial lung disease. Another point to note is that the general clinical picture linked to the antisynthetase syndrome is not specific for antisynthetase antibodies; patients with myositis-associated antibodies such as antipolymyositis-Scl and anti-U1RNP antibodies may also present with these features.

Antisignal recognition particle antibodies
Anti-SRP antibodies occur exclusively in polymyositis. They react with the signal recognition particle, a complex of RNA and protein involved in translocating newly synthesized proteins into the endoplasmic reticulum. Anti-SRP antibodies occur in about 5% of all adult patients with polymyositis and are associated with muscle inflammation of acute onset, severe degree, and refractoriness to therapy. Patients with anti-SRP antibodies are reported to have less intramuscular inflammation than do other patients with dermatomyositis or polymyositis.

Anti-Mi-2 antibodies
Anti-Mi-2 antibodies, targeted against a helicase involved in transcriptional activation almost always occur in patients with dermatomyositis, often in those with prominent cutaneous involvement. They are associated with classic cutaneous features of dermatomyositis, particularly erythroderma and the shawl sign. In comparison with patients with antisynthetase and anti-SRP antibodies, those with antibodies to Mi-2 usually have better prognosis.

Myositis-associated autoantibodies

Antinuclear antibodies (ANAs) are present in at least 80% of patients with dermatomyositis or polymyositis. Anti-Ro, anti-La, anti-Sm, or antiribonucleoprotein (anti-RNP) antibodies are found in some patients with polymyositis or dermatomyositis, the presence of such antibodies suggesting that the inflammatory myopathy is associated with another connective tissue disease, e.g. the presence of anti-Ro or anti-La antibodies would suggest the simultaneous presence (overlap) of Sjögren's syndrome. Similarly, anti-RNP antibodies are associated with the overlap of myositis with features of either SLE or systemic sclerosis, this clinical entity sometimes being termed 'mixed connective tissue disease'. Anti-Ku and anti-polymyositis-Scl antibodies occur in patients with polymyositis or dermatomyositis who have overlapping features of myositis and systemic sclerosis.

Diagnosis

Tissue biopsy remains the gold standard for diagnosing the inflammatory myopathies. Skin biopsy can sometimes obviate the need for muscle biopsy in patients with dermatomyositis. Both electromyography (EMG) and MRI studies may be valuable in the assessment of patients with possible polymyositis or dermatomyositis.

Muscle biopsy

The definitive test for establishing the diagnosis of inflammatory myopathy and excluding other causes of muscle weakness is muscle biopsy. The usual targets for muscle biopsy are the quadriceps or the deltoid, with proper processing of the sample being critical to the accuracy of its interpretation. The pathological features of muscle biopsies in patients with polymyositis and dermatomyositis are discussed above (see Pathology and pathophysiology).

Skin biopsy

In the proper clinical setting skin biopsies may be diagnostic in dermatomyositis. The skin lesions usually demonstrate mild epidermal atrophy, vacuolar changes in the basal keratinocyte layer, and a perivascular lymphoid infiltrate in the dermis. Assessments by both light microscopy and direct immunofluorescence are essential in diagnosis: immunofluorescence testing reveals an 'interface dermatitis' (deposition of complement components and immunoglobulin at the dermal–epidermal junction); membrane attack complex deposits are found along the dermal–epidermal junction and within the walls of dermal blood vessels.

Electromyography

EMG studies are abnormal in about 90% of patients with polymyositis or dermatomyositis. The principal role of EMG in the evaluation of neuromuscular disorders is in distinguishing weakness of myopathic origin from neuropathic conditions such as motor neuron disease, peripheral neuropathy (e.g. from vasculitis), and other disorders. However, the EMG findings of increased membrane irritability, increased insertional activity, fibrillation potentials, and complex repetitive discharges can be observed in a variety of myogenic processes, including infectious, toxic, or metabolic myopathies.

MRI

MRI can demonstrate areas of muscle inflammation (Fig. 19.11.7.5), oedema with active myositis, fibrosis, and calcification. It permits the assessment of large volumes of muscle tissue, can be repeated as a method of evaluating response to therapy, and may also be useful in selecting a muscle group for biopsy.

Differential diagnosis

Polymyositis and dermatomyositis must be distinguished from numerous disorders that cause subacute weakness, shown in Box 19.11.7.1. One particular point of diagnostic confusion relates to inclusion body myositis, a more indolent form of inflammatory myopathy associated with asymmetrical and distal motor weakness that may mimic polymyositis. Inclusion body myositis has distinctive pathological findings: 'rimmed vacuoles' distributed around the myocyte's edge, basophilic 'inclusion bodies' within these vacuoles, and filamentous inclusions within the cytoplasm. Inclusion body myositis is less responsive than polymyositis to treatment and cases of 'refractory polymyositis' often represent misdiagnoses of inclusion body myositis.

Treatment

Glucocorticoids, usually beginning with prednisone 1 mg/kg per day, remain the cornerstone of all initial treatment regimens for

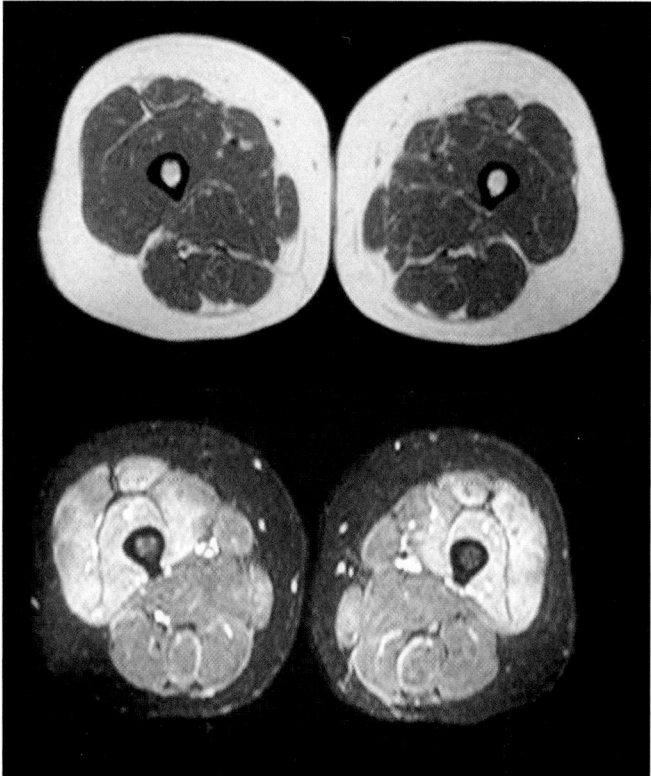

Fig. 19.11.7.5 MRI of the thighs in polymyositis: (upper) T_1 and (lower) STIR (short tau inversion recovery) sequencing demonstrates oedema in the anterior compartment of the muscles on the STIR sequences. This finding is compatible with active muscle inflammation.
(Courtesy of Dr Lisa Christopher.)

polymyositis and dermatomyositis. Decline of the creatine kinase level within 2 weeks of starting treatment may portend a good outcome, but improvement in muscle strength frequently lags behind and is sometimes not evident for up to 3 months. Patients should be treated with prednisone 1 mg/kg per day until the creatine kinase is normal (or nearly so), and then undergo a slow taper that does not exceed 10 mg/day per month.

Once the glucocorticoid taper has begun, creatine kinase levels are useful in gauging disease activity, but mild elevation of creatine kinase does not justify escalation in treatment, particularly if the patient's muscle strength continues to improve. Conversely, once treatment has begun, low creatine kinase levels do not guarantee inactive muscle disease. Dermatomyositis is particularly notorious for the finding of low or normal creatine kinase levels despite active muscle inflammation. Glucocorticoid myopathy is a common complication of treatment, and may be difficult to distinguish from active disease.

Many patients with polymyositis or dermatomyositis require additional immunosuppressive agents. Second agents should be started early (at the same time as glucocorticoid initiation) in patients with severe muscle disease, oesophageal or respiratory muscle weakness, interstitial lung disease, and other markers of aggressive disease. The preferred second agents remain either azathioprine (2 mg/kg per day) or methotrexate (25 mg/week). Cyclophosphamide may be preferred for patients who have severe interstitial lung disease at presentation or for the rare patient presenting with overt features of necrotizing vasculitis. Rituximab and

Box 19.11.7.1 Differential diagnosis of subacute weakness

Neurological

Inclusion body myositis, Guillain–Barré syndrome, myasthenia gravis, Eaton–Lambert syndrome, amyotrophic lateral sclerosis, muscular dystrophies (Duchenne, Becker, limb–girdle, fascioscapulohumeral)

Endocrine

Hyper- and hypothyroidism, Cushing's syndrome, Addison's disease.

Metabolic

Familial periodic paralysis, McArdle's disease, phosphofructokinase deficiency, adult acid maltase deficiency, mitochondrial myopathies.

Drugs

Alcohol, chloroquine, hydroxychloroquine, colchicine, penicillamine, corticosteroids, lipid-lowering agents, zidovudine.

Infections

Viral (echovirus), retroviral (HIV, HTLV-1), bacterial (staphylococci—pyomyositis), parasitic (trichinosis).

Rheumatic

Vasculitis, polymyalgia rheumatica, myositis associated with SLE, rheumatoid arthritis, or systemic sclerosis.

Other

Rhabdomyolysis, chronic graft-vs-host disease, rubella immunization.

intravenous immune globulin both show promise in the treatment of refractory disease. Finally, in addition to pharmacological treatments, physical therapy and rehabilitative medicine play important roles in patient recovery.

Prognosis

More prompt diagnoses, a broader range of therapies, and improved general medical care have improved the 5-year survival rate of patients with polymyositis or dermatomyositis to more than 80%. However, morbidity from both the diseases themselves and their treatments is high, and few patients emerge from treatment cured and unscathed. Several variables may contribute to worse outcomes or suboptimal therapeutic responses, including delay in diagnosis, the presence of severe myositis, dysphagia, pulmonary, or cardiac involvement, the diagnosis of inclusion body myositis, association with malignancy, and the presence of certain myositis-specific autoantibodies.

Likely future developments

The near future is likely to bring greater understanding of the molecular biology of the inflammatory myopathies, with elucidation of the role of myositis-specific autoantibodies in disease pathophysiology and phenotype, and insights into their implications for

prognosis. In addition, the role of rituximab and other biologic therapies will also be explored, with the anticipation of more effective and safer treatments for polymyositis and dermatomyositis.

Further reading

Bohan A, *et al.* (1977). A computer-assisted analysis of 153 patients with polymyositis and dermatomyositis. *Medicine*, **56**, 255.
Gerami P, *et al.* (2006). A systematic review of adult-onset clinically amyopathic dermatomyositis (dermatomyositis sine myositis): a missing link within the spectrum of the idiopathic inflammatory myopathies. *J Am Acad Dermatol*, **54**, 597.
Greenberg SA, Amato AA (2004). Uncertainties in the pathogenesis of dermatomyositis. *Curr Opin Neurol*, **13**, 356.
Hoogendijk JE, *et al.* (2004). 119th ENMC international workshop: trial design in adult idiopathic inflammatory myopathies, with the exception of inclusion body myositis, 10–12 October 2003, Naarden, The Netherlands. *Neuromusc Disord*, **14**, 337.
Sigurgeirsson B, *et al.* (1992). Risk of cancer in patients with dermatomyositis or polymyositis. *N Engl J Med*, **326**, 363.

19.11.8 Kawasaki's disease

Brian W. McCrindle

Essentials

Kawasaki's disease is an acute, self-limited, inflammatory vasculitis of unknown aetiology, with a peak incidence under 5 years of age.

Clinical features—the diagnosis is made in the presence of persistent fever for 5 days or more and at least four of the following five clinical signs: (1) nonpurulent conjunctivitis, (2) oropharyngeal inflammation, (3) cervical lymphadenopathy, (4) polymorphous exanthem, and (5) erythema of the palms and soles with subsequent desquamation. Incomplete presentations occur in approximately 25% of patients. The primary complications are cardiac, with coronary artery dilation and aneurysms evident in approximately 15 to 25% of untreated patients.

Management and prognosis—primary therapy consists of a single high dose of intravenous gammaglobulin, reducing the prevalence of coronary artery complications to approximately 4% if given within 10 days of the onset of fever. Persistent coronary artery lesions, with an ongoing risk of thrombosis and stenosis, are the predominant long-term morbidity. In adults, new presentations of myocardial ischemia with the associated finding of coronary artery aneurysms may suggest a previous episode of Kawasaki's disease during childhood.

Introduction

Kawasaki's disease is an acute, self-limited, inflammatory vasculitis, predominantly occurring in children under 5 years of age, complicated by coronary artery dilatation and aneurysms, with subsequent risk of thrombosis, stenosis, and cardiac ischaemia, and sudden death.

Historical perspective

Kawasaki's disease was first described in Japan in 1967 by Dr Tomisaku Kawasaki, a paediatrician. In his initial report he described the characteristic clinical features, but concluded that it was a self-limiting illness with no sequelae. Subsequently, it has been recognized that Kawasaki's disease is a systemic vasculitis with a predilection for the coronary arteries, resulting in dilatation and aneurysms. It has now been described world wide in all races, and has become the leading cause of acquired cardiac disease in children.

Aetiology, genetics, pathogenesis, and pathology

The aetiology of Kawasaki's disease is unknown. Some features suggest an infectious aetiology, including clinical similarities to infectious diseases, with a seasonal increase in incidence in winter to spring months and periodic epidemics, and recurrences being rare. Some features are consistent with a superantigen-mediated illness, whereas others suggest the presence of a conventional infection. Familial cases, although rare, do occur, and, together

---

Box 19.11.8.1 Epidemiological case definition of Kawasaki's disease

Classic clinical criteria[a]

Fever persisting at least 5 days[b]

Presence of at least four principal features:

- Changes in extremities
  - Acute—erythema of palms, soles; oedema of hands, feet
  - Subacute—periungual peeling of fingers, toes in weeks 2 and 3
- Polymorphous exanthem
- Bilateral bulbar conjunctival injection without exudate
- Changes in lips and oral cavity—erythema, lips cracking, strawberry tongue, diffuse injection of oral and pharyngeal mucosae
- Cervical lymphadenopathy (>1.5 cm diameter), usually unilateral

Exclusion of other diseases with similar findings[c]

Other clinical and laboratory findings

- Cardiovascular findings
  - Congestive heart failure, myocarditis, pericarditis, valvular regurgitation
  - Coronary artery abnormalities
  - Aneurysms of medium-sized noncoronary arteries
  - Raynaud's phenomenon
  - Peripheral gangrene
- Musculoskeletal system
  - Arthritis, arthralgia
- Gastrointestinal tract
  - Diarrhoea, vomiting, abdominal pain
  - Hepatic dysfunction
  - Hydrops of gallbladder

- Central nervous system
  - Extreme irritability
  - Aseptic meningitis
  - Sensorineural hearing loss
- Genitourinary system
  - Urethritis/meatitis
- Other findings
  - Erythema, induration at bacille Calmette–Guérin (BCG) inoculation site
  - Anterior uveitis (mild)
  - Desquamating rash in groin
- Laboratory findings in acute Kawasaki disease
  - Leukocytosis with neutrophilia and immature forms
  - Elevated erythrocyte sedimentation rate
  - Elevated C-reactive protein
  - Anaemia
  - Abnormal plasma lipids
  - Hypoalbuminaemia
  - Hyponatraemia
  - Thrombocytosis after week 1[d]
  - Sterile pyuria
  - Elevated serum transaminases
  - Elevated serum gammaglutamyl transpeptidase
  - Pleocytosis of cerebrospinal fluid
  - Leukocytosis in synovial fluid

[a] Patients with fever at least 5 days and less than four principal criteria can be diagnosed with Kawasaki's disease when coronary artery abnormalities are detected by two-dimensional echocardiography or angiography.

[b] In the presence of four or more principal criteria, diagnosis of Kawasaki's disease can be made on day 4 of illness. Experienced clinicians who have treated many patients with Kawasaki's disease may establish diagnosis before day 4

[c] See text.

[d] Some infants present with thrombocytopenia and disseminated intravascular coagulation.

From Newburger JW et al; Committee on Rheumatic Fever, Endocarditis and Kawasaki Disease; Council on Cardiovascular Disease in the Young; American Heart Association; American Academy of Pediatrics (2004), Diagnosis, treatment, and long-term management of Kawasaki disease: a statement for health professionals from the Committee on Rheumatic Fever, Endocarditis and Kawasaki Disease, Council on Cardiovascular Disease in the Young, American Heart Association. Circulation 110, 2747–71.

with marked differences in incidence according to race, suggest that some individuals may have a genetic predisposition.

The illness is characterized by a generalized systemic vasculitis. The coronary arteries are predominantly affected with dilatation and aneurysms, but other small- to medium-sized arteries may also be involved. Active inflammation with swelling and oedema of the endothelium and media is present acutely, with an initial influx of neutrophils followed by lymphocytes, mononuclear cells, and IgA plasma cells. Destruction of the internal elastic lamina leads to aneurysm formation. Resolution of active inflammation is followed by progressive fibrosis and intimal thickening, and stenoses may develop. Rupture occurs rarely in the acute stage. Thrombosis may be related to endothelial activation, thrombocytosis, and a hypercoagulable state in the acute stage, or chronically related to stasis within giant aneurysms.

Epidemiology

Although Kawasaki's disease has been reported world wide, the incidence remains highest in Japan and children of Japanese descent at about 110 cases per 100 000 children aged less than 5 years of age. The incidence is lowest in white people at less than a tenth of this rate. Although most cases occur in children aged less than 5 years, Kawasaki's disease has been reported in older children and adolescents. Boys are more commonly affected. Recurrence and familial occurrence are rare. Reported environmental factors have

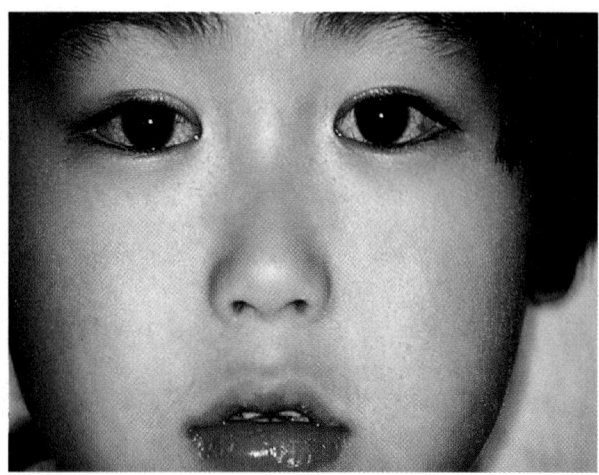

Fig. 19.11.8.1 Typical appearance of a patient with Kawasaki's disease. The picture is of a 5-year-old boy on the fourth day of illness: note the red eyes and red lips. (With acknowledgement to Dr T Kawasaki.)

been inconsistent, although a seasonal increase during the winter and early spring months is evident.

Prevention

Given that the aetiology remains unknown, prevention strategies are not available.

Table 19.11.8.1 Risk stratification and long-term management

Risk level	Pharmacological therapy	Physical activity	Follow-up and diagnostic testing	Invasive testing
I (no coronary artery changes at any stage of illness)	None beyond first 6–8 weeks	No restrictions beyond first 6–8 weeks	Cardiovascular risk assessment, counselling at 5-year intervals	None recommended
II (transient coronary artery ectasia disappears within first 6–8 weeks)	None beyond first 6–8 weeks	No restrictions beyond first 6–8 weeks	Cardiovascular risk assessment, counselling at 3- to 5-year intervals	None recommended
III (1 small–medium coronary artery aneurysm/major coronary artery)	Low-dose aspirin (3–5 mg/kg aspirin per day), at least until aneurysm regression documented	For patients <11 years old, no restriction beyond first 6–8 weeks; For patients 11–20 years old, physical activity guided by biennial stress test, evaluation of myocardial perfusion scan; contact or high-impact sports discouraged for patients taking antiplatelet agents	Annual cardiology folllow-up with echocardiogram + ECG. combined with cardiovascular risk assessment, counselling; biennial stress test/evaluation of myocardial perfusion scan	Angiography, if noninvasive test suggests ischaemia
IV (≥1 large or giant coronary artery aneurysm, or multiple or complex aneurysms in same coronary artery, without obstruction)	Long-term antiplatelet therapy and warfarin (target INR 20–25) or LMWH (target: antifactor Xa level 05–1.0 U/mL) should be combined in giant aneurysms	Contact or high-impact sports should be avoided because of risk of bleeding; other physical activity recommendations guided by stress test/evaluation of myocardial perfusion scan outcome	Biannual follow-up with echocardiogram + ECG; annual stress test/evaluation of myocardial perfusion scan	First angiography at 6–12 months or sooner if clinically indicated: repeated angiography if noninvasive test, clinical, or laboratory findings suggest ischaemia: elective repeat angiography under some circumstances (see text)
V (coronary artery obstruction)	Long-term low-dose aspirin: warfarin or LMWH if giant aneurysm persists: consider use of β-blockers to reduce myocardial oxygen consumption	Contact or high-impact sports should be avoided because of risk of bleeding; other physical activity recommendations guided by stress test/myocardial perfusion scan outcome	Biannual follow-up with echocardiogram + ECG; annual stress test/evaluation of myocardial perfusion scan	Angiography recommended to address therapeutic options

LMWH, low-molecular-weight heparin.

From Newburger JW et al; Committee on Rheumatic Fever, Endocarditis and Kawasaki Disease; Council on Cardiovascular Disease in the Young; American Heart Association; American Academy of Pediatrics (2004), Diagnosis, treatment, and long-term management of Kawasaki disease: a statement for health professionals from the Committee on Rheumatic Fever, Endocarditis and Kawasaki Disease, Council on Cardiovascular Disease in the Young, American Heart Association. Circulation 110, 2747–71. Table 1 p2764.

Clinical and laboratory features

Clinical and laboratory features are consistent with a generalized inflammatory process and are largely nonspecific (Box 19.11.8.1 and Fig. 19.11.8.1). The timely diagnosis therefore requires a high index of suspicion, but some features are more strongly suggestive of Kawasaki's disease and the doctor should be alert to these. The desquamation following the acute illness generally follows a characteristic pattern, beginning first in the periungual regions. Hydrops of the gallbladder occurs in about 15% of patients, with Henoch–Schonlein purpura usually easily excluded as the only other common cause. Thrombocytosis may become profound after the first week.

In addition to vasculitis, particularly coronary arteritis, cardiovascular involvement may be evident as a pancarditis, with valvulitis, myocarditis, and pericarditis with effusion. Rarely, patients may develop cardiovascular collapse or ventricular arrhythmias in the acute stage. Coronary artery changes are often evident by echocardiography at the time of diagnosis and are virtually diagnostic of Kawasaki's disease.

With the exception of arterial involvement, all abnormalities resolve without sequelae, although there have been rare reports of persistent sensorineural hearing loss.

Differential diagnosis

One of the challenges regarding the diagnosis of Kawasaki's disease rests in its similarities to a number of other childhood illnesses that are much more common. Viral infections, e.g. adenovirus, enterovirus, Epstein–Barr virus, and measles, and bacterial infections, e.g. scarlet fever, can have many clinical similarities to Kawasaki's disease. Toxin-mediated illness, e.g. staphylococcal scalded skin syndrome and toxic shock syndrome, also share similar clinical features. Although traditionally the presence of infection was presumed to exclude the diagnosis of Kawasaki's disease, many patients do indeed have concomitant infection.

Drug hypersensitivity reactions and Stevens–Johnson syndrome may be difficult to differentiate from Kawasaki's disease, given that many children are presumptively treated with antibiotics before the diagnosis of Kawasaki's disease is made. Other rarer conditions to be considered include Rocky Mountain spotted fever, leptospirosis, juvenile rheumatoid arthritis, and acrodynia.

Patients—particularly those who are younger or older than typical—may not manifest all of the clinical criteria simultaneously, so continued observation and repeated consideration of the diagnosis is required.

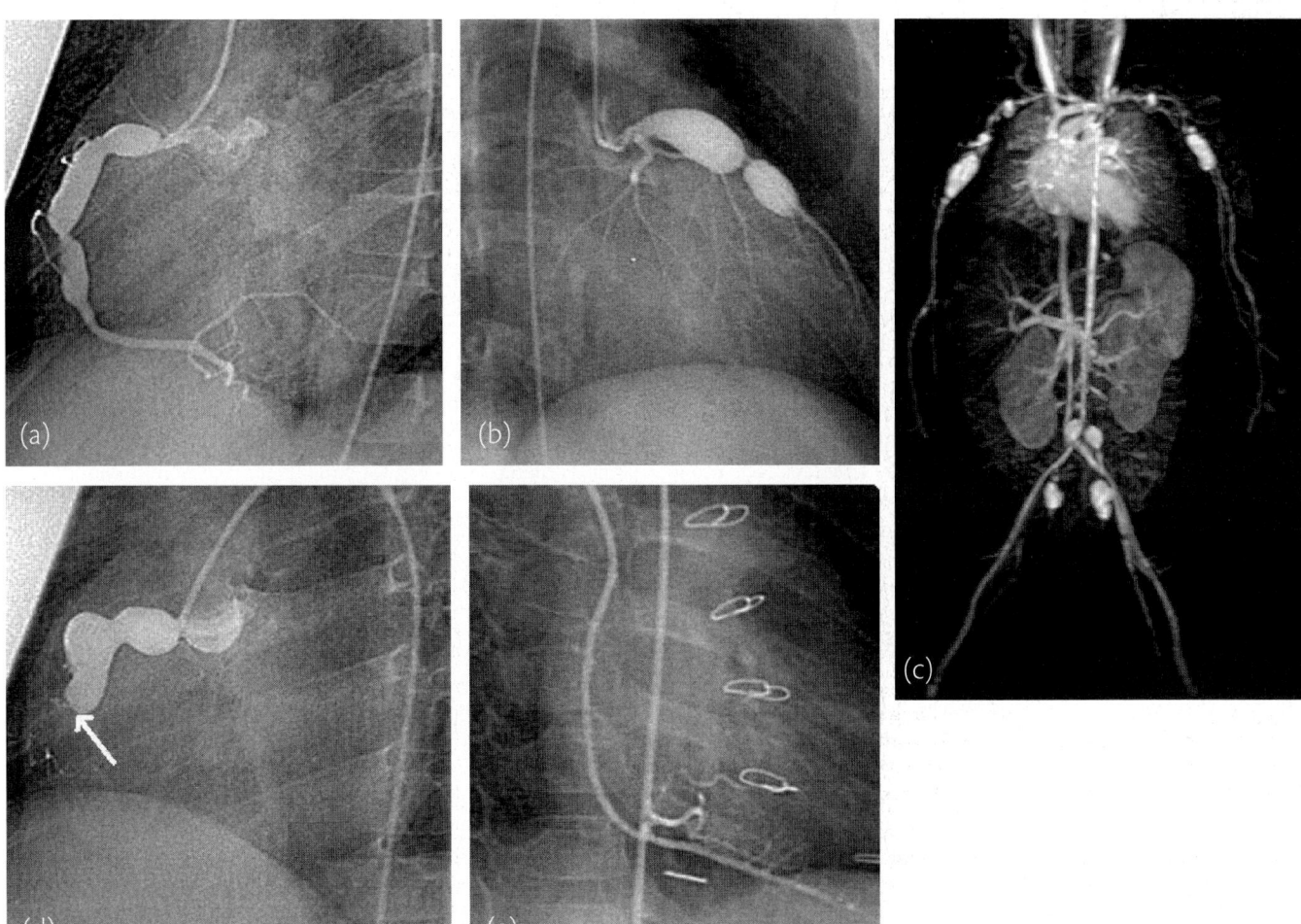

Fig. 19.11.8.2 Severe arterial involvement complicating Kawasaki's disease. (a) Multiple fusiform aneurysms along the length of the proximal right coronary artery. (b) A large fusiform and small saccular aneurysm of the proximal left anterior descending coronary artery branch. (c) Magnetic resonance angiogram showing aneurysmal arterial involvement in other small to medium-sized arteries.(d) Fusiform and saccular aneurysms of the right coronary artery with complete occlusion (arrow) of the distal exit of the aneurysm.(e) Successful reperfusion of the distal right coronary artery with placement of a right internal mammary artery bypass graft.

Evaluation of suspected incomplete Kawasaki disease (KD)

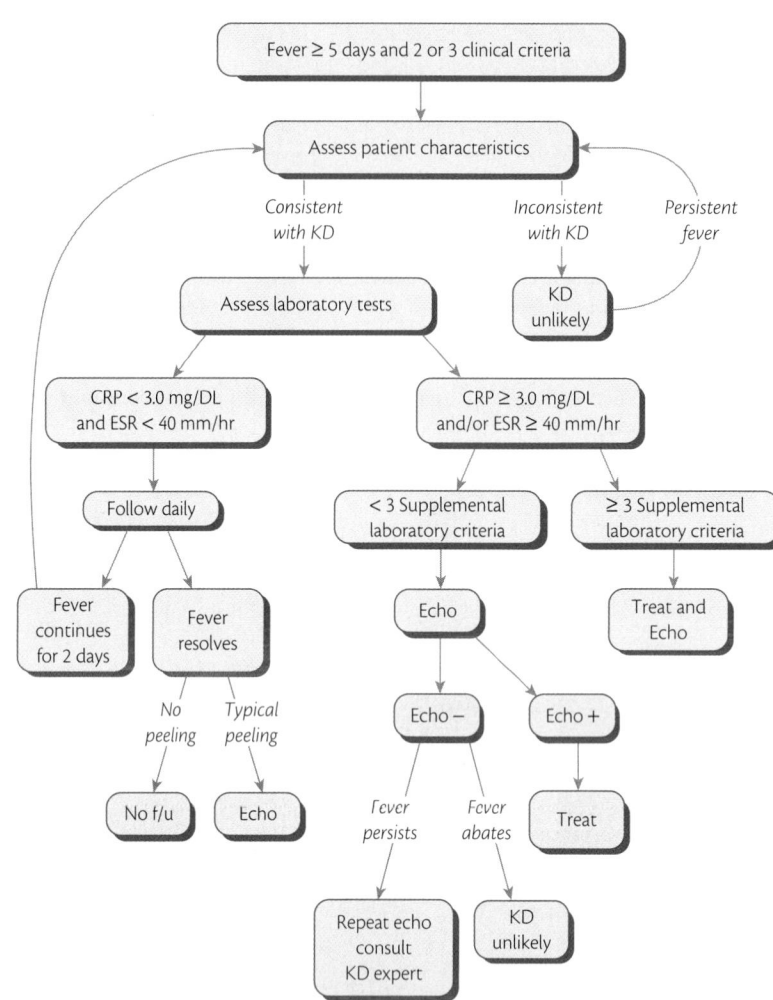

Fig.19.11.8.3 Evaluation of suspected incomplete Kawasaki's disease. CRP, C-reactive protein; DL, decilitre; Echo, echocardiography; ESR, erythrocyte sedimentation rate; KD, Kawasaki disease; mg, milligrams; mm, millimeters.
Reproduced from Newburger JW *et al*; Committee on Rheumatic Fever, Endocarditis and Kawasaki Disease; Council on Cardiovascular Disease in the Young; American Heart Association; American Academy of Pediatrics (2004), Diagnosis, treatment, and long-term management of Kawasaki disease. Circulation 110, 2747–71. Fig 1. With permission from Lippincott Williams and Wilkins.

Clinical investigation

There is no single 'diagnostic test' for Kawasaki's disease. Laboratory assessment is used to detect associated abnormalities (see Table 19.11.8.1) and exclude similar illnesses, as well as to provide additional evidence to support the diagnosis, particularly for patients with insufficient clinical criteria.

Echocardiography to detect early coronary abnormalities may provide strong evidence to support the diagnosis, as well as to identify those who may be evolving severe disease. It should be performed at the time of diagnosis, after 2 weeks, and at 6 to 8 weeks for patients with uncomplicated disease, but more frequently if severe coronary artery complications are evident. Quantitative measurements of coronary artery diameters are best related to body surface area-specific normal values for the definition of abnormalities. Echocardiography optimally images the proximal segments of the coronary arteries, with distal segments less well assessed. However, it is very rare for patients to have distal involvement without evidence of proximal abnormalities. For selected patients with severe coronary artery abnormalities, additional imaging may be required to determine the presence and extent of more distal involvement or involvement in other systemic arteries, either with magnetic resonance angiography or conventional coronary arteriography (Fig. 19.11.8.2).

Criteria for diagnosis

The diagnosis of Kawasaki's disease rests on meeting the classic clinical criteria. However, for patients early in their presentation or for those who do not have sufficient criteria, additional surveillance and laboratory testing may provide supportive evidence and identify those who require treatment, as shown in the algorithm in Fig. 19.11.8.3.

Treatment

In addition to supportive management, the mainstay of therapy is a single dose of 2 g/kg of intravenous gammaglobulin (IVIG), preferably given within the first 10 days from the onset of fever, ideally within 7 days. Timely treatment with IVIG reduces the risk of coronary artery complications to less than 4%. Patients presenting after 10 days should be given IVIG if they have persistent fever, evidence of ongoing inflammation, or evolving aneurysms. Patients are also usually given high-dose (anti-inflammatory) aspirin, at least until they are afebrile, and then low-dose (anti-platelet) aspirin for a period of 6 to 8 weeks.

Patients with persistent or recurrent fever after being given IVIG may benefit from an additional dose or treatment with pulse corticosteroids. Longer-term systemic anticoagulation is usually indicated

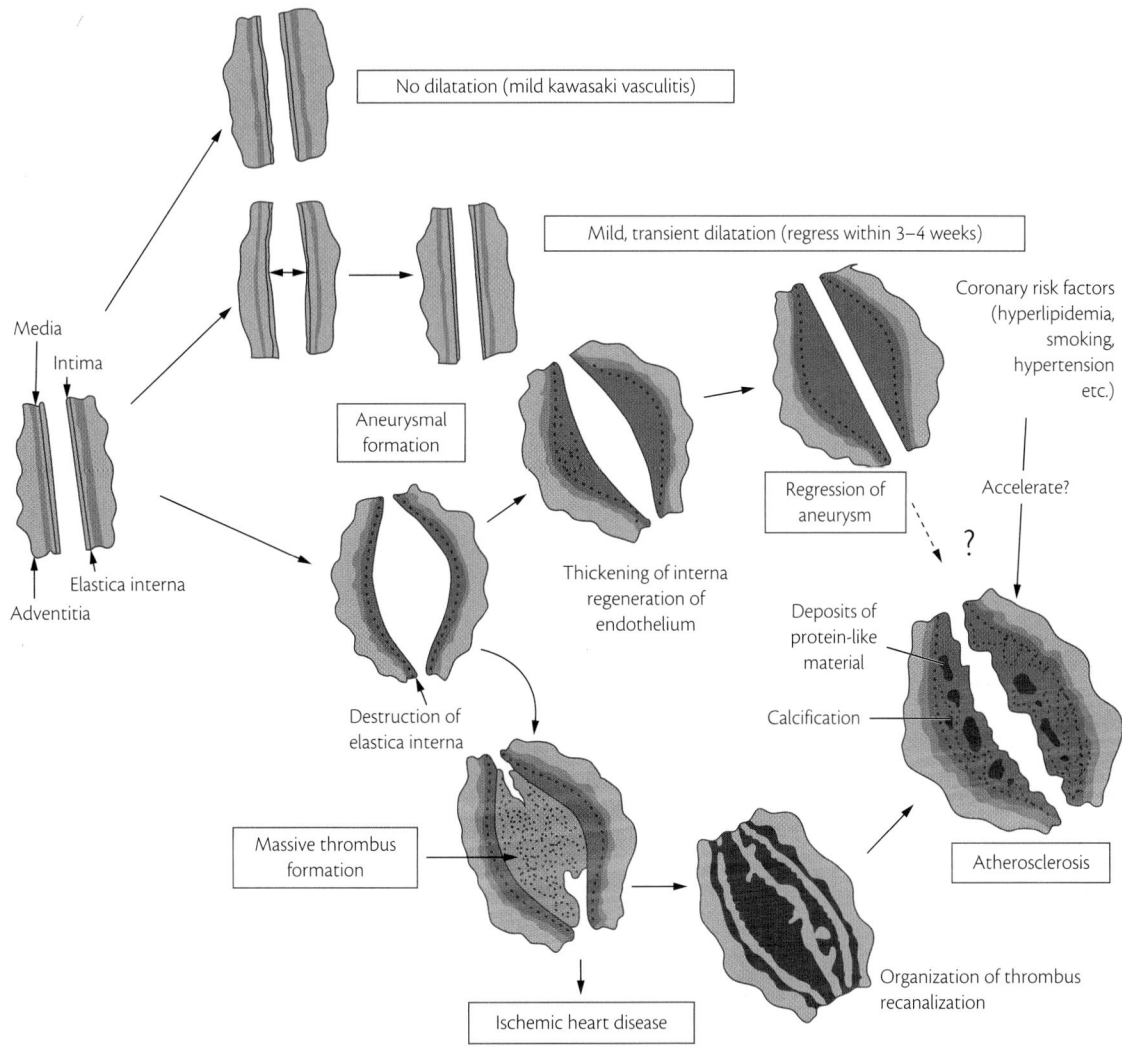

Fig. 19.11.8.4 Possible consequences of coronary artery involvement in Kawasaki's disease.
Reprinted from Progress in Pediatric Cardiology, 19, Hirohisa Kato, Cardiovascular complications in Kawasaki disease: coronary artery lumen and long-term consequences, 137-145, 2004, with permission from Elsevier.

for patients with multiple or large coronary artery aneurysms. Fibrinolytic agents may be necessary for patients who develop acute thromboses. Patients who develop coronary artery stenoses or occlusions may require catheter-based interventions or surgical revascularization (see Fig. 19.11.8.2). Rarely, cardiac transplantation has been performed for those with ischaemic cardiomyopathy or ventricular arrhythmias.

Prognosis and long-term management

Several studies have defined risk factors that identify patients at higher risk of developing coronary artery abnormalities. These may include male gender, age less than 1 year (more so if less than 6 months), higher C-reactive protein level, higher white blood cell or neutrophil count, thrombocytopenia, anaemia, low serum albumin level, and treatment delays or persistent or recurrent fever. However, the great majority of patients who have had Kawasaki's disease will have no or minimal coronary artery involvement, and are felt to have an excellent long-term prognosis. Screening and counselling about risk factors for atherosclerotic cardiovascular disease have been recommended, given the uncertainties concerning the ultra-long-term prognosis. In general, coronary artery involvement may show important regression over time, with a lesser degree of maximal abnormality predicting the earliest and more complete resolution (Fig. 19.11.8.4). Persistent abnormalities and risk of stenoses tend to be isolated to those patients with multiple or large aneurysms. For patients who have had important coronary artery complications, long-term surveillance, management, and prognosis are dependent on the ongoing risk of thrombosis and stenoses (Table 19.11.8.1). Rarely, previously healthy adult patients may present with myocardial ischaemia and a new diagnosis of coronary artery aneurysms, which may suggest a prior episode of undiagnosed Kawasaki disease during childhood.

Likely future developments

It is to be hoped that aetiological and pathophysiological mechanisms will be discovered, enabling preventive strategies, and also the development of alternative or additional therapies for preventing coronary artery abnormalities. Studies may also provide information relating to areas where prognosis or best treatment remains uncertain, e.g. the ultra-long-term prognosis for patients with no or minor coronary artery involvement, the best management of patients with persistent or recurrent fever, and the optimal anticoagulation regimen for patients with persistent coronary artery involvement.

Further reading

McCrindle BW, ed. (2004). Advances in Kawasaki disease. *Progr Pediatr Cardiol*, **19**, 91–206.

Newburger JW, *et al.* (1991). A single intravenous infusion of gamma globulin as compared with four infusions in the treatment of acute Kawasaki syndrome. *N Engl J Med*, **324**, 1633–9.

Newburger JW, *et al.* (2004). Diagnosis, treatment, and long-term management of Kawasaki disease: a statement for health professionals from the Committee on Rheumatic Fever, Endocarditis and Kawasaki Disease, Council on Cardiovascular Disease in the Young, American Heart Association. *Circulation*, **110**, 2747–71.

Parisi Q, *et al.* (2004). Clinical manifestations of coronary aneurysms in the adult as possible sequelae of Kawasaki disease during infancy. *Acta Cardiol*, **59**, 5–9.

Miscellaneous conditions presenting to the rheumatologist

Donncha O'Gradaigh

Essentials

Musculoskeletal symptoms may occur in a very wide range of diseases, or as a drug side effect. If the clinical picture is unusual, it is important that the physician keeps an open mind and reviews the history, signs, and investigation results carefully, looking for findings incongruent with 'common diagnoses'. Some of the more distinctive and important miscellaneous conditions that are likely to present to rheumatologists are the following.

Adult Still's disease—presents with high, spiking pyrexia, arthralgia, or arthritis, and a characteristic nonpruritic, maculopapular, salmon-pink rash. Commonly causes hepatosplenomegaly, generalized lymphadenopathy, and polyserositis (usually pericarditis and pleuritis). Diagnosis is primarily clinical: there are no specific laboratory features. Treatment is with nonsteroidal anti-inflammatory drugs (NSAIDs) and (in severe cases) steroids.

Pyoderma gangrenosum—a reactive neutrophilic dermatosis associated with ulcerative colitis, rheumatoid arthritis, and monoclonal gammopathies or other haematological malignancies. Produces painful ulcerative skin lesions, often associated with arthralgia/polyarthritis. Treatment includes corticosteroids, with ciclosporin or infliximab in resistant cases.

Sweet's syndrome—presents with tender red or purple raised nodules associated with fever and generalized myalgia and/or arthralgia.

Skin biopsy is diagnostic. Treatment is usually symptomatic, with symptoms resolving over 2 to 3 months.

Autoinflammatory disorders—a range of conditions presenting with periodic fevers and inflammation, with familial Mediterranean fever as the prototype, are caused by genetic mutations that affect pyrin function. Dramatic clinical responses can sometimes be obtained with soluble interleukin-1 receptor antagonist or anti-tumour necrosis factor α treatment.

Chronic regional pain syndrome—also known as algodystrophy, Sudeck's atrophy, and reflex sympathetic dystrophy—presents with pain, allodynia (pain in response to an innocuous stimulus), hyperalgesia (increased pain perception), and hyperpathia (an exaggerated delayed reaction), usually involving a single limb or body region, typically distal to the site of some (often trivial) traumatic event. Diagnosis is largely clinical. Treatment is with intensive physiotherapy; treatments for neuropathic/intractable pain are often given; high-dose bisphosphonates may be helpful.

Charcot's arthropathy—joint destruction is associated with neurological injury, most commonly due to diabetes. Gross proliferative osteoarthrosis is often seen radiologically. Pain-free joints rarely require treatment; painful joints can respond to intravenous bisphosphonate therapy, absence of weight-bearing, and a total contact cast.

Adult Still's disease

In 1971, Bywaters described a series of 14 adults with an illness very similar to the systemic onset type of juvenile idiopathic arthritis described by Still in 1897. Adult-onset Still's disease is found worldwide with an incidence of 1 to 3 per million, most commonly in the age range 16 to 35 years and affecting males and females equally in most populations. There is no consistent human leucocyte antigen (HLA) association.

Features common to both childhood- and adult-onset forms are the high, spiking pyrexia, arthralgia or arthritis, and a characteristic rash. The fever typically appears in the evening, and a patient with pyrexia of unknown origin should always be assessed at least once at the end of the day. Spikes in excess of 39°C are typical (and required in diagnostic criteria), although a return to

a normal temperature does not occur in 20%. Arthralgia is almost universal and may intensify during the febrile episodes. Distal interphalangeal joint involvement, seen in one in five patients, is useful to distinguish from other inflammatory arthropathies. The classic 'Still's rash' is a nonpruritic, maculopapular, salmon-pink rash on the trunk, thighs, and arms or axillae that appears transiently during the temperature spike (termed 'evanescent'). The rash may also appear on the face, palms, and soles, and at sites of skin trauma (Koebner's phenomenon) in a third of adults (Fig. 19.12.1). A (culture-negative) severe sore throat is relatively common in adults (although not a feature of the juvenile form).

Other common manifestations are hepatosplenomegaly with or without generalized lymphadenopathy, and polyserositis, of which pericarditis (in a third) and pleuritis are the most common.

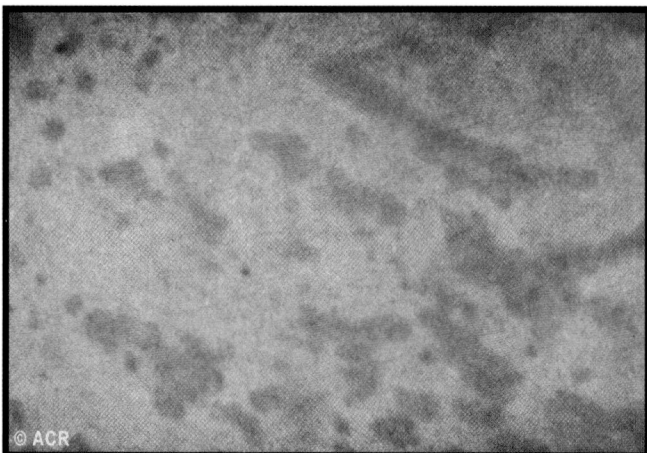

Fig. 19.12.1 The rash of Still's disease.

Rare features include sicca symptoms (dry eyes, mouth), myocarditis, restrictive lung disease, liver or renal failure, panophthalmitis or inflammatory orbital pseudotumour, epilepsy, intravascular coagulopathy or haemophagocytic syndrome, and amyloidosis.

Diagnosis is primarily clinical. The classic features may emerge only over a period of time, and the possibility of Still's disease may need to be reconsidered as symptoms progress. The differential diagnosis is wide, and while diagnostic criteria have been proposed they have poor sensitivity and specificity until infection (particularly infectious mononucleosis), neoplasia (lymphomas), and connective tissue diseases (such as polyarteritis nodosa and systemic rheumatoid vasculitis) have been excluded.

There are no specific laboratory features, but typical findings include elevated ESR and CRP, thrombocytosis, neutrophil leucocytosis (total leucocytes in excess of 15×10^9/litre) and a normochromic normocytic anaemia. Rheumatoid factor and antinuclear antibodies are negative in most cases. A serum ferritin more than $1000\,\mu$g/litre had sensitivity of 80% and specificity of 41% in a population with various rheumatological diseases: a low (less than 20%) fraction of glycosylated ferritin is more specific but not in general use.

Nonsteroidal anti-inflammatory drugs (NSAIDs) are the first-line treatment for fever and systemic features. If these agents fail, corticosteroids are required (two-thirds of cases), and should be initiated without delay in cases of myocarditis, pericardial tamponade, or other severe organ involvement. Doses of prednisolone in the range 0.5 to 1 mg/kg per day are usually given, and should be continued for 2 to 3 months after remission before gradually tapering the dose. In refractory cases with systemic features, or as steroid-sparing therapy, methotrexate is particularly useful. Salazopyrin, azathioprine, and intravenous immunoglobulin have also been used. The interleukin-1 receptor antagonist anakinra has emerged as the most valuable biologic therapy in resistant Still's disease.

Prognosis is variable. A chronic progressive arthritis is predicted by early arthritis (rather than arthralgia), particularly of the hip and shoulder, and occurs in 30 to 50% of cases, with ankylosis of the carpus and tarsus and involvement of the cervical spine and hips. Equal proportions of the remainder experience either a self-limiting course (lasting up to 1 year), or a polycyclic, relapsing and remitting course. The rash, fever, and serositis are typically less severe in subsequent relapses, and complete remissions up to 10 years after first presentation have been recorded.

Reactive haemophagocytic syndrome is a rare complication of systemic-onset juvenile arthritis, which has also been described in adult-onset Still's disease. Sharing many of its clinical features (fever, hepatosplenomegaly, lymphadenopathy), T-cell and macrophage activation and proliferation lead to phagocytosis of haematopoietic cells and cytokine activation. Diagnosis should be suspected when leucopenia and thrombocytopenia are found, the converse being more common in Still's disease. Diagnosis requires bone marrow biopsy. In most case series the condition has responded to corticosteroid, intravenous immunoglobulin, or anti-TNFα therapy as for adult-onset Still's disease itself.

Acne arthralgia

Patients may complain of myalgia, arthralgia, or swelling, typically involving the large joints. Most patients are male adolescents with aggressive acne. *Propionibacterium acnes* has been isolated from joint aspirates, but effusions are typically sterile and the arthritis is believed to be reactive rather than septic. Hydradenitis suppurativa, producing large abscesses in the axilla and groin, is also associated with a reactive type of large-joint oligoarthropathy. In both conditions, symptoms usually improve with treatment of the skin lesion.

A seronegative spondyloarthropathy syndrome of acne, palmoplantar pustulosis, hyperostosis (especially of the clavicles or sternum), and (sterile) osteomyelitis (SAPHO) is associated with enthesitis and an inflammatory polyarthritis that often includes the sacroiliac joints. As part of the spectrum of psoriatic arthritis, treatment with the anti-TNF-α antibodies infliximab, etanercept, and adalimumab is effective. See Chapter 19.6 for further discussion.

PAPA is a syndrome of pyogenic sterile arthritis, pyoderma gangrenosum, and acne, part of the spectrum of autoinflammatory disorders that is discussed later (see 'Familial Mediterranean fever').

Neutrophilic dermatoses

The neutrophilic dermatoses include pyoderma gangrenosum and Sweet's syndrome (acute febrile neutrophilic dermatosis). Erythema nodosum is part of this spectrum, but is discussed with sarcoidosis in Chapter 18.12.

Pyoderma gangrenosum is a reactive neutrophilic dermatosis associated with ulcerative colitis, rheumatoid arthritis, and monoclonal gammopathies or other haematological malignancies, which produces painful ulcerative skin lesions (Fig. 19.12.2). Lesions progress within 24 to 48 h from small papules to a 'cat's paw' appearance of adjacent ulcers, coalescing into the larger typical ulcer. Approximately 30% of patients describe arthralgia or a seronegative, progressive, erosive polyarthritis. Treatment includes corticosteroids, with addition of ciclosporin or use of infliximab (a TNFα chimeric antibody) in resistant cases.

Sweet's syndrome presents with tender red or purple raised nodules associated with fever and generalized myalgia and/or arthralgia (Fig. 19.12.3). Joint effusions may occur, and aspirates reveal high neutrophil counts. Sterile osteomyelitic foci have rarely been described. Skin biopsy is diagnostic (Fig. 19.12.3). Symptoms typically resolve over 2 to 3 months, requiring symptomatic treatment with an NSAID or intra-articular steroid. An association with acute

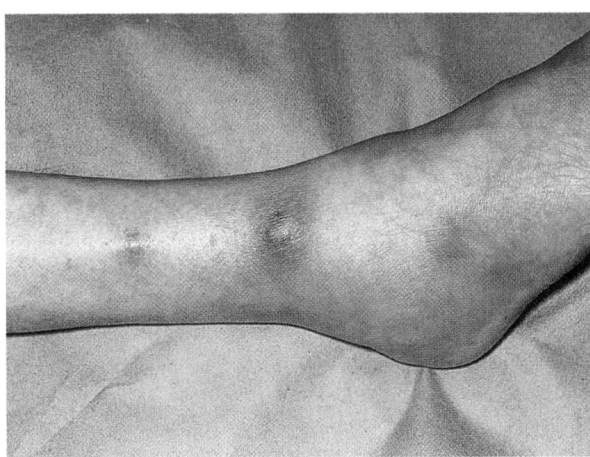

Fig. 19.12.2 Pyoderma gangrenosum.

myeloid (particularly premyelocytic) leukaemia is noted in about 15% of cases, and recombinant granulocyte colony-stimulating factor (rG-CSF) has also been implicated in a number of cases.

Panniculitis

Also called lupus erythematosus profundus, this is an unusual variation of cutaneous lupus characterized by recurrent inflammation of subcutaneous tissue, leading to fibrosis. Asymptomatic, firm, sharply defined, subcutaneous nodules or plaques appear on the proximal upper and lower limbs, buttocks, face, and scalp. Diagnosis requires a biopsy including the underlying fat. Histology reveals a nonspecific lobular panniculitis with necrobiosis of adipose tissue and fibrotic deposits. One in eight patients has systemic lupus erythematosus (SLE) at presentation, particularly generalized arthralgia and fatigue. A further 10 to 15% will develop SLE up to 10 years later. Skin and joint features are treated with hydroxychloroquine, although a steroid and dapsone are occasionally required for more florid panniculitis.

Multicentric reticulohistiocytosis

This is a rare systemic disease of unknown aetiology, although recent evidence suggests an association with human herpesvirus

(HHV) 8. Lipid-laden histiocytes and multinucleate giant cells infiltrate into various organs, principally skin and synovium. The condition presents most commonly in the fourth decade, with 40% having joint symptoms alone, 30% with isolated skin involvement, and 30% with both features. Light copper or red–brown nodules appear on the face and hands, but can appear anywhere, and may number from a few to several hundred. The spine and other joints may be involved. The use of bisphosphonates attenuates bony erosion and may have a direct, apoptotic effect on histiocytes, whereas the anti-TNF agents represent a major advance. Underlying malignancy is reported in 20 to 30% of cases.

Amyloidosis

Musculoskeletal features occur in three main settings. Dialysis-related amyloidosis is due to the accumulation of β_2-microglobulin. Synovitis usually involves large joints such as the hip and shoulder. MRI may show characteristic features, and joint fluid aspiration may identify amyloid deposits, particularly using the more sensitive combination of Congo red staining and immunocytochemistry. Symptomatic treatment with an NSAID is usually sufficient, considerations of the effect of NSAIDs on renal function being relevant only in those dialysis patients with substantial urine output, but the condition can be disabling and refractory. Significant improvement often follows transplantation. Cystic (lytic) bone lesions are typically painless, and present difficulties in the differential diagnosis. They may be complicated by a pathological fracture. Soft-tissue amyloid deposits usually present with entrapment neuropathies such as carpal tunnel syndrome.

In primary (AL) amyloidosis a symmetrical polyarthritis with synovitis and morning stiffness involves large and small joints. Radiological changes include osteoporosis and, less commonly, joint erosions. Diagnostic confusion can arise because frequently the erythrocyte sedimentation rate (ESR) is not significantly elevated. The synovitis is often described as 'pasty', and flexion contractures occur relatively early. The early appearance of carpal tunnel syndrome should also raise the suspicion of underlying amyloidosis. In addition to treatment addressing the underlying paraproteinaemia, joint symptoms may require therapy with a corticosteroid. Thalidomide, which decreases expression of the key

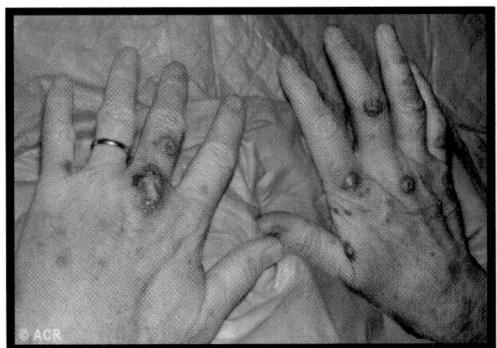

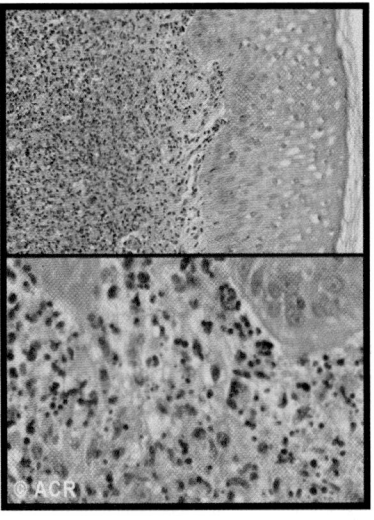

Fig. 19.12.3 Sweet's syndrome: the photo of the hands shows scattered pustular lesions characteristic of Sweet's syndrome. The low- and high-power views of a skin biopsy (stained with haematoxylin and eosin) from the same patient demonstrate the neutrophilic infiltration of the dermis that is characteristic of this condition. Nuclear debris is also present.

inflammatory cytokine TNFα and the downstream transcription factor NF-κB, has been effective in clinical studies.

A genetic basis has been identified in secondary (AA) amyloidosis, with the α/α genotype associated with clinical disease in white people, although rheumatological symptoms are uncommon in this form. Serum amyloid A (SAA)-activating transcription factor 1 (SAF-1) undergoes structural modification during inflammation, resulting in deposition of a truncated form of SAA in various organs. The Muckle–Wells syndrome of urticaria, deafness, arthritis, and amyloid nephropathy has recently been recognized as one of the autoinflammatory disorders discussed in the next section.

Autoinflammatory disorders

Familial Mediterranean fever (FMF) is the prototype of a group of disorders termed the 'autoinflammatory disorders', characterized by periodic fevers and inflammation without associated autoantibodies (Table 19.12.1; see also Chapter 12.12.2). Since the discovery of the genetic basis to a number of these conditions, a common mechanism is proposed related to alteration in regulation of the inflammatory cascade (Fig. 19.12.4). The understanding revealed by the genetic basis to these conditions has highlighted the therapeutic potential of the soluble interleukin-1 receptor antagonist (IL-1Ra) drug anakinra. Its use has led to dramatic therapeutic responses, including resolution of deafness in Muckle–Wells syndrome.

Familial Mediterranean fever

Familial Mediterranean fever is an autosomal recessive disorder in people of Armenian, Arab, and Sephardic Jewish descent. Presenting in childhood with episodes of fever and abdominal pain, synovitis occurs in 75% of cases. Monoarticular involvement of a knee or ankle, or symmetrical involvement of these joints, is the most common of the six patterns of joint involvement described. A symmetrical polyarthritis, indistinguishable from juvenile idiopathic arthritis, often causes diagnostic confusion, particularly as fever and abdominal pain are not uncommon in this condition. The pattern tends to be similar in subsequent episodes and, despite frequent florid synovitis, residual damage rarely occurs. Episodes typically last for less than 1 week, although more protracted attacks may persist for months. Treatment with colchicine has almost eliminated amyloidosis as a complication of this condition and it also reduces the frequency of symptom relapse. As mentioned above, the use of anakinra and anti-TNF biologic agents has achieved excellent results.

Several other periodic fever syndromes share the proposed mechanism and responsiveness to anti-TNF and anti-IL1Ra therapy (see Table 19.12.1).

Haematological disorders

Leukaemia, lymphoma, and uncommon lymphoproliferative disorders

Between 13 and 60% of patients with acute leukaemia will develop arthralgia or, less commonly, a frank arthritis. Monoarthritis, symmetrical polyarthritis, and a large joint oligoarthropathy are described. Diagnostic clues include a disproportionate amount of pain, fever, and weight loss, although in children the last may be mistaken for Still's disease.

Arthralgia is an uncommon feature of lymphomas, but 7 to 25% of patients with non-Hodgkin's lymphoma experience polyarthralgia, secondary gout, or hypertrophic pulmonary osteoarthropathy (see below) during the course of their disease.

Large granular lymphocyte syndrome is a monoclonal expansion of T cells associated with a variety of conditions including rheumatoid arthritis (in a third of cases). Both neutropenia and splenomegaly can occur, mimicking Felty's syndrome, and some consider the condition to be indistinguishable in every respect, including its management.

Human T-cell lymphotropic virus-1 (HTLV-1) is associated with the development of leukaemia or lymphoma, and may independently produce a symmetrical polyarthritis closely resembling rheumatoid arthritis.

Haemophilia

Prophylactic factor replacement between 2 and 18 years of age is cost-effective in preventing disabling joint complications. Without this, acute haemarthroses begin from around 5 years of age, causing recurring episodes of very painful and tender joint swelling, particularly in the hinge joints such as the knee, ankle, and elbow (presumably because these joints are less tolerant of angular or rotational strain). After only three or four episodes, haemosiderin deposition in synovium results in proliferation of synovial fibroblasts (with expression of the proto-oncogenes c-*myc* and *MDM2* noted *in vitro*), neovascularization, and activation of inflammatory cytokines.

Ultrasonography is useful in the differentiation of haemarthrosis from soft-tissue or subperiosteal haemorrhage. Early coagulation factor replacement, ice, joint immobilization, and elevation all reduce further bleeding. Joint aspiration may also be required (after adequate factor replacement). Rehabilitation is required to prevent contraction. Synovectomy by an intra-articular injection of radioactive isotope is a useful treatment in cases of chronic synovitis, but joint replacement continues to be needed where disabling secondary degenerative arthritis has occurred. Acute haemarthrosis due to disseminated intravascular coagulation should be similarly managed.

Cryoglobulinaemia

Cryoglobulins are immune complexes that precipitate spontaneously at low temperatures. Type I (25%) comprises a monoclonal immunoglobulin and is associated with lymphoproliferative disorders including myeloma and Waldenström's macroglobulinaemia. Type III accounts for 50% of cases, and is a complex of two polyclonal immunoglobulins, usually occurring as a paraneoplastic phenomenon. Type II (25%) complexes a monoclonal immunoglobulin, usually of IgM class, with a polyclonal anti-immunoglobulin typically of IgG type (i.e. a rheumatoid factor). Previously called mixed essential cryoglobulinaemia, it is now recognized that over 80% of patients with this condition have serological evidence of hepatitis C virus (HCV) infection. However, HCV is less likely to cause cryoglobulinaemic vasculitis among northern European populations and in North Americans than in southern Europeans, hence it is recognized that HCV is not sufficient to produce vasculitis. The virus induces a translocation t(14:18) in lymphocytes, which activates the antiapoptotic *BCL2*. In addition, a viral envelope protein E2 interacts with CD81 on B cells, reducing the threshold for B-cell production of immunoglobulins.

Table 19.12.1 Key features of the hereditary periodic fever syndromes

	FMF	HIDS	TRAPS (aka familial Hibernian fever)	PAPA	FCAS	Muckle–Wells syndrome	CINCA
Inheritance	Recessive	Recessive	Dominant	Dominant	Dominant	Dominant	Dominant
Predominant ancestries	Armenian, Arab, and Sephardic Jewish	Dutch, French, other European	Irish, Scottish	None	European	Northern European	None
Gene	MEFV	MVK	TNFRSF1A	PSTPIP1/CD2BP1	CIAS1/NALP3/PYPAF1	CIAS1/NALP3/PYPAF1	CIAS1/NALP3/PYPAF1
OMIM	249100	260920	142680	604416	120100	191900	607115
Protein	Pyrin	Mevalonate kinase	55-kDa TNF receptor	PSTPIP1/CD2BP1	Cryopyrin	Cryopyrin	Cryopyrin
Duration of episodes	1–3 days	3–7 days	>1 week	Variable	<24 h	24–48 h	Continuous, but with flares
Musculoskeletal features	Episodic monoarthritis + (see text)	Arthralgia, nonerosive polyarthritis	Severe migratory myalgia, arthralgia, nonerosive monoarthritis	Pyogenic sterile arthritis	Myalgias, polyarthralgias	Myalgias, arthralgias, large joint oligoarticular arthritis	Epiphyseal/patellar overgrowth, periosteal elevation, intermittent or chronic arthritis
Skin involvement	Erysipelas-like erythema	Nonspecific rash/eruptions	Migratory erysipelas-like rash overlying myalgias	Pyoderma gangrenosum, acne	Urticarial rash induced by cold	Urticarial rash	Urticarial rash
Other clinical features	Sterile peritonitis Pleurisy Pericardial effusion Scrotal pain	Abdominal pain/vomiting/diarrhoea Cervical lymphadenopathy Elevated IgD Elevated urinary mevalonate during attacks	Abdominal pain/peritonitis/diarrhoea/constipation Pleurisy Conjunctivitis/periorbital oedema Amyloid in 10%	Recurrent destructive inflammation in skin/joints/muscle	Nausea Headache Conjunctivitis	Abdominal pain Sensorineural deafness Conjunctivitis/episcleritis/optic disc oedema Amyloid in 10–50%	Abdominal symptoms rare Intellectual impairment Headache Sensorineural deafness Chronic aseptic meningitis Conjunctivitis/uveitis/papilloedema/blindness
Treatment	Colchicine prophylaxis Steroids for myalgia	NSAIDs/steroids for arthritis (anti-TNFα)	NSAIDs/steroids for attacks Anti TNFα prophylaxis	Steroids (anti-TNFα and IL-1 receptor antagonist)	Avoidance of cold IL-1 receptor antagonist NSAIDs	IL-1 receptor antagonist NSAIDs Steroids	IL-1 receptor antagonist (anti-TNFα)

CINCA, chronic infantile neurological cutaneous articular syndrome; FCAS, familial cold autoinflammatory syndrome; FMF, familial Mediterranean fever; HIDS, hyperimmunoglobulin D syndrome; NSAID, nonsteroidal anti-inflammatory drug; PAPA, pyogenic sterile arthritis, pyoderma gangrenosum, and acne; TNF, tumour necrosis factor; TRAPS, TNF-receptor associated periodic syndrome;

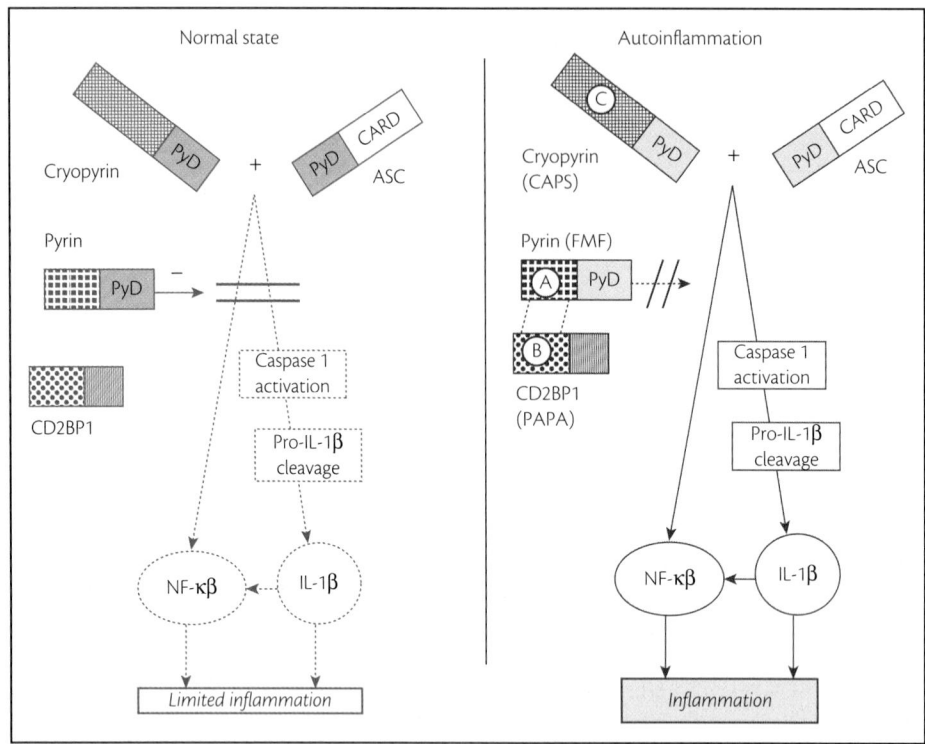

Fig. 19.12.4 Left panel: in the normal state proteins with a pyrin domain (PyD) regulate inflammation via interaction with the apoptotic speck-like protein containing the caspase recruitment domain (ASC), which induces increases in interleukin IL 1β and the transcription factor NF-κB. Pyrin normally acts to downregulate ASC-mediated inflammation. Right panel: autoinflammation can occur if: (a) mutations in pyrin reduce its inhibitory function (familial Mediterranean fever, FMF); (b) mutations in a pyrin-binding protein (CD2BP1) lead to pyrin being sequestered and prevented from working properly (pyoderma gangrenosum and acne or PAPA); or (c) there are gain-of-function mutations in cryopyrin-associated periodic syndromes (CAPS).

Precipitation of cryoglobulin leads to complement activation and vasculitis in small vessels. Complete vascular occlusion is less common. A classic triad of a palpable purpuric rash on the extremities, arthralgia, and muscle weakness is described. Joints are involved in 70% of patients in a relapsing and remitting pattern, affecting—in order of frequency—the hands, knees, ankles, and elbows. Inflammatory arthritis is uncommon and radiological changes do not occur. Other skin presentations include petechiae, urticaria, and acrocyanosis. Other organ involvement is frequently seen in addition to this triad, particularly glomerulonephritis.

Diagnosis requires meticulous attention to phlebotomy and laboratory techniques. A positive rheumatoid factor and raised ESR are supportive features, and urinalysis and microscopy, looking for an 'active sediment' (proteinuria, haematuria, and red cell casts), should always be carried out in patients presenting with purpura and arthralgia. A thorough search is required for underlying malignancy and for associated HCV infection.

Treatment is determined by the clinical presentation. Corticosteroids may suffice for arthralgia and mild skin involvement. In the presence of renal or more severe skin involvement, the addition of cyclophosphamide or the B-cell-depleting monoclonal antibody rituximab is recommended. Although cyclophosphamide does not result in an increase in HCV infection or hepatitis, rituximab increased viraemia twofold, and sequential therapy with antiviral drugs (interferon-α and ribavirin) may be necessary. However, the impact of a reduction in the viral load on the clinical manifestations of cryoglobulinaemic vasculitis is unclear, although a reduced risk of the lymphoproliferative disease is noted. Plasma exchange may be necessary to gain rapid control of disease in rapidly progressive glomerulonephritis or in the presence of a neuropathy.

POEMS

This term, coined by Bardwick in 1980, refers to an uncommon disorder that may present to any specialty, depending on the dominant feature in the spectrum of polyneuropathy, organomegaly, endocrinopathy, M-protein (i.e. a monoclonal paraproteinaemia), and skin abnormalities. Skin changes may resemble scleroderma. Radiographs show single (50% of cases) or multiple osteosclerotic lesions with unusual patterns of proliferative change, both of which are unexpected in myeloma. The diagnosis of POEMS should therefore be considered in those presenting with osteosclerotic lesions accompanied by paraproteinaemia, particularly when associated with peripheral neuropathy. Treatment is directed at the principal presenting features—bone lesions are rarely symptomatic unless they result in bone swelling or fracture. The paraproteinaemia may require melphalan and corticosteroid. Recently, the disorder has been related to altered expression of the vasogenic signal VEGF (vascular endothelial growth factor)—serum levels correlate with clinical course and response to therapy, and cases are reported of remission of POEMS after treatment with a VEGF-blocking monoclonal antibody, bevacizumab.

Hypogammaglobulinaemia

Primary hypogammaglobulinaemia is associated in 10 to 30% of patients with a nonerosive polyarthritis resembling rheumatoid arthritis. Features include morning stiffness, pain, and tender swelling in the peripheral joints. Subcutaneous nodules may appear. However, the rheumatoid factor is negative, histology reveals the absence of plasma cells, and permanent joint damage is rare. Most cases present between 2 and 5 years of age with infection. Synovitis may be transient or it may persist for many years, requiring symptomatic treatment. Intra-articular corticosteroid treatment is used, although these patients are somewhat more at risk of septic arthritis. In the absence of any intra-articular procedure, the rate of septic arthritis is approximately 20% over 20 years.

Sickle cell disease

Sickle cell crises commonly include bone pain, with 41% in a recent case series having at least one episode of avascular necrosis (50% hip, 40% vertebral). Vasodilator drugs have been used with varied results, and core decompression remains a contentious treatment for avascular necrosis in the orthopaedic literature. Avascular necrosis is less commonly associated with other haemoglobinopathies. Synovitis, frequently complicated by haemarthrosis, usually occurs during crises and is due to synovial infarction. The effusion is noninflammatory. Osteomyelitis may complicate avascular necrosis due to sickle cell disease, salmonella being particularly common, but septic arthritis is unusual. Hyperuricaemia and gout occur in 40% of adults with sickle cell disease, and is treated in the standard way. Less commonly, a hand-and-foot syndrome affects infants aged between 6 months and 2 years, dactylitis and periostitis producing symmetrical, tender, diffuse swelling and stiffness lasting several weeks.

Gastroenterological and metabolic conditions

Hepatitis

The common viral hepatitides caused by hepatitis A, B, and C viruses are associated with a serum sickness during their prodromal phase. Early morning stiffness and mild arthralgia, or—less commonly—inflammatory arthritis, affects the small joints of the hands and, in decreasing order of frequency, the knees, ankles, shoulders, wrists, and feet. The spine and hips are not usually affected. Symptoms typically resolve as hepatitis evolves. Less common features include a leucocytoclastic ('hypersensitivity') vasculitis in hepatitis A and an association with polyarteritis nodosa in hepatitis B. Hepatitis C is associated with cryoglobulinaemia (in 50%) and with antiphospholipid antibodies and thrombosis.

Enteropathies

Coeliac disease may result in osteoporosis or osteomalacia with bone pain and pathological fracture. Arthritis is uncommon, but can precede overt bowel symptoms by up to 3 years. Symmetrical involvement with swelling and stiffness can affect the lumbar spine, hips, knees, and shoulders. Dermatitis herpetiformis is more common among those with joint involvement. The joint manifestations resolve on changing to a gluten-free diet, and do not reappear on re-challenge with gluten.

Whipple's disease presents with fever and abdominal pain. Acute or subacute migratory polyarthritis may precede bowel symptoms by years, and typically involves the ankles, knees, shoulders, and elbows. Lymphadenopathy is a prominent feature. Duodenal biopsy shows periodic acid–Schiff-staining macrophages, and

the polymerase chain reaction detects the causative organism *Tropheryma whippelii*. Its presence within cells implies a mechanism similar to reactive arthritis, with a T-helper T_{H2}-dominant response and inability of the T_{H1} cellular immune response to clear the microbe from macrophages, which therefore perpetuate the inflammatory reaction.

Surgical procedures that bypass a section of (proximal) small bowel are associated with so-called 'bypass' arthritis. This ranges from a mono- or oligoarthropathy to a diffuse polyarthritis involving large and small joints. Tenosynovitis of the wrist is a particularly common feature. Treatment is symptomatic, though sulfasalazine is occasionally used as a disease-modifying therapy.

Wilson's disease

A disorder of copper metabolism, this condition typically presents in childhood with neurological problems. Some two-thirds of patients with Wilson's disease will develop musculoskeletal manifestations, half of them being symptomatic by 15 years of age. Features include arthritis (primary, attributed to copper deposition in synovium, or secondary, due to chondrocalcinosis), rhabdomyolysis, hypermobility (due to effects on collagen synthesis), and osteopenia. Radiological appearances are generally nonspecific, with joint space narrowing, sclerosis, and cyst formation. A fluffy periostitis at the greater trochanter and inferior aspect of the calcaneus, and corticated ossicles near affected joints (particularly the wrist), are characteristic but rare. Diagnosis requires measuring urinary 24-h copper excretion: ceruloplasmin may be elevated as part of an acute-phase response and therefore is of no diagnostic value in presentations with acute arthritis. Penicillamine is the mainstay of treatment for this condition and alleviates joint symptoms.

Ochronosis

Deficiency of the enzyme homogentisic acid dioxygenase results in an accumulation of this organic acid. Although a congenital disorder, symptoms rarely appear until the fourth decade. The classic clinical features of pigmentation of the ear and sclera, and urine darkening on standing (giving the alternative name alkaptonuria), allow easy diagnosis. Deposition also occurs in the synovium and may appear in joint fluid aspirate. Pain and swelling affect the large joints, and the thoracolumbar spine is also affected, producing pain and stiffness, but the lumbosacral spine is spared. Radiographs show chondrocalcinosis of the intervertebral discs with spondylosis that may progress to ankylosis. In the peripheral joints, radiological changes of degeneration appear, although osteophytes are often less marked than in other degenerative arthritides. Erosion may occur. Nitisinone is an inhibitor of an enzyme upstream of homogentisic acid, 4-hydroxyphenylpyruvate, with promising results in phase II trials.

Hyperlipidaemia

Articular symptoms can occur in a number of the hyperlipidaemias, particularly types II and IV. Joint manifestations typically precede diagnosis of the lipoprotein disorder. Xanthomas of tendons are a useful clue, but the clinical picture is otherwise nonspecific. Morning stiffness, pain, and tenderness are noted, but overt joint inflammation is uncommon. A migratory polyarthritis is occasionally described in type II hyperlipoproteinaemia, but oligoarthritis and tendonitis are more common. Tendon xanthomas may result in periarticular bone cyst formation. In two-thirds of patients, symptoms resolve with treatment of the lipid disorder, the remainder requiring symptomatic therapy.

Various other conditions

Musculoskeletal manifestations of HIV/AIDS

Rheumatological manifestations include serum sickness at seroconversion, pyomyositis, osteomyelitis (particularly in the setting of intravenous drug abuse), and a spectrum of presentations with acute arthropathy. Antiretroviral therapy, particularly zidovudine, may produce a polymyositis with ragged red fibres on muscle biopsy, whereas combination highly active antiretroviral therapy (HAART) is associated with a syndrome of autoimmune disorders including arthritis. CCR5, an important coreceptor for HIV located on T cells, is critical in a number of autoimmune disorders including rheumatoid arthritis. Very rare manifestations include a vasculitis that appears to be directly induced by the virus, and hypertrophic osteoarthropathy (see below) secondary to *Pneumocystis jiroveci* pneumonia. Arthritis or arthralgia occur in 1 to 25% of cases. Spondyloarthropathy with dactylitis and enthesitis is the most common. A severe, but self-limiting, large joint oligoarthritis has a predilection for the knees and ankles, resolving over 2 to 6 weeks and responding well to NSAIDs. A generalized articular syndrome is very short-lived although intensely painful, usually lasting only 24 h. Acute symmetrical polyarthritis is relatively uncommon and septic arthritis is rare.

Chronic regional pain syndrome

This is the preferred term for the disorders algodystrophy, Sudeck's atrophy, and reflex sympathetic dystrophy. Patients with chronic regional pain syndrome type 1 are those in whom a specific nerve injury is not identified. The dominant feature is pain, with allodynia (pain in response to an innocuous stimulus), hyperalgesia (increased pain perception), and hyperpathia (an exaggerated delayed reaction). Pain usually involves a single limb or body region, typically distal to the site of some (often trivial) traumatic event. Chronic regional pain syndrome may also follow myocardial infarction, stroke, pregnancy, or deep venous thrombosis. There is an association with HLA DR2. Other cardinal features relate to excessive activity of the sympathetic nervous system, with localized swelling, sweating, and piloerection in the early stages, the skin often appearing stretched and shiny. These manifestations subside, leading to a later chronic stage that is very resistant to therapy

Diagnosis is largely clinical, although diffuse osteopenia on plain radiography (comparing the symptomatic and normal limbs on the same film) and the absence of an acute-phase response are supportive. Bone scintigraphy offers the most reliable confirmation of the clinical impression. A three-phase scan is required, comparing the symptomatic and normal sides in the early blood phase (demonstrating hyperaemia in the affected part), bone pool phase (increased bone turnover), and delayed phase.

Intensive physiotherapy is the key element of treatment. Hypotheses of 'neurogenic inflammation' have supported the use of NSAIDs and free radical scavengers including *N*-acetylcysteine. Neuropathic medications with reported efficacy include pregabalin, amitriptyline, and tramadol. Lidocaine and clonidine may be used topically or via continuous epidural infusion (a late option).

Sympathetic nerve blocks (stellate ganglion or lumbar sympathetic chain) with long-acting anaesthetic and/or guanethidine are specialized techniques that are often quite effective in the short term, and may be useful to enable a patient to participate more fully in an exercise programme. High-dose bisphosphonates, either as intravenous pamidronate or as oral alendronate (40 mg daily for 8 weeks), have reduced pain and restored joint mobility in small studies.

Charcot's arthropathy

This joint destruction is associated with neurological injury. Originally described in tabes dorsalis, diabetes is now the most common cause, with 1 to 5% of those with diabetic neuropathy developing features of the condition. Attributing pain to ankle 'sprain' may result in significant delay in diagnosis. Radiologically, a gross proliferative osteoarthrosis is most commonly seen, but significant resorption of bone can also feature, and stress fractures occur in up to a third of patients. Pain-free joints rarely require treatment; moreover, orthopaedic procedures are associated with a high failure rate. Management of painful neuropathic joints is very difficult. Recent evidence points to activation of bone remodelling by cytokines released due to repetitive low-grade trauma, aggravated by free radicals, and advanced glycosylation end-products in diabetes. As such, bisphosphonate therapy (intravenously), non-weight bearing, and a total contact cast are recommended. Orthoses help to prevent stressing of related soft-tissue structures, and a broad range of analgesics, including agents such as amitriptyline and pregabalin, should be considered.

Tietze's syndrome/chostochondritis

Both conditions are of unknown aetiology, although a viral trigger has been proposed in Tietze's syndrome (chondropathia tuberosa). A single chostochondral joint (usually the second or third) is involved in 80% of patients. Coughing or deep breathing exacerbates paracentral chest pain. Tietze's syndrome is also associated with firm, tender lumps at the affected sites. Onset may be acute or more gradual, and the subsequent course is similarly variable, ranging from spontaneous remission to prolonged symptoms lasting for years. As these conditions typically affect middle-aged women, a visceral origin for the symptoms must not be overlooked. Local injection with lidocaine or a corticosteroid may provide symptomatic relief when necessary.

Miscellaneous disorders of synovium, bone, cartilage, and calcification

Synovium

Pigmented villonodular synovitis

Despite a growing number of cytogenetic abnormalities, the aetiology of pigmented villonodular synovitis as an inflammatory or neoplastic disorder remains uncertain. Three types are described. Giant-cell tumours of the tendon sheath occur most commonly in extensor tendons of the hand, although painless, large nodules may restrict movement. Treatment is by surgical excision, which allows histological confirmation of the diagnosis. Recurrence is rare.

Isolated nodular and true diffuse pigmented villonodular synovitis are intra-articular lesions occurring most commonly in the knee of adult men aged between 20 and 50 years. Pain, swelling, and a gradual reduction in the range of movement can continue for some years before the diagnosis is made. Aspiration of serosanguineous fluid in the absence of trauma should raise the suspicion, with MRI being the optimal imaging study. Intra-articular steroid administration gives effective but short-lived relief, and surgical excision is the treatment of choice. In the event of a recurrence (uncommon except in the diffuse form where it may occur in over 40% of cases), radioisotope synovectomy or radiotherapy may be used. In late stages, haemosiderin deposition and chronic inflammation can lead to destructive changes requiring arthroplasty.

Synovial (osteo-)chondromatosis (Reichel's syndrome)

A benign synovial proliferation, this is probably caused by reactive metaplasia secondary to osteoarthrosis, osteochondrosis, or other joint pathology. Most patients are men in their third to fifth decades. Typically monoarticular, usually in the knee, symptoms include joint swelling, locking, and giving way, suggestive of intra-articular loose bodies. Multiple (up to 200) calcified periarticular bodies of hyaline cartilage, 1 mm to 3 cm in size but usually uniform, fill the joint. Surgery is required to remove loose bodies. Malignant transformation to chondrosarcoma is rare.

Synovial haemangioma

A synovial haemangioma is a benign lesion comprising vascular and nonvascular tissue in an asymptomatic and well-localized intra-articular mass, most commonly in the knee (60%) or elbow (30%). Surgical excision is curative.

Lipomas are most commonly found in the thenar and hypothenar eminences, producing compressive symptoms. They may calcify or undergo fibrosis and infarction. Lipoma arborescens occurs particularly in the suprapatellar bursa, producing painless swelling. MRI changes are diagnostic and surgery is curative.

Some two-thirds of 'synovial sarcomas' arise in the thigh. The tissue of origin is mesenchymal, with differentiation to synovium. Prognosis is poor despite surgical excision and radiotherapy.

Bone and cartilage

Bone cysts may be symptomatic or arise as incidental findings, thereby causing diagnostic difficulty. Cysts may be aneurysmal (primary or secondary) or simple (also called unicameral), and can appear in children or adults. Simple cysts are rarely symptomatic or complicated by fracture, and management is expectant. Aneurysmal bone cysts are rare (1 per million), non-neoplastic, expansile lesions occurring principally in the metaphysis of long bones (50%), posterior part of the vertebrae (30%), or flat bones, particularly the pelvis. Most present with pain, swelling, or a pathological fracture at a mean age of 13 years. Radiological features that suggest the diagnosis include an eccentric location of a cyst containing fluid–fluid levels, and trabeculae that remain distinct within it. Management has evolved from the mainstay of curettage with bone grafting or implant of autologous marrow (rich in osteoblasts) to intralesional corticosteroid injection. However, recurrence rates are high (20 to 50%) and other options include embolization and radiotherapy. Secondary aneurysmal cysts complicate giant-cell tumours, chondroblastomas, and osteosarcomas, or they may develop from simple unicameral cysts.

Hereditary multiple exostoses are associated with mutations in one of three genes, *exostin 1, 2,* or *3*, on chromosome 8, 11, and 19 respectively, resulting in altered formation of the cartilage protein heparan sulphate.

Diffuse idiopathic skeletal hyperostosis

Presenting in middle age, and more commonly in men (2:1 male:female ratio), diffuse idiopathic skeletal hyperostosis (DISH, Forestier's disease), a condition of unknown aetiology, affects about 10% of men aged 65 years or over, and up to 58% of men with gout. Usually a radiological diagnosis, the criteria include the presence of new bone forming bridging osteophytes that span at least four adjacent thoracic vertebrae in the absence of degenerative disc disease or sacroileitis. The cortex is preserved, unlike the erosive process seen in the Romanus lesion of ankylosing spondylitis. New bone formation can occur at any site, although enthesial sites are especially common. Phalangeal tufting and an increase in the cortical thickness of the tubular bones of the hand and in the size of sesamoid bones are recognized. Symptoms include restriction in the range of movement, diffuse limb pain, and symptoms of nerve entrapment or myelopathy. Canal stenosis can occur in the lumbar spine. Fracture through bridging osteophytes may also produce pain. Hyperinsulinaemia is frequently associated and related features such as hypertension, type 2 diabetes, obesity, and hyperlipidaemia are more commonly seen in this group.

There is no medical treatment of proven value for established DISH. In the early stages, physical therapy may preserve the range of movement, and weight reduction is of value, both directly and in reducing hyperinsulinaemia. If oral hypoglycaemic agents are required, those that increase serum insulin levels should be avoided. Efforts to reduce heterotopic bone formation at sites of joint replacement have included radiotherapy and perioperative NSAIDs, with mixed results. Corticosteroid, given into joints or at enthesial sites, may also offer symptomatic relief.

Myositis ossificans

Calcification of muscle complicates an intramuscular haematoma after direct impact, occurring in 17 to 20% of such injuries. The anterior thigh and upper arm are the most common sites. Predictive signs at onset include local swelling, tenderness, and (particularly) reduced range of stretch in the involved muscle. A sympathetic knee effusion is described in up to half of those with myositis ossificans in the thigh. Diagnosis may be confirmed radiologically after 3 weeks. MRI will detect a haematoma very early, but to date has not identified specific features predictive of myositis ossificans. The classic 'rest, ice, compression, elevation' is appropriate in the acute setting, with NSAIDs where pain and swelling are particularly marked. Physical training should not resume until a full range of passive stretching is restored. Surgical debridement of ectopic calcification should be undertaken only if it interferes with limb function, and then only where bone is matured, as assessed by bone scintigraphy.

Fibrodysplasia (myositis) ossificans progressiva, by contrast, is a rare inherited disorder. It is characterized by abnormally short hallucles and ectopic calcification of striated muscle leading to disability as the neck, shoulders, spine, hips, and knees become progressively and relentlessly fixed. Additional variable features include fusion of the lateral masses in the lumbar spine, broad femoral necks, and widened metaphyses, as well as episodes of myositis, principally in the neck and upper paraspinal areas, preceding ossification. Histological misdiagnoses include sarcoma or rhabdomyosarcoma and juvenile fibromatosis. The disease appears to be due to a spontaneous genetic mutation in most cases, and prognosis is extremely variable. It has been difficult to evaluate therapeutic options for this reason, and no single measure is clearly of benefit, although there are theoretical grounds for the use of corticosteroids during episodes of myositis, bisphosphonates, and surgical debridement.

Ectopic calcification in renal disease

This is one aspect of renal osteodystrophy where painful calcification of soft tissue, particularly at sites of repeated trauma, occurs as a result of serum levels of calcium and phosphate exceeding their combined solubility. Careful monitoring of phosphate and calcium levels, particularly when vitamin D analogues are used, and early treatment of hyperparathyroidism are both important, because established calcification is usually intractable, although reversal after renal transplantation has been described.

Melorheostosis

This is a rare disorder of linear hyperostosis associated with fibrosis of the skin and soft tissue. Thickening of cortical bone appears in a linear fashion (akin to spilling wax on the side of a candle), usually involving one or several bones in the same (more commonly the lower) limb. Many cases are associated with skin changes in the dermatome corresponding to the origin (sclerotome) of the affected bone, resulting in joint contracture. Symptoms include joint pain, intermittent swelling, deformity, and nerve entrapment, usually presenting in the second decade of life. Surgical intervention is most successful.

Paraneoplastic presentations

Rheumatological presentations associated with malignancy include gout, poly- and dermatomyositis, necrotizing vasculitis and cryoglobulinaemia, systemic sclerosis, and the presentations of lymphoproliferative disorders mentioned above. There are two specific conditions: hypertrophic pulmonary osteoarthropathy and remitting, seronegative, symmetrical synovitis with pitting oedema (RS3PE). A seronegative polyarthritis without oedema and otherwise indistinguishable from rheumatoid arthritis may also occur.

Hypertrophic pulmonary osteoarthropathy is almost always associated with finger clubbing. Patients complain of pain and stiffness of the wrist and ankles, or of a more diffuse polyarthritis. Radiologically a proliferative periostitis is found, particularly at the diaphysis of wrists, ankles, and (less commonly) knees and elbows. Over 90% of cases have an intrathoracic malignancy, although infections or inflammatory conditions in pulmonary, cardiovascular, or gastrointestinal systems are seen. Primary hypertrophic pulmonary osteoarthropathy (pachydermoperiostitis) also occurs (5% of all cases). The cause of the condition remains unknown. The arthritis is typically coincident with the malignancy and resolves with treatment of the underlying disease. Radiotherapy (to the periostitis sites) and infusion of pamidronate have been successful in the treatment of resistant cases.

RS3PE was first described in 1985. Mostly affecting older men (mean age 71 years), a symmetrical polyarthritis involves the metacarpophalangeal and interphalangeal joints, wrists, and (less commonly) the elbows and shoulders. Tendon sheath involvement is quite common, and diffuse pitting oedema on the dorsum of the hands is characteristic. This condition has diverse clinical associations, but malignancy is detected in only 10% of cases. Resistance to corticosteroid treatment in this otherwise very responsive condition raises the possibility of malignancy, although in most cases the underlying disease is detected within weeks. In paraneoplastic presentations, symptoms mirror treatment and relapse of the tumour.

Drugs producing rheumatological presentations

Myalgia may occur on withdrawal of steroids, especially in those patients taking 10 mg prednisolone for at least 30 days. This is best managed by reintroducing the steroid with a more gradual reduction in dose (e.g. 1-mg steps every few days or weeks, depending on severity). Arthralgia and even arthritis are described as rare adverse effects of steroid therapy.

Muscle cramps or aching may also complicate therapy with digoxin, penicillamine, clofibrate, and the statins. Myositis and rhabdomyolysis are also recognized in patients prescribed this last group of drugs. The oral contraceptive is associated with a syndrome of persisting arthralgia, myalgia, morning stiffness, and even synovitis. Myopathy complicates statin and corticosteroid therapy, and chloroquine may cause neuromyopathy, particularly affecting the legs. Myasthenic weakness is an uncommon complication of penicillamine.

Hypersensitivity reaction is associated with penicillamine, sulphonamides, thiouracils, and allopurinol, to name but a few. Presentations vary, but typically include a small-vessel vasculitis and generalized arthralgia or arthritis.

Drug-induced systemic lupus erythematosus (SLE) is well recognized, although 10 times less common than classic SLE. It is characterized by the presence of antihistone antibodies, in distinction to the anti-DNA antibodies of classic SLE. Positive antinuclear antigen (ANA) antibodies are considerably more common than any clinical evidence of lupus. Other important distinctions from idiopathic SLE include resolution on withdrawal of the drug—renal and CNS involvement being rare, and rash uncommon—and older age of onset (50–60 years compared with a mean age of onset of 29 years in idiopathic SLE). Drug-induced SLE is uncommon among the black population, although this group accounts for 30% of idiopathic cases. The drugs associated with SLE include hydralazine and procainamide, with minocycline an important recent addition. TNF-blocking antibodies are associated with the emergence of ANA antibodies, and cases of clinical lupus are increasingly reported. These agents can be used safely by patients with idiopathic SLE, but oestrogen-containing contraceptives are generally regarded as being contraindicated. If a patient develops SLE, any concurrent medication should be withdrawn and the patient observed for a period. However, corticosteroids may be required where there is severe involvement. Antibodies may persist after satisfactory clinical resolution and are not of themselves an indication for continued treatment.

Isoniazid and phenobarbital have been associated with a shoulder–hand syndrome (discussed above as chronic regional pain syndrome). The mechanism of this association is unclear, though alteration in serotonin metabolism has been implicated.

Quinolone antibiotics can cause a tendinopathy. This may lead to rupture, most commonly of the Achilles tendon in elderly patients who are also taking corticosteroids.

Retinoids have been associated in recent years with a hyperostosis otherwise indistinguishable from DISH, discussed above.

This discussion of the associations between drugs and rheumatological presentations is far from complete, and the doctor should always consider drug therapy as a potential cause of new symptoms or signs.

Further reading

Bywaters EG (1971). Still's disease in the adult. *Ann Rheum Dis*, **30**, 121–33.

Ferri C, Mascia MT (2006). Cryoglobulinaemic vasculitis. *Curr Opin Rheumatol*, **18**, 54–63.

Keller JM (2005). New developments in ochronosis: a review of the literature. *Rheum Int*, **25**, 81–5.

Levin J, Werth VP (2006). Skin disorders with arthritis. *Best Prac Res Clin Rheumatol*, **20**, 809–26.

Phornphutkul, *et al.* (2002). Natural history of alkaptonuria. *N Engl J Med*, **347**, 2111–21.

Samuels J, Ozen S (2006). Familial Mediterranean fever and the other autoinflammatory syndromes: evaluation of the patient with recurrent fever. *Curr Opin Rheumatol*, **18**, 108–17.

Sharma A, Williams K, Raja SN (2006). Advances in treatment of complex regional pain syndrome: recent insights on a perplexing disease. *Curr Opin Anaesthesiol*, **19**, 566–72.

Index

Note: Numbers in italic refer to tables and/or illustrations separate from the text.

Species names for animals, plants, fungi and insects are listed by their Latin names, followed by their common name where appropriate.

Felty's syndrome 4307
hepatic involvement 2544
and rheumatoid arthritis 3589
female athlete triad 5376, *5376–7*
history 5376
incidence and aetiology 5376, *5376*
investigation and management 5377, *5377–8*
pathophysiology 5376, *5377*
skeletal effects 5377
femfibrozil 1670
femoral nerve neuropathy 5084
femoral vein cannulation 5510, *5511*
fenbrufen, adverse effects, hepatotoxicity *2532*
fenofibrate 1670
adverse effects, hepatotoxicity *2529*
fenoprofen
and asthma *3289*
rheumatoid arthritis *3594*
fenoterol
asthma 3302
COPD *3335*
fentanyl 3155, *3155*
palliative care 5422
feprazon, adverse effects, hepatotoxicity *2532*
ferpexide, adverse effects, hepatotoxicity *2529*
ferritin 4389
reference values *5435, 5444*
fertility *see* infertility
fetal alcohol syndrome *1468*, 2090, 5146
fetal programming 2083
fetal switch 4201
α-fetoprotein, reference values *5442*
fetus
adverse drug reactions 1468, 2187
effects of maternal diabetes 2138
growth and adult disease 2899
thyroid function 2142
fever of unknown origin 423
causes 423, *424–5*
common diseases 426
diagnostic spectrum 423
subpopulations 423
characteristics of 426
definition 423, *424*
drug-induced 426
factious 426
habitual hyperthermia 426
imaging techniques 426
immunocompromised host 435, *435*
prognosis 427
selective testing 427
therapeutic trials 427
watchful waiting 427
fever
acute pancreatitis 2564
cancer 382
dialysis patients 3941
feverfew, migraine prevention *4916*
fexofenadine 3282
fibrates 1670
fibreoptic bronchoscopy 3135
fibrillary glomerulonephropathies 4060
fibrillin 1 mutations, Marfan's syndrome 2838, *3779, 3781*
fibrinectin *1753*
fibrinogen titre *4196*
fibrinogen *1753, 4490, 4494*, 4494, *4503*
deficiency 4528
laboratory tests *4522, 4504*
plasma *4196*
pregnancy *2126*
reference values *5444*
fibrinolysis 416, 2601
meningitis 721
myocardial infarction *38*, 40, *42*
venous thromboembolism 3020
fibrinolytic system 4496, *4496–7*
Fibrinolytic Therapy Trialists' Collaborative Group 38
fibroadenoma of breast 1940, *1940*
fibroblast growth factor 2601
fibrodysplasia ossificans progressiva 3713, *3721*, 3765
clinical features *3731*, 3765, *3765–6*
differential diagnosis 3765
management 3766
pathophysiology 3765
fibrogenesis imperfecta ossium 3769
clinical features *3731*
fibroma, cardiac 2832
fibromatosis of breast 1941
fibropolycystic disease 2580
choledochal cyst 2582, *2582*
congenital hepatic fibrosis 2581
microhamartomas 2582
polycystic liver disease 2581, *2581*
fibrosing alveolitis
cryptogenic 3375
and rheumatoid arthritis 3588
systemic sclerosis 3673, *3673*
fibrous dysplasia 3720, *3721, 3761, 3762*
clinical features *3731*
monostotic 3762
polyostotic 3762
fibrous erionite pneumoconiosis 3423
Fick principle 2681, *2682*
fifth disease 608
filarial nephropathy 4088
clinical features 4088
management 4089
pathogenesis 4088
pathology 4088
filariasis 3085
cutaneous 1145
lymphatic 1153, *1154*
aetiology 1154
clinical features 1155, *1156–7*
diagnosis 1157
epidemiology and transmission 1155
Global Programme to Eliminate Lymphatic Filariasis 1158
mosquito vectors *1154*, 1155
pathogenesis 1155
treatment 1159
renal involvement 4075
see also individual conditions
Filifactor spp. *962*
Filler formula 3871
Filodes fulvidorsalis 1236
filoviruses 595, 1442
aetiology and genetics 596
areas of uncertainty 599
clinical features 598, *598–9*
diagnosis/differential diagnosis 599, *599*
epidemiology 597
future developments 600
pathogenesis/pathology 596
prevention 597
prognosis 599
treatment 599
finasteride
NNT *52*
skin disorders 4739
fine needle aspiration
bronchial 3220
thyroid cancer 1847
Finegoldia spp. *962*
fingers
boutonnière deformity 3587
clubbing *see* digital clubbing
dactylitis *3606*
swan-neck deformity 3587
fire smoke 3457
first-pass metabolism 1456
Fischoederius elongatus 1223
fish allergy 263
fish odour syndrome 4677
fish oils
in pregnancy 2090
Raynaud's phenomenon *3671*
fish poisoning 1346
carp gallbladder 1347
diagnosis and treatment 1347
gastrointestinal and neurotoxic syndromes 1346
prevention 1346
fish stings 1325, *1344, 1344–5*
clinical features 1345
epidemiology 1344, *1345*
incidence 1344
prevention 1345
treatment 1345
venom composition 1345
Fisher's syndrome 5034, 5037, 5090
fitness factors 411
FitzHugh-Curtis syndrome 944, *945*, 1260
flail chest 3510
flatbush diabetes 2008
flavin adenine dinucleotide 1487–8
flaviviruses 564
mosquito-borne 564–5
taxonomy *566*
tick-transmitted 565
see also individual viruses
Flavobacterium spp. *962*
flavoproteins 1490
flea-borne spotted fever 907
fleas 1225, *1232*, 1232
flecainide *2701*
adverse effects, hepatotoxicity *2532*
in renal failure *4179*
fleroxacin, typhoid fever *742*
Flexispira spp. *962*
Flexner, Abraham 11
flexor hallucis longus tendonitis *5382*
flies
blood-sucking 1226, *1226*
and hygiene 1236
FLIP protein 184
floods 121, 1440
flow-volume curves 3192, *3193*
expiration 3193, *3193*
inspiration 3193, *3193*
Flt-3, 4201
flucloxacillin *706*
adverse effects, hepatotoxicity *2533*
bacteraemia *703, 705*
endocarditis *704–5*
epidural abscess *702*
infective endocarditis *2817, 2818*
osteomyelitis *701*
pharmacokinetics *449*
pneumonia *702, 3238*
Raynaud's phenomenon *3671*
in renal failure *4185*
septic bursitis/arthritis *700*
spectrum of activity *446*
toxic shock syndrome *697*
urinary tract infection *702*
fluconazole
adverse effects, hepatotoxicity *2529*
in breast milk *1469*
candidiasis 1258
coccidioidomycosis 1022
cryptococcosis 1020
dermatophytoses 1002
disseminated candidosis 1013
drug interactions *1471*
oral candidiasis 2269
prophylactic *440*
in renal failure *4185*
flucytosine
fungal infections 1016–17
in renal failure *4185*
fludarabine 398
lymphoma *4320*
fludrocortisone suppression test 3064
fludrocortisone
congenital adrenal hyperplasia 1893
orthostatic hypotension *5063*
fluid balance
high altitude 1403
malaria 1079
pregnancy 2076
fluid replacement
acute renal trauma 3892
anaphylaxis 3112
critical illness 3118
diabetic ketoacidosis 2025
fluid restriction, heart failure 2720
fluid, requirements 1538, *1538*
flukes 1212
intestinal 1219
liver 1212
lung 1216
schistosomiasis 1202
flumazenil *1274*, 3156, 5265
hepatic encephalopathy 2502
flunarizine, migraine prevention *4916*
fluorescein angiography 5235
fluorescence bronchoscopy 3222
Fluorobacter spp. *962*
fluoroquinolone, pneumonia *3238*
fluorosis 3767
5-fluorouracil 398, 4736
adverse effects *400*
breast cancer *1937*
resistance *399*
fluoxetine
adverse effects *5313*
hyperprolactinaemia 2068
cataplexy *4833*
poisoning 1281
Raynaud's phenomenon *3671*